enzyme	-ASE
equal(ity)	IS(O)-
examination	-SCOPY, -OPSY
excess(ive)	-POLY-, HYPER- [Gk.], SUPER- [L.]
excision	-ECTOMY
extremity	-ACR-
eye	-OCUL- [L.], -OP(T)-, -OPHTHALM- [Gk.]
eyelid	-PALPEBR- [L.], -BLEPHAR- [Gk.]
face	-PROSOP-
false	-PSEUD-
far, end	-DIST- [L.], -TEL- [Gk.]
fast, quick	-TACHY-
fat (substance)	-STEAR-, -STEAT-, -LIP-
fat (tissue)	-ADIP-
faulty, bad	MAL- [L.] , DYS- [Gk.]
fear	-PHOB-
feces	-COPR-, -SCAT-
feel, touch	-TACT-, -PALP-
feeling, sensation	-ESTHE(T)-
female	-GYN(EC)-
fever	-FEBR- [L.], -PYRE(T)- [Gk.]
few	-OLIG- [Gk.], -PAUC- [L.]
finger (and toe)	-DIGIT- [L.], -DACTYL- [Gk.]
fingernail (and toenail)	-UNGU(I)- [L.], -ONYCH- [Gk.]
fixing, fixation	-PEXY
flat	-PLAN- [L.], -PLATY- [Gk.]
flesh	-SARC-, -CRE(AT)-
flow	-(R)RHE-
fold	-PLIC-
foot	-PED- [L.] ,-POD- [Gk.]
fore	-ANTER(I)-, ANTE- [L.], PRO- [Gk.]
forehead	-FRONT-
foreign	-XEN-, EX(O)-
form	-MORPH-
forming, formative, formation	-POIET-, -POIESIS
forward	PRO-, ANTE-, -ANTER(I)-
front	-ANTER(I)-
fungus	-MYC(ET)-
gall (bladder)	-CHOLE(CYST)-
gas	-AER- [L.,Gk.], -PNEUM(AT)- [Gk.]
gland	-ADEN-
glass(y)	-VITR- [L.], -HYAL- [Gk.]
good, well, normal	-EU-
green	-CHLOR- [Gk.], -VERD- [L.]
grow, increase	-CRESC- [L.], -AUX- [Gk.]
grow, vegetate	-PHYS-, -PHYT-
gum(s)	-GINGIV- [L.], -UL(E)- [Gk.]
hair	-PIL- [L.], -TRICH- [Gk.]
half	-HEMI- [Gk.], -SEMI- [L.]
hand	-MAN(U)- [L.], -CHEIR- [Gk.]
hard, harden	-DUR- [L.], -SCLER- [Gk.]
hasten	-OXY-
head	-CEPHAL- [Gk.], -CAPIT- [L.]
health(y)	-SAN- [L.], -HYGIE- [Gk.]
hear, hearing	-AUD(I)- [L.], -AC(O)U- [Gk.]
heart	-CARDI- [Gk.], -CORD- [L.]
heat	-CALOR(I)- [L.], -THERM- [Gk.]
heavy	-GRAV(I)- [L.], -BAR(Y)- [Gk.]
heel	-CALC-
height, promontory	-ACR-
hernia	-CELE
hidden	-CRYPT-
high	HYPER- [Gk.], SUPER- [L.]
hind, behind	-POSTER(I)-
hip, hipbone	-COX- [L.], -ISCH- [Gk.]
hollow	-CAV- [L.], -COEL-, -CEL- [Gk.]
hoof	-UNGUL-
horn, horny	-CORN- [L.], -KERAT-, -CERAT- [Gk.]
human	-HOMIN- [L.], -ANTHROP- [Gk.]

ill(ness)	See *disease*
incision	-TOMY
increase, grow	-CRESC- [L.], -AUX- [Gk.]
induce	-GOG-
inflammation	-ITIS
injure, i[illegible]	-TRAUMA(T)- [Gk.], -NOCI- [L.]
inner, d[illegible]	[illegible]ENT-
inside, [illegible]	[illegible]]
intesti[illegible]	[illegible]
iron	[illegible]Gk.]
island	[illegible]Gk.]
jaund[illegible]	[illegible]
jaw	[illegible]
—, upper	[illegible]
—, lower	-MANDIBUL-
joint	-ARTHR- [Gk.], -ARTICUL- [L.]
kill, destroy	-CID-
kidney	-REN- [L.], -NEPHR- [Gk.]
knee	-GEN(U)- [L.], -GON(Y)- [Gk.]
labor (in childbirth)	-TOC-, -LOCH(E/I)-
lack, lacking	-PEN-, A(N)-
large	-MEGA(L)-, -MACR- [Gk.], -MAGN- [L.]
last	-ULTIM-
layer	-LAMIN-
leg	-CRUR- [L.], -SKEL-, -SCEL- [Gk.]
lens	-PHAC-
less, below	INFRA-, SUB- [L.], HYP(O)- [Gk.]
life, live	-BI(O)- [Gk.], -VIT-, -VIV- [L.]
ligament	-DESM-
light (form of energy)	-PHOT-, -PHOS- [Gk.], -LUC- [L.]
light (not dark)	-CLAR-, -LUC-
light (not heavy)	-LEV-
like, alike, same	-HOM(O)-
-like	-OID
limb	-MEL(O)- [Gk.], -MEMBR- [L.]
lip	-LAB(I)- [L.], -CHEIL- [Gk.]
little, few	-OLIG- [Gk.], -PAUC- [L.]
little, small	-MICR- [Gk.], -PARV- [L.]
liver	-HEPAT-
local	-TOP-
loin	-LUMB-
long	-DOLICH-, -MACR-
love, affinity	-PHIL-
love, lust	-EROT-, -ERAST-
low	SUB- [L.], HYP(O)- [Gk.]
lower	-INFER(I)-
lung	-PNEUMON- [Gk.], -PULMON- [L.]
lust	-EROT-
man, male	-ANDR- [Gk.], -VIR- [L.]
man, human	-ANTHROP- [Gk.], -HOMIN- [L.]
many	-POLY- [Gk.], -MULT(I)- [L.]
marrow	-MEDULL- [L.], -MYEL- [Gk.]
mate, mating	-GAM(ET)- [Gk.], -CONJUG- [L.]
meal, dinner	-PRAND(I)-
medical	-IATR-
medicine, drug	-PHARMAC-
membrane	-MENING-
milk	-LAC(T)- [L.], -GALACT- [Gk.]
mind	-MENT- [L.], -PHREN- [Gk.]
mouth	-OR- [L.], -STOM(AT)- [Gk.]
movement	-KINES(I)-, -KINET-
much, many	-MULT(I)-, -PLUR- [L.], -POLY- [Gk.]
mucus	-MYX-, -BLENN-
muscle	-MY(O)-
nail (finger-, toe-)	-UNGU(I)- [L.], -ONYCH- [Gk.]
nape of the neck	-NUCH-
narrow, constricted	-STEN-
narrow, thin, fine	-LEPT- [Gk.], -TENU- [L.]

Continued on inside back cover

Blakiston's Gould Medical Dictionary

EDITORIAL BOARD

Blakiston's Gould Medical Dictionary

Fourth Edition

A modern comprehensive dictionary of the terms used in all branches of medicine and allied sciences; with illustrations and tables

McGraw-Hill Book Company
New York St. Louis San Francisco Auckland Bogotá Düsseldorf
Johannesburg London Madrid Mexico Montreal New Delhi
Panama Paris São Paulo Singapore Sydney Tokyo Toronto

Library of Congress Cataloging in Publication Data

Main entry under title:

Blakiston's Gould medical dictionary.

Based on Gould's medical dictionary.
1. Medicine—Dictionaries. I. Gennaro, Alfonso R. II. Gould, George Milbry, 1848–1922. Gould's medical dictionary. III. Title: Gould Medical dictionary.
[DNIM: 1. Dictionaries, Medical. W13.3 B637]
R121.B62 1979 610'.3 78-21929
ISBN 0-07-005700-1 (Text)
ISBN 0-07-005703-6 (Trade)

Blakiston's GOULD MEDICAL DICTIONARY

6 7 8 9 0 DODO 8 6

GOULD'S MEDICAL DICTIONARY
Fifth Edition, 1941
Fourth Edition, 1935
Third Edition, 1931
Second Edition, 1928
First Edition, 1926

A DICTIONARY OF MEDICAL TERMS—GOULD
First Edition, 1904

AN ILLUSTRATED DICTIONARY OF
MEDICINE, BIOLOGY, AND ALLIED SCIENCES—GOULD
First Edition, 1894

A NEW MEDICAL DICTIONARY—GOULD
First Edition, 1890

The vocabulary portion of this dictionary was set in Times Roman by Rocappi, Inc.
The appendix was set, also in Times Roman, by York Graphic Services, Inc.,
and the front matter was set by Precision Typographers, Inc.
The editors were J. Dereck Jeffers, Richard S. Laufer, Mark W. Cowell, and Robert I. Jones,
assisted by Isabelle Carmichael, Abe Krieger, and Benjamin Victor;
the designer was Merrill Haber; and
the production supervisor was Thomas J. LoPinto.
R. R. Donnelley & Sons Company was printer and binder.

CONTENTS

LIST OF CONTRIBUTORS

Don L. Allen, D.D.S.
Professor of Periodontics and Dean
University of Florida College of Dentistry
Gainesville, Florida

Tom P. Barden, M.D.
Professor of Obstetrics and Gynecology
University of Cincinnati College of Medicine
Cincinnati, Ohio

Alfred S. Berne, M.D.
Professor of Radiology
State University of New York
Upstate Medical Center
Attending Radiologist and Chief
Department of Radiology
Crouse-Irving Memorial Hospital
Syracuse, New York

Frederic W. Bruhn, B.S., M.D.
Chief, Pediatric Infectious Diseases
Walter Reed Army Medical Center
Washington, D.C.
Assistant Professor
Uniformed Services University of
The Health Sciences
Bethesda, Maryland

Henry N. Claman, M.D.
Professor of Medicine and of
Microbiology and Immunology
University of Colorado Medical School
Denver, Colorado

Alastair M. Connell, M.D., F.A.C.P., F.R.C.P.
Mark Brown Professor of Medicine
Professor of Physiology
Director, Division of Digestive Diseases
Department of Internal Medicine
University of Cincinnati Medical Center
Cincinnati, Ohio

Lawrence R. DeChatelet, Ph.D.
Professor of Biochemistry
Research Associate in Medicine
Bowman Gray School of Medicine of
Wake Forest University
Winston-Salem, North Carolina

Ralph E. Fishkin, D.O.
Clinical Assistant Professor
Psychiatry and Human Behavior
Thomas Jefferson University
Philadelphia, Pennsylvania

Warren W. Frost, D.V.M.
Director, Animal Care Facility
University of Colorado Medical Center
Denver, Colorado

Alfonso R. Gennaro, Ph.D.
Associate Dean for Science
Director, Department of Chemistry
Philadelphia College of Pharmacy and Science
Philadelphia, Pennsylvania

William Richard Green, M.D.
Professor of Ophthalmology and
Associate Professor of Pathology
Johns Hopkins University School of Medicine
Baltimore, Maryland

Paul A. Harper, M.D., M.P.H.
Professor Emeritus
Maternal and Child Health, Population Dynamics
Johns Hopkins School of Hygiene and Public Health
Baltimore, Maryland

Lawrence R. Hyman, M.D.
Assistant Professor
Pediatric Nephrology Division
Department of Pediatrics
Johns Hopkins University School of Medicine
Baltimore, Maryland

Judith B. Igoe, R.N., M.S.
Associate Professor
School of Nursing
Instructor, Department of Pediatrics
University of Colorado Medical Center
Denver, Colorado

David Jensen, Ph.D.
Physiologist and Author

Thomas H. Joyce III, M.D.
Professor, Department of Anesthesiology
University of Cincinnati
Cincinnati, Ohio

Edward H. Miller, M.D.
Professor and Director of Orthopaedic Surgery
University of Cincinnati Medical Center
Cincinnati, Ohio

Hyman B. Muss, M.D.
Associate Professor of Medicine
Department of Medicine
Bowman Gray School of Medicine of
Wake Forest University
Winston-Salem, North Carolina

Gerhard Nellhaus, M.D.
Pediatric Neurologist
Pacific State Hospital
Pomona, California

Audrey Hart Nora, M.D. M.P.H.
Director, Genetics
The Children's Hospital
Associate Clinical Professor of Pediatrics
University of Colorado Medical Center
Denver, Colorado

James J. Nora, M.D., M.P.H.
Professor of Pediatrics
Director of Pediatric Cardiology
University of Colorado Medical Center
Denver, Colorado

Richard B. Odom, M.D.
Chief, Dermatology Service
Letterman Army Medical Center
Presidio of San Francisco, California

Robert S. Pinals, M.D.
Professor, Department of Internal Medicine
State University of New York
Upstate Medical Center
Syracuse, New York

Robert W. Prichard, M.D.
Professor and Chairman
Department of Pathology
Bowman Gray School of Medicine of
Wake Forest University
Winston-Salem, North Carolina

Daniel D. Rabuzzi, M.D.
Professor, Department of Otolaryngology and
Communications Sciences
State University of New York
Upstate Medical Center
Syracuse, New York

Richard G. Sample, Ph.D.
Assistant Professor
Department of Pharmacology
Hahnemann Medical College and
Hospital of Philadelphia
Philadelphia, Pennsylvania

John J. Scocca, Ph.D.
Associate Professor
Department of Biochemistry
Johns Hopkins University School of Hygiene and
Public Health
Baltimore, Maryland

Richard W. Stander, M.D.
Director, Division of Education
The American College of Obstetricians and
Gynecologists
Chicago, Illinois

Richard George Wendel, M.D.
Assistant Clinical Professor of Surgery (Urology)
University of Cincinnati College of Medicine
Cincinnati, Ohio

Park Weed Willis III., M.D.
Professor of Medicine (Cardiology)
Department of Internal Medicine
University of Michigan
Ann Arbor, Michigan

John H. Wulsin, M.D.
Professor of Surgery
University of Cincinnati College of Medicine
Cincinnati, Ohio

John W. Vester, M.D.
Professor of Medicine
Professor of Clinical Biochemistry
University of Cincinnati College of Medicine
Director, Clinical Support Laboratory
Good Samaritan Hospital
Cincinnati, Ohio

Maurice Victor, M.D.
Professor of Neurology
Case-Western Reserve University
School of Medicine
Director, Neurology Service
Metropolitan General Hospital
Cleveland, Ohio

Leon Weiss, M.D.
Professor of Cell Biology
Chairman, Department of Animal Biology
School of Veterinary Medicine
University of Pennsylvania
Philadelphia, Pennsylvania

INDEX OF ANATOMICAL PLATES

Lexicographic Abbreviations and Symbols

accus.	accusative
adj.	adjective
adv.	adverb
alt.	alternate, alternative(ly)
Amer.	American
angl.	anglicized, anglicization
Ar.	Arabic
b.	born
BNA	Basle Nomina Anatomica
BR	British (Birmingham) Revision of BNA
ca.	*circa,* about
Cat.	Catalan
Cl.L.	Classical Latin
Colloq.	colloquial
com. n.	common noun (designating members of a biological taxonomic group having the corresponding proper name)
Cz.	Czech
D.	Dutch
d.	died
dial.	dialect, dialectal
dim.	diminutive
E.	English
erron.	erroneous, used erroneously to mean ...
F.	French
fem.	feminine
genit.	genitive
Gk.	Greek
Ger.	German
Gmc.	Germanic, i.e., Proto-Germanic, the prehistoric language ancestral to English, Dutch, German, Norse, Gothic, etc.
Hungar.	Hungarian
irreg.	irregular, irregularly
It.	Italian
Jap.	Japanese
L.	Latin
LG., LGer.	Low German
lit.	literal, literally
LL.	Late Latin, i.e., the Latin of the late Roman Empire
MD.	Middle Dutch
ME.	Middle English
MF.	Middle French
ML.	Medieval Latin
MLG., MLGer.	Middle Low German
mod.	modern
n.	noun
NA	Nomina Anatomica
NL.	New (Modern) Latin
nom.	nominative
obsc. orig.	of obscure origin
obsol.	obsolete
OE.	Old English
OF.	Old French
OL.	Old Latin, i.e., pre-Classical Latin
ON.	Old Norse
orig.	origin, original, originally
O.T.	Old Terminology (in anatomy)
part.	participle
pass.	passive
Per.	Persian
Pg.	Portuguese
pl.	plural
PNA	Paris Nomina Anatomica (the first version of the modern Nomina Anatomica)
Pol.	Polish
prep.	preposition
pron.	pronoun
q.v.	*quod vide,* which see
rel.	colaterally related, cognate
Russ.	Russian
sing., sg.	singular
Skr.	Sanskrit
Sp.	Spanish
Swed.	Swedish
syn.	synonym
tr.	"loan-translation," i.e., a native term used or coined in imitation of a given foreign term
unkn. orig.	of unknown origin
v.	verb
var.	variant
=	which is equivalent to, i.e., which is a transcription of, rendering of, variant of, or synonym of
←	which developed from
→	which developed into, became

Greek Alphabet with Transliterations

Greek letter		Name	Transliteration	Greek letter		Name	Transliteration
Α	α	alpha	a	Ν	ν	nu	n
Β	β	beta	b	Ξ	ξ	xi	x
Γ	γ	gamma	g; n before g, k, ch, x	Ο	o	omicron	o
Δ	δ	delta	d	Π	π	pi	p
Ε	ϵ	epsilon	e	Ρ	ρ	rho	r, rh
Ζ	ζ	zeta	z	Σ	σ	sigma	s
Η	η	eta	ē	Τ	τ	tau	t
Θ	θ	theta	th	Υ	υ	upsilon	y; u after vowel
Ι	ι	iota	i	Φ	ϕ	phi	ph
Κ	κ	kappa	k	Χ	χ	chi	ch
Λ	λ	lambda	l	Ψ	ψ	psi	ps
Μ	μ	mu	m	Ω	ω	omega	ō
					ʽ	''rough breathing''	h

Explanatory Notes

Arrangement of Entries

Alphabetical order The terms defined in this dictionary are set in boldface type and are arranged in one overall alphabetical order; that is, there are no subentries, and the spaces between words in phrases are disregarded. For example, phrases beginning with the word ''methyl'' are not all grouped together, but are interspersed with single words beginning with ''methyl-,'' depending strictly on what the next letter is: **methyl alcohol** comes before **methylate,** which comes before **methyl chloride. Methyl red test** is not to be looked up under **test**—since there are no subentries—but is to be found between **methyl red** and **methylrosaniline chloride.**

Some of the ''run-on'' entries constitute an exception to this rule of strict alphabetization. These terms are not defined independently but are appended to the definitions of the terms they are derived from (or otherwise closely related to):

> **opac·i·fy** (o·pas′i·fye) *v.* 1. to make opaque. 2. To become opaque.
> —**opac·i·fi·ca·tion** (o·pas″i·fi·kay′shun) *n.*

A run-on entry is used only if its alphabetical place as an independent entry would be very close to the entry it is appended to.

Two other minor exceptions to the rule of strict alphabetical order are names beginning with Mc or M', which are alphabetized as if spelled Mac... , and those beginning with St., which are alphabetized as if spelled out: Saint.

Homographs Where there are entries for two or more terms spelled exactly alike, a superscript numeral is prefixed to each of them to alert the reader to this fact:

[1]**mental,** *adj*. [L. *mentalis,* from *mens,* mind]. 1. Pertaining to the mind . . .
[2]**mental,** *adj*. [L. *ment*um, chin, + *-al*]. Pertaining to the chin.

On the other hand, differences involving typographic devices such as capital letters, italics, hyphens, and word spaces are regarded as differences in spelling, and entries so distinguished are not numbered:

Leishmania	**postmortem**	**keto-**
leishmania	**post mortem**	**keto**

In general, a term beginning with a capital letter precedes a similar term beginning with a small letter, and a term written as one word precedes a similar term written as two words. Sometimes, however, the more basic term precedes a secondary or derived version of it regardless of the way they are distinguished in punctuation or typography.

Nonalphabetical inclusions Some terms incorporate symbols, such as numerals and Greek letters, that are disregarded in the alphabetical placement; these terms are to be looked up as if the symbol were not there: **2-OS interval** comes right after **os interparietale,** and α-**globulin** comes right after **globulin** (but when spelled out as **alpha globulin,** it comes at its own place in the a's). This rule applies also to chemical prefixes such as *p*-, *o*-, *m*-, *d*-, *l*-, D-, and L-; for example, **p-aminohippuric acid** is entered in the a's, but when spelled out as **para-aminohippuric acid,** it comes at its own place in the p's.

Abbreviations and symbols in general—insofar as they consist of letters in the Roman alphabet—are entered at their own place in the alphabetical order. Various other symbols may be found in the Table of Medical Signs and Symbols in the Appendix.

Abbreviations used in the dictionary's own devices, such as *adj*. for "adjective," Gk. for "Greek," and Syn. for "synonym," are listed in the table on page xii.

Word Division

The centered dots in the boldface headwords are intended for one purpose only: to show where a word may be divided at the end of the line. Older systems of word division, still used in some dictionaries, purport to serve this function while at the same time marking all "syllable boundaries." Actually, not all syllable boundaries make acceptable division points, nor do all division points come at syllable boundaries.

The first or last letter of a word, for example, should not be split off even though it constitutes a syllable in itself: **ane·mia** (not **a·ne·mi·a**). In many cases this same principle applies within a complex word to the elements making it up: **poly·uria** (not **pol·y·u·ri·a**). In some cases, furthermore, the correct division comes between word elements in such a way that "syllable boundaries" are violated: **meth·yl·at·ed** (not **meth·y·la·ted**).

There are sometimes two or more acceptable ways of dividing a word, as for example **epi·neph·ri·ne·mia** or **epi·neph·rin·emia;** only one way, however, is shown for any entry.

In derivative terms that are not separately defined but are appended (run on) to main entries, center dots are usually inserted only from the point where the pronunciation (or the word division itself) departs from that of the main term (or from that of a preceding appended term): **nec·ro·bi·o·sis** (neck″ro·bye·o′sis) *n*. . . . —**necrobi·ot·ic** (·ot′ick) *adj*. Similarly in the case of plurals and other inflectional forms: **psy·cho·sis** (sigh·ko′sis) *n*., pl. **psycho·ses**(·seez) . . . .

In a series of homographs or of entries beginning with the same word, division points are shown only in the first entry:

[1]**men·tal**	**ar·cu·ate**	**Joh·ne's bacillus**
[2]**mental**	**arcuate artery**	**Johne's disease**

Foreign word divisions In Latin anatomical terms, the "native" Latin word divisions are shown: **zy·go·ma·ti·cus** (rather than **zy·go·mat·i·cus**), **pro·sta·ta** (rather than **pros·ta·ta**). This is the system used in Latin texts and also in the context of modern languages other than English. In an English context, however, it is also quite acceptable to divide the Latin words in the English way.

The division points shown for modern foreign names are generally those used in the language in question:

Al·ba·rrán (Spanish)
Bier·nac·ki (Polish)
Fa·vre (French)
Mor·ga·gni (Italian)

A few of the divisions allowable in the foreign language (especially in French) have been suppressed, however, as disconcerting or misleading in an English context: **Cal·mette** (rather than **Cal·met·te**).

Center dots in the parenthetic pronunciations have significance only for the phonetic spelling itself (see below), and do not necessarily coincide with the divisions shown in the boldface.

Pronunciation

In parentheses immediately after the boldface headwords, pronunciations are shown for single-word terms with the exception of (1) some of the ordinary words that any English-speaking person knows how to pronounce, (2) trademarks, and (3) alternate spellings and inflectional forms that are shown in the entry to which they are referred.

In a sequence of homographs that are pronounced alike, or of phrase entries involving one or more of the same words, the pronunciation of the repeated word is generally shown only in the first entry in which it occurs:

[1]**acrot·ic** (a·krot′ick) *adj.*
[2]**acrotic,** *adj.*

graaf·i·ian follicle (graf′ee·un)
graafian vessels

Lac·to·ba·cil·lus (lack″to·ba·sil′us) *n.*
Lactobacillus ac·i·doph·i·lus (as″i·dof′i·lus)

The pronunciations are based as far as possible on actual usage rather than on theoretical considerations, but there are many terms, especially some of the rarer ones, for which no standard pronunciation can be determined; in such cases one must simply have recourse to criteria of consistency or analogy.

For many terms, several alternative pronunciations are given, though these do not always exhaust the possibilities.

We have attempted to maintain consistency in the pronunciation of the many Latin entries that are not firmly established in English use. Vowels and consonants are generally given their fully anglicized values, so that Latin *ā* = "ay" (as in say), *ī* = "eye," *ē* and *ae* = "ee," *c* and *g* before *e* or *i* = "s" and "j," etc. Vowel length and accentuation, however, are modeled strictly on the Latin except where usage dictates otherwise. Thus latin *intestīnum* is pronounced "in·tes·tye′num" and not, by analogy to the English, "in·tes′ti·num." On the other hand, it would be useless to insist that a word like *apex* be pronounced "ap′ecks" on the grounds that the *a* in Latin is short, since its pronunciation in English is already well established as "ay′pecks."

With varying degrees of consistency, many English speakers favor the "continental" or "school" pronunciation of Latin vowels, approximating the Italian (or German) values of the letters: Latin *ā* = "ah," *ē* = "ay," *ī* = "ee," and *ae* = "eye" or "eh." These pronunciations are certainly more authentic and are better for purposes of international spoken communication, but they go against the norm established by a large body of uniformly anglicized pronunciations such as **nuclei:** "new′klee·eye" (not "nŏŏk′leh·ee") or **calcaneus:** "kal·kay′nee·us" (not "kal·kah′neh·ŏŏs"). To show both systems of pronunciation wherever variation might occur would increase the size and unwieldiness of thousands of Latin entries.

A different policy has been followed with the modern foreign names used in eponymic terms. Rather than give them broadly anglicized pronunciations we have used supplementary phonetic symbols for non-English sounds to show the authentic foreign pronunciations, as for example **Ehrlich** (e^{y}r′li^{k}h), **Quinquaud** (kæ^{n}·ko′). Many of the better known foreign names, of course, have more or less familiar anglicized pronunciations, and to impose an exotic foreign pronunciation on them in English contexts would be regarded as an affectation. Thus in the entry **Gram's stain** we show the pronunciation (gra^{h}m′) so that anyone who is interested can consult the pronunciation key and perhaps get some idea of how the name is pronounced in Danish; it is not recommended for actual use in the English phrase "Gram's stain."

Some names—foreign, English, and (especially) American—have been left unphoneticized because at press time we had not been able to ascertain their correct pronunciation. Others are left unphoneticized because their pronunciations were judged to be obvious to any English speaker.

The system of "phonetic spelling" used in this dictionary is meant to be usually interpretable at a glance by anyone familiar with the elementary principles of English spelling. However—English spelling being what it is—no such system can be entirely foolproof. The key that follows should resolve anything that might be puzzling to the reader at first glance.

PRONUNCIATION KEY 1: ENGLISH

Phonetic Spelling	*Examples*
a (+ consonant) = ă, "short a"	**fat, cathode** (kath′ode), **manic** (man′ick)

Note: The phonetic spelling "a" before a center dot indicates an ordinary "short a" in careful speech: **pathology** (pa·thol′uh·jee), but this may be reduced to an "uh" sound in more casual pronunciation: (puh·thol′uh·jee).

Phonetic Spelling	*Examples*
ă (before r) = "short a"	**carrot** (kăr′ut), **parasite** (păr′uh·site)
a...e = ā, "long a"	**same, face, vein** (vane), **hydrate** (high′drate)
ah = "broad a"	**father** (fah′~~th~~ur), **quality** (kwahl′i·tee) **far** (fahr), **artery** (ahr′tur·ee)
ai = ā, "long a"	**nail, faint, abatement** (uh·bait′munt) **dairy** (dair′ee)

Note: The phonetic spelling "air" often indicates a choice of pronunciations: **calcareous** (kal·kair′ee·us) (*or* kal·kerr′ee·us *or* kal·kăr′ee·us).

Phonetic Spelling	*Examples*
aw = "broad a" + "oo" *or* "short a" + "oo"	**now** (naw), **out** (awt), **caoutchouc** (kaw′chook)
aw	**law, fall** (fawl), **daughter** (daw′tur)
ay = ā, "long a"	**say, daisy** (day′zee), **later** (lay′tur)
e (+ consonant) = ĕ, "short e"	**get, said** (sed), **merry** (merr′ee)

Note: The phonetic spelling "e" before a center dot represents a choice of several sounds: **erythrocyte** (e·rith′ro·site) = (err·ith′ro·site *or* i·rith′ro·site *or* uh·rith′ro·site); **receptor** (re·sep′tur) = (ree·sep′tur *or* ri·sep′tur *or* ruh·sep′tur).

Note: A "silent e" is used (as in ordinary English spelling) after a consonant preceded by a, i, or o, to indicate the "long" sounds of these vowels. See a...e, i...e, o...e.

Phonetic Spelling		*Examples*
ee	= ē, "long e"	**see, ear** (eer), **fetal** (fee′tul), **machine** (muh·sheen′)
ew		**few, mute** (mewt), **beauty** (bew′tee) **new, duty** (dew′tee)

Note: After d, t, th, n, and l, the phonetic spelling "ew" represents a choice of pronunciations: **due** (dew) = (dyoo *or* doo).

eye	= ī, "long i"	**eye, island** (eye′lund)
g	"hard g" only	**get, give** (giv), **argue** (ahr′gew)

Note: See also ng and igh.

i	= ĭ, "short i"	**sit, physical** (fiz′i·kul) **irritate** (irr′i·tate)

Note: The phonetic spelling "i" in unaccented syllables often represents a reduced or obscure vowel approaching the "uh" sound rather than a clear short i: **hemolysis** (he·mol′i·sis), **polluted** (puh·lew′tid).

i...e	= ī, "long i"	**like, sign** (sine), **child** (chile′d)
igh	= ī, "long i"	**sigh, light, myositis** (migh″o·sigh′tis)
ng		**song, singer** (sing′ur)

Note: The "ng" sound in **singer** (sing′ur), **hangar** (hang′ur), is distinguished from the two-sound sequence in **finger** (fing′gur), **anger** (ang′gur), and from the still different sequence in **vanguard** (van′gahrd), **ungifted** (un·gif′tid).

o (+ consonant)	= ŏ, "short o"	**not, lock, follicle** (fol′i·kul) **foreign** (for′in), **coronary** (kor′uh·nerr·ee)

Note: In most kinds of American speech "short o" is pronounced the same as "broad a," so that **bother** rhymes with **father.** See ah.

o (end of syllable)	= ō, "long o"	**go, low** (lo), **motion** (mo′shun) **chlorine** (klo′reen)

Note: Before r, "long o" and "short o" are often interchangeable: **oral** (o′rul *or* or′ul).

o...e	= ō, "long o"	**bone, pore, roll** (role), **yolk** (yoke)
oh	= ō, "long o"	**post** (pohst), **methadone** (meth′uh·dohn)
oo		**too, pool, lose** (looz), **jejunum** (je·joo′num)
o͝o		**look** (lo͝ok), **pull** (po͝ol), **sugar** (sho͝og′ur)
s		**miss** (mis), **taste** (taist), **basic** (bay′sick)

Note: The phonetic spelling "s" never indicates the voiced ("z") sound: **music** (mew′zick), **plasma** (plaz′muh).

PRONUNCIATION KEY 1: ENGLISH (continued)

Phonetic Spelling	*Examples*
th (voiceless)	**thin, teeth, arithmetic** (uh·rith′me·tick)
~~th~~ (voiced)	**this** (~~th~~is), **teethe** (tee~~th~~), **rhythm** (ri~~th~~′um)
u =ŭ, "short u"	**nut, color** (kul′ur), **stomach** (stum′uck)
	burr (bur), **worst** (wurst), **fertile** (fur′til)
u (in unaccented syllables)	**nature** (nay′chur), **dorsal** (dor′sul)
uh	**America** (uh·merr′i·kuh), **psychology** (sigh·kol′uh·jee)
ue (used instead of "ew" in the syllable "sue")	**pseudocyst** (sue′do·sist = syoo′do· *or* soo′do·)
uy (used instead of "ye" after g)	**guiding** (guy′ding)
ye (after consonant and at end of syllable or before ′) = ī, "long i"	**dye, biceps** (bye′seps), **pint** (pye′nt)
zh	**fusion** (few′zhun), **measure** (mezh′ur), **rouge** (roozh)

Accents

A single accent (′) follows the most heavily stressed syllables of a word and a double accent (″) marks subordinate stresses: **hyperpigmentation** (high″pur·pig″men·tay′shun).

Note: Not all subordinate stresses are marked, since most of them are automatically determined either by the position of the main stress or by the sounds involved. In **parasite,** for example, the last syllable is pronounced with a subordinate stress, but the final accent mark (″) is left out as unhelpful and visually cluttering: (păr′uh·site). Before a main accent, however, most subordinate stresses are shown, because they help to establish the rhythm of the word at a glance.

PRONUNCIATION KEY 2: FOREIGN

Phonetic Spelling	*Examples*
a = the same as a^{h} (below): a sound between English "short a" and "broad a"	**Cajal** (ka·^{k}hal′), **Gehr·hardt** (gehr′hart)
æ = a sound between English "short a" and "short e"	**Svedberg** (sve^{y}d′bær^{y}), **Einthoven** (æynt′ho·vun)
æ^{n} = the same as æ but nasalized	**Marjolin** (mar·zho^{h}·læ^{n}′), **Guillain** (ghee·læ^{n}′)
a^{h} = a sound between English "short a" and "broad a"	**Pascal** (pa^{h}s·ka^{h}l′), **Mazzoni** (ma^{h}t·tso′nee), **Riga** (ree′ga^{h})
ah^{n} = "broad a" nasalized	**Chamberland** (shah^{n}·be^{h}r·lah^{n}′), **Vincent** (væ^{n}·sah^{n}′)
æw^{n} = the same as æw but nasalized (see æw in English section)	**São Paulo** (sæw^{n} pæw′loo)
^{c}h Used in some cases to show the palatal variant of ^{k}h. See ^{k}h (below)	**Böttcher** (bœt′^{c}hur)

Phonetic Spelling		*Examples*
^{e} (except after u; see u^{e})	= a short obscure vowel, or syllabification of a following consonant; often the same as the short u or uh (see English key)	**Hyrtl** (hirr′t^{e}l)
eh	= a lengthened version of English "short e"	**Breda** (breh′da^{h})
e^{h}	= "short e"	**Fouchet** (foo·she^{h}′), **Huschke** (hŏosh′ke^{h}), **Bernard** (be^{h}r·nahr′)

Note: In French, the phonetic spelling e^{h} at the end of a syllable may also be pronounced like e^{y} (see below): **Fouchet** (foo·she^{h}′ = also foo·she^{y}′).

^{eh}	See u^{eh}	
e^{y}	= a sound midway between eh and ee; comparable tothe English "long a" (as in late) but not a diphthong, i.e., with no "ee" glide at the end	**Fede** (fe^{y}′de^{h}), **Barré** (ba·re^{y}′), **Swediaur** (sve^{y}d′yaωwr)
gh	= the same as g; used sometimes to avoid possible confusion with the j sound	**Guillain** (ghee·læ^{n}′)
^{g}h	= a velar fricative like ^{k}h (see below) but softer	**van Bogaert** (va^{h}n bo′^{g}hært)
^{h}, h	Used in various combinations to modify the sound of a preceding letter (as in a^{h}, ^{c}h, e^{h}, gh, ^{g}h, i^{h}, ^{k}h, o^{h}). See these individual combinations.	
hh	Used after a vowel to show that an actual h sound is intended, not a modification of the vowel	**Behçet** (behh′chet)
i^{h}	A retracted ee sound; like oo without rounded lips	**Cyon** (tsi^{h}·o^{h}n′)
^{k}h	= A velar or palatal fricative; like k but without any stoppage of the air flow. In some types of Spanish pronunciation, it tends toward a simple h sound. In most pronunciations of German, it has a forward (palatal) quality after e or i and in certain other combinations—midway between the back ^{k}h as in *Bach* and an sh sound. (See also ^{c}h, above).	**Gil** (^{k}heel), **Cajal** (ka·^{k}hal′), **Gerlach** (ge^{h}r′la^{k}h), **Kocher** (ko^{k}h′ur), **Bekhterev** (be^{k}h′t^{y}e·r^{y}uf)

PRONUNCIATION KEY 2: FOREIGN (continued)

Phonetic Spelling		*Examples*
^{n}	Used to indicate nasalization of the preceding vowel; not a separate sound. See æ^{n}, ah^{n}, æw^{n}, œ^{n}, oh^{n}.	
œ	= like the "short e" sound but with rounded lips	**Loeffler** (lœf′lur), **Farabeuf** (fa·ra·bœf′)
œh	= like e^{y} but with rounded lips	**Froelich** (frœh′li^{k}h), **Dieulafoy** (dyœh·la·fwah′)
œ^{n}	= like œ but nasalized	**Brun** (brœ^{n})
o^{h}	= a sound between o and aw, usually short. Somewhat like British o in *cot*, but in French it tends toward the u in American *cut*. In Italian at the end of a stressed syllable, it is long.	**Golgi** (go^{h}l′jee), **Gottlieb** (go^{h}t′leep), **Bonnevie** (bo^{h}n·vee′), **de Toni** (de^{y}·to^{h}′nee)
oh^{n}	= a sound midway between o and o^{h}, nasalized	**Londe** (loh^{n}d), **Tenon** (tuh·noh^{n}′)
u^{e}	= like ee but with rounded lips; in German before a consonant in the same syllable, like "short i" but rounded.	**Dutemps** (du^{e}·tah^{n}′), **Büdinger** (bu^{e}′ding·ur), **Büngner** (bu^{e}ng′nur)
u^{eh}	= a sound midway between u^{e} and oo (in Swedish and Norwegian)	**Guldberg** (gu^{eh}l′bærg)
^{y} (except after e; see e^{y})	Indicates palatalization of a preceding consonant sound, i.e., modification of that sound by giving it a simultaneous "y" quality.	**Morgagni** (mor·gahn^{y}′ee), **Sémélaigne** (se^{y}·me^{y}·lehn^{y}′), **Castañeda** (ka^{h}s·ta^{h}·n^{y}e^{h}′tha^{h}), **Bekhteref** (be^{k}h′t^{y}e·r^{y}uf), **Kultschitzky** (kŏŏl^{y}·chit′skee), **Szent-Györgyi** (sen′d^{y}œr·d^{y}ee), **Dupuis** (du^{e}·pw^{y}ee′)
’	A glottal catch; a slight interruption of the air flow at the glottis as in the exclamation oh-oh! (o′’o). (Occurs in some Danish names.)	**Faber** (fah’′bur)

Many of the same phonetic spellings are used for the foreign names as for English, though in some cases the actual pronunciations differ considerably. For example:

ee	In a syllable closed by a consonant (and in French also finally) this sound is usually clipped short, not drawled or diphthongized as in English.	**Philippe** (fee·leep′), **Piccolo** (peek′ko·lo), **Petit** (puh·tee′), **Gil** (^{k}heel)

Phonetic Spelling		*Examples*
o, o...e, oh	A steady sound that does not vary in quality from beginning to end; not diphthongized like English long o; that is, it has no "w" glide at the end.	**Charcot** (shar·ko′), **Pautrier** (po·tree·e^{y}′), **Roth** (rote), **Ghon** (gohn)
l	After a vowel (in French, German, Italian, Spanish) it has a "light" or "bright" quality, the same as before a vowel; as in English *lee,* not as in English *eel.*	**Gilles** (zheel), **Heschl** (hesh′^{e}l), **Held** (helt)
r	Varies widely in different languages. In Italian, Spanish, Russian, and many other languages, it is trilled on the tip of the tongue; in Spanish and Italian between vowels it gets a single tap if single and a multiple trill if doubled.	**Casares** (ka·sah′res), **Albarrán** (al·ba·rra^{h}n′)

Plurals and Other Inflectional Forms

Plurals formed on a Latin or Greek pattern are generally shown for the nouns that have them: **ovum** (o′vum) *n.,* pl. **ova** (o′vuh); **bron·chus** (bronk′us) *n.,* pl. **bron·chi** (·eye); **ba·sis** (bay′sis) *n.,* pl. **ba·ses** (·seez). When there is a regular English plural used as well as the Latin or Greek one, both are usually shown: **gan·gli·on** (gang′glee·un) *n.,* pl. **gan·glia** (·glee·uh), **ganglions.**

Plurals are not explicitly given for every noun with a Latin or Greek ending, because for some of them the plural is rarely if ever encountered, or is encountered too seldom for there to be any specific usage established. Note, however, the following regular patterns:

Singular ending	*Plural ending*	*Examples*
-sis	**-ses** (·seez)	diagnosis: diagnoses myiasis: myiases hemolysis: hemolyses
-itis	**-itides** (·it′i·deez)	arthritis: arthritides dermatitis: dermatitides
-oma	**-omas** or **-omata**	adenoma: adenomas *or* adenomata

Sometimes a Latin or Greek-pattern plural is used much more than the singular, and is chosen to serve as the main entry. In that case, the singular is shown for it in the same way that a plural is shown for a singular entry: **oto·co·nia** (o″to·ko′nee·uh) *n.,* sing. **otoco·ni·um** (·nee·um). If no singular is used, as in the case of higher biological taxa, then the entry is marked "*n.pl.*" (noun plural).

Genitive (possessive) forms of Latin nouns are used in many of the Latin phrases defined in the dictionary, for example, *dentis* in the term **corona dentis** "crown of a tooth." The more important of these genitives are shown at the entries of the terms to which they belong:

dens (denz) *n.,* genit. **den·tis** (den′tis), pl. **den·tes** (·teez), genit. pl. **den·ti·um** (den′tee·um, den′shee·um) . . . TOOTH.

 For many nouns the genitive singular form is the same as the nominative plural, for example, *pili* "hairs" or "of a hair" (as in **arrector pili** "erector of a hair"), *vertebrae,* plural of *vertebra,* or genitive singular as in **arcus vertebrae** "arch of a vertebra, vertebral arch":

> **ver·te·bra** (vur'te·bruh) *n.*, pl. & genit. sing. **verte·brae** (·bree)
> **pi·lus** (pye'lus, pil'us) *n.*, pl. & genit. sing. **pi·li** (·lye)

For most Latin nouns ending in *-is,* the genitive singular coincides in form with the nominative singular, which is the headword form; these genitives are not explicitly indicated. Thus **ax·is** (ack'sis) *n.*, pl. **ax·es** (·seez), but in the phrase **dens axis,** for example, ("the dens of the axis"), *axis* is genitive.

Etymology

The material included in square brackets, just before the definition proper, is intended as a highly condensed account of how the meaning shown in the definition came to be represented by the form shown in the boldface headword. Broadly, two types of etymology are used: analytical and historical.

Analytical etymologies are applied mainly to terms coined in modern times from word elements usually already existing in English and other modern languages. These word elements are not usually glossed or explained where they occur in the etymologies, but are entered, etymologized, and defined at their own place in the dictionary:

> **mel·a·no·cyte** (mel'uh·no·site) *n.* [*melano-* + *-cyte*]. A fully differentiated melanin-containing cell; a cell that synthesizes melanosomes.
>
> **melan-, melano-** [Gk. *melas, melanos,* black, dark]. A combining form meaning (a) *black, dark;* (b) *pertaining to melanin.*
>
> **-cyte** [Gk. *kytos,* vessel, container, hollow]. A combining form meaning *cell.*

Historical etymologies in this dictionary are used mainly for those terms that have been acquired from other languages, as for example: **nerve,** *n.* [L. *nervus,* sinew, tendon; nerve], which is to say, "The English word *nerve* is an adaptation of the Latin word *nervus,* which originally and principally meant 'sinew' or 'tendon' but also came to be applied to what are now called nerves."

Some historical etymologies are more complicated: **pal·sy** (pawl'zee) *n.* [OF. *paralisie,* from L. *paralysis,* from Gk.]. This (with a couple of details added) means "The English word *palsy* derives from an earlier adaptation of the Old French *paralisie,* which developed from a variant of the Latin *paralysis,* which was adopted from Greek (παράλυσις)." The Greek form need not be shown explicitly in the etymology because its transliteration is the same as the Latin spelling given just before it.* (An analytical etymology of this original Greek word is given at the entry for *paralysis* itself: [Gk., from *para-,* beside, off, amiss, +*lysis,* loosening, dissolution].)

In some cases the intermediate steps in historical etymologies are left out, being merely routine stages in well-traveled routes of derivation: **car·di·ac** (kahr'dee·ack) *adj.* [Gk. *kardiakos*], which, more fully, would be shown as "[F. *cardiaque,* from L. *cardiacus,* from Gk. *kardiakos*]."

If the foreign source of a term is spelled (or transliterated) the same as the headword itself and also means substantially the same thing, then only a source-language label is needed within the brackets: **ab·do·men** (ab·do'mun, ab'do·mun) *n.* [L.]. If the source is spelled the same as the headword itself but its meaning is substantially different, then the source-language label is followed by an English gloss: **lens** (lenz) *n.* [L., lentil].

Verbs in Latin, Greek, and most other languages are cited in the infinitive form; Latin and Greek nouns are given in the nominative singular, and adjectives in the nominative singular masculine. When the usual citation form alone fails to show the stem form reflected in the headword, however, then for

* See Greek Alphabet with Transliterations.

nouns the genitive is usually also given, and for Latin verbs, the perfect participle: **mo·nad** (mo'nad) *n.* [Gk. *monas, monados,* unit]; **mar·gin** (mahr'jin) *n.* [L. *margo, marginis*]; **in·ject** (in·jekt') *v.* [*injicere, injectus,* to throw in].

Some terms, e.g., *headache, antidiabetic,* are not etymologized because their formation is obvious. Others, whose formation might not be obvious to everyone at first glance, become obvious in the light of their definitions, e.g., *myxochondrofibrosarcoma,* "a sarcoma whose parenchyma consists of anaplastic myxoid, chondroid, and fibrous elements."

In eponymic entries, the person whose name is incorporated in the term is identified within the etymological brackets: **Leyden's paralysis** [E. V. von *Leyden,* German neurologist, 1832–1910]. Where the name occurs again in a subsequent entry or in another part of the dictionary, the identification is reduced to the name alone:

Charcot-Leyden crystals [J. M. *Charcot,* French neurologist, 1825–1893; and E. V. von *Leyden*]

Charcot's joint [J. M. *Charcot*]

The bracketed notations "NA" and "BNA" identify Latin anatomical terms as ones listed in the current *Nomina Anatomica* and the earlier *Basle Nomina Anatomica,* respectively.

Definitions: Preferred Terms and Synonyms

The terms entered fall into two broad categories: (1) the so-called preferred terms, for which full-fledged definitions are given, and (2) their synonyms, which are defined by the preferred term set in small capital letters:

(1) **jaun·dice** . . . Yellowness of the skin, mucous membranes, and secretions; due to hyperbilirubinemia. Syn. *icterus.*

(2) **ic·ter·us** . . . JAUNDICE.

With certain exceptions, there is only one preferred term in any set of synonyms, and—style and context permitting—only the preferred term is used in definitions. This principle is important in maintaining a dictionary's consistency and efficiency.

Ideally, the preferred term of a set of synonyms is the one that is judged by the editorial board to be the best choice for general use. Actually there are many cases in which no clear-cut superiority of one term over another exists, or in which one term is superior in certain contexts but not in others. In such cases the choice of a preferred term must be to some extent arbitrary.

Entries for terms that have more than one meaning are divided into separate, numbered definitions or "senses":

pars intermedia . . . 1. The posterior portion of the adenohypophysis, between the pars distalis and the neurohypophysis . . . 2. The nervus intermedius; the intermediate part of the facial nerve.

If such a term has synonyms in one or another of its senses and is preferred over them, the synonyms are referred to the relevant sense of the preferred term by means of the sense number in parentheses:

intermediate lobe of the hypophysis. PARS INTERMEDIA (1).

If the preferred term is a homograph, references to it from synonyms use the appropriate prefixed numeral:

[1]**im·plant** (im·plant′) *v.* . . . To embed, set in.

[2]**im·plant** (im′plant) *n.* 1. A small tube or needle which contains radioactive material, placed in a tissue or tumor to deliver therapeutic doses of radiation. 2. A tissue graft placed in depth.

implantation graft. [2]IMPLANT (2).

The notation "[2]IMPLANT (2)" means that the second *implant* entry, in its second sense, is where the reader will find the meaning of *implantation graft.*

Cross References

The following cross-reference devices are the main ones used in this dictionary:

Abbreviated,	Standard abbreviations of this term are . . .
Adj.	The derived or corresponding adjective(s) is/are . . .
Comb. form	The combining form(s) corresponding to this term is/are . . .
Compare	Note the difference between this and. . . ; Not to be confused with . . .
Contr.	This term contrasts with or is complementary to . . .
NA	The official Latin (Nomina Anatomica) for this structure is . . .
Noun	The derived or corresponding noun(s) is/are . . .
See	This term is explained in (the entry or table mentioned)
See also	Further relevant information is given in (the entry, table, or plate mentioned)
Symbol,	Standard symbols for what this term denotes are . . .
Syn.	Important synonyms of this term are . . .
Vb.	The derived or corresponding verb(s) is/are . . .

Except for "See" references (which usually replace definitions altogether), cross references are appended at the end of definitions—or at the end of one of the numbered senses within definitions.

Blakiston's Gould Medical Dictionary

A

A 1. *In chemistry,* a symbol for argon. 2. *In molecular biology,* a symbol for adenine. 3. *In radiology,* symbol for area of heart shadow. 4. *In physics,* an abbreviation for *angstrom.*

A Symbol for absorbance.

A. Abbreviation for (a) *absolute;* (b) *anode.*

Å, A Abbreviation for *ångström, angstrom.*

A_2 The aortic valve closure component of the second heart sound.

a Symbol for absorptivity.

a. Abbreviation for (a) *accommodation;* (b) *ampere;* (c) *anode;* (d) *anterior;* (e) *aqua;* (f) *arteria.*

ā, āā [Gk. *ana,* of each]. Symbol meaning *the same quantity of each ingredient* in a prescription.

a, ab. A Latin preposition meaning *from,* as in *a tergo,* from behind, *a potu,* from drink, *ab igne,* from fire.

a-, ab-, abs- [L.]. A prefix meaning (a) *away from, outside of;* (b) *deviating from.*

a-, an- [Gk.]. A prefix meaning *un-, not, -less, lacking, lack of.*

A.A. Abbreviation for (a) *achievement age;* (b) *Alcoholics Anonymous.*

aaa disease [designation in the Ebers papyrus]. ANCYLOSTOMIASIS.

A.A.A.L.A.C. American Association for Accreditation in Laboratory Animal Care.

A.A.A.S. American Association for the Advancement of Science.

A.A.C.P. American Association of Colleges of Pharmacy.

A.A.D. American Academy of Dermatology.

A.A.D.S. American Association of Dental Schools.

A.A.E. American Association of Endodontists.

A.A.F.P. American Association of Family Physicians.

A.A.G.P. American Academy of General Practice.

A.A.I. American Association of Immunologists.

A.A.L.A.S. American Association for Laboratory Animal Science, formerly known as Animal Care Panel.

A.A.N. American Academy of Neurology.

A.A.O. American Association of Orthodontists.

A.A.O.P. American Academy of Oral Pathology.

A.A.O.R. American Academy of Oral Roentgenology.

A.A.O.S. American Academy of Orthopedic Surgeons.

A.A.P. (a) American Academy of Pediatrics; (b) American Academy of Pedodontics; (c) American Academy of Periodontology.

Aarane. Trademark for cromolyn sodium, a bronchial asthma inhibitor.

Ab Abbreviation for *antibody.*

ab-. 1. See *a-, ab-, abs-.* 2. A prefix designating *a cgs electromagnetic unit,* as abampere, abvolt.

abac·te·ri·al (ay″back·teer′ee·ul) *adj.* Without bacteria.

abacterial meningitis. ASEPTIC MENINGITIS.

Aba·die's sign (a·ba·dee′). 1. [J. *Abadie,* French neurologist, 1873–1946] Insensitivity to forceful pinching of the calcaneal tendon in tabes dorsalis. 2. [C. *Abadie,* French ophthalmologist, 1842–1932] Spasm of the levator palpebrae superioris muscle, occurring frequently in thyrotoxicosis but also seen normally, especially with tension and fatigue.

ab·alien·a·tion (ab·ay″lee·un·ay′shun) *n.* [L. *abalienare,* to separate, estrange]. Mental deterioration or derangement.

ab·am·pere (ab·am′peer) *n.* [*ab-* + *ampere*]. A cgs electromagnetic unit of current equivalent to 10 amperes.

A band [*a*nisotropic band]. The birefringent (doubly refractile) transverse band that forms the broad middle segment of each sarcomere in striated muscle fibrils, representing the zone occupied by thick myosin filaments interdigitated (except in the H zone) with the actin filaments. Contr. *I band.*

aban·don·ment, *n. In medical jurisprudence,* the withdrawal of a physician from the care of a patient, without reasonable notice of such withdrawal or without discharge from the case by the patient.

ab·ap·i·cal (ab·ap′i·kul) *adj.* [*ab-* + *apical*]. Away from or opposite the apex.

abap·tis·ton (ab″ap·tis′ton) *n.* [Gk., from *abaptistos,* unsinkable, from *baptizein,* to dip]. A conical trephine so designed that it will not slip through the bony opening and injure the underlying dura mater or brain.

abar·og·no·sis (ay·băr″og·no′sis) *n.* [*a-* + *barognosis*]. Loss or lack of the ability to estimate weight. Syn. *baragnosis.*

ab·ar·tic·u·lar (ab″ahr·tick′yoo·lur) *adj.* [*ab-* + *articular*]. Not connected with or situated near a joint.

abarticular gout. A form of gout in which structures other than the joints are involved.

ab·ar·tic·u·la·tion (ab″ahr·tick″yoo·lay′shun) *n.* [*ab-* + *articulation*]. 1. A diarthrodial joint. 2. A dislocation of a joint.

aba·sia (a·bay′zhuh, ·zee·uh) *n.* [*a-* + Gk. *basis,* step, + *-ia*]. Inability to walk despite the preservation of strength, coordination, and sensation in the legs. Contr. *astasia.* —**aba·sic** (·sick, ·zick) *adj.*

abasia-astasia. ASTASIA-ABASIA.

abasia trep·i·dans (trep′i·danz). TREMBLING ABASIA.

abat·ic (a·bat′ick) *adj.* Abasic; pertaining to or affected with abasia.

ab·at·tage, ab·a·tage (ab″uh·tahzh′) *n.* [F.]. 1. The slaughter of animals; specifically, the slaughter of diseased animals to prevent the infection of others. 2. The art of casting an animal preparatory to an operation.

ab·at·toir (ab″uh·twahr′) *n.* [F.]. A slaughterhouse or an establishment for the killing and dressing of animals.

ab·ax·i·al (ab·ack'see·ul) *adj.* [*ab-* + *axial*]. Not situated in the line of the axis of a structure.

Ab·be condenser (ahb'eh) [E. *Abbe,* German physicist, 1840-1905]. A system of lenses, attached to a microscope, for concentrating light on the object being examined.

Abbe-Zeiss cell [E. *Abbe* and C. *Zeiss*]. THOMA-ZEISS COUNTING CHAMBER.

Abbocillin. A trademark for certain preparations containing penicillin G.

Ab·bott's method [E. G. *Abbott,* U.S. orthopedist, 1871-1938]. A treatment of scoliosis by the application of a series of plaster jackets and bandages to achieve gradual overcorrection.

Abderhalden-Kaufmann-Lignac syndrome [E. *Abderhalden;* and G.O.E. *Lignac,* Dutch pediatrician, 20th century]. CYSTINOSIS.

Ab·der·hal·den reaction or **test** (ahp'dur·hahl·dun) [E. *Abderhalden,* Swiss pathologist, 1877-1946]. The appearance in the serum of an abnormal proteolytic enzyme active against a foreign protein; once thought to occur in pregnancy, cancer, schizophrenia, and various infections, thus serving as the basis of tests for those conditions.

ab·do·men (ab·do'mun, ab'do·mun) *n.,* pl. **abdomens, abdom·i·na** (·dom'i·nuh) [L.] [NA]. The large, inferior cavity of the trunk, extending from the brim of the pelvis to the diaphragm, bounded in front and at the sides by the lower ribs and abdominal muscles and behind by the vertebral column and the psoas and quadratus lumborum muscles. See also *abdominal regions.*

abdomen ob·sti·pum (ob·stye'pum) [L., bent, bowed]. An abdominal deformity, looking like severe constipation, resulting from congenitally short recti muscles.

abdomin-, abdomino-. A combining form meaning *abdomen, abdominal.*

ab·dom·i·nal (ab·dom'i·nul) *adj.* Of or pertaining to the abdomen. —**abdominal·ly** (·ee) *adv.*

abdominal angina. An acute attack of severe abdominal pain, commonly occurring after eating, and often recurrent and associated with weight loss, nausea, vomiting, and diarrhea. It is caused by narrowing or obstruction of the mesenteric arteries, primarily atherosclerotic in origin.

abdominal aorta. The abdominal continuation of the descending aorta. NA *aorta abdominalis.* See also Table of Arteries in the Appendix and Plates 5, 7, 8, 14.

abdominal aponeurosis. The wide, tendinous expanse by which the external oblique, internal oblique, and transverse muscles are inserted.

abdominal apoplexy. Infarction of an abdominal organ, usually the small intestine, resulting from vascular stenosis or occlusion.

abdominal cavity. The space within the body between the diaphragm and the pelvic floor, containing the abdominal viscera. NA *cavum abdominis.*

abdominal compression. Application of firm manual pressure for 10 seconds against a patient's abdomen following lumbar puncture to measure the rise and fall of cerebrospinal fluid pressure, to ensure its normal flow.

abdominal dropsy. ASCITES.

abdominal epilepsy. A seizure equivalent in which abdominal pain, a sense of nausea, and often headache are the most prominent symptoms.

abdominal fissure. CELOSOMA.

abdominal fistula. An opening through the abdominal wall which communicates with an abdominal viscus or space.

abdominal gestation. The form of extrauterine gestation in which the product of conception is located in the abdominal cavity.

abdominal hernia. VENTRAL HERNIA.

abdominal hysterectomy. Hysterectomy in which the removal is effected through an abdominal incision.

abdominal influenza. VIRAL GASTROENTERITIS.

abdominal inguinal ring. DEEP INGUINAL RING.

abdominal line. 1. Any line used in describing the surface of the abdomen, or indicating the boundary of an abdominal muscle. See also *abdominal regions.* 2. LINEA ALBA.

abdominal migraine. A syndrome of periodically recurring abdominal pain, nausea, vomiting, or diarrhea, replacing migraine headaches.

abdominal muscle deficiency syndrome. A congenital nonhereditary disorder characterized by partial or complete absence of abdominal muscles in association with anomalies of the gastrointestinal tract, urinary tract, and the extremities and cryptorchism. Syn. *prune-belly syndrome.*

abdominal nephrectomy. Nephrectomy performed through an abdominal incision.

abdominal nephrotomy. Nephrotomy performed through an abdominal incision.

abdominal paracentesis. Puncture of the abdominal wall with a trocar and cannula, usually for the relief of ascites.

abdominal phthisis. Peritoneal or intestinal tuberculosis.

abdominal pregnancy. Pregnancy with the fetus lying within the abdominal cavity.

abdominal ptosis. VISCEROPTOSIS.

abdominal reflex. Contraction of the abdominal muscles induced by stroking or scratching the overlying skin.

abdominal regions. The nine regions of the abdomen artificially delineated by two horizontal and two parasagittal lines. The horizontal lines are tangent to the cartilages of the ninth ribs and iliac crests, respectively, and the parasagittal lines are drawn vertically on each side from the middle of the inguinal ligament. The regions thus formed are: above, the right hypochondriac, the epigastric, and the left hypochondriac; in the middle, the right lateral or lumbar, the umbilical, and the left lateral or lumbar; and below, the right inguinal or iliac, the pubic or hypogastric, and the left inguinal or iliac. NA *regiones abdominis.*

abdominal respiration. Respiration caused by the contraction of the diaphragm and the elastic expansion and recoil of the abdominal walls. Contr. *thoracic respiration.*

abdominal retractor. A large, heavy instrument, often with a curved flange, to give greater retractive power during abdominal operations.

abdominal rib. 1. FLOATING RIB. 2. Ossification of an intersectio tendinea.

abdominal section. Incision into the abdominal cavity.

abdominal seizure equivalent. ABDOMINAL EPILEPSY.

abdominal testis. A testis that is undescended and remains in the abdominal cavity.

abdominal touch. Palpation of the abdomen for the diagnosis of intraabdominal conditions.

abdominal version. Manipulations to reposition the fetus or an abdominal viscus made exclusively through the external abdominal wall.

abdomino-. See *abdomin-.*

ab·dom·i·no·an·te·ri·or (ab·dom''i·no·an·teer'ee·ur) *adj.* [*abdomino-* + *anterior*]. *Obsol. In obstetrics,* designating a fetal position in which the belly is forward.

ab·dom·i·no·car·di·ac sign (ab·dom''i·no·kahr'dee·ack). LIVIERATO'S SIGN (1).

ab·dom·i·no·cen·te·sis (ab·dom''i·no·sen·tee'sis) *n.,* pl. **abdominocente·ses** (·seez) [*abdomino-* + *centesis*]. ABDOMINAL PARACENTESIS.

ab·dom·i·no·hys·ter·ec·to·my (ab·dom''i·no·hiss·tur·eck'tuh·mee) *n.* ABDOMINAL HYSTERECTOMY.

ab·dom·i·no·hys·ter·ot·o·my (ab·dom''i·no·hiss·tur·ot'uh·mee) *n.* Hysterotomy through an abdominal incision.

ab·dom·i·no·jug·u·lar reflux test (ab·dom''i·no·jug'yoo·lur). HEPATOJUGULAR REFLUX TEST.

ab·dom·i·no·per·i·ne·al (ab·dom''i·no·perr''i·nee'ul) *adj.* Pertaining to the abdominal and perineal regions.

ab·dom·i·no·pos·te·ri·or (ab·dom''i·no·pos·teer'ee·ur) *adj.* [*abdomino-* + *posterior*]. *Obsol. In obstetrics,* designating a fetal position in which the belly is toward the mother's back.

ab·dom·i·nos·co·py (ab·dom″i·nos′kuh·pee) *n.* [*abdomino-* + *-scopy*]. Diagnostic examination of the abdomen, externally by physical methods and internally by endoscopic methods.

ab·dom·i·no·tho·rac·ic (ab·dom″i·no·tho·ras′ick) *adj.* Pertaining to the abdominal and thoracic regions.

abdominothoracic arch. The lower boundary of the front of the thorax.

ab·dom·i·nous (ab·dom′i·nus) *adj.* Having a large abdomen.

ab·dom·i·no·uter·ot·o·my (ab·dom″i·no·yoo·tur·ot′uh·mee) *n.* [*abdomino-* + *uterotomy*]. *Obsol.* ABDOMINOHYSTEROTOMY.

ab·dom·i·no·ves·i·cal (ab·dom″i·no·ves′i·kul) *adj.* [*abdomino-* + *vesical*]. Pertaining to the abdomen and the urinary bladder.

abdominovesical pouch. A pouch formed by the reflection of the peritoneum from the anterior abdominal wall onto the distended urinary bladder; it contains the lateral and medial inguinal fossae.

ab·du·cens (ab·dew′sunz) *adj.* & *n.* 1. Of or pertaining to the abducens nerve. 2. ABDUCENS NERVE.

abducens nerve. The sixth cranial nerve, whose fibers arise from the nucleus in the dorsal portion of the pons near the internal genu of the facial nerve and run a long course to supply the lateral rectus muscle which rotates the eyeball outward. NA *nervus abducens.*

ab·du·cent (ab·dew′sunt) *adj.* [L. *abducens, abducentis,* from *ab-,* away, + *ducere,* to lead]. 1. Abducting. 2. ABDUCENS (1).

abducent nerve. ABDUCENS NERVE.

abducent nucleus. A nucleus lying under the floor of the fourth ventricle near the junction of the pons and medulla which gives origin to the abducent nerve.

abducent paralysis. Paralysis of the lateral rectus muscle of the eye due to a lesion of the sixth cranial nerve or its nucleus. The eye cannot be abducted and is convergent.

ab·duct (ab·dukt′) *v.* [L. *abducere,* to lead away]. To draw away from the median line or plane.

ab·duc·tion (ab·duck′shun) *n.* [L. *abductio,* from *abducere,* to lead away]. 1. A movement whereby one part is drawn away from the axis of the body or of an extremity. 2. *In ophthalmology,* (a) turning of the eyes outward from the central position by the lateral rectus muscles; (b) the turning of the eyes outward beyond parallelism under the artificial stimulus of base in prisms and expressed in terms of prism diopters, the measurement being the strongest prism power with which the eyes can maintain single vision at infinity.

abduction cap. An orthopedic appliance of canvas or leather to maintain abduction in cases of subdeltoid bursitis.

abduction paralysis. ABDUCTOR PARALYSIS.

ab·duc·tor (ab·duck′tur) *n.* [NL., from L. *abducere,* to lead away]. A muscle which, on contraction, draws a part away from the axis of the body or of an extremity. See also Table of Muscles in the Appendix.

abductor ac·ces·so·ri·us di·gi·ti mi·ni·mi (ack·se·so′ree·us dij′i·tye min′i·mye). A rare variant of the opponens digiti minimi (pedis) inserted into the base of the proximal phalanx of the little toe.

abductor cau·dae (kaw′dee). A muscle found in tailed animals, corresponding to the coccygeal muscle in man.

abductor di·gi·ti mi·ni·mi (dij′i·tye min′i·mye). The abductor muscle of the little finger or little toe. NA *musculus abductor digiti minimi.* See also Table of Muscles in the Appendix.

abductor digiti quin·ti (kwin′tye). ABDUCTOR DIGITI MINIMI.

abductor hal·lu·cis (hal′yoo·sis). A muscle of the medial side of the foot, inserted into the base of the first metatarsal. NA *musculus abductor hallucis.* See also Table of Muscles in the Appendix.

abductor hallucis lon·gus (long′gus). A rare muscle of the anterior region of the leg, inserted into the base of the first metatarsal.

abductor in·di·cis (in′di·sis). The first dorsal interosseous muscle of the hand.

abductor os·sis me·ta·tar·si quin·ti (oss′is met·uh·tahr′sigh kwin′tye). A variant slip of the abductor digiti minimi of the foot inserted into the tuberosity of the fifth metatarsal. See also Table of Muscles in the Appendix.

abductor paralysis. Paralysis of abduction, especially of the lateral rectus muscle of the eye. See also *abducens paralysis.*

abductor pol·li·cis bre·vis (pol′i·sis brev′is). The short abductor muscle of the thumb. NA *musculus abductor pollicis brevis.* See Table of Muscles in the Appendix.

abductor pollicis lon·gus (long′gus). The long abductor muscle of the thumb. NA *musculus abductor pollicis longus.* See Table of Muscles in the Appendix.

ab·em·bry·on·ic (ab″em″bree·on′ic) *adj.* [*ab-* + *embryonic*]. Away from or opposite the embryo.

ab·en·ter·ic (ab″en·terr′ick) *adj.* [*ab-* + *enteric*]. Affecting organs and structures outside the intestine.

Ab·er·crom·bie's degeneration [J. *Abercrombie,* Scottish physician, 1780–1844]. AMYLOID DEGENERATION.

Aberel. Trademark for tretinoin, a keratolytic.

ab·er·rant (uh·berr′unt) *adj.* [L. *aberrans,* from *ab-,* away, + *errare,* to wander]. Varying or deviating from the normal in form, structure, or course.

aberrant complex. An electrocardiographic deflection which varies in configuration from the normal because of ectopic impulse formation or abnormal conduction. Syn. *anomalous complex.*

aberrant ductules. DUCTULI ABERRANTES.

aberrant goiter. See *goiter.*

aberrant ureter. ECTOPIC URETER.

ab·er·ra·tion (ab″e·ray′shun) *n.* [L. *aberrare,* to wander, go astray]. 1. A deviation from the normal or the standard. 2. Any mild mental disorder. 3. *In biology,* an abnormal part or individual. 4. *In optics,* any imperfection in the refraction or the focalization of a lens.

ab·er·rom·e·ter (ab″e·rom′e·tur) *n.* An instrument for measuring aberration (4).

abeta·lipo·pro·tein·emia, abeta·lipo·pro·tein·ae·mia (ay″ bay″tuh·lip″o·pro·teen·ee′mee·uh) *n.* [*a-* + *β-lipoprotein* + *-emia*]. A disease entity due to almost total absence of *β*-lipoproteins, characterized by the presence in blood of acanthocytes, hypocholesterolemia, malabsorption of fat beginning in infancy, and later, ataxia, peripheral neuropathy, and frequent retinitis pigmentosa and muscular atrophy; an autosomal recessive hereditary trait. Syn. *Bassen-Kornzweig syndrome.*

abey·ance (a·bay′unce) *n.* [MF. *abeance,* expectation, desire]. 1. A cessation of activity or function. 2. A state of suspended animation.

ab·i·ent (ab′ee·unt) *adj.* [L. *abiens, abientis,* from *ab-,* away, + *ire,* to go]. Tending away from the source of a stimulus. Contr. *adient.*

Abi·es (ay′bee·eez, ab′ee·eez) *n.* [L.]. A genus of evergreen trees, the firs, belonging to the family Pinaceae.

Abies bal·sam·ea (bahl·sam′ee·uh). Balsam fir; the source of the oleoresin, known as fir balsam or Canada balsam, used as a microscopical mounting medium.

abi·et·ic (ay″bee·et′ick, ab″ee·et′ick) *adj.* Pertaining to the genus *Abies,* as abietic acid, which is present in the resin of *Abies* and other coniferous plants.

abietic acid. An acid, $C_{19}H_{29}COOH$, from the resin of various conifer species. The anhydride of the acid, or an isomeric form or modification of the anhydride, is the chief constituent of rosin.

abi·e·tin·ic acid (ay″bee·e·tin′ick, ab″ee·). ABIETIC ACID.

A bile. Bile collected from the common bile duct.

abio- [*a-,* without, un-, + *bio-*]. A combining form meaning (a) *nonliving;* (b) *nonviable.*

abio·gen·e·sis (ay″bye·o·jen′e·sis, ab″ee·o·) *n.* [*abio-* + *-gen-*

esis]. A theory that living organisms can originate from nonliving matter; spontaneous generation.

abio·ge·net·ic (ay″bye″o·je·net′ick, ab″ee·o·) *adj.* Characterized by or pertaining to abiogenesis.

abi·og·e·nous (ay″bye·oj′e·nus) *adj.* ABIOGENETIC.

abi·og·e·ny (ay″bye·oj′e·nee, ab″ee·) *n.* ABIOGENESIS.

abi·on·er·gy (ay″bye·on′ur·jee, ab″ee·) *n.* [*abio-* + *-ergy*]. ABIOTROPHY.

abi·o·sis (ay″bye·o′sis, ab″ee·) *n.* [*a-* + Gk. *biōsis*, way of life]. 1. Absence of life. 2. Nonviability. **—abi·ot·ic** (·ot′ick) *adj.*

abi·ot·ro·phy (ay″bye·ot′ruh·fee, ab″ee·) *n.* [*a-* + Gk. *biotroph*os, sustaining of life, + *-y*]. Loss of vitality such as to cause pathological deterioration and death of cells or tissue not associable with some mechanism such as infection or poisoning; or any condition presumed to be due to such a process, as baldness or Huntington's chorea; an old term introduced on the assumption that aging and degenerative disease represent the same defect of affected cells. **—abio·troph·ic** (ay″bye″o·trof′ick, ab″ee·o·trof′ick) *adj.*

ab·ir·ri·tant (ab·irr′i·tunt) *adj.* & *n.* [*ab-* + *irritant*]. 1. Tending to diminish irritation; soothing. 2. Pertaining to diminished sensitiveness. 3. An agent, such as a cream or powder, that relieves irritation. **—abirri·ta·tive** (·tuh·tiv) *adj.*; **abirri·tate** (·tate) *v.*

ab·ir·ri·ta·tion (ab·irr″i·tay′shun) *n.* [*ab-* + *irritation*]. Diminished tissue irritability; atony or asthenia.

ab·lac·ta·tion (ab″lack·tay′shun) *n.* [L. *ablactare*, to wean, from *ab-* + *lactare*, to give milk]. 1. The weaning of an infant. 2. The end of the period of mammary secretion.

ablas·tin (ay·blas′tin, ab·las′tin) *n.* [Gk. *ablast*os, not germinating, + *-in*]. An antibody-like substance, appearing in the blood of rats infected with trypanosomes, which inhibits reproduction of these organisms.

ab·late (ab·late′) *v.* [L. *auferre, ablatus*, to take away]. To remove, especially by cutting.

ab·la·tio (ab·lay′shee·o) *n.* [L.]. Detachment; removal; ablation.

ab·la·tion (ab·lay′shun) *n.* [L. *ablatio*, from *auferre*, to take away]. The removal of a part, as a tumor, by amputation, excision, or other mechanical means. **—ab·la·tive** (ab′luh·tiv, ab·lay′tiv) *adj.*

ablatio placentae. *Obsol.* ABRUPTIO PLACENTAE.

able·phar·ia (ay″blef·ăr′ee·uh, ab″lef·) *n.* [*a-* + *blephar-* + *-ia*]. A congenital defect marked by partial or total absence of the eyelids. **—ableph·a·rous** (ay·blef′uh·rus) *adj.*

ableph·a·ron (ay·blef′uh·ron) *n.* ABLEPHARIA.

ableph·a·ry (ay·blef′uh·ree) *n.* ABLEPHARIA.

ablep·sia (a·blep′see·uh) *n.* [Gk., blindness, from *blepsis*, sight, vision]. Loss or absence of vision.

ablep·sy (a·blep′see) *n.* ABLEPSIA.

ab·lu·ent (ab′lew·unt) *adj.* & *n.* [L. *abluere*, from *ab-*, away, + *lavare*, to wash]. 1. Detergent; cleansing. 2. A cleansing or washing agent, as a soap.

ab·lu·tion (uh·blew′shun) *n.* The act of washing or cleansing the body.

ab·mor·tal (ab·mor′tul) *adj.* [*ab-* + *mortal*]. Located or directed away from dead, dying, or injured tissue; applied particularly to electric currents generated in an injured organ, as a muscle.

ab·ner·val (ab·nur′vul) *adj.* [*ab-* + *nerve* + *-al*]. *Obsol.* Away from a nerve; denoting the direction of an electric current passing through muscle fibers away from the point of entrance of the nerve.

ab·neu·ral (ab·new′rul) *adj.* [*ab-* + *neural*]. *Obsol.* 1. Remote from the spinal or dorsal aspect; ventral. 2. Remote from the central nervous system. 3. ABNERVAL.

ab·nor·mal psychology. A branch of psychology dealing with mental processes and phenomena as well as abnormal behavior in pathologic states in subnormal as well as superior individuals and with special mental conditions such as dreams and hypnosis.

abnormal retinal correspondence. A condition found in concomitant strabismus, in which the patient, to avoid seeing double, makes the image formed at the extramacular area of the retina of the squinting eye "correspond" with the retinal image formed at the macula of the fixing eye. In the congruous or harmonious type of abnormal retinal correspondence, the subjective angle and the angle of anomaly are equal; in the incongruous or unharmonious type, the angles are unequal.

ABO blood group. That genetically determined blood group system defined by the agglutination reaction of erythrocytes exposed to the naturally occurring isoantibodies anti-A and anti-B and to similar antiserums. The serum of normal individuals contains isoantibodies against the antigens lacking in their erythrocytes, giving the following arrangement of antigens (isoagglutinogens) and antibodies:

Group (Landsteiner)	Erythrocyte Antigen (Agglutinogen)	Serum Antibody (Agglutinin)
O	A & B absent	anti-A, anti-B
A	A	anti-B
B	B	anti-A
AB	A,B	none

Subgroups of A are recognized and designated by subscripts, as A_1, A_2, etc.

ab·oma·si·tis (ab″o·muh·sigh′tis) *n.* [*abomas*um + *-itis*]. Inflammation of the abomasum.

ab·oma·sum (ab″o·may′sum) *n.*, pl. **aboma·sa** (·suh) [*ab-* + *omasum*]. The true digestive or glandular stomach of ruminants. Syn. *fourth stomach.*

ab·oma·sus (ab″o·may′sus) *n.*, pl. **aboma·si** (·sigh). ABOMASUM.

ab·orad (ab·o′rad) *adv.* & *adj.* [*abor*al + *-ad*]. Tending aborally; situated or directed away from the mouth.

ab·oral (ab·o′rul) *adj.* [*ab-* + *oral*]. Opposite to, or remote from, the mouth.

abort (uh·bort′) *v.* [L. *aboriri, abortus*, to be aborted, miscarried, from *ab-* + *oriri*, to come forth]. 1. To bring forth a nonviable fetus. 2. To terminate prematurely or stop in the early stages, as the course of a disease. 3. To check or fall short of maximal growth and development.

abort·ed systole. A premature cardiac systole, which produces no peripheral pulse wave because of minimal ventricular filling in the short preceding diastole.

abort·er, *n.* One who has undergone abortion, especially habitual or spontaneous abortion.

abor·ti·cide (uh·bor′ti·side) *n.* [*abort* + *-cide*]. 1. The killing of an unborn fetus. 2. An agent that destroys the fetus and produces abortion.

abor·tient (a·bor′shunt) *adj.* ABORTIFACIENT.

abor·ti·fa·cient (a·bor″ti·fay′shunt) *adj.* & *n.* [*abort* + *-facient*]. 1. Causing or inducing abortion. 2. A drug or agent inducing abortion.

abor·tin (a·bor′tin) *n.* [*abort*us + *-in*]. A broth filtrate of *Brucella abortus* used to elicit a reaction in patients with active brucellosis or in those who have recovered from the infection.

abortin reaction or **test.** The response in the skin to intracutaneous deposition of abortin. When positive, erythema and infiltration occur 1 to 3 days later, indicating active, or recovery from, brucellosis.

abor·tion (uh·bor′shun) *n.* [L. *abortio*, from *aboriri, abortus*, to be aborted, miscarried]. 1. The spontaneous or artificially induced expulsion of an embryo or fetus before it is viable. See also *miscarriage, premature delivery.* 2. The prematurely expelled product of conception; ABORTUS. 3. The checking or arrest of a process or disease before its development.

abor·tion·ist, *n.* A person who performs abortions, especially, one who performs them illegally.

abor·tive (uh·bor′tiv) *adj.* [L. *abortivus*]. 1. Prematurely born; undeveloped; immature; rudimentary. 2. Coming to an untimely end. 3. Checking the full development of a disease or cutting short its duration. 4. ABORTIFACIENT.

abortive poliomyelitis. A form of poliomyelitis characterized clinically by relatively mild symptoms which do not progress to central nervous system paralysis. Definite diagnosis rests upon isolation of the virus or serologic titer rise.

abortive typhoid. A form of typhoid fever characterized by an abrupt onset and subsidence of symptoms.

abor·tus (a·bor'tus) *n.*, pl. **abortuses** [L.]. An aborted fetus.

abortus bacillus. *BRUCELLA ABORTUS.*

abortus fever. A type of brucellosis caused by *Brucella abortus.*

abou·lia (a·boo'lee·uh) *n.* ABULIA.

abou·lo·ma·nia (a·boo"lo·may'nee·uh) *n.* ABULIA.

abra·chia (a·bray'kee·uh) *n.* [*a-* + *brachi-* + *-ia*]. Armlessness.

abra·chio·ceph·a·lia (a·bray"kee·o·se·fay'lee·uh) *n.* [*a-* + *brachio-* + *cephal-* + *-ia*]. Congenital absence of the head and arms.

abra·chio·ceph·a·lus (a·bray"kee·o·sef'uh·lus) *n.* [*a-* + *brachio-* + *cephalus*]. A headless and armless omphalosite.

abra·chi·us (a·bray'kee·us) *n.* [*a-* + *brachi-* + *-us*]. An armless individual.

abrad·ant (uh·bray'dunt) *n.* An abrasive.

abrade (uh·braid') *v.* [L. *abradere*, to scrape off, from *radere*, to scrape]. To rub or scrape away, to erode by friction.

abra·sion (uh·bray'zhun) *n.* [L. *abrasio*, from *abradere*, to scrape off]. 1. A spot denuded of skin, mucous membrane, or superficial epithelium by rubbing or scraping, as a corneal abrasion; an excoriation. 2. The mechanical wearing down of teeth, as from incorrect brushing, poorly fitting dental devices, or bruxism. Compare *attrition*, *dental erosion.*

abra·sive (uh·bray'siv, ·ziv) *adj.* & *n.* 1. Tending to abrade. 2. An agent or mechanical device used to scrape or rub off the external layers of a part; specifically, a substance such as carborundum, diamond chips, or pumice, used for grinding or polishing dental tissues or appliances.

abra·sor (uh·bray'zur) *n.* Any file or instrument used in the abrasion of a surface; a rasp.

ab·re·ac·tion (ab"ree·ack'shun) *n.* [*ab-* + *reaction*]. *In psychoanalysis,* the mental process by which repressed emotionally charged memories and experiences are brought to consciousness and relived with appropriate release. It may also occur in hypnosis and narcoanalysis.

ab·ric (ab'rick) *n.* FLOWERS OF SULFUR.

abridged A. O. color vision test. Abridged version of American Optical Company's charts, a group of pseudoisochromatic plates designed to detect color-vision deficiency.

Abri·ko·sov's or **Abri·ko·soff's tumor** (ah·bree·koh'suf) [A. I. *Abrikosov,* Russian pathologist, 1875–1955]. GRANULAR-CELL MYOBLASTOMA.

abro·sia (a·bro'zhuh, ·zee·uh) *n.* [Gk. *abrōsia*, from *a-* + *brōsis*, food, eating]. Abstinence from food; fasting.

ab·rup·tio (ab·rup'tee·o, ·shee·o) *n.* [L., from *ab-* + *rumpere, ruptus,* to break]. Abruption; a tearing away.

abruptio pla·cen·tae (pla·sen'tee). Premature separation of the placenta prior to delivery of the infant.

ab·scess (ab'sess) *n.* [L. *abscessus*, lit., withdrawal, from *ab(s)-*, away, off, + *cedere, cessus,* to go; tr. of Gk. *apostēma* (see *apostem*)]. A focus of suppuration within a tissue, organ, or region of the body. See also *microabscess, cold abscess.*

ab·sces·sus (ab·ses'us) *n.* [L.]. ABSCESS.

abscessus flat·u·o·sus (flat"yoo·o'sus). TYMPANITIC ABSCESS.

abscessus per de·cu·bi·tum (de·kew'bi·tum). WANDERING ABSCESS.

ab·scis·sa (ab·sis'uh) *n.* [L. *abscissum*, from *abscindere*, to cut off]. 1. The horizontal of the two coordinates used in plotting the interrelationship of two sets of data. Contr. *ordinate.* 2. *In optics,* the point where a ray of light crosses the principal axis.

ab·scis·sion (ab·sish'un, ab·sizh'un) *n.* [L. *abscissio*, from *abscindere*, to take away]. Removal of a part by cutting.

ab·scon·sio (ab·skon'see·o, ·shee·o) *n.* [L.]. A cavity, depression, or recess, either normal or pathologic; especially one in bone which conceals the head of a contiguous bone.

ab·scop·al (ab'sko·pul, ab·skop'ul) *adj.* [L. *ab*, off, away from, + *scopus*, mark, target, from Gk. *skopos*]. Occurring at a distance from the irradiated volume, but within the same organism; said of certain effects of radiation.

ab·sence, *n.* 1. Inattention to one's environment. 2. Temporary loss of consciousness, as in absence attacks or psychomotor seizures.

absence attack or **seizure.** A seizure characterized by a sudden transient lapse of consciousness, by a blank stare, as in a state of "suspended animation," sometimes accompanied by minor motor activities such as blinking of the eyes, smacking of lips, stereotyped hand movements and automatism, often occurring many times in succession; seen in petit mal epilepsy; associated with a typical three per second spike-and-wave pattern on the electroencephalogram. Syn. *petit mal seizure.* See also *minor motor seizure, psychomotor seizure.*

absence epilepsy. PETIT MAL EPILEPSY.

absence status. Absence attacks persisting for many minutes or even hours with no interval of normal mental activity between attacks.

ab·sen·tia epi·lep·ti·ca (ab·sen'shee·uh ep·i·lep'ti·kuh). ABSENCE ATTACK.

absent respiration. Inaudibility of respiratory sounds on auscultation of the chest.

abs. feb. Abbreviation for *absente febre;* in the absence of fever.

Ab·sid·ia (ab·sid'ee·uh) *n.* *MUCOR.*

ab·sinthe, ab·sinth (ab'sinth) *n.* [F.]. A green French liqueur composed of an alcoholic solution of absinthium, anise, and marjoram oils, and other aromatics.

ab·sinth·ism (ab'sinth·iz·um) *n.* A morbid state observed in acute or chronic abusers of absinthe, characterized by neuritis, hyperesthesia, and hallucinations. Acute excess may cause convulsions, psychotic manifestations, or paralysis.

ab·sin·thi·um (ab·sinth'ee·um) *n.* [L., from Gk. *apsinthion*]. Common wormwood; the leaves and tops of *Artemisia absinthium.* Has been used as an aromatic bitter, diaphoretic, anthelmintic, and flavoring agent.

ab·so·lute, *adj.* 1. Simple; pure; free from admixture. 2. Unlimited and unqualified. 3. Complete; entire; real. 4. *In physics,* derived from basic data, not arbitrary. Abbreviated, A.

absolute accommodation or **adjustment.** Accommodation of each eye considered individually.

absolute alcohol. DEHYDRATED ALCOHOL.

absolute blood count. The total number of each different type of leukocyte per unit volume of blood.

absolute cell increase. A rise in the number of leukocytes of a particular type per unit volume of blood. The absolute number of the cells of a given variety equals the total leukocyte count multiplied by the percentage of cells of that variety.

absolute constant. A constant that retains the same value under all circumstances.

absolute density. 1. The ratio of the mass of a substance to its volume. Compare *specific gravity.* 2. The light-absorbing power of the silver image in photographic materials.

absolute ether. Ether (3) containing no alcohol or water.

absolute field. The entire field of vision corresponding to the extreme extent of the intact retina.

absolute glaucoma. The completed glaucomatous process when the eyeball is hard and totally blind.

absolute humidity. The mass of water vapor per unit volume of air.

absolute hyperopia. Manifest hyperopia that cannot be corrected completely by accommodation, so that there is indistinct vision even for distance without corrective lenses.

absolute joule. JOULE (1).
absolute near point. The near point for either eye alone at which no effort at accommodation is made.
absolute refractory period. The refractory period during which no stimulus, however strong, can elicit a response.
absolute scotoma. Scotoma with perception of light entirely absent.
absolute temperature. Temperature reckoned from absolute zero.
absolute threshold. The lowest intensity, as measured under optimal experimental conditions, at which a stimulus is effective or perceived.
absolute zero. A temperature of approximately −273.2°C, or −459.7°F; the complete absence of heat.
ab·sorb, *v.* 1. In *physiology,* to take up or assimilate through a membrane or into a tissue, as products of digestion through gastrointestinal mucosa, or medicinal agents into the skin. 2. *In physics, radiology, and spectrophotometry,* to retain by conversion to another form, as radiant energy by conversion to heat or to some other form of molecular energy.
ab·sorb·able, *adj.* Capable of being absorbed.
absorbable cellulose. OXIDIZED CELLULOSE.
absorbable dusting powder. A biologically absorbable powder prepared from cornstarch by introducing certain ether linkages, and containing also 2% magnesium oxide; used as a surgeon's glove lubricant.
absorbable gelatin film. A sterile, non-antigenic, water-insoluble gelatin film prepared from a gelatin-formaldehyde; used both as a protective and as a temporary supportive structure in surgical membrane repair.
absorbable ligature. A ligature composed of degradable material, such as catgut, which can be absorbed by the tissues after enzymatic breakdown.
absorbable surgical suture. A sterile strand prepared from collagen derived from healthy mammals and capable of being absorbed by living tissue.
ab·sorb·ance (ub·sor'bunce) *n.* In applied spectroscopy, the negative logarithm, to the base 10, of transmittance. The term optical density has been used to express the absorbance of solutions. Symbol, *A.*
absorbed dose. *In radiology,* the amount of energy imparted by ionizing particles to a unit mass of irradiated material at a place of interest. Symbol, D. See also *rad.*
ab·sor·be·fa·cient (ab·sor"be·fay'shunt) *adj. & n.* [*absorb* + *-facient*]. 1. Causing or promoting absorption. 2. Any agent that promotes absorption.
ab·sorb·en·cy (ub·sor'bun·see) *n.* 1. The state or quality of being absorbent. 2. ABSORBANCE.
ab·sorb·ent (ub·sor'bunt, ub·zor'bunt) *adj. & n.* 1. Capable of absorbing fluids, gases, or light waves. 2. A drug, application, or dressing that promotes absorption of diseased tissues.
absorbent cotton. Cotton deprived of fatty matter so that it readily absorbs water.
ab·sorb·er, *n. In nuclear science,* any material that absorbs ionizing radiation.
ab·sorp·ti·om·e·ter (ab·sorp"shee·om'e·tur) *n.* 1. An instrument which determines the solubility of a gas, or the amount absorbed. 2. An apparatus which measures the thickness of a layer of fluid between two parallel sheets of plate glass in apparent apposition.
ab·sorp·tion (ub·sorp'shun, ·zorp') *n.* [L. *absorptio,* from *absorbere,* to swallow]. The state or process of being absorbed or the process of absorbing, as assimilation through a membrane or retention of radiant energy in a tissue by conversion to heat.
absorption atelectasis. OBSTRUCTIVE ATELECTASIS.
absorption band. A region of the absorption spectrum in which the absorptivity passes through a maximum or inflection.
absorption coefficient. A constant in the law of absorption for homogeneous radiations, $I_d = I_o e^{-\mu d}$, where I_o is the intensity of the radiation beam falling on an absorber of the thickness *d; e,* the base of the natural system of logarithms; I_d, the intensity of the beam after it emerges from the absorber; and μ, the linear absorption coefficient. μ divided by the density of the absorber is called the mass absorption coefficient.
absorption curve. *In radiobiology,* a curve showing variation in absorption of radiation as a function of wavelength.
absorption lens. A lens, used in eyeglasses, that selectively absorbs certain wavelengths of light and prevents these from reaching the retina.
absorption spectrum. 1. A spectrum of radiation which has passed through some selectively absorbing substance, as white light after it has passed through a vapor. Contr. *emission spectrum.* 2. ABSORPTION CURVE.
absorption test. The analysis of antigenic relationships and composition of bacterial cells and large molecules by reacting with a number of specific agglutinative or precipitating antibodies in succession and following the prior removal of the formed aggregates or precipitates by centrifugation. Useful in demonstrating shared and distinctive antigenic components of bacteria and other macromolecular structures.
ab·sorp·tive (ub·sorp'tiv) *adj.* Pertaining to absorption; absorbent.
ab·sorp·tiv·i·ty (ab"sorp·tiv'i·tee) *n. In spectrophotometry,* the ratio of the absorbance to the product of concentration and length of optical path; it is the absorbance per unit concentration and thickness (commonly 1 g of substance per 100 ml of solution, measured in a cell with an optical path of 1 cm). Symbol, *a.*
ab·sti·nence (ab'sti·nunce) *n.* Voluntary self-denial of or forbearance from indulgence of appetites, especially from food, alcoholic drink, or sexual intercourse.
abstinence delirium. Delirium occurring on withdrawal of alcohol or of a drug from one addicted to it.
abstinence syndrome. WITHDRAWAL SYNDROME.
ab·strac·tion (ab·strack'shun) *n.* [L. *abstractio,* from *abstrahere,* to draw away]. 1. Removal or separation of one or more ingredients from a compound, as an abstract from a crude drug. 2. Absorption of the mind; absent-mindedness; inattention to what goes on about oneself. 3. *In psychology,* isolation of a meaning or characteristic from a totality which is unique and inaccessible to comparison; may be performed by thinking, feeling, sensation, or intuition. 4. Bloodletting.
ab·u·leia (ab"yoo·lee'uh) *n.* ABULIA.
abu·lia (a·bew'lee·uh, a·boo'lee·uh) *n.* [Gk. *aboulia,* irresolution, indecision, from *boulē,* will, determination]. 1. *In psychiatry,* loss or defect of the ability to make decisions. See also *folie du doute.* 2. *In neurology,* failure in a conscious, alert, non-schizophrenic patient with intact motor capacity and understanding to respond adequately to internal or external stimuli by voluntary motor activity; in extreme cases may take the form of transient akinetic mutism; frequently associated with lesions of the frontal lobes. —**abu·lic** (·ick) *adj.*
abu·lo·ma·nia (a·bew"lo·may'nee·uh) *n.* ABULIA.
abut·ment (uh·but'munt) *n.* [OF. *abouter,* to fix the limits of]. A tooth used to support or stabilize a prosthetic appliance. —**abut,** *v.*
ab·volt (ab'vohlt) *n.* [*ab-* + *volt*]. A cgs electromagnetic unit of potential equivalent to 10^{-8} volt.
AC Abbreviation for (a) *air conduction;* (b) *alternating current;* (c) *anodic closure;* (d) *acromioclavicular.*
Ac 1. Symbol for actinium. 2. Abbreviation for *acetyl.*
ac, a.c., a-c Abbreviation for *alternating current.*
a.c. Abbreviation for *ante cibum;* before meals.
Aca·cia (uh·kay'shuh) *n.* A large genus of woody plants of the Leguminosae, found in warm regions, many being native to Africa and Australia.
acacia, *n.* The dried gummy exudate from the stems and

branches of *Acacia senegal* (Linné) Willdenow, or of some other African species of *Acacia,* occurring in translucent or somewhat opaque white to yellowish-white spheroidal tears; almost completely soluble in water. Consists of calcium, magnesium, and potassium salts of the polysaccharide arabic acid. Used as a suspending agent and, formerly, as a demulcent. Syn. *gum arabic, acacia gum.*

Acacia senegal. The most important of several African species of *Acacia* yielding gum arabic (acacia).

acal·ci·co·sis (ay·kal″si·ko′sis, uh·kal″) *n.* [*a-* + *calcic* + *-osis*]. The condition resulting from a diet continuously low in calcium.

acal·cu·lia (ay″kal·kew′lee·uh) *n.* [*a-* + L. *calcul*are, to calculate, + *-ia*]. Inability to learn or to do even the simplest arithmetical problems.

acamp·sia (ay·kamp′see·uh, uh·kamp′) *n.* [Gk. *akampsia,* inflexibility, from *kamptein,* to bend]. Inflexibility or rigidity of a joint or limb; ANKYLOSIS.

acanth-, acantho- [Gk. *akantha,* thorn]. A combining form meaning (a) *thorn, thorny;* (b) *spine, spiny;* (c) *prickle cell.*

acan·thes·the·sia, acan·thaes·the·sia (a·kanth″es·theezh′uh, ·theez′ee·uh) *n.* [*acanth-* + *esthesia*]. An abnormal sensation of being pricked with needles.

acan·thi·on, akan·thi·on (a·kanth′ee·on) *n.* [Gk. *akanthion,* a little thorn]. *In craniometry,* a point at the tip of the anterior nasal spine. **—acan·thi·al** (·ee·ul) *adj.*

acantho-. See *acanth-.*

acan·tho·am·e·lo·blas·to·ma (uh·kan″tho·am″e·lo·blas·to′muh) *n.* An ameloblastoma in which the cells are of the squamous or prickle-cell type.

Acan·tho·ceph·a·la (uh·kan″tho·sef′uh·luh) *n.pl.* [NL., from *acantho-* + Gk. *cephalē,* head]. A phylum of thorny-headed worms; adults are intestinal parasites of vertebrates, rarely of man. **—acanthocepha·lan** (·lun) *adj.*

acan·tho·ceph·a·li·a·sis (uh·kan″tho·sef″uh·lye′uh·sis) *n.* Infection by worms of the phylum Acanthocephala.

Acan·tho·chei·lo·ne·ma (uh·kan″tho·kigh″lo·nee′muh) *n.* [*acantho-* + *cheilo-* + *-nema*]. A genus of filariae.

acan·tho·chei·lo·ne·mi·a·sis (uh·kan″tho·kigh″lo·ne·migh′uh·sis) *n.* [*Acanthocheilonema* + *-iasis*]. DIPETALONEMIASIS.

acan·tho·cyte (uh·kan′tho·site) *n.* [*acantho-* + *-cyte*]. A malformed red blood cell characterized, in wet preparations, by projecting spines or spicules, giving the cell a thorny or burr-shaped appearance.

acan·tho·cy·to·sis (uh·kan″tho·sigh·to′sis) *n.* Large numbers of acanthocytes in the peripheral blood; characteristic of the congenital disorder abetalipoproteinemia.

acan·thoid (uh·kan′thoid) *adj.* [*acanth-* + *-oid*]. Resembling a spine; spinous.

acan·tho·ker·a·to·der·mia (uh·kan″tho·kerr″uh·to·dur′mee·uh) *n.* [*acantho-* + *keratodermia*]. Thickening of the horny layer of the skin of the hands or feet.

acan·tho·ker·a·to·ma (uh·kan″tho·kerr″uh·to′muh) *n.* KERATOACANTHOMA.

acan·thol·y·sis (ack″an·thol′i·sis, uh·kan″tho·lye′sis) *n.,* pl. **acantholy·ses** (·seez) [*acantho-* + *lysis*]. Loss of cohesion between epidermal cells or adnexal keratocytes due to degeneration of the intercellular cement substance or faulty formation of the intercellular bridges. Compare *acanthorrhexis.* **—acan·tho·lyt·ic** (uh·kan″tho·lit′ick) *adj.*

acantholysis bullosa. EPIDERMOLYSIS BULLOSA.

ac·an·tho·ma (ack″an·tho′muh) *n.,* pl. **acanthomas, acanthoma·ta** (·tuh) [*acanth-* + *-oma*]. 1. Any mass composed of the prickle-cell type of squamous cells; it may be benign or malignant, hyperplastic or neoplastic. 2. Well-differentiated squamous cell carcinoma.

acanthoma ad·e·noi·des cys·ti·cum (ad·e·noy′deez sis′ti·kum). TRICHOEPITHELIOMA.

acan·tho·pel·vis (uh·kan″tho·pel′vis) *n.* [*acantho-* + *pelvis*]. PELVIS SPINOSA.

acan·tho·pel·yx (uh·kan″tho·pel′icks) *n.* [*acantho-* + Gk. *pelyx,* bowl]. PELVIS SPINOSA.

Acan·tho·phis (a·kan′tho·fis) *n.* [*acanth-* + Gk. *ophis,* snake]. A genus of snakes of the family Elapidae.

Acanthophis ant·arc·ti·cus (ant·ahrk′ti·kus). The death adder of Australia and New Guinea which possesses a neurotoxic venom.

acan·thor·rhex·is (uh·kan″tho·reck′sis, ack″an·tho·) *n.* [*acantho-* + *-rrhexis*]. The process of rupture of the intercellular bridges of the prickle-cell layer of the epidermis due to increasing intercellular edema resulting from certain inflammatory conditions affecting the epidermis. Compare *acantholysis.*

ac·an·tho·sis (ack″an·tho′sis) *n.,* pl. **acantho·ses** (·seez) [*acanth-* + *-osis*]. Any abnormal condition of the prickle-cell layer of the epidermis, particularly hypertrophy. Compare *acanthoma.* **—acan·thot·ic** (·thot′ick) *adj.*

acanthosis nig·ri·cans (nig′ri·kanz, nigh′gri·). Hyperpigmentation of the body folds, especially of the axillae, associated with verrucous skin lesions at such sites. See also *benign acanthosis nigricans, malignant acanthosis nigricans, pseudo-acanthosis nigricans.*

acan·thro·cyte (uh·kan′thro·site) *n.* [*acanth-* + eryth*rocyte*]. ACANTHOCYTE.

acan·thro·cy·to·sis (uh·kan″thro·sigh·to′sis) *n.* ACANTHOCYTOSIS.

acap·nia (ay·kap′nee·uh) *n.* [NL., from Gk. *akapnos,* without smoke, from *kapnos,* smoke]. Subnormal concentration of carbon dioxide in the blood. Syn. *hypocapnia.* **—acap·ni·al** (·nee·ul) *adj.*

acap·su·lar (ay·kap′sue·lur) *adj. In biology,* without a capsule.

acar-, acari-, acaro- [Gk. *akari,* mite]. A combining form meaning (a) *mite;* (b) *itch.*

acar·a·cide (a·kăr′uh·side) *n.* ACARICIDE.

acar·dia (ay·kahr′dee·uh) *n.* [*acard*ius + *-ia*]. Congenital absence of the heart, usually in omphalosites. **—acar·di·ac** (·dee·ack) *adj. & n.*

acar·di·a·cus (ay″kahr·dye′uh·kus, ack″ahr·) *n.* [NL., acardiac]. An omphalosite completely lacking a heart.

acardiacus acephalus. An omphalosite without a head.

acardiacus amorphus. ANIDEUS.

acardiacus an·ceps (an′seps). ANIDEUS.

acar·dio·he·mia, acar·dio·hae·mia (ay·kahr″dee·o·hee′mee·uh, a·kahr″) *n.* [*a-* + *cardio-* + *hem-* + *-ia*]. Lack of blood in the heart.

acar·dio·tro·phia (ay·kahr″dee·o·tro′fee·uh, a·kahr″) *n.* [*a-* + *cardio-* + *troph-* + *-ia*]. Atrophy of the heart.

acar·di·us (a·kahr′dee·us, ay·kahr′) *n.* [Gk. *akardios,* heartless, from *kardia,* heart]. A parasitic twin that lacks a heart, usually an omphalosite.

acari. Plural of *acarus.*

acari-. See *acar-.*

acar·i·an (a·kăr′ee·un) *n.* ACARID.

ac·a·ri·a·sis (ack″uh·rye′uh·sis) *n.,* pl. **acaria·ses** (·seez). Any condition, usually a dermatitis, caused by an acarid or mite.

acar·i·cide (a·kăr′i·side) *n.* An agent that destroys acarids.

ac·a·rid (ack′uh·rid) *n.* [Gk. *akari*]. A tick or mite. **—acar·i·dan** (a·kăr′i·dun), **ac·a·rid·i·an** (ack″uh·rid′ee·un) *adj. & n.*

Ac·a·ri·na (ack″uh·rye′nuh, ·ree′nuh) *n.pl.* [NL., from Gk. *akari,* mite]. An order of Arachnida comprising the ticks and mites. Many species are important vectors of bacterial, protozoan, rickettsial, and spirochetal diseases. In addition, severe reactions may result from their bites.

ac·a·ri·no·sis (ack″uh·ri·no′sis, a·kăr″i·) *n.,* pl. **acarino·ses** (·seez) [*Acarina* + *-osis*]. ACARIASIS.

acar·i·o·sis (a·kăr″ee·o′sis) *n.,* pl. **acario·ses** (·seez) ACARIASIS.

acaro-. See *acar-.*

ac·a·ro·der·ma·ti·tis (ack″uh·ro·dur″muh·tye′tis) *n.* Any dermatitis caused by an acarid or mite.

acarodermatitis ur·ti·car·i·oi·des (ur″ti·kăr·ee·oy′deez). An urticarial and pruritic dermatitis resulting from contact with plant products infested with various species of mites.

ac·a·roid (ack′uh·roid) *adj.* [*acar-* + *-oid*]. Mitelike.

ac·a·ro·pho·bia (ack″uh·ro·fo·bee·uh, a·kăr″o·) *n.* [*acaro-* + *phobia*]. 1. Morbid fear of mites or of certain small animate or inanimate things, as worms or pins. 2. The delusion of being infested with parasites.
ac·a·ro·tox·ic (ack″uh·ro·tock′sick) *adj.* Poisonous or destructive to acarids.
acar·pous (ay·kahr′pus) *adj.* [Gk. *akarpos,* without fruit, from *karpos,* fruit]. 1. Having no elevations; not nodular. 2. Producing no fruit; sterile; barren.
Ac·a·rus (ack′uh·rus) *n.* [NL., from Gk. *akari,* mite]. A genus formerly including many kinds of mite, now limited to the cheese mites. **—acarus,** pl. **aca·ri** (·rye), *com. n.*
Acarus folliculorum. DEMODEX FOLLICULORUM.
Acarus scabiei. SARCOPTES SCABIEI.
acaryote. AKARYOTE.
acat·a·la·se·mia, acat·a·la·sae·mia (ay·kat″uh·lay·see′mee·uh) *n.* [*a-* + *catalase* + *-emia*]. Deficiency of the enzyme catalase in the blood. See also *acatalasia.*
acat·a·la·sia (ay″kat·uh·lay′zhuh, ·zee·uh) *n.* [*a-* + *catalase* + *-ia*]. A congenital absence of the enzyme catalase, a rare disease occurring mostly in the Japanese.
acat·a·lep·sia (ay·kat″uh·lep′see·uh) *n.* [Gk. *akatalēpsia,* inability to understand, from *katalēpsis,* grasping, seizure]. 1. Abnormal inability to understand. 2. Uncertainty in diagnosis. **—acatalep·tic** (·tick) *adj. & n.*
acat·a·lep·sy (ay·kat′uh·lep″see) *n.* ACATALEPSIA.
acat·a·ma·the·sia (a·kat″uh·muh·theezh′uh, ·theez′ee·uh) *n.* [*a-* + Gk. *katamathēsis,* thorough knowledge, + *-ia*]. *Obsol.* 1. Inability to understand conversation. 2. Pathologic blunting or deterioration of the senses, as in cortical deafness and blindness.
acat·a·pha·sia (ay·kat″uh·fay′zhuh, ·zee·uh) *n.* [*a-* + Gk. *kataphasis,* affirmation, + *-ia*]. SYNTACTIC APHASIA.
ac·a·tap·o·sis (ack″uh·tap′uh·sis) *n.* [*a-* + Gk. *kataposis,* swallowing]. *Obsol.* DYSPHAGIA.
ac·a·tas·ta·sia (ack″uh·tas·tay′zhuh, ·zee·uh) *n.* [Gk. *akatastasia,* disorder]. Irregularity; nonconformation to type; variation from the normal. **—acatas·tat·ic** (·tat′ick) *adj.*
ac·a·thex·ia (ack″uh·theck′see·uh) *n.* [*a-* + Gk. *kathexis,* retention, holding, + *-ia*]. Failure or inability to retain bodily secretions and excretions. **—aca·thec·tic** (·thek′tick) *adj.*
ac·a·thex·is (ack″uh·theck′sis) *n.* [*a-* + *cathexis*]. *In psychiatry,* lack of affect toward some thing or idea which unconsciously is very important to the individual.
acathisia. AKATHISIA.
acau·dal (ay·kaw′dul, a·kaw′dul) *adj.* [*a-* + *caudal*]. Tailless.
acau·date (ay·kaw′date, a·kaw′) *adj.* [*a-* + *caudate*]. Tailless.
Acc. An abbreviation for *accommodation.*
A.C.C. American College of Cardiology.
ac·cel·er·ans (ack·sel′ur·anz) *n.* [L., hastening]. *Obsol.* ACCELERATOR NERVE.
ac·cel·er·ant (ack·sel′ur·unt) *n.* ACCELERATOR (1).
accelerated hypertension. MALIGNANT HYPERTENSION.
accelerating fibers. Sympathetic nerve fibers which convey impulses that hasten the rapidity of the heatbeat and increase the force of the cardiac contractions.
ac·cel·er·a·tion, *n.* 1. Quickening, as of the pulse or the respiration. 2. Change of velocity (linear acceleration) or of direction of movement (centrifugal acceleration). See also *G.* 3. Advancement in physical growth beyond the norm for one's age and sex, applied particularly to bone age and height. 4. Advancement in intellectual growth or scholastic achievement beyond the average of one's age. 5. *In chemistry,* increase in the rate of a chemical reaction. **—ac·cel·er·ate,** *v.*
ac·cel·er·a·tor, *n.* 1. Any agent or part which quickens the speed of a function or process. 2. A machine, such as the betatron, cyclotron, linear accelerator, or synchrotron, that accelerates electrically charged atomic particles such as electrons, protons, deuterons, and alpha particles to nearly the speed of light. Syn. *atom smasher.* 3. CATALYST (2). **—ac·cel·er·a·to·ry** (ack·sel′ur·uh·tor″ee) *adj.*
accelerator globulin. FACTOR V. Abbreviated, AcG.
accelerator nerves. The cardiac sympathetic nerves, which when stimulated cause acceleration of the heart rate and increased cardiac contractile force.
accelerator uri·nae (yoor·eye′nee). BULBOSPONGIOSUS.
acceleratory reflex. Any reflex originating in the labyrinth of the inner ear in response to an increase or decrease in the rate of movement of the head. Syn. *kinetic reflex.*
ac·cel·er·in (ack·sel′ur·in) *n.* FACTOR VI.
ac·cel·er·om·e·ter (ack·sel″ur·om′e·tur) *n.* An instrument for measuring acceleration.
ac·cen·tu·a·tor (ack·sen′choo·ay″tur) *n.* A chemical substance which intensifies the action of a tissue stain.
ac·cep·tor (ack·sep′tur) *n.* A substance which accepts or combines with a product of a chemical reaction; applied especially to those substances which increase the rate of a reaction by acting as intermediaries in transferring another substance, such as hydrogen, from a reactant to the final product. See also *hydrogen acceptor.*
acceptor-control index. RESPIRATORY CONTROL INDEX.
ac·ces·sion (ack·sesh′un) *n.* An addition, as to a set of something.
ac·ces·sion·al (ack·sesh′un·ul) *adj.* Pertaining to an accession; additional.
accessional dentition. The eruption of those teeth which are not preceded by deciduous teeth; in man, the permanent molars.
ac·ces·so·ri·us (ack″ses·o′ree·us) *adj. & n.* [ML.]. 1. Accessory. 2. Quadratus plantae. See Table of Muscles in the Appendix. 3. ILIOCOSTALIS THORACIS.
accessorius ad flex·o·rem car·pi ra·di·a·lem (ad fleck·so′rum kahr′pye ray″dee·ay′lem). A variable additional slip of the flexor carpi radialis.
accessorius ad flex·o·rem di·gi·to·rum pro·fun·dum (ad fleck·so′rum dij·i·to′rum pro·fun′dum). An occasional additional slip of the flexor digitorum profundus, originating from the coronoid process of the ulna and usually associated with the tendons for the middle and index fingers.
accessorius ad flexorem pol·li·cis lon·gum (pol′i·sis long′gum). A variable extra part of the flexor pollicis longus.
accessorius of the gluteus minimus. An occasional slip of muscle lying under the gluteus minimus and inserted into the capsule of the hip joint.
ac·ces·so·ry (ack·ses′uh·ree) *adj. & n.* [ML. *accessorius,* from *accedere,* to be added]. Auxiliary, assisting; applied especially to a lesser organ or part which supplements a similar organ or part.
accessory auricle. CERVICAL AURICLE.
accessory canaliculi. The inconstant canals at the outer edge of the anterior condyloid foramen giving passage to veins.
accessory chromosome. MONOSOME.
accessory cuneate nucleus. A group of cells lying lateral to the main cuneate nucleus whose axons form the dorsal external arcuate fibers which reach the cerebellum by way of the inferior cerebellar peduncle. NA *nucleus cuneatus accessorius.*
accessory flocculus. PARAFLOCCULUS.
accessory ganglion. One of several vestigial ganglions associated with the embryonic dorsal roots of the vagus nerve and also with the hypoglossal nerve in certain mammals.
accessory gland. A mass of glandular tissue separate from the main body of a gland of similar structure.
accessory goiter. Aberrant goiter. See *goiter.*
accessory lacrimal gland. The palpebral part of a lacrimal gland. See also *Krause's gland, Rosenmueller's gland.*
accessory lobe of the parotid. A small, separate part of the parotid gland, usually found immediately above the duct.
accessory medial nucleus. A nucleus located at the edge of the central gray matter dorsomediad to the red nucleus in the upper midbrain.
accessory movement. SYNKINESIA.
accessory muscle. A muscle slip additional to the usual

components of a muscle, such as the scalenus minimus.

accessory nasal cartilages. Variable small plates of cartilage situated in each ala of the nose near the lateral margin of the lateral nasal cartilage. NA *cartilagines nasales accessoriae.*

accessory nasal sinus. PARANASAL SINUS.

accessory nerve. The eleventh cranial nerve, a motor nerve having both a bulbar origin along the lateral aspect of the medulla oblongata and a spinal origin from the upper five or six cervical segments. The bulbar part (internal ramus) runs with the vagus, sending motor fibers to the striate muscles of the larynx and pharynx. The spinal portion (external ramus) innervates the trapezius and sternocleidomastoid muscles. NA *nervus accessorius.* See also Table of Nerves in the Appendix.

accessory nucleus of the facial nerve. A small group of motor cells, dorsomedial to and functionally a part of the facial nucleus.

accessory nucleus of the oculomotor nerve. AUTONOMIC NUCLEUS OF THE OCULOMOTOR NERVE.

accessory olivary nucleus. See *dorsal accessory olivary nucleus, medial accessory olivary nucleus.*

accessory olive. ACCESSORY OLIVARY NUCLEUS.

accessory organs of the eye. ADNEXA OCULI.

accessory pancreas. A small mass of glandular structure similar to the pancreas and adjacent to it. NA *pancreas accessorium.*

accessory pancreatic duct. The proximal part of the dorsal pancreatic duct that usually persists. Syn. *duct of Santorini, Bernard's duct.* NA *ductus pancreaticus accessorius.*

accessory parotid gland. A small auxiliary parotid gland. NA *glandula parotis accessoria.*

accessory peroneal muscle. PERONEUS ACCESSORIUS.

accessory placenta. PLACENTA SUCCENTURIATA.

accessory process. A small tubercle situated at the back part of the base of the transverse process of the lumbar vertebrae. NA *processus accessorius vertebrarum lumbalium.*

accessory pterygoid. An occasional slip of muscle extending from the body of the sphenoid to the lateral pterygoid plate.

accessory root canal. A branching of a main tooth root canal.

accessory sign. A nonpathognomonic sign.

accessory spleen. A small mass of splenic tissue found either isolated or connected to the spleen by thin bands of splenic tissue. NA *lien accessorius.*

accessory stomach. ENTERIC CYST.

accessory suprarenal glands. Variable nodules that contain cortical or cortical and medullary suprarenal tissue. The nodules are usually small and are usually found near the main suprarenal glands. NA *glandulae suprarenales accessoriae.*

accessory symptom. A nonpathognomonic symptom. Syn. *assident symptom.*

accessory thyroid glands. Variable nodules of thyroid gland tissue that may be found anywhere from the base of the tongue to the upper mediastinum. NA *glandulae thyroideae accessoriae.*

ac·ci·dent, *n.* 1. *In legal medicine,* an event occurring to an individual without his expectation, and without the possibility of his preventing it at the moment of its occurrence. 2. An intercurrent or complicating symptom or event, not encountered in the regular course of a disease.

ac·ci·den·tal, *adj.* 1. Occurring outside the normal expectation. 2. Occurring by chance, or mischance.

accidental albuminuria. FALSE PROTEINURIA.

accidental bursa. An inconstant bursa due to friction or pressure.

accidental image. AFTERIMAGE.

ac·ci·den·tal·ism (ack″si·den′tul·iz·um) *n.* A system of medicine based on symptoms only, disregarding etiology or pathology.

accidental proteinuria. FALSE PROTEINURIA.

accidental symptom. A symptom present during the course of a disease but which has no relationship to the disease.

accident neurosis. TRAUMATIC NEUROSIS.

accident-prone, *adj.* Predisposed to accidents, due to psychological causes. —**accident-prone·ness,** *n.*

ac·cip·i·ter (ack·sip′i·tur) *n.* [L., hawk]. A facial bandage, no longer in general use, with tails radiating like the claws of a hawk.

ac·cli·ma·tion (ack″li·may′shun) *n.* ACCLIMATIZATION. —**ac·cli·mate** (ack′li·mate) *v.*

ac·cli·ma·ti·za·tion (a·klye″muh·ti·zay′shun) *n.* The process of adjusting to a strange or foreign climate, soil, or water, applied to plants, animals, and people. —**ac·cli·ma·tize** (a·klye′muh·tize) *v.*

ac·com·mo·da·tion, *n. In ophthalmology,* adjustment of the eye to variations in distance; the changes in the ciliary muscle and lens whereby the focus of light rays on the retina is maintained. Abbreviated, a., Acc. —**ac·com·mo·da·tive** (a·kom′uh·day″tiv) *adj.*

accommodation paralysis. Paralysis of the ciliary muscle of the eye.

accommodation phosphene. A subjective sensation of light produced by the sudden effort of accommodation, observed when a person is in the dark.

accommodation reflex. Constriction of the pupils, convergence of the eyes, and increased convexity of the lens when the eyes adjust for near vision. Syn. *near reflex.*

accommodative asthenopia. 1. Subnormal power of the function of accommodation. 2. The pain or discomfort resulting from strain or spasm of the ciliary muscle in accommodative effort.

accommodative esotropia or **strabismus.** In marked hyperopia, esotropia on accommodation if the amount of convergence is too great to be overcome by the available fusional amplitude. This may sometimes appear as esophoria for distant vision and esotropia for near vision; especially seen in young children. See also *intermittent convergent strabismus.*

accommodative spasm. SPASM OF ACCOMMODATION.

accomplishment quotient. ACHIEVEMENT QUOTIENT.

ac·cor·di·on, *adj.* Having folds resembling the bellows of an accordion, and consequently having distensibility or stretchability in excess of that due to elasticity alone.

accordion abdomen. A swelling of the abdomen attended with flattening of the arch of the diaphragm and increased respiration, not due to the presence of gas or a tumor and disappearing under anesthesia.

accordion graft. A full-thickness graft in which multiple slits are made so that the graft may be stretched to cover a large area.

ac·couche·ment (a·koosh·mah^n′, uh·koosh′munt) *n.* [F.]. PARTURITION.

accouchement for·cé (for·say′). Rapid delivery by manual dilation of the cervix followed by version or application of forceps and immediate extraction.

ac·cou·cheur (a·koo·shur′) *n.* [F.]. Obstetrician; a professionally trained person attending women in childbirth.

accoucheur's hand. A spasmodic cone-shaped deformity of the hand; characteristically seen in tetany.

ac·cou·cheuse (a·koo·shuhz′) *n.* [F.]. A female obstetrician; a midwife.

ac·cre·men·ti·tion (ack″ri·men·tish′un) *n.* [*ac(cre)-* as in accretion + *-(cre)ment* as in increment + *-ition* as in addition]. Increase and growth characterized by the addition of like tissue by simple fission, cellular division, and budding or gemmation. —**accrementi·tial** (·ul) *adj.*

ac·crete (a·kreet′) *v.* 1. To become attached by accretion. 2. To grow together.

ac·cre·tio cor·dis (a·kree′shee·o kor′dis). A serious form of adherent pericarditis with fibrous bands extending from the mediastinal surface of the parietal pericardium to the pleura, diaphragm, and chest wall.

ac·cre·tion (a·kree'shun) *n.* [L. *accretio*, from *accrescere*, to grow]. 1. Growth characterized by addition to the periphery, as in crystalline and certain organic compounds. 2. Adherence of parts normally separate. 3. A growing together; adhesion. 4. An accumulation of foreign matter, as about a tooth or within any cavity. —**accre·tive** (·tiv) *adj.*

accretion lines. Linear markings showing the addition of successive layers of enamel and dentin, seen in microscopic sections of a tooth; incremental lines.

ac·cro·chage (a·kro·shahzh') *n.* [F., hooking, engagement]. The transient synchronization of the inherently different rhythms of two cardiac impulse foci, as synchronization of the atrial and ventricular rhythms for a few beats in complete atrioventricular heart block.

A.C.D. American College of Dentists.

ACD solution [*a*cid + *c*itrate + *d*extrose]. An anticoagulant acid citrate dextrose solution; used to prevent coagulation of blood in collection and storage of whole blood for indirect transfusions.

-aceae [L. *-aceus*, of the nature of]. *In botany*, a suffix used in combination with the name of one of the principal genera to form the names of families of plants and bacteria. See also *-idae.*

Ace bandage. Trademark for woven cotton elastic bandage, obtainable in various widths, used especially on the extremities to provide gentle uniform pressure.

ac·e·bu·to·lol (as"e·bew'tuh·lol) *n.* (±)*N*-[3-Acetyl-4-[2-hydroxy-3-[(1-methylethyl)amino]propoxy]phenyl]butanamide, $C_{18}H_{28}N_2O_4$, an anti-adrenergic (β-receptor).

ace·cli·dine (a·see'kli·deen) *n.* 3-Acetoxyquinuclidine, $C_9H_{15}NO_2$, a parasympathomimetic agent.

ac·e·dap·sone (as"e·dap'sone) *n.* *N,N'*-(Sulfonyldi-4,1-phenylene)bisacetamide, $C_{16}H_{16}N_2O_4S$, an antimalarial and leprostatic drug.

ace·dia (a·see'dee·uh) *n.* [Gk. *akēdia*, apathy]. DEPRESSION (4).

acelia. ACOELIA.

acel·lu·lar (ay"sel'yoo·lur) *adj.* Without cells; not consisting of cells; not cellular.

acenaesthesia. ACENESTHESIA.

ac·e·naph·thene (as"e·naf'theen) *n.* 1,8-Ethylenenaphthalene, $C_{12}H_{10}$, a tricyclic solid hydrocarbon occurring in coal tar; used as an insecticide and fungicide, a dye intermediate, and in the manufacture of plastics.

ace·nes·the·sia, acoe·naes·the·sia (ay"see·nes·theezh'uh, ·theez'zee·uh, ay"sen·es·) *n.* [*a-* + *cenesthesia*]. Lack or loss of the normal awareness of one's own bodily parts or organs.

acen·o·cou·ma·rol (ay"sen·o·koo'muh·rol) *n.* 3-(α-Acetonyl-4-nitrobenzyl)-4-hydroxycoumarin, $C_{19}H_{15}NO_6$, an anticoagulant.

acen·tric (ay·sen'trick) *adj.* 1. Lacking a center. 2. Peripheral; eccentric. 3. Not arising centrally, as from a nerve center.

acentric chromosome. A chromosomal fragment without a centromere.

-aceous [L. *-aceus*]. A suffix meaning *pertaining to or characterized by.*

acephali. Plural of *acephalus.*

ace·pha·lia (ay"se·fay'lee·uh, as"e·) *n.* ACEPHALY.

ace·phal·ic (ay"se·fal'ick, as"e·) *adj.* [*a-* + *cephalic*]. ACEPHALOUS; headless or without a distinct head or headlike part.

acephalic gregarine. Any member of the Acephalina.

Aceph·a·li·na (ay·sef"uh·lye'nuh) *n.* A tribe of gregarines in which schizogony is lacking and in which the body of the trophozoite is not compartmentalized; includes the genus *Monocystis*, which inhabits the seminal vesicles of earthworms. Contr. *Cephalina.* —**aceph·a·line** (ay·sef'uh·line) *adj.*

aceph·a·lism (ay·sef'uh·liz·um, a·sef') *n.* ACEPHALY.

aceph·a·lo·bra·chia (ay·sef"uh·lo·bray'kee·uh, a·sef") *n.* [*a-* + *cephalo-* + *brachi-* + *-ia*]. Congenital absence of the head and arms.

aceph·a·lo·bra·chi·us (ay·sef"uh·lo·bray'kee·us, a·sef") *n.* [*a-* + *cephalo-* + *brachi-* + *-us*]. An omphalosite lacking head and arms.

aceph·a·lo·car·dia (ay·sef"uh·lo·kahr'dee·uh, a·sef") *n.* [*a-* + *cephalo-* + *cardi-* + *-ia*]. Congenital absence of the head and heart.

aceph·a·lo·car·di·us (ay·sef"uh·lo·kahr'dee·us, a·sef") *n.* [*a-* + *cephalo-* + *cardi-* + *-us*]. An omphalosite with neither head nor heart.

aceph·a·lo·chei·ria, aceph·a·lo·chi·ria (ay·sef"uh·lo·kigh'ree·uh, a·sef") *n.* [*a-* + *cephalo-* + *cheir-* + *-ia*]. Congenital absence of the head and hands.

aceph·a·lo·chei·rus, aceph·a·lo·chi·rus (ay·sef"uh·lo·kigh'rus, a·sef") *n.* [*a-* + *cephalo-* + *cheir-* + *-us*]. An omphalosite with neither head nor hands.

aceph·a·lo·cyst (ay·sef'uh·lo·sist, a·sef') *n.* [*a-* + *cephalo-* + *cyst*]. A sterile hydatid, without scolices or brood capsules, found in the human liver and other organs, representing aberrant development of the larval stage of *Echinococcus granulosus.*

aceph·a·lo·cys·tis rac·e·mo·sa (a·sef"uh·lo·sis'tis ras"e·mo'suh). HYDATIDIFORM MOLE.

aceph·a·lo·gas·ter (ay·sef"uh·lo·gas'tur, a·sef") *n.* [*a-* + *cephalo-* + *-gaster*]. An omphalosite without head, thorax, or abdomen, consisting only of a pelvis and legs.

aceph·a·lo·gas·te·ria (ay·sef"uh·lo·gas·teer'ee·uh, a·sef") *n.* [*acephalogaster* + *-ia*]. Congenital absence of the head, thorax, and upper part of the abdomen.

aceph·a·lo·po·dia (ay·sef"uh·lo·po'dee·uh, a·sef") *n.* [*a-* + *cephalo-* + *pod-* + *-ia*]. Congenital absence of the head and feet.

aceph·a·lo·po·di·us (ay·sef"uh·lo·po'dee·us, a·sef") *n.* An omphalosite with neither head nor feet.

acephalorachus. ACEPHALORRHACHUS.

aceph·a·lor·rha·chia (ay·sef"uh·lo·ray'kee·uh, a·sef") *n.* [*a-* + *cephalo-* + *rhachi-* + *-ia*]. Congenital absence of the head and vertebral column.

aceph·a·lor·rha·chus, aceph·a·lo·ra·chus (ay·sef"uh·lo·ray'kus, ·lor'uh·kus, a·sef") *n.* [*a-* + *cephalo-* + *rachi-* + *-us*]. An omphalosite with neither head nor vertebral column.

aceph·a·lo·sto·mia (ay·sef"uh·lo·sto'mee·uh, a·sef") *n.* [*a-* + *cephalo-* + *-stomia*]. A condition marked by congenital absence of the head, with a mouthlike aperture present at the upper part of the neck or chest.

aceph·a·los·to·mus (ay·sef"uh·los'tuh·mus, a·sef") *n.* An omphalosite exhibiting acephalostomia.

aceph·a·lo·tho·ra·cia (ay·sef"uh·lo·tho·ray'see·uh, a·sef") *n.* [*a-* + *cephalo-* + *thorac-* + *-ia*]. Congenital absence of the head and thorax.

aceph·a·lo·tho·rax (ay·sef"uh·lo·tho'racks, a·sef") *n.* [*a-* + *cephalo-* + *thorax*]. An omphalosite with neither head nor thorax.

aceph·a·lo·tho·rus (ay·sef"uh·lo·tho'rus, a·sef") *n.* ACEPHALOTHORAX.

aceph·a·lous (ay·sef'uh·lus) *adj.* Without a head; ACEPHALIC.

aceph·a·lus (ay·sef'a·lus, a·sef') *n.*, pl. **acepha·li** (·lye) [ML., from Gk. *akephalos*, headless]. Any one of a group of omphalositic monsters characterized by absence of the head.

acephalus acar·di·us (a·kahr'dee·us). ACEPHALOCARDIUS.

acephalus atho·rus (a·tho'rus). PSEUDOHEMIACARDIUS.

acephalus di·bra·chi·us (dye·bray'kee·us). An omphalosite without a head, but with two arms.

acephalus di·pus (dye'pus). A headless omphalosite with two feet.

acephalus mono·bra·chi·us (mon"o·bray'kee·us). An omphalosite lacking a head, with only one arm, and without lower extremities.

acephalus mono·pus (mon'o·pus). A headless omphalosite which has a single lower extremity and no arms.
acephalus pseu·do·acor·mus (sue''do·a·kor'mus). An omphalosite which lacks all but pelvis and lower extremities.
acephalus sym·pus (sim'pus). A headless omphalosite which has sympodia.
acephalus tho·rus acar·di·a·cus (tho'rus ay''kahr·dye'uh·kus). A headless omphalosite with thorax, but no heart.
aceph·a·ly (ay·sef'uh·lee, a·sef') *n.* [*a-* + *-cephaly*]. Absence of the head.
ac·e·pro·ma·zine (as''e·pro'muh·zeen) *n.* 1-[10-(Dimethylamino)propyl]-10*H*-phenothiazin-2-ylethanone, $C_{19}H_{22}N_2OS$, a veterinary tranquilizer usually employed as the maleate salt.
ac·er·ate (as'ur·ate) *adj.* [L. *acer*, sharp]. Sharp-pointed; ACICULAR.
acer·bi·ty (a·sur'bi·tee) *n.* [L. *acerbitas*, from *acerbus*, bitter, harsh]. Acidity combined with astringency.
acer·bo·pho·bia (a·sur''bo·fo'bee·uh) *n.* [L. *acerbus*, bitter, sour, + *-phobia*]. Morbid fear of sourness.
Acerdol. A trademark for calcium permanganate.
ac·ero·pho·bia (as''ur·o·fo'bee·uh) *n.* [L. *acer*, sharp, stinging, + *-phobia*]. ACERBOPHOBIA.
acer·vu·line (a·sur''vew·line, ·leen) *adj.* [L. *acervulus*, a little heap]. Agminated or aggregated, as certain mucous glands.
acer·vu·lus (a·sur'vew·lus) *n.* [L., diminutive of *acervus*, heap] [BNA]. BRAIN SAND.
aces·cent (a·ses'unt) *adj.* [L. *acescere*, to turn sour, from *acere*, to be sour]. 1. Acid, sour, or tart; ACIDULOUS. 2. Becoming sour. —**aces·cence** (·unce) *n.*
aces·o·dyne (a·ses'o·dine) *n.* [Gk. *akesōdynos*, from *akesis*, cure, + *odynē*, pain]. A pain-relieving agent; ANODYNE (2). —**ac·e·sod·y·nous** (as''e·sod'i·nus) *adj.*
ac·es·to·ma (as''es·to'muh) *n.* [Gk. *akesis*, healing, cure, + *-oma*]. Granulation tissue which becomes organized into scar tissue.
acet-, aceto-. A combining form meaning *connection with or derivation from acetic acid or acetyl.*
acetabula. Plural of *acetabulum.*
ac·e·tab·u·lar (as''e·tab'yoo·lur) *adj.* Pertaining to the acetabulum.
acetabular bone. OS ACETABULI.
acetabular fossa. A depression in the center of the acetabulum. NA *fossa acetabuli.*
acetabular lip or **labrum.** The fibrocartilaginous ring attached to the margin of the acetabulum. NA *labrum acetabulare.*
acetabular notch. A notch in the lower border of the acetabulum. NA *incisura acetabuli.*
ac·e·tab·u·lec·to·my (as''e·tab''yoo·leck'tuh·mee) *n.* Excision of the acetabulum.
ac·e·tab·u·lo·plas·ty (as''e·tab'yoo·lo·plas''tee) *n.* Any plastic operation on the acetabulum, especially an operation aimed at restoring or enlarging the acetabular cavity.
ac·e·tab·u·lum (as''e·tab'yoo·lum) *n.*, pl. **acetabu·la** (·luh) [L., vinegar cup, from *acetum*, vinegar]. 1. [NA] The cup-shaped depression on the outer aspect of the hipbone for the reception of the head of the femur. 2. The sucking cup of flukes.
ac·e·tal (as'e·tal'') *n.* [*acet-* + *al*cohol]. 1. 1,1-Diethoxyethane, $CH_3CH(OC_2H_5)_2$, formerly used as a hypnotic. 2. Generic name for products of the interaction of aldehydes and alcohol characterized by the presence of the $=C(OR)_2$ group.
ac·et·al·de·hyde (as''e·tal'de·hide, a·seet''al·de·hide) *n.* [*acet-* + *aldehyde*]. $CH_3.CHO$. A colorless liquid with a characteristic pungent odor. It results from the oxidation of ethyl alcohol or the reduction of acetic acid; a general narcotic. Syn. *acetic aldehyde, ethanal.*
acet·am·ide (a·set'uh·mide) *n.* Acetic acid amide, CH_3CONH_2, used industrially and in organic syntheses.
ac·et·ami·no·phen (as''e·tuh·mee'no·fen) *n.* *N*-Acetyl-*p*-aminophenol, $CH_3CONH.C_6H_4.OH$, an analgesic and antipyretic drug. Syn. *p-acetaminophenol.*
***p*-acet·ami·no·phe·nol** (a·set''uh·mee''no·fee'nol) *n.* ACETAMINOPHEN.
ac·et·an·i·lid (as''e·tan'i·lid) *n.* Acetylaniline, $C_6H_5NHCOCH_3$, an analgesic; prolonged use may lead to toxic symptoms.
ac·et·ar·sol (as''e·tahr'sol) *n.* ACETARSONE.
ac·et·ar·sone (as''e·tahr'sone) *n.* [*acet-* + *arsonic* acid]. 3-Acetylamino-4-hydroxyphenylarsonic acid, $C_8H_{10}AsNO_5$, a white or yellowish powder, slightly soluble in water. Used in the treatment of amebiasis and also in prophylaxis and treatment in certain cases of syphilis. Syn. *acetarsol.*
ac·e·tate (as'e·tate) *n.* Any salt or ester of acetic acid.
acet·a·zol·amide (a·set''uh·zo'luh·mide) *n.* 2-Acetylamino-1,3,4-thiadiazole-5-sulfonamide, $C_4H_6N_4O_3S_2$, a renal carbonic anhydrase inhibitor; employed as a diuretic and in the treatment of epilepsy and glaucoma.
acet·dia·mer·sul·fon·amides (a·set''dye''uh·merr·sul·fo'nuh·mide'z) *n.* Nonproprietary name for a mixture containing equal weights of sulfacetamide, sulfadiazine, and sulfamerazine.
ace·tic (a·see'tick) *adj.* [L. *acetum*, vinegar]. Pertaining to acetic acid.
acetic acid. 1. CH_3COOH, a colorless liquid with a pungent odor; the principal acid of vinegar. Syn. *ethanoic acid.* 2. An aqueous solution containing 36 to 37% CH_3COOH. It is occasionally used, when diluted, as an astringent and styptic. See also *diluted acetic acid, glacial acetic acid.*
acetic acid amide. ACETAMIDE.
acetic aldehyde. ACETALDEHYDE.
acetic anhydride. The anhydride of acetic acid, $(CH_3CO)_2O$; a colorless, mobile liquid having the odor of acetic acid. Used industrially and in organic syntheses.
acetic ether. ETHYL ACETATE.
acetic fermentation. Any process of fermentation resulting in the formation of acetic acid.
acetic thiokinase. An enzyme catalyzing the reaction between acetate and adenosine triphosphate to form acetyl coenzyme A.
Acetidine. Trademark for a combination of acetylsalicylic acid, phenacetin, and caffeine.
ace·ti·fi·ca·tion (a·see''ti·fi·kay'shun, a·set''i·) *n.* The production of acetic acid by acetic fermentation. —**ace·ti·fy** (a·see'ti·figh, a·set'i·figh) *v.*
ac·e·tim·e·ter (as''e·tim'e·tur) *n.* ACETOMETER.
ac·e·tin (as'e·tin) *n.* An ester formed by glycerin with one, two, or three molecules of acetic acid.
aceto-. See *acet-.*
ac·e·to·ace·tic acid (as''e·to·a·see'tick, a·see''to·a·see'tick). Acetylacetic acid, CH_3COCH_2COOH, a ketone acid produced in small amounts as a normal product of fat metabolism, but excessively when hepatic oxidation of fatty acids is markedly accelerated as in diabetic ketosis or starvation. Syn. *diacetic acid.*
acetoacetic ester. Ethyl acetoacetate, $CH_3COCH_2.COOC_2H_5$, a liquid used in the synthesis of many medicinals. Syn. *ethyl diacetate.*
Ace·to·bac·ter (a·see'to·back''tur, as''e·to·back'tur) *n.* [*aceto-* + *bacterium*]. A genus of aerobic bacteria of the family Pseudomonadaceae, possessing high oxidative powers and acid tolerance and capable of oxidizing various organic compounds to organic acids and other products, as ethyl alcohol to acetic acid. Important industrially in the production of vinegar. *Acetobacter aceti* is the principal and typical species.
ac·e·to·car·mine (as''e·to·kahr'min) *n.* A saturated solution of carmine in 45% acetic acid.
acetocarmine stain. 1. BELLING'S ACETOCARMINE STAIN. 2. SCHNEIDER'S ACETOCARMINE STAIN.
ac·e·to·hex·a·mide (as''e·to·heck'suh·mide) *n.* N-(*p*-Ace-

tylphenylsulfonyl)-N′-cyclohexylurea, $C_{15}H_{20}N_2O_4S$, an orally effective hypoglycemic compound.

acet·o·in (a·set′o·in) *n.* ACETYLMETHYLCARBINOL.

ac·e·tol·y·sis (as″e·tol′i·sis) *n.*, pl. **acetoly·ses** (·seez). A decomposition reaction, analogous to hydrolysis, of acetic acid or acetic anhydride with another substance. An acetyl radical may be attached to one of the breakdown products as part of the reaction.

ac·e·to·me·naph·thone (a·see″to·me·naf′thone, as″e·to·) *n.* Menadiol diacetate or 2-methyl-1,4-naphthohydroquinone diacetate, $C_{15}H_{14}O_4$, a vitamin K analogue used in the prevention and treatment of hypoprothrombinemia caused by a deficiency of vitamin K.

ac·e·tom·e·ter (as″e·tom′e·tur) *n.* A device for determining the amount of acetic acid present in a solution, as in vinegar. —**ac·e·to·met·ric** (as″e·to·met′rick) *adj.*

ac·e·to·mor·phine (a·see″to·mor′feen, as″e·to·) *n.* [*aceto-* + *morphine*]. HEROIN.

acetonaemia. KETONEMIA.

ac·e·ton·asth·ma (as″e·to·naz′muh) *n.* [*acetone* + *asthma*]. *Obsol.* Air hunger associated with ketonuria as in diabetic ketoacidosis. See also *diabetic acidosis.*

ac·e·tone (as′e·tone) *n.* [*acet-* + *-one*]. Dimethylketone or propanone, CH_3COCH_3; occurs normally in blood and urine in minute quantities which may become greatly increased in diabetics. Produced by synthesis for use as a solvent and industrial chemical.

acetone bodies. KETONE BODIES.

acetone chloroform. CHLOROBUTANOL.

ac·e·ton·emia, ac·e·to·nae·mia (as″e·to·nee′mee·uh) *n.* [*acetone* + *-emia*]. KETONEMIA. —**aceton·emic** (·nee′mick) *adj.*

ac·e·to·ni·trile (a·see″to·nigh′trile, ·tril, as″e·to·) *n.* [*aceto-* + *nitrile*]. Methyl cyanide, CH_3CN, an important solvent and reactant in organic synthesis.

ac·e·ton·uria (as″e·to·new′ree·uh) *n.* [*acetone* + *-uria*]. KETONURIA.

ace·ton·yl (a·see′to·nil, ·set′o·) *n.* [*acetone* + *-yl*]. The univalent radical CH_3COCH_2—, representing acetone less one atom of hydrogen.

ac·e·to·phen·a·zine (as″e·to·fen′uh·zeen) *n.* [*aceto-* + *phenothiazine*]. 2-Acetyl-10-{3-[4-(β-hydroxyethyl) piperazinyl]propyl} phenothiazine, $C_{23}H_{29}N_3O_2S$, a mild tranquilizing agent; used as the maleate salt.

ac·e·to·phe·net·i·din (a·see″to·fe·net′i·din, as″e·to·) *n.* [*aceto-* + *phenetidin*]. PHENACETIN.

acet·o·sal (a·set′o·sal) *n.* [*aceto-* + *salicylic*]. ASPIRIN.

ac·e·to·sul·fone sodium (as″e·to·sul′fone, a·see′to·). *N*-[[5-Amino-2-[(4-aminophenyl)sulfonyl]phenyl]sulfonyl]acetamide, monosodium salt, $C_{14}H_{14}N_3NaO_5S_2$, an antibacterial (leprostatic).

ace·tous (a·see′tus, as′e·) *adj.* [L. *acetosus*, from *acetum*, vinegar]. Pertaining to, resembling, forming, or containing vinegar or acetic acid.

acet·phe·nol·isa·tin (a·set″fee″nol·eye′suh·tin) *n.* [*acet-* + *phenol* + *isatin*]. 3,3-Bis(*p*-acetoxyphenyl)oxindole or diacetyldiphenolisatin, $C_{24}H_{19}NO_5$, a laxative.

ac·e·tri·zo·ate (as″e·trye·zo′ate) *n.* A salt of acetrizoic acid.

acet·ri·zo·ic acid (a·set″ri·zo′ick). 3-Acetylamino-2,4,6-triiodobenzoic acid, $C_9H_6I_3NO_3$, the sodium salt of which, sodium acetrizoate, is employed as a contrast medium.

ac·e·tu·rate (as″e·tew′rate) *n.* Any salt or ester of aceturic acid.

ac·e·tu·ric acid (as″e·tew′rick). *N*-Acetylglycine, $CH_3CONHCH_2COOH$, an acid sometimes employed to prepare stable salts of organic bases.

ace·tyl (a·see′til, as′e·til, ·teel) *n.* [*acet-* + *-yl*]. The univalent radical CH_3CO—, of acetic acid.

ac·e·tyl·ace·tic acid (as″e·til·a·see′tik). ACETOACETIC ACID.

ac·e·tyl·aden·y·late (as″e·til·a·den′i·late) *n.* [*acetyl* + *adenyl* + *-ate*]. The mixed anhydride formed by interaction of the carboxyl of acetic acid and the phosphate of adenylic acid.

a·cet·y·lase (a·set′i·lace, ·laze) *n.* [*acetyl* + *-ase*]. An enzyme that catalyzes the formation of *N*-acetylglutamate from glutamic acid and acetyl coenzyme A.

acet·y·la·tion (a·set″i·lay′shun, a·see″ti·) *n.* Introduction of an acetyl radical ($CH_3.CO$—) into the molecular structure of an organic compound, usually by reaction with acetic acid. —**acet·y·late** (a·set′i·late) *v.*

acet·y·la·tor (a·set′i·lay·tur) *n.* An individual as characterized by a rate of metabolic acetylation (as: slow acetylator, rapid acetylator).

ac·e·tyl-beta-meth·yl·cho·line (as″e·til·bay″tuh·meth·il·ko′leen) *n.* METHACHOLINE CHLORIDE.

ac·e·tyl·car·bro·mal (as″e·til·kahr′bro·mal, a·see″til·) *n.* [*acetyl* + *carbromal*]. *N*-Acetyl-*N*-bromodiethylacetylurea, $C_9H_{15}BrN_2O_3$, a sedative.

ac·e·tyl·cho·line (as″e·til·ko′leen, ·lin, a·see″til·) *n.* The acetic acid ester of choline, $(CH_3)_3N(OH)CH_2CH_2OCOCH_3$, a normal constituent of many body tissues. It is the chemical mediator of cholinergic nerve impulses; removal of acetyl by enzymatic hydrolysis, producing choline, inactivates it. Has been used in the treatment of a variety of diseases, but its effects are transient and variable.

ac·e·tyl·cho·lin·es·ter·ase (as″e·til·ko″lin·es′tur·ace, ·aze) *n.* Any enzyme, found in blood and various tissues, that catalyzes hydrolysis of acetylcholine but may also catalyze hydrolysis of noncholine esters.

acetyl coenzyme A. A compound in which an acetyl group is joined to coenzyme A by a thioester bond. It is an important metabolic intermediate, being an acetylating agent in a variety of reactions, providing energy for cell respiration, and also having other biochemical functions. Abbreviated, acetyl Co A. Syn. *active acetate.*

ac·e·tyl·cys·te·ine (as″e·til·sis′tee·een, ·sis·tee′in) *n.* [*acetyl* + *cysteine*]. *N*-Acetyl-L-cysteine, $C_5H_9NO_3S$, a mucolytic agent.

ac·e·tyl·dig·i·tox·in (as″e·til·dij″i·tock′sin) *n.* Digitoxin α-acetyl ester, $C_{43}H_{66}O_{14}$, a cardiac glycoside characterized by a relatively rapid onset and a short duration of action, compared with digitoxin.

acet·y·lene (a·set′i·leen) *n.* [*acetyl* + *-ene*]. A colorless gas, $CH\equiv CH$, with a characteristic, unpleasant odor; burns with a luminous, smoky flame. Has been used to determine cardiac output. Syn. *ethine, ethyne.*

acetylene series. A series of hydrocarbons, starting with acetylene, characterized by having a triple bond.

acetylene tetrachloride. TETRACHLOROETHANE.

acet·y·lide (a·set′i·lide, ·lid) *n.* A derivative of acetylene formed by replacing its hydrogen atoms by a metal, as cuprous acetylide, C_2Cu_2.

acet·y·li·za·tion (a·set″i·li·zay′shun) *n.* ACETYLATION.

ac·e·tyl·meth·yl·car·bi·nol (as″e·til·meth″il·kahr″bi·nol) *n.* [*acetyl* + *methyl* + *carbinol*]. 3-Hydroxy-2-butanone, $CH_3CHOHCOCH_3$, a product of bacterial fermentation in foodstuffs. Syn. *acetoin.*

acetylmethylcarbinol test or **reaction.** VOGES-PROSKAUER TEST.

acetyl number. The number of milligrams of potassium hydroxide required to combine with the acetic acid liberated by the saponification of 1 g of acetylated fat.

ace·tyl·sal·i·cyl·ic acid (a·see″til·sal″i·sil′ick, as″e·til·) ASPIRIN.

acetyl sulfisoxazole. N^1-(Acetyl-3,4-dimethyl-5-isoxazolyl)sulfanilamide, a derivative of sulfisoxazole practically insoluble in water and, hence, tasteless; has the actions of sulfisoxazole.

ac·e·tyl·sul·fon·a·mide (as″e·til·sul·fon′uh·mide, ·fo′nuh·mide) *n.* A sulfonamide in which the hydrogen atom of the NH_2 group, attached directly to the benzene ring, is replaced by an acetyl group; a conjugation which occurs in the liver of man and other species, except the canine. Harmful effects may be produced in the renal tubules and urinary tract by the precipitation of these compounds. This can be prevented if urine is kept alkaline.

ACG Abbreviation for *apexcardiogram.*

AcG Abbreviation for *accelerator globulin* (= FACTOR V).

Ac globulin. Accelerator globulin (= FACTOR V).

ach·a·la·sia (ack″uh·lay′zhuh, ·zee·uh) *n.* [*a-* + Gk. *chalasis,* relaxation, + *-ia*]. 1. Failure of relaxation of the lower esophagus at the cardiac sphincter with secondary dilatation of the upper esophagus. 2. *Obsol.* Generally, failure of relaxation of smooth muscle fibers in a tubular organ, for example at the cardiac or rectal sphincters in the intestinal tract, often resulting in dilatation of the tubular structure above (megaesophagus or megacolon).

Achard-Cas·taigne method or **test** (a·shahr′, kas·tehn^y′) [E. C. *Achard,* French physician, 1860–1944; and J. *Castaigne*]. METHYLENE BLUE TEST (1).

Achard-Thiers syndrome (tyair) [E. C. *Achard;* and J. *Thiers,* French physician, b.1885]. Diabetes mellitus in women with facial hirsutism, obesity, striae, hypertension, and amenorrhea; may represent a variant of Cushing's syndrome.

ache (ake) *n. & v.* 1. A dull, persisting pain of fixed location and of more or less constant or throbbing intensity. 2. Of a body part or region: to be the locus of such a pain.

achei·lia, achi·lia (a·kigh′lee·uh) *n.* [*a-* + *cheil-* + *-ia*]. A condition marked by congenital absence of the lips.

achei·lus, achi·lus (a·kigh′lus) *n.* An individual exhibiting acheilia. **—acheilous,** *adj.*

achei·ria, achi·ria (a·kigh′ree·uh) *n.* [Gk. *acheir,* handless (from *cheir,* hand) + *-ia*]. 1. Congenital absence of one or both hands. 2. Inability to indicate which side of the body was touched; a form of dyschiria. **—achei·rous** (·rus) *adj.*

achei·rus, achi·rus (a·kigh′rus) *n.* [Gk. *acheir,* handless, + *-us*]. An individual without hands.

achieve·ment age. *In psychology,* accomplishment expressed as equivalent to the age in years of the average child showing similar attainments; determined by standard tests. Abbreviated, A.A.

achievement quotient. *In psychology,* the ratio between achievement age, or actual level of scholastic performance, and mental age, or expected level of performance for age. Abbreviated, AQ.

Ach·il·lea (ack″i·lee′uh) *n.* [L., from Gk. *Achilleios,* of Achilles, who is said to have used the plant]. A genus of herbs of the family Compositae; the milfoil or yarrow. A composite-flowered herb.

Achilles bursa. The bursa lying between the calcaneal (Achilles) tendon and the calcaneus. NA *bursa tendinis calcanei, bursa tendinis Achillis.*

Achilles jerk or **reflex.** Plantar flexion of the foot, produced by contraction of the calf muscles and elicited by striking the tendon of the gastrocnemius and soleus muscles (calcaneal or Achilles tendon). Syn. *ankle jerk, triceps surae jerk.*

Achilles tendon [*Achilles,* Greek legendary hero vulnerable only in one heel]. CALCANEAL TENDON.

Achilles tendon reflex. ACHILLES JERK.

achil·lo·bur·si·tis (a·kil″o·bur·sigh′tis) *n.* [*Achilles* + *bursitis*]. Inflammation of the bursa of the calcaneal tendon.

achil·lo·dyn·ia (a·kil″o·din′ee·uh) *n.* [*Achilles* + *-odynia*]. Pain in the calcaneal tendon or its bursa.

ach·il·lor·rha·phy (ack″il·or′uh·fee) *n.* [*Achilles* + *-rrhaphy*]. Any suturing operation to repair the calcaneal tendon.

achil·lo·te·not·o·my (a·kil″o·te·not′uh·mee) *n.* [*Achilles* + *tenotomy*]. ACHILLOTOMY.

ach·il·lot·o·my (ack″i·lot′uh·mee) *n.* [*Achilles* + *-tomy*]. Surgical section of the calcaneal tendon.

achilus. ACHEILUS.

ACH index [*a*rm + *c*hest + *h*ip]. An index of nutrition based on measurements of arm girth, chest depth, and hip width.

achi·ral (ay·kye′rul) *adj.* Not chiral.

achiria. ACHEIRIA.

achlor·hy·dria (ay″klor·high′dree·uh, ack″lor·) *n.* [*a-* + *chlorhydria*]. The absence of hydrochloric acid in the stomach, even after stimulation with histamine. **—achlorhy·dric** (·drick) *adj.*

achlorhydric anemia. Anemia, usually hypochromic, associated with achlorhydria.

ach·luo·pho·bia (ack″loo·o·fo′bee·uh) *n.* [Gk. *achlus,* mist, dimness, + *-phobia*]. Morbid fear of darkness.

acho·lia (ay·ko′lee·uh, a·ko′) *n.* [*a-* + *chol-* + *-ia*]. 1. Absence or suppression of biliary secretion. 2. Any condition obstructing the flow of bile into the small intestine. 3. A mild temperament. **—achol·ic** (ay·kol′ick), **ach·o·lous** (ack′o·lus) *adj.*

ach·o·lu·ria (ack″o·lew′ree·uh, ay″ko·) *n.* [*a-* + *chol-* + *-uria*]. The absence of bilirubin in the urine. **—acholu·ric** (·rick) *adj.*

acholuric jaundice. Jaundice without demonstrable bilirubin in the urine.

achon·dro·pla·sia (a·kon″dro·play′zhuh, ·zee·uh, ay·kon″) *n.* [*a-* + *chondro-* + *-plasia*]. Abnormal osteogenesis resulting in the typical congenital dwarf, with disproportionately short extremities, relatively large head, depressed nasal bridge, stubby trident hands, and thoracolumbar kyphosis; due to disordered chondrification and ossification of the ends of the long bones beginning early in intrauterine life, with membrane bones developing normally; autosomal dominant, with most cases due to fresh mutation, both parents being normal. Syn. *chondrodystrophia fetalis.* **—achondro·plas·tic,** *adj.*

achon·dro·plast (a·kon′dro·plast, ay·kon′) *n. Informal.* ACHONDROPLASTIC DWARF.

achondroplastic dwarf. An individual affected with achondroplasia.

achon·dro·plas·ty (a·kon′dro·plas″tee, ay·kon′) *n.* ACHONDROPLASIA.

achor (ay′kor, ack′or) *n.* [Gk. *achōr,* dandruff]. Inflammatory and pustular eruption of hairy parts.

achor·dal (ay·kor′dul) *adj.* [*a-* + *chordal*]. ACHORDATE.

Achor·da·ta (ay″kor·day′tuh, ack″or·) *n.pl.* [*a-* + *Chordata*]. Animals without a notochord. **—achor·date** (ay·kor′date) *n. & adj.*

ach·o·re·sis (ack″o·ree′sis, ay″ko·) *n.* [*a-* + Gk. *chōrēsis,* capacity, from *chōra,* space, room]. Diminution in the usual volume of a hollow organ, as the stomach or urinary bladder.

Acho·ri·on (a·ko′ree·on) *n.* [NL., from Gk. *achōr,* scurf, dandruff]. *TRICHOPHYTON.*

Achorion gallinae. *TRICHOPHYTON GALLINAE.*

Achorion gypseum. *MICROSPORUM GYPSEUM.*

Achorion quinck·e·a·num (kwink″ee·ay′num). *TRICHOPHYTON MENTAGROPHYTES.*

Achorion schoenleinii. *TRICHOPHYTON SCHOENLEINII.*

Achor-Smith syndrome [R. W. P. *Achor,* U.S. physician, b. 1922; and L. A. *Smith,* U.S. physician, b. 1910]. Nutritional deficiency with hypokalemia.

achreo·cy·the·mia, achreo·cy·thae·mia (a·kree″o·sigh·theem′ee·uh) *n.* [Gk. *achroia,* paleness, + *cyt-* + *-hemia*]. *Obsol.* HYPOCHROMIC ANEMIA.

achres·tic (a·kres′tick) *adj.* [*a-* + Gk. *chrēstikos,* knowing how to use, from *chrēsthai,* to need, to use]. Pertaining to failure of use, as of a principle in the body.

achrestic anemia. *Obsol.* A megaloblastic, macrocytic anemia morphologically similar to pernicious anemia but unresponsive to liver extract therapy, possibly due in at least some cases to folic acid deficiency.

achro-, achroo- [Gk. *achroos,* from *a-* + *chroa,* complexion]. A combining form meaning *colorless.*

achroa·cyte (ay·kro′uh·site, a·kro′) *n.* [*a-* + Gk. *chroa,* complexion, + *-cyte*]. LYMPHOCYTE.

achroa·cy·to·sis (ay·kro″uh·sigh·to′sis, a·kro″) *n.* [*achroacyte* + *-osis*]. An increase in the number of lymphocytes in the blood; LYMPHOCYTHEMIA.

achroi·o·cy·the·mia, achroi·o·cy·thae·mia (a·kroy″o·sigh·

theem'ee·uh) *n. Obsol.* Achreocythemia (= HYPOCHROMIC ANEMIA).

achro·ma (ay·kro'muh, a·kro') *n.* [*a-* + Gk. *chrōma,* color, complexion]. ACHROMASIA.

achro·ma·cyte (ay·kro'muh·site, a·kro') *n.* [*achromat-* + *-cyte*]. A decolorized erythrocyte; a ghost or shadow corpuscle due to loss of hemoglobin.

achro·ma·sia (ack"ro·may'zhuh, ·zee·uh) *n.* [*a-* + *-chromasia*]. 1. Any condition, such as albinism, leukoderma, or vitiligo, in which there is discernible loss of normal color, usually of melanin, in the skin or in the iris. 2. *In histopathology,* failure of tissue or elements thereof to take stains in usual intensity. Syn. *achromia, achromatosis.*

achro·mat (ay'kro·mat, ack'ro·mat) *n.* [Gk. *achrōmatos,* colorless]. ROD-MONOCHROMAT.

achromat-, achromato-. A combining form meaning *achromatic, colorless.*

achro·mate (ay'kro·mate, ack'ro·mate) *n.* ROD-MONOCHROMAT.

achro·mat·ic (ay"kro·mat'ick) *adj.* [Gk. *achrōmatos,* colorless, + *-ic*]. 1. Without color. 2. Containing achromatin. 3. Not decomposing light into its constituent colors. 4. Staining with difficulty, as some cells or tissues.

achromatic fibrils. Fibrils of achromatic, nuclear, or cell substance forming lines which extend from pole to pole in a dividing nucleus, so as to form a spindle- or barrel-shaped figure.

achromatic figure. The spindle and asters in mitosis or meiosis.

achromatic lens. A double lens, each part made of such optical glass that the one neutralizes the dispersive effects of the other, without affecting the refraction.

achromatic objective. An objective corrected to bring two opposing colors to focus at the same point, by use of lens combinations containing glasses of differing refractive indices; they show moderate red and green fringes in oblique light.

achromatic spindle. ACHROMATIC FIGURE.

achro·ma·tin (ay·kro'muh·tin, a·kro') *n.* [*a-* + *chromatin*]. The faintly staining substance of the cell nucleus including the nuclear sap and euchromatin. —**achro·ma·tin·ic** (ay·kro"muh·tin'ick) *adj.*

achro·ma·tism (ay·kro'muh·tiz·um, a·kro') *n.* [*achromat-* + *-ism*]. 1. Absence of chromatic aberration. 2. Absence of color.

achromato-. See *achromat-.*

achro·mato·cyte (ay"kro·mat'o·site, a·kro'muh·to·) *n.* ACHROMACYTE.

achro·ma·tol·y·sis (ay·kro"muh·tol'i·sis) *n.,* pl. **achromatoly·ses** (·seez) [*achromato-* + *lysis*]. Dissolution of the achromatin of a cell.

achro·ma·to·phil (ay·kro'muh·to·fil", ay"kro·mat'o·fil) *n.* & *adj.* [*a-* + *chromatophil*]. Being or characterizing a microorganism or histologic element which does not stain readily.

achro·ma·to·phil·ia (ay·kro"muh·to·fil'ee·uh, ay"kro·mat"o·) *n.* [*achromatophil* + *-ia*]. The property of not staining readily. —**achromatophil·ic,** *adj.*

achro·ma·top·sia (a·kro"muh·top'see·uh) *n.* [*achromat-* + *-opsia*]. Total color blindness due to disease or injury of the retina, optic nerve, or pathway.

achro·ma·to·sis (a·kro"muh·to'sis, ack"ro·) *n.,* pl. **achromato·ses** (·seez) [*achromat-* + *-osis*]. ACHROMASIA.

achro·ma·tous (ay·kro'muh·tus, a·kro') *adj.* [Gk. *achrōmatos,* colorless, from *chrōma,* color, complexion]. Deficient in color; nonpigmented.

achro·ma·tu·ria (a·kro"muh·tew'ree·uh) *n.* [*achromat-* + *-uria*]. Lack of color in the urine.

achro·mia (a·kro'mee·uh, ay·) *n.* [*a-* + *chrom-* + *-ia*]. Absence of color.

achromia cutis. Absence of color in the skin. See also *leukoderma, vitiligo.*

achromia par·a·sit·i·ca (păr"uh·sit'i·kuh). The stage of tinea (pityriasis) versicolor in which the sites of infection of the skin with *Pityrosporum furfur* appear hypopigmented.

achro·mic (ay·kro'mick, a·kro') *adj.* [*a-* + *chrom-* + *-ic*]. Deficient in color; nonpigmented.

Achro·mo·bac·te·ra·ce·ae (ay·kro"mo·back·te·ray'see·ee) *n.pl.* [from *Achromobacter,* type genus]. A family of bacteria of the order Eubacteriales.

achro·mo·der·ma (a·kro"mo·dur'muh) *n.* [*a-* + *chromo-* + *-derma*]. Absence of color in the skin. See also *leukoderma, vitiligo.*

achro·mo·der·mia (a·kro"mo·dur'mee·uh) *n.* [*a-* + *chromo-* + *-dermia*]. ACHROMODERMA.

achro·mo·trich·ia (a·kro"mo·trick'ee·uh) *n.* [*a-* + *chromo-* + *-trichia*]. Loss or absence of pigment from hair; CANITIES.

achro·mous (a·kro'mus, ay·) *adj.* ACHROMIC.

Achromycin. A trademark for tetracycline, an antibiotic.

achroo-. See *achro-.*

ach·roo·am·y·loid (ack"ro·o·am'i·loid) *n.* [*achroo-* + *amyloid*]. Recently deposited amyloid which does not form a blue color with iodine.

ach·roo·cy·to·sis (ack"ro·o·sigh·to'sis, a·kro"o·) *n.* ACHROACYTOSIS.

ach·roo·dex·trin (ak"ro·o·decks'trin) *n.* [*achroo-* + *dextrin*]. A reducing dextrin formed by the action of the diastatic ferment of saliva or of acid upon starch. It is a modification of dextrin and may be precipitated by alcohol; it is not converted into sugar by ptyalin, nor colored by iodine.

Achú·ca·rro tannin silver stain (a·choo'ka·rro) [N. *Achúcarro,* Spanish histologist, 1881–1918]. A sequence tannic acid, diammine silver, and gold chloride process, used for staining astrocytes, glia, and nervous tissues.

achyl·ane·mia, achyl·anae·mia (ay·kigh"luh·nee'mee·uh, a·kigh") *n.* [*a-* + *chyl-* + *anemia*]. Hypochromic microcytic anemia due to iron deficiency and associated with achlorhydria.

achy·lia (ay·kigh'lee·uh, a·kigh') *n.* [*a-* + *chyl-* + *-ia*]. Absence of chyle. —**achy·lic** (·lick), **achy·lous** (·lus) *adj.*

achylia gas·tri·ca (gas'tri·kuh). Absence of gastric secretion of proteolytic enzymes and of hydrochloric acid, even after stimulation with histamine; frequently associated with gastric atrophy.

achylia pan·cre·at·i·ca (pan"kree·at'i·kuh). Pancreatic insufficiency; an absence of pancreatic juice resulting in fatty stools, malabsorption, and malnutrition.

achylic chloranemia. CHLOROSIS.

ach·y·lo·sis (ack"i·lo'sis) *n.* ACHYLIA.

achy·mia (ay·kigh'mee·uh, a·kigh') *n.* [*a-* + *chyme* + *-ia*]. Deficient formation of chyme. —**achy·mous** (·mus) *adj.*

acic·u·lar (a·sick'yoo·lur) *adj.* [from L. *acicula,* diminutive of *acus,* needle]. Needlelike; shaped like a needle.

ac·id (as'id) *adj.* & *n.* [L. *acidus,* from *acere,* to be sour]. 1. Sour. 2. A substance containing hydrogen replaceable by metals to form salts, and capable of dissociating in aqueous solution to form hydrogen ions (Arrhenius). 3. A substance, ionic or molecular, capable of yielding a proton to another substance (Brönsted and Lowry). This definition has the advantage over Arrhenius' in that it is applicable also to nonaqueous mediums. 4. A substance, ionic or molecular, capable of accepting a share in an electron pair, made available by a base, to form a coordinate covalent bond between the two substances (G. N. Lewis). This definition has the advantage over those of Arrhenius and of Brönsted and Lowry in being applicable also to substances which do not contain a proton (hydrogen ion). 5. Pertaining to or characteristic of an acid; ACIDIC (1). 6. *Slang.* LYSERGIC ACID DIETHYLAMIDE.

acid acriflavine. ACRIFLAVINE HYDROCHLORIDE.

acidaemia. ACIDEMIA.

acid alcohol. Alcohol containing various percentages of acid. In histologic techniques, a common mixture is 0.1% hydrochloric acid in 95% alcohol.

ac·id·am·i·nu·ria (as″id·am″i·new′ree·uh) *n.* AMINOACIDURIA.
acid anhydride. An oxide of a nonmetal, characterized by forming an acid with water.
acid-ash diet. A diet the redissolved ashed residue of which has a pH lower than 7.0. Such diets tend to reduce the pH of the urine.
acid-base balance or **equilibrium.** The state of dynamic equilibrium of acids and bases maintained in the body by physiologic processes such as respiration, elimination, and manufacture of buffers which keep the pH of the body constant. See also *acidosis, alkalosis.*
acid-base metabolism. Those physiologic activities which pertain to the relative concentrations of hydrogen and hydroxyl ions in the body.
acid carbonate. BICARBONATE.
acid cell. PARIETAL CELL.
ac·i·de·mia, ac·i·dae·mia (as″i·dee′mee·uh) *n.* [*acid* + *-emia*]. A decrease in blood pH below normal levels. Compare *acidosis.*
acid-fast, *adj.* Not decolorized by mineral acids after staining with aniline dyes; said of certain bacteria as well as some tissues and dyes.
acid-fast stains. Stains for certain bacteria (chiefly mycobacteria), hair cortex, ceroid and other lipofuscin pigments. Basic dyes and fluorochromes which resist decolorization by aqueous or alcoholic acid solutions are used.
acid-forming, *adj.* 1. Designating substances which produce acid in water. 2. *In nutrition,* designating those foods which yield an acid ash or residue when metabolized. Syn. *acidogenic.*
acid fuchsin. The disodium salt of the trisulfonic acid of rosaniline, $C_{20}H_{17}N_3Na_2O_9S_3$; a dye used as a biological stain.
acid glands. Glands which secrete acid, as the fundic glands of the stomach.
acid hematin method. A method for hemoglobin determination in which blood is diluted with 0.1 normal hydrochloric acid, and the color is compared with glass standards or with a standard hematin solution. Modifications of this are the Haden-Hausser method, the Wintrobe method, and the Sahli method.
acid hematins. Microcrystalline dark-brown pigments formed by the action of acids on hemoglobin.
acid·ic (a·sid′ick) *adj.* 1. Pertaining to or characteristic of an acid. 2. ACID-FORMING.
acid·i·fi·ca·tion (a·sid″i·fi·kay′shun) *n.* Conversion into an acid; process of becoming acid; addition of acid. —**acid·i·fy** (a·sid′i·figh) *v.;* **acid·i·fi·able** (a·sid″i·figh′uh·bul) *adj.*
acid·i·fi·er (a·sid′i·figh·ur) *n.* *In radiography and photography,* a weak organic acid, such as acetic acid, contained in or used prior to fixing solutions for the neutralization of developing solutions in order to arrest the developing process. See also *short stop.*
ac·i·dim·e·ter (as″i·dim′e·tur) *n.* An instrument for determining the degree of acidity of a liquid or the strength of an acid.
acid·i·met·ric (a·sid″i·met′rick, as″i·di·) *adj.* Pertaining to or involving acidimetry.
ac·i·dim·e·try (as″i·dim′e·tree) *n.* Measurement of the amount of free acid in a solution.
acid intoxication. A toxic condition of the body resulting from an excess of acids accumulated from within it or introduced from outside it.
ac·id·ism (as′i·diz·um) *n.* ACID INTOXICATION.
acid·i·ty (a·sid′i·tee) *n.* 1. The quality of being acid; sourness. 2. The state of being excessively acid. 3. The acid content of any substance.
acid magenta. ACID FUCHSIN.
acid maltase. A glucosidase found in the lysosomes which hydrolyzes maltose and other oligosaccharides to yield glucose residues, acting optimally at acid pH. Syn. *α-1,4 glucosidase, alpha-1,4 glucosidase.*
acid maltase deficiency. POMPE'S DISEASE.
acid number. The number of milligrams of potassium hydroxide required to neutralize the free fatty acids in 1 g of oil or fat, or to neutralize naturally occurring acids in 1 g of other substance, such as a resin.
acid·o·cyte (a·sid′o·site) *n. Obsol.* EOSINOPHIL LEUKOCYTE.
ac·i·do·cy·to·pe·nia (as″i·do·sigh″to·pee′nee·uh) *n.* [*acidocyte* + *-penia*]. *Obsol.* EOSINOPENIA.
ac·i·do·cy·to·sis (as″i·do·sigh·to′sis, a·sid″o·) *n.* [*acidocyte* + *-osis*]. *Obsol.* EOSINOPHILIA.
acid of sugar. OXALIC ACID.
ac·i·do·gen·ic (as″i·do·jen′ick) *adj.* ACID-FORMING.
ac·i·dom·e·ter (as″i·dom′e·tur) *n.* ACIDIMETER.
ac·i·do·pe·nia (as″i·do·pee′nee·uh) *n. Obsol.* EOSINOPENIA.
acid·o·phil (a·sid′o·fil) *adj. & n.* 1. ACIDOPHILIC. 2. An acidophilic cell, tissue element, or substance. 3. Specifically, an ALPHA CELL of the adenohypophysis. Contr. *basophil.*
acid·o·phile (a·sid′o·file) *adj. & n.* ACIDOPHIL.
acidophil granules. Granules that stain with acid dyes, especially eosin, acid fuchsin, or orange G.
acid·o·phil·ia (a·sid″o·fil′ee·uh) *n.* [*acid* + *-philia*]. Affinity for acid stains. Syn. *oxyphilia.* Contr. *basophilia.*
ac·i·do·phil·ic (as″i·do·fil′ick, a·sid″o·) *adj.* 1. Having an affinity for acid stains. Syn. *eosinophilic, oxyphilic.* Contr. *basophilic.* 2. Thriving in an acid medium; said especially of various microorganisms.
acidophilic adenoma. An adenoma whose parenchymal cells are eosinophilic, especially certain hypophyseal and sweat gland adenomas.
acidophilic erythroblast or **normoblast.** *Obsol.* NORMOBLAST (1).
ac·i·doph·i·lism (as″i·dof′i·liz·um) *n.* A condition of overabundance or overactivity of the acidophilic cells of the adenohypophysis.
acidophil leukocyte. *Obsol.* EOSINOPHIL LEUKOCYTE.
ac·i·doph·i·lous (as″i·dof′i·lus) *adj.* ACIDOPHILIC.
acidophilus milk. Milk inoculated with cultures of *Lactobacillus acidophilus;* has been used in various enteric disorders to provide a change of bacterial flora.
ac·i·do·re·sis·tant (as″i·do·re·zis′tunt) *adj.* Acid-resistant; not readily decolorized by acids; applied to certain microorganisms. Compare *acid-fast.* —**acidoresis·tance** (·tunce) *n.*
ac·i·do·sis (as″i·do′sis) *n.,* pl. **acido·ses** (·seez) [*acid* + *-osis*]. An abnormal state characterized by processes tending to increase the concentration of hydrogen ion in the body above the normal range or to increase the loss of base from the body. Physiological compensatory mechanisms act to return the lowered pH toward normal. Compare *acidemia.* See also *compensated acidosis, metabolic acidosis, respiratory acidosis.* —**aci·dot·ic** (·dot′ick) *adj.*
ac·i·dos·teo·phyte (as″i·dos′tee·o·fite) *n.* [Gk. *akis, akidos,* pointed object, + *osteophyte*]. A sharp-pointed bony projection or outgrowth; an osseous spicule.
acid oxide. An oxide of a nonmetal which produces an acid when combined with water; an acid anhydride.
acid phosphatase. An enzyme catalyzing release of phosphate ions from organic phosphates such as α- and β-glycerophosphates, optimally at about pH 4 to 5.
acid phosphate. A phosphate in which only one or two of the hydrogen atoms of phosphoric acid have been replaced by metals.
acid potassium tartrate. POTASSIUM BITARTRATE.
acid-resistant, *adj.* Not readily decolorized by acids; applied to certain microorganisms. Compare *acid-fast.*
acid salt. A salt that contains unreplaced hydrogen atoms of the acid from which the salt was formed, as $NaHCO_3$.
acid seromucoid. OROSOMUCOID.
acid tide. A period of increased excretion of acid radicals by the kidney 1 to 2 hours after a meal.
acid·u·late (a·sid′yoo·late) *v.* To render sour or acid in reaction; to pour acid into; to acidify. —**acidu·lant** (·lunt) *adj. & n.;* **acidu·lous** (·lus) *adj.*

Acidulin. Trademark for glutamic acid hydrochloride, a digestant.

ac·i·du·ria (as″i·dew′ree·uh) *n.* [*acid* + *-uria*]. The condition in which the urine is acid.

[1]**ac·i·du·ric** (as″i·dew′rick) *adj.* Exhibiting or pertaining to aciduria.

[2]**aciduric,** *adj.* [*acid* + L. *durare*, to endure, + *-ic*]. *Obsol.* Of bacteria: able to grow in an acid medium; acid-tolerant.

aciesis. Misspelling of *acyesis.*

ac·i·nal (as′i·nul) *adj.* ACINAR.

ac·i·nar (as′i·nur, ·nahr) *adj.* Of or pertaining to an acinus.

acinar cell. One of the cells lining an alveolus of a compound acinous gland. Syn. *acinous cell.*

ac·i·ne·sia (as″i·nee′zhuh, ·zee·uh) *n.* AKINESIA.

acini. Plural of *acinus.*

acin·ic (a·sin′ick) *adj.* ACINAR.

ac·i·no·tu·bu·lar (as″i·no·tew′bew·lur) *adj.* Consisting of tubular acini.

acinotubular gland. A gland with both tubular and saccular elements.

ac·i·nous (as′i·nus) *adj.* [L. *acinosus*, like grapes]. Resembling, consisting of, or pertaining to acini.

acinous cell. ACINAR CELL.

acinous gland. A gland in which the secretory endpieces have the form of an acinus.

a-c interval. The interval between the beginnings of the a and c waves of the jugular venous pulse, measuring the time between atrial and ventricular systole, normally less than 0.20 second.

ac·i·nus (as′i·nus) *n.*, pl. **ac·i·ni** (as′i·nigh) [L., berry, grape]. 1. A saccular terminal division of a compound gland having a narrow lumen, several of which combine to form a lobule. Compare *alveolus (4).* 2. The anatomic unit of the lung consisting of alveolar ducts and alveoli stemming from a terminal bronchiole.

Aciquel. Trademark for potassium glucaldrate, an antacid.

ackee. AKEE.

aclad·i·o·sis (a·klad″ee·o′sis) *n.* An uncommon fungus infection of the skin, caused by a species of *Acladium* and marked by ulceration.

A.C.L.A.M. American College of Laboratory Animal Medicine.

acla·sia (a·klay′zhuh, ·zee·uh) *n.* ACLASIS.

ac·la·sis (ack′luh·sis, a·klay′sis) *n.* [*a-* + Gk. *klasis*, breaking]. The blending of abnormally developed tissue with normal tissue.

aclas·tic (a·clas′tick) *adj.* [*a-* + *clastic*]. Not refracting.

acleis·to·car·dia (a·klye″sto·kahr′dee·uh, ay·klye″sto·) *n.* [*a-* + *cleisto-* + *-cardia*]. A condition in which the foramen ovale of the heart fails to close.

ac·mas·tic (ack·mas′tick) *adj.* [Gk. *akmastikos*, culminating, at its height]. ACMIC.

ac·me (ack′mee) *n.* [Gk. *akmē*]. 1. The highest point. 2. The crisis or critical stage of a disease.

ac·mic (ack′mick) *adj.* Pertaining to the acme of a disease. Contr. *epacmic, paracmic.*

ac·ne (ack′nee) *n.* [Byzantine Gk. *aknē*, probably from a copyist's error for *akmē*, skin eruption, lit. point, peak]. An inflammatory condition of the sebaceous glands common in adolescence and young adulthood, characterized by comedones which often become inflamed and form papules, pustules, nodules, and cysts, usually on the face, chest, and back. Syn. *acne vulgaris.* See also *keloid acne.*

acne ag·mi·na·ta (ag″mi·nay′tuh). LUPUS MILIARIS DISSEMINATUS FACIEI.

acne al·bi·da (al′bi·duh). ACNE MILIARIS.

acne ar·ti·fi·ci·a·lis (ahr·ti·fish·ee·ay′lis). An acneform eruption caused by exposure to tars, waxes, grease, or chlorinated hydrocarbons. See also *chloracne.*

acne atroph·i·ca (a·trof′i·kuh, ay·). ACNE VARIOLIFORMIS.

acne bacillus. *CORYNEBACTERIUM ACNES.*

acne ca·chec·ti·co·rum (ka·keck″ti·ko′rum). An acneform eruption seen in debilitated persons during long, wasting diseases, such as tuberculosis. The lesions occur on the trunk and legs, appearing as small, flat, dull-red papules and pustules.

acne co·ag·mi·na·ta (ko·ag″mi·nay′tuh). A pustular acneform eruption often seen after administering any of the halogens or their salts and among industrial workers exposed to hydrochloric acid, tar, tar vapor, oil, wax, or paraffin.

acne con·glo·ba·ta (kon·glo·bay′tuh). A severe and long-enduring form of acne, frequently affecting the lower part of the back, buttocks, and thighs in addition to the face and chest with abcesses, cysts, and sinuses as well as with the more common lesions of acne. Scarring, often hypertrophic and keloidal, is an inevitable consequence of healing.

acne cys·ti·ca (sis′ti·kuh). A form of acne in which the lesions are mainly cysts.

acne decalvans. FOLLICULITIS DECALVANS.

ac·ne·form (ack′ne·form) *adj.* Resembling acne.

acneform drug eruptions. Eruptions resembling acne and caused by certain drugs, principally iodides and bromides, but in some cases also caused by steroids.

ac·ne·gen (ack′ne·jen) *n.* [*acne* + *-gen*]. A substance that promotes acne. —**ac·ne·gen·ic** (ack″ne·jen′ick) *adj.*

ac·ne·ic (ack·nee′ick) *adj.* Of or pertaining to acne.

ac·ne·iform (ack·nee′i·form) *adj.* ACNEFORM.

acne in·du·ra·ta (in·dew·ray′tuh). A form of acne in which the lesions are mainly hard papules.

acne ker·a·to·sa (kerr·uh·to′suh). A rare form of acne consisting of soft, conical plugs of horn which become inflamed and form scars, usually at the angles of the mouth.

acne med·i·ca·men·to·sa (med″i·kuh·men·to′suh). An acneform drug eruption, caused by administration of certain drugs.

ac·ne·mia (ack·nee′mee·uh) *n.* [Gk. *aknēmos*, lacking the calf (from *knēmē*, calf) + *-ia*]. 1. Atrophy of the calves of the legs. 2. Congenital absence of the legs. —**acne·mous** (·mus) *adj.*

acne mil·i·a·ris (mil·ee·air′ris). A condition of the skin of the face, characterized by many milia.

acne ne·crot·i·ca (ne·krot′i·kuh). ACNE VARIOLIFORMIS.

acne necrotica mil·i·a·ris (mil″ee·air′is). A pruritic, papular, pustular, and scarring folliculitis of the scalp, with discrete and scattered lesions. Compare *folliculitis decalvans.*

acne neo·na·to·rum. (nee″o·nay·to′rum). Acneform eruption in a newborn in the nature of a nevoid anomaly, acne medicamentosa as from iodides or bromides ingested by the mother, or truly precocious acne.

acne pan·cre·at·i·ca (pan·kree·at′i·kuh). Small cysts in the pancreas due to obstruction of the smaller ducts.

acne pap·u·lo·sa (pap·yoo·lo′suh). A form of acne in which the lesions are mainly inflammatory papules.

acne pus·tu·lo·sa (pus·tew·lo′suh). A form of acne in which the lesions are mainly pustules.

acne ro·sa·cea (ro·zay′shee·uh, ro·zay′see·uh). A chronic dermatitis of the face, principally of the nose, paranasal areas, cheeks, and forehead, marked by telangiectasis, pustules, erythema, and a tendency to hypertrophy of the affected parts, especially the nose. Ophthalmic keratitis may occur.

acne scrof·u·lo·so·rum (skrof″yoo·lo·so′rum). An acneform process in those afflicted with tuberculosis of organs other than the skin. It is probably a tuberculid.

acne tar·si (tahr′sigh). An inflammatory affection of the large sebaceous glands of the eyelids (tarsal glands).

acne trop·i·ca (trop′i·kuh). A severe form of acne conglobata that occurs in hot, humid climates. The chest, parts of the abdomen, shoulders, arms, upper portion of the back, buttocks, and upper parts of thighs are commonly affected.

acne ur·ti·ca·ta (ur·ti·kay′tuh). A persistent condition, occurring especially in adult females with depressive illnesses, characterized by complaints of well-localized itching and a small wheal; actually the only lesions seen are deep excoriations on depigmented scars over the upper back and shoulder. Compare *acne urticata polycythemica.*

acne urticata poly·cy·the·mi·ca (pol″ee·sigh·thee′mi·kuh). A chronic, severely pruritic rash associated with polycythemia vera and characterized by pale red, wheal-like papules, occasionally surmounted by vesicles, appearing in crops on the face and extensor extremities and healing with residual scarring and hyperpigmentation.

acne va·ri·o·li·for·mis (văr″ee·o″li·for′mis). An uncommon acneform process affecting the brow and temporoparietal portion of the scalp at the hairline and sometimes beyond. The lesions are papulopustules that crust, ulcerate, and heal by scarring reminiscent of that of smallpox.

acne vul·ga·ris (vul·gair′is, ·găr′). ACNE.

ac·ni·tis (ack·nigh′tis) *n.* [*acne* + *-itis*]. *Obsol.* 1. PAPULONECROTIC TUBERCULID. 2. LUPUS MILIARIS DISSEMINATUS FACIEI.

A.C.N.M. American College of Nurse Midwifery.

ac·o·as·ma (ack″o·az′muh) *n.* ACOUSMA.

Ac·o·can·thera, Ac·o·kan·thera (ack″o·kan′thur·uh) *n.* [Gk. *akōkē,* point, + NL. *anthera,* anther]. An African genus of shrubs or trees of the Apocynaceae. Juices from the leaves and stems of several species contain a principle, acocantherin, similar to or identical with ouabain.

ac·o·can·ther·in (ack″o·kan′thur·in) *n.* [*Acocanthera* + *-in*]. OUABAIN.

Acodeen. Trademark for butamirate citrate, an antitussive.

acoe·lia, ace·lia (a·see′lee·uh, ay·) *n.* [*a-* + *coelom* + *-ia*]. Absence of a body cavity or coelom. —**acoe·li·ous** (·lee·us), **acoe·lom·ate** (·luh·mate), **acoe·lous** (·lus) *adj.*

acoenaesthesia. ACENESTHESIA.

A.C.O.G. American College of Obstetricians and Gynecologists.

Acokanthera. ACOCANTHERA.

ac·o·la·sia (ack″o·lay′zhuh, ·zee·uh) *n.* [Gk. *akolasia,* intemperance, from *kolazein,* to check, restrain]. Unrestrained self-indulgence; lust; intemperance. —**aco·las·tic** (·las′tick) *adj.*

aco·lous (ay·ko′lus, a·ko′lus) *adj.* [Gk. *akōlos,* from *kōlon,* limb]. Having no limbs.

aco·mous (ay·ko′mus, a·ko′) *adj.* [Gk. *akomos,* hairless, from *komē,* hair]. Bald. —**aco·mia** (·mee·uh) *n.*

Acon. Trademark for a water-dispersible preparation of vitamin A.

acon·a·tive (ay·kon′uh·tiv) *adj.* [*a-* + *conative*]. Having no wish or desire to make any physical or mental effort.

ac·o·nine (ack′o·neen, ·nin) *n.* An alkaloid, $C_{25}H_{41}NO_9$, obtained from aconitine but much less toxic.

acon·i·tase (a·kon′i·taze, ·tace) *n.* [*aconite* + *-ase*]. An enzyme of the citric acid cycle that catalyzes the breakdown of citric acid to *cis*-aconitic and isocitric acids.

ac·o·nite (ack′o·nite) *n.* [Gk. *akoniton,* wolf's bane]. A very poisonous drug obtained from the roots of *Aconitum napellus.* It has a bitter, pungent taste and leaves a sensation of numbness and tingling on the lips and tongue. Physiologically, it is a cardiac, respiratory, and circulatory depressant and produces sensory paralysis. The principal alkaloid is aconitine. Has been used as a diaphoretic, antipyretic, and diuretic.

ac·o·nit·ic acid (ack″o·nit′ick). 1,2,3-Propenetricarboxylic acid, $C_6H_6O_6$, representing citric acid minus a molecule of water; it occurs in two modifications, *cis-* and *trans-*. *cis-*Aconitic acid is an intermediate in the tricarboxylic acid cycle. Aconitic acid, presumably of *trans-* configuration, occurs in a number of plants, including species of *Aconitum,* beets, and sugar cane.

acon·i·tin (a·kon′i·tin) *n.* ACONITINE.

acon·i·tine (a·kon′i·teen, ·tin) *n.* An extremely poisonous alkaloid, $C_{34}H_{47}NO_{11}$, derived from *Aconitum napellus* and other species.

Ac·o·ni·tum (ack″o·night′um) *n.* [L.]. A genus of poisonous ranunculaceous plants, whose species are the source of aconite.

acon·ure·sis (a·kon″yoo·ree′sis) *n.* [Gk. *akōn,* involuntary, + *uresis*]. Involuntary urination.

acop·ro·sis (ay″kop·ro′sis, ack″o·pro′sis) *n.* [*acoprous* + *-osis*]. A deficiency or absence of feces in the intestine.

acop·rous (ay·kop′rus) *adj.* [Gk. *akopros,* from *kopros,* feces]. Devoid of fecal matter.

ac·o·rea (ack″o·ree′uh) *n.* [*a-* + Gk. *korē,* pupil, + *-ia*]. Absence of the pupil.

aco·ria, ako·ria (a·ko′ree·uh, ay·) *n.* [Gk. *akoria,* not eating to satiety, from *koros,* satiety]. A sensation of hunger not relieved even by a large meal, due to the absence of the feeling of satiety.

acor·mus (a·kor′mus, ay·) *n.* [*a-* + Gk. *kormos,* tree trunk]. An acardiac omphalosite lacking a trunk.

Acos·ta's disease [J. d'*Acosta,* Spanish missionary and author, 1539–1600]. ALTITUDE SICKNESS.

acos·tate (a·kos′tate, ay·) *adj.* [*a-* + *costate*]. Without ribs.

acou-, acouo- [Gk. *akouein,* to hear]. A combining form meaning *hearing.*

acou·es·the·sia, acou·aes·the·sia (a·koo″es·theezh′uh, ·theez′ee·uh, ack″oo·) *n.* [*acou-* + *esthesia*]. 1. The sense or faculty of hearing. 2. The ability to hear normally.

ac·ou·la·li·on (ack″oo·lay′lee·on) *n.* [*acou-* + Gk. *lalia,* talk, + *-on* (neuter suffix)]. An instrument used in teaching speech to deaf-mutes.

acou·me·ter (a·koo′me·tur) *n.* [*acou-* + *-meter*]. *Obsol.* AUDIOMETER. —**ac·ou·met·ric** (ack″oo·met′rick) *adj.*

ac·ou·om·e·ter (ack″oo·om′e·tur) *n.* *Obsol.* AUDIOMETER. —**acou·o·met·ric** (a·koo″o·met′rick, ack″oo·o·) *adj.*

acou·o·pho·nia (a·koo″o·fo′nee·uh) *n.* [*acouo-* + *-phonia*]. AUSCULTATORY PERCUSSION.

ac·ou·oph·o·ny (ack″oo·off′uh·nee) *n.* [*acouo-* + *-phony*]. AUSCULTATORY PERCUSSION.

acou·sia (a·koo′zhuh, ·zee·uh) *n.* [Gk. *akousia,* from *akousios,* unwilling, from *a-* + *ekousios,* willing]. An involuntary act.

-acousia, -acusia [Gk. *akousis,* hearing, + *-ia*]. A combining form meaning *condition of hearing.*

-acousis. See *-acousia.*

acous·ma (a·kooz′muh) *n.,* pl. **acousmas, acousma·ta** (·tuh) [Gk. *akousma,* something heard]. A simple auditory hallucination, as of buzzing or ringing.

acous·mat·ag·no·sis (a·kooz″muh·tag·no′sis) *n.* [Gk. *akousma, akousmatos,* something heard, + *a-* + *-gnōsis,* knowledge]. Inability to recognize sounds or understand spoken words; AUDITORY AGNOSIA.

acous·mat·am·ne·sia (a·kooz″muh·tam·nee′zhuh, ·zee·uh) *n.* [*acousma* + *amnesia*]. Inability to remember sounds.

acous·tic (uh·koos′tick) *adj.* [Gk. *akoustikos,* from *akouein,* to hear]. Pertaining to sound or hearing.

acoustic agraphia. Inability to write from dictation.

acoustic amnestic aphasia. An impairment in language capacity in which there is primarily a disturbed retention of syllables or words, as when a patient makes a mistake in the reproduction of three consecutive syllables or words of similar sound structure, losing their clear differentiation.

acoustic aphasia. AUDITORY APHASIA.

acoustic capsule. OTIC CAPSULE.

acoustic eminence. AREA VESTIBULARIS.

acoustic ganglion. The embryonic ganglionic mass which separates into spiral and vestibular ganglions.

acoustic image. An idea of something which has been heard.

acoustic meatus. See *external acoustic meatus, internal acoustic meatus.*

acoustic muscle reflex. A generalized jerking of the body in response to a loud, sudden noise.

acoustic nerve. VESTIBULOCOCHLEAR NERVE.

acoustic-nerve tumor. 1. Any tumor of the acoustic nerve. 2. Specifically, ACOUSTIC NEURILEMMOMA.

acoustic neurilemmoma. A benign tumor of the sheath of the eighth cranial nerve, usually growing at one cerebellopontine angle. Syn. *schwannoma.*

acoustic neuroma or **neurinoma.** ACOUSTIC NEURILEMMOMA.

acous·ti·co·fa·cial (uh·koos″ti·ko·fay′shul) *adj.* Pertaining jointly to the acoustic (vestibulocochlear) and facial nerves.

acousticofacial primordium or **ganglion.** The mass of neural crest tissue that differentiates into the ganglions of the vestibulocochlear and facial nerves.

acous·ti·co·mo·tor (uh·koos″ti·ko·mo′tur) *adj.* Pertaining to motor activity in response to a sound stimulus.

acousticomotor epilepsy. A form of reflex epilepsy in which seizures occur in response to sound stimuli, usually loud sudden noises; AUDIOGENIC EPILEPSY.

acous·ti·co·pal·pe·bral (uh·koos″ti·ko·pal′pe·brul) *adj.* [*acoustic* + *palpebral*]. Pertaining jointly to the vestibulocochlear nerve and to the eyelids.

acousticopalpebral reflex. AUDITORY-PALPEBRAL REFLEX.

acous·ti·co·pho·bia (uh·koos″ti·ko·fo′bee·uh) *n.* Morbid fear of sounds.

acoustic radiation. A large bundle of fibers in the posterior part of the internal capsule, running from the medial geniculate body to the superior and transverse temporal gyri. NA *radiatio acustica.*

acoustic reflex. 1. AURAL REFLEX. 2. AUDITORY-PALPEBRAL REFLEX.

acous·tics (uh·koos′ticks) *n.* The science of sound.

acoustic spots. The macula sacculi and the macula utriculi.

acoustic tetanus. Tetanus produced in a muscle-nerve preparation by rapidly repeated induction shocks, the period of which is determined by a tuning fork.

acoustic trauma. AUDITORY TRAUMA.

acoustic tubercle. AREA VESTIBULARIS.

ac·ou·tom·e·ter (ack″oo·tom′e·tur) *n. Obsol.* AUDIOMETER.

A.C.P. 1. American College of Physicians. 2. Animal Care Panel, now known as American Association for Laboratory Animal Science.

ac·quired, *adj.* Not present at birth but developed in an individual as a reaction to environment or through use or disuse. Contr. *congenital, hereditary, innate.*

acquired agammaglobulinemia. The depression of gamma globulin levels from previously normal to below 500 mg/dl which occurs equally in both sexes; may be primary without a clear underlying cause or secondary to a well-defined disease process leading to decreased synthesis or increased loss. In addition to greater susceptibility to bacterial infections, patients may develop symptoms of celiac syndrome and such diseases as systemic lupus erythematosus and other immunologic abnormalities.

acquired behavior. *In psychology,* the particular aspects of behavior that distinguish one individual from another or a child from an adult, ascribed primarily to experience rather than to heredity.

acquired character. A modification of the organism caused by an environmental factor or factors.

acquired drive. *In psychology,* a drive which is not part of the basic inherited makeup of the organism, but which was aroused and developed through experience.

acquired dysmenorrhea. SECONDARY DYSMENORRHEA.

acquired functional megacolon. IDIOPATHIC MEGACOLON.

acquired harelip. A cleft in the lip, caused by an accident, but giving the same appearance as congenital harelip.

acquired hemolytic anemia. Any anemia due to the action of an external agent or disease process upon normally constructed erythrocytes.

acquired hemolytic jaundice. Jaundice resulting from acquired hemolytic anemia.

acquired hernia. A noncongenital hernia resulting from strain or weight lifting, or as the direct result of operation or muscular weakening.

acquired hydromyelia. Cystic dilatation of the central canal of the spinal cord due to an acquired obstruction of cerebrospinal fluid circulation, as from a cerebellar tumor or injuries of the spinal cord.

acquired immunity. The enhanced resistance of a host to disease as a result of naturally acquired or artificially induced experience. Contr. *native immunity.* See also *active immunity, passive immunity.*

acquired multiple polyposis. POLYPOID ADENOMATOSIS.

acquired reflex. CONDITIONED REFLEX.

acquired teratism. A deformity which is the result of disease, violence, or operation.

acquired veil. *Obsol.* An obstruction or imperfection of voice due to exposure to cold, catarrhal conditions, overuse, or bad training.

acr-, acro- [Gk. *akros,* extreme; *akron,* extremity]. A combining form meaning (a) *extremity, tip, end;* (b) *height, promontory;* (c) *extreme, intense.*

ac·ral (ack′rul) *adj.* [*acr-* + *-al*]. Pertaining to the limbs or extremities.

ac·ra·mine yellow (ack′ruh·meen). AMINACRINE.

acra·nia (ay·kray′nee·uh, a·kra′) *n.* Partial or complete absence of the cranium at birth. —**acra·nial** (·nee·ul) *adj.;* **acra·ni·us** (·nee·us) *n.*

acra·sia (a·kray′zhuh, ·zee·uh) *n.* [Gk. *akrasia,* from *a-* + *kratos,* power, mastery]. Intemperance; lack of self-control.

acra·tia (a·kray′shee·uh) *n.* [Gk. *akratia*]. Impotence, loss of power.

acrat·ure·sis (uh·krat″yoo·ree′sis) *n.* [*acrat*ia + *uresis*]. Inability to urinate due to atony of the urinary bladder.

ac·re·mo·ni·o·sis (ack″re·mo″nee·o′sis) *n.* A fungus infection caused by *Acremonium potroni;* characterized by fever, gumma-like swellings, and perhaps keratitis.

-acria [*acr-* + *-ia*]. A combining form meaning *a condition of the extremities.*

ac·rid (ack′rid) *adj.* [L. *acer, acris,* sharp]. Pungent; irritating.

ac·ri·dine (ack′ri·deen, ·din) *n.* [*acrid* + *-ine*]. Dibenzo[*b,e*]pyridine, $C_{13}H_9N$, a constituent of coal tar. It is employed in the synthesis of various dyes, certain of which (acriflavine, diflavine, proflavine) are used as antiseptics. Mutations produced by acridine dyes, by virtue of their intercalation into molecules of deoxyribonucleic acid, have been employed by Crick as evidence of the triplet nature of the genetic code.

acridine stains. Dyes formed from acridine, including acriflavine and phosphine.

ac·ri·fla·vine (ack″ri·flay′veen, ·vin, ·flav′een, ·in) *n.* [*acri*dine + *flavine*]. 1. A mixture of 3,6-diamino-10-methylacridinium chloride and 3,6-diaminoacridine; a deep orange, granular powder, freely soluble in water. It is used chiefly as a local antiseptic, but has been administered intravenously in treating various infections. Syn. *neutral acriflavine.* 2. Basic acridine fluorochrome, C.I. No. 46000, used in a fluorescent Schiff reagent and as fluorochrome for elastic fibers.

acriflavine hydrochloride. A mixture of the hydrochlorides of 3,6-diamino-10-methylacridinium chloride and 3,6-diaminoacridine; a reddish-brown powder, freely soluble in water, used for the same purposes as acriflavine but more irritant because of its acid reaction. Syn. *acid acriflavine.*

ac·ri·sor·cin (ack″ri·zor′sin) *n.* 9-Aminoacridinium 4-hexylresorcinolate, $C_{13}H_{10}N_2.C_{12}H_{18}O_2$, used topically for treatment of tinea versicolor.

acrit·i·cal (ay·krit′i·kul, a·krit′) *adj.* 1. Without a crisis; not relating to a crisis. 2. Indeterminate, as regards prognosis.

ac·ri·to·chro·ma·cy (ack″ri·to·kro′muh·see) *n.* [Gk. *akritos,* undistinguishable, + Gk. *chrōma,* color]. 1. COLOR BLINDNESS. 2. ACHROMATOPSIA.

acro-. See *acr-.*

acroaesthesia. ACROESTHESIA.

ac·ro·ag·no·sis (ack″ro·ag·no′sis) *n.* [*acro-* + *a-* + *-gnosis*]. 1. Absence of sense of position, weight, shape, or even existence of a limb or limbs. 2. Loss of sensation in a limb.

ac·ro·an·es·the·sia, ac·ro·an·aes·the·sia (ack″ro·an″es·theezh′uh) *n.* Anesthesia of the extremities, from disease or after an anesthetic.

ac·ro·ar·thri·tis (ack″ro·ahr·thrigh′tis) *n.* Arthritis of the extremities.

ac·ro·as·phyx·ia (ack″ro·as·fick′see·uh) *n.* [*acro-* + *asphyxia*]. Intermittent digital cyanosis and pallor, precipitated by cold or emotion, with subsequent reactive hyperemia on rewarming; a manifestation of Raynaud's phenomenon.

ac·ro·atax·ia (ack″ro·a·tack′see·uh) *n.* [*acro-* + *ataxia*]. Incoordination of the muscles of the fingers and toes. Contr. *proximoataxia.*

ac·ro·blast (ack′ro·blast) *n.* [*acro-* + *-blast*]. A remnant of the Golgi apparatus.

ac·ro·brachy·ceph·a·ly (ack″ro·brack″ee·sef′uh·lee) *n.* [*acro-* + *brachy-* + *-cephaly*]. Congenital deformity of the skull, similar to oxycephaly, characterized by an abnormally high skull, greatly widened in the transverse diameter, and flattening of the head in the anteroposterior diameter. See also *craniofacial dysostosis.*

ac·ro·cen·tric (ack″ro·sen′trick) *adj.* [*acro-* + *centric*]. Of a chromosome: having the centromere closer to one end than to the center, resulting in one long and one very short arm. Contr. *metacentric, submetacentric, telocentric.*

ac·ro·ce·pha·lia (ack″ro·se·fay′lee·uh) *n.* [*acro-* + *-cephalia*]. OXYCEPHALY.

ac·ro·ce·phal·ic (ack″ro·se·fal′ick) *adj.* [*acro-* + *cephalic*]. OXYCEPHALIC.

ac·ro·ceph·a·lop·a·gus (ack″ro·sef·uh·lop′uh·gus) *n.*, pl. **acro-cephalopa·gi** (·guy, ·jye) [*acro-* + *cephalopagus*]. CRANIOPAGUS PARIETALIS.

ac·ro·ceph·a·lo·poly·syn·dac·ty·ly (ack″ro·sef″uh·lo·pol″ee·sin·dack′ti·lee) *n.* [*acrocephaly* + *poly-* + *syndactyly*]. A syndrome of acrocephaly, brachysyndactyly of the fingers, preaxial polydactyly, and syndactyly of the toes; classified as either type I (Noack's syndrome), an autosomal dominant trait, or type II (Carpenter's syndrome), an autosomal recessive trait further characterized by mental retardation, obesity, and hypogenitalism.

ac·ro·ceph·a·lo·syn·dac·tyl·ia (ack″ro·sef″uh·lo·sin″dack·til′ee·uh) *n.* ACROCEPHALOSYNDACTYLY.

ac·ro·ceph·a·lo·syn·dac·tyl·ism (ack″ro·sef″uh·lo·sin·dack′til·iz·um) *n.* ACROCEPHALOSYNDACTYLY.

ac·ro·ceph·a·lo·syn·dac·ty·ly (ack″ro·sef″uh·lo·sin·dack′ti·lee) *n.* [*acrocephaly* + *syndactyly*]. A form of craniosynostosis characterized by oxycephaly with syndactyly of the hands and feet and, often, malformation of other parts; variants are defined by anomalies present and mode of inheritance; markedly similar to craniofacial dysostosis, with which it may appear in the same patient. See also *Apert's syndrome.*

ac·ro·ceph·a·ly (ack″ro·sef′uh·lee) *n.* [*acro-* + *-cephaly*]. OXYCEPHALY.

ac·ro·chor·do·ma (ack″ro·kor·do′muh) *n.* CHORDOMA.

ac·ro·chor·don (ack″ro·kor′don) *n.* [Gk. *akrochordōn*, wart with a thin neck]. A cutaneous tag or fibroma pendulum.

ac·ro·ci·ne·sis (ack″ro·si·nee′sis) *n.* ACROKINESIS.

ac·ro·con·trac·ture (ack″ro·kun·track′chur) *n.* Contracture of the joints of the hands or feet.

ac·ro·cy·a·no·sis (ack″ro·sigh″uh·no′sis) *n.*, pl. **acrocyano·ses** (·seez). Symmetric mottled cyanosis of the hands and feet, associated with coldness and sweating; a vasospastic disorder accentuated by cold and emotion and relieved by warmth. Syn. *Crocq's disease.*

ac·ro·der·ma·ti·tis (ack″ro·dur″muh·tye′tis) *n.* [*acro-* + *dermatitis*]. Any inflammatory condition of the hands, arms, feet, or legs.

acrodermatitis chron·i·ca atroph·i·cans (kron′i·kuh a·trof′i·kanz). A characteristic, chronic, progressive inflammatory condition of the skin that tends to atrophy of the skin in a form that is likened to wrinkled cigarette paper.

acrodermatitis con·tin·ua (kon·tin′yoo·uh). A variant form of psoriasis resembling pustular psoriasis in all respects except that it arises without previous evidence of the disease. Syn. *Hallopeau's disease.*

acrodermatitis en·tero·path·i·ca (en″tur·o·path′i·kuh). A rare, sometimes familial disease of unknown cause appearing in the first year of life, and characterized by chronic, relapsing vesiculobullous dermatitis associated with mucous-membrane lesions, diarrhea, and alopecia. Syn. *Brandt syndrome, Danbolt-Closs syndrome.*

acrodermatitis hi·e·ma·lis (high″e·may′lis). Inflammatory changes in the skin of the hands and feet, attributable to winter weather; chapping.

acrodermatitis pus·tu·lo·sa per·stans (pus·tew·lo′suh pur′stanz). ACRODERMATITIS CONTINUA.

ac·ro·dol·i·cho·me·lia (ack″ro·dol″i·ko·mee′lee·uh) *n.* [*acro-* + *dolicho-* + *-melia*]. A condition in which the hands and feet grow disproportionately long or large.

ac·ro·dont (ack′ro·dont) *adj.* [*acr-* + *-odont*]. 1. Pertaining to a tooth which is ankylosed by its root to a bony eminence, and not inserted in a socket or alveolus. 2. Pertaining to an individual having teeth of this kind.

ac·ro·dyn·ia (ack″ro·din′ee·uh) *n.* [*acr-* + *-odynia*]. A syndrome seen in infancy and occasionally in older childhood, of extreme irritability alternating with periods of apathy, anorexia, pink itching hands and feet, scarlet tip of nose and cheeks, photophobia, profuse sweating, tachycardia, hypertension, and hypotonia, and frequently desquamation of the skin of the hands and feet. This condition is associated with ingestion of or contact with mercury, but also with inflammatory changes of obscure origin in the central nervous system. Syn. *Feer's disease, pink disease.*

ac·ro·ede·ma, ac·ro·oe·de·ma (ack″ro·e·dee′muh) *n.* [*acro-* + *edema*]. Persistent swelling of the hands or feet, due to any of numerous causes, such as peripheral neuropathy or trauma to the extremities.

ac·ro·es·the·sia, ac·ro·aes·the·sia (ack″ro·es·theezh′uh, ·theez′ee·uh) *n.* [*acro-* + *esthesia*]. Paresthesia or dysesthesia in the hands or feet.

ac·ro·ger·ia (ack″ro·jerr′ee·uh, ·jeer′ee·uh) *n.* [*acro-* + *ger-* + *-ia*]. A rare developmental defect of the dermis and subcutaneous fat which imparts a prematurely aged, thin, dry, transparent appearance to the skin of the hands and feet.

ac·rog·no·sis (ack″rog·no′sis) *n.* [*acro-* + *-gnosis*]. The general sensation of the physical existence of the extremities and of their parts.

ac·ro·hy·per·hi·dro·sis (ack″ro·high″pur·hi·dro′sis) *n.* [*acro-* + *hyperhidrosis*]. Excessive sweating of the hands or feet, or both.

ac·ro·hy·po·ther·my (ack″ro·high′po·thur″mee) *n.* [*acro-* + *hypothermy*]. Abnormal coldness of the extremities.

ac·ro·ker·a·to·sis (ack″ro·kerr″uh·to′sis) *n.* [*acro-* + *keratosis*]. Hyperkeratosis of the extremities, particularly of the hands and feet.

acrokeratosis ver·ru·ci·for·mis (ve·roo″si·for′mis). A genodermatosis marked by development of wart-like excrescences on the hands and feet and sometimes on adjacent areas.

ac·ro·ki·ne·sis (ak″ro·ki·nee′sis) *n.* [*acro-* + *kinesis*]. Excessive motion of the limbs, which may be the result of extrapyramidal motor disease or the side effect of psychotropic drugs.

acro·le·in (a·kro′lee·in) *n.* [*acrid* + L. *olere*, to smell, + *-in*]. Acrylic aldehyde, $CH_2{=}CHCHO$, a liquid of pungent odor resulting from decomposition of glycerin. Syn. *acrylic aldehyde.*

acrolein Schiff reaction. The ethylene group of acrolein condenses with tissue amino, sulfhydryl, and imidazole groups, giving rise to a positive Schiff aldehyde reaction at protein sites where these groups are abundant.

acrolein test. A test for glycerin and fats in which the suspected substance is heated with an equal quantity of potassium bisulfate. If glycerin or fats are present, acrolein is given off and is recognized by its characteristic irritating odor.

ac·ro·mac·ria (ack″ro·mack′ree·uh) *n.* [*acro-* + *macr-* + *-ia*]. ARACHNODACTYLY.

ac·ro·ma·nia (ack″ro·may′nee·uh) *n.* [*acro-* + *mania*]. A violent form of mania.

ac·ro·mas·ti·tis (ack″ro·mas·tye′tis) *n.* [*acro-* + *mastitis*]. Inflammation of the nipple.

ac·ro·me·ga·lia (ack″ro·me·gay′lee·uh) *n.* ACROMEGALY.

acro·me·gal·ic (ack″ro·me·gal′ick) *adj.* Pertaining to or exhibiting acromegaly.

acromegalic arthritis. A joint disease in acromegaly, characterized by initial hypertrophy and later degeneration of articular cartilage.

ac·ro·meg·a·loid (ack″ro·meg′uh·loid) *adj.* Resembling acromegaly.

ac·ro·meg·a·loid·ism (ack″ro·meg′uh·loy·diz·um) *n.* A state or condition of the body resembling acromegaly, but not caused by hyperpituitarism.

ac·ro·meg·a·ly (ack″ro·meg′uh·lee) *n.* [*acro-* + *-megaly*]. A chronic disease, usually of middle life, due to prolonged excessive secretion of adenohypophyseal growth hormone and characterized by overgrowth of bone, connective tissue, and viscera, especially enlargement of the acral parts of the body, as the hands, feet, face, head. May be due to an eosinophilic adenoma. Syn. *Marie's syndrome.*

ac·ro·mel·al·gia (ack″ro·me·lal′jee·uh) *n.* [*acro-* + *melalgia*]. ERYTHROMELALGIA.

ac·ro·mere (ack′ro·meer) *n.* [*acro-* + *-mere*]. The distal or outer segments of the retinal rods and cones.

ac·ro·meta·gen·e·sis (ack″ro·met″uh·jen′e·sis) *n.* [*acro-* + *meta-* + *-genesis*]. Undue growth of the extremities.

acro·mi·al (a·kro′mee·ul) *adj.* Pertaining to the acromion.

acromial angle. The subcutaneous bony point where the lateral border of the acromion becomes continuous with the spine of the scapula. NA *angulus acromialis.*

ac·ro·mic·ria (ack″ro·mick′ree·uh, ·migh′kree·uh) *n.* [*acro-* + *micr-* + *-ia*]. Underdevelopment of the extremities and of the skull as contrasted with visceral development.

acromicria con·gen·i·ta (kon·jen′i·tuh). *Obsol.* DOWN'S SYNDROME.

acro·mio·cla·vic·u·lar (a·kro″mee·o·kla·vick′yoo·lur) *adj.* Pertaining to the acromion and the clavicle.

acromioclavicular articulation or **joint.** The joint between the lateral end of the clavicle and the acromion of the scapula. NA *articulatio acromioclavicularis.* See also Table of Synovial Joints and Ligaments in the Appendix.

acromioclavicular ligament. The ligament connecting the lateral end of the clavicle and the nearby surface of the acromion of the scapula. NA *ligamentum acromioclaviculare.*

acro·mio·cor·a·coid (a·kro″mee·o·kor′uh·koid) *adj.* CORACOACROMIAL.

acro·mio·hu·mer·al (a·kro″mee·o·hew′mur·ul) *adj.* Pertaining to the acromion and the humerus.

acro·mi·on (a·kro′mee·on) *n.* [Gk. *akrōmion,* from *akron,* end, tip, + *ōmos,* shoulder] [NA]. The flat, somewhat triangular bony process formed by the lateral extension of the scapular spine, and situated just above the glenoid cavity. It articulates with the clavicle, and serves as a point of attachment for some of the fibers of the deltoid and trapezius muscles.

acro·mi·on·ec·to·my (a·kro″mee·on·eck′tuh·mee) *n.* Surgical removal of the acromion.

acromion process. ACROMION.

acro·mio·tho·rac·ic (a·kro″mee·o·tho·ras′ick) *adj.* Pertaining to the shoulder and thorax; thoracoacromial.

acrom·pha·lus (a·krom′fuh·lus) *n.* [*acr-* + *omphalus*]. 1. The center of the umbilicus, where the cord attaches. 2. Unusual prominence of the navel, often the first sign of an umbilical hernia. 3. Remains of the umbilical cord attached to the child.

ac·ro·myo·to·nia (ack″ro·migh″o·to′nee·uh) *n.* [*acro-* + *myotonia*]. Tonic muscular spasm of the hands or feet.

acro·my·ot·o·nus (ack″ro·migh·ot′o·nus) *n.* ACROMYOTONIA.

ac·ro·nar·cot·ic (ack″ro·nahr·kot′ick) *adj.* & *n.* [*acrid* + *narcotic*]. 1. Combining a local irritant effect, by acting directly on the peripheral nerves, with a general obtunding effect, by affecting the brain and vital centers in the cord. 2. An agent that has these effects.

ac·ro·neu·rop·a·thy (ack″ro·new·rop′uth·ee) *n.* Any neuropathy most evident in the more distal parts of the extremities, usually seen in hereditary sensory neuropathies or as a result of an inflammatory process, diabetes, vitamin deficiency (as in alcoholism or beriberi), or poisoning with arsenic, lead, or mercury. See also *polyneuritis.*

acro·neu·ro·sis (ack″ro·new·ro′sis) *n.* Any neurosis affecting the hands or feet, usually vasomotor in nature.

ac·ro·nine (ack′ro·neen) *n.* 3,12-Dihydro-6-methoxy-3,3,12-trimethyl-7*H*-pyrano[2,3-*c*] acridin-7-one, $C_{20}H_{19}NO_3$, an antineoplastic agent.

acron·y·chous (a·kron′i·kus) *adj.* [Gk. *akrōnychos,* from *akron,* extremity, tip, + *onyx,* nail]. Having claws, nails, or hooves.

ac·ro·nyx (ack′ro·nicks) *n.* [Gk. *akron,* end, edge, + *onyx,* nail]. An ingrowing nail.

acrooedema. ACROEDEMA.

ac·ro·os·te·ol·y·sis (ack′ro·os″tee·ol′i·sis) *n.* [*acro-* + *osteolysis*]. 1. Myelodysplasia with osseous lesions. 2. Loss of substance from the bones of the distal phalanges; may be familial or the result of occupational exposure to polyvinyl chloride.

ac·ro·pachy (ack′ro·pack″ee, a·krop′uh·kee) *n.* [Gk. *akropachēs,* thick at the end, + *-y*]. HYPERTROPHIC PULMONARY OSTEOARTHROPATHY.

ac·ro·pachy·der·ma (ack″ro·pack″ee·dur′muh) *n.* [*acro-* + *pachyderma*]. A syndrome characterized by abnormally small hands and feet with clubbing of the digits, and thickening of the skin over the face, scalp, and extremities, due to hypopituitarism. See also *hypertrophic pulmonary osteoarthropathy.*

ac·ro·pa·ral·y·sis (ack″ro·puh·ral′i·sis) *n.* Paralysis of the hands or feet.

ac·ro·par·es·the·sia, ac·ro·par·aes·the·sia (ack″ro·păr″es·theezh′uh, ·theez′ee·uh) *n.* [*acro-* + *paresthesia*]. A symptom complex associated with a variety of disorders of the peripheral nerves or posterior columns, characterized by tingling, pins-and-needles sensations, numbness or stiffness, and occasionally pain in the hands or feet or both. See also *carpal tunnel syndrome.*

ac·ro·pa·thol·o·gy (ack″ro·pa·thol′uh·jee) *n.* The pathology of the extremities, especially the morbid changes occurring in orthopedic diseases.

acrop·a·thy (a·krop′uth·ee) *n.* [*acro-* + *-pathy*]. Any abnormal condition of the extremities. —**ac·ro·path·ic** (ack″ro·path′ick) *adj.*

acrop·e·tal (a·krop′e·tul) *adj.* [*acro-* + L. *petere,* to seek]. Tending upward to a summit, applied to an inflorescence and to certain infections.

ac·ro·pho·bia (ack″ro·fo′bee·uh) *n.* [Gk. *akron,* height, promontory, + *-phobia*]. Morbid dread of being at a great height.

ac·ro·pig·men·ta·tion (ack″ro·pig″men·tay′shun) *n.* Increased melanin pigmentation of the distal parts of the extremities, particularly the knuckles. See also *acropigmentatio reticularis.*

ac·ro·pig·men·ta·tio re·tic·u·la·ris (ack″ro·pig·men·tay′shee·o re·tick″yoo·lair′is). A rare genodermatosis characterized by small brown, rough-surfaced, slightly depressed macules in a netlike pattern located on the extensor surfaces of the distal parts of the extremities.

ac·ro·pos·thi·tis (ack″ro·pos·thigh′tis) *n.* [Gk. *akroposthia,* tip of foreskin, from *posthē,* foreskin, + *-itis*]. Inflammation of the prepuce.

ac·ro·scle·ri·a·sis (ack″ro·skle·rye′uh·sis) *n.* [*acro-* + *scleriasis*]. ACROSCLEROSIS.
ac·ro·scle·ro·der·ma (ack″ro·skleer·o·dur′muh) *n.* [*acro-* + *scleroderma*]. A condition in which the skin of arms, hands, legs, and feet is palpably indurated. See also *scleroderma.*
ac·ro·scle·ro·sis (ack″ro·skle·ro′sis) *n.* [*acro-* + *sclerosis*]. A form of scleroderma affecting the fingers, characterized by Raynaud's phenomenon and ulceration. See also *sclerodactylia.*
ac·ro·sin (ack′ro·sin) *n.* [*acro*some + *-in*]. A proteolytic enzyme located in the acrosome of the spermatozoon, thought to be involved in the penetration of the egg by the spermatozoon.
ac·ro·som·al (ack″ro·so′mul) *adj.* Of or pertaining to an acrosome.
acrosomal granule. A large granule, formed by the coalescing of proacrosomal granules, present within the acrosomal vesicle in developing spermatids.
acrosomal system. The unique alteration of the Golgi complex in relation to developing spermatids.
acrosomal vesicle. The single membrane portion of the acrosomal system elaborated by the Golgi complex in developing spermatids.
ac·ro·some (ack′ro·sohm) *n.* [*acro-* + *-some*]. A dense granule of varying size and shape developed during spermiogenesis; located at the anterior pole of the nucleus and enclosed by the head and cap.
ac·ro·sphe·no·syn·dac·tyl·ia (ack″ro·sfee″no·sin″dack·til′ee·uh) *n.* [*acro-* + *spheno-* + *syndactylia*]. ACROCEPHALOSYNDACTYLY.
ac·ros·te·al·gia (ack″ros·tee·al′jee·uh) *n.* [*acr-* + *ostealgia*]. Pain in one or more of the bones of an extremity.
ac·ro·ter·ic (ack″ro·terr′ick) *adj.* [Gk. *akrōtēr*ion, extremity, + *-ic*]. Pertaining to the periphery or most distal parts, as the tips of the toes, fingers, or nose. —**ac·ro·te·ria** (ack″ro·teer′ee·uh) *n.pl.*
[1]**acrot·ic** (a·krot′ick) *adj.* [Gk. *akrotēs*, an extreme (from *akros*, extreme, outside, surface), + *-ic*]. Pertaining to the surface or periphery; specifically, to the glands of the skin.
[2]**acrotic,** *adj.* [*a-* + Gk. *krot*os, beat, + *-ic*]. Of the pulse, absent or imperceptible.
ac·ro·tism (ack′ro·tiz·um) *n.* [*a-* + Gk. *krot*os, beat, + *-ism*]. Absence or imperceptibility of the pulse.
ac·ro·tro·pho·neu·ro·sis (ack″ro·tro″fo·new·ro′sis) *n.* [*acro-* + *tropho-* + *neurosis*]. A trophic disturbance of the extremities caused by a nerve lesion.
acryl-, acrylo-. A combining form meaning *acrylic.*
acryl·ic (a·kril′ick) *adj.* & *n.* [*acr*olein + *-yl* + *-ic*]. 1. Of or pertaining to acrylic acid or its derivatives, or to an acrylic (2). 2. Any of various thermoplastic substances prepared by reaction and polymerization of sodium cyanide, acetone, methyl alcohol, and acid. They resemble clear glass, but are lighter in weight and permit passage of ultraviolet rays; used in making dental prostheses and artificial intraocular lenses. See also *methyl methacrylate.*
acrylic acid. Propenoic acid, $CH_2{=}CHCOOH$, used in the manufacture of plastics.
acrylic aldehyde. ACROLEIN.
acrylic resin. A synthetic resin, usually a polymer of methyl methacrylate. See also *acrylic (2).*
acrylo-. See *acryl-.*
ac·ry·lo·ni·trile (ack″ri·lo·nigh′tril, ·treel, ·trile) *n.* [*acrylo-* + *nitrile*]. Propene nitrile, $H_2C{=}CHCN$, used in the manufacture of synthetic rubber and plastics.
A.C.S. American College of Surgeons.
Actamer. Trademark for bithionol, a bacteriostatic agent.
Actase. A trademark for a preparation of human fibrinolysin used intravenously to accelerate intravascular dissolution of clots.
ACTH Abbreviation for *adrenocorticotropic hormone.*
Acthar. Trademark for a preparation of corticotropin.
ACTH test. Any of a number of procedures employing a challenge dose of adrenocorticotropic hormone to assess adrenocortical response.
Actidil. Trademark for triprolidine, an antihistaminic agent.
Actidione. Trademark for cycloheximide, an antibiotic.
actin-, actino- [Gk. *aktis, aktinos,* ray, beam; spoke]. A combining form meaning (a) *ray, radiant;* (b) *radiated structure.*
ac·tin (ack′tin) *n.* [L. *act*us, motion, + *-in*]. Protein constituent of the muscle fibril, occurring side by side with myosin and both participating in the muscle contractile mechanism. Actin can undergo a reversible transformation between a globular or monomeric (G-actin) and a fibrous or polymeric (F-actin) state.
acting in. Acting out which takes place in the therapeutic session or in relation to the therapist.
acting out. 1. *In psychiatry,* the expression of anxiety, emotional conflict, or feelings of love or hostility through such behavior as sexual promiscuity, stealing, fire setting, or other destructive or socially disapproved acts rather than through words; mostly seen in individuals with character disorders who are not aware of the relationship between their behavior and their conflicts or feelings. 2. Dramatization as play therapy. —**act out,** *v.*
ac·tin·ic (ack·tin′ick) *adj.* [*actin-* + *-ic*]. Pertaining to or designating radiant energy, especially that in the visible and ultraviolet spectrum, which produces marked chemical change.
actinic carcinoma. A basal cell or squamous cell carcinoma of the face and other exposed surfaces of the body, seen in persons who spend prolonged periods of time in direct sunlight.
actinic conjunctivitis. ACTINIC KERATOCONJUNCTIVITIS.
actinic dermatitis. ACTINODERMATITIS.
actinic dermatosis. A dermatosis due to exposure to sunlight. It may be urticarial, papular, or eczematous.
actinic keratoconjunctivitis. Inflammation of the conjunctiva and cornea with pain, photophobia, lacrimation, and smarting of the lids, caused by repeated flashes of bright light or ultraviolet radiation. See also *electric ophthalmia.*
actinic keratosis. A premalignant hyperkeratosis, thought to be caused by chronic exposure to sunshine.
ac·ti·nide (ack′ti·nide) *n.* Any of the group of related chemical elements starting with actinium and including thorium, palladium, uranium, neptunium, plutonium, americium, curium, berkelium, californium, einsteinium, fermium, mendelevium, nobelium, and lawrencium.
ac·tin·i·form (ack·tin′i·form) *adj.* [*actin-* + *-iform*]. Exhibiting radiate form or structure, such as the ray fungus or the sea anemone.
ac·ti·nism (ack′ti·niz·um) *n.* The production of chemical change by actinic radiation.
ac·tin·i·um (ack·tin′ee·um) *n.* [*actin-* + *-ium*]. Ac = 227. A radioactive element found in uranium ores, as pitchblende.
actino-. See *actin-.*
ac·ti·no·bac·il·lo·sis (ack″ti·no·bas″i·lo′sis) *n.,* pl. **actinobacil·lo·ses** (·seez) An actinomycosis-like disease of bovine and other domestic animals caused by *Actinobacillus lignieresii,* characterized by caseous abscesses in the tongue and cervical lymph nodes.
Ac·ti·no·ba·cil·lus (ack″ti·no·ba·sil′us) *n.* [*actino-* + *bacillus*]. A genus of the family Brucellaceae, composed of small, slender, gram-negative, nonmotile, nonsporulating rods. Formerly called *Malleomyces.*
Actinobacillus mal·lei (mal′ee·eye). *Obsol.* PSEUDOMONAS *MALLEI.*
ac·ti·no·chem·is·try (ack″ti·no·kem′is·tree) *n.* The branch of chemistry concerned with the reactions produced by actinic radiation.
ac·ti·no·der·ma·ti·tis (ack″ti·no·dur″muh·tye′tis) *n.* Dermatitis caused by exposure to sunlight, ultraviolet light, or x-rays.
ac·tino·gen (ack·tin′o·jen) *n.* [*actino-* + *-gen*]. Any substance

producing radiation. —**ac·ti·no·gen·ic** (ack″ti·no·jen′ick) *adj.;* **actino·gen·e·sis** (·jen′e·sis) *n.;* **actino·gen·ics** (·jen′icks) *n.*

ac·tino·graph (ack·tin′o·graf) *n.* 1. An instrument which records variations in the actinic strength of the sun's rays and hence permits the determination of proper time of exposure of a photographic plate; an exposure meter. 2. *Obsol.* RADIOGRAPH.

actinolite. ACTINOLYTE.

ac·ti·nol·o·gy (ack″ti·nol′uh·jee) *n.* [*actino-* + *-logy*]. 1. The homology existing between the successive segments, regions, or parts of a radially symmetric organ or organism. 2. Study of the chemical action and effects of light.

ac·tin·o·lyte (ack·tin′o·lite) *n.* [*actino-* + *-lyte*]. 1. A device which generates ultraviolet rays, as in actinotherapy. 2. Any substance which undergoes a rather marked change when exposed to light.

ac·ti·nom·e·ter (ack″ti·nom′e·tur) *n.* 1. An apparatus for determining the intensity of actinic rays. 2. A device which determines the degree of penetration of such rays. —**actinome·try** (·tree) *n.*

ac·ti·no·my·ce·li·al (ack″ti·no·migh·see′lee·ul) *adj.* 1. Pertaining to the mycelium of *Actinomyces.* 2. ACTINOMYCETIC.

Ac·ti·no·my·ces (ack″ti·no·migh′seez) *n.* [*actino-* + *-myces*]. A genus of microaerophilic bacteria, formerly classified as fungi, characterized by delicate branching mycelia which tend to fragment. Several species are responsible for actinomycosis. In tissues, granules may form, presenting in stained preparations eosinophilic clubs surrounding a central basophilic mass.

Actinomyces asteroides. NOCARDIA ASTEROIDES.

Actinomyces bo·vis (bo′vis). The species of bacteria causing actinomycosis in cattle.

Actinomyces is·ra·e·lii (iz·ray·ee′lee·eye). The species of bacteria causing actinomycosis in man.

Actinomyces madurae. NOCARDIA MADURAE.

Actinomyces somaliensis. NOCARDIA SOMALIENSIS.

Ac·ti·no·my·ce·ta·ce·ae (ack″ti·no·migh″se·tay′see·ee) *n.pl.* [from *Actinomyces*]. A family of the order Actinomycetales, including the genera *Nocardia* and *Actinomyces,* in which branching mycelium often fragments into shorter rod-shaped or spherical forms.

Ac·ti·no·my·ce·ta·les (ack″ti·no·migh″se·tay′leez) *n.pl.* A large order of microorganisms which includes a family essentially lacking mycelium, the Mycobacteriaceae, and three families in which true mycelium is produced, the Actinomycetaceae, Streptomycetaceae, and Actinoplanaceae.

ac·ti·no·my·cete (ack″ti·no·migh′seet, ·migh·seet′) *n.* An organism of the family Actinomycetaceae.

ac·ti·no·my·ce·tic (ack″ti·no·migh·see′tick) *adj.* Of or pertaining to an actinomycete.

ac·ti·no·my·ce·tin (ack″ti·no·migh·see′tin, ·migh′se·tin) *n.* [*actinomycete* + *-in*]. An antibacterial substance synthesized by several strains of *Actinomyces,* and effective against certain gram-negative and gram-positive organisms.

ac·ti·no·my·ce·tous (ack″ti·no·migh·see′tus) *adj.* Of or pertaining to an actinomycete.

ac·ti·no·my·cin (ack″ti·no·migh′sin) *n.* [*Actinomyces* + *-in*]. Any of an extensive family of polypeptide antibiotics, produced by various species of *Streptomyces,* believed to contain 3-amino-1,8-dimethylphenoxazonedicarboxylic acid as a common moiety. Specific members of the family are identified by roman numeral or letter designations, the latter often with numerical subscripts. Although toxicity limits general use of active members of this group of antibiotics, certain of them, as cactinomycin and dactinomycin, are of therapeutic interest because of antineoplastic activity.

actinomycin C. CACTINOMYCIN.

actinomycin D. DACTINOMYCIN.

ac·ti·no·my·co·ma (ack″ti·no·migh·ko′muh) *n.,* pl. **actinomycomas, actinomycoma·ta** (·tuh). A swelling produced by an organism of the genus *Actinomyces.*

ac·ti·no·my·co·sis (ack″ti·no·migh·ko′sis) *n.,* pl. **actinomyco·ses** (·seez). 1. A subacute or chronic granulomatous and suppurative infection of man, principally involving the orofacial, thoracic, and abdominal structures, chiefly caused by *Actinomyces israelii.* 2. A similar disease of animals such as cattle, caused by *Actinomyces bovis,* characterized by granulomatous lesions of the jaws.

ac·ti·no·my·cot·ic (ack″ti·no·migh·kot′ick) *adj.* Pertaining to or caused by actinomycosis.

ac·ti·no·my·co·tin (ack″ti·no·migh′ko·tin) *n.* An extract of cultures of *Actinomyces,* prepared like tuberculin and used in cases of actinomycosis.

ac·ti·non (ack′ti·non) *n.* Actinium emanation, a short-lived isotope of radon.

ac·ti·no·neu·ri·tis (ack″ti·no·new·rye′tis) *n.* Neuritis due to exposure to x-rays or radioactive substances.

ac·ti·no·phy·to·sis (ack″ti·no·figh·to′sis) *n.,* pl. **actinophyto·ses** (·seez) [*actino-* + *phytosis*]. BOTRYOMYCOSIS.

ac·ti·no·qui·nol (ack″ti·no·kwye′nole, ·kwin′ole) *n.* 8-Ethoxy-5-quinolinesulfoneic acid, $C_{11}H_{11}NO_4S$, an ultraviolet screening agent usually employed as the sodium salt.

ac·ti·no·rho·dine (ack″ti·no·ro′deen) *n.* An antibiotic substance, $C_{32}H_{26}O_{14}$, produced by *Streptomyces coelicolor.*

ac·ti·no·ru·bin (ack″ti·no·roo′bin) *n.* An antibiotic substance produced by a species of *Actinomyces* and named from its characteristic red mycelium; the substance is active against various organisms but is relatively toxic.

ac·ti·no·spec·to·cin (ack″ti·no·speck′to·sin) *n.* SPECTINOMYCIN.

ac·ti·no·ther·a·py (ack″ti·no·therr′uh·pee) *n.* Radiation therapy using light rays, most commonly ultraviolet. —**actino·ther·a·peu·tic** (·therr″uh·pew′tick) *adj.*

ac·tion current. The electric current accompanying membrane depolarization and repolarization in an excitable cell.

action of arrest. INHIBITION (1).

action potential. The complete cycle of electric changes in transmembrane potential occurring with depolarization and repolarization of an excitable cell as in nerve or muscle tissue.

action time. The duration of stimulation of the retina required to produce a visual sensation of maximum strength.

action tremor. A tremor which is present when the limbs are actively moved, or when they are actively maintained in certain positions, as when the arms are outstretched. Compare *intention tremor.*

activated charcoal. Charcoal that has been treated, as with steam and carbon dioxide or with other substances, to increase its adsorptive power. The medicinal grade is used to reduce hyperacidity, to adsorb toxins, and as an antidote against various poisons.

activated 7-dehydrocholesterol. CHOLECALCIFEROL.

activated resin. Resin that is either autopolymerizing or polymerized by ultraviolet light. Syn. *cold-curing resin.* Contr. *heat-curing resin.*

activated sleep. REM SLEEP.

activated water. Water containing ions, free atoms, radicals, and molecules in a highly reactive state; the transient result of passing ionizing radiation through it.

ac·ti·va·tion, *n.* 1. The process of activating or rendering active. 2. Stimulation of general cellular activity by the use of nonspecific therapy; plasma activation. 3. Stimulation of the ovum by the sperm or other agents causing cell division. 4. *In chemistry,* the transformation of any substance into a more reactive form, including the renewal of activity of a catalyst. 5. *In nuclear science,* the process of making a material radioactive by bombardment with neutrons, protons, or other nuclear particles. —**ac·ti·vate,** *v.;* **acti·vat·ed,** *adj.*

activation analysis. A method of chemical analysis by which a small amount of an element, otherwise difficult to identify and quantitatively determine, is made radioactive by bombardment with neutrons or other activating particles, and then qualitatively identified by observing the half-life of one or more of its radioisotopes and the characteristics of its radiations. Quantitative analysis is achieved through similar treatment of reference material containing a known amount of the element found to be present.
activation factor. FACTOR XII.
activation of enzymes. The means by which an enzyme that has little or no catalytic activity undergoes an increase in such activity; commonly, the presence of another substance of diverse nature is required.
activation product. FACTOR XII.
activation wave. The spread of electrical excitation over the heart.
ac·ti·va·tor, *n.* 1. An agent which is necessary to activate another substance as an agent, usually a metal ion, whose combination with a complete enzyme or its substrate activates the enzyme. Compare *coenzyme.* 2. A substance which stimulates the development of an embryonic structure. Syn. *inductor, organizer.* 3. An apparatus which charges water with radium emanations. 4. CATALYST. 5. A substance capable of causing the breakdown of an initiator by chemical means, rather than by the application of heat, in the polymerization of synthetic resins. 6. A myofunctional appliance that acts as a passive transmitter of force to accomplish orthodontic movement.
activator RNA. The RNA produced by the transcription of an integrator gene in the eukaryotic cell; by binding to a specific site elsewhere in the genome it initiates transcription of an adjacent structural gene.
ac·tive, *adj.* 1. Energetic, decisive, as active treatment. 2. Due to an intrinsic as distinguished from a passive force, as active hyperemia. 3. *In optics,* possessing the ability to rotate the plane of a polarized light beam. 4. *In psychoanalysis,* pertaining to masculine qualities in terms of the goal; also, pertaining to the endeavors of the analyst to influence the patient to produce material for analysis. 5. *In biochemistry,* pertaining to an actual or presumed derivative of a substance regarded as the participating form in biological reactions in which the parent compound itself does not exhibit full activity. 6. Causing or producing change.
active acetate. ACETYL COENZYME A.
active algolagnia. SADISM.
active anaphylaxis. A state of immediate hypersensitivity produced by the reintroduction of the antigen, presumed to result from the interaction of antigen and antibody fixed to tissues releasing pharmacologically active substances.
active center. ACTIVE SITE.
active electrode. A small electrode used for its exciting effect in a sharply localized area for stimulating muscles or nerves or recording potentials from muscles or nerves. See also *exploring electrode.*
active exercise. Exercise by voluntary effort of the patient.
active immunity. Immunity possessed by a host as the result of disease or unrecognized infection, or induced by immunization with microbes or their products or with other antigens. Contr. *passive immunity.*
active movement. Movement effected without any outside help.
active negativism. Doing the opposite of what a person is asked to do.
active site. 1. The portion of an enzyme, antibody, or other molecule, such as the combining site on an antibody molecule, that combines or reacts with other substances. 2. Specifically, the part of an enzyme to which the substrate or cofactor is linked in normal enzymic function.
active sleep. REM SLEEP.
active transport. Transport of a solute across a body membrane against a concentration gradient, i.e., from a region of low concentration to one relatively higher. Contr. *passive transport.*
active treatment. Vigorous management of a disease.
active tuberculosis. A clinically significant form of the disease, which is undergoing clinical or roentgenographic change and causing or capable of causing symptoms or disability; tubercle bacilli can usually be isolated.
ac·tiv·i·ty coefficient. *In physical chemistry,* the thermodynamic behavior of a substance. It is a measure of how the behavior of a given substance differs from its theoretical or ideal behavior.
ac·to·dig·in (ack″to·dij′in) *n.* 3β-(β-D-Glucopyranosyloxy)-14,23-dihydroxy-24-nor-5β,14β-chol-20(22)-en-21-oic acid, γ-lactone, $C_{29}H_{44}O_9$, a cardiotonic.
ac·to·my·o·sin (ack″to·migh′o·sin) *n.* A complex of the muscle proteins actin and myosin.
ac·tu·al cautery. A white-hot or red-hot iron used for cauterization.
acu- [L. *acus*]. A combining form meaning *needle.*
acuesthesia. ACOUESTHESIA.
acu·i·ty (a·kew′i·tee) *n.* [F. *acuité,* from L. *acutus,* sharp]. Sharpness; keenness of perception, as of vision or hearing.
acu·le·ate (a·kew′lee·ut, ·ate) *adj.* [L. *aculeatus,* from *aculeus,* a sting, prickle]. 1. *In botany,* armed with prickles, as the rose or other brier. 2. *In zoology,* having a sting.
acu·me·ter (a·kew′me·tur, a·koo′me·tur) *n. Obsol.* Acoumeter (= AUDIOMETER).
acu·mi·nate (a·kew′mi·nut, ·nate) *adj.* [L. *acuminatus,* from *acumen,* sharp point]. Sharp-pointed; conical; tapering to a point.
Acupan. A trademark for nefopam, an analgesic.
acu·pres·sure (ack′yoo·presh″ur) *n.* [*acu-* + *pressure*]. 1. A procedure to stop hemorrhage by compressing the artery with a needle inserted into the tissues upon either side. 2. SHIATSU.
acu·punc·ture (ack′yoo·punk″chur) *n.* [*acu-* + *puncture*]. 1. A method originating in China, used for relief of pain, in which fine needles inserted at certain points and along certain meridians are twirled rapidly. 2. Puncture of an organ or tissue with multiple fine needle points; used in the multipuncture method of smallpox vaccination.
acus (ay′kus) *n.* [L.]. A surgical needle.
acu·sec·tor (ack″yoo·seck′tur) *n.* [*acu-* + L. *sector,* a cutter]. An electric needle, operating on a high-frequency current, which cuts tissues like a scalpel. —**acusec·tion** (·shun) *n.*
-acusia. See *-acousia.*
acus·ti·cus (a·koos′ti·kus) *n.* [NL., acoustic]. VESTIBULOCOCHLEAR NERVE.
acute (uh·kewt′) *adj.* [L. *acutus,* sharp, from *acuere,* to sharpen (rel. to *acus,* needle)]. 1. Sharp; severe. 2. Having a rapid onset, a short course, and pronounced symptoms. Contr. *chronic, subacute.* 3. Sensitive, perceptive.
acute abdomen. A pathologic condition within the abdomen, requiring prompt surgical intervention.
acute abscess. An abscess associated with acute inflammation of the part in which it is formed.
acute alcoholism. Inebriety; drunkenness; a transient disturbance of mental and bodily functioning due to excessive alcohol intake.
acute angle-closure glaucoma. NARROW-ANGLE GLAUCOMA.
acute anterior poliomyelitis. PARALYTIC SPINAL POLIOMYELITIS.
acute appendicitis. A severe and rapidly developing attack of appendicitis, characterized by abdominal pain and tenderness usually in the right lower quadrant, and often by nausea, vomiting, fever, and leukocytosis.
acute arthritis. Acute inflammation of a joint, characterized by swelling, tenderness, heat, and redness.
acute articular rheumatism. Rheumatic fever with joint inflammation.
acute ascending myelitis. Inflammation of the spinal cord

beginning in the lower segments and progressing cephalad; may occur in spinal poliomyelitis, postvaccinal or postexanthematous myelitis, and rarely in *Herpesvirus simiae* and rabies infections.

acute ascending paralysis. GUILLAIN-BARRÉ DISEASE.

acute ataxia. Any ataxia of sudden onset, such as acute cerebellar ataxia.

acute bacterial endocarditis. Fulminant, rapidly progressive endocarditis, usually associated with a significant systemic infection, often by *Staphylococcus aureus.*

acute benign lymphoblastosis. *Obsol.* A misnomer for infectious mononucleosis (which does not involve lymphoblasts).

acute benign lymphocytic meningitis. *Obsol.* LYMPHOCYTIC CHORIOMENINGITIS.

acute berylliosis. An acute chemical pneumonia due to the inhalation of certain beryllium salts.

acute brachial neuritis or **radiculitis.** BRACHIAL NEURITIS.

acute brain syndrome. *In psychiatry,* any acute confusional state or delirium presumed to have a structural basis. Syn. *acute organic brain syndrome.* See also *organic brain syndrome.*

acute bronchitis. Acute inflammation of the bronchi due to infectious or irritant agents, characterized by cough with variable sputum production, fever, substernal soreness, and lung rales.

acute carcinoma or **carcinosis.** *Obsol.* INFLAMMATORY CARCINOMA.

acute care. INTENSIVE CARE.

acute cerebellar ataxia. A usually self-limited, benign cerebellar syndrome of sudden onset, with ataxia of stance and gait, dysmetria, intention tremor, dysarthria, nystagmus, adiadochokinesis, hypotonia, and occasionally fever, nausea, and vomiting, without evidence of an intracranial lesion or intoxication. Most common in childhood, may be related to a nonspecific respiratory or gastrointestinal illness or a viral infection.

acute chorea. 1. SYDENHAM'S CHOREA. 2. CHOREA GRAVIDARUM.

acute contagious conjunctivitis. CATARRHAL CONJUNCTIVITIS.

acute disseminated encephalomyelitis. A demyelinating disorder of the brain and spinal cord with widespread, variable neurologic symptoms, course, and outcome. It may be postinfectious or postvaccinal and may represent an immune-allergic response of the nervous system.

acute duodenal ileus. Obstruction of the lumen of the duodenum following operations or resulting from external pressure. Syn. *arteriomesenteric ileus, gastromesenteric ileus.*

acute erythremia. ERYTHREMIC MYELOSIS.

acute fibrinous enteritis. An acute inflammatory process associated with desquamation and fibrin deposition on the intestinal mucosa; not a clinical entity but a pathologic classification. Syn. *membranous enteritis.*

acute glomerulonephritis. An acute inflammatory disease involving the renal glomeruli, occurring principally as a sequel to infection with nephritogenic strains of group A beta-hemolytic streptococci, and variably characterized by hematuria, proteinuria, oliguria, azotemia, edema, hypertension, and hypocomplementemia occurring 7 to 14 days after infection; the mechanism is unknown but presumably involves glomerular deposits of immune complexes and activation of the complement system. See also *hemolytic streptococci.*

acute hallucinosis. The condition of having hallucinations, usually of sudden onset and lasting only a few weeks, accompanied by anxiety; commonly toxic in origin.

acute hematogenous osteomyelitis. See *acute osteomyelitis.*

acute hemorrhagic encephalitis or **leukoencephalitis.** *Obsol.* A syndrome of gross diffuse hemorrhage of the brain once thought a unitary disease entity but now known to represent acute necrotizing hemorrhagic encephalomyelitis, herpetic encephalitis, or pericapillary encephalorrhagia.

acute hemmorrhagic leukoencephalitis of Weston Hurst. ACUTE NECROTIZING HEMORRHAGIC ENCEPHALOMYELITIS.

acute hepatic porphyria of Watson. ACUTE INTERMITTENT PORPHYRIA.

acute idiopathic polyneuritis. GUILLAIN-BARRÉ DISEASE.

acute inclusion-cell encephalitis. HERPETIC ENCEPHALITIS.

acute infantile hemiplegia. Hemiplegia usually of sudden onset in an infant or child neurologically intact at birth, often ushered in or accompanied by fever, convulsions, and disturbances of consciousness; may be idiopathic or due to a wide variety of conditions. Syn. *hemiconvulsion-hemiplegia syndrome, Marie-Strufmpell encephalitis.* Compare *H.*H.E. syndrome.

acute infectious erythema. ERYTHEMA INFECTIOSUM.

acute infectious polyneuritis. GUILLAIN-BARRÉ DISEASE.

acute inflammation. Inflammation in which the onset is recent, progress is rapid, and the manifestations are pronounced.

acute inflammatory polyradiculoneuropathy. GUILLAIN-BARRÉ DISEASE.

acute intermittent porphyria. A metabolic disturbance of porphyrin metabolism, probably transmitted as a Mendelian dominant characteristic, affecting young adults or the middle-aged. Characterized clinically by periodic attacks of abdominal colic with nausea and vomiting, constipation, neurotic or psychotic behavior, and polyneuropathy. The urine contains excessive amounts of the porphyrin precursors δ-aminolevulinic acid and porphobilinogen. See also *porphyria.*

acute leukemia. A form of leukemia with rapid onset and progress if untreated, characterized by severe anemia, hemorrhagic manifestations, and susceptibility to infection; the predominant cells in the bone marrow and peripheral blood are blast forms.

acute myelitis. Any acute inflammation of the spinal cord, including transverse myelitis and the Guillain-Barré disease.

acute necrotizing encephalitis. HERPETIC ENCEPHALITIS.

acute necrotizing hemorrhagic encephalomyelitis. An acute disease mainly of children and young adults, usually preceded by a respiratory infection of indeterminate cause and characterized clinically by headache, fever, stiff neck, confusion, and signs of disease of one or both cerebral hemispheres and brainstem, and frequently by a fatal outcome; spinal fluid shows a polymorphonuclear pleocytosis and variable numbers of red cells, but normal glucose values. The destructive, hemorrhagic lesions of the brain are thought to represent the most fulminant form of demyelinative disease. Syn. *acute hemorrhagic leukoencephalitis of Weston Hurst.*

acute·ness (uh·kewt'nis) *n.* 1. The quality of being acute or sharp, as in perception, learning, or feeling. 2. Suddenness, brevity, or severity of an illness as contrasted with insidiousness and chronicity. 3. *In ophthalmology and audiology,* acuity; keenness of vision or of hearing.

acute neuronitis. GUILLAIN-BARRÉ DISEASE.

acute nonsuppurative hepatitis. INTERSTITIAL HEPATITIS.

acute obliterating bronchiolitis. BRONCHIOLITIS OBLITERANS.

acute organic brain syndrome or **disorder.** ACUTE BRAIN SYNDROME.

acute osteomyelitis. An inflammation of bone, either subperiosteal or affecting the medullary canal, of recent onset; usually severe, caused by bacteria, and hematogenous.

acute pelvic inflammatory disease. An acute inflammation of pelvic viscera, usually of bacterial, often gonococcal, origin. See also *pelvic inflammatory disease.*

acute pericarditis. An acute inflammation of the pericardium, characterized by serous, fibrinous, purulent, or hemorrhagic exudate.

acute peritonitis. Peritonitis with an abrupt onset and rapid course, characterized by abdominal pain, tenderness, vomiting, constipation, and fever; may be due to chemical irritation or bacterial infection, the latter being either primary or secondary.

acute perivascular myelinoclasis. ACUTE DISSEMINATED ENCEPHALOMYELITIS.

acute pharyngitis. A form of pharyngitis due to temperature changes, to the action of irritant substances, or to certain infectious causes, and characterized by pain on swallowing, by dryness, later by moisture, and often by hyperemia of the mucous membrane.

acute-phase reactant. Any of various proteins, such as C-reactive protein or fibrinogen, which are not antibodies but which appear in, or are increased in amount in, plasma during acute trauma or inflammatory reaction.

acute pyogenic meningitis. SUPPURATIVE MENINGITIS.

acute renal failure. Rapid decline in renal function followed by physiologic and biochemical abnormalities, as in acute tubular necrosis; generally due to damage of renal parenchyma by intrinsic disease or extrinsic factors.

acute respiratory disease. 1. A respiratory infection due to adenovirus, particularly types 4 and 7, occurring especially among military personnel, and characterized by fever, sore throat, cough, and malaise. Abbreviated, ARD. 2. Any acute infectious disease of the respiratory tract.

acute rheumatism. ACUTE RHEUMATIC FEVER.

acute rhinitis. Inflammation of the mucous membranes of the nose, usually marked by sneezing, nasal airway congestion, and discharge of watery mucus; CORYZA. See also *common cold.*

acute rhinitis of the newborn. Rhinitis in premature and full-term neonates from a variety of causes including maternal drug ingestion, chemical irritation, and infectious agents.

acute schizophrenic episode. A form of undifferentiated schizophrenia marked by the acute onset of symptoms, often associated with confusion, emotional turmoil, ideas of reference, dissociation, depression, or fear. In many cases there is recovery, while in others the disorganization progresses and takes on the characteristics of the catatonic, hebephrenic, or paranoid types of schizophrenia.

acute situational reaction. GROSS STRESS REACTION.

acute spasmodic laryngitis. SPASMODIC CROUP.

acute stress reaction. GROSS STRESS REACTION.

acute suppurative otitis media. Inflammation of the middle ear due to a pyogenic organism such as *Streptococcus pyogenes, Streptococcus pneumoniae, Hemophilus influenzae,* or *Staphylococcus aureus.*

acute suppurative synovitis. An acute, purulent synovitis, usually of infectious origin.

acute tonsillitis. Inflammation of the tonsils with sudden onset, pyrexia, constitutional symptoms, and intense sore throat, caused by a wide variety of infectious agents.

acute toxic encephalopathy. A syndrome of obscure origin affecting children, characterized by sudden onset of stupor or coma, convulsions, fever, decorticate or decerebrate postures and impaired respiratory and cardiovascular function; the cerebrospinal fluid is usually under increased pressure but is otherwise normal, and the brain shows only edema unless hypoxic changes supervene. Compare *Reye's syndrome.*

acute traumatic subdural hygroma. Collection of cerebrospinal fluid with a small admixture of blood in the subdural space following trauma, apparently caused by tears in the arachnoid membrane near the villi.

acute tubular necrosis. A retrogressive change in the kidneys associated with crushing injuries and other conditions producing shock, and sometimes accompanied by necrosis of distal and collecting tubules. Abbreviated, ATN. Syn. *lower nephron nephrosis.*

acute wasting paralysis. Rapidly evolving weakness and atrophy following an acute lower motor neuron lesion, as in paralytic spinal poliomyelitis, Guillain-Barré disease, and other lower motor neuron diseases.

acute yellow atrophy. Rapid, massive destruction of the liver, usually as a result of viral hepatitis.

acuti-. A combining form meaning *acute, acutely angled.*

acu·ti·cos·tal (a·kew″ti·kos′tul) *adj.* [*acuti-* + *costal*]. Having projecting ribs.

acuto-. A combining form meaning *acute.*

Acutran. Trademark for amphechloral, an anorexic drug.

A.C.V.M. American College of Veterinary Microbiologists.

A.C.V.P. American College of Veterinary Pathologists.

acy·a·no·blep·sia (ay·sigh″uh·no·blep′see·uh, a·sigh″) *n.* [*a-* + *cyano-* + *-blepsia*]. ACYANOPSIA.

acy·a·nop·sia (ay·sigh″uh·nop′see·uh, a·sigh″) *n.* [*a-* + *cyan-* + *-opsia*]. Inability to see blue colors.

acy·a·not·ic (ay·sigh″uh·not′ick) *adj.* Without cyanosis, as an acyanotic congenital cardiovascular defect.

acy·clia (ay·sigh′klee·uh, ay·sick′lee·uh) *n.* [*a-* + *cycl-* + *-ia*]. A state of arrested circulation of body fluids.

acy·clic (ay·sigh′klick, a·sick′lick) *adj.* 1. Not occurring in cycles; not characterized by a self-limited course; nonintermittent. 2. *In chemistry,* denoting organic compounds with an open-chain structure; ALIPHATIC. 3. *In botany,* not whorled.

ac·y·e·sis (as″ee·ee′sis, ay″sigh·ee′sis) *n.* [*a-* + *cyesis*]. 1. Sterility of the female. 2. Nonpregnancy. 3. Incapacity for natural delivery. —**acy·et·ic** (·et′ick) *adj.*

ac·yl (as′il, as′eel) *n.* [*acid* + *-yl*]. An organic radical derived by removal of a hydroxyl group (OH) from an organic acid, as RCO— derived from RCOOH.

Acylanid. Trademark for acetyldigitoxin, a cardiac glycoside.

ac·yl·a·tion (as″i·lay′shun) *n.* Introduction of an acyl radical into a compound.

acyl carrier protein. A small, heat-stable protein which serves as a carrier of acyl groups in the de novo synthesis of fatty acids. The acyl groups are esterified with a sulfhydryl residue on the protein's prosthetic group.

acy·o·blep·sia (as″ee·o·blep′see·uh, ay″sigh·o·) *n.* [*a-* + *cyano-* + *-blepsia*]. ACYANOPSIA.

acys·tia (ay·sis′tee·uh, a·sis′) *n.* [*a-* + *cyst-* + *-ia*]. Absence of the urinary bladder.

A d Abbreviation for *anisotropic disk* (= A DISK).

a.d. Abbreviation for *auris dextra;* right ear.

ad- [L.]. A prefix meaning (a) *to, toward;* (b) *near, beside;* (c) *addition to;* (d) *more intense.*

¹-ad [L. *ad,* to, toward]. *In anatomy and zoology,* an adverbial suffix meaning *-ward, toward.*

²-ad [Gk. *-as, -ados,* a noun suffix]. A suffix indicating (a) *a group or set made up of a* (specified) *number of members or units,* as triad, a group of three; (b) in chemistry, *an element or radical having a* (specified) *valence,* as monad (a univalent element or radical), tetrad (a quadrivalent element or radical); (c) in botany, *one of a larger category of plants including a* (specified) *genus,* as cycad, a plant related to the genus *Cycas.*

ADA American Dental Association; American Dietetic Association.

A.D.A.A. American Dental Assistants Association.

adac·rya (ay·dack′ree·uh, a·dack′) *n.* [*a-* + *dacry-* + *-ia*]. Absence or deficiency of tears.

adac·tyl·ia (ay″dack·til′ee·uh, a·dack·) *n.* [*a-* + *dactyl-* + *-ia*]. Congenital absence of fingers or toes, or both.

adac·ty·lism (ay·dack′ti·liz·um) *n.* ADACTYLIA.

adac·ty·lous (ay·dack′ti·lus) *adj.* [*a-* + *dactyl-* + *-ous*]. Lacking fingers or toes.

adac·ty·lus (ay·dack′ti·lus) *n.* [*a-* + *dactyl-* + *-us*]. An individual with congenital absence of fingers or toes, or both. —**adactyl,** *adj. & n.*

Adair Digh·ton syndrome [C. A. *Adair Dighton,* English otologist, b. 1885]. VAN DER HOEVE'S SYNDROME.

Adalin. Trademark for carbromal, a sedative.

ad·a·man·tine (ad″uh·man′teen, ·tine) *adj.* [Gk. *adamantinos,* of steel, like a diamond]. 1. Pertaining to dental enamel. 2. Very hard.

ad·a·man·ti·no·car·ci·no·ma (ad″uh·man″ti·no·kahr″si·no′muh) *n.* [*adamantine* + *carcinoma*]. A malignant ameloblastoma.

ad·a·man·ti·no·ma (ad″uh·man″ti·no′muh) *n.*, pl. **adamantinomas, adamantinoma·ta** (·tuh) [*adamantine* + *-oma*]. AMELOBLASTOMA.

ad·a·man·ti·no·ma·toid craniopharyngioma (ad″uh·man·ti·no′muh·toid). A craniopharyngioma with a cellular pattern resembling ameloblastoma.

ad·a·man·to·blast (ad″uh·man′to·blast) *n.* [*adamantine* + *-blast*]. AMELOBLAST.

ad·a·man·to·blas·to·ma (ad″uh·man″to·blas·to′muh) *n.* [*adamantoblast* + *-oma*]. AMELOBLASTOMA.

ad·a·man·to·ma (ad″a·man·to′muh) *n.* [*adamantine* + *-oma*]. AMELOBLASTOMA.

Adam·kie·wicz reaction (ah″dah[h]m·kyey′vich) [A. *Adamkiewicz,* Austrian pathologist, 1850–1921]. A reaction given by a protein containing tryptophan, being a violet color produced at the junction of a glacial acetic acid solution of the protein superimposed on concentrated sulfuric acid. The reaction is attributed to the presence of glyoxylic acid in the acetic acid.

Ad·am's apple [after *Adam,* who "ate the first apple" in the garden of Eden]. LARYNGEAL PROMINENCE.

ad·ams·ite (ad′um·zite, ·site) *n.* [R. *Adams,* U.S. chemist, 1889–1957]. 10-Chloro-5,10-dihydrophenarsazine, $C_{12}H_9AsClN$; a potential chemical warfare agent.

Adams' saw [W. *Adams,* English surgeon, 1820–1900]. A small, straight, long-handled saw, for osteotomy.

Adams-Stokes syndrome or **disease** [R. *Adams,* Irish physician, 1791–1875; and W. *Stokes*]. STOKES-ADAMS SYNDROME.

Adanon. Trademark for methadone, a narcotic analgesic used as the hydrochloride salt.

Ad·an·so·nia (ad″an·so′nee·uh) *n.* [M. *Adanson,* French naturalist, 1727–1806]. A genus of trees of the family Bombacaceae.

Adansonia dig·i·ta·ta (dij·i·tay′tuh). The baobab or calabash of Africa and India, the dried leaves of which are used by the natives as an antipyretic.

Adapin. Trademark for doxepin, an antidepressant drug.

ad·ap·ta·tion, *n.* 1. *In biology,* any change in structure, form, or habits of an organism enabling it to function adequately in a new or changed environment. 2. *In ophthalmology,* adjustment of the eye to varying intensities of light. See also *light adaptation, dark adaptation.* 3. In reflex action, decline in the frequency of impulses when a receptor is stimulated repeatedly, or cessation of continuous discharge at the same frequency by most receptors when subjected to a constant stimulus. 4. *In dentistry,* proper fitting of a denture or accurate adjustment of bands to teeth; close approximation of filling material to the walls of a tooth cavity. 5. *In psychiatry,* The process of adjustment by an individual to intrapsychic, interpersonal, or social conditions.

adaptation curve. A biphasic plot of the log units of brightness against the time (in minutes), which gives a characteristic slope for the normal course of dark adaptation.

adaptation disease. A biochemical or metabolic disorder due to physical or emotional stress, with a reversibility which may be effected spontaneously, therapeutically, or accidentally.

adaptation time. The interval between the onset of a steady and continuous stimulation of a receptor and the moment when no further change in sensory response occurs, as the time between exposure to darkness and attainment of maximal retinal sensitivity.

adapt·ed milk. MODIFIED MILK.

adapt·er, adap·tor, *n.* 1. A device which permits the fitting of one part of an instrument or apparatus to another, as a glass or rubber tube or metal collar. 2. An apparatus which converts the electric current to the form required in the various types of electrotherapy, or for a particular electric appliance.

adap·tive, *adj.* 1. Capable of adapting. 2. Showing a tendency toward adaptation.

adaptive behavior. Any behavior that helps an organism adjust to its environment. See also *adaptation (1, 5).*

adaptive colitis. IRRITABLE COLON.

adaptive enzyme. INDUCIBLE ENZYME.

adaptive hypertrophy. An increase in size which acts as a compensatory mechanism to adapt an organ or other structure (as the heart or a skeletal muscle) to increased functional requirements.

ad·ap·tom·e·ter (ad″ap·tom′e·tur) *n.* An instrument for measuring the time taken for retinal adaptation or for regeneration of the rhodopsin (visual purple); used to determine the minimum light threshold and to diagnose night blindness.

adaptor. ADAPTER.

ad·at·om (ad′at″um) *n.* An atom held on a surface by adsorption.

ad·ax·i·al (ad·ack′see·ul) *adj.* [*ad-* + *axial*]. On the side of, or directed toward, the axis of a structure.

ADC Abbreviation for *anodic duration contraction.*

add. Abbreviation for *adde* or *additur* in prescription writing.

ad·de (ad′ee) [L.]. Add; a direction used in prescription writing. Abbreviated, add.

ad·de·pha·gia (ad″e·fay′jee·uh) *n.* [variant of *adephagia*]. BULIMIA.

ad·der (ad′ur) *n.* [OE. *naedre*]. The common name of several genera of snakes, especially the *Vipera berus* of Britain and Europe, or of species of other genera of terrestrial snakes.

[1]**ad·dict** (ad′ikt) *n.* [L. *addictus,* given over, from *addicere,* to give up, to award, from *dicere,* to speak, say]. One who has become habituated to and dependent upon some practice, especially the use of alcohol or other drugs.

[2]**ad·dict** (uh·dikt′) *v.* To cause (an individual) to form an addiction. **—addict·ed,** *adj.*

ad·dic·tion (uh·dick′shun) *n.* Marked psychologic and physiologic dependence upon a substance, such as alcohol or other drug, which has gone beyond voluntary control. **—addic·tive,** *adj.*

ad·di·ment (ad′i·munt) *n.* [L. *addere,* to add]. *Obsol.* COMPLEMENT. **—ad·di·men·ta·ry** (ad″i·men′tuh·ree) *adj.*

Ad·dis and Shev·sky's test [T. *Addis,* U.S. internist, 1881–1949; and Marian C. *Shevsky*]. A concentration test for kidney function based upon the specific gravity of urine passed during the last 12 hours of a 24-hour period of fluid deprivation.

Addis count or **method** [T. *Addis*]. A technique for quantitative evaluation of the formed elements of urine, excluding squamous epithelial cells; the results are expressed as the numbers of a given element excreted per 24 hours.

Ad·di·so·ni·an (ad″i·so′nee·un) *adj.* Of or pertaining to Addison's disease or Addison's (pernicious) anemia.

Addisonian crisis. ADRENAL CRISIS.

Ad·di·son·ism (ad′i·sun·iz·um) *n.* [T. *Addison*]. 1. A syndrome sometimes present in pulmonary tuberculosis consisting of dark pigmentation of the skin, loss of weight and strength; somewhat resembles true Addison's disease. 2. ADDISON'S DISEASE (1).

Ad·di·son's anemia [T. *Addison,* English physician, 1793–1860]. PERNICIOUS ANEMIA.

Addison's disease or **syndrome** [T. *Addison*]. 1. Primary adrenocortical insufficiency, characterized by weakness, skin and mucous membrane pigmentation or bronzing, emaciation, hypotension, and gastrointestinal symptoms; usually idiopathic, possibly due to an autoimmune mechanism, but known causes include tuberculosis and, more rarely, metastatic tumor, amyloidosis, and hemochromatosis. Syn. *asthenia pigmentosa, melanoma suprarenale.* 2. PERNICIOUS ANEMIA.

Addison's keloid [T. *Addison*]. CIRCUMSCRIBED SCLERODERMA.

ad·di·tion *n.* A chemical reaction in which two elements or compounds unite without the loss or substitution of any atoms, or any loss of valence, as $H_2O + CO_2 = H_2CO_3$, $HCl + NH_3 = NH_4Cl$.

addition polymerization. Polymerization that does not involve elimination of a by-product.

addition product. A compound resulting from the direct union of two substances.

addition reaction. ADDITION.

ad·di·tur (ad'i·tur, ·toor) [L.]. Let there be added; a direction used in prescription writing. Abbreviated, add.

ad·du·cent (a·dew'sunt) *adj.* [L. *adducens, adducentis*]. Adducting.

¹ad·duct (a·dukt') *v.* [L. *adducere, adductus,* to draw to one's self, from *ad-* + *ducere,* to draw, pull, to lead]. 1. To draw toward the median line or plane of a body. 2. To turn the eyes inward from the central position.

²ad·duct (ad'ukt) *n.* [L. *adductus,* drawn together]. A complex resulting from chemical addition of two compounds.

ad·duc·tion (a·duck'shun) *n.* [ML. *adductio,* from L. *adducere,* to draw to one's self]. 1. Any movement whereby one part is brought toward another or toward the median line or plane of the body or part. 2. *In ophthalmology,* turning of the eyes inward from the central position, through contraction of the medial rectus muscles. This action may be voluntary, but usually is subconscious, following the stimulus of accommodation. See also *convergence-stimulus adduction.*

ad·duc·tor (a·duck'tur) *n.* Any muscle that draws a part toward the median line of the body or of a part. See also Table of Muscles in the Appendix.

adductor bre·vis (brev'is). The short adductor of the thigh. NA *musculus adductor brevis.* See also Table of Muscles in the Appendix.

adductor canal. A triangular fascial tunnel in the anterior region of the thigh bounded by the sartorius, vastus medialis, and adductor muscles; it extends from the femoral triangle to the adductor hiatus and gives passage to the femoral vessels, saphenous nerve, and nerve to the vastus medialis muscle. Syn. *Hunter's canal, subsartorial canal.* NA *canalis adductorius.*

adductor di·gi·ti se·cun·di (dij'i·tye se·kun'dye). A rare variant slip of muscle associated with the adductor hallucis and inserted into the lateral side of the base of the proximal phalanx of the second toe.

adductor hal·lu·cis (hal'yoo·sis). The adductor of the great toe. It has an oblique and a transverse head. NA *musculus adductor hallucis.* See also Table of Muscles in the Appendix.

adductor hallucis trans·ver·sus (trans·vur'sus). The transverse head of the adductor hallucis. NA *caput transversum musculi adductoris hallucis.* See also Table of Muscles in the Appendix.

adductor hiatus. A gap in the insertion of the adductor magnus into the femur, the level of transition between the femoral and popliteal vessels. NA *hiatus tendineus.*

adductor lon·gus (long'gus). The long adductor of the thigh. NA *musculus adductor longus.* See also Table of Muscles in the Appendix.

adductor mag·nus (mag'nus). The large adductor of the thigh. NA *musculus adductor magnus.* See also Table of Muscles in the Appendix.

adductor mi·ni·mus (min'i·mus). A variable portion of the adductor magnus of the thigh.

adductor pol·li·cis (pol'i·sis) [NA]. The adductor of the thumb. It has an oblique and a transverse head. NA *musculus adductor pollicis.* See also Table of Muscles in the Appendix.

adductor pollicis obli·quus (o·blye'kwus). The oblique head of the adductor pollicis. NA *caput obliquum musculi adductoris pollicis.*

adductor pollicis trans·ver·sus (trans·vur'sus). The transverse head of the adductor pollicis. NA *caput transversum musculi adductoris pollicis.*

adductor reflex of the foot. Contraction of the posterior tibial muscle resulting in adduction, inversion, and slight plantar flexion of the foot on stroking its inner border from the great toe to the heel. Syn. *Hirschberg's reflex.*

adductor reflex of the thigh. Contraction of the adductors of the thigh, produced by tapping the tendon of the adductor magnus with the thigh in abduction.

adductor tubercle. A small sharp projection on the upper medial margin of the medial epicondyle of the femur, where the tendon of the adductor magnus is inserted. NA *tuberculum adductorium.*

Ade·cid·u·a·ta (ay"de·sid"yoo·ay'tuh) *n.pl.* [NL., from *a-* + *deciduate*]. A division of mammals including those not having a deciduate placenta.

ade·lo·mor·phic (a·dee"lo·mor'fick, ad"e·lo·) *adj.* [Gk. *adēlos,* invisible, obscure (from *a-* + *dēlos,* visible) + *-morphic*]. Not clearly defined; formerly applied to certain cells in the gastric glands.

ade·lo·mor·phous (a·dee"lo·mor'fus, ad"e·lo·) *adj.* ADELOMORPHIC.

adelomorphous cell. CHIEF CELL (1).

adelph-, adelpho- [Gk. *adelphos,* brother]. A combining form meaning (a) *sibling;* (b) *twin, double, multiple;* (c) *grouping of like units.*

adel·pho·site (a·del'fo·site) *n.* [*adelpho-* + *-site*]. OMPHALOSITE.

adel·pho·tax·is (a·del"fo·tack'sis) *n.* [*adelpho-* + *taxis*]. The tendency of motile cells to arrange themselves into definite positions.

adel·pho·taxy (a·del'fo·tack"see) *n.* ADELPHOTAXIS.

-adelphus [Gk. *adelphos,* brother]. A combining form signifying *inferior duplicity in conjoined twins.*

aden-, adeno- [Gk. *adēn, adenos*]. A combining form meaning *gland, glandular.*

ad·e·nal·gia (ad"e·nal'jee·uh) *n.* [*aden-* + *-algia*]. A painful condition of a gland.

ad·e·nase (ad'e·nace, ·naze) *n.* [*aden*ine + *-ase*]. A deaminating enzyme that converts adenine to hypoxanthine.

ad·en·as·the·nia (ad"en·as·theen'ee·uh) *n.* [*aden-* + *asthenia*]. Functional deficiency of a gland.

aden·dric (ay·den'drick, a·den') *adj.* ADENDRITIC.

aden·dri·tic (ay"den·drit'ick, ad"en·) *adj.* Lacking dendrites, applied to certain spinal ganglion cells.

ad·e·nec·to·my (ad"e·neck'tuh·mee) *n.* [*aden-* + *-ectomy*]. The excision of a gland or lymph node.

ad·en·ec·to·pia (ad"en·eck·to'pee·uh) *n.* [*aden-* + *ectopia*]. Occurrence of a gland in an abnormal place.

Aden fever [*Aden,* South Arabia]. An acute viral febrile illness resembling dengue or sandfly fever.

ade·nia (a·dee'nee·uh) *n.* [*aden-* + *-ia*]. *Obsol.* A malignant lymphoma without leukemic blood changes.

aden·i·form (a·den'i·form) *adj.* [*aden-* + *-iform*]. Glandlike; shaped like a gland.

ad·e·nine (ad'i·neen, ·nin) *n.* [*aden-* + *-ine*]. 6-Aminopurine, $C_5H_5N_5$, a purine base occurring in RNA and DNA and important in energy storage and release as a component of adenosine triphosphate.

adenine arabinoside. 9-β-D-Arabinofuranosidoadenine, an antiviral agent possibly of value in the treatment of certain herpes virus infections. Syn. *ara-A, vidarabine.*

adenine riboside. ADENOSINE.

ad·e·ni·tis (ad"e·nigh'tis) *n.* [*aden-* + *-itis*]. Inflammation of a gland or lymph node.

Ade·ni·um (a·dee'nee·um) *n.* A genus of the family Apocynaceae, various species of which have provided arrow poisons for African natives, and from which glycosides have been obtained which have a digitalis-like action on the heart but cause tetanic convulsions.

adeno-. See *aden-.*

ad·e·no·ac·an·tho·ma (ad″e·no·ack″an·tho′muh) *n.* [*adeno-* + *acanthoma*]. An adenocarcinoma with foci of squamous cell differentiation, most commonly of endometrial origin.

ad·e·no·am·e·lo·blas·to·ma (ad″e·no·a·mel″o·blas·to′muh, ·am″e·lo·) *n.* [*adeno-* + *ameloblastoma*]. An ameloblastoma in which the epithelium exhibits a glandular structure and arrangement.

ad·e·no·an·gio·sar·co·ma (ad″e·no·an″jee·o·sahr·ko′muh) *n.* [*adeno-* + *angio-* + *sarcoma*]. A malignant mixed mesodermal tumor with foci of both glandular and vascular differentiation.

ad·e·no·can·croid (ad″e·no·kang′kroid) *n.* [*adeno-* + *cancroid*]. ADENOACANTHOMA.

ad·e·no·car·ci·no·ma (ad″e·no·kahr″si·no′muh) *n.* [*adeno-* + *carcinoma*]. 1. In histologic classification, a carcinoma in which the anaplastic parenchymal cells form glands. 2. In histogenetic classification, a carcinoma arising from the parenchyma of a gland.

ad·e·no·car·ci·no·ma·to·sis (ad″e·no·kahr″·si·no″muh·to′sis) *n.* Widespread involvement of the body by an adenocarcinoma.

ad·e·no·cele (ad′e·no·seel) *n.* [*adeno-* + *-cele*]. A cystic tumor containing adenomatous tissue.

ad·e·no·cel·lu·li·tis (ad″e·no·sel″yoo·lye′tis) *n.* [*adeno-* + *cellulitis*]. Inflammation of a gland and the surrounding tissue.

ad·e·no·chon·dro·ma (ad″e·no·kon·dro′muh) *n.* [*adeno-* + *chondr-* + *-oma*]. A tumor consisting of both glandular and cartilaginous tissue.

ad·e·no·cys·tic (ad″e·no·sis′tick) *adj.* [*adeno-* + *cystic*]. Containing glands, some or all of which form cystic spaces.

adenocystic disease. CYSTIC DISEASE OF THE BREAST.

ad·e·no·cys·to·car·ci·no·ma (ad″e·no·sis″to·kahr·si·no′muh) *n.* ADENOID CYSTIC CARCINOMA.

ad·e·no·cys·to·ma (ad″e·no·sis·to′muh) *n.* CYSTADENOMA.

adenocystoma lym·pho·ma·to·sum (lim·fo·muh·to′sum). WARTHIN'S TUMOR.

ad·e·no·cys·to·sar·co·ma (ad″e·no·sis″to·sahr·ko′muh) *n.* CYSTADENOSARCOMA.

ad·e·no·fi·bro·ma (ad″e·no·figh·bro′muh) *n.* FIBROADENOMA.

ad·e·no·fi·bro·sis (ad″e·no·figh·bro′sis) *n.* [*adeno-* + *fibrosis*]. 1. Fibrosis of a gland. 2. CYSTIC DISEASE OF THE BREAST.

ad·e·no·gen·e·sis (ad″e·no·jen′e·sis) *n.* [*adeno-* + *genesis*]. Development of a gland.

ad·e·no·gen·ic (ad″e·no·jen′ick) *adj.* ADENOGENOUS.

ad·e·nog·e·nous (ad″e·noj′e·nus) *adj.* [*adeno-* + *-genous*]. Originating from a gland.

ad·e·no·hy·per·sthe·nia (ad″e·no·high″pur·sthee′nee·uh) *n.* [*adeno-* + *hypersthenia*]. Excessive activity of glands.

adenohypersthenia gas·tri·ca (gas′tri·kuh). A condition in which the gastric juice is greatly increased or excessively acid.

ad·e·no·hy·poph·y·sis (ad″e·no·high·pof′i·sis) *n.* [*adeno-* + *hypophysis*]. The anterior, glandular part of the hypophysis, developing from somatic ectoderm of the posterior nasopharynx and secreting the following important hormones: prolactin, growth hormone, adrenocorticotropic hormone (ACTH), melanocyte-stimulating hormone (MSH), thyroid-stimulating hormone (TSH), follicle-stimulating hormone (FSH), and luteinizing hormone (LH); consists of a main body (the pars distalis), a tuberal part (the pars tuberalis), which extends upward on the anterior surface of the infundibulum, and the pars intermedia, located between the pars distalis and the neurohypophysis and sometimes classified as part of the neurohypophysis. Syn. *anterior pituitary, anterior lobe of the hypophysis.* NA alt. *lobus anterior hypophyseos.* Contr. *neurohypophysis.* See also Plate 26. —**adeno·hy·poph·y·se·al** (·high·pof″i·see′ul, ·high″po·fiz′ee·ul), **adeno·hy·po·phys·i·al** (·high″po·fiz′ee·ul) *adj.*

ad·e·noid (ad′e·noid) *adj.* & *n.* [Gk. *adenoeidēs,* glandular, from *adēn,* gland]. 1. Glandlike or glandular; especially, lymphoid. 2. Pertaining to the adenoids. 3. Hyperplastic lymphoid tissue often present in the nasopharynx, especially in children. Syn. *pharyngeal tonsil.* NA *tonsilla pharyngea.*

adenoid cystic carcinoma. A malignant tumor composed of nests and cords of small polygonal cells, often arranged in glandlike fashion around cores of mucoid material; found in the lower respiratory tract and salivary glands and occasionally in such other locations as the breast.

ad·e·noid·ec·to·my (ad″e·noy·deck′tuh·mee) *n.* Surgical removal of the adenoids.

adenoid facies. The characteristic open-mouthed and pinched-nose appearance associated with adenoid hypertrophy which interferes with nasal breathing.

ad·e·noid·ism (ad′e·noy·diz·um) *n.* A series of changes in respiration, facial contour, and tooth arrangement attributed to the presence of adenoids.

ad·e·noid·itis (ad″e·noy·dye′tis) *n.* Inflammation of the adenoids.

adenoid tissue. LYMPHATIC TISSUE.

ad·e·no·leio·myo·fi·bro·ma, ad·e·no·lio·myo·fi·bro·ma (ad″e·no·lye″o·migh″o·figh·bro′muh) *n.* [*adeno-* + *leiomyofibroma*]. ADENOMYOMA.

ad·e·no·leio·my·o·ma (ad″e·no·lye″o·migh·o′muh) *n.* [*adeno-* + *leiomyoma*]. ADENOMYOMA.

ad·e·no·li·po·ma (ad″e·no·li·po′muh) *n.* [*adeno-* + *lip-* + *-oma*]. A benign tumor with both glandular and adipose tissue elements.

ad·e·no·log·a·di·tis (ad″e·no·log″uh·dye′tis) *n.* [*adeno-* + Gk. *logades,* whites of the eyes, + *-itis*]. *Obsol.* 1. OPHTHALMIA NEONATORUM. 2. Inflammation of the glands and conjunctiva of the eyes.

ad·e·no·lym·phi·tis (ad″e·no·lim·figh′tis) *n.* LYMPHADENITIS.

ad·e·no·lym·pho·cele (ad″e·no·lim′fo·seel) *n.* [*adeno-* + *lympho-* + *-cele*]. Widening of the lymphatics and cystic dilatation of the lymph nodes, caused by an obstruction.

ad·e·no·lym·pho·ma (ad″e·no·lim·fo′muh) *n.* [*adeno-* + *lymphoma*]. Squamoid metaplasia of salivary gland tissue with hyperplasia of ectopic lymphoid tissue in the salivary gland.

ad·e·no·ma (ad″e·no′muh) *n.,* pl. **adenomas, adenoma·ta** (·tuh) [*aden-* + *-oma*]. A benign epithelial tumor whose parenchymal cells are similar to those composing the epithelium from which it arises; usually employed with tumors of the parenchyma of glands, but also applied to benign tumors of mucosal epithelium.

adenoma des·tru·ens (des′troo·enz). An adenoma with aggressive and destructive characteristics.

ad·e·no·ma·la·cia (ad″e·no·muh·lay′shuh, ·see·uh) *n.* [*adeno-* + *malacia*]. Abnormal softening of a gland.

adenoma ma·lig·num (ma·lig′num). MALIGNANT ADENOMA.

adenoma pseu·do·sar·co·ma·to·des (sue″do·sahr·ko″muh·to′deez). CYSTOSARCOMA PHYLLODES.

adenoma sebaceum PRINGLE'S ADENOMA SEBACEUM.

adenoma sub·stan·ti·ae cor·ti·ca·lis su·pra·re·na·lis (sub·stan′shee·ee kor·ti·kay′lis sue″pruh·re·nay′lis). CORTICAL ADENOMA.

adenoma su·do·rip·a·rum (sue″dor·ip′uh·rum). SWEAT GLAND ADENOMA.

ad·e·nom·a·toid (ad″e·nom′uh·toid, ·no′muh·toid) *adj.* Pertaining to or resembling an adenoma.

adenomatoid tumor. A rare, small, benign neoplasm of both male and female genital tracts, composed of varied stroma containing irregular spaces lined by cells which may resemble endothelium, epithelium, or mesothelium.

ad·e·no·ma·to·sis (ad″e·no″muh·to′sis) *n.,* pl. **adenomato·ses** (·seez). The occurrence of adenomas at several sites within an organ, as in the lung, or in several related organs, as in the endocrine system.

ad·e·nom·a·tous (ad″e·nom′uh·tus) *adj.* Pertaining to an adenoma.

adenomatous goiter. Nodular hyperplasia of the thyroid. Syn. *nodular goiter, multiple colloid adenomatous goiter.*

adenomatous sinusitis. GLANDULAR SINUSITIS.

ad·e·no·mere (ad′e·no·meer) *n.* [*adeno-* + *-mere*]. The terminal portion of a developing gland, which is ultimately responsible for its functioning.

ad·e·no·myo·hy·per·pla·sia (ad″e·no·migh″o·high·pur·play′zhuh) *n.* [*adeno-* + *myo-* + *hyperplasia*]. ISTHMIC NODULAR SALPINGITIS.

ad·e·no·my·o·ma (ad″e·no·migh·o′muh) *n.* [*adeno-* + *myoma*]. Endometriosis involving a leiomyoma, usually of the uterus. Syn. *adenoleiomyoma.*

ad·e·no·myo·me·tri·tis (ad″e·no·migh″o·me·trye′tis) *n.* [*adeno-* + *myometritis*]. Inflammatory thickening of the uterine wall, resembling an adenomyoma.

ad·e·no·myo·sal·pin·gi·tis (ad″e·no·migh″o·sal″pin·jye′tis) *n.* [*adeno-* + *myo-* + *salpingitis*]. ISTHMIC NODULAR SALPINGITIS.

ad·e·no·myo·sar·co·ma (ad″e·no·migh″o·sahr·ko′muh) *n.* [*adeno-* + *myo-* + *sarcoma*]. A malignant mixed mesodermal tumor composed of muscular and glandular elements.

ad·e·no·my·o·sis (ad″e·no·migh·o′sis) *n.* [*adeno-* + *my-* + *-osis*]. 1. Endometriosis involving muscular tissues such as the uterine wall or the uterine tube. 2. Any abnormal growth of glands and muscle fibers.

adenomyosis of the fallopian tube. ISTHMIC NODULAR SALPINGITIS.

ad·e·no·myxo·chon·dro·sar·co·ma (ad″e·no·mick″so·kon″dro·sahr·ko′muh) *n.* [*adeno-* + *myxo-* + *chondro-* + *sarcoma*]. A malignant mixed mesodermal tumor containing glandular, myxoid, and cartilaginous elements.

ad·e·no·myx·o·ma (ad″e·no·mick·so′muh) *n.* [*adeno-* + *myx-* + *-oma*]. A benign tumor containing glandular and myxoid elements, as mixed tumors of the salivary glands.

ad·e·no·myxo·sar·co·ma (ad″e·no·mick″so·sahr·ko′muh) *n.* [*adeno-* + *myxo-* + *sarcoma*]. A malignant mixed mesodermal tumor containing glandular and myxoid elements.

ad·e·non·cus (ad″e·nonk′us) *n.* [*aden-* + Gk. *onkos,* mass]. An enlargement or tumor of a gland.

ad·e·nop·a·thy (ad″e·nop′uth·ee) *n.* [*adeno-* + *-pathy*]. Any glandular disease, especially one characterized by swelling and enlargement of lymph nodes.

ad·e·no·phar·yn·gi·tis (ad″e·no·făr″in·jye′tis) *n.* [*adeno-* + *pharyngitis*]. Inflammation of the tonsils and pharynx.

ad·e·no·phleg·mon (ad″e·no·fleg′mon) *n.* [*adeno-* + *phlegmon*]. Suppurative inflammation of a gland.

ad·e·no·sal·pin·gi·tis (ad″e·no·sal″pin·jye′tis) *n.* [*adeno-* + *salpingitis*]. ISTHMIC NODULAR SALPINGITIS.

ad·e·no·sar·co·ma (ad″e·no·sahr·ko′muh) *n.* [*adeno-* + *sarcoma*]. A malignant mixed mesodermal tumor with glandular and supportive tissue elements.

adenosarcoma of the kidney. WILMS'S TUMOR.

ad·e·no·scle·ro·sis (ad″e·no·skle·ro′sis) *n.* [*adeno-* + *sclerosis*]. A hardening of a gland, with or without swelling.

ad·e·nose (ad′e·noce, ·noze) *adj.* [*aden-* + *-ose*]. Glandular; abounding in glands; glandlike.

aden·o·sine (a·den′o·seen, ·sin) *n.* Adenine riboside, $C_{10}H_{13}N_5O_4$, a nucleoside composed of one molecule each of adenine and D-ribose; one of the four main riboside components of ribonucleic acid.

adenosine di·phos·pha·tase (dye·fos′fuh·tace, ·taze). An enzyme catalyzing hydrolysis of adenosine diphosphate to adenosine monophosphate and phosphoric acid.

adenosine di·phos·phate (dye·fos′fate). $C_{10}H_{15}N_5O_{10}P_2$, a compound consisting one molecule each of adenine and D-ribose and one molecule of pyrophosphoric acid. It is an intermediate in the production of energy by the cell. Abbreviated, ADP. Syn. *adenosinediphosphoric acid, adenosine pyrophosphate.* See also *adenosine triphosphate.*

aden·o·sine·di·phos·pho·ric acid (a·den″o·seen·dye″fos·for′ick). ADENOSINE DIPHOSPHATE.

adenosine mono·phos·phate (mon″o·fos′fate). $C_{10}H_{14}N_5O_7P$, an ester composed of one molecule each of adenine, D-ribose, and phosphoric acid. Adenosine 5′-monophosphate, or muscle adenylic acid, is an intermediate in the release of energy for muscular and other types of cellular work. Adenosine 3′-monophosphate (yeast adenylic acid) is found in yeast. Abbreviated, AMP. Syn., *adenosinemonophosphoric acid, adenylic acid.* See also *cyclic adenosine monophosphate.*

aden·o·sine·mono·phos·pho·ric acid (a·den″o·seen·mon″o·fos·for′ick). ADENOSINE MONOPHOSPHATE.

adenosine 3′-phosphatase. An enzyme that liberates phosphoric acid from adenosine 3′-phosphate or yeast adenylic acid.

adenosine 5′-phosphatase. An enzyme that liberates phosphoric acid from adenosine 5′-phosphate or muscle adenylic acid.

adenosine phosphate. 5′-Adenylic acid, $C_{10}H_{14}N_5O_7P$, a nutrient.

adenosine py·ro·phos·phate (pye″ro·fos′fate). ADENOSINE DIPHOSPHATE.

adenosine tri·phos·pha·tase (trye·fos′fuh·tace, ·taze). An enzyme that catalyzes hydrolysis of adenosine triphosphate, especially one by which adenosine diphosphate and phosphate ion are formed, whereby free chemical energy for various cellular activities, including muscular contraction, is released.

adenosine tri·phos·phate (trye·fos′fate). $C_{10}H_{16}N_5O_{13}P_3$, a compound consisting of one molecule each of adenine and D-ribose with three molecules of phosphoric acid. Hydrolysis of it to similar esters containing one or two molecules of phosphoric acid is accompanied by release of energy for muscular and other types of cellular activity. Abbreviated, ATP. Syn. *adenosinetriphosphoric acid, adenylpyrophosphoric acid, adenylpyrophosphate.* See also *adenosine triphosphatase.*

aden·o·sine·tri·phos·pho·ric acid (a·den″o·seen·trye″fos·for′ick). ADENOSINE TRIPHOSPHATE.

ad·e·no·sis (ad″e·no′sis) *n.,* pl. **adeno·ses** (·seez) [*aden-* + *-osis*]. 1. Development of an excessive number of glandular elements without tumor formation. 2. Any glandular disease, especially of the lymph nodes.

adenosis of the breast. A form of mammary dysplasia characterized by excessive ductular and acinar proliferation.

ad·e·no·tome (ad′e·no·tome) *n.* [*adenoid* + *-tome*]. An instrument for removing the adenoids.

ad·e·not·o·my (ad″e·not′uh·mee) *n.* [*adeno-* + *-tomy*]. Incision of a gland.

ad·e·no·vi·rus (ad″e·no·vye′rus) *n.* [*adenoid* + *virus*]. A member of a large group of medium-sized, ether-resistant DNA viruses which may be pathogenic for the mucous membranes of the eye and the respiratory tract; associated with such syndromes as acute respiratory disease, pharyngoconjunctival fever, nonbacterial exudative pharyngitis, pneumonia, and sporadic and epidemic keratoconjunctivitis. Syn. *APC virus.*

Aden ulcer. A variety of tropical ulcer seen in Aden, South Arabia.

ad·e·nyl (ad′e·nil) *n.* The univalent radical $C_5H_4N_5$— present in adenine.

adenyl cy·clase (sigh′klace, ·klaze). An enzyme, bound to the plasma membrane of nearly all animal cells, that catalyzes the formation of a cyclic form of adenosine monophosphate.

ad·e·nyl·ic acid (ad″e·nil′ick). ADENOSINE MONOPHOSPHATE.

ad·e·nyl·py·ro·phos·pha·tase (ad″e·nil·pye″ro·fos′fuh·tace, ·taze) *n.* [*adenyl* + *pyrophosphatase*]. ADENOSINE TRIPHOSPHATASE.

ad·e·nyl·py·ro·phos·phate (ad″e·nil·pye″ro·fos′fate) *n.* [*adenyl* + *pyrophosphate*]. ADENOSINE TRIPHOSPHATE.

ad·e·nyl·py·ro·phos·pho·ric acid (ad″e·nil·pye″ro·fos·for′ick). ADENOSINE TRIPHOSPHATE.

ad·e·pha·gia (ad″e·fay′jee·uh) *n.* [Gk. *adēphagia*, gluttony, from *hadēn*, to one's fill, + *phagein*, to eat]. BULIMIA.

ad·eps (ad′eps) *n.*, pl. **adi·pes** (ad′i·peez) [L.]. 1. Lard, the purified omental fat of the hog; formerly used in ointments. 2. Animal fat.

adeps an·se·ri·nus (an″sur·eye′nus). Goose grease.

adeps ben·zo·i·na·tus (ben·zo·i·nay′tus). Lard containing 1% benzoin.

adeps la·nae (lay′nee). WOOL FAT.

adeps lanae hy·dro·sus (high·dro′sus). HYDROUS WOOL FAT.

adeps prae·pa·ra·tus (prep·uh·ray′tus). Purified hog fat.

adeps su·il·lus (sue·il′us). Hog lard.

ad·equal (ad·ee′kwul) *adj.* Nearly equal.

adequal cleavage. Cleavage producing almost equal blastomeres.

ad·e·quate contact. *In epidemiology*, that degree of contact between one person and another, such that if the first person is infectious and the other is susceptible, the latter will become infected.

adequate stimulus. Energy of a given type (mechanical, thermal, chemical, or electrical) having just sufficient intensity to evoke a response when applied for an adequate time to an excitable tissue. Energy of a different type may be sufficient to evoke a response either at lower intensity or only at higher intensity when applied to the same tissue. For example, rods and cones of the eye respond at a low threshold to electromagnetic vibrations between 400 and 800 mμ and respond only at a much higher threshold to mechanical stimuli.

ader·mia (ay·dur′mee·uh, a·) *n.* [*a-* + *-dermia*]. Absence or defect of the skin.

ader·min (ay·dur′min, a·) *n.* PYRIDOXINE.

ader·mo·gen·e·sis (ay·dur″mo·jen′e·sis) *n.* [*a-* + *dermo-* + *genesis*]. Imperfect development or regeneration of skin.

ADH Abbreviation for (a) *antidiuretic hormone;* (b) *alcohol dehydrogenase.*

A.D.H.A. American Dental Hygienists Association.

adhaesio. ADHESIO.

Ad·hat·o·da (ad·hat′o·duh) *n.* [Tamil]. A genus of plants of the family Acanthaceae. The fruit, leaves, and root of the East Indian plant *Adhatoda vasica*, or Malabar nut tree, are used in India as an expectorant and antispasmodic.

ad·he·pat·ic (ad″he·pat′ick) *adj.* [*ad-* + *hepatic.*] To the liver; (flowing) toward the liver.

ad·here (ad·heer′) *v.* [L. *adhaerere*, from *haerere*, to stick, be stuck]. 1. To stick or become stuck to another surface, as if by gluing. 2. To form an abnormal attachment to another organ or part. **—ad·her·ent,** *adj.;* **adher·ence,** *n.*

adherent placenta. A placenta that fails to separate from the uterine wall after childbirth. See also *placenta accreta, placenta increta, placenta percreta.*

ad·he·sio, ad·hae·sio (ad·hee′zee·o) *n.*, pl. **ad·he·si·o·nes, ad·hae·si·o·nes** (ad·hee″zee·o′neez) [L. *adhaesio*]. ADHESION.

adhesio in·ter·tha·la·mi·ca (in″tur·tha·lam′i·kuh) [NA]. A mass of gray matter that joins the surfaces of the adjacent thalami across the third ventricle, and which has no functional significance and is not always present.

ad·he·sion (ad·hee′zhun) *n.* [L. *adhaesio*, from *adhaerere*, to stick to]. 1. *In physics*, molecular force exerted between two surfaces in contact. 2. Abnormal fibrous union of an organ or part to another.

adhesion phenomenon. IMMUNE-ADHERENCE PHENOMENON.

adhesion test. The adhesion of trypanosomes, spirochetes, and other microorganisms to platelets in the presence of fresh homologous antiserum containing complement. Immune adherence may also be demonstrated with primate red blood cells and various microbial antigens.

ad·he·si·ot·o·my (ad·hee″zee·ot′uh·mee) *n.* *In surgery*, cutting or division of adhesions.

ad·he·sive (ad·hee′ziv) *adj.* & *n.* 1. Sticky; tenacious; tending to cling or stick. 2. Resulting in or attended with adhesion. 3. An adhesive substance. 4. ADHESIVE PLASTER.

adhesive arachnoiditis. CHRONIC ADHESIVE ARACHNOIDITIS.

adhesive bandage. A bandage composed of adhesive plaster or moleskin for immobilization or support of a part.

adhesive capsulitis. FROZEN SHOULDER.

adhesive pericardiomediastinitis. Fibrous adhesions between the pericardium and the mediastinum.

adhesive pericarditis. A form of pericarditis in which the two layers of serous pericardium tend to adhere by means of fibrous adhesions, usually the result of the organization of acute exudate.

adhesive peritonitis. Peritonitis characterized by the formation of fibrous bands between peritoneal surfaces.

adhesive plaster or **tape.** A composition having pressure-sensitive adhesive properties, spread evenly upon fabric, the back of which may be coated with a water-repellent film.

adhesive pleurisy. A form of fibrinous pleurisy in which fibrinous bands extend from the parietal to the visceral pleura.

adhesive serositis. FIBROUS ADHESION.

adhesive tenosynovitis. An inflammatory reaction of a tendon sheath which produces adhesions between tendon and tendon sheath.

adhesive vulvitis. Vulvitis associated with the sticking together of vulvar structures.

adi·ac·tin·ic (ay″dye·ack·tin′ick) *adj.* [*a-* + *diactinic*]. Impervious to, or not penetrated by, actinic rays.

adi·ad·o·cho·ki·ne·sis, adi·ad·o·ko·ki·ne·sis (ay″dye·ad″o·ko·ki·nee′sis, ad″ee·ad″o·ko·) *n.* [*a-* + *diadochokinesis*]. Inability to perform rapidly alternating movements, such as pronation and supination of the hands; seen in cerebellar disease and, in a milder form, in children with the minimal brain dysfunction syndrome.

adi·ad·o·ko·ci·ne·sis (ay″dye·ad″o·ko·si·nee′sis, ad″ee·ad″o·ko·) *n.* ADIADOCHOKINESIS.

adiadokokinesis. ADIADOCHOKINESIS.

Ad·i·an·tum (ad″ee·an′tum) *n.* [NL., from Gk. *adianton*, from *a-*, not, + *diantos*, wettable]. A genus of ferns, commonly called maidenhair. The north American species, *Adiantum capillus-veneris* and *A. pedatum*, have been used as remedies for coughs.

adi·a·pho·ret·ic (ay·dye″uh·fo·ret′ick) *adj.* & *n.* [*a-* + *diaphoretic*]. 1. Reducing, checking, or preventing perspiration; anhidrotic. 2. Any agent or drug that reduces, checks, or prevents perspiration. **—adiapho·re·sis** (·ree′sis) *n.*

a·di·as·to·le (ay″dye·as′tuh·lee, ad″eye·) *n.* Absence or imperceptibility of diastole.

adi·a·ther·mic (ay″dye·uh·thur′mick, ad″eye·uh·) *adj.* [*a-* + *diathermic*]. Impervious to radiant heat. **—adiather·mance, adiather·man·cy,** *n.*

adi·a·the·sic (ay″dye·uh·thees′ick, ·theez′ick) *adj.* ADIATHETIC.

adi·a·thet·ic (ay″dye·uh·thet′ick) *adj.* [*a-* + *diathetic*]. Without relation to any diathesis or constitutional tendency; applied to a symptom or disease.

adic·i·ty (a·dis′i·tee) *n.* [from the suffix *-ad*]. VALENCE.

ad·i·ent (ad′ee·unt) *adj.* [L. *adiens, adientis*, from *ad*, toward, + *ire*, to go]. Tending toward or approaching the source of a stimulus. Contr. *abient.*

Adie's pupil (ay′dee) [W. J. *Adie*, English physician, 1886–1935]. An abnormality of the pupil characterized by very slow adaptation and accommodation. The myotonic pupil will contract or dilate only after prolonged stimulation but is unusually sensitive to a 2.5% Mecholyl salt solution, which will not constrict a normal pupil. Syn. *Adie's tonic pupil, pseudo Argyll Robertson pupil.* See also *Adie's syndrome.*

Adie's syndrome [W. J. *Adie*]. Loss or impairment of pupillary constriction in reaction to light and slowness of constriction during accommodation, associated with loss of tendon reflexes in the legs.

Adie's tonic pupil. ADIE'S PUPIL.

adip-, adipo- [L. *adeps, adipis,* animal fat, lard]. A combining form meaning *fat, fats, fatty tissue.*

ad·i·pec·to·my (ad″i·peck′tuh·mee) *n.* Surgical removal of a mass of adipose tissue.

ad·i·phen·ine (ad″i·fen′een, a·dif′e·neen) *n.* 2-Diethylaminoethyl diphenylacetate, $C_{20}H_{25}NO_2$, an antispasmodic agent; used as the hydrochloride salt.

adip·ic (a·dip′ick) *adj.* [*adip-* + *-ic*]. Of or pertaining to fat.

adipic acid. Hexanedioic acid, $COOH(CH_2)_4COOH$, a dibasic acid obtained by oxidation of various fats.

adipo-. See *adip-*

ad·i·po·cele (ad′i·po·seel) *n.* [*adipo-* + *-cele*]. A true hernia with a hernial sac, containing only fatty tissue. Syn. *lipocele.*

ad·i·po·cel·lu·lar (ad″i·po·sel′yoo·lur) *adj.* [*adipo-* + *cellular*]. Made up of fat and connective tissue.

ad·i·po·cere (ad′i·po·seer) *n.* [*adipo-* + L. *cera,* wax]. A waxlike substance formed during decomposition of dead animal tissues (corpses) in the presence of moisture and in the absence of air, as under earth or water. It consists chiefly of fatty acids and their salts. —**ad·i·po·cer·a·tous** (ad″i·po·serr′uh·tus) *adj.*

ad·i·po·cyte (ad′i·po·site) *n.* [*adipo-* + *-cyte*]. LIPOCYTE.

ad·i·po·fi·bro·ma (ad″i·po·figh·bro′muh) *n.* LIPOFIBROMA.

ad·i·po·ki·net·ic (ad″i·po·ki·net″ick) *adj.* [*adipo-* + *kinetic*]. Pertaining to the mobilization of fats in the body.

adipokinetic action. The property, found in some hypophyseal preparations, of mobilizing free fatty acids from the depot fat stores of the body into the blood.

ad·i·po·ki·nin (ad″i·po·kigh′nin) *n.* [*adipo-* + *kinin*]. A polypeptide from the hypophysis of rabbits that produces an acute rise in serum fatty acid levels.

ad·i·pol·y·sis (ad″i·pol′i·sis) *n.* [*adipo-* + *-lysis*]. Cleavage or hydrolysis of fats during digestion, by fat-splitting enzymes. —**ad·i·po·lyt·ic** (ad″i·po·lit′ick) *adj.*

ad·i·po·ma (ad″i·po′muh) *n.* [*adip-* + *-oma*]. LIPOMA.

ad·i·po·ne·cro·sis (ad″i·po·ne·kro′sis) *n.* Necrosis of fatty tissue.

adiponecrosis neo·na·to·rum. (nee″o·nay·to′rum). Localized process of necrosis of fatty tissue occurring usually in large, well-nourished infants born after difficult labor, characterized by bluish-red lesions that become manifest 2 to 20 days after birth as deep subcutaneous indurations.

adiponecrosis sub·cu·ta·nea neonatorum (sub·kew·tay′nee·uh). ADIPONECROSIS NEONATORUM.

ad·i·po·pex·ia (ad″i·po·peck′see·uh) *n.* ADIPOPEXIS.

ad·i·po·pex·is (ad″i·po·peck′sis) *n.* [*adipo-* + *pexis*]. Fixation of fats; storage of fats. —**adipo·pec·tic** (·peck′tick), **adipo·pex·ic** (·peck′sick) *adj.*

ad·i·po·sa dys·tro·phia ge·ni·ta·lis (ad″i·po′suh dis·tro′fee·uh jen″i·tay′lis). ADIPOSOGENITAL DYSTROPHY.

ad·i·pose (ad′i·poce) *adj.* [*adip-* + *-ose*]. Fatty, fatlike, fat.

adipose capsule. FATTY CAPSULE OF THE KIDNEY.

adipose cell. FAT CELL.

adipose gland. See *brown fat.*

adipose gynandrism. SIMPSON'S SYNDROME in boys.

adipose gynism. SIMPSON'S SYNDROME in girls.

adipose organs. The fat lobules of adipose tissue regarded as distinct organs rather than simple tissue. Syn. *fat organs.*

adipose tissue. A form of connective tissue consisting of fat cells lodged in areolar tissue and arranged in lobules along the course of small blood vessels. See also *brown fat, white fat.*

adipose tumor. LIPOMA.

ad·i·po·sis (ad″i·po′sis) *n.* ADIPOSITY.

adiposis do·lo·ro·sa (do″luh·ro′suh). Extensive subcutaneous painful lipomas or diffuse accumulations of fat, occurring primarily during menopause. Syn. *Dercum's disease.*

adiposis he·pat·i·ca (he·pat′i·kuh). Fatty degeneration or infiltration of the liver.

adiposis or·cha·lis (or·kay′lis). ADIPOSOGENITAL DYSTROPHY.

adiposis tu·be·ro·sa sim·plex (tew·be·ro′suh sim′plecks). A disease resembling adiposis dolorosa, but marked by small subcutaneous fatty nodules which are painful or tender to the touch, and found mostly on the abdomen and extremities. Syn. *Anders' disease.*

ad·i·po·si·tis (ad″i·po·sigh′tis) *n.* [*adipose* + *-itis*]. Inflammation of the subcutaneous fatty tissue.

ad·i·pos·i·ty (ad″i·pos′i·tee) *n.* [from *adipose*]. 1. Corpulence; obesity. 2. An excessive accumulation of fat in the body, localized or general; fatty infiltration. Syn. *adiposis.*

ad·i·po·so·gen·i·tal (ad″i·po″so·jen′i·tul) *adj.* Involving both adipose tissue and genitalia.

adiposogenital dystrophy. Adiposity, retarded development of gonads, and occasionally diabetes insipidus; results from impaired function of the pituitary and hypothalamus; may be caused by craniopharyngioma, tumors of the hypophysis or other structures adjacent to the hypothalamus, trauma, basilar meningitis, or encephalitis. Syn. *Froelich's syndrome.*

ad·i·po·su·ria (ad″i·po·sue′ree·uh) *n.* [*adipose* + *-uria*]. The presence of fat in the urine; LIPURIA.

adip·sia (ay·dip′see·uh, a·dip′) *n.* [*a-* + Gk. *dipsa,* thirst, + *-ia*]. Absence of thirst; avoidance of drinking.

adip·sy (ay·dip′see, a·dip′see, ad′ip·see) *n.* ADIPSIA.

A disk. The transverse segment of a myofibril (or of a whole muscle fiber) which appears longitudinally as an A band.

ad·i·tus (ad′i·tus, a·dit′us) *n.,* pl. **aditus, adituses** [L., from *adire,* to enter, approach]. *In anatomy,* an entrance or inlet.

aditus ad an·trum (ad an′trum) [NA]. The opening between the attic of the tympanic cavity and the mastoid antrum.

aditus ad aquae·duc·tum ce·re·bri (ack·we·duck′tum serr′e·brye) [BNA]. The posterior portion of the third ventricle which is continuous with the cerebral aqueduct.

aditus glot·ti·dis inferior (glot′i·dis) [BNA]. The inferior entrance to the glottis; the space immediately below the true vocal folds.

aditus glottidis superior [BNA]. The superior entrance to the glottis; the space immediately above the vestibular folds.

aditus la·ryn·gis (la·rin′jis) [NA]. The entrance to the larynx, bounded anteriorly by the epiglottis, posteriorly by the upper ends of and the notch between the arytenoid and corniculate cartilages, and laterally by the aryepiglottic folds.

aditus or·bi·tae (or′bi·tee) [NA]. The margin of the orbit.

ad·just·able band. *In orthodontics,* a band provided with an adjusting screw or similar mechanism to permit alteration in size.

ad·just·ed death rate. STANDARDIZED DEATH RATE.

ad·just·ment, *n.* 1. *In biology,* changes undergone by a plant or animal better to adapt to its environment. 2. *In psychology,* the establishment of a relatively harmonious or functionally effective relationship between the individual, his inner self, and his environment. 3. The mechanism of a microscope which brings the objective into focus. 4. Chiropractic treatment aimed at reduction of subluxated vertebrae. 5. Modification of a completed dental restoration, appliance, or prosthesis.

adjustment reaction. A transient situational disturbance of personality occurring in reaction to some significant person, immediate event, or internal emotional conflict. The character of the reaction often varies with the age group.

adjustment reaction of adolescence. A transient situational personality disorder, frequently characterized by vacillations with reference to impulses and emotional tendencies, as well as disturbances in social conduct or sexual behavior, or the emergence of neurotic traits.

adjustment reaction of adult life. A transient situational personality disorder characterized by superficial maladjustment to a new or difficult environmental situation, and manifested by temporary anxiety, alcoholism, poor efficiency, or unconventional behavior. Syn. *adult situational reaction.* See also *gross stress reaction.*

adjustment reaction of childhood. A transient personality disorder in children from about age 4 to 12 years, manifested by such habit disturbances as enuresis, nail-biting, or thumb-sucking, by tantrums or such other disturbances of social conduct as truancy, stealing, or destructiveness, by excessive masturbation or sexual offenses, or by such neurotic traits as tics, stammering, somnambulism, overactivity, or phobias.

adjustment reaction of infancy. A transient personality disorder in the first years of life, frequently manifested by undue apathy or excitement and by feeding and sleeping difficulties.

adjustment reaction of late life. A transient situational personality disorder of adult life or even old age, which usually accentuates previous or precipitates latent disturbances.

ad·ju·vant (aj'oo·vunt) *adj. & n.* [L. *adjuvare,* to aid]. 1. Enhancing or administered to enhance the effectiveness of a treatment or substance. 2. Any adjuvant material. 3. *In immunology,* any substance that enhances the potency of an antigen which it accompanies.

adjuvant arthritis. Arthritis produced in rats by a single subcutaneous injection of Freund's adjuvant into the foot pad or tail; used as an experimental model for rheumatoid arthritis.

adjuvant elixir. GLYCYRRHIZA elixir.

Ad·le·ri·an (ad·leer'ee·un) *adj.* Pertaining to the doctrines and followers of Alfred Adler, Austrian psychiatrist, 1870–1937, founder of the school of individual psychology.

ad lib. Abbreviation for *ad libitum,* at pleasure; the amount desired.

ad·max·il·lary (ad·mack'si·lerr"ee) *adj.* Near or toward the maxilla.

admaxillary gland. ACCESSORY PAROTID GLAND.

ad·me·di·al (ad·mee'dee·ul) *adj.* Located near or approaching the median plane or central axis.

ad·me·di·an (ad·mee'dee·un) *adj.* ADMEDIAL.

ad·mi·nic·u·lum (ad"mi·nick'yoo·lum) *n.,* pl. **adminicu·la** (·luh) [L., support]. 1. A supporting structure. 2. A triangular fibrous expansion which extends from the superior pubic ligament to the posterior surface of the linea alba. NA *adminiculum lineae albae.*

adminiculum li·ne·ae al·bae (lin'ee·ee al'bee) [NA]. ADMINICULUM (2).

ad·mis·sion rate. The number of admissions to a medical unit, such as a clinic or hospital, per thousand of population, during a specific time period such as a year.

ad·mix·ture (ad·micks'chur) *n.* 1. The act, process, or product of mixing. 2. A substance added by mixing.

ad·na·sal (ad·nay'zul) *adj.* Pertaining to the nose; situated near the nose; toward the nose.

ad·nate (ad'nate) *adj.* [L. *adnatus,* connected by birth, from *ad-* + *natus,* born]. Congenitally attached or united.

ad nau·se·am (ad naw'zee·um, ·shee·um) [L.]. To the point of producing nausea.

ad·nexa (ad·neck'suh) *n.,* sing. **adnex·um** [L., connected parts, from *adnectere,* to connect to]. Accessory parts or appendages of an organ. Syn. *annexa.* **—adnex·al** (·sul) *adj.*

adnexal carcinoma. APPENDAGE-CELL CARCINOMA.

adnexa ocu·li (ock'yoo·lye). Appendages of the eye, as the lids and the lacrimal apparatus. NA *organa oculi accessoria.*

adnexa ute·ri (yoo'tur·eye). The uterine tubes and ovaries.

ad·nex·i·tis (ad"neck·sigh'tis) *n.* Inflammation of the adnexa uteri; SALPINGO-OOPHORITIS.

ad·nexo·gen·e·sis (ad·neck"so·jen'e·sis) *n.* [*adnexa* + *genesis*]. The forming of the extraembryonic membranes of the embryo.

Ad-Nil. Trademark for levamfetamine sulfate, an anorexigenic drug.

ad·o·les·cence, *n.* [L. *adolescentia,* from *adolescere,* to grow up, from *alescere,* to grow, from *alere,* to nourish]. The period of life extending from puberty to maturity. **—adoles·cent,** *adj. & n.*

adolescent crisis. IDENTITY CRISIS.

adolescent depression. Mild depression with anxiety seen in youth of both sexes whenever the problems of the identity crisis or of adult sexual behavior become acute or too stressful.

adolescent goiter. Diffuse enlargement of the thyroid of unknown cause, most frequently seen in girls during puberty.

adolescent kyphosis. SCHEURMANN'S DISEASE.

adolescent mammoplasia. Enlargement of the male breasts during adolescence; they later return to normal size.

adon·i·din (a·don'i·din) *n.* A mixture of glycosides and adonic acid derived from *Adonis vernalis,* a plant indigenous to Europe and Asia.

adon·in (a·don'in) *n.* A glycoside from *Adonis autumnalis.* It has powerful action as a heart stimulant.

Adon·is (a·don'is) *n.* A genus of European herbs belonging to the order Ranunculaceae. Certain species have been used for treatment of cardiac ailments.

ad·oral (ad·or'ul) *adj.* [*ad-* + *oral*]. Situated near the mouth; toward the mouth. **—adoral·ly,** *adv.*

ad·or·bit·al (ad·or'bi·tul) *adj.* Situated near the orbit; toward the orbit.

ADP Abbreviation for *adenosine diphosphate.*

A.D.P. Academy of Denture Prosthetics.

adren-, adreno-. A combining form meaning *adrenal.*

ad·re·nal (a·dree'nul) *adj. & n.* [*ad-* + *renal*]. 1. Situated adjacent to the kidney. 2. Pertaining to the adrenal glands. 3. ADRENAL GLAND.

adrenal apoplexy. Hemorrhage into the adrenal glands, usually part of the Waterhouse-Friderichsen syndrome.

adrenal cortex. The cortical portion of the adrenal gland.

adrenal cortical hyperplasia. ADRENOGENITAL SYNDROME.

adrenal cortical insufficiency. An acute or chronic failure of adrenal cortical secretion of glucocorticoid and mineralocorticoid hormones; the primary form is due to adrenal cortical disease and the secondary form to insufficient pituitary adrenocorticotropic hormone.

adrenal crisis. Acute adrenal failure; severe acute exacerbation of Addison's disease. Syn. *Addisonian crisis.*

adre·nal·ec·to·my (a·dree"nul·eck'tuh·mee) *n.* Surgical removal of an adrenal gland. **—adrenalecto·mize,** *v.*

adrenal gland. An endocrine gland located immediately above the superior pole of each kidney. It consists of a medulla that produces epinephrine and norepinephrine, and a cortex that is the source of many steroidal hormones involved in electrolyte and fluid balance, or in carbohydrate and protein metabolism. Syn. *suprarenal gland.* NA *glandula suprarenalis.* See also Plates 7, 8, 9, 14, 26.

adrenal hemorrhage syndrome. WATERHOUSE-FRIDERICHSEN SYNDROME.

adrenal hypernephroma. CORTICAL ADENOMA.

adrenal hypernephroma ma·lig·num (ma·lig'num). CORTICAL CARCINOMA.

Adrenalin. A trademark for epinephrine, the adrenal medullary hormone. Compare *adrenaline.*

adren·a·line (a·dren'uh·lin, ·leen) *n.* [*adrenal* + *-ine*]. *British Pharmacopoeia and Amer. colloq.* EPINEPHRINE. Compare *Adrenalin.*

adren·a·lin·emia, adren·a·lin·ae·mia (a·dren"uh·li·nee'mee·uh) *n.* [*adrenaline* + *-emia*]. The presence of epinephrine in the blood.

adren·a·lin·uria (a·dren"uh·li·nyoor'ee·uh) *n.* [*adrenaline* + *-uria*]. The presence of epinephrine in the urine.

adre·nal·ism (a·dree'nul·iz·um, a·dren''ul·iz·um) *n.* A condition due to dysfunction of the adrenal glands. See also *hyperadrenalism, hypoadrenalism.*

adre·nal·itis (a·dree''nul·eye'tis) *n.* Inflammation of the adrenal glands.

adrenal medulla. The medulla of the adrenal gland.

adrenal medullary hormone. Any hormone secreted by the medulla of the suprarenal gland, as epinephrine or norepinephrine.

adren·a·lone (a·dren'uh·lone) *adj.* 1-(3,4-Dihydroxyphenyl)-2-(methylamino)ethanone, $C_9H_{11}NO_3$, an ophthalmic adrenergic agent.

adrenal virilism syndrome. ADRENOGENITAL SYNDROME.

ad·ren·ar·che (ad''re·nahr'kee) *n.* [*adren-* + Gk. *archē*, beginning]. The time in the development of a child at which an increased output of adrenocortical hormones occurs, manifested by the appearance of pubic and axillary hair and increase in urinary steroid excretion. It usually occurs about the eighth or ninth year of life.

Adrenatrate. Trademark for epinephrine bitartrate, used in topical ophthalmic preparations.

ad·re·ner·gic (ad''re·nur'jick) *adj.* [*adren-* + *erg-* + *-ic*]. Of or pertaining to the type of chemical activity characteristic of epinephrine and epinephrine-like substances.

α-adrenergic. ALPHA ADRENERGIC.

β-adrenergic. BETA-ADRENERGIC.

adrenergic blocking agent. Any compound that selectively inhibits certain responses to adrenergic nerve activity and to norepinephrine and other sympathomimetic amines. On the basis of selective inhibition of the responses, the compounds may be classified as alpha- or beta-adrenergic blocking agents. Syn. *adrenolytic agent, sympatholytic agent.*

α-adrenergic blocking agent. ALPHA-ADRENERGIC BLOCKING AGENT.

β-adrenergic blocking agent. BETA-ADRENERGIC BLOCKING AGENT.

adrenergic nerve fibers. Nerve fibers which, upon stimulation, liberate norepinephrine at their terminations; include most of the postganglionic fibers of the sympathetic nervous system.

adrenergic receptor. See *alpha-adrenergic receptor, beta-adrenergic receptor.*

α-adrenergic receptor. ALPHA-ADRENERGIC RECEPTOR.

β-adrenergic receptor. BETA-ADRENERGIC RECEPTOR.

adre·nic (a·dree'nick, a·dren'ick) *adj.* Pertaining to the adrenal glands.

adrenic acid. 7,10,13,16-Docosatetraenoic acid, a fatty acid found esterified to cholesterol in the adrenal glands.

adre·nin (ad're·nin, a·dree'nin) *n.* EPINEPHRINE.

adre·nine (ad're·neen, a·dree'nin) *n.* EPINEPHRINE.

ad·re·ni·tis (ad''re·nigh'tis) *n.* ADRENALITIS.

adreno-. See *adren-*.

adre·no·chrome (a·dree'no·krome) *n.* [*adreno-* + *-chrome*]. A quinone-type oxidation product, $C_9H_9NO_3$, of epinephrine; occurs as red crystals.

adre·no·cor·ti·cal (a·dree''no·kor'ti·kul) *adj.* Pertaining to or derived from the adrenal cortex.

adrenocortical hormone. Any of the biologically active steroid hormones which have been isolated from the adrenal cortex.

adrenocortical obesity. BUFFALO OBESITY.

adrenocortical tumor of the ovary. An adrenocorticoid adenoma of the ovary.

adre·no·cor·ti·coid (a·dree''no·kor'ti·koid) *adj.* & *n.* 1. Pertaining to or resembling the adrenal cortex or the hormones secreted by it. 2. An adrenal cortical hormone.

adrenocorticoid adenoma of the ovary. One of a group of rare masculinizing tumors of the ovary, composed of cells resembling those of the adrenal cortex; characteristically causes defemination or virilism.

adre·no·cor·ti·co·mi·met·ic (a·dree''no·kor''ti·ko·migh·met'ick, ·mi·met'ick) *adj.* [*adrenocortic*al + *mimetic*]. Similar in activity or effect to an adrenal cortical steroid.

adre·no·cor·ti·co·tro·phic (a·dree''no·kor''ti·ko·tro'fick, ·trof'ick) *adj. Erron.* ADRENOCORTICOTROPIC.

adre·no·cor·ti·co·tro·phin (a·dree''no·kor''ti·ko·tro'fin) *n. Erron.* Adrenocorticotropin (= ADRENOCORTICOTROPIC HORMONE).

adre·no·cor·ti·co·tro·pic (a·dree''no·kor''ti·ko·tro'pick) *adj.* [*adrenocortic*al + *-tropic*]. Capable of stimulating or maintaining the growth and hormone-secretory function of the adrenal cortex.

adrenocorticotropic hormone. The adenohypophyseal hormone which stimulates and maintains the growth and hormone-secretory function of the adrenal cortex. Abbreviated, ACTH. Syn. *adrenocorticotropin.*

adrenocorticotropic hormone releasing factor. A substance, presumed to originate in the hypothalamus, which acts to release adrenocorticotropic hormone from the adenohypophysis.

adre·no·cor·ti·co·tro·pin (a·dree''no·kor''ti·ko·tro'pin) *n.* [*adreno-* + *corticotropin*]. ADRENOCORTICOTROPIC HORMONE.

Adreno-cortin. A trademark for an injectable extract of adrenal glands containing cortical steroids but substantially free of epinephrine.

adre·no·gen·i·tal (a·dree''no·jen'i·tul) *adj.* [*adreno-* + *genital*]. Pertaining to the adrenal glands and the gonads.

adrenogenital syndrome. A clinical condition associated with hypersecretion of androgenic hormones by adrenal cortical tissue or due to excess steroid hormone administration. It may be congenital or acquired; the acquired forms are due to adrenal hyperplasia or tumor. In the female, the congenital forms may result in pseudohermaphroditism and advanced physical growth, while the acquired forms may produce enlargement of the clitoris or virilism. In the male, the congenital forms manifest early enlargement of the penis and advanced somatic growth; in the acquired forms, these findings appear later; rarely, an adrenal tumor in the male produces feminization with gynecomastia. Compare *Cushing's syndrome, hyperaldosteronism.*

adre·no·leu·ko·dys·tro·phy (a·dree''no·lew''ko·dis'truh·fee) *n.* A metabolic encephalopathy of childhood, inherited as a sex-linked recessive trait and characterized by bronzing of the skin and other manifestations of Addison's disease combined with degeneration of the white matter in various parts of the cerebrum, brainstem, optic nerves, and sometimes the spinal cord; formerly considered a manifestation of Schilder's disease.

adre·no·lyt·ic (a·dree''no·lit'ick) *adj.* [*adreno-* + *-lytic*]. Inhibiting the function of adrenergic nerves or the physiologic responses to the action of epinephrine or norepinephrine.

adrenolytic agent. ADRENERGIC BLOCKING AGENT.

adre·no·med·ul·lary (a·dree''no·med'yoo·lerr·ee, ·me·dul'ur·ee) *adj.* Of or pertaining to the adrenal medulla.

adre·no·mi·met·ic (a·dree''no·mi·met'ick) *adj.* [*adreno* + *mimetic*]. SYMPATHOMIMETIC

adre·no·pause (a·dree'no·pawz) *n.* The hypothetical age at which production of certain adrenocortical hormones is reduced.

Adrenoscan. A trademark for radioactively labeled 19-iodocholesterol, a radiopaque.

Adrenosem. A trademark for carbazochrome, a systemic hemostatic.

adre·no·ste·rone (a·dree''no·ste·rone', ad''ren·os'te·rone) *n.* 4-Androstene-3,11,17-trione, $C_{19}H_{24}O_3$, a steroid hormone with androgenic properties; obtained from the adrenal cortex.

adre·no·sym·pa·thet·ic (a·dree''no·sim''puh·thet'ick) *adj.* Pertaining to the adrenal glands and the sympathetic nervous system.

adrenosympathetic syndrome. Episodes of paroxysmal hypertension, nervousness, tachycardia, palpitations, sweating, flushing or pallor, headache, nausea, vomiting, glycosuria, and chest and abdominal pain due to increased epinephrine and norepinephrine secretion, usually caused by pheochromocytoma, but at times by neuroblastoma or ganglioneuroma. Syn. *Page's syndrome.*

adre·no·trope (a·dree'no·trope) *n.* [*adreno-* + *-trope*]. A person with an adrenal type of endocrine diathesis.

adre·no·tro·phic (a·dree"no·tro'fick, ·trof'ick) *adj. Erron.* ADRENOTROPIC.

adre·no·tro·phin (a·dree"no·tro'fin) *n. Erron.* Adrenotropin (= ADRENOCORTICOTROPIC HORMONE).

adre·no·tro·pic (a·dree"no·tro'pick) *adj.* [*adreno-* + *-tropic*]. Having or pertaining to an effect on the adrenal gland, particularly the cortex.

adrenotropic hormone. ADRENOCORTICOTROPIC HORMONE.

adre·no·tro·pin (a·dree"no·tro'pin) *n.* ADRENOCORTICOTROPIC HORMONE.

ad·re·not·ro·pism (ad"re·not'ro·piz·um, a·dree"no·tro'piz·um) *n.* [*adreno-* + *-tropism*]. Dominance of the adrenal in the endocrine functions.

Adrestat. A trademark for carbazochrome, a systemic hemostatic.

Adriamycin. Trademark for doxorubicin hydrochloride.

Adrian-Bronk law [E. D. *Adrian,* English biologist, b. 1889; and D. W. *Bronk,* physiologist, b. 1897]. The frequency of discharge of a nerve is directly proportional to the intensity of the applied stimulus and to the number of individual neurons in the nerve.

Adrin. Trademark for an injectable preparation of epinephrine hydrochloride.

adro·mia (a·dro'mee·uh) *n.* [*a-* + *drom-* + *-ia*]. Complete failure of impulse conduction in muscle or nerve.

Adroyd. A trademark for oxymetholone, an anabolic steroid.

ad·sorb (ad·sorb') *v.* [*ad-* + L. *sorbere,* to suck up]. Of a substance: to attract and concentrate upon its surface, in a thin layer, molecules of a gas, liquid, or dissolved substance. —**adsorbed,** *adj.*

ad·sor·bate (ad·sor'bate, ad·zor'bate) *n.* Any substance that is adsorbed.

adsorbed diphtheria toxoid. A suspension of diphtheria toxoid precipitated or adsorbed by the addition of alum, aluminum hydroxide, or aluminum phosphate to a detoxified solution of the products of growth of the diphtheria baccillus, *Corynebacterium diphtheriae.*

adsorbed pertussis vaccine. A bacterial fraction or suspension of killed pertussis bacilli, precipitated or adsorbed by the addition of aluminum hydroxide or aluminum phosphate and resuspended.

adsorbed tetanus toxoid. A suspension of tetanus toxoid precipitated or adsorbed by the addition of alum, aluminum hydroxide, or aluminum phosphate to a detoxified solution of the products of growth of the tetanus bacillus, *Clostridium tetani.*

ad·sor·bent (ad·sor'bunt) *adj. & n.* 1. Adsorbing or having the capacity to adsorb. 2. Any adsorbent substance, such as activated charcoal or silica gel.

ad·sorp·tion (ad·sorp'shun) *n.* The process of adsorbing or of being adsorbed. —**adsorptive** (·tiv) *adj.*

ad·ster·nal (ad·stur'nul) *adj.* Situated near the sternum; toward the sternum.

A.D.T.A. American Dental Trade Association.

ad·ter·mi·nal (ad·tur'mi·nul) *adj.* [*ad-* + *terminal*]. Moving toward the end of a muscle; said of electric currents in muscular tissue.

ad·tor·sion (ad·tor'shun) *n.* [*ad-* + *torsion*]. A condition in which both eyes are turned toward the nose, and their vertical meridians converge above instead of being parallel. Compare *esotropia.*

adult, *adj. & n.* [L. *adultus,* from *adolescere,* to grow up]. 1. Mature; having attained full size, strength, and reproductive ability. 2. In human society: having attained the ability to handle personal affairs; of full legal age. 3. A full-grown and mature individual. 4. Of or pertaining to adults.

adult celiac disease. CELIAC SYNDROME.

adul·ter·ant (a·dul'tur·unt) *n.* Any substance that adulterates.

adul·ter·a·tion (a·dul"tur·ay'shun) *n.* [L. *adulterare,* to corrupt, from *ad-* + *alter,* other]. Admixture or substitution of inferior, impure, inert, or cheaper ingredients for gain, deception, or concealment. —**adul·ter·ate** (a·dul'tur·ate) *v.*

adult Fanconi syndrome [G. *Fanconi*]. A recessive heritable or acquired disorder of renal tubular function, beginning in adult life and characterized by any combination of proteinuria, aminoaciduria, renal glycosuria, hyperphosphaturia, hypophosphatemia, acidosis, and resultant severe osteomalacia. Cystinosis, however, does not occur. See also *Fanconi syndrome.*

adult hereditary chorea. HUNTINGTON'S CHOREA.

adult hypopituitarism. HYPOPITUITARISM.

adult polycystic disease. A form of polycystic disease inherited as an autosomal dominant trait, with progressive renal failure usually appearing in the fourth or fifth decade of life; hypertension is usually associated and hepatic cysts are often also present; there is a high incidence of cerebral arterial aneurysm.

adult progeria. WERNER'S SYNDROME.

adult rickets. OSTEOMALACIA.

adult situational reaction. ADJUSTMENT REACTION OF ADULT LIFE.

adult Still's disease [G. F. *Still*]. *Obsol.* FELTY'S SYNDROME. Compare *Still's disease.*

adult-type tuberculosis. CHRONIC TUBERCULOSIS.

adust (a·dust') *adj.* [L. *adustus,* burnt, scorched]. Affected by excess bodily heat, hence displaying signs of dehydration.

ad·vance, *v. In ophthalmology and surgery,* to perform an advancement.

ad·vance·ment, *n.* 1. A tenotomy followed by reattachment of the tendon at a more advanced point. 2. *In ophthalmology,* operative correction of strabismus, in which the muscle tendon opposite to the direction of the squint is removed at its insertion and sutured to the sclera anterior to the original attachment. See also *Lancaster's advancement.*

ad·ve·hent (ad'vee·unt, ad·vee'unt) *adj.* [L. *advehens, advehentis,* from *ad-* + *vehere,* to convey]. AFFERENT.

advehent vein. *In embryology,* the portion of the omphalomesenteric vein caudal to the liver and cranial to the transverse anastomoses; it becomes a branch of the portal vein.

ad·ven·ti·tia (ad"ven·tish'ee·uh) *n.* [short for NL. *tunica adventitia,* outer coat, from L. *adventicius,* coming from outside]. 1. The external covering of an organ derived from adjacent connective tissue. NA *tunica adventitia.* 2. Specifically, the outermost of the three coats of a blood vessel, consisting of connective tissue and elastic fibers. NA *tunica externa.* —**adven·ti·tial** (·tish'ul) *adj.*

adventitial cell. A phagocytic or fibroblastic cell situated on the outer surface of a lymph or blood vessel and with branches into the surrounding tissue.

adventitial neuritis. Neuritis affecting the nerve sheath.

ad·ven·ti·tious (ad"ven·tish'us) *adj.* 1. Accidental, foreign, acquired, as opposed to natural or hereditary. 2. Occurring in unusual or abnormal places. 3. Pertaining to the adventitia.

adventitious albuminuria. Proteinuria without detectable renal disease.

adventitious bursa. ACCIDENTAL BURSA.

adventitious cyst. A cavity associated with a foreign body or substance.

adventitious deafness. Loss of hearing after speech is established.

adventitious dentin. Secondary dentin formed in response to abnormal irritation.

adventitious embryony. Agamospermy in which the gametophyte stage is eliminated, the embryo arising from a sporophytic portion of the ovule.

adverse drug reaction. As defined by the Food and Drug Administration: a reaction that is noxious, unintended, and occurs at doses normally used in man for prophylaxis, diagnosis, or therapy of disease.

ad·ver·sive (ad·vur'siv) *adj.* [L. *advertere,* to turn toward]. Turning to one side; pertaining to rotation of the eyes, head, or trunk.

adversive seizure. CONTRAVERSIVE SEIZURE.

ady·nam·ia (ay"di·nam'ee·uh, ad"i·nay'mee·uh) *n.* [Gk., from *a-* + *dynamis,* power]. Loss of vital strength or muscular power; weakness; debility; ASTHENIA. **—ady·nam·ic** (·nam'ick) *adj.*

adynamia epi·sod·i·ca he·red·i·ta·ria (ep"i·sod'i·kuh he·red"i·tair'ee·uh). A form of periodic paralysis, usually with hyperkalemia and sometimes with minor degrees of myotonia. Syn. *Gamstorp's disease.* See also *periodic paralysis.*

adynamic ileus. General or regional failure of peristalsis due to inadequate intestinal muscular activity, resulting in intestinal obstruction.

ady·na·my (a·dye'nuh·mee) *n.* ADYNAMIA.

Aë·des (ay·ee'deez) *n.* [Gk. *aēdēs,* distasteful, unpleasant]. A genus of mosquitoes of the family Culicidae, of cosmopolitan distribution and including about 600 species, some of which are important vectors of human diseases, such as yellow fever, dengue, virus encephalitis, and certain filarial infections.

Aëdes ae·gyp·ti (ee·jip'tye). The principal vector of yellow fever and dengue. It breeds in urban areas.

ae·doe·o·ceph·a·lus (ee"dee·o·sef'uh·lus, ed"ee·o·) *n.* EDOCEPHALUS.

aedoeology. EDEOLOGY.

ae·lu·ro·phil·ia (e·lew"ro·fil'ee·uh) *n.* [Gk. *ailouros,* cat, + *-philia*]. GALEOPHILIA.

ae·lu·ro·pho·bia (e·lew"ro·fo'bee·uh) *n.* [Gk. *ailouros,* cat, + *-phobia*]. GALEOPHOBIA.

ae·lu·rop·sis (ee"lew·rop'sis, el"yoo·) *n.* [Gk. *ailouros,* cat, + *-opsis*]. Obliquity of the eye or of the palpebral fissure.

-aemia. See *-emia.*

aequator [BNA]. EQUATOR.

ae·quum (ee'kwum) *n.* [L., level, equal]. *Obsol.* The caloric intake necessary to maintain weight with normal physical activity. It varies with the individual's size and the nature of his activity.

aer-, aero- [Gk. *aēr, aeros,* air]. A combining form meaning (a) *air, aerial;* (b) *gas, gases.*

aeraemia. AEREMIA.

aer·ate (ay'ur·ate, air'ate) *v.* To charge with air or gas; to oxygenate, carbonate; to arterialize. **—aerat·ed** (·id) *adj.;* **aer·a·tor** (·ay·tur) *n.*

aer·a·tion (ay"ur·ay'shun, air"ay'shun) *n.* 1. Exposure to air. 2. Saturation of a fluid with air or a gas, as carbon dioxide. 3. The exchange of oxygen and carbon dioxide in the lungs.

aer·emia, aer·ae·mia (ay"ur·ee'mee·uh, air·) *n.* [*aer-* + *-emia*]. The presence of air in the blood. See also *decompression sickness.*

aer·en·ter·ec·ta·sia (ay"ur·en"tur·eck·tay'zhuh, ·zee·uh, air·en"tur·) *n.* [*aer-* + *enter-* + *ectasia*]. TYMPANITES; METEORISM.

aer fix·us (air fick'sus, ay'err) [NL., lit., fixed air]. CARBON DIOXIDE.

ae·ri·al conduction. AIR CONDUCTION.

aerial image. An image formed in space by use of a convex lens, as produced by indirect ophthalmoscopy.

aer·if·er·ous (ay"ur·if'ur·us, air") *adj.* [*aer-* + *-iferous*]. Conveying air, as the trachea, bronchi, and their branches.

aer·i·form (ay'ur·i·form, ay·eer') *adj.* Airlike; gaseous.

aero-. See *aer-.*

aero·at·e·lec·ta·sis (air"o·at"e·leck'tuh·sis, ay"ur·o·) *n.* [*aero-* + *atelectasis*]. A partial, reversible collapse of the lungs observed in aviators breathing 100% oxygen while flying at high altitudes.

Aero·bac·ter (ay"ur·o·back'tur, air'o·back"tur) *n.* [*aero-* + *bacter*ium]. ENTEROBACTER.

Aerobacter aerogenes. ENTEROBACTER AEROGENES.

aer·obe (ay"ur·obe, air"obe) *n.* [F. *aérobie,* from *aero-* + Gk. *bios,* life]. A microorganism which requires air or oxygen for the maintenance of life. The final hydrogen acceptor is molecular oxygen.

aer·o·bi·an (ay"ur·o'bee·un, air·) *adj.* AEROBIC (3).

aer·o·bic (ay"ur·o'bick, air·) *adj.* [*aerob*e + *-ic*]. 1. Utilizing oxygen. 2. Requiring air or free oxygen in order to live. 3. Pertaining to or produced by aerobes. 4. Of or pertaining to aerobics.

aerobic contraction. A type of muscular contraction in which oxygen is utilized.

aerobic metabolism. Metabolism utilizing oxygen as the ultimate proton acceptor, forming water as the end product.

aer·o·bics (ay"ur·o'bicks, air·) *n.* Exercise, or a system of exercise, such as bicycling or jogging, performed at a rate and intensity which allow aerobic rather than anaerobic metabolism to continue, thus promoting improvement of pulmonary and cardiovascular function.

aero·bi·ol·o·gy (ay"ur·o·bye·ol'uh·jee, air"o·) *n.* The science concerned with air-borne microbes, pollen, spores, dust, smoke, and other substances, as well as with their occurrence, characteristics, relation to human welfare, and control.

aero·bio·scope (ay"ur o·bye'o·skope, air"o·) *n.* [*aero-* + *bio-* + *-scope*]. An apparatus for collecting and filtering bacteria from the air to determine the bacterial content.

aero·bi·o·sis (ay"ur·o·bye·o'sis, air"o·) *n.* [*aero-* + *-biosis*]. Life that requires the presence of air, or molecular oxygen. **—aerobi·ot·ic** (·ot'ick) *adj.*

aero·cele (ay'ur·o·seel, air'o·) *n.* [*aero-* + *-cele*]. A swelling caused by the escape of air into an adventitious pouch usually connected with the trachea (tracheocele) or larynx (laryngocele); hence its size may vary with respiration or straining.

aero·col·pos (ay"ur·o·kol'pos, air"o·) *n.* [*aero-* + *-colpos*]. Distention of the vagina with air or gas.

aero·cys·tos·co·py (ay"ur·o·sis·tos'kuh·pee, air"o·) *n.* Examination of the interior of the urinary bladder with a cystoscope, the bladder being distended with air. **—aero·cys·to·scope** (·sis'tuh·skope) *n.*

aer·o·don·tal·gia (air"o·don·tal'jee·uh, ay"ur·o"don·) *n.* [*aer-* + *odontalgia*]. Pain occurring in the teeth of individuals exposed to decreased atmospheric pressure such as may occur from high-altitude ascent and in decompression chambers.

aero·duc·tor (air"o·duck'tur, ay"ur·o·) *n.* An apparatus to prevent asphyxia of the fetus when the aftercoming head is retained; no longer in common clinical use.

aero·em·bo·lism (air"o·em'bo·liz·um) *n.* 1. AIR EMBOLISM. 2. Embolism caused by the forcing of air bubbles from the alveoli into the pulmonary capillaries, due to expansion of air trapped in the lungs during rapid decompression; may occur, for example, when a diver using compressed air ascends rapidly and fails to exhale because of panic and glottal spasm. Compare *bends, decompression sickness.*

aero·em·phy·se·ma (air"o·em"fi·see'muh) *n.* [*aero-* + *emphysema*]. 1. The accumulation of gas bubbles in various tissues and organs; seen under conditions of decompression. 2. A form of chronic pulmonary emphysema resulting from repeated rapid decompression, as may occur in inadequately pressurized aircraft.

aero·gen (air'o·jen, ay'ur·o·) *n.* [*aero-* + *-gen*]. Any gas-producing microorganism.

aer·o·gen·e·sis (air"o·jen'e·sis, ay"ur·o·) *n.* [*aero-* + *genesis*]. Gas formation. **—aerogen·ic** (·ick), **aer·og·e·nous** (ay"ur·oj'e·nus) *adj.*

aero·gram (air'o·gram, ay'ur·o·) *n.* An x-ray film of an organ inflated with air; PNEUMOGRAM

aer·og·ra·phy (air·og'ruh·fee, ay''ur·) *n.* The description of air and its qualities.

Aerohalor. Trademark for a device to insufflate drugs into the respiratory tract.

aero·hy·drop·a·thy (air''o·high·drop'uth·ee, ay''ur·o·) *n.* [*aero-* + *hydropathy*]. AEROHYDROTHERAPY.

aero·hy·dro·ther·a·py (air''o·high''dro·therr''uh·pee, ay''ur·o·) *n.* [*aero-* + *hydrotherapy*]. The use of air and water in the treatment of disease.

aero·ion·iza·tion (air''o·eye'un·i·zay'shun, ay''ur·o·) *n.* [*aero-* + *ionization*]. The process of electrically charging particles (such as oil drops) suspended in the air, formerly used as an inhalation treatment for respiratory disease.

aero·iono·ther·a·py (air''o·eye''un·o·therr'uh·pee, ay''ur·o·) *n.* [*aero-* + *ion* + *therapy*]. Inhalation of air with electrically charged particles, used in the treatment of respiratory disease.

aer·om·e·ter (air·om'e·tur, ay''ur·) *n.* An instrument for determining the density of gases.

aero·neu·ro·sis (air''o·new·ro'sis, ay''ur·o·) *n.* A form of neurosis found in aviators, characterized by anxiety, restlessness, and various physical manifestations.

aero·oti·tis (air''o·o·tye'tis, ay''ur·o·) *n.* [*aero-* + *otitis*]. BAROTITIS.

aer·op·a·thy (ay''ur·op'uth·ee) *n.* Any pathologic condition brought about by changes in atmospheric pressure, as decompression sickness.

aero·pause (ay'ur·o·pawz, air'o·) *n.* That region of the earth's atmosphere, between the stratosphere and outer space, where its various functions (e.g., supplying breathing air and climate, filtrating cosmic factors, offering mechanical support) for man and aircraft begin to cease and conditions equivalent to outer space are gradually approached.

aero·peri·to·ne·um, aero·peri·to·nae·um (air''o·perr''i·tuh·nee'um, ay''ur·o·) *n.* PNEUMOPERITONEUM.

aero·peri·to·nia (air''o·perr''i·to'nee·uh, ay''ur·o·) *n.* [*aero-* + *peritoneum* + *-ia*]. PNEUMOPERITONEUM.

aero·pha·gia (ay''ur·o·fay'jee·uh, air''o·) *n.* [*aero-* + *-phagia*]. Spasmodic swallowing of air followed by noisy eructations.

aer·oph·a·gy (ay''ur·off'uh·jee) *n.* AEROPHAGIA.

aer·o·phil (air'o·fil, ay'ur·o·) *adj.* [*aero-* + *-phil*]. 1. Loving the open air. 2. AEROBIC (2).

aero·pho·bia (air''o·fo'bee·uh, ay''ur·o·) *n.* Morbid fear of drafts or of fresh air.

aero·phore (air'o·for, ay'ur·o·) *n.* [*aero-* + *-phore*]. 1. A device for inflating the lungs with air in any case of asphyxia. 2. An apparatus which purifies air for rebreathing, used by firemen and others.

aero·phyte (air'o·fite, ay'ur·o·) *n.* [*aero-* + *-phyte*]. EPIPHYTE.

aero·pi·eso·ther·a·py (air''o·pye·ee''so·therr'uh·pee, ay''ur·o·) *n.* [*aero-* + Gk. *piesis*, compression, + *therapy*]. Use of compressed or rarefied air in the treatment of disease.

Aeroplast. Trademark for vibesate, a film-forming surgical dressing.

aero·ple·thys·mo·graph (air''o·ple·thiz'mo·graf, ay''ur·o·) *n.* [*aero-* + Gk. *plēthysmos*, increase, filling, + *graph*]. An apparatus for registering graphically the volume of air inspired and expired.

aero·pleu·ra (air''o·ploor'uh, ay''ur·o·) *n.* [*aero-* + *pleura*]. PNEUMOTHORAX.

aer·o·scope (air'o·skope, ay'ur·o·) *n.* An instrument for the examination of air dust and for estimating the purity of the air.

aer·os·co·py (ay''ur·os'kuh·pee) *n.* Investigation of atmospheric conditions.

aero·si·al·oph·a·gy (ay''ur·o·sigh''ul·off'uh·jee, air''o·) *n.* [*aero-* + *sialo-* + *-phagy*]. The habit of constantly swallowing, and so taking air and saliva into the stomach.

aero·si·nus·itis (ay''ur·o·sigh''nuh·sigh'tis, air''o·) *n.* [*aero-* + *sinusitis*]. BAROSINUSITIS.

aer·o·sis (air·o'sis, ay'ur·) *n.* [*aer-* + *-osis*]. Formation of gas in any of the body tissues.

aero·sol (air'o·sol, ay'ur·o·) *n.* [*aero-* + *sol*]. 1. Atomized particles suspended in the air. 2. Any solution or compressed gas containing an agent for the treatment of the air to remove or destroy insects or microorganisms. 3. *In chemistry,* a colloid in which a gas is the dispersion medium.

Aerosol OT. Trademark for dioctyl sodium sulfosuccinate, a surface-active agent.

aero·space medicine. The branch of medicine that comprises areas of subject matter common to aviation medicine and space medicine.

Aerosporin. A trademark for polymyxin B sulfate, an antibiotic substance.

aero·stat·ics (air''o·stat'icks, ay''ur·o·) *n.* The branch of physics that treats of the properties of gases at rest, or in equilibrium.

aero·tax·is (air·o·tack'sis, ay''ur·o·) *n.*, pl. **aerotax·es** (·seez) [*aero-* + *taxis*]. The tendency of living organisms, especially aerobes and anaerobes, to be attracted or repelled, respectively, by oxygen or air.

aero·ther·a·peu·tics (air''o·therr''uh·pew'ticks, ay''ur·o·) *n.* A mode of treating disease by varying the pressure or the composition of the air breathed.

aero·ther·a·py (ay''ur o·therr'uh·pee, air''o·) *n.* AEROTHERAPEUTICS.

aero·ther·mo·ther·a·py (air''o·thur''mo·therr'uh·pee, ay''ur·o·) *n.* [*aero-* + *thermo-* + *-therapy*]. Treatment of disease with heated air.

aer·oti·tis (air''o·tye'tis, ay''ur·o·) *n.* [*aer-* + *otitis*]. BAROTITIS.

aerotitis media BAROTITIS MEDIA.

aero·to·nom·e·ter (air''o·to·nom'e·tur, ay''ur·o·) *n.* [*aero-* + *tonometer*]. An instrument for determining the tension of gases in the blood. —**aerotonome·try** (·tree) *n.*

aer·ot·ro·pism (air·ot'ro·piz·um, ay''ur·) *n.* [*aero-* + *tropism*]. 1. The inherent tendency of an aerobic organism to be attracted to a supply of air (positive aerotropism), as when various bacteria and protozoa collect about an air bubble; or (negative aerotropism) to be repelled by a supply of air. 2. *In botany,* the deviation of plant structures, such as roots, from the normal growth patterns because of the presence of air. —**aero·trop·ic** (air''o·trop'ick, ay''ur·o·) *adj.*

aero·tym·pa·nal (air''o·tim'puh·nul, ay''ur·o) *adj.* Pertaining to the air (specifically, that in the external auditory canal) and the tympanum.

aerotympanal conduction. AIR CONDUCTION.

aero·ure·thro·scope (air''o·yoo·ree'thruh·skope) *n.* A modified endoscope which permits viewing the urethra after it is inflated with air. —**aero·ure·thros·co·py** (·yoo''ree·thros'skuh·pee) *n.*

ae·ru·go (ee·roo'go) *n.* [L., from *aes, aeris,* copper]. 1. Rust of a metal. 2. Copper rust; VERDIGRIS.

Aes·cu·la·pi·an (es''kew·lay'pee·un) *adj.* [L. *Aesculapius,* after Gk. *Asklēpios,* Greek god of healing and medicine]. 1. Of or pertaining to the art of healing; medical; medicinal. 2. Specifically, pertaining to the practices of the Aesculapian sect of healers in ancient Greece and Asia Minor.

aesculetin. ESCULETIN.

aesculin. ESCULIN.

aesthesia. ESTHESIA.

aesthesio-. See *esthesio-*.

aesthesiology. ESTHESIOLOGY.

aesthesiometer. ESTHESIOMETER.

aesthesiophysiology. ESTHESIOPHYSIOLOGY.

aesthetic. ESTHETIC.

aestival. ESTIVAL.

aestivation. ESTIVATION.

aestivo-autumnal. ESTIVOAUTUMNAL.

aether. ETHER.

aethereal. ETHEREAL.

aetio-. See *etio-*.
aetiology. ETIOLOGY.
aetiopathogenesis. ETIOPATHOGENESIS.
aetioporphyrin. ETIOPORPHYRIN.
Afaxin. A trademark for oleovitamin A.
afe·brile (ay·feb′ril, ·feeb′) *adj.* [*a-* + *febrile*]. Without fever.
Afenil. Trademark for calcium chloride-urea, $CaCl_2 \cdot 4(NH_2)_2CO$, used intravenously in calcium therapy.
afe·tal, afoe·tal (ay·fee′tul, a·fee′tul) *adj.* Without a fetus.
¹af·fect (af′ekt) *n.* [L. *affectus*, from *afficere*, to influence]. 1. *In psychology*, the emotional aspect or feeling tone of a mental state, sensation, perception, or idea; affection as compared to cognition and conation in any mental process. 2. *In Freudian psychology*, the sum total of the various feelings which may be conscious or suppressed, accompanying or influencing a mental state or idea. 3. Psychic tension as manifested by certain bodily changes, such as perspiration, tachycardia, or blushing. 4. Class name for any emotion, feeling, mood, temperament. 5. A specific feeling or emotion, such as joy or sadness.
²af·fect (uh·fekt′) *v.* 1. To produce an effect upon. 2. To make an impression, as on the mind or emotions.
af·fect·a·bil·i·ty *n.* The capacity for responding to stimulation.
af·fec·tion, *n.* [L. *affectio*, condition, influence]. 1. Any pathologic state or condition. 2. *In psychology*, the emotional factor in consciousness. Contr. *cognition, conation.*
af·fec·tive (a·feck′tiv) *adj.* Pertaining to or involving affect or affection.
affective disorder or **psychosis**. Any major mental disorder which is characterized by episodes of extreme depression or elation, dominating the mental life of the patient and responsible for whatever loss of contact there is with the environment. The swings of mood are not precipitated by external events, and there is a strong hereditary component. Compare *psychotic depressive reaction.* See also *involutional psychosis, manic-depressive illness.*
affective identification. SYMPATHY.
affective insanity or **reaction**. AFFECTIVE DISORDER.
affective personality. CYCLOTHYMIC PERSONALITY.
affective-reaction psychosis. AFFECTIVE DISORDER.
affective sensibilities. VITAL SENSIBILITIES.
af·fec·tiv·i·ty (af″eck·tiv′i·tee) *n.* Susceptibility to emotional stimuli; emotionality.
af·fec·to·mo·tor (a·feck″to·mo′tur) *adj.* [*affect* + *motor*]. Exhibiting emotional disturbance and muscular activity.
af·fer·ent (af′ur·unt) *adj.* [L. *afferens*, from *ad-*, toward, + *ferre*, to carry]. Carrying toward; centripetal. Contr. *efferent.*
afferent anosmia. See *anosmia.*
afferent loop syndrome. Upper abdominal fullness and pain after meals, relieved by bilious vomiting; it is caused by impaired emptying of the proximal loop of a gastrojejunostomy.
afferent lymphatic. A vessel conveying lymph to a lymph node.
afferent motor aphasia. A form of motor aphasia resulting from lesions of the lower part of the postcentral region of the dominant cerebral hemisphere and characterized by a disorder of articulation attributed to disturbance of the kinesthetic (afferent) organization of motor acts.
afferent nerve. A nerve that transmits impulses from the periphery to the central nervous system; a sensory nerve.
afferent neuron. A neuron that conducts impulses to a nerve center; in the peripheral nervous system, that neuron which conducts impulses to nuclei in the central nervous system.
afferent tract or **pathway**. A nerve tract of the spinal cord conveying impulses toward the brain. Syn. *ascending tract.*
afferent veins. The veins that convey blood directly to an organ, as the portal vein.
af·fil·i·a·tion (a·fil″ee·ay′shun) *n.* [from L. *affiliare*, to adopt]. *In legal medicine*, imputing or fixing the paternity of a child.
af·fi·nal (a·figh′nul) *adj.* [L. *affinis*, neighboring, related by marriage]. 1. Connected through marriage. 2. Having the same origin.
af·fin·i·ty, *n.* [from L. *affinitas*, neighborhood, relation by marriage]. 1. An inherent relationship or selective tendency, often mutual, as an attraction, resemblance, kinship, or liking. 2. *In chemistry*, the force of attraction between atoms which causes them to enter into and maintain certain combinations. 3. *In immunology*, the attractive force between antigen and antibody. 4. *In biology*, the relationship between members of different species or more specialized groups which depends upon their resemblance in structure, implying a common origin.
affinity labeling. A method of labeling a molecule or the reactive portion of a molecule (such as the combining site of an antibody or the active site of an enzyme) by attaching a radioactive isotope or other labeling device to another molecule (such as a hapten, antigen, substrate, or cofactor) which has an affinity for that molecule or reactive site and may thus be expected to become bound to it.
af·fir·ma·tion, *n.* During autosuggestion, the stage in which the subject acquires a positive reactive tendency; facilitation of positive reaction tendency.
af·flux (af′lucks) *n.* [L. *affluere, affluxus*, to flow toward]. A sudden flow of blood or other fluid to a part. —**af·flu·ent** (af′lew·unt) *adj.;* **afflu·ence** (·unce) *n.*
af·flux·ion (a·fluck′shun) *n.* AFFLUX.
af·fu·sion (a·few′zhun) *n.* [L. *affundere, affusus*, to pour upon]. Pouring of water upon a part or upon the body, as in fever, to reduce temperature and calm nervous symptoms. Treating fevers by pouring cold water over the patient is called cold affusion.
afi·brin·o·gen·emia, afi·brin·o·gen·ae·mia (ay″figh·brin″o·jen·ee′mee·uh) *n.* [*a-* + *fibrinogen* + *-emia*]. Complete absence of fibrinogen in the blood. Compare *fibrinogenopenia.*
af·la·tox·in (af″luh·tock′sin) *n.* [*A*spergillus *fla*vus + *toxin*]. Any of a group of toxic, carcinogenic substances, chiefly affecting the liver, which are produced by strains of *Aspergillus flavus* and *A. parasiticus* and which may contaminate improperly stored peanuts or other foodstuffs.
Aflorone Acetate. A trademark for fludrocortisone acetate, a synthetic adrenocortical steroid.
afoetal. AFETAL.
African horse sickness. A highly infectious virus disease of horses and mules probably carried by mosquitoes; characterized by fever, systemic signs, and edema.
African lymphoma. BURKITT'S LYMPHOMA.
African tick-borne fever. Any of the tick-borne typhus fevers of Africa.
African trypanosomiasis. Any one of a number of trypanosomal infections of man and of animals occurring in Africa, including Gambian and Rhodesian trypanosomiasis (or sleeping sickness of man) and nagana of cattle. See also *trypanosomiasis.*
Afrin. Trademark for oxymetazoline, used as the hydrochloride salt as a vasoconstrictor to reduce swelling and congestion of the nasal mucosa.
af·ter·birth (af′tur·burth) *n.* The placenta and membranes expelled from the uterus following birth of the child. Syn. *secundines.*
af·ter·brain, *n.* MYELENCEPHALON.
af·ter·care, *n.* 1. Care or nursing of convalescents, especially that of mother and infant after childbirth or the postoperative treatment of surgical patients. 2. *In psychiatry*, the continuation of treatment and the rendering of other rehabilitative services in the community to a patient following a period of hospitalization in order to help him maintain and continue his adjustment.
af·ter·cat·a·ract, *n.* 1. A portion of lens substance or of lens

capsule retained after the extraction of an extracapsular cataract. 2. Any membrane in the area of the pupil following removal or absorption of the lens. See also *secondary cataract.*

af·ter·com·ing head. The head of the fetus in a breech presentation.

af·ter·cur·rent, *n.* An electric current induced in a muscle or nerve immediately following the "spike" potential.

af·ter·damp, *n.* A poisonous mixture of gases, containing principally carbon dioxide and nitrogen, found in coal mines after an explosion of inflammable gases.

af·ter·dis·charge, *n.* The discharge of impulses, as of a ganglion cell or neural circuit after the initial stimulus has ceased.

af·ter·ef·fect, *n.* A delayed response to a stimulus or agent, appearing only after the subsidence of the primary response.

af·ter·hear·ing, *n.* A sensation of hearing a sound after the stimulus which produces it has ceased; may be a symptom of some neuroses.

af·ter·im·age, *n.* A retinal impression that continues after the stimulus of the light or image has ceased to act. See also *negative afterimage, positive afterimage.*

afterimage test. *In ophthalmology,* a measurement of abnormal retinal correspondence in strabismus. The patient looks at a horizontal luminous filament first with the straight eye and then at a vertical one with the squinting eye. If the afterimages cross, correspondence is normal and binocular vision probably can be restored following correction of the strabismus.

af·ter·im·pres·sion, *n.* AFTERSENSATION.

af·ter·life·time, *n.* The duration of life of an insured person after a specified time.

af·ter·nys·tag·mus, *n.* Nystagmus that persists for some time after the stimulus producing optokinetic nystagmus is removed.

af·ter·pains, *n.* Pains from uterine contractions following delivery.

af·ter·per·cep·tion, *n.* Perception of an aftersensation.

af·ter·po·ten·tial, *n.* A small positive or negative wave that follows and is dependent on the main spike potential, seen in the oscillograph tracing of an action potential passing along a nerve.

af·ter·pres·sure, *n.* The sense of pressure that remains for a brief period after the removal of an object from the surface of the body.

af·ter·sen·sa·tion, *n.* A sensation continuing after the stimulus that produced it has ceased.

af·ter·sound, *n.* An auditory aftersensation.

af·ter·stain, *n.* COUNTERSTAIN.

af·ter·taste, *n.* A gustatory sensation continuing for some time after the stimulus provoking immediate taste has been removed.

af·ter·touch, *n.* The sensation that persists for a short time after contact with an object has ceased.

af·ter·treat·ment, *n.* AFTERCARE.

af·ter·vi·sion, *n.* Perception of an afterimage.

afunc·tion·al (ay·funk'shun·ul) *adj.* Without function; unable to function normally; lacking normal function.

afunctional occlusion. A malocclusion that will not allow mastication.

Ag [L. *argentum*]. 1. Symbol for silver. 2. *In immunology,* abbreviation for *antigen.*

AGA *In embryology,* abbreviation for *accelerated growth area.*

aga·lac·tia (ay"ga·lack'shee·uh, ·tee·uh) *n.* [Gk. *agalaktia,* from *gala, galaktos,* milk]. Nonsecretion or imperfect secretion of milk after childbrith. **—agalac·tous** (·tus) *adj.*

agalactia con·ta·gi·o·sa (kon·tay'jee·o·suh). An epidemic, contagious disease of sheep and goats caused by *Mycoplasma agalactiae,* characterized by mammitis, fever, keratoconjunctivitis, and arthritis.

aga·lax·ia (ay"ga·lack'see·uh, ag"uh·) *n.* [Gk. *agalax,* giving no milk, + *-ia*]. AGALACTIA.

aga·laxy (ag"uh·lack'see, ag'uh·lack"see) *n.* AGALACTIA.

ag·a·lor·rhea, ag·a·lor·rhoea (ag"uh·lo·ree'uh, a·gal"o·) *n.* [*a-* + Gk. *gala,* milk, + *-rrhea*]. A cessation of the flow of milk.

agam·ete (ay·gam'eet, ag'a·meet) *n.* [Gk. *agametos,* unmarried]. *In biology,* any unicellular organism which reproduces asexually.

aga·met·ic (ay"ga·met'ick, ag"uh·) *adj.* AGAMIC.

agam·ic (ay·gam'ick) *adj.* [Gk. *agamos,* unmarried, from *gamos,* marriage]. *In biology,* asexual; reproducing without union of sexual cells.

agam·ma·glob·u·li·ne·mia (ay·gam"uh·glob"yoo·li·nee'mee·uh) *n.* [*a-* + *gamma globulin* + *-emia*]. 1. Markedly reduced serum concentration of immunoglobulins. 2. Antibody-deficiency syndromes; specifically, congenital agammaglobulinemia, transient hypogammaglobulinemia, and acquired agammaglobulinemia. **—agammaglobuline·mic** (·mick) *adj.*

aga·mo·cy·tog·o·ny (ay·gam"o·sigh·tog'uh·nee, ag"uh·mo·) *n.* [*a-* + *gamo-* + *cyto-* + *-gony*]. AGAMOGENESIS.

Ag·a·mo·fi·lar·ia (ag"uh·mo·fi·lăr'ee·uh) *n.pl.* [*a-* + *gamo-* + *filaria*]. A group of filarial worms, with unknown stages of development and life cycle, rarely isolated from conjunctivas, eyelids, lips, and peritoneum of man.

aga·mo·gen·e·sis (ay·gam"o·jen'e·sis, ag"uh·mo·) *n.* [*a-* + *gamo-* + *genesis*]. 1. Asexual reproduction. 2. PARTHENOGENESIS. Syn. *agamogony, agamocytogony.* **—agamo·ge·net·ic** (·je·net'ick) *adj.*

aga·mog·o·ny (ag"uh·mog'uh·nee, ay"ga·) *n.* [*a-* + *gamo-* + *-gony*]. AGAMOGENESIS.

aga·mo·sper·my (ay·gam'o·spur"mee, ag'uh·mo·) *n.* [*a-* + *gamo-* + *sperm-* + *-y*]. Asexual seed production, a form of apomixis.

aga·mo·spore (ay·gam'o·spore, ag'uh·mo·) *n.* [*a-* + *gamo-* + *spore*]. *In biology,* an asexually produced spore.

aga·mous (ag'uh·mus) *adj.* [Gk. *agamos,* unmarried]. AGAMIC.

agan·gli·on·ic (ay·gang"glee·on'ick) *adj.* Having no ganglions; referring especially to the absence of the myenteric plexus cells of the colon.

aganglionic megacolon. HIRSCHSPRUNG'S DISEASE.

agan·gli·on·o·sis (ay·gang"glee·un·o'sis) *n.* 1. Absence of ganglion cells. 2. Congenital absence of the myenteric plexus ganglion cells seen in Hirschsprung's disease.

agar (ay'gahr, ag'ahr, ah'gahr) *n.* [Malay]. A solidifying agent consisting of a complex carbohydrate extracted from certain marine algae, as of the genus *Gelideum,* widely used as a base for bacteriologic media, as a hydrophilic colloid laxative, as a suspending agent, and as the basic ingredient of reversible hydrocolloid dental impression materials. See also *agarose.*

agar-agar, *n.* AGAR.

agar hanging block. *In bacteriology,* a small block of nutrient agar cut from a poured plate and placed on a cover glass, the surface next to the glass first having been touched with a loop from a young fluid culture or with a dilution from the same. It is examined upside down, the same as a hanging-drop culture.

agar·ic (a·găr'ick, ag'ur·ick) *n.* [Gk. *agarikon*]. 1. A fungus of the genus *Agaricus.* 2. The dried fruit body of the fungus *Polyporus officinalis,* formerly used for its anhidrotic action.

Agar·i·cus (a·gar'i·kus) *n.* A large genus of fungi.

Agaricus cam·pes·tris (kam·pes'tris). The common, nonpoisonous or edible mushroom.

agar plaque. A plug of agar, previously inoculated with an antibiotic producer, removed under sterile conditions, after incubation, and placed on an agar plate seeded with the test organisms, in order to measure the zone of inhibition which develops around the agar plug after further incubation.

agar plate. PLATE (3).

ag·a·rose (ag'uh·roce, ·roze) *n.* A polysaccharide obtained from agar used as a supporting medium for column chromatography and gel electrophoresis.

agar spot. A drop of seeded nutrient agar in a sterile Petri dish, used for the quantitative determination of antibiotic activity by subculturing in the presence of successive increments of antibiotics.

agar streak plate. Any agar plate on which microorganisms are streaked out for such determinations as purity or variation.

agar streak slant. Agar slanted in a test tube, on which bacteria are streaked.

agar wells. The holes made in seeded agar into which antibiotics may be introduced to determine the extent of the inhibition (of microorganisms) which results from the diffusion of the antibiotic from the well into the surrounding agar in the course of subsequent incubation.

agas·tric (ay·gas'trick, a·gas') *adj.* [*a-* + *gastric*]. Without an alimentary canal, as the tapeworms. **—agas·tria** (·tree·uh) *n.*

Aga·ve (a·gay'vee, a·gah'vee) *n.* [Gk. *agauos,* noble, brilliant]. A large genus of the family Amaryllidaceae, native North American plants.

Agave amer·i·ca·na (a·merr''i·kay'nuh, ·kan'uh). American aloe; the leaves of this plant have been used as a diuretic, antisyphilitic, and antiscorbutic.

-age. A suffix meaning (a) *cumulative result;* (b) *rate;* (c) *action or process.*

âge cri·tique (ahzh kree·teek) [F., lit., critical age]. CLIMACTERIC.

age·ne·sia (ay''je·nee'zhuh, ·zee·uh) *n.* AGENESIS.

agen·e·sis (ay·jen'e·sis) *n.* [*a-* + *genesis*]. 1. Lack of complete and normal development. 2. Congenital absence of an organ or part. 3. *Erron.* AGENNESIS.

age·nio·ce·pha·lia (ay·jee''nee·o·sef·ay'lee·uh, a·jen''ee·o·) *n.* [*a-* + *genio-* + *-cephalia*]. A minor degree of otocephalus, with the brain, cranial vault, and sense organs intact. **—agenio·ceph·a·lus** (·sef'uh·lus) *n.*

age·nio·ceph·a·ly (ay·jee''nee·o·sef'uh·lee, a·jen''ee·o·) *n.* AGENIOCEPHALIA.

agen·i·tal·ism (ay·jen'i·tul·iz·um) *n.* [*a-* + *genital* + *-ism*]. A symptom complex due to a deficiency of sex hormones, found in persons who lack testes or ovaries.

agen·ne·sis (aj''e·nee'sis, ay''je·) *n.* [*a-* + Gk. *gennēsis,* production, begetting]. Inability in a male to procreate, as through impotence or sterility.

agen·o·so·mia (ay·jen''o·so'mee·uh, a·jen'') *n.* [*a-* + *geno-* + *-somia*]. Defective development of the genitals.

agen·o·so·mus (ay·jen''o·so'mus, a·jen'') *n.* [*a-* + *geno-* + *-somus*]. A fetal monster with extrusion of the lower abdominal viscera because of a deficiency of the abdominal wall (celosoma); the genitalia are lacking or rudimentary.

agent, *n.* [L. *agens, agentis,* acting, active, from *agere,* to do, to act]. A substance or force which, by its action, effects changes.

age of consent. *In legal medicine,* the age at which a minor is considered capable of legally assenting to sexual intercourse or to marriage, varying from 13 years upward according to statute.

age·ra·sia (aj''e·ray'zee·uh) *n.* [Gk., eternal youth, from *a-* + *gēras,* old age, + *-ia*]. Vigorous, healthy old age.

ageu·sia (a·gew'zee·uh, ay·joo') *n.* [*a-* + *-geusia*]. Loss or impairment of the sense of taste. See also *central, conduction,* and *peripheral ageusia.* **—ageu·sic** (a·gew'zick) *adj.*

ageusic aphasia. Impairment in the ability to express in words thoughts related to the sense of taste.

ageus·tia (a·gew'stee·uh, a·joo') *n.* [Gk., fasting]. AGEUSIA.

ag·ger (ag'ur, aj'ur) *n.* [L., mound]. *In anatomy,* a projection, eminence, or mound.

agger na·si (nay'zigh) [NA]. An oblique ridge on the inner surface of the nasal process of the maxilla; the anterior part of the ethmoid crest.

ag·glom·er·ate (a·glom'ur·ut) *adj.* [L. *agglomeratus,* wound or clumped into a ball, from *glomus,* ball of thread]. Grouped or clustered into a mass. **—ag·glom·er·a·tion** (a·glom''ur·ay'shun) *n.*

ag·glu·ti·nate (a·gloo'ti·nate) *v.* [L. *agglutinare,* to glue, fasten, from *ad-* + *gluten,* glue]. 1. To fuse, cohere, adhere. 2. Of suspended particles or corpuscles: to aggregate, form clumps. 3. To cause to aggregate or form clumps. **—agglu·ti·na·tive** (·nuh·tiv) *adj.;* **aggluti·na·ble** (nuh·bul) *adj.;* **ag·glu·ti·na·tion** (a·gloo''ti·nay'shun) *n.*

agglutination of the vulva. VULVAR FUSION.

agglutination reaction. The clumping of particulate antigens, such as bacteria, erythrocytes, or yeasts, by antibody.

agglutination test. 1. A test in which an agglomeration or clumping of particles produces masses which may be seen either with the unaided eye or with the aid of a microscope. The test may be used for the identification of bacteria. 2. A test for the presence of specific antibodies in the blood serum of infected individuals which will produce clumping of the specific bacteria causing the infection.

ag·glu·ti·nin (a·gloo'ti·nin) *n.* [*agglutin*ate + *-in*]. An antibody occurring in a normal or immune serum which, when added to a suspension of its homologous, particulate antigen, causes the antigen elements to adhere to one another, forming clumps.

ag·glu·ti·no·gen (ag''lew·tin'o·jen, a·gloo'tin·o·jen) *n.* An antigen which, when injected into the animal body, stimulates the formation of a specific agglutinin. This, in turn, has the capacity to agglutinate the antigen.

ag·glu·ti·noid (a·gloo'ti·noid) *n. Obsol.* An agglutinin which can combine with its antigen but which has lost the ability to cause agglutination, thus becoming an incomplete antibody.

ag·glu·ti·no·phore (a·gloo'ti·no·fore) *n.* [*agglutin*in + *-phore*]. The factor present in an agglutinin which causes clumping; the antigen reactive site of the agglutinin.

ag·glu·ti·no·scope (ag''lew·tin'o·skope, a·gloo'ti·no·skope) *n.* An instrument used to observe the process of agglutination in a test tube and to facilitate the reading of the result.

[1]ag·gre·gate (ag're·gut) *adj. & n.* [L. *aggregatus,* from *aggregare,* to add to]. 1. Clumped, forming a group. 2. A clump, as the mass formed by certain antibodies and their homologous antigens.

[2]ag·gre·gate (ag're·gate) *v.* [L. *aggregare,* from *ad-* + *grex, gregis,* flock, crowd]. To gather into a mass; to clump.

aggregate follicles. An aggregation of lymph nodules situated in the mucous membrane of the lower part of the small intestine, opposite the mesenteric attachment. Syn. *Peyer's patches.* NA *folliculi lymphatici aggregati intestini tenuis.*

aggregate glands. AGGREGATE NODULES.

aggregate nodules. Groups of lymph nodules massed together in the wall of an organ, as in the mucosa of the small intestine. See also *aggregate follicles.*

ag·gre·ga·tion, *n.* Agmination; a massing together of materials; a congeries or collection of particles, parts, or bodies, usually of a similar nature.

ag·gres·sin (a·gres'in) *n.* A hypothetical soluble substance of bacterial origin which promotes infection by inhibiting host defenses.

ag·gres·sion, *n.* 1. *In psychiatry,* an act or attitude of hostility, commonly arising out of frustration or feelings of inferiority. See also *aggressive personality.* 2. *In psychoanalysis,* an innate, independent, instinctual disposition in man; it may be self- or outwardly destructive, may revert to the opposite, or may, when sublimated, serve to foster constructive, self-protective forms of adaptation and progressive self-assertion. **—ag·gres·sive,** *adj.*

aggressive behavior disorder. MINIMAL BRAIN DYSFUNCTION SYNDROME.

aggressive personality. An individual whose behavioral pattern is characterized by irritability, temper tantrums, and destructive attitudes and acts as dominant manifestations of frustration. Compare *passive-aggressive personality.*

aging-lung emphysema. Loss of elasticity of pulmonary tissue with alveolar dilatation seen with aging; an asymptomatic condition. See also *senile emphysema.*

aging pigment. LIPOFUSCIN.

agit. Abbreviation for L. *agita,* shake.

ag·i·tat·ed dementia. Dementia distinguished by great excitement, motor activity, and often continuous hallucinations.

agitated depression. A type of manic-depressive illness or involutional melancholia; characterized by marked restlessness, continual activity, despondency, and anxiety.

agitated paresis. General paresis characterized by sudden violent and destructive excitement.

agi·ta·tor cau·dae (aj·i·tay'tor kaw'dee) [L., wagger of the tail]. An occasional additional slip of the gluteus maximus muscle arising from the coccyx.

ag·i·to·graph·ia (aj''i·to·graf'ee·uh) *n.* [L. *agit*are, to drive, move hastily, + *-graphia*]. A condition characterized by excessive speed in writing, with unconscious omissions of letters, syllables, or words.

ag·i·to·la·lia (aj''i·to·lay'lee·uh) *n.* [L. *agit*are, to drive, move hastily, + *-lalia*]. AGITOPHASIA.

ag·i·to·pha·sia (aj''i·to·fay'zhuh, ·zee·uh) *n.* [L. *agit*are, to drive, move hastily, + *-phasia*]. A condition marked by excessive rapidity of speech, with sounds, syllables, or words unconsciously slurred, omitted, or distorted.

Ag·kis·tro·don (ag·kis'tro·don, ang·) *n.* [Gk. *ankistr*on, fish-hook, + *odōn,* tooth]. A genus of the Crotalidae.

Agkistrodon con·tor·trix (kon·tor'tricks). COPPERHEAD.

Agkistrodon pis·civ·o·rus (pi·siv'uh·rus). COTTONMOUTH MOCCASIN.

aglan·du·lar (ay·glan'dew·lur) *adj.* Having no glands; without glands.

ag·lia (ag'lee·uh) *n.* [Gk. *agliē,* incorrect form for *aigis,* speck in the eye]. A speck or spot upon the cornea or the sclera.

aglo·mer·u·lar (ay''glom·err'yoo·lur, ag''lom·) *adj.* Without glomeruli.

aglomerular kidney. 1. *In clinical medicine,* a kidney having a greatly diminished number of functioning glomeruli, found in congenital conditions such as aplasia of the kidney or in acquired conditions characterized by loss of glomeruli through progressive scarring. 2. A type of kidney normally found in some fishes in which glomeruli are entirely lacking; used in the study of renal physiology.

aglos·sia (ay·glos'ee·uh, a·glos') *n.* [*a-* + *-glossia*]. 1. Congenital absence of the tongue. 2. Loss of the ability to speak; mutism.

aglos·so·sto·mia (ay·glos''o·sto'mee·uh, a·glos'') *n.* [*a-* + *glosso-* + *-stomia*]. A condition in a monster in which the tongue is lacking and the mouth is imperforate.

aglos·sus (ay·glos'us, a·glos'us) *n.* [NL., from *a-* + Gk. *glōssa,* tongue]. An individual without a tongue.

aglu·cone (ay·gloo'kone, a·gloo') *n.* [*a-* + *gluc-* + *-one*]. 1. AGLYCONE. 2. The nonsugar portion of a glucoside.

ag·lu·ti·tion (ag''lew·tish'un) *n.* [*a-* + L. *glutire,* to swallow]. DYSPHAGIA.

agly·ce·mia, agly·cae·mia (ay''glye·see'mee·uh, ag''lye·) *n.* [*a-* + *glyc-* + *-emia*]. Absence of sugar in the blood.

agly·ce·mic, agly·cae·mic (ay''glye·see'mick, ag''lye·) *adj.* Having no sugar in the blood.

agly·cone (ay·glye'kone, a·glye'kone) *n.* [*a-* + *glyc-* + *-one*]. The nonsugar portion of a glycoside.

agly·cos·uria (ay·glye''ko·sue'ree·uh, a·glye'') *n.* [*a-* + *glycosuria*]. Absence of sugar in the urine.

agly·cos·uric (ay·glye''ko·sue'rick, a·glye''ko·) *adj.* Free from glycosuria; exhibiting no urinary sugar.

Ag·ly·pha (ag'li·fuh) *n.pl.* [Gk. *aglyphos,* uncarved, ungrooved]. A subdivision of the Colubridae family of snakes, distinguished from venomous varieties by the absence of grooved rear fangs. Contr. *Opisthoglypha, Proteroglypha, Solenoglypha.*

ag·ma·tine (ag'muh·teen, ·tin) *n.* Aminobutyl guanidine, $C_5H_{14}N_4$, an amine isolated from ergot and from herring spawn.

ag·mi·nate (ag'mi·nate) *adj.* [L. *agmen, agminis,* troop, swarm]. AGMINATED.

ag·mi·nat·ed (ag'mi·nay·tid) *adj.* Gathered into clumps or clusters; aggregate. —**ag·mi·na·tion** (ag''mi·nay'shun) *n.*

agminated nodules. AGGREGATE FOLLICLES.

ag·na·thia (ag·nayth'ee·uh) *n.* [*a-* + *gnath-* + *-ia*]. Absence or deficient development of the jaws. —**ag·na·thous** (ag'nuth·us) *adj.*

ag·na·tho·ceph·a·lus (ag·nay''tho·sef'uh·lus, ag''nuth·o·) *n.,* pl. **agnathocepha·li** (·lye) [*a-* + *gnatho-* + *-cephalus*]. A type of otocephalus in which the eyes are situated low on the face with approximation or fusion of the zygomas. —**agna·tho·ce·pha·lia** (·se·fay'lee·uh), **agnathoceph·aly** (·uh·lee) *n.*

ag·na·thus (ag'nuth·us, ag·nayth'us) *n.* An individual exhibiting agnathia.

ag·na·thy (ag'nuth·ee) *n.* AGNATHIA.

ag·nea, ag·noea (ag·nee'uh) *n.* [Gk. *agnoia,* lack of perception]. AGNOSIA.

ag·no·gen·ic (ag''no·jen'ick) *adj.* [Gk. *agnōtos,* unknown, + *-genic*]. Of unknown etiology. See also *cryptogenic.*

agnogenic myeloid metaplasia. Extramedullary hemopoiesis of unknown cause, characterized by hepatosplenomegaly and immature but not anaplastic cells in the peripheral blood.

ag·no·sia (ag·no'see·uh) *n.* [Gk. *agnōsia,* ignorance]. Loss or impairment of the ability to recognize features of the external world, as shapes, symbols, geometric relations, directions, or sounds, caused by lesion of the dominant cerebral hemisphere but not by any lesion affecting primary sensation or general intellectual function; in contrast to amorphosynthesis, agnosia affects equally the interpretation of stimuli received on either side of the body. Usually classified according to the sense or senses involved.

ag·nos·te·rol (ag·nos'te·rol, ·role) *n.* [L. *agnus,* lamb, + *sterol*]. A complex terpene alcohol, $C_{30}H_{47}OH$, found in wool fat. Formerly considered to be a sterol but now shown not to possess the structure characteristic of this group of compounds. See also *isocholesterol.*

ag·nos·tic (ag·nos'tick) *adj.* [Gk. *agnōst*os, unknown, unknowing, + *-ic*]. Pertaining to or characterized by agnosia.

agnostic alexia. Alexia caused by loss of the ability to recognize characters or their combinations. Compare *aphasic alexia.*

-agogue, -agog [Gk. *agōgos,* drawing forth, eliciting]. A combining form designating *a substance* (as a drug or other agent) *that induces or promotes secretion or expulsion.*

ag·om·phi·a·sis (ag''om·figh'uh·sis) *n.* [*a-* + Gk. *gomph*ios, molar, tooth, + *-iasis*]. 1. Looseness of the teeth. 2. Absence of teeth.

agom·phi·ous (a·gom'fee·us) *adj.* [Gk. *agomphios,* from *a-* + *gomphios,* molar, tooth]. Toothless.

ag·om·pho·sis (ag''om·fo'sis) *n.* [*a-* + *gomphosis*]. AGOMPHIASIS.

ago·nad·ism (ay·go'nad·iz·um) *n.* [*a-* + *gonad* + *-ism*]. Absence of the ovaries or testes, or their functions, and the resulting physiologic changes; it may be congenital or acquired. Compare *eunuchoidism.*

ag·o·nal (ag'uh·nul) *adj.* [*agony* + *-al*]. Pertaining to the period immediately preceding death; usually a matter of minutes but occasionally indicating a period of several hours.

agonal intussusception. Single or multiple areas of intussusception without clinical or pathological evidence of destruction or inflammation, sometimes found in the small intestine at the time of death.

ag·o·nist (ag'uh·nist) *n.* [Gk. *agōnistēs,* combatant, competitor, from *agōn,* contest]. 1. A contracting muscle engaged in the movement of a part and opposed by an antagonistic muscle. Syn. *protagonist.* 2. A substance capable of combining with an appropriate cellular receptor and producing a typical response for that particular substance.

ag·o·ny (ag'uh·nee) *n.* [L. *agonia,* from Gk. *agōnia,* struggle, anguish, from *agōn,* contest]. 1. Violent pain; extreme anguish, distress of mind. 2. The death struggle.

ag·o·ra·pho·bia (ag"o·ruh·fo'bee·uh) *n.* [Gk. *agora,* marketplace, forum, + *-phobia*]. Morbid fear of open places or spaces. Contr. *claustrophobia.*

-agra [Gk. *agra,* catch]. A combining form meaning *a seizure of pain.*

agram·ma·pha·sia (ay·gram"uh·fay'zhuh, a·gram") *n.* [*agrammatism* + *aphasia*]. AGRAMMATISM.

agram·ma·tism (ay·gram'uh·tiz·um, a·gram') *n.* A type of aphasia in which the patient is unable to frame a grammatical sentence, and though able to utter words, uses them without relation to their proper sequence or inflection.

agran·u·lar (ay·gran'yoo·lur) *adj.* Not granular; without granules.

agranular cortex. Cortex of the cerebrum which lacks a definite fourth cell layer, typical of areas in the frontal lobe.

agran·u·lo·cyte (ay·gran'yoo·lo·site, a·gran') *n.* A nongranular leukocyte. —**agran·u·lo·cyt·ic** (ay·gran"yoo·lo·sit'ick, a·gran") *adj.*

agran·u·lo·cy·the·mia, agran·u·lo·cy·thae·mia (a·gran"yoo·lo·sigh·theem'ee·uh, ay·gran") *n.* [*a-* + *granulocyte* + *-hemia*]. AGRANULOCYTOSIS (2).

agranulocytic angina. AGRANULOCYTOSIS (2).

agran·u·lo·cy·to·sis (a·gran"yoo·lo·sigh·to'sis, ay·gran") *n.* [*a-* + *granulocyte* + *-osis*]. 1. A decrease in the number of granulocytic leukocytes in the peripheral blood. 2. An acute febrile syndrome accompanied by fever, mucous membrane ulcers, and a decrease in granulocytes in the peripheral blood, often related to drug administration.

agran·u·lo·plas·tic (a·gran"yoo·lo·plas'tick, ay·gran") *adj.* [*a-* + *granuloplastic*]. 1. Not forming granular cells. 2. Forming nongranular cells only.

agran·u·lo·sis (a·gran"yoo·lo'sis, ay·gran") *n.* AGRANULOCYTOSIS (2).

agraph·es·the·sia (a·graf"es·theezh'uh, ay·) *n.* [*a-* + *graphesthesia*]. GRAPHANESTHESIA.

agraph·ia (ay·graf'ee·uh, a·graf') *n.* [*a-* + *-graphia*]. Loss of ability to write as a manifestation of aphasia.

A/G ratio. Abbreviation for *albumin-globulin ratio.*

agria. Feminine of *agrius.*

ag·ri·mo·ny (ag'ri·mo"nee) *n.* [L. *agrimonia,* from Gk. *argemōnē,* a kind of poppy]. Specifically, the root of *Agrimonia eupatoria,* a mild astringent.

ag·ri·us (ag'ree·us, ay'gree·us) *adj.,* fem. **ag·ria** (·ree·uh) [NL., from Gk. *agrios,* wild, harsh]. Severe; said of skin eruptions marked by enduring acute signs and symptoms.

Ag·ro·bac·te·ri·um (ag"ro·back·teer'ee·um) *n.* [Gk. *agros,* field, + *bacterium*]. A genus of gram-negative motile rods of the family Rhizobiaceae, principally found in the soil and on plant roots and stems, of which several species are pathogenic for plants. Includes the species *Agrobacterium tumefaciens.*

Agrobacterium tu·me·fa·ci·ens (tew"me·fay'shee·enz) [L., causing to swell]. A species of bacteria which causes crown gall, a cancerlike growth in plants, thus providing a model for research on mammalian cancer.

ag·ro·ma·nia (ag"ro·may'nee·uh) *n.* [Gk. *agros,* field, + *mania*]. An abnormal desire to live in the open country or in isolation.

agryp·net·ic (ag"rip·net'ick, ay"grip·) *adj.* [Gk. *agrypnētikos*]. AGRYPNOTIC.

agryp·nia (a·grip'nee·uh, ay·grip') *n.* [Gk., from *agrypnos,* sleepless, from *agrein,* to hunt, chase, + *hypnos,* sleep]. *Obsol.* INSOMNIA.

agryp·node (a·grip'node) *n.* [Gk. *agrypnōdēs,* making sleepless, from *agrypnos,* sleepless]. A pharmacologic agent or stimulus which induces wakefulness.

agryp·not·ic (ag"rip·not'ick, ay"grip·) *adj. & n.* [*agrypnia* + *-otic* as in hypnotic]. 1. Inducing, pertaining to, or characterized by insomnia. 2. AGRYPNODE.

agua·miel (ah"gwa·myel') *n.* [Sp., lit., honey water]. The sap of *Agave atrovirens* and *A. mexicana,* from which pulque, the fermented drink, is made. It is said to have diuretic, laxative, galactagogue, and nutrient properties.

ague (ay'gyoo) *n.* [OF., from L. *(febris) acuta,* acute (fever)]. 1. An attack of chills and fever; especially, a chill. 2. Specifically, an attack of malaria.

ague cake spleen. The enlarged spleen of chronic malaria.

ag·y·io·pho·bia (aj"ee·o·fo'bee·uh) *n.* [Gk. *agyia,* street, + *-phobia*]. Morbid fear of streets, as fear of crossing the street.

agy·ria (ay·jye'ree·uh, a·jye') *n.* [*a-* + *gyr-* + *-ia*]. Congenital absence of cerebral convolutions.

ah Symbol for hyperopic astigmatism.

A.H.A. 1. American Heart Association. 2. American Hospital Association.

AHF Abbreviation for *antihemophilic factor* (= FACTOR VIII).

AHG Abbreviation for *antihemophilic globulin* (= FACTOR VIII).

Ahu·ma·da–Del Cas·ti·llo syndrome (ah·oo·mah'tha, del·kas·tee'yo) [J. C. *Ahumada,* Argentinian, 20th century; and E. B. *Del Castillo*]. Galactorrhea and secondary amenorrhea unrelated to the termination of pregnancy.

aich·mo·pho·bia (ike"mo·fo'bee·uh) *n.* [Gk. *aichmē,* spear point, + *-phobia*]. Morbid dread of sharp or pointed objects, or of being touched by them or by a finger.

aidoio-. See *ede-.*

ail·ing, *adj.* Indisposed; in ill health; not well.

ail·ment, *n.* A disease; sickness; complaint; bodily infirmity.

ai·lu·ro·phil·ia (ay·lew"ro·fil'ee·uh, eye·lew"ro·) *n.* [Gk. *ailouros,* cat, + *-philia*]. GALEOPHILIA.

ai·lu·ro·pho·bia (ay·lew"ro·fo'bee·uh, eye·lew"ro·) *n.* [Gk. *ailouros,* cat, + *-phobia*]. GALEOPHOBIA.

A_2 influenza virus. ASIAN INFLUENZA VIRUS.

ai·nhum (eye·nyoon', eye'nyum) *n.* [Pg., from Yoruba *ayun*]. A tropical disease of unknown etiology, most common in blacks, in which a toe is slowly and spontaneously amputated by a fibrous ring.

air, *n.* 1. The mixture of gases that constitutes the earth's atmosphere, consisting of approximately 4 volumes of nitrogen and 1 volume of oxygen, with small amounts of carbon dioxide, ammonia, nitrates, organic matter, and the rare gases argon, neon, krypton, and xenon. By virtue of its oxygen content it is able to sustain respiration in aerobic organisms. The density of air at 0°C and standard sea-level pressure is roughly 1 kg/m^3. 2. *Obsol.* Any gas.

air bath. The therapeutic exposure of the naked body to air, usually warm or moist air.

air bed. A bed with an inflatable rubber mattress. Compare *alternating pressure pad.*

air-blast injury. ATMOSPHERIC BLAST INJURY.

air block. An air leak from the lung alveoli into the pulmonary connective tissue and mediastinum, which obstructs the normal inflow and outflow of air and obstructs pulmonary blood flow.

air-borne infection. The transfer of infection from one individual to another without direct contact between them by means of droplets of moisture containing the causative agent. Syn. *droplet infection.*

air·bra·sive (air·bray'siv) *adj.* [*air* + *abrasive*]. Pertaining to the technique of cutting tooth structure or of removing stain and calculus from tooth surfaces by use of a stream of abrasive powder, such as aluminum oxide or calcium magnesium carbonate, propelled at high speed through a fine nozzle by a compressed gas, such as carbon dioxide.

air cell. 1. Any anatomical compartment or cavity, often part of a partitioned larger space, which is filled with air, such as a pulmonary alveolus, a mastoid cell, or an ethmoid air cell. 2. PARANASAL SINUS. 3. (of the auditory tube:) See *cellulae pneumaticae tubae auditivae.*

air chamber. RELIEF CHAMBER.

air concussion. Aerial compression generated at the moment of detonation of a high explosive.

air conditioning. The process of modifying air by the control of its temperature and humidity and the removal of particulate matter.

air conduction. Transmission of sound vibrations to the eardrum through the external auditory canal. Abbreviated, A.C. Contr. *bone conduction.*

air conduction audiometry. Quantitative evaluation of hearing by introducing the stimulus through the air column in the external auditory canal.

air conduction hearing aid. An electronic hearing aid, the transmitter of which fits into the external auditory canal.

air conduction test. A test for hearing utilizing the transmission of sound through air.

air-contrast examination. A roentgenologic technique for coating the mucosa of a hollow viscus with a positive contrast agent (usually barium) and also distending it with gas (usually air). Syn. *double contrast examination.*

air cyst. A cyst containing air, seen especially in emphysema.

air cystometer. A device used to determine intravesical pressures and volumes while the urinary bladder is gradually filled with air or CO_2. —**air cystometry.**

air cystometrogram. A graphic recording of intravesical pressures and volumes used in air cystometry.

air dose. The roentgen dose measured at a point in air without scattering material.

air embolism. Air producing an obstruction in the heart or vascular system, usually resulting from surgery or trauma. Compare *aeroembolism.*

air-fluid level. A gas-fluid interface demonstrable by an x-ray beam parallel to it.

air hunger. The deep gasping respiration characteristic of severe diabetic acidosis and coma. Syn. *Kussmaul's respiration.*

air myelography. Radiographic examination of the spinal cord after injecting air into the subarachnoid space.

air passage. RESPIRATORY PASSAGE.

air pilots' disease. AERONEUROSIS.

airplane splint. A special type of splint that holds the arm in abduction with the forearm midway in flexion; generally of wire with an axillary strut and frequently incorporated in a plaster body support.

air pump. A pump used to exhaust the air from a chamber, or to force more air into a chamber already containing air.

air sac. A pulmonary alveolus; ALVEOLUS (2).

air sac disease. A severe inflammation of the pulmonary alveoli of poultry caused by *Mycoplasma gallisepticum* and complicated with coliform infection.

air·sick·ness, *n.* Motion sickness in aircraft flights.

air sinus. A cavity containing air within a bone; especially, a paranasal sinus.

air space. The space in tissues filled with air or other gases.

air swallowing. AEROPHAGIA.

air thermometer. A thermometer in which the expansive substance is air.

air tube. BRONCHUS.

air·way, *n.* 1. Any of several devices used to maintain a clear and unobstructed respiratory passage during general anesthesia. 2. RESPIRATORY PASSAGE.

aj·mal·i·cine (aj·mal'i·seen, ·sin) *n.* [after *Ajm*er, India, + *al*kaloid]. An alkaloid, $C_{21}H_{24}N_2O_3$, from *Rauwolfia serpentina.*

aj·ma·line (aj'muh·leen, ·lin) *n.* [after *Ajm*er, India, + *al*kaloid]. An alkaloid, $C_{20}H_{26}N_2O_2$, from *Rauwolfia serpentina;* rauwolfine.

aj·o·wan oil (aj'o·wahn). A volatile oil from the fruit of *Trachyspermum ammi;* contains thymol.

AK Above the knee; used to describe such an amputation in the leg. Contr. *BK.*

akanthesthesia, akanthaesthesia. ACANTHESTHESIA.

akanthion. ACANTHION.

akar·yo·cyte (ay·kăr'ee·o·site, a·kăr') *n.* [*a-* + *karyo-* + *-cyte*]. ERYTHROCYTE.

akar·y·o·ta (a·kăr''ee·o'tuh) *n.* AKARYOTE.

akar·y·ote (ay·kăr'ee·ote, a·kăr') *n.* & *adj.* [*a-* + Gk. *karyōtos,* nutlike]. 1. A nonnucleated cell. 2. NONNUCLEATED.

ak·a·this·ia, ac·a·this·ia (ack''uh·thiz'ee·uh) *n.* [*a-* + Gk. *kathisis,* sitting, + *-ia*]. 1. A condition in which one is compelled to change body positions frequently or to rise and pace the floor; the result of chronic ingestion of phenothiazine drugs. See also *tardive dyskinesia.* 2. *In psychiatry,* inability to sit down; intense anxiety about sitting.

ak·ee poisoning (ack''ee, a·kee') [Kru]. Acute, sometimes fatal, poisoning caused by eating the seeds or uncooked arils of the akee tree (*Blighia sapida* Koenig) found in tropical Africa and introduced in tropical America by slave traders.

aker·a·to·sis (a·kerr''uh·to'sis) *n.* [*a-* + *kerat-* + *-osis*]. A deficiency or absence of horny tissue, as of the nails.

akinaesthesia. AKINESTHESIA.

ak·i·ne·sia (ack''i·nee'zhuh, ·zee·uh) *n.* [Gk. *akinēsia,* from *kinēsis,* motion]. 1. Slowness of movement and underactivity (poverty of movement); characteristic of Parkinson's disease. 2. Any condition involving or characterized by immobility.

akinesia al·ge·ra (al'je·ruh, al·jeer'uh) [NL., from Gk. *algēros,* painful]. A form of hysteria characterized by painfulness associated with any kind of movements.

akinesia am·nes·ti·ca (am·nes'ti·kuh). Immobility from disuse of the muscles.

akinesia iri·dis (eye'ri·dis). Rigidity or immobility of the iris.

aki·ne·sic (ack''i·nee'zick, ·sick) *adj.* AKINETIC.

ak·i·ne·sis (ack''i·nee'sis) *n.* Immobility; AKINESIA.

akin·es·the·sia, akin·aes·the·sia (ay·kin''es·theezh'uh, ·theez'ee·uh, a·kin'') *n.* [*a-* + *kinesthesia*]. Loss of perception of position and movement; loss of deep sensation or muscle sense.

aki·net·ic (ack''i·net'ick, ay''ki·) *adj.* [*a-* + *kinetic*]. 1. Characterized by or affected with akinesia. 2. AMITOTIC.

akinetic epilepsy. A form of epilepsy characterized by akinetic seizures.

akinetic mutism. 1. A state in which the appearance of the patient, particularly that of the eyes, suggests consciousness, but in which the patient is in fact unconscious. 2. Any state in which the patient is conscious and alert but makes no voluntary movement; especially, PSEUDOCOMA. See also *abulia.*

akinetic seizure. An epileptic seizure marked by sudden loss of consciousness and motor power resulting in head nodding, body slumping, and often, a violent fall. The seizure is usually brief, and there may be no postictal confusion, stupor, or sleep.

Akineton. Trademark for biperiden, an antiparkinsonian drug.

Akis spi·no·sa (ay'kis spye·no'suh, ack'is). A beetle belonging to the family Tenebrionidae; an intermediate host for the cysticercoid of *Hymenolepis diminuta.*

ak·lo·mide (ack'lo·mide) *n.* 2-Chloro-4-nitrobenzamide, $C_7H_5ClN_2O_3$, a coccidiostatic drug.

ak·o·asm (ack'o·az·um) *n.* ACOUSMA.

akoria. ACORIA.

Akrinol. Trademark for acrisorcin.

Aku·rey·ri disease (ah'ku^e·ray·ri^h) [after *Akureyri,* a town in Iceland]. BENIGN MYALGIC ENCEPHALOMYELITIS.

Al Symbol for aluminum.

¹-al [L. *-alis*]. An adjective-forming suffix signifying *of or pertaining to; having the character of; appropriate to.*

²-al [*al*dehyde]. A suffix indicating *the presence of the aldehyde group.*

ala (ay'luh) *n.*, pl. & genit. sing. **alae** (ay'lee) [L.]. 1. A wing. 2. Any winglike process. 3. AXILLA.

ala au·ris (aw'ris). The auricle of the external ear.

al·a·bas·ter (al'uh·bas''tur) *n.* [L.]. A relatively hard, fine-grained form of gypsum or of calcite. —**al·a·bas·trine** (al''uh·bas'treen) *adj.*

ala ce·re·bel·li (serr·e·bel'eye). ALA LOBULI CENTRALIS.

ala ci·ne·rea (si·neer'ee·uh) [L., ashen, ash-gray] [BNA]. The trigone of the vagus nerve: the area in the floor of the fourth ventricle overlying the dorsal motor nucleus of the vagus nerve. Syn. *trigonum nervi vagi [NA], trigonum vagi, vagal triangle.*

ala cris·tae gal·li (kris'tee gal'eye) [NA]. ALAR PROCESS.

alae. Plural and genitive singular of *ala.*

ala eth·moi·da·lis (eth·moy·day'lis). ALAR PROCESS.

ala ilii (il'ee·eye). ALA OSSIS ILII.

ala la·te·ra·lis (lat·ur·ay'lis). 1. Either of the great wings of the sphenoid bone. 2. Either of the winglike lateral extensions of the frontal bone.

ala·lia (a·lay'lee·uh) *n.* [Gk. *alal*os, mute (from *a-* + *lal*ein, to talk) + *-ia*]. Impairment or loss of speech. Compare *mutism.* —**alal·ic** (a·lal'ick) *adj.*

ala lo·bu·li cen·tra·lis (lob'yoo·lye sen·tray'lis) [NA]. Either lateral extension of the central lobule of the cerebellum.

ala mag·na (mag'nuh) [L.]. The great wing of the sphenoid bone.

ala magna os·sis sphe·noi·da·lis (sfee''noy·day'lis) [BNA]. ALA MAJOR OSSIS SPHENOIDALIS.

ala major ossis sphenoidalis [NA]. The great wing of the sphenoid bone.

ala minor ossis sphenoidalis [NA]. The small wing of the sphenoid bone.

ala na·si (nay'zye) [NA]. The lower portion of the side of the nose; a wing of the nose.

al·a·nine (al'uh·neen, ·nin) *n.* α-Aminopropionic acid or 2-aminopropanoic acid, $CH_3CH(NH_2)COOH$. The L- form is a constituent of many proteins; it is classified as a nonessential amino acid. Syn. *α-alanine* (not to be confused with β-alanine, $CH_2NH_2CH_2COOH$, or 3-aminopropanoic acid), *lactamic acid, lactamine.*

alanine ami·no·trans·fer·ase (a·mee''no·trans'fur·ace, ·aze, am''i·no·). GLUTAMIC-PYRUVIC TRANSAMINASE.

L-alanine:2-oxoglutarate aminotransferase. GLUTAMIC-PYRUVIC TRANSAMINASE.

al·a·nyl (al'uh·nil) *n.* The univalent radical $CH_3CH(NH_2)CO$— of the amino acid alanine.

ala of the ilium. ALA OSSIS ILII.

ala of the sacrum. The flat, triangular surface of the bone extending outward from the base of the sacrum.

ala of the vomer. Either of the two lateral expansions of the superior border of the vomer. NA *ala vomeris.*

ala os·sis ilii (oss'is il'ee·eye) [NA]. The broad upward and lateral expansion of the iliac bone terminating in the iliac crest.

ala ossis ili·um (il'ee·um) [BNA]. ALA OSSIS ILII.

ala par·va os·sis sphe·noi·da·lis (pahr'vuh os'is sfee''noy·day'lis) [BNA]. ALA MINOR OSSIS SPHENOIDALIS.

alar (ay'lur) *adj.* [L. *alaris*]. 1. Of or pertaining to a wing or ala. 2. AXILLARY.

alar cartilages. The cartilages of the ala nasi. The major, or greater, alar cartilage (NA *cartilago alaris major*) is the curved fold of cartilage, connected to the inferior margin of the lateral nasal cartilage, whose crura form the anterior portion of the naris and which, together with its counterpart on the other side, forms the apex of the nose. The minor, or lesser, alar cartilages (NA *cartilagines alares minores*) are the small plates found in the fibrous tissue of the ala nasi.

alar lamina. ALAR PLATE.

alar ligament. 1. ALAR PLICA. 2. ALAR ODONTOID LIGAMENT.

alarm reaction. The sum of all nonspecific phenomena elicited by sudden exposure to stimuli, which affect large portions of the body and to which the organism is quantitatively or qualitatively not adapted; the first stage of the general adaptation syndrome, in which there is increased secretory activity of the anterior pituitary (adenohypophysis).

alar odontoid ligament. Either of the ligaments arising on each side of the apex of the odontoid process and connecting the axis with the skull. NA (pl.) *ligamenta alaria articulationis atlantoaxialis medianae.*

alar plate. The lateral wall of the neural tube dorsal to the sulcus limitans, associated with sensory nerves. Syn. *alar lamina.* NA *lamina alaris.*

alar plica. Any of the two fringelike folds of the synovial membrane of the knee joint, one on either side of the articular surface of the patella, converging posteriorly in the infrapatellar synovial fold. NA (pl.) *plicae alares.*

alar process. Either one of a pair of the processes of the anterior border of the crista galli of the ethmoid that articulates with the frontal bone. NA *ala cristae galli.*

alar scapula. WINGED SCAPULA.

ala·ryn·ge·al (ay''la·rin'jee·ul, ·jul) *adj.* Without a larynx; not involving the larynx.

alaryngeal speech. Speech developed after total laryngectomy, usually esophageal speech.

alas·trim (a·las'trim) *n.* [Pg., from *alastrar,* to spread, cover]. VARIOLA MINOR.

alastrim virus. The type of smallpox virus that causes variola minor, especially in man.

alate (ay'late) *adj.* [L. *alatus,* from *ala,* wing]. Winged, having wings.

ala tem·po·ra·lis (tem·po·ray'lis). The great wing of the sphenoid bone.

ala-tragus line. An imaginary line, drawn from the ala of the nose to the tragus of the ear, used in orientation of dental x-ray projection and as a reference line for complete denture construction.

ala·tus (ay·lay'tus) *n.* [L., winged]. An individual with marked backward projection of the scapulas. See also *winged scapula.*

ala ves·per·ti·li·o·nis (ves''pur·til·ee·o'nis) [L., wing of a bat]. *Obsol.* BROAD LIGAMENT OF THE UTERUS.

ala vo·me·ris (vo'mur·is) [NA]. ALA OF THE VOMER.

alb-, albo- [L. *albus*]. A combining form meaning *white, whitish.*

al·ba (al'buh) *n.* [short for *substantia alba*]. WHITE SUBSTANCE.

Albamycin. A trademark for novobiocin, an antibiotic.

Al·ba·rrán's gland (al''ba·rra^hn') [J. *Albarrán* y Domínguez, Cuban surgeon and urologist in France, 1860–1912]. SUBCERVICAL GLAND.

Albarrán's test [J. *Albarrán* y Domínguez]. POLYURIA TEST.

al·bas·pi·din (al·bas'pi·din) *n.* [*alb-* + *aspid*ium + *-in*]. An anthelmintic substance, $C_{25}H_{32}O_8$, extracted from aspidium (male fern).

Al·bee-Del·bet operation (awl'bee, del·be^h') [F. H. *Albee,* U.S. surgeon, 1876–1945; and P. *Delbet,* French surgeon, 1866–1924]. ALBEE'S OPERATION (2).

Albee fracture table [F. H. *Albee*]. An operating table designed to facilitate reduction of fractures and application of spicas and large casts.

Albee's operation [F. H. *Albee*]. 1. An operation for ankylosis of the hip, in which the surface of the femur and a corresponding area of the acetabulum are freshened and placed in contact. 2. A bone graft for an ununited fracture of the neck of the femur, the graft being passed through the trochanter into the head. Syn. *Albee-Delbet operation.* 3. A type of spinal fusion for tuberculous spondylitis, accomplished by transplanting a strong strip of bone from the tibia into the split spinous processes of several vertebrae.

Albee's saw [F. H. *Albee*]. An electrically operated, double rotary circular saw with adjustable blades, for use in preparing bone grafts.

al·ben·da·zole (al·ben'duh·zole) *n.* Methyl 5-(propylthio)-2-benzimidazolecarbamate, $C_{12}H_{15}N_3O_2S$, an anthelmintic agent.

Al·bers-Schön·berg's disease (al"bursshœhn'behrk) [H. E. *Albers-Schönberg,* German surgeon, 1865–1921]. OSTEOPETROSIS.

Al·bert's disease (al'behrt) [E. *Albert,* Austrian surgeon, 1841–1900]. 1. PAINFUL HEEL. 2. ACHILLODYNIA.

Albert's stain [H. *Albert,* U.S. bacteriologist, 1878–1930]. A stain used in a test for diphtheria bacilli. The cells are treated with a solution of toluidine blue and methyl green, then with a solution of iodine and potassium iodide. Diphtheria bacilli are stained light green, the metachromatic granules bluish-black, and the bars dark green to black.

al·bes·cent (al·bes'unt) *adj.* [L. *albescere,* to become white, from *albus,* white]. Whitish.

al·bi·cans (al'bi·kanz) *L. adj.,* pl. **al·bi·can·tia** (al'bi·kan"tee·uh) [L., from *albicare,* to whiten]. White; whitish.

al·bi·du·ria (al"bi·dew'ree·uh) *n.* [L. *albid*us, white, + *-uria*]. 1. Passage of very pale, almost colorless urine, of low specific gravity. 2. CHYLURIA.

al·bi·fac·tion (al"bi·fack'shun) *n.* [ML. *albificare,* to make white]. Act or process of blanching or rendering white.

al·bi·nism (al'bi·niz·um) *n.* [*albino* + *-ism*]. Hereditary absence of melanin pigment from the eyes or from the skin, hair, and eyes due to defective metabolism of the melanin precursor tyrosine; associated with several congenital ocular abnormalities and with visual defects and nystagmus.

al·bi·nis·mus (al"bi·niz'mus) *n.* ALBINISM.

al·bi·no (al·bye'no, al·bee'no) *n.* [Pg., from L. *albus,* white]. An individual affected with albinism. —**al·bi·not·ic** (al"bi·not'ick) *adj.*

al·bi·no·ism (al·bye'no·iz·um, al·bee') *n.* ALBINISM.

al·bi·nu·ria (al"bi·new'ree·uh) *n.* ALBIDURIA.

albo-. See *alb-*.

al·bo·ci·ne·re·ous (al"bo·si·neer'ee·us) *adj.* [*albo-* + *cinere*a + *-ous*]. Having both white and gray matter.

Albolene. Trademark for a brand of liquid petrolatum and certain products containing the same.

Albright-McCune-Sternberg syndrome [F. *Albright;* D. J. *McCune,* U.S. pediatrician, b. 1902; and W. H. *Sternberg,* U.S. pathologist, b. 1913]. ALBRIGHT'S SYNDROME.

Albright's syndrome [F. *Albright,* U.S. physician, 1900–1969]. The polyostotic form of fibrous dysplasia associated with large irregular melanotic macules arranged in a linear or segmental pattern tending to remain on one side of the midline of the body, and precocious puberty in females but only rarely in males. Syn. *Albright-McCune-Sternberg syndrome.*

Albucid. A trademark for sulfacetamide, a sulfonamide drug.

al·bu·gin·ea (al"bew·jin'ee·uh) *n.* [NL., albugineous]. TUNICA ALBUGINEA.

albuginea ocu·li (ock'yoo·lye). SCLERA.

albuginea ova·rii (o·vair'ee·eye). TUNICA ALBUGINEA OVARII.

albuginea penis. TUNICA ALBUGINEA PENIS.

albuginea testis. TUNICA ALBUGINEA TESTIS.

al·bu·gin·e·ous (al"bew·jin'ee·us) *adj.* [NL. *albugineus,* from L. *albugo,* whiteness]. 1. Whitish. 2. Belonging to a tunica albuginea.

al·bu·gi·ni·tis (al·bew"ji·nigh'tis, al"bew·ji·) *n.* Inflammation of a tunica albuginea.

al·bu·go (al·bew'go) *n.* [L., whiteness, from *albus,* white]. A white spot upon the cornea; a corneal opacity.

al·bu·men (al·bew'mun) *n.* [L., from *albus,* white]. 1. Egg white, consisting chiefly of albumin. 2. The stored food matter in a vegetable seed. 3. ALBUMIN.

al·bu·min (al·bew'min) *n.* [*album*en + *-in*]. One of a group of protein substances, the chief constituents of animal tissues. They are soluble in water, coagulable by heat, and composed of carbon, hydrogen, nitrogen, oxygen, and sulfur. Some varieties are named after their sources or characteristic reactions, such as acid albumin, alkali albumin, muscle albumin, ovum albumin, serum albumin, vegetable albumin. —**albu·mi·nous** (·mi·nus) *adj.*

albumin-, albumino-. A combining form meaning *albumin* or *albumen.*

al·bu·mi·nate (al·bew'mi·nate) *n.* Any compound of albumin with an acid or base; a product of the hydrolysis of albumin or globulin.

albumin-globulin ratio. The ratio of the albumin to the globulin concentration in blood serum. Normal value = 1.3 to 1.8. Values below 1.0 are said to be inverted and may be associated with various pathologic processes. Abbreviated, A/G ratio.

al·bu·mi·nif·er·ous (al·bew"mi·nif'ur·us) *adj.* Containing or yielding albumin.

al·bu·mi·nim·e·ter (al·bew"mi·nim'e·tur) *n.* ALBUMINOMETER. —**albuminime·try** (·tree) *n.*

albumino-. See *albumin-*.

al·bu·mi·no·cy·to·log·ic (al·bew"mi·no·sigh·to·loj'ick) *adj.* [*albumino-* + *cytologic*]. Referring to both the protein and cells (usually leukocytes) of a fluid; usually used in connection with the cerebrospinal fluid.

albuminocytologic dissociation. Elevated protein in cerebrospinal fluid without a corresponding rise in cell count, characteristic of the Guillain-Barré syndrome.

al·bu·mi·nog·e·nous (al·bew"mi·noj'e·nus) *adj.* Producing albumin.

al·bu·mi·noid (al·bew'mi·noid) *adj. & n.* 1. Resembling albumin; applied to certain protein derivatives having many of the characteristics of albumin. 2. SCLEROPROTEIN.

al·bu·mi·nol·y·sin (al·bew"mi·nol'i·sin) *n.* A lysin that causes dissolution of albumins. —**albuminoly·sis** (·sis) *n.*

al·bu·mi·nom·e·ter (al·bew"mi·nom'e·tur) *n.* [*albumino-* + *meter*]. An instrument for the quantitative estimation of protein in a fluid, as in urine. —**albuminome·try** (·tree) *n.*

al·bu·mi·nous (al·bew'mi·nus) *adj.* Resembling, pertaining to, or containing albumin or albumen.

albuminous degeneration. CLOUDY SWELLING.

albuminous gland. SEROUS GLAND.

al·bu·min·uret·ic (al·bew"min·yoo·ret'ick) *adj. & n.* [*albumin* + Gk. *ourētikos,* promoting urine]. 1. Causing proteinuria. 2. A drug that causes proteinuria.

al·bu·min·uria (al·bew"mi·new'ree·uh) *n.* [*albumin* + *-uria*]. The presence of albumin in the urine; may or may not be associated with renal parenchymal disease. —**albumin·uric** (·rick) *adj.*

albuminuria ac·e·ton·ica (as·e·ton'i·kuh). Proteinuria due to asphyxia.

albuminuria of adolescence. CYCLIC PROTEINURIA.

albuminuria par·cel·laire (par·se·lair'). PARTIAL ALBUMINURIA.

al·bu·mo·scope (al·bew'mo·skope) *n.* [*album*in + *-scope*]. HORISMASCOPE.

al·bu·mose (al'bew·moce, al·bew'moze) *n.* [*album*in + *-ose*]. An albuminous substance, among the first of the products of proteolysis, not coagulated by heat.

al·bu·mo·su·ria (al"bew·mo·sue'ree·uh) *n.* [*albumos*e + *-uria*]. The presence of Bence Jones protein in the urine.

Albumotope-LS. Trademark for aggregated radioiodinated I-131 serum albumin, used in lung scanning, especially for diagnosis of pulmonary embolism.

Albuspan. Trademark for normal human serum albumin.

al·bu·ter·ol (al·bew'tur·ole) *n.* α^1-[[(1,1-Dimethylethyl)amino]methyl]-4-hydroxy-1,3-benzenedimethanol,

$C_{13}H_{21}NO_3$, a bronchodilating agent, usually employed as the sulfate salt.

al·bu·to·in (al·bew'to·in) *n.* 3-Allyl-5-isobutyl-2-thiohydantoin, $C_{10}H_{16}N_2OS$, an anticonvulsant drug.

Al·ca·lig·e·nes fae·ca·lis (al"kuh·lij'e·neez fee·kay'lis) [NL., from *alkali* + Gk. *-genēs,* producing; *faecalis,* fecal]. An organism consisting of gram-negative motile rods belonging to the family Achromobacteraceae which turns litmus milk alkaline, does not attack carbohydrates, is commonly found in the intestinal tracts of vertebrates and in dairy products, and is only rarely pathogenic.

alcapton. ALKAPTON.

alcaptonuria. ALKAPTONURIA.

al·che·my (al'ke·mee) *n.* [ML. *alchimia,* from Ar. *al-kīmiyā,* probably from Gk. *chymeia,* from *chyma,* fluid]. The chemical science of the Middle Ages, which attempted to transmute base metals into gold and to find a remedy for all diseases.

al·clo·fen·ac (al·klo'fe·nack) *n.* 3-Chloro-4-(2-propenyloxy)-benzeneacetic acid, $C_{11}H_{11}ClO_3$, an anti-inflammatory agent.

al·cloxa (al·klock'suh) *n.* Chlorotetrahydroxy[(4,5-dihydro-2-hydroxy-5-oxo-1*H*-imidazol-4-yl)ureato]dialuminum, $C_4H_9Al_2ClN_4O_7$, an astringent, keratolytic agent.

Al·cock's canal [B. *Alcock,* Irish anatomist, 19th century]. PUDENDAL CANAL.

al·co·gel (al'ko·jel) *n.* An alcoholic, colloidal suspension with the dispersion medium a gel.

al·co·hol (al'kuh·hawl) *n.* [Early mod. E., spirit, distillate, orig. sublimate, fine powder, from ML., from Ar. *al-kuḥl,* (the) kohl, a dark powder (usually stibnite, Sb_2S_3) for outlining the eyes (rel. to *akḥal,* black)]. 1. A derivative of an aliphatic hydrocarbon that contains a hydroxyl (OH) group. Alcohols are classified on the basis of the number of hydroxyl groups present in the molecule, i.e., monohydric, dihydric, trihydric; or on the basis of the presence of a $—CH_2OH$ (primary alcohol), a $=CHOH$ (secondary alcohol), or a $\equiv COH$ (tertiary alcohol) group. 2. Specifically, ETHYL ALCOHOL. 3. Ethyl alcohol in a concentration of not less than 92.3 percent by weight or 94.9 percent by volume at 15.56° C.; a pharmaceutical solvent (USP).

al·co·hol·ase (al'ko·hol·ace, ·aze) *n.* ALCOHOL DEHYDROGENASE.

al·co·hol·ate (al'ko·hol·ate) *n.* 1. A molecular combination, analogous to a hydrate, of alcohol with any of various substances. 2. ALKOXIDE. 3. A preparation made with alcohol.

al·co·hol·a·ture (al"ko·hol'uh·chur) *n.* An alcoholic tincture.

alcohol bath. The sponging of the body with dilute alcohol for its soothing and cooling effect.

alcohol dehydrogenase. An enzyme capable of reversibly oxidizing ethanol to acetaldehyde. Nicotinamide adenine dinucleotide (NAD) is required, and other aliphatic alcohols of low molecular weight are likewise oxidized. Abbreviated, ADH. Syn. *alcoholase.*

alcohol formalin. A fixing fluid made up of 10 parts 37% formaldehyde and 95% alcohol to make 100 parts.

al·co·hol·ic (al"ko·hol'ick) *adj. & n.* 1. Pertaining to, containing, or producing alcohol. 2. An individual whose consumption of alcoholic beverages or other substances with similar effects results in his or her becoming habituated, dependent, or addicted, or interferes, or threatens to interfere, with his or her health, interpersonal relationships, or means of livelihood.

alcoholic cirrhosis. Laennec's cirrhosis associated with alcoholism.

alcoholic delirium. Delirium tremens associated with alcoholism.

alcoholic dementia or **insanity.** 1. A chronic form of Korsakoff's psychosis. 2. Dementia of indeterminate cause in an alcoholic.

alcoholic fermentation. Fermentation resulting in the conversion of carbohydrates into alcohol.

alcoholic myopathy. Any of several nonspecific disorders of skeletal muscles associated with alcoholism, such as hypopotassemia with vacuolar necrosis of muscle, or painful, swollen muscles accompanied by hyperpotassemia, myoglobinuria and renal damage.

alcoholic neuropathy or **neuritis.** The polyneuropathy that complicates alcoholism, probably due to a deficiency of B vitamins.

alcoholic paralysis. Paralysis resulting from polyneuropathy of chronic alcoholism.

alcoholic paranoia. ALCOHOL PARANOID STATE.

alcoholic psychosis. Any severe mental disorder associated with excessive ingestion of alcohol, as acute alcoholic hallucinosis, delirium tremens, Korsakoff's psychosis, or Wernicke's encephalopathy.

Alcoholics Anonymous. A fellowship of persons formerly addicted to alcohol who together through personal and group support seek to help other alcoholics to overcome their addiction. Abbreviated, A.A.

al·co·hol·ism (al'kuh·hol·iz·um) *n.* 1. ACUTE ALCOHOLISM. 2. CHRONIC ALCOHOLISM (1, 2, & 3).

al·co·hol·ize (al'ko·hol·ize) *v.* 1. To saturate or treat with alcohol. 2. To convert to alcohol. 3. [from ML. *alcohol,* fine powder, sublimate]. To convert to fine powder.

alcoholized iron. Finely powdered iron.

al·co·hol·om·e·ter (al"ko·hol·om'e·tur) *n.* A hydrometer or other instrument for determining the amount of alcohol in a liquid. **—alcoholome·try** (·tree) *n.*

al·co·holo·phil·ia (al"ko·hol"o·fil'ee·uh) *n.* A craving for alcoholic drinks or other intoxicants.

alcohol paranoid state. A paranoid state observed chiefly in chronic male alcoholics, characterized by excessive jealousy and delusions of the spouse's infidelity.

alcohol-soluble eosin. ETHYL EOSIN.

alcohol thermometer. A thermometer in which the expansive substance is alcohol.

al·co·hol·uria (al"ko·hol·yoo'ree·uh) *n.* [*alcohol* + *-uria*]. The presence of alcohol in urine.

al·co·hol·y·sis (al"ko·hol'i·sis) *n.,* pl. **alcoholy·ses** (·seez). A decomposition reaction, analogous to hydrolysis, of alcohol with another substance.

Alcopara. A trademark for bephenium hydroxynaphthoate, an anthelmintic.

al·co·sol (al'ko·sol) *n.* [*alco*hol + *sol*]. A colloidal solution in which alcohol is the dispersion medium.

al·cu·ro·ni·um chloride (al"kew·ro'nee·um). *N,N'*-Diallylnortoxiferinium dichloride, $C_{44}H_{50}Cl_2N_4O_2$, a muscle relaxant.

ald-, aldo-. A combining form meaning (a) *aldehyde;* (b) *related to an aldehyde.*

Aldactone. Trademark for spironolactone, a diuretic agent.

al·dar·ic acid (al·dăr'ick). A dicarboxylic sugar acid of the general formula $COOH(CHOH)_nCOOH$.

al·de·hyde (al'de·hide) *n.* [*al*cohol *dehyd*rogenatum, alcohol deprived of hydrogen]. A class of organic compounds intermediate between alcohols and acids, derived from their corresponding primary alcohols by oxidation and removal of two atoms of hydrogen, and converted into acids by the addition of an atom of oxygen. They contain the group —CHO.

aldehyde acid. Any substance containing both an aldehyde (—CHO) group and a carboxyl (—COOH) group.

aldehyde dehydrogenase. An enzyme which catalyzes the conversion of an aldehyde into its corresponding acid.

aldehyde fixative. *In histology and electron microscopy,* a glutaraldehyde, hydroxyadipaldehyde, other dialdehyde, or acrolein used as a fixing agent in place of, or in addition to, formaldehyde or osmic acid.

aldehyde mutase. An enzyme, occurring in liver and yeast, which catalyzes conversion of two molecules of acetaldehyde to one each of acetic acid and ethyl alcohol.

Alderlin. Trademark for pronethalol, a beta-adrenergic blocking agent.

Al·der's anomaly or **phenomenon** [A. *Alder,* German, 20th century]. Inclusions of deeply staining, azurophilic, toluidine-blue positive material in the cytoplasm of lymphocytes, granulocytes, and monocytes, often associated with mucopolysaccharidosis.

al·di·oxa (al″dye·ock′suh) *n.* Dihydroxy(4,5-dihydro-2-hydroxy-5-oxo-1*H*-imidazol-4-yl)ureato aluminum, $C_4H_7AlN_4O_5$, an astringent, keratolytic agent.

aldo-. See *ald-.*

al·do·bi·on·ic acid (al″do·bye·on′ick). An acid, $C_{12}H_{20}O_{12}$, produced by the hydrolysis of gum arabic and other gums, as well as of the specific carbohydrate of type 3 pneumococcus. Its components are D-glucuronic acid and D-galactose.

al·do·hex·ose (al″do·heck′soce) *n.* A hexose that contains an aldehyde group; examples are glucose, galactose, and mannose.

al·dol (al′dole, ·dol) *n.* 1. Beta-hydroxybutyric aldehyde, $CH_3CH(OH)CH_2CHO$, a condensation product of acetaldehyde. 2. One of a class of condensation products formed from an aldehyde.

al·dol·ase (al′do·lace, ·laze) *n.* [*aldol* + *-ase*]. An enzyme occurring in muscle and capable of splitting fructose 1,6-diphosphate into dihydroxyacetone phosphate and phosphoglyceraldehyde. Syn. *zymohexase.*

Aldomet. Trademark for methyldopa, an antihypertensive agent.

Aldomet Ester. Trademark for methyldopate, an antihypertensive drug; used as the hydrochloride salt.

al·don·ic acid (al·don′ick). Any of a group of monobasic sugar acids, having the general formula $CH_2OH(CHOH)_nCOOH$, obtained when the aldehyde group of an aldose is oxidized to carboxyl, without oxidizing the primary alcohol group.

al·do·pen·tose (al″do·pen′toce) *n.* A pentose containing an aldehyde group, such as arabinose, ribose, or xylose.

Aldor's test. VON ALDOR'S TEST.

al·dose (al′doce, al′doze) *n.* [*ald-* + *-ose*]. Any carbohydrate containing the aldehyde group —CHO.

al·do·side (al′do·side) *n.* A glycoside resulting from the condensation of an aldose and a compound containing a hydroxyl group.

al·do·ste·rone (al·dos′te·rone, al″do·ste·rone′, ·sterr′one, ·steer′one) *n.* [*aldo-* + *sterol* + *-one*]. 11β,21-Dihydroxy-3,20-diketo-4-pregnene-18-al, $C_{21}H_{28}O_5$, a potent adrenocortical hormone which, in very small amounts, maintains the life of adrenalectomized animals. It is a very potent regulator of the metabolism of sodium and potassium, many times more active than deoxycorticosterone in its effects on electrolyte metabolism, less effective in regulating carbohydrate metabolism. Formerly called *electrocortin.*

al·do·ste·ron·ism (al·dos′te·ro·niz·um, al″do·sterr′o·niz·um, al″do·ste·ro′niz·um) *n.* [*aldosterone* + *-ism*]. HYPERALDOSTERONISM.

al·do·ste·ro·no·ma (al·dos″te·ro·no′muh, al″do·sterr″o·no′muh) *n.* An aldosterone-producing tumor, usually a benign adenoma, composed of adrenal cortical cells; the principal cause of hyperaldosteronism.

al·do·tet·rose (al″do·tet′roce) *n.* A tetrose, such as threose, containing an aldehyde group.

al·dox·ime (al·dock′sim, ·seem) *n.* [*ald-* + *oxime*]. 1. The product derived from an aldehyde when the oxygen of the —CHO group is replaced by =NOH, forming the —CHNOH group. 2. Acetaldoxime, CH_3CHNOH.

Al·drich syndrome [R. A. *Aldrich,* U.S. pediatrician, b. 1917]. WISKOTT-ALDRICH SYNDROME.

al·drin (al′drin) *n.* [K. *Alder,* German chemist, b. 1907]. Common name for an insecticide containing not less than 95% 1,2,3,4,10,10-hexachloro-1,4,4a,5,8,8a-hexahydro-1,4,5,8-dimethanonaphthalene; the crystals are soluble in most organic solvents but insoluble in water. It is readily absorbed through the skin and is toxic.

alec·i·thal (a·les′i·thul, ay·) *adj.* [*a-* + *lecithal*]. Having little or no yolk, as the eggs of placental mammals.

alem·bic (a·lem′bick) *n.* [Ar. *al-anbīq,* the still, from Gk. *ambix,* cap of still]. A vessel that was formerly used for distillation.

Alep·po boil or **button** [after *Aleppo,* Syria]. A lesion of cutaneous leishmaniasis.

Alepsin. Trademark for phenytoin sodium, an anticonvulsant.

al·et·a·mine (al·et′uh·meen) *n.* α-Allylphenethylamine, $C_{11}H_{15}N$, an antidepressant; used as the hydrochloride salt.

al·e·tris (al′e·tris, a·lee′tris) *n.* The dried rhizome and roots of *Aletris farinosa,* colicroot. Formerly a popular remedy used in treating a variety of ailments.

aleu·ke·mia, aleu·kae·mia (al″yoo·kee′mee·uh) *n.* [*a-* + *leukemia*]. ALEUKEMIC LEUKEMIA. **—aleuke·mic, aleukae·mic** (·mick) *adj.*

aleukemic leukemia. A form of leukemia in which the total leukocyte count is normal or low, despite leukemic changes in the tissues and sometimes qualitative changes in the blood. Contr. *leukemic leukemia.*

aleu·kia he·mor·rha·gi·ca (a·lew′kee·uh hem″o·ray′ji·kuh). APLASTIC ANEMIA.

aleu·ko·cy·to·sis (ay·lew″ko·sigh·to′sis) *n.* [*a-* + *leukocyte* + *-osis*]. Severe leukopenia.

al·eu·rone (al′yoo·rone) *n.* [Gk. *aleuron,* meal, flour]. Small protein particles found in the endosperm of ripe seeds and in a special layer in a grain of wheat.

Aleu·tian disease (uh·lew′shun). A disease of mink characterized by hypergammaglobulinemia, glomerulonephritis, necrotizing arteritis, and accumulation of plasma cells in several organs, which is thought to be caused by a pronounced antibody response to viral antigens and has been used as a model for human viral diseases with immunologically mediated lesions; discovered in the Aleutian mink, a dark blue mutant of ranch-raised mink.

Al·ex·an·der's disease [W. S. *Alexander,* English neurologist, 20th century]. A rare degenerative disease of the central nervous system with onset in early infancy and a course of a few years, characterized clinically by lack of development, progressive spasticity, megalocephaly, and seizures, and pathologically by leukodystrophy and eosinophilic hyaline bodies at the pial surface and in the perivascular tissue.

Alexander's operation [W. *Alexander,* English surgeon, 1844–1919]. Suspension of the uterus by extraperitoneal shortening of the round ligaments.

alex·ia (a·leck′see·uh, ay·) *n.* [*a-* + *-lexia*]. Loss or impairment of ability to recognize or comprehend written or printed words as a manifestation of aphasia. Syn. *word blindness.* Compare *dyslexia.*

alex·i·dine (a·leck′si·deen) *n.* 1,1′-Hexamethylenebis[5-(2-ethylhexyl)biguanide], $C_{26}H_{56}N_{10}$, an antimicrobial agent.

alex·in (a·leck′sin) *n.* [Gk. *alexein,* to ward off, + *-in*]. COMPLEMENT.

alex·i·phar·mac (a·leck″si·fahr′mack) *n.* [Gk. *alexipharmakon,* from *alexein,* to ward off, + *pharmakon,* drug]. An antidote or defensive remedy against poison, venom, or infection.

aley·dig·ism (a·lye′dig·iz·um) *n.* [*a-* + *Leydig* cell + *-ism*]. Absence of interstitial cell function. Compare *hypoleydigism.*

Alez·zan·dri·ni's syndrome (a·le·san·dree′nee) [A. S. *Alezzandrini,* Argentinian ophthalmologist, 20th century]. A rare syndrome of unknown cause, appearing in late adolescence or early adult life, in which unilateral tapetoretinal degeneration with impairment of vision is followed by facial vitiligo and poliosis on the same side, and sometimes sensorineural hearing loss.

al·fa·do·lone (al·fuh·do'lone) *n.* 3α,21-Dihydroxy-5α-pregnane-11,20-dione, $C_{23}H_{34}O_5$, a component of Althesin, an anesthetic; usually employed as the 21-acetate.

al·fax·a·lone (al·fack'suh·lone) *n.* 3α-Hydroxy-5α-pregnane-11,20-dione, $C_{21}H_{32}O_3$, a component of Althesin, an anesthetic.

alg-, algio-, algo- [Gk. *algos,* pain]. A combining form meaning *pain* or *pertaining to pain.*

al·ga (al'guh) *n.,* pl. **al·gae** (al'jee) [L., seaweed]. A plant of the Algae. —**al·gal** (al'gul) *adj.*

Al·gae (al'jee) *n.pl.* One of the major divisions of the Thallophyta or primitive plants, including numerous marine plants, such as the seaweeds, rockweeds, freshwater pond scums, the stoneworts, and others. Because the algae can synthesize food, they are separated from the fungi which are saprophytic or parasitic.

alg·an·es·the·sia, alg·an·aes·the·sia (alg·an''es·theezh'uh, ·theez'ee·uh) *n.* [*alg-* + *anesthesia*]. ANALGESIA.

al·ge·don·ic (al''je·don'ick) *adj.* [Gk. *algēdōn,* pain, + *hēdonikos,* pleasant]. Pertaining to pleasure and pain, or to the pleasantness-unpleasantness of an experience. —**algedon·ics** (·icks) *n.*

al·gel·drate (al'jel·drate) *n.* Powdered hydrated aluminum hydroxide of the general formula $Al(OH)_3xH_2O$; used as an antacid.

al·ge·sia (al·jee'zee·uh) *n.* [Gk. *algēsis,* sense of pain, + *-ia*]. 1. Sensitivity to pain. 2. Excessive sensitivity to pain. —**alge·sic** (·sick) *adj.*

al·ge·sim·e·ter (al''je·sim'e·tur) *n.* [*algesia* + *meter*]. An instrument for determining the acuteness of the sense of pain by eliciting a measurable pain response. Syn. *algometer.*

al·ge·sim·e·try (al''je·sim'e·tree) *n.* [*algesia* + *-metry*]. Measurement of pain sensitivity by eliciting a quantitative, reproducible, and reliable response to a painful stimulus.

al·ge·si·om·e·ter (al·jee''zee·om'e·tur) *n.* ALGESIMETER.

al·ge·si·om·e·try (al·jee''zee·om'e·tree) *n.* ALGESIMETRY.

al·ges·the·sia, al·gaes·the·sia (al''jes·theezh'uh, ·theez'ee·uh) *n.* ALGESIA.

al·get·ic (al·jet'ick) *adj.* [Gk. *algēsis,* sense of pain, + *-ic*]. Pertaining to or producing pain.

-algia [Gk., from *algos,* pain, + *-ia*]. A combining form designating *a painful condition.*

al·gid (al'jid) *adj.* [L. *algidus,* from *algere,* to be cold]. 1. Cold or chilly. 2. Characterized by cold skin and hypotension, as algid malaria.

algid malaria. Falciparum malaria with gastrointestinal manifestations predominating, characterized by cold, clammy skin and hypotension.

algid pernicious fever. ALGID MALARIA.

algid stage. A condition occurring in cholera, falciparum malaria, and other diseases marked by extensive intestinal discharges, characterized by subnormal temperature, feeble flickering pulse, hypotension, and various neurologic symptoms.

al·gin (al'jin) *n.* [*alga* + *-in*]. SODIUM ALGINATE.

al·gi·nate (al'ji·nate) *n.* A salt of alginic acid extracted from marine kelp, believed to be a polymer of D-mannuronic acid. Certain such salts form viscous sols in water and may then react with calcium compounds to form an elastic, insoluble gel. See also *hydrocolloid.*

al·gin·ic acid (al·jin'ick). A gelatinous polysaccharide derived from marine algae of the *Fucus* type; it appears to consist entirely of D-mannuronic acid residues. The sodium salt produces with water a transparent mucilage, for which reason it is used as a suspending agent in pharmacy.

algio-. See *alg-.*

al·gio·mo·tor (al''jee·o·mo'tur) *adj.* [*algio-* + *motor*]. Causing pain on movement; causing painful spasm.

al·gio·mus·cu·lar (al''jee·o·mus'kew·lur) *adj.* [*algio-* + *muscular*]. Causing pain in the muscles.

Alglyn. Trademark for dihydroxyaluminum aminoacetate, an antacid.

algo-. See *alg-.*

al·go·ge·ne·sia (al''go·je·nee'zhuh) *n.* ALGOGENESIS.

al·go·gen·e·sis (al''go·jen'e·sis) *n.* [*algo-* + *-genesis*]. The source or origin of pain.

[1]**al·go·gen·ic** (al''go·jen'ick) *adj.* [L. *algor,* sensation of cold, + *-genic*]. Lowering the body temperature; producing cold or chill.

[2]**algogenic,** *adj.* [*algo-* + *-genic*]. Producing pain.

al·go·gram (al'go·gram) *n.* [*algo-* + *-gram*]. The record produced by an instrument for measuring pain.

al·go·lag·nia (al''go·lag'nee·uh) *n.* [*algo-* + Gk. *lagneia,* lust]. A sexual perversion in which the experiencing or inflicting of pain heightens sexual gratification or gives sexual pleasure without intercourse; masochism or sadism. —**algolag·nist** (·nist) *n.*

al·gom·e·ter (al·gom'e·tur) *n.* [*algo-* + *meter*]. ALGESIMETER.

al·go·pho·bia (al''go·fo'bee·uh) *n.* [*algo-* + *-phobia*]. Unreasonable or morbid dread of witnessing or of experiencing pain.

al·gor (al'gor) *n.* [L.]. Chill, coldness.

algor mor·tis (mor'tis) [L.]. Chill of death; the lowering of body temperature after death to the ambient temperature.

al·go·spasm (al'go·spaz·um) *n.* [*algo-* + *spasm*]. A painful spasm or cramp. —**al·go·spas·tic** (al''go·spas'tick) *adj.*

-algy. See *-algia.*

ali- [L. *ala*]. A combining form meaning (a) *wing;* (b) *shaped like a wing,* as the side parts of certain organs or structures.

al·i·ble (al'i·bul) *adj.* [L. *alibilis,* nutritive, from *alere,* to nourish]. Nutritive; absorbable and assimilable, as a food.

Al·i·bour water (al'i·boor). DALIBOUR WATER.

"Alice in Wonderland" syndrome. Depersonalization and hallucinations, especially Lilliputian hallucinations, observed with certain seizures, hypnagogic states, drugs, delirium, and schizophrenia.

al·i·cy·clic (al''i·sigh'click, ·sick'lick) *adj.* Having the properties of both aliphatic (open-chain) and cyclic (closed-chain) compounds.

Alidase. A trademark for hyaluronidase.

alien·a·tion (ay''lee·uh·nay'shun) *n.* [L. *alienatio,* from *alienus,* alien]. 1. *In forensic psychiatry,* mental derangement; insanity. 2. SELF-ALIENATION.

alien·ist (ail'yuh·nist, ay'lee·uh·nist) *n.* [F. *aliéniste,* from *aliéné,* insane]. 1. A psychiatrist. 2. Especially, a physician qualified in a court of law as an expert witness in the field of psychiatry. —**alien·ism** (·iz·um) *n.*

ali·es·ter·ase (al·i·es'tur·ace, ·aze) *n.* [L. *alius,* other, + *esterase*]. An esterase other than a true lipase or cholinesterase.

ali·form (al'i·form, ay'li·) *adj.* [*ali* + *-form*]. Shaped like a wing.

aligning power of the eye. VERNIER ACUITY.

alignment curve. The line of the dental arch; one following the mesiodistal diameters of the teeth in correct position.

al·i·ment (al'i·munt) *n.* [L. *alimentum,* from *alere,* to nourish]. Any food or nutritive substance.

al·i·men·ta·ry (al''i·men'tuh·ree) *adj.* [L. *alimentarius,* from *alimentum,* food]. 1. Nourishing, nutritious. 2. Of or pertaining to food and nutrition. 3. Pertaining to or caused by diet.

alimentary albuminuria. Albuminuria following the ingestion of a meal high in proteins.

alimentary azotemia. Elevation of the blood urea nitrogen secondary to the presence of a large amount of protein in the gastrointestinal tract, usually the result of hemorrhage.

alimentary bolus. BOLUS (2).

alimentary canal. The whole digestive tube from the mouth to the anus; the gastrointestinal tract. NA *canalis alimentarius.*

alimentary glycosuria. Glycosuria due to excessive ingestion of carbohydrates.

alimentary lipemia. Lipemia due to the ingestion of a high-fat diet.
alimentary system. The alimentary canal with its accessory glands.
alimentary tract or **tube.** ALIMENTARY CANAL.
al·i·men·ta·tion (al″i·men·tay′shun) *n.* Feeding; nourishment.
al·i·men·to·ther·a·py (al″i·men″to·therr′uh·pee) *n.* [*aliment* + *therapy*]. The treatment of disease by systematic feeding; dietary treatment.
ali·na·sal (al″i·nay′zul, ay″li·) *adj.* Pertaining to the ala nasi.
alip·a·mide (a·lip′uh·mide) *n.* 4-Chloro-3-sulfamoylbenzoic acid 2,2-dimethylhydrazide, $C_9H_{12}ClN_3O_3S$, a diuretic and antihypertensive agent.
al·i·phat·ic (al″i·fat′ick) *adj.* [Gk. *aleiphar, aleiphatos,* fat]. 1. Pertaining to a fat. 2. Belonging to or derived from the open-chain series of organic compounds; ACYCLIC (2).
aliphatic series. The series of organic compounds in which the linkages of successive carbon atoms are terminated, as in an open chain.
ali·quor·rhea (al″i·kwo·ree′uh, al″i·ko·, a·lye″kwo·) *n.* [*a-* + *liquor* + *-rrhea*]. Chronic deficiency of cerebrospinal fluid of unknown cause resulting in vomiting, confusion, weakness or paralysis, and hyperthermia.
al·i·quot (al′i·kwot, ·kwut) *n.* [L., some, several]. 1. A number which will divide a larger number without a remainder. 2. *In quantitative chemistry and pharmacy,* a definite known fraction of a larger sample, used to facilitate analysis.
ali·sphe·noid (al″i·sfee′noid) *adj.* & *n.* [*ali-* + *sphenoid*]. 1. Pertaining to the great wing of the sphenoid bone. 2. The bone that in adult life forms the main portion of the great wing of the sphenoid bone.
aliz·a·rin (a·liz′uh·rin) *n.* [F. *alizerine,* from obs. Sp. *alizari,* levantine madder, from Ar. *al-'uṣāra,* (the) juice, extract]. 1,2-Dihydroxyanthraquinone, $C_{14}H_8O_4$, an orange-red dyestuff originally isolated from madder, *Rubia tinctorum,* now made synthetically; insoluble in water but soluble in alkalies, in alcohol, and in ether; colors newly formed bone red in feeding experiments; used as a pH indicator, as a histochemical reagent for calcium, thallium, titanium, and zirconium, and industrially as an intermediate in the manufacture of dyestuffs.
alizarin carmine. ALIZARIN.
alizarin red S. 1,2-Dihydroxyanthraquinone-3-sulfonic acid sodium salt, variously used as a stain and reagent.
al·ka·le·mia, al·ka·lae·mia (al″kuh·lee′mee·uh) *n.* [*alkali* + *-emia*]. An elevation of blood pH above normal levels. Compare *alkalosis.*
al·ka·les·cent (al″kuh·les′unt) *adj.* Somewhat alkaline. —**al·kales·cence** (·unce) *n.*
al·ka·li (al′kuh·lye) *n.,* pl. **alka·lies, alka·lis** (·lize) [Ar. *al-qalī,* (the) ashes of saltwort, from *qala,* to fry]. 1. Essentially a hydroxide of an alkali metal. 2. A class of compounds that react with acids to form salts, turn red litmus blue, saponify fats, and form soluble carbonates. 3. Sometimes, a carbonate of alkali metals.
alkali albuminate. A compound of albumin and an alkali metal, usually in the form of a soluble powder, used as a culture medium.
alkali blue. Sodium triphenylrosaniline sulfonate; a dye.
alkali disease. Selenium poisoning in cattle.
alkalies. A plural of *alkali.*
alkali metal. Any of the metals lithium, sodium, potassium, rubidium, or cesium, belonging to group I in the periodic classification of chemical elements.
al·ka·lim·e·ter (al″kuh·lim′e·tur) *n.* An instrument for estimating the alkali in a substance. —**alka·li·met·ric** (·li·met′rick) *adj.;* **alka·lim·e·try** (·lim′e·tree) *n.*
al·ka·line (al′kuh·line, ·lin) *adj.* 1. Containing more hydroxyl than hydrogen ions. 2. Having the qualities of or pertaining to an alkali. Noun *alkalinity.*
alkaline air. *Obsol.* Free or volatile ammonia.
alkaline-ash diet. A diet used to raise the pH of the urine.
alkaline-earth metals. The divalent elements calcium, strontium, and barium. Some include magnesium in the group.
alkaline earths. The oxides of calcium, strontium, and barium, and sometimes including magnesium oxide.
alkaline hematin. A pigment suitable for hemoglobinometry made by diluting blood with 0.1 normal sodium hydroxide.
alkaline hematin method. Determination of hemoglobin in blood by photoelectric colorimetry of alkaline hematin.
alkaline incrusted cystitis. INCRUSTED CYSTITIS.
alkaline phosphatase. An enzyme liberating phosphate ions from various organic phosphates such as β-glycerophosphate with optimal activity in the pH range from 8.3 to 10.5.
alkaline tide. The temporary decrease in acidity of urine and body fluids after eating, attributed to the secretion of hydrochloric acid from the blood by the parietal cells of the stomach during gastric digestion.
al·ka·lin·i·ty (al″kuh·lin′i·tee) *n.* The quality of being alkaline.
al·ka·lin·ize (al′kuh·lin·ize) *v.* To render alkaline. —**al·ka·lin·iza·tion** (al″kuh·lin·i·zay′shun) *n.*
al·ka·li·nu·ria (al″kuh·li·new′ree·uh) *n.* Alkalinity of the urine.
alkali reserve. The components of blood that are capable of neutralizing acids, including sodium bicarbonate, phosphate salts and esters, and proteins.
alkalis. A plural of *alkali.*
al·ka·li·ther·a·py (al″kuh·lye·therr′uh·pee) *n.* 1. The use of alkalies in treating disease. 2. Administration of large doses of alkaline medication, as for peptic ulcer.
al·ka·lize (al′kuh·lize) *v.* ALKALINIZE. —**al·ka·li·za·tion,** *n.*
al·ka·loid (al′kuh·loid) *n.* [*alkali* + *-oid*]. A naturally occurring, basic, organic, nitrogenous compound, usually of plant origin; found generally as salts of organic acids, sometimes as free bases, esters, amides, or in glycosidic combination. Most are insoluble in water, soluble in organic solvents, and react with acids to form salts which are soluble in water and insoluble in organic solvents. Many alkaloids are medicinally valuable. —**al·ka·loi·dal** (al″kuh·loy′dul) *adj.*
al·ka·lo·sis (al″kuh·lo′sis) *n.,* pl. **alkalo·ses** (·seez) [*alkali* + *-osis*]. An abnormal state characterized by processes tending to decrease the concentration of hydrogen ion in the body below the normal range or to increase the loss of acid from the body; physiological compensatory mechanisms act to return the heightened pH toward normal. Syn. *baseosis.* Compare *alkalemia.* See also *compensated alkalosis, metabolic alkalosis, respiratory alkalosis.* —**alka·lot·ic** (·lot′ic) *adj.*
al·ka·lo·ther·a·py (al″kuh·lo·therr′uh·pee) *n.* ALKALITHERAPY.
al·kane (al′kane) *n.* [*alkyl* + *-ane*]. Any member of the paraffin series of hydrocarbons.
al·ka·net (al′kuh·net) *n.* [Sp. *alcaneta,* from *alcana,* from Ar. *al-ḥinnā',* (the) henna]. The root of the herb *Alkanna tinctoria,* which yields a red dye.
al·kan·nin, al·kan·in (al·kan′in) *n.* A valuable coloring matter obtained from alkanet.
al·kap·ton, al·cap·ton (al·kap′tun, ·tone) *n.* [*alkali* + Gk. *kaptein,* to gulp]. HOMOGENTISIC ACID.
al·kap·ton·uria, al·cap·ton·uria (al·kap″to·nyoo′ree·uh) *n.* [*alkapton* + *-uria*]. A hereditary defect of tyrosine metabolism, due to failure to synthesize active homogentisic acid oxidase in the liver, resulting in excessive excretion of homogentisic acid in the urine; characterized in middle life by darkening of connective tissue (ochronosis) and degenerative changes in joints, cartilage, and intervertebral disks; apparently transmitted, in most cases at least, by an autosomal recessive gene.
al·ka·ver·vir (al″kuh·vur′virr) *n.* [*alkaloid* + *Veratrum viride*]. A fraction of the alkaloids of *Veratrum viride* obtained

by a process involving selective extraction of the crude drug and selective precipitation of the alkaloids; used as a hypotensive.

al·ke·ken·gi (al″ke·ken′jee) *n.* [Ar. *al-kākanj,* (the) ground cherry]. The *Physalis alkekengi,* the winter cherry, or strawberry tomato; its leaves have been used as a diuretic.

al·kene (al′keen) *n.* [*alk*yl + *-ene*]. Any member of the series of unsaturated aliphatic hydrocarbons (ethylene series) having one double bond and represented by the general formula C_nH_{2n}.

alkene series. ETHYLENE SERIES.

Alkeran. Trademark for melphalan, an antineoplastic drug.

al·ker·mes (al·kur′meez, al′kur·meez) *n.* [F., from Ar. *al-qirmiz,* (the) kermes]. KERMES.

alk·ox·ide (al·kock′side, ·sid) *n.* [*alkoxy-* + *-ide*]. Any of a class of salts produced when the hydrogen atom of the hydroxyl group of an alcohol or phenol is replaced by a metal; specific salts are named for the particular alcohol involved, as sodium methoxide for CH_3ONa. Syn. *alcoholate.*

alk·oxy (al·kock′see) *adj.* Of or pertaining to alkoxyl.

alkoxy-. *In chemistry,* a combining form meaning *alkoxyl.*

alk·ox·yl (al·kock′sil) *n.* Any of a class of univalent radicals representing an aliphatic alcohol from which the hydrogen atom of the hydroxyl group is omitted; specific radicals are named for the particular alcohol involved, as methoxyl for CH_3O—.

al·kyl (al′kil, al′keel) *n.* [Ger. *Alk*ohol, alcohol, + *-yl*]. Any one of the univalent saturated hydrocarbon radicals of the general formula C_nH_{2n+1}; as methyl (CH_3), ethyl (C_2H_5), propyl (C_3H_7).

al·kyl·amine (al″kil·uh·meen′, al″kil·am′in) *n.* [*alkyl* + *amine*]. A substance having the constitution of ammonia in which an alkyl replaces hydrogen; one, two, or three hydrogen atoms of the ammonia molecule may be replaced, yielding primary (monalkylamines), secondary (dialkylamines), and tertiary (trialkylamines) alkylamines, respectively.

al·kyl·ate (al′ki·late) *v.* To introduce one or more alkyl radicals into a compound.

al·kyl·a·tion (al″ki·lay′shun) *n.* The introduction of one or more alkyl groups into an organic compound.

al·kyne (al′kine) *n.* [*alk*yl + *-yne*]. Any member of the series of unsaturated aliphatic hydrocarbons having a triple bond and represented by the general formula, C_nH_{2n-2}. Acetylene is the first hydrocarbon of the series, sometimes called the acetylene series.

all-, allo- [Gk. *allos,* other]. A combining form meaning (a) *other, different;* (b) *variant, alternate;* (c) *modified, altered;* (d) *deviant, abnormal;* (e) in chemistry, *an isomer, close relative, or variety of a compound;* (f) *the more stable of two isomers.*

al·la·ches·the·sia, al·la·chaes·the·sia (al″uh·kes·theezh′uh, ·theez′ee·uh) *n.* [Gk. *allachē,* elsewhere, + *esthesia*]. ALLESTHESIA.

allaestheia. ALLESTHESIA.

allant-, allanto-. A combining form meaning (a) *allantoic, allantoid, allantois;* (b) *derived from or related to allantoic acid or allantoin.*

al·lan·to·cho·ri·on (a·lan″to·ko′ree·on) *n.* The allantois and chorion fused together and thus forming a single structure; a chorion supplied by allantoic blood vessels. Syn. *chorion allantoideum.*

al·lan·to·en·ter·ic (a·lan″to·en·terr′ick) *adj.* [*allanto-* + *enteric*]. Pertaining to the allantois and the embryonic gut.

allantoenteric diverticulum. ALLANTOIC DIVERTICULUM.

allantoenteric duct. ALLANTOIC DUCT.

al·lan·to·gen·e·sis (a·lan″to·jen′e·sis) *n.* [*allanto-* + *genesis*]. The development of the allantois.

al·lan·to·ic (al″an·to′ick) *adj.* Pertaining to or contained in the allantois.

allantoic acid. An intermediate product, $C_4H_8N_4O_4$, in the degradation of purines, formed by the action of allantoinase on allantoin.

al·lan·to·ic·ase (al″an·to′i·kase) *n.* An enzyme involved in the degradation of purines in some animals, but not man, which converts allantoic acid to urea and glyoxylic acid.

allantoic bladder. A urinary bladder which develops as an evagination of the cloaca, homologous to the allantoic evagination.

allantoic circulation. UMBILICAL CIRCULATION.

allantoic cyst. Cystic dilatation of the urachus.

allantoic diverticulum. The endodermal diverticulum from the cloaca into the extraembryonic coelom in most amniotes, or into the body stalk in primates, which forms the epithelial lining of the allantois. Syn. *allantoenteric diverticulum.*

allantoic duct. The proximal part of the allantois opening into the cloaca. Syn. *allantoenteric duct.*

allantoic fluid. The fluid contents of the allantois.

allantoic sac. The distal enlarged part of the allantois, especially in Sauropsida. Syn. *allantoic vesicle.*

allantoic stalk. ALLANTOIC DUCT.

allantoic vein. UMBILICAL VEIN.

allantoic vesicle. ALLANTOIC SAC.

al·lan·toid (a·lan′toid) *adj.* [Gk. *allantoeidēs,* sausage-shaped, from *allas, allantos,* sausage]. Of or pertaining to the allantois.

Al·lan·toi·dea (al″an·toy′dee·uh) *n.pl.* [NL., from *allantois*]. *Obsol.* AMNIOTA. —**allantoi·de·an** (·dee·un) *adj.*

al·lan·toi·do·an·gi·op·a·gous (al″an·toy″do·an″jee·op′uh·gus) *adj.* [*allantoid* + *angio-* + *-pagus*]. OMPHALOANGIOPAGOUS.

al·lan·to·in (a·lan′to·in) *n.* [*allanto-* + *-in*]. 5-Ureidohydantoin, $C_4H_6N_4O_3$, a product of purine metabolism; found in allantoic fluid, amniotic fluid, fetal urine, and some plants. Used topically in suppurating wounds and ulcers to accelerate cell proliferation.

al·lan·to·in·ase (al″an·to′i·nace) *n.* An enzyme involved in the degradation of purines in some animals, but not man, which converts allantoin to allantoic acid.

al·lan·to·is (a·lan′to·is, ·toice) *n.,* pl. **al·lan·to·i·des** (al″an·to′i·deez, ·toy′deez) [NL., from Gk. *allantoeidēs,* allantoid, sausage-shaped, from *allas, allantos,* sausage]. An extraembryonic membrane arising as an outgrowth of the cloaca in amniotes. It functions as an organ of respiration and excretion in birds and reptiles and plays an important part in the development of the placenta in most mammals, its blood vessels forming the important pathways for the umbilical circulation.

al·las·so·ther·a·py (a·las″o·therr′uh·pee) *n.* [Gk. *allass*ein, to change, + *therapy*]. Treatment which requires changing the general biologic conditions of the individual.

al·lax·is (a·lack′sis) *n.* [Gk., exchange]. Metamorphosis; transformation.

al·le·go·ri·za·tion (al″e·gor″i·zay′shun) *n.* [from *allegory*]. 1. *In psychiatry,* the formation of neologisms. 2. CONDENSATION (6).

al·lel (a·lel′) *n.* ALLELE.

al·lele (a·leel′) *n.* [Ger. *Allel,* from Gk. *allēlōn,* one another, from *allos,* other]. One of a pair, or of a series, of variants of a gene having the same locus on homologous chromosomes. —**al·le·lic** (a·lee′lick) *adj.*

allelic complementation. An atypical and quantitatively incomplete kind of complementation sometimes occurring between two alleles, presumably because two defective proteins can interact to produce a functional unit.

allelo- [Gk. *allēlōn,* one another]. A combining form meaning (a) *reciprocal, complementary;* (b) *alternate, alternative.*

al·lelo·cat·a·lyt·ic (a·lel″o·kat″uh·lit′ick) *adj.* [*allelo-* + *catalytic*]. 1. Denoting two substances, each decomposing in the presence of the other; mutually catalytic or destructive. 2. Promoting reproduction, as when two or more unicellular organisms are placed in a drop of culture medium, reproduction proceeds more rapidly than when one organism is present. —**allelo·ca·tal·y·sis** (·kuh·tal'i·sis) *n.*

al·le·lo·morph (a·lee'lo·morf, a·lel'o·) *n.* 1. ALLELE. 2. *In chemistry,* one of two or more isomorphic substances that contain the same atoms and of the same valences but differing in the manner of their linkage. 3. *In chemistry,* the first of a mixture of isomers in a solution to separate or crystallize. —**al·le·lo·mor·phic** (a·lee"lo·mor'fick) *adj.;* **allelo·mor·phism** (·mor'fiz·um) *n.*

al·lelo·tax·is (a·lel"o·tack'sis, a·lee"lo·) *n.* [*allelo-* + *-taxis*]. The development of an organ or part from several different embryonic structures.

al·lelo·taxy (a·lel"o·tack'see, a·lee'lo·) *n.* ALLELOTAXIS.

al·lene (al'een) *n.* The gaseous hydrocarbon $CH_2{=}C{=}CH_2$. Syn. *propadiene.*

Al·len's test [E. V. *Allen,* U.S. anatomist, 1892–1943]. A test for radial or ulnar arterial occlusion, in which one of the arteries is compressed after blood has been forced out of the hand by making a tight fist; failure of blood to return to the hand when opened indicates that the artery not compressed has obstruction to blood flow.

Allen's tract. SOLITARY FASCICULUS.

Allen's treatment [F. M. *Allen,* U.S. physician, 20th century]. STARVATION TREATMENT (1).

al·len·the·sis (a·len'thi·sis) *n.* [*all-* + *enthesis*]. Introduction of foreign substances into the body.

Allercur. Trademark for clemizole, an antihistaminic agent used as the hydrochloride salt.

al·ler·gen (al'ur·jen) *n.* A substance capable of inducing an allergy. —**al·ler·gen·ic** (al"ur·jen'ick) *adj.;* **allergen·ic·i·ty** (·is'i·tee) *n.*

al·ler·gic (a·lur'jick) *adj.* Pertaining to or having an allergy.

allergic asthma. Asthma due to allergic mechanisms.

allergic balance. A state of equilibrium between the patient and his environment in which the total amount of noxious allergen does not exceed the patient's threshold of allergic tolerance.

allergic cataract. ATOPIC CATARACT.

allergic conjunctivitis. Conjunctivitis usually characterized by inflammation and lacrimation as an immunologic reaction.

allergic constitution. The inherited tendency to develop allergic states of the atopic variety.

allergic contact dermatitis. Allergic dermatitis due to contact of an allergenic substance with the skin.

allergic coryza. ALLERGIC RHINITIS.

allergic cystitis. A nonspecific inflammation of the urinary bladder, often without pus or bacteria in the urine, apparently caused by a local sensitivity reaction to one or more antigens.

allergic dermal-respiratory syndrome. A complex of atopic dermatitis and seasonal rhinitis and/or asthma.

allergic dermatitis. Dermatitis caused by sensitization and reexposure to an allergenic substance.

allergic eczema. Allergic dermatitis in the form of eczema.

allergic eczematous contact dermatitis. Allergic contact dermatitis, specifically the eczematous form.

allergic encephalomyelitis. EXPERIMENTAL ALLERGIC ENCEPHALOMYELITIS.

allergic granulomatosis. A form of polyarteritis nodosa in which allergic manifestations predominate.

allergic purpura. 1. Any purpura, thrombocytopenic or nonthrombocytopenic, which results from a presumed allergic reaction. Syn. *anaphylactoid purpura.* 2. HENOCH'S PURPURA. 3. SCHÖNLEIN'S PURPURA.

allergic reaction. The response elicited by an allergen after an allergic state has been established. It may be urticarial, eczematous, or tuberculin-type (infiltrative).

allergic rhinitis. Rhinitis which may be caused by any effective allergen, usually an inhalant such as pollen. See also *hay fever.*

allergic urticaria. Wheals caused by sensitization and reexposure to an allergenic substance, usually from ingestion, frequently from injection, rarely from inhalation or contact.

allergic vasculitis. Any of a group of syndromes, such as Henoch-Schönlein purpura or systemic lupus erythematosus, in which the principal underlying pathologic process is inflammation of blood vessels, particularly in the skin, kidneys, and joints; presumed to be due to deposition of antigen-antibody complexes in the vessel walls. Syn. *hypersensitivity angiitis.*

al·ler·gid (al'ur·jid, a·lur'jid) *n.* A lesion of nodular dermal allergid, based on a vasculitis.

al·ler·gist (al'ur·jist) *n.* A physician skilled in the diagnosis and treatment of allergic diseases.

al·ler·gi·za·tion (al"ur·ji·zay'shun) *n.* The process of inducing an allergic transformation.

al·ler·goid (al'ur·goid) *n.* A formalin-modified allergen used in hyposensitization therapy for allergic diseases.

al·ler·go·sis (al"ur·go'sis) *n.,* pl. **allergo·ses** (·seez) Any condition associated with an allergic state.

al·ler·gy (al'ur·jee) *n.* [Ger. *Allergie,* from *all-,* altered, from Gk. *allos,* other, + Gk. *ergon,* action]. A condition of acquired, specific alteration in biologic reactivity, initiated by exposure to an allergen and, after an incubation period, characterized by evocation of the altered reactivity upon reexposure to the same or a closely related allergen.

Al·les·che·ria (al"es·keer'ee·uh) *n.* A genus of fungi of the class Ascomycetes.

Allescheria boyd·ii (boy'dee·eye). The species regarded as one of the causes of mycetoma; it produces white or yellowish white granules. It is the perfect stage of *Monosporium apiospermum.*

al·les·the·sia, al·laes·the·sia (al"es·theezh'uh, ·theez'ee·uh) *n.* [*all-* + *esthesia*]. A disorder of discriminative sensation in which a stimulus is perceived as at a point on the body which is in fact remote from the point stimulated; usually associated with a lesion of the parietal lobe. Compare *allochiria.*

al·le·thrin (al'e·thrin) *n.* [*allyl* + py*rethrin*]. A liquid insecticidal chemical representing (±)-2-allyl-4-hydroxy-3-methyl-2-cyclopenten-1-one esterified with a mixture of *cis-* and *trans-dl-*chrysanthemum monocarboxylic acid.

al·li·cin (al'i·sin) *n.* The antibacterial, sulfur-containing principle obtained from common garlic (*Allium sativum*).

allied reflexes. Two separate reflexes elicited from widely separated regions of the body, producing common or reinforced protagonistic actions.

al·li·ga·tion (al"li·gay'shun) *n.* [L. *alligatio,* a binding together, from *ad-,* to, + *ligare,* to tie]. *In pharmacy,* the formula for solving problems concerning the mixing of solutions of different percentages; the rule of mixtures. If two substances when mixed retain the specific values of a property, the value of the mixture can be calculated from the equation $(aA + bB) / (a + b)$, where a and b are the proportions and A and B equal the respective values for the property.

al·li·ga·tor forceps. 1. A special type of forceps having long, slender angulated handles designed to be used with such instruments as an operating cystoscope or proctoscope. 2. A strong toothed forceps having a double lever, used in orthopedic surgery.

alligator-skin disease. A severe form of ichthyosis.

Al·ling·ham's operation (al'ing·um). 1. [Herbert W. *Allingham,* English surgeon, 1862–1904]. Inguinal colostomy just above the inguinal ligament. 2. [William *Allingham,* English surgeon, 1830–1908]. A type of rectal extirpation for cancer by an incision around the bowel into both ischiorectal fossae and back to the coccyx.

Al·lis's forceps [O. H. *Allis,* U.S. surgeon, 1836–1921]. A surgical forceps with fine, interlocking teeth which are adapted especially to securing and holding intestine, stomach wall, and other hollow viscera, without crushing them during surgical operations.

Allis's sign [O. H. *Allis*]. 1. When the hip is dislocated as in congenital acetabular dysplasia, the affected thigh is foreshortened when the level of the knees is viewed with both hips and knees flexed 90°. 2. When the neck of the femur is fractured, the fascia between the greater trochanter and the crest of the ilium is less tense than normally.

al·lit·er·a·tion (a·lit″ur·ay′shun) *n.* [*ad-* + L. *litera,* letter]. A form of dysphasia in which the patient chooses words with the same consonant sounds.

Al·li·um (al′ee·um) *n.* [L., garlic]. A genus of bulbous plants of the Liliaceae family, species of which include garlic, onion, leek, and chives.

allium, *n.* Any plant, bulb, or flower of the genus *Allium;* specifically, the bulb of garlic (*Allium sativum*); formerly used for the treatment of various ailments.

allo-. See *all-.*

al·lo·al·bu·mi·ne·mia, al·lo·al·bu·mi·nae·mia (al″o·al·bew″mi·nee′mee·uh) *n.* [*allo-* + *albumin* + *-emia*]. A condition, apparently inherited and which may not manifest any clinical abnormality, in which a variant of the common albumin is present in blood serum.

al·lo·bar·bi·tal (al″lo·bahr′bi·tol, ·tal) *n.* 5,5-Diallylbarbituric acid, $C_{10}H_{12}N_2O_3$, a sedative and hypnotic of intermediate to long duration of action. Syn. *diallylbarbituric acid.*

allochaesthesia. Allochesthesia (= ALLESTHESIA).

allocheiria. ALLOCHIRIA.

al·lo·chem·ic (al″o·kem′ick) *adj.* [*allo-* + *chem-* + *-ic*]. Pertaining to interactions (other than purely nutritional ones) involving chemicals by which organisms of one species affect the growth, health, behavior, or population of those of another species.

al·lo·ches·the·sia, al·lo·chaes·the·sia (al″o·kes·theez′ee·uh, ·theezh′uh) *n.* ALLESTHESIA.

al·lo·che·tia (al″o·kee′shee·uh, ·kee′tee·uh) *n.* ALLOCHEZIA.

al·lo·che·zia (al″o·kee′zee·uh) *n.* [*allo-* + Gk. *chezein*, to defecate, + *-ia*]. 1. The passage of feces from the body through an abnormal opening. 2. The passing of nonfecal matter from the bowels.

al·lo·chi·ria, al·lo·chei·ria (al″o·kigh′ree·uh, al″o·keer′ee·uh) *n.* [*allo-* + *chir-* + *-ia*]. A disorder of discriminative sensation in which a stimulus applied to one part of the body is perceived as if at a corresponding point on the opposite side; usually associated with a lesion of the parietal lobe. Compare *allesthesia.*

al·lo·cho·les·ter·ol (al″o·ko·les′tur·ole, ·ol) *n.* [*allo-* + *cholesterol*]. A sterol found in wool fat.

al·lo·cor·tex (al″o·kor′tecks) *n.* [*allo-* + *cortex*]. The areas or portions of the cerebral cortex where lamination is absent or incomplete, as the olfactory cortex, representing less developed or more primitive areas. Syn. *heterogenetic cortex, heterotypical cortex.*

al·loe·o·sis (al″ee·o′sis) *n.* [Gk. *alloiōsis,* alteration]. 1. A change; alterative effect; recovery from illness. 2. A change or alteration in the character of a constitution or a disease. **—alloe·ot·ic** (·ot′ick) *adj. & n.*

al·lo·erot·i·cism (al″o·e·rot′i·siz·um) *n.* ALLOEROTISM.

al·lo·er·o·tism (al″o·err′o·tiz·um) *n.* [*allo-* + *erotism*]. The tendency to seek sexual gratification from another. Contr. *autoerotism.*

al·lo·ge·ne·ic (al″o·je·nee′ick) *adj.* ALLOGENIC.

allogeneic homograft or **graft.** ALLOGRAFT.

al·lo·gen·ic (al″o·jen′ick) *adj.* [*allo-* + *-genic*]. Differing in genotype. Contr. *isogenic.*

allogenic transformation. *In bacterial genetics,* reciprocal transformation of two mutants to the wild type by the action of a transforming principle obtained from the other.

allogenic transplantation. ALLOGRAFT.

al·lo·graft (al″o·graft) *n.* [*allo-* + *graft*]. A tissue graft taken from a genetically nonidentical donor of the same species as the recipient. Syn. *homograft.* Compare *autograft.* Contr. *heterograft.*

al·lo·iso·leu·cine (al″o·eye″so·lew′seen) *n.* Either of the pair of stereoisomers, D-alloisoleucine and L-alloisoleucine, resulting from inversion of D- or L-isoleucine about one of the two asymmetric carbon atoms of the latter compounds. The L-form of alloisoleucine is found in the plasma of patients with maple syrup urine disease.

allometric equation. The power function, $y = bx^k$, to which many data in studies of relative growth conform. In the equation, y is a part, x the whole or another part of the organism, and b and k are constants.

al·lom·e·try (a·lom′e·tree) *n.* [*allo-* + *-metry*]. Variations in the relative size of a part, either in the course of an organism's growth or within a series of related organisms, or the measurement and study of such variations. See also *allomorphosis, heterauxesis.* **—al·lo·met·ric** (al″o·met′rick) *adj.*

al·lo·mor·phism (al″o·mor′fiz·um) *n.* [*allo-* + *morph-* + *-ism*]. The property possessed by certain substances of assuming a different crystalline form while remaining unchanged in chemical constitution. **—allo·mor·phic** (·mor′fick), **allomor·phous** (·fus) *adj.;* **al·lo·morph** (al′o·morf) *n.*

al·lo·mor·pho·sis (al″o·mor′fuh·sis, ·mor·fo′sis) *n.,* pl. **allomor·pho·ses** (·seez) [*allo-* + *morphosis*]. Allometric variation in a series of genetically different but related organisms, such as variation in relation of jaw length to skull length of the adult in a series of breeds of dogs. Contr. *heterauxesis.*

al·lo·path (al′o·path) *n.* [*allo-* + *-path*]. 1. A practitioner of allopathy (1). 2. As used by homeopaths: a regular medical practitioner.

al·lop·a·thist (a·lop′uh·thist) *n.* ALLOPATH.

al·lop·a·thy (a·lop′uth·ee) *n.* [*allo-* + *-pathy*]. 1. A system of medical treatment using remedies that produce effects upon the body differing from those produced by disease; the opposite of the homeopathic system. 2. As used by homeopaths: the regular medical profession. **—al·lo·path·ic** (al″o·path′ick) *adj.*

al·loph·a·sis (a·lof′uh·sis) *n.* [Gk., from *allo-* + *phasis,* utterance]. Incoherent, delirious speech.

al·lo·plasm (al′o·plaz·um) *n.* [*allo-* + *plasm*]. Functionally differentiated material derived from the protoplasm, such as flagella, cilia, or fibrils.

al·lo·plast (al′o·plast) *n.* [*allo-* + *-plast*]. *In biology,* a plastic compound of two or more tissues, as opposed to homoplast.

al·lo·plas·ty (al′o·plas″tee) *n.* [*allo-* + *-plasty*]. 1. A plastic operation in which material from outside the human body is utilized, such as stainless steel. Compare *heteroplasty.* 2. *In psychoanalysis,* the process whereby the libido of the growing individual directs its energies away from self and toward other individuals and objects as in acting out. **—al·lo·plas·tic** (al″o·plas′tick) *adj.*

al·lo·poly·ploid (al″o·pol′i·ploid) *adj. & n.* [*allo-* + *polyploid*]. 1. Having more than two complete sets of chromosomes derived from different species. 2. A hybrid with more than two complete sets of chromosomes derived from different species.

al·lo·poly·ploi·dy (al″o·pol′i·ploy″dee) *n.* The condition of having more than two complete sets of chromosomes derived from different species.

al·lo·preg·nane (al″o·preg′nane) *n.* 17-Ethylandrostane, $C_{21}H_{36}$, a saturated, solid, steroid hydrocarbon, a chemical and structural, but not biological, parent substance of adrenal cortical and certain other hormones. Syn. *5α-pregnane.*

al·lo·psy·chic (al″o·sigh′kick) *adj.* [*allo-* + *psychic*]. Pertaining to mental processes in their relation to the outside world. Contr. *autopsychic.*

al·lo·pu·ri·nol (al″o·pew′ri·nol) *n.* 1*H*-Pyrazolo[3,4-*d*]pyrimidin-4-ol, $C_5H_4N_4O$, a xanthine oxidase inhibitor which reduces the production of uric acid.

β-D-al·lo·py·ra·nose (al″o·pye′ruh·noce) *n.* [*allo-* + *pyranose*]. ALLOSE.

al·lo·rhyth·mia (al″o·rith′mee·uh) *n.* [*allo-* + *rhythm* + *-ia*]. An irregularity of cardiac rhythm. —**allorhyth·mic** (·mick) *adj.*

all-or-none law. The response of a single fiber of cardiac muscle, skeletal muscle, or nerve to an adequate stimulus is always maximal. The strength of response when a whole muscle or nerve trunk is stimulated depends upon the number of fibers stimulated.

all-or-nothing law. ALL-OR-NONE LAW.

al·lose (al′oce) *n.* An aldohexose sugar, $C_6H_{12}O_6$, stereoisomeric with D-glucose, prepared by synthesis; it is more exactly denoted as D-allose, or β-D-allopyranose.

al·lo·some (al′o·sohm) *n.* [*allo-* + *-some*]. 1. Originally, any chromosome distinguished from ordinary chromosomes (autosomes) by certain peculiarities of form, size, and behavior; usually a sex chromosome. Syn. *heterochromosome.* See also *accessory chromosome.* 2. A cytoplasmic inclusion introduced from without.

al·lo·ster·ic (al″o·steer′ick, ·sterr′) *adj.* [*allo-* + *steric*]. Pertaining to an alteration at one site that affects function at another site.

allosteric effector. A small molecule that produces an allosteric alteration in a protein. Syn. *modulator.*

allosteric protein. A protein with two independent specificities, one for function, as with the active site of an enzyme, and one for interaction with an inhibitor or an effector which thereby modifies the function of the active site.

allosteric site. An enzymic site, other than the active site, which noncompetitively binds molecules other than the substrate.

al·lo·syn·ap·sis (al″o·si·nap′sis) *n.*, pl. **allosynap·ses** (·seez) [*allo-* + *synapsis*]. A form of synapsis in hybrids, characterized by pairing between the chromosomes of both species. Syn. *allosyndesis.* Contr. *autosyndesis.*

al·lo·syn·de·sis (al″o·sin′de·sis) *n.* [*allo-* + *syndesis*]. ALLOSYNAPSIS.

al·lo·therm (al′o·thurm) *n.* [*allo-* + *-therm*]. An organism whose temperature is directly dependent upon that of its environment. —**allother·my** (·ee) *n.;* **al·lo·ther·mic** (al″o·thurm′ick) *adj.*

allotri-, allotrio- [Gk. *allotrios,* from *allos,* other]. A combining form meaning *strange, unusual, abnormal.*

al·lot·ri·o·don·tia (a·lot″ree·o·don′chee·uh) *n.* [*allotri-* + *-odontia*]. 1. The transplantation of teeth. 2. Occurrence of teeth in abnormal places, as in teratomas.

al·lot·rio·geu·sia (a·lot″ree·o·gew′zee·uh, ·joo′zee·uh) *n.* [*allotrio-* + *-geusia*]. 1. A perverted sense of taste. 2. Abnormal appetite.

al·lo·trio·lith (al″o·trye′o·lith, a·lot′ree·o·lith) *n.* [*allotrio-* + *-lith*]. A stone or calculus found in an unusual location, or of unusual composition.

al·lot·rio·pha·gia (a·lot″ree·o·fay′jee·uh) *n.* ALLOTRIOPHAGY.

al·lot·ri·oph·a·gy (a·lot″ree·off′uh·jee) *n.* [Gk. *allotriophagia,* eating the food of others, from *allotrio-* + *phagein,* to eat]. PICA.

al·lot·ri·uria (a·lot″ree·yoo′ree·uh) *n.* [*allotri-* + *-uria*]. Abnormality of the urine.

al·lo·trope (al′o·trope) *n.* [*allo-* + *-trope*]. One of the forms in which an element capable of assuming different forms may appear.

al·lo·troph·ic (al″o·trof′ick) *adj.* [*allo-* + *-trophic*]. Altered or modified so as to become less nutritious.

al·lo·trop·ic (al″o·trop′ick) *adj.* [*allo-* + *-tropic*]. 1. Pertaining to, or exhibiting, allotropy. 2. *In psychiatry,* characterizing a person who is preoccupied with what "other people" think, mean, or do.

al·lot·ro·pism (a·lot′ro·piz·um) *n.* ALLOTROPY.

al·lot·ro·py (a·lot′ruh·pee) *n.* [*allo-* + *-tropy*]. 1. The occurrence of an element in two or more distinct forms with differences in physical properties, as carbon, phosphorus, and sulfur. 2. Appearance in an unusual or abnormal form. 3. An attraction or tropism between different cells or structures, as between sperms and ova. 4. The manifestation of an allotropic personality.

al·lo·tryl·ic (al″o·tril′ick) *adj.* [*allotri-* + Gk. *hylē,* material, + *-ic*]. Caused by a strange or foreign principle or material.

al·lo·type (al′o·tipe) *n.* [*allo-* + *type*]. A genetically determined variant demonstrable by isoimmunization.

allox-. A combining form meaning *alloxan.*

al·lox·an (al′ock·san″, a·lock′sun) *n.* [*al*lantoin + *ox*alic + *-an*]. 2,4,5,6(1*H*,3*H*)-Pyrimidinetetrone, $C_4H_2N_2O_4$, obtainable by oxidation of uric acid. It has been found in the intestinal mucus during diarrhea and is used for the production of experimental diabetes through selective necrosis of the islets of Langerhans.

alloxan diabetes. Severe hyperglycemia and degeneration of the beta cells of the pancreas following the experimental administration of alloxan to animals.

al·lox·a·zine (a·lock′suh·zeen) *n.* [*allox-* + *azine*]. 1. The three-ring heterocylic compound pyrimido[4,5-*b*]quinoxaline-2,4(1*H*,3*H*)dione, $C_{10}H_6N_4O_2$. 2. Loosely, any derivative of alloxazine. 3. Sometimes, isoalloxazine and its derivatives.

al·lox·uria (al″ocks·yoo′ree·uh) *n.* [*allox-* + *-uria*]. The presence of purines in the urine. —**al·lox·ur** (al·ocks′ur, ·yoor), **al·lox·uric** (al″ocks·yoo′rick) *adj.*

all·spice, *n.* 1. PIMENTA. 2. Any of several other aromatic shrubs, such as the Carolina allspice, whose leaves have been used as an aromatic stimulant. It contains two toxic alkaloids.

al·lyl (al′il) *n.* [*all*ium + *-yl*]. The univalent radical $—CH_2CH{=}CH_2$ or $C_3H_5—$.

al·lyl·amine (al″il·am′in, ·a·meen′) *n.* 2-Propenylamine, C_3H_7N, a lacrimatory liquid with a strong ammoniacal odor; employed in the synthesis of medicinals.

al·lyl·ene (al′il·een) *n.* [*allyl* + *-ene*]. $HC{\equiv}CCH_3$, a gaseous hydrocarbon of the alkyne series. Syn. *methylacetylene, propyne.*

al·lyl·iso·bu·tyl·bar·bi·tu·ric acid (al″il·eye″so·bew″til·bahr″bi·tew′rick). BUTALBITAL.

al·lyl·iso·pro·pyl·bar·bi·tur·ic acid (al″il·eye″so·pro″pil·bahr″bi·tew′rick). APROBARBITAL.

allyl isosulfocyanate. ALLYL ISOTHIOCYANATE.

allyl isothiocyanate. C_3H_5NCS. Volatile oil of mustard, a colorless or pale yellow liquid, soluble in alcohol. Syn. *allyl mustard oil, allyl isosulfocyanate.*

allyl mustard oil. ALLYL ISOTHIOCYANATE.

***N*-al·lyl·nor·mor·phine** (al″il·nor·mor′feen) *n.* NALORPHINE.

allyl sulfide. $(C_3H_5)_2S$. A liquid of garlic-like odor, possibly present in garlic; has been used in cholera and tuberculosis.

al·ma·drate sulfate (al′muh·drate) *n.* Aluminum magnesium hydroxide oxide sulfate hydrate, $[(OH)_2AlOAl(OH)OMg]_2SO_4nH_2O$, an antacid.

Al·mén's reagent (ahl·meyn′) [A. T. *Almén,* Swedish physiologist, 1833–1903]. A solution of 5g tannic acid in 240 ml 50% alcohol to which is added 10 ml 25% acetic acid; used for detection in urine of nucleoprotein, with which it produces a precipitate.

al·mond (ah′mund, am′und, al′mund) *n.* [OF., from Gk. *amygdalē*]. The seed of *Prunus amygdalus,* a small tree widely cultivated in warm temperate regions of the world.

almond oil. The fixed oil from the kernels of varieties of *Prunus amygdalus* (*Amygdalus communis*); used as an emollient, a demulcent, and a nutrient. Syn. *sweet almond oil.*

alo·bar (ay·lo′bur, ·bahr) *adj.* [*a-* + *lobe* + *-ar*]. Not lobed; having no lobes.

alo·chia (a·lo′kee·uh) *n.* Absence of the lochia.

Al·oe (al′o·ee) *n.* [Gk. *aloē*]. A genus of liliaceous plants.

al·oe (al′o, al′o·ee) *n.* The dried juice of the leaves of *Aloe perryi, A. barbadensis, A. ferox,* and hybrids of this species with *A. africana* and *A. spicata.* A cathartic, its purgative properties are due to three pentosides (barbaloin, isobarbaloin, and beta-barbaloin) and to a resin. Syn. *aloes.*

al·oe-em·o·din (al'o em'o·din) *n.* 1,8-Dihydroxy-3-hydroxymethylanthraquinone, $C_{15}H_{10}O_5$, occurring in the free state and as glycoside in various species of aloe, also in rhubarb and in senna. It is an irritant cathartic.

al·oes (al'oze) *n.* ALOE.

alo·et·ic (al″o·et'ick) *adj.* Containing or pertaining to aloe.

alo·e·tin (al″o·ee'tin, ·et'in) *n.* 1. An aloe resin. 2. A yellow, crystalline principle obtainable from aloes.

alo·gia (a·lo'jee·uh) *n.* [Gk., irrationality; speechlessness, amazement, from *alogos,* speechless; irrational]. 1. Psychological or aphasic inability to speak. 2. Stupid or senseless behavior.

al·o·in (al'o·in) *n.* A mixture of active principles, chiefly barbaloin and iso-barbaloin, obtained from aloe. Used as laxative and purgative.

alon·i·mid (a·lon'i·mid) *n.* Spiro[naphthalene-1(4*H*),3′-piperidine]-2′,4,6′-trione, $C_{14}H_{13}NO_3$, a sedative and hypnotic agent.

al·o·pe·cia (al″o·pee'shee·uh, ·see·uh) *n.* [Gk. *alōpekia,* baldness, mange on foxes, from *alōpēx,* fox]. Loss of hair, usually from the scalp; may be partial or total, congenital, premature, or senile; baldness; CALVITIES. —**alope·cic** (·sick) *adj.*

alopecia ad·na·ta (ad·nay'tuh). ALOPECIA CONGENITALIS.

alopecia ar·e·a·ta (ăr″ee·ay'tuh, air″ee·ay'tuh). Loss of hair in circumscribed patches with little or no inflammation. The scalp and beard areas are usually involved.

alopecia cic·a·tri·sa·ta (sick″uh·tri·say'tuh). Circular and irregular patches of alopecia due to closely set points of inflammation and atrophy of the skin, causing permanent baldness of the area affected, usually the vertex. Syn. *pseudopelade.*

alopecia cir·cum·scrip·ta (sur″kum·skrip'tuh). ALOPECIA AREATA.

alopecia con·gen·i·ta·lis (kon·jen″i·tay'lis). An uncommon form of baldness apparent from birth, due to absence of hair follicles.

alopecia mu·ci·no·sa (mew″si·no'suh). Circumscribed patches of loss of hair, particularly on the face, attended by mucinous degeneration of the structure of the hair follicle; may be primary or a complication of malignant lymphoma.

alopecia pre·ma·tu·ra (pree″ma·tew'ruh). Baldness which occurs between puberty and middle life and resembles the senile type. The hair gradually thins and falls out in the male pattern, i.e., in frontal recession or on the vertex.

alopecia se·ni·lis (se·nigh'lis). Baldness which occurs in old age in the form of gradual thinning of the hair.

alopecia syph·i·lit·i·ca (sif″i·lit'i·kuh). Transient baldness occurring in the second stage of syphilis in the form of a "moth-eaten" appearance in the temporoparietal regions.

alopecia to·ta·lis (to·tay'lis). Complete baldness of the scalp, an extension of alopecia areata. Compare *alopecia universalis.*

alopecia uni·ver·sa·lis (yoo″ni·vur·say'lis). Loss of hair from all parts of the body, related to alopecia areata. Compare *alopecia totalis.*

Al·pers' disease [B. J. *Alpers,* U.S. neurologist, b. 1900]. PROGRESSIVE CEREBRAL POLIODYSTROPHY.

al·pha (al'fuh) *n.* [name of the letter A, α, first letter of the Greek alphabet]. The first of a series, or any particular member or subset of an arbitrarily ordered set; as in chemistry, often combined with the name of a compound to distinguish isomers or otherwise related substances. For many terms so designated, see under the specific noun. Symbol, α.

alpha-adrenergic, α-adrenergic. Of or pertaining to an alpha-adrenergic receptor.

alpha-adrenergic blocking agent, α-adrenergic blocking agent. Any agent, such as azapetine, phentolamine, and tolazoline, that combines with and causes blockade of the alpha-adrenergic receptor.

alpha-adrenergic receptor, α-adrenergic receptor. A postulated locus of action of adrenergic (sympathomimetic) agents at which primarily excitatory responses are elicited. Epinephrine is the most potent activator of this receptor. Contr. *beta-adrenergic receptor.*

alpha angle. The angle formed by intersection of the optic and visual axes at the nodal point of the eye. In myopia, the alpha angle is smaller than normal and the eye appears to converge; in hypermetropia, the angle is larger than normal and the eye appears to diverge.

alpha-blocking, α-blocking. Having the properties of an alpha-adrenergic blocking agent.

alpha cells. 1. Certain granular cells in the pancreatic islets. 2. Cells containing acidophil granules in the adenohypophysis.

alpha chain, α chain. The heavy chain of the IgA immunoglobulin molecule.

alpha chymotrypsin. A form of chymotrypsin.

Alphadrol. Trademark for fluprednisolone, an anti-inflammatory adrenocortical steroid.

alpha examination. ALPHA TEST.

alpha globulin, α-globulin. Any of the group of serum globulins having the greatest mobility on electrophoresis, including globulins that function in the transport of lipids, carbohydrates, thyroid hormone, and copper.

alpha-1,4 glucosidase. α-1,4 Glucosidase (= ACID MALTASE).

alpha granules. 1. The acidophil granules in the alpha cells of the adenohypophysis. 2. The acidophil granules in the cells of the pancreatic islets.

alpha helix, α-helix. A common spatial configuration of the polypeptide chains of proteins in which the chain assumes a helical form, 5.4 Å in pitch, 3.6 amino acids per turn, held together by hydrogen bonds between carbonyl and amino groups of different amino acids, and presenting the tertiary appearance of a hollow cylinder with radiating side groups.

alpha hemolysin, α-hemolysin. An exotoxin of *Staphylococcus aureus* that is hemolytic for rabbit red blood cells, dermonecrotic, and acutely lethal. Syn. *alpha lysin, necrotoxin.*

alpha hemolysis, α-hemolysis. Partial lysis of red cells on a blood agar medium, resulting in a green discoloration. Contr. *beta hemolysis.*

alpha-hemolytic, α-hemolytic. Causing alpha hemolysis; said of various bacteria, especially certain streptococci.

al·pha-hy·poph·a·mine (al'fuh high·pof'uh·meen, ·min) *n.* The oxytocin obtained from the posterior portion of the hypophysis.

alpha index. *In electroencephalography,* the percentage of time during which the electroencephalogram shows alpha rhythm.

alpha-iodine, *n.* THYROXINE.

alpha-lobeline, *n.* An alkaloid, $C_{22}H_{27}NO_2$, from lobelia; has been used as a respiratory stimulant.

alpha lysin. ALPHA HEMOLYSIN.

alpha methyldopa. METHYLDOPA.

al·pha·naph·thol (al″fuh·naf'thol) *n.* An isomer of betanaphthol; has been used as a local antiseptic and occasionally as an intestinal antiseptic.

al·pha-naph·thyl·thio·urea (al'fuh naf″thil·thigh″o·yoo·ree'uh) *n.* ANTU.

Alpha Omega Alpha. AΩA, the national medical honor society in the United States. Abbreviated, *AOA.*

alpha particle. A charged particle emitted from the nucleus of a radioactive atom, strongly ionizing, but weakly penetrating; a helium nucleus consisting of two protons and two neutrons, with a double positive charge and a mass of 4.0028 atomic mass units.

al·pha·pro·dine (al″fuh·pro'deen) *n.* *dl-α*-1,3-Dimethyl-4-

phenyl-4-propionoxypiperidine, $C_{16}H_{23}NO_2$, a synthetic narcotic used to relieve pain. Syn. *prisilidene.*

alpha rays. Positively charged helium nuclei emitted from radioactive substances. See also *alpha particle.*

alpha-receptor, α-receptor. ALPHA-ADRENERGIC RECEPTOR.

alpha rhythm. *In electroencephalography,* electrical oscillations or waves occurring at a rate of 8 to 13 per second. See also *Berger rhythm.*

alpha streptococci. A group of streptococci that causes alpha hemolysis. See also *viridans streptococci.*

alpha test. A series of eight types of intelligence tests designed for group application and for rapid scoring of soldiers able to read; first used by the U.S. Army in World War I.

alpha tocopherol, α-tocopherol. The most potent form of tocopherol.

alpha wave. See *alpha rhythm.*

al·phos (al'fos) *n.* [Gk., a kind of white "leprosy" or psoriasis]. 1. PSORIASIS. 2. LEPROSY.

al·pho·sis (al·fo'sis) *n.* [*alphos* + *-osis*]. LEUKODERMA.

al·pho·zone (al'fo·zone) *n.* Succinyl peroxide, $(HOOCCH_2CH_2CO)_2O_2$, used as a germicide in dilute aqueous solutions.

al·phus (al'fus) *n.* ALPHOS.

al·pine papilla (al·pine). A narrow and elongated papilla of the corium; seen in several skin diseases.

Al·port's syndrome [A. C. *Alport,* S. African physician, 1880–1959]. A hereditary syndrome characterized by variable degrees of renal failure often associated with progressive bilateral neurosensory hearing loss and occasionally with ocular abnormalities; thought to be transmitted as an autosomal dominant trait with variable penetrance, although in some families males are more frequently and severely affected than females, thus suggesting a sex linkage. Syn. *hereditary nephritis.*

al·pra·zo·lam (al·pray'zo·lam) *n.* 8-Chloro-1-methyl-6-phenyl-4*H*-1,2,4-triazole[4,3-*a*][1,4]benzodiazepine, $C_{17}H_{13}ClN_4$, a tranquilizer.

al·pre·no·lol (al·pren'o·lol) *n.* 1-(*o*-Allylphenoxy)-2-(isopropylamino)-2-propanol, $C_{15}H_{23}NO_2$, a beta-adrenergic receptor antagonist; used as the hydrochloride salt.

al·ser·ox·y·lon (al"sur·ock'si·lon) *n.* A fat-soluble alkaloidal fraction from the root of *Rauwolfia serpentina;* has the sedative, antihypertensive, and bradycrotic actions of reserpine and other alkaloids of the root.

Al·sto·nia (awl·sto'nee·uh) *n.* [C. *Alston,* Scottish physician, 1683–1760]. A genus of trees and shrubs of the Apocynaceae.

al·ter (awl'tur) *v.* [ML. *alterare,* from L. *alter,* other]. 1. To change or cause to become different in one or more characteristics. 2. To castrate.

al·ter·ant (awl'tur·unt) *adj. & n.* ALTERATIVE.

alteration ca·vi·taire (kav·i·tare') [F.]. Intracellular edema of epidermal cells, resulting in the formation of multilocular bullae.

al·ter·a·tive (awl'tur·uh·tive) *adj. & n.* 1. Changing; reestablishing healthy nutritive processes. 2. Any medicine that alters the processes of nutrition, restoring, in some unknown way, the normal functions of an organ or of the system. Arsenic, iodine, the iodides, mercury, and gold formerly were classed as alteratives.

al·ter ego (awl"tur ee'go) [L., lit., another "I"]. An individual so close to one's own character as to seem a second self.

al·ter·ego·ism (awl"tur·ee'go·iz·um, ·eg'o·iz·um) *n.* [*alter ego* + *-ism*]. Consideration or empathy for only those who are in the same situation as oneself.

Al·ter·nar·ia (awl"tur·nair'ee·uh, ·năr'ee·uh) *n.* A genus of fungi of the Dematiaceae family.

al·ter·nar·ic acid (awl"tur·nair'ick, ·năr'ick). An antibiotic substance derived from the fungus *Alternaria solani* that has negligible antibacterial activity but is inhibitory to some fungi.

al·ter·nate case method. The use of a drug or test on alternate patients with the same disease process, to determine the value of the drug or the test.

alternate hemianesthesia. CROSSED ANESTHESIA.

alternate hemiplegia. CROSSED PARALYSIS.

alternate host. INTERMEDIATE HOST.

alternate paired-case method. A method of investigating the efficacy of a drug or a test, by pairing patients with similar characteristics and extent of disease; one drug or test is used on one of the pair and compared with another drug or test used on the alternate of the pair.

al·ter·nat·ing calculus. A calculus composed of alternating layers of its constituents.

alternating current. Electric current that changes its direction with a characteristic frequency, commonly expressed in hertz (cycles per second). Abbreviated, AC. Contr. *direct current.*

alternating dominance of the eyes. Dominance of one eye at one time or for one function, alternating with that of the other eye for another time or function.

alternating hemiplegia. CROSSED PARALYSIS.

alternating hermaphroditism. LATERAL HERMAPHRODITISM.

alternating insanity or **psychosis.** MANIC-DEPRESSIVE ILLNESS.

alternating mydriasis. Mydriasis that, by normal light and convergence reaction, attacks first one eye and then the other; due to disorder of the central nervous system. Syn. *leaping mydriasis, springing mydriasis.*

alternating paralysis. CROSSED PARALYSIS.

alternating personality. *Obsol.* MULTIPLE PERSONALITY.

alternating pressure pad. An inflatable pad, used to prevent decubitus ulcers, that fits on top of a conventional mattress. The thickness of various segments of the pad changes at frequent intervals by means of an electrically operated pressure system.

alternating pulse. PULSUS ALTERNANS.

alternating strabismus. Strabismus in which either eye fixes alternately and the other eye deviates.

alternating sursumduction. A condition characterized by the upward movement of one eye while the other is fixed, seen in many normal individuals when fatigued or daydreaming, as well as in patients with strabismus.

alternating tremor. The involuntary rhythmic oscillations, averaging 4 hertz (cycles per second) with brief and equal pauses between cycles and an amplitude of 5 to 45°, produced by the regular sequential contractions of the agonistic and antagonistic muscles of a part (such as the head, hand, or a digit) and only in the waking state; due to a wide variety of lesions involving the basal ganglia, substantia nigra, and related pathways.

al·ter·na·tion, *n.* 1. The act or process of alternating or of performing alternately. 2. *In neurophysiology,* the phenomenon whereby only every other impulse is carried over the eighth cranial (vestibulocochlear) nerve when the exciting impulse is from 900 to 1800 hertz (cycles per second). Because of the refractory period of nerve impulses, the maximum frequency that can be carried by a nerve is about 900 hertz.

alternation of generations. *In biology,* the succession of asexual and sexual individuals in a life history, such as the alternation of polyp and medusa in the life cycle of many coelenterates.

al·ter·na·tor, *n.* An apparatus for converting direct current into alternating current.

Alt·hau·sen test (awlt'haow·zun) [T. L. *Althausen,* U.S. physician, b. 1897]. GALACTOSE TOLERANCE TEST.

al·thea (al·thee'uh) *n.* Marshmallow root. The peeled root of *Althaea officinalis,* a plant of the mallow family. It contains starch, gum, pectin, sugar, and asparagin. Has been used in the form of a decoction as a demulcent; also as a pill excipient.

Althesin. A trademark for a mixture of alfaxalone and alfadolone acetate used as an intravenous anesthetic.

al·thi·a·zide (al·thigh'uh·zide) *n.* 3-[(Allylthio)methyl]-6-chloro-3,4-dihydro-2*H*-1,2,4-benzothiadiazine-7-sulfonamide 1,1-dioxide, $C_{11}H_{14}ClN_3O_4S_3$, an antihypertensive drug.

alt. hor. Abbreviation for *alternis horis,* every other hour.

al·ti·tude alkalosis. Respiratory alkalosis resulting from hyperventilation during acclimatization to high altitude.

altitude sickness. A symptom complex resulting from the hypoxia encountered at high altitudes. The acute type is characterized by breathlessness, hyperventilation, lightheadedness, headache, malaise, irritability, and rarely by acute pulmonary edema. The chronic type (Monge's disease) usually occurs with acclimatization to altitudes above 15,000 feet and is manifested by polycythemia, vascular occlusions, gastrointestinal ulceration, and cardiac failure.

al·ti·tu·di·nal hemianopsia. HORIZONTAL HEMIANOPSIA.

altitudinal index. LENGTH-HEIGHT INDEX.

Alt·mann-Gersh method [R. *Altmann,* German histologist, 1852–1900; and I. *Gersh,* U.S. anatomist, b. 1907]. A method for fixing tissue by quickly freezing a specimen at -30°C and then dehydrating it.

Altmann's granules [R. *Altmann*]. MITOCHONDRIA.

al·tri·gen·der·ism (awl"tri·jen'dur·iz·um) *n.* [L. *alter,* other, + *gender* + *-ism*]. Nonerotic activities between members of opposite sexes; especially, the interest shown by a child in the late infantile period for members of the opposite sex.

al·trose (al'troce) *n.* An aldohexose sugar, $C_6H_{12}O_6$, stereoisomeric with D-glucose, prepared by synthesis; more exactly denoted as D-altrose or D-altropyranose.

Aludrine. A trademark for isoproterenol, a sympathomimetic amine used principally as a bronchodilator in the form of the hydrochloride salt.

Aludrox. Trademark for alumina and magnesia oral suspension.

al·um (al'um) *n.* [OF., from L. *alumen*]. 1. Any one of a class of double salts of general formula $M_2'SO_4.M_2'''(SO_4)_3.24H_2O$ or $M'M'''(SO_4)_2.12H_2O$, in which M' is a univalent metal or group, and M''' is a trivalent metal. 2. Ammonium alum, $AlNH_4(SO_4)_2.12H_2O$, or potassium alum, $AlK(SO_4)_2.12H_2O$, used as an astringent and emetic. 3. Exsiccated alum, a form deprived of most of its water of crystallization, used as an astringent.

alu·men (a·lew'min) *n.* ALUM.

alum hematoxylin. A dye lake of hematoxylin or hematein with potassium or ammonium aluminum sulfate, used in many formulas for the staining of nuclei and some other tissue elements.

alu·mi·na (a·lew'mi·nuh) *n.* [NL., from L. *alumen, aluminis,* alum]. Aluminum oxide, Al_2O_3, occurring naturally in many minerals, or prepared by chemical interaction.

alumina and magnesia oral suspension. A mixture of hydrated aluminum oxide and magnesium hydroxide employed as an antacid.

al·u·min·i·um (al"yoo·min'ee·um) *n.* ALUMINUM.

alu·mi·num (a·lew'mi·num) *n.* [NL., from *alumina,* aluminum oxide, from L. *alumen, aluminis,* alum]. Al = 26.9815. Valence, 3. A silver-white, light, ductile metal occurring abundantly in nature, chiefly in combination with silica and metallic oxides. It is soluble in acids and alkalies and, on exposure to air, takes on a coating of oxide. Because of its lightness (sp. gr. 2.7) and relative stability, it is used extensively for manufacturing and construction purposes. It readily forms alloys, some of which are of great importance. Powdered aluminum is variously used as a protective in treating ulcers and fissures, and has been used in treating silicosis.

aluminum acetate solution. A solution containing about 5.3% aluminum acetate, $Al(C_2H_3O_2)_3$; an astringent and antiseptic used after dilution with 10 to 40 parts of water as a gargle or a local application for ulcerative conditions. Syn. *Burow's solution.*

aluminum ammonium sulfate. Ammonium alum. See *alum* (2).

aluminum aspirin. Aluminum acetylsalicylate, $(CH_3COOC_6H_4COO)_2Al(OH)$, a water-insoluble, neutralized dosage form of aspirin.

aluminum chlor·hy·drox·ide (klor"high·drock'side). $Al(OH)_2Cl$, a water-soluble glassy solid; used as an antiperspirant.

aluminum chloride. $AlCl_3.6H_2O$. A white or yellow-white, deliquescent, crystalline powder, easily soluble in water; used as an astringent and antiseptic, especially in hyperhidrosis, applied as a 25% solution.

aluminum chlo·ro·hy·drate (klor"o·high'drate). ALUMINUM CHLORHYDROXIDE.

aluminum hydroxide. $Al(OH)_3$. A white, bulky, amorphous powder insoluble in water; a protective and astringent.

aluminum hydroxide gel. A white, viscous suspension of aluminum hydroxide equivalent to 4% Al_2O_3, used as gastric antacid, especially in the treatment of peptic ulcers. A dried aluminum hydroxide gel is used similarly.

aluminum oxide. Al_2O_3. A white, amorphous powder insoluble in water and, if it has been ignited, in acids; used for absorbing gases, water vapor, and in chromatographic analysis.

aluminum paste. A paste containing 10% powdered aluminum, 5% liquid petrolatum, and 85% zinc oxide ointment; used locally as a protective, especially around intestinal fistulas to protect surrounding skin against digestive action of intestinal fluids.

aluminum phosphate. $AlPO_4$. A white powder insoluble in water; used in the manufacture of dental and other cements and in ceramics.

aluminum phosphate gel. A white, viscous suspension containing 4.5% $AlPO_4$; used like aluminum hydroxide gel, but does not interfere with phosphate absorption.

aluminum potassium sulfate. Potassium alum. See *alum (2).*

aluminum silicate. Approximately $Al_2O_3.3SiO_2$. White powder or lumps; used for preparing dental cements and in ceramics.

aluminum sulfate. $Al_2(SO_4)_3.18H_2O$. A white, crystalline, odorless powder freely soluble in water; used in 5% solution as an astringent and antiseptic.

alum whey. A preparation obtained by boiling alum in milk and straining; formerly used as an astringent and internal hemostatic.

Alupent. Trademark for metaproterenol, a bronchodilator.

Alurate. A trademark for aprobarbital, a sedative and hypnotic.

alu·sia (a·lew'zee·uh) *n.* [Gk. *alysis,* distress (from *alyein,* to be distraught; to wander), + *-ia*]. HALLUCINATION.

al·ve·ar (al'vee·ur) *adj.* Of or pertaining to an alveus.

al·ve·at·ed (al'vee·ay·tid) *adj.* [L. *alveatus,* from *alveus,* a hollow, a trough]. Honeycombed; channeled; vaulted.

alvei. Plural of *alveus.*

alveol-, alveolo-. A combining form meaning *alveolus, alveolar.*

al·veo·la·bial (al"vee·o·lay'bee·ul) *n.* ALVEOLOLABIAL.

al·ve·o·lar (al·vee'uh·lur) *adj.* 1. Of or pertaining to an alveolus. 2. *In phonetics,* articulated with the tongue tip or blade touching, or forming a stricture at, the gums above the upper incisors, as the English consonant sounds t, d, n, s.

alveolar abscess. An abscess associated with an alveolar process and usually originating at the apex of a tooth or along a lateral surface of the root of a tooth. See also *periapical abscess, lateral root abscess.*

alveolar air. The air contained in the pulmonary alveoli and alveolar sacs.

alveolar angle. The angle formed between a line passing through a point beneath the nasal spine and the most prominent point of the lower edge of the alveolar process of the maxilla and the cephalic horizontal line.

alveolar arch. Either of the arches formed by the alveolar processes; the alveolar arch of the mandible (NA *arcus alveolaris mandibulae*) or the alveolar arch of the maxilla (NA *arcus alveolaris maxillae*).

alveolar artery. Any of the arteries supplying the teeth; the inferior alveolar artery (NA *arteria alveolaris inferior*), which provides branches to the the teeth of the mandible, the posterior superior alveolar artery (NA *arteria alveolaris superior posterior*), which supplies the molar and premolar teeth of the maxilla, or any of the anterior superior alveolar arteries (NA *arteriae alveolares superiores anteriores*), which supply the maxillary incisors and canines. Syn. *dental artery.* See also Table of Arteries in the Appendix.

alveolar bone. 1. The bone of the alveolar process, consisting of a thin cortical layer (the lamina dura or cribriform plate) which lines the tooth socket and is perforated by openings for blood vessels and nerves, an outer lamellar cortical plate which forms the outside of the process, and a small amount of cancellous bone in between. 2. Specifically, the thin layer of bone lining the tooth socket; LAMINA DURA (2). Syn. *cribriform plate.* Contr. *alveolar supporting bone.*

alveolar canals. 1. (of the maxilla:) The canals in the maxilla which transmit the posterior superior alveolar vessels and nerves to the upper molar teeth. NA *canales alveolares maxillae.* 2. The alveolar canals of the maxilla and the mandibular canal. Syn. *dental canals.*

alveolar cancer. 1. BRONCHIOLAR CARCINOMA. 2. A malignant tumor whose parenchymal cells form alveoli.

alveolar-capillary block syndrome. Arterial hypoxia due to alteration of the alveolar-capillary membrane by various disorders, hindering the diffusion of oxygen from the alveolar gas to capillary blood.

alveolar cell. 1. Any epithelial cell in the wall of a pulmonary alveolus. Compare *alveolar macrophage.* See also *great alveolar cell, squamous alveolar cell.* 2. Specifically, GREAT ALVEOLAR CELL. Contr. *pulmonary epithelial cell* (= SQUAMOUS ALVEOLAR CELL).

alveolar (cell) carcinoma. BRONCHIOLAR CARCINOMA.

alveolar crest. The most coronal aspect of the alveolar process.

alveolar duct. Any of the air passages in the lung branching from respiratory bronchioles and leading to alveolar sacs. NA (pl.) *ductuli alveolares.*

alveolar ectasia. Overdistention of pulmonary alveoli, as in compensatory emphysema.

alveolar eminence. Either one of two small protuberances situated on the outer surface of the mandible on either side of the midline and below the incisor teeth from which the mentalis muscle arises.

alveolar gland. A gland in which the secretory endpieces have a saccular form.

alveolar hypoventilation syndrome. PICKWICKIAN SYNDROME.

alveolar index. GNATHIC INDEX.

alveolar macrophage. A vigorously phagocytic cell, found in and on the surface of the pulmonary alveolar wall, which ingests inhaled particulate matter and microorganisms. Syn. *alveolar phagocyte, dust cell.* See also *heart-failure cell.*

alveolar mucosa. The vestibular mucous membrane between the attached gingiva and the fornix of the vestibule of the mouth.

alveolar nerve. Syn. *dental nerve.* See Table of Nerves in the Appendix.

alveolar osteitis. DRY SOCKET.

alveolar phagocyte. ALVEOLAR MACROPHAGE.

alveolar point. *In craniometry,* the midpoint on the anterior surface of the superior alveolar arch.

alveolar pore. One of the minute openings in the walls of the pulmonary alveoli, affording communication between neighboring alveoli.

alveolar pressure. Gas pressure within the pulmonary alveoli.

alveolar process. The ridge of bone, in each maxilla and in the mandible, containing the alveoli of the teeth; the alveolar process of the maxilla (NA *processus alveolaris maxillae*) or the alveolar process of the mandible (NA *pars alveolaris mandibulae*).

alveolar proteinosis. PULMONARY ALVEOLAR PROTEINOSIS.

alveolar ridge. 1. In the edentulous state, the bony remains of the alveolar process of the maxilla or mandible that formerly contained the teeth. 2. ALVEOLAR PROCESS.

alveolar sacs. The terminal groups of pulmonary alveoli; the branches of an alveolar duct. NA *sacculi alveolares.*

alveolar soft-part sarcoma. A poorly differentiated malignant tumor of the soft tissues whose component cells have an alveolar arrangement.

alveolar supporting bone. The cancellous bone and outer cortical plate of bone which support the teeth during mastication and which, together with the thin layer of bone lining the tooth sockets, constitute the bone of the alveolar process. Contr. *alveolar bone (2).* See also *alveolar bone (1).*

alveolar tumor. 1. BRONCHIOLAR CARCINOMA. 2. A tumor whose parenchymal cells form alveoli.

alveolar ventilation. Gas exchange between the inspired air and the blood in the alveoli of the lung; its rate per minute is calculated by the following equation: alveolar minute ventilation = (tidal volume − dead space) × respiratory rate.

alveolar vents. Communicating pores between neighboring alveoli in the lungs.

al·ve·o·late (al·vee'o·late) *adj.* [*alveol-* + *-ate*]. Pitted like a honeycomb. —**alveo·lat·ed** (·lay·tid) *adj.*

al·ve·o·lec·to·my (al″vee·o·leck'tuh·mee) *n.* Surgical removal of part of the alveolar process of the upper or lower jaw.

alveoli. Plural of *alveolus.*

alveoli den·ta·les (den·tay'leez) [NA]. The dental alveoli. See *alveolus (1).*

al·veo·lin·gual (al″vee·o·ling'gwul) *adj.* ALVEOLOLINGUAL.

alveoli pul·mo·nis (pul·mo'nis) [NA]. The alveoli of the lung. See *alveolus (2).*

alveoli pul·mo·num (pul·mo'num) [BNA]. ALVEOLI PULMONIS.

al·ve·o·li·tis (al″vee·o·lye'tis) *n.* Inflammation of alveoli or an alveolus. See also *dry socket.*

alveolitis sic·ca do·lo·ro·sa (sick'uh do·lo·ro'suh) [L., dry, painful]. DRY SOCKET.

alveolo-. See *alveol-.*

al·ve·o·lo·ba·sal (al·vee″uh·lo·bay'sul) *adj.* Pertaining to the alveolar portion of a jaw and to the denser basal portion of each jaw subjacent to the alveolar area which transmits pressure.

al·ve·o·lo·bas·i·lar (al·vee″uh·lo·bas'i·lur) *adj.* Pertaining to the alveolar point and the basion.

al·ve·o·lo·cap·il·lary (al·vee″uh·lo·kap'i·lerr·ee) *adj.* Of or pertaining to pulmonary alveoli and capillaries.

alveolocapillary membrane. The membrane, consisting of alveolar epithelium, capillary endothelium, and a basal lamina between them, that separates the pulmonary alveoli from the capillary lumina and through which respiratory gas exchange takes place.

al·ve·o·lo·cla·sia (al·vee″uh·lo·klay'zhuh, ·zee·uh) *n.* [*alveolo-* + *-clasia*]. A nonspecific breaking down of an alveolar process, causing loosening of the teeth. See also *periodontosis.*

al·ve·o·lo·con·dyl·ean (al·vee″uh·lo·kon·dil'ee·un) *adj. In craniometry,* pertaining to the anterior portion of the maxillary alveolus and the occipital condyles.

alveolocondylean plane. A plane tangent to the anteroinferior border of the maxillary alveolus and the inferior surface of the occipital condyles. Syn. *Broca's plane.*

al·ve·o·lo·den·tal (al·vee″uh·lo·den′tul) *adj.* [*alveolo-* + *dental*]. Pertaining to the teeth and their sockets.

al·ve·o·lo·la·bi·al (al·vee″uh·lo·lay′bee·ul) *adj.* Pertaining to the alveolar processes and the lips, or to the labial aspect of the alveolar process.

al·ve·o·lo·lin·gual (al·vee″uh·lo·ling′gwul) *adj.* Pertaining to the lingual aspects of the alveolar processes.

al·ve·o·lon (al·vee′o·lon) *n.* The point at which a straight line tangent to the posterior surfaces of the maxillary alveolar processes intersects the midline of the hard palate, or the median palatine suture. In many specimens this line will fall posterior to the tip of the posterior nasal spine. In these cases, the midline of the hard palate is to be prolonged until it intersects the line tangent to the posterior surfaces of the maxillary alveolar processes.

al·ve·o·lo·na·sal (al·vee″uh·lo·nay′zul) *adj.* Pertaining to the alveolar point and the nasion.

al·ve·o·lo·plas·ty (al·vee′uh·lo·plas″tee) *n.* Surgical alteration of the shape or size of the alveolar ridge to aid in the construction of dental prostheses.

al·ve·o·lo·sub·na·sal (al·vee″uh·lo·sub·nay′zul) *adj.* [*alveolo-* + *sub-* + *nasal*]. Pertaining to the alveolar portion of the maxilla that lies below the anterior bony aperture of the nose.

al·ve·o·lot·o·my (al″vee·o·lot′uh·mee) *n.* [*alveolo-* + *-tomy*]. Incision into a dental alveolus.

al·ve·o·lus (al·vee′o·lus) *n.*, pl. **alveo·li** (·lye) [L., diminutive of *alveus*]. A cavity, depression, pit, cell, or recess. Specifically: 1. A tooth socket; the cavity in which the root of a tooth is held in the alveolar process. NA (pl.) *alveoli dentales* (sing. *alveolus dentalis*). 2. An air cell of the lung; any of the numerous small pulmonary compartments in which the respiratory pathways terminate and through whose walls respiratory gases pass between air and blood. NA (pl.) *alveoli pulmonis* (sing. *alveolus pulmonis*). 3. A saclike termination of a racemose gland. Compare *acinus.*

al·veo·sub·na·sal (al″vee·o·sub·nay′zul) *adj.* ALVEOLOSUBNASAL.

alveosubnasal prognathism. The projection of the subnasal portion of the maxillary alveolus beyond the line of the facial profile.

al·ver·ine (al′vur·een) *n.* *N*-Ethyl-3,3′-diphenyldipropylamine, $C_{20}H_{27}N$, a smooth-muscle spasmolytic drug used as the citrate salt.

al·ve·us (al′vee·us) *n.*, pl. **al·vei** (·vee·eye) [L.]. 1. A trough, tube, or canal, as ducts and vessels of the body. 2. A cavity or excavation. Compare *alvus.*

alveus hip·po·cam·pi (hip″o·kam′pye) [NA]. A bundle of nerve fibers in the cerebral hemisphere investing the convexity of the hippocampus.

alvi. Plural of *alvus.*

al·vine (al′vine) *adj.* Of or pertaining to the alvus.

Alvinine. Trademark for biphenamine hydrochloride, a topical anesthetic with antibacterial and antifungal activity.

al·vi·no·lith (al·vye′no·lith, al′vi·) *n.* [*alvine* + *-lith*]. ENTEROLITH.

Alvodine. Trademark for piminodine, a synthetic narcotic analgesic used as the ethanesulfonate salt.

al·vus (al′vus) *n.*, pl. **al·vi** (·vye) [L.]. The abdomen with its contained viscera. Compare *alveus.*

alym·phia (ay·lim′fee·uh, a·lim′) *n.* Absence or deficiency of lymph.

alym·pho·cy·to·sis (ay·lim″fo·sigh·to′sis, a·lim″) *n.*, pl. **alymphocyto·ses** (·seez) [*a-* + *lymphocyte* + *-osis*]. 1. A marked decrease or an absence of lymphocytes in the blood. 2. SEVERE COMBINED IMMUNODEFICIENCY.

alym·pho·pla·sia (ay·lim″fo·play′zhuh, ·zee·uh) *n.* [*a-* + *lympho-* + *-plasia*]. Defective development of the lymphoid tissues; may be associated with defective thymic development. See also *thymic aplasia.*

Alypin. Trademark for amydricaine, a local anesthetic used as the hydrochloride salt.

alys·mus (a·liz′mus) *n.* [Gk. *alysmos*, disquiet, from *alyein*, to be restless]. Anxiety and restlessness which accompany physical disease.

al·y·so·sis (al″i·so′sis) *n.* [Gk. *alys*, boredom, + *-osis*]. Boredom.

Alz·hei·mer cell (ahlts′high·mur) [A. *Alzheimer*, German physician, and neuropathologist, 1864–1915]. An abnormal astrocyte, seen in hepatolenticular degeneration and in acquired hepatocerebral disease. Type I is a large astrocyte with dark nucleus and stainable cytoplasm seen near zones of necrosis. Type II is an astrocyte with large, pale, occasionally lobulated, sharply outlined nucleus, and sometimes intranuclear glycogen; cytoplasm is not usually seen.

Alzheimer's disease [A. *Alzheimer*]. A disease characterized by progressive dementia and diffuse cerebral cortical atrophy, and microscopically by the presence of argyrophil plaques, loss of neurons, and neurofibrillary tangles and granulovacuolar degeneration in the neurons that remain. These changes are also present in the basal ganglia. See also *presenile dementia.*

Alzheimer's plaque [A. *Alzheimer*]. ARGYROPHIL PLAQUE.

Alzinox. Trademark for dihydroxyaluminum aminoacetate, an antacid.

Am Symbol for americium.

A.M.A. American Medical Association.

amaas (ah′mahs) *n.* [Afrikaans]. VARIOLA MINOR.

am·a·cri·nal (am″uh·krye′nul) *adj.* AMACRINE.

am·a·crine (am′uh·krin, ·krine) *adj.* [*a-* + *macr-* + Gk. *is, inos*, fiber]. Having no long processes.

amacrine cell. A retinal cell which apparently lacks an axon; its body is in one of the lower rows of the inner nuclear layer, and its dendrite-like processes spread in the inner plexiform layer.

amad·i·none acetate (uh·mad′i·nohn). 17-(Acetoxy)-6-chloro-19-norpregna-4,6-diene-3,20-dione, $C_{22}H_{27}ClO_4$, a progestin.

amal·gam (uh·mal′gum) *n.* [ML. *amalgama*, probably from Gk. *malagma*, emollient, from *malassein*, to soften]. An alloy of mercury with any other metal or metals; used for restoring teeth and for making dental dies. See also *dental alloy, dental amalgam.*

amal·ga·mate (uh·mal′guh·mate) *v.* [from *amalgam*]. 1. To unite a metal in an alloy with mercury. 2. To unite two dissimilar substances. 3. To cover the zinc elements of a galvanic battery with mercury. —**amal·ga·ma·tion,** *n.*

amalgamation process. A method of extracting certain metals, especially gold and silver, from ores by alloying them with mercury.

amal·ga·ma·tor (uh·mal′guh·may″tur) *n.* An automatic device used for mixing mercury with a dental alloy to form an amalgam.

amalgam carrier. An instrument designed for carrying and introducing amalgam into the prepared cavity of a tooth.

amalgam plugger. CONDENSER (4).

am·an·din (uh·man′din, am′un·din) *n.* [F. *amandine*, from *amande*, almond]. A globulin contained in certain fruit kernels, such as sweet almonds and peach seeds.

Am·a·ni·ta (am″uh·nee′tah, ·nigh′tuh) *n.* [Gk. *amanitai*, a kind of fungus]. A genus of mushrooms belonging to the Agaricaceae.

Amanita mus·ca·ria (mus·kair′ee·uh, ·kăr′ee·uh) [L., from *musca*, fly]. A common poisonous mushroom; FLY AGARIC.

Amanita phal·loi·des (fa·loy′deez). A very poisonous species of mushroom; the source of amanita toxin and amanita hemolysin.

Amann's Viscol. A mixture of phenol, gum arabic, glycerin, and water, used as an aqueous mounting medium for histological sections.

aman·ta·dine (a·man′tuh·deen) *n.* 1-Adamantanamine, $C_{10}H_{17}N$, an antiviral compound often effective as a prophylactic agent against Asian influenza virus and of value in the treatment of parkinsonism; used as the water-soluble hydrochloride.

ama·ra (a·mahr'uh) *n.* [L. *amarus,* bitter]. BITTERS.

am·a·ranth (am'uh·ranth) *n.* [Gk. *amarantos,* never-fading, from *a-* + *marainein,* to wither]. 1. Any plant of the genus *Amaranthus.* An important cause of hay fever in North America west of Missouri and Iowa. 2. The trisodium salt of 1-(4-sulfo-1-naphthylazo)-2-naphthol-3,6-disulfonic acid, $C_{20}H_{11}N_2Na_3O_{10}S_3$, a dark red-brown powder used as a dye. Syn. *F.*D. & C. Red No. 2.

am·a·roid (am'uh·roid) *n.* [L. *amar*us, bitter, + *-oid*]. Any distinctly bitter vegetable extractive of definite chemical composition other than an alkaloid or a glycoside. The names of specific amaroids end in *-in* or *-inum.*

am·a·se·sis (am''uh·see'sis) *n.* [*a-* + Gk. *masēsis,* chewing]. Inability to chew.

amas·tia (a·mas'tee·uh, ay·mas') *n.* [*a-* + *mast-* + *-ia*]. Congenital absence of the breasts.

am·a·tho·pho·bia (am''uh·tho·fo'bee·uh) *n.* [Gk. *amathos,* sand, + *-phobia*]. A morbid fear of dust.

am·au·ro·sis (am''aw·ro'sis) *n.,* pl. **amauro·ses** (·seez) [Gk. *amaurōsis,* from *amauros,* dark, dim, blind]. Partial or total blindness, especially the type not associated with gross change or injury to the eye, such as that resulting from degenerative disease of the retina or optic nerve.

amaurosis fu·gax (few'gacks). Temporary blindness resulting from sudden acceleration, as in aerial flight, or from transient occlusion of the retinal arterioles.

amaurosis par·ti·a·lis fu·gax (pahr·shee·ay'lis few'gacks). Partial blindness associated with headache, vertigo, and scotomas. It is usually sudden and transitory.

am·au·rot·ic (am''aw·rot'ick) *adj. & n.* 1. Of or pertaining to amaurosis. 2. An individual affected with amaurosis.

amaurotic familial idiocy. Any of the lipidoses affecting the nervous system exclusively, classified according to time of onset as infantile or early infantile (TAY-SACHS DISEASE and SANDHOFF'S DISEASE), late infantile (BIELSCHOWSKY-JANSKÝ DISEASE), juvenile (SPIELMEYER-VOGT DISEASE), and adult or late juvenile (KUF'S DISEASE); characterized by dementia, motor paralysis, and except in the adult form, blindness.

amaxo·pho·bia (a·mack''so·fo'bee·uh) *n.* [Gk. *amax*a, wagon, + *-phobia*]. Morbid dread of being in, riding upon, or meeting any vehicle.

ama·zia (a·may'zee·uh) *n.* [*a-* + *maz-* + *-ia*]. AMASTIA.

amb-, ambi- [L.]. A prefix meaning *about, around.*

am·be·no·ni·um chloride (am''be·no'nee·um). N,N'-*bis*-2[(2-Chlorobenzyl) diethylammonium chloride]ethyloxamide, $C_{28}H_{42}Cl_4N_4$, a cholinesterase inhibitor used in the management of myasthenia gravis.

am·ber (am'bur) *n.* [Ar. *'anbar,* ambergris]. A fossil resin found in alluvial soils and lignite beds in various parts of the world, especially along the southern shores of the Baltic Sea.

am·ber·gris (am'bur·greece, ·gris) *n.* [MF. *ambre,* amber, + *gris,* gray]. An intestinal concretion of the sperm whale, *Physeter macrocephalus,* found floating on the sea, particularly in the southern hemisphere. It is usually gray in color with brown, white, or yellow streaks. It is used in perfumes, particularly as a fixative for floral odors, and has been used as a cordial and antispasmodic.

Amberlite. Trademark applied to a group of ion-exchange resins of the cation-exchange and anion-exchange type; certain of the purified resins are used medicinally. See also *carbacrylic resin, polyamine-methylene resin.*

amber mutation. A nonsense mutation in which the codon base sequence is UAG (uracil-adenine-guanine).

amber oil. A product of the dry distillation of amber; formerly used as rubefacient. Syn. *oleum succini.*

ambi-, ambo- [L.]. A combining form meaning *both.*

am·bi·dex·ter (am''bi·deck'stur) *n.* [L., from *ambi-*, both, + *dexter,* right]. An individual who can use either hand with equal facility.

am·bi·dex·ter·i·ty (am''bi·decks·terr'i·tee) *n.* [*ambi-* + *dexterity*]. The ability to use both hands with equal facility.

am·bi·dex·trous (am''bi·decks'trus) *adj.* [L. *ambidexter*]. Able to use both hands equally well. —**ambidex·trism** (·triz·um), **ambi·dex·tral·i·ty** (·decks·tral'i·tee) *n.*

am·bi·ent (am'bee·unt) *adj.* [L. *ambiens, ambientis,* from *ambire,* to go around]. 1. Moving about. 2. Surrounding, encompassing.

am·big·uo·spi·no·tha·lam·ic (am·big''yoo·o·spye''no·thuh·lam'ick) *adj.* Involving the ambiguous nucleus and adjacent spinothalamic tract.

ambiguospinothalamic paralysis. AVELLIS'S SYNDROME.

am·big·u·ous nucleus. AMBIGUUS NUCLEUS.

am·big·u·us (am·big'yoo·us) *adj.* [L.]. Of or pertaining to the nucleus ambiguus.

ambiguus nucleus. A column of cells lying in the lateral half of the reticular formation whose cells give origin to efferent fibers of the glossopharyngeal, vagus, and accessory nerves. Syn. *nucleus ambiguus [NA].*

am·bi·lat·er·al (am''bee·lat'ur·ul) *adj.* [*ambi-* + *lateral*]. Pertaining to or affecting both sides.

am·bi·le·vous, am·bi·lae·vous (am''bi·lee'vus) *adj.* [*ambi-* + *levo-* + *-ous*]. Clumsy in the use of both hands. Syn. *ambisinister.*

am·bi·oc·u·lar·i·ty (am''bee·ock·yoo·lerr'i·tee) *n.* [*ambi-* + *ocular* + *-ity*]. The ability to use both eyes equally well.

am·bi·o·pia (am''bee·o'pee·uh) *n.* [*ambi-* + *-opia*]. DIPLOPIA.

am·bi·sex·u·al (am''bee·seck'shoo·ul) *adj.* [*ambi-* + *sexual*]. 1. Common to both sexes. 2. Of undetermined or indeterminate sex. Compare *bisexual.* —**ambi·sex·u·al·i·ty** (·seck''shoo·al'i·tee) *n.*

am·bi·sin·is·ter (am''bi·sin'is·tur) *adj.* [*ambi-* + L. *sinister,* left]. AMBILEVOUS.

am·bi·ten·den·cy (am''bee·ten'din·see) *n.* [*ambi-* + *tendency*]. The state in which a trend in human behavior is accompanied by a corresponding countertrend, as a manic reaction arouses a depressive one.

am·biv·a·lence (am·biv'uh·lunce) *n.* [Ger. *Ambivalenz,* from *ambi-* + L. *valere,* to prevail]. 1. *In psychiatry,* the coexistence of two opposing drives, desires, attitudes, or emotions toward the same person, object, or goal. 2. Mixed feelings, such as love and hate, toward the same person; may be conscious, partly hidden from conscious awareness, or one side of the feelings may be unconscious. —**ambiv·a·lent** (·uh·lunt) *adj.*

am·biv·a·len·cy (am·biv'uh·lun·see) *n.* AMBIVALENCE.

am·bi·ver·sion (am''bi·vur'zhun) *n.* [*ambi-* + *version*]. A balance between introversion and extroversion.

am·bi·vert (am'bi·vurt) *n.* A personality type intermediate between extrovert and introvert.

ambly- [Gk. *amblys*]. A combining form meaning *obtuse, dull, faint.*

am·bly·acou·sia (am''blee·a·koo'zhuh, ·zee·uh) *n.* [*ambly-* + *-acousia*]. Defective hearing without any apparent organic basis.

am·bly·chro·ma·sia (am''bli·kro·may'zhuh, ·zee·uh) *n.* [*ambly-* + *-chromasia*]. A deficiency in nuclear chromatin which causes a cell to stain faintly. —**amblychro·mat·ic** (·mat'ick) *adj.*

Am·bly·om·ma (am''blee·om'uh) *n.* [*ambly-* + Gk. *omma,* eye]. A genus of hard-bodied ticks of the family Ixodidae. Several species act as vectors of rickettsial diseases of man and of heartwater fever of ruminants.

am·bly·ope (am'blee·ope) *n.* [Gk. *amblyōpos,* dim-sighted, from *ambly-* + *ōps, ōpos,* eye]. An individual with amblyopia.

am·bly·o·pia (am''blee·o'pee·uh) *n.* [Gk. *amblyōpia,* from *amblyōpos,* dim-sighted]. Dimness of vision, especially that not due to refractive errors or organic disease of the eye. It may be congenital or acquired. —**ambly·op·ic** (·op′ ick, ·o′pick) *adj.*

amblyopia al·bi·nis·mus (al·bi·niz′mus). Diminished vision with albinism.

amblyopia ex anopsia. Amblyopia from disuse or from nonuse, usually of one eye, as a result of uncorrected esotropia.

am·blyo·scope (am′blee·o·skope) *n.* [*amblyo*pia + *-scope*]. A device that presents a separate image of an artificial target to each eye; used in diagnosis and in some aspects of the treatment of disturbances of binocular vision.

Am·blys·to·ma (am·blis′to·ma) *n.* AMBYSTOMA.

ambo-. See *ambi-*.

am·bo·cep·tor (am′bo·sep″tur) *n.* [*ambo-* + re*ceptor*]. 1. *Obsol.* According to Ehrlich, an antibody present in the blood of immunized animals which contains two specialized elements: a cytophil group that unites with a cellular antigen, and a complementophil group that joins with the complement. 2. The anti-erythrocyte antibody in the complex of antibody and sheep erythrocytes used for determination of free complement in complement-fixation tests.

amboceptor unit. The smallest quantity of amboceptor in the presence of which a given quantity of red blood cells will be dissolved by an excess of complement.

Ambodryl. Trademark for bromodiphenhydramine, an antihistaminic agent used as the hydrochloride salt.

am·bo·my·cin (am″bo·migh′sin) *n.* An antibiotic, produced by *Streptomyces ambofaciens,* that possesses antineoplastic activity.

am·bon (am′bon) *n.* [Gk. *ambōn,* rim (of cup, of joint socket]. LABRUM GLENOIDALE.

am·bo·sex·u·al (am″bo·seck′shoo·ul) *adj.* AMBISEXUAL. —**ambo·sex·u·al·ity** (·seck″shoo·al′i·tee) *n.*

Am·boy·na or **Am·boi·na button** (am·boy′nuh) [after *Amboina,* Indonesia]. A skin lesion of yaws.

Am·bro·sia (am·bro′zhuh, ·zee·uh) *n.* [Gk., from *ambrosios,* immortal]. A genus of composite-flowered herbs. The common ragweed of North America, *Ambrosia artemisiifolia,* was used as a stimulant, tonic, antiperiodic, and astringent; properties of *A. trifida* are similar. The pollen of these two species is generally regarded as a frequent cause of hay fever.

am·bu·lance (am′bew·lunce) *n.* [F., field hospital, from *ambulant,* itinerant, from L. *ambulare,* to walk, travel]. 1. The staff and equipment of an army medical unit in the field. 2. In the United States, a vehicle for the transportation of the sick or wounded.

am·bu·lant (am′bew·lunt) *adj.* Moving, shifting; ambulatory.

ambulant blister. A blister that is shifted to different places.

am·bu·la·to·ry (am′bew·luh·tor″ee) *adj.* [L. *ambulatorius,* from *ambulare,* to move about, walk]. 1. Walking; of or for walking. 2. Able to walk; up and about; not bedridden. 3. Characterizing or pertaining to the conditions and treatment of ambulatory patients or of outpatients.

ambulatory automatism. A condition in which an epileptic patient, during a psychomotor seizure, walks around and is able to carry out some functions without being clearly conscious of either himself or his environment.

ambulatory plague. PESTIS MINOR.

ambulatory schizophrenia. A form of schizophrenia, usually of the simple but also of the schizoaffective type, in which the person so afflicted manages for the most part to avoid institutionalization.

ambulatory splint. A splint or brace used to maintain, or allow for, ambulatory traction.

ambulatory traction. Traction exerted by a walking splint or brace so that the pull is maintained upon the fractured limb or inflamed joint while the patient is up and about.

am·bu·phyl·line (am·bew′fi·leen) *n.* Theophylline aminoisobutanol, $C_7H_8N_4O_2.C_4H_{11}NO$, a diuretic and smooth-muscle relaxant drug.

am·bu·side (am′bew·side) *n.* *N*[1]-Allyl-4-chloro-6-[(3-hydroxy-2-butenylidene)amino]-*m*-benzenedisulfonamide, $C_{13}H_{16}ClN_3O_5S_2$, a diuretic agent.

am·bus·tion (am·bus′chun) *n.* [L. *ambustio,* from *amburere,* to burn, scorch, from *urere,* to burn]. A burn or scald.

Am·bys·to·ma (am·bis′to·muh) *n.* A genus of American salamander, used for experimental purposes. See also *axolotl.*

Amcill. Trademark for ampicillin, a semisynthetic penicillin antibiotic.

am·cin·a·fal (am·sin′uh·fal) *n.* (11β,16α)-9-Fluoro-11,21-dihydroxy-16,17-[(1-ethylpropylidene)bis(oxy)]pregna-1,4-diene-3,20-dione, $C_{26}H_{35}FO_6$, an anti-inflammatory agent.

am·cin·a·fide (am·sin′uh·fide) *n.* [11β,16α(*R*)]-9-Fluoro-11,21-dihydroxy-16,17-[1-phenylethylidene)bis(oxy)]-pregna-1,4-diene-3,20-dione, $C_{29}H_{33}FO_6$, an anti-inflammatory agent.

am·cin·o·nide (am·sin′o·nide) *n.* 9-Fluoro-11β,16α,17,21-tetrahydroxypregna-1,4-diene-3,20-dione cyclic acetal with cyclopentanone, 21-acetate, $C_{28}H_{35}FO_7$, a topical glucocorticoid. Formerly called *amcinopol.*

am·cin·o·pol (am·sin′o·pol, ·uh·pole) *n. Obsol.* AMCINONIDE.

Amdelate. A trademark for preparations of ammonium mandelate, a urinary antiseptic.

ameb-, amebo-. A combining form meaning (a) *ameba, amebic;* (b) *ameboid.*

ame·ba, amoe·ba (uh·mee′buh) *n.*, pl. **amebas, amoebas, amoe·bae** (·bee) [NL., from Gk. *amoibē,* change]. A protozoan belonging to the class Rhizopodea which moves by means of cytoplasmic extensions that are projected and retracted in response to external stimuli. Although many species are free-living, others are parasitic, principally in the intestinal tract of vertebrates and invertebrates.

ame·ba·cide (uh·mee′buh·side) *n.* AMEBICIDE.

am·e·bi·a·sis, am·oe·bi·a·sis (am″ee·bye′uh·sis) *n.* [*ameb-* + *-iasis*]. Infection, primarily colonic but also of the liver and other sites, with *Entamoeba histolytica.* See also *amebic dysentery, amebic abscess.*

amebiasis cu·tis (kew′tis). Ulceration of the skin due to amebas, especially in association with visceral amebiasis.

ame·bic, amoe·bic (uh·mee′bick) *adj.* Of, pertaining to, or caused by an ameba.

amebic abscess. A focus of liquefaction necrosis resulting from the histolytic action of amebas, usually *Entamoeba histolytica,* and differing from a true abscess by the absence of suppuration; occurs most often in the liver and the brain.

amebic colitis. Ulceration of the colon due to infection with *Entamoeba histolytica.*

amebic dysentery. Severe amebiasis, characterized by diarrhea (often containing mucus and blood), abdominal cramping, and fever. It is due to ulceration of the large intestine produced by *Entamoeba histolytica.*

amebic gangrene. Extensive destruction of the skin surrounding a drainage wound, following removal of an amebic abscess of the liver.

amebic granuloma. A massive, usually focal, involvement of the colon by *Entamoeba histolytica,* resulting in chronic proliferative inflammation that may be clinically confused with carcinomas. Syn. *ameboma.*

amebic hepatitis. A diffuse inflammation of the liver secondary to amebic colitis.

ame·bi·cide, amoe·bi·cide (a·mee′bi·side) *n.* [*ameb-* + *-cide*]. An agent fatal to amebas, especially to *Entamoeba histolytica.* —**ame·bi·ci·dal** (a·mee″bi·sigh′dul) *adj.*

ame·bo·cyte, amoe·bo·cyte (a·mee′bo·site) *n.* [*amebo-* + *-cyte*]. 1. Any ameboid cell. 2. A cell found in the coelomic fluid of echinoderms or among the tissues of various invertebrates. 3. LEUKOCYTE.

ame·boid, amoe·boid (a·mee′boid) *adj.* Resembling an ameba in form or in movement, as the leukocytes.

ameboid cell. A cell capable of changing its form and moving about like an ameba.

ameboid glioma. GLIOBLASTOMA MULTIFORME.

am·e·bo·ma, am·oe·bo·ma (am″ee·bo′muh) *n.* AMEBIC GRANULOMA.

ame·bu·la, amoe·bu·la (a·mee′bew·luh) *n.*, pl. **amebulas, ame·bu·lae** (·lee) [NL., diminutive of *ameba*]. Spores of protozoa and other organisms which are motile because of pseudopodial action.

ame·bu·ria, amoe·bu·ria (am″ee·bew′ree·uh) *n.* The presence of amebas in the urine.

ame·da·lin (a·mee′duh·lin) *n.* 1,3-Dihydro-3-methyl-3-[3-(methylamino)propyl]-1-phenyl-2*H*-indol-2-one, $C_{19}H_{22}N_2O$, an antidepressant normally employed as the hydrochloride.

amei·o·sis (am″eye·o′sis, ay″migh·) *n.* [*a-* + *meiosis*]. Aberrant meiosis, forming diploid spores or gametes.

amel-, amelo- [obs. E. *amel,* from OF. *esmail*]. A combining form meaning *enamel.*

amel·a·not·ic (ay·mel″uh·not′ick) *adj.* [*a-* + *melanotic*]. Containing no melanin or very small amounts of it.

amelanotic melanoma. A malignant melanoma without pigment production.

amel·eia (a·mel′ee·uh, am″e·lye′uh) *n.* [Gk., indifference, from *a-* + *melein,* to concern]. Apathy or indifference as part of a psychosis.

amel·ia (a·mel′ee·uh, ay·mee′lee·uh) *n.* [*a-* + *-melia*]. Congenital absence of the extremities.

amel·i·fi·ca·tion (a·mel″i·fi·kay′shun) *n.* [from *amel,* enamel]. The formation of dental enamel.

am·e·lo·blast (a·mel′o·blast, am′e·lo·) *n.* [*amelo-* + *-blast*]. An enamel cell; one of the columnar cells of the enamel organ, from which dental enamel is formed. Syn. *adamantoblast, ganoblast.* **—am·e·lo·blas·tic** (a·mel″o·blas′tick, am″e·lo·) *adj.*

ameloblastic odontoma. A neoplasm of epithelial and mesenchymal odontogenic tissue.

ameloblastic process. The cytoplasmic projection of an enamel-forming cell beyond the level of the terminal bar apparatus. Syn. *Tomes's process.*

ameloblastic sarcoma. AMELOBLASTOSARCOMA.

am·e·lo·blas·to·ma (am″e·lo·blas·to′muh, a·mel″o·) *n.* [*ameloblast* + *-oma*]. A tumor, found usually in the mandible, whose parenchyma is composed of epithelial cells resembling those of the enamel organ; locally aggressive and prone to recur. Syn. *adamantinoma, adamantoma.*

am·e·lo·blas·to·sar·co·ma (am″e·lo·blas″to·sahr·ko′muh) *n.* [*ameloblast* + *sarcoma*]. A malignant tumor derived from epithelial and mesenchymal odontogenic tissues.

am·e·lo·gen·e·sis (am″e·lo·jen′e·sis) *n.* [*amelo-* + *genesis*]. Histogenesis of the dental enamel.

amelogenesis im·per·fec·ta (im″pur·feck′tuh). An inherited condition of severe hypocalcification or hypoplasia of dental enamel.

am·e·lus (am′e·lus, a·mee′lus) *n.*, pl. **ame·li** (·lye) [*a-* + Gk. *melos,* limb]. An individual with congenital absence of all extremities.

ame·nia (a·mee′nee·uh) *n.* [*a-* + *men-* + *-ia*]. AMENORRHEA.

ameno·ma·nia, amoeno·ma·nia (a·men″o·may′nee·uh) *n.* [L. *amoen*us, pleasant, + *-mania*]. The manic phase of manic-depressive illness.

amen·or·rhea, amen·or·rhoea (a·men″o·ree′uh) *n.* [*a-* + *menorrhea*]. Absence of menstruation; characterized as primary if menarche has not occurred by 18 years of age; secondary if menstruation, once established, has not occurred for at least three months. **—amenor·rhe·al, amenor·rhoe·al** (·ree′ul) *adj.*

ament (ay′ment, am′ent) *n.* [L. *amens, amentis,* insane, from *a-*, away, + *mens,* mind]. A person suffering from severe mental subnormality, usually congenital.

amen·tia (a·men′shee·uh, ay·men′) *n.* [L., insanity, from *amens,* out of one's mind]. Subnormal mental development; especially, congenital mental deficiency; classified as undifferentiated or primary, or according to the known cause.

American eye fly. *HIPPELATES PUSIO.*

American hellebore. *VERATRUM VIRIDE.*

American mountain fever. COLORADO TICK FEVER.

American mucocutaneous leishmaniasis. A form of leishmaniasis due to *Leishmania braziliensis,* transmitted by sandflies of the genus *Phlebotomus,* and characterized by skin ulcers and ulceration and necrosis of the mucosa of the mouth and nose.

American Red Cross. A quasi-governmental agency and member of the International Red Cross, whose principal services are to the armed forces in peace and war, to the civilian population in disaster, and community services such as the teaching of first aid, life saving, maintenance of blood banks, and many other medically related volunteer services.

American spotted fever. ROCKY MOUNTAIN SPOTTED FEVER; an acute febrile illness caused by *Rickettsia rickettsii,* transmitted to man by ticks, with sudden onset of headache, chills, and fever; a characteristic exanthem occurs on the extremities and trunk.

American trypanosomiasis. CHAGAS' DISEASE.

American Type Culture Collection. An independent nonprofit organization, incorporated in Washington, D.C., devoted to the preservation of microbiologic and cell reference cultures and their distribution to the scientific community. Abbreviated, ATCC.

am·er·i·ci·um (am″ur·ish′ee·um, ·ee′shee·um) *n.* [after the *Americas*]. The radioactive element number 95; produced artificially. Symbol, Am.

am·er·is·tic (am″ur·is′tick) *adj.* [Gk. *ameristos,* undivided, from *a-* + *meros,* part]. Not segmented. **—am·er·ism** (·am′ ur·iz·um) *n.*

ame·si·al·i·ty (a·mee″zee·al′i·tee) *n.* [*a-* + *mesial*]. Shifting of a part, as the pelvis, to one side of the long axis of the body.

Am·e·tab·o·la (am″e·tab′o·luh) *n.pl.* [plural of *ametabolon*]. A group of insects with incomplete metamorphosis.

amet·a·bol·ic (ay·met″uh·bol′ick, am″e·tuh·) *adj.* AMETABOLOUS.

ame·tab·o·lon (am″e·tab′o·lon) *n.*, pl. **ametabo·la** (·luh) [Gk. neuter of *ametabolos,* unchanging]. An animal which develops without metamorphosis.

am·e·tab·o·lous (am″e·tab′uh·lus) *adj.* [Gk. *ametabolos,* unchanging, from *a-* + *metabolē,* change]. Lacking, or with minimal, metamorphosis; characterizing a mode of insect development in which the insect resembles the adult when it hatches from the egg, as in the silverfish and the springtail.

ameth·o·caine (am′e·tho·kane″, a·meth′o·) *n.* TETRACAINE.

Amethone. Trademark for amolanone, a local anesthetic used as the hydrochloride salt.

ame·tho·pter·in (a·meth″o·terr′in, am″e·thop′te·rin) *n.* A former name of methotrexate, an antineoplastic drug.

ame·tria (a·mee′tree·uh, a·met′ree·uh) *n.* [*a-* + *metr-* + *-ia*]. Congenital absence of the uterus. **—ame·trous** (·trus) *adj.*

ame·tro·he·mia, ame·tro·hae·mia (a·mee″tro·hee′mee·uh, a·met″ro·) *n.* [*a-* + *metro-* + *-hemia*]. *Obsol.* Deficiency in uterine blood supply.

am·e·tro·pia (am″e·tro′pee·uh) *n.* [Gk. *ametros,* without measure, + *-opia*]. Imperfect refractive ability due to defects of the media or the structures of the eye, which causes images to fail to focus directly upon the retina. See also *astigmatism, hyperopia, myopia, presbyopia.* **—ame·tro·pic** (·tro′ pick, ·trop′ick) *adj.*; **am·e·trope** (am′e·trope) *n.*

am·fo·nel·ic ac·id (am″fo·nel′ick). 7-Benzyl-1-ethyl-1,4-dihydro-4-oxo-1,8-naphthyridine-3-carboxylic acid, $C_{18}H_{16}N_2O_3$, a central nervous system stimulant.

am·i·an·thine (am″ee·an′theen) *adj.* AMIANTHOID.

amianthine degeneration. A retrogressive change in hyaline cartilage which produces an appearance resembling asbestos fibers.

am·i·an·thi·nop·sy (am″ee·an′thi·nop″see) *n.* [*am-* (irreg. for *an-*) + Gk. *ianthinos,* violet-colored, + *-opsy*]. Inability to see the color violet; inability to distinguish violet rays.

am·i·an·thoid (am″ee·an′thoid) *adj.* [Gk. *amianthos*, asbestos, + *-oid*]. Resembling asbestos; asbestoslike.

am·i·an·tho·sis (am″ee·an·tho′sis) *n.* [Gk. *amianthos*, asbestos, + *-osis*]. ASBESTOSIS.

Amicar. Trademark for the antifibrinolytic agent 6-aminohexanoic acid, an aminocaproic acid.

ami·cet·in (am″i·see′tin) *n.* An antibiotic substance, $C_{29}H_{42}N_6O_9$, isolated from cultures of a species of *Streptomyces* found in soil. It is markedly inhibitory to some organisms.

ami·clor·al (am″i·klor′al) *n.* A trichlorohydroxyethylglucose copolymer with glucose used as a veterinary food additive.

ami·cro·bic (ay″migh·kro′bick, am″eye·) *adj.* Pertaining to or characterized by absence of microorganisms.

ami·cron (ay·migh′kron, ay·mick′ron) *n.* [*a-* + *micron*]. A colloid particle, measuring about 10^{-7} cm or less than 5 nanometers in diameter, barely visible through the light microscope.

ami·crone (ay·migh′krone) *n.* AMICRON.

amic·u·lum (a·mick′yoo·lum) *n.*, pl. **amicu·la** (·luh) [L., a mantle or cloak, from *amicere*, to wrap]. A dense capsule of myelinated fibers surrounding the olivary nucleus.

ami·cy·cline (am″i·sigh′kleen) *n.* A tetracycline derivative of unspecified antibiotic action.

amid-, amido- [from *amide*]. A combining form designating (a) *a compound containing NH_2 united to an acid radical;* (b) *a compound containing the radical —CONH—*, as in proteins. Contr. *amino-*.

ami·dap·sone (am″i·dap′sone) *n.* [4-[(4-Aminophenyl)sulfonyl]phenyl]urea, $C_{13}H_{13}N_3O_3S$, an antiviral agent for poultry.

am·i·dase (am′i·dace, ·daze) *n.* [*amid-* + *-ase*]. Any enzyme catalyzing the hydrolysis of nonpeptide C=N linkages, generally with elimination of ammonia. Syn. *desamidase.*

am·ide (am′ide) *n.* [*ammonia* + *-ide*]. 1. Any organic compound containing the univalent radical $RCONH_2$, RCONHR, or $RCONR_2$, where R indicates an alkyl or aryl group. 2. A compound formed by the replacement of a hydrogen of ammonia by a metal, such as sodamide, $NaNH_2$.

am·i·deph·rine (am″i·def′reen) *n.* 3-(2-Methylamino-1-hydroxyethyl)methanesulfonanilide, $C_{10}H_{16}N_2O_3S$, an adrenergic drug; used as the mesylate (methanesulfonate) salt.

am·i·din (am′i·din) *n.* [F. *amidon*, starch, + *-in*]. The part of starch that is soluble in water; soluble starch.

am·i·dine (am·i·deen, ·din) *n.* Any compound containing the univalent radical $—C(NH_2)=NH$; any amide in which the oxygen is replaced by the divalent imide group, =NH.

amido-. See *amid-*.

ami·do·ben·zene (a·mee″do·ben′zeen, am″i·do·) *n.* ANILINE.

ami·do·ben·zol (a·mee″do·ben′zol, am″i·do·) *n.* ANILINE.

am·i·done hydrochloride (am′i·dohn). METHADONE hydrochloride.

ami·do·py·rine (a·mee″do·pye′reen ·rin, am″·i·do·) *n.* AMINOPYRINE.

am·i·dox·im (am″i·dock′sim) *n.* AMIDOXIME.

am·i·dox·ime (am″i·dock′seem) *n.* [*amid-* + *oxime*]. A compound containing the group $—C(NH_2)=NOH$; it is an amidine in which the hydrogen of the imide group has been replaced by an —OH; as acetamidoxime, $CH_3C(NH_2)=NOH$. Syn. *oxamidine.*

Amigen. A trademark for certain preparations of protein hydrolysate.

ami·ka·cin (am″i·kay′sin) *n.* A semisynthetic antibiotic, $C_{22}H_{43}N_5O_{13}$, derived from kanamycin, usually used as the sulfate salt.

Amikin. Trademark for amikacin, an antibiotic.

amil·o·ride (a·mil′o·ride) *n.* *N*-Amidino-3,5-diamino-6-chloropyrazinecarboxamide, $C_6H_8ClN_7O$, a natriuretic agent with marked potassium-sparing activity; used as the hydrochloride salt.

amim·ia (a·mim′ee·uh, ay·mim′) *n.* [*a-* + Gk. *mimos*, mime, actor, + *-ia*]. Loss of the ability to imitate and to communicate by gestures or signs.

am·in (am′in) *n.* AMINE.

amin-. See *amino-*.

ami·na·crine (a·mee′na·kreen) *n.* An amino derivative of acridine; of the several possible isomers, the 9-aminoacridine (or 5-aminoacridine in the British numbering system) possesses useful bacteriostatic and bactericidal powers. The hydrochloride, $C_{13}H_{10}N_2.HCl$, a yellow, crystalline powder, slightly soluble in water, is the form in which the compound is used. Syn. *aminoacridine.*

am·i·nate (am′i·nate) *v.* To introduce an amino group into a molecule; to form an amine. **—am·i·na·tion** (am″i·nay′shun) *n.*

amine (a·meen′, am′in) *n.* [*ammonia* + *-ine*]. Any member of the group of compounds formed by replacing one or more of the hydrogens of ammonia by one or more univalent hydrocarbon or other nonacidic organic radicals, such as RNH_2, RNHR′, and RN(R′)R″, where R, R′, and R″ may or may not represent the same radical. The amines are classified as primary, secondary, and tertiary depending on whether one, two, or three hydrogens are replaced.

amine oxidase. Monoamine oxidase, an enzyme which deaminates tyramine and tryptamine by oxidation to aldehyde, with liberation of ammonia.

Aminitrate phosphate. Trademark for trolnitrate phosphate, a vasodilator.

amino-, amin- [from *amine*]. A combining form meaning *pertaining to or containing the group NH_2 united to a radical other than an acid radical.* Contr. *amid-*.

ami·no·ace·tic acid (a·mee″no·a·see′tick). Aminoethanoic acid, NH_2CH_2COOH, a nonessential amino acid. It is a constituent of many proteins from which it may be obtained by hydrolysis. Has been used for treatment of muscular dystrophy and myasthenia gravis. Syn. *glycine.*

ami·no acid (a·mee′no, am′i·no). Any one of a large group of organic compounds of the general formula $RCH(NH_2)COOH$, R representing hydrogen or any organic radical. Naturally occurring amino acids have the NH_2 group in α position, and are usually of L- configuration. These compounds are amphoteric in reaction and represent the end products of protein hydrolysis. From amino acids, the body synthesizes its proteins. Ten of them that are essential to life cannot be synthesized by the human organism and must therefore be available in the diet: arginine, histidine, isoleucine, leucine, lysine, methionine, phenylalanine, threonine, tryptophan, and valine.

amino acid carboxylase. CARBOXYLASE (2).

amino acid decarboxylase. CARBOXYLASE (2).

ami·no·ac·i·dop·a·thy (am″i·no·as″i·dop′uth·ee, a·mee′no·) *n.* [*amino acid* + *-pathy*]. A specific defect in an enzymatic step in the metabolic pathway of one or more amino acids, or in a protein mediator necessary for the transport of certain amino acids into or out of cells.

amino acid oxidase. An enzyme capable of causing the oxidative deamination of amino acids.

D-amino acid oxidase. A flavoprotein enzyme present in animal tissues, responsible for the oxidative deamination of the D- or unnatural form of amino acids but not acting upon the L- or natural form.

L-amino acid oxidase. A flavoprotein enzyme present in animal tissues, responsible for oxidative deamination of the L- or natural form of amino acids but not acting upon the D- or unnatural form.

amino-acid tolerance test. A test based upon the theory that in liver disease there is a significant delay in the removal from the blood of injected amino acids.

ami·no·ac·id·uria (a·mee″no·as″i·dew′ree·uh) *n.* The presence of amino acids in the urine, especially in excess amounts, as in Fanconi syndrome.

ami·no·ac·ri·dine (a·mee″no·ack′ri·deen, ·din) *n.* AMINACRINE.

α-ami·no·adip·ic acid (al′fuh a·mee″no·a·dip′ick) [*amino-* + *adipic*]. A dibasic amino acid, $C_6H_{11}NO_4$, produced in the metabolism of lysine by liver homogenates, and also isolated from *Vibrio cholerae.*

amino alcohol. Any of a group of compounds containing both an alcoholic hydroxyl group and an amino group.

ami·no·ben·zene (a·mee″no·ben′zeen) *n.* ANILINE.

***p*-ami·no·ben·zene·ar·son·ic acid** (păr″uh·a·mee″no·ben″zeen·ahr·son′ick). ARSANILIC ACID.

ami·no·ben·zene·sul·fon·a·mide (a·mee″no·ben″zeen·sul·fon′uh·mide) *n.* SULFANILAMIDE.

ami·no·ben·zo·ate (a·mee″no·ben′zo·ate) *n.* A salt or ester of an aminobenzoic acid.

ami·no·ben·zo·ic acid (a·mee″no·ben·zo′ick). 1. An acid, $NH_2C_6H_4COOH$, occurring as ortho-, meta-, and para-isomers. 2. PARA-AMINOBENZOIC ACID.

4-ami·no·ben·zo·yl·gly·cine (a·mee″no·ben″zo·il·glye′sin, ·seen). *p*-AMINOHIPPURIC ACID.

ami·no·ca·pro·ic acid (a·mee″no·ka·pro′ick) [*amino-* + *caproic*]. Hexanoic acid (caproic acid) with an amino substituent. 2-Aminohexanoic acid, also called α-aminocaproic acid, $CH_3(CH_2)_3CHNH_2COOH$, is norleucine, an amino acid occurring in many proteins. 6-Aminohexanoic acid, often designated simply aminocaproic acid, $CH_2NH_2(CH_2)_4COOH$, is used as an antifibrinolytic agent in the treatment of excessive bleeding from systemic hyperfibrinolysis and urinary fibrinolysis.

α-aminocaproic acid. NORLEUCINE.

amino diabetes. FANCONI SYNDROME.

2-ami·no·eth·ane·sul·fon·ic acid (a·mee″no·eth″ane·sul·fon′ick). TAURINE.

2-ami·no·eth·a·nol (a·mee″no·eth′uh·nol) *n.* ETHANOLAMINE.

4-ami·no·fo·lic acid (a·mee″no·fo′lick). AMINOPTERIN.

Aminoform. Trademark for methenamine, a urinary tract antiseptic.

ami·no·glu·cose (a·mee″no·gloo′koce) *n.* GLUCOSAMINE.

2-aminoglucose. GLUCOSAMINE.

α-ami·no·glu·tar·ic acid (al′fuh a·mee″no·gloo·tăr′ick). GLUTAMIC ACID.

ami·no·glu·teth·i·mide (am″i·no·gloo·teth′i·mide, a·mee″no·) *n.* 2-(*p*-Aminophenyl)-2-ethylglutarimide, $C_{13}H_{16}NO_2$, an anticonvulsant drug.

ami·no·gly·co·side (a·mee″no·glye′ko·side) *n.* [*amino* + *glycoside*]. Any of a group of bacterial antibiotics, including gentamicin, kanamycin, neomycin, and streptomycin, which act by inhibiting bacterial protein synthesis and which contain an inositol ring substituted with one or two amino or guanido groups and with one or more sugars, including one or more aminosugars.

2-aminoheptane. TUAMINOHEPTANE.

2-ami·no·hex·a·no·ic acid (a·mee″no·heck″suh·no′ick). NORLEUCINE.

***p*-ami·no·hip·pu·ric acid** (păr″uh·a·mee″no·hi·pew′rick). *p*-Aminobenzoylaminoacetic acid, $NH_2C_6H_4CONHCH_2COOH$, used as the sodium salt in kidney function tests. Syn. *4-aminobenzoylglycine.*

α-ami·no·hy·dro·cin·nam·ic acid (al′fuh a·mee″no·high″dro·si·nam′ick). PHENYLALANINE.

2-amino-3-hy·droxy·bu·ta·no·ic acid (·high·drock″see·bew″tuh·no′ick). THREONINE.

α-amino-β-hy·droxy·bu·tyr·ic acid (·high·drock″si·bew·tirr′ick). THREONINE.

2-amino-3-hy·droxy·pro·pa·no·ic acid (·high·drock″see·pro″puh·no′ick). SERINE.

α-amino-β-hy·droxy·pro·pi·on·ic acid (·high·drock″see·pro″pee·on′ick). SERINE.

α-amino-3-in·dole·pro·pi·on·ic acid (·in″dole·pro″pee·on′ick). TRYPTOPHAN.

α-amino·iso·ca·pro·ic acid (al′fuh a·mee′no eye″so·ka·pro′ick). LEUCINE.

α-amino·iso·va·ler·ic acid (al′fuh a·mee″no·eye″so·va·lerr′ick). VALINE.

δ-ami·no·lev·u·lin·ic acid (del′tuh a·mee″no·lev″yoo·lin′ick). $HOOC(CH_2)_2COCH_2NH_2$, an intermediate in the biosynthesis of porphyrins and heme; a precursor of porphobilinogen, with which it is found in the urine in some forms of porphyria.

ami·no·lip·id (a·mee″no·lip′id, am″i·no·) *n.* [*amino-* + *lipid*]. A fatty acid ester of an alcohol containing nitrogen in the amino form.

2-amino-3-mer·cap·to·pro·pa·no·ic acid (·mur·kap″to·pro″puh·no′ick). CYSTEINE.

ami·no·meth·an·am·i·dine (a·mee″no·meth″an·am′i·deen, ·din) *n.* GUANIDINE.

2-amino-3-meth·yl·bu·ta·no·ic acid (·meth″il·bew″tuh·no′ick). VALINE.

ami·no·met·ra·dine (a·mee″no·met′ruh·deen) *n.* 1-Allyl-3-ethyl-6-aminotetrahydropyrimidinedione, $C_9H_{13}N_3O_2$, an orally effective nonmercurial diuretic. TM *Mincard.*

ami·no·pent·a·mide (a·mee″no·pent′uh·mide) *n.* 4-Dimethylamino-2,2-diphenylvaleramide, $C_{19}H_{24}N_2O$, a parasympatholytic agent with predominantly atropine-like pharmacologic action; used as the sulfate salt.

ami·no·pep·ti·dase (a·mee″no·pep′ti·dace, ·daze) *n.* An enzyme occurring in intestinal mucosa, yeast, and certain bacteria. It catalyzes hydrolysis of polypeptides at the end having a free amino group, producing an amino acid and a smaller peptide which may undergo further hydrolysis under the influence of the enzyme.

α-amino-β-phen·yl·pro·pi·on·ic acid (al′fuh a·mee′no bay′tuh fen″il·pro″pee·on′ick). PHENYLALANINE.

am·i·noph·er·ase (am″i·nof′ur·ace, ·aze) *n.* [*amino-* + Gk. *pherein*, to carry, + *-ase*]. TRANSAMINASE.

ami·no·phyl·line (a·mee″no·fil′een, am″i·nof′i·leen, ·in) *n.* Theophylline ethylenediamine, $(C_7H_8N_4O_2)_2$-$C_2H_4(NH_2)_2.xH_2O$, occurring as white or slightly yellowish granules or powder, soluble in water. It has the action and uses of theophylline, modifying blood flow, relaxing bronchial and other smooth musculature, and producing diuresis.

ami·no·poly·pep·ti·dase (a·mee″no·pol″i·pep′ti·dace, ·daze, am″i·no·) *n.* [*amino-* + *polypeptide* + *-ase*]. A proteolytic enzyme occurring in yeast, intestinal mucosa, kidney spleen, and liver. Its action is the cleavage of polypeptides which contain either a free amino group or a basic nitrogen atom carrying at least one hydrogen atom.

2-ami·no·pro·pa·no·ic acid (a·mee″no·pro″puh·no′ick). ALANINE.

α-ami·no·pro·pi·on·ic acid (al′fuh a·mee″no·pro″pee·on′ick). ALANINE.

β-ami·no·pro·pio·ni·trile, beta-aminopropionitrile (bay′tuh a·mee″no·pro″pee·o·nigh′trile, ·tril) *n.* $H_2NCH_2CH_2CN$, a potent inhibitor of the lysyl oxidases of bone and connective tissue, preventing cross-linking between tropocollagen molecules.

ami·no·pter·in (a·mee″no·terr′in, am″i·nop′te·rin) *n.* 4-Aminopteroylglutamic acid or 4-aminofolic acid, $C_{19}H_{20}N_8O_5$, a folic acid antagonist.

ami·no·pu·rine (a·mee″no·pew′reen, am″i·no·) *n.* A purine in which one or more hydrogens are replaced by amino groups, as in adenine (6-aminopurine) and in 2-aminopurine, which functions as a mutagen by acting as an adenine analogue.

ami·no·py·rine (a·mee″no·pye′reen ·rin) *n.* 4-Dimethylamino-2,3-dimethyl-1-phenyl-3-pyrazolin-5-one, $C_{13}H_{17}N_3O$, an antipyretic and analgesic that may cause agranulocytosis on continued use. Syn. *amidopyrine.*

amin·o·rex (a·min′o·recks) *n.* 4,5-Dihydro-5-phenyl-2-oxazoline, $C_9H_{10}N_2O$, an anorexic agent.

ami·no·sa·lic·y·late (a·mee″no·sa·lis′i·late) *n.* A salt or ester of an aminosalicylic acid.

ami·no·sal·i·cyl·ic acid (a·mee″no·sal″i·sil′ick). 1. An acid, $NH_2C_6H_3OHCOOH$, occurring as ortho-, meta-, and para-isomers. 2. PARA-AMINOSALICYLIC ACID.

ami·no·suc·ci·nam·ic acid (a·mee″no·suck″si·nam′ick, am″i·no·). ASPARAGINE.

amino sugar. Any of a class of sugars in which one or more hydroxyl groups have been replaced by amino groups, as, for example, glucosamine and galactosamine.

ami·no·su·ria (a·mee″no·sue′ree·uh, am″i·no·) *n.* [irreg., from *amino-* + *-uria*]. The presence of amines in the urine.

ami·no·tol·u·ene (a·mee″no·tol′yoo·een) *n.* TOLUIDINE.

α-ami·no·va·ler·ic acid (al′fuh a·mee″no·va·lerr′ick). NORVALINE.

α-amino-*n*-valeric acid. NORVALINE.

am·i·nu·ria (am″i·new′ree·uh) *n.* AMINOSURIA.

Amipaque. A trademark for metrizamide, a radiopaque diagnostic aid.

am·i·phen·a·zole (am″i·fen′uh·zole) *n.* 2,4-Diamino-5-phenylthiazole, $C_9H_9N_3S$, an antagonist to respiratory depression caused by large doses of narcotics; used as the hydrochloride salt. Syn. *DAPT.*

am·i·quin·sin (am″i·kwin′sin) *n.* 4-Amino-6,7-dimethoxyquinoline, $C_{11}H_{12}N_2O_2$, an antihypertensive drug; used as the hydrochloride salt.

am·iso·met·ra·dine (am″eye·so·met′ruh·deen) *n.* 6-Amino-3-methyl-1-(2-methylallyl)uracil, $C_9H_{13}N_3O_2$, an orally effective nonmercurial diuretic.

am·i·thi·o·zone (am″i·thigh′o·zone) *n.* *p*-Formylacetanilid thiosemicarbazone or *p*-acetylaminobenzaldehyde thiosemicarbazone, $C_{10}H_{12}N_4OS$; has been employed for treatment of tuberculosis, leprosy, and lupus vulgaris. Syn. *thiacetazone.*

ami·to·sis (am″i·to′sis, ay″migh·to′sis) *n.* [*a-* + *mitosis*]. Aberrant reproduction; reproduction by direct nuclear cleavage or simple fission. —**ami·tot·ic** (·tot′ick) *adj.*

am·i·trip·ty·line (am″i·trip′ti·leen) *n.* 10,11-Dihydro-*N,N*-dimethyl-5*H*-dibenzo[*a,d*]cycloheptene-$\Delta^{5,\gamma}$-propylamine, $C_{20}H_{23}N$, an antidepressant drug; used as the hydrochloride salt.

amm-, ammo- [Gk. *ammos*]. A combining form meaning *sand.*

am·me·ter (am′ee·tur, am′mee·tur) *n.* [*am*pere + *meter*]. A type of galvanometer in which the electric current is measured directly in amperes.

am·mine (a·meen′, am′een) *n.* A complex cation formed by union of a metal with one or more molecules of ammonia, as diammine silver or tetrammine copper. Compare *amine.*

am·mism (am′iz·um) *n.* [Gk. *ammos,* sand]. AMMOTHERAPY.

ammo-. See *amm-.*

am·moi·din (a·moy′din) *n.* The methyl ether of 8-hydroxy-4′,5′,6,7-furocoumarin, $C_{12}H_8O_4$, obtained from the fruits of the herb *Ammi majus.* When given internally or applied externally, followed by exposure to sunlight, it induces normal pigmentation in patients with leukodermic areas. The substance is identical with xanthotoxin and methoxsalen.

am·mo·nate (am′o·nate) *n.* A compound containing ammonia of crystallization, analogous to one containing water of crystallization.

am·mo·na·tion (am″o·nay′shun) *n.* A process of combining a compound with ammonia. —**am·mo·nate** (am′o·nate) *v.*

am·mo·ne·mia, am·mo·nae·mia (am″o·nee′mee·uh) *n.* [*ammonia* + *-emia*]. Excessive amounts of ammonia or its compounds in the blood; may be accompanied by symptoms such as hypothermia, hypotension, and disordered states of consciousness. See also *hyperammonemia.*

am·mo·nia (uh·mo′nyuh) *n.* [NL., from SAL *AMMONIAC*, q.v.]. A colorless, pungent gas, NH_3, very soluble in water, a very small portion combining with it to form ammonium hydroxide. The ammonia of commerce is produced synthetically from nitrogen and hydrogen or obtained by the destructive distillation of nitrogenous organic matter. It is used as a detergent, a saponifying agent, in refrigeration, and for other industrial applications.

am·mo·ni·ac (uh·mo′nee·ack) *n.* [Gk. *ammōniakon*]. A gum resin from a Persian umbelliferous plant, *Dorema ammoniacum,* which has been employed in chronic bronchitis as a stimulating expectorant and counterirritant.

am·mo·ni·a·cal (am″o·nigh′uh·kul) *adj.* Pertaining to ammonia.

ammoniacal fermentation. Fermentation giving rise to ammoniacal gas and carbon dioxide, which combine to form ammonium carbonate.

ammoniaemia. Ammoniemia (= AMMONEMIA).

ammonia rash. DIAPER RASH.

am·mo·ni·at·ed (a·mo′nee·ay·tid) *adj.* Saturated or combined with ammonia.

ammoniated mercury. Ammoniated mercuric chloride, $HgNH_2Cl$; a topically applied anti-infective agent. Syn. *white precipitate.*

ammonia water. A 10% solution of ammonia in water.

am·mo·ni·emia, am·mo·ni·ae·mia (a·mo″nee·ee′mee·uh) *n.* AMMONEMIA.

am·mo·ni·fi·ca·tion (a·mon″i·fi·kay′shun, a·mo″ni·) *n.* The production of ammonia by bacterial action.

am·mo·ni·um (a·mo′nee·um) *n.* [from *ammonia*]. The univalent radical NH_4^+. It exists only as an ion in combination with an anion.

ammonium alum. ALUM (2).

ammonium bifluoride. $NH_4F.HF$, solutions of which are germicidal and have been used for treating pyorrhea alveolaris.

ammonium biphosphate. AMMONIUM PHOSPHATE, MONOBASIC.

ammonium bromide. NH_4Br, formerly used as a sedative and somnifacient.

ammonium carbonate. A compound of ammonium acid carbonate, NH_4HCO_3, and ammonium carbamate, NH_2COONH_4, in varying proportions. It is a stimulant expectorant and reflex stimulant.

ammonium chloride. NH_4Cl. Used as a saline expectorant, diuretic, and systemic and urinary acidifier.

ammonium dihydrogen phosphate. AMMONIUM PHOSPHATE, MONOBASIC.

ammonium hydroxide. NH_4OH. A weakly ionizing base formed to a slight extent when ammonia (NH_3) is dissolved in water. The term is frequently applied, not correctly, to aqueous solutions of ammonia. Compare *diluted ammonia solution, strong ammonia solution.*

ammonium hypophosphite. $NH_4PH_2O_2$. Has been used in treating bronchitis and laryngitis.

ammonium iodide. NH_4I. Has been used in treating asthma and in chronic bronchitis when the exudate is fibrinous.

ammonium mandelate. $C_6H_5CH(OH)COONH_4$. Used as a urinary antiseptic.

ammonium muriate. AMMONIUM CHLORIDE.

ammonium oxalate. $(NH_4)_2C_2O_4.H_2O$. Used as an analytical reagent.

ammonium persulfate. $(NH_4)_2S_2O_8$. A disinfectant and deodorizer, applied in 0.5 to 2.0% solution.

ammonium phosphate, dibasic. $(NH_4)_2HPO_4$. Has been used medicinally. Syn. *secondary ammonium phosphate, diammonium hydrogen phosphate.*

ammonium phosphate, monobasic. $(NH_4)H_2PO_4$. Has been used medicinally. Syn. *primary ammonium phosphate, ammonium biphosphate, ammonium dihydrogen phosphate.*

ammonium pic·ro·car·mi·nate (pick″ro·kahr′mi·nate). The ammonium salts of a mixture or complex of picric acid and carmine (1).

ammonium salicylate. $C_6H_4OHCOONH_4$. Has been used as an antirheumatic and antipyretic.

ammonium sulfate. $(NH_4)_2SO_4$. Used as a protein precipitant.

am·mo·ni·uria (a·mo″nee·yoo′ree·uh) *n.* An excess of ammonia in the urine.

am·mo·nol·y·sis (am″o·nol′i·sis) *n.* Any interaction of ammonia with another substance in which the ammonia functions similarly to water in hydrolysis.

Ammon's horn [The Egyptian god *Ammon,* represented with a ram's head]. HIPPOCAMPUS.

am·mo·ther·a·py (am″o·therr′uh·pee) *n.* [Gk. *ammos*, sand, + *therapy*]. Sand baths in the treatment of disease; no longer in general use. Syn. *arenation.*

am·ne·mon·ic (am″ne·mon′ick) *adj.* [*a-* + *mnemonic*]. Pertaining to impairment or loss of memory.

amnemonic agraphia. Inability to write connected or meaningful sentences, even though able to write letters and words.

amnemonic aphasia. *Obsol.* AMNESIC APHASIA.

am·ne·sia (am·nee′zhuh, ·zee·uh) *n.* [Gk. *amnēsia,* forgetfulness, from *a-* + *memnēsthai,* to remember]. Loss or impairment of retentive memory.

am·ne·sic (am·nee′zick, ·sick) *adj.* Of, pertaining to, or suffering from amnesia.

amnesic amimia. *Obsol.* A condition in which gestures or signs can be made but their proper meanings cannot be remembered.

amnesic amusia. *Obsol.* A form of aphasia in which a patient is able to recognize a tune but is unable to name it.

amnesic aphasia. A form of aphasia in which the patient is unable to find specific words, particularly to name or describe objects, resulting in hesitant and fragmentary speech.

amnesic colorblindness. COLOR APHASIA.

am·nes·tic (am·nes′tick) *adj.* [Gk. *amnēstia*, forgetfulness (= *amnēsia*), + *-ic*]. AMNESIC.

amnestic aphasia. AMNESIC APHASIA.

amnestic apraxia. *Obsol.* A form of apraxia in which actions can be imitated but not performed on command.

amnestic color dysnomia. A specific defect in naming colors due to loss of memory of color names, despite preservation of other aspects of language function.

amnestic-confabulatory syndrome. A syndrome observed in organic brain syndromes, characterized by retro- and anterograde amnesia, defects in retention and recall of ideas or facts, disorientation, and confabulation, seen in varying degrees of severity, usually due to senile sclerosis, Korsakoff's syndrome, electroshock therapy, or bilateral prefrontal lobotomy.

amnestic syndrome. AMNESTIC-CONFABULATORY SYNDROME.

amnia. A plural of *amnion.*

amnio-. A combining form meaning *amnion, amnionic.*

am·nio·car·di·ac (am″nee·o·kahr′dee·ack) *adj.* [*amnio-* + *cardiac*]. Of or pertaining to the embryonic coelom and the developing heart.

amniocardiac vesicle. In lower vertebrates (e.g., birds), that part of the coelom which lies below and lateral to the developing heart in its early stages and is destined to form the pericardial cavity.

am·nio·cen·te·sis (am″nee·o·sen·tee′sis) *n.* [*amnio-* + *centesis*]. Puncture of the intrauterine amniotic sac through the abdominal wall with a trochar and cannula to obtain a sample of amniotic fluid; used in prenatal diagnosis of certain chromosomal disorders, such as Down's syndrome, and many hereditary metabolic diseases, and to study fetal maturation in late pregnancy.

am·nio·cho·ri·al (am″nee·o·ko′ree·ul) *adj.* Pertaining to the amnion and the chorion.

am·nio·em·bry·on·ic (am″nee·o·em″bree·on′ick) *adj.* Pertaining to the embryo and the amnion.

amnioembryonic rudiment. The inner cell mass of the early blastocyst from which the amnion and the blastoderm differentiate. Syn. *intrachorionic rudiment.*

amnioembryonic vesicle. The early amnion.

am·nio·gen·e·sis (am″nee·o·jen′e·sis) *n.* [*amnio-* + *genesis*]. The development or formation of the amnion.

am·ni·og·ra·phy (am″nee·og′ruh·fee) *n.* Radiography of the uterine contents after injection of a radiopaque substance into the amniotic sac. —**am·nio·gram** (am′nee·o·gram) *n.*

am·ni·on (am′nee·on) *n.,* pl. **amnions, am·nia** (·nee·uh) [Gk.]. The innermost of the fetal membranes forming a fluid-filled sac for the protection of the embryo. Its thin, translucent wall is composed of an inner layer of ectoderm and an outer layer of mesoderm continuous with the embryonic somatopleure at the umbilicus. After the second month of development, it obliterates the extraembryonic coelom, forms a sheath about the umbilical cord, and fuses loosely with the chorionic mesoderm.

am·ni·on·ic (am″nee·on′ick) *adj.* AMNIOTIC.

amnionic fold. AMNIOTIC FOLD.

am·ni·o·ni·tis (am″nee·o·nigh′tis) *n.* AMNIOTITIS.

am·ni·or·rhea, am·ni·or·rhoea (am″nee·o·ree′uh) *n.* [*amnio-* + *-rrhea*]. The premature escape or discharge of the amniotic fluid.

am·ni·or·rhex·is (am″nee·o·reck′sis) *n.* [*amnio-* + *-rrhexis*]. Rupture of the amnion.

am·ni·os (am′nee·os) *n.* [Gk.]. AMNION.

Am·ni·o·ta (am″nee·o′tuh) *n.pl.* A group comprising those vertebrates with an amnion and allantois: mammals, birds, and reptiles. Contr. *Anamniota.* —**am·ni·ote** (am′nee·ote) *adj. & n.*

am·ni·ot·ic (am″nee·ot′ick) *adj.* Of or pertaining to the amnion.

amniotic adhesions. Collagenous adhesions between the amnion and the fetus, usually resulting in fetal malformation.

amniotic amputation. Amputation of a portion of the fetus, usually an extremity, supposedly due to constriction by an amniotic adhesion or band.

amniotic band. A band of amniotic epithelium adherent to the fetus or to the umbilical cord.

amniotic cavity. The fluid-filled cavity of the amnion.

amniotic cyst. An accumulation of amniotic fluid between the amniotic folds as a result of adhesive folds or of traumatic dissection during parturition.

amniotic ectoderm. The internal epithelium lining the amnion and continuous with the epidermis of the embryo at the umbilicus.

amniotic fluid. The transparent, almost colorless, fluid contained within the amniotic sac surrounding the fetus, composed of albumin, urea, creatinine, water, various salts, and cells.

amniotic fluid embolism. A rare type of embolism seen in the mother following delivery, in which multiple emboli containing cellular elements from the amniotic fluid are widely disseminated, the clinical picture resembling that seen in fat embolism. See also *amniotic fluid syndrome.*

amniotic fluid syndrome. Obstetric shock and frequently sudden death due to massive intravenous infusion of amniotic fluid causing pulmonary edema and pulmonary embolic changes. The major complication is hemorrhage due to disseminated intravascular coagulation.

amniotic fold. One of the folds of the blastoderm that unite over the embryo to form amnion and chorion in sauropsidans and many mammals.

amniotic raphe. The point of fusion of the amniotic folds over the embryo in sauropsidans and certain mammals.

amniotic ring. The ring found by the attached margin of the amnion at the umbilicus.

amniotic sac. The fluid-filled sac formed by the amnion.

am·ni·o·ti·tis (am″nee·o·tye′tis) *n.* [*amniotic* + *-itis*]. Inflammation of the amnion.

am·nio·tome (am′nee·o·tome) *n.* [*amnio-* + *-tome*]. An instrument for puncturing the fetal membranes.

am·ni·ot·o·my (am″nee·ot′uh·mee) *n.* [*amnio-* + *-tomy*]. Rupture of the fetal membranes.

amo·bar·bi·tal (am″o·bahr′bi·tal, ·tol) *n.* 5-Ethyl-5-isoamylbarbituric acid, $C_{11}H_{18}N_2O_3$, a hypnotic and sedative, used as such and also as the sodium derivative, which is water-soluble.

am·o·di·a·quine (am″o·dye′uh·kween, ·kwin) *n.* 4-(7-Chloro-4-quinolylamino)-α-diethylamino-*o*-cresol, $C_{20}H_{22}ClN_3O$, an antimalarial drug; used as the dihydrochloride salt.

Amodril. Trademark for levamfetamine succinate, an anorexigenic drug.

Amoe·ba (a·mee′buh) *n.* ENTAMOEBA.

amoeba. AMEBA.

amoebiasis. AMEBIASIS.

amoebic. AMEBIC.

amoebicide. AMEBICIDE.

Amoe·bi·dae (a·mee′bi·dee) *n.pl.* A family of the Rhizopoda.

amoebocyte. AMEBOCYTE.

amoeboid. AMEBOID.

amoeboma. AMEBOMA.

amoebula. AMEBULA.

amoeburia. AMEBURIA.

amoenomania. AMENOMANIA.

amok. AMUCK.

amo·la·none (a·mo′luh·nohn) *n.* 3-(β-Diethylaminoethyl)-2-oxo-3-phenyl-2,3-dihydrobenzofuran, $C_{20}H_{23}NO_2$, a drug with anticholinergic and local anesthetic actions; used as the hydrochloride salt for topical anesthesia of the lower urinary tract.

amor (am′or) *n.* [L.]. Love.

amo·ra·lia (am″o·ray′lee·uh, ay″mo·) *n.* [*amoral* + *-ia*]. Sociopathic personality disturbance.

amor in·sa·nus (in·say′nus). EROTOMANIA.

amor les·bi·cus (lez′bi·kus). LESBIANISM; female homosexuality.

amorph (ay′morf, am′orf) *n.* [*a-* + *-morph*]. A mutation in which the mutant allele does not act at all. Compare *hypomorph.*

amor·phia (a·mor′fee·uh) *n.* [Gk., formlessness]. AMORPHISM.

amor·phic (a·mor′fick) *adj.* AMORPHOUS.

amor·phin·ism (ay·mor′fi·niz·um, a·mor′) *n.* [*a-* + *morphine* + *-ism*]. The withdrawal syndrome resulting when morphine is withheld from an addict.

amor·phism (a·mor′fiz·um) *n.* The state or quality of being amorphous.

amor·pho·syn·the·sis (ay·mor″fo·sin′the·sis, a·) *n.* [*a-* + *morpho-* + *synthesis*]. Imperception or neglect of one side of the body and the external space on that side; interpreted as a defect in spatial summation and attributed to a lesion in the contralateral parietal lobe. Compare *agnosia.*

amor·phous (a·mor′fus) *adj.* [Gk. *amorphos,* from *a-* + *morphē,* form]. 1. Formless, shapeless. 2. *In biology,* without visible differentiation in structure. 3. *In chemistry,* not crystalline.

amorphous fetus. ANIDEUS.

amorphous insulin. The form of insulin obtained in commercial processes in the absence of added zinc or certain other metal ions; a prompt-acting insulin. Syn. *unmodified insulin.*

amor·phus (a·mor′fus) *n.* [NL., from Gk. *amorphos,* formless]. ANIDEUS.

amorphus glob·u·lus (glob′yoo·lus). ANIDEUS.

amor sui (soo′ee, soo′eye) [L.]. Love of self; vanity.

amo·tio (a·mo′shee·o, a·mo′tee·o) *n.* [L., from *amovere,* to remove, take away]. Detachment.

amotio ret·i·nae (ret′i·nee) [L.]. *Obsol.* DETACHMENT OF THE RETINA.

amo·ti·va·tion·al (ay″mo·ti·vay′shun·ul) *adj.* Pertaining to lack of motivation.

amotivational syndrome. *In psychology,* general apathy, mental confusion, and lack of goals, as sometimes observed in student dropouts; association with habitual marijuana use has been proposed but found not to be significant.

amox·a·pine (a·mock′suh·peen) *n.* 2-Chloro-11-(1-piperazinyl)dibenz[*b,f*][1,4]oxazepine, $C_{17}H_{16}ClN_3O$, an antidepressant.

amox·i·cil·lin (a·mock″si·sil′in) *n.* 4-Thia-1-azabicyclo [3.2.0]heptane-2-carboxylic acid, $C_{16}H_{19}N_3O_5S$, a semisynthetic penicillin antibiotic.

Amoxil. Trademark for amoxicillin, a semisynthetic penicillin antibiotic.

AMP Abbreviation for *adenosine monophosphate.*

amp An abbreviation for (a) *ampere;* (b) *amperage.*

am·per·age (am′peer″ij, am′pur·ij) *n.* The number of amperes passing in a given electric circuit. Abbreviated, amp.

am·pere (am′peer, am·peer′) *n.* [A. M. *Ampère,* French physicist, 1775-1836]. The unit of electric current defined by the Conférence Génerale des Poids et Mesures as the steady current which when flowing in straight parallel wires, infinite in length and of negligible cross section, 1 meter apart in free space, will produce a force between the wires of 2×10^{-7} meter-kilogram-second (mks) unit (newton) per meter of length. It is equivalent to the current produced by one volt through a resistance of one ohm. Abbreviated, a., amp.

am·pere·me·ter (am′peer·mee·tur) *n.* AMMETER.

amph-. See *amphi-.*

am·phe·chlor·al (am″fe·klor′al) *n.* α-Methyl-*N*-(2,2,2-trichloroethylidene)phenethylamine, $C_{11}H_{12}Cl_3N$, a sympathomimetic drug used as an anorexic agent.

am·phe·rot·o·ky (am″fur·ot′uh·kee) *n.* [Gk. *amphoteros,* both, + *tokos,* offspring]. Production of both sexes in a single parthenogenetic brood. —**ampheroto·kous** (·kus), **amphe·roto·kal** (·kul) *adj.*

am·phet·a·mine (am·fet′uh·meen, ·min) *n.* [*a*lpha + *me*thyl + *ph*enyl + *e*thyl + *amine*]. 1. Racemic 1-phenyl-2-aminopropane, $C_6H_5CH_2CHNH_2CH_3$, a colorless, volatile, mobile liquid. Formerly used as a nasal vasoconstrictor, by inhalation. Various salts have been used as central nervous system stimulants. 2. In common usage, amphetamine sulfate, dextroamphetamine sulfate, and methamphetamine hydrochloride, all of which act as central nervous system stimulants.

amphi-, amph- [Gk. (rel. to L. *ambi-*)]. A prefix signifying (a) *both, of both kinds,* (b) *on both sides, about, around;* (c) in chemistry, *having substituents in the 2 and 6 positions of two symmetrical 6-membered fused rings.*

am·phi·ar·thro·sis (am″fee·ahr·thro′sis) *n.,* pl. **am·phi·ar·thro·ses** (·seez) [*amphi-* + *arthrosis*] [BNA]. An articulation of contiguous bony surfaces which are connected by either fibrocartilage or an interosseous ligament, and permitting only slight motion. —**amphiar·throt·ic** (·throt′ick) *adj.*

am·phi·as·ter (am′fee·as″tur) *n.* [*amphi-* + *aster*]. The achromatic figure in mitosis, consisting of two asters connected by a spindle. Formerly called *diaster.*

Am·phib·ia (am·fib′ee·uh) *n.pl.* [Gk., pl. of *amphibion* (*zōon*), amphibious (animal)]. A class of vertebrates which includes the salamanders and newts, frogs and toads, the tropical Apoda, and certain extinct orders; distinguished by scaleless skin, paired limbs with toes, gills in at least larval stages, lungs in most orders, and a three-chambered heart. —**amphibia,** *com. n.pl.;* **amphib·i·an** (·ee·un) *adj. & n.*

am·phib·i·ous (am·fib′i·us) *adj.* [Gk. *amphibios,* from *amphi-,* both, + *bios,* life]. Capable of living both on land and in water.

am·phi·blas·tic (am″fi·blas′tick) *adj.* [*amphi-* + *-blastic*]. *In biology,* forming unequal segments.

am·phi·blas·tu·la (am″fi·blas′tew·luh) *n.* [*amphi-* + *blastula*]. 1. A ciliated larval stage of many sponges. 2. A blastula produced by amphiblastic cleavage.

am·phi·bles·tro·des (am″fi·bles·tro′deez) *n.* [Gk. *amphiblēstroeidēs* (*chitōn*), net-like (membrane), retina, from *amphiblēstron,* net]. *Obsol.* RETINA.

am·phi·bol·ic (am″fi·bol′ick) *adj.* [Gk. *amphibolos,* ambiguous]. 1. Uncertain, wavering. 2. Having both an anabolic and a catabolic function; said of certain metabolic pathways.

amphibolic stage. The stage of a disease intervening between its height and its decline; the stage of uncertain prognosis.

am·phib·o·lous (am·fib′uh·lus) *adj.* AMPHIBOLIC.

am·phi·coe·lous, am·phi·ce·lous (am″fi·see′lus) *adj.* [Gk. *amphikoilos,* from *amphi-* + *koilos,* hollow]. Biconcave; applied to the centrum of the vertebra of certain fishes.

am·phi·cra·nia (am″fi·kray′nee·uh) *n.* [*amphi-* + *-crania*]. Headache affecting both sides of the head. Contr. *hemicrania.*

am·phi·cre·at·i·nine (am″fi·kree·at′i·neen, ·nin) *n.* [*amphi-* + *creatinine*]. One of the tissue leucomaines of the creatinine type.

am·phi·cyte (am′fi·site) *n.* [*amphi-* + *-cyte*]. SATELLITE CELL (1).

am·phi·des·mic (am″fi·dez′mick) *adj.* AMPHIDESMOUS.

am·phi·des·mous (am″fi·dez′mus) *adj.* [*amphi-* + *desm-* + *-ous*]. Furnished with a double ligament.

am·phi·er·o·tism (am″fee·err′o·tiz·um) *n.* [*amphi-* + *erotism*]. *Obsol.* 1. A condition in which one can conceive of one's self as being either male or female or both at the same time. 2. Sexual attraction to both males and females.

am·phi·gas·tru·la (am″fi·gas′troo·luh) *n.* [*amphi-* + *gastrula*]. A gastrula having blastomeres of different size in the two hemispheres as a result of total unequal cleavage.

am·phi·gen·e·sis (am″fi·jen′e·sis) *n.* [*amphi-* + *genesis*]. 1. Sexual reproduction. Syn. *amphigony.* 2. BISEXUALITY (1). —**amphi·ge·net·ic** (·je·net′ick) *adj.*

am·phi·gen·ic (am″fi·jen′ick) *adj.* AMPHIGENOUS.

am·phig·e·nous (am·fij′e·nus) *adj.* [Gk. *amphigenēs,* of doubtful gender, from *amphi-* + *genos,* kind, gender]. BISEXUAL (1).

am·phig·o·ny (am·fig′uh·nee) *n.* [*amphi-* + *-gony*]. Sexual reproduction.

am·phi·kar·y·on (am″fi·kăr′ee·on) *n.* [*amphi-* + *karyon*]. A diploid nucleus.

am·phi·mix·is (am″fi·mick′sis) *n.,* pl. **amphimix·es** (·eez) [*amphi-* + Gk. *mixis,* mixing]. 1. *In genetics,* interbreeding; heterozygosis. 2. *In psychoanalysis,* urethral, oral, and anal erotism combined.

amphi·mor·u·la (am″fi·mor′yoo·luh) *n.,* pl. **amphimoru·lae** (·lee) [*amphi-* + *morula*]. A morula resulting from unequal segmentation, the cells of the hemispheres being unlike in size. Syn. *unequal stereoblastula.*

am·phi·ox·us (am″fee·ock′sus) *n.* [NL., from *amphi-* + Gk. *oxys,* sharp]. A lancelet, *Amphioxus lanceolata,* a primitive marine chordate belonging to the subphylum Cephalochorda, regarded by many as a connecting link between the invertebrates and vertebrates.

am·phi·path (am′fi·path) *n.* [*amphi-* + *-path,* having an affinity for (from Gk. *pathos,* feeling)]. AMPHIPHILE. —**am·phi·path·ic** (am″fi·path′ick) *adj.*

am·phi·phile (am′fi·file) *n.* [*amphi-* + *-phile*]. A compound that possesses both a hydrophilic and a lipophilic chemical group, by virtue of which it tends to be miscible with water and with hydrocarbons. —**am·phi·phil·ic** (am″fi·fil′ick) *adj.*

Am·phi·sto·ma·ta (am″fi·sto′muh·tuh) *n.pl.* [NL., from *amphi-* + Gk. *stomata,* mouths]. A suborder of trematode worms, distinguished by a prominent posterior ventral sucking disk.

am·phi·tene (am′fi·teen) *n.* [*amphi-* + *-tene*]. ZYGOTENE.

am·phit·o·ky (am·fit′uh·kee) *n.* [*amphi-* + Gk. *tokos,* offspring]. AMPHEROTOKY. —**amphito·kal** (·kul) *adj.*

am·phit·ri·chate (am·fit′ri·kit, ·kate) *adj.* AMPHITRICHOUS.

am·phit·ri·chous (am·fit′ri·kus) *adj.* [*amphi-* + *trich-* + *-ous*]. Having flagella at both ends.

ampho- [Gk. *amphō*]. A combining form meaning *both.*

am·pho·di·plo·pia (am″fo·di·plo′pee·uh) *n.* [*ampho-* + *diplopia*]. Double vision affecting each of the eyes.

Amphogel. Trademark for aluminum hydroxide gel, an antacid.

am·pho·lyte (am′fo·lite) *n.* AMPHOTERIC ELECTROLYTE.

am·pho·my·cin (am″fo·migh′sin) *n.* An antibiotic substance produced by *Streptomyces canus.*

am·pho·phil (am′fo·fil) *adj. & n.* [*ampho-* + *-phil*]. 1. AMPHOPHILIC. 2. A cell whose cytoplasm stains with both acidic and basic dyes.

amphophil granules. Granules staining with both acid and basic dyes.

am·pho·phil·ic (am″fo·fil′ick) *adj.* [*ampho-* + *-philic*]. Having an affinity for both basic and acidic dyes.

am·phoph·i·lous (am·fof′i·lus) *adj.* AMPHOPHILIC.

am·pho·ric (am·fo′rick) *adj.* [Gk. *amphorikos,* like an amphora]. Resembling the sound produced by blowing across the mouth of an empty jar or bottle; used to describe respiration or resonance.

amphoric resonance. A low-pitched, hollow sound, resembling tympanitic resonance, obtained by auscultation over a pneumothorax or large pulmonary cavity.

amphoric respiration or **breathing.** Respiration characterized by amphoric resonance on auscultation. Compare *cavernous respiration.*

am·pho·ter·ic (am″fo·terr′ick) *adj.* [Gk. *amphoteros,* each of two]. Having both acidic and basic properties; capable of behaving either as a weak acid or a weak base, as aluminum hydroxide, $Al(OH)_3 \rightleftharpoons H_3AlO_3$.

amphoteric electrolyte. An electrolyte that can act as either an acid or a base.

amphoteric element. An element whose oxide in aqueous solution has the ability to act either as an acid or as a base.

am·pho·ter·i·cin B (am″fo·terr′i·sin) *n.* An antibiotic substance, $C_{46}H_{73}NO_{20}$, produced by strains of *Streptomyces nodosus*; active against fungi. Used for treatment of deep-seated mycotic infections.

amphoteric reaction. The reaction of a compound as an acid or base depending upon the substrate.

amphoteric salt. A salt that has both acidic and basic properties.

am·pho·ter·ism (am″fo·terr′iz·um, am·fot′ur·iz·um) *n.* The quality of being amphoteric.

am·phot·ero·di·plo·pia (am·fot″ur·o·di·plo′pee·uh) *n.* [Gk. *amphoteros,* each of two, + *diplopia*]. AMPHODIPLOPIA.

am·pi·cil·lin (am″pi·sil′in) *n.* α-Aminobenzyl penicillin, $C_{16}H_{19}N_3O_4S$, a semisynthetic penicillin that is well absorbed when taken orally and is acid resistant. It is more effective than penicillin G against certain gram-negative bacteria.

am·pli·fi·ca·tion, *n.* 1. *In microscopy,* the enlargement of the visual area, as amplification 200×, or 200 diameters. 2. The magnification of sound. 3. *In electricity,* the increase of electric current in either voltage or amperage, as of a transformer. —**am·pli·fy,** *v.*

am·pli·fi·er, *n.* 1. Any device that enlarges, magnifies, or increases the size, strength, or power of an object or force. 2. The concavo-convex lens between the objective and ocular of a microscope. 3. Any device that increases the amplitude or power level of an electrical signal by using one or more electron tubes or solid-state devices which derive energy from a power supply.

am·pli·tude, *n.* [L. *amplitudo,* breadth, from *amplus,* broad]. Range: extent, as of a vibration or oscillation, represented as the greatest value of a quantity which varies periodically.

am·poule (am′pool) *n.* AMPUL.

am·pro·tro·pine (am″pro·tro′peen, ·pin) *n.* 3-Diethylamino-2,2-dimethylpropyl tropate, $C_{18}H_{29}NO_3$, a parasympatholytic agent employed as an antispasmodic; used as the phosphate salt.

am·pul, am·pule (am′pul, am′pyool, am′pool) *n.* [L. *ampulla,* flask, bottle]. 1. A container, commonly made of glass and capable of being hermetically sealed, intended to hold sterile preparations usually intended for parenteral use. 2. Any of a class of preparations consisting of a sealed container holding a medicament. Such preparations are now more commonly known as injections.

am·pul·la (am·pul'uh, am·pŏŏl'uh) *n.*, pl. **ampul·lae** (·lee) [L., small flask or bottle] [NA]. The dilated extremity of a canal or duct, as of the mammary ducts and semicircular canals.

ampulla ca·na·li·cu·li la·cri·ma·lis (kan·uh·lick'yoo·lye lack·ri·may'lis) [NA]. AMPULLA OF THE LACRIMAL DUCT.

ampulla duc·tus de·fe·ren·tis (duck'tus def·e·ren'tis) [NA]. AMPULLA OF THE DUCTUS DEFERENS.

ampulla ductus la·cri·ma·lis (lack·ri·may'lis) [BNA]. Ampulla canaliculi lacrimalis (= AMPULLA OF THE LACRIMAL DUCT).

ampullae mem·bra·na·ce·ae (mem·bruh·nay'see·ee) [NA]. MEMBRANOUS AMPULLAE.

ampullae os·se·ae (os'ee·ee) [NA]. OSSEOUS AMPULLAE.

ampulla he·pa·to·pan·cre·a·ti·ca (hep''uh·to·pan·kree·at'i·kuh) [NA]. HEPATICOPANCREATIC AMPULLA.

ampulla lac·ti·fe·ra (lack·tif'e·ruh). The dilatation of a milk duct near its opening on the nipple.

ampulla mem·bra·na·cea anterior (mem·bruh·nay'see·uh) [NA]. The anterior membranous ampulla. See *membranous ampullae.*

ampulla membranacea la·te·ra·lis (lat·e·ray'lis) [NA]. The lateral membranous ampulla. See *membranous ampullae.*

ampulla membranacea posterior [NA]. The posterior membranous ampulla. See *membranous ampullae.*

ampulla membranacea superior [BNA]. AMPULLA MEMBRANACEA ANTERIOR.

ampulla of the ductus deferens. The dilated distal end of the ductus deferens just before its junction with the duct of the seminal vesicle. NA *ampulla ductus deferentis.* See also Plate 25.

ampulla of the gallbladder. A dilatation sometimes present where the gallbladder empties into the cystic duct.

ampulla of the lacrimal duct. A slight dilatation of the lacrimal duct beyond the punctum. NA *ampulla canaliculi lacrimalis.*

ampulla of the rectum. The dilated terminal portion of the rectum just proximal to the anal canal. NA *ampulla recti.*

ampulla of the uterine tube. The dilated portion of the uterine tube near its fimbriated end. NA *ampulla tubae uterinae.*

ampulla of the vagina. The dilated upper end of the vagina, where it joins the cervix of the uterus.

ampulla of Va·ter (fah'tur) [A. *Vater,* German anatomist, 1684–1751]. HEPATICOPANCREATIC AMPULLA.

ampulla os·sea anterior (os'ee·uh) [NA]. The anterior osseous ampulla. See *osseous ampullae.*

ampulla ossea la·te·ra·lis (lat·e·ray'lis) [NA]. The lateral osseous ampulla. See *osseous ampullae.*

ampulla ossea posterior [NA]. The posterior osseous ampulla. See *osseous ampullae.*

ampulla ossea superior [BNA]. AMPULLA OSSEA ANTERIOR.

ampulla phre·ni·ca (fren'i·kuh). A pouchlike dilatation of the esophagus which may occasionally be present just above the diaphragm.

am·pul·lar (am·pul'ur, ·pŏŏl', am'puh·lur) *adj.* Pertaining to or resembling an ampulla.

ampulla rec·ti (reck'tye) [NA]. AMPULLA OF THE RECTUM.

ampullar pregnancy. Gestation in the outer portion of the uterine tube.

am·pul·lary (am'pul·err''ee) *adj.* AMPULLAR.

ampullary aneurysm. A small saccular aneurysm; it is most common in the arteries of the brain. See also *berry aneurysm.*

ampullary sulcus. The external transverse groove on each membranous ampulla for the entrance of the ampullary nerve. NA *sulcus ampullaris.*

am·pul·late (am'puh·late, am·pŏŏl'ate) *adj.* Having or shaped like an ampulla.

ampulla tu·bae ute·ri·nae (tew'bee yoo·te·rye'nee) [NA]. AMPULLA OF THE UTERINE TUBE.

am·pul·lu·la (am·pul'yoo·luh) *n.*, pl. **ampullu·lee** (·lee) [L., dim. of *ampulla*]. A minute ampulla, as in the lymphatic or lacteal vessels.

am·pu·tate (am'pew·tate) *v.* [L. *amputare, amputatus,* from *putare,* to prune]. To cut off all or part of an extremity, digit, organ, or projecting part of the body.

amputating knife. A long, pointed, single- or double-edged instrument, used for amputations.

amputating ulcer. A penetrating ulcer encircling a part, such as a toe, leading ultimately to loss of the distal portion.

am·pu·ta·tion (am''pew·tay'shun) *n.* [L. *amputatio,* from *amputare,* to amputate]. 1. Surgical removal of all or a part of a limb, a projecting part or process, or an organ of the body. 2. Traumatic or spontaneous loss of a limb, part, or organ.

amputation appliance. A prosthesis for an amputated limb.

amputation by transfixion. An amputation performed by thrusting an amputating knife through a limb and cutting the flaps from within out.

amputation flap. A simple, broad-based flap which needs no advancement, and is shaped to provide proper contour of the part to be covered.

amputation neuroma. A benign, tumorlike mass of proliferating proximal nerve fibers and fibrous tissue, which sometimes occurs in the stump of a severed nerve.

amputation stump. The rounded and shaped distal portion of an amputated limb or organ.

am·pu·tee (am''pew·tee') *n.* One who has had major amputation of one or more limbs.

am·py·zine (am'pi·zeen) *n.* (Dimethylamino)pyrazine, $C_6H_9N_3$, a central stimulant drug; used as the sulfate salt.

am·quin·ate (am·kwin'ate) *n.* Methyl 7-(diethylamino)-4-hydroxy-6-propyl-3-quinolinecarboxylate, $C_{18}H_{24}N_2O_3$, an antimalarial drug.

amuck (uh·muck') *adv.* [Malay *amok,* furious attack]. In a state of frenzy, often with homicidal tendencies.

amu·sia (a·mew'zee·uh) *n.* [Gk. *amousia,* unmusicalness, lack of harmony]. Loss or impairment of the ability to produce or comprehend music or musical sounds, caused by lesion of the cerebrum but not by lesion affecting primary sensory, motor, or general intellectual function.

am·y·cho·pho·bia (am''i·ko·fo''bee·uh) *n.* [Gk. *amychē,* scratch, skin wound, + *-phobia*]. Morbid fear of being lacerated, scratched, or clawed.

am·y·dri·a·sis (am''i·drye'uh·sis) *n.* [*a-* + *mydriasis*]. Pupillary contraction. Contr. *mydriasis.*

amyd·ri·caine (a·mid'ri·kane) *n.* 2-Benzoxy-2-dimethylaminomethyl-1-dimethylaminobutane, $C_{16}H_{26}N_2O_2$; has been used as a local anesthetic, in the form of the hydrochloride salt.

amy·el·en·ceph·a·lus (ay·migh''e·len·sef'uh·lus) *n.* [*a-* + *myel-* + *encephal-* + *-us*]. A fetus having neither brain nor spinal cord. —**amyelen·ce·phal·ic** (·se·fal'ick) *adj.;* **amyelen·ceph·a·lia** (·se·fay'lee·uh) *n.*

amy·e·lia (am''eye·ee'lee·uh, ·el'ee·uh, ay''migh·) *n.* [*a-* + *myel-* + *-ia*]. Congenital partial or complete absence of the spinal cord. —**amy·el·ic** (·el'ick, ·ee'lick) *adj.*

amy·e·li·nat·ed (ay·migh'e·li·nay''tid, a·migh') *adj.* UNMYELINATED.

amy·e·lin·ic (ay·migh''e·lin'ick) *adj.* [*a-* + *myelinic*]. UNMYELINATED.

amyelinic neuroma. A traumatic neuroma composed of unmyelinated fibers.

amy·e·lon·ic (a·migh''e·lon'ick, ay·migh'') *adj.* [*a-* + *myelon* + *-ic*]. 1. Without bone marrow. 2. Without a spinal cord; amyelic.

amy·e·lus (a·migh'e·lus) *n.* [*a-* + *myel-* + *-us*]. An individual with partial or complete absence of the spinal cord. —**amye·lous,** *adj.*

amygdal-, amygdalo-. A combining form meaning (a) *amygdaloid body;* (b) *tonsil, tonsillar;* (c) *almond, of almonds.*

amyg·da·la (a·mig'duh·luh) *n.*, pl. **amygda·lae** (·lee) [L., almond, from Gk. *amygdalē*]. AMYGDALOID BODY.

amyg·da·lase (a·mig'duh·lace, ·laze) *n.* [Gk. *amygdalē*, almond, + *-ase*]. EMULSIN.

am·yg·dal·ic acid (am″ig·dal'ick). MANDELIC ACID.

amyg·da·lin (a·mig'duh·lin) *n.* [Gk. *amygdalē*, almond, + *-in*]. A glycoside, $C_{20}H_{27}NO_{11}$, of mandelonitrile and gentiobiose, occurring in bitter almond and other sources. In the presence of water, the enzyme emulsin causes its hydrolysis into glucose, benzaldehyde, and hydrocyanic acid.

amygdalo-. See *amygdal-.*

amyg·da·loid (a·mig'duh·loid) *adj.* [Gk. *amygdaloeidēs,* from *amygdalē,* almond]. Shaped like an almond.

amygdaloid body. An almond-shaped mass of gray matter situated in the lateral wall and roof of the inferior horn of the lateral ventricle. NA *corpus amygdaloideum.*

amyg·da·loid·ec·to·my (a·mig″duh·loy·deck'tuh·mee) *n.* [*amygdaloid* + *-ectomy*]. AMYGDALOTOMY.

amygdaloid nucleus. AMYGDALOID BODY.

amygdaloid tubercle. A prominence in the wall of the inferior horn of the lateral ventricle overlying the amygdaloid body.

amyg·da·lo·lith (a·mig'duh·lo·lith, am″ig·dal'o·lith) *n.* [*amygdalo-* + *-lith*]. *Rare.* TONSILLAR CALCULUS.

amyg·da·lot·o·my (a·mig″duh·lot'uh·mee) *n.* [*amygdalo-* + *-tomy*]. Surgical destruction of the amygdaloid body.

am·yl (am'il, ay'mil) *n.* [*amyl-* + *-yl*]. 1. PENTYL. 2. Any mixture of several pentyl radicals. 3. Any five-carbon chain of unknown structure. —**amyl·ic** (a·mil'ick) *adj.*

amyl-, amylo- [Gk. *amylon*]. A combining form meaning *starch.*

am·y·la·ceous (am″i·lay'shus) *adj.* [*amyl-* + *-aceous*]. Containing starch; starchlike.

amyl alcohol. 1. Any of eight isomeric alcohols of the composition $C_5H_{11}OH$, variously denominated. 2. Commercial amyl alcohol consisting predominantly of isoamyl alcohol (3-methyl-1-butanol); the primary constituent of fusel oil.

am·y·lase (am″i·lace, ·laze) *n.* [*amyl-* + *-ase*]. Any of two general types of enzymes that accelerate hydrolysis of starch and glycogen to produce different carbohydrate derivatives. α-Amylase (alpha amylase) occurs in malt, in certain molds and bacteria, and in saliva and pancreatic juice; it produces dextrins as hydrolysis products. A concentrated preparation of this enzyme, obtained from nonpathogenic bacteria, is used medicinally as an anti-inflammatory drug. β-Amylase (beta amylase) occurs in grains, in malt, and in vegetables; it produces maltose.

Amylcaine. A former trademark for naepaine, a local anesthetic, used as the hydrochloride. See also *Amylsine.*

amyl·ene (am'i·leen, ay'mi·leen) *n.* [*amyl-* + *-ene*]. A liquid hydrocarbon, C_5H_{10}, having anesthetic properties but too toxic and flammable to use.

amylene hydrate. Tertiary amyl alcohol, $C_2H_5(CH_3)_2COH$. A narcotic substance; rarely used by itself, but employed as a solvent for and synergist with the basal anesthetic tribromoethanol.

amyl nitrite. Isoamyl nitrite, $C_5H_{11}ONO$. A yellowish liquid, having an ethereal, fruity odor and a pungent, aromatic taste; used by inhalation to relax arterial spasms and of especial value in angina pectoris. Its action is immediate but fleeting.

amyl nitrite test. 1. A test to determine the extent of arteriolar spasticity versus arteriolar sclerosis by measuring the fall in diastolic blood pressure on inhalation of amyl nitrite. 2. A test to determine the origin of heart murmurs by changing the heart rate, peripheral arterial resistance, and venous return.

amylo-. See *amyl-.*

am·y·lo·bar·bi·tone (am″i·lo·bahr'bi·tone) *n.* British name for amobarbital.

am·y·lo·clast (am'i·lo·klast) *n.* [*amylo-* + Gk. *klastos,* broken]. An enzyme that catalyzes hydrolysis of starch. —**am·y·lo·clas·tic** (am″i·lo·klas'tick) *adj.*

am·y·lo·dex·trin (am″i·lo·decks'trin) *n.* [*amylo-* + *dextrin*]. SOLUBLE STARCH.

am·y·lo·dys·pep·sia (am″i·lo·dis·pep'see·uh) *n.* [*amylo-* + *dyspepsia*]. Inability to digest starchy foods.

am·y·loid (am'i·loid) *n.* [*amyl-* + *-oid*]. A complex protein deposited in tissues, characterized physically by its hyaline gross structure and fibillar ultrastructure, and chemically by special staining reactions. It is composed, in part, of proteins very similar to or identical with immunoglobulins or their fragments.

amyloid bodies. Microscopic, concentrically laminated, hyaline bodies occurring in the acini of the prostate, in the meninges, in diseased lungs, and occasionally in other sites; staining like amyloid with metachromatic aniline dyes. Syn. *corpora amylacea.*

amyloid degeneration. A retrogressive change characterized by the replacement or distortion of normal structures by material having the waxy appearance and staining properties of amyloid.

amyloid disease. AMYLOIDOSIS.

amyloid kidney. A kidney in which amyloid has been deposited.

amyloid liver. A liver in which amyloid has been deposited.

am·y·loi·do·sis (am″i·loy·do'sis) *n.* Deposition of amyloid in various organs or tissues of the body. See also *primary amyloidosis, secondary amyloidosis.*

amyloidosis cu·tis (kew'tis). The presence of amyloid in the skin in the clinical form of pruritic papules or plaques; it is not necessarily associated with systemic amyloidosis.

amyloid tumor. A nonneoplastic nodule situated usually on a vocal fold, a few millimeters in diameter, spherical, and often pedunculated. Made up principally of a hyaline acidophilic substance which has staining reactions like primary amyloid. Less often found in the wall of the urinary bladder and rarely in other sites.

am·y·lol·y·sis (am″i·lol'i·sis) *n.* [*amylo-* + *-lysis*]. The digestion of starch, or its conversion into maltose. —**amy·lo·lyt·ic** (·lo·lit'ick) *adj.*

amylolytic enzyme. An enzyme that hydrolyzes starch to dextrin and maltose, as ptyalin or pancreatic amylase.

am·y·lo·mal·tase (am″i·lo·mawl'tace, ·taze) *n.* A bacterial enzyme that converts maltose to amylose and glucose.

am·y·lo·pec·tin (am″i·lo·peck'tin) *n.* [*amylo-* + *pectin*]. The outer, almost insoluble, highly branched polysaccharide of starch granules. It stains violet with iodine. Contr. *amylose.*

am·y·lo·pec·ti·no·sis (am″y·lo·peck″ti·no'sis) *n.* [*amylopectin* + *-osis*]. Glycogenosis caused by a defect of amylo-(1,4→1,6)-transglucosidase (branching enzyme), with storage of glycogen having branches longer than normal in the liver, kidney, heart, muscle, and reticuloendothelial system, and diminished response to glucagon and epinephrine. Syn. *Andersen's disease, brancher deficiency glycogenosis, type IV of Cori.*

am·y·lo·phos·pho·ryl·ase (am″i·lo·fos·for'il·ace, ·aze) *n.* [*amylo-* + *phosphorylase*]. An enzyme catalyzing synthesis of amylose from glucose 1-phosphate.

am·y·lo·plast (am'i·lo·plast) *n.* [*amylo-* + *-plast*]. A granule in the protoplasm of a plant cell that forms starch by photosynthesis.

am·y·lop·sin (am″i·lop'sin) *n.* [*amylo-* + *-psin* (as in trypsin)]. PANCREATIC AMYLASE.

am·y·lose (am'i·loce, ·loze) *n.* [*amyl-* + *-ose*]. The inner, relatively soluble, unbranched or linear polysaccharide of starch granules. It stains blue with iodine. Contr. *amylopectin.*

am·y·lo·su·crase (am″i-lo·soo′krace, ·kraze) *n.* A bacterial enzyme that converts sucrose to amylose and fructose.

amylo- (1,4→1,6)-trans·glu·co·sy·lase (trans·gloo·ko′si·lace, ·gloo′ko·) *n.* An enzyme involved in the conversion of amylose to glycogen. Syn. *brancher enzyme.*

am·y·lum (am′i·lum) *n.* [L., from Gk. *amylon,* neuter of *amylos,* fine-ground]. STARCH (1).

amy·lu·ria (am″i·lew′ree·uh) *n.* [*amyl-* + *-uria*]. The presence of starch in the urine.

amyo·es·the·sia, amyo·aes·the·sia (ay·migh″o·es·theezh′uh, ·theez′ee·uh, a·migh″) *n.* [*a-* + *myo-* + *esthesia*]. State of being without muscle sense; lack of the sense of motion, weight, and position.

amyo·es·the·sis, amyo·aes·the·sis (ay·migh″o·es·thees′is, a·migh″) *n.* AMYOESTHESIA.

amyo·pla·sia (ay·migh″o·play′zhuh, ·zee·uh) *n.* [*a-* + *myo-* + *-plasia*]. Lack of muscle formation and development. —**amyo·plas·tic** (·plas′tick) *adj.*

amyoplasia con·gen·i·ta (kon·jen′i·tuh). Arthrogryposis multiplex due to congenital muscle deficiency.

amyo·sta·sia (ay·migh″o·stay′zhuh, ·zee·uh, a·migh″) *n.* [*a-* + *myo-* + Gk. *stasis,* standing, stoppage, + *-ia*]. A tremor of the muscles, causing difficulty in standing, often seen in diseases involving the basal ganglia. —**amyo·stat·ic** (·stat′ick) *adj.*

amyostatic syndrome. 1. Any extrapyramidal disorder. 2. HEPATOLENTICULAR DEGENERATION.

amyo·tax·ia (ay·migh″o·tack′see·uh, a·migh″o·) *n.* [*ataxia* + *myo-*]. Ataxia or incoordination due to difficulties in controlling voluntary movements. —**amyotax·ic** (·sick) *adj.*

amy·o·taxy (ay·migh′o·tack″see) *n.* AMYOTAXIA.

amyo·to·nia (ay·migh″o·to′nee·uh) *n.* [*a-* + *myo-* + *-tonia*]. Lack of muscular tone; floppiness.

amyotonia con·gen·i·ta (kon·jen′i·tuh). *Obsol.* Pronounced muscular flaccidity and weakness in infancy, due to a variety of causes. Compare *myotonia congenita.* See also *floppy-infant syndrome, infantile spinal muscular atrophy, benign congenital hypotonia.*

amyo·tro·phia (ay·migh″o·tro′fee·uh, a·migh″o·) *n.* Amyotrophy (= MUSCULAR ATROPHY).

amyotrophia spi·na·lis pro·gres·si·va (spye·nay′lis pro·gre·sigh′vuh). 1. Progressive muscular atrophy secondary to loss of spinal innervation. 2. INFANTILE SPINAL MUSCULAR ATROPHY.

amyotrophic lateral sclerosis. An idiopathic degenerative disease of the upper and lower motor neurons, with onset chiefly in middle age, characterized by motor weakness and spastic limbs associated with muscular atrophy, fasciculations, and fibrillations, and with bulbar and pseudobulbar palsy. Pathologically, there is a loss of neurons in the anterior horns of the spinal cord and in the bulbar nuclei and degeneration of the corticospinal and corticobulbar tracts.

amyotrophic syphilitic myelitis. Syphilitic meningomyelitis resulting in muscle wasting.

amy·ot·ro·phy (am″eye·ot′ruh·fee, ay″migh·) *n.* [*atrophy* + *myo-*]. MUSCULAR ATROPHY. —**amyo·troph·ic** (ay·migh″o·trof′ick, ·tro′fick, a·migh″o·) *adj.*

Am·y·ris (am′i·ris) *n.* A genus of tropical trees and shrubs producing fragrant resins and gums, such as elemi.

Amytal. Trademark for amobarbital, a sedative and hypnotic.

amyx·ia (a·mick′see·uh, ay·mick′) *n.* [*a-* + *myx-* + *-ia*]. Absence or deficiency of mucous secretion.

amyx·or·rhea, amyx·or·rhoea (a·mick″so·ree′uh, ay·mick″) *n.* [*a-* + *myxo-* + *-rrhea*]. Absence of the normal flow of mucous secretion.

An., an. Abbreviation for *anode.*

-an. *In chemistry,* a suffix that indicates *a sugarlike substance, a glycoside, or a gum.*

an-. See *a-.*

ANA Abbreviation for *nuclear antibody.*

A. N. A. 1. American Nurses Association. 2. American Neurological Association.

ana (an′uh) [Gk.]. So much of each. Symbol, ā, āā.

ana- [Gk.]. A prefix meaning (a) *up, upward, upper;* (b) *back, backward;* (c) *again, anew;* (d) in chemistry, *having substituents in the 1 and 5 positions of two symmetrical 6-membered fused rings.*

anab·a·sine (a·nab′uh·seen, ·sin) *n.* 2-(3-Pyridyl)piperidine, $C_{10}H_{14}N_2$, a liquid alkaloid from the Russian herb *Anabasis aphylla* and from *Nicotiana glauca,* with effects similar to those of nicotine; used as an insecticide.

an·a·bi·ot·ic (an″uh·bye·ot′ick) *adj. & n.* [Gk. *anabiōsis,* revival, from *anabioun,* to come to life again]. 1. Apparently lifeless but capable of being revived. 2. Any agent used to effect restoration or revival. —**anabi·o·sis** (·o′sis) *n.*

an·a·bol·er·gy (an″uh·bol′ur·jee) *n.* [*anabolic* + *-ergy*]. The work performed or energy used in anabolic processes.

anab·o·lin (a·nab′o·lin) *n.* Any substance formed during the anabolic process.

anab·o·lism (a·nab′uh·liz·um) *n.* [Gk. *anabolē,* buildup, prelude, from *ana-,* up, + *ballein,* to throw]. Synthetic or constructive metabolism; especially, the conversion of simple nutritive compounds into complex living matter. Contr. *catabolism.* —**an·a·bol·ic** (an″uh·bol′ick) *adj.*

an·a·camp·tics (an″uh·kamp′ticks) *n.* [Gk. *anakamptein,* to bend back]. The study of reflection of light or of sound. —**anacamp·tic** (·tick) *adj.*

An·a·car·di·a·ce·ae (an″uh·kahr″dee·ay′see·ee) *n.pl.* A family of plants, found mostly in the tropics, reported to cause dermatitis on contact, including poison ivy, poison oak.

anacatadidymus. ANAKATADIDYMUS.

ana·ce·li·a·del·phus (an″uh·see″lee·uh·del′fus) *n.* [*ana-* + *celi-* + *-adelphus*]. A paired monstrosity united by the thorax or upper part of the abdomen. —**anaceliadelphous,** *adj.*

an·acid·i·ty (an″uh·sid′i·tee) *n.* [*an-* + *acidity*]. 1. The absence of normal acidity. 2. ACHLORHYDRIA.

anac·la·sis (a·nack′luh·sis) *n.* [Gk. *anaklasis,* from *ana-,* back, + *klan,* to break, deflect]. Reflection or refraction of light or sound. —**an·a·clas·tic** (an″uh·klas′tick) *adj.*

anac·li·sis (a·nack′li·sis) *n.* [Gk. *anaklisis,* a reclining position; a back to lean against, from *ana-,* back, + *klinein,* to lean]. The state of being emotionally dependent upon others; specifically, in psychoanalysis, the state in which the satisfaction of the sex libido is conditioned by some other instinct, such as hunger; used especially in reference to the dependence of an infant on a mother or mother surrogate for his sense of well-being. —**ana·clit·ic** (an″uh·klit′ick) *adj.*

anaclitic depression. *In child psychiatry,* an acute and striking impairment of an infant's physical, social, and intellectual development which sometimes occurs following a sudden separation from a loving parent figure. See also *hospitalism.*

anaclitic object choice. *In psychoanalysis,* the conscious or unconscious choice of a love object, resembling the person upon whom the individual was dependent for emotional support or comfort in infancy.

an·ac·me·sis (an·ack′me·sis, an″ack·mee′sis) *n.* [*an-* + *acme* + *-esis*]. Maturation arrest in the granulocytic cells of the bone marrow.

an·acou·sia, an·acu·sia (an″uh·koo′zhuh, ·zee·uh) *n.* [*an-* + Gk. *akousis,* hearing, + *-ia*]. Complete deafness.

anac·ro·a·sia (an·ack″ro·ay′zee·uh, ·zhuh) *n.* [*an-* + Gk. *akroasis,* hearing, listening, attention, + *-ia*]. AUDITORY APHASIA.

an·a·crot·ic (an″uh·krot′ick) *adj.* [Gk. *ana,* up, + *krotos,* beat]. Pertaining to the upstroke or ascending limb of a pressure wave. Contr. *catacrotic.*

anacrotic incisura or **notch.** ANACROTIC SHOULDER.

anacrotic pulse. A palpable twice-beating arterial pulse with both pulses occurring during systole before the second heart sound; the first impulse is due to accentuation of the normal anacrotic shoulder; seen best in the carotid artery in cases of aortic stenosis.

anacrotic shoulder. A pause or notch in the ascending limb of the arterial pulse-wave tracing at the time of maximal left ventricular ejection; it is prominent in cases of aortic stenosis.

anac·ro·tism (a·nack'ruh·tiz·um) *n.* [*anacrotic* + *-ism*]. The condition in which one or more notches or waves occur on the ascending limb of the arterial pulse tracing.

anacusia. ANACOUSIA.

an·a·cu·sis, an·a·cou·sis (an''uh·koo'sis) *n.* [*an-* + Gk. *akousis*, hearing]. ANACOUSIA.

an·a·de·nia (an''uh·dee'nee·uh) *n.* [*an-* + *aden-* + *-ia*]. 1. Deficiency of glandular activity. 2. Absence of glands.

an·a·did·y·mus (an''uh·did'i·mus) *n.* [*ana-* + *-didymus*]. A monster showing inferior duplicity but union above, as a dipygus. **—anadidymous,** *adj.*

ana·dip·sia (an''uh·dip'see·uh) *n.* [*ana-* + Gk. *dipsa*, thirst, + *-ia*]. POLYDIPSIA.

Anadrol. A trademark for oxymetholone, an anabolic steroid.

anaedeous. ANEDEOUS.

anaemia. ANEMIA.

anaemic. ANEMIC.

an·aer·obe (an'air·obe, an·air'obe, ·ay'ur·obe) *n.* [*an-* + *aerobe*]. A microorganism that will grow in the absence of molecular oxygen. The final hydrogen acceptors are such compounds as nitrates, sulfates, and carbonates (anaerobic respiration) or organic compounds (fermentation).

an·aer·o·bi·ase (an·air''o·bye'ace, ·aze) *n.* A proteolytic enzyme which acts under anaerobic conditions and is present in a number of anaerobes.

an·aer·o·bic (an''air·o'bick) *adj.* [*an-* + *aerobic*] 1. Not utilizing oxygen. 2. Growing best in an oxygen-free atmosphere. 3. Of or pertaining to an anaerobe.

anaerobic contraction. A phase of muscular contraction utilizing no molecular oxygen.

anaerobic metabolism. Metabolism carried on in the absence of molecular oxygen.

an·aero·bi·o·sis (an''air·o·bye·o'sis, an·ay''ur·o·) *n.* [*an-* + *aero-* + *-biosis*]. Life sustained in the absence of molecular oxygen. See also *anaerobe.* **—anaerobi·ot·ic** (·ot'ick) *adj.*

an·aero·gen·ic (an''air·o·jen'ick, an·ay''ur·o·) *adj.* [*an-* + *aerogenic*]. Not gas-producing.

an·aero·phyte (an·air'o·fite, an·ay'ur·o·, an'air·o·) *n.* [*an-* + *aero-* + *-phyte*]. A plant capable of living without a direct supply of oxygen.

anaesth... See *anesth....*

an·a·gen (an'uh·jen) *n.* [*ana-* + *-gen*esis]. The early, productive phase of the hair cycle in a follicle, in which a new hair is synthesized. Contr. *catagen, telogen.*

ana·gen·e·sis (an''uh·jen'e·sis) *n.* [NL., from Gk. *anagennēsis*]. *Obsol.* Reparation or reproduction of tissues; regeneration.

an·a·ges·tone (an''uh·jes'tone) *n.* 17-Hydroxy-6-methylpregn-4-en-20-one, $C_{22}H_{33}O_2$, a progestational steroid; used as the acetate ester.

an·a·go·ge (an''uh·go'jee, an'uh·go''jee) *n.* [Gk. *anagōgē*, lifting up, spiritual uplift]. Spiritual, moral, or idealistic phases of thought.

an·a·gog·ic (an''uh·goj'ick) *adj.* [Gk. *anagōgios*, spiritually uplifting, mystical]. 1. Pertaining to spiritual, moral, or idealistic thoughts. 2. *In psychoanalysis,* pertaining to the efforts of the subconscious to achieve such thoughts; also, pertaining to dream material which expresses such ideas, as contrasted with that representing the sexual forces of the unconscious.

an·a·go·gy (an'uh·go''jee, ·goj''ee) *n.* ANAGOGE.

ana·kata·did·y·mus (an''uh·kat''uh·did'i·mus) *n.* [*ana-* + *kata-* + *-didymus*]. Conjoined twins exhibiting both inferior and superior duplicity. **—anakatadidymous,** *adj.*

anakh·re (a·nack'reh) *n.* GOUNDOU.

an·a·ku·sis (an''uh·koo'sis, ·kew'sis) *n. Rare.* ANACOUSIA.

anal (ay'nul) *adj.* 1. Pertaining to or situated near the anus. 2. *In psychoanalytic theory,* pertaining to the anal stage. See also *anal character, anal erotism.*

an·al·bu·min·emia, an·al·bu·min·ae·mia (an''al·bew''mi·nee'mee·uh) *n.* [*an-* + *albumin* + *-emia*]. 1. A hereditary disorder in which the synthesis of plasma albumin is impaired. 2. Deficiency or absence of plasma albumin.

anal canal. The terminal portion of the large intestine extending from the rectum to the anus. NA *canalis analis.*

anal character. A type of personality in which anal erotic traits dominate beyond the period of childhood.

anal columns. Vertical folds of the mucous membrane of the anal canal. Syn. *rectal columns.* NA *columnae anales.*

anal crypt. One of the small cul-de-sacs between the anal columns. Syn. *anal sinus, rectal sinus.* NA (pl.) *sinus anales* (sing. *sinus analis*).

an·a·lep·tic (an''uh·lep'tick) *adj. & n.* [Gk. *analēptikos*, restorative, from *ana-*, up, + *lambanein*, to take]. 1. Stimulating the central nervous system. 2. Restorative; hastening convalescence. 3. A drug or other agent whose most prominent action is analeptic, such as one used to restore consciousness after fainting, anesthesia, or coma.

anal erotism. Localization of libido in the anal zone.

Analexin. Trademark for phenyramidol, an analgesic drug used as the hydrochloride salt.

anal fissure. An elongated break in the anal mucosa, frequently causing itching, pain, and bleeding, that tends to persist because of repeated trauma from passage of hard feces, infection, and sphincter spasm. The lesion may be associated with a sentinel pile.

anal fistula. A sinus opening from the anorectal area into the connective tissue about the rectum or discharging externally.

an·al·ge·sia (an''al·jee'zee·uh) *n.* [Gk. *analgēsia*, from *an-* + *algos*, pain]. Insensibility to painful stimuli without loss of consciousness.

analgesia al·ge·ra (al'je·ruh, al·jeer'uh) [NL., from Gk. *algēros*, painful]. Spontaneous pain in a part that is insensitive to painful stimuli.

analgesia do·lo·ro·sa (do·lo·ro'suh). ANALGESIA ALGERA.

an·al·ge·sic (an''al·jee'zick, ·jee'sick) *adj. & n.* [*analgesia* + *-ic*]. 1. Relieving pain. 2. Not affected by pain. 3. A drug that relieves pain. **—an·al·ge·sist** (an''al·jee'zist) *n.*; **an·al·gize** (an'al·jize) *v.*

analgesic panaris. Painless lesions of the fingers, as in Morvan's disease.

Analgesine. Trademark for antipyrine, an analgesic and antipyretic.

an·al·get·ic (an''al·jet'ick) *adj.* [Gk. *analgētos*, painless, insensible to pain, from *an-* + *algos*, pain]. ANALGESIC.

an·al·gia (an·al'jee·uh) *n.* [*an-* + *-algia*]. ANALGESIA. **—anal·gic** (·jick) *adj.*

anal gland. Any gland of the anal region.

anal hillock. ANAL TUBERCLE.

an·al·ler·gic (an''uh·lur'jick) *adj.* [*an-* + *allergic*]. Not producing allergy, anaphylaxis, or hypersensitivity.

anal membrane. *In embryology,* the dorsal part of the cloacal membrane caudal to the urorectal septum.

anal mound. *In embryology,* a mound produced by the anterior median union of the anal tubercles.

an·a·logue, an·a·log (an'uh·log) *n.* [F., from Gk. *analogos*, conformable, proportionate]. 1. An organ or part having the same function as another but differing in structure and origin, as the wing of an insect and the wing of a bird. 2. One of a group of compounds with similar electronic structure, but with different atoms, as an isologue. 3. A chemical compound which resembles a metabolically active substance structurally, but may differ functionally by being either inactive or opposite in effect. 4. (*In attributive use*) Functioning by the use of a similar object or structure as a model; specifically, of a computer: representing numerical values by physical quantities, such as lengths or voltages, so as to allow the manipulation of numerical data over a continuous range of values. Contr. *digital* (4).

anal·o·gy (uh·nal'uh·jee) *n.* [Gk. *analogia,* proportion, correspondence]. 1. Resemblance in two or more attributes between two things which differ in other respects. 2. *In biology,* a similarity in function without correspondence in structure and origin. —**analo·gous** (·gus) *adj.*

anal papilla. Any of the small elevations occasionally present on the free margins of the anal valves or at the bases of the anal columns. Syn. *papilla of Morgagni.*

anal pit. PROCTODEUM.

anal plate. ANAL MEMBRANE.

anal reflex. Contraction of the external anal sphincter in response to stroking or pricking the skin or mucous membrane in the perianal region. Syn. *wink response.*

anal ring. A ring-shaped ridge about the embryonic anal orifice produced by growth and fusion of the anal tubercles.

anal sinus. 1. PROCTODEUM. 2. ANAL CRYPT.

anal sphincter. Either of the sphincter ani muscles.

anal stage. *In psychoanalysis,* the stage of development, from 9 or 12 months of age to as late as 36 months, during which the child becomes concerned with his excreta. See also *anal character, anal erotism.*

anal triangle. A triangle with the base between the two ischial tuberosities and the apex at the coccyx.

anal tubercle. One of a pair of eminences lateral to the anal opening in the embryo.

anal valves. Valvelike folds in anal mucous membrane which join together the lower ends of the anal columns. NA *valvulae anales.*

anal·y·sand (a·nal'i·sand) *n.* A person being psychoanalyzed.

anal·y·sis (a·nal'i·sis) *n.*, pl. **analy·ses** (·seez) [Gk., dissolving, resolution, from *analyein,* to dissolve]. 1. The determination of the nature, properties, or composition of a substance. 2. The resolution of a compound body into its constituent parts. 3. *In psychiatry,* PSYCHOANALYSIS. —**an·a·lyt·ic** (an''uh·lit'ick), **analyt·i·cal** (·i·kul) *adj.*

an·a·lyst (an'uh·list) *n.* 1. A person who performs analyses to determine the properties of a substance. 2. *In psychiatry,* one who analyzes the psyche; usually, one who adheres to Freudianism; a psychoanalyst.

analytical chemistry. The branch of chemistry concerned with the detection (qualitative analysis) and determination (quantitative analysis) of substances.

analytical ultracentrifuge. An ultracentrifuge which is equipped with instrumentation to permit optical observation of the sedimentation of substances in solution.

analytic psychiatry. The school of psychiatry based on psychoanalytic theories originally developed by Sigmund Freud.

analytic psychology. The school of psychology that regards the libido not as an expression of the sex instinct, but of the will to live; the unconscious mind is thought to express certain archaic memories of race. Individuals are differentiated as extroverts and introverts, and the personality is said to be made up of an outer-directed persona and a soul or anima. Syn. *Jungian psychology.*

analytic rule. *In psychoanalysis,* a rule for patients in therapy requiring free associations to be voiced, unedited and unselected, in the order of their occurrence. Syn. *fundamental rule.*

an·a·lyz·er (an'uh·lye''zur) *n.* 1. An analyst. 2. Any apparatus or instrument for determining a given component, whether chemical, as in an autoanalyzer, or electrical frequency, as in electroencephalography. 3. A functional neurological unit consisting of an afferent nerve pathway and its central connections, allowing differentiation of stimuli. 4. In a polariscope, the Nicol prism which exhibits the properties of light after polarization. 5. An apparatus for recording the excursions of tremor movements.

an·am·ne·sis (an''am·nee'sis) *n.*, pl. **anamne·ses** (·seez) [Gk. *anamnēsis,* recall, reminiscence, from *ana-,* back, + *mimnēskein,* to remind]. 1. Memory, recall. 2. Information gained from the patient and others regarding his medical history.

an·am·nes·tic (an''am·nes'tick) *adj.* [Gk. *anamnēstikos,* easily recalled]. 1. Of or pertaining to anamnesis. 2. Aiding memory. 3. Pertaining to a quickened immunologic response, as in an anamnestic reaction.

anamnestic reaction or **response.** The heightened immunologic response of an organism to a specific antigen to which the organism has previously responded.

An·am·ni·o·ta (an·am''nee·o'tuh) *n.pl.* A group of vertebrates having no amnion; includes the fishes and the amphibia. Contr. *Amniota.*

an·am·ni·ot·ic (an·am''nee·ot'ick) *adj.* Without an amnion; pertaining to the Anamniota.

ana·mor·pho·sis (an''uh·mor'fuh·sis, ·mor·fo'sis) *n.*, pl. **ana·morpho·ses** (·seez) [Gk. *amamorphōsis,* a forming anew]. 1. The tendency toward increasing complication and differentiation of animate systems. 2. *In optics,* the process by which a distorted image is corrected by means of a curved mirror.

an·an·a·ba·sia (an·an''uh·bay'zhuh) *n.* [*an-* + Gk. *anabasis,* ascent, + *-ia*]. Neurotic inability to ascend to heights.

an·an·a·phy·lax·is (an·an''uh·fi·lack'sis) *n.* [*an-* + *anaphylaxis*]. ANTIANAPHYLAXIS.

Ananase. Trademark for the proteolytic enzyme preparation bromelains or plant protease concentrate.

an·an·a·sta·sia (an·an''uh·stay'zhuh, ·zee·uh) *n.* [*an-* + Gk. *anastasis,* the act of standing up, rising, + *-ia*]. Neurotic inability to rise from a sitting posture, or stand up.

anancastia. ANANKASTIA.

an·an·dria (an·an'dree·uh) *n.* [Gk., from *an-* + *anēr, andros,* man, + *-ia*]. Lack of virility; impotence.

an·an·gio·pla·sia (an·an''jee·o·play'zhuh, ·zee·uh) *n.* [*an-* + *angio-* + *-plasia*]. Congenital narrowing of the caliber of the blood vessels.

an·an·gio·plas·tic (an·an''jee·o·plas'tick) *adj.* [*an-* + *angio-* + *-plastic*]. Characterized by defective development of the vascular system.

an·an·kas·tia, an·an·cas·tia (an''un·kas'tee·uh, an''ang·) *n.* [Gk. *anankastos,* forced, constrained, + *-ia*]. 1. OBSESSIVE-COMPULSIVE NEUROSIS. 2. Any psychopathologic condition in which the individual feels forced to act, think, or feel against his will. —**anankas·tic, anancas·tic** (·tick) *adj.*

anankastic personality. OBSESSIVE-COMPULSIVE PERSONALITY.

an·a·pei·rat·ic (an''uh·pye·rat'ick) *adj.* [Gk. *anapeirai,* exercises (from *peira,* trial, attempt), + *-ic*]. Designating a condition which results from overuse of a muscle or group of muscles, as a cramp.

anapeiratic paralysis. A neurosis in which the subject believes he is paralyzed from excessive use of his limbs.

ana·phase (an'uh·faze) *n.* [*ana-* + *phase*]. 1. The stage of mitosis between the metaphase and telophase, in which the daughter chromosomes move apart toward the poles of the spindle, to form the amphiaster. 2. A late stage of the first (anaphase I) or second (anaphase II) meiotic division.

an·a·phia (an·ay'fee·uh) *n.* [*an-* + Gk. *haphē,* touch, + *-ia*]. Defective or absent sense of touch. Adj. *anaptic.*

an·a·pho·re·sis (an''uh·fo·ree'sis) *n.* [*ana-* + *-phoresis*]. 1. Diminished activity of the sweat glands. Contr. *diaphoresis.* 2. IONTOPHORESIS. —**anapho·ret·ic** (·ret'ick) *adj.*

ana·pho·ria (an''uh·for'ee·uh) *n.* [*ana-* + *-phoria*]. A tendency toward upward turning of an eye and of its visual axis when the other eye is covered.

an·aph·ro·dis·ia (an·af''ro·diz'ee·uh) *n.* [Gk., from *an-* + *aphrodisia*]. Reduction or impairment of sexual desire.

an·aph·ro·dis·i·ac, (an·af'ro·diz'ee·ack) *adj.* & *n.* [*an* + *aphro-*

disiac]. 1. Allaying sexual desire. 2. An agent that allays sexual desire.

ana·phy·lac·tic (an″uh·fi·lack′tick) *adj.* 1. Pertaining to the production or state of anaphylaxis. 2. Increasing sensitivity.

anaphylactic antibody. The antibody concerned in anaphylaxis; usually of the IgE class.

anaphylactic reaction. ANAPHYLAXIS (2).

anaphylactic shock. Shock occurring as all or part of a severe anaphylactic reaction; may be preceded by acute respiratory distress. See also *anaphylaxis.*

ana·phy·lac·tin (an″uh·fi·lack′tin) *n.* ANAPHYLACTIC ANTIBODY.

ana·phy·lac·to·gen (an″uh·fi·lack′to·jen) *n.* [*anaphylactic* + *-gen*]. Any substance capable of producing a state of anaphylaxis. —**anaphy·lac·to·gen·ic** (·lack″to·jen′ick) *adj.*

ana·phy·lac·toid (an″uh·fi·lack′toid) *adj.* [*anaphylactic* + *-oid*]. Of, pertaining to, or resembling anaphylactoid shock. Compare *anaphylactic.*

anaphylactoid purpura. ALLERGIC PURPURA (1).

anaphylactoid shock, crisis, or **reaction.** A syndrome resembling anaphylactic shock but independent of antigen-antibody reactions and produced by the injection of a variety of substances, including certain colloids such as peptones, into the body.

ana·phyla·tox·in (an″uh·fil″uh·tock′sin) *n.* [*anaphylaxis* + *toxin*]. A polypeptide or combination of polypeptides cleaved from C5 and C3 components of complement which may release histamine from mast cells and therefore simulates some of the phenomena of anaphylaxis. Syn. *serotoxin.*

ana·phy·lax·is (an″uh·fi·lack′sis) *n.*, pl. **anaphylax·es** (·seez) [*ana-* + Gk. *phylaxis,* guarding, protection, from *phylax,* guard]. 1. A state of immediate hypersensitivity following sensitization to a foreign protein, drug, or other substance, usually through the parenteral route. The responsible antibody is amost always of the IgE class. 2. The clinical manifestation of such a state, occurring in immediate response to reintroduction of the specific antigen, variably characterized by pruritic urticaria, edema, respiratory distress (due to bronchial constriction), pulmonary hyperemia, and shock, and ranging in severity from mild to quickly fatal. Adj. *anaphylactic.*

ana·phylo·tox·in (an″uh·fil″o·tock′sin) *n.* ANAPHYLATOXIN.

an·a·pla·sia (an″uh·play′zhuh, ·zee·uh) *n.* [Gk. *anaplasis,* remodeling, re-formation, + *-ia*]. The assumption by a cell of morphologic characteristics not indigenous in normal derivatives of the inner cell mass of the embryo and correlated with the appearance of the functional characteristics of cancer. Often equated with assumption of embryonal characteristics, but differing from embryonal cells both morphologically and functionally.

anap·la·sis (a·nap′luh·sis) *n.* [Gk., modeling, remodeling]. *Obsol.* The stage of normal development and growth in an individual.

An·a·plas·ma (an″uh·plaz′muh) *n.* A genus of blood parasites (order Rickettsiales, family Anaplasmataceae) found in the erythrocytes of cattle and other ruminants; formerly thought to be protozoans. See also *anaplasmosis.*

an·a·plas·mo·sis (an″uh·plaz·mo′sis) *n.* A disease of cattle and other ruminants characterized by anemia and icterus, due to parasitization of the red blood cells by *Anaplasma.*

an·a·plas·tic (an″uh·plas′tick) *adj.* 1. Pertaining to or affected with anaplasia; cancerous. 2. Pertaining to anaplasty.

anaplastic surgery. ANAPLASTY.

an·a·plas·ty (an′uh·plas″tee) *n.* [Gk. *anaplastos,* remodeled, restored, + *-y*]. Plastic surgery for the restoration of lost or absent parts.

an·a·ple·ro·sis (an″uh·ple·ro′sis) *n.*, pl. **anaplero·ses** (·seez) [Gk. *anaplērōsis,* a filling up, from *plērēs,* full]. The restoration or repair of a wound or lesion in which there has been a loss of substance.

ana·poph·y·sis (an″uh·pof′i·sis) *n.*, pl. **anapophy·ses** (·seez) [*ana-* + *apophysis*]. An accessory process of a lumbar or thoracic vertebra, corresponding to the inferior tubercle of the transverse process of a typical thoracic vertebra.

an·ap·tic (an·ap′tick) *adj.* [*an-* + Gk. *haptikos,* sensitive to touch]. Pertaining to or characterized by anaphia.

an·a·rith·mia (an″uh·rith′mee·uh) *n.* [*an-* + Gk. *arithmein,* to count, + *-ia*]. Inability to count due to a parietal lobe lesion.

an·ar·thria (an·ahr′three·uh) *n.* [Gk. *anarthros,* inarticulate, weak, disjointed, + *-ia*]. Loss of speech due to a defect in articulation. —**anar·thric** (·thrick) *adj.*

anarthria cen·tra·lis (sen·tray′lis). *Obsol.* Partial aphasia due to a lesion in the central nervous system.

anarthria lit·e·ra·lis (lit·e·ray′lis). Stammering.

an·a·sar·ca (an″uh·sahr′kuh) *n.* [NL., from *ana-* + Gk. *sarx, sarkos,* flesh]. Generalized edema; an accumulation of interstitial fluid in the subcutaneous connective tissue and the serous cavities of the body. —**anasar·cous** (·kus) *adj.*

anasarca hys·ter·i·cum (hi·sterr′i·kum). A transient swelling, generally of the abdomen, in a hysterical individual.

anasarcous sound. A moist bubbling sometimes heard on auscultation over edematous skin.

an·a·schis·tic (an″uh·skis′tick, ·shis′tick) *adj.* [*ana-* + *schist-* + *-ic*]. Splitting longitudinally in meiosis; applied to bivalents and tetrads. Contr. *diaschistic.*

an·a·stal·sis (an″uh·stahl′sis, ·stal′sis) *n.* [Gk., from *ana-* + *stalsis,* checking, staunching]. 1. REVERSED PERISTALSIS. 2. Styptic action. —**anastal·tic** (·tick) *adj.*

anas·ta·sis (a·nas′tuh·sis) *n.*, pl. **anasta·ses** (·seez) [Gk., causing to stand, resurrection]. Recovery; convalescence. —**an·a·stat·ic** (an″uh·stat′ick) *adj.*

an·as·tig·mat·ic (an″uh·stig·mat′ick, an·as″tig·) *adj.* [*an-* + *astigmatic*]. Free from astigmatism; corrected for astigmatism, said especially of photographic objectives which are also corrected for spherical and chromatic aberration.

anas·to·mo·sis (a·nas″tuh·mo′sis) *n.*, pl. **anastomo·ses** (·seez) [Gk. *anastomōsis,* an opening, outlet, from *stoma,* mouth]. 1. An intercommunication of blood or lymph vessels by natural anatomic arrangement (as the arterial arches in the palm of the hand between the radial and ulnar arteries) or by collateral channels around a joint (as at an elbow) whereby pathways for the blood supply to a peripheral part are maintained after interruption to the chief arterial supply. Anastomoses between small peripheral vessels are constant. 2. A surgical communication made between the blood vessels (as between the portal vein and the inferior vena cava) or between two hollow organs or by two parts of the same organ (as between the jejunum and stomach, the hepatic duct and small intestine, or the ureter and colon). 3. An intermingling of fibers from two nerves, or from joining the cut ends of a nerve. —**anasto·mot·ic** (·mot′ick) *adj.*; **anas·to·mose** (a·nas′tuh·moze) *v.*

anastomosis ar·te·rio·ve·no·sa (ahr·teer″ee·o·vee·no′suh) [NA]. ARTERIOVENOUS ANASTOMOSIS.

anastomotic aneurysm. CIRSOID ANEURYSM (2).

anastomotic arch. An arch uniting two veins or arteries.

anastomotic operation. A surgical procedure whereby two hollow organs, vessels, or ducts are joined by suture so that their contents may flow from one to the other.

anastomotic ulcer. An ulcer at the suture line between the stomach and jejunum, usually following gastroenterostomy for peptic ulcer disease.

an·as·tral (an·as′trul) *adj.* [*an-* + *astral*]. Without an aster; pertaining to an achromatic figure without asters.

anastral mitosis. Mitosis occurring without the formation of asters.

anat. Abbreviation for *anatomic, anatomical, anatomy.*

anat·a·bine (a·nat′uh·been, ·bin) *n.* 2-(3-Pyridyl)-1,2,3,6-tetrahydropyridine, $C_{10}H_{12}N_2$, a minor alkaloid of tobacco.

an·a·tom·ic (an″uh·tom′ick) *adj.* [Gk. *anatomikos*]. 1. Pertaining to anatomy. 2. Structural.

anatomic age. Age as judged by body development.
an·a·tom·i·cal (an"uh·tom'i·kul) *adj.* ANATOMIC.
anatomical dead space. The space in the trachea, bronchi, and air passages in general which contains air that does not reach the alveoli during respiration, the total volume of air in these conduits being about 140 ml. See also *physiological dead space.*
anatomical snuffbox. ANATOMIST'S SNUFFBOX.
anatomic conjugate. CONJUGATA VERA.
anatomic conjugate diameter. INTERNAL CONJUGATE DIAMETER.
anatomic crown. The portion of a tooth covered with enamel.
anatomic dead space. ANATOMICAL DEAD SPACE.
anatomic injection. Filling the vessels of a cadaver or of an organ with preservative or coagulating solutions for purposes of dissection.
anatomic lobule of the liver. A polygonal prism with the central vein running through the center of its long axis, with branches of the portal vein, the interlobular bile ducts, branches of the hepatic artery, and lymph vessels running in the periphery. Contr. *physiologic lobule of the liver.*
anatomic neck. The constricted portion of the humerus, just below the articular surface, serving for the attachment of the capsular ligament.
an·a·tom·i·co·clin·i·cal (an·uh·tom"i·ko·klin'i·kul) *adj.* Relating anatomic and clinical considerations, such as the pathologic anatomy and the symptoms of a disease.
anatomic position. *In human anatomy,* the attitude of a person standing erect with arms at the sides and palms forward; presupposed in anatomical discourse using directional terms based on posture, such as anterior, posterior.
anatomic rigidity. *Obsol.* Rigidity of the cervix uteri which, though neither edematous nor tender, is not wholly effaced in labor, but retains its length and dilates only to a certain extent.
anatomic root. The part of a human tooth covered by cementum. NA *radix dentis.* Contr. *clinical root.*
anatomic tooth. An artificial tooth that more or less duplicates the anatomic form of a natural one.
anatomic tubercle. TUBERCULOSIS VERRUCOSA.
anat·o·mist (uh·nat'uh·mist) *n.* A person who specializes or is skilled in anatomy.
anatomist's snuffbox. A hollow, triangular space on the dorsum of the hand at the base of the metacarpal of the thumb, when it is extended. It is formed on the sides by the tendons of the long and short extensor muscles of the thumb. Syn. *tabatiesre anatomique.*
anat·o·my (uh·nat'uh·mee) *n.* [Gk. *anatomē,* dissection, from *anatemnein,* to dissect, from *temnein,* to cut]. 1. The science or branch of morphology which treats of the structure of animals or plants and the relation of their parts. 2. The structure of an organism or of one of its parts. 3. Dissection of the various parts of a plant or animal.
ana·tox·in (an"uh·tock'sin) *n.* [*ana-* + *toxin*]. TOXOID.
ana·tri·crot·ic (an"uh·trye·krot'ick) *adj.* [*ana-* + *tricrotic*]. Of a pulse wave, characterized by three notches on the ascending limb.
ana·tri·cro·tism (an"uh·trye'kro·tiz·um) *n.* A condition of having an anatricrotic contour, as on an arterial pulse wave.
[1]**an·atroph·ic** (an"uh·trof'ick) *adj.* [*an-* + *atrophic*]. Correcting or preventing atrophy.
[2]**ana·troph·ic** (an"uh·trof'ick) *adj.* [Gk. *anatrophē*, nurture, feeding, + *-ic*]. Nourishing.
ana·tro·pia (an"uh·tro'pee·uh) *n.* [*ana-* + *-tropia*]. A tendency of the eyes to turn upward when at rest.
an·au·dia (an·aw'dee·uh) *n.* [Gk., speechlessness, from *an-* + *audē*, speech, voice, + *-ia*]. APHONIA.
Anavar. Trademark for oxandrolone, an anabolic steroid.
ana·ven·in (an"uh·ven'in) *n.* [*ana-* + *venin*]. A venom which has been altered by physical or chemical agents that eliminate its toxic property but make little or no change in its antigenic qualities.
an·az·o·lene (an·az'o·leen) *n.* 4-Hydroxy-5-[[4-(phenylamino)-5-sulfo-1-naphthalenyl]azo]-2,7-naphthalenedisulfonic acid, $C_{26}H_{17}N_3O_{10}S_3$, usually employed as the disodium salt; a diagnostic aid used in the determination of blood volume and cardiac output.
an·az·o·tu·ria (an·az"o·tew'ree·uh) *n.* [*an-* + *azot-* + *-uria*]. An absence or deficiency of nitrogenous elements in the urine, affecting chiefly urea.
ancestral cell. Any formative cell, as a myeloblast, lymphoblast, blastomere.
Ancef. Trademark for cefazolin sodium, a semisynthetic cephalosporin.
an·chor (ank'ur) *v.* 1. To secure or fasten; to fix firmly. 2. *In psychology,* to relate to a point of reference, as a person, a situation, or an idea.
an·chor·age (ank'ur·ij) *n.* 1. The fixation of a floating or displaced viscus, whether by a natural process or by surgical means. 2. A tooth, the teeth, or an extraoral base used for resistance in applying an orthodontic force.
anchor band. A band applied to one tooth as an anchor to aid in moving a second tooth.
anchoring villus. One of the placental villi with ends attached to the exposed surface of the decidua basalis by basal ectoderm.
anchyl-, anchylo-. See *ankyl-.*
an·chy·lops (ang'ki·lops) *n.* [Gk. *ankylos*, curved, + *-ops,* eye]. *Obsol.* An abscess at the inner angle of the eye.
Ancillin. Trademark for diphenicillin, a semisynthetic penicillin.
An·cis·tro·don (an·sis'tro·don) *n.* *AGKISTRODON.*
Ancobon. A trademark for flucytosine, an antifungal.
an·co·ne·us (ang·ko'nee·us, ang"ko·nee'us) *n.*, pl. **anco·nei** (·nee·eye) [NL., from Gk. *ankōn,* elbow]. A small triangular muscle at the back of the elbow joint. NA *musculus anconeus.* See also Table of Muscles in the Appendix.
anconeus in·ter·nus (in·tur'nus). EPITROCHLEO-OLECRANONIS.
an·co·noid (ang'ko·noid) *adj.* [Gk. *ankōnoeidēs,* curved, from *ankōn,* elbow]. Resembling the elbow.
ancyl-, ancylo-. See *ankyl-.*
An·cy·los·to·ma (an"si·los'tuh·muh, ang"ki·) *n.* [*ankylo-* + *-stoma*]. A genus of hookworms.
Ancylostoma amer·i·ca·num (a·merr"i·kay'num). *NECATOR AMERICANUS.*
Ancylostoma bra·zil·i·en·se (bra·zil"ee·en'see). A species of hookworm that infects cats and dogs; instances of human infestation, producing larva migrans or creeping eruption, have been reported in South America, Africa, and the Orient.
Ancylostoma ca·ni·num (ka·nigh'num). A common species of parasite of dogs and cats but rarely of man, found particularly in the Northern Hemisphere.
Ancylostoma du·o·de·na·le (dew"o·de·nay'lee). The species of nematode also known as the Old World hookworm; a major cause of hookworm infection, principally of man.
An·cy·lo·sto·mat·i·dae (an"si·lo·sto·mat'i·dee, ang"ki·) *n.pl.* A family of hookworms of the superfamily Strongyloidea, characterized by oral cutting organs. The hookworms of man of the genera *Ancylostoma* and *Necator* belong to this family.
an·cy·lo·sto·mi·a·sis (an"si·lo·sto·migh'uh·sis, ang"ki·) *n.*, pl. **ancylostomia·ses** (·seez) [*ancylostoma* + *-iasis*]. Hookworm infection; more specifically infection by *Ancylostoma duodenale, A. braziliense,* or *A. caninum.* Syn. *hookworm disease.*
An·der·nach's ossicles (ahn'dur·nah^{k}h) [J. Guenther von *Andernach,* German physician, 1487–1574]. SUTURAL BONES.
An·dersch's ganglion [C. S. *Andersch,* German anatomist, 18th century]. INFERIOR GANGLION (1).

An·ders' disease [J. M. *Anders,* U.S. physician, 1854–1936]. ADIPOSIS TUBEROSA SIMPLEX.

An·der·sen's disease [Dorothy H. *Andersen,* U.S. pediatrician and pathologist, 1901–1963]. 1. AMYLOPECTINOSIS. 2. CYSTIC FIBROSIS OF THE PANCREAS.

Andersen's syndrome [Dorothy H. *Andersen*]. CYSTIC FIBROSIS OF THE PANCREAS.

An·der·son-Fa·bry disease [W. *Anderson,* English dermatologist, 19th century; and J. *Fabry*]. ANGIOKERATOMA CORPORIS DIFFUSUM UNIVERSALE.

Anderson splint [R. *Anderson,* U.S. orthopedist, 1891–1971]. A splint, used in fracture of the femur, which employs the principle of countertraction of the well leg.

andr-, andro- [Gk. *anēr, andros,* man]. A combining form signifying *man, male, masculine.*

an·dra·nat·o·my (an″druh·nat′uh·mee) *n.* [*andr-* + *anatomy*]. 1. Human anatomy. 2. Human male anatomy.

andrei-, andreio- [Gk. *andreios,* masculine, pertaining to men]. See *andr-.*

an·dreio·blas·to·ma (an″dree·o·blas·to′muh, an″drye·) *n.* [*andreio-* + *blastoma*]. ANDROBLASTOMA.

an·drei·o·ma (an″dree·o·muh, an″drye·) *n.* [*andrei-* + *-oma*]. ANDROBLASTOMA.

An·drews' operation [E. W. *Andrews,* U.S. surgeon, 1856–1927]. A technique for repair of inguinal hernia, a modification of the Bassini method.

an·dri·at·rics (an″dree·at′ricks) *n.* [*andr-* + *-iatrics*]. A branch of medicine dealing with disorders peculiar to men, especially of the genitalia.

an·dri·a·try (an·drye′uh·tree) *n.* ANDRIATRICS.

andro-. See *andr-.*

an·dro·blas·to·ma (an″dro·blas·to′muh) *n.* [*andro-* + *blastoma*]. A testicular or ovarian tumor composed of stromal cells; it may be very primitive, or differentiated into Sertoli cells resembling those of the normal testis, and may be hormonally inactive or may produce feminization or masculinization.

an·dro·ga·lac·tor·rhea (an″dro·guh·lack″to·ree′uh) *n.* [*andro-* + *galactorrhea*]. ANDROGALACTOZEMIA.

an·dro·ga·lac·to·ze·mia (an″dro·ga·lack″to·zee′mee·uh) *n.* [*andro-* + *galacto-* + Gk. *zēmia,* loss]. The secretion of milk from the male breast.

an·dro·gam·one (an″dro·gam′ohn) *n.* [*andro-* + *gamone*]. A gamone present in a spermatozoon.

an·dro·gen (an′dro·jin) *n.* [*andro-* + *-gen*]. A hormone that promotes the development and maintenance of male secondary sex characteristics and structures. Contr. *estrogen.* See also *androsterone, testosterone.* **—an·dro·gen·ic** (an″dro·jen′ick) *adj.*

an·dro·gen·e·sis (an″dro·jen′e·sis) *n.* [*andro-* + *genesis*]. Activation of the egg by the sperm followed by development of the egg without the participation of the egg nucleus.

androgenic hilar-cell tumor. ADRENOCORTICOID ADENOMA OF THE OVARY.

an·dro·gen·ic·i·ty (an″dro·je·nis′i·tee) *n.* The ability to exert androgenic effects.

androgenic zone. The hypertrophic, inner zone of the fetal adrenal cortex, which involutes rapidly after birth. Syn. *boundary zone, fetal cortex, x zone.*

an·drog·e·nous (an·droj′e·nus) *adj.* [*andro-* + *-genous*]. Giving birth to males.

an·dro·gyne (an′dro·jine, ·jin) *n.* [Gk. *androgynos,* hermaphroditic, from *anēr, andros,* man, + *gynē,* woman]. 1. A female pseudohermaphrodite. 2. A person exhibiting androgynoid characteristics. **—an·drog·y·nous** (an·droj′i·nus) *adj.*

an·dro·gy·ne·i·ty (an″dro·ji·nee′i·tee) *n.* ANDROGYNY.

an·dro·gy·nic (an″dro·jye′nick, ·jin′ick) *adj.* ANDROGYNOID.

an·drog·y·nism (an·droj′i·niz·um) *n.* ANDROGYNY.

an·drog·y·noid (an·droj′i·noid) *adj.* [*androgyne* + *-oid*]. 1. Hermaphroditic; showing the characteristics of both sexes. 2. Of doubtful sex.

an·drog·y·nus (an·droj′i·nus) *n.* ANDROGYNE.

an·drog·y·ny (an·droj′i·nee) *n.* 1. HERMAPHRODITISM. 2. The condition of being an androgyne.

an·droid (an′droid) *adj.* [*andr-* + *-oid*]. 1. Resembling the male. 2. Specifically, of a pelvis: having a shape typical of that of the male, with a deeper cavity than is usual in the female and an inlet which is wedge-shaped, having a narrowed anterior portion. Contr. *anthropoid, gynecoid, platypellic.*

Androline. A trademark for testosterone.

an·drol·o·gy (an·drol′uh·jee) *n.* [*andro-* + *-logy*]. The science of diseases of the male sex, especially of those of the male reproductive organs.

an·dro·ma·nia (an″dro·may′nee·uh) *n.* [*andro-* + *-mania*]. NYMPHOMANIA.

an·drom·edo·tox·in (an·drom″e·do·tock′sin) *n.* A toxic principle, $C_{31}H_{50}O_{10}$, found in *Andromeda (Pieris) japonica* and other ericaceous plants. It has potent hypotensive action, and causes convulsions, labored respiration, and cardiac paralysis.

an·dro·mor·phous (an″dro·mor′fus) *adj.* [Gk. *andromorphos*]. Having the form of a man.

an·droph·i·lous (an″drof′i·lus) *adj.* [*andro-* + *-philous*]. ANTHROPOPHILIC.

an·dro·pho·bia (an″dro·fo′bee·uh) *n.* [*andro-* + *-phobia*]. Pathologic fear or dislike of men.

an·dro·stane (an′dro·stane) *n.* A saturated, solid, steroid hydrocarbon, $C_{19}H_{32}$, the parent substance of androgenic hormones.

an·dro·stene·di·ol (an″dro·steen′dye·ole, ·dee·ole) *n.* Any one of three isomeric derivatives, $C_{19}H_{30}O_2$, of androstane characterized by the presence of two alcohol groups and an unsaturated linkage (C═C).

an·dro·stene·di·one (an″dro·steen′dye·ohn, ·dee·ohn) *n.* Any one of three isomeric derivatives, $C_{19}H_{26}O_2$, of androstane characterized by the presence of two ketone groups and an unsaturated linkage (C═C).

an·dro·ster·one (an·dros′te·rone) *n.* 3α-Hydroxy-17-androstanone, $C_{19}H_{30}O_2$, an androgenic steroid isolated from male urine. Compare *epiandrosterone.*

-ane. A suffix designating *a saturated aliphatic carbon compound.*

Anectine Chloride. A trademark for succinylcholine chloride, a skeletal-muscle relaxant.

ane·de·ous, anae·de·ous (a·nee′dee·us) *adj.* [*an-* + *ede-* + *-ous*]. Lacking external genital organs.

anelectrotonic current. A hyperpolarizing current produced at the anode during passage of electricity through an irritable tissue. See also *anelectrotonus.*

an·elec·trot·o·nus (an″e·leck·trot′uh·nus) *n.* [*ana-* + *electrotonus*]. The reduced irritability of a nerve or muscle at the positive pole during passage of an electric current, caused by hyperpolarization of the cell membrane. Contr. *catelectrotonus.* **—anelec·tro·ton·ic** (·tro·ton′ick) *adj.*

ane·mia, anae·mia (uh·nee′mee·uh) *n.* [Gk. *anaimia,* lack of blood, from *an-* + *haima,* blood, + *-ia*]. A reduction below normal in erythrocytes, hemoglobin, or hematocrit. See also *aplastic anemia, hemolytic anemia, hypochromic microcytic anemia, myelophthisic anemia, sickle cell anemia.*

anemia pseu·do·leu·ke·mi·ca (sue″do·lew·kee′mi·kuh). VON JAKSCH'S ANEMIA.

anemia pseudoleukemica in·fan·tum (in·fan′tum). VON JAKSCH'S ANEMIA.

ane·mic, anae·mic (uh·nee′mick) *adj.* Affected with, pertaining to, or characteristic of anemia.

anemic infarct. WHITE INFARCT.

anemic murmur. A hemic murmur, presumably due to an increased velocity of blood flow, that may be heard in patients with anemia.

anemic necrosis. Death of tissue following a decrease in blood flow or oxygen content below a critical level.

Anem·o·ne (a·nem'uh·nee) *n.* [Gk. *anemōnē*, windflower]. A genus of the Ranunculaceae, most of the species of which have active medicinal and poisonous qualities.

anem·o·nin (a·nem'uh·nin) *n.* A crystalline constituent, $C_{10}H_8O_4$, of *Anemone pulsatilla* and other members of the Ranunculaceae; has been used as an antispasmodic, sedative, and anodyne.

ane·mo·pho·bia (an"e·mo·fo'bee·uh, a·nee'mo·) *n.* [Gk. *anemos*, wind, + *-phobia*]. Morbid dread of drafts or of winds.

an·en·ce·pha·lia (an·en"se·fay'lee·uh, an"en·) *n.* ANENCEPHALY. —**anence·phal·ic** (·fal'ick) *adj. & n.*

an·en·ceph·a·lus (an"en·sef'uh·lus) *n.*, pl. **anencepha·li** (·lye) A fetus showing partial or complete anencephaly. —**anencepha·lous**, *adj.*

an·en·ceph·a·ly (an"en·sef'uh·lee) *n.* [*an-* + *-encephaly*]. Absence of the cerebrum, cerebellum, and flat bones of the skull in a fetus.

an·en·ter·ous (an·en'tur·us) *adj.* [*an-* + *enter-* + *-ous*]. *In biology*, having no intestine, as a tapeworm.

aneph·ric (ay·nef'rick, a·) *adj.* [*a-* + *nephr-* + *-ic*]. 1. Lacking one or both kidneys as a congenital or acquired defect. 2. Having suffered complete and permanent loss of kidney function.

an·ep·ia (an·ep'ia) *n.* [Gk. *anepēs*, speechless (from *epos*, word, speech) + *-ia*]. Inability to speak.

an·ep·i·plo·ic (an·ep"i·plo'ick) *adj.* [*an-* + *epiploic*]. Having no epiploon or omentum.

an·er·ga·sia (an"ur·gay'zhuh, ·zee·uh) *n.* [Gk., unemployment, idleness, from *ergasia*, work, function]. 1. Lack of purposeful functioning. 2. ORGANIC BRAIN SYNDROME. —**aner·gas·tic** (·gas'tick) *adj.*

an·er·gic (an·ur'jick) *adj.* Pertaining to or exhibiting anergy.

anergic stupor. Stupor with marked decrease in spontaneous movements.

an·er·gy (an'ur·jee) *n.* [*an-* + *-ergy*]. Absence of reaction to a specific antigen or allergen.

an·er·oid (an'ur·oid) *adj.* [*a-* + Gk. *nēros*, water, + *-oid*]. Working without a fluid, as an aneroid barometer.

aneroid barometer. A barometer in which changes of pressure are indicated by the collapsing or bulging tendency of a thin, corrugated cover of a partially evacuated metallic box.

an·eryth·ro·blep·sia (an"e·rith"ro·blep'see·uh) *n.* [*an-* + *erythro-* + *-blepsia*]. ANERYTHROPSIA.

an·eryth·ro·cyte (an"e·rith'ro·site) *n.* [*an-* + *erythrocyte*]. An erythrocyte without hemoglobin.

an·eryth·ro·pla·sia (an"e·rith"ro·play'zhuh, ·zee·uh, an·err"i·thro·) *n.* [*an-* + *erythroplasia*]. Inadequate formation of erythrocytes.

an·eryth·rop·sia (an"e·rith·rop'see·uh, an·err"ith·) *n.* [*an-* + *erythr-* + *-opsia*]. Impaired color perception of red; PROTANOPIA.

an·es·the·ki·ne·sia, an·aes·the·ki·ne·sia (an·es"thi·ki·nee'zee·uh, ·zhuh, ·kigh·nee') *n.* ANESTHEKINESIS.

an·es·the·ki·ne·sis, an·aes·the·ki·ne·sis (an·es"thi·ki·nee'sis, ·kigh·nee') *n.* [*an-* + *esthe*sia + *kinesis*]. Sensory and motor paralysis, combined.

an·es·the·sia, an·aes·the·sia (an"es·theezh'uh, ·theez'ee·uh) *n.* [Gk. *anaisthēsia*, insensibility, from *an-* + *aisthēsis*, perception, sensation, + *-ia*]. 1. Insensibility, general or local, induced by anesthetic agents, hypnosis, or acupuncture. 2. Loss of sensation, of neurogenic or psychogenic origin.

anesthesia do·lo·ro·sa (do"lo·ro'suh). Intractable pain experienced in an area of hypesthesia, usually combined with motor paralysis.

an·es·the·sim·e·ter, an·aes·the·sim·e·ter (an·es"thi·zim'e·tur) *n.* 1. An instrument that measures the amount of an anesthetic administered in a given time. 2. An instrument that determines the amount of pressure necessary to produce a sensation of touch.

Anesthesin. A trademark for ethyl *p*-aminobenzoate, a local anesthetic.

an·es·the·si·ol·o·gist, an·aes·the·si·ol·o·gist (an"es·theez"ee·ol'uh·jist) *n.* A physician who is a specialist in anesthesiology. Compare *anesthetist.*

an·es·the·si·ol·o·gy, an·aes·the·si·ol·o·gy (an"es·theez"ee·ol'uh·jee) *n.* The art and science of administering local and general anesthetics to produce the various types of anesthesia.

an·es·the·si·om·e·ter, an·aes·the·si·om·e·ter (an"es·theez"ee·om'e·tur) *n.* ANESTHESIMETER.

an·es·thet·ic, an·aes·thet·ic (an"es·thet'ick) *adj. & n.* [Gk. *anaisthētos*]. 1. Causing anesthesia. 2. Insensible to touch, pain, or other stimulation. 3. A drug that produces local or general loss of sensibility.

anesthetic ether. ETHER (3).

anesthetic index. On a body-weight basis, the amount of anesthetic agent required to produce respiratory arrest divided by the amount required to produce surgical anesthesia.

anesthetic leprosy. TUBERCULOID LEPROSY.

an·es·the·tist, an·aes·the·tist (an·es'thi·tist) *n.* A person, not necessarily a physician, who administers anesthetics. Compare *anesthesiologist.*

an·es·the·tize, an·aes·the·tize (an·es'thi·tize) *v.* To place under the influence of an anesthetic; to induce anesthesia; to render anesthetic. —**an·es·the·ti·za·tion, an·aes·the·ti·za·tion** (an·es"thi·ti·zay'shun), **an·es·the·ti·zer, an·aes·the·ti·zer** (an·es'thi·tye"zur) *n.*

an·es·the·tom·e·ter, an·aes·the·tom·e·ter (an·es"thi·tom'e·tur) *n.* ANESTHESIMETER.

an·es·trum, an·oes·trum (an·es'trum) *n.* ANESTRUS.

an·es·trus, an·oes·trus (an·es'trus) *n.* [*an-* + *estrus*]. Cessation of ovarian function, transient or permanent, in female animals, depending on seasonal changes, pregnancy, lactation, age, or pathologic conditions. Compare *diestrus.* —**anestrous,** *adj.*

Anethaine. Trademark for tetracaine hydrochloride, a local anesthetic.

an·e·thole (an'e·thole) *n.* 1-Methoxy-4-propenylbenzene, $C_{10}H_{12}O$, the chief constituent of anise and fennel oils; used as a flavoring agent and carminative.

ane·thum (a·nee'thum) *n.* [L., from Gk. *anēthon*]. The dried fruit of *Anethum graveolens*, indigenous to southern Europe; has been used as a carminative and for flavoring. Syn. *dill.*

an·e·to·der·ma (an"e·to·dur'muh) *n.* [Gk. *anetos*, slack, + *derma*]. Dermatosis of unknown cause that may start as inflamed macules that later become atrophied. In the Jadassohn type, the atrophy is marked by wrinkling and depression; in the Schweninger and Buzzi type, the atrophy is marked by protrusion. In both types, a sense of herniation is appreciated by palpation of the lesions.

an·eu·ploid (an'yoo·ploid, an·yoo'ploid) *adj.* [*an-* + *euploid*]. Having an uneven multiple of the basic number of chromosomes. Contr. *euploid.* —**aneu·ploidy** (·ploy"dee) *n.*

aneu·ria (a·new'ree·uh) *n.* [*a-* + *neur-* + *-ia*]. Lack of nervous energy. —**aneu·ric** (·rick) *adj.*

an·eu·rin (an'yoo·rin) *n.* [*a-* + *neur-* + *-in*]. THIAMINE.

aneurine hydrochloride. The British Pharmacopoeia name for thiamine hydrochloride.

aneurism. ANEURYSM.

an·eu·rysm (an'yoo·riz·um) *n.* [Gk. *aneurysma*, from *eurys*, wide]. A localized, abnormal dilatation of an artery, or laterally communicating blood-filled sac, which typically progresses in size, manifests expansile pulsation, and has a bruit. It is often associated with pain, pressure symptoms, erosion of contiguous parts, and hemorrhage.

an·eu·rys·mal (an"yoo·riz'mul) *adj.* Of or pertaining to an aneurysm.

aneurysmal bone cyst. A subperiosteal tumor which bulges the periosteum, usually showing a rim of calcification.

aneurysmal giant-cell tumor. ANEURYSMAL BONE CYST.

aneurysmal phthisis. Compression of major bronchi with

consequent atelectasis, pneumonitis, and bronchiectasis by aneurysms of the descending thoracic aorta.

aneurysmal varix. An arteriovenous aneurysm in which the blood flows directly into adjacent veins, causing them to be dilated, tortuous, and pulsating.

an·eu·rys·mat·ic (an″yoo·riz·mat′ick) *adj.* ANEURYSMAL.

an·eu·rys·mec·to·my (an″yoo·riz·meck′tuh·mee) *n.* Excision of an aneurysm.

aneurysm needle. A needle fixed on a handle, half curved and at a right angle to the handle, with an eye at the point; used for passing a ligature about a vessel.

an·eu·rys·mo·plasty (an″yoo·riz′mo·plas″tee) *n.* Restoration of an artery in the treatment of aneurysm; reconstructive endoaneurysmorrhaphy.

an·eu·rys·mor·rha·phy (an″yoo·riz·mor′uh·fee) *n.* [*aneurysm* + *-rrhaphy*]. Repair of an aneurysm by means of obliterative suture of the sac.

an·eu·rys·mot·o·my (an″yoo·riz·mot′uh·mee) *n.* Incision of an aneurysm for the purpose of suturing or to promote granulation.

an·eu·rys·mus (an″yoo·riz′mus) *n.* ANEURYSM.

an·eu·tha·na·sia (an″yoo·thuh·nay′zhuh, ·zee·uh) *n.* [*an-* + *euthanasia*]. A painful or difficult death.

an·frac·tu·os·i·ty (an·frack″chew·os′i·tee) *n.* [from *anfractuous*]. 1. Any one of the furrows or sulci between the cerebral convolutions. 2. Any spiral turn or winding.

an·frac·tu·ous (an·frack′chew·us) *adj.* [L. *anfractuosus,* from *anfractus,* turn, winding, from *frangere,* to break]. Winding, turning, sinuous.

angei-. See *angi-.*

an·gei·al (an·jye′ul) *adj.* [*angei-* + *-al*]. VASCULAR.

an·gel·i·ca (an·jel′i·kuh) *n.* An aromatic plant of the genus *Angelica,* especially *Angelica archangelica.* The fruit, roots, and rhizomes were formerly used, chiefly in household medicine, as a carminative, diuretic, and emmenagogue. The seeds were supposed to have antimalarial properties.

an·gel·ic acid (an·jel′ick). *cis*-2-Methyl-2-butenoic acid, $C_5H_8O_2$, a constituent of the roots of *Angelica archangelica;* has been used in the treatment of rheumatism.

an·ge·lique (an″je·leek′) *n.* [F.]. ANGELICA.

angel's scapula or **wing.** WINGED SCAPULA.

An·ger camera [H. O. *Anger,* U.S. electrical engineer, b. 1920]. A direct-viewing radiation imaging apparatus; the system locates the site of a gamma-ray interaction by comparison of pulses produced by an array of photomultiplier tubes looking at a scintillator.

angi-, angio- [Gk. *angeion*]. A combining form meaning *vessel, vascular.*

an·gi·ec·ta·sia (an″jee·eck·tay′zhuh, ·zee·uh) *n.* ANGIECTASIS.

an·gi·ec·ta·sis (an″jee·eck′tuh·sis) *n.,* **angiecta·ses** (·seez) [*angi-* + *ectasis*]. Abnormal dilatation of a blood vessel. See also *telangiectasis.* —**angi·ec·tat·ic** (·eck·tat′ick) *adj.*

an·gi·ec·tid (an″jee·eck′tid) *n.* [*angiec*tasis + *-id*]. An abnormal intradermal venous dilatation, consisting of a circumscribed conglomerate mass of venules, which causes a frequently tense and tender elevation of the skin.

an·gi·ec·to·my (an″jee·eck′tuh·mee) *n.* [*angi-* + *-ectomy*]. Excision of all or part of a blood vessel; an arteriectomy or a venectomy.

an·gi·ec·to·pia (an″jee·eck·to′pee·uh) *n.* [*angi-* + *ectopia*]. Displacement or abnormal position of a blood vessel. —**angiec·top·ic** (·top′ick) *adj.*

an·gi·itis (an″jee·eye′tis) *n.,* pl. **angi·it·i·des** (·it′i·deez) [*angi-* + *-itis*]. Inflammation of a blood or lymph vessel.

an·gi·na (an′ji·nuh, an·jye′nuh) *n.* [L., from *angere,* to strangle]. 1. A spasmodic, cramplike, oppressive pain or attack. 2. Specifically, ANGINA PECTORIS. 3. Any of various diseases marked by attacks of choking or suffocation, especially an affection of the throat. 4. *Obsol.* Sore throat.

angina ab·do·mi·nis (ab·dom′i·nis). ABDOMINAL ANGINA.

angina cor·dis (kor′dis). ANGINA PECTORIS.

angina cru·ris (kroo′ris) [L., of the leg]. INTERMITTENT CLAUDICATION.

angina de·cu·bi·tus. (de·kew′bi·tus, ·tooce) [L., of recumbency]. Angina pectoris occurring when the patient is in the recumbent position.

angina hy·per·cy·a·not·i·ca (high″pur·sigh·uh·not′i·kuh). HYPERCYANOTIC ANGINA.

an·gi·nal (an′ji·nul, an·jye′nul) *adj.* Of or pertaining to angina, usually angina pectoris.

anginal syndrome. ANGINA PECTORIS.

angina no·tha (no′thuh) [L., from Gk. *nothos,* illegitimate, spurious]. ANGINA PECTORIS VASOMOTORIA.

angina pec·to·ris (peck′to·ris). Paroxysmal retrosternal or precordial pain, often radiating to the left shoulder and arm, due to inadequate blood and oxygen supply to the heart, characteristically precipitated by effort, cold, or emotion and relieved by nitroglycerin.

angina pectoris va·so·mo·to·ria (vay″so·mo·to′ree·uh, vas″o·). *Obsol.* Angina pectoris due to vasomotor disorders, without primary heart disease. See also *vasovagal attack (of Gowers).*

an·gi·noid (an′ji·noid) *adj.* Resembling angina.

an·gi·no·pho·bia (an″ji·no·fo′bee·uh, an·jye″no·) *n.* Abnormal fear of angina pectoris.

an·gi·nose (an″ji·noce, ·noze) *adj.* Pertaining to angina or angina pectoris.

an·gi·nous (an′ji·nus) *adj.* ANGINOSE.

angio-. See *angi-.*

an·gio·blast (an′jee·o·blast) *n.* [*angio-* + *-blast*]. 1. Special primordium derived from extraembryonic endoderm, which gives rise to the blood cells and blood vessels in the early embryo. 2. That part of the mesenchyme, especially extraembryonic, from which the first blood cells and blood vessels arise. 3. A vasoformative cell of the mesenchyme. —**an·gio·blas·tic** (an″jee·o·blas′tick) *adj.*

angioblastic meningioma. A meningioma containing large numbers of blood vessels of differing size and shape.

an·gio·blas·to·ma (an″jee·o·blas·to′muh) *n.,* pl. **angioblastomas, angioblastoma·ta** (·tuh) [*angio-* + *blastoma*]. 1. A blood-vessel tumor, usually described as invasive or malignant. 2. The development of blood-vessel-like spaces in a cellular tumor of mesodermal type.

an·gio·car·dio·gram (an″jee·o·kahr′dee·o·gram) *n.* [*angio-* + *cardio-* + *-gram*]. A radiograph of the heart and great vessels after the intravascular injection of a radiopaque medium.

an·gio·car·di·og·ra·phy (an″jee·o·kahr″dee·og′ruh·fee) *n.* [*angio-* + *cardio-* + *-graphy*]. Radiographic examination of the thoracic vessels and the heart chambers after the intravascular injection of radiopaque material. —**angiocar·dio·graph·ic** (·dee·o·graf′ick) *adj.*

an·gio·car·di·op·a·thy (an″jee·o·kahr″dee·op′uth·ee) *n.* [*angio-* + *cardio-* + *-pathy*]. Any disease of the heart and blood vessels.

an·gio·cav·er·no·ma (an″jee·o·kav″ur·no′muh) *n.* [*angio-* + *cavernoma*]. CAVERNOUS ANGIOMA.

an·gio·cav·ern·ous (an″jee·o·kav′ur·nus) *adj.* Pertaining to cavernous angioma.

an·gio·chei·lo·scope (an″jee·o·kigh′lo·scope) *n.* [*angio-* + *cheilo-* + *-scope*]. An instrument which magnifies the capillary circulation of the lips, permitting direct observation.

an·gio·cho·li·tis (an″jee·o·ko·lye′tis) *n.* CHOLANGITIS.

an·gio·chon·dro·ma (an″jee·o·kon·dro′muh) *n.* [*angio-* + *chondroma*]. A benign tumor containing both vascular and cartilaginous elements; sometimes applied to certain hamartomas and sometimes to certain benign cartilaginous tumors with a prominent vascular stroma or capsule.

Angio-Conray. Trademark for sodium iothalamate, a roentgenographic contrast medium.

an·gio·der·ma·ti·tis (an″jee·o·dur″muh·tye′tis) *n.* [*angio-* + *dermat-* + *-itis*]. Inflammation of the blood vessels of the skin.

an·gio·di·a·ther·my (an″jee·o·dye′uh·thur″mee) *n.* Obliteration of blood vessels by diathermy.

an·gio·dys·tro·phia (an″jee·o·dis·tro′fee·uh) *n.* ANGIODYSTROPHY.

an·gio·dys·tro·phy (an″jee·o·dis′truh·fee) *n.* [*angio-* + *dystrophy*]. Defective nutrition of the blood vessels.

an·gio·ec·ta·sia (an″jee·o·eck·tay′zhuh, ·zee·uh) *n.* [*angio-* + *ectasia*]. Varices or dilated tufts of capillaries in the skin; usually seen in older people as red or purplish areas on the skin of the trunk. Syn. *senile ectasia.*

an·gio·ede·ma (an″jee·o·e·dee′muh) *n.* [*angio-* + *edema*]. An acute, transitory, localized, painless swelling of the subcutaneous tissue or submucosa of the face, hands, feet, genitalia, or viscera. It may be hereditary or caused by a food or drug allergy, an infection, or by emotional stress. Syn. *angioneurotic edema.* See also *hereditary angioedema.*

an·gio·el·e·phan·ti·a·sis (an″jee·o·el″e·fan·tye′uh·sis) *n.* [*angio-* + *elephantiasis*]. Nodular or lobulated masses of vascular tumors (angiomas), especially of the subcutaneous tissues, which commonly bleed on pressure, may pulsate, and sometimes are erectile.

an·gio·en·do·the·li·o·ma (an″jee·o·en″do·theel″ee·o′muh) *n.* [*angio-* + *endothelioma*]. 1. A tumor thought to arise from the endothelium of blood vessels rather than from reticuloendothelial cells. 2. EWING'S SARCOMA.

an·gio·fi·bro·blas·to·ma (an″jee·o·figh″bro·blas·to′muh) *n.* An angioma with fibroblastic tissue between the vascular structures.

an·gio·fi·bro·ma (an″jee·o·figh·bro′muh) *n.*, pl. **angiofibromas, angiofibroma·ta** (·tuh) [*angio-* + *fibroma*]. A fibroma rich in blood vessels or lymphatics, usually forming a pedunculated skin tag.

an·gio·gen·e·sis (an″jee·o·jen′e·sis) *n.* [*angio-* + *-genesis*]. The development of the blood vessels. **—angio·gen·ic** (·jen′ick) *adj.*

an·gio·gli·o·ma (an″jee·o·glye·o′muh) *n.* [*angio-* + *glioma*]. A glioma which is rich in blood vessels.

an·gio·gli·o·ma·to·sis (an″jee·o·glye·o″muh·to′sis) *n.* [*angioglioma* + *-osis*]. The presence of numerous foci of proliferating capillaries and neuroglia.

an·gio·gram (an′jee·o·gram) *n.* [*angio-* + *-gram*]. A radiographic visualization of a blood vessel or vessels after intravascular injection of a radiopaque medium.

an·gi·og·ra·phy (an″jee·og′ruh·fee) *n.* [*angio-* + *-graphy*]. 1. Determination of the arrangement of blood or lymph vessels without dissection, as by capillaroscopy, fluoroscopy, or radiography. 2. *In radiology,* the visualization of blood vessels by injection of a nontoxic radiopaque substance.

an·gio·he·mo·phil·ia, an·gio·hae·mo·phil·ia (an″jee·o·hee″mo·fil′ee·uh) *n.* VASCULAR HEMOPHILIA.

an·gio·hy·per·to·nia (an″jee·o·high″pur·to′nee·uh) *n.* [*angio-* + *hypertonia*]. *Obsol.* VASOCONSTRICTION.

an·gio·hy·po·to·nia (an″jee·o·high″po·to′nee·uh) *n.* [*angio-* + *hypotonia*]. *Obsol.* VASODILATATION.

an·gi·oid (an′jee·oid) *adj.* [*angi-* + *-oid*]. 1. Linear. 2. Resembling a blood or lymph vessel.

angioid streaks. The brown, gray, black, or red flat serrated streaks radiating out from the optic disk in the ocular fundus, usually seen in patients with pseudoxanthoma elasticum and less commonly with Paget's disease.

an·gio·im·mu·no·blas·tic lymphadenopathy (an″jee·o·im″yoo·no·blas′tick). IMMUNOBLASTIC LYMPHADENOPATHY.

an·gio·ker·a·to·ma (an″jee·o·kerr″uh·to′muh) *n.*, pl. **angiokeratoma·ta** (·tuh) [*angio-* + *keratoma*]. A small, vascular tumor topped by hyperkeratosis.

angiokeratoma cor·po·ris dif·fu·sum (kor′po·ris di·few′sum). ANGIOKERATOMA CORPORIS DIFFUSUM UNIVERSALE.

angiokeratoma corporis diffusum uni·ver·sa·le (yoo·ni·vur·say′lee). An inherited disorder of glycolipid metabolism, due to a deficiency of a ceramide-trihexosidase-cleaving enzyme; characterized clinically by a "critical phase" in childhood and adolescence of periodic fevers, pain, and acroparesthesia, transient proteinuria, and usually the appearance of the typical angiokeratomas over the trunk, buttocks, and genitalia; a "quiescent phase" during early maturity of asymptomatic proteinuria, hypohidrosis and anhidrosis, hypertension, and edema; and an "accelerated phase" with central nervous system disturbances and renal and cardiac failure in middle life; transmitted as a sex-linked recessive trait with full expression in the hemizygous male and occasionally partial penetrance in the heterozygous female. Abnormalities of the conjunctiva, cornea, lens, and retina may be observed. Syn. *Fabry's disease.*

angiokeratoma For·dyce (for′dice) [J. A. *Fordyce*]. A common characteristic condition of small, vascular tumors commonly situated on the scrotum. Hyperkeratosis is not particularly evident.

angiokeratoma Mi·bel·li (mee·bel′lee) [V. *Mibelli,* Italian dermatologist, 1860–1910]. A progressive condition, beginning at puberty, in which small, vascular, verrucous growths develop on the backs of the fingers and toes and over the knees.

an·gio·ki·ne·sis (an″jee·o·ki·nee′sis) *n.* [*angio-* + *kinesis*]. VASOMOTION.

an·gio·li·po·ma (an″jee·o·li·po′muh) *n.* [*angio-* + *lipoma*]. A lipoma with prominent blood vessels.

an·gio·lith (an′jee·o·lith) *n.* [*angio-* + *-lith*]. A calculus in a blood vessel. See also *arteriolith, phlebolith.* **—an·gio·lith·ic** (an″jee·o·lith′ick) *adj.*

an·gi·ol·o·gy (an″jee·ol′uh·jee) *n.* [*angio-* + *-logy*]. 1. The scientific study and body of knowledge of the blood vessels and the lymphatic system. 2. The lymphatic and blood vessel systems.

an·gio·lu·poid (an″jee·o·lew′poid) *n.* [*angio-* + *lupoid*]. A form of cutaneous sarcoidosis characterized by blue-red nodules and telangiectasia, usually on the nose or adjacent areas of the face.

angiolupoid of Brocq and Pau·tri·er (po·tree·e^y′) [L. A. J. *Brocq* and L. M. *Pautrier*]. ANGIOLUPOID.

an·gi·ol·y·sis (an″jee·ol′i·sis) *n.* [*angio-* + *-lysis*]. Obliteration of a blood vessel during embryonal, fetal, or postnatal life; by progressive fibrosis, or by thrombosis followed by organization and cicatrization, as obliteration of the ductus arteriosus.

an·gi·o·ma (an″jee·o′muh) *n.*, pl. **angiomas, angioma·ta** (·tuh) [*angi-* + *-oma*]. A hamartomatous tumor composed of blood vessels or lymphatic vessels; a hemangioma or lymphangioma. **—angi·om·a·tous** (·om′uh·tus) *adj.*

angioma ar·te·ri·a·le ra·ce·mo·sum (ahr·teer·ee·ay′lee ras·e·mo′sum). A complex meshwork of small blood vessels near or attached to an artery.

angioma in·fec·ti·o·sum (in·feck″shee·o′sum). ANGIOMA SERPIGINOSUM.

an·gio·ma·la·cia (an″jee·o·ma·lay′shuh, ·see·uh) *n.* [*angio-* + *malacia*]. Softening of the blood vessels.

angioma pig·men·to·sum atroph·i·cum (pig·men·to′sum a·trof′i·kum). XERODERMA PIGMENTOSUM.

angioma se·ni·le (se·nigh′lee). PAPILLARY VARIX.

angioma ser·pi·gi·no·sum (sur·pij·i·no′sum). A rare dysplasia of small blood vessels marked by a serpiginous progression of the condition.

an·gi·o·ma·to·sis (an″jee·o″muh·to′sis) *n.*, pl. **angiomato·ses** (·seez) [*angioma* + *-osis*]. A pathologic state of the blood vessels marked by the formation of multiple angiomas.

angiomatosis ret·i·nae (ret′i·nee). Hemangioma of the retina. See also *Hippel-Lindau disease.*

an·gi·om·a·tous (an″jee·om′uh·tus) *adj.* Of, pertaining to, or resembling angiomas.

an·gio·meg·a·ly (an″jee·o·meg′uh·lee) *n.* [*angio-* + *-megaly*]. Enlargement of the blood vessels, especially of the eyelids.

an·gi·om·e·ter (an″jee·om′e·tur) *n.* [*angio-* + *-meter*]. An instrument formerly used for measuring the diameter or tension of a blood vessel.

an·gio·myo·li·po·ma (an″jee·o·migh″o·li·po′muh) *n.* [*angio-* + *myo-* + *lipoma*]. A benign hamartomatous tumor with muscular, vascular, and adipose tissue elements.

an·gio·my·o·ma (an″jee·o·migh·o′muh) *n.* [*angio-* + *myoma*]. A uterine leiomyoma with a prominent vascular component.

an·gio·myo·neu·ro·ma (an″jee·o·migh″o·new·ro′muh) *n.* [*angio-* + *myo-* + *neuroma*]. GLOMUS TUMOR.

an·gio·my·op·a·thy (an″jee·o·migh·op′uth·ee) *n.* [*angio-* + *myopathy*]. Any disorder involving the muscular portion of the blood vessels.

an·gio·myo·sar·co·ma (an″jee·o·migh″o·sahr·ko′muh) *n.* [*angio-* + *myo-* + *-sarcoma*]. A sarcoma with differentiation into muscular cells and development of primitive vascular structures; a variety of malignant mixed mesodermal tumor.

an·gio·neu·rec·to·my (an″jee·o·new·reck′tuh·mee) *n.* [*angio-* + *neur-* + *-ectomy*]. Excision of blood vessels and nerves.

an·gio·neu·ro·ma (an″jee·o·new·ro′muh) *n.* [*angio-* + *neuroma*]. A benign tumor composed of vascular tissue and nerve fibers.

an·gio·neu·ro·my·o·ma (an″jee·o·new″ro·migh·o′muh) *n.* [*angio-* + *neuro-* + *myoma*]. GLOMUS TUMOR.

an·gio·neu·ro·sis (an″jee·o·new·ro′sis) *n.*, pl. **angioneuro·ses** (·seez) [*angio-* + *neurosis* (2)]. A disorder of the vasomotor nerves. —**angioneu·rot·ic** (·rot′ick) *adj.*

angioneurotic edema. ANGIOEDEMA.

an·gio·no·ma (an″jee·o·no′muh) *n.* [*angio-* + Gk. *nomē*, ulcer]. Ulceration of a blood vessel.

an·gio·os·teo·hy·per·tro·phy (an″jee·o·os″tee·o·high·pur′truh·fee) *n.* [*angio-* + *osteo-* + *hypertrophy*]. KLIPPEL-TRÉNAUNAY-WEBER SYNDROME.

an·gio·pa·ral·y·sis (an″jee·o·puh·ral′i·sis) *n.* [*angio-* + *paralysis*]. VASOMOTOR PARALYSIS. —**angio·par·a·lyt·ic** (·păr″uh·lit′ick) *adj.*

an·gio·pa·re·sis (an″jee·o·pa·ree′sis, ·păr′e·sis) *n.* [*angio-* + *paresis*]. Partial vasomotor paralysis.

an·gi·op·a·thy (an″jee·op′uth·ee) *n.* [*angio-* + *-pathy*]. Any disease of the vascular system. See also *angiitis.*

an·gio·pha·co·ma·to·sis (an″jee·o·fa·ko″muh·to′sis, ·fack″o·) *n.* [*angio-* + *phacomatosis*]. HIPPEL-LINDAU DISEASE.

angiophacomatosis re·ti·nae et ce·re·bel·li (ret′i·nee et serr·e·bel′eye). HIPPEL-LINDAU DISEASE.

an·gio·pla·nia (an″jee·o·play′nee·uh) *n.* [*angio-* + Gk. *planos*, wandering, + *-ia*]. ANGIECTOPIA.

an·gio·pla·ny (an′jee·o·play″nee) *n.* ANGIECTOPIA.

an·gio·plas·ty (an′jee·o·plas″tee) *n.* [*angio-* + *-plasty*]. Plastic surgery of injured or diseased blood vessels.

an·gio·poi·e·sis (an″jee·o·poy·ee′sis) *n.*, pl. **angiopoie·ses** (·seez) [*angio-* + *-poiesis*]. The formation of blood vessels in new tissue. —**angiopoi·et·ic** (·et′ick) *adj.*

an·gio·pres·sure (an′jee·o·presh″ur) *n.* The production of hemostasis without ligation, by angiotribe, hemostat, or other pressure.

an·gio·re·tic·u·lo·ma (an″jee·o·re·tick″yoo·lo′muh) *n.* [*angio-* + *reticul-* + *-oma*]. Hemangioblastoma, usually of the cerebellum.

an·gio·ret·i·nog·ra·phy (an″jee·o·ret″i·nog′ruh·fee) *n.* [*angio-* + *retino-* + *-graphy*]. Visualization of the blood vessels of the retina after injection of a nontoxic radiopaque or fluorescing substance.

an·gi·or·rha·phy (an″jee·or′uh·fee) *n.* [*angio-* + *-rrhaphy*]. Suture of a blood vessel.

an·gi·or·rhex·is (an″jee·o·reck′sis) *n.*, pl. **angiorrhex·es** (·seez) [*angio-* + *-rrhexis*]. Rupture of a blood vessel.

an·gio·sar·co·ma (an″jee·o·sahr·ko′muh) *n.* [*angio-* + *sarcoma*]. A sarcoma in which anaplastic cells form vascular spaces.

an·gio·scle·ro·sis (an″jee·o·skle·ro′sis) *n.* [*angio-* + *sclerosis*]. Hardening and thickening of the walls of the blood vessels. —**angioscle·rot·ic** (·rot′ick) *adj.*

angiosclerotic paroxysmal myasthenia. VENOUS CLAUDICATION.

an·gio·scope (an′jee·o·skope) *n.* [*angio-* + *-scope*]. An instrument, such as a specialized microscope, for examining capillary vessels.

an·gio·sco·to·ma (an″jee·o·sko·to′muh) *n.* [*angio-* + *scotoma*]. A visual-field disturbance caused by entoptic shadows of retinal blood-vessels and other structures.

an·gi·o·sis (an″jee·o′sis) *n.* ANGIOPATHY.

an·gio·spasm (an′jee·o·spaz·um) *n.* [*angio-* + *spasm*]. A localized, intermittent contracture of a blood vessel. —**an·gio·spas·tic** (an″jee·o·spas′tick) *adj.*

angiospastic anesthesia. Loss of sensibility due to ischemia in an area produced by spasm or occlusion of the blood vessels.

angiospastic syndrome. 1. ACROPARESTHESIA. 2. ANGIONEUROSIS. 3. RAYNAUD'S PHENOMENON.

an·gio·sperm (an′jee·o·spurm) *n.* [*angio-* + *sperm*]. A plant whose seeds are protected by a pericarp.

an·gio·stax·is (an″jee·o·stack′sis) *n.* [*angio-* + *staxis*]. The oozing of blood, as seen in hemophilia.

an·gio·ste·no·sis (an″jee·o·ste·no′sis) *n.* [*angio-* + *stenosis*]. Narrowing of the lumen of a blood vessel.

an·gi·os·te·o·sis (an″jee·os·tee·o′sis) *n.* [*angi-* + *osteosis*]. Ossification of blood vessels.

an·gio·tel·ec·ta·sia (an″jee·o·tel″eck·tay′zhuh, ·zee·uh) *n.* [*angio-* + *tel-* + *ectasia*]. TELANGIECTASIS. —**angiotelec·tat·ic** (·tat′ick) *adj.*

an·gio·tel·ec·ta·sis (an″jee·o·tel·eck′tuh·sis) *n.* TELANGIECTASIS.

an·gio·ten·ic (an″jee·o·ten′ick) *adj.* [*angio-* + Gk. *ten-* (from *teinein*, to stretch) + *-ic*]. Caused or marked by distention of the blood vessels.

an·gio·ten·sin (an″jee·o·ten′sin) *n.* [*angio*tonin + hyper*tensin*]. An octapeptide, produced in circulating plasma by interaction of the enzyme renin and the alpha$_2$-globulin angiotensinogen. It appears to be the pressor-vasoconstrictor and aldosterone-stimulating component of the renal pressor system. Used as a pressor agent in hypotensive states. Sometimes called angiotensin II, to distinguish it from its physiologically inactive decapeptide precursor angiotensin I. The 2-8 heptapeptide fragment of angiotensin II, sometimes called angiotensin III, is also found in human and other plasma and is known to stimulate aldosterone secretion. Formerly called *angiotonin, hypertensin.*

angiotensin amide. The synthetic 1-L-asparaginyl-5-L-valyl peptide analogue of angiotensin II. It is a powerful vasoconstrictor and vasopressor.

an·gio·ten·sin·ase (an″jee·o·ten′si·nace) *n.* 1. Any of various peptidases in tissues and plasma which degrade angiotensin II. 2. Originally, the enzyme converting angiotensin I to angiotensin II.

an·gio·ten·sin·o·gen (an″jee·o·ten·sin′o·jen) *n.* The plasma globulin on which renin acts to produce angiotensin. Syn. *hypertensinogen.*

an·gio·throm·bo·sis (an″jee·o·throm·bo′sis) *n.* Blood vessel thrombosis. —**angiothrombot·ic** (·bot′ick) *adj.*

an·gi·ot·o·my (an″jee·ot′uh·mee) *n.* [*angio-* + *-tomy*]. Incision into a blood vessel.

an·gio·ton·ic (an″jee·o·ton′ick) *adj.* [*angio-* + *tonic*]. Tending to increase vascular tension.

an·gio·to·nin (an″jee·o·to′nin) *n.* An early name for angiotensin II.

an·gio·tribe (an′jee·o·tribe) *n.* [*angio-* + *-tribe*]. A clamp with powerful jaws for crushing arteries embedded in tissue.

an·gio·troph·ic (an″jee·o·trof′ick) *adj.* [*angio-* + *trophic*]. Pertaining to nutrition of blood vessels.

an·gi·tis (an·jye′tis) *n.* ANGIITIS.

-angium [NL., from Gk. *angeion*, vessel, container]. A combining form designating *a containing or supporting structure.*

an·gle alpha. ALPHA ANGLE.

angle bisection technique. A technique for the roentgenographic exposure of intraoral films, by which the beam of radiation is directed at right angles to an imaginary plane which bisects the angle formed by the long axis of the tooth being examined and the plane of the film. See also *Cieszynski's rule of isometry.*

angle board. A device used to facilitate the establishment of reproducible angular relationships between a patient's head or body and the plane of an x-ray film.

angle-closure glaucoma. NARROW-ANGLE GLAUCOMA.

angle of anomaly. The degree of shift from the normal to the abnormal retinal correspondence observed in squint.

angle of aperture. *In optics,* the angle included between two lines joining the opposite points of the periphery of a lens and the focus.

angle of a rib. An angle of the body of a rib at the attachment of the iliocostalis muscle and the point at which the rib bends laterally. NA *angulus costae.*

angle of circulatory efficiency. The angle of elevation of a limb at which normal color returns after ischemia or blanching from circulatory stasis in the affected structure.

angle of convergence. The angle between the two visual axes when the eyes are turned inward. See also *meter-angle.*

angle of elevation. *In optics,* the angle made by the visual plane with its primary position when moved upward or downward.

angle of incidence. *In optics,* the acute angle between a ray, incident upon a surface, and the perpendicular to the surface at the point of incidence.

angle of inclination of the pelvis. 1. INCLINATION OF THE PELVIS. 2. The angle formed by the anterior wall of the pelvis with the anteroposterior diameter of the pelvic inlet. 3. The angle formed by the pelvis with the general line of the trunk or by the plane of the outlet of the pelvis with the horizon.

angle of Lou·is (Fr. loo·ee') [A. *Louis,* French surgeon, 1723–1792]. ANGLE OF THE STERNUM.

angle of Lud·wig (Ger. loot'vikh) [D. *Ludwig,* German anatomist, 1625–1680]. ANGLE OF THE STERNUM.

angle of polarization. The angle of reflection at which light is most completely polarized.

angle of Qua·tre·fages (ka·truh·fahzh') [J. L. A. de *Quatrefages* de Bréau, French anthropologist, 1810–1892]. PARIETAL ANGLE.

angle of reflection. The angle that a reflected ray of light makes with a line drawn perpendicular to the point of incidence.

angle of refraction. The angle formed by a refracted ray of light with the perpendicular at the point of refraction.

angle of Rolando [L. *Rolando*]. ROLANDIC ANGLE.

angle of supination. The extent to which the forearm is capable of being supinated from a position of full pronation; about 180°.

angle of Sylvius. SYLVIAN ANGLE.

angle of the anterior chamber. ANTERIOR CHAMBER ANGLE.

angle of the eye. The inner canthus of the eye.

angle of the iris. ANTERIOR CHAMBER ANGLE.

angle of the jaw. ANGLE OF THE MANDIBLE.

angle of the lips. ANGLE OF THE MOUTH.

angle of the mandible. The junction of the base of the body of the mandible with the posterior border of its ramus. NA *angulus mandibulae.*

angle of the mouth. The angle formed by the union of the lips at each extremity of the oral opening. NA *angulus oris.*

angle of the pubes. SUBPUBIC ANGLE.

angle of the sternum. The angle between the manubrium and the body of the sternum. NA *angulus sterni.*

angle-recession glaucoma. A form of secondary glaucoma.

Angle's classification [E. H. *Angle,* U.S. orthodontist, 1855–1930]. A classification of occlusion based on the mediodistal (anteroposterior) relationship of the upper and lower jaws. There are three classes, with several types and divisions, which are defined primarily by the occlusal relationship of the mesiobuccal cusp of the upper first permanent molar to the teeth of the lower arch.

angles of the scapula. The three angles of the triangular scapula: the inferior angle of the scapula, the lateral angle of the scapula, and the superior angle of the scapula.

An·gli·cus sudor (ang'gli·kus). ENGLISH SWEATING FEVER.

an·go·phra·sia (ang''go·fray'zhuh, ·zee·uh) *n.* [L. *ang*ere, to strangle, + *phras*is (from Gk.), speech, diction, + *-ia*]. *Obsol.* A halting, choking, and drawling type of speech occurring in general paralysis.

an·gor (ang'gor) *n.* [L., anguish]. 1. Extreme distress. 2. ANGINA (1).

angor an·i·mi (an'i·migh). A sense of imminent death.

angor noc·tur·nus (nock·tur'nus). PAVOR NOCTURNUS.

angor pec·to·ris (peck'to·ris). ANGINA PECTORIS.

ang·strom, ång·ström (ang'strum, awng'strem) *n.* [A. J. *Ångström,* Swedish physicist, 1814–1874]. 1. An angstrom unit; a unit of length equal to 10^{-8} cm ($^1/_{100}$ millionth of a centimeter); used for measuring wavelengths, as of visible light, x-rays, and radium radiation. Abbreviated, A, Å. 2. Sometimes defined as the wavelength of the red line of the cadmium spectrum divided by 6438.4696, and then called the international angstrom.

angstrom unit. ANGSTROM. Abbreviated, A.U., Å.U.

An·guil·lu·la (ang·gwil'yoo·luh) *n.* [NL., dim. of L. *anguilla,* eel]. *STRONGYLOIDES.*

an·guil·lu·li·a·sis (ang''gwi·lew·lye'uh·sis) *n.* [*Anguillul*a + *-iasis*]. STRONGYLOIDIASIS.

an·guil·lu·lo·sis (ang''gwi·lew·lo'sis) *n.* [*Anguillul*a + *-osis*]. STRONGYLOIDIASIS.

an·gu·lar (ang'gew·lur) *adj.* [L. *angularis*]. 1. Of, pertaining to, or forming an angle. 2. Pertaining to or situated near an angle. 3. Describing or pertaining to a type of chemical structure in which a component ring or group forms an angle rather than a straight alignment.

angular aperture. Diameter of a microscope objective measured by the angle made by lines from the most divergent rays capable of entering the objective from the focal point.

angular artery. The terminal part of the facial artery, supplying the lacrimal sac, orbicularis oculi, and nose. NA *arteria angularis.*

angular blepharitis. Blepharitis involving the medial angle of the eye with blocking of the puncta lacrimalia.

angular cheilitis. An acute or chronic inflammation of the skin and contiguous labial mucous membrane at the angles of the mouth, of variable and frequently mixed etiology.

angular cheilosis. 1. Cheilosis affecting the angles of the lips. 2. Specifically, ANGULAR CHEILITIS.

angular curvature. A deformity of the spine resulting from tuberculosis of the vertebrae. Syn. *Pott's curvature.*

angular gyrus. A cerebral convolution which forms the posterior portion of the inferior parietal lobule and arches over the posterior end of the superior temporal sulcus. NA *gyrus angularis.*

angular movement. The movement—backward or forward, inward or outward—that may take place between two bones.

angular notch or **incisure.** A notch in the lesser curvature of the stomach formed at the junction of its body and the pyloric portion. NA *incisura angularis.*

angular nucleus. SUPERIOR VESTIBULAR NUCLEUS.

angular spine. SPHENOID SPINE.

angular stomatitis. PERLÈCHE.

angular sulcus. ANGULAR NOTCH.

an·gu·lat·ed catheter. A catheter with its leading end or beak bent so as to facilitate its passage.

an·gu·la·tion (ang''gew·lay'shun) *n.* 1. The formation of an abnormal angle in a hollow organ (as of the intestine or ureter), often becoming the site of an obstruction. 2. A deviation from the normal long axis, as in a fractured bone healed out of line. —**an·gu·late** (ang'gew·late) *v.*

anguli. Plural and genitive singular of *angulus.*

an·gu·lus (ang'gew·lus) *n.*, pl. & genit. sing. **angu·li** (·lye) [L.]. Angle, corner.

angulus acro·mi·a·lis (a·kro·mee·ay'lis) [NA]. ACROMIAL ANGLE.

angulus cos·tae (kos'tee) [NA]. ANGLE OF A RIB.

angulus inferior sca·pu·lae (skap'yoo·lee) [NA]. INFERIOR ANGLE OF THE SCAPULA.

angulus in·fra·ster·na·lis (in·fruh·stur·nay'lis) [NA]. COSTAL ANGLE.

angulus iri·dis (eye'ri·dis) [BNA]. Angulus iridocornealis (= IRIDOCORNEAL ANGLE).

angulus iri·do·cor·ne·a·lis (eye"ri·do·kor·nee·ay'lis) [NA]. IRIDOCORNEAL ANGLE.

angulus la·te·ra·lis sca·pu·lae (lat·e·ray'lis skap'yoo·lee) [NA]. LATERAL ANGLE OF THE SCAPULA.

angulus man·di·bu·lae (man·dib'yoo·lee) [NA]. ANGLE OF THE MANDIBLE.

angulus ma·stoi·de·us os·sis pa·ri·e·ta·lis (mas·toy'dee·us oss'is pa·rye·e·tay'lis) [NA]. MASTOID ANGLE.

angulus oc·ci·pi·ta·lis os·sis pa·ri·e·ta·lis (ock·sip·i·tay'lis oss'is pa·rye·e·tay'lis) [NA]. The posterior superior angle of the parietal bone.

angulus ocu·li la·te·ra·lis (ock'yoo·lye lat·e·ray'lis) [NA]. LATERAL ANGLE OF THE EYE.

angulus oculi me·di·a·lis (mee·dee·ay'lis) [NA]. MEDIAL ANGLE OF THE EYE.

angulus oris (o'ris) [NA]. ANGLE OF THE MOUTH.

angulus pa·ri·e·ta·lis alae mag·nae (pa·rye·e·tay'lis ay'lee mag'nee) [BNA]. MARGO PARIETALIS ALAE MAJORIS.

angulus posterior py·ra·mi·dis (pi·ram'i·dis) [BNA]. MARGO POSTERIOR PARTIS PETROSAE.

angulus pu·bis (pew'bis) [BNA]. ANGULUS SUBPUBICUS (= SUBPUBIC ANGLE).

angulus sphe·noi·da·lis os·sis pa·ri·e·ta·lis (sfee·noy·day'lis oss'is pa·rye·e·tay'lis) [NA]. The anteroinferior angle of the parietal bone, which articulates with the great wing of the sphenoid bone.

angulus ster·ni (stur'nigh) [NA]. ANGLE OF THE STERNUM.

angulus sub·pu·bi·cus (sub·pew'bi·kus) [NA]. SUBPUBIC ANGLE.

angulus superior py·ra·mi·dis (pi·ram'i·dis) [BNA]. MARGO SUPERIOR PARTIS PETROSAE.

angulus superior sca·pu·lae (skap'yoo·lee) [NA]. SUPERIOR ANGLE OF THE SCAPULA.

anhaematopoiesis. ANHEMATOPOIESIS.

anhaematosis. Anhematosis (= ANHEMATOPOIESIS).

anhaemolytic. ANHEMOLYTIC.

anhaemopoiesis. Anhemopoiesis (= ANHEMATOPOIESIS).

an·hal·a·mine (an·hal'uh·meen, ·min) *n.* [*Anhal*onium + *amine*]. 6,7-Dimethoxy-8-hydroxy-1,2,3,4-tetrahydroisoquinoline, $C_{11}H_{15}NO_3$, an alkaloid from mescal buttons.

an·ha·line (an'huh·leen, ·lin) *n.* *p*-(2-Dimethylaminoethyl)phenol, $C_{10}H_{15}NO$, an alkaloid from mescal buttons. It is identical with hordenine found in barley.

an·ha·lon·i·dine (an"huh·lon'i·deen, ·din) *n.* 1,2,3,4-Tetrahydro-6,7-dimethoxy-1-methyl-8-isoquinolinol, $C_{12}H_{17}NO_3$, an alkaloid from mescal buttons.

an·ha·lo·nine (an"huh·lo'neen, ·nin, an·hal'o·) *n.* An alkaloid, $C_{12}H_{15}NO_3$, from mescal buttons.

An·ha·lo·ni·um (an"huh·lo'nee·um) *n. Obsol.* LOPHOPHORA.

an·he·do·nia (an"he·do'nee·uh) *n.* [*an-* + Gk. *hēdonē*, pleasure, + *-ia*]. *In psychology,* overall or chronic absence of pleasure in acts which normally give pleasure.

an·he·ma·to·poi·e·sis, an·hae·ma·to·poi·e·sis (an·hem"uh·to·poy·ee'sis, an·hee"muh·to·) *n. Obsol.* Lack or failure of hematopoiesis. —**anhematopoi·et·ic** (·et'ick) *adj.*

an·he·ma·to·sis, an·hae·ma·to·sis (an"hee"muh·to'sis, an"hem"uh·) *n.* [*an-* + *hematosis*]. ANHEMATOPOIESIS.

an·he·mo·lyt·ic, an·hae·mo·lyt·ic (an"hee"mo·lit'ick, an"hem"o·) *adj.* Not hemolytic; not destructive of blood corpuscles.

an·he·mo·poi·e·sis, an·hae·mo·poi·e·sis (an·hee"mo·poy·ee'sis) *n.* [*an-* + *hemopoiesis*]. ANHEMATOPOIESIS. —**anhemo·poi·et·ic** (·et'ick) *adj.*

an·hi·dro·sis (an"hi·dro'sis, an"high·) *n.*, pl. **anhidro·ses** (·seez) [*an-* + *hidrosis*]. Deficiency or absence of sweat secretion. —**anhi·drot·ic** (·drot'ick) *adj.*

anhydr-, anhydro- [Gk. *anydros,* waterless, from *an-* + *hydōr,* water]. A combining form meaning (a) *waterless, lacking fluid;* (b) *an anhydride of a compound.*

anhydraemia. ANHYDREMIA.

an·hy·drase (an·high'drace, ·draze) *n.* [*anhydr-* + *-ase*]. Any enzyme catalyzing a reaction involving removal of water.

an·hy·dra·tion (an"high·dray'shun) *n.* DEHYDRATION.

an·hy·dre·mia, an·hy·drae·mia (an"high·dree'mee·uh) *n.* [*an-* + *hydr-* + *-emia*]. A decreased amount of water in the blood plasma.

an·hy·dride (an·high'dride) *n.* [*an-* + *hydride*]. A compound resulting from the abstraction of water from a substance.

Anhydrite. A trademark for anhydrous calcium sulfate.

anhydro-. See *anhydr-.*

an·hy·dro·git·a·lin (an·high"dro·jit'uh·lin, ·ji·tay'lin) *n.* [*anhydro-* + *gitalin*]. GITOXIN.

an·hy·dro·hy·droxy·pro·ges·ter·one (an·high"dro·high·drock"see·pro·jes'tur·ohn) *n.* ETHISTERONE.

Anhydron. Trademark for cyclothiazide, an orally effective diuretic and antihypertensive drug.

an·hy·dro·sug·ar (an·high"dro·shoog'ur) *n.* Any monosaccharide of the empirical formula $C_n(H_2O)_{n-1}$.

an·hy·drous (an·high'drus) *adj.* [Gk *anydros,* waterless, from *an-* + *hydōr,* water]. *In chemistry,* characterized by absence of water, especially of water of crystallization.

anhydrous lanolin. WOOL FAT.

an·hyp·no·sis (an"hip·no'sis) *n.* [*an-* + *hypn-* + *-osis*]. Sleeplessness; insomnia.

ani·a·ci·no·sis (a·nigh"uh·si·no'sis, ay·nigh") *n.* [*a-* + *niacin* + *-osis*]. PELLAGRA.

an·i·an·thi·nop·sy (an"ee·an'thi·nop"see, an"eye·) *n.* [*an-* + Gk. *ianthinos*, violet-colored, + *-opsy*]. Inability to recognize violet tints.

an·ic·ter·ic (an"ick·terr'ick) *adj.* [*an-* + *icteric*]. Without jaundice.

an·id·e·us (a·nid'ee·us) *n.* [NL., from Gk. *aneideos,* formless, from *an-* + *eidos,* form]. The lowest form of omphalosite, in which the parasitic fetus is a shapeless mass of flesh covered with skin. Syn. *acardiacus amorphus, amorphus, amorphus globulus, holocardius amorphus.* —**anid·i·an, anid·e·an** (·ee·un), **an·i·dous** (an·eye'dus) *adj.*

an·i·dox·ime (an"i·dock'seem) *n.* The *o*-[[(4-methoxyphenyl)amino]carbonyl]oxime of 3-diethylamino-1-phenyl-1-propanone, $C_{21}H_{27}N_3O_3$, an analgesic agent.

an·i·ler·i·dine (an"i·lerr'i·deen) *n.* Ethyl 1-(4-aminophenethyl)-4-phenylisonipecotate, $C_{22}H_{28}N_2O_2$, an analgesic related to meperidine; used as the hydrochloride and phosphate salts.

an·i·lide (an'i·lide, an'i·lid) *n.* 1. Any member of the group of compounds containing the radical $C_6H_5NH—$. They may be formed by the action of an acid chloride or acid anhydride on aniline. 2. Sometimes, a compound having the group $NH_2C_6H_4—$.

ani·linc·tus (ay"ni·link'tus) *n.* [NL., from *anus* + L. *linguere, linctus,* to lick]. ANILINGUS.

an·i·line (an'i·leen, ·lin, ·line) *n.* [Ar. *an-nīl,* indigo (from Skr. *nīla,* dark blue), + *-ine*]. Phenylamine or aminobenzene, $C_6H_5NH_2$, a colorless liquid with a faint, characteristic odor, obtained from coal tar and other nitrogenous substances or prepared by the reduction of nitrobenzene. It is slightly soluble in water, miscible with alcohol and ether, and forms soluble, crystallizable salts with acids. Various derivatives constitute the aniline dyes or coal tar colors. See also *anilide.*

aniline black. NIGRANILINE.

aniline blue, W. S. An acid aniline dye of the triphenylmethane series, a mixture of trisulfonates of diphenyl rosaniline and triphenyl pararosaniline; used to stain collagenous fibers and as a general stain, usually a 0.2 to 1.0% solution of aniline blue in water or in 90% alcohol.

aniline carcinoma. Carcinoma of the urinary bladder, frequent among workers in the aniline dye industry.

aniline-fuchsin-methyl green method. A modification of Altmann's stain for mitochondria using methyl green as the counterstain instead of picric acid. The mitochondria are stained red against a green background.

aniline oil. A solvent consisting of a mixture of aniline, toluidine, xylidine, and other products resulting from the distillation of coal; used in histologic technique.

ani·lin·gus (ay″ni·ling′gus) *n.* [NL., from *an*us + L. *ling*ere, to lick]. The erotic practice of applying the mouth to the anus.

an·i·lin·ism (an′i·li·niz·um) *n.* ANILISM.

an·il·ism (an′il·iz·um) *n.* [*anil*ine + *-ism*]. The syndrome characterized by methemoglobinemia, cyanosis, headache, gastrointestinal manifestations, weakness, dyspnea, and syncope; due to aniline poisoning by vapor inhalation or skin absorption.

anil·i·ty (a·nil′i·tee) *n.* [L. *anilitas,* from *anilis,* old-womanish, from *anus,* old woman]. 1. Senility; imbecility. 2. The state or condition of being like an old woman. **—an·ile** (an′ile) *adj.*

anil·o·pam (a·nil′o·pam, an′i·lo·pam) *n.* (−)-4-[2-(1,2,4,5-Tetrahydro-8-methoxy-2-methyl-3*H*-3-benzazepin-3-yl)ethyl]benzenamine, $C_{20}H_{26}N_2O$, an analgesic agent; usually used as the dihydrochloride.

an·i·ma (an′i·muh) *n.* [L. breath, vital principle, soul]. 1. The soul; the vital principle. 2. The active principle of a drug or medicine. 3. According to Jung, the inner personality or the soul, as opposed to the outer character or persona, which an individual presents to the world; also, the more feminine aspect of the inner self. Contr. *animus (2).*

an·i·mal charcoal. Charcoal derived from roasting animal bones and other tissue; largely used as a decolorizing agent. Syn. *bone black.*

an·i·mal·cule (an″i·mal′kewl) *n.* [NL. *animalculum*]. A minute or microscopic animal; a protozoan.

an·i·mal·cu·lum (an″i·mal′kew·lum) *n.,* pl. **animalcu·la** (·luh) [NL., dim. of L. *animal*]. ANIMALCULE.

animal dextrin. GLYCOGEN.

animal diastase. Any of the amylolytic enzymes of animals, such as ptyalin or amylopsin.

animal magnetism. The hypothetical force or spiritlike effluvium emanating from certain men, as from certain metals, to others and capable of healing through mesmerism.

animal pole. 1. The formative pole of an ovum distinguished by having more cytoplasm and pigment. 2. In the mammalian blastocyst, the pole containing the inner cell mass. Syn. *apical pole, germinal pole.* Contr. *vegetal pole.*

animal protection tests. Tests designed to protect animals against specific infection or intoxication by the administration of the homologous antibodies.

animal protein factor. VITAMIN B_{12}. Abbreviated, APF.

animal starch. GLYCOGEN.

an·i·mas·tic (an″i·mas′tick) *adj.* [ML. *animasticus,* from L. *anima,* soul]. Pertaining to the psyche or soul.

an·i·ma·tism (an′i·muh·tiz·um) *n.* The attribution of personality (not soul) to the animate and inanimate phenomena of nature, frequently a part of hallucinations and simple schizophrenia.

an·i·mism (an′i·miz·um) *n.* 1. The belief that all animals, inanimate objects, and natural phenomena possess conscious souls; a characteristic of many primitive religions. 2. The theory that all the phenomena of nature are the product of an immaterial, activating soul or spirit, the anima mundi (soul of the world).

an·i·mus (an′i·mus) *n.* [L., spiritual principle, spirit]. 1. A spirit or feeling of hatred or hostility. 2. According to Jung, the masculine as compared with the feminine aspect of the inner self. Contr. *anima (3).*

an·ion (an′eye·on) *n.* [Gk. *aniōn,* going up, from *anienai,* to go up]. An ion carrying one or more negative charges, and migrating to the anode on electrolysis, usually shown with negative superscript, as Cl^- (chloride), SO_4^{2-} (sulfate), PO_4^{3-} (phosphate). Contr. *cation.* **—an·ion·ic** (an″eye·on′ick) *adj.*

anion exchange resin. A highly polymerized synthetic organic compound containing amine groups; the basic form has the property of withdrawing acid from a liquid medium in which the resin is placed, and for this reason is utilized as a gastric antacid to control symptoms in simple hyperacidity and in peptic ulcer. See also *polyamine-methylene resin.*

anionic detergent. A detergent, such as soap or salts of sulfated alcohols, in which the cleansing action is inherent in the anion.

an·irid·ia (an″eye·rid′ee·uh, an″i·rid′ee·uh) *n.* [*an-* + *irid-* + *-ia*]. Absence or defect of the iris; specifically, congenital hypoplasia of the iris, usually bilateral and transmitted as a dominant autosomal trait.

anis-, aniso- [Gk. *anisos,* from *an-* + *isos,* equal, even]. A combining form meaning *unequal, unsymmetrical, dissimilar.* Contr. *is-, iso-.*

ani·sa·ki·a·sis (an″i·sa·kigh′uh·sis, a·nis″uh·) *n.* Intestinal infection by the nematode *Anisakis marina,* usually due to ingestion of undercooked herring; characterized by eosinophilic granulomas in the intestine, sometimes followed by perforation of the intestinal wall.

Ani·sa·kis ma·ri·na (an″i·sah′kis ma·ree′nuh). A nematode whose mature forms parasitize marine mammals and whose larval forms infect herring. See also *anisakiasis.*

an·is·al·de·hyde (an″is·al′de·hide) *n.* [*anise* + *aldehyde*]. *p*-Methoxybenzaldehyde, $CH_3OC_6H_4CHO$, used in organic syntheses and perfumery. Syn. *anisic aldehyde.*

an·ise (an′is) *n.* [Gk. *anison*]. The dried ripe fruit of *Pimpinella anisum*; has been used as a mild aromatic carminative. Syn. *anise seed, aniseed.* **—anis·ic** (a·nis′ick, a·nee′sick) *adj.*

an·i·seed (an′i·seed) *n.* [*anise* + *seed*]. ANISE.

aniseed oil. ANISE OIL.

an·is·ei·kom·e·ter (an″is·eye·kom′e·tur) *n.* [*anis-* + Gk. *eikōn,* image, + *-meter*]. A device for measuring the inequality of size when the two retinal images differ. Syn. *eikonometer.*

an·is·ei·ko·nia (an″is·eye·ko′nee·uh) *n.* [*anis-* + Gk. *eikōn,* image, + *-ia*]. A condition in which the image size seen by one eye is different from that seen by the other. Contr. *iseikonia.* **—anisei·kon·ic** (·kon′ick) *adj.*

anise oil. The volatile oil from anise or star anise; a flavoring agent. Formerly used as a carminative and expectorant.

anisic acid. *p*-Methoxybenzoic acid, $CH_3OC_6H_4COOH$; has been used as an antiseptic, antipyretic, and antirheumatic.

anisic aldehyde. ANISALDEHYDE.

an·i·sin·di·one (an″i·sin·dye′ohn) *n.* 2-(*p*-Methoxyphenyl)indane-1,3-dione, $C_{16}H_{12}O_3$, a synthetic anticoagulant drug.

aniso-. See *anis-.*

an·iso·chro·ma·sia (an·eye″so·kro·may′zhuh, ·zee·uh, an″i·so·) *n.* [*aniso-* + *-chromasia.*]. Decreased staining of the inner portion of erythrocytes, associated with lack of hemoglobin.

an·iso·chro·mat·ic (an·eye″so·kro·mat′ick) *adj.* ANISOCHROMIC.

an·iso·chro·mia (an·eye″so·kro′mee·uh, an″i·so·) *n.* [*aniso-* + *-chromia*]. 1. Variation in the intensity of staining of erythrocytes due to differences in hemoglobin content. 2. HETEROCHROMIA. **—anisochro·mic** (·mick) *adj.*

an·iso·co·ria (an·eye″so·ko′ree·uh) *n.* [*aniso-* + Gk. *korē,* pupil, + *-ia*]. Inequality in the diameter of the pupils.

an·iso·cy·to·sis (an·eye″so·sigh·to′sis, an″i·so·) *n.* [*aniso-* + *cyt-* + *-osis*]. Inequality in the size of erythrocytes.

an·iso·dac·ty·lous (an·eye″so·dack′ti·lus, an″i·so·) *adj.* [*aniso-* + *dactyl-* + *-ous*]. Having digits of unequal length. —**anisodactylus,** *n.*

an·iso·dont (an·eye′so·dont) *adj.* [*anis-* + *-odont*]. Possessing irregular teeth of unequal length.

an·isog·a·my (an″eye·sog′uh·mee) *n.* [*aniso-* + *-gamy*]. The conjugation of gametes having unequal size but the same general morphology. —**anisoga·mous** (·mus) *adj.*

an·isog·na·thous (an″eye·sog′nuth·us) *adj.* [*aniso-* + *gnath-* + *-ous*]. Having jaws which do not match, one being considerably wider than the other, especially in the molar region.

an·iso·gyn·e·co·mas·tia (an″i·so·jin″e·ko·mas′tee·uh) *n.* [*aniso-* + *gynecomastia*]. Unequal enlargement of the male breast due to unilateral glandular hyperplasia.

an·iso·kary·o·sis (an·eye″so·kăr·ee·o′sis) *n.* [*aniso-* + *kary-* + *osis*]. Significant variation in nuclear size among cells of the same type.

an·iso·ko·nia (an″i·so·ko′nee·uh) *n.* ANISEIKONIA.

an·is·ole (an′i·sole) *n.* Methyl phenyl ether, $C_6H_5OCH_3$, used in perfumery and organic syntheses.

an·iso·me·lia (an·eye″so·mee′lee·uh) *n.* [*aniso-* + *-melia*]. An inequality between corresponding limbs. —**an·isom·e·lous** (an″eye·som′e·lus) *adj.*

an·iso·me·ria (an·eye″so·merr′ree·uh) *n.* [*aniso-* + *mer-* + *-ia*]. Irregularity between the successive segments of organs or parts. —**aniso·mer·ic** (·merr′ick) *adj.*

an·iso·me·tro·pia (an·eye″so·me·tro′pee·uh) *n.* [Gk. *anisometros*, incommensurate, + *-opia*]. A difference in the refraction of the two eyes. —**anisome·trop·ic** (·trop′ick) *adj.;* **aniso·met·rope** (·met′rope) *n.*

an·iso·mor·phic (an·eye″so·mor′fick) *adj.* [*aniso-* + *morph-* + *-ic*]. HETEROMORPHOUS.

anisomorphic gliosis. HETEROMORPHOUS GLIOSIS.

an·iso·mor·phous (an·eye″so·mor′fus) *adj.* [*aniso-* + *morph-* + *-ous*]. HETEROMORPHOUS.

an·iso·my·cin (an·eye″so·migh′sin) *n.* An antibiotic substance, $C_{14}H_{19}NO_4$, isolated from cultures of species of *Streptomyces,* active against *Trichomonas vaginalis* and *Entamoeba histolytica.*

an·iso·nu·cle·o·sis (an·eye″so·new·klee·o′sis, an″i·so·) *n.* [*aniso-* + *nucle-* + *-osis*]. Variation in nuclear size within a group of cells of the same general type.

an·iso·pia (an″eye·so′pee·uh) *n.* [*anis-* + *-opia*]. ANISOMETROPIA.

an·iso·poi·kilo·cy·to·sis (an·eye″so·poy″ki·lo·sigh·to′sis) *n.* [*aniso-* + *poikilocytosis*]. Variation of size and shape, especially in erythrocytes.

an·iso·sphyg·mia (an″i·so·sfig′mee·uh) *n.* [*aniso-* + *sphygm-* + *-ia*]. *Obsol.* Inequality of arterial pulsation in symmetric vessels, as the two radial or dorsalis pedis arteries.

an·iso·sthen·ic (an″i·so·sthen′ick) *adj.* [Gk. *anisosthenēs*, from *aniso-* + *sthenos,* strength]. Not of equal power, said of pairs of muscles.

an·iso·ton·ic (an·eye″so·ton′ick) *adj.* [*an-* + *isotonic*]. Characterized by unequal osmotic pressure.

an·iso·trop·ic (an″eye″so·trop′ick) *adj.* [*an-* + *isotropic*]. 1. Having different values of a property (as refractive index, tensile strength, elasticity, electrical or heat conductivity, or rate of solution) in different directions, especially in a crystal. 2. *In biology,* responding differently to the same external stimulus in different parts of an organism. 3. In an ovum, possessing a predetermined axis or axes. Noun *anisotropy.*

anisotropic band. A BAND.

anisotropic disk. A DISK.

an·iso·tro·pine methylbromide (an″eye″so·tro′peen). 8-Methyltropinium bromide 2-propylvalerate, $C_{17}H_{32}BrNO_2$, a parasympatholytic agent.

an·isot·ro·py (an″eye·sot′ruh·pee) *n.* The property or quality of being anisotropic.

ani·su·ria (an″i·sue′ree·uh) *n.* [*anis-* + *-uria*]. A condition characterized by alternate polyuria and oliguria.

ani·trog·e·nous (ay″nigh·troj′e·nus, an″eye·) *adj.* [*a-* + *nitrogenous*]. Nonnitrogenous.

Anitsch·kow cell or **myocyte** (ah·neech′kuf) [N. N. *Anitschkow,* Russian pathologist, 1885–1964]. A cardiac histiocyte having a characteristic bar of chromatin with fibrils radiating toward the nuclear membrane, normally present in connective tissue of the heart and coronary vessels; it proliferates in rheumatic inflammation and is seen in Aschoff nodules.

An·kis·tro·don (ang·kis′tro·don) *n.* AGKISTRODON.

an·kle, *n.* [ON. *ankula* (rel. to Gk. *ankylē* and *ankōn,* elbow, L. *angulus,* corner, angle, and *uncus,* hook)]. 1. The region of juncture between the foot and leg. 2. The joint between the distal ends of the tibia and fibula proximally and the talus distally. It is a hinge joint or ginglymus. NA *articulatio talocruralis.* See also Table of Synovial Joints and Ligaments in the Appendix.

ankle bone. TALUS.

ankle clonus. Clonic contractions of the calf muscles in response to sudden pressure against the sole of the foot, with the leg extended, or to tapping the calcaneal tendon; seen in corticospinal tract disorders.

ankle drop. DROPPED FOOT.

ankle jerk or **reflex.** ACHILLES JERK.

ankle mortise. The space in the ankle joint, between the lateral and medial malleoli, occupied by the talus.

ankyl-, ankylo- [Gk. *ankylos,* crooked, curved]. A combining form meaning (a) *crooked, crookedness, bent;* (b) *adhesion, growing together of parts.*

an·ky·lo·bleph·a·ron (ank″i·lo·blef′uh·ron) *n.* [*ankylo-* + *blepharon*]. The adhesion of the edges of the eyelids to each other.

an·ky·lo·chei·lia, an·ky·lo·chi·lia (ank″i·lo·kigh′lee·uh) *n.* [*ankylo-* + *cheil-* + *-ia*]. Adhesion of the lips to each other.

an·ky·lo·col·pos, an·ky·lo·kol·pos (ank″i·lo·kol′pos) *n.* [*ankylo-* + *-colpos*]. Atresia of the vagina or the vulva.

an·ky·lo·dac·tyl·ia (ank″i·lo·dack·til′ee·uh) *n.* [*ankylo-* + *-dactylia*]. A deformity resulting from the adhesion of fingers or toes to one another.

an·ky·lo·dac·ty·ly (ank″i·lo·dack′ti·lee) *n.* ANKYLODACTYLIA.

an·ky·lo·glos·sia (ank″i·lo·glos′ee·uh) *n.* [*ankylo-* + *-glossia*]. TONGUE-TIE.

ankylokolpos. ANKYLOCOLPOS.

an·ky·losed (ank′i·loazd, ·loast) *adj.* [from *ankylosis*]. 1. Stiff; firmly united; bound down with adhesions. 2. Designating a joint immobilized by some pathologic or operative process within or outside the capsule. —**an·ky·lose** (ank′i·loze, ·loce) *v.*

ankylosing spondylitis. A chronic progressive arthritis of young men, of unknown etiology, affecting mainly the spinal and sacroiliac joints, leading to fusion and deformity. Syn. *rheumatoid spondylitis.* See also *rheumatoid arthritis.*

an·ky·lo·sis (ank″i·lo′sis) *n.,* pl. **ankylo·ses** (·seez) [Gk. *ankylōsis,* from *ankyloun,* to bend, crook]. Stiffness or fixation of a joint.

an·ky·lo·sto·mi·a·sis (ank″i·lo·sto·migh′uh·sis) *n.* ANCYLOSTOMIASIS.

An·ky·los·to·mum (ank″i·los′to·mum) *n.* ANCYLOSTOMA.

an·ky·lo·tome (ank′i·lo·tome, ang·kil′o·) *n.* [*ankylo-* + *-tome*]. A knife for operating on tongue-tie.

an·ky·lot·o·my (ank″i·lot′uh·mee) *n.* [*ankylo-* + *-tomy*]. An operation for the relief of tongue-tie.

an·la·ge (ahn′lah·guh) *n.,* pl. **anla·gen** (·gun) [Ger., arrangement, laying on]. 1. The undifferentiated embryonic cells or tissue from which an organ or part develops; a rudiment. Syn. *primordium, blastema.* 2. *In genetics,* the hereditary predisposition for a given trait (such as a talent or disorder) or even for the entire genotype of an individual.

An·nam ulcer (a·nam′) [after *Annam* (Vietnam)]. A variety of tropical ulcer seen in Vietnam.

an·nat·to (ah·nah′to, a·nat′o) *n.* [a Cariban name of the tree]. A coloring matter obtained from the pulp surrounding the seeds of the *Bixa orellana.*

an·neal (a·neel′) *v.* [OE. *anǣlan,* from *an,* on, + *ǣlan,* to kindle]. 1. To apply a regulated process of heating and cooling to glass or metal to relieve internal stress induced by manufacturing processes or heat. Compare *temper.* 2. *In dentistry,* to heat gold foil to render it cohesive.

annealing lamp. A heating device used by dentists for annealing gold foil.

annectant. ANNECTENT.

an·nec·tent, an·nec·tant (a·neck′tunt) *adj.* [L. *annectens,* from *ad-,* to, + *nectere,* to bind, connect]. Linking, joining, or binding together, as annectent convolutions.

annectent gyri. The many short bridges of gray substance that may connect neighboring gyri across intervening fissures. NA *gyri annectentes.*

an·ne·lid (an′e·lid) *adj. & n.* 1. Of or pertaining to the phylum Annelida. 2. An annelid worm.

An·nel·i·da (a·nel′i·duh) *n.pl.* [NL., from L. *anellus,* a little ring]. A phylum of segmented worms including the earthworms, marine and freshwater worms, and leeches.

an·ne·lism (an′e·liz·um) *n.* [L. *anel*lus, small ring, + *-ism*]. The state of being ringed; a ringed structure.

an·nex·a (a·neck′suh) *n.pl.* ADNEXA.

an·nex·i·tis (an″eck·sigh′tis) *n.* ADNEXITIS.

an·ni·hi·la·tion radiation. The production of two photons when an electron and a positron unite and are annihilated.

an·ni·ver·sa·ry reaction. *In psychiatry,* the occurrence of marked anxiety symptoms or their defensive expressions, on specific dates, such as the anniversary of the death of a parent, which often represent a symbolic reenactment of an earlier important loss or bereavement.

an·not·to (a·not′o) *n.* [Galibi]. ANNATTO.

an·nu·lar (an′yoo·lur) *adj.* [L. *annularis,* from *anulus,* ring]. Forming a ring; ring-shaped.

annular cartilage. 1. Any ring-shaped cartilage. 2. CRICOID CARTILAGE.

annular cataract. A peripheral ring-shaped lens opacity.

annular hernia. UMBILICAL HERNIA.

annular keratitis. MARGINAL KERATITIS.

annular ligament. 1. (of the radius:) A strong band in the proximal radioulnar joint, encircling the head of the radius and attached to the anterior and posterior margins of the radial notch of the ulna, thus holding the head of the radius against the ulna. NA *ligamentum anulare radii.* 2. (of the stapedial base:) A ring of elastic fibers encircling the base of the stapes and binding it to the rim of the vestibular window. NA *ligamentum anulare stapedis.*

annular pancreas. An anomalous form of the pancreas encircling the duodenum.

annular placenta. A placenta extending around the interior of the uterus in the form of a belt.

annular scleritis. Inflammation of the sclera at the limbus.

annular scotoma. A partial or complete area of blindness in the form of a ring. Syn. *ring scotoma.*

annular stricture. A ringlike obstruction produced by a contracture which involves the entire circumference of a canal or the intestine.

annular synechia. Adherence of the entire pupillary margin of the iris to the lens or the vitreous body. Compare *posterior synechia.*

annular thrombus. A thrombus involving the whole circumference of a vessel but not occluding it.

An·nu·la·ta (an″yoo·lay′tuh) *n.pl.* ANNELIDA.

an·nu·late (an′yoo·late) *adj. & n.* [L. *annulatus,* from *anulus,* ring]. 1. Characterized by, made up of, or surrounded by, rings. 2. ANNELID.

an·nu·let (an′yoo·let) *n.* [dim. from L. *annulus,* ring]. A narrow colored ring on the surface of or around some organs.

annuli. Plural of *annulus.*

an·nu·lo·cyte (an′yoo·lo·site) *n.* [*annul*ar + *-cyte*]. A markedly hypochromic erythrocyte, in which the central portion is inconspicuous, giving the appearance of a red ring.

an·nu·lo·plas·ty (an′yoo·lo·plas·tee) *n.* [*annul*us + *-plasty*]. Surgical correction of the deformed annulus surrounding a diseased mitral or tricuspid cardiac valve.

an·nu·lose (an′yoo·loce) *adj.* Possessing rings.

an·nu·lo·spi·ral (an″yoo·lo·spye′rul) *adj.* [*annul*ar + *spiral*]. Afferent nerve endings, with bandlike branches winding around the muscle fiber, found in muscle spindles.

an·nu·lot·o·my (an″yoo·lot′uh·mee) *n.* [*annul*us + *-tomy*]. Surgical division of a ring, usually an annulus of a cardiac valve.

an·nu·lus (an′yoo·lus) *n.*, pl. **annu·li** (·lye). ANULUS; a ring or ringlike structure.

annulus cru·ra·lis (kroo·ray′lis). FEMORAL RING.

annulus fe·mo·ris (fem′o·ris) [BNA]. Anulus femoralis (= FEMORAL RING).

annulus fi·bro·car·ti·la·gi·ne·us mem·bra·nae tym·pa·ni (figh″bro·kahr·ti·la·jin′ee·us mem·bray′nee tim′puh·nigh) [BNA]. Anulus fibrocartilagineus membranae tympani (= FIBROUS RING (4)).

annulus fi·bro·sus (figh·bro′sus). FIBROUS RING.

annulus fibrosus fi·bro·car·ti·la·gi·nis in·ter·ver·te·bra·lis (figh″bro·karh·ti·laj′i·nis in″tur·vur·te·bray′lis) [BNA]. Anulus fibrosus disci intervertebralis (= FIBROUS RING (1)).

annulus in·gui·na·lis ab·do·mi·na·lis (ing·gwi·nay′lis ab·dom·i·nay′lis) [BNA]. Anulus inguinalis profundus (= DEEP INGUINAL RING).

annulus inguinalis sub·cu·ta·ne·us (sub·kew·tay′nee·us) [BNA]. Anulus inguinalis superficialis (= SUPERFICIAL INGUINAL RING).

annulus iri·dis major (eye′ri·dis) [BNA]. Anulus iridis major (= GREATER RING OF THE IRIS).

annulus iridis minor [BNA]. Anulus iridis minor (= LESSER RING OF THE IRIS).

annulus mi·grans (migh′granz). A disease of the tongue marked by red patches with yellow borders which spread over its dorsal surface and sometimes over its margins and under surface.

annulus of Zinn [J. G. *Zinn*]. LIGAMENT OF ZINN.

annulus ova·lis (o·vay′lis). The rounded or oval margin of the foramen ovale of the heart. NA *limbus fossae ovalis.*

annulus ten·di·ne·us com·mu·nis [Zinni] (ten·din′ee·us kom·yoo′nis) [BNA]. Anulus tendineus communis (= LIGAMENT OF ZINN).

annulus tym·pa·ni·cus (tim·pan′i·kus) [BNA]. Anulus tympanicus (= TYMPANIC RING).

annulus ure·thra·lis (yoo″re·thray′lis) [BNA]. URETHRAL RING.

¹ano-. A combining form meaning *anus, anal.*

²ano- [Gk. *anō*]. A combining form meaning *up, upper, upward.*

an·o·chro·ma·sia (an″o·kro·may′zhuh, ·zee·uh) *n.* [*ano-* + *-chromasia*]. 1. Concentration of hemoglobin about the periphery of erythrocytes with the centers pale; a condition noted in certain types of anemia. 2. Absence of the usual staining reaction in a cell or tissue; ACHROMASIA (2).

ano·ci·as·so·ci·a·tion (a·no″see·uh·so″see·ay′shun) *n.* [*a-* + *noci-* + *association*]. An anesthetic procedure designed to minimize surgical shock, fear, and postoperative neuroses by excluding most of the painful and harmful stimuli. Syn. *anocithesia.* See also *Crile's theory.*

ano·ci·a·tion (a·no″see·ay′shun) *n.* ANOCIASSOCIATION.

ano·ci·the·sia (a·no″si·theezh′uh, ·theez′ee·uh) *n.* [*a-* + *noci-* + *esthesia*]. ANOCIASSOCIATION.

ano·coc·cyg·e·al (ay″no·kock·sij′ee·ul) *adj.* Pertaining to the anus and the coccyx.

anococcygeal body. The intermingled mass of muscular and fibrous tissue between the anal canal and the coccyx.

anococcygeal ligament. A dense band of connective tissue which connects the tip of the coccyx with the external sphincter of the anus. NA *ligamentum anococcygeum.*

anococcygeal plexus. A nerve plexus formed from the anterior branches of the fifth sacral and coccygeal nerves and part of the anterior branch of the fourth sacral nerve.

ano·cu·ta·ne·ous (ay″no·kew·tay′nee·us) *adj.* [*ano-* + *cutaneous*]. Pertaining to the anus and the skin.

anocutaneous line. The junction between skin and mucous membrane at the anus.

an·o·dal (an·o′dul) *adj.* ANODIC.

an·ode (an′ode) *n.* [Gk. *anodos,* ascent, from *anō,* up, + *hodos,* way]. The positive pole of a galvanic battery or other electric device. Abbreviated, A., a., An., an. Contr. *cathode.*

anode block. HYPERPOLARIZATION BLOCK.

anode excitation. Excitation of the nerve at the anode when the hyperpolarization block is removed.

ano·derm (ay′no·durm) *n.* [*ano-* + *-derm*]. The specialized epidermis of the anal canal between the external perianal skin and the internal rectal mucosa.

an·o·der·mous (an″o·dur′mus) *adj.* [*an-* + *derm-* + *-ous*]. Lacking skin.

an·od·ic (a·nod′ick, a·no′dick) *adj.* Pertaining to an anode; ELECTROPOSITIVE (1).

anodic block. HYPERPOLARIZATION BLOCK.

anodic oxidation. An electrochemical process by which certain articles are given a thin coating of metallic oxide, usually for the purpose of retarding corrosion, by immersing them as the anodes in an oxidizing electrolyte bath.

an·od·mia (an·od′mee·uh) *n.* [*an-* + Gk. *odmē,* smell, + *-ia*]. ANOSMIA.

an·odon·tia (an″o·don′chee·uh) *n.* [Gk. *anodōn, anodontos,* toothless, + *-ia*]. Absence of teeth; may be congenital or acquired.

an·o·dyne (an′o·dine) *adj.* & *n.* [Gk. *anōdynos,* from *an-* + *odynē,* pain]. 1. Relieving pain. 2. A drug that eases or allays pain.

an·o·dyn·ia (an″o·din′ee·uh, ·dye′nee·uh) *n.* [Gk. *anōdynia,* from *an-* + *odynē,* pain, + *-ia*]. Absence of pain. **—an·od·i·nous** (an·od′i·nus) *adj.*

an·o·e·sia (an″o·ee′zhuh, ·zee·uh) *n.* [Gk. *anoēsia,* lack of understanding, from *a-* + *noēsis,* understanding, + *-ia*]. Severe mental subnormality.

anoestrum. Anestrum (= ANESTRUS).

anoestrus. ANESTRUS.

an·o·et·ic (an″o·et′ick) *adj.* [Gk. *anoētos,* noncognitive, from *a-* + *noētos,* cognitive]. 1. Not entirely conscious; pertaining to the fringe of consciousness. 2. Affected with, or of the nature of, anoesia or mental subnormality.

ano·gen·i·tal (ay″no·jen′i·tul) *adj.* Pertaining to the anus and the genital organs.

anogenital band. PERINEAL RAPHE.

anoia (a·noy′uh) *n.* [Gk., lack of understanding, from *a-* + *noos,* mind, + *-ia*]. Severe mental subnormality.

anom·a·lad (a·nom′uh·lad) *n.* [*anomaly* + *-ad* (as in triad, tetrad)]. A pattern of development initiated by a single structural defect which subsequently leads to associated secondary defects.

anom·a·lo·scope (a·nom′uh·lo·skope) *n.* [*anomalous* + *-scope*]. An instrument used for the detection of color blindness.

anom·a·lous (a·nom′uh·lus) *adj.* [Gk. *anōmalos,* uneven, irregular, from *an-* + *homalos,* even, normal]. Abnormal, irregular.

anomalous atrial bands. CHIARI'S NETWORK.

anomalous beat. A heart beat abnormally conducted in the ventricles.

anomalous complex. ABERRANT COMPLEX.

anomalous correspondence. ABNORMAL RETINAL CORRESPONDENCE.

anomalous pulmonary venous drainage. Drainage of one or more of the pulmonary veins into a structure other than the left atrium (usually the right atrium or the superior vena cava).

anom·a·ly (a·nom′uh·lee) *n.* [Gk. *anōmalia,* irregularity]. Any deviation from the usual; any organ or part existing in an abnormal form, structure, or location. For representative anomalies, see Table of Representative Monstrosities and Anomalies (Terata) in the Appendix.

an·o·mer (an′o·mur) *n.* [*ano-* + *-mer*]. A stereoisomer, such as α- and β-D-glucose, whose sole configurational difference is in the steric arrangement about carbon atom 1. **—an·o·mer·ic** (an″o·merr′ick) *adj.*

ano·mia (a·no′mee·uh) *n.* [*a-* + Gk. *onoma,* name, + *-ia*]. Loss of ability to name objects; a type of amnesic aphasia. **—an·om·ic** (a·nom′ick) *adj.*

anomic aphasia. ANOMIA.

an·o·mous (an·o′mus) *adj.* [Gk. *anōmos,* from *an-* + *ōmos,* shoulder]. Without shoulders.

an·onych·ia (an″o·nick′ee·uh) *n.* [*an-* + *onych-* + *-ia*]. Absence of the nails.

anon·y·ma (a·non′i·muh) *n.* [NL., innominate, from Gk. *anōnymos,* nameless]. BRACHIOCEPHALIC TRUNK.

ano·op·sia (an″o·op′see·uh) *n.* [*ano-* + *-opsia*]. Strabismus in which the eye is turned upward; HYPERTROPIA; SUPRAVERGENCE.

ano·pel·vic (ay″no·pel′vick) *adj.* Pertaining to the anus and the pelvis.

anopelvic version. *Obsol.* Manipulation of the pelvis of the fetus with a finger in the mother's rectum.

ano·per·i·ne·al (ay″no·perr″i·nee′ul) *adj.* Pertaining to the anus and the perineum.

Anoph·e·les (a·nof′e·leez) *n.* [Gk. *anōphelēs,* harmful]. A genus of mosquitoes including the obligatory biologic vectors of malaria, and vectors in filariasis and some of the arbovirus encephalitides.

Anopheles al·bi·man·us (al″bi·man′us). A species of mosquito native to tropical America, characterized by white hind feet; a common malarial vector.

Anopheles ar·gy·ri·tar·sis (ahr″ji·ri·tahr′sis, ahr·jirr″i·). A South American species of mosquito; a vector of malaria.

Anopheles cru·ci·ans (kroo′shee·anz). A species of mosquito that carries the malarial parasite, found in the United States, Mexico, and Cuba; infrequently molests man.

Anopheles cu·li·ci·fa·ci·es (kew″li·si·fay′shee·eez). A species of mosquito common to Arabia, India, and Siam; the most important vector of malaria in India.

Anopheles dar·lin·gi (dahr·ling′guy). A species of mosquito found in Brazil and British Guiana, highly anthropophilic and a malarial vector.

Anopheles gam·bi·ae (gam′bee·ee). An important vector of malaria of Africa, also responsible for a major outbreak of malaria in Brazil upon the accidental transport of the vector to South America.

Anopheles hyr·ca·nus (hur·kay′nus). A species of mosquito found from South Europe to China and Japan. An important vector of malaria and filariasis.

Anopheles mac·u·li·pen·nis (mack″yoo·li·pen′is). The type species of the genus, found throughout Europe and many other parts of the world; it is an active malarial vector.

Anopheles quad·ri·mac·u·la·tus (kwah″dri·mack·yoo·lay′tus). A species of mosquito that is the chief vector of human malaria in the United States.

anoph·e·li·cide (a·nof′e·li·side) *n.* An agent that destroys mosquitoes of the genus *Anopheles.*

anoph·e·li·fuge (a·nof′e·li·fewj) *n.* An agent that prevents the bite or attack of mosquitoes of the genus *Anopheles.*

Anoph·e·li·ni (a·nof″e·lye′nigh) *n.pl.* A tribe of the subfamily Culicinae of mosquitoes, including three genera, of which *Anopheles* is important as a vector of malaria.

ano·pho·ria (an″o·fo′ree·uh) *n.* [Gk. *anōphoros*, borne upwards, + *-ia*]. HYPERPHORIA.

an·oph·thal·mia (an″off·thal′mee·uh) *n.* ANOPHTHALMOS (1).

an·oph·thal·mos (an″off·thal′mos) *n.* [Gk., eyeless, from *an-* + *ophthalmos*, eye]. 1. Congenital absence of one or both eyes. 2. An individual born without one or both eyes.

an·o·pia (an·o′pee·uh) *n.* [*an-* + *-opia*]. Absence of sight, especially when due to a lesion of the visual pathways. 2. ANOPSIA.

ano·plas·ty (ay′no·plas·tee) *n.* Plastic surgery or repair of the anus or anal canal.

An·o·plu·ra (an″o·ploo′ruh) *n.pl.* [NL., from Gk. *anoplos*, unarmed, + *oura*, tail]. An order of the Insecta; parasitic, sucking insects without wings; lice.

an·op·sia (an·op′see·uh) *n.* [*an-* + *-opsia*]. 1. Failure to use visual capacity. 2. ANOOPSIA.

an·or·chia (an·or′kee·uh) *n.* ANORCHISM.

an·or·chi·dism (an·or′ki·diz·um) *n.* ANORCHISM.

an·or·chism (an·or′kiz·um, an′or·) *n.* [*anorchus* + *-ism*]. Absence of the testes. —**anor·chous** (·kus) *adj.*

an·or·chus (an·or′kus) *n.* [NL., from Gk. *anorchos*, without testicles, castrated, from *an-* + *orchis*, testicle]. An individual showing congenital absence of the testes.

ano·rec·tal (ay″no·reck′tul) *adj.* Pertaining to the anus and the rectum. —**anorec·tum** (·tum) *n.*

anorectal abscess. An abscess of the perirectal adipose tissue near the anus. Syn. *perirectal abscess.*

anorectal junction or **line.** LINEA SINUOSA ANALIS.

anorectal syndrome. Soreness, itching, burning, and redness of the rectum and redness of the anus, occurring after administration by mouth of vitamin B complex together with certain broad-spectrum antibiotics.

an·orec·tic (an″o·reck′tick) *adj.* & *n.* [Gk. *anorektos*, without appetite, from *orexis*, appetency, desire]. 1. Characterized by or causing anorexia. 2. Any agent that causes anorexia.

ano·rec·to·plas·ty (ay″no·reck′to·plas″tee) *n. In surgery,* repair or reconstruction of the anus and rectum.

an·orec·tous (an″o·reck′tus) *adj.* Without appetite; characterized by anorexia.

an·oret·ic (an″o·ret′ick) *adj.* & *n.* ANORECTIC.

an·orex·ia (an″o·reck′see·uh) *n.* [Gk., from *an-* + *orexis*, appetite, + *-ia*]. Absence of appetite. Adj. & n. *anorectic.*

anorexia ner·vo·sa (nur·vo′suh). A syndrome of unknown cause characterized by profound aversion to food, leading to emaciation and sometimes serious nutritional deficiencies; usually seen in young women.

an·orex·i·ant (an″o·reck′see·unt) *adj.* & *n.* 1. Causing depression of appetite. 2. An agent that depresses appetite.

an·orex·ic (an″o·reck′sick) *adj.* & *n.* ANORECTIC.

an·orex·i·gen·ic (an″o·reck″si·jen′ick) *adj.* [*anorexia* + *-genic*]. Causing depression of appetite.

an·or·gas·mia (an″or·gaz′mee·uh) *n.* ANORGASMY.

an·or·gas·my (an″or·gaz′mee) *n.* [*an-* + *orgasm* + *-y*]. A condition, usually psychic, in which there is a failure to reach a climax during coitus.

an·or·thog·ra·phy (an″or·thog′ruh·fee) *n.* [*an-* + *orthography*]. *Obsol.* Inability to write correctly.

an·or·tho·pia (an″or·tho′pee·uh) *n.* [*an-* + *orth-* + *-opia*]. 1. *In optometry,* a defect in vision in which straight lines do not seem straight, and parallelism or symmetry is not properly perceived. 2. Squinting; obliquity of vision. See also *strabismus.*

ano·scope (ay′no·skope) *n.* An instrument for examining the lower rectum and anal canal. —**anos·copy** (ay·nos′kuh·pee) *n.*

an·os·mat·ic (an″oz·mat′ick) *adj.* ANOSMIC.

an·os·mia (an·oz′mee·uh) *n.* [Gk. *anosmos*, without smell (from *an-* + *osmē*, odor), + *-ia*]. Absence of the sense of smell due to organic or psychological factors; organic forms are characterized as afferent when due to loss of olfactory nerve conductivity, central when due to cerebral disease, obstructive when due to obstruction of nasal fossae, and peripheral when due to diseases of the peripheral ends of the olfactory nerves.

an·os·mic (an·oz′mick) *adj.* Of or pertaining to anosmia.

anosmic aphasia. Impairment in the ability to express in words thoughts related to the sense of smell.

ano·sog·no·sia (a·no″sog·no′zhuh, ·zee·uh) *n.* [*a-* + *noso-* + *gnosis* + *-ia*]. Inability to recognize, or denial, on the part of the patient that he is hemiplegic.

ano·spi·nal (ay″no·spye′nul) *adj.* Pertaining to the anus and the spinal cord.

anospinal center. *Obsol.* An area including certain segments of the spinal cord, particularly the second, third, and fourth sacral segments, a lesion of which results in disturbed function of the anal sphincter.

an·os·teo·pla·sia (an·os″tee·o·play′zhuh) *n.* [*an-* + *osteo-* + *-plasia*]. CLEIDOCRANIAL DYSOSTOSIS.

an·os·to·sis (an″os·to′sis) *n.* [*an-* + *ostosis*]. Defective development of bone.

an·o·tia (an·o′shuh, ·shee·uh) *n.* [*an-* + *ot-* + *-ia*]. Congenital absence of the pinnae or external ears.

ano·tro·pia (an″o·tro′pee·uh) *n.* [*ano-* + *-tropia*]. *In optometry,* HYPERTROPIA.

an·o·tus (an·o′tus) *n.* An individual showing congenital absence of the ears (anotia). —**anotous,** *adj.*

ano·ves·i·cal (ay″no·ves′i·kul) *adj.* [*ano-* + *vesical*]. Pertaining to the anus and the urinary bladder.

an·ovu·lar (an·o′vew·lur, ·ov′yoo·) *adj.* Not associated with ovulation.

anovular menstruation. Menstruation not preceded by the release of an ovum.

an·ovu·la·to·ry (an·o′vew·luh·to″ree) *adj.* 1. ANOVULAR. 2. Suppressing ovulation.

an·ox·emia, an·ox·ae·mia (an″ock·see′mee·uh) *n.* [*an-* + *ox-* + *-emia*]. Subnormal blood oxygen content. —**anox·emic, anox·ae·mic** (·mick) *adj.*

anoxemia test. HYPOXEMIA TEST.

anoxemic albuminuria. ALBUMINURIA ACETONICA.

anoxemic erythrocytosis. Secondary polycythemia due to hypoxia.

an·ox·ia (an·ock′see·uh) *n.* [*an-* + *ox-* + *-ia*]. Extreme deficiency of oxygen in tissues; severe hypoxia. —**anox·ic** (·sick) *adj.*

anoxic encephalopathy. HYPOXIC ENCEPHALOPATHY.

anoxic headache. A generalized and sometimes throbbing headache caused by the extreme vasodilation with cerebral hypoxia, as at high altitudes.

Anrep effect. Increase in myocardial contractility due to increase in aortic pressure; a form of homeometric autoregulation of the heart.

an·sa (an′suh) *n.*, pl. & genit. sing. **an·sae** (·see) [L., handle]. A loop.

ansa cer·vi·ca·lis (sur″vi·kay′lis) [NA]. A nerve loop in the cervical plexus which supplies the infrahyoid muscles; formed at the side of the neck by fibers derived from the first, second, and third cervical nerves. See also *inferior root of the ansa cervicalis, superior root of the ansa cervicalis.*

Ansadol. A trademark for salicylanilide, a fungistatic agent.

ansae. Plural and genitive singular of *ansa.*

ansae ner·vi spi·na·lis (nur′vye spye·nay′lis) [NA]. Loops of nerve fibers connecting anterior spinal nerves.

ansae ner·vo·rum spi·na·li·um (nur·vo′rum spye·nay′lee·um) [BNA]. ANSAE NERVI SPINALIS.

ansa hy·po·glos·si (high″po·glos′eye). ANSA CERVICALIS.

ansa len·ti·cu·la·ris (len·tick″yoo·lair′is) [NA]. A bundle of efferent fibers from the globus pallidus, passing around the medial border of the internal capsule to join the fasciculus lenticularis.

ansa len·ti·for·mis (len·ti·for′mis). ANSA LENTICULARIS.

ansa ner·vi hy·po·glos·si (nur′vye high·po·glos′eye) [BNA]. ANSA CERVICALIS.

ansa of Vieus·sens (vyœ·sah^{n}ss′) [R. *Vieussens*]. ANSA SUBCLAVIA.

ansa pe·dun·cu·la·ris (pe·dunk″yoo·lair′is) [NA]. Fibers from the medial and basal surface of the thalamus passing below the lenticular nucleus and radiating to the cortex of the temporal lobe and insula.

ansa sa·cra·lis (sa·kray′lis). A loop joining the coccygeal ganglion with the sympathetic trunks of the two sides.

ansa sub·cla·via (sub·klay′vee·uh) [NA]. A loop, between the inferior and middle cervical ganglions of the sympathetic chain, passing around the subclavian artery.

an·sate (an′sate) *adj.* [L. *ansatus,* from *ansa,* handle]. Having a handle; handle-shaped; loop-shaped, ANSIFORM.

ansa vi·tel·li·na (vit″e·lye′nuh). VITELLINE ANSA.

¹an·ser·ine (an′sur·ine, ·in) *adj.* [L. *anserinus,* from *anser,* goose]. 1. Pertaining to or like a goose. 2. Designating an extremity with unduly prominent tendons because of muscle wasting.

²an·ser·ine (an′sur·een, ·in) *n.* *N*-β-Alanyl-1-methyl-L-histidine, $C_{10}H_{16}N_4O_3$, a dipeptide found in muscles of birds, reptiles, and fishes.

anserine bursa. A bursa beneath the pes anserinus, the conjoined tendons of insertion of the gracilis, sartorius, and semitendinosus muscles.

anserine skin. GOOSEFLESH.

an·si·form (an′si·form) *adj.* Loop-shaped; ANSATE.

ansiform lobule. A lobule of the posterior lobe of the cerebellum, extending from the superior surface of the hemisphere around the posterior border to the inferior surface; the inferior and superior semilunar lobules collectively. Syn. *lobulus ansiformis.*

Ansolysen Tartrate. Trademark for pentolinium tartrate.

Anspor. Trademark for cephradine, a semisynthetic cephalosporin.

ant-. See *anti-.*

-ant [L. *-ans, -antis,* participle ending of *a*-stem verbs]. Suffix denoting *an agent or thing that promotes a specific action.*

Antabuse. Trademark for disulfiram, a substance used in the treatment of alcoholism.

ant·ac·id (ant·as′id) *n.* A substance that neutralizes acids or relieves acidity.

an·tag·o·nism (an·tag′uh·niz·um) *n.* [from *antagonize*]. Opposition; the mutually opposing or resisting action seen between organisms (antibiosis), muscles, functions, disease, and drugs; or between drugs and functions; or between drugs and disease. —**an·tag·o·nis·tic** (an·tag″uh·nis′tick) *adj.*

an·tag·o·nist (an·tag′uh·nist) *n.* [Gk. *antagōnistēs,* competitor, opponent]. 1. A drug that opposes the effects of another by physiological or chemical action or by a competitive mechanism for the same receptor sites. 2. ANTAGONISTIC MUSCLE. 3. ANTAGONISTIC TOOTH.

antagonistic action. 1. Counteraction; opposition. 2. The effect of an opposing agent or principle, such as a muscle or a drug.

antagonistic muscle. A muscle acting in opposition to another (the agonist), as the triceps, which extends the elbow, in opposition to the biceps, which flexes the elbow.

antagonistic reflexes. Reflexes in response to different stimuli which elicit opposing effects, as the flexion and extension of a limb with resulting dominance of the stronger reflex. The nociceptive reflexes usually predominate.

antagonistic tooth. A tooth that meets another tooth or teeth of the opposite dental arch during mastication or in occlusion.

an·tag·o·nize (an·tag′uh·nize) *v.* [Gk. *antagōnizesthai,* to oppose, from *anti-* + *agōn,* contest]. 1. To neutralize the effects of a substance, such as a drug or chemical; to counteract. 2. To act in opposition to, as certain muscles.

ant·al·gic (ant·al′jick) *adj.* [*ant-* + *alg-* + *-ic*]. 1. Countering pain. 2. Pertaining to a position, attitude, or posture in order to avoid pain.

ant·al·ka·line (ant·al′ka·line, ·lin) *adj. & n.* 1. Neutralizing alkalies. 2. An agent that neutralizes alkalies.

Antallergan. Trademark for pyrilamine maleate, an antihistaminic drug.

ant·aph·ro·dis·i·ac (ant″af″ro·diz′ee·ack) *adj. & n.* ANAPHRODISIAC.

an·taz·o·line (an·taz′o·leen) *n.* 2-(*N*-Benzylanilinomethyl)-2-imidazoline, $C_{17}H_{19}N_3$, an antihistaminic agent; used as the hydrochloride and phosphate salt.

an·te (an′tee, an′teʰ). A Latin preposition meaning *before.*

ante- [L.]. A prefix meaning *before, preceding, in front of, prior to, anterior to.*

an·te·au·ral (an″tee·aw′rul) *adj.* [*ante-* + *aural*]. Situated in front of the ear.

an·te·bra·chi·al (an″te·bray′kee·ul) *adj.* Of or pertaining to the forearm or antebrachium.

an·te·bra·chi·um (an″te·bray′kee·um) *n.,* pl. **antebra·chia** (·kee·uh) [*ante-* + *branchium*] [NA]. FOREARM.

an·te ci·bum (an″tee sib′um, see′bum) [L.]. Before meals, used in prescription writing. Abbreviated, a.c.

an·te·cu·bi·tal (an″te·kew′bi·tul) *adj.* [*ante-* + *cubital*]. Situated in front of the elbow.

antecubital fossa. The depression in front of the elbow. NA *fossa cubitalis.*

antecubital space. The triangular space in front of the elbow, often used as the site of venipuncture.

an·te·cur·va·ture (an″te·kur′vuh·chur) *n.* A forward curvature.

an·te·flex·ion (an″te·fleck′shun) *n.* [*ante-* + *flexion*]. A bending forward.

anteflexion of the uterus. A condition in which the fundus of the uterus is bent excessively forward on the cervix.

an·te·grade (an′te·grade) *adj.* ANTEROGRADE.

an·te·hy·poph·y·sis (an″te·high·pof′i·sis, ·hi·pof′i·sis) *n.* [*ante-* + *hypophysis*]. ADENOHYPOPHYSIS.

ante mor·tem (mor′tum) *adv. phrase* [L.]. Before death, as: 1 hr ante mortem. Compare *antemortem (adj.).* Contr. *post mortem.*

an·te·mor·tem (an″tee·mor′tum) *adj.* [from the adv. phrase *ante mortem*]. Before death.

antemortem statement. A declaration made immediately before death, which, if made with the consciousness of impending death, is legally considered an exception to the hearsay rule of the law of evidence.

antemortem thrombus. An intravascular blood clot that occurs before death.

an·te·nar·i·al (an″te·nair′ee·ul) *adj.* [*ante-* + *narial*]. Situated in front of the nostrils.

an·te·na·tal (an″tee·nay′tul) *adj.* [*ante-* + *natal*]. Occurring or existing before birth; prenatal.

an·ten·na (an·ten′uh) *n.,* pl. **anten·nae** (·ee), **antennas** [L., sailyard]. One of the lateral paired appendages at the side of the anterior segment of the head of arthropods.

Antepar. A trademark for piperazine citrate, an anthelmintic.

an·te·pa·ri·e·tal (an″tee·puh·rye′e·tul) *adj.* In front of the parietal lobe of the brain.

an·te·par·tal (an″tee·pahr′tul) *adj.* ANTEPARTUM.

ante par·tum (pahr′tum) *adv. phrase* [L.]. Before delivery, as: 12 hrs ante partum. Compare *antepartum (adj.).* Contr. *post partum.*

an·te·par·tum (an″tee·pahr′tum) *adj.* [from the adv. phrase *ante partum*]. Before delivery. Compare *ante partum.* Contr. *intrapartum, postpartum.*

antepartum hemorrhage. Bleeding from the uterus before delivery.

Antergan. Trademark for *N*-benzyl-*N′*,*N′*-dimethyl-*N*-phenylethylenediamine, an antihistaminic substance used as the hydrochloride salt.

an·te·ri·ad (an·teer′ee·ad) *adv. In anatomy,* forward; in a posterior-to-anterior direction. Compare *ventrad.*

an·te·ri·or (an·teer′ee·ur) *adj.* [L.]. *In anatomy* (with reference to the human or animal body as poised for its usual manner of locomotion): fore, in front; situated or advanced relatively far in the direction of normal locomotion. Compare *ventral.* Contr. *posterior,* —*anterior·ly, adv.*

anterior adductor space. THENAR SPACE (2).

anterior asynclitism. Biparietal obliquity; the lateral inclination of the fetal head at the superior pelvic strait, which brings the sagittal suture nearer to the sacral promontory. Syn. *Naegele's obliquity.*

anterior atlantoocipital ligament. ANTERIOR ATLANTOOCCIPITAL MEMBRANE.

anterior atlantooccipital membrane. A dense membrane extending from the anterior (ventral) surface and cranial margin of the anterior arch of the atlas to the anterior border of the foramen magnum and inferior surface of the basilar part of the occipital bone. NA *membrana atlantooccipitalis anterior.*

anterior axial embryonic cataract. A congenital cataract in which a small opacity is located in the central zone of the lens, but vision is usually not affected; inherited as a dominant trait.

anterior border ring. SCHWALBE'S LINE.

anterior brain vesicle. PROSENCEPHALON.

anterior cardinal veins. The paired primary veins of the anterior part of the embryo; they unite with the posterior cardinal veins to form the common cardinal veins.

anterior central gyrus. PRECENTRAL GYRUS.

anterior centriole. The centriole that gives rise to the axial filament of the spermatozoon.

anterior cerebellar lobe. A median unpaired structure including all that part of the cerebellum which lies on the rostral side of the primary fissure.

anterior cerebellar notch. A broad, flat depression on the anterior margin of the upper surface of the cerebellum, between the two hemispheres.

anterior chamber. The space between the cornea and the iris. NA *camera anterior bulbi.*

anterior chamber angle. The angle marking the periphery of the anterior chamber of the eye, formed by the attached margin of the iris and the junction of the sclera and cornea and functioning as a drainage route for aqueous humor. Syn. *filtration angle, iridocorneal angle.* NA *angulus iridocornealis.*

anterior chamber drainage angle. ANTERIOR CHAMBER ANGLE.

anterior choroiditis. Inflammation involving the periphery of the choroid.

anterior ciliary artery. NA (pl.) *arteriae ciliares anteriores.* See *ciliary artery.*

anterior clinoid process. A prominent process that juts backward from the medial extremity of the lesser wing of the sphenoid bone behind the optic canal. NA *processus clinoideus anterior.*

anterior column. A division of the longitudinal columns of gray matter in the spinal cord. NA *columna anterior medullae spinalis.*

anterior column cells. Generally, all cells located in the anterior horn of the spinal cord; especially, those in the anterior horn of the spinal cord whose axons project peripherally and to other levels of the cord. See also *anterior horn cell.*

anterior commissure. A rounded cord of nerve fibers placed in front of the columns of the fornix, connecting olfactory centers and parts of the temporal cortex of the cerebral hemispheres. It has an anterior and a posterior part. NA *commissura anterior cerebri.*

anterior communicating artery. A short trunk connecting the two anterior cerebral arteries. NA *arteria communicans anterior cerebri.*

anterior compartment. ANTERIOR TIBIAL COMPARTMENT.

anterior compartment syndrome. ANTERIOR TIBIAL COMPARTMENT SYNDROME.

anterior condylar canal. HYPOGLOSSAL CANAL.

anterior cornual syndrome. PROGRESSIVE SPINAL MUSCULAR ATROPHY.

anterior corticospinal tract. Fibers of the corticospinal tract which, without decussating, descend directly in the anterior funiculus, normally to the upper thoracic region. NA *tractus corticospinalis anterior, tractus pyramidalis anterior.*

anterior cranial fossa. The most elevated in position of the three fossae into which the internal base of each side of the skull (right and left) is divided. It lodges the frontal lobe of the brain and is formed by the orbital part of the frontal bone, the cribriform plate of the ethmoid bone, and the lesser wing of the sphenoid bone. NA *fossa cranii anterior.*

anterior cubital region. The triangular area distal to the elbow, bounded above by a line joining the two humoral epicondyles, medially by the pronator teres muscle, and laterally by the brachioradialis muscle. NA *regio cubiti anterior.*

anterior curvature. KYPHOSIS.

anterior deformity. LORDOSIS.

anterior embryotoxon. A congenital defect of the eye characterized by an opaque ring in the corneal stroma extending almost to the limbus and resembling an arcus senilis, but evident at or shortly after birth. It may be hereditary or occur in association with blue sclera syndrome, megalocornea, aniridia, or hypercholesterolemia. Syn. *arcus juvenilis.*

anterior ethmoid foramen. A canal between the ethmoid and frontal bones, giving passage to the nasal branch of the ophthalmic nerve and anterior ethmoid vessels. NA *foramen ethmoidale anterius.*

anterior focal point. The anterior conjugate focus. See *conjugate foci.*

anterior fontanel. The membranous area at the point of union of the frontal, sagittal, and coronal sutures, which closes usually during the second year. NA *fonticulus anterior.*

anterior forceps. The U-shaped bundles from the radiation of the corpus callosum that are distributed to the frontal pole of the cerebral hemisphere. NA *forceps minor.*

anterior gluteal line. A line on the lateral aspect of the ilium beginning at the anterior extremity of the iliac crest and curving downward and backward to the upper part of the greater sciatic notch. NA *linea glutea anterior.*

anterior guide. That part of an articulator on which the anterior guide pin rests to maintain the vertical dimension of occlusion; it influences the degree of separation of the casts in eccentric relationships.

anterior horn. The anterior column of gray matter as seen in a cross section of the spinal cord. NA *cornu anterius medullae spinalis.*

anterior horn cell. A large multipolar nerve cell in the anterior horn of the spinal cord whose axon constitutes an efferent fiber innervating a muscle. These cells are the most likely to be affected by the virus causing paralytic spinal poliomyelitis.

anterior hypothalamic area. The anterior medial part of the hypothalamus, lying lateral to the periventricular nucleus and posterior to the preoptic nuclei.

anterior hypothalamic decussation or **commissure.** A bundle of nerve fibers in the dorsal part of the supraoptic commissures, which in part consists of pallidohypothalamic fibers and in part probably connects the hypothalamic regions of the two sides. Syn. *Ganser's commissure.* See also *commissurae supraopticae.*

anterior hypothalamic nucleus. A mass of poorly differentiated cells in the anterior hypothalamic area.

anterior inferior iliac spine. A projection on the anterior border of the ilium. NA *spina iliaca anterior inferior.*

anterior interventricular sulcus. A groove situated on the sternocostal surface of the heart, separating the ventricles. NA *sulcus interventricularis anterior.*

anterior lateral fontanel. ANTEROLATERAL FONTANEL.

anterior ligament of the malleus. A band connecting the neck and anterior process of the malleus to the anterior wall of the tympanic cavity near the petrotympanic fissure, with some fibers continuing through the fissure to the sphenoid bone. NA *ligamentum mallei anterius.*

anterior limb of the internal capsule. The portion of the internal capsule that lies between the caudate and lentiform nuclei.

anterior lingual gland. One of the paired compound tubuloalveolar mixed glands close behind the tip of the tongue. The ducts open at the margin of the fimbriated folds. Syn. *Blandin's gland.* NA *glandula lingualis anterior.*

anterior lobe of the hypophysis. ADENOHYPOPHYSIS. NA *lobus anterior hypophyseos.*

anterior longitudinal cardiac sulcus. ANTERIOR INTERVENTRICULAR SULCUS.

anterior longitudinal ligament. A broad fibrous band running from the atlas to the sacrum on the anterior side of the vertebral column and attached to the anterior surface of each vertebral body, serving with the posterior longitudinal ligament and the intervertebral disks to secure the joints between the vertebral bodies. NA *ligamentum longitudinale anterius.*

anterior mallear fold. 1. A fold on the external surface of the tympanic membrane stretching from the mallear prominence to the tympanic sulcus of the temporal bone, forming the lower anterior border of the pars flaccida. NA *plica mallearis anterior membranae tympani.* 2. A fold of mucous membrane on the inner aspect of the tympanic membrane over the anterior process of the malleus. NA *plica mallearis anterior tunicae mucosae cavi tympani.*

anterior malleolar fold. ANTERIOR MALLEAR FOLD.

anterior median fissure. A groove extending the entire length of the spinal cord in the midline anteriorly, and incompletely dividing it into two symmetrical parts. NA *fissura mediana anterior medullae spinalis.*

anterior median nucleus. A vertical plate of small cells, in front of and ventral to the Edinger-Westphal nucleus, which perhaps represents the rostral continuation of the latter.

anterior mediastinum. The division of the mediastinum that contains the internal thoracic vessels, loose areolar tissue, lymphatic vessels, and a few lymph nodes. NA *mediastinum anterius.*

anterior medullary velum. SUPERIOR MEDULLARY VELUM.

anterior nasal spine. A median, sharp process formed by the forward prolongation of the two maxillas at the lower margin of the anterior aperture of the nose. NA *spina nasalis anterior maxillae.*

anterior neck triangle. The triangle bounded in front by the median line of the neck, behind by the anterior margin of the sternocleidomastoid, and above by the lower border of the body of the mandible and a line extending from the angle of the mandible to the mastoid process; it is divided into the inferior carotid, superior carotid, submandibular, and suprahyoid triangles.

anterior neuropore. A neuropore at the cephalic end of the neural tube.

anterior nuclei of the thalamus. Nuclear masses located in the anterior part of the thalamus. NA *nuclei anteriores thalami.*

anterior obturator tubercle. An occasional projection on the obturator crest of the superior ramus of the pubis; the anterior margin of the obturator groove. NA *tuberculum obturatorium anterius.*

anterior palatine foramen. INCISIVE FOSSA (1).

anterior perforated space. ANTERIOR PERFORATED SUBSTANCE.

anterior perforated substance. A depressed area of gray matter at the base of the brain, rostral to the optic tract, containing numerous small foramens transmitting arteries to the basal ganglions. Syn. *olfactory area.* NA *substantia perforata anterior.*

anterior pillar of the fauces. PALATOGLOSSAL ARCH.

anterior pillar of the fornix. COLUMN OF THE FORNIX.

anterior pituitary. ADENOHYPOPHYSIS.

anterior pituitary gonadotropin. Any of the gonad-stimulating hormones produced by the anterior lobe of the hypophysis, including follicle-stimulating hormone, luteinizing hormone, and prolactin or luteotropic hormone.

anterior pituitary-like factor, hormone, principle, or **substance.** CHORIONIC GONADOTROPIN.

anterior polar cataract. An opacity, which may vary in size, of the central anterior capsule of the lens; usually congenital and often inherited as a regular or irregular dominant trait.

anterior poliomyelitis. PARALYTIC SPINAL POLIOMYELITIS.

anterior process of the malleus. A long, delicate process that passes from the neck of the malleus forward toward the petrotympanic fissure, to which it is connected by the anterior ligament of the malleus. Formerly called *long process of the malleus, processus gracilis.* NA *procesus anterior mallei.*

anterior rhinoscopy. Examination of the nares by means of a rhinoscope.

anterior rhizotomy. Surgical division of the anterior motor nerve roots within the dura mater.

anterior root. VENTRAL ROOT.

anterior sacral foramen. One of the eight foramens (four on each side) on the anterior surface of the sacrum, connecting with the sacral canal, and giving passage to the anterior branches of the sacral nerves. NA (pl.) *foramina sacralia pelvina* (sing. *foramen sacrale pelvinum*).

anterior sacral plexus. A venous plexus that connects the sacral intervertebral veins with the lumbar and pelvic veins. NA *plexus venosus sacralis.*

anterior sclerotomy. Sclerotomy through the sclera anterior to the ciliary body and into the anterior chamber of the eye.

anterior spinal paralysis or **poliomyelitis.** PARALYTIC SPINAL POLIOMYELITIS.

anterior spinocerebellar tract. A tract of nerve fibers that arise from cells of posterior column of the same and opposite sides, and ascend in the lateral funiculus of the spinal cord to reach the cerebellum by way of the superior cerebellar peduncle. NA *tractus spinocerebellaris anterior.*

anterior spinothalamic tract. A tract of nerve fibers that arise from cells in the posterior column, cross in the anterior white commissure, ascend in the anterior funiculus, and terminate in the thalamus; it conducts impulses from touch and pressure stimuli. NA *tractus spinothalamicus anterior.*

anterior staphyloma. Thinning and ectasia of the cornea, with the iris adhering to the corneoscleral limbus.

anterior superior hemorrhagic polioencephalitis. WERNICKE'S ENCEPHALOPATHY.

anterior superior iliac spine. The projection formed by the anterior extremity of the iliac crest. NA *spina iliaca anterior superior.*

anterior superior polioencephalitis. WERNICKE'S ENCEPHALOPATHY.

anterior symblepharon. Symblepharon that occurs when the edge of an eyelid is adherent.

anterior synechia. Adhesion between the iris and the transparent cornea.

anterior thalamic peduncle. See *thalamic peduncles.*

anterior tibial compartment. The compartment of muscles in the lower leg which is bounded by fascial planes anterior to the interosseous membrane of the leg.

anterior tibial compartment syndrome or **anterior tibial syndrome.** Pain, swelling, and ultimate necrosis of muscles within the anterior tibial compartment due to extravasated fluid, seen after local trauma, arterial occlusion, or cannulation of the femoral artery. Syn. *anterior compartment syndrome.* See also *shin splints.*

anterior tubercle. A tubercle at the anterior part of the extremity of the transverse process of certain cervical vertebrae. NA *tuberculum anterius vertebrarum cervicalium.*

anterior urethritis. Inflammation of the part of the urethra situated anterior to the inferior layer of the urogenital diaphragm.

anterior white commissure. WHITE COMMISSURE (1).

antero-. A combining form meaning *anterior, forward, from front to.*

an·tero·col·lis (an"tur·o·kol'is) *n.* [*antero-* + tortic*ollis*]. Forward flexion in torticollis.

an·tero·dor·sal (an"tur·o·dor'sul) *adj.* [*antero-* + *dorsal*]. *In embryology,* pertaining to the dorsal aspect of the head region.

an·tero·ex·ter·nal (an"tur·o·ecks·tur'nul) *adj.* [*antero-* + *external*]. Situated in front to the outer side.

an·tero·grade (an'tur·o·grade) *adj.* [*antero-* + *-grade,* from L. *gradi,* to step, walk]. 1. Proceeding forward. 2. Concerning events following the onset of the condition, as anterograde amnesia. Contr. *retrograde.*

anterograde amnesia or **memory.** Loss of ability to form new memories or to learn. Contr. *retrograde amnesia.*

an·tero·in·fe·ri·or (an"tur·o·in·feer'ee·ur) *adj.* [*antero-* + *inferior*]. Situated in front and below.

an·tero·in·te·ri·or (an"tur·o·in·teer'ee·ur) *adj.* [*antero-* + *interior*]. Situated in front and internally.

an·tero·in·ter·nal (an"tur·o·in·tur'nul) *adj.* [*antero-* + *internal*]. Situated in front to the inner side.

an·tero·lat·er·al (an"tur·o·lat'ur·ul) *adj.* [*antero-* + *lateral*]. In front and to one side; from the front to one side.

anterolateral fasciculus of Gowers. GOWERS' TRACT.

anterolateral fontanel. The membranous space between the parietal, frontal, great wing of the sphenoid, and temporal bones; usually closes by 3 months of age.

anterolateral spinal sulcus. A broad, shallow groove on the anterolateral surface of the spinal cord, corresponding to the line of the origin of the ventral nerve roots.

anterolateral sulcus of the medulla oblongata. The continuation cephalad of the anterolateral spinal sulcus, from which emerge the roots of the hypoglossal nerves. NA *sulcus lateralis anterior medullae oblongatae.*

an·tero·me·di·al (an"tur·o·mee'dee·ul) *adj.* [*antero-* + *medial*]. In front and toward the midline.

an·tero·me·di·an (an"tur·o·mee'dee·un) *adj.* [*antero-* + *median*]. In front and in the midline.

an·tero·me·si·al (an"tur·o·mee'zee·ul) *adj.* ANTEROMEDIAL.

an·tero·pa·ri·e·tal (an"tur·o·pa·rye'e·tul) *adj.* [*antero-* + *parietal*]. Forward and parietal, as the anteroparietal area of the cranium.

an·tero·pi·tu·i·tary (an"tur·o·pi·tew'i·terr"ee) *adj.* [*antero-* + *pituitary*]. Pertaining to the adenohypophysis.

an·tero·pos·te·ri·or (an"tur·o·pos·teer'ee·ur) *adj.* [*antero-* + *posterior*]. Extending from before backward; pertaining to both front and back.

anteroposterior diameter. 1. In measuring the pelvic inlet, the line which joins the sacrovertebral angle and pubic symphysis. See also *internal conjugate diameter, external conjugate diameter.* 2. In measuring the pelvic outlet, the distance between the lower margin of the symphysis pubis and the tip of the sacrum or the tip of the coccyx. Syn. *sacropubic diameter, coccygeopubic diameter.*

an·tero·su·pe·ri·or (an"tur·o·sue·peer'ee·ur) *adj.* [*antero-* + *superior*]. Situated in front and above.

an·tero·trans·verse (an"tur·o·trans·vurce') *adj.* Pertaining to the anterior and transverse portion of a structure.

anterotransverse diameter. The line joining the tips of the great wings of the sphenoid.

an·te·ver·sion (an"te·vur'zhun) *n.* [*ante-* + *version*]. A tipping, tilting, or displacement forward of an organ or part, especially of the uterus. —**ante·vert** (·vurt') *v.;* **ante·vert·ed** (·vur'tid) *adj.*

anth-, antho- [Gk. *anthos,* flower]. A combining form meaning *flower, floral, flowerlike.*

Anthalazine. Trademark for piperazine phosphate, an anthelmintic.

ant·he·lix (ant·hee'licks) *n.* [NA]. The curved ridge of the pinna just anterior to the helix and following through most of the course of the helix.

ant·hel·min·thic (ant"hel·min'thick, an"thel·) *adj. & n.* ANTHELMINTIC.

ant·hel·min·tic (ant"hel·min'tick, an"thel·) *adj. & n.* [*ant-* + *heminth* + *-ic*]. 1. Destructive or eliminative of intestinal worms. 2. A remedy for intestinal worms.

an·thel·my·cin (an"thel·migh'sin) *n.* An antibiotic substance, produced by *Streptomyces longissimus,* that has anthelmintic activity.

an·the·lone (an'the·lone) *n.* UROGASTRONE.

an·the·ma (an·theem'uh, anth'e·muh) *n.,* pl. **anthema·ta** (·tuh), **anthemas** [Gk. *anthēma,* from *anthein,* to bloom]. 1. EXANTHEMA. 2. Any skin eruption.

an·the·mis (anth'e·mis) *n.* [Gk., camomile]. English or Roman camomile. The flower heads of *Anthemis nobilis;* has been used in coughs and spasmodic infantile complaints, and as a stomachic tonic.

an·ther (an'thur) *n.* [Gk. *anthēros,* flowery, blooming]. *In biology,* that part of the stamen which contains pollen.

Anthiomaline. Trademark for antimony lithium thiomalate, an antiprotozoal agent.

Anthisan. A trademark for pyrilamine maleate, an antihistaminic substance.

antho-. See *anth-.*

an·tho·cy·a·nin (an"tho·sigh'uh·nin) *n.* [*antho-* + *cyan-* + *-in*]. Any of a class of glycosides comprising the soluble coloring matter of blue, red, and violet flowers, and the reds and purples of autumn leaves. Contr. *xanthophyll.*

an·tho·cy·a·nin·uria (an"tho·sigh"a·nin·yoo'ree·uh) *n.* [*anthocyanin* + *-uria*]. BEETURIA.

An·tho·my·ia (an"tho·migh'ee·uh, ·migh'uh) *n.* [*antho-* + *-myia*]. A genus of flies which, depositing their ova on food, especially on vegetable material, cause intestinal myiasis.

Anthony's bacterial capsule stain [E. E. *Anthony,* U.S. bacteriologist, b. 1906]. Cells appear dark blue and capsules blue violet when air-dried smears are stained with crystal violet solution and then treated with copper sulfate solution.

an·tho·pho·bia (an"tho·fo'bee·uh) *n.* [*antho-* + *phobia*]. An abnormal dislike or fear of flowers.

anthr-, anthra-. A combining form denoting *the presence of the anthracene nucleus.*

anthrac-, anthraco-. [Gk. *anthrax, anthrakos,* charcoal, carbuncle]. A combining form meaning (a) *coal, charcoal, carbon;* (b) *anthrax.*

an·thra·ce·mia, an·thra·cae·mia (an"thruh·see'mee·uh) *n.* 1. Bacteremia or septicemia caused by *Bacillus anthracis.* 2. An increase in the level of carbon monoxide in the blood, due to carbon monoxide poisoning.

an·thra·cene (an'thruh·seen) *n.* [*anthrac-* + *-ene*]. $C_{14}H_{10}$, a tricyclic solid hydrocarbon obtained by distillation from coal tar and other carbon compounds.

an·thra·ci·dal (an"thruh·sigh'dul) *adj.* Lethal for *Bacillus anthracis.*

anthraco-. See *anthrac-.*

an·thra·co·gram (an"thruh·ko·gram) *n.* [*anthraco-* + *-gram*]. A photograph or diagram showing the distribution of mineral material in an incompletely incinerated section of a tissue or organ.

an·thra·coid (an'thruh·koid) *adj.* [*anthrac-* + *-oid*]. 1. Resembling carbon. 2. Resembling anthrax.

an·thra·co·ne·cro·sis (an"thruh·ko·ne·kro'sis) *n.* [*anthraco-* + *necrosis*]. A focus of blackened necrotic tissue.

an·thra·co·sil·i·co·sis (an″thruh·ko·sil·i·ko′sis) *n.* [*anthraco-* + *silicosis*]. Pneumoconiosis characterized by deposition of carbon and silicon, the pathologic effects being those of silicon dioxide.

an·thra·co·sis (an″thruh·ko′sis) *n.*, [Gk. *anthrakōsis,* carbonization, charring]. Pigmentation, particularly of the lungs, by carbon particles; usually harmless. —**anthra·cot·ic** (·kot′ick) *adj.*

an·thra·lin (an′thruh·lin) *n.* [*anthr-* + *-al* + *-in*]. 1,8-Dihydroxyanthranol, $C_{14}H_{10}O_3$, used externally for treatment of various skin diseases. Syn. *dithranol (Brit.).*

an·thra·my·cin (an″thruh·migh′sin) *n.* (*E*)-3-(5,10,11,11a-Tetrahydro-9,11-dihydroxy-8-methyl-5-oxo-1*H*-pyrrolo-[2,1-c][1,4]benzodiazepin-2-yl)-2-propenamide, $C_{16}H_{17}N_3O_4$, an antineoplastic agent.

an·thra·nil·ic acid (an″thruh·nil′ick). *o*-Aminobenzoic acid, $NH_2C_6H_4COOH$, an important intermediate in many syntheses.

an·thra·nol (an′thruh·nol, ·nole) *n.* 9-Hydroxyanthracene, $C_{14}H_{10}O$, derivatives of which are used medicinally. See also *anthralin, anthrarobin.*

an·thra·qui·none (an″thruh·kwi·nohn′, ·kwin′ohn) *n.* [*anthra-* + *quinone*]. 9,10-Dioxoanthracene, $C_{14}H_8O_2$. Derivatives of it occur in aloe, cascara sagrada, rhubarb, and senna and are responsible for the cathartic action.

an·thra·ro·bin (an″thruh·ro′bin) *n.* [*anthr-* + *araroba* + *-in*]. 3,4-Dihydroxyanthranol, $C_{14}H_{10}O_3$; used externally for treatment of skin diseases.

an·thrax (an′thraks) *n.*, pl. **an·thra·ces** (an′thruh·seez) [Gk., coal, charcoal, carbuncle]. 1. An acute infectious disease of cattle and sheep, transmissible to man and caused by *Bacillus anthracis.* 2. A carbuncle or malignant pustule.

anthrax bacillus. *BACILLUS ANTHRACIS.*

anthrax polypeptide. The capsular substance of *Bacillus anthracis,* consisting of a polypeptide of D-glutamic acid, and possessing antiphagocytic properties.

anthrax vaccine. Attenuated cultures or antigenic preparations of anthrax bacilli used to immunize against the disease.

an·throne (an′throne) *n.* 9,10-Dihydro-9-oxoanthracene, $C_{14}H_{10}O$; used in the determination of sugar in body fluids.

anthrop-, anthropo- [Gk. *anthrōpos*]. A combining form meaning *human being.*

an·thro·pho·bia (an″thro·fo′bee·uh) *n.* ANTHROPOPHOBIA.

an·thro·po·bi·ol·o·gy (an″thruh·po·bye·ol′uh·jee) *n.* The biologic study of man and the anthropoid apes.

an·thro·po·gen·e·sis (an″thruh·po·jen′e·sis) *n.*, pl. **anthropo·gene·ses** (·seez) [*anthropo-* + *-genesis*]. 1. The evolution (phylogenesis) of the human species. 2. The development (ontogenesis) of the human organism. —**anthropo·ge·net·ic** (·je·net′ick) *adj.*

an·thro·pog·e·ny (an″thro·poj′e·nee) *n.* ANTHROPOGENESIS. —**anthro·po·gen·ic** (·po·jen′ick) *adj.*

an·thro·poid (an′thruh·poid) *adj.* [Gk. *anthrōpoeidēs,* manlike, of human form]. 1. Pertaining to the Anthropoidea. Contr. *prosimian.* 2. Characteristic of anthropoid apes. 3. Specifically, of a pelvis: resembling that of the great apes, being long, narrow, and oval, with the anteroposterior diameter greater than the transverse. Contr. *android, gynecoid, platypellic.*

anthropoid ape. 1. Any of the true or hominoid apes, as distinct from various large monkeys sometimes called apes. 2. GREAT APE.

An·thro·poi·dea (an″thro·poy′dee·uh) *n.pl.* The suborder of Primates that includes monkeys, apes, and humans. Contr. *Prosimii.*

anthropoid thinking. PRIMITIVE THINKING.

an·thro·pol·o·gy (an″thruh·pol′uh·jee) *n.* [*anthropo-* + *-logy*]. The scientific study of humanity. See *cultural anthropology, physical anthropology.*

an·thro·pom·e·ter (an″thro·pom′e·tur) *n.* [*anthropo-* + *meter*]. A somatometric caliper used in taking the larger measurements of the human body.

anthropometric identification. BERTILLON SYSTEM.

an·thro·pom·e·try (an″thro·pom′e·tree) *n.* [*anthropo-* + *-metry*]. The scientific measurement of the human body, its various parts, and the skeleton; often used in serial and comparative studies and in systems of identification. —**anthro·po·met·ric** (·po·met′rick) *adj.*; **anthro·pom·e·trist** (·pom′e·trist) *n.*

an·thro·po·mor·phic (an″thruh·po·mor′fick) *adj.* [Gk. *anthrōpomorphos,* from *anthrōpos,* man, + *morphē,* form]. 1. Manlike; having a human form. 2. Of or pertaining to anthropomorphism.

an·thro·po·mor·phism (an″thruh·po·mor′fiz·um) *n.* The attribution of human properties to nonhuman objects.

an·thro·poph·a·gy (an″thro·pof′uh·jee) *n.* [Gk. *anthrōpophagia,* from *anthrōpos,* man, + *phagein,* to eat]. 1. Cannibalism. 2. Sexual perversion leading to rape, mutilation, and cannibalism.

an·thro·po·phil·ic (an″thruh·po·fil′ick) *adj.* [*anthropo-* + *-philic*]. Showing a preference for human beings over animals; man-loving. Syn. *androphilous.*

an·thro·po·pho·bia (an″thruh·po·fo′bee·uh) *n.* [*anthropo-* + *phobia*]. Pathologic fear of people or society.

an·thro·po·so·ma·tol·o·gy (an″thruh·po·so″muh·tol′uh·jee) *n.* [*anthropo-* + *somatology*]. The science of the development, structure, and functions of the human body.

ant·hy·drop·ic (ant″high·drop′ick) *adj.* & *n. Obsol.* ANTIHYDROPIC.

ant·hyp·not·ic (ant″hip·not′ick) *adj.* & *n.* [*ant-* + *hypnotic*]. 1. Tending to induce wakefulness or prevent sleep. 2. An agent that tends to induce wakefulness or prevent sleep.

anti-, ant- [Gk.]. A prefix meaning (a) *against, opposed to, counter;* (b) *combating, inhibiting, preventing, counteracting, neutralizing;* (c) *alleviating;* (d) *situated opposite;* (e) (italicized) in chemistry, *the stereoisomeric form of certain compounds* (as aldoximes) *in which substituent atoms or groups are in trans- relationship.* Contr. *syn-.*

an·ti·ac·id (an″tee·as′id) *n.* ANTACID.

an·ti·ad·re·ner·gic (an″tee·ad″re·nur′jick) *adj.* Inhibiting, counteracting, or modifying adrenergic action.

an·ti·ag·glu·ti·nin (an″tee·uh·gloo′ti·nin) *n.* A substance having the power of neutralizing the corresponding agglutinin.

an·ti·ag·gres·sin (an″tee·uh·gres′in) *n.* An antibody that neutralizes an aggressin produced by microorganisms.

an·ti·al·bu·mate (an″tee·al′bew·mate) *n.* [*anti-* + *albumin* + *-ate*]. A product resulting from the incomplete digestion of albumin formed during gastric digestion.

an·ti·al·bu·min (an″tee·al·bew′min, ·al′bew·min) *n.* An antibody to albumin.

an·ti·al·bu·mi·nate (an″tee·al·bew′mi·nate) *n.* ANTIALBUMATE.

an·ti·alex·in (an″tee·a·leck′sin) *n.* [*anti-* + *alexin*]. ANTICOMPLEMENT.

an·ti·ame·bic, an·ti·amoe·bic (an″tee·uh·mee′bick) *adj.* & *n.* 1. Counteracting infection with amebas. 2. A drug or other agent active in the treatment of infection with amebas.

an·ti·am·y·lase (an″tee·am′i·lace, ·laze) *n.* A substance that neutralizes the action of amylase.

an·ti·ana·phy·lax·is (an″tee·an″uh·fi·lack′sis) *n.*, pl. **antiana·phylax·es** (·seez). A condition in which a sensitized animal (e.g., a guinea pig) is refractory to anaphylaxis because of a saturation or exhaustion of fixed antibodies, or because of an excess of free antibodies which prevents the antigen from making contact with the fixed antibodies.

an·ti·an·dro·gen (an″tee·an′dro·jin) *adj.* & *n.* 1. Inhibiting or modifying androgen activity. 2. A compound that inhibits or modifies the action of an androgen in any way.

antianemia factor or **principle.** A substance counteracting or preventing anemia; usually the specific substance in liver (vitamin B_{12}) used in treating pernicious anemia. See also *intrinsic factor.*

an·ti·ane·mic, an·ti·anae·mic (an″tee·uh·nee′mick) *adj. & n.* 1. Preventing or correcting anemia. 2. A substance used in the treatment or prevention of anemia.

an·ti·an·thrax (an″tee·an′thraks) *adj.* Combating anthrax or the anthrax bacillus.

antianthrax polypeptide. A lysine-containing basic polypeptide occurring in serum, leukocytes, and tissues, which has anthracidal activity.

antianthrax serum. A serum prepared by immunizing horses against anthrax bacilli or anthrax antigens; used in the treatment of human anthrax.

an·ti·an·ti·body (an″tee·an′ti·bod″ee) *n.* An antibody to an antibody.

an·ti·ar·ach·nol·y·sin (an″tee·ăr″ack·nol′i·sin, an″tee·uh·rack·) *n.* [*anti-* + *arachnolysin*]. An antivenin counteracting spider venom.

an·ti·a·rin (an′tee·uh·rin, an″tee·air′in) *n.* An alkaloid from the gum-resinous exudate known as upas antiar, obtained from the East Indian tree *Antiaris toxicaria,* or deadly upas tree. It is a violent poison, causing vomiting, evacuation, irregular heart action, prostration, and death.

an·ti·a·ris (an″tee·ahr′is, ·air′is) *n.* An arrow poison produced from the resinous exudate of the upas tree of the East Indies. Its action is similar to that of curare.

an·ti·ar·rhyth·mic (an″tee·a·rith′mick) *adj.* Preventing or effective against arrhythmia.

an·ti·ar·thrit·ic (an″tee·ahr·thrit′ick) *adj. & n.* 1. Tending to relieve the symptoms of arthritis. 2. An agent that tends to relieve arthritic pain.

an·ti·asth·mat·ic (an″tee·az·mat′ick) *adj. & n.* 1. Preventing or relieving asthmatic attacks. 2. An agent that prevents or checks asthmatic attacks.

an·ti·bac·te·ri·al (an″tee·back·teer′ee·ul) *adj. & n.* 1. Preventing the growth of bacteria or destroying bacteria by physical and chemical agents. 2. An agent that prevents or hinders the growth of or destroys bacteria.

antibacterial immunity. Immunity due to an antagonism to the growth and development of microorganisms in a tissue or organism. Syn. *antiblastic immunity.*

antibacterial spectrum. ANTIBIOTIC SPECTRUM.

Antibason. Trademark for methylthiouracil, a thyroid inhibitor.

an·ti·beri·beri (an″tee·berr·i·berr′ee) *adj.* Tending to relieve or cure beriberi.

antiberiberi vitamin. VITAMIN B_1.

an·ti·bi·o·sis (an″tee·bye·o′sis) *n.* [*anti-* + *-biosis*]. 1. An association between organisms of different species that is harmful to at least one of them; specifically, an association between organisms of ecologically competing species in which one party harms or inhibits the other, most typically by production of a chemical substance, as in the case of various microorganisms. Compare *symbiosis.* 2. The field of therapy utilizing antibiotics.

an·ti·bi·ot·ic (an″tee·bye·ot′ick) *adj. & n.* [*anti-* + *biotic*]. 1. Pertaining to antibiosis. 2. Of or pertaining to the products of certain organisms (as penicillin) used against infections caused by other organisms. 3. An antibiotic substance.

antibiotic sensitivity. The lowest concentration of an antibiotic (expressed numerically) capable of suppressing the growth of a microorganism under standardized conditions.

antibiotic spectrum. The range of activity of an antibiotic against different microorganisms. Syn. *antibacterial spectrum, antimicrobial spectrum.*

an·ti·blas·tic (an″tee·blas′tick) *adj.* [*anti-* + *-blastic*]. Antagonistic to growth of microorganisms in a tissue or organism.

antiblastic immunity. ANTIBACTERIAL IMMUNITY.

an·ti·body (an′ti·bod″ee) *n.* [tr. (ca. 1900) of Ger. *Antikörper,* from *Körper,* body]. One of a class of substances, natural or induced by exposure to an antigen, which have the capacity to react with specific or closely related antigens. In the serum, they occur within the immunoglobulins. Abbreviated, Ab.

antibody-deficiency syndromes. The heterogeneous defects of production of antibody, usually associated with a diminution in the concentration in the serum of one or more immunoglobulins. Included in this grouping are transient hypogammaglobulinemia, congenital and acquired agammaglobulinemias, congenital and acquired dysgammaglobulinemias, and hereditary thymic aplasias.

anti·bot·u·li·nus (an″tee·bot″yoo·lye′nus) *adj.* Combating *Clostridium botulinum* or neutralizing botulinum toxin.

antibotulinus serum. An antitoxin prepared in animals that have been immunized by botulinus toxoid.

an·ti·bra·chi·um (an″ti·bray′kee·um) *n.* [BNA]. *Erron.* ANTEBRACHIUM. **—antibrachi·al** (·ul) *adj.*

an·ti·car·cin·o·gen (an″tee·kahr·sin′o·jen) *n.* An agent that opposes the action of carcinogens.

an·ti·ca·rio·gen·ic (an″tee·kăr″ee·o·jen′ick) *adj.* [*anti-* + *cariogenic*]. Having the quality of being able to prevent or inhibit decay, especially dental decay.

an·ti·cat·a·lyst (an″tee·kat′uh·list) *n.* Any substance that retards the action of a catalyst by acting directly upon it.

an·ti·cat·a·lyz·er (an″tee·kat′uh·lye·zur) *n.* ANTICATALYST.

an·ti·ca·thex·is (an″tee·ka·theck′sis) *n.* [*anti-* + *cathexis*]. A condition in which an emotional charge is released from one impulse and shifted to an impulse of an opposite nature, as when unconscious hate appears as conscious love. Syn. *counterinvestment.*

an·ti·cath·ode, an·ti·kath·ode (an″tee·kath′ode) *n.* The metal plate or target of a Crookes or x-ray tube. It is situated opposite the cathode and is struck by the cathode rays, giving rise to the x-rays.

an·ti·ceph·a·lin (an″tee·sef′uh·lin) *n.* A coagulation inhibitor in plasma or tissues that blocks the acceleratory effects of partial thromboplastins.

an·ti·chei·rot·o·nus, an·ti·chi·rot·o·nus (an″ti·kigh·rot′uh·nus) *n.* [NL., from Gk. *anticheir,* thumb, + *tonos,* tension]. Forcible and steady inflexion of the thumb, sometimes seen before or during an epileptic seizure.

an·ti·chlor (an′tee·klor) *n.* SODIUM THIOSULFATE.

an·ti·cho·les·ter·emic (an″tee·ko·les″tur·ee′mick) *adj.* [*anti-* + *cholesteremia* + *-ic*]. Having an action that reduces the level of cholesterol in the blood.

an·ti·cho·lin·er·gic (an″tee·ko″lin·ur′jick, ·kol″in·) *adj.* Pertaining to, acting as, or caused by a cholinergic blocking agent.

an·ti·cho·lin·es·ter·ase (an″tee·ko″lin·es′tur·ace, ·aze) *n.* A substance which inhibits the enzyme activity of cholinesterase.

an·tic·i·pa·tion, *n.* The apparent progressively earlier clinical onset of a hereditary disease in successive generations, as affirmed by Mott's law of anticipation.

an·ti·co·ag·u·lant (an″tee·ko·ag′yoo·lunt) *adj. & n.* 1. Preventing or retarding coagulation, especially of blood. 2. A substance, such as heparin or bishydroxycoumarin, that prevents or retards clotting of blood. **—anticoagu·la·tive** (·luh·tiv) *adj.*

an·ti·co·ag·u·lat·ed blood (an″tee·ko·ag′yoo·lay·tid). Blood that has been kept fluid by the addition of an anticoagulant.

an·ti·co·don (an″tee·ko′don) *n.* [*anti-* + *codon*]. The nucleotide triplet in a transfer ribonucleic acid molecule which pairs with a messenger ribonucleic acid codon during translation.

an·ti·col·la·gen·ase (an″tee·kol′uh·je·nace, ·naze) *n.* An antibody capable of neutralizing collagenase found in the commercial preparations of *Clostridium perfringens* antitoxin.

an·ti·com·ple·ment (an″tee·kom′ple·munt) *n.* A substance capable of neutralizing, inhibiting, or destroying a complement. Syn. *antialexin.* **—anti·com·ple·men·ta·ry** (·kom″ple·men′tuh·ree) *adj.*

an·ti·con·cep·tive (an″tee-kun-sep′tiv) *adj.* CONTRACEPTIVE.

anti·con·cus·sion plug (an″tee-kun-kush′un). A device fitted into the external auditory meatus and worn, wherever there is exposure to detonations, as in battle during artillery fire, to protect the eardrums from injury.

an·ti·con·vul·sant (an″tee-kun-vul′sunt) *adj.* & *n.* 1. Tending to prevent or arrest seizures. 2. A therapeutic agent that prevents or arrests seizures.

anti·con·vul·sive (an″tee-kun-vul′siv) *adj.* Of or pertaining to an action or to a therapeutic agent that prevents or allays seizures.

an·ti·cus (an-tye′kus) *adj.* [L., front, foremost]. ANTERIOR; in front of.

anticus reflex. PIOTROWSKI'S ANTERIOR TIBIAL REFLEX.

an·ti·cu·tin (an″tee-kew′tin) *n.* [*anti-* + *cut*is + *-in*]. Any substance capable of specifically inhibiting or reducing the capacity of an antigen to produce a reaction in the skin of a sensitized subject.

an·ti·de·pres·sant (an″tee-de-pres′unt) *adj.* & *n.* 1. Tending to prevent or alleviate depression. 2. Any drug used for the treatment of depression. Two classes of such drugs are of major importance: (a) certain dibenzazepine derivatives (tricyclic antidepressants), such as imipramine and amitriptyline; (b) monoamine oxidase inhibitors, such as isocarboxazid and tranylcypromine.

an·ti·de·pres·sion (an″tee-de-presh′un) *adj.* ANTIDEPRESSANT (1).

an·ti·de·pres·sive (an″tee-de-pres′iv) *adj.* ANTIDEPRESSANT (1).

an·ti·di·a·bet·ic (an″tee-dye″uh-bet′ick) *adj.* & *n.* 1. Having an action that alleviates diabetes. 2. An agent used for treatment of diabetes.

antidiabetic hormone. INSULIN.

an·ti·di·ar·rhe·al, anti·di·ar·rhoe·al (an″tee-dye″uh-ree′ul) *adj.* Preventing or overcoming diarrhea.

an·ti·di·ure·sis (an″tee-dye″yoo-ree′sis) *n.* [*anti-* + *diuresis*]. The suppression of the excretion of urine.

an·ti·di·uret·ic (an″tee-dye′yoo-ret′ick) *adj.* & *n.* [*anti-* + *diuretic*]. 1. Opposing, diminishing, or preventing the excretion of urine. 2. An agent that suppresses excretion of urine.

antidiuretic hormone. The pressor principle, a peptide hormone, of the posterior pituitary; used in medicine primarily for its antidiuretic effect. Abbreviated, ADH. Syn. *vasopressin, beta-hypophamine.*

an·ti·dote (an′ti-dote) *n.* [Gk. *antidotos,* from *antididonai,* to give as a remedy, from *didonai,* to give]. Any agent administered to prevent or counteract the action of a poison. **—anti·dot·al** (-doat′ul) *adj.*

an·ti·do·ta·ri·um (an″ti-do-tair′ee-um) *n.,* pl. **antidota·ria** [ML.]. A hospital formulary of the Middle Ages, typified by the twelfth-century Antidotarium of Salerno, which was used as a guide to the compounding of drugs prescribed by Salernitan physicians.

an·ti·drom·ic (an″ti-drom′ick) *adj.* [Gk. *antidrom*ein, to run in a contrary direction, from *anti-* + *dromos,* running, course]. Conducting nerve impulses in a direction opposite to the normal. Contr. *orthodromic.* **—antidrom·i·cal·ly,** *adv.*

antidromic inhibition. RECURRENT INHIBITION.

an·ti·dys·en·ter·ic (an″tee-dis″in-terr′ick) *adj.* & *n.* 1. Tending to combat dysentery. 2. An agent for preventing, relieving, or curing dysentery.

antidysenteric serum. A polyvalent antiserum prepared generally in horses against a variety of species of *Shigella,* but disappointing in the therapy of shigellosis.

an·ti·ec·ze·mat·ic (an″tee-eck-se-mat′ick, -eg-ze-) *n.* A drug or other agent used for alleviation of eczema.

anti-egg-white-injury factor. BIOTIN.

an·ti·emet·ic (an″tee-e-met′ick) *adj.* & *n.* [*anti-* + *emetic*]. 1. Relieving or preventing nausea and vomiting. 2. An agent that prevents or relieves nausea and vomiting.

an·ti·en·zyme (an″tee-en′zime) *n.* 1. Any agent or substance that inhibits or prevents the action of an enzyme, such as an antibody or another enzyme. Syn. *antiferment.* 2. Specifically, an antibody formed in reaction to the injection of an enzyme.

an·ti·ep·i·lep·tic (an″tee-ep″i-lep′tick) *adj.* & *n.* 1. Suppressing or controlling epileptic seizures. 2. A therapeutic agent for suppression or control of epileptic seizures.

an·ti·er·y·sip·e·loid (an″tee-err-i-sip′e-loid) *adj.* Preventing or relieving erysipeloid.

antierysipeloid serum. A serum prepared in horses subjected to increasing subcutaneous injections of live cultures of *Erysipelothrix rhusiopathiae,* now generally superseded in the treatment of erysipeloid by antibiotics.

an·ti·es·tro·gen (an″tee-es′tro-jin) *adj.* & *n.* 1. Inhibiting or modifying estrogen action. 2. A compound that inhibits or modifies the action of an estrogen.

an·ti·fe·brile (an″tee-fee′bril, -feb′ril) *adj.* & *n.* [*anti-* + *febrile*]. 1. Relieving or reducing fever. 2. An agent used to relieve or reduce fever.

Antifebrin. Trademark for acetanilid, an analgesic.

an·ti·fer·ment (an″tee-fur′ment) *n.* 1. An agent that prevents fermentation. 2. ANTIENZYME. **—anti·fer·men·ta·tive** (-fur-men′tuh-tiv) *adj.*

an·ti·fet·ish·ism (an″tee-fet′ish-iz-um) *n.* [*anti-* + *fetish* + *-ism*]. Sexual aversion based on an exaggerated dislike of some characteristic of potential sex partners; thought to serve commonly as a defense mechanism of latent homosexuals. **—antifetish·is·tic,** *adj.*

an·ti·fi·bri·nol·y·sin (an″tee-figh″bri-nol′i-sin) *n.* Any substance that inhibits the proteolytic action of fibrinolysin. See also *antiplasmin.* **—antifibri·no·lyt·ic** (-no-lit′ick) *adj.*

an·ti·fi·bro·ma·to·gen·ic (an″tee-figh-bro″muh-to-jen′ick) *adj.* [*anti-* + *fibroma* + *-genic*]. Acting to prevent the formation of fibromas or fibrous connective tissue.

an·ti·fi·lar·i·al (an″tee-fi-lăr′ee-ul) *adj.* & *n.* 1. Combating filaria. 2. Any drug or agent useful in treating infections caused by filaria.

an·ti·flat·u·lent (an″tee-flat′yoo-lunt) *adj.* & *n.* 1. Tending to prevent flatulence or gastric distress. 2. A drug or agent that prevents flatulence or gastric distress.

an·ti·flux (an′ti-flucks) *n.* [*anti-* + *flux*]. A substance, such as graphite, used to limit the flow of solder.

Antiformin. Trade name for a strongly alkaline solution of sodium hypochlorite, used as a disinfectant and as a reagent for the concentration of tubercle bacilli in sputum.

an·ti·fun·gal (an″tee-fung′gul) *adj.* & *n.* 1. Suppressing or destroying fungi, or effective against fungal infections. 2. Any agent useful in treating fungal infections. Syn. *antimycotic.*

an·ti·ga·lac·tic (an″tee-guh-lack′tick) *adj.* & *n.* [*anti-* + *galactic*]. 1. Lessening the flow of milk. 2. A drug or agent that lessens the flow of milk.

an·ti·gen (an′ti-jin) *n.* [*anti*body + *-gen*]. Any substance eliciting an immunologic response, such as the production of antibody specific for that substance. Abbreviated, Ag. See also *ABO blood group.* **—anti·gen·ic** (-jen′ick) *adj.*

antigen-antibody reaction. The specific combination of an antigen and its antibody.

an·ti·ge·ne·mia (an″ti-je-nee′mee-uh) *n.* The presence of an antigen in the blood.

antigenic determinant. An antigen molecule component that determines the reactive specificity of the antigen; specifically, an epitope, or site whose structure is such as to allow the attachment of certain antibody molecules. See also *combining site.*

an·ti·ge·nic·i·ty (an″ti-je-nis′i-tee) *n.* The capacity to produce an immune response; the state or quality of being an antigen.

an·ti·ger·mi·nal (an″ti-jur′mi-nul) *adj.* Opposite the germinal (animal) pole.

antigerminal pole. VEGETAL POLE.

an·ti·glob·u·lin (an″tee·glob′yoo·lin) *n.* A naturally occurring or artificially induced antibody that reacts with globulin, usually gamma globulin.

antiglobulin serum. An immune serum containing antibodies to one or more globulins, usually immunoglobulins; used in the antiglobulin test.

antiglobulin test. A test originally developed for the detection of Rh antibodies. It depends on the fact that the antibodies coating the erythrocytes consist of human serum globulins. A potent precipitating rabbit anti-human serum is used. It will detect human globulin coating any particle (e.g., erythrocytes, brucella organisms). Syn. *Coombs' test, direct developing test, Race-Coombs test.*

an·ti·grav·i·ty (an″tee·grav′i·tee) *adj.* Resisting or opposing the force of gravity.

antigravity muscles. Muscles, chiefly extensors, the contractions of which support the body against the force of gravity, as in standing.

antigravity reflexes. Reflexes which, through contraction of the extensor muscles, support the body against the force of gravity.

anti-gray-hair factor. PARA-AMINOBENZOIC ACID.

anti-g suit (an″tee·jee′). A suit worn to avoid the deleterious effects of rapid changes in velocity and direction of flight, consisting of rubber bladders which, when rapidly inflated, exert pressure over the abdomen and lower extremities, thus preventing venous pooling there and lowering of arterial pressure in the head. Syn. *g suit.*

antihaemolysin. ANTIHEMOLYSIN.

antihaemolytic. ANTIHEMOLYTIC.

antihaemorrhagic. ANTIHEMORRHAGIC.

antihaemorrhoidal. ANTIHEMORRHOIDAL.

an·ti·he·lix (an″ti·hee′licks) *n.* ANTHELIX.

an·ti·hel·min·thic (an″tee·hel·min′thick) *adj. & n.* ANTHELMINTIC.

an·ti·hel·min·tic (an″tee·hel·min′tick) *adj. & n.* ANTHELMINTIC.

an·ti·he·mol·y·sin, an·ti·hae·mol·y·sin (an″tee·hee·mol′i·sin) *n.* A substance that prevents or inhibits hemolysis.

an·ti·he·mo·lyt·ic, anti·hae·mo·lyt·ic (an″ti·hee″mo·lit′ick, ·hem″o·) *adj.* 1. Pertaining to an antihemolysin. 2. Acting to prevent hemolysis.

an·ti·he·mo·phi·lic factor (an″tee·hee″mo·fil′ick) FACTOR VIII. Abbreviated, AHF.

antihemophilic globulin. FACTOR VIII. Abbreviated, AHG.

an·ti·hem·or·rhag·ic, an·ti·haem·or·rhag·ic (an″tee·hem″o·raj′ick) *adj. & n.* 1. Checking hemorrhage. 2. An agent that prevents or arrests hemorrhage.

antihemorrhagic vitamin. VITAMIN K.

an·ti·hem·or·rhoi·dal, anti·haem·or·rhoi·dal (an″tee·hem″uh·roy′dul) *adj. & n.* 1. Preventing or relieving hemorrhoids. 2. A drug or agent that prevents or relieves hemorrhoids.

anti·hi·drot·ic (an″tee·hi·drot′ick, ·high·drot′ick) *adj. & n.* [*anti-* + *hidrotic*]. 1. Diminishing or preventing the secretion of sweat. 2. A drug or agent that diminishes or prevents the secretion of sweat.

an·ti·his·ta·mine (an″tee·hiss′tuh·meen, ·min) *n.* A substance capable of preventing, counteracting, or diminishing the pharmacologic effects of histamine. **—anti·his·ta·min·ic** (·hiss″tuh·min′ick) *adj. & n.*

an·ti·hor·mone (an″tee·hor′mone) *n.* A substance formed in blood that antagonizes the action of a hormone, particularly a polypeptide or protein hormone which may have an antigenic action in producing the antihormone.

an·ti·hy·a·lu·ron·i·dase (an″tee·high″uh·lew·ron′i·dace, ·daze) *n.* An antienzyme that destroys hyaluronidase.

an·ti·hy·drop·ic (an″tee·high·drop′ick) *adj. & n.* [*anti-* + *hydropic*]. 1. Relieving edematous or dropsical conditions. 2. A drug or agent that prevents or relieves edematous or dropsical conditions.

an·ti·hy·per·ten·sive (an″tee·high″pur·ten′siv) *adj. & n.* [*anti-* + *hypertensive*]. 1. Counteracting elevated blood pressure. 2. A drug that counteracts elevated blood pressure.

an·ti·hyp·not·ic (an″tee·hip·not·ick) *adj. & n.* [*anti-* + *hypnotic*]. 1. Tending to prevent sleep. 2. Any agent that tends to prevent sleep.

Antihypo. A trademark for potassium percarbonate.

an·ti-in·fec·tion (an″tee·in·feck′shun) *adj.* Useful in preventing infection.

an·ti-in·fec·tive (an″tee·in·feck′tiv) *adj. & n.* 1. Tending to counteract or prevent infection. 2. A substance that counteracts infection.

an·ti-in·flam·ma·to·ry (an″tee·in·flam′uh·tor·ee) *adj. & n.* 1. Combating inflammation. 2. Any agent that combats inflammation.

antikathode. ANTICATHODE.

an·ti·ke·to·gen (an″tee·kee′to·jen) *n.* A substance that prevents formation of ketone bodies; an antiketogenic substance.

an·ti·ke·to·gen·e·sis (an″tee·kee″to·jen′e·sis) *n.* [*anti-* + *ketogenesis*]. Prevention of the production of ketone bodies, as by the utilization of carbohydrate rather than fatty acids. **—antiketogen·ic** (·ick) *adj.*

an·ti·leu·ke·mic, an·ti·leu·kae·mic (an″tee·lew·kee′mick) *adj.* Suppressing or controlling leukemia or its symptoms.

an·ti·lew·is·ite (an″tee·lew′i·sight) *n.* [*anti-* + *lewisite*]. DIMERCAPROL.

an·ti·li·pase (an″tee·lye′pace, ·paze, ·lip′ace, ·aze) *n.* A substance inhibiting or counteracting a lipase.

an·ti·lip·fan·o·gen (an″tee·lip·fan′o·jen) *n.* A substance in blood serum which opposes the formation of fat granules from lipfanogens.

an·ti·lipo·trop·ic (an″tee·lip″o·tro′pick, ·trop′ick) *adj.* [*anti-* + *lipotropic*]. Having the property of deflecting methyl groups from choline synthesis, thus causing abnormal deposition of fats or interfering with their removal.

an·ti·lu·et·ic (an″tee·lew·et′ick) *adj. & n.* [*anti-* + *luetic*]. ANTISYPHILITIC.

an·ti·lym·pho·cyt·ic (an″tee·lim″fo·sit′ick) *adj.* Inhibiting or suppressing the proliferation of lymphocytes.

antilymphocytic globulin. Globulin removed from the serum of a subject immunized against the lymphocytes of the same species (homologous antilymphocytic globulin) or of a different species (heterologous antilymphocytic globulin).

antilymphocytic serum. A specially prepared serum containing antibodies against lymphocytes, used especially in prevention of rejections against transplanted organs.

an·ti·ly·sin (an″tee·lye′sin) *n.* Antibody to lysin which destroys the latter.

an·ti·ly·sis (an″tee·lye′sis) *n.*, pl. **antily·ses** (·seez) The process of destruction of a lysin by its antilysin.

an·ti·lyt·ic (an″tee·lit′ick) *adj. & n.* 1. Pertaining to an antilysin or to antilysis. 2. Destroying lysin or preventing its action. 3. A substance that destroys lysin or prevents its action.

an·ti·ma·lar·i·al (an″tee·muh·lăr′ee·ul) *adj. & n.* 1. Preventing or suppressing malaria. 2. A drug that prevents or suppresses malaria.

an·ti·mat·ter, *n.* Matter composed of the elementary counterparts or antiparticles of ordinary matter.

an·ti·mel·lin (an″tee·mel′in) *n.* A glycoside from the bark of *Eugenia jambolana* or jambul.

an·ti·me·nin·go·coc·cic (an″tee·me·ning″go·kock′sick) *adj.* Effective against meningococci; ANTIMENINGOCOCCUS.

antimeningococcic or **antimeningococcus serum.** A serum obtained from the blood of an animal immunized with cultures of the several groups of meningococci (*Neisseria meningitidis*). It has been supplanted by chemotherapeutic agents.

an·ti·me·nin·go·coc·cus (an″tee·me·ning″go·kock′us) *adj.* Effective against meningococci; ANTIMENINGOCOCCIC.

an·ti·men·or·rhag·ic (an″tee·men·o·ray′jick, ·raj′ick) *adj. & n.*

[*anti-* + *menorrhagic*]. 1. Tending to reduce menstrual flow. 2. A medication or method for controlling profuse prolonged menstrual flow.

an·ti·mer (an'ti·mur) *n.* [*anti-* + *-mer*]. ENANTIOMORPH.

an·ti·mere (an'ti·meer) *n.* [*anti-* + *-mere*]. 1. Any one of the segments of the body that is bounded by planes typically at right angles to the long axis of the body. 2. A segment exhibiting bilateral symmetry with respect to the longitudinal axis.

an·ti·mes·en·ter·ic (an''tee·mes''in·terr'ick) *adj.* Of or pertaining to the part of the intestine opposite the mesenteric attachment.

an·ti·me·tab·o·lite (an''tee·me·tab'o·lite) *n.* A substance having a molecular structure similar to an essential metabolite but inhibiting or opposing its action. The mechanism of antagonism is considered to be a competition between antimetabolite and metabolite for a specific enzyme in an organism.

an·ti·me·tro·pia (an''tee·me·tro'pee·uh) *n.* [*anti-* + *metr-* + *-opia*]. A condition characterized by opposing states of refraction in the two eyes, as the existence of myopia in one eye and of hypermetropia in the other.

an·ti·mi·cro·bi·al (an''tee·migh·kro'bee·ul) *adj.* & *n.* 1. Destroying microbes; inhibiting, suppressing, or preventing their growth. 2. An agent that destroys microbes or suppresses or prevents their growth.

antimicrobial spectrum. ANTIBIOTIC SPECTRUM.

Antiminth. Trademark for pyrantel pamoate, an anthelmintic.

an·ti·mo·ni·al (an''ti·mo'nee·ul) *adj.* & *n.* 1. Pertaining to or containing antimony. 2. A pharmacologic preparation containing antimony.

antimonial powder. ANTIMONY POWDER.

an·ti·mo·nic (an''ti·mo'nick, ·mon'ick) *adj.* Containing antimony in the pentavalent state.

an·ti·mo·ni·ous (an''ti·mo'nee·us) *adj.* ANTIMONOUS.

an·ti·mo·nous (an''ti·mo'nus) *adj.* Containing antimony in the trivalent state.

an·ti·mo·ny (an'ti·mo''nee) *n.* [ML. *antimonium*, perh. from alteration of *althimodium*, from Ar. *al-uthmud*]. Sb = 121.75. A metallic, crystalline element possessing a bluish-white luster. Found native as the sulfide, Sb_2S_3, and the oxide; it is a constituent of many minerals. Used commercially chiefly for making alloys where its property of expanding on solidification is of considerable value. The actions of antimony compounds resemble those of arsenic, but they are less toxic. They produce nausea, emesis, enteritis, and nephritis. The nauseant action is used in expectorant and diaphoretic mixtures; they were formerly employed to produce circulatory depression in fever, and for catharsis and emesis. Certain complex antimony compounds are valuable antiprotozoan agents.

antimony butter. ANTIMONY TRICHLORIDE.

an·ti·mo·nyl (an'ti·mo·nil) *n.* SbO, the univalent radical of antimonous compounds.

antimony lithium thiomalate. Approximately $C_{12}H_9Li_6O_{12}S_3Sb.9H_2O$, used for treatment of filariasis, trypanosomiasis, lymphogranuloma, and schistosomiasis.

antimony potassium tartrate. $2KSbOC_4H_4O_6.H_2O$, used as an antiprotozoal agent and, rarely, as an expectorant and emetic. Syn. *tartar emetic.*

antimony powder. An antimonial powder consisting of antimony trioxide (Sb_2O_3) and calcium phosphate; formerly employed as a diaphoretic, an emetic in large doses, and a cathartic. Syn. *James's powder, pulvis antimonialis.*

antimony sodium tartrate. $NaSbOC_4H_4O_6$, used for the same purposes as antimony potassium tartrate but more soluble in water.

antimony sodium thioglycollate. $C_4H_4NaO_4S_2Sb$, a trivalent antimony compound used for the treatment of schistosomiasis, leishmaniasis, filariasis, and granuloma inguinale.

antimony test. An old test for kala azar in which a solution of a pentavalent antimony compound is stratified beneath a mixture of blood and potassium acetate. A flocculent precipitate forms immediately in advanced cases of kala azar, but may take as long as 15 minutes in new cases. Syn. *Chopra's test.*

antimony thioglycollamide. $Sb(SCH_2CONH_2)_3$, a trivalent antimony compound used for the same purposes as antimony sodium thioglycollate.

antimony trichloride. $SbCl_3$, a deliquescent solid that fumes in air and is strongly caustic; used as a reagent.

an·ti·my·cin A (an''ti·migh'sin). An antibiotic substance, $C_{28}H_{40}N_2O_9$, isolated from a *Streptomyces* species and possessing also insecticidal and miticidal activity.

an·ti·my·cot·ic (an''tee·migh·kot'ick) *adj.* & *n.* [*anti-* + *mycotic*]. ANTIFUNGAL.

an·ti·nar·cot·ic (an''tee·nahr·kot'ick) *adj.* & *n.* 1. Preventing narcosis. 2. Any antinarcotic substance, such as the morphine antagonists nalorphine and naloxone.

an·ti·nau·se·ant (an''tee·naw'zee·unt) *adj.* & *n.* 1. Tending to prevent or alleviate nausea. 2. An agent used to prevent or alleviate nausea.

an·ti·neo·plas·tic (an''tee·nee''o·plas'tick) *adj.* Inhibiting or destroying neoplastic cells or tumors.

antineoplastic virus. Any virus capable of inhibiting or destroying neoplastic cells or tumors.

an·ti·neo·plas·ton (an''tee·nee''o·plas'ton) *n.* Any of certain substances extracted from urine which are known to promote regression in neoplastic cells in vitro and which may function similarly in vivo.

an·ti·neu·ral·gic (an''tee·new·ral'jick) *adj.* Alleviating neuralgia.

an·ti·neu·rit·ic (an''tee·new·rit'ick) *adj.* & *n.* 1. Effective in relieving or preventing neuritis or neuropathy. 2. An agent or drug used to prevent or relieve neuritis or neuropathy, such as vitamin B_1 or thiamine.

antineuritic vitamin. VITAMIN B_1.

an·ti·neu·tri·no (an''tee·new·tree'no) *n.* The antiparticle of the neutrino; its properties are identical with those of the neutrino, but it has opposite spin and momentum.

an·ti·neu·tron (an''tee·new'tron) *n.* The antiparticle of the neutron; its properties are identical with those of the neutron, but it has opposite magnetic moment.

an·tin·i·on (an·tin'ee·on) *n.* [*ant-* + *inion*]. *In craniometry,* the point in the sagittal plane farthest removed from the inion. —**antini·al** (·ul) *adj.;* **antini·ad** (·ad) *adv.*

an·ti·no·ci·cep·tive (an''tee·no''si·sep'tiv) *adj.* [*anti-* + *nociceptive*]. ANALGESIC.

an·ti·nu·cle·ar (an''tee·new'klee·ur) *adj.* [*anti-* + *nuclear*]. Of an antibody: reacting with components of cell nuclei.

antinuclear antibody or **factor.** An antibody against DNA, nucleoprotein, or other components of cell nuclei; present in most cases of systemic lupus erythematosus.

an·ti·obe·sic (an''tee·o·bee'sick) *adj.* & *n.* [*anti-* + *obese* + *-ic*]. 1. Tending or intended to prevent or combat obesity. 2. An agent or drug used to prevent or combat obesity.

an·ti·odon·tal·gic (an''tee·o·don·tal'jick) *adj.* [*anti-* + *odontalgic*]. Relieving or preventing toothache.

an·ti·op·so·nin (an''tee·op'so·nin) *n.* A substance that retards or destroys the action of an opsonin.

an·ti·ox·i·dant (an''tee·ock'si·dunt) *n.* Any substance that delays or prevents the process of oxidation.

an·ti·par·a·lyt·ic (an''tee·păr''uh·lit'ick) *adj.* Alleviating paralysis.

an·ti·par·a·sit·ic (an''tee·păr''uh·sit'ick) *adj.* & *n.* 1. Inhibiting or destroying parasites. 2. An agent that destroys or inhibits parasites.

an·ti·par·kin·son (an''tee·pahr'kin·sun) *adj.* ANTIPARKINSONIAN.

an·ti·par·kin·so·nian (an''tee·pahr''kin·so'nee·un) *adj.* [*anti-* + *parkinsonian*]. Alleviating the symptoms of parkinsonism.

an·ti·par·kin·son·ism (an″tee·pahr′kin·sun·iz·um) *adj.* ANTIPARKINSONIAN.

an·ti·par·ti·cle (an″tee·pahr′ti·kul) *n.* A particle of the same mass and magnitude of other properties as an elementary particle (as the proton, electron, neutron, or neutrino), but opposite in charge, spin, momentum, or other property. Interaction of an elementary particle with its counterpart antiparticle results in annihilation of both. All elementary particles are supposed to have corresponding antiparticles. See also *antineutrino, antineutron, antiproton, positron.*

an·ti·pel·lag·ra (an″tee·pe·lag′ruh) *adj.* Preventing or curing pellagra.

an·ti·pep·sin (an″tee·pep′sin) *n.* A hypothetical antienzyme or a substance which inhibits the action of pepsin.

an·ti·pep·tone (an″tee·pep′tone) *n.* A variety of peptone not acted upon by trypsin.

an·ti·pe·ri·od·ic (an″tee·peer″ee·od′ick) *adj. & n.* 1. Lessening the intensity of or preventing attacks of a periodic disease, as of malaria. 2. A medicinal agent for the treatment of a periodic disease, especially malaria.

an·ti·per·i·stal·sis (an″tee·perr″i·stahl′sis, ·stal′sis) *n.* REVERSED PERISTALSIS. **—antiperistal·tic** (·tick) *adj.*

anti-pernicious-anemia factor. VITAMIN B_{12}.

anti-pernicious-anemia liver factor. VITAMIN B_{12}.

an·ti·per·son·nel (an″tee·pur″suh·nel′) *adj.* Designed to wound, obstruct, or kill military personnel.

an·ti·phage (an′ti·faje) *adj.* Counteracting bacteriophages.

antiphage serum. A serum produced against a particular bacteriophage.

an·ti·phago·cyt·ic (an″tee·fag″o·sit′ick) *adj.* Preventing phagocytosis.

an·ti·phlo·gis·tic (an″tee·flo·jis′tick) *adj. & n.* [*anti-* + *phlogistic*]. 1. Counteracting, reducing, or preventing inflammation or fever. 2. An agent that subdues or reduces inflammation or fever.

an·ti·phone (an′ti·fone) *n.* [*anti-* + *-phone*]. A device worn in the auditory meatus, intended to protect the wearer from noise.

an·ti·phthi·ri·ac, an·ti·phthei·ri·ac (an″tee·thigh′ree·ack) *adj. & n.* [*anti-* + Gk. *phtheir,* louse]. 1. Effective against lice or the conditions caused by them. 2. An agent used to combat louse infestation.

an·ti·plas·min (an″tee·plaz′min) *n.* Any substance that inhibits either activation or action of the proteolytic activity of plasmin; specifically, a naturally occurring substance or chemical that inhibits the lytic action of plasmin on fibrin.

an·ti·plas·tic (an″tee·plas′tick) *adj.* 1. Unfavorable to granulation or to the healing process. 2. Preventing or checking plastic exudation. Compare *aplastic.*

an·ti·pneu·mo·coc·cic (an″tee·new″mo·kock′sick) *adj.* [*anti-* + *pneumococcic*]. Inhibiting or destructive to *Streptococcus pneumoniae.*

antipneumococcic serum–type specific. ANTIPNEUMOCOCCUS SERUM, TYPE SPECIFIC.

an·ti·pneu·mo·coc·cus (an″tee·new″mo·kock′us) *adj.* ANTIPNEUMOCOCCIC.

antipneumococcus serum, type specific. An antiserum prepared from the blood of horses or rabbits that have been immunized with cultures of specific types of pneumococci; effective in the therapy of pneumococcal infection with the homologous type, but essentially abandoned in favor of the use of antibiotics.

an·tip·o·dal (an·tip′uh·dul) *adj.* [*antipodes* + *-al*]. Situated directly opposite.

an·ti·pode (an′ti·pode) *n.*, pl. **an·tip·o·des** (an·tip′o·deez) [Gk. *antipous, antipodos,* with the feet opposite]. 1. A thing or quality that is the exact opposite of another. 2. A chemical compound that has an opposite spatial arrangement of its atoms as compared with an otherwise identical compound. Compare *enantiomorph.* 3. (plural) Parts of the earth that are diametrically opposite.

an·ti·pres·sor (an″tee·pres′ur) *adj.* [*anti-* + *pressor*]. Preventing or counteracting the blood pressure-raising activity of some modality.

an·ti·pro·throm·bin (an″tee·pro·throm′bin) *n.* A substance that directly or indirectly reduces prothrombin activity, such as bishydroxycoumarin or heparin.

an·ti·pro·ton (an″tee·pro′ton) *n.* The antiparticle of the proton; it is equal in mass but opposite in charge to the proton.

an·ti·pro·to·zo·al (an″tee·pro·tuh·zo′ul) *adj.* ANTIPROTOZOAN.

an·ti·pro·to·zo·an (an″tee·pro·tuh·zo′un) *adj.* Preventing or inhibiting growth of protozoa, or destroying them.

an·ti·pru·rit·ic (an″tee·proo·rit′ick) *adj. & n.* [*anti-* + *pruritic*]. 1. Relieving or preventing itching. 2. A medicinal agent that relieves or prevents itching.

an·ti·pso·ri·at·ic (an″tee·so″ree·at′ick) *adj.* Tending to relieve the symptoms of psoriasis.

an·ti·pyo·gen·ic (an″tee·pye″o·jen′ick) *adj.* [*anti-* + *pyogenic*]. Preventing or inhibiting suppuration.

an·ti·py·re·sis (an″tee·pye·ree′sis) *n.* The treatment of fever with antipyretic agents.

an·ti·py·ret·ic (an″tee·pye·ret′ick) *adj. & n.* [*anti-* + *pyretic*]. 1. Reducing or preventing fever. 2. A medicinal or other agent that reduces or prevents fever.

an·ti·py·rine (an″ti·pye′rin, ·reen, ·pye·reen′) *n.* 2,3-Dimethyl-1-phenyl-3-pyrazolin-5-one, $C_{11}H_{12}N_2O$, an antipyretic and analgesic. Syn. *phenazone.* See also *Auralgan.*

antipyrine salicylate. An equimolecular interaction product of antipyrine and salicylic acid, $C_{18}H_{18}N_2O_4$; used as an antipyretic and analgesic.

an·ti·py·rino·ma·nia (an″tee·pye″rin·o·may′nee·uh) *n.* [*antipyrine* + *-mania*]. A condition similar to morphinism, due to excessive use of antipyrine. It is marked by nervous excitement.

an·ti·rab·ic (an″tee·rab′ick, ·ray′bick) *adj.* Preventing rabies, as the Pasteur treatment.

an·ti·ra·chit·ic (an″tee·ra·kit′ick) *adj. & n.* [*anti-* + *rachitic*]. 1. Preventing or counteracting development of rickets. 2. An agent for the prevention or cure of rickets.

antirachitic vitamin. VITAMIN D.

an·ti·ren·net (an″tee·ren′it) *n.* ANTIRENNIN.

an·ti·ren·nin (an″tee·ren′in) *n.* An antibody capable of neutralizing the milk-curdling action of rennin.

an·ti·re·tic·u·lar (an″tee·re·tick′yoo·lur) *adj.* [*anti-* + *reticular*]. Pertaining to a factor operating against the reticuloendothelial system.

anti-Rh agglutinin. An acquired antibody against any antigen of the Rh group.

an·ti·rheo·scope (an″tee·ree′o·skope) *n.* [Gk. *antirroia,* back current, + *-scope*]. A device for investigating vertigo of ocular origin.

an·ti·rheu·mat·ic (an″tee·roo·mat′ick) *adj. & n.* 1. Preventing or allaying rheumatism. 2. An agent that prevents or allays rheumatism.

anti-Rh serum. 1. A serum containing antibodies against one or more of the Rh antigens. 2. A serum containing antibodies against $Rh_o(D)$ antigens.

an·ti·ri·bo·fla·vin (an″tee·rye″bo·flay′vin, ·flav′in) *n.* Any compound that interferes with the biochemical action of riboflavin.

an·ti·ri·cin (an″tee·rye′sin, ·ris′in) *n.* The antibody to ricin.

an·ti·sca·bet·ic (an″tee·ska·beet′ick, ·ska·bet′ick) *adj. & n.* 1. Effective against the *Sarcoptes scabiei,* which causes scabies. 2. An agent effective in the treatment of scabies.

an·ti·sca·bi·et·ic (an″tee·skay″bee·et′ick) *adj. & n.* ANTISCABETIC.

an·ti·schis·to·so·mal (an″tee·shis″to·so′mul, ·skis″) *adj. & n.* 1. Counteracting schistosomiasis. 2. A medicinal agent used to treat schistosomiasis.

an·ti·scor·bu·tic (an″tee·skor·bew′tick) *adj. & n.* [*anti-* + *scorbutic*]. 1. Preventing or curing scurvy. 2. An agent that prevents or cures scurvy.

antiscorbutic acid. ASCORBIC ACID.

antiscorbutic vitamin. ASCORBIC ACID.

an·ti·seb·or·rhe·ic (an″tee·seb″o·ree′ick) *adj. & n.* 1. Combating seborrhea. 2. An agent effective in the treatment of seborrhea.

an·ti·se·cre·to·ry (an″tee·se·kree′tuh·ree) *adj.* Inhibiting the action of secretory glands.

an·ti·sep·sis (an″ti·sep′sis) *n.* Prevention of sepsis or poisoning by the destruction of microorganisms or their exclusion from the body tissues and fluids, or by preventing or checking their growth and multiplication.

an·ti·sep·tic (an″ti·sep′tick) *adj. & n.* [*anti-* + *septic*]. 1. Stopping or inhibiting growth of bacteria. 2. Any one of a large group of organic and inorganic compounds which stops or inhibits the growth of bacteria without necessarily killing them, thus checking putrefaction.

antiseptic surgery. The application of antiseptic methods in surgery and in the treatment of infected wounds. Compare *aseptic surgery.*

antisera. A plural of *antiserum.*

an·ti·se·ro·to·nin (an″tee·see″ro·to′nin) *adj.* Inhibiting or modifying serotonin activity.

an·ti·se·rum (an′tee·seer″um, ·serr″um) *n.*, pl. **antiserums, antise·ra** (·uh). Any serum of man or animals containing antibodies, either natural or acquired, as by immunization or disease.

an·ti·si·al·a·gogue, an·ti·si·al·a·gog (an″tee·sigh·al′uh·gog) *n.* [*anti-* + *sial-* + *-agogue*]. An agent that diminishes or checks salivation.

an·ti·si·al·ic (an″tee·sigh·al′ick) *adj. & n.* [*anti-* + *sialic*]. 1. Diminishing or checking salivation. 2. An agent that diminishes or checks salivation.

anti·small·pox vaccine. SMALLPOX VACCINE.

an·ti·so·cial (an″tee·so′shul) *adj.* Characterizing a sociopathic state marked by the refusal to accept the obligations and restraints imposed by society.—**anti·so·ci·al·i·ty** (·so″shee·al′i·tee) *n.*

antisocial personality. *In psychiatry,* an individual whose behavioral patterns are basically unsocialized, bringing him constantly into conflict with other people or society. Such a person feels no guilt, does not profit from experience or punishment, maintains no loyalties nor identifies with any authority or code, is frequently callous, hedonistic, emotionally immature, and irresponsible, and usually rationalizes this behavior so that it appears warranted and reasonable. Compare *dyssocial behavior, psychopath.*

an·ti·spas·mod·ic (an″tee·spaz·mod′ick) *adj. & n.* 1. Relieving or preventing spasms of smooth muscle. 2. An agent that relieves or prevents spasms of smooth muscle. Syn. *spasmolytic.*

an·ti·spas·tic (an″tee·spas′tick) *adj. & n.* [*anti-* + *spastic*]. 1. Relieving or preventing spasms of skeletal muscle or spasticity. 2. An agent that relieves or prevents spasms of skeletal muscle or spasticity.

an·ti·spi·ro·che·tic, an·ti·spi·ro·chae·tic (an″tee·spye″ro·kee′tick, ·ket′ick) *adj. & n.* 1. Arresting the growth and development of spirochetes. 2. An agent that arrests the growth and development of spirochetes.

an·ti·staph·y·lol·y·sin (an″tee·staf″i·lol′i·sin, ·staf″i·lo·lye′sin) *n.* [*anti-* + *staphylolysin*]. The specific antibody which neutralizes the hemolytic, dermonecrotic, and lethal effects of staphylococcal alpha lysin, or toxin.

an·ti·ste·ril·i·ty (an″tee·ste·ril′i·tee) *adj.* Combating sterility.

antisterility vitamin. VITAMIN E.

an·ti·ster·num (an″tee·stur′num) *n.* [*anti-* + *sternum*]. The part of the back opposite the breast.

anti·stiff·ness factor. A fat-soluble substance, involved in calcium and phosphorus metabolism, present in green vegetables, raw cream, and raw sugar-cane juice. Animals deprived of the factor develop muscular degeneration and stiffness, calcinosis, and histologic lesions of collagen necrosis.

Antistine. Trademark for antazoline, an antihistaminic agent used as the hydrochloride and phosphate salt.

an·ti·strep·to·coc·cic (an″tee·strep″to·cock′sick) *adj.* Antagonistic to or preventing the growth of streptococci.

an·ti·strep·to·dor·nase (an″tee·strep″to·dor′nace) *n.* An antibody capable of neutralizing streptodornase.

an·ti·strep·to·he·mo·ly·sin, an·ti·strep·to·hae·mo·ly·sin (an″tee·strep″to·he·mol′i·sin, ·hee″mo·lye′sin) *n.* [*anti-* + *strepto-* + *hemolysin*]. ANTISTREPTOLYSIN.

anti·strep·to·ki·nase (an″tee·strep″to·kigh′nace) *n.* An antibody present in the serum which prevents the activation of plasminogen by streptokinase. It may develop in serum following infection with hemolytic streptococci or by injections of streptokinase for therapeutic reasons.

an·ti·strep·tol·y·sin (an″tee·strep·tol′i·sin, ·strep″to·lye′sin) *n.* The specific antibody to streptolysin of group A hemolytic streptococci, useful in the diagnosis of recent streptococcal infection and such sequellae as rheumatic fever.

an·ti·su·dor·al (an″tee·sue′dur·ul) *n.* ANTISUDORIFIC.

an·ti·su·dor·if·ic (an″tee·sue″duh·rif′ick) *adj. & n.* [*anti-* + *sudorific*]. 1. Checking excretion of sweat. 2. An agent that checks excretion of sweat.

an·ti·syph·i·lit·ic (an″tee·sif″i·lit′ick) *adj. & n.* 1. Active against syphilis. 2. An agent effective in the treatment of syphilis.

an·ti·te·tan·ic (an″tee·te·tan′ick) *adj.* Effective against tetanus.

antitetanic serum. TETANUS ANTITOXIN.

an·ti·the·nar (an″ti·theen′ahr, ·ur) *n.* HYPOTHENAR.

an·ti·ther·mic (an″tee·thur′mick) *adj.* [*anti-* + *thermic*]. Cooling; ANTIPYRETIC.

an·ti·throm·bin (an″tee·throm′bin) *n.* A substance that inhibits the activity of thrombin; may be naturally occurring in blood, a chemical agent, or a physical agent.

an·ti·throm·bo·plas·tin (an″tee·throm″bo·plas′tin) *n.* A substance capable of inhibiting the clot-accelerating effect of thromboplastins.

an·ti·thy·roid (an″tee·thigh′roid) *adj.* Opposing the action of thyroid hormone or having an action against the thyroid gland.

an·ti·tox·ic (an″tee·tock′sick) *adj.* [*anti-* + *toxic*]. 1. Effective against poison. 2. Of or pertaining to an antitoxin.

antitoxic unit. The amount of antitoxin which neutralizes a given amount of toxin relative to the standard.

an·ti·tox·i·gen (an″tee·tock′si·jen) *n.* Any antigen, or toxin, which promotes antitoxin elaboration.

an·ti·tox·in (an″tee·tock′sin) *n.* 1. An antibody elaborated in the body, capable of neutralizing a given toxin (bacterial, plant, or animal toxin). 2. A sterile solution of one or more antibodies for a specific toxin, generally prepared from blood serum or plasma of an animal or human immunized against the toxin; used to counteract the same toxin in humans or other animals.

an·ti·tox·in·o·gen (an″tee·tock·sin′o·jen) *n.* ANTITOXIGEN.

an·ti·trag·i·cus (an″ti·traj′i·kus) *n.* A vestigial slip of muscle associated with the antitragus. NA *musculus antitragicus.* See also Table of Muscles in the Appendix.

an·ti·tra·gus (an″ti·tray′gus) *n.* [NA]. The projection of the pinna just opposite and posterior to the tragus. —**anti·trag·ic** (·traj′ick) *adj.*

an·ti·trich·o·mo·nal (an″tee·trick″o·mo′nul) *adj.* TRICHOMONACIDAL.

an·ti·tris·mus (an″tee·triz′mus) *n.* [*anti-* + *trismus*]. A condition of tonic spasm in which the mouth is forced open and cannot be closed.

an·ti·trope (an′ti·trope) *n.* [*anti-* + *-trope*]. Either one of a pair of symmetrical organs.

an·ti·try·pa·no·so·mal (an″tee·tri·pan″o·so′mul) *adj.* [*anti-* + *Trypanosoma* + *-al*]. TRYPANOCIDAL.

an·ti·tryp·sin (an″tee·trip′sin) *n.* An antibody inhibiting the action of trypsin.

antitrypsin test. A test based on the ability of blood serum to inhibit the action of trypsin. It is said to be of value in the diagnosis of carcinoma, nephritis, and other conditions.

an·ti·tryp·tase (·trip'tace, ·taze) *n.* ANTITRYPSIN.

an·ti·tu·ber·cu·lous (an"tee·tew·bur'kew·lus) *adj.* Directed or acting against tuberculosis.

an·ti·tus·sive (an"tee·tus'iv) *adj. & n.* [*anti-* + *tussive*]. 1. Decreasing or relieving the amount and severity of coughing. 2. An agent that reduces the amount and severity of coughing.

an·ti·ty·phoid (an"tee·tigh'foid) *adj. & n.* 1. Counteracting or preventing typhoid fever. 2. An antityphoid serum.

an·ti·ul·cer·a·tive (an"tee·ul'sur·uh·tiv) *adj. & n.* 1. Preventing or combating ulceration. 2. A substance used to prevent or combat ulceration.

an·ti·ure·ase (an"ti·yoor'ee·ace, ·aze) *n.* An antibody to urease.

an·ti·ven·ene (an"tee·ven'een) *n.* ANTIVENIN.

an·ti·ve·ne·re·al (an"tee·ve·neer'ee·ul) *adj.* Preventing or curing venereal disease.

an·ti·ven·in (an"tee·ven'in) *n.* 1. An antitoxin to a venin. 2. An antitoxic serum prepared by immunizing animals against the venom of snakes, insects, or other animals.

an·ti·ven·om (an"tee·ven'um) *n.* ANTIVENIN.

Antivert. Trademark for meclizine hydrochloride, an antinauseant.

an·ti·vi·ral (an"tee·vye'rul) *adj.* Antagonistic to, weakening, or destroying a virus.

an·ti·vi·rot·ic (an"tee·vye·rot'ick) *n.* A substance that is detrimental to viruses and can be used to treat virus diseases.

an·ti·vir·u·lin (an"tee·virr'yoo·lin) *n.* The antibody-like substance elaborated in animals injected with rabies virus, inactivating the pathogenicity of the virus.

an·ti·vi·rus (an"tee·vye'rus, an'tee·vye"rus) *n.* Any substance, antibody or otherwise, capable of neutralizing the activity of a virus.

an·ti·vi·ta·min (an"tee·vye'tuh·min) *n.* Any substance that prevents the normal metabolic functioning of vitamins; a vitamin-destroying enzyme, or a chemical substance that renders the vitamin unabsorbable or ineffective.

an·ti·viv·i·sec·tion (an"tee·viv"i·seck'shun) *n. & adj.* Opposition to, or opposed to, vivisection or animal experimentation. —**antivivisection·ist,** *n.*

an·ti·xen·ic (an"ti·zen'ick) *adj.* [*anti-* + *xen-* + *-ic*]. Pertaining to the reaction which occurs when a foreign substance is introduced into living tissue.

an·ti·xe·roph·thal·mic (an"tee·zeer"off·thal'mick) *adj.* Preventing xerophthalmia.

antixerophthalmic vitamin. VITAMIN A.

an·ti·xe·rot·ic (an"tee·ze·rot'ick) *adj.* [*anti-* + *xerotic*]. Preventing dryness of the skin.

an·ti·zy·mot·ic (an"tee·zye·mot'ick) *adj. & n.* [*anti-* + *zymotic*]. 1. Preventing or checking fermentation or enzymic action. 2. An agent that checks or prevents fermentation or enzymic action.

ant·lo·pho·bia (ant"lo·fo'bee·uh) *n.* [Gk. *antlos*, flood, + *-phobia*]. A morbid fear of floods.

An·ton's syndrome [G. *Anton,* Czechoslovakian neuropsychiatrist, 1858-1933]. Denial of blindness by a patient with bilateral occipital lesions; usually accompanied by confabulation, with the patient claiming to see objects in the blind fields.

antr-, antro-. A combining form meaning *antrum, antral.*

antra. A plural of *antrum.*

an·tra·cele (an'truh·seel) *n.* ANTROCELE.

an·tral (an'trul) *adj.* Pertaining to an antrum.

antral fistula. A fistula communicating with an antrum or cavity in bone.

an·trec·to·my (an·treck'tuh·mee) *n.* Surgical removal of an antrum or its walls, especially the pyloric antrum or the mastoid antrum.

Antrenyl Bromide. Trademark for oxyphenonium bromide, an anticholinergic agent.

an·tri·tis (an·trye'tis) *n.* 1. Inflammation of an antrum, for example, the pyloric antrum. 2. *Obsol.* Specifically, inflammation of the antrum of Highmore (= MAXILLARY SINUS); maxillary sinusitis.

antro-. See *antr-.*

an·tro·at·ti·cot·o·my (an"tro·at"i·kot'uh·mee) *n.* [*antro-* + *attic* + *-tomy*]. *In surgery,* the opening of the mastoid antrum and the attic of the tympanum.

an·tro·cele (an'tro·seel) *n.* [*antro-* + *-cele*]. A saclike accumulation of fluid in the maxillary sinus.

an·tro·na·sal (an"tro·nay'zul) *adj.* [*antro-* + *nasal*]. Pertaining to the maxillary sinus and the nasal cavity.

ant·ro·phose (an'tro·foze) *n.* [*antro-* + *phose*]. A phose having its origin in the central ocular mechanism.

an·tro·scope (an'tro·skope) *n.* [*antro-* + *-scope*]. An instrument for examining the maxillary sinus. —**an·tros·co·py** (an·tros'kuh·pee) *n.*

an·tros·to·my (an·tros'tuh·mee) *n.* [*antro-* + *-stomy*]. Surgical opening of an antrum for drainage.

an·trot·o·my (an·trot'uh·mee) *n.* [*antro-* + *-tomy*]. ANTROSTOMY.

an·tro·tym·pan·ic (an"tro·tim·pan'ick) *adj.* Pertaining to the mastoid antrum and the tympanic cavity.

an·trum (an'trum) *n.*, pl. **an·tra** (·truh) [L., cave, hollow, from Gk. *antron*]. 1. Any of various anatomic cavities or dilatations, such as: mastoid antrum, cardiac antrum, pyloric antrum. 2. *Obsol.* Specifically, the antrum of Highmore (= MAXILLARY SINUS).

antrum car·di·a·cum (kahr·dye'uh·kum) [BNA]. CARDIAC ANTRUM.

antrum ma·stoi·de·um (mas·toy'dee·um) [NA]. MASTOID ANTRUM.

antrum of Highmore [N. *Highmore,* English anatomist and physician, 1613-1685]. MAXILLARY SINUS.

antrum of the ear. MASTOID ANTRUM.

antrum of the testis. MEDIASTINUM TESTIS.

antrum of the uterine tube. A saclike dilatation of the uterine tube about an inch from the fimbriated extremity; regarded by some as occurring only in pregnancy.

antrum py·lo·ri·cum (pi·lor'i·kum) [NA]. PYLORIC ANTRUM.

antrum tym·pa·ni·cum (tim·pan'i·kum) [BNA]. Antrum mastoideum (= MASTOID ANTRUM).

Antrypol. Trademark for suramin sodium, an antitrypanosomal and antifilarial agent.

ANTU. [*a*lpha*n*apthyl *t*hio*u*rea]. 1-(1-Naphthyl)-2-thiourea, $C_{11}H_{10}N_2S$, a rodenticide.

Antuitrin-growth. Trademark for a preparation of growth hormone extracted from the adenohypophysis.

Antuitrin-S. Trademark for a preparation of chorionic gonadotropin obtained from human pregnancy urine.

Anturane. Trademark for sulfinpyrazone.

anu·bis baboon (a·new'bis) [*Anubis,* an ancient Egyptian god represented as a jackal]. OLIVE BABOON.

anu·cle·ar (ay·new'klee·ur, a·new') *adj.* Without a nucleus; applied to an erythrocyte.

anu·cle·ate (ay·new'klee·ate) *adj.* Lacking a nucleus.

anu·cle·o·lar (ay"new·klee'o·lur, an"yoo·) *adj.* Without a nucleolus.

anuli. Plural of *anulus.*

anuli fi·bro·si cor·dis (fye·bro'sigh kor'dis) [NA]. The dense fibrous rings surrounding the atrioventricular, aortic, and pulmonary trunk openings of the heart; FIBROUS RINGS (2).

anu·lus (an'yoo·lus) *n.*, pl. **anu·li** (·lye) [L., ring, finger ring, dim. of *anus,* ring]. A ring of tissue about an opening.

anulus con·junc·ti·vae (kon·junk·tye'vee) [NA]. CONJUNCTIVAL RING.

anulus fe·mo·ra·lis (fem·o·ray'lis) [NA]. FEMORAL RING.

anulus fi·bro·car·ti·la·gi·ne·us mem·bra·nae tym·pa·ni (fye"bro·kahr·ti·la·jin'ee·us mem·bray'nee tim'puh·nigh) [NA]. FIBROUS RING (3).

anulus fi·bro·sus dis·ci in·ter·ver·te·bra·lis (fye·bro'sus dis'kigh in·tur·vur·te·bray'lis) [NA]. FIBROUS RING (1).

anulus in·gui·na·lis pro·fun·dus (ing·gwi·nay'lis pro·fun'dus) [NA]. DEEP INGUINAL RING.

anulus inguinalis su·per·fi·ci·al·is (sue''pur·fish·ee·ay'lis) [NA]. SUPERFICIAL INGUINAL RING.

anulus iri·dis major (eye'ri·dis) [NA]. GREATER RING OF THE IRIS.

anulus iridis minor [NA]. LESSER RING OF THE IRIS.

anulus ten·di·ne·us com·mu·nis (ten·din'ee·us kom·yoo'nis) [NA]. LIGAMENT OF ZINN.

anulus tym·pa·nic·us (tim·pa'ni·kus) [NA]. TYMPANIC RING.

anulus um·bi·li·ca·lis (um·bil·i·kay'lis) [NA]. UMBILICAL RING.

an·ure·sis (an''yoo·ree'sis) *n.*, pl. **anure·ses** (·seez) [*an-* + *uresis*]. ANURIA. —**anu·ret·ic** (·ret'ick) *adj.*

an·uria (an·yoo'ree·uh) *n.* [*an-* + *-uria*]. Suppression or arrest of urinary output, resulting from impairment of renal function (secretory type) or from obstruction in the urinary tract (excretory type). —**anu·ric** (·rick) *adj.*

an·u·rous (a·new'rus) *adj.* [*an-* + Gk. *oura*, tail, + *-ous*]. Without a tail; applied to frogs and toads.

an·u·ry (an'yoo·ree) *n.* ANURIA.

anus (ay'nus) *n.* [L., orig., ring] [NA]. The termination of the rectum; the outlet of the alimentary canal. See also Plates 14, 23, 25. Adj. *anal.*

anus vag·i·na·lis (vaj·i·nay'lis). ATRESIA ANI VAGINALIS.

anus ves·i·ca·lis (ves·i·kay'lis). An anomaly in which the anus is imperforate, the rectum opening into the urinary bladder.

anus vul·vo·vag·i·na·lis (vul''vo·vaj·i·nay'lis). An anomaly in which the anal opening communicates with the vulva.

an·vil (an'vil) *n.* INCUS.

anx·i·e·tas tib·i·a·rum (ang·zye'i·tas tib''ee·air'um). RESTLESS LEGS.

anx·i·e·ty (ang·zye'i·tee) *n.* [L. *anxietas,* from *angere,* to press, distress]. A feeling of apprehension, uncertainty, or tension stemming from the anticipation of an imagined or unreal threat, sometimes manifested by tachycardia, palpitation, sweating, disturbed breathing, trembling, or even paralysis. See also *anxiety neurosis.*

anxiety attack. A feeling of impending death or physical collapse, acute panic or crisis. See also *anxiety neurosis.*

anxiety hysteria. A neurosis characterized by the presence of persistent and realistically unwarranted apprehensiveness in relation to a specific object or situation. See also *phobic neurosis.*

anxiety neurosis, reaction, or **state.** A psychoneurotic disorder characterized by diffuse anxious expectation not restricted to definite situations, persons, or objects; emotional instability; irritability; apprehensiveness and a sense of fatigue; caused by incomplete repression of emotional problems, and frequently associated with somatic symptoms. See also *psychophysiologic disorders.*

AOA Abbreviation for *Alpha Omega Alpha.*

AORN Association of Operating Room Nurses.

aort-, aorto-. A combining form meaning *aorta, aortic.*

aor·ta (ay·or'tuh) *n.*, L. pl. & genit. sing. **aor·tae** (·tee) [NL., from Gk. *aortē,* literally, something hung, suspended] [NA]. The large vessel arising from the left ventricle and distributing, by its branches, arterial blood to every part of the body. It ends by bifurcating into the common iliacs at the fourth lumbar vertebra. The portion extending from the heart to the third thoracic vertebra is divided into an ascending, an arch, or transverse part, and a descending part. The thoracic portion extends to the diaphragm; the abdominal, to the bifurcation. See also Table of Arteries in the Appendix and Plates 5, 8.

aorta ab·do·mi·na·lis (ab·dom''i·nay'lis) [NA]. ABDOMINAL AORTA.

aorta ascen·dens (a·sen'denz) [NA]. ASCENDING AORTA.

aorta de·scen·dens (de·sen'denz) [NA]. DESCENDING AORTA.

aor·tal (ay·or'tul) *adj.* AORTIC.

aor·tal·gia (ay''or·tal'jee·uh) *n.* [*aort-* + *-algia*]. Pain in the region of the aorta, usually due to the pressure of an aneurysm against surrounding tissues.

aorta of Val·sal·va [A. M. *Valsalva*]. AORTIC SINUS.

aorta tho·ra·ca·lis (tho·ra·kay'lis) [BNA]. Aorta thoracica (= THORACIC AORTA).

aorta tho·ra·ci·ca (tho·ras'i·kuh) [NA]. THORACIC AORTA.

aor·tic (ay·or'tick) *adj.* Of or pertaining to the aorta.

aortic aneurysm. An aneurysm of the aorta, which may cause severe pressure symptoms and eventually may rupture.

aortic arches. 1. Six pairs of embryonic vascular arches encircling the pharynx in the visceral arches. In mammals, the left fourth arch becomes a part of the systemic circulatory system and the sixth pair becomes incorporated in the pulmonary circulation. 2. (sing.) ARCH OF THE AORTA.

aortic arch syndrome or **arteritis.** Partial or total thrombotic obliteration of the major branches of the aortic arch secondary to inflammatory changes of varied etiology, usually encountered in young women. Pulses are impalpable in the head, neck, and arms, and there is evidence of cerebral, cardiac, and arm ischemia.

aortic area. The second right interspace near the sternum, where aortic sounds and murmurs are often best heard.

aortic atresia. An uncommon congenital anomaly of the aortic orifice associated with hypoplasia of the ascending aorta and the left ventricle; there is severe congestive heart failure and cyanosis; the prognosis is invariably poor.

aortic bodies. Chemoreceptive clusters of nerve-associated epithelioid cells adjacent to the subclavian arteries near the aortic arch, identical to the carotid bodies and like them not a part of the paraganglion system. Syn. *glomera aortica.*

aortic-body tumor. A benign tumor resembling a carotid-body tumor but occurring at the aortic arch.

aortic bulb. BULB OF THE HEART.

aortic hiatus. An opening behind the median arcuate ligament of the diaphragm giving passage to the aorta. NA *hiatus aorticus.*

aortic insufficiency or **incompetence.** AORTIC REGURGITATION.

aortic isthmus. A constriction of the fetal aorta between the left subclavian artery and the ductus arteriosus. NA *isthmus aortae.*

aortic murmur. 1. A murmur due to aortic valve disease. 2. A murmur heard at the aortic area or over the abdominal aorta.

aor·ti·co·pul·mo·nary (ay''or·ti·ko·pul'mo·nerr·ee) *adj.* Pertaining to the aorta and the pulmonary system.

aorticopulmonary septum. The partition formed by growth of the truncoconal ridges and separating the aorta from the pulmonary trunk in the developing heart.

aor·ti·co·pul·mon·ic (ay·or''ti·ko·pul·mon'ick) *adj.* Pertaining to the aorta and the pulmonary artery.

aor·ti·co·re·nal (ay·or''ti·ko·ree'nul) *adj.* [*aortic* + *renal*]. Near the aorta and kidney.

aorticorenal ganglia. The outlying portions of the celiac ganglion, near the origin of each renal artery. NA *ganglia aorticorenalia.*

aortic plexus. A fine network of visceral nerves surrounding the aorta; continuous around both the thoracic and abdominal portions of the aorta through the aortic hiatus.

aortic regurgitation. Backflow of blood from the aorta into the left ventricle through or around an abnormal or prosthetic aortic valve.

aortic septum. AORTICOPULMONARY SEPTUM.

aortic sinus. One of the pouch-like dilatations of the aorta opposite the cusps of the semilunar valves. Syn. *aorta of Valsalva.* NA *sinus aortae.*

aortic stenosis. A narrowing of the aortic valve orifice, the aortic outflow tract, or of the aorta itself.

aortic triangle. *Rare.* A triangle seen on the left anterior oblique roentgenogram of the heart, formed inferiorly by the upper border of the aortic arch, posteriorly by the upper thoracic spine, and anteriorly by the left subclavian artery.

aortic valve. A valve consisting of three semilunar cusps situated at the junction of the aorta and the left ventricle of the heart. NA *valva aortae.*

aortic vestibule. The space within the left ventricle adjoining the root of the aorta.

aortic window. A radiolucent area on the left anterior oblique and lateral roentgenogram of the chest, below the aortic arch and above and behind the cardiopericardial silhouette.

aor·ti·tis (ay″or·tye′tis) *n.* Inflammation of the aorta.

aorto-. See *aort-.*

aor·to·ca·val (ay·or″to·kay′vul) *adj.* Pertaining to or involving the aorta and vena cava (as: aortocaval fistula).

aor·to·gram (ay·or′to·gram) *n.* The film made by aortography.

aor·tog·ra·phy (ay″or·tog′ruh·fee) *n.* Roentgenography of the aorta after the intravascular injection of radiopaque material. —**aor·to·graph·ic** (ay·or″to·graf′ick) *adj.*

aor·to·il·i·ac (ay·or″to·il′ee·ack) *adj.* [*aorto-* + *iliac*]. Pertaining to the abdominal aorta and the iliac arteries.

aortoiliac steal syndrome. Mesenteric vascular insufficiency due to reflux redistribution of blood from the mesenteric to the iliofemoral system; seen with aortoiliac reconstructive surgical procedures or lumbar sympathectomy in patients with marginal mesenteric blood supply. See also *steal syndrome.*

aor·to·re·no·gram (ay·or″to·ree′no·gram) *n.* A radiographic depiction of the aorta and kidneys through the use of contrast medium injected into the aorta.

aor·tot·o·my (ay″or·tot′uh·mee) *n.* [*aorto-* + *-tomy*]. Cutting or opening the aorta.

A.O.T.A. American Occupational Therapy Association.

Ao·tus (ay·o′tus) *n.* [Gk. *aōtos,* earless]. A monotypic genus of the Cebidae. See also *douroucouli.*

AP. An anteroposterior projection of x-rays, i.e., passing from front to back of an anatomic part.

ap-, aph-, apo- [Gk.]. A prefix meaning (a) *away from, from;* (b) *deprived, separated;* (c) *derived from, related to* (especially in names of chemical compounds).

A.P.A. American Physiotherapy Association; American Psychiatric Association.

apal·les·the·sia, apal·laes·the·sia (a·pal″es·theezh′uh, ·theez′ee·uh) *n.* [*a-* + *pallesthesia*]. Loss of the ability to perceive vibrations. Syn. *pallanesthesia.*

apan·crea (ay·pan′kree·uh, ay·pang′) *n.* Absence of the pancreas. —**apan·cre·at·ic** (·kree·at′ick) *adj.*

ap·an·dria (ap·an′dree·uh) *n.* [*ap-* + *andr-* + *-ia*]. Pathologic dislike of the male sex.

ap·an·thro·pia (ap″an·thro′pee·uh) *n.* [Gk. *apanthrōpia,* from *ap-* + *anthrōpos,* man, + *-ia*]. ANTHROPOPHOBIA.

ap·an·thro·py (ap·an′thro·pee) *n.* ANTHROPOPHOBIA.

apar·a·lyt·ic (ay″păr″uh·lit′ick, a·păr″) *adj.* Without paralysis.

ap·ar·thro·sis (ap″ahr·thro′sis) *n.,* pl. **aparthro·ses** (·seez) [Gk. *aparthrōsis,* articulation]. *Obsol.* DIARTHROSIS.

apas·tia (a·pas′tee·uh) *n.* [Gk., fast, fasting, from *a-* + *-pastos* (from *pateisthai,* to eat), + *-ia*]. Abstinence from food; seen in mental disorders. —**apas·tic** (·tick) *adj.*

ap·a·thism (ap′uh·thiz·um) *n.* [*apathy* + *-ism*]. Slowness in reacting to any stimuli. Contr. *erethism (2).*

ap·a·tite (ap′uh·tite) *n.* [Gk. *apatē,* deceit (since it has been mistaken for other minerals), + *-ite*]. A type of mineral having the formula $[Ca_3(PO_4)_2]_3.CaX_2$, where X_2 may be CO_3, $(OH)_2$, Cl_2, F_2, O, or SO_4. The inorganic component of bones and teeth contains a form of apatite.

ap·at·ro·pine (ap·at′ro·peen, ·pin) *n.* APOATROPINE.

A patterns or **syndromes.** See *A-V patterns.*

ap·a·zone (ap′uh·zone) *n.* 5-(Dimethylamino)-9-methyl-2-propyl-1*H*-pyrazolo[1,2-α][1,2,4]-benzotriazine-1,3(2*H*)-dione, $C_{16}H_{20}N_4O_2$, an anti-inflammatory agent.

APC A therapeutic formulation of aspirin, phenacetin, and caffeine.

APC virus [*a*deno-*p*haryngeal-*c*onjunctival]. ADENOVIRUS.

ape, *n.* 1. Any nonhuman primate of the superfamily Hominoidea, including chimpanzees, gorillas, orangutans, gibbons, and siamangs. 2. Loosely, any of various large primates including certain tailless monkeys, as the Barbary ape.

ape fissure. A fissure of the human brain which corresponds with that present in an ape as the lunate sulcus.

ape hand. A deformity of the hand such that the thumb is turned out and the hand flattened, caused by wasting of the abductor indicis, thenar and hypothenar, interossei and lumbrical muscles; seen in progressive spinal muscular atrophy or lesions of the median and ulnar nerve.

apei·ro·pho·bia (a·pye″ro·fo′bee·uh) *n.* [Gk. *apeiros,* boundless (from *peras* or *peiras,* end, limit), + *-phobia*]. A morbid fear of infinity.

apel·lous (a·pel′us) *adj.* [*a-* + *pell-* + *-ous*]. 1. Skinless; not cicatrized, applied to wounds. 2. Without a prepuce; circumcised.

Apelt's test (ah′pult) [F. *Apelt,* German physician, 1877–1911]. NONNE-APELT TEST.

ap·en·ter·ic (ap″en·terr′ick) *adj.* [*ap-* + *enteric*]. ABENTERIC.

ape·ri·ent (a·peer′ee·unt) *adj.* & *n.* [L. *aperiens, aperientis,* from *aperire,* to open]. LAXATIVE.

ape·ri·od·ic (ay″peer″ee·od′ick, a·peer″) *adj.* Devoid of periodicity or rhythm.

aperi·os·te·al (ay″perr″ee·os′tee·ul) *adj.* Without periosteum.

aperiosteal amputation. An amputation in which the bone is divided through a circumferential zone denuded of all periosteum.

aper·i·stal·sis (ay·perr″i·stal′sis, ·stahl′sis, a·perr″) *n.* 1. Absence of peristalsis. 2. Specifically, ACHALASIA.

aper·i·tive (a·perr′i·tiv) *adj.* & *n.* 1. Stimulating the appetite; a stimulant to the appetite. 2. LAXATIVE. Compare *aperient.*

ap·er·tom·e·ter (ap″ur·tom′e·tur) *n.* An optic device for determining the angle of aperture of microscopic objectives.

Apert's syndrome (a·pehr′) [E. *Apert,* French pediatrician, 1868–1940]. The typical form of acrocephalosyndactyly, distinguished by osseous and soft-tissue syndactyly of the middle three fingers.

aper·tu·ra (ap″ur·tew′ruh) *n.,* pl. **apertu·rae** (·ree) [L.]. Aperture; opening.

apertura aque·duc·tus coch·le·ae (ack″we·duck′tus cock′lee·ee). The opening of the aqueduct of the cochlear canaliculus on the petrous portion of the temporal bone.

apertura ex·ter·na aque·duc·tus ves·ti·bu·li (ecks·tur′nuh ack·we·duck′tus ves·tib′yoo·lye) [NA]. The external opening of the aqueduct of the vestibule.

apertura externa ca·na·li·cu·li coch·le·ae (kan·uh·lick′yoo·lye kock′lee·ee) [NA]. The external opening of the cochlear canaliculus in the posterior wall of the jugular fossa of the temporal bone.

apertura inferior canaliculi tym·pa·ni·ci (tim·pan′i·sigh) [BNA]. The inferior opening of the tympanic canaliculus on the inferior surface of the petrous portion of the temporal bone between the jugular fossa and the opening of the carotid canal.

apertura la·te·ra·lis ven·tri·cu·li quar·ti (lat·ur·ay′lis ven·trick′yoo·lye kwahr′tye) [NA]. LATERAL APERTURE OF THE FOURTH VENTRICLE.

apertura me·di·a·lis ven·tri·cu·li quar·ti (mee·dee·ay′lis ven·trick′yoo·lye kwahr′tye) [BNA]. Apertura mediana ventriculi quarti (= MEDIAN APERTURE OF THE FOURTH VENTRICLE).

apertura me·di·a·na ven·tri·cu·li quar·ti (mee·dee·ay′nuh ven·trick′yoo·lye kwahr′tye) [NA]. MEDIAN APERTURE OF THE FOURTH VENTRICLE.

apertura pelvis inferior [NA]. INFERIOR PELVIC APERTURE.

apertura pelvis superior [NA]. SUPERIOR PELVIC APERTURE.

apertura pi·ri·for·mis (pirr″i·form′is) [NA]. One of the two anterior nasal openings of the skull.

apertura si·nus fron·ta·lis (sigh′nus fron·tay′lis) [NA]. The opening of a frontal sinus.

apertura sinus sphe·noi·da·lis (sfee·noy·day′lis) [NA]. The opening of a sphenoid sinus.

apertura superior ca·na·li·cu·li tym·pa·ni·ci (kan·uh·lick′yoo·lye tim·pan′i·sigh) [BNA]. The upper opening of the tympanic canaliculus into the cavity of the middle ear.

apertura tho·ra·cis inferior (tho·ray′sis) [NA]. The inferior boundary of the thoracic cavity.

apertura thoracis superior [NA]. The superior opening of each thoracic cavity, bounded by the first thoracic vertebra, the first rib, and the manubrium of the sternum.

apertura tym·pa·ni·ca ca·na·li·cu·li chor·dae (tim·pan′i·kuh kan·uh·lick′yoo·lye kor′dee) [BNA]. APERTURA TYMPANICA CANALICULI CHORDAE TYMPANI.

apertura tympanica canaliculi chordae tym·pa·ni (tim′puh·nigh) [NA]. The opening of the canaliculus for the chorda tympani into the tympanic cavity.

ap·er·ture (ap′ur·chur) *n.* [L. *apertura,* from *aperire,* to expose, open]. 1. An opening; orifice. 2. *In optics,* the diameter of the exposed portion of a lens, designated as the ratio of the focal length to this diameter, as f4, in which the aperture is 1 inch and the focal length is 4 inches.

Apestrin. Trademark for a preparation of chorionic gonadotropin obtained from human pregnancy urine.

apex (ay′pecks) *n.*, genit. **api·cis** (ap′i·sis), L. pl. **api·ces** (ap′i·seez) [L.]. 1. The tip or top of anything; point or extremity of a cone. 2. *In optics,* the junction of the two refractive sides of a prism. 3. *In craniometry,* the highest point in the transverse vertical section of the vault of a skull oriented on the Frankfort horizontal plane, the plane of section passing through the poria. 4. The radicular end of a tooth.

apex au·ri·cu·lae (aw·rick′yoo·lee) [NA]. A small pointed tubercle occasionally seen on the upper margin of the auricle; it is thought to correspond to the apex of the ear in lower mammals.

apex auriculae (Darwini) [C. R. *Darwin*] [BNA]. APEX AURICULAE.

apex beat. APEX IMPULSE.

apex ca·pi·tis fi·bu·lae (kap′i·tis fib′yoo·lee) [NA]. The apex of the head of the fibula.

apex ca·pi·tu·lae fibulae (ka·pit′yoo·lee) [BNA]. APEX CAPITIS FIBULAE.

apexcardiogram, apex cardiogram. A graphic recording of ultra-low-frequency precordial chest-wall movements. Abbreviated, ACG.

apex car·ti·la·gi·nis ary·te·noi·de·ae (kahr·ti·laj′i·nis ăr″i·te·noy′dee·ee) [NA]. The upper extremity of the arytenoid cartilage.

apex co·lum·nae pos·te·ri·o·ris (ko·lum′nee pos″teer·ee·o′ris) [BNA]. APEX CORNUS POSTERIORIS MEDULLAE SPINALIS.

apex cor·dis (kor′dis) [NA]. APEX OF THE HEART.

apex cor·nus pos·te·ri·o·ris me·dul·lae spi·na·lis (kor′nooce pos·teer·ee·o′ris me·dul′ee spye·nay′lis) [NA]. The extremity of the posterior gray column or horn of the spinal cord. See also *substantia gelatinosa.*

apex cus·pi·dis (kus′pi·dis) [NA]. The tip or apex of a cusp of a tooth.

apex impulse. The point of maximum outward movement of the cardiac left ventricle during systole, normally localized in the fifth left intercostal space in the midclavicular line. Syn. *left ventricular thrust.*

apex lin·guae (ling′gwee) [NA]. The tip of the tongue.

apex murmur. A murmur heard best over the apex of the heart. Syn. *apical murmur.*

apex na·si (nay′zye) [NA]. The tip of the nose.

apex of the head of the fibula. The pointed proximal extremity of the fibula. NA *apex capitis fibulae.*

apex of the heart. The lowest and leftmost point of the heart represented by the left ventricle. It is usually described as being behind the fifth left intercostal space 8 to 9 cm (in the adult) from the midsternal line. NA *apex cordis.*

apex of the lung. The upper extremity of the lung behind the border of the first rib. NA *apex pulmonis.*

apex os·sis sa·cri (oss′is say′krye, sack′rye) [NA]. The caudal end of the sacrum.

apex par·tis pe·tro·sae os·sis tem·po·ra·lis (pahr′tis pe·tro′see oss′is tem·po·ray′lis) [NA]. The medial portion of the petrous part of the temporal bone.

apex pa·tel·lae (pa·tel′ee) [NA]. The inferior blunt tip of the patella.

apex pro·sta·tae (pros′ta·tee) [NA]. The caudal portion of the prostate gland.

apex pul·mo·nis (pul·mo′nis) [NA]. APEX OF THE LUNG.

apex py·ra·mi·dis os·sis tem·po·ra·lis (pi·ram′i·dis oss′is tem·po·ray′lis) [BNA]. APEX PARTIS PETROSAE OSSIS TEMPORALIS.

apex ra·di·cis den·tis (rad′i·sis den′tis, ray·dye′sis) [NA]. The apex of the root of a tooth.

apex su·pra·re·na·lis (glan·du·lae dex·trae) (sue″pruh·re·nay′lis glan′dew·lee decks′tree) [BNA]. The upper extremity of the right adrenal gland.

apex ve·si·cae uri·na·ri·ae (ve·sigh′see yoo·ri·nair′ee·ee) [NA]. The portion of the urinary bladder to which the median umbilical ligament is attached.

APF Abbreviation for *animal protein factor* (= VITAMIN B_{12}).

Ap·gar score or **rating** [Virginia *Apgar,* U.S. anesthesiologist, b. 1909]. A quantitative estimate of the condition of an infant 1 to 5 minutes after birth, derived by assigning points to the quality of heart rate, respiratory effort, color, muscle tone, and reflexes; expressed as the sum of these points, the maximum or best score being 10.

aph-. See *ap-.*

A.P.H.A. American Public Health Association.

A.Ph.A. American Pharmaceutical Association.

apha·cia (a·fay′shee·uh, ·see·uh) *n.* APHAKIA.

apha·gia (a·fay′jee·uh) *n.* [*a-* + *-phagia*]. Inability to swallow, either of organic or psychic origin.

aphagia al·ge·ra (al·jeer′uh, al′je·ruh) [NL., from Gk. *algēros,* painful]. Inability or refusal to swallow because of pain.

apha·kia (a·fay′kee·uh) *n.* [*a-* + *phak-* + *-ia*]. The condition in which the lens is absent from the dioptric system. —**apha·kic** (·kick), **apha·ki·al** (·kee·ul) *adj.*

aphakic eye. An eye deprived of its crystalline lens.

apha·lan·gia (af″uh·lan′jee·uh, ay″fa·) *n.* [*a-* + *phalang-* + *-ia*]. Loss or absence of fingers or toes.

apha·lan·gi·a·sis (af″uh·lan·jye′uh·sis, ay″fal·an·) *n.* APHALANGIA.

aph·al·ge·sia (af″al·jee′zee·uh) *n.* [NL., from Gk. *haphē,* touch, + *algesia*]. A hysterical state wherein pain is induced by contact with a harmless object that has symbolic significance for the patient.

aphan·i·sis (a·fan′i·sis) *n.* [Gk. disappearance, obliteration, from *aphanizein,* to do away with]. *In psychoanalysis,* extinction of sexuality in the individual, as opposed to the fear of castration.

apha·sia (ay·fay′zhuh, a·fay′zhuh, ·zee·uh) *n.* [Gk., speechlessness, from *a-* + *phasis,* utterance, + *-ia*]. Loss or impairment of the reception or use of language caused by lesion of the cerebrum but not by any lesion affecting primary sensation, motility of the vocal musculature or its subjection to voluntary control, or general intellectual function; includes alexia, the agnosias affecting linguistic abilities, the apraxias limited to spoken and written language, and other disorders. Compare *anarthria, dysarthria.*

apha·sic (ay·fay′zick, a·fay′zick) *adj. & n.* 1. Of, pertaining to, or afflicted with aphasia. 2. A person afflicted with aphasia.

aphasic alexia. Alexia in which characters and their combinations can be recognized and classified but in which the language they represent is not fully understood. Compare *agnostic alexia.*

aphasic seizure. Transient cessation of speech as a manifestation of an abnormal electrical discharge usually from the temporal lobe.

apha·si·ol·o·gy (a·fay″zee·ol′uh·jee) *n.* The study of aphasia.

aph·e·lot·ic (af″e·lot′ick) *adj.* Of or pertaining to aphelxia.

aphelx·ia (a·felk′see·uh) *n.* [*ap-*, away, + Gk. *helxis*, dragging, attraction, + *-ia*]. 1. Absentmindedness; inattention or indifference to external impressions. 2. Daydreaming.

aphe·mia (a·fee′mee·uh) *n.* [*a-* + *-phemia*]. PURE WORD MUTENESS.

aph·e·pho·bia (af″e·fo′bee·uh) *n.* [Gk. *haphē*, touch, + *-phobia*]. Pathologic fear of physical contact with people or objects.

aphe·re·sis (af″e·ree′sis) *n.* [Gk. *aphairesis*, removal, from *aphairein*, to take away]. PHERESIS.

aphi·lan·thro·py (ay″fi·lan′thruh·pee, af″i·lan′thruh·pee) *n.* [*a-* + *philanthropy*]. ASOCIALITY.

Aph·i·o·chae·ta (af″ee·o·kee′tuh) *n.* A genus of flies of the family Phoridae. The species *Aphiochaeta ferruginea* and *A. scalaris* produce intestinal myiasis, widely distributed in the tropics.

apho·nia (a·fo′nee·uh, ay·fo′nee·uh) *n.* [Gk. *aphōnia*, speechlessness, from *phōnē*, voice]. 1. Loss of speech due to a peripheral lesion, as in laryngeal paralysis or vocal cord tumor. 2. Hysterical loss of the power of speech. 3. Voicelessness. —**aph·o·nous** (af′uh·nus), **aphon·ic** (a·fon′ick) *adj.*

aphonia par·a·no·i·ca (păr″uh·no′i·kuh). The stubborn silence encountered in certain mental disorders.

aphose (ay′foze, a·foze′, af′oze) *n.* [*a-* + *phose*]. A subjective dark spot or shadow in the field of vision. Contr. *phose.*

aphra·sia (a·fray′zhuh, ·zee·uh) *n.* [*a-* + Gk. *phrasis*, expression, phrase, text, + *-ia*]. 1. Loss of ability to utter connected words or phrases. 2. Refusal to speak; APHONIA PARANOICA.

aphre·nia (a·free′nee·uh) *n.* [*a-* + Gk. *phrēn*, mind, + *-ia*]. DEMENTIA.

aph·ro·dis·i·ac (af″ro·diz′ee·ack) *adj.* & *n.* [Gk. *aphrodisiakos*, sexual, erotic, from *aphrodisia*, sexual pleasures, from *Aphroditē*, goddess of love]. 1. Stimulating the sexual appetite; erotic. 2. An agent that stimulates, or is purported to stimulate, sexual passion or power.

aph·ro·dis·io·ma·nia (af″ro·diz′ee·o·may′nee·uh) *n.* [*aphrodisia* + *mania*]. Exaggerated sexual interest and excitement; EROTOMANIA (1).

aph·ro·ne·sia (af″ro·nee′zhuh, ·zee·uh) *n.* [Gk. *aphronēsis*, folly (from *aphrōn*, senseless, foolish), + *-ia*]. DEMENTIA.

aphro·nia (a·fro′nee·uh) *n.* [Gk. *aphrōn*, senseless (from *phronein*, to understand) + *-ia*]. Lack of practical judgment or of good sense.

aph·tha (af′thuh) *n.*, pl. **aph·thae** (af′thee) [L., from Gk., thrush]. 1. A white painful oral ulcer of unknown cause. 2. APHTHOUS STOMATITIS.

aphtha epi·zo·ot·i·ca (ep″ee·zo·ot′i·kuh). FOOT-AND-MOUTH DISEASE.

aphthae trop·i·cae (trop′i·kee, ·see). Small white, painful mouth ulcerations which may occur in patients with tropical sprue.

aphtha ser·pens (sur′penz). NOMA.

aph·thenx·ia (af·thenk′see·uh) *n.* [*a-* + Gk. *phthenxis*, utterance, + *-ia*]. *Obsol.* A form of aphasia in which speech sounds are poorly enunciated.

aph·thoid (af′thoid) *adj.* APHTHOUS.

aph·thon·gia (af·thon′jee·uh) *n.* [*a-* + Gk. *phthongos*, sound, + *-ia*]. A rare form of anarthria caused by spasm of the muscles of speech, which occurs in professional speakers and is analogous to writer's cramp; an occupational neurosis.

aph·tho·sis (af·tho′sis) *n.* [*aphtha* + *-osis*]. A degenerative disease of mucous membrane with the development of ulcers. See also *aphtha.*

aph·thous (af′thus) *adj.* Pertaining to, affected with, or resembling aphthae.

aphthous fever. FOOT-AND-MOUTH DISEASE.

aphthous stomatitis. Inflammation of the oral mucosa, characterized by the presence of small, painful ulcerations.

aphthous ulcer. CANKER SORE.

api-, apio- [L. *apis*]. A combining form meaning *bee.*

apic-, apici-, apico-. A combining form meaning *apex, apical.*

api·cal (ap′i·kul, ay′pi·kul) *adj.* 1. At or pertaining to the apex. 2. Situated relatively near the apex.

apical abscess. PERIAPICAL ABSCESS.

apical dental ligament. A fibrous cord extending from the summit of the dens of the axis to the occipital bone near the anterior margin of the foramen magnum. Syn. *apical odontoid ligament, suspensory ligament.* NA *ligamentum apicis dentis.*

apical foramen. The passage at the end of the root of a tooth for the vessels and nerves of the dental pulp. NA *foramen apicis dentis.*

apical granuloma. PERIAPICAL GRANULOMA.

apical murmur. APEX MURMUR.

apical odontoid ligament. APICAL DENTAL LIGAMENT.

apical pole. ANIMAL POLE.

api·cec·to·my (ay″pi·seck′tuh·mee, ap″i·) *n.* [*apic-* + *-ectomy*]. 1. Removal of the apex of a tooth root. Syn. *apicoectomy.* 2. Exenteration of the air cells of the apex of the petrous pyramid.

api·ce·ot·o·my (ay″pi·see·ot′uh·mee, ap″i·) *n.* APICOECTOMY.

apices. Plural of *apex.*

apici-. See *apic-.*

api·ci·tis (ap″i·sigh′tis, ay″pi·) *n.* [*apic-* + *-itis*]. Inflammation of an apex of a part or organ.

apico-. See *apic-.*

api·co·ec·to·my (ap″i·ko·eck′tuh·mee) *n.* [*apico-* + *-ectomy*]. Removal of the apex of a tooth root. Syn. *apicectomy.*

api·col·y·sis (ap″i·kol′i·sis) *n.*, pl. **apicoly·ses** (·seez) [*apico-* + *-lysis*]. Artificial collapse of the apex of a lung by separation of the parietal pleura from the chest wall; formerly used in the treatment of pulmonary tuberculosis with apical cavities.

api·co·pos·te·ri·or (ap″i·ko·pos·teer′ee·ur) *adj.* Apical and posterior; used to designate the uppermost segment of the superior lobe of the left lung, sometimes considered to be two segments, the apical and the posterior.

api·cot·o·my (ap″i·kot′uh·mee, ay″pi·) *n.* [*apico-* + *-tomy*]. APICECTOMY.

api·ec·to·my (ap″ee·eck′tuh·mee, ay″pee·) *n.* APICECTOMY.

apio-. See *api-.*

api·ol (ay′pee·ol, ·ole, ap′ee·) *n.* [L. *apium*, parsley, + *-ol*]. 1-Allyl-2,5-dimethoxy-3,4-methylenedioxybenzene, $C_{12}H_{14}O_4$, a constituent of parsley oil; has been used as an antipyretic and emmenagogue. Syn. *parsley camphor.*

api·ole (ay′pee·ole, ap′ee·ole) *n.* APIOL.

apio·pho·bia (ay″pee·o·fo′bee·uh, ap″ee·o·) *n.* APIPHOBIA.

apio·ther·a·py (ay″pee·o·therr′uh·pee, ap″ee·o) *n.* [*apio-* + *therapy*]. Treatment of disease with bee venom.

api·pho·bia (ay″pi·fo′bee·uh, ap″i·) *n.* [*api-* + *-phobia*]. Morbid terror of bees and their sting.

Apis (ay′pis) *n.* [L., bee]. A genus of bees of the family Apidae.

Apis mel·lif·era (me·lif′ur·uh) [L., honey-producing, from *mel*, honey]. The honeybee.

Api·um (ay′pee·um, ap′ee·um) *n.* [L., parsley]. A genus of herbs of the carrot family.

Apium gra·ve·o·lens (grav″ee·o′lenz, gra·vee′o·) [L., strong-smelling]. Celery. See *celery fruit.*

A.P.L. Trademark for a brand of chorionic gonadotropin.

apla·cen·tal (ay″pla·sen′tul, ap″luh·) *adj.* Without a placenta.

ap·la·nat·ic (ap″luh·nat′ick) *adj.* [Gk. *aplanēs*, straight, unwavering]. Corrected for spherical aberration, as an aplanatic focus or an aplanatic lens. —**apla·na·sia** (·nay′zhuh, ·zee·uh), **aplan·a·tism** (a·plan′uh·tiz·um) *n.*

aplanatic lens. A lens corrected for spherical aberration. Syn. *rectilinear lens.*

apla·sia (a·play'zhuh, ·zee·uh) *n.* [*a-* + *-plasia*]. 1. Defective development or production of a tissue or organ. Compare *hypoplasia.* 2. In the somatotype, a physique in which the whole body or a region of the body is poorly developed.

aplasia ax·i·a·lis ex·tra·cor·ti·ca·lis con·gen·i·ta (ack·see·ay'lis eck"struh·kor·ti·kay'lis kon·jen'i·tuh). PELIZAEUS-MERZBACHER DISEASE.

aplas·tic (ay·plas'tick, a·plas'tick) *adj.* [*a-* + *plastic*]. 1. Structureless; formless. 2. Incapable of forming new tissue. 3. Of or pertaining to aplasia. 4. Designating an inflammation with little or no production of granulation tissue.

aplastic anemia. 1. Anemia resulting from failure of cell production in the bone marrow, associated with marrow hypoplasia, hyperplasia, or dysplasia. 2. A clinical syndrome characterized by decrease in all formed elements of the peripheral blood and all their bone-marrow precursors, with associated manifestations of anemia, bleeding, and infection. NA *aleukia hemorrhagica, atrophic anemia.*

apleu·ria (a·ploor'ee·uh, ay·ploor') *n.* [*a-* + *pleur-* + *-ia*]. Congenital ecostatism or absence of the ribs.

ap·nea, ap·noea (ap'nee·uh, ap·nee'uh) *n.* [*a-* + *-pnea*]. The cessation or suspension of breathing. Compare *asphyxia.* —**ap·ne·ic, ap·noe·ic** (ap·nee'ick) *adj.*

apnea va·gi (vay'guy, ·jye). Temporary cessation of respiration due to vagal stimulation.

apnea ve·ra (veer'uh). Apnea from failure of stimulation of the medullary respiratory center, due to a decreased P_{CO_2}.

ap·neu·ma·to·sis (ap·new"muh·to'sis) *n.* [*a-* + *pneumat-* + *-osis*]. ATELECTASIS.

ap·neu·mia (ap·new'mee·uh) *n.* [*a-* + *pneum-* + *-ia*]. Congenital absence of the lungs.

ap·neu·sis (ap·new'sis) *n.*, pl. **apneu·ses** (·seez) [*a-* + Gk. *pneusis,* breathing]. A state of maintained contraction of the inspiratory muscles due to prolonged tonic discharge of inspiratory medullary neurons.

ap·neus·tic (ap·new'stick) *adj.* Pertaining to or exhibiting apneusis.

apnoea. APNEA.

apo-. See *ap-.*

apo·at·ro·pine (ap"o·at'ro·peen, ·pin) *n.* [*apo-* + *atropine*]. Atropyltropeine, $C_{17}H_{21}NO_2$, an alkaloid in belladonna; also obtained by splitting water from atropine.

ap·o·cam·no·sis (ap"o·kam·no'sis) *n.* [Gk. *apokamnein,* to be exhausted, tired out (from *kamnein,* to toil, be weary), + *-osis*]. Intense and readily induced fatigue, as in myasthenia gravis.

apo·car·te·re·sis (ap"o·kahr"te·ree'sis) *n.* [Gk. *apokarterēsis,* from *karterēsis,* endurance, holding out, from *karteros,* steadfast, obstinate]. Suicide by self-starvation.

apo·chro·mat·ic (ap"o·kro·mat'ick) *adj.* [*apo-* + *chromatic*]. Without or free from chromatic and spherical aberration.

apo·clei·sis (ap"o·klye'sis) *n.* [Gk. *apokleisis,* a shutting up]. Aversion to eating.

apo·co·de·ine (ap"o·ko'dee·een, ·in, ·ko'deen) *n.* An alkaloid, $C_{18}H_{19}NO_2$, derived from codeine; has been used as an expectorant, emetic, and cathartic.

apo·crine (ap'o·krin) *adj.* [*apo-* + *-crine*]. 1. Designating a type of secretion in which the secretion-filled free end of a gland cell is pinched off, leaving the nucleus and most of the cytoplasm to recover and repeat the process. Contr. *holocrine, merocrine.* 2. Of or pertaining to the apocrine glands.

apocrine carcinoma. A tumor composed of anaplastic cells resembling those of apocrine epithelium; the term is often applied to extramammary Paget's carcinoma. See also *Paget's disease (3).*

apocrine glands. Glands producing sweat of a characteristic odor; larger and more deeply situated than the ordinary sweat glands, and found in the axillary, mammary, anal, and genital areas. Contr. *eccrine glands.*

ap·o·cy·nam·a·rin (ap"o·si·nam'uh·rin) *n.* A bitter principle obtained from *Apocynum androsaemifolium;* probably identical with the aglycone of cymarin. It is emetic and diuretic.

ap·o·cyn·e·in (ap"o·sin'ee·in, ·sigh'nee·in) *n.* A cardioactive glycoside from apocynum.

apoc·y·nin (a·pos'i·nin) *n.* 4-Hydroxy-3-methoxyacetophenone, $C_9H_{10}O_3$, a constituent of apocynum.

apoc·y·num (a·pos'i·num) *n.* [Gk. *apokynon,* dog's-bane]. The dried rhizome and roots of *Apocynum cannabinum* or of *A. androsaemifolium.* Contains cymarin, a glycoside closely related to many glycosides of the digitalis group. The physiologic actions of apocynum are similar to those of digitalis. Syn. *black Indian hemp, Canada hemp.*

ap·o·dal (ap'o·dul) *adj.* [*a-* + *pod-* + *-al*]. Without feet; lacking feet.

apo·de·mi·al·gia (ap"o·dee"mee·al'jee·uh) *n.* [Gk. *apodēmia,* life abroad, being away from home (from *dēmos,* district, country), + *-algia*]. An abnormal dislike of home life, with a desire for wandering; wanderlust.

apo·dia (ay·po'dee·uh, a·pod') *n.* [Gk., lack of feet, from *apous, apodos,* lacking feet]. Congenital absence of feet.

ap·o·dous (ap'o·dus) *adj.* [Gk. *apous, apodos,* lacking feet]. APODAL.

apo·en·zyme (ap"o·en'zime, ·zim) *n.* The purely protein part of an enzyme which, with the coenzyme, forms the complete enzyme or holoenzyme.

apo·fer·ri·tin (ap"o·ferr'i·tin) *n.* A protein in the intestinal mucosa having the property of binding and storing iron as ferritin.

ap·o·gam·ia (ap"o·gam'ee·uh) *n.* APOGAMY.

apog·a·my (a·pog'uh·mee) *n.* [*apo-* + *-gamy*]. The asexual production of a sporophyte from a gametophyte.

apo·lar (ay·po'lur) *adj.* [*a-* + *polar*]. Having no poles, as of nerve processes.

ap·o·mict (ap'o·mikt) *n.* An individual or species that is produced by or that reproduces by apomixis. —**apo·mic·tic** (·mick'tick) *adj.*

ap·o·mix·ia (ap"o·mick'see·uh) *n.* APOMIXIS.

ap·o·mix·is (ap"o·mick'sis) *n.*, pl. **apomix·es** (·seez) [*apo-* + Gk. *mixis,* mixing, intercourse]. Asexual reproduction, which may be vegetative (vegetative apomixis) or may involve seed production (agamospermy).

apo·mor·phine (ap"o·mor'feen, ·fin) *n.* An alkaloid, $C_{17}H_{17}NO_2$, derived from morphine by abstraction of a molecule of water. The hydrochloride salt is used as an emetic.

ap·o·myt·to·sis (ap"o·mi·to'sis) *n.* [Gk. *apomyttesthai,* to blow the nose, (from *myxa,* mucus, phlegm), + *-osis*]. Any disease marked by stertorous respiration or sneezing.

ap·o·neu·ror·rha·phy (ap"o·new·ror'uh·fee) *n.* [*aponeurosis* + *-rrhaphy*]. Suturing of an aponeurosis, as of the abdominal wall.

ap·o·neu·ro·sis (ap"o·new·ro'sis, a·pon"yoo·) *n.*, pl. **aponeuro·ses** (·seez) [Gk. *aponeurōsis,* from *neuron,* tendon, sinew] [NA]. An expanded tendon consisting of a fibrous or membranous sheet, serving as a means of attachment for flat muscles at their origin or insertion, or as a fascia to enclose or bind a group of muscles. —**aponeu·rot·ic** (·rot'ick) *adj.*

aponeurosis epi·cra·ni·a·lis (ep"i·kray"nee·ay'lis) [NA alt.]. GALEA APONEUROTICA.

aponeurosis lin·guae (ling'gwee) [NA]. The fibrous connective-tissue framework of the tongue to which are attached the various intrinsic and extrinsic muscles of the tongue.

aponeurosis mus·cu·li bi·ci·pi·tis bra·chii (mus'kew·lye bye·sip'i·tis bray'kee·eye) [NA]. A sheet of connective tissue that serves as a partial attachment of the biceps brachii muscle into the deep fascia of the ulnar side of the forearm.

aponeurosis of insertion. An aponeurosis that serves as an insertion for a muscle.

aponeurosis of investment. An aponeurosis that binds or encloses a group of muscles.

aponeurosis of origin. An aponeurosis that serves as the origin of a muscle.

aponeurosis of the occipitofrontalis muscle. GALEA APONEUROTICA.

aponeurosis of the soft palate. A thin, firm, fibrous layer attached above to the hard palate and becoming gradually thinner toward the free margin of the velum.

aponeurosis pal·ma·ris (pal·mair'is) [NA]. PALMAR APONEUROSIS.

aponeurosis plan·ta·ris (plan·tair'is) [NA]. PLANTAR APONEUROSIS.

ap·o·neu·ro·si·tis (ap″o·new″ro·sigh'tis) *n.* Inflammation of an aponeurosis.

ap·o·neu·rot·o·my (ap″o·new·rot'uh·mee) *n.* [*aponeurosis* + *-tomy*]. Incision of an aponeurosis.

apon·ia (a·pon'ee·uh) *n.* [Gk., from *ponos,* work, toil; pain]. 1. Abstention from work; nonexertion. 2. Absence of pain.

apoph·y·sate (a·pof'i·sate) *adj.* Provided with an apophysis.

apoph·y·se·al (a·pof″i·see'ul, ap″o·fiz'ee·ul) *adj.* Of or pertaining to an apophysis.

ap·o·phys·i·al (ap″o·fiz'ee·ul) *adj.* APOPHYSEAL.

apoph·y·sis (a·pof'i·sis) *n.*, pl. **apophy·ses** (·seez) [Gk., from *apo-,* from, off, + *physis,* growth] [NA]. A process, outgrowth, or projection of some part or organ, as of a bone.

apoph·y·si·tis (a·pof″i·sigh'tis) *n.* Inflammation of an apophysis.

ap·o·plec·tic (ap″o·pleck'tick) *adj.* [Gk. *apoplēktikos*]. Of or pertaining to apoplexy. Compare *apoplectiform.*

apoplectic dementia. Dementia due to a cerebrovascular accident.

ap·o·plec·ti·form (ap″o·pleck'ti·form) *adj.* Resembling apoplexy. Compare *apoplectic.*

apoplectiform myelitis. *Obsol.* Disease of the spinal cord of sudden onset.

ap·o·plexy (ap'o·pleck″see) *n.* [Gk. *apoplēxia,* from *apo-* + *plēssein,* to strike]. 1. CEREBROVASCULAR ACCIDENT. 2. Gross hemorrhage into or infarction of any organ. Adj. *apoplectic.*

apo·pnix·is (ap″o·pnick'sis) *n.* [Gk. *apopnigein, apopnix-,* to choke, suffocate, from *pnix, pnigos,* choking, suffocation]. GLOBUS HYSTERICUS.

apo·pro·tein (ap″o·pro'tee·in, ·teen) *n.* The protein portion of a conjugated protein, exclusive of the prosthetic group.

apop·to·sis (ap″op·to'sis, ap″o·) *n.* [Gk. *apoptōsis,* a falling off or away, from *ptōsis,* a fall, from *piptein,* to fall]. Orderly deletion of cells from a given population by means of cell breakdown into membrane-bound fragments (apoptotic bodies) followed either by shedding from an epithelial surface or by phagocytosis. **—apop·tot·ic** (·tot'ick) *adj.*

apoptotic bodies. The membrane-bound cell fragments produced by apoptosis.

apo·qui·nine (ap″o·kwye'nine, ·kwi·neen') *n.* An alkaloid, $C_{19}H_{22}N_2O_2$, obtained by demethylation of quinine.

ap·or·rhip·sis (ap″o·rip'sis) *n.* [Gk., from *aporrhiptein,* to throw off]. The inappropriate discarding of clothing or throwing off of bedclothes; seen in delirium and in some mental disorders.

apo·sia (a·po'zhuh, ·zee·uh) *n.* [*a-* + Gk. *posis,* drinking, + *-ia*]. ADIPSIA.

apo·sid·er·in (ap″o·sid'ur·in) *n.* [*apo-* + *sider-* + *-in*]. The colorless to brown glycoprotein matrix remaining after natural or artificial removal of iron from hemosiderin.

ap·o·si·tia (ap″o·sish'ee·uh, ·sit'ee·uh) *n.* [Gk., from *sitos,* food]. Aversion to or loathing of food. See also *anorexia nervosa.* **—apo·sit·ic** (·sit'ick) *adj.*

ap·o·some (ap'o·sohm) *n.* [*apo-* + *-some*]. *Obsol.* A cytoplasmic cellular inclusion produced by the cell itself.

apos·po·ry (a·pos'puh·ree) *n.* [*apo-* + Gk. *spora,* seed, + *-y*]. Apogamy involving the replacement of spores by unspecialized cells not undergoing meiosis.

apos·ta·sis (a·pos'tuh·sis) *n.*, pl. **aposta·ses** (·seez) [Gk., from *apo-,* away, + *stasis,* standing]. 1. The end or crisis of an attack of disease; termination of a disease by crisis. 2. ABSCESS.

ap·o·stem (ap'o·stem) *n.* [Gk. *apostēma,* abscess, lit. removal, withdrawal, from *aphistanai,* to withdraw, stand apart, from *ap-,* away, + *histanai,* to set, stand]. ABSCESS.

ap·o·ste·ma (ap″o·stee'muh) *n.* [Gk.]. Apostem (= ABSCESS).

apos·thia (a·pos'thee·uh) *n.* [*a-* + Gk. *posthē,* foreskin, + *-ia*]. Congenital absence of the prepuce.

apoth·e·caries' weight (a·poth'e·kair″eez). A system of weights and measures once used in compounding medicines. The troy pound of 5760 grains is the standard. It is subdivided into 12 ounces. The ounce is subdivided into 8 drachms, the drachm into 3 scruples, and the scruple into 20 grains. For fluid measure the quart of 32 fluidounces is subdivided into 2 pints, the pint into 16 fluidounces, the fluidounce into 8 fluidrachms, and the fluidrachm into 60 minims. See also Table of Medical Signs and Symbols and Tables of Weights and Measures in the Appendix.

apoth·e·cary (a·poth'e·kerr″ee) *n.* [L. *apothecarius,* storekeeper, from Gk. *apothēkē,* storehouse]. 1. A pharmacist; one who prepares and distributes medicinal products, particularly those dispensed on the prescription of a licensed medical practitioner. 2. PHARMACY (2).

ap·ous (ap'us) *adj.* [Gk., from *a-* + *pous,* foot]. APODAL.

apo·zy·mase (ap″o·zye'mace, ·maze) *n.* The protein component of a zymase.

ap·pal·laes·the·sia (a·pal″es·theezh'uh, ·theez'ee·uh) *n.* [*ap-* + *pallaesthesia*] APALLESTHESIA.

ap·pa·ra·tus (ap″uh·ray'tus, ·rat'us) *n.*, pl. **apparatus** [L., provision, equipment, from *apparare,* to prepare for]. 1. A collection of instruments or devices used for a special purpose. 2. *In anatomy,* the system or group or organs or parts of organs performing a certain function; a physical mechanism.

apparatus di·ges·to·ri·us (dye″jes·to'ree·us) [NA]. DIGESTIVE SYSTEM.

apparatus la·cri·ma·lis (lack″ri·may'lis) [NA]. All the organs associated with the production and flow of tears.

apparatus re·spi·ra·to·ri·us (re·spye″ruh·to'ree·us, res″pi·) [NA]. RESPIRATORY SYSTEM.

apparatus uro·ge·ni·ta·lis (yoo″ro·jen·i·tay'lis) [NA]. UROGENITAL SYSTEM.

ap·par·ent anemia. PSEUDOANEMIA.

apparent movement. AUTOKINETIC PERCEPTION.

apparent position. *In ophthalmology,* the position in space to which the mind projects a visual image.

apparent strabismus. A subjective strabismus in which the alpha angle is seen as too large or too small according to the degree of myopia or hyperopia.

append-, appendo-. See *appendic-, appendico-.*

ap·pend·age (uh·pen'dij) *n.* 1. Anything appended, usually of minor importance. 2. A limb or limblike structure.

appendage-cell carcinoma. Carcinoma of the skin containing elements resembling skin appendages. Syn. *adnexal carcinoma.*

appendages of the eye. The eyelashes, eyebrows, eyelids, lacrimal gland, lacrimal sac and ducts, and conjunctiva.

ap·pen·dec·to·my (ap″en·deck'tuh·mee) *n.* [*append-* + *-ectomy*]. 1. Excision of the vermiform appendix. 2. Excision of any specified appendix or appendage.

appendic-, appendico-. A combining form meaning *appendix.*

ap·pen·di·cal (a·pen'di·kul) *n.* APPENDICEAL.

ap·pen·di·ceal (ap″en·dis'ee·ul, ·dish″ee·ul, a·pen″di·see'ul) *adj.* Of or pertaining to the vermiform appendix.

appendiceal abscess. An abscess in the vermiform appendix and adjacent tissue, usually following acute suppurative appendicitis.

appendiceal neuroma. Hyperplasia of nerve fibers in an atrophic vermiform appendix.

ap·pen·di·cec·to·my (a·pen″di·seck′tuh·mee) *n.* [*appendic-* + *-ectomy*]. APPENDECTOMY.

appendices. Plural of *appendix.*

appendices epi·plo·i·cae (ep·i·plo′i·see) [NA]. Fatty projections of the serous coat of the large intestine.

appendices epo·o·pho·ri (ep·o·off′o·rye). Appendices vesiculosae (= VESICULAR APPENDICES).

appendices ve·si·cu·lo·sae (ve·sick·yoo·lo′see), sing. **appendix vesiculosa** [NA]. VESICULAR APPENDICES.

ap·pen·di·cial (ap″en·dish′ul) *adj.* APPENDICEAL.

ap·pen·di·ci·tis (a·pen″di·sigh′tis) *n.* Inflammation of the vermiform appendix.

appendicitis oblit·er·ans (o·blit′ur·anz). OBLITERATIVE APPENDICITIS.

ap·pen·di·clau·sis (a·pen″di·klaw′sis) *n.* [*appendic-* + blend of L. *clausus,* closed, and Gk. *klēisis,* closure]. Obstruction or obliteration of the vermiform appendix, producing the clinical features of acute appendicitis.

appendico-. See *appendic-.*

ap·pen·di·co·en·ter·os·to·my (a·pen″di·ko·en·tur·os′tuh·mee) *n.* [*appendico-* + *enterostomy*]. The establishment of an artificial opening between the appendix and small intestine.

ap·pen·di·co·lith (a·pen′di·ko·lith″) *n.* A fecalith in the appendiceal lumen, usually calcified enough to be radiologically visible.

ap·pen·di·cos·to·my (a·pen″di·kos′tuh·mee) *n.* [*appendico-* + *-stomy*]. An operation to bring the vermiform appendix through the abdominal wall and cut off its tip, so as to provide for external drainage and irrigation of the bowel.

ap·pen·dic·u·lar (ap″en·dick′yoo·lur) *adj.* 1. Of or pertaining to an appendage. 2. APPENDICEAL.

appendicular artery. The branch of the ileocolic artery supplying the vermiform appendix. NA *arteria appendicularis.*

appendicular asynergy. Faulty coordination of the limbs, especially of the hands and feet.

appendicular muscle. A muscle inserted on the upper or lower extremity.

appendicular skeleton. The skeleton of the pectoral and pelvic girdles and limbs.

ap·pen·dic·u·late (ap″en·dick′yoo·lut, ·late) *adj.* Possessing or forming one or more appendages.

ap·pen·dix (a·pen′dicks) *n.*, pl. **appen·di·ces** (·di·seez) [L., from *appendere,* to hang to, from *pendere,* to hang]. 1. An appendage. 2. VERMIFORM APPENDIX.

appendix au·ri·cu·la·ris (aw·rick″yoo·lair′is). AURICLE (2).

appendix epi·di·dy·mi·dis (ep″ee·di·dim′i·dis) [NA]. A small appendage on the head of the epididymis consisting of vestigial mesonephric tubules or ducts.

appendix fi·bro·sa he·pa·tis (figh·bro′suh hep′uh·tis) [NA]. A variable fibrous band at the left extremity of the left lobe of the liver.

appendix of the laryngeal ventricle. SACCULE OF THE LARYNX.

appendix tes·tis (tes′tis) [NA]. A remnant of the cranial part of the paramesonephric duct, attached to the testis. See also *hydatid of Morgagni, vesicular appendix.*

appendix ven·tri·cu·li la·ryn·gis (ven·trick′yoo·lye la·rin′jis) [BNA]. Sacculus laryngis (= SACCULE OF THE LARYNX).

appendix ver·mi·for·mis (vur·mi·for′mis) [NA]. VERMIFORM APPENDIX.

appendo-. See *appendic-, appendico-.*

ap·per·cep·tion (ap″ur·sep′shun) *n.* [NL. *apperceptio* (Leibnitz), from L. *ad-* + *perceptio,* gathering, comprehension]. Consciousness of the relation of new events, situations, or sensations to the individual's own emotions, past experiences, and memories. —**appercep·tive** (·tiv) *adj.*

ap·per·son·a·tion (a·pur″suh·nay′shun) *n.* APPERSONIFICATION.

ap·per·son·i·fi·ca·tion (ap″ur·son″i·fi·kay′shun) *n.* [*ad-* + *personification*]. *In psychiatry,* unconscious identification with another, sometimes famous, person in part or in whole.

ap·pe·tite (ap′e·tite) *n.* [L. *appetitus,* from *appetere,* to desire, seek]. 1. Any natural desire or craving to satisfy a physical or psychic need. 2. Specifically, a desire for food, not necessarily prompted by hunger.

appetite center. FEEDING CENTER.

ap·pe·tiz·er (ap′e·tye″zur) *n.* A food, medicine, or aperitif taken before a meal to stimulate the appetite.

ap·pla·nate (ap′la·nate) *adj.* [ML. *applanatus,* flattened, from *ad-* + *planus,* flat]. Horizontally flattened. —**ap·pla·na·tion** (ap″la·nay′shun) *n.*

applanation tonometry. A method of determining the intraocular pressure by measuring the force required to flatten a small area of cornea. Compare *indentation tonometry.*

ap·pli·ca·tor (ap′li·kay″tur) *n.* An instrument used in making local applications.

ap·plied anatomy. Anatomy as a factor in diagnosis and treatment.

applied chemistry. A branch of chemistry that emphasizes the practical rather than the theoretical aspects of the science.

applied psychology. 1. A branch of psychology which emphasizes practical rather than theoretical objectives. See also *clinical psychology.* 2. The interpretation of data in history, literature, and other such fields according to psychologic principles. 3. The application of the principles of psychology to such areas as business, medicine, or education.

ap·pli·qué form (ap″li·kay′). Young *Plasmodium falciparum,* found as a blister on the margin of the red blood cell just under the cell membrane.

ap·pose (a·poze′) *v.* [F. *aposer*]. To place next to one another; to juxtapose.

ap·po·si·tion (ap″o·zish′un) *n.* [ML. *appositio,* from L. *apponere,* to place next to]. 1. The act of fitting together; the state of being fitted together; juxtaposition. 2. The laying on of successive layers, as in bone or tooth formation.

ap·pre·hen·sion (ap″re·hen′shun) *n.* [L. *apprehensio,* from *apprehendere,* to grasp, seize]. 1. The act of mentally grasping a fact; thus it lies somewhere between mere perception and full understanding or comprehension. 2. Suspicion or fear; a foreboding about a future event, usually an unfavorable one.

ap·proach, *n. In surgery,* the manner of securing access to a joint, cavity, part, or organ by a suitable incision through the overlying or neighboring structures.

ap·prox·i·mal (a·prock′si·mul) *adj.* [L. *approximare,* to draw near to, + *-al*]. Situated close or near; contiguous; next to each other.

[1]**ap·prox·i·mate** (uh·prock′si·mut) *adj.* APPROXIMAL.

[2]**ap·prox·i·mate** (uh·prock′si·mate) *v.* To bring together, bring near. —**ap·prox·i·ma·tion,** *n.*

aprac·tag·no·sia (ay·prack″tag·no′see·uh, a·prack″) *n.* [*apractic* + *agnosia*]. A perceptual disorder involving the visual and motor elements in the spatial disposition of an action, in which the patient is unable to arrange objects, figures, or lines according to a two-dimensional or three-dimensional plan.

aprac·tic (ay·prack′tick, a·prack′) *adj.* [Gk. *apraktos,* inactive, idle, impotent]. Pertaining to or marked by apraxia.

apractic aphasia. MOTOR APHASIA.

ap·ra·my·cin (ap″ruh·migh′sin) *n.* An antibiotic produced by *Streptomyces tenebrarius.*

aprax·ia (ay·prack′see·uh, a·prack′) *n.* [Gk., inaction, from *praxis,* action]. Loss or impairment of the ability to perform a learned motor act due to lesion of the cerebral hemispheres but not to any lesion affecting mobility or the patient's desire to perform the act, or causing involuntary movement; presumably represents a disconnection of the cortical motor areas from the cortical areas in which the decision to perform a motor act is made. —**aprax·ic** (·sick), **aprac·tic** (·prack′tick) *adj.*

AP reactant. Abbreviation for *acute-phase reactant.*

Apresoline. Trademark for hydralazine.

apricot kernel oil. PERSIC OIL.

aprin·dine (a·prin'deen) *n.* *N*-(2,3-Dihydro-1*H*-inden-2-yl)-*N'*,*N'*-diethyl-*N*-phenyl-1,3-propanediamine, $C_{22}H_{30}N_2$, an antiarrhythmic, cardiac depressant.

ap·ro·bar·bi·tal (ap"ro·bahr'bi·tal, ·tol) *n.* 5-Allyl-5-isopropylbarbituric acid, $C_{10}H_{14}N_2O_3$, a sedative and hypnotic having an intermediate duration of action.

aproc·tia (ay·prock'shee·uh, a·prock') *n.* [*a-* + *proct-* + *-ia*]. IMPERFORATE ANUS. —**aproc·tous** (·tus) *adj.*

apro·sex·ia (ap"ro·seck'see·uh, ay"pro·seck') *n.* [Gk., want of attention, from *prosexis,* attention]. A mental disturbance consisting in inability to fix attention upon a subject.

aprosexia nasalis. The symptom complex consisting of headache, listlessness, easy fatigability, inattention, and other behavioral manifestations sometimes seen in chronic hypertrophic rhinitis, sinusitis, and adenoiditis, possibly related to the low-grade chronic infection and anemia frequently present.

apro·so·pia (ap"ro·so'pee·uh, ay"pros·o'pee·uh) *n.* [*a-* + *pro-sop-* + *-ia*]. Congenital absence of part or all of the face. —**apros·o·pous** (ay·pros'o·pus) *adj;* **aprosopus,** *n.*

apro·ti·nin (ay·pro'ti·nin, a·) *n.* A polypeptide, extracted from animal tissues, that inhibits various proteinases and may be administered prophylactically or therapeutically for such effect.

ap·sel·a·phe·sia (ap·sel"uh·fee'zhuh, ·zee·uh) *n.* [*a-* + Gk. *psēlaphēsis,* touching, palpation, + *-ia*]. Loss of the tactile sense.

ap·si·thu·rea (ap"si·thew'ree·uh) *n.* Apsithyria; HYSTERICAL APHONIA.

ap·si·thy·ria (ap"si·thigh'ree·uh) *n.* [*a-* + Gk. *psithyrizein,* to whisper, + *-ia*]. HYSTERICAL APHONIA.

ap·sych·ia (ap·sick'ee·uh, ap·sigh'kee·uh, ay·sick', a·sigh') *n.* [Gk., from *a-* + *psychē,* life, spirit, consciousness, + *-ia*]. Loss of consciousness; a faint or swoon.

A.P.T.A. American Physical Therapy Association.

Aptine. Trademark for alprenolol.

ap·ti·tude (ap'ti·tewd) *n.* [L. *aptitudo,* fitness, from *aptus,* fit, apt]. A natural ability or inclination to learn or understand.

aptitude test. Any set of selected and standardized tests to provide an estimate of an individual's ability in a particular field or profession.

Apt test [L. *Apt,* U.S. pediatrician, b. 1922]. A test to differentiate maternal from fetal blood in a newborn child's stomach by exposing a hemolysate of the stomach content to a weakly alkaline solution; if it is fetal hemoglobin, the solution remains pink.

ap·ty·a·lia (ap"tye·ay'lee·uh, ap"ti·) *n.* APTYALISM.

ap·ty·a·lism (ap·tye'u·liz·um, ay·tye') *n.* [*a-* + *ptyalism*]. Deficiency or absence of saliva.

APUD cell. Acronym for a cell possessing the capability of *a*mine *p*recursor *u*ptake and *d*ecarboxylation and of synthesizing and secreting polypeptide hormones. It originates in the neural crest and is found in diverse tissues.

apud·o·ma (ay"puh·do'muh) *n.* APUD TUMOR.

APUD tumor. A benign or malignant tumor which is composed of APUD cells and which may cause secondary clinical effects by secreting polypeptide hormones. Syn. *apudoma.*

apus (ay'pus) *n.* [Gk. *apous,* footless, from *pous,* foot]. An individual lacking feet or the entire lower extremities.

apy·e·tous (a·pye'uh·tus) *adj.* [irreg., from *a-* + Gk. *py-* + *-ous*]. Nonsuppurative; nonpurulent; without pus.

apyk·no·mor·phous, (a·pick"no·mor'fus, ay·) *adj.* Not pyknomorphous; characterizing a condition in which the stained elements of a cell are not packed closely together.

ap·y·rase (ap'i·race, ·raze) *n.* [*a*denyl*pyro*phosphat*ase*]. Any enzyme that hydrolyzes adenosine triphosphate with liberation of phosphate and energy and that is believed to be associated with actomyosin activity.

apy·rene (ay·pye'reen) *adj.* [Gk. *apyrēnos,* pitless, stoneless, from *pyrēn,* fruit stone]. Of sperm cells, having no nucleus, due to degeneration of chromosomes. Contr. *oligopyrene, eupyrene.*

apy·rex·ia (ay"pye·reck'see·uh, ap"eye·) *n.* [Gk., from *pyressein,* to be feverish]. Absence of fever. —**apyrex·i·al** (·see·ul), **apy·ret·ic** (·ret'ick) *adj.*

AQ Abbreviation for *achievement quotient.*

aq. Abbreviation for *aqua,* water.

ÂQRS *In electrocardiography,* the symbol for the mean manifest electrical axis of the QRS complex, measured in degrees and microvolt seconds.

aq·ua (ack'wuh, ay'kwuh, ah'kwuh) *n.,* pl. **aq·uae** (·wee), **aquas** [L.]. Water; especially medicated water, as aromatic waters, saturated solutions of volatile oils, or other volatile substances in water. Abbreviated, a., aq.

aquae·duc·tus (ack"we·duck'tus) *n.* [BNA]. Aqueductus (= AQUEDUCT).

Aquamephyton. Trademark for an aqueous colloidal solution of phytonadione used to prevent or treat hemorrhage caused by hypoprothrombinemia.

aq·ua·pho·bia (ack"wuh·fo'bee·uh) *n.* [*aqua* + *-phobia*]. HYDROPHOBIA (2).

aqua re·gia (ree'jee·uh). NITROHYDROCHLORIC ACID.

Aquasol A. Trademark for a water-dispersible preparation of vitamin A.

Aquatag. Trademark for benzthiazide, a diuretic and antihypertensive agent.

aq·ue·duct (ack'we·dukt) *n.* [L. *aquaeductus,* from *aquae,* of water, + *ductus,* leading]. A canal for the passage of fluid; any canal. —**aq·ue·duc·tal** (ack"we·duck'tul) *adj.*

aqueductal atresia. AQUEDUCTAL STENOSIS.

aqueductal forking. Failure of development of the cerebral aqueduct (aqueductal stenosis) and replacement by multiple ependymal-lined channels, most of which do not communicate with the ventricles.

aqueductal gliosis. Proliferation of periaqueductal glia and glial protrusion into the cerebral aqueduct, the walls of which have been denuded of ependyma.

aqueductal stenosis. Narrowing of the cerebral aqueduct from multiple causes, congenital or acquired, leading to hydrocephalus.

aqueduct of Fal·lo·pi·us (fa·lo'pee·us) [G. *Fallopius*]. FACIAL CANAL.

aqueduct of Syl·vi·us (sil'vee·us) [F. *Sylvius,* Dutch physician, 1614–1672]. CEREBRAL AQUEDUCT.

aqueduct of the cochlea. A canal which establishes a communication between the perilymphatic space of the osseous labyrinth and the subarachnoid space and transmits a vein for the cochlea. NA *ductus perilymphaticus, aqueductus cochleae.*

aqueduct of the vestibule. A canal of the vestibule of the ear, running from the vestibule and opening on the back of the petrous portion of the temporal bone and containing the endolymphatic duct and a small vein. NA *aqueductus vestibuli.*

aqueduct stenosis. AQUEDUCTAL STENOSIS.

aque·duc·tus (ack"we·duck'tus) *n.* [L. *aquaeductus*]. AQUEDUCT.

aqueductus ce·re·bri (serr'e·brye) [NA]. CEREBRAL AQUEDUCT.

aqueductus coch·le·ae (kock'lee·ee). [NA alt]. AQUEDUCT OF THE COCHLEA. NA alt. *ductus perilymphaticus.*

aqueductus ves·ti·bu·li (ves·tib'yoo·lye) [NA]. 1. AQUEDUCT OF THE VESTIBULE. 2. ENDOLYMPHATIC DUCT (1).

aque·ous (ay'kwee·us, ack'wee·us) *adj.* & *n.* [ML. *aqueus,* from L. *aqua,* water]. 1. Watery; in, of, or with water. 2. AQUEOUS HUMOR.

aqueous chamber of the eye. The anterior and posterior chambers collectively.

aqueous flare. *In ophthalmology,* the Tyndall effect or light scattering as the light traverses the anterior chamber of the eye in inflammatory conditions, due to increased protein concentration in the aqueous humor caused by dilatation of blood vessels.

aqueous humor. A clear, watery secretion product of the ciliary epithelium. It fills the anterior and posterior chambers of the eye. NA *humor aquosus.*

Aquex. Trademark for clopamide, an antihypertensive drug.

Aquinone. A trademark for menadione (vitamin K_3).

aquo- [L. *aqua*]. A combining form denoting (a) *presence of water in a complex ion*, called aquo ion; (b) *derivation from water*, as an aquo acid or aquo base.

aq·uo·co·bal·a·min (ack″wo·ko·bawl′uh·min) *n.* Vitamin B_{12b}; cyanocobalamin (vitamin B_{12}) in which the cyanide ligand coordinated to cobalt is replaced by a water molecule.

Ar 1. A symbol for argon. 2. A symbol for the aryl group.

ar-. In chemistry, a combining form meaning *aromatic.*

-ar [L. *-aris* (variant of *-alis* → E. *-al*)]. An adjective-forming suffix meaning (a) *of or pertaining to*; (b) *like, having the character of.*

ara-A. ADENINE ARABINOSIDE.

arab-, arabo-. A combining form meaning (a) *related to arabinose;* (b) *having the stereochemical arrangement of atoms or groups of atoms in arabinose.*

ar·a·ban (ăr′uh·ban) *n.* [*arab-* + *-an*]. A pentosan, $(C_5H_{10}O_5)_n$, found in certain gums and pectins; a polymer of arabinose.

ar·a·bic acid (ăr′uh·bick, a·rab′ick). A polysaccharide; the chief constituent of acacia (gum arabic), in which it occurs in the form of calcium, magnesium, and potassium salts. Syn. *arabin.*

ar·a·bin (ăr′uh·bin, a·rab′in) *n.* ARABIC ACID.

arab·i·nose (a·rab′i·noce, ăr′uh·bi·noce″) *n.* [*arabin* + *-ose*]. $CHO(CHOH)_3CH_2OH$; an aldopentose which exists in two structural configurations, differentiated as L-arabinose and D-arabinose. The L- sugar, also called pectinose, pectin sugar, gum sugar, is widely distributed in plants, usually as a component of a complex polysaccharide. D-Arabinose may be obtained by degradation of dextrose (D-glucose).

ar·a·bin·o·syl cytosine. (ăr″uh·bin′o·sil). CYTARABINE.

arab·i·tol (a·rab′i·tol, ·tole, ăr′uh·bi·tol″) *n.* $CH_2OH(CHOH)_3CH_2OH$; an alcohol derived from arabinose.

ara-C. CYTARABINE.

arach·ic acid (a·rack′ick, a·ray′kick). ARACHIDIC ACID.

ar·a·chid·ic (ăr″uh·kid′ick) *adj.* Pertaining to the peanut, *Arachis hypogaea.*

arachidic acid. $CH_3(CH_2)_{18}COOH$; a solid fatty acid from peanut oil.

ar·a·chi·don·ic acid (a·rack″i·don′ick, a·ray″ki·, ăr″uh·ki·). 5,8,11,14-Eicosatetraenoic acid, $C_{20}H_{32}O_2$, an unsaturated fatty acid occurring in animal phosphatides and certain fats.

ara·chis oil (ăr′uh·kis, a·ray′kis) [*Arachis* (*hypogaea*), the peanut]. PEANUT OIL.

arachn-, arachno- [Gk. *arachnēs*, spider]. A combining form meaning (a) *spider, spiderlike;* (b) *arachnoid.*

arach·ne·pho·bia (uh·rack″ne·fo′bee·uh) *n.* [*arachn-* + *phobia*]. Morbid fear of spiders.

arach·nid (uh·rack′nid) *n.* A member of the class Arachnida.

Arach·ni·da (a·rack′ni·duh) *n.pl.* [NL., from Gk. *arachnēs*, spider]. A large class of the Arthropoda which includes scorpions, spiders, mites, and ticks. They are wingless, usually lack antennae, and, as adults, have four pairs of legs.

arach·nid·ism (uh·rack′nid·iz·um) *n.* [*arachnid* + *-ism*]. A condition produced by the bite of a poisonous spider; spider venom poisoning.

ar·ach·ni·tis (ar″ack·nigh′tis) *n.* ARACHNOIDITIS.

arachno-. See *arachn-.*

arach·no·dac·ty·ly (uh·rack″no·dack′ti·lee) *n.* [*arachno-* + *-dactyly*]. A condition in which the fingers, and sometimes the toes, are abnormally long and thin; seen in Marfan's syndrome and in homocystinuria. Syn. *spider fingers.*

arach·no·gas·tria (uh·rack″no·gas′tree·uh) *n.* [*arachno-* + *-gastria*]. The protuberant abdomen of an emaciated person with ascites. Syn. *spider belly.*

arach·noid (uh·rack′noid) *n.* [Gk. *arachnoeidēs*, cobweblike, from *arachnē*, spider's web]. The arachnoid membrane; the central of the three meninges covering the brain (arachnoidea encephali) and spinal cord (arachnoidea spinalis). It is very fine and delicate in structure, following the pia mater into each sulcus and around each convolution, but separated from it by the subarachnoid space. The two membranes are often considered as one, the piarachnoid. **—arachnoid, arach·noi·dal** (ăr″ack·noy′dul) *adj.*

arachnoidal granulations. ARACHNOID GRANULATIONS.

arach·noi·dea (ăr″ack·noy′dee·uh) *n.* [NL., short for *membrana* (or *meninx*) *arachnoidea*]. ARACHNOID.

arachnoidea en·ce·pha·li (en·sef′uh·lye) [NA]. The arachnoid of the brain.

ar·ach·noi·de·an (ăr″ack·noy′dee·un) *adj.* ARACHNOID, ARACHNOIDAL.

arachnoidea spi·na·lis (spye·nay′lis) [NA]. The arachnoid of the spinal cord.

arachnoid fibroblastoma. MENINGIOMA.

arachnoid granulations. Prolongations of the arachnoid layer of the cerebral meninges through the dura mater into the superior sagittal sinus and into the parasinoidal sinuses. NA *granulationes arachnoideales.*

arach·noid·ism (uh·rack′noid·iz·um) *n.* ARACHNIDISM.

arach·noid·itis (uh·rack′noy·dye′tis) *n.* [*arachnoid* + *-itis*]. Inflammation of the piarachnoid of the spinal cord and brain.

arachnoiditis of the cerebral hemispheres. Thickening and opacity of the piarachnoid of the brain, either in response to disease of the meninges or underlying brain, or having no discernible cause or associated symptoms.

arachnoiditis os·sif·i·cans (os·if′i·kanz). Compression of the spinal cord due to bony deposits in the arachnoid.

arachnoid membrane. ARACHNOID.

arachnoid sheath. A delicate partition lying between the pial sheath and the dural sheath of the optic nerve.

arach·noid-ure·ter·os·to·my (a·rack′noid yoo·ree″tur·os′tuh·mee) *n.* A one-stage operation for the relief of progressive hydrocephaly, no longer used, in which cerebrospinal fluid is shunted from the upper lumbar subarachnoid space into a ureter.

arachnoid villi. ARACHNOID GRANULATIONS.

arach·no·ly·sin (uh·rack″no·lye′sin, ăr″ack·nol′i·sin) *n.* [*arachno-* + *lysin*]. A substance contained in the spider *Epeira diadema*, which causes hemolysis of erythrocytes.

arach·no·the·li·o·ma (uh·rack″no·theel·ee·o′muh) *n.* [*arachno-* + endo*thelioma*]. MENINGIOMA.

Aralen. Trademark for chloroquine, an antimalarial and antiamebic.

Ara·lia (a·ray′lee·uh) *n.* A genus of aromatic plants of the family Araliaceae.

Aralia rac·e·mo·sa (ras″e·mo′suh). American spikenard, the dried rhizome and roots of which were formerly used as a stimulant and diaphoretic.

Aramine. Trademark for metaraminol, a sympathomimetic amine used as the bitartrate salt.

Aran-Du·chenne disease or **syndrome** (a·rahⁿ′, dueᵉ·shen′) [F. A. *Aran*, French physician, 1817–1861; and G. B. A. *Duchenne*]. PROGRESSIVE SPINAL MUSCULAR ATROPHY.

ara·ne·ism (a·ray′nee·iz·um) *n.* [L. *aranea*, spider, + *-ism*]. ARACHNIDISM.

ara·ne·ous (a·ray′nee·us) *adj.* [L. *araneosus*, from *aranea*, spider, spider's web]. Resembling a cobweb.

ar·a·no·tin (ăr″uh·no′tin) *n.* An antiviral agent, $C_{20}H_{18}N_2O_7S_2$, produced by the fungus *Arachniotus aureus* (Eidam) Schroeter.

Aran·tius' ligament (a·ran'chee·us) [J. C. *Arantius* (*Aranzio*), Italian anatomist and physician, 1530–1589]. LIGAMENTUM VENOSUM.

Arantius' ventricle [J. C. *Arantius*]. The terminal depression of the median sulcus of the fourth ventricle immediately ventral to the obex.

ara·phia (a·ray'fee·uh) *n.* [*a-* + Gk. *raphē*, seam, + *-ia*]. DYSRAPHISM.

ara·ro·ba (ahr''uh·ro'buh, ăr''uh·ro'buh) *n.* [Pg., from Tupi]. An oxidation product of resin deposited in the wood of the trunk of *Andira araroba.* From it is obtained chrysarobin, a complex mixture of reduction products of chrysophanol. It has been used in skin affections. Syn. *Goa powder.*

Ara's test. TAKATA-ARA TEST.

ar·ba·pros·til (ahr''buh·pros'til) *n.* (15*R*)-15-Methylprostaglandin E_2, $C_{21}H_{34}O_5$, an antisecretory, anti-ulcer agent.

ar·bo·re·ous (ahr·bo'ree·us) *adj.* ARBORESCENT.

ar·bo·res·cent (ahr''bo·res'unt) *adj.* [L. *arborescens, arborescentis,* becoming a tree, from *arbor,* tree]. Branched like a tree; resembling a tree in appearance.

ar·bo·ri·za·tion (ahr''bo·ri·zay'shun) *n.* [from L. *arbor,* tree]. 1. A conformation or arrangement resembling the branching of a tree. 2. DENDRITE. 3. FERNING. **—ar·bo·rize** (ahr'bo·rize) *v.*

arborization block. A delay in cardiac conduction in the terminal fibers of the Purkinje network. See also *intraventricular heart block.*

arborization test. FERN TEST.

ar·bor·vi·rus (ahr''bor·vye'rus, ahr''bur·) *n.* ARBOVIRUS.

ar·bor·vi·tae (ahr''bur·vye'tee) *n.* [L., tree of life]. A tree or shrub of the genus *Thuja* or the related genus *Thujopsis.*

arbor vitae. 1. [BNA] ARBOR VITAE CEREBELLI. 2. A series of ridges and folds of the mucosa within the uterine cervix. NA *plicae palmatae.* 3. ARBORVITAE.

arbor vitae ce·re·bel·li (serr·e·bel'eye) [NA]. The arborescent appearance of the white substance in a sagittal section of the cerebellum.

arborvitae oil. CEDAR LEAF OIL.

ar·bo·vi·rus (ahr''bo·vye'rus) *n.* [*ar*thropod-*bo*rne + *virus*]. Any one of over 200 RNA viruses biologically transmitted between susceptible vertebrate hosts by blood-sucking arthropods.

arbovirus encephalitis. Any encephalitis or encephalomyelitis caused by an arbovirus, such as eastern equine encephalomyelitis and St. Louis encephalitis.

ar·bu·tin (ahr'bew·tin, ahr·bew'tin) *n.* [from L. *arbutus,* strawberry tree, + *-in*]. A bitter glycoside from the *Arctostaphylos uva-ursi,* or bearberry. See also *uva-ursi.*

ar·cade (ahr·kade') *n.* [F.]. A series of arches; used especially of blood vessels.

ar·ca·num (ahr·kay'num) *n.*, pl. **arca·na** (·nuh) [L., from *arcanus,* closed, secret]. A medicine compounded from a secret formula.

ar·ca·tu·ra (ahr''kuh·tew'ruh) *n.* [NL., from L. *arcus,* a bow, an arch]. A condition of horses marked by the excessive outward curvature of the forelegs.

arc de cer·cle (ărk duh sehrk'l) [F., arc or segment of a circle]. A pathologic posture in which there is extreme bending of the body forward or backward; sometimes seen in hysteria.

arch, *n.* [OF. *arche,* from L. *arcus,* bow, arch]. A structure or an anatomic part having a curved outline resembling that of an arc or a bow.

arch-, archi- [Gk. *archē,* beginning, origin]. A prefix meaning (a) *chief, first;* (b) in anatomy and biology, *primitive, original, ancestral.*

ar·cha·ic (ahr·kay'ick) *adj.* [Gk. *archaikos,* old-fashioned]. *In psychiatry,* designating elements, largely unconscious, in the psyche which are remnants of man's prehistoric past, and which reappear in dreams and other symbolic manifestations; used primarily in analytic psychology. **—ar·cha·ism** (ahr'kay·iz·um) *n.*

archaic-paralogical thinking. PRIMITIVE THINKING.

archaic repression. PRIMARY REPRESSION.

archaic thinking. PRIMITIVE THINKING.

arch bar. ARCH WIRE.

ar·che·go·ni·um (ahr''ke·go'nee·um) *n.*, pl. **archego·nia** (·nee·uh) [NL., from Gk. *archegonos,* original, primal]. *In botany,* the structure which produces the egg in bryophytes and pteridophytes.

arch·en·ceph·a·lon (ahr''ken·sef'uh·lon) *n.*, pl. **archencepha·la** (·luh) [*arch-* + *encephalon*]. The portion of the primitive brain anterior to the notochord, from which the forebrain and midbrain have developed. **—archen·ce·phal·ic** (·se·fal'ick) *adj.*

arch·en·ter·on (ahr·ken'tur·on) *n.*, pl. **archen·tera** (·tur·uh) [*arch-* + *enteron*]. The embryonic alimentary cavity of the gastrula, lined by endoderm. Syn. *archigaster, coelenteron, gastrocoel, primitive gut.* **—arch·en·ter·ic** (ahr''ken·terr'ick) *adj.*

ar·cheo·ki·net·ic (ahr''kee·o·ki·net'ick, ·kigh·net'ick) *adj.* [Gk. *archaios,* ancient, + *kinetic*]. Pertaining to a phylogenetically ancient or primitive type of motor function, represented in mammals by the peripheral and ganglionic nervous systems. Contr. *paleokinetic, neokinetic.*

ar·che·py·on (ahr·ke·pye'on, ahr·kep'ee·on) *n.* [*arch-* + Gk. *pyon,* pus]. Caseated or thickened pus.

arches of the foot. See *longitudinal arch of the foot, transverse arch of the foot.*

ar·che·type (ahr'ke·tipe) *n.* [Gk. *archetypon,* from *archē,* origin, + *typos,* impression, image]. 1. A basic model; prototype. 2. *In comparative anatomy,* an ideal, generalized structural pattern of one of the main kinds of organisms, assumed to be the form of the original ancestor of the group. 3. *In analytic and Jungian pyschology,* a mental remnant or primordial urge, largely unconscious, of man's prehistoric past, which reappears in symbolic form in dreams, works of art, various impulses, or symptomatic acts.

archi-. See *arch-.*

ar·chi·coele, ar·chi·coel (ahr'ki·seel) *n.* [*archi-* + *-coele*]. BLASTOCOELE.

ar·chi·gas·ter (ahr'ki·gas''tur) *n.* [*archi-* + *-gaster*]. ARCHENTERON.

ar·chi·gas·tru·la (ahr''ki·gas'troo·luh) *n.* [*archi-* + *gastrula*]. A primitive ciliated type of gastrula formed largely by simple invagination.

archinephric duct. PRONEPHRIC DUCT.

ar·chi·neph·ron (ahr''ki·nef'ron) *n.* [*archi-* + *nephron*]. PRONEPHROS. **—archineph·ric** (·rick) *adj.*

ar·chi·pal·li·um (ahr''ki·pal'ee·um) *n.* [*archi-* + *pallium*]. The olfactory pallium or the olfactory cerebral cortex; the rhinencephalon; the oldest part of the cerebral cortex. **—archipalli·al** (·ul) *adj.*

ar·chi·plasm (ahr'ki·plaz·um) *n.* ARCHOPLASM.

ar·chi·sleep (ahr'ki·sleep) *n.* [*archi-* + *sleep*]. *Obsol.* REM SLEEP.

ar·chi·stome (ahr'ki·stome) *n.* [*archi-* + *-stome*]. BLASTOPORE.

ar·chi·tec·ton·ic (ahr''ki·teck·ton'ick) *adj.* [Gk. *architektonikos,* architectural]. Pertaining to the structural arrangement or architectural construction of an organ or part. **—architecton·ics** (·icks) *n.*

archo- [Gk. *archos,* rectum]. *Obsol.* A combining form meaning *rectal.*

arch of the aorta. The transverse portion of the aorta between its ascending and descending portions. NA *arcus aortae.* See also Table of Arteries in the Appendix and Plates 5, 7.

ar·cho·plasm (ahr'ko·plaz·um) *n.* [Gk. *archōn,* ruler, + *-plasm*]. The protoplasmic matter from which the centrosomes, asters, and spindle fibers are derived and of which they are composed. **—ar·cho·plas·mic** (ahr''ko·plaz'mick) *adj.*

ar·cho·plas·ma (ahr''ko·plaz'muh) *n.* ARCHOPLASM.

ar·chos (ahr'kos) *n.* [Gk.]. *Obsol.* ANUS.

ar·chu·sia (ahr·kew'zee·uh, ·choo') *n.* [Gk. *archē*, beginning, + *ousia*, essence]. A hypothetical cellular substance, possibly a vitamin B, which aids the migration, growth, and reproduction of cells.

arch wire. A wire that is fitted along either side of the dental arch for stabilization of the teeth or to provide a basis for orthodontic movement.

ar·ci·form (ahr'si·form) *adj.* ARCUATE.

arc·ta·tion (ahrk·tay'shun) *n.* [L. *arctare, artare*, to draw or press close together]. Contracture of an opening or canal; STENOSIS.

arc·tic hysteria or **madness.** PIBLOKTO.

ar·cu·al (ahr'kew·ul) *adj.* ARCUATE.

ar·cu·ate (ahr'kew·ate) *adj.* [L. *arcuatus*]. Arched; curved; bow-shaped.

arcuate artery. 1. (of the foot:) A slightly curved branch of the dorsal pedal artery which originates near the first metatarsal joint, crosses the foot over the bases of the metatarsal bones giving off the second, third, and fourth dorsal metatarsal arteries, and anastomoses with the lateral tarsal and lateral plantar arteries. NA *arteria arcuata pedis.* 2. (of the kidney:) Any of the arteries within the substance of the kidney which are branches of the interlobar arteries and follow an arched course parallel to the greater curvature of the kidney. NA (pl.) *arteriae arcuatae renis.*

arcuate eminence. A rounded protuberance on the anterior aspect of the petrosal portion of the temporal bone, marking the location of the superior semicircular canal. NA *eminentia arcuata.*

arcuate fasciculus. Long association fibers of the cerebrum that form a ventral part, connecting the superior and middle frontal convolutions with the temporal lobe, and a dorsal part (fasciculus longitudinalis superior), connecting the upper and caudal portions of the frontal lobe with the occipital and parietal portions of the temporal lobe.

arcuate fiber. One of a number of bow-shaped or arched nerve fibers in the brain. See also *external arcuate fibers, internal arcuate fibers.*

arcuate ligament. 1. (of the knee:) ARCUATE POPLITEAL LIGAMENT. 2. (of the pubis:) ARCUATE PUBIC LIGAMENT. 3. (of the diaphragm:) See *lateral arcuate ligament, medial arcuate ligament.* See also *median arcuate ligament.*

arcuate line. 1. The iliac portion of the iliopectineal line. NA *linea arcuata ossis ilii.* 2. An arched thickening of the obturator fascia from which the iliococcygeal portion of the levator ani muscle arises. NA *arcus tendineus musculi levatoris ani.*

arcuate nucleus. 1. Any of the irregular small flattened cellular masses in the medulla oblongata ventral to the pyramids. NA (pl.) *nuclei arcuati.* 2. POSTEROMEDIAL VENTRAL NUCLEUS OF THE THALAMUS.

arcuate popliteal ligament. The ligament which is attached to the head of the fibula and arches over the tendon of the popliteus muscle and blends with the capsule of the knee joint. Syn. *arcuate ligament of the knee.* NA *ligamentum popliteum arcuatum.*

arcuate pubic ligament. The arched inferior portion of the capsule of the articulation between the two pubic bones. Syn. *subpubic ligament.* NA *ligamentum arcuatum pubis.*

arcuate scotoma. A form of Bjerrum's scotoma.

arcuate vein. Any of the arched veins at the bases of the renal pyramids, accompanying the arcuate arteries of the kidney. NA (pl.) *venae arcuatae renis.*

ar·cu·a·tion (ahr''kew·ay'shun) *n.* [L. *arcuatio*, from *arcuare*, to bend like a bow]. Curvature, especially of a bone.

ar·cu·a·to·floc·cu·lar tract (ahr''kew·ay''to·flock'yoo·lur). STRIAE MEDULLARES VENTRICULI QUARTI.

ar·cus (ahr'kus) *n.*, pl. & genit. sing. **ar·cus** (ahr'koos) [L.]. 1. ARCH. 2. A discernible arc or ring, as corneal arcus. See also *arcus juvenilis, arcus senilis.*

arcus al·ve·o·la·ris man·di·bu·lae (al·vee·o·lair'is man·dib'yoo·lee) [NA]. The alveolar arch of the mandible. See *alveolar arch.*

arcus alveolaris max·il·lae (mack·sil'ee) [NA]. The alveolar arch of the maxilla. See *alveolar arch.*

arcus anterior at·lan·tis (at·lan'tis) [NA]. The anterior arch of the atlas.

arcus aor·tae (ay·or'tee) [NA]. ARCH OF THE AORTA.

arcus car·ti·la·gi·nis cri·coi·de·ae (kahr·ti·laj'i·nis kri·koy'dee·ee) [NA]. The anterior portion of the cricoid cartilage.

arcus cos·ta·lis (kos·tay'lis) [NA]. COSTAL ARCH.

arcus cos·ta·rum (kos·tair'um) [BNA]. Arcus costalis. (= COSTAL ARCH).

arcus den·ta·lis inferior (den·tay'lis) [NA]. The inferior dental arch; dental arch of the lower teeth.

arcus dentalis superior [NA]. The superior dental arch; dental arch of the upper teeth.

arcus glos·so·pa·la·ti·nus (glos''o·pal·uh·tye'nus) [BNA]. Arcus palatoglossus. (= PALATOGLOSSAL ARCH).

arcus ilio·pec·ti·ne·us (il''ee·o·peck·tin'ee·us) [NA]. The band of fascia between the lacuna musculorum and the lacuna vasorum.

arcus ju·ve·ni·lis (joo·ve·nigh'lis). A congenital opaque ring in the corneal stroma resembling an arcus senilis but evident at or shortly after birth; ANTERIOR EMBRYOTOXON.

arcus lip·i·dus (lip'i·dus). ARCUS SENILIS.

arcus lum·bo·cos·ta·lis la·te·ra·lis (lum·bo·kos·tay'lis lat·e·ray'lis) [BNA]. Ligamentum arcuatum laterale (= LATERAL ARCUATE LIGAMENT).

arcus lumbocostalis me·di·a·lis (mee·dee·ay'lis) [BNA]. Ligamentum arcuatum mediale (= MEDIAL ARCUATE LIGAMENT).

arcus pa·la·ti·ni (pal·uh·tye'nigh) [BNA]. PALATAL ARCHES.

arcus pa·la·to·glos·sus (pal''uh·to·glos'us) [NA]. PALATOGLOSSAL ARCH.

arcus pa·la·to·pha·ryn·ge·us (pal''uh·to·fa·rin'jee·us) [NA]. PALATOPHARYNGEAL ARCH.

arcus pal·ma·ris pro·fun·dus (pal·mair'is pro·fun'dus) [NA]. DEEP PALMAR ARCH.

arcus palmaris su·per·fi·ci·a·lis (sue''pur·fish·ee·ay'lis) [NA]. SUPERFICIAL PALMAR ARCH.

arcus pal·pe·bra·lis inferior (pal·pe·bray'lis) [NA]. The inferior palpebral arch; the arterial arcade in the lower eyelid.

arcus palpebralis superior [NA]. The superior palpebral arch; the arterial arcade in the upper eyelid.

arcus pe·dis lon·gi·tu·di·na·lis (ped'is lon''ji·tew·di·nay'lis) [NA]. LONGITUDINAL ARCH OF THE FOOT.

arcus pedis trans·ver·sa·lis (trans·vur·say'lis) [NA]. TRANSVERSE ARCH OF THE FOOT.

arcus pha·ryn·go·pa·la·ti·nus (fa·rin''go·pal·uh·tye'nus) [BNA]. Arcus palatopharyngeus (= PALATOPHARYNGEAL ARCH).

arcus plan·ta·ris (plan·tair'is) [NA]. PLANTAR ARTERIAL ARCH.

arcus posterior at·lan·tis (at·lan'tis) [NA]. The posterior arch of the atlas.

arcus pu·bis (pew'bis) [NA]. PUBIC ARCH.

arcus se·ni·lis (se·nigh'lis). An opaque ring at the edge of the cornea, seen in many individuals of middle age and especially old age; due to lipoid deposits in the stroma. Syn. *gerotoxon, arcus lipidus.* Compare *arcus juvenilis.*

arcus senilis len·tis (len'tis). An opaque ring in the equator of the crystalline lens; it sometimes occurs in the aged.

arcus su·per·ci·li·a·ris (sue''pur·sil·ee·air'is) [NA]. SUPRAORBITAL RIDGE.

arcus tar·se·us inferior (tahr'see·us) [BNA]. ARCUS PALPEBRALIS INFERIOR.

arcus tarseus superior [BNA]. ARCUS PALPEBRALIS SUPERIOR.

arcus ten·di·ne·us (ten·din'ee·us) [NA]. TENDINOUS ARCH.

arcus tendineus fas·ci·ae pel·vis (fash'ee·ee pel'vis) [NA]. The tendinous arch of the pelvic fascia. See *tendinous arch.*

arcus tendineus mus·cu·li le·va·to·ris ani (mus'kew·lye lev·uh·to'ris ay'nigh) [NA]. The tendinous arch of the levator ani. See *tendinous arch.*

arcus tendineus musculi so·lei (so'lee·eye) [NA]. The tendinous arch of the soleus muscle. See *tendinous arch.*

ar·cus ve·no·si di·gi·ta·les (ahr'koos ve·no'sigh dij·i·tay'leez) [BNA]. A series of communicating venous branches across the dorsal aspect of the proximal ends of the finger.

arcus ve·no·sus dor·sa·lis pe·dis (ve·no'sus dor·say'lis ped'is) [NA]. A venous arch on the dorsal aspect of the foot covering the back of the metatarsal bones.

arcus venosus ju·gu·li (jug'yoo·lye) [NA]. JUGULAR VENOUS ARCH

arcus venosus pal·ma·ris pro·fun·dus (pal·mair'is pro·fun'dus) [NA]. A venous arch which accompanies the deep palmar arterial arch.

arcus venosus palmaris su·per·fi·ci·a·lis (sue''pur·fish·ee·ay'lis) [NA]. A venous arch which accompanies the superficial palmar arterial arch.

arcus venosus plan·ta·ris (plan·tair'is) [NA]. A venous arch which accompanies the plantar arterial arch.

arcus ver·te·brae (vur'te·bree) [NA]. VERTEBRAL ARCH.

arcus vo·la·ris pro·fun·dus (vo·lair'is pro·fun'dus) [BNA]. Arcus palmaris profundus (= DEEP PALMAR ARCH).

arcus volaris su·per·fi·ci·a·lis (sue''pur·fish·ee·ay'lis) [BNA]. Arcus palmaris superficialis (= SUPERFICIAL PALMAR ARCH).

arcus volaris ve·no·sus pro·fun·dus (ve·no'sus pro·fun'dus) [BNA]. ARCUS VENOSUS PALMARIS PROFUNDUS.

arcus volaris venosus su·per·fi·ci·a·lis (sue''pur·fish·ee·ay'lis) [BNA]. ARCUS VENOSUS PALMARIS SUPERFICIALIS.

arcus zy·go·ma·ti·cus (zye·go·mat'i·kus) [NA]. ZYGOMATIC ARCH.

arc-welder's disease or **nodulation.** SIDEROSIS (2).

ARD Abbreviation for *acute respiratory disease.*

ar·dent pulse. A pulse beat with a quick, full wave which seems to strike the finger at a single point.

area (air'ee·uh, ăr'ee·uh) *n.*, L. pl. & genit. sing. **are·ae** (air'ee·ee) [L., piece of level ground]. 1. A limited extent of surface; a region. 2. A field or system of intellectual activity or study. 3. A structural or functional part of the cerebral cortex.

area acu·sti·ca (a·koos'ti·kuh) [BNA]. AREA VESTIBULARIS.

area Cel·si (sel'sigh). [A. C. *Celsus,* Roman physician, 1st century A.D.]. ALOPECIA AREATA.

area cen·tra·lis (sen·tray'lis). The area of the retina in the center of which is the fovea centralis and which has the greatest concentration of cones and more than one layer of ganglion cells.

area cho·roi·dea (ko·roy'dee·uh). A thin-walled part of the embryonic brain, the site of the future choroid plexus of the third ventricle.

area coch·le·ae (kock'lee·ee) [NA]. The anterior inferior portion of the lateral end of the internal acoustic meatus overlying the cochlea.

area cri·bro·sa me·dia (kri·bro'suh mee'dee·uh). AREA VESTIBULARIS INFERIOR.

area cribrosa pa·pil·lae re·na·lis (pa·pil'ee re·nay'lis) [NA]. The surface onto which the papillary ducts of a renal pyramid open into a minor calix.

area cribrosa superior. AREA VESTIBULARIS SUPERIOR.

areae. L. plural and genitive singular of *area.*

areae gas·tri·cae (gas'tri·see) [NA]. GASTRIC AREAS.

area em·bry·o·na·lis (em·bree·o·nay'lis). EMBRYONIC DISK.

area ger·mi·na·ti·va (jur''mi·nuh·tye'vuh). EMBRYONIC DISK.

area in·ter·con·dy·la·ris an·te·ri·or ti·bi·ae (in''tur·kon·di·lair'is an·teer'ee·or tib'ee·ee) [NA]. The region between the proximal articular surfaces of the tibia.

area intercondylaris posterior tibiae [NA]. The deep notch between the condyles of the tibia.

area ner·vi fa·ci·a·lis (nur'vye fay·shee·ay'lis) [NA]. The area at the lateral end of the internal acoustic meatus where the facial nerve leaves the meatus and enters the facial canal.

area nu·da (new'duh) [NA]. BARE AREA OF THE LIVER.

area opa·ca (o·pay'kuh). The opaque peripheral area of the blastoderm of birds and reptiles which is continuous with the yolk and surrounds the area pellucida.

area para·ter·mi·na·lis (păr''uh·tur·mi·nay'lis). A space on the medial aspect of the embryonic cerebral hemisphere.

area par·ol·fac·to·ria (Bro·cae) (păr''ol·fack·to'ree·uh) (bro'see, bro'kee) [BNA]. Area subcallosa (= PAROLFACTORY AREA).

area pel·lu·ci·da (pe·lew'si·duh). The central transparent area of the blastoderm of birds and reptiles overlying the subgerminal cavity.

area pos·tre·ma (pos·tree'muh). A narrow zone on the lateral wall of the fourth ventricle, separated from the ala cinerea by the funiculus separans.

area sub·cal·lo·sa (sub·kal·o'suh) [NA]. PAROLFACTORY AREA.

are·a·tus (air''ee·ay'tus) *adj.*, f. **area·ta** [NL., from *area*]. Occurring in patches.

area vas·cu·lo·sa (vas·kew·lo'suh). The inner vascular zone of the area opaca; it consists of three layers.

area ves·ti·bu·la·ris (ves·tib''yoo·lair'is) [NA]. An area in the lateral angle of the floor of the fourth ventricle overlying the nuclei of the vestibular nerve.

area vestibularis inferior [NA]. The posterior inferior portion of the lateral end of the internal acoustic meatus where the fibers of the vestibular nerve pass through the bone to the saccule.

area vestibularis superior [NA]. The posterior superior portion of the lateral end of the internal acoustic meatus where the fibers of the vestibular nerve pass through the bone to the utricle and ampullae of the anterior and lateral semicircular ducts.

area vi·tel·li·na (vit·e·lye'nuh). The outer nonvascular zone of the area opaca; it consists of ectoderm and endoderm.

Are·ca (a·ree'kuh, ăr'e·kuh) *n.* [NL., from Pg., from Malayalam *aṭekka*]. A small genus of palm trees of tropical Asia and the Malay Archipelago; areca palm.

Areca catechu. A species of *Areca* cultivated in India, the Malay Archipelago, and the East Indies; betel-nut palm. The dried ripe seeds contain several alkaloids, the most important being arecoline.

are·co·line (a·ree'ko·leen, ·lin, a·reck'o·) *n.* Methyl 1,2,5,6-tetrahydro-1-methylnicotinate, $C_8H_{13}NO_2$, a liquid alkaloid from the seeds of *Areca catechu.* It is a parasympathomimetic agent; formerly used in human medicine but now used only as a veterinary anthelmintic and cathartic.

are·flex·ia (ay''re·fleck'see·uh) *n.* Absence of reflexes.

are·gen·er·a·tion (ay''re·jen''ur·ay'shun) *n.* [*a-* + *regeneration*]. Failure of tissue to regenerate after disease or injury. —**are·gen·er·a·tive** (ay''re·jen'ur·uh·tiv), **aregenera·to·ry** (·to''ree) *adj.*

aregeneratory anemia. PRIMARY REFRACTORY ANEMIA.

ar·e·na·ceous (ăr''e·nay'shus) *adj.* [L. *arenaceus,* from *arena,* sand]. Sandy.

ar·e·na·tion (ăr''e·nay'shun) *n.* [from L. *arena,* sand]. 1. A sand bath. 2. Sand baths in the treatment of disease; no longer in general use. Syn. *ammotherapy.*

are·na·vi·rus (ăr''e·nuh·vye'rus, a·ree''nuh·) *n.* [L. *arena,* sand, + *virus*]. Any of a group of RNA viruses having characteristic fine granules in their virions, as seen in electron micrographs, as well as a group-specific antigen; the virus of lymphocytic choriomeningitis is the prototype of the group.

ar·ene (ăr'een) *n.* [*ar*omatic + *-ene*]. Any aromatic hydrocarbon; any hydrocarbon in which at least one benzene ring is present.

are·no·vi·rus (ăr''e·no·vye'rus) *n.* ARENAVIRUS.

are·o·la (a·ree'o·luh) *n.*, L. pl. **areo·lae** (·lee), [L., dim. of *area,* area]. 1. Any minute interstice or space in a tissue. 2. A colored or pigmented ring surrounding some central point or space, as a nipple or pustule. 3. The part of the iris enclosing the pupil. —**areo·lar** (·lur) *adj.*

areola mam·mae (mam'ee) [NA]. The pigmented area surrounding the nipple of the breast. This enlarges during pregnancy, producing the second areola. Syn. *areola papillaris, mammary areola.* See also Plate 24.

areola pa·pil·la·ris (pap"i·lair'is). AREOLA MAMMAE.

areolar glands. Glands in the areola about the nipple in the female breast. They are intermediate in character between mammary glands and apocrine sweat glands. NA *glandulae areolares.*

areolar glands of Montgomery. MONTGOMERY'S GLANDS.

areolar tissue. A form of loose connective tissue composed of cells and delicate collagenous and elastic fibers interlacing in all directions.

Arfonad camphorsulfonate. Trademark for trimethaphan camsylate.

ar·gam·bly·o·pia (ahr·gam"blee·o'pee·uh) *n.* [Gk. *argos,* idle, + *amblyopia*]. *In optometry,* amblyopia from disuse or from nonuse, usually of one eye, as a result of uncorrected esotropia. Syn. *amblyopia ex anopsia.*

Ar·gas (ahr'gas) *n.* [NL., perhaps from Gk. *argos,* living without labor]. A genus of ticks of the Argasidae.

Ar·gas·i·dae (ahr·gas'i·dee) *n.pl.* A family of soft-bodied ticks.

Argas per·si·cus (pur'si·kus). A species of tick primarily ectoparasitic on birds and occasionally man; the vector of avian spirochetosis.

argent-, argento- [L., *argentum*]. A combining form meaning *silver, containing silver.*

ar·gen·taf·fin, ar·gen·taf·fine (ahr·jen'tuh·fin) *adj.* [*argent-* + *affinity*]. Reducing silver of its own innate capacity, without aid of light or subsequently applied developers or reducing agents. Compare *argyrophil.*

argentaffin carcinoma. CARCINOID.

argentaffin cells. Cells having an affinity for silver salts and therefore capable of being stained by them.

argentaffin fibers. RETICULAR FIBERS.

ar·gen·taf·fi·no·ma (ahr·jen"tuh·fi·no'muh, ahr"jen·taf"i·no'muh) *n.* [*argentaffin* + *-oma*]. CARCINOID.

argentaffinoma syndrome. CARCINOID SYNDROME.

argentaffin tumor. CARCINOID.

ar·gen·tic (ahr·jen'tick) *adj.* [*argent-* + *-ic*]. Containing silver in its higher, bivalent state (Ag^{2+}).

argento-. See *argent-.*

ar·gen·to·phil, ar·gen·to·phile (ahr·jen'to·fil) *adj.* [*argento-* + *-phil*]. Stainable by impregnation with silver salts; ARGYROPHIL.

argentophil fibers. RETICULAR FIBERS.

ar·gen·to·phil·ic (ahr·jen"to·fil'ick) *adj.* ARGYROPHIL.

ar·gen·tous (ahr·jen'tus) *adj.* [*argent-* + *-ous*]. Containing silver in its lower, univalent state (Ag^{+}).

ar·gen·tum (ahr·jen'tum) *n.* [L.]. SILVER.

ar·gi·am·bly·o·pia (ahr"jee·am"blee·o'pee·uh) *n.* ARGAMBLYOPIA.

ar·gil·la·ceous (ahr"ji·lay'shus) *adj.* [L. *argillaceus,* from *argilla,* white clay]. Claylike; composed of clay.

ar·gi·nase (ahr'ji·nace, ·naze) *n.* [*arginine* + *-ase*]. An enzyme, found in liver and other tissues, that catalyzes hydrolysis of L-arginine to ornithine and urea.

ar·gi·nine (ahr'ji·neen, ·nin) *n.* [*argent-* (first isolated in combination with silver atoms) + *-ine*]. 1-Amino-4-guanidovaleric acid, $C_6H_{14}N_4O_2$, the L-form of which is an amino acid component of animal and vegetable proteins; while nitrogen equilibrium can be maintained in its absence for a short period, it appears to be a dietary essential for humans. The glutamate and hydrochloride salts are used therapeutically as ammonia detoxicants.

arginine glutamate. The L(+)-arginine salt of L(+)-glutamic acid, $C_{11}H_{23}N_5O_6$, used in the treatment of ammonia intoxication due to hepatic failure.

arginine hydrochloride. L(+)-Arginine hydrochloride, $C_6H_{14}N_4O_2.HCl$, used intravenously to lower blood ammonia levels in patients with encephalopathies associated with ammoniacal azotemia.

arginine phosphate. PHOSPHOARGININE.

ar·gi·ni·no·suc·cin·ic acid (ahr"ji·nee"no·suck·sin'ick). An intermediate compound, $C_{10}H_{18}N_4O_6$, in the synthesis of arginine, formed by the enzymatic condensation of citrulline and aspartic acid.

ar·gi·ni·no·suc·cin·ic·ac·id·u·ria (ahr"ji·nee"no·suck·sin'ick as"i·dew'ree·uh) *n.* [*argininosuccinic acid* + *-uria*]. A recessively inherited metabolic disorder in which there is a deficiency of argininosuccinase with high concentration of argininosuccinic acid in blood, cerebrospinal fluid, and urine as well as ammonia intoxication; manifested clinically by mental retardation, friable and tufted hair, ataxia, convulsions, vomiting, often a refusal to eat proteins, and hepatomegaly.

ar·gi·nyl (ahr'ji·nil) *n.* The univalent radical, $H_2NC(:NH)NHCH_2CH_2CH_2CH(NH_2)CO—$, of the amino acid arginine.

Argivene. Trademark for arginine hydrochloride.

ar·gol (ahr'gol) *n.* [Norman French *argoil,* unkn. orig.]. The crust, consisting largely of crude potassium bitartrate (tartar), deposited on the inside of wine casks during fermentation.

ar·gon (ahr'gon) *n.* [Gk. *argos,* idle, + *-on*]. An inert gaseous element, atomic weight 39.948, present in the atmosphere. It may be obtained by fractionation of liquid air. Symbol, Ar.

Ar·gonz–Del Castillo syndrome. AHUMADA–DEL CASTILLO SYNDROME.

Ar·gyll Rob·ert·son pupil or **sign** (ahr·gile') [D. M. C. L. *Argyll Robertson,* Scottish physician, 1837–1909]. A pupil which constricts on accommodation but not to light; usually bilateral and seen in syphilis of the central nervous system, in miosis, and occasionally in other diseases.

argyr-, argyro- [Gk. *argyros*]. A combining form meaning *silver.*

ar·gyr·ia (ahr·jirr'ee·uh, ahr·jye'ree·uh) *n.* [*argyr-* + *-ia*]. A dusky-gray or bluish discoloration of the skin and mucous membranes produced by the prolonged administration or application of silver preparations. Syn. *argyrosis.* —**argyr·ic** (·ick) *adj.*

Argyrol. Trademark for a preparation somewhat similar to mild silver protein used as a nonirritating antiseptic in infections of the mucous membranes.

ar·gy·ro·len·tis (ahr·jye"ro·len'tis, ahr"ji·ro·) *n.* [*argyro-* + L. *lentis,* of the lens]. A condition of the lens of the eye seen rarely in prolonged silver intoxication, characterized by a golden sheen to the anterior lens capsule.

ar·gy·ro·phil, ar·gy·ro·phile (ahr·jye'ro·fil, ahr'ji·ro·) *adj.* [*argyro-* + *-phil*]. Stainable by impregnation with silver salts, followed by light or photographic development or both. Compare *argentaffin.*

ar·gy·ro·phil·ia (ahr·jye"ro·fil'ee·uh, ahr"ji·ro) *n.* The property of being argyrophil(ic).

ar·gy·ro·phil·ic (ahr·jye"ro·fil'ick, ahr"ji·ro·) *adj.* ARGYROPHIL.

argyrophil plaque. A microscopic, extracellular lesion of the cerebral gray matter, marking an area of active neuronal degeneration, staining readily with silver, and consisting of particles of neuronal debris surrounding a core of coagulation necrosis that frequently contains amyloid material; a major pathologic feature of Alzheimer's disease.

ar·gy·ro·sid·er·o·sis (ahr"ji·ro·sid"ur·o'sis) *n.* [*argyro-* + *siderosis*]. A form of pneumoconiosis caused by inhalation of iron oxide mixed with silver; seen in arc welders, silver polishers, and workers in iron and steel factories.

ar·gy·ro·sis (ahr"ji·ro'sis) *n.* ARGYRIA.

arhinencephalia. ARRHINENCEPHALIA.

arhinia. ARRHINIA.

arhythmia. ARRHYTHMIA.

Arias-Ste·lla cells (ar″yas·teh'l^{y}ah, ar″yas·es·tey'yah) [J. *Arias-Stella,* Peruvian pathologist, b. 1924]. Endometrial columnar cells with hyperchromatic nuclei displaying both proliferative and secretory activity under the influence of trophoblastic tissue; an atypical pattern of endometrium associated with ectopic pregnancy.

ari·bo·fla·vin·o·sis (ay·rye″bo·flay·vi·no'sis) *n.* [*a-* + *riboflavin* + *-osis*]. Dietary deficiency of riboflavin, associated with the syndrome of angular cheilosis and stomatitis, corneal vascularity, nasolabial seborrhea, and genitorectal dermatitis.

ar·i·cine (ăr'i·seen, ·sin) *n.* An alkaloid, $C_{22}H_{26}N_2O_4$, obtained from several varieties of cinchona bark.

aristo- [Gk. *aristos*]. A combining form meaning *best.*

Aristocort. A trademark for the glucocorticoid triamcinolone and certain of its derivatives.

Aristoderm. A trademark for the glucocorticoid triamcinolone acetonide.

aris·to·gen·ics (a·ris″to·jen'icks) *n.* [*aristo-* + *-genic* + *-s*]. *Obsol.* EUGENICS; specifically, positive eugenics. **—aristogenic,** *adj.*

Aristol. A trademark for thymol iodide, a topical antiseptic.

Aris·to·lo·chia (a·ris″to·lo'kee·uh) *n.* [Gk. *aristolocheia,* from *aristo-* + *locheia,* childbirth]. A genus of herbs or shrubs of the Aristolochiaceae; many species have been used medicinally.

Aristolochia re·tic·u·la·ta (re·tick″yoo·lay'tuh, ·lah'tuh). Texas snakeroot. See also *serpentaria.*

Aristolochia serpentaria. Virginia snakeroot. See also *serpentaria.*

Aristospan. Trademark for triamcinolone hexacetonide, a glucocorticoid steroid.

ar·ith·met·ic mean, (ăr″ith·met'ick). The result obtained by the addition of a series of quantities and division by the number of such quantities.

arith·mo·ma·nia (a·rith″mo·may'nee·uh) *n.* [Gk. *arithmos,* number, + *mania*]. A morbid impulse to count objects; a preoccupation with numbers.

Ar·i·zo·na bacteria. Lactose-fermenting Enterobacteriaceae, biochemically and serologically related to the *Salmonella,* capable of producing illness in man, other mammals, and in fowl; frequently carried by reptiles.

Ar·kan·sas stone (ahr'kun·saw) [after *Arkansas,* U.S.]. A fine, very smooth sharpening stone used for maintaining precision cutting edges of dental instruments.

ar·kyo·chrome (ahr'kee·o·krome″) *n.* [Gk. *arkys, arkyos,* net, + *-chrome*]. A nerve cell in which the stainable portion of the cytoplasm is in the form of a network.

Arlef. Trademark for flufenamic acid.

Arlidin. Trademark for nylidrin.

Arlt's trachoma [C. F. von *Arlt,* Bohemian ophthalmologist, 1812–1887]. GRANULAR TRACHOMA.

arm, *n.* [Gmc. (rel. to L. *armus* and to Gk. *harmos,* shoulder joint)]. 1. *In anatomy,* the upper extremity from the shoulder to the elbow. 2. Popularly, the arm and the forearm. 3. That portion of the stand connecting the body or tube of a microscope with the pillar. 4. *In prosthodontics,* part of a clasp or other retaining or stabilizing device of a removable prosthesis.

ar·ma·men·tar·i·um (ahr'muh·men·tair'ee·um) *n.,* pl. **armamentar·ia** (·ee·uh), [L., armory, arsenal]. All the books, journals, medicines, instruments, and laboratory and therapeutic equipment possessed by a physician, surgeon, or medical institution to assist in the practice of medicine.

Ar·man·ni-Eb·stein lesion (ar·ma^{h}n'nee, ep'shtine) [L. *Armanni,* Italian pathologist, 1839–1903; and W. *Ebstein*]. Glycogen vacuolation of the terminal straight portion of the renal proximal convoluted tubules, seen in diabetic glomerulosclerosis.

armed bougie. A bougie having a caustic attached to the tip.

Ar·me·nian disease. FAMILIAL MEDITERRANEAN FEVER.

Ar·mil·li·fer (ahr·mil'li·fur) *n.* [NL., from L. *armilla,* bracelet, + *ferre,* to carry, bear]. A genus of pentastomes (tongue worms) normally parasitic of reptiles, whose larvae have been found in the liver, lungs, and spleen of man. The medically important species are *Armillifer armillatus* and *A. moniliformis.*

arm-lung time test. A test in which the time is measured from the injection of ether into a vein of the arm until the odor of ether appears in the breath; used as a measurement of the velocity of blood flow; a circulation time test.

ar·mored heart. A heart with calcification of the pericardium, usually secondary to pericarditis.

arm·pit, *n.* AXILLA.

arm-tongue time test. A test in which the time is measured from the injection of a substance into an arm vein until the taste of it is noticed in the mouth; used as a measurement of the velocity of blood flow; a circulation time test.

Ar·neth's count or **classification** (ahr'net) [J. *Arneth,* German physician, 1873–1955]. A system of dividing peripheral blood granulocytes into five classes according to the number of nuclear lobes, the least mature cells being tabulated on the left, giving rise to the terms "shift to left" and "shift to right" as an indication of granulocytic immaturity or hypermaturity, respectively.

Arneth's formula, index, or **method** [J. *Arneth*]. ARNETH'S COUNT.

ar·ni·ca (ahr'ni·kuh) *n.* The dried flower heads of the *Arnica montana.* A counterirritant, arnica was formerly popularly used as a tincture for sprains, bruises, and surface wounds.

Ar·nold-Chia·ri syndrome or **malformation** (ahr'no^{h}lt, kyah'ree) [J. *Arnold,* German pathologist, 1835–1915; and H. *Chiari*]. A group of congenital anomalies at the base of the brain characteristically including an extension of the cerebellar tissue and a displacement of the medulla and inferior part of the fourth ventricle into the cervical canal; may or may not be accompanied by a meningomyelocele. Syn. *cerebellomedullary malformation syndrome.*

Ar·nold's neuralgia (ahr'no^{h}lt) [F. *Arnold,* German anatomist, 1803–1890]. A rare and ill-defined form of paroxysmal suboccipital pain that shifts to the crown of the head or, less frequently, to the shoulder. Syn. *auriculotemporal neuralgia.*

Ar·nold sterilizer (ahr'nuld) [W. E. *Arnold,* U.S. inventor, 19th century]. An apparatus for generating steam at 100°C, used to kill vegetative forms of bacteria after 15 to 30 minutes of exposure. See also *fractional sterilization.*

Ar·noux's sign (ar·noo') [E. *Arnoux,* French obstetrician, b. 1871]. In twin pregnancy the double and quadruple rhythmic sounds of the two fetal hearts beating in and then out of unison.

ar·o·mat·ic (ăr″o·mat'ick) *adj. & n.* [Gk. *arōmatikos,* from *arōma,* spice]. 1. Having a spicy odor. 2. Characterized by a fragrant, spicy taste and odor, as cinnamon, ginger, or an essential oil. 3. Any aromatic plant or substance, as a medicine or drug. 4. Designating any carbon compound originating from benzene, C_6H_6, or containing at least one benzene ring or similar unsaturated heterocyclic ring, as pyridine. 5. Any aromatic organic compound.

aromatic acid. Any acid derived from benzene or containing a benzene or other aromatic ring.

aromatic alcohol. Any alcohol containing a benzene or other aromatic ring.

aromatic ammonia spirit. A flavored, hydroalcoholic solution of ammonia and ammonium carbonate having an aromatic, pungent odor; used as a reflex stimulant.

aromatic bitters. Medicinal preparations that combine the properties of aromatics with those of simple bitters.

aromatic elixir. A pleasant-tasting vehicle prepared from compound orange spirit, syrup, and alcohol.

aromatic series. The series of organic compounds derived from benzene and characterized by the presence of a number of carbon atoms arranged in the form of a closed chain with conjugate double bonds.

aromatic water. WATER (2).

arous·al reaction (uh·row'zul). The electrical change from cerebral cortical rhythms characteristic of a sleeping or anesthetized animal to rhythms resembling those recorded during the waking condition, produced by stimulation of parts of the ascending reticular activating system, and leading to physical signs of arousal in the animal.

Arquel. A trademark for meclofenamic acid, an anti-inflammatory agent.

ar·rec·tor (a·reck'tur) *n.*, pl. **ar·rec·to·res** (ar"eck·to'reez) [NL., from L. *arrigere,* to set up, from *ad-* + *regere,* to direct]. An erector muscle.

arrector pi·li (pye'lye), pl. **arrectores pi·lor·um** (pi·lo'rum). Any of the minute, fan-like, involuntary muscles attached to the hair follicles which, by contraction, erect the hair and cause so-called goose-flesh. Syn. *pilomotor muscle.* NA (pl.) *musculi arrectores pilorum.* See also Table of Muscles in the Appendix.

ar·rest (uh·rest') *v. & n.* 1. To interrupt or check. 2. To render inactive. 3. An interruption or stoppage, as of a bodily, developmental, or pathological process.

ar·rest·ed development. Failure of an organism to carry out its normal growth processes, stopping at an initial or intermediate stage of the process; used particularly in reference to psychological development.

arrhen-, arrheno- [Gk. *arrhēn*]. A combining form meaning *male.*

ar·rhe·no·blas·to·ma (ăr"e·no·blas·to'muh, a·ree"no·) *n.* [*arrheno-* + *blastoma*]. An ovarian tumor, sometimes malignant, whose cells reproduce to varying degrees the appearance of immature testicular tubules, the less differentiated forms being masculinizing.

ar·rhe·no·ma (ăr"e·no'muh) *n.* [*arrhen-* + *-oma*]. ARRHENOBLASTOMA.

ar·rhe·no·no·ma (ăr"e·no·no'muh) *n.* ARRHENOBLASTOMA.

ar·rhe·no·to·cia (ăr"e·no·to'see·uh, ·shee·uh, a·ree"no·) *n.* ARRHENOTOKY.

ar·rhe·not·o·ky (ăr"e·not'uh·kee) *n.* [Gk. *arrhenotokia,* the bearing of male children, from *arrhēn,* male, + *tokos,* childbirth]. *In zoology,* the parthenogenetic production of male individuals exclusively. —**arrhenoto·kous** (·kus) *adj.*

ar·rhin·en·ce·pha·lia, arhin·en·ce·pha·lia (ăr"in·en·se·fay'lee·uh, ay·rye"nen·) *n.* [*a-* + *rhinencephal*on + *-ia*]. A form of partial anencephalia in which there is partial or total absence of the rhinencephalon and malformation of the nose.

ar·rhin·en·ceph·a·ly (a·rin"en·sef'uh·lee, ay·rye"nen·) *n.* ARRHINENCEPHALIA.

ar·rhi·nia, arhi·nia (a·rin'ee·uh, a·rye'nee·uh) *n.* [Gk. *arrhinos,* noseless, + *-ia*]. Congenital absence of the nose.—**arrhi·nic** (·nick) *adj.*

ar·rhyth·mia, arhyth·mia (a·rith'mee·uh) *n.* [Gk. *arrhythmos,* unrhythmical, + *-ia*]. An alteration or abnormality of normal cardiac rhythm. —**arrhyth·mic, arhyth·mic** (·mick) *adj.*

ar·rhyth·mo·gen·ic (a·rith"mo·jen'ick) *adj.* Producing arrhythmia.

ar·row·root, *n.* [from its use by American Indians to absorb arrow poison from wounds]. A variety of starch derived from *Maranta arundinacea,* a plant of the West Indies and southern United States.

ar·sa·nil·ic acid (ahr"suh·nil'ick). *p*-Aminobenzenearsonic acid, $NH_2C_6H_4AsO(OH)_2$, the starting compound for the synthesis of many useful medicinal arsenicals.

arsen-, arseno-. A combining form designating (a) *a compound containing arsenic;* (b) *a compound containing the —As:As— group.*

ar·se·nate (ahr'se·nate) *n.* Any salt or ester of arsenic acid.

ar·se·nic (ahr'se·nick, ahrs'nick) *n.* [Gk. *arsenikon,* yellow orpiment, from Ar. *az-zirnīkh,* from Pers. *zirnīkh,* from *zar,* gold]. As = 74.9216. 1. A brittle, usually steel-gray element of both metallic and nonmetallic properties. It exists in four allotropic modifications, the most important of which is the gray, or so-called metallic, arsenic. It sublimes readily, the vapor having a garlicky odor. Its salts have been used in medicine for their tonic effect, for ability to increase the hematinic effect of iron, in skin diseases, in certain pulmonary diseases, for destruction of protozoan parasites, and as caustics. 2. ARSENIC TRIOXIDE.

ar·sen·ic (ahr·sen'ick) *adj.* Of, pertaining to, or containing arsenic.

arsenic acid. Orthoarsenic acid, H_3AsO_4; used in the manufacture of medicinal and insecticidal arsenates.

ar·sen·i·cal (ahr·sen'i·kul) *adj. & n.* 1. Of, pertaining to, caused by, or containing arsenic. 2. A drug, fungicide, or insecticide the effect of which depends on its arsenic content.

arsenical carcinoma. A carcinoma of the skin following prolonged ingestion or exposure to arsenical compounds.

arsenical keratosis. Hyperkeratosis, usually of the palms and soles, due to arsenic in the body as a result of ingestion or injection.

arsenical paralysis. ARSENICAL POLYNEUROPATHY.

arsenical polyneuropathy. Polyneuropathy with paresthesia, sensory deficits, and muscle weakness seen in the later stages of arsenic poisoning, and often associated with hyperpigmentation of the skin, palmar and plantar hyperkeratosis, white transverse lines (Mees' lines) on the nails, and sometimes signs and symptoms of encephalopathy.

arsenical tremor. A tremor seen in arsenic poisoning.

arsenic trioxide. Arsenous oxide, As_2O_3, the principal form in which inorganic arsenic was used medicinally. Syn. *arsenous acid, white arsenic.*

ar·se·nide (ahr'se·nide) *n.* [*arsen-* + *-ide*]. A compound of arsenic with another element in which the arsenic is negatively charged.

ar·se·ni·ous (ahr·see'nee·us) *adj.* ARSENOUS.

ar·se·nite (ahr'se·nite) *n.* [*arsen-* + *-ite*]. A salt of arsenous acid.

ar·sen·iu·ret (ahr·sen'yoo·ret) *n.* [*arsenic* + *-uret*]. *Obsol.* ARSENIDE.

ar·sen·iu·ret·ted (ahr·sen'yoo·ret"id) *adj.* Combined with arsenic so as to form an arsenide.

arseno-. See *arsen-.*

ar·se·no·cho·line (ahr"se·no·ko'leen) *n.* A choline analogue which contains arsenic in place of nitrogen. It can be incorporated into lecithins for prevention of the fatty liver of choline deficiency.

ar·se·no·ther·a·py (ahr"se·no·therr'uh·pee) *n.* Treatment of disease by means of arsenical drugs.

ar·se·nous (ahr'se·nus, ahr·see'nous) *adj.* [*arsen-* + *-ous*]. Containing arsenic in the positive trivalent form.

arsenous acid. ARSENIC TRIOXIDE.

arsenous oxide. ARSENIC TRIOXIDE.

ar·sen·ox·ide (ahr"se·nock'side) *n.* 3-Amino-4-hydroxyphenylarsine oxide, $C_6H_6AsNO_2$; a metabolic product of arsphenamine which accounts for its activity. See also *oxophenarsine hydrochloride.*

ar·sine (ahr·seen', ahr'seen, ahr'sin) *n.* Hydrogen arsenide, or arsenous hydride, AsH_3. A poisonous gas with a garlicky odor.

ar·sin·ic acid (ahr·sin'ick). Any acid of the type of RHAs(:O)OH or of RR'As(:O)OH, where R is any hydrocarbon radical and R' is the same or a different hydrocarbon radical.

ar·son·ic acid (ahr·son'ick). Any acid of the type of $RAs(:O)(OH)_2$, where R is any hydrocarbon radical.

ar·son·val·iza·tion (ahr"sun·val"i·zay'shun) *n.* [J. A. d'*Arsonval*]. D'ARSONVALIZATION.

ars·phen·a·mine (ahrs·fen'uh·meen, ·min) *n.* [*arsenic* + *phen-* + *amine*]. Diaminodihydroxyarsenobenzene dihydrochloride, $C_{12}H_{12}As_2N_2O_2.2HCl.2H_2O$. The antisyphilitic, effective also in other protozoal infections, first prepared by Ehrlich in 1909. It has been superseded by other organic arsenicals and by antibiotics. Syn. *Ehrlich's 606.*

ars·thi·nol (ahrs'thi·nol, nole) *n.* The cyclic 3-hydroxypropylene ester of 3-acetamido-4-hydroxydithiobenzenearsonous acid, $C_{11}H_{14}AsNO_3S_2$, a trivalent arsenical; effective against intestinal amebiasis and yaws.

Artane. Trademark for trihexyphenidyl, an antispasmodic drug used as the hydrochloride salt.

artefact. ARTIFACT.

ar·te·graft (ahr'te·graft) *n.* An arterial graft consisting of a segment of bovine carotid artery with the enzyme ficin and dialdehyde starch.

Ar·te·mis·ia (ahr"te·miz'ee·uh) *n.* [after *Artemis,* Greek goddess of forest and hills]. A genus of widely distributed plants of the Compositae. Various members have been used in folk medicine, including absinthium and santonica. Because the pollens of these plants are wind-borne, they are among the more important causes of hay fever, especially in the Mountain and Pacific states.

ar·ter·ec·to·my (ahr"tur·eck'tuh·mee) *n.* ARTERIECTOMY.

ar·ter·e·nol (ahr·teer'e·nole, ahr"tur·en'ol) *n.* NOREPINEPHRINE.

arteri-, arterio-. A combining form meaning *artery, arterial.*

ar·te·ria (ahr·teer'ee·uh) *n.*, pl. & genit. sing. **arte·ri·ae** (·ee·ee) [L.]. ARTERY. Abbreviated, a.

arteria ace·ta·bu·li (as·e·tab'yoo·lye) [BNA]. Ramus acetabularis arteriae obturatoriae (= the acetabular branch of the obturator artery).

arteria al·ve·o·la·ris inferior (al·vee·o·lair'is) [NA]. The inferior alveolar artery. See *alveolar artery.*

arteria alveolaris superior posterior [NA]. The posterior superior alveolar artery. See *alveolar artery.*

arteria an·gu·la·ris (ang·gew·lair'is) [NA]. ANGULAR ARTERY.

arteria ano·ny·ma (a·non'i·muh) [BNA]. Truncus brachiocephalicus (= BRACHIOCEPHALIC TRUNK).

arteria ap·pen·di·cu·la·ris (ap"en·dick·yoo·lair'is) [NA]. APPENDICULAR ARTERY.

arteria ar·cu·a·ta pe·dis (ahr·kew·ay'tuh ped'is) [NA]. The arcuate artery of the foot. See *arcuate artery.*

arteria as·cen·dens ileo·co·li·ca (a·sen'denz il"ee·o·ko'li·kuh) [NA]. The ascending branch of the ileocolic artery.

arteria au·di·ti·va in·ter·na (aw·di·tye'vuh in·tur'nuh) [BNA]. Arteria labyrinthi (= LABYRINTHINE ARTERY).

arteria au·ri·cu·la·ris posterior (aw·rick"yoo·lair'is) [NA]. The posterior auricular artery. See Table of Arteries in the Appendix.

arteria auricularis pro·fun·da (pro·fun'duh) [NA]. The deep auricular artery. See Table of Arteries in the Appendix.

arteria ax·il·la·ris (ack·si·lair'is) [NA]. The axillary artery. See Table of Arteries in the Appendix.

arteria ba·si·la·ris (bas·i·lair'is) [NA]. BASILAR ARTERY.

arteria bra·chi·a·lis (bray·kee·ay'lis) [NA]. BRACHIAL ARTERY.

arteria brachialis su·per·fi·ci·a·lis (sue"pur·fish·ee·ay'lis) [NA]. A variant superficial vessel arising from a high division of the brachial artery.

arteria buc·ca·lis (buh·kay'lis) [NA]. BUCCAL ARTERY.

arteria buc·ci·na·to·ria (buck·si·nuh·to'ree·uh) [BNA]. Arteria buccalis (= BUCCAL ARTERY).

arteria bul·bi pe·nis (bul'bye pee'nis) [NA]. The artery of the bulb of the penis. See Table of Arteries in the Appendix.

arteria bulbi ure·thrae (yoo·ree'three) [BNA]. Arteria bulbi penis. See *bulb of penis* in Table of Arteries in the Appendix.

arteria bulbi ves·ti·bu·li (ves·tib'yoo·lye) [NA]. Artery of the bulb of the vestibule of the vagina. See Table of Arteries in the Appendix.

arteria ca·na·lis pte·ry·goi·dei (ka·nay'lis terr·i·goy'dee·eye) [NA]. The artery of the pterygoid canal. See Table of Arteries in the Appendix.

arteria ca·ro·tis com·mu·nis (ka·ro'tis, ka·rot'is kom·yoo'nis) [NA]. COMMON CAROTID ARTERY.

arteria carotis ex·ter·na (eck·stur'nuh) [NA]. EXTERNAL CAROTID ARTERY.

arteria carotis in·ter·na (in·tur'nuh) [NA]. INTERNAL CAROTID ARTERY.

arteria cau·dae pan·cre·a·tis (kaw'dee pan·kree'uh·tis) [NA]. A branch of the splenic (lienal) artery to the tail of the pancreas.

arteria ce·ca·lis anterior (see·kay'lis) [NA]. The anterior cecal branch of the ileocolic artery.

arteria cecalis posterior [NA]. The posterior cecal branch of the ileocolic artery.

arteria cen·tra·lis re·ti·nae (sen·tray'lis ret'i·nee) [NA]. The central artery of the retina.

arteria ce·re·bel·li inferior anterior (serr·e·bel'eye) [NA]. The anterior inferior cerebellar artery. See Table of Arteries in the Appendix.

arteria cerebelli inferior posterior [NA]. The posterior inferior cerebellar artery. See Table of Arteries in the Appendix.

arteria cerebelli superior [NA]. The superior cerebellar artery. See Table of Arteries in the Appendix.

arteria ce·re·bri anterior (serr'e·brye) [NA]. The anterior cerebral artery. See Table of Arteries in the Appendix.

arteria cerebri me·dia (mee'dee·uh) [NA]. The middle cerebral artery. See Table of Arteries in the Appendix.

arteria cerebri posterior [NA]. The posterior cerebral artery. See Table of Arteries in the Appendix.

arteria cer·vi·ca·lis ascen·dens (sur·vi·kay'lis a·sen'denz) [NA]. The ascending cervical artery. See Table of Arteries in the Appendix.

arteria cervicalis pro·fun·da (pro·fun'duh) [NA]. The deep cervical artery. See Table of Arteries in the Appendix.

arteria cervicalis su·per·fi·ci·a·lis (sue"pur·fish·ee·ay'lis) [NA]. The superficial cervical artery. See Table of Arteries in the Appendix.

arteria cho·ri·oi·dea (ko·ree·oy'dee·uh) [BNA]. Arteria choroidea anterior. See *choroid* in Table of Arteries in the Appendix.

arteria cho·roi·dea anterior (ko·roy'dee·uh) [NA]. The anterior choroid artery. See Table of Arteries in the Appendix.

arteria cir·cum·flexa fe·mo·ris la·te·ra·lis (sur·kum·fleck'suh fem'o·ris lat·e·ray'lis) [NA]. The lateral femoral circumflex artery. See Table of Arteries in the Appendix.

arteria circumflexa femoris me·di·a·lis (mee·dee·ay'lis) [NA]. The medial femoral circumflex artery. See Table of Arteries in the Appendix.

arteria circumflexa hu·me·ri anterior (hew'mur·eye) [NA]. The anterior humeral circumflex artery. See Table of Arteries in the Appendix.

arteria circumflexa humeri posterior [NA]. The posterior humeral circumflex artery. See Table of Arteries in the Appendix.

arteria circumflexa ilii pro·fun·da (il'ee·eye pro·fun'duh) [NA]. The deep iliac circumflex artery. See Table of Arteries in the Appendix.

arteria circumflexa ilii su·per·fi·ci·a·lis (sue"pur·fish·ee·ay'lis) [NA]. The superficial iliac circumflex artery. See Table of Arteries in the Appendix.

arteria circumflexa sca·pu·lae (skap'yoo·lee) [NA]. The circumflex scapular artery. See Table of Arteries in the Appendix.

arteria coe·li·a·ca (see·lye'uh·kuh) [BNA]. Truncus celiacus (= CELIAC TRUNK).

arteria co·li·ca dex·tra (ko'li·kuh decks'truh) [NA]. The right colic artery. See Table of Arteries in the Appendix.

arteria colica me·dia (mee'dee·uh) [NA]. The middle colic artery. See Table of Arteries in the Appendix.

arteria colica si·nis·tra (si·nis'truh) [NA]. The left colic artery. See Table of Arteries in the Appendix.

arteria col·la·te·ra·lis me·dia (ko·lat"e·ray'lis mee'dee·uh) [NA]. MIDDLE COLLATERAL ARTERY.

arteria collateralis ra·di·a·lis (ray·dee·ay'lis) [NA]. RADIAL COLLATERAL ARTERY.

arteria collateralis ul·na·ris inferior (ul·nair'is) [NA]. The inferior ulnar collateral artery. See *ulnar collateral artery.*

arteria collateralis ulnaris superior [NA]. The superior ulnar collateral artery. See *ulnar collateral artery.*

arteria co·mi·tans ner·vi is·chi·a·di·ci (kom'i·tanz nur'vye is·kee·ad'i·sigh) [NA]. The companion artery of the sciatic nerve; SCIATIC ARTERY.

arteria com·mu·ni·cans an·te·ri·or ce·re·bri (kom·yoo'ni·kanz an·teer'ee·or serr'e·brye) [NA]. ANTERIOR COMMUNICATING ARTERY.

arteria communicans posterior cerebri [NA]. POSTERIOR COMMUNICATING ARTERY.

arteria co·ro·na·ria dex·tra (kor·o·nair'ee·uh deck'struh) [NA]. The right coronary artery. See Table of Arteries in the Appendix.

arteria coronaria si·nis·tra (si·nis'truh) [NA]. The left coronary artery. See Table of Arteries in the Appendix.

arteria cre·mas·te·ri·ca (krem·as·terr'i·kuh) [NA]. CREMASTERIC ARTERY.

arteria cys·ti·ca (sis'ti·kuh) [NA]. CYSTIC ARTERY.

arteria de·fe·ren·ti·a·lis (def"e·ren"shee·ay'lis) [BNA]. Arteria ductus deferentis (= DEFERENTIAL ARTERY).

arteria dor·sa·lis cli·to·ri·dis (dor·say'lis kli·tor'i·dis) [NA]. The dorsal artery of the clitoris. See Table of Arteries in the Appendix.

arteria dorsalis na·si (nay'zye) [NA]. The dorsal nasal artery. See Table of Arteries in the Appendix.

arteria dorsalis pe·dis (ped'is) [NA]. The dorsal pedal artery. See Table of Arteries in the Appendix.

arteria dorsalis pe·nis (pee'nis) [NA]. Dorsal artery of the penis. See Table of Arteries in the Appendix.

arteria duc·tus de·fe·ren·tis (duck'toos def"e·ren'tis) [NA]. DEFERENTIAL ARTERY.

arteriae. Plural and genitive singular of *arteria.*

arteriae al·ve·o·la·res su·pe·ri·o·res an·te·ri·o·res (al·vee·o·lair'eez sue·peer·ee·o'reez an·teer·ee·o'reez) [NA]. The anterior superior alveolar arteries. See *alveolar artery.*

arteriae ar·ci·for·mes (ahr·si·for'meez) [BNA]. Arteriae arcuatae renis. See *arcuate artery.*

arteriae ar·cu·a·tae re·nis (ahr·kew·ay'tee ree'nis) [NA]. Arcuate arteries of the kidney. See *arcuate artery.*

arteriae bron·chi·a·les (brong·kee·ay'leez) [BNA]. The arteries that supply the bronchi. They are quite variable in origin, course, and distribution. The commonest origin is from the thoracic aorta.

arteriae ce·re·bri (serr'e·brye) [NA]. The cerebral arteries. See Table of Arteries in the Appendix.

arteriae ci·li·a·res an·te·ri·o·res (sil·ee·air'eez an·teer·ee·o'reez) [NA]. The anterior ciliary arteries. See *ciliary artery.*

arteriae ciliares pos·te·ri·o·res bre·ves (pos·teer·ee·o'reez brev'eez) [NA]. The short posterior ciliary arteries. See *ciliary artery.*

arteriae ciliares posteriores lon·gae (long'ghee, lon'jee) [NA]. The long posterior ciliary arteries. See *ciliary artery.*

arteriae con·junc·ti·va·les an·te·ri·o·res (kon·junk·ti·vay'leez an·teer·ee·o'reez) [NA]. The anterior conjunctival arteries. See Table of Arteries in the Appendix.

arteriae conjunctivales pos·te·ri·o·res (pos·teer·ee·o'reez) [NA]. The posterior conjunctival arteries. See Table of Arteries in the Appendix.

arteriae di·gi·ta·les dor·sa·les ma·nus (dij·i·tay'leez dor·say'leez man'oos) [NA]. The dorsal digital arteries of the hand. See Table of Arteries in the Appendix.

arteriae digitales dorsales pe·dis (ped'is) [NA]. The dorsal digital arteries of the foot. See Table of Arteries in the Appendix.

arteriae digitales pal·ma·res com·mu·nes (pal·mair'eez kom·yoo'neez) [NA]. The common palmar digital arteries. See Table of Arteries in the Appendix.

arteriae digitales palmares pro·pri·ae (pro'pree·ee) [NA]. The proper palmar digital arteries. See Table of Arteries in the Appendix.

arteriae digitales plan·ta·res com·mu·nes (plan·tair'eez kom·yoo'neez) [NA]. The common plantar digital arteries. See Table of Arteries in the Appendix.

arteriae digitales plantares pro·pri·ae (pro'pree·ee) [NA]. The proper plantar digital arteries. See Table of Arteries in the Appendix.

arteriae digitales vo·la·res com·mu·nes (vo·lair'eez kom·yoo'neez) [BNA]. Arteriae digitales palmares communes (= the common palmar digital arteries).

arteriae digitales volares pro·pri·ae (pro'pree·ee) [BNA]. Arteriae digitales palmares propriae (= the proper palmar digital arteries).

arteriae epi·scle·ra·les (ep"i·skle·ray'leez) [NA]. The episcleral arteries. See Table of Arteries in the Appendix.

arteriae gas·tri·cae bre·ves (gas'tri·see brev'eez) [NA]. The short gastric arteries. See Table of Arteries in the Appendix.

arteriae he·li·ci·nae pe·nis (hel·i·sigh'nee pee'nis) [NA]. The helicine arteries of the penis; the small coiled arteries that empty into the spaces of the corpora cavernosa.

arteriae ile·ae (il'ee·ee) [BNA]. Arteriae ilei (= the ileal arteries).

arteriae ilei (il'ee·eye) [NA]. The ileal arteries. See Table of Arteries in the Appendix.

arteriae in·ter·cos·ta·les pos·te·ri·o·res I et II (in·tur·kos·tay'leez pos·teer·ee·o'reez) [NA]. Posterior intercostal arteries I, II. See Table of Arteries in the Appendix.

arteriae intercostales posteriores III–XI [NA]. Posterior intercostal arteries III–XI. See Table of Arteries in the Appendix.

arteriae in·ter·lo·ba·res re·nis (in·tur·lo·bair'eez ree'nis) [NA]. INTERLOBAR ARTERIES OF THE KIDNEY.

arteriae in·ter·lo·bu·la·res he·pa·tis (in"tur·lob·yoo·lair'eez hep'uh·tis) [NA]. The interlobular arteries of the liver. See *interlobular artery.*

arteriae interlobulares re·nis (ree'nis) [NA]. The interlobular arteries of the kidney. See *interlobular artery.*

arteriae in·tes·ti·na·les (in·tes·ti·nay'leez) [BNA]. INTESTINAL ARTERIES.

arteriae je·ju·na·les (je·joo·nay'leez) [NA]. The jejunal arteries. See Table of Arteries in the Appendix.

arteriae la·bi·a·les an·te·ri·o·res pu·den·di mu·li·e·bris (lay·bee·ay'leez an·teer·ee·o'reez pew·den'dye mew·lee·ee'bris) [BNA]. Rami labiales anteriores arteriae femoralis (= the anterior labial branches of the femoral artery).

arteriae labiales pos·te·ri·o·res pu·den·di mu·li·e·bris (pos·teer·ee·o'reez pew·den'dye mew·lee·ee'bris) [BNA]. Rami labiales posteriores arteriae pudendae internae (= the posterior labial branches of the internal pudendal artery).

arteriae lum·ba·les (lum·bay'leez) [NA]. The lumbar arteries. See Table of Arteries in the Appendix.

arteriae me·di·as·ti·na·les an·te·ri·o·res (mee"dee·as·ti·nay'leez an·teer·ee·o'reez) [BNA]. Rami mediastinales aortae thoracicae internae (= the mediastinal branches of the internal thoracic artery.

arteriae me·ta·car·pe·ae dor·sa·les (met·uh·kahr'pee·ee dor·say'leez) [NA]. The dorsal metacarpal arteries. See Table of Arteries in the Appendix.

arteriae metacarpeae pal·ma·res (pal·mair'eez) [NA]. The palmar metacarpal arteries. See Table of Arteries in the Appendix.

arteriae metacarpeae vo·la·res (vo·lair'eez) [BNA]. Arteriae metacarpeae palmares (= the palmar metacarpal arteries).

arteriae me·ta·tar·se·ae dor·sa·les (met·uh·tahr'see·ee dor·say'leez) [NA]. The dorsal metatarsal arteries. See Table of Arteries in the Appendix.

arteriae metatarseae plan·ta·res (plan·tair'eez) [NA]. The plantar metatarsal arteries. See Table of Arteries in the Appendix.

arteriae na·sa·les pos·te·ri·o·res, la·te·ra·les, et sep·ti (na·say'leez pos·teer·ee·o'reez lat·e·ray'leez et sep'tye) [NA]. The posterior, lateral, and septal nasal arteries. See Table of Arteries in the Appendix.

arteriae nu·tri·ci·ae hu·me·ri (new·trye'see·ee, new·trish'ee·ee hew'mur·eye) [NA]. Nutrient arteries of the humerus.

arteriae nutriciae pel·vis re·na·lis (pel'vis re·nay'lis) [BNA]. Nutrient arteries of the renal *pelvis.*

arteriae oe·so·pha·ge·ae (ee·so·faj'ee·ee) [BNA]. Rami esophagei aortae thoracicae (= the esophageal branches of the thoracic aorta).

arteriae pa·la·ti·nae mi·no·res (pal·uh·tye'nee mi·no'reez) [NA]. The lesser palatine arteries. See Table of Arteries in the Appendix.

arteriae pal·pe·bra·les la·te·ra·les (pal·pe·bray'leez lat·e·ray'leez) [NA]. The lateral palpebral arteries. See *palpebal artery.*

arteriae palpebrales me·di·a·les (mee·dee·ay'leez) [NA]. The medial palpebral arteries. See *palpebral artery.*

arteriae pan·cre·a·ti·co·du·o·de·na·les in·fe·ri·o·res (pan·kree·at"i·ko·dew·o·de·nay'leez in·feer·ee·o'reez) [NA]. The inferior pancreaticoduodenal arteries. See Table of Arteries in the Appendix.

arteriae per·fo·ran·tes (pur·fo·ran'teez) [NA]. PERFORATING ARTERIES.

arteriae phre·ni·cae in·fe·ri·o·res (fren'i·see in·feer·ee·o'reez) [NA]. The inferior phrenic arteries. See Table of Arteries in the Appendix.

arteriae phrenicae su·pe·ri·o·res (sue·peer·ee·o'reez) [NA]. The superior phrenic arteries. See Table of Arteries in the Appendix.

arteria epi·gas·tri·ca inferior (ep·i·gas'tri·kuh) [NA]. The inferior epigastric artery. See Table of Arteries in the Appendix.

arteria epigastrica su·per·fi·ci·a·lis (sue"pur·fish·ee·ay'lis) [NA]. The superficial epigastric artery. See Table of Arteries in the Appendix.

arteria epigastrica superior [NA]. The superior epigastric artery. See Table of Arteries in the Appendix.

arteriae pu·den·dae ex·ter·nae (pew·den'dee ecks·tur'nee) [NA]. The external pudendal arteries. See Table of Arteries in the Appendix.

arteriae re·cur·ren·tes ul·na·res (reck·ur·en'teez ul·nair'eez) [BNA]. Plural of *arteria recurrens ulnaris.*

arteriae re·nis (ree'nis) [NA]. Renal arteries, as a group.

arteriae re·tro·du·o·de·na·les (ret"ro·dew·o·de·nay'leez) [NA]. Retroduodenal branches of the gastroduodenal artery.

arteriae sa·cra·les la·te·ra·les (sa·kray'leez lat·e·ray'leez) [NA]. The lateral sacral arteries. See Table of Arteries in the Appendix.

arteriae scro·ta·les an·te·ri·o·res (skro·tay'leez an·teer·ee·o'reez) [BNA]. Rami scrotales anteriores arteriae femoralis (= the anterior scrotal branches of the femoral artery).

arteriae scrotales pos·te·ri·o·res (pos·teer·ee·o'reez) [BNA]. Rami scrotales posteriores arteriae pudendae internae (= the posterior scrotal branches of the internal pudendal artery).

arteriae sig·moi·de·ae (sig·moy'dee·ee) [NA]. The sigmoid arteries. See Table of Arteries in the Appendix.

arteriae su·pra·du·o·de·na·les su·pe·ri·o·res (sue"pruh·dew·o·de·nay'leez sue·peer·ee·o'reez) [NA]. Variable small arteries supplying the first part of the duodenum; when present they usually arise from the gastroduodenal artery.

arteriae su·ra·les (sue·ray'leez) [NA]. The sural arteries. See Table of Arteries in the Appendix.

arteriae tar·se·ae me·di·a·les (tahr'see·ee mee·dee·ay'leez) [NA]. The medial tarsal arteries. See Table of Arteries in the Appendix.

arteriae tem·po·ra·les pro·fun·dae (tem·po·ray'leez pro·fun'dee) [NA]. The deep temporal arteries. See Table of Arteries in the Appendix.

arteria eth·moi·da·lis anterior (eth·moy·day'lis) [NA]. The anterior ethmoid artery. See Table of Arteries in the Appendix.

arteria ethmoidalis posterior [NA]. The posterior ethmoid artery. See Table of Arteries in the Appendix.

arteriae thy·mi·cae (thigh'mi·see) [BNA]. Rami thymici arteriae thoracicae internae (= the thymic branches of the internal thoracic artery).

arteriae ve·si·ca·les in·fe·ri·o·res (ves·i·kay'leez in·feer·ee·o'reez) [BNA]. Plural of arteria vesicalis inferior.

arteriae vesicales su·pe·ri·o·res (sue·peer·ee·o'reez) [NA]. The superior vesical arteries. See Table of Arteries in the Appendix.

arteria fa·ci·a·lis (fay·shee·ay'lis) [NA]. FACIAL ARTERY.

arteria fe·mo·ra·lis (fem·o·ray'lis) [NA]. FEMORAL ARTERY.

arteria fi·bu·la·ris (fib·yoo·lair'is) [NA alt.]. PERONEAL ARTERY. NA alt. *arteria peronea.*

arteria fron·ta·lis (fron·tay'lis) [BNA]. Arteria supratrochlearis (= the supratrochlear artery).

arteria gas·tri·ca dex·tra (gas'tri·kuh decks'truh) [NA]. The right gastric artery. See Table of Arteries in the Appendix.

arteria gastrica si·nis·tra (si·nis'truh) [NA]. The left gastric artery. See Table of Arteries in the Appendix.

arteria gas·tro·du·o·de·na·lis (gas"tro·dew·o·de·nay'lis) [NA]. The gastroduodenal artery. See Table of Arteries in the Appendix.

arteria gas·tro·epi·plo·i·ca dex·tra (gas"tro·ep·i·plo'i·kuh decks'truh) [NA]. The right gastroepiploic artery. See Table of Arteries in the Appendix.

arteria gastroepiploica si·nis·tra (si·nis'truh) [NA]. The left gastroepiploic artery. See Table of Arteries in the Appendix.

arteria ge·nu in·fe·ri·or la·te·ra·lis (jen'yoo in·feer'ee·or lat·e·ray'lis) [BNA]. Arteria genus inferior lateralis. See *genicular* in Table of Arteries in the Appendix.

arteria genu inferior me·di·a·lis (mee·dee·ay'lis) [BNA]. Arteria genus inferior medialis. See *genicular* in Table of Arteries in the Appendix.

arteria genu me·dia (mee'dee·uh) [BNA]. Arteria genus media. See *genicular* in Table of Arteries in the Appendix.

arteria ge·nus de·scen·dens (jen'oos de·sen'denz) [NA]. The descending genicular artery. See Table of Arteries in the Appendix.

arteria genus inferior la·te·ra·lis (lat·e·ray'lis) [NA]. The lateral inferior genicular artery. See Table of Arteries in the Appendix.

arteria genus inferior me·di·a·lis (mee·dee·ay'lis) [NA]. The medial inferior genicular artery. See Table of Arteries in the Appendix.

arteria genus me·dia (mee'dee·uh) [NA]. The middle genicular artery. See Table of Arteries in the Appendix.

arteria genus superior la·te·ra·lis (lat·e·ray'lis) [NA]. The lateral superior genicular artery. See Table of Arteries in the Appendix.

arteria genus superior me·di·a·lis (mee·dee·ay'lis) [NA]. The medial superior genicular artery. See Table of Arteries in the Appendix.

arteria ge·nu su·pe·ri·or la·te·ra·lis (jen'yoo sue·peer'ee·or lat·e·ray'lis) [BNA]. Arteria genus superior lateralis. See *genicular* in Table of Arteries in the Appendix.

arteria genu superior me·di·a·lis (mee·dee·ay'lis) [BNA]. Arteria genus superior medialis. See *genicular* in Table of Arteries in the Appendix.

arteria genu su·pre·ma (sue·pree'muh) [BNA]. Arteria genus descendens. See *genicular* in Table of Arteries in the Appendix.

arteria glu·taea inferior (gloo·tee'uh) [BNA]. Arteria glutea inferior. See *gluteal* in Table of Arteries in the Appendix.

arteria glutaea superior [BNA]. Arteria glutea superior. See *gluteal* in Table of Arteries in the Appendix.

arteria glu·tea inferior (gloo'tee·uh, gloo·tee'uh) [NA]. The inferior gluteal artery. See Table of Arteries in the Appendix.

arteria glutea superior [NA]. The superior gluteal artery. See Table of Arteries in the Appendix.

arteria hae·mor·rhoi·da·lis inferior (hem″o·roy·day′lis) [BNA]. Arteria rectalis inferior. See *rectal* in Table of Arteries in the Appendix.

arteria haemorrhoidalis me·dia (mee′dee·uh) [BNA]. Arteria rectalis media. See *rectal* in Table of Arteries in the Appendix.

arteria haemorrhoidalis superior [BNA]. Arteria rectalis superior. See *rectal* in Table of Arteries in the Appendix.

arteria he·pa·ti·ca (he·pat′i·kuh) [BNA]. Arteria hepatica communis (= COMMON HEPATIC ARTERY).

arteria hepatica com·mu·nis (kom·yoo′nis) [NA]. COMMON HEPATIC ARTERY.

arteria hepatica pro·pria (pro′pree·uh) [NA]. PROPER HEPATIC ARTERY.

arteria hy·a·loi·dea (high·uh·loy′dee·uh) [NA]. HYALOID ARTERY.

arteria hy·po·gas·tri·ca (high·po·gas′tri·kuh) [BNA]. Arteria iliaca interna. See *iliac* in Table of Arteries in the Appendix.

arteria ileo·co·li·ca (il·ee·o·ko′li·kuh) [NA]. The ileocolic artery. See Table of Arteries in the Appendix.

arteria ili·a·ca com·mu·nis (i·lye′uh·kuh kom·yoo′nis) [NA]. The common iliac artery. See Table of Arteries in the Appendix.

arteria iliaca ex·ter·na (ecks·tur′nuh) [NA]. The external iliac artery. See Table of Arteries in the Appendix.

arteria iliaca in·ter·na (in·tur′nuh) [NA]. The internal iliac artery. See Table of Arteries in the Appendix.

arteria ilio·lum·ba·lis (il·ee·o·lum·bay′lis) [NA]. The iliolumbar artery. See Table of Arteries in Appendix.

arteria in·fra·or·bi·ta·lis (in″fra·or·bi·tay′lis) [NA]. The infraorbital artery. See Table of Arteries in the Appendix.

arteria in·ter·cos·ta·lis su·pre·ma (in″tur·kos·tay′lis sue·pree′muh) [NA]. The highest intercostal artery. See Table of Arteries in the Appendix.

arteria in·ter·os·sea anterior (in·tur·os′ee·uh) [NA]. The anterior interosseous artery. See Table of Arteries in the Appendix.

arteria interossea com·mu·nis (kom·yoo′nis) [NA]. The common interosseous artery. See Table of Arteries in the Appendix.

arteria interossea dor·sa·lis (dor·say′lis) [BNA]. Arteria interossea posterior. See *interosseous* in Table of Arteries in the Appendix.

arteria interossea posterior [NA]. The posterior interosseous artery. See Table of Arteries in the Appendix.

arteria interossea re·cur·rens (re·kur′enz) [NA]. The recurrent interosseous artery. See Table of Arteries in the Appendix.

arteria interossea vo·la·ris (vo·lair′is) [BNA]. Arteria interossea anterior. See *interosseous* in Table of Arteries in the Appendix.

ar·te·ri·al (ahr·teer′ee·ul) *adj.* Of or pertaining to an artery.

arteria la·bi·a·lis inferior (lay·bee·ay′lis) [NA]. The inferior labial artery. See Table of Arteries in the Appendix.

arteria labialis superior [NA]. The superior labial artery. See Table of Arteries in the Appendix.

arteria la·by·rin·thi (lab·i·rin′thigh) [NA]. LABYRINTHINE ARTERY.

arteria la·cri·ma·lis (lack·ri·may′lis) [NA]. The lacrimal artery. See Table of Arteries in the Appendix.

arterial arc of Rio·lan (ryo^h·lah^n′) [J. *Riolan*, French anatomist, 1580–1637]. An occasional artery situated in the posterior abdominal wall which forms a connection between the superior mesenteric artery and a branch of the inferior mesenteric artery.

arteria la·ryn·gea inferior (la·rin′jee·uh) [NA]. The inferior laryngeal artery. See Table of Arteries in the Appendix.

arteria laryngea superior [NA]. The superior laryngeal artery. See Table of Arteries in the Appendix.

arterial blood. The blood in the vascular system from the point of origin of the small venules in the lungs to the capillary beds in tissues where oxygen is released and carbon dioxide taken up; includes the blood in the pulmonary veins. Contr. *venous blood.*

arterial bridge. A segment of vein or a synthetic graft used to bridge a gap in an injured or diseased artery.

arterial bulb. BULB OF THE HEART.

arterial capillary. PRECAPILLARY.

arterial cerebral circle. ARTERIAL CIRCLE OF THE CEREBRUM.

arterial circle of the cerebrum. The arterial anastomosis at the base of the brain, formed in front by the anterior communicating artery joining together the anterior cerebral arteries; laterally by the internal carotid arteries and the posterior communicating arteries joining them with the posterior cerebral arteries; and behind by the posterior cerebral arteries branching from the basilar artery. NA *circulus arteriosus cerebri.*

arterial diastole. The phase of the arterial pressure pulse following arterial systole.

arterial headache. Vascular headache of the migraine type.

arterial hypertension. Abnormally elevated blood pressure in the arterial side of the circulatory system.

arteria li·e·na·lis (lye·e·nay′lis) [NA]. The lienal or splenic artery. See Table of Arteries in the Appendix.

arteria li·ga·men·ti te·re·tis ute·ri (lig·uh·men′tye te·ree′tis yoo′tur·eye) [NA]. The artery of the round ligament of the uterus. See Table of Arteries in the Appendix.

arteria lin·gua·lis (ling·gway′lis) [NA]. The lingual artery. See Table of Arteries in the Appendix.

ar·te·ri·al·iza·tion (ahr·teer″ee·ul·i·zay′shun) *n.* 1. The process of making or becoming arterial; the change from venous blood into arterial. 2. VASCULARIZATION. —**ar·te·ri·al·ize** (ahr·teer′ee·uh·lize) *v.*

arterial murmur. A sound made by arterial blood flow.

arterial nephrosclerosis. Renal atrophy and scarring characterized by coarse granulation of the parenchymal surface and by glomerular, tubular, and interstitial alterations associated with arteriosclerotic changes in the large and medium-sized renal arteries. Syn. *benign nephrosclerosis, senile arteriosclerotic nephrosclerosis.*

arteria lo·bi cau·da·ti (lo′bye kaw·day′tye) [NA]. The artery of the caudate lobe of the liver; there is one from the right branch of the proper hepatic artery and one from the left branch of the proper hepatic artery.

arterial pressure. Hydrostatic pressure of the blood within an arterial lumen.

arterial systole. The highest phase of the arterial pressure pulse, consequent upon ejection of blood from the heart.

arterial transfusion. Transfusion of blood by intraarterial injection.

arterial ulcer. Ulceration due to arterial insufficiency or occlusion.

arteria lum·ba·lis ima (lum·bay′lis eye′muh) [NA]. The lowest lumbar artery. See Table of Arteries in the Appendix.

arteria mal·le·o·la·ris an·te·ri·or la·te·ra·lis (mal·ee·o·lair′is an·teer′ee·or lat·e·ray′lis) [NA]. The anterior lateral malleolar artery. See Table of Arteries in the Appendix.

arteria malleolaris anterior me·di·a·lis (mee·dee·ay′lis) [NA]. The anterior medial malleolar artery. See Table of Arteries in the Appendix.

arteria malleolaris posterior la·te·ra·lis (lat·e·ray′lis) [BNA]. Ramus malleolaris lateralis arteriae peroneae, pl. rami malleolares laterales arteriae peroneae (= the lateral malleolar branches of the peroneal artery).

arteria malleolaris posterior me·di·a·lis (mee·dee·ay′lis) [BNA]. Ramus malleolaris medialis arteriae tibialis posterioris, pl. rami malleolares mediales arteriae tibialis posterioris (= the medial malleolar branches of the posterior tibial artery).

arteria mam·ma·ria interna (ma·mair′ee·uh) [BNA]. Arteria thoracica interna. See *thoracic* in Table of Arteries in the Appendix.

arteria mas·se·te·ri·ca (mas·e·terr'i·kuh) [NA]. The masseteric artery. See Table of Arteries in the Appendix.

arteria max·il·la·ris (mack·si·lair'is) [NA]. The maxillary artery. See Table of Arteries in the Appendix.

arteria maxillaris ex·ter·na (ecks·tur'nuh) [BNA]. Arteria facialis. (= FACIAL ARTERY).

arteria maxillaris in·ter·na (in·tur'nuh) [BNA]. Arteria maxillaris. See *maxillary* in Table of Arteries in the Appendix.

arteria me·di·a·na (mee·dee·ay'nuh) [NA]. The median artery. See Table of Arteries in the Appendix.

arteria me·nin·gea anterior (me·nin'jee·uh) [NA]. The anterior meningeal artery. See Table of Arteries in the Appendix.

arteria meningea me·dia (mee'dee·uh) [NA]. The middle meningeal artery. See Table of Arteries in the Appendix.

arteria meningea posterior [NA]. The posterior meningeal artery. See Table of Arteries in the Appendix.

arteria men·ta·lis (men·tay'lis) [NA]. The mental artery. See Table of Arteries in the Appendix.

arteria me·sen·te·ri·ca inferior (mes·en·terr'i·kuh) [NA]. The inferior mesenteric artery. See Table of Arteries in the Appendix.

arteria mesenterica superior [NA]. The superior mesenteric artery. See Table of Arteries in the Appendix.

arteria mus·cu·lo·phre·ni·ca (mus''kew·lo·fren'i·kuh) [NA]. The musculophrenic artery. See Table of Arteries in the Appendix.

arteria nu·tri·cia fe·mo·ris inferior (new·trye'see·uh, new·trish'ee·uh fem·o·ris) [BNA]. The inferior nutrient artery of the femur.

arteria nutricia femoris superior [BNA]. The superior nutrient artery of the femur.

arteria nutricia fi·bu·lae (fib'yoo·lee) [BNA]. The nutrient artery of the fibula.

arteria nutricia hu·me·ri (hew'mur·eye) [BNA]. Nutrient artery of the humerus; singular of NA *arteriae nutriciae humeri.*

arteria nutricia ti·bi·ae (tib'ee·ee) [BNA]. The nutrient artery of the tibia.

arteria ob·tu·ra·to·ria (ob·tew·ruh·to'ree·uh) [NA]. The obturator artery. See Table of Arteries in the Appendix.

arteria obturatoria ac·ces·so·ria (ack·se·so'ree·uh) [NA]. A variable accessory obturator artery arising as a branch of the inferior epigastric artery.

arteria oc·ci·pi·ta·lis (ock·sip·i·tay'lis) [NA]. The occipital artery. See Table of Arteries in the Appendix.

arteria oph·thal·mi·ca (off·thal'mi·kuh) [NA]. The ophthalmic artery. See Table of Arteries in the Appendix.

arteria ova·ri·ca (o·vair'i·kuh) [NA]. OVARIAN ARTERY.

arteria pa·la·ti·na ascen·dens (pal·uh·tye'nuh a·sen'denz) [NA]. The ascending palatine artery. See Table of Arteries in the Appendix.

arteria palatina de·scen·dens (de·sen'denz) [NA]. The descending palatine artery. See Table of Arteries in the Appendix.

arteria palatina major [NA]. The greater palatine artery. See Table of Arteries in the Appendix.

arteria pan·cre·a·ti·ca dor·sa·lis (pan''kree·at'i·kuh dor·say'lis) [NA]. DORSAL PANCREATIC ARTERY.

arteria pancreatica inferior [NA]. INFERIOR PANCREATIC ARTERY.

arteria pancreatica mag·na (mag'nuh) [NA]. The great pancreatic artery; the largest pancreatic branch of the splenic artery, principally supplying the tail of the pancreas.

arteria pan·cre·a·ti·co·du·o·de·na·lis inferior (pan·kree·at''i·ko·dew·o·de·nay'lis) [BNA]. Singular of NA arteriae pancreaticoduodenales inferiores. (= the inferior pancreaticoduodenal arteries).

arteria pancreaticoduodenalis superior [NA]. The superior pancreaticoduodenal artery. See Table of Arteries in the Appendix.

arteria pe·nis (pee'nis) [BNA]. Artery of the penis.

arteria per·fo·rans pri·ma (pur'fo·ranz prye'muh) [BNA]. The first perforating artery, a branch of the deep femoral artery.

arteria perforans se·cun·da (se·kun'duh) [BNA]. The second perforating artery, a branch of the deep femoral artery.

arteria perforans ter·tia (tur'shuh) [BNA]. The third perforating artery, a branch of the deep femoral artery.

arteria pe·ri·car·di·a·co·phre·ni·ca (perr·i·kahr·dye'uh·ko·fren'i·kuh) [NA]. The pericardiacophrenic artery. See Table of Arteries in the Appendix.

arteria pe·ri·ne·a·lis (perr·i·nee·ay'lis) [NA]. The perineal artery. See Table of Arteries in the Appendix.

arteria pe·ri·nei (perr·i·nee'eye) [BNA]. Arteria perinealis. See *perineal* in Table of Arteries in the Appendix.

arteria pe·ro·nea (perr·o·nee'uh) [NA]. PERONEAL ARTERY. NA alt. *arteria fibularis.*

arteria pha·ryn·gea ascen·dens (fa·rin'jee·uh a·sen'denz) [NA]. The ascending pharyngeal artery. See Table of Arteries in the Appendix.

arteria phre·ni·ca inferior (fren'i·kuh) [BNA]. Singular of NA *arteriae phrenicae inferiores* (= the inferior phrenic arteries).

arteria plan·ta·ris la·te·ra·lis (plan·tair'is lat·e·ray'lis) [NA]. The lateral plantar artery. See Table of Arteries in the Appendix.

arteria plantaris me·di·a·lis (mee·dee·ay'lis) [NA]. The medial plantar artery. See Table of Arteries in the Appendix.

arteria pop·li·tea (pop·lit'ee·uh) [NA]. The popliteal artery. See Table of Arteries in the Appendix.

arteria prin·ceps pol·li·cis (prin'seps pol'i·sis) [NA]. The principal artery of the thumb. See Table of Arteries in the Appendix.

arteria pro·fun·da bra·chii (pro·fun'duh bray'kee·eye) [NA]. The deep brachial artery. See Table of Arteries in the Appendix.

arteria profunda cli·to·ri·dis (kli·tor'i·dis) [NA]. The deep artery of the clitoris. See Table of Arteries in the Appendix.

arteria profunda fe·mo·ris (fem'o·ris) [NA]. The deep femoral artery. See Table of Arteries in the Appendix.

arteria profunda lin·guae (ling'gwee) [NA]. The deep lingual artery. See Table of Arteries in the Appendix.

arteria profunda pe·nis (pee'nis) [NA]. The deep artery of the penis. See Table of Arteries in the Appendix.

arteria pu·den·da in·ter·na (pew·den'duh in·tur'nuh) [NA]. The internal pudendal artery. See Table of Arteries in the Appendix.

arteria pul·mo·na·lis (pul·mo·nay'lis) [BNA]. Truncus pulmonalis (= PULMONARY TRUNK).

arteria pulmonalis dex·tra (decks'truh) [NA]. The right pulmonary artery. See Table of Arteries in the Appendix.

arteria pulmonalis si·nis·tra (si·nis'truh) [NA]. The left pulmonary artery. See Table of Arteries in the Appendix.

arteria ra·di·a·lis (ray·dee·ay'lis) [NA]. The radial artery. See Table of Arteries in the Appendix.

arteria radialis in·di·cis (in'di·sis) [NA]. The radial artery of the index finger. See Table of Arteries in the Appendix.

ar·te·ri·arc·tia (ahr·teer''ee·ahrk'shee·uh, ·tee·uh) *n.* [NL., from *arteri-* + L. *arct*are, to press together, + *-ia*]. *Rare.* Vasoconstriction or stenosis of an artery.

arteria rec·ta·lis inferior (reck·tay'lis) [NA]. The inferior rectal artery. See Table of Arteries in the Appendix.

arteria rectalis me·dia (mee'dee·uh) [NA]. The middle rectal artery. See Table of Arteries in the Appendix.

arteria rectalis superior [NA]. The superior rectal artery. See Table of Arteries in the Appendix.

arteria re·cur·rens ra·di·a·lis (re·kur'enz ray·dee·ay'lis) [NA]. The radial recurrent artery. See Table of Arteries in the Appendix.

arteria recurrens ti·bi·a·lis anterior (tib·ee·ay'lis) [NA]. The anterior recurrent tibial artery. See Table of Arteries in the Appendix.

arteria recurrens tibialis posterior [NA]. The posterior recurrent tibial artery. See Table of Arteries in the Appendix.

arteria recurrens ul·na·ris (ul·nair'is) [NA]. The recurrent ulnar artery. See Table of Arteries in the Appendix.

arteria re·na·lis (re·nay'lis) [NA]. The renal artery. See Table of Arteries in the Appendix.

arteria sa·cra·lis la·te·ra·lis (sa·kray'lis lat·e·ray'lis) [BNA]. Singular of NA *arteriae sacrales laterales.* See *sacral* in Table of Arteries in the Appendix.

arteria sacralis me·dia (mee'dee·uh) [BNA]. Arteria sacralis mediana. See *sacral* in Table of Arteries in the Appendix.

arteria sacralis me·di·a·na (mee·dee·ay'nuh) [NA]. The median sacral artery. See Table of Arteries in the Appendix.

arteria sca·pu·la·ris de·scen·dens (skap·yoo·lair'is de·sen'denz) [NA]. The descending scapular artery. See Table of Arteries in the Appendix.

arteria scapularis dor·sa·lis (dor·say'lis). [NA alt]. The decending scapular artery. NA alt. *arteria scapularis descendens.*

arteria seg·men·ti an·te·ri·o·ris (seg·men'tye an·teer·ee·o'ris) [NA]. Anterior segmental branch of the renal artery.

arteria segmenti anterioris in·fe·ri·o·ris (in·feer·ee·o'ris) [NA]. Anterior inferior segmental branch of the renal artery.

arteria segmenti anterioris su·pe·ri·o·ris (sue·peer·ee·o'ris) [NA]. Anterior superior segmental branch of the renal artery.

arteria segmenti in·fe·ri·o·ris (in·feer·ee·o'ris) [NA]. Inferior segmental branch of the renal artery.

arteria segmenti la·te·ra·lis (lat·e·ray'lis) [NA]. Lateral segmental branch of the left branch of the proper hepatic artery.

arteria segmenti me·di·a·lis (mee·dee·ay'lis) [NA]. Medial segmental branch of the left branch of the proper hepatic artery.

arteria segmenti pos·te·ri·o·ris (pos·teer·ee·o'ris) [NA]. 1. Posterior segmental branch of the right branch of the proper hepatic artery. 2. Posterior segmental branch of the renal artery.

arteria segmenti su·pe·ri·o·ris (sue·peer·ee·o'ris) [NA]. Superior segmental branch of the renal artery.

ar·te·ri·a·sis (ahr"te·rye'uh·sis) *n.*, pl. **arteria·ses** (·seez) [*arteri-* + *-iasis*]. *Rare.* Degeneration of an artery.

arteria sper·ma·ti·ca ex·ter·na (spur·mat'i·kuh ecks·tur'nuh) [BNA]. Arteria cremasterica (= CREMASTERIC ARTERY).

arteria spermatica in·ter·na (in·tur'nuh) [BNA]. Internal spermatic artery; the ovarian or the testicular artery.

arteria sphe·no·pa·la·ti·na (sfee"no·pal·uh·tye'nuh) [NA]. The sphenopalatine artery. See Table of Arteries in the Appendix.

arteria spi·na·lis anterior (spye·nay'lis) [NA]. The anterior spinal artery. See Table of Arteries in the Appendix.

arteria spinalis posterior [NA]. The posterior spinal artery. See Table of Arteries in the Appendix.

arteria ster·no·clei·do·mas·toi·dea (stur"no·klye·do·mas·toy'dee·uh) [BNA]. Ramus sternocleidomastoideus arteriae occipitalis, pl. rami sternocleidomastoidei arteriae occipitalis (= the sternocleidomastoid branches of the occipital artery).

arteria sty·lo·mas·toi·dea (stye"lo·mas·toy'dee·uh) [NA]. The stylomastoid artery. See Table of Arteries in the Appendix.

arteria sub·cla·via (sub·klay'vee·uh) [NA]. The subclavian artery. See Table of Arteries in the Appendix.

arteria sub·cos·ta·lis (sub·kos·tay'lis) [NA]. The subcostal artery. See Table of Arteries in the Appendix.

arteria sub·lin·gua·lis (sub·ling·gway'lis) [NA]. The sublingual artery. See Table of Arteries in the Appendix.

arteria sub·men·ta·lis (sub·men·tay'lis) [NA]. The submental artery. See Table of Arteries in the Appendix.

arteria sub·sca·pu·la·ris (sub·skap·yoo·lair'is) [NA]. The subscapular artery. See Table of Arteries in the Appendix.

arteria su·pra·or·bi·ta·lis (sue"pruh·or·bi·tay'lis) [NA]. The supraorbital artery. See Table of Arteries in the Appendix.

arteria su·pra·re·na·lis inferior (sue"pruh·re·nay'lis) [NA]. The inferior suprarenal artery. See Table of Arteries in the Appendix.

arteria suprarenalis me·dia (mee'dee·uh) [NA]. The middle suprarenal artery. See Table of Arteries in the Appendix.

arteria suprarenalis superior [NA]. The superior suprarenal artery. See Table of Arteries in the Appendix.

arteria su·pra·sca·pu·la·ris (sue"pruh·skap·yoo·lair'is) [NA]. The suprascapular artery. See Table of Arteries in the Appendix.

arteria su·pra·tro·chle·a·ris (sue"pruh·trock·lee·air'is) [NA]. The supratrochlear artery. See Table of Arteries in the Appendix.

arteria tar·sea la·te·ra·lis (tahr'see·uh lat·e·ray'lis) [NA]. The lateral tarsal artery. See Table of Arteries in the Appendix.

arteria tem·po·ra·lis me·dia (tem·po·ray'lis mee'dee·uh) [NA]. The middle temporal artery. See Table of Arteries in the Appendix.

arteria temporalis pro·fun·da anterior (pro·fun'duh) [BNA]. The anterior deep temporal artery.

arteria temporalis profunda posterior [BNA]. The posterior deep temporal artery.

arteria temporalis su·per·fi·ci·a·lis (sue"pur·fish·ee·ay'lis) [NA]. The superficial temporal artery. See Table of Arteries in the Appendix.

arteria tes·ti·cu·la·ris (tes·tick·yoo·lair'is) [NA]. TESTICULAR ARTERY.

arteria tho·ra·ca·lis la·te·ra·lis (tho·ra·kay'lis lat·e·ray'lis) [BNA]. Arteria thoracica lateralis. See *thoracic* in Table of Arteries in the Appendix.

arteria thoracalis su·pre·ma (sue·pree'muh) [BNA]. Arteria thoracica suprema. See *thoracic* in Table of Arteries in the Appendix.

arteria tho·ra·ci·ca in·ter·na (tho·ras'i·kuh in·tur'nuh) [NA]. The internal thoracic artery. See Table of Arteries in the Appendix.

arteria thoracica la·te·ra·lis (lat·e·ray'lis) [NA]. The lateral thoracic artery. See Table of Arteries in the Appendix.

arteria thoracica su·pre·ma (sue·pree'muh) [NA]. The highest thoracic artery. See Table of Arteries in the Appendix.

arteria tho·ra·co·acro·mi·a·lis (tho"ruh·ko·a·kro·mee·ay'lis) [NA]. The thoracoacromial artery. See Table of Arteries in the Appendix.

arteria tho·ra·co·dor·sa·lis (tho"ruh·ko·dor·say'lis) [NA]. The thoracodorsal artery. See Table of Arteries in the Appendix.

arteria thy·re·oi·dea ima (thigh·ree·oy'dee·uh eye'muh) [BNA]. Arteria thyroidea ima. See *thyroid* in Table of Arteries in the Appendix.

arteria thyreoidea inferior [BNA]. Arteria thyroidea inferior. See *thyroid* in Table of Arteries in the Appendix.

arteria thyreoidea superior [BNA]. Arteria thyroidea superior. See *thyroid* in Table of Arteries in the Appendix.

arteria thy·roi·dea ima (thigh·roy'dee·uh eye'muh) [NA]. The lowest thyroid artery. See Table of Arteries in the Appendix.

arteria thyroidea inferior [NA]. The inferior thyroid artery. See Table of Arteries in the Appendix.

arteria thyroidea superior [NA]. The superior thyroid artery. See Table of Arteries in the Appendix.

arteria ti·bi·a·lis anterior (tib·ee·ay'lis) [NA]. The anterior tibial artery. See Table of Arteries in the Appendix.

arteria tibialis posterior [NA]. The posterior tibial artery. See Table of Arteries in the Appendix.

arteria trans·ver·sa col·li (trans·vur'suh kol'eye) [NA]. The transverse cervical artery. See Table of Arteries in the Appendix.

arteria transversa fa·ci·ei (fay·shee·ee'eye, fay'shee·eye) [NA]. The transverse facial artery. See Table of Arteries in the Appendix.

arteria transversa sca·pu·lae (skap'yoo·lee) [BNA]. Arteria suprascapularis. See *suprascapular* in Table of Arteries in the Appendix.

arteria tym·pa·ni·ca anterior (tim·pan'i·kuh) [NA]. The anterior tympanic artery. See Table of Arteries in the Appendix.

arteria tympanica inferior [NA]. The inferior tympanic artery. See Table of Arteries in the Appendix.

arteria tympanica posterior [NA]. The posterior tympanic artery. See Table of Arteries in the Appendix.

arteria tympanica superior [NA]. The superior tympanic artery. See Table of Arteries in the Appendix.

arteria ul·na·ris (ul·nair'is) [NA]. The ulnar artery. See Table of Arteries in the Appendix.

arteria um·bi·li·ca·lis (um·bil·i·kay'lis) [NA]. The umbilical artery. See Table of Arteries in the Appendix.

arteria ure·thra·lis (yoo·ree·thray'lis) [NA]. The urethral artery. See Table of Arteries in the Appendix.

arteria ute·ri·na (yoo·tur·eye'nuh) [NA]. UTERINE ARTERY.

arteria va·gi·na·lis (vaj·i·nay'lis) [NA]. The vaginal artery. See Table of Arteries in the Appendix.

arteria ver·te·bra·lis (vur·te·bray'lis) [NA]. The vertebral artery. See Table of Arteries in the Appendix.

arteria ve·si·ca·lis inferior (ves·i·kay'lis) [NA]. The inferior vesical artery. See Table of Arteries in the Appendix.

arteria vesicalis superior [BNA]. Singular of NA *arteriae vesicales superiores* (= the superior vesical arteries).

arteria vo·la·ris in·di·cis ra·di·a·lis (vo·lair'is in'di·sis ray·dee·ay'lis) [BNA]. Arteria radialis indicis. See *radial* in Table of Arteries in the Appendix.

arteria zy·go·ma·ti·co·or·bi·ta·lis (zye·go·mat''i·ko·or·bi·tay'lis) [NA]. The zygomaticoorbital artery. See Table of Arteries in the Appendix.

ar·te·ri·ec·ta·sia (ahr·teer''ee·eck·tay'zhuh, ·zee·uh) *n.* ARTERIECTASIS.

ar·te·ri·ec·ta·sis (ahr·teer''ee·eck'tuh·sis) *n.* [*arteri-* + *ectasis*]. Arterial dilatation.

ar·te·ri·ec·to·my (ahr·teer''ee·eck'tuh·mee) *n.* [*arteri-* + *-ectomy*]. Excision of an artery or portion of an artery. Compare *endarterectomy.*

ar·te·ri·ec·to·pia (ahr·teer''ee·eck·to'pee·uh) *n.* [*arteri-* + *ectopia*]. Displacement or abnormality of the course of an artery.

arterio-. See *arteri-*.

ar·te·rio·ar·te·ri·al (ahr·teer''ee·o·ahr·teer'ee·ul) *adj.* Connecting, or both originating and ending in, arteries.

arterioarterial embolization. ATHEROEMBOLIZATION.

ar·te·rio·cap·il·lary (ahr·tee''ree·o·kap'i·lăr·ee) *n.* PRECAPILLARY.

arteriocapillary fibrosis. Fibrosis of small arteries and arterioles, with variable degrees of hyalinization and reduction in the size of the lumens, a manifestation of arteriolosclerosis.

arteriocapillary fibrosis of Gull and Sutton [W. W. *Gull* and H. G. *Sutton*]. ARTERIOCAPILLARY FIBROSIS.

ar·te·rio·fi·bro·sis (ahr·teer''ee·o·figh·bro'sis) *n.* An increment of fibrous connective tissue in the walls of arteries; endarteritis obliterans.

ar·te·rio·gram (ahr·teer'ee·o·gram) *n.* 1. A roentgenogram of an artery after injection with a contrast material. 2. A tracing of the arterial pulse.

ar·te·rio·graph (ahr·teer'ee·o·graf) *n.* An instrument which graphically presents the pulse.

ar·te·ri·og·ra·phy (ahr·teer''ee·og'ruh·fee) *n.* 1. Graphic presentation of the pulse; sphygmography. 2. Roentgenography of the arteries after the intravascular injection of a radiopaque substance. —**ar·te·rio·graph·ic** (ahr·teer''ee·o·graf'ick) *adj.*

ar·te·ri·o·la (ahr·teer''ee·o'luh, ahr''te·rye'o·luh) *n.*, pl. & genit. sing. **arterio·lae** (·lee) [NL.]. ARTERIOLE.

arteriolae rec·tae (reck'tee) [NA]. STRAIGHT ARTERIOLES.

arteriola ma·cu·la·ris inferior (mack·yoo·lair'is) [NA]. The arteriole supplying the inferior portion of the macula of the retina.

arteriola macularis superior [NA]. The arteriole supplying the superior portion of the macula of the retina.

arteriola me·di·a·lis re·ti·nae (mee·dee·ay'lis ret'i·nee) [NA]. The arteriole supplying the central portion of the retina.

arteriola na·sa·lis re·ti·nae inferior (na·say'lis ret'i·nee) [NA]. The arteriole supplying the lower portion of the nasal part of the retina.

arteriola nasalis retinae superior [NA]. The arteriole supplying the superior portion of the nasal part of the retina.

ar·te·ri·o·lar (ahr·teer''ee·o'lur) *adj.* Of or pertaining to an arteriole.

arteriolar capillary. PRECAPILLARY.

arteriola rec·ta (reck'tuh). Singular of NA *arteriolae rectae;* STRAIGHT ARTERIOLE.

arteriolar nephrosclerosis. Renal atrophy and scarring characterized by fine granulation of the parenchymal surface and by glomerular, tubular, and interstitial alterations associated with arteriosclerotic changes of the afferent arterioles.

arteriolar sclerosis. ARTERIOLOSCLEROSIS.

arteriola tem·po·ra·lis re·ti·nae inferior (tem·po·ray'lis ret'i·nee) [NA]. The arteriole to the inferior portion of the temporal part of the retina.

arteriola temporalis retinae superior [NA]. The arteriole to the superior portion of the temporal part of the retina.

ar·te·ri·ole (ahr·teer'ee·ole) *n.* [NL. *arteriola,* dim. of *arteria*]. Any of the minute, smallest arterial branches which, together with the precapillaries, comprise the intermediate vessels between the larger arteries and the capillaries; arterioles have a relatively thick muscular wall and are responsible in large part for peripheral resistance in the vasculature and the effects thereof on rate of blood flow.

ar·te·rio·lith (ahr·teer'ee·o·lith) *n.* [*arterio-* + *-lith*]. A calculus in an artery. —**ar·te·rio·lith·ic** (ahr·teer''ee·o·lith'ick) *adj.*

ar·te·ri·o·li·tis (ahr·teer''ee·o·lye'tis) *n.* Inflammation of arterioles.

ar·te·ri·o·lo·ne·cro·sis (ahr·teer·ee·o''lo·ne·kro'sis) *n.* Degeneration of the arterioles resulting in necrosis. —**arteriolo·ne·crot·ic** (·ne·krot'ick) *adj.*

ar·te·ri·o·lop·a·thy (ahr·teer''ee·o·lop'uth·ee) *n.* [*arteriole* + *-pathy*]. Any disease of arterioles.

ar·te·ri·o·lo·scle·ro·sis (ahr·teer·ee·o''lo·skle·ro'sis) *n.*, pl. **arte·riolosclero·ses** (·seez) [*arteriole* + *sclerosis*]. Thickening of arterioles, usually due to hyalinization or fibromuscular hyperplasia. —**arterioloscle·rot·ic** (·rot'ick) *adj.*

ar·te·rio·ma·la·cia (ahr·teer''ee·o·ma·lay'shee·uh) *n.* [*arterio-* + *malacia*]. Softening of an arterial wall.

ar·te·rio·mes·en·ter·ic (ahr·teer''ee·o·mes''en·terr'ick) *adj.* Pertaining to the arteries in the mesentery.

arteriomesenteric ileus. ACUTE DUODENAL ILEUS.

ar·te·rio·ne·cro·sis (ahr·teer''ee·o·ne·kro'sis) *n.* Necrosis of an artery or arteries.

ar·te·ri·op·a·thy (ahr·teer''ee·op'uth·ee) *n.* [*arterio-* + *-pathy*]. Any diseased state of arteries.

ar·te·rio·pla·nia (ahr·teer''ee·o·play'nee·uh) *n.* [*arterio-* + *-plania*]. A condition in which an anomaly is present in the course of an artery.

ar·te·rio·plas·ty (ahr·teer'ee·o·plas''tee) *n.* [*arterio-* + *-plasty*]. An operation for aneurysm in which the artery is reconstructed by using the aneurysmal walls to restore its continuity. —**ar·te·rio·plas·tic** (ahr·teer''ee·o·plas·tick) *adj.*

ar·te·rio·pres·sor (ahr·teer''ee·o·pres'ur) *adj.* Causing increased blood pressure in the arteries. See also *vasopressor.*

ar·te·rio·punc·ture (ahr·teer'ee·o·punk''chur) *n.* Insertion of a needle into an artery, or surgical division or opening of an artery, chiefly for the abstraction of blood.

ar·te·rio·re·nal (ahr·teer''ee·o·ree'nul) *adj.* Pertaining to the renal arteries.

ar·te·ri·or·rha·phy (ahr·teer″ee·or′uh·fee) *n.* [*arterio-* + *-rrhaphy*]. Suture of an artery.

ar·te·ri·or·rhex·is (ahr·teer″ee·o·reck′sis) *n.*, pl. **arteriorrhex·es** (·seez) [*arterio-* + *-rrhexis*]. Rupture of an artery.

ar·te·rio·scle·ro·sis (ahr·teer″ee·o·skle·ro′sis) *n.*, pl. **arterioscle·ro·ses** (·seez) [*arterio-* + *sclerosis*]. Any of various proliferative and degenerative changes in arteries, not necessarily related to each other, resulting in thickening of the walls, loss of elasticity, and in some instances, calcium deposition. —**arterioscle·rot·ic** (·rot′ick) *adj.*

arteriosclerosis oblit·er·ans (o·blit′ur·anz). Arteriosclerosis with proliferation of the intima to the extent of obstructing the lumen. See also *endarteritis obliterans.*

arteriosclerotic dementia. Impairment of cognitive functions due to the effects of atherosclerotic occlusion and ischemic infarction, usually multiple, of the brain. Syn. *atherosclerotic psychosis.*

arteriosclerotic gangrene. A dry gangrene of the extremities, due to failure of the terminal circulation in persons afflicted with arteriosclerosis. Syn. *senile gangrene.*

arteriosclerotic psychosis. ARTERIOSCLEROTIC DEMENTIA.

ar·te·rio·spasm (ahr·teer′ee·o·spaz·um) *n.* Spasm of an artery. —**ar·te·rio·spas·tic** (ahr·teer″ee·o·spas′tick) *adj.*

ar·te·rio·ste·no·sis (ahr·teer″ee·o·ste·no′sis) *n.*, pl. **arterioste·no·ses** (·seez) [*arterio-* + *stenosis*]. Narrowing of the caliber of an artery.

ar·te·ri·os·to·sis (ahr·teer″ee·os·to′sis) *n.* [*arteri-* + *ostosis*]. Calcification of an artery.

ar·te·rio·strep·sis (ahr·teer″ee·o·strep′sis) *n.*, pl. **arteriostrep·ses** (·seez) [*arterio-* + Gk. *strepsis,* a twisting]. The twisting of an artery for the purpose of staying a hemorrhage.

ar·te·rio·tome (ar·teer′ee·o·tome) *n.* A knife for use in arteriotomy.

ar·te·ri·ot·o·my (ahr·teer″ee·ot′uh·mee) *n.* [*arterio-* + *-tomy*]. Incision or opening of an artery.

ar·te·rio·ve·nous (ahr·teer″ee·o·vee′nus) *adj.* Both arterial and venous; involving an artery and a vein or an arteriole and a venule.

arteriovenous anastomosis. A modified vessel which connects an arteriole and a venule without the intervention of capillaries. Such structures are numerous in the palm, the sole, and the pulp of terminal digital phalanges. NA *anastomosis arteriovenosa.*

arteriovenous fistula or **aneurysm.** Abnormal direct communication, single or multiple, between an artery and a vein without interposition of capillaries; it may be congenital or acquired.

arteriovenous shunt. A surgically created arteriovenous fistula. Syn. *AV shunt.* See also *Scribner shunt.*

ar·te·rio·ver·sion (ahr·teer″ee·o·vur′zhun) *n.* [*arterio-* + *version*]. A method of arresting hemorrhage by turning arteries inside out.

ar·te·rio·vert·er (ahr·teer″ee·o·vur′tur) *n.* An instrument used to perform arterioversion.

ar·te·ri·tis (ahr″te·rye′tis) *n.* [*arteri-* + *-itis*]. Inflammation of an artery. See also *endarteritis, periarteritis.*

arteritis deformans. ENDARTERITIS DEFORMANS.

arteritis obliterans. ENDARTERITIS OBLITERANS.

ar·te·ry (ahr′tur·ee) *n.* [L. *arteria,* from Gk. *artēria,* orig., air vessel: trachea, bronchus; artery (conceived as an air vessel)]. A vessel conveying blood away from the heart. It is composed of three coats: the intima (interna), the media, and the adventitia (externa). In comparison to veins, arteries have a thick wall and small lumen. For arteries listed by name, see Table of Arteries in the Appendix. See also Plates 7, 8.

artery flap. VASCULAR FLAP.

artery forceps. A forceps, usually self-locking and with scissors handles, used for seizing and compressing an artery.

arthr-, arthro- [Gk. *arthron* (rel. to Gk. ar*ariskein,* to fit, join, and to L. *ar*tus, joint)]. A combining form meaning *joint.*

ar·thral·gia (ahr·thral′jee·uh) *n.* [*arthr-* + *-algia*]. Pain affecting a joint. —**arthral·gic** (·jick) *adj.*

arthralgia hys·ter·i·ca (his·terr′i·kuh). Pain in the joints, of psychogenic origin.

arthralgia sat·ur·ni·na (sat·ur·nigh′nuh). Musculoskeletal pain, seen in lead poisoning.

ar·threc·to·my (ahr·threck′tuh·mee) *n.* [*arthr-* + *-ectomy*]. Excision of a joint.

ar·thres·the·sia (ahr″thres·theezh′uh, ·theez′ee·uh) *n.* [*arthr-* + *esthesia*]. Sensory perception of movements of a joint.

ar·thri·flu·ent (ahr″thri·floo′unt, ahr·thrif′loo·unt) *adj.* [*arthr-* + L. *fluens, fluent*is, flowing (from *fluere,* to flow)]. Flowing from a joint.

arthrifluent abscess. A migrating abscess having its origin in a diseased joint.

ar·thrit·ic (ahr·thrit′ick) *adj.* & *n.* [Gk. *arthritikos,* gouty]. 1. Pertaining to or affected by arthritis. 2. An individual affected with arthritis.

arthritic erythema. HAVERHILL FEVER.

arthritides. Plural of *arthritis.*

ar·thri·tis (ahr·thrigh′tis) *n.*, pl. **ar·thrit·i·des** (·thrit′i·deez) [Gk. *arthritis* (*nosos*), (disease) of the joints, from *arthron,* joint]. Inflammation of a joint.

arthritis de·for·mans (de·for′manz). RHEUMATOID ARTHRITIS.

arthritis deformans juvenilis. OSTEOCHONDRITIS DEFORMANS JUVENILIS.

arthritis fun·go·sa (fung·go′suh). FUNGOUS ARTHRITIS.

arthritis ure·thrit·i·ca (yoo″re·thrit′i·kuh). REITER'S SYNDROME.

arthro-. See *arthr-.*

ar·thro·cele (ahr′thro·seel) *n.* [*arthro-* + *-cele*]. 1. Any swollen joint. 2. Hernia of the synovial membrane through a joint capsule.

ar·thro·cen·te·sis (ahr″thro·sen·tee′sis) *n.*, pl. **arthrocente·ses** (·seez) [*arthro-* + *centesis*]. Incision into or puncture through a joint capsule to relieve an effusion.

ar·thro·chon·dri·tis (ahr″thro·kon·drye′tis) *n.* [*arthro-* + *chondritis*]. *Obsol.* OSTEOCHONDRITIS (1).

ar·thro·cla·sia (ahr″thro·klay′zhuh, ·zee·uh) *n.* [*arthro-* + *-clasia*]. The breaking down of an ankylosis in order to produce free movement of a joint.

ar·thro·cla·sis (ahr″thro·klay′sis, ahr·throck′luh·sis) *n.*, pl. **arthrocla·ses** (·seez) [*arthro-* + *-clasis*]. ARTHROCLASIA.

ar·thro·de·sia (ahr″thro·dee′zhuh, ·zee·uh) *n.* ARTHRODESIS.

ar·thro·de·sis (ahr″thro·dee′sis, ahr·throd′e·sis) *n.*, pl. **arthrode·ses** (·seez) [*arthro-* + *-desis*]. Fusion of a joint by removing the articular surfaces and securing bony union. Syn. *operative ankylosis.*

ar·thro·dia (ahr·thro′dee·uh) *n.*, pl. **arthro·di·ae** (·dee·ee) [NL., from Gk. *arthrōdia,* from *arthrōdēs,* well-jointed, articulated]. GLIDING JOINT. —**arthro·di·al** (·dee·ul) *adj.*

ar·thro·dyn·ia (ahr″thro·din′ee·uh) *n.* [*arthr-* + *-odynia*]. ARTHRALGIA. —**arthrodyn·ic** (·ick) *adj.*

ar·thro·dys·pla·sia (ahr″thro·dis·play′zhuh, ·zee·uh) *n.* [*arthro-* + *dysplasia*]. A condition, usually inherited, in which the patellas are rudimentary, the heads of the radii dislocated, and the nails generally absent. See also *nail-patella syndrome.*

ar·thro·em·py·e·sis (ahr″thro·em·pye·ee′sis) *n.* [*arthro-* + *empyesis*]. PYARTHROSIS.

ar·thro·en·dos·co·py (ahr″thro·en·dos′kuh·pee) *n.* [*arthro-* + *endoscopy*]. ARTHROSCOPY.

ar·thro·erei·sis (ar″thro·e·rye′sis) *n.* [*arthro-* + Gk. *ereisis,* propping, shoring up]. Surgical limitation of the mobility of a joint.

ar·thro·gram (ahr′thro·gram) *n.* [*arthro-* + *-gram*]. A roentgenogram of a joint space after injection of contrast media.

ar·throg·ra·phy (ahr·throg′ruh·fee) *n.* [*arthro-* + *-graphy*]. Roentgenography of a joint space after the injection of positive or negative (or both positive and negative) contrast media.

ar·thro·gry·po·sis (ahr″thro·gri·po′sis) *n.* [*arthro-* + *gryposis*].

Retention of a joint in a fixed position due to muscular contraction or to extracapsular or intracapsular adhesions.

arthrogryposis mul·ti·plex con·gen·i·ta (mul'ti·plecks kon·jen'i·tuh). A syndrome, congenital in origin, characterized by deformity and ankylosis of joints, usually in flexion, with limitation of motion, muscular atrophy, and contractures; may be neurogenic or rarely myogenic.

arthrogryposis syndrome. ARTHROGRYPOSIS MULTIPLEX CONGENITA.

ar·thro·ka·tad·y·sis (ahr"thro·ka·tad'i·sis) *n.* [*arthro-* + Gk. *katadysis,* a going down]. Intrapelvic protrusion of the acetabulum from thinning and eburnation of the pelvic wall; of undetermined etiology. Syn. *Otto's pelvis.*

ar·thro·lith (ahr'thro·lith) *n.* [*arthro-* + *-lith*]. A calcareous or gouty deposit within a joint.

ar·thro·li·thi·a·sis (ahr"thro·li·thigh'uh·sis) *n.*, pl. **arthrolithiases** (·seez). [*arthrolith* + *-iasis*]. GOUT.

ar·throl·o·gy (ahr·throl'uh·jee) *n.* [*arthro-* + *-logy*]. 1. The science and body of knowledge of the joints. 2. The system of joints.

ar·throl·y·sis (ahr·throl'i·sis) *n.* [*arthro-* + *-lysis*]. Surgical freeing of an ankylosed joint.

ar·throm·e·ter (ahr·throm'e·tur) *n.* [*arthro-* + *-meter*]. An instrument for measuring and recording the extent of movement in a joint. —**arthrome·try** (·tree) *n.*

ar·thron·cus (ahr·thronk'us) *n.* [NL., from *arthr-* + Gk. *onkos,* mass]. 1. A joint tumor. 2. Swelling of a joint.

ar·thro·on·y·cho·dys·pla·sia (ahr"thro·on"i·ko·dis·play'zhuh, ·zee·uh) *n.* [*arthro-* + *onycho-* + *dysplasia*]. NAIL-PATELLA SYNDROME.

ar·thro·os·teo·on·y·cho·dys·pla·sia (ahr"thro·os"tee·o·on"i·ko·dis·play'zhuh) *n.* [*arthro-* + *osteo-* + *onycho-* + *dysplasia*]. NAIL-PATELLA SYNDROME.

arthropathic psoriasis. PSORIATIC ARTHROPATHY.

ar·throp·a·thy (ahr·throp'uth·ee) *n.* [*arthro-* + *-pathy*]. 1. Any joint disease. 2. CHARCOT'S JOINT. —**ar·thro·path·ic** (ahr"thro·path'ick) *adj.*

ar·thro·phyte (ahr'thro·fight) *n.* [*arthro-* + *-phyte*]. An abnormal growth occurring within a joint; a joint mouse.

ar·thro·plas·ty (ahr'thro·plas"tee) *n.* [*arthro-* + *-plasty*]. 1. Reconstruction, by natural modification or artificial replacement, of a diseased, damaged, or ankylosed joint. 2. The making of an artificial joint. —**ar·thro·plas·tic** (ahr"thro·plas'tick) *adj.*

ar·thro·pod (ahr'thro·pod) *n.* A member of the Arthropoda.

Ar·throp·o·da (ahr·throp'o·duh) *n.pl.* [*arthro-* + *-poda*]. The largest phylum of the animal kingdom; includes the crustacea, insects, myriopods, arachnids, and related forms. The members are bilaterally symmetrical, having a limited number of segments, a chitinous exoskeleton, and jointed appendages. —**arthropo·dal, arthropo·dan,** *adj.*

arthropod-borne virus. ARBOVIRUS.

ar·thror·rha·gia (ahr"thro·ray'jee·uh) *n.* [*arthro-* + *-rrhagia*]. Hemorrhage into a joint.

ar·thro·scle·ro·sis (ahr"thro·skle·ro'sis) *n.* [*arthro-* + *sclerosis*]. The hardening or stiffening of a joint or joints.

ar·thro·scope (ahr'thro·skope) *n.* [*arthro-* + *-scope*]. An instrument used for the visualization of the interior of a joint.

ar·thros·co·py (ahr·thros'kuh·pee) *n.* [*arthro-* + *-scopy*]. Examination of the interior of a joint with an arthroscope.

ar·thro·sis (ahr·thro'sis) *n.*, pl. **arthro·ses** (·seez) [Gk. *arthrōsis,* jointing, articulation]. 1. An articulation or joint; a suture. 2. A degenerative process in a joint.

ar·thro·spore (ahr'thro·spore) *n.* [*arthro-* + *spore*]. A fungal spore formed by the segmentation of the hyphae, resulting in the formation of rectangular, thick-walled cells.

ar·thros·to·my (ahr·thros'tuh·mee) *n.* [*arthro-* + *-stomy*]. An incision into a joint, as for drainage.

ar·thro·tome (ahr'thro·tome) *n.* [*arthro-* + *-tome*]. A stout knife used in joint surgery; a cartilage knife.

ar·throt·o·my (ahr·throt'uh·mee) *n.* [*arthro-* + *-tomy*]. An incision into a joint.

ar·thro·tro·pia (ahr"thro·tro'pee·uh) *n.* [*arthro-* + *trop-* + *-ia*]. Torsion or twisted condition of a limb.

ar·throus (ahr'thrus) *adj.* [*arthr-* + *-ous*]. Pertaining to a joint or joints; jointed.

Ar·thur performance scale [G. A. *Arthur,* U.S. psychologist, 20th century]. A test to measure general mental ability, most widely used with children and adolescents, which emphasizes manipulation, rather than language items which can be largely eliminated where linguistic or cultural factors play a role, as in aphasia, in educationally deprived children, or in those with a bilingual background.

Ar·thus' phenomenon or **reaction** (ar·tuᵉss') [N. M. *Arthus,* French physiologist, 1862–1945]. A generalized or local anaphylactic reaction, the result of the union of antigen and antibody within the tissues, manifested by local edema and inflammation.

ar·tic·u·lar (ahr·tick'yoo·lur) *adj.* & *n.* [L. *articularis,* from *articulus,* joint]. 1. Pertaining to an articulation, or to a muscle or ligament associated with it. 2. A bone of the lower jaw of fishes, amphibians, and reptiles which articulates with the quadrate bone to form the mandibular joint. Its homologue in man is the malleus.

articular bone. ARTICULAR (2).

articular calculus. An arthritic calculus.

articular capsule. JOINT CAPSULE.

articular cartilage. Cartilage that covers the articular surfaces of bones. See also Plate 2.

articular corpuscles. The tactile corpuscles in a joint capsule. NA *corpuscula articularia.*

articular disk. A disk of fibrocartilage, dividing the joint cavity of certain joints. NA *discus articularis.*

ar·tic·u·la·re (ahr·tick"yoo·lair'ee) *n.* [L., short for *os articulare,* articular bone]. ARTICULAR (2).

articular eminence. ARTICULAR TUBERCLE.

articular fracture. A fracture that also involves the articular surface of a bone.

articularis gen·us (ahr·tick"yoo·lair'is jen'us, jen'oos). A small muscle arising from the distal fourth of the anterior surface of the femur and inserted into the capsule of the knee joint. NA *musculus articularis genus.* See also Table of Muscles in the Appendix.

articular muscle. A muscle that is attached or inserted onto a joint capsule. NA *musculus articularis.*

articular process. See *inferior articular process, superior articular process.*

articular tubercle. The projection upon the zygomatic process of the temporal bone which marks the anterior boundary of the mandibular fossa. Syn. *articular eminence.* NA *tuberculum articulare ossis temporalis.*

¹ar·tic·u·late (ahr·tick'yoo·lut) *adj.* [L. *articulatus,* jointed]. 1. Divided into joints. 2. Expressed or expressing oneself in concatenations of discrete symbols, as in human speech. 3. Expressed or expressing oneself coherently and fluently.

²ar·tic·u·late (ahr·tick'yoo·late) *v.* [L. *articulare, articulatus,* from *articulus,* joint]. 1. To unite by one or more joints. 2. To produce ordered and coordinated speech sounds; to enunciate. 3. To express (thoughts, feelings) in connected discourse. 4. *In dentistry,* to position or adjust artificial teeth. See also *articulator.*

ar·tic·u·lat·ing paper. A carbon paper on which the patient bites, to show the relationship of the teeth in occlusion.

ar·ti·cu·la·tio (ahr·tick"yoo·lay'shee·o) *n.*, pl. **articu·la·ti·o·nes** (·lay"shee·o'neez) [L.] 1. [NA] ARTICULATION. 2. [BNA, PNA] Junctura synovialis (= SYNOVIAL JOINT).

articulatio acro·mio·cla·vi·cu·la·ris (a·kro"mee·o·kla·vick"yoo·lair'is) [NA]. ACROMIOCLAVICULAR ARTICULATION.

articulatio at·lan·to·ax·i·a·lis la·te·ra·lis (at·lan"to·ack·see·ay'lis lat·e·ray'lis) [NA]. LATERAL ATLANTOAXIAL JOINT.

articulatio atlantoaxialis me·di·ana (mee·dee·ay'nuh) [NA]. MEDIAN ATLANTOAXIAL JOINT.

articulatio at·lan·to·epi·stro·phi·ca (at·lan''to·ep·i·strof'i·kuh) [BNA]. Articulatio atlantoaxialis mediana. (= MEDIAN ALTANTOAXIAL JOINT).

articulatio at·lan·to·oc·ci·pi·ta·lis (at·lan''to·ock·sip·i·tay'lis) [NA]. ATLANTOOCCIPITAL JOINT.

articulatio cal·ca·neo·cu·boi·dea (kal·kay''nee·o·kew·boy'dee·uh) [NA]. CALCANEOCUBOID ARTICULATION.

articulatio ca·pi·tis cos·tae (kap'i·tis kos'tee) [NA]. The joint between the head of a rib and its corresponding vertebral bodies.

articulatio ca·pi·tu·li (ka·pit'yoo·lye) [BNA]. ARTICULATIO CAPITIS COSTAE.

articulatio car·po·me·ta·car·pea pol·li·cis (kahr''po·met·uh·kahr'pee·uh pol'i·sis) [NA]. The carpometacarpal articulation of the thumb. See *carpometocarpal articulation.*

articulatio co·chle·ar·is (kock·lee·air'is) [BNA]. A variety of hinge joint or ginglymus in which there is some lateral movement.

articulatio com·po·si·ta (kom·poz'i·tuh) [NA]. A joint between more than two bones.

articulatio con·dy·la·ris (kon·di·lair'is) [NA]. CONDYLAR JOINT.

articulatio cos·to·trans·ver·sa·ria (kos''to·trans·vur·sair'ee·uh) [NA]. The joint between the tubercle of a rib and the transverse process of the corresponding vertebra.

articulatio co·ty·li·ca (kot·il'i·kuh) [NA alt.]. SPHEROID ARTICULATION. NA alt. *articulatio spheroidea.*

articulatio cox·ae (kock'see) [NA]. HIP JOINT.

articulatio cri·co·ary·te·noi·dea (krye''ko·ăr·i·tee·noy'dee·uh) [NA]. CRICOARYTENOID ARTICULATION.

articulatio cri·co·thy·re·oi·dea (krye''ko·thigh·ree·oy'dee·uh) [BNA]. Articulatio cricothyroidea. (= CRICOTHYROID ARTICULATION).

articulatio cri·co·thy·roi·dea (krye''ko·thigh·roy'dee·uh) [NA]. CRICOTHYROID ARTICULATION.

articulatio cu·bi·ti (kew'bi·tye) [NA]. The elbow joint. See *elbow.*

articulatio cu·neo·na·vi·cu·la·ris (kew''nee·o·na·vick·yoo·lair'is) [NA]. CUNEOCLAVICULAR ARTICULATION.

articulatio el·lip·soi·dea (el·ip·soy'dee·uh) [NA]. A form of ball-and-socket joint in which the articular surfaces are ovoid in shape.

articulatio ge·nu (jen'yoo) [BNA]. Articulatio genus. See *knee.*

articulatio ge·nus (jen'us, jen'oos) [NA]. The knee joint. See *knee.*

articulatio hu·me·ri (hew'mur·eye) [NA]. SHOULDER JOINT.

articulatio hu·me·ro·ra·di·a·lis (hew''mur·o·ray·dee·ay'lis) [NA]. HUMERORADIAL ARTICULATION.

articulatio hu·me·ro·ul·na·ris (hew''mur·o·ul·nair'is) [NA]. HUMEROULNAR ARTICULATION.

articulatio in·cu·do·mal·le·a·ris (ing·kew''do·mal·ee·air'is) [NA]. INCUDOMALLEAR ARTICULATION.

articulatio in·cu·do·mal·le·o·la·ris (ing·kew''do·mal·ee·o·lair'is) [BNA]. Articulatio incudomallearis (= INCUDOMALLEAR ARTICULATION).

articulatio in·cu·do·sta·pe·dia (ing·kew''do·stay·pee'dee·uh) [NA]. INCUDOSTAPEDIAL ARTICULATION.

articulatio man·di·bu·la·ris (man·dib·yoo·lair'is) [BNA]. Articulatio temporomandibularis (= TEMPOROMANDIBULAR ARTICULATION).

articulatio ma·nus (man'oos, man'us) [BNA]. Singular of NA *articulationes manus.*

articulatio me·dio·car·pea (mee·dee·o·kahr'pee·uh) [NA]. MEDIOCARPAL ARTICULATION.

ar·tic·u·la·tion (ahr·tick''yoo·lay'shun) *n.* [F., from L. *articulatio,* from *articulare,* to articulate, from *articulus,* q.v.]. 1. The production of ordered and coordinated speech sounds. Compare *phonation.* 2. The junction of two or more bones or skeletal parts. The articulations include the fibrous joints (syndesmoses, sutures, and gomphoses), cartilaginous joints (synchondroses and symphyses), and synovial joints (the movable joints). Syn. *joint.* NA *articulatio, junctura ossium.* 3. The positioning of artificial teeth. 4. OCCLUSION.

articulationes. Plural of *articulatio.*

articulationes ca·pi·tu·lo·rum cos·ta·rum (ka·pit·yoo·lo'rum kos·tair'um) [BNA]. Plural of NA *articulatio capitis costae.*

articulationes car·po·me·ta·car·pe·ae (kahr''po·met·uh·kahr'pee·ee) [NA]. CARPOMETACARPAL ARTICULATIONS.

articulationes cos·to·chon·dra·les (kos''to·kon·dray'leez) [NA]. The cartilaginous joints occurring between a costal cartilage and the distal end of its appropriate rib.

articulationes cos·to·ver·te·bra·les (kos''to·vur·te·bray'leez) [NA]. The joints between the ribs and the vertebrae.

articulationes di·gi·to·rum ma·nus (dij·i·to'rum man'oos, man'us) [BNA]. Articulationes interphalangeae manus.

articulationes digitorum pe·dis (ped'is) [BNA]. ARTICULATIONES INTERPHALANGEAE PEDIS.

articulationes in·ter·car·pe·ae (in·tur·kahr'pee·ee) [NA]. INTERCARPAL ARTICULATIONS.

articulationes in·ter·chon·dra·les (in''tur·kon·dray'leez) [NA]. The joints between the costal cartilages.

articulationes interchondrales cos·ta·rum (kos·tay'rum) [BNA]. ARTICULATIONES INTERCHONDRALES.

articulationes in·ter·me·ta·car·pe·ae (in''tur·met·uh·kahr'pee·ee) [NA]. INTERMETACARPAL ARTICULATIONS.

articulationes in·ter·me·ta·tar·se·ae (in''tur·met·uh·tahr'see·ee) [NA]. INTERMETATARSAL ARTICULATIONS.

articulationes in·ter·pha·lan·ge·ae ma·nus (in·tur·fa·lan'jee·ee man'oos, man'us) [NA]. The interphalangeal articulations of the hand; the joints between the phalanges of the fingers.

articulationes interphalangeae pe·dis (ped'is) [NA]. The interphalangeal articulations of the foot; the joints between the phalanges of the toes.

articulationes in·ter·tar·se·ae (in·tur·tahr'see·ee) [NA]. INTERTARSAL ARTICULATIONS.

articulationes ma·nus (man'oos, man'us) [NA]. The articulations of the hand; the various named joints of the hand and wrist. See also Table of Synovial Joints and Ligaments in the Appendix.

articulationes me·ta·car·po·pha·lan·ge·ae (met·uh·kahr''po·fa·lan'jee·ee) [NA]. METACARPOPHALANGEAL ARTICULATIONS.

articulationes me·ta·tar·so·pha·lan·ge·ae (met·uh·tahr''so·fa·lan'jee·ee) [NA]. METATARSOPHALANGEAL ARTICULATIONS.

articulationes os·si·cu·lor·um au·di·tus (os·ick·yoo·lo'rum aw·dye'toos, ·tus) [NA]. The joints between the bones of the middle ear cavity.

articulationes pe·dis (ped'is) [NA]. The articulations of the foot; the various named joints of the foot and the ankle. See also Table of Synovial Joints and Ligaments in the Appendix.

articulationes ster·no·cos·ta·les (stur''no·kos·tay'leez) [NA]. STERNOCOSTAL ARTICULATIONS.

articulationes tar·so·me·ta·tar·se·ae (tahr''so·met·uh·tahr'see·ee) [NA]. TARSOMETATARSAL ARTICULATIONS.

articulation of the pisiform bone. PISIFORM ARTICULATION.

articulatio os·sis pi·si·for·mis (oss'is pye·si·for'mis) [NA]. The articulation of the pisiform bone; PISIFORM ARTICULATION.

articulatio pe·dis (ped'is). A joint of the foot; singular of articulationes pedis.

articulatio pla·na (play'nuh) [NA]. GLIDING JOINT.

articulatio ra·dio·car·pea (ray''dee·o·kahr'pee·uh) [NA]. The radiocarpal articulation; WRIST JOINT.

articulatio ra·dio·ul·na·ris dis·ta·lis (ray''dee·o·ul·nair'is dis·tay'lis) [NA]. The distal radioulnar articulation. See *elbow.*

articulatio radioulnaris prox·i·ma·lis (prock·si·may'lis) [NA]. The proximal radioulnar articulation. See *elbow.*

articulatio sa·cro·ili·a·ca (sack·ro·i·lye'uh·kuh, say·kro·) [NA]. SACROILIAC ARTICULATION.

articulatio sel·la·ris (se·lair'is) [NA]. SADDLE JOINT.

articulatio sim·plex (sim'plecks) [NA]. SIMPLE ARTICULATION.

articulatio sphe·roi·dea (sfeer·oy'dee·uh) [NA]. SPHEROID ARTICULATION; ball-and-socket joint.

articulatio ster·no·cla·vi·cu·la·ris (stur"no·kla·vick·yoo·lair'is) [NA]. STERNOCLAVICULAR ARTICULATION.

articulatio sub·ta·la·ris (sub·tay·lair'is) [NA]. SUBTALAR ARTICULATION.

articulatio ta·li trans·ver·sa (tay'lye trans·vur'suh) [BNA]. Articulatio tarsi transversa (= TRANSVERSE TARSAL ARTICULATION).

articulatio ta·lo·cal·ca·nea (tay"lo·kal·kay'nee·uh) [BNA]. Articulatio subtalaris (= SUBTALAR ARTICULATION).

articulatio ta·lo·cal·ca·neo·na·vi·cu·la·ris (tay"lo·kal·kay"nee·o·na·vick·yoo·lair'is) [NA]. TALOCALCANEONAVICULAR ARTICULATION.

articulatio ta·lo·cru·ra·lis (tay"lo·kroo·ray'lis) [NA]. The talocrural articulation; ANKLE JOINT.

articulatio ta·lo·na·vi·cu·la·ris (tay"lo·na·vick·yoo·lair'is) [BNA]. TALONAVICULAR ARTICULATION.

articulatio tar·si trans·ver·sa (tahr'sigh trans·vur'suh) [NA]. TRANSVERSE TARSAL ARTICULATION.

articulatio tem·po·ro·man·di·bu·la·ris (tem"po·ro·man·dib·yoo·lair'is) [NA]. TEMPOROMANDIBULAR ARTICULATION.

articulatio ti·bio·fi·bu·la·ris (tib"ee·o·fib·yoo·lair'is). 1. [NA] TIBIOFIBULAR ARTICULATION (2). 2. [NA alt.]. TIBIOFIBULAR SYNDESMOSIS. NA alt. *syndesmosis tibiofibularis.*

articulatio tro·choi·dea (tro·koy'dee·uh) [NA]. PIVOT JOINT.

ar·tic·u·la·tor (ahr·tick'yoo·lay"tur) *n.* An instrument used in dentistry for holding casts of the jaws or teeth in proper relation during the construction of artificial dentures. It may be adjusted so as to duplicate the mandibular movements of the patient.

ar·tic·u·lus (ahr·tick'yoo·lus) *n.*, pl. **articu·li** (·lye) [L., joint, division, dim. of *artus,* joint (rel. to Gk. *ar*thron)]. 1. A joint; a knuckle. 2. A segment; a part; a limb.

ar·ti·fact, ar·te·fact (ahr'ti·fakt) *n.* [L. *arte,* by skill, + *factum,* made]. *In science and medicine,* an artificial or extraneous feature accidentally or unavoidably introduced into an object of observation and which may simulate a natural or relevant feature of that object.

ar·ti·fi·cial abortion. INDUCED ABORTION.

artificial antigen. Any laboratory-made or modified antigen, not occurring naturally; including conjugated antigens, such as azoproteins, antigens modified by other chemical or physical treatment, and specially synthesized polypeptides.

artificial anus. An opening made surgically from the lumen of the bowel to the external surface of the body to permit expulsion of feces.

artificial catalepsy. Catalepsy induced by hypnosis.

artificial crown. A metallic, porcelain, or plastic substitute that replaces all or most of the crown of a tooth.

artificial denture. A prosthesis that replaces missing natural teeth.

artificial eye. Glass, celluloid, rubber, or plastic made to resemble the front of the eye, and worn in the socket to replace a lost one, or over a blind eye for cosmetic effect.

artificial fecundation. Fertilization by artificial insemination.

artificial feeding. 1. The introduction of food into the body by means of artificial devices. 2. The nourishing of an infant of nursing age by any means other than breast milk.

artificial fever. Purposefully produced fever for therapeutic benefit, as by the induction of malaria, by the injection of foreign protein, or by means of a fever cabinet.

artificial glycosuria. Glycosuria resulting from puncture of the floor of the fourth ventricle in the inferior part of the medulla.

artificial insemination. The instrumental injection of semen into the vagina or uterus to induce pregnancy; insemination without coitus.

artificial lung. IRON LUNG.

artificial pneumothorax. PNEUMOTHORAX (2).

artificial respiration. The maintenance of breathing by artificial ventilation, in the absence of normal spontaneous respiration. Most effective methods include mouth-to-mouth breathing for emergencies and the use of a respirator for prolonged application.

artificial salt. A mixture of salts simulating the composition of salts naturally present in well-known mineral springs, especially those in Europe.

artificial stone. A specially calcined gypsum product that is harder than plaster of paris; used in dentistry. See also *calcium sulfate. Densite, Hydrocal.*

artificial tetanus. Muscle spasm produced by a drug.

ar·tis·tic anatomy. That branch of anatomy which treats of the external form of man and animals, their osseous and muscular systems, and their relation to painting and sculpture.

ary·epi·glot·tic (ăr"ee·ep"i·glot'ick) *adj.* [*ary*tenoid + *epiglottic*]. Pertaining to the arytenoid cartilage and the epiglottis.

aryepiglottic fold. A fold of mucous membrane in each lateral wall of the aditus laryngis, which extends from the arytenoid cartilage to the epiglottis. NA *plica aryepiglottica.*

ary·epi·glot·ti·cus (ăr"ee·ep"i·glot'i·kus) *n.* The continuation of the oblique arytenoid muscle. See also Table of Muscles in the Appendix.

ary·epi·glot·tid·e·an (ăr"ee·ep"i·glot·id'ee·un) *adj.* ARYEPIGLOTTIC.

ar·yl (ăr'il) *n.* [*ar*omatic + *-yl*]. An organic radical derived from an aromatic hydrocarbon by the removal of one hydrogen atom, as phenyl (C_6H_5—) from benzene.

ar·yl·ar·so·nate (ăr"il·ahr'so·nate) *n.* Any aromatic organic salt of arsenic, as arsphenamine.

ar·yl·ene (ăr'i·leen) *n.* [*aryl* + *-ene*]. Any bivalent radical derived from an aromatic hydrocarbon by removal of a hydrogen atom from each of two carbon atoms of the nucleus, as phenylene (C_6H_4=) from benzene.

ar·y·te·no·epi·glot·tic (ăr"i·tee"no·ep·i·glot'ick, a·rit"e·no·) *adj.* ARYEPIGLOTTIC.

ary·te·no·epi·glot·ti·cus (ăr"i·tee"no·ep·i·glot'i·kus) *n.* ARYEPIGLOTTICUS.

ar·y·te·noid (ăr"i·tee'noid, a·rit'e·noid) *adj.* [Gk. *arytainoeidēs,* ladle-shaped, from *arytaina,* ladle, cup]. 1. Resembling the mouth of a pitcher. 2. Pertaining to the arytenoid cartilages and muscles.

arytenoid cartilage. One of two cartilages of the back of the larynx resting on the cricoid cartilage and regulating, by means of the attached muscles, the tension of the vocal folds. NA *cartilago arytenoidea.*

ar·y·te·noid·ec·to·my (ăr·i·tee"noy·deck'tuh·mee) *n.* [*arytenoid* + *-ectomy*]. Removal of an arytenoid cartilage.

ar·y·te·noi·di·tis (ăr"i·tee"noy·dye'tis, a·rit"e·noy·) *n.* [*arytenoid* + *-itis*]. Inflammation of the arytenoid cartilages or muscles.

arytenoid muscles. See Table of Muscles in the Appendix.

ar·y·te·noi·do·pexy (ăr"i·te·noy'do·peck"see) *n.* [*arytenoid* + *-pexy*]. Surgical fixation of the arytenoid cartilages or muscles.

ary·vo·ca·lis (ăr"i·vo·kay'lis) *n.* A portion of the vocalis muscle inserted into the vocal fold.

As Symbol for arsenic.

As. Abbreviation for *astigmatism; astigmatic.*

a.s. Abbreviation for *auris sinistra,* left ear.

as·a·fet·i·da, as·a·foet·i·da (as"uh·fet'i·duh) *n.* [ML., from Per. *azā,* mastic, + L. *foetidus,* stinking]. An oleo-gum-resin obtained from the rhizomes and roots of species of *Ferula.* It occurs as soft yellow-brown masses and has a bitter taste and a persistent offensive odor due to a volatile oil consisting largely of a mercaptan. It has been used as a carminative and psychic sedative.

asa·phia (a·say'fee·uh) *n.* [Gk., indistinctness, from *a-* + *saphēs*, distinct, + *-ia*]. Indistinct speech associated with cleft palate.

asar·cia (a·sahr'shee·uh, ·see·uh) *n.* [Gk. *asarkia*, from *a-* + *sarx, sarkos*, flesh, + *-ia*]. Emaciation; leanness.

as·a·rum (as'uh·rum, a·săr'um) *n.* [L., from Gk. *asaron*, hazelwort]. The dried rhizome and roots of *Asarum canadense*, formerly used as a carminative and bitter aromatic flavor. Syn. *Canada snakeroot, wild ginger.*

as·bes·tos (as·bes'tus, az·) *n.* [Gk., lit., unquenchable, from *a-* + *sbestos*, quenched, from *sbennynai*, to quench]. A calcium-magnesium silicate mineral of flexible or elastic fibers; the best nonconductor of heat.

asbestos bodies. Long, slender cylinders with a transparent capsule composed of protein and a core of altered asbestos fiber; found in the lungs, air passages, sputum, and feces of patients with asbestosis and of many apparently normal people.

as·bes·to·sis (as''bes·to'sis, az·) *n.*, pl. **asbesto·ses** (·seez) [*asbestos* + *-osis*]. Diffuse interstitial pulmonary fibrosis due to the prolonged inhalation of asbestos dust.

asbestos transformation. A change in cartilage, especially of the hyaline type, often associated with advanced age, which leads to a softening of the tissue and to the formation of spaces in it.

as·ca·ri·a·sis (as''kuh·rye'uh·sis) *n.*, pl. **ascaria·ses** (·seez) [*Ascaris* + *-iasis*]. 1. Infection by a nematode of the genus *Ascaris*. 2. Specifically, infection of the human intestine, with a short migratory phase, by *Ascaris lumbricoides*, with occasional involvement of other organs, as the stomach or liver; heavy infection may cause bronchopneumonia, abdominal pain, and, occasionally, intestinal obstruction.

as·car·i·cide (as·kăr'i·side) *n.* [*ascarid* + *-cide*]. A medicine that kills ascarids.

as·ca·rid (as'kuh·rid) *n.*, pl. **ascarids, as·car·i·des** (as·kăr'i·deez). A worm of the family Ascaridae.

As·car·i·dae (as·kăr'i·dee) *n.pl.* [NL.]. A family of nematode worms, which includes the genera *Ascaris* and *Toxocara*.

As·ca·rid·i·dae (as·ka·rid'i·dee) *n.pl.* [NL.]. ASCARIDAE.

as·car·i·dole, as·car·i·dol (as·kăr'i·dol, ·dole) *n.* [*ascarid* + *-ole*]. 1,4-Peroxido-*p*-menthene-2, $C_{10}H_{16}O_2$, an unsaturated terpene peroxide; the principal and active constituent of chenopodium oil. Used as an anthelmintic.

As·ca·ris (as'kuh·ris) *n.* [Gk., an intestinal worm]. A genus of intestinal nematodes of the family Ascaridae.

Ascaris equorum. *PARASCARIS EQUORUM.*

Ascaris lum·bri·coi·des (lum·bri·koy'deez). A species of roundworm causing ascariasis in man and (var. *suis*) in swine.

Ascaris meg·a·lo·ceph·a·la (meg''uh·lo·sef'uh·luh). *PARASCARIS EQUORUM.*

Ascaris mys·tax (mis'tacks) [Gk., moustache]. *TOXOCARA CATI.*

Ascaris su·um (sue'um). *ASCARIS LUMBRICOIDES* var. *suis.*

as·cend·ing, *adj.* 1. Taking an upward course; rising. 2. In the nervous system, AFFERENT; conducting impulses or progressing up the spinal cord or from peripheral to central.

ascending aorta. The first part of the aorta. NA *aorta ascendens.* See also Table of Arteries in the Appendix and Plate 5.

ascending colon. The portion of the colon that extends from the cecum to the hepatic flexure. NA *colon ascendens.* See also Plate 13.

ascending degeneration. Secondary or wallerian degeneration of the myelin sheath and axons of sensory tracts progressing cranially from the point of injury in the spinal cord.

ascending frontal gyrus. PRECENTRAL GYRUS.

ascending limb. 1. The portion of a renal tubule which extends from the bend in the loop of Henle to the distal convoluted portion. 2. An upward slope in a graphic wave, representing increase, as of pressure, volume, or velocity.

ascending lumbar vein. An ascending vein of the posterior abdominal wall, becoming the hemiazygos vein on the left side and the azygos vein on the right. NA *vena lumbalis ascendens.*

ascending mesocolon. The ascending portion of the mesentery connecting the colon with the posterior abdominal wall. NA *mesocolon ascendens.*

ascending paralysis. GUILLAIN-BARRÉ SYNDROME.

ascending parietal gyrus. POSTCENTRAL GYRUS.

ascending poliomyelitis. A form of paralytic poliomyelitis beginning in the lower limbs and progressing upward, sometimes affecting the muscles of respiration and deglutition with fatal result.

ascending polyneuritis. GUILLAIN-BARRÉ SYNDROME.

ascending tract. AFFERENT TRACT.

Asch·heim-Zon·dek reaction (ahsh'hime, tsohn'deck) [S. *Aschheim*, German gynecologist, b. 1878; and B. *Zondek*, German gynecologist in Israel, 1891–1966]. Follicular growth and luteinization are produced by substances in the urine of pregnant women, whereas the urine following oophorectomy and the menopause contains only the follicle growth-stimulating substance. See also *Aschheim-Zondek test.*

Aschheim-Zondek test [S. *Aschheim* and B. *Zondek*]. A test for pregnancy in which the subcutaneous injection of urine from a pregnant woman into an immature mouse will cause the mouse ovaries to enlarge, with hyperemia, hemorrhage, and maturation of the ovarian follicles.

Asch·ner's phenomenon (ahsh'nur) [B. *Aschner*, Austrian gynecologist, b. 1883]. OCULOCARDIAC REFLEX.

Asch·off cell (ahsh'ohf) [K. A. L. *Aschoff*, German pathologist, 1866–1942]. The characteristic cell of the Aschoff body in rheumatic fever; a large, elongated cell with one or more vesicular nuclei, having a central mass of chromatin from which fibrils radiate toward the nuclear membrane.

Aschoff's bodies or **nodules** [K. A. L. *Aschoff*]. A myocardial granuloma specific for the carditis associated with rheumatic fever, located in the vicinity of a blood vessel, consisting of a central eosinophilic zone surrounded by roughly parallel rows of Anitschkow cells, Aschoff cells, lymphocytes, plasma cells, neutrophils, mast cells, and fibrocytes.

Asch's operation [M. J. *Asch*, U.S. otolaryngologist, 1833–1902]. An operation, no longer in use, to correct deviation of the nasal septum through a cruciate incision over the deflection.

asci. Plural of *ascus.*

as·ci·tes (a·sigh'teez) *n.*, pl. **ascites** [Gk. *askitēs*, a kind of dropsy, from *askos*, bag]. The accumulation of serous fluid in the peritoneal cavity, most commonly encountered with heart failure and portal hypertension. Syn. *abdominal dropsy, hydroperitoneum.* —**as·cit·ic** (a·sit'ick) *adj.*

ascites ad·i·po·sus (ad·i·po'sus). Milky fluid in the peritoneal cavity due to lipid-containing cells, probably resulting from lymphatic obstruction, and usually associated with cancer or tuberculosis.

ascites chy·lo·sus (kigh·lo'sus). Chyle in the peritoneal cavity due to rupture of the lacteals. Syn. *chylous ascites.*

ascites sac·ca·tus (sa·kay'tus). A form of ascites in which the effusion is prevented by adhesions or inflammatory exudate from entering the general peritoneal cavity.

ascites vag·i·na·lis (vaj''i·nay'lis). A collection of liquid within the sheath of the rectus abdominis muscle.

ascites vul·ga·ti·or (vul·gay'tee·or). A form of ascites apparently due to diseased kidneys, and preceded by scanty, highly colored urine.

as·cle·pi·as (as·klee'pee·us) *n.* [Gk. *asklēpias*, swallow-wort, after *Asklēpios*, god of healing]. The root of *Asclepias tuberosa*, a plant of the order Asclepiadaceae. It has been used as an emetic, cathartic, diaphoretic, and expectorant; formerly popular in the treatment of pleurisy.

asco-. A combining form meaning *ascus.*

as·co·carp (as'ko·kahrp) *n.* [*asco-* + *-carp*]. The developed fruit of Ascomycetes, or ascus-producing structure.

as·co·car·pic (as"ko·kahr'pick) *adj.* ASCOCARPOUS.

as·co·car·pous (as"ko·kahr'pus) *adj.* Of or pertaining to an ascocarp.

as·co·go·nid·i·um (as"ko·go·nid'ee·um) *n.*, pl. **ascogonid·ia** (·ee·uh) [*asco-* + *gonidium*]. A portion of the female sex organ in ascomycetous fungi which, after fertilization, develops into asci.

As·co·li test (ah'sko·lee) [A. *Ascoli,* Italian serologist, 1877–1957]. A precipitin test for the detection of soluble anthrax antigens in which a saline solution extract of suspected tissue is superimposed on anthrax antiserum; a precipitate forming at the junction of the liquids is a positive test.

Ascoli treatment [A. *Ascoli*]. A treatment for malaria with intravenous epinephrine in conjunction with antimalarial drugs, once thought to eradicate malarial parasites in the spleen by causing splenic contraction.

As·co·my·ce·tes (as"ko·migh·see'teez) *n.pl.* [*asco-* + *mycetes*]. One of the four large classes of fungi in which the ultimate reproductive spores are produced internally in an ascus. —**ascomyce·tous** (·tus) *adj.*

ascor·bate (uh·skor'bate) *n.* A salt of ascorbic acid.

ascor·bic acid (uh·skor'bick) [*a-* + *scorbutus* + *-ic*]. The enol form of 3-oxo-L-gulofuranolactone, $C_6H_8O_6$, occurring in significant amounts in citrus fruits, the systemic lack of which eventually leads to scurvy. It is a white or slightly yellowish crystalline powder, fairly stable when dry, but in aqueous solution rapidly destroyed by the oxygen of the air. Ascorbic acid functions in various oxidation-reduction reactions of the tissues and is essential for normal metabolism. Syn. *vitamin C.* See Table of Chemical Constituents of Blood in the Appendix.

ascorbic acid oxidase. A copper-containing enzyme found in plants, but not in animals, which catalyzes the oxidation of ascorbic acid to dehydroascorbic acid.

ascor·byl palmitate (as·kor'bil). L-Ascorbic acid 6-palmitate, $C_{22}H_{38}O_7$, a pharmaceutical antioxidant and food preservative.

as·co·spore (as'ko·spore) *n.* A spore produced in an ascus.

as·cus (as'kus) *n.*, pl. **as·ci** (ass'eye, as'kigh) [Gk. *askos,* wineskin, belly, bladder]. The characteristic spore case of the Ascomycetes; usually consisting of a cell containing eight spores.

A.S.D.C. American Society of Dentistry for Children.

-ase [from diast*ase*]. A suffix which is attached to the name of a biochemical substance to designate an *enzyme* that catalyzes reactions with that substance.

Asellacrin. A trademark for somatropin, a growth stimulant.

Asel·li's glands (ah·sel'lee) [G. *Aselli,* Italian physician and anatomist, 1581–1626]. Lymph nodes at the base of the mesentery near the pancreas, receiving lymph from the intestine.

as·e·ma·sia (as"e·may'zee·uh) *n.* [*a-* + Gk. *sēmasia,* signal, indication, meaning]. *Obsol.* ASYMBOLIA.

ase·mia (a·see'mee·uh) *n.* [*a-* + Gk. *sēma,* sign, + *-ia*]. *Obsol.* ASYMBOLIA.

asep·sis (ay·sep'sis, a·sep'sis) *n.* [*a-* + *sepsis*]. Exclusion of microorganisms. —**asep·tic** (·tick) *adj.*

aseptic meningitis. Meningeal inflammation produced by one of numerous agents, predominantly viral, characterized by meningeal irritation with cerebrospinal fluid showing an increase in white blood cells (usually mononuclear); normal glucose, usually normal protein, and bacteriologic sterility. Compare *suppurative meningitis.* See also *lymphocytic choriomeningitis.*

aseptic necrosis. Necrosis without infection.

aseptic peritonitis. CHEMICAL PERITONITIS.

aseptic surgery. Operative procedure in the absence of germs, everything coming in contact with the wound being sterile; a system of surgical techniques and practices designed to exclude all infectious microorganisms from the wound. Compare *antiseptic surgery.*

asex·u·al (ay·seck'shoo·ul, a·seck') *adj.* 1. Not involving the distinction between male and female. 2. Characterizing reproduction without sexual union. —**asexual·ly** (·lee) *adv.*

asexual dwarf. A dwarf with deficient sexual development.

asexual spore. A spore formed without previous fusion of nuclear material, as in fungi.

ash, *n.* The incombustible mineral residue that remains when a substance is incinerated.

A.S.H.A. American School Health Association.

Ash·er·man's syndrome [J. G. *Asherman,* Czechoslovakian gynecologist in Israel, b. 1889]. Intrauterine adhesions with associated amenorrhea, usually following vigorous curettage. Syn. *traumatic amenorrhea, traumatic intrauterine synechiae..*

Ash·hurst's splint [J. *Ashhurst,* U.S. surgeon, 1839–1900]. A splint with a footpiece, used after leg fractures or excision of the knee joint.

Ash·man's phenomenon [R. *Ashman,* 20th century]. *In electrocardiography,* aberrant conduction of the ventricular beat ending a short cycle preceded by a long cycle; seen in atrial fibrillation and other arrhythmias.

asi·a·lia (ay"sigh·ay'lee·uh, ay"sigh·al'ee·uh) *n.* [*a-* + *sial-* + *-ia*]. Deficiency or failure of the secretion of saliva.

Asian influenza virus. A subtype of influenza virus A, designated A_2, first recovered from an influenza epidemic in Hong Kong and Singapore in 1957.

asi·at·i·co·side (ay"zee·at'i·ko·side) *n.* An antibiotic substance derived from Madagascar varieties of the perennial umbelliferous herb *Centella asiatica* (*Hydrocotyle asiatica*); it is active against *Mycobacterium tuberculosis* in animals, but is toxic.

asid·er·o·sis (ay·sid"ur·o'sis) *n.* [*a-* + *sider-* + *-osis*]. An abnormal decrease in the iron reserves of the body. —**asider·ot·ic** (·ot'ick) *adj.*

asiderotic anemia. IRON-DEFICIENCY ANEMIA.

As·ken·stedt's method. A test for indican in the urine, using precipitation with mercuric chloride followed by Obermayer's reagent and extraction with chloroform.

As·kle·pios (as·klee'pee·os). Greek god of healing; as Roman god of medicine, *Aesculapius.*

Ask-Up·mark kidney [E. *Ask-Upmark,* 20th century]. A type of segmental renal hypoplasia characterized by a misshapen kidney bearing a discrete transverse groove in the cortex, which overlies an absent renal pyramid and a calyx with a dilated tip. Histologically, the parenchyma beneath the grooves contains thyroidlike tubules, thickened arteries, and no glomeruli. The lesion is usually unilateral and is associated with hypertension.

aso·cial (ay·so'shul) *adj.* 1. Withdrawn from, not interested in other people and their activities nor in the realities of one's environment. 2. Indifferent toward accepted social standards, customs, and rules. Compare *antisocial, dyssocial.* —**aso·ci·al·i·ty** (ay·so"shee·al'i·tee) *n.*

aso·ma (a·so'muh, ay·) *n.*, pl. **asomas, asoma·ta** (·tuh) [*a-* + Gk. *sōma,* body]. A placental parasite (omphalosite) with an ill-formed head and only a rudimentary body. —**aso·mous** (·mus) *adj.*

aso·nia (a·so'nee·uh) *n.* [*a-* + L. *son*us, sound, + *-ia*]. 1. TONE DEAFNESS. 2. A type of amusia in which the patient is no longer able to distinguish between one musical tone and another.

asp, *n.* [Gk. *aspis*]. 1. A small venomous snake, *Vipera aspis,* found in Africa and the Near East. 2. The horned viper, *Cerastes cornutus.*

as·pal·a·so·ma (as·pal"uh·so'muh) *n.* [Gk. *aspalax,* blind rat, + *-soma*]. Median or lateral eventration of the lower abdomen, having three distinct openings for the urinary bladder, the rectum, and the genital organs; a celosoma limited to the lower abdomen.

as·par·a·gin (as·păr'uh·jin) *n.* ASPARAGINE.

as·par·a·gin·ase (as·păr'uh·ji·nace, ·naze) *n.* An enzyme, present in liver and other animal tissues as well as in plants, yeast, and bacteria, which catalyzes hydrolysis of asparagine to asparaginic acid and ammonia; has antileukemic activity.

as·par·a·gine (as·păr'uh·jeen, ·jin) *n.* [*asparagus* + *-ine*]. α-Aminosuccinamic acid, the β-amide of asparaginic or aspartic acid, $C_4H_8N_2O_3$, a nonessential amino acid occurring in many proteins. Syn. *asparamide, aminosuccinamic acid.*

as·par·a·gin·ic acid (as·păr"uh·jin'ick). ASPARTIC ACID.

as·par·a·gi·nyl (as·păr'uh·ji·nil) *n.* The univalent radical, $NH_2COCH_2CH(NH_2)CO$—, of asparagine, the monamide of aspartic acid.

as·par·am·ide (as·păr'uh·mide, as"păr·am'ide) *n.* ASPARAGINE.

as·par·tase (as·pahr'tace, ·taze) *n.* An enzyme, present in several bacteria, which catalyzes the conversion of aspartic acid to fumaric acid and ammonia.

as·par·tame (as·pahr'tame) *n.* The 1-methyl ester of *N*-α-aspartylphenylalanine, $C_{14}H_{18}N_2O_5$, a noncarbohydrate sweetener.

as·par·tate ami·no·trans·fer·ase (as·pahr'tate a·mee"no·trans'fur·ace). GLUTAMIC-OXALOACETIC TRANSAMINASE.

L-aspartate:2-oxoglutarate aminotransferase. GLUTAMIC-OXALOACETIC TRANSAMINASE.

as·par·tic acid (as·pahr'tick). Aminosuccinic acid, $COOHCH(NH_2)CH_2COOH$, a hydrolysis product of asparagine and of many proteins. Syn. *asparaginic acid.*

as·par·to·cin (as·pahr'to·sin) *n.* An antibiotic, produced by *Streptomyces griseus* var. *spiralis,* active against gram-positive bacteria.

as·par·to·ki·nase (as·pahr"to·kigh'nace) *n.* [*aspartic* + *kinase*]. An allosteric enzyme that catalyzes the reaction of aspartic acid with adenosine triphosphate to give aspartyl phosphate. The reaction constitutes the first step in the *de novo* synthesis of pyrimidines.

as·par·to·yl (as·pahr'to·il) *n.* The divalent radical, —$COCH_2CH(NH_2)CO$—, of aspartic acid.

as·par·tyl (as·pahr'til) *n.* The univalent radical, $COOHCH_2CH(NH_2)CO$—, of aspartic acid.

as·par·tyl·gly·cos·am·i·nu·ria (as·pahr"til·glye"ko·sam·i·new'ree·uh) *n.* An inborn error of metabolism associated with mental retardation in which there is an excessive urinary excretion of 2-acetamido-1-(beta-L-aspartamido)-1,2-deoxyglucose, a component of certain glycoproteins.

aspartyl phosphate. 4-Phosphoaspartic acid, $H_2O_3PCOCH_2$-$CHNH_2COOH$, an intermediate in the biosynthetic pathway for pyrimidines.

β-aspartyl phosphate. ASPARTYL PHOSPHATE.

aspas·tic (ay·spas'tick) *adj.* Not spastic; not characterized by spasm.

aspe·cif·ic (ay"spe·sif'ick) *adj.* Nonspecific; not a specific.

as·pect, *n.* [L. *aspectus,* view, sight, appearance, from *ad-* + *specere,* to look]. 1. The part or side that faces in a particular direction. 2. The particular appearance, as of a face.

As·per·gil·la·ce·ae (as"pur·ji·lay'see·ee) *n.pl.* A family of fungi and molds which includes the genera *Aspergillus* and *Penicillium.*

as·per·gil·lic acid (as"pur·jil'ick). 2-Hydroxy-3-isobutyl-6-(1-methylpropyl)pyrazine 1-oxide, $C_{12}H_{20}N_2O_2$, an antibiotic substance produced by *Aspergillus flavus.*

as·per·gil·lin (as"pur·jil'in) *n.* A pigment obtained from the spores of *Aspergillus niger.*

as·per·gil·lo·ma (as"pur·ji·lo'muh) *n.* [*aspergillus* + *-oma*]. A mass of mycelial elements of *Aspergillus fungus,* forming a spheroidal mass within a fibrous-walled lung cavity which is usually continuous with a bronchus; not a true tumor; the main type of fungus ball seen in the lung.

as·per·gil·lo·sis (as"pur·ji·lo'sis, as·pur") *n.,* Primary or secondary infection by any of various species of *Aspergillus,* especially *A. fumigatus.* The most common site of human infection is the lung where, after inhalation of spores, aspergillomas may form in preexisting cavities or bronchiectases, the fungus sometimes invading contiguous tissues or disseminating hematogenously to other organs.

As·per·gil·lus (as"pur·jil'us) *n.* [NL., from *aspergill*]. A genus of fungi of the family Aspergillaceae, in which the conidiophore is swollen into a head from which radiate numerous sterigmata bearing chains of conidia, and sometimes producing secondary sterigmata bearing in turn chains of conidia. Generally saprophytic, but plant and animal infections occur. The species *Aspergillus fumigatus* is the most common invader of plants and animals; *A. flavus* and *A. parasiticus* produce aflatoxins. See also *aflatoxin.* —**aspergillus,** pl. **aspergil·li** (·eye) *com. n.*

as·per·lin (as'pur·lin) *n.* An antibiotic, $C_{10}H_{12}O_5$, produced by *Aspergillus nidulans,* with antibacterial and antineoplastic activities.

asper·ma·tism (ay·spur'muh·tiz·um, a·spur') *n.* [*a-* + *spermat-* + *-ism*]. 1. Nonemission of semen, whether owing to nonsecretion or to nonejaculation. 2. Defective secretion of semen or lack of formation of spermatozoa. —**asper·mat·ic** (ay"spur·mat'ick) *adj.*

asper·ma·to·gen·e·sis (ay·spur"ma·to·jen'e·sis) *n.* [*a-* + *spermatogenesis*]. Failure of spermatozoa to mature.

asper·mia (ay·spur'mee·uh, a·spur') *n.* ASPERMATISM. —**asper·mous** (·mus) *adj.*

as·per·ous (as'pur·us) *adj.* [L. *asper,* rough, + *-ous*]. Uneven; having a surface with distinct, minute elevations.

as·phyx·ia (as·fick'see·uh) *n.* [Gk., stopping of the pulse, from *a-* + *sphyxis,* pulse, + *-ia*]. Systemic oxygen deficiency and carbon dioxide accumulation, usually due to impaired respiration, leading to loss of consciousness. Compare *apnea, suffocation.* —**asphyx·i·al** (·see·ul) *adj.*

asphyxia liv·i·da (liv'i·duh). Asphyxia neonatorum associated with cyanotic skin, strong pulse, and active reflexes. Syn. *blue asphyxia.*

asphyxia ne·o·na·to·rum (nee"o·nay·to'rum). Asphyxia of the newborn.

as·phyx·i·ant (as·fick'see·unt) *adj.* & *n.* 1. Producing asphyxia. 2. An agent capable of producing asphyxia. —**asphyxi·ate** (·ate) *v.*

asphyxia pal·li·da (pal'i·duh). Asphyxia neonatorum attended by a slow, weak pulse, abolished reflexes, and a very pale skin.

aspid-, aspido- [Gk. *aspis, aspidos*]. A combining form meaning *shield.*

as·pid·i·um (as·pid'ee·um) *n.* [NL., from Gk. *aspidion,* little shield]. The rhizome and stipes of European aspidium or male fern, *Dryopteris filix-mas,* or of American aspidium or marginal fern, *D. marginalis;* both are sources of aspidium oleoresin, used for expelling tapeworm.

as·pi·do·sper·ma (as"pi·do·spur'muh) *n.* [*aspido-* + Gk. *sperma,* seed]. The dried bark of *Aspidosperma quebracho-blanco* containing the alkaloids aspidospermine, quebrachine, and others; it has been used as a respiratory stimulant in asthmatic and cardiac dyspnea. Syn. *quebracho.*

as·pi·do·sper·mine (as"pi·do·spur'meen, ·min) *n.* An alkaloid, $C_{22}H_{30}N_2O_2$, from quebracho (aspidosperma); has been used as a respiratory stimulant.

as·pi·ra·tion (as"pi·ray'shun) *n.* [L. *aspiratio,* from *aspirare,* to breathe upon]. 1. *Obsol.* Breathing, especially breathing in. 2. The drawing of foreign matter or other material in the upper respiratory tract into the lungs with the breath. 3. The withdrawal by suction of fluids or gases from a cavity, as with an aspirator. 4. In speech, the expulsion of breath as in the pronunciation of h or after an initial p or t in English. —**as·pi·rate** (as'pi·rate) *v.*

aspiration pneumonia. Pneumonia due to inhalation into the bronchi of a foreign body, gastric contents, or infected material from the upper respiratory tract, usually occurring during periods of depressed consciousness.

as·pi·ra·tor (as'pi·ray"tur) *n.* A negative pressure apparatus for withdrawing fluids from cavities.

as·pi·rin (as'pi·rin, as'prin) *n.* [*acetyl* + *spira*eic (=salicylic) + *-in*]. Acetylsalicylic acid, $C_6H_4O(COCH_3)COOH$, a white crystalline powder hydrolyzing in moist air to acetic and salicylic acids. An analgesic, antipyretic, and antirheumatic.

As·pis cor·nu·tus (as'pis kor·new'tus). *CERASTES CORNUTUS.*

asple·nia (a·splee'nee·uh) *n.* [*a-* + *splen-* + *-ia*]. Acquired or congenital absence of the spleen.

asplenia syndrome. IVEMARK SYNDROME.

aspo·ro·gen·ic (ay·spo"ro·jen'ick, as"po·ro·) *adj.* [*a-* + *sporogenic*]. 1. Producing no spores. 2. Reproduced without spores.

aspo·rog·e·nous (as"po·roj'e·nus, ay"spo·) *adj.* ASPOROGENIC.

aspo·rous (a·spo'rus, ay·spor'us) *adj.* [*a-* + *spor-* + *-ous*]. Without spores; especially without the resistant phase, as in the case of many bacteria.

aspor·u·late (ay·spor'yoo·late, a·spor') *adj.* Producing no spores.

As·sam fever (a·sam') [*Assam,* state in northeastern India]. KALA AZAR.

as·sas·sin bug. Any of various bloodsucking bugs of the family Reduviidae which prey primarily on other insects but which also attack humans and other mammals, inflicting a painful bite that is toxic in some species; *Triatoma, Panstrongylus,* and related genera include vectors of Chagas' disease. Syn. *kissing bug.*

as·say (ass'ay, a·say') *n.* & *v.* [OF. (var. of *essay*), trial, test, from L. *exagium,* a weighing (rel. to *exigere,* to weigh, measure, test)]. 1. The testing or analyzing of a substance to determine its potency or the proportion of one or more constituents. 2. The recorded result of an assay. 3. To perform an assay (on). 4. The substance to be assayed.

as·si·dent (as'i·dunt) *adj.* [L. *assidere,* to sit by, from *ad-* + *sedere,* sit]. Usually, but not always, accompanying a disease.

assident symptom. A nonpathognomonic symptom. Syn. *accessory symptom.*

as·sim·i·la·tion (a·sim"i·lay'shun) *n.* [L. *assimilatio,* from *assimilare,* to liken, to make like, from *ad-* + *similis,* like]. 1. Absorption of a substance by tissues, cells, or organs. 2. Specifically, absorption of nutrients and other substances by the cells of the body after ingestion and digestion. 3. *Obsol.* ANABOLISM. 4. *In psychology,* mental reception of impressions, and their assignment by the consciousness to their proper place; mental assimilation. 5. A psychic process by which an unpleasant fact, having been faced, is integrated into a person's previous experience. 6. The abnormal fusion of bones, as the fusion of the transverse processes of the last lumbar vertebra with the lateral masses of the first sacral vertebra, or the atlas with the occipital bone. **—as·sim·i·late** (a·sim'i·late) *v.;* **as·sim·i·la·ble** (a·sim'i·luh·bul) *adj.*

Ass·mann focus (a^h^ss'ma^h^n) [H. *Assmann,* German internist, 1882–1950]. A roentgenologically demonstrated early focus of pulmonary tuberculosis; it is an ill-defined acute exudative and caseous lesion in the infraclavicular or subapical area of the lung.

as·so·ci·ate *n.* 1. *In psychology,* any item or phenomenon mentally linked with another. 2. A person with whom one is grouped by some common trait, experience, or interest. **—associ·ate** (·ate) *v.*

as·so·ci·at·ed automatic movement. SYNKINESIS.

associate degree nurse. A technical nurse holding a degree in nursing from an accredited 2-year college program.

associated movements. 1. Synergic, coincident, or consensual movements of muscles other than the leading ones, as swinging of the arms in walking. 2. In the normal infant, movements of one limb tending to be accompanied by similar involuntary movements of the opposite limb, a phenomenon which disappears as coordination and muscle power are increased. Persistence of such or similar movements, or return thereof in states of cortical dysfunction, is pathologic. See also *mirror movements.*

as·so·ci·a·tion *n.* 1. *In chemistry,* the correlation or aggregation of substances or functions. 2. *In psychology,* a mental linking, as that of objects, persons, or events with ideas, thoughts, or sensations.

association area. Any area of the cerebral cortex connected with the primary sensory and motor areas by association fibers, and usually homotypical in structure; concerned with the higher mental activities, such as the integration, interpretation, and memory storage of various stimuli, and the ability to carry out complex tasks, such as speaking, reading, or writing. Contr. *projection area.*

association cell. AMACRINE CELL.

association cortex. Cerebral cortex belonging to the association areas or to an association area. Often in phrases such as association visual cortex, association motor cortex, etc. See also *association area.*

association fibers. Nerve fibers situated just beneath the cortical substance and connecting the adjacent cerebral gyri. NA *fibrae arcuatae cerebri.*

association of ideas. The mental link established between two similar ideas or two ideas of simultaneous occurrence.

association test. 1. *In psychology,* any test designed to determine the nature of the mental or emotional link between a stimulus and a response. 2. Commonly, a test used to determine the nature, or to measure the speed, of the response with a word given by a subject to a word offered him. The response is determined by previous experience and may reveal a great deal about the subject's past, personality, and attitudes.

association time. *In psychology,* the time required to establish a response to a given stimulus in an association test.

association word. The verbal stimulus or verbal response in an association test.

as·so·cia·tive (a·so'shee·uh·tiv, a·so'see·, ·ay"tiv) *adj.* Pertaining to or based upon association.

associative facilitation. *In psychology,* the effect of previous associations in making it easier to establish new ones.

associative inhibition or **interference.** 1. *In psychology,* the blocking or weakening of a mental link when one part of it is linked to a new association. 2. Difficulty in establishing a new association because of previous ones.

associative learning. *In psychology,* the principle that items experienced together are mentally linked, so that they tend to reinforce one another.

associative memory. 1. *In psychology,* the recalling of some item, thought, or event previously experienced by thinking of something linked with it, in order for the present idea to invoke the former associations. 2. The process of recalling by association.

associative reaction. A response in an association test.

associative thinking. 1. *In psychology,* the mental process whereby a subject brings to bear on a thought at hand all relevant present factors. 2. *In psychiatry,* FREE ASSOCIATION.

as·so·nance (as'uh·nunce) *n.* [F., from L. *assonare,* to echo, answer with a sound]. A pathologic tendency to employ alliteration.

as·sort·a·tive mating (a·sor'tuh·tiv). Nonrandom mating based on phenotypic similarity. Contr. *disassortative mating.*

As·ta·cus (as'tuh·kus) *n.* [NL., from Gk. *astakos,* crayfish]. A genus of crustaceans comprising the crayfish. The species *Astacus japonicus* and *A. similis* are important second intermediate hosts of the *Paragonimus westermanii.*

asta·sia (a·stay'zhuh, ·zee·uh) *n.* [Gk., unsteadiness, from *a-* + *stasis,* standing, + *-ia*]. Inability to stand despite the preservation of strength, coordination, and sensation in the legs. Contr. *abasia.* —**astat·ic** (a·stat'ick) *adj.*

astasia-abasia. Inability to walk or stand despite retained strength, coordination, and sensation in the legs; usually a symptom of hysteria, sometimes of bilateral frontal lobe disease.

astatic epilepsy or **seizure.** AKINETIC SEIZURE.

as·ta·tine (as'tuh·teen, ·tin) *n.* [Gk. *astatos*, unstable, + *-ine*]. At = 210. Element number 85, prepared in 1940 by bombarding bismuth with alpha particles. It is radioactive and forms no stable isotopes.

aste·a·to·sis (a·stee"uh·to'sis, as"tee·) *n.* [*a-* + *steat-* + *-osis*]. A dermatosis in which sebum is deficient in amount or quality, resulting in dryness, scaliness, or fissuring of the skin.

aster-, astero- [Gk. *astēr, asteros*]. A combining form meaning *star, star-shaped.*

as·ter (as'tur) *n.* [Gk. *astēr,* star]. The radiating structure made up of microtubules, surrounding the centriole of a cell, seen at the beginning of mitosis. —**as·tral** (·trul) *adj.*

aster·eo·cog·no·sy (a·sterr"ee·o·kog'no·see, ay·steer") *n.* ASTEREOGNOSIS.

aster·e·og·no·sis (a·steer"ee·og·no'sis, ay·sterr") *n.*, [*a-* + *stereognosis*]. Inability to recognize the size, shape, or texture of objects, even though the primary senses (tactile, painful, thermal, vibratory) are intact or relatively intact. Syn. *tactile amnesia.*

as·te·ri·on (as·teer'ee·on) *n.*, pl. **aste·ria** (·ree·uh) [Gk. *aster-* + *-ion*]. *In craniometry,* the meeting point of the lambdoid, parietomastoid, and occipitomastoid sutures.

as·te·rix·is (as"te·rick'sis) *n.* [noun from Gk. *astēriktos,* unsupported, unstable, from *a-* + *stērinx,* prop, support]. A motor disturbance characterized by intermittent lapses of postural tone, producing flapping movements of the outstretched hands; seen with such conditions as hepatic coma, uremia, and respiratory acidosis. Syn. *flapping tremor.* —**aste·ric·tic** (·rick'tick) *adj.*

aster·nal (ay·stur'nul, a·stur'nul) *adj.* 1. Not joined to the sternum. 2. Without a sternum.

asternal ribs. FALSE RIBS.

aster·nia (ay·stur'nee·uh, a·stur') *n.* [*a-* + *stern-* + *-ia*]. Absence of the sternum.

astero-. See *aster-.*

as·ter·oid (as'tur·oid) *adj.* [Gk. *asteroeidēs,* starlike, from *astēr,* star]. Star-shaped.

asteroid body. Any star-shaped structure such as is found in the cytoplasm of giant cells in sarcoidosis or berylliosis or in a number of fungous infections, actinomycosis, and nocardiosis.

asteroid hyalitis. Inflammation of the vitreous body in which calcium soaps form, giving rise to crystalline opacities.

asthen-, astheno- [Gk. *asthenēs,* weak, from *a-* + *sthenos,* strength]. A combining form meaning *weak, weakness.*

as·the·nia (as·theen'ee·uh) *n.* [Gk. *astheneia,* from *asthenēs,* weak]. Absence or loss of strength; weakness; ADYNAMIA.

asthenia cru·rum par·es·thet·i·ca (kroo'rum păr·es·thet'i·kuh). RESTLESS LEGS.

asthenia pig·men·to·sa (pig·men·to'suh). ADDISON'S DISEASE.

asthenia uni·ver·sa·lis con·gen·i·ta (yoo"ni·vur·say'lis kon·jen'i·tuh). A psychophysiologic disorder characterized by many gastrointestinal as well as vasomotor disturbances.

as·then·ic (as·thenn'ick) *adj.* [Gk. *asthenikos*]. 1. Of or pertaining to asthenia. 2. See *asthenic type.*

asthenic personality. A personality disorder marked by chronic easy fatigability, low energy, lack of enthusiasm, inability to enjoy one's self, and hypersensitivity to physical and emotional stress. See also *neurasthenic neurosis.*

asthenic type. A physical type marked by a tall, slender, flat-chested, angular form, and poor muscular development.

as·the·no·bi·o·sis (as"thi·no·bye·o'sis) *n.* [*astheno-* + *biosis*]. A biologic state of reduced activity closely allied to hibernation or estivation, yet not induced by climate, temperature, or humidity.

as·the·no·co·ria (as"thi·no·ko'ree·uh) *n.* [*astheno-* + *cor-* + *-ia*]. A sluggish or slow pupillary reaction to light, seen in hypoadrenocorticism.

as·the·nol·o·gy (as"thi·nol'uh·jee) *n.* [*astheno-* + *-logy*]. The theory that anatomic and functional anomalies are associated with constitutional weakness or debility.

as·the·nom·e·ter (as"the·nom'e·tur) *n.* 1. A type of dynamometer used to detect and measure asthenia. 2. An instrument for measuring muscular asthenopia.

as·the·no·pho·bia (as"thi·no·fo'bee·uh) *n.* [*astheno-* + *-phobia*]. Morbid fear of weakness.

as·the·no·pia (as"thi·no'pee·uh) *n.* [*asthen-* + *-opia*]. Any of the symptoms dependent on fatigue of the ciliary or the extraocular muscles, such as pain around the eyes, headache, photophobia, dimness or blurring of vision, nausea, vertigo, and twitching of the eyelids; eyestrain. —**asthe·nop·ic** (·nop'ick) *adj.;* **as·the·nope** (as'thi·nope) *n.*

as·the·no·sper·mia (as"thi·no·spur'mee·uh) *n.* [*astheno-* + *-spermia*]. Weakness or loss of vitality of the spermatozoa.

as·the·nox·ia (as"thi·nock'see·uh) *n.* [*asthen-* + *ox-* + *-ia*]. A condition of insufficient oxidation of waste products, as ketosis from insufficient oxidation of fatty acids.

asth·ma (az'muh) *n.* [Gk.]. A disease characterized by an increased responsiveness of the trachea and bronchi to various stimuli (often allergens) and manifested by widespread airway narrowing that changes in severity either spontaneously or as a result of therapy; present as episodic dyspnea, cough, and wheezing.

asthma crystals. CHARCOT-LEYDEN CRYSTALS.

asth·mat·ic (az·mat'ick) *adj. & n.* [Gk. *asthmatikos*]. 1. Pertaining to, caused by, or affected with asthma. 2. An individual chronically affected with asthma.

asthmatic bronchitis. Asthmatic signs and symptoms associated with apparent bronchial infection.

asthma weed. LOBELIA.

astig·ma·graph (a·stig'muh·graf) *n.* An instrument for detecting astigmatism.

as·tig·mat·ic (as"tig·mat'ick) *adj.* 1. Of, pertaining to, or affected with astigmatism. 2. Pertaining to an apparatus for detecting astigmatism. 3. Pertaining to a means (as lenses) to correct astigmatism.

astigmatic band. In refraction, an apparent band of light seen under retinoscopy when one of the chief meridians is neutralized.

astig·ma·tism (a·stig'muh·tiz·um) *n.* [*a-* + Gk. *stigma, stigmatos,* mark, spot, + *-ism*]. A congenital or acquired defect of vision which results from irregularity in the curvature of one or more refractive surfaces (cornea, anterior and posterior surfaces of the lens) of the eye. When such a condition occurs, rays emanating from a point are not brought into focus at one point on the retina, but appear to spread as a line in various directions depending upon the curvature. Abbreviated, As.

astig·ma·tom·e·ter (a·stig"muh·tom'e·tur) *n.* ASTIGMOMETER.

as·tig·mat·o·scope (as"tig·mat'uh·skope) *n.* ASTIGMOSCOPE.

as·tig·mic (a·stig'mick) *adj.* ASTIGMATIC.

as·tig·mom·e·ter (as"tig·mom'e·tur) *n.* An instrument which measures the degree of astigmatism. —**astigmome·try** (·tree) *n.*

astig·mo·scope (a·stig'muh·skope) *n.* An instrument for detecting and measuring astigmatism. —**as·tig·mos·copy** (as"tig·mos'kuh·pee) *n.*

astom·a·tous (a·stom'uh·tus, ·sto'muh·) *adj.* [*a-* + *stomat-* + *-ous*]. 1. Without a mouth or stoma. 2. *In botany,* without stomas.

asto·mia (a·sto'mee·uh) *n.* [*a-* + *-stomia*]. Congenital absence of the mouth.

as·to·mous (as'to·mus) *adj.* [Gk. *astomos,* from *a-* + *stoma,* mouth]. ASTOMATOUS.

astr-, astro- [Gk. *astron*, star]. A combining form meaning (a) *pertaining to the stars;* (b) *resembling a star.*

Astrafer. Trademark for dextriferron.

as·trag·a·lec·to·my (as·trag″uh·leck′to·mee) *n.* [*astragal*us + *-ectomy*]. Excision of the talus.

as·trag·a·lus (as·trag′a·lus) *n.*, pl. **astraga·li** (·lye) [L., from Gk. *astragalos*, a term applied to various small bones, and to dice (made from such bones)]. TALUS. —**astraga·lar** (·lur) *adj.*

Astragalus, *n.* [L., from Gk. *astragalos*, milk vetch]. A genus of leguminous plants some varieties of which yield gum tragacanth.

as·tral (as′trul) *adj.* [L. *astralis*, from Gk. *astron*, star]. 1. Of or pertaining to stars. 2. Of or pertaining to an aster.

astral mitosis. Mitosis characterized by the presence of an achromatic spindle complex formed by centrioles and related asters. This is the only type present in animal cells.

astral rays. The radiating structures of an aster.

as·tra·pho·bia (as″truh·fo′bee·uh) *n.* ASTRAPOPHOBIA.

as·tra·po·pho·bia (as″truh·po·fo′bee·uh) *n.* [Gk. *astrapē*, lightning, + *-phobia*]. Morbid fear of lightning and thunderstorms.

as·trin·gent (a·strin′junt) *adj. & n.* [L. *a(d)stringens, a(d)stringentis*, from *a(d)stringere*, to bind, draw together, from *ad-* + *stringere, strictus*, to tie, tighten]. 1. Producing contractions; capable of or tending to shrink or pucker tissues or mucous membranes. 2. An agent that produces contraction or shrinkage of organic tissues or that arrests hemorrhages, diarrhea, or other discharges. —**astrin·gen·cy** (·jun·see) *n.*

astringent bitters. Medical preparations that are astringent and also have the properties of simple bitters.

astro-. See *astr-*.

as·tro·blast (as′tro·blast) *n.* [*astro-* + *-blast*]. A primitive cell that develops into an astrocyte.

as·tro·blas·to·ma (as″tro·blas·to′muh) *n.* A glioma intermediate in differentiation between glioblastoma multiforme and astrocytoma.

as·tro·cyte (as′tro·site) *n.* [*astro-* + *-cyte*]. A many-branched stellate neuroglial cell, attached to the blood vessels of the brain and spinal cord by perivascular feet. —**as·tro·cyt·ic** (as″tro·sit′ick) *adj.*

astrocytic glioma. ASTROCYTOMA.

as·tro·cy·to·ma (as″tro·sigh·to′muh) *n.*, pl. **astrocytomas, astrocytoma·ta** (·tuh) A benign glial tumor made up of well-differentiated astrocytes.

astrocytoma gi·gan·to·cel·lu·la·re (jye·gan″to·sel″yoo·lair′ee). GLIOBLASTOMA MULTIFORME.

astrocytoma, grade 1. ASTROCYTOMA.

astrocytoma, grade 2. ASTROBLASTOMA.

astrocytoma, grades 3 and 4. GLIOBLASTOMA MULTIFORME.

as·tro·cy·to·sis (as″tro·sigh·to′sis) *n.* An increase both in the number and the size of astrocytes.

as·trog·lia (as·trog′lee·uh) *n.* Neuroglia composed of astrocytes.

as·trog·li·o·ma (as·trog″lee·o′muh) *n.* [*astroglia* + *-oma*]. ASTROCYTOMA.

as·tro·gli·o·sis (as″tro·glye·o′sis) *n.* [*astroglia* + *-osis*]. 1. ASTROCYTOSIS. 2. Enlargement and excessive production of astrocytic fibers.

as·troid (as′troid) *adj.* [*astr-* + *-oid*]. Star-shaped.

as·tro·ma (as·tro′muh) *n.* ASTROCYTOMA.

as·tro·pho·bia (as″tro·fo′bee·uh) *n.* Morbid fear of the stars and celestial space.

as·tro·phys·ics (as″tro·fiz′icks) *n.* A branch of science dealing with the application of physical laws to astronomical bodies.

as·tro·sphere (as′tro·sfeer) *n.* [*astro-* + *sphere*]. The collective radiations of fibrillar cytoplasm which extend from the centrosphere during cell division.

as·y·go·ag·na·thus (as″i·go·ag′nuth·us) *n.* AZYGOAGNATHUS.

asyl·la·bia (as″i·lay′bee·uh, ay″si·) *n.* [*a-* + Gk. *syllabē*, syllable, + *-ia*]. A form of motor aphasia in which individual letters are recognized, but the formation of syllables and words is difficult or impossible.

asy·lum (uh·sigh′lum) *n.* [L., from Gk. *asylon*, sanctuary]. An institution for the support, safekeeping, cure, or education of those incapable of caring for themselves.

asym·bo·lia (as″im·bo′lee·uh) *n.* [*a-* + *symbol* + *-ia*]. An aphasia in which there is an inability to understand or use acquired symbols, such as speech, writing, or gestures, as means of communication.

asym·bo·ly (a·sim′bo·lee) *n.* ASYMBOLIA.

asym·met·ric (as″i·met′rick, ay″si·) *adj.* [Gk. *asymmetros*, incommensurable, disproportionate]. Pertaining to or exhibiting asymmetry.

asym·met·ri·cal (ay″si·met′rick·al, as″i·) *adj.* ASYMMETRIC.

asymmetric carbon atom. A carbon atom which lacks either a plane or center of symmetry; of significance in determining optical activity and certain biological properties.

asym·me·try (ay·sim′i·tree, a·sim′) *n.* [Gk. *asymmetria*, disproportion, from *a-* + *symmetria*, symmetry]. 1. *In anatomy and biology*, lack of similarity or correspondence of the organs and parts on each side of an organism. 2. *In chemistry*, absence of symmetry in the arrangement of the atoms and radicals within a molecule.

asym·phy·tous (a·sim′fi·tus) *adj.* [Gk. *asymphytos*, from *a-* + *symphytos*, grown together]. Distinct; not grown together.

asymp·to·mat·ic (ay″simp″tuh·mat′ick, a·simp″to·) *adj.* Symptomless; exhibiting or producing no symptoms.

asymptomatic neurosyphilis. Syphilitic infection of the central nervous system diagnosed by pathologic findings in the cerebrospinal fluid in an individual with no clinical symptoms or abnormal signs on neurologic examination. The newer serologic tests for syphilis are almost always positive.

as·ymp·tot·ic (as″im·tot′ick) *adj.* [Gk. *asymptōtos*, from *a-* + *syn-*, together, + *ptōtos*, fallen, falling]. Of or pertaining to a straight line which an indefinitely extended curve continually approaches as a limit, that is, reaches only at infinity.

asymptotic wish fulfilment. 1. A psychological state wherein the patient has found the neurotic expression which would resolve his conflicts or compensate for them, but wherein his ego is strong enough to compel him to postpone indefinitely putting the neurotic solution into effect (Freud). 2. The gratification of a desire in a substitute, "almost-but-not-quite" way.

asyn·ap·sis (ay″si·nap′sis) *n.* [*a-* + *synapsis*]. Failure of homologous chromosome pairs to fuse during meiosis.

asyn·chro·nism (ay·sing′kro·niz·um, a·sing′) *n.* Absence of synchronism; disturbed coordination.

asyn·cli·tism (ay·sing′kli·tiz·um, a·sing′) *n.* [*a-* + *synclitism*]. A somewhat lateral tilting of the fetal head at the superior strait of the pelvis.

asyn·de·sis (a·sin′de·sis) *n.*, pl. **asynde·ses** (·seez) [*a-* + *syndesis*]. 1. SYNTACTIC APHASIA. 2. ASYNAPSIS. —**asyn·det·ic** (as″in·det′ick, ay″sin·) *adj.*

asyn·ech·ia (ay″si·neck′ee·uh, as″i·) *n.* [*a-* + *synechia*]. Absence of continuity in structure.

asy·ner·gia (as″i·nur′jee·uh, ay″si·) *n.* DYSSYNERGIA.

asyn·er·gy (ay·sin′ur·jee, a·sin′) *n.* [*a-* + *synergy*]. DYSSYNERGIA. —**asy·ner·gic** (ay″si·nur′jick, as″i·) *adj.*

asy·ne·sia (as″i·nee′zee·uh) *n.* [Gk., from *a-* + *syne*tos, intelligent, + *-ia*]. Stupidity; loss or disorder of mental power. —**asy·net·ic** (·net′ick) *adj.*

asy·no·dia (as″i·no′dee·uh) *n.* [*a-* + Gk. *synod*os, meeting, concourse, coming together, + *-ia*]. Nonsimultaneous orgasm in sexual intercourse.

asyn·tax·ia (ay″sin·tack′see·uh, as″in·) *n.* [Gk., disorder, from *syntaxis*, arrangement, organization]. Failure of orderly embryonic development.

asyntaxia dor·sa·lis. (dor·say′lis). Failure of the neural tube to close.

asys·tem·at·ic (ay·sis″te·mat′ick) *adj.* 1. ASYSTEMIC. 2. Without a system or orderly arrangement.

asys·tem·ic (ay″sis·tem′ick, as″is·) *adj.* [*a-* + *systemic*]. Diffuse or generalized; not restricted to a specific system or to one organ system.

asys·to·le (ay·sis′to·lee, a·sis′) *n.* [*a-* + *systole*]. Absence of contraction of the heart, especially of the ventricles. —**asys·tol·ic** (·tol′ick) *adj.*

asys·to·lia (ay″sis·to′lee·uh, as″is·) *n.* ASYSTOLE.

At Symbol for astatine.

A t, Ât *In electrocardiography*, symbol for the mean manifest direction and magnitude of repolarization of the myocardium determined algebraically and measured in degrees and microvolt seconds.

A.T.10 [*anti*tetany]. DIHYDROTACHYSTEROL.

Atabrine. A trademark for quinacrine.

atac·tic (a·tack′tick) *adj.* [Gk. *ataktos*, irregular]. Irregular; incoordinate; ataxic.

atac·ti·form (a·tack′ti·form) *adj.* Ataxialike; mildly ataxic.

atac·til·ia (ay″tack·til′ee·uh, at″ack·) *n.* [*a-* + *tactile* + *-ia*]. Loss of tactile sense.

at·a·rac·tic (at″uh·rack′tick) *adj.* & *n.* [Gk. *ataraktos*, calm, undisturbed, + *-ic*]. 1. Of or pertaining to ataraxy; tranquilizing. 2. A drug capable of promoting tranquility; a tranquilizer.

at·ar·al·ge·sia (at″ăr·al·jee′zee·uh) *n.* [*ataraxic* + *algesia*]. A combination of sedation and analgesia.

Atarax. Trademark for hydroxyzine hydrochloride.

at·a·rax·ia (at″uh·rack′see·uh) *n.* ATARAXY.

at·a·rax·ic (at″uh·rack′sick) *adj.* & *n.* [*ataraxy* + *-ic*]. 1. Promoting tranquility, tranquilizing. 2. A drug capable of promoting tranquility; a tranquilizer.

at·a·raxy (at′uh·rack″see) *n.* [Gk. *ataraxia*, from *ataraktos*, undisturbed, from *a-* + *tarassein*, to disturb]. A state of complete equanimity, mental homeostasis, or peace of mind.

atav·ic (a·tav′ick, at′uh·vick) *adj.* [L. *atavus*, ancestor, + *-ic*]. Not resembling either parent, but similar to a grandparent or more remote ancestor.

at·a·vism (at′uh·viz·um) *n.* [L. *atavus*, ancestor, + *-ism*]. The reappearance of remote ancestral characteristics in an individual. —**ata·vis·tic** (at″uh·vis′tick) *adj.*

atax·apha·sia (a·tack″suh·fay′zhuh, ·zee·uh) *n.* [Gk. *ataxia*, disorder, + *aphasia*]. SYNTACTIC APHASIA.

atax·ia (a·tack′see·uh) *n.* [Gk., disorder, from *a-* + *taxis*, arrangement, order, + *-ia*]. Incoordination of voluntary muscular action, particularly of the muscle groups used in activities such as walking or reaching for objects; due to any interference with the peripheral or central nervous system pathways involved in balancing muscle movements. See also *cerebellar ataxia*. —**atax·ic** (a·tack′sick) *adj.*

ataxia cor·dis (kor′dis). *Obsol.* ATRIAL FIBRILLATION.

atax·i·a·graph (a·tack′si·uh·graf) *n.* A device for recording the degree of ataxia.

atax·i·am·e·ter (a·tack″see·am′e·tur) *n.* ATAXIAGRAPH.

ataxi·apha·sia (a·tack″see·uh·fay′zhuh, ·zee·uh) *n.* [Gk. *ataxia*, disorder, + *aphasia*]. SYNTACTIC APHASIA.

ataxia-telangiectasia. An inherited disorder characterized by onset of progressive cerebellar ataxia in infancy or childhood; oculocutaneous telangiectasia; frequently, recurrent infections of the lungs and sinuses; and often, defects in cellular immunity and in the immunoglobulin system; and a propensity for the development of malignant disease. Syn. *Louis-Bar syndrome.*

ataxic amimia. *Obsol.* Inability to make gestures because of loss of muscle power and coordination.

ataxic aphasia. *Obsol.* MOTOR APHASIA.

ataxic gait. A clumsy and uncertain gait in which the legs are far apart, and when taking a step, the leg is lifted abruptly and too high and then is brought down so that the whole sole of the foot strikes the ground at once; seen usually in patients with lesions of the posterior column of the spinal cord, as in tabes dorsalis.

ataxic paraplegia. SUBACUTE COMBINED DEGENERATION OF THE SPINAL CORD.

ataxic speech. CEREBELLAR SPEECH.

ataxic tremor. INTENTION TREMOR.

atax·io·phe·mia (a·tack″see·o·fee′mee·uh) *n.* ATAXOPHEMIA.

atax·io·pho·bia (a·tack″see·o·fo′bee·uh) *n.* [Gk. *ataxia*, disorder, + *-phobia*]. A morbid fear of untidiness or disorder.

ataxo·phe·mia (a·tack″so·fee′mee·uh) *n.* [*ataxia* + *-phemia*]. Incoherence; faulty coordination of speech muscles.

ATCC Abbreviation for *American Type Culture Collection.*

-ate [L. *-atus*, participial ending of a-stem verbs]. A suffix meaning (a) *having the form or character of;* (b) in chemistry, *a salt or ester of certain acids with a name ending in -ic*, as carbonate, citrate, *or a compound derived from a* (specified) *compound*, as alcoholate.

Atebrin. A trademark for quinacrine.

atel-, atelo- [Gk. *atelēs*, incomplete, from *a-* + *telos*, end]. A combining form meaning *imperfect or incomplete.*

at·e·lec·ta·sis (at″e·leck′tuh·sis) *n.*, pl. **atelecta·ses** (·seez) [*atel-* + Gk. *ektasis*, extension]. A state of incomplete expansion of the lungs, because of their failure to expand at birth or the collapse of pulmonary alveoli soon after; collapse of a portion of a lung. —**ate·lec·tat·ic** (·leck·tat′ick) *adj.*

atelectasis of the newborn. Incomplete expansion of the lungs at birth and for the first few days of life.

atelectatic rale. CREPITANT RALE.

atel·ei·o·sis (a·tel″eye·o′sis, at″e·lye·o′sis) *n.*, pl. **ateleio·ses** (·seez) [Gk. *ateleia*, incompleteness, + *-osis*]. PITUITARY DWARFISM. —**atelei·ot·ic** (·ot′ick) *adj.*

at·el·en·ce·pha·lia (at″el·en·se·fay′lee·uh) *n.* [*atel-* + *-encephalia*]. Imperfect development of the brain.

at·el·en·ceph·a·ly (a·tel″en·sef′uh·lee, at″el·) *n.* ATELENCEPHALIA.

At·e·les (at′e·leez) *n.* [Gk. *atelēs*, incomplete, unfinished (referring to lack of thumb)]. A genus of the Cebidae comprising the spider monkeys.

ate·lia (a·tee′lee·uh) *n.* [Gk. *ateleia*, incompleteness, from *a-* + *telos*, end, + *-ia*]. 1. Lack of, or deficiency in, development. 2. PITUITARY DWARFISM. —**ate·lic** (·lick) *adj.*

atel·i·o·sis (a·tel″ee·o′sis, ·eye·o′sis, a·tee″lee·) *n.*, pl. **atelio·ses** (·seez) [Gk. *ateleia*, incompleteness, + *-osis*]. PITUITARY DWARFISM. —**ateli·ot·ic** (·ot′ick) *adj.*

at·e·lo·car·dia (at″e·lo·kahr′dee·uh) *n.* [*atelo-* + *-cardia*]. An imperfect or undeveloped state of the heart.

at·e·lo·ceph·a·lous (at″e·lo·sef′uh·lus) *adj.* [*atelo-* + *cephal-* + *-ous*]. Having the skull or head more or less imperfectly developed.

at·e·lo·chei·lia (at″e·lo·kigh′lee·uh) *n.* [*atelo-* + *cheil-* + *-ia*]. Defective development of the lip.

at·e·lo·chei·ria (at″e·lo·kigh′ree·uh) *n.* [*atelo-* + *cheir-* + *-ia*]. Defective development of the hand.

at·e·lo·en·ce·pha·lia (at″e·lo·en″se·fay′lee·uh) *n.* ATELENCEPHALIA.

at·e·lo·glos·sia (at″e·lo·glos′ee·uh) *n.* [*atelo-* + *-glossia*]. Congenital defect in the tongue.

at·e·log·na·thia (at″e·log·nath′ee·uh, ·nayth′ee·uh) *n.* [*atelo-* + *gnath-* + *-ia*]. Imperfect development of a jaw, especially of the lower jaw.

at·e·lo·ki·ne·sia (at″e·lo·kigh·nee′zhuh, ·zee·uh) *n.* [Gk. *atelēs*, endless, + *kinēsis*, motion, + *-ia*]. TREMOR.

at·e·lo·mit·ic (at″e·lo·mit′ick) *adj.* [*a-* + *telo-* + *mit-* + *-ic*]. Nonterminal; applied to the spindle-fiber attachment of chromosomes.

at·e·lo·my·e·lia (at″e·lo·migh·ee′lee·uh) *n.* [*atelo-* + *myel-* + *-ia*]. Congenital defect of the spinal cord.

at·e·lo·po·dia (at″e·lo·po′dee·uh) *n.* [*atelo-* + *-podia*]. Defective development of the foot.

at·e·lo·pro·so·pia (at″e·lo·pro·so′pee·uh) *n.* [*atelo-* + *prosop-* + *-ia*]. Incomplete facial development.

at·e·lo·ra·chid·ia, at·e·lor·rha·chid·ia (at″e·lo·ra·kid′ee·uh) *n.*

[*atelo-* + *-rachidia*]. Imperfect development of the spinal column, as in spina bifida.

at·e·lo·sto·mia (at''e·lo·sto'mee·uh) *n.* [*atelo-* + *-stomia*]. Incomplete development of the mouth.

ate·pho·bia (at''e·fo'bee·uh) *n.* [Gk. *atē*, ruin, + *-phobia*]. Morbid fear of catastrophe.

athe·lia (a·theel'ee·uh) *n.* [*a-* + *thel-* + *-ia*]. Absence of the nipples.

athero- [Gk. *athērē*, gruel, porridge]. A combining form meaning (a) *fatty degeneration;* (b) *atheroma.*

ath·ero·cheu·ma (ath''ur·o·kew'muh) *n.*, pl. **atherocheumas, atherocheuma·ta** (·tuh) [*athero-* + Gk. *cheuma*, stream, flow]. ATHEROMATOUS ABSCESS.

ath·ero·em·bo·li·za·tion (ath''ur·o·em''bo·li·zay'shun) *n.* Embolism formation in which atheromatous intima breaks off within an artery and lodges in distal small branches. Syn. *arterioarterial embolization.*

ath·ero·gen·e·sis (ath''ur·o·jen'e·sis) *n.* [*athero-* + *genesis*]. The development of atherosclerosis. **—atherogen·ic** (·ick) *adj.*

atherogenic index. The ratio of the relationship between two major lipoprotein groups, S_f 0-12 and S_f 12-400; claimed to be a measure of susceptibility to coronary atherosclerosis.

ath·er·o·ma (ath''ur·o'muh) *n.*, pl. **atheromas, atheroma·ta** (·tuh) [Gk., from *athērē*, gruel]. 1. An atherosclerotic plaque in an artery. 2. SEBACEOUS CYST. **—ather·om·a·tous** (·om'uh·tus) *adj.*

ath·er·o·ma·to·sis (ath''ur·o''muh·to'sis) *n.*, [*atheroma* + *-osis*]. ATHEROSCLEROSIS.

atheromatous abscess. The pultaceous, poorly cellular material of an atherosclerotic plaque. Not a true abscess. Syn. *atherocheuma.*

atheromatous degeneration. A retrogressive change, with the deposition of lipids in the degenerated tissue.

ath·ero·scle·ro·gen·ic (ath''ur·o·sklerr''o·jen·ick) *adj.* [*atherosclerosis* + *-genic*]. 1. Produced by or due to atherosclerosis. 2. Producing atherosclerosis.

ath·ero·scle·ro·sis (ath''ur·o''skle·ro'sis) *n.*, pl. **atherosclero·ses** (·seez) [*athero-* + *sclerosis*]. A variable combination of changes in the intima of arteries (as distinct from arterioles) consisting of the focal accumulation of lipids, complex carbohydrates, blood and blood products, fibrous tissue, and calcium deposits, and associated with medial changes.

atherosclerosis obliterans. ARTERIOSCLEROSIS OBLITERANS.

ath·ero·scle·rot·ic (ath''ur·o·skle·rot'ick) *adj.* Of or pertaining to atherosclerosis.

ath·e·toid (ath'e·toid) *adj.* & *n.* 1. Pertaining to or resembling athetosis; affected with athetosis. 2. An individual with athetosis.

athe·to·sic (ath''e·to'sick) *adj.* ATHETOID.

ath·e·to·sis (ath''e·to'sis) *n.*, pl. **atheto·ses** (·seez) [Gk. *athetos*, without position, out of place, + *-osis*]. Involuntary movements characterized by recurrent, slow, wormlike, and more or less continual change of position of the fingers, toes, hands, feet, and other parts of the body; usually the result of one or more lesions of the basal ganglia, particularly their central connections and the putamen; seen chiefly in cerebral palsy and kernicterus, as well as after encephalitis, toxic encephalopathies, and cerebrovascular accidents.

ath·e·tot·ic (ath''e·tot'ick) *adj.* ATHETOID.

athi·a·min·o·sis (ay·thigh''uh·mi·no'sis) *n.* [*a-* + *thiamine* + *-osis*]. Thiamine deficiency. See also *beriberi.*

Athi·o·rho·da·ce·ae (ay·thigh''o·ro·day'see·ee) *n.pl.* A family of photosynthetic nonsulfur purple bacteria.

ath·lete's foot. TINEA PEDIS.

athlete's heart. Cardiac enlargement, without underlying heart disease, seen in trained athletes.

ath·let·ic type. A physique characterized by good muscular development, leanness, flat abdomen, and broad chest.

atho·rus (a·tho'rus) *n.* [NL., from *a-* + *thorax* + *-us*]. A rare type of acephalus in which only parts of abdomen, pelvis, and lower limbs are present.

athrep·sia (a·threp'see·uh) *n.* [Gk. *athreptos*, ill-nourished (from *threpsis*, nourishment) + *-ia*]. 1. MARASMUS. 2. MALNUTRITION. 3. ATHREPTIC IMMUNITY. **—athrep·tic** (·tick) *adj.*

athreptic immunity. Immunity resulting from the failure of an infecting organism to find the necessary conditions for the production of infection.

athy·mic (ay·thigh'mick, a·) *adj.* [Gk. *athymos*, fainthearted, passionless, from *a-* + *thymos*, spirit]. 1. Lacking the thymus. 2. Without feeling.

athy·rea (ay·thigh'ree·uh, a·) *n.* ATHYREOSIS.

athy·re·o·sis (ay·thigh''ree·o'sis, a·) *n.*, pl. **athyreo·ses** (·seez) [*a-* + *thyreo-* + *-osis*]. Inadequate or absent secretion of thyroid hormone, producing the clinical picture of cretinism in infancy and of myxedema in children and adults. See also *Gull's disease.*

athy·re·ot·ic (ay·thigh''ree·ot'ick, a·) *adj.* Pertaining to athyreosis.

athy·roid·ism (ay·thigh'roy·diz·um) *n.* [*a-* + *thyroid* + *-ism*]. ATHYREOSIS.

athy·ro·sis (ay''thigh·ro'sis, ath''eye·ro'sis) *n.* ATHYREOSIS.

atlant-, atlanto- [Gk. *atlas, atlantos*]. A combining form meaning *atlas, atlantal.*

at·lan·tal (at·lan'tul) *adj.* Pertaining to the atlas.

at·lan·to·ax·i·al (at·lan''to·ack'see·ul) *adj.* [*atlanto-* + *axial*]. Pertaining to the atlas and the axis or epistropheus.

atlantoaxial joint. See *lateral atlantoaxial joint, median atlantoaxial joint.*

atlantoaxial ligament. See *lateral atlantoaxial* in Table of Synovial Joints and Ligaments in the Appendix.

at·lan·to·bas·i·la·ris in·ter·nus (at·lan''to·bas''i·lair'is in·tur'nus). A rare variant of the longus capitis muscle arising from the anterior tubercle of the atlas and inserted into the basilar part of the occipital bone.

at·lan·to·epi·stroph·ic (at·lan''to·ep·i·strof'ick) *adj.* [*atlanto-* + *epistrophic*]. ATLANTOAXIAL.

at·lan·to·oc·cip·i·tal (at·lan''to·ock·sip'i·tul) *adj.* Pertaining to the atlas and the occipital bone.

atlantooccipital joint. Either of the two joints between the occiput and the atlas. NA *articulatio atlantooccipitalis.* See also Table of Synovial Joints and Ligaments in the Appendix.

atlantoocipital ligament. See Table of Synovial Joints and Ligaments in the Appendix.

atlantooccipital membrane. See *anterior atlantooccipital membrane, posterior atlantooccipital membrane.*

at·las (at'lus) *n.* [Gk., the giant *Atlas*, represented bearing the world on his shoulders] [NA]. The first cervical vertebra, articulating with the occipital bone of the skull and with the axis. See also Table of Bones in the Appendix.

atlas assimilation. PLATYBASIA.

atlo-. See *atlant-, atlanto-.*

at·lo·ax·oid (at''lo·ack'soid) *adj.* ATLANTOAXIAL.

at·lo·did·y·mus (at''lo·did'i·mus) *n.* [*atlo-* + *-didymus*]. DICEPHALUS MONAUCHENOS.

atm Abbreviation for *atmosphere.*

atm-, atmo- [Gk. *atmos*, steam, vapor]. A combining form denoting (a) *vapor;* (b) *gas, air.*

at·mol·y·sis (at·mol'i·sis) *n.*, pl. **atmoly·ses** (·seez) [*atmo-* + *lysis*]. A method of separating mixed gases or vapors by means of diffusion through a porous substance.

at·mom·e·ter (at·mom'e·tur) *n.* [*atmo-* + *meter*]. An instrument that measures the amount of water evaporated from a given surface in a given time, to determine the humidity of the atmosphere.

at·mo·sphere (at'muh·sfeer) *n.* [*atmo-* + *sphere*]. 1. The gaseous envelope overlying the solid or liquid surface of a planet. See also *troposphere, stratosphere, ionosphere.* 2. Any gaseous medium in relation to objects immersed in it or exposed to it. 3. A standard unit of gas pressure based on the average pressure of the earth's atmosphere at sea level, equal to 1.01325 × 10^5 newtons/m^2 (1013.250 mb), which is equivalent to 760 mmHg, 1.0332 kg/cm^2, or 14.696 lb/in^2. Abbreviated, atm. —**at·mo·spher·ic** (at″muh·sferr′ick, ·sfeer′ick) *adj.*

atmospheric blast injury. Blast injury resulting from the transmission of the shock wave of an explosion through air.

atmospheric pressure. The pressure, expressed in various units, exerted by the atmosphere due to its weight. See also *atmosphere* (3).

ATN Abbreviation for *acute tubular necrosis.*

ato·cia (a·to′shee·uh, ·see·uh) *n.* [Gk. *atokia,* from *a-* + *tok*os, childbirth, + *-ia*]. *Obsol.* Sterility of the female.

ato·lide (ay′to·lide) *n.* 2-Amino-4′-(diethylamino)-*o*-benzotoluidide, $C_{18}H_{23}N_3O$, an anticonvulsant.

at·om (at′um) *n.* [Gk. *atomos,* indivisible, from *a-* + *tomos,* cut, piece]. The smallest particle of an element capable of existing individually or in combination with one or more atoms of the same or another element. It consists of a relatively heavy inner core, or nucleus, with a positive electric charge, and a number of lighter planetary particles, with negative charges, revolving or vibrating continuously around the nucleus in a vast empty space. The positive heavy particles in the nucleus are called protons, and the orbital particles are called electrons. The number of protons or of electrons in an electrically neutral atom is given by its atomic number. In addition to protons, the nucleus also contains neutrons, which are neutral particles resulting from the combination of a proton and an electron. The sum of protons and neutrons in the nucleus is called the mass number of the atom, or its mass or atomic weight. All atoms are constructed of these three fundamental building stones. —**atomic** (uh·tom′ick) *adj.*

atomic clock. A device that uses the vibrations of atomic nuclei or of molecules to measure time intervals, especially short intervals, with high precision.

atomic disintegration. The disintegration of atoms, either naturally, as in natural radioactivity, or artificially, as by the bombardment of atomic nuclei with protons, deuterons, alpha particles, neutrons, or photons, whereby new atoms are formed and more or less energy is liberated. Practically all elements have been disintegrated by artificial means. Generally the product differs only slightly from the original, but some atoms, as uranium of atomic weight 235, undergo fission into two atoms of approximately equal weight with release of much energy. See also *radioisotope.*

atomic energy. Energy released in reactions involving the nucleus of an atom, as by fission of a heavy nucleus or fusion of light nuclei, hence more specifically called nuclear energy.

atomic fission. NUCLEAR FISSION.

atomic heat. The specific heat of an element multiplied by its atomic weight.

at·o·mic·i·ty (at″uh·mis′i·tee) *n.* VALENCE.

atomic mass. The mass of an element measured on an arbitrary scale and expressed relatively to mass 12 for carbon.

atomic nucleus. The small, positively charged core of an atom that contains, except for ordinary hydrogen, protons and neutrons.

atomic number. The positive charge on the nucleus of an atom conferred by and equal to the number of protons in the nucleus and also equal to the number of electrons outside the nucleus of a neutral atom. Each element has a characteristic atomic number. Symbol, Z.

atomic pile reactor. NUCLEAR REACTOR.

atomic weight. A number representing the relative weight of an atom of an element compared with the carbon isotope of mass 12 as standard. It is the mean value of the isotopic weights of an element. Abbreviated, at. wt.

at·om·iza·tion (at″um·i·zay′shun) *n.* The mechanical process of breaking up a liquid into a fine spray.

at·om·ize (at′uh·mize) *v.* 1. To reduce to very small particles. 2. To convert a liquid or solid to a fine spray or minute particles. 3. To subject to atomic bombardment or attack.

at·om·iz·er (at′uh·migh·zur) *n.* A device for converting a liquid into a fine spray; used in medicine for inhalation therapy. Syn. *vaporizer.*

atom smasher. ACCELERATOR (3).

ato·nia (a·to′nee·uh) *n.* [Gk., from *a-* + *ton*os, tone, + *-ia*]. Absence of tonus.

aton·ic (a·ton′ick) *adj.* [*a-* + *tonic*]. Characterized by atonia.

atonic bladder. Markedly diminished or absent tonus of the detrusor muscle of the urinary bladder. See also *neurogenic bladder.*

atonic diplegia. HYPOTONIC DIPLEGIA.

atonic "drop" epilepsy. AKINETIC EPILEPSY.

atonic epilepsy. AKINETIC EPILEPSY.

ato·nic·i·ty (a·to·nis′i·tee) *n.* 1. Lack of tone. 2. HYPOTONICITY.

atonic seizure. AKINETIC SEIZURE.

atonic ulcer. An indolent or slow-healing ulcer.

at·o·ny (at′uh·nee) *n.* ATONIA.

ato·pen (at′o·pen) *n.* [*atop*ic + allerg*en*]. An antigen or allergen of the sort involved in atopic conditions such as seasonal rhinitis and asthma.

Atophan. Trademark identifying the original cinchophen.

atop·ic (ay·top′ick, a·top′ick) *adj.* [Gk. *atopos,* unusual, untoward, out of place, from *a-* + *topos,* place]. 1. Pertaining to atopy or to an atopen. 2. ECTOPIC.

atopic cataract. A cataract appearing in young persons who have had chronic and usually severe atopic dermatitis. Syn. *allergic cataract.*

atopic dermatitis or **eczema.** An intensely pruritic, frequently chronic, exematous dermatitis that occurs in persons of atopic constitution and characteristically involves the face and antecubital and popliteal fossae.

atopic dermatitis cataract. ATOPIC CATARACT.

atopic reagin. REAGIN.

atop·og·no·sia (a·top″og·no′see·uh, ay·) *n.* [*a-* + *topognos*is + *-ia*]. Lack of ability to locate a sensation accurately.

atop·og·no·sis (a·top″og·no′sis, ay·) *n.* ATOPOGNOSIA.

at·o·py (at′uh·pee) *n.* [Gk. *atopia,* unusualness, singularity, from *atopos,* out of place]. A genetically determined disorder in which there is an increased capacity to form reagin antibodies and to acquire certain allergic diseases, especially asthma, hay fever, urticaria, and atopic dermatitis.

atox·ic (ay·tock′sick, a·tock′sick) *adj.* [*a-* + *toxic*]. Not venomous; not poisonous.

ATP Abbreviation for *adenosine triphosphate.*

ATPase Abbreviation for *adenosine triphosphatase.*

atra·che·lia (ay″tra·kee′lee·uh, at″ra·) *n.* [*atrachel*ous + *-ia*]. The condition of having little or no neck.

atra·che·lo·ceph·a·lus (a·track″e·lo·sef′uh·lus, at″ruh·kee″lo·) *n.* [*a-* + *trachelo-* + *-cephalus*]. A monster with head and neck absent or poorly developed.

atra·che·lous (ay·track′e·lus, at″ruh·kee′lus) *adj.* [Gk. *atrachēlos,* from *a-* + *trachēlos,* neck]. Having little or no neck.

atrans·fer·ri·ne·mia (ay·trans·ferr″i·nee′mee·uh) *n.* [*a-* + *transferrin* + *-emia*]. Lack of plasma transferrin, resulting in low plasma iron and severe iron deficiency anemia; probably inherited as an autosomal recessive trait.

atrau·mat·ic (ay″traw·mat′ick) *adj.* Not productive of trauma.

Atrax (ay′traks) *n.* A genus of Australian poisonous spiders related to the American tarantulas. They are similar to the black widow in effect, and treatment for their bite is similar.

atre·mia (a·tree′mee·uh) *n.* [*a-* + Gk. *trem*ein, to tremble, + *-ia*]. Hysterical inability to walk, stand, or sit without general discomfort and trembling, all movements being readily and smoothly executed in the recumbent position. Syn. *Neftel's disease.*

atre·sia (a·tree'zhuh, ·zee·uh) *n.* [*a-* + *-tresia*]. Closure, imperforation, or congenital absence of a normal opening or canal, as of the anus, vagina, auditory meatus, or pupil. Adj. *atresic, atretic.*

atresia ani vag·i·na·lis (ay'nye vaj"i·nay'lis). An anomaly in which there is imperforate anus, the rectum opening into the vagina. Syn. *anus vaginalis.*

atresia fol·lic·u·li (fol·ick'yoo·lye). The blighting of an ovarian follicle with deterioration of the ovum before maturation. The atresic follicle is characterized by a small cystic space, lined with thinned follicle cells, which subsequently progresses to complete obliteration.

atresia of iter. AQUEDUCTAL STENOSIS.

atresia vul·vae (vul'vee). VULVAR FUSION.

atre·sic (a·tree'zick) *adj.* ATRETIC; pertaining to or characterized by atresia.

atresic teratism. A deformity in which the natural openings are occluded.

atret-, atreto- [Gk. *atrētos,* from *a-,* not, + *trētos,* perforated]. A combining form meaning *imperforate, imperforation.*

atre·tic (a·tret'ick) *adj.* [Gk. *atrētos,* imperforate, from *a-* + *trētos,* perforated]. Pertaining to or characterized by atresia.

atretic follicle. An involuted or degenerated ovarian follicle. Syn. *corpus atreticum.*

atre·to·ceph·a·lus (a·tree"to·sef'uh·lus) *n.* [*atreto-* + *-cephalus*]. A monster with imperforate nostrils or mouth.

atre·to·cor·mus (a·tree"to·kor'mus) *n.* [*atreto-* + Gk. *kormos,* trunk]. An individual having one or more of the body openings imperforate.

atre·to·cys·tia (a·tree"to·sis'tee·uh) *n.* [*atreto-* + *cyst-* + *-ia*]. Atresia of the urinary bladder.

atre·to·gas·tria (a·tree"to·gas'tree·uh) *n.* [*atreto-* + *-gastria*]. Imperforation of the cardiac or pyloric orifice of the stomach.

atre·to·le·mia (a·tree"to·lee'mee·uh) *n.* [*atreto-* + Gk. *laimos,* gullet, + *-ia*]. Imperforation of the esophagus or pharynx.

atre·to·me·tria (a·tree"to·mee'tree·uh) *n.* [*atreto-* + *metr-* + *-ia*]. Atresia of the uterus.

at·re·top·sia (at"re·top'see·uh) *n.* [*atret-* + *-opsia*]. Imperforation of the pupil.

atre·tor·rhin·ia (a·tree"to·rin'ee·uh, ·rye'nee·uh) *n.* [*atreto-* + *rhin-* + *-ia*]. Nasal atresia.

atre·to·sto·mia (a·tree"to·sto'mee·uh) *n.* [*atreto-* + *-stomia*]. Imperforation of the mouth.

atret·ure·thria (a·tret"yoo·ree'three·uh) *n.* [*atret-* + *urethr-* + *-ia*]. Imperforate urethra.

atri-, atrio-. A combining form meaning *atrium, atrial.*

atria. Plural of *atrium.*

atri·al (ay'tree·ul) *adj.* Of or pertaining to an atrium.

atrial appendectomy. Excision of an auricular appendage of a cardiac atrium as part of an operation for the relief of mitral stenosis.

atrial beat. A WAVE (2).

atrial diastole. The interval during which the cardiac atria dilate and fill with blood.

atrial fibrillation. A cardiac arrhythmia characterized by rapid, irregular atrial impulses and ineffective atrial contractions; the heartbeat varies from 60 to 180 per minute and is grossly irregular in intensity and rhythm.

atrial flutter. A cardiac arrhythmia due to an abnormality of atrial excitation; the atria beat regularly at about 300 per minute and the ventricles respond at a submultiple of the atrial rate, usually about 150 per minute.

atrial gallop. A low-pitched heart sound, which occurs in presystole just after atrial contraction, just prior to the first heart sound.

atrial kick. Atrial contribution to ventricular filling resulting from atrial systole; absent with atrial fibrillation; the atrial kick increases the end diastolic fiber length of the ventricle, resulting in increased myocardial contractility.

atrial rhythm. Cardiac rhythm originating in an ectopic focus in the atrial musculature.

atrial septum. INTERATRIAL SEPTUM.

atrial standstill. Absence of atrial contractions for one or more cardiac cycles.

atrial tachycardia. A rapid regular tachycardia with a rate of 140 to 220 per minute, originating from an ectopic focus in the atrium. Episodes may be paroxysmal.

atrich·ia (a·trick'ee·uh) *n.* [Gk. *atrichos,* hairless (from *thrix,* hair), + *-ia*]. Any condition, congenital or acquired, in which hair is substantially gone. Compare *alopecia.*

atrich·o·sis (at"ri·ko'sis) *n.* ATRICHIA.

atrichosis con·ge·ni·ta·lis (kon·jen·i·tay'lis). Absence or failure of development of hair from birth.

at·ri·chous (at'ri·kus) *adj.* [Gk. *atrichos,* hairless, from *a-* + *thrix,* hair]. Of bacteria, having no flagella.

atrio-. See *atri-.*

atrio·fem·o·ral (ay"tree·o·fem'uh·rul) *adj.* 1. Of or pertaining to a cardiac atrium and a femoral artery. 2. Specifically, connecting an atrium to a femoral artery (by way of an iliac artery or, occasionally, the distal aorta), as in a left atriofemoral bypass.

atrio·sep·tal (ay"tree·o·sep'tul) *adj.* Pertaining to a cardiac atrium and the interatrial septum.

atrio·sep·to·pexy (ay"tree·o·sep'to·peck"see) *n.* [*atrio-* + *septo-* + *-pexy*]. Operation on the atrial septum of the heart for closure of a defect.

atrio·sep·tos·to·my (ay"tree·o·sep·tos'tuh·mee) *n.* The creation by surgical or mechanical means of an opening in the interatrial septum of the heart.

atri·ot·o·my (ay"tree·ot'uh·mee) *n.* Surgical opening into an atrium of the heart.

atrio·ven·tric·u·lar (ay"tree·o·ven·trick'yoo·lur) *adj.* Pertaining to the atria and the ventricles of the heart. Abbreviated, AV.

atrioventricular band. ATRIOVENTRICULAR BUNDLE.

atrioventricular block. A cardiac conduction abnormality in which transmission of the excitatory impulse from the cardiac atrium to the ventricle through the AV node is slowed or stopped. Three degrees of severity are recognized: first degree (prolonged atrioventricular conduction), second degree (partial atrioventricular block), and third degree (complete atrioventricular block). Syn. *heart block.*

atrioventricular bundle. A band of specialized conduction tissue of the heart which arises from the atrioventricular node. It divides into two branches which descend on either side of the interventricular septum and ramify among the muscle fibers of the ventricles, transmitting contraction impulses to the ventricles. Syn. *bundle of His.* NA *fasciculus atrioventricularis.*

atrioventricular dissociation with interference. INTERFERENCE DISSOCIATION.

atrioventricular heart block. ATRIOVENTRICULAR BLOCK.

atrioventricular interval. The interval between atrial and ventricular contractions.

atrio·ven·tric·u·la·ris com·mu·nis (ay"tree·o·ven·trick·yoo·lair'is com·yoo'nis). A congenital malformation of the heart in which the atrial and ventricular septa and the endocardial cushions have failed to fuse; there is a single atrioventricular valve ring with deformity of the valve leaflets and large atrial and ventricular septal defects, resulting functionally in a two-chambered heart. Syn. *common atrioventricular canal, complete endocardial cushion defect.*

atrioventricular node. A small mass of interwoven conducting tissue beneath the right atrial endocardium anterior to the coronary sinus; branches of the conducting system entering the ventricles originate here. NA *nodus atrioventricularis.*

atrioventricular rhythm. JUNCTIONAL RHYTHM.

atrioventricular sulcus. CORONARY SULCUS.

atrioventricular tachycardia. JUNCTIONAL TACHYCARDIA.

atrioventricular valves. The mitral and tricuspid valves of the heart.

atri·um (ay'tree·um) *n.*, pl. **atria** (ay'tree·uh), genit. sing. **atrii** (ay'tree·eye) [L., hall, atrium]. 1. The first chamber on either side of the heart, which receives the blood from the veins. NA *atrium cordis.* See also Plate 5. 2. The part of the tympanic cavity of the ear below the head of the malleus. 3. The end of an alveolar duct.

atrium cor·dis (kor'dis) [NA]. An atrium of the heart.

atrium cordis dex·trum (decks'trum). The right atrium of the heart.

atrium cordis si·nis·trum (si·nis'trum). The left atrium of the heart.

atrium dex·trum (decks'trum) [NA]. The right atrium of the heart.

atrium me·a·tus me·dii (mee·ay'tus mee'dee·eye) [NA]. A depression in the lateral nasal wall anterior to the middle meatus.

atrium of infection. The point of entrance of bacteria, as in infectious disease.

atrium si·nis·trum (si·nis'trum) [NA]. The left atrium of the heart.

atrium va·gi·nae (va·jye'nee). VESTIBULE OF THE VAGINA.

at·ro·lac·ta·mide (at"ro·lack'tuh·mide) *n.* α-Hydroxy-α-phenylpropionamide, $C_9H_{11}NO_2$, an anticonvulsant used experimentally in epilepsy.

Atromid-S. Trademark for clofibrate.

At·ro·pa (at'ro·puh) *n.* [NL., from Gk. *Atropos,* one of the Fates]. A genus of herbs of the Solanaceae; the source of belladonna and atropine.

atro·phia (a·tro'fee·uh) *n.* ATROPHY.

atroph·ic (a·trof'ick, a·tro'fick) *adj.* Pertaining to or characterized by atrophy.

atrophic anemia. APLASTIC ANEMIA.

atrophic arthritis. RHEUMATOID ARTHRITIS.

atrophic chronic acrodermatitis. ACRODERMATITIS CHRONICA ATROPHICANS.

atrophic cirrhosis. LAENNEC'S CIRRHOSIS.

atrophic gastritis. Chronic gastritis with diffuse mucosal inflammation and varying degrees of mucosal atrophy.

atrophic glossitis. HUNTER'S GLOSSITIS.

atrophic papulosquamous dermatitis. DEGOS' DISEASE.

atrophic pharyngitis. Chronic pharyngitis attended by atrophy of the mucous membrane.

atrophic rhinitis. 1. A disease of uncertain etiology affecting young swine, causing chronic atrophy of the turbinate bones and deformity of the face. 2. OZENA.

atrophic sclerosis. ULEGYRIA.

atrophic thrombosis. MARANTIC THROMBOSIS.

atrophic vaginitis. Inflammation of the mucous membrane of the vagina, usually occurring after the menopause.

at·ro·phied (at'ruh·feed) *adj.* Affected with atrophy.

at·ro·pho·der·ma (at"ruh·fo·dur'muh) *n.* Atrophy of the skin.

atrophoderma of Pa·si·ni and Pie·ri·ni (pa·zee'nee, pye^h·ree'nee) [A. *Pasini* and L. E. *Pierini,* Italian, 20th century]. Patches of depression and hyperpigmentation of the skin, usually on the back in females.

atrophoderma re·tic·u·la·tum (re·tick"yoo·lay'tum). FOLLICULITIS ULERYTHEMATOSA RETICULATA.

atrophoderma ver·mic·u·la·ris (vur·mick"yoo·lair'is). FOLLICULITIS ULERYTHEMATOSA RETICULATA.

at·ro·phy (at'ruh·fee) *n.* & *v.* [Gk. *atrophia,* lack of nourishment, atrophy, from *a-* + *trophē,* nourishment]. 1. An acquired local reduction in the size of a cell, tissue, organ, or region of the body, which may be physiologic or pathologic. 2. To undergo such reduction.

at·ro·pine (at'ro·peen, ·pin) *n.* [*Atropa* + *-ine*]. *dl*-Hyoscyamine or *dl*-tropyl tropate, $C_{17}H_{23}NO_3$, an alkaloid obtained from *Atropa belladonna* and other solanaceous plants. It is a parasympatholytic agent used principally for its spasmolytic effect on smooth muscle and for its action in diminishing secretions.

atropine methylbromide. Methylatropine bromide, $C_{17}H_{23}NO_3.CH_3Br$, a dosage form of atropine.

atropine methylnitrate. Methylatropine nitrate, $C_{17}H_{23}NO_3.CH_3NO_3$, a dosage form of atropine.

atropine oxide. The 8-oxide derivative of atropine with anticholinergic properties; used as the hydrochloride salt.

atropine sulfate. $(C_{17}H_{23}NO_3)_2.H_2SO_4.H_2O$. The most frequently used salt of atropine.

at·ro·pin·iza·tion (at"ro·pin·i·zay'shun) *n.* 1. The bringing under the influence of, or treating with, atropine. 2. The administration of belladonna or atropine until physiologic effects become manifest. —**at·ro·pin·ize** (at'ro·pi·nize) *v.*

at·ro·scine (at'ro·seen, ·sin) *n.* [*Atropa* + hyo*scine*]. $C_{17}H_{21}NO_4.H_2O$. *dl*-Scopolamine. An alkaloid from several species of the Solanaceae. Has been used as a mydriatic.

A.T.S. Antitetanus serum.

attached gingiva. The portion of the gingiva firmly attached to the tooth and to the periosteum of the alveolar bone.

at·tach·ment *n.* 1. The place where one organ is fixed to another, such as the origin or the insertion of a muscle in a bone. 2. A component of a partial denture which retains and stabilizes it by frictional retention to a natural tooth or abutment. 3. Development of an interpersonal bond or commitment, as of a mother for her child.

attachment apparatus. The tissues that retain a tooth in its socket; the alveolar bone proper, the cementum, and the periodontal ligament.

attachment plaque. The plate of dense cellular material forming each half of a desmosome.

at·tar (at'ur) *n.* [Per. *'aṭar,* from Ar. *'iṭr,* perfume]. Any of the fragrant volatile oils.

attar of rose. ROSE OIL.

at·tend·ing nurse. 1. PUBLIC HEALTH NURSE. 2. A nurse responsible for the care of a patient or a group of patients for a given period of time or for specific activities.

attending physician. A physician who is a member of a hospital staff and regularly attends patients at the hospital.

attending staff. 1. The physicians and surgeons who are members of a hospital staff, and regularly attend their patients at the hospital. Syn. *visiting staff.* 2. The physicians and surgeons who, as members of a hospital staff, have the specific obligation of supervising and teaching house staff, fellows, and sometimes medical students.

attending surgeon. A surgeon associated with the responsible staff of a hospital, visiting the patients at specific times, performing major surgical operations, and supervising the postoperative care through directions to the house surgeon.

at·ten·tion disorder. MINIMAL BRAIN DYSFUNCTION SYNDROME.

attention hypothesis. *In psychology,* the hypothesis that attention tends to be selectively, automatically, and irresistibly drawn toward the area of greatest personal interest or concern and that therefore a person is selectively attracted to those whose character makeup most fits his own inner needs, whether healthy or neurotic.

attention span. 1. The period of time an individual can actively attend to or concentrate upon one thing; used particularly with respect to learning processes, active play, and work. 2. *In psychology,* the number of objects or impressions that can be reported after a brief period of observation, usually 0.1 second.

at·ten·u·at·ed virus. A virus whose disease-producing ability has been lessened by heat, chemicals, and other means.

at·ten·u·a·tion (a·ten"yoo·ay'shun) *n.* [L. *attenuare,* to thin, lessen, from *tenuis,* thin]. 1. A thinning, weakening, or diluting; especially a reduction of the virulence of a virus or pathogenic microorganism, as by successive culture, repeated inoculation, or exposure to light, heat, air, or a weakening agent. 2. *In radiology,* the process by which a beam of radiation is reduced in energy when passing through some material. —**at·ten·u·ate** (a·ten'yoo·ate) *v.*

at·tic (at'ick) *n.* [F. *attique,* Attic (in architecture)]. Part of the tympanic cavity situated above the atrium of the ear. It contains the incus and the head of the malleus. Syn. *epitympanum.*

attic disease. Chronic suppurative inflammation of the attic of the tympanic cavity; often resulting from cholesteatoma.

at·tic·itis (at"ick·eye'tis) *n.* [*attic* + *-itis*]. Inflammation of the lining membrane of the attic of the middle ear.

at·ti·co·an·trot·o·my (at"i·ko·an·trot'uh·mee) *n.* [*attic* + *antro-* + *-tomy*]. Surgical opening of the attic and mastoid air cells.

at·ti·co·mas·toid (at"i·ko·mas'toid) *adj.* Pertaining to the attic and the mastoid.

at·ti·cot·o·my (at"i·kot'uh·mee) *n.* [*attic* + *-tomy*]. Surgical opening of the attic of the tympanum.

at·ti·tude (at'i·tewd) *n.* [F., from L. *aptitudo,* fitness]. 1. Posture; the position of the body and limbs. 2. A consistent predisposition, or readiness, which is acquired and generally characterized by its affective aspects, to respond to an object, idea, or person in a certain way.

attitude of the fetus. The relation of the fetal members to one another in utero.

at·tol·lens au·rem (a·tol'enz aw'rem) [L., lifting the ear]. The superior auricular muscle. See Table of Muscles in the Appendix.

at·ton·i·ty (a·ton'i·tee) *n.* [L. *attonitus,* stunned]. A state of stupor with complete or partial immobility; occurs most frequently in the catatonic type of schizophrenia, but also in severe depressive illnesses.

at·trac·tion sphere. ASTROSPHERE.

at·tra·hens au·rem (at'ra·henz aw'rem) [L., drawing the ear forward]. The anterior auricular muscle. See Table of Muscles in the Appendix.

at·tri·tion (a·trish'un) *n.* [L. *attritio,* from *ad-,* on, + *terere,* to rub]. 1. An abrasion, rubbing, or chafing of the skin or any surface. 2. A functional wearing away by the forces of usage; as of tooth structure by mastication. Compare *abrasion, erosion.*

attrition murmur. A murmur heard in pericarditis, presumably due to friction between the visceral and parietal pericardium.

at. wt. Abbreviation for *atomic weight.*

A-type cancer cells. Cells from well-nourished portions of tumors; they have small nucleoli and abnormally active protein formation. Contr. *B-type cancer cells.*

atyp·ia (ay·tip'ee·uh) *n.* [NL., from *a-* + *type* + *-ia*]. *In exfoliative cytology,* cellular variations from normal which fall short of anaplasia.

atyp·i·cal (ay·tip'i·kul) *adj.* Not typical; irregular.

atypical amyloidosis. PARA-AMYLOIDOSIS.

atypical child. 1. A child with minimal brain dysfunction syndrome. 2. An autistic child.

atypical coloboma. A coloboma located in a part of the eye other than inferiorly or at the optic disk.

atypical facial neuralgia. Persistent severe pain in the face, head, and neck for which no cause can be found; usually observed in young women and unresponsive to analgesic medications.

atypical lymphocyte. Any lymphocyte differing from the normal but not anaplastic; often applied to cells seen in infectious mononucleosis and in other viral infections.

atypical mycobacteria. Mycobacteria other than *Mycobacterium tuberculosis* and *M. bovis* capable of causing human disease. Unlike the typical species, they are nonpathogenic for guinea pigs, and the infections are not communicable but are acquired by contamination from the environment. See also *Runyon groups.*

atypical pneumonia. PRIMARY ATYPICAL PNEUMONIA.

atypical verrucous endocarditis. LIBMAN-SACHS ENDOCARDITIS.

Au [L. *au*rum]. Symbol for gold.

A.U., Å.U. An abbreviation for *angstrom unit* (= ANGSTROM), sometimes written A.u., Å.u., a.u., å.u.

A.U.A. American Urological Association.

Aub-Du Bois standards (awb, doo·boiz') [J. C. *Aub,* U.S. physician, 1890–1973; and E. F. *Du Bois,* U.S. physiologist, 1882–1959]. A table of normal basal metabolic rates expressed as calories per square meter per hour, and given for each sex and age group.

Au·ber·ger blood group (o·behr·zheʸ'). A blood group characterized by the presence of an erythrocyte antigen demonstrable by reaction with anti-Au^a antibody prepared from the serum of a patient named Auberger who developed the antibody after receiving multiple transfusions.

Au·bert's phenomenon (o·behr') [H. *Aubert,* German physiologist, 1826–1892]. The optical illusion in which a vertical line inclines to one side as the head is inclined to the opposite side.

Auch·me·ro·my·ia (awk"me·ro·migh'ee·uh) *n.* [Gk. *auchmēros,* dirty, + *-myia*]. A genus of Diptera found in Africa.

Auchmeromyia lu·te·o·la (lew·tee'o·luh) [L., yellowish]. A species of fly whose larvae (Congo floor maggots) feed on blood and cause myiasis.

au·di·mut·ism (aw"dee·mew'tiz·um) *n.* [*audio-* + *mutism*]. Muteness not associated with deafness.

au·dio (aw'dee·o) *adj.* [from the combining form *audio-*]. Pertaining to sound or to hearing.

audio- [L. *audire,* to hear]. A combining form meaning (a) *auditory, hearing;* (b) *sound.*

audio analgesia. The technique of using sound to allay pain associated with operative procedures.

au·dio·epi·lep·tic seizure (aw"dee·o·ep"i·lep'tick). AUDIOGENIC SEIZURE.

audio frequency. Any one of the frequencies that fall within the normal range of human hearing.

au·dio·gen·ic (aw"dee·o·jen'ick) *adj.* [*audio-* + *-genic*]. Caused or induced by sound.

audiogenic epilepsy, seizure, or **convulsion.** A form of reflex epilepsy induced by sound, usually a loud, sudden noise. Syn. *acousticomotor epilepsy.*

au·dio·gram (aw'dee·o·gram) *n.* A graphic record showing the variations of auditory acuity of an individual over the normal frequency range, as indicated by an audiometer.

au·di·ol·o·gy (aw"dee·ol'uh·jee) *n.* [*audio-* + *-logy*]. The science of hearing.

au·di·om·e·ter (aw"dee·om'e·tur) *n.* An instrument, such as a pure tone audiometer or a speech or phonograph audiometer, for measuring hearing acuity. —**au·dio·met·ric** (aw"dee·o·met'rick) *adj.*

audiometric curve. AUDIOGRAM.

au·di·om·e·trist (aw"dee·om'e·trist) *n.* A person skilled in the use of an audiometer.

au·di·om·e·try (aw"dee·om'e·tree) *n.* The quantitative and qualitative evaluation of a person's hearing by the use of an audiometer.

audio-ocular reflex. Movement of the eyes toward the source of a sudden sound.

au·dio·vis·u·al (aw"dee·o·vizh'yoo·ul) *adj.* [*audio-* + *visual*]. Of, pertaining to, or using both sound and sight, especially in teaching and learning methods.

au·di·phone (aw'di·fone) *n.* [*audio-* + *-phone*]. DENTIPHONE.

audit-, audito-. A combining form meaning *auditory.*

au·di·tion (aw·dish'un) *n.* [L. *auditio,* from *audire,* to hear]. 1. The process of hearing. 2. The sense of hearing.

au·di·tive (aw'di·tiv) *adj.* AUDITORY.

au·di·tog·no·sis (aw"di·tog·no'sis) *n.,* pl. **auditogno·ses** (·seez) [*audito-* + *gnosis*]. 1. The ability to perceive and interpret sounds. 2. In physical diagnosis, the use of percussion and auscultation.

audito-oculogyric reflex. AUDIO-OCULAR REFLEX.

au·di·to·psy·chic (aw″di·to·sigh′kick) *adj.* Pertaining to the auditory association area.
au·di·to·ry (aw′di·tor″ee) *adj.* [L. *auditorius,* from *auditus,* (sense of) hearing]. Pertaining to the act or the organs of hearing.
auditory acuity test. The determination of the threshold of a person's hearing by the use of various instruments and techniques, such as an audiometer, recorded word list, or tuning forks.
auditory agnosia. Failure to recognize sounds in general in the absence of deafness.
auditory alternans. AUSCULTATORY ALTERNANS.
auditory amnesia. AUDITORY APHASIA.
auditory aphasia. A form of sensory or receptive impairment of language capacity with lack of comprehension of the spoken word in the absence of deafness.
auditory association area. The cortical association area just inferior to the auditory projection area, related to it anatomically and functionally by association fibers; Brodmann's area 42.
auditory aura. An acoustic sensation that sometimes ushers in an epileptic seizure, in particular any seizure originating in the temporal lobe.
auditory bulla. TYMPANIC BULLA.
auditory canal. Acoustic meatus. See *external acoustic meatus, internal acoustic meatus.*
auditory capsule. OTIC CAPSULE.
auditory center. The auditory projection area and auditory association area together.
auditory cortex. AUDITORY PROJECTION AREA.
auditory field. The area within which a given sound is audible.
auditory meatus. Acoustic meatus. See *external acoustic meatus, internal acoustic meatus.*
auditory memory span. The number of unrelated speech sounds (syllables, numerals, words) a person is able to recall and to repeat in order after having heard them once at the rate of one per second.
auditory nerve. VESTIBULOCOCHLEAR NERVE.
auditory-palpebral reflex. Reflex closing of the eyes in response to a sudden loud noise; may be demonstrated on one side. Syn. *auropalpebral reflex, acousticopalpebral reflex.*
auditory percussion. AUSCULTATORY PERCUSSION.
auditory pit. The embryonic invagination of the auditory placode that later becomes the otocyst or auditory vesicle. Syn. *otic pit.*
auditory placode. The dorsolateral ectodermal anlage of the internal ear. Syn. *otic placode.*
auditory projection area. The cortical receptive center for auditory impulses, located in the transverse temporal gyri. Syn. *Brodmann's area 41, auditosensory area, auditory cortex.*
auditory radiation. ACOUSTIC RADIATION.
auditory receptive aphasia. AUDITORY APHASIA.
auditory receptive center. AUDITORY PROJECTION AREA.
auditory reflex. 1. Any reflex that involves an auditory mechanism. 2. Specifically, AUDITORY-PALPEBRAL REFLEX.
auditory seizure. Episodic sounds heard by the patient as a manifestation of abnormal electrical discharges from an auditory area in the cerebral cortex; the sounds are usually fairly crude and unorganized, such as hissing or ringing, but may be complex patterns of speech or a musical phrase; they may occur alone or as the precursor of a psychomotor or generalized seizure.
auditory sensory aphasia. AUDITORY APHASIA.
auditory stalk. The temporary epithelial connection between auditory vesicle and superficial ectoderm. Syn. *placodal stalk.*
auditory teeth. Microscopic elevations on the surface of the vestibular lip of the internal spiral sulcus of the cochlear duct. NA *dentes acustici.*
auditory threshold. The minimum perceptible sound, usually measured in decibels.
auditory training. The training of a person with impaired hearing in the full use of the hearing that he has available.
auditory trauma. Impairment of hearing due to degeneration in the inner ear produced by extremely loud or prolonged sounds; may be temporary or permanent.
auditory tube. The canal, lined by mucous membrane, with partly bony, partly cartilaginous support, connecting the pharynx with the tympanic cavity on each side. Syn. *eustachian tube, pharyngotympanic tube.* NA *tuba auditiva.* See also Plates 12, 20.
auditory verbal agnosia. Failure to recognize ordinary words in a spoken language with which the patient is familiar; the patient's reaction is like that of an individual listening to a foreign language with which he is very slightly familiar.
auditory vesicle. The vesicular anlage of the inner ear. Syn. *otocyst, otic vesicle.*
au·di·to·sen·so·ry (au″di·to·sen′suh·ree) *adj.* Pertaining to the auditory projection area.
auditosensory area. AUDITORY PROJECTION AREA.
Au·en·brug·ger's sign (aw′un·broog″ur) [L. J. *Auenbrugger,* Austrian physician, 1722–1809]. A sign of pericardial effusion in which there is bulging of the epigastrium.
Au·er·bach's ganglia (aw′ur·bahkh) [L. *Auerbach,* German anatomist, 1828–1897]. Nerve cell bodies in the myenteric plexus.
Auerbach's plexus [L. *Auerbach*]. MYENTERIC PLEXUS.
Auer bodies [J. *Auer,* U.S. physician, 1875–1948]. Large granules, globules, or slender rods of azurophilic substance, which are peroxidase-positive and give positive reactions for protein, found in the cytoplasm of myeloblasts, myelocytes, occasionally in older granulocytes, monoblasts, monocytes, and histiocytes in acute leukemia.
aug·men·ta·tion mammoplasty. A plastic surgical procedure in which the size and shape of the breasts are altered by implantation of autologous or artificial materials.
aug·ment·ed unipolar limb lead. *In electrocardiography,* a unipolar limb lead producing electrocardiographic waves 50 percent greater than the actual potential from that limb. Symbol, aV. Syn. *Goldberger limb lead.*
aug·men·tor (awg·men′tur) *n.* An agent that increases or accelerates the action of auxetics, though it is unable to initiate cell division when used alone.
augmentor fibers. ACCELERATING FIBERS.
augmentor nerves. ACCELERATOR NERVES.
aug·na·thus (awg·nayth′us) *n.* [Gk. *au,* again, further, + *-gnathus*]. A rare anomaly in which a second lower jaw is parasitic on that of the host.
Au·jesz·ky's disease (aw′yes·kee) [A. *Aujeszky,* Hungarian physician, 1869–1933]. PSEUDORABIES.
au·lo·pho·bia (aw″lo·fo′bee·uh) *n.* [Gk. *aulos,* flute, + *phobia*]. A morbid fear of flutes.
au·lo·phyte (aw′lo·fight) *n.* [Gk. *aulos,* pipe, tube, hollow, + *-phyte*]. A symbiotic plant; one that lives within another, but not as a parasite.
aur-, auri-, auro- [L. *auris*]. A combining form meaning *ear.*
au·ra (aw′ruh) *n.,* pl. **auras, au·rae** (·ree) [L., from Gk., breeze, aura]. A premonitory sensation or warning experienced at the beginning of a seizure, which the patient remembers and which indicates the location of the discharging focus.
aura asth·mat·i·ca (az·mat′i·kuh). A sensation of tightness in the chest, or other subjective phenomena which forewarns the patient of an asthmatic attack.
aura cur·so·ria (kur·so′ree·uh). CURSIVE EPILEPSY.
aurae. A plural of *aura.*
aura hys·ter·i·ca (his·terr′i·kuh). Any warning sensation which supposedly occasionally introduces a hysterical attack.

¹au·ral (aw'rul) *adj.* [L. *auris*, ear, + *-al*]. Pertaining to the ear; AUDITORY.
²aural, *adj.* Pertaining to an aura.
aural calculus. Inspissated and sometimes calcified cerumen in the external acoustic meatus.
aural forceps. A dressing forceps used in aural surgery.
Auralgan. Trademark for a solution of antipyrine and benzocaine; used for treatment of otitis media.
aural reflex. Any reflex that involves an auditory mechanism. See also *auditory reflex.*
aural speculum. A small, hollow instrument with an expanded end inserted in the ear for examination of the external auditory meatus and the tympanic membrane.
aural syringe. A syringe for flushing out excessive cerumen from the external auditory meatus.
au·ra·mine O (aw'ruh·meen). A basic aniline dye of the diphenylmethane series used in fluorescence microscopy.
auramine-rhodamine stain. A mixture of auramine and rhodamine dyes used for staining tubercle bacilli.
au·ran·o·fin (aw·ran'o·fin) *n.* (1-Thio-β-D-glucopyranosato)(triethylphosphine)gold 2,3,4,6-tetracetate, $C_{20}H_{34}AuO_9PS$, an antiarthritic agent.
au·ran·ti·am·a·rin (aw·ran"tee·am'uh·rin) *n.* [*aurantium* + L. *amarus*, bitter, + *-in*]. A bitter glycoside, $C_{22}H_{31}O_{15}$, obtained from orange peel.
aur·an·ti·a·sis (aw"ran·tye'uh·sis) *n.* [NL. *aurantium*, orange (as if from L. *aurum*, gold), + *-iasis*]. CAROTENOSIS.
aurantiasis cu·tis (kew'tis). Any condition in which the skin appears golden in color, usually caused by excessive ingestion of carotene.
au·ran·ti·um (au·ran'shee·um) *n.* [NL., from F. or E. *orange*]. Orange.
au·rate (aw'rate) *n.* A salt of auric acid.
Aurcoloid-198. A trademark for a solution of colloidal gold containing radioactive gold 198.
Aureomycin. Trademark for chlortetracycline.
Aureotope-Au 198. A trademark for a solution of colloidal gold containing radioactive gold 198.
aures. Plural of *auris.*
auri- [L. *aurum*]. A combining form designating (a) *gold;* (b) in chemistry, *the presence of gold in the trivalent or auric state.*
auri-. See *aur-*.
au·ric (aw'rick) *adj.* [*aurum* + *-ic*]. 1. Pertaining to or containing gold. 2. *In chemistry,* pertaining to compounds of trivalent gold.
auric acid. $HAuO_2$, an amphoteric substance which behaves feebly as an acid to form salts with strong bases.
auric bromide. GOLD BROMIDE.
au·ri·cle (aw'ri·kul) *n.* [L. *auricula,* dim. of *auris,* ear]. 1. The pinna of the ear; the projecting part of the external ear. 2. An appendage to an atrium of the heart; auricular appendage. NA *auricula atriii.* 3. Any ear-shaped structure or appendage. 4. ATRIUM.
au·ric·u·la (aw·rick'yoo·luh) *n.*, pl. **auricu·lae** (·lee). AURICLE.
auricula atrii (ay'tree·eye) [NA]. AURICLE (2).
auricula cor·dis (kor·dis) [BNA]. Auricula atrii (= AURICLE (2)).
auricula dex·tra (decks'truh) [NA]. The auricle of the right atrium of the heart.
au·ric·u·lar (aw·rick'yoo·lur) *adj. & n.* 1. Pertaining to or shaped like an auricle. 2. ATRIAL. 3. An auricular muscle.
auricular appendage or **appendix.** AURICLE (2).
auricular cartilage. The cartilage of the pinna of the ear. NA *cartilago auriculae.*
au·ric·u·lare (aw·rick"yoo·lair'ee, ·lahr'ay) *n.*, pl. **auricu·la·ria** (·lair'ee·uh) [NL.]. *In craniometry,* a point on the root of the zygomatic process of the temporal bone lying perpendicularly above the center of the external auditory meatus.
auricular fibrillation. ATRIAL FIBRILLATION.
auricular flutter. ATRIAL FLUTTER.
au·ri·cu·la·ris (aw·rick"yoo·lair'is) *n.*, pl. **auricula·res** (·reez) [L.]. An auricular muscle.
auricular ligament. Any of the three extrinsic ligaments fixing the cartilage of the auricle to the skull: the anterior auricular ligament (NA *ligamentum auriculare anterius*), connecting the tragus and helical spine to the zygomatic arch, the posterior auricular ligament (NA *ligamentum auriculare posterius*), connecting the eminence of the concha to the mastoid process, or the superior auricular ligament (NA *ligamentum auriculare superius*), connecting the helical spine to the bony external acoustic meatus. NA (pl.) *ligamenta auricularia.*
auricular muscle. See Table of Muscles in the Appendix.
auricular point. The central point of the external acoustic meatus.
auricular tachycardia. ATRIAL TACHYCARDIA.
auricular training. AUDITORY TRAINING.
auricular tube. EXTERNAL ACOUSTIC MEATUS.
auricular tubercle. 1. (of Darwin:)A blunt tubercle projecting from the upper free margin of the helix toward the center of the auricle. Syn. *Darwin's tubercle.* NA *tuberculum auriculae.* 2. *In embryology,* any of the six tubercles on the hyoid and mandibular arches which form the auricle of the ear.
auricula si·nis·tra (si·nis'truh) [NA]. The auricle of the left atrium of the heart.
auriculo-. A combining form meaning *auricle, auricular.*
au·ric·u·lo·breg·mat·ic (aw·rick"yoo·lo·breg·mat'ick) *adj.* Pertaining to the auricle (1) and the bregma.
auriculobregmatic line. A line passing from the auricular point to the bregma, dividing the preauricular from the postauricular part of the cranium.
au·ric·u·lo·fron·ta·lis (aw·rick"yoo·lo·fron·tay'lis) *n.* A portion of the anterior auricular muscle.
au·ric·u·lo·pal·pe·bral (aw·rick"yoo·lo·pal'pe·brul, ·pal·pee'brul) *adj.* [*auriculo-* + *palpebral*]. Pertaining to the auricle (1) and the eyelids.
auriculopalpebral reflex. Closure of the eyelids in response to noxious stimuli applied to the top part of the auditory meatus.
au·ric·u·lo·pres·sor (aw·rick"yoo·lo·pres'ur) *adj.* [*auriculo-* + *pressor*]. Tending to raise atrial pressure.
auriculopressor reflex. Tachycardia secondary to a rise in right atrial pressure. Compare *Bainbridge effect.*
au·ric·u·lo·tem·po·ral (aw·rick"yoo·lo·tem'puh·rul) *adj.* Pertaining to the auricle (1) and to the temporal region.
auriculotemporal neuralgia. ARNOLD'S NEURALGIA.
auriculotemporal syndrome. Local redness and sweating of the cheek with pain anterior to the tragus, produced during mastication of food or tasting; following a suppuration and fistulation of the parotid gland. Syn. *Frey's syndrome.*
au·ric·u·lo·ven·tric·u·lar (aw·rick"yoo·lo·ven·trick'yoo·lur) *adj.* ATRIOVENTRICULAR.
au·ris (aw'ris) *n.*, pl. **au·res** (·reez), genit. pl. **au·ri·um** (aw'ree·um) [L.] [NA]. EAR.
auris dex·tra (decks'truh). The right ear. Abbreviated, a.d.
auris ex·ter·na (ecks·tur'nuh) [NA]. EXTERNAL EAR.
auris in·ter·na (in·tur'nuh) [NA]. INTERNAL EAR.
auris me·dia (mee'dee·uh) [NA]. MIDDLE EAR.
auris si·nis·tra (si·nis'truh). The left ear. Abbreviated, a.s.
au·rist (aw'rist) *n.* A specialist in diseases of the ear.
¹auro- [L. *aurum*]. A combining form designating (a) *gold;* (b) in chemistry, *the presence of gold in the univalent or aurous state.*
²auro-. See *aur-*.
au·ro·pal·pe·bral (aw"ro·pal'pe·brul, ·pal·pee'brul) *adj.* [*auro-* + *palpebral*]. Pertaining to the ear and the eyelids.
auropalpebral reflex. AUDITORY-PALPEBRAL REFLEX.
au·ro·ra·pho·bi·a (aw·ro"ruh·fo'bee·uh) *n.* [*aurora* borealis + *-phobia*]. A morbid fear of northern lights.
Auroscan. Trademark for gold Au-198 injection.
au·ro·ther·a·py (aw"ro·therr'uh·pee) *n.* [*auro-* + *therapy*].

The administration of gold salts in the treatment of disease.

auro·thio·glu·cose (aw″ro·thigh″o·gloo′koce) *n.* [*auro-* + *thio-* + *glucose*]. A compound of gold with thioglucose, $C_6H_{11}AuO_5S$, used for the treatment of rheumatoid arthritis; administered in oil suspension.

au·rous (aw′rus) *adj.* [*aurum* + *-ous*]. 1. Pertaining to gold and its compounds. 2. *In chemistry,* pertaining to compounds of univalent gold.

au·rum (aw′rum) *n.* [L.]. GOLD.

aus·cul·ta·tion (aws″kul·tay′shun) *n.* [L. *auscultatio,* listening, from *auscultare,* to listen to (rel. to L. *auris* and Gk. *ous,* ear)]. The perception and interpretation of sounds arising from various organs, especially the heart, lungs, and pleura, to aid in the determination of their physical condition. —**aus·cul·ta·to·ry** (aws·kul′tuh·to·ree) *adj.;* **aus·cult** (aws·kult′), **aus·cul·tate** (aws′kul·tate) *v.;* **aus·cult·able** (aws·kult′uh·bul) *adj.*

auscultation tube. *In otology,* an instrument for listening to the forced passage of air into the middle ear of a patient.

auscultatory alternans. Alternation of the intensity of heart sounds or murmurs, reflecting alternation of force of ventricular contraction in ventricular failure.

auscultatory gap. In measuring blood pressure by the auscultatory method, a zone of silence occurring 10 to 30 mm below the true level of systolic pressure and continuing for 20 to 40 mm downward toward the diastolic level. The reason for the absence of Korotkov sounds is unknown.

auscultatory percussion. Auscultation of the sounds produced by percussion. Syn. *auditory percussion.*

Aus·tin and Van Slyke's method. A method for determination of chlorides in whole blood, using picric acid to precipitate the proteins, silver nitrate to precipitate the chlorides, and titration with starch and potassium iodide.

Austin Flint murmur [*Austin Flint,* U.S. physician, 1812–1886]. A late diastolic rumbling apical murmur, heard in severe aortic regurgitation, probably resulting from expulsion of blood from the left atrium into the dilated left ventricle.

Austin Moore's pins [*Austin* T. *Moore,* U.S. orthopedist, b. 1899]. Large metal pins with threaded ends for holding nuts, used for maintaining position in intracapsular fractures of the femur.

Aus·tra·lian antigen. HEPATITIS-ASSOCIATED ANTIGEN.

Australian X disease. MURRAY VALLEY ENCEPHALITIS.

Aus·tra·lor·bis (aws″truh·lor′bis) *n.* [L. *australis,* south, + *orbis,* circle]. A genus of snails that may serve as intermediate hosts for blood flukes (*(Schistosoma* sp.).

aut-, auto- [Gk. *autos*]. A combining form meaning *self, one's own, spontaneous, independent.*

au·ta·coid (aw′tuh·koid) *n.* [*aut-* + Gk. *akos,* remedy, + *-oid*]. Any member of a group of substances of diverse chemical structure that occur normally in the body and have a wide range of intense pharmacological activities, such as serotonin, histamine, bradykinin, and angiotensin.

au·te·cic, au·toe·cic (aw·tee′sick) *adj.* AUTECIOUS.

au·te·cious, au·toe·cious (aw·tee′shus) *adj.* [*aut-* + Gk. *oikia,* house, + *-ous*]. Applied to parasitic fungi that pass through all the stages of their existence in the same host.

au·te·me·sia (aw·te·mee′shuh, ·see·uh) *n.* [*aut-* + *emesis* + *-ia*]. 1. Idiopathic vomiting. 2. Vomiting at will by certain psychiatric patients.

au·thor·i·tar·i·an character. *In psychology,* a personality who asks unquestioning subordination and obedience, but who is intolerant of weakness in others, rejects members of groups other than his own, is very rigid, and requires all issues to be decided in black and white, yet may accept superior authority in a servile way. See also *ecomania.*

au·tism (aw′tiz·um) *n.* [*aut-* + *-ism*]. 1. A tendency in one's thinking where all material, including objective reality, is given meaning unduly influenced by personal desires or needs; an interest in daydreaming and fantasy. 2. A form of behavior and thinking observed in young children, in which the child seems to concentrate upon himself or herself without regard for reality; often appears as excessive shyness, fearfulness, or aloofness and later as withdrawal and introspection. Intellect is not impaired. It may be an early manifestation or part of the childhood type of schizophrenia. See also *autistic child.*

au·tis·tic (aw·tis′tick) *adj.* 1. Pertaining to or characterized by autism. 2. Descriptive of behavior, particularly seen in the autistic child, in which there is little or no attempt at verbal communication, disregard for other people and animate objects, excessive playing with one's body such as spinning about, and often a preoccupation with bright or pointed inanimate objects; sometimes also seen in children who are emotionally deprived, perceptually handicapped, or mentally retarded, or who lack sensory stimulation.

autistic child. A child who does not relate to his environment, especially not to people, and whose overall functioning is immature and often appears retarded. See also *infantile autism, childhood type of schizophrenia, symbiotic psychosis.*

autistic gesture. A muscular automatism involving more muscles than a tic.

autistic thinking. AUTISM.

auto-. See *aut-.*

au·to·ag·glu·ti·na·tion (aw″to·uh·gloo″ti·nay′shun) *n.* 1. Agglutination which occurs without the addition of a specific antiserum. 2. Agglutination of the blood cells of an individual by his own serum.

au·to·ag·glu·ti·nin (aw″to·uh·gloo′ti·nin) *n.* An agglutinin contained in the serum of an individual which causes an agglutination of his own cells.

au·to·al·ler·gi·za·tion (aw″to·al″ur·ji·zay′shun) *n.* [*auto-* + *allergization*]. AUTOSENSITIZATION.

au·to·am·pu·ta·tion (aw″to·am″pew·tay′shun) *n.* Spontaneous amputation, as of a diseased organ, growth, or appendage.

au·to·anal·y·sis (aw″to·uh·nal′i·sis) *n.,* pl. **autoanaly·ses** (·seez). Analysis of one's own mental disorder; employed as a psychotherapeutic method.

Autoanalyzer. Trademark for an instrument in which chemical and other analyses are done automatically as the fluid-borne unknown substance is mixed with reagents in a continuously-flowing stream which passes through appropriate environmental and analytical modules.

au·to·an·am·ne·sis (aw″to·an″am·nee′sis) *n.,* pl. **autoanamne·ses** (·seez) [*auto-* + *anamnesis*]. A medical or psychiatric history obtained solely from the patient.

au·to·an·ti·bi·o·sis (aw″to·an″tee·bye·o′sis) *n.* [*auto-* + *antibiosis*]. The self-inhibition of a culture medium as a result of the previous growth of the organism in the medium.

au·to·an·ti·body (aw″to·an′ti·bod″ee) *n.* 1. An antibody produced by an organism to its own tissues. 2. *In hematology,* an antibody contained in the serum of an individual that causes agglutination or lysis of his erythrocytes.

au·to·au·di·ble (aw″to·aw′di·bul) *adj.* Audible to one's self; applied to heart sounds or cephalic bruits.

au·to·ca·tal·y·sis (aw″to·ka·tal′i·sis) *n.,* pl. **autocataly·ses** (·seez) [*auto-* + *catalysis*]. The process by which a chemical reaction is accelerated by one or more products of the reaction acting as catalysts. —**auto·cat·a·lyst** (·kat′uh·list) *n.;* **auto·cat·a·lyt·ic** (·kat″uh·lit′ick) *adj.*

au·to·ca·thar·sis (aw″to·ka·thahr′sis) *n.* [*auto-* + *catharsis*]. Psychotherapy by encouraging the patient to write out or paint his experiences or impressions and thus rid himself of his mental complexes.

au·to·cho·le·cys·to·du·o·de·nos·to·my (aw″to·ko″le·sis″to·dew″o·de·nos′tuh·mee) *n.* [*auto-* + *cholecyst* + *duodeno-* + *-stomy*]. The spontaneous formation of an opening between the gallbladder and duodenum, secondary to adhesions between the two organs; the opening may permit passage of gallstones into the duodenum.

au·to·cho·le·cys·to·trans·verse·co·los·to·my (aw″to·ko″le·sis″ to·trans·vurs″ko·los′tuh·mee) *n.* [*auto-* + *cholecyst* + *transverse* + *colo-* + *-stomy*]. The spontaneous formation of an opening between the gallbladder and the transverse colon, secondary to adhesions between the two organs; the opening may permit passage of gallstones into the transverse colon.

au·toch·tho·nous (aw·tock′thuh·nus) *adj.* [Gk. *autochthonos*, from *auto-* + *chthōn*, land]. 1. Formed or originating in the place where found, as a clot. 2. Native; aboriginal.

autochthonous idea. An idea originating in the unconscious, which to the patient seems literally to have come from the outside.

au·toc·la·sis (aw·tock′luh·sis) *n.*, pl. **autocla·ses** (·seez) [*auto-* + *-clasis*]. A breaking up of a part due to causes developed within itself.

au·to·clave (aw′to·klave) *n.* & *v.* [F., self-locking, from *auto-* + L. *clavis*, key]. 1. An apparatus for sterilizing objects by steam under pressure. 2. To sterilize in an autoclave.

au·to·con·den·sa·tion (aw″to·kon″den·say′shun) *n.* [*auto-* + *condensation*]. An electrotherapeutic method of applying high-frequency currents in which the patient or affected part constitutes one plate of a capacitor.

au·to·con·duc·tion (aw″to·kun·duck′shun) *n.* [*auto-* + *conduction*]. An electrotherapeutic method of applying high-frequency currents by induction. The patient or part is placed within a large solenoid which acts as the secondary of a transformer.

au·to·cy·to·tox·in (aw″to·sigh″to·tock′sin) *n.* [*auto-* + *cytotoxin*]. A cell toxin produced against the cells of one's own body.

au·to·dep·i·la·tion (aw″to·dep″i·lay′shun) *n.* [*auto-* + *depilation*]. TRICHOLOGIA (2).

au·to·di·ges·tion (aw″to·di·jes′chun) *n.* Digestion of the stomach walls by gastric juice, as in disease of the stomach or after death. Compare *autolysis.*

au·to·echo·la·lia (aw″to·eck″o·lay′lee·uh) *n.* [*auto-* + *echolalia*]. Stereotypy in which the patient continually repeats some word or phrase of his own and perseverates on words said meaningfully; seen in neuropathologic states such as Pick's disease. Compare *verbigeration.*

au·to·echo·prax·ia (aw″to·eck″o·prack′see·uh) *n.* [*auto-* + *echopraxia*]. Stereotypy in which the patient continually repeats some action he has previously experienced; a form of perseveration.

autoecic. Autecic (= AUTECIOUS).

autoecious. AUTECIOUS.

au·to·ec·ze·ma·ti·za·tion (aw″to·eck·zee″muh·ti·zay′shun) *n.* Autosensitization dermatitis characterized by eczematization.

au·to·emas·cu·la·tion (aw″to·e·mas″kew·lay′shun) *n.* [*auto-* + *emasculation*]. Self-inflicted amputation of the external genitalia, a rare psychotic act.

au·to·ep·i·la·tion (aw″to·ep″i·lay′shun) *n.* [*auto-* + *epilation*] *Obsol.* Spontaneous loss of hair.

au·to·erot·i·cism (aw″to·e·rot′i·siz·um) *n.* AUTOEROTISM.

au·to·er·o·tism (aw″to·err′o·tiz·um) *n.* [*auto-* + *erotism*]. Self-gratification from sexual instinct, including satisfaction from masturbation and from the individual's own oral, anal, and visual sources and fantasies. Compare *narcissism.* Contr. *alloerotism.* —**auto·erot·ic** (·e·rot′ick) *adj.*

au·to·fel·la·tio (aw″to·fe·lay′shee·o) *n.* Fellatio practiced upon oneself.

au·to·flu·o·ro·scope (aw″to·floo″ur·uh·scope) *n.* [*auto-* + *fluoroscope*]. A direct-viewing radiation imaging apparatus similar to the Anger camera but with the single scintillator replaced by a mosaic of many scintillator cells.

au·to·flu·o·ros·co·py (aw″to·floo·uh·ros′kuh·pee) *n.* Examination with the autofluoroscope.

au·tog·a·my (aw·tog′uh·mee) *n.* [*auto* + *-gamy*]. 1. *In botany*, self-fertilization. 2. A form of inbreeding marked by conjugation of closely related cells or nuclei. —**autoga·mous** (·mus) *adj.*

au·to·gen·e·sis (aw″to·jen′e·sis) *n.* ABIOGENESIS. —**auto·ge·net·ic** (·je·net′ick) *adj.*

au·to·gen·ic (aw″to·jen′ick) *adj.* AUTOGENOUS.

au·tog·e·nous (aw·toj′e·nus) *adj.* [Gk. *autogenēs*, self-produced; kindred (from *auto-* + *genos*, kind, race), + *-ous*]. 1. Self-generated. 2. Arising within the organism; applied to toxins, pathologic states, or vaccines.

autogenous graft. AUTOGRAFT.

autogenous inhibition. A reflex relaxation referred to the point of stimulation.

autogenous vaccine. A vaccine made from a culture of microorganisms obtained from the patient himself.

au·to·graft (aw′to·graft) *n.* [*auto-* + *graft*]. Any tissue removed from one part of an individual's body and applied to another part. Compare *homograft.*

au·tog·ra·phism (aw·tog′ruh·fiz·um) *n.* [*auto-* + *graph-* + *-ism*]. DERMOGRAPHIA.

au·to·he·mag·glu·ti·na·tion, au·to·hae·mag·glu·ti·na·tion (au″to·heem″uh·gloo·ti·nay′shun) *n.* [*auto-* + *hem-* + *agglutination*]. Agglutination of an individual's erythrocytes by his own plasma.

au·to·he·mol·y·sin, au·to·hae·mol·y·sin (au″to·hee·mol′i·sin) *n.* [*auto-* + *hemo-* + *lysin*]. A substance in an individual's plasma which produces lysis of his own erythrocytes.

au·to·he·mol·y·sis, au·to·hae·mol·y·sis (aw″to·hee·mol′i·sis) *n.* Hemolysis of an individual's erythrocytes by his own serum.

au·to·he·mo·ther·a·py, au·to·hae·mo·ther·a·py (aw″to·hee″mo·therr′uh·pee) *n.* [*auto-* + *hemotherapy*]. Treatment of disease with the patient's own blood, withdrawn by venipuncture and reinjected intramuscularly.

au·to·hy·drol·y·sis (aw″to·high·drol′i·sis) *n.* Spontaneous hydrolysis.

au·to·hyp·no·sis (aw″to·hip·no′sis) *n.* Self-induced hypnosis. —**autohyp·not·ic** (·not′ick) *adj.*

au·to·hyp·no·tism (aw″to·hip′nuh·tiz·um) *n.* The practice of autohypnosis.

au·to·im·mu·ni·ty (aw″to·i·mew′ni·tee) *n.* [*auto-* + *immunity*]. A condition in which an immune response is directed against a constituent of an organism's own body. —**auto·im·mune** (·i·mewn′) *adj.*

au·to·im·mu·ni·za·tion (aw″to·im″yoo·ni·zay′shun) *n.* The production or development of an autoimmunity.

au·to·in·fec·tion (aw″to·in·feck′shun) *n.* Infection by an organism existing within the body or transferred from one part of the body to another.

au·to·in·fu·sion (aw″to·in·few′zhun) *n.* [*auto-* + *infusion*]. AUTOTRANSFUSION (1).

au·to·in·oc·u·la·bil·i·ty (aw″to·i·nock″yoo·luh·bil′i·tee) *n.* The potential for autoinoculation.

au·to·in·oc·u·la·tion (aw″to·i·nock″yoo·lay′shun) *n.* Inoculation in one part of the body by an organism present in another part; self-inoculation.

au·to·in·tox·i·cant (aw″to·in·tock′si·kunt) *n.* [*auto-* + *intoxicant*]. A poison originating within the body.

au·to·in·tox·i·ca·tion (aw″to·in·tock″si·kay′shun) *n.* [*auto-* + *intoxication*]. Poisoning by metabolic products elaborated within the body; generally, toxemia of pathologic states.

au·to·iso·ly·sin (aw″to·eye″so·lye′sin, ·eye·sol′i·sin) *n.* [*auto-* + *isolysin*]. An antibody that dissolves the erythrocytes of the individual from whom it was obtained, as well as of others of the same species.

au·to·ki·ne·sis (aw″to·ki·nee′sis) *n.* [*auto-* + *kinesis*]. Voluntary movement. —**autoki·net·ic** (·net′ick) *adj.*

autokinetic perception or **phenomenon.** The illusion of movement of an object in space, usually vague and perceived differently by different observers; may be due to displacement of the eyes or head or to successive stimulation of adjacent retinal points by momentary stationary lights.

au·tol·o·gous (aw·tol'uh·gus) *adj.* [*auto-* + *-logous* as in homologous]. Derived from, or from a part of, the same organism; autogenous. Compare *homologous.*

au·tol·y·sate (aw·tol'i·sate) *n.* That which results from or is produced by autolysis.

au·tol·y·sin (aw·tol'i·sin, aw"to·lye'sin) *n.* A substance that produces autolysis.

au·tol·y·sis (aw·tol'i·sis) *n.* [*auto-* + *lysis*]. 1. Self-digestion of tissues within the living body. 2. The chemical splitting-up of the tissue of an organ by the action of an enzyme peculiar to it. 3. The hemolytic action of the blood serum or plasma of an animal upon its own cells. —**au·to·lyt·ic** (aw"to·lit'ick) *adj.;* **au·to·lyze** (aw'to·lize) *v.*

autolytic enzyme. An enzyme producing autolysis or digestion of the cell in which it exists, usually at the death of the cell.

automat-, automato- [Gk. *automatos*]. A combining form meaning *automatic, spontaneous, initiatory.*

automata. A plural of *automaton.*

au·to·mat·ic (aw"to·mat'ick) *adj.* [Gk. *automatos,* self-acting, spontaneous]. 1. Performed without the influence of the will; spontaneous. 2. Self-regulatory, self-propelled.

automatic bladder. REFLEX BLADDER.

automatic obedience. COMMAND AUTOMATISM.

automatic writing. 1. *In psychology,* a dissociative phenomenon in which an individual writes material while his attention is distracted and consciously unaware of what he writes; used occasionally for experimental purposes, for testing the relative disassociative capacity of a patient, and as a means of access to unconscious data. 2. The writing that follows the suggestions made to a patient while he is in a hypnotic trance.

au·tom·a·tin (aw·tom'uh·tin) *n.* [*automat-* + *-in*]. 1. A hypothetical substance in the heart which normally initiates myocardial contraction. 2. An extract of bovine heart muscle, used therapeutically in various circulatory disorders.

au·to·ma·tin·o·gen (aw"to·ma·tin'o·jen) *n.* [*automatin* + *-gen*]. A hypothetical substance in the heart and muscles which, through the action of potassium, is converted to automatin.

au·tom·a·tism (aw·tom'uh·tiz·um) *n.* [F. *automatisme,* from Gk. *automatismos,* that which happens by itself]. 1. Performance of normally voluntary acts without apparent volition, as in somnambulism and in hysterical and epileptic states. 2. *In biology,* independent activity of cells and tissues, as the beating of a heart freed from its nervous connections.

au·tom·a·ti·za·tion (aw·tom"uh·ti·zay'shun) *n.* *In psychiatry,* automatic obedience to infantile impulses.

automato-. See *automat-.*

au·to·mat·o·gen (aw"to·mat'o·jen) *n.* AUTOMATINOGEN.

au·tom·a·ton (aw·tom'uh·ton) *n.,* pl. **automatons, automa·ta** (·tuh) [neuter noun form of Gk. *automatos,* automatic]. 1. A person who acts in an involuntary or mechanical manner. 2. A robot or mechanism designed to follow programmed instructions.

au·to·my·so·pho·bia (aw"to·migh"so·fo'bee·uh) *n.* [*auto-* + *mysophobia*]. Abnormal dread of personal uncleanliness.

au·to·ne·phrec·to·my (aw"to·ne·freck'tuh·mee) *n.* [*auto-* + *nephrectomy*]. The complete or nearly complete loss of renal parenchyma and function secondary to complete ureteral obstruction or to an inflammatory disease such as tuberculosis. Compare *renal autoamputation.*

au·to·no·ma·sia (aw"to·no·may'zhuh, ·zee·uh) *n.* [*aut-* + Gk. *onomasia,* expression, naming, from *onoma,* name]. AMNESIC APHASIA.

au·to·nom·ic (aw"tuh·nom'ick) *adj.* [*autonomy* + *-ic*]. Normally independent of volition; specifically, pertaining to the involuntary or autonomic nervous system.

autonomic center. Any center of the brain or spinal cord regulating visceral functions by way of the parasympathetic and thoracolumbar outflows.

autonomic epilepsy. CONVULSIVE EQUIVALENT.

autonomic imbalance. Absence of normal equilibrium between actions of the sympathetic and parasympathetic nervous systems.

autonomic nerve. A nerve of the autonomic nervous system.

autonomic nervous system. An aggregation of ganglions, nerves, and plexuses through which the viscera, heart, blood vessels, smooth muscles, and glands receive their motor innervation. It is divided into the craniosacral or parasympathetic system, and the thoracicolumbar or sympathetic system. NA *systema nervosum autonomicum.*

autonomic neuron. A neuron that is a component of the autonomic nervous system.

autonomic nucleus of the oculomotor nerve. The group of nerve cells that give rise to the parasympathetic fibers of the oculomotor nerve. Syn. *Edinger-Westphal nucleus.* NA *nucleus autonomicus nervi oculomotorii, nucleus accessorius nervi oculomotorii.*

autonomic plexus. Any plexus of branches of autonomic nerves surrounding an organ or vessel, each such plexus being named from its associated structure, as coronary plexus, enteric plexus. NA (pl.) *plexus autonomici.*

autonomic sensibilities. VITAL SENSIBILITIES.

au·ton·o·mous (aw·ton'uh·mus) *adj.* [Gk. *autonomos* from *auto-* + *nomos,* law]. Independent in origin, action, or function; self-governing.

autonomous bladder. A paralytic condition of the urinary bladder characterized by loss of voluntary and reflex micturition, seen in patients with destructive lesions of the lumbosacral spinal cord or of both sensory and motor roots of the sacral plexus.

autonomous potentials. Continuous potentials arising spontaneously from neurons in the absence of stimulation.

au·to·oph·thal·mo·scope (aw"to·off·thal'muh·skope) *n.* An ophthalmoscope for examining one's own eyes.

au·to·oph·thal·mos·co·py (aw"to-off·thal·mos'kuh·pee) *n.* [*auto-* + *ophthalmoscopy*]. A phenomenon in which the retinal vessels become entoptically visible.

au·to-ox·i·da·tion (aw"to·ock'si·day·shun) *n.* 1. Spontaneous oxidation by atmospheric oxygen, without added oxidant. 2. A reaction in which two molecules of a substance react in such a way that one is oxidized and the other reduced. Syn. *auto-oxidation-reduction.*

auto-oxidation-reduction. AUTO-OXIDATION (2).

au·top·a·thy (aw·top'uth·ee) *n.* [Gk. *autopatheia,* primary affection]. IDIOPATHY. —**auto·path·ic** (aw"to·path'ick) *adj.*

au·to·pha·gia (aw"to·fay'jee·uh) *n.* [*auto-* + *-phagia*]. 1. Self-consumption; emaciation. 2. The biting or eating of one's own flesh.

au·toph·a·gy (aw·tof'uh·jee) *n.* AUTOPHAGIA.

au·to·phil·ia (aw"to·fil'ee·uh) *n.* [*auto-* + *-philia*]. NARCISSISM.

au·to·pho·bia (aw"to·fo'bee·uh) *n.* [*auto-* + *-phobia*]. A pathologic dread of one's self or of being alone.

au·to·pho·nia (aw"to·fo'nee·uh) *n.* AUTOPHONY.

au·to·phono·ma·nia (aw"to·fon"o·may'nee·uh, ·fo"no·) *n.* [*auto-* + *phonomania*]. Suicidal mania.

au·toph·o·ny (aw·tof'o·nee) *n.* [*auto-* + *phon-* + *-y*]. A condition in some middle ear and auditory tube diseases in which an individual's voice seems more resonant to himself.

aut·oph·thal·mo·scope (awt"off·thal'muh·skope) *n.* AUTO-OPHTHALMOSCOPE.

aut·oph·thal·mos·co·py (awt"off·thal·mos'kuh·pee) *n.* AUTO-OPHTHALMOSCOPY.

au·to·plas·tic (aw"to·plas'tick) *adj.* 1. Of or pertaining to autoplasty or to an autograft. 2. *In psychiatry,* pertaining to the indirect internal modification and adaptation of impulses prior to their outward expression, as found in neuroses.

au·to·plas·ty (aw'to·plas"tee) *n.* [*auto-* + *-plasty*]. Repair of a defect by grafting tissue taken from another area of the same body. Compare *homoplasty*. —**auto·plast** (·plast) *n.*

au·to·pneu·mo·nec·to·my (aw″to·new″mo·neck′tuh·mee) *n.* [*auto-* + *pneumonectomy*]. Obstruction or occlusion of a main bronchus, rendering one lung functionless.

au·to·po·lym·er·iz·ing resin (aw″to·pol′i·mur·eye″zing, ·pol·im′ur·). A resin that is polymerized by a chemical activator and an initiator without the use of external heat. Syn. *self-curing resin.*

au·to·poly·ploi·dy (aw″to·pol′i·ploy·dee) *n.* [*auto-* + *polyploidy*]. The state of having more than two complete sets of chromosomes derived from one species.

au·to·pro·throm·bin (aw″to·pro·throm′bin) *n.* [*auto-* + *prothrombin*]. Any one of a group of substances that may result from the conversion of prothrombin to thrombin under specific circumstances. Several autoprothrombins have been described, and some have clot-promoting activity. The exact relationship of the autoprothrombins to the clotting factors demonstrated by other methods is not clear.

au·to·pro·tol·y·sis (aw″to·pro·tol′i·sis) *n.* [*auto-* + *proton* + *-lysis*]. The process by which a molecule transfers a proton (hydrogen ion) to another identical molecule, as in the ionization of water: $2H_2O \rightarrow H_3O^+ + OH^-$.

au·top·sy (aw′top·see) *n.* [Gk. *autopsia*, seeing with one's own eyes, from *aut-* + *opsis*, sight, seeing]. A medical examination of the body after death to confirm or correct the clinical diagnosis, to ascertain the cause of death, to improve understanding of disease processes and aid medical teaching. Syn. *necropsy, postmortem.*

au·to·psy·chic (aw″to·sigh′kick) *adj.* Pertaining to self-consciousness or to ideas relating to the individual's own personality. Contr. *allopsychic.*

au·to·psy·cho·sis (aw″to·sigh·ko′sis) *n.* [*auto-* + *psychosis*]. A mental derangement in which the patient's ideas about himself are distorted.

au·to·ra·dio·gram (aw″to·ray′dee·o·gram) *n.* RADIOAUTOGRAPH.

au·to·ra·dio·graph (aw″to·ray′dee·o·graf) *n.* RADIOAUTOGRAPH.

au·to·ra·di·og·ra·phy (aw″to·ray″dee·og′ruh·fee) *n.* RADIOAUTOGRAPHY.

au·to·reg·u·la·tion (aw″to·reg·yoo·lay′shun) *n.* The process of adjustments whereby a physiologic system, usually an organ or a vascular bed, is able to maintain its own normal state by varying some factor such as blood flow or nutrient concentration to match its needs in the face of internal or external changes and stresses. See also *homeometric autoregulation, heterometric autoregulation.*

au·to·re·in·fu·sion (aw″to·ree·in·few′zhun) *n.* [*auto-* + *reinfusion*]. AUTOTRANSFUSION (2).

au·to·sen·si·ti·za·tion (aw″to·sen″si·ti·zay′shun) *n.* Sensitization to a constituent of an organism's own body.

autosensitization dermatitis. An inflammatory condition of the skin, usually eczematous in form, and thought to be caused by products of an already damaged epidermis after sensitization to those products.

au·to·sex·ing (aw″to·seck′sing) *n.* The determination of sex in animals by such genetic traits as feather color and other characteristics at birth or hatching.

au·to·site (aw′to·site) *n.* [Gk. *autositos*, bringing one's own provisions, from *auto-* + *sitos*, food]. That member of an unequal twin monster which is capable of independent existence, and which nourishes the other twin (the parasite). The latter may be a complete fetus or accessory body parts attached to the autosite or to the placenta. —**au·to·sit·ic** (aw″to·sit′ick) *adj.*

autosomal recessive alymphocytic agammaglobulinemia. SWISS TYPE AGAMMAGLOBULINEMIA.

au·to·some (aw′to·sohm) *n.* [*auto-* + *-some*]. A non-sex-determining chromosome; any chromosome other than the X and Y chromosomes. —**auto·so·mal** (aw″to·so′mul) *adj.*

au·to·sple·nec·to·my (aw″to·sple·neck′tuh·mee) *n.* [*auto-* + *splen-* + *-ectomy*]. Destruction of most or all of the splenic tissue by a disease process, usually sickle cell anemia.

au·to·sug·gest·ibil·i·ty (aw″to·sug·jes″ti·bil′i·tee) *n.* Susceptibility to autosuggestion.

au·to·sug·ges·tion (aw″to·sug·jes′chun) *n.* 1. The acceptance of a thought or idea, predominantly from within one's own mind, which induces some mental or physical action or change. 2. The persistence in consciousness of impressions gained while in a hypnotic state. Syn. *self-suggestion.* See also *traumatic suggestion.*

au·to·syn·de·sis (aw″to·sin′de·sis) *n.* [*auto-* + *syndesis*]. In hybrids, the pairing of chromosomes derived from the same parent. Contr. *allosynapsis.*

au·to·syn·noia (aw″to·si·noy′uh) *n.* [*auto-* + Gk. *synnoia*, meditation]. A state of introversion in which the subject is so concentrated in his thoughts or hallucinations that he loses all interest in the outside world.

au·to·tech·ni·con (aw″to·teck′ni·kon) *n.* An electrically timed machine for the automatic fixation, dehydration, and impregnation of tissue specimens, and for staining sections.

au·tot·o·my (aw·tot′uh·mee) *n.* [*auto-* + *-tomy*]. 1. A mechanism by means of which many organisms are able to cast off parts of their body. 2. Self-division; FISSION (2). 3. A surgical operation performed on one's own body.

au·to·top·ag·no·sia (aw″to·top·ag·no′zhuh, ·zee·uh) *n.* [*auto-* + *topagnosia*]. Loss of ability to identify or orient parts of one's own body; a defect in appreciation or awareness of the body scheme, seen in lesions involving the angular gyrus or thalamoparietal pathways. Syn. *somatotopagnosia.*

au·to·trans·form·er (aw″to·trans·for′mur) *n.* A step-down transformer used extensively in varying the voltage to the primary windings of a high-voltage x-ray transformer.

au·to·trans·fu·sion (aw″to·trans·few′zhun) *n.* [*auto-* + *transfusion*]. 1. Compression of the extremities and abdomen to increase venous return, raise blood pressure, and perfuse vital organs. Syn. *autoinfusion.* 2. Reinfusion of the patient's own blood, as during hemorrhage or surgery. Syn. *autoreinfusion.*

au·to·trans·plan·ta·tion (aw″to·trans″plan·tay′shun) *n.* The operation of transplanting to a part of the body tissue taken from another area in the same body. —**auto·trans·plant** (·trans′plant) *n.*

au·to·troph (aw′to·trof, ·trofe) *n.* [*auto-* + *-troph*]. A bacterium able to grow in an inorganic environment by using carbon dioxide as its sole source of carbon for anabolic metabolism. Contr. *heterotroph.* See also *chemotroph, phototroph.* —**au·to·tro·phic** (aw″to·tro′fick, ·trof′ick) *adj.*

au·to·tro·phant (aw′to·tro″funt) *n.* AUTOTROPH.

au·to·trophe (aw′to·trofe, aw″to·trofe′) *n.* AUTOTROPH.

au·to·vac·ci·na·tion (aw″to·vack″si·nay′shun) *n.* Revaccination of an individual, using vaccine obtained from his own body.

au·to·vac·cine (aw″to·vack′seen) *n.* AUTOGENOUS VACCINE.

au·tox·i·da·tion (aw·tock″si·day′shun) *n.* AUTO-OXIDATION.

au·tum·nal fever (au·tum′nul). PRETIBIAL FEVER.

aux-, auxo- [Gk. *auxē*, growth, increase]. A combining form meaning (a) *growth;* (b) *increase;* (c) in biochemistry, *accelerating or stimulating.*

auxano- [Gk. *auxanein*, to increase]. A combining form meaning *growth.*

aux·ano·gram (awk·san′o·gram) *n.* A pure plate culture of microorganisms prepared by auxanography.

aux·a·nog·ra·phy (awk″suh·nog′ruh·fee) *n.* [*auxano-* + *-graphy*]. A method for ascertaining the nutrient medium most suited to the growth requirements of a particular strain of microorganisms. —**aux·a·no·graph·ic** (awk″suh·no·graf′ick) *adj.*

-auxe [Gk. *auxē*, growth, increase]. A combining form meaning *hypertrophy, enlargement.*

aux·e·sis (awk·see′sis) *n.*, pl. **auxe·ses** (·seez) [Gk. *auxēsis*, growth, increase]. 1. An increase in size or bulk; growth. 2. Growth in size by cell expansion without cell division; hypertrophy.

aux·et·ic (awk·set'ick) *adj. & n.* [Gk. *auxētikos,* promoting growth]. 1. Of or pertaining to auxesis. 2 Stimulating growth. 3. A hypothetical substance that excites cell reproduction; an agent that causes proliferation of human cells, especially leukocytes.

aux·il·ia·ry (awg·zil″ee·ur·ee) *n.* ADMINICULUM.

aux·in (awk'sin) *n.* [*aux-* + *-in*]. Indoleacetic acid, a plant growth hormone formed from tryptophan.

aux·i·om·e·ter (awk″see·om'e·tur) *n.* AUXOMETER.

auxo-. See *aux-.*

auxo·bar·ic (awk″so·băr'ick) *adj.* [*auxo-* + *bar-* + *-ic*]. Denoting increased pressure, especially relating to a rise in pressure in the cardiac ventricles during the isovolumetric and early ejection phases.

auxo·car·dia (awk″so·kahr'dee·uh) *n.* [*auxo-* + *-cardia*]. 1. The normal increase of the volume of the heart during diastole. Contr. *miocardia.* 2. Cardiac enlargement from hypertrophy or dilatation.

auxo·chrome (awk'so·krome) *n.* [*auxo-* + *-chrome*]. 1. That which increases color. 2. A chemical group which, added to a chromophore group, will produce a dye. 3. Increase or development of color. —**auxo·chro·mous** (awk″so·kro'mus) *adj.*

auxo·cyte (awk'so·site) *n.* [*auxo-* + *-cyte*]. A spermatocyte, oocyte, or sporocyte during its early growth period.

auxo·drome (awk'so·drome) *n.* A standard schedule of development. See also *Wetzel's grid.*

aux·om·e·ter (awk·som'e·tur) *n.* [*auxo-* + *-meter*]. A device for measuring the magnifying power of lenses.

auxo·ton·ic (awk″so·ton'ick) *adj.* [*auxo-* + *tonic*]. Contracting against increasing tension or resistance.

auxo·tro·phic (awk″so·trof'ick, ·tro'fick) *adj.* [*auxo-* + *-trophic*]. Differing from the wild-type, or prototrophic, strain of an organism by an additional nutritional requirement. —**auxo·troph** (awk'so·trof, ·trofe) *n.*

AV Abbreviation for (a) *atrioventricular*; (b) *arteriovenous.*

Av. Abbreviation for *avoirdupois.*

aV Symbol for augmented unipolar limb lead.

av·a·lanche (av'uh·lanch) *n.* [F.]. The phenomenon or process, encountered when ionizing emanations are being measured, whereby an ion produces another ion by collision, and these ions in turn produce other ions by further collisions, until a rush of ions and accompanying electrons results.

aval·vu·lar (ay·val'vew·lur, a·val') *adj.* [*a-* + *valvular*]. Lacking any structure for temporarily closing a passage or an opening.

avas·cu·lar (ay·vas'kew·lur) *adj.* [*a-* + *vascular*]. 1. Pertaining to inadequate blood supply. 2. Lacking blood vessels.

avas·cu·lar·ize (ay·vas'kew·lur·ize, a·vas') *v.* To render a part bloodless, as by compression or bandaging. —**avas·cu·lar·iza·tion** (ay·vas″kew·lur·i·zay'shun) *n.*

avascular necrosis. Necrosis due to inadequate blood flow.

Avazyme. A trademark for a preparation of the proteolytic enzyme chymotrypsin, proposed for use in the treatment of soft tissue inflammation and edema.

AV block. ATRIOVENTRICULAR BLOCK.

Avel·lis's syndrome or **paralysis** (ah·vel'is) [G. *Avellis,* German otolaryngologist, 1864-1916]. Ipsilateral paralysis of the soft palate, pharynx, and larynx and the laryngeal muscles due to a lesion of the ambiguus nucleus and tractus solitarius on that side with contralateral loss of pain and temperature sense due to involvement of the spinothalamic tract adjacent to the lesion.

Ave·na (a·vee'nuh) *n.* [L., oats]. A genus of plants; the grain of *Avena sativa,* one of the most important species, is the oat.

Aventyl. Trademark for nortriptyline, an antidepressant and tranquilizing drug used as the hydrochloride salt.

av·er·age, *n. & adj.* 1. The figure arrived at by adding together several quantities and dividing by the number of quantities; arithmetic mean. 2. Usual, typical; median.

average deviation. MEAN DEVIATION.

average dose. A dose which may be expected ordinarily to produce the therapeutic effect for which the ingredient or preparation is most commonly employed.

average life. Mean radioactive life; the average of the individual lives of all the atoms of a radioactive substance (1.443 times the radioactive half-life).

average localization law. Visceral pain is most accurately localized in the least mobile viscera.

aver·sion therapy (a·vur'zhun). *In psychiatry,* any form of treatment that involves applying some painful experience or punishment to a well-established behavior, inducing a motivational conflict between the desire for acting in a certain way and the fear of the unpleasant consequences; applied particularly to the treatment of alcoholism or sexual deviation; a form of conditioning.

aver·sive therapy (a·vur'siv). AVERSION THERAPY.

Avertin. Trademark for tribromoethanol.

Avertin with amylene hydrate. Trademark for tribromoethanol solution; used for basal anesthesia by rectal administration and for control of certain convulsive conditions. Syn. *bromethol (Brit.).*

Aves (ay'veez) *n.pl.* [L., plural of *avis,* bird]. The class of vertebrates that comprises the birds.

AV heart block. ATRIOVENTRICULAR BLOCK.

avi·an (ay'vee·un) *adj.* [L. *avis,* bird]. Of, pertaining to, or caused by birds.

avian diphtheria. AVIAN POX.

avian encephalomyelitis. A viral disease of chickens, characterized by tremor and ataxia.

avian epidemic blindness. OCULAR LYMPHOMATOSIS.

avian influenza. An acute respiratory disease of domestic and wild birds caused by any of a group of distinct myxoviruses. See also *fowl plague.*

avian leukosis complex. A group of viral diseases of birds characterized by proliferation of immature leukocytes.

avian malaria. Malaria of birds and poultry due to numerous species of the genus *Plasmodium.*

avian molluscum. AVIAN POX.

avian Paget's disease. OSTEOPETROTIC LYMPHOMATOSIS.

avian pneumoencephalitis. NEWCASTLE DISEASE.

avian pox. A disease of birds caused by poxviruses of the fowl, turkey, pigeon, and canary subgroups, characterized by inflammation and hyperplasia of the epidermis followed by scab formation and desquamation, and diphtheritic membranes in the upper respiratory and digestive tracts.

avian pseudoplague. NEWCASTLE DISEASE.

avian tuberculosis. A form of tuberculosis affecting fowl, caused by *Mycobacterium tuberculosis* var. *avium,* characterized by tubercles composed primarily of epithelioid cells. Various mammals including, rarely, humans may be infected.

avi·a·tion medicine. The branch of medicine that deals with problems peculiar to aviation, including selection, support, and treatment of the flier, assistance in designing aircraft and related equipment to meet human physiologic requirements, adaptation to varying conditions of flight, and the problems involved in the transport of the sick and wounded. Compare *space medicine.*

avi·a·tor's ear. Barotitis media aquired in aviation.

av·i·din (av'i·din) *n.* A biotin-inactivating protein in raw egg white.

avid·i·ty (a·vid'i·tee) *n.* [L. *avidus,* eager, greedy]. 1. *In immunology,* the rate of neutralization of antigen, such as toxin, by antibody. 2. The firmness of union of antibody to antigen.

Avinar. Trademark for uredepa.

AV interval. ATRIOVENTRICULAR INTERVAL.

avir·u·lent (ay·virr'yoo·lunt, a·virr') *adj.* Without virulence.

avi·ta·min·osis (ay·vye"tuh·mi·no'sis, a·vye", ay"vi·tam"i·no'sis) *n.*, pl. **avitamin·oses** (·no'seez) [*a-* + *vitamin* + *-osis*]. Any disease resulting from deficiency of a vitamin.

avitaminosis C. SCURVY.

Avlosulfon. Trademark for dapsone.

AV nicking [*a*rterio*v*enous]. The nicking of a retinal vein by pressure from the artery.

AV node. ATRIOVENTRICULAR NODE.

avo·ca·lia (ay·vo·kay'lee·uh, av"o·) *n.* [*a-* + *vocal* + *-ia*]. A form of motor amusia characterized chiefly by the loss of the ability to sing.

Avo·ga·dro's number (ah"vo·gah'dro) [A. *Avogadro*, Italian physicist, 1776–1856]. The number of molecules of a substance in one gram-molecular weight; it is 6.06 × 10^{23}.

avoid·ance *n.* *In psychiatry,* a conscious or unconscious defense mechanism through which the individual seeks to escape anxiety, conflict, danger, fear, and pain. Efforts at avoidance may be physical as well as psychologic.

av·oir·du·pois (av"ur·duh·poiz') *n.* [ME. *avoir de pois,* from OF. *avoir,* goods, + *pois,* weight]. The English system of weights and measures. Abbreviated, Av. See also Tables of Weights and Measures in the Appendix.

avoirdupois ounce. The sixteenth part of the avoirdupois pound, or 437.5 grains (28.35 grams). Abbreviated, oz. See also Tables of Weights and Measures in the Appendix.

avoirdupois pound. Sixteen avoirdupois ounces, or 7,000 grains; equivalent to 1.2153 troy pounds. Symbol, lb. See also Table of Weights and Measures in the Appendix.

avo·par·cin (ay"vo·pahr'sin) *n.* An antibiotic obtained from *Streptomyces candidus.*

Avosyl. A trademark for mephenesin.

A-V patterns or **syndromes.** Significant alterations in the degree of either exotropia or esotropia when the patient looks up or down. An A pattern shows more divergence in down gaze or more convergence in up gaze; in the V pattern, the reverse holds, with more divergence in up gaze rather than in down gaze.

AV shunt. ARTERIOVENOUS SHUNT.

avul·sion (a·vul'shun) *n.* [L. *avulsio,* from *avellere,* to tear away]. A forcible tearing or wrenching away of a part, as a polyp, a nerve, or a limb.

avulsion fissure. The separation of the tibial tuberosity, due to violent action of the patellar tendon.

avulsion fracture. The tearing off of a bony prominence, as a tuberosity, by the forcible pull of its tendinous or muscular attachments.

avulsion of the bulb. Forcible separation of the eyeball by tearing the muscles, the tendons, and the optic nerve.

A wave. Abbreviation for *alpha wave.*

a wave. 1. The positive-pressure wave in the atrial or venous pulse, produced by atrial contraction. 2. The atrial wave of the apex cardiogram representing the outward motion of the cardiac apex which results from additional ventricular filling produced by atrial contraction. Syn. *atrial beat.*

ax. Abbreviation for *axis.*

ax-, axo-. A combining form denoting (a) *axis;* (b) *axon or axis cylinder.*

axan·thop·sia (ay"zan·thop'see·uh) *n.* [*a-* + *xanth-* + *-opsia*]. YELLOW BLINDNESS.

Ax·en·feld's intrascleral nerve loop (a^h^k'sun·felt) [K. T. P. P. *Axenfeld,* German ophthalmologist, 1867–1930]. An anomalous loop of the ciliary nerve in the scleral layer of the eyeball.

Axenfeld's syndrome [K. T. P. P. *Axenfeld*]. A syndrome of posterior embryotoxon, iris abnormalities, and glaucoma; inherited as an autosomal dominant trait.

axen·ic (ay·zen'ick, ay·zee'nick) *adj.* [*a-* + *xen-* + *-ic*]. 1. Not contaminated by any foreign organisms, hence a pure culture, as of protozoa. 2. Of or pertaining to germ-free animals.

axe·roph·thol (ay"ze·rof'thol, ack"se·rof'thol) *n.* [*a-* + *xerophth*almia]. VITAMIN A.

axes. Plural of *axis.*

axi-, axio-. A combining form meaning *axis, axial.*

ax·i·al (ack'see·ul) *adj.* 1. Of or pertaining to an axis. 2. *In dentistry,* relating to or parallel with the long axis of a tooth. —**axial·ly** (·ee) *adv.*

axial accumulation. AXIAL STREAMING.

axial artery. The first main artery to a developing limb bud.

axial asynergy. TRUNCAL ATAXIA.

axial current. The faster-moving current along the axis or center of a vascular lumen, carrying in the bloodstream, especially in the smaller arteries, a preponderance of erythrocytes over the slower, plasma-rich, outer current.

axial fiber. 1. The axis cylinder of a nerve fiber. 2. The central spiral filament, probably contractile, of the flagellum of the spermatozoon.

axial filament. The central contractile fibril of a cilium or flagellum which arises from a centriole or blepharoplast.

axial fusiform cataract. SPINDLE CATARACT.

axial hyperopia. Hyperopia due to abnormal shortness of the anteroposterior diameter of the eye, the refractive power being normal.

axial illumination. Illumination by light conveyed in the direction of the optical axis of the objective and ocular of the microscope.

axial light. Light rays that are parallel to each other and to the optic axis.

axial mesoderm. PARAXIAL MESODERM.

axial muscle. A muscle attached to the vertebral column.

axial neuritis. 1. A form of neuritis that affects the central part of a nerve. 2. *In ophthalmology,* the selective involvement of the papillomacular bundle.

axial plate. PRIMITIVE STREAK.

axial skeleton. The skeleton of the head and trunk.

axial stream. The central, faster-moving portion of the bloodstream in a vessel. See also *axial current.*

axial streaming. The accumulation of erythrocytes in the axial stream. Syn. *axial accumulation.*

axial tomography. Sectional radiography in which a series of cross-sectional images along an axis is combined to constitute a three-dimensional scan. See also *computed tomography.*

axial walls. Walls of a prepared cavity in a tooth, which are parallel with its long axis.

ax·i·a·tion (ack"see·ay'shun) *n.* The formation or development of axial structures, such as the notochord and neural tube.

ax·if·u·gal (ack·sif'yoo·gul) *adj.* AXOFUGAL.

ax·i·lem·ma (ack"si·lem'uh) *n.* AXOLEMMA.

ax·il·la (ack·sil'uh) *n.*, pl. & genit. sing. **axil·lae** (·ee) [L.] The region between the arm and the thoracic wall, bounded anteriorly by the pectoralis major muscle, and posteriorly by the latissimus dorsi muscle; the armpit. NA *fossa axillaris.*

ax·il·lary (ack'si·lerr"ee) *adj.* Of or pertaining to the axilla.

axillary arch. An occasional muscle slip in the axilla connecting the latissimus dorsi or teres major with the pectoralis major.

axillary fossa. AXILLA.

axillary glands. The axillary lymph nodes.

axillary nerve. See Table of Nerves in the Appendix.

axillary paralysis. Paralysis of the axillary nerve resulting in the loss of function of the deltoid muscle; usually due to fracture or dislocation of the humerus, or to pressure from a crutch.

axillary plexus. The plexus of lymph nodes and lymphatic vessels in the axilla.

axillary plica. A fold of skin and muscle which bounds the axilla anteriorly (plica axillaris anterior) and posteriorly (plica axillaris posterior).

axillary region. A region upon the lateral aspect of the thorax, extending from the axilla to a line drawn from the lower border of the mammary region to that of the scapular region. NA *regio axillaris.*

axillary vein thrombosis. PAGET-SCHROETTER'S SYNDROME.

ax·il·lo·sub·cla·vi·an (ack"si·lo·sub·klay'vee·un) *adj.* Pertaining to the axilla and the subclavian areas.

axillosubclavian vein. The axillary vein and its extension, the subclavian vein, considered as one vessel.

axio-. See *axi-.*

ax·io·buc·co·lin·gual (ack"see·o·buck"o·ling'gwul) *adj.* Pertaining to the long axis and the buccal and lingual surfaces of a tooth.

axiobuccolingual plane. A plane parallel with the long axis of a tooth, passing through both the buccal and lingual surfaces.

ax·io·la·bio·lin·gual (ack"see·o·lay"bee·o·ling'gwul) *adj.* Pertaining to the long axis and the labial and lingual surfaces of a tooth.

axiolabiolingual plane. A plane parallel with the long axis of an incisor tooth and passing through its labial and lingual surfaces.

ax·ip·e·tal (ack·sip'e·tul) *adj.* AXOPETAL.

Axiquel. Trademark for valnoctamide.

ax·is (ack'sis) *n.*, pl. **ax·es** (·seez) [L.]. 1. An imaginary line passing through the center of a body; also the line about which a rotating body turns. 2. [NA] The second cervical vertebra. Syn. *epistropheus.* See also Table of Bones in the Appendix.

axis bul·bi ex·ter·nus (bul'bye ecks·tur'nus) [NA]. An imaginary line passing through the anterior and posterior poles of the eyeball.

axis bulbi in·ter·nus (in·tur'nus) [NA]. An imaginary line passing through the anterior pole of the eyeball to a point on the retina just deep to the posterior pole of the eyeball.

axis cylinder. AXON.

axis cylinder process. AXON.

axis deviation. *In electrocardiography,* variation of the mean electrical axis of the heart beyond the normal range. See also *left axis deviation, right axis deviation.*

axis len·tis (len'tis) [NA]. An imaginary line passing through the anterior and posterior poles of the lens.

axis ocu·li ex·ter·na (ock'yoo·lye ecks·tur'nuh) [BNA]. AXIS BULBI EXTERNUS.

axis oculi in·ter·na (in·tur'nuh) [BNA]. AXIS BULBI INTERNUS.

axis op·ti·ca (op'ti·kuh) [BNA]. Axis opticus (= OPTIC AXIS).

axis op·ti·cus (op'ti·kus) [NA]. OPTIC AXIS.

axis pel·vis (pel'vis) [NA]. PELVIC AXIS.

axis traction. Traction in the axis or direction of a channel, as of the pelvis, through which the fetus is to be drawn.

axis-traction forceps. An obstetric forceps, the so-called high forceps instrument, equipped with a mechanism to permit rotation of the fetal head and traction in the line of the pelvic axis.

axis uteri (yoo'tur·eye). 1. The long diameter of the uterus. 2. An imaginary line passing transversely through the uterus near its junction with the cervix, on which it is said to turn in retroversion.

axo-. See *ax-.*

axo·den·drit·ic (ack"so·den·drit'ick) *adj.* [*axo-* + *dendritic*]. Pertaining to an axon and to dendrites.

axodendritic synapse. A type of synapse in which the end-feet of the axon of one neuron are in contact with the dendrites of another neuron.

axo·fu·gal (ack"so·few'gul, ack·sof'yoo·gul) *adj.* [*axo-* + *-fugal*]. Pertaining to nerve impulses transmitted from the cell body to the periphery.

ax·og·e·nous (ack·soj'e·nus) *adj.* [*axo-* + *-genous*]. Originating in an axon.

ax·oid (ack'soid) *adj.* [*ax-* + *-oid*]. 1. Pivot-shaped. 2. Pertaining to the second cervical joint.

ax·oi·de·an (ack·soy'dee·un) *adj.* AXOID.

axo·lem·ma (ack"so·lem'uh) *n.* [*axo-* + *-lemma*]. The plasma membrane surrounding the axon of a neuron, and reaching deep to the myelin sheath. Syn. *axilemma.*

ax·o·lotl (ack'suh·lot"ul) *n.* [Nahuatl]. Any of the salamanders of the genus *Ambystoma,* which retain gills for respiration in the adult stage.

ax·o·mat·ic (ack"so·mat'ick) *adj.* [*ax-* + *somatic*]. Pertaining to an axon and the cell body of a neuron.

axomatic synapse. A type of synapse in which the end-feet of the axon of one neuron are in contact with the cell body of another neuron.

ax·om·e·ter (ack·som'e·tur) *n.* An instrument for adjusting spectacles to the axes of the eyes.

ax·on (acks'on) *n.* [Gk. *axōn,* axis]. The efferent process of a nerve cell. Syn. *neurit, axis cylinder process.* **—ax·o·nal** (ack'suh·nul) *adj.*

axonal reaction. The sequence of changes whereby a nerve cell body seeks to restore the integrity of its axon when it has been interrupted by injury or disease; best seen in the anterior horn cells of the spinal cord, the larger sensory neurons, and the motor nuclei of the cranial nerves, the changes include swelling of the nerve cell body, chromatolysis so that the Nissl granules are no longer stained by basic aniline dyes, and swelling and peripheral displacement of the nucleus. Syn. *primary degeneration of Nissl.* See also *central chromatolysis.*

ax·on·a·prax·is (ack"son·uh·prack'sis) *n.* [*axon* + *a-* + *praxis*]. NEURAPRAXIA.

ax·one (ack'sone) *n.* AXON.

ax·o·ne·ma (ack'so·nee'muh) *n.* AXONEME.

ax·o·neme (ack'so·neem) *n.* [*axo-* + *-neme*]. The axial filament of the flagellum of a protozoan.

axon hillock. The conically shaped part of a nerve cell body from which the axon originates.

axono- [Gk. *axōn, axonos,* axis]. A combining form meaning (a) *axis;* (b) *axon.*

ax·o·nom·e·ter (ack"so·nom'e·tur) *n.* [*axono-* + *-meter*]. An instrument used for locating the axis of astigmatism, or for determining the axis of a cylindrical lens.

ax·on·ot·me·sis (ack"suh·not·mee'sis) *n.* [*axono-* + Gk. *tmēsis,* cutting]. Injury to a nerve, as from severe compression which damages the nerve fibers, causing motor and sensory deficits without completely severing the nerve, so that recovery may occur.

axon reaction. AXONAL REACTION.

axon reflex. A response occurring without involvement of a nerve cell body or a synapse (hence not a true reflex), which results from a stimulus applied to a terminal branch of a sensory nerve and gives rise to an impulse that ascends to a collateral branch of the same nerve fiber, down which it is conducted antidromically to an effector organ; believed to be important in the local regulation of blood vessel caliber, especially in the skin.

ax·op·e·tal (ack·sop'e·tul) *adj.* [*axo-* + *-petal*]. Pertaining to nerve impulses transmitted along an axon toward the cell body.

axo·plasm (ack'so·plaz·um) *n.* Undifferentiated cytoplasm, neuroplasm, of the axon in which neurofibrils are embedded.

aya·huas·co (ah"yuh·wahs'ko) *n.* [Sp., from Quechua]. *Banisteria caapi,* a Brazilian plant containing banisterine.

Aya·la's test, index, or **quotient** (a·yah'lah) [A. G. *Ayala,* Italian neurologist, 1878–1943]. A manometric estimate of the volume of the cerebrospinal fluid reservoir, obtained from the formula QF/I, where Q is the amount in milliliters of cerebrospinal fluid removed, I the initial or opening pressure, and F the final or closing pressure. The normal quotient is 5.5 to 6.5; a value above 7.0 suggests a large reservoir, as in communicating hydrocephalus or cerebral atrophy; a value below 5.0 indicates a small reservoir, as in cerebral edema, an expanding intracranial lesion, or subarachnoid block.

Ayer·za's syndrome or **disease** (a·yerr'sah) [A. *Ayerza,* Argentinian physician, 1861-1918]. Intense cyanosis, polycythemia, heart failure due to chronic pulmonary insufficiency, and sclerosis of the pulmonary vascular bed.

Ayfivin. Trademark for bacitracin, an antibiotic.

ayp·nia (ay·ip'nee·uh) *n.* [Gk., from *a-* + *hypnos*, sleep, + *-ia*]. INSOMNIA.

Az Symbol for azote.

az-, aza-, azo- [*azo*te]. A combining form indicating *the presence of nitrogen in a compound.*

az·a·bon (az'uh·bon, ay'zuh·bon) *n.* 3-Sulfanilyl-3-azabicyclo[3.2.2]nonane, $C_{14}H_{20}N_2O_2S$, a central stimulant drug.

aza·cos·ter·ol (ay''zuh·kos'tur·ole) *n.* (3β,17β)-17-[[3-(Dimethylamino)propyl]methylamino]androst-5-en-3-ol, $C_{25}H_{44}N_2O$, an avian chemosterilant; used as the hydrochloride salt.

az·a·cy·clo·nol (az''uh·sigh'klo·nol) *n.* α,α-Diphenyl-4-piperidinemethanol, $C_{18}H_{21}NO$, used as the hydrochloride salt for control of psychotic symptoms.

az·a·gua·nine (az''uh·gwah'neen) *n.* 8-Azaguanine; guanine in which the —CH= group in position 8 is replaced by —N=. It interferes with the growth of certain mouse tumors, possibly because a nucleic acid containing 8-azaguanine functions as an antimetabolite for a corresponding nucleic acid containing guanine.

aza·na·tor (az'uh·nay·tur, ay'zuh·) *n.* 5-(1-Methyl-4-piperidinylidene)-5H-[1]benzopyrano[2,3-b]pyridine, $C_{18}H_{18}N_2O$, a bronchodilator; usually used as the maleate salt.

az·a·per·one (az'uh·pur·ohn'') *n.* 4'-Fluoro-4-[4-(2-pyridyl)-1-piperazinyl]butyrophenone, $C_{19}H_{22}FN_3O$, a tranquilizer.

azap·e·tine (az·ap'uh·teen, ay·zap') *n.* 6-Allyl-6,7-dihydro-5*H*-dibenz[*c,e*]azepine, $C_{17}H_{17}N$, an adrenergic blocking agent; used as the phosphate salt for treatment of certain peripheral vascular diseases.

az·a·ri·bine (az''uh·rye'been, ay''zuh·) *n.* 2-(β-D-Ribofuranosyl)-*as*-triazine-3,5(2*H*,4*H*)-dione 2',3',5'-triacetate, $C_{14}H_{17}N_3O_9$, an orally effective antipsoriatic agent.

az·a·ser·ine (az''uh·seer'een) *n.* *O*-Diazoacetyl-L-serine, $C_5H_7N_3O_4$, an antibiotic produced by a *Streptomyces* species and also synthesized; used in treating leukemia, but of doubtful value.

az·at·a·dine (a·zat'uh·deen) *n.* 6,11-Dihydro-11-(1-methyl-4-piperidylidene)-5*H*-benzo[5,6]cyclohepta[1,2,-*b*]pyridine, $C_{20}H_{22}N_2$, an antihistaminic drug; used as the maleate salt.

az·a·thi·o·prine (az''uh·thigh'o·preen) *n.* 6-[(1-Methyl-4-nitroimidazol-5-yl)thio]purine, $C_9H_7N_7O_2S$, a derivative of mercaptopurine used experimentally in the treatment of leukemia and as a suppressive drug in diseases produced by altered immune mechanisms.

azed·a·rach (a·zed'uh·rack) *n.* [Per. *āzād dira^kht*, free, or noble, tree]. The dried bark of the root of *Melia azedarach*, an Asiatic tree naturalized in the southern United States. Preparations of it have been used as an anthelmintic against nematodes.

az·e·la·ic acid (az''e·lay'ick) [*az-* + *ela*io- + *-ic*]. Nonanedioic acid, $COOH(CH_2)_7COOH$, obtained by oxidation of certain acids in oils and fats; derivatives are used as plasticizers.

azeo·trope (ay'zee·o·trope, a·zee'o·trope) *n.* [*a-* + Gk. *zein*, to boil, + *-trope*]. The particular composition of a mixture of two or more substances exhibiting a minimum or a maximum boiling point for all possible mixtures of the particular substances, and thereby having a constant boiling point. —**azeo·trop·ic** (ay''zee·o·trop'ick) *adj.*

azeotropic mixture. AZEOTROPE.

aze·pin·a·mide (az''e·pin'uh·mide, ay''ze·) *n.* 1-[(*p*-Chlorophenyl)sulfonyl]-3-(hexahydro-1*H*-azepin-1-yl)urea, $C_{13}H_{18}ClN_3O_3S$, an orally effective hypoglycemic agent.

aze·te·pa (az''e·tee'puh, ay''ze·) *n.* *p,p*-Bis(1-aziridinyl)-*N*-ethyl-*N*-(1,3,4,-thiadiazol-2-yl)phosphinic amide, $C_8H_{14}N_5OPS$, an antineoplastic compound.

azi-. A prefix indicating *the presence of the group* N_2.

az·ide (az'ide, ·id, ay'zide) *n.* [*az-* + *-ide*]. A compound containing the univalent $—N_3$ group.

az·ine (az'een, ay'zeen) *n.* [*az-* + *-ine*]. Any of a class of heterocyclic compounds containing six atoms in the ring, at least one of which is nitrogen. The number of nitrogen atoms is distinguished by prefixes, as *mono*azine, *di*azine, *tri*azine.

azo (az'o, ay'zo) *adj.* [from the combining form *az(o)-*]. *In chemistry,* of or pertaining to a compound containing the group —N:N— united to two hydrocarbon groups.

azo-. See *az-.*

azo·ben·zene (az''o·ben'zeen, ay''zo·) *n.* [*azo-* + *benzene*]. Benzeneazobenzene, $C_6H_5N{:}NC_6H_5$; used in organic synthesis.

azo·car·mine G (az''o·karh'min, ·mine) *n.* A sodium salt of the disulfonic acid derivative of phenylrosinduline; used in some methods for staining connective tissue and as a plasma stain.

Azochloramid. Trademark for chloroazodin.

azo dyes. A group of synthetic organic dyes derivable from azobenzene, containing the chromophore—N:N—.

azo·li·mine (a·zo'li·meen) *n.* 2-Imino-3-methyl-1-phenyl-4-imidazolidinone, $C_{10}H_{11}N_3O$, a diuretic.

azo·lit·min (az''o·lit'min, ay''zo·) *n.* [*azo-* + *lit*mus + *-in*]. A dark-red coloring matter obtained from litmus and used as an indicator, especially in routine bacteriologic work with milk.

azo·o·sper·ma·tism (ay·zo''o·spur'muh·tizm, az''o·) *n.* AZOOSPERMIA.

azo·o·sper·mia (ay·zo''o·spur'mee·uh, az''o·) *n.* [Gk. *azōos*, lifeless, + *sperm* + *-ia*]. Absence of live spermatozoa in the semen.

azo·pro·tein (az''o·pro'tee·in, ·pro'teen, ay''zo·) *n.* [*azo-* + *protein*]. One of a group of synthetic antigens formed by coupling proteins with diazonium compounds.

Azor·e·an disease (ay·zor'ee·un, a.zor') [*Azores* Islands]. An incompletely characterized progressive degenerative disease of the central nervous system occurring in people living in, or descended from families immigrated from, the Azores Islands; inherited as an autosomal dominant trait.

azo·ru·bin S (az''o·roo'bin) *n.* A red azo dye that has been used intravenously in a test for liver function; delayed appearance of the dye in the duodenal fluid signifies hepatic damage.

Azosulfamide. A trademark for disodium 2-(4'-sulfamylphenylazo)-7-acetamido-1-hydroxynaphthalene-3,6-disulfonate, an antibacterial agent.

azot-, azoto- [*azote*]. A combining form meaning *nitrogen, nitrogenous.*

azote (az'ote, ay'zote) *n.* [F., from Gk. *azōos*, lifeless]. An early name for nitrogen. Symbol, Az. —**azot·ic** (a·zot'ick) *adj.*

az·o·te·mia, az·o·tae·mia (az''o·tee'mee·uh) *n.* [*azot-* + *-emia*]. The presence of excessive amounts of nitrogenous compounds in the blood. —**azo·tem·ic** (·tem'ick) *adj.*

azotemic osteodystrophy. Those bony alterations occurring as a complication of renal failure or Fanconi's syndrome; includes osteomalacia, osteosclerosis, and osteitis fibrosa cystica.

azotic acid. NITRIC ACID.

azot·i·fi·ca·tion (a·zot''i·fi·kay'shun) *n.* [from *azote*]. Fixation of atmospheric nitrogen.

Az·o·to·bac·ter (az''uh·to·back'tur, a·zo'to·back''tur) *n.* [*azoto-* + *-bacter*]. A genus of soil and water bacteria capable of fixing atmospheric nitrogen. See also *nitrogen fixers.*

az·o·tom·e·ter (az''o·tom'e·tur, ay''zo·) *n.* [*azoto-* + *-meter*]. A device for gasometrically measuring the nitrogen content of compounds in solution. —**azotome·try** (·tree) *n.*

az·o·to·my·cin (az''o·to·migh'sin, ay·zo''to·migh'sin) *n.* An antibiotic substance, produced by *Streptomyces ambofaciens,* that has antineoplastic activity.

az·o·tor·rhea, az·o·tor·rhoea (az″uh·to·ree′uh, ay·zo″to·) *n.* [*azoto-* + *-rrhea*]. Excessive amounts of nitrogenous material in the urine; or in the feces, as seen in malabsorption syndromes.

az·o·tu·ria (az″o·tew′ree·uh, ay″zo·) *n.* [*azot-* + *-uria*]. 1. An increase of the nitrogenous substances in the urine. 2. A disease of horses associated with necrosis of cramped skeletal muscle and myoglobinuria. Syn. *Monday morning disease of horses.* —**azo·tu·ric** (·tew′rick) *adj.*

az·ul (az′yool, a·sool′) *n.* [Sp., blue, from the late-stage hyperpigmentation in the disease]. PINTA.

azu·lene (az′yoo·leen) *n.* Cyclopentacycloheptene, $C_{10}H_8$, intensely blue leaflets or plates; it occurs in certain volatile oils.

Azulfidine. Trademark for sulfasalazine, an antibacterial.

azure (azh′ur, ay′zhur) *n.* [OF., OSp. *(l′)azur,* (the) azure, from Ar. *lāzaward,* lapis lazuli, from Per. *lāzhward*]. A basic thiazine dye; used in blood and connective-tissue stains.

azure A. A dimethylthionine made usually by oxidative demethylation of methylene blue. A valuable basic dye used for staining nuclei, ribonucleic acid, acid mucopolysaccharides, and bacteria. Used also in stain mixtures as a general tissue stain.

azure A carbacrylic resin. AZURESIN.

azure B. Trimethylthionine, made by demethylation of methylene blue. A basic thiazine dye used extensively in blood stains and as a tissue stain for nucleic acids.

azure C. Monomethylthionine, usually made by oxidative demethylation of methylene blue. A basic thiazine dye used as a tissue stain for nucleic acids and mucopolysaccharides.

azure II-eosin. GIEMSA STAIN.

az·u·res·in (az″yoo·rez′in, azh″ur·ez′in) *n.* A complex combination of the blue dye azure A and a carbacrylic cationic exchange resin, used as a diagnostic aid for the detection of gastric anacidity without intubation. Syn. *azure A carbacrylic resin.*

azu·ro·phil (a·zhoor′o·fil, azh′ur·o·) *adj.* [*azure* + *-phil*]. Staining purplish red with Giemsa, Wright, Leishman, and similar blood stains, contrasting with the darker red-purple of nuclei and the light blue of cytoplasms; characteristic of certain cytoplasmic granules in leukocytes.

azu·ro·phile (azh′ur·o·file, ·fil, a·zhoor′o·) *adj.* AZUROPHIL.

azu·ro·phil·ia (azh″ur·o·fil′ee·uh, a·zhoor″o·) *n.* The property of being azurophil. —**azurophil·ic** (·ick) *adj.*

az·y·go·ag·na·thus (az″i·go·ag′nuth·us) *n.* [*a-* + *zygoma* + *agnathus*]. A form of otocephaly in which there is no mandible and the zygomas are absent or vestigial.

az·y·gog·ra·phy (az″i·gog′ruh·fee) *n.* Radiographic visualization of the azygos vein after injection of opaque contrast material, usually into an adjacent rib or the spinous process of an adjacent vertebra.

az·y·gos (az′i·gos, a·zye′gos) *n.* [Gk., unpaired, from *a-* + *zygon,* yoke]. An unpaired anatomic structure.

azygos line veins. MEDIAL SYMPATHETIC VEINS.

azygos lobe. A variable, partially separate portion of the upper medial part of the superior lobe of the right lung. When present, it is isolated from the main part of the lobe by a deep groove occupied by the azygos vein.

azygos uvu·lae (yoo′vew·lee). UVULAE; the muscle of the uvula. See also Table of Muscles in the Appendix.

azygos vein. An unpaired vein of the posterior body wall beginning in the right lumbar region, ascending in the right thoracic wall, and finally emptying into the superior vena cava. NA *vena azygos.* See also Table of Veins in the Appendix.

az·y·gous (az′i·gus, a·zye′gus) *adj.* [Gk. *azygos,* from *a-* + *zygon,* yoke]. Unpaired.

azym·ia (a·zye′mee·uh, a·zym′ee·uh) *n.* [Gk. *azymos,* unleavened, + *-ia*]. The absence of an enzyme or ferment.

azym·ic (a·zye′mick, a·zym′ick) *adj.* [Gk. *azymos,* from *a-* + *zymē,* leaven]. 1. Not rising from a fermentation; unfermented. 2. Not containing enzymes.

B

B Symbol for boron.

Ba Symbol for barium.

Baastrup's disease. Mutual compression of the spinous processes of adjacent vertebrae.

Bab·bitt metal [I. *Babbitt,* U.S. inventor, 1799–1862]. An alloy of tin, antimony, and copper formerly used extensively in making dies and counterdies in dental laboratory procedures.

Bab·cock-Levy test [H. *Babcock,* U.S. psychologist, d. 1952; and Lydia *Levy,* U.S. physiologist, 20th century]. An examination designed to measure intellectual deterioration by testing vocabulary, general information, symbol substitution, and the copying of designs with respect to correctness, speed, and accuracy; useful in determining deterioration of cognitive functions.

Babcock's operation [W. W. *Babcock,* U.S. surgeon, 1872–1963]. Extirpation of varicose segments of the saphenous vein by inserting a bulb-tipped probe or stripper and drawing the vein out. See also *Jackson-Babcock operation.*

Babcock test [S. M. *Babcock,* U.S. agricultural chemist, 1843–1931]. A test for determining the percentage content of butterfat in milk, cream, or ice cream by centrifuging a mixture of equal quantities of the specimen and sulfuric acid.

Ba·beş-Ernst bodies (bah'be^y^sh, ehrnst) [V. *Babeş,* Rumanian microbiologist, 1854–1926; and P. *Ernst,* German pathologist, 1859–1937]. Metachromatic granules in bacteria.

Ba·be·sia (ba·bee'zhuh, ·zee·uh) *n.* [V. *Babeş*]. A genus of intracellular, nonpigmented sporozoa which invade the red blood cells of cattle, sheep, horses, rodents, dogs, and monkeys but rarely of man. Members of this genus are oval or pear-shaped.

Babesia bi·gem·i·na (bye·jem'i·nuh). The species of *Babesia* that causes Texas fever of cattle; commonly transmitted by ticks of the genus *Boophilus,* now usually by *Boophilus microplus.*

Babesia bo·vis (bo'vis). A species of *Babesia* found in European countries which is slightly smaller than *B. bigemina* and transmitted by the ticks *Ixodes ricinus* and *Haemaphysalis punctata;* the cause of a disease similar to Texas fever.

Babesia ca·nis (kay'nis, kan'is). The species of *Babesia* that causes canine babesiosis, a disease transmitted by ticks.

Babesia equi (eck'wye). The species of *Babesia* that causes equine biliary fever in horses, mules, and donkeys.

Babesia ovis (o'vis). The etiologic agent of babesiosis of sheep.

bab·e·si·a·sis (bab"e·sigh'uh·sis) *n.*, pl. **babesia·ses** (·seez) [*Babesia* + *-iasis*]. BABESIOSIS.

ba·be·si·o·sis (ba·bee"see·o'sis) *n.*, pl. **babesio·ses** (·seez) [*Babesia* + *-osis*]. A febrile, hemolytic disease, primarily observed in animals and rarely in man, caused by infection with *Babesia.* Syn. *piroplasmosis.*

Babeş' nodules or **tubercles** [V. *Babeş*]. Microglial proliferation described in cases of rabies.

Ba·bin·ski-Froeh·lich disease (F. ba·bæ^n·skee', Pol. ba·bin' skee) [J. F. F. *Babinski,* French neurologist, 1857–1932; and A. *Froehlich*]. ADIPOSOGENITAL DYSTROPHY.

Babinski-Na·geotte syndrome (na^h·zho^ht') [J. F. F. *Babinski* and J. *Nageotte,* French pathologist, 1866–1948]. A medullary syndrome caused by lesions in the distribution of the vertebral artery involving usually the nucleus ambiguus, solitary fasciculus, descending root of the trigeminal nerve, restiform body, sympathetic pathways, pyramidal tract, medial lemniscus, and often also the hypoglossal nucleus; characterized clinically by ipsilateral paralysis of the soft palate, pharynx, and larynx, sometimes of the tongue, hemianesthesia of the face, Horner's syndrome, and cerebellar hypotonia and ataxia, together with spastic hemiplegia as well as loss of position sense on the opposite side.

Babinski phenomenon or **reflex** [J. F. F. *Babinski*]. 1. BABINSKI SIGN (1). 2. BABINSKI'S PRONATION PHENOMENON. 3. TRUNK-THIGH SIGN OF BABINSKI.

Babinski's combined flexion phenomenon [J. F. F. *Babinski*]. TRUNK-THIGH SIGN OF BABINSKI.

Babinski sign [J. F. F. *Babinski*]. 1. Extension of the great toe when the lateral aspect of the sole is stroked sharply. After infancy this reflex is abnormal and indicates disturbance of the corticospinal tract. Syn. *extensor plantar reflex or response.* 2. BABINSKI'S PLATYSMA SIGN. 3. BABINSKI'S REINFORCEMENT SIGN. 4. TRUNK-THIGH SIGN OF BABINSKI.

Babinski's platysma sign [J. F. F. *Babinski*]. Failure of the platysma to contract on the paretic side, with an exaggerated contraction of the platysma on the unaffected side, when the mouth is opened against resistance; seen in hemiplegia involving the muscles of facial expression. Syn. *platysma phenomenon.*

Babinski's pronation phenomenon [J. F. F. *Babinski*]. Pronation of the paretic arm occurs (a) if the palms of the hands are held in approximation with the thumbs upward and then are shaken or jarred; (b) if the arms are actively abducted with the forearms in supination; or (c) if the arms are passively abducted with the forearms in supination and then suddenly released.

Babinski's reinforcement sign [J. F. F. *Babinski*]. In hemiplegia, when the patient sits so that his legs hang free, forceful pulling of the flexed fingers of one side against those of the other results in extension of the leg on the paretic side.

Babinski's syndrome [J. F. F. *Babinski*]. 1. Syphilitic aortic insufficiency or aortic aneurysm, tabes dorsalis, and Argyll Robertson pupils. 2. BABINSKI-NAGEOTTE SYNDROME. 3. ADIPOSOGENITAL DYSTROPHY.

Babinski-Vaquez syndrome [J. F. F. *Babinski* and L. H. *Vaquez*]. BABINSKI-NAGEOTTE SYNDROME.

ba·boon, *n.* [F. *babuin*]. Any of the large, terrestrial African monkeys of the genera *Papio, Mandrillus,* and *Theropithecus.* Because of their size and some anatomic similarities to man, baboons of the genus *Papio* have been used in cardiovascular studies, organ transplantation, and other types of surgical research.

ba·by, *n.* An infant; a child up to about one year of age when walking and first words usually are achieved.

bac·ca·lau·re·ate nurse. In the United States, a nurse holding a bachelor's degree in nursing from a university or collegiate program accredited by the National League for Nursing.

Bac·cel·li's sign (bahch·el'lee) [G. *Baccelli,* Italian physician, 1832–1916]. A sign of pleural effusion in which whispered voice sounds are heard over the chest.

bac·ci·form (back'si·form) *adj.* [L. *bacca*, berry, + *-form*]. Berry-shaped.

Bach·mann's bundle [J. G. *Bachmann,* U.S. physiologist, b. 1877]. An anterior interatrial myocardial band.

Bach·man test [G. W. *Bachman,* U.S. parasitologist, b. 1890]. An intradermal test for trichinosis made from an extract of the larvae of *Trichinella.*

Bach·tia·row's sign (bakh·tee·ah'rof). Extension and slight abduction of the thumb on stroking the patient's forearm down along the radius with the thumb and forefinger, indicative of reflex hyperactivity.

ba·cill (ba·sil') *n.* A short rodlike lozenge.

bacill-, bacilli-, bacillo-. A combining form meaning *bacillus.*

Bac·il·la·ce·ae (bas''i·lay'see·ee) *n.pl.* A family of Eubacteriales comprising the genera *Bacillus* and *Clostridium.*

bacillaemia. BACILLEMIA.

ba·cil·lar (bas'i·lur, ba·sil'ur) *adj.* BACILLARY.

bac·il·lary (bas'i·lerr''ee) *adj.* 1. Pertaining to bacilli or to a bacillus. 2. Consisting of or containing rods.

bacillary dysentery. Any of a group of infectious diseases caused by invasion of the colon, primarily by pathogenic bacteria of the genus *Shigella,* characterized by the frequent passage of blood-stained stools or of exudate consisting of blood and mucus, and often accompanied by tenesmus, abdominal cramps, and fever. Syn. *shigellosis.* Compare *amebic dysentery.*

bacillary white diarrhea. PULLORUM DISEASE.

bac·il·le·mia, bac·il·lae·mia (bas''i·lee'mee·uh) *n.* [*bacill-* + *-emia*]. The presence of bacilli in the blood.

bacilli-. See *bacill-.*

ba·cil·li·form (ba·sil'i·form) *adj.* Having the shape or appearance of a bacillus; rod-shaped.

bacillo-. See *bacill-.*

ba·cil·lo·pho·bia (ba·sil''o·fo'bee·uh) *n.* [*bacillo-* + *-phobia*]. BACTERIOPHOBIA.

bac·il·lu·ria (bas''i·lew'ree·uh) *n.* The presence of bacilli in the urine.

Ba·cil·lus (ba·sil'us) *n.* [L., small staff]. A genus of rod-shaped, gram-positive bacteria capable of producing endospores, belonging to the family Bacillaceae; *Bacillus subtilis* is a prototype.

bacillus, *n.*, pl. **bacil·li** (·eye) [L.]. 1. Any rod-shaped bacterium. 2. *Obsol.* Any member of the class Schizomycetes.

Bacillus acidophilus. LACTOBACILLUS ACIDOPHILUS.

Bacillus aer·og·e·nes cap·su·la·tus (ay·ur·oj'e·neez kap·sue·lay'tus). CLOSTRIDIUM PERFRINGENS.

Bacillus aert·rycke (ărt'rye·keh). SALMONELLA TYPHIMURIUM.

Bacillus ag·ni (ag'nigh). CLOSTRIDIUM PERFRINGENS B.

Bacillus an·thra·cis (an'thruh·sis). An aerobic spore-forming species pathogenic to man, although in nature it is primarily a pathogen of cattle and horses; the cause of anthrax.

Bacillus bifidus. LACTOBACILLUS BIFIDUS.

Bacillus bot·u·li·nus (bot''yoo·lye'nus). CLOSTRIDIUM BOTULINUM.

Bacillus bo·vi·sep·ti·cus (bo·vi·sep'ti·kus). PASTEURELLA MULTOCIDA.

Bacillus brev·is (brev'is). A group of bacilli, widely distributed in soil, from which gramicidin, gramicidin S, and tyrocidine, powerful broad-spectrum antibiotic agents, have been extracted.

bacillus Cal·mette-Gué·rin (kal·met', gey·ræn') [L. C. A. *Calmette;* and C. *Guérin,* French bacteriologist, 1872–1961]. A strain of *Mycobacterium tuberculosis* var. *bovis,* attenuated by extended cultivation on a medium containing bile; used in vaccines for immunization against tuberculosis. Abbreviated, BCG.

Bacillus coli. ESCHERICHIA COLI.

Bacillus diphtheriae. CORYNEBACTERIUM DIPHTHERIAE.

Bacillus dysenteriae. SHIGELLA DYSENTERIAE.

Bacillus enteritidis. SALMONELLA ENTERITIDIS.

Bacillus er·y·sip·e·la·tos-su·is (err''i·sip''e·lay'tos soo'is). ERYSIPELOTHRIX RHUSIOPATHIAE.

Bacillus fecalis alcaligenes. ALCALIGENES FECALIS.

Bacillus fu·si·for·mis (few''zi·for'mis). FUSOBACTERIUM FUSIFORME.

Bacillus gas·troph·i·lus (gas·trof'i·lus). LACTOBACILLUS ACIDOPHILUS.

Bacillus hof·man·nii (hof·man'ee·eye). CORYNEBACTERIUM PSEUDODIPHTHERITICUM.

Bacillus influenzae. HEMOPHILUS INFLUENZAE.

Bacillus lac·tis aer·og·e·nes (lack'tis ay·ur·oj'e·neez). ENTEROBACTER AEROGENES.

Bacillus lac·u·na·tus (lack''yoo·nay'tus). MORAXELLA LACUNATA.

Bacillus leprae. MYCOBACTERIUM LEPRAE.

Bacillus mallei. PSEUDOMONAS MALLEI.

Bacillus mes·en·ter·i·cus (mes''en·terr'i·kus). BACILLUS PUMILUS.

Bacillus mu·co·sus cap·su·la·tum (mew·ko'sus kap·sue·lay'tum). KLEBSIELLA PNEUMONIAE.

Bacillus oe·de·ma·ti·ens (ee''de·may'shee·enz). CLOSTRIDIUM NOVYI.

Bacillus oe·de·ma·tis ma·lig·ni (ee·dee'muh·tis ma·lig'nye). CLOSTRIDIUM NOVYI.

Bacillus para·bot·u·li·nus (păr''uh·bot''yoo·lye'nus). CLOSTRIDIUM BOTULINUM C.

Bacillus para·ty·pho·sus A (păr''uh·tye·fo'sus). SALMONELLA PARATYPHI A.

Bacillus paratyphosus B. SALMONELLA SCHOTTMUELLERI.

Bacillus perfringens. CLOSTRIDIUM PERFRINGENS.

Bacillus pertussis. BORDETELLA PERTUSSIS.

Bacillus pestis. YERSINIA PESTIS.

Bacillus poly·myxa (pol''ee·mick'suh). An aerobic, spore-forming, gram-negative, sugar-fermenting rod, widely distributed in water, soil, milk, and decaying vegetables; the source of polymyxin.

Bacillus pro·dig·i·o·sus (pro·dij·ee·o'sus). SERRATIA MARCESCENS.

Bacillus proteus. PROTEUS VULGARIS.

Bacillus pu·mi·lus (pew'mi·lus). Aerobic spore-forming encapsulated bacteria. Syn. *Bacillus mesentericus.*

Bacillus pyo·cy·a·ne·us (pye''o·sigh·ay'nee·us). PSEUDOMONAS AERUGINOSA.

Bacillus sub·ti·lis (sub'ti·lis, sub·tye'lis). The type species of the genus *Bacillus,* which infects human beings only rarely; the source of subtilin.

Bacillus sui·sep·ti·cus (soo·i·sep'ti·kus). PASTEURELLA MULTOCIDA.

Bacillus tetani. CLOSTRIDIUM TETANI.

Bacillus tuberculosis. MYCOBACTERIUM TUBERCULOSIS.

Bacillus whit·mo·ri (whit·mo'rye). PSEUDOMONAS PSEUDOMALLEI.

Bacillus xerosis. CORYNEBACTERIUM XEROSIS.

bac·i·tra·cin (bas''i·tray'sin) *n.* [*bacillus* + Margaret *Tracy,*

U.S., 20th century, from whose tissues the substance was isolated, + *-in*]. A polypeptide antibiotic produced by an organism belonging to the *licheniformis* group of *Bacillus subtilis.* It is active against many gram-positive organisms, as streptococci, staphylococci, and pneumococci, and certain gram-negative cocci, as gonococci and meningococci, but ineffective against most gram-negative organisms.

back, *n.* 1. Dorsum; the posterior aspect. 2. The posterior part of the trunk from the neck to the pelvis.

back·ache, *n.* Pain in the lower lumbar or lumbosacral region of the back.

back·bone, *n.* VERTEBRAL COLUMN.

back·cross, *n.* A crossbreeding between a parental strain and its hybrid offspring from a previous crossbreeding.

back·ground radiation. Radiation arising from a source other than the one directly under consideration or study, such as cosmic rays, environmental radiation, or radioactive material that may be in the vicinity.

back·ing, *n.* A metal support used to attach a facing in the construction of a dental prosthesis.

back injury. Any injury to the muscles of the back or to the spinal column, such as a sprain, concussion, twist, fracture, or damage to an intervertebral disk; frequently associated with pain which may be due to lesions of fascia, muscles, bones, or ligaments, or to specific neurologic symptoms and findings due to injury of the spinal cord or nerve roots.

back mutation. A mutation that reverses a mutant to its original form.

back pressure. In the cardiovascular system, the pressure increase, engorgement, and dilatation proximal to a narrowed heart valve or blood vessel or caused by failure of the ventricle adequately to pump and to eject blood. See also *backward failure.*

back reflex. Contraction of the erector spinae muscle when the paravertebral lumbar and sacral areas are tapped with the patient in the prone position.

back·rest, *n.* Any device used to support the back in a sitting or semireclining position.

back·scat·ter, *n.* Radiation that is deflected by a scattering process at angles greater than 90° to the original direction of the beam of radiation.

back·ward failure. Heart failure in which symptoms result predominantly from elevation of venous pressure behind the failing ventricle, e.g., engorgement of the lung due to failure of the left ventricle.

back·ward·ness, *n.* 1. Retarded physical or mental development or both due to any extrinsic cause, as general illness, social or sensory deprivation. 2. Educational retardation not due to intrinsic mental deficiency.

backward progression or **titubation.** RETROPULSION (2).

bac·lo·fen (back'lo·fen) *n.* 4-Amino-3-(4-chlorophenyl)butanoic acid, $C_{10}H_{12}ClNO_2$, a muscle relaxant.

ba·con spleen. A spleen with areas of amyloid deposits, having the appearance of fried bacon on the cut surface.

-bacter. A combining form meaning *a bacterial organism.*

bac·ter·emia, bac·ter·ae·mia (back"te·ree'mee·uh) *n.* [*bacteri-* + *-emia*]. The presence of living bacteria in the blood. Compare *pyemia, septicemia.*

bac·ter·emic, bac·ter·ae·mic (back"te·ree'mick) *adj.* Pertaining to or having bacteremia.

bacteremic shock. 1. Any shock state occurring during bacteremia. 2. The shock state occurring in the course of bacteremia caused by gram-negative bacteria, characterized by severe hypotension and generalized circulatory failure, and simulated in laboratory animals by the injection of endotoxin derived from gram-negative bacteria.

bacteri-, bacterio-. A combining form meaning *bacteria, bacterial.*

bac·te·ria (back·teer'ee·uh) *n.*, sing. **bacte·ri·um** (·ee·um) [Gk. *baktērion,* staff]. Microscopic unicellular prokaryotic organisms which generally divide by transverse binary fission, possess rigid cell walls, and exhibit three principal forms: round or coccal, rodlike or bacillary, and spiral or spirochetal. Also included are *Mycoplasma* lacking cell walls and the Actinomycetales in which some forms are filamentous and branching. Genetic recombination occurs. Bacteria may be partially or totally aerobic or anaerobic; they may or may not be motile, capsulated, or spore-forming. They may possess diverse biochemical and enzymatic activities, are widely prevalent in nature and in relation to plants and animals, and may be saprophytic or pathogenic.

Bac·te·ri·a·ce·ae (back·teer"ee·ay'see·ee) *n.pl.* [*Bacteri*um- + *-aceae*]. *Obsol.* SCHIZOMYCETES.

bac·te·ri·ae·mia (back·teer"ee·ee'mee·uh) *n.* Bacteriemia (= BACTEREMIA).

bac·te·ri·al (back·teer'ee·ul) *adj.* Pertaining to, consisting of, or caused by bacteria.

bacterial allergy. Delayed hypersensitivity induced by a bacterium.

bacterial antagonism. The adverse effect produced by one species of microorganism upon the growth and development of another.

bacterial endocarditis. A prolonged, febrile, grave bacterial infection of the endocardium or the heart valves, or both, characterized by fever, heart murmur, splenomegaly, embolic phenomena, and bacteremia. Syn. *subacute bacterial endocarditis.* Compare *acute bacterial endocarditis.*

bacterial enzyme. An enzyme existing in, or produced by, bacteria.

bacterial phase variation. The occurrence of the H or flagellar antigens of *Salmonella* and other organisms in a relatively more specific phase (phase 1) and a relatively less specific phase (phase 2).

bacterial plaque. See *dental plaque.*

bacterial polysaccharide. A substance of polysaccharide nature elaborated by bacteria. Such substances are of particular importance in immunologic phenomena, since they usually possess antigenic properties.

bacterial protein. Any protein formed by bacteria.

bacterial spectrum. ANTIBIOTIC SPECTRUM.

bacterial vaccine. An emulsion of bacteria, killed, living, or attenuated, used for the purpose of stimulating the immune response of a patient to infection by the same organism.

bacterial variation. A hereditary deviation from the modal form of a particular bacterium with regard to any property such as morphology, biochemical reaction, pigment production, colonial characteristic, virulence, or toxigenicity. See also *colony.*

bac·te·ri·cide (back·teer'i·side) *n.* [*bacteri-* + *-cide*]. An agent that destroys bacteria. —**bac·te·ri·cid·al** (back·teer"i·sigh' dul) *adj.*

bac·te·ri·cid·in (back·teer"i·sigh'din) *n.* [*bactericide* + *-in*]. An antibody that in the presence of complement kills bacteria.

bac·ter·id (back'tur·id) *n.* [*bacteri-* + *-id*]. A pustular eruption on the hands and feet believed to be caused by sensitization to bacterial products from a focus of infection.

bac·te·ri·e·mia, bac·te·ri·ae·mia (back·teer"ee·ee'mee·uh) *n.* BACTEREMIA.

bac·ter·in (back'tur·in) *n.* BACTERIAL VACCINE.

bacterio-. See *bacteri-.*

bac·te·rio·chlo·ro·phyll (back·teer"ee·o·klor'o·fil) *n.* A pigment, similar in structure and function to green plant chlorophyll, found in the photosynthetic nonsulfur purple bacteria *Athiorhodaceae* and sulfur purple bacteria *Thiorhodaceae.*

bac·te·rio·cid·in (back·teer"ee·o·side'in) *n.* BACTERICIDIN.

bac·te·rio·cin (back·teer'ee·o·sin) *n.* [*bacterio-* + *-cin* (as in *colicin*)]. Any of the proteins (such as colicins) produced by various strains of bacteria which are lethal for certain other strains closely related to them.

bac·te·ri·oc·la·sis (back·teer″ee·ok′luh·sis) *n.*, pl. **bacterioclases** (·seez) [*bacterio-* + *-clasis*]. The destruction or fragmentation of bacteria, a phenomenon similar to bacteriolysis by bacteriophage.

bac·te·rio·er·y·thrin (back·teer″ee·o·err′i·thrin) *n.* [*bacterio-* + *erythrin*]. A red pigment present in certain bacteria.

bac·te·rio·flu·o·res·cein (back·teer″ee·o·floo″uh·res′ee·in) *n.* [*bacterio-* + *fluorescein*]. A fluorescent coloring matter produced by the action of certain bacteria.

bac·te·rio·gen·ic (back·teer″ee·o·jen′ick) *adj.* [*bacterio-* + *-genic*]. 1. Caused by bacteria. 2. Of bacterial origin.

bac·te·ri·og·e·nous (back·teer″ee·oj′e·nus) *adj.* [*bacterio-* + *-genous*]. BACTERIOGENIC.

bac·te·rio·he·mol·y·sin, bac·te·rio·hae·mol·y·sin (back·teer″ee·o·hee·mol′i·sin) *n.* [*bacterio-* + *hemolysin*]. Any bacterial product or toxin, such as staphylolysin, streptolysin, tetanolysin, or hemolysins of *Clostridium perfringens*, that releases hemoglobin from red blood cells in vitro, but that may or may not be active in vivo.

bac·te·ri·oid (back·teer′ee·oid) *adj.* & *n.* 1. Resembling a bacterium. 2. A structure or organism resembling a bacterium.

bac·te·ri·ol·o·gist (back·teer″ee·ol′uh·jist) *n.* A person who specializes in bacteriology.

bac·te·ri·ol·o·gy (back·teer″ee·ol′uh·jee) *n.* The science and study of bacteria. —**bacte·ri·o·log·ic** (·ee·o·loj′ick), **bacterio·log·i·cal** (·i·kul) *adj.*

bac·te·rio·ly·sin (back·teer″ee·o·lye′sin) *n.* [*bacterio-* + *lysin*]. A specific antibody which, together with other substances, is capable of causing the dissolution of the homologous bacterium.

bac·te·ri·ol·y·sis (back·teer″ee·ol′i·sis) *n.*, pl. **bacterioly·ses** (·seez) [*bacterio-* + *lysis*]. The intracellular or extracellular dissolution of bacteria. See also *immune bacteriolysis*. —**bacte·rio·lyt·ic** (·ee·o·lit′ick) *adj.*

Bac·te·rio·ne·ma (back·teer″ee·o·nee′muh) *n.* [*bacterio* + *-nema*]. A genus of bacteria, gram-positive, nonsporeforming, nonmotile, facultative anaerobes of the family Actinimycetaceae, having a fermentative metabolism which produces from carbohydrates the end products carbon dioxide and lactic, formic, acetic, propionic, and succinic acids; found normally in the oral cavity of man and other primates, especially in dental calculus and plaque.

bac·te·rio·op·so·nin (back·teer″ee·o·op′so·nin) *n.* BACTERIOPSONIN. —**bacterio·op·son·ic** (·op·son′ick) *adj.*

bac·te·rio·phage (back·teer′ee·o·faij, ·fahzh) *n.* [*bacterio-* + *-phage*]. One of a group of viruses infecting bacteria, sometimes resulting in lysis of the bacterial cell. —**bac·te·rio·phag·ic** (·back·teer″ee·o·faj′ick) *adj.*; **bacteri·oph·a·gy** (·off′uh·jee) *n.*

bac·te·rio·pho·bia (back·teer″ee·o·fo′bee·uh) *n.* A morbid dread of bacteria or other microorganisms.

bac·te·rio·pro·tein (back·teer″ee·o·pro′tee·in) *n.* Any one of a number of protein substances contained in bacteria.

bac·te·ri·op·so·nin (back·teer″ee·op′so·nin) *n.* An opsonin which acts upon bacteria, as distinguished from one affecting erythrocytes. —**bacteri·op·son·ic** (·op·son′ick) *adj.*

bac·te·ri·o·sis (back·teer″ee·o′sis) *n.* Any disease of bacterial origin.

bac·te·ri·os·ta·sis (back·teer″ee·os′tuh·sis, ·o·stay′sis) *n.*, pl. **bacteriosta·ses** (·seez) [*bacterio-* + *stasis*]. Arrest or hindrance of the growth of bacteria.

bac·te·rio·stat (back·teer′ee·o·stat) *n.* [*bacterio-* + *-stat*]. Any agent which arrests or hinders the growth of bacteria.

bac·te·rio·stat·ic (back·teer″ee·o·stat′ick) *adj.* Arresting or hindering the growth of bacteria.

bacteriostatic spectrum. ANTIBIOTIC SPECTRUM.

bacteriostatic water for injection. Sterile water for injection containing one or more suitable bacteriostatic agents. See also *sterile water for injection, water for injection.*

bac·te·rio·ther·a·py (back·teer″ee·o·therr′uh·pee) *n.* The treatment of disease by the introduction of bacteria or their products into the system. —**bacterio·ther·a·peu·tic** (·therr·uh·pew′tick) *adj.*

bac·te·rio·tox·in (back·teer″ee·o·tock′sin) *n.* 1. A toxin that destroys bacteria. 2. A toxin produced by bacteria. —**bacteriotox·ic** (·sick) *adj.*

bac·te·rio·trop·ic (back·teer″ee·o·trop′ick) *adj.* [*bacterio-* + *-tropic*]. *Obsol.* Rendering bacteria susceptible to phagocytosis.

bac·te·ri·ot·ro·pin (back·teer″ee·ot′ro·pin) *n.* [*bacterio-* + *tropin*]. *Obsol.* An opsonin aiding the phagocytic action of certain cells, as leukocytes.

bac·te·ri·stat·ic (back·teer″i·stat′ick) *adj.* BACTERIOSTATIC.

Bac·te·ri·um (back·teer′ee·um) *n.* [NL., from Gk. *baktērion*, small staff]. *Obsol.* A genus of bacteria.

bacterium. Singular of *bacteria.*

Bacterium aerogenes. ENTEROBACTER AEROGENES.

Bacterium al·ka·les·cens (al″kuh·les′enz). A biotype of the alkalescens-dispar group of *Escherichia coli;* formerly classified as *Shigella.*

Bacterium am·big·u·um (am·big′yoo·um). SHIGELLA AMBIGUA.

Bacterium avi·sep·ti·cum (ay″vi·sep′ti·kum). PASTEURELLA MULTOCIDA.

Bacterium bo·vi·sep·ti·cum (bo″vi·sep′ti·kum). PASTEURELLA MULTOCIDA.

Bacterium cholerae-suis. SALMONELLA CHOLERAESUIS.

Bacterium coli. ESCHERICHIA COLI.

Bacterium dis·par (dis′pahr). A biotype of *Escherichia coli*, formerly classified as *Shigella.*

Bacterium dysenteriae. SHIGELLA DYSENTERIAE.

Bacterium enteritidis. SALMONELLA ENTERITIDIS.

Bacterium flexneri. SHIGELLA FLEXNERI.

Bacterium fried·län·de·ri (freed·len′duh·rye). KLEBSIELLA PNEUMONIAE.

Bacterium fu·si·for·mis (few″zi·for′mis). FUSOBACTERIUM FUSIFORME.

Bacterium lac·tis aer·og·e·nes (lack′tis ay″ur·oj′e·neez). ENTEROBACTER AEROGENES.

Bacterium monocytogenes. LISTERIA MONOCYTOGENES.

Bacterium para·dys·en·ter·i·ae (păr″uh·dis·en·terr′ee·ee). SHIGELLA FLEXNERI.

Bacterium para·ty·pho·sum A (păr″uh·tigh·fo′sum). SALMONELLA PARATYPHI A.

Bacterium paratyphosum B. SALMONELLA SCHOTTMÜLLERI.

Bacterium paratyphosum C. SALMONELLA HIRSCHFELDII.

Bacterium pneumoniae. KLEBSIELLA PNEUMONIAE.

Bacterium shi·gae (shee′ghee). SHIGELLA DYSENTERIAE.

Bacterium sonnei. SHIGELLA SONNEI.

Bacterium sui·pes·ti·fer (soo·i·pes′ti·fur). SALMONELLA CHOLERAESUIS.

Bacterium sui·sep·ti·cum (soo·i·sep′ti·kum). PASTEURELLA MULTOCIDA.

Bacterium tu·la·ren·se (too″luh·ren′see). FRANCISELLA TULARENSIS.

Bacterium typhimurium. SALMONELLA TYPHIMURIUM.

Bacterium ty·pho·sum (tye·fo′sum). SALMONELLA TYPHOSA.

bac·te·ri·uria (back·teer″ee·yoo′ree·uh) *n.* The presence of bacteria in the urine.

bac·ter·oid (back′tur·oid) *adj.* & *n.* 1. Resembling a bacterium. 2. A bacterium modified in form or structure.

Bac·te·roi·da·ce·ae (back″tur·oy·day′see·ee) *n.pl.* A family of bacteria of the order Eubacteriales; the type genus is *Bacteroides.*

Bac·ter·oi·des (back·tur·oy′deez) *n.* A genus of obligate anaerobic, nonsporogenous gram-negative bacilli with rounded ends, which may be normal inhabitants of the genital, intestinal, and respiratory tracts, but may also cause severe infections.

Bacteroides frag·i·lis (fraj′i·lis). A species of *Bacteroides* which is a dominant member of the normal colonic flora and on occasion is capable of causing severe infections such as peritonitis, empyema, abscesses, urinary tract infection, and septicemia.

Bacteroides fun·di·li·for·mis (fun″di·li·for′mis). SPHAEROPHORUS NECROPHORUS.

Bacteroides me·lan·i·no·gen·i·cus (me·lan″i·no·jen′i·kus). A species of *Bacteroides* found in the mouth, urine, feces, abdominal wounds, puerperal sepsis, or focal kidney infections. In culture, melanin pigment is produced.

Bacteroides pneumosintes. DIALISTER PNEUMOSINTES.

bac·ter·uria (back″tur·yoo′ree·uh) *n.* BACTERIURIA.

bael (bel, bale) *n.* ²BEL.

bael·fruit (bel′froot, bale′froot) *n.* ²BEL.

Baer's treatment [W. S. *Baer,* U.S. orthopedist, 1872–1931]. 1. In an ankylosed joint, the adhesions are broken and sterile oil is injected into the joint to prevent re-formation of adhesions. 2. MAGGOT THERAPY.

ba·gas·sco·sis (bag″uh·sko′sis) *n.* BAGASSOSIS.

ba·gasse (ba·gas′) *n.* [F.]. The fibrous, dusty material in sugarcane after the juice has been extracted.

bagasse disease. BAGASSOSIS.

ba·gas·so·sis (bag″uh·so′sis) *n.*, pl. **bagasso·ses** (·seez) [*bagasse* + *-osis*]. A pneumoconiosis due to inhalation of the dust of bagasse, characterized clinically by dyspnea, malaise, fever, and diffuse bronchopneumonia.

Bagh·dad boil [after *Baghdad,* Iraq]. CUTANEOUS LEISHMANIASIS.

Baghdad spring anemia [after *Baghdad,* Iraq]. A form of acute hemolytic anemia thought to be caused by acquired sensitivity to inhaled pollens of certain plants native to the Middle East.

bag of waters. The fetal membranes and amniotic fluid which serve during pregnancy to protect the fetus. See also *amnion.*

Ba·hia ulcer (ba·ee′uh) [after *Bahia* (*Baía*), Brazil]. A skin ulcer occurring in American mucocutaneous leishmaniasis.

Bail·lar·ger's bands, layers, lines, striae, or **stripes** (bye·yar·zhey′) [J. G. F. *Baillarger,* French neurologist, 1809–1890]. STRIPES OF BAILLARGER.

Baillarger's principle [J. G. F. *Baillarger*]. Patients with aphasia who have lost the power of voluntary speech may retain certain automatic expressions and swear words, usually employed inappropriately and indiscriminately.

Baillarger's sign [J. G. F. *Baillarger*]. Inequality of the pupils seen in general paresis.

Bain·bridge effect or **reflex** [F. A. *Bainbridge,* English physiologist, 1874–1921]. Acceleration of the heart rate due to rise of pressure in the right atrium under certain conditions. Not a true reflex; the increased rate is caused by direct mechanical deformation of the pacemaker fibers. See also *intrinsic cardiac rate regulation.*

Ba·ker's cyst [W. M. *Baker,* English surgeon, 1839–1896]. 1. A synovial cyst in the popliteal space arising from the semimembranosus bursa or the knee joint and, in the latter case, frequently associated with intraarticular abnormality in the knee. 2. A herniation of synovial membrane from the joint.

baker's stigmas. Corns on the fingers from kneading dough.

baking soda. SODIUM BICARBONATE.

BAL Abbreviation or acronym for *British antilewisite* (= DIMERCAPROL).

balan-, balano- [Gk. *balanos,* acorn]. A combining form meaning *glans, balanic.*

bal·anced anesthesia. Anesthesia produced by pharmacologically active doses of two or more agents or methods of anesthesia, each of which contributes to the total desired effect.

balanced occlusion, articulation, or **bite.** Occlusion of the teeth that presents harmonious relationships of occluding surfaces in centric and eccentric positions within the functional range, such as during mastication or in swallowing; *in prosthodontics,* it is developed to provide stability of prostheses; *in periodontics,* the term is related to the endurance or tolerance of the periodontal membrane in occlusal function.

balanced polymorphism. A form of genetic equilibrium (segregational equilibrium) in which loss of two alleles via mortality of their recessive homozygotes is in balance owing to a selective advantage of heterozygous individuals.

balanced suspension. A system of splints, slings, ropes, pulleys, and weights to suspend the lower extremity as an adjunct to fracture treatment or following an operation.

balanced traction. Balanced suspension used in conjunction with traction, usually skeletal, in the treatment of lower extremity fractures or following an operation.

balanced translocation. A translocation occurring when the individual or gamete contains no more or less than the normal diploid or haploid genetic material.

ba·lan·ic (ba·lan′ick) *adj.* [*balan-* + *-ic*]. Of or pertaining to the glans of the penis or of the clitoris.

balanic hypospadias. The commonest, usually mild, form of hypospadias, in which the urethral opening is at the site of the frenulum, which is usually rudimentary or absent.

bal·a·nit·ic (bal″uh·nit′ick) *adj.* 1. Of or pertaining to balanitis. 2. *Erron.* BALANIC.

bal·a·ni·tis (bal″uh·nigh′tis) *n.* [*balan-* + *-itis*]. 1. Inflammation of the glans penis or glans clitoridis. 2. BALANOCHLAMYDITIS.

balanitis xe·rot·i·ca ob·lit·er·ans (ze·rot′i·kuh ob·lit′ur·anz). A chronic, progressive, atrophic, sclerosing disease of the penile skin which may eventuate in urethral stenosis.

balano-. See *balan-.*

bal·a·no·chlam·y·di·tis (bal″uh·no·klam″i·dye′tis) *n.* [*balano-* + *chlamyd-* + *-itis*]. Inflammation of the glans and prepuce of the clitoris. Compare *balanitis.*

bal·a·no·plas·ty (bal′uh·no·plas″tee) *n.* [*balano-* + *-plasty*]. Plastic surgery of the glans penis.

bal·a·no·pos·thi·tis (bal″uh·no·pos·thigh′tis) *n.* [*balano-* + *posthitis*]. Inflammation of the glans penis and of the prepuce.

bal·a·no·pre·pu·tial (bal″uh·no·pre·pew′shul) *adj.* [*balano-* + *preputial*]. Pertaining to the glans penis and the prepuce.

bal·a·nor·rha·gia (bal″uh·no·ray′juh, ·jee·uh) *n.* [*balano-* + *-rrhagia*]. Hemorrhage from the glans penis.

bal·a·nor·rhea, bal·a·nor·rhoea (bal″uh·no·ree′uh) *n.* [*balano-* + *-rrhea*]. Purulent balanitis.

bal·an·tid·i·al (bal″an·tid′ee·ul) *adj.* Of or pertaining to protozoans of the genus *Balantidium.*

bal·an·ti·di·a·sis (bal″an·ti·dye′uh·sis) *n.*, pl. **balantidia·ses** (·seez) [*Balantid*ium + *-iasis*]. An infection of the large intestine with *Balantidium coli,* varying in severity from mild colitis to acute dysentery.

Bal·an·tid·i·um (bal″an·tid′ee·um) *n.* [NL., from Gk. *balantidion,* little bag]. A genus of ciliated, parasitic protozoans.

Balantidium co·li (ko′lye). A common parasite of hogs; occasionally infects man, causing severe dysentery.

bal·an·ti·do·sis (bal″an·ti·do′sis) *n.* BALANTIDIASIS.

bal·a·nus (bal′uh·nus) *n.* [Gk. *balanos,* acorn, glans]. The glans of the penis or of the clitoris.

Balarsen. Trademark for arsthinol, a trivalent organic arsenical employed in the treatment of intestinal amebiasis and yaws.

Bal·bia·ni rings (bal·bya·nee′) [E. G. *Balbiani,* French embryologist, 1823–1899]. Large localized swellings of chromonemata of polytene chromosomes, similar in appearance to lampbrush chromosomes. See also *chromosome puff.*

bald·ness, *n.* Absence of hair; ALOPECIA; CALVITIES.

Bal·duz·zi's sign (bahl·doot′tsee). Bilateral or contralateral response to eliciting the adductor reflex of the foot.

Bald·win operation [J. F. *Baldwin,* U.S. gynecologist, 1850–1936]. The formation of an artificial vagina by transplantation of a loop of intestine between the urinary bladder and rectum.

Bal·dy-Web·ster operation [J. M. *Baldy,* U.S. gynecologist, 1860–1934; and J. C. *Webster*]. A uterine suspension in which the round ligaments are brought backward through an incision in the broad ligaments and plicated on the posterior aspect of the uterus.

Bal·four's operation (bal'foor) [D. C. *Balfour,* U.S. surgeon, 1882–1963]. A modification of Polya's operation, designed to avoid kinking of the intestinal loop.

Ba·lint's syndrome (bah'lint). Impairment of oculomotor function due to bilateral lesions of the occipital lobes. It consists of any or all of the following: an inability to turn the eyes to a point in the visual field, despite the fact that eye movements are full; a failure to touch or grasp an object offered to the patient (optic ataxia of an arm); and a defect in visual attention.

Bal·kan frame [after the *Balkan* countries, where first used]. An overhead quadrilateral frame, supported by uprights fastened to the bedposts; used to suspend immobilized fractured limbs and to apply continuous traction by weights and pulleys; also used to facilitate mobility of patients under treatment for fracture.

Balkan grippe. Q FEVER.

ball, *n.* 1. *In anatomy,* any globular part. 2. *In veterinary medicine,* a pill or bolus.

Bal·lance's operation [C. A. *Ballance,* English surgeon, 1856–1936]. Anastomosis of the hypoglossal nerve with the facial nerve to alleviate posttraumatic or postoperative permanent facial paralysis.

Ballance's sign [C. A. *Ballance*]. A sign for rupture of the spleen in which the dullness in the right flank will shift with position, but not that on the left.

ball-and-socket joint. A type of synovial joint, such as that of the hip or shoulder, in which the rounded head of one bone lodges in a concave surface on the other. Syn. *spheroid articulation.* NA *articulatio spheroidea.*

Bal·let's sign (ba·leh') [G. *Ballet,* French physician, 1853–1916]. Partial or complete immobility of the eye from paralysis of one or more extrinsic ocular muscles; seen in thyroid ophthalmopathy.

Bal·lin·gall's disease [G. *Ballingall,* English surgeon, 1780–1855]. MYCETOMA.

bal·lism (bal'iz·um) *n.* [Gk. *ballismos,* a jumping about]. Jerky, swinging, or flinging movements of the arms and legs, as seen in extrapyramidal disorders such as Sydenham's chorea.

bal·lis·mus (ba·liz'mus) *n.* BALLISM.

bal·lis·tic (ba·lis'tick) *adj.* [L. *ballista,* projectile-throwing engine, from Gk. *ballein,* to throw]. 1. Associated with or activated by a sudden physical impulse. 2. Pertaining to missiles or projectiles.

ballisto-. A combining form meaning *ballistic.*

bal·lis·to·car·dio·gram (ba·lis''to·kahr'dee·o·gram) *n.* The record made by a ballistocardiograph, consisting of a series of consecutive waves termed H, I, J, K, L, M, N, etc. Abbreviated, BCG.

bal·lis·to·car·dio·graph (ba·lis''to·kahr'dee·o·graf) *n.* [*ballisto- + cardiograph*]. An instrument that records the recoil movements of the body resulting from cardiac contraction and the impact produced thereon by the ejection of blood from the ventricles.

bal·lis·to·pho·bia (ba·lis''to·fo'bee·uh) *n.* [*ballisto- + -phobia*]. Morbid fear of projectiles or missiles.

ball mill. An apparatus employing tumbling balls or pebbles to break up or pulverize various materials.

bal·lonne·ment (bal·on·mah$^{n'}$) *n.* [F.]. BALLOONING.

bal·loon·ing, *n.* Surgical distention of any body cavity by air or other means for examination or therapeutic purposes.

ballooning degeneration. 1. Swelling and rounding of the cells of the lower layers of the epithelium, seen in certain virus eruptions of the skin. 2. Swelling and rounding of neurons in the so-called storage diseases, particularly Tay-Sachs disease, due to the crowding of the cytoplasm of the nerve cells with fine particles of a complex material composed of lipid, protein, and carbohydrate.

bal·lotte·ment (ba·lot·mah$^{n'}$, ba·lot'munt) *n.* [F., tossing, shaking]. A diagnostic maneuver used to palpate a floating object or deeply placed movable organ or tumor. By judicious pushing and rebound (direct ballottement), or by sudden counterpressure (indirect ballottement), the displaced object is made to impinge on the containing wall, the impact being felt by the palpating fingers or hand.

ball probang. A probang having an ivory bulb attached to one end.

Ball's operation [C. B. *Ball,* Irish surgeon, 1851–1916]. 1. A method of iliac colostomy. 2. Inguinal herniorrhaphy in which the twisted stump of the sac is made fast in the ring. 3. Division of the nerve filaments supplying the perianal region for the relief of pruritis.

ball thrombus. A rounded thrombus found in the heart, especially in an atrium.

ball-valve action. The alternate blocking and opening of a narrow passage by a floating object acting as a valve, as a gallstone in the common bile duct.

ball-valve thrombus. BALL THROMBUS.

balm (bahm) *n.* [OF. *basme,* from L. *balsamum*]. 1. BALSAM. 2. Any substance which heals, relieves, or soothes pain.

bal·ne·ol·o·gy (bal''nee·ol'uh·jee) *n.* [L. *balne*um, bath, + *-logy*]. The science of baths and their therapeutic uses. See also *balneotherapy.*

bal·neo·ther·a·py (bal''nee·o·therr'uh·pee) *n.* [*balne*um + *therapy.*]. Therapeutic use of baths.

Ba·ló's concentric sclerosis or **disease** (bah^{h}l'o) [J. *Baló,* Hungarian neurologist, b. 1896]. CONCENTRIC SCLEROSIS.

Baló's encephalitis peri·ax·i·a·lis con·cen·tri·ca (perr''ee·ack·see·ay'lis kon·sen'tri·kuh) [J. *Baló*]. CONCENTRIC SCLEROSIS.

bal·sam (bawl'sum) *n.* [L. *balsamum,* from Gk. *balsamon*]. 1. The resinous, aromatic, liquid, or semisolid substance obtained from certain trees by natural exudation or by artificial extraction and consisting chiefly of resins and volatile oils containing esters of cinnamic and benzoic acids. See also *Canada balsam.* 2. Sometimes, a substance which is not a true balsam in that it contains no cinnamic or benzoic acid, as copaiba. **—bal·sam·ic** (bawl·sam'ick) *adj.*

balsam of Peru. PERUVIAN BALSAM.

balsam tree. The balsam fir, *Abies balsamea,* which yields Canada balsam.

Bal·ser's fat necrosis (bah^{h}l'zur) [W. *Balser,* German physician, 19th century]. The fat necrosis associated with acute pancreatitis.

Bal·thaz·ar Foster murmur. FOSTER'S RULE.

bam·ber·my·cins (bam''bur·migh'sinz) *n.* An antibiotic substance obtained principally from *Streptomyces bambergiensis* and consisting primarily of moenomycin A and C.

bam·boo spine. The vertebral column as it appears radiographically in advanced ankylosing spondylitis, with ossification of outer layers of the fibrous rings.

ba·meth·an (bay'meth·an, bam'eth·an) *n.* α-[(Butylamino)-methyl]-*p*-hydroxybenzyl alcohol, $C_{12}H_{19}NO_2$, a vasodilator; used as the sulfate salt.

bam·i·fyl·line (bam''i·fil'een) *n.* 8-Benzyl-7-[2-[ethyl(2-hydroxyethyl)amino]ethyl]theophylline, $C_{20}H_{27}N_5O_3$, a bronchodilator; used as the hydrochloride salt.

Ban·croft's filariasis [J. *Bancroft,* English physician, 1836–1894]. WUCHERERIASIS.

band, *n.* 1. That which binds. 2. *In zoology,* a stripe. 3. *In anatomy,* a ligament or long slender bundle of fibers; also, a disk of a striated muscle fiber as seen in its longitudinal section. 4. *In dentistry,* a metal strip encircling and fitted to a tooth. See also *orthodontic band.*

ban·dage (ban'dij) *n.* [F., from *bande,* a strip]. A strip of gauze, muslin, flannel, or other material, usually in the form of a roll, of various widths and lengths, but sometimes triangular or tailed, used to hold dressing in place, to apply pressure, to immobilize a part, to support a dependent or injured part, to obliterate tissue cavities, or to check hemorrhage.

bandage shears. Strong shears for cutting bandages, with the blades usually bent at an angle to the shaft, and with a blunted tip to protect the patient.

band·box resonance. TYMPANITIC RESONANCE (2).

band cell. A developmental stage of a granular leukocyte, found in the circulating blood, intermediate between the metamyelocyte and the adult segmented form. The nucleus is bandlike and the cytoplasm and granules are those of the corresponding adult cell.

band keratopathy or **keratitis.** Deposition of calcium in the superficial corneal stroma and Bowman's membrane seen in chronic intraocular inflammatory disease (as in Still's disease) and in systemic disorders in which hypercalcemia is a feature. Syn. *kearatite en bandelette.*

Ban·dl's ring (bahn′dᵉl) [Ludwig *Bandl,* Austrian gynecologist, b. 1842]. PATHOLOGIC RETRACTION RING.

band of Gia·co·mi·ni (jah″ko·mee′nee) [C. *Giacomini,* Italian anatomist, 1841–1898]. A narrow band of fibers connecting the uncus and dentate gyrus.

Bandol. Trademark for carbiphene, an analgesic used as the hydrochloride salt.

bands of Pic·co·lo·mi·ni (peek·ko·loʰ′mee·nee) [A. *Piccolomini*]. STRIAE MEDULLARES VENTRICULI QUARTI.

bang, *n.* [Hindi]. BHANG.

Bang's disease (bahng) [B. L. F. *Bang,* Danish physician, 1848–1932]. A disease of cattle caused by *Brucella abortus.*

bang·ung·ut (bahng·ōōng′ōōt) *n.* [Tagalog, nightmare]. The occurrence, described initially and chiefly in the Philippines, of sudden and unexplained death during the night in a previously healthy young man; various causes have been postulated.

ban·i·ster·ine (ban″i·sterr′een, ·in, ba·nis′tuh·reen, ·rin) *n.* An alkaloid, $C_{13}H_{12}N_2O$, from ayahuasco, *Banisteria caapi,* which has been employed in encephalitis lethargica. See also *harmine.*

ban·jo splint (ban′jo). A hand splint usually made of wire in the shape of a banjo or racket, attached to the forearm and sometimes incorporated in plaster. Generally used for the attachment of rubber-band traction devices for comminuted fractures and overriding of phalangeal bones.

bank, *n.* A reserve stock of body fluids and parts usually maintained at a hospital or other medical facility.

Banminth. Trademark for pyrantel, an anthelmintic; used as the tartrate salt.

Banthine bromide. Trademark for methantheline bromide, an anticholinergic drug.

Ban·ting·ism (ban′ting·iz·um) *n.* [W. *Banting,* English undertaker and coffinmaker, 1797–1878]. *Obsol.* Dieting for obesity, mainly by restricting intake of carbohydrates and fats.

Ban·ti's syndrome or **disease** (bahn′tee) [G. *Banti,* Italian pathologist, 1852–1925]. 1. Portal hypertension, congestive splenomegaly, and hypersplenism due to an obstructive lesion in the splenic vein, portal vein, or intrahepatic veins. 2. Originally, a primary disease of the spleen.

bap·ti·sia (bap·tizh′uh, ·tiz′ee·uh) *n.* [NL., from Gk. *baptisis,* dipping, baptism]. The dried root of *Baptisia tinctoria,* indigo broom or yellow wild indigo, formerly used medicinally.

bap·ti·tox·ine (bap″ti·tock′sin, ·seen) *n.* CYTISINE.

¹bar, *n.* [OF. *barre*]. 1. A band or stripe. 2. A fetal or visceral arch. 3. That part of the horse's upper jaw which has no teeth. 4. That portion of the wall of a horse's hoof reflected sharply anteriorly onto the sole from each buttress. The two bars are separated by the frog. 5. A segment of metal connecting two or more components of a removable partial denture.

²bar, *n.* [Gk. *baros,* weight]. A unit of atmospheric pressure representing one megadyne per square centimeter.

bar-, baro- [Gk. *baros,* weight, heaviness]. A combining form meaning (a) *weight, pressure;* (b) *atmospheric pressure.*

baraesthesia. BARESTHESIA.

baraesthesiometer. BARESTHESIOMETER.

bar·ag·no·sis (băr″ag·no′sis) *n.* [*bar-* + *a-* + *gnosis*]. ABAROGNOSIS.

Baralyme. Trade name for a mixture of barium and calcium hydroxide; used to absorb carbon dioxide in closed anesthesia.

Bá·rány's pointing test (bah′rahnʸ) [R. *Bárány,* Austrian physician, 1876–1936]. The patient points with finger or toe at a fixed object alternately with eyes open and closed. Constant failure of the limb to return to the former position indicates a unilateral cerebellar lesion.

Bárány's test [R. *Bárány*]. CALORIC TEST.

bar·ba (bahr′buh) *n.* [L.]. The beard.

bar·ba ama·ril·la (bahr′buh am″uh·ril′uh, ah·mah·ree′yah) [Sp., yellow beard]. *BOTHROPS ATROX.*

barb·al·o·in (bahr·bal′o·in) *n.* [after *Bar*bados + *aloin*]. The pentoside chiefly responsible for the purgative action of aloe. See also *aloin.*

Bar·ba·ry ape (bahr′buh·ree) [after *Barbary,* the Mediterranean coastal regions of Africa]. The tailless North African monkey *Macaca sylvanus.*

bar·bei·ro (bahr·bay′roo) *n.* [Pg., lit., barber]. ASSASSIN BUG.

barbeiro fever. CHAGAS' DISEASE.

Bar·be·rio's test (bar·beh′ryo) [Michele *Barberio,* Italian physician, b. 1872]. A test for semen in which a drop of spermatic fluid or an aqueous extract of spermatic stain, when treated with a saturated aqueous solution of picric acid, shows a precipitate of yellow refractile crystals.

bar·ber·ry (bahr′bur·ee) *n.* BERBERIS.

bar·ber's itch. Folliculitis of the beard.

Barber's method. Isolation of a single microorganism by the use of a mechanically operated pipet under a microscopic field.

barbiero. Misspelling of BARBEIRO.

bar·bi·tal (bahr′bi·tol, ·tal) *n.* [*barbit*uric + *-al*]. 5,5-Diethylbarbituric acid or diethylmalonylurea, $C_8H_{12}N_2O_3$, a white crystalline powder; a long-acting hypnotic and sedative. Syn. *barbitone, diethylbarbituric acid.*

bar·bi·tal·ism (bahr′bi·tol·iz·um) *n.* [*barbital* + *-ism*]. BARBITURISM.

barbital sodium. The sodium derivative, water-soluble, of barbital. Syn. *sodium barbital, soluble barbital.*

bar·bi·tone (bahr′bi·tone) *n.* BARBITAL.

bar·bi·tu·ism (bahr′bi·tew″iz·um, bahr·bitch′oo·iz·um) *n.* BARBITURISM.

bar·bi·tu·rate (bahr·bitch′oo·rate, bahr″bi·tewr′ate) *n.* [*barbituric* + *-ate*]. Any derivative of barbituric acid, $C_4H_4N_2O_3$ formed by the substitution of an aliphatic or aromatic group on a carbon or nitrogen atom in the acid. Barbiturates are used as hypnotic and sedative drugs. Modifications in their structure influence the power and rapidity of their effects. The depressant effects of these drugs are exerted upon the higher centers of the brain.

bar·bi·tu·ric acid (bahr″bi·tewr′ick). Malonylurea, $C_4H_4N_2O_3$, the parent compound of the barbiturates.

bar·bi·tu·rism (bahr′bi·tewr·iz·um, bahr·bitch′oor·iz·um) *n.* [*barbitur*ate + *-ism*]. Physiologic, pathologic, and psychologic changes produced by ingestion of barbiturates in excess of therapeutic amounts; may be acute or chronic.

bar·bo·tage (bahr·bo·tahzh′) *n.* [F., from *barboter,* to dabble]. A method of spinal anesthesia in which part of the anesthetic solution is injected into the subarachnoid space; spinal fluid is then aspirated into the syringe and reinjected. This procedure may be repeated several times before the entire content of the syringe is finally injected. In this way, the anesthetic agent is more widely diffused, though the anesthesia is frequently spotty.

Bar·coo rot or **disease** (bahr·koo′) [after *Barcoo* River, Australia]. VELD SORE.

Bar·de·le·ben's operation (bahr′de·leʸ·bun) [A. von *Bardeleben*, German surgeon, 1861-1914]. An operation formerly used for double harelip with protruding maxilla in which the vomer is divided subperiosteally before reduction of the deformity.

Bar·den·heu·er's operation (bahr′dun·hoy·ur) [B. *Bardenheuer*, German surgeon, 1839-1913]. Fixation of a floating spleen in an extraperitoneal pocket.

Bar·det-Biedl syndrome (bar·deʰ′, bee′dul) [G. *Bardet*, French physician, b. 1885; and A. *Biedl*, Austrian physician, 1869-1933]. LAURENCE-MOON-BIEDL SYNDROME.

Bard-Pic syndrome (baʰr, peek) [L. *Bard*, Swiss physician, 1857-1930; and A. *Pic*, French physician, 1863-1943]. Progressive jaundice and cachexia, associated with cancer of the head of the pancreas.

Bard's sign [L. *Bard*]. Increased oscillations of the eyeballs when the examiner's finger is moved from right to left and back, seen in organic nystagmus; in congenital nystagmus the oscillations stop under the same conditions.

bare area of the liver. A triangular area on the superior surface of the liver devoid of peritoneum, enclosed by the coronary ligament. NA *area nuda*.

Bä·ren·sprung's disease (behr′un·shproong) [F. W. F. von *Bärensprung*, German dermatologist, 1822-1864]. TINEA CRURIS.

bar·es·the·sia, bar·aes·the·sia (băr″es·theezh′uh, ·theez′ee·uh) *n.* [*bar-* + *esthesia*]. Perception of weight or pressure; PRESSURE SENSE.

bar·es·the·si·om·e·ter, bar·aes·the·si·om·e·ter (băr″es·theez″ee·om′e·tur) *n.* [*bar-* + *esthesiometer*]. An instrument for estimating the sensitivity of the weight or pressure sense.

Bar·foed's reagent [C. T. *Barfoed*, Swedish physician, 1815-1899]. A solution of crystallized copper acetate and acetic acid; used in the detection of monosaccharides.

Barfoed's test [C. T. *Barfoed*]. A copper reduction test for glucose in urine.

bar·i·at·rics (băr″ee·at′ricks) *n.* [*bar-* (as if Gk. *baros*, weight, could refer to obesity) + *-iatrics*]. The branch of medicine concerned with the prevention and treatment of obesity. —**bariatric,** *adj.*

bar·i·to·sis (băr″i·to′sis) *n.* A pneumoconiosis due to the inhalation of barium dust.

bar·i·um (băr′ee·um) *n.* [Gk. *barys*, heavy, + *-ium*]. Ba = 137.34. A metal belonging to the alkaline earths and occurring in nature only in the form of divalent compounds. All its soluble salts are poisonous. See also Table of Elements in the Appendix.

barium carbonate. $BaCO_3$; a white, heavy powder, almost insoluble in water, used as a reagent.

barium chloride. $BaCl_2 \cdot 2H_2O$; a water-soluble salt used to precipitate sulfate ions. A violent stimulant of all smooth muscles; has been used to increase the force of cardiac contraction in atrioventricular dissociation (Stokes-Adams syndrome).

barium hydroxide. $Ba(OH)_2 \cdot 8H_2O$; a water-soluble base, used as a chemical reagent.

barium sulfate. $BaSO_4$; a water-insoluble salt, employed as an opaque radiographic contrast medium.

bark, *n.* 1. The covering of the wood of exogenous trees; all tissues outside the cambium. 2. CINCHONA.

Bar·ker's operation [A. E. J. *Barker*, English surgeon, 1850-1916]. 1. Excision of the talus. 2. Excision of the hip, using an anterior approach.

bar·ley, *n.* Any cereal grass of the genus *Hordeum*, order Graminales; used as food, and also in the preparation of malt.

barley water. A decoction of pearl barley prepared by boiling with water; used as demulcent and food for children with diarrhea.

Bar·low's disease [T. *Barlow*, English physician, 1845-1945]. INFANTILE SCURVY.

Barlow's syndrome [J. B. *Barlow*, South African physician, 20th century]. An apical systolic murmur, systolic click, and an electrocardiogram of inferior ischemia, in association with mitral regurgitation due to mitral valve prolapse. Syn. *electrocardiographic-auscultatory syndrome.*

barn, *n.* A unit expressing the probability of a specific nuclear reaction occurring, stated in terms of cross-sectional area. It is equivalent to 10^{-24} sq cm.

Barns·dale bacillus. MYCOBACTERIUM ULCERANS.

baro-. See *bar-*.

baro·cep·tor (băr″o·sep′tur) *n.* [*baro-* + *receptor*]. BARORECEPTOR.

bar·o·don·tal·gia (băr″o·don·tal′jee·uh) *n.* [*bar-* + *odontalgia*]. AERODONTALGIA.

bar of the bladder. The transverse ridge joining the openings of the ureters on the inner surface of the urinary bladder; it forms the posterior boundary of the trigone. NA *plica interureterica.*

bar·og·no·sis (băr″og·no′sis) *n.*, pl. **barogno·ses** (·seez) [*baro-* + *gnosis*]. The ability to estimate weight; the perception of weight.

baro·graph (băr′o·graf) *n.* [*baro-* + *-graph*]. A self-registering barometer.

baro·ma·crom·e·ter (băr″o·ma·krom′e·tur) *n.* [*baro-* + *macro-* + *meter*]. An apparatus to measure the weight and length of infants.

ba·rom·e·ter (ba·rom′e·tur) *n.* [*baro-* + *meter*]. An instrument that measures atmospheric pressure; commonly a capillary tube sealed at one end, filled with mercury, and inverted in a mercury reservoir. At sea level the height of the mercury column normally stands at 760 mm, or 30 inches, rising or falling directly as the atmospheric pressure. —**ba·rom·e·try** (ba·rom′e·tree) *n.*

baro·met·ric (băr·o·met′rick) *adj.* Of, pertaining to, or indicated by a barometer or barometry.

barometric pressure. The pressure of the atmosphere, as indicated by a barometer.

baro-oti·tis (băr″o·o·tye′tis) *n.* BAROTITIS.

baro·pac·er (băr′o·pay″sur) *n.* [*baro-* + *pace* (as in *pacemaker*) + *-er*]. An electronic device, typically implanted in the neck, which continuously stimulates the branch of the glossopharyngeal nerve innervating the carotid sinus; used experimentally in treatment of hypertension. —**baro·pace,** *v.*

baro·pho·bia (băr″o·fo′bee·uh) *n.* [*baro-* + *-phobia*]. A morbid fear of the pull of gravity.

baro·re·cep·tor (băr″o·re·sep′tur) *n.* [*baro-* + *receptor*]. 1. A nerve ending, located largely in the walls of the carotid sinus and of the aortic arch, sensitive to stretching induced by changes of blood pressure within the vessels or direct pressure from without. It generates afferent impulses conducted to medullary centers to cause reflex vasodilatation and fall of blood pressure, as by increase of systemic pressure and a reflex rise in systemic arterial pressure when blood pressure within the carotid sinus and aortic arch is suddenly raised. 2. Any peripheral receptor sensitive to mechanical deformation.

baro·scope (băr′o·skope) *n.* [*baro-* + *-scope*]. A sensitive barometer.

baro·si·nus·itis (băr″o·sigh″nus·eye′tis) *n.* [*baro-* + *sinusitis*]. Inflammation of the sinuses, characterized by edema and hemorrhage, caused by changes in atmospheric pressure.

Ba·ros·ma (ba·roz′muh, ·ros′muh) *n.* [NL., from Gk. *barys*, heavy, + *osmē*, odor]. A genus of strong-scented plants of the Rutaceae, native to the Cape of Good Hope and vicinity, several species of which yield the buchu of commerce.

ba·ros·min (ba·roz′min, ·ros′min) *n.* 1. A glycoside obtained from buchu and other sources. Syn. *diosmin.* 2. A concentrate prepared from buchu.

Barosperse. A trademark for barium sulfate, a radiologic contrast medium.

bar·o·tal·gia (băr″o·tal′jee·uh) *n.* [*bar-* + *otalgia*]. Pain arising in the middle ear caused by a difference of air pressure between the middle ear and the surrounding atmosphere.

bar·o·ti·tis (băr″o·tye′tis) *n.* [*bar-* + *otitis*]. Inflammation of the ear, or a part of it, caused by changes in atmospheric pressure.

barotitis ex·ter·na (ecks·tur′nuh). An acute or chronic, traumatic ear condition resulting in inflammation of the external auditory canal and tympanic membrane, caused by a pressure differential between the external auditory canal and the middle ear; it is usually associated with imperforate plugging of the external ear.

barotitis me·dia (mee′dee·uh). Inflammation or bleeding in the middle ear due to a difference between air pressure in the middle ear and external atmospheric pressure (as during airplane descent, in diving, or in a hyperbaric chamber), producing pain, tinnitus, and, occasionally, diminution in hearing and vertigo. Syn. *otic barotrauma, aerotitis media.*

baro·trau·ma (băr″o·traw′muh) *n.*, pl. **barotrauma·ta** (·tuh) [*baro-* + *trauma*]. Injury of certain organs, especially the auditory tube and the middle ear, due to a change in atmospheric pressure or water pressure.

Ba·rra·quer's disease (Sp. ba·rra·kehr′, Cat. buh·rruh·keʸ′) [J. A. *Barraquer* Roviralta, Spanish physician, b. 1852]. PROGRESSIVE LIPODYSTROPHY.

Barraquer-Si·mons disease (zee′monss) [J. A. *Barraquer* Roviralta; and A. *Simons,* German physician, b. 1879]. PROGRESSIVE LIPODYSTROPHY.

Barraquer's operation [I. *Barraquer,* Spanish ophthalmologist, b. 1884]. PHACOERYSIS.

Barr body [M. L. *Barr,* Canadian anatomist, b. 1908]. SEX CHROMATIN.

bar·rel chest. A large thorax rounded in cross section, which may be normal in certain types of stocky build, or may indicate increased vital capacity as in certain peoples indigenous to high altitudes, or may be a sign of pulmonary emphysema. See also *emphysematous chest.*

bar·ren, *adj.* [OF. *baraigne*]. Of a female, STERILE (1).

Barr-Epstein virus. EPSTEIN-BARR VIRUS.

Bar·ré's sign (ba·reʸ′) [J. A. *Barré,* French neurologist, b. 1880]. The patient lies prone and his legs are flexed at the knees to an angle of 90°. If there is disease of the corticospinal tracts, the patient is unable to hold his legs flexed.

Barré's syndrome [J. A. *Barré*]. GUILLAIN-BARRÉ DISEASE.

Bar·rett's esophagus or **syndrome** [N. *Barrett,* British physician, 20th century]. Ectopic gastric mucosa in the lower esophagus, frequently leading to ulceration and stricture.

Barrett's ulcer [N. *Barrett*]. Ulcer of the esophagus arising from ectopic gastric mucosa. See also *Barrett's esophagus.*

Bartholin abscess. An abscess of the excretory duct of Bartholin's gland.

Bar·tho·lin cyst (bar′to·leen) [C. *Bartholin,* Danish anatomist, 1655–1738]. A cyst resulting from chronic bartholinitis, containing a clear fluid which replaces the suppurative exudate.

bar·tho·lin·itis (bahr″to·li·nigh′tis) *n.* [*Bartholin*'s gland + *-itis*]. Inflammation of the major vestibular glands.

Bartholin's duct [C. *Bartholin*]. 1. The duct of a major vestibular gland at the vaginal introitus. 2. The duct of a major sublingual gland.

Bartholin's gland [C. *Bartholin*]. Either of the major vestibular glands. NA *glandula vestibularis major.* See *vestibular glands.*

Barth's hernia (bart) [J. B. P. *Barth,* Alsatian physician, 1806–1877]. Incarceration of small intestinal loops between a persistent vitelline duct and the abdominal wall.

Bar·ton·el·la (bahr″tun·el′uh) *n.* [A. L. *Barton,* Peruvian physician, 20th century]. A genus of the Rickettsiales (family Bartonellaceae) which multiply in fixed tissue cells and parasitize erythrocytes, consisting of minute, pleomorphic rods and cocci which invade erythrocytes and endothelium in man. They occur without an intermediate host in man and in arthropod vectors are found only as *Bartonella bacilliformis,* the causative agent of bartonellosis.

bar·ton·el·li·a·sis (bahr″tun·el·eye′uh·sis) *n.* BARTONELLOSIS.

bar·ton·el·lo·sis (bahr″tun·el·o′sis) *n.* [*Bartonella* + *-osis*]. An arthropod-borne infection caused by *Bartonella bacilliformis,* presenting two clinical types of disease: a severe form (Oroya fever), characterized by fever, a rapidly developing macrocytic anemia, and frequently by intercurrent infections with high mortality; and a benign form (verruga peruana), characterized by a verrucous eruption of hemangioma-like nodules and by negligible mortality.

Bar·ton's forceps [J. R. *Barton,* U.S. surgeon, 1794–1871]. An obstetric forceps with a hinge in one handle.

Barton's operation [J. R. *Barton*]. Intertrochanteric osteotomy for ankylosis of the hip.

Bart's hemoglobin. An abnormal hemoglobin, composed of four gamma peptide chains, which is considered the fetal equivalent of hemoglobin H; it is associated with erythrocytic sickling.

Bart·ter's syndrome [F. C. *Bartter,* U.S. physician, b. 1914]. Hypokalemic alkalosis, hyperaldosteronism with normal blood pressure, hyperplasia of the juxtaglomerular apparatus, dwarfism, and sometimes an abnormal renin response to angiotensin; of unknown cause.

bary- [Gk. *barys*]. A combining form meaning (a) *heavy;* (b) *deep, low.*

bary·pho·nia (băr″i·fo′nee·uh) *n.* [*bary-* + *-phonia*]. *Rare.* A heavy or deep quality of voice.

ba·ry·ta (ba·rye′tuh, băr′i·tuh) *n.* Barium oxide, BaO.

baryta water. An aqueous solution of barium hydroxide.

ba·ry·tes (ba·rye′teez, băr′i·teez) *n.* [Gk. *barytēs,* heaviness]. BARYTA.

B. A. S. British Anatomical Society.

ba·sal (bay′sul) *adj.* [*base* + *-al*]. 1. Fundamental; basic. 2. Indicating the lowest or least, as basal metabolic rate; deepest, as basal layer. 3. Pertaining to the initial unconscious state as induced by basal anesthesia.

basal anesthesia. A preliminary, usually incomplete anesthesia requiring supplementation. Thus, narcosis may be induced by injection of appropriate drugs, whereupon relatively small amounts of inhalation anesthetics are needed to produce surgical anesthesia.

basal angle. The angle between the sphenoid and clivus in the lateral projection.

basal body. A minute granule at the base of a cilium or flagellum, derived from the centriole and producing the cilium or flagellum.

basal bone. 1. *In prosthodontics,* the osseous tissue of the mandible and maxillae excepting the rami and processes; that which provides a stable base for the support of artificial dentures. 2. *In orthodontics,* the fixed bony framework that limits the movement of teeth in the establishment of a stable occlusion.

basal cell. One of the cells of the deepest layer of a stratified epithelium.

basal cell carcinoma. A tumor composed of embryonal cells resembling those of the basal cell layer of the skin. It is locally invasive but rarely metastasizes.

basal cell layer. The deepest layer of cells in the germinative layer of a stratified epithelium.

basal cell nevus syndrome. The occurrence, often familial, of multiple basal cell carcinomas and cysts of the jaws together with such miscellaneous defects as scoliosis, bifid ribs, and mesenteric cysts. It may be an autosomal dominant trait.

basal cell tumor of the ovary. GRANULOSA CELL TUMOR.

basal cistern. The subarachnoid space at the base of the brain, divided by the optic chiasma into the cistern of the chiasma and the interpeduncular cistern.

basal conditions. The set of conditions regarded as necessary for accurate measurement of basal metabolism; specifically, consciousness and complete rest in a fasting (12 to 18 hours) subject in a warm atmosphere.

basal decidua. DECIDUA BASALIS.

basal drainage. Removal of cerebrospinal fluid from the basal cistern.

basal ectoderm. That part of the trophoblast covering the eroded uterine surface of the placental sinuses, continuous with the tips of the chorionic villi; it partly disappears in late pregnancy.

basal fissure. DECIDUAL FISSURE.

basal ganglia. The caudate and lenticular nuclei, claustrum, subthalamic nucleus, and substantia nigra.

basal ganglionic paralysis. Weakness due to a lesion of the basal ganglions, as in paralysis agitans.

basal granule. BASAL BODY.

ba·sal·i·o·ma (bay·sal″ee·o′muh) *n.* BASAL CELL CARCINOMA.

Basaljel. A trademark for basic aluminum carbonate employed as a gastric antacid.

basal lamina. A thin noncellular layer of ground substance, recognizable by electron microscopy, which lies immediately beneath epithelial surfaces; the uppermost layer of the basement membrane. Syn. *basement lamina.*

basal layer. 1. The nondeciduate stratum basale of the endometrium, containing the blind ends of the uterine glands. 2. BASAL CELL LAYER.

basal layer of Weil. ZONE OF WEIL.

basal membrane. A sheet of tissue which forms the outer layer of the choroid and lies immediately under the pigment layer of the retina. It consists of a feltwork of elastic fibers and a thin homogenous layer lying next to the pigmented cells of the retina. NA *lamina basalis choroideae.*

basal metabolic rate. The quantity of energy expended per unit of time under basal conditions; usually expressed as large calories (Cal) per square meter of body surface per hour. Abbreviated, B.M.R.

basal metabolism. The minimum amount of energy expenditure necessary to sustain life, measured when the subject is conscious and at complete rest in a warm atmosphere 12 to 18 hours after the intake of food. See also *basal metabolic rate.*

basal neck fracture. A common fracture of the neck of the femur located in the extracapsular position at the distal portion of the neck parallel to the intertrochanteric line.

ba·sal·oid (bay′sul·oid) *adj.* Resembling a basal cell of the skin.

basal olfactory fasciculus. A diffuse system of nerve fibers that arise in the basal olfactory nuclei, pass beneath the head of the caudate nucleus, give terminal or collateral fibers to the tuber cinereum and mamillary body (olfactohypothalamic tract), and continue to the tegmentum of the midbrain (olfactotegmental tract), some reaching the medulla and spinal cord.

basal olfactory nuclei. A collective name applied to the gray substance of the olfactory tract, olfactory trigone, olfactory area, gyrus paraterminalis, and parolfactory area.

basal plate of the cranium. A cartilaginous plate of the embryonic cranium representing the fused parachordal plates of lower forms. It is the predecessor of the occipital bone.

basal plate of the gravid uterus. That part of the decidua basalis incorporated into the placenta, including its covering of basal ectoderm from the trophoblast.

basal plate of the neural tube. The lateral wall of the neural tube ventral to the sulcus limitans; motor in function. NA *lamina basalis.*

basal ridge. A bandlike ridge of enamel on the lingual surface of an incisor or canine tooth, arising from the neck of the tooth toward its crown. NA *cingulum.*

basal seat. DENTURE FOUNDATION.

basal surface. *In dentistry,* the surface of an artificial denture that rests upon and is in intimate contact with the denture foundation.

basal temperature. The temperature of the healthy body after a sufficient period of rest, usually obtained in the fasting state before arising after at least 8 hours of relaxed sleep.

basal vein. A vein located at the base of the brain. NA *vena basalis.* See also Table of Veins in the Appendix.

bas·cu·la·tion (bas″kew·lay′shun) *n.* [F. *basculer,* to seesaw]. Replacing a retroverted uterus by pressing upward on the fundus and downward on the cervix.

base, *n.* [MF., from L. *basis,* from Gk.]. 1. The lowest part of a body or any of its parts, or the foundation upon which anything rests. 2. The principal ingredient of a substance or compound. 3. *In chemistry,* (1) a compound which yields hydroxyl ions (OH^-) in aqueous solution and which reacts with an acid to produce a salt and water; (2) a proton acceptor: a substance capable of taking up protons such as a purine or pyrimidine; or (3) a substance having an electron pair which may be shared by another substance which lacks such a pair, and is therefore called an acid, to form a coordinate covalent bond between the two substances. Contr. *acid.*

base analogue. An analogue of one of the purine or pyrimidine bases normally found in ribonucleic or deoxyribonucleic acid.

baseball finger. Luxation of a distal phalanx with rupture of the distal portion of the extensor tendon, resulting in a drop of the phalanx; caused by an injury when catching a baseball.

base curve. *In optics,* the standard curve on the back of a toric lens. The front surface is so ground that, in combination with the base curve, the desired optical strength is obtained.

bas·e·doid (bas′e·doid) *adj.* [*Basedow*'s disease + *-oid*]. Designating an atypical form of thyroid disease, not hyperthyroidism.

bas·e·dow·oid (bas′e·do·woid) *adj.* BASEDOID.

Ba·se·dow's disease (bah′ze·do) [K. A. von *Basedow,* German physician, 1799–1854]. GRAVES' DISEASE.

base hospital. An army hospital within the lines of communication, comparatively well-equipped and staffed to receive and care for sick and wounded returned from field hospitals.

base line. *In craniometry,* a line running backward from the infraorbital ridge through the middle of the external auditory meatus, and prolonged to the middle line of the head posteriorly.

Ba·sel·la (ba·sel′uh) *n.* A genus of plants of the Basellaceae. *Basella rubra,* Malabar nightshade, is an esculent herb cultivated throughout India, where the juice of the leaves is used for respiratory diseases of infants.

base material. Any material, such as acrylic resin, metal, shellac, or vulcanite, used to make an artificial permanent or temporary denture base.

base·ment lamina. BASAL LAMINA.

basement membrane. The delicate, noncellular layer on which an epithelium is seated. It may contain reticular fibers and can be selectively stained with silver stains.

base of the brain. The undersurface of the brain; FACIES INFERIOR CEREBRI.

base of the heart. The general area occupied by the roots of the great vessels and the portion of the wall of the heart between them. NA *basis cordis.*

base of the skull. The floor of the skull, containing the anterior, middle, and posterior cranial fossae.

ba·se·o·sis (bay″see·o′sis) *n.,* pl. **baseo·ses** (·seez) [*base* + *-osis*]. ALKALEMIA.

base pair. A pair of nucleotides in a nucleic acid; one of the pair must always be a purine while the nucleotide of the complementary chain must always be a pyrimadine. In base pairing, guanine is paired with cytosine while adenine is paired with thymine or uracil.

base·plate, *n.* A form which is a negative reproduction of the edentulous jaw made by either adapting a material such as shellac to cast or fabricating an acrylic resin form to the edentulous cast; upon the baseplate, an occlusal wax rim is developed which is used to help establish jaw relationships and in which the artificial teeth are initially set.

base ratio. The ratio of molar quantities of the bases found in deoxyribonucleic acid or ribonucleic acid.

bases. Plural of *basis* and of *base.*

bas-fond (bah·fohn′) *n.* [F., bottom]. FUNDUS; specifically, the depressed area in the posterior wall of the urinary bladder just behind and above the trigone. It enlarges and deepens when there is obstruction to urination. In the male, it is also described as the postprostatic pouch.

Bash·am's mixture [W. R. *Basham,* English physician, 1804–1877]. IRON AND AMMONIUM ACETATE SOLUTION.

Bash·ford carcinoma 63. A poorly differentiated transplantable carcinoma originally found as a spontaneous tumor in the breast of a noninbred mouse.

basi-, basio-. A combining form meaning (a) *basion, basial;* (b) *base, basis, basilar;* (c) *basic.*

ba·si·al (bay′see·ul) *adj.* Of or relating to the basion.

ba·si·al·ve·o·lar (bay″see·al·vee′uh·lur) *adj.* Pertaining to the basion and the alveolar point.

ba·si·bran·chi·al (bay″see·brank′ee·ul) *n.* [*basi-* + *branchial*]. A copula or unpaired skeletal element uniting the sides or ventral ends of each branchial arch skeleton.

ba·si·breg·mat·ic axis (bay″see·breg·mat′ick). The line connecting the basion and bregma.

ba·sic (bay′sick) *adj.* 1. Pertaining to the base or basis; fundamental. 2. *In chemistry,* of or pertaining to a base.

basic anhydride. An oxide of a metal; it forms a base with water.

basic fuchsin. A mixture of rosaniline and pararosaniline hydrochlorides, dyes of the triphenylmethane group; available also as the acetate salts. Used as a germicide, as an ingredient of the antifungal preparation Castellani's paint, as a bacterial and histologic stain, and as a chemical reagent. Syn. *magenta.*

ba·si·chro·ma·tin (bay″see·kro′muh·tin) *n.* [*basi-* + *chromatin*]. That portion of the chromatin stained by basic aniline dyes. It represents tightly coiled DNA, inactive in transcription of the genetic code. Syn. *heterochromatin.* Contr. *euchromatin.*

ba·sic·i·ty (ba·sis′i·tee, bay·) *n.* 1. The quality of being basic. 2. Of an acid: the fact of having a given number of replaceable hydrogen atoms, as monobasic, dibasic.

basic oxide. An oxide of a metal which produces a base when combined with water.

ba·si·cra·ni·al (bay″see·kray′nee·ul) *adj.* [*basi-* + *cranial*]. Pertaining to the base of the skull.

basicranial axis. A line connecting the basion to the midpoint of the sphenoethmoid suture.

basic salt. A salt capable of further reaction with acid because of the presence of hydroxyl or other basic groups.

basic stain. A dye in which the cation is colored and does the staining. Basic stains are the common stains for chromatin in nuclei, for nucleoproteins, for mucins, and for calcium-salt deposits in tissues.

basidi-, basidio-. A combining form meaning *basidial, basidium.*

basidia. Plural of *basidium.*

ba·sid·i·al (bay·sid′ee·ul) *adj.* Pertaining to or consisting of basidia.

basidio-. See *basidi-.*

Ba·sid·i·ob·o·lus (ba·sid″ee·ob′o·lus) *n.* [NL., from *basidio-* + Gk. *bolos,* throw, casting]. A genus of Phycomycetes. See also *phycomycosis.*

ba·sid·io·ge·net·ic (ba·sid″ee·o·je·net′ick) *adj.* [*basidio-* + *genetic*]. *In biology,* produced on a basidium.

ba·sid·io·my·cete (ba·sid″ee·o·migh·seet′) *n.* A fungus of the class Basidiomycetes.

Ba·sid·io·my·ce·tes (ba·sid″ee·o·migh·see′teez) *n.pl.* [*basidio-* + *mycetes*]. A large class of fungi comprising genera which produce spores upon basidia. It includes the smuts, rusts, mushrooms, puffballs, and their allies.

ba·sid·io·phore (ba·sid′ee·o·fore) *n.* [*basidio-* + *-phore*]. A branch or a portion of a thallus bearing a basidium.

ba·sid·io·spore (ba·sid′ee·o·spore) *n.* A spore of the Basidiomycetes, formed by a basidium.

ba·sid·i·um (ba·sid′ee·um) *n.*, pl. **basid·ia** (·ee·uh) [NL., from Gk. *basidion,* dim. of *basis,* step, base]. *In botany,* the cell which produces basidiospores.

ba·si·fa·cial (bay″see·fay′shul) *adj.* [*basi-* + *facial*]. Pertaining to the lower portion of the face.

basifacial axis. A line joining the subnasal point and the midpoint of the sphenoethmoid suture.

ba·si·hy·al (bay″see·high′ul) *n.* [*basi-* + *hy-* + *-al*]. One of a series of bones forming the hyoid arch; in man it forms the body of the hyoid bone. See also *ceratohyal.*

bas·i·lar (bas′i·lur) *adj.* Of or pertaining to the base or basis of a structure or organ.

basilar arachnoiditis. A form of chronic adhesive arachnoiditis more or less limited to the base of the brain.

basilar artery. An artery lodged in the basilar sulcus and formed by the union of the two vertebral arteries. NA *arteria basilaris.* See also Table of Arteries in the Appendix.

basilar artery insufficiency syndrome. The clinical picture of insufficient blood flow through the basilar artery, characterized by a variable degree and duration of diplopia, vertigo, dysarthria, dysphagia, numbness, and weakness of one side of the face or body, blindness, and depressed consciousness; may be due to occlusion of the basilar or vertebral arteries, and ineffective collateral circulation.

basilar cartilage. The cartilage in the foramen lacerum.

basilar fibers. Specialized connective-tissue fibers in the basilar membrane of the cochlea.

basilar impression. Protrusion of the upper cervical spine into the base of the skull.

basilar insufficiency. BASILAR ARTERY INSUFFICIENCY SYNDROME.

basilar membrane. The membranous portion of the spiral lamina of the cochlea, extending from the extremity of the osseous spiral lamina to the lateral wall, and forming the fibrous base upon which the spiral organ (of Corti) rests. NA *lamina basilaris.*

basilar meningitis. Inflammation of the meninges affecting chiefly the base of the brain, with collection of exudate predominantly in the basal cisterns.

basilar neck fracture. BASAL NECK FRACTURE.

basilar papilla. SPIRAL ORGAN (OF CORTI).

basilar plexus. A venous plexus over the basilar part of the occipital bone, connecting the two inferior petrosal sinuses and the marginal and internal vertebral plexuses. NA *plexus basilaris.* See also Table of Veins in the Appendix.

basilar process. A strong, quadrilateral plate of bone forming the anterior portion of the occipital bone, in front of the foramen magnum.

basilar sinus. BASILAR PLEXUS.

basilar sulcus. A groove along the median line of the ventral surface of the pons lodging the basilar artery. NA *sulcus basilaris pontis.*

basilar suture. A suture formed by the junction of the basilar process of the occipital bone with the posterior surface of the body of the sphenoid.

basilar vertebra. The last lumbar vertebra.

ba·si·lat·er·al (bay″si·lat′ur·ul) *adj.* Both basilar and lateral.

ba·sil·ic vein (ba·sil′ick) [ML. *vena basilica*, from Ar. *bāsilīq* (Avicenna), apparently from Gk. *basilikos*, royal]. The large superficial vein of the arm on the medial side of the biceps brachii muscle. NA *vena basilica.* See also Table of Veins in the Appendix.

basilo-. A combining form meaning *base, basilar.*

bas·i·lo·breg·mat·ic (bas″i·lo·breg·mat′ick, ba·sil″o·) *adj.* Pertaining to the base of the skull and bregma.

bas·il oil (baz′il). A volatile oil from the Indian plant, *Ocimum basilicum*, the common basil; consists principally of *l*-linalool and methyl cinnamate.

bas·i·lo·men·tal (bas″i·lo·men′tul, ba·sil″o·) *adj.* [*basilo-* + *mental*]. Pertaining to the base of the skull and to the chin.

bas·i·lo·pha·ryn·ge·al (bas″i·lo·fa·rin′jee·ul, ba·sil″o·) *adj.* Pertaining to the basilar part of the occipital bone and to the pharynx.

bas·i·lo·sub·na·sal (bas″i·lo·sub·nay′zul, ba·sil″o·) *adj.* BASINASAL.

ba·si·na·sal (bay″see·nay′zul) *adj.* Pertaining to the basion and nasion.

basio-. See *basi-*.

ba·sio·al·ve·o·lar (bay″see·o·al·vee′uh·lur) *adj.* Pertaining to the basion and to the alveolar point.

ba·sio·breg·mat·ic (bay″see·o·breg·mat′ick) *adj.* Pertaining to the basion and bregma.

basiobregmatic line. The line joining the basion and bregma.

ba·si·oc·cip·i·tal (bay″see·ock·sip′i·tul) *adj.* Pertaining to the basilar part of the occipital bone.

basioccipital bone. 1. In many of the lower vertebrate animals and in embryonic mammals, the separate bone forming the median posterior part of the central axis of the skull. 2. In the human adult, the basilar part of the occipital bone.

ba·si·on (bay′see·on) *n.* [L. *basis*, base, + *-ion*]. *In craniometry*, the point on the anterior margin of the foramen magnum where the midsagittal plane of the skull intersects the plane of the foramen magnum.

ba·sio·tribe (bay′see·o·tribe″) *n.* An instrument used for basiotripsy.

ba·sio·trip·sy (bay′see·o·trip″see) *n.* [*basio-* + *-tripsy*]. Crushing or perforating the fetal head to facilitate delivery.

ba·si·pha·ryn·ge·al (bay″si·fa·rin′jee·ul) *adj.* [*basi-* + *pharyngeal*]. Pertaining to the posterior part of the body of the sphenoid bone (base of the sphenoid) and to the pharynx.

basipharyngeal canal. A small passage occasionally present between the ala of the vomer and vaginal process of the sphenoid. NA *canalis vomerovaginalis.*

ba·si·pho·bia (bay″si·fo′bee·uh) *n.* BASOPHOBIA.

ba·si·pre·sphen·oid (bay″see·pree·sfee′noid) *adj.* Pertaining to the basisphenoid and presphenoid bones.

basipresphenoid bone. Any one of the ossification centers from which the presphenoid part of the sphenoid bone develops.

ba·si·rhi·nal, ba·sir·rhi·nal (bay″si·rye′nul) *adj.* Designating a cerebral fissure located at the base of the rhinencephalon.

ba·sis (bay′sis) *n.*, pl. **ba·ses** (·seez) [L., from Gk., step, base]. A base, foundation, or fundamental part; the part opposite the apex.

basis car·ti·la·gi·nis ary·te·noi·de·ae (kahr·ti·laj′i·nis ăr″i·te·noy′dee·ee) [NA]. The base of the arytenoid cartilage; it contains the area of articulation with the cricoid cartilage.

basis ce·re·bri (serr′e·brye) [BNA]. FACIES INFERIOR CEREBRI.

basis coch·le·ae (kock′lee·ee) [NA]. The base of the cochlea; the portion abutting on the internal acoustic meatus.

basis cor·dis (kor′dis) [NA]. BASE OF THE HEART.

basis cra·nii ex·ter·na (kray′nee·eye ecks·tur′nuh) [NA]. The external aspect of the base of the skull.

basis cranii in·ter·na (in·tur′nuh) [NA]. The internal aspect of the base of the skull.

basis glan·du·lae su·pra·re·na·lis (glan′dew·lee sue″pruh·re·nay′lis) [BNA]. FACIES RENALIS GLANDULAE SUPRARENALIS.

basis lin·guae (ling′gwee). ROOT OF THE TONGUE.

basis man·di·bu·lae (man·dib′yoo·lee) [NA]. The base of the mandible; the rounded inferior margin of the body of the mandible.

basis mo·di·o·li (mo·dye′o·lye) [NA]. The base of the modiolus; the portion abutting on the internal acoustic meatus.

basis na·si (nay′zye) [BNA]. The base of the nose; the portion above the upper lip which contains the two external nasal openings.

basis os·sis me·ta·car·pa·lis (oss′is met″uh·kahr·pay′lis) [NA]. The base of a metacarpal bone; the proximal end which articulates with the appropriate carpal bone.

basis ossis me·ta·tar·sa·lis (met″uh·tahr·say′lis) [NA]. The base of a metatarsal bone; the proximal end which articulates with the appropriate tarsal bone.

basis ossis sa·cri (say′krye, sack′rye) [NA]. The base of the sacrum; the cranial surface.

basis os·si·um me·ta·car·pa·li·um (oss′ee·um met″uh·kahr·pay′lee·um) [BNA]. BASIS OSSIS METACARPALIS.

basis ossium me·ta·tar·sa·li·um (met″uh·tahr·say′lee·um) [BNA]. BASIS OSSIS METATARSALIS.

basis pa·tel·lae (pa·tel′ee) [NA]. The base of the patella; the proximal border.

basis pe·dun·cu·li ce·re·bri (pe·dunk′yoo·lye serr′e·brye) [BNA]. Crus cerebri (= CRUS OF THE CEREBRUM).

basis pha·lan·gis di·gi·to·rum ma·nus (fa·lan′jis dij″i·to′rum man′oos, man′us) [NA]. The base of a phalanx of the hand; the proximal end.

basis phalangis digitorum pe·dis (ped′is) [NA]. The base of a phalanx of the foot; the proximal end.

ba·si·sphe·noid (bay″see·sfee′noid) *n.* [*basi-* + *sphenoid*]. The lower part of the sphenoid bone, which embryonically developed as a separate bone.

basis pros·ta·tae (pros′tuh·tee) [NA]. The base of the prostate gland; the portion in contact with the lower part of the urinary bladder.

basis pul·mo·nis (pul·mo′nis) [NA]. The base of a lung; the diaphragmatic surface.

basis py·ra·mi·dis re·na·lis (pi·ram′i·dis re·nay′lis) [NA]. The base of a renal pyramid; the portion of a renal pyramid which is directed toward the surface of a kidney.

basis sta·pe·dis (stay′pe·dis) [NA]. The base of the stapes; the portion which articulates with the vestibular (oval) window.

ba·si·syl·vi·an (bay″see·sil′vee·un) *n.* [*basi-* + *sylvian*]. The transverse basilar portion or stem of the lateral cerebral sulcus of the cerebral hemisphere.

ba·si·tem·po·ral (bay″see·tem′po·rul) *adj.* [*basi-* + *temporal*]. Pertaining to the lower part of the temporal bone.

ba·si·ver·te·bral (bay″see·vur′te·brul) *adj.* [*basi-* + *vertebral*]. Pertaining to the centrum of a vertebra.

bas·ket, *n.* 1. See *basket cells.* 2. A condensation of intracellular neurofibrils seen in Alzheimer's disease.

basket cells. The cells of the cerebellar cortex, the axons of which give off sprays of small branches, which enclose the somata of adjoining Purkinje cells as though in a series of baskets.

basket implant. A fenestrated, acrylic framework designed to be embedded in the eye socket after enucleation, for use as a prosthesis for an artificial eye.

Basle Nomina Anatomica. A list of anatomic terms (in Latin) adopted in Basle, Switzerland, in 1895. Abbreviated, BNA. See also *Nomina Anatomica.*

baso-. A combining form meaning (a) *base, basic;* (b) *basal.*

ba·so·phil (bay′so·fil) *adj.* & *n.* [*baso-* + *-phil*]. 1. BASOPHILIC. 2. A basophilic substance, cell, or tissue element. 3. Specifically, a beta cell of the adenohypophysis.

basophil adenoma. BASOPHILIC ADENOMA.

basophil cell. A cell in which basic dyes stain granules in the cytoplasm or all of the cytoplasm.

ba·so·phile (bay'so·file, ·fil) *n.* & *adj.* BASOPHIL.

basophil granules. Granules staining with basic dyes, especially those of the methylene blue series, or hematoxylin.

basophil granulocyte. BASOPHIL LEUKOCYTE.

ba·so·phil·ia (bay''so·fil'ee·uh) *n.* [*basophil* + *-ia*]. 1. An increased number of basophils in the circulating blood. 2. Stippling of the red cells with basic staining granules, representing a degenerative condition as seen in severe anemia, leukemia, malaria, lead poisoning, and other toxic states. 3. An affinity for basic dyes.

ba·so·phil·ic (bay''so·fil'ick) *adj.* [*basophil* + *-ic*]. Susceptible to staining by basic rather than by acid dyes. Contr. *acidophilic.*

basophilic adenoma. An adenoma of the hypophysis made up of basophil cells. See also *Cushing's syndrome.*

basophilic degeneration. 1. MUCOUS DEGENERATION. 2. BASOPHILIA (2).

basophilic erythroblast (of Fer·ra·ta) (fe·rrah'tah). BASOPHILIC NORMOBLAST.

basophilic leukemia. A granulocytic leukemia in which the predominating cells belong to the basophilic series.

basophilic normoblast. A nucleated red blood cell with coarse, condensed nuclear chromatin, no nucleoli, and a moderate amount of deep blue cytoplasm without hemoglobin.

basophilic tumor of the pituitary. BASOPHILIC ADENOMA.

ba·soph·i·lism (bay·sof'i·liz·um) *n.* BASOPHILIA.

basophil leukocyte. A leukocyte containing granules that contain histamine and heparin and stain deep purple (basic dye) with Wright's stain. The nucleus often shows no distinct lobulation.

ba·so·philo·cyt·ic (bay''so·fil·o·sit'ick) *adj.* [*basophil* + *cyt-* + *-ic*]. BASOPHILIC.

basophilocytic leukemia. BASOPHILIC LEUKEMIA.

ba·soph·i·lous (bay·sof'i·lus) *adj.* BASOPHILIC.

ba·so·pho·bia (bay''so·fo'bee·uh, bas''o·) *n.* [Gk. *basis*, step, + *phobia*]. A morbid fear of walking or standing erect, without muscular impairment. —**basopho·bic** (·bick) *adj.;* **basopho·bi·ac** (·bee·ack) *n.*

ba·so·plasm (bay'so·plaz·um) *n.* The portion of the cytoplasm which readily takes a basic stain.

ba·so·squa·mous (bay''so·skway'mus) *adj.* Pertaining to or composed of basal and squamous cells.

basosquamous carcinoma. A malignant growth of skin, composed of both basal and squamous cells.

bass deafness (bace). Deafness to notes low in pitch, while higher notes are heard.

Bas·sen-Korn·zweig syndrome. ABETALIPOPROTEINEMIA.

Bas·set's operation (ba·seh') [A. *Basset,* French surgeon, 1882–1951]. Radical extirpation of carcinoma of the vulva, including dissection of superficial and deep inguinal nodes.

bas·si·net (bas''i·net') *n.* [F., dim. of *bassin,* basin]. 1. An infant's crib or bed; a wicker basket with a hood at one end, used as a cradle. 2. An infant's crib or bed in a hospital as representative of the services and equipment needed to care for one infant in an obstetrical or pediatric unit.

Bas·si·ni operation (bahs·see'nee) [E. *Bassini,* Italian surgeon, 1844–1924]. A basic hernioplasty in which the inguinal ligament and conjoined tendon are sutured behind the spermatic cord.

bas·so·rin (bas'o·rin) *n.* [*Bassora*, after *Basra,* Iraq, + *-in*]. A water-insoluble constituent of tragacanth and certain other gums.

Bas·tian-Bruns law or **sign** (bas'chun, bas'tyun; broonss) [H. C. *Bastian,* English neurologist, 1837–1925; and L. von *Bruns*]. A complete transverse lesion of the spinal cord above the lumbar enlargement causes complete loss of tendon reflexes of the lower extremities.

Bastian's law. BASTIAN-BRUNS LAW.

bast sheath. PHLOEM SHEATH.

bath, *n.* 1. A washing or immersion for cleansing purpose. 2. A bathing place or room. 3. Any yielding medium such as air, vapor, sand, or water, in which the body is wholly or partially immersed for therapeutic purposes. It may be designed to cleanse, soothe, stimulate, irritate, heat, or cool.

bath-, batho- [Gk. *bathos*]. A combining form meaning (a) *depth;* (b) *downward, lower.*

bath·es·the·sia, bath·aes·the·sia (bath''es·theezh'uh, ·theez'ee·uh) *n.* [*bath-* + *esthesia*]. Deep sensation; muscle, tendon, and joint sensation and pressure sensibility.

bathing-trunk nevus. A congenital anomaly in the clinical form of pigmentation, papules, nodules, and hair in a conglomeration that resembles bathing trunks when located on the lower part of body. Histologically, the lesion consists of ordinary melanocytes.

bath·mo·trop·ic (bath''mo·trop'ick) *adj.* Of or pertaining to bathmotropism; pertaining to any stimulus that increases or lessens the excitability of muscular tissue, especially cardiac tissue.

bath·mot·ro·pism (bath·mot'ruh·piz·um) *n.* [Gk. *bathmos*, step, degree, + *-tropism*]. Influence on the excitability of muscle tissue, used especially in reference to cardiac musculature.

batho-. See *bath-.*

batho·chrome (bath'o·krome) *n.* [*batho-* + *-chrome*]. An atom or a group of atoms that have the effect when introduced into a molecule or ion of displacing the absorption maximum of its spectrum to a lower frequency (greater wavelength). Contr. *hypsochrome.* —**batho·chro·mic** (bath''o·kro'mick) *adj.*

batho·pho·bia (bath''o·fo'bee·uh) *n.* [*batho-* + *-phobia*]. Morbid fear of depths.

bath·ro·ceph·a·ly (bath''ro·sef'uh·lee) *n.* [Gk. *bathron*, platform, scaffold, + *-cephaly*]. A condition in which the skull has a shelflike projection at the squamosal suture of the occipital bone.

bathy- [Gk. *bathys*]. A combining form meaning *deep, low.*

bathy·car·dia (bath''i·kahr'dee·uh) *n.* [*bathy-* + *-cardia*]. An anatomic variant in which the heart is in a lower position than usual within the thorax.

bathy·chrome (bath'i·krome) *n.* BATHOCHROME. —**bathy·chro·mic** (bath·i·kro'mick) *adj.*

bathy·es·the·sia, bathy·aes·the·sia (bath''ee·es·theezh'uh, ·theez'ee·uh) *n.* BATHESTHESIA.

bato·pho·bia (bat''o·fo'bee·uh) *n.* [Gk. *batos*, passable, + *-phobia*]. 1. Dread of passing high objects, as fear of passing near a high building or of going through a deep valley. 2. Morbid fear of being on something of great height.

ba·tra·chi·an (ba·tray'kee·un) *adj.* [Gk. *batrachos,* frog]. Froglike. See also *frog position.*

Bat·son's plexus. VERTEBRAL VENOUS SYSTEM.

bat·ta·rism (bat'uh·riz·um) *n.* Battarismus; stammering.

bat·ta·ris·mus (bat''uh·riz'mus) *n.* [Gk. *battarismos*]. Stammering.

Batten-Bielschowsky-Spielmeyer-Janský disease [F. E. *Batten,* English neurologist, 1865–1918; M. *Bielschowsky,* W. *Spielmeyer,* and J. *Janský*]. BIELSCHOWSKY-JANSKÝ DISEASE.

Bat·ten-Ma·you disease (may'oo) [F. E. *Batten,* and M. S. *Mayou,* English ophthalmologist, 1876–1934]. SPIELMEYER-VOGT DISEASE.

bat·tered-child syndrome. A clinical condition in young children due to serious physical abuse, generally from a parent or foster parent, and a significant cause of childhood disability and death. See also *child abuse.*

bat·tery, *n.* [F. *batterie,* from *battre,* to beat]. 1. A device which converts chemical to electrical energy. 2. A series of two or more pieces of apparatus connected so as to augment their effects, as a battery of boilers, prisms, or galvanic cells. 3. A group or series of things or procedures used similarly or for common purpose, as tests given to a subject for the purpose of diagnosis of disease or of psychological analysis. 4. The unlawful beating of another.

bat·tle·dore (bat'ul·dore) *n.* A paddle or something shaped like a paddle.

battledore hand. The large hand of acromegaly.

battledore placenta. A placenta in which the insertion of the umbilical cord is at the margin.

bat·tle fatigue. WAR NEUROSIS.

Bat·tle's sign [W. H. *Battle,* English surgeon, 1855–1936]. Ecchymosis over the mastoid, or blood behind the tympanic membrane, seen in fractures of the base of the skull.

bat·yl alcohol (bat'il). 3-(Octadecyloxy)-1,2-propanediol, $C_{21}H_{44}O_3$, a crystalline alcohol isolated from shark-liver oil and yellow marrow.

Bau·de·loque's diameter (bo·dlo^h^k') [J. L. *Baudeloque,* French obstetrician, 1746–1810]. EXTERNAL CONJUGATE DIAMETER.

Bau·er's test. GALACTOSE TOLERANCE TEST.

Bau·hin's valve (bo·æn') [G. *Bauhin,* Swiss anatomist, 1560–1624]. ILEOCECAL VALVE.

Bau·mès' sign (bo·mess') [J. B. J. *Baumès,* French physician, 1756–1828]. Retrosternal pain in angina pectoris.

Baum·gar·ten's syndrome [W. *Baumgarten,* U.S. physician, 1873–1945]. CRUVEILHIER-BAUMGARTEN SYNDROME.

Ba·u·ru ulcer (bah·oo·roo') [after *Bauru,* Brazil]. A skin ulcer occurring in American mucocutaneous leishmaniasis.

baux·ite (bawk'site) *n.* [F., from *Les Baux,* France]. A naturally occurring mixture of hydrous aluminum oxides and aluminum hydroxides; the principal source of aluminum.

bauxite fume pneumoconiosis. A type of pulmonary fibrosis observed in the abrasive manufacturing industry and among aluminum workers.

bay·ber·ry (bay'bur·ee, ·berr·ee) *n.* The wax myrtle, *Myrica cerifera* or *M. pennsylvanica.* The dried bark of the root was formerly used as an astringent.

bay·cu·ru (bye·koo'roo) *n.* [Tupi]. The root of a Brazilian plant, *Limonium brasiliensis,* used by the natives as a discutient in glandular swellings and as an astringent gargle.

Bayer 205. The trade name under which suramin sodium was originally introduced.

Baygon. A trademark for *o*-isopropoxyphenol methylcarbamate, $C_{11}H_{15}NO_3$, a widely used insecticide for roach control.

Bayle's disease (be^h^l) [A. L. J. *Bayle,* French physician, 1799–1858]. GENERAL PARALYSIS.

bay oil. The volatile oil from leaves of *Pimenta racemosa;* contains eugenol. A perfume oil.

Baz·ett formula or **index** (baz'it) [H. C. *Bazett,* U.S. physiologist, 1885–1950]. A formula for correction for the heart rate in computing the Q-T interval of the electrocardiogram: K (corrected Q-T interval) = observed Q-T interval/ $\sqrt{\text{cycle length in seconds}}$, normal for K being 0.36 to 0.42.

Ba·zin's disease (ba·zæn') [A. P. E. *Bazin,* French dermatologist, 1807–1878]. ERYTHEMA INDURATUM.

B bile. Bile from the gallbladder.

B cell. B LYMPHOCYTE.

BCG Abbreviation for (a) *bacillus Calmette-Guérin;* (b) *ballistocardiogram* or *ballistocardiograph.*

BCG vaccine [*b*acillus *C*almette-*G*uérin]. A vaccine made from cultures of attenuated bovine tubercle bacilli, used to obtain immunity against tuberculosis.

b.d. Abbreviation for *bis die,* twice a day; used in prescriptions.

B. D. A. British Dental Association.

bdel·li·um (del'ee·um) *n.* [L., from Gk. *bdellion*]. A resinous gum exuding from various species of *Commiphora.* It resembles myrrh and has been used similarly.

Bdel·lo·nys·sus (del''o·nis'us) *n.* [NL., from Gk. *bdella,* leech, + *nyssein,* to sting]. A genus of small parasitic mites. Syn. *Liponyssus.*

Bdellonyssus ba·co·ti (bah·ko'tee). The common rat mite; this species will attack man, producing an uncomfortable dermatitis, and is thought to be a vector of endemic typhus. Syn. *Liponyssus bacoti, Ornithonyssus bacoti.*

bde·lyg·mia (de·lig'mee·uh) *n.* [Gk., nausea]. A morbid loathing of food.

b.d.s. Abbreviation for *bis die sumendum,* to be taken twice a day (= b.i.d.).

Be Symbol for beryllium.

bead·ed, *adj.* 1. Having or formed into, beads. 2. *In bacteriology,* indicating the nonuniform appearance of certain organisms such as *Corynebacterium diphtheriae* when stained.

beaded hair. MONILETHRIX.

beaded lizard. *Heloderma horridum,* a venomous lizard of Mexico related to the Gila monster.

beading of the ribs. RACHITIC ROSARY.

beaked pelvis. A pelvis in which the pubic bones are compressed laterally so as to approach each other, and are pushed forward; a condition seen in osteomalacia.

beam, *n. In radiology and radiobiology,* a directed stream of particles, such as electrons or photons.

bear·ber·ry, *n.* UVA URSI.

Beard's disease [G. M. *Beard,* U.S. physician, 1839–1883]. NEURASTHENIA.

bear·er protein. *Obsol.* APOENZYME.

bear·ing down. 1. The feeling of weight or pressure in the pelvis in pregnancy and certain diseases. 2. Contraction of abdominal muscles during labor, either as a reflex of uterine contractions or in a conscious effort to expel the fetus.

bearing-down pain. 1. A feeling of distress with a sensation of dragging of the pelvic organs; occurs in pelvic inflammatory disease. 2. (usually plural) Pains accompanying bearing down in labor.

beat, *n.* An impulse, throb, or pulsation, as of the heart and blood vessels.

beat·ing, *n. In massage,* percussion movements in which the half-closed fists are brought down alternately in a rapid succession of blows. Movement is largely from the wrist.

Beau's lines (bo) [J. H. S. *Beau,* French physician, 1806–1865]. Transverse depressions seen on the fingernails after an exhausting disease.

bea·ver·tail liver. A liver with a large flat left lobe, suggesting resemblance to the tail of a beaver.

be·bee·rine (be·bee'reen, ·rin) *n.* [*bebeeru* + *-ine*]. The *d-* form of an alkaloid, $C_{36}H_{38}N_2O_6$, from the root of *Cissampelos pareira* or from *Ocotea rodioei* (*Nectandra*). The *l-* form of the alkaloid is curine. Syn. *chondodendrine, pelosine.*

be·bee·ru (be·bee'roo) *n.* [Sp.and Pg. *bibiru*]. A common name for the tropical South American tree *Ocotea rodioei.*

be·can·thone (be·kan'thone) *n.* 1-[[2-[Ethyl(2-hydroxy-2-methylpropyl) amino]ethyl]amino]-4-methylthioxanthen-9-one, $C_{22}H_{28}N_2O_2S$, an antischistosomal compound; used as the hydrochloride salt.

Bechterew. See *Bekhterev.*

Beck·er's disease. COLLAGENOSIS.

Beck's operation [C. S. *Beck,* U.S. surgeon, 1894–1971]. 1. An operation of the pericardium in order to improve the myocardial circulation. See also *cardiomyopexy, cardiopericardiopexy.* 2. Revascularization of the heart by diverting arterial blood into the coronary sinus and its tributaries.

Beck's triad [C. S. *Beck*]. 1. Low arterial blood pressure, high venous pressure, and a quiet heart in acute cardiac compression. 2. Ascites, high venous pressure, and a quiet heart in chronic cardiac compression.

Beck·with-Wie·de·mann syndrome [J. B. *Beckwith,* U.S. pathologist, b. 1933]. Macroglossia, omphalocele, and gigantism; sometimes with the addition of neonatal hypoglycemia, microcephaly, port-wine nevus, and other abnormalities.

bec·lo·meth·a·sone (beck″lo·meth′uh·sone) *n.* 9-Chloro-11β,17,21-trihydroxy-16β-methylpregna-1,4-diene-3,20-dione, $C_{22}H_{29}ClO_5$, a glucocorticoid steroid usually employed as the dipropionate ester.

Bec·que·rel ray (beck·rel′) [A. H. *Becquerel,* French physicist, 1852–1908]. An early term for any emanation from a radioactive substance. The emanations are now known as alpha particles, beta particles, and gamma rays.

bed, *n. In anatomy,* a matrix (as a nail bed) or a network (as a capillary bed).

bed bath. A bath given to a patient in bed.

bed·bug, *n.* A blood-sucking wingless bug, *Cimex lectularius,* which lives and lays its eggs in the crevices of bedsteads, upholstered furniture, and walls. It is apparently not a vector of pathogenic organisms, although it has been suspected.

bed·fast, *adj.* [*bed* + *-fast,* fixed]. BEDRIDDEN.

Bed·nar's aphthae (bed′nahr) [A. *Bednar,* Austrian pediatrician, 1816–1888]. Superficial, transient traumatic erosions on the posterior hard palate in newborn infants; may be due to sucking on the tongue or having the mouth wiped. Secondary infection may occur. Compare *cachectic aphthae.*

bed net. Mosquito netting suspended over the bed, its edges being tucked in about the mattress to prevent the entrance of insects.

bed·pan, *n.* A shallow, suitably shaped receptacle, serving to receive the urine and feces of a person confined to bed.

bed rest. 1. A device to support patients in bed. 2. The keeping of a patient in bed for therapeutic purposes.

bed·rid·den, *adj.* Confined to bed.

Bed·so·nia (bed·so′nee·uh) *n.* CHLAMYDIA.

bed·sore, *n.* DECUBITUS ULCER.

bed traction. Any form of traction in which the patient is of necessity confined to bed.

beef tapeworm. *TAENIA SAGINATA.*

beer-drinkers' cardiomyopathy. Congestive heart failure and nonspecific cardiomyopathy presumed due to cobalt added to beer; encountered among patients consuming large quantities of beer and reversible to some extent after abstinence from beer containing cobalt.

Beer's dye test. A test for renal function in which methylene blue, given orally or intravenously, is normally cleared after many hours. In chronic pyelonephritis, coincident with rupture of the dye-stained abscesses, the urine becomes blue periodically after original clearance is reached.

Beer's law ($be^{y}r$) [A. *Beer,* German physicist, 1825–1863]. The transmittance of light through a stable solution is an exponential function of the product of the concentration of solute and the length of path in the solution.

beer test. A test in which the patient drinks a quantity of beer or other alcoholic drink in order to encourage reactivation of a chronic gonorrhea.

bees·wax, *n.* Wax obtained from honeycombs. See also *yellow wax.*

bee·tle, *n.* [OE. *bitula,* from *bītan,* to bite]. Any insect of the order Coleoptera distinguished by a leathery integument, mandibulate mouth parts, and two pairs of wings: the front pair, which are horny and nonfunctional as organs of flight, and under these the hind pair, which are functional and folded when the insect is at rest.

beetle disease. SCARABIASIS.

beet sugar. Sucrose from sugar beets.

beet·uria (bee·tew′ree·uh) *n.* [*beet* + *-uria*]. Red discoloration of the urine as a result of eating beets.

Bee·vor's sign [C. E. *Beevor,* English neurologist, 1854–1908]. 1. On sitting up from the recumbent position, the umbilicus is displaced upward because of paralysis of the inferior portion of the rectus abdominis muscles. 2. Overaction of antagonistic muscles seen in the paralysis of hysterical neurosis.

be·hav·ior, be·hav·iour (be·hay′vyur) *n.* 1. The sum total of responses of an organism to internal and external stimuli; loosely, anything an organism does. 2. Observable activity directly correlated with psychic processes. —**behavior·al, behaviour·al** (·ul) *adj.*

behavioral science. Any science, such as psychology, social anthropology, or sociology, employing observational and experimental methods in studying the actions and conduct of human beings or animals within their physical and social environment.

be·hav·ior·ism, be·hav·iour·ism (be·hay′vyur·iz·um) *n.* A school of psychology, concerned with observable, tangible, and measurable data, such as behavior and human activities, but excluding ideas and emotions as purely subjective phenomena.

be·hav·ior·is·tic (be·hay″vyur·is′tick) *adj.* 1. Of or pertaining to behaviorism. 2. BEHAVIORAL.

behavioristic therapy. BEHAVIOR THERAPY.

behavior reflex. CONDITIONED REFLEX.

behavior therapy. *In psychiatry,* an approach to the treatment of overt disturbed human behavior and emotions, regarded as evidence of faulty learning and as maladaptive and undesirable conditioned responses, by dealing with the symptoms themselves through extinguishing the undesirable conditioned responses and establishing desirable ones according to the principles of modern learning theory.

Beh·çet's disease or **syndrome** (behh′chet) [H. *Behçet,* Turkish dermatologist, 1889–1948]. A multisystem disease of unknown cause, seen particularly in young males, characterized by recurrent pyoderma, mucous membrane ulceration, iridocyclitis with hypopyon, arthralgia, thrombophlebitis, and neurologic abnormalities.

be·hen·ic acid (be·hen′ick). Docosanoic acid, $CH_3(CH_2)_{20}COOH$; a waxy solid isolated from many fats and oils.

Behre's test. A test for acetone in which vapor from hot urine containing acetone reacts with salicylic aldehyde and sodium hydroxide to produce a pink to rose color.

Bei·gel's disease (bye′gul) [H. *Beigel,* German physician, 1830–1879]. PIEDRA.

bej·el (bej′ul) *n.* [Ar. *bajal*]. An infectious nonvenereal treponemal disease, occurring principally in children in the Middle East; the infecting organism is undistinguishable from *Treponema pallidum.*

Bé·késy audiometry [G. von *Békésy,* U.S. physiologist, b. 1899]. A specialized audiometric technique using continuous and interrupted tones to aid in determining the site of a lesion in the auditory system.

Bekh·te·rev-Men·del reflex ($be^{k}h't^{y}e \cdot r^{y}uf$) [V. M. *Bekhterev,* Russian neurologist, 1857–1927; and K. *Mendel*]. 1. Plantar flexion of the toes in a patient with corticospinal tract disease, elicited by tapping or stroking the dorsum of the foot over the cuboid bone or the fourth or fifth metatarsals. A normal person exhibits slight dorsoflexion of the toes or no response. 2. CARPOPHALANGEAL REFLEX (1).

Bekhterev's arthritis or **disease** [V. M. *Bekhterev*]. ANKYLOSING SPONDYLITIS.

Bekhterev's deep reflex [V. M. *Bekhterev*]. In corticospinal tract disease, sudden release of one foot bent firmly but passively in the plantar direction may result in dorsiflexion of the foot with flexion of the knee and hip.

Bekhterev's fibers or **layer** [V. M. *Bekhterev*]. KAES'S LAYER.

Bekhterev's nucleus [V. M. *Bekhterev*]. SUPERIOR VESTIBULAR NUCLEUS.

Bekhterev's reaction [V. M. *Bekhterev*]. In tetany, repetition of the minimum strength of electric current necessary to initiate muscular contraction will cause tetanic contraction unless the strength is diminished at every interruption of current or change in density.

Bekhterev's reflex [V. M. *Bekhterev*]. 1. BEKHTEREV-MENDEL REFLEX (1). 2. CARPOPHALANGEAL REFLEX (1). 3. BEKHTE-

REV'S DEEP REFLEX. 4. HYPOGASTRIC REFLEX. 5. NASAL REFLEX. 6. PARADOXICAL PUPILLARY REFLEX.

Bekhterev's sign [V. M. *Bekhterev*]. 1. BEKHTEREV'S REFLEX. 2. Loss of automatic movements of the face with retention of voluntary movement. 3. Anesthesia of the skin bounding the popliteal fossa, sometimes seen in tabes dorsalis.

¹bel, *n.* [A. G. *Bell,* U.S. inventor, 1847–1922]. A unit frequently used to measure the intensity of sound, commonly the intensity above the normal threshold of hearing. See also *decibel.*

²bel, *n.* [Hindi]. The dried, half-ripe fruit of *Aegle marmelos,* or baelfruit of India. It has been used as a remedy for chronic diarrhea and dysentery. The ripe fruit is slightly laxative. Syn. *belae fructus, Bengal quince.*

bel·ae fruc·tus (bel'ee fruck'tus). ²BEL.

belch, *n. & v.* 1. The eruption of gas from the stomach through the mouth. 2. To erupt gas from the stomach through the mouth.

Belgian Congo anemia. KASAI.

bell, *n.* In the jargon of sports medicine, the dazed state following a blow to the head.

bel·la·don·na (bel''uh·don'uh) *n.* [It., fine lady]. Deadly nightshade. A perennial plant, *Atropa belladonna,* of the order Solanaceae, indigenous to southern Europe and Asia and cultivated in the United States. Its properties are due chiefly to its content of hyoscyamine, which under certain conditions is racemized to atropine. Both leaves and root are employed, in various dosage and application forms. It is used as an antispasmodic, as a cardiac and respiratory stimulant, to check secretions (such as sweat and milk), and as an anodyne. See also *atropine.*

bel·la·don·nine (bel''uh·don'een, ·in) *n.* [*belladonna* + *-ine*]. An alkaloid, $C_{34}H_{42}N_2O_4$, found in solanaceous plants such as belladonna and hyoscyamus.

bell-crowned, *adj.* Pertaining to a tooth with a crown that is large near the occlusal surface and tapers sharply toward the neck.

belle in·dif·fé·rence (bel aeⁿ·dee·fay·rahⁿce') [F., total unconcern]. *In psychiatry,* the inappropriate lack of concern for their disabilities and the implications thereof, characteristic of certain patients with the conversion type of hysterical neurosis.

Belle·vue scale [*Bellevue* Hospital, New York City]. WECHSLER-BELLEVUE INTELLIGENCE SCALE.

Bel·ling's acetocarmine stain. Acetocarmine to which an iron salt is added; used for chromosomes.

Bell-Magendie law [C. *Bell* and F. *Magendie*]. BELL'S LAW.

bel·lones (be·lohnz') *n.* [Sp.]. Partial nasal obstruction in horses due to polyps in the posterior nares and sometimes associated with roaring.

bellows sound or **murmur.** An endocardial murmur that sounds like a bellows.

Bell's disease [C. *Bell,* Scottish surgeon and physiologist, 1774–1842]. BELL'S PALSY.

Bell's law [C. *Bell*]. 1. The ventral roots of the spinal cord are motor and the dorsal roots sensory in function. 2. In a reflex arc, the nerve impulse can be conducted in one direction only.

Bell's mania [L. V. *Bell,* U.S. physician, 1806–1862]. The acute excitement seen in the manic type of manic-depressive illness.

Bell's muscle [C. *Bell*]. MUSCLE OF BELL.

bell sound. COIN SOUND.

Bell's palsy or **paralysis** [C. *Bell*]. Peripheral paralysis or weakness of muscles innervated by the facial nerve, of unknown cause.

Bell's phenomenon or **sign** [C. *Bell*]. When the eyelids are forcibly closed, the eyes are turned sharply upward, due to the reflex association of the superior rectus with the orbicularis muscle; in peripheral facial palsy or paralysis, the attempt to close the eye on the affected side is accompanied by the turning of the eyeball upward, and the lid that is meant to close opens widely.

Bell's spasm [C. *Bell*]. 1. FACIAL HEMISPASM. 2. POSTPARALYTIC FACIAL SPASM.

bell tympany. COIN SOUND.

bel·ly, *n.* [OE. *baelig,* bag, skin]. 1. The abdominal cavity or abdomen. 2. Of a muscle: the most prominent, fleshy, central portion.

belly button. UMBILICUS.

belly of a muscle. The most prominent, fleshy, central portion of a muscle. NA *venter musculi.*

bel·o·ne·pho·bia (bel''o·ne·fo'bee·uh) *n.* [Gk. *belonē,* needle, + *-phobia*]. A morbid dread of pins and needles, and of sharp-pointed objects in general.

bel·ox·a·mide (bel·ock'suh·mide) *n.* *N*-(Benzyloxy)-*N*-(3-phenylpropylacetamide), $C_{18}H_{21}NO_2$, an anticholesteremic agent.

bem·e·gride (bem'e·gride, ·grid) *n.* 3-Ethyl-3-methylglutarimide, $C_8H_{13}NO_2$, an analeptic used in the management of acute barbiturate intoxication.

ben·ac·ty·zine (ben·ack'ti·zeen) *n.* 2-Diethylaminoethylbenzilate, $C_{20}H_{25}NO_3$, an anticholinergic compound employed as a tranquilizer in the management of neuroses; used as the hydrochloride salt.

Ben·a·cus (ben'uh·kus) *n.* A genus of water bugs.

Benacus gris·cus (gris'kus). A species of *Benacus* known as the giant water bug which inflicts a bite that is painful, but not poisonous, to human beings.

Benadryl. Trademark for diphenhydramine, an antihistaminic agent used as the hydrochloride salt.

ben·a·pry·zine (ben''uh·prye'zeen) *n.* 2-(Ethylpropylamino)ethyl benzilate, $C_{21}H_{27}NO_3$, an anticholinergic agent, usually used as the hydrochloride salt.

ben·a·zo·line (ben·ay'zo·leen) *n.* 2-[(2-Methylbenzo[*b*]thien-3-yl)methyl]-2-imidazoline, $C_{13}H_{14}N_2S$, a vasoconstrictor employed as a nasal decongestant; used as the hydrochloride salt.

Bence Jones cylinders [H. *Bence Jones,* English physician, 1813–1873]. Cylindrical material from the seminiferous tubules which occasionally appears in the urine.

Bence Jones protein [H. *Bence Jones*]. An abnormal protein, usually consisting of immunoglobulin light chains, found in the urine of some patients with myeloma.

Bence Jones protein test [H. *Bence Jones*]. A precipitate appearing when urine is heated to 50 to 60°C, disappearing at the boiling point, and reappearing on cooling indicates the presence of Bence Jones protein.

bench surgery. Surgery performed on an organ (such as a kidney) that has been removed from the body, to be reimplanted immediately after the operation. Syn. *ex vivo surgery.*

Ben·da's test (bæⁿ·dah') [R. *Benda,* French physician, b. 1896]. Injection of epinephrine causes in normal persons an outpouring of young cells from the spleen and marrow into the blood, but not in persons with anemia; the number of monocytes, however, may rise.

ben·da·zac (ben'duh·zack) *n.* [(1-Benzyl-1*H*-indazol-3-yl)oxy]acetic acid, $C_{16}H_{14}N_2O_3$, an anti-inflammatory drug.

Ben·der gestalt test [Lauretta *Bender,* U.S. neuropsychiatrist, b. 1897]. A diagnostic and experimental psychological test in which the subject reproduces a series of nine simple designs. Deviations from the originals are interpreted in terms of gestalt laws of perception and organization; especially useful in the diagnosis of visual-motor deficits.

bending reflex. Passive palmar flexion of the wrist results normally in flexion of the elbow; in frontal lobe lesions the associated response in the proximal muscles may be greatly increased.

Bendopa. Trademark for levodopa, an antiparkinsonian agent.

ben·dro·flu·me·thi·a·zide (ben''dro·floo''me·thigh'uh·zide) *n.*

3-Benzyl-3,4-dihydro-6-(trifluoromethyl)-2*H*-1,2,4-benzothiadiazine-7-sulfonamide 1,1-dioxide, $C_{15}H_{14}F_3N_3O_4S_2$, an orally effective diuretic and antihypertensive agent.

bends, *n.* [from the writhing and arching of the back in pain]. The dull, throbbing, progressive, shifting pain of the muscles, bones, and joints in decompression sickness.

Ben·e·dict and Franke's method [S. R. *Benedict*, U.S. chemist, 1884–1936]. A test for uric acid in urine in which diluted urine is treated with arsenophosphotungstic acid reagent and sodium cyanide and the blue color compared with a standard uric acid solution similarly treated.

Benedict and Hitch·cock's reagent [S. R. *Benedict*]. A phosphate reagent used for blood uric acid testing.

Benedict and New·ton's method [S. R. *Benedict*]. A blood protein precipitation method employing tungstomolybdic acid.

Benedict and Theis's method [S. R. *Benedict*]. A test for inorganic phosphates in which a trichloroacetic acid filtrate of serum is treated with molybdic acid and reduced with hydroquinone sulfite reagent.

Benedict's method [S. R. *Benedict*]. 1. Glucose in the urine is estimated by titrating the urine with Benedict's quantitative reagent. 2. Sulfur in the urine is estimated by adding urine to Benedict's sulfur reagent. 3. A test for uric acid in which a tungstic acid blood filtrate is mixed with acid lithium chloride and silver nitrate.

Benedict's picrate method [S. R. *Benedict*]. A test for glucose in urine in which color produced by picric acid reduction is compared with permanent inorganic standards which represent definite concentrations of sugar.

Benedict's solution [S. R. *Benedict*]. An easily reduced solution containing copper sulfate; used in urine tests for glucose and other reducing substances.

Benedict's test [S. R. *Benedict*]. A qualitative test for glucose and other reducing sugars, the presence of which is established by reduction of a blue cupric salt in alkaline solution with formation of a green, yellow, or red precipitate. May also be performed quantitatively.

Benedict's uric acid reagent [S. R. *Benedict*]. A solution of sodium tungstate and of arsenic, phosphoric, and hydrochloric acids; used for determining blood uric acid.

Be·ne·dikt's syndrome (beʸ'ne·dikt) [M. *Benedikt*, Austrian physician, 1835–1920]. Ipsilateral oculomotor paralysis and contralateral cerebellar ataxia, tremor, and corticospinal tract signs, caused by a lesion of the midbrain involving the oculomotor and red nuclei. Involvement of the cerebral peduncle causes contralateral hemiparesis, and extension to the medial lemniscus, contralateral loss of position and tactile sensation.

Benemid. Trademark for probenecid, a uricosuric agent.

Bengal quince. ²BEL.

be·nign (be·nine') *adj.* [L. *benignus*, kind]. Not malignant.

benign acanthosis nigricans. Acanthosis nigricans due to a hereditary factor.

be·nig·nant (be·nig'nant) *adj.* BENIGN.

benign congenital hypotonia. A term devised by Walton to designate a condition of infants who manifest limp and flabby limbs and delay in sitting up and walking and who improve gradually, some completely and others incompletely.

benign hemangioendothelioma. HEMANGIOENDOTHELIOMA (1).

benign intracranial hypertension. PSEUDOTUMOR CEREBRI.

benign juvenile melanoma. JUVENILE MELANOMA.

benign leprosy. TUBERCULOID LEPROSY.

benign lymphocytic choriomeningitis or **meningitis.** LYMPHOCYTIC CHORIOMENINGITIS.

benign lymphogranulomatosis. SARCOIDOSIS.

benign lymphoma. *Obsol.* A misnomer for nodular lymphoma.

benign M-component hypergammaglobulinemia. The increased concentration in serum of M-component in individuals with no clinical disease, as seen particularly in advanced age, or with benign skin disease such as lichen myxedematosis.

benign migratory glossitis. Chronic glossitis characterized by local areas of inflammation and atrophy of filiform papillae. Such areas may change shape or location. Syn. *geographic tongue, wandering rash, glossitis areata exfoliativa.*

benign mucosal pemphigoid. A skin disease of unknown cause in which bullae and areas of epithelial loss occur on the orificial mucous membranes, especially those of the mouth and eyes; scarring may follow. Syn. *cicatricial pemphigoid.*

benign myalgic encephalomyelitis. Fatigue, headache, intense muscle pain, slight or transient muscle weakness and mental disturbances, but usually normal cerebrospinal fluid findings, occurring in epidemics and thought to be viral in origin. Syn. *Akureyri disease, epidemic neuromyasthenia, Iceland disease.*

benign nephrosclerosis. ARTERIAL NEPHROSCLEROSIS.

benign osteoblastoma. OSTEOBLASTOMA (1).

benign paroxysmal peritonitis. FAMILIAL MEDITERRANEAN FEVER.

benign paroxysmal vertigo (of childhood). A variety of vestibular neuronitis, occurring in young children, characterized by sudden onset, brief duration of instability which may be so severe as to immobilize the child, normal hearing and absence of tinnitus, but frequently nystagmus, pallor, sweating, and vomiting during the attacks, which are recurrent but which cease spontaneously after a period of a few months or years. Caloric tests show disordered vestibular function in the form of unilateral or bilateral moderate, severe, or complete paresis.

benign prolinuria. A defect in renal tubular reabsorption resulting in the presence of large amounts of proline, hydroxyproline, and glycine in the urine, found in association with many disease states. It may be harmless. See also *glycinuria, hyperprolinemia, Joseph's syndrome.*

benign recurrent endothelial-leukocytic meningitis. MOLLARET'S MENINGITIS.

benign recurrent meningitis. MOLLARET'S MENINGITIS.

benign reticulosis. CAT-SCRATCH DISEASE.

benign tertian malaria. VIVAX MALARIA.

Benison. A trademark for the 17-benzoate ester of betamethasone, a synthetic glucocorticoid.

ben·ne oil (ben'ee). SESAME OIL.

Ben·nett angle [N. G. *Bennett*, English dental surgeon, 1870–1947]. The angle formed by the sagittal plane and the path of the advancing condyle during lateral mandibular movement as viewed in the horizontal plane.

Bennett movement [N. G. *Bennett*]. The bodily lateral movement or lateral shift of the mandible resulting from the movements of the condyles along the lateral inclines of the mandibular fossae in lateral jaw movement.

Bennett's cells [J. H. *Bennett*, English obstetrician, 1816–1891]. Large fat-filled cells found in degenerated ovarian cysts.

Bennett's fracture [E. H. *Bennett*, Irish surgeon, 1837–1907]. An oblique and usually unstable fracture of the base of the thumb metacarpal extending from the radial metaphyseal flare to the middle of the carpometacarpal articular surface.

Benn·hold's test [H. *Bennhold*, German physician, b. 1893]. CONGO RED TEST.

Benoquin. A trademark for monobenzone, a melanin pigment-inhibiting agent.

be·nor·ter·one (be·nor'tur·ohn) *n.* 17β-Hydroxy-17-methyl-*B*-norandrost-4-en-3-one, $C_{19}H_{28}O_2$, a steroid with antiandrogen activity.

ben·ox·i·nate (ben·ock'si·nate) *n.* 2-Diethylaminoethyl 4-amino-3-butoxybenzoate, $C_{17}H_{28}N_2O_3$, a surface anesthetic agent useful in ophthalmology; used as the hydrochloride salt.

Benoxyl. A trademark for benzoyl peroxide, employed as an antiseptic.

ben·per·i·dol (ben·perr'i·dol) *n.* 1-{1-[3-(*p*-Fluorobenzoyl)-propyl]-4-piperidyl}-2-benzimidazolinone, $C_{22}H_{24}FN_3O_2$, a tranquilizer.

ben·sa·lan (ben'suh·lan) *n.* 3,5-Dibromo-*N*-(*p*-bromobenzyl)salicylamide, $C_{14}H_{10}Br_3NO_2$, a germicide.

ben·ton·ite (ben'tun·ite) *n.* [after Fort *Benton,* Montana]. A native, colloidal, hydrated aluminum silicate. It swells in water and is useful in the preparation of pastes and lotions and as a suspending agent for insoluble medicaments in mixtures and emulsions.

Bentyl. Trademark for dicyclomine, a spasmolytic agent used as the hydrochloride salt.

ben·ure·stat (ben·yoor'e·stat) *n.* 2-(*p*-Chlorobenzamido)-acetohydroxamic acid, $C_9H_9ClN_2O_3$, a urease inhibitor.

benz-, benzo-. A combining form meaning (a) *benzene;* (b) *presence of the benzene ring.*

benz·al·de·hyde (ben·zal'de·hide) *n.* [*benz-* + *aldehyde*]. C_6H_5CHO. A colorless liquid, used as a flavoring agent and in the synthesis of drugs or perfumes.

benz·al·ko·ni·um chloride (ben"zal·ko'nee·um) [*benz-* + *alkyl* + *ammonium*]. A mixture of alkyl dimethylbenzylammonium chlorides of the general formula $C_6H_5CH_2N(CH_3)_2RCl$, in which R represents a mixture of alkyl radicals from C_8H_{17} to $C_{18}H_{37}$. A white or yellowish white powder or in gelatinous pieces; soluble in water. It is an effective surface disinfectant which is germicidal for many pathogenic, nonsporulating bacteria and fungi.

benz·an·thra·cene (ben·zan'thruh·seen) *n.* [*benz-* + *anthracene*]. 1,2-Benzanthracene, $C_{18}H_{12}$, a hydrocarbon occurring in coal tar which has carcinogenic activity.

Benzapas. Trademark for calcium benzoylpas, an antituberculous drug.

ben·za·thine penicillin G (ben'zuh·theen). *N,N'*-Dibenzylethylenediamine dipenicillin G, a penicillin of low water solubility that yields effective blood levels of the antibiotic for a prolonged period after injection and is relatively stable in the stomach after oral administration.

benz·az·o·line (benz·az'o·lin, ·leen) *n.* TOLAZOLINE.

Benzedrex. Trademark for propylhexedrine, a volatile sympathomimetic used by inhalation as a vasoconstrictor to relieve nasal congestion.

Benzedrine. A trademark for amphetamine, a central nervous system stimulant used mainly as the sulfate salt.

ben·zene (ben'zeen, ben·zeen') *n.* [*benzoin* + *-ene*]. An aromatic hydrocarbon, C_6H_6, obtained chiefly as a by-product in the manufacture of coke. It is a clear, colorless, highly flammable liquid of characteristic odor, miscible with many organic liquids. It is extensively used as a solvent and in synthesis. Inhalation of its fumes may be toxic. Syn. *benzol.*

ben·zene car·box·yl·ic acid. (ben"zeen·kahr"bock·sil'ick). BENZOIC ACID.

benzene hexachloride. The designation commonly, though incorrectly, applied to commerical mixtures of stereoisomers of 1,2,3,4,5,6-hexachlorocyclohexane ($C_6H_6Cl_6$), employed as insecticides. The gamma isomer, a purified grade of which is called lindane, is of greatest entomological and medical interest. Abbreviated, BHC.

benzene ring. The arrangement of atoms in benzene whereby six carbon atoms are joined in a hexagonal ring by a bonding structure which is a hybrid between single and double bonds. See also *resonance (3).*

ben·zes·trol (ben·zes'trol) *n.* [*benz-* + *estrogen* + *-ol*]. 4,4'-(1,2-Diethyl-3-methyltrimethylene)diphenol, $C_{20}H_{26}O_2$, in the isomeric form having greatest estrogenic activity; orally effective as an estrogen.

ben·ze·tho·ni·um chloride (ben"ze·tho'nee·um). Benzyldimethyl {2-[2-(*p*-1,1,3,3-tetramethylbutylphenoxy)ethoxy]ethyl}ammonium chloride, $C_{27}H_{42}ClNO_2$, a local anti-infective cationic detergent employed as a germicide and antiseptic.

ben·zet·i·mide (ben·zet'i·mide) *n.* 2-(1-Benzyl-4-piperidyl)-2-phenylglutarimide, $C_{23}H_{26}N_2O_2$, an antiparkinson drug used as the hydrochloride salt.

benz·hex·ol (benz·heck'sol) *n.* TRIHEXYPHENIDYL.

ben·zi·dine (ben'zi·deen) *n.* *p*-Diaminodiphenyl, $NH_2C_6H_4C_6H_4NH_2$, formerly used as a reagent for the detection of blood and in certain other tests depending on the presence of peroxidase. Generally replaced because of demonstrated carcinogenicity.

ben·zi·lo·ni·um bromide (ben"zi·lo'nee·um). 1,1-Diethyl-3-hydroxypyrrolidinium bromide benzilate, $C_{22}H_{28}BrNO_3$, an anticholinergic agent.

benz·im·id·az·ole (benz"im·id'uh·zole) *n.* [*benz-* + *imidazole*]. 1. The dicyclic compound $C_7H_6N_2$, representing the fusion of a benzene and an imidazole ring. 2. Any derivative of the preceding.

ben·zin, ben·zine (ben'zin, ben'zeen, ben·zeen') *n.* [*benz-* + *-in*]. A mixture mainly of aliphatic hydrocarbons obtained in the fractional distillation of petroleum. See also *petroleum ether, ligroin.*

benz·in·do·py·rine (benz"in·do·pye'reen) *n.* 1-Benzyl-3-[2-(4-pyridyl)ethyl]indole, $C_{22}H_{20}N_2$, a tranquilizer; used as the hydrochloride salt.

benzo-. See *benz-.*

ben·zo·ate (ben'zo·ate) *n.* [*benzo-* + *-ate*]. Any salt or ester of benzoic acid, as sodium benzoate or ethyl benzoate.

ben·zo·caine (ben'zo·kane) *n.* [*benzo-* + *-caine*]. ETHYL AMINOBENZOATE.

benz·oc·ta·mine (benz·ock'tuh·meen) *n.* *N*-Methyl-9,10-ethanoanthracene-9(10*H*)-methylamine, $C_{18}H_{19}N$, a muscle relaxant and sedative; used as the hydrochloride salt.

ben·zo·depa (ben"zo·dep'uh) *n.* Benzyl [bis(1-aziridinyl)-phosphinyl]carbamate, $C_{12}H_{16}N_3O_3P$, an antineoplastic compound.

ben·zo·di·az·e·pine (ben"zo·dye·az'e·peen) *n.* Any of a class of structurally related compounds, as chlordiazepoxide, diazepam, and oxazepam, having sedative, anticonvulsant, and skeletal muscle relaxant properties; used for treatment of anxiety and various other purposes.

ben·zo·di·ox·ane, ben·zo·di·ox·an (ben"zo·dye·ock"san) *n.* [*benzo-* + *dioxane*]. 1. Either of two isomeric dicyclic substances, $C_8H_8O_2$, identified as 1,3-benzodioxane and 1,4-benzodioxane, respectively. 2. A generic term for any derivative of the preceding, as piperoxan, which is 2-(1-piperidylmethyl)-1,4-benzodioxane, an adrenergic blocking agent.

benzodioxane test. A test for pheochromocytoma in which a benzodioxane derivative, functioning as an adrenergic blocking agent, is injected intravenously; hypotensive effect for 10 minutes or longer is characteristic of pheochromocytoma.

ben·zo·ic acid (ben·zo'ick). Benzenecarboxylic acid, C_6H_5COOH, white scales or needles; used as a preservative and mild antiseptic.

benzoic aldehyde. BENZALDEHYDE.

ben·zoin (ben'zoin, ·zo·in, ben·zo'in) *n.* [MF. *benjoin,* from Ar. *lubān jāwī,* Javanese frankincense]. A balsamic resin obtained from *Styrax benzoin, S. tonkinensis,* and other species of *Styrax.* It is used as a stimulating expectorant, as an inhalant in respiratory tract inflammations, and as an external antiseptic and protective. Syn. *gum benjamin, gum benzoin.* —**ben·zoi·nat·ed** (ben·zo'i·nay"tid) *adj.*

benzoin flowers. Benzoic acid, especially that obtained by sublimation from benzoin.

ben·zol, ben·zole (ben'zole) *n.* [*benz-* + *-ol*]. BENZENE.

ben·zo·na·tate (ben·zo'nuh·tate) *n.* ω-Methoxypoly(ethyleneoxy)ethyl-*p*-butylaminobenzoate, $C_{30}H_{53}NO_{11}$, an antitussive drug.

ben·zo·ni·trile (ben"zo·nigh'tril, ·treel) *n.* [*benzo-* + *nitrile*].

Phenyl cyanide, C_6H_5CN, a colorless, flammable liquid; used in organic synthesis.

ben·zo·phe·none (ben″zo·fe·nohn′) *n.* [*benzo-* + *-phenone*]. Diphenyl ketone, $(C_6H_5)_2CO$, a crystalline solid; used in organic synthesis.

ben·zo·qui·none (ben″zo·kwi·nohn′) *n.* QUINONE (1).

ben·zo·qui·non·i·um chloride (ben″zo·kwi·no′nee·um). 2,5-*bis*(3-Diethylaminopropylamino)benzoquinone-*bis*-benzyl chloride, $C_{34}H_{50}Cl_2N_4O_2$, a skeletal-muscle relaxant.

Benzosol. A trademark for guaiacol benzoate.

ben·zo·sul·fi·mide (ben″zo·sul′fi·mide, ·mid) *n.* [*benzo-* + *sulf-* + *imide*]. SACCHARIN.

benz·ox·i·quine (ben·zock′si·kwin) *n.* 8-Quinolinol benzoate (ester), $C_{16}H_{11}NO_2$, a disinfectant.

ben·zo·yl (ben′zo·il, ·eel) *n.* [*benzo-* + *-yl*]. The univalent radical C_6H_5CO, derived from benzoic acid.

benzoyl chloride. C_6H_5COCl, a pungent liquid; used in organic synthesis and as a reagent, and formerly as a local application to ulcerating surfaces.

benzoyl coenzyme A. An intermediate compound in the formation of hippuric acid from benzoic acid and coenzyme A.

ben·zo·yl·ec·go·nine (ben″zo·il·eck′go·neen, ·nin) *n.* [*benzoyl* + *ecgonine*]. An alkaloidal constituent, $C_{16}H_{19}NO_4$, of certain varieties of coca leaves; also produced by boiling an aqueous solution of cocaine.

ben·zo·yl·gly·cine (ben″zo·il·glye′seen, ·sin) *n.* [*benzoyl* + *glycine*]. HIPPURIC ACID.

benzoyl green. MALACHITE GREEN.

ben·zo·yl·guai·a·col (ben″zo·il·gwye′uh·kol) *n.* [*benzoyl* + *guaiacol*]. GUAIACOL BENZOATE.

ben·zo·yl·meth·yl·ec·go·nine (ben″zo·il·meth″il·eck′go·neen, ·nin) *n.* COCAINE.

ben·zo·yl·pas calcium (ben″zo·il′paz). Calcium 4-benzamidosalicylate, $C_{28}H_{20}CaN_2O_8 \cdot 5H_2O$, a tuberculostatic agent.

benzoyl peroxide. $(C_6H_5CO)_2O_2$, a crystalline solid; used in organic synthesis and by topical application in skin diseases and burns as a keratolytic.

benz·phet·a·mine (benz·fet′a·meen) *n.* *N*-Benzyl-*N*,α-dimethylphenethylamine, $C_{17}H_{21}N$, an anorexigenic drug; used as the hydrochloride salt.

benz·py·rene (benz·pye′reen) *n.* [*benz-* + *pyrene*]. A carcinogenic hydrocarbon, $C_{20}H_{12}$, occurring in coal tar. Used as a flurochrome for fats.

benz·pyr·in·i·um bromide (benz″pye·rin′ee·um). 1-Benzyl-3-hydroxypyridinium bromide dimethylcarbamate, $C_{15}H_{17}BrN_2O_2$, a cholinergic agent having the actions and uses of neostigmine.

benz·quin·a·mide (benz·kwin′uh·mide) *n.* *N,N*-Diethyl-1,3,-4,6,7,11b-hexahydro-2-hydroxy-9,10-dimethoxy-2*H*-benzo[*a*]quinolizine-3-carboxamide acetate, $C_{22}H_{32}N_2O_5$, a tranquilizer.

benz·thi·a·zide (benz·thigh′uh·zide) *n.* 3-[(Benzylthio)methyl]-6-chloro-2*H*-1,2,4-benzothiadiazine-7-sulfonamide 1,1-dioxide, $C_{15}H_{14}ClN_3O_4S_3$, an orally effective diuretic and antihypertensive agent.

benz·tro·pine (benz·tro′peen) *n.* 3-Diphenylmethoxytropane, $C_{21}H_{25}NO$, a parasympatholytic drug with anticholinergic, antihistaminic, and local anesthetic activity; used as the mesylate (methanesulfonate) in the symptomatic treatment of parkinsonism.

ben·zyd·a·mine (ben·zid′uh·meen) *n.* 1-Benzyl-3-[3-(dimethylamino) propoxy]-1*H*-indazole, $C_{19}H_{23}N_3O$, an analgesic and antipyretic agent, usually used as the hydrochloride.

ben·zyl (ben′zil, ·zeel) *n.* [*benz-* + *-yl*]. The univalent radical $C_6H_5CH_2$—.

benzyl alcohol. Phenylmethyl alcohol, $C_6H_5CH_2OH$, a colorless liquid; employed as a local anesthetic on mucous membranes and as a bacteriostatic agent. Syn. *phenylcarbinol.*

benzyl benzoate. $C_6H_5CH_2CO_2CH_2C_6H_5$, a colorless, oily liquid; used as a scabicide.

benzyl bromide. $C_6H_6CH_2Br$. A colorless liquid; has been used as a lacrimator in chemical warfare.

benzyl cinnamate. A constituent of cinnamein from Peruvian balsam.

ben·zyl·i·dene (ben·zil′i·deen) *n.* [*benzyl* + *-idene*]. The divalent radical C_6H_5CH=.

ben·zyl·par·a·ben (ben″zil·păr′uh·ben) *n.* Benzyl *p*-hydroxybenzoate, $C_{14}H_{12}O_3$, used as a preservative for medicinal agents.

be·phen·i·um hy·droxy·naph·tho·ate (be·fen′ee·um high·drock′see·naf′tho·ate). Benzyldimethyl(2-phenoxyethyl)-ammonium 3-hydroxy-2-naphthoate(1:1), $C_{28}H_{29}NO_4$, an anthelmintic used in the treatment of hookworm.

ber·ber·ine (bur′bur·een, ·in) *n.* An alkaloid, $C_{20}H_{19}NO_5$, found in berberis and many other plants. Used as a reagent for staining blood protozoa and tubercle bacilli.

ber·ber·is (bur′bur·is) *n.* [NL., from Ar. *barbārīs*]. The dried rhizome and roots of various shrubs of the genus *Mahonia;* formerly used as a bitter tonic. The chief constituents are berberine and resin. Syn. *barberry.*

ber·ga·mot oil (bur′guh·mot). A volatile oil from the rind of the fresh fruit of *Citrus bergamia,* containing linalyl acetate; used as a perfume and insecticide.

Ber·ga·ra-Wartenberg sign. WARTENBERG'S SIGN (1).

Berg·en·hem's operation (bær′yen·heym) [B. L. *Bergenhem,* Swedish surgeon, b. 1898]. Implantation of the ureters into the rectum, for relief of exstrophy of the urinary bladder.

Ber·ge·ron-He·noch chorea or **disease** (behr·zhe·rohn′, hey′ nokh) [E. J. *Bergeron,* French physician, 1817–1900; and E. *Henoch*]. BERGERON'S CHOREA.

Bergeron-Henoch electric chorea. BERGERON'S CHOREA.

Bergeron's chorea or **disease** [E. J. *Bergeron*]. A rare form of movement disorder in children, characterized by sudden involuntary contractions of groups of muscles as if stimulated by an electric shock; probably not chorea by myoclinic epilepsy. Syn. *Bergeron-Henoch chorea.*

Ber·ger rhythm or **wave** (behr′gur) [H. *Berger,* German neuropsychiatrist, 1873–1941]. *In electroencephalography,* the bilateral posterior alpha rhythm of substantially constant frequency of 8 to 13 hertz, inhibited by visual stimuli and mental attention.

Ber·ger's operation (behr·zhey′) [P. *Berger,* French surgeon, 1845–1908]. Interscapulothoracic amputation at the shoulder girdle.

Ber·ger's sign (behr′gur) [E. *Berger,* Austrian ophthalmologist, 1855–1926]. An elliptically shaped pupil seen in early neurosyphilis.

Bergh's test. VAN DEN BERGH'S TEST.

Berg·mann's astrocytes or **glia** (behrk′mahn) [G. H. *Bergmann,* German physician, 1781–1861]. Astrocytes of a special type interspersed among the Purkinje cells of the cerebellum, which, when Purkinje cells are destroyed, undergo hyperplasia and form a dense band.

Bergmann's cords or **conductors** [G. H. *Bergmann*]. STRIAE MEDULLARES VENTRICULI QUARTI.

Bergmann's incision. VON BERGMANN'S INCISION.

Berg·meis·ter's papilla (behrk′mye·stur) [O. *Bergmeister,* Austrian ophthalmologist, 1845–1918]. A preretinal or papillary veil consisting of a conical mass of glial elements representing rudimentary developmental tissue that has failed to reabsorb.

Ber·go·nié-Tri·bon·deau law (behr·gohn·nyey′, tree·bohn·do′) [J. A. *Bergonié,* French physician, 1857–1925; and L. M. F. A. *Tribondeau,* French physician, 1872–1918]. The radiosensitivity of cells varies directly with their reproductive capacity and inversely with their degree of differentiation.

beri·beri (berr′ee·berr′ee) *n.* [Singhalese, from *beri,* weakness]. A disease of the heart and peripheral nerves, with or without edema (wet and dry forms); prevalent in the orient among people subsisting on a diet of polished rice and in the occident among alcoholics; due to nutritional deficiency, mainly of vitamin B_1 (thiamine).

beriberi heart disease. High-output cardiac failure with cardiomegaly and edema, attributable to thiamine deficiency resulting in a marked decrease in peripheral resistance and disordered myocardial metabolism.

Ber·ke·feld filter (behr'ke·felt) [W. *Berkefeld,* German manufacturer, 1836–1897]. A filter, graded V (coarse), N (normal), and W (fine), of diatomaceous earth designed to retain bacteria and spores and to allow the recovery of viruses in the filtrate.

berke·li·um (burk'lee·um) *n.* [after *Berkeley,* California]. Chemical element No. 97, Bk = 247.07, produced artificially in minute amounts.

Ber·lin's disease (behr·leen') [R. *Berlin,* German ophthalmologist, 1833–1897]. COMMOTIO RETINAE.

ber·lock dermatitis (bur'lock) [Ger. *Berlocke,* trinket, charm]. BERLOQUE DERMATITIS.

ber·loque dermatitis (bur·lock') [F. *breloque,* trinket, charm]. A skin eruption appearing as droplet-shaped red patches, especially on the face and neck, sometimes followed by brown pigmentation; caused by perfume and other liquid cosmetics containing the photosensitizing chemical bergapten.

Ber·nard-Hor·ner syndrome (behr·nahr') [C. *Bernard,* French physiologist, 1813–1878; and J. F. *Horner*]. HORNER'S SYNDROME.

Bernard's canal or **duct** [C. *Bernard*]. ACCESSORY PANCREATIC DUCT.

Bernard's granular layer [C. *Bernard*]. The inner granular zone of the acinar cells of the pancreas.

Bernard-Sou·lier syndrome (sool·yey') [J. *Bernard,* French hematologist, 20th century; and J.-P. *Soulier,* French hematologist, 20th century]. A coagulation disorder characterized by a hemorrhagic diathesis, prolonged bleeding time, abnormal prothrombin consumption, thrombocytopenia, and large, morphologically abnormal platelets.

Bernard's puncture [C. *Bernard*]. The experimental needling of the floor of the third cerebral ventricle, rendering an animal temporarily diabetic.

Bernard's syndrome [C. *Bernard*]. HORNER'S SYNDROME.

Bern·hardt-Roth syndrome (behrn'hart, roht) [M. *Bernhardt,* German neurologist, 1844–1915; and V. K. *Roth,* Russian neurologist, 1848–1916]. MERALGIA PARESTHETICA.

Bernhardt's paresthesia [M. *Bernhardt*]. MERALGIA PARESTHETICA.

Bern·heim's syndrome (behr·nem') [*Bernheim,* French physician, 20th century]. Obstruction to right ventricular outflow with right ventricular failure, presumed to be due to bulging of a hypertrophied interventricular septum into the right ventricular cavity; seen in patients with severe left ventricular hypertrophy.

Bernheim's therapy [H. *Bernheim,* French physician, 1840–1919]. Hypnotism in the treatment of neuroses.

Ber·noul·li's principle (Ger. behr·noo'lee, F. behr·noo·yee') [J. *Bernoulli,* Swiss mathematician, 1654–1705]. The lateral pressure of a fluid passing through a tube of varying diameter is least at the most constricted part, where velocity is greatest, and is most at the widest part, where velocity is least.

Bern·reu·ter personality inventory [R. G. *Bernreuter,* U.S. psychologist, b. 1901]. A test for older children and adults based on questions to be answered "yes" or "no," designed to measure neurotic tendency, self-sufficiency, introversion, dominance, sociability, and confidence.

Bern·stein's theory [F. *Bernstein,* U.S. biochemist, b. 1878]. The theory that the ABO blood group antigens are determined by a set of three allelic genes, those for A and B being dominant over that for O and codominant with each other.

berry aneurysm. A small, thin-walled aneurysm that protrudes from the arteries of the arterial circle of the cerebrum or its major branches, usually located at bifurcations and branches, and attributed to developmental defects in the media and elastica. Syn. *saccular aneurysm.*

Ber·ti·el·la (bur"tee·el'uh) *n.* [P. *Bert,* French physiologist, 1833–1886]. A genus of tapeworm parasites.

Bertiella mu·cro·na·ta (mew"kro·nay'tuh). A species of tapeworm parasitic to man, found in the intestine.

Bertiella stu·de·ri (stew'de·rye). A species of tapeworm found in primates, including man.

ber·til·lon·age (bur"til·uh·nahzh', berr"tee·yo·nahzh') *n.* [F.]. BERTILLON SYSTEM.

Ber·til·lon system (behr·tee·yohn') [A. *Bertillon,* French criminologist, 1853–1914]. A system for identifying persons by the use of selected measurements of various parts of the body; now largely superseded by the use of fingerprints.

be·ryl·li·o·sis (berr·il"ee·o'sis) *n.,* pl. **beryllio·ses** (·seez) [*beryllium* + *-osis*]. An acute pneumonia or a chronic granulomatous pneumoconiosis due to the inhalation of certain beryllium salts.

be·ryl·li·um (be·ril'ee·um) *n.* [NL., from Gk. *bēryllos,* beryl]. Be = 9.0122. A divalent metallic element occurring chiefly as beryllium aluminum silicate or beryl. Formerly called *glucinum.*

be·ryth·ro·my·cin (be·rith"ro·migh'sin) *n.* 12-Deoxyerythromycin, an antiamebic agent.

bes·i·clom·e·ter (bes"i·klom'e·tur) *n.* [F. *besicles,* spectacles, + *-meter*]. An instrument used by opticians for measuring the forehead to obtain the proper width for spectacle frames.

Bes·nier-Boeck disease (bey·nyey') [E. *Besnier,* French dermatologist, 1831–1909; and C. P. M. *Boeck*]. SARCOIDOSIS.

Besnier-Boeck-Schaumann disease [E. *Besnier,* C. P. M. *Boeck,* and J. N. *Schaumann*]. SARCOIDOSIS.

bes·noi·ti·o·sis (bez·noy"tee·o'sis) *n.* A chronic debilitating disease of cattle and horses originally thought to be caused by the organism *Globidium besnoiti* but now believed to be caused by a protozoan of the genus *Besnoitia.*

bes·ti·al·i·ty (bes"tee·al'i·tee) *n.* [L. *bestialis,* from *bestia,* beast]. 1. Behavior resembling that of an animal. 2. Sexual relations between human beings and animals.

Best's disease or **macular degeneration** [F. *Best,* German physician, 1871–1965]. A form of heredofamilial (usually autosomal dominant) macular degeneration appearing in early childhood, characterized by yellowish or reddish-yellow, sharply demarcated macular lesions which evolve to a partially pigmented atrophic scar, and loss of central acuity. Syn. *infantile macular degeneration, vitelliruptive macular degeneration.*

be·syl·ate (be'sil·ate) *n.* Any salt or ester of benzenesulfonic acid, $C_6H_5SO_3H$; a benzenesulfonate.

Be·ta (bee'tuh) *n.* [L., beet]. A genus of herbs comprising the beets.

be·ta (bay'tuh, bee'tuh) *n.* [name of the letter B, β, second letter of the Greek alphabet]. The second of a series, or any particular member or subset of an arbitrarily ordered set; in chemistry, often combined with the name of a compound to indicate (1) the second of two isomers, or (2) the position of a substituent on the second carbon atom from a functional group. For many terms beginning with *beta-*, see under the specific noun. Symbol, β.

beta-adrenergic, β-adrenergic. Of or pertaining to a beta-adrenergic receptor.

beta-adrenergic blocking agent, β-adrenergic blocking agent. Any agent, such as propranolol, that combines with and causes blockade of the beta-adrenergic receptor.

beta-adrenergic receptor, β-adrenergic receptor. A locus of action of adrenergic (sympathomimetic) agents at which primarily inhibitory responses are elicited. Isoproterenol is the most potent activator of this receptor. Contr. *alpha-adrenergic receptor.*

beta-aminopropionitrile. β-AMINOPROPIONITRILE.

beta angle. The angle formed between the radius fixus and a line joining the bregma and hormion.

beta-blocking, β-blocking. Having the properties of a beta-adrenergic blocking agent.

beta cells. 1. Cells in the pancreatic islets in which the cytoplasm contains alcohol-soluble granules. 2. Cells containing basophil granules in the adenohypophysis.

Beta-Chlor. Trademark for chloral betaine, a hypnotic and sedative drug.

be·ta·cism (bee'tuh·siz·um, bay') *n.* [Gk. *bēta*, name of letter *β*, + *-ism*]. Overuse of the sound of "b" in speech, or conversion of other sounds into it.

Betadine. Trademark for a complex of polyvinylpyrrolidone and iodine (povidone-iodine) used locally as an anti-infective agent.

be·ta·eu·caine (bay"tuh·yoo'kane) *n.* EUCAINE.

beta examination. BETA TEST.

beta globulin, β-globulin. Any of a group of serum globulins intermediate between alpha and gamma globulins in electrophoretic mobility, including globulins that function in the transport of lipids, carbohydrates, hormones, and iron, and a small fraction of antibodies or immunoglobulins.

beta granules. Granules of the beta cells of the adenohypophysis or of the pancreatic islets.

beta hemolysin, β-hemolysin. A phospholipase released by some strains of *Staphylococcus aureus* which lyses human and sheep red blood cells when refrigerated after prior incubation at 37°C.

beta hemolysis, β-hemolysis. Complete lysis of red blood cells around a colony on a blood agar medium, resulting in a clear zone around the colony. Contr. *alpha hemolysis.*

beta-hemolytic, β-hemolytic. Causing beta hemolysis; said of various bacteria, especially certain streptococci.

beta-hemolytic streptococcal pharyngitis. Inflammation of the pharynx caused by *Streptococcus pyogenes,* Lancefield group A streptococci; a major cause of acute sore throat or exudative pharyngitis.

be·ta·his·tine (bay"tuh·his'teen) *n.* 2-[2-(Methylamino)ethyl]pyridine, $C_8H_{12}N_2$, a histamine-like drug used as the dihydrochloride to reduce frequency of vertiginous episodes in Ménière's syndrome, and as a vasodilator.

be·ta-hy·poph·a·mine (bay"tuh·high·pof'uh·meen, ·min) *n.* ANTIDIURETIC HORMONE.

be·ta·ine (bay'tuh·een, ·in, be·tay'een, ·in) *n.* [L. *beta,* beet, + *-ine*]. 1. Carboxymethyltrimethylammonium hydroxide anhydride, $(CH_3)_3NCH_2COO$; a crystalline substance occurring in sugar beets or prepared synthetically. It is an active methyl donor in the synthesis of choline and creatine, and may be useful in preventing hepatic cirrhosis; used as the hydrochloride salt. 2. Any one of a group of organic compounds in which the proton donor and acceptor sites are parts of the same molecule; considered as internal salts of quaternary ammonium bases. Syn. *lycine, oxyneurine, trimethylglycine.*

betaine aldehyde. An oxidation product of choline.

beta-keto·hy·droxy·bu·tyr·ic acid (bay"tuh·kee"to·high·drock"see·bew·tirr'ick). ACETOACETIC ACID.

Betalin S A trademark for thiamine hydrochloride.

beta lysin. A thermostable bactericidal serum constituent; similar to leukin and obtained from granulocytes and perhaps from blood platelets. The relation of this factor to immunity is not clear.

be·ta·meth·a·sone (bay"tuh·meth'uh·sone) *n.* 9α-Fluoro-16β-methylprednisolone, $C_{22}H_{29}FO_5$, a synthetic glucocorticoid with potent anti-inflammatory action; isomeric with dexamethasone.

be·ta·mi·cin (bay"tuh·migh'sin) *n.* A streptamine derivative, $C_{19}H_{38}N_4O_{10}$, an antibacterial agent usually used as the sulfate salt.

be·ta·naph·thol (bay"tuh·naf'thol) *n.* β-Hydroxynaphthalene, $C_{10}H_7OH$, a white crystalline powder; used locally as a parasiticide and, formerly, as a vermifuge and intestinal antiseptic.

beta·naph·thyl (bay"tuh·naf'thil) *n.* The radical $C_{10}H_7$—, from betanaphthol.

beta oxidation. Oxidation of the carbon atom which is in the beta position with reference to some functional group. In fatty acid catabolism, the carbon atom beta to the carboxyl group is oxidized, and a two-carbon unit is removed.

Betapar. A trademark for meprednisone.

beta particle. *In nuclear science,* a radiation from certain radioactive materials, identical with the electron or its positively charged counterpart, the positron.

Betapen VK. A trademark for penicillin V potassium.

Betaprone. Trademark for propiolactone, a disinfectant.

beta rays. Electrons emitted from certain radioactive elements. See also *beta particle.*

beta-receptor, β-receptor. BETA-ADRENERGIC RECEPTOR.

beta rhythm. *In electroencephalography,* low potential fast waves of more than 13 (usually 18 to 30) hertz, present in many normal adults and seen most frequently in the precentral region.

beta streptococci. Streptococci belonging to 13 groups, A to O, each of which is distinguished by a specific carbohydrate, and which generally produce a complete hemolysis on blood agar. Group A streptococci are responsible for most streptococcal diseases of man.

beta test. A group intelligence test, designed for soldiers who were illiterate or unable to read English, using signs and pictures; first used by the U.S. Army in World War I.

be·ta·to·pic (bay"tuh·to'pick) *adj.* [*beta* particle + *-topic* as in isotopic]. Of or pertaining to two atoms that differ by one in atomic number, so that by expulsion of a beta particle from the nucleus of the atom of an element of lower atomic number it is converted to an atom of the element having an atomic number greater by one unit.

be·ta·tron (bay'tuh·tron, bee'tuh·tron) *n.* [*beta* particle + *-tron*]. An apparatus for accelerating electrons, by magnetic induction, to energies equivalent to millions of electron volts.

beta wave. See *beta rhythm.*

be·ta·zole (bay'tuh·zole) *n.* 3-(2-Aminoethyl)pyrazole, $C_5H_9N_3$, an analogue of histamine; used as the dihydrochloride salt in diagnostic tests of gastric secretion.

be·tel (bee'tul, bet'ul) *n.* [Pg., from Malayalam *vet̤t̤ila*]. An astringent masticatory stimulant used in southeast Asia, prepared by mixing the nut of the catechu palm, *Areca catechu,* with quicklime and wrapping in a leaf of *Piper betle.* Its habitual use stains the teeth black.

betel-nut carcinoma. A squamous cell carcinoma usually on the inside of the cheek; observed in persons who chew betel.

betel oil. The volatile oil from betel leaves; used as a local stimulant.

bête rouge (bet roozh), pl. **bêtes rouges** [F., lit., red bug, red beast]. CHIGGER.

be·thane·chol chloride (be·thane'kole). Carbamylmethylcholine chloride, $C_7H_{17}ClN_2O_2$, a cholinergic drug not destroyed by cholinesterase.

be·than·i·dine (be·than'i·deen) *n.* 1-Benzyl-2,3-dimethylguanidine, $C_{10}H_{15}N_3$, an antihypertensive drug; used as the sulfate.

Bet·ten·dorff 's test [A. J. H. M. *Bettendorff,* German chemist, 1839–1902]. A test for arsenic in which the suspected liquid is mixed with hydrochloric acid; stannous chloride solution and a piece of tinfoil are added. A brown color or precipitate indicates the presence of arsenic.

Bet·u·la (bet'yoo·luh, bech'oo·luh) *n.* [L.]. A genus of northern deciduous hardwood trees comprising the birches.

betula oil. The volatile oil from the bark of *Betula lenta;* chemically methyl salicylate.

be·tween·brain, *n.* DIENCEPHALON.

Betz cell [V. A. *Betz,* Russian anatomist, 1834–1894]. A giant pyramidal cell of the fifth layer of the motor cortex.

bev, BEV Abbreviation for *billion electron volts.*

Bev·an's operation [A. D. *Bevan,* U.S. surgeon, 1861–1943]. 1. Cholecystectomy through a vertical incision along the outer border of the rectus muscle. 2. An operation for undescended testicle, in which the testicle is brought down and fastened in the scrotum.

bev·a·tron (bev'uh·tron) *n.* [*b*illion *e*lectron *v*olts + *-tron*]. PROTON-SYNCHROTRON.

be·zoar (bee'zor, bee'zo·ur) *n.* [Ar. *bāzahr,* from Per. *pād-zahr,* protecting against poison]. A concretion found in the stomach or intestine of some animals, especially ruminants, most commonly composed of ingested hair; may form a cast of the stomach large enough to cause obstruction. Also found in some children and adults who pluck their own or a doll's hair and ingest it, usually a highly neurotic trait. Formerly believed to have magic medicinal properties.

Be·zold-Brücke effect (bey'tsohlt, bruek'eh) [A. von *Bezold,* German physiologist, 1836–1868; and E. W. R. von *Brücke*]. The shift of perceived hue toward either yellow or blue when the intensity of illumination of the retina by light of a given wavelength is increased. Three wavelengths, however (404 nm, 478 nm, 573 nm), are always perceived as the same hue regardless of the amount of retinal illuminance.

Bezold-Ja·risch reflex (yah'rish) [A. von *Bezold* and A. *Jarisch*]. BEZOLD REFLEX.

Bezold reflex [A. von *Bezold*]. Hypotension and bradycardia mediated by receptors primarily in the left ventricle via the vagus nerve, occurring in response to veratrine and probably to myocardial infarction.

Bezold's abscess [F. *Bezold,* German otologist, 1842–1908]. A deep neck abscess secondary to perforation of the mastoid process from acute or chronic mastoiditis.

Bezold's sign [F. *Bezold*]. Swelling below the apex of the mastoid process; considered a sign of mastoiditis.

BHA Abbreviation for *butylated hydroxyanisole.*

bhang (bang, bahng) *n.* [Hindi]. Stems and leaves of the hemp plant as used in India for infusion in beverages and for smoking; a form of cannabis comparable to marijuana. See also *cannabis.*

BHC Abbreviation for the insecticide *benzene hexachloride.*

BHT Abbreviation for *butylated hydroxytoluene.*

Bi Symbol for bismuth.

bi- [L. *bis,* twice]. A prefix meaning (a) *two, twice, double;* (b) in anatomy, *connection with* or *relation to each of two symmetrically paired parts;* (c) in chemistry, *presence of two atoms* or *equivalents* (of a component) or *presence* (of this component) *in double the usual proportion* or *in double the proportion of the other component.*

bi·al·am·i·col (bye·al·am'i·kol) *n.* 6,6′-Diallyl-α,α′-bis(diethylamino)-4,4′-bi-*o*-creosol, $C_{28}H_{40}N_2O_2$, an antiamebic drug; used as the dihydrochloride salt.

Bi·al's reagent (bee'ahl) [M. *Bial,* German physician, 1870–1908]. A solution of 30% hydrochloric acid, 10% ferric chloride solution, and orcinol; used in the detection of pentose.

Bial's test [M. *Bial*]. A test for pentose in which glucose must be removed from the urine by fermentation before adding Bial's reagent; if pentose is present, a green flocculent precipitate of furfural is formed.

bi·ased error. Nonrandom error; systematic error.

biased sample. A sample that is not representative of its field.

bi·astig·ma·tism (bye''uh·stig'muh·tiz·um) *n.* [*bi-* + *astigmatism*]. A condition of the eye in which both corneal and lenticular astigmatism exist, and are corrected separately by crossed cylinders.

bi·au·ric·u·lar (bye''aw·rick'yoo·lur) *adj.* [*bi-* + *auricular*]. Pertaining to both external ears.

biauricular line. The line separating the anterior from the posterior portion of the skull; it extends from one external auditory meatus over the vertex to the other.

bi·ax·i·al (bye·ack'see·ul) *adj.* [*bi-* + *axial*]. Furnished with two axes.

biaxial joint. A synovial joint in which movement is around two transverse axes at right angles to each other, as a condylar joint or a saddle joint.

bi·bal·lism (bye·bal'iz·um) *n.* Ballism involving the limbs on both sides, indicative of lesions in both subthalamic nuclei.

biblio- [Gk. *biblion,* book, from *biblos,* papyrus]. A combining form meaning *book.*

bib·lio·clast (bib'lee·o·klast) *n.* [*biblio-* + *-clast*]. A person who mutilates or destroys books.

bib·lio·klep·to·ma·nia (bib''lee·o·klep''to·may'nee·uh) *n.* [*biblio-* + *kleptomania*]. A morbid desire to steal books.

bib·lio·ma·nia (bib''lee·o·may'nee·uh) *n.* [*biblio-* + *mania*]. An abnormal or intense desire to collect books, especially curious and rare ones.

bib·lio·pho·bia (bib''lee·o·fo'bee·uh) *n.* [*biblio-* + *phobia*]. A morbid fear or hatred of books.

bib·lio·ther·a·py (bib''lee·o·therr'uh·pee) *n.* [*biblio-* + *therapy*]. 1. Reading, especially of books, in the treatment of mental disorders. 2. Generally, the reading of books for mental health.

bibo (bib'o) *n.* TAMPAN.

bi·cap·i·tate (bye·kap'i·tate) *adj.* [*bi-* + *capitate*]. Having two heads; dicephalous.

bi·car·bon·ate (bye·kahr'buh·nate) *n.* [*bi-* + *carbonate*]. A salt of carbonic acid characterized by the radical HCO_3.

bi·car·dio·gram (bye·kahr'dee·o·gram) *n.* [*bi-* + *cardiogram*]. The summated electrocardiogram yielded by the atria and ventricles beating normally; no longer in use.

bi·ceph·a·lous (bye·sef'uh·lus) *adj.* DICEPHALOUS.

bi·ceps (bye'seps) *n.,* pl. **biceps·es** (·iz) [L., two-headed]. A muscle having two heads, as the biceps brachii, the biceps femoris. See also Table of Muscles in the Appendix.

biceps femoris reflex. EXTERNAL HAMSTRING REFLEX.

biceps jerk or **reflex.** Contraction of the biceps brachii muscle with flexion at the elbow when its tendon is struck.

bi·chlo·ride (bye·klo'ride) *n.* 1. Any compound containing two atoms of chlorine, especially a salt having two chloride atoms. 2. MERCURY BICHLORIDE.

bi·chro·mate (bye·kro'mate) *n.* DICHROMATE.

Bicillin. A trademark for benzathine penicillin G, an antibiotic.

bi·cip·i·tal (bye·sip'i·tul) *adj.* [L. *biceps, bicipitis,* two-headed, + *-al*]. 1. Two-headed. 2. Pertaining to a muscle having two heads.

bicipital aponeurosis. A fibrous expansion of the tendon of insertion of the biceps brachii muscle into the fascia of the upper medial portion of the forearm.

bicipital groove. INTERTUBERCULAR SULCUS.

bicipital muscle. A muscle having two heads or attachments of origin.

bicipital ridge. Either one of the crests of bone delimiting the intertubercular sulcus.

bi·cip·i·to·ra·di·al (bye·sip''i·to·ray'dee·ul) *adj.* Pertaining to the biceps brachii and the radial tuberosity.

bicipitoradial bursa. A synovial bursa between the distal portion of the radial tuberosity and the tendon of the biceps brachii muscle. Syn. *bursa bicipitoradialis [NA].*

BiCNU. Trademark for carmustine (BCNU), an antineoplastic.

bi·con·cave (bye''kon'kave, ·kon·kave') *adj.* Bounded by two concave surfaces.

biconcave lens. A negative or minus, thick-edged lens, having concave spherical surfaces upon its opposite sides; used in the correction of myopia.

bi·con·vex (bye''kon'vecks, ·kon·vecks') *adj.* Bounded by two convex surfaces.

biconvex lens. A positive or plus, thin-edged lens, having two convex surfaces; used in the correction of hyperopia.

bi·cor·nate (bye·kor′nate) *adj.* BICORNUATE.

bi·cor·nu·ate (bye·kor′new·ate) *adj.* [*bi-* + *cornu* + *-ate*]. Having two horns.

bicornuate uterus. UTERUS BICORNIS.

bi·cor·nu·ous (bye·kor′new·us) *adj.* BICORNUATE.

bi·cou·dé catheter (bee·koo·day′) [F., double elbow]. An angulated catheter with the tip or leading end bent at two points to form a double elbow.

bi·cus·pid (bye·kus′pid) *adj.* & *n.* [*bi-* + L. *cuspis, cuspidis,* point]. 1. Having two cusps, as bicuspid teeth, or as the mitral valve of the heart. 2. A bicuspid tooth; in the human dentition, a premolar.

bicuspid valve. MITRAL VALVE.

b.i.d. Abbreviation for *bis in die;* twice daily.

bi·dac·ty·ly (bye·dack′ti·lee) *n.* [*bi-* + *-dactyly*]. Congenital absence of all fingers or toes except the first and fifth. Syn. *lobster-claw deformity.*

Bid·der's ganglion [F. H. *Bidder,* German anatomist, 1810–1894]. A collection of nerve cells in the frog's heart.

bi·der·mo·ma (bye″dur·mo′muh) *n.* [*bi-* + *derm-* + *-oma*]. TERATOMA.

Bie·brich scarlet (bee′brikh) [after *Biebrich,* Germany]. A red acid azo dye used as a plasma stain, as a muscle and cytoplasm stain in selective collagen staining methods, and as a reagent for basic protein at high pH levels.

Biedl-Bar·det syndrome (bee′dul, bar·deh′) [A. *Biedl,* Czechoslovakian physiologist, 1869–1933; and G. *Bardet,* French physician, b. 1885]. LAURENCE-MOON-BIEDL SYNDROME.

bi·elec·trol·y·sis (bye″e·leck·trol′i·sis) *n.,* pl. **bielectroly·ses** (·seez) [*bi-* + *electrolysis*]. The electrolysis of two substances, one at each pole.

Biel·schow·sky-Jan·ský disease (beel·shohf′skee, yahn′skee) [M. *Bielschowsky,* German neuropathologist, 1869–1940; and J. *Janský,* Czechoslovakian physician, 1873–1921]. A hereditary disorder of lipid metabolism manifesting itself between 2 and 4 years of age by convulsions, extrapyramidal disorders of movement, spasticity, and rapidly progressive dementia and blindness due to retinal degeneration. Syn. *late infantile amaurotic familial idiocy.* See also *amaurotic familial idiocy.*

Bielschowsky's disease [M. *Bielschowsky*]. BIELSCHOWSKY-JANSKÝ DISEASE.

Bielschowsky's sign [M. *Bielschowsky*]. In paresis of the superior oblique muscle of the eyeball, tilting the patient's head toward the side of the paralyzed eye produces hypertropia and increased vertical diplopia.

Bielschowsky strabismus [M. *Bielschowsky*]. Strabismus due to hyperfunction of the inferior oblique muscle of the eyeball.

Bier·mer's anemia or **disease** (beer′mur) [A. *Biermer,* German physician, 1827–1892]. PERNICIOUS ANEMIA.

Bier·nac·ki's sign (birr·nats′kee) [E. A. *Biernacki,* Polish physician, 1866–1911]. Insensitivity to pressure over the ulnar nerve, as seen in tabes dorsalis.

Bier's block (beer) [A. K. G. *Bier,* German surgeon, 1861–1949]. 1. A method of producing anesthesia in a limb by intravenous injections of local anesthetic (originally ½% cocaine or procaine) after the part has been rendered bloodless by elevation and constriction. 2. An early technique of spinal anesthesia using cocaine.

Bier spots [A. K. G. *Bier*]. Spots or blanched areas in the skin due to diminution of blood supply.

Bier's suction [A. K. G. *Bier*]. A first-aid treatment for snakebite which employs suction tubes over the wound to draw out the venom.

Biett's disease (byet) [L. T. *Biett,* Swiss physician, 1781–1840]. LUPUS ERYTHEMATOSUS.

bi·fid (bye′fid) *adj.* [L. *bifidus,* from *bi-* + *findere,* to split]. Divided into two parts; cleft.

bifid foot. CLEFT FOOT.

bifid pelvis. A congenital anomaly of the renal pelvis in which there are two major calyxes.

bifid skull. CRANIUM BIFIDUM.

bifid spine. SPINA BIFIDA.

bifid tongue. A tongue the anterior portion of which is cleft in the median line.

bifid uvula. CLEFT UVULA.

bi·fo·cal (bye·fo′kul) *adj.* Having two foci; applied to a system of lenses or spectacles.

bi·fo·cals, *n. pl.* 1. A pair of lenses for spectacles, each one having a part that corrects for distant vision and another that corrects for close vision. See also *cement bifocals, one-piece bifocals.* 2. The spectacles containing such lenses.

bi·fron·tal (bye·frun′tul) *adj.* Pertaining to both frontal bones, or both frontal lobes of the brain, or subdivisions thereof.

bifurcate ligament. A dorsal ligament of the foot attached posteriorly to the calcaneus, dividing anteriorly into the calcaneocuboid ligament (NA *ligamentum calcaneocuboideum*), which is attached to the cuboid, and the calcaneonavicular ligament (NA *ligamentum calcaneonaviculare*), attached to the navicular. NA *ligamentum bifurcatum.*

bi·fur·ca·tio (bye″fur·kay′shee·o) *n.,* pl. **bifur·ca·ti·o·nes** (·kay·shee·o′neez) [NL.]. BIFURCATION.

bi·fur·ca·tion (bye″fur·kay′shun) *n.* [F., from L. *bifurcus,* two-pronged, from *furca,* pitchfork]. 1. Division into two branches. 2. The site of a division into two branches. —**bi·fur·cate** (bye′fur·kate) *adj.* & *v.*

bifurcationes. Plural of *bifurcatio.*

bifurcation of the trachea. The point at which the trachea terminates by dividing into the two primary bronchi, their openings separated by the carina of the trachea. NA *bifurcatio tracheae.*

bi·fur·ca·tio tra·che·ae (bye·fur·kay′shee·o tray′kee·ee) [NA]. BIFURCATION OF THE TRACHEA.

Big·e·low's lithotrite [H. J. *Bigelow,* U.S. surgeon, 1818–1890]. An instrument with jaws, inserted through the urethra, for crushing large stones in the urinary bladder.

Bigelow's method [H. J. *Bigelow*]. A procedure for reducing dislocation of the hip, using the iliofemoral or Y ligament as a fulcrum.

bi·gem·i·nal (bye·jem′i·nul) *adj.* [L. *bigeminus,* from *geminus,* twin]. Occurring in pairs; double; twin.

bigeminal pregnancy. Twin pregnancy; gestation with two fetuses.

bigeminal pulse. A pulse characterized by paired beats in close proximity, with a longer interval between the pairs; the normal first beat is greater in amplitude than the second or premature beat.

bigeminal rhythm. An arrhythmia in which every alternate heartbeat occurs prematurely.

bi·gem·i·ny (bye·jem′i·nee) *n.* [*bigemin*al + *-y*]. 1. The condition of occurring in pairs. 2. BIGEMINAL RHYTHM.

big·head, *n.* Any of various diseases of animals resulting in edema or bony enlargement of the head, specifically: 1. An acute photosensitization in sheep, caused by ingestion of certain plants, commonly affecting the face and ears, which become thickened and pendulous. 2. An acute infectious disease of young rams, caused by *Clostridium novyi* and characterized by swelling of the head; first described in Australia.

big heel. Painful enlargement of the calcaneus, of unknown etiology, but possibly due to yaws; occurring mainly in Africa and Taiwan.

big liver disease. VISCERAL LYMPHOMATOSIS.

bi·go·ni·al (bye·go′nee·ul) *adj.* Pertaining to or indicating both sides of the gonium, or lower jaw.

bigonial arc. *In craniometry,* a measurement around the anterior margin of the mandible.

bi·is·chi·al (bye·is′kee·ul) *adj.* Pertaining to the two ischial tuberosities.

biischial diameter. TRANSVERSE DIAMETER OF THE PELVIC OUTLET.

Bikele's sign. Resistance to passive extension of the elbow when the arm is elevated at the shoulder; seen in conditions resulting in irritated nerve roots, as with brachial plexus neuritis or in meningitis.

bi·labe (bye'labe) *n.* [*bi-* + *-labe*]. A surgical instrument for removing foreign bodies from the urinary bladder through the urethra.

bi·lam·i·nar (bye·lam'i·nur) *adj.* [*bi-* + *laminar*]. Formed of or having two layers.

bilaminar blastoderm. BILAMINAR BLASTODISK.

bilaminar blastodisk. A two-layered embryonic disk before mesoderm formation. See also *gastrula.*

bi·lat·er·al (bye·lat'ur·ul) *adj.* [*bi-* + *lateral*]. Pertaining to two sides; pertaining to or affecting both sides of the body. —**bilateral·ism** (·iz·um) *n.;* **bilateral·ly** (·ee) *adv.*

bilateral astereognosis. TACTILE AGNOSIA.

bilateral cleavage. Cleavage in a single plane producing equal parts.

bilateral electroconvulsive therapy. Electroshock therapy with the electrodes applied against both cerebral hemispheres.

bilateral harelip. DOUBLE HARELIP.

bilateral hermaphroditism. The form of human hermaphroditism in which there is either an ovotestis on each side or a separate ovary and testis on each side.

bilateral strabismus. ALTERNATING STRABISMUS.

bilateral subtotal ablation of the frontal cortex. FRONTAL GYRECTOMY.

bilateral symmetry. Symmetry with respect to a median plane; the property of having two lateral halves that correspond in a mirror-image spatial arrangement.

bi·lay·er (bye'lay·ur) *n.* A layer two molecules thick, such as that formed on the surface of the aqueous phase by phospholipids in aqueous solution.

bile, *n.* [L. *bilis*]. A bitter, alkaline, greenish-yellow to golden-brown fluid, secreted by the liver and poured into the duodenum. It contains bile salts, cholesterol, lecithin, fat, various pigments, and mucin. Functionally, it aids in the emulsification, digestion, and absorption of fats and in the alkalinization of the intestines.

bile acid. Any one of the naturally occurring free acids of bile or those formed by the conjugation of glycine or taurine with a cholic acid, forming glycocholic and taurocholic acids, respectively.

bile canaliculi. The intercellular channels in hepatic cords that convey bile toward the interlobular bile ducts.

bile cyst. CHOLEDOCHUS CYST.

bile duct. The cystic, hepatic, or common duct or any of the ducts of the liver connecting with the hepatic duct.

bile-duct hamartoma. VON MEYENBURG COMPLEX.

bile nephrosis. Histopathologic abnormality consisting of swollen renal tubular cells and bile casts in association with Laennec's cirrhosis. Azotemia may or may not be present. The significance of these changes is not known.

bile papilla. MAJOR DUODENAL PAPILLA.

bile pigment. Any of the substances responsible for the color of bile, principally bilirubin and biliverdin, both derived from hemoglobin.

bile salts. Sodium salts of the bile acids, normally present in bile.

bile solubility. The property possessed by pneumococci of dissolving in bile.

bile solubility test. A test for identifying pneumococci based on the fact that they dissolve in bile or bile salts.

Bil·har·zia (bil·hahr'zee·uh) *n.* [T. M. *Bilharz,* German parasitologist, 1825–1862]. *SCHISTOSOMA.*

bil·har·zi·a·sis (bil''hahr·zye'uh·sis) *n.* [*Bilharz*ia + *-iasis*]. SCHISTOSOMIASIS.

bili-. A combining form meaning (a) *bile, biliary;* (b) *derived from bile.*

bil·i·ary (bil'ee·air''ee) *adj.* 1. Of or pertaining to bile, or involving the bile duct or biliary tract. 2. Conveying bile.

biliary calculus. A solid mass formed within the biliary system, composed of bile salts, calcium, bilirubin, and cholesterol in various proportions.

biliary cirrhosis. Cirrhosis due to extrahepatic bile duct obstruction or chronic intrahepatic inflammatory disease with bile duct obstruction; clinical manifestations include jaundice, pruritus, hepatosplenomegaly, xanthomatosis, and steatorrhea.

biliary colic. Pain caused by the passage of a gallstone in the bile duct.

biliary duct. BILE DUCT.

biliary dyskinesia or **dyssynergia.** Upper abdominal discomfort or pain similar to biliary colic, believed to originate in the biliary tract but not associated with demonstrated biliary pathology.

biliary intralobular canal. A bile canaliculus in a hepatic cord.

biliary stasis. Abnormal stagnation of bile flow in biliary capillaries and ducts.

biliary system. BILIARY TRACT.

biliary tract or **tree.** The entire hepatic duct system, including hepatic ducts, gallbladder, cystic duct, and common bile duct.

bil·i·cy·a·nin (bil''i·sigh'uh·nin) *n.* [*bili-* + *cyan-* + *-in*]. A blue pigment obtained by the interaction of an ammoniacal solution of bilirubin and zinc chloride.

bil·i·fla·vin (bil''i·flav'in, ·flay'vin, bye''li·) *n.* [*bili-* + *flavin*]. A yellow coloring matter derivable from biliverdin.

bil·i·fus·cin (bil''i·fus'in) *n.* [*bili-* + L. *fus*cus, dark, + *-in*]. A normal fecal pigment (or possibly two isomeric substances) analogous to mesobilifuscin but having two vinyl groups in place of the two ethyl groups of mesobilifuscin.

bi·lig·u·late (bye·lig'yoo·late) *adj.* [*bi-* + L. *ligula,* little tongue]. Formed like two tongues or having two tongue-like processes.

bil·i·hu·min (bil''i·hew'min) *n.* [*bili-* + *humin*]. An insoluble residue left after treating gallstones with various solvents.

Bili-Labstix. A trademark for reagent strips employed in urinalysis.

bil·i·leu·kan (bil''i·lew'kan) *n.* A colorless precursor of bilifuscin.

bil·i·neu·rine (bil''i·new'reen, ·rin) *n.* CHOLINE.

bil·ious (bil'yus) *adj.* [L. *biliosus*]. 1. Pertaining to bile. 2. Designating disorders arising from an excess of bile.

bilious dyspepsia. Indigestion attributed to impaired secretion of bile. See also *biliousness.*

bilious headache. 1. Headache associated with biliousness. 2. MIGRAINE.

bil·ious·ness (bil'yus·nis) *n.* A symptom complex combining varying degrees of malaise, headache, bloating, and constipation; traditionally, but probably erroneously, attributed to disorders of biliary flow.

bil·i·pra·sin (bil''i·pray'sin) *n.* [*bili-* + Gk. *prasinos,* green]. An intermediate bile pigment formed in the oxidation of bilirubin to biliverdin. Syn. *choleprasin.*

bil·i·pur·pu·rin (bil''i·pur'pew·rin) *n.* [*bili-* + *purpurin*]. CHOLEHEMATIN.

bil·i·ru·bin (bil''i·roo'bin) *n.* [*bili-* + L. *rub*er, red, + *-in*]. $C_{33}H_{36}N_4O_6$. Orange-red crystals or powder. The principal pigment of bile, formed by reduction of biliverdin, normally present in feces and found in the urine in obstructive jaundice. It is insoluble in water. See also Table of Chemical Constituents of Blood in the Appendix.

bil·i·ru·bin·ate (bil''i·roo'bi·nate) *n.* A salt of bilirubin.

bilirubin clearance test. A test for liver function based upon the ability of the liver to remove injected bilirubin from the blood.

bil·i·ru·bi·ne·mia, bil·i·ru·bi·nae·mia (bil''i·roo''bi·nee'mee·uh) *n.* [*bilirubin* + *-emia*]. 1. The presence of bilirubin in the blood; jaundice. 2. HYPERBILIRUBINEMIA.

bil·i·ru·bin·glo·bin (bil″i-roo′bin-glo″bin) *n.* A transitional stage in the production of bilirubin from hemoglobin. It is the substance which remains after the removal of iron from the hemoglobin.

bil·i·ru·bi·nu·ria (bil″i-roo-bi-new′ree-uh) *n.* The presence of bilirubin in the urine. Normally it occurs in small amounts and is increased in obstructive jaundice.

bil·i·uria (bil″i-yoo′ree-uh) *n.* [*bili-* + *-uria*]. The presence of bile salts in the urine.

bil·i·ver·din (bil″i-vur′din) *n.* [*bili-* + *verd-* + *-in*]. $C_{33}H_{34}N_4O_6$; a dark-green bile pigment, formed in the body from hemoglobin, but largely reduced in the liver to bilirubin. Biliverdin may also be obtained by oxidizing bilirubin.

Bill·roth's cords (bil′rote) [C.A.T. *Billroth,* Austrian surgeon, 1829–1894]. RED PULP.

Billroth's operation [C. A. T. *Billroth*]. 1. Pylorectomy with end-to-end anastomosis of the upper portion of the stomach to the duodenum. Syn. *Billroth I operation.* 2. Partial gastric resection, with closure of the duodenal stump and gastrojejunostomy. Syn. *Billroth II operation.*

bi·lo·bate (bye-lo′bate) *adj.* Having, or divided into, two lobes.

bilobate scrotum. A congenital failure of the lateral halves of the scrotum to fuse at the line of the median raphe, resulting in a separate pouch for each testis.

bi·lobed, *adj.* BILOBATE.

bilobed placenta. DUPLEX PLACENTA.

bi·loc·u·lar (bye-lock′yoo-lur) *adj.* [*bi-* + *loculus* + *-ar*]. Having two cells, compartments, or chambers.

bilocular bladder. A sacculated urinary bladder having two pouches.

bilocular heart. COR BILOCULARE.

bilocular stomach. HOURGLASS STOMACH.

bi·loc·u·late (bye-lock′yoo-late) *adj.* BILOCULAR.

Bilopaque. A trademark for tyropanoate sodium, an oral radiopaque agent.

bi·man·u·al (bye-man′yoo-ul) *adj.* [*bi-* + *manual*]. Pertaining to or performed by both hands.

bimanual palpation. 1. Employment of two examining hands in physical examination. 2. *In gynecology,* the palpation of the pelvic organs with one hand on the lower abdomen and the fingers of the other hand inserted in the vagina or rectum.

bimanual version. Manipulation through the abdominal wall with one hand with the aid of one or more fingers of the other within the vagina.

bin- [L. *bini*]. A combining form meaning (a) *two, two at a time;* (b) in chemistry, *bi-*.

bin·an·gle (bin′ang-gul) *n.* [*bin-* + *angle*]. A dental instrument having offsetting blades at either end of the shank.

bi·na·ry (bye′nuh-ree, bye′nerr-ee) *adj.* [L. *binarius*]. 1. Dichotomous; divided or dividing in two. 2. Containing or consisting of two components or things. 3. *In chemistry,* compounded of two elements. 4. *In anatomy,* separating into two branches or parts.

binary fission. Cell division in which first the nucleus, then the cytoplasm divide into two equal parts, producing two daughter cells; common in somatic cell reproduction and as a form of asexual reproduction in such unicellular organisms as protozoa and bacteria. Contr. *multiple fission.*

bi·na·sal (bye-nay′zul) *adj.* Pertaining to both nasal visual fields.

binasal hemianopsia. Blindness on the nasal side of the visual field of both eyes, usually due to disease of the outer sides of the optic chiasma.

bin·au·ral (bin-aw′rul) *adj.* [*bin-* + *aural*]. 1. Pertaining to or having two ears. 2. Involving the use of both ears.

binaural stethoscope. A stethoscope with earpieces for insertion into both ears of the user, and connected by flexible tubing to the chest piece.

bin·au·ric·u·lar (bin-aw-rick′yoo-lur) *adj.* BIAURICULAR.

binauricular arc. A measurement from the center of one auditory meatus to the other, directly upward across the top of the head.

binauricular axis. *In craniometry,* the imaginary line joining the two auricular points.

bind, *v. In chemistry,* to unite with, as in the combination of two substances having affinity.

bind·er, *n.* 1. A wide bandage or girdle worn to support the abdomen or breasts after childbirth or operations, as an obstetric or abdominal binder. 2. A substance, such as gelatin or glucose, used to impart cohesiveness to the powdered ingredients of tablet formulations on compression.

Bi·net age (bee-neh′) [A. *Binet,* French psychologist, 1857–1911]. Mental age as estimated by the Binet-Simon intelligence scale.

Binet's formula [A. *Binet*]. Children under 9 years of age whose mental development is retarded by 2 years are probably mentally deficient; and children of 9 years or older, retarded by 3 years are definitely deficient.

Binet-Si·mon intelligence scale or **test** (see-mohn′) [A. *Binet;* and T. *Simon,* French psychologist, 1873–1961]. A method of estimating the relative mental development of a child between 3 and 12 years of age and expressing it as an intelligence quotient, the mental age being divided by the chronological age. Originally devised for French children, it has been adapted to many cultures, such as the Stanford revision for the United States.

Bing-Neel syndrome [J. *Bing* and A. V. *Neel,* Scandinavian physicians, 20th century]. Hyperglobulinemia and increased viscosity of the blood, with impairment of articulation through small cerebral and retinal vessels and manifestations of diffuse central nervous system disturbance.

Bing's sign [R. *Bing,* German neurologist, 20th century]. Extension of the great toe, elicited by pricking the dorsum of the foot with a pin; seen in corticospinal tract disease; a variant of the Babinski sign (1).

bi·ni·ra·my·cin (bi-neer″uh-migh′sin) *n.* An antibiotic produced by a variant strain of *Streptomyces bikiniensis.*

bin·oc·u·lar (bi-nock′yoo-lur, bye-nock′) *adj. & n.* [*bin-* + *ocular*]. 1. Of or pertaining to both eyes or to the use of both eyes at once. 2. An instrument with two eyepieces for use with both eyes at once.

binocular accommodation. Simultaneous accommodation of both eyes.

binocular diplopia. The most common type of diplopia; due to a derangement of muscular balance of the two eyes; the images of an object are thrown upon noncorresponding points of the retina.

binocular false projection. ABNORMAL RETINAL CORRESPONDENCE.

binocular loupe. A binocular magnifier, consisting of a combination of lenses in an optical frame, worn like spectacles, providing depth perception.

binocular microscope. A microscope having two eyepieces, one for each eye, so that the object is seen with both eyes.

binocular objectives. Low-powered paired objectives for stereoscopic vision in dissecting microscopes.

binocular parallax. The angle of convergence of the visual axes.

binocular perception. Seeing with two eyes so that only one visual image is appreciated, i.e., the two retinal images are fused.

binocular rivalry. RETINAL RIVALRY.

binocular vision. The faculty of using both eyes synchronously, without diplopia.

bi·no·mi·al (bye-no′mee-ul) *n.* [ML. *binomius,* having two names]. 1. A botanical or zoological name consisting of two terms, the first designating the genus, the second the species. 2. A mathematical expression consisting of two variable terms.

bin·otic (bin-o′tick) *adj.* [*bin-* + *otic*]. BINAURAL.

bin·ox·ide (bin·ock′side, bye·nock′) *n.* DIOXIDE.

Bin·swang·er's disease, dementia, or **encephalopathy** (bin′ svaʰng·ur) [O. *Binswanger,* German neurologist, 1859–1929]. Chronic progressive subcortical encephalopathy of later life, characterized pathologically by a patchy demyelination of the cerebral white matter, due presumably to arteriosclerosis of small blood vessels.

bi·nu·cle·ar (bye·new′klee·ur) *adj.* BINUCLEATED.

bi·nu·cle·ate (bye·new′klee·ate) *adj.* BINUCLEATED.

bi·nu·cle·at·ed (bye·new′klee·ay·tid) *adj.* Having two nuclei.

binucleated cell. A cell, most commonly found in liver, whose nucleus has undergone mitosis without a division of the cytoplasm.

bio- [Gk. *bios,* life, lifetime]. A combining form meaning (a) *life; pertaining to living organisms or vital phenomena;* (b) *biological.*

bio·acous·tics (bye″o·uh·koos′ticks) *n.* [*bio-* + *acoustics*]. The scientific study of the sounds produced by and affecting living organisms, especially with regard to communicative function.

bio·as·say (bye″o·as′ay) *n.* [*bio-* + *assay*]. A method of determining the potency of a substance by comparing its effects on living material quantitatively with those of a standard substance. Syn. *biological assay.*

bio·au·tog·ra·phy (bye″o·aw·tog′ruh·fee) *n.* [*bio-* + *auto-* + *-graphy*]. A technique similar to radioautography in which the growth response of specific microorganisms (rather than radioactivity) is used for detection of a compound or compounds on a paper chromatogram. —**bio·au·to·graph·ic** (bye″o·aw·to·graf′ick) *adj.*

bio·avail·abil·i·ty (bye″o·uh·vale″uh·bil′i·tee) *n.* [*bio-* + *availability*]. PHYSIOLOGICAL AVAILABILITY.

bi·ob·jec·tive (bye″ub·jeck′tiv) *adj.* Having two objective lenses.

bio·cat·a·lyst (bye″o·kat′uh·list) *n.* ENZYME; a biochemical catalyst.

bi·oc·cip·i·tal (bye·ock·sip′i·tul) *adj.* Pertaining to the right and left occipital lobes of the brain, or both occipital bones, or subdivisions thereof.

bio·ce·no·sis (bye″o·se·no′sis) *n.,* pl. **bioceno·ses** (·seez) [NL., from *bio-* + Gk. *koinōsis,* sharing]. A group of different types of organisms living together in the same environment. See also *biotope.*

bio·chem·is·try (bye″o·kem′is·tree) *n.* [*bio-* + *chemistry*]. The chemistry of living tissues or of life; physiological or biological chemistry. —**biochem·i·cal** (·i·kul) *adj.*

bio·chem·or·phic (bye″o·ke·mor′fick) *adj.* [*bio-* + *chem-* + *-morphic*]. Noting the relationship between chemical structure and biologic activity; pertaining to biochemorphology.

bio·chem·or·phol·o·gy (bye″o·kem″or·fol′uh·jee) *n.* [*bio-* + *chem-* + *morphology*]. The science dealing with the chemical structure of foods and drugs and their reactions on living organisms.

bio·chrome (bye′o·krome) *n.* [*bio-* + *-chrome*]. Pigment synthesized in the metabolic processes of living organisms.

bio·cli·mat·ics (bye″o·klye·mat′icks) *n.* BIOCLIMATOLOGY.

bio·cli·ma·tol·o·gy (bye″o·klye″muh·tol′uh·jee) *n.* [*bio-* + *climatology*]. The study of the effect of climate on life.

bi·o·cy·tin (bye″o·sigh′tin) *n.* A complex of biotin and lysine occurring in yeast and possibly in other natural products.

bi·o·cy·tin·ase (bye″o·sigh′ti·nace, ·naze) *n.* An enzyme present in liver and blood which hydrolyzes biocytin into biotin and lysine.

bio·dy·nam·ics (bye″o·dye·nam′icks) *n.* The study of the dynamic processes manifested in the behavior of organisms.

bio·elec·tric (bye″o·e·leck′trick) *adj.* Of or pertaining to bioelectricity.

bio·elec·tric·i·ty (bye″o·e·leck·tris′i·tee) *n.* Electric phenomena occurring in living tissues; effects of electric currents upon living tissues.

bioelectric potential. The difference of electric potential between the inside and the outside of a cell.

bio·en·er·get·ics (bye″o·en″ur·jet′icks) *n.* The science of the transformation of energy in biologic functions.

bio·equiv·a·lence (bye″o·e·kwiv′uh·lunce) *n.* Equivalent physiological availability of a drug in two or more dosage forms.

bio·eth·ics (bye″o·eth′icks, bye′o·eth·icks) *n.* The ethical principles, or the discipline formulating such principles, which govern the uses of biological and medical technology, especially as they bear directly on the treatment of human life.

bio·feed·back (bye″o·feed′back) *n.* The technique of providing an individual with ongoing sensory awareness of the state of one or more of his body processes, through such means as monitoring devices which produce visual displays or tones of varying pitch, in order to facilitate the exercise of conscious control over normally involuntary or unconscious body functions.

bio·fla·vo·noid (bye″o·flav′o·noid, ·flay′vo·noid) *n.* [*bio-* + *flavonoid*]. Any flavone compound or derivative having biological or pharmacological activity, such as vitamin P.

bio·gen·e·sis (bye″o·jen′e·sis) *n.* [*bio-* + *genesis*]. 1. The doctrine that living things are produced only from living things. Contr. *abiogenesis.* 2. Loosely, both ontogeny and phylogeny. —**bio·ge·net·ic** (·je·net′ick), **bi·og·e·nous** (bye·oj′ e·nus) *adj.*

biogenetic law. RECAPITULATION THEORY.

bi·og·e·ny (bye·oj′e·nee) *n.* BIOGENESIS.

bio·haz·ard (bye′o·haz″urd) *n.* A biological hazard to life or health, especially one constituted by the presence of dangerous microorganisms, as in experimentation on genetic recombination.

bio·ki·net·ics (bye″o·ki·net′icks, ·kigh·net′icks) *n.* The kinetics of life; the science of the movements of or within living organisms.

biol. Abbreviation for *biology.*

bi·o·log·ic (bye″uh·loj′ick) *adj. & n.* 1. Of or pertaining to biology or to living organisms and their products. 2. BIOLOGICAL (2).

bi·o·log·i·cal (bye″uh·loj′i·kul) *adj. & n.* 1. BIOLOGIC (1). 2. A product of biologic origin used in the diagnosis, prevention, or treatment of disease. Included are serums, vaccines, antitoxins, and antigens.

biological agent. Any of certain classifications of microorganisms, or any toxic substance derived from living organisms, that can produce death or disease in man, animals, and growing plants.

biological assay. BIOASSAY.

biological assaying. BIOLOGICAL STANDARDIZATION.

biological availability. The extent to which the active ingredient of a food, nutrient, or drug can be absorbed and made available to the body in a physiologic state. Syn. *physiologic availability.*

biological chemistry. BIOCHEMISTRY.

biological criminology. *In criminology,* the study of the criminal with respect to body build and genetic makeups.

Biological Stain Commission. A nonprofit corporation organized by the several national scientific societies concerned with the quality of dyes available for staining and other biological purposes. The Commission's laboratory tests various dyes and issues certification labels authorized to be affixed to bottles containing dye from batches meeting Commission standards. Such dyes are designated as Certified or Commission Certified.

biological standardization. The standardization of drugs or biological products by their pharmacologic action on animals.

biological variation. Inherent differences between individuals who, for most purposes, are considered to be within a homogeneous group.

biological warfare. *In military medicine,* tactics and techniques of conducting warfare by use of biological agents.

biologic or **biological half-life.** HALF-LIFE (3).

biologic history. The life history of any organism.

biologic test. A precipitin test for blood, meat, and similar protein-containing substances.

biologic therapy. Treatment with biologicals.

bi·ol·o·gist (bye·ol'uh·jist) *n.* A person specializing in biology.

bi·ol·o·gy (bye·ol'uh·jee) *n.* [*bio-* + *-logy*]. The science of life, including microbiology, botany, zoology, and all their branches.

bio·lu·mi·nes·cence (bye''o·lew''mi·nes'unce) *n.* [*bio-* + *luminescence*]. Luminescence caused by living organisms; PHOSPHORESCENCE (1).

bio·ma·te·rial (bye''o·muh·teer'ee·ul) *n.* 1. Any material employed in a prosthetic device, such as a skeletal component, heart valve, or pacemaker, which is implanted in or is otherwise in contact with the tissues of a living organism. 2. (pl. form, *biomaterials*:) The branch of applied science concerned with the selection and evaluation of such materials, especially from the standpoints of durability and degree of tolerance by host tissues.

bio·math·e·mat·ics (bye''o·math''e·mat'icks) *n.* Mathematics applied to or concerned with biologic phenomena.

bio·me·chan·ics (bye''o·me·kan'icks) *n.* 1. The mechanics of the living organism, especially of the levers and arches of the skeleton, and the forces applied to them by the muscles and by gravity. 2. The science in which physical and engineering principles are applied to biological systems such as the musculoskeletal, cardiovascular, or central nervous system.

bio·med·i·cal (bye''o·med'i·kul) *adj.* Pertaining to both biology and medicine.

biomedical engineering. The branch of engineering that deals with the design of materials and machines used in medicine.

bi·om·e·ter (bye·om'e·tur) *n.* [*bio-* + *meter*]. An instrument for measuring the amount of carbon dioxide given off by a microorganism or tissue.

bi·o·met·rics (bye''o·met'ricks) *n.* BIOSTATISTICS.

bi·om·e·try (bye·om'e·tree) *n.* [*bio-* + *-metry*]. 1. BIOSTATISTICS. 2. Calculation of the expectancy of life, for life insurance purposes.

bio·mi·cros·co·py (bye''o·migh·kros'kuh·pee) *n.* Microscopic study of living cell structures. —**bio·mi·cro·scope** (·migh'kruh·scope) *n.*; **bio·mi·cro·scop·ic** (·migh''kro·skop'ick) *adj.*

bi·on·ics (bye·on'icks) *n.* The science concerned with developing electronic, mathematical, or physical models which simulate parallel phenomena found in living systems, as the vertebrate nervous system for cybernetic engineering.

bio·phar·ma·ceu·tics (bye''o·fahr·muh·sue'ticks) *n.* The study of the interrelationships of absorption, distribution, metabolism, storage, and excretion of drugs with the physicochemical properties of body tissues, drugs, and drug dosage forms.

bi·o·phore (bye'o·fore) *n.* [*bio-* + *-phore*]. A hypothetical vital unit in Weismann's theory of the architecture of the germ plasm, varying in complexity from that of a molecule to that of a cell, and with manifold properties and functions depending upon biologists' conceptions. —**bi·o·phor·ic** (bye''o·for'ick) *adj.*

bio·pho·tom·e·ter (bye''o·fo·tom'e·tur) *n.* [*bio-* + *photometer*]. An instrument designed to measure the rate and degree of dark adaptation.

bio·phys·ics (bye''o·fiz'icks) *n.* [*bio-* + *physics*]. The physics of life processes. 2. Application of the methods of physics in biological studies.

bi·op·la·sis (bye·op'luh·sis) *n.* [*bio-* + Gk. *plasis,* moulding, conformation]. ANABOLISM. —**bi·o·plas·tic** (bye''o·plas'tick) *adj.*

bio·plasm (bye'o·plaz·um) *n.* [*bio-* + *-plasm*]. Living protoplasmic substance, as distinguished from inclusions and by-products of protoplasmic activity. —**bio·plas·mic** (bye''o·plaz'mick) *adj.*

bi·op·sy (bye'op·see) *n.* & *v.* [*bio-* + *-opsy*]. 1. The excision, for diagnostic study, of a piece of tissue from a living body. 2. The tissue so excised. 3. To perform a biopsy on.

bio·psy·chic (bye''o·sigh'kick) *adj.* [*bio-* + *psychic*]. Pertaining to mental phenomena as they apply to biology; pertaining or relating to the mind or thinking in life.

bio·psy·cho·log·i·cal (bye''o·sigh''kuh·loj'i·kul) *adj.* PSYCHOBIOLOGICAL.

bio·psy·chol·o·gy (bye''o·sigh·kol'uh·jee) *n.* PSYCHOBIOLOGY.

biopsy needle. A hollow needle designed to obtain, by puncture, small amounts of tissue for microscopic examination and diagnosis.

biopsy punch. CUTISECTOR.

bi·op·ter·in (bye·op'tur·in) *n.* [*bio-* + *pterin*]. 1-(2-Amino-4-hydroxy-6-pteridinyl)-1,2-propanediol, $C_9H_{11}N_5O_3$, a probable intermediate in the synthesis of folic acid; occurs in yeast and in human urine.

bi·op·tome (bye·op'tome) [*biopsy* + *-tome*]. An instrument for obtaining biopsy specimens, especially one which can be passed through a catheter.

bi·or·bi·tal (bye·or'bi·tul) *adj.* Of or pertaining to both orbits.

biorbital angle. *In optics,* the angle formed by the intersection of the axes of the orbits.

bio·rhythm (bye'o·rith''um) *n.* Any regular, cyclic, biologically regulated pattern of change or fluctuation in an organism, such as the menstrual cycle or regular periodic variations in body temperature, blood pressure, or mood.

bi·os I (bye'os). INOSITOL.

bios IIb. BIOTIN.

bi·ose (bye'oce) *n.* [*bi-* + *-ose*]. DISACCHARIDE.

-biosis [Gk. *biōsis*]. A combining form meaning *a* (specified) *way of life.*

bio·sta·tis·tics (bye''o·sta·tis'ticks) *n.* [*bio-* + *statistics*]. 1. The application of statistical principles and methods in biology. 2. Specifically, statistical analysis of vital and demographic data.

bi·os·ter·ol (bye·os'tur·ol, ·ole) *n.* VITAMIN A.

bio·syn·the·sis (bye''o·sin'thi·sis) *n.,* pl. **biosynthe·ses** (·seez) [*bio-* + *synthesis*]. 1. The synthesis of a substance in living matter. 2. The formative reactions which take place during metabolism, as of enzymes or amino acids. —**bio·syn·thet·ic** (·sin·thet'ick) *adj.*

bi·o·ta (bye·o'tuh) *n.* [Gk. *biotē,* way of life]. The flora and fauna, collectively, of a region.

bio·te·lem·e·try (bye''o·te·lem'e·tree) *n.* [*bio-* + *telemetry*]. Telemetry in which the results of measurements of certain vital functions of a subject are transmitted electronically to a distant receiving station and there are indicated or recorded.

bi·ot·ic (bye·ot'ick) *adj.* [Gk. *biōtikos*]. 1. Pertaining to life or living matter. 2. Pertaining to biota.

biotic potential. Soil yield in terms of living growth useful to man.

bi·ot·ics (bye·ot'icks) *n.* The science of vital activities.

bi·o·tin (bye'o·tin, bye·ot'in) *n.* *cis*-Hexahydro-2-oxo-1*H*-thieno[3,4]imidazoline-4-valeric acid, $C_{10}H_{16}N_2O_3S$, a member of the vitamin B complex, present in small amounts in plant and animal tissues. It counteracts the injury syndrome caused by egg white; probably essential for man. Syn. *vitamin H, coenzyme R, bios IIb.* See also *egg-white injury.*

biotin carboxylase. An enzyme which condenses bicarbonate with biotin to form carboxybiotin.

bio·tope (bye'o·tope) *n.* [*bio-* + Gk. *topos,* place]. An area exhibiting the same environmental characteristics and supporting the same types of inhabitants (flora and fauna) throughout. See also *biocenosis.*

bio·trans·for·ma·tion, *n.* The chemical changes that a compound, especially a drug, undergoes in a living system.

Biot's breathing, respiration, or **sign** (byo) [C. *Biot,* French physician, b. 1878]. Grossly irregular breathing, each breath varying in rate and depth; seen with lesions of the medulla or with medullary compression from increased intracranial pressure.

bio·type (bye'o·tipe) *n.* 1. A group of individuals all of which have the same genotype. 2. SOMATOTYPE. —**bio·typ·ic** (bye″o·tip'ick) *adj.*

bio·ty·pol·o·gy (bye″o·tye·pol'uh·jee) *n.* [*biotype* + *-logy*]. The systematic study of body types correlated with physiologic and psychologic aspects, as constitutional variations and inadequacies.

bi·ovu·lar (bye·o'vyoo·lur) *adj.* [*bi-* + *ovular*]. Pertaining to or derived from two ova.

biovular twins. FRATERNAL TWINS.

B.I.P. Abbreviation for *bismuth iodoform paste.*

bip·a·ra (bip'uh·ruh) *n.*, pl. **biparas, bipa·rae** (·ree) [*bi-* + *-para*]. A woman who has borne two children at different labors.

bi·pa·ri·etal (bye″puh·rye'e·tul) *adj.* 1. Pertaining to both parietal bones. 2. Pertaining to the right or left parietal lobes of the brain, or subdivisions thereof.

biparietal diameter. The distance from one parietal eminence to the other.

biparietal obliquity. ANTERIOR or POSTERIOR ASYNCLITISM.

bip·a·rous (bip'uh·rus) *adj.* [*bi-* + *-parous*]. 1. Producing two offspring at a birth. 2. Having given birth twice.

bi·par·tite (bye·pahr'tite) *adj.* Divided into, or consisting of, two parts or divisions.

bipartite placenta. A placenta with two divisions.

bipartite uterus. UTERUS SEPTUS.

bi·ped (bye'ped) *n.* [*bi-* + *-ped*]. An animal that normally walks and stands on two feet. Contr. *quadruped.* —**bi·ped·al** (bye″ped'ul) *adj.*

bi·ped·i·cled flap (bye·ped'i·kuld). A pedicle flap that remains attached at both ends.

bi·pen·nate (bye·pen'ate) *adj.* [*bi-* + *pennate*]. Having the appearance of a feather with barbs on both sides of the shaft, as certain muscles. Contr. *unipennate.*

bipennate muscle. A muscle whose fibers are inserted on two sides of a central tendon. NA *musculus bipennatus.*

bi·pen·ni·form (bye·pen'i·form) *adj.* BIPENNATE.

bi·per·i·den (bye·perr'i·den) *n.* α-(Bicyclo[2.2.1]hept-5-en-2-yl)-α-phenyl-1-piperidinepropanol, $C_{21}H_{29}NO$, used as the hydrochloride or lactate salt as an anticholinergic agent for treatment of parkinsonism.

Biphenabid. A trademark for probucol, an anticholesteremic.

bi·phen·a·mine (bye·fen'uh·meen) *n.* 2-(Diethylamino)ethyl 2-hydroxy-3-biphenylcarboxylate, $C_{19}H_{23}NO_3$, a topical anesthetic with antibacterial and antifungal activity, normally employed as the hydrochloride salt.

bi·phen·yl (bye·fen'il) *n.* $C_6H_5C_6H_5$, a compound found in coal tar.

bi·phos·phate (bye·fos'fate) *n.* A salt of phosphoric acid in which one of the three hydrogen atoms of the acid is replaced by a base.

bi·po·lar (bye·po'lur) *adj.* 1. Having or involving two poles; specifically, having negative and positive poles or leads. 2. Pertaining to a neuron having an afferent and efferent process.

bipolar axis. *In electrocardiography,* the electrical axis determined from standard limb leads.

bipolar cells of the retina. Bipolar cells of the inner nuclear layer of the retina, connected with the rods and cones of the retina externally and ramifying internally in the middle of the molecular layer.

bi·po·lar·i·ty (bye″po·lăr'i·tee) *n.* [*bi-* + *polarity*]. 1. The condition of having two processes extending from opposite poles, as a nerve cell. 2. The use of two electrodes in stimulation of muscle or nerve, or in recording bioelectric potentials.

bipolar limb lead. STANDARD LIMB LEAD.

bipolar nerve cell. A nerve cell having two prolongations of the cytoplasm, as in the vestibular ganglion of the eighth cranial nerve.

bipolar pressure. Pressure on the two ends of a bone. It is used in differentiating fractures from contusions, producing pain in the case of the former.

bipolar version. Manipulation of both the pelvis and the vertex of the fetus.

bi·po·ten·ti·al·i·ty (bye″po·ten″shee·al'i·tee) *n.* The capacity of developing into two different types of tissues.

bipotentiality of the gonad. Bisexual organization of the indifferent gonad; the medullary part is thought capable of forming the testis, and the cortex of forming the ovary.

bipp, *n.* [*b*ismuth subnitrate *i*odoform *p*etrolatum *p*aste]. A dressing for wounds, composed of bismuth subnitrate 1 part, iodoform 2 parts, petrolatum 1 part. Syn. *bismuth iodoform paste.*

birch, *n.* Any tree of the genus *Betula.* Birch tar, or the tarry oil of *Betula pendula,* has been used in certain skin diseases. The bark of *B. lenta,* the sweet birch, yields a fragrant volatile oil, which consists, like that of *Gaultheria procumbens,* almost entirely of methyl salicylate.

bird-breeder's lung. A pulmonary hypersensitivity reaction to antigens in bird excreta, characterized by cough, fever, dyspnea, and weight loss; seen usually in pigeon and parakeet (budgerigar) fanciers.

bird face. A face characterized by a receding chin and beak-like appearance of the nose; the result of mandibular hypoplasia (micrognathia).

bird-headed dwarfism. A congenital disorder, possibly due to various causes, characterized by low birth weight, marked but proportionate shortness of stature, a proportionately small head, hypoplasia of the maxilla and mandible with beak-like protrusion of the nose, mental retardation, and a variety of other skeletal, cutaneous, and genital anomalies. Syn. *Seckel's syndrome.*

bird louse. MALLOPHAGA.

bird pox. AVIAN POX.

bird pox diphtheria. AVIAN POX.

Bird's disease [G. *Bird,* English physician, 1814–1854]. OXALURIA.

bi·re·frac·tive (bye″re·frack'tiv) *adj.* Doubly refractive; characterized by birefringence.

bi·re·frin·gence (bye″re·frin'junce) *n.* The property of having more than one refractive index, according to the direction of the traversing light. It is possessed by all except isometric crystals, by transparent substances that have undergone internal strains (e.g., glass), and by substances that have different structures in different directions (e.g., fibers). Syn. *double refraction.* See also *flow birefringence.* —**birefrin·gent** (·junt) *adj.*

birth, *n.* [ON. *byrdhr*]. In viviparous species, the offspring's emergence from the womb of the mother.

birth canal. The channel formed by the uterus and vagina which conveys the fetus through the pelvic canal during parturition.

birth certificate. A legal form on which the date and place of birth, name and sex of child, names of parents, and other pertinent information are recorded.

birth control. Any means used to help control reproduction, such as methods of facilitating, timing, or preventing conception, sexual abstinence or alternatives, abortion, sterilization, and artificial insemination. Compare *contraception.*

birth injury. Any injury suffered by a neonate during parturition, such as fracture of a bone, subluxation of a joint, injury to peripheral nerves, or intracranial hemorrhage.

birth·mark, *n.* A congenital skin lesion, usually either a vascular hamartoma or pigmented nevus, but possibly of another nature.

birth membranes. The two fetal membranes, inner amnion

and outer chorion, which enclose the amniotic fluid. A portion of the chorion contributes to the placenta.

birth palsy or **paralysis**. 1. Any paralysis due to injury sustained during birth. 2. CEREBRAL PALSY. 3. BRACHIAL BIRTH PALSY.

birth rate. The proportion of births in a given year and area to the midyear population of that area, usually expressed as the number of live births per thousand of population.

birth registration area. The territory from which the United States Bureau of the Census collects birth records. Since 1933, this has been the entire United States.

birth trauma. 1. *In psychiatry*, the hypothesis which relates the development of anxiety and neurosis to the universal psychic shock of being born. 2. BIRTH INJURY.

bis- [L. *bis*, twice]. A prefix meaning (a) *twice, both;* (b) in chemistry, *the doubling of a complex expression.*

bis·a·bol (bis'uh·bol) *n.* A kind of myrrh from a species of trees of East Africa, genus *Commiphora,* used largely in finer grades of myrrh.

bis·a·co·dyl (bis''uh·ko'dil, ·ack'o·dil) *n.* Bis(*p*-acetoxyphenyl)-2-pyridylmethane, $C_{22}H_{19}NO_4$, a laxative drug.

bisacodyl tan·nex (tan'ecks). A water-soluble complex of bisacodyl and tannic acid, employed as a cathartic.

Bisch·off's test (bish'off) [C. A. *Bischoff*, German chemist, 1855–1908]. Bile acids when heated with dilute sulfuric acid and sucrose produce a red color.

Biscumarol. A trademark for dicumarol (= BISHYDROXYCOUMARIN).

bi·sect (bye·sekt') *v.* [*bi-* + L. *secare, sectus,* to cut]. To cut into two roughly equal parts.

bisected brain syndrome. SPLIT BRAIN.

bi·sec·tion (bye·seck'shun) *adj.* [*bi-* + *section*]. A cutting into two nearly equal parts.

bisection technique. ANGLE BISECTION TECHNIQUE.

bi·sex·ous (bye·seck'sus) *adj.* HERMAPHRODITIC.

bi·sex·u·al (bye·seck'shoo·ul) *adj.* [*bi-* + *sexual*]. 1. Exhibiting both homosexual and heterosexual behavior, or attracted sexually to both males and females. 2. HERMAPHRODITIC.

bi·sex·u·al·i·ty (bye·secks''yoo·al'i·tee, bye·seck''shoo·) *n.* [*bi-* + *sexuality*]. 1. The condition of being equally attracted sexually to males and females. 2. HERMAPHRODITISM.

bis·fer·i·ens pulse (bis·ferr'ee·enz, bis·feer') [L., striking, beating twice]. A pulse characterized by two palpable waves or beats during systole, an initial percussion wave, and a second tidal wave. Compare *anacrotic pulse, dicrotic pulse.*

bis·fer·i·ous (bis·ferr'ee·us, bis·feer') *adj.* [*bis-* + L. *ferire,* to strike]. Having two peaks or beats. See also *bisferiens pulse.*

bis·hy·droxy·cou·ma·rin (bis''high·drock''see·koo'muh·rin) *n.* [*bis-* + *hydroxy-* + *coumarin*]. 3,3'-Methylenebis(4-hydroxycoumarin), $C_{19}H_{12}O_6$, originally isolated from spoiled sweet clover, eating of which caused hemorrhagic disease in cattle. It occurs as a white crystalline powder, practically insoluble in water; used as an anticoagulant. Syn. *dicoumarin, dicoumarol, melitoxin.*

Bis·kra button [after *Biskra,* Algeria]. CUTANEOUS LEISHMANIASIS.

bis·muth (biz'muth) *n.* [Ger. *Wismut*]. Bi = 208.980. A white, crystalline metal with a reddish tint. Its insoluble salts are employed chiefly because of their protective action on mucous membranes; the salts are also feebly antiseptic. Various compounds of bismuth, soluble and insoluble, have been employed for the treatment of syphilis.

bismuth and emetine iodide. A reddish-orange salt, practically insoluble in water; used in the treatment of amebic colitis.

bismuth carbonate. BISMUTH SUBCARBONATE.

bis·mu·thia (biz·mewth'ee·uh, ·muth'ee·uh) *n.* A blue discoloration of skin and mucous membranes resulting from administration of bismuth compounds.

bismuth iodoform paste. BIPP. Abbreviated, B.I.P.

bis·muth·o·sis (biz''muth·o'sis) *n.* Chronic bismuth poisoning.

bis·mutho·tar·trate (biz''muth·o·tahr'trate) *n.* A salt of tartaric acid in which a bismuthyl (BiO) radical replaces the hydroxyl hydrogen of one or both of the secondary alcohol groups in the tartaric acid component of the salt.

bismuth potassium tartrate. A water-soluble salt containing 60 to 64% bismuth; has been used as an antisyphilitic, by intramuscular injection.

bismuth salicylate. 1. A mixture of salicylic acid and bismuth subsalicylate. 2. Loosely, BISMUTH SUBSALICYLATE.

bismuth sodium tartrate. A water-soluble salt formerly used as an antisyphilitic.

bismuth sodium triglycollamate. A double salt of sodium bismuthyl triglycollamate and sodium triglycollamate, approximately $C_{24}H_{28}BiN_4Na_7O_{25}$; very soluble in water. Effective orally in the management of certain forms of syphilis and also in some cases of lupus erythematosus, lichen planus, and scleroderma.

bismuth subcarbonate. Approximately $2(BiO)_2CO_3.H_2O$; a white salt, insoluble in water; used as a protective in gastrointestinal diseases as well as for local application.

bismuth subgallate. Approximately $C_6H_2(OH)_3COO\text{-}Bi(OH)_2$; a bright yellow powder, practically insoluble in water. Has been used externally as a dusting powder, sometimes internally in treating enteritis. Syn. *dermatol.*

bismuth subnitrate. Approximately $4BiNO_3(OH)_2.BiO(OH)$; a white powder, practically insoluble in water. Used like bismuth subcarbonate but yields some nitrite ion in the intestines.

bismuth subsalicylate. Approximately $C_6H_4(OH)COOBiO$; a white powder, practically insoluble in water. Its antiseptic action is superior to that of other basic bismuth salts. Used in the treatment of enteritis, and has been used as an antisyphilitic.

bismuth tribromphenate. Approximately $BiOH.(C_6H_2Br_3O)_2.Bi_2O_3$; a yellow powder, practically insoluble in water. Used as an antiseptic, both internally and externally.

bismuth tribromphenol. BISMUTH TRIBROMPHENATE.

bis·muth·yl (biz'muth·il, ·eel) *n.* [*bismuth* + *-yl*]. The univalent radical BiO.

bismuthyl gly·co·lo·yl·ar·sa·nil·ate (glye·ko''lo·il·ahr''suh·nil'ate). The chemical name for glycobiarsol, an amebicide.

bis·o·brin (bis'o·brin) *n.* *meso*-1,1'-Tetramethylenebis[1,2,3,4-tetrahydro-6,7-dimethoxyisoquinoline], $C_{26}H_{36}N_2O_4$, a fibrinolytic agent used as the lactate salt.

bi·son neck. Excess adiposity of the neck, as seen in Cushing's syndrome. See also *buffalo obesity.*

bis·ox·a·tin (bis·ock'suh·tin) *n.* 2,2-Bis(*p*-hydroxyphenyl)-2*H*-1,4-benzoxazin-3(4*H*)-one, $C_{20}H_{15}NO_4$, a cathartic; used as the diacetate ester.

bi·spi·nous diameter (bye·spye'nus). The distance between the spines of the ischia.

bis·sa (bis'uh) *n.* A disease of man and sheep, common in Egypt; characterized by the production of edema; due to ingestion of the bisse plant by sheep and of mutton by man.

bissabol. BISABOL.

bissinosis. BYSSINOSIS.

bis·tort (bis'tort) *n.* [*bis-* + L. *torquere, tortus,* to twist]. The rhizome of the herbaceous plant *Polygonum bistorta.* It contains tannin, and has been used as astringent.

bis·tou·ry (bis'too·ree) *n.* [F. *bistouri,* from It. *pistorino,* of Pistoia]. A long, narrow knife, either straight or curved and sharp-pointed or probe-pointed, designed for cutting from within outward; formerly used to open abscesses, enlarge sinuses or fistulas, or cut constrictions in strangulated hernias.

Bistrimate. A trademark for bismuth sodium triglycollamate.

bi·sul·fide (bye·sul'fide, ·fid) *n.* [*bi-* + *sulfide*]. A binary compound containing two atoms of sulfur. Syn. *disulfide.*

bi·sul·fite (bye·sul'fite) *n.* [*bi-* + *sulfite*]. Any compound containing the radical HSO_3; an acid sulfite.

bi·tar·trate (bye·tahr'trate) *n.* [*bi-* + *tartrate*]. A salt of tartaric acid characterized by the radical $HC_4H_4O_6$, representing tartaric acid wherein one hydrogen has been replaced. Syn. *acid tartrate.*

bite, *v.* & *n.* 1. To seize or grasp with the teeth or to puncture with the mouthparts. 2. The forcible closure of the lower against the upper teeth; the measure of force exerted by such closure as recorded in pounds by gnathodynamometer. 3. A skin puncture produced by the teeth or mouth parts of an insect or animal. 4. INTEROCCLUSAL RECORD.

bite block. 1. A device used to hold the jaws open while operating in or through the oral cavity. 2. A device used to hold a film in position in intraoral radiography. 3. OCCLUSION RIM.

bite guard. An appliance worn on the teeth to relieve excessive occlusal forces; usually used in the treatment of bruxism or occlusal trauma.

bi·tem·po·ral (bye·tem'pur·ul) *adj.* 1. Pertaining to both temples. 2. Pertaining to both temporal lobes of the brain, or both temporal bones, or subdivisions thereof. 3. Pertaining to both temporal fields of vision.

bitemporal diameter. The distance between the extremities of the coronal suture.

bitemporal hemianopsia. Blindness on the temporal side of the visual field, due to disease of the central parts of the optic commissure.

bite plate. OCCLUSION RIM.

bite·wing, *n.* A type of dental x-ray film having a central fin or wing upon which the teeth can close to hold the film in place.

bi·thi·o·nol (bye·thigh'o·nol) *n.* 2,2′-Thiobis(4,6-dichlorophenol), $C_{12}H_6Cl_4O_2S$, a crystalline powder, insoluble in water. Has been used as bacteriostatic agent in soap formulations.

bi·thi·o·nol·ate (bye·thigh'uh·no·late) *n.* 2,2′-Thiobis(4,6-dichlorophenol), $C_{12}H_6Cl_4O_2S$, a topical anti-infective, usually used as the disodium salt.

Bi·thyn·ia (bi·thin'ee·uh) *n.* [after *Bithynia,* Asia Minor]. A genus of snails whose species serve as intermediate hosts of the trematodes of man. The species *Bithynia tentaculata* of eastern Europe is the host of the cat liver fluke, *Opisthorchis felineus; B. fuchsiana* and *B. longicornis* of China are hosts of *Clonorchis sinensis.*

Bi·tis (bye'tis) *n.* A genus of venomous snakes of the Viperidae.

Bitis ga·bon·i·ca (ga·bon'i·kuh). The Gaboon viper of equatorial Africa; has a powerful neurotoxic venom.

Bitis la·che·sis (la·kee'sis). The large-headed puff adder; a species found from South Africa to southern Arabia; has a hemotoxic venom.

Bitis na·si·cor·nis (nay"zi·kor'nis). The rhinoceros viper of equatorial Africa; has a hemotoxic venom.

bi·tol·te·rol (bye·toal'te·role) *n.* 4-[2-(*tert*-Butylamino)-1-hydroxyethyl]-*o*-phenylene di-*p*-toluate, $C_{28}H_{31}NO_5$, a bronchodilator.

Bi·tôt's spots (bee·to') [P. A. *Bitôt,* French surgeon, 1822–1888]. XEROSIS CONJUNCTIVAE.

bitter almond oil. The volatile oil from the dried ripe kernel of *Prunus amygdalus* var. *amara* or from other kernels containing amygdalin. It contains principally benzaldehyde, partly combined with hydrocyanic acid. Sometimes used as a flavor.

bit·ter·ling (bit'ur·ling) *n.* [Ger.]. A small European fish now common around New York; also, one of a different species common in Japan and used for human pregnancy tests.

bitterling test. A test for pregnancy performed by placing a female bitterling in a quart of fresh water containing two teaspoonsful of the patient's urine. Enlargement of the ovipositor indicates a positive test.

bitter orange oil. A volatile oil from the fresh peel of the fruit of *Citrus aurantium;* used as flavor.

bitter principle. AMAROID.

bit·ters, *n.* A medicinal substance used for its bitter taste, chiefly to increase appetite or as a tonic.

bit·ter·sweet, *n.* DULCAMARA.

Bitt·ner milk factor. MILK FACTOR.

bi·tu·ber·al (bye·tew'bur·ul) *adj.* BIISCHIAL.

bi·tu·ber·ous (bye·tew'bur·us) *adj.* Having or pertaining to two tubers or tuberosities, especially ischial tuberosities.

bituberous diameter. BIISCHIAL DIAMETER.

bi·tu·men (bi·tew'mun, bye-, bit'yoo·mun) *n.* [L.]. Any one of a group of native solid or semisolid hydrocarbons.

bi·urate (bye·yoo'rate) *n.* An acid salt of uric acid.

bi·u·ret (bye"yoo·ret', bye'yoo·ret) *n.* Carbamylurea, $NH_2CONHCONH_2$, obtained by heating urea.

biuret reaction. A reaction given by compounds which contain acid amide groups in close proximity, as by biuret or by proteins. A red-violet to blue-violet color is produced on adding a cupric sulfate solution to an alkaline solution of the specimen.

bi·va·lence (bye·vay'lunce) *n.* 1. The state of being bivalent. 2. AMBIVALENCE. —**biva·len·cy** (·lun·see) *adj.*

bi·va·lent (bye·vay'lunt, biv'uh·lunt) *adj.* & *n.* [*bi-* + *valent*]. 1. Able to combine with or displace two atoms of hydrogen or their equivalent; having a valence of 2. Syn. *divalent.* 2. Double or paired. 3. AMBIVALENT. 4. BIVALENT CHROMOSOME.

bivalent chromosome. A structure formed by the association of homologous chromosomes in the zygotene and pachytene stages of meiosis and serving as source of the tetrad in diplotene.

bi·valve (bye'valv) *n.* & *v.* [*bi-* + *valve*]. 1. A mollusk with double shells, as a clam or oyster. 2. To section a solid organ incompletely, as if opening a clam or oyster. —**bi·val·vu·lar** (·val'vew·lur) *adj.*

bi·ven·ter (bye·ven'tur) *n.* & *L. adj.* [NL., from *bi-* + *venter*]. 1. DIGASTRIC MUSCLE. 2. Having two bellies, as a muscle; DIGASTRIC. —**bi·ven·tral,** *adj.*

biventral lobule. PARAMEDIAN LOBULE.

bi·ven·tric·u·lar (bye"ven·trick'yoo·lur) *adj.* Involving both cardiac ventricles.

bi·zy·go·mat·ic (bye·zye"go·mat'ick) *adj.* Of or pertaining to the two zygomatic bones.

Biz·zo·ze·ro nodules (beedz·oʰdz'e·ro) [G. *Bizzozero,* Italian physician, 1846–1901]. Small nodular thickenings of the intercellular bridges of the cells of the epidermis.

Bizzozero's blood platelet [G. *Bizzozero*]. *Obsol.* ACHROMACYTE.

Bjer·rum's screen (byerr'o͝om) [J. P. *Bjerrum,* Danish ophthalmologist, 1827–1892]. A 1 meter square screen that is used at a distance of 1 meter to plot accurately the central field of vision.

Bjerrum's sign or **scotoma** [J. P. *Bjerrum*]. An arcuate visual field defect extending from the blind spot around the macula, considered to be pathognomic of simple glaucoma.

Bk Symbol for berkelium.

BK Below the knee; used to describe such an amputation in the leg. Contr. *AK.*

black ape. A crested, nearly tailless monkey, *Macaca nigra,* found on the island of Celebes. A significant number of these monkeys have a spontaneous diabetic syndrome very similar to human diabetes mellitus.

black balsam. PERUVIAN BALSAM.

black cancer. A malignant melanoma.

black cardiac. A patient with the severe cyanosis of Ayerza's syndrome.

black cataract. A cataract in which the color of the lens, having gradually changed from the yellow of nuclear sclerosis to amber and reddish brown, has turned almost black.

black cohosh. CIMICIFUGA.

black·damp, *n.* A mixture of carbon dioxide and other gases which collects in mines and deep shafts; it supports neither respiration nor combustion. Syn. *chokedamp.*

Black Death. BLACK PLAGUE.

black disease. Necrotic hepatitis of sheep, resulting from interaction of an anaerobic bacterium, *Clostridium novyi,* and immature flukes, *Fasciola hepatica,* in the liver.

black draft. An infusion of senna with magnesium sulfate; a purgative.

black eye. Ecchymosis of the skin surrounding the eye as the result of trauma.

black fever. KALA AZAR.

black fly. *SIMULIUM.*

black, hairy tongue. A tongue with a brown, furlike patch on the dorsum, due to hypertrophied filiform papillae and the presence of pigment.

black haw. *VIBURNUM PRUNIFOLIUM.*

black·head, *n.* 1. COMEDO. 2. HISTOMONIASIS, a disease of poultry sometimes marked by a cyanotic condition of the head.

black Indian hemp. APOCYNUM.

black induration. Fibrosis, especially of the lung, due to anthracosis.

black jaundice. An extreme degree of jaundice; specifically, septicemia with acute hemolytic anemia and hemoglobinuria of the newborn. See also *Winckel's disease.*

black·leg, *n.* A febrile, generally fatal, infectious disease of cattle and sheep, characterized by diffuse, crepitating swelling in the muscles of the back and legs, usually caused by *Clostridium chauvei,* but sometimes by *C. septicum* or *C. novyi.* Syn. *black quarter, emphysematous gangrene.*

black light. WOOD'S LIGHT.

black measles. HEMORRHAGIC MEASLES.

black mustard. The finely ground seeds of the herb *Brassica nigra,* used as an emetic and locally as a counterirritant application.

black·out, *n.* 1. Temporary loss or diminution of vision and consciousness produced by transient cerebral and retinal ischemia; in aviation, it usually results from strong acceleration in a plane parallel with the long axis of the body. Compare *syncope.* 2. A period during alcoholic intoxication for which the patient demonstrates no memory upon detoxication.

black plague. A form of plague, epidemic in Europe and Asia in the 14th century; so called because of extensive skin hemorrhages.

black quarter. BLACKLEG.

Black's classification [G. V. *Black,* U.S. dentist, 1836–1915]. A system of classification of dental cavities by location.

black sickness. KALA AZAR.

black snake. 1. A poisonous snake, *Pseudechis porphyriacus,* of Australia. 2. Any of several nonpoisonous North American snakes.

Black's test [O. F. *Black,* U.S. chemist, 1867–1933]. A test for β-hydroxybutyric acid in which Black's reagent (ferric chloride, ferrous chloride, water) and hydrogen peroxide are added to an extract of urine which has been treated with plaster of Paris, ether, hydrochloric acid, and barium carbonate. The development of a rose color is a positive test.

black·tongue, *n.* A disease of dogs similar to pellagra, due to a deficiency of niacin. Compare *black, hairy tongue.*

black vomit. Dark vomited matter, consisting of digested blood and gastric contents.

black·wa·ter fever. A complication of falciparum malaria, characterized by intravascular hemolysis, hemoglobinuria, tachycardia, high fever, and a poor prognosis.

black widow. *Latrodectus mactans,* a poisonous black spider with some red or yellow markings, found in most warm parts of the world. Its bite has been fatal in about 5 per cent of the reported cases. The body of the female is about half an inch long and, in the usual North American varieties, has a red hourglass figure on the underside of its globose abdomen. The male is smaller and does not bite.

blad·der, *n.* 1. A membranous sac serving for the reception of fluids or gases, as the swim bladder of some fishes. 2. A hollow organ which serves as a reservoir for urine or bile, as the urinary bladder or gallbladder. Comb. form *vesic(o)-, cyst(o)-.*

bladder bar. BAR OF THE BLADDER.

bladder diverticulum. A congenital or acquired outpouching of the urinary bladder wall, lacking a normal complement of bladder muscle.

bladder hernia. The protrusion of any part of the urinary bladder through any opening in the abdominal wall.

bladder injury. 1. Damage to the urinary bladder through penetration of the abdominal wall, vagina, rectum, buttock, hernial sac, or by accidental injury during abdominal operation or hernioplasty. 2. Rupture of the urinary bladder, either intraperitoneal or extraperitoneal, from fracture of the pelvis, pressure or injury over a distended organ, or occasionally unrelieved retention in an atonic bladder. Extraperitoneal rupture results in extravasation of urine into the retropubic space.

bladder training. Establishing the control of urination as a habit during infancy or early childhood.

bladder triangle. TRIGONE (2).

bladder worm. The larval stage of a tapeworm; CYSTICERCUS.

blade, *n.* 1. The cutting portion of a surgical knife or of surgical scissors. 2. One of the two arms or limbs of forceps.

Blair-Brown graft [V.P. *Blair,* U.S. surgeon, b. 1871; and J. B. *Brown,* U.S. surgeon, b. 1899]. INTERMEDIATE SPLIT GRAFT.

Blair-Brown knife [V. P. *Blair* and J. B. *Brown*]. A knife specially designed to cut skin for grafts; gauges regulate accurately the thickness of the grafts.

Blake·more's tube [A. H. *Blakemore,* U.S. surgeon, b. 1897]. A specially designed, triple-lumened tube, with sausage-shaped balloon tip, used to control acute hemorrhage from esophageal varices by tamponage.

Blalock-Taussig operation [A. *Blalock,* U.S. surgeon, 1899–1964; and Helen B. *Taussig*]. A surgical anastomosis between the subclavian artery and pulmonary artery, designed to circumvent pulmonary stenosis and increase pulmonary blood flow; used primarily in palliation of tetralogy of Fallot.

blanc fixe (blahnk ficks). BARIUM SULFATE.

blanch, *v.* [MF. *blanchir*]. To become or to make pale.

bland, *adj.* [L. *blandus,* caressing, flattering]. 1. Smooth or soothing. 2. Not irritating. 3. Not infected.

bland diet. A diet free of roughage, spices, or other irritating ingredients.

bland infarct. An infarct free from infection.

Blandin-Nuhn gland. Blandin's gland (= ANTERIOR LINGUAL GLAND).

Blan·din's glands (blah^{n}·dæ$^{n'}$) [P. F. *Blandin,* French surgeon, 1798–1849]. ANTERIOR LINGUAL GLANDS.

bland necrosis. ASEPTIC NECROSIS.

Bland-White-Gar·land syndrome [E. F. *Bland,* U.S. physician, b. 1901; P. D. *White,* U.S. physician, b. 1886; and J. *Garland,* U.S. physician, b. 1893]. Anomalous origin of the left coronary artery from the pulmonary artery, resulting in angina pectoris and myocardial infarction in young children.

Blan·for·dia (blan·for'dee·uh) *n.* *ONCOMELANIA.*

blast-, blasto- [Gk. *blastos,* germ]. A combining form meaning (a) *bud;* (b) *budding;* (c) *germ;* (d) *the early stages of the embryo.*

-blast [Gk. *blastos,* germ]. A combining form meaning (a) *a sprout, shoot,* or *germ;* (b) in biology, *a formative cell, a germ layer,* or *a formative constituent of living matter.*

blast cell [from the combining form *-blast*]. The least differentiated member of a line of blood-forming elements which can be clearly identified as a member of that line.

blast-cell leukemia. STEM-CELL LEUKEMIA.

blas·te·ma (blas·tee'muh) *n.*, pl. **blastemas, blastema·ta** (·tuh) [Gk. *blastēma*, offspring, offshoot]. 1. The formative cellular matrix from which an organ, tissue, or part is derived; ANLAGE (1). 2. A small bud of competent cells from which begins the regeneration of an organ or appendage. 3. The budding or sprouting part of a plant. 4. The hypothetical formative lymph or fluid from which cells or organs are formed. —**blas·te·mal** (·mul), **blas·te·mat·ic** (·te·mat'ick), **blas·tem·ic** (blas·tem'ick) *adj.*

-blastic [Gk. *blastikos*, budding, sprouting]. A combining form meaning *germinating, arising, growing.*

blastin (blas'tin) *n.* A substance which nourishes or stimulates cell growth and activity.

blast injury or **syndrome.** Trauma to the viscera and to the central nervous system caused by rapid changes in the environmental pressure, as in bomb explosions; usually manifested by pulmonary hemorrhage, intestinal rupture, rupture of the eardrums, and shock. The brain and meninges may show diffuse and focal hemorrhages.

blasto-. See *blast-*.

blastocele. BLASTOCOELE.

blas·to·chyle (blas'to·kile) *n.* [*blasto-* + *chyle*]. The fluid in the blastocoele.

blas·to·coele, blas·to·coel (blas'to·seel) *n.* [*blasto-* + *-coele*]. The central cavity of the blastula or blastocyst.

blas·to·cyst (blas'to·sist) *n.* [*blasto-* + *cyst*]. 1. BLASTULA. 2. The modified mammalian blastula consisting of trophoblast, inner cell mass, and blastocoele.

Blas·to·cys·tis hom·i·nis (blas''to·sis'tis hom'i·nis). A nonpathogenic fungus inhabiting the intestine of man and other animals.

blas·to·derm (blas'to·durm) *n.* [*blasto-* + *-derm*]. *In embryology:* 1. The cellular disk of blastomeres derived from the blastodisk of meroblastic ova. 2. The primitive germ layer or epithelium of a blastula or blastocyst from which the primary germ layers are derived. 3. By extension, the germinal membrane after the formation of the several germ layers. —**blas·to·der·mal** (blas''to·dur'mul), **blastoder·mic** (·mick) *adj.*

blastodermic membrane. BLASTODERM (3).

blastodermic vesicle. BLASTOCYST (2).

blas·to·disk, blas·to·disc (blas'to·disk) *n.* [*blasto-* + *disk*]. 1. The uncleaved cytoplasmic disk capping the embryonic pole of meroblastic ova. 2. The embryonic or germinal disk of mammals.

blas·to·gen·e·sis (blas''to·jen'e·sis) *n.*, pl. **blastogene·ses** (·seez) [*blasto-* + *-genesis*]. 1. The early development of the embryo during cleavage and the formation of the germ layers. See also *organogenesis.* 2. Weismann's theory of origin and development from germ plasm, in contradistinction to pangenesis, as postulated by Darwin. 3. Reproduction by budding. —**blastogen·ic** (·ick), **blasto·ge·net·ic** (·je·net'ick) *adj.*

blas·tog·e·ny (blas·toj'e·nee) *n.* [*blasto-* + *-geny*]. 1. BLASTOGENESIS. 2. The germ history of an organism (Haeckel); a division of ontogeny.

blas·to·ki·ne·sis (blas''to·ki·nee'sis, ·kigh·nee'sis) *n.* [*blasto-* + *kinesis*]. A process of cephalocaudal reversal in the egg of insects and certain cephalopods.

blas·to·ki·nin (blas''to·kigh'nin) *n.* [*blasto-* + *kinin*]. A protein fraction, first isolated from the pregnant rabbit uterus, believed capable of inducing and regulating blastocyst development in the mammalian uterus.

blas·tol·y·sis (blas·tol'i·sis) *n.*, pl. **blastoly·ses** (·seez) [*blasto-* + *lysis*]. Dissolution of a blastoderm or germ cell.

blas·to·ma (blas·to'muh) *n.*, pl. **blastomas, blastoma·ta** (·tuh) [*blast-* + *-oma*]. A tumor whose parenchymal cells have certain embryonal characteristics, as fibroblastoma or chondroma. —**blas·tom·a·tous** (·tom'uh·tus) *adj.*

blastoma epen·dy·ma·le (e·pen''di·may'lee). EPENDYMOMA.

blas·tom·a·to·gen·ic (blas·tom''uh·to·jen'ick) *adj.* [*blastoma* + *-genic*]. Pertaining to factors or agents which excite cellular multiplication resulting in neoplastic growth.

blas·to·mere (blas'to·meer) *n.* [*blasto-* + *-mere*]. Any one of the cells into which the fertilized ovum divides. Syn. *cleavage cell, segmentation cell.*

Blas·to·my·ces (blas''to·migh'seez) *n.* [*blasto-* + *-myces*]. A genus of fungi pathogenic to man.

Blastomyces bra·sil·i·en·sis (bra·zil''ee·en'sis). A species of fungus that is the causative agent of South American blastomycosis. It reproduces in tissue and in culture at 37°C by multiple-budding cells and thereby differs from the singly budding cells of *Blastomyces dermatitidis.*

Blastomyces der·ma·tit·i·dis (dur''ma·tit'i·dis). A species of fungus that is the causative agent of North American blastomycosis. The organism is spheroid and budding in tissues; it produces aerial hyphae in culture.

blas·to·my·cete (blas''to·migh·seet', ·migh'seet) *n.* A fungus of the genus *Blastomyces.*

Blas·to·my·ce·tes (blas''to·migh·seet'eez) *n.pl.* [*blasto-* + *mycetes*]. A group of pathogenic fungi which includes the genus *Blastomyces.*

blas·to·my·ce·tic (blas''to·migh·see'tick) *adj.* Pertaining to or caused by the budding fungi of the genus *Blastomyces.*

blastomycetic dermatitis. A skin disease, such as blastomycosis or erosio interdigitale blastomycetica, caused by one of the yeast-like fungi.

blas·to·my·cin (blas''to·migh'sin) *n.* [*Blastomyces* + *-in*]. A sterile, standardized liquid concentrate of soluble growth products elaborated by the fungus *Blastomyces dermatitidis;* used in skin tests for the diagnosis of blastomycosis.

blas·to·my·co·sis (blas''to·migh·ko'sis) *n.*, pl. **blastomyco·ses** (·seez) [*blasto-* + *mycosis*]. Any disease caused by yeast-like fungi, especially species of *Blastomyces.* See also *North American blastomycosis, South American blastomycosis.*

blas·to·neu·ro·pore (blas''to·new'ro·pore) *n.* The temporary aperture in certain embryos formed by the coalescence of the blastopore and neuropore.

blas·to·pore (blas'to·pore) *n.* [*blasto-* + *-pore*]. The external opening of the archenteron in a gastrula. The avian and mammalian primitive streaks have been regarded by some as closed blastopores; hence the primitive pit, or the opening into the notochordal canal, may be considered a remnant of a blastopore. —**blas·to·por·ic** (blas''to·por'ick) *adj.*

blastoporic canal. NOTOCHORDAL CANAL.

blas·to·sphere (blas'to·sfeer) *n.* [*blasto-* + *sphere*]. 1. BLASTULA. 2. BLASTOCYST.

blas·to·spore (blas'to·spore) *n.* [*blasto-* + *spore*]. A spore formed by budding in the asexual reproduction of fungi; a type of thallospore. —**blas·to·spor·ic** (blas''to·spor'ick) *adj.*

blas·tot·o·my (blas·tot'uh·mee) *n.* [*blasto-* + *-tomy*]. The separation of blastomeres or groups of blastomeres, either naturally or artificially.

blas·tu·la (blas'tew·luh) *n.*, pl. **blastulas, blastu·lae** (·lee) [NL., dim. of Gk. *blastos*, bud]. A spherical mass consisting of a central cavity surrounded by a single layer of cells produced by the cleavage of the ovum; frequently modified by the presence of yolk. —**blastu·lar** (·lur) *adj.;* **blas·tu·la·tion** (blas''tew·lay'shun) *n.*

Bla·tel·la (bla·tel'uh) *n.* [NL., dim. of L. *blatta*, cockroach]. A genus of cockroaches.

Blatella ger·man·i·ca (jur·man'i·kuh). A species of cockroach which can serve as the intermediate host of *Hymenolepis diminuta.*

Blat·ta (blat'uh) *n.* [L., cockroach]. A genus of cockroaches of the family Blattidae. The species *B. orientalis*, the oriental cockroach, has been incriminated as an intermediate host of *Hymenolepis diminuta.*

Blaud's pills (blo) [P. *Blaud*, French physician, 1774–1858]. FERROUS CARBONATE PILLS.

BLB mask. BOOTHBY-LOVELACE-BULBULIAN MASK.

bleaching powder. CHLORINATED LIME.

bleb, *n.* A localized collection of fluid, as serum or blood, in the epidermis. Compare *blister, bulla, vesicle.*

bleed, *v.* 1. To lose blood from a blood vessel, either to the outside or the inside of the body. 2. To draw blood from a person.

bleed·er, *n.* 1. A person subject to frequent hemorrhages, as a hemophiliac. 2. A blood vessel which has escaped closure by cautery or ligature during a surgical procedure. 3. A blood vessel from which there is persistent uncontrolled bleeding.

bleed·ing, *n.* 1. The escape of blood from the vessels. 2. PHLEBOTOMY.

bleeding ear. NAMBI UVU.

bleeding time. The time required for bleeding to cease from a puncture wound, usually of the ear lobe or ball of the finger, under standardized conditions. The normal value varies with the method. See also *Duke method, Ivy method.*

blem·ma·trope (blem'uh·trope) *n.* [Gk. *blemma,* a glance, + *-trope*]. An apparatus for showing the various positions of the eye in its orbit.

blend·ing, *n.* The mutual solubilization of two normally immiscible solvents by the addition of a colloidal electrolyte.

blending inheritance. The apparent fusion in the progeny of the separate characteristics of the parents, now explained in Mendelian terms as dependent upon several pairs of genes.

blenn-, blenno- [Gk. *blenna*]. A combining form meaning *mucus, mucous.*

blen·noph·thal·mia (blen''off·thal'mee·uh) *n.* [*blenn-* + *ophthalmia*]. CATARRHAL CONJUNCTIVITIS.

blen·nor·rha·gia (blen''o·ray'jee·uh) *n.* [*blenno-* + *-rrhagia*]. 1. An excessive mucous discharge. 2. GONORRHEA.

blen·nor·rhea, blen·nor·rhoea (blen''o·ree'uh) *n.* [*blenno-* + *-rrhea*]. BLENNORRHAGIA. **—blennor·rhe·al, blen-nor·rhoe·al** (·ree'ul) *adj.*

Blenoxane. Trademark for bleomycin sulfate, an antineoplastic.

ble·o·my·cin sulfate (blee''o·migh'sin). A mixture of cytotoxic glycopeptide antibiotics obtained from a strain of *Streptomyces verticillus* and used as an antineoplastic.

Bleph. A trademark for the sodium salt of sulfacetamide.

blephar-, blepharo- [Gk. *blepharon*]. A combining form meaning *eyelid.*

blephara. Plural of *blepharon.*

bleph·ar·ad·e·ni·tis (blef''ur·ad''e·nigh'tis) *n.* [*blephar-* + *adenitis*]. Inflammation of the tarsal glands.

bleph·a·ral (blef'uh·rul) *adj.* [*blephar-* + *-al*]. Pertaining to the eyelids.

bleph·a·rec·to·my (blef''uh·reck'tuh·mee) *n.* [*blephar-* + *-ectomy*]. Excision of a part or the whole of an eyelid.

bleph·ar·ede·ma (blef'ur·e·dee'muh) *n.* [*blephar-* + *edema*]. Swelling or edema of the eyelids.

bleph·a·re·lo·sis (blef''uh·re·lo'sis) *n.*, pl. **blepharelo·ses** (·seez) [*blephar-* + Gk. *eilein,* to roll, + *-osis*]. ENTROPION.

bleph·a·rism (blef'uh·riz·um) *n.* [*blephar-* + *-ism*]. Spasm of the eyelids causing rapid repetitive involuntary winking.

blepharitides. Plural of *blepharitis.*

bleph·a·ri·tis (blef''uh·rye'tis) *n.*, pl. **blepha·rit·i·des** (·rit''i·deez) [*blephar-* + *-itis*]. Inflammation of the eyelids.

blepharitis an·gu·la·ris (ang''gew·lair'is). ANGULAR BLEPHARITIS.

blepharitis cil·i·a·ris (sil''ee·air'is). MARGINAL BLEPHARITIS.

blepharitis gan·grae·no·sa (gang''gre·no'suh). GANGRENOUS BLEPHARITIS.

blepharitis mar·gi·na·lis (mahr''ji·nay'lis). MARGINAL BLEPHARITIS.

blepharitis par·a·sit·i·ca (păr''uh·sit'i·kuh). PARASITIC BLEPHARITIS.

blepharitis sim·plex (sim'plecks). SIMPLE BLEPHARITIS.

blepharitis squa·mo·sa (skway·mo'suh). SQUAMOUS BLEPHARITIS.

blepharitis ul·ce·ro·sa (ul''se·ro'suh). ULCERATIVE BLEPHARITIS.

blepharo-. See *blephar-.*

bleph·a·ro·ad·e·ni·tis (blef''uh·ro·ad''e·nigh'tis) *n.* BLEPHARADENITIS.

bleph·a·ro·ad·e·no·ma (blef''uh·ro·ad''e·no'muh) *n.* [*blepharo-* + *adenoma*]. *Obsol.* An adenoma of the eyelid.

bleph·a·ro·ath·er·o·ma (blef''uh·ro·ath''ur·o'muh) *n.* [*blepharo-* + *atheroma*]. A sebaceous, epidermal, or dermoid cyst of the eyelid.

bleph·a·ro·blen·nor·rhea, bleph·a·ro·blen·nor·rhoea (blef''uh·ro·blen''o·ree·uh) *n.* [*blepharo-* + *blennorrhea*]. Conjunctivitis with a purulent discharge.

bleph·a·ro·chal·a·sis (blef''uh·ro·kal'uh·sis) *n.* [*blepharo-* + Gk. *chalasis,* a slackening]. A redundance of the skin of the eyelids, seen in both sexes under the age of 20. Starting with an intermittent, painless angioneurotic edema and redness, repeated attacks result in loss of skin elasticity, subcutaneous atrophy, and capillary proliferation.

bleph·a·ro·chrom·hi·dro·sis (blef''uh·ro·krome''hi·dro'sis) *n.* [*blepharo-* + *chromhidrosis*]. Colored sweat of the eyelids, usually of a bluish tint.

bleph·a·ro·clei·sis (blef''uh·ro·klye'sis) *n.* [*blepharo-* + *-cleisis*]. ANKYLOBLEPHARON.

bleph·a·roc·lo·nus (blef''uh·rock'lo·nus) *n.* [*blepharo-* + *clonus*]. Intermittent spasm, often merely fasciculation, of the orbicularis oculi muscle, especially the lower lid. Compare *blepharospasm.*

bleph·a·ro·con·junc·ti·vi·tis (blef''uh·ro·kun·junk''ti·vye'tis) *n.* [*blepharo-* + *conjunctivitis*]. Inflammation of both the eyelids and the conjunctiva.

bleph·a·ro·di·as·ta·sis (blef''uh·ro·dye·as'tuh·sis) *n.* [*blepharo-* + *diastasis*]. Excessive separation of the eyelids; inability to close the eyelids completely.

bleph·a·ro·dys·chroia (blef''uh·ro·dis·kroy'uh) *n.* [*blepharo-* + *dyschroia*]. Discoloration of the eyelid from nevus or from any other cause.

[1]**bleph·ar·oe·de·ma** (blef''ur·e·dee'muh) *n.* [*blephar-* + *oedema*]. BLEPHAREDEMA.

[2]**bleph·a·ro·ede·ma** (blef''uh·ro·e·dee'muh) *n.* [*blepharo-* + *edema*]. BLEPHAREDEMA.

bleph·a·ro·me·las·ma (blef''uh·ro·me·laz'muh) *n.* [*blepharo-* + Gk. *melasma,* black spot]. Seborrhea nigricans occurring on the eyelid.

bleph·a·ron (blef'uh·ron) *n.*, pl. **blepha·ra** (·ruh) [Gk.]. EYELID.

bleph·a·ron·cus (blef''uh·ronk'us) *n.* [*blephar-* + Gk. *onkos,* a mass]. A tumor or swelling of the eyelid.

bleph·a·ro·pa·chyn·sis (blef''uh·ro·pa·kin'sis) *n.* [*blepharo-* + *pachynsis*]. Abnormal thickening of the eyelid.

bleph·a·ro·phi·mo·sis (blef''uh·ro·figh·mo'sis) *n.* [*blepharo-* + *phimosis*]. A rare condition characterized by diminution of both dimensions of the palpebral fissure; may be congenital or acquired.

bleph·a·roph·ry·plas·ty (blef''uh·rof'ri·plas''tee) *n.* [*blephar-* + *ophrys* + *-plasty*]. Plastic surgery of the eyebrow and eyelid. **—blepha·roph·ry·plas·tic** (·rof''ri·plas'tick) *adj.*

bleph·a·ro·phy·ma (blef''uh·ro·figh'muh) *n.* [*blepharo-* + *phyma*]. A tumor of, or outgrowth from, the eyelid.

bleph·a·ro·plast (blef'uh·ro·plast) *n.* [*blepharo-* + *plast*]. 1. A basal body from which a cilium or flagellum grows. 2. A centriole which forms such basal bodies.

bleph·a·ro·plas·ty (blef'uh·ro·plas''tee) *n.* [*blepharo-* + *-plasty*]. An operation for the restoration of any part of the eyelid. **—bleph·a·ro·plas·tic** (blef''uh·ro·plas'tick) *adj.*

bleph·a·ro·ple·gia (blef''uh·ro·plee'jee·uh) *n.* [*blepharo-* + *-plegia*]. Paralysis of an eyelid.

bleph·a·rop·to·sis (blef''uh·rop·to'sis) *n.* [*blepharo-* + *ptosis*]. Ptosis of the upper eyelid.

bleph·a·ro·py·or·rhea, bleph·a·ro·py·or·rhoea (blef''uh·ro·

pye·o·ree'uh) *n.* [*blepharo-* + *pyorrhea*]. A flow of pus from the eyelid.

bleph·a·ror·rha·phy (blef"uh·ror'uh·fee) *n.* [*blepharo-* + *-rrhaphy*]. Repair by suturing of a cut or lacerated eyelid.

bleph·a·ro·spasm (blef'uh·ro·spaz·um) *n.* [*blepharo-* + *spasm*]. Spasm of the orbicularis oculi muscle; in particular, tonic or persistent spasm as is present with foreign bodies or inflammatory conditions of the eye; occasionally psychogenic. Compare *blepharoclonus.*

bleph·a·ro·sphinc·ter·ec·to·my (blef"uh·ro·sfink"tur·eck'tuh·mee) *n.* [*blepharo-* + *sphincter* + *-ectomy*]. An operation to lessen the pressure of the upper lid upon the cornea.

bleph·a·ro·stat (blef'uh·ro·stat) *n.* [*blepharo-* + *-stat*]. An instrument for holding the eyelids apart during operations upon the eyes or lids.

bleph·a·ro·ste·no·sis (blef"uh·ro·ste·no'sis) *n.* [*blepharo-* + *stenosis*]. BLEPHAROPHIMOSIS.

bleph·a·ro·sym·phy·sis (blef"uh·ro·sim'fi·sis) *n.*, pl. **blepharo-symphy·ses** (·seez) [*blepharo-* + *symphysis*]. BLEPHAROSYNECHIA.

bleph·a·ro·syn·ech·ia (blef"uh·ro·si·neck'ee·uh, ·si·nee'kee·uh, ·sin"e·kigh'uh) *n.*, pl. **blepharosynech·i·ae** (·ee·ee) [*blepharo-* + *synechia*]. Adhesion or growing together of the eyelids.

bleph·a·rot·o·my (blef"uh·rot'uh·mee) *n.* [*blepharo-* + *-tomy*]. Incision into the eyelid.

-blepsia [Gk. *blepsis*, sight, seeing, + *-ia*]. A combining form meaning *a condition of sight or vision.*

Bles·sig-Iva·nov cystoid degeneration of the retina [R. *Blessig,* Russian ophthalmologist, 1830–1878; and V. P. *Ivanov,* Russian ophthalmologist, b. 1861]. Cystic spaces at the periphery of the retina; a form of mucoid degeneration. See also *cystoid degeneration of the retina.*

blight, *n.* A fungus disease of plants.

blight·ed ovum. A fertilized ovum in which development has been severely retarded to produce a relatively hydramniotic sac containing a small amorphous mass or no fetal tissue.

blind, *adj.* 1. Without sight; deprived of sight. 2. Performed without the knowledge of specific facts which usually guide such a process or operation, as a blind test (in drug trials) or a blind abdominal exploration. 3. Hidden, difficult to discover, locate, identify; obscure. 4. Closed at one end, as a blind gut, pouch, or fistula.

blind abscess. An abscess which does not point on a surface.

blind boil. A boil that does not form a core; a nonsuppurating boil.

blind experiment. An experiment in which, to ensure objectivity, either the subject or the observer (single-blind), or both (double-blind), does not know which of several forms of treatment the subject is receiving.

blind fistula. A type of fistula which has only one opening, externally on the skin or internally upon the mucosal surface.

blind gut. CECUM.

blind headache. MIGRAINE.

blinding filaria. *ONCHOCERCA VOLVULUS.*

blind-loop syndrome. The existence of bypassed segments or diverticula in the small intestine, postsurgical or congenital in origin, resulting in stasis, abnormal bacterial flora, diarrhea, weight loss, multiple vitamin deficiency, and megaloblastic anemia.

blind·ness, *n.* Loss or absence of vision; inability to see. See also *amaurosis.*

blind pouch. CUL-DE-SAC.

blind spot. The physiologic scotoma in the visual field, temporal to the fixation point, representing the entrance of the optic nerve, where the rods and cones are absent. Syn. *Mariotte's blind spot, punctum cecum.*

blind test. BLIND EXPERIMENT.

blink *v.* & *n.* 1. To close and open the eyes quickly; may be voluntary, spontaneous, of central origin, or a reflex response. 2. A single quick closure and opening of the eyes.

blink reflex or **response.** Involuntary blinking of both eyes in response to almost any stimulus about the face that suddenly compresses the muscle or underlying bone.

blis·ter, *n.* & *v.* 1. A vesicle resulting from the exudation of serous fluid between the epidermis and dermis. 2. The agent by which the blister is produced. 3. To cause a blister to be formed.

blister gas. *In military medicine,* a gas or finely dispersed liquid used for casualty effect; it injures the eyes and lungs and blisters the skin. Compare *vesicant.*

bloat, *n.* 1. Puffiness; swelling; distention; edema; turgidity from any cause. 2. *In veterinary medicine,* an abnormal accumulation of gas in the stomach or intestines, resulting in distention of the abdomen. Syn. *wind colic, tympany.*

Bloch's method for dopa oxidase (blo^{k}h) [B. *Bloch,* Swiss dermatologist, 1878–1933]. A histochemical method based on conversion of dihydroxyphenylalanine to melanin on exposure to tissue containing dopa oxidase. Leukocytes and melanoblasts turn black due to their dopa oxidase content. See also *dopa reaction.*

Bloch-Sulz·ber·ger syndrome [B. *Bloch; and M. B. Sulzberger,* U.S. dermatologist, b. 1895]. INCONTINENTIA PIGMENTI.

block, *n.* 1. Any obstruction of a passage or opening. 2. Any form of interference with the normal propagation of an impulse, as in heart or nerve block or regional anesthesia. 3. *In histology,* a paraffin or celloidin mass in which a slice of tissue is embedded to facilitate the cutting of thin sections by a microtome. 4. *In psychiatry,* BLOCKING.

blockade reaction. *In histochemistry,* the prevention of access of a color-producing identifying reagent to sites where it normally reacts by preoccupation or destruction of the responsible chemical end groups by another non-color-producing reaction.

Blockain. Trademark for propoxycaine, a local anesthetic used as the hydrochloride salt.

block anesthesia. Anesthesia produced by injecting an anesthetic solution into the nerve trunks supplying the operative field, or infiltrating close to the nerves, or by a wall of anesthetic solution injected about the field so that painful impulses will not reach the brain.

block design test. *In psychology,* a performance test using drawings or model sets of blocks of increasing complexity of color and arrangement; used as a test of intelligence and to distinguish between organic and functional brain disorders.

block·ing, *n.* 1. Interference with the propagation of nerve currents in a given direction. 2. *In psychiatry,* a sudden difficulty in remembering or an interruption of a train of thought, sometimes followed by an abrupt change of subject; usually due to unconscious emotional factors. 3. The cutting of tissue and organ specimens into pieces of proper size for histologic study. 4. The fastening of embedded histologic specimens onto an apparatus for microtome processing.

α-blocking. ALPHA-BLOCKING.

β-blocking. BETA-BLOCKING.

blocking antibody. A thermostable antibody, usually of the IgG class, sometimes produced in both allergic (atopic) and nonallergic individuals as a response to specific immunization which is believed to prevent the union of antigen (atopen, allergen) and reagin. Clinical tolerance in allergy following various desensitizing procedures may depend upon the titer of this antibody.

blocking group. In peptide synthesis, a group that is reacted with a free amino or carboxyl group on an amino acid to prevent its taking part in subsequent formation of peptide bonds.

block vertebrae. A congenital defect in which two or more vertebral bodies are joined without intervening disk or cartilage; frequently associated with Klippel-Feil syndrome.

Blocq's disease [P. O. *Blocq,* French physician, 1860–1896]. ASTASIA-ABASIA.

Blond·lot's rays (blohⁿ·lo′) [P. R. *Blondlot,* French physicist, 1849–1930]. N-RAYS.

blood, *n.* [Gmc.]. The fluid tissue which circulates through the heart, arteries, capillaries, and veins, supplies oxygen and nutrients to the other tissues of the body, and removes from them carbon dioxide and waste products of metabolism. It is made up of plasma and cellular elements. The latter consists of erythrocytes, leukocytes, and blood platelets. NA *sanguis.* Comb. form *hem(o)-, hemat(o)-.* See also Plate 5 and Table of Chemical Constituents of Blood in the Appendix.

blood agar. A solid culture medium containing agar and blood, used for growing certain organisms.

blood albumin. SERUM ALBUMIN.

blood-aqueous barrier. A functional barrier between the blood and aqueous humor.

blood bank. An organization or facility which procures, and stores under refrigeration, whole blood kept fluid by anticoagulants. In addition, blood banks usually recruit blood donors, bleed them, test donor and recipient for immunologic compatibility, provide one or more components of blood, and in some cases, infuse blood.

blood bicarbonate. The amount of bicarbonate present in the blood, indicating the alkali reserve.

blood blister. A blister that contains blood.

blood-brain barrier. The functional barrier between the brain capillaries and the brain tissue which allows some substances from the blood to enter the brain rapidly while other substances either enter slowly or not at all. See also *blood-cerebrospinal-fluid barriers.*

blood calculus. A calculus situated in a blood vessel, derived from a thrombus and infiltrated with salts of calcium, as an arteriolith or phlebolith.

blood cell. Any of the cells or corpuscles that constitute elements of the circulating blood; an erythrocyte or a leukocyte.

blood-cerebrospinal-fluid barriers. The functional barriers between the blood supplying the central nervous system, including its covering membranes, and the cerebrospinal fluid. See also *blood-brain barrier.*

blood clot. A semisolid gel resulting from polymerization of fibrin and which may contain other blood elements trapped in fibrin network. Compare *thrombus.*

blood-clotting factor. COAGULATION FACTOR. See also *factor I to factor XIII.*

blood corpuscle. BLOOD CELL; especially, an erythrocyte.

blood-cortical barrier. BLOOD-BRAIN BARRIER.

blood count. The determination of the number of erythrocytes or leukocytes per cubic millimeter of blood.

blood culture. The inoculation of microbiologic media with blood for the isolation and identification of microorganisms.

blood cyst. A cyst filled with blood.

blood disk. ERYTHROCYTE.

blood dop·ing. The withdrawal, preservation, and subsequent infusion of one's own blood after the original loss has been made up by the body; occasionally done by athletes on the assumption that it will augment the oxygen-carrying capacity of the blood by increasing the red cell mass above normal.

blood dust of Mül·ler (muᵉl′ur) [J. *Müller*]. HEMOCONIA.

blood dyscrasia. Any abnormal condition of the formed elements of blood or of the constituents required for clotting.

blood fluke. Any of various flukes that inhabit the circulatory system of man or animals. See also *schistosomiasis.*

Blood·good's operation [J. C. *Bloodgood,* U.S. surgeon, 1867–1935]. Transplantation of the rectus muscle or its sheath for the cure of inguinal hernia when the conjoined tendon is obliterated.

blood grouping. Determination of an individual's blood group by laboratory tests; blood typing. See also *cross matching, antiglobulin test.*

blood groups. Immunologically distinct, genetically determined classes of human erythrocytes, depending on specific antigens (agglutinogens) in the erythrocytes for which the groups are named, and antibodies (agglutinins) in the serum. When incompatible bloods are mixed, agglutination results, which may be followed by hemolysis. Blood groups are of great importance in blood transfusions, hemolytic disease of the newborn (erythroblastosis fetalis), in medicolegal problems, anthropology, and genetics. In a broader sense, may include immunological inherited differences in leukocytes, platelets, hemoglobins, haptoglobins, and Gm serum groups. In the Standard or Universal grouping (Landsteiner's), the isoagglutinogens, A and B, can be lacking, or one or both be present in a given individual; the serum contains those isoagglutinins (anti-A or α, anti-B or β antibodies) which react upon the isoagglutinogens not present in the individual's erythrocytes. Thus:

Antigens on cells	O	A	B	AB
Antibodies in serum	anti-A anti-B	anti-B	anti-A	

Group A has been split into various subgroups (A_1, A_2, etc.). Moss's grouping IV, II, III, I, and Janský's I, II, III, IV are equivalent to the Standard grouping. Commonly involved in erythroblastosis fetalis and in transfusion reactions are the

Rh/Hr groups

Fischer-Race's nomenclature	Weiner's nomenclature
C	rh′
D	Rh_o
E	rh″
c	hr′
d (postulated)	Hr_o
e	hr″

Other groups include the following systems: MNSs, P, Lutheran, Kell, Lewis, Duffy, Kidd, Diego, Sutter, Xg, I, and others. New groups are still being determined. Blood groups have been found in other animal species. See also *ABO blood group.*

blood island or **islet.** One of the masses of condensed splanchnic mesenchyme in the wall of the yolk sac that gives rise to the primitive erythrocytes of the embryo and to the vascular plexus of the yolk sac.

blood lacuna. Any one of the cavities containing maternal blood in the early syncytiotrophoblast before the development of the true villi; they become the intervillous spaces of the placenta.

blood lake. HEMATOMA.

blood·less amputation. An amputation in which, owing to control, but little blood is lost, or, because of crushing or other circumstance, the circulation has ceased within the field of operation.

bloodless fold of Treves (treevz) [F. *Treves,* English surgeon, 1853–1923]. ILEOCECAL FOLD.

bloodless operation. A surgical procedure performed with little or no significant loss of blood.

bloodless phlebotomy. PHLEBOSTASIS.

blood·let·ting, *n.* PHLEBOTOMY.

blood mole. A mass of coagulated blood and retained fetal membranes and placenta, sometimes found in the uterus after an abortion. Syn. *carneous mole.*

blood pack·ing. BLOOD DOPING.

blood patch. Blood, usually 10–15 ml, drawn from the patient and injected into the epidural space to provide fibrin clot, sealing a rent in the dura; an infrequent technique in treating post-spinal puncture headache.

blood plague. NAMBI UVU.

blood plaque. BLOOD PLATELET.

blood plasma. The fluid portion of blood.

blood platelet. A spheroidal or ovoid light-gray body found in blood, about 1.0 to 2.5 μm in diameter, and numbering about 300,000 per cubic millimeter; an essential part of the hemostatic mechanism.

blood poisoning. SEPTICEMIA.

blood pressure. The pressure exerted by the circulating blood on the walls of the vessels or of the heart, especially the arterial pressure as measured by sphygmomanometry. Abbreviated, B.P.

blood pump. 1. A device for pumping blood rapidly into an artery or vein. 2. The apparatus for propelling the blood in an extracorporeal circulatory system.

blood quotient. The result obtained by dividing the quantity of hemoglobin in the blood by the number of erythrocytes, expressed in each case as a percentage of the normal amount.

blood relationship. A relationship by birth; CONSANGUINITY.

blood relative. A person related to another by a common ancestor.

blood·root, *n.* SANGUINARIA.

blood·stream, *n.* [*blood* + *stream*]. The flow of blood in its circulation through the body.

blood substitute. A substance, or combination of substances, used in place of blood, such as dextran, polyvinylpyrrolidone, plasma, albumin, gelatin, or certain electrolyte solutions.

blood sugar. The carbohydrate of the blood, chiefly glucose.

blood test. 1. A serologic test for syphilis. 2. BLOOD COUNT. 3. A test for detection of blood, usually one based on the peroxidase activity of blood, as the benzidine test or guaiac test.

blood type. The specific reaction pattern found when blood is tested by its reactions to antiserums for the various blood groups. See also *blood groups.*

blood typing. BLOOD GROUPING.

blood urea nitrogen. Nitrogen in the form of urea found in whole blood or serum; normal range is 8 to 20 mg per 100 ml. Its content is used to evaluate kidney function. Abbreviated, BUN.

blood vessel. Any of the tubular channels that convey the blood in its circulation through the body; an artery, vein, or capillary.

bloody sweat. HEMATHIDROSIS.

Bloom's syndrome [D. *Bloom,* U.S. dermatologist, b. 1892]. A hereditary disorder, transmitted as an autosomal recessive trait and appearing predominantly in children of Jewish ancestry; characterized by short stature, hypoplasia of the facial bones, a telangiectatic erythematous rash involving the face and sometimes other areas, sensitivity to sunlight, and an increased risk of leukemia.

Blount-Bar·ber syndrome [W. P. *Blount,* U.S. orthopedist, b. 1900; and J. R. *Barber,* Canadian orthopedist, 20th century]. OSTEOCHONDROSIS DEFORMANS TIBIAE.

blow·fly, *n.* A fly belonging to the family Calliphoridae.

blue baby. A newborn child suffering from cyanosis due either to pulmonary disease and inadequate oxygenation of the blood, as in congenital atelectasis, or to a congenital malformation of the heart or great vessels with significant shunting of venous blood to the arterial side.

blue blindness. A rare form of tritanopia in which there is inability to distinguish blue. See also *yellow blindness.*

blue bloater. A patient with chronic bronchitis, alveolar hypoventilation, cyanosis, hypercapnia, and cor pulmonale. Contr. *pink puffer.*

blue·bot·tle fly. A fly belonging to the family Calliphoridae.

blue cohosh. CAULOPHYLLUM.

blue-diaper syndrome. A familial condition seen in infants involving abnormal tryptophan metabolism, with resultant conversion to indican and other indole derivatives by the intestinal flora, causing blue discoloration of the diapers.

blue-dome cyst. A breast cyst occurring in mammary dysplasia and characterized by the blue color imparted to light passing through the exposed portion of the cyst. See also *cystic disease of the breast.*

blue dot cataract. PUNCTATE CATARACT.

blue drum. A distinct blue appearance of the tympanic membrane. It may be due to congenital prominence of the jugular bulb or to blood or blood-tinged fluid behind the drum, as in hemotympanum.

blue-eye, *n.* BUNG-EYE.

blue-fabric lesion. Incrustation of the fibrous connective and reticular tissues of the spleen with calcium salts and hemosiderin, producing the appearance of blue cloth in sections stained with hematoxylin and eosin.

blue kidney. Renal hemosiderosis without splenic or hepatic hemosiderosis, resulting from severe intravascular hemolysis.

blue line. LEAD LINE.

blue milk. Milk which develops a bluish tint due to contamination with *Pseudomonas aeruginosa.*

blue nevus. A nevus composed of spindle-shaped pigmented melanocytes usually in the middle and lower two-thirds of the dermis.

blue phlebitis. PHLEGMASIA CERULEA DOLENS.

blue pus. Pus having a blue-green color because of the pigments liberated by the multiplication of *Pseudomonas aeruginosa.*

blue-pus microbe. *PSEUDOMONAS AERUGINOSA.*

blue rubber bleb nevus. A type of hemangioma of the skin, usually multiple and associated with hemangiomas of the gastrointestinal tract and mucous membranes.

blue-sclera syndrome. A congenital, often hereditary, condition of unknown cause in which the scleras are deep indigo blue, sometimes fading with age; often associated with osteogenesis imperfecta and deafness, but may occur in the absence of bone fragility.

blue sclerotics. BLUE-SCLERA SYNDROME.

blue spot. Any of various kinds of localized bluish discoloration of the skin, such as Mongolian spot, blue nevus, or macula cerulea.

blue·stone, *n.* COPPER SULFATE.

blue sweat. Perspiration that has a blue color; may occur in copper workers, or when *Pseudomonas pyocyanea* secretes pyocyanin pigment into sweat.

blue tetrazolium. 3,3′-(3,3′-Dimethoxy-4,4′-biphenylene)-bis[2,5-diphenyl-2*H*-tetrazolium chloride], $C_{40}H_{32}Cl_2N_8O_2$, variously used as a reagent for reducing substances. See also *tetrazolium salts.*

blue·tongue, *n.* An epizootic disease of sheep characterized by acute inflammation of the gastrointestinal, respiratory, and muscular systems; the causative agent is an arthropod-borne double-stranded RNA virus.

blue velvet. 1. A mixture of concentrated paregoric, elixir of terpin hydrate, codein, and tripelennamine. 2. Amytal sodium and Pyribenzamine (tripelennamine).

blue vitriol. COPPER SULFATE.

Blum·berg's sign (bloom′behrk) [M. *Blumberg,* German surgeon, 1873–1955]. The production of pain by sudden release of pressure of the examiner's hand from the abdomen; rebound tenderness, a sign of peritoneal inflammation.

Blu·me·nau's nucleus (bloo·me·naow′, Ger. bloom′e·naow) [L. V. *Blumenau,* Russian neurologist, 1862–1931]. The lateral part of the cuneate nucleus.

Blu·mer's shelf [G. A. *Blumer,* U.S. physician, 1858–1940]. A pathological finding observed on rectal examination, due to a thickening of the peritoneum of the rectouterine pouch which produces a shelflike projection into the rectum. The thickening may be due to an inflammatory or neoplastic process.

blun·der·buss pelvis. ANTHROPOID PELVIS.

blunt dissection. *In surgery,* the exposure of structures or separation of tissues without cutting. Contr. *sharp dissection.*

blunt hook. An instrument for exercising traction upon the fetus in an arrested breech presentation.

blunt retractor. A toothed retractor, with rounded teeth to avoid injury to tissues.

blush, *n.* A reddening of the skin, usually involuntary and caused by embarrassment or sudden emotion; FLUSH (1).

B lymphocyte [*b*ursa-dependent]. A lymphocyte which originates as a stem cell from bone marrow, differentiating in the bursa of Fabricus in birds and at an analogous but unknown site in mammals, and which bears immunoglobin receptors for antigen on its surface. Stimulation of its surface by antigen triggers its further differentiation into the plasma cell, which is responsible for production of circulating antibody. Syn. *B cell.* Contr. *T lymphocyte.*

Blyth's test [A. W. *Blyth,* English physician, 1845–1921]. A test for lead in water by which the addition of a 1% alcohol tincture of cochineal to water containing lead results in the formation of a precipitate.

B. M. A. British Medical Association.

B.M.R. Abbreviation for *basal metabolic rate.*

BNA Abbreviation for *Basle Nomina Anatomica.* See also *NA.*

board of health. An official board in a municipality, state, or province, responsible for maintaining public health through sanitation and providing a limited range of clinical and laboratory services.

Bo·a·ri's operation (bo·ah'ree) [A. *Boari,* Italian surgeon, 19th century]. *Obsol.* Transplantation of the ductus deferens into the urethra for the relief of male sterility.

Boas-Oppler bacillus [I. I. *Boas* and B. *Oppler*]. LACTOBACILLUS OF BOAS-OPPLER.

Bo·as' point (bo'ahs) [I. I. *Boas,* German physician, 1858–1938]. A point of tenderness at the left of the twelfth thoracic vertebra, sometimes found in patients with gastric ulcer.

Boas' reagent [I. I. *Boas*]. A solution of resorcinol, sugar, and alcohol, used in testing for free hydrochloric acid.

Boas' sign [I. I. *Boas*]. A sign of cholecystitis in which there is an area of hyperesthesia over the lower right rib cage posteriorly.

Boas' test [I. I. *Boas*]. 1. In intestinal atony, a splashing sound can be obtained by succussion after the injection of a relatively small quantity (200 to 300 ml) of water into the empty colon. 2. A glass rod dipped in an alcohol, resorcinol, and sucrose solution is applied to a drop of the filtrate from the stomach; a deep scarlet streak is produced if hydrochloric acid is present in the gastric contents.

boat conformation. A relatively unstable configuration of hexagonal ring compounds of the cyclohexane type in which two opposite ring atoms (1 and 4 position) both lie above (or below) the plane formed by the other four ring atoms. Contr. *chair conformation.*

bobble-head doll syndrome. A movement disorder seen in children with noncommunicating hydrocephalus, characterized by rhythmic to-and-fro bobbing of the head and shoulder, and reminiscent of dolls with weighted heads set on a coiled spring who nod continuously.

Bo·broff's operation (bah·brohf') [F. V. *Bobroff,* Russian surgeon, b. 1858]. Osteoplastic closure of spina bifida.

Boch·da·lek's foramen (bokh'da·leck) [V. A. *Bochdalek,* Bohemian anatomist, 1801–1883]. FORAMEN OF BOCHDALEK.

Bochdalek's ganglion [V. A. *Bochdalek*]. A gangliform enlargement, or pseudoganglion, at the junction of the middle and anterior branches of the superior dental plexus.

Bochdalek's lumbocostal triangle [Victor *Bochdalek,* Bohemian anatomist, 1835–1868]. LUMBOCOSTAL TRIANGLE OF BOCHDALEK.

Bock·hart's impetigo (bohk'hart) [M. *Bockhart,* German physician, d. 1921]. IMPETIGO FOLLICULARIS.

Bo·dan·sky's method [A. *Bodansky,* U.S. biochemist, 1896–1941]. A test for serum phosphatase in which the difference between inorganic phosphate before and after incubation with sodium glycerophosphate substrate indicates a measure of phosphatase activity.

Bodansky unit [A. *Bodansky*]. The amount of phosphatase required to liberate 1 mg of phosphorus as the phosphate ion from a sodium glycerophosphate substrate during the first hour of incubation at 37°C and pH 8.6.

Bodian staining method [D. *Bodian,* U.S. neuroanatomist, b. 1910]. A silver impregnation method for the demonstration of nerve fibers and endings in paraffin sections, in which protargol activated by metallic copper is used.

Bo·do (bo'do) *n.* A genus of flagellate protozoa found in feces, urine, and ulcerations, but thought to be of little or no pathologic importance.

body, *n.* 1. The animal frame with its organs. 2. The largest and primarily central part of an organ, as the body of the uterus. 3. A mass of matter. 4. A small organ, as the carotid body. See also *corpus, corpuscle.*

body agnosia. AUTOTOPAGNOSIA.

body cavity. The peritoneal, pleural, and pericardial cavities, and that of the tunica vaginalis testis. See also *coelom.*

body cells. SOMATIC CELLS.

body fluid. Liquid (as blood, tears, or urine) obtained from or present in the body of an organism.

body fold. One of the various folds formed by the rapid growth of the embryonic area.

body image. In psychology, the conscious and unconscious concepts, which may differ from each other, each person has of his own physical self as an object in and bound by space, including body parts, shape, posture, and motion. Syn. *body schema.*

body-image agnosia. AUTOTOPAGNOSIA.

body louse. The louse *Pediculus humanus corporis,* a vector of disease and the cause of pediculosis corporis.

body mechanics. The sum of the mechanical relationships among the various systems of the body, especially among the skeletal, muscular, and visceral systems, or the scientific study and manipulation of these relationships.

body of High·more [N. *Highmore,* English physician, 1613–1685]. MEDIASTINUM TESTIS.

body of Ret·zi·us (rets'ee·ōōs) [A. A. *Retzius,* Swedish anatomist, 1796–1860]. A condensed cytoplasmic mass with pigment granules found at the lower end of the hair cells of the spiral organ (of Corti).

body of the ischium. The portion of the ischium which enters into the formation of the acetabulum and terminates below in the ischial tuber.

body-righting reflex. A righting reflex initiated by asymmetric stimulation of pressure receptors on the surface of the body. It may be a body-righting reflex acting on the head, which tends to keep the head orientated in relation to the surface with which the body is in contact, or it may be acting on the body, which ensures orientation of the body in space or in relation to the surface with which it is in contact.

body schema. BODY IMAGE.

body segment. A somite, or a division of the body derived from an embryonic somite.

body sense. Impressions from somatic structures which orient with regard to the body or its parts in space or which concern contacts or degrees of contact.

body snatching. Unauthorized removal of a corpse from the grave.

body stalk. The extraembryonic mesoderm connecting the chorion and the caudal region of the amnioembryonic vesicle. It forms a path for the allantoic blood vessels and the connective tissue of the future umbilical cord.

body surface area. The area covered by a person's skin

expressed in square meters, calculated from the formula $S = 0.007184 \times W^{0.425} \times H^{0.725}$, where S = surface area in square meters, W = body weight in kilograms, and H = height in centimeters. Nomograms constructed from this formula are used clinically to estimate body surface area, as for fluid requirements and drug dosages. An average newborn has a surface area of about 0.2 m²; a child weighing 30 kg, about 1 m²; and an adult weighing 70 kg, about 1.76 m².

body type. SOMATOTYPE.

body-weight ratio. Body weight in grams divided by height in centimeters.

Boeck's sarcoid (bœhk) [Caesar P. M. *Boeck,* Norwegian dermatologist, 1845–1917]. SARCOIDOSIS.

Boeck's scabies [Carl W. *Boeck,* Norwegian dermatologist, 1808–1875]. SCABIES CRUSTOSA.

Boer·haa·ve syndrome (boor'hah·vuh) [H. *Boerhaave,* Dutch physician, 1668–1738]. Complete rupture of the esophagus, followed by emptying of gastric content into the mediastinum, with eventual entrance into a pleural cavity, usually the left; painful swallowing is often present. Compare *Mallory-Weiss syndrome.*

Boer·ner-Lu·kens test. A complement fixation test for syphilis.

Boet·ti·ger method. A colorimetric method for glycogen based on the color development through the action of diphenylamine or glycogen.

Bo·gros' space (boʰ·gro') [A. J. *Bogros,* French anatomist, 1786–1823]. RETROINGUINAL SPACE.

Böh·ler's splint (bœh'lur) [L. *Böhler,* Austrian surgeon, b. 1885]. A wire extension splint used in the treatment of fractured fingers.

Böh·mer's hematoxylin (bœh'mur). An alum hematoxylin stain.

Bohr effect [N. H. D. *Bohr,* Danish physicist, 1885–1962]. The influence or effect exerted by carbon dioxide upon the dissociation of oxygen from hemoglobin and some related compounds.

Bohr magneton [N. H. D. *Bohr*]. The magnetic moment of a paramagnetic molecule, equal to that of one unpaired electron.

boil, *n.* FURUNCLE.

boil·er·mak·ers' deafness. Hearing loss resulting from working among loud noises; usually affects high frequency sounds first. See also *auditory trauma.*

boiling point. The temperature at which a liquid has a vapor pressure equal to the barometric or external pressure.

Boi·vin antigen. ENDOTOXIN.

bo·lan·di·ol (bo''lan·dye'ole) *n.* Estr-4-ene-3β,17β-diol, $C_{18}H_{28}O_2$, an anabolic steroid, usually employed as the dipropionate ester.

bo·las·ter·one (bo·las'tur·ohn) *n.* 7α,17-Dimethyltestosterone, $C_{21}H_{32}O_2$, an anabolic steroid.

bol·de·none (bol·deen'ohn, bol'de·nohn) *n.* 17β-Hydroxyandrosta-1,4-dien-3-one, $C_{19}H_{26}O_2$, an anabolic steroid; used as the undecylenate ester.

bol·do (bol'do, bul'do) *n.* [Sp., from Araucanian]. The dried leaves of the boldu tree, *Peumus boldus,* formerly used as an aromatic stimulant and diuretic.

bole, *n.* A translucent, soft variety of clay formerly much used in medicine—internally as an astringent, externally as an absorbent.

bol·e·nol (bol'e·nol, ·nole) *n.* 19-Nor-17α-pregn-5-en-17-ol, $C_{20}H_{32}O$, an anabolic steroid.

Bo·len test. A blood test in which differences in the appearance of a retracted clot are supposed to differentiate between normal and cancerous individuals.

Bo·ley gauge. A vernier-type measuring instrument calibrated to the metric system, often used in making dental measurements.

Bolles' splint. A splint used in the treatment of fracture of the coronoid process of the ulna.

Bol·ling·er's granules (boʰl'ing·ur) [O. *Bollinger,* German pathologist, 1843–1909]. The yellow sulfurlike granules of actinomycosis seen originally in actinomycosis of cattle.

bol·man·ta·late (bol·man'tuh·late) *n.* 17β-Hydroxyestr-4-en-3-one adamantane-1-carboxylate, $C_{29}H_{40}O_3$, an anabolic steroid.

bo·lom·e·ter (bo·lom'e·tur) *n.* [Gk. *bolē,* ray, + *-meter*]. A device for measuring minute differences in radiant heat. Syn. *thermic balance.*

Bol·ton cranial base. A triangular base formed by the Bolton nasion plane and lines joining the center of sella turcica with the Bolton point and the nasion.

Bolton nasion plane. A line passing through the Bolton point and the nasion on the lateral radiograph. It marks the junction of the face and cranium.

Bolton point. *In craniometry,* a point in the median line midway between the postcondylar notches on the occipital bone, the posterior termination of the Bolton nasion plane. It is located as the most superior point in the profile of the postcondylar notches when viewed in the lateral radiograph.

Bolton registration point. The center of the Bolton cranial base, a point midway on a perpendicular from the Bolton nasion plane to the center of sella turcica.

Bolt·worth skate. A non-weight-bearing device, mobile in all directions, with a wide base, usable when the leg is in plaster, after such surgical procedures as arthroplasty of the hip joint.

bo·lus (bo'lus) *n.* [L. *bolus,* clod, large pill, from Gk. *bolos,* lump, clod]. 1. A large pill. 2. The rounded mass of food prepared by the mouth for swallowing. Syn. *alimentary bolus.* 3. BOLE. 4. *In angiography,* a rapidly injected volume of radiographic contrast medium.

Bom·bay blood [after *Bombay,* India]. Variants of the ABO blood group, first described in 1952; presumed to be caused by rare genes modifying the expression of the common A and B genes, in which the propositus behaves as Group O, but the agglutination expected of normal group O cells with anti-H serum is lacking, and a strong anti-H antibody is present in the serum. Mating of two apparent nonsecretors may give rise to a secretor.

bomb calorimeter. An apparatus for measuring the heat of combustion, as of foods and fuel.

Bonamine. Former trademark for meclizine, an antinauseant used as the hydrochloride salt. Now designated *Bonine.*

bond, *n.* The linkage or adhesive force between atoms, as in a compound, usually effected by the transfer of one or more electrons from one atom to another, or by the sharing, equally or unequally, of one or more pairs of electrons by two atoms.

bon·duc (bon'dook) *n.* [Ar. *bunduq,* hazelnut]. The seeds of a tropical plant, *Caesalpinia crista;* formerly used as a tonic and antiperiodic.

Bon·dy operation (boʰn'dee) [G. *Bondy,* German otologist, 20th century]. MODIFIED RADICAL MASTOIDECTOMY.

bone, *n.* [Gmc.]. 1. A supportive rigid connective tissue consisting of an abundant matrix of collagen fibers impregnated with minerals which are chiefly calcium compounds, enclosing many much-branched cells, the osteocytes. The body of each osteocyte occupies an ovoid space, the lacuna; its branches lie in minute, branching tubules, the canaliculi. See also *endosteum, hydroxyapatite, ossein, ossification, osteogenesis, osteoid, periosteum.* 2. An element or individual member of the skeleton, as the femur, the parietal bone. NA *os.* Comb. form *osse(o)-, ossi-, ost-, oste(o)-.* For bones listed by name, see Table of Bones in the Appendix. See also Plate 1. **—bony,** *adj.*

bone absorption. The resorption of bone. See also *osteoclasis.*

bone age. Age as judged roentgenologically from bone development; it is compared with the normal ossification for that chronologic age.

bone ash. The white mineral constituents that remain after calcination or incineration of bone.

bone black. ANIMAL CHARCOAL.

bone cell or **corpuscle.** A cell in a lacuna of bone. Syn. *osteocyte.*

bone conduction. Transmission of sound vibrations to the middle and internal ear via the bones of the skull. Contr. *air conduction.*

bone conduction audiometry. Evaluation of sensorineural hearing level by introducing the stimulus directly to the skin over the mastoid process of the temporal bone.

bone conduction hearing aid. An electronic hearing aid, the transmitter of which is held against the skin over the mastoid process.

bone conduction test. The testing of hearing threshold by placing a tuning fork or audiometer oscillator directly against a bone of the skull, usually the mastoid process.

bone-cutting forceps. A double-jointed or single-jointed, powerful, heavy-bladed cutting forceps, with great power derived from the leverage exerted by the long handles.

bone cyst. A cyst occurring in bone, as the result of a pathologic change. See also *osteitis fibrosa cystica.*

bone graft. A graft composed of bone; may be cortical, cancellous, or medullary; used to repair bone defects, to afford support, or to supply osteogenic tissue.

bone-holding forceps. A forceps with heavy jaws and long handles, for use in holding bone during an operation.

bone inlay. A bone graft fitted into the two fragments and lying across a fracture or filling a gap between the fragments, to promote healing.

bone-marrow transfusion. A transfusion into a bone-marrow cavity, usually of the sternum, femur, or tibia.

bone nippers. 1. RONGEUR. 2. A small bone-trimming forceps.

bone of Ber·tin (behr·tæⁿ') [J. *Bertin,* French anatomist, 1712–1781]. CONCHA SPHENOIDALIS.

bone oil. An oil obtained by destructive distillation of bone or deer's horn; formerly used as an antispasmodic. Syn. *Dippel's oil.*

bone on·lay. A strip of transplanted bone laid across a fracture to encourage or strengthen union, and held in position by wires, pins, screws, or other devices.

bone peg. A peg or screw fashioned of beef bone, used in bone operations to secure immobility.

bone reflex. A reflex presumed to be elicited by stimulus applied to a bone, but actually due to the stretching of a muscle tendon as it is inserted into the bone.

bone seeker. A radioisotope that tends to lodge in the bones when it is introduced into the body, as strontium 90 which behaves chemically like calcium.

bone·set, *n.* 1. An herb of the genus *Eupatorium,* used in making a therapeutic tea. 2. A blunt surgical instrument used with a mallet to impact a bone graft or fragment.

bone·set·ter, *n.* One who specializes in setting bones, especially an uneducated empiric, and often a pretender to hereditary skill in the business.

bone wax. A waxy material used for packing bone, especially during skull operations, for the arrest of bone bleeding.

Bonine. Trademark for meclizine, an antinauseant drug used as the hydrochloride salt.

Bon·jean's ergotin. An aqueous ergot extract.

Bonne·vie-Ull·rich syndrome (boʰn·vee', o͝ol'rikh) [K. *Bonnevie,* 1872–1950; and O. *Ullrich,* German physician, 1894–1957]. GONADAL DYSGENESIS.

Bon·nier's syndrome (boʰn·yeʸ') [P. *Bonnier,* French otolaryngologist, 1861–1918]. A lesion of the lateral vestibular nucleus and adjacent pathways in the medulla oblongata, resulting in paroxysmal vertigo, nystagmus, symptoms of involvement of cranial nerves IX and X (glossopharyngeal paralysis) and sometimes III and V, contralateral hemiplegia, tachycardia, pallor, and frequently generalized weakness and somnolence.

Bon·will triangle [W. G. A. *Bonwill,* U.S. dentist, 1833–1899]. An equilateral triangle bounded by lines from the contact point of the lower central incisors, or the medial line of the residual ridge of the mandible, to the condyle on either side and from one condyle to the other.

bony ankylosis. Complete fixation of a joint due to fusion of the bones.

bony crater. A concavity in the cancellous portion of the mandibular or maxillary alveolar process resulting from the spread of inflammation in periodontal disease.

bony heart. A heart with calcareous patches.

bony labyrinth. OSSEOUS LABYRINTH.

boo·mer·ang leg (boo'mur·ang). SABER SHIN.

boom·slang (boom'slang) *n.* [Afrikaans *boom,* tree, + *slang,* snake]. *Dispholidus typus,* a rear-fanged, venomous, colubrid snake of Africa.

Bo·oph·i·lus (bo·off'i·lus) *n.* [NL., from Gk. *bous,* ox, cattle, + *philos,* fond of]. A genus of ticks.

Boophilus an·nu·la·tus (an"yoo·lay'tus). A cattle tick that carries *Babesia bigemina;* once the commonest carrier in the United States.

Boophilus mi·cro·plus (migh'kro·plus). A cattle tick that carries *Babesia bigemina;* now the commonest carrier.

booster dose. That portion of an immunizing agent given at a later period to stimulate effects of a previous dose of the same agent. See also *immunization.*

Booth·by-Love·lace-Bul·bul·ian mask. An apparatus used in the administration of oxygen; the mask is fitted with an inspiratory-expiratory valve and a rebreathing bag.

boot-shaped heart. *In radiology,* the abnormal cardiac configuration associated with the marked right ventricular hypertrophy seen in tetralogy of Fallot and with left ventricular dilatation and hypertrophy usually secondary to aortic regurgitation.

bor-, boro-. A combining form meaning *boron.*

bo·rac·ic acid (bo·ras'ick). BORIC ACID.

bor·age (bur'ij, borr'ij) *n.* [OF., from LL. *borrago,* from *burra,* rough hair]. The plant *Borago officinalis,* formerly used as a demulcent and diaphoretic.

bo·rate (bo'rate) *n.* Any salt of boric acid.

bo·rax (bo'racks) *n.* [ML., from Ar. *būraq,* from Per. *būrah*]. SODIUM BORATE.

bor·bo·ryg·mus (bor"bo·rig'mus) *n.,* pl. **borboryg·mi** (·migh) [Gk. *borborygmos*]. The rumbling noise caused by flatus gurgling through fluid in the intestines.

Bor·deaux mixture (bor·do') [after *Bordeaux,* France]. A fungicide prepared from copper sulfate, calcium oxide, and water.

bor·der·line, *adj.* 1. Pertaining to any phenomenon or datum not easily classifiable in such categories as normal or abnormal. 2. Describing an individual whose mentality or emotional status is near the dividing line between normal and abnormal.

borderline leprosy. DIMORPHOUS LEPROSY.

borderline mental retardation. Subnormal intellectual functioning in which the intelligence quotient is approximately 68 to 85, resulting primarily in impairment of school achievement in the regular educational process.

borderline personality organization. BORDERLINE SYNDROME.

borderline state or **psychosis.** *In psychiatry,* a diagnostic term to describe situations when it is difficult to determine whether a patient's symptoms are chiefly neurotic or psychotic, particularly when the symptoms shift from one pattern to another and are severe, including much acting out and schizophrenic-like behavior.

borderline syndrome. *In psychiatry,* an impairment of ego function noted in individuals who harbor a residue of repressed anger and who cannot relate meaningfully to or love other people, and who in consequence develop nonpsychotic but deviant mechanisms, such as withdrawal, impulsiveness, splitting, projective identification, or passive compliance at the price of real involvement, to maintain a precarious mental equilibrium. Syn. *borderline personality organization.*

Bor·de·tel·la (bor·de·tel'uh) *n.* [J. J. B. V. *Bordet,* Belgian bacteriologist, 1870–1961]. A genus of gram-negative bacteria, formerly included in the genus *Hemophilus.*

Bordetella bron·chi·sep·ti·ca (bronk"i·sep'ti·kuh). A small gram-negative rod-shaped bacterium, a secondary invader in canine distemper, a cause of respiratory infection in small animals such as guinea pigs and rabbits, and rarely responsible for a human infection resembling whooping cough. Syn. *Hemophilus bronchiseptica.*

Bordetella para·per·tuss·is (păr·uh·pur·tuss'is) A gram-negative bacterium, resembling *B. pertussis,* that is the etiologic agent of parapertussis. Syn. *Hemophilus parapertussis.*

Bordetella per·tus·sis (pur·tuss'is) A gram-negative rod-shaped bacterium that is the cause of whooping cough. Syn. *Hemophilus pertussis.*

Bor·det-Gen·gou agar or **plate** (bor·de$^{h'}$, zhah^{n}·goo') [J.J.B.V. *Bordet;* and O. *Gengou,* French bacteriologist, 1875–1957]. A bacteriological growth medium specifically designed for the isolation of *Bordetella* species.

Bordet-Gengou bacillus. *BORDETELLA PERTUSSIS.*

Bordet's test [J. J. B. V. *Bordet*]. A serum test for blood, meat, and similar protein-containing substances.

Bord·ley-Rich·ards method. A test for uric acid adapting Folin's method to capillary-tube colorimetry.

bo·ric acid (bo'rick). H_3BO_3. Colorless scales, crystals, or white crystalline powder, soluble in water. Used as a mild antiseptic on mucous membranes. Serious or fatal poisoning resulting from transcutaneous absorption may occur. Syn. *boracic acid, orthoboric acid.*

bor·ne·ol (bor'nee·ol) *n.* [after *Borneo* + *-ol*]. 2-Hydroxycamphane, $C_{10}H_{17}OH$, a terpene alcohol in trees of the genus *Dryobalanops,* and occurring also as a constituent of certain volatile oils; used in the preparation of perfumes and incense.

Born·holm disease (born·hol'm') [after *Bornholm,* Denmark]. EPIDEMIC PLEURODYNIA.

bor·nyl (bor'nil, ·neel) *n.* [after *Borneo* + *-yl*]. The univalent $—C_{10}H_{17}$ radical representing borneol without the hydroxyl group.

boro-. See *bor-.*

bo·ro·cit·ric acid (bo"ro·sit'rick). A combination of boric and citric acids formerly used as a solvent for urates and phosphates in urinary calculi.

bo·ro·glyc·er·ide (bo"ro·glis'ur·ide, ·id) *n.* BOROGLYCERIN.

bo·ro·glyc·er·in (bo"ro·glis'ur·in) *n.* An interaction product of boric acid and glycerin.

boroglycerin glycerite. A viscid, yellowish liquid prepared by heating together boric acid and glycerin. Has been used for antiseptic effect.

bo·ron (bo'ron, bor'on) *n.* [*bor*ax + *-on* as in carbon]. B = 10.81. A nonmetallic element of the aluminum group; it is the characteristic element of boric acid, the borates, metaborates, and perborates.

bo·ro·sal·i·cyl·ic acid (bo"ro·sal"i·sil'ick). A mixture of boric and salicylic acids which has been used externally like salicylic acid.

Bor·rel·ia (bo·ree'lee·uh, bo·rel'ee·uh) *n.* [A. *Borrel,* French bacteriologist, 1876–1936]. A genus of large, coarsely coiled spirochetes, of many species, parasitic in man and other warm-blooded animals, and including the causative agents of relapsing fever.

Borrelia buc·ca·lis (buh·kay'lis). A spirochete found in the mouth, of no proven pathogenicity. Syn. *Treponema buccale.*

Borrelia dut·to·nii (dut·o'nee·eye). The spirochete that causes tick-borne relapsing fever.

Borrelia re·cur·ren·tis (ree"kur·en'tis). The spirochete that causes louse-borne relapsing fever.

Borrelia re·frin·gens (re·frin'jenz). A nonpathogenic spirochete found on the external genitalia of both sexes. Syn. *Treponema refringens.*

Borrelia vin·cen·tii (vin·sent'ee·eye). An anaerobic spirochete found in the normal oral cavity and in conjunction with a fusiform bacillus associated with Vincent's angina. Syn. *Treponema vincentii.*

bor·rel·i·din (bo·rel'i·din) *n.* An antibiotic substance produced by *Streptomyces rochei;* active against species of *Borrelia* in experimental animals.

boss, *n.* [OF. *boce*]. A rounded or knoblike protuberance, as on the side of a bone or tumor.

bos·se·lat·ed (bos'e·lay·tid) *adj.* With a knoblike protuberance, or boss.

bos·se·la·tion (bos"e·lay'shun) *n.* The condition of having bosses or of becoming bosselated.

boss·ing, *n.* BOSSELATION.

Bos·ton exanthema. An exanthematous illness with fever, sore throat, headache, and abdominal pain caused by an echovirus (type 16).

Boston's sign [L. N. *Boston,* U.S. physician, 1871–1931]. An eye sign of hyperthyroidism in which the upper lid descends in a jerky rather than a smooth motion, following the downward motion of the eye.

bot, *n.* The larva of a botfly, especially of the species infecting the horse and related animals. Bots infect the cavities of the facial bones, the stomach and intestine, and the subcutaneous connective tissue, causing severe damage.

Bo·tal·lo's duct (bo·ta^{h}l'lo) [L. *Botallo,* Italian anatomist, 1530–1600]. DUCTUS ARTERIOSUS.

bo·tan·ic (buh·tan'ick) *adj.* [Gk. *botanikos,* from *botanē,* herb, pasture]. 1. Of or pertaining to plants. 2. Of or pertaining to botany. —**botan·i·cal** (·i·kul) *adj.*

bot·a·ny (bot'uh·nee) *n.* [*botanic* + *-y*]. The branch of biology dealing with plants. —**bot·a·nist** (bot'uh·nist) *n.*

bot·fly, *n.* A fly of the family Oestridae, Gastrophilidae, or Cuterebridae, whose larvae are parasitic in cavities and tissues of animals and sometimes of man.

Both respirator [E. T. *Both,* British engineer, 20th century]. An artificial respirator, similar to Drinker's respirator, but made of wood.

bothri-, bothrio-. A combining form meaning *bothrium.*

bothria. Plural of *bothrium.*

bo·thrid·i·um (bo·thrid'ee·um) *n.,* pl. **bothrid·ia** (·ee·uh). BOTHRIUM.

Both·rio·ceph·a·lus (both"ree·o·sef'uh·lus) *n.* [*bothrio-* + *-cephalus*]. *DIPHYLLOBOTHRIUM.*

Bothriocephalus **anemia.** TAPEWORM ANEMIA.

both·ri·oid (both'ree·oid) *adj.* [*bothri-* + *-oid*]. Pitted; foveolated; covered with pitlike marks.

both·ri·on (both'ree·on) *n.* [Gk., small pit]. BOTHRIUM.

both·ri·um (both'ree·um) *n.,* pl. **both·ria** (·ree·uh) [NL; from Gk. *bothrion,* small pit]. A grooved sucker, such as is seen on the head of the tapeworm *Diphyllobothrium latum.*

bo·throp·ic (bo·throp'ick) *adj.* Pertaining to or produced by a pit viper of the genus *Bothrops.*

bothropic antivenin. Polyvalent serum for the venom of pit vipers of the genus *Bothrops.*

Bo·throps (bo'throps) *n.* [Gk. *bothros,* pit, + Gk. *ōps,* face, eye]. A genus of pit vipers, Crotalidae, found chiefly in Central and South America.

Bothrops al·ter·na·ta (ahl·tur·nay'tuh). A venomous snake of South America.

Bothrops at·rox (at'rocks, ay'trocks). A pit viper, the fer-de-lance, having a powerful hemotoxic venom; the commonest cause of snakebite in Panama.

Bothrops jararaca. JARARACA.

Bothrops neu·wie·dii (new·weed'ee·eye). The white-tailed jararaca.

Bothrops num·mi·fer (num'i·fur). The jumping pit viper.

bo·tog·e·nin (bo·toj'e·nin) *n.* A steroidal sapogenin obtained from the Mexican yam *Dioscorea mexicana;* a possible source for synthesis of other steroids.

bot·ry·oid (bot'ree·oid) *adj.* [Gk. *botryoeidēs,* from *botrys,* bunch of grapes]. Resembling in shape a bunch of grapes, due to many rounded prominences.

botryoid sarcoma or **tumor.** SARCOMA BOTRYOIDES.

bot·ryo·my·co·sis (bot"ree·o·migh·ko'sis) *n.,* pl. **botryomyco·ses** (·seez) [Gk. *botrys,* bunch of grapes, + *mycosis*]. 1. A bacterial infection, usually staphylococcal, in which the organisms as seen in tissues form groups resembling actinomycotic colonies. 2. Specifically, a chronic infectious disease of horses and, rarely, of cattle; characterized by dense fibrous tissue containing multiple suppurating foci of staphylococci. —**botryomy·cot·ic** (·kot'ick) *adj.*

Bo·try·tis (bo·trye'tis) *n.* [NL., from Gk. *botrys,* bunch of grapes]. A genus of soil fungi belonging to the order Moniliales and parasitic for a number of plants.

bots, *n.* Infection with botfly larvae. See also *bot.*

Bött·cher's cells (bœt'ᶜhur) [A. *Böttcher,* German anatomist, 1831–1889]. CELLS OF BÖTTCHER.

bot·tle jaw. Submandibular edema of sheep and cattle due to hypoproteinemia.

bottle nose. A nasal deformity resulting from acne rosacea.

bottle sound. AMPHORIC RESPIRATION.

bot·u·li·form (bot'yoo·li·form) *adj.* [L. *botulus,* sausage, + *-iform*]. Sausage-shaped.

bot·u·lin (bot'yoo·lin) *n.* The neurotoxin produced by *Clostridium botulinum,* which causes botulism. —**bot·u·li·nal** (bot"yoo·lye'nul) *adj.*

bot·u·li·num (bot"yoo·lye'num) *n.* A member of the species *Clostridium botulinum,* which causes botulism.

bot·u·li·nus (bot"yoo·lye'nus) *n.* [short for *Bacillus botulinus,* a former name of the organism]. BOTULINUM.

bot·u·lism (bot'yoo·liz·um) *n.* Poisoning of man and animals by a group of immunologically distinct types of *Clostridium botulinum,* acquired by man generally by the ingestion of improperly canned or preserved food. The clinical syndrome results from the action of a potent neurotoxin at the myoneural junction, and is characterized by diplopia, dysphagia, muscle weakness, and respiratory failure.

bou·ba (boo'buh) *n.* 1. YAWS. 2. AMERICAN MUCOCUTANEOUS LEISHMANIASIS.

Bou·chard's nodes (boo·shahr') [J. C. *Bouchard,* French physician, 1837–1915]. Bony enlargement of the proximal interphalangeal joints, seen in osteoarthritis.

Bou·chet-Gsell disease (boo·shehⁿ', ksel). SWINEHERD'S DISEASE.

Bou·gain·ville rheumatism [after *Bougainville,* Solomon Islands]. EPIDEMIC TROPICAL ACUTE POLYARTHRITIS.

bou·gie (boo·zhee', boo'zhee) *n.* [F., candle]. 1. A slender cylindrical instrument of rubber, waxed silk, or other material, for introduction into the body passages, as the urethra, anus, or other canal. It may be plain or tipped, angled or straight, being intended for use in exploration, in dilatation of strictures, as a guide for the passage of other instruments, or for the induction of labor. 2. A suppository, particularly for insertion into the urethra.

bougie à boule (ah bool) [F.]. A bulbous or bulb-tipped bougie.

bou·gie·nage. BOUGINAGE.

bou·gi·nage, bou·gie·nage (boo"zhee·nahzh') *n.* Introduction of a bougie into an orifice or tubular organ.

Bouil·laud's disease or **syndrome** (booy·yo') [J. B. *Bouillaud,* French physician, 1796–1881]. RHEUMATIC FEVER.

bouil·lon (boo"yon', bo͝ol'yon) *n.* [F.]. BROTH.

Bouin's fixative (bwæⁿ) [P. *Bouin,* French anatomist, 1870–1962]. A 75:25:5 mixture of picric acid, formaldehyde, and acetic acid; used in histologic procedures.

Bouin's picroformol acetic fixative [P. *Bouin*]. BOUIN'S FIXATIVE.

Bou·len·ge·ri·na (boo·len"je·ree'nuh) *n.* A genus of aquatic cobras inhabiting the rain forests of tropical Africa, possessing predominantly neurotoxic venom.

bou·lim·ia (boo·lim'ee·uh) *n.* BULIMIA.

bouncing Bet. *SAPONARIA OFFICINALIS.*

bound, *adj.* United in chemical or physical combination.

bound·a·ry zone. ANDROGENIC ZONE.

Bourbanal. A trademark for ethyl vanillin.

bour·donne·ment (boor·dun·mahn') *n.* [F., a buzzing]. A buzzing or humming sound heard during auscultation, or heard subjectively from any cause. The former is thought to be due to the contraction of muscle fibrils.

Bourne method. 1. A histochemical method for alkaline phosphatase based on the action of the enzyme on glycerophosphate and calcium chloride to produce calcium phosphate and the staining of the latter with alizarin sulfonate. 2. A histochemical method for ascorbic acid based on reduction of silver nitrate by ascorbic acid. 3. A histochemical method for sulfhydryl groups using acetic acid, nitroprusside, ammonium sulfate, and ammonium hydroxide to obtain purplish-blue color.

Bour·ne·ville's disease (boor·nᵉ·veel') [D. M. *Bourneville,* French neurologist, 1840–1909]. TUBEROUS SCLEROSIS.

Bour·quin-Sher·man unit [Anne *Bourquin,* U.S. chemist, b. 1897; and H. C. *Sherman,* U.S. chemist, 1875–1955]. The amount of riboflavin which, when fed daily to rats, will give an average gain of 3 g a week during a test period of 4 to 8 weeks in excess of gains in control rats without riboflavin.

bou·stro·phe·don·ic (boos"tro·fe·don'ick) *adj.* [Gk. *boustrophēdon,* turning like oxen in plowing]. Pertaining to the writing of alternate lines in opposite directions.

boustrophedonic imaging. Scanning in which the detector that records isotopic emissions moves in alternating opposite directions in a descending series of horizontal lines.

bou·ton·neuse fever (boo·ton·uhz') [F., pimply]. The prototype of the tick-borne typhus fevers of Africa, widely distributed in Africa and the Mediterranean, Caspian, and Black Sea basins; in which infection caused by *Rickettsia conori* is transmitted by the bite of ixodid ticks, with dogs and rodents as animal hosts. Clinically, characterized by a necrotic initial lesion (tache noire), headache, fever, rash, and, generally, a favorable prognosis.

bou·ton·niere deformity (boo·ton·yair'). BUTTONHOLE DEFORMITY.

bou·tons ter·mi·naux (boo·tohn' terr·mee·no') [F.]. END FEET.

Bou·ve·ret's syndrome (boo·vrehⁿ') [L. *Bouveret,* French physician, 1850–1929]. Paroxysmal atrial tachycardia.

Bo·ve·ri's test (bo·veh'ree) [P. *Boveri,* Italian neurologist, 1879–1932]. A test in which 1 ml of 1:1000 potassium permanganate is layered over an equal amount of cerebrospinal fluid. If the latter contains an excess of globulins, a yellow ring will appear at the line of junction of the two fluids.

bo·vine (bo'vine) *adj.* [L. *bovinus,* from *bos, bovis,* ox, cow]. 1. Cattlelike. 2. Relating to or derived from a cow or ox.

bovine face. FACIES BOVINA.

bovine heart. COR BOVINUM.

bovine malignant catarrh. An infectious disease of cattle characterized by inflammation of eyes and nostrils, erosion of the oral mucosa, and neurologic signs.

bovine piroplasmosis. TEXAS FEVER.

bovine pleuropneumonia. A disease of cattle characterized by extensive pulmonary consolidation and pleural effusion, caused by *Mycoplasma mycoides.*

bovine smallpox. VACCINIA.

bovine tuberculosis. A form of tuberculosis in cattle caused by *Mycobacterium bovis* and transmitted to man and other animals by consumption of raw milk from infected cattle.

Bow·ditch effect (baʊw'dich) [H. P. *Bowditch,* U.S. physiologist, 1840–1911]. Increase in myocardial contractility due to increase in pulse rate; a form of homeometric autoregulation of the heart.

Bowditch law or **phenomenon** [H. P. *Bowditch*]. The all-or-none law as applied to the heart: any threshold or suprathreshold stimulus to the myocardium will produce a maximal contractile response.

bow·el (baow'ul) *n.* [OF. *boel,* from L. *botellus,* a sausage]. INTESTINE.

bowel movement. 1. The evacuation of feces; an act of defecation. 2. The feces evacuated by defecation; a stool.

bowel training. The establishing of regular habits of defecation during early childhood.

Bow·en's disease or **epithelioma** [J. T. *Bowen,* U.S. dermatologist, 1857-1941]. 1. Intraepithelial squamous cell carcinoma of the skin, forming distinctive plaques. 2. A similar carcinoma occurring in mucous membranes.

Bow·ie's ethyl violet–Biebrich scarlet stain. A neutral stain made from ethyl violet and Biebrich scarlet; used for staining pepsinogen granules in sections of stomach.

bow·leg, *n.* Lateral curvature of the lower extremities.

Bow·man's capsule [W. *Bowman,* English anatomist, 1816-1892]. GLOMERULAR CAPSULE.

Bowman's glands [W. *Bowman*]. Serous glands found in the olfactory mucous membrane.

Bowman's membrane [W. *Bowman*]. A thin membrane that separates the corneal epithelium from the substantia propria of the cornea.

bow·man's root. *Gillenia trifoliata.* See *Gillenia.*

box·er's ear. A hematoma of the external ear. See also *cauliflower ear.*

boxer's encephalopathy. PUNCH-DRUNK STATE.

box·i·dine (bock'si·deen) *n.* 1-[2-[[4'-(Trifluoromethyl)-4-biphenylyl]oxy]ethyl]pyrrolidine, $C_{19}H_{20}F_3NO$, a hypocholesteremic drug; it also blocks synthesis of adrenal steroids.

Boy·den's sphincter [E. A. *Boyden,* U.S. anatomist, b. 1886]. SPHINCTER OF THE COMMON BILE DUCT.

Boyd's types of *Shigella* [J. S. K. *Boyd,* English bacteriologist, 20th century]. A subgroup of the genus *Shigella,* including 15 principal serotypes, originally recognized in India, but now known to occur throughout the world.

Boyle's law [R. *Boyle,* English physicist, 1627-1691]. At any given temperature the volume of a given mass of gas varies in inverse proportion to the pressure exerted upon it.

Boze·man's catheter [N. *Bozeman,* U.S. surgeon, 1825-1905]. TWO-WAY CATHETER.

B.P. Abbreviation for (a) *blood pressure* (b) *British Pharmacopoeia.*

B.P.C. British Pharmaceutical Codex.

BR British or Birmingham Revision (of BNA terminology).

Br Symbol for bromine.

brace, *n.* [L. *brachium,* arm]. An apparatus that gives support to any movable part of the body, intended for permanent use, in contradistinction to a splint; may assist in locomotion, and is frequently attached to clothing, as to shoes; sometimes jointed to permit flexion.

brachi-, brachio- [L. *brachium*]. A combining form meaning (a) *arm;* (b) *brachial.*

brachia. Plural of *brachium.*

brachia ce·re·bel·li (serr·e·bel'eye). CEREBELLAR PEDUNCLES.

bra·chi·al (bray'kee·ul) *adj.* [L. *brachialis,* from *brachium,* arm]. Of or pertaining to an arm or a structure like an arm.

brachial artery. An artery which originates as a continuation of the axillary artery and terminally branches into the radial and ulnar arteries, distributing blood to the various muscles of the arm, the shaft of the humerus, the elbow joint, the forearm, and the hand. NA *arteria brachialis.* See also Plate 7 and Table of Arteries in the Appendix.

brachial-basilar insufficiency syndrome. SUBCLAVIAN STEAL SYNDROME.

brachial birth palsy. Paralysis of the arm due to injury of the brachial plexus during birth. See also *lower brachial plexus paralysis, upper brachial plexus paralysis.*

brachial block. Interscalene, supraclavicular, or axillary injection of a local anesthetic agent to produce neural blockade of the brachial plexus.

brachial bulb. CERVICAL ENLARGEMENT.

bra·chi·al·gia (bray"kee·al'juh, ·jee·uh, brack"ee·) *n.* [*brachi-* + *-algia*]. Pain in the arm often related to a lesion of the brachial plexus.

brachialgia stat·i·ca par·es·thet·i·ca (stat'i·kuh păr·es·thet'i·kuh). Paresthesia of an arm developing at night due to positional pressure on the brachial plexus.

bra·chi·a·lis (bray"kee·ay'lis, brack"ee·) *n.* [L.]. A muscle lying under the biceps brachii and covering the front of the elbow joint. NA *musculus brachialis.* See also Table of Muscles in the Appendix.

brachial neuritis. NEURALGIC AMYOTROPHY.

brachial palsy or **paralysis.** Paralysis of an arm. See also *brachial birth palsy.*

brachial plexus. A plexus of nerves located in the neck and axilla and composed of the anterior rami of the lower four cervical and first thoracic nerves. NA *plexus brachialis.* See also Plate 16.

brachial plexus neuralgia. Severe paroxysmal pain, manifested in the neck, shoulder, arm, and hand, in the distribution of any of the branches of the brachial plexus without objective sensory or motor changes; frequently of obscure cause.

bra·chi·form (bray'ki·form) *adj.* [*brachi-* + *-form*]. Arm-shaped.

brachio-. See *brachi-.*

bra·chio·ce·phal·ic (bray"kee·o·se·fal'ick) *adj.* [*brachio-* + *cephalic*]. Pertaining to the arm and the head.

brachiocephalic artery. BRACHIOCEPHALIC TRUNK.

brachiocephalic trunk. The largest branch of the arch of the aorta which divides into the right common carotid and right subclavian arteries; the innominate artery. NA *truncus brachiocephalicus.*

bra·chio·cyl·lo·sis (bray"kee·o·si·lo'sis) *n.* [*brachio-* + Gk. *kyllōsis,* deformation, clubbing]. Curvature of the humerus.

bra'chio·fa·cial (bray"kee·o·fay'shul) *adj.* [*brachio-* + *facial*]. Pertaining to the arm and the face.

bra·chio·ra·di·a·lis (bray"kee·o·ray"dee·ay'lis) *adj.* & *n.* [*brachio-* + *radialis*]. 1. Pertaining to the arm and radius. 2. The brachioradialis muscle. NA *musculus brachioradialis.* See Table of Muscles in the Appendix.

brachioradialis reflex. A stretch reflex due to contraction of the brachioradialis muscle, with flexion and supination of the forearm and occasionally flexion of the fingers on percussion of the styloid process or lower third of the lateral surface of the radius while the forearm is held in semiflexion and semipronation. Syn. *periosteoradial reflex, radial reflex, supinator reflex.*

bra·chi·ot·o·my (bray"kee·ot'uh·mee) *n.* [*brachio-* + *-tomy*]. *In surgery and obstetrics,* the cutting or removal of an arm.

bra·chi·um (bray'kee·um, brack'ee·um) *n.,* genit. **bra·chii** (·kee·eye), pl. **bra·chia** (·uh) [L., from Gk. *brachion*] [NA]. 1. The arm, especially the upper arm. 2. Any armlike structure.

brachium col·li·cu·li in·fe·ri·o·ris (kol·ick'yoo·lye in·feer·ee·o'ris) [NA]. BRACHIUM OF THE INFERIOR COLLICULUS.

brachium colliculi su·pe·ri·o·ris (sue·peer·ee·o'ris) [NA]. BRACHIUM OF THE SUPERIOR COLLICULUS.

brachium conjunctivum (ce·re·bel·li) (serr·e·bel'eye) [BNA]. Pedunculus cerebellaris superior (= SUPERIOR CEREBELLAR PEDUNCLE).

brachium of the inferior colliculus. A strand of fibers from the inferior colliculus together with fibers of the lateral lemniscus ending in the medial geniculate body. NA *brachium colliculi inferioris.*

brachium of the superior colliculus. A strand of optic fibers which continue beyond the lateral geniculate body to end in the optic stratum of the superior colliculus and in the pretectal areas. NA *brachium colliculi superioris.*

brachium pon·tis (pon'tis) [BNA]. Pedunculus cerebellaris medius (= MIDDLE CEREBELLAR PEDUNCLE).

brachium qua·dri·ge·mi·num in·fe·ri·us (kwah·dri·jem'i·num in·feer′ee·us) [BNA]. Brachium colliculi inferioris (= BRACHIUM OF THE INFERIOR COLLICULUS).

brachium quadrigeminum su·pe·ri·us (sue·peer′ee·us) [BNA]. Brachium colliculi superioris (= BRACHIUM OF THE SUPERIOR COLLICULUS).

Brach·mann–de Lange syndrome. CORNELIA DE LANGE SYNDROME (1).

Bracht-Wäch·ter bodies (brah^{k}ht, ve^{k}h′tur) [E. F. E. *Bracht,* German pathologist, b. 1882; and H. J. G. *Wächter,* German physician, b. 1878]. 1. Perivascular myocardial microabscesses, encountered in acute bacterial endocarditis. 2. Lesions seen in the hearts of rabbits with experimentally induced bacteremia.

brachy- [Gk. *brachys* (rel. to L. *brevis*)]. A combining form meaning *short.*

brachy·car·dia (brack″ee·kahr′dee·uh) *n.* [*brachy-* + *-cardia*]. BRADYCARDIA.

brachy·ce·pha·lia (brack″ee·se·fay′lee·uh) *n.* [*brachy-* + *-cephalia*]. Shortness of the head, the cephalic index being 81.0 to 85.4. —**brachyce·phal·ic** (·fal′ick), **brachy·ceph·a·lous** (·sef′uh·lus) *adj.*

brachy·ceph·a·lism (brack″ee·sef′uh·liz·um) *n.* BRACHYCEPHALIA.

brachy·ceph·a·ly (brack″ee·sef′uh·lee) *n.* BRACHYCEPHALIA.

brachy·chei·lia, brachy·chi·lia (brack″ee·kigh′lee·uh) *n.* [*brachy-* + *cheil-* + *-ia*]. Abnormal shortness of the lip.

bra·chych·i·ly (bra·kick′il·ee) *n.* BRACHYCHEILIA.

brachy·chi·rous, brachy·chei·rous (brack″ee·kigh′rus) *adj.* [*brachy-* + *cheir-* + *-ous*]. Having short hands. —**brachychi·ria** (·ree·uh), **brachychi·rism** (·riz·um) *n.*

brachy·cra·ni·al (brack″ee·kray′nee·ul) *adj.* [*brachy-* + *cranial*]. Having a cranial index between 80.0 and 84.9.

brachy·dac·tyl·ia (brack″ee·dack·til′ee·uh) *n.* [*brachy-* + *-dactylia*]. Abnormal shortness of the fingers or toes. —**brachydactyl·ic** (·ick), **brachy·dac·ty·lous** (·dack′ti·lus) *adj.*

brachy·dac·ty·ly (brack″ee·dack′ti·lee) *n.* BRACHYDACTYLIA.

brachy·glos·sal (brack″ee·glos′ul) *adj.* [*brachy-* + *glossal*]. Having a short tongue. —**brachyglos·sia** (·ee·uh) *n.*

brachy·gnath·ous (brack″ee·nath′us) *adj.* [*brachy-* + *-gnathous*]. Having an abnormally short lower jaw. —**brachy·gna·thia** (·nayth′ee·uh), *n.;* **brachygnathus,** *n.*

brachy·ker·kic (brack″ee·kur′kick) *adj.* [*brachy-* + Gk. *kerkis,* shuttle, radius]. Pertaining to or having a forearm disproportionately shorter than the upper arm.

brachy·mei·o·sis (brack″ee·migh·o′sis) *n.,* pl. **brachymeio·ses** (·seez) [*brachy-* + *meiosis*]. The third division, i.e., the second reduction division, in the ascus of Ascomycetes.

brachy·met·a·po·dy (brack″ee·met′a·po·dee) *n.* [*brachy-* + *meta-* + *-pody*]. A condition in which the metatarsals are shorter than the average.

brachy·mor·phic (brack″ee·mor′fick) *adj.* [*brachy-* + *-morphic*]. Characterized by a stature shorter than usual.

brachy·mor·phy (brack′i·mor″fee) *n.* [*brachy-* + *-morphy*]. Short stature.

brachy·pel·lic (brack″ee·pel′ick) *adj.* [*brachy-* + *-pellic*]. Pertaining to or having an oval type of pelvis in which the transverse diameter exceeds the anteroposterior diameter by not more than 3 cm.

brachy·pel·vic (brack″ee·pel′vick) *adj.* BRACHYPELLIC.

brachy·pha·lan·gia (brack″ee·fa·lan′jee·uh) *n.* [*brachy-* + *phalang-* + *-ia*]. A condition in which the phalanges are abnormally short. —**brachypha·lan·gous** (·lang′gus) *adj.*

brachy·pha·lan·gy (brack″ee·fa·lan′jee) *n.* BRACHYPHALANGIA.

brachy·po·dous (brack″ee·po′dus, bra·kip′o·dus) *adj.* [*brachy-* + *pod-* + *-ous*]. *In biology,* possessing a short foot or stalk.

brachy·pro·sop·ic (brack″ee·pro·sop′ick, ·so′pick) *adj.* [*brachy-* + *prosopic*]. Having a short face.

brachy·rhin·ia (brack″ee·rin′ee·uh) *n.* [*brachy-* + *rhin-* + *-ia*]. Abnormal shortness of the nose.

brachy·rhyn·chus (brack″ee·ring′kus) *n.* [*brachy-* + Gk. *rhynchos,* snout]. Abnormal shortness of maxilla and nose; usually associated with cyclopia or cebocephalia, but occasionally occurring alone.

brachy·skel·ic (brack″ee·skel′ick) *adj.* [*brachy-* + Gk. *skelos,* leg]. Characterized by abnormal shortness of the legs.

brachy·sta·sis (brack″ee·stay′sis) *n.* [*brachy-* + *stasis*]. A process in which a muscle does not relax to its former length following a contraction and maintains its original degree of tension in its new state. —**brachy·stat·ic** (·stat′ick) *adj.*

brachystatic contraction. BRACHYSTASIS.

brachy·ther·a·py (brack″ee·therr′uh·pee) *n.* Close-range irradiation.

brachy·uran·ic (brack″ee·yoo·ran′ick) *adj.* [*brachy-* + *uran-* + *-ic*]. Having a palatomaxillary index above 115.

brack·et, *n.* [from MF. *braguette,* codpiece]. A metal lug soldered to an orthodontic band by means of which other parts of an appliance, such as an arch wire, rubber band, or ligature, may be attached to the band.

bracket table. A tray that is an integral part of the dental operating unit on which various instruments and materials are arranged for convenience.

Brack·ett's operation [E. G. *Brackett,* U.S. orthopedist, 1860–1944]. Surgical repair of fracture of the femoral neck, in which fragments are fixed in the hollowed-out head of the femur, and the greater trochanter is transplanted upward to the site of the fracture.

Brad·ford frame [E. H. *Bradford,* U.S. orthopedist, 1848–1926]. A canvas-covered, rectangular, gas-pipe frame, devised originally for handling children with tuberculous disease of the spine, but extended later to the care of joint disease and for immobilization after operations, in adults as well as in children.

Bradosol bromide. Trademark for the antiseptic domiphen bromide.

brad·sot (brad′sot) *n.* BRAXY.

brady- [Gk. *bradys*]. A combining form meaning *slow.*

brady·ar·thria (brad″ee·ahr′three·uh) *n.* [*brady-* + *arthr-,* articulation, + *-ia*]. BRADYLALIA.

brady·aux·e·sis (brad″ee·awk·see′sis) *n.* [*brady-* + *auxesis*]. A type of relative growth in which a part grows at a slower rate than the whole organism or another part.

brady·car·dia (brad″ee·kahr′dee·uh) *n.* [*brady-* + *-cardia*]. Slowness of the heartbeat; a heart rate of less than 60 per minute for a human adult or 120 per minute for a fetus.

brady·ci·ne·sis (brad″ee·si·nee′sis) *n.* BRADYKINESIA.

brady·crot·ic (brad″ee·krot′ick) *adj.* [*brady-* + *-crotic*]. Characterized by a slowness of the pulse.

brady·di·as·to·le (brad″ee·dye·as′to·lee) *n.* [*brady-* + *diastole*]. Prolongation of the diastolic interval beyond normal limits.

brady·di·as·to·lia (brad″ee·dye·as·to′lee·uh) *n.* BRADYDIASTOLE.

brady·glos·sia (brad″ee·glos′ee·uh) *n.* [*brady-* + *-glossia*]. Slowness of speech, due to difficulty in tongue movement. See also *bradylalia.*

brady·ki·ne·sia (brad″ee·ki·nee′zhuh, ·zee·uh, ·kigh·nee′) *n.* [*brady-* + *-kinesia*]. Slowness and poverty of movement, as in disorders affecting the extrapyramidal system and in the catatonic type of schizophrenia. —**bradyki·net·ic** (·net′ick) *adj.*

brady·ki·ne·sis (brad″ee·ki·nee′sis) *n.* BRADYKINESIA.

brady·ki·nin (brad″ee·kigh′nin, ·kin′in) *n.* [*brady-* + Gk. *kinein,* to move, + *-in*]. A polypeptide containing 9 amino acid residues, released from the plasma alpha globulin bradykininogen (kallidinogen) by a kallikrein. It derives its name from its effect in slowly developing contraction of isolated guinea pig ileum. A potent vasodilator, it also increases capillary permeability and produces edema. Syn. *kallidin-9.*

brady·ki·nin·o·gen (brad″ee·ki·nin′o·jen, ·kigh·nin′o·jen) *n.* [*bradykinin* + *-gen*]. An alpha globulin present in blood plasma which serves as the precursor for bradykinin and the substrate for kallikreins. Bradykininogen appears to be identical with kallidinogen.

brady·la·lia (brad″ee·lay′lee·uh) *n.* [*brady-* + *-lalia*]. 1. Slow or labored speech due to central nervous system disturbance, as in Sydenham's chorea or other extrapyramidal motor disorders. 2. The slow speech observed in certain depressive illnesses.

brady·lex·ia (brad″ee·leck′see·uh) *n.* [*brady-* + *-lexia*]. Abnormal slowness in reading, due to either a central nervous system disturbance or an inadequate reading ability.

brady·pha·sia (brad″ee·fay′zhuh, ·zee·uh) *n.* [*brady-* + *-phasia*]. BRADYLALIA.

brady·phre·nia (brad″ee·free′nee·uh) *n.* [*brady-* + *-phrenia*]. Sluggish mental activity; may be due to organic causes or symptomatic of a depressive illness or reaction.

brady·pnea (brad″ee·nee′ah) *n.* [*brady-* + *-pnea*]. An abnormally slow rate of breathing.

brady·pra·gia (brad″ee·pray′jee·uh) *n.* [*brady-* + Gk. *prassein, prag-*, to do, + *-ia*]. Abnormally slow action, especially physical activity.

brady·prax·ia (brad″ee·prack′see·uh) *n.* [*brady-* + *-praxia*]. BRADYPRAGIA.

brady·rhyth·mia (brad″ee·rith′mee·uh) *n.* [*brady-* + *rhythm* + *-ia*]. 1. Slowing of the heart or pulse rate; BRADYCARDIA. 2. *In electroencephalography,* slowing of the brain wave rate below that expected for age and normal physiologic state, as awake, asleep, or drowsy; often, delta rhythm and slow-wave complexes.

brady·sper·ma·tism (brad″ee·spur′muh·tiz·um) *n.* [*brady-* + *spermat-* + *-ism*]. Slow or delayed ejaculation of semen during intercourse.

brady·sper·mia (brad″ee·spur′mee·uh) *n.* BRADYSPERMATISM.

brady·tel·eo·ki·ne·sia (brad″ee·tel″ee·o·ki·nee′zee·uh) *n.* BRADYTELEOKINESIS.

brady·tel·eo·ki·ne·sis (brad″ee·tel″ee·o·ki·nee·sis, ·teel″ee·o·) *n.* [*brady-* + *teleo-* + *kinesis*]. The type of incoordination in which a movement is halted before completion, then completed slowly and irregularly; seen in cerebellar disease.

Bragard's sign. The production of sciatic pain by dorsiflexion of the foot during the raising of a straightened leg.

braid·ism (bray′diz·um) *n.* [J. *Braid,* British physician, 1795–1860]. Hypnotism, due not to animal magnetism, but to the power of concentration of attention.

braid·ist (bray′dist) *n.* [J. *Braid*]. A hypnotist.

braille (brail) *n.* [L. *Braille,* French teacher of the blind and inventor, 1809–1852]. A compact alphabet and set of numbers and scientific and musical symbols adapted for the blind, using raised dots or points arranged in two six-dot vertical columns.

Brails·ford-Morquio syndrome [J. F. *Brailsford,* British radiologist, 20th century; and L. *Morquio*]. MORQUIO'S SYNDROME.

brain, *n.* [OE. *braegen*←Gmc. *bragna-* (rel. to Gk. *bregma,* sinciput)]. That part of the central nervous system contained in the cranial cavity, consisting of the cerebrum, cerebellum, pons, and medulla oblongata. NA *encephalon.* See also Plates 17, 18.

brain aneurysm. Any aneurysm of the cerebral blood vessels, usually of the arterial circle of the cerebrum.

brain axis. BRAINSTEM.

brain·case, *n.* The portion of the skull containing the brain; NEUROCRANIUM.

brain cavity. The cavity of one of the embryonic brain vesicles.

brain clip. DURA CLIP.

brain concussion. 1. Violent shaking or agitation of the brain and the transient paralysis of nervous function therefrom. 2. Immediate abolition of consciousness, transient in nature, usually due to a blunt, nonpenetrating injury which causes a change in the momentum of the head.

brain damage. 1. BRAIN INJURY. 2. Loosely, CEREBRAL PALSY. 3. Loosely, MINIMAL BRAIN DYSFUNCTION SYNDROME.

brain-damaged child. A child who sustained some injury or insult to his nervous system before, during, or after birth and who usually has some impairment of perception or intellect, behavioral difficulties (especially undirected hyperkinetic behavior), and clumsiness or deficits in fine motor coordination. Speech problems and mild to major neurological abnormalities may be present. Causes are multiple and include hypoxia, infections, physical trauma, and toxins.

brain death. An irreversible abolition of all brain function. The following requirements for brain death are generally agreed upon: unresponsiveness to all stimuli, absence of spontaneous respiration and of pupillary, oculocephalic, vestibuloocular, and gag reflexes, and an electroencephalogram recorded for 30 minutes or longer at 24-hour intervals, showing no electrical activity over two microvolts at maximum gain despite stimulation with sound and pain-producing stimuli.

brain·ed·ness (bray′nid·nis) *n.* CEREBRAL DOMINANCE.

brain fever. Meningitis or encephalitis.

brain-injured child. BRAIN-DAMAGED CHILD.

brain injury. 1. Any form of trauma to the brain, whether of infectious, mechanical (metabolic and toxic), or vascular origin, and resulting in a variety of pathologic changes. The clinical manifestations are highly variable, depending on the nature, extent, site, and duration of the injury. 2. Any one of the forms of cerebral dysfunction due to injury sustained before, during, or shortly after birth. See also *cerebral palsy, minimal brain dysfunction syndrome.*

brain needle. A biopsy needle used in neurosurgery.

brain·pan, *n.* CRANIUM.

brain purpura. PERICAPILLARY ENCEPHALORRHAGIA.

brain sand. Psammoma bodies in the pineal body; corpora arenacea.

Brain's reflex [W. R. *Brain,* English neurologist, 1895–1966]. Extension of the paralyzed flexed arm when a patient with hemiplegia leans forward to assume the quadrupedal or "all-fours" position.

brain·stem, *n.* The portion of the brain remaining after the cerebral hemispheres and cerebellum have been removed. See also Plates 17, 18.

brainstem activating system. RETICULAR ACTIVATING SYSTEM.

brainstem epilepsy, fit, or **seizure.** Intermittent exaggerations of decerebrate postures, simulating the tonic phase of a tonic-clonic convulsion; not related to epilepsy.

brain sugar. GALACTOSE.

brain syndrome. ORGANIC BRAIN SYNDROME.

brain vesicles. The primary embryonic subdivisions of the brain.

brain·wash·ing, *n.* The systematic psychologic intervention into and perversion of an individual's thoughts and mental organization in order to break down his own standards of values and induce behavior radically different from that expected as a result of his earlier upbringing, but conforming to a pattern set forth by the person or organization practicing the psychologic attack. Syn., *menticide.*

brain wave. A fluctuation in the spontaneous electrical activity of the brain observed with amplification as in an electroencephalogram. Regular frequencies of brain waves are classified as alpha, beta, gamma, delta, or theta rhythms. See also *spike.*

brak·ing pipet. A micropipet in which a brake is inserted between the mouthpiece and the tip. The brake is a constriction which limits the flow of air and permits finer control of fluid movement.

branched-chain ketoaciduria. MAPLE-SYRUP URINE DISEASE.

branch·er deficiency glycogenosis. AMYLOPECTINOSIS.

brancher enzyme. Amylo-(1,4→1,6)-transglucosylase, an enzyme involved in the conversion of amylose to glycogen.

branchi-, branchio- [Gk. *branchia,* gills]. A combining form meaning (a) *gill;* (b) *branchial.*

bran·chia (brang'kee·uh) *n.,* pl. **bran·chi·ae** (·kee·ee) [L., from Gk.]. ²GILL.

bran·chi·al (brang'kee·ul) *adj.* 1. Pertaining to the branchiae or gills. 2. By extension, pertaining to the embryonic visceral arches.

branchial arch. 1. One of the posthyoid gill arches in lower vertebrates. 2. Any of the visceral arches in embryos of higher vertebrates.

branchial carcinoma. BRANCHIOGENIC CARCINOMA.

branchial cleft. 1. One of the slitlike openings between the gills, as in fishes. 2. VISCERAL CLEFT.

branchial cleft cyst. BRANCHIAL CYST.

branchial cyst. A cyst due to anomalous development of the embryonal visceral pouches or grooves.

branchial duct. The tubular second or fourth visceral groove opening into the cervical sinus of the embryo.

branchial fistula. LATERAL FISTULA OF THE NECK.

branchial groove. VISCERAL GROOVE.

branchial inclusion cyst. BRANCHIAL CYST.

branchial pouch. PHARYNGEAL POUCH.

III–IV branchial pouch syndrome. THYMIC APLASIA.

branch·ing, *n. In nuclear science,* the occurrence of two or more processes by which atoms of a radioactive nuclide can undergo decay.

branching enzyme. BRANCHER ENZYME.

branchio-. See *branchi-.*

bran·chio·gen·ic (brang"kee·o·jen'ick) *adj.* [*branchio-* + *-genic*]. Produced or developed from a branchial or visceral cleft or arch.

branchiogenic carcinoma. A squamous cell carcinoma arising from the epithelium of a branchial cyst or other branchial apparatus remnants.

branchiogenic cyst. BRANCHIAL CYST.

bran·chi·og·e·nous (brang"kee·oj'e·nus) *adj.* BRANCHIOGENIC.

bran·chi·o·ma (brang"kee·o·muh) *n.,* pl. **branchiomas, branchi·oma·ta** (·tuh) [*branchi-* + *-oma*]. BRANCHIOGENIC CARCINOMA.

bran·chio·mere (brang'kee·o·meer) *n.* [*branchio-* + *-mere*]. A segment of the visceral mesoderm which develops into a branchial or visceral arch.

bran·chi·om·er·ism (brang"kee·om'ur·iz·um) *n.* Serial arrangement of the visceral arches or branchiomeres.

bran·chio·mo·tor (brang"kee·o·mo'tur) *adj.* Pertaining to muscles arising from the branchial arches.

branchiomotor nucleus of the facial nerve. FACIAL NUCLEUS.

Brandt syndrome [T. E. *Brandt*]. ACRODERMATITIS ENTEROPATHICA.

bran·dy, *n.* [D. *brandewijn,* from *brant,* distilled, + *wijn,* wine]. 1. The product of the distillation of fermented grape juice; it contains 48 to 54%, by volume, C_2H_5OH, ethyl alcohol. 2. The product of the distillation of a fermented fruit juice, as cherry, peach, or apricot brandy.

Bran·ham's sign [H. H. *Branham,* U.S. surgeon, 19th century]. The closure of an arteriovenous fistula by digital compression causes slowing of the pulse, a rise in diastolic pressure, and disappearance of the cardiac murmur.

bran·ny, *adj.* Resembling broken and separated coats of grain, such as wheat or oats; scaly.

brash, *n.* [MF. *breche,* breach]. 1. PYROSIS. 2. Any eruption. 3. An attack of illness.

brasilin. BRAZILIN.

brass chills. METAL FUME FEVER.

brass founder's ague. METAL FUME FEVER.

Bras·si·ca (bras'i·kuh) *n.* [L., cabbage]. A genus of herbaceous plants that includes the cabbages, cauliflowers, turnips, mustards, and others. See also *mustard, mustard oil, black mustard.*

Brat·ton and Mar·shall's method. A colorimetric method for sulfonamides in blood and urine based upon the amount of purplish red azo dye formed by the coupling of diazotized sulfanilamide with *N*-(1-naphthyl) ethylenediamine dihydrochloride.

Brau·er's operation (braow'ur) [L. *Brauer,* German surgeon, 1865–1951]. Cardiolysis for relief of adherent pericardium.

Brau·ne's ring (braow'neʰ) [C. W. *Braune,* German anatomist, 1831–1892]. PHYSIOLOGIC RETRACTION RING.

Braun's test (braown) [C. H. *Braun,* German physician, 1847–1911]. A test in which sodium hydroxide and picric acid produce a deep red color in the presence of glucose.

brawny, *adj.* [MF. *braon,* fleshy part, muscle]. 1. Fleshy; muscular. 2. Thick or hard, as brawny edema.

brawny trachoma. A late stage of trachoma in which the conjunctiva is thickened due to scarring and chronic inflammatory cell infiltration.

Brax·ton Hicks contraction [J. *Braxton Hicks,* English gynecologist, 1823–1897]. Irregular and usually painless uterine contractions that occur with increasing frequency throughout pregnancy.

Braxton Hicks sign [J. *Braxton Hicks*]. A sign of pregnancy after the third month in which intermittent uterine contractions can be detected.

Braxton Hicks version [J. *Braxton Hicks*]. Manipulation by the bimanual method to bring the fetal head into the pelvis. This has been advocated in treatment of placenta previa and prolapsed cord.

braxy (brack'see) *n.* An infectious toxemia of sheep caused by *Clostridium septicum,* characterized by focal infection of the abomasum and sudden death; seen mainly in Scotland, Norway, and Iceland.

bra·ye·ra (bra·yair'uh) *n.* [*Brayer,* French physician 19th century]. The dried panicles of the pistillate flowers of *Hagenia abyssinica,* the kussotree. Has been used as an anthelmintic against tapeworms. Syn. *cusso, kousso, kusso.*

bra·zal·um stain (bra·zal'um). A nuclear stain made by the formula for hemalum, but by using brazilin instead of hematoxylin.

bra·zier's disease (bray'zhurz). Poisoning from zinc.

Bra·zil·ian spotted fever. Rocky Mountain spotted fever in South America.

Brazilian trypanosomiasis. CHAGAS' DISEASE.

braz·i·lin, bras·i·lin (braz'i·lin) *n.* A yellow crystalline compound, $C_{16}H_{14}O_5$, from *Caesalpinia echinata* (Brazilwood) or certain other redwood trees; used as a dye.

bread-and-butter pericardium. A peculiar appearance produced in fibrinous pericarditis by the rubbing of the two surfaces of the membrane over each other.

bread-crumbing tremor. PILL-ROLLING TREMOR.

bread sugar. DEXTROSE.

breakage-fusion-bridge cycle. A chromosomal sequence found in the gametophyte and endosperm of corn, initiated by a chromosomal break and fusion of broken ends of the duplicated chromosome to give a dicentric, which in anaphase forms a bridge broken by subsequent cell division. The process then recurs at the next cell division.

break·bone fever. DENGUE.

break·ing point. The point at which one can no longer inhibit one's respiration voluntarily, and the respiratory reflexes initiate breathing once again.

break·through bleeding. The prolonged and excessive bleeding caused by shedding of the endometrium at irregular times in the menstrual cycle among women taking hormonal contraceptives.

breast, *n.* 1. The front of the chest. 2. One of the mammary glands.

breast·bone, *n.* STERNUM.

breast-fed, *adj.* Nursed at a woman's breast.

breast milk. Milk from a woman's breast.

breast-milk jaundice. Intense jaundice with increased unconjugated bilirubin, seen in breast-fed infants during the second to fourth week of life as a result of a steroid substance in the breast milk which inhibits glucuronyl transferase activity in the infant.

breast pump. A pump for removing milk from a lactating breast.

breath, *n.* 1. The air inhaled or exhaled during respiration. 2. A single act of respiration.

breath alcohol method. A method for rapidly measuring the concentration of alcohol in the expired air of an individual to determine whether or not he is intoxicated.

Breathalyzer. Trademark for an instrument used to determine whether or not a person is alcoholically intoxicated.

breathe, *v.* To inhale and exhale air alternately; RESPIRE (1).

breath-holding attack or **spell.** A benign nonepileptic phenomenon observed in children, usually between 6 months and 4 years of age, almost always precipitated by a slight injury, anger, frustration, fear, or the desire for attention, in which the child holds his breath, becoming hypoxic and cyanotic, and rarely pale, and then briefly opisthotonic and unconscious, after which breathing is resumed automatically. Occasionally the opisthotonic phase may be followed by a brief generalized seizure. Syn. *reflex hypoxic crisis.*

breath-holding test. 1. Measurement of the pressor response to forced exhalation with closed glottis against a measured resistance. See also *Valsalva's maneuver.* 2. Measurement of the length of time a person can hold his breath voluntarily. See also *breaking point.*

breath sounds. Respiratory sounds heard on auscultation of the lungs.

Bre·da's disease (breh'da) [A. *Breda,* Italian dermatologist, 1850–1933]. YAWS.

breech, *n.* BUTTOCKS.

breech presentation. The presentation of the fetal buttocks and/or the feet first at the cervix. See also *complete breech presentation, frank breech presentation.*

breeder reactor. 1. A nuclear reactor that creates more fissionable fuel than it consumes. 2. A nuclear reactor that produces the same kind of fissionable fuel that it consumes, regardless of the amount.

breg·ma (breg'muh) *n.,* pl. **bregma·ta** (·tuh) [Gk., sinciput (rel. to Gmc. *bragna-* → E. *brain*)]. *In craniometry,* the junction of the coronal and sagittal sutures. **—breg·mat·ic** (breg·mat'ick) *adj.*

bregmatic space. ANTERIOR FONTANEL.

breg·ma·to·dym·ia (breg″muh·to·dim'ee·uh) *n.* [*bregma* + *-dymia*]. CRANIOPAGUS PARIETALIS.

breg·ma·to·lamb·doid arc (breg″muh·to·lam·doid). *In craniometry,* a measurement along the sagittal suture from the bregma to the lambda.

Breh and Gaebler's method. A test for potassium in which potassium is precipitated from a chloride-free blood filtrate as potassium silver cobaltinitrite which is measured colorimetrically.

brei (brye) *n.* [Ger., pap, pulp]. Mush; soupy mixture; tissue ground to a pulp.

Bremer's test [L. *Bremer,* U.S. physician, 1844–1914]. A test for diabetes in which a peripheral blood film is prepared in the usual way, dried in a hot-air oven, and stained with methylene blue and eosin. The erythrocytes of diabetics stain green-yellow, those of nondiabetics brown.

brems·strah·len (brem'strah·lun) *n.* [Ger. lit., braking-radiation]. The secondary photon radiation produced by the interaction of energized electrons and the atomic nuclei of the material through which they pass.

brems·strah·lung (brem'strah·lung) *n.* BREMSSTRAHLEN.

bren·ner·o·ma (bren″ur·o'muh) *n.* BRENNER TUMOR.

Bren·ner tumor [F. *Brenner,* German pathologist, b. 1877]. A solid or cystic tumor of the ovaries, composed of cords or nests of polyhedral epithelial cells separated by an abundant connective-tissue stroma; generally benign and having no known endocrine activity.

brepho·plas·tic (bref″o·plas'tick) *adj.* [Gk. *brephos,* fetus, + *-plastic*]. Designating embryonic, fetal, or newborn tissues which are used for transplantation to fetal, young, or adult animals.

Brethine. Trademark for terbutaline sulfate, a bronchodilator.

bre·tyl·i·um tosylate (bre·til'ee·um). *N-o*-Bromobenzyl-*N*-ethyl-*N,N*-dimethylammonium *p*-toluenesulfonate, $C_{11}H_{17}BrN{\cdot}C_7H_7SO_3$; a hypotensive drug of variable effectiveness.

Breu·er reflex (broy'ur) [J. *Breuer,* Austrian psychiatrist, 1842–1925]. HERING-BREUER REFLEX.

Breus's mole (broyce) [C. *Breus,* Austrian obstetrician, 1852–1914]. A type of missed abortion in which the patient expels, or has removed surgically, a small chorionic vesicle surrounded by blood clot, placenta, and decidual tissue. Syn. *subchorial tuberous hematoma of the decidua.*

Breutsch's disease. RHEUMATIC BRAIN DISEASE.

brevi- [L. *brevis* (rel. to Gk. *brachys*)]. A combining form meaning *short.*

brev·i·col·lis (brev″i·kol'is) *n.* [NL., from *brevi-* + L. *collum,* neck]. A deformity characterized by shortness of the neck and limitation of head movements and sometimes of the facial muscles.

brevi·lin·e·al (brev″i·lin'ee·ul) *adj.* [*brevi-* + *lineal*]. Pertaining to a body type which is shorter and broader than normal.

brevi·ra·di·ate (brev″i·ray'dee·ut, ·ate) *adj.* [*brevi-* + *radiate*]. Having short processes.

breviradiate cell. A variety of neuroglial cells which have short processes.

Brevital. Trademark for methohexital, an ultrashort-acting barbiturate used as the sodium derivative.

Brevital Sodium. Trademark for sodium methohexital, an ultrashort-acting barbiturate; used intravenously as a basal and general anesthetic.

Brew·er's infarcts [G. E. *Brewer,* U.S. surgeon, 1861–1939]. Conical reddened areas in the kidney, occurring in acute unilateral hematogenous pyelonephritis, which resemble ischemic infarcts.

Brewer's kidney [G. E. *Brewer*]. Multiple small cortical abscesses occurring in acute hematogenous pyelonephritis.

brewer's yeast. Dried cells of *Saccharomyces cerevisiae,* as used in the brewing of beer; a natural source of protein and vitamin B complex. Syn. *dried yeast.*

bribe, *n. In psychoanalysis,* a compromise in which the ego accepts the symptoms of a neurosis and, in turn, placates the superego by suffering.

Brick·er's loop [E. M. *Bricker,* U.S. surgeon, b. 1908]. ILEAL CONDUIT.

bridge, *n.* 1. *In anatomy,* any ridge or spanlike structure. 2. A partial denture supported by one or more teeth. See also *bridgework.* 3. In electricity, an apparatus for measuring the resistance of a conductor.

bridge coloboma. A form of coloboma affecting the iris, in which the cleft is separated from the pupil by a bridging strand of iris or by persistent pupillary membrane.

bridge flap. A tubed flap that remains attached at both ends and in the middle.

bridge of the nose. The prominence formed by the junction of the nasal bones.

bridge·work, *n.* 1. An appliance made of artificial crowns of teeth to replace missing natural teeth. Such crowns are connected to natural teeth or roots for anchorage by means of a bridge. A fixed bridge is one which is permanently fastened to its abutments; a removable bridge is one which, though held firmly in place, may be removed by the wearer. 2. The technique of making bridges.

bridg·ing graft. A graft that connects the cut ends of arteries, bones, or nerves where there is loss of substance and the divided ends cannot be approximated.

bri·dle, *n.* 1. A band or filament stretching across the lumen of a passage, or from side to side of an ulcer, scar, or abscess. 2. FRENUM.

bridle stricture. A membranous fold or band stretched across a canal, such as the urethra, causing partial obstruction.

Briggs' bag [J. E. *Briggs,* U.S. surgeon, 1869–1942]. A distensible rubber bag, no longer widely used, for the control of bleeding after suprapubic prostatectomy.

Briggs law. *In legal medicine,* a statute enacted in Massachusetts, in 1921, requiring a person who has committed certain crimes, or the same crime more than once, to undergo a psychiatric examination by experts in order to determine whether that individual suffers from a mental illness of such severity as to affect his responsibility and to require treatment in a mental hospital.

bright-field microscopy. Microscopy utilizing transillumination of the specimen with light rays in the optical axis of the microscope. Contr. *dark-field microscopy.*

bright·ness, *n.* The attribute of sensation by which an observer is aware of different luminances.

Bright's disease [R. *Bright,* English physician, 1789–1858]. CHRONIC GLOMERULONEPHRITIS.

Bright's murmur [R. *Bright*]. CORIACEOUS STREPITUS; a pericardial friction rub.

bril·liance, *n. In color optics,* BRIGHTNESS. —**bril·liant** (·yunt) *adj.*

brilliant cresyl blue. A basic dye, having highly metachromatic properties; chiefly used for the supravital staining of blood to demonstrate the reticulocytes.

brilliant green. A basic dye of the triphenylmethane series used in culture media and as a stain.

brilliant vital red. VITAL RED.

Brill's disease [N. E. *Brill,* U.S. physician, 1860–1925]. Recrudescent louse-borne typhus caused by *Rickettsia prowazekii* and characterized by headache, fever, malaise, and rash.

Brill-Sym·mers disease [N. E. *Brill;* and D. *Symmers,* U.S. pathologist, 1879–1957]. NODULAR LYMPHOMA.

Brill-Zins·ser disease [N. E. *Brill;* and H. *Zinsser,* U.S. bacteriologist, 1878–1940]. BRILL'S DISEASE.

brim of the pelvis. The margin of the inlet of the pelvis.

brim·stone, *n.* Native sulfur.

brin·ase (brin'ace, ·aze) *n.* A fibrinolytic enzyme derived from *Aspergillus nidulans.*

brine, *n.* Salt water; a strong saline solution; specifically, a strong solution of sodium chloride.

bri·no·lase (brye'no·lace, ·laze) *n.* A fibrinolytic enzyme obtained from *Aspergillus oryzae.*

Brin·ton's disease [W. *Brinton,* English physician, 1823–1867]. Gastric carcinoma of the linitis plastica type.

Bri·quet's ataxia (bree·keh') [P. *Briquet,* French physician, 1796–1881]. Ataxia as a manifestation of hysterical neurosis.

Briquet's syndrome [P. *Briquet*]. HYSTERIA (1).

bris·ket, *n.* The ventral aspect of the thorax of cattle.

brisket disease. A disease of cattle grazing at high altitudes, characterized by pulmonary hypertension and right heart failure; a counterpart of altitude sickness in man.

Bris·saud-Ma·rie syndrome (bree·so') [E. *Brissaud,* French physician, 1852–1909; and P. *Marie*]. Unilateral spasm of the lips and tongue as a manifestation of hysterical neurosis.

Brissaud's disease or **syndrome** [E. *Brissaud*]. 1. Facial spasm on one side with paralysis of the opposite extremities. 2. BRISSAUD'S INFANTILISM.

Brissaud's infantilism. Infantilism seen as a consequence of hypofunction of the thyroid gland.

Brissaud's reflex [E. *Brissaud*]. Contraction of the tensor of the fascia lata on stimulation of the sole of the foot.

Bristamycin. A trademark for erythromycin stearate, an antibiotic.

bris·tle probang. A probang having on the end a sheath of bristles or horsehair that can be made to spread like an umbrella as the instrument is drawn out.

Brit·ish antilewisite. DIMERCAPROL. Abbreviated, BAL.

British gum. DEXTRIN.

British thermal unit. In general, the heat required to raise the temperature of one pound of water one degree Fahrenheit. Because of variation of the specific heat of water with temperature, the reference temperature must be specified. For the interval 60 to 61°F, a BTU is equivalent to 1054.54 joules. The international table BTU, which is independent of temperature, is equivalent to 1055.06 joules.

brittle bones. OSTEOGENESIS IMPERFECTA.

broach, *n.* [OF. *broche*]. Any one of a variety of finely tapered instruments used in endodontics for removing the contents of the dental pulp chamber and canals and inserting treatment materials; the basic types are barbed and smooth.

Broad·bent's apoplexy [William H. *Broadbent,* English physician, 1835–1907]. A cerebrovascular accident in which a hemorrhage in the cerebral substance eventually breaks into one of the lateral ventricles.

Broadbent's inverted sign [W. H. *Broadbent*]. Pulsations synchronous with ventricular systole seen on the left posterolateral chest wall; thought due to aneurysmal left atrial dilatation, but probably reflects left ventricular hypertrophy.

Broadbent's law [W. H. *Broadbent*]. Upper motor neuron lesions produce a milder form of paralysis in those muscles generally concerned with bilateral contractions than in those which act unilaterally.

Broadbent's sign [Walter *Broadbent,* English physician, 1868–1951]. Systolic retraction of the eleventh and twelfth left ribs and interspaces posteriorly, due to pericardial adhesions to the diaphragm; a sign of adhesive pericarditis.

broad-beta disease [from the characteristic broad beta band on electrophoresis]. Hyperlipoproteinemia type 3. See *hyperlipoproteinemia.*

broad ligament of the uterus. A fold of peritoneum which extends laterally from the uterus to the pelvic wall on each side. NA *ligamentum latum uteri.*

broad-spectrum antibiotic. An antibiotic effective in the treatment of various infections caused by different types of microorganisms.

broad tapeworm. *DIPHYLLOBOTHRIUM LATUM.*

Bro·ca's angle (broh·kah') [P. P. *Broca,* French surgeon and anthropologist, 1824–1880]. PARIETAL ANGLE.

Broca's aphasia [P. P. *Broca*]. A classical division of aphasia, including those aphasic syndromes involving primarily the production rather than the reception of language; characterized generally by slow and laborious speech, telegraphic speech, and agraphia, with relatively intact comprehension. The lesion responsible is in opercular and insular cortex adjacent to Broca's area (Brodmann's area 44) or subjacent white matter. Syn. *motor aphasia, expressive aphasia, executive aphasia.*

Broca's area [P. P. *Broca*]. Brodmann's area 44, situated in the left hemisphere at the posterior end of the third (inferior) frontal convolution; responsible for the executive or motor aspects of speech in most persons.

Broca's band [P. P. *Broca*]. A diagonal strip of gray matter in the posterior part of the anterior perforated substance, extending from the inferior medial surface of a cerebral hemisphere to the region of the amygdaloid body.

Broca's center, convolution, or **gyrus** [P. P. *Broca*]. BROCA'S AREA.

Broca's parolfactory area [P. P. *Broca*]. PAROLFACTORY AREA.

Broca's plane [P. P. *Broca*]. ALVEOLOCONDYLEAN PLANE.

Broca's point [P. P. *Broca*]. AURICULAR POINT.

Brock operation [R. C. *Brock,* English surgeon, b. 1903]. Pulmonary valvotomy for pulmonary valve stenosis.

Brock's syndrome [R. C. *Brock*]. MIDDLE LOBE SYNDROME.

Brocq's disease [L. A. J. *Brocq,* French dermatologist, 1856–1928]. 1. PARAPSORIASIS EN PLAQUES. 2. ALOPECIA CICATRISATA.

bro·cre·sine (bro·kree′zeen) *n.* α-(Aminoxy)-6-bromo-*m*-cresol, $C_7H_8BrNO_2$, an inhibitor of histidine decarboxylase.

Bro·ders' classification [A. C. *Broders,* U.S. pathologist, 1885–1964]. A system in which tumors are divided into four grades, the prognosis supposedly becoming less favorable as the grade increases. Grade I tumors are chiefly composed of cells resembling adult cells; grade IV tumors, of markedly anaplastic cells; and grades II and III tumors are intermediate in appearance.

Bro·die's abscess [B. C. *Brodie,* English surgeon, 1783–1862]. A chronic metaphyseal abscess, usually seen in the tibia of young adults.

Brodie's serocystic disease [B. C. *Brodie*]. CYSTOSARCOMA PHYLLODES.

Brodie's tumor [B. C. *Brodie*]. CYSTOSARCOMA PHYLLODES.

Brod·mann's areas (brohd′mahnn) [K. *Brodmann,* German neurologist, 1868–1918]. Numbered regions of the cerebral cortex originally differentiated by histologic criteria, now used to identify cortical functions: *areas 1, 2, 3,* the somesthetic area; *area 4,* the motor area; *area 4S,* between areas 4 and 6, a lesion of which causes spasticity of the muscles innervated by it; *areas 5, 7,* the somesthetopsychic area; *area 6,* the premotor area; *area 8,* the adjacent superior part of the frontal cortex, a region involved with eye movement and pupillary change; *area 17,* the visual projection area; *areas 18, 19,* the visuopsychic area; *area 41,* the auditory projection area; *area 42,* the auditopsychic area; *area 44,* Broca's area.

Brodmann's map [K. *Brodmann*]. The map of areas of the human cerebral cortex, differentiated by their cellular patterns. The numbers assigned to these areas are still used for convenient reference.

broken wind. HEAVES.

brom-, bromo- [Gk. *brōmos*]. A combining form meaning (a) *a bad smell;* (b) in chemistry, *the presence of bromine.*

bro·mate (bro′mate) *n.* A salt of bromic acid.

bro·ma·to·ther·a·py (bro″muh·to·therr′uh·pee) *n.* [Gk. *brōma, brōmatos,* food, + *therapy*]. DIETOTHERAPY.

bro·ma·to·tox·in (bro″muh·to·tock′sin) *n.* [Gk. *brōma, brōmatos,* food, + *toxin*]. Any poison generated in food by the growth of microorganisms.

bro·ma·to·tox·ism (bro″muh·to·tock′siz·um) *n.* [*bromatotoxin* + *-ism*]. Poisoning with infected or contaminated food.

bro·maz·e·pam (bro·maz′e·pam, bro·may′ze·pam) *n.* 7-Bromo-1,3-dihydro-5-(2-pyridyl)-2*H*-1,4-benzodiazepin-2-one, $C_{14}H_{10}BrN_3O$, a psychotherapeutic drug.

bro·ma·zine (bro′muh·zeen) *n.* BROMODIPHENHYDRAMINE.

brom·chlor·e·none (brom·klor′e·nohn) *n.* 6-Bromo-5-chloro-2-benzoxazolinone, $C_7H_3BrClNO_2$, a local anti-infective agent.

brom·cre·sol green (brom·kree′sol). BROMOCRESOL GREEN.

bromcresol purple. BROMOCRESOL PURPLE.

bro·me·lains (bro′me·lainz) *n.* PLANT PROTEASE CONCENTRATE.

bro·me·lin (bro′me·lin) *n.* A protein-digesting enzyme from pineapple.

brom·eth·ol (brom·eth′ol) *n.* TRIBROMOETHANOL SOLUTION.

brom·hex·ine (brome·heck′seen) *n.* 3,5-Dibromo-N^{α}-cyclohexyl-N^{α}-methyltoluene-α,2-diamine, $C_{14}H_{20}$-Br_2N_2, an expectorant and mucolytic drug; used as the hydrochloride salt.

brom·hi·dro·si·pho·bia (brome″hi·dro″si·fo′bee·uh) *n.* [*bromhidrosis* + *phobia*]. Morbid dread of offensive smells, with hallucinations as to the perception of them.

brom·hi·dro·sis (brome″hi·dro′sis, brom″hi·) *n.* [*brom-* + *hidrosis*]. Excretion of sweat with an unpleasant odor. Syn. *osmidrosis, fetid perspiration.*

bro·mic acid (bro′mick). An unstable acid, $HBrO_3$, known only in aqueous solution; it forms stable salts, called bromates.

bro·mide (bro′mide, ·mid) *n.* [*brom-* + *-ide*]. Any binary salt in which univalent bromine is the anion, as sodium bromide, NaBr. The bromides are used medicinally to check the convulsions of epilepsy and tetanus, as analgesics, and as sedatives.

bromide poisoning. BROMISM.

bro·mi·dro·sis (bro″mi·dro′sis) *n.* BROMHIDROSIS.

bro·min·ate (bro′min·ate) *v.* To treat with bromine.

brom·in·di·one (brom″in·dye′ohn) *n.* 2-(*p*-Bromophenyl)-1,3-indandione, $C_{15}H_9BrO_2$, an anticoagulant drug.

bro·mine (bro′meen, ·min) *n.* [F. *brome,* from Gk. *brōmos,* bad smell]. Br = 79.904. A reddish-brown liquid which, at ordinary temperatures, gives off a heavy, suffocating vapor. It is a very active escharotic and disinfectant. See also Table of Elements in the Appendix.

bromine acne. The acneform eruption that may ensue following ingestion of bromine.

bromine poisoning. BROMISM.

bro·min·ism (bro′min·iz·um) *n.* BROMISM.

bro·mism (bro′miz·um) *n.* [*brom*ide + *-ism*]. A disease state caused by the prolonged or excessive administration of bromide compounds; it is characterized by headache, drowsiness, lethargy, dysarthria, often mania with psychotic behavior and acneform skin lesions.

brom·iso·val·um (brom″eye·so·val′um) *n.* (α-Bromoisovaleryl) urea, $C_6H_{11}BrN_2O_2$, a sedative and hypnotic.

bromo-. See *brom-.*

bro·mo·ac·et·an·i·lid (bro″mo·as″e·tan′i·lid) *n.* *p*-Monobromoacetanilid, C_8H_8BrNO; has been used as an analgesic and antipyretic.

bro·mo·cam·phor (bro″mo·kam′fur) *n.* MONOBROMATED CAMPHOR.

bro·mo·cre·sol green (bro″mo·kree′sol). Tetrabromo-*m*-cresolsulfonphthalein, an indicator used for determination of hydrogen-ion concentration.

bromocresol purple. Dibromo-*o*-cresolsulfonphthalein, an indicator used for determination of hydrogen-ion concentration.

bro·mo·crip·tine (bro″mo·krip′teen) *n.* 2-Bromoergocryptine, $C_{32}H_{40}BrN_5O_5$, a prolactin inhibitor.

bro·mo·de·oxy·uri·dine (bro″mo·dee·ock″see·yoo′ri·deen) *n.* A mutagenic base analogue of thymidine. See also *bromouracil.*

bro·mo·der·ma (bro″mo·dur′muh) *n.* [*bromo-* + *-derma*]. An eruption due to ingestion of bromides.

bro·mo·di·eth·yl·ace·tyl·urea (bro″mo·dye·eth″il·as″e·til·yoo·ree′uh, a·see″til·) *n.* CARBROMAL.

bro·mo·di·phen·hy·dra·mine (bro″mo·dye·fen·high′druh·meen) *n.* $C_{17}H_{20}BrNO$, an antihistamine; used as the hydrochloride salt. Syn. *bromazine.*

bro·mo·form (bro′mo·form) *n.* Tribromomethane, $CHBr_3$, a heavy colorless, mobile liquid, slightly soluble in water. Has been used as a sedative but is toxic.

bro·mo·hy·per·hi·dro·sis (bro″mo·high″pur·hi·dro′sis, ·high·dro′sis) *n.* [*bromo-* + *hyperhidrosis*]. The excessive secretion of malodorous sweat.

bro·mo·hy·per·i·dro·sis (bro″mo·high″pur·i·dro′sis) *n.* BROMOHYPERHIDROSIS.

bro·mo·ma·nia (bro″mo·may′nee·uh) *n.* [*bromo-* + *-mania*]. Psychosis from the excessive use of bromides.

bro·mo·men·or·rhea, bro·mo·men·or·rhoea (bro″mo·men″o·ree′uh) *n.* [*bromo-* + *menorrhea*]. Disordered menstruation marked by offensive odor.

bro·mo·phe·nol blue (bro″mo·fee′nol). Tetrabromophenolsulfonphthalein, an indicator used for determination of hydrogen-ion concentration.

bro·mop·nea, bro·mop·noea (bro″mop·nee′uh, bro″mo·nee′uh) *n.* [*bromo-* + Gk. *pnoia,* breath]. HALITOSIS.

bro·mo·thy·mol blue (bro″mo·thigh′mol). Dibromothymolsulfonphthalein, an indicator used for determination of hydrogen-ion concentration.

bro·mo·ura·cil (bro″mo·yoo′ruh·sil) *n.* [*bromo-* + *-uracil*]. 5-Bromouracil, a base analogue of thymine which can be incorporated in the latter's position in deoxyribonucleic acid and which can cause mutation by converting an adenine-thymine base pair to a guanine-cytosine pair. Its deoxyriboside is bromodeoxyuridine.

bro·mox·a·nide (bro·mock'suh·nide) *n.* 4'-Bromo-3-*tert*-butyl-α',α',α'-trifluoro-5-nitro-2,6-cresoto-*o*-toluidide, $C_{19}H_{18}BrF_3N_2O_4$, an anthelmintic agent.

brom·per·i·dol (brome·perr'i·dole) *n.* 4-[4-(*p*-Bromophenyl)-4-hydroxypiperidino]-4'-fluorobutyrophenone, $C_{21}H_{23}BrFNO_2$, a tranquilizer.

brom·phen·ir·a·mine (brome"fen·irr'uh·meen) *n.* *dl*-2-*p*-Bromo-α-[2-(dimethylamino)ethyl]benzyl}pyridine, $C_{16}H_{19}BrN_2$, an antihistaminic drug; used as the maleate salt.

brom·phe·nol blue (brom·fee'nol). BROMOPHENOL BLUE.

Bromsulphalein. Trademark for sodium sulfobromophthalein, a diagnostic aid for evaluation of liver function. Abbreviated, BSP.

Bromsulphalein test. A test based upon the ability of the liver to remove injected Bromsulphalein from the blood. Delayed removal indicates hepatic dysfunction.

Bromtetragnost. A trademark for sulfobromophthalein sodium.

brom·thy·mol blue (brom·thigh'mol). BROMOTHYMOL BLUE.

Bromural. A trademark for bromisovalum, a sedative and hypnotic.

bronch-, broncho-. A combining form meaning *bronchus, bronchial.*

bronch·ad·e·ni·tis (bronk·ad"e·nigh'tis) *n.* [*bronch-* + *adenitis*]. Inflammation of the bronchial lymph nodes.

bronchi-, bronchio-. A combining form meaning *bronchial.*

bronchi. Plural and genitive singular of *bronchus.*

bron·chi·al (bronk'ee·ul) *adj.* Of, pertaining to, or involving the bronchi or their branches.

bronchial asthma. ASTHMA.

bronchial breath sounds. The tubular, blowing, harsh sound of bronchial respiration.

bronchial bud. One of the outgrowths of the embryonic bronchi responsible for the continued growth and branching of the bronchial tree.

bronchial calculus. A concretion of mucus or exudate, infiltrated with mineral salts, situated in the bronchial tree.

bronchial cartilage. Plates of cartilage, in some instances very minute, found in the bronchial tubes.

bronchial cyst. BRONCHOGENIC CYST.

bronchial fistula. 1. An abnormal tract communicating between the pleural cavity and a bronchus, usually associated with empyema. 2. An abnormal tract leading from a bronchus to a cutaneous opening, the result of gangrene or abscess of the lung.

bronchial glands. 1. The mixed glands of the mucous membrane of the bronchi. NA *glandulae bronchiales.* 2. The chain of lymph nodes along the bronchi.

bronchial pneumonia. BRONCHOPNEUMONIA.

bronchial respiration. On auscultation, tubular blowing breath sounds normally heard over the larynx, trachea, and larger bronchi; heard over the lungs in any disease process producing pulmonary consolidation, sounds are louder, longer, and higher pitched in expiration than in inspiration.

bronchial septum. The carina of the trachea. See *carina.*

bronchial spasm. BRONCHOSPASM.

bronchial stenosis. BRONCHOSTENOSIS.

bronchial tree. The arborization of the bronchi of the lung, considered as a structural and functional unit.

bronchial tube. BRONCHUS.

bron·chi·ec·ta·sis (bronk"ee·eck'tuh·sis) *n.*, pl. **bronchiecta·ses** (·seez) [*bronchi-* + *ectasis*]. Saccular or tubular dilatation of one or more bronchi, usually due to bronchial obstruction and infection, and accompanied by cough, mucopurulent sputum, hemoptysis, and recurrent pneumonia. —**bronchi·ec·tat·ic** (·eck·tat'ick) *adj.*

bronchi lo·ba·res (lo·bair'eez [NA]. LOBAR BRONCHI.

bron·chio·gen·ic (bronk"ee·o·jen'ick) *adj.* BRONCHOGENIC.

bronchiolar carcinoma. A well-differentiated adenocarcinoma of the lung, either focal or multicentric, and of disputed origin, characterized by tall columnar, mucus-producing cells which spread over the pulmonary alveoli.

bron·chi·ole (bronk'ee·ole) *n.* [NL. *bronchiolum,* dim. of *bronchium*]. One of the small (1 mm or less in diameter) subdivisions of the bronchi. See also *respiratory bronchiole.* —**bron·chi·o·lar** (brong·kigh'o·lur) *adj.*

bron·chi·o·lec·ta·sis (bronk"ee·o·leck'tuh·sis) *n.*, pl. **bronchio·lecta·ses** (·seez) [*bronchiole* + *ectasis*]. Dilatation of bronchioles. See also *bronchiectasis.*

bronchioli. Plural of *bronchiolus.*

bronchioli re·spi·ra·to·rii (res"pi·ruh·tor'ee·eye, re·spye"ruh·) [NA]. RESPIRATORY BRONCHIOLES.

bron·chi·ol·itis (bronk"ee·o·lye'tis) *n.* Inflammation of the bronchioles; most often caused by respiratory syncytial virus in infants. Syn. *capillary bronchitis.*

bronchiolitis fi·bro·sa oblit·e·rans (figh·bro'suh o·blit'ur·anz). BRONCHIOLITIS OBLITERANS.

bronchiolitis oblit·e·rans (o·blit'ur·anz). Bronchiolitis characterized by the organization of exudate in the bronchioles with fibrotic obliteration of the lumen; may be due to inhalation of nitrogen dioxide or other irritating fumes.

bron·chi·o·lo·al·ve·o·lar (brong"kee·o"lo·al·vee'uh·lur, brong·kye"o·) *adj.* Pertaining to the pulmonary alveoli and bronchioles.

bronchioloalveolar cell carcinoma. A malignant tumor composed of cells having features of both alveolar cells and bronchiolar epithelium, usually appearing as a small peripheral lung tumor.

bron·chi·o·lus (brong·kigh'o·lus) *n.*, pl. **bronchio·li** (·lye) [NA]. BRONCHIOLE.

bron·chio·spasm (bronk'ee·o·spaz·um) *n.* BRONCHOSPASM.

bronchi seg·men·ta·les (seg"men·tay'leez) [NA]. SEGMENTAL BRONCHI.

bron·chi·tis (bron·kigh'tis, brong·kigh'tis) *n.*, pl. **bron·chit·i·des** (·kit'i·deez) [*bronch-* + *-itis*]. Inflammation of the mucous membrane of the bronchi. —**bron·chit·ic** (·kit'ick) *adj.*

bronchitis con·vul·si·va (kon·vul·sigh'vuh). *Obsol.* PERTUSSIS.

bron·chi·um (bronk'ee·um) *n.*, pl. **bron·chia** (·ee·uh) [L., from Gk. *bronchion,* bronchus]. A subdivision of a bronchus which is larger than a bronchiole.

broncho-. See *bronch-.*

bron·cho·bil·i·ary (bronk"o·bil'ee·air"ee) *adj.* Pertaining to a bronchus and the biliary tract.

bronchobiliary fistula. An abnormal communication between a bronchus and the biliary tract, usually as a result of hepatic abscess or trauma.

bron·cho·can·di·di·a·sis (bronk"o·kan·di·dye'uh·sis) *n.* [*broncho-* + *candidiasis*]. BRONCHOMONILIASIS.

bron·cho·cav·ern·ous (bronk"o·kav'ur·nus) *adj.* Bronchial and cavernous.

bronchocavernous respiration. A form of respiration intermediate in character between bronchial and cavernous respiration, heard over a pulmonary cavity with adjacent pulmonary consolidation.

bron·cho·cele (bronk'o·seel) *n.* [*broncho-* + *-cele*]. A localized dilatation of a bronchus.

bron·cho·co·lic (bronk"o·kol'ic, ·ko'lick) *adj.* Pertaining to a bronchus and the colon.

bronchocolic fistula. An abnormal communication between a bronchus and the colon, usually as a result of empyema or subphrenic abscess.

bron·cho·con·stric·tion (bronk"o·kun·strick'shun) *n.* [*broncho-* + *constriction*]. Constriction of the pulmonary air passages. —**bronchoconstric·tive** (·tiv) *adj.*

bron·cho·con·stric·tor (bronk"o·kun·strik'tur) *n.* [*broncho-* + *constrictor*]. Any substance which decreases the caliber of the pulmonary air passages.

bron·cho·dil·a·ta·tion (bronk"o·dil"uh·tay'shun, ·dye"luh·tay'shun) *n.* [*broncho-* + *dilatation*]. The widening of the caliber of the pulmonary air passages by the use of drugs or surgical instruments.

bron·cho·di·la·tor (bronk″o·dye·lay′tur, ·di·lay′tur) *n.* [*broncho-* + *dilator*]. 1. Any drug which has the property of increasing the caliber of the pulmonary air passages. 2. An instrument used for this purpose.

bron·cho·ede·ma (bronk″o·e·dee′muh) *n.* [*broncho-* + *edema*]. Swelling of the bronchial epithelium which may produce airway obstruction.

bron·cho·esoph·a·ge·al, bron·cho-oesoph·a·ge·al (bronk″o·e·sof″uh·jee′ul) *adj.* Pertaining to a bronchus and the esophagus.

bronchoesophageal fistula. An abnormal communication between a bronchus and the esophagus; may be congenital or acquired.

bronchoesophageal muscle. A small inconstant bundle of smooth muscle connecting the esophagus and the left main bronchus. NA *musculus bronchoesophageus.* See also Table of Muscles in the Appendix.

bron·cho·esoph·a·gol·o·gy (bronk″o·e·sof″uh·gol′uh·jee) *n.* [*broncho-* + *esophago-* + *-logy*]. The field of medicine specializing in disorders of the esophagus and bronchial tree.

bron·cho·esoph·a·gos·co·py, bron·cho-oesoph·a·gos·co·py (bronk″o·e·sof″uh·gos′kuh·pee) *n.* [*broncho-* + *esophagoscopy*]. Visual examination of the interior of the larger tracheobronchial tubes and the esophagus with the aid of an instrument.

bron·cho·gen·ic (bronk″o·jen′ick) *adj.* [*broncho-* + *-genic*]. 1. Arising in a bronchus or in the bronchi. 2. *In embryology,* capable of forming the bronchi.

bronchogenic carcinoma. Any of several cellular types of carcinoma arising from the bronchi; usually squamous-cell and found in the segmental bronchi, with adenocarcinoma and poorly differentiated carcinoma less common and of different distribution.

bronchogenic cyst. Cysts having the structure of bronchial walls, usually occurring in the superior mediastinum.

bronchogenic tuberculosis. Drainage of a caseous tuberculous lesion into the bronchial lumen with dissemination of tuberculosis to new areas of the lung.

bron·chog·e·nous (brong·koj′e·nus) *adj.* BRONCHOGENIC.

bronchogenous tuberculosis. BRONCHOGENIC TUBERCULOSIS.

bron·cho·gram (bronk′o·gram) *n.* [*broncho-* + *-gram*]. Radiograph of the bronchial tree made after the introduction of a radiopaque substance.

bron·chog·ra·phy (brong·kog′ruh·fee) *n.* [*broncho-* + *-graphy*]. Radiographic visualization of the bronchial tree after the introduction of a radiopaque contrast material. —**bron·cho·graph·ic** (bronk″o·graf′ick) *adj.*

bron·cho·lith (bronk′o·lith) *n.* [*broncho-* + *-lith*]. A calculus or concretion in the bronchial tree.

bron·cho·li·thi·a·sis (bronk″o·li·thigh′uh·sis) *n.*, pl. **broncholithia·ses** (·seez) [*broncho-* + *lithiasis*]. A condition characterized by the formation of calculi in the bronchi.

bron·chol·o·gy (brong·kol′uh·jee) *n.* [*broncho-* + *-logy*]. The branch of medicine dealing with the study and treatment of diseases of the bronchial tree.

bron·cho·me·di·as·ti·nal trunk (bronk″o·mee″dee·as·tye′nul) [*broncho-* + *mediastinal*]. One of two collecting lymph vessels, right and left, receiving lymph from the heart, lungs, thorax, and upper surface of the liver. The one on the right empties into the right lymphatic duct or into the angle of junction of the right subclavian and internal jugular veins; the one on the left empties into the thoracic duct or independently into the angle of junction of the left subclavian and internal jugular veins. NA *truncus bronchomediastinalis.*

bron·cho·mon·i·li·a·sis (bronk″o·mon·i·lye′uh·sis) *n.*, pl. **bronchomonilia·ses** (·seez) [*broncho-* + *moniliasis*]. A bronchial disease caused by infection with species of *Candida,* usually *C. albicans.*

bron·cho·mo·tor (bronk′o·mo′tur) *adj.* [*broncho-* + *motor*]. Pertaining to the neuromuscular mechanisms which control the caliber of the pulmonary air passages.

bron·cho·my·co·sis (bronk″o·migh·ko′sis) *n.*, pl. **bronchomyco·ses** (·seez) [*broncho-* + *mycosis*]. A fungous disease of the bronchial tree.

broncho-oesophageal. BRONCHOESOPHAGEAL.

broncho-oesophagology. BRONCHOESOPHAGOLOGY.

broncho-oesophagoscopy. BRONCHOESOPHAGOSCOPY.

bron·chop·a·thy (brong·kop′uth·ee) *n.* [*broncho-* + *-pathy*]. Any abnormality in a bronchus.

bron·choph·o·ny (brong·kof′uh·nee) *n.* [*broncho-* + *-phony*]. The clear resonant voice sounds normally heard on auscultation over a large bronchus; heard in disease over an area of pulmonary consolidation. See also *pectoriloquy.*

bron·cho·plas·ty (bronk′o·plas·tee) *n.* [*broncho-* + *-plasty*]. *In surgery,* repair of a bronchial defect.

bron·cho·pleu·ral (bronk″o·ploor′ul) *adj.* Pertaining to a bronchus and the pleural cavity, as bronchopleural fistula.

bron·cho·pneu·mo·nia (bronk″o·new·mo′nyuh) *n.* [*broncho-* + *pneumonia*]. Pulmonary inflammation with exudation into the alveoli, concentrated about the bronchi, which are also involved; occurs principally in childhood and old age; due to a variety of causative organisms.

bron·cho·pneu·mo·ni·tis (bronk″o·new″mo·nigh′tis) *n.* [*broncho-* + *pneumonitis*]. BRONCHOPNEUMONIA.

bron·cho·pul·mo·nary (bronk″o·pul′mo·nerr″ee) *adj.* [*broncho-* + *pulmonary*]. Pertaining to both the bronchi and the lungs.

bronchopulmonary dysplasia. An apparently dose-related consequence of oxygen therapy in newborns with respiratory distress syndrome, identified during life by overinflated lungs, heavy linear and curvilinear densities mixed with areas of lobular emphysema distributed throughout the lungs on chest roentgenograms, excessive shedding of normal epithelial cells on exfoliative cytology, and marked bronchiolar and alveolar damage at autopsy.

bronchopulmonary segment. Any of the subdivisions of a pulmonary lobe, each bounded by connective-tissue septa and supplied by a segmental bronchus; named, according to location within the lobe, as follows: (of the superior lobe of the right lung:) apical, posterior, anterior; (of the superior lobe of the left lung:) apicoposterior, anterior, superior lingular, inferior lingular; (of the middle lobe of the right lung:) lateral, medial; (of the inferior lobe of the right or the left lung:) apical (or superior), subapical (or subsuperior), basal medial (or cardiac), basal anterior, basal lateral, basal posterior. NA (pl.) *segmenta bronchopulmonalia.*

bron·chor·rha·phy (brong·kor′uh·fee) *n.* [*broncho-* + *-rrhaphy*]. The suturing of a bronchus.

bron·chor·rhea, bron·chor·rhoea (bronk″o·ree′uh) *n.* [*broncho-* + *-rrhea*]. Excessive discharge of mucus from the bronchial mucous membranes. —**bronchor·rhe·al** (·ree′ul) *adj.*

bron·cho·scope (bronk′o·skope) *n.* & *v.* [*broncho-* + *-scope*]. 1. An instrument for the visual examination of the interior of the bronchi. 2. To examine with a bronchoscope. —**bron·cho·scop·ic** (bronk″o·skop′ick) *adj.;* **bron·chos·co·py** (brong·kos′kuh·pee) *n.*

bronchoscopic position. Supine position of the patient with hyperextension of the neck, aligning the larynx and trachea to permit introduction of a bronchoscope.

bron·cho·spasm (bronk′o·spaz·um) *n.* [*broncho-* + *spasm*]. Temporary narrowing of the bronchi due to violent, involuntary contraction of the smooth muscle of the bronchi.

bron·cho·spi·ro·che·to·sis, bron·cho·spi·ro·chae·to·sis (bronk″o·spye″ro·kee·to′sis) *n.* [*broncho-* + *spirochetosis*]. Hemorrhagic chronic bronchitis, associated with spirochetal organisms. Syn. *Castellani's disease.*

bron·cho·spi·rog·ra·phy (bronk″o·spye·rog′ruh·fee) *n.* [*broncho-* + *spiro-* + *-graphy*]. The graphic recording of the functional capacity of the lungs.

bron·cho·spi·rom·e·ter (bronk″o·spye·rom′e·tur) *n.* A spirometer connected to an intrabronchial catheter, designed to measure the functional capacity of a single lung or lung segment.

bron·cho·spi·rom·e·try (bronk″o·spye·rom′e·tree) *n.* [*broncho-* + *spirometry*]. The determination of various aspects of the functional capacity of the lungs, a single lung, or a lung segment.

bron·cho·ste·no·sis (bronk″o·ste·no′sis) *n.*, pl. **bronchosteno·ses** (·seez) [*broncho-* + *stenosis*]. Narrowing of the lumen of one or more bronchi.

bron·chos·to·my (brong·kos′tuh·mee) *n.* [*broncho-* + *-stomy*]. Fistulization of a bronchus through the chest wall.

bron·chot·o·my (brong·kot′uh·mee) *n.* [*broncho-* + *-tomy*]. Incision into a bronchus.

bron·cho·ve·sic·u·lar (bronk″o·ve·sick′yoo·lur) *adj.* [*broncho-* + *vesicular*]. Pertaining to the bronchi and the pulmonary alveoli.

bronchovesicular respiration. A form of respiration intermediate between bronchial and vesicular; heard over areas of patchy pulmonary consolidation; inspiration and expiration are equal in duration.

bron·chus (bronk′us) *n.*, pl. & genit. sing. **bron·chi** (·eye) [Gk. *bronchos,* trachea, throat]. 1. [NA] One of the primary branches of the trachea or such of its branches within the lung as contain cartilage in their walls. See also *primary bronchus, secondary bronchus.* 2. [BNA] Bronchus principalis (= PRIMARY BRONCHUS).

bronchus lin·gu·la·ris inferior (ling·gew·lair′is) [NA]. The lower bronchus of the lingula of the upper lobe of the left lung.

bronchus lingularis superior [NA]. The upper bronchus of the lingula of the upper lobe of the left lung.

bronchus lo·ba·ris (lo·bair′is) [NA]. LOBAR BRONCHUS.

bronchus lobaris in·fe·ri·or dex·ter (in·feer′ee·or decks′tur) [NA]. The right lower lobar bronchus, ventilating the lower lobe of the right lung.

bronchus lobaris inferior si·nis·ter (si·nis′tur) [NA]. The left lower lobar bronchus, ventilating the lower lobe of the left lung.

bronchus lobaris me·di·us dex·ter (mee′dee·us decks′tur) [NA]. The right middle lobar bronchus, ventilating the middle lobe of the right lung.

bronchus lobaris superior dexter [NA]. The right superior lobar bronchus, ventilating the upper lobe of the right lung.

bronchus lobaris superior si·nis·ter (si·nis′tur) [NA]. The left superior lobar bronchus, ventilating the upper lobe of the left lung.

bronchus prin·ci·pa·lis (prin·si·pay′lis) [NA]. PRIMARY BRONCHUS; either of the two bronchi, right (bronchus principalis dexter) and left (bronchus principalis sinister), which originate in the bifurcation of the trachea.

bronchus seg·men·ta·lis (seg·men·tay′lis) [NA]. SEGMENTAL BRONCHUS.

bronchus segmentalis an·te·ri·or lo·bi su·pe·ri·o·ris dex·tri (an·teer′ee·or lo′bye sue·peer·ee·o′ris decks′trye) [NA]. The bronchus of the anterior segment of the upper lobe of the right lung.

bronchus segmentalis anterior lobi superioris si·nis·tri (si·nis′trye) [NA]. The bronchus of the anterior segment of the upper lobe of the left lung.

bronchus segmentalis api·ca·lis lo·bi in·fe·ri·o·ris dex·tri (ap·i·kay′lis lo′bye in·feer·ee·o′ris decks′trye) [NA]. The bronchus of the apical segment of the lower lobe of the right lung. NA alt. *bronchus segmentalis superior lobi inferioris dextri.*

bronchus segmentalis apicalis lobi inferioris si·nis·tri (si·nis′trye) [NA]. The bronchus of the apical segment of the lower lobe of the left lung. NA alt. *bronchus segmentalis superior lobi inferioris sinistri.*

bronchus segmentalis apicalis lobi su·pe·ri·o·ris dex·tri (sue·peer·ee·o′ris decks′trye) [NA]. The bronchus of the apical segment of the upper lobe of the right lung.

bronchus segmentalis api·co·pos·te·ri·or lo·bi su·pe·ri·o·ris si·nis·tri (ap″i·ko·pos·teer′ee·or lo′bye sue·peer·ee·o′ris si·nis′trye) [NA]. The bronchus of the apical posterior segment of the upper lobe of the left lung.

bronchus segmentalis ba·sa·lis an·te·ri·or lo·bi in·fe·ri·o·ris dex·tri (ba·say′lis an·teer′ee·or lo′bye in·feer·ee·o′ris decks′trye) [NA]. The bronchus of the anterior basal segment of the lower lobe of the right lung.

bronchus segmentalis basalis anterior lobi inferioris si·nis·tri (si·nis′trye) [NA]. The bronchus of the anterior basal segment of the lower lobe of the left lung.

bronchus segmentalis basalis la·te·ra·lis lo·bi in·fe·ri·o·ris dex·tri (lat·e·ray′lis lo′bye in·feer·ee·o′ris decks′trye) [NA]. The bronchus of the lateral basal segment of the lower lobe of the right lung.

bronchus segmentalis basalis lateralis lobi inferioris si·nis·tri (si·nis′trye) [NA]. The bronchus of the lower lateral segment of the lower lobe of the left lung.

bronchus segmentalis basalis me·di·a·lis lo·bi in·fe·ri·o·ris dex·tri (mee·dee·ay′lis lo′bye in·feer·ee·o′ris decks′trye) [NA]. The bronchus of the medial basal segment of the lower lobe of the right lung. NA alt. *bronchus segmentalis cardiacus lobi inferioris dextri.*

bronchus segmentalis basalis medialis lobi inferioris si·nis·tri (si·nis′trye) [NA]. The bronchus of the medial basal segment of the lower lobe of the left lung. NA alt. *bronchus segmentalis cardiacus lobi inferioris sinistri.*

bronchus segmentalis basalis posterior lo·bi in·fe·ri·o·ris dex·tri (lo′bye in·feer·ee·o′ris decks′trye) [NA]. The bronchus of the posterior basal segment of the lower lobe of the right lung.

bronchus segmentalis basalis posterior lobi inferioris si·nis·tri (si·nis′trye) [NA]. The bronchus of the posterior basal segment of the lower lobe of the left lung.

bronchus segmentalis car·di·a·cus lo·bi in·fe·ri·o·ris dex·tri kahr·dye′uh·kus lo′bye in·feer·ee·o′ris decks′trye) [NA alt.]. The bronchus of the cardiac segment of the lower lobe of the right lung (= BRONCHUS SEGMENTALIS BASALIS MEDIALIS LOBI INFERIORIS DEXTRI).

bronchus segmentalis cardiacus lobi inferioris si·nis·tri (si·nis′trye) [NA alt.]. The bronchus of the cardiac segment of the lower lobe of the left lung (= BRONCHUS SEGMENTALIS BASALIS MEDIALIS LOBI INFERIORIS SINISTRI).

bronchus segmentalis la·te·ra·lis lo·bi me·dii dex·tri (lat·e·ray′lis lo′bye mee′dee·eye decks′trye) [NA]. The bronchus of the lateral segment of the middle lobe of the right lung.

bronchus segmentalis me·di·a·lis lo·bi me·dii dex·tri (mee·dee·ay′lis lo′bye mee′dee·eye decks′trye) [NA]. The bronchus of the medial segment of the middle lobe of the right lung.

bronchus segmentalis posterior lo·bi su·pe·ri·o·ris dex·tri (lo′bye sue·peer·ee·o′ris decks′trye) [NA]. The bronchus of the posterior segment of the upper lobe of the right lung.

bronchus segmentalis sub·api·ca·lis lo·bi in·fe·ri·o·ris dex·tri (sub·ap·i·kay′lis lo′bye in·feer·ee·o′ris decks′trye) [NA]. The bronchus of the subapical segment of the lower lobe of the right lung. NA alt. *bronchus segmentalis subsuperior lobi inferioris dextri.*

bronchus segmentalis subapicalis lobi inferioris si·nis·tri (si·nis′trye) [NA]. The bronchus of the subapical segment of the lower lobe of the left lung. NA alt. *bronchus segmentalis subsuperior lobi inferioris sinistri.*

bronchus segmentalis sub·su·pe·ri·or lo·bi in·fe·ri·o·ris dex·tri (sub·sue·peer′ee·or lo′bye in·feer·ee·o′ris decks′trye) [NA alt.]. The bronchus of the subsuperior segment of the lower lobe of the right lung (= BRONCHUS SEGMENTALIS SUBAPICALIS LOBI INFERIORIS DEXTRI).

bronchus segmentalis subsuperior lobi inferioris si·nis·tri (si·nis′trye) [NA alt.]. The bronchus of the subsuperior segment of the lower lobe of the left lung (= BRONCHUS SEGMENTALIS SUBAPICALIS LOBI INFERIORIS SINISTRI).

bronchus segmentalis superior lo·bi in·fe·ri·o·ris dex·tri (lo′ bye in·feer·ee·o′ris decks′trye) [NA alt.]. The bronchus of the superior segment of the lower lobe of the right lung (= BRONCHUS SEGMENTALIS APICALIS LOBI INFERIORIS DEXTRI).

bronchus segmentalis superior lobi inferioris si·nis·tri (si·nis′ trye) [NA alt.]. The bronchus of the superior segment of the lower lobe of the left lung (= BRONCHUS SEGMENTALIS APICALIS LOBI INFERIORIS SINISTRI).

Bronkephrine. A trademark for ethylnorepinephrine, a bronchodilator.

Brøn·sted and Low·ry substance (brœn′steth, laow′ree) [J. N. *Brønsted* (*Brönsted*), Danish chemist, 1879–1947; and T. M. *Lowry*]. ACID (3).

bron·to·pho·bia (bron″to·fo′bee·uh) *n.* [Gk. *brontē*, thunder, + *-phobia*]. A morbid fear of thunder.

bronze diabetes. HEMOCHROMATOSIS.

brood capsule or **cyst.** A stalked vesicle that develops from the germinative epithelium of an echinococcus cyst. Brood capsules may detach from the mother cyst, become enlarged, and produce brood capsules and scolices within themselves to form daughter cysts.

brooding mania. A psychoneurotic disorder characterized by an impulse to prolonged and anxious meditation. See also *melancholia.*

brood membrane. The internal germinative layer of the hydatid cyst of *Echinococcus granulosus,* which on proliferation gives rise to scolices, brood capsules, or daughter cysts. Syn. *endocyst, inner germinal layer.*

Brooke's tumor or **epithelioma** [H. A. G. *Brooke,* English dermatologist, 1854–1919]. TRICHOEPITHELIOMA.

broom-tops, *n.* SCOPARIUS.

Bro·phy's operation [T. W. *Brophy,* U.S. oral surgeon, 1848–1928]. A repair of cleft palate, closed by means of wire tension sutures reinforced by lead plates.

broth, *n.* A liquid nutritive medium for the culture of microorganisms, prepared from finely chopped lean meat or dehydrated meat extract.

brow, *n.* 1. The upper anterior portion of the head; FOREHEAD. 2. SUPRAORBITAL RIDGE; EYEBROW (1).

brow ague. *Obsol.* Neuralgia of the first division of the trigeminal nerve.

brown atrophy. A form of atrophy in which the atrophic organ is of a deeper brown than normal because of an increase of pigment; observed in the heart, skeletal muscles, and liver.

Browne-McHar·dy's dilator [D. C. *Browne,* U.S. physician, b. 1898; and G. G. *McHardy,* U.S. physician, b. 1910]. An esophageal dilator.

Browne's sign. CRICHTON-BROWNE'S SIGN.

brown fat. The cytochrome-pigmented adipose tissue found in rodents, hibernating animals, and various other mammals including human embryos and newborn, consisting of multilocular fat cells; formerly thought to be glandular tissue because of its extensive vascularization and lobular organization and still widely referred to as adipose gland or hibernating gland. Contr. *white fat.*

Brown·ian motion or **movement** [R. *Brown,* Scottish botanist, 1773–1858]. The ceaseless erratic motion of very small particles suspended in a liquid or gas, caused by unequal impact of the surrounding molecules of liquid or gas on the suspended particles. Syn. *pedesis.*

brown induration. Pulmonary hemosiderosis and fibrosis resulting from chronic, passive hyperemia of the lung, usually the result of left ventricular failure or mitral stenosis.

brown mixture. COMPOUND OPIUM AND GLYCYRRHIZA MIXTURE.

Brown-Pearce tumor. A poorly differentiated transplantable carcinoma which arose in the area of a scar of a syphilitic lesion of a rabbit's scrotum.

brown recluse. A poisonous spider, *Loxosceles reclusa,* of south central United States. See also *loxoscelism.*

Brown's ataxia. SANGER BROWN'S ATAXIA.

Brown-Sé·quard's syndrome or **paralysis** (broon seʸ·kwar′, seʸ·kar′) [C. E. *Brown-Séquard,* French physiologist, 1817–1894]. Contralateral loss of pain and thermal sensation and ipsilateral affection of proprioception and corticospinal tract function; due to a lesion confined to one-half of the spinal cord.

brown snake. A venomous snake, *Pseudechis scutellatus,* of New Guinea and Australia.

Brown's sheath syndrome [H. W. *Brown,* U.S. ophthalmologist, b. 1898]. Inability to move the eye upward and inward, usually unilateral, due to congenital or acquired shortening of the anterior tendon sheath of the superior oblique muscle.

Brown's test [G. E. *Brown,* U.S. physician, 20th century]. COLD PRESSOR TEST.

brown sugar. Partially refined cane sugar.

brown-tail caterpillar rash or **dermatitis.** BROWN-TAIL RASH.

brown-tail rash. A common form of dermatitis caused by the brown-tail moth, *Euproctis chrysorrhea.*

brown tumor. A tumorlike lesion of bone, seen in patients with hyperparathyroidism, histologically resembling the giant-cell tumor of bone.

brow presentation. Presentation of the brow of the fetus at the cervix.

Bru·cel·la (broo·sel′uh) *n.* [D. *Bruce,* British physician, 1855–1931]. A genus of small, gram-negative, nonmotile, short bacilli or coccobacilli which are not acid-fast and do not form endospores; the cause of brucellosis, infectious abortion in cattle, and other animal diseases. —**brucella,** pl. **brucel·lae** (·ee) *com. n.;* **brucel·lar** (·ur) *adj.*

Brucella abor·tus (a·bor′tus). The causative agent of infectious abortion in cattle; can also affect other species including humans.

Brucella can·is (kan′is). The causative organism of infectious abortion in dogs.

Bru·cel·la·ce·ae (broo″se·lay′see·ee) *n.pl.* A large family of gram-negative rod-shaped bacteria which includes *Brucella, Pasteurella, Francisella, Hemophilus,* and *Bordetella;* pathogenic to man and animals.

Brucella mel·i·ten·sis (mel″i·ten′sis). A causative agent of brucellosis in goats, sheep, and cattle, which can be transmitted to man.

Brucella ovis (o′vis). The causative organism of chronic epididymitis in rams.

Brucella su·is (sue′is). The causative agent of infectious abortion in hogs; can also affect other species including humans.

Brucella tu·la·ren·sis (tew″luh·ren′sis). *FRANCISELLA TULARENSIS.*

brucella vaccine. A vaccine obtained from *Brucella melitensis,* used in the prevention of brucellosis in animals and possibly man.

Brucellergen. Trademark for a suspension of *Brucella* nucleoproteins used in the intradermal test for the diagnosis of brucellosis.

Brucellergen reaction. A skin reaction produced by the intradermal injection of antigen processed from *Brucella abortus.*

bru·cel·li·a·sis (broo″se·lye′uh·sis) *n.,* pl. **brucellia·ses** (·seez) [*brucella* + *-iasis*]. BRUCELLOSIS.

Brucellin. Trademark for a culture filtrate from species of *Brucella;* used in the diagnosis, prophylaxis, and treatment of brucellosis.

bru·cel·lo·sis (broo″se·lo′sis) *n.,* pl. **brucello·ses** (·seez) [*Brucella* + *-osis*]. An infectious disease due to organisms of the genus *Brucella,* transmitted to man from other species. The acute illness is characterized by fever, sweating, weakness, and aching without localizing findings; the same manifestations may persist for months or years in the chronic illness.

Bruch's membrane (broo͝kh) [K. W. L. *Bruch*, German anatomist, 1819–1884]. BASAL MEMBRANE.

bruc·ine (broo'seen, ·sin) *n.* [D. *Bruce*]. $C_{23}H_{26}N_2O_4$. A poisonous alkaloid found in various species of *Strychnos;* a white crystalline powder with a bitter taste. Has been used chiefly as a simple bitter; appears to be depressant to peripheral motor and sensory nerves.

brucine method. A test for determination of nitrates, based on the development of a yellow color by brucine in the presence of nitrates and concentrated sulfuric acid.

Brücke's line (brueck'eh) [E. W. R. von *Brücke*, Austrian physiologist, 1819–1892]. The doubly refractive dark band of a striated muscle fiber.

Brücke's muscle [E. W. R. von *Brücke*]. The meridional portion of the ciliary muscle.

Brücke's tunic or **tunica** [E. W. R. von *Brücke*]. The retinal layers deep to the rods and cones.

Bruck's disease (broo͝k) [A. *Bruck*, German physician, b. 1865]. A disease of bone characterized by multiple fractures, ankyloses, and muscle atrophy.

Bru·dzin·ski's cheek sign (broo·jyin'skee) [J. *Brudzinski*, Polish physician, 1874–1917]. A sign of meningeal irritation in which pressure on both cheeks just below the zygomatic arch causes flexion of both elbows and rapid lifting of the arms.

Brudzinski's contralateral leg signs [J. *Brudzinski*]. Signs of meningeal irritation in which (a) passive flexion of one thigh is accompanied by flexion of the opposite hip and knee; and (b) when one leg and thigh are flexed and the other extended, lowering of the flexed limb is followed by flexion of the contralateral one.

Brudzinski's neck sign [J. *Brudzinski*]. A sign of meningeal irritation in which passive flexion of the head is followed by flexion of both thighs and legs.

Brudzinski's signs [J. *Brudzinski*]. Signs of meningeal irritation, especially of meningitis. See also *Brudzinski's cheek sign, Brudzinski's contralateral leg signs, Brudzinski's neck sign, Brudzinski's symphysis sign.*

Brudzinski's symphysis sign [J. *Brudzinski*]. A sign of meningeal irritation in which pressure on the symphysis pubis is followed by flexion of both lower extremities.

Brug·ia (broo͝g'ee·uh, broo'jee·uh) *n.* [S. L. *Brug*, Dutch parasitologist, 1879–1946]. A genus of filarial nematodes.

Brugia ma·la·yi (may·lay'eye, ·ee). A species of filaria infecting man by mosquito bite, endemic in the Far East. See also *Malayan filariasis.*

Brugsch's syndrome (broo͝ksh) [K. L. T. *Brugsch*, German physician, b. 1878]. ACROPACHYDERMA.

bruis·a·bil·i·ty (brooz''uh·bil'i·tee) *n.* The readiness with which bruising occurs in response to trauma.

bruise (brooz) *n. & v.* 1. An injury producing capillary hemorrhage below an unbroken skin; contusion. 2. To inflict a bruise or bruises on a person or a part; to contuse. 3. To hurt or wound psychologically.

bruisse·ment (brwees·mahn') *n.* [F., rustling noise]. A purring sound heard on auscultation.

bruit (broo·ee') *n.* [F., noise, din]. 1. Formerly, any abnormal noise in the body heard on auscultation. 2. Specifically, a murmur or other sound related to the circulation, heard over a part, such as arteriovenous bruit, carotid bruit, cephalic bruit, systolic bruit, or thyroid bruit.

bruit d'ai·rain (dair·an') [F., brazen sound]. COIN SOUND.

bruit de ca·non (duh ka·nohn') [F.]. CANNON SOUND.

bruit de cuir neuf (duh kweer nuhf) [F., sound of new leather]. CORIACEOUS STREPITUS.

bruit de dia·ble (duh dyab'l) [F., humming top sound]. A continuous humming murmur, heard particularly over the jugular veins; a jugular venous hum.

bruit de Roger. ROGER MURMUR.

Brun·hil·de virus. POLIOMYELITIS VIRUS, type 1.

Brun·ner's glands (broo͝n'ur) [J. C. *Brunner*, Swiss anatomist, 1653–1727]. DUODENAL GLANDS.

Bruns' ataxia (broonss) [L. von *Bruns*, German neurologist, 1858–1916]. 1. Decomposition of upright stance and gait, with a tendency to fall or stagger backwards, due to bilateral lesion of frontal lobes. 2. Slowness and incoordination of limbs on one side, mimicking cerebellar ataxia, and due to a lesion of the contralateral frontal lobe.

Brun·schwig's operation [A. *Brunschwig*, U.S. surgeon, 1901–1969]. 1. DUODENOPANCREATECTOMY. 2. Complete pelvic exenteration for advanced pelvic cancer. 3. Radical hysterectomy and pelvic lymph node excision for cancer of the cervix.

Bruns' frontal lobe ataxia. BRUNS' ATAXIA.

Bruns' law or **sign** [L. von *Bruns*]. BASTIAN-BRUNS LAW.

Brun's sign (brœn) [L. *Brun*, French physician, 20th century]. HAND SIGN OF BRUN.

Bruns' syndrome [L. von *Bruns*]. Paroxysmal headache, vertigo, vomiting, and sometimes falling when the position of the head is suddenly changed; originally thought to be due to cysticercosis of the fourth ventricle, now known to be caused by other lesions of the third and fourth ventricles that intermittently obstruct the flow of spinal fluid.

Brun·ton's rule [T. L. *Brunton*, English pharmacologist, 1844–1916]. A rule to determine dosage of medicine for children; specifically, dose = child's age in years, multiplied by adult dose, divided by 25.

brush border. The free cell surface modifications, consisting of microvilli, of such cells as those of the proximal tubule of the kidney.

brush burn. FRICTION BURN.

brush electrode. A wire brush used in some electrostatic machines to apply faradic current over a large area of the body surface.

Brush·field's spots [T. *Brushfield*, English physician, 1858–1937]. Speckled white or very light yellow, clearly defined pinpoints seen on the irides of children with Down's syndrome, which disappear if later the color of the iris changes to brown; rarely seen in normal infants, but their absence may serve to rule out suspected cases of mongolism.

Brushy Creek fever. PRETIBIAL FEVER.

Bru·ton's agammaglobulinemia. CONGENITAL AGAMMAGLOBULINEMIA.

brux·ism (bruck'siz·um) *n.* [Gk. *brychein, bryx-*, to gnash the teeth]. Grinding or gnashing of the teeth; an unconscious habit often occurring in sleep, but sometimes during mental or physical concentration or strain, or in disturbed or retarded children.

bruxo·ma·nia (bruck''so·may'nee·uh) *n.* [*bruxism* + *mania*]. Bruxism as a manifestation of a psychoneurotic disorder.

Bry·ant's line [T. *Bryant*, English surgeon, 1828–1914]. The vertical line of the iliofemoral triangle.

Bryant's operation [T. *Bryant*]. Lumbar colostomy made between the last rib and the iliac crest, with permanent fixation of the bowel.

Bryant's sign [T. *Bryant*]. When the humerus is dislocated, the anterior and posterior boundaries of the axillary fossa are lowered.

Bryant's triangle [T. *Bryant*]. ILIOFEMORAL TRIANGLE.

bryg·mus (brig'mus) *n.* [Gk. *brygmos*, biting]. BRUXISM.

bry·o·nia (brigh·o'nee·uh) *n.* [L., from Gk. *bryōnia*]. The root of the bryony plant, *Bryonia alba* or *B. dioica*, which contains the glycosides bryonin and bryonidin. Has been used as an irritant emetic, drastic cathartic, and vesicant.

bry·on·i·din (brigh·on'i·din) *n.* A glycoside from the plant *Bryonia alba.*

bry·o·nin (brigh'o·nin) *n.* A glycoside from *Bryonia alba.*

bryo·phyte (brigh'o·fite) *n.* [Gk. *bryon*, moss, + *-phyte*]. A division of the plant kingdom that includes liverworts and mosses. —**bryo·phyt·ic** (brigh''o·fit'ick) *adj.*

BSP, B.S.P. Abbreviation for *Bromsulphalein,* a trademark for sulfobromophthalein sodium.

BTPS [*b*ody *t*emperature, *p*ressure, *s*aturation]. A set of standard conditions for measuring gas volume: body temperature, ambient pressure, and saturation with water vapor at that temperature and pressure.

Btu, BTU Abbreviation for *British thermal unit.*

B-type cancer cells. Cells from poorly nourished portions of tumors, which show enlargement of the nucleolar apparatus but no evidence of protein synthesis. Contr. *A-type cancer cells.*

bu·aki disease (boo·ack'ee). A deficiency disease of the Congo region of Africa, characterized by skin depigmentation, anemia, and edema.

bu·bas (boo'bahss) *n.* [Pg.]. 1. YAWS. 2. AMERICAN MUCOCUTANEOUS LEISHMANIASIS.

bubas bra·zil·i·en·sis (bra·zil"ee·en'sis). AMERICAN MUCOCUTANEOUS LEISHMANIASIS.

bu·bo (boo'bo, bew'bo) *n.* [L., from Gk. *boubōn,* groin, bubo]. Any inflammatory enlargement of lymph nodes, usually those of the groin or axilla; commonly associated with chancroid, lymphogranuloma venereum, and plague.

bu·bon·ad·e·ni·tis (bew"bon·ad"e·nigh'tis) *n.* [Gk. *boubōn,* groin, + *adenitis*]. Inflammation of an inguinal lymph node.

bu·bon·al·gia (bew"bon·al'jee·uh) *n.* [Gk. *boubōn,* groin, + *-algia*]. Pain in the inguinal region.

bu·bon·ic (bew·bon'ick) *adj.* [Gk. *boubōn,* groin, bubo, + *-ic*]. Of, pertaining to, or affected with buboes.

bubonic plague. Plague characterized by lymph-node swelling, caused by *Yersinia pestis* infection.

bu·bono·cele (bew·bon'o·seel) *n.* [Gk. *boubōnokēlē,* from *boubōn,* groin, + *kēlē,* swelling]. INCOMPLETE INGUINAL HERNIA.

bu·bon·u·lus (bew·bon'yoo·lus) *n.*, pl. **bubonu·li** (·lye) [L., small bubo]. Focal suppurative lymphangitis, especially on the dorsum of the penis.

bu·cai·nide (bew·kay'nide) *n.* 1-Hexyl-4-(*N*-isobutylbenzimidoyl)piperazine, $C_{21}H_{35}N_3$, an antiarrhythmic agent usually used as the dimaleate salt.

bu·car·dia (bew·kahr'dee·uh, boo·kahr') *n.* [Gk. *bous,* ox, + *-cardia*]. COR BOVINUM.

buc·ca (buck'uh) *n.*, pl. **buc·cae** (·ee, ·see) [NA]. CHEEK. —**buc·cal** (·ul) *adj.*

bucca ca·vi oris (kav'eye o'ris). The inner surface of the cheek.

buccal artery. The branch of the maxillary artery that supplies the buccinator muscle and the mucous membrane of the cheek. NA *arteria buccalis.*

buccal fat pad. SUCKING PAD.

buccal glands. The mixed glands of the mucous membrane of the cheek. NA *glandulae buccales.*

buccal hiatus. TRANSVERSE FACIAL CLEFT.

buccal nerve. The sensory branch of the mandibular nerve to the cheek. NA *nervus buccalis.* See also Table of Nerves in the Appendix.

buccal occlusion. Occlusion occurring when a premolar or a molar tooth is situated lateral to the line of occlusion.

buccal raphe. The scarlike vestige of the union of the parts of the cheek derived, respectively, from the maxillary and mandibular processes.

buccal torus. An inconstant slight ridge along the buccal raphe.

buc·ci·na·tor (buck'si·nay"tur) *n.* [L., trumpeter]. The muscular foundation of the cheek. NA *musculus buccinator.* See also Table of Muscles in the Appendix.

buccinator artery. BUCCAL ARTERY.

buccinator crest. An inconstant ridge running forward from the base of the coronoid process of the mandible, giving origin to fibers of the buccinator muscle.

buccinator nerve. BUCCAL NERVE.

bucco-. A combining form meaning *cheek, buccal.*

buc·co·ax·i·al (buck"o·ack'see·ul) *adj.* Pertaining to the buccal and axial walls of a dental cavity.

buc·co·cer·vi·cal (buck"o·sur'vi·kul) *adj.* [*bucco-* + *cervical*]. 1. Pertaining to the cheek and the neck. 2. Pertaining to the buccal surface and neck of a tooth.

buc·co·dis·tal (buck"o·dis'tul) *adj.* Pertaining to the buccal and distal walls of a dental cavity.

buc·co·fa·cial (buck"o·fay'shul) *adj.* [*bucco-* + *facial*]. Pertaining to the outer surface of the cheek.

buccofacial obturator. Any mechanical device for closing an opening through the cheek into the mouth.

buc·co·gin·gi·val (buck"o·jin'ji·vul, ·jin·jye'vul) *adj.* [*bucco-* + *gingival*]. Pertaining to the cheek and the gums.

buccogingival lamina. VESTIBULAR LAMINA.

buc·co·la·bi·al (buck"o·lay'bee·ul) *adj.* [*bucco-* + *labial*]. Pertaining to the cheek and the lip.

buc·co·lin·gual (buck"o·ling'gwul) *adj.* [*bucco-* + *lingual*]. Pertaining to the cheek and the tongue.

buc·co·me·si·al (buck"o·mee'zee·ul, ·mes'ee·ul) *adj.* Pertaining to the buccal and mesial walls of a dental cavity.

buc·co·na·sal (buck"o·nay'zul) *adj.* [*bucco-* + *nasal*]. Pertaining to the cheek and nose.

bucconasal membrane. *In embryology,* a thin epithelial membrane formed at the site of a primary choana by the apposition of stomodeal and olfactory epithelia. It ruptures during the seventh week.

buc·co·oc·clu·sal (buck"o·uh·kloo'zul) *adj.* Pertaining to the buccal and occlusal surfaces of a tooth.

buc·co·pha·ryn·ge·al (buck"o·fa·rin'jee·ul) *adj.* [*bucco-* + *pharyngeal*]. Pertaining to the cheek and the pharynx.

buccopharyngeal area. The part of the embryonic disk anterior to the head process and devoid of mesoderm; the anlage of the buccopharyngeal membrane.

buccopharyngeal membrane. The membrane separating stomodeum and pharynx, composed of ectoderm and endoderm. It ruptures in embryos of 2.5 mm.

buc·co·pha·ryn·ge·us (buck"o·fa·rin'jee·us) *n.* [NL.]. The portion of the superior constrictor muscle of the pharynx that arises from the pterygomandibular raphe. NA *pars buccopharyngea musculi constrictoris pharyngis superioris.*

buc·co·pulp·al (buck"o·pulp'ul) *adj.* Pertaining to the buccal and pulpal walls of a dental cavity.

buc·co·ver·sion (buck"o·vur'zhun) *n.* [*bucco-* + *version*]. The condition of a tooth being out of the line of normal occlusion in the buccal direction.

buc·cu·la (buck'yoo·luh) *n.*, pl. **buccu·lae** (·lee) [L., small cheek]. The fleshy fold beneath the chin which forms what is called a double chin.

bu·chu (bew'kew, boo'koo) *n.* [Zulu *bucu*]. The leaves of several species of *Barosma,* which contain a volatile oil. Formerly used as a diuretic.

bucked knees. *In veterinary medicine,* anterior deviation of the carpus in a horse, resulting in constant partial flexion of the knee.

Buck's extension [G. *Buck,* U.S. surgeon, 1807–1877]. Traction by means of adhesive straps applied to the skin of the lower extremity.

Buck's fascia [G. *Buck*]. The deep fascia of the penis.

Buck's operation [G. *Buck*]. Correction of bony ankylosis of the knee by removal of a wedge of bone including the patella and portions of the condyles.

buck tooth. A protruding front tooth.

Bucky diaphragm (bŏŏk'ee) [G. P. *Bucky,* German roentgenologist, 1880–1963]. A radiographic device that reduces the amount of scattered radiation reaching the film, consisting of a moving grid of thin parallel strips of lead alternating with radiolucent material arranged on the radius of curvature of a cylinder whose center is at the focal spot of the x-ray tube.

Buclamase. A trademark for a preparation of the anti-inflammatory enzyme α-amylase.

bu·cli·zine (bew'kli·zeen) *n.* 1-(*p-tert*-Butylbenzyl-4-chloro-α-phenylbenzyl)piperazine, $C_{28}H_{33}ClN_2$, an antihistaminic, antinauseant, and sedative drug; used as the dihydrochloride salt.

buc·ne·mia (buck-nee'mee-uh) *n.* [Gk. *bous*, ox, + *knēmē*, shin, + *-ia*]. Any diffuse, tense swelling of the leg, as elephantiasis or phlegmasia alba dolens.

Bucospan. A trademark for scopolamine butylbromide.

bu·cry·late (bew'kri-late) *n.* Isobutyl 2-cyanoacrylate, $C_8H_{11}NO_2$, employed in surgery as a tissue adhesive.

bud, *n.* 1. *In embryology,* a protuberance or outgrowth which is the primordium of an appendage or an organ. 2. *In anatomy,* an organ or structure shaped like the bud of a plant. 3. *In mycology,* GEMMA; a cell arising by extrusion, as in yeasts.

Budd-Chia·ri syndrome (kyah'ree) [G. *Budd,* English physician, 1808–1882; and H. *Chiari*]. Hepatic vein occlusion due to idiopathic thrombosis, tumor, or other causes, resulting in hepatosplenomegaly, jaundice, ascites, and portal hypertension.

bud·ding, *n. In biology,* a form of asexual reproduction occurring in the lower animals and plants, in which the parent organism develops projections which develop into new individuals.

Budd's cirrhosis or **jaundice** [G. *Budd*]. ACUTE YELLOW ATROPHY.

Budd's disease [G. *Budd*]. Chronic hepatomegaly without jaundice, attributed to intestinal intoxication.

Bü·ding·er-Lud·loff-Lä·wen disease (buᵉ'ding-ur, lood'loff, leʸ' vun) [K. *Büdinger,* Austrian surgeon, b. 1867; K. *Ludloff,* German orthopedic surgeon, b. 1864; and A. *Läwen,* German surgeon, b. 1876]. Pathologic fracture of the patellar cartilage.

Bueng·ner's bands (buᵉng'nur) [O. von *Buengner,* German neurologist, 1858–1905]. Syncytial tubes of proliferating Schwann cells found in the proximal segment of an injured but regenerating peripheral nerve.

Buer·ger's disease (buᵉr'gur) [L. *Buerger,* U.S. physician, 1879–1943]. Thrombosis with organization and a variable degree of associated inflammation in the arteries and veins of the extremities, occasionally of the viscera, progressing to fibrosis about these structures and associated nerves, and complicated by ischemic changes in the parts supplied; a disease of young and middle-aged tobacco-smoking males. Syn. *thromboangiitis obliterans.*

Buer·gi's hypothesis (buᵉr'ghee) [E. *Buergi,* Swiss pharmacologist, b. 1872]. Drugs possessing identical pharmacologic action summate their therapeutic effects when administered simultaneously; potentiation occurs only if the two agents have different pharmacologic activity.

bu·fa·gin (bew'fuh-jin) *n.* Any one of several cardioactive steroid genins present in the skin secretions of toads, as bufotalin and bufotoxin.

bu·fa·lin (bew'fuh-lin) *n.* A cardioactive steroid aglycone, closely related to bufotalin, present in the skin secretions of toads.

buf·fa·lo hump. A deposition of adipose tissue in the interscapular area of patients with Cushing's syndrome, due to hypercortisolism.

buffalo obesity. The obesity usually seen in Cushing's syndrome, confined chiefly to the trunk, face, and neck.

buf·fer, *n.* & *v.* 1. A substance which, when present in a solution or added to it, resists change of hydrogen-ion concentration when either acid or alkali is added. 2. To treat with a buffer.

buffer action. The action exhibited by certain chemical substances which, when added to a fluid, tend to maintain its reaction (pH) within narrow limits even when acid or base is added in not excessive amounts.

buffer capacity. The ability of a buffer to resist changes in pH upon the addition of acid or base, defined as the amount, in gram-equivalents per liter, of strong acid or base required to change the pH of the buffer by one pH unit.

buffer salt. The salt of a weak acid and strong base, or of a strong acid and a weak base which, in solution, tends to resist a change in reaction upon addition of acid or alkali, respectively.

buffer solution. A solution prepared from a weak acid and a salt of the weak acid, or a weak base and a salt of the weak base, which resists any appreciable change in pH on the addition of small amounts of acid or alkali or by dilution with water.

buffy coat. The layer of white cells and platelets which forms between the erythrocytes and plasma when fluid blood is centrifuged.

Bu·fo (bew'fo) *n.* [L.]. A genus of toads, the secretions of certain species of which have physiologic or diagnostic importance. —**bufo,** *com. n.*

bufo reaction. A biologic pregnancy test: when urine containing chorionic gonadotropic hormone from a pregnant woman is injected into a male toad, spermatozoa migrate from the testes to the urinary bladder and can be demonstrated in the toad's urine.

bu·for·min (bew-for'min) *n.* 1-Butylbiguanide, $C_6H_{15}N_5$, an orally effective hypoglycemic agent.

bu·fo·tal·in (bew''fo-tal'in) *n.* [*bufo* + digi*talin*]. A cardioactive steroid aglycone, $C_{26}H_{36}O_6$, present in the skin secretions of toads.

bu·fo·ten·i·dine (bew''fo-ten'i-deen) *n.* The betaine form of bufotenin; a component of the secretion of the skin glands of the toad *Bufo vulgaris.*

bu·fo·ten·in, bu·fo·ten·ine (bew''fo-ten'in, -een) *n.* 5-Hydroxy-*N,N*-dimethyltryptamine, $C_{12}H_{16}N_2O$, a component of the secretion of the skin glands of the toad *Bufo vulgaris.* It causes hypertension and strong and lasting vasoconstriction.

bufo·tox·in (bew''fo-tock'sin) *n.* [*bufo* + *toxin*]. A suberylarginine ester of bufotalin, $C_{40}H_{60}N_4O_{10}$; the principal toxin present in the skin secretions of toads and lizards.

bug, *n.* 1. An insect of the order Hemiptera or suborder Heteroptera. 2. Loosely, any insect or other small arthropod.

bug·gery (bug'ur-ee) *n.* [F. *bougre,* from ML. *Bulgarus,* Bulgar, heretic, sodomite]. SODOMY.

Buie's operation [L. A. *Buie,* U.S. surgeon, b. 1890]. Hemorrhoidectomy under caudal anesthesia with the patient in a prone position.

Buist's method (byoost) [R. C. *Buist,* Scottish obstetrician, 1860–1939]. Artificial respiration for asphyxia neonatorum, by alternately turning the infant from stomach to back.

bulb, *n.* [L. *bulbus,* onion, from Gk. *bolbos,* bulbous plant]. 1. An oval or circular expansion of a cylinder or tube. 2. MEDULLA OBLONGATA.

bul·bar (bul'bur, bul'bahr) *adj.* 1. Of or pertaining to a bulb, or a bulb-shaped structure or part. 2. Pertaining to or involving the medulla oblongata. 3. Of or pertaining to the eyeball.

bulbar anesthesia. Loss of sensation due to a lesion in the medulla oblongata, or pons.

bulbar apoplexy. A cerebrovascular accident involving the substance of the medulla oblongata or pons, causing a variety of neurologic disturbances depending upon the extent of the lesion, and including paralysis of one or both sides of the body, inability to swallow, talk, move the tongue or lips, and dyspnea.

bulbar ataxia. Incoordination due to a disturbance of cerebellar pathways by a lesion in the pons or medulla oblongata.

bulbar conjunctiva. The mucous membrane covering the anterior third of the eyeball, from the junction with the eyelids to the margin of the cornea. NA *tunica conjunctiva bulbi.*

bulbar paralysis. 1. A clinical syndrome due to involvement of the nuclei of the last four or five cranial nerves, characterized principally by paralysis or weakness of the muscles which control swallowing, talking, movement of the tongue and lips, and sometimes respiratory paralysis. 2. PROGRESSIVE BULBAR PARALYSIS.

bulbar plexus. A nerve plexus found in the embryo surrounding the bulb of the heart.

bulbar poliomyelitis. PARALYTIC BULBAR POLIOMYELITIS.

bulbar septum. AORTICOPULMONARY SEPTUM.

bulbar speech. The thick slurred speech occurring when the nuclei of the medulla concerned with speech are damaged or when there is injury to both corticobulbar tracts.

bulbar swelling. One of the endocardial ridges of the embryonic bulb of the heart.

bulbar tractotomy. MEDULLARY TRACTOTOMY.

bulbi. Plural and genitive singular of *bulbus.*

bulbo-. A combining form meaning *bulb, bulbar.*

bul·bo·atri·al (bul″bo·ay′tree·ul) *adj.* Pertaining to the bulb of the heart and atrium of the heart.

bulboatrial crest. A ridge on the internal surface of the embryonic heart corresponding to the external bulboatrial groove. See also *bulboventricular crest.*

bul·bo·cap·nine (bul″bo·kap′neen, ·nin) *n.* An alkaloid, $C_{19}H_{19}NO_4$, in the tubers of the plants *Bulbocapnus cavus.* The phosphate and the hydrochloride have been used in certain diseases of the nervous system, as parkinsonism, chorea, and ataxic conditions.

bul·bo·cav·er·no·sus (bul″bo·kav·ur·no′sus) *n.*, pl. **bulbocav·erno·si** (·sigh) [*bulbo-* + L. *cavernosus,* hollow]. BULBOSPONGIOSUS.

bulbocavernosus reflex. PENILE REFLEX.

bulb of the corpus cavernosum urethrae. BULB OF THE PENIS.

bulb of the eye. EYEBALL.

bulb of the heart. The anterior division of the embryonic heart within the pericardial cavity. Its proximal part is incorporated into the right ventricle; its distal part forms the aortic and pulmonary valve region of the heart. NA *bulbus aortae.*

bulb of the penis. The expanded proximal portion of the corpus spongiosum of the penis. NA *bulbus penis.*

bulb of the posterior horn. An eminence on the superior part of the medial wall of the posterior horn of the lateral ventricle, overlying the occipital part of the occipital radiation of the corpus callosum. NA *bulbus cornus posterioris.*

bulb of the urethra. The portion of the male urethra surrounded by the bulb of the penis.

bulb of the vestibule. Either one of the paired masses of erectile tissue located on either side of the vestibule of the vagina, homologous to the bulb of the penis. NA *bulbus vestibuli vaginae.*

bul·bo·mem·bra·nous (bul″bo·mem′bruh·nus) *adj.* Pertaining to the bulbar and membranous portion of the urethra.

bul·bo·nu·cle·ar (bul″bo·new′klee·ur) *adj.* [*bulbo-* + *nuclear*]. Pertaining to the medulla oblongata and its nerve nuclei.

bul·bo·spi·nal (bul″bo·spye′nul) *adj.* [*bulbo-* + *spinal*]. Pertaining to the medulla oblongata and the spinal cord.

bulbospinal poliomyelitis. PARALYTIC BULBAR POLIOMYELITIS and PARALYTIC SPINAL POLIOMYELITIS.

bul·bo·spon·gi·o·sus (bul″bo·spon″jee·o′sus) *n.*, pl. & genit. sing. **bulbospongio·si** (·sigh) [*bulbo-* + L. *spongiosus,* spongy]. A muscle encircling the bulb and adjacent, proximal parts of the penis in the male and encircling the orifice of the vagina and covering the lateral parts of the vestibular bulbs in the female. Syn. *bulbocavernosus.* NA *musculus bulbospongiosus.* See also Table of Muscles in the Appendix.

bulbospongiosus reflex. PENILE REFLEX.

bul·bo·ure·thral (bul″bo·yoo·ree′thrul) *adj.* Pertaining to the bulb of the penis and the urethra.

bulbourethral gland. Either of the compound tubular glands situated in the urogenital diaphragm, anterior to the prostate gland. NA *glandula bulbourethralis.* See also Plate 25.

bulbourethral septum. A partial median fibrous septum of the urethral bulb.

bul·bous (bul′bus) *adj.* Having or containing bulbs; bulb-shaped; swollen; terminating in a bulb.

bul·bo·ven·tric·u·lar (bul″bo·ven·trick′yoo·lur) *adj.* Pertaining to the bulb of the heart and the ventricle of the heart.

bulboventricular crest. A ridge on the internal surface of the embryonic ventricles corresponding to the external bulboventricular sulcus. It later becomes the bulboatrial crest.

bulboventricular fold. A transverse fold between the bulb of the heart and ventricle, which disappears when the proximal part of the bulb is incorporated into the right ventricle.

bulboventricular loop. The U-shaped or S-shaped loop of the embryonic heart involving chiefly the bulb of the heart and ventricle.

bulboventricular sulcus. The groove formed by the loop of the embryonic cardiac tube in the pericardial cavity.

bulb suture. A technique employed where, after resection, the nerve cannot be sutured without undue tension. The neighboring joint is flexed and the untrimmed nerve ends are laid side by side, with as much overlap as possible, and united by strong sutures; the wound is closed, and gradual extension is then effected with elongation of the nerve. This may be followed by secondary suture.

bul·bus (bul′bus) *n.*, pl. & genit. sing. **bul·bi** (·bye) [L., onion]. BULB.

bulbus aor·tae (ay·or′tee) [NA]. BULB OF THE HEART.

bulbus ar·te·ri·o·sus (ahr·teer·ee·o′sus). BULB OF THE HEART.

bulbus cor·dis (kor′dis). BULB OF THE HEART.

bulbus cor·nu pos·te·ri·o·ris (kor′new pos·teer·ee·o′ris) [BNA]. Bulbus cornus posterioris (= BULB OF THE POSTERIOR HORN).

bulbus cor·nus pos·te·ri·o·ris (kor′nus pos·teer·ee·o′ris) [NA]. BULB OF THE POSTERIOR HORN.

bulbus oc·u·li (ock′yoo·lye) [NA]. EYEBALL.

bulbus ol·fac·to·ri·us (ol·fack·to′ree·us) [NA]. OLFACTORY BULB.

bulbus penis [NA]. BULB OF THE PENIS.

bulbus pi·li (pye′lye) [NA]. The bulb of a hair; the expanded proximal end of the root of a hair.

bulbus ure·thrae (yoo·ree′three) [BNA]. BULB OF THE URETHRA.

bulbus ve·nae ju·gu·la·ris in·fe·ri·or (vee′nee jug·yoo·lair′is in·feer′ee·or) [NA]. INFERIOR BULB OF THE INTERNAL JUGULAR VEIN.

bulbus venae jugularis superior [NA]. SUPERIOR BULB OF THE INTERNAL JUGULAR VEIN.

bulbus ve·sti·bu·li va·gi·nae (ves·tib′yoo·lye va·jye′nee) [NA]. BULB OF THE VESTIBULE.

bu·le·sis (bew·lee′sis) *n.* [Gk. *boulēsis,* will]. The will, or an act of the will.

bu·lim·a·rex·ia (bew·lim″uh·reck′see·uh) *n.* [*bulimia* + Gk. *arexis,* prevention, counteracting, + *-ia*]. A neurotic disorder characterized by alternate gorging and self-emptying by vomiting, fasting, or self-induced diarrhea. Most frequently seen in young affluent women and thought to be associated with low self-esteem and fear of failure and rejection. Differs from anorexia nervosa in the regularity and frequency of eating binges. —**bulimarex·ic** (·sick) *adj.*

bu·lim·ia (bew·lim′ee·uh, boo·) *n.* [Gk. *boulimia,* from *bous,* ox, + *limos,* hunger]. An insatiable appetite and excessive food intake; seen in psychotic states and in the Kleine-Levin syndrome and with bilateral ablation of the temporal lobes.

bu·lim·ic (bew·lim′ick) *adj.* Pertaining to or affected with bulimia.

Bu·li·nus (bew·lye′nus) *n.* A genus of freshwater snails, whose species serve as the intermediate hosts for *Schistosoma haematobium.*

bul·la (bŏŏl′uh, bul′uh) *n.*, pl. **bul·lae** (·ee) [L.]. 1. A large bleb or blister either within or beneath the epidermis and filled with lymph or serum. 2. *In anatomy*, a rounded, thin-walled bony prominence.

bulla eth·moi·da·lis ca·vi na·si (eth·moy·day'lis kay'vye nay'zye) [NA]. A rounded prominence in the lateral wall of the middle nasal meatus, overlying large ethmoid air cells.

bulla ethmoidalis os·sis eth·moi·da·lis (os'is eth·moy·day'lis) [NA]. A rounded prominence of the ethmoid labyrinth, enclosing large middle ethmoid air cells.

bul·late (bo͝ol'ate, bul'ate) *adj.* 1. Blistered; marked by bullae. 2. Inflated, bladderlike, vesiculate. —**bul·la·tion** (bo͝ol·ay'shun, bul·) *n.*

bulla tym·pa·ni (tim'puh·nigh). TYMPANIC BULLA.

bulla tym·pan·i·ca (tim·pan'i·kuh). TYMPANIC BULLA.

bulldog forceps. A short spring forceps used to occlude or compress a blood vessel temporarily.

bul·lec·to·my (bul·eck'tuh·mee) *n.* [*bulla* + *-ectomy*]. Excision of a bulla, especially bullae of the lungs.

bullet forceps. An instrument for extracting bullets.

bullet lens. SPHEROPHAKIA.

Bul·lis fever [after Camp *Bullis*, Texas]. A mild, tick-borne, presumably rickettsial disease characterized by lymphadenopathy, leukopenia, and rash.

bull·neck diphtheria. *Obsol.* Severe nasopharyngeal diphtheric infection with swelling of the submandibular areas and anterior neck due to cervical lymph node enlargement.

bul·lous (bo͝ol'us, bul') *adj.* Pertaining to or characterized by bullae.

bullous dermatosis. A condition of the skin marked by bullae, as in erythema multiforme, dermatitis herpetiformis, and pemphigus vulgaris.

bullous emphysema. An obstructive type of pulmonary emphysema, characterized by replacement of normal lung tissue by large, air-containing, cystlike structures.

bullous fever. The fever that accompanies pemphigus.

bullous impetigo. A type of impetigo caused by *Staphylococcus aureus* and characterized by bullae, seen usually in children. The lesions develop particularly in the axillae, groins, intergluteal areas, and in the creases of fat.

bullous keratitis. KERATITIS BULLOSA.

bullous pemphigoid. A chronic skin disease characterized by large bullae occurring over a wide area and having a tendency to heal without scarring; may represent an autoimmune disease.

Buminate. A trademark for salt-poor normal human serum albumin.

Bum·ke's anxiety pupil (bo͞om'keh) [O. C. E. *Bumke*, German neurologist, 1877–1950]. A transient state of mydriasis, with impaired pupillary responses to light and accommodation, observed in anxious and psychoneurotic individuals who have no other ocular or cerebral abnormalities.

bumper fracture. A fracture of the leg from collision with the bumper of an automobile; usually associated with a common peroneal nerve injury.

BUN Abbreviation for *blood urea nitrogen.*

bu·nam·i·dine (bew·nam'i·deen) *n.* *N,N*-Dibutyl-4-(hexyloxy)-1-naphthamidine, $C_{25}H_{38}N_2O$, an anthelmintic; used as the hydrochloride salt.

bu·nam·io·dyl sodium (bew''nam·eye'o·dil). Sodium 3-(3-butyrylamino-2,4,6-triiodophenyl)-2-ethylacrylate, $C_{15}H_{15}I_3NaO_3$, formerly used as a roentgenographic contrast medium.

bun·dle, *n. In biology,* a fascicular grouping of elementary tissues, as nerve fibers or muscle fibers. See also *fasciculus.*

bundle bone. Bone traversed by coarse collagenous fibers (Sharpey's perforating fibers), as where tendons or ligaments are affixed.

bundle branch block. Delay or block of conduction through either of the branches of the bundle of His, causing one ventricle to be activated and contract before the other.

bundle H1 of Forel. THALAMIC FASCICULUS.

bundle of His [W. *His*, Jr., German physiologist, 1863–1934]. ATRIOVENTRICULAR BUNDLE.

bundle of Kent [A. F. S. *Kent*, English physiologist, 1863–1958]. A bridge of muscular tissue joining the atria and ventricles at the right margin of the septum. It is considered an anomalous or aberrant atrioventricular bundle which, in some cases, may conduct impulses.

α-bun·ga·ro·tox·in (bung''guh·ro·tock'sin) *n.* [*Bungarus* + *toxin*]. A neurotoxin from snake venom which blocks neuromuscular transmission by binding to acetylcholine receptors on motor end plates; used experimentally to identify and label acetylcholine receptors.

Bun·ga·rus (bung'guh·rus, bung·gahr'us) *n.* [Telegu *baṅgāru*, golden]. A genus of venomous snakes found in southern Asia, commonly known as the kraits.

Bungarus can·di·dus (kan'di·dus). The common or Indian krait; especially dangerous because of its extremely virulent venom.

bung-eye, *n.* An eye disease of Australian aborigines, probably habronemic ophthalmomyiasis.

Büngner's bands. BUENGNER'S BANDS.

bun·ion (bun'yun) *n.* A swelling of a bursa of the foot, especially of the metatarsophalangeal joint of the great toe; associated with a thickening of the adjacent skin and a forcing of the great toe into adduction (hallux valgus).

bun·ion·ec·to·my (bun''yun·eck'tuh·mee) *n.* [*bunion* + *-ectomy*]. Excision of a bunion; plastic repair of the first metatarsophalangeal joint.

bun·ion·ette (bun''yun·et') *n.* Enlargement of the metatarsophalangeal joint of the little toe in a fashion resembling a small bunion.

Bun·nell's test. PAUL-BUNNELL TEST.

bu·no·dont (bew'no·dont) *adj.* [Gk. *bounos*, mound, hill, + *-odont*]. Provided with rounded or conical cusps, applied to molar teeth. Contr. *lophodont.*

bu·no·lol (bew'nuh·lol) *n.* (±)-5-[3-(*tert*-Butylamino)-2-hydroxypropoxy]-3,4-dihydro-1(2*H*)-naphthalenone, $C_{17}H_{25}NO_3$, an antiadrenergic agent (β-receptor), usually employed as the hydrochloride salt.

Bun·sen absorption coefficient (bo͞on'zun) [R. W. E. von *Bunsen*, German chemist, 1811–1899]. A quantitative expression of gas solubility; the ratio of the volume which would be occupied by the dissolved gas at standard conditions to the volume of the solvent under the experimental conditions.

Bunsen-Roscoe law. LAW OF BUNSEN-ROSCOE.

Bunsen solubility coefficient [R. W. E. von *Bunsen*]. The volume of a gas, measured at 0°C and one atmosphere of pressure, dissolved by a unit volume of liquid when the liquid is equilibrated with the gas under one atmosphere of pressure at a specified temperature.

Bu·nyam·ve·ra (boo''nyam·veer'uh). BUNYAMWERA.

Bu·nya·mwe·ra group (boo''nya·mwehr'uh). A group of immunologically related arboviruses which are transmitted by mosquitoes; may cause headache, fever, and myalgia in man.

Bunyamwera supergroup. A family of immunologically related genera of arboviruses which includes the Bunyamwera group, C group, and California group.

Bunyamwera virus. A virus isolated from *Aëdes* mosquitoes in Uganda and pathogenic for various animals including man.

buph·thal·mia (bewf·thal'mee·uh) *n.* [NL., from Gk. *bouphthalmos*, ox-eye, a kind of fish (from *bous*, ox, + *ophthalmos*, eye)]. Progressive enlargement of the infant cornea and eye due to increased intraocular pressure from congenital or secondary glaucoma. —**buphthal·mic,** *adj.*

buph·thal·mos, buph·thal·mus (bewf·thal'mus) *n.* BUPHTHALMIA.

bu·pic·o·mide (bew·pick'uh·mide) *n.* 5-Butylpicolinamide, $C_{10}H_{14}N_2O_3$, an antihypertensive agent.

bu·piv·a·caine (bew·piv'uh·kayn) *n.* 1-Butyl-2',6'-pipecoloxylidide, $C_{18}H_{28}N_2O$, a long-acting local anesthetic of the amide type; an analog of mepivacaine.

bu·pro·pi·on (bew·pro'pee·on) *n.* (±)-2-(*tert*-Butylamino)-3'-chloropropiophenone, $C_{13}H_{18}ClNO$, an antidepressant substance usually employed as the hydrochloride salt.

bu·quin·o·late (bew·kwin'o·late) *n.* 4-Hydroxy-6,7-bis-(2-methylpropoxy)-3-quinolinecarboxylic acid, ethyl ester, $C_{20}H_{27}NO_5$, employed as a coccidiostat for poultry.

bur, burr, *n.* 1. *In botany,* a rough, prickly shell or case. 2. EAR LOBE. 3. A rotary cutting instrument in any one of various shapes and having numerous fine cutting blades; used in the dental handpiece in the preparation of teeth for restoration. 4. *In surgery,* an instrument similar in form to a dental bur, but larger, designed for surgical operations upon the bones. See also *burr cell.*

bu·ra·mate (bew'ruh·mate) *n.* 2-Hydroxyethyl benzylcarbamate, $C_{10}H_{13}NO_3$, an anticonvulsant and tranquilizer.

bur·bot (bur'but) *n.* [MF. *bourbotte,* from OF. *bourbe,* mud]. A freshwater fish of the genus *Lota,* allied to the cod, which serves as the intermediate host of the tapeworm *Diphyllobothrium latum* in North America.

burbot liver oil. The oil, containing vitamins A and D, extracted from the liver of the burbot, *Lota maculosa.*

Burchard's test. LIEBERMANN-BURCHARD TEST.

Bur·dach's nucleus (boor'dakh) [K. F. *Burdach,* German anatomist and physiologist, 1776–1847]. CUNEATE NUCLEUS.

Bur·dwan fever (bur·dwahn') [after *Burdwan,* India]. KALA AZAR.

bu·ret, bu·rette (bew·ret') *n.* [F.]. A graduated glass tube, commonly having a stopcock, used in volumetric analysis for measuring volumes of liquids.

Bür·ger-Grütz disease (buer'gur, gruets). FAMILIAL FAT-INDUCED HYPERLIPEMIA.

Bur·gun·dy pitch [F. *poix de Bourgogne*]. The resinous exudation from the stem of *Picea abies;* formerly used, in plaster form, as a rubefacient.

bur·ied suture. A suture completely covered by, and not involving, the skin.

bu·rim·a·mide (bew·rim'uh·mide) *n.* 1-(4-Imidazol-4-ylbutyl)-3-methyl-2-thiourea, $C_9H_{16}N_4S$, an experimental H_2-receptor blocking agent.

Bur·kitt's lymphoma or **tumor** [D. P. *Burkitt,* Uganda physician, 20th century]. A malignant lymphoma usually occurring in children, typically involving the retroperitoneal area and the mandible, but sparing the peripheral lymph nodes, bone marrow, and spleen.

Bur·ma boil. Oriental sore; a lesion of cutaneous leishmaniasis.

burn, *v.* & *n.* 1. To oxidize or be oxidized by fire or equivalent means. 2. To cause, or to be the locus of, a sensation of heat. 3. The tissue reaction or injury resulting from application of heat, extreme cold, caustics, radiation, friction, or electricity; classified as simple hyperemic (first degree), vesicant (second degree), destructive of skin and underlying tissues (third degree).

Bur·nett's syndrome [C. H. *Burnett,* U.S. physician, b. 1901]. MILK-ALKALI SYNDROME.

burning feet syndrome. The sensation of burning and other paresthesias and dysesthesias of the feet and, rarely, of the hands; observed in the aged and in alcoholic and diabetic neuropathy, and in other neuropathies of obscure etiology.

burning tongue. GLOSSODYNIA.

bur·nish·er, *n.* An instrument for condensing and smoothing and polishing the surface of a dental filling or inlay.

burn·out, *n.* The elimination of an invested wax pattern from a mold by means of dry heat preparatory to a casting procedure.

burnt alum. EXSICCATED ALUM.

Bu·row's solution (boo'ro) [K. A. *Burow,* German surgeon, 1809–1874]. ALUMINUM ACETATE SOLUTION; used topically as an astringent.

burr. BUR.

burr cell. A poikilocyte, having one or more spiny projections along its periphery, found in the blood of patients with uremia, as a rare congenital anomaly, in chronic liver disease, and sometimes in other states. See also *acanthocyte.*

bur·row, *n.* A cuniculus, passage, gallery, or tunnel in the skin that houses a metazoal parasite, particularly the mite that causes scabies.

bur·sa (bur'suh) *n.,* L.pl. & genit. sing. **bur·sae** (·see) [ML., bag, purse, from Gk. *byrsa,* wineskin, hide]. 1. A small sac lined with synovial membrane and filled with fluid interposed between parts that move upon each other. NA *bursa synovialis.* See also Plate 2. 2. A diverticulum of the abdominal cavity.

bursa an·se·ri·na (an"sur·eye'nuh) [NA]. ANSERINE BURSA.

bursa bi·ci·pi·to·gas·tro·cne·mi·a·lis (bye·sip"i·to·gas"tro·k'nee·mee·ay'lis) [BNA]. GASTROCNEMIUS BURSA.

bursa bi·ci·pi·to·ra·di·a·lis (bye·sip"i·to·ray·dee·ay'lis) [NA]. BICIPITORADIAL BURSA.

bursa cu·bi·ta·lis in·ter·os·sea (kew·bi·tay'lis in·tur·os'ee·uh) [NA]. The interosseus cubital bursa; a synovial bursa between the tendon of the biceps brachii muscle and the ulna and neighboring muscles.

bursae sub·ten·di·ne·ae mus·cu·li sar·to·rii (sub·ten·din'ee·ee mus'kew·lye sahr·to'ree·eye) [NA]. The subtendinous bursas of the sartorius muscle; the synovial bursas between the tendon of the sartorius muscle and the tendons of the semitendinosus and gracilis muscles, and usually communicating with the anserine bursa.

bursae tro·chan·te·ri·cae mus·cu·li glu·tei me·dii (tro·kan·terr'i·see mus'kew·lye gloo'tee·eye mee'dee·eye) [NA]. The trochanteric bursas of the gluteus medius muscle. See *trochanteric bursa.*

bursa ili·a·ca sub·ten·di·nea (i·lye'uh·kuh sub·ten·din'ee·uh) [BNA]. Bursa subtendinea iliaca (= ILIAC SUBTENDINOUS BURSA).

bursa ilio·pec·ti·nea (il"ee·o·peck·tin'ee·uh) [NA]. ILIOPECTINEAL BURSA.

bursa in·fra·hy·oi·dea (in·fruh·high·oy'dee·uh) [NA]. SUBHYOID BURSA.

bursa in·fra·pa·tel·la·ris pro·fun·da (in"fruh·pat·e·lair'is pro·fun'duh) [NA]. INFRAPATELLAR BURSA.

bursa is·chi·a·di·ca mus·cu·li glu·tei max·i·mi (is"kee·ad'i·kuh mus'kew·lye gloo'tee·eye mack'si·migh) [NA]. The ischial bursa of the gluteus maximus muscle. See *ischial bursa.*

bursa ischiadica musculi ob·tu·ra·to·rii in·ter·ni (ob·tew·ruh·to'ree·eye in·tur'nigh) [NA]. The ischial bursa of the obturator internus muscle. See *ischial bursa.*

bursa mu·co·sa (mew·ko'suh) [BNA]. Bursa synovialis (= BURSA (1)).

bursa mucosa sub·cu·ta·nea (sub·kew·tay'nee·uh) [BNA]. BURSA SYNOVIALIS SUBCUTANEA.

bursa mucosa sub·fas·ci·a·lis (sub·fash"ee·ay'lis) [BNA]. BURSA SYNOVIALIS SUBFASCIALIS.

bursa mucosa sub·mus·cu·la·ris (sub·mus"kew·lair'is) [BNA]. BURSA SYNOVIALIS SUBMUSCULARIS.

bursa mucosa sub·ten·di·nea (sub·ten·din'ee·uh) [BNA]. BURSA SYNOVIALIS SUBTENDINEA.

bursa mus·cu·li co·ra·co·bra·chi·a·lis (mus'kew·lye kor"uh·ko·bray·kee·ay'lis) [NA]. A synovial bursa between the tendon of the coracobrachialis muscle, the subscapularis muscle, and the coracoid process.

bursa musculi gas·tro·cne·mii la·te·ra·lis (gas"tro·k'nee'mee·eye lat·e·ray'lis) [BNA]. BURSA SUBTENDINEA MUSCULI GASTROCNEMII LATERALIS.

bursa musculi gastrocnemii me·di·a·lis (mee·dee·ay'lis) [BNA]. BURSA SUBTENDINEA MUSCULI GASTROCNEMII MEDIALIS.

bursa musculi la·tis·si·mi dor·si (la·tis'i·migh dor'sigh) [BNA]. BURSA SUBTENDINEA MUSCULI LATISSIMI DORSI.

bursa musculi ob·tu·ra·to·rii in·ter·ni (ob"tew·ruh·to'ree·eye in·tur'nigh) [BNA]. BURSA ISCHIADICA MUSCULI OBTURATORII INTERNI.

bursa musculi pop·li·tei (pop·lit'ee·eye) [BNA]. RECESSUS SUBPOPLITEUS.

bursa musculi sar·to·rii pro·pria (sahr·to'ree·eye pro'pree·uh) [BNA]. Any of the bursae subtendineae musculi sartorii.

bursa musculi se·mi·mem·bra·no·si (sem"i·mem·bruh·no'sigh) [NA]. A large double synovial bursa. One part lies between the semimembranosus muscle, the medial head of the gastrocnemius muscle, and the knee joint and usually communicates with the cavity of the knee joint. The other part lies between the semimembranosus muscle and the medial condyle of the tibia.

bursa musculi ster·no·hy·oi·dei (stur"no·high·oy'dee·eye) [BNA]. Bursa infrahyoidea (= SUBHYOID BURSA).

bursa musculi sub·sca·pu·la·ris (sub·skap"yoo·lair'is) [BNA]. Bursa subtendinea musculi subscapularis (= SUBSCAPULAR BURSA).

bursa of Fa·bri·ci·us (fah·bree'see·us) [J. C. *Fabricius*, Danish entomologist, 19th century]. A cloacal lymphoepithelial organ in birds which receives hematopoietic stem cells from the bone marrow and induces their differentiation to B lymphocytes.

bursa of the omentum. OMENTAL BURSA.

bursa omen·ta·lis (o·men·tay'lis) [NA]. OMENTAL BURSA.

bursa ova·ri·ca. (o·vair'i·kuh) [BNA]. OVARIAN BURSA.

bursa pha·ryn·gea (fa·rin'jee·uh) [NA]. PHARYNGEAL BURSA.

bursa prae·pa·tel·la·ris sub·cu·ta·nea (pree·pat·e·lair'is sub·kew·tay'nee·uh) [BNA]. Bursa subcutanea prepatellaris (= SUBCUTANEOUS PREPATELLAR BURSA).

bursa praepatellaris sub·fas·ci·a·lis (sub·fash·ee·ay'lis) [BNA]. Bursa subfascialis prepatellaris (= SUBFASCIAL PREPATELLAR BURSA).

bursa praepatellaris sub·ten·di·nea (sub·ten·din'ee·uh) [BNA]. Bursa subtendinea prepatellaris (= SUBTENDINOUS PREPATELLAR BURSA).

bursa sub·acro·mi·a·lis (sub"a·kro"mee·ay'lis) [NA]. SUBACROMIAL BURSA.

bursa sub·cu·ta·nea acro·mi·a·lis (sub"kew·tay'nee·uh a·kro"mee·ay'lis) [NA]. A synovial bursa in the subcutaneous tissue overlying the acromion.

bursa subcutanea ole·cra·ni (o"le·kray'nigh) [NA]. OLECRANON BURSA.

bursa subcutanea pre·pa·tel·la·ris (pree·pat·e·lair'is) [NA]. SUBCUTANEOUS PREPATELLAR BURSA.

bursa subcutanea tro·chan·te·ri·ca (tro·kan·terr'i·kuh) [NA]. A synovial bursa in the subcutaneous tissue overlying the greater trochanter of the femur.

bursa sub·del·toi·dea (sub"del·toy'dee·uh) [NA]. SUBDELTOID BURSA.

bursa sub·fas·ci·a·lis pre·pa·tel·la·ris (sub·fash·ee·ay'lis pree·pat·e·lair'is) [NA]. SUBFASCIAL PREPATELLAR BURSA.

bursa sub·ten·di·nea ili·a·ca (sub·ten·din'ee·uh i·lye'uh·kuh) [NA]. ILIAC SUBTENDINOUS BURSA.

bursa subtendinea mus·cu·li gas·tro·cne·mii la·te·ra·lis (mus'kew·lye gas"tro·k'nee'mee·eye lat·e·ray'lis) [NA]. The lateral gastrocnemius bursa. See *gastrocnemius bursa.*

bursa subtendinea musculi gastrocnemii me·di·a·lis (mee·dee·ay'lis) [NA]. The medial gastrocnemius bursa. See *gastrocnemius bursa.*

bursa subtendinea musculi la·tis·si·mi dor·si (la·tis'i·migh dor'sigh) [NA]. A synovial bursa between the tendons of the latissimus dorsi and the teres major muscles.

bursa subtendinea musculi ob·tu·ra·to·rii in·ter·ni (ob"tew·ruh·to'ree·eye in·tur'nigh) [NA]. A narrow, elongated bursa between the tendon of the obturator internus muscle and the capsule of the hip joint, occasionally communicating with the ischial bursa of the obturator internus.

bursa subtendinea musculi sub·sca·pu·la·ris (sub·skap·yoo·lair'is) [NA]. SUBSCAPULAR BURSA.

bursa subtendinea pre·pa·tel·la·ris (pree·pat·e·lair'is) [NA]. SUBTENDINOUS PREPATELLAR BURSA.

bursa sy·no·vi·a·lis (si·no·vee·ay'lis) [NA]. A synovial bursa; BURSA (1).

bursa synovialis sub·cu·ta·nea (sub·kew·tay'nee·uh) [NA]. Any synovial bursa located in subcutaneous tissue, usually over a prominence of bone. Each may be given a specific name from the underlying structure, as olecranon or prepatellar bursa. Some are constant, but many are inconstant, and some are rarely seen.

bursa synovialis sub·fas·ci·a·lis (sub·fash·ee·ay'lis) [NA]. Any synovial bursa situated between a band of deep fascia and an underlying structure, as the subfascial prepatellar bursa.

bursa synovialis sub·mus·cu·la·ris (sub·mus·kew·lair'is) [NA]. Any synovial bursa situated between a muscle and some underlying structure. Each may be given a specific name from the overlying muscle, as the subdeltoid bursa. There is considerable variation in the presence, size, and extent of such bursas.

bursa synovialis sub·ten·di·nea (sub·ten·din'ee·uh) [NA]. Any synovial bursa situated between a tendon and an underlying prominence usually of bone. Each may be given a specific name from the overlying muscle tendon, as the anserine bursa, beneath the pes anserinus, or the gastrocnemius bursas.

bursa ten·di·nis Achil·lis (ten'di·nis a·kil'is) [NA alt.]. ACHILLES BURSA. NA alt. *bursa tendinis calcanei.*

bursa tendinis cal·ca·nei (kal·kay'nee·eye) [NA]. ACHILLES BURSA. NA alt. *bursa tendinis Achillis.*

bursa tro·chan·te·ri·ca mus·cu·li glu·taei me·dii anterior (tro·kan·terr'i·kuh mus'kew·lye gloo'tee·eye mee'dee·eye) [BNA]. A small bursa separating the tendon of the gluteus medius muscle from the lateral surface of the greater trochanter; one of the trochanteric bursas of the gluteus medius. See also *trochanteric bursa.*

bursa trochanterica musculi glu·tei ma·xi·mi (gloo'tee·eye mack'si·migh) [NA]. The trochanteric bursa of the gluteus maximus muscle. See *trochanteric bursa.*

bursa trochanterica musculi glutei mi·ni·mi (min'i·migh) [NA]. The trochanteric bursa of the gluteus minimus muscle. See *trochanteric bursa.*

bur·sec·to·my (bur·seck'tuh·mee) *n.* [*bursa* + *-ectomy*]. Surgical removal of a bursa.

Bur·ser·a·ce·ae (bur"sur·ay'see·ee) *n.pl.* [*Bursera,* type genus]. A family of aromatic resinous trees and shrubs.

bur·si·tis (bur·sigh'tis) *n.* Inflammation of a bursa.

bur·so·lith (bur'so·lith) *n.* [*bursa* + *-lith*]. A calculus formed within a bursa.

Bu·ru·li ulcer (buh·roo'lee) [after *Buruli* County, along the Nile in Uganda]. A rapidly spreading skin ulcer due to *Mycobacterium ulcerans.*

Bury's disease [J. S. *Bury,* English physician, 1852–1944]. ERYTHEMA ELEVATUM DIUTINUM.

Busch·ke's disease or **scleredema** (bŏŏsh'ke^h) [A. *Buschke,* German dermatologist, 1868–1943]. SCLEREDEMA ADULTORUM.

bush·mas·ter, *n. Lachesis mutua,* a pit viper found in South America and southern Central America. It may attain a length of 11 or 12 feet and produces a powerful hemotoxic venom.

bu·spi·rone (bew·spye'rone) *n.* *N*-[{4-[4-(2-Pyrimidinyl)-1-piperazinyl]butyl}]-1,1-cyclopentanediacetimide, $C_{21}H_{31}N_5O_2$, a tranquilizer usually used as the hydrochloride salt.

Bus·quet's disease (bu^{e}ss·ke^h') [P. *Busquet,* French physician, b. 1866]. Periostitis resulting in dorsal metatarsal exostoses.

Bus·se-Busch·ke's disease (bŏŏs'e^h, bŏŏsh'ke^h) [D. *Busse,*

German physician, 1867–1922; and A. *Buschke*]. CRYPTOCOCCOSIS.

bu·sul·fan (bew·sul'fan) *n.* 1,4-Butanediol dimethanesulfonate, $C_6H_{14}O_6S_2$, a neoplastic suppressant used in the treatment of chronic granulocytic leukemia.

but-, buto-. A combining form meaning *a substance or compound containing a group of four carbon atoms.*

bu·ta·bar·bi·tal (bew"tuh·bahr'bi·tol, ·tal) *n.* 5-Ethyl-5-*sec*-butylbarbituric acid, $C_{10}H_{16}N_2O_3$, a sedative and hypnotic of intermediate duration of action; used as the sodium derivative.

bu·ta·caine (bew'tuh·kane) *n.* 3-Di-*n*-butylaminopropyl-*p*-aminobenzoate, $C_{18}H_{30}N_2O_2$, a local anesthetic used as the sulfate salt.

bu·tac·e·tin (bew·tas'e·tin) *n.* 4'-*tert*-Butoxyacetanilide, $C_{12}H_{17}NO_2$, an analgesic and antidepressant drug.

bu·ta·cla·mol (bew·tuh·klay'mole) *n.* (±)-3α-*tert*-Butyl-2,3,-4,4aβ,8,9,13bα,14-octahydro-1*H*-benzo[6,7]cyclohepta[1,2,3-de]pyrido[2,1-*a*]isoquinolin-3-ol, $C_{25}H_{31}NO$, a tranquilizer normally employed as the hydrochloride salt.

bu·ta·di·ene (bew"tuh·dye'een) *n.* 1,3-Butadiene, $CH_2{=}CHCH{=}CH_2$, a gaseous hydrocarbon derived from petroleum and used in the manufacture of synthetic rubber and many other substances.

bu·tal·bi·tal (bew·tal'bi·tol, ·tal) *n.* 5-Allyl-5-isobutylbarbituric acid, $C_{11}H_{16}N_2O_3$, a sedative and hypnotic with intermediate duration of action. Syn. *allylbarbituric acid, allylisobutylbarbituric acid.*

bu·tam·ben (bew·tam'ben) *n.* BUTYL *p*-AMINOBENZOATE.

bu·ta·mi·rate (bew·tuh·migh'rate) *n.* 2-[2-(Diethylamino)-ethoxy]ethyl 2-phenylbutyrate, $C_{18}H_{29}NO_3$, an antitussive agent usually used as the citrate salt.

bu·tane (bew'tane) *n.* [*but-* + *-ane*]. The hydrocarbon $CH_3CH_2CH_2CH_3$, a colorless flammable gas occurring in natural gas and in solution in crude petroleum.

bu·ta·no·ic acid (bew"tuh·no'ick). BUTYRIC ACID.

bu·ta·nol (bew'tuh·nol) *n.* BUTYL ALCOHOL.

bu·ta·per·a·zine (bew"tuh·perr'uh·zeen) *n.* 1-[10-[3-(4-Methyl-1-piperazinyl)propyl]phenothiazin-2-yl]-1-butanone, $C_{24}H_{31}N_3OS$, a tranquilizer usually employed as the maleate salt.

Butaphyllamine. Trademark for ambuphylline, a diuretic and smooth muscle relaxant drug.

Butazolidin. Trademark for phenylbutazone, a drug with anti-inflammatory, analgesic, and antipyretic properties.

Butch·er's saw [R. G. H. *Butcher*, Irish surgeon, 1819–1891]. A saw in which the blade can be fixed at any angle.

bu·tene (bew'teen) *n.* [*but-* + *-ene*]. A four-carbon aliphatic hydrocarbon containing one double bond; two isomers are known: 1-butene or α-butylene, $CH_3CH_2CH{=}CH_2$; 2-butene, or β-butylene, $CH_3CH{=}CHCH_3$. Both are gases occurring in oil or coal gas.

bu·ten·yl (bew'te·nil) *n.* [*butene-* + *-yl*]. The unsaturated radical C_4H_7, of which there are three isomeric forms: 1-butenyl is $CH_3CH_2CH{=}CH{-}$; 2-butenyl is $CH_3CH{=}CHCH_2{-}$; 3-butenyl is $CH_2{=}CHCH_2CH_2{-}$.

Butesin. A trademark for butyl *p*-aminobenzoate, a local anesthetic.

bu·te·thal (bew'te·thal) *n.* 5-*n*-Butyl-5-ethylbarbituric acid, $C_{10}H_{16}N_2O_3$, a sedative and hypnotic of intermediate duration of action.

bu·teth·amine (bew·teth'uh·meen) *n.* 2-Isobutylaminoethyl *p*-aminobenzoate, $C_{13}H_{20}N_2O_2$, a local anesthetic; used as the formate and hydrochloride salts.

Butethanol. A trademark for tetracaine, a local anesthetic.

bu·thi·a·zide (bew·thigh'uh·zide) *n.* 6-Chloro-3,4-dihydro-3-isobutyl-2*H*-1,2,4-benzothiadiazine-7-sulfonamide 1,1-dioxide, $C_{11}H_{16}ClN_3O_4S_2$, a diuretic and antihypertensive drug.

Bu·thus (bewth'us) *n.* A genus of scorpions of the Mediterranean area and Manchuria.

Buthus co·ci·ta·nus (ko"si·tay'nus). A poisonous scorpion found in North Africa; its bite is occasionally fatal.

Buthus ita·li·cus (i·tal'i·kus). A poisonous black scorpion found in northern Africa and southern Europe.

Buthus mar·ten·si (mahr·ten'sigh). A poisonous scorpion of Manchuria.

bu·tir·o·sin (bew·tirr'o·sin) *n.* An antibacterial mixture of streptamine glycosides obtained from *Bacillus circulans*, usually used as the sulfate dihydrate, $C_{21}H_{41}N_5O_{12}\cdot 2H_2SO_4\cdot 2H_2O$.

Butisol. A trademark for butabarbital, a sedative and hypnotic used as the sodium derivative.

But·ler and Tut·hill's method (Weinbach's modification). A test for sodium in which it is precipitated from a blood filtrate as uranyl zinc sodium acetate which is titrated with sodium hydroxide.

But·ler's solution. A hypotonic solution of the electrolytes of plasma, containing 30 mEq per liter sodium, 25 mEq per liter chloride, 20 mEq per liter potassium, 20 mEq per liter lactate, and 5 mEq per liter phosphorus.

Butoben. A trademark for butyl *p*-hydroxybenzoate, a preservative.

bu·to·nate (bew'tuh·nate) *n.* O,O-Dimethyl(2,2,2-trichloro)-1-(butyryloxyethyl)phosphonate, $C_8H_{14}Cl_3O_5P$, an anthelmintic agent.

bu·to·py·ro·nox·yl (bew"to·pye"ro·nock'sil) *n.* Butyl mesityl oxide, $C_{12}H_{18}O_4$, a yellowish liquid, insoluble in water; used as an insect repellent and toxicant.

bu·tor·pha·nol (bew·tor'fuh·nole) *n.* (−)-17-(Cyclobutylmethyl)morphinan-3,14-diol, $C_{21}H_{29}NO_2$, an analgesic, antitussive agent.

bu·tox·a·mine (bew·tock'suh·meen) *n.* α-[1-(*tert*-Butylamino)ethyl]-2,5-dimethoxybenzyl alcohol, $C_{15}H_{25}NO_3$, a compound with hypoglycemic and hypolipemic activities; used as the hydrochloride salt.

bu·trip·ty·line (bew·trip'ti·leen) *n.* (±)-10,11-Dihydro-*N,N*,β-trimethyl-5*H*-dibenzo[*a,d*]cycloheptene-5-propylamine, $C_{21}H_{27}N$, an antidepressant drug; used as the hydrochloride salt.

butt, *v.* 1. *In prosthodontics,* to place directly against the tissues covering the alveolar ridge. 2. To bring any two square-ended surfaces into contact.

but·ter, *n.* [L. *butyrum*, from Gk. *boutyron*, from *bous*, cow, + *tyros*, cheese]. 1. The fatty part of milk, obtained by rupturing the fat globules by churning or mechanical agitation. 2. Various vegetable fats having the consistency of butter. 3. Certain anhydrous chlorides having the appearance or consistency of butter.

but·ter·fly, *n.* 1. An adhesive dressing used to hold wound edges together in place of a suture. 2. A piece of paper so arranged over the air passages of an anesthetized patient that it will indicate whether or not he is breathing. 3. A type of intravenous needle with wings.

butterfly rash. Any skin lesion across the nose and the malar eminences, as in systemic lupus erythematosus, dermatomyositis, tuberous sclerosis, or seborrheic dermatitis.

butterfly vertebra. A congenital biconcave appearance of a vertebral body in the AP view due to lack of or incomplete fusion of the left and right halves. Syn. *cleft vertebra.*

but·ter·milk, *n.* The milk that remains after churning butter.

but·ter·nut bark. JUGLANS.

butter yellow. *p*-Dimethylaminoazobenzene, $C_6H_5N{=}NC_6H_4N(CH_3)_2$, a yellow crystalline powder; used to color fats and in the preparation of Töpfer's reagent.

but·tock (but'uck) *n.* One of the two fleshy parts of the body posterior to the hip joints.

but·ton, *n.* [MF. *bouton*]. The residual mass of metal in a dental casting procedure.

but·ton·hole, *n.* *In surgery,* a small, straight opening into an organ or part.

buttonhole deformity or **dislocation.** A protrusion or partial protrusion of the joint of a finger through a defect in the extensor aponeurosis. Syn. *boutonniere deformity.*

buttonhole fracture. PUNCTURE FRACTURE.

buttonhole incision. A small, straight cut made into an organ or cavity.

buttonhole method of cardiac massage. An open-chest method previously used for resuscitation after the heart has stopped beating.

button suture. A mattress suture that includes a button on either side of the wound to prevent cutting of the skin by the suture.

but·tress, *n.* 1. A support or prop. 2. A thickening of the sole of a horse's hoof between the frog and the posterior end of the bar.

bu·tyl (bew'til) *n.* [*but-* + *-yl*]. The univalent hydrocarbon radical, C_4H_9. It occurs as normal butyl, $CH_3CH_2CH_2CH_2$—, abbreviated *n*-butyl; iso-butyl, $(CH_3)_2CHCH_2$—, abbreviated *i*-butyl; secondary butyl, $CH_3CH_2(CH_3)CH$—, abbreviated *sec*-butyl; and tertiary butyl, $(CH_3)_3C$, abbreviated *tert*-butyl.

butyl alcohol. Normal butyl alcohol, $CH_3CH_2CH_2CH_2OH$; used as a solvent, as a denaturant for ethyl alcohol, and in synthesis. Syn. *butanol.*

butyl *p*-aminobenzoate. Normal butyl *p*-aminobenzoate, $NH_2C_6H_4COOC_4H_9$. A crystalline powder, almost insoluble in water; used as a local anesthetic. Syn. *butamben.*

bu·tyl·at·ed (bew'ti·lay·tid) *adj.* Characterizing a compound to which the butyl group has been attached, usually by replacement of a hydrogen atom.

butylated hy·droxy·an·is·ole (high·drock"see·an'i·sole). *tert*-Butyl-4-methoxyphenol, $C_{11}H_{16}O_2$, used as an antioxidant in cosmetics and pharmaceuticals which contain oils or fats. Abbreviated, BHA.

butylated hy·droxy·tol·u·ene (high·drock"see·tol'yoo·een). 2,6-Di-*tert*-butyl-*p*-cresol, $C_{15}H_{24}O$, used as an antioxidant in cosmetics and pharmaceuticals which contain oils or fats. Abbreviated, BHT.

bu·tyl·ene (bew'til·een) *n.* BUTENE.

butyl *p*-hydroxybenzoate. $HOC_6H_4COOC_4H_9$. A white, crystalline powder, very slightly soluble in water; used as preservative of medicinals and foods.

bu·tyl·i·dene (bew·til'i·deen) *n.* The divalent radical $CH_3(CH_2)_2CH$=.

Butyn. A trademark for butacaine, a local anesthetic; used as the sulfate salt.

butyr-, butyro-. A combining form meaning *butyric.*

bu·tyr·a·ceous (bew"ti·ray'shus) *adj.* Resembling butter; containing or yielding butterlike substances.

bu·tyr·ate (bew'ti·rate) *n.* [*butyr-* + *-ate*]. A salt or an ester of butyric acid.

bu·tyr·ic (bew·tirr'ick) *adj.* [L. *butyrum*, butter, + *-ic*]. Pertaining to, or derived from, butter.

butyric acid. Butanoic acid, $CH_3CH_2CH_2COOH$, a viscid liquid having a rancid smell. It occurs in butter as a glyceride and is found also in various plant and animal tissues.

butyric fermentation. Fermentation resulting in the conversion of sugars, starches, and milk into butyric acid.

bu·tyr·in (bew'ti·rin) *n.* [*butyr-* + *-in*]. Glyceryl tributyrate, $(C_3H_7COO)_3C_3H_5$, a constituent of butterfat. Syn. *tributyrin.*

bu·tyr·in·ase (bew'ti·ri·nace) *n.* An enzyme that hydrolyzes butyrin, found in the blood serum.

butyro-. See *butyr-.*

bu·tyro·cho·lin·es·ter·ase (bew"ti·ro·ko"li·nes'tur·ace, ·aze) *n.* PSEUDOCHOLINESTERASE.

bu·tyr·oid (bew"ti·roid) *adj.* [*butyr-* + *-oid*]. Buttery; having the consistency of butter.

bu·tyr·yl (bew'ti·ril) *n.* [*butyr-* + *-yl*]. The radical $CH_3CH_2CH_2CO$— of butyric acid.

bux·ine (buck'seen, ·sin) *n.* [L. *buxus*, box-tree, + *-ine*]. An alkaloid, $C_{19}H_{21}NO_3$, from the leaves of the boxwood, *Buxus sempervirens.*

buzz, *n.* A term used in sports medicine to describe ringing in the ears following a blow on the head.

Buz·zard's reflex [J. *Buzzard*, English neurologist, 1831–1919]. 1. The knee jerk, reinforced by voluntary pressing of the toes against the floor at the time the patellar tendon is struck. 2. RIDDOCH'S MASS REFLEX.

B virus. *HERPESVIRUS SIMIAE.*

Bwam·ba fever. A mild febrile disease due to an arbovirus, probably mosquito-borne, occurring in Uganda and characterized by headache, generalized pains, and conjunctivitis.

Bwamba virus. An arbovirus isolated from cases of fever in Uganda.

By·ers-Ban·ker disease (bigh'urz, bank'ur) [R. K. *Byers*, U.S. pediatrician, b. 1896, and B. Q. *Banker*, U.S. neuropathologist, b. 1922]. A heredofamilial form of progressive spinal muscular atrophy which becomes clinically manifest in late infancy or early childhood and progresses more slowly than infantile spinal muscular atrophy, permitting survival into adolescence or even adulthood; probably inherited as an autosomal recessive trait. See also *progressive spinal muscular atrophy.*

By·ler disease [*Byler*, an Amish kindred]. An autosomal recessive disease characterized clinically by foul-smelling stools, repeated episodes of jaundice, hepatosplenomegaly, small stature, and death during the first decade; the basic defect is intrahepatic cholestasis.

by·pass, *n.* A surgically created detour between two points in a physiologic pathway, as in the vascular or gastrointestinal systems, often to circumvent obstruction or to place the circumvented portion at rest. Compare *shunt.*

bys·si·no·sis (bis"i·no'sis) *n.*, pl. **byssino·ses** (·seez) [Gk. *byssinos*, flaxen, linen, + *-osis*]. A pneumoconiosis due to inhalation of high concentrations of the dust of cotton, linen, or other plant fibers used industrially; wheezing and dyspnea are most prominent when the patient returns to work on Monday after a Sunday holiday. The essentially irreversible chronic stage, occurring most frequently in long-time textile workers, is characterized by severe airway obstruction and impaired elastic recoil due to chronic bronchitis and emphysema. Syn. *Monday morning fever.*

bys·soid, (bis'oid) *adj.* [Gk. *byssos*, flax, linen, + *-oid*]. Cottonlike, made up of delicate threads.

bys·so·phthi·sis (bis"o·thigh'sis, ·tis'is) *n.* [Gk. *byssos*, flax, linen, + *phthisis*]. BYSSINOSIS.

By·wa·ters' syndrome [E. G. L. *Bywaters*, British physician, b. 1910]. 1. ACUTE TUBULAR NECROSIS. 2. CRUSH SYNDROME.

C

C *In chemistry,* a symbol for carbon. *In molecular biology,* a symbol for cytosine.

C Abbreviation for (a) *complement;* (b) formerly, *curie.*

C. Abbreviation for (a) *cuspid* or *canine* of the second dentition; (b) *Celsius, centigrade;* (c) *closure;* (d) *contraction;* (e) *cylinder, cylindrical lens.*

C., c. Abbreviation for (a) *calorie;* (b) *cathode;* (c) *centigrade;* (d) *centimeter;* (e) *congius;* (f) *hundredweight.*

C′ Symbol for complement.

c. Abbreviation for (a) *cum,* with; (b) *centum,* one hundred; (c) *cuspid* or *canine* of the primary dentition.

CA Abbreviation for *chronological age.*

Ca 1. Symbol for calcium. 2. Abbreviation for *cancer.*

ca. Abbreviation for *cathode.*

cab·bage, *n.* [*CABG*]. Coronary artery bypass graft, a surgical procedure for blockage of a coronary artery.

cabbage goiter. A goiter produced experimentally by the feeding of cabbage to rabbits and other animals.

CABG (kab′ij). Acronym for coronary artery bypass graft, a surgical procedure for blockage of a coronary artery.

cab·i·net bath. A hot-air or steam bath in which all but the patient's head is enclosed within a box heated by electric elements.

ca·ble graft. *In neurosurgery,* the placing together of several sections of nerve to be transplanted, to bridge a gap in a nerve larger than the sections available for the grafting.

Cab·ot splint [A. T. *Cabot,* U.S. surgeon, 1852–1912]. A posterior wire splint with a footpiece at a right angle, designed for the treatment of fractures of the leg where traction is not required.

Cabot's rings [R. C. *Cabot,* U.S. physician, 1868–1939]. RING BODIES.

cac-, caco- [Gk. *kakos,* bad]. A combining form meaning *bad, diseased, defective, deformed, vitiated.*

ca·cao (ka·kay′o, ka·kah′o) *n.* [Sp., from Nahuatl *cacahuatl,* cacao beans]. Seeds from *Theobroma cacao* from which cacao butter, chocolate, and cocoa are prepared.

cacao butter. THEOBROMA OIL.

-cace [Gk. *kakē,* badness]. A combining form meaning *a bad, diseased, deformed, or vitiated condition.*

cac·er·ga·sia (kack″ur·gay′zhuh, ·zee·uh, kas″ur·) *n.* [*cac-* + *ergasia*]. *Obsol.* Defective mental or physical function.

cac·es·the·sia, cac·aes·the·sia (kack″es·theezh′uh, ·theez′ee·uh) *n.* [*cac-* + *esthesia*]. Any disagreeable sensation. **—caces·the·sic, cacaes·the·sic** (·theez′ick) *adj.*

ca·chec·tic (ka·keck′tick) *adj.* Pertaining to or characterized by cachexia.

cachectic aphthae. Ulcerous lesions appearing beneath the tongue, along the inner cheeks and palates; seen in debilitated, severely undernourished individuals, particularly children, with poor oral hygiene. Syn. *Riga's aphthae.* Compare *Bednar's aphthae.*

cachectic infantilism. Infantilism, or dwarfism, due to chronic malnutrition, infection, or emotional deprivation.

ca·chet (ka·shay′, kash′ay) *n.* [F., from *cacher,* to hide]. Two circles of wafer (rice paper) sealed together and enclosing medication; the resulting dosage form may be swallowed after moistening with water.

ca·chex·ia (ka·keck′see·uh) *n.* [Gk. *kachexia,* bad condition]. Severe generalized weakness, malnutrition, and emaciation. Adj. *cachectic.*

cachexia ex·oph·thal·mi·ca (eck″sof·thal′mi·kuh). Cachexia associated with thyrotoxicosis.

cachexia hy·po·phys·i·o·pri·va (high″po·fiz″ee·o·prye′vuh). 1. Cachexia associated with hypopituitarism. 2. SIMMONDS' DISEASE.

cachexia stru·mi·pri·va (stroo″mi·prye′vuh). POSTOPERATIVE MYXEDEMA.

cachexia thy·ro·pri·va (thigh″ro·prye′vuh). POSTOPERATIVE MYXEDEMA.

cach·in·na·tion (kack″i·nay′shun) *n.* [L. *cachinnare,* to laugh loudly]. Immoderate laughter, as in hysteria or certain psychoses.

ca·chou (kah·shoo′) *n.* [F., from Pg. *cachu*]. An aromatic pill or tablet for deodorizing the breath.

caco-. See *cac-.*

caco·de·mo·nia (kack″o·de·mo′nee·uh) *n.* [Gk. *kakodaimonia,* from *kakodaimon,* evil spirit]. A psychotic, usually schizophrenic, disorder in which the patient believes he is possessed by or of an evil spirit.

caco·de·mo·no·ma·nia (kack″o·dee″muh·no·may′nee·uh, ·de·mo″no·) *n.* CACODEMONIA.

cac·o·dyl (kack′o·dil) *n.* 1. The organic arsenical radical As—. 2. Tetramethyldiarsenic, $(CH_3)_2As{=}As(CH_3)_2$, a liquid with an extremely offensive odor.

cac·o·dyl·ate (kack″o·dil′ate) *n.* A salt of cacodylic acid. The sodium, calcium, and iron salts have been used in medicine.

cac·o·dyl·ic acid (kack″o·dil′ick). DIMETHYLARSINIC ACID.

cac·o·geu·sia (kack″o·gyoo′see·uh, ·joo′see·uh) *n.* [*caco-* + *-geusia*]. A bad taste not due to food, drugs, or other matter; frequently a part of the aura in psychomotor epilepsy.

cac·o·pho·nia (kack″o·fo′nee·uh) *n.* CACOPHONY.

ca·coph·o·ny (ka·kof′uh·nee) *n.* [Gk. *kakophōnia*]. An abnormally harsh or discordant voice or sound. **—caco·phon·ic** (kack·o·fon′ick) *adj.*

ca·cos·mia (ka·koz′mee·uh) *n.* [Gk. *kakosmia,* bad smell, from *osmē,* smell]. Unpleasant, imaginary odors, particularly putrefactive odors; commonly reported as the aura in uncinate epilepsy.

cac·ti·no·my·cin (kack″ti·no·migh′sin) *n.* A mixture of antibiotics, now rarely used, produced by *Streptomyces chrysomallus,* that consists mainly of actinomycin C_2 and actinomycin C_3 with some dactinomycin, and that has antineoplastic activity. Syn. *actinomycin C.*

ca·dav·er (kuh·dav′ur) *n.* [L., from *cadere,* to fall]. A dead body, especially that of a human being; a corpse. —**cadaver·ic** (·ick) *adj.*

cadaveric lividity. LIVOR MORTIS.

cadaveric reaction. *In electromyography,* the total loss of electrical response in the affected muscles, as in the acute stage of periodic paralysis.

cadaveric rigidity. RIGOR MORTIS.

cadaveric spasm. Early or, at times, immediate appearance of rigor mortis; seen after death from certain causes. The muscle spasm actually causes movements of the limbs.

ca·dav·er·ine (ka·dav′ur·een, ·in) *n.* [*cadaver* + *-ine*]. Pentamethylenediamine, $NH_2(CH_2)_5NH_2$, a ptomaine formed by the action of the *Vibrio comma* on protein.

ca·dav·er·ous (kuh·dav′ur·us) *adj.* Resembling a cadaver; of a deathly pallor.

cad·dy stools (kad′ee). Feces that resemble fine, dark, sandy mud; seen with yellow fever.

cade oil (kade). JUNIPER TAR.

cad·mi·um (kad′mee·um) *n.* [NL., from Gk. *kadmeia,* calamine]. Cd = 112.40. A bluish-white metal used as a constituent of alloys and in electroplating.

cadmium sulfide. CdS. A light-yellow or orange powder, insoluble in water; used as a shampoo for treatment of seborrheic dermatitis and as a pigment.

ca·du·ca (ka·dew′kuh) *n.* [L. *caducus,* fallen, falling, from *cadere,* to fall]. DECIDUA.

ca·du·ce·us (ka·dew′see·us) *n.* [L., herald's staff]. 1. The symbol or insignia of medicine, consisting of the staff of Asclepius about which a single serpent is coiled. 2. In the Medical Corps of the United States Army, a symbol consisting of a staff with two formal wings at the top and two serpents entwined about the remainder.

ca·du·cous (ka·dew′kus) *adj.* [L. *caducus,* fallen, falling]. *In botany,* characterizing floral parts that drop off very early or easily, as compared with persistent ones.

caec-, caeco-. CEC-, CECO-.

caeca. CECA.

caecal. CECAL.

caecectomy. CECECTOMY.

cae·ci·tas (see′si·tas) *n.* [L.]. Blindness.

caecitis. CECITIS.

caecocele. CECOCELE.

caecocolic. CECOCOLIC.

caecocolostomy. CECOCOLOSTOMY.

caecoileostomy. CECOILEOSTOMY.

caecopexy. CECOPEXY.

caecoplication. CECOPLICATION.

caecoptosis. CECOPTOSIS.

caecorrhaphy. CECORRHAPHY.

caecosigmoidostomy. CECOSIGMOIDOSTOMY.

caecostomy. CECOSTOMY.

caecotomy. CECOTOMY.

caecum. CECUM.

caecum cu·pu·la·re (kew″pew·lair′ee) [BNA]. Cecum cupulare (= CUPULAR CECUM).

caecum ve·sti·bu·la·re (ves·tib″yoo·lair′ee) [BNA]. Cecum vestibulare (= VESTIBULAR CECUM).

caenogenesis. CENOGENESIS.

caeruloplasmin. CERULOPLASMIN.

Caes·al·pin·ia (sez″al·pin′ee·uh, ses″al·) *n.* [A. *Cesalpino,* Italian botanist and physician, 1519–1603]. A genus of tropical trees of the family Leguminosae. Several species have been used medicinally.

caesarean. CESAREAN.

ca·fard (ka·fahr′, kaf′ahrd) *n.* [F., low spirits, the "blues"]. A subacute depressive illness characterized by attacks of severe depression and irritability.

café au lait spots (ka·fay′o lay′) [F., coffee with milk]. Light brown patches of the skin, seen especially in neurofibromatosis and in polyostotic fibrous dysplasia.

Cafergot. Trademark for a mixture of caffeine and ergotamine used in treatment of migraine.

caf·fe·ic acid (ka·fee′ick). 3,4-Dihydroxycinnamic acid, $C_9H_8O_4$, occurring in conjugated form in coffee and other plants.

caf·feine (kaf′ee·in, ka·feen′) *n.* [Ger. *Kaffein,* from *Kaffe,* coffee]. An alkaloid, $C_8H_{10}N_4O_2$, chemically 1,3,7-trimethylxanthine, found in the leaves and beans of the coffee tree, in tea, and in guarana, the roasted pulp of the fruit of *Paullinia sorbilis,* or prepared synthetically. Occurs as long needles, slightly soluble in cold water. It is a cerebral, circulatory, and renal stimulant. See also *coffee.*

caffeine and sodium benzoate. A mixture of approximately equal parts of caffeine and sodium benzoate. It is a form of caffeine especially suited for subcutaneous injection.

caffeine-withdrawal headache. A vascular headache due to cranial artery dilatation resulting from abrupt caffeine withdrawal after prolonged excessive administration; the headache is generalized, throbbing, often accompanied by nausea, rhinorrhea, and lethargy, and may be terminated by caffeine or amphetamines.

caf·fein·ism (kaf′een·iz·um) *n.* A toxic condition due to the excessive ingestion of coffee or other caffeine-containing substances.

Caf·fey's disease or **syndrome** [J. *Caffey,* U.S. pediatrician, b. 1895]. INFANTILE CORTICAL HYPEROSTOSIS.

caged-ball prosthesis. An artificial cardiac valve consisting of a plastic or metal ball within a cage formed of metal struts.

caged-lens prosthesis. A prosthetic cardiac valve consisting of a freely floating lens-shaped disk in the valve cage.

ca·hin·ca (ka·hink′uh) *n.* [Tupi]. The dried roots of *Chiococca alba,* and other species of *Chiococca,* a genus of shrubs of tropical America. It has been used as a diuretic, purgative, tonic, and emetic.

ca·in·ca (ka·ink′uh) *n.* CAHINCA.

-caine [Ger. Kokain]. A combining form designating *a local anesthetic compound or substance.*

cai·no·pho·bia (kigh″no·fo′bee·uh, kay″no·) *n.* [Gk. *kainos,* new, + *phobia*]. NEOPHOBIA.

cais·son disease (kay′sun). DECOMPRESSION SICKNESS.

Ca·jal's cell (ka·khal′) [S. Ramón y *Cajal,* Spanish neurologist, 1852–1934]. ASTROCYTE.

Cajal's gold-sublimate method [S. Ramón y *Cajal*]. A method for staining astrocytes in which sections are impregnated with gold sublimate.

Cajal's interstitial nucleus [S. Ramón y *Cajal*]. The nucleus of the medial longitudinal fasciculus.

Cajal's silver methods [S. Ramón y *Cajal*]. Methods based upon silver impregnations reduced by a photographic developer such as hydroquinone. There are many variations; some have a high selectivity for certain cells of the nervous system, others for various types of nerve fibers.

caj·e·put oil, caj·u·put oil (kaj′uh·put). The volatile oil distilled from leaves and twigs of species of *Melaleuca;* contains 50 to 65% of eucalyptol. Has been used as a stimulating expectorant, anthelmintic, and externally as a rubefacient and antiparasitic.

caj·e·put·ol, caj·u·put·ol (kaj′uh·puh·tol″) *n.* EUCALYPTOL.

caked, *adj.* Compressed, tense, or hardened, due to engorgement or induration.

caked bag. In cows, inflammation of an udder.

caked breast. PUERPERAL MASTITIS.

caked kidney. CAKE KIDNEY.

cake kidney. A form of crossed renal ectopia in which there is congenital fusion of both kidneys into a solid, irregularly lobate mass. The ureter of the displaced kidney crosses the midline before draining distally. Syn. *clump kidney, lump kidney.*

Cal Abbreviation for *Calorie* (= KILOCALORIE).

cal Abbreviation for *calorie.*

Cal·a·bar bean (kal'uh·bahr) [after *Calabar,* Nigeria]. The poisonous seed of a leguminous vine, *Physostigma venenosum,* of Africa. See also *physostigmine.*

Calabar swellings [after *Calabar,* Nigeria]. Edematous, painful, subcutaneous swellings occurring in different parts of the body of natives of Calabar and other parts of West Africa, probably due to an allergic reaction to *Loa loa* infection.

cal·a·mine (kal'uh·mine, ·min) *n.* [ML. *calamina,* from L. *cadmia,* from Gk. *kadmeia*]. 1. Native zinc carbonate. 2. Prepared calamine: zinc oxide with a small amount of ferric oxide; a pink powder, insoluble in water, used as a local application in the treatment of skin diseases. It is also used to impart a "flesh color" to ointments, washes, and powders.

cal·a·mus (kal'uh·mus) *n.* [L., a reed]. The rhizome of the plant, *Acorus calamus,* that contains a volatile oil and a bitter principle. The root is aromatic, stomachic, and tonic, and has been used as an ingredient of many popular bitters.

calamus scrip·to·ri·us (skrip·to'ree·us) [BNA]. The inferior part of the rhomboid fossa; so named because it is shaped like a penpoint.

calc-, calci-, calco- [L. *calx, calcis,* lime]. A combining form meaning (a) *calcium;* (b) *calcium salts.*

calcaemia. CALCEMIA.

calcane-, calcaneo-. A combining form meaning *calcaneus, calcaneal.*

cal·ca·ne·al (kal·kay'nee·ul) *adj.* Pertaining to the heel or to the calcaneus.

calcaneal apophysis. The epiphysis of the posterior part of the calcaneus.

calcaneal spur. Calcific healing of a chronic avulsion injury of the plantar fascia from the calcaneus.

calcaneal sulcus. The groove along the medial aspect of the calcaneus adjacent to the posterior articular surface lodging the interosseous talocalcaneal ligament. NA *sulcus calcanei.*

calcaneal tendon. The common tendon of the gastrocnemius and soleus muscles inserted into the heel. NA *tendo calcaneus.*

calcaneal tuberosity. The posterior extremity of the calcaneus. NA *tuber calcanei.*

cal·ca·ne·an (kal·kay'nee·un) *adj.* CALCANEAL.

calcaneo-. See *calcane-.*

calca·neo·as·trag·a·lar (kal·kay"nee·o·as·trag'uh·lur) *adj.* [*calcaneo-* + *astragalar*]. TALOCALCANEAL.

cal·ca·neo·ca·vus (kal·kay"nee·o·kay'vus) *n.* [*calcaneo-* + *cavus*]. TALIPES CALCANEOCAVUS.

cal·ca·neo·cu·boid (kal·kay"nee·o·kew'boid) *adj.* Pertaining to the calcaneus and the cuboid.

calcaneocuboid articulation. The joint between the calcaneus and the cuboid. NA *articulatio calcaneocuboidea.* See also Table of Synovial Joints and Ligaments in the Appendix.

calcaneocuboid ligament. The part of the bifurcate ligament that connects the calcaneus and the cuboid. NA *ligamentum calcaneocuboideum.* See also *dorsal calcaneocuboid ligament, plantar calcaneocuboid ligament.*

cal·ca·ne·o·dyn·ia (kal·kay"nee·o·din'ee·uh) *n.* [*calcane-* + *-odynia*]. Pain in the heel, or calcaneus.

cal·ca·neo·fib·u·lar (kal·kay"nee·o·fib'yoo·lur) *adj.* Pertaining to the calcaneus and the fibula.

calcaneofibular ligament. A ligament of the ankle joint attached to the lower end of the fibula and the lateral surface of the calcaneus. NA *ligamentum calcaneofibulare.*

cal·ca·neo·na·vic·u·lar (kal·kay"nee·o·na·vick'yoo·lur) *adj.* Pertaining to the calcaneus and the navicular.

calcaneonavicular ligament. The part of the bifurcate ligament that connects the calcaneus and the navicular. NA *ligamentum calcaneonaviculare.*

cal·ca·neo·val·gus (kal·kay"nee·o·val'gus) *n.* [*calcaneo-* + *valgus*]. TALIPES CALCANEOVALGUS.

cal·ca·ne·um (kal·kay'nee·um) *n.,* genit. sing. **calca·nei** (·nee·eye), pl. **calca·nea** (·nee·uh) [L., short for *os calcaneum,* heel bone] [BR]. CALCANEUS.

cal·ca·ne·us (kal·kay'nee·us) *n.,* pl. & genit. sing. **calca·nei** (·nee·eye) [L., from *calx,* heel]. 1. [NA] The heel bone. NA alt. *os calcis.* See Table of Bones in the Appendix. 2. TALIPES CALCANEUS.

calcaneus apophysitis. Epiphysitis of the heel bone, or calcaneus.

cal·ca·no·dyn·ia (kal·kay"no·din'ee·uh, kal"kuh·no·) *n.* CALCANEODYNIA.

cal·car (kal'kahr) *n.,* pl. **cal·car·ia** (kal·kăr'ee·uh) [L., a spur, from *calx,* heel]. Any spur or spurlike point. **—cal·ca·rate** (kal'kuh·rate) *adj.*

calcar avis (ay'vis) [L., bird's spur] [NA]. A ridge in the wall of the posterior horn of the lateral ventricle, caused by the inward bulging of the floor of the calcarine fissure.

cal·car·e·ous (kal·kair'ee·us) *adj.* [L. *calcarius,* of lime]. 1. Pertaining to or of the nature of limestone. 2. Having a chalky appearance or consistency. 3. Containing calcium.

calcareous chondrodystrophy. CHONDRODYSTROPHIA CALCIFICANS CONGENITA.

calcareous degeneration or **infiltration.** Deposition of salts of calcium in degenerate or necrotic tissue.

calcar fe·mo·ra·le (fem"o·ray'lee). A plate of compact bone projecting almost vertically from the femoral shaft upward into the neck toward the greater trochanter; it is well seen in radiographs.

cal·ca·rine (kal'kuh·rin, ·reen) *adj.* Pertaining to or like a calcar.

calcarine area. VISUAL PROJECTION AREA.

calcarine fissure. CALCARINE SULCUS.

calcarine sulcus. A sulcus on the medial aspect of the occipital lobe of the cerebrum, between the lingual gyrus and the cuneus. NA *sulcus calcarinus.*

cal·car·i·uria (kal·kair"ee·yoo'ree·uh) *n.* [L. *calcari*us, of lime, + *-uria*]. The presence of calcium salts in the urine.

cal·ce·mia, cal·cae·mia (kal·see'mee·uh) *n.* [*calc-* + *-emia*]. HYPERCALCEMIA.

calci-. See *calc-.*

cal·ci·bil·ia (kal"si·bil'ee·uh) *n.* [*calci-* + *bili-* + *-ia*]. Calcium in the bile.

cal·cic (kal'sick) *adj.* Of or pertaining to lime or calcium.

cal·ci·co·sis (kal"si·ko'sis) *n.,* pl. **calcico·ses** (·seez) [*calci-* + *-osis*]. A form of pneumoconiosis due to the inhalation of marble (calcium carbonate) dust.

cal·cif·a·mes (kal·sif'uh·meez) *n.* [*calci-* + L. *fames,* hunger]. Abnormal desire to eat calcium-containing materials; a form of pica.

cal·ci·fe·di·ol (kal"si·fe·dye'ol) *n.* 25-Hydroxycholecalciferol, $C_{27}H_{44}O_2$, a calcium regulator.

cal·cif·er·ol (kal·sif'ur·ol) *n.* Vitamin D_2, obtained by irradiation of ergosterol; 1 mg represents 40,000 units of vitamin D activity.

cal·cif·er·ous (kal·sif'ur·us) *adj.* [*calci-* + *-ferous*]. Containing calcium carbonate.

cal·cif·ic (kal·sif'ick) *adj.* Forming, causing, or involving deposition of a calcium salt.

cal·ci·fi·ca·tion (kal"si·fi·kay'shun) *n.* The deposit of calcareous matter within the tissues of the body.

calcified cartilage. A cartilage in which a calcareous deposit is contained in the matrix.

calcified fetus. LITHOPEDION.

calcified tumor of skin. 1. Any cutaneous neoplasm containing calcium. 2. PILOMATRICOMA.

cal·ci·fy (kal'si·figh) *v.* To deposit mineral salts as in calcification. **—calci·fied** (·fide) *adj.*

calcifying epithelioma of Mal·herbe (mal·e^h^rb′) [A. *Malherbe*]. PILOMATRICOMA.

calcifying giant-cell tumor. CHONDROBLASTOMA.

cal·cig·er·ous (kal·sij′ur·us) *adj.* [*calci-* + *-gerous*]. Containing a calcium salt.

cal·cim·e·ter (kal·sim′e·tur) *n.* An apparatus for determining the amount of calcium in the blood.

cal·ci·na·tion (kal″si·nay′shun) *n.* The process of expelling volatile matter by heating, especially carbon dioxide and water from inorganic compounds, but in some cases involving also the combustion of organic matter. —**cal·cine** (kal′sine) *v.*; **cal·cined** (kal′sine′d) *adj.*

calcined magnesia. Magnesium oxide prepared by ignition of the carbonate.

cal·ci·nol (kal′si·nole) *n.* CALCIUM GLUCONATE.

cal·ci·no·sis (kal″si·no′sis) *n.*, pl. **calcino·ses** (·seez) [*calci-* + *-osis*]. 1. The deposition of calcium salts in tissues. 2. Sometimes specifically, CALCINOSIS CUTIS.

calcinosis cu·tis (kew′tis). The deposition of calcium salts in the skin and subcutaneous tissues without detectable injury of the affected parts or without hypercalcemia.

calcinosis cutis cir·cum·scrip·ta (sur″kum·skrip′tuh). Nodular calcification in the skin and subcutaneous tissues; seen frequently in the extremities, particularly the hands, in scleroderma.

calcinosis cutis universalis. CALCINOSIS UNIVERSALIS.

calcinosis uni·ver·sa·lis (yoo″ni·vur·say′lis). Widespread calcified plaques that tend to ulcerate and heal slowly, and involve subcutaneous tissues, muscles, tendons, and nerve sheaths; seen especially in children and young adults and associated with such disorders as dermatomyositis, scleroderma, and Raynaud's disease. Etiology is unknown, but serum calcium, phosphorus, and alkaline phosphatase levels are normal.

cal·ci·pe·nia (kal″si·pee′nee·uh) *n.* [*calci-* + *-penia*]. Calcium deficiency.

cal·ci·phy·lax·is (kal″si·fi·lack′sis) *n.* [*calci-* + *phylaxis*]. A type of experimentally induced calcification in which a hypersensitive state is induced by certain substances (e.g., parathyroid hormone), followed after a critical period by administration of a challenging substance (e.g., metal salts).

cal·cis (kal′sis) *n.* [L.]. 1. Genitive of *calx;* of the heel. 2. Os calcis (= CALCANEUS (1)).

cal·cite (kal′site) *n.* A mineral form of calcium carbonate.

cal·ci·to·nin (kal″si·to′nin) *n.* A single-chain polypeptide hormone consisting of 32 amino acids, apparently existing as several active fractions; secreted by the parafollicular cells of the thyroid gland in mammals and by the ultimobranchial bodies in birds, reptiles, amphibians and fish. The hormone lowers both plasma calcium and phosphate by inhibiting bone resorption without augmenting calcium accretion. It also causes increased renal excretion of phosphate, calcium, chloride, sodium, and magnesium. Syn. *thyrocalcitonin.*

cal·ci·um (kal′see·um) *n.* [L. *calx, calcis*, limestone, + *-ium*]. Ca = 40.08. A brilliant, silver-white metal, characterized by strong affinity for oxygen. It is an abundant and widely distributed element.

calcium acetate. A white, amorphous powder, $Ca(C_2H_3O_2)_2$, soluble in water; has been used medicinally as a source of calcium.

calcium acetylsalicylate. A white powder, $(CH_3COOC_6H_4\text{-}COO)_2Ca.2H_2O$, readily soluble in water; used as an antirheumatic and analgesic.

calcium aminosalicylate. A white crystalline powder, $(NH_2C_6H_3(OH)COO)_2Ca$, freely soluble in water; used as a tuberculostatic drug. Syn. *calcium para-aminosalicylate.*

calcium arsenate. A white powder, $Ca_3(AsO_4)_2$, slightly soluble in water; used as an insecticide.

calcium balance. The relationship within the body between the net intake and elimination of calcium.

calcium benzoate. White powder or crystals, $(C_6H_5COO)_2\text{-}Ca.3H_2O$; has been used medicinally as a source of calcium and benzoate ions.

calcium ben·zo·yl·pas (ben·zo′il·pas″). Calcium 4-benzamidosalicylate, $C_{28}H_{20}CaO_8$; an antituberculous drug.

calcium bromide. A white granular salt, $CaBr_2$, very deliquescent and very soluble in water; has been employed as a sedative and antiepileptic.

calcium cacodylate. A white, granular powder $[(CH_3)_2\text{-}AsO_2]_2Ca.H_2O$, very soluble in water; has been used for the same purposes as sodium cacodylate.

calcium carb·as·pi·rin (kahrb·as′pi·rin). Calcium acetylsalicylate-urea complex, $C_{19}H_{18}CaN_2O_9$; a water-soluble analgesic.

calcium carbide. A gray, crystalline solid, CaC_2, decomposed by water to yield acetylene.

calcium carbonate. Any of the forms of $CaCO_3$, including chalk, marble, and whiting. Used as an antacid.

calcium chloride. $CaCl_2.2H_2O$. White, deliquescent fragments or granules, soluble in water; used medicinally for the effects of calcium ion.

calcium creosotate. A mixture of the calcium compounds of creosote, representing about 50% creosote; has been used as an expectorant and intestinal antiseptic.

calcium cyanamide. CaNCN. Gray lumps or powder. Reacts with water to produce ammonia. Used in fertilizers.

calcium cyclamate. The calcium salt of cyclamic acid, employed as a sweetening agent.

calcium disodium edathamil. CALCIUM DISODIUM EDETATE.

calcium disodium ede·tate (ed′e·tate). Calcium disodium (ethylenedinitrilo) tetraacetate or calcium disodium ethylenediaminetetraacetate, $C_{10}H_{12}CaN_2Na_2O_8.xH_2O$, a white, crystalline powder, freely soluble in water. A metal complexing agent used for diagnosis and treatment of lead poisoning.

Calcium Disodium Versenate. Trademark for calcium disodium edetate.

calcium EDTA (ee·dee·tee·ay). CALCIUM DISODIUM EDETATE.

calcium fluoride. A white powder, CaF_2, insoluble in water; has been recommended for prevention of caries.

Calcium folinate SF. A trademark for leucovorin calcium.

calcium glu·bi·o·nate (gloo·bye′uh·nate). Calcium D-gluconate lactobionate, monohydrate, $C_{18}H_{32}CaO_{19}.H_2O$, a calcium replenishing agent.

calcium gluconate. A white crystalline or granular powder, $[CH_2OH(CHOH)_4COO]_2Ca.H_2O$, soluble in water; used medicinally for the effects of calcium.

calcium glycerophosphate. $CaC_3H_5(OH)_2PO_4$. A white crystalline powder, soluble in water; used as a calcium and phosphate dietary supplement.

calcium gout. CALCINOSIS.

calcium hydrate. CALCIUM HYDROXIDE.

calcium hydroxide. Slaked lime, $Ca(OH)_2$, the active ingredient of lime water.

calcium hypochlorite. $Ca(ClO)_2$. A principal ingredient of chlorinated lime; used as an antiseptic, disinfectant, and bleaching agent.

calcium hypophosphite. A white, crystalline powder, $Ca(PH_2O_2)_2$, freely soluble in water; has been used medicinally for the effects of calcium and hypophosphite ions.

calcium hyposulfite. CALCIUM THIOSULFATE.

calcium iodide. A white powder, $CaI_2.6H_2O$, soluble in water; has been used like potassium iodide.

calcium iodobehenate. A white or yellowish powder, containing principally $Ca(C_{22}H_{42}IO_2)_2$, insoluble in water. In the body, it slowly liberates iodide ions, for which effect it is used.

calcium iodostearate. A cream-colored powder, $Ca(C_{18}H_{34}IO_2)_2$, insoluble in water, containing approximately 27% iodine; formerly used as a prophylactic against goiter.

calcium ipo·date (eye′po·date). The calcium salt of 3-(dimethylaminomethyleneamino)-2,4,6-triiodohydrocinnamic acid; administered orally for radiographic visualization of the biliary system. See also *sodium ipodate.*

calcium lactate. A white powder, $Ca(C_3H_5O_3)_2.5H_2O$, soluble in water; used medicinally for the effects of calcium ion.

calcium lactophosphate. A mixture of calcium lactate, calcium acid lactate, and calcium acid phosphate; soluble in water; formerly used therapeutically as a source of calcium.

calcium leucovorin. The calcium salt of folinic acid (2); used as an antidote for folic acid antagonists.

calcium levulinate. A white crystalline powder, $Ca(CH_3COCH_2COO)_2.2H_2O$, very soluble in water; used medicinally for the effects of calcium ion.

calcium mandelate. A white powder, $Ca(C_6H_5CHOHCOO)_2$, slightly soluble in water. Used medicinally for the effect of mandelic acid as a urinary antiseptic.

calcium oxalate. CaC_2O_4; a white, crystalline powder, practically insoluble in water. A form in which calcium is precipitated in certain pathological conditions and in analyses for the element.

calcium oxide. CaO. Lime; quicklime; burnt lime. Used industrially but not medicinally.

calcium pantothenate. A white powder, $Ca(C_9H_{16}NO_5)_2$, soluble in water; employed for the effect of dextrorotatory pantothenic acid, one of the B-complex vitamins. It is supplied in dextrorotatory and racemic forms, the latter having half the activity of the former. See also *vitamin B complex.*

calcium para-aminosalicylate. CALCIUM AMINOSALICYLATE.

calcium perborate. A white powder, approximately $Ca(BO_3)_2.7H_2O$, soluble in water; used in dentifrices.

calcium permanganate. Violet crystals, $Ca(MnO_4)_2.4H_2O$, readily soluble in water; an antiseptic, disinfectant, and deodorizer.

calcium peroxide. A cream-colored powder, CaO_2, practically insoluble in water; has been used as antacid and antiseptic in gastric and intestinal disorders.

calcium phenolsulfonate. A water-soluble powder, $Ca(C_6H_4OHSO_3)_2$; has been used as an intestinal antiseptic and astringent.

calcium phosphate. Any one of three salts, differing in the proportion of calcium and phosphate: monobasic calcium phosphate, $CaH_4(PO_4)_2.H_2O$, a deliquescent and strongly acid powder; dibasic calcium phosphate, $CaHPO_4.2H_2O$, used as a calcium and phosphorus dietary supplement; tribasic calcium phosphate, $Ca_3(PO_4)_2$, used as an antacid.

calcium phytate. The calcium salt of the hexaphosphate ester of inositol. The insolubility of this salt may prevent normal absorption of dietary calcium.

calcium poly·car·bo·phil (pol″ee·kahr′bo·fil). The calcium salt of a polycarboxylic, cross-linked hydrophilic resin, employed as a cathartic.

calcium propionate. $Ca(C_3H_5O_2)_2$. A white powder, soluble in water; used to prevent molding of bread.

calcium saccharate. A white powder, $CaC_6H_8O_8.4H_2O$, practically insoluble in water; used as a stabilizer for injections of calcium gluconate.

calcium D-saccharate. CALCIUM SACCHARATE.

calcium salicylate. A white, crystalline powder, $Ca(C_6H_4OHCOO)_2.2H_2O$, soluble in water; has been used as a source of salicylate.

calcium santonate. A white, crystalline powder, $Ca(C_{15}H_{19}O_4)_2$, insoluble in water; has been used as an anthelmintic.

calcium santoninate. CALCIUM SANTONATE.

calcium sulfate. $CaSO_4$, occurring naturally as the dihydrate gypsum which, when partially or completely dehydrated (calcined) by heating, constitutes plaster of Paris.

calcium sulfide. When pure, CaS, occurring as colorless crystals. Crude calcium sulfide, formerly official, was used both externally and internally for the treatment of various skin diseases; at present, used as depilatory. Sulfurated lime and liver of lime are terms occasionally applied to crude calcium sulfide. A solution of calcium sulfides (di-, penta-) known as sulfurated lime solution (Vleminckx's solution) is used in treating various skin diseases.

calcium sulfite. A white powder, $CaSO_3.2H_2O$, slightly soluble in water; a preservative and antiseptic.

calcium sulfocarbolate. CALCIUM PHENOLSULFONATE.

calcium thiosulfate. White crystals, $CaS_2O_3.6H_2O$, soluble in water; has been used as an internal antiseptic.

calcium tungstate. $CaWO_4$. A constituent of the mineral scheelite, but usually prepared by precipitation; used in preparing screens of fluoroscopes and in manufacturing fluorescent paints.

calcium un·dec·y·le·nate (un·des′i·le·nate). $Ca(C_{11}H_{19}O_2)_2$, an antifungal agent.

cal·ci·uria (kal″see·yoo′ree·uh) *n.* 1. Calcium in the urine. 2. HYPERCALCINURIA.

calco-. See *calc-.*

cal·co·glob·u·lin (kal″ko·glob′yoo·lin) *n.* [*calco-* + *globulin*]. A combination of calcium with protein such as is found in calcospherites, probably representing an early stage in the process of laying down calcium salts in teeth and bone.

cal·co·sphe·rite, cal·co·sphae·rite (kal″ko·sfeer′ite) *n.* [*calco-* + L. *sphaera*, sphere, + *-ite*]. One of the granules or globules formed in tissues like bone and shell by a loose combination of protein and blood-borne calcium salts.

cal·co·spher·ule (kal″ko·sfeer′yool, ·sfeer′ool) *n.* [*calco-* + *spherule*]. 1. A minute sphere, a combination of protein and calcium, found in certain diseased tissues. 2. Specifically, MICHAELIS-GUTMANN BODY.

cal·cu·lary (kal′kew·lerr·ee) *adj.* Of or pertaining to a calculus or to calculi.

cal·cu·lo·gen·e·sis (kal″kew·lo·jen′e·sis) *n.*, pl. **calculogene·ses** (·seez) [*calculus-* + *-genesis*]. The origin or development of calculi.

cal·cu·lo·sis (kal″kew·lo′sis) *n.* [*calculus* + *-osis*]. The presence of a calculus or an abnormal concretion.

cal·cu·lus (kal′kew·lus) *n.*, pl. **calcu·li** (·lye) [L., pebble, stone, dim. of *calx*, stone, limestone, from Gk. *chalix*, pebble, gravel]. A solid concretion composed chiefly of mineral substances and salts found in ducts, passages, hollow organs, cysts, and on the surfaces of teeth. Organic materials such as cells and mucus may form a centrum or nidus and may be dispersed as a matrix for the mineral deposits, as salts of calcium, of uric acid, or of bile acids. —**calculous,** *adj.*

calculus fel·le·us (fel′ee·us). GALLSTONE.

Caldecort. A trademark for calcium undecylenate, an antifungal agent.

Cald·well-Luc operation (luᵉk) [G. W. *Caldwell,* U.S. surgeon, 1866–1946; and H. *Luc,* French laryngologist, 1855–1925]. An opening made through the canine fossa into the maxillary sinus.

Caldwell's projection [E. W. *Caldwell,* U.S. radiologist, 1870–1918]. A PA x-ray projection of the skull taken with the forehead and nose positioned on the film and the central ray projected 23° caudally in relation to a theoretical line from the meatus of the eye and the glabella. Designed to demonstrate the orbits, the cranial vault, and the frontal sinuses.

cal·e·fa·cient (kal″e·fay′shunt) *adj.* & *n.* [L. *calefacere,* to warm]. 1. Warming; causing a sensation of warmth. 2. A medicine, externally applied, that causes a sensation of warmth.

ca·len·du·la (ka·len′dyoo·luh) *n.* [L. *calendae,* first day of the month, when the plant was supposed to blossom]. 1. A plant of the genus *Calendula,* of the Compositae. 2. The dried ligulate floret of plants of this genus, especially *C. officinalis.*

cal·en·tu·ra (kal″en·tew′ruh) *n.* [Sp., heating, fever]. In the Philippine Islands, an epidemic disease of horses, possibly of trypanosomal origin.

calf (kaf) *n.,* pl. **calves** (kavz) [ON. *kālfi*]. The thick, fleshy part of the back of the leg, formed by the gastrocnemius and soleus muscles and overlying tissues. NA *regio cruris posterior.*

calf bone. FIBULA.

CALGB Cancer and Acute Leukemia Group B, an international cooperative group dedicated to clinical cancer research.

cal·i·ber, cal·i·bre (kal′i·bur) *n.* [MF. *calibre,* from Ar. *qālib,* shoemaker's last, from Gk. *kalapous*]. The diameter of a cylindrical or round body, as an artery.

cal·i·bra·tion (kal″i·bray′shun) *n.* 1. The specification and measurements of the properties or performance of a device, so that it may be used for subsequent measuring procedures. 2. The measurement of the caliber of a tube, or the determination or rectification of the graduations on a tube, pipet, or balance weights. —**cal·i·bra·tor** (kal′i·bray·tur) *n.;* **cal·i·brate** (kal′i·brate) *v.*

calibre. CALIBER.

cal·i·ce·al (kal″i·see′ul) *adj.* Of or pertaining to a calix.

caliceal diverticulum. A congenital or acquired outpouching or sac arising from a renal calix.

cal·i·cec·ta·sis (kal″i·seck′tuh·sis, kay″li·) *n.,* pl. **calicecta·ses** (·seez) [*calix* + *ectasis*]. Dilatation of a renal calix.

cal·i·cec·to·my (kal″i·seck′tuh·mee, kay″li·) *n.* [*calix* + *-ectomy*]. Removal of a calix of the renal pelvis.

calices. Plural of *calix.*

calices re·na·les (re·nay′leez), sing. **calix rena·lis** [NA]. RENAL CALICES.

calices renales ma·jo·res (ma·jo′reez) [NA]. The major calices of the kidney. See *renal calix.*

calices renales mi·no·res (mi·no′reez) [NA]. The minor calices of the kidney. See *renal calix.*

ca·lic·i·form (ka·lis′i·form) *adj.* Shaped like a calix.

caliculi. Plural of *caliculus.*

ca·li·cu·lus (ka·lick′yoo·lus) *n.,* pl. **calicu·li** (·lye) [L., dim. of *calix,* cup]. A small cuplike structure.

caliculus gu·sta·to·ri·us (gus″tuh·tor′ee·us), pl. **caliculi gustato·rii** (·ee·eye) [NA]. TASTE BUD.

caliculus oph·thal·mi·cus (off·thal′mi·kus) [NA]. OPTIC CUP.

Cal·i·for·nia disease. COCCIDIOIDOMYCOSIS.

California encephalitis. Encephalitis in man caused by California virus; characterized by insidious onset of fever, headache, and mild to severe neurological symptoms.

California encephalitis virus. An arbovirus of the California group which has been isolated from rabbits, squirrels, and field mice but whose natural reservoir is unknown. The species of mosquito responsible for its transmission to man has not been definitely identified.

California group. A group of immunologically related arboviruses that includes the California encephalitis virus.

California virus. CALIFORNIA ENCEPHALITIS VIRUS.

cal·i·for·ni·um (kal″i·for′nee·um) *n.* [after *California,* U.S.A.]. Cf = 249. A radioactive element discovered by bombarding an isotope of curium with alpha particles.

Calioben. A trademark for calcium iodobehenate.

cal·i·per (kal′i·pur) *n.* [alteration of *caliber*]. 1. A curved and hinged instrument with adjustable legs or jaws for measuring the thickness and the outside or inside diameters of objects. 2. Any type of such an instrument, as a micrometer caliper.

caliper splint. A splint designed for the leg, consisting of two metal rods from a posterior thigh band or a padded ischial ring to a metal plate attached to the sole of the shoe at the instep.

cal·i·sa·ya (kal″i·say′uh) *n.* [Sp.]. Cinchona bark, especially that of *Cinchona calisaya.*

cal·is·then·ics (kal″iss·then′icks) *n.* [Gk. *kal*los, beauty, + *sthenos,* strength]. A system of, or the practice of, light gymnastics by various rhythmic movements of the body; intended to develop the muscles and graceful carriage.

ca·lix (kay′licks, kal′icks) *n.,* pl. **ca·li·ces** (kal′i·seez, kay′li·seez) [L., cup, goblet]. 1. A cuplike structure. 2. Specifically, RENAL CALIX. 3. (Of an ovum:) The wall of the graafian follicle from which the ovum has escaped. Compare *calyx.*

Cal·kins method [L. A. *Calkins,* U.S. obstetrician, 1894–1960]. Delay of placental delivery until the uterus assumes a globular shape indicative of placental detachment from the uterine lining.

Cal·lan·der's amputation [C. L. *Callander,* U.S. surgeon, 1892–1947]. Amputation at the knee joint preserving long anterior and posterior flaps; the patella is removed, and the resulting fossa receives the femoral stump.

Call-Ex·ner bodies [F. von *Call,* Austrian physician, 1844–1917; and S. *Exner*]. Minute rosettelike groupings of cells occurring in the granulosa membrane of the ovarian follicle either before or after formation; also sometimes seen in granulosa cell tumors.

cal·li·pe·dia (kal″i·pee′dee·uh) *n.* [Gk. *kallipais, kallipaidos,* having beautiful children, + *-ia*]. 1. The desire to give birth to a beautiful child. 2. The superstition that if a pregnant woman concentrates upon having a beautiful child or looks at representations of one, her baby will be beautiful.

Cal·liph·o·ra (kal·if′o·ruh) *n.* [Gk. *kallos,* beauty, + *phoros,* bearing]. A genus of flies that feeds chiefly on animal refuse. The maggots of these flies cause myiasis.

Calliphora vom·i·to·ria (vom″i·tor′ee·uh). The common blowfly or blue bottle; may deposit ova in neglected wounds of man and other mammals.

Cal·li·phor·i·dae (kal″i·for′i·dee) *n.pl.* [from *Calliphora,* type genus]. A family of the Diptera which includes many large blue, green, or copper-colored species, commonly called bluebottle, greenbottle, and blowflies. They normally deposit their eggs or larvae in the decaying flesh of dead animals but may be secondary invaders of neglected wounds and sores. —**cal·liph·o·rid** (ka·lif′uh·rid) *adj. & n.*

Cal·li·thric·i·dae (kal″i·thris′i·dee) *n.pl.* CALLITRICHIDAE.

Cal·li·thrix (kal′i·thricks) *n.* [L., a kind of monkey, from Gk. *kallithrix,* having beautiful hair or mane]. A genus of the Callitrichidae comprising the typical marmosets.

Cal·li·trich·i·dae (kal″i·trick′i·dee) *n.pl.* [Gk. *kallitrichos,* producing luxuriant hair]. A family of Anthropoidea comprising the marmosets and tamarins.

Cal·li·tro·ga (kal″i·tro′guh) *n.* [NL., from *Calliphoridae* + Gk. *trōgein,* to gnaw, eat]. A genus of flies of the Calliphoridae; the screwworm flies.

Callitroga amer·i·ca·na (a·merr″i·kah′nuh, ·kay′nuh). *CALLITROGA HOMINIVORAX.*

Callitroga hom·i·ni·vo·rax (hom″i·ni·vo′racks). The screwworm, an obligate parasite of warm-blooded animals, including man, in tropical and subtropical regions of the Western Hemisphere. The ova are deposited by the adult fly on unbroken living tissue, and the larvae, hatched in less than half a day, enter the skin and produce suppurative lesions. Syn. *Callitroga americana.*

Callitroga ma·cel·la·ria (mas″e·lair′ee·uh). A species of calliphorid fly whose larvae feed on dead and moribund tissue of cattle, horses, and sheep.

cal·lo·ma·nia (kal″o·may′nee·uh) *n.* [Gk. *kallos,* beauty, + *mania*]. A delusional state characterized by a belief in one's own beauty.

cal·lo·sal (ka·lo′sul) *adj.* [*callosum* + *-al*]. Pertaining to the corpus callosum.

callosal demyelinating encephalopathy. MARCHIAFAVA-BIGNAMI DISEASE.

callosal gyrus. CINGULATE GYRUS.

callosal sulcus. The groove separating the corpus callosum from the overlying cingulate gyrus. NA *sulcus corporis callosi.*

cal·lose (kal'oce, ·oze) *n.* A polysaccharide (β,1,3-glucan) from bean extracts.

cal·los·i·tas (ka·los'i·tas) *n.* [L.]. CALLOSITY.

cal·los·i·ty (ka·los'i·tee) *n.* [L. *callositas*]. A circumscribed area of skin thickened by hypertrophy of the horny layer of the epidermis, caused by friction or pressure. Syn. *callus.*

cal·lo·so·mar·gin·al (ka·lo''so·mahr'ji·nul) *adj.* Pertaining to the callosal and marginal gyri of the brain.

callosomarginal fissure or **sulcus.** CINGULATE SULCUS.

cal·lo·sum (ka·lo'sum) *n.*, pl. **callo·sa** (·suh). CORPUS CALLOSUM.

cal·loused ulcer. HYPERKERATOTIC ULCER.

cal·lus (kal'us) *n.* [L.]. 1. A callosity, especially of the palm or sole. 2. New growth of incompletely organized bony tissue surrounding the bone ends in fracture; a part of the reparative process. —**callous,** *adj.*

calm·a·tive (kahl'muh·tiv) *adj. & n.* SEDATIVE.

Cal·mette's vaccine [L. C. A. *Calmette,* French bacteriologist, 1863–1933]. BCG VACCINE.

Calmette test [L. C. A. *Calmette*]. A tuberculin test in which dilute tuberculin is applied to the conjunctiva; now rarely used.

cal·o·mel (kal'o·mel) *n.* [Gk. *kalos,* beautiful, + *melas,* black]. Mercurous chloride, HgCl. A white powder, insoluble in water; formerly used as a cathartic and diuretic, now used, in ointment form, as a local antibacterial.

calomel electrode. An electrode consisting of calomel, mercury, and potassium chloride solution; used as a standard, as in determining hydrogen-ion concentration, because it develops a constant potential.

cal·or (kal'or, kay'lor) *n.* [L.]. Heat; one of the four classic signs of inflammation: calor, rubor, tumor, dolor.

cal·o·ra·di·ance (kal''o·ray'dee·unce) *n.* [L. *calor,* heat, + *radiance*]. Emission of heat rays ranging from 250 to 55,000 nm.

cal·o·res·cence (kal''o·res'unce) *n.* The conversion of invisible heat rays into luminous heat rays.

calori- [L. *calor*]. A combining form meaning *heat.*

ca·lo·ric (ka·lo'rick) *adj.* Pertaining to a calorie, calories, or to heat.

caloric test. With the patient's head tilted 30° forward from the horizontal, the external auditory meatuses are irrigated in turn for 30 seconds with water at 30°C and 44°C, with a pause of at least 5 minutes between irrigations. In normal persons, cold water induces a slight tonic deviation to the side being irrigated, followed, after about 20 seconds by nystagmus with the fast component to the opposite side. Irrigation with warm water induces nystagmus to the same side. If the vestibular nerve or labyrinth is destroyed as the result of disease, no nystagmus is produced upon testing the diseased side.

Cal·o·rie, Cal·o·ry (kal'uh·ree) *n.* [F., from L. *calor,* heat]. KILOCALORIE.

cal·o·rie, cal·o·ry, *n.* Any one of several heat units that represent the quantity of heat required to raise the temperature of 1 g water by 1°C but that differ slightly from each other in the specific 1° interval of temperature selected. The units are also defined in equivalent mechanical energy units, the equivalents for one calorie ranging from 4.1816 to 4.2045 joules. Syn. *small calorie, gram calorie.* Compare *Calorie, kilocalorie.*

cal·o·rif·ic (kal''o·rif'ick) *adj.* Heat-producing; pertaining to heat or calories.

ca·lo·ri·ge·net·ic (ka·lor''i·je·net'ick) *adj.* CALORIGENIC.

ca·lo·ri·gen·ic (ka·lor''i·jen'ick, kal''or·i·) *adj.* [*calori-* + *-genic*]. Heat-producing; applied to certain foods and hormones.

calorigenic action. 1. SPECIFIC DYNAMIC ACTION. 2. The total heat liberated by a food or food constituent when metabolized by the body.

cal·o·rim·e·ter (kal''o·rim'e·tur) *n.* [*calori-* + *-meter*]. An instrument for measuring the heat production of an individual or a physical system under standard conditions. See also *bomb calorimeter.*

calorimetric equivalent. The amount of heat necessary to raise the temperature of the calorimeter one degree Celsius.

cal·o·rim·e·try (kal''o·rim'e·tree) *n.* [*calori-* + *-metry*]. The determination of the total heat produced or released by an individual or a physical system by use of a calorimeter. —**cal·o·ri·met·ric** (kal''o·ri·met'rick) *adj.*

Calory. Calorie (= KILOCALORIE).

calory. CALORIE.

Ca·lot's triangle (ka·lo') [J. F. *Calot,* French surgeon, 1861–1944]. TRIANGLE OF CALOT.

ca·lum·ba (ka·lum'buh) *n.* The dried root of *Jateorrhiza palmata,* native to East Africa and Madagascar; contains alkaloids and the bitter glycoside columbin. Has been used as a simple bitter.

Calurin. Trademark for calcium carbaspirin, a water-soluble analgesic.

cal·u·ster·one (kal·yoo'ste·rone) *n.* 7β,17α-Dimethyltestosterone, $C_{21}H_{32}O_2$, an antineoplastic agent.

cal·var·ia (kal·vair'ee·uh) *n.*, pl. & genit. sing. **calvar·i·ae** (·ee·ee) [L., skull, from *calva,* scalp] [NA]. The upper part of the skull; the skullcap. —**calvar·i·al** (·ee·ul) *adj.*

calvarial hyperostosis. HYPEROSTOSIS FRONTALIS INTERNA.

cal·var·i·um (kal·vair'ee·um) *n.* CALVARIA.

Cal·vé's disease (kal·vey') [J. *Calvé,* French orthopedist, 1895–1954]. 1. Osteochondrosis of the vertebrae. 2. Osteochondrosis of the head of the femur.

Calvé's vertebra plana [J. *Calvé*]. VERTEBRA PLANA.

cal·vi·ti·es (kal·vish'ee·eez) *n.* [L.]. Loss of hair, especially on the crown of the head; alopecia, baldness.

¹calx (kalks) *n.* [L., lime]. CALCIUM OXIDE; lime.

²calx, *n.*, genit. sing. **cal·cis** (kal'sis), pl. **cal·ces** (kal'seez) [L.] [NA]. HEEL.

cal·y·can·thine (kal''i·kan'theen) *n.* An alkaloid, $C_{22}H_{26}N_4$, found in several species of plants of *Calycanthus* and elsewhere, having strychnine-like action.

calyceal. CALICEAL.

calycectasis. CALICECTASIS.

calycectomy. CALICECTOMY.

calyces. A plural of *calyx.*

calyces renales [BNA]. Calices renales (= RENAL CALICES).

calyces renales ma·jo·res (ma·jo'reez) [BNA]. Calices renales majores. See *renal calix.*

calyces renales mi·no·res (mi·no'reez) [BNA]. Calices renales minores. See *renal calix.*

calyciform. CALICIFORM.

ca·lyc·i·nal (ka·lis'i·nul) *adj.* CALYCINE.

ca·ly·cine (kay'li·seen, kal'i·) *adj.* Pertaining to or resembling a calyx.

calyculi. Plural of *calyculus.*

calyculi gus·ta·to·rii (gus·tuh·to'ree·eye) [BNA]. Caliculi gustatorii (= TASTE BUDS).

calyculus. CALICULUS.

Ca·lym·ma·to·bac·te·ri·um gran·u·lo·ma·tis (ka·lim''uh·to·back·teer'ee·um gran·yoo·lo'muh·tis). A gram-negative coccobacillus that is responsible for the venereal disease granuloma inguinale. Syn. *Donovania granulomatis, Klebsiella granulomatis.*

ca·lyx (kay'licks, kal'icks) *n.*, pl. **calyxes, caly·ces** (kal'i·seez, kay'li·) [ML., from Gk. *kalyx,* shell, pod, calyx]. 1. The outer sheath of a flower or bud, formed by the sepals. 2. CALIX.

cam·ben·da·zole (kam·ben'duh·zole) *n.* Isopropyl 2-(4-thiazolyl)-5-benzimidazolecarbamate, $C_{14}H_{14}N_4O_2S$, an anthelmintic agent.

cam·bi·um (kam'bee·um) *n.*, pl. **cam·bia** (·bee·uh) [L., exchange]. A layer of tissue formed between the wood and the bark of exogenous plants.

cambium layer. The cellular layer of the periosteum.

cam·bo·gia (kam·bo'jee·uh) *n.* GAMBOGE.

cam·el curve. The occurrence of two febrile peaks separated by a period of normal temperature, as may be encountered in poliomyelitis with a fever in the prodromal stage, followed by several days of normalcy, and then by the onset of the sustained febrile course.

ca·me·ra (kam'e·ruh) *L. n.,* pl. & genit. sing. **came·rae** (·ree). *In anatomy,* a chamber or compartment.

camera anterior bul·bi (bul'bye) [NA]. ANTERIOR CHAMBER of the eyeball.

cam·era lu·ci·da (lew'si·duh). An optical device used to project onto paper the image of an object so that an accurate drawing can be made.

camera ocu·li an·te·ri·or (ock'yoo·lye an·teer'ee·or) [BNA]. Camera anterior bulbi (= ANTERIOR CHAMBER).

camera oculi posterior [BNA]. Camera posterior bulbi (= POSTERIOR CHAMBER).

camera posterior bul·bi (bul'bye) [NA]. POSTERIOR CHAMBER of the eyeball.

camera sep·ti lu·ci·di (sep'tye lew'si·dye). CAVITY OF THE SEPTUM PELLUCIDUM.

camera vi·trea bul·bi (vit'ree·uh bul'bye) [NA]. VITREOUS CHAMBER.

cam·i·sole (kam'i·sole) *n.* [F.]. A canvas shirt with very long sleeves; used as a straitjacket.

Cam·midge test or **reaction** [P. J. *Cammidge,* English physician, b. 1872]. A test supposed to ascertain diagnosis of pancreatitis or pancreatic malignancy, in which one of two urine specimens is treated with mercuric chloride; both are then treated with hydrochloric acid and subjected to the phenylhydrazine test; a difference in residue indicates pancreatic disease.

Camoform. Trademark for bialamicol, an antiamebic drug used as the dihydrochloride salt.

Camolar. Trademark for cycloguanil, an antimalarial drug used as the pamoate salt.

camomile. CHAMOMILE.

Camoquin. Trademark for amodiaquine, an antimalarial drug used as the dihydrochloride salt.

Camp·bell's operation [W. C. *Campbell,* U.S. orthopedist, 1880–1941]. 1. A method of onlay bone grafting for ununited fracture. 2. An operation for relief of recurrent dislocation of the patella in which a flap of the joint capsule is passed through a tunnel in the quadriceps femoris above.

Cam·per's fascia (kahm'pur) [P. *Camper,* Dutch physician, 1722–1789]. The superficial, loose, fat-containing layer of the superficial fascia of the anterior abdominal wall.

Camper's line [P. *Camper*]. FACIAL LINE.

cam·pes·ter·ol (kam·pes'tur·ol) *n.* A sterol, $C_{28}H_{48}O$, occurring in small amounts in the fixed oil from rape seed, soybean, and wheat germ.

camp fever. EPIDEMIC TYPHUS.

camph-, campho-. A combining form meaning *camphor.*

cam·phene (kam'feen) *n.* [*camph-* + *-ene*]. A terpene hydrocarbon, $C_{10}H_{16}$, occurring in several volatile oils.

campho-. See *camph-.*

cam·phor (kam'fur) *n.* [Malay *kāpūr*]. A ketone, $C_{10}H_{16}O$, obtained from the volatile oil of *Cinnamomum camphora,* a tree indigenous to eastern Asia, or produced synthetically. It is a mild irritant and antiseptic and has been used as a carminative and stimulant. —**camphor·at·ed** (·ay·tid), **cam·phor·ic** (kam·for'ick) *adj.*

cam·pho·ra·ceous (kam''fo·ray'shus) *adj.* Resembling or containing camphor.

camphor and soap liniment. A preparation containing hard soap, camphor, rosemary oil, alcohol, and water; a rubefacient embrocation.

cam·phor·ate (kam'fo·rate) *n.* [*camphor* + *-ate*]. A salt of camphoric acid.

camphorated chloral. A liquid prepared from equal parts of chloral hydrate and camphor; has been used as a counterirritant and anodyne.

camphorated menthol. A liquid mixture of equal parts of menthol and camphor; has been used externally as a counterirritant and anodyne.

camphorated oil. CAMPHOR LINIMENT.

camphorated opium tincture. A hydroalcoholic solution of opium containing also anise oil, benzoic acid, camphor, and glycerin; used as an antiperistaltic drug in treating diarrheas. Syn. *paregoric.*

camphor flowers. Camphor obtained by sublimation.

cam·phor·ic acid (kam·for'ick). A dibasic acid, $C_{10}H_{16}O_4$, obtained by oxidation of camphor; formerly used to control the night sweats of pulmonary tuberculosis.

camphor ice. A cosmetic preparation of camphor, spermaceti, white beeswax, and a vegetable oil.

cam·phor·ism (kam'fur·iz·um) *n.* Camphor poisoning characterized by gastritis and symptoms of an acute organic brain syndrome, including convulsions and coma.

camphor liniment. A solution of camphor in cottonseed oil; a counterirritant embrocation.

camphor oil. A volatile oil obtained from the camphor tree, *Cinnamomum camphora;* has been used as a rubefacient.

cam·phoro·ma·nia (kam''fur·o·may'nee·uh) *n.* An abnormal craving for camphor.

camphor spirit. A solution of camphor in alcohol.

camphor water. A saturated solution of camphor in distilled water; used as a vehicle and an ingredient of eyewashes.

cam·pim·e·ter (kam·pim'e·tur) *n.* [L. *campus,* field, + *-meter*]. An instrument for measuring the field of vision. See also *perimeter.* —**campime·try** (·tree) *n.*

camp·to·cor·mia (kamp''to·kor'mee·uh) *n.* [Gk. *kamptein,* to bend, + *kormos,* trunk, + *-ia*]. A static deformity of hysterical origin characterized by a forward flexion of the trunk.

camp·to·dac·ty·ly (kamp''to·dack'ti·lee) *n.* [Gk. *kamptein,* to bend, + *-dactyly*]. A condition in which one or more fingers are constantly flexed at one or both phalangeal joints.

cam·syl·ate (kam'sil·ate) *n.* Any salt or ester of camphorsulfonic acid, $C_{10}H_{15}OSO_2OH$; a camphorsulfonate.

Ca·mu·ra·ti-Eng·el·mann disease (kah''moo·rah'tee, eng'ul·mahnn). PROGRESSIVE DIAPHYSEAL DYSPLASIA.

Can·a·da balsam. A turpentine gathered from the natural blisters of the bark of the tree *Abies balsamea;* used as a mounting medium by microscopists.

Canada-Cronkhite syndrome. CRONKHITE-CANADA SYNDROME.

Canada hemp. APOCYNUM.

Canada snakeroot. ASARUM.

Canada turpentine. CANADA BALSAM.

Ca·na·dian crutch. A lightweight crutch so constructed that the weight of the body is transmitted to it through the extended arm and palm of the hand that grasps the horizontal handle.

can·a·dine (kan'uh·deen, ·din) *n.* Tetrahydroberberine, $C_{20}H_{21}NO_4$, a colorless alkaloid from the plant *Hydrastis canadensis.*

ca·nal (kuh·nal') *n.* [L. *canalis,* channel, from *canna,* reed]. Any tubular channel; DUCT.

canales. Plural of *canalis.*

canales al·ve·o·la·res max·il·lae (al·vee·o·lair'eez mack·sil'ee) [NA]. The alveolar canals of the maxilla. See *alveolar canals.*

canales di·plo·i·ci (di·plo'i·sigh) [NA]. Spaces in the diploë occupied by the diploic veins.

canales lon·gi·tu·di·na·les mo·di·o·li (lon''ji·tew·di·nay'leez mo·dye'o·lye) [NA]. Small passages in the modiolus which transmit vessels and nerves.

canales pa·la·ti·ni (pal·uh·tye'nigh) [BNA]. PALATINE CANALS.

canales palatini mi·no·res (mi·no'reez) [NA]. The lesser palatine canals. See *palatine canals.*

canales se·mi·cir·cu·la·res os·sei (sem''ee·sur·kew·lair'eez os'ee·eye) [NA]. OSSEOUS SEMICIRCULAR CANALS.

can·a·lic·u·lar (kan″uh·lick′yoo·lur) *adj.* Of or pertaining to a canaliculus.

canalicular abscess. A mammary abscess that communicates with a milk duct.

canalicular apparatus. GOLGI APPARATUS.

canalicular scissors. Delicate scissors, one blade of which is probe-pointed; used for slitting the lacrimal canaliculus.

canaliculi. Plural of *canaliculus.*

canaliculi ca·ro·ti·co·tym·pa·ni·ci (ka·rot″i·ko·tim·pan′i·sigh) [NA]. CAROTICOTYMPANIC CANALS.

canaliculi den·ta·les (den·tay′leez) [NA]. DENTINAL TUBULES.

canaliculi la·cri·mo·les (lack·ri·may′leez) [NA]. Plural of *canaliculus lacrimalis;* LACRIMAL CANALICULI.

canaliculi vas·cu·lo·si (vas·kew·lo′sigh). HAVERSIAN CANALS.

can·a·lic·u·lo·plas·ty (kan·uh·lick′yoo·lo·plas″tee) *n.* [*canaliculus* + *-plasty*]. Plastic repair of a canaliculus, especially that leading from the punctum to the lacrimal sac.

can·a·lic·u·lus (kan″uh·lick′yoo·lus) *n.*, pl. **canalicu·li** (·lye) [L., dim. of *canalis*]. 1. A small canal; especially that leading from the lacrimal punctum to the lacrimal sac of the eye. 2. Any one of the minute canals opening into the lacunas of bone. —**cana·lic·u·la·tion** (·lick″yoo·lay′shun), **canalicu·li·za·tion** (·li·zay′shun) *n.*

canaliculus chor·dae tym·pa·ni (kor′dee tim′puh·nigh) [NA]. A small canal in the petrous portion of the temporal bone for the passage of the chorda tympani nerve.

canaliculus coch·le·ae (kock′lee·ee) [NA]. The passageway in the temporal bone which transmits the perilymphatic duct and a small vein.

canaliculus la·cri·ma·lis (lack·ri·may′lis) [NA]. LACRIMAL CANALICULUS.

canaliculus mas·toi·de·us (mas·toy′dee·us) [NA]. MASTOID CANALICULUS.

canaliculus tym·pa·ni·cus (tim·pan′i·kus) [NA]. TYMPANIC CANALICULUS.

can·a·line (kan′uh·leen, ·lin) *n.* [*Canavalia* + *-ine*]. 2-Amino-4-(aminoxy)butyric acid, $NH_2OCH_2CH_2CH(NH_2)COOH$, an amine found in jack beans, where it is formed from arginine.

ca·na·lis (ka·nay′lis) *n.*, pl. **cana·les** (·leez) [L.]. CANAL.

canalis ad·duc·to·ri·us (a·duck·to′ree·us) [NA]. ADDUCTOR CANAL.

canalis ali·men·ta·ri·us (al″i·men·tair′ee·us) [NA]. ALIMENTARY CANAL.

canalis ana·lis (ay·nay′lis) [NA]. ANAL CANAL.

canalis ba·si·pha·ryn·ge·us (bay″see·fa·rin′jee·us) [BNA]. Canalis vomerovaginalis (= BASIPHARYNGEAL CANAL).

canalis ca·ro·ti·cus (ka·rot′i·kus) [NA]. CAROTID CANAL.

canalis car·pi (kahr′pye) [NA]. CARPAL TUNNEL.

canalis cen·tra·lis (sen·tray′lis) [NA]. CENTRAL CANAL OF THE SPINAL CORD.

canalis cer·vi·cis ute·ri (sur′vi·sis yoo′te·rye) [NA]. CANAL OF THE CERVIX OF THE UTERUS.

canalis con·dy·la·ris (kon″di·lair′is) [NA]. CONDYLAR CANAL.

canalis con·dy·loi·de·us (kon″di·loy′dee·us) [BNA]. Canalis condylaris (= CONDYLAR CANAL).

canalis fa·ci·a·lis (fay″shee·ay′lis) [NA]. FACIAL CANAL.

canalis fe·mo·ra·lis (fem″o·ray′lis) [NA]. FEMORAL CANAL.

canalis hy·a·loi·de·us (high″uh·loy′dee·us) [NA]. HYALOID CANAL.

canalis hy·po·glos·si (high″po·glos′eye) [NA]. HYPOGLOSSAL CANAL.

canalis in·ci·si·vus (in·si·sigh′vus) [NA]. INCISIVE CANAL.

canalis in·fra·or·bi·ta·lis (in″fruh·or·bi·tay′lis) [NA]. INFRAORBITAL CANAL.

canalis in·gui·na·lis (ing″gwi·nay′lis) [NA]. INGUINAL CANAL.

canalis man·di·bu·lae (man·dib′yoo·lee) [NA]. MANDIBULAR CANAL.

canalis mus·cu·lo·tu·ba·ri·us (mus″kew·lo·tew·bair′ee·us) [NA]. MUSCULOTUBAL CANAL.

canalis na·so·la·cri·ma·lis (nay″so·lack·ri·may′lis) [NA]. NASOLACRIMAL CANAL.

canalis nu·tri·ci·us (new·tris′ee·us) [NA]. HAVERSIAN CANAL.

canalis ob·tu·ra·to·ri·us (ob″tew·ruh·to′ree·us) [NA]. OBTURATOR CANAL.

canalis op·ti·cus (op′ti·kus) [NA]. OPTIC CANAL.

canalis pa·la·ti·nus major (pal″uh·tye′nus) [NA]. The greater palatine canal. See *palatine canals.*

canalis pa·la·to·va·gi·na·lis (pal″uh·to·vaj·i·nay′lis) [NA]. PHARYNGEAL CANAL.

canalis pha·ryn·ge·us (fa·rin′jee·us) [BNA]. Canalis palatovaginalis (= PHARYNGEAL CANAL).

canalis pte·ry·goi·de·us (terr″i·goy′dee·us) [NA]. PTERYGOID CANAL.

canalis pte·ry·go·pa·la·ti·nus (terr″i·go·pal·uh·tye′nus) [BNA]. PTERYGOPALATINE CANAL. See also *palatine canals.*

canalis pu·den·da·lis (pew″den·day′lis) [NA]. PUDENDAL CANAL.

canalis py·lo·ri·cus (pi·lor′i·kus) [NA]. PYLORIC CANAL.

canalis ra·di·cis den·tis (rad′i·sis den′tis) [NA]. ROOT CANAL.

canalis sa·cra·lis (sa·kray′lis) [NA]. SACRAL CANAL.

canalis se·mi·cir·cu·la·ris an·te·ri·or (sem″ee·sur·kew·lair′is an·teer′ee·or) [NA]. The anterior semicircular canal of the bony labyrinth of the inner ear. See *osseous semicircular canals.*

canalis semicircularis la·te·ra·lis (lat·e·ray′lis) [NA]. The lateral semicircular canal of the bony labyrinth of the inner ear. See *osseous semicircular canals.*

canalis semicircularis pos·te·ri·or (pos·teer′ee·or) [NA]. The posterior semicircular canal of the bony labyrinth of the inner ear. See *osseous semicircular canals.*

canalis semicircularis superior [BNA]. CANALIS SEMICIRCULARIS ANTERIOR.

canalis spi·na·lis (spye·nay′lis) [BNA]. Canalis vertebralis (= VERTEBRAL CANAL).

canalis spi·ra·lis coch·le·ae (spi·ray′lis cock′lee·ee) [NA]. OSSEOUS COCHLEAR CANAL.

canalis spiralis mo·di·o·li (mo·dye′o·lye) [NA]. SPIRAL CANAL OF THE MODIOLUS.

canalis ven·tri·cu·li (ven·trick′yoo·lye) [NA]. GASTRIC CANAL.

canalis ver·te·bra·lis (vur″te·bray′lis) [NA]. VERTEBRAL CANAL.

canalis vo·me·ro·va·gi·na·lis (vom″ur·o·vaj·i·nay′lis) [NA]. BASIPHARYNGEAL CANAL.

ca·nal·iza·tion (ka·nal″i·zay′shun, kan″ul·i·zay′shun, ·eye·zay′shun) *n.* 1. The formation of new channels in tissues, as the formation of new blood vessels in a thrombus. 2. A system of wound drainage without tubes. —**ca·nal·ize** (ka·nal′ize, kan′ul·ize) *v.*

canalized fibrinoid. The layered fibrinoid material having a striated or canalized appearance, found especially on the chorionic plate during the last half of pregnancy.

canal of Corti [A. *Corti*]. TUNNEL OF CORTI.

canal of Nuck [A. *Nuck*]. In the female, the vaginal process of peritoneum passing into the inguinal canal.

canal of the cervix of the uterus. The portion of the uterine cavity situated in the cervix, extending from the isthmus to the ostium of the uterus. Syn. *cervical canal.* NA *canalis cervicis uteri.* See also Plate 23.

canal of the chorda tympani. CANALICULUS CHORDAE TYMPANI.

canal of the greater petrosal nerve. A canal opening into the hiatus of the facial canal for the passage of the greater (superficial) petrosal nerve.

canal of the lesser petrosal nerve. An opening in the petrous portion of the temporal bone for the passage of the lesser (superficial) petrosal nerve. Syn. *superior tympanic canaliculus.*

canals of Pe·tit (puh·tee′) [F. P. du *Petit,* French physician, 1664–1771]. ZONULAR SPACES.

Can·a·val·ia (kan″uh·val′yuh) *n.* [NL.]. A genus of tropical herbs having long pods with seeds or beans, which are used as a source of urease; jack beans.

can·a·van·ine (kan·av'uh·neen, kan"uh·van'een) *n.* An amino acid, $C_5H_{12}N_4O_3$, from jack beans; it is a potent inhibitor of bacterial growth by its competition with L-arginine.

Can·a·van's disease or **spongy degeneration** (kan'uh·vun) [M. M. *Canavan,* U.S. anatomist, 1879–1953]. SPONGY DEGENERATION OF INFANCY.

can·cel·late (kan'se·late) *adj.* CANCELLOUS.

can·cel·lat·ed (kan'se·lay·tid) *adj.* CANCELLOUS.

can·cel·lous (kan'se·lus) *adj.* [L. *cancelli*, lattice, + *-ous*]. Characterized by reticulated or latticed structure, as the spongy tissue of bones or, in botany, certain leaves consisting largely of veins. —**can·cel·la·tion** (kan·se·lay'shun) *n.*

cancellous bone. A form of bone in which the matrix is arranged in a network of rods, plates, or tubes (the trabeculae), with spaces between filled with marrow. NA *substantia spongiosa.*

can·cer (kan'sur) *n.* [L., crab]. 1. A malignant tumor. 2. Any disease characterized by malignant tumor formation or proliferation of anaplastic cells. See also *carcinoma, sarcoma.*

cancer en cui·rasse (ahn kwi·ras'). 1. Widely infiltrating carcinoma of the skin of the thorax, usually arising in mammary carcinoma. 2. Widespread carcinoma of the pleura.

can·cer·i·ci·dal (kan"sur·i·sigh'dul) *adj.* [*cancer* + *-cidal*]. Able to kill the cells of a malignant tumor.

can·cer·i·gen·ic (kan"sur·i·jen'ick) *adj.* CARCINOGENIC.

cancer milk. A milky fluid that can be expressed or scraped from the cut surface of certain carcinomas, especially those of the mammary gland.

cancer nest. A small group of cancer cells.

cancer oc·cul·tus (o·kul'tus). Carcinoma manifest first by the appearance of metastasis.

can·cero·gen (kan'sur·o·jen) *n.* CARCINOGEN. —**can·cero·gen·ic** (kan"sur·o·jen'ick) *adj.*

can·cer·ol·o·gy (kan"sur·ol'uh·jee) *n. Obsol.* The study and science of cancer. Compare *oncology.* —**cancerolo·gist,** *n.*

can·cero·pho·bia (kan"sur·o·fo'bee·uh) *n.* CARCINOPHOBIA.

can·cer·ous (kan'sur·us) *adj.* Of or pertaining to cancer; like a cancer.

cancerous goiter. A carcinoma of the thyroid gland.

can·cer·pho·bia (kan"sur·fo'bee·uh) *n.* CARCINOPHOBIA.

can·croid (kang'kroid) *n. & adj.* [L. *cancr-*, cancer, + *-oid*]. 1. SQUAMOUS CELL CARCINOMA. 2. Of or pertaining to squamous cell carcinoma.

cancroid corpuscle. An epithelial pearl of a squamous cell carcinoma.

can·crum oris (kang'krum or'is). Noma of the mouth.

can·de·la (kan·dee'luh) *n.* [L., candle, from *candere,* to shine]. The new unit of luminous intensity, of such magnitude that a black-body radiator at the temperature at which pure platinum solidifies has a luminous intensity of 60 candelas per square centimeter. Abbreviated, cd.

Candeptin. Trademark for candicidin, an antibiotic active against *Candida albicans.*

can·di·ci·din (kan"di·sigh'din) *n.* A polyene antibiotic, produced by a soil actinomycete similar to *Streptomyces griseus,* which is fungistatic and fungicidal; highly effective against *Candida albicans.* Used primarily for local treatment of candidal vaginitis.

Can·di·da (kan'di·duh) *n.* [L. *candidus,* white]. A genus of yeastlike, opportunistically pathogenic fungi. Syn. *Monilia.* —**can·di·dal** (·dul) *adj.*

Candida al·bi·cans (al'bi·kanz). A fungus of low pathogenicity that inhabits the mucous membranes; produces thrush and other types of candidiasis; THRUSH FUNGUS.

can·di·di·a·sis (kan"di·dye'uh·sis) *n.,* pl. **candidia·ses** (·seez) [*Candida* + *-iasis*]. A condition produced by infection with a fungus of the genus *Candida,* usually *C. albicans;* involving various parts of the body, as skin, mucous membrane, nails, bronchi, lungs, heart, vagina, and gastrointestinal tract, and rarely, occurrence of septicemia. See also *thrush, intertrigo, onychomycosis, paronychomycosis, perlesche, erosio interdigitalis blastomycetica.*

can·di·did (kan'di·did) *n.* A sterile grouped vesicular lesion of the hands or body resulting from hypersensitivity to a focus of *Candida* infection.

can·di·du·ria (kan"di·dew'ree·uh) *n.* The presence of candidal organisms in the urine.

can·di·ru (kan'di·roo) *n.* [Pg., from Tupi *candérú*]. A minute catfish of South America, which is attracted to the salt in urine and may enter the urethra of unprotected bathers.

can·dle, *n.* The unit of intensity of light, variously defined in terms of light sources; replaced by *candela.*

canebrake yellow fever. BLACKWATER FEVER.

ca·nel·la (ka·nel'uh) *n.* [dim. of L. *canna,* reed]. The bark of the tree, *Canella winterana,* native to the West Indies, dried and without the cork layer; popularly used as an aromatic tonic. Syn. *white cinnamon.*

ca·nes·cine (ka·nes'een) *n.* DESERPIDINE.

cane sugar. Sucrose from sugar cane.

ca·nic·o·la fever (ka·nick'o·luh). The form of leptospirosis in man caused by infection with *Leptospira canicola.*

Can·i·dae (kan'i·dee) *n. pl.* The dog family of the order Carnivora, including the typical canines (wolves, coyotes, jackals, domestic dogs) and foxes, together with divergent forms such as the Asiatic wild dogs and African hunting dogs.

ca·nine (kay'nine) *adj. & n.* [L. *caninus,* from *canis,* dog]. 1. Pertaining to or resembling dogs. 2. A member of the dog family. 3. Pertaining to a canine tooth. 4. CANINE TOOTH.

canine babesiosis. A disease of dogs caused by infection of the erythrocytes by protozoa of the genus *Babesia;* characterized by fever, anemia, and icterus.

canine distemper. A pantropic virus disease occurring among animals of the family Canidae and certain other carnivores such as mink and racoons; may be characterized by respiratory, enteric, or neurological symptoms.

canine eminence. A prominence on the outer side of the maxilla, corresponding to the root of the canine tooth.

canine fossa. A depression on the external surface of the maxilla, above and to the outer side of the socket of the canine tooth. NA *fossa canina.*

canine laugh. RISUS SARDONICUS.

canine leptospirosis. STUTTGART DISEASE.

canine piroplasmosis. CANINE BABESIOSIS.

canine spasm. RISUS SARDONICUS.

canine teeth. Sharp tearing teeth of mammals, located between the incisors and premolars. In the human dentition, also called *cuspids.* NA *dentes canini.*

canine transmissible venereal tumor. A tumor usually found on or near the external genitalia of dogs which can be naturally transmitted by coition; also the first neoplasm to be experimentally transmitted from animal to animal.

canine typhus. STUTTGART DISEASE.

canine venereal tumor. CANINE TRANSMISSIBLE VENEREAL TUMOR.

canine yellow fever. NAMBI UVU.

ca·ni·nus (kay·nigh'nus, ka·) *n.,* pl. **cani·ni** (·nye) [L.]. LEVATOR ANGULI ORIS.

ca·ni·ti·es (ka·nish'ee·eez) *n.* [L.]. Grayness or whiteness of the hair. Syn. *poliosis.*

canities un·gui·um (ung'gwee·um) [L., whiteness of the nails]. LEUKONYCHIA.

can·ker (kang'kur) *n.* [L. *cancer,* a crab]. 1. An ulceration, especially one of the mouth and lips; also a gangrenous ulcer or gangrenous stomatitis. 2. APHTHOUS STOMATITIS; THRUSH. 3. A disease of the horn-forming membrane of horse's hoofs, leading to destruction of the cells and loss of the horn-secreting function. 4. Granulomatous inflammation of the external ears, particularly of dogs and rabbits.

canker rash. SCARLET FEVER.

can·ker·root, *n.* Usually, the root of *Coptis groenlandica* (gold thread).

canker sore. A small ulceration of the mucous membrane of the mouth.

can·na·bi·di·ol (kan''uh·bi·dye'ol) *n.* A constituent of cannabis which, on isomerization to a tetrahydrocannabinol, exhibits to a great degree the activity of cannabis.

can·na·bin (kan'uh·bin) *n.* A resinous substance from Indian hemp; it has the characteristic activity of cannabis.

can·na·bi·nol (ka·nab'i·nol) *n.* A substance, $C_{21}H_{26}O_2$, resulting from spontaneous dehydrogenation of tetrahydrocannabinol in cannabis. Though commonly considered physiologically inactive, cannabinol has some of the characteristic activity of cannabis.

can·na·bis (kan'uh·bis) *n.* [L., from Gk. *kannabis* (rel. to Gmc. *khanipiz* → E. *hemp*)]. The flowering or fruiting tops of the pistillate hemp plant, *Cannabis sativa,* of which there are two varieties, Indian and American, the former being the more potent. The active constituents have been shown to be tetrahydrocannabinols. Cannabis is classified as a hallucinogen. In large doses it produces mental exaltation, intoxication, and a sensation of double consciousness in some individuals. It is important as an intoxicant, but has no rational therapeutic use. Bhang, ganga, charas, kif, hashish, and marijuana are among the various names by which the drug and certain preparations of it are known.

can·na·bism (kan'uh·biz·um) *n.* Poisoning resulting from excessive or habitual use of cannabis.

can·ni·bal·ism (kan'i·bul·iz·um) *n.* [*cannibal* + *-ism*]. 1. The eating of one's own kind, frequently observed in the postpartum rabbit or rat. 2. Specifically, the eating of human flesh by human beings. —**can·ni·bal·is·tic** (kan''i·bul·is'tick) *adj.*

can·non·ball, *n. In radiology,* a sharply defined, round, homogeneous, dense shadow in the lung, commonly produced by metastatic carcinoma or by a granuloma.

cannon bone. The functional and complete metacarpal or metatarsal bone in the leg of a hoofed quadruped, especially of the horse. Contr. *splint bone.*

Cannon's law of denervation [W. B. *Cannon,* U.S. physiologist, 1871–1945]. When in a series of efferent neurons a unit is destroyed, an increased irritability to the physiologic neurotransmitter develops in the isolated structure or structures, the effects being maximal in the part directly denervated.

cannon sound. An accentuated first heart sound heard in complete heart block when atrial systole occurs slightly before ventricular systole.

Cannon's point or **ring** [W. B. *Cannon*]. An inconstant focal area of apparent narrowing or contraction of the transverse colon, seen radiographically during barium enema examination, but of no clinical significance. Presumed to be a point of overlap between nerve plexuses or vascular supply.

cannon wave. A large positive venous pulse wave that occurs when the right atrium contracts against a tricuspid valve closed by right ventricular systole or cannot empty into the right ventricle for any other reason (tumor, stenosis, congenital abnormality, thrombus).

can·nu·la (kan'yoo·luh) *n.,* pl. **cannulas, cannu·lae** (·lee) [L., small reed]. An artificial tube of various sizes and shapes often fitted with a trocar for insertion into a tube or cavity of the body, as an artery or the trachea. —**cannu·lar** (·lur), **cannu·late** (·late) *adj.*

can·nu·late (kan'yoo·late) *v.* To insert a cannula into a body cavity or hollow organ. —**can·nu·la·tion** (kan''yoo·lay'shun) *n.*

can·nu·lize (kan'yoo·lize) *v.* CANNULATE. —**can·nu·li·za·tion** (kan''yoo·li'zay'shun) *n.*

can·ren·o·ate potassium (kan·ren'o·ate). The potassium salt of 17-hydroxy-3-oxo-17α-pregna-4,6-diene-21-carboxylate, $C_{22}H_{29}KO_4$, an aldosterone antagonist.

can·re·none (kan're·nohn) *n.* 17-Hydroxy-3-oxo-17α-pregna-4,6-diene-21-carboxylic acid γ-lactone, $C_{22}H_{28}O_3$, an aldosterone antagonist.

canth-, cantho-. A combining form meaning *canthus, canthal.*

can·thal (kan'thul) *adj.* Of or pertaining to a canthus.

can·tha·ri·a·sis (kan''thuh·rye'uh·sis) *n.,* pl. **cantharia·ses** (·seez) [*cantharis* + *-iasis*]. The presence in the body of coleopterous insects or their larvae, or disease states arising from their presence.

can·thar·i·des (kan·thăr'i·deez) *n. pl.* [Gk. *kantharides,* pl. of *kantharis,* a kind of beetle]. The dried insects, *Cantharis vesicatoria,* yielding cantharidin; has been used externally as a rubefacient and vesicant.

can·thar·i·din (kan·thăr'i·din) *n.* The active principle, $C_{10}H_{12}O_4$, of cantharides and other insects; formerly used topically as a counterirritant.

can·thar·i·dism (kan·thăr'i·diz·um) *n.* Cantharidin poisoning caused by absorption, sometimes of toxin from the blister produced by local application of cantharidin.

can·tha·ris (kan'thuh·ris). Singular of *cantharides.*

can·thec·to·my (kan·theck'tuh·mee) *n.* [*canth-* + *-ectomy*]. Excision of a canthus.

canthi. Plural of *canthus.*

can·thi·tis (kan·thigh'tis) *n.* Inflammation of a canthus. See also *angular blepharitis.*

cantho-. See *canth-.*

can·thol·y·sis (kan·thol'i·sis) *n.,* pl. **cantholy·ses** (·seez) [*cantho-* + *-lysis*]. Canthotomy with section of the lateral palpebral ligament.

can·tho·plas·ty (kan'tho·plas''tee) *n.* [*cantho-* + *-plasty*]. 1. Increasing the length of the palpebral fissure by slitting the outer canthus. 2. Any plastic restoration of a canthal defect.

can·thor·rha·phy (kan·thor'uh·fee) *n.* [*cantho-* + *-rrhaphy*]. *In plastic surgery,* shortening of the palpebral fissure by suture of the canthus.

can·thot·o·my (kan·thot'uh·mee) *n.* [*cantho-* + *-tomy*]. Surgical division of a canthus.

can·thus (kanth'us) *n.,* pl. **can·thi** (·eye) [Gk. *kanthos*]. Either of the two angles formed by the junction of the eyelids, designated outer or lateral, and inner or medial. Syn. *palpebral angle.*

Cantil. Trademark for mepenzolate bromide, an anticholinergic.

can·ti·le·ver bridge (kan'ti·lee''vur). A bridge fixed at one end and with either no support or with a lug resting on the adjoining tooth at the other end.

caou·tchouc (kaow'chook, F. kaow·choo') *n.* [F., rubber]. The terpene hydrocarbon substance dispersed in the milky juice that exudes upon incision of a number of tropical trees belonging to the families Euphorbiaceae, Artocarpaceae, and Apocynaceae. When pure, caoutchouc is nearly white, soft, elastic, and glutinous; it is soluble in organic solvents.

cap. Abbreviation for (a) *capiat;* let him take; (b) *capsula;* a capsule.

cap, *n.* A covering or coverlike structure; a tegmen. See also *pulp cap.*

ca·pac·i·tance (ka·pas'i·tunce) *n.* The quantity of electricity which a condenser (capacitor) or other structure can hold per volt of electric pressure applied.

ca·pac·i·tor (ka·pas'i·tur) *n.* An instrument for holding or storing charges of electricity; CONDENSER (3).

Capastat. A trademark for capreomycin, an antibiotic.

Cape aloe. Aloe obtained from the plant *Aloe ferox,* and hybrids of this species with *A. africana* and *A. spicata.*

cap·e·line bandage (kap'uh·lin). A bandage resembling a cap or hood, suitable for the head, shoulder, or amputation stump.

Cap·gras' syndrome (kap·grah') [J. M. *Capgras,* French psychiatrist, 1873–1950]. A psychotic state in which the subject believes that a person well known to him is a double or imposter and is not to be trusted.

cap·il·lar·ec·ta·sia (kap″i·lăr″eck·tay′zee·uh, ·zhuh) *n.* [*capillary* + *ectasia*]. Dilatation of the capillaries.

ca·pil·la·ri·a·sis (ka·pil″uh·rye′uh·sis, kap″i·luh·) *n.* Infection by nematodes of the genus *Capillaria.* See also *intestinal capillariasis.*

cap·il·lar·i·os·co·py (kap″i·lăr·ee·os′kuh·pee) *n.* CAPILLAROSCOPY.

cap·il·lar·i·tis (kap″i·lăr·eye′tis) *n.* [*capillary* + *-itis*]. A progressive pigmentary disorder of skin with dilatation, but not inflammation, of superficial capillaries, not associated with any systemic complications and running a benign self-limited course.

cap·il·lar·i·ty (kap″i·lăr′i·tee) *n.* 1. CAPILLARY ATTRACTION. 2. Elevation or depression of liquids in capillary tubes due to the surface tension of the liquid.

cap·il·la·ros·co·py (kap″i·lăr·os′kuh·pee) *n.* [*capillary* + *-scopy*]. Microscopical examination of the cutaneous capillaries for diagnosis.

cap·il·lary (kap′i·lair″ee) *adj.* & *n.* [L. *capillaris*, from *capillus*, hair]. 1. Of or pertaining to a hair, to a hairlike filament, or to a tube with a minute bore. 2. A minute blood vessel connecting the smallest ramifications of the arteries with those of the veins or one of the smallest lymph vessels. NA *vas capillare.*

capillary action. 1. CAPILLARY ATTRACTION. 2. CAPILLARITY.

capillary angioma. An angioma whose vessels are of capillary size and structure.

capillary attraction. The surface force which draws aqueous liquids into and along the lumen of a capillary tube.

capillary bed. The capillaries, collectively, of a given area or organ.

capillary bronchitis. BRONCHIOLITIS.

capillary drain. A drain of horsehair or silkworm gut used to keep a wound open for a short period.

capillary hemangioma. A benign vascular tumor composed largely of capillaries.

capillary pulse. Pulsation sometimes observable at the arterial end of skin capillaries, best seen as alternate blanching and flushing of the nailbeds; occurs in aortic regurgitation and high-cardiac-output states.

capillary resistance test. 1. TOURNIQUET TEST. 2. DALLDORF TEST.

capillary respirometry. A microrespirometric method in which changes in the volume of gases in a capillary tube connecting a chamber filled with a respiring sample with a chamber containing only media and reagents are measured. The capillary tube contains an index droplet, the displacement of which serves to determine the changes in gas volume.

capillary tube. A tube with a minute lumen.

capillary tube colorimetry. Colorimetry employing capillary tubes in which reagents are placed, mixed, and read by means of a colorimeter.

cap·il·li·ti·um (kap″i·lish′ee·um) *n.*, pl. **capilli·tia** (·ee·uh) [L., the hair]. One of the protoplasmic threads that form a network in the spore capsule of *Myxomycetes.*

cap·il·lo·ve·nous (kap″i·lo·vee′nus) *adj.* [*capillary* + *venous*]. 1. Pertaining to a junctional vessel between a capillary and a venule. 2. Pertaining to the capillaries and first subpapillary venous plexus of the skin.

ca·pil·lus (ka·pil′us) *n.*, pl. **capil·li** (·eye) [L.]. A hair; specifically, a hair of the head.

cap·i·stra·tion (kap″i·stray′shun) *n.* [L. *capistratus*, masked]. 1. PHIMOSIS. 2. PARAPHIMOSIS.

capita. Plural of *caput.*

cap·i·tal operation. An operation that may threaten life; a grave, serious, or major operation.

cap·i·tate (kap′i·tate) *adj.* [L. *capitatus*, headed]. *In biology,* having a head or a headlike termination; head-shaped.

capitate bone. The largest of the carpal bones. NA *os capitatum.* See also Table of Bones in the Appendix.

cap·i·ta·tum (kap″i·tay′tum) *n.*, pl. **capita·ta** (·tuh) [L.]. CAPITATE BONE.

cap·i·tel·lum (kap″i·tel′um) *n.*, pl. **capitel·la** (·uh) [L., dim. of *caput*]. A small head or rounded process of bone. —**capitel·lar** (·ur) *adj.*

ca·pit·u·lum (ka·pit′yoo·lum) *n.*, genit. sing. **capitu·li** (·lye), pl. **capitu·la** (·luh) [L., dim. of *caput*]. The small eminence on the distal end of the humerus, which articulates with the radius. —**capitu·lar** (·lur) *adj.*

capitulum cos·tae (kos′tee) [BNA]. CAPUT COSTAE.

capitulum fi·bu·lae (fib′yoo·lee) [BNA]. CAPUT FIBULAE.

capitulum hu·me·ri (hew′mur·eye) [NA]. The eminence on the distal surface of the lateral condyle of the humerus for articulation with the head of the radius.

capitulum mal·lei (mal′ee·eye) [BNA]. CAPUT MALLEI.

capitulum man·di·bu·lae (man·dib′yoo·lee) [BNA]. CAPUT MANDIBULAE.

capitulum os·si·um me·ta·car·pa·li·um (os′ee·um met″uh·kahr·pay′lee·um) [BNA]. CAPUT OSSIS METACARPALIS.

capitulum ossium me·ta·tar·sa·li·um (met″uh·tahr·say′lee·um). CAPUT OSSIS METATARSALIS.

capitulum ra·dii (ray′dee·eye) [BNA]. CAPUT RADII.

capitulum San·to·ri·nii (san″to·ree′nee·eye) [G. D. *Santorini*]. A small elevation at the apex of the arytenoid cartilage.

capitulum sta·pe·dis (stay′pe·dis) [BNA]. CAPUT STAPEDIS.

capitulum ul·nae (ul′nee) [BNA]. CAPUT ULNAE.

Ca·pi·vac·cius' ulcer (kahn″pee·vahnch′us, kap″i·vach′us) [G. *Capivaccio*, Italian surgeon, 16th century]. Gastric ulcer complicated by cancer.

Capla. Trademark for mebutamate, an antihypertensive agent.

Cap·lan's syndrome [A. *Caplan*, British physician, 20th century]. Massive anthracosilicotic nodular fibrosis of the lung in patients with rheumatoid arthritis.

-capnia [Gk. *kapnos*, smoke, + *-ia*]. A combining form signifying *the presence of carbon dioxide.*

cap·o·ben·ic acid (kap·o·ben′ick). 6-(3,4,5-Trimethoxybenzamido)hexanoic acid, $C_{16}H_{23}NO_6$, an antiarrhythmic agent.

capped elbow. Inflammatory swelling of the subcutaneous bursa over the olecranon process of a horse.

capped hock. Inflammatory swelling of the subcutaneous bursa over the calcaneal tuberosity of a horse.

Capps's pleural reflex [J. A. *Capps*, U.S. physician, 1872–1964]. PLEURAL SHOCK.

cap·rate (kap′rate) *n.* Any salt or ester of capric acid.

cap·reo·my·cin (kap″ree·o·migh′sin) *n.* An antibiotic produced by *Streptomyces capreolus*, usually used as the sulfate salt.

cap·ric acid (kap′rick). Decanoic acid, $CH_3(CH_2)_8COOH$, a solid fatty acid occurring as a glyceride in butter and other animal fats.

ca·pril·o·quism (ka·pril′o·kwiz·um) *n.* [L. *caper*, goat, + *loqui*, to speak, + *-ism*]. EGOPHONY.

ca·pri·lo·qui·um (ka·pri·lo′kwee·um) *n.* Capriloquism; EGOPHONY.

cap·ro·ate (kap′ro·ate) *n.* Any salt or ester of caproic acid.

Caprocid. A trademark for aminocaproic acid, an antifibrinolytic agent.

Caprocin. A trademark for capreomycin sulfate.

ca·pro·ic acid (ka·pro′ick). Hexanoic acid, $CH_3(CH_2)_4COOH$, a liquid fatty acid occurring as a glyceride in butter and other animal fats.

cap·ro·in (kap′ro·in) *n.* Any of the caproic acid esters of glycerin.

cap·ry·late (kap′ri·late) *n.* Any salt or ester of caprylic acid.

ca·pryl·ic acid (ka·pril′ick). Octanoic acid, $CH_3(CH_2)_6COOH$, a solid fatty acid occurring in butter, coconut oil, and other fats and oils.

cap·sa·i·cin (kap·say′i·sin) *n.* 8-Methyl-*N*-vanillyl-6-nonenamide, $C_{18}H_{27}NO_3$, the pungent principle of capsicum.

cap·san·thin (kap·san'thin) *n.* A carotenoid pigment, $C_{40}H_{58}O_3$, in capsicum.

Capsebon. Trademark for a suspension of cadmium sulfide used as a therapeutic shampoo for seborrheic dermatitis of the scalp.

cap·si·cum (kap'si·kum) *n.* The dried fruit of *Capsicum frutescens* (bush red pepper) or of several other varieties (tabasco or Louisiana long or short peppers). Its characteristic pungent constituent is capsaicin. Various preparations of capsicum have been used for local counterirritant action and, internally, for tonic and carminative effects.

cap·sid (kap'sid) *n.* The protein coat surrounding the nucleic acid of viruses, formed in a helical or icosahedral shape by a regular arrangement of capsomers.

cap·so·mer (kap'so·mur) *n.* [*capsid* + *-mer*]. The structural subunit of the capsid of a virus, consisting of one or several kinds of polypeptide chains.

cap·so·mere (kap'so·meer) *n.* CAPSOMER.

capsul-, capsulo-. A combining form meaning *capsule.*

cap·su·la (kap'sue·luh) *n.*, pl. & genit. sing. **capsu·lae** (·lee) [L.]. CAPSULE.

capsula adi·po·sa re·nis (ad·i·po'suh ree'nis) [NA]. FATTY CAPSULE OF THE KIDNEY.

capsula ar·ti·cu·la·ris (ahr·tick''yoo·lair'is) [NA]. JOINT CAPSULE.

capsula articularis acro·mio·cla·vi·cu·la·ris (a·kro''mee·o·kla·vick''yoo·lair'is) [NA]. The capsule of the acromioclavicular joint.

capsula articularis ar·ti·cu·la·ti·o·nis ra·dio·car·pe·ae (ahr·tick''yoo·lay·shee·o'nis ray''dee·o·kahr'pee·ee) [NA]. The capsule of the wrist joint.

capsula articularis articulationis tar·si trans·ver·sae (tahr'sigh trans·vur'see) [NA]. The capsule of the transverse tarsal joint.

capsula articularis articulationis tem·po·ro·man·di·bu·la·ris (tem''puh·ro·man·dib''yoo·lair'is) [NA]. The capsule of either temporomandibular joint.

capsula articularis ar·ti·cu·la·ti·o·num ver·te·bra·rum (ahr·tick''yoo·lay·shee·o'num vur·te·bray'rum) [NA]. The capsule of any synovial vertebral joint, that is, the joint between any two articular processes.

capsula articularis at·lan·to·axi·a·lis la·te·ra·lis (at·lan''to·ack·see·ay'lis lat·e·ray'lis) [NA]. The capsule of either lateral joint between the atlas and axis.

capsula articularis atlantoaxialis me·di·ana (mee·dee·ay'nuh) [NA]. The capsule of the joint between the atlas and dens of the axis.

capsula articularis at·lan·to·oc·ci·pi·ta·lis (at·lan''to·ock·sip·i·tay'lis) [NA]. The capsule of either joint between the atlas and occipital bone.

capsula articularis cal·ca·neo·cu·boi·de·ae (kal·kay''nee·o·kew·boy'dee·ee) [NA]. The capsule of the calcaneocuboid joint.

capsula articularis ca·pi·tis cos·tae (kap'i·tis kos'tee) [NA]. The capsule of the joint of the head of a rib with a vertebra.

capsula articularis car·po·me·ta·car·pea pol·li·cis (kahr''po·met·uh·kahr'pee·uh pol'i·sis) [NA]. The capsule of the carpometacarpal joint of the thumb.

capsula articularis cos·to·trans·ver·sa·ri·ae (kos''to·trans·vur·sair'ee·ee) [NA]. The capsule of any one of the joints between the tubercle of a rib and the corresponding transverse process of a vertebra.

capsula articularis cox·ae (kock'see) [NA]. The capsule of the hip joint.

capsula articularis cri·co·ary·te·noi·dea (krye''ko·ăr''i·tee·noy'dee·uh) [NA]. The capsule of either arytenoid cartilage with the cricoid cartilage.

capsula articularis cri·co·thy·re·oi·dea (krye''ko·thigh·ree·oy'dee·uh) [BNA]. CAPSULA ARTICULARIS CRICOTHYROIDEA.

capsula articularis cri·co·thy·roi·dea (krye''ko·thigh·roy'dee·uh) [NA]. The capsule of either inferior horn of the thyroid cartilage with the cricoid cartilage.

capsula articularis cu·bi·ti (kew'bi·tye) [NA]. The capsule of the elbow joint.

capsula articularis ge·nus (jen'oos) [NA]. The capsule of the knee joint.

capsula articularis hu·me·ri (hew'mur·eye) [NA]. The capsule of the shoulder joint.

capsula articularis man·di·bu·lae (man·dib'yoo·lee) [BNA]. CAPSULA ARTICULARIS ARTICULATIONIS TEMPOROMANDIBULARIS.

capsula articularis ma·nus (man'oos) [NA]. The capsule of the combined wrist and intercarpal joints.

capsula articularis os·sis pi·si·for·mis (oss'is pye·si·for'mis) [NA]. The capsule of the joint between the pisiform and hamate bones.

capsula articularis ra·dio·ul·na·ris dis·ta·lis (ray''dee·o·ul·nair'is dis·tay'lis) [NA]. The capsule of the distal radioulnar joint.

capsula articularis ster·no·cla·vi·cu·la·ris (stur''no·kla·vick·yoo·lair'is) [NA]. The capsule of the sternoclavicular joint.

capsula articularis ster·no·cos·ta·lis (stur''no·kos·tay'lis) [NA]. The capsule of the joint between the sternum and either first rib.

capsula articularis sub·ta·la·ris (sub·tay·lair'is) [NA]. The capsule of the joint between the talus and calcaneus, or the subtalar joint.

capsula articularis ta·lo·cal·ca·nea (tay''lo·kal·kay'nee·uh) [BNA]. CAPSULA ARTICULARIS SUBTALARIS.

capsula articularis ta·lo·cru·ra·lis (tay''lo·kroo·ray'lis) [NA]. The capsule of the ankle joint.

capsula articularis ta·lo·na·vi·cu·la·ris (tay''lo·na·vick·yoo·lair'is) [BNA]. The capsule of the joint between the talus and the navicular bone.

capsula articularis ti·bio·fi·bu·la·ris (tib''ee·o·fib·yoo·lair'is) [NA]. The capsule of the tibiofibular joint.

capsulae. Plural and genitive singular of *capsula.*

capsulae ar·ti·cu·la·res at·lan·to·epi·stro·phi·cae (ahr·tick''yoo·lair'eez at·lan''to·ep·i·strof'i·see) [BNA]. The capsules of joints between the atlas and axis.

capsulae articulares ca·pi·tu·li cos·tae (ka·pit'yoo·lye kos'tee) [BNA]. The capsules of the joint of the head of a rib with a vertebra.

capsulae articulares car·po·me·ta·car·pe·ae (kahr''po·met·uh·kahr'pee·ee) [NA]. The capsules of the carpometacarpal joints of the four medial digits.

capsulae articulares di·gi·to·rum ma·nus (dij·i·to'rum man'oos) [BNA]. The capsules of the joints of the digits of the hand.

capsulae articulares digitorum pe·dis (ped'is) [BNA]. The capsules of the joints of the digits of the foot.

capsulae articulares in·ter·me·ta·car·pe·ae (in·tur·met·uh·kahr'pee·ee) [NA]. Capsules of the intermetacarpal joints.

capsulae articulares in·ter·me·ta·tar·se·ae (in·tur·met·uh·tahr'see·ee) [NA]. Capsules of the intermetatarsal joints.

capsulae articulares in·ter·pha·lan·ge·a·rum ma·nus (in·tur·fa·lan·jee·ay'rum man'oos) [NA]. The capsules of the interphalangeal joints of the hand.

capsulae articulares interphalangearum pe·dis (ped'is) [NA]. The capsules of the interphalangeal joints of the foot.

capsulae articulares me·ta·car·po·pha·lan·ge·ae (met·uh·kahr''po·fa·lan'jee·ee) [NA]. The capsules of the metacarpophalangeal joints.

capsulae articulares meta·tar·so·pha·lan·ge·ae (met·uh·tahr''so·fa·lan'jee·ee) [NA]. The capsules of the metatarsophalangeal joints.

capsulae articulares tar·so·me·ta·tar·se·ae (tahr''so·met·uh·tahr'see·ee) [NA]. The capsules of the tarsometatarsal joints.

capsula ex·ter·na (ecks·tur'nuh) [NA]. EXTERNAL CAPSULE.

capsula fi·bro·sa glan·du·lae thy·roi·de·ae (fi·bro'suh glan' dew·lee thigh·roy'dee·ee) [NA]. The fibrous investment of the thyroid gland.

capsula fibrosa (Glis·so·ni) (gli·so'nigh) [BNA]. CAPSULA FIBROSA PERIVASCULARIS.

capsula fibrosa pe·ri·vas·cu·la·ris (perr''i·vas·kew·lair'is) [NA]. The stroma of the liver including the fibrous investment over the surface of the liver and the connective tissue surrounding the vessels and duct system within the liver.

capsula fibrosa re·nis (ree'nis) [NA]. FIBROUS CAPSULE OF THE KIDNEY.

capsula glo·me·ru·li (glo·merr'yoo·lye) [NA]. GLOMERULAR CAPSULE.

capsula in·ter·na (in·tur'nuh) [NA]. INTERNAL CAPSULE.

capsula len·tis (len'tis) [NA]. CAPSULE OF THE LENS.

capsula nu·clei den·ta·ti (new'klee·eye den·tay'tye) [BNA]. A layer of gray matter surrounding the dentate nucleus.

cap·su·lar (kap'sue·lur) *adj.* Pertaining to, resembling, or within a capsule.

capsular ankylosis. An ankylosis due to cicatricial thickening or shortening of the joint capsule.

capsular cataract. Cataract due to opacity of the lens capsule or capsular remnants following surgery or trauma.

capsular cell. SATELLITE CELL (1).

capsular hemiplegia or **paralysis.** Hemiplegia without aphasia or sensory or emotional disturbances, due to a lesion in the contralateral internal capsule.

capsular ligament. JOINT CAPSULE.

capsular polysaccharide. A polysaccharide found in the capsule of a bacterium, as of a pneumococcus, determining its type specificity and its degree of virulence. It may act as a hapten or complete antigen.

capsular pseudocirrhosis. Fibrous thickening of the capsule with extension into the subjacent liver.

capsular thrombosis syndrome. CAPSULAR HEMIPLEGIA.

cap·sule (kap'sool, ·syool) *n.* [L. *capsula,* small box]. 1. A membranous investment of a part. 2. An envelope surrounding certain organisms. 3. A soluble shell, usually made of gelatin, for administering medicines. 4. *In physiology,* an instrument used for the optical recording of pressure changes or vibrations, as pressure pulses or heart sounds. It consists of a cylindrical chamber closed on one end by a thin membrane to which is glued a small mirror. Pressure changes cause movement of the membrane and deflections of a beam of light which is reflected to a photokymograph.

cap·su·lec·to·my (kap''sue·leck'tuh·mee) *n.* [*capsul-* + *-ectomy*]. Excision of a capsule.

capsule of a nerve cell. The portion of the neurilemma which covers a ganglion cell.

capsule of the kidney. The fat-containing connective tissue encircling the kidney. It consists of an inner fibrous capsule and an outer adipose capsule (the perirenal fat).

capsule of the lens. A transparent, structureless membrane enclosing the lens of the eye. NA *capsula lentis.*

cap·su·li·tis (kap''sue·ligh'tis) *n.* Inflammation of a capsule, as that of the liver (perihepatitis), a joint (knee or ankle), or the labyrinth (otosclerosis).

capsulo-. See *capsul-.*

cap·su·lo·len·tic·u·lar (kap''sue·lo·len·tick'yoo·lur) *adj.* [*capsulo-* + *lenticular*]. Pertaining to the capsule and the lens of the eye.

capsulolenticular cataract. A cataract involving the lens nucleus or cortex and capsule.

cap·su·lo·plas·ty (kap'sue·lo·plas''tee) *n.* An operation for plastic repair of a joint capsule.

cap·su·lor·rha·phy (kap''sue·lor'uh·fee) *n.* [*capsulo-* + *-rrhaphy*]. Suture of a capsule; especially suture of a joint capsule to repair a rent or to prevent dislocation.

cap·su·lo·tha·lam·ic (kap''sue·lo·thuh·lam'ick) *adj.* Pertaining to or involving the internal capsule and the thalamus.

capsulothalamic syndrome. Hemianesthesia, partial hemiplegia, and emotional instability, usually due to a hemorrhagic lesion in the contralateral thalamus and internal capsule.

cap·sul·o·tome (kap'sue·luh·tome) *n.* [*capsulo-* + *-tome*]. CYSTOTOME.

cap·su·lot·o·my (kap''sue·lot'uh·mee) *n.* [*capsulo-* + *-tomy*]. 1. Incision into a joint capsule. 2. Incision of the lens capsule or lens capsular remnants. See also *cystotomy (2).*

cap·ta·mine (kap'tuh·meen) *n.* 2-(Dimethylamino)ethanethiol, $C_4H_{11}NS$, a compound with cutaneous depigmenting activity; used as the hydrochloride salt.

cap·ta·tion (kap·tay'shun) *n.* [L. *captatio,* from *captare,* to seize]. The first or light stage of hypnotism.

cap·ti·va·tion (kap·ti·vay'shun) *n.* CAPTATION.

cap·to·di·ame (kap''to·dye'ame) *n.* 2-[*p*-(Butylthio)-α-phenylbenzylthio]-*N,N*-dimethylethylamine, $C_{21}H_{29}NS_2$, a mild sedative; used as the hydrochloride salt.

cap·ture, *n.* [L. *captura,* from *capere,* to take]. *In nuclear physics,* any process in which the nucleus of an atom acquires an additional elementary particle.

cap·u·chin monkey (kap'yoo·shin, ka·pew'chin) [F., from It. *cappuccino,* hood]. Any monkey of the genus *Cebus.*

cap·u·ride (kap'yoo·ride) *n.* (2-Ethyl-3-methylvaleryl)urea, $C_9H_{18}N_2O_2$; a hypnotic drug.

ca·put (kap'ut) *n.,* genit. **ca·pi·tis** (kap'i·tis), pl. **capi·ta** (·tuh) [L. (rel. to Gmc. **haubud-* →E. *head*)]. HEAD.

caput an·gu·la·re mus·cu·li qua·dra·ti la·bii su·pe·ri·o·ris (ang·gew·lair'ee mus'kew·lye kwah·dray'tye lay'bee·eye sue·peer·ee·o'ris) [BNA]. Musculus levator labii superioris alaeque nasi (= LEVATOR LABII SUPERIORIS ALAEQUE NASI).

caput bre·ve mus·cu·li bi·ci·pi·tis bra·chii (brev'ee mus'kew·lye bye·sip'i·tis bray'kee·eye) [NA]. The short head of the biceps muscle of the arm which arises from the supraglenoid tubercle of the scapula.

caput breve musculi bicipitis fe·mo·ris (fem'o·ris) [NA]. The short head of the biceps muscle which arises from the distal portion of the linea aspera.

caput cos·tae (kos'tee) [NA]. The head of a rib.

caput de·for·ma·tum (dee·for·may'tum). Osteochondrosis of the head of the femur.

caput epi·di·dy·mi·dis (ep''ee·di·dim'i·dis) [NA]. HEAD OF THE EPIDIDYMIS.

caput fe·mo·ris (fem'o·ris) [NA]. The head of the femur.

caput fi·bu·lae (fib'yoo·lee) [NA]. The head of the fibula, the portion which articulates with the lateral condyle of the tibia.

caput ga·le·a·tum (gal''ee·ay'tum). A child's head that emerges at birth covered with the caul.

caput hu·me·ra·le mus·cu·li ex·ten·so·ris car·pi ul·na·ris (hew·mur·ay'lee mus'kew·lye ecks·ten·so'ris kahr'pye ul·nair'is) [NA]. The humeral head of the extensor carpi ulnaris muscle.

caput humerale musculi fle·xo·ris car·pi ul·na·ris (fleck·so'ris kahr'pye ul·nair'is) [NA]. The humeral head of the flexor carpi ulnaris muscle which arises from the medial epicondyle of the humerus.

caput humerale musculi flexoris di·gi·to·rum sub·li·mis (dij·i·to'rum sub·lye'mis) [BNA]. CAPUT HUMEROULNARE MUSCULI FLEXORIS DIGITORUM SUPERFICIALIS.

caput humerale musculi pro·na·to·ris te·re·tis (pro·nuh·to'ris te·ree'tis) [NA]. The humeral head of the pronator teres muscle which arises from the medial epicondyle of the humerus.

caput hu·me·ri (hew'mur·eye) [NA]. The head of the humerus which articulates with the glenoid cavity of the scapula.

caput hu·me·ro·ul·na·re mus·cu·li flex·o·ris di·gi·to·rum su·per·fi·ci·a·lis (hew''mur·o·ul·nair'ee mus'kew·lye fleck·so'ris dij·i·to'rum sue''pur·fish·ee·ay'lis) [NA]. The humeroulnar head of the muscle which arises from the medial epicondyle of the humerus and the proximal part of the ulna.

caput in·fra·or·bi·ta·le mus·cu·li qua·dra·ti la·bii (in''fruh·or·

bi·tay'lee mus'kew·lye kwah·dray'tye lay'bee·eye) [BNA]. Musculus levator labii superioris (= LEVATOR LABII SUPERIORIS).

caput la·te·ra·le mus·cu·li gas·tro·cne·mii (lat·e·ray'lee mus'kew·lye gas"tro·k'nee'mee·eye) [NA]. The lateral head of the gastrocnemius muscle which arises from the back of the lateral condyle of the femur.

caput laterale musculi tri·ci·pi·tis bra·chii (trye·sip'i·tis bray'kee·eye) [NA]. The lateral head of the triceps brachii muscle which arises from the posterolateral surface of the humerus lateral to the groove for the radial nerve.

caput lon·gum mus·cu·li bi·ci·pi·tis bra·chii (long'gum mus'kew·lye bye·sip'i·tis bray'kee·eye) [NA]. The long head of the muscle which arises from the supraglenoid tubercle of the scapula.

caput longum musculi bicipitis fe·mo·ris (fem'o·ris) [NA]. The long head of the muscle which arises from the tuberosity of the ischium.

caput longum musculi tri·ci·pi·tis bra·chii (trye·sip'i·tis bray'kee·eye) [NA]. The long head of the triceps brachii muscle which arises from the infraglenoid tubercle of the humerus.

caput mal·lei (mal'ee·eye) [NA]. The head of the malleus.

caput man·di·bu·lae (man·dib'yoo·lee) [NA]. The head of the mandible, the proximal portion of each condylar process which articulates, respectively, with the right and left temporal bones.

caput me·di·a·le mus·cu·li gas·tro·cne·mii (mee·dee·ay'lee mus'kew·lye gas"tro·k'nee'mee·eye) [NA]. The medial head of the gastrocnemius muscle which arises from the back of the medial condyle of the femur.

caput mediale musculi tri·ci·pi·tis bra·chii (trye·sip'i·tis bray'kee·eye) [NA]. The medial head of the triceps brachii muscle which arises from the posterior aspect of the humerus medial to the groove for the radial nerve.

caput me·du·sae (me·dew'see). Dilatation of the periumbilical venous plexus, with blood flowing away from the umbilicus; seen with portal hypertension.

caput mus·cu·li (mus'kew·lye) [NA]. The head of a muscle.

caput nu·clei cau·da·ti (new'klee·eye kaw·day'tye) [NA]. The head of the caudate nucleus.

caput ob·li·quum mus·cu·li ad·duc·to·ris hal·lu·cis (ob·lye'kwum mus'kew·lye a·duck·to'ris hal'yoo·sis) [NA]. The oblique head of the adductor hallucis muscle. See Table of Muscles in the Appendix.

caput obliquum musculi adductoris pol·li·cis (pol'i·sis) [NA]. The oblique head of the adductor pollicis muscle which arises from the capitate bone and adjacent portions of the second and third metacarpals. See also Table of Muscles in the Appendix.

caput ob·sti·pum (ob'sti·pum). TORTICOLLIS.

caput os·sis me·ta·car·pa·lis (oss'is met"uh·kahr·pay'lis) [NA]. The head of a metacarpal bone, the distal end.

caput ossis me·ta·tar·sa·lis (met"uh·tahr·say'lis) [NA]. The head of a metatarsal bone, the distal end.

caput pan·cre·a·tis (pan·kree'uh·tis) [NA]. The head of the pancreas, the portion lying within the concavity of the duodenum.

caput pha·lan·gis ma·nus (fa·lan'jis man'oos) [NA]. The head of any phalanx of the digits of the hand, the distal end of each one.

caput phalangis pe·dis (ped'is) [NA]. The head of any phalanx of the digits of the foot, the distal end of each one.

caput pro·fun·dum mus·cu·li flex·o·ris pol·li·cis bre·vis (pro·fun'dum mus'kew·lye fleck·so'ris pol'i·sis brev'is) [NA]. The deep head of the flexor pollicis brevis muscle.

caput qua·dra·tum (kwah·dray'tum). A deformity of the head in rickets, manifested by a flattened top and sides, with projecting occiput and prominent frontal bosses.

caput ra·di·a·le mus·cu·li flex·o·ris di·gi·to·rum su·per·fi·ci·a·lis (ray·dee·ay'lee mus'kew·lye fleck·so'ris dij·i·to'rum sue"pur·fish·ee·ay'lis) [NA]. The radial head of the muscle which arises from a small area in the volar aspect of the proximal part of the radius.

caput ra·dii (ray'dee·eye) [NA]. The head of the radius.

caput sta·pe·dis (sta·pee'dis) [NA]. The head of the stapes, the portion which articulates with the long crus of the incus.

caput suc·ce·da·ne·um (suck"se·day'nee·um). Swelling of the presenting part of the head of the fetus, produced during labor, and resulting in edema and varying degrees of hemorrhage of the scalp.

caput su·per·fi·ci·a·le mus·cu·li flex·o·ris pol·li·cis bre·vis (sue"pur·fish·ee·ay'lee mus'kew·lye fleck·so'ris pol'i·sis brev'is) [NA]. The superficial head of the flexor pollicis brevis muscle.

caput ta·li (tay'lye) [NA]. The head of the talus, which articulates with the navicular.

caput trans·ver·sum mus·cu·li ad·duc·to·ris hal·lu·cis (trans·vur'sum mus'kew·lye a·duck·to'ris hal'yoo·sis) [NA]. The transverse head of the adductor hallucis muscle; ADDUCTOR HALLUCIS TRANSVERSUS.

caput transversum musculi adductoris pol·li·cis (pol'i·sis) [NA]. The transverse head of the adductor pollicis muscle which arises from the ridge on the palmar surface of the third metacarpal.

caput ul·nae (ul'nee) [NA]. The head of the ulna, the distal end.

caput ul·na·re mus·cu·li ex·ten·so·ris car·pi ul·na·ris (ul·nair'ee mus'kew·lye ecks·ten·so'ris kahr'pye ul·nair'is) [NA]. The ulnar head of the extensor carpi ulnaris muscle.

caput ulnare musculi flex·o·ris car·pi ul·na·ris (fleck·so'ris kahr'pye ul·nair'is) [NA]. The ulnar head of the muscle which arises from the medial margin of the ulna.

caput ulnare musculi pro·na·to·ris te·re·tis (pro"nay·to'ris te·ree'tis) [NA]. The ulnar head of the muscle which arises from the coronoid process of the ulna.

caput zy·go·ma·ti·cum mus·cu·li qua·dra·ti la·bii su·pe·ri·o·ris (zye·go·mat'i·kum mus'kew·lye kwah·dray'tye lay'bee·eye sue·peer"ee·o'ris) [BNA]. Musculus zygomaticus minor. See *zygomatic* in the Table of Muscles in the Appendix.

CAR Abbreviation for *conditioned avoidance response.*

Ca·ra·bel·li's cusp or **tubercle** (kah·rah·bel'ee) [G. C. *Carabelli,* Austrian dentist, 1787–1842]. The fifth cusp occurring on the mesiolingual surface of upper first molar teeth, always bilateral; it is not always present.

car·a·mel (kăr'uh·mul) *n.* A pharmaceutical coloring aid composed of burnt sugar which has partially carbonized.

car·am·i·phen (kahr·am'i·fen) *n.* 1-Phenylcyclopentanecarboxylic acid 2-diethylaminoethyl ester, $C_{18}H_{27}NO_2$, a parasympatholytic drug; used as the hydrochloride salt in the treatment of parkinsonism.

car·a·pace (kăr'uh·pace) *n.* [F.]. A chitinous or bony shield covering the entire back or a portion of the back of certain animals.

ca·ra·te (ka·rah'teh) *n.* [Quechua]. PINTA.

car·a·way (kăr'a·way) *n.* [Ar. *karawyā,* from Gk. *karon*]. The dried fruit of *Carum carvi;* the characteristic odor and taste are imparted by volatile oil. Has been used as a stomachic and carminative.

caraway oil. The volatile oil distilled from the fruit of *Carum carvi;* contains 50 to 60% carvone. Used as a flavor.

carb-, carbo- [L. *carbo,* coal, charcoal]. A combining form meaning (a) *carbon;* (b) *carbonic;* (c) *carboxyl.*

car·ba·chol (kahr'buh·kole, ·kol) *n.* Carbamoylcholine chloride, $C_6H_{15}ClN_2O_2$, a choline ester with potent parasympathomimetic action; now employed primarily as a miotic in the local treatment of glaucoma.

car·ba·cryl·a·mine resins (kahr"buh·kril'uh·meen). A mixture of the cation exchangers carbacrylic resin and potassium carbacrylic resin and the anion exchanger polyamine-methylene resin; used as an adjunct to increase fecal excretion of sodium.

car·ba·cryl·ic resin (kahr"buh·kril'ick). The hydrogen form of cross-linked polyacrylic polycarboxylic cation exchange resins. Such a resin is useful clinically for its ability to remove sodium from intestinal fluid by a process of exchange with hydrogen in the resin; absorption of potassium by the resin is compensated for by inclusion of some potassium carbacrylate while the acidity resulting from liberation of hydrogen ion is neutralized with polyamine-methylene resin. See also *carbacrylamine resins.*

car·ba·dox (kahr'buh·docks) *n.* Methyl 3-(2-quinoxalinyl-methylene)carbazate N^1,N^4-dioxide, $C_{11}H_{10}N_4O_4$, an antibacterial agent.

car·ba·mate (kahr'buh·mate, kahr·bam'ate) *n.* A salt of carbamic acid; it contains the univalent radical NH_2COO. See also *urethan.*

car·bam·az·e·pine (kahr''bam·az'e·peen) *n.* 5*H*-Dibenz[*b,f*]azepine-5-carboxamide, $C_{15}H_{12}N_2O$, an anticonvulsant drug.

car·bam·ic acid (kahr·bam'ick). Aminoformic acid, NH_2COOH, the monoamide of carbonic acid; occurs only in the form of salts and esters; the latter are known as urethanes.

car·bam·ide (kahr·bam'ide, kahr'buh·mide) *n.* UREA.

car·bam·i·dine (kahr·bam'i·deen, ·din) *n.* GUANIDINE.

carb·ami·no compound (kahr''buh·mee'no, kahr·bam'i·no). A type of compound formed by the combination of carbon dioxide with a free amino group in an amino acid or a protein. Carbaminohemoglobin, which plays an important role in carbon dioxide transport by the blood, is a carbamino compound formed by the combination of hemoglobin and carbon dioxide.

carb·ami·no·he·mo·glo·bin, carb·ami·no·hae·mo·glo·bin (kahr''buh·mee''no·hee'muh·glo''bin) *n.* [*carb-* + *amino* + *hemoglobin*]. Hemoglobin united with carbon dioxide.

car·bam·o·yl (kahr·bam'o·il) *n.* CARBAMYL.

car·bam·yl (kahr·bam'il) *n.* The univalent radical NH_2CO— of carbamic acid, NH_2COOH.

car·bam·y·la·tion (kahr·bam''i·lay'shun) *n.* The process of adding a carbamyl group (NH_2CO—) to an amino group by interaction with carbamyl phosphate.

carbamyl phosphate $NH_2COOPO_3H_2$. A transfer form for the carbamyl group (NH_2CO—), as in the synthesis of citrulline from ornithine.

car·bam·yl·urea (kahr·bam'il·yoo·ree'uh) *n.* BIURET.

carb·an·i·on (kahrb·an'eye·on) *n.* An organic ion carrying a negative charge at a carbon atom. Contr. *carbonium.*

car·ban·tel (kahr'ban''tel) *n.* 1-(*p*-Chlorophenyl)-3-valerimidoylurea, $C_{12}H_{16}ClN_3O$, an anthelmintic, usually used as the lauryl sulfate salt, $C_{24}H_{42}ClN_3O_5S$.

car·bar·sone (kahr·bahr'sone) *n.* *p*-Ureidobenzenearsonic acid, $C_7H_9AsN_2O_4$, a pentavalent arsenical formerly used in the treatment of intestinal amebiasis and *Trichomonas* vaginitis.

car·ba·sus (kahr'buh·sus) *n.* [L., from Gk. *karpasos,* flax]. Gauze; thin muslin used in surgery.

carbasus ab·sor·bens (ab·sor'benz). Absorbent gauze.

carbasus absorbens ad·hae·si·va (ad·hee·sigh'vuh). Adhesive absorbent gauze.

carbasus absorbens ster·i·lis (sterr'i·lis). Sterile absorbent gauze.

carbasus car·bo·la·ta (kahr·bo·lay'tuh). Carbolated gauze.

carbasus io·do·for·ma·ta (eye·o''do·for·may'tuh). Iodoform gauze.

car·baz·o·chrome (kahr·baz'o·krome) *n.* Adrenochrome monosemicarbazone, $C_{10}H_{12}N_4O_3$; used in the form of a complex with sodium salicylate as a systemic hemostatic in capillary bleeding.

car·ba·zole (kahr'buh·zole) *n.* Diphenylenimine, $C_{12}H_9N$, a reagent for sugars.

car·ben·i·cil·lin (kahr·ben''i·sil'in) *n.* α-Carboxybenzylpenicillin, $C_{17}H_{18}N_2O_6S$, a semisynthetic penicillin with a wide spectrum of activity against gram-negative bacteria, especially *Pseudomonas;* administered parenterally, as the disodium salt.

carbenicillin indanyl sodium. An ester of the monosodium salt of carbenicillin and 2,3-dihydroindan-5-ol.

carbenicillin phenyl sodium. The phenyl ester of the monosodium salt of carbenicillin.

car·be·nox·o·lone (kahr·be·nock'suh·lone) *n.* 3β-Hydroxy-11-oxoolean-12-en-30-oic acid hydrogen succinate, $C_{34}H_{50}O_7$, an antibacterial usually used as the disodium salt.

car·be·ta·pen·tane (kahr·bay''tuh·pen'tane) *n.* 2-(Diethylaminoethoxy)ethyl 1-phenylcyclopentyl-1-carboxylate, $C_{20}H_{31}NO_3$, an antitussive drug; used as the citrate salt.

carb·he·mo·glo·bin, carb·hae·mo·glo·bin (kahrb''hee'muh·glo''bin) *n.* CARBAMINOHEMOGLOBIN.

car·bi·do·pa (kahr·bi·do'puh) *n.* (−)-L-α-Hydrazino-3,4-dihydroxy-α-methylhydrocinnamic acid monohydrate, $C_{10}H_{14}N_2O_4 \cdot H_2O$, an antihypertensive agent.

car·bi·nol (kahr'bi·nol) *n.* METHYL ALCOHOL.

car·bin·ox·a·mine (kahr''bin·ock'suh·meen) *n.* 2-[*p*-Chloro-α-(2-dimethylaminoethoxy)benzyl]pyridine, $C_{16}H_{19}ClN_2O$, an antihistaminic drug; used as the maleate salt.

car·bi·phene (kahr'bi·feen) *n.* 2-Ethoxy-*N*-methyl-*N*-[2-(methylphenethylamino)ethyl]-2,2-diphenylacetamide, $C_{28}H_{34}N_2O_2$, an analgesic; used as the hydrochloride salt.

Carbitol. 1. Trademark for diethylene glycol monoethyl ether, $C_6H_{14}O_3$, used principally as a solvent. 2. Trademark for various ethers of diethylene glycol, the specific ether being indicated by a qualifying adjective, such as methyl or butyl.

carbo-. See *carb-.*

car·bo·ben·zoxy chloride (kahr''bo·ben·zock'see). Benzyl chloroformate, $C_8H_7ClO_2$, used in peptide synthesis to combine with and protect amino groups.

Carbocaine. Trademark for mepivacaine, a local anesthetic; used as the hydrochloride salt.

car·bo·clor·al (kahr''bo·klor'al) *n.* Ethyl (2,2,2-trichloro-1-hydroxyethyl)carbamate, $C_5H_8Cl_3NO_3$, a hypnotic.

car·bo·cy·clic (kahr''bo·sigh'click, ·sick'lick) *adj.* [*carbo-* + *cyclic*]. *In chemistry,* pertaining to compounds of the closed-chain type in which all the ring atoms are carbon. See also *heterocyclic, homocyclic.*

car·bo·cys·teine (kahr·bo·sis'teen) *n.* *S*-(Carboxymethyl)cysteine, $C_5H_9NO_4S$, a mucolytic agent.

Carbogen. Trademark for mixture of 95% oxygen and 5% carbon dioxide used as a respiratory stimulant.

car·bo·he·mo·glo·bin, car·bo·hae·mo·glo·bin (kahr''bo·hee'muh·glo''bin) *n.* CARBAMINOHEMOGLOBIN.

car·bo·hy·drase (kahr''bo·high'drace, ·draze) *n.* [*carbohydr*ate + *-ase*]. An enzyme capable of converting higher carbohydrates into simple sugars.

car·bo·hy·drate (kahr''bo·high'drate) *n.* [*carbo-* + *hydrate*]. An organic substance belonging to the class of compounds represented by the sugars, dextrins, starches, and celluloses; it contains carbon, hydrogen, and oxygen. Formerly it was believed that hydrogen and oxygen were always present in the proportion found in water; but this is not always the case. The carbohydrates form a large class of organic compounds; they may be further classified into monosaccharides, disaccharides, trisaccharides, oligosaccharides, and polysaccharides.

carbohydrate-induced hyperlipemia. 1. FAMILIAL HYPERBETA- AND HYPERPREBETALIPOPROTEINEMIA. 2. FAMILIAL HYPERPREBETALIPOPROTEINEMIA.

carbohydrate-induced hypertriglyceridemia. CARBOHYDRATE-INDUCED HYPERLIPEMIA.

car·bo·hy·drat·u·ria (kahr·bo·high''dray·tew'ree·uh) *n.* The presence of an abnormally large proportion of carbohydrates in the urine; glycosuria.

carbol-. A combining form meaning *phenol.*

carbol-aniline fuchsin stain. A reagent for Negri bodies, which are stained crimson by treatment with a solution containing phenol, aniline, and basic fuchsin and afterward with a solution of methylene blue. Syn. *Goodpasture's stain.*

car·bo·late (kahr'bo·late) *n. & v.* 1. PHENATE. 2. To impregnate with phenol.

carbol-fuchsin solution. A solution of phenol, basic fuchsin, and resorcinol in a solvent medium of acetone, alcohol, and water; used topically as an antifugal preparation. Syn. *Castellani's paint.*

carbol-fuchsin stain. A solution containing phenol and basic fuchsin, used for staining tubercle bacilli and other acid-fast bacteria.

car·bol·ic acid (kahr·bol'ick). PHENOL.

car·bo·li·gase (kahr''bo·lye'gace, ·gaze) *n.* An enzyme in animal and plant tissue which converts pyruvic acid to acetylmethylcarbinol.

car·bo·lism (kahr'buh·liz·um) *n.* [*carbol*ic + *-ism*]. Phenol poisoning.

car·bo·lize (kahr'bo·lize) *v.* CARBOLATE (2).

car·bo·lu·ria (kahr''bo·lew'ree·uh) *n.* [*carbol*ic + *-uria*]. The presence of phenol in the urine, producing a dark discoloration.

car·bo·mer (kahr'bo·mur) *n.* A polymer of acrylic acid, cross-linked with a polyfunctional agent, that is used for preparing suspensions and as an emulsifying agent.

carbomer 934P. Official name for carbomer.

car·bo·my·cin (kahr''bo·migh'sin) *n.* [*carbo-* + *-mycin*]. An antibiotic substance, $C_{42}H_{67}NO_{16}$, produced by selected strains of *Streptomyces halstedii.* Possesses inhibitory activity especially against gram-positive bacteria, but is also active against certain rickettsiae and large viruses. It has been used to treat patients who have become resistant to penicillin and other antibiotics.

car·bon (kahr'bun) *n.* [L. *carbo,* charcoal]. C = 12.011. A nonmetallic element widely distributed in nature. Its three allotropic forms are exemplified by the diamond, graphite, and charcoal. It occurs in all organic compounds; the ability of its atoms to link to each other affords an innumerable variety of combinations. See also Table of Elements in the Appendix.

car·bo·na·ceous (kahr''buh·nay'shus) *adj.* Of, pertaining to, consisting of, or yielding carbon.

carbon arc lamp. A source of therapeutic light produced by an electric arc between carbon electrodes. It contains a mixture of wavelengths from 2200 to 40,000 angstroms. The intensity of wavelengths may be altered by impregnation of the carbon electrodes with different salts.

[1]car·bon·ate (kahr'buh·nate, ·nut) *n.* [*carbon* + *-ate*]. The divalent radical CO_3; any salt or ester containing this radical, as salts or esters of carbonic acid.

[2]car·bon·ate (kahr'buh·nate) *v.* To charge with carbon dioxide.

carbon bisulfide. CARBON DISULFIDE.

carbon black. Finely divided carbon obtained by the incomplete combustion of natural gas, animal tissues, oils, wood, or other organic substances.

carbon cycle. The cyclic process of carbon in living organisms, consisting of the photosynthesis of carbohydrate from carbon dioxide, the metabolic reactions of carbohydrates, fats, and proteins in plants and animals, and the ultimate conversion of the carbon of these compounds to carbon dioxide.

carbon dioxide. CO_2, an odorless, colorless, noncombustible gas; a waste product of aerobic metabolism excreted via the blood in the pulmonary capillaries into the lung alveoli. It is an essential component of the blood buffer system and the prime physiologic stimulant of the respiratory center in the medulla oblongata. See also Table of Chemical Constituents of Blood in the Appendix.

carbon dioxide absorption anesthesia. CLOSED ANESTHESIA.

carbon dioxide acidosis. RESPIRATORY ACIDOSIS.

carbon dioxide snow. Solid carbon dioxide used medicinally as an escharotic and commercially as a refrigerant. Syn. *dry ice.*

carbon dioxide therapy. 1. *In psychiatry,* a form of shock treatment in which carbon dioxide is administered by inhalation until profound physiologic changes, including convulsions, occur. 2. *In dermatology,* the application of solid carbon dioxide to lesions for purposes of extirpation by deep freezing.

carbon disulfide. A colorless or slightly yellow, highly flammable liquid, CS_2; has been used externally as a counterirritant. A solvent of wide application.

car·bon·ic acid (kahr·bon'ick). A feebly ionizing acid, H_2CO_3, formed when carbon dioxide is dissolved in water.

carbonic acid gas. CARBON DIOXIDE.

carbonic anhydrase. An enzyme containing zinc, found in erythrocytes and in tissues, which catalyzes the reaction $H_2O + CO_2 \rightleftharpoons H_2CO_3$. In the transport of CO_2 in the body, the reaction proceeds to the right in the tissues and to the left in the lungs, and in each instance is catalyzed by carbonic anhydrase.

car·bo·ni·um (kahr·bo'nee·um) *n.* An organic ion positively charged at a carbon atom in consequence of electron deficiency. Contr. *carbanion.*

car·bon·iza·tion (kahr''bun·i·zay'shun) *n.* 1. Decomposition of organic compounds by heat in the absence of air, driving off the volatile matter and leaving the carbon. 2. Charring. —**car·bon·ize** (kahr'bun·ize) *v.*

carbon monoxide. A colorless, odorless, poisonous gas, CO, resulting from the combustion of carbonaceous compounds in an insufficient supply of oxygen. It combines firmly with hemoglobin, preventing subsequent union with oxygen. See also *carboxyhemoglobin.*

car·bon·om·e·ter (kahr''bun·om'e·tur) *n.* An apparatus for measuring the amount of carbon dioxide in a room or in exhaled breath. —**carbonome·try** (·tree) *n.*

carbon tetrachloride. Tetrachloromethane, CCl_4, a colorless, nonflammable liquid, active as an anthelmintic, especially against hookworm. Used as a fire extinguisher, a solvent, and an insecticide.

carbon tetrachloride method. A method for separating pollen in which partially dried staminate flowers are soaked in carbon tetrachloride and gently beaten with a pestle to loosen the pollen from the anthers. This is strained through muslin, which passes only the carbon tetrachloride and pollen. The desired pollen is then obtained by passing the suspension through a fine filter.

car·bon·uria (kahr''buh·new'ree·uh) *n.* The presence of carbon compounds in the urine, particularly carbon dioxide.

car·bon·yl (kahr'bon·il, ·eel) *n.* [*carbon* + *-yl*]. The divalent organic radical CO.

carbonyl chloride. PHOSGENE.

Carbopol. A trademark for carbomer.

Carbo-Resin. Trademark for a sodium-excreting composition of carbacrylamine resins.

Carborundum. A trademark for silicon carbide, SiC, a substance of extreme hardness.

Carbose D. A trademark for carboxymethylcellulose sodium.

Carbowax. Trademark for certain polyethylene glycols, of the general formula $HOCH_2(CH_2OCH_2)_xCH_2OH$, having a molecular weight above 1000. They are waxlike solids, soluble in water and in many organic solvents; employed in some ointment bases, also for embedding and sectioning of tissue for certain histologic studies.

Carboxide. Trademark for a mixture of ethylene oxide and carbon dioxide used as a fumigant.

car·boxy·bi·o·tin (kahr·bock''see·bye'o·tin) *n.* The form of biotin that has carbon dioxide bonded to it during intermediary metabolism and in decarboxylation reactions.

car·boxy·he·mo·glo·bin, car·boxy·hae·mo·glo·bin (kahr·bock''see·hee'mo·glo''bin, ·hem'o·glo''bin) *n.* [*carb-* + *oxy-* + *hemoglobin*]. The compound formed with hemoglobin by carbon monoxide in the blood. The hemoglobin thus bound is unavailable for oxygen transport because its reaction with carbon monoxide is reversible only at an extremely slow rate.

car·boxy·he·mo·glo·bi·ne·mia, car·boxy·hae·mo·glo·bi·nae·mia (kahr·bock″see·hee″mo·glo″bi·nee′mee·uh) *n.* [*carboxyhemoglobin* + *-emia*]. The presence in the blood of carboxyhemoglobin, or of excessive carboxyhemoglobin, with or without clinical evidence of poisoning.

car·box·yl (kahr·bock′sil) *n.* [*carb-* + *ox-* + *-yl*]. The group COOH characteristic of organic acids. The hydrogen can be replaced by metals, forming salts.

car·box·yl·ase (kahr·bock′sil·ace, ·aze) *n.* [*carboxyl* + *-ase*]. 1. Any of a group of enzymes catalyzing the addition of CO_2 to appropriate acceptors; nearly all have biotin as a prothetic group. 2. Formerly, DECARBOXYLASE.

car·box·yl·ic acid (kahr″bock·sil′ick). An acid containing the COOH group.

Carboxymethocel. Trademark for the sodium salt of carboxymethylcellulose.

car·boxy·meth·yl·cel·lu·lose (kahr·bock″see·meth″il·sel′yoo·loce) *n.* A polycarboxymethyl ether of cellulose, available as the sodium salt, a white powder dispersible in water to form viscous solutions useful for their thickening, suspending, and stabilizing properties; when in the form of a negatively charged resin, it is used as a cation exchanger in ion-exchange chromatography. Abbreviated, CM-cellulose.

car·boxy·myo·glo·bin (kahr·bock″see·migh′o·glo″bin) *n.* [*carb-* + *oxy-* + *myoglobin*]. A relatively rare compound formed by generation of a covalent bond between carbon monoxide and myoglobin. Compare *carboxyhemoglobin.*

car·boxy·pep·ti·dase (kahr·bock″see·pep′ti·dace, ·daze) *n.* [*carb-* + *oxy-* + *peptidase*]. An enzyme, widely distributed but found especially in pancreatic juice, capable of catalyzing hydrolysis of polypeptides at the terminus having a free carboxyl group, producing an amino acid and a smaller peptide which may undergo further hydrolysis under the influence of the enzyme.

car·boxy·poly·pep·ti·dase (kahr·bock″see·pol″ee·pep′ti·dace, ·daze) *n.* CARBOXYPEPTIDASE.

car·bro·mal (kahr′bro·mal, kahr·bro′mul) *n.* Bromodiethylacetylurea, $C_7H_{13}BrN_2O_2$, a white, crystalline powder, very slightly soluble in water; used as a sedative and mild hypnotic.

car·bun·cle (kahr′bunk·ul) *n.* [L. *carbunculus,* tumor]. An extensive, deep-seated, spreading, stubborn infection, usually staphylococcal, of skin and underlying tissues, usually situated on the back of the neck or on the back, with numerous irregular intercommunicating and coalescing abscesses, some of which discharge through multiple external openings. —**car·bun·cu·lar** (kahr·bunk′yoo·lur) *adj.*

car·bun·cu·lo·sis (kahr·bunk″yoo·lo′sis) *n.* A condition characterized by the formation of carbuncles in rapid succession or simultaneously.

car·bu·ter·ol (kahr·byoo′tur·ol) *n.* [5-[2-(*tert*-Butylamino)-1-hydroxyethyl]-2-hydroxyphenyl]urea, $C_{13}H_{21}N_3O_3$, a bronchodilator usually employed as the hydrochloride.

car·byl·a·mine (kahr″bil·uh·meen′) *n.* ISOCYANIDE.

carbylamine reaction. A test for primary amines, in which a characteristic unpleasant odor of an isocyanide is evolved on heating the amine with chloroform and an alcoholic solution of potassium hydroxide.

Carcholin. A trademark for carbachol.

carcin-, carcino- [Gk. *karkinos,* lit., crab]. A combining form meaning *cancer.*

carcino-. See *carcin-.*

car·ci·no·cy·the·mia (kahr″si·no·sigh·thee′mee·uh) *n.* [*carcino-* + *cyt-* + *-hemia*]. The presence of large numbers of carcinoma cells in the peripheral blood, at times giving the appearance of leukemia.

car·ci·no·em·bry·on·ic (kahr″si·no·em·bree·on′ick) *adj.* Pertaining to or characteristic of both embryos and carcinomas.

carcinoembryonic antigen. A glycoprotein present in malignant endodermal tissue, fetal colonic mucosa, and in the blood plasma of patients with cancer of the gastrointestinal tract. Useful in monitoring response to gastrointestinal cancer therapy, since tumor-related plasma levels tend to correlate with tumor mass. Abbreviated, CEA.

car·ci·no·fe·tal (kahr″si·no·fee′tul) *adj.* Pertaining to or characteristic of both carcinomas and fetuses. Compare *carcinoembryonic, oncofetal.*

car·ci·no·gen (kahr′si·no·jen, kahr·sin′o·jen) *n.* [*carcino-* + *-gen*]. Any agent or substance which produces cancer, accelerates the development of cancer, or acts upon a population to change its total frequency of cancer in terms of numbers of tumors or distribution by site and age. —**car·ci·no·gen·ic** (kahr″si·no·jen′ick) *adj.;* **carcino·ge·nic·i·ty** (·je·nis′i·tee) *n.*

car·ci·no·gen·e·sis (kahr″si·no·jen′e·sis) *n.* [*carcino-* + *-genesis*]. Origin or production of cancer. —**carcino·ge·net·ic** (·je·net′ick) *adj.*

car·ci·noid (kahr′si·noid) *n.* [*carcin-* + *-oid*]. A tumor arising from the argentaffin cells of the gastrointestinal tract or sometimes from a bronchus, which occasionally metastasizes, producing the carcinoid syndrome.

car·ci·noid·o·sis (kahr″si·noy·do′sis) *n.* CARCINOID SYNDROME.

carcinoid syndrome. Skin flushing, diarrhea, wheezing, and fibrosis of the right-sided cardiac structures; resulting from metastasis of a carcinoid tumor to the liver, and high levels of blood serotonin. Syn. *carcinoidosis.*

car·ci·no·ma (kahr″si·no′muh) *n.*, pl. **carcinomas, carcinoma·ta** (·tuh) [Gk. *karkinōma,* cancer, from *karkinos,* lit., crab]. A malignant tumor whose parenchyma is composed of anaplastic epithelial cells. Contr. *sarcoma.* See also *adenocarcinoma, basal cell carcinoma, carcinoma simplex, intermediate-cell carcinoma, squamous cell carcinoma.*

carcinoma bron·chi·o·lo·rum (brong″kee·o·lo′rum). BRONCHIOLAR CARCINOMA.

carcinoma in situ. A growth disturbance of epithelial surfaces in which normal cells are replaced by anaplastic cells that show no behavioral characteristics of cancer, such as invasion and metastasis.

carcinoma mu·co·cel·lu·la·re ova·rii (mew″ko·sel·yoo·lair′ee o·vair′ee·eye). KRUKENBERG'S TUMOR.

carcinoma oc·cul·ta (o·kul′tuh). A carcinoma which remains unsuspected until metastases occur.

carcinoma sim·plex (sim′plecks). A carcinoma in which differentiation is absent or poor; usually a cylindrical-cell carcinoma, but may be derived from epidermis or other lining epithelium.

carcinoma sub·stan·ti·ae cor·ti·ca·lis su·pra·re·na·lis (sub·stan′chee·ee kor·ti·kay′lis sue″pruh·re·nay′lis). An adrenal cortical carcinoma.

car·ci·nom·a·toid (kahr″si·nom′uh·toid, ·no′muh·toid) *adj.* & *n.* 1. Resembling a carcinoma. 2. *In experimental oncology,* epithelial proliferation in induced papillomas without invasion of adjacent tissue.

car·ci·no·ma·toi·des al·ve·o·ge·ni·ca mul·ti·cen·tri·ca (kahr″si·no″muh·toy′deez al″vee·o·jen′i·kuh mul″ti·sen′tri·kuh). BRONCHIOLAR CARCINOMA.

car·ci·nom·a·to·pho·bia (kahr″si·nom″uh·to·fo′bee·uh) *n.* CARCINOPHOBIA.

car·ci·no·ma·to·sis (kahr″si·no″muh·to′sis) *n.* [*carcinoma* + *-osis*]. Widespread dissemination of carcinoma throughout the body.

car·ci·nom·a·tous (kahr″si·nom′uh·tus) *adj.* Pertaining to or having the characteristics of a carcinoma.

carcinomatous cerebellar degeneration. A nonmetastatic effect of carcinoma taking the form of a diffuse degeneration of the cerebellar cortex and deep cerebellar nuclei, often accompanied by affection of brainstem nuclei and posterior and lateral colums of the spinal cord, and by pleocytosis.

carcinomatous dermatitis. Reddening of the skin, usually of the breast, associated with a carcinoma. See also *inflammatory carcinoma.*

carcinomatous mastitis. A variety of breast cancer which clinically resembles inflammation.

carcinomatous myelopathy. A rare effect of carcinoma on the spinal cord, independent of metastases or neoplastic compression; characterized by subacute degeneration of the posterior and lateral columns and often associated with cerebellar degeneration.

carcinomatous myopathy. Nonmetastatic affection of muscle, taking the form of polymyostitis, dermatomyostitis, or myasthenic syndrome in association with carcinoma, most often of the lung.

carcinomatous neuropathy or **polyneuropathy.** A subacute or chronic sensory or sensorimotor polyneuropathy, occurring as a remote effect of carcinoma and characterized pathologically by a noninflammatory degeneration of the peripheral nerves and dorsal root ganglia and roots and by an elevation of cerebrospinal fluid protein.

car·ci·no·pho·bia (kahr″si·no·fo′bee·uh) *n.* [*carcino-* + *-phobia*]. Obsessive or hypochondriacal fear of cancer.

car·ci·no·sar·co·ma (kahr″si·no·sahr·ko′muh) *n.* A tumor having the characteristics of carcinoma and sarcoma; a malignant mixed mesodermal tumor. Compare *collision tumor.*

car·ci·no·sis (kahr″si·no′sis) *n.*, pl. **carcino·ses** (·seez) [Gk. *karkinōsis,* development of cancer]. CARCINOMATOSIS.

car·da·mom (kahr′duh·mum, ·mom) *n.* [Gk. *kardamōmon*]. The dried, ripe fruit or seed of *Elettaria cardamomum,* a plant of the ginger family of China and the East Indies. Contains a volatile oil, which imparts a characteristic odor and flavor. Has been used as a carminative and stomachic.

cardamom oil. The volatile oil distilled from the seeds of *Elettaria cardamomum;* used as a flavor.

Car·den's amputation [H. D. *Carden,* English surgeon, b. 1872]. A single-flap operation cutting through the condyles of the femur just above the articular surface.

cardi-, cardio- [Gk. *kardia*]. A combining form meaning (a) *heart, cardiac;* (b) *cardial.*

car·dia (kahr′dee·uh) *n.*, pl. **car·di·ae** (·dee·ee), **cardias** [NL., from Gk. *kardia,* heart]. The esophageal orifice and adjacent area of the stomach. See also *cardiac orifice.* Adj. *cardiac, cardial.*

-cardia [*cardi-* + *-ia*]. A combining form designating *a state or condition of the heart.*

car·di·ac (kahr′dee·ack) *adj. & n.* [Gk. *kardiakos,* from *kardia,* heart]. 1. Of or pertaining to the heart. 2. Of or pertaining to the cardia of the stomach. 3. A person with heart disease.

cardiac albuminuria. Proteinuria associated with heart failure.

cardiac aneurysm. Ballooning of a weakened portion of the heart wall, sometimes occurring after coronary occlusion.

cardiac angina. ANGINA PECTORIS.

cardiac antrum. A dilatation sometimes found in the abdominal portion of the esophagus.

cardiac apnea. The temporary period of suspended breathing in Cheyne-Stokes respiration.

cardiac arrest. The cessation of cardiac output and effective circulation either because of ventricular asystole or of ventricular fibrillation.

cardiac asthma. Paroxysmal dyspnea and wheezing, often during sleep, due to left ventricular cardiac failure.

cardiac atrophy. Atrophy of the heart observed especially in chronic, wasting diseases.

cardiac axis. A line passing through the center of the base and apex of the heart.

cardiac catheter. A long flexible tube of inert material designed to be inserted into the heart, usually by way of a peripheral artery or vein, for diagnostic or therapeutic purposes.

cardiac chamber. CHAMBER OF THE HEART.

cardiac cirrhosis. Progressive fibrosis of hepatic central lobular structures as well as of portal spaces, the result of chronic congestive heart failure.

cardiac compression. Cardiac restriction with inability to fill completely, due to pericardial fibrosis or calcification. See also *cardiac tamponade, constrictive pericarditis.*

cardiac cycle. The complete series of events occurring in the heart during systole and diastole.

cardiac diuretic. A substance, such as digitalis, which produces diuresis by increasing the efficiency of the heart in patients with cardiac edema.

cardiac dropsy. CARDIAC EDEMA.

cardiac dyspnea. Dyspnea due to cardiac failure.

cardiac edema. Edema due to the increased capillary and venous pressure of cardiac failure; it is most marked in the dependent parts of the body, particularly the ankles upon standing.

cardiac failure. HEART FAILURE.

cardiac ganglia. Ganglia of the superficial cardiac plexus, located between the aortic arch and the bifurcation of the pulmonary artery. NA *ganglia cardiaca.*

cardiac glands. 1. The glands of the cardia of the stomach. 2. Glands occurring in the esophagus which clearly resemble the glands seen in the cardia of the stomach.

cardiac glycogen storage disease. POMPE'S DISEASE.

cardiac impulse. 1. APEX IMPULSE. 2. Any impulse of the heart transmitted through the chest wall so that it can be seen or felt by an examiner.

cardiac incisure. 1. The angle between the fundus of the stomach and the esophagus. NA *incisura cardiaca ventriculi.* 2. The notch on the anterior border of the left lung occupied by the heart within the pericardium. NA *incisura cardiaca pulmonis sinistri.*

cardiac index. The volume per minute of cardiac output per square meter of body surface area. The normal resting average is 2.2 liters.

cardiac infundibulum. That part of the right ventricle derived from the proximal part of the bulbus cordis of the embryonic heart; the anterosuperior part of the ventricle communicating with the pulmonary trunk.

cardiac massage. Rhythmic compression of the heart, either directly or through the closed chest, in the effort to maintain an effective circulation in cardiac asystole or ventricular fibrillation.

cardiac murmur. Any adventitious sounds or noises heard in the region of the heart, generally classified according to their area of origin and time of occurrence in the cardiac cycle.

cardiac muscle. MYOCARDIUM.

cardiac muscle fibers. The distinctive fibers of cardiac muscle which are characterized by having disks in the myofibrils and by having centrally placed nuclei.

cardiac nerve. See Table of Nerves in the Appendix.

cardiac neurosis. NEUROCIRCULATORY ASTHENIA.

cardiac notch. CARDIAC INCISURE (2).

car·dí·a·co ne·gro (kahr·dee′a·ko neh′gro, kahr·dye′uh·ko) [Sp.]. BLACK CARDIAC.

cardiac orifice. The opening between the esophagus and the stomach. NA *ostium cardiacum.*

cardiac output. The blood volume in liters ejected per minute by the left ventricle.

cardiac plexus. A network of visceral nerves situated at the base of the heart. The superficial part lies beneath the arch of the aorta just anterior to the right pulmonary artery. The deep part of the cardiac plexus lies anterior to the bifurcation of the trachea between it and the arch of the aorta. Each portion contains nerve fibers of both sympathetic and vagal origin. NA *plexus cardiacus.*

cardiac reserve. The ability of the heart to increase its output in the face of increased physiologic demands, as during exercise.

cardiac resuscitation. Restoration of heartbeat after cardiac arrest or fibrillation, by the prompt employment of such measures as cardiac massage, artificial respiration, stimulating drugs, or (when indicated) defibrillation.

cardiac skeleton. SKELETON OF THE HEART.

cardiac souffle. CARDIAC MURMUR.

cardiac sounds. HEART SOUNDS.

cardiac sphincter. The area of high tone in the lower esophagus; an important component of the mechanism of gastroesophageal continence.

cardiac standstill. CARDIAC ARREST.

cardiac tamponade. Compression of the heart by fluid within the pericardium, which hinders venous return, restricts the heart's ability to fill, and produces increased systemic and pulmonary venous pressure and decreased cardiac output. See also *cardiac compression.*

cardiac tonic. A tonic that strengthens the heart muscle.

cardiac tube. The embryonic heart.

car·di·al (kahr'dee·ul) *adj.* [*cardi-* + *-al*]. Of or pertaining to the cardia.

car·di·al·gia (kahr''dee·al'jee·uh) *n.* [*cardi-* + *-algia*]. 1. Pain in the region of the heart. 2. HEARTBURN.

car·di·am·e·ter (kahr''dee·am'e·tur) *n.* [*cardia* + *-meter*]. An apparatus for determining the position of the cardiac orifice of the stomach.

car·di·a·neu·ria (kahr''dee·a·new'ree·uh) *n.* [*cardi-* + *a-* + *neur-* + *-ia*]. *Rare.* Lack of tone in the heart.

car·di·asth·ma (kahr''dee·az'muh) *n.* CARDIAC ASTHMA.

cardia ven·tri·cu·li (ven·trick'yoo·lye). The cardiac portion of the stomach, an indefinite area of the stomach adjacent to the esophagus; CARDIA.

car·di·cen·te·sis (kahr''di·sen·tee'sis) *n.*, pl. **cardicente·ses** (·seez). CARDIOCENTESIS.

Cardidigin. A trademark for digitoxin, a cardiac stimulant.

car·di·ec·ta·sis (kahr''dee·eck'tuh·sis) *n.*, pl. **cardiecta·ses** (·seez) [*cardi-* + *ectasis*]. Dilatation of the heart.

car·di·ec·to·my (kahr''dee·eck'tuh·mee) *n.* [*cardi-* + *-ectomy*]. *Rare.* Excision of the cardiac end of the stomach.

Cardilate. A trademark for erythrityl tetranitrate, a vasodilator and antihypertensive.

car·di·nal eye movements. The eight principal movements of the eye from the primary position gazing straight ahead: to the left, to the right, up, up and to the right or left, down, and down to the right or left.

cardinal flower. A common name for several species of *Lobelia,* chiefly *L. cardinalis.*

cardinal ligament. The lower portion of the broad ligament which is firmly united to the supravaginal portion of the cervix.

cardinal vein. Any one of the common cardinal veins.

cardio-. See *cardi-.*

car·dio·ac·cel·er·a·tor (kahr''dee·o·ack·sel'uh·ray''tur) *adj.* & *n.* [*cardio-* + *accelerator*]. 1. Quickening the action of the heart. 2. An agent which quickens the action of the heart. —**cardioac·cel·er·a·tion** (·sel''ur·ay'shun) *n.*

cardioaccelerator center. 1. SPINAL CARDIOACCELERATOR CENTER. 2. Any one of the three postulated higher centers. The precise locations of these centers are not known; they are thought to be in the floor of the fourth ventricle, in the posterior hypothalamic region, and in the motor and premotor areas of the cerebral cortex.

car·dio·ac·tive (kahr''dee·o·ack'tiv) *adj.* Affecting the heart.

car·dio·an·gi·ol·o·gy (kahr''dee·o·an''jee·ol'uh·jee) *n.* [*cardio-* + *angiology*]. The branch of medicine that is concerned with the heart and blood vessels.

car·dio·aor·tic (kahr''dee·o·ay·or'tick) *adj.* [*cardio-* + *aortic*]. Pertaining to the heart and the aorta.

cardioaortic interval. CARDIOARTERIAL INTERVAL.

car·dio·ar·te·ri·al (kahr''dee·o·ahr·teer'ee·ul) *adj.* [*cardio-* + *arterial*]. Pertaining to the heart and the arteries.

cardioarterial interval. The interval between the apex impulse and the arterial pulsation, measuring the speed of propagation of the pulse wave.

car·dio·asth·ma (kahr''dee·o·az'muh) *n.* CARDIAC ASTHMA.

car·dio·au·di·to·ry (kahr''dee·o·aw'di·tor''ee) *adj.* [*cardio-* + *auditory*]. Pertaining to the heart and the sense of hearing.

cardioauditory syndrome. A recessively inherited defect characterized by sensory deafness, mutism, prolonged QT interval on the electrocardiogram, recurrent syncope, and sudden death, the latter two usually due to ventricular arrhythmia. Syn. *Jervell and Lange-Nielson's syndrome, surdocardiac syndrome.*

car·dio·cele (kahr'dee·o·seel) *n.* [*cardio-* + *-cele*]. Hernia of the heart.

car·dio·cen·te·sis (kahr''dee·o·sen·tee'sis) *n.*, pl. **cardiocente·ses** (·seez) [*cardio-* + *centesis*]. Puncture of a chamber of the heart for diagnosis or therapy.

car·dio·ci·net·ic (kahr''dee·o·si·net'ick) *adj.* CARDIOKINETIC.

car·dio·cir·rho·sis (kahr''dee·o·sirr·o'sis) *n.* CARDIAC CIRRHOSIS.

car·dio·cla·sia (kahr''dee·o·klay'zhuh, ·zee·uh) *n.* CARDIORRHEXIS.

car·di·oc·la·sis (kahr''dee·ock'luh·sis) *n.*, pl. **cardiocla·ses** (·seez) [*cardio-* + *-clasis*]. CARDIORRHEXIS.

car·dio·di·la·tor (kahr''dee·o·dye·lay'tur) *n.* [*cardio-* + *dilator*]. An instrument for dilating the esophageal opening of the stomach.

car·dio·di·o·sis (kahr''dee·o·dee·o'sis, ·dye·o'sis) *n.*, pl. **cardiodio·ses** (·seez) [*cardio-* + Gk. *diōsis,* a forcing open]. Dilatation of the cardiac end of the stomach by means of an instrument passed through the esophagus.

car·dio·dy·nam·ics (kahr''dee·o·dye·nam'icks) *n.* [*cardio-* + *dynamics*]. Kinetic mechanisms by means of which the heartbeat insures the circulation of the blood from the heart to the periphery and back to the heart. —**cardiody·nam·ic** (·ick) *adj.*

car·di·o·dyn·ia (kahr''dee·o·din'ee·uh) *n.* [*cardi-* + *-odynia*]. CARDIALGIA (1).

car·dio·esoph·a·ge·al (kahr''dee·o·e·sof''uh·jee'ul) *adj.* [*cardio-* + *esophageal*]. Pertaining to the stomach and the esophagus, usually to their junction.

cardioesophageal relaxation. A lack of tone of the cardiac sphincter, usually associated with chalasia (2).

car·dio·fa·cial syndrome (kahr''dee·o·fay'shul). The association between congenital heart disease and unilateral facial weakness involving only the lip depressors.

car·dio·gen·e·sis (kahr''dee·o·jen'e·sis) *n.*, pl. **cardiogene·ses** (·seez) [*cardio-* + *-genesis*]. Development of the embryonic heart.

car·dio·gen·ic (kahr''dee·o·jen'ick) *adj.* [*cardio-* + *-genic*]. 1. Pertaining to the development of the heart. 2. Having origin in the heart or produced by the heart.

cardiogenic area. The region in the splanchnic mesoderm anterior to the embryonic disk where the heart first appears in development. See also *cardiogenic plate.*

cardiogenic plate. An area of splanchnic mesoderm at the cephalic margin of the embryonic area below the coelom that gives rise to the endothelial tubes of the embryonic heart.

cardiogenic shock. Shock due to impairment of cardiac output, associated with inadequate peripheral circulatory compensatory response.

Cardiografin. A trademark for meglumine diatrizoate in an injectable dosage form suitable for angiocardiography and aortography.

car·dio·gram (kahr'dee·o·gram) *n.* 1. ELECTROCARDIOGRAM. 2. A record of cardiac pulsation made by a cardiograph.

car·dio·graph (kahr'dee·o·graf) *n.* [*cardio-* + *graph*]. 1. ELECTROCARDIOGRAPH. 2. An instrument which records cardiac pulsation and movement as transmitted through the chest wall. —**car·dio·graph·ic** (kahr″dee·o·graf′ick) *adj.*

car·di·og·ra·phy (kahr″dee·og′ruh·fee) *n.* [*cardio-* + *-graphy*]. Analysis of cardiac action by instrumental means, especially by tracings which record its movements.

Cardio-green. A trademark for indocyanine green, a diagnostic aid.

car·dio·he·pat·ic (kahr″dee·o·he·pat′ick) *adj.* [*cardio-* + *hepatic*]. Pertaining to the heart and the liver.

cardiohepatic angle. The angle formed by the junction of the upper border of hepatic dullness with the right lateral border of cardiac dullness.

cardiohepatic triangle. The triangular region in the right fifth intercostal space separating the heart and the upper surface of the liver.

car·di·oid (kahr′dee·oid) *adj.* [*cardi-* + *-oid*]. Like a heart.

car·dio·in·hib·i·to·ry (kahr″dee·o·in·hib′i·tor·ee) *adj.* [*cardio-* + *inhibitory*]. Diminishing, restraining, or suppressing the heart's action, as the cardioinhibitory fibers which pass to the heart through the vagus nerves.

cardioinhibitory center. The dorsal motor nucleus of the vagus nerve from which arise inhibitory fibers to the heart.

car·dio·ki·net·ic (kahr″dee·o·ki·net′ick) *adj. & n.* [*cardio-* + *kinetic*]. 1. Stimulating the action of the heart. 2. An agent that stimulates the action of the heart.

car·dio·ky·mog·ra·phy (kahr″dee·o·kigh·mog′ruh·fee) *n.* [*cardio-* + *kymography*]. A method for recording changes in the size of the heart by kymographic means. See also *kymography, radiokymography.*

car·dio·lip·in (kahr″dee·o·lip′in) *n.* [*cardio-* + *lipin*]. A phospholipid composed of two molecules of phosphatidic acid esterified to a single glycerol molecule. Essential for the reactivity of beef heart antigens in the serologic test for syphilis.

car·dio·lith (kahr′dee·o·lith) *n.* [*cardio-* + *-lith*]. A cardiac concretion.

car·di·ol·o·gist (kahr″dee·ol′uh·jist) *n.* A specialist in the diagnosis and treatment of disorders of the heart.

car·di·ol·o·gy (kahr″dee·ol′uh·jee) *n.* [*cardio-* + *-logy*]. The study of the heart and its functions.

car·di·ol·y·sis (kahr″dee·ol′i·sis) *n.*, pl. **cardioly·ses** (·seez) [*cardio-* + *lysis*]. 1. Resection of the precordial ribs and sternum to free the heart and its adherent pericardium from the anterior chest wall, to which they are bound by adhesions, as in adhesive mediastinopericarditis. 2. Cardiac degeneration or destruction.

car·dio·ma·la·cia (kahr″dee·o·ma·lay′shee·uh) *n.* [*cardio-* + *malacia*]. Pathologic softening of the heart musculature.

car·dio·me·ga·lia gly·co·gen·i·ca dif·fu·sa (kahr″dee·o·me·gay′lee·uh glye·ko·jen′i·kuh di·few′zuh). POMPE'S DISEASE.

car·dio·meg·a·ly (kahr″dee·o·meg′uh·lee) *n.* [*cardio-* + *-megaly*]. Enlargement of the heart.

car·dio·mel·a·no·sis (kahr″dee·o·mel″uh·no′sis) *n.*, pl. **cardio·melano·ses** (·seez) [*cardio-* + *melanosis*]. Deposition of pigment in the heart muscle.

car·dio·mel·ic (kahr″dee·o·mel′ick, mee′lick) *adj.* [*cardio-* + *mel-* + *-ic*]. Pertaining to or involving the heart and the limbs.

cardiomelic syndrome. HOLT-ORAM SYNDROME.

car·dio·men·su·ra·tor (kahr″dee·o·men′shoo·ray′tur) *n.* [*cardio-* + L. *mensurator,* from *mensurare,* to measure]. An instrument for the detection of cardiac enlargement by direct correlation of the transverse diameter of the heart with body weight and height.

car·di·o·men·to·pexy (kahr″dee·o·men′to·peck″see) *n.* [*cardi-* + *omento-* + *-pexy*]. The operation of bringing vascular omentum through the diaphragm and attaching it to the heart for improving cardiac vascularization.

car·di·om·e·ter (kahr″dee·om′e·tur) *n.* [*cardio-* + *-meter*]. An experimental apparatus which envelops the ventricles of a heart, recording their changes in volume, hence force of contraction, during a cardiac cycle.

car·di·om·e·try (kahr″dee·om′e·tree) *n.* [*cardio-* + *-metry*]. The measurement of the size of the heart, or of the force exerted with each contraction.

car·dio·my·op·a·thy (kahr″dee·o·migh·op′uth·ee) *n.* [*cardio-* + *myo-* + *-pathy*]. Any disease of the myocardium; myocardiopathy.

car·dio·myo·pex·y (kahr″dee·o·migh′o·peck″see) *n.* [*cardio-* + *myo-* + *-pexy*]. The operation of suturing living muscular tissue, generally from the pectoral region to the abraded surface of the heart, to provide improved vascularization of the heart.

car·dio·my·ot·o·my (kahr″dee·o·migh·ot′uh·mee) *n.* [*cardio-* + *myo-* + *-tomy*]. An operation for stenosis of the cardiac sphincter; consists of freeing the esophagus from the diaphragm and pulling it into the abdominal cavity, where the constricting muscle is divided anteriorly and posteriorly without dividing the mucous coat.

car·dio·nec·tor (kahr″dee·o·neck′tur) *n.* [*cardio-* + L. *nector,* joiner]. All those structures within the heart which regulate the heartbeat, consisting of the sinoatrial node, the atrioventricular node, and the atrioventricular bundle.

car·dio·neph·ric (kahr″dee·o·nef′rick) *adj.* [*cardio-* + *nephric*]. Pertaining to the heart and the kidneys.

car·dio·neu·ral (kahr″dee·o·new′rul) *adj.* [*cardio-* + *neural*]. Pertaining to the innervation of the heart.

car·dio·pal·u·dism (kahr″dee·o·pal′yoo·diz·um) *n.* [*cardio-* + *paludism*]. Malarial cardiomyopathy, usually due to *Plasmodium falciparium,* and characterized by heart failure.

car·dio·path (kahr′dee·o·path) *n.* [*cardio-* + *-path*]. A person with heart disease; CARDIAC (3). —**car·dio·path·ic** (kahr″dee·o·path′ick) *adj.*

car·dio·path·ia (kahr″dee·o·path′ee·uh) *n.* CARDIOPATHY.

car·dio·pa·thol·o·gy (kahr″dee·o·pa·thol′uh·jee) *n.* [*cardio-* + *pathology*]. Pathology of the heart.

car·di·op·a·thy (kahr″dee·op′uth·ee) *n.* [*cardio-* + *-pathy*]. Any disease or disorder of the heart.

car·dio·peri·car·dio·pexy (kahr″dee·o·perr″i·kahr′dee·o·peck″see) *n.* [*cardio-* + *pericardio-* + *-pexy*]. An operation for coronary artery disease, designed to increase collateral circulation and blood flow of the myocardium by the production of adhesive pericarditis.

car·dio·peri·car·di·tis (kahr″dee·o·perr″i·kahr·dye′tis) *n.* [*cardio-* + *pericarditis*]. *Rare.* MYOPERICARDITIS.

car·dio·pho·bia (kahr″dee·o·fo′bee·uh) *n.* [*cardio-* + *phobia*]. Abnormal fear of heart disease.

car·dio·phone (kahr′dee·o·fone) *n.* [*cardio-* + *-phone*]. An instrument which makes the heart sounds audible.

car·dio·plas·ty (kahr′dee·o·plas″tee) *n.* Plastic surgery of the cardiac sphincter, as for cardiospasm.

car·dio·ple·gia (kahr″dee·o·plee′jee·uh) *n.* [*cardio-* + *-plegia*]. 1. Paralysis of the heart, or cardiac arrest, as from direct trauma or blow. 2. Elective, temporary cardiac arrest, usually by drugs, as in the course of cardiac surgery.

car·dio·pneu·mat·ic (kahr″dee·o·new·mat′ick) *adj.* [*cardio-* + *pneumatic*]. Pertaining to bodily events in which both the cardiovascular and the pulmonary systems participate.

car·dio·pneu·mo·graph (kahr″dee·o·new″mo·graf) *n.* An instrument designed for graphically recording cardiopneumatic movements. —**cardio·pneu·mog·ra·phy** (·new·mog′ruh·fee) *n.*

car·di·op·to·sia (kahr″dee·op·to′shuh, ·see·uh) *n.* CARDIOPTOSIS.

car·di·op·to·sis (kahr″dee·op·to′sis, kahr″dee·o·to′sis) *n.*, pl. **cardiopto·ses** (·seez) [*cardio-* + *ptosis*]. Downward displacement of the heart; prolapse of the heart.

car·dio·pul·mo·nary (kahr″dee·o·pŏŏl′muh·nerr·ree) *adj.* [*cardio-* + *pulmonary*]. Pertaining to the heart and lungs.

cardiopulmonary murmur. A murmur produced by the impact of the heart against the lungs, or in airways intermittently narrowed and compressed by the beating heart.

cardiopulmonary-obesity syndrome. PICKWICKIAN SYNDROME.

cardiopulmonary resuscitation. A prescribed sequence of steps including the establishment of a clear open airway, closed-chest cardiac massage, and drug treatments designed to reestablish normal breathing following cardiac arrest. Abbreviated, CPR.

car·dio·pul·mon·ic (kahr″dee·o·pŏŏl·mon′ick) *adj.* CARDIOPULMONARY.

car·dio·punc·ture (kahr″dee·o·punk′chur) *n.* [*cardio-* + *puncture*]. CARDIOCENTESIS.

car·dio·py·lo·ric (kahr″dee·o·pye·lo′rick, ·pi·lo′rick) *adj.* Pertaining to both the cardiac and the pyloric portions of the stomach.

car·dio·ra·di·ol·o·gy (kahr″dee·o·ray″dee·ol′uh·jee) *n.* A subspecialty of radiology dealing with the roentgenology of cardiac disease. —**cardiora·dio·log·ic** (·dee·o·loj′ick) *adj.*

car·dio·re·nal (kahr″dee·o·ree′nul) *adj.* [*cardio-* + *renal*]. Pertaining to the heart and kidneys.

car·dio·re·spi·ra·to·ry (kahr″dee·o·res′pi·ruh·tor″ee, ·re·spye′ruh·tor″ee) *adj.* [*cardio-* + *respiratory*]. Of or pertaining to the heart and the respiratory system.

cardiorespiratory murmur. CARDIOPULMONARY MURMUR.

car·di·or·rha·phy (kahr″dee·or′uh·fee) *n.* [*cardio-* + *-rrhaphy*]. Suturing of the heart muscle.

car·di·or·rhex·is (kahr″dee·o·reck′sis) *n.*, pl. **cardiorrhex·es** (·seez) [*cardio-* + *-rrhexis*]. Rupture of the heart.

car·di·os·chi·sis (kahr″dee·os′ki·sis) *n.*, pl. **cardioschi·ses** (·seez) [*cardio-* + *-schisis*]. Division of adhesions between the heart and the chest wall in adhesive pericarditis.

car·dio·scope (kahr′dee·o·skope) *n.* 1. An instrument for the examination or visualization of the interior of the cardiac chambers. 2. An instrument which, by means of a cathode-ray oscillograph, projects an electrocardiographic or a phonocardiographic record on a luminous screen.

car·dio·spasm (kahr′dee·o·spaz·um) *n.* [*cardio-* + *spasm*]. ACHALASIA (1).

car·dio·ste·no·sis (kahr″dee·o·ste·no′sis) *n.* [*cardio-* + *stenosis*]. 1. Constriction of the heart, especially of the conus arteriosus pulmonalis. 2. The development of such a constriction.

car·dio·sym·phy·sis (kahr″dee·o·sim′fi·sis) *n.*, pl. **cardiosym·phy·ses** (·seez) [*cardio-* + *symphysis*]. ADHESIVE PERICARDIOMEDIASTINITIS.

car·dio·ta·chom·e·ter (kahr″dee·o·ta·kom′e·tur) *n.* [*cardio-* + *tacho-* + *meter*]. 1. An instrument that counts the total number of heartbeats over long periods of time. 2. An instrument that continuously computes and displays the heart rate of an individual in beats per minute.

car·dio·ther·a·py (kahr″dee·o·therr′uh·pee) *n.* [*cardio-* + *therapy*]. Treatment of heart disease.

car·di·ot·o·my (kahr″dee·ot′uh·mee) *n.* [*cardio-* + *-tomy*]. Dissection or incision of the heart or the cardiac end of the stomach.

car·dio·ton·ic (kahr″dee·o·ton′ick) *adj.* & *n.* [*cardio-* + *tonic*]. 1. Increasing the contractility of the cardiac muscle; generally applied to the effect of digitalis and related drugs. 2. An agent that increases the contractility of the cardiac muscle.

car·dio·tox·ic (kahr″dee·o·tock′sick) *adj.* [*cardio-* + *toxic*]. Having a poisonous effect on the heart.

car·dio·vas·cu·lar (kahr″dee·o·vas′kew·lur) *adj.* [*cardio-* + *vascular*]. Pertaining to the heart and blood vessels. Abbreviated, CV.

cardiovascular failure. Circulatory failure or heart failure.

cardiovascular surgery. Surgery pertaining to the heart and major blood vessels.

cardiovascular syphilis. One of the complications of late syphilis, characterized primarily by aortitis, with aortic dilatation and aneurysm; aortic valvulitis producing aortic regurgitation; coronary ostial stenosis and rarely myocarditis.

cardiovascular system. The complex circuit of chambers and channels, including the heart, arteries, capillaries, and veins, by which the blood is propelled and conveyed throughout the body.

car·dio·vec·tog·ra·phy (kahr″dee·o·veck·tog′ruh·fee) *n.* VECTORCARDIOGRAPHY.

car·dio·ver·sion (kahr″dee·o·vur′zhun) *n.* [*cardio-* + *version*]. Electrical reversion of cardiac arrhythmias to normal sinus rhythm, formerly using alternating current, but now employing direct current. See also *defibrillation.*

car·dio·ver·ter (kahr″dee·o·vur′tur) *n.* The apparatus used for cardioversion, consisting of monitors, as electrocardiograph read-out and pacing equipment.

car·di·peri·car·di·tis (kahr″dee·perr″i·kahr·dye′tis) *n.* Cardiopericarditis (= MYOPERICARDITIS).

car·di·tis (kahr·dye′tis) *n.* [*cardi-* + *-itis*]. Inflammation of the heart.

-cardium [NL., from Gk. *kardia*, heart]. A combining form designating *a structural layer of the heart or a membrane associated with the heart.*

Cardrase. Trademark for ethoxzolamide, a diuretic drug.

car·e·bar·ia (kăr″e·băr′ee·uh) *n.* [Gk. *karēbaria*, heaviness in the head]. Unpleasant head sensations, such as pressure or heaviness.

car·ene (kăr′een) *n.* A dicyclic liquid hydrocarbon, $C_{10}H_{16}$, classed as a terpene, found in turpentine obtained from several *Pinus* species. Several isomers, differing in the position of a double bond, exist.

Carfusin. A trademark for carbol-fuchsin solution.

Car·i·ca (kăr′i·kuh) *n.* [L., dried fig]. A genus of trees of the family Caricaceae.

Carica pa·pa·ya (pa·pah′yuh). The papaw tree of tropical America; contains in its leaves and fruit the proteolytic enzyme papain (papayotin) and other enzymes, and the alkaloid carpaine; the leaves also contain the glycoside carposide. The dried latex and leaves are used as a digestant.

car·ies (kair′eez) *n.* [L., decay]. A molecular death of bone or teeth, corresponding to ulceration in the soft tissues. See also *dental caries.*

caries of the spine. Tuberculous osteitis of the bodies of the vertebrae and intervertebral fibrocartilages, producing curvature of the spine.

caries sic·ca (sick′uh). A form of tuberculous caries characterized by absence of suppuration, obliteration of the cavity of a joint, and sclerosis and concentric atrophy of the articular extremities of the bones.

ca·ri·na (ka·ree′nuh, ka·rye′nuh) *n.*, L. pl. & genit. sing. **cari·nae** (·nee) [L., keel]. 1. Any keel-like structure. 2. (of the trachea:) The anteroposterior cartilaginous ridge in the bifurcation of the trachea which separates the openings of the two primary bronchi. NA *carina tracheae.* —**cari·nal** (·nul), **car·i·nate** (kăr′in·ate) *adj.*

carinal cyst. A bronchogenic cyst attached at the ridge demarcating the trachea from its bifurcation (carina).

Carinamide. A trademark for *p*-(benzylsulfonamido)benzoic acid, $C_{14}H_{13}NO_4S$, which inhibits tubular excretion of penicillin and has been used in conjunction with the antibiotic to maintain therapeutic blood levels of the latter.

carina na·si (nay′zye). A narrow, cleftlike space between the agger nasi and the inner surface of the dorsum nasi.

carinate abdomen. A keel-shaped belly, prominent in the middle and receding at the sides, with a sharply convex contour.

carinate breast. PIGEON BREAST.

carina tra·che·ae (tray′kee·ee) [NA]. The carina of the trachea; CARINA (2).

carina ure·thra·lis va·gi·nae (yoo·re·thray′lis va·jye′nee) [NA]. URETHRAL CARINA.

cario-. A combining form meaning *caries.*

car·io·gen·ic (kăr″ee·o·jen′ick) *adj.* [*cario-* + *-genic*]. Conducive to the development of dental caries.

car·io·stat·ic (kăr″ee·o·stat′ick) *adj.* [*cario-* + *-static*]. Having the quality of preventing or inhibiting carious activity.

car·i·ous (kair'ee·us) *adj.* 1. Pertaining to or affected with caries of the teeth. 2. Rotting or decaying.

car·iso·pro·dol (kahr·eye''so·pro'dol) *n.* *N*-Isopropyl-2-methyl-2-propyl-1,3-propanediol dicarbamate, $C_{12}H_{24}N_2O_4$, a congener of meprobamate with mephenesin-like action; used as a muscle relaxant.

Carls·bad salt [after *Carlsbad* (Karlovy Vary), Czechoslovakia]. A mineral salt mixture from the Carlsbad springs, whose waters have been used for their supposed curative properties, or a similar synthetic salt.

Carl Smith's disease [*Carl* H. *Smith,* U.S. hematologist, 1895–1971]. INFECTIOUS LYMPHOCYTOSIS.

Car·man's meniscus sign [R. D. *Carman,* U.S. physician, 1875–1926]. MENISCUS SIGN.

car·man·ta·dine (kahr·man'tuh·deen) *n.* 1-(1-Adamantyl)-2-azetidinecarboxylic acid, $C_{14}H_{21}NO_2$, an antiparkinsonian agent.

Carmethose. A trademark for sodium carboxymethylcellulose, a synthetic colloid.

car·min·a·tive (kahr·min'uh·tiv) *adj. & n.* [ML. *carminare,* to card, comb out]. 1. Having the power to relieve flatulence and colic. 2. A substance, usually an aromatic drug, used as a carminative agent.

car·mine (kahr'min, ·mine) *n.* [ML. *carminium,* from Ar. *qirmiz,* kermes]. 1. CARMINE DYE. 2. The color of carmine dye. —**car·min·ic** (kahr·min'ick) *adj.*

carmine cell. A modified alpha cell of the adenohypophysis which stains deep red with azocarmine; ordinary acidophils are stained orange.

carmine dye. A bright-red coloring matter prepared from cochineal, the active staining principle being carminic acid; of use in staining in toto, for staining tissues in bulk which are later sectioned; used as a specific stain for glycogen and for mucus and as a counterstain for blue vital dyes.

carminic acid. The red coloring principle of cochineal.

car·mus·tine (kahr'mus·teen) *n.* 1,3-Bis(2-chloroethyl)-1-nitrosourea, $C_5H_9Cl_2N_3O_2$, an antineoplastic agent.

car·nau·ba (kahr·naw'buh) *n.* [Pg.]. The root of *Copernicia cerifera,* a wax-producing palm tree of tropical America; has been used as an alterative.

carnauba wax. The wax obtained from the leaf of *Copernicia cerifera;* occasionally used in dermatologic formulations.

car·ne·ous (kahr'nee·us) *adj.* [L. *carneus,* from *caro,* flesh]. Of, pertaining to, or resembling flesh.

carneous degeneration. RED DEGENERATION.

carneous mole. BLOOD MOLE.

car·ni·da·zole (kahr·nigh'duh·zole) *n.* Methyl [2-(2-methyl-5-nitroimidazol-1-yl)-ethyl]thiocarbamate, $C_8H_{12}N_4O_3S$, an antiprotozoal.

car·ni·fi·ca·tion (kahr''ni·fi·kay'shun) *n.* [L. *caro, carnis,* flesh]. Alteration of tissue so that it resembles flesh (i.e., skeletal muscle); often used in reference to lung tissue alteration.

car·ni·tine (kahr'ni·teen) *n.* α-Amino-β-hydroxybutyric acid trimethylbetaine, $C_7H_{15}NO_3$, a constituent of striated muscle and liver; identical with vitamin B_T.

Car·niv·o·ra (kahr·niv'uh·ruh) *n.pl.* [NL.]. An order of mainly carnivorous and predatory mammals comprising the Canidae (dog family), Ursidae (bears), Procyonidae (raccoons, kinkajous, pandas), Mustelidae (weasels, skunks, badgers, otters), Viverridae (civets, genets, mongooses), Hyaenidae (hyenas), and Felidae (cat family).

car·ni·vore (kahr'ni·vore) *n.* A member of the order Carnivora.

car·niv·o·rous (kahr·niv'uh·rus) *adj.* [L. *carnivorus,* from *caro, carnis,* flesh, + *vorare,* to devour]. Entirely or primarily meat-eating; subsisting on animal flesh, especially that of vertebrates.

car·no·sine (kahr'no·seen, ·sin) *n.* β-Alanylhistidine, $C_9H_{14}N_4O_3$, a dipeptide component of muscle tissue.

car·no·sin·emia (kahr''no·si·nee'mee·uh) *n.* [*carnosine* + *-emia*]. An inborn error of amino acid metabolism in which there are abnormally high levels of carnosine in serum and urine, even when sources of this dipeptide are excluded from the diet, as well as high concentrations of homocarnosine in cerebrospinal fluid; manifested clinically by progressive neurologic deficit with severe mental retardation and seizures.

car·no·sin·uria (kahr''no·sin·yoo'ree·uh) *n.* [*carnosine* + *-uria*]. CARNOSINEMIA.

car·ob (kăr'ub) *n.* [Ar. *kharrūbah*]. A tree of the Near East, *Ceratonia siliqua,* whose pods yield carob gum, used in various pharmaceutical and cosmetic preparations.

Ca·ro·li's disease (ka·roh·lee') [J. *Caroli,* French physician, 20th century]. Multiple communicating cysts of the biliary tree.

Caronamide. An early form of the trademark Carinamide.

carotenaemia. CAROTENEMIA.

car·o·tene (kăr'o·teen) *n.* [L. *carota,* carrot, + *-ene*]. Any of three isomeric hydrocarbons, of the formula $C_{40}H_{56}$, distinguished by the prefixed symbols α-, β-, and γ-. All are synthesized by plants, the α- and β-isomers being the more abundant. When pure they are red or purple crystalline solids, the color being due to the presence of a series of conjugated ethylenic linkages. The carotenes are precursors of vitamin A, β-carotene yielding two molecules of vitamin A, the others one molecule.

car·o·ten·emia, car·o·te·nae·mia (kăr''o·te·nee'mee·uh) *n.* The presence of carotene in the circulating blood. Syn. *hypercarotenemia.*

ca·rot·e·noid, ca·rot·i·noid (ka·rot'i·noid) *n. & adj.* [*carotene* + *-oid*]. 1. One of a group of plant pigments occurring in carrots, tomatoes, and other vegetables, and in fruits and flowers. Chemically, carotenoids are unsaturated hydrocarbons of high molecular weight containing a series of conjugated ethylenic linkages or derivatives of such hydrocarbons. 2. Pertaining to or characteristic of a carotenoid.

car·o·te·no·sis, car·o·ti·no·sis (kăr''o·ti·no'sis) *n.,* pl. **carotino·ses** (·seez) [*carotene* + *-osis*]. Pigmentation of the skin due to carotene and carotenoids in the tissues.

ca·rot·ic (ka·rot'ick) *adj.* [Gk. *karōtikos,* stupefying]. *Obsol.* Characterized by or pertaining to stupor or coma.

ca·rot·i·co·cli·noid (ka·rot''i·ko·klye'noid) *adj.* Pertaining to an internal carotid artery and a clinoid process of the sphenoid bone.

ca·rot·i·co·tym·pan·ic (ka·rot''i·ko·tim·pan'ick) *adj.* Pertaining to the carotid canal and the tympanum.

caroticotympanic canals. Two or three short canals extending from the carotid canal to the tympanic cavity; they give passage to branches of the internal carotid plexus. NA *canaliculi caroticotympanici.*

caroticotympanic nerves. NA *nervi caroticotympanici.* See Table of Nerves in the Appendix.

ca·rot·id (ka·rot'id) *adj. & n.* [Gk. *karōtides,* carotid arteries]. 1. Pertaining to a carotid artery or nerve. 2. CAROTID ARTERY.

carotid aneurysm. An aneurysm of the carotid artery.

carotid arteriography. Radiography of the carotid artery after the injection of radiopaque material.

carotid artery. 1. The common carotid artery or either of its branches, the external and internal carotid arteries. 2. Specifically, the common carotid artery, the principal artery on either side of the neck. See also *common carotid artery, external carotid artery, internal carotid artery.*

carotid artery insufficiency syndrome. Contralateral weakness and numbness, aphasia, and ipsilateral monocular blindness due to atherosclerosis or other lesion causing obstruction of an internal carotid artery or one of its major branches.

carotid artery syndrome. CAROTID ARTERY INSUFFICIENCY SYNDROME.

carotid body. Any one of several irregular epithelioid masses situated at or near the bifurcation of the carotid artery, and innervated by the intercarotid or sinus branch of the glossopharyngeal nerve. NA *glomus caroticum.*

carotid-body reflex. A reflex initiated by changes in blood oxygen content, acting on chemoreceptors in the carotid body; marked hypoxia increases respiratory rate, blood pressure, and heart rate. See also *chemoreceptor.*

carotid-body tumor. A benign tumor, sometimes locally invasive, at the bifurcation of the common carotid artery, composed of nests of ovoid or polygonal cells having a rich cytoplasm and small vesicular or dense nuclei, in a vascular fibrous stroma duplicating the histologic structure of the carotid body.

carotid canal. A canal in the petrous portion of the temporal bone; it gives passage to the internal carotid artery. NA *canalis caroticus.*

carotid-cavernous fistulous aneurysm. An aneurysm in the carotid artery at the point where it traverses the cavernous sinus. It is most often the result of a head injury, but a few arise spontaneously. Cephalic bruit and exophthalmos are two common symptoms.

carotid ganglion. A small enlargement sometimes found in the internal carotid plexus.

carotid gland. CAROTID BODY.

carotid groove. The groove lodging the cavernous sinus and the internal carotid artery; it lies lateral to the sella turcica, from the foramen lacerum to the medial side of the anterior clinoid process. NA *sulcus caroticus.*

carotid nerves. Sympathetic nerves, from the superior cervical ganglion, which innervate the smooth muscles and glands of the head. See also *external carotid nerve, internal carotid nerve.*

ca·rot·i·do·sym·pa·tho·atri·al reflex (ka·rot″i·do·sim″puh·tho·ay′tree·ul). A reflex elicited by carotid sinus hypotension in which reflex sympathetic stimulation increases atrial contractility.

ca·rot·i·do·va·go·atri·al reflex (ka·rot″i·do·vay″go·ay′tree·ul). A reflex elicited by carotid sinus hypotension which decreases inhibitory vagal influences on the atria and increases atrial contractility.

ca·rot·i·do·ven·tric·u·lar reflex (ka·rot″id·o·ven·trick′yoo·lur). A reflex elicited by carotid sinus hypotension in which reflex sympathetic stimulation of the ventricle increases ventricular contractility.

carotid plexus. 1. Any of the networks of sympathetic nerve fibers surrounding the carotid arteries. See also *common carotid plexus, external carotid plexus, internal carotid plexus.* 2. Specifically, INTERNAL CAROTID PLEXUS.

carotid ridge. The sharp ridge between the inferior aperture of the carotid canal and the jugular fossa.

carotid sheath. The fibrous sheath about the carotid arteries and associated structures. NA *vagina carotica fasciae cervicalis.*

carotid sinus. 1. A slight dilatation of the common carotid artery at its bifurcation, the walls of which are innervated by the intercarotid or sinus branch of the glossopharyngeal nerve. It is concerned with the regulation of systemic blood pressure. NA *sinus caroticus.* 2. An extension of the cavernous sinus into the carotid canal.

carotid sinus hypersensitivity. Susceptibility to carotid sinus syncope.

carotid sinus massage or **pressure.** Carotid sinus stimulation by intermittent finger pressure, designed to enhance vagal tone and slow the heart rate or terminate an arrythmia.

carotid sinus reflex. A neural reflex arising from stimulation of pressure-sensitive mechano-receptors in the carotid sinus. Carotid sinus hypotension, with decreased stretch of these receptors, results in vasoconstriction, venoconstriction, bradycardia, and increased cardiac contractility. See also *baroreceptor.*

carotid sinus syncope or **syndrome.** Profound hypotension and bradycardia following carotid sinus stimulation, with resultant dizziness, fainting or convulsions, and occasionally other neurologic symptoms.

carotid triangle. SUPERIOR CAROTID TRIANGLE.

carotid tubercle. A prominence of the sixth cervical vertebra on the anterior part of its transverse process, against which the common carotid artery can be compressed. NA *tuberculum caroticum vertebrae cervicalis VI.*

ca·rot·i·dyn·ia (ka·rot″i·din′ee·uh) *n.* CAROTODYNIA.

car·o·tin (kăr′o·tin) *n.* CAROTENE.

carotinemia. CAROTENEMIA.

carotinoid. CAROTENOID.

carotinosis. CAROTENOSIS.

ca·ro·tis (ka·rot′is, ·ro′tis) *n.* [NL., sing. of *carotides,* from Gk. *karōtides*]. CAROTID ARTERY.

ca·rot·o·dyn·ia (ka·rot″o·din′ee·uh) *n.* [*carot*id + *-odynia*]. Cervicofacial pain or migraine or both associated with pain and tenderness of the carotid artery at its bifurcation and swelling of the overlying tissues.

-carp [Gk. *karpos*]. A combining form meaning *fruit.*

carp-, carpo-. A combining form meaning *carpus, carpal.*

car·pa·ine (kahr′pay·een, ·in) *n.* An alkaloid, $C_{14}H_{25}NO_2$, from the leaves of *Carica papaya.*

car·pal (kahr′pul) *adj. & n.* 1. Pertaining to the wrist or carpus. 2. CARPAL BONE.

carpal arches. CARPAL RETE.

carpal bone. Any of the eight wrist bones between the metacarpals and the radius and ulna. NA *os carpi, pl.* ossa carpi. See also Table of Bones in the Appendix.

carpal canal. CARPAL TUNNEL.

carpal ligament. See *extensor retinaculum of the wrist, flexor retinaculum of the wrist, radiate carpal ligament, palmar carpal ligament.*

carpal rete. An arterial anastomosis between branches of the ulnar and radial arteries in the region of the wrist; there are dorsal and volar sets of channels.

carpal tunnel. The space between the flexor retinaculum of the wrist and the carpal bones, through which pass the tendons of the long flexors of the fingers and the long flexor of the thumb and the median nerve. NA *canalis carpi.*

carpal tunnel syndrome. A symptom complex due to compression of the median nerve within the carpal tunnel, characterized by disturbances of sensation in the area of the skin supplied by the median nerve, pain on sharp flexion of the wrist, edema of the fingers, tense and shiny skin, and atrophy of the thenar muscles.

car·pec·to·my (kahr·peck′tuh·mee) *n.* [*carp-* + *-ectomy*]. Excision of a carpal bone or bones.

Car·pen·ter's syndrome [G. *Carpenter,* English physician, 1859–1910]. See *acrocephalopolysyndactyly.*

car·phen·a·zine (kahr·fen′uh·zeen) *n.* 1-{10-(3-[-(2-Hydroxyethyl)-1-piperazinyl]propyl)phenothiazin-2-yl}-1-propanone, $C_{24}H_{31}N_3O_2S$, a tranquilizer; used as a maleate salt.

car·pho·lo·gia (kahr″fo·lo′jee·uh) *n.* CARPHOLOGY.

car·phol·o·gy (kahr·fol″uh·jee) *n.* [Gk. *karphologia,* from *karphos,* bit or scrap, as of wool, + *legein,* to collect or pick]. Aimless picking and plucking at bedclothes, seen in delirious states, fevers, and exhaustion. Syn. *floccillation.*

carpo-. See *carp-.*

car·po·meta·car·pal (kahr″po·met·uh·kahr′pul) *adj.* Pertaining to the carpal and the metacarpal bones.

carpometacarpal articulation. 1. Any of the joints between the distal row of carpal bones (trapezium, trapezoid, capitate, hamate) and the bases of the metacarpals. 2. (of the fingers:) Any of the joints between the distal row of carpal bones and the bases of the four medial metacarpals. NA (pl.) *articulationes carpometacarpeae.* See also Table of Synovial Joints and Ligaments in the Appendix. 3. (of the thumb:) The saddle joint between the trapezium and the base of the first metacarpal. NA *articulatio carpometacarpea pollicis.*

carpometacarpal ligament. Any of the ligaments of the carpometacarpal articulations of the fingers, including the dorsal carpometacarpal ligaments (NA (pl.) *ligamenta carpometacarpea dorsalia*), connecting the trapezium, trapezoid, and hamate to the base of the second metacarpal, the capitate to the third metacarpal, the hamate and capitate to the fourth, and the capitate to the fifth; the palmar carpometacarpal ligaments (NA (pl.) *ligamenta carpometacarpea palmaria*), connecting the trapezium to the second metacarpal, the trapezium, capitate, and hamate to the third, and the hamate to the fourth and fifth; and the interosseous carpometacarpal ligaments, connecting the contiguous angles of the capitate and hamate to the third and fourth metacarpals.

carpometacarpal reflex. CARPOPHALANGEAL REFLEX.

car·po·ped·al (kahr'po·ped'ul) *adj.* [*carpo-* + *ped-* + *-al*]. Affecting the wrists and feet, or the fingers and toes.

carpopedal spasm. A spasm of the hands and feet, or of the thumbs and great toes; associated with tetany.

car·po·pha·lan·ge·al (kahr''po·fa·lan'jee·ul, ·fa·lan·jee'ul) *adj.* [*carpo-* + *phalangeal*]. Pertaining to the wrist and the phalanges.

carpophalangeal reflex. 1. Percussion of the dorsal aspect of the carpal and metacarpal areas is followed by flexion of the fingers; a variation of the finger flexor reflex. 2. Percussion of the extensor tendons of the flexed wrist is followed by its reflex extension.

car·pro·fen (kahr'pro·fen) *n.* (±)-6-Chloro-α-methyl-9*H*-carbazole-2-acetic acid, $C_{15}H_{12}ClNO_2$, an anti-inflammatory agent.

Carpule. Trademark for a glass cartridge containing a sterile solution of a drug which is loaded into a specially designed syringe and is ready for hypodermic injection.

car·pus (kahr'pus) *n.*, pl. & genit. sing. **car·pi** (·pye) [NL., from Gk. *karpos,* wrist] [NA]. 1. The group of eight bones between the metacarpals and the radius and ulna. 2. The part of the upper limb containing the eight carpal bones; WRIST (1). See also Table of Synovial Joints and Ligaments in the Appendix. Adj. *carpal.*

car·ra·geen (kăr'uh·jeen) *n.* See *Chondrus crispus.*

Car·rel-Da·kin treatment (ka·rel') [A. *Carrel,* French surgeon, 1873–1944; and H. D. *Dakin*]. The frequent and regularly repeated irrigation of open wounds with Dakin's solution.

Carrel flask [A. *Carrel*]. A vessel with a slanting or horizontal neck, used in tissue culture.

Carrel-Lind·bergh pump [A. *Carrel* and C. A. *Lindbergh*]. A perfusion apparatus for keeping organs alive outside the body.

car·ri·er, *n.* 1. A well person or one convalescing from an infectious disease who shows no signs or symptoms of the disease but who harbors and eliminates the microorganism, and so spreads the disease. 2. An individual who bears a mutant gene without manifesting its phenotypic expression, usually applied to those heterozygous for a severe recessive gene. 3. A quantity of a naturally occurring element added to a minute amount of pure isotope, especially one that is radioactive, to facilitate chemical handling of the isotope. 4. A compound capable of reversible oxidation-reduction, which thus acts as a hydrogen carrier. 5. A device, as an instrument, for holding something while it is being carried or is being used.

carrier-free, *adj. In radiochemistry,* pertaining to or characterizing a radioactive isotope in which none of the stable forms of the isotope is present.

car·ri·on (kăr'ee·un) *n.* [OF. *caroigne,* from L. *caro,* flesh]. The putrefying flesh of animal carcasses.

Ca·rrión's disease (ka·rryoʰn') [D. A. *Carrión,* Peruvian medical student, 1859–1885]. BARTONELLOSIS.

car·ron oil (kăr'un). A mixture of equal parts of linseed oil and lime water; used in the treatment of burns.

Carr-Price test [F. H. *Carr,* English chemist, b. 1871; and E. A. *Price*]. A test for vitamin A performed with antimony trichloride, which with vitamin A produces a blue color that may be quantitatively measured.

carrying angle. The angle between the longitudinal axis of the forearm and that of the arm when the forearm is extended.

car sickness. Motion sickness from riding in an automobile or similar road vehicle.

Cars·well's grapes [R. *Carswell,* English physician, 1793–1857]. Pulmonary tubercles.

car·taz·o·late (kahr·taz'o·late) *n.* Ethyl 4-(butylamino)-1-ethyl-1*H*-pyrazolo[3,4-*b*]pyridine-5-carboxylate, $C_{15}H_{22}N_4O_2$, an antidepressant.

Car·ter's operation [W. W. *Carter,* U.S. otolaryngologist and plastic surgeon, 1869–1950]. 1. A rhinoplasty in which a portion of rib and its cartilage is used to form a new bridge for the nose. 2. Submucous resection for deflection of the nasal septum.

Car·te·sian (kahr·tee'zhun) *adj.* Pertaining to methods, theories, or doctrines originated by or associated with René Descartes (Cartesius), French scientist and philosopher, 1596–1650.

Cartesian diver manometry. A micromanometric technique for the gasometric determination of isolated enzymes and the metabolic activity of minute quantities of tissue.

Cartesian diver method. Any method that measures pressure changes at a gas-liquid interface by determining the variations in position of a gas-filled tube floating in the liquid.

Car·tha·mus (kahr'thuh·mus) *n.* A genus of Eurasian herbs of the family Carduaceae.

Carthamus tinc·to·ri·us (tink·tor'ee·us). Safflower; American or bastard saffron. The dried flowers are used in making an infusion used popularly as a diaphoretic. The fixed oil from the seed, which contains unsaturated acid glycerides, has been used in regimens for lowering the serum cholesterol level.

car·ti·lage (kahr'ti·lij) *n.* [L. *cartilago*]. Gristle; a white, semiopaque, nonvascular connective tissue composed of a highly polymerized matrix containing nucleated cells which lie in cavities or lacunas of the matrix. When boiled, cartilage yields chondrin.

cartilage bone. 1. Bone preceded during development by a mass of hyaline cartilage which it largely replaces. 2. A bone which has been preceded by a cartilaginous primordium.

cartilage capsule. The more basophil matrix next to or near a cartilage lacuna.

cartilage corpuscle. *Rare.* CHONDROCYTE.

cartilage graft. A cartilage autograft or homograft, commonly used for replacing damaged or destroyed cartilage, or to replace bone loss.

cartilage-hair hypoplasia. A genetic disorder, reported among certain Amish people in the United States and Canada, characterized by dwarfism due to hypoplasia of cartilage and abnormally short, thin, and sparse hair; inherited as an autosomal recessive with reduced penetrance.

cartilage of San·to·ri·ni (saʰn·to·ree'nee) [G. D. *Santorini*]. CORNICULATE CARTILAGE.

cartilage of Wris·berg (vriss'behrk) [H. A. *Wrisberg*]. CUNEIFORM CARTILAGE.

cartilagines. Plural of *cartilago.*

cartilagines ala·res mi·no·res (ay·lair'eez mi·no'reez) [NA]. The minor alar cartilages. See *alar cartilages.*

cartilagines la·ryn·gis (la·rin'jis) [NA]. LARYNGEAL CARTILAGES.

cartilagines na·sa·les ac·ces·so·ri·ae (na·say'leez ack·se·so'ree·ee) [NA]. ACCESSORY NASAL CARTILAGES.

cartilagines na·si (nay'zye) [NA]. Cartilages of the nose.

cartilagines se·sa·moi·de·ae na·si (ses''uh·moy'dee·ee nay'zye) [BNA]. Cartilagines alares minores (= minor alar cartilages). See *alar cartilages.*

cartilagines tra·che·a·les (tray″kee-ay′leez) [NA]. Cartilages of the trachea.
car·ti·la·gin·i·fi·ca·tion (kahr″ti-la-jin″i-fi-kay′shun) *n.* A change into cartilage; chondrification.
car·ti·lag·i·nous (kahr″ti-laj′i-nus) *adj.* Pertaining to or consisting of cartilage.
cartilaginous septum of the nose. The angular cartilage plate forming the anterior part of the nasal septum. NA *cartilago septi nasi.*
cartilaginous skeleton. Cartilage that is the precursor of most of the bony skeleton.
car·ti·la·go (kahr″ti-lay′go) *n.*, genit. **carti·la·gi·nis** (-laj′i-nis), pl. **carti·la·gi·nes** (-laj′i-neez) [L.]. CARTILAGE.
cartilago ala·ris major (ay-lair′is) [NA]. Major alar cartilage. See *alar cartilages.*
cartilago ar·ti·cu·la·ris (ahr-tick″yoo-lair′is) [NA]. ARTICULAR CARTILAGE.
cartilago ary·te·noi·dea (ăr″i-te-noy′dee-uh) [NA]. ARYTENOID CARTILAGE.
cartilago au·ri·cu·lae (aw-rick′yoo-lee) [NA]. AURICULAR CARTILAGE.
cartilago cor·ni·cu·la·ta (kor-nick″yoo-lay′tuh) [NA]. CORNICULATE CARTILAGE.
cartilago cos·ta·lis (kos-tay′lis) [NA]. COSTAL CARTILAGE.
cartilago cri·coi·dea (kri-koy′dee-uh) [NA]. CRICOID CARTILAGE.
cartilago cu·ne·i·for·mis (kew-nee-i-for′mis) [NA]. CUNEIFORM CARTILAGE.
cartilago epi·glot·ti·ca (ep-i-glot′i-kuh) [NA]. EPIGLOTTIC CARTILAGE. See also *epiglottis.*
cartilago epi·phy·si·a·lis (ep″i-fiz-ee-ay′lis) [NA]. EPIPHYSEAL PLATE (2).
cartilago me·a·tus acu·sti·ci (mee-ay′toos a-koos′ti-sigh) [NA]. The cartilage of the external acoustic meatus; it is a continuation of the auricular cartilage in the wall of the lateral part of the external auditory canal.
cartilago na·si la·te·ra·lis (nay′zye lat-e-ray′lis) [NA]. LATERAL NASAL CARTILAGE.
cartilago sep·ti na·si (sep′tye nay′zye) [NA]. CARTILAGINOUS SEPTUM OF THE NOSE.
cartilago se·sa·moi·dea (ses″uh-moy′dee-uh) [NA]. SESAMOID CARTILAGE.
cartilago thy·re·oi·dea (thigh-ree-oy′dee-uh) [BNA]. Cartilago thyroidea (= THYROID CARTILAGE).
cartilago thy·roi·dea (thigh-roy′dee-uh) [NA]. THYROID CARTILAGE.
cartilago tri·ti·cea (tri-tis′ee-uh) [NA]. TRITICEOUS CARTILAGE.
cartilago tu·bae au·di·ti·vae (tew′bee aw-di-tye′vee) [NA]. The cartilage of the auditory tube.
cartilago vo·me·ro·na·sa·lis (vom″e-ro-na-say′lis) [NA]. VOMERONASAL CARTILAGE.
car·um (kăr′um) *n.* [Gk. *karon*]. CARAWAY.
car·un·cle (kăr′ung-kul, ka-runk′ul) *n.* [L. *caruncula*, a little piece of flesh]. 1. Any small, fleshy, red mass or nodule. 2. Specifically, LACRIMAL CARUNCLE. —**ca·run·cu·lar** (ka-runk′yoo-lur), **caruncu·late** (-late), **caruncu·la·ted** (-lay-tid) *adj.*
ca·run·cu·la (ka-runk′yoo-luh) *n.*, pl. **caruncu·lae** (-lee) [L.]. CARUNCLE.
carunculae hy·me·na·les (high″me-nay′leez) [NA]. HYMENAL CARUNCLES.
caruncula la·cri·ma·lis (lack-ri-may′lis) [NA]. LACRIMAL CARUNCLE.
caruncula sub·lin·gua·lis (sub″ling-gway′lis) [NA]. SUBLINGUAL CARUNCLE.
ca·rus (kair′us) *n.* [Gk. *karos*, deep sleep]. *Obsol.* Profound lethargy, stupor, or coma.
car·va·crol (kahr′vuh-krol) *n.* 2-Hydroxy-*p*-cymene, $C_{10}H_{14}O$, isomeric with thymol. It occurs in several volatile oils and is actively germicidal.
Car·val·lo's sign. A sign of tricuspid regurgitation in which the systolic murmur is augmented by inspiration.
car·vone (kahr′vone) *n.* A terpene ketone, $C_{10}H_{14}O$, found in the volatile oils of caraway, dill, fennel, and spearmint; used as a flavor.
cary-, caryo-. See *kary-.*
caryenchyma. KARYENCHYMA (= NUCLEAR SAP).
caryo-. See *kary-.*
caryochrome. KARYOCHROME (= KARYOCHROME CELL).
car·y·o·phyl·lus (kăr″ee-o-fil′us) *n.* [NL., from Gk. *karyophyllon*]. CLOVE.
CAS Chemical Abstracts Service.
Ca·sal's collar or **necklace** (ka-sahl′) [G. *Casal*, Spanish physician, 1681–1759]. The erythematous pigmented skin lesions on the neck in pellagra.
cas·an·thra·nol (kas-an′thruh-nol) *n.* A purified mixture of anthranol glycosides derived from *Cascara sagrada;* used as a cathartic.
Ca·sa·res Gil's stain (ka-sah′res kheel). A method of staining flagella in which carbolfuchsin is used to stain smears which have been treated with a special mordant composed of tannic acid, hydrated aluminum chloride, zinc chloride, basic fuchsin, and alcohol (60%).
casava. CASSAVA.
cas·ca bark (kas′kuh). The bark of *Erythrophleum guineense,* an African tree. See also *erythrophleine.*
cas·cade (kas-kade′) *v. & n.* [F., from It. *cascare*, to fall]. 1. To spill over, usually rapidly, as over terraces. 2. To be built up in stages, as an electrical process. 3. A structure or a process involving such spilling over or building up.
cascade generator. A generator in which the transformers are arranged in a cascaded series with separate insulation for the production of high voltages. Used in x-ray therapy.
cascade stomach. *In radiology,* a variant of the normal gastric contour, in which the upper posterior wall is pushed forward, giving the stomach the appearance of a glass retort; the cardia fills first, with subsequent spilling over into the pyloric segment.
cas·cara (kas-kăr′uh) *n.* [Sp. *cáscara*, bark]. CASCARA SAGRADA.
cascara sa·gra·da (sah-grah′duh). The bark of *Rhamnus purshiana,* the chief constituents of which are anthraquinone derivatives; an irritant cathartic.
cas·ca·ril·la (kas″kuh-ril′uh) *n.* [Sp., dim. of *cáscara*]. The bark of *Croton eluteria,* native to the Bahama Islands; an aromatic bitter.
cas·ca·ril·lin (kas″kuh-ril′in) *n.* The bitter principle, $C_{12}H_{18}O_4$, of cascarilla.
cas·ca·rin (kas′kuh-rin) *n.* A glycosidal cathartic fraction isolated from cascara sagrada.
case-, caseo-. A combining form meaning (a) *casein;* (b) *caseous.*
ca·se·ase (kay′see-ace, -aze) *n.* [*case-* + *-ase*]. An enzyme from bacterial cultures which digests albumin and casein.
¹ca·se·ate (kay′see-ate) *n.* 1. LACTATE. 2. CASEINATE.
²caseate, *v.* To undergo caseation necrosis.
ca·se·a·tion (kay″see-ay′shun) *n.* 1. The precipitation of casein during the coagulation of milk. 2. CASEATION NECROSIS.
caseation necrosis. A type of tissue death resulting in loss of all cellular outlines and the gross appearance of crumbly cheeselike material; seen typically in tuberculosis.
case fatality rate. The proportion of fatal cases of a specific disease, usually expressed as the number of deaths from the disease per 100 persons affected.
case history. An account of a particular case of disease or other medically significant condition, including all relevant or possibly relevant parts of the patient's medical history.
ca·se·ic acid (kay′see-ick, ka-see′ick). LACTIC ACID.
ca·se·i·form (kay′see-i-form) *adj.* Like cheese or casein.
ca·sein (kay′seen, -see-in) *n.* [L. *caseus*, cheese, + *-in*]. A

protein obtained from milk by the action of rennin or acids.

ca·sein·ate (kay·see'nate, ·see'i·nate) *n.* A compound of casein and a metal.

ca·sein·o·gen (kay·seen'o·jen, kay″see·in'o·jen) *n.* A compound protein of milk, yielding casein when acted upon by digestive enzymes; the precursor of casein, analogous to fibrinogen and myosinogen (myogen).

caseo-. See *case-*.

ca·seo·cal·cif·ic (kay″see·o·kal·sif'ick) *adj.* Possessing areas both of caseation and of calcification.

ca·se·ous (kay'see·us) *adj.* [L. *case*us, cheese, + *-ous*]. 1. Resembling, or having the nature or consistency of, cheese. 2. Characterized by caseation necrosis.

caseous abscess. An abscess in which the necrotic material has a cheesy appearance, usually tuberculous.

caseous degeneration. CASEATION NECROSIS.

caseous fermentation. Fermentation resulting in the conversion of milk into cheese.

caseous pneumonic tuberculosis. Exudative tuberculosis of the lung which has undergone a characteristic type of necrosis, simulating cheese in its gross appearance.

Case's pad sign. A roentgenologic appearance of a smooth localized pressure deformity, usually on the inferior surface of the pyloric antrum or duodenal bulb, accentuated by the prone position. Originally considered indicative of a mass in the region of the pancreas.

case·work, *n.* The task of professional social workers or psychiatric social workers who, through personal counseling and the aid of various social services, seek to help individuals and their families with their personal and social problems.

case·worm, *n.* *ECHINOCOCCUS.*

Cas·i·mi·roa (kas″i·mi·ro'uh, kas″i·mirr'o·uh) *n.* [*Casimiro* Gómez de Ortega, Spanish botanist, 1740–1818]. A genus of plants belonging to the Rutaceae.

Casimiroa ed·u·lis (ed'yoo·lis). A species of *Casimiroa* found in Mexico. The leaves have been used as an anthelmintic.

Ca·so·ni's test (ka·zo'nee) [T. *Casoni*, Italian physician, 1880–1933]. A test for echinococcus disease in which sterile hydatid fluid from echinococcic cysts of lung or liver of sheep is injected intracutaneously. An urticarial wheal surrounded by a zone of erythema appearing rapidly and an area of erythema and edema lasting 2 to 3 days is indicative of echinococcus disease.

cas·sa·va, ca·sa·va (ka·sah'vuh) *n.* [Taino *caçabi*]. 1. Any of several plants of the genus *Manihot*. 2. The starch obtained from rhizomes of *M. esculenta* and *M. aipi;* a nutrient and the source of tapioca.

Cas·ser's (Cas·se·rio's) fontanel [J. *Casserio*, Italian anatomist, 1561–1616]. POSTEROLATERAL FONTANEL.

Cas·sia (cash'uh, cash'ee·uh) *n.* [Gk. *kasia*]. A genus of the Leguminosae, several species of which provide senna.

cassia, *n.* An old name, still used commercially, for the coarser varieties of cinnamon.

cassia bark. A variety of cinnamon native to China.

Cassia fistula. PURGING CASSIA.

cassia oil. CINNAMON OIL.

cast, *n. & v.* 1. A mass of fibrous material, protein coagulum, or exudate that has taken the form of some cavity in which it has been molded; classified according to the source, as bronchial, intestinal, nasal, esophageal, renal, tracheal, urethral, or vaginal. 2. An accurate reproduction in form of an object, structure, or part in some plastic substance which has taken form in an impression or mold. 3. PLASTER OF PARIS CAST. 4. *Colloq.* Of the eye: STRABISMUS. 5. To produce a specific form by pouring metal or plaster into a prepared mold. 6. *In veterinary medicine,* to throw an animal on its side for restraint.

Cas·taigne method (kas·tehnʸ') [J. *Castaigne*, French physician, 1860–1944]. METHYLENE BLUE TEST (1).

Cas·ta·ñe·da's rat-lung method (kahˢs″tahⁿ·nʸehʸ'thah) [M. R. *Castañeda*, Mexican virologist]. The use of the rat lung, following intranasal inoculation with species of *Rickettsia*, as a source of the microorganisms for the production of vaccines.

Castañeda vaccine [M. R. *Castañeda*]. A vaccine against typhus fever prepared by Casteñeda's rat-lung method.

Ca·stel·lani's disease (kahʰ″stel·lah'nee) [A. *Castellani*, Italian pathologist, 1879–1971]. BRONCHOSPIROCHETOSIS.

Castellani's paint [A. *Castellani*]. CARBOL-FUCHSIN SOLUTION.

Cas·tel method. 1. A histochemical method for arsenic using copper acetate to obtain a green salt of arsenic. 2. A histochemical method for bismuth based on treating tissue with a solution of brucine sulfate, sulfuric acid, and potassium iodide to obtain red granules.

cas·tile soap (kas·teel') [after *Castile*, Spain]. A hard soap usually prepared from sodium hydroxide and olive oil. Much commercial castile soap contains coconut oil soap to increase its lathering quality.

cast·ing, *n.* 1. *In dentistry,* the act of forcing molten metal into a suitable mold. 2. The object or product formed by the casting. 3. *In veterinary medicine,* the act of throwing an animal on its side for restraint.

cas·tor (kas'tur) *n.* CASTOREUM.

castor bean. The seed of *Ricinus communis,* from which castor oil is obtained.

cas·to·re·um (ka·sto'ree·um) *n.* [L. *castorium*, from *castor*, beaver]. Dried preputial glands and their secretion, obtained from the beaver, *Castor fiber.* It is a reddish-brown substance with a strong odor; formerly used in hysteria, its action resembling that of musk.

castor oil. The fixed oil obtained from the seed of *Ricinus communis;* the oil contains glycerides of ricinoleic acid which impart cathartic activity.

castor xylene. A mixture composed of castor oil, 1 part, and xylene, 3 parts; used for clearing or clarifying collodion or celloidin of objects embedded in them.

cas·tra·tion (kas·tray'shun) *n.* [L. *castrare*, to castrate]. ORCHIECTOMY; the excision of one or both testes or ovaries; taken as evidence of hypersecretion of follicle-stimulating or luteinizing hormone or both. —**cas·trat·ed** (kas'tray·tid) *adj.;* **cas·trate** (kas'trate) *n. & v.*

castration anxiety. 1. Anxiety due to the fantasied fear of loss of the genitals or injury to them; may be provoked by events which have symbolic significance, such as loss of a tooth, an object, or a job, or a humiliating experience. 2. Fear of a young boy that he will lose his penis.

castration cells. Enlarged beta cells of the pars distalis of the hypophysis, showing vacuolization and eccentric displacement of the nucleus following castration.

castration complex. 1. Castration anxiety occurring after childhood, associated primarily with fear of loss of the genital, especially the male, organ. 2. The symptoms of the fear of the loss of any pleasure-giving body part (or excretion) or of even the fear that every pleasure will be followed by loss and pain. 3. In the female, the fantasy of once having had a penis but of having lost it.

cas·tro·phre·nia (kas″tro·free'nee·uh) *n.* [*castr*ate + *-phrenia*]. A morbid fear or delusion, occasional in schizophrenic patients, that their thoughts are being sucked out of their brains by enemies.

cas·u·is·tics (kazh″oo·is'ticks, kaz″yoo·) *n.* The study of individual cases as a means of arriving at the general history of a disease.

CAT Abbreviation for (a) *Children's Apperception Test;* (b) *computed axial tomography* or *computer-assisted tomography.*

cat-, cata-, cath- [Gk. *kata*, down]. A prefix meaning (a) *downward;* (b) *in accordance with;* (c) *against, back;* (d) *completely.*

cata-. See *cat-*.

cata·ba·si·al (kat″uh·bay'see·ul, ·zee·ul) *adj.* [*cata-* + *basial*].

Pertaining to or denoting a skull in which the basion is lower than the opisthion.

ca·tab·a·sis (ka·tab'uh·sis) *n.*, pl. **cataba·ses** (·seez) [Gk. *katabasis*, descent]. The stage of abatement of a disease. —**cat·a·bat·ic** (ka·tuh·bat'ick) *adj.*

cata·bi·o·sis (cat''uh·bye·o'sis) *n.*, pl. **catabio·ses** (·seez) [*cata-* + *-biosis*]. 1. CATABOLISM. 2. Physiologic aging or senescence of a cell or group of cells. Compare *necrobiosis.* —**catabi·ot·ic** (·ot'ick) *adj.*

catabiotic force. The energy derived from the breakdown of food or body tissues.

ca·tab·o·lism (ka·tab'uh·liz·um) *n.* [Gk. *katabolē*, throwing down]. The degradative or destructive phase of metabolism concerned with the breaking down by the body of complex compounds, often with liberation of energy. Compare *anabolism, biosynthesis.* —**cat·a·bol·ic** (kat·uh·bol'ick) *adj.*

ca·tab·o·lite (ka·tab'o·lite) *n.* Any product of catabolism.

ca·tab·o·lize (ka·tab'o·lize) *v.* To transform by catabolism; to subject to catabolism.

cata·caus·tic (kat·uh·kaws'tick) *n.* [*cata-* + *caustic*]. *In optics*, a curve formed by the reflection of rays of light. Syn. *catacaustic curve.*

cat·a·clei·sis (kat''uh·klye'sis) *n.*, pl. **cataclei·ses** (·seez) [Gk. *katakleisis*, a closing]. *Obsol.* Closure of the eyelids by adhesion or by spasm.

cata·clo·nus (kat''uh·klo'nus) *n.* [*cata-* + *clonus*]. *Obsol.* Rhythmic convulsive movements which are of functional or hysterical nature rather than expressions of true epilepsy. —**cata·clon·ic** (·klon'ick) *adj.*

cat·a·cous·tics (kat''uh·koos'ticks) *n.* [*cat-* + *acoustics*]. The science of reflected sound; echolocation.

cata·crot·ic (kat''uh·krot'ick) *adj.* [*cata-* + *-crotic*]. 1. Designating the descending limb of the arterial pulse wave. 2. Characterized by catacrotism. Contr. *anacrotic.*

cat·ac·ro·tism (ka·tack'ro·tiz·um) *n.* A condition in which the descending, or catacrotic, limb of the arterial pulse wave is characterized by a notch, wave, or irregularity.

catadidymus. KATADIDYMUS.

cata·di·op·tric (kat''uh·dye·op'trick) *adj.* [*cata-* + *dioptric*]. Pertaining to both reflection and refraction of light rays.

cat·a·gelo·pho·bia (kat''uh·jel''o·fo'bee·uh) *n.* [Gk. *katagelōs*, derision, + *phobia*]. Abnormal fear of ridicule.

cat·a·gen (kat'uh·jin) *n.* [*cata-* + *-gen*esis]. The brief transitional period between growth and quiescence in a hair follicle. Contr. *anagen, telogen.*

cat·a·lase (kat'uh·lace, ·laze) *n.* [*catal*ysis + *-ase*]. An enzyme found in tissues, capable of decomposing hydrogen peroxide to water and molecular oxygen.

cat·a·lep·sis (kat''uh·lep'sis) *n.* CATALEPSY.

cat·a·lep·sy (kat'uh·lep''see) *n.* [Gk. *katalēpsis*, a seizing]. A state of markedly diminished responsiveness, usually trancelike, in which there is a loss of voluntary motion and a peculiar plastic rigidity of the muscles, by reason of which they retain for an exceedingly long time any position in which they are placed. The condition may occur in organic or psychologic disorders, especially in hysteria and in schizophrenia, and under hypnosis. —**ca·ta·lep·tic** (kat''uh·lep'tick) *adj.* & *n.*

cat·a·lep·ti·form (kat''uh·lep'ti·form) *adj.* CATALEPTOID.

cat·a·lep·tize (kat''uh·lep'tize) *v.* To provoke catalepsy.

cat·a·lep·toid (kat''uh·lep'toid) *adj.* [*catalept*ic + *-oid*]. Resembling catalepsy.

Ca·tal·pa (kuh·tal'puh) *n.* [Creek *kutuhlpa*]. A genus of American and Asiatic trees of the Bignoniaceae. The seeds of *Catalpa bignonioides* and *C. speciosa*, of North America, have been used in the treatment of asthma.

ca·tal·y·sis (ka·tal'i·sis) *n.*, pl. **cataly·ses** (·seez) [Gk. *katalysis*, dissolution]. The process of change in the velocity of a chemical reaction through the presence of a substance which apparently remains chemically unaltered throughout the reaction. The velocity may be increased, in which case the process is described as positive catalysis, or it may be decreased, in which case the process is described as negative catalysis.

cat·a·lyst (kat'uh·list) *n.* 1. A substance having the power to produce catalysis. 2. A substance which alters the velocity of a chemical reaction. Its concentration at the beginning of the reaction is equal to its concentration at the end. See also *biocatalyst, enzyme.* —**cat·a·lyt·ic** (kat''uh·lit'ick) *adj.*

cat·a·lyze (kat'uh·lize) *v.* [F. *catalyser*]. 1. To act as a catalyst. 2. To influence a chemical reaction by means of a catalyst. —**cat·a·ly·za·tion** (kat''uh·li·zay'shun) *n.*

cat·a·lyz·er (kat'uh·lye·zur) *n.* CATALYST.

cat·a·me·nia (kat''uh·mee'nee·uh) *n.* [Gk. *katamēnia*]. MENSTRUATION. —**catame·ni·al** (·nee·ul) *adj.*

catamenial dermatitis. DERMATITIS DYSMENORRHEICA.

catamenial epilepsy. Seizures which occur in association with menstruation.

cat·am·ne·sis (kat''am·nee'sis) *n.*, pl. **catamne·ses** (·seez) [*cata-* + Gk. *mnēsis*, remembering]. The follow-up medical history of a patient after an initial examination or an illness. Compare *anamnesis.* —**catam·nes·tic** (·nes'tick) *adj.*

cat·a·pasm (kat'uh·paz·um) *n.* [Gk. *katapasma*, powder]. A dry powder to be sprinkled upon the skin or upon a sore.

cata·pha·sia (kat''uh·fay'zhuh, ·zee·uh) *n.* [Gk. *kataphas*is, affirmation, + *-ia*]. A form of stereotypy in which the patient keeps repeating the same word or series of words.

cat·a·pha·sis (kat''uh·fay'sis) *n.* CATAPHASIA.

ca·taph·o·ra (ka·taf'o·ruh) *n.* [Gk. *kataphora*]. *Obsol.* 1. Marked somnolence with periods of partial wakefulness. 2. SEMICOMA.

cata·pho·re·sis (kat''uh·fo·ree'sis, ·for'e·sis) *n.* [*cata-* + *-phoresis*]. ELECTROPHORESIS. —**catapho·ret·ic** (·ret'ick) *adj.*

cata·pho·ria (kat''uh·for'ee·uh) *n.* [Gk. *kataphor*os, inclined downward, + *-ia*]. A tendency of the visual axes of both eyes to incline below the horizontal plane.

cata·phor·ic (kat''uh·for'ick) *adj.* 1. Pertaining to cataphoresis. 2. Pertaining to cataphora.

cata·phy·lax·is (kat''uh·fi·lack'sis) *n.* [*cata-* + *phylaxis*]. 1. Movement and transportation of leukocytes and antibodies to the site of an infection. 2. The overcoming of bodily resistance to infection. —**cata·phy·lac·tic** (·fi·lack'tick) *adj.*

cata·pla·sia (kat''uh·play'zhuh, ·zee·uh) *n.* [*cata-* + *-plasia*]. 1. The stage of decline of life. 2. Degenerative changes affecting cells and tissues, especially reversion to an earlier or embryonic type of cell or tissue. 3. Application of a plaster or coating.

ca·tap·la·sis (ka·tap'luh·sis) *n.*, pl. **catapla·ses** (·seez) [Gk. *kataplasis*, application of a poultice]. CATAPLASIA.

cat·a·plasm (kat'uh·plaz·um) *n.* [Gk. *kataplasma*]. A poultice, of various substances and usually applied when hot.

cat·a·plexy (kat'uh·pleck''see) *n.* [Gk. *kataplēxis*, amazement, from *kataplēssein*, to strike down]. Temporary paralysis of the cranial and somatic musculature brought on by bouts of laughter, anger, or other emotional states; part of the clinical tetrad of narcolepsy, cataplexy, sleep paralyses, and hypnagogic hallucinations.—**cat·a·plec·tic** (kat'uh·pleck'tick) *adj.*

Catapres. A trademark for clonidine hydrochloride, an antihypertensive.

cat·a·ract (kat'uh·rakt) *n.* [L. *cataracta*, portcullis, from Gk. *katarraktēs*]. Partial or complete opacity of the crystalline lens or its capsule. See also *immature cataract, incipient cataract, mature cataract, membranous cataract, sutural cataract.* —**cat·a·rac·tous** (kat''uh·rack'tus) *adj.*

ca·ta·rac·ta cen·tra·lis pul·ve·ru·len·ta (kat''uh·rack'tuh sen·tray'lis pul''ve·rew·len'tuh). EMBRYONAL NUCLEAR CATARACT.

cataracta co·ro·na·ria (kor·o·nair'ee·uh). CORONARY CATARACT.

cataracta neu·ro·der·mat·i·ca (dur·mat'i·kuh). ATOPIC CATARACT.

cataract needle. A needle used for operating upon a cataract or its capsule.

cataract spoon. A small spoon-shaped instrument used to remove the lens in cataract operations.

ca·tarrh (ka·tahr′) *n.* [Gk. *katarrhous,* from *katarrhein,* to flow down]. Inflammation of mucous membranes, especially those of the air passages, associated with mucoid exudate. —**catarrh·al** (·ul) *adj.*

catarrhal conjunctivitis. A usually acute inflammation of the conjunctiva with smarting of the eyes, heaviness of the lids, photophobia, and excessive mucous or mucopurulent secretion, due to a variety of contagious organisms such as those of the genera *Hemophilus* and *Staphylococcus,* but sometimes becoming chronic as a sequela of the acute form or because of irritation from polluted atmosphere or allergic factors. Syn. *pinkeye.*

catarrhal croup. SPASMODIC CROUP.

catarrhal fever. *Obsol.* 1. COMMON COLD. 2. HERPETIC FEVER.

catarrhal jaundice. INFECTIOUS HEPATITIS.

catarrhal ophthalmia. Hyperemia of the conjunctiva with a mucopurulent secretion.

catarrhal otitis media. SEROUS OTITIS MEDIA.

catarrhal pharyngitis. ACUTE PHARYNGITIS.

cat·ar·rhine (kat′uh·rine) *adj.* [Gk. *katarrhin,* hook-nosed, from *kata,* down, + *rhis, rhinos,* nose]. Having the nostrils close together and pointing forward and downward; a characteristic of human beings, apes, and Old World monkeys, in contrast to the New World monkeys. Contr. *platyrrhine.*

cat·a·stal·sis (kat″uh·stal′sis, ·stahl′sis) *n.* [Gk. *katastaltikos,* from *katastellein,* to check]. A downward-moving wave of contraction occurring in the gastrointestinal tract during digestion. There is no preceding wave of inhibition.

cat·a·state (kat′uh·state) *n.* [Gk. *katastatos,* settled down]. Any result or product of catabolism.

cat·a·stroph·ic reaction. Marked anxiety, agitation, aggressiveness, unreasoning and unreasonable behavior, and autonomic disturbances in response to a threatening situation or severe shock; observed particularly in brain-injured individuals such as those who suddenly are affected with motor aphasia.

catathermometer. KATATHERMOMETER.

cata·thy·mia (kat″uh·thigh′mee·uh) *n.* [*cata-* + *-thymia*]. The existence of a complex in the unconscious mind which is heavily charged with affect or feeling so as to produce a pronounced effect in consciousness.

cata·to·nia (kat″uh·to′nee·uh) *n.* [*cata-* + *-tonia*]. A phase or type of schizophrenia in which the patient seems to lack the will to talk or move and stands or sits in one position, assumes fixed postures, and resists attempts to activate motion or speech. A benign stupor which frequently may be punctuated by violent outbursts, hallucinosis, and panic. —**cata·ton·ic** (kat″uh·ton′ick) *adj.* & *n.*

catatonic type of schizophrenia. A form of schizophrenia characterized by disturbances in motor behavior, one type marked chiefly by withdrawal and generalized inhibition (stupor, mutism, negativism, and waxy flexibility) and the other by excitement and frenzied motor activity.

cata·tro·pia (kat″uh·tro′pee·uh) *n.* [*cata-* + *-tropia*]. A strabismus characterized by the downward deviation of either eye while the other eye fixes.

cat-bite fever. CAT-SCRATCH DISEASE.

catch·ment area. A geographic area for whose inhabitants a health facility, such as a hospital or mental health center, has the responsibility. See also *community medicine, community psychiatry.*

cat ear. CAT'S-EAR.

cat·e·chin (kat′e·chin, ·kin) *n.* An acid substance, $C_{15}H_{14}O_6$, from gambir (pale catechu) and other sources. An amorphous yellow powder, soluble in water; used in dyeing and tanning.

cat·e·chol (kat′i·chole, ·kole, ·kol) *n.* PYROCATECHOL.

cat·e·chol·a·mine (kat″i·kol′uh·meen, ·min) *n.* Any one of a group of sympathomimetic amines containing a catechol moiety, including especially epinephrine, norepinephrine (levarterenol), and dopamine.

cat·e·chu (kat′e·choo, ·koo) *n.* [Malay *kăchū*]. An extract prepared from the wood of *Acacia catechu,* a native tree of the East Indies, containing about 25% catechutannic acid and hence a powerful astringent; formerly used as a remedy for diarrhea of children and as a gargle and mouthwash. See also *gambir.*

cat·e·chu·ic acid (kat″e·choo′ick, ·kew′ick). CATECHIN.

cat·e·gor·i·cal hemisphere. The cerebral hemisphere specialized to subserve the functions involved in language; DOMINANT HEMISPHERE. Contr. *representational hemisphere.*

cat·elec·trot·o·nus (kat″e·leck·trot′uh·nus) *n.* [*cata-* + *electrotonus*]. The increased irritability of a nerve or muscle at the negative pole during passage of an electric current, caused by partial depolarization of the resting transmembrane potential of the irritable tissue. Contr. *anelectrotonus.* —**catelec·tro·ton·ic** (·tro·ton′ick) *adj.*

cat·e·nat·ing (kat′e·nay·ting) *adj.* [L. *catena,* chain]. Connected with a group or series of other signs and symptoms.

cat·er·pil·lar dermatitis, rash, or **urticaria.** An eruption due to the highly irritating or sensitizing substances on hairs of the larvae of certain Lepidoptera, characterized first by erythematous macules and then by wheals.

caterpillar flap. A narrow tubed flap that is advanced end-over-end to reach its ultimate destination.

caterpillar hair ophthalmia. OPHTHALMIA NODOSA.

cat flea. *CTENOCEPHALIDES FELIS.*

cat·gut, *n.* A suture and ligature material made from the submucosa of sheep's intestine, cleansed, treated, and twisted. Sterilized and put up aseptically in glass tubes, in sizes from 00000 to 8. Varieties are: plain (untreated), chromicized (treated with chromic trioxide), and iodized (immersed in a solution of iodine and potassium iodide).

cathaeresis. CATHERESIS.

ca·thar·sis (ka·thahr′sis) *n.,* pl. **cathar·ses** (·seez) [Gk. *katharsis,* a cleansing]. 1. PURGATION. 2. *In psychoanalysis,* the healthful and therapeutic release of tension and anxiety by "talking out" and emotionally reliving repressed incidents and honestly facing the cause of the difficulty.

ca·thar·tic (ka·thahr′tick) *adj.* & *n.* [Gk. *kathartikos,* from *katharein,* to clean]. 1. Producing catharsis; causing evacuation of the bowels. 2. A medicine used to produce evacuations of the bowels; a purgative.

cathartic acid. An active principle from several species of *Cassia.*

ca·thect (ka·thekt′) *v.* [Gk. *kathektikos,* capable of holding or retaining]. *In psychiatry,* to charge ideas with affect or feeling. See also *cathexis.*

ca·thec·tic (ka·theck′tick) *adj.* Of or pertaining to cathexis.

ca·thec·ti·cize (ka·theck′ti·size) *v.* CATHECT.

ca·thep·sin (ka·thep′sin) *n.* [Gk. *kathepsein,* to boil down, + *-in*]. Any one of several proteolytic enzymes present in tissue, catalyzing the hydrolysis of high molecular weight proteins to proteoses and peptones, and having an optimum pH between 4 and 5. It is believed that after death the tissues become acid, and cathepsin produces autolysis (proteolysis).

ca·ther·e·sis, ca·thaer·e·sis (ka·therr′e·sis, ka·theer′, kath″e·ree′sis) *n.* [Gk. *kathairesis,* a pulling down, reducing]. *Obsol.* 1. Prostration or weakness induced by medication. 2. A mild caustic action.

cath·e·ret·ic (kath″e·ret′ick) *adj.* & *n.* [Gk. *kathairetikos,* reducing]. *Obsol.* 1. Reducing; weakening; prostrating. 2. Mildly caustic. 3. A mild caustic.

cath·e·ter (kath′e·tur) *n.* [Gk. *kathetēr,* from *kathienai,* to send down]. A hollow tube of metal, glass, hard or soft rubber, silicone, rubberized silk, or plastic for introduction into a cavity through a narrow canal, for the purpose of discharging the fluid contents of a cavity or for establishing the patency of a canal; specifically, one intended to be passed into the bladder through the urethra for the relief of urinary retention.

catheter fever. A febrile episode ascribed to the passage or retention of a catheter.

catheter gauge. A metal sheet having circular holes punched in it which fit exactly certain catheters or sounds.

cath·e·ter·ism (kath'e·tur·iz·um) *n.* The habitual use of a catheter.

catheter·ize (kath'e·tur·ize) *v.* 1. To insert a catheter. 2. To withdraw urine by means of a urethral catheter. —**cath·eter·iza·tion** (·i·zay'shun) *n.*

catheter life. Constant employment of catheterization by persons who are unable to void urine naturally or who can evacuate only a portion of the bladder contents because of high residual urine.

cath·e·tero·stat (kath'e·tur·o·stat'', ka·theet'ur·o·) *n.* [*catheter* + *-stat*]. A stand for holding and sterilizing catheters.

catheter pacemaker. A temporary or permanent device inserted in the tip of an intracardiac catheter, designed to stimulate the heart electrically.

ca·thex·is (ka·theck'sis) *n.*, pl. **cathex·es** (·seez) [Gk. *kathexis,* holding]. *In psychoanalysis,* the conscious or unconscious investment of an object or idea with psychic energy, i.e., with feelings and meanings. It may be qualitatively defined by terms, such as ego, object, libidinal, instinctual, or erotic. Adj. *cathectic.*

cathisophobia. KATHISOPHOBIA.

cath·ode (kath'ode) *n.* [Gk. *kathodos,* the way down, descent]. The negative electrode or pole of an electric circuit. Abbreviated, C., ca., K., ka. Contr. *anode.*

cathode ray. Streams of electrons emitted from the cathode in low-pressure electrical discharge tubes, such as a Crookes tube or cathode-ray tube, and accelerated by a potential applied at the anode. Beams of cathode rays may be deflected by electric or magnetic fields; when they impinge on a suitable screen, they produce fluorescence, as in an oscilloscope.

cathode-ray oscillograph. An instrument in which a pencil of electrons, striking a fluorescent screen, will trace a graph of any two variables that have been converted into electric equivalents. Its virtue is absence of mechanical inertia, and hence the ability to record changes of extreme rapidity with absolute accuracy. Abbreviated, CRO.

cathode-ray oscilloscope. OSCILLOSCOPE.

ca·thod·ic (ka·thod'ick) *adj.* 1. Pertaining to a cathode; electronegative. 2. Proceeding downward; efferent or centrifugal, as a nerve current or nerve impulse.

Cathomycin. A trademark for novobiocin, an antibiotic.

cat·ion (kat'eye·on) *n.* [Gk. *katiōn,* from *katienai,* to go down]. A positive ion moving toward, or being evolved at, the cathode in electrolytic cells or discharge tubes. Contr. *anion.* —**cat·ion·ic** (kat''eye·on'ick) *adj.*

cation exchange resin. 1. A highly polymerized synthetic organic compound consisting of a large nondiffusible anion and a simple diffusible cation, which latter can be exchanged for a cation in the medium in which the resin is placed. 2. *In medicine,* such a resin, often modified to avoid disturbance in the balance of other physiologically important ions; used to remove sodium ions from the body in treating conditions resulting from abnormal retention of sodium. See also *carbacrylamine resins, carbacrylic resin, potassium carbacrylate.*

cationic detergent. A detergent, such as a quaternary ammonium salt, in which the cleansing action is inherent in the cation.

cat·lin (kat'lin) *n.* CATLING.

cat·ling, *n.* A long, double-edged amputation knife especially adapted to the dividing of tissues between close-lying bones.

cat method. A method of assay for digitalis.

ca·top·tric (ka·top'trick) *adj.* [Gk. *katoptrikos,* in a mirror, reflected, from *katoptron,* mirror]. Of or pertaining to catoptrics.

ca·top·trics (ka·top'tricks) *n.* [*catoptric* + *-s*]. The branch of physics dealing with the principles of reflected light.

catoptric test. The diagnosis of cataract by means of the reflection of the Purkinje images from the cornea and lens capsules.

ca·top·tro·scope (ka·top'tro·skope) *n.* [Gk. *katoptr*ic + *-scope*]. An instrument for examining objects by reflected light from mirrors.

CAT scan. A radiographic scan by computed (axial) tomography.

cat-scratch antigen. Sterilized pus from an infected lymph node or a bubo of a known case of cat-scratch disease, used in an intradermal skin test.

cat-scratch disease or **fever.** A usually self-limited disease clinically manifested by fever, regional or generalized lymphadenitis, and occasionally aseptic meningoencephalitis; probably due to a virus transmitted by a scratch from an animal with sheathed claws, most often a cat.

cat's-ear. A deformity of the human ear causing it to resemble somewhat a cat's ear; characterized by abnormal enlargement and folding forward of the superior part of the helix. Syn. *cat ear.*

cat's-eye pupil. An elongated, slitlike pupil.

Cat·tell infant intelligence scale or **test** (ka·tel') [R. B. *Cattell,* English psychologist, b. 1905]. A modification of the revised Stanford-Binet test adapted for children from 2 to 30 months of age.

cat test. The induction of vomiting and other signs in cats following the administration of filtrates of staphylococcal cultures suspected of being enterotoxigenic and responsible for staphylococcal food poisoning.

cattle grub. The larva of those species of botfly infecting cattle. See also *bot.*

cattle plague. RINDERPEST.

cat unit. The amount of digitalis that will kill a cat when injected intravenously, calculated per kilogram of the animal.

Cau·ca·sian (kaw·kay'zhun) *n.* [after the *Caucasus,* in Asia]. A member of a white-skinned race of people.

caud-, caudo-. A combining form meaning *caudal, tail.*

cau·da (kaw'duh) *n.*, pl. & genit. sing. **cau·dae** (·dee) [L.]. 1. TAIL. 2. A structure resembling or analogous to a tail; a tail-like appendage.

cauda ce·re·bel·li (serr·e·bel'eye). *Obsol.* VERMIS.

cau·dad (kaw'dad) *adv.* [*caud-* + *-ad*]. Toward the tail; caudally; in human anatomy, downward. Contr. *cephalad.*

cauda epi·di·dy·mi·dis (ep''ee·di·dim'i·dis) [NA]. TAIL OF THE EPIDIDYMIS.

cauda equi·na (e·kwye'nuh) [NA]. The roots of the sacral and coccygeal nerves, collectively; so called because of their resemblance to a horse's tail.

cauda equina syndrome. Pain, combined variously with sphincteric disturbances and an asymmetric, atrophic, areflexic paralysis and sensory loss in the distribution of the lumbosacral roots; due to compression of the cauda equina. Compare *conus medullaris syndrome.*

cauda he·li·cis (hel'i·sis) [NA]. An appendage of the cartilage of the ear at the union of the helix and anthelix.

cau·dal (kaw'dul) *adj.* 1. Of, pertaining to, or involving the cauda. 2. Directed toward the tail or cauda; in human anatomy, inferior. Contr. *cranial.*

caudal anesthesia. Anesthesia induced by intermittent or continuous injection of the anesthetic into the sacral canal.

caudal flexure. A flexure of the caudal end of the embryo.

caudal genital fold. EPIGONAL FOLD.

caudal medullary rest. A remnant of the medullary coccygeal vesicle that normally disappears about the sixth fetal month, but may give rise to sacrococcygeal cysts or fistulas.

caudal medullary vestige. COCCYGEAL VESTIGE.
caudal mesonephros. 1. The caudal part of the mesonephros, associated with the gonad, that does not undergo complete degeneration. 2. The part of the mesonephros caudal to the genital mesonephros, the tubules of which form the paradidymis or paroophoron. See also *paragenitalis.*
caudal regression syndrome. A spectrum of anomalies with varying degree of developmental failure in the lower lumbar, sacral, and coccygeal vertebrae; especially sacral agenesis; often associated with neurologic defects.
caudal sheath. MANCHETTE.
cauda nu·clei cau·da·ti (new'klee·eye kaw·day'tye) [NA]. The tail of the caudate nucleus.
cauda pan·cre·a·tis (pan·kree'uh·tis) [NA]. The tail of the pancreas, which has the largest amount of islet tissue and is most frequently the site of islet-cell tumors.
cauda stri·a·ti (strye·ay'tye). The narrow, posterior portion of the caudate nucleus.
cau·date (kaw'date) *adj.* [ML. *caudatus,* from L. *cauda*]. Having a tail or a tail-like appendage. —**cau·da·tion** (kaw·day'shun) *n.*
caudate lobe. The tailed lobe of the liver that separates the right extremity of the transverse fissure from the commencement of the fissure for the inferior vena cava. NA *lobus caudatus.* See also Plate 13.
caudate nucleus. An elongated arched gray mass which projects into and forms part of the lateral wall of the lateral ventricle; part of the corpus striatum. NA *nucleus caudatus.*
caudate process. 1. The elevated portion of the liver extending from the caudate lobe to the undersurface of the right lobe. NA *processus caudatus hepatis.* 2. The lower end of one of the divisions of the anthelix of the external ear.
cau·da·tum (kaw·day'tum) *n.*, pl. **cauda·ta** (·tuh) [L.]. CAUDATE NUCLEUS.
caudo-. See *caud-.*
cau·do·ceph·al·ad (kaw''do·sef'ul·ad) *adv.* [*caudo-* + *cephalad*]. In the direction from the tail toward the head.
caul, *n.* [OF. *cale*]. 1. A portion or all of the fetal membranes covering the head and carried out in advance of it in labor. 2. GREATER OMENTUM.
caul-, cauli-, caulo- [Gk. *kaulos*]. A combining form meaning *stem.*
cauli-. See *caul-.*
cau·li·flow·er ear. Thickening and irregularity of the auricle following repeated blows; seen in pugilists. See also *boxer's ear.*
cauliflower excrescence. A tumor or other lesion with an irregular corrugated surface resembling a cauliflower.
cau·line (kaw'lin, ·line) *adj. In biology,* pertaining to a stem.
caulo-. See *caul-.*
cau·lo·phyl·line (kaw''lo·fil'een, ·in) *n.* *N*-Methylcytisine, $C_{12}H_{16}N_2O$, an alkaloid from caulophyllum.
cau·lo·phyl·lum (kaw''lo·fil'um) *n.* The dried rhizome and roots of *Caulophyllum thalictroides,* containing the alkaloid caulophylline, glycosides, and saponins. It produces intermittent contractions of the gravid uterus and is also said to possess diuretic and anthelmintic properties.
cau·lo·ple·gia (kaw''lo·plee'jee·uh, ·juh) *n.* [*caulo-* + *-plegia*]. *Obsol.* Paralysis affecting the penis.
cau·mes·the·sia, cau·maes·the·sia (kaw''mes·theezh'uh, ·theez'ee·uh) *n.* [Gk. *kauma,* burning heat, + *esthesia*]. The sensation of burning up with heat, when the temperature of neither the patient nor the environment is high.
cau·sal·gia (kaw·sal'jee·uh) *n.* [Gk. *kausos,* fever, + *-algia*]. 1. A syndrome, described by Weir Mitchell, which develops after penetrating wounds with partial injury of the medial, ulnar, or sciatic nerve. It is characterized by a sensation of severe burning pain in the hand or foot, the skin of which becomes smooth and shiny, or scaly and discolored, accompanied by profuse sweating of the involved part, particularly under conditions of emotional stress. 2. Any burning pain in the affected part following a nerve injury.—**causal·gic** (·jick) *adj.*
causalgia syndrome or **causalgic syndrome.** CAUSALGIA (1).
caus·al treatment. Treatment directed against the cause of a disease rather than against its symptoms.
caus·tic (kaws'tick) *adj. & n.* [Gk. *kaustikos,* from *kaiein,* to burn]. 1. Very irritant; burning; capable of destroying tissue. 2. A substance that destroys tissue. 3. *In optics,* a curve to which the rays of light reflected or refracted by another curve are tangent. See also *catacaustic, diacaustic.*
caustic alkali. The hydroxide of an alkali element; commonly, potassium or sodium hydroxide.
caustic bougie. ARMED BOUGIE.
caustic pencil or **stick.** A molded pencil, stick, or cone of silver nitrate.
caustic potash. POTASSIUM HYDROXIDE.
caustic soda. SODIUM HYDROXIDE.
cau·ter·ant (kaw'tur·unt) *adj. & n.* CAUSTIC; ESCHAROTIC.
cau·ter·ize (kaw'tur·ize) *v.* 1. To apply a cautery or a caustic to. 2. To destroy (tissue) by the application of a cauterizing agent or by cautery. —**cau·ter·i·za·tion** (kaw''tur·i·zay'shun) *n.*
cau·tery (kaw'tur·ee) *n.* [Gk. *kautērion,* branding iron]. A device to coagulate or destroy tissue by a chemical or by heat. See also *electrocautery.*
cautery knife. A knife to produce cautery, usually with an insulated handle and heated by electricity or in a flame.
cautery pneumonectomy. The removal of a lung by cautery.
cautery surgery. The use of cautery in surgical procedures, usually applied to benign and malignant growths of the skin.
ca·va (kay'vuh, kav'uh) *adj. & n.*, pl. **ca·vae** (·vee) [L.]. 1. Feminine of L. *cavus,* hollow. 2. Plural of L. *cavum,* cavity. 3. VENA CAVA. —**ca·val** (·vul) *adj.*
caval mesentery or **fold.** An embryonic mesentery, separated from the primitive mesentery of the stomach by the mesenteric recess, in which develops a part of the inferior vena cava and the caudate lobe of the liver.
cav·al·ry bone. RIDER'S BONE.
cav·al·ry·man's osteoma. RIDER'S BONE.
caval valve. The semilunar valve in the right atrium of the heart between the orifice of the inferior vena cava and the right atrioventricular orifice. NA *valvula venae cavae inferioris.*
cav·a·scope (kav'uh·skope) *n.* An instrument for examining a body cavity.
cave of Meck·el [J. F. *Meckel,* Elder]. CAVUM TRIGEMINALE.
ca·ve·o·la (ka·vee'o·luh) *n.*, pl. **caveo·lae** (·lee) [NL., from L. *cavea,* cavity]. 1. A very small cavity or recess. 2. Specifically, CAVEOLA INTRACELLULARIS.
caveola in·tra·cel·lu·la·ris (in''truh·sel''yoo·lair'is), pl. **caveolae intracellula·res** (·reez). One of the small vesicular invaginations of the plasma membrane of a cell (as for example in some capillary endothelium) connected to the surface by a narrower neck. Sometimes the surface invaginations may pinch off by constriction of their necks and move into the cytoplasm as a spherical vesicle.
cav·ern, *n.* [L. *caverna*]. A cavity or hollow, specifically: 1. A pathologic cavity in the lung due to necrosis of its tissues. 2. The cavity of a dilated bronchus.
ca·ver·na (ka·vur'nuh) *n.*, pl. **caver·nae** (·nee) [L.]. A cavity or hollow space.
cavernae cor·po·ris spon·gi·o·si pe·nis (kor'po·ris spon·jee·o'sigh pee'nis) [NA]. The cavities of the corpus spongiosum of the penis.
cavernae cor·po·rum ca·ver·no·so·rum pe·nis (kor'po·rum kav''ur·no·so'rum pee'nis) [NA]. The cavities of the corpora cavernosa of the penis.
cav·er·ni·tis (kav''ur·nigh'tis) *n.* [*cavern* + *-itis*]. Inflammation of the corpora cavernosa. See also *Peyronie's disease.*
cav·er·no·ma (kav''ur·no'muh) *n.*, pl. **cavernomas, cavernoma·**

ta (·tuh) [*cavern* + *-oma*]. A benign cavernous tumor; CAVERNOUS HEMANGIOMA.

cav·er·no·si·tis (kav″ur·no·sigh′tis) *n.* CAVERNITIS.

cav·er·nos·to·my (kav″ur·nos′tuh·mee) *n.* [*cavern* + *-stomy*]. The drainage of a pulmonary abscess or cavity through the chest wall.

cav·er·no·sum (kav″ur·no′sum) *n.*, pl. **caverno·sa** (·suh) [L. *cavernosus*, full of hollows]. CORPUS CAVERNOSUM.

cav·ern·ous (kav′ur·nus) *adj.* Having hollow spaces.

cavernous angioma. An angioma in which the vascular spaces are large or cystic, like the erectile tissue of the penis.

cavernous body. CORPUS CAVERNOSUM.

cavernous groove. CAROTID GROOVE.

cavernous hemangioma. A benign vascular tumor made up of large, thin-walled vascular channels.

cavernous lymphangioma. HYGROMA.

cavernous optic atrophy. Severe degeneration of the optic nerve with connective tissue replacement, excavation of the disc, and depression of the lamina cribrosa; usually due to glaucoma.

cavernous plexus. 1. A sympathetic nerve plexus in the cavernous sinus surrounding the internal carotid artery, formed by fibers from the internal carotid nerve. 2. (of the penis or clitoris:) A nerve plexus in the corpus cavernosum. 3. (pl.: of the nasal conchae:) Venous plexuses found in the mucous membrane overlying the nasal conchae. NA *plexus cavernosi concharum.*

cavernous rale. A hollow, metallic sound heard in advanced tuberculosis, caused by the expansion and contraction of a pulmonary cavity during respiration.

cavernous respiration. A peculiar hollow, blowing, resonant breathing sound heard over lung cavities. See also *amphoric respiration.*

cavernous sinus. An irregularly shaped sinus of the dura mater, located on the side of the body of the sphenoid bone, and extending from the superior orbital fissure in front to the apex of the petrous bone behind. NA *sinus cavernosus.*

cavernous sinus–neuralgia syndrome. GODTFREDSEN'S SYNDROME.

cavernous sinus syndrome. Proptosis, edema of the conjunctiva and eyelids, and palsy of the muscles supplied by the third, fourth, and sixth cranial nerves, due to partial or total occlusion of the cavernous sinus by thrombus, tumor, or arteriovenous aneurysm.

cavernous sinus thrombosis. Inflammation of a cavernous sinus with thrombus formation.

cavernous tissue. ERECTILE TISSUE.

cavernous urethra. The portion of the urethra contained in the corpus spongiosum penis. Syn. *penile urethra.*

Ca·via (kay′vee·uh) *n.* [Carib *cabiai*, capybara]. The genus of cavies, including the guinea pig.

cav·i·ar spots (kav′ee·ahr). Phlebectasia of the tongue, producing small red-brown smooth papules.

cav·i·tary (kav′i·terr·ee) *adj.* 1. Of or pertaining to a cavity. 2. Characterized by cavitation.

ca·vi·tas (kav′i·tas) *n.*, genit. **ca·vi·ta·tis** (kav″i·tay′tis), pl. **cavita·tes** (kav″i·tay′teez) [L.]. A cavity.

cavitas gle·noi·da·lis (glen″oy·day′lis) [NA]. GLENOID CAVITY.

cavitas pul·pae (pul′pee). PULP CAVITY.

cav·i·tate (kav′i·tate) *v.* 1. To form a cavity. 2. To produce cavitation.

cav·i·ta·tion (kav″i·tay′shun) *n.* 1. The formation of a cavity or cavities in an organ or tissue, usually as a result of disease. 2. The process of amnion formation in man and certain mammals. 3. Reduction of the hydrodynamic pressure within a liquid, as by subjecting it to ultrasonic vibration, to a value below the vapor pressure, so that spaces or cavities form in it momentarily.

Ca·vi·te fever (ka·vee′tay) [after *Cavite*, Philippine Islands]. DENGUE.

cav·i·ty (kav′i·tee) *n.* [MF. *cavité*, from L. *cavitas*]. 1. A hole or hollow space. 2. The lesion produced by dental caries.

cavity of the larynx. The hollow space in the larynx that is continuous with that in the pharynx and extends downward to the trachea. NA *cavum laryngis.*

cavity of the septum pellucidum. A cavity in the septum pellucidum found occasionally between its two glial layers, extending from the genu of the corpus callosum anteriorly to the anterior limb and to the columns of the fornix posteriorly. NA *cavum septi pellucidi.*

cavity of the uterus. The space within the uterus lined with endometrium; the size depends upon the state of the uterus. NA *cavum uteri.*

cavity preparation. The removal of carious tooth substance and the proper shaping of a cavity to receive and retain a filling material.

ca·vo·gram (kay′vo·gram) *n.* [vena *cava* + *-gram*]. A radiographic depiction of the vena cava, inferior or superior.

ca·vog·ra·phy (kay·vog′ruh·fee) *n.* Radiographic demonstration of the vena cava, either superior or inferior.

ca·vo·sur·face (kay″vo·sur′fus) *adj.* Of, pertaining to, or designating the wall of a cavity and the surface of a tooth.

cavosurface angle. The angle formed by the meeting of a cavity wall with the surface of the tooth.

cavosurface bevel. That portion of the enamel wall of a cavity which is cut back at an obtuse angle to the tooth surface in order to remove short and friable enamel rods at the cavity margin.

ca·vo·val·gus (kay″vo·val′gus) *n.* Talipes calcaneocavus combined with talipes valgus.

ca·vo·va·rus (kay″vo·vair′us) *n.* Talipes cavus combined with talipes calcaneovarus.

ca·vum (kay′vum) *n.*, genit. **ca·vi** (kay′vye), pl. **ca·va** (·vuh) [L.]. *In anatomy,* a cavity or chamber.

cavum ab·do·mi·nis (ab·dom′i·nis) [NA]. ABDOMINAL CAVITY.

cavum ar·ti·cu·la·re (ahr·tick″yoo·lair′ee) [NA]. JOINT CAVITY.

cavum con·chae (kong′kee) [NA]. The inferior part of the concha of the ear.

cavum co·ro·na·le (kor·o·nay′lee) [NA]. The portion of the pulp cavity lying within the crown of a tooth; PULP CHAMBER.

cavum den·tis (den′tis) [NA]. PULP CAVITY.

cavum epi·du·ra·le (ep″i·dew·ray′lee) [NA]. EPIDURAL SPACE.

cavum hy·a·loi·de·um (high·uh·loy′dee·um). VITREOUS CHAMBER.

cavum in·fra·glot·ti·cum (in·fruh·glot′i·kum) [NA]. The cavity of the larynx immediately below the vocal folds.

cavum la·ryn·gis (la·rin′jis) [NA]. CAVITY OF THE LARYNX.

cavum me·di·a·sti·na·le an·te·ri·us (mee·dee·as″ti·nay′lee an·teer′ee·us) [BNA]. The anterior mediastinal area; it is only a potential cavity.

cavum mediastinale pos·te·ri·us (pos·teer′ee·us) [BNA]. The posterior mediastinal area; it is only a potential cavity.

cavum me·dul·la·re (med·yoo·lair′ee) [NA]. The medullary space of a bone.

cavum Mon·roii (mon·ro′ee·eye) [A. *Monro*, Scottish anatomist]. The most rostral part of the third ventricle.

cavum na·si (nay′zye) [NA]. NASAL CAVITY.

cavum oris (o′ris) [NA]. ORAL CAVITY.

cavum oris pro·pri·um (pro′pree·um) [NA]. The portion of the oral cavity lying inside the upper and lower rows of teeth.

cavum pel·vis (pel′vis) [NA]. PELVIC CAVITY.

cavum pe·ri·car·dii (perr·i·kahr′dee·eye) [NA]. PERICARDIAL CAVITY.

cavum pe·ri·to·nei (perr″i·to·nee′eye) [NA]. PERITONEAL CAVITY.

cavum pha·ryn·gis (fa·rin′jis) [NA]. The cavity of the pharynx.

cavum pleu·rae (ploo'ree) [NA]. PLEURAL CAVITY.
cavum pleu·ro·peri·car·di·a·co·peri·to·ne·a·le (ploo"ro·perr·i·kahr·dye"a·ko·perr"i·to·nee·ay'lee). The embryonic coelom.
cavum pleu·ro·peri·car·di·a·le (ploo"ro·perr"i·kahr·dee·ay'lee). The pleural and pericardial part of the coelom.
cavum psal·te·rii (sahl·teer'ee·eye). A small cavity occasionally present above the commissure of the fornix. It may communicate with the cavity of the septum pellucidum.
cavum sep·ti pel·lu·ci·di (sep'tye pe·lew'si·dye) [NA]. CAVITY OF THE SEPTUM PELLUCIDUM.
cavum sub·arach·noi·de·a·le (sub"uh·rack·noy·dee·ay'lee) [NA]. SUBARACHNOID SPACE.
cavum sub·du·ra·le (sub·dew·ray'lee) [BNA]. SUBDURAL SPACE.
cavum tho·ra·cis (tho·ray'sis) [NA]. THORACIC CAVITY.
cavum tri·ge·mi·na·le (trye·jem·i·nay'lee) [NA]. The pocket between the two layers of dura mater occupied by the trigeminal ganglion.
cavum tym·pa·ni (tim'puh·nigh) [NA]. TYMPANIC CAVITY.
cavum ute·ri (yoo'tur·eye) [NA]. CAVITY OF THE UTERUS.
cavum ve·li in·ter·po·si·ti (vee'lye in·tur·poz'i·tye). A small extension of the subarachnoid space occasionally present within the velum interpositum.
cavum Ver·gae (vur'jee, ·ghee) [A. *Verga*, Italian anatomist, 1811–1895]. A caudal extension of the cavity of the septum pellucidum from the fornix to the splenium of the corpus callosum.
ca·vus (kay'vus) *adj. & n.* [L.]. 1. Hollow, concave. 2. PES CAVUS OR TALIPES CAVUS.
ca·vy (kay'vee) *n.* [NL. *Cavia*]. Any of several short-tailed, rough-haired rodents from the family Caviidae; usually, a guinea pig.
cay·enne pepper (kay·en', kigh·en'). CAPSICUM.
cayenne-pepper spot. PAPILLARY VARIX.
Ca·ze·nave's disease (kah^nz·nahv') [P. L. A. *Cazenave*, French dermatologist, 1795–1877]. PEMPHIGUS FOLIACEUS.
Cb Symbol for columbium (= NIOBIUM).
CBC Complete blood count.
CBG Abbreviation for *corticosteroid-binding globulin.*
C bile. Bile from the hepatic duct.
CB lead. *In electrocardiography,* a precordial exploring electrode placed at the cardiac apex, paired with an indifferent electrode in the back near the angle of the scapula; a bipolar lead.
C body. A spherical structure found around the microvilli of the columnar absorptive cells of human colonic mucosa; it is 20–80 nm in diameter and surrounded by a membrane; origin from R bodies has been suggested.
CBS Abbreviation for *chronic brain syndrome.*
C. C. Commission Certified; indicating that a sample of the dye so marked has been submitted to the Biological Stain Commission and has been found by the Commission to meet its standards for the dye.
cc An abbreviation for *cubic centimeter* (= c^3).
C carbohydrate. A carbohydrate found in pneumococci.
CCK Abbreviation for *cholecystokinin.*
CCK-PZ Abbreviation for *cholecystokinin-pancreozymin.*
CCNU [. . .*c*hloroethyl. . .*c*ycloethyl. . .*n*itros*u*rea]. 1-(2-Chloroethyl)-3-cyclohexyl-1-nitrosourea, $C_9H_{16}ClN_3O_2$, an antineoplastic. Syn. *lomustine.*
CCU Coronary care unit or cardiac care unit.
Cd Symbol for cadmium.
cd Abbreviation for *candela.*
CDC Abbreviation for *Center for Disease Control* (formerly: *Communicable Disease Center*).
Ce Symbol for cerium.
CEA Abbreviation for *carcinoembryonic antigen.*
ce·as·mic (see·az'mick) *adj.* [Gk. *keazein*, ke*keasm*enos, to split, sever]. Characterized by embryonic fissures after birth.
ceasmic teratism. A deformity in which parts that should be united remain in their primitive, fissured state.
Ce·bi·dae (see'bi·dee) *n.pl.* [From *Cebus,* type genus]. A family of Anthropoidea comprising the New World monkeys proper. See also *Ceboidea.* Contr. *Callitrichidae.*
Cebione. A trademark for ascorbic acid.
ce·bo·ce·pha·lia (see"bo·se·fay'lee·uh) *n.* [Gk. *kēbos*, monkey, + *-cephalia*]. A condition, related to incipient cyclopia, in which there is absence or marked defect of the nose, with, however, two orbital cavities and two eyes, the region between the eyes being narrow and flat.
ce·bo·ceph·a·lus (see"bo·sef'uh·lus) *n.* An individual showing cebocephalia. —**cebo·ce·phal·ic** (·se·fal'ick), **cebocephalous,** *adj.*
ce·bo·ceph·a·ly (see"bo·sef'uh·lee) *n.* CEBOCEPHALIA.
Ce·boi·dea (se·boy'dee·uh) *n.pl.* The superfamily of Anthropoidea comprising all New World nonhuman primates. Contr. *Cercopithecoidea.*
Ce·bus (see'bus) *n.* [Gk. *kēbos*, a kind of African monkey]. A genus of medium-sized South and Central American monkeys with semiprehensile tails.
cec-, caec, ceco-, caeco-. A combining form meaning *cecum.*
ceca. Plural of *cecum.*
ce·cal, cae·cal (see'kul) *adj.* Of or resembling a cecum.
cecal appendage. VERMIFORM APPENDIX.
cecal foramen. FORAMEN CECUM.
cecal fossa. A fold of peritoneum forming a pouch upon the surface of the right iliopsoas muscle, and extending to the apex of the cecum.
cecal plica. A fold of peritoneum, the unfused portion of the ascending mesocolon, which forms the right boundary of the cecal fossa.
ce·cec·to·my, cae·cec·to·my (see·seck'tuh·mee) *n.* [*cec-* + *-ectomy*]. Excision of the cecum.
ceci-. See *cec-.*
ce·ci·tis, cae·ci·tis (see·sigh'tis) *n.* [*cec-* + *-itis*]. Inflammation of the cecum.
ceco-. See *cec-.*
ce·co·cele, cae·co·cele (see'ko·seel) *n.* [*ceco-* + *-cele*]. Herniation of the cecum.
ce·co·co·lic, cae·co·co·lic (see"ko·ko'lick, ·kol'ick) *adj.* [*ceco-* + *colic*]. Pertaining to the cecum and the colon.
ce·co·co·los·to·my, cae·co·co·los·to·my (see"ko·ko·los'tuh·mee) *n.* [*ceco-* + *colostomy*]. The formation of an anastomosis between the cecum and some part of the colon.
ce·co·il·e·os·to·my, cae·co·il·e·os·to·my (see"ko·il"ee·os'tuh·mee) *n.* [*ceco-* + *ileo-* + *-stomy*]. The formation of an anastomosis between the cecum and the ileum.
Cecon. A trademark for ascorbic acid.
ce·co·pexy, cae·co·pexy (see'ko·peck"see) *n.* [*ceco-* + *-pexy*]. Fixation of the cecum by a surgical operation.
ce·co·pli·ca·tion, cae·co·pli·ca·tion (see"ko·pli·kay'shun) *n.* [*ceco-* + *plication*]. An operation for the relief of dilated cecum, consisting in taking tucks or folds in the wall.
ce·cop·to·sis, cae·cop·to·sis (see"kop·to'sis) *n.*, pl. **cecopto·ses, caecopto·ses** (·seez) [*ceco-* + *ptosis*]. Downward displacement of the cecum.
ce·cor·rha·phy, cae·cor·rha·phy (see·kor'uh·fee) *n.* [*ceco-* + *-rrhaphy*]. Suture of the cecum.
ce·co·sig·moid·os·to·my, cae·co·sig·moid·os·to·my (see"ko·sig"moid·os'tuh·mee) *n.* [*ceco-* + *sigmoidostomy*]. The establishment of an anastomosis between the cecum and sigmoid colon.
ce·cos·to·my, cae·cos·to·my (see·kos'tuh·mee) *n.* [*ceco-* + *-stomy*]. The establishment of a permanent artificial opening into the cecum.
ce·cot·o·my, cae·cot·o·my (see·kot'uh·mee) *n.* [*ceco-* + *-tomy*]. Incision into the cecum.
ce·cum, cae·cum (see'kum) *n.*, pl. **ce·ca, cae·ca** (·kuh) [L. *(intestinum) caecum,* from *caecus,* blind]. 1. [NA] The large blind pouch or cul-de-sac in which the large intestine begins. See also Plate 13. 2. The blind end of any of various

tubular structures. See also *cupular cecum, vestibular cecum.*

cecum cu·pu·la·re (kew·pew·lair'ee) [NA]. CUPULAR CECUM.

cecum ves·ti·bu·la·re (ves·tib·yoo·lair'ee) [NA]. VESTIBULAR CECUM.

ce·dar (see'dur) *n.* [Gk. *kedros*]. Any of various trees of the genera *Cedrus, Juniperus,* and *Thuja.*

cedar leaf oil. A volatile oil from the leaves of the American arborvitae or white cedar, *Thuja occidentalis,* containing ketones, chiefly thujone and fenchone. Formerly used in menstrual disorders, occasionally as a counterirritant.

cedar oil. A transparent oil obtained from the red cedar, *Juniperus virginiana;* used as clearing agent in histology and with oil-immersion lenses.

Cedilanid. Trademark for crystalline lanatoside C, a cardioactive glycoside from *Digitalis lanata.* See also *digoxin.*

Cedilanid-D. Trademark for deslanoside, or desacetyl lanatoside C, a cardioactive glycoside.

ce·drene (see'dreen) *n.* A volatile liquid hydrocarbon, $C_{15}H_{24}$, found in red cedar oil (*Juniperus virginiana*), clove oil, and cubeb oil.

ce·dron (see'dron) *n.* The seeds of the tree *Simaba cedron,* formerly considered to have antimalarial activity.

CeeNU. A trademark for lomustine, an antineoplastic agent.

Ceepryn chloride. Trademark for cetylpyridinium chloride, an antiseptic and detergent.

cef·a·drox·il (sef''uh·drock'sil) *n.* (6*R*,7*R*)-7-[(*R*)-2-amino-2-(*p*-hydroxyphenyl)acetamido]-3-methyl-8-oxo-5-thia-1-azabicyclo[4.2.0]oct-2-ene-2-carboxylic acid, $C_{16}H_{17}N_3O_5S$, an antibacterial agent of the cephalosporin type with a mechanism of action similar to the penicillins.

Cefadyl. A trademark for cephapirin sodium.

cef·a·man·dole (sef''uh·man'dole) *n.* $C_{18}H_{18}N_6O_5S_2$, an antibiotic of the cephalosporin type.

cefamandole naf·ate (naf'ate). The formate ester of cefamandole.

ce·faz·o·lin (se·faz'o·lin) *n.* $C_{14}H_{14}N_8O_4S_3$, an antibiotic of the cephalosporin type, usually used as the sodium salt.

ce·fox·i·tin (se·fock'si·tin) *n.* $C_{16}H_{17}N_3O_7S_2$, an antibiotic of the cephalosporin type.

cel-. See (a) *coel-;* (b) *celi-.*

Ce·las·trus (se·las'trus) *n.* [Gk. *kēlastros,* holly]. A genus of trees and shrubs of the family Celastraceae.

Celastrus scan·dens (skan'denz). The American bittersweet of North America; has been used as a cathartic, diuretic, and alterative.

Celbenin. A trademark for the sodium salt of methicillin, a semisynthetic penicillin antibiotic.

¹-cele [Gk. *kēlē*]. A combining form meaning (a) *tumor;* (b) *hernia;* (c) *pathologic swelling.*

²-cele. See *-coele.*

Cel·e·bes ape (sel'e·beez) [after *Celebes,* an island in Indonesia]. BLACK APE.

cel·ery fruit. The dried, ripe fruit of the celery plant *Apium graveolens,* containing a volatile oil; used as a stimulant and a condiment.

Celestone. Trademark for betamethasone, a synthetic glucocorticoid.

celi-, coeli-, celio-, coelio- [Gk. *koilia*]. A combining form meaning *abdomen* or *belly.*

ce·li·ac, coe·li·ac (see'lee·ack) *adj.* [Gk. *koiliakos,* from *koilia,* belly]. Abdominal; pertaining to the abdomen.

celiac artery. CELIAC TRUNK.

celiac axis. CELIAC TRUNK.

celiac disease. CELIAC SYNDROME.

celiac ganglia. The collateral sympathetic ganglia lying in the celiac plexus near the origin of the celiac artery. NA *ganglia celiaca.*

celiac infantilism. PANCREATIC INFANTILISM.

celiac plexus. A large nerve plexus lying in front of the aorta around the origin of the celiac trunk. It is formed by fibers from the splanchnic and vagus nerves and is distributed to the abdominal viscera. NA *plexus celiacus.*

celiac rickets. Rickets resulting from lack of absorption of vitamin D and loss of calcium in the stool, associated with the celiac syndrome.

celiac syndrome or **disease.** One of the malabsorption syndromes characterized by malnutrition, abnormal stools, and varying degrees of edema, skeletal disorders, peripheral neuropathy, and anemia. Abnormalities of the small intestinal villi and the response to a gluten-free diet are diagnostic. See also *infantile celiac disease.*

celiac trunk. The short, thick artery arising from the anterior (ventral) aspect of the abdominal aorta between the two crura of the diaphragm. It usually divides into the hepatic, splenic, and left gastric arteries. NA *truncus celiacus.* See also Plate 8.

ce·li·a·del·phus, coe·li·a·del·phus (see''lee·uh·del'fus) *n.* [*celi-* + *-adelphus*]. OMPHALOPAGUS.

ce·li·ec·ta·sia, coe·li·ec·ta·sia (see''lee·eck·tay'zhuh, ·zee·uh) *n.* [*celi-* + *ectasia*]. Abnormal distention of the abdominal cavity.

celio-. See *celi-.*

ce·lio·col·pot·o·my, coe·lio·col·pot·o·my (see''lee·o·kol·pot'uh·mee) *n.* [*celio-* + *colpotomy*]. The opening of the abdomen through the vagina, for the removal of a tumor or other body.

ce·lio·en·ter·ot·o·my, coe·lio·en·ter·ot·o·my (see''lee·o·en''tur·ot'uh·mee) *n.* [*celio-* + *enterotomy*]. The opening of the intestine through an incision in the abdominal wall.

ce·lio·gas·trot·o·my, coe·lio·gas·trot·o·my (see''lee·o·gas·trot'uh·mee) *n.* [*celio-* + *gastrotomy*]. The opening of the stomach through an abdominal incision.

ce·li·o·ma, coe·li·o·ma (see''lee·o'muh) *n.,* [*celi-* + *-oma*]. *Rare.* MESOTHELIOMA.

ce·lio·my·o·mec·to·my, coe·lio·my·o·mec·to·my (see''lee·o·migh''o·meck'tuh·mee) *n.* [*celio-* + *myomectomy*]. The removal of a myoma (of the uterus) through an abdominal incision.

ce·lio·para·cen·te·sis, coe·lio·para·cen·te·sis (see''lee·o·păr''uh·sen·tee'sis) *n.,* [*celio-* + *paracentesis*]. Tapping, or paracentesis, of the abdomen.

ce·li·or·rha·phy, coe·li·or·rha·phy (see''lee·or'uh·fee) *n.* [*celio-* + *-rrhaphy*]. Suture of the abdominal wall.

ce·lio·scope, coe·lio·scope (see'lee·uh·skope) *n.* CELOSCOPE.

ce·li·os·co·py, coe·li·os·co·py (see''lee·os'kuh·pee) *n.* [*celio-* + *-scopy*]. PERITONEOSCOPY.

ce·li·ot·o·my, coe·li·ot·o·my (see''lee·ot'uh·mee) *n.* [*celio-* + *-tomy*]. *In surgery,* the opening of the abdominal cavity.

ce·li·tis, coe·li·tis (see·lye'tis) *n.* [*cel-* + *-itis*]. Any inflammatory condition of the abdomen.

cell-, cello-. A combining form meaning *cellulose.*

cell, *n.* [L. *cella,* cubicle, compartment (rel. to Gmc. *ᵏhallo* → E. *hall* and to Gmc. *ᵏhul-* → E. *hole, hollow*)]. 1. A highly integrated, constantly changing system that is the structural and functional unit of the living organism, and that has the ability to assimilate, grow, reproduce, and respond to stimuli. 2. An apparatus, consisting of electrodes and an electrolyte solution, for converting chemical into electrical energy or the reverse. 3. A compartment; particularly, a hollow space in a bone.

cel·la (sel'uh) *n.,* pl. **cel·lae** (·ee) [L., compartment, chamber]. The central part of the lateral ventricle of the brain, extending from the interventricular foramen to the splenium of the corpus callosum.

cel·la·bu·rate (sel''uh·bew'rate) *n.* Cellulose acetate butyrate employed as an enteric coating for tablets.

Cel·la·no blood group [*Cellano,* the patient in whom it was first seen]. At first thought to be a distinct blood group, but now recognized as belonging to the Kell blood group.

Cellase 1000. Trademark for cellulase (2), used as an inflammation counteractant.

cell axis. An imaginary line passing through the nucleus and the central apparatus of a cell.
cell biology. A comprehensive discipline which includes cytology, cytogenetics, molecular biology, cellular physiology, and the ultrastructure of cells.
cell body. The portion of a neuron that contains the nucleus and its surrounding cytoplasm and from which the axon and dendrites extend. See also *perikaryon.*
cell-color ratio. The ratio between the percentage of erythrocytes in blood and the percentage of hemoglobin.
cell cone. PEARL (1).
cell division. A biological process by which two or more cells are formed from one, usually by mitosis, meiosis, or amitosis.
cell doctrine. CELL THEORY.
celle claire [F.]. CLEAR CELL (2, 3).
cell juice. CYTOCHYLEMA.
cell mass. *In embryology,* a group of cells forming the primordium of an organ or of an organism.
cell-mediated immunity. Immunity which is maintained primarily by T lymphocytes rather than by the freely circulating antibody characteristic of humoral immunity; seen in immune response to viruses, fungi, and certain bacterial infections, in rejection of foreign tissue and of tumors, and in delayed hypersensitivity.
cell membrane. PLASMA MEMBRANE.
cell nest. An isolated mass of epithelial cells surrounded by connective tissue, as in carcinoma.
cello-. See *cell-.*
cel·lo·bi·ose (sel″o·bye′oce, ·oze) *n.* A disaccharide, $C_{12}H_{22}O_{11}$, formed by the partial hydrolysis of cellulose. On hydrolysis it yields two molecules of glucose.
cel·lo·dex·trin (sel″o·decks′trin) *n.* Any of a mixture of dextrin-like substances resulting from partial hydrolysis of cellulose by acids.
cell of Betz [V. A. *Betz*]. BETZ CELL.
cell of origin. A nerve cell body of the ganglion or nucleus from which a nerve fiber originates.
cell of termination. A nerve cell whose dendrites receive impulses from the axon of another cell or cells.
cel·loi·din (se·loy′din) *n.* One of many cellulose nitrates or cellulose acetates; used for embedding tissues in histologic technique. See also *pyroxylin.*
Cellophane. Trademark for a nonpermeable, transparent cellulose derivative used to maintain moisture in, or to protect, a surgical dressing or other substances.
Cellosize. A trademark for hydroxyethyl cellulose, a thickener and suspending agent for pharmaceutical preparations.
Cellothyl. A trademark for methylcellulose.
cell plate. The equatorial thickening of the spindle fibers from which the intercellular septum arises in the division of plant cells. It is vestigial in some animals.
cell rest. FETAL REST.
cell sap. HYALOPLASM.
cells of Bött·cher (bœt′ᶜhur) [A. *Böttcher*]. Dark polyhedral cells between the basilar membrane and the cells of Claudius.
cells of Ca·jal (ka·ᵏhal′) [S. Ramón y *Cajal*]. ASTROCYTES.
cells of Clau·dius (klaow′dyo͞os, angl. klaw′dee·us) [F. M. *Claudius,* German anatomist, 1822–1869]. Clear polygonal cells of varying heights, above the basilar membrane of the cochlear duct and beyond the cells of Hensen.
cells of Dei·ters (dye′turss) [O. F. K. *Deiters,* German anatomist, 1834–1863]. 1. The outer phalangeal cells of the spiral organ (of Corti). 2. Large nerve cells in the lateral vestibular nucleus of the medulla oblongata.
cells of Gian·nuz·zi (jaʰn·noot′tsee) [G. *Giannuzzi,* Italian anatomist, 1839–1876]. DEMILUNE.
cells of Hen·sen (hen′zun) [V. *Hensen,* German pathologist, 1835–1924]. Tall cells with a small base and enlarged upper part outside the outer phalangeal cells of the spiral organ (of Corti).
cells of Kul·tschitz·sky (ko͞olʸ·chits′kee) [N. *Kultschitzsky*]. The argentaffin cells of the intestinal glands.
cells of Meynert [T. H. *Meynert*]. SOLITARY CELLS OF MEYNERT.
cells of Pa·neth (pah′net) [J. *Paneth,* German physician, 1857–1890]. PANETH CELLS.
cells of Schwann. SCHWANN CELLS.
cells of van Ge·huch·ten (vaʰn ᵍhe·hœᵏh′tun) [A. *van Gehuchten,* Belgian neurologist, 1861–1914]. GOLGI CELLS, type II.
cell theory. The theory that the cell is the unit of organic structure and that cell formation is the essential process of life and its phenomena.
cellul-, celluli-, cellulo-. A combining form meaning *cell, cellular.*
cel·lu·la (sel′yoo·luh) *n.,* pl. **cellu·lae** (·lee) [L.]. Any small enclosed space; CELLULE (1).
cellulae an·te·ri·o·res (an·teer·ee·o′reez) [NA]. The anterior ethmoidal cells. See *ethmoidal cells.*
cellulae eth·moi·da·les (eth·moy·day′leez) [NA]. ETHMOIDAL CELLS.
cellulae ma·stoi·de·ae (mas·toy′dee·ee) [NA]. MASTOID CELLS.
cellulae me·diae (mee′dee·ee) [NA]. The middle ethmoidal cells. See *ethmoidal cells.*
cellulae pneu·ma·ti·cae tu·bae au·di·ti·vae (new·mat′i·see tew′bee aw·di·tye′vee) [NA]. Air cells related to the bony portion of the auditory tube.
cellulae pneumaticae tu·ba·ri·ae (tew·bair′ee·ee) [BNA]. CELLULAE PNEUMATICAE TUBAE AUDITIVAE.
cellulae pos·te·ri·o·res (pos·teer·ee·o′reez) [NA]. The posterior ethmoidal cells. See *ethmoidal cells.*
cellulae tym·pa·ni·cae (tim·pan′i·see) [NA]. Small spaces which are subdivisions of the middle ear cavity.
cel·lu·lar (sel′yoo·lur) *adj.* Pertaining to or consisting of cells.
cellular immunology. The study of the cells which mediate immune responses, such as lymphocytes and macrophages.
cellular infiltration. 1. Passage of cells into tissues in the course of acute, subacute, or chronic inflammation. 2. Migration or invasion of cells of neoplasms.
cellular pathology. The study of changes in cells as the basis of disease.
cellular physiology. Physiology of individual cells, as compared with entire tissues or organisms.
cellular sheath. *Obsol.* EPINEURIUM.
cel·lu·lase (sel′yoo·lace, ·laze) *n.* 1. Any of several enzymes, found in bacteria and other lower organisms, capable of catalyzing the hydrolysis of cellulose to cellobiose. 2. A concentrate of cellulose-splitting enzymes, derived from *Aspergillus niger,* used as an inflammation counteractant.
cel·lule (sel′yool) *n.* [F., from L. *cellula,* small storeroom]. 1. A small cell. 2. CELL.
cellule claire [F.]. CLEAR CELL (2, 3).
celluli-. See *cellul-.*
cel·lu·lif·u·gal (sel″lew·lif′yoo·gul) *adj.* [*celluli-* + *-fugal*]. Moving away from a cell body.
cel·lu·lin (sel′yoo·lin) *n.* CELLULOSE.
cel·lu·li·tis (sel″yoo·lye′tis) *n.* [*cellule* + *-itis*]. A diffuse inflammation of connective tissue, especially of subcutaneous tissue.
cellulo-. See *cellul-.*
Celluloid. Trademark for a tough, flammable synthetic thermoplastic composed of cellulose nitrate and camphor or other plasticizer; formerly used in surgery and dentistry.
Celluloid jacket. A jacket made principally of Celluloid, fashioned over a plaster mold of the patient's body.
cel·lu·lo·sa (sel″yoo·lo′suh) *adj.* Pertaining to a cellular coat.
cel·lu·lose (sel′yoo·loce) *n.* $(C_6H_{10}O_5)_n$. The principal carbohydrate constituent of the cell membranes of all plants. Absorbent cotton is one of the purest forms of cellulose;

commercially, wood is the principal source of it. Pure cellulose is a white, amorphous mass, insoluble in most of the common solvents.

cellulose acetate phthalate. A substance prepared by heating together phthalic anhydride and cellulose acetate; used for enteric coating of tablets and capsules.

cellulose ether. A product resulting from the reaction of a caustic alkali derivative of cellulose and an alkyl ester of an organic acid. An important compound of this type is methyl cellulose.

Cellulose gum. A trademark for carboxymethylcellulose sodium.

cell wall. In bacteria, fungi, most algae, and all higher plants, the more or less rigid envelope, exterior to the plasma membrane, which encloses and shapes the cell.

celo-. See *coel-, coelo-.*

celom. COELOM.

celomic. COELOMIC.

Celontin. Trademark for methsuximide, an anticonvulsant.

ce·lo·scope, coe·lo·scope (see'lo·skope) *n.* [*celo-* + *-scope*]. An instrument for illuminating and examining a cavity of the body.

ce·lo·so·ma, coe·lo·so·ma (see"lo·so'muh) *n.* [*celo-* + *soma*]. A congenital body cleft, with eventration; associated with various anomalies of the extremities, of the genitourinary apparatus, of the intestinal tract, and even of the whole trunk. Syn. *abdominal fissure.*

ce·lo·so·mia, coe·lo·so·mia (see"lo·so'mee·uh) *n.* CELOSOMA

ce·lo·so·mus, coe·lo·so·so·mus (see"lo·so'mus) *n.*, pl. **celoso·mi, coeloso·mi** (·migh). An individual with celosoma.

ce·lo·the·li·o·ma, coe·lo·the·li·o·ma (see"lo·theel"ee·o'muh) *n.* [*celo-* + *theli-* + *-oma*]. *Rare.* MESOTHELIOMA.

Cels. An abbreviation for *Celsius.*

Cel·si·us (sel'see·us) *adj.* [A. *Celsius,* Swedish astronomer, 1701–1744]. Pertaining to or designating the centigrade temperature scale in which 0° is set at the freezing point of water and 100° at the boiling point. Abbreviated, C. Contr. *Fahrenheit.* See also Table of Thermometric Equivalents in the Appendix.

ce·ment (se·ment') *n.* [L. *caementum,* a rough stone]. 1. Any plastic material capable of becoming hard and of binding together the objects that are contiguous to it. 2. Any material used for filling cavities in teeth, seating crowns or inlays, or for protecting the dental pulp from harmful stimuli. 3. CEMENTUM.

cement bifocals. Bifocals in which greater refractive power is obtained by cementing a wafer onto the front or back of the lens.

ce·ment·i·cle (se·men'ti·kul) *n.* A calcified body found free in the connective tissue of the periodontal membrane, or fused with the cementum of a tooth.

ce·ment·i·fi·ca·tion (se·men"ti·fi·kay'shun) *n.* CEMENTOGENESIS.

cement kidney. *Obsol.* A calcified kidney.

cement line. The optically demonstrable interface between older bone matrix and more recently formed matrix.

ce·men·to·blast (se·men'to·blast) *n.* [*cementum* + *-blast*]. A cell that takes part in the formation of the dental cementum.

ce·men·to·blas·to·ma (se·men"to·blas·to'muh) *n.* [*cementum* + *blastoma*]. A cementoma with prominent cellular components.

ce·men·to·den·ti·nal (se·men"to·den'ti·nul) *adj.* Pertaining to the cementum and dentin of a tooth.

ce·men·to·enam·el (se·men"to·e·nam'ul) *adj.* Pertaining to the cementum and enamel of a tooth.

cementoenamel junction. The junction between the enamel and the cementum of a tooth.

ce·men·to·gen·e·sis (se·men"to·jen'e·sis) *n.* [*cementum* + *genesis*]. Formation of the cementum.

ce·men·to·ma (see"men·to'muh, sem"en·) *n.*, pl. **cementomas, cementoma·ta** (·tuh) [*cementum* + *-oma*]. A benign dysontogenetic tumor composed of odontogenic, cementum-producing connective tissue.

ce·men·to·path·ia (se·men"to·path'ee·uh) *n.* [*cementum* + *-pathia*]. Pathologic degeneration of the cementum surrounding a tooth; formerly thought to account for noninflammatory periodontal destruction (periodontosis).

ce·men·to·sis (see"men·to'sis) *n.*, pl. **cementoses** (·seez) [*cementum* + *-osis*]. HYPERCEMENTOSIS.

cement substance. INTERCELLULAR CEMENT.

ce·men·tum (se·men'tum) *n.*, pl. **cemen·ta** (·tuh) [L. *caementum,* rough stone] [NA]. The bony tissue that covers the root of a tooth, in man, and may cover parts of the crown of a tooth in certain animals, such as the ungulates.

C.E. mixture. An inhalation anesthetic composed of a mixture of chloroform and ether; now rarely used.

[1]cen-, caen-, ceno-, caeno- [Gk. *kainos,* new]. A combining form meaning *new, recent.*

[2]cen-, coen-, ceno-, coeno- [Gk. *koinos*]. A combining form meaning (a) *general;* (b) *common.*

cen·a·del·phus, coen·a·del·phus (sen"uh·del'fus) *n.* [*cen-* + *-adelphus*]. DIPLOPAGUS.

Cendevax. A trademark for live rubella virus vaccine.

ce·nes·the·sia, coe·naes·the·sia (see"nes·theezh'uh, ·theez'ee·uh, sen"es·) *n.* [*cen-* + *esthesia*]. The general sense of bodily existence, the sum of the multiple stimuli coming from the various parts of the body, and hence the basis for feelings of health or sickness. Compare *cenesthopathy.* **—cenes·thet·ic, coenaes·thet·ic** (·thet'ick) *adj.*

ce·nes·thop·a·thy (see"nes·thop'uth·ee) *n.* [*cen-* + *esthesia* + *-pathy*]. The general feeling of discomfort or fatigue in illness as a result of multiple stimuli from various parts of the body; it may be accompanied by a mild form of depersonalization. Compare *cenesthesia.*

ceno-. See *cen-.*

cenocyte. COENOCYTE.

ce·no·gen·e·sis, cae·no·gen·e·sis (see"no·jen'e·sis, sen"o·) *n.* [*ceno-,* new, + *-genesis*]. The development of structures during ontogeny in adaptive response to the embryonic, larval, or fetal mode of life. Compare *palingenesis.* See also *recapitulation theory.* **—ceno·ge·net·ic, caeno·ge·net·ic** (·je·net'ick) *adj.*

Cenolate. A trademark for sodium ascorbate.

ceno·pho·bia (sen"o·fo'bee·uh, see"no·) *n.* KENOPHOBIA.

ce·no·site (see'no·site, sen'o·) *n.* COINOSITE.

cen·sor, *In psychoanalysis,* that part of the unconscious self, composed of the superego and parts of the ego, which acts as a guard, as in dreams, to keep repressed material from emerging into consciousness. See also *censorship.*

cen·sor·ship, *n. In psychoanalysis,* the restrictions imposed upon a pure instinctual impulse by counterforces in the unconscious and conscious levels of the mind before it discharges itself upon the environment.

cen·tau·ry (sen'taw·ree) *n.* [Gk. *kentaurion,* from the centaur Chiron]. 1. A popular name for various plants of the genus *Centaurium.* 2. The dried flowering plant of *Centaurium umbellatum.* Centaury possesses the bitter properties of the gentians and has been used as a stomachic.

cen·ter, cen·tre, *n.* 1. The midpoint of any surface or body. 2. A nucleus or collection of nuclei, or even a relatively imprecisely defined anatomic region in the brain, brainstem, or spinal cord subserving a particular function. See also *area, nucleus.*

Center for Disease Control. An agency of the United States government, located in Atlanta, Georgia, which plans, conducts, coordinates, supports, and evaluates national programs for the prevention and control of communicable and vector-borne diseases and other preventable conditions, including those related to malnutrition. Abbreviated, CDC. Formerly called *Communicable Disease Center.*

cen·ter·ing, cen·tring (sen'tur·ing) *n.* 1. *In microscopy,* arrangement of an object or an accessory so that its center coincides with the optical axis of the microscope. 2. *In* *optics,* placing of the lens before the eye or in a spectacle frame so that the visual axis passes through the optical center of the lens. The decentering of the lens produces a prism effect. —**cen·ter, cen·tre,** *n. & v.*

center of curvature. *In ophthalmology,* the center of the sphere of which a lens curvature is the segment.

center of ossification. A region at which bone first appears in cartilage or membrane.

center of rotation. *In ophthalmology,* the point around which the eyeball rotates under the action of the extrinsic muscles.

cen·te·sis (sen·tee'sis) *n.,* pl. **cente·ses** (·seez) [Gk. *kentēsis,* pricking]. Puncture; perforation.

centi- [L. *centum,* hundred]. A combining form meaning (a) *hundredth part;* (b) *hundred.*

cen·ti·bar (sen'ti·bahr) *n.* [*centi-* + *-bar*]. One one-hundredth of a bar; a unit of atmospheric pressure.

cen·ti·grade (sen'ti·grade) *adj.* [*centi-* + L. *gradus,* step]. Designating a temperature scale based on a given interval divided into 100 degrees; specifically, CELSIUS.

cen·ti·gram (sen'ti·gram) *n.* [*centi-* + *gram*]. The hundredth part of a gram, equal to 0.1543 grain. Abbreviated, cg. See also Table of Weights and Measures in the Appendix.

cen·ti·li·ter, cen·ti·li·tre (sen'ti·lee"tur) *n.* [*centi-* + *liter*]. The hundredth part of a liter, equal to 0.6102 cubic inch. Abbreviated, cl. See also Table of Weights and Measures in the Appendix.

cen·ti·me·ter, cen·ti·me·tre (sen'ti·mee"tur, son'ti·) *n.* [*centi-* + *-meter*]. The hundredth part of a meter, equal to 0.3937 (about $^2/_5$) inch. Abbreviated, cm. See also Table of Weights and Measures in the Appendix.

centimeter-gram-second system. The system based upon the use of the centimeter, gram, and second as units of length, mass, and time, respectively. Abbreviated, CGS system.

cen·ti·nor·mal (sen"ti·nor'mul) *adj.* [*centi-* + *normal*]. Having one one-hundredth of the normal strength, said of a solution containing one one-hundredth of a gram equivalent of the solute in 1 liter of solution.

cen·ti·pede (sen'ti·peed) *n.* [L. *centipeda,* from *centum,* hundred, + *pes, pedis,* foot]. Any myriapod of the class Chilopoda, with a pair of legs on each segment of the body except the last two. The claws of the first body segment have openings at the tips for expulsion of neurotoxic venom. The bite of centipedes of temperate climates seldom produces more than mild, local symptoms in man; that of tropical species causes necrotic lesions as well as general symptoms of lymphangitis, vomiting, fever, and headache.

cen·ti·poise (sen'ti·poiz) *n.* [*centi-* + *poise*]. A unit of viscosity equal to 1/100 of a poise. It is the viscosity of water at 20°C. Abbreviated, cp.

centr-, centro-. A combining form meaning *center, central.*

centra. A plural of *centrum.*

[1]**cen·trad** (sen'trad) *n.* [*cent-* + *rad*ian]. An angular measure, one one-hundredth of a radian; about 0.57°.

[2]**centrad,** *adv.* [*centr-* + *-ad*]. Toward the center, or toward the median line.

cen·trage (sen'trij) *n.* [*centr-* + *-age*]. A condition in which the centers of all the refracting surfaces of the eye are in one straight line.

cen·tral (sen'trul) *adj.* 1. Situated at or near the center. 2. Basic, fundamental. 3. Of or pertaining to the central nervous system. 4. Of or pertaining to the centrum (2).

central ageusia. Loss or impairment of taste due to a lesion in the cerebral centers for taste.

central amputation. An amputation in which the flaps are joined so that the suture line runs across the end of the stump.

central anesthesia. Anesthesia due to a lesion of the central nervous system.

central angiospastic retinopathy. CENTRAL SEROUS RETINOPATHY.

central anosmia. See *anosmia.*

central aphasia. CONDUCTION APHASIA.

central-bearing device. *In prosthodontics,* a mechanical device that provides a central point of bearing, or support, between the upper and lower occlusion rims; consisting of a contacting point, attached to one occlusion rim, and a plate, attached to the other, on which the point rests or moves.

central blindness. 1. CENTRAL SCOTOMA. 2. CORTICAL BLINDNESS.

central body. 1. CENTROSOME. 2. Sometimes, CENTRIOLE.

central canal of the spinal cord. The small tube, containing cerebrospinal fluid and lined by ependyma, that extends through the center of the spinal cord from the conus medullaris to the lower part of the fourth ventricle. It represents the embryonic neural tube. NA *canalis centralis.*

central cell. CHIEF CELL (1).

central choroiditis. Choroiditis in which the exudate is in the region of the macula lutea.

central chromatolysis. Dissolution of cytoplasmic Nissl substance in the center of the body of a neuron; the first event in chromatolysis.

central cirrhosis. CARDIAC CIRRHOSIS.

central core disease. A familial disorder of muscle, characterized by the presence in the majority of muscle fibers of cores within which mitochondria are absent and the myofibrils appear abnormal. Clinically, the patients present as floppy infants, but the muscle weakness appears to be stationary or only very slowly progressive.

central deafness. Deafness due to a lesion involving the auditory pathways or auditory centers of the brain.

central enchondroma. ENCHONDROMA.

Central European encephalitis. RUSSIAN TICK-BORNE ENCEPHALITIS.

central excitatory state. A relatively prolonged state in which excitatory influences overbalance inhibitory influences in the spinal cord, possibly due to activity in reverberating circuits or prolonged effects of synaptic mediators, resulting in irradiation of excitatory impulses to many somatic areas of the spinal cord but also to autonomic areas, as may occur in chronic paraplegia. Contr. *central inhibitory state.*

central fissure. CENTRAL SULCUS.

central fovea. FOVEA CENTRALIS.

central gelatinous substance. SUBSTANTIA GRISEA CENTRALIS MESENCEPHALI.

central giant-cell tumor. GIANT-CELL TUMOR (1).

central gray substance. SUBSTANTIA GRISEA CENTRALIS MESENCEPHALI.

central illumination. *In microscopy,* illumination produced by the rays of light reflected from the mirror passing perpendicularly through the object.

central inhibitory state. A relatively prolonged state in which inhibitory influences overbalance excitatory ones in the spinal cord, possibly due to reverberating circuits or prolonged effects of synaptic mediators. Contr. *central excitatory state.*

central light. AXIAL LIGHT.

central lobule. A lobule of the superior vermis of the cerebellum. NA *lobulus centralis.*

central magnocellular nucleus. NUCLEUS PROPRIUS OF THE POSTERIOR HORN.

central medial nucleus of the thalamus. The large, flask-shaped, deeply staining cells which, together with the rhomboid nucleus, make up the adhesio interthalamica and the immediately adjacent thalamic area. NA *nucleus centralis medialis.*

central necrosis. 1. Necrosis of the liver around the central vein. 2. Death of tissue in the middle of a mass of cells.

central nervous system. The structures of the nervous system supported by astrocytes and oligodendroglia rather than by fibroblasts and enclosed by the piarachnoid; includes the brain, spinal cord, olfactory bulb, and optic nerve. Abbreviated, CNS. NA *systema nervosum centrale.*

central neurogenic hyperventilation. Increased rate and depth of respiration, seen in comatose patients with lesions of the lower midbrain–upper pontine tegmentum.

central nucleus of the thalamus. A mass of cells in the medial part of the thalamus lying lateral to the medial and posterior ventral nuclei and partly embedded in the internal medullary lamina. Syn. *centrum medianum.* NA *nucleus centromedianus thalami.*

central paralysis. Paralysis due to a lesion or lesions of the brain or spinal cord.

central pneumonia. Pneumonia with consolidation near the hilus or in the interior of a lobe, producing few signs and symptoms until the lesion extends to the periphery of the lung.

central pontine myelinolysis. A syndrome of unknown etiology, observed in association with alcoholism, malnutrition, gross electrolytic disturbances, and other debilitating states, characterized pathologically by a symmetric focus of demyelination in the center of the basis pontis, and clinically by the acute evolution of quadriparesis and pseudobulbar palsy.

central pulverulent cataract. EMBRYONAL NUCLEAR CATARACT.

central punctate retinitis. A form of diabetic retinopathy.

central retinal artery. A branch of the ophthalmic artery, which in the distal part of its course runs in the center of the optic nerve and branches to form the four major retinal arterioles. NA *arteria centralis retinae.*

central scotoma. Blindness in the central area of the visual field, or involving the normal point of fixation, caused by a lesion and dysfunction of the macular region of the eye.

central serous retinopathy. A condition characterized by edema and hyperemia of the retina, occurring in adult life and more often in men, in which there is an abrupt onset of blurred vision and central scotoma. Funduscopic examination reveals a wet-appearing raised macula with a surrounding ring-shaped reflex and slight hyperpigmentation, usually only in one eye. Etiology is unknown, but multiple factors, including allergies, may play a role. Although self-limited, the condition is often recurrent.

central spindle. A central group of fibers extending between the asters, in contrast to the peripheral ones attached to chromosomes.

central stop diaphragm. *In microscopy,* a diaphragm having a circular slit just within its margin, the center remaining opaque.

central sulcus. 1. A groove situated about the middle of the lateral surface of the cerebral hemisphere, separating the frontal from the parietal lobe. NA *sulcus centralis.* 2. (of the insula:) A deep groove crossing backward and upward on the surface of the insula, dividing it into a larger, anterior portion, occupied by the short gyri of the insula, and a smaller, posterior portion, occupied by the long gyrus of the insula. NA *sulcus centralis insulae.*

central tegmental tract. Nerve fibers that arise in the red nucleus and reticular formation and end in the olivary nucleus. NA *tractus tegmentalis centralis.*

central tendon. The aponeurosis in the center of the diaphragm. NA *centrum tendineum.*

central vein of the suprarenal gland. The vein that receives blood from all the vessels of the cortex and medulla of the suprarenal gland. NA *vena centralis glandulae suprarenalis.*

central veins of the liver. The veins in the center of the liver lobules into which the sinusoids empty. NA *venae centrales hepatis.*

central venous pressure. The pressure representative of the filling pressure of the right ventricle, measured peripherally or centrally, corrected for the hydrostatic pressure between the heart and the point of measurement; used to monitor fluid replacement, as in shock or severe burns. Abbreviated, CVP.

central vertigo. CEREBRAL VERTIGO.

central vision. Vision with the eye turned directly toward the object so that the image falls upon the macula lutea, providing the most acute vision. Syn. *direct vision, macular vision.* See also *macular sparing.*

cen·tra·phose (sen'truh·foze) *n.* [*centr-* + *aphose*]. A subjective sensation of darkness originating in the visual center.

cen·tra·zene (sen'truh·zeen) *n.* 1,4-Dimethyl-1,4-diphenyl-2-tetrazene, $C_{14}H_{16}N_4$, an antineoplastic drug.

centre. CENTER.

cen·tren·ce·phal·ic (sen''tren·se·fal'ick) *adj.* [*centr-* + *encephalic*]. Pertaining to or designating the neuron systems that are symmetrically connected with both cerebral hemispheres and that serve to coordinate their functions. These circuits are located in the higher brainstem and include the thalamus with the diencephalon, mesencephalon, and rhombencephalon.

centrencephalic epilepsy or **seizure.** Any epilepsy in which the epileptogenic discharge originates in the central integrating system of the higher brainstem, with electroencephalographic abnormalities consequently appearing simultaneously over both cerebral hemispheres. Included are generalized seizures, absence attacks, myoclonic epilepsy, akinetic seizures, and certain types of psychomotor seizures and other automatisms.

centri-. A combining form meaning *center.*

cen·tric (sen'trick) *adj.* [Gk. *kentrikos,* of the center]. Pertaining to a center, as opposed to peripheral.

-centric. A combining form meaning (a) *with a center or centers* (of a specified kind or number); (b) *with* (something) *at its center.*

centric fusion. A process in which two acrocentric chromosomes join to produce a metacentric chromosome. The actual mechanism in some, if not all, cases involves a reciprocal translocation with loss of one centromere and its very small chromosome arms.

cen·tric·i·put (sen·tris'i·put) *n.* [*centri-* + L. *caput,* head]. The part of the head situated between the sinciput and the occiput; the midhead. —**cen·tri·cip·i·tal** (sen''tri·sip'i·tul) *adj.*

centric occlusion. The maximum, unstrained, occlusal contact relationship of the teeth; associated with centric relation of the mandible to the maxilla.

centric relation. The condition in which the mandibular condyles rest unstrained in their most posterior position in the mandibular fossae and from which position all mandibular movements are initiated.

cen·trif·u·gal (sen·trif'yoo·gul) *adj.* [*centri-* + *-fugal*]. 1. Acting or proceeding in a direction away from a center or axis. 2. Efferent; moving outward from a nerve center. Contr. *centripetal.*

centrifugal conductibility. The ability to transmit centrifugal impulses from the nervous centers to the periphery.

cen·trif·u·gal·iza·tion (sen·trif''yoo·gul·i·zay'shun) *n.* CENTRIFUGATION.

cen·trif·u·ga·tion (sen·trif''yoo·gay'shun) *n.* Separation of a substance, e.g., a suspension of particulate matter, into components of different densities by means of a centrifuge.

cen·tri·fuge (sen'tri·fewj) *n.* & *v.* [*centri-* + *-fuge*]. 1. An apparatus for separating substances of different densities by centrifugal force. 2. To separate into components of different densities by means of a centrifuge.

centrifuge microscope. A high-speed centrifuge provided with windows which permit microscopical observation of the material being sedimented. See also *ultracentifuge.*

cen·tri·lob·u·lar (sen''tri·lob'yoo·lur) *adj.* [*centri-* + *lobular*]. In the central portion of a lobule, usually of the liver.

centrilobular emphysema. Emphysema involving primarily the central portion of the secondary lobule of the lung.

centrilobular necrosis. Necrosis of the liver around the central vein.

Centrine. Trademark for aminopentamide, a parasympatholytic drug used as the sulfate salt.

centring. CENTERING.

cen·tri·ole (sen'tree·ole) *n.* [*centri-* + *-ole*]. A minute oval composed of microtubules, representing a nucleation center of microtubule formation; usually found in the centrosome and frequently considered to be the division center of the cell.

cen·trip·e·tal (sen·trip'e·tul) *adj.* [*centri-* + L. *pet*ere, to seek, + *-al*]. 1. Acting or proceeding toward the center from the periphery. 2. Afferent; moving toward a nerve center. Contr. *centrifugal.*

centripetal conductibility. The ability to transmit centripetal impulses from the periphery to the nervous centers.

centro-. See *centr-.*

cen·tro·ac·i·nar (sen"tro·as'i·nur) *adj.* [*centro-* + *acinar*]. Of or pertaining to the specialized cells in the central part of pancreatic acini.

centroacinar cells. The cells of the intercalated ducts of the pancreas which, in certain planes of section, appear surrounded by the zymogenic cells of the pancreatic acini.

cen·tro·cyte (sen'tro·site) *n.* [*centro-* + *-cyte*]. A cell containing single and double granules of various sizes.

cen·tro·des·mose (sen"tro·dez'moce, ·moze) *n.* [*centro-* + Gk. *desmos,* band]. The primary band which connects the centrosomes and gives rise to the central spindle in cell division.

cen·tro·des·mus (sen"tro·dez'mus) *n.* CENTRODESMOSE.

cen·tro·don·tous (sen"tro·don'tus) *adj.* [Gr. *kentr*on, sharp point, + *odont-* + *-ous*]. Furnished with sharp-pointed teeth.

cen·tro·dor·sal (sen"tro·dor'sul) *adj.* Central and dorsal.

centrodorsal nucleus. NUCLEUS PROPRIUS OF THE POSTERIOR HORN.

cen·tro·lec·i·thal (sen"tro·les'i·thul) *adj.* [*centro-* + *lecithal*]. Having the yolk in the center, as insect eggs.

cen·tro·me·di·an (sen"tro·mee'dee·un) *adj.* Central and median.

centromedian nucleus of the thalamus. CENTRAL NUCLEUS OF THE THALAMUS.

cen·tro·mere (sen'tro·meer) *n.* [*centro-* + *-mere*]. The constriction in a chromosome where it is attached to a spindle fiber. Syn. *kinetochore.*

centroparietal thalamic peduncle. See *thalamic peduncles.*

cen·tro·phose (sen'tro·foze) *n.* [*centro-* + *phose*]. A subjective sensation of light originating in the visual centers.

cen·tro·some (sen'tro·sohm) *n.* [*centro-* + *-some*]. The centrosphere together with the centriole or centrioles.

cen·tro·sphere (sen'tro·sfeer) *n.* [*centro-* + *sphere*]. The specialized area of the cytoplasm in which the centriole is located and from which the astral fibers (astrospheres) extend during cell division; the Golgi apparatus often surrounds it.

cen·tro·the·ca (sen"tro·theek'uh) *n.* [*centro-* + *theca*]. IDIOSOME.

cen·trum (sen'trum) *n.*, pl. **centrums, cen·tra** (·truh) [L.]. 1. The center or middle part. 2. The body of a vertebra, exclusive of the bases of the arches.

centrum me·di·a·num (mee·dee·ay'num). CENTRAL NUCLEUS OF THE THALAMUS.

centrum ova·le (o·vay'lee). The medullary center; the central white matter seen on making a section of the brain at the level of the upper surface of the corpus callosum.

centrum se·mi·ova·le (sem"ee·o·vay'lee) [BNA]. CENTRUM OVALE.

centrum ten·di·ne·um (ten·din'ee·um) [NA]. CENTRAL TENDON.

centrum tendineum pe·ri·nei (perr·i·nee'eye) [NA]. PERINEAL BODY.

Cen·tru·roi·des (sen"troo·roy'deez) *n.* A genus of Scorpionida, the true scorpions. Some species with seriously poisonous bites are the *Centruroides suffusus* (the durango) and the *C. noxius,* found from the southern United States to Panama, and the *C. sculpturatus,* found in Arizona.

cenurosis. COENUROSIS.

cenurus. COENURUS.

Cepacol. A trademark for cetylpyridinium chloride.

ceph·a·ce·trile (sef'uh·see'trile) *n.* $C_{13}H_{13}N_3O_6S$, an antibiotic of the cephalosporin type, usually employed as the sodium salt.

ceph·a·e·line (sef·ay'e·leen) *n.* Desmethylemetine, $C_{28}H_{38}N_2O_4$, an alkaloid of ipecac having emetic activity.

cephal-, cephalo- [Gk. *kephalē*]. A combining form meaning *head.*

ceph·a·lad (sef'ul·ad) *adv.* [*cephal-* + *-ad*]. Toward the head.

ceph·a·lal·gia (sef"uh·lal'jee·uh) *n.* [*cephal-* + *-algia*]. Headache. —**cephalal·gic** (·jick) *adj.*

ceph·a·lal·gy (sef'uh·lal"jee) *n.* CEPHALALGIA.

Ceph·a·lan·thus (sef"uh·lan'thus) *n.* A genus of plants of the Rubiaceae. *Cephalanthus occidentalis* is the common buttonbush of North America; its bitter bark has been used as laxative and tonic and in periodic fevers and paralysis. The bark contains cephalein, a crystalline acid principle, cephaletin, a bitter principle, and a toxic glycoside, cephalanthin.

ceph·a·lea (sef"uh·lee'uh) *n.* [Gk. *kephalaia,* inveterate headache]. A severe headache. See also *cephalea attonita.*

cephalea at·to·ni·ta (a·ton'i·tuh). A severe headache, especially with intolerance of light and sound, as seen with certain infectious diseases.

ceph·a·lex·in (sef"uh·leck'sin) *n.* 7-(D-α-Amino-α-phenylacetamido)-3-methyl-3-cephem-4-carboxylic acid, $C_{16}H_{17}N_3O_4S$, a semisynthetic cephalosporin C antibiotic with an antibacterial spectrum similar to that of cephalothin.

ce·phal·gia (se·fal'jee·uh) *n.* CEPHALALGIA.

ceph·al·he·ma·to·ma (sef"ul·hee·muh·to'muh) *n.* [*cephal-* + *hematoma*]. A collection of blood beneath the pericranium, forming a tumorlike swelling.

ceph·al·hy·dro·cele (sef"ul·high'dro·seel) *n.* [*cephal-* + *hydrocele*]. Effusion of cerebrospinal fluid beneath the scalp in fractures of the skull.

-cephalia. See *-cephaly.*

ce·phal·ic (se·fal'ick) *adj.* [Gk. *kephalikos,* from *kephalē,* head]. Pertaining to the head.

cephalic aura. An aura often described as a feeling of diffuse heaviness, fullness, or pressure of the head.

cephalic flexure. MESENCEPHALIC FLEXURE.

cephalic ganglionated plexus. The four parasympathetic ganglia (the ciliary, pterygopalatine, otic, and submandibular) in close topographic relation to the branches of the fifth cranial nerve, and connected by fine nerve filaments with the superior cervical ganglion of the sympathetic nervous system.

cephalic index. The ratio of the greatest width of the head, taken wherever it may be found in a horizontal plane perpendicular to the sagittal plane, × 100, to the greatest length, taken in the sagittal plane between glabella and opisthocranion. Its values are classified as:

dolichocephalic	x-75.9
mesocephalic	76.0-80.9
brachycephalic	81.0-85.4
hyperbrachycephalic	85.5-x

cephalic presentation. Presentation in which any part of the head is the presenting part.

cephalic tetanus. Tetanus occasionally observed following head injuries, involving individually or in combination the muscles supplied by the facial, trigeminal, oculomotor, or hypoglossal nerves. The disease tends to spread rapidly, with seizures.

cephalic vein. [ML. *vena cephalica,* from Ar. *qīfāl* (Avicenna), perhaps from Gk. *kephalikos,* cephalic (the vein was thought to drain blood from the head)]. A superficial vein located on the lateral side of the arm which drains blood from the radial side of the hand and forearm into the axillary vein. NA *vena cephalica.* See also Table of Veins in the Appendix.

cephalic version. Turning of the fetus to establish a cephalic presentation.

ceph·a·lin (sef'uh·lin) *n.* [*cephal-* + *-in*]. A phospholipid in which phosphatidic acid is esterified to an ethanolamine base. Syn. *phosphatidyl ethanolamine.*

Ceph·a·li·na (sef"uh·lye'nuh) *n.* A tribe of gregarines in which schizogony is lacking and in which the body of the trophozoite is divided into two or three chambers; includes the genera *Gregarina* and *Lankesteria,* which inhabit insects and other invertebrates. Contr. *Acephalina.* —**ceph·a·line** (sef'uh·line) *adj.*

cephalin-cholesterol flocculation test. A test for liver function which measures the capacity of serum of persons with hepatic disease to flocculate a colloidal suspension of cephalin cholesterol-complex. The result is expressed from 0 to 4 plus.

ceph·a·li·tis (sef"uh·lye'tis) *n.* [*cephal-* + *-itis*]. ENCEPHALITIS.

ceph·a·li·za·tion (sef"uh·li·zay'shun) *n. In biology,* concentration of important organs at the head region of the body.

cephalo-. See *cephal-.*

ceph·a·lo·cau·dal (sef"uh·lo·kaw'dul) *adj.* [*cephalo-* + *caudal*]. *In anatomy,* relating to the long axis of the body, head to tail.

ceph·a·lo·cele (sef'uh·lo·seel) *n.* [*cephalo-* + *-cele*]. Hernia of the brain; protrusion of a mass of the cranial contents. See also *encephalocele.*

ceph·a·lo·cen·te·sis (sef"uh·lo·sen·tee'sis) *n.,* pl. **cephalocente·ses** (·seez) [*cephalo-* + *centesis*]. *In surgery,* puncture of the cranium.

ceph·a·lo·chord (sef"uh·lo·kord) *n.* The cephalic portion of the notochord.

Ceph·a·lo·chor·da (sef"uh·lo·kor'duh) *n.pl.* [*cephalo-* + *chorda*]. The subphylum of Chordata represented by amphioxus.

ceph·a·lo·di·pro·so·pus (sef"uh·lo·dye·pro'so·pus, ·dye"pro·so'pus) *n.* [*cephalo-* + *diprosopus*]. An individual having attached to its head a more or less incomplete parasitic head; a form of dicephalus parasiticus or diprosopus parasiticus.

ceph·a·lo·dym·ia (sef"uh·lo·dim'ee·uh) *n.* [*cephalo-* + *-dymia*]. CRANIOPAGUS.

ceph·a·lo·dyn·ia (sef"uh·lo·din'ee·uh) *n.* [*cephal-* + *-odynia*]. Headache.

ceph·a·lo·gen·e·sis (sef"uh·lo·jen'e·sis) *n.,* pl. **cephalogene·ses** (·seez) [*cephalo-* + *genesis*]. The origin and development of the primordia of the head.

ceph·a·lo·gly·cin (sef"uh·lo·glye'sin) *n.* 7-(D-α-Aminophenylacetamido) cephalosporanic acid, $C_{18}H_{19}N_3O_6S$, a semisynthetic antibiotic derived from cephalosporin C.

ceph·a·lo·graph (sef'uh·lo·graf) *n.* [*cephalo-* + *-graph*]. An instrument for diagrammatically recording the size and form of the head.

ceph·a·log·ra·phy (sef"uh·log'ruh·fee) *n.* [*cephalo-* + *-graphy*]. A method of diagrammatically recording the size and form of the head.

ceph·a·lo·gy·ric (sef"uh·lo·jye'rick) *adj.* [*cephalo-* + *gyr-* + *-ic*]. Pertaining to or causing rotation of the head.

ceph·a·lo·hem·a·to·cele, ceph·a·lo·haem·a·to·cele (sef"uh·lo·hem'uh·to·seel") *n.* [*cephalo-* + *hematocele*]. A hematocele beneath the scalp, communicating with a dural sinus.

ceph·a·lo·he·ma·to·ma, ceph·a·lo·hae·ma·to·ma (sef"uh·lo·hee"muh·to'muh) *n.* CEPHALHEMATOMA.

ceph·a·loid (sef'uh·loid) *adj.* [*cephal-* + *-oid*]. Resembling the head; head-shaped.

ceph·a·lom·e·lus (sef"uh·lom'e·lus) *n.,* pl. **cephalome·li** (·lye) [*cephalo-* + *-melus*]. An individual having a supernumerary limb attached to the head.

ceph·a·lo·me·nia (sef"uh·lo·mee'nee·uh) *n.* [*cephalo-* + *men-* + *-ia*]. Vicarious menstruation through the nose.

ceph·a·lo·men·in·gi·tis (sef"uh·lo·men"in·jye'tis) *n.* [*cephalo-* + *meningitis*]. Inflammation of the meninges of the brain. See also *meningitis.*

ceph·a·lom·e·ter (sef"uh·lom'e·tur) *n.* [*cephalo-* + *-meter*]. *In craniometry,* an instrument for measuring the head.

cephalometric axis. Y AXIS.

ceph·a·lom·e·try (sef"uh·lom'e·tree) *n.* [*cephalo-* + *-metry*]. 1. *In plastic surgery,* use of the cephalometer for comparison with casts in facial reconstruction. 2. *In orthodontics,* a procedure utilizing anatomical tracings of lateral head plates identifying anatomical points, planes, and angles to assay the patient's growth or evaluate treatment. —**cepha·lo·met·ric** (·lo·met'rick) *adj.*

ceph·a·lo·nia (sef"uh·lo'nee·uh) *n.* [Gk. *kephalōn,* plant with a bulb (from *kephalē,* head), + *-ia*]. Macrocephaly with hypertrophy of the brain.

cephalo-oculocutaneous telangiectasia. ATAXIA-TELANGIECTASIA.

ceph·a·lo·or·bi·tal (sef"uh·lo·or'bi·tul) *adj.* [*cephalo-* + *orbital*]. Pertaining to the cranium and orbits.

ceph·a·lop·a·gus (sef"uh·lop'uh·gus) *n.,* pl. **cephalopa·gi** (·guy, ·jye) [*cephalo-* + *-pagus*]. CRANIOPAGUS. —**cephalop·agous,** *adj.*

cephalopagus oc·cip·i·ta·lis (ock·sip"i·tay'lis). CRANIOPAGUS OCCIPITALIS.

cephalopagus pa·ri·e·ta·lis (pa·rye"e·tay'lis). CRANIOPAGUS PARIETALIS.

ceph·a·lop·a·gy (sef"uh·lop'uh·jee) *n.* [*cephalo-* + *-pagy*]. CRANIOPAGY.

ceph·a·lop·a·thy (sef"uh·lop'uth·ee) *n.* [*cephalo-* + *-pathy*]. ENCEPHALOPATHY.

ceph·a·lo·pel·vic (sef"uh·lo·pel'vick) *adj.* Pertaining to the head of the fetus and the pelvis of the mother.

cephalopelvic disproportion. A disparity between the size of the head of the fetus and the opening in the maternal pelvis; usually, excessive size of the fetal head in relation to the maternal pelvis. Abbreviated, CPD.

ceph·a·lo·pha·ryn·ge·us (sef"uh·lo·fa·rin'jee·us) *L. adj.* [*cephalo-* + *pharyngeus*]. Of or pertaining to the cranium and pharynx.

cephalopharyngeus muscle. A portion of the superior constrictor muscle of the pharynx.

ceph·a·lo·ple·gia (sef"uh·lo·plee'jee·uh) *n.* [*cephalo-* + *-plegia*]. Paralysis of the muscles about the head and face.

ceph·a·lo·pod (sef'uh·lo·pod) *n.* [*cephalo-* + *-pod*]. A mollusk of the class Cephalopoda, such as an octopus, squid, or cuttlefish.

ceph·a·lor·i·dine (sef"uh·lor'i·deen) *n.* A semisynthetic antibiotic, $C_{19}H_{17}N_3O_4S_2$, that differs from cephalothin in having a pyridine substituent in place of an acetoxy group, and in being more soluble in water; the antibacterial spectrum is similar to that of cephalothin but cephaloridine causes less pain on intramuscular injection.

ceph·a·los·co·py (sef"uh·los'kuh·pee) *n.* [*cephalo-* + *-scopy*]. Auscultation of the head.

ceph·a·lo·spor·in (sef"uh·lo·spor'in) *n.* Any one group of diverse antibiotic substances, produced by certain species of *Cephalosporium.* Cephalosporin C, structurally related to the penicillins, has moderate antibacterial activity; its semisynthetic derivatives cephalothin, cephaloridine, and cephaloglycin are more active. Cephalosporin N is identical with penicillin N and synnematin B. Cephalosporins P_1 to P_5 are steroid derivatives.

ceph·a·lo·spo·ri·o·sis (sef"uh·lo·spor·ee·o'sis) *n.,* pl. **cephalo·sporio·ses** (·seez). An infection caused by a species of *Cephalosporium.*

Ceph·a·lo·spo·ri·um (sef"uh·lo·spor'ee·um) *n.* A genus of fungi which are similar to *Aspergillus* or *Penicillum* in spore formation and to *Sporotrichum* in appearance. They are common allergens and contaminants and constitute one of the genera responsible for mycetoma.

ceph·a·lo·thin (sef″uh·lo·thin) *n.* Sodium 7-(thiophene-2-acetamido)cephalosporanate, $C_{16}H_{15}N_2NaO_6S_2$, a bactericidal antibiotic which is active against many gram-positive and gram-negative organisms. See also *cephaloridine.*

ceph·a·lo·tho·rac·ic (sef″uh·lo·tho·ras′ick) *adj.* [*cephalo-* + *thoracic*]. 1. Pertaining to the head and thorax. 2. Designating those arthropods having the head joined to the thorax.

cephalothoracic lipodystrophy. PROGRESSIVE LIPODYSTROPHY.

ceph·a·lo·tho·ra·co·il·i·op·a·gus (sef″uh·lo·tho″ruh·ko·il″ee·op′uh·gus) *n.* [*cephalo-* + *thoraco-* + *iliopagus*]. SYNADELPHUS.

ceph·a·lo·tho·ra·cop·a·gus (sef″uh·lo·thor″uh·kop′uh·gus) *n.*, pl. **cephalothoracopa·gi** (·guy, ·jye) [*cephalo-* + *thoracopagus*]. Conjoined twins (diplopagi) united by their heads, necks, and thoraxes.

cephalothoracopagus asym·me·tros (a·sim′e·tros). CEPHALOTHORACOPAGUS MONOSYMMETROS.

cephalothoracopagus di·bra·chi·us (dye·bray′kee·us). THORADELPHUS.

cephalothoracopagus di·sym·me·tros (dye·sim′e·tros). Conjoined twins in which the single head exhibits two equal opposite faces.

cephalothoracopagus mono·sym·me·tros (mon·o·sim′e·tros). Conjoined twins with fused thoraxes and a single head that bears two opposite faces, one incomplete.

ceph·a·lo·tome (sef′uh·lo·tome) *n.* [*cephalo-* + *-tome*]. An instrument for performing cephalotomy on a fetus.

ceph·a·lot·o·my (sef″uh·lot′uh·mee) *n.* [*cephalo-* + *-tomy*]. The opening or division of the head of a fetus to facilitate delivery.

ceph·a·lo·trac·tor (sef″uh·lo·track′tur) *n.* [*cephalo-* + *tractor*]. OBSTETRIC FORCEPS.

ceph·a·lo·tribe (sef′uh·lo·tribe) *n.* [*cephalo-* + *-tribe*]. An instrument for crushing the head of a fetus.

ceph·a·lo·trid·y·mus (sef″uh·lo·trid′i·mus) *n.* [*cephalo-* + *tridymus*]. TRICEPHALUS.

ceph·a·lo·trip·sy (sef′uh·lo·trip″see) *n.* [*cephalo-* + Gk. *tripsis*, rubbing]. *In obsterics,* the crushing of the fetal head when delivery is otherwise impossible.

ceph·a·lo·trip·tor (sef″uh·lo·trip′tur) *n.* CEPHALOTRIBE.

ceph·a·lo·tro·pic (sef″uh·lo·tro′pick, ·trop′ick) *adj.* [*cephalo-* + *-tropic*]. Characterizing a drug or other agent that has an affinity for brain tissue or modifies brain physiology. Compare *psychotropic.*

ceph·a·lo·try·pe·sis (sef″uh·lo·trye·pee′sis, ·tri·pee′sis) *n.* [*cephalo-* + Gk. *trypēsis,* boring]. Trephining of the skull.

ceph·a·lox·ia (sef″uh·lock′see·uh) *n.* [*cephal-* + Gk. *loxos*, oblique, + *-ia*]. TORTICOLLIS.

-cephalus [Gk. *-kephalos,* -headed, from *kephalē,* head]. A combining form designating (a) an individual with a specified *abnormality of the head,* or the abnormality itself; (b) in biological taxonomy, an organism with a specified *kind of head.*

-cephaly [*cephal-* + *-y*]. A combining form designating a *condition* or *characteristic of the head.*

ceph·a·pi·rin (sef″uh·pye′rin) *n.* $C_{17}H_{17}N_3O_6S_2$, an antibiotic of the cephalosporin type, usually used as the sodium salt.

ceph·ra·dine (sef′ruh·deen) *n.* A cephalosporin-type antibiotic, $C_{16}H_{19}N_3O_4S$, of unspecified action.

CER Abbreviation for *conditioned escape response.*

cer-, cero- [L. *cera*]. A combining form meaning (a) *wax;* (b) *resembling wax.*

ce·ra (seer′uh, serr′uh) *n.* [L.]. Wax obtained from plants or made by insects; consists of monohydric, high molecular weight alcohols and/or their esters, fatty acids, hydrocarbons, and possibly other substances, depending on the source. **—ce·ra·ceous** (se·ray′shus) *adj.*

cera al·ba (al′buh) [L.]. WHITE WAX.

cera fla·va (flay′vuh) [L.]. YELLOW WAX.

cer·am·ide (serr·am′ide) *n.* The sphingosine-fatty acid portion of a cerebroside.

cer·a·sin (serr′uh·sin) *n.* [Gk. *kerasos*, bird-cherry]. 1. A resin from the bark of cherry, peach, and plum trees. 2. CERASINOSE. 3. KERASIN.

cer·a·si·nose (serr′uh·si·noce, se·ras′i·noce) *n.* [*cerasin* + *-ose*]. A carbohydrate found in the gum of the cherry tree.

Ce·ras·tes cor·nu·tus (se·ras′teez kor·new′tus) [Gk. *kerastēs,* horned, from *keras,* horn]. The horned viper of the African deserts. Its venom is predominantly hemotoxic.

cerat-, cerato- [Gk. *keras, keratos*]. A combining form meaning *horn, horny.* Compare *kerat-.*

ce·rate (seer′ate, serr′ate) *n.* [L. *ceratum*, from *cera*, wax]. *In pharmacy,* an unctuous preparation consisting of wax mixed with oils, fatty substances, or resins, and of such a consistency that at ordinary temperatures it can be spread readily on linen or muslin, and yet so firm that it will not melt or run when applied to the skin. **—ce·rat·ed** (seer′ay·tid, serr′) *adj.*

cerato-. See *cerat-.*

cer·a·to·cri·coid (serr″uh·to·krye′koid) *n.* [*cerato-* + *cricoid*]. A variable slip of the posterior cricoarytenoid muscle, extending from the cricoid cartilage to the inferior cornu of the thyroid cartilage. NA *musculus ceratocricoideus.*

cer·a·to·hy·al (serr″uh·to·high′ul) *n.* [*cerato-* + *hyal*]. 1. The lesser cornu of the hyoid bone. See *cornua of the hyoid bone.* 2. One of a series of bones forming the hyoid arch of which only the basihyal is found in man as the hyoid bone, the ceratohyal and epihyal bones being represented by the stylohyoid ligament and styloid process of the temporal bone. A varying number of elements are found in many mammals other than man.

Cer·a·to·ni·a (serr″uh·to′nee·uh) *n.* [Gk. *keratonia,* carob tree]. A genus of trees of the Leguminosae, whose single species, *Ceratonia siliqua,* the carob, is native to the regions about the Mediterranean. The falcate fleshy beans, carob pods, of this tree are rich in sugar and have been used as a demulcent.

cer·a·to·pha·ryn·ge·us (serr″uh·to·fa·rin′jee·us) *n.* [*cerato-* + *pharyngeus*]. The portion of the middle constrictor of the pharynx arising from the cornu of the hyoid bone. NA *pars ceratopharyngea musculi constrictoris pharyngis medii.*

Cer·a·to·phyl·lus (serr″uh·to·fil′us) *n.* [*cerato-* + Gk. *phyllon*, leaf]. A genus of fleas.

Ceratophyllus fas·ci·a·tus (fash·ee·ay′tus). The common rat flea of the United States and Europe; a vector of typhus fever and a host of *Hymenolepis diminuta.*

Cer·a·to·po·gon·i·dae (serr″uh·to·po·gon′i·dee) *n.pl.* [from *Ceratopogon* (type genus), from *cerato-* + Gk. *pōgōn,* beard]. A widespread family of very small bloodsucking gnats or midges. See also *Culicoides.* **—cerato·po·go·nid** (·po′guh·nid) *adj. & n.*

cer·car·ia (sur·kăr′ee·uh) *n.*, pl. **cercar·i·ae** (·ee·ee) [Gk. *kerkos,* tail]. Any trematode worm in its second stage of larval life. **—cercar·i·al** (·ee·ul) *adj.*; **cercari·an** (·un) *adj. & n.*

cercarial dermatitis. SCHISTOSOME DERMATITIS.

cer·clage (sair·klahzh′) *n.* [F., encirclement]. *In orthopedics,* application of wire or metal band encircling a bone; a method of osteosynthesis in oblique and certain comminuted fractures.

Cer·co·ce·bus (sur″ko·see′bus) *n.* [Gk. *kerkos*, tail, + *kēbos,* a kind of African monkey]. A genus of the Cercopithecidae comprising the mangabeys.

Cer·co·mo·nas (sur″ko·mo′nas, sur·kom′o·nas) *n.* A genus of coprozoic flagellates.

Cercomonas in·tes·ti·na·lis (in·tes″ti·nay′lis). *Obsol.* 1. *CHILOMASTIX MESNILI.* 2. *GIARDIA LAMBLIA.*

Cer·co·pi·the·ci·dae (sur″ko·pith·ee′si·dee) *n.pl.* [from *Cercopithecus,* type genus]. A family of Anthropoidea comprising the Old World monkeys. See also *Cercopithecoidea.*

Cer·co·pith·e·coi·dea (sur″ko·pith″e·koy′dee·uh) *n.pl.* The superfamily of Anthropoidea comprising the Old World monkeys. Contr. *Ceboidea, Hominoidea.*

Cer·co·pi·the·cus (sur″ko·pith·ee′kus, ·pith′e·kus) *n.* [Gk. *kerkopithēkos,* a long-tailed monkey]. A genus of the Cercopithecidae comprising the guenons and their allies.

Cercopithecus ae·thi·ops (eeth′ee·ops). A widespread species (or species group) of small, partially ground-dwelling African monkeys; the vervets or green monkeys.

ce·rea flex·i·bil·i·tas (seer′ee·uh fleck″si·bil′i·tas) [L.]. WAXY FLEXIBILITY.

cerebell-, cerebelli-, cerebello-. A combining form meaning *cerebellum, cerebellar.*

cer·e·bel·lar (serr″e·bel′ur) *adj.* Pertaining to or involving the cerebellum.

cerebellar apoplexy. Any cerebrovascular accident involving the cerebellum, usually a cerebellar hemorrhage.

cerebellar ataxia. 1. Muscular incoordination due to disease of the cerebellum or its central connections. 2. Any of the degenerative cerebellar ataxias of genetic or uncertain origin, which may include olivopontocerebellar ataxia, Marie's hereditary cerebellar ataxia, dyssynergia cerebellaris progressiva, and other uncommon forms. See also *hemisphere syndrome, vermis syndrome.*

cerebellar epilepsy or **fit.** BRAINSTEM EPILEPSY.

cerebellar–foramen magnum herniation. TONSILLAR HERNIATION.

cerebellar fossae. Two shallow, concave recesses on the lower part of the inner surface of the occipital bone for the reception of the hemispheres of the cerebellum.

cerebellar gait. A wide-based, unsteady, irregular, lateral reeling gait due to disease or dysfunction of the cerebellum or cerebellar pathways.

cerebellar peduncle. Any of the stalks of white matter consisting of large nerve fiber bundles running between a hemisphere of the cerebellum and the medulla oblongata, pons, and other parts of the brain. See also *inferior, middle,* and *superior cerebellar peduncle.*

cerebellar pressure cone. The downward displacement of the inferior mesial parts of the cerebellar hemispheres (ventral paraflocculi or tonsillae) through the foramen magnum, the result of a sharp pressure gradient between intracranial and intraspinal pressures, as in posterior fossa tumors or general brain swelling, and frequently causing death from medullary compression. See also *tentorial pressure cone.*

cerebellar rigidity. The opisthotonic position sometimes observed in patients with large midline cerebellar lesions and probably due to compression of the brainstem.

cerebral spastic diplegia. SPASTIC DIPLEGIA (2).

cerebellar speech. The slow, slurred, and jerky speech seen in cerebellar disorders; may be intermittent and explosive or syllabic and singsong in character. See also *scanning speech.*

cerebellar stalk. CEREBELLAR PEDUNCLE.

cerebellar tonsil. The tonsilla of the cerebellum. See *tonsilla* (1).

cerebelli-. See *cerebell-.*

cer·e·bel·li·form (serr″e·bel′i·form) *adj.* Resembling the cerebellum.

cer·e·bel·lif·u·gal (serr″e·be·lif′yoo·gul) *adj.* [*cerebelli-* + *-fugal*]. Tending away from the cerebellum.

cer·e·bel·lip·e·tal (serr″e·be·lip′i·tul) *adj.* [*cerebelli-* + L. *petere,* to seek, + *-al*]. Tending toward the cerebellum.

cer·e·bel·li·tis (serr″e·be·lye′tis) *n.* Inflammation of the cerebellum.

cerebello-. See *cerebell-.*

cer·e·bel·lo·bul·bar (serr″e·bel″o·bul′bur) *adj.* [*cerebello-* + *bulbar*]. Pertaining to or involving the cerebellum and the medulla oblongata.

cerebellobulbar tract. FASTIGIOBULBAR TRACT.

cer·e·bel·lof·u·gal (serr″e·be·lof′yoo·gul) *adj.* CEREBELLIFUGAL.

cerebellofugal degeneration. DYSSYNERGIA CEREBELLARIS PROGRESSIVA.

cerebellofugal degeneration ataxia. Ataxia as the main manifestation of dyssynergia cerebellaris progressiva.

cer·e·bel·lo·med·ul·lary (serr″e·bel″o·med′yoo·lair·ee) *adj.* [*cerebello-* + *medullary*]. Pertaining to or involving the cerebellum and the medulla oblongata.

cerebellomedullary cistern. A large subarachnoid space formed by the arachnoid stretching across from the inferior surface of the cerebellum to the dorsal surface of the medulla oblongata. NA *cisterna cerebellomedullaris.*

cerebellomedullary malformation syndrome. ARNOLD-CHIARI SYNDROME.

cer·e·bel·lo·pon·tine (serr″e·bel″o·pon′teen) *adj.* Pertaining to or involving the cerebellum and the pons.

cerebellopontine angle. A region bounded laterally by the petrous portion of the temporal bone, medially by the cerebellum and brainstem, below by the floor of the posterior fossa of the skull, and above by the tentorium cerebelli. An area in which tumors frequently occur.

cerebellopontine angle tumor. An acoustic neurilemmoma occupying its usual site in one cerebellopontine angle.

cerebellopontine-angle tumor syndrome. Tinnitus, impairment and loss of hearing, ipsilateral paralysis of the sixth and seventh cranial nerves, involvement of the trigeminal (fifth cranial) nerve, vertigo and nystagmus, and signs of cerebellar disturbances, such as vomiting and ataxia due to a neurilemmoma or other tumor in the area of the cerebellopontine angle. See also *acoustic nerve tumor.*

cer·e·bel·lo·ret·i·nal (serr″e·bel″o·ret′i·nul) *adj.* [*cerebello-* + *retinal*]. Pertaining to the cerebellum and the retina.

cerebelloretinal angiomatosis. HIPPEL-LINDAU DISEASE.

cer·e·bel·lo·ru·bral (serr″e·bel″o·roo′brul) *adj.* [*cerebello-* + L. *ruber,* red]. Pertaining to the tract of the superior cerebellar peduncle running from the dentate nucleus to the red nucleus.

cerebellorubral fiber. A fiber of the superior cerebellar peduncle terminating in the red nucleus.

cer·e·bel·lo·ru·bro·spi·nal (serr″e·bel″o·roo″bro·spye′nul) *adj.* Pertaining to the cerebellum, the red nucleus, and the spinal cord.

cer·e·bel·lo·spi·nal (serr″e·bel″o·spye′nul) *adj.* Pertaining to the cerebellum and the spinal cord, a descending fiber tract.

cer·e·bel·lo·tha·lam·ic (serr″e·bel″o·tha·lam′ick) *adj.* [*cerebello-* + *thalamic*]. Pertaining to the cerebellum and the thalamus.

cerebellothalamic fiber. A fiber of the superior cerebellar peduncle terminating in the thalamus.

cer·e·bel·lo·ves·tib·u·lar (serr″e·bel″o·ves·tib′yoo·lur) *adj.* Pertaining to the cerebellum and the vestibular nuclei.

cerebellovestibular tract. Efferent fibers arising in the fastigial nuclei and ending in the ipsilateral vestibular nuclei; part of the fastigiobulbar tract.

cer·e·bel·lum (serr″e·bel′um) *n.,* genit. sing. **cerebel·li** (·eye), pl. **cerebel·la** (·luh) [ML., dim. of *cerebrum*] [NA]. The inferior part of the brain lying below the cerebrum and above the pons and medulla oblongata, consisting of two lateral lobes and a middle lobe. See also Plates 17, 18.

cerebr-, cerebri-, cerebro-. A combining form meaning *cerebrum, cerebral, brain.*

cer·e·bral (serr′e·brul, se·ree′brul) *adj.* Pertaining to or involving the cerebrum.

cerebral accident. CEREBROVASCULAR ACCIDENT.

cerebral adiposity. *Obsol.* Obesity due to disease of the brain, especially of the hypothalamus and hypophysis.

cerebral akinesia. Loss of motion associated with a cerebral lesion.

cerebral allergy. Symptoms of cerebral disturbances associated with a definitively established allergy.

cerebral anthrax. The encephalopathy sometimes complicating intestinal or pulmonary anthrax in which the organisms invade the brain.

cerebral apophysis. PINEAL BODY.

cerebral apoplexy. CEREBROVASCULAR ACCIDENT.

cerebral aqueduct. The elongated, slender cavity of the midbrain which connects the third and fourth ventricles. NA *aqueductus cerebri.* See also Plate 18.

cerebral blast concussion or **syndrome.** Blast injury causing no external skull trauma, but rendering the patient unconscious, due to diffuse or focal cerebral and meningeal hemorrhages; observed chiefly in soldiers exposed to nearby explosions.

cerebral blindness. CORTICAL BLINDNESS.

cerebral blood flow. The rate, in milliliters per minute, at which blood flows through the brain, measured by the rate of diffusion of inert gases (nitrous oxide, krypton) into the brain. Approximate value of cerebral blood flow in normal persons is 750 ml per minute. See also *Kety method.*

cerebral bulb. *Obsol.* MEDULLA OBLONGATA.

cerebral cavities. VENTRICLES OF THE BRAIN.

cerebral compression. Increased intracranial pressure due to any space-taking lesion such as tumors, hematomas, or abscesses.

cerebral concussion. BRAIN CONCUSSION.

cerebral cortex. The cortex of the cerebrum. See *cortex* (3, 4).

cerebral cortex reflex. Contraction of the pupil when, in a darkened room, a patient's attention is directed to a light visible to the peripheral portion of his retina.

cerebral cranium. The portion of the skull containing the brain; the brain case; neurocranium.

cerebral croup. *Obsol.* SPASMODIC CROUP.

cerebral deafness. CENTRAL DEAFNESS.

cerebral death. BRAIN DEATH.

cerebral dominance. The normal tendency for one cerebral hemisphere, usually the left, to be better developed in certain functions, especially speech and handedness.

cerebral dysrhythmia. Any abnormal electrical rhythm of the brain as revealed by the electroencephalogram. The brain waves may be too fast, too slow, or may alternate between the two types. Dysrhythmia is frequently associated with an epileptiform condition.

cerebral fossae. Two shallow, concave recesses on the upper part of the internal surface of the occipital bone for the reception of the occipital lobes of the cerebrum.

cerebral gigantism. A syndrome of unknown cause, characterized by markedly accelerated growth in height and gain in weight, especially in infancy, acromegalic features, typical facies and high-arched palate, nonprogressive neurologic dysfunctions with mental retardation, and occasionally a dilated ventricular system on pneumoencephalography. Growth hormone levels are not increased.

cerebral hemianesthesia. Anesthesia affecting one side of the body due to a lesion in the contralateral internal capsule or in the lenticular nucleus or their central connections.

cerebral hemiplegia. Paralysis of one side of the body resulting from a lesion on the opposite side of the brain.

cerebral hernia. A protrusion of the brain through an acquired opening in the skull, as a result of operation, injury, or disease.

cerebral impotence. PSYCHIC IMPOTENCE.

cerebral infantile lipidosis. INFANTILE AMAUROTIC FAMILIAL IDIOCY.

cerebral localization. 1. Assignment or determination of a certain area of the brain as the region exercising control over a given physiologic act or faculty. 2. Assignment or determination of an area of the brain as the site of a lesion.

cerebral malaria. Acute neurologic and mental disturbances, not readily explained by severe fever or metabolic derangements, in a patient with confirmed malaria, usually due to infection with *Plasmodium falciparum.*

cerebral metabolic rate. The rate at which oxygen is consumed in the brain, calculated by multiplying the rate of cerebral blood flow by the difference in oxygen content between the arterial blood and the blood in the internal jugular vein.

cerebral palsy. Popularly, any of a group of congenital diseases, usually nonprogressive and dating from infancy or early childhood, characterized by a major disorder of motor function.

cerebral paralysis. 1. Any paralysis due to a lesion of the brain. 2. CEREBRAL PALSY.

cerebral paraplegia. Paralysis of both legs due to a bilateral cerebral lesion, as in such conditions as meningioma of the falx or thrombosis of the superior sagittal sinus. See also *cerebral palsy.*

cerebral peduncle. One of two large bands of white matter containing descending axons of upper motor neurons which emerge from the underside of the cerebral hemispheres to approach each other as they enter the rostral border of the pons. Between the peduncles, which form the ventral part of the mesencephalon, lies the interpeduncular fossa. NA *pedunculus cerebri.*

cerebral pseudotumor. PSEUDOTUMOR CEREBRI.

cerebral respiration. *Obsol.* The slow, deep respiration seen with increased intracranial pressure. Contr. *central neurogenic hyperventilation.*

cerebral rheumatism. RHEUMATIC BRAIN DISEASE.

cerebral spastic diplegia. SPASTIC DIPLEGIA (2).

cerebral spastic infantile paralysis. SPASTIC DIPLEGIA (1).

cerebral spasticity. Spasticity due to organic disease of the brain; the extent depends on the underlying lesion.

cerebral tetanus. CEPHALIC TETANUS.

cerebral thrombosis. 1. Thrombosis occurring in a cerebral blood vessel. 2. Cerebral infarction secondary to thrombotic occlusion of a cerebral blood vessel.

cerebral vascular accident. CEREBROVASCULAR ACCIDENT.

cerebral ventricles. VENTRICLES OF THE BRAIN.

cerebral vertigo. Vertigo that has its origin in the cerebral cortex, and more specifically in the temporoparietal cortex bordering the Sylvian fissure.

cerebral vesicles. The paired lateral outpouchings of the telencephalon which become the cerebral hemispheres.

cer·e·bra·tion (serr″e·bray′shun) *n.* Mental activity; thinking.

cerebri-. See *cerebr-.*

cer·e·bric acid (serr′e·brick, se·reb′rick). A fatty acid from brain tissue.

ce·re·bri·form (se·ree′bri·form) *adj.* [*cerebr-* + *-iform*]. Resembling the brain.

cer·e·brif·u·gal (serr″e·brif′yoo·gul) *adj.* [*cerebri-* + *-fugal*]. Of nerve fibers or impulses: efferent with respect to the cerebral cortex; transmitting or transmitted from the brain to the periphery.

cer·e·brin·ic acid (serr″e·brin′ick). CEREBRIC ACID.

cer·e·brip·e·tal (serr″e·brip′e·tul) *adj.* [*cerebri-* + L. *petere*, to seek, + *-al*]. Of nerve fibers or impulses: afferent with respect to the cerebral cortex; transmitting or transmitted from the periphery to the brain.

cer·e·bri·tis (serr″e·brye′tis) *n.* [*cerebr-* + *-itis*]. 1. ENCEPHALITIS. 2. Inflammation of the cerebrum.

cerebro-. See *cerebr-.*

cer·e·bro·cer·e·bel·lar (serr″e·bro·serr″e·bel′ur) *adj.* Pertaining to the cerebrum and the cerebellum.

cerebrocerebellar atrophy. Any degenerative disease of the central nervous system characterized by cerebellar signs in combination with such cerebral disturbances as loss of intellect, seizures, extrapyramidal signs, or loss of vision or hearing.

cer·e·bro·cor·ti·cal (serr″e·bro·kor′ti·kul) *adj.* [*cerebro-* + *cortical*]. Pertaining to or involving the cerebral cortex.

cer·e·bro·cu·prein (serr″e·bro·kew′preen, ·pree·in) *n.* A water-soluble copper-containing protein isolated from brain.

cer·e·bro·hep·a·to·re·nal syndrome (serr″e·bro·hep″uh·to·ree′nul). A hereditary disorder characterized by abnormal craniofacial development, marked generalized hypotonia, cortical renal cysts, hepatomegaly with intrahepatic biliary cirrhosis, macrogyria, polymicrogyria, and sudanophilic leukodystrophy; and sometimes including low birth weight, congenital heart disease, and ophthalmic, skeletal, and genital anomalies. Syn. *Zellweger's syndrome.*

cer·e·broid (serr'e·broid) *adj.* [*cerebr-* + *-oid*]. Brainlike.

cer·e·bro·mac·u·lar (serr"e·bro·mack'yoo·lur) *adj.* [*cerebro-* + *macular*]. Pertaining to or involving the brain and the macula of the eye.

cerebromacular degeneration. CEREBRORETINAL DEGENERATION.

cer·e·bro·ma·la·cia (serr"e·bro·ma·lay'shuh, ·see·uh) *n.* [*cerebro-* + *malacia*]. ENCEPHALOMALACIA.

cer·e·bro·med·ul·lary (serr"e·bro·med'yoo·lerr"ee) *adj.* [*cerebro-* + *medullary*]. Pertaining to the brain and spinal cord.

cer·e·bron (serr"e·bron) *n.* PHRENOSIN.

cer·e·bron·ic acid (serr"e·bron'ick). A 24-carbon hydroxyacid occurring in the cerebroside phrenosin.

cerebro-ocular renal disease. OCULOCEREBRORENAL SYNDROME.

cer·e·bro·path·ia psy·chi·ca tox·e·mi·ca (serr"e·bro·path'ee·uh sigh'ki·kuh tock·see'mi·kuh). KORSAKOFF'S SYNDROME.

cer·e·bro·pon·tile (serr"e·bro·pon'tile) *adj.* CEREBROPONTINE.

cer·e·bro·pon·tine (serr"e·bro·pon'tine) *adj.* [*cerebro-* + *pontine*]. Pertaining to the cerebrum and the pons.

cer·e·bro·ret·i·nal (serr"e·bro·ret'i·nul) *adj.* [*cerebro-* + *retinal*]. Of, pertaining to, or involving the brain and the retina.

cerebroretinal degeneration. Any of a group of hereditary degenerative diseases affecting chiefly the ganglion cells of brain, retina, and intestine, and manifested by progressive dementia and retinal changes. The principal forms are the infantile, late infantile, juvenile, and late juvenile forms of amaurotic familial idiocy, the infantile form of Gaucher's disease, and Niemann-Pick disease.

cer·e·bro·scle·ro·sis (serr"e·bro·skle·ro'sis) *n.* Sclerosis of cerebral tissue.

cer·e·brose (serr'e·broce, ·broze) *n.* GALACTOSE.

cer·e·bro·side (serr'e·bro·side) *n.* [*cerebrose* + *-ide*]. Any lipid, found in brain and other tissues, containing one molecule each of sphingosine, galactose (or occasionally glucose), and a fatty acid as the structural components. Syn. *galactolipid, glycolipid, glycospingoside.* See also *galactosphingoside, glucosphingoside.*

cerebroside lipidosis. GAUCHER'S DISEASE.

cerebroside sulfatase deficiency. METACHROMATIC LEUKODYSTROPHY.

cer·e·bro·spi·nal (serr"e·bro·spye'nul) *adj.* [*cerebro-* + *spinal*]. Pertaining to the brain and the spinal cord.

cerebrospinal axis. CENTRAL NERVOUS SYSTEM.

cerebrospinal fever. CEREBROSPINAL MENINGITIS.

cerebrospinal fluid. The fluid within the cerebral ventricles and between the arachnoid membrane and pia mater of the brain and spinal cord. Abbreviated, CSF.

cerebrospinal meningitis. Inflammation of the meninges of the brain and spinal cord; usually suppurative meningitis. See also *aseptic meningitis.*

cerebrospinal nerve. Any nerve taking origin from the brain or spinal cord.

cerebrospinal nervous system. *Obsol.* The brain, spinal cord, and cranial and spinal nerves; formerly sometimes thought to constitute a unity as distinct from the sympathetic (= autonomic) system.

cerebrospinal otorrhea. Drainage of cerebrospinal fluid from the ear, usually the result of a posterior fossa basilar skull fracture, rarely from erosion of the petrous portion of the temporal bone caused by tumor.

cerebrospinal rhinorrhea. Leakage of cerebrospinal fluid from the nose, usually the result of a fracture of the frontal bone with associated tearing of the dura mater and arachnoid.

cerebrospinal sclerosis. MULTIPLE SCLEROSIS.

cer·e·bro·ten·di·nous (serr"e·bro·ten'di·nus) *adj.* [*cerebro-* + *tendinous*]. Pertaining to the brain and the tendons.

cerebrotendinous xanthomatosis. A familial degenerative disease characterized clinically by cataracts, xanthomas of the Achilles tendon, and a neurologic disorder involving pathways in the spinal cord, brainstem, and cerebellum; pathologically xanthomatous lesions have been found not only in the tendons and white matter of the cerebellum, but also in the lungs; thought to be transmitted as an autosomal recessive trait.

cer·e·bro·to·nia (serr"e·bro·to'nee·uh) *n.* [*cerebro-* + *-tonia*]. The behavioral counterpart of component III (ectomorphy) of the somatotype, manifested predominantly by extreme awareness of the external environment as well as of the internal self, with tendencies toward inhibition of bodily enjoyment and activity (the viscerotonic and somatotonic expressions).

cer·e·bro·vas·cu·lar (serr"e·bro·vas'kew·lur) *adj.* [*cerebro-* + *vascular*]. Pertaining to the blood vessels or blood supply of the brain.

cerebrovascular accident. A symptom complex resulting from cerebral hemorrhage or from embolism or thrombosis of the cerebral vessels, characterized by alterations in consciousness, seizures, and development of focal neurologic deficits. Syn. *stroke (informal).*

cer·e·brum (serr'e·brum, se·ree'brum) *n.*, genit. sing. **cere·bri** (·brye), pl. **cere·bra** (·bruh) [L.] [NA]. The largest portion of the brain, occupying the whole upper part of the cranium, and consisting of the right and left hemispheres; the endbrain; telencephalon. See also Plates 16, 17, 18.

cer·e·lose (serr'e·loce, ·loze) *n.* DEXTROSE.

Če·ren·kov radiation (che·r^yen·ko^hff') [A. *Čerenkov,* Soviet physicist, b.1904]. Visible light emitted when charged particles pass through a transparent material at a velocity greater than that of light in the material. It can be seen, for example, as a blue glow in the water around the fuel elements of pool reactors.

ce·re·ous (seer'e·us) *adj.* [L. *cereus,* from *cera,* wax]. Made of wax.

cer·e·sin (serr'e·sin, seer'e·sin) *n.* A naturally occurring solid mixture of hydrocarbons somewhat resembling white beeswax; used as an impression compound.

cer·e·sine (serr'e·seen, seer'e·seen, ·sin) *n.* CERESIN.

Cerespan. A trademark for papaverine.

ce·ric (seer'ick) *adj.* Pertaining to or containing the tetravalent form of cerium.

ce·ri·um (seer'ee·um) *n.* [from *Ceres,* an asteroid]. Ce = 140.12. One of the rare-earth metals. It forms two series of salts, cerous and ceric.

cerium oxalate. A mixture of the oxalates of cerium, neodymium, praseodymium, lanthanum, and other associated elements; occurs as a white or slightly pink powder, insoluble in water; has been used in treating vomiting of pregnancy.

cero-. See *cer-.*

Cer-o-cillin. Trademark for penicillin O, a biosynthetic penicillin useful for patients sensitive to penicillin G.

ce·roid (seer'oid) *n.* [*cer-* + *-oid*]. Any of a variety of yellow to brown acid-fast pigments, insoluble in lipid solvents, representing end products of peroxidation of unsaturated fatty acids; they occur in many tissues, and in a variety of physiologic and pathologic states.

ce·rot·ic acid (se·rot'ick). *n*-Hexacosanoic acid, $C_{26}H_{52}O_2$, a saturated fatty acid found in certain waxes.

ce·rous (seer'us) *adj.* [*cerium* + *-ous*]. Of, pertaining to, or containing the trivalent salt of cerium.

cer·ti·fi·able (sur"ti·figh'uh·bul) *adj. In law and medicine,* indicating a person who by reason of a mental disorder needs guardianship, or requires commitment to a mental hospital or institution.

cer·ti·fi·ca·tion (sur"ti·fi·kay'shun) *n.* 1. The issuing of a guarantee by a person or organization authorized to do so. 2. A statement by an officially recognized and legally constituted body, such as a medical board, that a person or institution has met or complied with certain standards of excellence. 3. The issuance upon a prescribed form by a licensed medical practitioner as to the occurrence and cause of death. 4. The legal process whereby a judicial authority acting on factual and medical evidence declares a person legally insane. See also *commitment.* —**cer·ti·fy,** *v.*

certified color. In the United States, any coloring agent which is officially certified to meet specifications for use in foods, drugs, and cosmetics as determined by federal statute.

certified stain. Any specific batch of a dye that is certified by the Biological Stain Commission as complying with chemical and functional specifications established by the Commission for the dye.

ce·ru·lean (se·roo'lee·un) *adj.* Sky-blue; azure.

ce·ru·lean cataract (se·roo'lee·un). PUNCTATE CATARACT.

ce·ru·lo·plas·min, cae·ru·lo·plas·min (se·roo''lo·plaz'min, seer''oo·lo·) *n.* [L. *caeruleus*, dark blue, + *plasmin*]. A plasma protein (alpha$_2$-globulin) that contains eight atoms of copper, probably in covalent linkage. It represents at least 90% of copper normally in plasma, and is estimated by its oxidase ability; blood values range from about 32 to 38 mg per 100 ml, but are usually markedly decreased in hepatolenticular degeneration.

ce·ru·men (se·roo'mun) *n.* [NL., from L. *cera,* wax]. A secretion of specialized glands of the external auditory meatus; earwax. —**ceru·mi·nous** (·mi·nus) *adj.*

Cerumenex. A trademark for a solution of polyethylene glycol and a surfactant, used to facilitate removal of ear wax by irrigation.

ce·ru·mi·no·sis (se·roo''mi·no'sis) *n.* [*cerumen* + *-osis*]. An excessive secretion of cerumen.

ceruminous glands. The specialized glands of the external auditory meatus which secrete the watery component of the cerumen. NA *glandulae ceruminosae.*

cervic-, cervico-. A combining form meaning *neck, cervix, cervical.*

cer·vi·cal (sur'vi·kul) *adj.* 1. Of or pertaining to the neck or the neck region of the body. 2. Pertaining to the cervix or neck of a part or organ, as of a tooth or of the uterus.

cervical adenitis. Inflammation of lymph nodes in the neck.

cervical ansa. ANSA CERVICALIS.

cervical arch. One of the second to sixth visceral arches forming part of the cervical region.

cervical artery. Any one of the arteries found in the neck. See Table of Arteries in the Appendix.

cervical auricle. Accessory auricle; a projection of the skin, sometimes containing cartilage, found over the sternocleidomastoid muscle; a developmental anomaly of the region around the second visceral groove.

cervical canal. The portion of the uterine cavity situated in the cervix, extending from the isthmus to the ostium of the uterus. NA *canalis cervicis uteri.* See also Plate 23.

cervical conization. Removal of a cone of tissue around the ostium uteri, the apex of the cone extending up the endocervical canal.

cervical cyst. BRANCHIAL CYST.

cervical diverticulum. An incomplete fistula in the cervical region, derived from a pharyngeal pouch (internal) or a visceral groove (external).

cervical duct. The temporary, external duct of the cervical vesicle formed as the cervical sinus is closed over by the opercular process of the hyoid arch.

cervical enlargement. A thickening of the spinal cord from the level of the third cervical to the second thoracic vertebra, maximal at the sixth cervical vertebra, the level of attachment of the nerves of the brachial plexus. NA *intumescentia cervicalis.*

cervical fascia. DEEP CERVICAL FASCIA.

cervical fissure. A congenital fissure of the neck.

cervical fistula. An open communication between the pharynx and the surface of the neck arising by retention of a visceral groove and pouch with perforation of their closing plate.

cervical flexure. A flexure of the embryonic brain, concave ventrally, occurring at the junction of hindbrain and spinal cord.

cervical ganglion. 1. Any of the ganglia, inferior, middle (NA *ganglion cervicale medium*), or superior (NA *ganglion cervicale superius*), on the sympathetic trunk in the neck. See also Plate 15. 2. GANGLION OF THE CERVIX UTERI.

cervical glands. The lymph nodes of the neck.

cervical intumescence. CERVICAL ENLARGEMENT.

cer·vi·ca·lis as·cen·dens (sur·vi·kay'lis a·sen'denz). ILIOCOSTALIS CERVICIS.

cervical line. The line about the neck of a tooth at the junction of enamel and cementum.

cervical myalgic headache. MUSCLE-CONTRACTION HEADACHE.

cervical os. OSTIUM UTERI.

cervical plexus. A plexus in the neck formed by the anterior branches of the upper four cervical nerves. NA *plexus cervicalis.*

cervical plug. MUCOUS PLUG (1).

cervical posterior plexus. A nerve plexus derived from the posterior branches of the first, second, and third cervical nerves lying beneath the semispinalis muscle. Syn. *posterior cervical plexus of Cruveilhier.*

cervical pregnancy. A rare condition in which the impregnated ovum is implanted in the cervical canal, where it develops until the uterus expels it.

cervical punch. CERVICAL PUNCH BIOPSY CLAMP.

cervical punch biopsy clamp. An instrument for the performance of biopsy of the cervix of the uterus.

cervical radicular syndrome. CERVICOBRACHIAL NEURITIS.

cervical ribs. Occasional riblike processes of the cervical vertebrae.

cervical rib syndrome. Sensory, motor, or vascular symptoms in one or both upper extremities due to compression of the brachial plexus and subclavian artery in the neck by a rudimentary or fully developed cervical rib or an anomalous first thoracic rib. See also *scalenus anterior syndrome, Wright's syndrome.*

cervical sinus. A triangular depression caudal to the hyoid arch containing the posterior visceral arches and grooves; it is obliterated superficially by the growth of the hyoid arch and forms the cervical vesicle.

cervical spine. Loosely, the spinous process of a cervical vertebra.

cervical sympathetic paralysis. HORNER'S SYNDROME.

cervical threads. Plastic threads attached to an intrauterine contraceptive device to facilitate removal and also to determine if the device is still in place.

cervical tubercle. A prominence at the junction of the upper part of the neck of the femur and the greater trochanter. It marks the beginning of the intertrochanteric line.

cervical vertebrae. The vertebrae of the neck. NA *vertebrae cervicales.*

cervical vesicle. The cervical sinus after it is obliterated superficially by growth of the hyoid arch.

cervical viscera. The cervical portions of the digestive and respiratory tracts, and the thyroid and parathyroid glands.

cer·vi·cec·to·my (sur''vi·seck'tuh·mee) *n.* [*cervic-* + *-ectomy*]. Excision of the cervix of the uterus.

cer·vi·ci·tis (sur''vi·sigh'tis) *n.* [*cervic-* + *-itis*]. Inflammation of the cervix of the uterus.

cervico-. See *cervic-.*

cer·vi·co·au·ral (sur''vi·ko·aw'rul) *adj.* CERVICOAURICULAR.

cer·vi·co·au·ric·u·lar (sur''vi·ko·aw·rick'yoo·lur) *adj.* [*cervico-* + *auricular*]. Pertaining to the neck and the ear.

cer·vi·co·ax·il·lary (sur''vi·ko·ack''si·lerr·ee) *adj.* [*cervico-* + *axillary*]. Pertaining to the neck and the axilla.

cervicoaxillary canal. The region bounded anteriorly by the clavicle, posteriorly by the scapula, and medially by the thoracic wall, together with their attached muscles.

cer·vi·co·bra·chi·al (sur″vi·ko·bray′kee·ul, ·brack′ee·ul) *adj.* [*cervico-* + *brachial*]. Pertaining to the neck and the upper extremity or member.

cer·vi·co·bra·chi·al·gia (sur″vi·ko·bray″kee·al′jee·uh, ·brack″ee·) *n.* [*cervico-* + *brachialgia*]. A neuralgia in which pain extends from the cervical region to the arms or fingers. See also *brachial neuritis.*

cervicobrachial neuritis. Irritation and chronic inflammation of the lower cervical and first thoracic nerves, seen in middle-aged or elderly persons, and attributed to narrowing of the cervical intervertebral canal by protruded disk material; characterized by neuralgia, alterations in sensation, muscle weakness, and atrophy in the corresponding dermatomes. Compare *neuralgic amyotrophy.*

cervicobrachial syndrome. SCALENUS ANTERIOR SYNDROME.

cer·vi·co·buc·cal (sur″vi·ko·buck′ul) *adj.* [*cervico-* + *buccal*]. Pertaining to the buccal surface of the neck of a molar or premolar tooth.

cer·vi·co·col·pi·tis (sur″vi·ko·kol·pye′tis) *n.* [*cervico-* + *colpitis*]. Inflammation of the uterine cervix and the vagina.

cer·vi·co·dyn·ia (sur″vi·ko·din′ee·uh) *n.* [*cervic-* + *-odynia*]. Pain or neuralgia of the neck.

cer·vi·co·fa·cial (sur″vi·ko·fay′shul) *adj.* [*cervico-* + *facial*]. Pertaining to both the neck and the face.

cer·vi·co·la·bi·al (sur″vi·ko·lay′bee·ul) *adj.* Pertaining to the cervical portion of the labial surface of an incisor or canine tooth.

cer·vi·co·lin·gual (sur″vi·ko·ling′gwul) *adj.* Pertaining to the lingual surface of a tooth at or near the cervix.

cer·vi·co·pu·bic (sur″vi·ko·pew′bick) *adj.* Pertaining to the cervix of the uterus and the pubic bone.

cervicopubic muscle. A few strands of smooth muscle found in the pelvic fascia extending between the cervix of the uterus and the pubic bone.

cer·vi·co·rec·tal (sur″vi·ko·reck′tul) *adj.* Pertaining to the cervix of the uterus and the rectum.

cervicorectal muscle. A few strands of smooth muscle found in the pelvic fascia between the cervix of the uterus and the rectum.

cer·vi·co·tho·ra·cic (sur″vi·ko·tho·ras′ick) *adj.* [*cervico-* + *thoracic*]. Pertaining to the neck and the thorax.

cervicothoracic ganglion. STELLATE GANGLION.

cervicothoracic outlet syndrome. SCALENUS ANTERIOR SYNDROME.

cervicothoracic plexus. The cervical and brachial plexuses considered together.

cer·vi·co·uter·ine (sur″vi·ko·yoo′tur·ine) *adj.* Of or pertaining to the cervix of the uterus.

cervicouterine canal. CERVICAL CANAL.

cer·vi·co·va·gi·nal (sur″vi·ko·va·jye′nul, ·vaj′i·nul) *adj.* Pertaining to the cervix of the uterus and to the vagina.

cer·vi·co·vag·i·ni·tis (sur″vi·ko·vaj″i·nigh′tis) *n.* Inflammation of the cervix of the uterus and the vagina.

cer·vi·co·ves·i·cal (sur″vi·ko·ves′i·kul) *adj.* [*cervico-* + *vesical*]. Pertaining to the cervix of the uterus and urinary bladder.

cervicovesical muscle. A few strands of smooth muscle found in the pelvic fascia between the cervix of the uterus and the urinary bladder.

cer·vix (sur′vicks) *n.*, genit. sing. **cer·vi·cis** (sur′vi·sis), pl. **cer·vi·ces** (sur′vi·seez) [L.]. A constricted portion or neck. Adj. *cervical.*

cervix co·lum·nae pos·te·ri·o·ris gri·se·ae (ko·lum′nee pos·teer″ee·o′ris griz′ee·ee) [BNA]. The constricted portion of the posterior column of gray matter in the spinal cord.

cervix den·tis (den′tis) [NA alt.]. The neck of a tooth. NA alt. *collum dentis.*

cervix ob·sti·pa (ob·stye′puh). TORTICOLLIS.

cervix of the uterus. The cylindrical lower portion of the uterus between the isthmus and the ostium. NA *cervix uteri.* See also Plate 23.

cervix ute·ri (yoo′tur·eye) [NA]. CERVIX OF THE UTERUS.

cervix ve·si·cae (ve·sigh′kee, ·see) [NA]. NECK OF THE BLADDER.

ce·ryl (seer′il) *n.* The univalent radical $C_{26}H_{53}$ of the alcohol component of certain waxes.

ce·sar·e·an, cae·sar·e·an (se·zair′ee·un) *adj.* [Julius *Caesar*, who was thought to be so delivered]. Pertaining to a cesarean section.

cesarean hysterectomy. A hysterectomy performed immediately after a cesarean section. Compare *radical cesarean section.*

cesarean section. Delivery of the fetus through an abdominal and uterine incision.

Ce·sa·ris-De·mel bodies (cheh′zah·rees deh′mel) [A. *Cesaris-Demel,* Italian pathologist, 1866–1938]. Leukocytic bodies observed in certain types of anemia.

ce·si·um (see′zee·um) *n.* [L. *caesius,* bluish gray]. Cs = 132.905. A member of the alkali group of elements, which includes sodium, potassium, lithium, and rubidium. Cesium forms a number of salts in which its valence is 1. The physiologic actions of cesium are similar to those of potassium. Several of its salts have been used medicinally, largely experimentally.

Ces·tan-Che·nais syndrome (ses·tah^{n}′, shuh·neh^{h}′) [R. *Cestan,* French neurologist, 1872–1934; and L. J. *Chenais.*]. Unilateral paralysis of the soft palate and vocal cord with ipsilateral Horner's syndrome and contralateral hemiplegia and hemianesthesia, due to occlusion of the vertebral artery.

Cestan's sign [R. *Cestan*]. LEVATOR SIGN.

Cestan's syndrome. CESTAN-CHENAIS SYNDROME.

Ces·to·da (ses·to′duh) *n. pl.* [L. *cestus,* girdle, belt]. A subclass of Platyhelminthes that includes the tapeworms.

ces·tode (ses′tode) *adj. & n.* 1. Of or pertaining to the Cestoda. 2. One of the Cestoda.

ces·to·di·a·sis (ses″to·dye′uh·sis) *n.*, pl. **cestodia·ses** (·seez) [*cestode* + *-iasis*]. Infection with tapeworms.

ces·toid (ses′toid) *adj.* 1. Resembling a tapeworm. 2. Caused by or consisting of tapeworms.

ce·ta·ce·um (se·tay′shee·um, ·see·um) *n.* [L. *cetus,* whale]. SPERMACETI.

cet·al·ko·ni·um chloride (set″al·ko′nee·um, seet″). Cetyldimethylbenzylammonium chloride, $C_{25}H_{46}ClN$, a local anti-infective compound.

Cetavlon. Trademark for cetrimide, an antiseptic detergent.

cetic acid. PALMITIC ACID.

ce·tin (see′tin) *n.* Cetyl palmitate or cetyl cetylate, $C_{32}H_{64}O_2$, the chief constituent of spermaceti. —**ce·tic** (·tick), **ce·tin·ic** (se·tin′ick) *adj.*

Cetomacrogol. A trademark for polyethyleneglycol 1000 monocetyl ether, employed in ointment vehicles for medicinal agents.

ce·to·phen·i·col (see″to·fen′i·kol) *n.* D-*threo*-*N*-[*p*-acetyl-β-hydroxy-α-(hydroxymethyl)phenethyl]-2, 2-dichloroacetamide, $C_{13}H_{15}Cl_2NO_4$, an antibacterial agent.

Ce·trar·ia (se·trair′ee·uh) *n.* [L. *caetra,* short Spanish shield]. A genus of lichens. See *Iceland moss.*

ce·tri·mide (see′tri·mide) *n.* Chiefly tetradecyltrimethylammonium bromide, $C_{17}H_{38}BrN$, with some dodecyl-trimethylammonium and hexadecyl-trimethylammonium bromides. An antiseptic detergent.

ce·tyl (see′til, set′il) *n.* The univalent radical $C_{16}H_{33}$, compounds of which occur in beeswax, spermaceti, and other waxes. Syn. *hexadecyl.*

cetyl alcohol. Hexadecanol, $C_{16}H_{33}OH$; white, waxy crystals, insoluble in water. Used as an ingredient of washable ointment bases.

cetyl ce·tyl·ate (see′ti·late). CETIN.

cetyl pal·mi·tate (pal′mi·tate). CETIN.

ce·tyl·pyr·i·din·i·um chloride (see″til·pirr″i·din′ee·um). A quaternary ammonium compound, $C_{21}H_{40}ClNO$; used as a topical antiseptic and detergent.

cev·a·dil·la (sev″uh·dil′uh) *n.* [Sp. *cebadilla*]. SABADILLA.

cev·a·dine (sev'uh·deen) *n.* An alkaloid, $C_{32}H_{49}NO_9$, from the sabadilla seed and veratrum viride. Syn. *veratrine.*

Cevalin. A trademark for ascorbic acid.

ce·ve·ra·trum alkaloids (see"ve·ray'trum). A subdivision of alkaloids derived from the 12 known species of *Veratrum;* the other group is known as jerveratrum and is devoid of therapeutic activity.

cev·ine (sev'een, ·in, see'veen, ·vin) *n.* An alkaloid, $C_{27}H_{43}NO_8$, found in sabadilla seed and veratrum. See also *veracevine.*

ce·vi·tam·ic acid (sev"i·tam'ick, see"vi·). ASCORBIC ACID.

Cey·lon sickness [after *Ceylon* (Sri Lanka)]. BERIBERI.

Cf Symbol for californium.

CF lead. *In electrocardiography,* a precordial exploring electrode paired with an indifferent electrode on the left leg.

CFT Abbreviation for *complement-fixation test.*

cg Abbreviation for *centigram.*

CGD Abbreviation for *chronic granulomatous disease.*

C genes. Genes coding for the constant regions of immunoglobin molecules. Contr. *V genes.*

CGS Abbreviation for centimeter-gram-second, a system of measurement based on the centimeter as the unit of length, the gram as the unit of mass, and the second as the unit of time.

Chad·dock's reflex or **sign** [C. G. *Chaddock,* U.S. neurologist, 1861–1936]. 1. A great-toe reflex elicited by scratching the skin around the lateral malleolus, seen in pyramidal tract lesions. 2. Flexion of the wrist and extension and fanning of the fingers caused by irritation of the ulnar aspect of the lower forearm in hemiplegia.

chaeromania. Cheromania (= AMENOMANIA).

chae·to·min, che·to·min (kee·to'min) *n.* An antibiotic substance, isolated from cultures of several species of the genus *Chaetomium,* active in vitro against a variety of microorganisms.

Chae·to·mi·um (kee·to'mee·um) *n.* [Gk. *chaitōma,* plume]. A genus of soil fungi belonging to the order Sphaeriales of which several species may act as allergens.

chafe, *v.* [OF. *chaufer,* from L. *calefacere,* to make warm]. To irritate the skin, usually by friction.

Cha·gas-Cruz disease (shah'gus, krooss) [C. *Chagas* and O. G. *Cruz*]. CHAGAS' DISEASE.

Chagas' disease [C. *Chagas,* Brazilian physician, 1879–1934]. A disease caused by the hemoflagellate *Trypanosoma cruzi,* transmitted by various bugs of the family Reduviidae. It occurs in the Western Hemisphere, especially is South and Central America, and affects mainly children and young adults. The acute disease is characterized by fever, edema, exanthemas, lymphadenopathy, and occasionally meningoencephalitis; chronic manifestations are cardiomyopathy with heart failure and arrhythmia, megaesophagus, and megacolon. Syn. *American trypanosomiasis.*

cha·gas·ic (sha·gaz'ick) *adj.* Pertaining to Chagas' disease.

Cha·gres fever (chah'gres) [after the *Chagres* River, Panama]. 1. Fever with headache and malaise caused by sandfly-borne arboviruses, endemic in Panama. 2. *Obsol.* A malignant form of malaria that affected workers in Panama in the nineteenth century.

α chain. ALPHA CHAIN.

γ chain. GAMMA CHAIN.

δ chain. DELTA CHAIN.

ε chain. EPSILON CHAIN.

κ chain. Kappa chain. See *light chain.*

λ chain. Lambda chain. See *light chain.*

μ chain. MU CHAIN.

chain ligature. A ligature used by tying broad pedicles in sections, the whole mass being constricted in sections by a chain of interlocking ligatures.

chain reaction. 1. *In chemistry,* a reaction that once initiated propagates itself by interactions of the reactants with active intermediate products such as atoms or free radicals. 2. *In nuclear science,* a reaction that stimulates its own repetition, as when a fissionable nucleus absorbs a neutron and fissions, releasing more than one additional neutron; the neutrons in turn can be absorbed by other fissionable nuclei, releasing more neutrons.

chain reflex. A series of consecutive reflexes, each of which is initiated by the preceding one, resulting in an integrated action.

chain saw. *In surgery,* a saw with teeth that are linked together like a chain.

chain-stitch suture. A suture made with the sewing machine stitch.

chair conformation. The usual and relatively stable configuration of hexagonal ring compounds of the cyclohexane type, in which the two opposite ring atoms (1 and 4 position) lie on opposite sides of the plane formed by the middle four ring atoms. Contr. *boat conformation.*

cha·la·sia (ka·lay'zee·uh) *n.* [Gk. *chalasis,* loosening, + *-ia*]. 1. Relaxation of a sphincter, as of the cardiac sphincter of the esophagus. 2. Specifically, a condition of unknown cause, frequently occurring in infants, rarely in adults, characterized by regurgitation immediately after feeding when supine. Barium examination reveals free reflux from the stomach into the esophagus with absence or decrease in esophageal peristalsis. It may be associated with esophagitis and hiatus hernia.

cha·la·za (ka·lay'zuh) *n.,* pl. **chala·zae** (·zee), **chalazas** [Gk., hailstone, hard lump]. 1. One of the two spiral opalescent cords formed as a prolongation of the dense albumen about the yolk toward the blunt and the narrow ends of the avian egg. 2. *In botany,* the place where the seed coats unite with the nucellus in the seed or ovule.

cha·la·zi·on (ka·lay'zee·on, kay·lay') *n.,* pl. **chala·zia** (·zee·uh) [Gk.]. A chronic granulomatous inflammation of the eyelid occurring as the result of blockage of a tarsal gland.

cha·la·zo·der·mia (ka·lay"zo·dur'mee·uh) *n.* [Gk. *chalasis,* loosening, + *-dermia*]. DERMATOLYSIS.

chalc-, chalco- [Gk. *chalkos,* copper]. A combining form meaning (a) *copper;* (b) *brass.*

chal·ci·tis (kal·sigh'tis) *n.* CHALKITIS.

chalco-. See *chalc-.*

chal·co·sis (kal·ko'sis) *n.* [*chalc-* + *-osis*]. A deposit of copper particles in the lungs or in other tissues. See also *chalkitis.*

chal·i·co·sis (kal"i·ko'sis) *n.,* pl. **chalico·ses** (·seez) [Gk. *chalix, chalikos,* gravel, + *-osis*]. A pneumoconiosis common among stonecutters, caused by inhalation of dust.

chalk-. See *chalc-.*

chalk (chawk) *n.* [L. *calx,* lime]. $CaCO_3$. An impure, native form of calcium carbonate. —**chalky** (chaw'kee) *adj.*

chalk gout. TOPHACEOUS GOUT.

chal·ki·tis (kal·kigh'tis) *n.* [Gk. *chalkos,* copper, + *-itis*]. Ocular inflammation resulting from hypersensitivity to brass; usually follows rubbing the eyes after handling brass.

chalko-. See *chalc-.*

chalk·stone, *n.* A gouty deposit of sodium urate in the hands or feet; TOPHUS.

chalky calculus. A calculus made up principally of salts of calcium.

chal·lenge, *n. & v.* 1. The administration of a substance for the purpose of evoking and assessing the response; specifically, the administration of an antigen for the purpose of evoking an immune response, usually a secondary response. 2. To administer such an antigen or other substance.

cha·lone (kay'lone, kal'ohn) *n.* [Gk. *chalōn,* slackening, from *chalan,* to slacken]. Any of various tissue-specific substances of uncertain composition, present in various tissues, that inhibit mitosis and may be a factor in maintaining balance between cell production and cell loss in tissues.

cha·lyb·e·ate (ka·lib'ee·ut) *adj. & n.* [Gk. *chalyps, chalybos,* steel, + *-ate*]. 1. Containing iron; having the color or taste of iron. 2. A medicinal preparation containing iron.

chamae-. See *chame-.*

chamaecephaly. CHAMECEPHALY.
chamaeconch. CHAMECONCH.
chamaeconcha. Chameconcha (= CHAMECONCH).
chamaeconchous. Chameconchous (= CHAMECONCH).
chamaecranial. CHAMECRANIAL.
chamaeprosopic. CHAMEPROSOPIC.
cham·aer·rhine (kam'e·rine) *adj.* [*chamae-* + *-rrhine*]. 1. *In somatometry,* having a broad and flat nose with a height-breadth index of 85.0 or more. 2. *In craniometry,* having a wide apertura piriformis with a nasal index of 51.0 or more.
cham·az·u·lene (kam·az'yoo·leen) *n.* [*cham*omile + *azulene*]. A hydrocarbon, $C_{15}H_{18}$, responsible for the blue color of oil of chamomile.
cham·ber (chaim'bur) *n.* [OF. *chambre,* from L. *camera,* vaulted chamber]. 1. *In anatomy,* a small cavity or space, as of an eye or the heart. 2. An apparatus in which material to be investigated is enclosed.
chamber angle. ANTERIOR CHAMBER ANGLE.
Cham·ber·lain's line [W. E. *Chamberlain,* U.S. radiologist, b.1892]. *In radiology,* on lateral radiograph of the skull, a straight line drawn from the posterior lip of the foramen magnum to the posterior border of the hard palate. If the dens extends significantly above this line, basilar impression may be diagnosed.
Chamberlain's projection [W. E. *Chamberlain*]. TOWNE'S PROJECTION.
chamber of the heart. An atrium or a ventricle of the heart.
chame-, chamae- [Gk. *chamai,* on the ground]. A combining form meaning *low.*
cham·e·ceph·a·lus, cham·ae·ceph·a·lus (kam"e·sef'uh·lus) *n.,* pl. **chamecepha·li** (·lye) [*chame-* + *-cephalus*]. An individual with a flat head.
cham·e·ceph·a·ly, cham·ae·ceph·a·ly (kam"e·sef'uh·lee) *n.* [*chame-* + *-cephaly*]. *In somatometry,* a condition of the head in which the length-height index, or the ratio of the height of the head to its greatest length, is 57.6 or less. A condition in which the vault of the head is low and receding. —**chame·ce·phal·ic, chamae·cephal·ic** (·se·fal'ick), **cham·e·ceph·a·lous, cham·ae·ceph·a·lous** (kam"e·sef'uh·lus) *adj.*
cham·e·conch, cham·ae·conch (kam'ee·konk") *adj.* [*chame-* + *Gk. konchē,* shell, shell-like cavity]. *In craniometry,* designating orbits the index of which (the ratio of orbital height to orbital breadth) is 75.9 or less.
cham·e·con·cha, cham·ae·con·cha (kam"e·konk'uh) *adj.* CHAMECONCH.
cham·e·con·chous, cham·ae·con·chous (kam"e·konk'us) *adj.* CHAMECONCH.
cham·e·cra·ni·al, cham·ae·cra·ni·al (kam"e·kray'nee·ul) *adj.* [*chame-* + *cranial*]. *In craniometry,* designating skulls with a length-height index of 69.9 or less.
cham·e·pro·sop·ic, cham·ae·pro·sop·ic (kam"e·pro·sop'ick, ·pro·so'pick) *adj.* [*chame-* + *prosopic*]. *In craniometry,* designating a facial skeleton that is relatively low and broad, with a total facial index of 74.9 or less. The index is the ratio of morphologic facial height, or distance from nasion to gnathion, to bizygomatic width.
cham·fer (cham'fur) *n.* [MF. *chanfreint,* beveled edge]. A form of gingival marginal finish given to the preparation of a tooth for a crown restoration; it is a shallow curve from an axial wall to the cavosurface; a covelike margination.
cham·o·mile, cam·o·mile (kam'o·mile) *n.* [Gk. *chamaimēlon*]. 1. ANTHEMIS. 2. MATRICARIA.
chan·cre (shank'ur) *n.* [F., from L. *cancer*]. A lesion, usually an ulcer, formed at the site of primary inoculation; generally, the initial lesion of syphilis or chancroid, or of such diseases as sporotrichosis and tularemia.
chancre re·dux (ree'ducks). A syphilitic lesion which is a recurrent ulcer at the site of a previous syphilitic chancre.
chan·croid (shank'roid) *n.* [*chancre* + *-oid*]. An acute localized venereal disease caused by *Haemophilus ducreyi,* characterized by ulceration at the site of inoculation and by painful enlargement and suppuration of regional lymph nodes. —**chan·croi·dal** (shang·kroy'dul) *adj.*
change of life. CLIMACTERIC.
ch'ang shan (chang'shan) *n.* [Chinese]. A medicinal herb, probably originating from *Dichroa febrifuga,* long used in China as an antimalarial. The isomeric alkaloids α-dichroine, β-dichroine, and γ-dichroine, as well as the isomer alkaloids febrifugine and isofebrifugine, have been reported as constituents.
chan·nel, *n.* [OF. *chanel,* from L. *canalis*]. A canal.
Cha·os cha·os (kay'os kay'os) [L.]. A species of saprophytic ameba.
Chaoul therapy (shaowl) [H. *Chaoul,* German radiologist, b.1887]. CONTACT RADIATION THERAPY.
Chaoul tube [H. *Chaoul*]. A special x-ray tube designed to be used at very short target-skin distance for superficial therapy.
Chap·man bag [J. *Chapman,* English physician, 1821-1894]. An elongated ice bag designed for application to the spine.
chapped, *adj.* Designating areas of skin cracked, roughened, and sometimes reddened by exposure to cold. —**chap,** *v.*
Cha·put's method (sha·pue') [H. *Chaput,* French surgeon, 1857-1919]. A method of treating chronic osteomyelitis by curetting the cavity and filling it with fat taken from the abdomen or thigh.
char·ac·ter, *n. In biology,* any structural or functional property of an organism.
character analysis. Psychoanalytic therapy aimed at the character defenses.
character defense. *In psychiatry,* the concept that personality traits serve as unconscious defense mechanisms.
character disorder. A pattern of behavior and emotional response, such as acting out, that is socially disapproved or unacceptable with little evidence of anxiety or other symptoms seen in neuroses. Compare *character neurosis.* See also *personality disorder.*
character impulse disorder. MINIMAL BRAIN DYSFUNCTION SYNDROME.
character neurosis. Disturbed behavioral patterns and emotional responses similar to those seen in a character disorder, except that the neurotic conflicts are expressed in socially acceptable though exaggerated ways not easily recognized as symptoms.
char·ac·ter·ol·o·gy (kăr"uck·tur·ol'uh·jee) *n.* The study and defining of personality based on such physical attributes as the shape and color of body parts and the distribution of fat. Compare *psychognosis (3), somatotype.*
char·as (chahr'us, chur'us) *n.* [Hindi *caras*]. Cannabis resin, especially as used for smoking.
char·bon (shahr'bon) *n.* [F.]. ANTHRAX.
char·coal, *n.* The residue, largely amorphous carbon, obtained by incomplete combustion (destructive distillation) of animal or vegetable matter.
Char·cot-Bött·cher crystalloid (shar·ko', bœt'chur) [J.M. *Charcot,* French neurologist, 1825-1893; and A. *Böttcher*]. A crystal-like structure, often needle-shaped, found near the nucleus of some human Sertoli cells. They may be up to several micrometers long and are composed of densely-packed 150 Å filaments. Their origin and function are unknown.
Charcot-Bou·chard aneurysm (boo·shahr') [J.M. *Charcot;* and C.J. *Bouchard*]. One of the microaneurysms on small arteries in the brain which can cause cerebral hemorrhage in hypertension.
Charcot-Leyden crystals [J. M. *Charcot,* and E. V. von *Leyden*]. Colorless, pointed, often needlelike crystals occurring in the sputum in bronchial asthma and in the feces in amebic colitis and other ulcerative diseases of the colon.
Charcot-Marie-Tooth disease [J. M. *Charcot,* P. *Marie,* and H. H. *Tooth*]. PERONEAL MUSCULAR ATROPHY.
Charcot's arthritis, arthropathy, or **arthrosis** [J. M. *Charcot*]. CHARCOT'S JOINT.
Charcot's cirrhosis [J. M. *Charcot*]. BILIARY CIRRHOSIS.

Charcot's disease [J. M. *Charcot*]. 1. CHARCOT'S JOINT. 2. PERONEAL MUSCULAR ATROPHY. 3. AMYOTROPHIC LATERAL SCLEROSIS.

Charcot's intermittent fever [J. M. *Charcot*]. Intermittent fever due to intermittent biliary obstruction and cholangitis, usually due to stones.

Charcot's joint [J. M. *Charcot*]. A neuropathic arthropathy in which articular cartilage and subjacent bone degenerate while hypertrophic changes occur at the joint edges and present an irregular deformity with instability of the joint. Most commonly seen in diabetic polyneuritis, syringomyelia, and tabes dorsalis.

Charcot's laryngeal vertigo [J. M. *Charcot*]. Vertigo or fainting accompanying severe coughing. See also *cough syncope.*

Charcot's syndrome [J. M. *Charcot*]. INTERMITTENT CLAUDICATION.

Charcot's zone [J. M. *Charcot*]. HYSTEROGENIC ZONE.

Charcot triad [J. M. *Charcot*]. Nystagmus, intention tremor, and staccato speech, occurring in multiple sclerosis due to brainstem involvement.

char·la·tan (shahr'luh·tun) *n.* [It. *ciarlatano*]. 1. One who claims to have more knowledge or skill than he really has. 2. *In medicine,* a quack. —**charlatan·ism** (·iz·um) *n.*

char·ley horse. A contused or severely strained muscle, particularly the quadriceps, in athletes.

Char·lin's syndrome [C. *Charlin,* b.1886]. NASOCILIARY NEURALGIA.

Charl·ton blanching test [W. *Charlton,* German physician, b.1889]. SCHULTZ-CHARLTON BLANCHING TEST.

char·pie (shahr'pee) *n.* [F.]. Scraped lint.

char·ta (kahr'tuh) *n.*, pl. **char·tae** (·tee) [L.]. 1. A strip of paper impregnated, or coated, with a medicinal substance, applied externally. 2. A paper, suitably folded, containing a single dose or portion of medicinal powder to be used internally or externally.

char·treus·in (shahr·trooz'in) *n.* An antibiotic substance forming greenish-yellow crystals, isolated from cultures of *Streptomyces chartreusis;* it is active against certain gram-positive organisms and mycobacteria.

char·tu·la (kahr'tew·luh) *n.*, pl. **chartu·lae** (·lee) [dim. of *charta*]. A small paper, suitably folded, containing a single dose of a medicinal powder.

Chas·sai·gnac's tubercle (sha·seh·nyahk') [E. P. M. *Chassaignac,* French surgeon, 1804–1879]. The carotid tubercle on the transverse process of the sixth cervical vertebra.

Chas·tek paralysis [S. J. *Chastek,* U.S. fox breeder, 20th century]. A dietary disease of silver foxes, characterized clinically by anorexia, ataxia, paralysis of the limbs, abnormal sensitivity to pain, and convulsions, and pathologically by symmetrical foci of degeneration in the thalamus, colliculi, brainstem nuclei, and folia of the cerebellar vermis; caused by a thiamine-splitting enzyme, thiaminase, contained in raw fish viscera added to the diet.

Chauf·fard-Min·kow·ski syndrome (sho·fahr', ming·kohf'skee) [A. M. E. *Chauffard,* French physician, 1855–1932; and O. *Minkowski,* Lithuanian pathologist, 1851–1931]. HEREDITARY SPHEROCYTOSIS.

Chauffard-Still disease or **syndrome** [A. M. E. *Chauffard* and G. F. *Still*]. STILL'S DISEASE.

Chaulmestrol. A trademark for ethyl chaulmoograte, a drug used in the treatment of leprosy.

chaul·moo·gra oil (chol·moo'gruh) [Bengali *cāulmugrā*]. A yellow oil expressed from the seeds of *Taraktogenos kurzii, Hydnocarpus wightiana* or *H. anthelmintica,* trees of Burma and India. It contains chaulmoogric, gynocardic, and hydnocarpic acids; used in the treatment of leprosy. See also *hydnocarpus oil.*

chaul·moo·grate (chol·moo'grate) *n.* An ester of chaulmoogric acid.

chaul·moo·gric acid (chol·moo'grick). 13-(2-Cyclopenten-l-yl)tridecanoic acid, $C_{18}H_{32}O_2$, an unsaturated crystalline acid obtained from chaulmoogra and hydnocarpus oils.

chav·i·cine (chav'i·seen) *n.* A yellowish, oily substance, $C_{17}H_{19}NO_3$; one of the active constituents of black pepper. It appears to be a stereoisomer of piperine.

chav·i·col (chav'i·kol) *n.* *p*-Allylphenol, $C_9H_{10}O$, a constituent of the volatile oil from leaves of *Chavica betel.*

chay (chay, chye) *n.* [Malayalam *cāya-vĕr*]. 1. The East Indian plant *Oldenlandia umbellata.* 2. The root of *O. umbellata* which yields a madder-like dye.

chaya (chay'uh, chye'uh) *n.* CHAY.

CHD Congenital heart disease; coronary heart disease.

ChE Abbreviation for *cholinesterase.*

Chea·dle's disease [W. B. *Cheadle,* English pediatrician, 1836–1910]. INFANTILE SCURVY.

check bite. A plastic impression of the teeth, serving as a guide for alignment in an articulator; used in orthodontics and dental prosthetics. It consists of bites taken in hard wax or soft modeling compound, which record centric, eccentric, and protrusive occlusion.

check ligament. 1. A thickening of the orbital fascia running from the insertion of the medial rectus muscle to the medial orbital wall (medial check ligament) or from the insertion of the lateral rectus muscle to the lateral orbital wall (lateral check ligament). 2. ALAR ODONTOID LIGAMENT.

check·up, *n.* A medical examination; may be a general physical examination or involve a specific organ or system, such as vision, hearing, or the cardiovascular system.

Ché·diak-Hi·gashi anomaly, disease, or **syndrome** [M. *Chédiak,* 20th century; and O. *Higashi*]. An autosomal, recessively inherited disorder characterized by deeply staining, coarse peroxidase-positive granules in the cytoplasm of neutrophils and eosinophils; associated with albinism, hepatosplenomegaly, lymphadenopathy, and recurrent skin infections. When albinism is absent, the condition is called the Steinbrinck type.

cheek, *n.* The side of the face; composed of skin, mucous membrane, and the fat, connective tissue, and muscles intervening. NA *bucca.*

cheek·bone, *n.* ZYGOMATIC BONE.

cheese fly. A fly of the genus *Piophila.*

cheese skippers. The larvae of the cheese fly *Piophila casei.*

cheese·wash·er's disease. Mild chronic interstitial pneumonitis, probably associated with mold sensitivity.

cheesy (cheez'ee) *adj.* Of the nature of cheese; CASEOUS.

cheesy abscess. CASEOUS ABSCESS.

cheil-, cheilo- [Gk. *cheilos*]. A combining form meaning *lip.*

chei·lal·gia (kigh·lal'juh, ·jee·uh) *n.* [*cheil-* + *-algia*]. Pain in the lips.

chei·lec·to·my (kigh·leck'tuh·mee) *n.* [*cheil-* + *-ectomy*]. Excision of a portion of the lip.

cheil·ec·tro·pi·on (kyle"eck·tro'pee·on) *n.* [*cheil-* + *ectropion*]. Eversion of the lips.

chei·li·tis, chi·li·tis (kigh·lye'tis) *n.* [*cheil-* + *-itis*]. Inflammation of the lips.

cheilitis ac·tin·i·ca (ack·tin'i·kuh). A form of cheilitis in which the lips are irritated by sunlight; usually seen in persons whose skin is sensitive to light.

cheilitis ex·fo·li·a·ti·va (ecks·fo"lee·uh·tye'vuh). Persistent peeling of the lips.

cheilitis glan·du·la·ris (glan"dew·lair'is). GLANDULAR CHEILITIS.

cheilitis glandularis apos·te·ma·to·sa (a·pos"te·ma·to'suh). GLANDULAR CHEILITIS.

cheilitis ven·e·na·ta (ven"e·nay'tuh). Contact dermatitis of the lips, often caused by sensitization to allergens in lipsticks, toothpastes, or woodwind instruments.

cheilo-. See *cheil-.*

chei·lo·an·gio·scope (kigh"lo·an'jee·o·skope) *n.* [*cheilo-* + *angio-* + *-scope*]. An apparatus for observing the circulation of the capillaries of the human lip.

chei·lo·gnatho·pal·a·tos·chi·sis (kigh"lo·nath"o·pal·uh·tos'ki·sis) *n.* [*cheilo-* + *gnatho-* + *palatoschisis*]. Unilateral or bilateral cleft of the upper lip, alveolar process, and palate.

chei·lo·gnatho·pros·o·pos·chi·sis (kigh″lo·nath″o·pros·o·pos′ki·sis) *n.* [*cheilo-* + *gnatho-* + *prosoposchisis*]. Oblique facial cleft involving also the upper lip and upper jaw.

chei·lo·gnatho·ura·nos·chi·sis (kigh″lo·nath″o·yoor″uh·nos′ki·sis) *n.* [*cheilo-* + *gnatho-* + *uranoschisis*]. A cleft which involves the upper lip, alveolar process, and palate.

chei·lo·plas·ty (kigh′lo·plas″tee) *n.* [*cheilo-* + *-plasty*]. Any plastic operation upon the lip.

chei·lor·rha·phy (kigh·lor′uh·fee) *n.* [*cheilo-* + *-rrhaphy*]. Suture of a cut or lacerated lip.

chei·los·chi·sis (kigh·los′ki·sis) *n.*, pl. **cheiloschi·ses** (·seez) [*cheilo-* + *-schisis*]. HARELIP.

chei·los·co·py (kigh·los′kuh·pee) *n.* [*cheilo-* + *-scopy*]. Microscopic observation of the circulation in the blood vessels of the lip.

chei·lo·sis (kigh·lo′sis) *n.*, pl. **cheilo·ses** (·seez) [*cheil-* + *-osis*]. A disorder of the lips often due to a deficiency of riboflavin, characterized by fissures, especially at the angles of the lips.

chei·lo·sto·ma·to·plas·ty (kigh″lo·sto′ma·to·plas″tee) *n.* [*cheilo-* + *stomato-* + *-plasty*]. Plastic repair of the lips and mouth.

chei·lot·o·my (kigh·lot′uh·mee) *n.* [*cheilo-* + *-tomy*]. Excision of a part of the lip.

chei·ma·pho·bia (kigh″muh·fo′bee·uh) *n.* [Gk. *cheima*, winter, + *phobia*]. Abnormal fear of cold or winter.

cheir-, cheiro- [Gk. *cheir*]. A combining form meaning *hand.*

chei·rag·ra, chi·rag·ra (kigh·rag′ruh) *n.* [*cheir-* + *-agra*]. 1. Gout of the hand associated with twisting and deformity of the fingers. 2. Any painful condition of the hand.

chei·ral·gia, chi·ral·gia (kigh·ral′juh, ·jee·uh) *n.* [*cheir-* + *-algia*]. Pain in the hand.

cheiralgia par·es·thet·i·ca (păr″es·thet′i·kuh). Numbness and pain in the part of the hand supplied by the superficial branch of the radial nerve.

cheirapsy. CHIRAPSY.

cheir·ar·thri·tis, chir·ar·thri·tis (kigh″rahr·thrigh′tis) *n.* [*cheir-* + *arthritis*]. Inflammation of the joints of the hands and fingers.

cheiro-. See *cheir-*.

chei·ro·kin·es·thet·ic, chei·ro·kin·aes·thet·ic (kigh″ro·kin″es·thet′ick) *adj.* [*chiro-* + *kinesthetic*]. Pertaining to the subjective perception of the motions of the hand, particularly in writing.

chei·rol·o·gy, chi·rol·o·gy (kigh·rol′uh·jee) *n.* [*cheiro-* + *-logy*]. 1. A method of communicating with deaf-mutes by means of the hands. 2. The study of the hand.

chei·ro·meg·a·ly, chi·ro·meg·a·ly (kigh″ro·meg′uh·lee) *n.* [*cheiro-* + *-megaly*]. Enlargement of one or both hands, not due to disease of the hypophysis. See also *pseudoacromegaly.*

chei·ro·plas·ty, chi·ro·plas·ty (kigh′ro·plas″tee) *n.* [*cheiro-* + *-plasty*]. Plastic operation on the hand.

chei·ro·pom·pho·lyx (kigh″ro·pom′fo·licks) *n.* [*cheiro-* + *pompholyx*]. An ill-defined, inflammatory, pruritic skin disease confined to the hands and feet, characterized by vesicles or blebs on the palms and sides of the fingers.

chei·ro·spasm, chi·ro·spasm (kigh′ro·spaz·um) *n.* [*cheiro-* + *spasm*]. WRITER'S CRAMP.

chek·an (check′an) *n.* CHEKEN.

chek·en (check′en) *n.* [Araucan *chequeñ*]. The leaves of *Eugenia cheken*, a South American shrub; formerly used in the treatment of bronchitis.

che·late (kee′late) *adj., n., & v.* 1. Having the ring-type structure formed in chelation. 2. A compound formed by chelation. 3. To bind (a metal ion) with a chelating agent. **—che·lat·ed,** *adj.*

che·lat·ing agent. Any compound, usually organic, having two or more points of attachment at which an atom of a metal may be joined or coordinated in such a manner as to form a ring-type structure.

che·la·tion (ke·lay′shun) *n.* [*chela*, crab's or lobster's claw (from Gk. *chēlē*), suggested by the way in which the metal atom is "gripped" by the organic groups]. 1. A type of interaction between an organic compound (having two or more points at which it may coordinate with a metal) and the metal so as to form a ring-type structure. 2. A type of interaction, shown by organic compounds having both a carbonyl (CO) group and a hydroxyl (OH) group, in which by hydrogen bond formation involving generally two such molecules, but sometimes only one, a ring-type structure is produced.

chel·e·ryth·rine (kel″e·rith′reen, ·rin, kel·err′ith·) *n.* An alkaloid, $C_{21}H_{19}NO_5$, from chelidonium, sanguinaria, and other plants.

chel·i·do·nine (kel′i·do·neen, ·nin) *n.* A crystalline alkaloid, $C_{20}H_{19}NO_5$, of chelidonium.

chel·i·do·ni·um (kel″i·do′nee·um) *n.* [Gk. *chelidonion*, celandine]. The leaves and stems of *Chelidonium majus*, a drastic cathartic and, externally, irritant.

Chel-Iron. A trademark for ferrocholinate, a hematinic.

chellin. KHELLIN.

cheloid. KELOID.

Chel·sea pen·sion·er [after *Chelsea* hospital for invalid soldiers, London]. Compound confection of guaiac; contains guaiac resin, rhubarb, potassium bitartrate, nutmeg, sublimed sulfur, and clarified honey. A traditional remedy in England for rheumatism and gout.

chem-, chemi-, chemico-, chemio-, chemo- [Gk. *chēmeia*, alchemy]. A combining form meaning *chemical, chemistry.*

chemi-. See *chem-*.

chem·i·cal (kem′i·kul) *adj. & n.* 1. Of or pertaining to chemistry. 2. A substance of determinate chemical composition, especially such as may be produced or used in laboratory or industrial processes.

chemical action. The molecular change produced in any substance through the action of heat, light, electricity, or another chemical.

chemical affinity. AFFINITY (2).

chemical agent. *In military medicine*, a solid, liquid, or gas which through its chemical properties produces lethal, injurious, or irritant effects; a screening or colored smoke, or an incendiary agent. War gases, smokes, and incendiaries are the three main groups.

chemical antidote. An antidote that converts a poison to an insoluble compound or to some other harmless derivative.

chemical attraction. AFFINITY (2).

chemical burn. A burn produced by caustics (acid or alkaline), irritant gases, or other chemical agents.

chemical cauterization. A procedure in which a caustic substance is used to destroy tissue.

chemical embryology. Investigation of the development of an organism on a physicochemical basis.

chemical meningitis. Aseptic meningitis, usually resulting from subarachnoid injection of foreign materials such as gases or chemical compounds.

chemical pathology. The study of diseased structures and processes by the application of chemical methods.

chemical peritonitis. Inflammation of the peritoneum due primarily to the irritating effects of a variety of chemical substances, either introduced from without or present as a result of disease or trauma. It occurs in both acute and chronic forms.

chemical rays. Solar rays that produce chemical change.

chemical reflex. A reflex initiated by hormones or other chemical substances in the blood. Syn. *humoral reflex.*

chemical sense. Perception of chemical agents in the neighborhood of, or in contact with, the body; as smell, taste, and the detection of irritating chemicals on the mucous membranes.

chemical stimulus. A stimulus due to, or produced by, chemical means.

chemical warfare. The use in war of toxic gases, incendiary mixtures, and other chemicals, for defensive or offensive purposes.

chemical warfare agent. Any agent used in chemical warfare, especially toxic gas. See also *war gas.*

chemico-. See *chem-.*

chem·i·co·bi·o·log·i·cal (kem″i·ko·bye″uh·loj′i·kul) *adj.* BIOCHEMICAL.

chem·i·co·cau·tery (kem″i·ko·kaw′tur·ee) *n.* Cauterization by means of chemical agents.

chemi·lu·mi·nes·cence (kem″i·lew·mi·nes′unce) *n.* [*chemi-* + *luminescence*]. Light produced by means of a chemical reaction and entirely independent of any heat involved. Syn. *cold light.*

chem·i·no·sis (kem″i·no′sis) *n.* [*chemi-* + alteration of *-nosus,* from Gk. *nosos,* disease]. Any disease produced by a chemical agent.

chemio-. See *chem-.*

chem·i·o·taxis (kem″ee·o·tack′sis) *n.* CHEMOTAXIS.

chem·ist (kem·ist) *n.* [F. *chimiste,* from ML. *(al)chimista,* alchemist]. A person skilled in chemistry.

chem·is·try (kem′is·tree) *n.* [*chemist* + *-ry*]. The science of the structure of matter and the composition of substances, their properties, transformation, analysis, synthesis, and manufacture.

chemo-. See *chem-.*

che·mo·cep·tor (kee″mo·sep″tur, kem″o·) *n.* CHEMORECEPTOR.

che·mo·co·ag·u·la·tion (kee″mo·ko·ag″yoo·lay′shun, kem″o·) *n.* [*chemo-* + *coagulation*]. The precipitation of proteins or colloids in a jellylike, soft mass by means of chemical agents.

che·mo·dec·to·ma (kee″mo·deck·to′muh, kem″o·) *n.*, pl. **chemodectomas, chemodectoma·ta** (·tuh) [*chemo-* + Gk. *dektikos,* receptive, + *-oma*]. Any tumor whose parenchymal cells resemble those of chemoreceptor organs, such as the carotid body, and form cell balls.

che·mo·dif·fer·en·ti·a·tion (kee″mo·dif·e·ren″shee·ay′shun, kem″o·) *n.* [*chemo-* + *differentiation*]. According to Huxley, the period in a cell before it displays any overt signs of specialization.

che·mo·nu·cle·ol·y·sis (kee″mo·new″klee·ol′i·sis, kem″o·) *n.* [*chemo-* + *nucleo-* + *-lysis*]. The dissolution of extruded nucleus pulposus by injection of a proteolytic enzyme, such as chymopapain.

che·mo·pal·li·dec·to·my (kee″mo·pal″i·deck′tuh·mee, kem″o·) *n.* [*chemo-* + globus *pallid*us + *-ectomy*]. The destruction of the globus pallidus by a chemical substance, usually ethyl alcohol, in the treatment of movement disorders.

che·mo·pro·phy·lax·is (kee″mo·pro″fi·lack′sis, kem″o·) *n.*, pl. **chemoprophylax·es** (·seez) [*chemo-* + *prophylaxis*]. Prevention of disease by the administration of a chemotherapeutic agent.

che·mo·re·cep·tor (kee″mo·re·sep″tur, kem″o·) *n.* 1. One of the side chains or receptors of molecules in a living cell, presumed to have the power of fixing chemical substances in the same way that bacterial toxins are fixed. 2. A sensory end organ capable of reacting to a chemical stimulus.

che·mo·re·flex (kee″mo·ree′flecks, kem″o·) *n.* CHEMICAL REFLEX.

che·mo·sis (ke·mo′sis) *n.*, pl. **chemo·ses** (·seez) [Gk. *chēmōsis,* condition of the eyes, where the cornea swells like a cockleshell, *chēmē*]. Swelling of the conjunctiva. —**che·mot·ic** (·mot′ick) *adj.*

chemo·stat (kem′o·stat) *n.* [*chemo-* + *-stat*]. A device for keeping bacterial cultures growing exponentially at a constant population size and at a controlled rate of growth by having a constant delivery of fresh medium and an overflow siphon.

che·mo·sur·gery (kee″mo·sur′jur·ee, kem″o·) *n.* [*chemo-* + *surgery*]. 1. Removal of diseased or unwanted tissue by the application of chemicals. 2. The fixation in situ of malignant, gangrenous, infected, or other tissue by chemical means to facilitate the use of frozen sections in maintaining microscopic control over the extent of an excision.

che·mo·syn·the·sis (kee″mo·sin′thuh·sis, kem″o·) *n.* Chemical synthesis utilizing energy supplied by the reacting substances, as opposed to photosynthesis, in which radiant energy is utilized. —**chemo·syn·thet·ic** (·sin·thet′ick) *adj.*

chemosynthetic autotroph. CHEMOTROPH.

che·mo·tax·is (kee″mo·tack′sis, kem″o·) *n.*, pl. **chemotax·es** (·seez) [*chemo-* + *-taxis*]. 1. The response of organisms to chemical stimuli; attraction toward a substance is positive and repulsion is negative chemotaxis. 2. CHEMOTROPISM. —**chemo·tac·tic** (tack′tick) *adj.*

che·mo·taxy (kee″mo·tack″see, kem″o·) *n.* [*chemo-* + *-taxy*]. CHEMOTAXIS.

che·mo·thal·a·mot·o·my (kee″mo·thal″uh·mot′uh·mee, kem″o·) *n.* [*chemo-* + *thalamotomy*]. The destruction of a portion of the thalamus, usually the ventral nucleus, by a chemical substance such as ethyl alcohol, in the treatment of movement disorders.

che·mo·ther·a·peu·tic (kee″mo·therr″uh·pew′tick, kem″o·) *adj.* Of or pertaining to chemotherapy.

chemotherapeutic index. The relationship existing between the toxicity of a compound for the body and the toxicity for parasites. Kolmer represents it as follows:

$$\text{C.I.} = \frac{\text{maximal tolerated dose per kg body wt}}{\text{minimal curative dose per kg body wt}}$$

che·mo·ther·a·py (kee″mo·therr′uh·pee, kem″o·) *n.* Prevention or treatment of disease by chemical agents.

che·mo·troph (kee′mo·trof, kem′o·) *n.* [*chemo-* + *-troph*]. An autotrophic bacterium able to oxidize an inorganic compound (as of iron, sulfur, or nitrate) specific to a particular species to secure energy for anabolic metabolism. —**che·mo·troph·ic** (kee″mo·trof′ick, kem″o·) *adj.*

che·mot·ro·pism (ke·mot′ro·piz·um) *n.* [*chemo-* + *-tropism*]. 1. Attraction of cells by chemical substances. 2. *In immunology,* the positive attraction of phagocytes to microorganisms, cellular debris, and areas of inflammation.

chem·ur·gy (kem′ur·jee) *n.* Chemistry as applied specifically to the development of derivatives from raw materials, especially from agricultural products, for industry, e.g., the manufacture of paints from soybean oil, or fire extinguishers from licorice root.

Che·nais syndrome (shuh·neh′) [L. J. *Chenais,* French physician, 1872–1950]. CESTAN-CHENAIS SYNDROME.

che·no·de·oxy·cho·lic acid (kee″no·dee·ock″si·ko′lick). 3,7-Dihydroxycholanic acid, $C_{23}H_{37}(OH)_2COOH$. One of the four bile acids isolated from human bile.

Che·no·po·di·um (kee″no·po′dee·um) *n.* [Gk. *chēn,* goose, + *podion,* little foot]. A genus of herbs of the family Chenopodiaceae.

chenopodium oil. A volatile oil from *Chenopodium ambrosioides* var. *anthelminticum,* containing over 65% ascaridol, $C_{10}H_{16}O_2$, which imparts anthelmintic activity to the oil.

Cherenkov radiation. ČERENKOV RADIATION.

che·ro·ma·nia, chae·ro·ma·nia (kerr″o·may′nee·uh, keer″o·) *n.* [Gk. *chairein,* to rejoice, + *mania*]. AMENOMANIA.

che·ro·pho·bia (kerr″o·fo′bee·uh, keer″o·) *n.* [*chairein,* to rejoice, + *phobia*]. A morbid fear of gaiety or happiness.

cher·ry, *n.* The fruit of any of a number of species of the genus *Prunus,* trees having typical globose drupes; family, Rosaceae.

Cher·ry and Cran·dall's test. A test for lipase in which pancreatic lipase in serum is allowed to act on a substrate of olive oil, lipase then being determined by the amount of fatty acid liberated.

cherry juice. A pharmaceutical flavor expressed from the ripe fruit of *Prunus cerasus,* the sour cherry.

cherry-red spot. A bright red area seen in the macular region in such conditions as the infantile and juvenile forms of amaurotic familial idiocy, Niemann-Pick disease, and Gaucher's disease, as a result of the accumulation of metabolic products within the ganglion cells; the foveola is free of ganglion cells thus allowing visualization of the redness of the choroid.

cher·ub·ism (cherr'ub·iz·um, cherr'yoo·biz·um) *n.* [*cherub* + *-ism*]. The characteristic facies of familial multilocular cystic disease or familial fibrous swelling of the jaws, marked by protuberance of the cheeks and jaws with upturned eyes.

Ches·el·den operation (chez'il·din) [W. *Cheselden,* English surgeon, 1688–1752]. Creation of an artificial pupil by iridotomy.

chest, *n.* [L. *cista,* from Gk. *kistē,* basket]. The front of the thorax.

chest lead. PRECORDIAL LEAD.

chetomin. CHAETOMIN.

Che·va·lier Jack·son's operation [*Chevalier Jackson,* U.S. laryngologist, 1865–1958]. VENTRICULOCORDECTOMY.

Chè·vre·mont-Com·baire method (shev·ruh·mohⁿ', kohⁿ·behr'). A histochemical method for riboflavin based on reduction of riboflavin to leucoriboflavin and reoxidation to red granules of rhodoflavin.

Cheyne-Stokes respiration (chain) [J. *Cheyne,* Scottish physician, 1777–1836; and W. *Stokes*]. Periodic breathing characterized by intervals of hyperpnea which alternate with intervals of apnea; rhythmic waxing and waning of respiration; occurs most commonly in older patients with heart failure and cerebrovascular disease.

CHF Abbreviation for *congestive heart failure.*

Chia·ri-From·mel syndrome or **disease** (kyah'ree) [H. *Chiari,* Austrian pathologist, 1851–1916; and R. *Frommel*]. Postpartum galactorrhea with low levels of urinary gonadotropin associated with pituitary adenoma, with or without acromegaly.

Chiari's malformation [H. *Chiari*]. ARNOLD-CHIARI SYNDROME.

Chiari's network [H. *Chiari*]. Fine fibers stretching across the right atrium, and attaching to the openings of the vena cava and coronary sinus, and the crista terminalis.

Chiari's syndrome [H. *Chiari*]. 1. ARNOLD-CHIARI SYNDROME. 2. BUDD-CHIARI SYNDROME. 3. CHIARI-FROMMEL SYNDROME.

chi·asm (kigh'az·um) *n.* CHIASMA.

chi·as·ma (kigh·az'muh) *n.,* pl. **chiasma·ta** (·tuh), **chiasmas** [Gk., a cross- or X-shaped object, from *chi,* name of the letter χ]. A crossing; specifically: 1. OPTIC CHIASMA. 2. *In genetics,* the crossing of two chromatids in meiotic prophase, thought to be a physical manifestation of genetic crossing-over. —**chias·mal** (·mul), *adj.*

chiasmal arachnoiditis. OPTICOCHIASMATIC ARACHNOIDITIS.

chiasmal recess. OPTIC RECESS.

chiasma op·ti·cum (op'ti·kum) [NA]. OPTIC CHIASMA.

chiasma syndrome or **chiasmal syndrome.** A group of symptoms due to a lesion in the optic chiasma and marked by impaired vision, headache, vertigo, and limitation of the visual field.

chiasmata. A plural of *chiasma.*

chiasma ten·di·num (ten'di·num) [NA]. The site of the passage of the tendons of the flexor digitorum profundus muscle between the tendons of the flexor digitorum superficialis muscle; there is one for each of the fingers.

chi·as·mat·ic (kigh''az·mat'ick) *adj.* Pertaining to or resembling a chiasma.

chiasmatic groove or **sulcus.** The variable groove of the sphenoid bone, situated between the optic canals, anterior to the tuberculum sellae. NA *sulcus chiasmatis.*

chick antidermatitis factor. PANTOTHENIC ACID.

chick·en breast. PIGEON BREAST.

chicken cholera. FOWL CHOLERA.

chicken-fat clot. A blood clot formed after death, consisting of a light-yellow upper portion and an accumulation of erythrocytes in its dependent portion.

chicken mite. *DERMANYSSUS GALLINAE.*

chick·en·pox, *n.* An acute, contagious disease, principally of childhood, caused by the varicella virus, characterized by a superficial eruption of macular transparent vesicles which appear in successive crops on different parts of the body.

chi·cle·ro ulcer (chi·kleh'ro) [Sp., chicle gatherer]. A lesion of American cutaneous leishmaniasis caused by infection with *Leishmania mexicana.*

chief agglutinin. The specific agglutinin developed as the result of immunization, exceeding the concentration (titer) of related or "group" agglutinins.

chief cell. 1. The predominant, slightly basophilic pyramidal, granular cell of the gastric glands in the fundic region of the stomach. Zymogen granules, consisting of pepsinogen, are present. Occasionally, these cells are present in the cardiac portion of the stomach. Syn. *adelomorphous cell, central cell, peptic cell.* 2. CHROMOPHOBE CELL. 3. The principal cell of the parathyroid gland, often divided into dark chief cells and light chief cells.

chief surgeon. 1. The surgeon-in-charge of a hospital or of a surgical team. 2. *In U.S. Army medicine,* the senior medical officer assigned to a general headquarters or to an expeditionary force as a staff officer.

chig·ger (chig'ur) *n.* [West African origin]. A larval mite of the genus *Trombicula* or *Eutrombicula;* the attachment of the common chigger to the skin causes severe inflammatory lesions in warm-blooded animals, including man.

chig·oe, chig·o (chig'o) *n.* [Carib]. A flea of the species *Tunga penetrans.*

chi·kun·gu·nya (chick''ŏŏng·gŏŏn'yuh) *n.* [Yao (Bantu), lit., that which bends up, in reference to joint pains and stiffness]. A dengue-like disease caused by a group A togavirus, characterized especially by high fever, headache, rigor, and severe arthralgia.

chil-. See *cheil-.*

Chi·lai·di·ti's syndrome. The presence in an x-ray film of interposed bowel loops between the liver and diaphragm when the patient is upright. There are usually no clinical signs or symptoms, but the condition has sometimes been associated with abdominal pain, distention, and nocturnal vomiting, with absent liver dullness or liver mass in the midabdomen or in the right lower quadrant.

chil·blain, *n.* Hyperemia and swelling of the skin, due to cold, and followed by severe itching or burning; vesicles and bullae may form, and these may lead to ulceration.

child, *n.* 1. An individual who has not reached the age of puberty. 2. An individual between the toddling stage and adolescence.

child abuse. Treatment of a child by a parent or guardian characterized by intentional acts that result in physical injury, toleration of conditions that injure the child or threaten the child's health, or illegal sexual acts upon the child. Legal definitions vary from state to state.

child-abuse syndrome. BATTERED-CHILD SYNDROME.

child analysis. *In psychiatry,* modified psychoanalytic treatment as applied to the problems of a child, to remove obstacles to healthy personality development.

child·bear·ing period. The time of life, from puberty until prior to the menopause, during which a woman is capable of reproduction.

child·bed, *n.* The condition of a woman in labor; PARTURITION.

childbed fever. PUERPERAL FEVER.

child·birth, *n.* Giving birth to a child; human parturition.

child health associate. A physician's assistant with a baccalaureate degree specializing in pediatrics.

child·hood aphasia. Any impairment or loss of the use of language occurring in a child who had previously acquired language in a normal manner.

childhood progeria. HUTCHINSON-GILFORD SYNDROME.

childhood type of schizophrenia. A condition characterized by schizophrenic or schizophrenic-like symptoms, occurring before puberty, which may vary from the more differentiated forms because of the immaturity of the patient. It may be manifested by grossly immature behavior, failure to develop a separate identity from the mother, marked withdrawal, and introspection, and may include infantile autism.

childhood-type tuberculosis. PRIMARY TUBERCULOSIS.

chil·dren's apperception test. *In psychology,* a thematic apperception test devised for clinical work with children aged 3 to 10, and consisting of 10 pictures of animals in various situations. The stories made up by the child about the pictures may reveal the dynamics of his interpersonal relationships, drives, and defenses. Abbreviated, CAT.

Children's Bureau. A disbanded division of the Social Security Administration of the United States which was concerned with the health and welfare of the whole child. It provided grants to the states for maternal and child health, and made available to national, state, and local organizations its publications and information service. Its responsibilities are now carried out by the Office of Child Development.

Chi·le niter [after *Chile,* South America]. SODIUM NITRATE.

Chile saltpeter [after *Chile,* South America]. SODIUM NITRATE.

chilitis. CHEILITIS.

chill, *n.* 1. A sensation of cold accompanied by involuntary shivering or shaking and skin pallor. 2. A respiratory illness due to exposure to cold or damp.

chilo-. See *cheil-.*

Chi·lo·mas·tix (kigh″lo·mas′ticks) *n.* [*chilo-* + Gk. *mastix,* whip, scourge]. A genus of flagellates parasitic in man and other animals.

Chilomastix mes·nili (mes·nil′eye). The species of *Chilomastix* found in the intestine of man.

chi·lopa (ki·lop′uh) *n.* ONYALAI.

Chi·lop·o·da (ki·lop′o·duh) *n. pl.* [*chilo-* + *poda*]. The centipedes; a division of the arthropod group Myriapoda.

chi·me·ra, chi·mae·ra (kigh·meer′uh, ki·meer′uh) *n.* [Gk. *chimaira,* a mythological composite monster]. 1. A plant composed of two genetically distinct types of tissue resulting from somatic mutation, segregation, or from artificial fusion, as in graft hybrids; mosaic. 2. A compound embryo produced by grafting approximately equal halves of two embryos, usually of different species or strains. 3. An animal rendered immunologically tolerant to tissue of another species by prior viable cell transplants from that species. 4. *In genetics,* an individual whose tissues are composed of two genetically different cell lines derived from different zygotes, as, for example, is usually found for the blood cells of dizygotic cattle twins. Compare *mosaic (2).*

chi·mer·ism (ki·meer′iz·um, kigh′mur·iz·um) *n.* [*chimera* + *-ism*]. The presence of two distinct cell types in a given individual, each of which is derived from a different zygote.

chim·ney-sweeps' carcinoma. A squamous cell carcinoma of the scrotum.

chim·pan·zee (chim″pan·zee′, chim·pan′zee) *n.* [Kongo *chimpenzi*]. An African ape of the genus *Pan* (principally *P. troglodytes*). See also *pygmy chimpanzee.*

chin-, chino- [Ger. *Chinin*]. A combining form meaning *quinine.*

chin, *n.* [OE. *cinn*←Gmc. *kinnuz* (rel. to Gk. *genys*)]. The lower part of the face, at or near the symphysis of the lower jaw. NA *mentum.* Comb. form *geni(o)-, mento-.*

CHINA Acronym for chronic infectious neuropathic (or neurotropic) agent. See *china virus.*

Chi·na clay. KAOLIN.

Chinacrin. A trademark for quinacrine, an antimalarial used as the hydrochloride salt.

china virus [*ch*ronic *i*nfectious *n*europathic (*n*eurotropic) *a*gent]. Any of the transmissible agents (presumably viruses) causing "slow" infections of the nervous system.

chinch, *n.* [Sp. *chinche,* bedbug, from L. *cimex*]. A bug of the family Cimicidae.

chin cough. WHOOPING COUGH.

Chi·nese gelatin. AGAR.

Chinese restaurant syndrome. Sensation of burning, pressure about the face and chest, and often headache, produced in susceptible individuals by the ingestion of monosodium L-glutamate, often used in Chinese and other food to enhance flavors.

chi·ni·o·fon (ki·nigh′o·fon, kin′ee·o·fon) *n.* A mixture of 7-iodo-8-hydroxyquinoline-5-sulfonic acid, its sodium salt, and sodium bicarbonate; a canary yellow powder, soluble in water. Formerly used as an amebicide in the treatment of dysentery.

chino-. See *chin-.*

chi·noi·dine (ki·noy′deen, ·din) *n.* A mixture of amorphous alkaloids obtained in the manufacture of quinine. Has been employed as an inexpensive febrifuge, but has only slight antimalarial action.

Chinosol. A trademark for the bactericide 8-hydroxyquinoline sulfate (oxyquinoline sulfate).

chin reflex. JAW JERK.

chin-sternum-heart syndrome. A form of traumatic cardiac injury occurring in parachute jumpers who hit the ground violently in the upright position, after partial opening of the parachute; the chin strikes the sternum, which strikes the heart.

chi·on·ablep·sia (kye″on·a·blep′see·uh) *n.* [Gk. *chiōn,* snow, + *ablepsia*]. SNOW BLINDNESS.

chi·o·na·blep·sy (kye″o·nuh·blep′see) *n.* SNOW BLINDNESS.

chi·o·nan·thus (kigh″o·nan′thus) *n.* The dried bark of the root of the fringe tree, *Chionanthus virginicus.* Has been used as a bitter tonic, diuretic, and aperient.

chi·o·no·pho·bia (kigh″uh·no·fo′bee·uh) *n.* [Gk *chiōn,* snow, + *phobia*]. Abnormal fear of snow.

chip fracture. A minor fracture involving a bony process.

chir-, chiro-. See *cheir-, cheiro-.*

chiragra. CHEIRAGRA.

chi·ral (kigh′rul) *adj.* [*chir-* + *-al*]. Being right- or left-handed; said of an asymmetrical molecule or crystal. See also *enantiomorph.* —**chi·ral·i·ty** (kigh·ral′i·tee) *n.*

chiralgia. CHEIRALGIA.

chi·rap·sia (kigh·rap′see·uh) *n.* [Gk. *kheirapsia,* from *kheir,* hand, + h*apsis,* touch, + *-ia*]. Friction with the hand; MASSAGE.

chi·rap·sy, chei·rap·sy (kigh′rap·see) *n.* [Gk. *kheirapsia,* handling, massage]. The marking of a child in utero with the image of an object longed for and touched by the mother; a magical belief.

chirarthritis. CHEIRARTHRITIS.

chi·ra·ta (chi·rah′tuh, kigh·ray′tuh) *n.* The dried green gentian of northern India, *Swertia chirayita;* has been used as a bitter tonic.

chi·ris·mus (kigh·riz′mus) *n.* [Gk. *kheirismos,* manipulation, handling]. 1. Spasm of the hand. 2. A form of massage.

chiro-. See *cheir-.*

chirokinesthetic. CHEIROKINESTHETIC.

chirology. CHEIROLOGY.

chiromegaly. CHEIROMEGALY.

chiroplasty. CHEIROPLASTY.

chi·rop·o·dist (kigh·rop′o·dist, ki·rop′) *n.* [Gk. *kheiropodēs,* having chapped feet, + *-ist*]. PODIATRIST.

chi·rop·o·dy (kigh′rop′o·dee, ki·rop′) *n.* [*chiropodist* + *-y*]. PODIATRY.

chiropompholyx. CHEIROPOMPHOLYX.

chi·ro·prac·tic (kigh″ro·prack′tick) *n.* [*chiro-* + Gk. *praktikos,* from *prassein,* to do]. A system of therapeutics based upon the theory that disease is caused by abnormal function of the nervous system; attempts to restore normal function are made through manipulation and treatment of the structures of the body, especially those of the spinal column. —**chi·ro·prac·tor** (kigh′ro·prack″tur) *n.*

chi·ro·prac·tor (kigh′ro·prack″tur) *n.* A practitioner of chiropractic.

chirospasm. Cheirospasm (= WRITER'S CRAMP).

chi·rur·geon (kigh·rur′jun) *n.* [Gk. *cheirourgos,* working by hand]. SURGEON.

chi·rur·gery (kigh·rur'je·ree) *n.* SURGERY. —**chirur·gic** (·jick), **chirur·gi·cal** (·ji·kul) *adj.*

chi-square test. A test used to determine whether an observed series of frequencies differ between themselves, or from a series of frequencies expected according to some hypothesis, to a greater degree than may be expected to occur by chance.

chi·tin (kigh'tin) *n.* [Gk. *chitōn*, tunic, + *-in*]. The structural material of skeletons of arthropods, with few exceptions occurring only in invertebrates. It is a condensation product of acetylglucosamine molecules, as cellulose is a condensation product of glucose molecules. —**chitin·ous** (·us) *adj.*

chi·to·bi·ose (kigh"to·bye'oce, ·oze) *n.* A partial hydrolysis product of chitin; it contains two acetylglucosamine molecules linked in the same manner as the two glucose molecules of cellobiose.

chi·to·sa·mine (kigh·to"suh·meen') *n.* GLUCOSAMINE.

Chi·tral fever (chi·trahl') [after *Chitral*, Pakistan]. PHLEBOTOMUS FEVER.

chit·tam bark, chit·tem bark (chit'um). CASCARA SAGRADA.

chlamyd-, chlamydo- [Gk. *chlamys, chamydos*]. A combining form meaning *mantle.*

Chla·myd·ia (kla·mid'ee·uh) *n.* [L., from Gk. *chlamydion*, short mantle]. A genus of gram-negative bacteria (family Chlamydiaceae), readily filtrable, obligate intracellular parasites which are the causative agents of the psittacosis-lymphogranuloma-trachoma group of infections. Formerly called *Bedsonia.* —**chlamydia,** pl. **chlamyd·i·ae** (·ee·ee), *com. n.;* **chlamyd·i·al** (·ee·ul) *adj.*

Chla·myd·i·a·ce·ae (kla·mid"ee·ay'see·ee) *n. pl.* A family of obligate intracellular parasites, intermediate between true viruses and the rickettsiae and gram-negative bacteria, which includes the single genus *Chlamydia.* Formerly called *Chlamydozoaceae.*

Chlamydia psit·ta·ci (sit'uh·sigh). The species of *Chlamydia* which causes psittacosis in man and many clinical and subclinical diseases in other animals and in birds. Formerly called *Chlamydozoon psittaci, Miyagawanella psittaci.*

Chlamydia tra·cho·ma·tis (tra·ko'muh·tis). The species of *Chlamydia* that includes the causative agents of trachoma, inclusion conjunctivitis, lymphogranuloma venereum, and a large proportion of nongonococcal urethritis in man, and pneumonitis in laboratory mice.

chlamydo-. See *chlamyd-.*

Chlam·y·do·bac·te·ri·a·ce·ae (klam"i·do·back·teer"ee·ay'see·ee) *n. pl.* A family of nonpathogenic water-inhabiting organisms composed of cells in chains surrounded by a sheath that may or may not be impregnated with iron or manganese.

chlam·y·do·spore (klam'i·do·spore) *n.* [*chlamydo-* + *spore*]. A thick-walled spore of certain fungi; it is not produced on a basidium but represents a transformed vegetative cell.

Chlam·y·do·zo·a·ce·ae (klam"i·do·zo"ay'cee·ee) *n. pl.* CHLAMYDIACEAE.

Chlam·y·do·zo·on (klam"i·do·zo'on) *n.* [*chlamydo-* + Gk. *zōon*, animal]. *CHLAMYDIA.*

chlo·as·ma (klo·az'muh) *n.*, pl. **chloasma·ta** (·tuh) [Gk., greenness]. 1. Patchy hyperpigmentation located chiefly on the forehead, temples, cheeks, nipples, and median line of the abdomen. The condition may become marked during pregnancy, menstruation, functional derangements of the uterus, or in ovarian disorders and tumors. 2. *Obsol.* Patchy tan-brown-black hyperpigmentation, especially on the brow and cheeks; of unknown cause, but may be due to the action of sunshine upon perfume or to endocrinopathy.

chloasma grav·i·da·rum (grav"i·dair'um). CHLOASMA (1).

chloasma he·pat·i·cum (he·pat'i·kum). Spots of skin hyperpigmentation speciously attributed to hepatic dysfunction.

chloasma ute·ri·num (yoo"te·rye'num). CHLOASMA (1).

chlo·phe·di·a·nol (klo"fe·dye'uh·nol) *n.* α-(2-Dimethylaminoethyl)-*o*-chlorobenzhydrol, $C_{17}H_{20}ClNO$, an antitussive drug; used as the hydrochloride salt.

chlor-, chloro- [Gk. *chlōros*, greenish yellow]. A combining form meaning (a) *green, pale green;* (b) *chlorine;* (c) in chemistry, *having chlorine as a substitute for hydrogen.*

chlor·ac·ne (klor·ack'nee) *n.* [*chlor-* + *acne*]. An acneform eruption caused by chlorinated hydrocarbons.

chloraemia. CHLOREMIA.

chlo·ral (klo'ral, klor'ul) *n.* 1. Trichloroacetaldehyde, CCl_3CHO, a colorless, caustic liquid of pungent odor. 2. CHLORAL HYDRATE.

chlo·ral·am·ide (klor"ul·am'ide, ·id) *n.* CHLORALFORMAMIDE.

chloral betaine. A chloral hydrate-betaine adduct, $C_2H_3Cl_3O_2.C_5H_{11}NO_2$, used as a hypnotic and sedative drug.

chloral camphor. A fluid prepared by mixing equal parts of camphor and chloral; has been used externally as a local anodyne.

chlo·ral·form·am·ide (klor"ul·form·am'ide, ·id, ·form'uh·mide, ·mid) *n.* A crystalline solid, $C_3H_4Cl_3NO_2$; has been used as a hypnotic.

chloral hydrate. 2,2,2-Trichloro-1,1-ethanediol, $CCl_3CH(OH)_2$, colorless or white crystals which are very soluble in water; used as a rapid somnifacient, an anticonvulsant, and as an ingredient of anodyne liniments.

chlo·ral·ize (klor'ul·ize) *v.* To put under the influence of chloral.

chloral menthol. The liquid resulting from interaction of equal parts of chloral hydrate and menthol; has been used as counterirritant and local anesthetic.

chlo·ra·lose (klor'uh·loce, ·loze) *n.* An interaction product, $C_8H_{11}Cl_3O_6$, of chloral (anhydrous) and glucose (dextrose); has been used as a hypnotic.

chlo·ral·ure·thane (klo"rul·yoor'e·thane) *n.* CARBOCLORAL.

chlor·am·bu·cil (klor·am'bew·sil) *n.* 4-{*p*-[Bis(2-chloroethyl)-amino]phenyl}butyric acid, $C_{14}H_{19}Cl_2NO_2$, a nitrogen mustard derivative used as an antineoplastic drug.

chlor·am·ine (klor'uh·meen) *n.* CHLORAMINE-T.

chloramine-T, *n.* Sodium *p*-toluenesulfonchloramide, $CH_3C_6H_4SO_2N(Na)Cl.3H_2O$. A white or faintly yellow crystalline powder, unstable in air; a topical antiseptic.

chlor·am·phen·i·col (klor"am·fen'i·kol) *n.* D(−)-*threo*-2,2-Dichloro-*N*-[β-hydroxy-α-(hydroxymethyl)-*p*-nitrophenethyl] acetamide, $C_{11}H_{12}Cl_2N_2O_5$, an antibiotic substance produced by *Streptomyces venezuelae* Burkholder, and also synthetically. It is effective against a variety of gram-positive and gram-negative organisms, such as *Mycoplasma* and *Rickettsia;* it may produce serious blood dyscrasias.

chlor·ane·mia, chlor·anae·mia (klor"uh·nee'mee·uh) *n.* [*chlor-* + *anemia*]. CHLOROSIS (1).

chlo·rate (klo'rate, klor'ate) *n.* A salt of chloric acid; the radical ClO_3^-.

Chlorazene. A trademark for the antiseptic substance chloramine-T.

chlor·ben·side (klor·ben'side) *n.* Bis(*p*-chlorobenzyl)sulfide, $C_{14}H_{12}Cl_2S$, a miticide.

chlor·bu·ta·nol (klor·bew'tuh·nol) *n.* CHLOROBUTANOL.

chlor·bu·tol (klor·bew'tol) *n.* CHLOROBUTANOL.

chlor·cre·sol (klor·kree'sol) *n.* CHLOROCRESOL.

chlor·cy·cli·zine (klor·sigh'kli·zeen) *n.* 1-(*p*-Chloro-α-phenylbenzyl)-4-methylpiperazine, $C_{18}H_{21}ClN_2$, an antihistaminic agent; used as the hydrochloride salt.

chlor·dan (klor'dan) *n.* CHLORDANE.

chlor·dane (klor'dane) *n.* 1,2,4,5,6,7,8,8-Octachloro-2,3,3a,4,7,7a-hexahydro-4,7-methanoindene, $C_{10}H_6Cl_8$, an insecticide.

chlor·dan·to·in (klor·dan'to·in) *n.* 5-(1-Ethylpentyl)-3-[(trichloromethyl)thio]hydantoin, $C_{11}H_{17}Cl_3N_2O_2S$, an antifungal drug, applied locally.

chlor·di·az·ep·ox·ide (klor"dye·az·ep·ock'side) *n.* 7-Chloro-2-(methylamino)-5-phenyl-3*H*-1,4-benzodiazepine 4-oxide,

$C_{16}H_{14}ClN_3O$, a tranquilizer; used as the hydrochloride salt.

chlo·rel·lin (klo·rel'in) *n.* A substance produced by certain algae, notably species of *Chlorella,* which inhibits the growth of various gram-positive and gram-negative bacteria.

chlor·e·mia, chlor·ae·mia (klor·ee'mee·uh) *n.* [*chlor-* + *-emia*]. 1. CHLOROSIS (1). 2. An excess of chlorides in the blood.

chlor·eph·i·dro·sis (klor"ef·i·dro'sis) *n.* [*chlor-* + *ephidrosis*]. A condition characterized by greenish perspiration.

Chloresium. A trademark for certain medicinal products containing chlorophyll.

Chlor-ethamine. Trademark for ethylenediamine dihydrochloride, a urine acidifier.

Chloretone. A trademark for chlorobutanol, an antibacterial preservative.

chlor·gua·nide (klor·gwah'nide) *n.* CHLOROGUANIDE.

chlor·hex·i·dine (klor·heck'si·deen) *n.* 1,1'-Hexamethylenebis[5-(*p*-chlorophenyl)biguanide], $C_{22}H_{30}Cl_2N_{10}$, a topical antiseptic agent generally used as the dihydrochloride salt.

chlor·hy·dria (klor·high'dree·uh) *n.* [*chlor-* + *hydr-* + *-ia*]. The presence of hydrochloric acid in the stomach.

Chlorhydrol. A trademark for aluminum chlorhydroxide, an antiperspirant.

chlo·ric acid (klo'rick, klor'ick). $HClO_3$. An acid known only in solution and in the form of its salts (chlorates).

chlo·ride (klo'ride, klor'ide) *n.* A salt of hydrochloric acid; a binary compound containing Cl^-.

chloride shift. The reversible exchange of chloride and bicarbonate ions between erythrocytes and plasma to effect transport of carbon dioxide and maintain ionic equilibrium during respiration.

chloride space. A theoretical volume of body fluid containing all the body chloride at a concentration equal to that in a plasma ultrafiltrate.

chlo·rid·uria (klo"ri·dew'ree·uh) *n.* An excess of chlorides in the urine.

chlo·ri·nate (klo'ri·nate, klor'i·) *v.* 1. To treat or combine with chlorine, as for disinfecting sewage or drinking water. 2. To introduce chlorine atoms into (molecules of a compound). —**chlo·ri·nat·ed** (klo'ri·nay·tid) *adj.;* **chlo·ri·na·tion** (klo"ri·nay'shun) *n.*

chlorinated lime. The product of the chlorination of lime; consists chiefly of calcium hypochlorite and calcium chloride. Employed as a disinfectant.

chlor·in·da·nol (klor·in'duh·nol) *n.* 7-Chloro-4-indanol, C_9H_9ClO, a spermatocidal agent.

chlo·rine (klo'reen, ·rin, klor'een) *n.* [*chlor-* + *-ine*]. Cl = 35.453. A greenish yellow gas of suffocating odor and very irritant. A powerful germicide in the presence of moisture with which it forms hypochlorous and hydrochloric acids, the former decomposing with the liberation of nascent oxygen. It has been used by inhalation in the treatment of acute coryza.

chlor·i·son·da·mine chloride (klor"i·son'duh·meen). 4,5,6,7-Tetrachloro-2-(2-dimethylaminoethyl)isoindoline dimethylchloride, $C_{14}H_{20}Cl_6N_2$, a ganglionic blocking agent used for management of hypertension.

chlo·rite (klo'rite, klor'ite) *n.* A salt containing the radical ClO_2^-, derived from chlorous acid.

chlor·mad·i·none (klor·mad'i·nohn) *n.* 6-Chloro-17-hydroxypregna-4,6-diene-3,20-dione, $C_{21}H_{27}ClO_3$, an orally effective progestogen used, as the acetate ester, in combination with an estrogen for sequential control of ovulation to prevent conception.

chlor·mer·o·drin (klor·merr'o·drin) *n.* 3-(Chloromercuri)-2-methoxypropylurea, $C_5H_{11}ClHgN_2O_2$, an orally effective mercurial diuretic.

chlormerodrin Hg 197. Chlormerodrin in which the mercury atom has been replaced by radioactive Hg-197, used as a diagnostic aid in renal function determination.

chlormerodrin Hg 203. Chlormerodrin in which the mercury atom has been replaced by radioactive Hg-203, used as a diagnostic aid in renal function determination.

chlor·mez·a·none (klor·mez'uh·nohn) *n.* 2-(*p*-Chlorophenyl)tetrahydro-3-methyl-4*H*-1,3-thiazin-4-one-1,1-dioxide, $C_{11}H_{12}ClNO_3S$, a tranquilizer.

chloro-. See *chlor-.*

chlo·ro·ac·e·to·phe·none (klor"o·as"e·to·fee'nohn) *n.* C_8H_7ClO. A white solid used as a lacrimator in chemical warfare. It has an odor resembling that of apple blossoms. See also *war gas.*

chlo·ro·ane·mia, chlo·ro·anae·mia (klor"o·uh·nee'mee·uh) *n.* [*chloro-* + *anemia*]. CHLOROSIS (1).

chlo·ro·az·o·din (klor"o·az'o·din) *n.* α,α'-Azobis(chloroformamidine), $C_2H_4Cl_2N_6$, yellow needles or flakes, very slightly soluble in water; used as a topical antiseptic.

Chlorobenzilate. A trademark for ethyl 4,4'-dichlorobenzilate, $C_{14}H_{10}Cl_2O_3$, an acaricide.

chlo·ro·bu·ta·nol (klor"o·bew'ta·nol) *n.* 1,1,1-Trichloro-2-methyl-2-propanol, $C_4H_7Cl_3O$, white crystals, slightly soluble in water. Formerly used as a sedative and hypnotic, and externally as a local anesthetic and antiseptic. Now used as an antibacterial preservative in various solutions. Syn. *chlorbutol, acetone-chloroform.*

chlo·ro·cre·sol (klor"o·kree'sol) *n.* Parachlorometacresol, C_7H_7ClO, colorless crystals, slightly soluble in water; used for the sterilization and preservation of injections and, to some extent, as a surgical antiseptic.

chlo·ro·cru·o·rin (klor"o·kroo'uh·rin) *n.* Any of several iron-porphyrin proteins of extremely high molecular weight and containing a corresponding large number of iron atoms; found in some invertebrates. Dilute solutions of chlorocruorins are green; concentrated solutions are red.

chlo·ro·form (klor'uh·form) *n.* Trichloromethane, $CHCl_3$, heavy, colorless liquid having a characteristic ethereal odor. The commercial article contains up to 2% by volume of alcohol. It is used as an organic solvent and, medicinally, as an anesthetic, anodyne, and antispasmodic. Externally it is irritant. —**chlo·ro·form·ic** (klor"uh·form'ick) *adj.*

chloroformic digitalin. FRENCH DIGITALIN.

chlo·ro·form·ism (klor'uh·form·iz·um) *n.* 1. Habitual use of chloroform for its narcotic effect. 2. Symptoms produced by this use of the drug.

chlo·ro·form·iza·tion (klor"uh·for·mi·zay'shun) *n.* 1. The act of administering chloroform as an anesthetic. 2. The anesthetic effect from the inhalation of chloroform.

chloroform liniment. A solution of chloroform in camphor and soap liniment; used as a local irritant.

chlo·ro·gua·nide (klor"o·gwah'nide) *n.* 1-(*p*-Chlorophenyl)-5-isopropylbiguanide, $C_{11}H_{16}ClN_5$, an antimalarial drug; used as the hydrochloride salt. Syn. *proguanil.*

chlo·ro·labe (klor'o·labe) *n.* [*chloro-* + *-labe*]. One of two cone pigments of the normal eye. The substance absorbs light most actively in the green portion of the spectrum. Contr. *erythrolabe.* See also *iodopsin.*

chlo·ro·leu·ke·mia (klor"o·lew·kee'mee·uh) *n. Obsol.* GRANULOCYTIC SARCOMA.

chlo·ro·lym·pho·ma (klor"o·lim·fo'muh) *n.* [*chloro-* + *lymphoma*]. *Obsol.* GRANULOCYTIC SARCOMA.

chlo·ro·ma (klo·ro'muh) *n.*, pl. **chloromas, chloroma·ta** (·tuh) [*chlor-* + *-oma*]. GRANULOCYTIC SARCOMA.

Chloromycetin. Trademark for the antibiotic substance chloramphenicol.

chlo·ro·my·e·lo·ma (klor"o·migh"e·lo'muh) *n.*, pl. **chloromyelomas, chloromyeloma·ta** (·tuh) [*chloro-* + *myeloma*]. *Obsol.* GRANULOCYTIC SARCOMA.

chlo·ro·per·cha (klor"o·pur'chuh) *n.* Solution of gutta-percha in chloroform; used in dentistry for nonconducting cavity linings, pulp cappings, and for filling the roots of pulpless teeth.

chlo·ro·phe·nol (klor"o·fee'nol) *n.* Monochlorophenol, HOC_6H_4Cl. The *o-* variety is a colorless liquid; the *m-* and *p*-isomers are crystalline. *p*-Chlorophenol is used as a topical antiseptic.

chlo·ro·phen·o·thane (klor″o·fen′o·thane) *n.* 1,1,1-Trichloro-2,2-bis(*p*-chlorophenyl)ethane, $C_{14}H_9Cl_5$, white powder or crystals, insoluble in water; an insecticide. Used medicinally as a pediculicide. Commonly known as DDT. Syn. *dicophane.*

chlo·ro·phyll, chlo·ro·phyl (klor′uh·fil) *n.* [*chloro-* + Gk. *phyllon,* leaf]. The green coloring matter responsible for photosynthesis in plants. It consists of chlorophyll a, $C_{55}H_{72}MgN_4O_5$, and chlorophyll b, $C_{55}H_{70}MgN_4O_6$. Used as a coloring agent and, medicinally, in the treatment of various lesions, and as a deodorant.

chlo·ro·phyl·lase (klor″o·fil′ace, ·aze) *n.* An enzyme that splits or hydrolyzes chlorophyll.

chlo·ro·pia (klor·o′pee·uh) *n.* [*chlor-* + *-opia*]. CHLOROPSIA.

chlo·ro·pic·rin (klor″o·pick′rin) *n.* Trichloronitromethane, CCl_3NO_2, a colorless, odorous liquid used as an insecticide, as a lacrimatory and emetic chemical warfare agent, and to block sulfhydryl reactions in histochemistry. Syn. *chlorpicrin.*

Chlo·rop·i·dae (klo·rop′i·dee) *n. pl.* OSCINIDAE.

chlo·ro·plast (klor′o·plast) *n.* [*chloro-* + *-plast*]. An organelle bearing the chlorophyll of plant cells. Compare *chromoplast.*

chlo·ro·plas·tid (klor″o·plas′tid) *n.* [*chloro-* + *plastid*]. CHLOROPLAST.

chlo·ro·plas·tin (klor″o·plas′tin) *n.* [*chloro-* + *plastin*]. The cytoplasm in chloroplasts.

chlo·ro·pro·caine (klor″o·pro′kane) *n.* 2-(Diethylamino)ethyl 4-amino-2-chlorobenzoate, $C_{13}H_{19}ClN_2O_2$, a local anesthetic agent similar in structure and action to procaine but with more rapid onset of action and greater anesthetic potency; also used as the hydrochloride salt.

chloroprocaine penicillin. A crystalline salt of 2-chloroprocaine and penicillin O, similar to procaine penicillin G, especially useful for patients who are allergic to penicillin G.

chlo·rop·sia (klo·rop′see·uh) *n.* [*chlor-* + *-opsia*]. A defect of vision in which all objects appear green. It occurs occasionally in digitalis poisoning.

chlo·ro·pu·rine (klor″o·pew′reen, ·rin) *n.* 6-Chloropurine, $C_5H_3ClN_4$, the chlorine analogue of 6-aminopurine or adenine. It inhibits experimental sarcoma, possibly through ability to block a metabolic step in conversion of adenine to guanine.

chlo·ro·quine (klor′o·kween) *n.* 7-Chloro-4-(4-diethylamino-1-methylbutylamino)quinoline, $C_{18}H_{26}ClN_3$, principally an antimalarial and antiamebic; used as the diphosphate salt.

chlo·ro·sar·co·ma (klor″o·sahr·ko′muh) *n.* [*chloro-* + *sarcoma*]. GRANULOCYTIC SARCOMA.

chlo·ro·sis (klo·ro′sis) *n.*, pl. **chloro·ses** (·seez) [*chlor-* + *-osis*]. 1. A form of hypochromic microcytic anemia, most common in young women, characterized by a marked reduction of hemoglobin in the blood, with but a slight diminution in number of red cells. 2. *In zoology,* green tissue pigmentation in frogs and other lower vertebrates due to accumulation of biliverdin.

chlorosis ru·bra (roo′bruh). Anemia without pallor, due to dilatation of peripheral vessels.

chlo·ro·stig·ma (klor″o·stig′mah) *n.* A South American plant, *Chlorostigma stuckertianum* (Asclepiadaceae), which contains an alkaloid, chlorostigmine, which has been used to stimulate the secretion of milk.

chlo·ro·then (klo′ro·then) *n.* 2-[(5-Chloro-2-thenyl)(2-dimethylaminoethyl)amino]pyridine, $C_{14}H_{18}ClN_3S$, an antihistaminic drug; used as the citrate or hydrochloride salt.

chlo·ro·thi·a·zide (klor″o·thigh′uh·zide) *n.* 6-Chloro-2*H*-1,2,4-benzothiadiazine-7-sulfonamide 1,1-dioxide, $C_7H_6ClN_3O_4S_2$, an orally effective diuretic and antihypertensive drug. Also used intravenously as the sodium salt.

chlo·ro·thy·mol (klor″o·thigh′mol) *n.* Monochlorothymol, $C_{10}H_{13}ClO$, a white, crystalline powder, almost insoluble in water; used as a germicide.

chlo·rot·ic (klo·rot′ick) *adj.* Affected by or pertaining to chlorosis.

chlorotic anemia. An iron-deficiency anemia occurring in chlorosis.

chlo·ro·tri·an·i·sene (klor″o·trye·an′i·seen) *n.* Chlorotris(*p*-methoxyphenyl)ethylene, $C_{23}H_{21}ClO_3$, a synthetic estrogen.

chlo·rous acid (klo′rus, klor′us). $HClO_2$; an acid which has not been isolated, but salts of which, called chlorites, are known.

chlo·ro·vi·nyl·di·chlo·ro·ar·sine (klor″o·vye″nil·dye″klor·o·ahr′seen) *n.* $ClCH{=}CHAsCl_2$. Lewisite; a potent lacrimator, lung irritant, and vesicant, developed for use as a chemical warfare agent. It is systemically toxic because of its arsenic content. See also *war gas.*

chlo·ro·xy·le·nol (klor″o·zye′le·nole, ·nol) *n.* 2-Chloro-5-hydroxy-1,3-dimethylbenzene, C_8H_9ClO; a creamy-white, crystalline powder used as an antiseptic in ointment form or in oil solution.

Chlorpactin XCB. A trademark for oxychlorosene, a topical anti-infective.

chlor·phen·e·sin (klor·fen′e·sin) *n.* 3-(*p*-Chlorophenoxy)propane-1,2-diol, $C_9H_{11}ClO_3$, a local antibacterial and antifungal agent.

chlorphenesin carbamate. 3-(*p*-Chlorophenoxy)-2-hydroxypropyl carbamate, $C_{10}H_{12}ClNO_4$, a skeletal-muscle relaxant drug.

chlor·phen·ir·amine (klor″fen·irr′a·meen) *n.* 2-[*p*-Chloro-α-(2-dimethylaminoethyl)benzyl] pyridine, $C_{16}H_{19}ClN_2$, an antihistaminic drug; used as the maleate salt.

chlor·phe·nol (klor·fee′nol) *n.* CHLOROPHENOL.

chlor·phen·ox·amine (klor″fen·ock′suh·meen) *n.* 2-[(*p*-Chloro-α-methyl-α-phenylbenzyl)oxy]-*N,N*-dimethylethylamine, $C_{18}H_{22}ClNO$, an anticholinergic, usually used as the hydrochloride.

chlor·phen·ter·mine (klor·fen′tur·meen) *n.* *p*-Chloro-α,α-dimethylphenethylamine, $C_{10}H_{14}ClN$, an anorexigenic drug; used as the hydrochloride salt.

chlor·pic·rin (klor·pick′rin) *n.* CHLOROPICRIN.

chlor·prom·a·zine (klor·prom′uh·zeen) *n.* 2-Chloro-10-(3-dimethylaminopropyl)phenothiazine, $C_{17}H_{19}ClN_2S$, an antipsychotic agent with sedative and antiemetic effects; used chiefly as the hydrochloride salt.

chlor·pro·pa·mide (klor·pro′puh·mide) *n.* 1-[(*p*-Chlorophenyl)sulfonyl]-3-propylurea, $C_{10}H_{13}ClN_2O_3S$, an orally effective hypoglycemic drug.

chlor·pro·phen·pyr·id·a·mine (klor″pro·fen·pirr·id′uh·meen) *n.* CHLORPHENIRAMINE.

chlor·pro·thix·ene (klor″pro·thick′seen) *n.* 2-Chloro-9-(3-dimethylaminopropylidene)thiaxanthene, $C_{18}H_{18}ClNS$, an antipsychotic agent with antiemetic activity.

chlor·quin·al·dol (klor″kwin·al′dol) *n.* 5,7-Dichloro-8-hydroxyquinaldine, $C_{10}H_7Cl_2NO$, a topically applied keratoplastic, antibacterial, and antifungal drug.

chlor·tet·ra·cy·cline (klor″tet·ruh·sigh′kleen) *n.* An antibiotic substance, $C_{22}H_{23}ClN_2O_8$, biosynthesized by the actinomycete *Streptomyces aureofaciens;* a yellow, crystalline powder. It is a broad-spectrum antibiotic, acting against many gram-positive and gram-negative bacteria and also against rickettsiae and certain viruses. Used mainly as the hydrochloride salt.

chlor·thal·i·done (klor·thal′i·dohn) *n.* 2-Chloro-5-(1-hydroxy-3-oxo-1-isoindolinyl)benzenesulfonamide, $C_{14}H_{11}ClN_2O_4S$, an orally effective diuretic and antihypertensive drug.

chlor·thy·mol (klor·thigh′mol) *n.* CHLOROTHYMOL.

Chlor-Trimeton. Trademark for chlorpheniramine, an antihistaminic drug used as the maleate salt.

Chlorylen. Trademark for trichloroethylene, an analgesic inhalant.

chlor·zox·a·zone (klor·zock'suh·zone) *n.* 5-Chloro-2-benzoxazolinone, $C_7H_4ClNO_2$, a skeletal-muscle relaxant.

cho·a·na (ko·ay'nuh, ko·ah'nuh) *n.*, pl. **choa·nae** (·nee) [Gk. *choanē*, funnel]. 1. A funnel-like opening. 2. Either of the posterior nasal orifices. —**choa·nal** (·nul) *adj.*

chocolate cyst. 1. Any cyst filled with degenerated blood. 2. The ovarian lesion characteristic of endometriosis.

choke, *v.* 1. To prevent access of air to the lungs by compression or obstruction of the trachea or larynx. 2. To suffer partial or complete suffocation from mechanical obstruction by a foreign body or external pressure, or from laryngeal spasm caused by an irritating gas or liquid.

choke·damp, *n.* BLACKDAMP.

choked disk. PAPILLEDEMA.

chokes, *n.* A clinical manifestation of decompression sickness caused by free gas bubbles lodged in the pulmonary capillaries, and characterized by severe dyspnia, a nonproductive paroxysmal cough, and deep substernal pain precipitated by deep inspiration or by inhalation of tobacco smoke.

choking gas. *In military medicine,* a casualty gas, such as phosgene, that causes irritation and inflammation of the bronchial tubes and lungs.

chol-, chole-, cholo- [Gk. *cholē*]. A combining form meaning *bile* or *gall.*

cholaemia. CHOLEMIA.

cholaemic. CHOLEMIC.

cho·la·gogue, cho·la·gog (ko'luh·gog, kol'uh·) *n.* [Gk. *kholagōgos*]. Any agent that promotes the flow of bile. See also *cholecystagogue.*

cho·lal·ic acid (ko·lal'ick, ko·lay'lick). CHOLIC ACID (1).

chol·amine (kol'uh·meen) *n.* ETHANOLAMINE.

Cholan-DH. A trademark for dehydrocholic acid, a choleretic.

cho·lane (ko'lane, kol'ane) *n.* [*chol-* + *-ane*]. A tetracyclic hydrocarbon, $C_{24}H_{42}$, which may be considered as the parent substance of sterols, hormones, bile acids, and digitalis aglycones.

chol·an·e·re·sis (ko·lan''e·ree'sis, ko''lan·err'e·sis) *n.* [*cholan*ic + Gk. *erēsis*, removal]. An increase in the output or elimination of cholic acid, its conjugates and their salts, such as sodium taurocholate and sodium glycocholate.

cholangi-, cholangio- [*chol-* + *angi-*]. A combining form meaning *bile duct, biliary passage.*

chol·an·gi·ec·ta·sis (ko·lan''jee·eck'tuh·sis) *n.*, pl. **cholangiecta·ses** (·seez) [*cholangi-* + *ectasis*]. A dilatation of extrahepatic or intrahepatic biliary passages.

cholangio-. See *cholangi-.*

chol·an·gio·car·ci·no·ma (ko·lan''jee·o·kahr''si·no'muh) *n.* [*cholangio-* + *carcinoma*]. Carcinoma of the bile ducts.

chol·an·gio·en·ter·os·to·my (ko·lan''jee·o·en''tur·os'tuh·mee) *n.* [*cholangio-* + *enterostomy*]. *In surgery,* an anastomosis between a bile duct and the intestine.

chol·an·gio·gas·tros·to·my (ko·lan''jee·o·gas·tros'tuh·mee) *n.* [*cholangio-* + *gastrostomy*]. *In surgery,* the formation of an anastomosis between a bile duct and the stomach.

chol·an·gio·gen·e·sis (ko·lan''jee·o·jen'e·sis) *n.* Bile duct formation.

chol·an·gio·gram (ko·lan'jee·o·gram) *n.* The x-ray film produced by means of cholangiography.

chol·an·gi·og·ra·phy (ko·lan''jee·og'ruh·fee) *n.* [*cholangio-* + *-graphy*]. Radiography of the bile ducts.

chol·an·gi·ole (ko·lan'jee·ole) *n.* [*cholangi-* + *-ole*, diminutive suffix]. A small intrahepatic bile duct.

chol·an·gi·o·lit·ic (ko·lan''jee·o·lit'ick) *adj.* [*cholangiolit*is + *-ic*]. Pertaining to inflammation of the bile ducts, especially the small branches.

cholangiolitic cirrhosis. Biliary cirrhosis in which the smallest bile radicles are the principal seat of disease.

cholangiolitic hepatitis. CHOLESTATIC HEPATITIS.

chol·an·gi·o·li·tis (ko·lan''jee·o·lye'tis) *n.*, pl. **cholangio·lit·i·des** (·lit'i·deez) [*cholangiol*e + *-itis*]. Inflammation of the bile ducts within the liver.

chol·an·gi·o·ma (ko·lan''jee·o'muh) *n.*, pl. **cholangiomas, cholangioma·ta** (·tuh) [*cholangi-* + *-oma*]. CHOLANGIOCARCINOMA.

chol·an·gi·os·to·my (ko·lan''jee·os'tuh·mee) *n.* [*cholangio-* + *-stomy*]. *In surgery,* the drainage of any of the bile ducts by means of abdominal incision and penetration into the hepatic, cystic, or common bile duct.

chol·an·gi·ot·o·my (ko·lan''jee·ot'uh·mee) *n.* [*cholangio-* + *-tomy*]. Incision into any of the bile ducts, usually for removal of a calculus.

cholangitic cirrhosis. A form of biliary cirrhosis involving the larger intrahepatic bile ducts, accompanied by fibrosis and inflammation.

chol·an·gi·tis (kol''an·jye'tis, ko''lan·) *n.*, pl. **cholan·git·i·des** [*cholang*i- + *-itis*]. Inflammation of the biliary ducts. —**cholan·git·ic** (·jit'ick) *adj.*

cho·lan·ic acid (ko·lan'ick). The hydroxyl-free, steroid parent substance, $C_{24}H_{40}O_2$, of the unconjugated bile acids, the most important of which are cholic acid (1) and deoxycholic acid.

chol·ano·poi·e·sis (ko·lan''o·poy·ee'sis) *n.*, pl. **cholanopoie·ses** (·seez) [*cholan*ic + *-poiesis*]. The synthesis of cholic acid, or of its conjugates, or of natural bile salts.

chol·ano·poi·et·ic (ko·lan''o·poy·et'ick) *adj.* [*cholan*ic + *-poietic*]. Having the property of increasing the synthesis of cholic acid.

cho·late (ko'late) *n.* Any salt of cholic acid.

chole-. See *chol-.*

cho·le·bil·i·ru·bin (kol''e·bil''i·roo'bin, ko''le·) *n.* [*chole-* + *bilirubin*]. 1. Bilirubin after passage through the hepatic cells. 2. The form of bilirubin present in bile and blood in hepatocellular or obstructive jaundice, giving a positive reaction to the direct van den Bergh test.

Cholebrine. A trademark for iocetamic acid, a radiopaque agent.

cho·le·cal·cif·er·ol (kol''e·kal·sif'ur·ol, ko''le·) *n.* Vitamin D_3, prepared from 7-dehydrocholesterol. Syn. *activated 7-dehydrocholesterol.*

cho·le·chrom·e·re·sis (kol''e·kro·me·ree'sis, ko''le·) *n.* [*chole-* + *chrom-* + Gk. *erēsis*, removal]. Increased output or elimination of bile pigment.

cho·le·chro·mo·poi·e·sis (kol''e·kro''mo·poy·ee'sis, ·ko''le·) *n.* [*chole-* + *chromo-* + *-poiesis*]. The synthesis of bile pigments.

cho·le·cy·a·nin (kol''e·sigh'uh·nin, ko''le·) *n.* BILICYANIN.

cho·le·cyst (kol'e·sist, ko'le·) *n.* [*chole-* + *-cyst*]. GALLBLADDER. —**chole·cys·tic** (·sis'tick) *adj.*

cho·le·cyst·a·gogue (kol''e·sist'uh·gog, ko''le·) *n.* [*cholecyst* + *-agogue*]. An agent or agency that causes or promotes the evacuation of the gallbladder, by stimulating contraction of its musculature, or by relaxation of the sphincter of Oddi; a cholecystokinetic agent.

cho·le·cys·tal·gia (kol''e·sis·tal'juh, ·jee·uh, ko''le·) *n.* [*cholecyst* + *-algia*]. BILIARY COLIC.

cho·le·cys·tec·ta·sia (kol''e·sis·teck·tay'zhuh, ·zee·uh, ko''le·) *n.* [*cholecyst* + *ectasia*]. Distention or dilatation of the gallbladder.

cho·le·cys·tec·to·my (kol''e·sis·teck'tuh·mee, ko''le·) *n.* [*cholecyst* + *-ectomy*]. Excision of the gallbladder and cystic duct.

cho·le·cyst·en·ter·or·rha·phy (kol''e·sist·en''tur·or'uh·fee, ko''le·) *n.* [*colecyst* + *enterorrhaphy*]. The suturing of the gallbladder to the small intestine.

cho·le·cyst·en·ter·os·to·my (kol''e·sist·en''tur·os'tuh·mee) *n.* [*cholecyst* + *enterostomy*]. *In surgery,* the formation of an anastomosis between the gallbladder and the small intestine.

cho·le·cys·tis (ko''le·sis'tis, kol''e·) *n.* [NL., from Gk. *cholē*, bile, + *kystis*, bladder]. GALLBLADDER.

cho·le·cys·ti·tis (ko''le·sis·tye'tis, kol''e·) *n.*, pl. **cholecys·tit·i·des** (·tit'i·deez) [*cholecyst* + *-itis*]. Inflammation of the gallbladder.

cho·le·cys·to·co·lon·ic (kol''e·sis''to·ko·lon'ick, ko''le·) *adj.*

[*cholecyst* + *colonic*]. Pertaining to the gallbladder and the colon.

cho·le·cys·to·co·los·to·my (kol″e·sis″to·ko·los′tuh·mee) *n.* [*cholecyst* + *colostomy*]. *In surgery,* the formation of an anastomosis between the gallbladder and some portion of the upper colon.

cho·le·cys·to·cu·ta·ne·ous (kol″e·sis″to·kew·tay′nee·us) *adj.* [*cholecyst* + *cutaneous*]. Pertaining to the gallbladder and skin, usually to a fistula connecting them.

cho·le·cys·to·du·o·de·nal (kol″e·sis″to·dew″o·dee′nul, ·dew·od′e·nul) *adj.* [*cholecyst* + *duodenal*]. Pertaining to the gallbladder and duodenum.

cho·le·cys·to·du·o·de·no·co·lic (ko″le·sis″to·dew·od′e·no·ko′lick) *adj.* [*cholecyst* + *duodeno-* + *colic*]. Pertaining to the gallbladder, duodenum, and colon.

cho·le·cys·to·du·o·de·nos·to·my (kol″e·sis″to·dew″o·de·nos′tuh·mee) *n.* [*cholecyst* + *duodenostomy*]. *In surgery,* the formation of an anastomosis between the gallbladder and the duodenum.

cho·le·cys·to·elec·tro·co·ag·u·lec·to·my (kol″e·sis″to·e·leck″tro·ko·ag·yoo·leck′tuh·mee) *n.* [*cholecyst* + *electro-* + *coagulate* + *-ectomy*]. Electrosurgical obliteration of the gallbladder.

cho·le·cys·to·en·ter·os·to·my (kol″e·sis″to·en″tur·os′tuh·mee) *n.* [*cholecysto-* + *enterostomy*]. The surgical creation of a connection between the gallbladder and the small intestine.

cho·le·cys·to·gas·tric (kol″e·sis″to·gas′trick) *adj.* [*cholecyst* + *gastric*]. Pertaining to the gallbladder and stomach, usually to a fistula between these organs.

cho·le·cys·to·gas·tros·to·my (kol″e·sis″to·gas·tros′tuh·mee) *n.* [*cholecyst* + *gastrostomy*]. *In surgery,* formation of an anastomosis between the gallbladder and the stomach.

cho·le·cys·to·gram (kol″e·sis′to·gram, ko″le·) *n.* [*cholecyst* + *-gram*]. A radiograph of the gallbladder.

cho·le·cys·tog·ra·phy (kol″e·sis·tog′ruh·fee, ko″le·) *n.* [*cholecyst* + *-graphy*]. Radiography of the gallbladder after ingestion or intravenous injection of a radiopaque substance excreted in bile. —**chole·cys·to·graph·ic** (·sis″to·graf′ick) *adj.*

cho·le·cys·to·il·e·os·to·my (kol″e·sis″to·il·ee·os′tuh·mee) *n.* [*cholecyst* + *ileostomy*]. *In surgery,* the formation of an anastomosis between the gallbladder and the ileum.

cho·le·cys·to·je·ju·nos·to·my (kol″e·sis″to·jee″joo·nos′tuh·mee) *n.* [*cholecyst* + *jejunostomy*]. *In surgery,* the formation of an anastomosis between the gallbladder and the jejunum.

cho·le·cys·to·ki·net·ic (kol″e·sis″to·ki·net′ick) *adj.* [*cholecyst* + *kinetic*]. Possessing the property of causing or promoting gallbladder contraction. See also *cholecystagogue.*

cho·le·cys·to·ki·nin (kol″e·sis″to·kigh′nin, ko″le·) *n.* [*cholecyst* + Gk. *kin*ein, to move, + *-in*]. A hormone, produced by the upper intestinal mucosa, which causes contraction of the gallbladder and secretion of pancreatic enzymes; now known to be identical with the substance formerly called pancreozymin. Abbreviated, CCK.

cholecystokinin-pancreozymin. CHOLECYSTOKININ. Abbreviated, CCK-PZ.

cho·le·cys·to·li·thi·a·sis (kol″e·sis″to·li·thigh′uh·sis, ko″le·) *n.* [*cholecyst* + *lithiasis*]. The presence of one or more gallstones in the gallbladder.

cho·le·cys·to·li·thot·o·my (kol″e·sis″to·li·thot′uh·mee, ko″le·) *n.* [*cholecyst* + *lithotomy*]. *In surgery,* removal of gallstones from the gallbladder.

cho·le·cys·to·pexy (kol″e·sis′to·peck″see, ko″le·) *n.* [*cholecyst* + *-pexy*]. Suture of the gallbladder to the abdominal wall.

cho·le·cys·tor·rha·phy (kol″e·sis·tor′uh·fee, ko″le·) *n.* [*cholecyst* + *-rrhaphy*]. Suture of the gallbladder, especially to the abdominal wall.

cho·le·cys·tos·to·my (kol″e·sis·tos′tuh·mee, ko″le·) *n.* [*cholecyst* + *-stomy*]. *In surgery,* the establishment of an opening into the gallbladder, usually for external drainage of its contents.

cho·le·cys·tot·o·my (kol″e·sis·tot′uh·mee, ko″le·) *n.* [*cholecyst* + *-tomy*]. Incision into the gallbladder to remove gallstones.

cho·le·doch (ko′le·dock) *adj.* [Gk. *cholēdochos,* containing bile]. CHOLEDOCHAL.

cho·le·doch·al (ko·led′uh·kul, ko″le·dock′ul) *adj.* [*choledoch* + *-al*]. Pertaining to the common bile duct.

choledochal cyst. CHOLEDOCHUS CYST.

cho·led·o·chec·ta·sia (ko·led″o·keck·tay′zhuh, ·zee·uh) *n.* [*choledoch* + *ectasia*]. Dilatation of the common bile duct.

cho·led·o·chec·to·my (ko·led″o·keck′tuh·mee) *n.* [*choledoch* + *-ectomy*]. Excision of a part of the common bile duct.

choledochi. Plural and genitive singular of *choledochus.*

cho·led·o·chi·tis (ko·led″o·kigh′tis) *n.* [*choledoch* + *-itis*]. Inflammation of the common bile duct.

cho·led·o·cho·cu·ta·ne·ous (ko·led″uh·ko·kew·tay′nee·us) *adj.* [*choledoch* + *cutaneous*]. Pertaining to the gallbladder and skin, usually to a fistula between them.

cho·led·o·cho·cys·tos·to·my (ko·led″uh·ko·sis·tos′tuh·mee) *n.* [*choledocho-* + *cystostomy*]. *In surgery,* an anastomosis between the common bile duct and the gallbladder.

cho·led·o·cho·do·chor·rha·phy (ko·led″uh·ko·do·kor′uh·fee) *n.* [*choledoch* + chole*doch* + *-rrhaphy*]. *In surgery,* uniting the ends of a divided common bile duct, usually over an indwelling catheter.

cho·led·o·cho·du·o·de·nos·to·my (ko·led″uh·ko·dew″o·de·nos′tuh·mee) *n.* [*choledoch* + *duodenostomy*]. *In surgery,* the establishment of a passage between the common bile duct and the duodenum.

cho·led·o·cho·en·ter·os·to·my (ko·led″uh·ko·en″tur·os′tuh·mee) *n.* [*choledoch* + *enterostomy*]. *In surgery,* the establishment of a passage between the common bile duct and the small intestine.

cho·led·o·cho·gas·tros·to·my (ko·led″uh·ko·gas·tros′tuh·mee) *n.* [*choledoch* + *gastrostomy*]. *In surgery,* the formation of an anastomosis between the common bile duct and the stomach.

cho·led·o·cho·je·ju·nos·to·my (ko·led″uh·ko·jee″joo·nos′tuh·mee) *n.* [*choledocho-* + *jejuno-* + *-stomy*]. *In surgery,* an anastomosis between the common bile duct and the jejunum.

cho·led·o·cho·li·thi·a·sis (ko·led″uh·ko·li·thigh′uh·sis) *n.* [*choledoch* + *lithiasis*]. The presence of calculi in the common bile duct.

cho·led·o·cho·li·thot·o·my (ko·led″uh·ko·li·thot′uh·mee) *n.* [*choledoch* + *lithotomy*]. *In surgery,* removal of a calculus by incision of the common bile duct.

cho·led·o·cho·litho·trip·sy (ko·led″uh·ko·lith′o·trip″see) *n.* [*choledoch* + *lithotripsy*]. *In surgery,* the crushing of a gallstone in the common bile duct without opening the duct.

cho·led·o·cho·plas·ty (ko·led′uh·ko·plas″tee) *n.* [*choledoch* + *-plasty*]. A plastic operation upon the common bile duct.

cho·led·o·chor·rha·phy (ko·led″o·kor′uh·fee) *n.* [*choledoch* + *-rrhaphy*]. *In surgery,* the repair of the divided common bile duct.

cho·led·o·chos·to·my (ko·led″o·kos′tuh·mee) *n.* [*choledoch* + *-stomy*]. *In surgery,* the draining of the common bile duct through the abdominal wall.

cho·led·o·chot·o·my (ko·led″o·kot′uh·mee) *n.* [*choledoch* + *-tomy*]. An incision into the common bile duct.

cho·led·o·chus (ko·led′o·kus) *n.*, pl. & genit. sing. **choledo·chi** (·kye) [NL., from Gk. *cholēdochos,* from *cholē,* bile, + *dochos,* containing]. COMMON BILE DUCT.

choledochus cyst. Congenital cystic dilatation of the common bile duct, usually due to its constriction close to the hepaticopancreatic ampulla, clinically manifested at times varying from shortly after birth to later in childhood by pain, abdominal tumor, hepatic enlargement, cirrhosis, and jaundice. Exacerbations and remissions are common. Syn. *bile cyst.*

Choledyl. Trademark for oxtriphylline, a drug with actions characteristic of theophylline.

cho·le·glo·bin (kol″e·glo′bin, ko″le·) *n.* [*chole-* + *globin*].

Combined native protein (globin) and open-ring iron-porphyrin, which is bile pigment hemoglobin; a precursor of biliverdin. Syn. *verdoglobin.*

cho·le·gogue (ko'le·gog, kol'e·) *n.* CHOLAGOGUE.

cho·le·hem·a·tin, cho·le·haem·a·tin (ko''le·heem'uh·tin, kol''e·) *n.* [*chole-* + *hematin*]. Pigment found in the bile and biliary concretions of ruminants; identical with phylloerythrin.

cho·le·ic (ko·lay'ick, ko·lee'ick) *adj.* [*chole-* + *ic*]. Pertaining to bile.

choleic acid. Any one of the several stable molecular compounds formed by deoxycholic acid with other substances, especially fatty acids.

cho·le·lith (ko'le·lith, kol''e·) *n.* [*chole-* + *-lith*]. BILIARY CALCULUS; GALLSTONE. —**cho·le·lith·ic** (ko''le·lith'ick) *adj.*

cho·le·li·thi·a·sis (ko''le·li·thigh'uh·sis, kol''e·) *n.*, pl. **choleli·thia·ses** (·seez) [*chole-* + *lithiasis*]. The presence of, or a condition associated with, calculi in the gallbladder or in a bile duct.

cho·le·li·thot·o·my (ko''le·li·thot'uh·mee, kol''e·) *n.* [*chole-* + *lithotomy*]. Incision for the removal of gallstones.

cho·lem·e·sis (ko·lem'e·sis) *n.*, pl. **choleme·ses** (·seez) [*chol-* + *emesis*]. Vomiting of bile.

cho·le·mia, cho·lae·mia (ko·lee'mee·uh) *n.* [*chol-* + *-emia*]. 1. HEPATIC ENCEPHALOPATHY. 2. HEPATIC COMA. 3. The presence of bile in the blood.

cho·le·mic, cho·lae·mic (ko·lee'mick, ·lem'ick) *adj.* Pertaining to, resulting from, or caused by cholemia.

cholemic nephrosis. BILE NEPHROSIS.

cho·le·poi·e·sis (kol''e·poy·ee'sis, ko''le·) *n.* [*chole-* + *-poiesis*]. The process of formation of bile by the liver.

cho·le·poi·et·ic (kol''e·poy·et'ick, ko''le·) *adj. & n.* [*chole-* + *-poietic*]. 1. Stimulating the processes or a process concerned in the formation of bile. 2. A cholepoietic agent.

cho·le·pra·sin (ko''le·pray'sin, kol''e·) *n.* [*chole-* + Gk. *prasinos,* leek-green]. BILIPRASIN.

cho·le·pyr·rhin (ko''le·pirr'in, kol''e·) *n.* [*chole-* + Gk. *pyrrhos,* red, tawny, + *-in*]. *Obsol.* BILIRUBIN.

chol·era (kol'ur·uh) *n.* [L., from Gk.]. 1. A specific infectious disease of man caused by *Vibrio cholerae.* A soluble toxin produced in the intestinal tract by the vibrio alters the permeability of the mucosa and causes a profuse, watery diarrhea with fluid and electrolyte depletion; occurs endemically and epidemically in Asia. 2. *Obsol.* Any of various conditions characterized by profuse vomiting and diarrhea.

cholera-blue pigment. A color base obtained by dissolving cholera-red in concentrated sulfuric acid and then neutralizing with caustic soda.

chol·era·gen (kol'ur·uh·jen) *n.* The heat-labile protein enterotoxin, produced by *Vibrio cholerae,* which acts on the intestinal epithelial cells, causing the characteristic depletion of intestinal fluid and electrolytes in cholera.

chol·er·a·ic (kol''ur·ay'ick) *adj.* Pertaining to, resembling, or having characteristics of cholera.

cholera mor·bus (mor'bus). *Obsol.* Any acute severe gastroenteritis.

cholera nos·tras (nos'tras) [L., of our country, native]. SALMONELLOSIS.

cholera-red pigment. A color base found in cultures of cholera bacilli, which upon addition of mineral acids, gives a violet color. On rendering the solution alkaline and shaking it with benzene, the cholera-red is obtained in brownish-red lamellas. Distillation of cholera-red with zinc dust gives indole.

cholera-red reaction. A nonspecific test for the *Vibrio cholerae* in which a pink color develops upon the addition of 8 drops of sulfuric acid to a 24-hour growth of the organism in 10 ml of peptone broth; the test is dependent on the production of indole and the reduction of nitrate.

cholera sic·ca (sick'uh) [L., dry]. Cholera in which death occurs before there has been vomiting or diarrhea.

cholera sid·er·ans (sid'ur·anz) [L., fulminant, sudden]. CHOLERA SICCA.

cholera vaccine. A sterile suspension of killed cholera vibrios (*Vibrio cholerae*), of strains selected for high antigenic efficiency, in isotonic sodium chloride solution or other suitable diluent which may contain an antimicrobial agent. Vaccine-induced immunity is incomplete and short-lived.

cho·le·re·sis (ko''le·ree'sis, kol''e·) *n.*, pl. **cholere·ses** (·seez) [*chol-* + Gk. *erēsis,* removal]. Increased secretion of bile by the liver.

cho·le·ret·ic (ko''le·ret'ick, kol''e·) *adj. & n.* 1. Pertaining to or stimulating choleresis. 2. Any substance that stimulates choleresis.

choleretic diarrhea. Diarrhea due to excess bile in the colon, usually resulting from resection or disease of the terminal ileum.

chol·er·ic (kol'ur·ick) *adj.* [L. *cholericus,* bilious]. Easily angered; irritable.

chol·er·i·form (kol'ur·i·form) *adj.* Resembling cholera.

choler·oid (kol'ur·oid) *adj.* CHOLERIFORM.

chol·ero·ma·nia (kol''ur·o·may'nee·uh) *n.* [*cholera* + *mania*]. 1. The acute organic brain disorder seen during the course of cholera. 2. CHOLEROPHOBIA.

chol·ero·pho·bia (kol''ur·o·fo'bee·uh) *n.* [*cholera* + *phobia*]. Abnormal fear of cholera.

chol·er·rha·gia (kol''e·ray'jee·uh, ·ko''le·) *n.* [*chole-* + *-rrhagia*]. A copious flow of bile.

cho·les·tane (kol'es·tane, ko·les') *n.* [*cholesterol* + *-ane*]. $C_{27}H_{48}$; a fully saturated hydrocarbon derivative of cyclopentanophenanthrene containing in addition two methyl groups (at carbon atoms 10 and 13) and a C_8H_{17} aliphatic group (at carbon atom 17). It may be considered a parent hydrocarbon from which many sterols, including cholesterol, are derived.

cho·les·ta·nol (ko·les'tuh·nole, ·nol) *n.* 1. Cholestan-3β-ol, or 3β-hydroxycholestane, $C_{27}H_{47}OH$, occurring in various tissues; it represents cholesterol in which the double bond is saturated. Syn. *dihydrocholesterol.* 2. Any hydroxyl derivative of cholestane of the general formula $C_{27}H_{47}OH$.

cho·le·sta·sis (ko''le·stay'sis) *n.* [*chole-* + *-stasis*]. Stoppage or slowing of flow in biliary channels, especially in the small intrahepatic branches. —**chole·stat·ic** (·stat'ick) *adj.*

cholestatic cirrhosis. Cirrhosis secondary to biliary obstruction.

cholestatic hepatitis. Hepatitis due to obstruction of the small intrahepatic bile channels by bile of altered and presumably more viscous composition.

cho·les·te·a·to·ma (ko·les''tee·uh·to'muh) *n.*, pl. **cholesteatomas, cholesteatoma·ta** (·tuh) [*chole-* + *steatoma*]. An epidermal inclusion cyst of the middle ear or mastoid bone, sometimes in the external ear canal, brain, or spinal cord. True cholesteatoma is rare and of congenital origin. Syn. *pearly tumor.* See also *pseudocholesteatoma.* —**cholestea·tom·a·tous** (·tom'uh·tus) *adj.*

cholesteatoma of the ovary. A teratoma with epidermal inclusion cysts.

cho·les·te·a·to·sis (ko·les''tee·uh·to'sis) *n.*, pl. **cholesteato·ses** (·seez) [*chole-* + *steatosis*]. The presence of an abundance of cholesterol or its esters in a focus of degeneration or necrosis, usually the intima of the aorta.

cho·les·tene (kol'es·teen, ko·les'teen) *n.* Any of several hydrocarbons of the formula $C_{27}H_{46}$, resulting from introduction of a double bond in cholestane; the position of the double bond characterizes specific cholestenes. Cholest-5-ene is the immediate parent hydrocarbon of cholesterol.

cho·les·te·nol (ko·les'te·nol) *n.* Any hydroxyl derivative of a cholestene, having the general formula $C_{27}H_{45}OH$. An important cholestenol is cholesterol.

cholesteraemia. Cholesteremia (= CHOLESTEROLEMIA).

cho·les·ter·ase (ko·les'tur·ace) *n.* An enzyme, present in blood and other tissues, that hydrolyzes cholesterol esters to form cholesterol and fatty acids.

cho·les·ter·emia, cho·les·ter·ae·mia (ko·les″tur·ee′mee·uh) *n.* CHOLESTEROLEMIA.

cho·les·ter·in (ko·les′tur·in) *n.* CHOLESTEROL.

cho·les·ter·in·uria (ko·les″tur·i·new′ree·uh) *n.* The presence of cholesterol in the urine.

cho·les·ter·ol (ko·les′tur·ol) *n.* [*chole-* + *sterol*]. Cholest-5-en-3β-ol, $C_{27}H_{45}OH$, an unsaturated monohydric alcohol of the class of sterols; a constituent of all animal fats and oils, of bile, gallstones, nervous tissue, egg yolk, and blood, and sometimes found in foci of fatty degeneration. It is a white, crystalline substance, insoluble in water. It is important in metabolism and a derivative can be activated to form a vitamin D. See also Table of Chemical Constituents of Blood in the Appendix.

cho·les·ter·ol·emia, cho·les·ter·ol·ae·mia (ko·les″tur·ol·ee′mee·uh) *n.* [*cholesterol* + *-emia*]. 1. The presence of cholesterol in the blood. 2. HYPERCHOLESTEROLEMIA.

cho·les·ter·ol·er·e·sis (ko·les″tur·ol·err′e·sis) *n.* [*cholesterol* + Gk. *erēsis,* removal]. An increased elimination of cholesterol in the bile.

cho·les·ter·olo·poi·e·sis (ko·les″tur·ol·o·poy·ee′sis) *n.* [*cholesterol* + *-poiesis*]. The synthesis of cholesterol.

cho·les·ter·ol·o·sis (ko·les″tur·ol·o′sis) *n.* A condition marked by an abnormal deposition of cholesterol, as in mucosa of the gallbladder.

cho·les·ter·o·sis (ko·les″tur·o′sis) *n.* CHOLESTEROLOSIS.

cho·les·ter·yl (ko·les′tur·il) *n.* $C_{27}H_{45}$. The radical of cholesterol.

cho·les·tyr·a·mine (ko·les′ti·ruh·meen) *n.* A strongly basic anion exchange resin having a demonstrated affinity for bile acids; used in adjunctive therapy in the management of patients with elevated cholesterol levels.

cho·le·ver·din (kol″e·vur′din, ko″le·) *n.* BILIVERDIN.

cho·lic (ko′lick, kol′ick) *adj.* CHOLEIC.

cholic acid. 1. 3,7,12-Trihydroxycholanic acid, $C_{24}H_{40}O_5$, one of the unconjugated bile acids. In bile it occurs as the sodium salt of the conjugated taurocholic or glycocholic acid. Syn. *cholalic acid.* 2. Any one of the several unconjugated bile acids which are hydroxy derivatives of cholanic acid.

cho·lin (ko′lin) *n.* CHOLINE.

cho·line (ko′leen, ·lin, kol′een, ·in) *n.* (β-Hydroxyethyl)trimethylammonium hydroxide, $(CH_3)_3N(OH)CH_2CH_2OH$, a liquid base widely distributed in nature as a component of lecithin and other phospholipids. An insufficient supply of choline or other lipotropic factors in the diet may result in accumulation of fat in the liver and other body dysfunctions. As a drug, choline has an effect similar to that of parasympathetic stimulation. Various salts of choline are used as lipotropic agents. See also *acetylcholine.*

cho·line·acet·y·lase (ko″leen·a·set′i·lace, ·laze) *n.* An enzyme obtained from brain which catalyzes the synthesis of acetylcholine in the presence of adenosine triphosphate as an energy source.

choline kinase. An enzyme that catalyzes the reaction between choline and adenosine triphosphate to yield phosphocholine and adenosine diphosphate. This is the first step in a pathway for the biosynthesis of phosphatidylcholine, a major component of membranes and transport lipoproteins, in many animal tissues.

cho·line·mi·met·ic (ko″leen·mi·met′ick) *adj.* CHOLINOMIMETIC.

choline oxidase. An enzyme catalyzing the oxidation of choline.

cho·lin·er·gic (ko″lin·ur′jick, kol″in·) *adj.* [*choline* + *erg-* + *-ic*]. Pertaining to or designating the type of chemical activity characteristic of acetylcholine or of agents which mimic the actions of acetylcholine. See also *parasympatholytic, parasympathomimetic.*

cholinergic blocking agent. Any agent which blocks the action of acetylcholine or acetylcholine-like substances, i.e., which blocks the action of cholinergic nerves.

cholinergic crisis. Marked muscular weakness and respiratory paralysis, due to the presence of excess amounts of acetylcholine; usually seen in patients with myasthenia gravis as a result of overmedication with anticholinesterase drugs. Compare *myasthenic crisis.*

cholinergic fibers. CHOLINERGIC NERVES.

cholinergic nerves. Those nerves which, upon stimulation, release a cholinergic substance (acetylcholine) at their terminations; they include all autonomic preganglionic nerves (sympathetic and parasympathetic), postganglionic parasympathetic nerves, somatic motor nerves to skeletal muscles, and fibers to sweat glands and certain blood vessels.

cholinergic urticaria. Small, relatively nonpruritic wheals, provoked by heat generated by exercise or emotion. Thought to be caused by acetycholine or a metabolic abnormality.

cho·lin·es·ter·ase (ko″li·nes′tur·ace, ·aze) *n.* Any enzyme found in blood and in various other tissues that catalyzes hydrolysis of choline esters, including acetylcholine. Abbreviated, ChE.

cho·li·no·gen·ic (ko″li·no·jen′ick) *adj.* [*choline* + *-genic*]. CHOLINERGIC.

cholinogenic dermatosis. A dermatosis, usually urticarial or erythematous, produced by efferent cholinergic impulses via the autonomic nervous system.

cholinogenic urticaria. CHOLINERGIC URTICARIA.

cho·li·no·lyt·ic (ko″li·no·lit′ick) *adj.* [*choline* + *-lytic*]. ANTICHOLINERGIC.

cho·li·no·mi·met·ic (ko″li·no·mi·met′ick) *adj.* [*choline* + *mimetic*]. Having an action similar to that of acetylcholine.

cholo-. See *chol-.*

chol·o·chrome (kol′o·krome) *n.* [*cholo-* + *-chrome*]. BILE PIGMENT.

Cholografin. Trademark for iodipamide, a roentgenographic contrast medium for intravenous cholangiography and cholecystography used as the methylglucamine (meglumine) or sodium salt.

cho·lo·lith (kol′o·lith, ko′luh·) *n.* [*cholo-* + *lith*]. GALLSTONE. —**cho·lo·lith·ic** (kol″o·lith′ick, ko″lo·) *adj.*

cho·lo·li·thi·a·sis (kol″o·li·thigh′uh·sis, ko″lo·) *n.* CHOLELITHIASIS.

chol·or·rhea (kol·o·ree′uh, ko″luh·) *n.* [*cholo-* + *-rrhea*]. Profuse secretion of bile.

cho·lo·tho·rax (ko″lo·tho′racks, kol″o·) *n.* [*cholo-* + *thorax*]. Bile in the pleural cavities.

Choloview. A trademark for iodoxamic acid, a radiographic contrast agent.

Choloxin. Trademark for dextrothyroxine sodium, an anticholesteremic agent.

chol·uria (ko·lew′ree·uh) *n.* [*chol-* + *-uria*]. The presence of bile in the urine.

Choman's method for nickel [B. R. *Choman,* U.S. bacteriologist, b. 1926]. Fresh frozen sections are treated with ammonia fumes and then 1% dimethylglyoxime in 95% alcohol. Red acicular crystals develop.

chon·do·den·drine (kon″do·den′drin) *n.* BEBEERINE.

Chon·do·den·dron (kon″do·den′dron) *n.* A genus of South American climbing plants of the Menispermaceae. *Chondodendron tomentosum* is the source of pareira.

chondr-, chondri-, chondro- [Gk. *chondros*]. A combining form meaning *cartilage, cartilaginous.*

chon·dral (kon′drul) *adj.* [*chondr-* + *al*]. Cartilaginous; pertaining to cartilage.

chon·drec·to·my (kon·dreck′tuh·mee) *n.* [*chondr-* + *-ectomy*]. *In surgery,* the excision of cartilage.

chondri-. See *chondr-.*

chondrification center. A region at which cartilage is first formed.

chon·dri·fy (kon′dri·figh) *v.* To convert into cartilage; to become cartilage or cartilaginous. —**chon·dri·fi·ca·tion** (kon″dri·fi·kay′shun) *n.*

chon·dri·gen (kon″dri·jen) *n.* [*chondri-* + *-gen*]. The protein of cartilage which is converted by boiling into chondrin; similar to collagen.

chon·drin (kon'drin) *n.* [*chondr-* + *-in*]. A protein material obtained by boiling cartilage; primarily gelatin obtained from the collagen component of the cartilage.

chondrin balls. Isogenous cell groups in cartilage and their surrounding basophil matrix.

chondrio- [Gk. *chondrion,* small grain]. A combining form meaning *chondriosome, mitochondrion.*

chon·drio·cont (kon'dree·o·kont) *n.* [*chondrio-* + Gk. *kontos,* pole]. A filamentous or rod-shaped mitochondrion.

chon·drio·ki·ne·sis (kon"dree·o·kigh·nee'sis) *n.,* pl. **chondrio-kine·ses** (·seez) [*chondrio-* + *kinesis*]. Division of the mitochondrial complex during karyokinesis.

chon·dri·o·ma (kon·dree·o'muh) *n.,* pl. **chondriomas, chondri-oma·ta** (·tuh). CHONDRIOME.

chon·dri·ome (kon'dree·ome) *n.* [*chrondrio-* + *-ome*]. A generic term for mitochondria regardless of shape.

chon·drio·mite (kon'dree·o·mite) *n.* [*chondrio-* + Gk. *mitos,* thread]. A thread-shaped mitochondrion.

chon·drio·some (kon'dree·o·sohm) *n.* [*chondrio-* + *-some*]. A general term for all forms of mitochondria and other cytoplasmic bodies of the same nature. —**chon·drio·som·al** (kon"dree·o·so'mul) *adj.*

chon·dri·tis (kon·dry'tis) *n.* [*chondr-* + *-itis*]. Inflammation of a cartilage.

chondro-. See *chondr-.*

chon·dro·al·bu·mi·noid (kon"dro·al·bew'mi·noid) *n.* [*chondro-* + *albuminoid*]. An insoluble protein component of cartilage matrix similar to elastin.

chon·dro·an·gio·path·ia cal·ca·rea seu punc·ta·ta (kon"dro·an"jee·o·path'ee·uh kal·kair'ee·uh siw punk·tay'tuh). CHONDRODYSTROPHIA CALCIFICANS CONGENITA.

chon·dro·blast (kon'dro·blast) *n.* [*chondro-* + *-blast*]. A cartilage-forming cell.

chon·dro·blas·to·ma (kon"dro·blas·to'muh) *n.* [*chondro-* + *blastoma*]. A rare chondrocytic tumor of young males, usually involving the epiphyses; it is locally aggressive but does not metastasize.

chon·dro·cal·ci·no·sis (kon"dro·kal"si·no'sis) *n.* [*chondro-* + *calcinosis*]. 1. Deposition of calcium salts in cartilaginous tissues. 2. PSEUDOGOUT SYNDROME.

chon·dro·cal·syn·ovi·tis (kon"dro·kal·sin"o·vye'tis) *n.* [*chondro-* + *calc-* + *synovitis*]. 1. Deposition of calcium salts in cartilage and synovial tissues. 2. PSEUDOGOUT SYNDROME.

chon·dro·cla·sis (kon"dro·klay'sis) *n.,* pl. **chondrocla·ses** (·seez) [*chondro-* + *-clasis*]. 1. Crushing of a cartilage. 2. Resorption of cartilage.

chon·dro·clast (kon'dro·klast) *n.* [*chondro-* + *-clast*]. A cell concerned in the resorption of cartilage.

chon·dro·cos·tal (kon"dro·kos'tul) *adj.* [*chondro-* + *costal*]. Pertaining to the ribs and their cartilages.

chon·dro·cra·ni·um (kon"dro·kray'nee·um) *n.* [*chondro-* + *cranium*]. The embryonic cartilaginous cranium.

chon·dro·cyte (kon'dro·site) *n.* [*chondro-* + *-cyte*]. A cartilage cell. —**chon·dro·cyt·ic** (kon"dro·sit'ick) *adj.*

chon·dro·der·ma·ti·tis (kon"dro·dur"muh·tye'tis) *n.* [*chondro-* + *dermatitis*]. Inflammation of cartilage and overlying skin.

chondrodermatitis no·du·la·ris he·li·cis (nod·yoo·lair'is hel'i·sis). Painful nodules of the ear, usually seen on the rim of the ear in men. Frostbite has often preceded their occurrence.

chon·dro·dys·pla·sia (kon"dro·dis·play'zhuh, ·zee·uh) *n.* [*chondro-* + *dysplasia*]. ENCHONDROMATOSIS.

chondrodysplasia punc·ta·ta (punk·tay'tuh, ·tah'tuh). CHONDRODYSTROPHIA CALCIFICANS CONGENITA.

chon·dro·dys·tro·phia (kon"dro·dis·tro'fee·uh) *n.* CHONDRODYSTROPHY.

chondrodystrophia cal·cif·i·cans con·gen·i·ta (kal·sif'i·kanz kon·jen'i·tuh). An inherited (autosomal recessive) disease characterized by shortness of the neck and limbs, kyphoscoliosis, flat nose and widely separated eyes, and sometimes associated with cataracts and mental retardation. Syn. *Conradi's disease.*

chondrodystrophia fe·ta·lis (fee·tay'lis). ACHONDROPLASIA.

chondrodystrophia fetalis cal·ca·rea (kal·kair'ee·uh). CHONDRODYSTROPHIA CALCIFICANS CONGENITA.

chondrodystrophia fetalis cal·cif·i·cans (kal·sif'i·kanz). CHONDRODYSTROPHIA CALCIFICANS CONGENITA.

chondrodystrophia fetalis hy·po·plas·ti·ca (high"po·plas'ti·kuh). CHONDRODYSTROPHIA CALCIFICANS CONGENITA.

chondrodystrophia hy·per·plas·ti·ca (high·pur·plas'ti·kuh). MULTIPLE HEREDITARY EXOSTOSES.

chondrodystrophia hy·po·plas·ti·ca (high"po·plas'ti·kuh). 1. Undeveloped cartilage, showing little or no proliferation. 2. ACHONDROPLASIA.

chondrodystrophia ma·la·cia (ma·lay'shuh, ·see·uh). Cartilage similar to chondrodystrophia hypoplastica (1) except that the cartilage is soft.

chondrodystrophic dwarf. ACHONDROPLASTIC DWARF.

chon·dro·dys·tro·phy (kon"dro·dis'truh·fee) *n.* [*chondro-* + *dystrophy*]. One of a group of disorders characterized by a defect in the formation of bone from cartilage, congenital in origin. —**chondro·dys·tro·phic** (·dis·tro'fick) *adj.*

chon·dro·ec·to·der·mal (kon"dro·eck"to·dur'mul) *adj.* [*chondro-* + *ectodermal*]. Pertaining to cartilage developed from ectoderm, as certain branchial arch cartilages from the neural crest.

chondroectodermal dysplasia. A rare congenital disorder characterized by enchondromatosis, ectodermal dysplasia, bilateral polydactyly, polymetacarpalism, dental dysplasia, and sometimes congenital heart disease. Syn. *Ellis-van Creveld syndrome.*

chon·dro·epi·troch·le·a·ris (kon"dro·ep"i·trock·lee·air'is) *L. adj.* [*chondro-* + *epitrochlearis*]. Pertaining to rib cartilages and the region above the trochlea of the humerus.

chondroepitrochlearis muscle. CHONDROHUMERALIS MUSCLE.

chon·dro·fi·bro·ma (kon"dro·figh·bro'muh) *n.* [*chondro-* + *fibroma*]. A fibroma containing cartilaginous tissue.

chon·dro·fi·bro·sar·co·ma (kon"dro·figh"bro·sahr·ko'muh) *n.* [*chondro-* + *fibrosarcoma*]. A type of malignant mixed mesodermal tumor containing fibrosarcomatous and chondrosarcomatous components.

chon·dro·gen (kon'dro·jen) *n.* CHONDRIGEN.

chon·dro·gen·e·sis (kon"dro·jen'uh·sis) *n.* [*chondro-* + *-genesis*]. Formation of cartilage. —**chondro·ge·net·ic** (·je·net'ick), **chondro·gen·ic** (·jen'ick) *adj.*

chondrogenic zone. The layer of cartilage formation under the deep face of the perichondrium.

chon·drog·e·nous (kon·droj'e·nus) *adj.* [*chondro-* + *-genous*]. Producing cartilage.

chon·dro·glos·sus (kon"dro·glos'us) *L. adj.* [*chondro-* + Gk. *glōssa,* tongue]. Pertaining to the cartilaginous tip of the hyoid bone and the tongue.

chondroglossus muscle. A variable portion of the hyoglossus muscle. NA *musculus chondroglossus.* See also Table of Muscles in the Appendix.

chon·dro·hu·me·ra·lis (kon"dro·hew·mur·ay'lis) *L. adj.* [NL., from *chondro-* + *humeral*]. Pertaining to the cartilages of the ribs and the humerus.

chondrohumeralis muscle. An occasional slip of muscle found in the axillary fascia.

chon·droid (kon'droid) *adj.* [*chondr-* + *-oid*]. Resembling cartilage.

chondroid tissue. A form of cartilage which remains in an embryonic state of development.

chon·dro·it·ic acid (kon"dro·it'ick). CHONDROITIN SULFATE.

chon·dro·i·tin (kon·dro'i·tin) *n.* A complex nitrogenous substance which, in the form of chondroitin sulfate, occurs combined with protein as chondromucoid, a constituent of cartilage.

chondroitin sulfate. A compound which on hydrolysis yields sulfuric acid, acetic acid, chondrosamine, and glucuronic acid; the prosthetic group of the glycoprotein chondromucoid; heparin has a similar chemical structure. Syn. *chondroitic acid, chondroitin sulfuric acid.*

chondroitin sulfate B. DERMATAN SULFATE.

chon·dro·i·tin·sul·fu·ric acid (kon·dro″i·tin·sul·few′rick). CHONDROITIN SULFATE.

chon·dro·lipo·sar·co·ma (kon″dro·lip″o·sahr·ko′muh) *n.* [*chondro-* + *liposarcoma*]. A malignant mixed mesodermal tumor composed of liposarcomatous and chondrosarcomatous elements.

chon·dro·ma (kon·dro′muh) *n.*, pl. **chondromas, chondroma·ta** (·tuh) [*chondr-* + *-oma*]. A benign tumor composed of cartilage (either hyaline cartilage or fibrocartilage); may grow from bone, cartilage, or other tissue. See also *ecchondroma, enchondroma.*

chon·dro·ma·la·cia (kon″dro·ma·lay′shuh, ·see·uh) *n.* [*chondro-* + *malacia*]. Softening of a cartilage.

chon·dro·ma·to·sis (kon″dro·muh·to′sis) *n.* [*chondroma* + *-osis*]. The presence of multiple chondromas.

chon·drom·a·tous (kon·drom′uh·tus) *adj.* 1. Of or pertaining to a chondroma. 2. *Erron.* CARTILAGINOUS.

chon·dro·mere (kon′dro·meer) *n.* [*chondro-* + *-mere*]. A cartilaginous segment of the embryonic vertebral column.

chon·dro·meta·pla·sia (kon″dro·met·uh·play′zhuh, ·zee·uh) *n.* [*chondro-* + *metaplasia*]. 1. Metaplasia of cartilage. 2. Cartilaginous metaplasia of synovial structures.

chon·dro·mu·coid (kon″dro·mew′koid) *n.* [*chondro-* + *mucoid*]. A mucoid found in cartilage; a glycoprotein in which chondroitin sulfate is the prosthetic group.

chon·dro·myxo·he·man·gio·en·do·the·lio·sar·co·ma (kon″dro·mick″so·he·man″jee·o·en·do·theel″ee·o·sahr·ko′muh) *n.* [*chondro-* + *myxo-* + *hemangio-* + *endothelio-* + *sarcoma*]. A malignant mixed mesodermal tumor containing chondrosarcomatous, myxosarcomatous, and angiosarcomatous elements.

chon·dro·myx·oid (kon″dro·mick′soid) *adj.* [*chondro-* + *myxoid*]. Composed of cartilaginous and myxoid elements.

chondromyxoid fibroma. A benign bone tumor whose parenchyma is composed of embryonal cartilage cells which differentiate into fibrous, myxoid, and cartilaginous foci in various combinations.

chon·dro·myx·o·ma (kon″dro·mick·so′muh) *n.* [*chondro-* + *myxoma*]. A benign connective-tissue tumor with cartilaginous and mucinous compounds.

chon·dro·myxo·sar·co·ma (kon″dro·mick″so·sahr·ko′muh) *n.* [*chondro-* + *myxosarcoma*]. A sarcoma whose parenchyma is composed of anaplastic myxoid and chondroid elements.

chon·dro·os·teo·dys·tro·phy (kon″dro·os″tee·o·dis′truh·fee) *n.* [*chondro-* + *osteo-* + *dystrophy*]. MORQUIO'S SYNDROME.

chon·dro·os·te·o·ma (kon″dro·os″tee·o′muh) *n.* [*chondro-* + *osteoma*]. 1. OSTEOCHONDROMA. 2. EXOSTOSIS CARTILAGINEA.

chon·dro·os·teo·sar·co·ma (kon″dro·os″tee·o·sahr·ko′muh) *n.* [*chondro-* + *osteosarcoma*]. A malignant mixed mesodermal tumor containing chondrosarcomatous and osteosarcomatous elements, and following the clinical course of osteosarcoma.

chon·drop·a·thy (kon·drop′uth·ee) *n.* [*chondro-* + *-pathy*]. Any disease involving cartilage.

chon·dro·pha·ryn·ge·us (kon″dro·fa·rin′jee·us) *L. adj.* [*chondro-* + NL. *pharyngeus,* pharyngeal]. Pertaining to the cartilaginous tip of the hyoid bone and pharynx.

chondropharyngeus muscle. The portion of the middle constrictor of the pharynx which arises from the stylohyoid ligament. NA *pars chondropharyngea musculi constrictoris pharyngis medii.*

chon·dro·phyte (kon′dro·fite) *n.* [*chondro-* + *-phyte*]. A hypertrophic cartilaginous outgrowth.

chon·dro·plast (kon′dro·plast) *n.* [*chondro-* + *-plast*]. CHONDROBLAST.

chon·dro·plas·ty (kon′dro·plas″tee) *n.* [*chondro-* + *-plasty*]. A plastic operation on cartilage.

chon·dro·po·ro·sis (kon″dro·po·ro′sis) *n.*, pl. **chondroporo·ses** (·seez) [*chondro-* + *porosis*]. Thinning of cartilage by the enlargement of its lacunae; occurs preceding the process of endochondral osteogenesis.

chon·dro·pro·tein (kon″dro·pro′tee·in) *n.* [*chondro-* + *protein*]. A protein occurring normally in cartilage.

chon·dro·sa·mine (kon·dro′sa·meen) *n.* 2-Amino-D-galactose, a structural unit of chondroitin sulfate. Syn. *galactosamine.*

chon·dro·sar·co·ma (kon″dro·sahr·ko′muh) *n.* [*chondro-* + *sarcoma*]. A malignant tumor composed of anaplastic chondrocytes; it may occur as a central or peripheral tumor of bone. —**chondrosar·co·ma·tous** (·ko′muh·tus) *adj.*

chondrosarcoma myx·o·ma·to·des (mick″so·muh·to′deez). CHONDROMYXOSARCOMA.

chon·dro·sin (kon′dro·sin) *n.* A disaccharide, representing a molecule each of glucuronic acid and chondrosamine, produced by the hydrolysis of chondroitin sulfate.

chon·dro·sis (kon·dro′sis) *n.*, pl. **chondro·ses** (·seez) [*chondr-* + *-osis*]. Formation of cartilage.

chon·dro·ster·nal (kon″dro·stur′nul) *adj.* [*chondro-* + *sternal*]. Pertaining to the costal cartilages and to the sternum.

chon·dro·tome (kon′dro·tome) *n.* [*chondro-* + *-tome*]. An instrument for cutting cartilage.

chon·drot·o·my (kon·drot′uh·mee) *n.* [*chondro-* + *-tomy*]. *In surgery,* the division of a cartilage.

Chon·drus (kon′drus) *n.* A small genus of red algae of the Gigartinaceae.

Chondrus cris·pus (kris′pus). A species of red algae; the dried bleached plant, called carrageen or Irish moss, yields carrageenin, a mucilaginous principle, proteins, and salts of iodine, chlorine, and bromine. It is demulcent and somewhat nutrient; used as an emulsifying agent.

cho·ne·chon·dro·ster·non (ko″nee·kon·dro·stur′non) *n.* [Gk. *kōnos,* cone, + *chondro-* + Gk. *sternon,* chest]. FUNNEL CHEST.

chop amputation. Amputation by a circular cut through the soft parts and bone without provision for flaps.

Cho·part's amputation (shoʰ·pahr′) [F. *Chopart,* French surgeon, 1743–1795]. An amputation of the foot consisting of a disarticulation of the tarsal bones, leaving only the talus and calcaneus.

Chopart's joint [F. *Chopart*]. The articulation of the calcaneus and talus with the remaining tarsal bones.

Chopra's test. ANTIMONY TEST.

Choranid. A trademark for chorionic gonadotropin.

chord-, chordo- [Gk. *chordē,* gut, string]. A combining form meaning (a) *cord;* (b) *notochord.*

chor·da (kor′duh) *n.*, pl. & genit. sing. **chor·dae** (·dee) [L., from Gk. *chordē,* string]. 1. A cord, tendon, or nerve trunk. 2. The chorda dorsalis (= NOTOCHORD). —**chor·dal** (·dul), **chor·date** (·date) *adj.*

chor·da·blas·to·pore (kor″duh·blas′to·pore) *n.* [*chorda* + *blastopore*]. A term applied to the primitive pit to indicate its supposed homology to a blastopore.

chorda dor·sa·lis (dor·say′lis). NOTOCHORD.

chordae ten·di·ne·ae (ten·din′ee·ee) [NA]. TENDINOUS CORDS.

chordae Wil·li·sii (wil·is′ee·eye). Fibrous bands crossing through the dural sinuses.

chorda gu·ber·na·cu·lum (gew·bur·nack′yoo·lum). The part of the genital ligament that develops in the inguinal crest and adjacent body wall. It forms a part of the gubernaculum testis in the male, and a part of the round ligament of the uterus in the female.

chordal canal. NOTOCHORDAL CANAL.

chor·da·meso·blast (kor″duh·mez′o·blast, ·mee′so·blast) *n.* [*chorda* + *mesoblast*]. The middle germ layer before segregation into notochord and mesoblast.

chor·da·meso·derm (kor″duh·mez′o·durm, ·mee′so·durm) *n.* [*chorda* + *mesoderm*]. The embryonic area in a blastula or early gastrula destined to form the notochord and mesoderm. It occupies the region of the dorsal blastoporic lip and is thus the organizer.

chorda obli·qua mem·bra·nae in·ter·os·se·ae an·te·bra·chii (o·blye′kwuh mem·bray′nee in·tur·os′ee·ee an·tee·bray′kee·

ee) [NA]. An oblique cord of fibrous tissue passing from the tuberosity of the ulna to the tuberosity of the radius.

chorda saliva. Saliva produced by stimulation of the chorda tympani.

Chor·da·ta (kor·day'tuh, ·dah'tuh) *n.pl.* [NL., from *chorda*]. A phylum of the animal kingdom whose members are characterized by having at some stage in their development a notochord, a tubular central nervous system lying dorsal to the notochord, and lateral clefts in the walls of the pharynx.

chor·date (kor'date) *adj.* & *n.* [*chord-* + *-ate*]. 1. Possessing a notochord; belonging or pertaining to the phylum Chordata. 2. A member of the phylum Chordata.

chorda tym·pa·ni (tim'puh·nigh) [NA]. A nerve that originates from the facial nerve, traverses the tympanic cavity, and joins the lingual branch of the mandibular nerve. See also Table of Nerves in the Appendix and Plate 15.

chor·dee (kor·dee') *n.* [F. *cordée*, corded]. A curvature of the penis with concavity downward; an accompaniment of hypospadias, occasionally caused by scar tissue resulting from urethral infection or trauma. —**chor·de·ic** (·dee'ick) *adj.*

chordeic penis. CHORDEE.

chord·en·ceph·a·lon (kord''en·sef'uh·lon) *n.* [*chord-* + *encephalon*]. The portion of the central nervous system of vertebrates whose development is induced by the notochord; the mesencephalon, rhombencephalon, and spinal cord; it is segmental and divided into alar and basal plates.

chor·di·tis (kor·dye'tis) *n.* [*chord-* + *-itis*]. 1. Inflammation of a spermatic cord. 2. Inflammation of a vocal fold.

chorditis fi·bri·no·sa (figh''bri·no'suh). Acute laryngitis with deposition of fibrin on the vocal folds.

chorditis no·do·sa (no·do'suh). SINGER'S NODE.

chorditis tu·be·ro·sa (tew''be·ro'suh). SINGER'S NODE.

chordo-. See *chord-*.

chor·do·blas·to·ma (kor''do·blas·to'muh) *n.* [*chordo-* + *-blastoma*]. A malignant chordoma.

chor·do·car·ci·no·ma (kor''do·kahr''si·no'muh) *n.* [*chordo-* + *carcinoma*]. CHORDOMA.

chor·do·ep·i·the·li·o·ma (kor''do·ep''i·theel·ee·o'muh) *n.* [*chordo-* + *epithelioma*]. CHORDOMA.

chor·doid (kor'doid) *adj.* [*chord-* + *-oid*]. Resembling the notochord or notochordal tissue.

chordoid tumor. CHORDOMA.

chor·do·ma (kor·do'muh) *n.*, pl. **chordomas, chordoma·ta** (·tuh) [*chord-* + *-oma*]. A locally aggressive tumor composed of embryonal notochordal cells and large (physaliphorous) and small vacuolated cells. It occurs anywhere along the vertebral column, usually in the sacrococcygeal region or the base of the skull.

chor·dot·o·my (kor·dot'uh·mee) *n.* [*chordo-* + *-tomy*]. Surgical division of certain tracts of the spinal cord, e.g., the lateral spinothalamic tract for relief of pain.

cho·rea (ko·ree'uh) *n.* [Gk. *choreia*, dance]. 1. Widespread, arrhythmic, involuntary movements of a forcible, rapid, jerky type and of brief duration; seen in Sydenham's and Huntington's chorea.—**chore·al** (·ul), **chore·ic** (·ick), **cho·re·at·ic** (ko''ree·at'ick) *adj.*

chorea-athetosis-agitans syndrome. 1. Any extrapyramidal disorder. 2. HUNTINGTON'S CHOREA.

chorea grav·i·da·rum (grav·i·dair'um). Sydenham's chorea occurring during or aggravated by pregnancy.

chorea in·sa·ni·ens (in·say'nee·enz). *Obsol.* Delirious or hypomanic excitement occasionally observed in Sydenham's chorea.

chorea minor. SYDENHAM'S CHOREA.

choreic abasia. Inability to walk due to choreic spasm of muscles in the lower extremities.

cho·re·i·form (ko·ree'i·form) *adj.* Resembling chorea.

choreiform syndrome (of Prechtl) (prekh'tel). A form or component of the minimal brain dysfunction syndrome in children, manifested by jerky, ticlike twitching of the face, trunk, and extremities, readily inhibited when attention is called to it, as well as restless, uncontrolled behavior, and poor school performance.

cho·reo·ath·e·toid (ko''ree·o·ath'e·toid) *adj.* Pertaining to choreoathetosis.

cho·reo·ath·e·to·sis (ko''ree·o·ath''e·to'sis) *n.* A condition characterized by both choreiform and athetoid movements. See also *paroxysmal choreoathetosis.*

chori-, chorio-. A combining form meaning (a) *chorion;* (b) *choroid.*

cho·ri·al (ko'ree·ul) *adj.* CHORIONIC.

chorio-. See *chori-.*

cho·rio·ad·e·no·ma (ko''ree·o·ad·e·no'muh) *n.* [*chorio-* + *adenoma*]. A tumor intermediate in malignancy between hydatidiform mole and choriocarcinoma.

chorioadenoma des·tru·ens (des'troo·enz). CHORIOADENOMA.

cho·rio·al·lan·to·ic (ko''ree·o·al''an·to'ick) *adj.* Pertaining to the chorion and to the allantois or to the chorioallantois.

chorioallantoic graft. A graft of tissue onto the chorioallantoic membrane of the hen's egg, which furnishes a favorable environment for growth.

chorioallantoic membrane. In Sauropsida, a vascular extraembryonic membrane formed by fusion of the allantois and chorion.

cho·rio·al·lan·to·is (ko''ree·o·a·lan'to·is, ·a·lan'toice) *n.* [*chorio-* + *allantois*]. The membrane formed by the union of chorion and allantois in birds and certain mammals and vascularized by the allantoic blood vessels. That of chicks is used for the culture of viruses in the preparation of vaccines. Compare *placenta.*

cho·rio·am·ni·on·ic (ko''ree·o·am''nee·on'ick) *adj.* Pertaining to the chorion and the amnion.

cho·rio·am·nio·ni·tis (ko''ree·o·am''nee·o·nigh'tis) *n.* [*chorio-* + *amnion* + *-itis*]. Inflammation of the fetal membranes.

cho·rio·an·gi·o·ma (ko''ree·o·an·jee·o'muh) *n.* [*chorio-* + *angioma*]. The most common tumor of the placenta, composed of fetal blood vessels, connective tissue, and trophoblast; it is benign.

cho·rio·an·gi·op·a·gus (ko''ree·o·an''jee·op'uh·gus) *n.*, pl. **chorioangiopa·gi** (·guy, ·jye) [*chorio-* + *angio-* + *-pagus*]. 1. One of identical twins. 2. OMPHALOSITE.

chorioangiopagus pa·ra·sit·i·cus (păr''uh·sit'i·kus). A placental parasitic twin; OMPHALOSITE.

cho·rio·blas·to·sis (ko''ree·o·blas·to'sis) *n.*, pl. **chorioblasto·ses** (·seez) [*chorio-* + *blast-* + *-osis*]. Abnormal proliferation of cells of the chorion.

cho·rio·cap·il·la·ris (ko''ree·o·kap''i·lair'is) *n.* [*chorio-* + L. *capillaris*, from *capillus*, hair]. The network of capillaries over the inner portion of the choroid coat of the eye. —**chorio·cap·il·lary** (kap'i·lerr''ee) *adj.*

choriocapillary lamina or **layer.** The inner layer of the choroid, consisting of a capillary plexus. NA *lamina choroidocapillaris.*

cho·rio·car·ci·no·ma (ko''ree·o·kahr''si·no'muh) *n.* [*chorio-* + *carcinoma*]. A highly malignant tumor composed of cytotrophoblast and syncytial trophoblast, found most commonly in the uterus and testis, and more rarely in an ovary or other site.

cho·rio·cele (ko'ree·o·seel) *n.* [*chorio-* + *-cele*]. A hernial protrusion of the choroid coat of the eye.

cho·rio·ep·i·the·li·o·ma (ko''ree·o·ep''i·theel·ee·o'muh) *n.* [*chorio-* + *epithelioma*]. CHORIOCARCINOMA.

cho·rio·gen·e·sis (ko''ree·o·jen'e·sis) *n.*, pl. **choriogene·ses** (·seez) [*chorio-* + *genesis*]. The development of the chorion.

cho·ri·oid (ko'ree·oid) *adj.* & *n.* CHOROID.

cho·ri·oi·dea (ko''ree·oy'dee·uh) *n.* [BNA]. Choroidea (= CHOROID).

chorioid plexus. CHOROID PLEXUS.

cho·ri·o·ma (ko''ree·o'muh) *n.*, pl. **choriomas, chorioma·ta** (·tuh) [*chori-* + *-oma*]. 1. Any benign tumor of chorionic elements. 2. CHORIOCARCINOMA. See also *chorioadenoma, hydatidiform mole.*

cho·rio·men·in·gi·tis (ko''ree·o·men''in·jye'tis) *n.* [*chorio-* + *meningitis*]. LYMPHOCYTIC CHORIOMENINGITIS.

cho·ri·on (ko'ree·on) *n.* [Gk.]. The outermost of the fetal membranes, consisting of an outer trophoblastic epithelium lined internally by extraembryonic mesoderm. Its villous portion, vascularized by allantoic blood vessels, forms the fetal part of the placenta.

chorion al·lan·toi·de·um (al"an·toy'dee·um). ALLANTOCHORION.

chorion avil·lo·sum (av"i·lo'sum) [NL., non-villous]. CHORION LAEVE.

cho·ri·on·ep·i·the·li·o·ma (ko"ree·on·ep"i·theel·ee·o'muh) *n.* [*chorion* + *epithelioma*]. CHORIOCARCINOMA.

chorion fron·do·sum (fron·do'sum). 1. The villous part of the chorion which forms the fetal placenta. 2. The entire chorion until the third month of development, when the chorion laeve develops.

cho·ri·on·ic (ko"ree·on'ick) *adj.* Of or pertaining to the chorion.

chorionic carcinoma. *Rare.* CHORIOCARCINOMA.

chorionic circulation. UMBILICAL CIRCULATION.

chorionic cyst. An uncommon cyst of the placenta, arising in the chorionic plate, usually near the umbilical cord bulging toward the fetus. Histologically, it is lined by cells of trophoblastic origin.

chorionic gonadotropin. The water-soluble gonadotropic substance, originating in chorionic tissue, obtained from the urine of pregnant women. It is also secreted by choriocarcinomas.

chorionic gonadotropic hormone. CHORIONIC GONADOTROPIN.

chorionic plate. The chorionic membrane of the placental region, formed externally by the trophoblastic layer and internally by a fibrous lining layer of mesoderm.

chorionic vesicle. The gestation sac covered by chorionic villi and containing the embryo.

chorionic villus. A villus of the chorion or of the placenta.

cho·ri·o·ni·tis (kor"ee·o·nigh'tis) *n.* [*chorion* + *-itis*]. 1. Placental inflammation. 2. *Obsol.* SCLERODERMA.

chorion lae·ve (lee'vee) [L., smooth]. The smooth membranous part of the chorion devoid of prominent villi.

chorion om·pha·loi·de·um (om·fa·loy'dee·um). OMPHALOCHORION.

chorion vil·lo·sum (vi·lo'sum). CHORION FRONDOSUM.

cho·rio·ret·i·nal (ko"ree·o·ret'i·nul) *adj.* Pertaining to the choroid and retina.

cho·rio·ret·i·ni·tis (ko"ree·o·ret"i·nigh'tis) *n.* Inflammation of the choroid and retina.

cho·rio·ret·i·nop·a·thy (ko"ree·o·ret"i·nop'uth·ee) *n.* [*chorio-* + *retino-* + *-pathy*]. Disease involving both the choroid and retina.

chor·i·sis (kor'i·sis) *n.*, pl. **chori·ses** (·seez) [Gk. *chōrisis*, separation]. *In botany*, the splitting of an organ into parts, each of which forms a perfect organ.

chorist-, choristo- [Gk. *chōristos*, separable]. A combining form meaning *separated, misplaced.*

choristo-. See *chorist-*.

cho·ris·to·blas·to·ma (ko·ris"to·blas·to'muh) *n.* [*choristo-* + *blastoma*]. A true tumor originating in a choristoma.

cho·ris·to·ma (kor"i·sto'muh) *n.*, pl. **choristomas, choristoma·ta** (·tuh) [*chorist-* + *-oma*]. A benign tumor composed of elements foreign to the tissue where the tumor is found; it may arise through developmental displacement of tissue from one place to another, or from metaplasia; e.g., a mass of normal bone marrow cells in the adrenal gland.

cho·roid (kor'oid, ko'roid) *adj.* & *n.* [Gk. *choroeidēs (chorioeidēs) chitōn*, chorion-like tunic]. 1. Designating or pertaining to a delicate vascular membrane or structure. 2. The pigmented vascular tunic of the eye, continuous with the ciliary body anteriorly, and lying between the sclera and the retina; the choroid membrane. NA *choroidea.* See also Plate 19.

choroid-, choroido-. A combining form meaning *choroid.*

cho·roi·dal (ko·roy'dul) *adj.* Of or pertaining to the choroid.

choroidal hemorrhage. Bleeding of the vessels of the choroid of the eye; may be seen by ophthalmoscopic examination.

choroid artery. See Table of Arteries in the Appendix.

choroid coloboma. A developmental defect in the choroid of the eyeball, consisting of a persistent fissure, associated with decreased vision in the overlying retina; may also involve retinal pigment epithelium, retina, and sclera.

cho·roi·dea (ko·roy'dee·uh) *n.* [NA]. CHOROID (2).

cho·roid·e·re·mia (ko"roid·e·ree'mee·uh) *n.* [*choroid* + Gk. *erēmia*, absence]. Atrophy of the choroid; transmitted as an autosomal recessive trait.

choroid fissure. 1. The ventral fissure in the optic cup and the optic stalk of the embryo. 2. The line of invagination of the tela choroidea of the lateral ventricles of the brain. NA *fissura choroidea.*

cho·roid·itis (ko"roy·dye'tis) *n.* [*choroid* + *-itis*]. Inflammation of the choroid of the eye. See also *anterior choroiditis, central choroiditis, diffuse choroiditis, exudative choroiditis, metastatic choroiditis.*

choroiditis gut·ta·ta (guh·tay'tuh). Familial degeneration of the macula combined with characteristically grouped hyaline bodies. Syn. *Tay's choroiditis.*

choroid membrane or **coat.** CHOROID (2).

choroido-. See *choroid-*.

cho·roi·do·cy·cli·tis (ko·roy"do·sick·ligh'tis, ·sigh·kligh'tis) *n.* [*choroido-* + *cyclitis*]. Inflammation of the choroid and ciliary body.

cho·roi·do·iri·tis (ko·roy"do·eye·rye'tis, ·i·rye'tis) *n.* [*choroido-* + *iritis*]. Inflammation of the choroid and iris.

cho·roi·do·ret·i·ni·tis (ko·roy"do·ret"i·nigh'tis) *n.* [*choroido-* + *retinitis*]. CHORIORETINITIS.

choroid plexus. One of the longitudinal, lobulated, invaginated processes, consisting of a vascular plexus and a covering of ependyma, which project into each of the ventricles of the brain; specifically, the choroid plexus of the third ventricle (NA *plexus choroideus ventriculi tertii*), the choroid plexus of the fourth ventricle (NA *plexus choroideus ventriculi quarti*), or the choroid plexus of either lateral ventricle (NA *plexus choroideus ventriculi lateralis*).

cho·ro·ma·nia (kor"o·may'nee·uh) *n.* [Gk. *choros*, dance, + *mania*]. *Obsol.* 1. CHOREA INSANIENS. 2. SALTATORY SPASM.

choy, *n.* CHAY.

choya (choy'uh) *n.* CHAY.

chre·ma·to·pho·bia (kree"muh·to·fo'bee·uh) *n.* [Gk. *chrēmata*, money, + *phobia*]. Abnormal fear of money.

Chris·tel·ler method. A histochemical method for gold using stannous chloride to localize gold.

Chris·ten·sen-Krab·be disease [E. *Christensen* and K. H. *Krabbe*]. PROGRESSIVE CEREBRAL POLIODYSTROPHY.

Chris·tian disease or **syndrome** [H. A. *Christian*, U.S. physician, 1876–1951]. HAND-SCHÜLLER-CHRISTIAN DISEASE.

Christian Science. A religious sect and system of healing through prayer and the triumph of mind over matter.

Christian Science practitioner. One who practices the spiritual healing of illnesses according to the teachings of Mary Baker Eddy.

Christian-Weber disease [H. A. *Christian* and F. P. *Weber*]. WEBER-CHRISTIAN DISEASE.

Christ·mas disease [S. *Christmas*, English boy, 20th century, in whom the factor was first discovered]. A hemophilioid disease resulting from a hereditary deficiency of the procoagulant factor IX. Syn. *hemophilia B.*

Christmas factor [S. *Christmas*]. FACTOR IX.

-chroia [Gk. *chrōs*, color, + *-ia*]. A combining form meaning *coloration.*

chrom-, chromo- [Gk. *chrōma*]. A combining form meaning (a) *color, colored;* (b) *pigment, pigmented;* (c) *chromium.*

chromaesthesia. CHROMESTHESIA.

chro·maf·fin (kro'muh·fin, kro·maf'in) *adj.* [*chrom-* + L. *affinis*, having affinity for]. Describing or pertaining to the reaction of certain tissue constituents, as catecholamines and some other phenolic substances, in being oxidized to a yellow or brown compound on fixation with a dichromate. Certain cells of the adrenal medulla, of paraganglions, and of some other tissues react positively.

chromaffin bodies. Small chromaffin cell masses on either side of the abdominal aorta.

chromaffin cells. Cells of tissues, such as the adrenal medulla, that give a positive chromaffin reaction.

chro·maf·fino·blas·to·ma (kro·maf″in·o·blas·to′muh) *n.* [*chromaffin* + *blastoma*]. *Obsol.* PHEOCHROMOCYTOMA.

chro·maf·fi·no·ma (kro″muh·fi·no′muh, kro·maf″i·) *n.* [*chromaffin* + *-oma*]. PHEOCHROMOCYTOMA.

chro·maf·fi·nop·a·thy (kro·maf″i·nop′uth·ee) *n.* Any diseased or pathologic condition in chromaffin tissue, as in the adrenals or elsewhere.

chromaffin tumor. PHEOCHROMOCYTOMA.

Chromalbin. A trademark for chromated Cr 51 serum albumin.

chro·ma·phil (kro′muh·fil). *adj. & n.* CHROMOPHIL.

chro·ma·phobe (kro′muh·fobe). *adj. & n.* CHROMOPHOBE.

chro·ma·sia (kro·may′zhuh, ·zee·uh) *n.* Color effect produced by chromatic aberration in the functioning of lenses.

-chromasia [NL., from Gk. *chrōma,* color]. A combining form designating *a condition or property involving color or color perception.*

chromat-, chromato- [Gk. *chrōma, chrōmatos*]. A combining form meaning (a) *color;* (b) *pigment, pigmentation;* (c) *chromatin.*

chro·mate (kro′mate) *n.* [*chrom-* + *-ate*]. Any salt of chromic acid.

chromated Cr 51 serum albumin. Blood serum albumin labeled with radioactive chromium used for the detection and measurement of gastrointestinal protein loss or placental localization.

chro·ma·te·lop·sia (kro″mat·e·lop′see·uh) *n.* [*chrom-* + Gk. *atelēs,* imperfect, + *-opsia*]. COLOR BLINDNESS.

chro·ma·te·lop·sis (kro″mat·e·lop′sis) *n.* [*chrom-* + Gk. *atelēs,* imperfect, + *opsis,* sight]. COLOR BLINDNESS.

chromate method. A histochemical method for lead based on precipitation of yellow lead chromate.

chro·mat·ic (kro·mat′ick) *adj.* [Gk. *chrōmatikos*]. 1. Of or pertaining to color, especially to hue, or to hue and saturation together. 2. Readily stainable; pertaining to readily stainable constituents in cells.

chromatic aberration. Unequal refraction of different parts of the spectrum, producing indistinct images surrounded by a halo of colors.

chromatic audition. The induction of subjective color sensations by certain sounds, such as yellow by "u" sounds. See also *chromesthesia.*

chromatic dispersion. *In physics,* splitting of a beam of white light into different wavelengths or frequencies, and consequently into different colors.

chromatic figure. The chromosomes or the pattern formed by the chromosomes in meiosis or mitosis.

chro·mat·ic·ness, *n.* A characteristic of color consisting of hue and saturation taken together; the quality of color rather than its intensity.

chromatic vision. Vision pertaining to the color sense.

chro·ma·tid (kro′muh·tid) *n.* [*chromat-* + *-id*]. One of the two bodies, sister chromosomes, resulting from the longitudinal splitting of a chromosome, in preparation for mitosis; especially, one of the four parts of a tetrad, formed by the longitudinal splitting of synaptic mates, in preparation for meiosis.

chro·ma·tin (kro′muh·tin) *n.* [*chromat-* + *-in*]. The chromosomal DNA-containing material in a nucleus that readily stains with nuclear stains, as in the Feulgen reaction.

chromatin bodies. CHROMOSOMES.

chromatin-negative, *adj.* Lacking a sex chromatin body, as in gonial cells in both sexes and in somatic cells of individuals with only one X chromosome.

chromatin-positive, *adj.* Possessing a sex chromatin body in the nucleus of somatic cells, and therefore having more than one X chromosome, as in the normal female type and in the Klinefelter syndrome.

chromatin reticulum. Diffuse appearance of chromonemal precursor substance as seen during interphase.

chro·ma·tism (kro′muh·tiz·um) *n.* [*chromat-* + *-ism*]. 1. A hallucination in which colored lights are seen. 2. Abnormal pigment deposits.

chromato-. See *chromat-.*

chro·ma·to·der·ma·to·sis (kro″muh·to·dur″muh·to′sis) *n.*, pl. **chromatodermato·ses** (·seez) [*chromato-* + *dermatosis*]. Any condition of the skin marked by a lasting change of color.

chro·ma·to·dys·o·pia (kro″muh·to·dis·o′pee·uh) *n.* [*chromato-* + *dys-* + *-opia*]. COLOR BLINDNESS.

chro·ma·tog·e·nous (kro″muh·toj′e·nus) *adj.* [*chromato-* + *-genous*]. Producing color.

chro·mato·gram (kro·mat′o·gram, kro′muh·to·) *n.* [*chromato-* + *-gram*]. *In chromatography,* the porous solid matrix (column, paper, thin layer) after the separation procedure has been applied and the matrix treated with a suitable developing agent to indicate the location of the separated components of the mixture submitted to chromatographic treatment.

chromatographic analysis. Separation of chemical constituents by any procedure of chromatography.

chro·ma·tog·ra·phy (kro″muh·tog′ruh·fee) *n.* [*chromato-* + *-graphy*]. The procedure by which a mixture of substances is separated by fractional extraction or adsorption or ion exchange on a porous solid (as a column of aluminum oxide, or cellulose) by means of one or more flowing liquid or gaseous solvents, especially by the process of partition chromatography. The principal types of chromatography are: column, gas, paper, liquid, and thin-layer. —**chro·mato·graph** (kro·mat′o·graf, kro′muh·to·) *v.;* **chro·mato·graph·ic** (kro·mat″o·graf′ick, kro″muh·to·) *adj.*

chro·ma·toid (kro′muh·toid) *adj.* [*chromat-* + *-oid*]. Pertaining to or resembling chromatin.

chromatoid bodies. Hematoxylin-staining spicules and irregular masses, having a negative Feulgen reaction, found in amebic cysts.

chro·ma·tol·o·gy (kro″muh·tol′uh·jee) *n.* [*chromato-* + *-logy*]. The science of colors.

chro·ma·tol·y·sis (kro″muh·tol′i·sis) *n.*, pl. **chromatoly·ses** (·seez) [*chromato-* + *-lysis*]. Dissolution of the cytoplasmic Nissl substance of the body of a neuron; usually occurs as part of the axonal reaction.—**chroma·to·lyt·ic** (·to·lit′ick) *adj.*

chro·ma·to·mere (kro·mat′o·meer, kro′muh·to·) *n.* [*chromato-* + *-mere*]. The part or parts of a platelet colored brightly with stains of the Romanovsky type.

chro·ma·tom·e·ter (kro″muh·tom′e·tur) *n.* [*chromato-* + *-meter*]. 1. An instrument for measuring intensity of color. 2. A chart of colors arranged in a way that allows it to be used as a color scale.

chro·ma·tom·e·try (kro″muh·tom′e·tree) *n.* [*chromato-* + *-metry*]. The measurement of degree of color or of color perception.

chro·ma·to·path·ia (kro″muh·to·path′ee·uh) *n.* CHROMATOPATHY.

chro·ma·top·a·thy (kro″muh·top′uth·ee) *n.* [*chromato-* + *-pathy*]. Any abnormality of color of skin.

chro·ma·to·phane (kro·mat′o·fane, kro′muh·to·) *n.* [*chromato-* + *-phane*]. Highly colored oil droplets in the visual cells of certain animals, as in birds.

chro·ma·to·phil (kro′muh·to·fil, kro·mat″o·) *adj. & n.* CHROMOPHIL.

chro·ma·to·phil·ia (kro″muh·to·fil′ee·uh) *n.* [*chromato-* + *-philia*]. An affinity for stains.

chro·ma·to·pho·bia (kro″muh·to·fo′bee·uh) *n.* CHROMOPHOBIA.

chro·ma·to·phore (kro·mat′o·fore, kro′muh·to·) *n.* [*chromato-* + *-phore*]. 1. *In botany,* a colored plastid. 2. *In zoology,* a pigmented, branched connective-tissue cell.

chro·ma·to·phor·ic (kro″muh·to·for′ick) *adj.* [*chromato-* + *-phoric*]. Of or pertaining to a chromatophore.

chro·ma·to·phor·o·ma (kro″muh·to·fo·ro′muh) *n. Rare.* [*chromato-* + *-phor* + *-oma*]. MELANOMA.

chro·ma·to·phoro·troph·ic (kro″muh·to·for″o·trof′ick) *adj. Erron.* CHROMATOPHOROTROPIC.

chro·ma·to·phoro·tro·pic (kro″muh·to·for″o·tro′pick, trop′ick) *adj.* [*chromatophore* + *-tropic*]. Influencing or affecting chromatophores.

chromatophorotropic hormone. INTERMEDIN.

chro·ma·toph·o·rous (kro″muh·tof′o·rus) *adj.* [*chromato-* + *-phorous*]. 1. Containing pigment or pigment cells. 2. CHROMATOPHORIC.

chro·ma·to·plasm (kro·mat′o·plaz·um, kro′muh·to·) *n.* The substance of the chromatophores as distinguished from the other cell substances, such as nucleoplasm, cytoplasm, metaplasm.

chro·ma·to·plast (kro·mat′o·plast, kro′muh·to·) *n.* [*chromato-* + *-plast*]. CHROMATOPHORE.

chro·ma·to·pseu·dop·sis (kro″muh·to·sue·dop′sis) *n.* [*chromato-* + *pseud-* + Gk. *opsis*, sight]. COLOR BLINDNESS.

chro·ma·top·sia (kro″muh·top′see·uh) *n.* [*chromat-* + *-opsia*]. A disorder of visual sensation in which color impressions are disturbed or arise subjectively, with objects appearing colored unnaturally or colorless objects as colored; may be due to disturbance of the optic centers, to psychic disturbances, or to drugs.

chro·ma·top·sy (kro′muh·top″see) *n.* CHROMATOPSIA.

chro·mat·op·tom·e·ter (kro″muh·top·tom′e·tur) *n.* CHROMOPTOMETER.

chro·mat·op·tom·e·try (kro″muh·top·tom′e·tree) *n.* CHROMOPTOMETRY.

chro·ma·to·sis (kro″muh·to′sis) *n.*, pl. **chromato·ses** (·seez) [*chromat-* + *-osis*]. 1. PIGMENTATION. 2. A pathologic process or pigmentary disease characterized by a deposit of coloring matter in a locality where it is usually not present, or in excessive quantity in regions where pigment normally exists.

chro·ma·tu·ria (kro″muh·tew′ree·uh) *n.* [*chromat-* + *-uria*]. Abnormal coloration of the urine.

-chrome [Gk. *chrōma*, color]. A combining form meaning *colored.*

chrome (krome) *n.* [Gk. *chrōma*, color]. Chromium or one of its ores or compounds.

chrome alum. Chromium potassium sulfate, $CrK(SO_4)_2.12H_2O$.

chrome alum, ammonium. Chromium ammonium sulfate, $CrNH_4(SO_4)_2.12H_2O$.

chrome green. 1. Chromic oxide, Cr_2O_3, a green pigment. 2. A mixture of chrome yellow and Prussian blue.

chrome hematoxylin. A stain for lipofuscins, containing equal parts of 1% aqueous hematoxylin and 2% aqueous chrome alum.

1,2-chro·mene (-kro′meen) *n.* 1,2-Benzopyran, the parent substance of many plant pigments.

chrom·es·the·sia, chrom·aes·the·sia (kro″mes·theezh′uh, ·theez′ee·uh) *n.* [*chrom-* + *esthesia*]. The association or perception of colors together with the sensation of hearing, especially of certain words, and of smell, taste, or touch.

chrome ulcer. An ulcer due to the action of chrome salts; seen in tanners and others who work with chromium.

chrome yellow. LEAD CHROMATE.

chrom·het·ero·tro·pia (krome·het″ur·o·tro′pee·uh) *n.* [*chrom-* + *heterotropia*]. HETEROCHROMIA.

chrom·hi·dro·sis (krome″hi·dro′sis, ·high·dro′sis) *n.* [*chrom-* + *hidrosis*]. The secretion of colored sweat.

-chromia [*chrom-* + *-ia*]. A combining form designating (a) *a state of pigmentation;* (b) *a state involving color perception.*

chro·mic (kro′mick) *adj.* [*chrom-* + *-ic*]. 1. Of or pertaining to chromium. 2. Designating compounds containing the trivalent form of chromium.

chromic acid. CHROMIUM TRIOXIDE.

chromic anhydride. CHROMIUM TRIOXIDE.

chro·mi·cize (kro′mi·size) *v.* To impregnate or treat with chromic acid or a chromium salt.

chromic trioxide. CHROMIUM TRIOXIDE.

chro·mid·i·al (kro·mid′ee·ul) *adj.* Of or pertaining to chromidia.

chromidial substance. CHROMOPHIL SUBSTANCE.

chro·mid·i·um (kro·mid′ee·um) *n.*, pl. **chromid·ia** (·ee·uh). One of the chromatic substances found in the cytoplasm.

chro·mi·dro·sis (kro″mi·dro′sis) *n.* CHROMHIDROSIS.

Chromitope sodium. A trademark for sodium chromate Cr 51 injection.

chro·mi·um (kro′mee·um) *n.* [NL., from *chrome*]. Cr = 51.996. A hard, bright, silvery metal; largely used as a protective plating for other metals and in the manufacture of alloys characterized by strength and resistance to corrosion. It forms chromous and chromic salts.

chromium release test. A method of assessing the ability in vitro of antiserum or cells to lyse target cells, which are labeled with radioactive ^{51}Cr; release of ^{51}Cr after addition of serum or cells is taken as a measure of their cytotoxicity.

chromium trioxide. Dark, purplish-red crystals, CrO_3, very soluble in water. Used as an astringent, caustic, and germicide. Syn. *chromic acid.*

chromo-. See *chrom-.*

Chro·mo·bac·te·ri·um (kro″mo·back·teer′ee·um) *n.* [*chromo-* + *bacterium*]. A genus of nonpathogenic bacteria of the Rhizobiaceae including aerobic forms which produce a violet, chromoparic pigment, soluble in alcohol but not in chloroform.

chro·mo·blast (kro′mo·blast) *n.* [*chromo-* + *-blast*]. CHROMATOPHORE.

chro·mo·blas·to·my·co·sis (kro″mo·blas″to·migh·ko′sis) *n.*, pl. **chromoblastomyco·ses** (·seez) [*chromo-* + *blastomycosis*]. An infection of the skin characterized principally by the development of verrucous lesions, caused by various fungi, including *Hormodendrum pedrosoi, H. compactum, H. dermatitidis, Cladosporium carrionii,* and *Phialophora verrucosa.*

chro·mo·cen·ter (kro′mo·sen″tur) *n.* [*chromo-* + *center*]. 1. A structural peculiarity of the salivary gland chromosomes in *Drosophila;* the fused mass of heterochromatin of all the chromosomes with six armlike extensions of euchromatin. 2. An irregular mass of chromatin, often confused with a nucleolus because of similarity in staining properties.

chro·mo·crin·ia (kro·mo·krin′ee·uh) *n.* [*chromo-* + Gk. *krinein*, to separate, + *-ia*]. The secretion or excretion of colored material.

chro·mo·cys·tos·co·py (kro″mo·sis·tos′kuh·pee) *n.* [*chromo-* + *cystoscopy*]. Cystoscopy and inspection of the orifices of the ureters after the administration of a substance that will stain the urine.

chro·mo·cyte (kro′mo·site) *n.* [*chromo-* + *-cyte*]. Any colored cell.

chro·mo·dac·ry·or·rhea, chro·mo·dac·ry·or·rhoea (kro″mo·dack″ree·o·ree′uh) *n.* [*chromo-* + *dacryo-* + *-rrhea*]. The flow of colored tears from the Harderian glands in rats. This oily, thick secretion contains large amounts of porphyria resulting in "blood-caked whiskers."

chro·mo·der·ma·to·sis (kro″mo·dur″muh·to′sis) *n.* CHROMATODERMATOSIS.

chro·mo·gen (kro′mo·jen) *n.* [*chromo-* + *-gen*]. Any substance which, under suitable conditions, is capable of producing color. See also *chromophore.*

chro·mo·gen·e·sis (kro″mo·jen′e·sis) *n.* [*chromo-* + *-genesis*]. The production of pigments or coloring matter, as by bacterial action. —**chromogen·ic** (·ick) *adj.*

chro·mo·lip·id (kro″mo·lip′id) *n.* LIPOCHROME.

chro·mo·lip·oid (kro″mo·lip′oid) *n.* [*chromo-* + *lipoid*]. LIPOCHROME.

chro·mo·mere (kro′mo·meer) *n.* [*chromo-* + *-mere*]. 1. One of the beadlike chromatin granules arranged in a linear series in a chromosome. 2. CHROMATOMERE.

chro·mom·e·try (kro·mom'e·tree) *n.* CHROMATOMETRY.

chro·mo·my·co·sis (kro''mo·migh·ko'sis) *n.*, pl. **chromomycoses** (·seez) [*chromo-* + *mycosis*]. CHROMOBLASTOMYCOSIS.

chro·mo·nar (kro'mo·nahr) *n.* Ethyl [[3-[2-(diethylamino)-ethyl]-4-methyl-2-oxo-2*H*-1-benzopyran-7-yl]oxy]acetate, $C_{20}H_{27}NO_5$, a coronary vasodilator; used as the hydrochloride salt.

chro·mo·ne·ma (kro''mo·nee'muh) *n.*, pl. **chromonema·ta** (·tuh) [*chromo-* + *-nema*]. A longitudinal subdivision of a chromosome. —**chromone·mal** (·mul) *adj.*

chro·mo·nu·cle·ic acid (kro''mo·new·klee'ick). DEOXYRIBONUCLEIC ACID.

chrom·onych·ia (kro''mo·nick'ee·uh) *n.* [*chrom-* + *onych-* + *-ia*]. Abnormal coloration of a nail or nails.

chro·mo·par·ic (kro''mo·păr'ick) *adj.* [*chromo-* + L. *parere*, to produce, + *-ic*]. Concerning excretion of pigment formed within cells into the surrounding medium.

chro·mop·a·rous (kro·mop'uh·rus) *adj.* [*chromo-* + *-parous*]. CHROMOPARIC.

chro·mo·pexy (kro'mo·peck''see) *n.* [*chromo-* + *-pexy*]. A type of ultraphagocytosis in which the absorbed colloid is a chromogen.—**chro·mo·pec·tic** (kro''mo·peck'tick) *adj.*

chro·mo·phane (kro'mo·fane) *n.* CHROMATOPHANE.

chro·mo·phil (kro'mo·fil) *adj.* & *n.* [*chromo-* + *-phil*]. 1. Taking a deep stain. 2. A cell that takes a deep stain. —**chro·mo·phil·ic** (kro''mo·fil'ick), **chro·moph·i·lous** (kro·mof'i·lus) *adj.*

chromophil cells. The alpha and beta cells of the adenohypophysis.

chro·mo·phile (kro'mo·file, ·fil) *n.* & *adj.* CHROMOPHIL.

chromophil granules. Small basophilic granules in nerve cells. Syn. *Nissl bodies.*

chromophil substance. A nucleoprotein in the cytoplasm of many cells staining deeply with basic dyes. Syn. *chromidial substance.*

chromophil tumor. PHEOCHROMOCYTOMA.

chro·mo·phobe (kro'mo·fobe) *adj.* & *n.* [*chromo-* + *-phobe*]. 1. Not staining easily. 2. A cell that does not stain easily. 3. Specifically, CHROMOPHOBE CELL.

chromophobe adenoma or **tumor.** An adenoma of the adenohypophysis made up of chromophobe cells, neither basophilic nor acidophilic.

chromophobe cell. One of the faintly staining cells of the adenohypophysis, thought to give rise to alpha cells and beta cells.

chro·mo·pho·bia (kro''mo·fo'bee·uh) *n.* [*chromo-* + *phobia*]. 1. Abnormal fear or dislike of colors or of certain colors. 2. *In histology,* staining little or not at all, said of intracellular granules or of certain cells.

chro·mo·pho·bic (kro''mo·fo'bick) *adj.* [*chromo-* + *phobic*]. Not stainable; not readily absorbing color.

chro·mo·phore (kro'mo·fore) *n.* [*chromo-* + *-phore*]. 1. An atom or group of atoms or electrons in a molecule which is chiefly responsible for a spectral absorption band. 2. CHROMATOPHORE.

chro·mo·phor·ic (kro''mo·for'ick) *adj.* [*chromo-* + *-phoric*]. 1. Pertaining to cells, such as bacteria or hemoglobin, which produce pigments and retain them within the cell. 2. Of or pertaining to a chromophore.

chro·moph·o·rous (kro·mof'uh·rus) *adj.* [*chromo-* + *-phorous*]. CHROMOPHORIC.

chro·mo·phose (kro'mo·foze) *n.* [*chromo-* + Gk. *phōs*, light]. A subjective sensation of a spot of color in the eye.

chro·mo·phy·to·sis (kro''mo·figh·to'sis) *n.* [*chromo-* + *phytosis*]. TINEA VERSICOLOR.

chro·mo·plasm (kro'mo·plaz·um) *n.* [*chromo-* + *plasm*]. The network of a nucleus which is easily stained.

chro·mo·plast (kro'mo·plast) *n.* [*chromo-* + *-plast*]. 1. Any cell bearing pigment, as in the choroid of the eye or in the skin. 2. *In protozoology,* certain colored plastids. Compare *chloroplast.*

chro·mo·plas·tid (kro''mo·plas'tid) *n.* CHROMOPLAST.

chro·mo·pro·tein (kro''mo·pro'tee·in) *n.* Any protein containing a chromophoric group, such as hematin.

chro·mop·sia (kro·mop'see·uh) *n.* CHROMATOPSIA.

chrom·op·tom·e·ter (kro''mop·tom'e·tur) *n.* [*chrom-* + *optometer*]. An instrument for determining the extent of development of color vision. —**chromoptome·try** (·tree) *n.*

chro·mos·co·py (kro·mos'kuh·pee) *n.* [*chromo-* + *-scopy*]. The determination of the color of objects.

chromosomal aberration. A variation from the normal in structure or number of the chromosomes for a given species.

chro·mo·some (kro'muh·sohm) *n.* [*chromo-* + *-some*]. Any one of the separate, deeply staining bodies, commonly rod-, J- (or L-), or V-shaped, which arise from the nuclear network during mitosis and meiosis. They carry the hereditary factors (genes), and are present in constant number in each species. In man, there are 46 in each cell, except in the mature ovum and sperm where the number is halved. A complete set of 23 is inherited from each parent. —**chro·mo·so·mal** (kro''muh·so'mul) *adj.*

chromosome coil. A spiral formed between two or more chromonemata.

chromosome complement. The normal diploid chromosome set of the somatic cells of a species.

chromosome mapping. The process of locating genes on chromosomes. See also *cytologic mapping, genetic mapping.*

chromosome puff. Chromatic material accumulating at a restricted site on a chromosome, especially in dipteran salivary gland cells, thought to reflect functional activity of the gene at that site during differentiation.

chro·mo·tricho·my·co·sis (kro''mo·trick''o·migh·ko'sis) *n.* [*chromo-* + *trichomycosis*]. TRICHOMYCOSIS AXILLARIS.

chro·mo·trope (kro'mo·trope) *n.* [*chromo-* + *-trope*]. 1. A tissue component that stains metachromatically when treated with a metachromatic dye. 2. Any of several dyes, differentiated by numerical suffixes.

chro·mous (kro'mus) *adj.* [*chrom-* + *-ous*]. Designating compounds containing the bivalent form of chromium.

chron-, chrono- [Gk. *chronos*]. A combining form meaning *time.*

chro·nax·ie, chro·naxy (kro'nack·see) *n.* [Gk. *chronos*, time, + *axia*, value]. The duration of time that a current of twice the rheobasic (galvanic threshold) intensity must flow in order to excite the tissue being tested. Chronaxie is related to irritability and is used in testing for irritability changes in nerve and muscle.

chro·nax·im·e·ter (kro''nack·sim'e·tur) *n.* A device for measuring chronaxie.

chron·ic (kron'ick) *adj.* [L. *chronicus*, from Gk. *chronikos*, temporal]. Long-continued; of long duration or frequent recurrence. Contr. *acute, subacute.* —**chro·nic·i·ty** (kro·nis'i·tee) *n.*

chronic abscess. A persistent abscess, usually occurring in the musculoskeletal system.

chronic acholuric jaundice. HEREDITARY SPHEROCYTOSIS.

chronic adhesive arachnoiditis. Local or generalized thickening of the arachnoid due to inflammation from infection, noxious agents, hemorrhage, trauma, or congenital anomalies. Commonly involved are the spinal cord, posterior fossa around the cerebellum, and the optic chiasma. Symptoms and signs vary with the site and extent of the adhesions.

chronic alcoholism. 1. Chronic excessive use of alcoholic drinks such as to interfere with the drinker's health, interpersonal relations, or means of livelihood. 2. Addiction to alcohol. 3. Medical and psychiatric diseases caused by chronic excessive use of alcohol.

chronic anal ulcer triad. Hypertrophied anal papillae, anal ulcer, and sentinel pile.

chronic anterior poliomyelitis. *Obsol.* PROGRESSIVE SPINAL MUSCULAR ATROPHY.

chronic appendicitis. Recurring attacks of right-sided abdominal pain without definite signs and symptoms of acute appendicitis. The appendix when removed may show little or no pathologic change.

chronic aseptic meningitis. Chronic nonbacterial meningitis of unknown cause. See also *Mollaret's meningitis.*

chronic brain syndrome. *In psychiatry,* any chronic cerebral disorder presumed to have a structural basis. See also *organic brain syndrome.*

chronic bronchitis. A clinical disorder characterized by excessive mucous secretion in the bronchial tree and manifested by chronic productive cough.

chronic cardiac compression. CONSTRICTIVE PERICARDITIS.

chronic carrier. One who harbors an infectious organism for a prolonged period, but presents no symptoms of disease.

chronic catarrhal enteritis. Enteritis due to passive hyperemia in which the mucosa is thickened and covered by mucus and, in cases of long standing, is associated with atrophy.

chronic catarrhal laryngitis. The most common form of laryngitis, consisting of a hypertrophic and an atrophic stage; characterized by hoarseness, pain, dryness of the throat, dysphagia, and cough.

chronic congestive splenomegaly. A syndrome characterized by portal hypertension, splenomegaly, gastrointestinal hemorrhage, leukopenia, anemia, and thrombocytopenia.

chronic conjunctivitis. Prolonged inflammation of the conjunctiva usually with follicular or pupillary hyperplasia.

chronic cystic mastitis. CYSTIC DISEASE OF THE BREAST.

chronic dental fluorosis. Hypoplasia and discoloration of the teeth, resulting from the continued use, during the formative period of the tooth, of water containing large amounts of fluorine. Syn. *mottled enamel.*

chronic desquamative gingivitis. A chronic, basically degenerative, condition of the gingivae characterized by a diffuse atrophy of the epithelium.

chronic discoid lupus erythematosus. A chronic skin disease characterized by well-defined erythematous patches, often resulting in scarring, chiefly on the areas of the face where flushing commonly occurs; systemic symptoms are absent and the LE test is negative.

chronic endemic dental fluorosis. CHRONIC DENTAL FLUOROSIS.

chronic familial granulomatosis. CHRONIC GRANULOMATOUS DISEASE.

chronic familial icterus or **jaundice.** HEREDITARY SPHEROCYTOSIS.

chronic fibroid tuberculosis. Slowly progressive pulmonary tuberculosis with extensive fibrosis and mild symptoms.

chronic glandular cystitis. Chronic inflammation of the urinary bladder characterized by papillary or bleb-like projections on the vesical mucosa, chiefly in the region of the trigone; similar to cystitis cystica.

chronic glomerulonephritis. Glomerulonephritis characterized clinically by variable duration and progressive renal insufficiency. Pathologically there is progressive interstitial fibrosis with chronic inflammatory cells, tubular atrophy, and glomerulosclerosis. Syn. *Bright's disease.*

chronic granulomatous disease. A disorder, thought to be X-linked, in which phagocytic ingestion of bacteria is normal but bactericidal action is impaired; characterized by lymphadenopathy, hepatosplenomegaly, rash, pneumonia, anemia, leukocytosis, and hypergammaglobulinemia. Abbreviated, CGD.

chronic hemorrhagic osteomyelitis. GIANT-CELL TUMOR (1).

chronic hyperplastic perihepatitis. POLYSEROSITIS.

chronic hypochromic anemia. IRON-DEFICIENCY ANEMIA.

chronic idiopathic jaundice. *Obsol.* DUBIN-JOHNSON SYNDROME.

chronic idiopathic steatorrhea. Longstanding malabsorption for which no etiology is found.

chronic infantile lobar sclerosis. PELIZAEUS-MERZBACHER DISEASE.

chronic infectious arthritis. RHEUMATOID ARTHRITIS.

chronic infectious neuropathic agent. Any one of the transmissible agents, usually viral, that produces latent, chronic, or slow infection of the central nervous system. Acronym, CHINA. See also *slow infection.*

chronic intermittent juvenile jaundice. *Obsol.* GILBERT'S SYNDROME.

chronic interstitial hepatitis. *Obsol.* LAENNEC'S CIRRHOSIS.

chronic interstitial pancreatitis of infancy. CYSTIC FIBROSIS OF THE PANCREAS.

chronic intussusception. Intussusception occurring gradually without acute symptoms.

chronic leukemia. A form of leukemia in which the expected duration of life is 1 to 20 years or more. The cell types are usually the more mature forms of the specific blood series (granulocytic, lymphocytic, or monocytic). The onset is usually insidious, with few early symptoms.

chronic mountain sickness. Monge's disease. See *altitude sickness.*

chronic murine pneumonia. A widespread lung disease of rats, of uncertain etiology but thought to be due to *Mycoplasma pulmonis* and a virus.

chronic nonleukemic myelosis. A myeloproliferative disorder.

chronic organic brain disorder. CHRONIC BRAIN SYNDROME.

chronic parenchymatous salpingitis. Chronic interstitial inflammation and thickening of the muscular coat of the uterine tube.

chronic pharyngitis. A form of pharyngitis that is generally the result of repeated acute attacks and is associated with hypertrophic pharyngitis or atrophic pharyngitis.

chronic polyarthritis. RHEUMATOID ARTHRITIS.

chronic progressive hereditary chorea. HUNTINGTON'S CHOREA.

chronic progressive nonhereditary chorea. SENILE CHOREA.

chronic proximal spinal muscular atrophy. WOHLFART-KUGELBERG-WELANDER DISEASE.

chronic pseudomembranous bronchitis. Chronic bronchial inflammation with formation of a pseudomembrane.

chronic pulmonary emphysema. EMPHYSEMA (1).

chronic renal failure. Progressive renal insufficiency and uremia, due to irreversible and progressive renal, glomerular, tubular, or interstitial disease.

chronic rhinitis. Rhinitis usually due to repeated attacks of acute rhinitis, producing in the early stages hypertrophic rhinitis and in the later stages atrophic rhinitis, and the presence of dark, offensive-smelling crusts (ozena).

chronic sclerosing osteomyelitis. GARRÉ'S OSTEOMYELITIS.

chronic serous arachnoiditis. CHRONIC ADHESIVE ARACHNOIDITIS.

chronic serous synovitis. HYDRARTHROSIS.

chronic serpiginous ulcer. MOOREN'S ULCER.

chronic simple glaucoma. OPEN-ANGLE GLAUCOMA.

chronic spinal muscular atrophy. PROGRESSIVE SPINAL MUSCULAR ATROPHY.

chronic superficial glossitis. MOELLER'S GLOSSITIS.

chronic traumatic encephalopathy. PUNCH-DRUNK STATE.

chronic tuberculosis. Tuberculosis resulting from progression of the primary lesion or reactivation of previously dormant foci, and rarely from exogenous reinfection. Syn. *adult-type tuberculosis.*

chronic vegetating salpingitis. Excessive hypertrophy of the mucosa of the uterine tube.

chronic X-linked granulomatosis. CHRONIC GRANULOMATOUS DISEASE.

chrono-. See *chron-.*

chrono·graph (kron'o·graf) *n.* [*chrono-* + *-graph*]. An instrument for recording small intervals of time in physiologic and psychophysical experiments.

chron·o·log·ic (kron"uh·loj'ick) *adj.* [*chrono-* + *log-* + *-ic*]. 1. Arranged in time sequence. 2. Reckoned in terms of dates (years, months, days).

chron·o·log·i·cal (kron"uh·loj'i·kul) *adj.* CHRONOLOGIC.

chronological age. The actual time elapsed since the birth of a living individual, as distinguished from anatomic, physiologic, developmental, or mental age. Abbreviated, CA.

chro·nom·e·try (kro·nom'e·tree) *n.* [*chrono-* + *-metry*]. The measuring of time.

chrono·pho·bia (kron''o·fo'bee·uh) *n.* [*chrono-* + *phobia*]. An abnormal fear of time.

chrono·scope (kron'uh·skope) *n.* [*chrono-* + *-scope*]. An instrument for measuring short intervals of time.

chrono·tro·pic (kron''o·trop'ick, tro'pick) *adj.* [*chrono-* + *-tropic*]. Having an effect on or influencing the cardiac rate.

chrys-, chryso- [Gk. *chrysos*, gold]. A combining form meaning *gold, golden yellow*, or *yellow*.

chrys·a·lis (kris'uh·lis) *n.*, pl. **chry·sal·i·des** (kri·sal'uh·deez) [L. *chrysallis*, gold-colored pupa of butterflies]. The pupa of an insect, especially during the stage in which it is enclosed in a cocoon.

chrys·a·ro·bin (kris''uh·ro'bin) *n.* [*chrys-* + ar*aroba* + *-in*]. A substance obtained from Goa powder, deposited in the wood of *Andira araroba*, a Brazilian tree. It is a brown to orange-yellow powder; chemically, it is largely a complex mixture of reduction products of chrysophanic acid, emodin, and the methyl ether of the latter. Used in the treatment of skin diseases.

chrys·a·zin (kris'uh·zin) *n.* DANTHRON.

chry·si·a·sis (kri·sigh'uh·sis) *n.*, pl. **chrysia·ses** (·seez) [*chrys-* + *-iasis*]. A permanent pigmentation of the skin caused by the parenteral use of gold preparations; may be reticular in type, but is usually patchy; exaggerated by exposure to sunlight.

chryso-. See *chrys-*.

chryso·cy·a·no·sis (kris''o·sigh''uh·no'sis) *n.*, pl. **chrysocyano·ses** (·seez) [*chryso-* + *cyanosis*]. A bluish discoloration of the skin caused by intracutaneous deposition of some gold salts.

chryso·der·ma (kris''o·dur'muh) *n.* [*chryso-* + *derma*]. CHRYSIASIS.

Chryso·my·ia (kris''o·migh'yuh) *n.* [*chryso-* + *-myia*]. A genus of blowflies.

Chrysomyia bez·zia·na (bez·ee·ay'nuh). A species of fly which produces wound myiasis; found in Africa, parts of Asia, Australia, and the Philippines.

chrys·o·phan (kris'o·fan) *n.* A glycoside, $C_{16}H_{18}O_8$, found in rhubarb.

chrys·o·phan·ic acid (kris''o·fan'ick). CHRYSOPHANOL.

chry·soph·a·nol (kri·sof'uh·nol) *n.* 1,8-Dihydroxy-3-methylanthraquinone, $C_{15}H_{10}O_4$, a constituent of rhubarb, aloes, cascara, of species of *Rhamnus*, and of chrysarobin.

Chry·sops (krye'sops) *n.* [Gk. *chrysōps*, gold-colored]. A genus of small tabanid, biting flies, abundant in temperate and tropical America and Africa; certain species transmit diseases to man and animals. *Chrysops discalis*, the western deer fly, transfers *Pasteurella tularensis*, which causes tularemia. *C. silacea* and *C. dimidiata* are intermediate hosts of *Loa loa*.

chryso·ther·a·py (kris''o·therr'uh·pee) *n.* [*chryso-* + *therapy*]. The use of gold compounds in the treatment of disease.

chthono·pha·gia (thon''o·fay'juh, ·jee·uh) *n.* [Gk. *chthōn*, earth, + *-phagia*]. GEOPHAGY.

chtho·noph·a·gy (tho·nof'uh·jee) *n.* GEOPHAGY.

Church·ill-Cope reflex [E. D. *Churchill*, U.S. surgeon, b. 1895; and O. J. *Cope*, U.S. surgeon, b. 1902]. Reflex increase in respiratory rate as a result of distension of the pulmonary vascular bed.

Churg-Strauss syndrome [J. *Churg*, U.S. pathologist, b. 1910; and L. *Strauss*, 20th century]. A type of necrotizing vasculitis involving small arteries and veins, accompanied by fever, eosinophilia, extravascular granulomas, and frequent involvement of skin, lungs, and peripheral nerves; it occurs in asthmatic patients.

chur·rus (chur'us) *n.* CHARAS.

Chvos·tek's sign (khvos'teck) [F. *Chvostek*, Austrian surgeon, 1835–1884]. A sign of facial nerve hyperirritability in which tapping of the face in front of the ear produces spasm of the ipsilateral facial muscles; an important sign in tetany and hypocalcemic states, and seen in other conditions, including anxiety states.

chyl-, chyli-, chylo-. A combining form meaning *chyle*.

chylaemia. CHYLEMIA.

chyl·an·gi·o·ma (kigh·lan''jee·o'muh) *n.* [*chyl-* + *angioma*]. 1. Retention of chyle in lymphatic vessels with dilatation of the latter. 2. A lymphangioma containing chyle.

chyle (kile) *n.* [Gk. *chylos*, juice]. A milk-white emulsion of fat globules in lymph formed in the small intestine during digestion. —**chy·lous** (kigh'lus) *adj.*

chyle corpuscle. Any cell suspended in chyle.

chy·le·mia, chy·lae·mia (kigh·lee'mee·uh) *n.* [*chyl-* + *-emia*]. The presence of chyle in the blood.

chyle varix. A varix of a lymphatic vessel which transports chyle; may be seen in filariasis.

chyli-. See *chyl-*.

chy·li·dro·sis (kigh''li·dro'sis) *n.* [*chyl-* + *hidrosis*]. Milkiness of the sweat.

chylo-. See *chyl-*.

chy·lo·cele (kigh'lo·seel) *n.* [*chylo-* + *-cele*]. Accumulation of chyle in the tunica vaginalis of the testis.

chy·lo·der·ma (kigh''lo·dur'muh) *n.* [*chylo-* + *-derma*]. Accumulation of chyle in the thickened skin and enlarged lymphatic vessels, usually due to filariasis.

chy·loid (kigh'loid) *adj.* Resembling chyle.

chy·lo·me·di·as·ti·num (kigh''lo·mee''dee·as·tye'num) *n.* The presence of chyle in the mediastinum.

chy·lo·mi·cron (kigh''lo·migh'kron) *n.*, pl. **chylomi·cra** (·kruh), **chylomicrons** [*chylo-* + *micron*]. An extremely small particle of lipid, observed in blood after ingestion of fat, and consisting primarily of triglyceride.

chy·lo·mi·cro·ne·mia (kigh''lo·migh''kro·nee'mee·uh) *n.* An excess of chylomicrons in the blood, usually due to a deficiency of lipoprotein lipase.

chy·lor·rhea, chy·lor·rhoea (kigh''lo·ree'uh) *n.* [*chylo-* + *-rrhea*]. 1. An excessive flow of chyle. 2. Diarrhea characterized by a milky color of the feces due to the rupture of small intestinal lymphatics. 3. Release of chyle from rupture or other injury of the thoracic duct.

chy·lo·sis (kigh·lo'sis) *n.*, pl. **chylo·ses** (·seez) [*chyle* + *-osis*]. The conversion of food into chyle, followed by absorption of the chyle.

chy·lo·tho·rax (kigh''lo·tho'racks) *n.* [*chylo-* + *thorax*]. An accumulation of chyle in the thoracic cavity.

chy·lous (kigh'lus) *adj.* Pertaining to or involving chyle.

chylous ascites. ASCITES CHYLOSUS.

chylous cyst. A cyst found in lymphatics, containing chyle.

chy·lu·ria (kigh·lew'ree·uh) *n.* [*chyl-* + *-uria*]. The presence of chyle or lymph in the urine, usually due to a fistulous communication between the urinary and lymphatic tracts or to lymphatic obstruction.

chy·lus (kigh'lus) *n.*, genit. **chy·li** (·lye) [NA]. CHYLE.

Chymar. A trademark for chymotrypsin.

Chymase. A trademark for chymotrypsin.

chyme (kime) *n.* [Gk. *chymos*, juice]. 1. Strictly: the viscid, fluid contents of the stomach consisting of food that has undergone gastric digestion, and has not yet passed into the duodenum. 2. Loosely: any digesta in the stomach or small intestine. —**chy·mous** (kigh'mus) *adj.*

chy·mo·pa·pa·in (kigh''mo·pa·pay'in) *n.* [Gk. *chymos*, juice, + *papain*]. Any one of several proteolytic enzyme fractions obtained from papaya.

chy·mo·sin (kigh'mo·sin) *n.* [F. *chymosine*]. RENNIN.

chy·mo·sin·o·gen (kigh''mo·sin'o·jen) *n.* [*chymosin* + *-gen*]. The precursor of chymosin or rennin.

chy·mo·tryp·sin (kigh''mo·trip'sin) *n.* [*chymo-* + *trypsin*]. A proteolytic enzyme found in the intestine and formed from the chymotrypsinogen of the pancreatic juice by the action of trypsin. It acts simultaneously with trypsin to hydrolyze proteins and protein digestion products to polypeptides and amino acids. Chymotrypsin of bovine origin, obtainable in α-, β-, and γ-forms, differs in solubility and other properties. The enzyme is used to reduce soft-tissue inflammation and edema; the α- form is employed in zonulysis.

chy·mo·tryp·sin·o·gen (kigh″mo·trip·sin′o·jen) *n.* [*chymotrypsin* + *-gen*]. The precursor, occurring in pancreatic juice, of the enzyme chymotrypsin.

chy·mus (kigh′mus) *n.* [BNA]. CHYME.

Ci Abbreviation for *curie.*

C. I. Abbreviation for (a) *color index;* (b) *chemotherapeutic index.*

Ciac·cio's fixatives (chaʰt′cho) [C. *Ciaccio,* Italian pathologist, 1877–1956]. Mixtures containing 2 to 5% potassium bichromate and 10 to 20% formalin with a little added formic or acetic acid; used to render unsaturated fats insoluble, permitting histologic identification.

ci·biso·tome (sigh·bis′o·tome, si·bis′) *n.* [Gk. *kibisis,* pouch, + *-tome*]. CYSTOTOME (2).

ci·bo·pho·bia (sigh″bo·fo′bee·uh) *n.* [L. *cibus,* food, + *phobia*]. Abnormal aversion to food, or to eating.

cic·a·tri·cial (sick″uh·trish′ul) *adj.* [F. *cicatrice,* scar, + *-al*]. Pertaining to or like a scar.

cicatricial ectropion. Ectropion due to contraction of scar tissue from accidental or surgical trauma; may involve one or both eyelids.

cicatricial entropion. Entropion due to scar tissue on the inner side of the lid; affects the upper lid most commonly.

cicatricial hypertrophy. Overgrowth of connective tissue in a scar; increase in scar tissue.

cicatricial pemphigoid. BENIGN MUCOSAL PEMPHIGOID.

cicatricial stenosis. Constriction, as of a duct, due to scar-tissue formation.

cic·a·tric·u·la (sick″uh·trick′yoo·luh) *n.*, pl. **cicatricu·lae** (·lee) [L., diminutive of *cicatrix,* scar]. A little scar.

cic·a·trix (sick′uh·tricks) *n.*, pl. **cic·a·tri·ces** (sick″uh·trye′seez), **cicatrixes** [L.]. The fibrous connective tissue which follows healing of a wound or loss of substance due to infection. Typically soft and red when new, it tends to become avascular, hard, and contracted when old; SCAR.

cic·a·tri·zant (sick″uh·trye′zunt, si·kat′ri·zunt) *adj.* & *n.* 1. Promoting cicatrization. 2. A medicinal agent that promotes cicatrization.

cic·a·tri·za·tion (sick″uh·tri·zay′shun) *n.* Formation of a cicatrix or scar. —**cic·a·trize** (sick′uh·trize) *v.*

cicatrized infarct. An infarct in which the necrotic mass is replaced or encapsulated by fibrous connective tissue.

cic·er·ism (sis′ur·iz·um) *n.* [L. *cicer,* chick-pea, + *-ism*]. An animal disease produced experimentally that corresponds to human lathyrism; it is due to toxic action of certain legumes.

cic·lo·pir·ox (sick″lo·peer′ocks) *n.* 6-Cyclohexyl-1-hydroxy-4-methyl-2(1*H*)-pyridinone, $C_{12}H_{17}NO_2$, an antifungal agent usually used as the olamine (ethanolamine) salt, $C_{14}H_{24}N_2O_3$.

ci·clo·pro·fen (sigh″klo·pro′fen) *n.* α-Methylfluorene-2-acetic acid, $C_{16}H_{14}O_2$, an anti-inflammatory agent.

Ci·cu·ta (si·kew′tuh) *n.* [L.]. A genus of the Umbelliferae including water hemlocks; many species are poisonous.

cic·u·tism (sick′yoo·tiz·um) *n.* [*Cicuta* + *-ism*]. Poisoning with water hemlock, *Cicuta virosa;* marked by dilatation of the pupils, cyanosis of the face, convulsions, and coma.

cic·u·tox·in (sick″yoo·tock′sin) *n.* A poisonous principle in certain plants of the genus *Cicuta.* Its actions are similar to those of picrotoxin.

CID Abbreviation for *cytomegalic inclusion disease.*

ci·dal (sigh′dul) *adj.* [by generalization from words ending in *-cidal* such as bactericidal, vermicidal]. *Informal.* Lethal, destructive (for some specified kind of organism or cell).

-cide [L. *-cida,* from *caedere,* to kill]. A combining form meaning (a) *killer;* (b) *killing.*

Cidex. A trademark for glutaraldehyde, a disinfectant.

ci·dox·e·pin (sigh·dock′se·pin) *n.* 3-Dibenz[*b,e*]oxepin-11(6*H*)-ylidene-*N,N*-dimethyl-1-propanamine, $C_{19}H_{21}NO$, an antidepressant.

Cie·szyn·ski's rule of isometry (chʸe·shin′skee) [A. *Cieszynski,* Polish dentist and physician, b. 1882]. The normal x-ray beam is directed perpendicularly to a plane which lies midway between the plane of the tooth desired and the plane of the film.

cig·a·rette drain. A drain of gauze surrounded by rubber tissue, rubber dam, or split rubber tubing.

Cignolin. A trademark for anthralin, a drug used externally in the treatment of skin diseases.

ci·gua·te·ra (see″gwuh·terr′uh) *n.* [American Sp. *cigua,* sea snail]. A serious and sometimes fatal disease caused by ingestion of a variety of tropical marine fishes.

ci·gua·tox·in (see″gwuh·tock′sin) *n.* [*cigua* + *toxin*]. A substance with anticholinesterase activity present in fishes that cause ciguatera and believed to be the principle responsible for the disease.

cili-, cilio- [L. *cilium,* eyelid]. A combining form meaning (a) *cilia;* (b) *ciliary.*

cil·ia (sil′ee·uh) *n. pl.*, sing. **cil·i·um** (·ee·um) [L.] 1. [NA] EYELASHES. 2. The threadlike cytoplasmic processes of cells which beat rhythmically, thereby causing the locomotion of certain aquatic organisms or propelling fluids over surfaces covered by ciliated cells.

cil·i·ary (sil′ee·uh·ree, ·err″ee) *adj.* 1. Pertaining to or resembling an eyelid or eyelash. 2. Pertaining to the ciliary body or its component structures. 3. Pertaining to or resembling cilia.

ciliary artery. Any of the many branches of the ophthalmic and lacrimal arteries which supply the choroid, the ciliary body, and the iris. The posterior ciliary arteries arise from the ophthalmic artery and pass through the sclera near the optic nerve, with the several short posterior ciliary arteries (NA *arteriae ciliares posteriores breves*) supplying the choroid and the two long posterior ciliary arteries (NA *arteriae ciliares posteriores longae*) passing between the sclera and the choroid to the ciliary body, where they anastomose with the anterior ciliary arteries. The several anterior ciliary arteries (NA *arteriae ciliares anteriores*) derive from the lacrimal artery and the ophthalmic artery, give off episcleral and conjunctival branches, pierce the sclera near the cornea, and anastomose with the long posterior ciliary arteries in the greater arterial circle of the iris, which supplies the ciliary body and the iris.

ciliary blepharitis. MARGINAL BLEPHARITIS.

ciliary body. A wedge-shaped thickening in the middle layer (vascular tunic) of the eyeball, anterior to the choroid and posterior to the iris, consisting of the ciliary ring, the ciliary muscle, and, on the internal surface, the ciliary crown, which bears the ciliary processes. NA *corpus ciliare.*

ciliary canal. The spaces of the iridocorneal angle.

ciliary crown. The anterior portion of the inner surface of the ciliary body, bearing the ciliary processes. NA *corona ciliaris.*

ciliary disk. CILIARY RING.

ciliary ganglion. The ganglion at the back of the orbit; from it arise postganglionic parasympathetic fibers to the ciliary muscle and the constrictor muscle of the iris. NA *ganglion ciliare.*

ciliary glands. Modified sweat glands of the eyelids. NA *glandulae ciliares.*

ciliary hypocyclosis. Hypocyclosis due to weakness of the ciliary muscle.

ciliary margin. The peripheral border of the iris. NA *margo ciliaris.*

ciliary movement. The unidirectional, rhythmic, lashing movement of cilia, as on the epithelium of the respiratory tract and in certain microorganisms.

ciliary muscle. The muscular band which is located in the anterior outer portion of the ciliary body overlying the ciliary crown and whose contraction effects accommodation for near vision by relaxing the zonular fibers attached to the ciliary processes, thus allowing the lens to become more convex. NA *musculus ciliaris.* See also Table of Muscles in the Appendix.

ciliary nerves. See Table of Nerves in the Appendix.

ciliary neuralgia. Neuralgic pain of the eye, brow, or temple. See also *histamine cephalalgia.*

ciliary plicae. The small folds between the ciliary processes. NA *plicae ciliares.*

ciliary processes. The radiating folds, located on the anterior internal surface of the ciliary body with their free anterior ends projecting toward the lens, which serve as attachments for the zonular fibers and secrete most of the aqueous humor. NA *processus ciliares.*

ciliary reflex. The normal constriction of the pupil in accommodation of the eye.

ciliary region. The zone around the cornea of the eye, corresponding to the position of the ciliary body.

ciliary ring. The minutely grooved band which forms the thin posterior portion of the ciliary body; an anterior continuation of the choroid just posterior to the ciliary crown. NA *orbiculus ciliaris.*

ciliary staphyloma. A staphyloma in the region of the ciliary body.

ciliary zone. GREATER RING OF THE IRIS.

ciliary zonule. The suspensory structure for the lens of the eye, consisting of filaments (zonular fibers) attached to the capsule of the lens in the region of the equator and radiating outward to the ciliary body. Syn. *zonule of Zinn.* NA *zonula ciliaris.*

Cil·i·a·ta (sil″ee·ay′tuh) *n. pl.* A class of Protozoa characterized by the presence of cilia. The only important human ciliate is the intestinal parasite *Balantidium coli.*

cil·i·ate (sil′ee·ate) *n.* A protozoan possessing cilia.

cil·i·at·ed (sil′ee·ay·tid) *adj.* Possessing cilia.

ciliated cell. A cell provided with cilia.

ciliated epithelium. A form of epithelium in which the cells bear vibratile filaments or cilia on their free surfaces.

cilio-. See *cili-.*

cil·io·cy·to·pho·ria (sil″ee·o·sigh″to·for′ee·uh) *n.* [*cilio-* + *cyto-* + *-phoria*]. Massive destruction of the ciliated bronchial epithelium associated with certain infections, especially virus pneumonia.

cil·io·scle·ral (sil″ee·o·skleer′ul) *adj.* [*cilio-* + *scleral*]. Pertaining to the ciliary body and the sclera of the eye.

cil·io·spi·nal (sil″ee·o·spye′nul) *adj.* Pertaining to the ciliary body and the spinal cord.

ciliospinal center. The sympathetic nervous center in the eighth cervical and first three thoracic segments of the spinal cord; the origin of cervical sympathetic nerves that innervate the dilator muscle of the pupil of the eye.

ciliospinal reflex. Dilatation of the ipsilateral pupil on pinching the skin on one side of the neck.

cilium. Singular of *cilia*; EYELASH.

cilium in·ver·sum (in·vur′sum). Ingrowing of an eyelash due to cogenital malposition of the follicle.

Cilloral. A trademark for penicillin G potassium.

cil·lo·sis (si·lo′sis) *n.* [L. *cill*ere, to agitate, + *-osis*]. A spasmodic trembling of the eyelid. —**cil·lot·ic** (·lot′ick) *adj.*

ci·met·i·dine (sigh·met′i·deen) *n.* 1-Cyano-2-methyl-3-[2-[[(5-methylimidazol-4-yl)methyl]thio]ethyl]guanidine, $C_{10}H_{16}N_6S$, an antagonist to histamine H_2 receptors.

Ci·mex (sigh′mecks) *n.* [L., bug]. A genus of bedbugs and similar insects of the family Cimicidae, species of which are parasitic to man and vectors of disease.

Cimex he·mip·te·rus (he·mip′te·rus). An important bloodsucking species of *Cimex* parasitic to man; the oriental bedbug.

Cimex lec·tu·la·rius (leck″tew·lair′ee·us) [ML., from L. *lectus,* bed]. The common bedbug.

Cimex ro·tun·da·tus (ro″tun·day′tus). *CIMEX HEMIPTERUS.*

Ci·mic·i·dae (sigh·mis′i·dee) *n. pl.* [NL., from *Cimex,* type genus]. A family of wingless bloodsucking insects of the order Hemiptera, ectoparasites of mammals and birds; the bedbugs and their allies.

cim·i·cif·u·ga (sim″i·sif′yoo·guh) *n.* [NL., bugbane]. The dried rhizome and roots of *Cimicifuga racemosa;* cohosh bugbane. It contains cimicifugin, or macrotin, a resin. The drug has been used in chronic rheumatism, chorea, and tinnitus. Syn. *black cohosh.*

cim·i·cif·u·gin (sim″i·sif′yoo·jin) *n.* The resin from cimicifuga.

cin·an·ser·in (sin·an′sur·in) *n.* 2′-[[3-(Dimethylamino)propyl] thio] cinnamanilide, $C_{20}H_{24}N_2OS$, an inhibitor of serotonin; used as the hydrochloride salt.

Cinaphyl. A trademark for theophylline sodium glycinate.

cin·cham·i·dine (sin·kam′i·deen, ·din) *n.* HYDROCINCHONIDINE.

cin·cho·caine (sin′ko·kane) *n.* British name for the local anesthetic substance dibucaine.

cin·cho·na (sing·ko′nuh) *n.* [Countess of *Chinchon,* Peru, 17th century]. The dried bark of the stem or root of *Cinchona succirubra* or its hybrids, known as red cinchona, or of *C. ledgeriana, C. calisaya,* or hybrids of these with other species of *Cinchona,* known as calisaya bark or yellow cinchona. The trees are natives of South America. Cinchona contains more than 20 alkaloids, the most important being quinine, quinidine, cinchonine, and cinchonidine. Cinchona has the physiologic action and therapeutic uses of its chief alkaloid, quinine. It is also an astringent, bitter, and stomachic tonic. Syn. *Peruvian bark, Jesuits' bark.* —**cin·chon·ic** (sing·kon′ick) *adj.;* **cin·chon·i·za·tion** (sing·kon″i·zay′shun) *n.;* **cin·chon·ize** (sing′kon·ize) *v.*

cin·chon·a·mine (sing″kon·am′een, ·in, sing·kon′uh·meen, ·min) *n.* An alkaloid, $C_{19}H_{24}N_2O$, of cuprea bark.

cin·chon·i·dine (sing·kon′i·deen, ·din) *n.* An alkaloid, $C_{19}H_{22}N_2O$, from cinchona; it resembles quinine in its actions.

cin·cho·nine (sing′ko·neen, ·nin) *n.* An alkaloid, $C_{19}H_{22}N_2O$, derived from cinchona. It is similar to quinine in therapeutic effects, but less active.

cin·cho·nism (sing′ko·niz·um) *n.* The adverse systemic effect of cinchona or its alkaloids when given in full doses or the toxic effects of excessive use of these drugs. The symptoms include anorexia, nausea, vomiting, diarrhea, vertigo, tinnitus, headache, and visual disturbances.

cin·cho·phen (sing′ko·fen) *n.* 2-Phenylcinchoninic acid, $C_{16}H_{11}NO_2$, a white powder, almost insoluble in water. It has been used as a uricosuric agent, but it may cause severe toxic effects, including hepatitis.

cin·cho·tan·nic acid (sing″ko·tan′ick). CINCHOTANNIN.

cin·cho·tan·nin (sing″ko·tan′in) *n.* The characteristic tannin of cinchona; it exists as a glycoside.

cinc·ture (sink′chur) *n.* [L. *cinctura*]. A girdle or belt.

cincture sensation. A sensation of constriction around the body. See also *zonesthesia.*

cine- [Gk. *kinēma,* movement]. A combining form meaning *motion picture.* See also *kine-.*

cine (sin′ee) *adj.* Motion-picture, cinematic.

cine·an·gio·car·dio·gram (sin″ee·an″jee·o·kahr″dee·o·gram) *n.* [*cine-* + *angiocardiogram*]. An angiocardiogram recorded with x-ray motion-picture technique.

cine·an·gio·car·di·og·ra·phy (sin″ee·an″jee·o·kahr″dee·og′ruh·fee) *n.* [*cine-* + *angiocardiography*]. The use of a motion-picture camera to record fluoroscopic images of the heart and great vessels after injection of radiopaque contrast material.

cine-angiogram, *n.* An angiogram recorded with x-ray motion-picture technique.

cine coronary arteriography. Motion-picture radiologic study of the coronary arteries by injection of radiopaque contrast material.

cine·esoph·a·go·gram (sin″ee·e·sof′uh·go·gram) *n.* [*cine-* + *esophagogram*]. An esophagogram recorded by x-ray motion-picture technique.

cine·flu·o·rog·ra·phy (sin″e·floo″ur·og′ruh·fee) *n.* [*cine-* +

fluorography]. The motion-picture recording of fluoroscopic images.

cin·e·mat·ic (sin″e·mat′ick) *adj.* 1. Of or pertaining to motion pictures. 2. KINEMATIC.

cin·e·ole, cin·e·ol (sin′ee·ole, ·ol) *n.* EUCALYPTOL.

cin·e·plas·tic (sin″e·plas′tick) *adj.* KINEPLASTIC.

cin·e·plas·ty (sin′e·plas″tee) *n.* KINEPLASTY.

cine·ra·di·og·ra·phy (sin″e·ray″dee·og′ruh·fee) *n.* [*cine-* + *radiography*]. CINEROENTGENOGRAPHY.

ci·ne·rea (si·neer′ee·uh) *n.* [L. *cinereus,* ash-colored]. The gray substance of the brain or spinal cord.

cine·roent·gen·og·ra·phy (sin″e·rent″gen·og′ruh·fee) *n.* [*cine-* + *roentgenography*]. The depiction of the anatomic structure of an organ, usually in motion, by x-ray motion-picture technique.

cin·ges·tol (sin·jes′tol) *n.* 19-Nor-17α-pregn-5-en-20-yn-17-ol, $C_{20}H_{28}O$, a progestational steroid.

cin·gu·lar (sing′gew·lur) *adj.* CINGULATE.

cin·gu·late (sing′gew·late, ·lut) *adj.* 1. Of or pertaining to a cingulum. 2. Having a zone or girdle, usually of transverse bands or marks.

cingulate fissure. CINGULATE SULCUS.

cingulate gyrus. The convolution that lies immediately above the corpus callosum on the medial aspect of each cerebral hemisphere. Syn. *gyrus cinguli [NA], callosal gyrus.*

cingulate sulcus. A sulcus on the medial aspect of the cerebral hemisphere separating the superior frontal gyrus and paracentral lobule from the cingulate gyrus below; it terminates by dividing into subparietal and marginal portions. NA *sulcus cinguli.*

cin·gu·lec·to·my (sing″gew·leck′tuh·mee) *n.* [*cingulum* + *-ectomy*]. Surgical removal under direct vision of a portion of the cingulate gyrus, usually Brodmann's area 24 and immediately adjacent tissue.

cin·gu·lot·o·my (sing″gew·lot′uh·mee) *n.* The interruption of fibers of the white matter of the cingulate gyrus by means of stereotactic application of heat or cold.

cin·gu·lo·trac·to·my (sing″gew·lo·track′tuh·mee) *n.* [*cingulum* + *tract* + *-tomy*]. The surgical incision of the projections of the cingulate gyrus to the thalamus. It is used rarely, in control of psychotic disorders.

cin·gu·lum (sing′gew·lum) *n.,* genit. **cingu·li** (·lye), pl. **cingu·la** (·luh) [L.]. 1. A girdle or zone. 2. *Obsol.* HERPES ZOSTER. 3. [NA] A bundle of association fibers running in the cingulate gyrus of the brain from the anterior perforated substance to the hippocampal gyrus. 4. [NA] BASAL RIDGE.

cingulum ex·tre·mi·ta·tis in·fe·ri·o·ris (eck·strem″i·tay′tis in·feer·ee·o′ris) [BNA]. Cingulum membri inferioris. (= PELVIC GIRDLE).

cingulum extremitatis su·pe·ri·o·ris (sue·peer·ee·o′ris) [BNA]. Cingulum membri superioris (= SHOULDER GIRDLE).

cingulum mem·bri in·fe·ri·o·ris (mem′brye in·feer·ee·o′ris) [NA]. PELVIC GIRDLE.

cingulum membri su·pe·ri·o·ris (sue·peer·ee·o′ris) [NA]. SHOULDER GIRDLE.

cin·gu·lum·ot·o·my (sing″gew·luh·mot′uh·mee) *n.* CINGULOTOMY.

cin·na·mal·de·hyde (sin″uh·mal′de·hide) *n.* Cinnamic aldehyde, $C_6H_5CH{=}CHCHO$, the chief constituent of cinnamon oil and prepared synthetically. A flavoring agent.

cin·na·med·rine (sin″a·med′reen) *n.* 2-(Cinnamylmethylamino)-1-phenyl-1-propanol, $C_{19}H_{23}NO$, a compound with uterine antispasmodic activity.

cin·nam·e·in (si·nam′ee·in, sin″uh·mee′in) *n.* Benzyl cinnamate, $C_{16}H_{14}O_2$, a constituent of Peruvian and tolu balsams.

cin·na·mene (sin′uh·meen, sin·am′een) *n.* STYROL.

cin·nam·ic acid (si·nam′ick). 3-Phenylpropenoic acid, $C_6H_5CH{=}CHCOOH$, occurring in Peruvian and tolu balsams, storax, and some benzoin resins. It has been used in treating tuberculosis.

cinnamic alcohol. CINNAMYL ALCOHOL.

cinnamic aldehyde. CINNAMALDEHYDE.

cin·na·mon (sin′uh·mun) *n.* [Gk. *kinnamōmon*]. The dried bark of several species of *Cinnamomum,* native to Ceylon and China, the latter variety being known in commerce under the name of cassia. *Cinnamomum loureirii,* Saigon cinnamon, and *C. zeylanicum,* Ceylon cinnamon, are commonly used. It contains a volatile oil, and is used as a carminative and aromatic stimulant, and as a spice.

cinnamon oil. The volatile oil obtained from the leaves and twigs of *Cinnamomum cassia.* Its chief constituent is cinnamaldehyde. A flavor, carminative, and local stimulant. Syn. *cassia oil.*

cin·nam·yl alcohol (si·nam′il). 3-Phenyl-2-propen-1-ol, $C_6H_5CH{=}CHCH_2OH$, a crystalline alcohol occurring in Peruvian balsam and storax. Used in perfumery. Syn. *cinnamic alcohol.*

cin·nar·i·zine (si·năr′i·zeen) *n.* 1-Cinnamyl-4-(diphenylmethyl)piperazine, $C_{26}H_{28}N_2$, an antihistaminic drug.

cin·ox·a·cin (si·nock′suh·sin) *n.* 1-Ethyl-1,4-dihydro-4-oxo[1,3]dioxolo[4,5-*g*]cinnoline-3-carboxylic acid, $C_{12}H_{10}N_2O_5$, an antibacterial agent.

cin·per·ene (sin′pur·een) *n.* 2-(1-Cinnamyl-4-piperidyl)-2-phenylglutarimide, $C_{25}H_{28}N_2O_2$, a tranquilizer.

cin·ta·zone (sin′tuh·zone) *n.* 2-Pentyl-6-phenyl-1*H*-pyrazolo[1,2-a]cinnoline-1,3(2*H*)-dione, $C_{22}H_{22}N_2O_2$, an anti-inflammatory agent.

cin·tri·a·mide (sin·trye′uh·mide) *n.* 3,4,5,-Trimethoxycinnamamide, $C_{12}H_{15}NO_4$, a tranquilizer.

cir·ca·di·an (sur·kay′dee·un) *adj.* [L. *circa,* around, + *dies,* day]. Manifested or recurring in cycles of about 24 hours. Contr. *infradian, ultradian.*

cir·ci·nate (sur′si·nate) *adj.* [L. *circinatus,* from *circinare,* to make round]. Having a circular outline or a ring formation.

circinate retinopathy. A lesion seen in a number of conditions in which vascular inadequacy is present, characterized by a complete or incomplete ring of lipids deposited in the deeper layers of the retina, usually in the area centralis.

circinate syphilitic erythema. TERTIARY CIRCINATE ERYTHEMA.

cir·cle, *n.* [L. *circulus*]. 1. A ring; a line, every point on which is equidistant from a point called the center. 2. A ringlike anastomosis of arteries or veins.

circle of diffusion. The imperfect image formed by incomplete focalization, the position of the true focus not having been reached by some of the rays of light, or else having been passed.

circle of Hal·ler [A. von *Haller*]. VASCULAR CIRCLE OF THE OPTIC NERVE.

circle of Wil·lis [T. *Willis*]. ARTERIAL CIRCLE OF THE CEREBRUM.

circle of Zinn [J. G. *Zinn*]. VASCULAR CIRCLE OF THE OPTIC NERVE.

cir·cuit (sur′kit) *n.* [L. *circuitus,* from *circumire,* to go around]. A path or course which, when not interrupted, returns upon itself, such as the path of a circulating fluid in a system of tubes, or the path of nerve impulses in reflex arcs.

cir·cu·lar (sur′kew·lur) *adj.* [L. *circularis,* from *circulus,* circle]. 1. Ring-shaped. 2. Pertaining to a circle. 3. Marked by alternations of despondency and excitation, as in a manic-depressive illness.

circular amputation. An operation performed with the use of a flap by circular sweeps or incisions around the limb vertical to the long axis of the bone.

circular bandage. A bandage that is wound about the limb or part.

circular enterorrhaphy. The suturing of two completely divided sections of an intestine.

circular folds. The shelflike folds of the mucous membrane of the small intestine. NA *plicae circulares.*

circular insanity or **dementia.** Manic-depressive illness of the circular type.
circular ligament. PERIODONTAL LIGAMENT.
circular plicae. CIRCULAR FOLDS.
circular sinus. A sinus consisting of the two cavernous sinuses and their communications across the median line by means of the anterior and posterior intercavernous sinuses, all of which surround the hypophysis.
circular sulcus. A limiting furrow surrounding the base of the insula, separating it from the operculum. NA *sulcus circularis insulae.*
circular suture. A suture that is applied to the entire circumference of a divided part, as the intestine.
cir·cu·la·tion (sur″kew·lay′shun) *n.* [L. *circulatio*]. Passage in a circuit, as the circulation of the blood. See also Plates 5, 6. —**cir·cu·la·to·ry** (sur′kew·luh·tor″ee) *adj.*
circulation of Ser·ve·tus (sur·vee′tus) [M. *Servetus,* Spanish physician, 1511–1553]. PULMONARY CIRCULATION.
circulation time. The rate of blood flow; the time required for blood to flow from one part of the body to another, as from arm to lung or arm to tongue, or to pass through the whole circulatory system.
circulation time test. 1. ARM-LUNG TIME TEST. 2. ARM-TONGUE TIME TEST.
circulatory failure. Inadequacy of the cardiovascular system to fulfill its function of providing transport of nutritive and other substance to and from the tissue cells; it may be caused by cardiac or peripheral conditions. See also *backward failure, cardiac failure, forward failure.*
cir·cu·lus (sur′kew·lus) *n.,* pl. & genit. sing. **circu·li** (·lye) [L.]. CIRCLE (2).
circulus ar·te·ri·o·sus ce·re·bri (ahr·teer″ee·o′sus serr′e·brye) [NA]. ARTERIAL CIRCLE OF THE CEREBRUM.
circulus arteriosus hal·leri (hal′e·rye) [A. von *Haller*]. VASCULAR CIRCLE OF THE OPTIC NERVE.
circulus arteriosus iri·dis major (eye′ri·dis) [NA]. GREATER ARTERIAL CIRCLE OF THE IRIS.
circulus arteriosus iridis minor [NA]. LESSER ARTERIAL CIRCLE OF THE IRIS.
circulus arteriosus (Wil·li·sii) (wil·is′ee·eye) [T. *Willis*] [BNA]. Circulus arteriosus cerebri (= ARTERIAL CIRCLE OF THE CEREBRUM).
circulus ar·ti·cu·la·ris vas·cu·lo·sus (ahr·tick″yoo·lair′is vas·kew·lo′sus) [NA]. The vascular anastomosis around any joint.
circulus vas·cu·lo·sus ner·vi op·ti·ci (vas·kew·lo′sus nur′vye op′ti·sigh) [NA]. VASCULAR CIRCLE OF THE OPTIC NERVE.
circum- [L.]. A prefix meaning *around, about, on all sides, surrounding.*
cir·cum·anal (sur″kum·ay′nul) *adj.* [*circum-* + *anal*]. Periproctal; surrounding the anus.
circumanal glands. The sebaceous and apocrine glands in the skin about the anus.
cir·cum·are·o·lar (sur″kum·uh·ree′o·lur) *adj.* Around an areola, especially of the breast.
cir·cum·ar·tic·u·lar (sur″kum·ahr·tick′yoo·lur) *adj.* [*circum-* + *articular*]. Around a joint.
cir·cum·ci·sion (sur″kum·sizh′un) *n.* [L. *circumcisio,* from *circumcidere,* to cut around]. The removal of the foreskin; excision of the prepuce. —**cir·cum·cise** (sur′kum·size) *v.*
cir·cum·cor·ne·al (sur″kum·kor′nee·ul) *adj.* [*circum-* + *corneal*]. Around or about the cornea.
cir·cum·duc·tion (sur″kum·duck′shun) *n.* [L. *circumductio,* from *circumducere,* to lead around]. The movement of a limb in such a manner that its distal part describes a circle, the proximal end being fixed.
cir·cum·fe·ren·tia (sur·kum″fur·en′shee·uh) *n.* [L.]. Circumference.
circumferentia ar·ti·cu·la·ris ra·dii (ahr·tick″yoo·lair′is ray′dee·eye) [NA]. The articular surface of the head of the radius.
circumferentia articularis ul·nae (ul′nee) [NA]. The articular surface of the head of the ulna.
cir·cum·fer·en·tial (sur·kum″fur·en′shul) *adj.* Pertaining to the circumference; encircling.
circumferential cartilage. The fibrocartilaginous rim about certain articulations.
circumferential lamella. A thin layer of bone deposited under the periosteum or endosteum.
cir·cum·flex (sur′kum·flecks) *adj.* [L. *circumflexus,* from *circumflectere,* to bend about]. Bending around; designating a number of arteries having a winding course.
circumflex artery. See Table of Arteries in the Appendix.
circumflex nerve. The axillary nerve. See Table of Nerves in the Appendix.
circumflex paralysis. AXILLARY PARALYSIS.
cir·cum·in·su·lar (sur″kum·in′sue·lur) *adj.* [*circum-* + *insular*]. Surrounding the insula of the cerebral cortex.
cir·cum·len·tal (sur″kum·len′tul) *adj.* [*circum-* + NL. *lens, lentis,* lens, + *-al*]. Surrounding a lens.
circumlental space. The interspace between the ciliary body and the equator of the lens.
cir·cum·lin·ear (sur″kum·lin′ee·ur) *adj.* Around a line.
cir·cum·lo·cu·tion (sur″kum·lo·kew′shun) *n.* [L. *circumlocutio,* from *circum,* around, + *loqui,* to speak]. A roundabout way of speaking; the use of several words to express the idea of a single one; may be volitional or due to partial aphasia. —**circum·loc·u·to·ry** (·lock′yoo.to·ree) *adj.*
cir·cum·ne·vic (sur″kum·nee′vick) *adj.* [*circum-* + *nevus* + *-ic*]. Surrounding a nevus.
circumnevic vitiligo. HALO NEVUS.
cir·cum·nu·cle·ar (sur″kum·new′klee·ur) *adj.* [*circum-* + *nuclear*]. Surrounding a nucleus; PERINUCLEAR.
cir·cum·oral (sur″kum·or′ul) *adj.* [*circum-* + *oral*]. Surrounding the mouth.
cir·cum·pen·nate (sur″kum·pen′ate) *adj.* [*circum-* + *pennate*]. Of muscles, exhibiting a structure in which the muscle fibers are inserted into the tendon in a pattern resembling an open fan. Contr. *pennate, unipennate, bipennate.*
cir·cum·po·lar·iza·tion (sur″kom·po″lur·i·zay′shun) *n.* [*circum-* + *polarization*]. The rotation of a ray of polarized light.
cir·cum·pulp·ar (sur″kum·pulp′ur) *adj.* [*circum-* + *pulpar*]. Surrounding the pulp of a tooth.
circumpulpar dentin. The major part of the dentin which lies next to the pulp.
cir·cum·scribed (sur′kum·skrye′bd) *adj.* Enclosed within narrow limits by an encircling boundary.
circumscribed aneurysm. An aneurysm, either true or false, in which the contents are still within the arterial wall though there may be rupture of one or more of its coats.
circumscribed cerebral atrophy. [1]PICK'S DISEASE.
circumscribed hypertrophic proctitis. A well-demarcated annular lesion of the rectal mucosa confined to the region of the sphincteric ring, characteristically exhibiting thick folds and deep sulci and causing severe pain with bleeding on defecation.
circumscribed myxedema. Circumscribed deposition of mucinous material in the pretibial skin, occurring during thyrotoxicosis or treatment for thyrotoxicosis. Syn. *pretibial myxedema.*
circumscribed peritonitis. LOCALIZED PERITONITIS.
circumscribed pyocephalus. A brain abscess.
circumscribed scleroderma. Scleroderma in which the changes are limited to local areas of the skin and associated subcutaneous tissue. Syn. *morphea.*
circumscribed vaginitis. Inflammation of the mucosa of the vagina, which is enclosed in or confined to a limited area of the vagina.
circumstantial evidence. Evidence that is beyond actual demonstration, but that tends to prove the principal fact inferentially by establishing a set of limiting circumstances.
cir·cum·stan·ti·al·i·ty (sur″kum·stan″shee·al′i·tee) *n.* *In psychiatry,* indulging in many irrelevant and unnecessary

details when answering a simple question because of too little selective suppression.

cir·cum·ton·sil·lar (sur″kum·ton′si·lur) *adj.* PERITONSILLAR.

cir·cum·val·late (sur″kum·val′ate) *adj.* [L. *circumvallatus,* from *circumvallare,* to surround with a wall]. Surrounded by a trench, as the vallate papillae of the tongue.

circumvallate papilla. VALLATE PAPILLA.

circumvallate placenta. A placenta in which an overgrowth of decidua parietalis separates the placental margin from the chorionic membranous plate, resulting in the formation of a thick white ring about the circumference of the placenta and reduction in distribution of fetal blood vessels to the placental periphery.

cir·cum·vas·cu·lar (sur″kum·vas′kew·lur) *adj.* [*circum-* + *vascular*]. Surrounding a blood vessel, or other vessel; perivascular.

cir·cus (sur′kus) *adj.* [L., circle]. Characterized by circular movements.

circus movement. 1. Rapid, circular movements or somersaults, produced by injury on one side to some part of the posture-controlling mechanisms of the nervous system, as the vestibular apparatus or the cerebral peduncles. 2. A rolling gait with circumduction as seen in certain basal ganglion disorders. 3. A theory of the mechanism of atrial flutter and fibrillation in which a circular unidirectional excitation wave travels around and around the atrium and reenters the same pathway to initiate another contraction cycle, because the atrial tissue is no longer refractory to stimulation when the original impulse reaches its starting point.

ci·ro·le·my·cin (si·ro″le·migh′sin) *n.* An antibiotic substance, produced by *Streptomyces bellus* var. *cirolerosis* var. *nova,* that has antineoplastic and antibacterial activities.

cir·rho·sis (si·ro′sis) *n.*, pl. **cirrho·ses** (·seez) [Gk. *kirrhos,* orange-colored, + *-osis*]. 1. Any diffuse fibrosis which destroys the normal lobular architecture of the liver with destruction and regeneration of hepatic parenchymal cells. 2. Interstitial inflammation of any tissue or organ. —**cir·rhot·ic** (si·rot′ick) *adj.*

cir·rus (sirr′us) *n.*, pl. **cir·ri** (·eye) [L., curl]. *In zoology,* a slender, flexible appendage, such as the hairlike appendages on worms and insects, especially the protruding male genital organ of cestodes.

cirs-, cirso- [Gk. *kirsos*]. A combining form meaning *swollen vein, varix, varicose.*

cir·sec·to·my (sur·seck′tuh·mee) *n.* [*cirs-* + *-ectomy*]. Excision of a varix or a portion thereof.

cirso-. See *cirs-.*

cir·soid (sur′soid) *adj.* [*cirs-* + *-oid*]. Resembling a varix or dilated vein.

cirsoid aneurysm. 1. A tortuous lengthening and dilatation of a part of an artery. Syn. *racemose aneurysm.* 2. A dilatation of a group of vessels (arteries, veins, and capillaries), the whole forming a pulsating subcutaneous tumor, occurring most often in the scalp. Syn. *anastomotic aneurysm.*

cir·som·pha·los (sur·som′fuh·los) *n.*, pl. **cirsompha·li** (·lye) [*cirs-* + *omphalos*]. Dilated veins around the umbilicus.

cis- [L.]. A prefix meaning (a) *on this side, on the same side;* (b) *in chemistry, having certain atoms or groups of atoms on the same side of a molecule;* usually restricted to cyclic compounds with two stereogenic atoms. Symbol, Z. Contr. *trans-.*

cis·sa (sis′uh) *n.* [Gk. *kissa,* craving for strange food]. PICA.

Cis·sam·pe·los (si·sam′puh·los) *n.* [Gk. *kissos,* ivy, + *ampelos,* vine]. A genus of climbing plants of the Menispermaceae. *Cissampelos pareira,* the false pareira of tropical America, has been used as a tonic and diuretic.

cis·tern (sis′turn) *n.* [L. *cisterna,* cistern]. 1. A reservoir. 2. A large subarachnoid space.

cis·ter·na (sis·tur′nuh) *n.*, pl. **cister·nae** (·nee) [L.]. 1. CISTERN. 2. CISTERNA CHYLI.

cisterna am·bi·ens (am′bee·enz) [BNA]. Cisterna venae magnae cerebri (= CISTERN OF THE GREAT CEREBRAL VEIN).

cisterna ce·re·bel·lo·me·dul·la·ris (serr·e·bel″o·med″yoo·lair′is) [NA]. CEREBELLOMEDULLARY CISTERN.

cisterna chi·as·ma·tis (kigh·az′muh·tis) [NA]. CISTERN OF THE CHIASMA.

cisterna chy·li (kigh′lye) [NA]. The saclike beginning of the thoracic duct, located between the crura of the diaphragm at the level of the last thoracic vertebra.

cisterna cor·po·ris cal·lo·si (kor′po·ris kal·o′sigh). CISTERN OF THE CORPUS CALLOSUM.

cisternae sub·arach·noi·da·les (sub″uh·rack″noy·day′leez) [BNA]. CISTERNAE SUBARACHNOIDEALES.

cisternae sub·arach·noi·de·a·les (sub″uh·rack·noy″dee·ay′leez) [NA]. The subarachnoid spaces collectively.

cisterna fos·sae la·te·ra·lis ce·re·bri (fos′ee lat·e·ray′lis serr′e·brye) [NA]. CISTERN OF THE LATERAL CEREBRAL FOSSA.

cisterna in·ter·pe·dun·cu·la·ris (in″tur·pe·dunk″yoo·lair′is) [NA]. INTERPEDUNCULAR CISTERN.

cis·ter·nal (sis·tur′nul) *adj.* Of or pertaining to a cistern or cisterna.

cisterna la·mi·nae ter·mi·na·lis (lam′i·nee tur·mi·nay′lis). A small extension of the cistern of the chiasma lying anterior to the lamina terminalis.

cisternal arachnoiditis. Chronic adhesive arachnoiditis with thickening of the arachnoid in the posterior cranial fossa and enlargement of the basilar cisterns, causing obstructive hydrocephalus.

cisternal puncture. Puncture of the cisterna magna with a hollow needle, for diagnostic or therapeutic purposes.

cisterna mag·na (mag′nuh). CEREBELLOMEDULLARY CISTERN.

cisterna pe·ri·lym·pha·ti·ca (perr″ee·lim·fat′i·kuh). The portion of the vestibule of the ear lying just within the oval window and filled with perilymph which communicates with the subarachnoid spaces via the aqueduct of the cochlea.

cisterna pon·tis (pon′tis). PONTINE CISTERN.

cisterna ve·nae mag·nae ce·re·bri (vee′nee mag′nee serr′e·brye) [BNA]. CISTERN OF THE GREAT CEREBRAL VEIN.

cistern of the chiasma. The subarachnoid space below and in front of the optic chiasma. NA *cisterna chiasmatis.*

cistern of the corpus callosum. The subarachnoid space between the arachnoid, which is in contact with the inferior border of the falx cerebri, and the corpus callosum.

cistern of the great cerebral vein. The cistern containing the great cerebral vein, formed by the arachnoid stretching over the transverse cerebral fissure from the splenium of the corpus callosum to the superior surface of the cerebellum.

cistern of the lateral cerebral fossa. The subarachnoid space of the temporal pole formed by the arachnoid stretching across the lateral sulcus. NA *cisterna fossae lateralis cerebri.*

cistern of the Sylvian fissure. CISTERN OF THE LATERAL CEREBRAL FOSSA.

cis·tern·og·ra·phy (sis″tur·nog′ruh·fee) *n.* [*cistern* + *-graphy*]. *In radiology,* the visualization of the subarachnoid cisterns of the posterior fossa by means of special contrast media.

cis-trans effect (sis tranz). *In genetics,* a phenomenon whereby two separate mutant genes produce a phenotypic effect when located on homologous chromosomes (trans) but not when located on the same chromosome (cis), indicating that they belong to the same functional unit (cistron) and are allelic.

cis·tron (sis′tron) *n.* The portion of genetic material (DNA) that codes, and is responsible for the synthesis of, a protein or a polypeptide chain; classified according to their genetic response in the cis-trans effect.

cis·ves·ti·tism (sis·ves′ti·tiz·um) *n.* [*cis-* + L. *vestire,* to clothe]. The practice of dressing in clothes suitable to the sex, but not the age, occupation, or position of the wearer, as in the case of a civilian impersonating a military person.

Citanest. Trademark for prilocaine, a local anesthetic used as the hydrochloride salt.

ci·ten·a·mide (si·ten'uh·mide) *n.* 5*H*-Dibenzo[*a,d*]cycloheptene-5-carboxamide, $C_{16}H_{13}NO$, an anticonvulsant agent.

cit·ra·con·ic acid (sit''ruh·kon'ick). Methylmaleic acid, $C_5H_6O_4$, a dicarboxylic acid obtained on heating citric acid.

cit·ral (sit'ral) *n.* 3,7-Dimethyl-2,6-octadienal, $C_{10}H_{16}O$, an aldehyde in oils of lemon, orange, and lemon grass; occurs as a mixture of two geometric isomers, known as geranial and neral. A yellow liquid of strong lemon odor; used as a flavor.

cit·ra·min (sit'ruh·min) *n.* Methenamine anhydromethylenecitrate, $C_{13}H_{20}N_4O_7$; has been used as a urinary antiseptic.

cit·rate (sit'rate, sigh''trate) *n. & v.* 1. Any salt or ester of citric acid. 2. To treat with a citrate or citric acid.

citrate condensing enzyme. CITRATE SYNTHASE.

citrated caffeine. A mixture of equal parts of caffeine and citric acid, the latter increasing the solubility of caffeine in water.

citrated ferrous chloride. A mixture of ferrous chloride and citric acid, used as a hematinic.

citrated whole human blood. Human blood, withdrawn aseptically, which may contain either citrate ion or heparin as an anticoagulant.

citrate-phosphate-dextrose. An anticoagulant-preservative solution used in blood transfusions.

citrate synthase. An enzyme, present in large variety of animal, plant, and bacterial cells, that catalyzes condensation of acetyl coenzyme A with oxaloacetate to form citrate, in the first step of the citric acid cycle. Syn. *citric synthase, citrate condensing enzyme, citric condensing enzyme, citrogenase, condensing enzyme, oxaloacetate transacetase.*

cit·ric acid (sit'rick). 2-Hydroxy-1,2,3-propanetricarboxylic acid, $C_6H_8O_7$, widely distributed in plant and animal tissues; may be obtained from citrus fruits. White crystals or powder; very soluble in water. Used as an acidulant in pharmaceutical preparations, beverages, and confectionery. In the body, it is oxidized to carbon dioxide and water.

citric acid cycle. A cyclic series of enzyme-catalyzed reactions whereby acetate produced in the metabolism of fats, carbohydrates, and proteins is oxidized to carbon dioxide and water with release of energy. Entering the cycle via acetyl coenzyme A, the acetate successively forms citric and other carboxylic acids and also certain dicarboxylic acids in the course of its oxidation. The cycle is the common pathway for converting foodstuffs to energy. Syn. *tricarboxylic acid cycle, Krebs cycle.*

citric condensing enzyme. CITRATE SYNTHASE.

citric synthase. CITRATE SYNTHASE.

cit·rin (sit'rin) *n.* A crystalline substance, said to be a mixture of hesperidin, quercitrin, and eriodictyol glycoside, isolated from lemon juice. It combats the increased permeability of capillary walls, such as occurs in scurvy and certain other diseases. See also *vitamin P.*

cit·rine ointment (sit'reen, ·rin). An ointment of mercuric nitrate.

cit·ri·nin (sit'ri·nin) *n.* 4,6-Dihydro-8-hydroxy-3,4,5-trimethyl-6-oxo-3*H*-2-benzopyran-7-carboxylic acid, $C_{13}H_{14}O_5$, an antibiotic produced by *Penicillium citrinum* and *Aspergillus niveus;* forms yellow crystals.

cit·ro·gen·ase (sit''ro·jen'ace, ·aze, si·troj'en·ace, ·aze) *n.* CITRATE SYNTHASE.

cit·ron (sit'run) *n.* [MF., from L. *citrus*]. The tree, *Citrus medica,* or its fruit. The fruit rind is used in conserves.

cit·ro·nel·lal (sit''ro·nel'al) *n.* A mixture of stereoisomeric aldehydes, of the formula $C_{10}H_{18}O$, in citronella oil and other volatile oils.

cit·ro·nel·la oil (sit''ruh·nel'uh). A yellowish-green volatile oil obtained chiefly from the sweet-scented citronella grass. It consists largely of geraniol and citronellal; an insect repellant.

ci·tro·vo·rum factor (si·tro'vo·rum). A growth factor for *Leuconostoc citrovorum,* found in liver and green vegetables; a member of the vitamin B complex closely related, if not identical, to folinic acid (2).

ci·trul·lin (si·trul'in) *n.* A resinoid from *Citrullus colocynthis;* used as a cathartic in veterinary practice.

ci·trul·line (sit'rul·een, si·trul') *n.* δ-Ureidonorvaline, $C_6H_{13}N_3O_3$, an amino acid, first isolated from watermelon, involved in the formation, in the liver, of urea from ammonia and carbon dioxide; it is an intermediate between ornithine and arginine, two other amino acids involved in producing urea.

ci·trul·lin·emia, ci·trul·lin·ae·mia (sit''rul·in·ee'mee·uh, si·trul'') *n.* [*citrulline* + *-emia*]. An inborn error of amino acid metabolism in which there is a deficiency in argininosuccinic acid synthetase in the liver, an excessive amount of citrulline in blood, urine, and cerebrospinal fluid, and ammonia intoxication; manifested clinically by failure to thrive, vomiting, irritability, seizures, mental retardation, cortical atrophy, and disturbances of liver function.

Ci·trul·lus (si·trul'us) *n.* A genus of melon-bearing vines native to Africa. See also *citrullin, colocynth.*

Cit·rus (sit'rus) *n.* [L.]. A genus of trees of the Rutaceae. From this genus come the orange, lemon, citron, lime, and bergamot.

cit·to·sis (si·to'sis) *n.* [Gk. *kitta,* craving for strange food, + *-osis*]. PICA.

Ci·vatte's poikiloderma (see·vat') [A. *Civatte,* French dermatologist, 1877–1956]. RETICULATED PIGMENTED POIKILODERMA.

Ci·vi·ni·ni's spine (chee·vee·nee'nee) [F. *Civinini,* Italian anatomist, 1805–1844]. A small process on the lateral pterygoid plate.

Cl Symbol for chlorine.

cl Abbreviation for *centiliter.*

Cl. Abbreviation for *Clostridium.*

Cla·do·nia (kla·do'nee·uh) *n.* [Gk. *kladōn,* branch]. A genus of lichens. *Cladonia rangiferina,* reindeer moss, has been used medicinally as a stomachic and pectoral, and as a food.

Clad·o·spo·ri·um (klad''o·spo'ree·um) *n.* [NL., from Gk. *klados,* branch, + *spore*]. A genus of darkly pigmented fungi, including saprophytic and pathogenic species, in which conidiophores produce conidia in branched chains, called the Cladosporium type of sporulation (formerly called Hormodendrum type). *Cladosporium carrioni* is one of the fungi causing chromoblastomycosis; *C. mansonii* causes tinea nigra in Asia, and *C. werneckii,* in the Americas. *Cladosporium trichoides* (*C. bantianum*) causes brain and lung abscesses.

clair·voy·ance (klair·voy'unce) *n.* [F., from *clair,* clear, + *voir,* to see]. The direct awareness, with no help from sense impressions, of events taking place in the outside world. See also *extrasensory perception, psi phenomena.*

Clamoxyl. A trademark for clamoxyquin.

clam·ox·y·quin (klam·ock'si·kwin) *n.* 5-Chloro-7-[3-(diethylamino)propylaminomethyl]-8-quinolinol, $C_{17}H_{24}ClN_3O$, an antiamebic drug; used as the dihydrochloride salt.

clamp, *n.* An instrument for holding and compressing vessels or hollow organs to prevent hemorrhage or the escape of contents during the progress of an operation. See also *clip, forceps.*

clang association [Ger. *Klang,* sound]. Association of words or of ideas with words because of their similarity in sound; seen in psychoses, particularly in manic-depressive illness and schizophrenia.

clap, *n.* [OF. *clapoir*]. *Slang.* GONORRHEA.

clap·ping, *n. In massage,* percussion movements in which the cupped palms are brought down alternately in a rapid succession of blows. The movement of the hands is chiefly from the wrist.

Cla·ra cell (klah'rah) [M. *Clara,* Austrian histologist, 20th century]. A cell, present in terminal bronchioles, in which the cytoplasm contains numerous mitochondria.

cla·rif·i·cant (kla·rif'i·kunt) *n.* An agent used to clarify turbid liquids.

clar·i·fy (klăr'i·fye) *v.* To remove the turbidity of a liquid or a naturally transparent substance by allowing the suspended matter to subside, by adding a clarificant or substance that precipitates suspended matter, or by moderate heating. —**clarify·ing,** *adj.*; **clar·i·fi·ca·tion** (klăr"i·fi·kay'shun) *n.*

clarifying agent. CLARIFICANT. Compare *clearing agent.*

Clarke-Had·field syndrome [C. *Clarke;* and G. *Hadfield,* English pathologist, b. 1889]. PANCREATIC INFANTILISM.

Clarke's column [J. A. L. *Clarke,* English physician, 1817–1880]. THORACIC NUCLEUS.

Clarke's dorsal nucleus [J. A. L. *Clarke*]. THORACIC NUCLEUS.

Clark's body area rule [A. *Clark,* U.S. pharmacologist, 20th century]. A rule to determine dosage of medicine for children; specifically, dose = body surface area of child, multiplied by adult dose, divided by body surface area of adult (or 1.7 m^2).

Clark's rule [A. *Clark*]. A rule to determine dosage of medicine for children; specifically, dose = child's weight in pounds, multiplied by adult dose, divided by 150.

Clark's sign [Alonzo *Clark,* U.S. physician, 1807–1887]. A sign of incipient peritonitis in which there is obliteration of liver dullness on percussion, due to tympanites.

Clark technique. A radiographic technique utilized in dentistry to aid in the location of impacted teeth.

Clark test. Carcinoma of the endometrium may be suspected when profuse bleeding occurs following withdrawal of a probe from the uterine canal.

-clasia. See *-clasis.*

-clasis [Gk. *klasis*]. A combining form meaning *breaking, breaking up.*

clas·mato·cyte (klaz·mat'o·site, klaz'muh·to·) *n.* [Gk. *klasma, klasmatos,* fragment, + *-cyte*]. A macrophage of connective tissue. —**clas·mato·cyt·ic** (klaz·mat"o·sit'ick, klaz"muh·to·) *adj.*

clasmatocytic lymphoma. *Obsol.* RETICULUM-CELL SARCOMA.

clas·mo·cy·to·ma (klaz"mo·sigh·to'muh) *n.* [Gk. *klasma,* fragment, + *-cytoma*]. *Obsol.* RETICULUM-CELL SARCOMA.

clasp, *n.* 1. A component of a removable partial denture; it serves as a retentive device by encircling a tooth. 2. *In surgery,* any apparatus to keep tissues together, especially bony structures.

clasp-knife phenomenon, rigidity, or **spasticity.** A form of the stretch reflex in which resistance of a muscle to passive extension is followed by sudden relaxation, like the snapping of a clasp-knife blade; seen especially in spastic hemiparesis.

classic epidemic typhus. EPIDEMIC TYPHUS.

classic typhus. EPIDEMIC TYPHUS.

-clast [Gk. *-klastēs,* -breaker, destroyer]. A combining form meaning *something* (as an instrument) *that breaks.*

clas·tic (klas'tick) *adj.* [Gk. *klastos,* broken]. Breaking up into fragments; causing division.

clastic anatomy. The study of anatomy by means of models in which the different layers can be removed to show the position and relations of the structures underneath.

clas·to·thrix (klas'to·thricks) *n.* [Gk. *klastos,* broken, + *thrix,* hair]. TRICHORRHEXIS NODOSA.

-clasty [*-clast* + *-y*]. A combining form meaning *breaking, breaking up.*

Clat·wor·thy's sign [H. W. *Clatworthy,* Jr., U.S. surgeon, b. 1917]. In a patient with portal hypertension, roentgenographic demonstration of anterior displacement of the duodenum as a result of retroperitoneal edema due to incomplete development of venous collaterals.

Claude's syndrome (klode) [H. C. J. *Claude,* French neuropsychiatrist, 1869–1945]. Ipsilateral oculomotor paresis with contralateral ataxia and hemichorea, caused by a lesion in the central portion of one red nucleus.

clau·di·ca·tion (klaw·di·kay'shun) *n.* [L. *claudicatio,* from *claudicare,* to limp]. 1. Lameness or limping. 2. Specifically, INTERMITTENT CLAUDICATION.

claus·tro·phil·ia (klaws"tro·fil'ee·uh) *n.* [L. *claustrum,* bar, lock, confinement, + *-philia*]. An abnormal desire to shut doors and windows and be shut up in a confined space.

claus·tro·pho·bia (klaws"tro·fo'bee·uh) *n.* [L. *claustrum,* enclosure, confinement, + *phobia*]. An abnormal fear of being in a small room or in a confined space, such as a railway compartment. Contr. *agoraphobia.*

claus·trum (klaws'trum) *n.,* pl. **claus·tra** (·truh) [L., a lock or bar]. 1. A barrier, as a membrane partially closing an opening, or one bearing a resemblance to a barrier. 2. [NA] The layer of gray matter between the insula of the cerebral cortex and the lenticular nucleus. —**claus·tral** (·trul) *adj.*

clau·su·ra (klaw·sue'ruh) *n.* [L., closing, barrier]. ATRESIA.

cla·va (klay'vuh) *n.,* pl. **cla·vae** (·vee) [L., club]. One of the two ovoid eminences in the caudal end of the fourth ventricle, representing continuations of the fasciculus gracilis. Subjacent to the clava is the gracilis nucleus. NA *tuberculum nuclei gracilis.* —**cla·val** (·vul) *adj.*

clav·a·cin (klav'uh·sin) *n.* An antibiotic substance, $C_7H_6O_4$, produced in cultures of several different fungi. Syn. *clavatin, claviformin, patulin.*

cla·vate (klay'vate) *adj.* Club-shaped.

clav·a·tin (klav'uh·tin) *n.* CLAVACIN.

Clav·i·ceps (klav'i·seps) *n.* [L. *clava,* club, + *-ceps,* from *caput,* head]. A genus of fungi. The sclerotium of *Claviceps purpurea,* developed on plants of rye, *Secale cereale,* is the source of ergot.

clav·i·cle (klav'i·kul) *n.* [L. *clavicula,* bolt, fastener, from *clavis,* key]. A bone of the shoulder girdle articulating medially with the sternum and laterally with the acromion of the scapula; the collarbone. NA *clavicula.* See also Table of Bones in the Appendix and Plates 1, 13. —**cla·vic·u·lar** (kla·vick'yoo·lur) *adj.*

clav·i·cot·o·my (klav"i·kot'uh·mee) *n.* [*clavicle* + *-tomy*]. Surgical section of the clavicle.

cla·vi·cu·la (kla·vick'yoo·luh) *n.,* pl. & genit. sing. **clavicu·lae** (·lee) [NA]. CLAVICLE.

clavicular notch. A depression on each superior lateral aspect of the upper end of the sternum for articulation with the clavicles. NA *incisura clavicularis.*

cla·vic·u·late (kla·vick'yoo·late) *adj.* Having a clavicle.

cla·vic·u·lec·to·my (kla·vick"yoo·leck'tuh·mee) *n.* [*clavicula* + *-ectomy*]. *In surgery,* removal of the clavicle, performed in some cases of thyroid cancer or other tumors, osteomyelitis of the clavicle, and limitation of arm motion where the shoulder joint has become fused.

clav·i·for·min (klav"i·for'min) *n.* CLAVACIN.

clavi·pec·to·ral (klav"i·peck'tuh·rul) *adj.* Pertaining to the clavicle and the chest.

clavipectoral fascia. The portion of the deep fascia of the pectoral region which is attached above to the clavicle and coracoid process and which surrounds the subclavius and pectoralis minor muscles. NA *fascia clavipectoralis.*

cla·vus (klay'vus) *n.,* pl. **cla·vi** (·vye) [L., nail]. 1. A corn; a cone-shaped, circumscribed hyperplasia of the horny layer of the epidermis, in which there is an ingrowth as well as an outgrowth of horny substance forming epidermal thickenings, chiefly about the toes; caused by friction or pressure. 2. A severe headache described as the sensation of a nail being driven into the head.

claw foot. TALIPES CAVUS.

claw hand. A deformity, resulting from paralysis of the ulnar and/or median nerve, in which there is hyperextension of the proximal phalanges of the fingers and flexion of the terminal two phalanges, abduction of the fifth finger, and flattening of the hand. It is also seen as an end result of Volkmann's contracture.

Clay·brook's sign [E. B. *Claybrook,* U.S. surgeon, 1871–1931]. A sign for rupture of an abdominal viscus in which the heart and respiratory sounds are clearly heard over the abdominal area.

clay pipe cancer. Carcinoma of the lip and tongue, presumably due to the stem of a clay pipe.

cla·zo·lam (klay'zo·lam) *n.* 2-Chloro-5,9,10,14b-tetrahydro-5-methylisoquino[2,1-*d*][1,4]benzodiazepin-6(7*H*)-one, $C_{18}H_{17}ClN_2O$, a minor tranquilizer.

clear·ance, *n.* The removal of a substance from the blood by the kidneys. See also *clearance test (1).*

clearance test. 1. A test of the excretory efficiency of the kidneys based upon the amount of blood cleared of a substance in 1 minute as determined by the ratio of the substance in the blood to the amount excreted in the urine during a fixed time. 2. A test for liver function based on the ability of the liver to remove a substance from the blood.

clear cell. 1. A nonstaining light chief cell of the parathyroid. Syn. *water-clear cell.* 2. An epidermal cell considered to be of neural origin which has a small, darkly stained nucleus and clear, slightly basophilic cytoplasm in sections stained with hematoxylin and eosin. 3. The parenchymal cell of most renal-cell carcinomas and occasionally of tumors of the parathyroid and ovary. Syn. *celle claire, cellule claire.* See also *nevus cell, melanocyte.*

clear cell carcinoma. RENAL CELL CARCINOMA.

clear·ing, *n.* 1. The displacement of alcohol or other dehydrating agent from tissue blocks by a paraffin solvent, preparatory to paraffin infiltration and embedding of histologic specimens. 2. The displacement of dehydrating agent from a stained section by an essential oil, xylene, or other liquid, to increase the clarity and transparency and prepare the section for mounting in a resinous mounting medium.

clearing agent. *In microscopy,* a substance used to render tissues transparent for mounting.

cleav·age (klee'vij) *n.* 1. The linear clefts in the skin indicating the general direction of the fibers and to a certain extent governing the arrangement of lesions in skin diseases. 2. An early stage of the process of development between fertilization and the blastula, when the embryo consists of a mass of dividing cells, the blastomeres. 3. The process or act of splitting or producing a cleft.

cleavage cavity. BLASTOCOELE.

cleavage cell. BLASTOMERE.

cleavage lines. Lines plotted on the skin to indicate the direction of tension. These lines lie in the direction in which the skin stretches least and are perpendicular to the direction of greatest stretch. Thus, linear scars following the direction of skin tension usually spread little, whereas scars crossing cleavage lines have an opposite tendency.

cleavage nucleus. The nucleus of the ovum which controls or initiates cleavage. It may be syngamic, parthenogenetic, or androgenic.

cleavage plane. 1. The area in a cell or developing ovum where cell division takes place. See also *cleavage.* 2. Any plane in the body along which organs or structures may be separated with minimal damage.

cleavage spindle. A spindle formed during cleavage of the ovum or blastomeres.

cleft, *adj. & n.* 1. Divided. 2. A fissure; especially one of embryonic origin.

cleft cheek. TRANSVERSE FACIAL CLEFT.

cleft foot. A congenital deformity in which the cleft between adjacent toes extends into the metatarsal region.

cleft hand. A congenital deformity of the hand in which the cleft between adjacent fingers extends into the metacarpal region.

cleft lip. HARELIP.

cleft palate. A congenital defect due to failure of fusion of embryonic facial processes resulting in a fissure through the palate. This may be complete, extending through both hard and soft palates into the nose, or any degree of incomplete, or partial, cleft. Often associated with harelip.

cleft sternum. A congenital fissure of the sternum.

cleft tongue. BIFID TONGUE.

cleft uvula. A congenital condition in which the uvula is split into two halves because of the failure of the posterior palatine folds to unite.

cleft vertebra. BUTTERFLY VERTEBRA.

cleid-, cleido- [Gk. *kleis, kleidos,* key, collarbone]. A combining form meaning *clavicle, clavicular.*

cleido-. See *cleid-.*

clei·do·cos·tal (klye"do·kos'tul) *adj.* [*cleido-* + *costal*]. Pertaining to the ribs and the clavicle.

clei·do·cra·ni·al (klye"do·kray'nee·ul) *adj.* [*cleido-* + *cranial*]. Pertaining to the clavicle and the cranium.

cleidocranial dysostosis, dysplasia, or **dystrophia.** A congenital complex consisting of poor tooth formation, incomplete ossification of the skull, malformation of the palatine arch, and more or less aplasia of the clavicles. Other bones may also be involved. The head is often large and brachicephalic, and there is shortness without dwarfism; may be due to a dominant genetic factor.

clei·do·hu·mer·al (klye"do·hew'mur·ul) *adj.* [*cleido-* + *humeral*]. Pertaining to the clavicle and the humerus.

clei·do·hy·oid (klye"do·high'oid) *adj.* [*cleido-* + *hyoid*]. Pertaining to the clavicle and the hyoid bone.

clei·do·ic (klye·do'ick, klye'do·ick) *adj.* [Gk. *kleido*un, to lock up, + *-ic*]. Isolated from the environment; self-contained.

clei·do·mas·toid (klye"do·mas'toid) *adj.* [*cleido-* + *mastoid*]. Pertaining to the clavicle and the mastoid process.

clei·do·oc·cip·i·tal (klye"do·ock·sip'i·tul) *adj.* [*cleido-* + *occipital*]. Pertaining to the clavicle and the occiput.

cleidooccipital muscle. A variable portion of the sternocleidomastoid extending from the occipital bone to the clavicle.

clei·do·scap·u·lar (klye"do·skap'yoo·lur) *adj.* [*cleido-* + *scapular*]. Pertaining to the clavicle and the scapula.

clei·do·ster·nal (klye"do·stur'nul) *adj.* [*cleido-* + *sternal*]. Pertaining to the clavicle and the sternum.

clei·dot·o·my (klye·dot'uh·mee) *n.* [*cleido-* + *-tomy*]. *In obstetrics,* section of the clavicles when the shoulders of the fetus are too broad to pass; an operation performed when the head is delivered, and the child dead.

-cleisis [Gk. *kleisis*]. A combining form meaning *closure, occlusion.*

cleist-, cleisto-, clist-, clisto- [Gk. *kleistos*]. A combining form meaning *closed.*

cleisto-. See *cleist-.*

clei·thro·pho·bia (klye"thro·fo'bee·uh) *n.* [Gk. *kleithron*, bar, + *phobia*]. CLAUSTROPHOBIA.

clem·as·tine (klem'us·teen) *n.* (+)-2-[2-[(*p*-Chloro-α-methyl-α-phenylbenzyl)oxy]ethyl]-1-methylpyrrolidine, $C_{21}H_{26}ClNO$, an antihistaminic drug.

clem·i·zole (klem'i·zole) *n.* 1-(4-Chlorobenzyl)-2-(pyrrolidinylmethyl)-1,3-benzimidazole, $C_{19}H_{20}ClN_3$, an antihistaminic agent; used as the hydrochloride salt.

Cleocin. A trademark for clindamycin, an antibiotic.

cle·oid (klee'oid) *n.* [Gk. *kleis*, key, + *-oid*]. A clawlike instrument used in carving or trimming dental restorations.

cleptomania. KLEPTOMANIA.

cleptophobia. KLEPTOPHOBIA.

Clé·ram·bault-Kan·din·sky complex or **syndrome** (kleʸ·rahⁿ·bo', kaʰn·dʸin'skee) [G. de *Clérambault,* French psychiatrist, 1872–1934; and V. C. *Kandinsky,* Russian psychiatrist, 1825–1889]. In certain psychoses, a state in which the patient feels that his mind is being controlled by another person or an outside influence.

click, *n.* A single or multiple extra heart sound, occurring in systole. See also *ejection click, systolic click.*

clicking rale. A weak, sticky sound heard during inspiration, accompanying the early stages of pulmonary tuberculosis, and caused by air passing through soft material in the smaller bronchi.

cli·din·i·um bromide (kli·din'ee·um). 3-Hydroxy-1-methylquinuclidinium bromide benzilate, $C_{22}H_{26}BrNO_3$, an anticholinergic drug.

clier. CLYER.

cli·ma·co·pho·bia (klye″muh·ko·fo′bee·uh) *n.* [Gk. *klimax, klimakos*, ladder, + *phobia*]. An abnormal fear of steps or staircases.

cli·mac·ter·ic (klye·mack′tur·ick, klye″mack·terr′ick) *n. & adj.* [Gk. *klimaktēr*, a critical point in life, lit., rung of a ladder, from *klimax*, ladder]. 1. A period of life at which the bodily system was believed to undergo marked changes, usually between the ages of 40 to 50; the period in which menopause occurs. See also *male climacteric.* 2. Of or pertaining to this period of life.

climacteric arthritis. MENOPAUSAL ARTHRITIS.

climacteric insanity, melancholia, or **psychosis.** An involutional psychotic disorder occurring at the menopause or at the corresponding age period in men.

cli·mac·te·ri·um (klye″mack·tirr′ee·um) *n.*, pl. **climacte·ria** (·ee·uh) [NL.]. CLIMACTERIC.

cli·mac·tic (klye·mack′tick) *adj.* Of or pertaining to a climax.

cli·mat·ic bubo. LYMPHOGRANULOMA VENEREUM.

cli·ma·tol·o·gy (klye″muh·tol′uh·jee) *n. In medicine*, the study of climate in relation to health and disease.

cli·ma·to·ther·a·py (klye″muh·to·therr′uh·pee) *n.* The treatment of disease by means of a suitable climate.

cli·max, *n.* [Gk. *klimax*, ladder]. 1. The height of a disease; the period of greatest intensity. 2. ORGASM.

climb·ing fibers of the cerebellum. Afferent fibers entering the cerebellar cortex from the white matter, probably through the middle cerebellar peduncle to synapse directly with the dendrites of the Purkinje cells.

clin-, clino- [Gk. *klinein*, to lean]. A combining form meaning (a) *inclination;* (b) *declination;* (c) *clinoid.*

clin·da·my·cin (klin″duh·migh′sin) *n.* 7(*S*)-Chloro-7-deoxylincomycin, $C_{18}H_{33}ClN_2O_5S$, a derivative of the antibiotic lincomycin that has antibacterial and antiparasitic activities.

clin·ic (klin′ick) *n.* [Gk. *klinikos*, from *klinē*, bed]. 1. Medical instruction given at the bedside or in the presence of the patient whose symptoms are studied and whose treatment is considered. 2. A place where such instruction is given. 3. A gathering of instructors, students, and patients for the study and treatment of disease. 4. A place where medical care is given to ambulant patients who live at home. 5. A form of group practice in which several physicians work in cooperative association.

clin·i·cal (klin′i·kul) *adj.* 1. Pertaining to bedside treatment or to a clinic. 2. Pertaining to the symptoms and course of a disease as observed by the physician, in opposition to the anatomic changes found by the pathologist, or to a theoretical or experimental approach.

clinical analysis. 1. Thorough examination of symptoms, lesions, and history to determine the nature of a disease and its cause. 2. Examination of body fluids and tissues for the diagnosis of diseases.

clinical chemistry. The science and practice of the chemical analysis of body tissues to diagnose disease.

clinical crown. The portion of a tooth above the gingival attachment. Contr. *anatomic crown.*

clinical diagnosis. A diagnosis based upon the history and physical examination of the patient, without the aid of laboratory tests.

clinical equivalents. Those chemical equivalents which provide the same therapeutic effects when administered in equal amounts.

clinical immunology. The study of immunological processes and immunologically mediated diseases in patients.

clinical jaundice. Icterus with obvious yellowing of the skin, sclera, and episclera.

clinical medicine. 1. The study of disease of the living patient. 2. The instruction of medical students from living patients.

clinical nurse specialist. A professional nurse with highly developed knowledge and skills in the care of patients within some specialty; ordinarily holds a master's degree in the nursing specialty.

clinical oncology. The study of naturally occurring tumors in patients. Contr. *experimental oncology.*

clinical-pathological conference. A teaching exercise in which a selected example of a disease process is presented by a clinician who does not know the diagnosis, but attempts to make one from the clinical record, while detailing his reasoning to the audience. A pathologist then presents the examination either of autopsy material or of tissue removed at surgery, usually making a definitive diagnosis. Another discussion of interesting points in differential diagnosis, pathogenesis, or treatment follows. Abbreviated, CPC.

clinical pathology. The diagnosis of disease by laboratory methods.

clinical pharmacy. The division of pharmacy concerned principally with the appropriate use of drugs by patients whether prescribed by the physician or self-administered. It involves drug selection and surveillance, and is concerned with patient response, adverse reactions, and the avoidance of undesirable drug interactions in the patient.

clinical psychologist. A psychologist with a graduate degree, usually a Ph.D. who has had additional supervised postdoctoral training, who specializes in clinical psychology.

clinical psychology. A branch of applied psychology which specializes, often in collaboration with physicians and psychiatrists in a medical or mental health setting, in the evaluation and treatment of mental, behavioral, and neurologic disorders, as well as research into psychological aspects of such disorders.

clinical record. A group of forms used by a physician, clinic, or hospital to record a patient's medical history. It covers the results of physical examination, laboratory findings, admission diagnosis, progress of the disease, medications used, consultations, operations performed, and final diagnosis and disposition.

clinical root. The part of a tooth apically from the gingival sulcus. Contr. *anatomic root.*

clinical surgery. Surgery on patients, as opposed to experimental or animal surgery; the application of surgical knowledge to the care of patients.

clinical thermometer. A thermometer used to ascertain the body temperature, so constructed that the maximum reading remains stationary after removal of the thermometer from the patient.

cli·ni·cian (kli·nish′un) *n.* 1. A physician whose opinions, teachings, and treatment are based upon experience with living patients. 2. A clinical instructor. 3. One who practices medicine.

clinico-. A combining form meaning *clinical.*

clin·i·co·hem·a·to·log·ic, clin·i·co·haem·a·to·log·ic (klin″i·ko·hem″uh·to·loj′ick, ·hee″muh·to·) *adj.* [*clinico-* + *hematologic*]. Pertaining to both the clinical evaluation of a patient and examination of his blood.

clin·i·co·pa·thol·o·gy (klin″i·ko·pa·thol′uh·jee) *n.* CLINICAL PATHOLOGY.

clin·i·co·ra·dio·log·ic (klin″i·ko·ray″dee·o·loj′ick) *adj.* CLINICOROENTGENOLOGIC.

clin·i·co·roent·gen·o·log·ic (klin″i·ko·rent″ghin·o·loj′ick) *adj.* Pertaining to the correlation between clinical and roentgenologic examinations of a patient. Syn. *clinicoradiologic.*

clin·i·my·cin (klin″i·migh′sin) *n.* 7(*S*)-Chloro-7-deoxylincomycin, $C_{18}H_{33}ClN_2O_5S$, a derivative of lincomycin with antiparasitic activity.

Clinitest reagent tablet. A trademark for a reagent tablet used to determine the quantity of reducing sugars in urine.

Clinium. Trademark for lidoflazine, a coronary vasodilator.

clino-. See *clin-.*

cli·no·ceph·a·lism (klye″no·sef′uh·liz·um) *n.* CLINOCEPHALY.

cli·no·ceph·a·lus (klye″no·sef′uh·lus) *n.*, **clinocepha·li** (·lye) [*clino-* + *-cephalus*]. An individual having a clinocephalic skull.

cli·no·ceph·a·ly (klye″no·sef′uh·lee) *n.* [*clino-* + *-cephaly*]. A congenital defect of the skull in which the upper surface is concave or saddle-shaped. —**clino·ce·phal·ic** (·se·fal'ick), **clino·ceph·a·lous** (·sef'uh·lus) *adj.*

cli·no·dac·tyl·ism (klye"no·dack'til·iz·um) *n.* [*clino-* + *dactyl-* + *-ism*]. A congenital defect consisting of abnormal bending of fingers or toes. —**clinodacty·lous** (·us) *adj.*

cli·no·dac·ty·ly (klye"no·dack'ti·lee) *n.* [*clino-* + *-dactyly*]. CLINODACTYLISM.

cli·noid (klye'noid) *adj.* [Gk. *klinē*, bed, + *-oid*]. Resembling a bed.

clinoid process. See *anterior clinoid process, middle clinoid process, posterior clinoid process.*

cli·nom·e·ter (klye·nom'i·tur, kli·nom') *n.* CLINOSCOPE.

cli·no·scope (klye'no·skope) *n.* [*clino-* + *-scope*]. An instrument for measuring the torsion of the eyes when gazing at a fixed object with the axes of vision presumably parallel.

cli·ox·a·nide (klye·ock'suh·nide) *n.* 4'-Chloro-3,5-diiodosalicylanilide acetate, $C_{15}H_{10}ClI_2NO_3$, an anthelmintic.

clip, *n.* A device or appliance used in surgery to grip skin or other tissue to secure apposition, to control hemorrhage, or to assist in localization by radiography. Compare *clamp, forceps.*

clipped speech. Speech in which each word is cut short.

cli·pro·fen (klye·pro'fen) *n.* 3-Chloro-4-(2-thenoyl)hydratropic acid, $C_4H_{11}ClO_3S$, an anti-inflammatory agent.

clis·e·om·e·ter (klis"ee·om'e·tur, kliz"ee·) *n.* [Gk. *klisis*, inclination, + *meter*]. An instrument for measuring the degree of inclination of the pelvic axis.

clist-. See *cleist-.*

Clistin. Trademark for carbinoxamine, an antihistaminic drug used as the maleate salt.

clisto-. See *cleist-.*

clit·i·on (klit'ee·on) *n.* [Gk. *klitos*, slope, + *-ion*]. *In craniometry,* a point where the median sagittal plane meets the center of the uppermost margin of the dorsum sellae.

clit·o·ral (klit'uh·rul) *adj.* Of or pertaining to the clitoris.

clit·o·ral·gia (klit"o·ral'juh, ·jee·uh, klye"to·) *n.* [*clitoris* + *-algia*]. Pain referred to the clitoris.

clitorid-, clitorido- [Gk. *kleitoris, kleitoridos*]. A combining form meaning *clitoris.*

clit·o·ri·dauxe (klit"o·ri·dawk'see, klye"to·ri·) *n.* [*clitorid-* + *-auxe*]. Hypertrophy of the clitoris.

clit·o·rid·e·an (klit"o·rid'ee·un, klye"to·) *adj.* CLITORAL.

clit·o·ri·dec·to·my (klit"o·ri·deck'tuh·mee) *n.* [*clitorid-* + *-ectomy*]. Excision of the clitoris.

clit·o·ri·di·tis (klit"o·ri·dye'tis) *n.* [*clitorid-* + *-itis*]. Inflammation of the clitoris.

clitorido-. See *clitorid-.*

clit·o·ri·dot·o·my (klit"o·ri·dot'uh·mee) *n.* [*clitorido-* + *-tomy*]. Incision of the clitoris.

clit·o·ris (klit'o·ris, klye'to·ris) *n.*, genit. sing. **cli·to·ri·dis** (kli·to'ri·dis), L. pl. **cli·to·ri·des** (kli·to'ri·deez) [Gk. *kleitoris*] [NA]. A small erectile organ of the female external genitalia measuring about 2 cm in length and located at the anterior junction of the labia minora; homologous to the penis in the male, but lacking a corpus spongiosum and urethral passage. Adj. *clitoral.*

clitoris crisis. A paroxysm of sexual excitement occurring in women suffering from tabes dorsalis.

clit·o·rism (klit'o·riz·um, klye'to·) *n.* 1. Enlargement or hypertrophy of the clitoris. 2. TRIBADISM. 3. A condition of painful and persistent erection of the clitoris; analogous to priapism in the male.

clit·o·ri·tis (klit"o·rye'tis, klye"to·) *n.* [*clitoris* + *-itis*]. Inflammation of the clitoris.

clit·o·ro·ma·nia (klit"uh·ro·may'nee·uh, klye"tuh·ro·) *n.* [*clitoris* + *mania*]. NYMPHOMANIA.

clit·o·ro·meg·a·ly (klit"uh·ro·meg'uh·lee) *n.* [*clitoris* + *-megaly*]. A pathologically large clitoris.

clit·o·rot·o·my (klit"o·rot'uh·mee) *n.* CLITORIDOTOMY.

clit·or·rha·gia (klit"o·ray'jee·uh) *n.* [*clitoris* + *-rrhagia*]. Hemorrhage from the clitoris.

cli·vus (klye'vus) *n.*, pl. **cli·vi** (·vye) [L., hill]. 1. A slope. 2. [NA] The slanting dorsal surface of the body of the sphenoid bone between the sella turcica and the basilar process of the occipital bone.

clivus mon·ti·cu·li (mon·tick'yoo·lye). DECLIVE OF THE CEREBELLUM.

CL lead. *In electrocardiography,* a precordial (chest) exploring electrode paired with an electrode on the left arm.

clo (klo) *n.* An arbitrary quantitative unit of the thermal insulation value of clothing. *In aviation medicine,* 1 clo is the amount of clothing required to maintain in comfort a resting-sitting human adult male whose metabolic rate is approximately 50 kilogram calories per square meter of body surface per hour, when the environmental temperature is 70° F (21.1° C), and humidity is less than 50%. In terms of absolute thermal insulation units, 1 clo is 0.18° C per square meter per kilogram calorie per hour.

clo·a·ca (klo·ay'kuh) *n.*, pl. **cloa·cae** (·see) [L., sewer]. 1. In the early embryo, the entodermal chamber common to the hindgut and allantois; later to the hindgut and urogenital duct or sinus. 2. In Anamniota, Sauropsida, and aplacental mammals, a common chamber for the rectum and urogenital orifices. —**cloa·cal** (·kul) *adj.*

cloacal duct. The caudal part of the cloaca before the urorectal septum completely divides the rectum and urogenital sinus.

cloacal hillock. GENITAL TUBERCLE.

cloacal membrane. A delicate membrane of ectoderm and endoderm separating the embryonic hindgut from the external or ectodermal cloaca.

cloacal passage. CLOACAL DUCT.

cloacal plate. CLOACAL MEMBRANE.

cloacal septum. URORECTAL SEPTUM.

cloacal tubercle. GENITAL TUBERCLE.

clo·a·co·gen·ic (klo"uh·ko·jen'ick, klo·ay"ko·) *adj.* [*cloaca* + *-genic*]. Originating in vestigial remnants of the embryonic cloaca, as: cloacogenic cancer.

clo·ba·zam (klo'buh·zam) *n.* 7-Chloro-1-methyl-5-phenyl-1*H*-1,5-benzodiazepine-2,4(3*H*,5*H*)-dione, $C_{16}H_{13}ClN_2O_2$, a minor tranquilizer.

clo·cor·to·lone (klo·kor'tuh·lone) *n.* 9-Chloro-6α-fluoro-11β,21-dihydroxy-16α-methylpregna-1,4-diene-3,20-dione, $C_{22}H_{28}ClFO_4$, a glucocorticoid; used as the 21-acetate ester.

clo·dan·o·lene (klo·dan'o·leen) *n.* 1-[[5-(3,4-Dichlorophenyl)furfurylidene]amino]hydantoin, $C_{14}H_9Cl_2N_3O_3$, a skeletal muscle relaxant.

clo·da·zon (klo'duh·zone) *n.* 5-Chloro-1-[3-(dimethylamino)-propyl]-3-phenyl-2-benzimidazolinone, $C_{18}H_{20}ClN_3O$, an antidepressant agent usually employed as the hydrochloride and monohydrate.

clo·faz·i·mine (klo·faz'i·meen) *n.* 3-(*p*-Chloroanilino)-10-(*p*-chlorophenyl)-2,10-dihydro-2-(isopropylimino)phenazine, $C_{27}H_{22}Cl_2N_4$, a tuberculostatic and leprostatic drug.

clo·fi·brate (klo·figh'brate) *n.* Ethyl 2-(*p*-chlorophenoxy)-2-methylpropionate, $C_{12}H_{15}ClO_3$, an anticholesteremic drug.

clo·flu·car·ban (klo"floo·kahr'ban) *n.* 4,4'-Dichloro-3-(trifluoromethyl)carbanilide, $C_{14}H_{19}Cl_2F_3N_2O$, an antifungal and antibacterial agent usually incorporated into disinfectant and deodorant soaps.

clo·ges·tone (klo·jes'tone) *n.* 6-Chloro-3β,17-dihydroxypregna-4,6-dien-20-one, $C_{21}H_{29}ClO_3$, a progestational steroid; used as the diacetate ester.

clo·ma·cran (klo'muh·kran) *n.* 2-Chloro-9-[3-(dimethylamino)propyl]acridan, $C_{18}H_{21}ClN_2$, a tranquilizer; used as the phosphate salt.

clo·me·ges·tone (klo"me·jes'tone) *n.* 6-Chloro-17-hydroxy-16α-methylpregna-4,6-diene-3,20-dione, $C_{22}H_{29}ClO_4$, a progestational steroid; used as the 17-acetate ester.

clo·meth·er·one (klo·meth'ur·ohn) *n.* 6α-Chloro-16α-methylpregn-4-ene-3,20-dione, $C_{22}H_{31}ClO_2$, a steroid with antiestrogen activity.

Clomid. Trademark for clomiphene, a drug that induces ovulation.

clo·min·o·rex (klo·min′o·recks) *n.* 2-Amino-5-(*p*-chlorophenyl)-2-oxazoline, $C_9H_9ClN_2O$, an anorexigenic drug.

clo·mi·phene (klo′mi·feen) *n.* 2-[*p*-(2-Chloro-1,2-diphenylvinyl)phenoxy]triethylamine, $C_{26}H_{28}ClNO$, a drug that induces ovulation and is used, as the citrate salt, for the treatment of infertility associated with anovulation.

clo·mip·ra·mine (klo·mip′ruh·meen) *n.* 3-Chloro-5-[3-(dimethylamino)propyl]-10,11-dihydro-5*H*-dibenz[*b,f*]azepine, $C_{19}H_{23}ClN_2$, an antidepressant agent usually used as the hydrochloride.

clonal selection theory. *In immunology,* the theory that lymphocytes are precommitted to respond to a very limited number of antigens (perhaps only one) by virtue of corresponding antigen-specific receptors on their surfaces.

clo·na·ze·pam (klo·nay′ze·pam) *n.* 5-(*o*-Chlorophenyl)-1,3-dihydro-7-nitro-2*H*-1,4-benzodiazepin-2-one, $C_{15}H_{10}ClN_3O_3$, an anticonvulsant.

clone, *n.* [Gk. *klōn,* twig, slip]. 1. A group of individuals of like genetic constitution obtained by asexual reproduction from a single original individual. Reproduction may occur by continued fission, as in bacteria or protozoa; by continued budding, as in hydras; or by propagation from cuttings, as in plants. See also *pure line.* 2. A group of cells derived from a single cell by repeated mitoses. **—clo·nal** (klo′nul) *adj.*

clo·nic (klo′nick, klon′ick) *adj.* Pertaining to clonus; characterized by rapid involuntary alternate muscular contractions and relaxations, applied especially to generalized seizures. Contr. *tonic (2).*

clon·i·co·ton·ic (klon″i·ko·ton′ick) *adj.* TONIC-CLONIC.

clonic-tonic, *adj.* TONIC-CLONIC.

clo·ni·dine (klo′ni·deen) *n.* 2-(2,6-Dichloroanilino)-2-imidazoline, $C_9H_9Cl_2N_3$, an antihypertensive drug; used as the hydrochloride salt.

clo·ni·trate (klo·nigh′trate) *n.* 3-Chloro-1,2-propanediol dinitrate, $C_3H_5ClN_2O_6$, a coronary vasodilator.

clo·nix·e·ril (klo·nick′se·ril) *n.* 2,3-Dihydroxypropyl 2-(3-chloro-*o*-toluidino)-nicotinate, $C_{16}H_{17}ClN_2O_4$, an analgesic.

clo·nix·in (klo·nick′sin) *n.* 2-(3-Chloro-*o*-toluidino)nicotinic acid, $C_{13}H_{11}ClN_2O_2$, an analgesic.

clo·nor·chi·a·sis (klo″nor·kigh′uh·sis) *n.* [*Clonorchi*s + *-iasis*]. An infection caused by *Clonorchis sinensis,* characterized by hepatic lesions produced by adult worms in the biliary passages.

clo·nor·chi·o·sis (klo·nor″kee·o′sis) *n.*, pl. **clonorchio·ses** (·seez) [*Clonorchi*s + *-osis*]. CLONORCHIASIS.

Clo·nor·chis (klo·nor′kis, klon·or′kis) *n.* [Gk. *klōn,* twig, + *orchis*]. A genus of flukes indigenous to the Orient.

Clonorchis si·nen·sis (si·nen′sis). The most common of the liver flukes, having as definitive hosts man or other mammals.

clo·nus (klo′nus) *n.* [Gk. *klonos,* turmoil]. A series of rapid rhythmic contractions of a muscle occurring in response to maintained passive stretch of the muscle, as ankle clonus, patellar clonus. Compare *tonus.* Adj. *clonic.* **—clo·nic·i·ty** (klo·nis′i·tee) *n.*

C-loop. A surgically constructed loop of bowel in the shape of the letter C.

clo·pam·ide (klo·pam′ide) *n.* 4-Chloro-*N*-(2,6-dimethylpiperidino)-3-sulfamoylbenzamide, $C_{14}H_{20}ClN_3O_3S$, an antihypertensive drug.

Clopane. Trademark for cyclopentamine, a sympathomimetic amine used as the hydrochloride salt.

clo·pen·thix·ol (klo″pen·thick′sol) *n.* 4-[3-(2-Chlorothioxanthen-9-ylidene)propyl]-1-piperazineethanol, $C_{22}H_2$-ClN_2OS, a tranquilizer.

clo·per·i·done (klo·perr′i·dohn) *n.* 3-[3-[4-(*m*-Chlorophenyl)-1-piperazinyl]propyl]-2,4-(1*H*,3*H*)-quinazolinedione, $C_{21}H_{23}ClN_4O_2$, a sedative and tranquilizer; used as the hydrochloride salt.

clo·pi·dol (klo′pi·dole) *n.* 3,5-Dichloro-2,6-dimethyl-4-pyridinol, $C_7H_7Cl_2NO$, a poultry coccidiostat.

clo·pim·o·zide (klo·pim′o·zide) *n.* 1-[1-[4,4-Bis(*p*-fluorophenyl)butyl]-4-piperidyl]-5-chloro-2-benzimidazolinone, $C_{28}H_{28}ClF_2N_3O$, a neuroleptic or major tranquilizer of long duration.

clo·pi·rac (klo′pi·rack) *n.* 1-(*p*-Chlorophenyl)-2,5-dimethylpyrrole-3-acetic acid, $C_{14}H_{14}ClNO_2$, an anti-inflammatory agent.

clo·pred·nol (klo·pred′nole) *n.* 6-Chloro-11β,17,21-trihydroxypregna-1,4,6-triene-3,20-dione, $C_{21}H_{25}ClO_5$, a glucocorticoid steroid agent.

Clo·quet's canal (kloh·keh′) [J. G. *Cloquet,* French anatomist, 1790–1883]. HYALOID CANAL.

Cloquet's ganglion [J. G. *Cloquet*]. A plexiform intermingling of fibers of the two nasopalatine nerves in the incisive canal. It is not a true ganglion.

Cloquet's node or **gland** [J. G. *Cloquet*]. The highest deep inguinal lymph node situated in the femoral ring.

Clorarsen. A trademark for dichlorophenarsine hydrochloride.

clor·a·zep·ic acid (klor″uh·zep′ick). 7-Chloro-2,3-dihydro-2,2-dihydroxy-5-phenyl-1*H*-1,4-benzodiazepine-3-carboxylic acid, $C_{16}H_{13}ClN_2O_4$, a tranquilizer; used as the dipotassium salt.

clor·eth·ate (klor·eth′ate, klor′eth·ate) *n.* Bis(2,2,2-trichloroethyl) carbonate, $C_5H_4Cl_6O_3$, a sedative and hypnotic.

clor·ex·o·lone (klor·eck′so·lone) *n.* 6-Chloro-2-cyclohexyl-3-oxo-5-isoindolinesulfonamide, $C_{14}H_{17}ClN_2O_3S$, a diuretic drug.

clor·o·phene (klor′o·feen) *n.* 4-Chloro-α-phenyl-*o*-cresol, $C_{13}H_{11}ClO$, a disinfectant.

clor·pren·a·line (klor·pren′uh·leen) *n.* *o*-Chloro-α-[(isopropylamino)methyl]benzyl alchohol, $C_{11}H_{16}ClNO$, a bronchodilator drug; used as the hydrochloride salt.

clor·ter·mine (klor·tur′meen) *n.* *o*-Chloro-α,α-dimethylphenethylamine, $C_{10}H_{14}ClN$, an anorexiant drug; used as the hydrochloride salt.

closed anesthesia. Inhalation anesthesia with complete rebreathing of the anesthetic gases. Soda-lime generally is used to absorb the excess carbon dioxide.

closed bite. An extreme overbite in which the lower incisors and canines are posterior to the upper, almost touching the gum line when the jaws are closed.

closed-chain, *adj.* Pertaining to or designating an organic compound in which the carbon (or substituent) atoms are bonded so as to form a closed ring. See also *carbocyclic.*

closed-chest cardiac massage. Cardiac massage in the unopened chest by rhythmic compression of the heart between the sternum and vertebral column. Contr. *open-chest cardiac massage.*

closed-circuit anesthesia. Anesthesia produced by an anesthetizing apparatus in which explosive agents used in anesthesia are prevented from coming in contact with sparks or flames.

closed circulation theory. The theory that in the spleen blood moves directly from the arteries of the ellipsoids, through capillaries, into the venous sinusoids. Blood escapes into the pulp through openings in the walls of the sinusoids. Contr. *open circulation theory.*

closed fracture. SIMPLE FRACTURE.

closed gland. *Obsol.* ENDOCRINE GLAND.

closed hospital. A hospital in which only physicians who are members of the hospital staff may practice.

closed pneumothorax. A pneumothorax which does not communicate with the lung and has no opening through the chest wall.

closed reduction. Reduction of a fractured bone, performed without making a surgical incision.

closed tuberculosis. INACTIVE TUBERCULOSIS.

closing plate. Any epithelial membrane, usually bilaminar, closing a potential orifice; especially one separating a visceral groove and pouch.

clo·sir·a·mine (klo·sirr′uh·meen) *n.* 8-Chloro-11-[2-(dimethylamino)ethyl]-6,11-dihydro-5*H*-benzo[5,6]cyclohepta[1,2-*b*]pyridine, $C_{18}H_{21}ClN_2$, an antihistaminic agent usually used as the aceturate (*N*-acetyglycine) salt.

Clos·trid·i·um (klos·trid'ee·um, klo·strid') *n.* [NL., dim. from Gk. *klōstēr,* spindle]. A genus of anaerobic spore-bearing bacteria of ovoid, spindle, or club shape; widely distributed in nature. —**clostridium,** pl. **clostrid·ia,** *com. n.;* **clostridi·al,** *adj.*

Clostridium bot·u·li·num (bot''yoo·lye'num). A species of *Clostridium* that produces a very powerful toxin in food which when ingested may cause toxemia. The species includes types A, B, E, and F, the principal causes of human botulism; type Cβ, the cause of forage poisoning of cattle in Australia; and type D, the cause of lamzietke in cattle in Africa.

***Clostridium botulinum* A.** A type of the species that produces botulism in man and limberneck in chickens, found predominantly in the Rocky Mountain and Pacific Coast states and in English soils.

***Clostridium botulinum* B.** A type that produces botulism in man and limberneck in chickens, found most commonly in the Mississippi Valley, Great Lakes region, and Atlantic Coast states.

***Clostridium botulinum* Cα.** A type that causes paralysis in chickens and produces botulism in wild ducks.

Clostridium chau·voei (sho·vo'eye). A species of *Clostridium* that is the principal cause of blackleg in cattle and occasionally sheep, goats, and swine.

Clostridium his·to·lyt·i·cum (his·to·lit'i·kum). A species of *Clostridium* that is gram-positive, anaerobic, saccharolytic and proteolytic, and forms terminal oval spores; may produce invasive infection of wounds.

Clostridium no·vyi (no'vee·eye). A species of *Clostridium* that includes a type A found in gas gangrene, and types B and C which produce a strong soluble toxin.

Clostridium para·bot·u·li·num equi (păr''uh·bot·yoo·lye'num eck'wye). *CLOSTRIDIUM BOTULINUM* type D.

Clostridium per·frin·gens (pur·frin'jenz). A species of plump, nonmotile, gram-positive rod, occurring in chains and singly, that produces a variety of toxins and is the most important cause of gas gangrene as well as the cause of dysentery of sheep. The species includes type A, the principal cause of gas gangrene in man; type B, the cause of lamb dysentery; type C, the cause of struck in sheep; types D and E, the cause of enterotoxemia of sheep.

Clostridium sep·ti·cum (sep'ti·kum). A species of *Clostridium* sometimes found in gas gangrene, in braxy of sheep, malignant edema of cattle, and also in some cases of blackleg in cattle.

Clostridium spo·rog·e·nes (spo·roj'e·neez). A species of *Clostridium* frequently found as a contaminant in deep wounds; it is generally considered to be nonpathogenic but may cause foul odor in such wounds.

Clostridium tet·a·ni (tet'uh·nigh). A species of *Clostridium* that causes tetanus and is present in soil and in human and animal intestines; characterized by spherical terminal spores and the production of tetanus toxin, a potent exotoxin.

Clostridium wel·chii (wel'chee·eye). *CLOSTRIDIUM PERFRINGENS.*

clo·sure, n. 1. The act of completing or closing an electric circuit. Abbreviated, C. 2. The closing of a wound by suture.

clo·syl·ate (klo'sil·ate) *n.* Any salt or ester of *p*-chlorobenzenesulfonic acid, $ClC_6H_4SO_2OH$; a *p*-chlorobenzenesulfonate.

clot, *n. & v.* 1. The semisolid mass that forms as the result of coagulation, as of blood or lymph. Syn. *coagulum.* 2. To form a clot; to coagulate.

clo·thi·a·pine (klo·thigh'uh·peen) *n.* 2-Chloro-11-(4-methyl-1-piperazinyl)dibenzo[*b,f*][1,4]thiazepine, $C_{18}H_{18}ClN_3S$, a tranquilizer.

clo·thix·a·mide (klo·thick'suh·mide) *n.* 4-[3-(2-Chlorothioxanthen-9-ylidene)propyl]-*N*-methyl-1-piperazinepropionamide, $C_{24}H_{28}ClN_3OS$, a tranquilizer; used as the maleate salt.

clot retraction. The contraction or shrinkage of a blood clot resulting in the extrusion of serum. A function of blood platelets within the fibrin network.

clot-retraction time. The length of time required under standard conditions, for the appearance or completion of clot retraction.

clo·trim·a·zole (klo·trim'uh·zole) *n.* 1-[(2-Chlorophenyl)diphenylmethyl]-1*H*-imidazole, $C_{22}H_{17}ClN_2$, a broad-spectrum antifungal agent demonstrating activity against dermatophytes.

clot·ting time. The length of time required, under standard conditions, for shed blood to coagulate.

cloud chamber. An apparatus for studying ionizing rays. When nuclear particles, such as alpha particles, are shot into a chamber containing supersaturated water vapor, the particle produces gas ions, each of which condenses a droplet of water, thus marking the path of the particle.

cloud·ed, *adj.* 1. Unclear, disordered, as of mental or sensory processes. 2. Blurred, indistinct.

Cloud·man melanoma S91. A transmissible malignant melanoma which arose spontaneously at the base of the tail of a female DBA mouse.

cloudy swelling. A retrogressive change in the cytoplasm of parenchymatous cells, whereby the cell enlarges and the outline becomes irregular. These changes lead to gross swelling of the organ and obscuring of its usual features.

clove, *n.* The dried flower bud of *Eugenia caryophyllata;* contains volatile oil and caryophyllin, a lactone. Clove is stimulant; it has been used in nausea and vomiting and to correct flatulence.

clove-hitch knot. A knot formed of two contiguous loops, placed around an object, such as a limb, the ends of the cord parallel and extending in opposite directions. This knot remains firm only so long as traction is applied.

clove oil. The volatile oil from clove; contains eugenol. It is a local anesthetic, a powerful germicide, and a local irritant.

clo·ver·leaf deformity. Roentgenologically, a disfigured duodenal bulb, having roughly the appearance of a three-leaf clover; due to contraction of scar tissue following, or associated with, chronic duodenal ulcer.

cloverleaf nail. An intramedullary nail which in cross section is shaped like a clover leaf; used particularly for internal fixation of fractures of the femur.

cloverleaf skull deformity syndrome. Intrauterine synostosis of the coronal and lambdoidal sutures associated with hydrocephalus, possibly secondary to platybasia. There is a grotesque trilobed skull, downward displacement of the ears, exophthalmos, secondary corneal damage, beak nose, prognathism, and frequently other associated skeletal deformities.

clown·ism, *n.* An emotional display with grotesque contortions; seen in certain neuroses, such as hysteroepilepsy.

clox·a·cil·lin (klock''suh·sil'in) *n.* 3-(*o*-Chlorophenyl)-5-methyl-4-isoxazolylpenicillin, $C_{19}H_{18}ClN_3O_5S$, a semisynthetic penicillin antibiotic; used as the sodium salt.

clox·y·quin (klock'si·kwin) *n.* 5-Chloro-8-quinolinol, C_9H_6ClNO, an antibacterial agent.

clo·za·pine (klo'zuh·peen) *n.* 8-Chloro-11-(4-methyl-1-piperazinyl)-5*H*-dibenzo[*b,e*][1,4]diazepine, $C_{18}H_{19}ClN_4$, a sedative.

CLSH Abbreviation for *corpus luteum-stimulating hormone* (= LUTEINIZING HORMONE).

clubbed, *adj.* Characterizing an extremity or structure that is gnarled, misshapen, or bulbous.

clubbed finger. A finger with bulbous enlargement of the terminal phalanx, a curved nail, and with or without osseous change.

club·bing, *n.* The condition of having a clubbed part or structure.

club·foot, *n.* A congenital malformation, either single or bilateral, in which the forefoot is inverted and rotated, accompanied by shortening of the calcaneal tendon and contracture of the plantar fascia. See also *talipes.*

club·hand, *n.* A congenital deformity of the hand characterized by one of the following distortions: (a) palmar displacement with or without radial or ulnar deviation; (b) dorsal displacement with or without radial or ulnar deviation. The deformity may be due to contracture of ligaments and muscles, or it may be caused by defective development of the radius, ulna, or carpal bones. The most common form of clubhand is caused by defective development of the radius, producing radial and palmar distortion.

club moss. LYCOPODIUM.

club motor. A plastic motor whose point of attachment is to a prepared knob of tissue.

clump kidney. CAKE KIDNEY.

clumsy child syndrome. MINIMAL BRAIN DYSFUNCTION SYNDROME.

clu·ne·al (kloo'nee·ul) *adj.* [*clunes* + *-al*]. Pertaining to the buttocks.

clu·nes (kloo'neez) *n. pl.* [L.] [NA alt.]. BUTTOCKS. NA alt. *nates.*

clu·pan·o·don·ic acid (kloo·pan''o·don'ick). Docosapentaenoic acid, acid $C_{22}H_{34}O_2$, an unsaturated acid obtained from certain fish oils.

clu·pe·ine (kloo'pee·een, ·in) *n.* A protamine, having a molecular weight of approximately 4400, obtained from herring roe.

Clu·sia (kloo'zhuh, ·zee·uh) *n.* [C. de *Lécluse,* French botanist, 1526–1609]. A genus of plants of the Guttiferae, many species of which yield a gum resin called West Indian balsam.

clus·ter, *n.* A number of similar things considered as a group because of their relation to each other or simultaneity of occurrence.

cluster headache. A type of headache that occurs predominantly in males, characterized by intense, unilateral orbital pain, lasting 30 to 60 minutes and recurring, usually nightly, for several weeks, followed by complete freedom for months or years; formerly attributed to release of histamine. Syn. *paroxysmal nocturnal cephalgia, migrainous neuralgia, Horton's headache.*

Clute's incision [H. M. *Clute,* U.S. surgeon, 1890–1946]. An abdominal incision for repair of diaphragmatic hernia.

clut·ter·ing, *n.* A developmental disorder of speech characterized by an uncontrollably hurried delivery resulting in dysrhythmia and the omission of phonetic segments.

Clut·ton's joints [H. H. *Clutton,* English surgeon, 1850–1909]. Symmetrical bilateral hydrarthrosis of the knees occurring in congenital syphilis.

cly·er, cli·er (kligh'ur) *n.* [D. *klier,* gland]. A scrofulous tumor in cattle, produced by tuberculous infection.

cly·sis (klye'sis) *n.,* pl. **cly·ses** (·seez) [Gk. *klysis,* from *klyzein,* to wash]. 1. Administration of an enema; cleansing by means of an enema. 2. Subcutaneous or intravenous administration of fluids.

Clysodrast. A trademark for bisacodyl tannex.

clys·ter (klis'tur) *n.* [Gk. *klystēr*]. ENEMA.

Cm Symbol for curium.

cm Abbreviation for *centimeter.*

CM-cellulose. Abbreviation for *carboxymethylcellulose.*

CMP Abbreviation for *cytidine monophosphate* (= CYTIDYLIC ACID).

cnemic index. The ratio of the mediolateral (transverse) diameter of the diaphysis of the tibia (distance between the medial margin and the interosseous crest × 100) to the dorsoventral (sagittal) diameter (distance between the crista anterior and the facies posterior), both diameters taken at the level of the nutrient foramen. Values of the index are classified as platycnemic, x-64.9; mesocnemic, 65.0-69.9; eurycnemic, 70.0-x.

cne·mis (nee'mis) *n.,* pl. **cnem·i·des** (nem'i·deez) [Gk. *knēmē*]. The shin or tibia. —**cne·mic** (nee'mick) *adj.*

Cni·dar·ia (nigh·dăr'ee·uh) *n. pl.* [NL., from Gk. *knidē,* nettle, sea-nettle]. COELENTERATA.

CNS Abbreviation for *central nervous system.*

Co Symbol for cobalt.

co- [L.]. A prefix meaning (a) *with, together, jointly, mutual;* (b) *to the same degree.*

CoA Abbreviation for *coenzyme A.*

co·ac·er·vate (ko·as'ur·vate, ko''a·sur'vate) *n.* [L. *coacervare,* to heap up]. The product formed when two hydrophilic colloids of opposite sign are mixed and form a stable particle which may form a separate phase. —**co·ac·er·va·tion** (ko·as''ur·vay'shun) *n.*

co·ad·ap·ta·tion (ko''ad·ap·tay'shun) *n.* [*co-* + *adaptation*]. Correlated variation in two mutually dependent organs.

coagula. Plural of *coagulum.*

co·ag·u·la·ble (ko·ag'yoo·luh·bul) *adj.* Capable of coagulating or being coagulated. —**co·ag·u·la·bil·i·ty** (ko·ag''yoo·luh·bil'i·tee) *n.*

co·ag·u·lant (ko·ag'yoo·lunt) *adj. & n.* 1. Causing the formation of a clot or coagulum. 2. An agent that causes formation of a clot or coagulum.

co·ag·u·lase (ko·ag'yoo·lace, ·laze) *n.* [*coagul*ate + *-ase*]. A protein elaborated by cultures of *Staphylococcus aureus* which reacts with prothrombin or a closely related substance of plasma (the coagulase reacting factor) to cause plasma coagulation by converting fibrinogen to fibrin.

coagulase test. A test to determine the potential pathogenicity of staphylococci. Cultures of *Staphylococcus aureus* elaborate a protein, coagulase, which clots human or rabbit plasma in the presence of anticoagulants, but cultures of *Staphylococcus epidermidis* do not.

co·ag·u·late (ko·ag'yoo·late) *v.* [L. *coagulare*]. To change, or cause to change, from a fluid to a gelatinous or semisolid state, especially by agglutination of colloidal particles.

co·ag·u·lat·ed proteins. A class of protein derivatives produced by heating solutions of various proteins. Coagulation of protein is believed to involve a preliminary denaturation which is followed by precipitation.

co·ag·u·lat·ing enzyme. An enzyme, such as renin, that converts soluble proteins into insoluble products.

co·ag·u·la·tion (ko·ag''yoo·lay'shun) *n.* The change from a fluid to a gelatinous or semisolid state, especially by agglutination of colloidal particles.

coagulation factor. Any factor in the blood or plasma that contributes to the coagulation of blood. For specific factors, see *factor I* to *factor XIII.*

coagulation necrosis. A variety of necrosis characterized by cell death in situ with preservation of cell form and arrangement; most frequent in infarction. Contr. *liquefaction necrosis.*

coagulation time. CLOTTING TIME.

coagulation vitamin. VITAMIN K.

co·ag·u·la·tive (ko·ag'yoo·lay''tiv) *adj.* 1. Having the nature of coagulation. 2. Associated with coagulation.

co·ag·u·lo·grams (ko·ag'yoo·lo·gramz) *n. Colloq.* A series of tests that indicate changes that occur during blood coagulation and fibrinolysis.

co·ag·u·lop·a·thy (ko·ag''yoo·lop'·uh·thee) *n.* Any disorder of blood coagulation.

co·ag·u·lum (ko·ag'yoo·lum) *n.,* pl. **coagu·la** (·luh) [L.]. The semisolid mass that forms as the result of coagulation. Syn. *clot.*

coagulum pyelolithotomy. Removal of calculi from the renal collecting system using clotted blood or blood products to entrap the calculi.

Coak·ley's operation [C. G. *Coakley,* U.S. laryngologist, 1862–1934]. Removal of the anterior sinus wall and curettage of the sinus cavity, for relief of sinusitis; no longer in use.

co·a·lesce (ko·uh·less') *v.* [L. *coalescere*]. 1. To unite or bring together previously separate parts or things. 2. To grow together or unite by growth.

co·a·les·cence (ko″uh·les′unce) *n.* The union of two or more parts or things previously separate. —**coales·cent** (·unt) *adj.*

coal min·er's disease. ANTHRACOSILICOSIS.

coal oil. KEROSENE OIL.

coal tar. A by-product in the destructive distillation of coal; a black, viscid fluid. Among the products obtained from coal tar by distillation are anthracene, benzene, naphtha, creosote, phenol, and pitch. From the basic oil of coal tar are manufactured the aniline or coal-tar colors or dyes. Preparations of coal tar are employed locally to relieve itching and in the treatment of certain skin diseases.

co·ap·ta·tion (ko″ap·tay′shun) *n.* [L. *coaptatio*]. The proper union or adjustment of displaced parts, such as the ends of a fractured bone or the lips of a wound. —**co·apt** (ko·apt′) *v.;* **coapt·ing,** *adj.*

coaptation splint. A series of narrow splints of uniform size placed parallel to one another and held by adhesive plaster or leather, used to envelop a limb, such as the upper arm or thigh, where uniform and complete support is desired in the area covered.

coapting suture. A suture that brings the divided skin edges accurately together.

co·arct (ko·ahrkt′) *v.* [L. *coarctare*, to confine, crowd]. To narrow or constrict (especially, the lumen of a blood vessel). —**coarct·ed,** *adj.*

co·arc·tate (ko·ahrk′tate) *adj. & v.* [L. *coarctatus*]. 1. Crowded together. 2. COARCT.

coarctate retina. The condition caused by an effusion of liquid between the retina and the choroid; it gives the retina a funnel shape.

co·arc·ta·tion (ko″ahrk·tay′shun) *n.* Narrowing or stricture of a vessel, as the aorta, or of a canal.

co·arc·tot·o·my (ko″ahrk·tot′uh·mee) *n.* [*coarct*ation + *-tomy*]. The cutting of a stricture.

coarse nodular cirrhosis. Fibrosis of the liver with large regenerative nodules, often the sequel of severe necrosis resulting from viral hepatitis.

coarse, *adj.* Involving movement through a relatively wide range. Said of tremors and other involuntary oscillatory movement of skeletal muscle. Contr. *fine.*

co·ar·tic·u·la·tion (ko″ahr·tick″yoo·lay′shun) *n.* [*co-* + *articulation*]. SYNOVIAL JOINT.

coat, *n.* A cover or membrane covering a part or substance.

coat·ing, *n.* A covering or layer of a substance, as of a wound or the tongue, or of a capsule or tablet.

coat-sleeve amputation. An amputation in which one long skin flap, like a coat sleeve, is left to enclose the stump.

Coats's disease [G. *Coats,* English ophthalmologist, 1876–1915]. RETINITIS EXUDATIVA.

co·bal·a·min (ko·bawl′uh·min) *n.* [*cobal*t + vita*min*]. 1. Generic name for members of the vitamin B_{12} family, as cyanocobalamin and hydroxocobalamin. 2. The portion of the molecule of crystalline vitamin B_{12} (cyanocobalamin), exclusive of the cyano group, occurring in all vitamin B_{12} analogues.

co·balt (ko′bawlt) *n.* [Ger. *Kobold*]. Co = 58.9332. A hard, gray, ductile metal used in alloys. It is a component of cyanocobalamin; lack of the element may result in anemia. It appears to effect more complete utilization of iron in hemoglobin synthesis. Polycythemia has been produced in animals by administration of cobalt. Larger doses of soluble salts are emetic, due to local irritant effect. See also Table of Elements in the Appendix.

cobalt 60. A radioactive isotope of cobalt, the radiation from which is employed in the treatment of cancer. This isotope, of atomic weight 60, has a half-life of 5.27 years and emits beta and gamma rays.

co·bal·ti·ni·trite (ko″bawl·ti·nigh′trite) *n.* Any complex salt containing cobalt and nitrite in an anion of the composition $[Co(NO_2)_6]^{-3}$.

cobaltinitrite reaction for potassium. A reaction that demonstrates presence of potassium in biological specimens and other materials by the formation of birefringent crystals of potassium cobaltinitrite by interaction of the substance being tested with a solution containing sodium cobaltinitrite.

co·bal·tous (ko·bawl′tus) *adj.* [*cobalt* + *-ous*]. Pertaining to, or containing cobalt in the bivalent state.

co·ba·mide (ko′buh·mide) *n.* Any of the class of physiologically active compounds with a dimethylbenzimidazoyl nucleus, characteristic of cyanocobalamin.

cob·bler's chest. FUNNEL CHEST.

cob·ble·stone nevus. An anomaly of dermal connective tissue that produces a clinical appearance of cobbled paving stones on the overlying cutaneous surface.

Cobefrin. Trademark for nordefrin, a vasoconstrictor used as the hydrochloride salt.

Cobione. A trademark for cyanocobalamin.

co·bra (ko′bruh) *n.* [Pg. *cobra* (*de capello*), (hooded) snake]. Any one of several species of snakes of the genus *Naja* and related genera.

cobra head sign. In cystography, a radiolucent halo that appears around the stenotic internal orifice of the ureter, caused by dilatation of its intramural portion; seen in ureterocele. Syn. *spring onion sign.*

cobra lec·i·thid (les′i·thid). A hemolytic compound (lecithinase) formed by cobra venom and the lecithin of the host cells.

co·bra·ly·sin (ko″bruh·lye′sin, ko·bral′i·sin) *n.* [*cobra* + *lysin*]. The hemolytic toxin of cobra venom. It is a lecithinase destroyed by heat and neutralized by antivenin.

co·ca (ko′kuh) *n.* [Sp., from Quechua *kuka*]. The leaves of the shrubs *Erythroxylon coca, E. truxillense,* or *E. novogranatense,* containing cocaine and other alkaloids.

co·caine (ko·kane′) *n.* [*coca* + *-ine*]. Methylbenzoylecgonine, $C_{17}H_{21}NO_4$, an alkaloid obtained from the leaves of *Erythroxylon coca* and other species of *Erythroxylon;* occurs as colorless to white crystals, or white, crystalline powder; slightly soluble in water. For most purposes the hydrochloride is preferred to the base. The base is used in ointments and oily solution because of its greater solubility in fatty vehicles. —**cocain·ist** (·ist) *n.;* **cocain·ize** (·ize) *v.*

cocaine bug. Paresthesia caused by cocaine poisoning, commonly described as insects crawling on the skin.

cocaine hydrochloride. The hydrochloride of the alkaloid cocaine; occurs as colorless crystals, or as white, crystalline powder; very soluble in water. Locally cocaine is a paralyzant to the peripheral ends of the sensory nerves, to a lesser degree to the motor nerves, and stimulating to the muscular coats of blood vessels. Systemically it is stimulant to all parts of the central nervous system. The most important use of cocaine is as a local application to mucous membranes, either for the purpose of contracting blood vessels or of lessening sensation. Continued use internally causes addiction. See also *cocainism.*

cocaine nitrate. A salt, similar to cocaine hydrochloride, useful in formulations in which chloride ion may provide chemical incompatibility (as with silver salts).

co·cain·ism (ko·kain′iz·um, ko·kay′in·iz·um) *n.* 1. The habitual use of or addiction to cocaine. 2. The mental and systemic disturbances resulting from the habitual use of cocaine. See also *cocainomania.*

co·caino·ma·nia (ko·kain″o·may′nee·uh, ko·kay″in·o·) *n.* [*cocaine* + *mania*]. 1. The habit of using cocaine. 2. Mental derangement due to cocaine addiction. —**cocainoma·ni·ac** (·nee·ack) *n.*

co·car·box·yl·ase (ko″kahr·bock′sil·ace, ·aze) *n.* Thiamine pyrophosphate, the coenzyme or prosthetic component of carboxylase; catalyzes decarboxylation of various α-keto acids, as pyruvic and α-ketoglutaric.

co·car·ci·no·gen (ko″kahr′si·no·jen, ·kahr·sin′o·) *n.* [*co-* + *carcinogen*]. A noncarcinogenic agent which augments the carcinogenic process.

co·car·ci·no·gen·e·sis (ko″kahr″si·no·jen′e·sis) *n.* The induction of a tumor with the participation of a cocarcinogen.

cocc-, cocci-, cocco- [Gk. *kokkos*]. A combining form meaning (a) *grain, seed;* (b) *coccus.*

coc·cal (kock′ul) *adj.* Pertaining to or caused by a coccus.

cocci. Plural of *coccus.*

cocci-. See *cocc-.*

coccidi-, coccidio-. A combining form meaning *coccidium, coccidia.*

coccidia. Plural of *coccidium.*

Coc·cid·ia (kock·sid′ee·uh) *n. pl.* An order or group of cell parasites of the class Sporozoa; common in many vertebrates and invertebrates but rare in man.

coc·cid·i·al (kock·sid′ee·ul) *adj.* Pertaining to or caused by coccidia.

coccidio-. See *coccidi-.*

coc·cid·i·oi·dal (kock·sid″i·oy′dul) *adj.* Pertaining to, or caused by fungi of the genus *Coccidioides.*

coccidioidal granuloma. PROGRESSIVE COCCIDIOIDOMYCOSIS.

Coc·cid·i·oi·des (kock·sid″ee·oy′deez) *n.* [*coccidi-* + L. *-oides*, from Gk. *eidos*, form]. A genus of parasitic fungi found in soil and pathogenic for many animals, characterized by branching mycelia with arthrospores on artificial cultivation and by endosporulating spherules in tissues.

Coccidioides im·mi·tis (i·migh′tis). The causative agent of coccidioidomycosis. The organism is spheroid, nonbudding, and endosporulating in the tissues; it produces branching, septate, aerial hyphae and arthrospores in culture.

coc·cid·i·oi·din (kock·sid″ee·oy′din) *n.* [*Coccidioides* + *-in*]. The sterile filtrate of cultures of *Coccidioides immitis* grown on a synthetic medium, used as a skin-testing material for the detection of delayed hypersensitivity to the infection and as the antigen in complement-fixation and precipitin tests.

coc·cid·i·oi·do·my·co·sis (kock·sid″ee·oy″do·migh·ko′sis) *n.* [*Coccidioides* + *mycosis*]. An infection or disease endemic in southwestern United States, Mexico, and some areas of South America, generally acquired by inhalation of the spores of *Coccidioides immitis.* See also *disseminated coccidioidomycosis, primary coccidioidomycosis.*

coc·cid·i·oi·do·sis (kock·sid″ee·oy·do′sis) *n.*, [*Coccidioides* + *-osis*]. COCCIDIOIDOMYCOSIS.

coc·cid·i·o·sis (kock·sid″ee·o′sis) *n.* [*coccidi-* + *-osis*]. A usually self-limited intestinal infection by a coccidium, *Isospora hominis* or *I. belli*, characterized by watery, mucoid diarrhea; most common in the tropics.

coc·cid·io·stat (kock·sid′ee·o·stat) *n.* [*coccidio-* + *-stat*]. Any agent that arrests or hinders the growth of a pathogenic coccidium to a degree sufficient for prophylactic or therapeutic treatment of disease caused by the organism.

coc·cid·io·stat·ic (kock·sid″ee·o·stat′ick) *adj.* [*coccidio-* + *-static*]. Arresting or hindering the growth of coccidia.

coc·cid·i·um (kock·sid′ee·um) *n.*, pl. **coccid·ia** (·uh) [NL., diminutive of *coccus*]. Any organism of the order Coccidia.

cocco-. See *cocc-.*

coc·co·ba·cil·lary (kock″o·bas′i·lerr·ee) *adj.* Of or pertaining to a coccobacillus.

coc·co·ba·cil·li·form (kock″ko·ba·sil′i·form) *adj.* Resembling a coccobacillus.

coccobacilliform coryza. INFECTIOUS CORYZA.

coc·co·ba·cil·lus (kock″o·ba·sil′us) *n.*, pl. **coccobacil·li** (·eye). A short, thick, oval bacillus; in appearance, midway between the coccus and the bacillus.

coc·co·gen·ic (kock″o·jen′ick) *adj.* COCCOGENOUS.

coc·cog·e·nous (kock·oj′e·nus) *adj.* [*cocco-* + *-genous*]. Produced by cocci.

coc·coid (kock′oid) *adj.* Pertaining to or resembling a coccus.

coc·cu·lin (kock′yoo·lin) *n.* [*cocculus* + *-in*]. PICROTOXIN.

coc·cu·lus (kock′yoo·lus) *n.* The dried fruit of *Anamirta cocculus;* a convulsant poison which has been used externally against lice. See also *picrotoxin.*

coc·cus (kock′us) *n.*, pl. **coc·ci** (·sigh, ·eye) [Gk. *kokkos*, grain, seed]. A bacterium whose greatest diameter is not more than twice its shortest.

Coccus, *n.* A genus of small insects that is the source of cochineal.

coccy-. A combining form meaning *coccyx.*

coc·cy·al·gia (kock″see·al′juh, ·jee·uh) *n.* [*coccy-* + *-algia*]. COCCYGODYNIA.

coc·cy·ceph·a·lus (kock″si·sef′uh·lus) *n.*, pl. **coccycepha·li** (·lye) [Gk. *kokkyx*, cuckoo, + *-cephalus*]. An individual with a beaked process for a head. —**coccycephalous,** *adj.*

coc·cy·dyn·ia (kock″si·din′ee·uh) *n.* COCCYGODYNIA.

coccyg-, coccygo-. A combining form meaning *coccyx.*

coc·cyg·e·al (kock·sij′ee·ul) *adj.* Pertaining to or involving the coccyx.

coccygeal body. CORPUS COCCYGEUM.

coccygeal fistula. SACROCOCCYGEAL FISTULA.

coccygeal foveola. A persistent depression near the tip of the coccyx at the site of the terminal attachment of the embryonic neural tube to the dermis. NA *foveola coccygea.*

coccygeal ganglion. The terminal ganglion formed by the fusion of the caudal ends of the sympathetic trunks of both sides, situated in front of the coccyx. NA *ganglion impar.*

coccygeal glabella. A minute hairless area located in the coccygeal region at the vortex of the hair whorls. It may become a small pit, the coccygeal foveola.

coccygeal gland or **glomus.** CORPUS COCCYGEUM.

coccygeal nerve. Either of the last pair of spinal nerves, supplying the skin in the region of the coccyx. NA *nervus coccygeus.* See also *coccygeal plexus.*

coccygeal neuralgia. COCCYGODYNIA.

coccygeal plexus. A plexus formed by the union of the anterior branches of the coccygeal nerve and the fifth sacral nerve with a communicating filament from the fourth sacral nerve. NA *plexus coccygeus.*

coccygeal sinus. COCCYGEAL FOVEOLA.

coccygeal vestige. A remnant of the saccular termination of the embryonic neural tube located in the integument near the tip of the coccyx; derived from the medullary coccygeal vesicle.

coc·cy·gec·to·my (kock″si·jeck′tuh·mee) *n.* [*coccyg-* + *-ectomy*]. Surgical excision of the coccyx.

coccygeo-. A combining form meaning (a) *coccygeal;* (b) *coccygeus.*

coc·cy·geo·fe·mo·ra·lis (kock·sij″ee·o·fem·o·ray′lis) *L. adj.* Pertaining to the coccyx and femur.

coccygeofemoralis muscle. A variant of the gluteus maximus muscle extending from the coccyx to the linea aspera of the femur or from the sacrotuberous ligament to the fascia of the thigh.

coc·cyg·eo·pu·bic (kock·sij″ee·o·pew′bick) *adj.* Pertaining to the coccyx and the pubes.

coccygeopubic diameter. ANTEROPOSTERIOR DIAMETER (2).

coc·cyg·e·us (cock·sij′ee·us) *n.*, pl. **coccyg·ei** (·ee·eye). One of the muscles of the pelvic diaphragm. NA *musculus coccygeus.* See also Table of Muscles in the Appendix.

coccygeus dorsalis. SACROCOCCYGEUS DORSALIS.

coccygeus ventralis. SACROCOCCYGEUS VENTRALIS.

coccygo-. See *coccyg-.*

coc·cy·go·dyn·ia (kock″si·go·din′ee·uh) *n.* [*coccyg-* + *-odynia*]. Pain in the region of the coccyx.

coc·cyx (kock′sicks) *n.*, genit. sing. **coccy·gis** (·jis), L. pl. **coc·cy·ges** (kock′si·jees, kock·sigh′jeez), [Gk. *kokkyx*]. The last bone of the vertebral column, formed by the union of four rudimentary vertebrae. NA *os coccygis.* See also Plates 1, 14, 23.

Co·chin-Chi·na diarrhea [Cochin China (= southern Vietnam)]. TROPICAL SPRUE.

coch·i·neal (kotch″i·neel′, kotch′i·neel) *n.* [Sp. *cochinilla*]. The dried female insects, *Coccus cacti*, enclosing the young larvae. On extracting the insects with an aqueous solution of alum, a dark purplish solution representing an aluminum lake of the coloring principle carminic acid is obtained; the solution has been used for coloring medicinal preparations.

coch·lea (kock'lee·uh) *n.*, L. pl. & genit. sing. **coch·le·ae** (·lee·ee) [L., snail, from Gk. *kochlos*, shellfish] [NA]. The portion of the petrous part of the temporal bone which houses the membranous and osseous labyrinths, i.e., the essential organs of hearing. It describes 2½ turns about a central pillar called the modiolus or columella, thus forming the spiral canal of the cochlea, which is about 1½ inches in length. Projecting outward from the modiolus there is a thin, bony plate, the osseous spiral lamina, which divides the canal into the scala vestibuli and the scala tympani. —**coch·le·ar** (kock'lee·ur) *adj.*

cochlear aqueduct. AQUEDUCT OF THE COCHLEA.

cochlear articulation. SCREW ARTICULATION.

cochlear canal. COCHLEAR DUCT.

cochlear duct. The endolymph-filled, triangular (in cross section) canal between the scala tympani and scala vestibuli; it contains the spiral organ (of Corti). NA *ductus cochlearis.* See also Plate 20.

cochlear fenestra. COCHLEAR WINDOW.

cochlear ganglion. SPIRAL GANGLION OF THE COCHLEA.

coch·le·ar·i·form (kock"lee·ăr'i·form) *adj.* [*cochlear* + *-iform*]. Shaped like the shell of a snail.

cochleariform process. The curved terminal portion of the bony semicanal for the tensor tympani muscle forming a pulley over which the tendon of the muscle plays. NA *processus cochleariformis.*

cochlear nerve. The cochlear part of the vestibulocochlear nerve. NA *pars cochlearis nervi octavi.* See also Table of Nerves in the Appendix.

cochlear nuclei. Nuclear masses in which the fibers of the cochlear nerve terminate. These are the ventral cochlear and the dorsal cochlear nuclei located, respectively, ventral and dorsal to the inferior cerebellar peduncle (restiform body). NA *nuclei cochleares, ventralis et dorsalis.*

cochlear recess. An elliptic pit below the oval window of the vestibule, forming part of the cochlea. It contains small foramens for the passage of nerves from the duct of the cochlea. NA *recessus cochlearis vestibuli.*

cochlear reflex. AUDITORY REFLEX.

cochlear window. A round opening in the medial wall of the middle ear, closed by the secondary tympanic membrane. Syn. *round window.* NA *fenestra cochlea.* See also Plate 20.

cochlear zone. The membranous part of the spiral lamina or lamina basilaris.

coch·leo·or·bic·u·lar (kock"lee·o·or·bick'yoo·lur) *adj.* Pertaining to the cochlea and the orbicular muscles.

cochleoorbicular reflex. AUDITORY-PALPEBRAL REFLEX.

coch·leo·pal·pe·bral (kock'lee·o·pal'pe·brul) *adj.* Pertaining to the cochlea and the palpebral muscles.

cochleopalpebral reflex. AUDITORY-PALPEBRAL REFLEX.

coch·leo·ves·tib·u·lar (kock"lee·o·ves·tib'yoo·lur) *adj.* Pertaining to the cochlea and the vestibule of the ear.

Coch·lio·my·ia (kock"lee·o·migh'yuh) *n.* [Gk. *kochlios*, a spiral, + *-myia*]. *CALLITROGA.*

Cochliomyia americana. *CALLITROGA HOMINIVORAX.*

Cochliomyia hominivorax. *CALLITROGA HOMINIVORAX.*

Cochliomyia macellaria. *CALLITROGA MACELLARIA.*

co·cil·la·na (ko"si·lay'nuh, ·lan'uh) *n.* [American Sp.] The bark of the tree *Guarea rusbyi.* Used as a nauseating expectorant.

Cock·ayne's syndrome [E. A. *Cockayne*, English physician, 1880–1956]. Dwarfism, retinal atrophy, deafness, photosensitive dermatitis, beaklike nasal deformity, microcephaly and retardation, and slowly progressive signs of upper motor neuron and cerebellar dysfunction, probably an autosomal recessive trait.

cock·le·burr crystals. Dark-yellow or brown crystals of ammonium urate occurring in alkaline urine.

cock·roach, *n.* [Sp. *cucaracha*]. An insect of the genus *Blatella, Blatta,* or *Periplaneta.*

cock·up splint. A splint for immobilizing the hand in hyperextension during healing of a wound or fracture.

co·co (ko'ko) *n.* YAWS.

co·coa, co·co (ko'ko) *n.* CACAO.

cocoa butter. THEOBROMA OIL.

Coco Diazine. A trademark for sulfadiazine, an antibacterial.

co·con·scious (ko·kon'shus) *n. & adj.* [*co-* + *conscious*]. 1. *In psychiatry,* a dissociated mental state coexisting with a person's consciousness, but without his awareness, though it is psychodynamically active and may account for various normal and abnormal mental phenomena. 2. In or of such a state. See also *foreconscious.* —**coconscious·ness,** *n.*

co·co·nut oil. The fixed oil in the fruit of the coconut palm, *Cocos nucifera.* Used chiefly in soap manufacture for its high lathering quality.

cocto- [L. *coquere, coctus,* to cook]. A combining form meaning *boiled, modified by heat, at boiling point.*

coc·to·an·ti·gen (kock"to·an'ti·jin) *n.* [*cocto-* + *antigen*]. Any antigen subjected to high temperature, such as 70°C for 1 hour, as used in the preparation of antisera for the identification of meat and fish products.

coc·to·im·mu·no·gen (kock"to·i·mew'no·jen) *n.* [*cocto-* + *immuno-* + *-gen*]. COCTOANTIGEN.

coc·to·la·bile (kock"to·lay'bil, ·bile) *adj.* [*cocto-* + *labile*]. Destroyed or altered by heating to 100° C.

coc·to·pre·cip·i·tin (kock"to·pre·sip'i·tin) *n.* [*cocto-* + *precipitin*]. A precipitin produced in an animal by immunization with a boiled antigen, such as serum protein.

coc·to·sta·bile (kock"to·stay'bil, ·bile) *adj.* [*cocto-* + *stabile*]. Able to withstand the temperature of boiling water without change.

coc·to·sta·ble (kock"to·stay'bul) *adj.* COCTOSTABILE.

cod, *n.* Any of various fish of the family Gadidae, especially the common cod, *Gadus morrhua.* See also *cod-liver oil.*

co·da·mine (ko'duh·meen) *n.* An opium alkaloid, $C_{20}H_{25}NO_4$.

co·de·car·box·yl·ase (ko"dee·kahr·bock'sil·ace, ·aze) *n.* Pyridoxal phosphate; the prosthetic component of the enzyme which catalyses decarboxylation of L-amino acids, as well as of certain transaminating enzymes, in which latter case it is commonly referred to as cotransaminase.

co·de·hy·dro·gen·ase I (ko"dee·high'dro·je·nace, ·naze). NICOTINAMIDE ADENINE DINUCLEOTIDE.

codehydrogenase II. NICOTINAMIDE ADENINE DINUCLEOTIDE PHOSPHATE.

co·de·ia (ko·dee'yuh) *n.* CODEINE.

co·deine (ko'deen, ko'dee·een, ko·dee'in) *n.* [Gk. *kōdeia*, poppyhead, + *-ine*]. Methylmorphine, $C_{18}H_{21}NO_3$, an alkaloid of opium, resembling morphine in action, but weaker; an analgesic, antitussive, and antidiarrheal.

codeine phosphate. $C_{18}H_{21}NO_3.H_3PO_4.1\frac{1}{2}H_2O$, the codeine salt most soluble in water (1 g in 2.5 ml).

codeine sulfate. $(C_{18}H_{21}NO_3)_2.H_2SO_4.5H_2O$; 1 g dissolves in 30 ml of water.

cod-liver oil. 1. The partially destearinated fixed oil obtained from fresh livers of *Gadus morrhua* and other species of the family Gadidae. Contains vitamins A and D, for the effects of which the oil is used medicinally. 2. A nondestearinated cod-liver oil of the same vitamin potency as cod-liver oil; used chiefly for administration to animals.

Cod·man's triangle [E. A. *Codman*, U.S. surgeon, 1869–1940]. The little trumpet-shaped cuff of reactive periosteal bone which surrounds the upper limit of a bone tumor or infection and which appears in an x-ray as a triangular space beneath the uplifted periosteal edge. This signifies subperiosteal, extracortical involvement.

Codman's tumor [E. A. *Codman*]. CHONDROBLASTOMA.

co·dom·i·nant (ko·dom'i·nunt) *adj.* [*co-* + *dominant*]. Of or pertaining to two alleles which are both expressed in a heterozygote.

co·don (ko'don) *n.* [*code* + *-on*]. An informational unit of genetic material composed of three nucleotides of DNA or RNA.

co·dox·ime (ko·dock'seem) *n.* Dihydrocodeinone *O*-(carboxymethyl)oxime, $C_{20}H_{24}N_2O_5$, an antitussive drug.

co·ef·fi·cient (ko''e·fish'unt) *n.* [*co-* + *efficient*]. 1. Multiplier. 2. A figure indicating the degree of physical or chemical alteration characteristic of a given substance under stated conditions.

coefficient of correlation. A measure of the degree of association between two characteristics in a series of observations. Its value ranges from −1, representing perfect negative correlation, to +1, representing perfect positive correlation.

coefficient of inbreeding. A mathematical index (symbol, *F*), with values between zero and unity, which for individuals expresses the probability that two genes at a locus are identical by descent and which for a population expresses the degree of nonrandom mating in comparison with a base population whose inbreeding coefficient is defined as zero. Thus, a child of a marriage of second cousins has a coefficient $F = 1/16$, and a population with a fraction *c* of cousin marriages and no other consanguinity has a coefficient of *c*/16.

coefficient of light extinction. The amount of light of a specific wavelength absorbed by a 1.0% solution of a substance in a layer 1.0 cm thick.

coefficient of refraction. The quotient of the sine of the angle of refraction into the sine of the angle of incidence.

coefficient of solubility of a gas. The amount of a gas which is dissolved at a given temperature in 1 ml of a liquid, when the pressure of gas on the liquid is 760 mm Hg.

coefficient of variation. The standard deviation of a series of observations expressed as a per cent of the mean of the series.

coel-, coelo- [Gk. *koilos*]. A combining form meaning *concave, hollow, cavity.*

-coele [Gk. *koilia*, cavity]. A combining form designating *a chamber, a ventricle, or a normal cavity of the body.*

Coe·len·ter·a·ta (se·len''tur·ay'tuh) *n. pl.* [NL., from Gk. *koilia*, cavity, + *enteron*, intestine]. A phylum of primitive metazoans, including hydras, jellyfishes, corals, and sea anemones, which are radially symmetrical and whose only internal space is a digestive cavity; typified by alternate generations of asexual polyps and sexual medusae. Syn. *Cnidaria.* —**coe·len·ter·ate** (se·len'tur·ut, ·ate) *n. & adj.*

coe·len·ter·on (se·len'tur·on) *n.*, pl. **coelen·tera** (·tur·uh) [*coel-* + *enteron*]. 1. The entodermal gut cavity in diploblastic animals. 2. ARCHENTERON.

coeli-. See *celi-.*

coeliac. CELIAC.

coeliadelphus. Celiadelphus (= OMPHALOPAGUS).

coeliectasia. CELIECTASIA.

coelio-. See *celi-.*

coeliocolpotomy. CELIOCOLPOTOMY.

coelioenterotomy. CELIOENTEROTOMY.

coeliogastrotomy. CELIOGASTROTOMY.

coelioma. Celioma (= MESOTHELIOMA).

coeliomyomectomy. CELIOMYOMECTOMY.

coelioparacentesis. CELIOPARACENTESIS.

coeliorrhaphy. CELIORRHAPHY.

coelioscope. Celioscope (= CELOSCOPE).

coelioscopy. Celioscopy (= PERITONEOSCOPY).

coeliotomy. CELIOTOMY.

coelitis. CELITIS.

coelo-. See *coel-.*

coe·lom, ce·lum (see'lum) *n.*, pl. **coeloms, coe·lo·ma·ta** (se·lo'muh·tuh, se·lom'uh·tuh) [Gk. *koilōma*, cavity]. The embryonic body cavity formed in the lateral mesoderm, which subsequently becomes divided into pericardial, pleural, and peritoneal cavities in developing mammals. —**coe·lom·ic, ce·lom·ic** (se·lom'ick) *adj.*

coelomic cleft. The fissure in the lateral mesoderm which forms the coelomic cavity and divides the mesoderm into somatic and visceral layers.

coelomic pouch. One of a series of evaginations from the wall of the archenteron of lower vertebrates that form the mesodermal somites of the embryo.

coe·los·chi·sis, ce·los·chi·sis (see·los'ki·sis) *n.* [*coelo-* + *-schisis*]. GASTROSCHISIS.

coeloscope. CELOSCOPE.

coelosoma. CELOSOMA.

coelosomia. Celosomia (= CELOSOMA).

coelosomus. CELOSOMUS.

coelothelioma. Celothelioma (= MESOTHELIOMA).

coen-. See *cen-.*

coenadelphus. Cenadelphus (= DIPLOPAGUS).

coenaesthesia. CENESTHESIA.

coenesthesia. CENESTHESIA.

coeno-. See *cen-.*

coe·no·cyte, ce·no·cyte (see'no·site, sen'o·) *n.* [*coeno-* + *-cyte*]. A multinucleate mass of protoplasm which has arisen as a result of nuclear division but without cytoplasmic division; seen in the vegetative bodies of some algae and fungi, as the plasmodium of slime molds. —**coe·no·cyt·ic** (see''no·sit'ick) *adj.*

coe·nu·ri·a·sis (see''new·rye'uh·sis) *n.* COENUROSIS.

coe·nu·ro·sis, ce·nu·ro·sis (see''new·ro'sis) *n.*, pl. **coenuro·ses, cenuro·ses** (·seez) [*coenurus* + *-osis*]. Involvement of the central nervous system by the larval stage of the dog tapeworm, *Multiceps multiceps.* The lesions usually consist of many budding vesicles at the base of the brain.

coe·nu·rus, ce·nu·rus (se·new'rus) *n.*, pl. **coenu·ri, cenu·ri** (·rye) [*coen-* + *-urus*, from Gk. *oura*, tail]. The bladderworm stage of the dog tapeworm, *Multiceps multiceps*, characterized by having multiple heads invaginated from the wall into the bladder cavity.

co·en·zyme (ko·en'zime) *n.* [*co-* + *enzyme*]. A nonprotein substance which, in combination with an apoenzyme, forms a complete enzyme, or holoenzyme; prosthetic group of an enzyme. Syn. *cofactor.* Compare *activator (1).*

coenzyme I. NICOTINAMIDE ADENINE DINUCLEOTIDE.

coenzyme II. NICOTINAMIDE ADENINE DINUCLEOTIDE PHOSPHATE.

coenzyme A. A nucleotide composed of adenylic acid, pantothenic acid, 2-mercaptoethylamine, and phosphoric acid which in the presence of a suitable enzyme can transfer an acyl group, as acetyl, from one substance to another. Abbreviated, CoA.

coenzyme Q. UBIQUINONE.

coenzyme R. BIOTIN.

coercive force. The magnetic force required to remove the magnetic induction in a previously magnetized material.

coeur en sa·bot (kur ahn sa·bo') [F.]. BOOT-SHAPED HEART.

co·fac·tor (ko'fack·tur) *n.* 1. Any factor operating in conjunction with a principal factor. 2. COENZYME.

COFAL test. A complement fixation test used to detect the presence of group-specific protein antigens of avian leukosis/sarcoma viruses.

co·fer·ment (ko·fur'ment) *n.* [*co-* + *ferment*]. COENZYME.

cof·fee, *n.* [It. *caffè*, from Turkish, from Ar. *qahwah*]. The dried and roasted ripe seeds of various species of *Coffea*, including *C. arabica, C. liberica,* and *C. robusta.* An infusion is stimulant because of its content of caffeine and, possibly, a volatile oil, caffeol.

cof·fee·ber·ry, *n.* CASCARA SAGRADA.

coffee-grounds vomit. Vomit consisting of altered blood in the contents of the stomach.

Cof·fey's operation [R. C. *Coffey*, U.S. surgeon, 1869–1933]. Implantation of the ureters into the sigmoid obliquely through the bowel wall so as to obtain a valvelike effect and minimize the danger of ascending infection.

cof·fin, *n.* In the anatomy of the horse, the hollow portion of the hoof.

coffin bone. The distal or third phalanx of a horse's foot.

coffin joint. The joint between the second and third phalanges of a horse's foot; the distal interphalangeal joint.

coffin-lid crystals. TRIPLE PHOSPHATE CRYSTALS.

Co·gan's syndrome [D. G. *Cogan*, U.S. neuroophthalmolo-gist, b. 1908]. 1. Vertigo, tinnitus, progressive bilateral deafness, pain in the eyes, photophobia and impaired vision, usually in young adults; associated with interstitial keratitis not due to syphilis, but possibly a form of vasculitis. 2. The congenital form of ocular motor apraxia.

Cogentin. Trademark for benztropine, a parasympatholytic drug used as the mesylate (methanesulfonate) salt in the symptomatic treatment of paralysis agitans.

Cogesic. Trademark for prodilidine, an analgesic used as the hydrochloride salt.

Cog·gins test. An immunodiffusion technique used to detect the presence of antibodies in the serum of horses with infectious equine anemia.

cog·nate vascular bed. A region normally supplied by a specified artery. Contr. *collateral vascular bed.*

cog·ni·tion (kog·nish'un) *n.* [L. *cognitio,* from *cognoscere,* to know]. *In psychology,* the conscious faculty or process of knowing, of becoming, or being aware of thoughts or perceptions, including understanding and reasoning. Contr. *affection, conation.* —**cog·ni·tive** (kog'ni·tiv) *adj.*

cog·wheel respiration. INTERRUPTED RESPIRATION.

cogwheel rigidity. A special type of extrapyramidal rigidity in which passive stretching of muscle, as for instance in the dorsiflexion of the hand, yields a rhythmically jerky resistance, as though the limb were being pulled over a ratchet; probably this represents a tremor which is masked by rigidity in an attitude of repose, but emerges during manipulation.

co·hab·i·ta·tion (ko·hab''i·tay'shun) *n.* [*co-* + L. *habitare,* to dwell]. The living together as, or as if, husband and wife.

co·here (ko·heer') *v.* [L. *cohaere*]. To stick together. —**co·her·ent,** *adj.*

co·her·ence (ko·heer'unce) *n.* [L. *cohaerentia,* from *cohaerere,* to stick together]. Reasonable connectedness of thought shown in speech, writing, or other activities.

coherent smallpox. A form of smallpox in which the pustules coalesce but retain their individuality.

co·he·sion (ko·hee'zhun) *n.* [L., from *cohaerere,* to stick, cling]. The attractive force between the same kind of molecules, i.e., the force which holds the molecules of a substance together. —**cohe·sive** (·siv) *adj.*

cohesive bandage. A type of bandage that has the property of sticking to itself, but not to other substances.

Cohn·heim's theory [J. F. *Cohnheim,* German pathologist, 1839–1884]. The theory that groups of embryonic cells, or rests, remain behind during development, later giving rise to neoplasms.

Cohn method. CORPER AND COHN METHOD.

co·ho·ba snuff (ko·ho'buh, ko·hob'uh). A powder derived from the seeds of *Piptadenia peregrina* which contains N,N-dimethyltryptamine and is used in Haiti for its hallucinogenic effects.

co·hort (ko'hort) *n. In statistics,* a group of individuals sharing some common characteristic, often age and sex.

co·hosh (ko'hosh, ko·hosh') *n.* [Algonquian]. An American Indian name for several medicinal plants, as black cohosh (*Cimicifuga racemosa*), blue cohosh (*Caulophyllum thalictroides*), and red cohosh (*Actaea spicata*).

coil gland. SWEAT GLAND.

coin lesion. A discrete spherical mass shadow on radiographs of the lung.

coi·no·site (koy'no·site, ko·in'o·) *n.* [Gk. *koinos,* common, + *-site*]. An animal parasite capable of separating itself from its host at will; a free, commensal organism.

coin sound. In pneumothorax, a clear ringing note produced by striking a coin, placed flat upon the chest, with the edge of another coin.

coital reflex. GENITAL REFLEX.

co·i·tion (ko·ish'un) *n.* [L. *coitio,* from *coire,* to go together]. COITUS.

co·i·to·pho·bia (ko''i·to·fo'bee·uh) *n.* [*coitus* + *phobia*]. Abnormal dread or aversion to coitus.

co·i·tus (ko'i·tus) *n.* [L., from *coire,* to go together]. The act of sexual union; copulation. —**coi·tal** (·tul) *adj.*

coitus in·ter·rup·tus (in·tur·up'tus). Sexual intercourse in which the penis is withdrawn and the semen discharged outside the vagina.

coitus res·er·va·tus (rez''ur·vay'tus). Deliberately prolonged coitus without discharge of semen.

col-, coli-, colo-. A combining form meaning *colon.*

col (kol) *n.* [F., from L. *collum,* neck]. A valleylike depression between the facial and lingual gingival papillae; it conforms to the shape of the interproximal surface of the tooth.

Colace. A trademark for dioctyl sodium sulfosuccinate.

co·la nut. KOLA.

co·la·tion (ko·lay'shun) *n.* [L. *colare,* to strain]. The act of filtering or straining.

col·a·to·ri·um (kol''uh·tor'ee·um) *n.,* pl. **colato·ria** (·ee·uh) [L.]. *In pharmacy,* a sieve, colander, or strainer.

col·a·ture (kol'uh·choor) *n.* [L. *colatura*]. 1. *In pharmacy,* a liquid that has been subjected to colation. 2. COLATION.

col·chi·cine (kol'chi·seen, ·sin, kol'ki·) *n.* [*colchicum* + *-ine*]. An alkaloid, $C_{22}H_{25}NO_6$, of colchicum; a pale yellow, exceedingly bitter powder, freely soluble in water. Employed in the treatment of gout. It speeds up the evolutionary processes in plants by doubling chromosome numbers.

col·chi·cin·iza·tion (kol''chi·sin·i·zay'shun) *n.* Treatment with colchicine.

col·chi·cum (kol'chi·kum, kol'ki·kum) *n.* [L., from Gk. *kolchikon*]. The corm and seed of the plant *Colchicum autumnale,* the properties of which are due to the alkaloid colchicine. It has been used in the treatment of acute gout and some forms of rheumatism.

cold, *n.* 1. The comparative lack of heat. 2. The COMMON COLD: a mild, acute, contagious, upper respiratory viral infection of short duration, characterized by coryza, watering of the eyes, cough, and occasionally, fever.

cold abscess. An abscess not associated with the usual signs of inflammation, such as redness, swelling, and heat.

cold agglutination phenomenon. The agglutination of human group O erythrocytes at 0 to 4°C, but not at body temperature, due to the adsorption on the surface of the red cells of 19S gamma globulins, and occurring in primary atypical pneumonia, certain viral disease, acquired hemolytic anemia, trypanosomiasis, blackwater fever, and other unidentifiable states.

cold agglutination test. A test to demonstrate the cold agglutination phenomenon.

cold agglutinin. An agglutinin in serum which produces maximum clumping of erythrocytes at 4°C and none at 37°C. See also *cold agglutination phenomenon.*

cold-blood·ed, *adj.* Poikilothermic; without ability to regulate the body temperature; said of fishes, reptiles, and amphibians whose temperatures remain close to that of the environment. Contr. *warm-blooded.*

cold cautery. Cauterization by extreme cold, as by carbon dioxide snow.

cold cream. A type of cosmetic cream of varying composition.

cold-curing resin. ACTIVATED RESIN.

cold emission. Emission of electrons from an unheated cathode under the influence of a very strong electric field.

cold freckle. LENTIGO.

cold-growing. Of bacteria: PSYCHROPHILIC.

cold hemagglutination. A phenomenon caused by the presence of cold agglutinin.

cold hemagglutinin. COLD AGGLUTININ.

cold hemolysin. A hemolysin active at temperatures lower than 37°C, usually most active at 4°C.

cold injury. Trauma to the body resulting from exposure to very low temperatures; may be a freezing or nonfreezing injury.

cold light. CHEMILUMINESCENCE.

cold pressor test. A rise in blood pressure is observed after the immersion of one hand in ice water for 1 minute. Individuals showing an excessive rise in blood pressure or an unusual delay in return to normal blood pressure are thought likely to develop essential hypertension.

cold sore. HERPES FACIALIS.

cold spots. Areas on the surface of the skin overlying the nerve endings that are stimulated by low temperatures.

cold urticaria. A form of physical allergy elicitable by exposure to cold.

cole-, coleo- [Gk. *koleon*, sheath, scabbard]. A combining form meaning (a) *sheath;* (b) *vagina.*

co·lec·to·my (ko·leck'tuh·mee) *n.* [*col-* + *-ectomy*]. Excision of all or a portion of the colon.

Colectril. Trademark for amiloride, a potassium-sparing natriuretic agent used as the hydrochloride salt.

co·le·i·tis (ko''lee·eye'tis, kol''ee·) *n.* [*cole-* + *-itis*]. VAGINITIS.

Cole·man-Shaf·fer diet [W. *Coleman*, U.S. physician, 1869–1948; and P. A. *Shaffer*, U.S. biochemist, 1881–1960]. A high-calorie, frequent-feeding diet for the treatment of typhoid fever.

coleo-. See *cole-.*

co·leo·cele (ko'lee·o·seel'', kol'ee·o·) *n.* [*coleo-* + *-cele*]. A vaginal tumor or hernia.

co·leo·cys·ti·tis (ko''lee·o·sis·tye'tis) *n.* [*coleo-* + *cystitis*]. Inflammation of the vagina and urinary bladder.

Co·le·op·te·ra (ko''lee·op'tur·uh, kol''ee·) *n. pl.* [Gk. *koleopteros*, sheath-winged]. The order of insects that comprises the beetles. **—coleopter·ous** (·us) *adj.*

co·le·op·to·sis (ko''lee·op·to'sis) *n.*, pl. **coleopto·ses** (·seez) [*coleo-* + *ptosis*]. Prolapse of the vaginal wall.

co·le·ot·o·my (ko''lee·ot'uh·mee) *n.* [*coleo-* + *-tomy*]. COLPOTOMY.

co·les (ko'leez) *n.* [L. *colis, caulis*, stem]. PENIS.

coles fe·mi·ni·nus (fem''i·nigh'nus). CLITORIS.

Colestid. A trademark for colestipol, an antihyperlipemic agent.

co·les·ti·pol (ko·les'ti·pole) *n.* A copolymer of tetraethylenepentamine with 1-chloro-2, 3-epoxypropane. The polymer is highly insoluble and therefore is normally used as the hydrochloride salt, in which approximately 20 percent of the amine nitrogen atoms are protonated; used as an antihyperlipemic agent.

Co·ley's toxin or **fluid** [W. B. *Coley*, U.S. surgeon, 1862–1936]. A preparation of bacterial toxins once used in the treatment of cancer.

coli-. See *col-.*

co·li·bac·il·le·mia, coli·bac·il·lae·mia (ko''lee·bas''i·lee'mee·uh) *n.* [*colibacil*lus + *-emia*]. The presence of *Escherichia coli* in the blood.

co·li·bac·il·lo·sis (ko''lee·bas''i·lo'sis) *n.* [*colibacil*lus + *-osis*]. Infection with *Escherichia coli.*

co·li·bac·il·lu·ria (ko''lee·bas''i·lew'ree·uh) *n.* [*colibacil*lus + *-uria*]. The presence of *Escherichia coli* in the urine.

co·li·ba·cil·lus (ko''lee·ba·sil'us) *n.*, pl. **colibacil·li** (·eye). The colon bacillus, *Escherichia coli.*

[1]col·ic (kol'ick) *n.* [Gk. *kōlikos*]. 1. Acute paroxysmal abdominal pain usually due to smooth muscle contraction, obstruction, or twisting. 2. In early infancy paroxysms of pain, crying, and irritability, due to such causes as swallowing air, overfeeding, intestinal allergy, and emotional factors. Adj. *colicky.*

[2]co·lic (ko'lick) *adj.* Of or pertaining to the colon.

co·li·ca (ko'li·kuh) *n.* COLIC ARTERY.

colic angle. The angle formed by the junction of abdominal and umbilical colon in the fetus.

colic artery. Any one of the three arteries that supply the colon. See also Table of Arteries in the Appendix.

co·li·cin (ko'li·sin, kol'i·) *n.* [(*E.*)*coli* + *-c-* (as in *-cide*) + *-in*]. Any of various bacteriocins active against particular strains of *Escherichia coli* or of other Enterobacteriaceae.

co·li·cine (ko'li·seen, kol'i·) *n.* COLICIN.

colic intussusception. Intussusception involving the colon only.

col·icky (kol'i·kee) *adj.* 1. Of, pertaining to, resembling, or causing colic. 2. Suffering from or caused by colic.

colic valve. ILEOCECAL VALVE.

[1]co·li·form (ko'li·form) *adj.* [*coli-* + *form*]. 1. Pertaining to or resembling the colon-aerogenes group.

[2]coliform, *adj.* [L. *col*um, sieve, + *form*]. Sievelike, cribriform; ETHMOID.

co·li·gran·u·lo·ma (ko''lee·gran''yoo·lo'muh) *n.* [*coli-* + *granuloma*]. HJÄRRE'S DISEASE.

co·li group (ko'lye). COLON-AEROGENES GROUP.

colinearity. COLLINEARITY.

co·li·phage (ko'li·faje) *n.* A bacteriophage of *Escherichia coli.*

co·lis·ti·meth·ate sodium (ko·lis''ti·meth'ate). Pentasodium colistinmethanesulfonate, $C_{58}H_{105}N_{16}Na_5O_{28}S_5$; a water-soluble derivative of colistin suitable for intramuscular injection.

co·lis·tin (ko·lis'tin, kol'is·tin) *n.* A basic polypeptide antibiotic obtained from *Bacillus colistinus;* closely related chemically and in antibacterial range to polymyxin B. It has largely been replaced by other antibiotics with less toxicity.

co·li·tis (ko·lye'tis) *n.* [*col-* + *-itis*]. Inflammation of the colon.

colitis pol·yp·o·sa (pol''i·po'suh). COLONIC PSEUDOPOLYPS.

co·li·uria (ko''lee·yoo'ree·uh) *n.* COLIBACILLURIA.

coll-, colla-, collo- [Gk. *kolla*, glue]. A combining form meaning (a) *collagen;* (b) *colloid.*

colla-. See *coll-.*

col·la·cin (kol'uh·sin) *n.* A substance found in colloid degeneration of the skin.

col·la·gen (kol'uh·jin) *n.* [*colla-* + *-gen*]. The albuminoid substance of the white fibers of connective tissues, cartilage, and bone. It is converted into gelatin by boiling. **—col·la·gen·ic** (kol''uh·jen'ick), **col·lag·e·nous** (kuh·laj'e·nus) *adj.*

col·la·gen·ase (kol'uh·je·nace, ·naze) *n.* [*collagen* + *-ase*]. A proteolytic enzyme which hydrolyzes collagen; one of the major exotoxins of *Clostridium perfringens* type A. It attacks the collagen of subcutaneous tissues and muscles and thus may contribute to the spread of gas gangrene. Syn. *kappa toxin.*

collagen disease. Any of various clinical syndromes characterized by widespread alterations of connective tissue, including inflammation and fibrinoid degeneration, as in rheumatic fever, rheumatoid arthritis, polyarteritis, systemic lupus erythematosus, generalized scleroderma, or dermatomyositis.

col·la·gen·iza·tion (kol''uh·je·nye·zay'shun, kol·aj''e·) *n.* The replacement of normal elements of a given area by collagenous connective tissue.

col·la·gen·o·sis (kol''uh·je·no'sis, kol·aj''e·no'sis) *n.*, pl. **collageno·ses** (·seez) [*collagen* + *-osis*]. 1. An African cardiopathy characterized by heart failure and visceral infarction with endocardial fibrosis and sclerosis, and mural thrombosis. 2. COLLAGEN DISEASE.

collagenous fibers. The flexible, fibrillar, nonelastic, connective-tissue fibers which are the commonest type. They make up the main mass of such structures as the corium, fasciae, tendons, ligaments, aponeuroses, periostea, and capsules of organs, and form also the fibrillar component of the intercellular substance (matrix) of bone and cartilage.

col·lapse, *v. & n.* [L. *collabi, collapsus*, to fall together]. 1. To cave in or be deflated. 2. To cause to cave in or be deflated. 3. Extreme depression, exhaustion, or prostration from physical or psychogenic causes. 4. SHOCK. 5. An abnormal sagging of an organ or the obliteration of its cavity.

collapse therapy. The treatment of pulmonary tuberculosis by any surgical procedure designed to decrease lung volume, such as artificial pneumothorax, extrapleural thoracoplasty, or interruption of the phrenic nerve.

collaps·ing pulse. A pulse characterized by an extremely rapid downstroke or descent from the peak. See also *Corrigan's pulse.*

col·lar, *n.* [L. *collare,* from *collum,* neck]. A supportive or protective band around a neck.

col·lar·bone, *n.* CLAVICLE.

col·lar·ette (kol″ur·et′) *n.* A ring or collar of scales following involution of some blisters.

collar of Ve·nus. A rarely seen, mottled, marblelike skin of the neck occurring in syphilis.

col·lat·er·al (kuh·lat′ur·ul) *adj. & n.* [ML. *collateralis,* from L. *latus, lateris,* side]. 1. Accessory or secondary; not direct or immediate. 2. A side branch, as of a vessel or a nerve fiber.

collateral artery. Any of the four branches of the brachial and deep brachial arteries which descend through a portion of the upper arm and terminate by anastamosis near the elbow joint. See also *middle collateral artery, radial collateral artery, ulnar collateral artery.*

collateral circulation. The circulation established for an organ or a part through anastomotic communicating channels, when the original direct blood supply is obstructed or abolished.

collateral eminence. A ridge on the floor of the lateral ventricle, corresponding to the depth of the collateral sulcus of the temporal lobe. NA *eminentia collateralis.*

collateral fibers. The delicate lateral branches of the axon of a neuron.

collateral fissure. COLLATERAL SULCUS.

collateral ganglion. Any of the ganglions of the sympathetic nervous system located in the mesenteric nervous plexuses around the abdominal aorta and its larger visceral branches.

collateral inheritance. The appearance of characters in collateral members of a family, as when an uncle and a niece show the same character, inherited by the related individuals from a common ancestor.

collateral ligament. Either of the ligaments, two to a joint, on the sides of the metacarpophalangeal joints (NA (pl.) *ligamenta collateralia articulationum metacarpophalangearum*), the metatarsophalangeal joints (NA (pl.) *ligamenta collateralia articulationum metatarsophalangearum*), and the interphalangeal joints of the hand (NA (pl.) *ligamenta collateralia articulationum interphalangearum manus*) and the foot (NA (pl.) *ligamenta collateralia articulationum interphalangearum pedis*). See also *fibular, radial, tibial,* and *ulnar collateral ligament.*

collateral respiration. The passage of air between lobules within the same lobe of a lung, allowing ventilation of a lobule whose bronchiole is obstructed.

collateral sulcus. A furrow on the medial aspect of the cerebrum, between the subcalcarine and subcollateral gyri, corresponding to the collateral eminence. NA *sulcus collateralis.*

collateral trigone. A triangular area at the junction of the posterior and inferior horns of the lateral ventricles. NA *trigonum collaterale.*

collateral vascular bed. A region supplied by various arteries in the vicinity. Contr. *cognate vascular bed.*

col·lect·ing tubules. The ducts conveying the urine from the renal tubules (nephrons) to the minor calices of the renal pelvis. NA *tubuli renales recti.*

collecting vein. A vein formed by the confluence of several sublobular veins of the liver.

col·lec·tive unconscious. *In analytic psychology,* the portion of the unconscious which theoretically is inherited and common to mankind.

col·lec·tor, *n.* An instrument, variously modified, used in bronchoesophagology to collect secretions for bacteriological and cytological examination.

col·lege, *n.* [L. *collegium,* society]. 1. An organized society or body of persons having common professional training and interests. 2. An institution of higher learning.

Col·les' fascia (kol′eez, kol′is) [A. *Colles,* Irish surgeon, 1773–1843]. The deep layer of the superficial fascia of the perineum.

Colles' fracture [A. *Colles*]. A fracture of the radius and ulna about 1 inch above the wrist with dorsal displacement of the distal fragment, creating a silver-fork deformity.

Colles' law [A. *Colles*]. A child with congenital syphilis, whose mother has no clinical evidence of the disease, does not infect the mother.

Colles' ligament [A. *Colles*]. The lateral extension of the falx inguinalis.

Col·let-Si·card syndrome (koʰ·leʰ′, see·kahʳ′) [F.-J. *Collet,* French otolaryngologist, b. 1870; and J.A. *Sicard*]. Paralysis of the muscles innervated by the ninth, tenth, eleventh, and twelfth cranial nerves; may follow a fracture of the floor of the posterior cranial fossa.

col·lic·u·li·tis (kol·ick″yoo·lye′tis) *n.* [*collicul*us + *-itis*]. Inflammation of the colliculus seminalis.

col·lic·u·lo·ru·bral (kol·ick″yoo·lo·roo′brul) *adj.* [*collicul*us + *rubral*]. Pertaining to the superior colliculus and the red nucleus.

colliculorubral tract. TECTORUBRAL TRACT.

col·lic·u·lus (kol·ick′yoo·lus) *n.,* pl. & genit. sing. **collicu·li** (·lye) [L., from *collis,* hill]. A small eminence.

colliculus ab·du·cen·tis (ab″dew·sen′tis). FACIAL COLLICULUS.

colliculus car·ti·la·gi·nis ary·te·noi·de·ae (kahr·ti·laj′i·nis ăr″i·tee·noy′dee·ee) [NA]. A small eminence found on the ventral (anterior) margin and ventrolateral surface of the arytenoid cartilage.

colliculus fa·ci·a·lis (fay″shee·ay′lis), pl. **colliculi facia·les** (·leez) [NA]. FACIAL COLLICULUS.

colliculus inferior, pl. **colliculi in·fe·ri·o·res** (in·feer·ee·o′reez) [NA]. INFERIOR COLLICULUS.

colliculus se·mi·na·lis (sem″i·nay′lis, see″mi·) [NA]. An elevation of the posterior wall of the prostatic portion of the urethra; on it opens the prostatic utricle; the ejaculatory ducts and numerous ducts of the prostate gland open on either side into the prostatic sinus.

colliculus superior, pl. **colliculi su·pe·ri·o·res** (sue·peer·ee·o′reez) [NA]. SUPERIOR COLLICULUS.

colliculus ure·thra·lis (yoo″re·thray′lis). COLLICULUS SEMINALIS.

col·li·dine (kol′i·deen, ·din) *n.* Any of three derivatives of pyridine of the composition $C_8H_{11}N$: α-collidine is 4-ethyl-2-methylpyridine; β-collidine is 3-ethyl-4-methylpyridine; γ-collidine is 2,4,6-trimethylpyridine. All are liquids obtained from coal tar.

col·li·ga·tive (kol′i·gay″tiv, kuh·lig′uh·tiv) *adj.* [L. *colligare,* to bind together, from *ligare,* to bind]. *In physical chemistry,* pertaining to those properties of matter that depend on the number of particles (molecules or ions) but do not depend on their chemical nature, for example, the pressure of a volume of a (perfect) gas.

col·li·ma·tor (kol′i·may″tur) *n.* [from NL. *collimare,* from a misreading of L. *collineare,* to bring into a straight line, from *con-,* with, together, + *linea,* line]. 1. The diaphragm of a spectroscope, the purpose of which is to provide a beam of parallel rays of light by means of a small slit at the focus of its lens. 2. A fixed telescope for adjusting the optical axis of an instrument, as a photomicrographic camera. 3. A diaphragm or system of diaphragms made of an absorbing material, designed to define the dimensions and direction of a beam of radiation.

col·lin·e·ar (ko·lin′ee·ur) *adj.* [*com-* + *linear*]. *In optics,* lying in the same straight line.

col·lin·ear·i·ty (ko·lin″ee·ăr′i·tee) *n.* The relationship between informational nucleotide residues in a molecule of DNA and amino acid residues in the corresponding molecule of protein; there is a correspondence in the sequence of mutational sites in DNA, as judged by recombination analysis, and in the sequence of amino acid alterations in protein.

Col·lin·so·nia (kol″in·so′nee·uh) *n.* [P. *Collinson,* English botanist, 1694–1768]. A genus of Lamiaceae, the mint family.

Col·lip unit [J. B. *Collip,* Canadian biochemist and physician, 1892–1965]. A dosage unit of parathyroid extract, representing 1/100th of the amount of extract which will produce a rise of 5 mg per 100 ml in the serum calcium level of a 20-kg dog within a period of 15 hours.

col·li·qua·tion (kol″i·kway′shun) *n.* [F., from L. *liquare,* to liquefy, melt]. The breakdown of tissue, usually necrotic, so that it becomes liquefied.

col·liq·ua·tive (kol·ick′wuh·tiv, kol′i·kway″tiv) *adj.* Marked by profuse or excessive fluid discharges.

colliquative albuminuria. Proteinuria seen in the course of and during convalescence from severe fevers.

colliquative necrosis. LIQUEFACTION NECROSIS.

colliquative softening. A condition in which the affected tissues liquefy.

col·li·sion, *n. In obstetrics,* a complication which occurs occasionally when twins are small and when their presenting parts attempt to enter the superior strait at the same time.

collision tumor. A tumor in which a sarcoma is thought to invade a carcinoma, or vice versa.

col·li·tis (kol·eye′tis) *n.* [L. *coll*um, neck, + *-itis*]. TRIGONITIS.

collo-. See *coll-.*

col·lo·di·on (kol·o′dee·on) *n.* [Gk. *kollōdēs,* glutinous]. A dressing for wounds made by dissolving pyroxylin in ether and alcohol.

col·loid (kol′oid) *n.* [*coll-* + *-oid*]. 1. A state of subdivision of matter in which the individual particles are of submicroscopic size and consist either of single large molecules, as of proteins, or aggregates of smaller molecules; such particles, collectively referred to as the dispersed phase, occur more or less uniformly distributed in a dispersion medium. The dimension of a colloid particle, arbitrarily fixed, is between 1 and 100 nanometers. 2. A substance in the colloid state. 3. The clear, gelatinous, eosinophilic, stored secretion of the thyroid gland; also other collections of gelatinous material, as the secretion of the intermediate lobe of the hypophysis. —**col·loi·dal** (kuh·loy′dul, kol·oy′dul) *adj.*

colloidal gold test. The precipitation by abnormal cerebrospinal fluid of colloidal gold from suspensions of various concentrations; formerly used in the diagnosis of neurosyphilis and other central nervous system diseases.

colloidal osmotic pressure. ONCOTIC PRESSURE.

colloidal solution. A macroscopically homogeneous system consisting of either single, large molecules or aggregations of smaller molecules (the dispersed phase) suspended in a liquid (the continuous phase). See also *sol.*

colloid carcinoma. MUCINOUS CARCINOMA.

colloid chemistry. Study of the properties developed by substances in the colloidal state of subdivision.

colloid cyst. A cyst containing gelatinous material whose consistency approaches that of thyroid gland colloid.

colloid degeneration. Abnormal production of colloid.

colloid goiter. A diffuse, lumpy goiter in which many of the follicles are abnormally distended with colloid; often associated with iodine deficiency.

colloid milium. A rare skin disease characterized by the presence, especially on the face and hands, of minute, shining, flat or slightly raised lesions of a pale lemon or bright lemon color. It is a form of colloid degeneration of the skin, affecting persons of middle or advanced age.

col·loi·do·cla·sia (kuh·loy″do·klay′zee·uh, ·zhuh) *n.* [*colloid* + *-clasia*]. A breaking up of the physical equilibrium of the colloids in the living body, producing anaphylactoid shock; attributed to entrance into the bloodstream of unchanged (undigested) colloids. —**colloido·clas·tic** (·klas′tick) *adj.*

col·loi·do·cla·sis (kuh·loy″do·klay′sis) *n.,* pl. **colloidocla·ses** (·seez). COLLOIDOCLASIA.

colloidoclastic shock. COLLOIDOCLASIA.

col·loi·do·pexy (kuh·loy′do·peck″see) *n.* Phagocytosis of foreign colloidal material.

col·loid·oph·a·gy (kol″oy·dof′uh·jee) *n.* [*colloid* + *-phagy*]. Invasion and ingestion of colloid by macrophages, as in the thyroid gland.

colloid osmotic pressure. ONCOTIC PRESSURE.

colloid ovarian cystoma. PSEUDOMUCINOUS CYSTADENOMA.

colloid ovarian tumor. PSEUDOMUCINOUS CYSTADENOMA.

col·lo·ne·ma (kol″o·nee′muh) *n.,* pl. **collonemas, collonema·ta** (·tuh) [*collo-* + *-nema*]. A lipoma with extensive mucoid degeneration.

col·lum (kol′um) *L. n.,* genit. sing. **col·li** (·eye), pl. **col·la** (·luh) [NA]. NECK.

collum ana·to·mi·cum hu·me·ri (an·uh·tom′i·kum hew′mur·eye) [NA]. ANATOMIC NECK of the humerus.

collum chi·rur·gi·cum hu·me·ri (ki·rur′ji·kum hew′mur·eye) [NA]. SURGICAL NECK of the humerus.

collum cos·tae (kos′tee) [NA]. The neck of a rib.

collum den·tis (den′tis) [NA]. The neck of a tooth.

collum dis·tor·tum (dis·tor′tum). TORTICOLLIS.

collum fe·mo·ris (fem′o·ris) [NA]. The neck of the femur.

collum fol·li·cu·li pi·li (fol·ick′yoo·lye pye′lye) [BNA]. The neck of a hair follicle.

collum glan·dis (glan′dis) [NA]. The neck of the penis; the constriction at the base of the glans.

collum mal·lei (mal′ee·eye) [NA]. The neck of the malleus.

collum man·di·bu·lae (man·dib′yoo·lee) [NA]. The neck of the mandible; there is a right and a left one.

collum ra·dii (ray′dee·eye) [NA]. The neck of the radius.

collum sca·pu·lae (skap′yoo·lee) [NA]. The neck of the scapula.

collum ta·li (tay′lye) [NA]. The neck of the talus.

collum ve·si·cae fel·le·ae (ve·sigh′kee fel′ee·ee) [NA]. NECK OF THE GALLBLADDER.

col·lu·nar·i·um (kol″yoo·năr′ee·um) *n.,* pl. **collunar·ia** (·ee·uh) [L. *coll*uere, to wash out, + *nar*is]. A solution intended to be used in the nose.

col·lu·to·ri·um (kol″yoo·to′ree·um) *n.,* pl. **colluto·ria** (·ree·uh) [NL., from L. *colluere,* to rinse out]. A mouthwash.

col·lu·to·ry (kol′yoo·tor·ee) *n.* COLLUTORIUM.

col·lyr·i·um (kuh·lirr′ee·um) *n.,* pl. **collyr·ia** (·ee·uh), **collyriums** [Gk. *kollyrion,* eye salve]. A preparation for local application to the eye, usually a wash or lotion.

colo-. See *col-.*

col·o·bo·ma (kol″uh·bo′muh) *n.,* pl. **coloboma·ta** (·tuh), **colobomas** [Gk. *kolobōma,* from *koloboun,* to mutilate]. 1. Any congenital, pathologic, or operative defect, especially of the eye; occurring most commonly in the iris, ciliary body, or choroid, usually as a cleft placed inferiorly. 2. One or more congenital fissures of the eyelid or eyelids, usually the upper. —**coloboma·tous** (·tus) *adj.*

coloboma au·ris (aw′ris). A developmental malformation of the external ear caused by defect of the hyomandibular groove with resulting cleft between the tragus and antitragus.

coloboma of the optic nerve. A coloboma caused by partial closure or nonclosure of the fetal fissure of the optic stalk.

coloboma of the retina. A coloboma caused by partial closure or nonclosure of the fetal fissure of the optic cup; usually associated with a similar defect in the choroid.

coloboma pal·pe·brae (pal′pe·bree, pal·pee′bree) [L., of the eyelid]. COLOBOMA (2).

co·lo·ce·cos·to·my (ko″lo·see·kos′tuh·mee) *n.* [*colo-* + *cecostomy*]. CECOCOLOSTOMY.

co·lo·co·lic (ko″lo·ko′lick) *adj.* Pertaining to or between two parts of the colon, as: colocolic anastomosis.

co·lo·co·los·to·my (ko″lo·ko·los′tuh·mee) *n.* [*colo-* + *colostomy*]. An anastomosis between two noncontinuous segments of the colon in order to short-circuit the lumen around inoperable obstructing tumors or to prepare for later resection.

col·o·cynth (kol′o·sinth) *n.* [Gk. *kolokynthis*]. The dried pulp of the unripe but full-grown fruit of *Citrullus colocynthis;* a drastic cathartic.

co·lo·cys·to·plas·ty (ko″lo·sis′to·plas·tee) *n.* [*colo-* + *cysto-* + *-plasty*]. An operation in which a segment of the colon is sutured to the urinary bladder to increase bladder capacity.

Cologel. A trademark for methylcellulose.
co·logne spirit (kuh·lone'). ETHYL ALCOHOL.
cologne water. A solution of certain volatile oils in alcohol and water used as a toilet water or perfume.
co·lo·hep·a·to·pexy (ko"lo·hep'uh·to·peck"see) *n.* [*colo-* + *hepatopexy*]. Fixation of the colon to the liver to form adhesions.
Co·lom·bian spotted fever [after *Colombia,* South America]. Rocky Mountain spotted fever in South America.
co·lom·bo (ko·lom'bo) *n.* CALUMBA.
co·lon (ko'lun) *n.* [Gk. *kolon*] [NA]. The part of the large intestine beginning at the cecum and terminating at the end of the sigmoid flexure. In the various parts of its course it is known as ascending colon, transverse colon, descending colon, and sigmoid colon; the last is sometimes divided into the iliac colon and the pelvic colon. See also Plates 8, 10, 13, 14.
colon-aerogenes group. A group of non-spore-forming gram-negative aerobic bacilli of the genera *Escherichia* and *Aerobacter,* which when found in water is evidence of fecal contamination.
colon as·cen·dens (a·sen'denz) [NA]. ASCENDING COLON.
colon bacillus. *ESCHERICHIA COLI.*
colon des·cen·dens (de·sen'denz) [NA]. DESCENDING COLON.
co·lo·ni·al (kuh·lo'nee·ul) *adj.* Of, pertaining to, or existing as a colony.
colonial spirit. METHYL ALCOHOL.
co·lon·ic (ko·lon'ick) *adj.* Of or pertaining to the colon.
colonic pseudopolyps. Polypoid masses composed of granulation tissue projecting from the luminal surface of the colon; frequently associated with ulcerative colitis.
co·lon·o·scope (ko·lon'uh·skope) *n.* A flexible fiberoptic instrument passed per anum, used for examination of the luminal surface of the colon.
co·lon·os·co·py (ko"luh·nos'kuh·pee) *n.* The procedure of examining the colon with a colonoscope. **—colonosco·pist,** *n.*
colon sig·moi·de·um (sig·moy'dee·um) [NA]. SIGMOID COLON.
colon trans·ver·sum (trans·vur'sum) [NA]. TRANSVERSE COLON.
col·o·ny (kol'uh·nee) *n.* [L. *colonia*]. 1. *In bacteriology,* a group or mass of microorganisms in a culture, derived from a single cell. Variations in bacterial structure or antigenic composition are often expressed in the form of the colony, as smooth, rough, dwarf. 2. *In cell biology,* a group of cells in culture or in certain experimental tissues, as spleen colony, a cluster of hematopoietic cells derived from stem cells administered to an irradiated animal.
colony counter. A device for counting bacterial colonies; usually consists of an illuminated transparent plate, divided into spaces of known area, over which a petri dish containing the colonies is placed.
co·lo·pexy (kol'o·peck"see, ko'lo·) *n.* [*colo-* + *-pexy*]. *Obsol.* The suturing of the sigmoid flexure to the abdominal wall.
co·lo·pho·ny (kol'o·fo"nee, ko·lof'uh·nee) *n.* [Gk. *kolophōnia,* of Colyphon]. ROSIN.
co·lo·proc·tos·to·my (ko"lo·prock·tos'tuh·mee) *n.* [*colo-* + *procto-* + *-stomy*]. The formation of a new passage between the colon and the rectum.
co·lop·to·sia (ko"lop·to'zee·uh) *n.* COLOPTOSIS.
co·lop·to·sis (ko"lop·to'sis) *n.*, pl. **colopto·ses** (·seez) [*colo-* + *ptosis*]. Prolapse or displacement of the colon.
Col·o·ra·do tick fever. A nonexanthematous acute viral disease of man occurring in the western United States and transmitted by a bite of the tick *Dermacentor andersoni;* characterized by short course, intermittent fever, leukopenia, and occasionally meningoencephalitis.
color amblyopia. PARTIAL COLOR BLINDNESS.
color aphasia. Color dysnomia as a manifestation of aphasia.
color blindness. Inability to perceive one or more, or rarely all, colors. **—color-blind,** *adj.*
color dysnomia. An inability to name colors despite retained ability to match them and discriminate among them; may be due to an expressive aphasia or to a specific defect in recalling the names of colors and not associated with other defects of linguistic function.
color gustation. A form of synesthesia in which color sensations accompany the sensation of taste.
color hearing. A form of synesthesia in which sensations of color are associated with different sounds.
col·or·im·e·ter (kul"ur·im'e·tur) *n.* An instrument for determining color intensity, as for measuring the hemoglobin in blood. See also *photoelectric colorimeter.*
col·or·i·met·ric (kul"ur·i·met'rick) *adj.* Of or pertaining to a colorimeter or to colorimetry. **—colorimet·ri·cal·ly** (·ri·kuh·lee) *adv.*
col·or·im·e·try (kul"ur·im'e·tree) *n.* [*color* + *-metry*]. 1. The science of determining colors. 2. Chemical analysis by the use of a colorimeter.
color index. The amount of hemoglobin per erythrocyte relative to normal, obtained by the following formula: C.I. = (percent normal hemoglobin concentration/percent normal erythrocyte count. Different laboratories use different normal values in this formula. Compare *Colour Index.*
color name aphasia. An inability to find the names of colors, associated with parietal lesions.
co·lor·rha·phy (ko·lor'uh·fee) *n.* [*colo-* + *-rrhaphy*]. Suture of the colon.
color scotoma. Color blindness limited to a part of the visual field; may exist without interruption of the field for white light.
color sense. *In ophthalmology,* the faculty of distinguishing light of various wavelengths.
color threshold test. A lantern type test of the ability of color-vision-deficient individuals to identify colored light signals at intensities ranging from the normal chromatic thresholds to 100 times as great; used chiefly in psychology.
color vision test. See *abridged A.* O. color vision test, color threshold test, Ishihara's test.
co·lo·scope (ko'luh·skope) *n.* COLONOSCOPE.
co·lo·sig·moid·os·to·my (ko"lo·sig"moid·os'tuh·mee) *n.* [*colo-* + *sigmoido-* + *-stomy*]. An anastomosis between the sigmoid and some other part of the colon.
co·los·to·my (ko·los'tuh·mee) *n.* [*colo-* + *-stomy*]. The formation of an artificial anus in the anterior abdominal wall or loin. The opening into the colon may be anywhere depending on the location of the diseased condition, as cecostomy or sigmoidostomy.
colostomy bag. A rubber bag worn as a belt, especially constructed to receive the intestinal excreta from a colostomy opening.
col·os·tra·tion (kol"us·tray'shun) *n.* [L. *colostratio,* from *colostrum*]. Any disorder of infants caused by colostrum, such as a diarrheal reaction.
co·los·tror·rhea, co·los·tror·rhoea (ko·los"tro·ree'uh) *n.* [*colostrum* + *-rrhea*]. Profuse discharge of colostrum.
co·los·trum (ko·los'trum) *n.* [L.] [BNA]. The first milk from the mother's breasts after the birth of the child. It is laxative, and assists in the expulsion of the meconium. Contains greater quantities of lactalbumin and lactoprotein than later milk.
colostrum corpuscle or **body.** One of the phagocytic cells of the mammary glands, found in the colostrum, containing fat globules. These corpuscles are present for the first 2 weeks after parturition and may again appear when the milk is diminishing. After the third day, the globules are freed by the bursting of cells to form the true milk.
colostrum test. A pregnancy test in which 0.02 ml of equal parts of human colostrum and saline solution is injected intradermally. No areola or a slight areola (less than 1 inch in diameter) indicates a positive test.
co·lot·o·my (ko·lot'uh·mee) *n.* [*colo-* + *-tomy*]. Incision of the colon; may be abdominal, lateral, lumbar, or iliac, according to the region of entrance.

Col·our Index. A comprehensive publication of the Society of Dyers and Colourists, Bradford, Yorkshire, and the American Association of Textile Chemists and Colorists. The second edition 1956-58, with Supplement 1963, lists a large number of industrially used as well as older dyestuffs, pigments, and stains. Each substance is uniquely identified by Colour Index (C.I.) number specifying particular chemical materials.

-colous [L. *col*ere, to cultivate, inhabit, + *-ous*]. A combining form meaning *inhabiting, growing in.*

colp-, colpo- [Gk. *kolpos*]. A combining form meaning *vagina, vaginal.*

col·pal·gia (kol·pal'jee·uh) *n.* [*colp-* + *-algia*]. Pain in the vagina.

col·pa·tre·sia (kol''pa·tree'zhuh, ·zee·uh) *n.* [*colp-* + *atresia*]. Occlusion or atresia of the vagina.

col·pec·ta·sia (kol''peck·tay'zhuh, ·zee·uh) *n.* [*colp-* + *ectasia*]. Dilatation of the vagina.

col·pec·to·my (kol·peck'tuh·mee) *n.* [*colp-* + *-ectomy*]. Excision of the vagina.

col·pe·de·ma (kol''pe·dee'muh) *n.* [*colp-* + *edema*]. Edema of the vagina.

col·peu·ryn·ter (kol''pew·rin'tur) *n.* [*colp-* + Gk. *eurynein*, to make wide]. An inflatable bag or sac formerly used for dilating the vagina.

col·peu·rys·is (kol''pew·ris·is, kol·pew'ris·is) *n.* Dilatation of the vagina, especially that effected by means of the colpeurynter.

col·pi·tis (kol·pye'tis) *n.* [*colp-* + *-itis*]. Inflammation of the vagina.

colpo-. See *colp-*.

col·po·cele (kol'po·seel) *n.* [*colpo-* + *-cele*]. A hernia in the vagina.

col·po·clei·sis (kol''po·klye'sis) *n.*, pl. **colpoclei·ses** (·seez) [*colpo-* + *-cleisis*]. Closure of the vagina by suturing.

col·po·hy·per·pla·sia cys·ti·ca (kol''po·high·pur·play'zhuh sis'ti·kuh). EMPHYSEMATOUS VAGINITIS.

col·po·per·i·neo·plas·ty (kol''po·perr''i·nee'o·plas''tee) *n.* [*colpo-* + *perineo-* + *-plasty*]. Plastic surgery of the perineum and vagina.

col·po·per·i·ne·or·rha·phy (kol''po·perr''i·nee·or'uh·fee) *n.* [*colpo-* + *perineo-* + *-rrhaphy*]. Suture of a cut or lacerated vagina and perineum.

col·po·pexy (kol'po·peck''see) *n.* [*colpo-* + *-pexy*]. Fixation of the vagina by suturing it to a surrounding structure.

col·po·plas·ty (kol'po·plas''tee) *n.* [*colpo-* + *-plasty*]. Plastic repair of the vagina.

col·por·rha·phy (kol·por'uh·fee) *n.* [*colpo-* + *-rrhaphy*]. Suture of the vagina for repair.

col·por·rhex·is (kol''po·reck'sis) *n.*, pl. **colporrhex·es** (·seez) [*colpo-* + *-rrhexis*]. Traumatic separation of the cervix of the uterus from its vaginal attachments.

-colpos [Gk. *kolpos*, vagina, womb]. A combining form meaning *vagina.*

col·po·scope (kol'po·skope) *n.* [*colpo-* + *-scope*]. An instrument for the visual examination of the vagina and cervix; a vaginal speculum. **—col·po·scop·ic** (kol''po·skop'ick) *adj.*; **col·pos·co·py** (kol·pos'kuh·pee) *n.*

col·pot·o·my (kol·pot'uh·mee) *n.* [*colpo-* + *-tomy*]. Incision of the vagina.

Colprone. Trademark for medrogestone, a progestational steroid.

Colprosterone. A trademark for progesterone.

colts·foot, *n.* An herb, *Tussilago farfara*, of the aster family; its leaves have been used as a demulcent and bitter, and sometimes for treatment of chronic cough.

Co·lu·bri·dae (ko·lew'bri·dee) *n. pl.* [NL., from L. *coluber, colubri*, snake]. A family of snakes, most of which are nonpoisonous. The fangs (in the species that have them) are fixed, grooved, and in the rear of the mouth. See also *boomslang*. **—col·u·brid** (kol'yoo·brid) *adj.* & *n.*

Col·um·bacz fly (kol'um·bahts) [after *Golubac (Hungar. Kolumbácz)*, Yugoslavia]. *SIMULIUM COLUMBACZENSE.*

co·lum·bi·an spirit (kuh·lum'bee·un). METHYL ALCOHOL.

Columbia-SK virus. A strain of virus belonging to the picornavirus group and responsible for encephalomyocarditis, with the natural reservoir in rodents, but capable of infecting a wide range of hosts, including man.

co·lum·bin (ko·lum'bin) *n.* A bitter glycoside in calumba.

co·lum·bi·um (ko·lum'bee·um) *n.* [after *Columbia*, South Carolina]. NIOBIUM.

col·u·mel·la (kol''yoo·mel'uh) *n.*, pl. **columel·lae** (·lee) [NL., small column]. 1. The septum of the nasal vestibule, the medial boundary of the nostrils. 2. The modiolus or central axis of the cochlea of the human ear. 3. A bone in land Amphibia, many reptiles, and birds which takes the place of the ossicles of the ear in man.

col·umn (kol'um) *n.* & *v.* [L. *columna*]. 1. A supporting pillar; a pillar-shaped structure. 2. To place tampons in the vagina to support a prolapsed uterus. **—co·lum·nar** (ko·lum'nur) *adj.*

co·lum·na (ko·lum'nuh) *n.*, pl. **colum·nae** (·nee) [L.]. COLUMN.

columna anterior me·dul·lae spi·na·lis (me·dul'ee spye·nay'lis) [NA]. ANTERIOR COLUMN.

columnae ana·les (ay·nay'leez) [NA]. ANAL COLUMNS.

columnae car·ne·ae (kahr'nee·ee). TRABECULAE CARNEAE.

columnae gri·se·ae (griz'ee·ee) [NA]. COLUMNS OF THE GRAY MATTER.

columnae rec·ta·les (reck·tay'leez) [BNA]. Columnae anales (= ANAL COLUMNS).

columnae re·na·les (ree·nay'leez) [NA]. RENAL COLUMNS.

columnae ru·ga·rum (roo·gair'um) [NA]. COLUMNS OF THE VAGINA.

columna for·ni·cis (for'ni·sis) [NA]. COLUMN OF THE FORNIX.

columna la·te·ra·lis me·dul·lae spi·na·lis (lat·e·ray'lis me·dul'ee spye·nay'lis) [NA]. LATERAL COLUMN.

columna na·si (nay'zye). COLUMELLA (1).

columna posterior me·dul·lae spi·na·lis (me·dul'ee spye·nay'lis) [NA]. POSTERIOR COLUMN.

columnar cell. An epithelial cell in which the height is markedly greater than the width.

columnar-cell carcinoma. ADENOCARCINOMA.

columnar epithelium. Epithelium that is distinguished by elongated, prismatic, or columnar cells.

columna ru·ga·rum anterior (roo·gair'um) [NA]. The anterior column of the vagina. See *columns of the vagina.*

columna rugarum posterior [NA]. The posterior column of the vagina. See *columns of the vagina.*

columna ver·te·bra·lis (vur·te·bray'lis) [NA]. VERTEBRAL COLUMN.

column chromatography. Chromatography in which the porous solid is packed into a tube and separation is achieved either by adsorption, using a single solvent or a mixture of miscible solvents, or by partition, using two immiscible solvents.

co·lum·ni·za·tion (kol·um''ni·zay'shun, kol''um·ni·) *n. Obsol.* Placement of tampons in the vagina to support a prolapsed uterus.

column of Ber·tin (behr·tæ^n') [E. J. *Bertin*, French anatomist, 1712-1781]. RENAL COLUMN.

column of Bur·dach (bŏŏr'dak̲h) [K. F. *Burdach*, German anatomist, 1776-1847]. CUNEATE FASCICULUS.

column of Goll [F. *Goll*]. FASCICULUS GRACILIS MEDULLAE SPINALIS.

column of the fornix. One of the two anterior, arched pillars of the fornix, terminating in the mammillary bodies. NA *columna fornicis.*

columns of Morgagni. ANAL COLUMNS.

columns of the gray matter. Divisions of the longitudinal column of gray matter in the spinal cord: the anterior column, the lateral column, and the posterior column. NA *columnae griseae.*

columns of the vagina. Two median, longitudinal ridges formed by the rugae of the vagina: that of the anterior wall (*columna rugarum anterior*) and that of the posterior wall (*columna rugarum posterior*). NA *columnae rugarum.*

Coly-Mycin M. A trademark for colistimethate sodium, an antibacterial.

Coly-Mycin S. A trademark for colistin sulfate, an antibacterial.

col·za oil (kol'zuh). RAPE OIL.

com-, con-, cor- [L., from *cum,* with]. A prefix meaning *with, jointly, together.*

¹co·ma (ko'muh) *n.* [Gk. *kōma,* deep sleep]. A state in which the patient is incapable of sensing or responding, either to external stimuli or to inner needs.

²coma [Gk. *komē,* hair; tail of a comet]. *In optics and ophthalmology,* a blurred part of an image resulting from spherical aberration.

com·a·tose (kom'uh·toce, ·toze, ko'muh·) *adj.* In a condition of coma; resembling coma.

coma vigil (ko'muh vij'il) [L., wakeful coma]. PSEUDOCOMA.

co·ma vi·gile (kohⁿ·mahʰ vee·zheel') [Fr., wakeful coma]. PSEUDOCOMA.

Combantrin. A trademark for pyrantel pamoate.

combat fatigue, exhaustion, or **neurosis.** WAR NEUROSIS.

comb disease. FAVUS OF FOWLS.

combined anesthesia. 1. Anesthesia produced by a combination of anesthetics, such as chloroform, ether, and nitrous oxide, or by a combination of methods. 2. Anesthesia produced by anesthetics plus somnifacient drugs. See also *balanced anesthesia.*

combined aphasia. The presence of two or more types of aphasia in the same individual.

combined fat- and carbohydrate-induced hyperlipemia. FAMILIAL HYPERCHYLOMICRONEMIA WITH HYPERPREBETALIPOPROTEINEMIA.

combined flexion of the trunk and thigh sign. TRUNK-THIGH SIGN OF BABINSKI.

combined gynecography. Gynecography together with hysterosalpingography.

combined pelvimetry. A combination of external and internal pelvimetry.

combined sclerosis. SUBACUTE COMBINED DEGENERATION OF THE SPINAL CORD.

combined system disease. Any intrinsic disease of the spinal cord affecting the posterior and lateral columns. See also *subacute combined degeneration of the spinal cord.*

combined version. BIMANUAL VERSION.

comb·ing (ko'ming) *n.* The radial arrangement of elongated cells around vessels or vascular spaces, seen particularly in spindle-cell sarcomas.

combining site. The portion of an antibody molecule that combines with an antigenic determinant. See also *Fab fragment.*

Com·by's sign (kohⁿ·bee') [J. *Comby,* French pediatrician, 1853–1947]. Stomatitis of the buccal mucosa, sometimes with whitish-yellow patches, appearing before the Koplik's spots in measles.

com·e·do (kom'e·do, ko·mee') *n.,* pl. **com·e·do·nes** (kom''e·do'neez) [L., maggot (to which a blackhead expressed from the skin was likened), lit., glutton, from *comedere,* to devour, from *edere,* to eat]. A collection of sebaceous material and keratin retained in the hair follicle and excretory duct of the sebaceous gland, the surface covered with a black dot due to oxidation of sebum at the follicular orifice. It is the primary lesion of acne vulgaris; usually found on the face, chest, and back, and more commonly occurring during adolescence.

comedo adenocarcinoma. COMEDOCARCINOMA.

com·e·do·car·ci·no·ma (kom''e·do·kahr''si·no'muh) *n.* [*comedo* + *carcinoma*]. A type of adenocarcinoma of the breast in which the ducts are filled with cells, which, when expressed from the cut surface, resemble comedos.

comedones. Plural of *comedo.*

co·mes (ko'meez) *n.,* pl. **com·i·tes** (kom'i·teez) [L., companion]. *In anatomy,* an artery which accompanies a nerve, or a vein which accompanies an artery.

com·frey (kum'free) *n.* [OF. *confirie*]. A plant of the genus *Symphytum;* the root of the common comfrey, *S. officinale,* has been used as a demulcent, astringent, and bitter drug, and was a common ingredient of formulations for treatment of cough.

comma bacillus. *VIBRIO CHOLERAE.*

command automatism. *In psychiatry,* the compulsive or automatic obedience and carrying out by an individual of suggestions or requests made by others.

commander's balsam. COMPOUND BENZOIN TINCTURE.

comma tract (of Schultze). A tract, comma-shaped in cross section, located in the dorsal funiculus of the spinal cord and made up of the descending branches of the dorsal root fibers. NA *fasciculus interfascicularis, fasciculus semilunaris.*

com·mem·o·ra·tive sign (kuh·mem'o·ruh·tiv). A sign due to a previous disease.

com·men·sal·ism (kuh·men'sul·iz·um) *n.* [L. *commensalis,* from *com-,* together, + *mensa,* table]. A more or less intimate association between organisms of different species, without injury to either organism and with some benefit, such as nourishment and protection, to one; as the association of the small crab and the oyster in whose mantle cavity it lives. See also *symbiosis.* —**commensal,** *n. & adj.*

commercial amyl alcohol. AMYL ALCOHOL (2).

com·mi·nute (kom'i·newt) *v. & adj.* [L. *comminuere* to lessen]. 1. *In chemistry,* to pulverize; to divide into fine particles. 2. *In surgery,* to fracture a bone so that it is shattered into several pieces. 3. Shattered, pulverized. —**comminut·ed** (·id) *adj.;* **com·mi·nu·tion** (kom''i·new'shun) *n.*

comminuted fracture. A fracture in which there is splintering or fragmentation of the bone.

Com·miph·o·ra (kom·if'uh·ruh) *n.* [Gk. *kommi,* gum, + *phoros,* bearing]. A genus of shrubs and trees of the Burseraceae, found in Africa and the East Indies. Various species yield myrrh and bdellium.

Commission Certified stain. A stain which has been certified by the Biological Stain Commission. Abbreviated, C.C.

com·mis·su·ra (kom''i·shoor'uh, ·syoor'uh, ·soor'uh) *n.,* pl. & genit. sing. **commissu·rae** (·ee) [L.]. COMMISSURE.

commissura al·ba me·dul·lae spi·na·lis (al'buh me·dul'ee spye·nay'lis) [NA]. WHITE COMMISSURE (1).

commissura anterior alba medullae spinalis [BNA]. Commissura alba medullae spinalis (= WHITE COMMISSURE (1)).

commissura anterior ce·re·bri (serr'e·brye) [NA]. ANTERIOR COMMISSURE.

commissura anterior gri·sea me·dul·lae spi·na·lis (griz'ee·uh me·dul'ee spye·nay'lis) [BNA]. The anterior gray commissure of the spinal cord. See *gray commissure of the spinal cord.*

commissurae su·pra·op·ti·cae (sue''pruh·op'ti·see) [NA]. In the human brain, the combined ventral supraoptic decussation (of Gudden), the dorsal or superior supraoptic decussation (of Meynert), and the anterior hypothalamic decussation (of Ganser).

commissura for·ni·cis (for'ni·sis) [NA]. COMMISSURE OF THE FORNIX.

commissura ha·be·nu·la·rum (ha·ben''yoo·lair'um) [NA]. HABENULAR COMMISSURE.

commissura hip·po·cam·pi (hip''o·kam'pye) [BNA]. Commissura fornicis (= COMMISSURE OF THE FORNIX).

commissura inferior (Guddeni) [BNA]. VENTRAL SUPRAOPTIC DECUSSATION.

com·mis·sur·al (kom·ish'ur·ul, kom''i·shoor'ul) *adj.* Pertaining to or having the properties of a commissure.

commissura la·bi·o·rum anterior (lay''bee·or'um) [NA]. The anterior junction of the labia majora.

commissura labiorum oris (o'ris) [NA]. The junction of the upper and lower lip on either side of the mouth.

commissura labiorum posterior [NA]. An indefinite ridge connecting the posterior extremities of the labia majora.

commissural cell. A nerve cell of the gray matter of the spinal cord, the axon of which passes through one of the commissures and enters the white matter of the other side of the cord.

commissural fibers. Fibers joining an area of the cortex of one cerebral hemisphere to a similar area of the other.

commissural nucleus. A collection of nerve cells in the medulla oblongata formed by the junction of the nuclei of the solitary tract at the posterior end of the fourth ventricle.

commissural nucleus of the accessory nerve. COMMISSURAL NUCLEUS.

commissural nucleus of the alae cinereae. COMMISSURAL NUCLEUS.

commissural nucleus of the medulla oblongata (of Cajal). COMMISSURAL NUCLEUS.

commissural nucleus of the solitary fasciculus. COMMISSURAL NUCLEUS.

commissural nucleus of the vagus nerve. COMMISSURAL NUCLEUS.

commissura mol·lis (mol'is) [L., soft]. ADHESIO INTERTHALAMICA.

commissura pal·pe·bra·rum·la·te·ra·lis (pal·pe·brair'um lat·e·ray'lis) [NA]. The lateral junction of the upper and lower eyelids.

commissura palpebrarum me·di·a·lis (mee·dee·ay'lis) [NA]. The medial junction of the upper and lower eyelids.

commissura posterior ce·re·bri (serr'e·brye) [NA]. POSTERIOR COMMISSURE OF THE CEREBRUM.

commissura posterior me·dul·lae spi·na·lis (me·dul'ee spye·nay'lis) [BNA]. The posterior gray commissure of the spinal cord. See *gray commissure of the spinal cord.*

commissura superior (Meynerti) [BNA]. DORSAL SUPRAOPTIC DECUSSATION.

com·mis·sure (kom'i·shur, ·syoor) *n.* [L. *commissura,* a joining together]. 1. Strands of nerve fibers uniting like structures in the two sides of the brain or spinal cord. 2. The region of union of such structures as the lips, eyelids, labia majora, or cardiac valves.

commissure of Forel [A. H. *Forel*]. SUPRAMAMILLARY DECUSSATION.

commissure of the fornix. The transverse part of the fornix, uniting the crura. NA *commissura fornicis.*

com·mis·su·ro·spi·nal (kom·ish''oo·ro·spye'nul) *adj.* Pertaining to the posterior commissure of the spinal cord and the spinal cord.

commissurospinal tract. Descending nerve fibers arising from the nucleus of the posterior commissure and entering the medial longitudinal fasciculus.

com·mis·sur·ot·o·my (com''i·shur·ot'uh·mee) *n.* [*commissure* + *-tomy*]. 1. Surgical destruction of a commissure, usually the anterior commissure, particularly in the treatment of certain psychiatric disorders. 2. Surgical division of a stenosed cardiac valve.

com·mit·ment, *n. In legal medicine,* the obligatory hospitalization or institutionalization of a patient in need of treatment, particularly for a mental disorder. Compare *certification (4).*

common atrioventricular canal. ATRIOVENTRICULARIS COMMUNIS.

common bile duct. The duct formed by the union of the cystic and the hepatic ducts. NA *ductus choledochus.*

common cardinal veins. Paired primary veins located in the septum transversum, connecting the anterior and posterior cardinal veins with the sinus venosus. Syn. *ducts of Cuvier.*

common carotid artery. An artery that originates on the right from the brachiocephalic trunk and on the left from the arch of the aorta, and has external and internal carotid, rarely superior thyroid, ascending pharyngeal, and even vertebral branches. It distributes blood to the region of the neck and head. NA *arteria carotis communis.*

common carotid plexus. A network of sympathetic nerve fibers surrounding the common carotid artery, formed by branches of the superior cervical ganglion. NA *plexus caroticus communis.*

common cold. A mild, acute, contagious upper respiratory viral infection of short duration, characterized by coryza, watering of the eyes, cough, and, occasionally, fever.

common hepatic artery. The hepatic artery to the point just distal to the branching off of the right gastric and gastroduodenal arteries. NA *arteria hepatica communis.* See also Table of Arteries in the Appendix.

common hepatic duct. The common duct formed by the union of the left hepatic duct, which drains the left and caudate lobes of the liver, and the right hepatic duct, which drains the right and quadrate lobes of the liver. NA *ductus hepaticus communis.* See also Plate 13.

common interclinoid foramen. A canal formed by an anomalous process connecting the anterior, middle, and posterior clinoid processes of the sphenoid bone.

common pharyngobranchial duct. The medial part of the fourth pharyngeal pouch forming a common duct for the ultimobranchial body (fifth pouch) and the lateral part of the fourth pouch.

common reference lead. In an electrical recording system, as in electroencephalography, the inactive or indifferent electrode to which the active electrodes are connected.

common vent. CLOACA.

com·mo·tio (kuh·mo'shee·o) *n.* [L.]. A concussion; shock.

commotio cer·e·bri (serr'i·brye). BRAIN CONCUSSION.

commotio ret·i·nae (ret'i·nee). Dysfunction of the retina from a blow on or near the eye; characterized by sudden blindness, but little or no ophthalmoscopic evidence of any lesion. The sight is usually regained, and its loss is supposedly due to disturbance of the retinal elements.

commotio spi·na·lis (spye·nay'lis). CONCUSSION OF THE SPINAL CORD.

com·mu·ni·ca·ble (kuh·mew'ni·kuh·bul) *adj.* Transmissible from one source to another.

communicable disease. 1. An infectious disease transmissible from one source (either an animal or a person) to another, directly or indirectly (as via a vector). 2. Often, CONTAGIOUS DISEASE. Compare *infectious disease.*

Communicable Disease Center. Former name of the Center for Disease Control.

com·mu·ni·cans (kom·yoo'ni·kanz) *L. adj.* Communicating; connecting.

com·mu·ni·cate, *v.* [L. *communicare,* to share, impart]. *In anatomy,* to join or to form an unbroken passage from one place to another; ANASTOMOSE. —**com·mu·ni·ca·tion,** *n.*

com·mu·ni·cat·ed insanity. FOLIE À DEUX.

com·mu·ni·cat·ing arteries. The anterior and posterior communicating arteries of the cerebrum. See Table of Arteries in the Appendix.

communicating hydrocele. Hydrocele in which the fluid-filled tunica vaginalis is patent, connecting directly with the peritoneal cavity.

communicating hydrocephalus. A form of hydrocephalus in which there is communication between the ventricles and the spinal subarachnoid space; usually caused by obliteration of the cerebral subarachnoid space, the result of meningitis or subarachnoid hemorrhage. Contr. *obstructive hydrocephalus.*

community health nurse. A qualified nurse working for a public health official or agency to assist in safeguarding the health of people in the home, community health clinic, or designated district, and who gives instruction and care to people at home.

community medicine. Health care for all members of a community, emphasizing preventive medicine and early diagnosis as well as therapy.

community mental health center. Any facility or group of facilities that is based within the community, for the prevention and treatment of mental illness.

community psychiatry. The diagnosis and treatment of mental and emotional disorders within a patient's own community, employing all resources and techniques available there.

com·mu·ta·tor (kom′yoo·tay″tur) *n.* RHEOTROPE.

comp. Abbreviation for *compositus,* compound.

com·pac·ta (kom·pack′tuh) *n.* Substantia compacta (= COMPACT BONE).

compact bone. Osseous tissue in which marrow spaces are replaced by cylindrical, concentrically laminated haversian systems, each with an axial vascular channel, the haversian canal. NA *substantia compacta.*

compact layer. STRATUM COMPACTUM.

companion artery of the sciatic nerve. SCIATIC ARTERY.

companionate marriage. A form of marriage for sexual companionship without legal obligation, economic responsibility, or desire for children.

com·par·a·scope (kum·păr′uh·scope) *n.* An apparatus attached to two microscopes for the simultaneous comparison of two different specimens.

com·par·a·tive anatomy. Investigation and comparison of the anatomy of different orders of animals or of plants, one with another.

comparative embryology. Investigation and comparison of the embryology of different orders of animals or of plants, one with another.

comparative pathology. Investigation and comparison of disease in various animals, including man, to arrive at resemblances and differences which may clarify disease as a phenomenon of nature.

comparative physiology. The comparative study of the physiology of different animals and plants, or the comparison of analogous physiologic mechanisms in different species.

com·pa·ra·tor (kom′puh·ray″tur, kum·păr′uh·tur) *n.* A type of colorimeter in which a place is provided for a standard solution or solutions to be visually compared with an unknown solution under similar lighting conditions.

com·pat·i·bil·i·ty, *n.* [L. *compati,* to have compassion]. 1. Congruity; the power of a drug or a drug substance in a medicine to mix with another without deleterious chemical change or loss of therapeutic power. 2. In blood grouping, (a) in vitro, no interaction between two bloods; (b) in vivo, no reaction whatsoever from the injection of a blood found to be compatible by laboratory tests. 3. HISTOCOMPATIBILITY. 4. The ability to exist together in harmony. —**com·pat·i·ble,** *adj.*

compatibility testing. CROSS MATCHING.

Compazine. Trademark for prochlorperazine, an antiemetic and tranquilizing drug used as the base and the edisylate (ethanedisulfonate) and maleate salts.

com·pen·sate, *v.* [L. *compensare,* to balance]. To correct a function that has been adversely affected. —**com·pen·sat·ing,** *adj.*

compensated acidosis. Acidosis in which the physiologic compensatory mechanisms are able to restore a normal pH of about 7.4.

compensated alkalosis. Alkalosis in which the physiologic compensatory mechanisms are able to restore a normal pH of about 7.4.

compensating curve. The anteroposterior and lateral curvature in the alignment of the occluding surfaces and incisal edges of artificial teeth, used to develop balanced occlusion.

compensating ocular. A lens that compensates for axial aberration of the objective lens.

compensating operation. *In ophthalmology,* tenotomy of the associated antagonist in cases of diplopia from paresis of one of the ocular muscles.

com·pen·sa·tion, *n.* 1. The process of counterbalancing a lack or a defect of a bodily or physiologic function.

compensation neurosis. A neurotic reaction motivated by the uncontrollable desire to receive a monetary award for damages or injuries or some other secondary gain; a common complication in traumatic neurosis. See also *secondary gain.*

com·pen·sa·to·ry (kum·pen′suh·to″ree) *adj.* Making up for a loss, counteracting an extreme.

compensatory curvature. In spinal curvature, a secondary curve, occurring as the result of the efforts of the trunk to maintain its upright position.

compensatory emphysema. Simple nonobstructive overdistention of lung segments or an entire lung in adaptation to collapse, destruction, or removal of lung tissue.

compensatory hypertrophy. 1. Hypertrophy in response to destruction or injury in the opposite paired organ or in another part of the same organ. 2. Hypertrophy, as of skeletal or cardiac muscles, in response to habitual vigrous exercise.

compensatory pause. *In cardiology,* a long interval immediately following a premature beat, compensating by its length for the prematurity of the beat; caused by a second impulse arriving when the previously excited myocardial tissue is still in a refractory state.

com·pe·tence, *n.* [L. *competentia,* agreement]. 1. *In legal medicine,* the possession of qualifications, capacity, soundness of mind, or other legally acceptable standards to perform certain acts and to take responsibility for them. 2. *In genetics,* the property whereby a cell is able to be transformed by a molecule of transforming DNA.

com·pet·i·tive inhibition. 1. *In physiology,* inhibition of the passage of an impulse through a neuron due to the dominance thereof by a stronger impulse. 2. *In biochemistry,* the reversible continuing competition between a substrate and a structurally similar inhibitor for the same receptor site on an enzyme molecule. Contr. *noncompetitive inhibition, uncompetitive inhibition.*

competitive inhibitor. *In biochemistry,* a compound similar in structure to a substrate or coenzyme that competes with the substrate or coenzyme for the same active receptor site on an enzyme molecule.

com·plaint, *n.* A disease or ailment.

Complamin. Trademark for xanthinol niacinate, a peripheral vasodilator.

com·ple·ment (kom′ple·munt) *n.* [L. *complementum,* from *complere,* to complete]. Any one of a group of at least nine factors, designated C1, C2, etc., that occurs in the serum of normal animals that enters into various immunologic reactions, is generally absorbed by combinations of antigen and antibody, and with the appropriate antibody, may lyse erythrocytes, kill or lyse bacteria, enhance phagocytosis and immune adherence, and exert other effects. Complement activity is destroyed by heating the serum at 56°C for 30 minutes. Abbreviated, C.

com·ple·men·tal (kom″ple·men′tul) *adj.* Adding to, enhancing, perfecting, or completing something.

complemental air. The amount of air that can still be inhaled after a normal inspiration. Syn. *inspiratory reserve volume.*

complemental space. The portion of the pleural cavity, just above the attachments of the diaphragm, which is not filled with lung during ordinary inspiration.

com·ple·men·ta·ry (kom″ple·men′tuh·ree) *adj.* 1. COMPLEMENTAL. 2. Of or pertaining to complement.

complementary colors. Two colors which, when combined as light rays, produce white.

complementary emphysema. COMPENSATORY EMPHYSEMA.

complementary replacement. RETINAL RIVALRY.

com·ple·men·ta·tion (kom″ple·men·tay′shun) *n.* *In genetics,* the phenomenon whereby two different mutants, each expressed phenotypically in a haploid organism such as bacteriophage, bacterium, or mold, can produce a fully wild phenotype when they occur together in a cell (e.g., mixed infection, partial heterozygosis, or heterokaryon formation). In these and in ordinarily diploid organisms, complementation may be expected if the two mutants occur in different genes, but not if they occur in the same gene, and is therefore useful in defining the gene as a unit of function.

complement fixation. The entering of complement into combination with an antigen-antibody aggregate so that it is not available for subsequent reaction in the indicator systems of hemolysis or bacteriolysis. The basis of the Wassermann test and other serologic tests.

complement-fixation reaction. An antigen-antibody combination with complement.

complement-fixation test. A test based on the complement-fixation reaction in which antigen uniting with its antibody combines with the complement and thus inactivates or fixes it. Abbreviated, CFT.

com·ple·men·toid (kom″ple·men′toid) *n.* A complement which through the agency of heat has lost its capacity for causing lysis but still retains its binding property with the amboceptor.

com·ple·men·to·phil (kom″ple·men′to·fil) *n.* [*complement* + *-phil*]. According to Ehrlich, the haptophore group of the antibody (amboceptor) by means of which it combines with the complement.

com·plete abortion. Abortion in which all the products of conception are shed or expelled, including fetus, placenta, and (if not already removed at curettage) decidua.

complete antibody. An antibody that is detectable by standard serologic procedures, saline active, such as agglutination or precipitation.

complete breech presentation. A breech presentation in which buttocks and feet appear first. Syn. *double breech presentation.*

complete disinfectant. A disinfectant that destroys the spores as well as the vegetating cells.

complete dislocation. A dislocation in which there is complete separation of the joint surfaces.

com·plet·ed test. A test for *Escherichia coli* in water in which organisms from typical colonies of a confirmed test are transferred to lactose broth and agar slants. The formation of gas in the lactose broth and the demonstration of gram-negative non-spore-forming bacilli in the agar culture indicate a positive test.

complete endocardial cushion defect. ATRIOVENTRICULARIS COMMUNIS.

complete fracture. A fracture in which the continuity of the entire bone is destroyed.

complete heart block. Complete atrioventricular block. See *atrioventricular block.*

complete hernia. A hernia in which the hernial sac and its contents have escaped through the opening; applied especially to inguinal hernias where the sac and its contents are to be found in the scrotum or labium majus.

complete laryngotomy. Incision of the larynx through its whole length.

complete ophthalmoplegia. Paralysis of both the extrinsic and the intrinsic muscles of the eye, with divergent strabismus, ptosis, dilated fixed pupils, and loss of accommodation.

complete segmentation. HOLOBLASTIC CLEAVAGE.

com·plex (kom′plecks) *n.* [L. *complexus,* encompassing, interweaving, surrounding]. 1. *In psychoanalysis,* a group of associated ideas with strong emotional tone, which have been transferred by the conscious mind into the unconscious, and which influence the personality. 2. A combination of signs and symptoms or related factors; a symptom complex. See also *syndrome.* 3. *In electrocardiography,* a deflection corresponding to a phase of the cardiac cycle.

com·plex infection. Simultaneous infection by more than one organism.

complex periodontitis. PERIODONTITIS COMPLEX.

complex salt. A salt containing a cation, or anion, or both, composed of several elements, as $[Cu(NH_3)_4]SO_4$ and $K_4[Fe(CN)_6]$.

com·plex·us (kom·pleck′sus) *n.* [L.]. The semispinalis capitis muscle. See Table of Muscles in the Appendix.

com·pli·ance, *n.* 1. The extension or displacement of a substance under unit load. 2. Specifically, the volume change produced in the lungs by a given change in pressure, measured at the peak of tidal volume when there is no air flow. 3. The degree of distensibility of elastic structures, such as blood vessels, the heart, or lungs, with low compliance equivalent to stiffness, and high compliance to marked distensibility.

com·pli·cat·ed cataract. Cataract secondary to intraocular disease.

complicated fracture. A fracture associated with injury of the surrounding soft parts, which will complicate treatment, or recovery, or both.

com·pli·cat·ing disease. A secondary or independent disease superimposed upon one already existing.

com·pli·ca·tion (kom″pli·kay′shun) *n.* [L. *complicare,* to fold together]. An accidental condition or second disease occurring in the course of a primary process.

Compocillin-V. Trademark for hydrabamine phenoxymethyl penicillin or hydrabamine penicillin V.

Compocillin-VK. Trademark for potassium phenoxymethyl penicillin or potassium penicillin V.

com·pos·ite flap. COMPOUND FLAP.

composite odontoma. A tumor composed of various histologic elements of the tooth germ.

com·po·si·tion, *n.* [L. *compositio,* a putting together]. 1. The constitution of a mixture. 2. The kind and number of atoms contained in the molecule of a compound.

com·pos men·tis (kom′pus men′tis) [L.]. Of sound mind.

com·pound, *adj. & n.* 1. Composed of parts that are entities in their own right. 2. Complicated; multiple. 3. A substance composed of two or more elements chemically combined in definite proportion.

compound 1080. SODIUM FLUOROACETATE.

compound A (Kendall's). DEHYDROCORTICOSTERONE.

compound aneurysm. An aneurysm in which one or more coats of an artery are ruptured and the others merely dilated.

compound articulation. A synovial joint in which more than two bones are involved.

compound B (Kendall's). CORTICOSTERONE.

compound benzoin tincture. A tincture prepared from benzoin, aloe, storax, tolu balsam, and alcohol; used as an inhalant in bronchitis by steam vaporization; as an antiseptic and protective application to chapped hands, minor wounds; and occasionally as a stimulating expectorant in chronic bronchitis. Syn. *Turlington's balsam.*

compound C (Kendall's). Allopregnane-$3\alpha,11\beta,17\alpha,21$-tetrol-20-one, a steroidal constituent of the adrenal cortex.

compound cyst. MULTILOCULAR CYST.

compound D (Kendall's). Allopregnane-$3\beta,11\beta,17\alpha,20\beta,21$-pentol, a steroidal constituent of adrenal cortex.

compound dislocation. A dislocation in which there is a communication with the joint from inside or outside, through a wound.

compound E (Kendall's). CORTISONE.

compound effervescent powders. SEIDLITZ POWDERS.

compound ether spirit. A solution containing ethyl oxide, ethereal oil, and alcohol. Has been used as an anodyne and antispasmodic.

compound eye. The organ of vision formed of several closely grouped prismatic eyes (ommatidia) as in most arthropods.

compound F (Kendall's). HYDROCORTISONE.

compound F (Wintersteiner's). CORTISONE.

compound Fa6 (Reichstein's). CORTISONE.

compound flap. A pedicle flap that is lined with skin or mucous membrane, as for repair of a cheek or the nose, or that contains other tissue, such as bone or cartilage.

compound fracture. A fracture in which the point of fracture is in contact with the external surface of the body. Contr. *simple fracture.*

compound G-11. HEXACHLOROPHENE.

compound gland. A gland which has a branching system of ducts.

compound glycyrrhiza mixture. COMPOUND OPIUM AND GLYCYRRHIZA MIXTURE.
compound granule cell. A rounded phagocytic microglial cell with cytoplasm distended by globules of lipid and other debris.
compound iodine solution. STRONG IODINE SOLUTION.
compound microscope. A microscope that consists of two or more lenses or lens systems, of which one, the objective lens, placed near the object, gives a large and inverted real image; the other, the ocular lens, acting like a simple microscope, gives an enlarged virtual image of the real image.
compound myopic astigmatism. Astigmatism in which both meridians are myopic, but one more so than the other.
compound nevus. A common pigmented mole consisting of areas of melanocytes in both the dermoepidermal and the intracutaneous zones.
compound opium and glycyrrhiza mixture. A preparation containing camphorated opium tincture, glycyrrhiza fluidextract, antimony potassium tartrate, alcohol, glycerin, and water. A nauseating expectorant. Syn. *brown mixture.*
compound ovarian tumor. An ovarian teratoma.
compound presentation. Prolapse of an extremity of the fetus alongside the presenting part.
compound Q (Reichstein's). DEOXYCORTICOSTERONE
compound rosin cerate. DESHLER'S SALVE.
compound sodium borate solution. DOBELL'S SOLUTION.
compound tincture of camphor. PAREGORIC.
comprehensive medical care. The provision of health services to meet all medical needs, preventive and therapeutic, for individuals seeking medical care.
com·press (kom'press) *n.* [L. *compressus,* from *comprimere,* to press together]. A folded cloth or pad of other soft material, wet or dry, hot or cold, applied firmly to a part.
compressed-air illness or **sickness.** DECOMPRESSION SICKNESS.
com·pres·sion (kum·presh'un) *n.* 1. The state of being compressed. 2. The act of pressing or squeezing together.
compression anuria. Anuria associated with the crush syndrome.
compression atelectasis. Collapse of part or all of a lung due to pressure by extrinsic factors such as pleural effusion or tumor.
compression atrophy. PRESSURE ATROPHY.
compression cone. A device that applies external pressure to the body during radiography; usually used in conjunction with fluoroscopy to compress a barium-filled viscus to demonstrate the mucosal pattern of a local portion of the gastrointestinal tract.
compression cyanosis. Severe cyanosis of the head, neck, and upper arm when the superior vena cava is compressed, as in severe, prolonged compression of the chest.
compression diaphragm. COMPRESSION CONE.
compression fracture. A fracture in which a surface of a bone is driven toward another bony surface; commonly found in vertebral bodies.
compression neuritis. Neuritis caused by compression of a nerve.
compression paralysis. Paralysis caused by pressure on a nerve.
compression thrombosis. A thrombosis due to compression of a vessel, as by a tumor.
compression-traction syndrome. SCALENUS ANTERIOR SYNDROME.
compression syndrome. CRUSH SYNDROME.
com·pres·sor (kum·pres'ur) *n.* 1. An instrument for compressing an artery or other part. 2. A muscle having a compressing function. See Table of Muscles in the Appendix.
compressor bul·bi pro·pri·us (bul'bye pro'pree·us). The portion of the bulbospongiosus muscle in the male which ensheathes the bulb of the corpus spongiosum penis.
compressor hemi·sphe·ri·cum bul·bi (hem''i·spheer'i·kum bul'bye). A portion of the bulbospongiosus muscle in the male underlying the compressor bulbi proprius and ensheathing the bulb of the corpus spongiosum penis and proximal part of the penile urethra.
compressor la·bii (lay'bee·eye). The portion of the orbicularis oris muscle in which the bundles of fibers pass obliquely from the skin surrounding the mouth toward the mucous membrane; these fibers are said to flatten the lips.
compressor na·ris (nair'is). A muscle of facial expression. It is triangular in shape and lies along the side of the nose above the wing; the transverse part of the nasalis muscle. NA *pars transversa musculi nasalis.*
compressor na·si (nay'zye). COMPRESSOR NARIS.
compressor ra·di·cis pe·nis (rad'i·sis pee'nis). A portion of the bulbospongiosus muscle in the male passing around the root of the penis.
compressor ure·thrae (yoo·ree'three). SPHINCTER URETHRAE.
compressor va·gi·nae (va·jye'nee). The bulbospongiosus muscle in the female.
compressor ve·nae dor·sa·lis (vee'nee dor·say'lis). A variable portion of the bulbospongiosus muscle which unites with its fellow of the opposite side in a tendon that passes over the dorsal vein of the penis.
Comp·ton effect or **collision** [A. H. *Compton,* U.S. physicist, 1892–1954]. The increase in wavelength of electromagnetic radiation when scattered by matter, as by an elastic collision between a photon and an atomic electron such that the photon loses energy (with increase in wavelength) and the electron gains energy.
Compton electron [A. H. *Compton*]. RECOIL ELECTRON.
com·pul·sion, *n.* [L. *compulsio,* from *compellere,* to *compel*]. 1. An irresistible impulse. 2. *In psychiatry,* an impulse to do something against the conscious will of the individual at the time it is done, and usually stemming from an obsession. 3. An unwanted, insistent, repetitive, and intrusive urge to carry out an act which is against the conscious wishes or standards of the individual, and representative of hidden, wholly unacceptable wishes or ideas. Failure to perform the act brings out overt anxiety.
compulsion neurosis. OBSESSIVE-COMPULSIVE NEUROSIS.
com·pul·sive, *adj.* Pertaining to, caused by, or characteristic of a compulsion. —**compulsive·ness,** *n.;* **compulsive·ly,** *adv.*
compulsive laughter. Laughter that is without cause and mirthless as seen in certain psychoses, especially schizophrenia; the patient usually does not know he is laughing.
compulsive personality. OBSESSIVE-COMPULSIVE PERSONALITY.
compulsive ritual. *In psychiatry,* a series of acts performed repetitively under compulsion; failure to carry out the acts results in tension and anxiety.
compulsive swearing syndrome. GILLES DE LA TOURETTE DISEASE.
com·put·ed axial tomography. COMPUTED TOMOGRAPHY. Abbreviated, CAT.
computed tomography. A method of imaging in which a computer is used to reconstruct the anatomic features registered by axial tomography. Abbreviated, CT.
com·put·er-assisted tomography. COMPUTED TOMOGRAPHY. Abbreviated, CAT.
com·put·er·ized tomography. COMPUTED TOMOGRAPHY.
co·mus (ko'mus) *n.* [Gk. *komē,* luminous tail of a comet]. A crescentic patch of yellow near the optic disk; seen in high myopia.
con-. See *com-.*
con-. See *cono-.*
Conadil. Trademark for sulthiame, an anticonvulsant drug.
co·na·ri·um (ko·nair'ee·um) *n.,* pl. **cona·ria** (·ee·uh) [Gk. *kōnarion,* small cone]. PINEAL BODY.
co·na·tion (ko·nay'shun) *n.* [L. *conari,* to try]. The exertive power of the mind, including will and desire, as expressed in a conscious tendency to act. Contr. *affection, cognition.* —**co·na·tive** (kon'uh·tiv, ko'nuh·tiv) *adj.*
con·can·a·val·in A (kon·kan''uh·val'in, ·vay'lin) [*con-* + *Can-*

*aval*ia + *-in*]. A mitogenic glycoprotein prepared from jack bean meal.

Con·ca·to's disease (kohng·kah'to) [L. M. *Concato,* Italian physician, 1825–1882]. POLYSEROSITIS.

con·cave (kon'kave, kon·kave') *adj.* [L. *concavus,* hollow]. Possessing a curved, depressed surface. Contr. *convex.* **—con·cav·i·ty** (kon·kav'i·tee) *n.*

concave lens. BICONCAVE LENS.

concave mirror. A mirror with a concave reflecting surface.

con·ca·vo-con·vex (kon·kay"vo·kon'vecks, ·kon·vecks') *adj.* Bounded by a concave surface on one side and a convex surface on the other.

con·cealed hernia. A hernia that is not evident by ordinary manual examination.

concealed penis. A congenital anomaly in which the penis, in this condition usually only rudimentary, is hidden within the scrotum or perineal skin.

con·ceive, *v.* [L. *concipere,* to take in]. To become pregnant.

con·cen·trat·ed scarlet fever antitoxin. SCARLET FEVER STREPTOCOCCUS ANTITOXIN.

con·cen·tra·tion, *n.* 1. The bringing together, or collection within a limited area, of some entity, as of certain cells in a brain center or nucleus. 2. The fixing and limiting of a person's attention of an object, idea, field of endeavor, or aspect thereof. 3. The process of increasing the strength of a solution by evaporating the solvent, or of increasing the potency of a pharmacologically active substance by eliminating inactive constituents. 4. The relative content, variously expressed, of a component of a solution or other mixture of two or more substances.

concentration ratio. The ratio of the concentration of a substance in one place to its concentration in another, as the ratio of the concentration of a substance in the urine to its concentration in the blood.

concentration test. A test of kidney function based upon the normal ability of the kidneys to concentrate or dilute urine. See also *Addis and Shevky's test, Fishberg's test, Lashmet and Newburgh's test, Mosenthal test, Volhard's and Fahr's test.*

con·cen·tric (kun·sen'trick) *adj.* Having a common center.

concentric atrophy. Atrophy, as of an organ or a structure, beginning on the outside and proceeding inward.

concentric demyelination. CONCENTRIC SCLEROSIS.

concentric lamella. One of the plates of bone making up the haversian systems in compact bone.

concentric sclerosis. A form of cerebral demyelinative disease, characterized by the occurrence of alternating bands of destruction and preservation of myelin in a series of concentric rings; probably a variant of Schilder's disease. Syn. *Baló's encephalitis periaxialis concentrica.*

con·cept, *n. In psychology,* the image or notion formed by the mind of an action or object. **—con·cep·tu·al,** *adj.*

concept formation. CONCEPTION (2).

con·cep·tion, *n.* 1. *In biology,* the fertilization of the ovum by the spermatozoon, occurring in the human female usually about the twelfth to fifteenth day after the first day of menstrual flow. 2. *In psychology,* the act of mentally forming ideas, especially abstract ideas; the process of conceiving ideas and of forming concepts. **—conception·al, concep·tive,** *adj.*

con·cep·tus (kon·sep'tus) *n.,* pl. **conceptuses** [L.]. That which is conceived; an embryo or fetus.

con·cer·ti·na effect (kon"sur·tee'nuh). An electrocardiographic finding in the Wolff-Parkinson-White syndrome; the PR interval progressively shortens as the QRS complex widens, then progressively lengthens as the QRS complex narrows.

conch-, concho-. A combining form meaning *concha.*

con·cha (kong'kuh) *n.,* pl. & genit. sing. **con·chae** (·kee) [L., from Gk. *konchē*]. A shell; a shell-like organ, as the hollow part of the external ear. See also *nasal concha.*

concha au·ri·cu·lae (aw·rick'yoo·lee) [NA]. The hollow of the external ear.

conchal crest. A crest on the medial surface of the maxilla and the palatine bone, for articulation with the inferior concha. NA *crista conchalis maxillae.*

conchal process. DESCENDING PROCESS.

concha na·sa·lis inferior (nay·say'lis) [NA]. The inferior nasal concha. See *nasal concha.*

concha nasalis me·dia (mee'dee·uh) [NA]. The middle nasal concha. See *nasal concha.*

concha nasalis superior [NA]. The superior nasal concha. See *nasal concha.*

concha nasalis su·pre·ma (sue·pree'muh) [NA]. The supreme nasal concha. See *nasal concha.*

concha nasalis suprema (San·to·ri·ni) (san·to·ree'nee) [BNA]. The bone of the supreme nasal concha.

concha sphe·noi·da·lis (sfee"noy·day'lis) [NA]. A thin bony plate forming one lateral half of the anterior and inferior surface of the body of the sphenoid. Each originally forms as a hollow ossicle containing the rudiment of a sphenoid sinus. In the adult skull, the concha becomes fused with the remainder of the sphenoid and with the ethmoid and palatine bones.

con·chi·tis (kong·kigh'tis) *n.* [*conch-* + *-itis*]. Inflammation of a concha.

concho-. See *conch-.*

con·cho·tome (kong'ko·tome) *n.* [*concho-* + *-tome*]. An instrument for the surgical removal of the conchae.

con·cli·na·tion (kon"kli·nay'shun) *n.* ADTORSION.

con·com·i·tant (kon·kom'i·tunt) *adj.* [L. *concomitari,* to accompany]. Accompanying.

concomitant strabismus. Strabismus in which the angle of deviation is the same in all gazes and with either eye fixing.

concomitant symptoms. Accessory phenomena occurring in connection with the essential phenomena of a disease.

con·cor·dance (kun·kor'dunce) *n.* [ML. *concordantia,* concord]. *In genetics,* a similarity of the members of a twin pair with respect to a particular trait. Contr. *discordance.*

con·cre·ment (kong'kre·munt) *n.* [L. *concrementum,* from *concrescere,* to grow together]. CONCRETION.

con·cres·cence (kon·kres'unce) *n.* 1. A growing together of the roots of two teeth. 2. A process by which the formative embryonic cells of the germ ring converge and fuse at the blastopore to form the axial part of the embryo during gastrulation.

concrete thinking. *In psychology and psychiatry,* mental processes characterized by literalness and the tendency to be bound to the most immediate and obvious sense impressions, as well as a lack of generalization and abstraction. Thus, an individual who is asked in what way a pear and a banana are alike may answer concretely, "they are both yellow," or "soft," instead of "they are both fruits." See also *primitive thinking.*

con·cre·tio cor·dis (kon·kree'shee·o kor'dis). Adhesive calcific pericarditis with complete or incomplete obliteration of the pericardial space.

con·cre·tion (kon·kree'shun) *n.* 1. Solidification, calculus formation. 2. A calculus or deposit. 3. Parts normally separate, as the fingers.

con·cret·iz·ing (kon'kre·tye"zing) *n.* The process of illustrating, applying, or proving an abstraction by means of a concrete situation.

con·cur·rent (kun·kur'unt) *adj.* [L. *concurrens,* from *con-,* together, + *currere,* to run]. Occurring at the same time.

concurrent infection. Simultaneous existence of two or more forms of infection.

con·cus·sion (kun·kush'un) *n.* [L. *concussio*]. 1. The state of being shaken; a severe shaking or jarring of a part, as by an explosion, or a violent blow. 2. The morbid state resulting from such a jarring. 3. BRAIN CONCUSSION.

concussion cataract. A soft cataract due to an explosion or some other concussion.

concussion of the labyrinth. Deafness, tinnitus, or vertigo from a blow or an explosion; may be transient or permanent.

concussion of the spinal cord. A condition caused by severe shock of the spinal column, with or without appreciable lesions of the cord; usually leading to functional disturbances analogous to railway spine.

con·den·sate (kon·den'sate) *n. In chemistry,* a substance, usually a liquid, obtained by condensation.

con·den·sa·tion (kon"den·say'shun) *n.* 1. The act of making more compact or dense. 2. The changing of a gaseous substance to a liquid, or a liquid to a solid. 3. *In chemistry,* the union of two or more molecules by the linking of carbon chains and the formation of more complex carbon chains, usually with elimination of small molecules such as NH_3, H_2O. See also *polymerization.* 4. The pathologic hardening, with or without contraction, of a soft organ or tissue. 5. The act of condensing a mass of amalgam or gold foil in the insertion of dental restorations in order to achieve accurate adaptation to cavity walls, to express excess mercury from amalgam, and to secure a more solid filling. 6. *In psychopathology,* a psychic mechanism whereby one idea becomes the symbolic expression of many incompatible, repressed ideas; the meaning of this symbol may not be clear to the conscious mind or to others. —**con·dense,** *v.*

condensation polymerization. CONDENSATION (3).

con·densed milk. Milk that is partially evaporated and enriched by the addition of sugar.

con·dens·er, *n.* 1. A lens or combination of lenses used in microscopy for gathering and concentrating rays of light. 2. An apparatus for condensing gases or vapors. 3. An apparatus for the accumulation of electricity. 4. One of a number of instruments with a blunt end, usually serrated; used to condense amalgam or gold-foil filling material into a dental cavity.

condenser points. Instruments used for packing gold foil or amalgam into prepared cavities in teeth.

con·dens·ing diaphragm. A diaphragm containing lenses for converging the light rays.

condensing enzyme. CITRATE SYNTHASE.

condensing osteitis. A form of osteitis usually involving both marrow and periosteum and resulting in the filling of the medullary cavity with a dense bony mass; new bone usually forms on the surface, so that the bone becomes heavier and denser than normal.

con·di·tion, *v.* To establish, by training or repeated exposure, a specific response to a particular stimulus.

con·di·tion·al, *adj.* Subject to or depending on a condition.

conditional lethal. A mutant gene, such as an auxotroph, whose lethality or lack of it is a function of environmental conditions.

con·di·tioned, *adj.* Determined or established by a condition or conditioning.

conditioned avoidance response. *In psychology,* a conditioned reflex that prevents the occurrence of a painful or unpleasant stimulus. Abbreviated, CAR. Compare *conditioned escape response.*

conditioned escape response. *In psychology,* a conditioned reflex that terminates a painful stimulus, or separates the organism from it. Abbreviated, CER. Compare *conditioned avoidance response.*

conditioned hemolysis. A phenomenon observed in hemagglutination tests for Chagas' disease in which red blood cells previously absorbed with a polysaccharide fraction of *Trypanosoma cruzi* are hemolyzed by contact with the serum of the same patient.

conditioned reflex or **response.** An automatic response to a stimulus which did not previously evoke the response; produced by repeatedly pairing a stimulus which normally does not produce a natural physiologic response with a second stimulus which normally produces a specific and innate response.

conditioned stimulus. A stimulus to which a conditioned reflex has been developed. Abbreviated, CS.

con·di·tion·ing, *n.* 1. *In psychology,* the process of attaching a new stimulus to an old response or a new response to an old stimulus; the process of establishing one or more conditioned reflexes. 2. The development of better physiologic condition through physical exercise.

con·dom (kon'dum) *n.* [Dr. *Conton,* English physician, 18th century, said to be the inventor]. A sheath of thin rubber, plastic, or skin worn over the penis during copulation for preventing conception or infection.

condom drainage appliance. A sheath of rubber or plastic worn over the penis and connected to a bag to afford urinary drainage in the incontinent patient.

con·duct (kun·duckt') *v.* [L. *conducere*]. 1. To transmit, as through a channel or through nerve fibers. 2. To possess the quality or ability needed for conduction.

con·duc·tance (kun·duck'tunce) *n.* The ability to conduct electrical or thermal energy; in electrical measurements the reciprocal of resistance. See also *mho.*

con·duc·ti·bil·i·ty, *n.* 1. The capacity for being conducted. 2. CONDUCTIVITY; conducting power.

con·duct·ing artery. An artery of large caliber and elastic walls, as the aorta, common carotid artery, or subclavian artery.

con·duc·tion, *n.* [L. *conductio,* bringing together]. The passage or transfer of electrons, heat, sound, or any form of mass or energy through suitable media, or of nerve and muscle impulses through those tissues. —**con·duc·tiv·i·ty,** *n.*

conduction ageusia. Loss or impairment of taste due to a lesion in the nervous pathways between their peripheral origin and their central centers.

conduction aphasia. Aphasia due to interruption of association fibers connecting cortical centers, a concept prominent in nineteenth and early twentieth century schemes for classification of the aphasias, in which it included the syndromes of transcortical motor, transcortical sensory, subcortical motor, and subcortical sensory aphasia.

conduction deafness. Deafness due to disease or a defect of the external or middle ear, or both; frequently caused by a lesion of the tympanic membrane or of the ossicles.

conduction syndrome. DISCONNECTION SYNDROME.

con·duc·tom·e·try (kon"duck·tom'e·tree) *n.* The determination of the quantity of material present in a mixture by measurement of its effect on the electrical conductivity of the mixture. —**con·duc·to·met·ric** (kun·duck"to·met'rick) *adj.*

con·duc·tor, *n.* 1. A body or substance that transmits energy by direct molecular transfer; applied to carriers of heat, electric currents, and sound. 2. An instrument serving as a guide for the surgeon's knife.

conductor so·no·rus of Bergmann (so·no'rus) [G. H. *Bergmann*]. *Obsol.* STRIAE MEDULLARES VENTRICULI QUARTI.

con·du·pli·ca·to cor·po·re (kon·dew"pli·kay'to kor'po·ree) [L.]. With the body doubled on itself; said of a position of the fetus.

con·du·ran·gin (kon"dew·ran'jin, ·rang'ghin) *n.* A mixture of glycosides from condurango bark; formerly used as a stomachic and astringent in chronic dyspepsia.

con·du·ran·go (kon"dew·rang'go) *n.* [Am. Sp.]. The dried bark of the vine *Marsdenia cundurango;* has been used as a bitter and astringent stomachic.

condyl-, condylo-. A combining form meaning *condyle.*

con·dy·lar (kon'di·lur) *adj.* Pertaining to or associated with a condyle.

condylar articulation. CONDYLAR JOINT.

condylar axis. A line through the two mandibular condyles around which the mandible may rotate during a part of the opening movement.

condylar canal. A small canal occasionally present in the floor of the condylar fossa for the passage of a vein from the transverse sinus. NA *canalis condylaris.*

condylar foramen. CONDYLAR CANAL.

condylar fossa. Either of two small pits on the lower surface of the basilar part of the occipital bone, one situated behind each occipital condyle. NA *fossa condylaris.*

condylar guide. The part of a dental articulator that produces simulated movements of the condyles in the temporomandibular joints.

condylar joint. A form of synovial joint in which an ovoid articular surface or condyle of one bone is received into an elliptical articular surface. NA *articulatio condylaris.*

condylar process. The posterior process on the upper border of the ramus of the mandible. NA *processus condylaris.*

con·dy·lar·thro·sis (kon″di·lahr·thro′sis) *n.,* pl. **condylarthro·ses** (·seez) [*condyl-* + *arthrosis*]. CONDYLAR JOINT.

con·dyle (kon′dile, ·dil) *n.* [Gk. *kondylos,* knuckle, joint]. Any rounded eminence such as occurs in the joints of many of the bones, especially the femur, humerus, and mandible. See also *dextrocondylism, infracondylism, levocondylism.*

con·dy·lec·to·my (kon″di·leck′tuh·mee) *n.* [*condyl-* + *-ectomy*]. Excision of a condyle.

condyli. Plural and genitive singular of *condylus.*

con·dyl·i·on (kon·dil′ee·on) *n.* [Gk. *kondylion,* dim. of *kondylos*]. *In craniometry,* a point either at the medial or at the lateral tip of a condyle of the mandible.

condylo-. See *condyl-.*

con·dy·loid (kon′di·loid) *adj.* CONDYLAR.

condyloid articulation or **joint.** CONDYLAR JOINT.

condyloid emissary vein. An inconstant venous channel passing through the occipital bone above each condyle and connecting the sigmoid sinus with the vertebral or a deep cervical vein. NA *vena emissaria condylaris.*

condyloid foramen. CONDYLAR CANAL.

condyloid fossa. CONDYLAR FOSSA.

condyloid process. CONDYLAR PROCESS.

condyloid tubercle. A protuberance on the condyle of the mandible to which the temporomandibular ligament attaches.

con·dy·lo·ma (kon″di·lo′muh) *n.,* pl. **condylomas, condyloma·ta** (·tuh) [Gk. *kondylōma,* knob]. A wartlike growth or tumor, usually near the anus or pudendum. —**condy·lom·a·tous** (·lom′uh·tus, ·lo′muh·tus) *adj.*

condyloma acu·mi·na·tum (a·kew″mi·nay′tum), *pl.* **condylo·ma·ta acumina·ta.** A soft, warty nodule occurring on the mucosal surfaces of the female genitals, the glans penis, or around the anus; it is of viral origin.

condyloma la·tum (lay′tum). A syphilitic papule characteristic of secondary syphilis, where two surfaces of skin come into opposition; often warty and vegetative, very infectious, and usually teeming with *Treponema pallidum.*

con·dy·lot·o·my (kon″di·lot′uh·mee) *n.* [*condylo-* + *-tomy*]. OSTEOTOMY; especially, a division through the condyles of a bone.

con·dy·lus (kon′di·lus) *n.,* pl. & genit. sing. **condy·li** (·lye) [Gk. *kondylos,* knuckle] [NA]. CONDYLE.

condylus hu·me·ri (hew′mur·eye) [NA]. The condyle of the humerus; the entire distal end.

condylus la·te·ra·lis fe·mo·ris (lat·e·ray′lis fem′o·ris) [NA]. The lateral condyle of the femur; the lateral part of the distal articulating surface of the femur.

condylus lateralis ti·bi·ae (tib′ee·ee) [NA]. The lateral condyle of the tibia; the lateral portion of the upper articulating surface of the tibia with the femur.

condylus me·di·a·lis fe·mo·ris (mee·dee·ay′lis fem′o·ris) [NA]. The medial condyle of the femur; the medial portion of the distal articulating surface of the femur.

condylus medialis ti·bi·ae (tib′ee·ee) [NA]. The medial condyle of the tibia; the medial portion of the proximal articulating surface of the tibia with femur.

condylus oc·ci·pi·ta·lis (ock·sip″i·tay′lis) [NA]. The occipital condyle; either articulating surface of the occipital bone with the corresponding right and left superior articulation of the atlas.

cone, *n. & v.* [Gk. *kōnos*]. 1. A solid body having a circle for its base and terminating in a point. 2. The mechanical element of the tooth crown; a term used by physical anthropologists in relation to the evolutionary development of teeth. 3. One of the light-receptive, flask-shaped cells which, with the associated rods, forms an outer layer, the neuroepithelial layer of the retina. Contr. *rod* (2). 4. To make cone-shaped. 5. To cut and remove tissue in a rotary movement.

cone cell. CONE (3).

cone fiber. One of the fibers of the retinal cones.

cone-monochromat, *n.* An individual said to have, besides rods, only one of three types of cones in his retina, seeing all wavelengths of light as one hue, such as green or blue; compared to rod-monochromats, such persons are rare and show no secondary visual symptoms.

cone·nose or **cone·nosed bug.** A bug of the genus *Triatoma.* See also *assassin bug.*

cone of light. 1. The triangular reflection of light whose apex is at the tip of the malleus and whose base is formed at the junction of the eardrum with the tympanic ring. Syn. *Politzer's cone.* 2. The bundle of light rays entering the pupil and forming the retinal image.

cone opsin. The protein moiety located in the cones of the retina which, under the influence of light, forms iodopsin with retinene$_1$ and cyanopsin with retinene$_2$. Syn. *photopsin.*

cone pigment. IODOPSIN or CHLOROLABE.

Conestron. Trademark for a preparation of naturally occurring, water-soluble, conjugated estrogens of equine origin.

co·nex·us (ko·neck′sus) *n.* CONNEXUS.

con·fab·u·la·tion (kon·fab″yoo·lay′shun) *n.* [L. *confabulatio,* a discoursing together]. The fabrication of ready answers and fluent recitals of fictitious experiences in compensation for actual gaps in memory; seen primarily as a component of the amnestic syndrome.

con·fec·tion, *n.* [L. *confectio,* preparation]. *In pharmacy,* a soft mass of a vegetable drug mixed with sugar, syrup, or honey.

confidential communication. PRIVILEGED COMMUNICATION.

con·fi·den·ti·al·i·ty, *n. In medicine,* the relationship between a patient and his physician or any other member of a health care team, based on the assumption that all information will remain private and will be used only for his treatment and given out only with the patient's consent. See also *privileged communication.*

con·fig·u·ra·tion, *n.* [L. *configuratio,* shaping]. Arrangement in space of atoms or groups of atoms of a molecule that can be changed only by breaking and making bonds. Compare *conformation.* —**configuration·al,** *adj.*

con·fine·ment, *n.* 1. Restraint. 2. Lying-in, childbirth; parturition.

con·flict, *n. In psychiatry,* the clash of pure instinct with various psychic forces in its attempt to discharge its energies without modification, or between opposing forces within the psyche, as wishes.

con·flu·ence (kon′floo·unce) *n.* 1. A flowing together or merging of streams. 2. A uniting, as of neighboring lesions like vesicles and pustules.

con·flu·ens si·nu·um (kon′floo·enz sin′yoo·um) [NA]. Confluence of the sinuses; the dilated junction of the superior sagittal, the straight, the occipital, and the transverse sinuses of the dura mater. See also Plate 17.

con·flu·ent (kon′floo·unt) *adj.* [L. *confluens,* from *con-,* together, + *fluere,* to flow]. 1. Running together; merged. Contr. *discrete.* 2. *In anatomy,* coalesced or blended; applied to two or more bones originally separate, but subsequently formed into one.

confluent kidney. Congenital fusion of two kidneys.

confluent smallpox. A severe form of smallpox in which the pustules spread and run together.

con·fo·cal (kon·fo′kul) *adj.* [*con-* + *focal*]. Having the same focus. See also *parfocal.*

con·for·ma·tion (kon″for·may′shun) *n.* [L. *conformatio,* symmetrical forming]. Any arrangement in space of atoms or groups of atoms of a molecule that can arise by rotation about a single bond and that is capable of finite existence. —**conformation·al,** *adj.*

conformational analysis. Study of the physical and chemical properties of a compound in relation to its geometry and the relative amounts of its conformational isomers.

conformational isomer. Any of two or more isomers with different conformations that have energetically favorable states allowing finite existence of the isomers.

con·form·er, *n.* CONFORMATIONAL ISOMER.

con·fron·ta·tion, *n.* 1. Any method for approximating the visual fields without special equipment, commonly by bringing an object from the periphery into the patient's field of vision, and the patient indicating when he first sees the object. 2. The bringing together of a patient with another person, or confronting a patient with certain facts, for diagnostic or therapeutic purposes.

con·fu·sion, *n.* [L. *confusio,* from *confundere,* to confuse]. 1. A state of mental bewilderment. 2. *In neurology,* disorientation as to time, place, or person; sometimes accompanied by disturbed consciousness. 3. A mixing or confounding. —**confusion·al** *adj.*

confusion colors. A set of colors so chosen that they cannot be distinguished by one who is color-blind.

confusion letters. In testing vision, type letters, such as C, G, O, or F, P, T, liable to be mistaken for one another.

cong. An abbreviation for *congius.*

con·ge·la·tion (kon″je·lay′shun) *n.* [L. *congelatio,* from *congelare,* to congeal, from *gelare,* to freeze]. 1. The effect of intense cold on the animal economy or any organ or part. See also *frostbite.* 2. COAGULATION.

con·ge·ner (kon′je·nur) *n.* [L., of the same race or kind, from *cum,* with, + *genus,* descent, stock, kind]. 1. An organism, structure, or substance allied by origin, nature, or function to another. 2. A species of organism belonging to the same genus as another. —**con·gen·er·ous** (kon·jen′ur·us), **con·ge·ner·ic** (kon″je·nerr′ick) *adj.*

con·gen·i·tal (kun·jen′i·tul) *adj.* [L. *congenitus*]. Existing before or at birth, though not necessarily detected at that time. Compare *familial, genetic, hereditary.* Contr. *acquired.*

congenital achromia. ALBINISM.

congenital acromicria. DOWN'S SYNDROME.

congenital adrenal hyperplasia. The congenital form of the adrenogenital syndrome; secondary to exzyme deficiencies related to a mutant autosomal recessive gene.

congenital agammaglobulinemia. A congenital deficiency (in serum) of immunoglobulins, characterized clinically by increased susceptibility to bacterial infections; may be (a) a sex-linked recessive trait, affecting male infants, resulting in a failure to produce antibodies with undue susceptibility to bacterial infections usually in the second half-year of life, but with delayed hypersensitivity relatively intact and a tendency to develop symptoms similar to those seen in collagen diseases; (b) sporadic, affecting both sexes, with immunoglobulin levels somewhat higher than those seen in the sex-linked form; or (c) a part of combined immune deficiency.

congenital agraphia. DEVELOPMENTAL AGRAPHIA.

congenital alexia. DEVELOPMENTAL ALEXIA.

congenital alopecia. ALOPECIA CONGENITALIS.

congenital amaurosis. Total blindness existing at birth when no change can be seen in the eye to account for it.

congenital amaurotic familial idiocy. Tay-Sachs disease manifest at birth, formerly distinguished from Tay-Sachs disease by some writers.

congenital amputation. An amputation that occurs in the uterus as the result of some pathologic or accidental process; thought most often to be related to amniotic bonds or adhesions.

congenital anemia of the newborn. ERYTHROBLASTOSIS FETALIS.

congenital aneurysm. An aneurysm due to a developmental defect.

congenital aphasia. DEVELOPMENTAL APHASIA.

congenital aplastic anemia. A hereditary disorder, transmitted as an autosomal recessive, characterized by hypoplasia of all bone marrow elements, abnormal skin pigmentation, various skeletal anomalies including short stature, hypoplasia of the spleen, and sometimes genitourinary anomalies and mental retardation. Syn. *Fanconi's anemia.* Compare *congenital hypoplastic anemia.*

congenital aregenerative anemia. CONGENITAL APLASTIC ANEMIA.

congenital atelectasis. ATELECTASIS OF THE NEWBORN.

congenital cerebral palsy. CEREBRAL PALSY.

congenital chorea. A form of cerebral palsy manifested by chorea, and usually also by athetosis. See also *choreoathetosis.*

congenital cloaca. Generally, any malformation in which the rectum opens into the genitourinary tract.

congenital contracture. Deformity resulting from contractures originating in utero. See also *arthrogryposis multiplex congenita.*

congenital cyanosis. Cyanosis due to a congenital lesion of the heart or of the great vessels, or to atelectasis of the lungs.

congenital deaf-mutism. Inability to speak, due to congenital deafness or loss of hearing before establishment of speech.

congenital deformity of the foot. TALIPES.

congenital disease. Any disorder present at birth; may be hereditary or acquired in utero. Compare *familial disease, hereditary disease.*

congenital dislocation (of the hip). A potentially crippling abnormality, commonly involving one or both hip joints. Though present at birth, it is often discovered only after the child starts to walk.

congenital diverticulum. An outpouching of a hollow organ or viscus present at birth, as an esophageal diverticulum, an intestinal diverticulum, or a diverticulum ilei.

congenital double athetosis. STATUS MARMORATUS.

congenital dyslexia. DEVELOPMENTAL DYSLEXIA.

congenital dysmenorrhea. PRIMARY DYSMENORRHEA.

congenital edema. 1. SCLEREMA NEONATORUM. 2. MILROY'S DISEASE.

congenital elephantiasis. A rare anomaly due to maldevelopment of the lymphatic channels.

congenital facial diplegia. MÖBIUS' SYNDROME.

congenital familial nonhemolytic jaundice. CRIGLER-NAJJAR SYNDROME.

congenital fibrous ankylosis. Fibrosis affecting many of the joints; due to a variety of causes manifested as clubfoot and extension of knees and ankles.

congenital fracture. INTRAUTERINE FRACTURE.

congenital glaucoma. Glaucoma occurring in infants and children, usually transmitted as an autosomal recessive trait, resulting from incomplete or faulty development of the anterior chamber angle structures. May also occur as a primary or secondary glaucoma in association with numerous conditions such as oculocerebrorenal syndrome, rubella syndrome, neurofibromatosis, Sturge-Weber disease, aniridia, and Axenfeld's syndrome.

congenital harelip. Congenital fissure of the upper lip, due to failure of fusion of embryonic facial processes, often associated with cleft palate. The fissure may be of varying degrees, from a notch at the vermilion border to complete separation between the median nasal process and the maxillary process, the cleft extending into the nostril.

congenital heart block. Heart block due to defective development of the conduction system.

congenital hemiplegia. Spastic hemiplegia present at or shortly after birth. See also *cerebral palsy.*

congenital hemolytic anemia. HEREDITARY SPHEROCYTOSIS.

congenital hemolytic jaundice or **icterus.** HEREDITARY SPHEROCYTOSIS.

congenital hernia. A hernia present in fetal life and existing at birth, as an inguinal hernia in which the processus vaginalis remains patent, leading to the early descent of intestine into the scrotum, or a diaphragmatic hernia in which abdominal organs have passed into the thoracic cavity.

congenital hydrocele. The presence at birth of excessive fluid in the tunica vaginalis surrounding the testis, causing abnormal swelling.

congenital hydrocephalus. Hydrocephalus present at or shortly after birth; may be of the obstructive or communicating type and due to various causes.

congenital hydromyelia. Usually a diffuse dilatation of the central canal of the spinal cord with atrophy, mainly of the gray matter.

congenital hyperbilirubinemia. Excessive bilirubin in the serum from any of various hereditary defects, as in Gilbert's syndrome or Crigler-Najjar syndrome.

congenital hypoplastic anemia. Progressive normochromic, normocytic anemia appearing in early infancy, resulting from deficient erythropoiesis in the marrow while production of leukocytes and platelets is normal. Although there is a significant familial incidence, no clear genetic basis has been established. Syn. *Diamond-Blackfan anemia or syndrome, constitutional erythroid hypoplasia.* Compare *congenital aplastic anemia.*

congenital hypothyroidism. A form of infantile hypothyroidism.

congenital ichthyosiform erythroderma. ERYTHRODERMA ICHTHYOSIFORME CONGENITUM.

congenital ichthyosis. ICHTHYOSIS CONGENITA.

congenital iridodialysis. A cleft in the periphery of the iris which is present at birth.

congenital jaundice. 1. Jaundice present at or very shortly after birth. 2. Specifically, CONGENITAL OBLITERATIVE JAUNDICE.

congenital laryngeal stridor. Noisy, hoarse, or crowing respiratory sounds in newborns and infants, usually on inspiration; may be present transiently or persist due to a flabby epiglottis or malformations or tumors of the larynx or trachea.

congenital leukokeratosis mu·co·sae oris. (mew·ko'see o'ris). NEVUS SPONGIOSUS ALBUS.

congenital lysine intolerance. An inborn error of metabolism in which there is a deficiency of lysine dehydrogenase, excessive amounts of lysine and arginine in the blood, and periodic ammonia intoxication; clinically manifested by mental retardation. See also *hyperlysinemia.*

congenital megacalycosis. Enlarged, clubbed minor calices without impairment of renal function; sometimes confused with the changes seen in chronic pyelonephritis.

congenital megacolon. HIRSCHSPRUNG'S DISEASE.

congenital myasthenia. A frequently familial form of myasthenia, with onset in infancy or early childhood, usually with ptosis and extraocular muscle palsies, and a progressive course similar to the myasthenia seen in adults. See also *neonatal myasthenia.*

congenital myotonia. MYOTONIA CONGENITA.

congenital myxedema. CRETINISM.

congenital nephrotic syndrome. Nephrotic syndrome developing within the first six months of life. In Finnish families, the disease is thought to be inherited as an autosomal recessive trait.

congenital nystagmus. Nystagmus, present at birth or noted in early life, usually lateral and usually involving both eyes; may be hereditary or due to causes which prevent the development of fixation, including central nervous system lesions, albinism, high myopia, and congenital cataracts. May be associated with head nodding or turning.

congenital obliterative jaundice. Congenital jaundice from primary biliary atresia.

congenital oculoacousticocerebral degeneration. NORRIE'S DISEASE.

congenital oculofacial paralysis. MÖBIUS' SYNDROME.

congenital palmoplantar hyperkeratosis. KERATOSIS PALMARIS ET PLANTARIS.

congenital pancreatic steatorrhea. CYSTIC FIBROSIS OF THE PANCREAS.

congenital papilledema. PSEUDOPAPILLEDEMA.

congenital paramyotonia. PARAMYOTONIA CONGENITA.

congenital poikiloderma. ROTHMUND-THOMSON SYNDROME.

congenital poikiloderma vasculare atrophicans. FOCAL DERMAL HYPOPLASIA SYNDROME.

congenital polycystic disease. A hereditary disease in which the parenchyma of the kidney and less frequently that of the liver and pancreas are replaced to a variable extent by multiple cysts.

congenital porphyria. ERYTHROPOIETIC PORPHYRIA.

congenital pterygium. EPITARSUS.

congenital ptosis. PROGRESSIVE EXTERNAL OPHTHALMOPLEGIA.

congenital retrocele. RETROCELE.

congenital rubella syndrome. RUBELLA SYNDROME.

congenital scoliosis. Scoliosis due to a congenital defect in the development of the spine, such as a hemivertebra.

congenital sensory neuropathy. HEREDITARY SENSORY RADICULAR NEUROPATHY.

congenital spastic paraplegia. Spastic paralysis of the legs in infants, due to a congenital lesion of the brain. See also *cerebral palsy, spastic diplegia.*

congenital stippled epiphyses. CHONDRODYSTROPHIA CALCIFICANS CONGENITA.

congenital syphilis. Infection of a fetus with *Treponema pallidum* by placental transfer from the mother, usually after the fourth month of pregnancy.

congenital thyroid aplasia. CRETINISM.

congenital torticollis. Shortening and fibrosis of the sternomastoid muscle beginning in the first months of life, resulting in inclination of the head to one side. Compare *spasmodic torticollis.*

congenital universal muscular hypoplasia. BENIGN CONGENITAL HYPOTONIA.

congenital urethral valve. Modified folds of the mucous membrane of the prostatic urethra which may give rise to urinary obstruction.

congenital wryneck. CONGENITAL TORTICOLLIS.

con·ge·ries (kon'je·reez) *n.* [L., from *congerere,* to bring together]. Aggregation; agglomeration.

con·ges·tion, *n.* 1. An abnormal accumulation of fluid within the vessels of an organ or part; usually blood, but occasionally bile or mucus. 2. HYPEREMIA. —**con·gest·ed, con·ges·tive,** *adj.*

congestive cirrhosis. CARDIAC CIRRHOSIS.

congestive dysmenorrhea. Painful menstruation due to an intense congestion of the pelvic viscera.

congestive glaucoma. NARROW-ANGLE GLAUCOMA.

congestive heart failure. A state in which circulatory congestion exists as a result of heart failure.

con·gi·us (kon'jee·us) *n.,* pl. **con·gii** (kon'jee·eye) [L.]. An apothecaries' measure equal to a gallon. Abbreviated, C., c., cong.

con·glo·bate (kon·glo'bate) *adj.* [L. *conglobatus,* from *globus,* ball, sphere]. Forming a rounded mass.

¹con·glom·er·ate (kun·glom'uh·rate) *v.* [L. *conglomerare,* to roll together]. 1. To gather or accumulate into a mass. 2. To form into a mass.

²con·glom·er·ate (kon·glom'uh·rut) *adj.* 1. Massed together; aggregated. 2. A mass or aggregate of heterogeneous composition. — **con·glom·er·a·tion** (kun·glom''uh·ray'shun) *n.*

conglomerate gland. *Obsol.* ACINOUS GLAND.

conglomerate tubercle. A large lesion of tuberculosis formed by the growth and fusion of miliary tubercles.

con·glu·tin (kon·gloo'tin) *n.* [L. *conglutinare,* to glue together]. A simple protein of the globulin type; found in lupines, almonds, beans, and seeds of various leguminous plants.

con·glu·ti·nant (kon·gloo'ti·nunt) *adj.* Adhesive; promoting union, as of the edges of a wound.

con·glu·ti·na·tion (kon·gloo''ti·nay'shun) *n.* Abnormal union of two contiguous surfaces or bodies.

conglutination phenomenon. When treated with conglutinin, a firm clumping of particles such as red blood cells or bacteria occurs in the presence of antibody and nonhemolytic complement.

conglutination test. An antigen-antibody reaction in which a conglutinin is added.

con·glu·ti·nin (kon·gloo'ti·nin) *n.* [L. *conglutin*are, to glue together, + *-in*]. A nonspecific substance in the serums of certain animal species; it causes or aids in the agglomeration or lysis of certain cells or particles previously sensitized with antiserum and complement. Commonly found in bovine serums.

Con·go (kong'go). *n.* CONGO RED.

Congo floor maggot. The larva of the fly *Auchmeromyia luteola.*

Congo red. Sodium diphenyldiazo-bis-α-naphthylamine sulfonate, $C_{32}H_{22}N_6Na_2O_6S_2$, a dye used as a pH indicator, as a test for amyloidosis, for determination of blood volume, as a histologic stain, and for other diagnostic tests.

Congo red test. A test for amyloidosis in which Congo red is injected intravenously. In normal persons, 30% of the dye disappears from the blood within an hour, but in amyloid disease 40 to 100% disappears.

con·gru·ence (kon·groo'unce) *n.* [L. *congruentia*]. The quality or state of agreement or coinciding in some limited aspect of two or more otherwise different objects or data. —**con·gru·ent** (·unt) *adj.*

congruent articulation. An articulation in which the surfaces correspond in form and curvature.

con·hy·drine (kon·high'dreen, ·drin) *n.* 2-(α-Hydroxypropyl)-piperidine, $C_8H_{17}NO$, an alkaloid of conium.

coni. Plural and genitive singular of *conus.*

coni-, conio-, koni-, konio- [Gk. *konia*]. A combining form meaning *dust.*

con·i·cal (kon'i·kul) *adj.* [Gk. *kōnikos*]. Resembling or shaped like a cone.

conical cornea. KERATOCONUS.

conical papilla. A variant form of filiform papilla.

conical trephine. A trephine with a truncated, cone-shaped crown, and provided with oblique ridges on its outer surface to stop its progress as soon as the bone is penetrated.

co·nic·e·ine (ko·nis'ee·een, ·in, kon"i·see'in, ko'ni·seen) *n.* Either of two isomeric alkaloids, $C_8H_{15}N$, in conium. β-Coniceine is 2-propenylpiperidine; α-coniceine is 2-propyl-1,4,5,6-tetrahydropyridine.

conidi-, conidio-. A combining form meaning *conidium.*

conidia. Plural of *conidium.*

co·nid·io·phore (ko·nid'ee·o·fore) *n.* [*conidio-* + *-phore*]. The mycelial structure of a fungus which bears conidia.

co·nid·io·spore (ko·nid'ee·o·spore) *n.* [*conidio-* + *spore*]. CONIDIUM.

co·nid·i·um (ko·nid'ee·um) *n.*, pl. **conid·ia** (·ee·uh) [NL., diminutive of Gk. *konis,* dust.]. An asexual spore cut from a fungus filament. —**conidi·al** (·ul) *adj.*

coni epi·di·dy·mi·dis (ep"ee·di·dim'i·dis) [NA alt.]. LOBULES OF THE EPIDIDYMIS. NA alt. *lobuli epididymidis.*

co·ni·ine (ko'nee·een, ·in, ko'neen) *n.* [*coni*um + *-ine*]. 2-Propylpiperidine, $C_8H_{17}N$, an alkaloid of conium.

conio-. See *coni-.*

co·ni·om·e·ter (ko"nee·om'e·tur) *n.* KONIMETER.

co·ni·o·sis (ko"nee·o'sis) *n.*, pl. **conio·ses** (·seez) [*coni-* + *-osis*]. A disease or morbid condition due to inhalation of dust.

co·nio·spo·ri·o·sis (ko"nee·o·spo"ree·o'sis) *n.*, pl. **coniosporio·ses** (·seez). Acute pneumonitis from inhalation of spores of the fungus *Coniosporium corticale;* occurring among lumbermen stripping maple bark.

coni tu·bu·lo·si (tew"bew·lo'sigh) *n.* RENAL PYRAMIDS.

co·ni·um (ko·nigh'um, ko'nee·um) *n.* [Gk. *kōneion,* hemlock]. Poison hemlock, *Conium maculatum,* the fruit and leaves of which were formerly used medicinally in the treatment of spasmodic disorders. The activity of the plant is due to alkaloids which produce motor paralysis.

coni vas·cu·lo·si (vas"kew·lo'sigh). LOBULES OF THE EPIDIDYMIS.

con·i·za·tion (kon"i·zay'shun) *n.* Excision of a cone of tissue, or a reaming out, as of a diseased endocervix.

con·joined, *adj.* Coming or brought together.

conjoined manipulation. The use of both hands in obstetric or gynecologic procedure, one being in the vagina and the other on the abdomen. See also *bimanual palpation* (2).

conjoined ramus. In the adult pelvis, the united inferior ramus of the pubis and ramus of the ischium.

conjoined tendon or **muscle.** FALX INGUINALIS.

conjoined twins. Equal or unequal uniovular twins, united.

con·joint, *adj.* 1. Conjoined. 2. Pertaining to or done by two or more things in combination.

con·ju·gal (kon'juh·gul) *adj.* [L. *conjugalis,* from *conjux,* spouse]. Of or pertaining to marriage or to husband and wife.

conjugal cancer. Cancer in both husband and wife, occurring simultaneously or successively.

con·ju·ga·ta (kon"joo·gay'tuh) *n.*, pl. **conjuga·tae** (·tee) [NA]. Conjugate diameter; ANTEROPOSTERIOR DIAMETER of the pelvic inlet.

conjugata ve·ra (veer'uh) [L., true conjugate]. The distance from the middle of the sacral promontory to the posterior surface of the symphysis pubis. See also *obstetric conjugate.*

con·ju·gate (kon'joo·gut, kon'juh·gate) *adj.* & *n.* [L. *conjugatus,* yoked together, connected]. 1. Coupled, conjoint, acting together. 2. Joined together but opposite in some characteristic, as a conjugate acid and base so related that when the acid loses a proton it is thereby converted to the base. 3. A substance formed by the union of two compounds. 4. CONJUGATE DIAMETER.

con·ju·gat·ed antigen. An antigen modified chemically, as by acylation, or by the attachment of a hapten by a diazo or a peptide linkage to free amino groups on a protein.

conjugated bile acid. Bile acid combined with another substance such as glycine or taurine.

conjugate deviation. 1. The movement of both eyes in parallel, or the turning of the eyes in such a way that their visual axes remain parallel. 2. The forced and persistent turning of the eyes and head toward one side, usually toward the side of the lesion; observed with some disorders of the central nervous system. Compare *skew deviation.*

conjugated glucuronate. GLUCURONIDE.

conjugate diameter. Any of a number of diameters of the pelvis; especially, ANTEROPOSTERIOR DIAMETER (1).

conjugated protein. A protein combined with a nonprotein group, other than a salt of a simple protein.

conjugate foci. Two interchangeable points at corresponding distances from a lens; the focal point of the image and the point of the object.

conjugate gaze. The act of looking with the eyes coordinated in the same direction.

conjugate gaze paralysis, palsy, or **defect.** Lack of coordinate movements of the eyes, such as inability of both eyes to track concomitantly a moving object laterally or vertically.

con·ju·ga·tion, *n.* 1. The process in lower organisms, analogous to fertilization, involving the fusion of gametes, or the temporary union of individuals with exchange of nuclear material. 2. *In chemistry,* a specific structure in organic compounds exhibited by alternating single and double bonds between successive carbons atoms. 3. *In biochemistry,* the reaction by which an organic compound foreign to the body combines with a substance naturally available in the body to produce the elimination form of the foreign compound.

conjugation nucleus. SEGMENTATION NUCLEUS.

con·junc·ti·va (kon"junk·tye'vuh) *n.*, pl. & genit. sing. **con·juncti·vae** (·vee) [L. *conjunctivus,* serving to connect]. The mucous membrane covering the anterior portion of the eyeball, reflected upon the lids and extending to their free edges. NA *tunica conjunctiva.* See also *bulbar conjunctiva, palpebral conjunctiva.* —**conjuncti·val** (·vul) *adj.*

conjunctival corpuscle. An encapsulated tactile nerve ending located in the conjunctiva.

conjunctival cyst. A cystic structure in the substantia propria of the conjunctiva.

conjunctival fornix. FORNIX OF THE CONJUNCTIVA.

conjunctival glands. 1. Mucosal glands in the eyelid, particularly behind the superior tarsal plate. Syn. *Wolfring's glands.* NA *glandulae conjunctivales.* 2. ACCESSORY LACRIMAL GLANDS.

conjunctival reflex. Closure of the eyelids induced by touching the conjunctiva. Syn. *lid reflex.*

conjunctival ring. A ring of denser tissue marking the attachment of the bulbar conjunctiva to the corneoscleral limbus. NA *anulus conjunctivae.*

conjunctival sac. The potential space between the bulbar and palpebral layers of conjunctiva. NA *saccus conjunctivae.*

conjunctival test or **reaction.** A test for allergy in immediate (atopic) hypersensitivity, in which the antigen is instilled into the conjunctival sac. A positive test consists of hyperemia of the conjunctival vessels, with itching and lacrimation.

con·junc·ti·vi·tis (kun·junk″ti·vye′tis) *n.* [*conjunctiva* + *-itis*]. Inflammation of the conjunctiva.

conjunctivitis ca·tar·rha·lis aes·ti·va (kat″ahr·ay′lis es·tye′vuh). VERNAL CONJUNCTIVITIS.

conjunctivitis granulosa. TRACHOMA.

conjunctivitis med·i·ca·men·to·sa (med″i·kuh·men·to′suh). 1. ALLERGIC CONJUNCTIVITIS. 2. PRIMARY IRRITANT CONJUNCTIVITIS.

conjunctivitis no·do·sa (no·do′suh). OPHTHALMIA NODOSA.

con·junc·ti·vo·plas·ty (kon″junk·tye′vo·plas·tee) *n.* Plastic surgery of the conjunctiva.

con·nec·tive tissue. Any of the tissues of the body that support the specialized elements or parenchyma; particularly adipose, areolar, osseous, cartilaginous, elastic, fibrous connective, and lymphatic tissues.

con·nec·tor, *n.* The part of a dental bridge or prosthetic appliance that unites two or more components.

Con·nell suture [F. G. *Connell,* U.S. surgeon, 1875–1968]. A type of suture in enterorrhaphy, using only one row of continuous inverting through-and-through stitches.

con·nex·us (kon·eck′sus) *n.* [L.]. A connecting structure; a connection.

connexus in·ter·ten·di·ne·us (in·tur·ten·din′ee·us) *n.* [NA]. Any narrow oblique band interconnecting the tendons of the extensor digitorum communis muscle on the back of the hand.

connexus in·ter·tha·la·mi·cus (in″tur·thuh·lam′i·kus). ADHESIO INTERTHALAMICA.

Conn's syndrome [J. W. *Conn,* U.S. physician, 20th century]. Hyperaldosteronism due to an adrenal tumor. Syn. *primary aldosteronism.*

cono-, con- [Gk. *kōnos*]. A combining form meaning *cone.*

co·noid (ko′noid) *adj.* [Gk. *kōnoeidēs,* conical]. Conelike.

conoid cervix. Malformation of the cervix of the uterus characterized by a conical shape and elongation, with constriction of the ostium uteri.

conoid ligament. A dense conical band of fibers attached by its apex to the base of the coracoid process medial to the trapezoid ligament and by its base to the conoid tubercle on the undersurface of the clavicle; a part of the coracoclavicular ligament. NA *ligamentum conoideum.*

conoid process. CONOID TUBERCLE.

conoid tubercle. A rough elevation on the inferior surface on the acromial end of the clavicle to which the conoid portion of the coracoclavicular ligament is attached. NA *tuberculum conoideum.*

Con·ol·ly's system [J. *Conolly,* Irish physician in England, 1794–1866]. The humane treatment of the insane, using no restraints such as chains.

Co·no·rhi·nus (ko″no·rye′nus) *n.* [NL., from Gk. *kōnos,* cone, + *rhis, rhinos,* nose]. *PANSTRONGYLUS.*

Con·ra·di's disease or **syndrome** (koʰn·rah′dee) [E. *Conradi,* German physician, 20th century]. CHONDRODYSTROPHIA CALCIFICANS CONGENITA.

Conray. Trademark for meglumine iothalamate, a radiographic contrast medium for intravenous urography.

con·san·guin·i·ty (kon″sang·gwin′i·tee) *n.* [L. *consanguinitas,* from *sanguis,* blood]. 1. The relationship arising from common close ancestors; blood relationship. 2. INBREEDING; consanguineous mating. —**consanguin·e·ous** (·ee·us) *adj.*

con·science (kon′shunce) *n.* [L. *conscientia,* from *conscire,* to know, be conscious]. 1. The moral, self-critical part of one's self wherein have developed and reside standards of behavior and performance and value judgments. 2. The conscious superego.

con·scious (kon′shus) *adj. & n.* [L. *conscius,* from *con-* + *scire,* to know]. 1. Aware of one's own existence, of one's own mental states, and of the impressions made upon one's senses; able to take cognizance of sensations. 2. *In psychiatry,* the part of the psyche which is the object of immediate attention or awareness, as opposed to the subconscious and the unconscious.

con·scious·ness (kon′shus·nis) *n.* The state or fact of being conscious.

con·sec·u·tive aneurysm. An aneurysm following rupture of all the arterial coats, with infiltration of surrounding tissues with blood.

consecutive angiitis. Inflammation of vessels by extension from adjacent tissues.

consecutive insanity. A psychosis following a systemic disease or an injury.

con·sen·su·al (kun·sen′shoo·ul, kon·sens′yoo·ul) *adj.* [L. *consensus,* agreement, + *-al*]. 1. Of or pertaining to involuntary excitation by stimulation of another part. 2. Pertaining to or caused by involuntary movement accompanying voluntary movements.

consensual action. *In psychology,* involuntary actions accompanied by awareness and sensations of the act.

consensual eye reflex. CONSENSUAL LIGHT REFLEX.

consensual light reflex. The concurrent contraction of the shaded pupil when the other one is exposed to a bright light.

consensual reaction. 1. A reaction that is independent of the will. 2. CROSSED REFLEX.

consensual reflex. CROSSED REFLEX.

consensual validation. *In psychology,* the determination that a phenomenon is real, and not an illusion, by agreement among several persons as to what they perceived, or the confirmation of one's own evaluations or observations by those of others.

con·sent, *n.* [OF., from L. *consentire,* to agree, from *sentire,* to feel]. An implicit or explicit acquiescence in a proposed course of medical action by a patient or one who can legally bind him. In emergencies, consent is implied by law. See also *informed consent.*

con·ser·va·tive, *adj.* 1. Aiming at the preservation and restoration of injured parts. 2. Aiming at treatment by careful observation, limited or well-established therapy; not radical, experimental, or innovative.

conservative surgery. Measures directed to the preservation rather than the removal of a part.

conservative treatment. 1. Treatment which is entirely expectant and abstains from any interference until absolutely necessary. 2. *In surgery,* preservation rather than excision or physiologic alteration.

con·sis·tence, *n.* CONSISTENCY.

con·sis·ten·cy, *n.* 1. The degree of density, firmness, viscosity, or resistance to movement of matter. 2. Agreement, constancy, or compatibility of a patient's history, signs, or symptoms of a disease.

con·sol·i·dant (kun·sol′i·dunt) *adj. & n.* 1. Tending to heal or promoting the healing of wounds or fractures; favoring cicatrization. 2. An agent that promotes healing or cicatrization.

con·sol·i·da·tion, *n.* [L. *consolidare,* to make firm.]. The process of becoming firm or solid, as a lung in pneumonia. **—con·sol·i·date,** *v.*

con·so·nat·ing (kon'so·nay"ting) *adj.* [L. *consonare, consonatus,* to sound together, sound loudly, to echo]. Loud, clear, and resonant, as though reinforced by sympathetic vibrations.

consonating rale. A moderately coarse rale which sounds unusually loud and clear, being reinforced by transmission through an area of consolidated lung.

con·sper·gent (kun·spur'junt) *n.* [L. *conspergere,* to sprinkle]. A dusting powder, such as starch or lycopodium, often used on pills or suppositories to prevent their sticking to each other.

con·stant, *n.* 1. *In physics,* a property which remains numerically the same, and which may serve as a unit of measurement. 2. *In mathematics,* a quantity, having a definite and fixed value in a certain stage of investigation. See also *absolute constant.*

constant region. The region of an immunoglobulin molecule which remains invariable from molecule to molecule within an immunoglobulin class. Contr. *variable region.*

con·stel·la·tion (kon"ste·lay'shun) *n.* [L. *constellatio,* a collection of stars]. *In psychiatry,* a group of allied thoughts held together by a common emotional experience around a nuclear idea.

con·sti·pa·tion (kon"sti·pay'shun) *n.* [L. *constipatio,* from *constipare,* to press closely together]. A condition in which the bowels are evacuated at long intervals or with difficulty; costiveness. **—con·sti·pate** (kon'sti·pate) *v.*

con·sti·tu·tion, *n.* [L. *constitutio,* from *constituere,* to fix]. 1. GENOTYPE. 2. The total individuality of the person, including his inherited qualities and the cumulative effects of his reactions to all the environmental factors which influenced his physical and emotional development. 3. *In chemistry,* the arrangement of atoms to form a molecule. **—con·sti·tute,** *v.*

con·sti·tu·tion·al (kon"sti·tew'shun·ul) *adj.* 1. Having to do with or inherent in the structure of body or mind. 2. Forming the composition of something.

constitutional aplastic anemia. CONGENITAL APLASTIC ANEMIA.

constitutional disease. 1. An inherent disease, owing to the individual's inherited genotypic characteristics. 2. A disease involving the entire body, as contrasted to a disease confined to one part.

constitutional erythroid hypoplasia. CONGENITAL HYPOPLASTIC ANEMIA.

constitutional formula. A formula that indicates the relation to each other of various radicals and atoms in a compound. It does not show the linkage of each atom.

constitutional hepatic dysfunction. GILBERT'S SYNDROME.

constitutional hyperbilirubinemia. GILBERT'S SYNDROME.

constitutional infantile anemia. CONGENITAL APLASTIC ANEMIA.

constitutional jaundice. A familial nonhemolytic nonobstructive jaundice. See also *Dubin-Johnson syndrome, Rotor syndrome, Crigler-Najjar syndrome, Gilbert's syndrome.*

constitutional medicine. The branch of medicine which deals with the relation between a patient's constitution and his susceptibility to disease.

constitutional reaction. 1. Any general, systemic, nonlocal reaction to a stimulus. 2. Any immediate or delayed systemic response to administration of a substance, as anaphylactic shock and serum sickness resulting from immunization, or the aftereffect of a histamine releaser.

constitutional symptom. A symptom produced by the effect of the disease on the whole body.

con·sti·tu·tive enzyme. An enzyme whose concentration in a cell is constant and is not influenced by substrate concentration. Contr. *inducible enzyme.*

constitutive mutation. A mutation that results in a fixed, unregulated production of an enzyme.

con·stric·tion, *n.* [L. *constrictio,* from *constringere,* to bind together]. A contraction or narrowing.

constriction ring. PHYSIOLOGIC RETRACTION RING.

con·stric·tive, *adj.* Tending to constrict; causing constriction.

constrictive pericarditis. Pericardial inflammation and fibrosis which results in squeezing of the heart and restriction of return blood flow as well as cardiac contraction. Syn. *Pick's disease.*

con·stric·tor, *n.* Any muscle that contracts or tightens any part of the body.

constrictor muscles of the pharynx. See Table of Muscles in the Appendix.

constrictor ra·di·cis pe·nis (rad'i·sis pee'nis, ra·dye'sis). A portion of the bulbospongiosus muscle, a few fibers encircling the root of the penis.

constrictor va·gi·nae (va·jye'nee). The bulbospongiosus muscle in the female.

constructional apraxia. APRACTAGNOSIA.

constructive aggression. Aggressiveness which is self-protective and preservative and represents a realistic response to threats by other people.

Consulid. A trademark for sulfachlorpyridazine.

con·sult, *v.* To hold a consultation; to confer, as with a consultant or an expert.

con·sul·tant, *n.* *In medicine,* a consulting physician; one summoned by the physician in attendance to give counsel in a case; usually, a specialist.

con·sul·ta·tion, *n.* *In medicine,* a deliberation between two or more physicians concerning the diagnosis and the proper method of treatment in a case.

consulting staff. A body of physicians, surgeons, and other specialists of a hospital who serve primarily as consultants to the attending staff.

con·sump·tion *n.* [L. *consumptio,* from *consumere,* to consume]. 1. Using up; depletion. 2. TUBERCULOSIS. **—consump·tive** (·tiv) *adj.*

consumption coagulopathy. DISSEMINATED INTRAVASCULAR COAGULATION.

consumptive albuminuria. COLLIQUATIVE ALBUMINURIA.

consumptive's weed. *ERIODICTYON.*

con·tact, *n.* [L. *contactum,* from *contingere,* to touch]. 1. Direct or indirect exposure to a source of infection, usually to a person affected with a contagious disease. 2. A person who has been exposed to a contagious disease. 3. A touching or connection. **—con·tac·tile** (kon·tack'til), **contac·tu·al** (·choo·ul) *adj.*

contact action. CATALYSIS.

con·tac·tant (kon·tack'tunt) *n.* An allergen that induces sensitization and evokes the response of that sensitization by direct contact with the skin or mucous membranes.

contact areas. The areas on the proximal surfaces of teeth which touch adjacent teeth.

contact bed. A large open basin containing a layer of coke or cinders, used for purifying sewage by bringing it into contact with bacteria, which set up rapid decomposition and destruction of the organic matter. See also *septic tank.*

contact cancer. A cancer occurring on a surface, as on a lip, that has been in contact with a cancer of the opposing surface.

contact dermatitis. A dermatitis resulting either from the primary irritant effect of a substance or from sensitization to a substance coming in contact with the skin.

contact factor. FACTOR XII.

contact inhibition. The restraint in cell growth and division which normally follows contact between animal tissue cells, but which is lacking in cancer cells.

contact lens. A lens for the correction of refractive errors, consisting of a plastic shell, the concavity of which is in contact with the globe of the eye; a layer of liquid is interposed between the lens and the cornea.

contact points. CONTACT AREAS.

contact radiation therapy. *In radiology,* relatively low-voltage, superficial therapy, delivered by an x-ray tube having an extremely short target-skin distance and capable of delivering large doses per minute.

contact ratio. In pulsed ultrasonic therapy, the ratio of the duration of an impulse of energy to that of the interval between impulses.

contact reflex. A reflex flexion at the knee and hip with elevation of the leg resulting from gentle stimulation of the dorsum of the foot.

contact test. PATCH TEST.

contact therapy. CONTACT RADIATION THERAPY.

contact ulcer. Superficial ulceration on the edge of the cartilaginous portion of the vocal folds; often caused by abuse of the voice or chronic aspiration.

con·ta·gion (kun·tay'jun) *n.* [L. *contagio,* from *contingere,* to touch]. 1. The process whereby disease spreads from one person to another, by direct or indirect contact. 2. The microbe or virus which serves to transmit disease. Compare *infection.* **—conta·gious,** *adj.;* **contagious·ness,** *n.*

contagious anthrax. ANTHRAX (1).

contagious disease. 1. An infectious disease communicable by contact with one suffering from it, with his bodily discharge, or with an object touched by him. 2. Often, COMMUNICABLE DISEASE. Compare *infectious disease.*

contagious epithelioma. AVIAN POX.

contagious pustular dermatitis. ORF.

contagious pustular stomatitis. A highly contagious virus disease of the lips, gums, and nares of horses.

con·tam·i·na·tion, *n.* [L. *contaminatio,* from *contaminare,* to bring into contact]. 1. Soiling with infectious or other harmful agents. 2. *In psychiatry,* the fusion of words, resulting in a neologism; often the first step in the process of condensation (6). 3. *In radiobiology,* the presence of radioactive material in an area where it is unwanted or harmful. **—con·tam·i·nate,** *v.;* **contami·nant,** *n.*

con·tem·pla·tio (kon"tem·play'shee·o) *n.* [L., a viewing]. CATALEPSY.

con·tem·pla·tive (kun·tem'pluh·tiv) *n.* [L. *contemplari,* to contemplate]. *In psychopathology,* one who habitually induces orgasm through fantasy.

con·tent (kon'tent) *n.* [L. *contentum,* from *continere,* to contain]. 1. That which is contained; especially in psychology. See also *latent content, manifest content.* 2. The amount or proportion (as of an element or substance) present or yielded.

content uniformity. An official test to insure uniform concentration of active ingredients in individual tablets, capsules, and those dry-filled powders used for reconstitution as liquid preparations.

con·ti·nence (kon'ti·nunce) *n.* [L. *continentia,* from *continere,* to hold back, refrain]. 1. Self-restraint, especially in regard to sexual intercourse. 2. Control of bladder or bowel function. 3. The proper functioning of any sphincter or other structure of the gastrointestinal tract so as to prevent regurgitation or premature emptying. **—conti·nent** (·nunt) *adj.*

con·tin·gen·cy table. A two-way frequency table showing the frequency of occurrence of classifications of one variable for specified classification of the other variable.

con·tin·u·ous bath or **tub.** A bathtub in which a patient is restrained and immersed in water at 32 to 37°C (90 to 98°F) for hours at a time; sometimes used for its sedative effect on agitated patients.

continuous caudal anesthesia or **analgesia.** The maintaining of anesthesia by the insertion of a caudal needle or plastic catheter through the caudal hiatus into the sacrum for serial intermittent injections of the anesthetic agent.

continuous current. A current passing through a circuit in one direction.

continuous drainage. Constant emptying of a viscus, usually the urinary bladder by a retained catheter or tube.

continuous epilepsy. STATUS EPILEPTICUS.

continuous loop wiring. A procedure for reduction and immobilization of jaw fractures by the use of a long strand of wire wound around several selected teeth in each fragment.

continuous medium or **phase.** DISPERSION MEDIUM.

continuous murmur. A murmur lasting throughout both phases of the cardiac cycle, or starting in systole and continuing into diastole.

continuous sacral anesthesia. Induction of anesthesia by means of a caudal needle that is inserted into the second posterior sacral foramen and attached to an apparatus for periodic injections of the anesthetic agent.

continuous spectrum. A spectrum without sudden variations, representing a continuous variation of wavelengths from one end to the other.

continuous spinal anesthesia. The maintaining of anesthesia by means of a spinal needle that is left in place so that the anesthetic drug can be administered periodically as needed.

continuous suture. A suturing in which the suture material is continued from one end of the wound to the other; may be of several types.

continuous tremor. A form of tremor which resembles that of parkinsonism, but which may be remittent, and may be diminished or arrested by voluntary effort.

continuous tub. CONTINUOUS BATH.

continuous variations. A series of minute variations.

con·tour, *n.* 1. The line or surface that bounds, defines, or terminates a figure. 2. The surface shape of a dental restoration designed to restore functional anatomy of the tooth.

con·toured, *adj.* Having an irregular but smoothly undulating surface, like that of a relief map; said of a bacterial culture.

contour lines of Owen [R. *Owen*]. Accentuated incremental lines in the dentin of a tooth which result from disturbances in the mineralization process; seen in ground sections.

contra- [L. *contra*]. A prefix meaning (a) *against, contrary;* (b) *opposite.*

con·tra-an·gles, *n. pl.* Two or more bends in the shaft or shank of an instrument which place the distal or working end in line with the axis of the handle or proximal end. **—contra·an·gled,** *adj.*

con·tra·cep·tion (kon"truh·sep'shun) *n.* [*contra-* + *conception*]. Prevention of conception, as a means of birth control.

con·tra·cep·tive (kon"truh·sep'tiv) *adj. & n.* 1. Preventing or tending to prevent conception. 2. An agent which prevents conception, such as medicated jelly in the vagina, a condom, a cervical pessary or diaphragm, or a systemically acting steroid that inhibits ovulation.

con·tract (kun·trakt') *v.* [L. *contrahere,* to draw together]. 1. To draw the parts together; shrink. 2. To acquire by contagion or infection.

contracted foot. TALIPES CAVUS.

contracted kidney. The shriveled condition of a kidney at the end stage of chronic glomerulonephritis, nephrosclerosis, or chronic pyelonephritis.

contracted pelvis. A pelvis having one or more major diameters reduced in size, interfering with parturition.

con·trac·tile (kon·track'til, ·tile) *adj.* Having the power or tendency to contract.

contractile vacuole. A vacuole in the cytoplasm of certain protozoa, which rhythmically and gradually increases in size and then collapses.

con·trac·til·i·ty (kon"track·til'i·tee) *n.* The property of shortening upon the application of a stimulus.

con·trac·tion (kun·track'shun) *n.* Shortening, especially of the fibers of muscle tissue.

contraction ring (of Bandl, Lusk, Schroeder, or **White).** RETRACTION RING.

contract practice. Partial or complete medical service furnished to an individual, or a group of individuals, by a physician, or a group of physicians, for compensation that has been mutually agreed upon.

con·trac·ture (kun·track'chur) *n.* [L. *contractura*, from *contrahere*, to draw together]. 1. Shortening, as of muscle or scar tissue, producing distortion or deformity or abnormal limitation of movement of a joint. 2. Retarded relaxation of muscle, as when it is injected with veratrine.

con·tra·fis·su·ra (kon"truh·fi·shoor'uh) *n.* [*contra-* + *fissura*]. Cranial fissure or fracture produced by a blow upon the skull at a point distant from, or opposite to, the lesion. See also *contrecoup, coup-contrecoup injury.*

con·tra·in·di·cant (kon"truh·in'di·kunt) *n.* CONTRAINDICATION.

con·tra·in·di·ca·tion (kon"truh·in"di·kay'shun) *n.* A symptom, indication, or condition in which a remedy or a method of treatment is inadvisable or improper. —**contra·in·di·cate** (·in'di·kate) *v.*

con·tra·lat·er·al (kon"truh·lat'ur·ul) *adj.* [*contra-* + *lateral*]. Situated on, affecting, or pertaining to the opposite side of the body. Contr. *ipsilateral.*

contralateral hemiplegia. A paralysis of one side of the body due to a lesion of the opposite side of the brain or brainstem.

contralateral reflex. A reflex elicited in response to a stimulus applied to the other side of the body; CROSSED REFLEX.

Contrapar. A trademark for gloxazone, an anaplasmodastat.

con·trar·i·ness (kon·trair'ee·nis) *n.* NEGATIVISM.

con·trast, *n.* The visual differentiability of variations in photographic or film densities produced on a radiograph by structural composition of the object or objects radiographed.

contrast bath. The alternate immersion of the hands or feet in hot and cold water.

con·tra·stim·u·lant (kon"truh·stim'yoo·lunt) *adj.* & *n.* 1. Counteracting stimulation; depressing; sedative. 2. Any agent that counteracts stimulation; a sedative.

con·tra·stim·u·lus (kon"truh·stim'yoo·lus) *n.* Anything that counteracts the effects of a stimulus.

contrast medium. A substance that, due to a difference in its absorption of x-rays from all or local surrounding tissues, permits radiographic demonstration of a space or organ.

contrast stain. A staining method in which two or more elements of tissue appear as contrasting colors by using a sequence of dyes or a combination of dyes of differing colors.

contrast test. A test performed or reaction elicited in one area and contrasted with the response of another area to simultaneous and identical application of excitant.

con·tra·sug·gest·ibil·i·ty (kon"truh·sug·jest"i·bil'i·tee) *n.* NEGATIVISM.

con·tra·ver·sion (kon"truh·vur'zhun) *n.* [*contra-* + *version*]. A turning away from or in the opposite direction. —**contra·ver·sive** (·siv) *adj.*

contraversive seizure. Deviation of the eyes, the head and eyes, and rarely of the whole body to the side opposite an epileptogenic lesion; may occur without loss of consciousness or during the tonic phase of a generalized convulsion; most commonly due to a lesion in Brodmann's area 6 or 8, but occasionally to lesions in the temporal or occipital lobe.

con·tre·coup (kohn"truh·koo') *n.* [F., counterblow]. Injury of a part opposite to that struck, due to transmission of the shock, especially when the force is exerted against an organ or part containing fluid, as the skull, stomach, intestine, or urinary bladder. See also *contrafissura, coup-contrecoup injury.*

con·trec·ta·tion (kon"treck·tay'shun) *n.* [L. *contrectatio*, from *contrectare*, to touch]. 1. The impulse to approach and caress a person of the opposite sex. 2. Foreplay preparatory to coition.

contributory negligence. Failure to exercise ordinary care, or performance of a voluntary act which a reasonable person ordinarily would not do, which is believed to have contributed to resultant injury.

con·trol, *n.* [F. *contrôle*, from MF. *contrerolle*, counter-roll, counter-register]. 1. A standard by which to check observations, and insure the validity of their results. 2. A patient or subject, human or animal, or a group of patients or subjects, selected to participate in an experimental situation, as the trial of a drug, under the same experimental conditions as a similar individual or group except for omission or exclusion of the variable, e.g., drug, being investigated.

control animal. An animal serving as a check or standard of comparison in experimental studies. See also *control.*

control experiment. An experiment used to check or verify other experiments, using conditions identical except for one factor.

controlled association. *In psychology*, a procedure for eliciting a relevant response to a given stimulus, as asking an examinee to name the opposite of a particular word.

controlled substances. In the United States, those substances specifically identified as having potential for abuse and mentioned in the Controlled Substances Act of 1970.

contused wound. A wound produced by a blunt instrument or weapon.

con·tu·sion (kon·tew'zhun) *n.* [L. *contusio*, from *contundere*, to crush]. 1. An injury usually caused by a blow in which the skin is not broken; BRUISE. —**con·tuse** (kon·tewz') *v.*; **con·tused** (·tewzd') *adj.*

co·nus (ko'nus) *n.*, pl. & genit. sing. **co·ni** (·nigh) [L., from Gk. *kōnos*]. 1. CONE. 2. A crescentic patch of atrophic choroid tissue near the optic disk, most common in myopia.

conus ar·te·ri·o·sus (ahr·teer"ee·o'sus) [NA]. The cone-shaped eminence of the right ventricle of the heart from which the pulmonary trunk arises. NA alt. *infundibulum.* See also Plate 5.

conus arteriosus pul·mo·na·lis (pul·mo·nay'lis). CONUS ARTERIOSUS.

conus elas·ti·cus la·ryn·gis (e·las'ti·kus la·rin'jis) [NA]. The elastic upper part of the cricothyroid membrane.

conus me·dul·la·ris (med"yoo·lair'is) [NA]. The conelike termination of the spinal cord, the pia mater of which continues as the filum terminale.

conus medullaris syndrome. Sudden symmetric saddle area sensory loss, mild-to-moderate lower extremity motor and reflex deficit, marked bowel and bladder dysfunction, and impotence; due to compression of the end of the spinal cord. Compare *cauda equina syndrome.*

conus ter·mi·na·lis (tur"mi·nay'lis). CONUS MEDULLARIS.

conus tu·bu·lo·si (tew"bew·lo'sigh). *Obsol.* RENAL PYRAMID.

con·va·les·cence (kon"vuh·les'unce) *n.* [L. *convalescere*, to grow strong]. 1. The stage of gradual recovery of strength and health after an illness or injury. 2. The period of time spent in recovery. —**convales·cent** (·unt) *adj.* & *n.*

convalescent serum. The serum of the blood a patient recovering from an infectious disease; may be injected for prophylaxis of a particular infection in a susceptible individual, or used in diagnosis of a particular infection when the serum shows an appropriate titer rise.

con·val·lar·ia (kon"va·lair'ee·uh) *n.* [NL., from L. *convallis*, valley]. The dried rhizome and roots of *Convallaria majalis*, the lily of the valley. It contains several cardioactive glycosides of variable activity.

con·vec·tion (kun·veck'shun) *n.* [L. *convectio*, from *convehere*, to bring together]. A transmission or carrying, as of heat.

convection current. A current of a liquid or gas heated to a temperature above that of the surrounding medium; it rises to the surface or boundary because of its lesser density, and thus the entire fluid or gas circulates until it acquires the same temperature.

con·ve·nience form. The alteration of basic dental cavity preparation form to facilitate instrumentation and insertion of the restorative material.

con·ven·tion·al diathermy. A process of electrotherapy by which an alternating electric current of moderately high frequency, 500 to 3000 kilohertz per second, at wavelengths of 600 to 100 meters, is run through the body surface to produce local heat in the underlying tissues.

con·ver·gence (kun·vur'junce) *n.* [L. *convergere*, to incline together]. 1. Inclination or direction toward a common point, center, or focus, as of the axes of vision upon the near point. 2. CONCRESCENCE. 3. The coming together of a group of afferent nerves upon a motoneuron of the ventral horn of the spinal cord. —**conver·gent** (·junt) *adj.*

convergence center. The medial group of cells of the oculomotor nucleus.

convergence defect, insufficiency, or **paralysis.** Inability to direct the visual axes of the two eyes toward each other, due to weakness of the extraocular muscles involved; usually of central nervous system origin, but sometimes precipitated by fatigue.

convergence near point. RELATIVE NEAR POINT.

convergence-stimulus adduction. Adduction of the eyes brought about by fixing the gaze on an object placed at the near point.

convergent strabismus. ESOTROPIA.

converging lens. A double convex or planoconvex lens that focuses rays of light.

con·ver·sion (kun·vur'zhun) *n.* [L. *conversio*, from *convertere*, to turn around]. 1. *In psychiatry,* a defense mechanism whereby unconscious emotional conflict is transformed into physical disability, the affected part always having symbolic meaning pertinent to the nature of the conflict. See also *conversion type of hysterical neurosis.* 2. *In obstetrics,* an alteration in the presentation of the fetus to facilitate delivery.

conversion hysteria. 1. CONVERSION TYPE OF HYSTERICAL NEUROSIS. 2. DISSOCIATIVE TYPE OF HYSTERICAL NEUROSIS.

conversion reaction. CONVERSION TYPE OF HYSTERICAL NEUROSIS.

conversion type of hysterical neurosis. The form of hysterical neurosis in which the impulse causing anxiety is converted into functional symptoms of the special senses or voluntary nervous system, and may include anesthesia (anosmia, blindness, or deafness), paralysis (paresis, aphonia, monoplegia, or hemiplegia), or dyskinesias (tic, tremor, akinesia) and ataxia. The patient often shows a lack of concern (belle indifférence) for his deficits, which may provide him with secondary gains by the attention and sympathy obtained or by relieving him of responsibilities.

con·ver·tin (kon·vur'tin) *n.* FACTOR VII.

con·vex (kon'veks, kun·veks') *adj.* [L. *convexus*]. Rounded, as a swelling of round or spherical form on the external surface; gibbous. Contr. *concave.* —**con·vex·i·ty** (kon·veck'si·tee) *n.*

convex lens. BICONVEX LENS.

convex mirror. A mirror with a convex reflecting surface.

con·vexo-con·cave (kon·veck"so·kon'kave, ·kun·kave') *adj.* Having one convex and one concave surface.

convexo-concave lens. A lens having a convex and a concave surface, which would not meet if continued. Its properties are those of a convex lens of the same focal distance.

con·vexo-con·vex (kon·veck"so·kon'vecks, ·kun·vecks') *adj.* Having two convex surfaces; BICONVEX.

con·vo·lut·ed (kon"vo·lew'tid) *adj.* [L. *convolutus*, from *convolvere*, to enfold]. Folded in curves or contorted windings; coiled, as tubules.

convoluted gland. SWEAT GLAND.

convoluted tubules. 1. The contorted tubules of the testis. 2. The parts of the renal tubule which lie in the cortex, as the proximal and distal convoluted portions of the nephron. NA *tubuli renales contorti.*

con·vo·lu·tion (kon"vo·lew'shun) *n.* A fold, twist, or coil of any organ, especially any one of the prominent convex parts of the brain, separated from each other by depressions or sulci. See also *gyrus.* —**convolution·al,** *adj.*

convolutional atrophy. 1. Degeneration or atrophy primarily of the gray or white matter (or both) of the cerebral convolutions. 2. Shrinkage of the cerebral gyri and deepening of the sulci obvious on gross inspection of the outside of a brain, not necessarily representing atrophy primarily of the convolutions.

convolutional cerebral atrophy. CONVOLUTIONAL ATROPHY.

convolutional impressions or **markings.** Areas of decreased bone density in the shape of the subjacent cerebral convolutions, observed on the inner surface of the cranium, usually in cases of chronic abnormally high intracranial pressure. Syn. *digital markings or impressions.* NA *impressiones digitatae.*

con·vol·vu·lin (kon·vol'view·lin) *n.* A glycosidal resin from the roots of jalap; a cathartic.

con·vul·sant (kun·vul'sunt) *n.* A medicine that causes convulsions.

con·vul·sion (kun·vul'shun) *n.* [L. *convulsio*, from *convellere*, to tear loose]. An involuntary general paroxysm of muscular contraction, which may be tonic or clonic or tonic followed by clonic. See also *generalized seizure.* —**convulsive,** *adj.*

con·vul·sion·ary (kun·vul'shun·err·ee) *n.* CONVULSANT.

con·vul·sio par·ti·cu·la·ris (kon·vul'shee·o pahr·tick"yoo·lair'is). SPASMODIC TORTICOLLIS.

con·vul·siv·ant (kon·vul'siv·unt) *n.* CONVULSANT.

convulsive equivalent. A form of epilepsy, especially in children, characterized by recurrent paroxysms of autonomic and sometimes behavioral disturbances, usually without specific systemic or intracranial disease, but with frequent abnormalities on the electroencephalogram, and responding to adequate anticonvulsant therapy. Common symptoms include headache, abdominal pain, nausea, vomiting, pallor, flushing, dizziness, faintness, sweating, fever, chills, and temper outbursts; postictal drowsiness and sleep of varying duration may follow. Other forms of epilepsy may be present. Syn. *seizure equivalent.*

convulsive reflex. Incoordinated convulsive muscular contractions.

convulsive state. STATUS EPILEPTICUS.

convulsive tic. FACIAL HEMISPASM.

convulsive tremor. PARAMYOCLONUS MULTIPLEX.

Con·way-Byrne diffusion method. A microcolorimetric method for ammonia and nitrogen based on diffusion of ammonia from an alkalinized solution to a standard acid solution followed by titration.

Conway cell. A standard microdiffusion vessel consisting of two concentric petri dish-like containers having the same floor. The outer wall is higher than the inner, and it is sealed with a square glass plate. A standard absorbing fluid, placed in the inner chamber, absorbs by simple gaseous diffusion the volatile substance placed in the outer chamber. It is used clinically in the determination of gases in body fluids, as alcohol in blood.

Conway method. A method for chloride based on the oxidation of chloride to chlorine by acid permanganate, displacement of iodide by chlorine, and estimation of iodine liberated by titration or colorimetry.

Cooke-Pon·der method. A method for classifying leukocytes by making a differential neutrophil count in which five different types of cells are classified according to the number of nuclear lobes.

cool·ant (kool'unt) *n.* REFRIGERANT.

Coo·ley's anemia or **disease** [T. B. *Cooley*, U.S. physician, 1871-1945]. Thalassemia major. See *thalassemia.*

Cooley's trait [T. B. *Cooley*]. Thalassemia minor. See *thalassemia.*

Coo·lidge tube [W. D. *Coolidge*, U.S. physical chemist, 1873-1977]. A highly evacuated x-ray tube, equipped with a hot-filament cathode and a tungsten anode.

Coo·mas·sie Blue. Trademark for sodium anazolene, a stain and diagnostic aid.

Coombs serum [R. R. A. *Coombs*, British immunologist, b. 1921]. ANTIGLOBULIN SERUM.

Coombs' test [R. R. A. *Coombs*]. ANTIGLOBULIN TEST.

Coons's fluorescent antibody method [A. J. *Coons*, U.S. immunologist, b. 1912]. 1. Direct method: A technique of detecting antigen-antibody reactions in which smears or sections containing antigen are examined under the fluorescence microscope after treatment with solutions of fluorescein-labeled specific antibody. 2. Indirect or double-layer technique: Unlabeled specific antibody is used first as in (1), followed by treatment with fluorescent antibody against gamma globulin. 3. "Sandwich" technique for detecting antibody: The section is first treated with dilute solution of antigen and the excess is washed off. Then fluorescent antibody is applied to the section.

Coo·per's disease [A. P. *Cooper*, English surgeon, 1768–1841]. CYSTIC DISEASE OF THE BREAST.

Cooper's fascia [A. P. *Cooper*]. CREMASTERIC FASCIA.

Cooper's hernia [A. P. *Cooper*]. RETROPERITONEAL HERNIA.

Cooper's ligament [A. P. *Cooper*]. 1. A fold of the transversalis fascia attached to the iliopectineal eminence and pubic spine. 2. A group of arching fibers connecting the base of the olecranon with the coronoid process on the medial aspect of the elbow joint.

Cooper's method [A. P. *Cooper*]. WHITE'S METHOD.

Cooper's suspensory ligaments [A. P. *Cooper*]. Suspensory ligaments of the breast. See *suspensory ligament (6)*.

co·or·di·nate covalent bond. A bond consisting of a pair of electrons shared by two atoms and thus joining them, both electrons being contributed by one of the atoms.

co·or·di·nat·ed reflex. A coordinated reaction of several muscles in orderly progression.

coordinate valence. Covalence in which one atom or ion contributes both electrons of the pair, and the other atom or ion supplies no electrons.

co·or·di·na·tion (ko·or″di·nay′shun) *n.* [L. *coordinatio*, from *co-* + *ordinare*, to put in order]. 1. The harmonious activity and proper sequential action of those parts which cooperate in the performance of any function. 2. *In neurology*, the combination of nervous impulses in motor centers to ensure cooperation of the appropriate muscles in a reaction or reflex. 3. *In chemistry*, the joining of an ion or molecule to a metal ion by a nonionic valence bond to form a complex ion or molecule. See also *ligand*.

coot·ie (koo′tee) *n.* [Malay *kutu*]. *Slang.* BODY LOUSE.

co·pai·ba (ko·pay′buh, ko·pye′buh) *n.* [Sp. and Pg., of Tupian origin]. The oleoresin obtained from trees of *Copaifera* species (Leguminosae), native to South America. Has been used as stimulant, diuretic, diaphoretic, and expectorant; formerly was used in gonorrhea.

copaiba balsam. COPAIBA.

co·pal (ko′pal) *n.* Any of various resins obtained from certain trees of the Leguminosae, Dipterocarpaceae, and Coniferae, some of which may be used to prepare dental cavity varnishes.

cope, *n.* [L. *cappa*, cloak]. The upper or cavity side of a denture flask.

Co·pen·ha·gen method. HOLGER NIELSEN METHOD.

co·pe·pod (ko′pe·pod) *n.* [Gk. *kōpē*, oar, + *-pod*]. Any of various small freshwater or saltwater crustaceans, some of which are intermediate hosts to worms parasitic in man.

cop·ing (ko′ping) *n.* A thin metal cap fitted to a prepared tooth to provide retention and support for an artificial crown.

Cop·lin jar [W. M. L. *Coplin*, U.S. physician, 1864–1928]. A boxlike glass vessel with perpendicular grooves for holding microscopical slides apart during staining.

copo·dys·ki·ne·sia (kop″o·dis·ki·nee′zhuh) *n.* [Gk. *kopos*, fatigue, + *dyskinesia*]. *Obsol.* FATIGUE SPASMS.

co·poly·mer (ko·pol′i·mur) *n.* [*co-* + *polymer*]. The product resulting from copolymerization.

co·po·lym·er·iza·tion (ko″pol·im″ur·i·zay′shun) *n.* A polymerization which involves two or more distinct molecular species. —**co·po·lym·er·ize** (ko″pol·im′ur·ize) *v.*

cop·per, *n.* [L. *cyprum*, metal of Cyprus]. Cu = 63.546. A reddish-brown, malleable metal, various salts of which have been used as astringents in inflammation of mucous membranes, as emetics, and, externally, as caustics. In certain nutritional anemias, particularly in infants, copper appears to enhance absorption of iron.

copper amalgam. An amalgam in which copper is the principal ingredient; formerly believed to possess germicidal qualities when used as a dental filling material.

cop·per·as (kop′ur·us) *n.* [OF. *couperose*]. FERROUS SULFATE.

copper citrate. $Cu_2C_6H_4O_7$. Cupric citrate; possesses the astringent and antiseptic properties of copper salts and has been used in the treatment of conjunctivitis and trachoma.

copper enzyme. One of the copper-containing enzymes, as tyrosinase and dopa oxidase.

cop·per·head, *n.* A pit viper, *Agkistrodon contortrix*, found in the eastern half of the United States, that attains a length of about 3 feet; its bite is common but seldom fatal except in children.

Copper 7. Trademark for a plastic intrauterine contraceptive device shaped like the numeral 7 and wrapped with copper wire.

copper sulfate. $CuSO_4.5H_2O$. Cupric sulfate, blue crystals or powder, soluble in water, used as an emetic, tonic, and astringent.

copper sulfate method. A test for specific gravity and hemoglobin in which drops of plasma or whole blood are put into a graded series of copper sulfate solutions of known specific gravity. Line charts are used for the conversion of plasma or whole blood gravities into hemoglobin or protein concentrations.

Copper T. Trademark for a T-shaped plastic intrauterine contraceptive device wound with copper wire.

copper un·dec·y·len·ate (un·des′i·le·nate). $[CH_2{=}CH(CH_2)_8COO]_2Cu$. Used locally as a fungicide.

copper wire artery. The change to orange of the normal bright-red color of the retinal arterioles; seen in arteriolar sclerosis.

copr-, copro- [Gk. *kopros*]. A combining form meaning *feces, dung.*

co·pra itch. Acarodermatitis urticarioides from handling copra infested with mites. See also *Tyroglyphus*.

copra oil. COCONUT OIL.

co·pre·cip·i·ta·tion (ko″pre·sip″i·tay′shun) *n.* Precipitation of a contaminant with a desired precipitate even though the solubility constant of the contaminant has not been exceeded. This phenomenon is usually due to adsorption. —**co·pre·cip·i·tate** (ko″pre·sip′i·tate) *v.*

cop·rem·e·sis (kop·rem′i·sis) *n.*, pl. **copreme·ses** (·seez) [*copr-* + *emesis*]. Vomiting of fecal matter.

copro-. See *copr-*.

cop·ro·an·ti·body (kop″ro·an′ti·bod·ee) *n.* [*copro-* + *antibody*]. Intestinal antibody found in the stool.

cop·roc·tic (kop·rock′tick) *adj.* Relating to feces; fecal.

cop·ro·cul·ture (kop′ro·cul″ture) *n.* [*copro-* + *culture*]. Microbiologic culture of the feces.

cop·ro·ex·am·i·na·tion (kop″ro·eg·zam·i·nay′shun) *n.* [*copro-* + *examination*]. Any type of laboratory examination of feces.

cop·ro·lag·nia (kop″ro·lag′nee·uh) *n.* [*copro-* + Gk. *lagneia*, salaciousness]. Sexual perversion in which pleasure is obtained from the idea, sight, or handling of feces.

cop·ro·la·lia (kop″ro·lay′lee·uh, ·lal′ee·uh) *n.* [*copro-* + *-lalia*]. The repetitious, usually involuntary utterance of obscene words, primarily those referring to feces and fecal subjects, and to coitus; a symptom of such psychotic disorders as the Gilles de la Tourette syndrome and certain organic brain syndromes.

cop·pro·lalo·ma·nia (kop″ro·lal″o·may′nee·uh) *n.* COPROLALIA.

cop·ro·lith (kop'ro·lith) *n.* [*copro-* + *-lith*]. 1. A hard mass of fecal matter in the bowels. 2. Fossilized feces.

cop·roph·a·gy (kop·rof'uh·jee) *n.* [*copro-* + *-phagy*]. Eating of feces. —**coproph·a·gous** (·gus) *adj.*

cop·ro·phe·mia (kop"ro·fee'mee·uh) *n.* [*copro-* + Gk. *phēmē*, speech, + *-ia*]. Obscene speech.

cop·ro·phil·ia (kop"ro·fil'ee·uh) *n.* [*copro-* + *-philia*]. An abnormal interest in fecal matter, seen in certain psychoses. See also *coprolagnia.*

cop·roph·i·lous (kop·rof'i·lus) *adj.* [*copro-* + *-philous*]. Growing upon fecal matter; said of certain bacteria.

cop·ro·pho·bia (kop"ro·fo'bee·uh) *n.* [*copro-* + *phobia*]. 1. An abnormal fear of fecal matter. 2. The fear of or aversion to bowel movements.

cop·ro·phra·sia (kop"ro·fray'zee·uh) *n.* [*copro-* + *-phrasia*]. The abnormal interjection of obscene words into speech. See also *coprolalia.*

cop·ro·por·phy·rin (kop"ro·por'fi·rin) *n.* [*copro-* + *porphyrin*]. Any of four isomeric, metal-free porphyrins, characterized by having four methyl groups and four propionic acid residues ($—CH_2CH_2COOH$) as substituent groups; first isolated from feces in congenital porphyria. One or more coproporphyrins occur also in normal urine, in larger amounts in urine in certain diseased states, and also following administration of certain drugs.

cop·ro·por·phy·rin·uria (kop"ro·por"fi·ri·new'ree·uh) *n.* The excretion of an abnormal amount of coproporphyrin in urine.

cop·ro·stane (kop'ro·stane) *n.* A steroid hydrocarbon, $C_{27}H_{48}$, isomeric with cholestane, differing from the latter in the manner of juncture of two of the component rings (the A and B rings). Syn. *pseudocholestane.*

co·pros·ta·nol (ko·pros'tuh·nol) *n.* COPROSTEROL.

co·pros·ter·ol (ko·pros'tur·ol) *n.* [*copro-* + *sterol*]. A sterol, $C_{27}H_{48}O$, excreted in feces; apparently derived from cholesterol, but structurally related to coprostane rather than to cholestane.

cop·ro·zo·ic (kop"ro·zo'ick) *adj.* [*copro-* + *-zoic*]. Living in feces, as protozoans found in fecal matter.

Cop·tis, *n.* A genus of herbs of the Ranunculaceae, the crowfoot family. *Coptis groenlandica,* or goldthread, has been used as a simple bitter tonic.

cop·u·la (kop'yoo·luh) *n.*, pl. **copulas, copu·lae** (·lee) [L., link]. 1. A median swelling of the pharyngeal floor uniting the hyoid arches in the embryo, the future root of the tongue. 2. The body of the hyoid.

cop·u·la·tion (kop"yoo·lay'shun) *n.* [L. *copulare,* to bind]. COITUS.

copy choice. A hypothetical mechanism for genetic crossing-over, by which a new chromosome is synthesized as a copy of an existing one to some point and of the homologous existing chromosome from there on.

copy error. A mistake in nucleotide selection during DNA synthesis, a phenomenon regarded as a major cause of spontaneous mutation.

co·quilles (ko·keel', F. koʰ·keeʸ') *n. pl.* [F., shells]. A variety of dark eyeglasses curved like shells.

cor, *n.*, genit. **cor·dis** (kor'dis) [L. (rel. to Gk. *kardia* and to Gmc. *ᵏhert-* → E. *heart*)] [NA]. HEART.

cor-, core-, coro- [Gk. *korē*]. A combining form meaning *pupil* (of the eye).

cor-. See *com-.*

cor·a·cid·i·um (kor"a·sid'ee·um) *n.*, pl. **coracid·ia** (·ee·uh) [Gk. *korakidion,* a small hook]. The ciliated larval stage of the fish tapeworm, *Diphyllobothrium latum.*

coraco-. A combining form meaning *coracoid, coracoid process.*

cor·a·co·acro·mi·al (kor"uh·ko·a·kro'mee·ul) *adj.* Of, pertaining to, or involving the coracoid and the acromion processes.

coracoacromial ligament. A triangular ligament joining the coracoid process to the acromion. NA *ligamentum coracoacromiale.*

cor·a·co·bra·chi·a·lis (kor"uh·ko·bray'kee·ay'lis, ·brack"ee·ay'lis) *n.* [L.]. A muscle of the upper and medial part of the arm, arising from the coracoid process of the scapula. NA *musculus coracobrachialis.* See also Table of Muscles in the Appendix.

coracobrachialis bre·vis (brev'is). A variable part of the coracobrachialis muscle.

coracobrachialis superior. CORACOBRACHIALIS BREVIS.

cor·a·co·cla·vic·u·lar (kor"uh·ko·kla·vick'yoo·lur) *adj.* Pertaining to the coracoid process of the scapula and the clavicle.

coracoclavicular ligament. A strong band of connective tissue between the coracoid process of the scapula and the clavicle; it consists of two parts, the conoid and trapezoid ligaments.

cor·a·co·hu·mer·al (kor"uh·ko·hew'mur·ul) *adj.* Pertaining to the coracoid process of the scapula and the humerus.

coracohumeral ligament. The broad, strong band passing from the lateral edge of the coracoid process of the scapula to the greater tubercle of the humerus. NA *ligamentum coracohumerale.*

cor·a·coid (kor'uh·koid) *adj.* & *n.* [Gk. *korakoeidēs,* raven-like]. 1. Having the shape of a crow's beak. 2. CORACOID PROCESS.

coracoid process. A beak-shaped process of the scapula. NA *processus coracoideus.* See also Plate 1.

coracoid tuberosity. The conoid tubercle together with the trapezoid line.

coral calculus. A calculus that is branched, as in the formation of staghorn coral.

cor·al·li·form cataract (kor·al'i·form). An unusual form of congenital cataract in which the opacities are grouped toward the center of the lens so that they resemble a piece of coral, and extend from the anterior to the posterior capsule.

coral snake. Any of several small, brightly colored elapid snakes of the genera *Micrurus, Micruroides,* and *Leptomicrurus,* whose venom is neurotoxic.

coral ulcer. An ulcer produced by silica-headed darts from coral, injected into wounds in coral lacerations.

Coramine. A trademark for nikethamide, a respiratory stimulant.

cor bi·au·ric·u·la·re (bye"aw·rick"yoo·lair'ee). COR TRILOCULARE BIATRIUM.

cor bi·loc·u·la·re (bye·lock"yoo·lair'ee). A congenital malformation of the heart in which there is only one atrium and one ventricle, with a common atrioventricular valve, due to failure of development of the interatrial and interventricular septums. Syn. *bilocular heart.*

cor bi·ven·tric·u·la·re (bye"ven·trick"yoo·lair'ee). COR TRILOCULARE BIVENTRICULARE.

cor bo·vi·num (bo·vye'num) [L., lit., bovine]. A greatly enlarged heart, particularly referring to the left ventricular hypertrophy associated with aortic regurgitation.

cord, *n.* [Gk. *chordē,* string]. 1. Any stringlike body. 2. A column of cells.

cor·date (kor'date) *adj.* Heart-shaped.

cordate pelvis. A pelvis with a heart-shaped inlet.

cord bladder. Dysfunction of the urinary bladder, due to a lesion in the spinal cord.

cord blood. Blood obtained from the umbilical cord.

cor·dec·to·my (kor·deck'tuh·mee) *n.* [*cord* + *-ectomy*]. Excision of a cord, as removal of a vocal fold.

cor·dial (kor'jul, kor'dee·ul) *n.* 1. A preparation which supposedly stimulates the heart and is invigorating. 2. A pleasantly flavored alcoholic liqueur which supposedly aids digestion.

cor·di·form (kor'di·form) *adj.* [*cord* + *-iform*]. Cordate; shaped like a heart.

cor·di·tis (kor·dye'tis) *n.* Inflammation of the spermatic cord; FUNICULITIS.

corditis no·do·sa (no·do'suh). A nodular lesion of the membranous portion of the vocal folds, commonly found in singers, public speakers, and those working around irritating gases.

cor·do·pexy (kor'do·peck"see) *n.* [*cord* + *-pexy*]. The suturing of a vocal fold to a new support to relieve the stenosis resulting from bilateral abduction paralysis.

cordotomy. CHORDOTOMY.

Cordran. Trademark for flurandrenolide, an anti-inflammatory glucocorticoid.

Cor·dy·lo·bia (kor"di·lo'bee·uh) *n.* A genus of African blowflies.

Cordylobia an·thro·poph·a·ga (an·thro·pof'uh·guh). A species of blowfly whose first-stage larvae penetrate the skin of mammals and produce boil-like lesions. Syn. *tumbu fly.*

cordy pulse (kor'dee). HIGH-TENSION PULSE.

core-. See *cor-*.

core, *n.* & *v.* 1. A metal casting or fabrication, usually with a post in the root canal, designed to retain an artificial tooth crown. 2. A sectional record, usually made of a gypsum material, of the relationships of various parts of a dental prosthesis such as teeth, metallic restorations, or copings. 3. The central mass of necrotic matter in a boil. 4. To cut away or ream out the central portion of a structure, as the cervix uteri.

cor·e·cli·sis (kor"e·klye'sis) *n.*, pl. **corecli·ses** (·seez) [*core-* + Gk. *kleisis,* a closing]. Pathologic closure or obliteration of the pupil.

cor·ec·ta·sis (kor·eck'tuh·sis) *n.*, pl. **corecta·ses** (·seez) [*cor-* + *ectasis*]. Dilatation of the pupil.

cor·ec·tome (kor·eck'tome) *n.* [*cor-* + *-ectome*]. IRIDECTOME.

cor·ec·to·pia (kor"eck·to'pee·uh) *n.* [*cor-* + *ectopia*]. Displacement of the pupil; an abnormality in which the pupil is not in the center of the iris.

cor·e·di·al·y·sis (kor"e·dye·al'i·sis) *n.*, pl. **coredialy·ses** (·seez) [*core-* + *dialysis*]. Production of an artificial pupil at the ciliary border of the iris.

core disease. CENTRAL CORE DISEASE.

co·rel·y·sis (ko·rel'i·sis) *n.*, pl. **corely·ses** (·seez) [*core-* + *-lysis*]. The detachment of iritic adhesions to the lens or cornea.

cor·e·om·e·ter (kor"e·om'e·tur) *n.* [*core-* + *-meter*]. PUPILLOMETER.

cor·eo·plas·ty (kor'ee·o·plas"tee) *n.* [*core-* + *-plasty*]. Any operation for forming an artificial pupil.

cor·e·plas·ty (kor'e·plas"tee) *n.* COREOPLASTY.

core polymerase. RNA polymerase without the sigma factor.

co-re·pres·sor (ko"re·pres'ur) *n.* A metabolite capable of activating the repressor produced by a regulator gene.

cor·e·ste·no·ma (kor"e·ste·no'muh) *n.* [*core-* + Gk. *stenōma,* a narrow place]. An abnormal narrowing of the pupil.

co·ri·a·ceous (ko·ree·ay'shus) *adj.* [L. *coriaceus,* from *corium,* hide]. 1. Like leather in texture or quality. 2. Of or pertaining to leather.

coriaceous strepitus. An auscultatory sound resembling the creaking of leather, heard in pericarditis or in pleurisy.

co·ri·an·der (ko"ree·an'dur) *n.* [Gk. *koriannon*]. The dried ripe fruit of *Coriandrum sativum* (Umbelliferae). Aromatic, carminative, and stimulant, but used mainly to give flavor to certain medicinal preparations.

coriander oil. The volatile oil from coriander, containing chiefly *d*-linalool. Used as a flavor.

co·ri·an·drol (ko"ree·an'drol) *n.* *d*-Linalool, $C_{10}H_{18}O$, the chief constituent of coriander oil.

Co·ri·ar·ia (ko"ree·ăr'ee·uh) *n.* [L., from *corium,* leather]. A genus of poisonous shrubs of a wide geographic distribution.

Cori cycle (kor'ee) [C. F. *Cori,* b. 1896, and Gerty T. *Cori,* 1896–1957, U.S. biochemists]. A series of enzymatic reactions which purport to show the mode of conversion of lactic acid (formed during muscular activity from glycogen) to glucose in the liver, and its subsequent anabolism to glycogen in muscle.

Cori ester [C. F. *Cori* and Gerty T. *Cori*]. GLUCOSE 1-PHOSPHATE.

Cori's glycogenoses [C. F. *Cori* and Gerty T. *Cori*]. The glycogenoses as classified by the Coris.

Cori's limit dextrinosis [C. F. *Cori* and Gerty T. *Cori*]. LIMIT DEXTRINOSIS.

co·ri·um (ko'ree·um) *n.* [L., hide, skin] [NA]. DERMIS.

cork·screw artery. One of the smaller, tortuous, retinal arterioles in the posterior portion of the retina, seen as a congenital abnormality and in hypertension.

cor·meth·a·sone (kor·meth'uh·sone) *n.* 6,6,9-Trifluoro-11β,17,21-trihydroxy-16α-methylpregna-1,4-diene-3,20-dione, $C_{22}H_{27}F_3O_4$, a topical anti-inflammatory agent usually used as the 21-acetate ester ($C_{24}H_{29}F_3O_6$).

corn, *n.* [L. *cornu,* horn]. CLAVUS (1).

corne-, corneo-. A combining form meaning (a) *corneum, corneous;* (b) *cornea, corneal.*

cor·nea (kor'nee·uh) *n.* [short for L. *cornea tunica,* horny covering] [NA]. The transparent anterior portion of the eyeball, its area occupying about one-sixth the circumference of the globe. It is continuous with the sclera, and is nourished from the looped blood vessels at its peripheral border. See also Plate 19. —**cor·ne·al** (·nee·ul) *adj.*

cornea gut·ta·ta (guh·tay'tuh). A degenerative condition of the posterior surface of the cornea with wartlike thickenings of Descemet's membrane, resembling Hassall-Henle bodies but larger and axially as well as peripherally located; may progress to Fuch's dystrophy.

corneal arcus. An opaque ring in the corneal stroma; ARCUS JUVENILIS or ARCUS SENILIS.

corneal astigmatism. Astigmatism due to defective curvature or refractive surface of the cornea.

corneal corpuscle. A fibroblast of the substantia propria of the cornea.

corneal graft or **transplant.** Corneal tissue, usually human, transplanted into a defective cornea to provide a clear window.

corneal infiltrate. An opacity of the cornea resulting from infiltration of fluids or cells or from scar tissue caused by such infiltration as a consequence of injury or disease.

corneal microscope. A high-power lens used to examine the cornea and iris in the living patient.

corneal pannus. Extension of vessels into the cornea from the limbus.

corneal plexus. A nerve plexus of the cornea, derived from the ciliary nerves and divided into three parts: an annular corneal plexus about the periphery of the cornea; a subepithelial corneal plexus beneath the corneal epithelium; and intraepithelial corneal plexus.

corneal reflex. Reflex closure of the eyelids when the cornea is touched.

corneal spaces. Spaces in the interstitial cement substance between the lamellas of the substantia propria of the cornea.

corneal spot. LEUKOMA (1).

corneal steatosis. Deposits of fat in the cornea.

corneal trephine. A small cutting trephine used to remove a circular section of the cornea in keratoplasty.

Cor·ne·lia de Lange's syndrome (lahng'uh) [*Cornelia de Lange,* Dutch pediatrician, 20th century]. 1. A complex of congenital malformations characterized by microbrachycephalia; peculiar facies; anomalies of the limbs, ranging from mild syndactyly to gross micromelia with or without phocomelia, hirsutism, and other abnormalities; and mild to usually severe mental and physical retardation. The cause is obscure, but abnormal dermatoglyphic and chromosomal patterns have been reported. 2. A complex of congenitally large muscles, giving the infant the appearance of a midget wrestler, together with mental retardation and, sometimes, spasticity or extrapyramidal disturbances.

Cor·nell-Coxe performance-ability scale [Ethel L. *Cornell,* U.S. psychologist, b. 1892; and W. W. *Coxe,* U.S. psychologist, b. 1886]. *In clinical psychology,* a nonverbal test of intelligence used as a supplement to the Stanford-Binet test or alone in cases with speech or language difficulty; included are such tests as picture arrangement, memory for design, and cube construction.

Cornell Medical Index [after *Cornell University*]. A medical history form, which can be checked by clerks, designed to save the physician's time; useful for large-volume work.

Cornell response. A variant of Babinski's phenomenon, elicited by scratching the dorsum of the foot along the inner side of the extensor tendon of the great toe. See also *great-toe reflex.*

Cornell unit of riboflavin. One Cornell unit of riboflavin = 1 microgram of riboflavin, defined by the growth effect on chicks.

corneo-. See *corne-.*

cor·neo·bleph·a·ron (kor″nee·o·blef′uh·ron) *n.* [*corneo-* + *blepharon*]. Adhesion of the surface of the eyelid to the cornea.

cor·neo·man·dib·u·lar (kor″nee·o·man·dib′yoo·lur) *adj.* Pertaining to the cornea and the mandible.

corneomandibular reflex. Deflection of the lower jaw to one side when, with the subject's mouth open, the cornea of the opposite eye is irritated.

cor·neo·oc·u·lo·gy·ric (kor″nee·o·ock″yoo·lo·jye′rick) *adj.* [*corneo-* + *oculogyric*]. Pertaining to movements of the eye as a consequence of stimulation of the cornea.

corneooculogyric reflex. A variant of the conjunctival reflex, consisting of a contralateral or upward deviation of the eyes in response to stimulation of the conjunctiva or cornea, with associated contraction of the orbicularis oculi.

cor·neo·pter·y·goid (kor″nee·o·terr′i·goid) *adj.* Pertaining to the cornea and the pterygoid process.

corneopterygoid reflex. CORNEOMANDIBULAR REFLEX.

cor·neo·scle·ra (kor″nee·o·skleer′uh) *n.* The sclera and the cornea considered as forming one tunic. —**corneoscle·ral** (·ul) *adj.*

corneoscleral limbus. The circumference of the cornea at its junction with the sclera. NA *limbus corneae.*

cor·ne·ous (kor′nee·us) *adj.* [L. *corneus*]. Horny or hornlike.

cor·ne·um (kor′nee·um) *n.* STRATUM CORNEUM.

cor·nic·u·late (kor·nick′yoo·lut) *adj.* [L. *corniculatus,* in the form of a horn]. Furnished with horns or horn-shaped appendages.

corniculate cartilage. The cartilaginous nodule on the tip of an arytenoid cartilage. NA *cartilago corniculata.*

corniculate tubercle. A rounded eminence on each side of the entrance to the laryngeal cavity lying over the corniculate cartilage. NA *tuberculum corniculatum.*

cor·nic·u·lum (kor·nick′yoo·lum) *n.*, pl. **cornicu·la** (·luh) [L., little horn]. A small cornu or hornlike process.

corniculum la·ryn·gis (la·rin′jis). CORNICULATE CARTILAGE.

cor·ni·fi·ca·tion (kor″ni·fi·kay′shun) *n.* The degenerative process by which the cells of a stratified squamous epithelium are converted into dead, horny squames as in the epidermis and such epidermal derivatives as hair, nails, feathers. —**cor·ni·fied** (kor′ni·fide) *adj.*

corn·meal agar. A culture medium which favors the production of mycelia and chlamydospores by the yeast *Candida albicans.*

cor·noid (kor′noid) *adj.* [L. *cornu*, horn, + *-oid*]. Resembling horn.

cornoid lamella. A horn plug penetrating the epidermis and having a central column of parakeratotic cells, microscopically diagnostic of porokeratosis.

corn oil. The fixed oil from the embryo of the seed of *Zea mays.* Used as a therapeutic nutrient and as a solvent and vehicle for injectable medicaments, especially hormones.

corn·starch, *n.* The granules separated from the grain of *Zea mays;* occurring as irregular, angular, white masses or as fine powder; insoluble in cold water and alcohol. Used as a demulcent, a dusting powder, in enemas, in various dermatologic formulations, and as a disintegrator for tablets.

corn sugar. GLUCOSE.

corn syrup. A transparent syrup obtained by partial hydrolysis of cornstarch; contains dextrins, maltose, and dextrose.

cor·nu (kor′new) *n.*, genit. **cor·nus** (kor′noos, ·nus), pl. **cor·nua** (·new·uh) [L.]. A horn; a horn-shaped process or excrescence. —**cornu·al** (·ul) *adj.*

cornua coc·cy·gea (cock·sigh′jee·uh, ·sij′ee·uh) [BNA]. Plural of *cornu coccygeum.*

cornual pregnancy. 1. Gestation occurring in one horn of a uterus bicornis. 2. INTERSTITIAL PREGNANCY.

cornu Am·mo·nis (am·o′nis). Ammon's horn (= HIPPOCAMPUS).

cornu an·te·ri·us me·dul·lae spi·na·lis (an·teer′ee·us me·dul′ee spye·nay′lis) [NA]. ANTERIOR HORN; the anterior column of gray matter as seen in a cross section of the spinal cord. See also *cornua of the gray matter.*

cornu anterius ven·tri·cu·li la·te·ra·lis (ven·trick′yoo·lye lat·e·ray′lis) [NA]. The anterior cornu of the lateral ventricle. See *cornua of the lateral ventricle.*

cornua of the falciform margin. Medial prolongations of the falciform margin of the fossa ovalis in the fascia lata: the superior cornu (NA *cornu superius marginis falciformis*) and the inferior cornu (NA *cornu inferius marginis falciformis*).

cornua of the gray matter. Divisions of the columns of the gray matter in the spinal cord as seen in cross section: the anterior horn (NA *cornu anterius medullae spinalis*), the lateral horn (NA *cornu laterale medullae spinalis*), and the posterior horn (NA *cornu posterius medullae spinalis*).

cornua of the hyoid bone. Segments of the hyoid bone: the greater cornu (NA *cornu majus ossis hyoidei*) projects backward from the lateral border of the body. The lesser cornu (NA *cornu minus ossis hyoidei*) projects upward from the angle of junction of the body and the greater cornu.

cornua of the lateral ventricle. Prolongations of the lateral ventricle of the cerebral hemisphere: the anterior cornu (NA *cornu anterius ventriculi lateralis*) extends into the frontal lobe; the inferior cornu (NA *cornu inferius ventriculi lateralis*) extends into the temporal lobe; the posterior cornu (NA *cornu posterius ventriculi lateralis*) extends into the occipital lobe. See also Plate 17.

cornua of the thyroid cartilage. Processes of the thyroid cartilage: the prolongation of its posterior border upward on either side is the superior cornu (NA *cornu superius cartilaginis thyroideae*). The prolongation downward on either side is the inferior cornu (NA *cornu inferius cartilaginis thyroideae*).

cornua sa·cra·lia (sa·kray′lee·uh) [BNA]. Plural of *cornu sacrale.*

cornu cer·vi (sur′vye) [L.]. HARTSHORN (1).

cornu coc·cy·ge·um (kock·sigh′jee·um, ·sij′ee·um) [NA]. CORNU OF THE COCCYX.

cor·nu·com·mis·sur·al nuclei (kor″new·kom·ish′oo·rul). Two cell columns extending the length of the spinal cord and occupying the medial margin of the dorsal and ventral horn. These nuclei probably relay impulses across the midline.

cornu cu·ta·ne·um (kew·tay′nee·um) [L.]. CUTANEOUS HORN.

cornu in·fe·ri·us car·ti·la·gi·nis thy·roi·de·ae (in·feer′ee·us kahr·ti·laj′i·nis thigh·roy′dee·ee) [NA]. The inferior cornu of the thyroid cartilage. See *cornua of the thyroid cartilage.*

cornu inferius fos·sae ova·lis (fos′ee o·vay′lis) [BNA]. CORNU INFERIUS MARGINIS FALCIFORMIS.

cornu inferius mar·gi·nis fal·ci·for·mis (mahr′ji·nis fal·si·for′mis) [NA]. The inferior cornu of the falciform margin. See *cornua of the falciform margin.*

cornu inferius ven·tri·cu·li la·te·ra·lis (ven·trick′yoo·lye lat·e·ray′lis) [NA]. The inferior cornu of the lateral ventricle. See *cornua of the lateral ventricle.*

cornu la·te·ra·le me·dul·lae spi·na·lis (lat·e·ray′lee me·dul′ee spye·nay′lis) [NA]. LATERAL HORN; the lateral column of gray matter as seen in a cross section of the spinal cord. See also *cornua of the gray matter.*

cornu ma·jus os·sis hy·oi·dei (may'jus os'is high·oy'dee·eye) [NA]. The greater cornu of the hyoid bone. See *cornua of the hyoid bone.*

cornu mi·nus os·sis hy·oi·dei (migh'nus os'is high·oy'dee·eye) [NA]. The lesser cornu of the hyoid bone. See *cornua of the hyoid bone.*

cornu of the coccyx. Either of the paired, large superior articular processes of the first coccygeal vertebra, articulating with the cornu of the sacrum. NA *cornu coccygeum.*

cornu of the sacrum. Either of the paired inferior articular processes of the fifth sacral vertebra. NA *cornu sacrale.*

cornu of the uterus. Either lateral prolongation of the uterine cavity into which an oviduct opens.

cornu pos·te·ri·us me·dul·lae spi·na·lis (pos·teer'ee·us me·dul'ee spye·nay'lis) [NA]. POSTERIOR HORN; the posterior column of gray matter as seen in cross section of the spinal cord. See also *cornua of the gray matter.*

cornu posterius ven·tri·cu·li la·te·ra·lis (ven·trick'yoo·lye lat·e·ray'lis) [NA]. The posterior cornu of the lateral ventricle. See *cornua of the lateral ventricle.*

cornu sa·cra·le (sa·kray'lee) [NA]. CORNU OF THE SACRUM.

cornu su·pe·ri·us car·ti·la·gi·nis thy·roi·de·ae (sue·peer'ee·us kahr·ti·laj'i·nis thigh·roy'dee·ee) [NA]. The superior cornu of the thyroid cartilage. See *cornua of the thyroid cartilage.*

cornu superius fos·sae ova·lis (fos'ee o·vay'lis) [BNA]. CORNU SUPERIUS MARGINIS FALCIFORMIS.

cornu superius mar·gi·nis fal·ci·for·mis (mahr'ji·nis fal·si·for'mis) [NA]. The superior cornu of the falciform margin. See *cornua of the falciform margin.*

coro-. See *cor-.*

cor·o·cli·sis, cor·o·clei·sis (kor"o·klye'sis) *n.* CORECLISIS.

co·rol·la (ko·rol'uh) *n.* [L., small garland]. The petals of a flower.

co·rom·e·ter (ko·rom'e·tur) *n.* [*coro-* + *-meter*]. PUPILLOMETER.

coron-, corono-. A combining form meaning *coronal.*

co·ro·na (ko·ro'nuh) *n.*, pl. & genit. sing. **coro·nae** (·nee) [L.]. 1. A crown. 2. CORONA RADIATA.

corona ca·pi·tis (kap'i·tis). The crown of the head; the top of the head.

corona ci·li·a·ris (sil·ee·air'is) [NA]. CILIARY CROWN.

corona cli·ni·ca (klin'i·kuh) [NA]. CLINICAL CROWN; the part of a tooth exposed to the oral cavity.

corona den·tis (den'tis) [NA]. CROWN OF A TOOTH.

corona glan·dis pe·nis (glan'dis pee'nis) [NA]. The posterior border of the glans penis.

cor·o·nal (kor'o·nul, ko·ro'nul) *adj.* [L. *coronalis,* from *corona,* crown]. 1. Of or pertaining to a corona or crown, especially the crown of the head, as: coronal suture. 2. Of or pertaining to the coronal suture, as: coronal plane. 3. Situated relatively near the crown, especially the crown of a tooth.

cor·o·na·le (kor"o·nah'lee, ·nay'lee) *n.* [L., neuter of *coronalis,* pertaining to a crown]. 1. *Obsol.* FRONTAL BONE. 2. The point on the coronal suture intersected by the greatest frontal diameter.

co·ro·na·lis (kor·o·nay'lis) *L. adj.* Coronal; pertaining to the coronal plane.

coronal plane. FRONTAL PLANE (1), especially one in the head.

coronal section. A section in a vertical and frontal plane making a 90° angle with the sagittal plane of the head.

coronal suture. The union of the frontal with the parietal bones transversely across the vertex of the skull. NA *sutura coronalis.*

co·ron·a·men (ko·ron'uh·men) *n.* CORONET (2).

corona ra·di·a·ta (ray"dee·ay'tuh) [NA]. 1. A radiating mass of white nerve fibers extending from the internal capsule to the cerebral cortex. 2. A zone of granulosa cells surrounding the zona pellucida of the ovum, which persists for some time after ovulation.

cor·o·nary (kor'uh·nerr"ee) *adj. & n.* [L. *coronarius,* from *corona,* garland]. 1. Of or pertaining to vessels, nerves, or attachments that encircle a part or an organ. 2. Pertaining to or involving the coronary arteries. 3. *Colloq.* A coronary thrombosis or occlusion with myocardial infarction; a "heart attack."

coronary artery. See Table of Arteries in the Appendix.

coronary bone. The small pastern or second phalanx of a horse's foot.

coronary cataract. A cataract which may be congenital or develop in early life, in which club-shaped opacities are arranged like a wreath or crown in the periphery of the cortex near the equator of the lens. Vision is usually not affected.

coronary chemoreflex. BEZOLD REFLEX.

coronary circulation. The circulation of the blood through the coronary blood vessels of the heart.

coronary cushion. The matrix of the upper edge of the hoof in solipeds.

coronary failure syndrome. CORONARY INSUFFICIENCY.

coronary insufficiency or **failure.** Prolonged precordial pain or discomfort without conventional evidence of myocardial infarction; subendocardial ischemia due to a disparity between coronary blood flow and myocardial needs.

coronary ligament 1. (of the liver:) A reflection of the peritoneum between the liver and the diaphragm surrounding the bare area of the liver. NA *ligamentum coronarium hepatis.* See also *triangular ligament.* 2. (of the knee:) A thick inner portion of the capsule of the knee joint which attaches the medial and lateral menisci to the tibia.

coronary occlusion. Complete blockage of a branch of the arterial system that supplies blood to the heart muscle.

coronary plexus. A continuation of the cardiac plexus of autonomic fibers, divided into a larger posterior part which accompanies the left coronary artery and is distributed chiefly to the left atrium and ventricle and a smaller anterior part which follows the right coronary artery and is distributed to the right atrium and ventricle.

coronary reflex. INTERCORONARY REFLEX.

coronary sinus. A venous sinus that drains most of the cardiac veins, opens into the right atrium, and is located in the lower part of the coronary sulcus of the heart. It is derived from the transverse portion of the embryonic sinus venosus. NA *sinus coronarius.* See also Plate 5.

coronary stenosis. Narrowing of a coronary artery without complete blockage.

coronary sulcus. A groove on the external surface of the heart separating the atria from the ventricles, containing the trunks of the nutrient vessels of the heart. Syn. *atrioventricular sulcus.* NA *sulcus coronarius.*

coronary thrombosis. Formation of a thrombus in a coronary artery of the heart.

coronary T wave. *In electrocardiography,* deep arrow-shaped symmetrical inversion of the T wave, seen in myocardial infarction.

coronary valve. A semicircular fold of the endocardium of the right atrium at the orifice of the coronary sinus. NA *valvula sinus coronarii.*

corona seb·or·rhe·i·ca (seb"o·ree'i·kuh). Seborrheic dermatitis manifest by greasy scaling largely at the hairline frontally.

corona ven·e·ris (ven'e·ris). CROWN OF VENUS.

corona virus. A medium-sized (80 to 160 nm) enveloped RNA virus associated with upper respiratory tract disease in humans. So called because on electron microscopy the virion appears to be surrounded by a crown of projections with bulbous tips.

co·ro·ne (ko·ro'nee) *n.* [Gk. *korōnē,* something hooked, curved]. *Obsol.* The coronoid process of the mandible.

cor·o·ner (kor'uh·nur) *n.* [Anglo-French *corouner,* a local officer of the crown]. A legal officer, now usually a physician, of a municipality or county whose duty it is to hold inquests regarding sudden, violent, or unexplained deaths.

coroner's jury. A jury that attends a coroner's inquest, to determine the cause of a death.

cor·o·net (kor'o·net, kor·o·net') *n.* [OF. *coronete,* dim. of *corona*]. 1. *In biology,* a crowning circle of hairs. 2. The lowest part of the pastern at its junction with a horse's hoof.

co·ro·ni·on (ko·ro'nee·on) *n.*, pl. **coro·nia** (·nee·uh). *In craniometry,* the point at the tip of the coronoid process of the mandible. If the tip is divided into two, the measuring point is to be located on the anterior division.

cor·o·ni·tis (kor"o·nigh'tis) *n.* [*corone*t + *-itis*]. Inflammation of the coronet of a horse's hoof.

corono-. See *coron-*.

cor·o·no·bas·i·lar (kor"uh·no·bas'i·lur, kuh·ro'no·) *adj.* Of or pertaining to the coronal suture and the basilar aspect of the skull.

co·ro·no·fa·cial (kuh·ro"no·fay'shul, kor"uh·no·) *adj.* [*corono-* + *facial*]. Of or pertaining to the crown of the head and to the face.

cor·o·noid (kor'o·noid) *adj.* [Gk. *korōnē,* crow, crow's beak, + *-oid*]. Curved like a beak, as the coronoid process of the ulna or of the mandible.

coronoid fossa. A depression in the humerus into which the apex of the coronoid process of the ulna fits in extreme flexion of the forearm. NA *fossa coronoidea.*

coronoid process. 1. A thin, flattened process projecting from the anterior portion of the upper border of the ramus of the mandible and serving for the insertion of the temporal muscle. NA *processus coronoideus mandibulae.* 2. A triangular projection from the upper end of the ulna, forming the lower part of the radial notch. NA *processus coronoideus ulnae.*

co·ros·co·py (ko·ros'ko·pee) *n.* [*coo-* + *-scopy*]. RETINOSCOPY.

Cor·per and Cohn method. A method for detecting tubercle bacilli in sputum in which sputum is treated with oxalic acid and centrifuged; the supernatant fluid is then cultured for tubercle bacilli.

corpora. Plural of *corpus.*

corpora albicantia. Plural of *corpus albicans.*

corpora amy·la·cea (am·i·lay'see·uh) [L.]. AMYLOID BODIES.

corpora Aran·tii (a·ran'shee·eye) [G. C. *Arantius*]. NODULES OF THE SEMILUNAR VALVES.

corpora are·na·cea (ăr·e·nay'see·uh). Psammoma bodies in the pineal body; brain sand.

corpora bi·ge·mi·na (bye·jem'i·nuh). OPTIC LOBES.

corpora ca·ver·no·sa (kav·ur·no'suh). Plural of *corpus cavernosum.*

corpora he·mor·rha·gi·ca (hem·o·raj'i·kuh). Plural of *corpus hemorrhagicum.*

cor·po·ra ni·gra (kor'puh·ruh nye'gruh). Small black nodules on the irides of horses and cattle, sometimes as large as 1 cm in diameter; have been mistaken for neoplasms. Syn. *granula iridis.*

corpora pa·ra·aor·ti·ca (păr"uh·ay·or'ti·kuh) [NA]. PARA-AORTIC BODIES.

corpora qua·dri·ge·mi·na (kwah·dri·jem'i·nuh). The inferior and superior colliculi collectively. See also *lamina tecti.* See also Plate 18.

corpora res·ti·for·mia (res"ti·for'mee·uh). Plural of *corpus restiforme.*

cor pseu·do·tri·loc·u·la·re (sue"do·trye·lock"yoo·lair'ee). A congenital malformation of the heart in which there are three functioning chambers, the fourth being rudimentary, as seen with tricuspid atresia.

corps ronds (kor rohⁿ) [F., round bodies]. The large round dyskeratotic cells in the upper epidermis, found in Darier's disease and familial benign pemphigus.

cor pul·mo·na·le (pul"mo·nay'lee). Acute right heart strain or chronic right ventricular hypertrophy with or without heart failure resulting from disease states which affect the function and/or structure of the lungs and cause pulmonary hypertension. Syn. *pulmonary heart disease.*

cor·pus (kor'pus) *n.*, genit. **cor·po·ris** (kor'po·ris), pl. **cor·po·ra** (kor'po·ruh) [L.]. BODY.

corpus adi·po·sum buc·cae (ad"i·po'sum buck'ee, ·see) [NA]. SUCKING PAD.

corpus adiposum fos·sae is·chio·rec·ta·lis (fos'ee is"kee·o·reck·tay'lis) [NA]. The mass of fat in the ischiorectal fossa.

corpus adiposum in·fra·pa·tel·la·re (in"fra·pat"e·lair'ee) [NA]. The mass of adipose tissue situated just distal to the patella.

corpus adiposum or·bi·tae (or'bi·tee) [NA]. The fat body of the orbital cavity; fatty connective tissue filling the space between the eyeball, optic nerve, ocular muscles, and lacrimal glands, and supporting the orbital vessels and nerves.

corpus al·bi·cans (al'bi·kanz), pl. **cor·po·ra al·bi·can·tia** (kor'po·ruh al·bi·kan'tee·uh, ·chee·uh) [NA]. The white, fibrous scar in an ovary; produced by the involution of a corpus luteum.

corpus albicans cyst. A cystic corpus luteum remnant.

corpus amyg·da·loi·de·um (a·mig"duh·loy'dee·um) [NA]. AMYGDALOID BODY.

corpus atre·ti·cum (a·tret'i·kum). ATRETIC FOLLICLE.

corpus cal·ca·nei (kal·kay'nee·eye) [BNA]. The body of the calcaneus.

corpus cal·lo·sum (ka·lo'sum) [NA]. The great transverse commissure connecting the cerebral hemispheres; a broad, arched band of white matter at the bottom of the longitudinal fissure of the cerebrum.

corpus callosum radiation. A fiber tract of the corpus callosum fibers to the medullary center of each cerebral hemisphere. NA *radiatio corporis callosi.*

corpus can·di·cans (kan'di·kanz). CORPUS ALBICANS.

corpus ca·ver·no·sum (kav"ur·no'sum) pl. **cor·po·ra ca·ver·no·sa** (kor'po·ruh kav·ur·no'suh) [L., cavernous body]. Either of the two cylinders of erectile tissue, right and left, separated proximally to form the crura and united distally, which constitute the greater part of the penis in the male (NA *corpus cavernosum penis*) and of the clitoris in the female (NA *corpus cavernosum clitoridis*).

corpus cavernosum cli·to·ri·dis (kli·tor'i·dis) [NA]. The corpus cavernosum of the clitoris.

corpus cavernosum–corpus spongiosum shunt. A surgical procedure for treatment of priapism in which a window is created between the corpora cavernosa of the penis to facilitate drainage of blood.

corpus cavernosum penis (pee'nis) [NA]. The corpus cavernosum of the penis. See also Plate 25.

corpus cavernosum–saphenous vein shunt. A surgical procedure for treatment of priapism in which the saphenous vein is sutured to the corpus cavernosum to afford venous drainage.

corpus cavernosum ure·thrae (yoo·ree'three) [BNA]. CORPUS SPONGIOSUM PENIS.

corpus ce·re·bel·li (serr"e·bel'eye). The cerebellum exclusive of the flocculonodular lobe.

corpus ci·li·a·re (sil"ee·air'ee) [NA]. CILIARY BODY.

cor·pus·cle (kor'pus·ul) *n.* [L. *corpusculum,* dim. of *corpus*]. 1. A small rounded body. 2. An encapsulated sensory nerve end organ. 3. A cell, especially a blood cell.

corpuscle of Golgi [C. *Golgi*]. A specialized encapsulated sensory nerve end organ on a tendon in series with muscle fibers.

corpuscle of Vater-Pacini. PACINIAN CORPUSCLE.

corpus cli·to·ri·dis (kli·tor'i·dis) [NA]. The body of the clitoris.

corpus coc·cy·ge·um (kock·sij'ee·um) [NA]. A small arteriovenous anastomotic body associated with the median sacral artery.

corpus cos·tae (kos'tee) [NA]. The body of a rib, the portion distal to the tubercle.

corpuscula. Plural of *corpusculum.*

Cortrosyn. A trademark for cosyntropin, an adrenocorticotropic hormone.

corpuscula ar·ti·cu·la·ria (ahr·tick"yoo·lair'ee·uh) [NA]. ARTICULAR CORPUSCLES.

corpuscula bul·boi·dea (bul·boy′dee·uh) [NA]. Thin laminated capsules of connective tissue, each surrounding a core of terminal nerve fibers.

corpuscula ge·ni·ta·lia (jen″i·tay′lee·uh) [NA]. GENITAL CORPUSCLES.

corpuscula la·mel·lo·sa (lam·e·lo′suh) [NA]. LAMELLAR CORPUSCLES.

corpuscula ner·vo·rum ar·ti·cu·la·ria (nur·vo′rum ahr·tick″yoo·lair′ee·uh) [BNA]. Corpuscula articularia (= ARTICULAR CORPUSCLES).

corpuscula nervorum ge·ni·ta·lia (jen″i·tay′lee·uh) [BNA]. Corpuscula genitalia (= GENITAL CORPUSCLES).

corpuscula nervorum ter·mi·na·lia (tur″mi·nay′lee·uh) [BNA]. CORPUSCULA NERVOSA TERMINALIA.

corpuscula ner·vo·sa ter·mi·na·lia (nur·vo′suh tur″mi·nay′lee·uh) [NA]. The corpuscles surrounding terminal nerve fibers.

cor·pus·cu·lar (kor·pus′kew·lur) *adj.* Of or pertaining to a corpuscle or corpuscles.

corpuscular radiation. Subatomic particles such as electrons, protons, neutrons, deuterons, or alpha particles, traveling at high velocities.

corpuscula re·nis (ree′nis) [NA]. RENAL CORPUSCLES.

corpuscula tac·tus (tack′tus) [NA]. TACTILE CORPUSCLES.

cor·pus·cu·lum (kor·pus′kew·lum) *n.*, pl. **corpuscu·la** (·luh) [L., dim. of *corpus*]. CORPUSCLE.

corpusculum ar·ti·cu·la·re mo·bi·le (ahr·tick″yoo·lair′ee mo′bi·lee). ARTHROLITH.

corpus de·lic·ti (de·lick′tye) [L., the body of the crime]. The existing facts necessary to establish proof that a crime has been committed.

corpus epi·di·dy·mi·dis (ep″ee·di·dim′i·dis) [NA]. The body of the epididymis, the middle portion.

corpus fe·mo·ris (fem′o·ris) [NA]. The shaft of the femur.

corpus fi·bro·sum (figh·bro′sum), pl. **corpora fibro·sa**. The scarlike structure in the ovary which represents the end result of an atretic follicle. It has a small central cicatrix surrounded by a narrow zone of hyalinized tissue, and is usually smaller than the corpus albicans.

corpus fi·bu·lae (fib′yoo·lee) [NA]. The shaft of the fibula.

corpus for·ni·cis (for′ni·sis) [NA]. The body of the fornix, the middle portion.

corpus ge·ni·cu·la·tum (je·nick″yoo·lay′tum). GENICULATE BODY.

corpus geniculatum la·te·ra·le (lat″e·ray′lee) [NA]. LATERAL GENICULATE BODY.

corpus geniculatum me·di·a·le (mee″dee·ay′lee) [NA]. MEDIAL GENICULATE BODY.

corpus glan·du·lae bul·bo·ure·thra·lis (glan′dew·lee bul″bo·yoo·re·thray′lis) [BNA]. The body of the bulbourethral gland.

corpus glandulae su·do·ri·fe·rae (sue″do·rif′e·ree) [NA]. The coiled portion of a sweat gland, the secretory portion.

corpus glan·du·la·re pro·sta·tae (glan·dew·lair′ee pros′tuh·tee) [BNA]. SUBSTANTIA GLANDULARIS PROSTATAE.

corpus he·mor·rha·gi·cum (hem″o·raj′i·kum). A collapsed graafian follicle containing blood; an early phase of a corpus luteum.

corpus hu·me·ri (hew′mur·eye) [NA]. The shaft of the humerus.

corpus in·cu·dis (ing·kew′dis, ing′kew·dis) [NA]. The portion of the incus which articulates with the malleus.

corpus lin·guae (ling′gwee) [NA]. The large anterior portion of the tongue.

corpus lu·te·um (lew′tee·um) pl. **corpora lu·tea** [NA]. The yellow endocrine body formed in the ovary in the site of a ruptured graafian follicle. The large pale corpus luteum of pregnancy is called a true corpus luteum; the smaller dark corpus luteum of menstruation is called a false corpus luteum. See also Plate 23.

corpus luteum cyst. Cystic distention of a corpus luteum.

corpus luteum–stimulating hormone. LUTEINIZING HORMONE. Abbreviated, CLSH.

corpus Luy·sii (lew·ee′see·eye) [J. B. *Luys*, French physician, 1828–1898]. SUBTHALAMIC NUCLEUS.

corpus ma·mil·la·re (mam″i·lair′ee) [NA]. MAMILLARY BODY.

corpus mam·mae (mam′ee) [NA]. The main mass of a mammary gland.

corpus man·di·bu·lae (man·dib′yoo·lee) [NA]. The horseshoe-shaped horizontal portion of the mandible.

corpus max·il·lae (mack·sil′ee) [NA]. The pyramidal portion of the maxilla which surrounds the maxillary sinus.

corpus me·dul·la·re ce·re·bel·li (med·yoo·lair′ee serr·e·bel′eye) [NA]. The inner white matter of the cerebellum.

corpus nu·clei cau·da·ti (new′klee·eye kaw·day′tye) [NA]. The portion of the caudate nucleus lying in the floor of the central portion of the lateral ventricle.

corpus os·sis hy·oi·dei (os′is high·oy′dee·eye) [NA]. The central portion of the hyoid bone.

corpus ossis ilii (il′ee·eye) [NA]. The portion of the iliac bone which enters into the formation of the acetabulum.

corpus ossis ili·um (il′ee·um) [BNA]. CORPUS OSSIS ILII.

corpus ossis is·chii (is′kee·eye) [NA]. The portion of the ischium which enters into the formation of the acetabulum and terminates below in the tuber of the ischium.

corpus ossis me·ta·car·pa·lis (met″uh·kahr·pay′lis) [NA]. The shaft of a metacarpal bone.

corpus ossis me·ta·tar·sa·lis (met″uh·tahr·say′lis) [NA]. The shaft of a metatarsal bone.

corpus ossis pu·bis (pew′bis) [NA]. The portion of a pubic bone which articulates with its fellow of the opposite side.

corpus ossis sphe·noi·da·lis (sfee″noy·day′lis) [NA]. The central portion of the sphenoid bone; the sphenoid air sinuses are located within this portion.

corpus os·si·um me·ta·car·pa·li·um (os′ee·um met″uh·kahr·pay′lee·um) [BNA]. CORPUS OSSIS METACARPALIS.

corpus ossium me·ta·tar·sa·li·um (met″uh·tahr·say′lee·um) [BNA]. CORPUS OSSIS METATARSALIS.

corpus pan·cre·a·tis (pan·kree′uh·tis) [NA]. The portion of the pancreas extending from the head, on its right, ending in the tail on its left.

corpus pa·pil·la·re co·rii (pap·i·lair′ee kor′ee·eye) [BNA]. STRATUM PAPILLARE CORII.

corpus pe·nis (pee′nis) [NA]. The shaft of the penis.

corpus pha·lan·gis di·gi·to·rum ma·nus (fa·lan′jis dij·i·to′rum man′oos, man′us) [NA]. The shaft of any phalanx of the digits of the hand.

corpus phalangis digitorum pe·dis (ped′is) [NA]. The shaft of any phalanx of the digits of the foot.

corpus pi·ne·a·le (pin″ee·ay′lee) [NA]. PINEAL BODY.

corpus pon·to·bul·ba·re (pon″to·bul·bair′ee). A nuclear mass caudal to the dorsal cochlear nucleus, receiving fibers from the pons and sending fibers to the cerebellum.

corpus qua·dri·ge·mi·na (kwah·dri·jem′i·nuh) [BNA]. CORPORA QUADRIGEMINA.

corpus ra·dii (ray′dee·eye) [NA]. The shaft of the radius.

corpus res·ti·for·me (res″ti·for′mee) [BNA]. Pedunculus cerebellaris inferior (= INFERIOR CEREBELLAR PEDUNCLE).

corpus re·ti·cu·la·re co·rii (re·tick·yoo·lair′ee ko′ree·eye) [BNA]. Stratum reticulare (= RETICULAR LAYER).

corpus spon·gi·o·sum pe·nis (spon″jee·o′sum pee′nis) [NA]. The cylinder of erectile tissue surrounding the penile urethra.

corpus spongiosum ure·thrae mu·li·e·bris (yoo·ree′three mew·lee·ee′bris [BNA]. The corpus spongiosum of the female urethra; actually there is no erectile tissue about the female urethra, but there are some veins coursing longitudinally in the submucosa.

corpus ster·ni (stur′nigh) [NA]. The body of the sternum.

corpus stri·a·tum (strye·ay′tum) [NA]. The caudate and lenticular nuclei together with the internal capsule which separates them.

corpus ta·li (tay′lye) [NA]. The body of the talus, the central portion.

corpus ti·bi·ae (tib′ee·ee) [NA]. The shaft of the tibia.

corpus tra·pe·zoi·de·um (trap″e·zoy′dee·um) [NA]. TRAPEZOID BODY.

corpus ul·nae (ul′nee) [NA]. The shaft of the ulna.

corpus un·guis (ung′gwis) [NA]. The distal, exposed portion of a fingernail or a toenail.

corpus ute·ri (yoo′tur·eye) [NA]. The body of the uterus, the portion between the cervix and the fundus.

corpus ven·tri·cu·li (ven·trick′yoo·lye) [NA]. The body of the stomach, the large central portion.

corpus ver·te·brae (vur′te·bree) [NA]. The body of a vertebra, the central, short column of bone.

corpus ve·si·cae fel·le·ae (ve·sigh′see fel′ee·ee) [NA]. The body of the gallbladder, the portion between the fundus and the neck.

corpus vesicae uri·na·ri·ae (yoo·re·nair′ee·ee) [NA]. The body of the urinary bladder, the portion between the fundus and the trigone.

corpus ve·si·cu·lae se·mi·na·lis (ve·sick′yoo·lee sem″i·nay′lis, see″mi·) [BNA]. The body of a seminal vesicle, the main portion of each gland.

corpus vi·tre·um (vit′ree·um) [NA]. VITREOUS BODY.

corpus Wolf·fi (wolf′eye) [BNA]. MESONEPHROS.

cor·rect·ed transposition of the great arteries or **vessels.** A form of congenital heart disease in which the aorta occupies the anterior position usually occupied by the pulmonary artery, while the pulmonary artery lies behind it. The aorta, however, arises from a right ventricle which carries arterial blood and the pulmonary artery from a left ventricle carrying venous blood.

cor·rec·tive (ko·reck′tiv) *adj.* & *n.* 1. Intended or designed to correct or to modify favorably. 2. A substance used to modify or make more pleasant the action of the principal ingredients of a prescription.

corrective orthodontics. The management of malocclusion wherein appliance therapy is principally responsible for the changes accomplished.

corrective therapy. 1. *In physical medicine,* a medically supervised program of physical exercise and activities for the purpose of improving or maintaining the health of the patient through individual or group participation. 2. Specifically, techniques designed to conserve and increase neuromuscular strength and skill, to reestablish or improve ambulation, to improve habits of personal health, and to promote relaxation by adjustment to physical and mental stresses.

cor·re·lat·ed atrophy. Atrophy secondary to the removal or destruction of other parts of the body, as atrophy of bone and muscle following amputation of an extremity.

cor·re·la·tion (kor″e·lay′shun) *n.* [ML. *correlatio,* from *com-,* with, + *relatio,* relation]. *In biometry,* the degree of association between two characteristics in a series of observations, usually expressed as the coefficient of correlation. —**cor·re·late** (kor′e·late) *v.;* **cor·rel·a·tive** (ko·rel′uh·tiv) *adj.*

correlative differentiation. DEPENDENT DIFFERENTIATION.

cor·re·spond·ing retinal areas or **points.** The retinal area of each eye which has an identical direction in the opposite retina. See also *retinal correspondence.*

Cor·ri·gan's pulse [D. J. *Corrigan,* Irish physician, 1802–1880]. A pulse characterized by a rapid forceful ascent (water-hammer quality) and rapid downstroke or descent (collapsing quality); seen with aortic regurgitation and hyperkinetic circulatory states.

Corrigan's respiration [D. J. *Corrigan*]. *Obsol.* A shallow rapid blowing respiration seen often in the presence of fever.

cor·rin ring (kor′in). The porphyrin-like ring that forms the central structure of vitamin B_{12}, in which two of the pyrrole rings are linked directly rather than through a methene bridge.

cor·ro·sion preparation. A preparation in which the vessels, ducts, or cavities of organs are filled by a fluid that will harden and preserve the shape of the vessel or cavity after the organ itself is corroded, digested, or destroyed.

cor·ro·sive, *adj.* & *n.* 1. Tending to eat or wear away, especially by chemical action. 2. A substance that destroys organic tissue either by direct chemical means or by causing inflammation and suppuration.

corrosive gastritis. An acute inflammation of the stomach caused by corrosive poisons.

corrosive sublimate. MERCURY BICHLORIDE.

cor·ru·ga·tor (kor′oo·gay″tur) *n.* [L. *corrugare,* to wrinkle]. That which wrinkles, as the corrugator supercilii muscle.

corrugator cu·tis ani (kew′tis ay′nigh). A thin layer of smooth muscle arranged radially around the anus in the subcutaneous tissue.

corrugator su·per·cil·ii (sue″pur·sil′ee·eye). A muscle of facial expression located beneath the medial portion of each eyebrow. NA *musculus corrugator supercilii.* See also Table of Muscles in the Appendix.

cor·set, *n.* [OF., dim. of *cors,* body]. *In surgery,* a removable appliance embracing the trunk from pelvis to chest; used for correction of deformities, for support of injured bones and muscles of the spine or thorax, or in control of ventral hernia.

corset liver. A liver with a fibrotic groove on the anterior surface at the costal margin, said to be produced by compression of the liver by a rib from tight corset stays.

Cortate. A trademark for deoxycorticosterone (acetate), a salt-regulating adrenocortical hormone.

Cortef. A trademark for hydrocortisone, an anti-inflammatory glucocorticoid.

cor·tex (kor′tecks) *n.,* pl. **cor·ti·ces** (·ti·seez) [L., bark]. 1. The bark of an exogenous plant. 2. [NA] The peripheral portion of an organ, situated just beneath the capsule. 3. *In neuroanatomy,* the external gray layer of the brain, as: cerebral cortex, cerebellar cortex. 4. *In neurology,* a functional area of the cerebral cortex, as: auditory cortex, motor cortex. Comb. form *cortic(o)-.*

cortex ce·re·bel·li (serr″e·bel′eye) [NA]. The cortex of the cerebellum.

cortex ce·re·bri (serr′e·brye) [NA]. The cortex of the cerebrum.

cortex glan·du·lae su·pra·re·na·lis (glan′dew·lee sue″pruh·re·nay′lis) [NA]. The cortex of the adrenal gland.

cortex len·tis (len′tis) [NA]. The softer, external portion of the lens of the eye.

cortex no·di lym·pha·ti·ci (no′dye lim·fat′i·sigh) [NA]. The cortex of a lymph node, the peripheral portion containing lymph nodules.

cortex re·nis (ree′nis) [NA]. The cortex of a kidney.

cortic-, cortico-. A combining form meaning *cortex, cortical.*

cor·ti·cal (kor′ti·kul) *adj.* Of or pertaining to a cortex.

cortical adenoma. A benign neoplasm composed principally of cells resembling those of the adrenal cortex, but with little or no tendency to form acini.

cortical arch. The renal substance that stretches from one column to another and surrounds the base of a pyramid.

cortical blindness. Loss of visual sensation, including light and dark, together with loss of reflex blinking to bright illumination or threatening gestures, but with intact pupillary reflexes, normal ocular motility, and normal retinoscopy; due to disturbances of cerebral visual centers.

cortical bone. The compact bone next to the surface of a bone.

cortical carcinoma. A carcinoma composed mainly of cells resembling those of the adrenal cortex.

cortical cataract. A cataract due to the loss of transparency of the outer layers of the lens.

cortical cords. The secondary cordlike invaginations of the germinal epithelium of the embryonic gonad that differentiate into primary follicles and oogonia.

cortical deafness. Deafness due to bilateral lesions of Heschl's gyri.

cortical degeneration. 1. Any degenerative disease of the central nervous system involving primarily gray matter.

2. GENERAL PARALYSIS. 3. The degeneration of the cortex of any organ.

cortical hormone. ADRENOCORTICAL HORMONE.

cortical potential. ELECTROCORTICAL POTENTIAL.

cortical rays. MEDULLARY RAYS.

cortical sinus. A lymph sinus in the cortex of a lymph node.

cor·ti·cate (kor'ti·kate) *adj.* [L. *corticatus*, covered with bark]. Having a bark or cortex.

cortices. Plural of *cortex.*

cor·ti·cif·u·gal (kor"ti·sif'yoo·gul) *adj.* [*cortic-* + *-fugal*]. Conducting away from the cortex. Contr. *corticipetal.*

cor·ti·cin (kor'ti·sin) *n.* A hypothetical morphogenetic inductor secreted by the cortical component of a developing embryonic vertebrate gonad which inhibits differentiation of the medullary gonadal component, resulting in development of an ovary. See also *medullarin.*

cor·ti·cip·e·tal (kor"ti·sip'e·tul) *adj.* [*cortic-* + *-petal*]. Conducting toward the cortex. Contr. *corticifugal.*

cortico-. See *cortic-.*

cor·ti·co·bul·bar (kor"ti·ko·bul'bur) *adj.* [*cortico-* + *bulbar*]. Pertaining to the cerebral cortex and the medulla oblongata.

corticobulbar tract. Fibers of the pyramidal system that originate in the motor cortex, pass through the internal capsule, and terminate in the motor nuclei of the cranial nerves. NA *fibrae corticonucleares.*

cor·ti·co·col·lic·u·lar (kor"ti·ko·kol·ick'yoo·lur) *adj.* Pertaining to the cerebral cortex and a colliculus.

corticocollicular tract. Part of the posterior commissure; nerve fibers that arise in the cerebral cortex and go to the stratum zonale of the midbrain.

cor·ti·co·ge·nic·u·late (kor"ti·ko·je·nick'yoo·lut) *adj.* Pertaining to the cerebral cortex and a geniculate body.

corticogeniculate tract. Nerve fibers arising in the calcarine area of the cerebral cortex and ending in the lateral geniculate body.

cor·ti·co·hy·po·tha·lam·ic (kor"ti·ko·high"po·thuh·lam'ick) *adj.* Pertaining to the cerebral cortex and the hypothalamus.

corticohypothalamic tracts. Nerve fibers that arise in the premotor and posterior orbital areas and end directly in the hypothalamus. NA *tractus corticohypothalamici.*

cor·ti·coid (kor'ti·koid) *n.* CORTICOSTEROID.

cor·ti·co·med·ul·lary (kor"ti·ko·med'yoo·lerr·ee) *adj.* Pertaining to the cortex and the medulla of an organ, as those of the kidney, or to the cerebral cortex and the medulla oblongata.

cor·ti·co·mes·en·ce·phal·ic (kor"ti·ko·mez·en"se·fal'ick) *adj.* Pertaining to the cerebral cortex and the mesencephalon.

cor·ti·co·ni·gral (kor"ti·ko·nigh'grul) *adj.* [*cortico-* + *nigral*]. Pertaining to the cerebral cortex and the substantia nigra.

corticonigral tract. A component of the extrapyramidal system; fibers arise principally from Brodmann's areas 4 and 6 of the cortex, with some contribution from temporal and parietal lobes, and pass through the stratum intermedium of the cerebral peduncle to synapse with the cells of the substantia nigra.

cor·ti·co·nu·cle·ar (kor"ti·ko·new'klee·ur) *adj.* [*cortico-* + *nuclear*]. Pertaining to the cerebral cortex and the motor nuclei of the cranial nerves.

corticonuclear tract. CORTICOBULBAR TRACT.

cor·ti·co·pal·li·dal (kor"ti·ko·pal'i·dul) *adj.* [*cortico-* + *pallidal*]. Pertaining to the cerebral cortex and the globus pallidus.

corticopallidal tract. Nerve fibers that arise in the premotor area of the cerebral cortex and end in the globus pallidus.

cor·ti·co·pon·tile (kor"ti·ko·pon'tile) *adj.* CORTICOPONTINE.

cor·ti·co·pon·tine (kor"ti·ko·pon'teen) *adj.* [*cortico-* + *pontine*]. Pertaining to the cerebral cortex and the pons.

corticopontine fibers. Fibers arising from the cortex of the frontal lobe and from the parietal, temporal, and portions of the occipital lobe, and descending uncrossed to the pontine nuclei. NA *fibrae corticopontinae.*

corticopontine tract. Collectively, the fibers of the frontopontine, temporopontine, parietopontine, and occipitopontine tracts which descend from the cortex, pass through the internal capsule, and terminate in the pontine nuclei. NA *tractus corticopontinus.*

cor·ti·co·pon·to·cer·e·bel·lar (kor"ti·ko·pon"to·serr·e·bel'ur) *adj.* [*cortico-* + *ponto-* + *cerebellar*]. 1. Connecting the cerebral cortex with the cerebellum by way of the pons, as: corticopontocerebellar pathway. 2. Pertaining to any neurologic function or disorder involving this connection pathway.

cor·ti·co·ru·bral (kor"ti·ko·roo'brul) *adj.* [*cortico-* + *rubr-* + *-al*]. Pertaining to the cerebral cortex and the red nucleus.

corticorubral fiber. A fiber going from the premotor cortex to the red nucleus.

corticorubral tract. A component of the extrapyramidal system; fibers arise principally from Brodmann's areas 4 and 6 with some contribution from areas 3 and 5 of the parietal lobe of the cortex, pass through the posterior limb of the internal capsule, and enter the superior radiation of the red nucleus.

cor·ti·co·spi·nal (kor"ti·ko·spye'nul) *adj.* Pertaining to the brain cortex and the spinal cord.

corticospinal tracts. Efferent tracts that descend from the motor cortex through the internal capsule, cerebral peduncles, pons, and medulla, where they undergo incomplete decussation to form the lateral and anterior corticospinal tracts. They are concerned in finely coordinated voluntary movements. NA *fibrae corticospinales.*

cor·ti·co·ste·roid (kor"ti·ko·steer'oid, ·sterr'oid, kor"ti·kos'tur·oid) *n.* [*cortico-* + *steroid*]. Any steroid which has certain chemical or biological properties characteristic of the hormones secreted by the adrenal cortex. Syn. *corticoid.*

corticosteroid-binding globulin. TRANSCORTIN.

cor·ti·cos·ter·one (kor"ti·kos'tur·ohn) *n.* 4-Pregnene-11,21-diol-3,20-dione, $C_{21}H_{30}O_4$, a steroid hormone occurring in the adrenal cortex. It influences carbohydrate and electrolyte metabolism and muscular efficiency and protects against stress.

cor·ti·co·stri·ate (kor"ti·ko·strye'ate) *adj.* [*cortico-* + *striate*]. Pertaining to nerve fibers arising in the cerebral cortex and terminating in the corpus striatum.

corticostriate fibers. Fibers transmitting impulses from the cerebral cortex to the corpus striatum; part of the extrapyramidal system.

corticostriate radiation. Fibers running between the corpus striatum and the cerebral cortex. NA *radiatio corporis striati.*

cor·ti·co·stri·a·to·spi·nal (kor"ti·ko·strye"uh·to·spye'nul) *adj.* Pertaining to nervous pathways involving the cerebral cortex, corpus striatum, and spinal cord.

corticostriatospinal degeneration. CREUTZFELDT-JAKOB DISEASE (1).

cor·ti·co·strio·ni·gral (kor"ti·ko·strye"o·nigh'grul) *adj.* [*cortico-* + *stria* + *nigr-* + *-al*]. Pertaining to the cerebral cortex, the corpus striatum, and substantia nigra.

corticostrionigral system. EXTRAPYRAMIDAL SYSTEM.

cor·ti·co·tha·lam·ic (kor"ti·ko·thuh·lam'ick) *adj.* Pertaining to the cerebral cortex and the thalamus.

corticothalamic fasciculus. A nerve fiber tract from the cerebral cortex to various thalamic nuclei. See also *fasciculi corticothalamici.*

corticothalamic fibers. Projections from various areas of the cerebral cortex into the thalamus; apparently have an inhibitory or sensitizing influence on sensory relay nuclei in the thalamus.

corticothalamic tract. The nerve fibers running from the cerebral cortex to the thalamus. See also *thalamocortical fibers.*

cor·ti·co·troph·in (kor"ti·ko·trof'in, ·tro'fin) *n.* CORTICOTROPIN. —**corticotroph·ic** (·ick) *adj.*

corticotropic hormone. ADRENOCORTICOTROPIC HORMONE.

cor·ti·co·tro·pin (kor"ti·ko·tro'pin) *n.* A hormonal preparation having adrenocorticotropic activity derived from the adenohypophysis of certain domesticated animals. —**cor·tico·tro·pic** (·trop'ick, ·tro'pick) *adj.*

Cortifan. A trademark for hydrocortisone, an anti-inflammatory glucocorticoid.

cor·tin (kor'tin) *n.* An extract of adrenal cortex that contains several hormones; has been used in treating adrenal cortical hypofunction.

cor·ti·sol (kor'ti·sol) *n.* HYDROCORTISONE.

cor·ti·sone (kor'ti·sone) *n.* 17-Hydroxy-11-dehydrocorticosterone, $C_{21}H_{28}O_5$, a glucogenic adrenocortical steroid produced commercially by synthesis; used, as the acetate, chiefly for substitution therapy in adrenal insufficiency, and in acute infections, in shock, in allergic states, and in the collagen diseases. Syn. *Kendall's compound E, Wintersteiner's compound F, Reichstein's substance Fa.*

cortisone acetate. The monoacetate ester of cortisone, a crystalline powder, practically insoluble in water; the form in which cortisone is used therapeutically.

Cor·ti's teeth [A. *Corti,* Italian anatomist, 1822–1888]. AUDITORY TEETH.

cor·tiv·a·zol (kor·tiv'uh·zole) *n.* 11*β*,17,21-Trihydroxy-6,16*α*-dimethyl-2'phenyl-2'*H*-pregna-2,4,6-trieno [3,2-*c*]-pyrazol-20-one, $C_{30}H_{36}N_2O_3$, a glucocorticoid usually used as the 21-acetate ($C_{32}H_{38}N_2O_5$).

cor·to·dox·one (kor''to·dock·sone) *n.* 17,21-Dihydroxypregn-4-ene-3,20-dione, $C_{21}H_{30}O_4$, a steroid with anti-inflammatory activity.

Cortogen. A trademark for cortisone, the glucogenic adrenocortical steroid.

cor·tol (kor'tol) *n.* A metabolite, $C_{21}H_{36}O_5$, of hydrocortisone (cortisol).

cor·to·lone (kor'to·lone) *n.* A metabolite, $C_{21}H_{34}O_5$, of cortisone.

Cortone. A trademark for cortisone, the glucogenic adrenocortical steroid.

cor tri·atri·a·tum (trye·ay''tree·ay'tum). A congenital cardiac anomaly assuming one of several types, with the shared feature of having three chambers preceding the ventricles: (a) division of the left atrium by a septum separating the mitral valve from the pulmonary vein openings; (b) three atria, the left receiving the pulmonary veins, the middle receiving the superior vena cava, the right receiving the inferior vena cava; (c) a third atrium lying between the septum primum and septum secundum, receiving the left superior vena cava and emptying into the coronary sinus.

cor tri·au·ri·cu·la·re (trye''aw·rick''yoo·lair'ee). A congenital cardiac anomaly in which failure of resorption of the common pulmonary vein leads to the formation of an appendage projecting into the left atrium to take a position close to the mitral valve.

Cortril. A trademark for hydrocortisone, an anti-inflammatory glucocorticoid.

cor tri·lo·cu·la·re (trye·lock''yoo·lair'ee). A three-chambered heart; in humans, a congenital anomaly in which there is either a single atrium or a single ventricle. Syn. *trilocular heart.*

cor triloculare bi·atri·um (bye·ay'tree·um). A congenital cardiac anomaly consisting of absence of the ventricular septum; the two atria communicate with a common single ventricle.

cor triloculare bi·ven·tri·cu·la·re (bye''ven·trick''yoo·lair'ee). A congenital cardiac anomaly due to failure of development of the interatrial septum; the heart is composed of a single atrium and two ventricles.

cor triloculare mon·atri·a·tum (mon·ay''tree·ay'tum). COR TRILOCULARE BIVENTRICULARE.

Cortrophin Zinc ACTH. A trademark for sterile corticotropin zinc hydroxide suspension.

Cortrosyn. A trademark for cosyntropin, an adrenocorticotropic hormone.

cor·us·ca·tion (kor''us·kay'shun) *n.* [L. *coruscare,* to glitter]. The subjective sensation of light flashes.

cor vil·lo·sum (vi·lo'sum). Fibrinous pericarditis in which fibrin projects from the pericardial surface in villous processes.

co·ryd·a·lis (ko·rid'uh·lis) *n.* [Gk. *korydalos,* crested lark]. The tuber of *Dicentra canadensis,* squirrel corn, or of *D. cucullaria,* Dutchman's-breeches, containing several alkaloids, including corydaline, isocorydine, and protopine; has been used as a tonic and alterative.

cor·ym·bi·form (kor·im'bi·form) *adj.* [L. *corymbus,* a cluster, + *-iform*]. Designating a form of syphilid with a large lenticular papule in the center of an irregular group of papules.

Cor·y·ne·bac·te·ri·um (kor''i·ne·back·teer'ee·um, ko·rye''ne·) *n.* [Gk. *korynē,* club, + *bacterium*]. A genus of slender, aerobic, nonmotile, non-spore-forming, gram-positive bacteria of which *Corynebacterium diphtheriae* is the type species; varying from slightly curved to club-shaped and branching forms; showing irregular staining. This genus includes a large group of diphtheroid bacilli, such as *C. acnes,* and *C. pyogenes,* mainly saprophytic and morphologically similar to *C. diphtheriae;* found in normal tissues and secretions as well as in pathologic conditions; probably not causative. —**corynebacterium,** pl. **corynebacte·ria,** *com. n.*

Corynebacterium diph·the·ri·ae (dif·theer'ee·ee). The causative organism of diphtheria; the varieties *gravis, mitis,* and *intermedius* have been described; produces a potent exotoxin. Syn. *Bacillus diphtheriae.*

Corynebacterium hof·man·nii (hof·man'ee·eye). *CORYNEBACTERIUM PSEUDODIPHTHERITICUM.*

Corynebacterium pseu·do·diph·the·rit·i·cum (sue''do·dif·the·rit'i·kum). A species with morphology similar to *Corynebacterium diphtheriae,* but nonpathogenic, having its habitat in normal throats.

Corynebacterium xe·ro·sis (ze·ro'sis). A species found in the keratin layer in xerosis conjunctivae, in chronic conjunctivitis, and also in normal eyes.

co·ry·za (ko·rye'zuh) *n.* [Gk. *koryza,* nasal mucus]. Inflammation of the mucous membranes of the nose, usually marked by sneezing, nasal airway congestion, and discharge of watery mucus; acute rhinitis. See also *common cold.*

cosm-, cosmo- [Gk. *kosmos,* order, world, universe]. A combining form meaning (a) *universe, universal;* (b) *pertaining to outer space.*

Cosmegen. Trademark for dactinomycin, an antibiotic useful in the treatment of various tumors.

cos·met·ic (koz·met'ick) *adj. & n.* [Gk. *kosmētikos,* skilled in ordering, from *kosmos,* order]. 1. Serving or intended to improve appearance. 2. A preparation applied to the skin or its appendages to alter its appearance, to protect it, to beautify, or to promote attractiveness.

cos·mic ray. A very penetrating radiation originating outside the earth's atmosphere, capable of producing ionization in passing through air or other matter. Primary cosmic rays probably consist of atomic nuclei, mainly protons, having energies up to 10^{15} electron volts; they are absorbed in the upper atmosphere. Secondary cosmic rays are produced when primary rays interact with nuclei and electrons in the earth's atmosphere; these consist mainly of mesons, protons, neutrons, electrons, and photons.

cos·mo·tron (koz'mo·tron) *n.* [cosmo- + *-tron*]. PROTON-SYNCHROTRON.

cost-, costi-, costo-. A combining form meaning *rib, costal.*

cos·ta (kos'tuh) *n.,* pl. & genit. sing. **cos·tae** (·tee) [L.] [NA]. RIB. —**cos·tal** (·tul) *adj.*

costae fluc·tu·an·tes (fluck''tew·an'teez). FLOATING RIBS.

costae spu·ri·ae (spew'ree·ee) [NA]. FALSE RIBS.

costae ve·rae (veer'ee) [NA]. TRUE RIBS.

costal angle. The angle formed by the right and left costal cartilages at the xiphoid process. NA *angulus infrasternalis.*

costal arch. The arch of the ribs. NA *arcus costalis.*

costal cartilage. The cartilage occupying the interval between the ribs and the sternum or adjacent cartilages. NA *cartilago costalis.*

costal fossae. The inferior and superior facets on the bodies of the vertebrae where articulation occurs with the heads of the ribs. NA *fovea costalis inferior and fovea costalis superior.*

costal fovea. COSTAL FOSSA.

cos·tal·gia (kos·tal'jee·uh) *n.* [*cost-* + *-algia*]. Intercostal neuralgia; pain in the ribs.

costal groove. COSTAL SULCUS.

cos·ta·lis (kos·tay'lis) *L. adj.* Of or pertaining to the ribs.

costalis muscle. ILIOCOSTALIS THORACIS.

costal notch. Any of the facets on the lateral border of the sternum for articulation with the costal cartilages. NA *incisura costalis.*

costal pleura. The portion of the parietal pleura which lines the bony wall of the thoracic cavity. NA *pleura costalis.*

costal process. 1. An embryonic rib primordium, the ventrolateral outgrowth of the caudal, denser half of a sclerotome. 2. An anterior or ventral projection on the lateral part of a cervical vertebra; it corresponds to the central end of a rib of the thoracic region.

costal respiration. Respiration effected primarily by intercostal muscles moving the thoracic cage. Contr. *diaphragmatic respiration.*

costal sulcus. The groove along the inferior aspect of the rib for the intercostal vessels and nerves. NA *sulcus costae.*

costal tubercle. A roughened elevation found on the dorsal margin of a rib at the junction of the neck and body. It articulates with the tip of the transverse process of the corresponding vertebra. NA *tuberculum costae.*

costal tuberosity. A rough area on the undersurface of the medial end of the clavicle, which gives attachment to the costoclavicular ligament. NA *impressio ligamenti costoclavicularis.*

cos·tate (kos'tate) *adj.* Ribbed; furnished with ribs or connecting structures.

cos·tec·to·my (kos·teck'tuh·mee) *n.* [*cost-* + *-ectomy*]. Excision of a rib or a part of one.

Cos·ten's syndrome [J. B. *Costen,* U.S. otolaryngologist, 1895–1962]. Malfunction of the temporomandibular joint, originally thought to be secondary to dental malocclusion with associated neuralgia and ear symptoms; now considered part of the myofacial pain-dysfunction syndrome.

costi-. See *cost-.*

cos·ti·car·ti·lage (kos''ti·kahr'ti·lij) *n.* COSTAL CARTILAGE.

cos·ti·form (kos'ti·form) *adj.* [*cost-* + *-iform*]. Rib-shaped.

cos·tive (kos'tiv) *adj. & n.* [OF. *costivé,* from L. *constipare, constipatus,* to press together]. 1. Causing, pertaining to, or characterized by constipation. 2. An agent that decreases intestinal motility. **—costive·ness** (·nus) *n.*

costo-. See *cost-.*

cos·to·ar·tic·u·lar (kos''to·ahr·tick'yoo·lur) *adj.* [*costo-* + *articular*]. Pertaining to a rib and a joint.

costoarticular line. A line drawn between the sternoclavicular articulation and the tip of the eleventh rib.

cos·to·car·ti·lage (kos''to·kahr'ti·lij) *n.* COSTAL CARTILAGE.

cos·to·cer·vi·cal (kos''to·sur'vi·kul) *adj.* [*costo-* + *cervical*]. Pertaining to the ribs and the neck.

cos·to·cer·vi·cal·is (kos''to·sur''vi·kay'lis) *L. adj.* Pertaining to the ribs and the neck.

costocervicalis muscle. ILIOCOSTALIS CERVICIS.

costocervical trunk. A main branch of the subclavian artery. It gives off the deep cervical artery and continues as the highest intercostal artery. NA *truncus costocervicalis.* See also Plate 8.

cos·to·chon·dral (kos''to·kon'drul) *adj.* [*costo-* + *chondral*]. Pertaining to the ribs and their cartilages.

cos·to·chon·dri·tis (kos''to·kon·drye'tis) *n.* [*costo-* + *chondritis*]. Inflammation of a costal cartilage.

cos·to·cla·vic·u·lar (kos''to·kla·vick'yoo·lur) *adj.* [*costo-* + *clavicular*]. Pertaining to the ribs and the clavicle.

costoclavicular ligament. The ligament between the first rib and the clavicle. NA *ligamentum costoclaviculare.*

costoclavicular line. PARASTERNAL LINE.

costoclavicular syndrome. Pain in an arm, with loss of sensation, muscle weakness and wasting distally, and frequently obliteration of the radial pulse, due to compression of the subclavian artery and the brachial plexus between the clavicle and first rib.

cos·to·co·lic (kos''to·ko'lick) *adj.* [*costo-* + *colic*]. Pertaining to the ribs and the colon.

costocolic fold. PHRENICOCOLIC LIGAMENT.

cos·to·cor·a·coid (kos''to·kor'uh·koid) *adj.* [*costo-* + *coracoid*]. Pertaining to the ribs and the coracoid process.

costocoracoid membrane or **ligament.** A dense layer of fascia extending between the subclavius muscle and the pectoralis minor, and forming the anterior portion of the sheath of the axillary vessels.

costocoracoid muscle. A variable muscle arising from one or more ribs and inserted into the coracoid process.

cos·to·di·a·phrag·mat·ic (kos''to·dye''uh·frag·mat'ick) *adj.* [*costo-* + *diaphragmatic*]. Pertaining to the ribs and the diaphragm.

costodiaphragmatic recess. A bilateral space between the reflection of the costal pleura upon the diaphragm into which the inferior edge of the lung advances on inspiration. NA *recessus costodiaphragmaticus pleurae.*

cos·to·lum·bar (kos''to·lum'bahr, ·bur) *adj.* Pertaining to the ribs and the lumbar region or loins; lumbocostal.

cos·to·me·di·as·ti·nal (kos''to·mee''dee·uh·stye'nul) *adj.* [*costo-* + *mediastinal*]. Pertaining to the ribs and the mediastinum.

costomediastinal recess. A bilateral space between the reflection of the costal pleura upon the anterior mediastinum into which the border of the lung advances on inspiration. NA *recessus costomediastinalis pleurae.*

costomediastinal sinus. COSTOMEDIASTINAL RECESS.

cos·to·phren·ic (kos''to·fren'ick) *adj.* [*costo-* + *phrenic*]. Pertaining to the ribs and the diaphragm.

costophrenic angle. The angle formed by the ribs and diaphragm.

cos·to·pneu·mo·pexy (kos''to·new'mo·peck''see) *n.* [*costo-* + *pneumo-* + *-pexy*]. A surgical operation in which a lung is attached to a rib.

cos·to·scap·u·lar (kos''to·skap'yoo·lur) *adj.* [*costo-* + *scapular*]. Of or pertaining to the ribs and the scapula; scapulocostal.

cos·to·ster·nal (kos''to·stur'nul) *adj.* [*costo-* + *sternal*]. Pertaining to a rib and the sternum.

cos·to·tome (kos'tuh·tome) *n.* [*costo-* + *-tome*]. Heavy curved shears or forceps with a hooked limb against which the knife blade acts; used for rib resection.

cos·tot·o·my (kos·tot'uh·mee) *n.* [*costo-* + *-tomy*]. *In surgery,* the division of a rib.

cos·to·trans·verse (kos''to·trans·vurce') *adj.* [*costo-* + *transverse*]. Pertaining to a rib and the transverse process of a vertebra; applied to the joint between them and to the ligaments joining them.

cos·to·trans·ver·sec·to·my (kos''to·trans''vur·seck'tuh·mee) *n.* [*costotransverse* + *-ectomy*]. Excision of part of a rib and a transverse process of a vertebra.

costotransverse ligament. The ligament which connects the back of the neck of a rib to the corresponding transverse process. NA *ligamentum costotransversarium.* See also *lateral costotransverse ligament, superior costotransverse ligament.*

cos·to·ver·te·bral (kos''to·vur'te·brul) *adj.* [*costo-* + *vertebral*]. Pertaining to a rib and the vertebral column; applied to the joints between them.

cos·to·xiph·oid (kos''to·zif'oid) *adj.* [*costo-* + *xiphoid*]. Pertaining to the ribs and the xiphoid cartilage.

costoxiphoid ligaments. Ligaments extending from the xiphoid process to the seventh costal cartilage. NA *ligamenta costoxiphoidea.*

co·syn·tro·pin (ko″sin·tro′pin) *n.* Synthetic corticotropin.

¹cot, *n.* FINGER COT.

²cot, *n.* [Hindi *khāṭ,* from Dravidian]. A small bed.

co·tar·nine (ko·tahr′neen, ·nin) *n.* [from *narcotine,* by transposition of letters]. An alkaloid, $C_{12}H_{15}NO_4$, obtained by oxidation of narcotine. Cotarnine chloride has been used as a hemostatic in uterine hemorrhage and hemoptysis.

Cotazym. Trademark for pancrelipase, a lipolytic enzyme preparation.

cot death. Crib death (= SUDDEN INFANT DEATH SYNDROME).

Cothera. Trademark for dimethoxanate, an antitussive drug used as the hydrochloride salt.

co·throm·bo·plas·tin (ko·throm″bo·plas′tin) *n.* [*co-* + *thromboplastin*]. FACTOR V.

Cotinazin. A trademark for isoniazid, an antituberculosis drug.

cot·i·nine (kot′i·neen) *n.* *l*-1-Methyl-5-(3-pyridyl)-2-pyrrolidinone, $C_{10}H_{12}N_2O$, a psychic stimulant; used as the fumarate salt.

co·to (ko′to) *n.* [Sp. *cotocoto,* from Quechua]. Coto bark; the bark of a tree native to Bolivia, *Aniba coto.* It has been used in treatment of diarrhea and for the night sweats of pulmonary tuberculosis.

co·trans·am·i·nase (ko″trans·am′i·nace, ·naze) *n.* Pyridoxal phosphate, the prosthetic component of certain transaminating enzymes, as well as of the enzyme carboxylase which catalyzes decarboxylation of L-amino acids, in which latter case it is commonly referred to as codecarboxylase.

cot·ton, *n.* [Ar. *quṭn*]. The hairs of the seed of cultivated varieties of *Gossypium herbaceum* or of other species of *Gossypium.*

cotton-ball metastasis. CANNONBALL METASTASIS.

cot·ton·mouth, *n.* COTTONMOUTH MOCCASIN.

cottonmouth moccasin. A swamp-dwelling pit viper, *Agkistrodon piscivorus,* found in southern United States. Syn. *water moccasin.*

cotton oil. COTTONSEED OIL.

cotton red A, B, or **C.** CONGO RED.

cotton-root bark. GOSSYPIUM.

cottonseed oil. The fixed oil from the seed of cultivated species of *Gossypium.*

Cotton's fracture [F. J. *Cotton,* U.S. surgeon, 1869–1938]. TRIMALLEOLAR FRACTURE.

Cotton's position [F. J. *Cotton*]. Immobilization of the wrist in slight flexion with the hand everted on the forearm, used in treatment of fractures of the lower end of the radius.

cotton wool. Raw or absorbent cotton.

cotton-wool exudates. Fluffy, white, superficial lesions in the retina from microinfarction of the nerve fiber layer; seen in hypertensive retinopathy and collagen vascular diseases.

cot·y·le·don (kot″i·lee′don) *n.* [Gk. *kotylēdōn,* any cup-shaped hollow]. 1. Any one of the groups of villi separated by smooth chorion characteristic of the ruminant semiplacenta. 2. Any one of the rounded lobules bounded by placental septums into which the uterine surface of a discoid placenta is divided. 3. The primary or seed leaf in the phanerogamic embryo. —**coty·le·don·ary** (·lee′duh·nerr″ee) *adj.*

cotyledonary villi. Villi grouped in rosettes and separated by smooth chorion, as in cotyledonary placentas of ruminants.

cot·y·loid (kot′i·loid) *adj.* [Gk. *kotyloeidēs*]. Cup-shaped.

cotyloid bone. OS ACETABULI.

cotyloid cavity. ACETABULUM.

cotyloid foramen. A notch in the acetabulum converted into a foramen by a ligament; it gives passage to vessels and nerves.

couch grass. TRITICUM.

couch·ing, *n.* RECLINATION.

cou·dé catheter (koo·day′) [F., bent]. An angulated catheter with the tip or leading end bent at one point only to form an elbow or coudé tip.

cough (kof) *v.* & *n.* 1. To expel air suddenly and violently from the lungs after deep inspiration and closure of the glottis; a protective reflex caused by irritation of the laryngeal, tracheal, or bronchial mucosa. 2. A single instance of such an expulsion of air. 3. A condition, transient or chronic, in which persistent irritation of respiratory mucosa gives rise to episodes of coughing.

cough plates. A dish of nutrient medium intended for inoculation by having the patient cough directly onto the medium; chiefly used in the diagnosis of whooping cough.

cough syncope. Fainting following a severe episode of coughing.

cou·lomb (koo·lom′, koo′lom) *n.* [C. A. de *Coulomb,* French physicist, 1736–1806]. 1. The unit of electric quantity; the quantity of electricity transferred by a current of 1 ampere in 1 second. 2. The unit of charge in the meter-kilogram-second (mks) system, being the charge that accumulates in a capacitor if a current of 1 ampere flows into the capacitor for 1 second.

Coumadin. Trademark for warfarin, an anticoagulant used as the sodium derivative.

cou·ma·rin (koo′muh·rin) *n.* [Tupi *cumarú,* tonka-bean tree]. 1,2-Benzopyrone, $C_9H_6O_2$, widely distributed in the vegetable kingdom, including the tonka bean. Has been used for its odorous quality, as in imitation vanilla extracts, and for concealing odors, but as continued ingestion may produce hemorrhage its use as a food flavor has been prohibited.

Coun·cil·man bodies or **cells** [W. T. *Councilman,* U.S. pathologist, 1854–1933]. Oxyphilic inclusion bodies occurring in the cytoplasm of liver cells in yellow fever and certain other viral diseases, presumably zones of cytoplasmic coagulation necrosis surrounding virus particles.

count, *n.* [L. *computum,* computation]. The number obtained by reckoning the units of a series or collection, as blood count, the number of blood cells per unit volume of blood.

counter- [L. *contra*]. A prefix meaning (a) *against, opposing;* (b) *opposite;* (c) *offsetting, counteracting;* (d) *contrastive, complementary;* (e) *reactive, retaliatory.*

count·er, *n.* An apparatus designed to facilitate counting. See also *Geiger-Mufller counter, scintillation counter.*

coun·ter·ac·tion (kaown″tur·ack′shun) *n.* The action of a drug or agent opposed to that of some other drug or agent.

coun·ter·die (kaown′tur·dye) *n.* [*counter-* + *die*]. The opposite or reverse image of a die, made of metal or other substance of suitable hardness; used together with the die to form or swage some material in the fabrication of a dental restoration.

coun·ter·ex·ten·sion (kaown″tur·ecks·ten′shun) *n.* [*counter-* + *extension*]. Traction made in a direction opposite to that in which traction is made by another force.

coun·ter·fis·sure (kaown′tur·fish″ur) *n.* CONTRAFISSURA.

coun·ter·in·di·ca·tion (kaown″tur·in·di·kay′shun) *n.* CONTRAINDICATION.

coun·ter·in·vest·ment (kaown″tur·in·vest′munt) *n.* [*counter-* + *investment*]. ANTICATHEXIS.

coun·ter·ir·ri·tant (kaown″tur·irr′i·tunt) *n.* [*counter-* + *irritant*]. An agent that produces inflammation of the skin for the relief of a more deep-seated inflammation. —**counter·ir·ri·ta·tion** (·irr″i·tay′shun) *n.*; **counter·ir·ri·tate** (·irr′i·tate) *v.*

coun·ter·open·ing (kaown′tur·o″pun·ing) *n.* [*counter* + *opening*]. A second incision into an abscess or cavity, made opposite to the first, for purposes of drainage.

coun·ter·pho·bia (kaown″tur·fo′bee·uh) *n.* [*counter-* + *-phobia*]. The seeking out or preference for the same situation of which a phobic person was, or still is, afraid, as a result of the pleasure derived from having conquered or conquering the anxiety produced by that situation. —**counter·pho·bic** (·bick) *adj.*

coun·ter·poi·son (kaown′tur·poy″zun) *n.* A poison that counteracts another poison.

coun·ter·pres·sure (kaown'tur·presh''ur) *n.* Manipulation to counterbalance pressure by exercising force in the opposite direction.

coun·ter·pul·sa·tion (kaown''tur·pul·say'shun) *n.* 1. Pulsation against something. 2. *In cardiology,* the use of a mechanical device to propel blood through the arteries at a time when the heart is in diastole.

coun·ter·punc·ture (kaown'tur·punk''chur) *n.* COUNTEROPENING.

coun·ter·shock (kaown'tur·shock'') *n.* [*counter-* + *shock*]. 1. A phase of the alarm reaction or first phase of the general adaptation syndrome. 2. An electric shock administered through two electrodes on the chest, to convert the cardiac rhythm from atrial or ventricular fibrillation to normal sinus rhythm.

coun·ter·stain (kaown'tur·stain'') *n.* 1. A second general stain applied before or after the principal stain, to afford better contrast and to color other tissue elements beside the one demonstrated by the principal stain. 2. To apply a counterstain.

coun·ter·stroke (kaown'tur·stroke'') *n.* CONTRECOUP.

coun·ter·trac·tion (kaown'tur·track''shun) *n. In surgery,* a traction which offsets another, as in reducing fractures.

coun·ter·trans·fer·ence (kaown''tur·trans'fur·unce) *n.* [*counter-* + *transference*]. *In psychiatry,* the conscious or unconscious emotional reaction of the therapist to the patient, which may interfere with psychotherapy.

coun·ter·trend (kaown'tur·trend'') *n. In psychiatry,* an opposing, contrary, but often reciprocal or complementary drive, desire, or trend.

counting cell. COUNTING CHAMBER.

counting chamber. An apparatus with a ruled chamber of fixed depth used for counting cells in a fluid; especially, that in which diluted blood is placed for counting the erythrocytes, leukocytes, and platelets.

coup-con·tre·coup injury (koo' kohn'truh·koo'') [F.]. Bruising of the surface of the brain beneath the point of impact (coup injury) and the more extensive lacerations and contusions on the opposite side of the brain (contrecoup injury). See also *contrafissura, contrecoup.*

cou·pled beat. BIGEMINAL RHYTHM.

cou·pling (kup'ling) *n.* The phase of gene linkage in which two different mutant genes are located on the same chromosome and therefore are inclined to be inherited either together or not at all in the next generation.

court plaster. A solution of isinglass made with alcohol, glycerin, and hot water spread on silk and allowed to dry; used to hide blemishes or to close small wounds.

cou·vade (koo·vahd') *n.* [F., from *couver,* to brood, incubate]. A custom among certain primitive peoples whereby the husband goes through mock labor while his wife is giving birth.

couvade syndrome. The psychophysiologic manifestations of anxiety, but occasionally of denial and repression of anxiety, in the husbands of pregnant women, which mimic such common complaints of gravid females as abdominal pains, nausea, and vomiting.

Cou·ve·laire uterus (koo·v^e·lair') [A. *Couvelaire,* French obstetrician, 1873–1948]. A pregnant uterus with a bluish, purplish, coppery coloration, and woody consistency due to premature separation of the placenta with interstitial myometrial hemorrhage.

Cour·voi·sier's law (koor·vwa^{h}z·ye^y') [J. *Courvoisier,* French surgeon, 1843–1918]. In jaundice due to obstruction of the common bile duct by gallstones, the gallbladder is often contracted; a distended gallbladder suggests obstruction from other causes, e.g., carcinoma of the pancreas.

co·va·lence (ko·vay'lunce) *n.* [*co-* + *valence*]. A bond between two atoms in which both of the atoms concerned contribute the electron or electrons; normal covalence. —**cova·lent** (·lunt) *adj.*

cove-plane T wave. CORONARY T WAVE.

cov·er glass. *In microscopy,* the thin slip of glass covering the object mounted on the slide.

cover slip. COVER GLASS.

cover test. *In ophthalmology,* a test for extraocular muscle defects in which the patient fixates on a target in different directions of gaze while one eye is covered; the position of that eye is noted on removal of the cover. If, on uncovering, an eye shifts outward, for example, its position under cover was inward.

cover-uncover test. *In ophthalmology,* a test for the evaluation of visual acuity in individuals, such as infants or mental retardates, for whom testing with a Snellen chart using pictures is not feasible, in which one eye is covered while the other is fixed on some target. If an eye moves consistently upon covering the other, poor alignment or amblyopia may exist.

cow, *n. Informal.* A radioisotope generator producing short-lived daughter nuclides which are eluted (milked) as required.

cow·age, cow·hage (kow'ij) *n.* [Hindi *kavānch, kavāch*]. 1. The tropical woody vine *Mucuna pruriens (Stizolobium pruritum),* the pods of which have hairs that cause severe itching. 2. A preparation of the hairs of *Mucuna pruriens,* usually with honey, formerly used as a vermifuge and counterirritant.

Cow·dria ru·mi·nan·ti·um (kaow'dree·uh roo''mi·nan'chee·um). An obligatory intracytoplasmic parasite resembling rickettsia, transmitted by ticks; the etiologic agent of heartwater fever of sheep, goats, and cattle.

cow gait. A swaying movement due to knock-knee.

cow-horn stomach. STEERHORN STOMACH.

Cow·ie's test. GUAIAC TEST.

cow·itch (kaow'ich) *n.* COWAGE.

Cow·ling's rule. A rule to determine the dosage of medicines for children; specifically, the age of the child in years at next birthday and multiplied by the adult dose, divided by 24. Compare *Young's rule.*

cow·per·i·tis (kaow''pur·eye'tis, koo''pur·) *n.* [*Cowper*'s glands + *-itis*]. Inflammation of the bulbourethral glands.

Cow·per's cyst (koo'pur, kaow'pur) [W. *Cowper,* English surgeon, 1666–1709]. A retention cyst of the bulbourethral glands.

Cowper's glands [W. *Cowper*]. BULBOURETHRAL GLANDS.

Cowper's ligament [W. *Cowper*]. The part of the fascia lata attached to the pubic crest.

cow·pox, *n.* [*cow* + *pox*]. VACCINIA.

cox- [L. *coxa*]. A combining form meaning *hip, hip joint.*

coxa (kock'suh) *n.,* pl. & genit. sing. **cox·ae** (·see) [L.] [NA]. HIP. —**cox·al** (·sul) *adj.*

cox·al·gia (kock·sal'jee·uh) *n.* [*cox-* + *-algia*]. Pain in the hip joint; especially, disease of the hip. —**coxal·gic** (·jick) *adj.*

coxalgic pelvis. An obliquely contracted pelvis, due to unequal pressure of the femora in unilateral disease of the hip in early life.

cox·al·gy (kock'sal''jee) *n.* COXALGIA.

coxa mag·na (mag'nuh). Enlargement of the hip due to degenerative joint disease of the head and neck of the femur.

coxa pla·na (play'nuh). OSTEOCHONDRITIS DEFORMANS JUVENILIS.

cox·ar·thri·tis (kock''sahr·thrye'tis) *n.* [*cox-* + *arthritis*]. COXITIS.

cox·ar·throc·a·ce (kocks''ahr·throck'uh·see) *n.* [*cox-* + *arthro-* + *-cace*]. A fungoid inflammation of the hip joint.

cox·ar·thro·lis·thet·ic pelvis (kocks·ahr''thro·lis·thet'ick). [*cox-,* hip, + *arthr-,* joint, + Gk. *olisthētikos,* from *olisthēsis,* dislocation]. A unilateral or bilateral transversely contracted pelvis, resulting from softening about the acetabulum with projection of the head of the femur into the pelvic cavity.

coxa val·ga (val'guh). A condition, the reverse of coxa vara, in which the angle between the neck and the shaft of the femur is increased above 140°.

coxa va·ra (vair'uh). A condition in which the neck of the femur is bent downward sufficiently to cause symptoms; this bending may reach such an extent that the neck forms, with the shaft, a right angle or less, instead of the normal angle of 120 to 140°.

Cox·i·el·la (kock"see·el'uh) *n.* [H. R. *Cox,* U.S. bacteriologist, b. 1907]. A genus of the family Rickettsiaceae, which includes the causative agent of Q fever.

Coxiella bur·ne·tii (bur·net'ee·eye). The species of *Coxiella* which is the etiologic agent of Q fever.

cox·i·tis (kock·sigh'tis) *n.*, pl. **cox·it·i·des** (kock·sit'i·deez) [*cox-* + *-itis*]. Inflammation of the hip joint.

coxitis co·ty·loi·dea (kot"i·loy'dee·uh). Coxitis confined principally to the acetabulum.

cox·odyn·ia (kock"so·din'ee·uh) *n.* [*cox-* + *-odynia*]. Pain in the hip; COXALGIA.

Cox·sack·ie disease (kok·sak'ee, kuk·) [after *Coxsackie,* N.Y., home of patient in whom virus was found]. A variety of clinical syndromes resulting from infection with the Coxsackie viruses. The clinical entities include herpangina, exanthematous febrile diseases, aseptic meningitis, a disease mimicking poliomyelitis, myocarditis, pericarditis, and pleurodynia.

Coxsackie virus. Any of a group of antigenically distinct picornaviruses; the cause of Coxsackie disease in humans and found experimentally to induce destruction of striated muscle, paralysis, and death in infant mice.

Cox's yolk-sac method [H. R. *Cox*]. The inoculation of rickettsiae into the yolk sac of the chick embryo, making available large amounts of rickettsial antigen for vaccines and for serologic tests.

Cox vaccine [H. R. *Cox*]. A vaccine against epidemic typhus, prepared from *Rickettsia prowazeki* cultivated on the yolk-sac membrane of the chick embryo.

co·zy·mase (ko·zye'mace, ·maze) *n.* NICOTINAMIDE ADENINE DINUCLEOTIDE.

Coz·zo·li·no's zone (ko^ht"tso·lee'no). FISSULA ANTE FENESTRAM.

cp Abbreviation for *centipoise.*

C.P. Chemically pure.

CPC Abbreviation for *clinical-pathological conference.*

CPD Abbreviation for (a) *cephalopelvic disproportion;* (b) *citrate-phosphate-dextrose.*

CPK Abbreviation for *creatine phosphokinase* (= CREATINE KINASE).

CPR Abbreviation for *cardiopulmonary resuscitation.*

cps Cycle(s) per second (= HERTZ).

CR Abbreviation for *conditioned reflex* or *response.*

Cr Symbol for chromium.

crab louse. *PHTHIRIUS PUBIS.*

crab orchard salt. MAGNESIUM SULFATE; named after a locale in Kentucky where it was obtained.

Crab·tree effect [H. G. *Crabtree,* English biochemist, 20th century]. The inhibition of cellular respiration produced by high concentrations of glucose.

crab yaws. Yaws with hyperkeratosis and fissuring of the soles of the feet, resulting in the peculiar gait that gives rise to the name.

cracked heel. 1. GREASE HEEL. 2. Hyperkeratosis and the formation of fissures of the soles, usually caused by *Nocardia keratolytica;* most often seen in parts of Asia and Africa.

cracked nipple. A nipple in which the epidermis is broken and fissured.

cracked-pot resonance, note, or **sound.** A characteristic clinking sound, elicited by percussion over a pulmonary cavity communicating with a bronchus, especially when the percussion is forcible and the patient's mouth is open. Compare *cranial cracked-pot sound.*

crackling rale. SUBCREPITANT RALE.

cra·dle, *n.* 1. A small bed for a baby. 2. A frame of wicker, wood or wire, used to prevent the bedclothes from coming in contact with a fractured or injured part.

cradle cap. Heavy, greasy crusts on the scalp of an infant; seborrheic dermatitis of infants.

cradle pessary. A cradle-shaped pessary once commonly used in the correction of uterine displacements.

craft neurosis. OCCUPATIONAL NEUROSIS.

Crä·mer method (kre^y'mur). A histochemical method for nitrate based on the interaction of nitron to give a birefringent insoluble salt.

cramp, *n.* 1. Painful, involuntary contraction of a muscle, such as occurs at night in normal individuals in a foot or leg, or in swimmers. 2. Any cramplike pain, as of the intestine. 3. Spasm of certain muscles, which may be intermittent, as in tetany, or occupational, resulting from their excessive use. 4. *Colloq.* (usually pl.) DYSMENORRHEA.

Cran·dall's test. CHERRY AND CRANDALL'S TEST.

crane fly. A dipteran insect of the genus *Tipulidae.*

crani-, cranio- [Gk. *kranion,* skull]. A combining form meaning *cranium, cranial.*

-cranía [*cran*ium + *-ia*]. A combining form designating (a specified) *kind or condition of the skull or head.*

crania. A plural of *cranium.*

cra·ni·ad (kray'nee·ad) *adv.* [*crani-* + *-ad*]. Toward the cranium or head.

cra·ni·al (kray'nee·ul) *adj.* 1. Of or pertaining to the cranium or the skull. 2. Directed toward the head; in human anatomy, superior. Contr. *caudal.*

cranial arteritis. GIANT-CELL ARTERITIS (1).

cranial capacity. The volume of the cranial cavity.

cranial cavity. The hollow of the skull.

cranial cracked-pot sound. The change in sound on percussion of the skull where there is widening of the sutures; a diagnostic sign, after early infancy, of increased intracranial pressure. Compare *cracked-pot resonance.* See also *Macewen's sign.*

cranial diameters of the fetus. FETAL CRANIAL DIAMETERS.

cranial flexure. A flexure of the embryonic brain.

cranial fossa. Any of the three depressions in the floor of the interior of the skull. See also *anterior cranial fossa, middle cranial fossa, posterior cranial fossa.*

cranial gaps. Occasional congenital fissures of the skull.

cranial genital fold. PROGONAL FOLD.

cranial index. The ratio of the greatest width of the cranium, taken wherever it may be found on the parietal bones or on the squama temporalis in a horizontal plane perpendicular to the sagittal plane, × 100, to the greatest length, taken in the sagittal plane between glabella and opisthocranion. Values of the index are classified as:

ultradolichocranial	*x*-64.9
hyperdolichocranial	65.0-69.9
dolichocranial	70.0-74.9
mesocranial	75.0-79.9
brachycranial	80.0-84.9
hyperbrachycranial	85.0-89.9
ultrabrachycranial	90.0-*x*

cranial length. The measurement from the glabella to the opisthocranion.

cranial mesonephros. The part of the mesonephros, anterior to the gonad, that degenerates during development.

cranial nerve aplasia. NUCLEAR APLASIA.

cranial nerve palsy or **paralysis.** Paralysis of the parts of the body controlled by the cranial nerves, usually caused by, and accompanying, some other disorder.

cranial nerves. Nerves arising directly from the brainstem and making their exit to the periphery via openings in the skull: I, olfactory; II, optic; III, oculomotor; IV, trochlear; V, trigeminal; VI, abducent; VII, facial (including nervus intermedius); VIII, vestibulocochlear (cochlear and vestibular); IX, glossopharyngeal; X, vagus; XI, accessory; XII, hypoglossal. Usually described and numbered as 12 pairs, the first two are not true nerves but nerve-fiber tracts of the brain; the caudal 10 pairs originate from nuclei in the brainstem, except for that part of XI which has a spinal root. NA *nervi craniales.*

cranial puncture. VENTRICULAR PUNCTURE.

cranial reflex. Any reflex whose paths are connected directly with the brain by cranial nerves.

cranial sutures. The sutures between the bones of the cranium. NA *suturae cranii.*

cranial vault. CALVARIA.

cra·ni·ec·to·my (kray″nee·eck′tuh·mee) *n.* [*crani-* + *-ectomy*]. *In surgery,* removal of strips or pieces of the cranial bones.

cranio-. See *crani-.*

cra·nio·ba·sal length (kray″nee·o·bay′sul). The measurement from the nasion to the Bolton point.

cra·nio·buc·cal (kray″nee·o·buck′ul) *adj.* Pertaining to the cranium and the buccal cavity.

craniobuccal pouch. In the embryo, a diverticulum from the buccal cavity from which the anterior lobe of the hypophysis is developed. Syn. *Rathke's pouch.*

cra·nio·car·po·tar·sal (kray″nee·o·kahr″po·tahr′sul) *adj.* Pertaining to the cranium and the carpal and tarsal bones.

craniocarpotarsal dysplasia. Microstomia, deep-set eyes, flattening of the midface, colobomatous changes in the nostrils, kyphoscoliosis, talipes equinovarus, and ulnar deviation of the fingers without bony alteration; inherited as an autosomal dominant.

cra·nio·cele (kray′nee·o·seel) *n.* [*cranio-* + *-cele*]. ENCEPHALOCELE.

cra·nio·cer·e·bral (kray″nee·o·serr′e·brul) *adj.* Pertaining to the cranium and the cerebral hemispheres.

cra·nio·cer·vi·cal (kray″nee·o·sur′vi·kul) *adj.* [*cranio-* + *cervical*]. Of or pertaining to the cranium and the neck.

cra·ni·oc·la·sis (kray″nee·ock′luh·sis) *n.*, pl. **cranioclа·ses** (·seez) [*cranio-* + *-clasis*]. The operation of breaking the fetal head by means of the cranioclast.

cra·nio·clast (kray′nee·o·klast) *n.* [*cranio-* + *-clast*]. Heavy forceps for crushing the fetal head.

cra·nio·clas·ty (kray′nee·o·klas″tee) *n.* [*cranio-* + *-clasty*]. CRANIOCLASIS.

cra·nio·clei·do·dys·os·to·sis (kray″nee·o·klye″do·dis″os·to′sis) *n.* CLEIDOCRANIAL DYSOSTOSIS.

cra·nio·did·y·mus (kray″nee·o·did′i·mus) *n.*, pl. **craniodidy·mi** (·migh) [*cranio-* + *-didymus*]. CRANIOPAGUS.

cra·nio·fa·cial (kray″nee·o·fay′shul) *adj.* Of or pertaining to the cranium and the face.

craniofacial axis. The axis through the bones forming the base of the skull.

craniofacial dysostosis. A malformation inherited as an autosomal dominant trait and characterized by premature closure of the coronal and/or sagittal sutures, leading to associated anomalies such as malformed auditory canals and ears, high narrow palate, crowded malaligned upper teeth, and moderate mental retardation. Syn. *Crouzon's disease.* See also *acrocephalosyndactyly.*

cra·nio·fe·nes·tria (kray″nee·o·fe·nes′tree·uh) *n.* [*cranio-* + L. *fenestra*, window, + *-ia*]. A congenital bony defect involving the total thickness of the skull. See also *craniolacunia.*

cra·nio·graph (kray′nee·o·graf) *n.* [*cranio-* + *-graph*]. An instrument for recording the outlines of the skull.

cra·ni·og·ra·phy (kray″nee·og′ruh·fee) *n.* [*cranio-* + *-graphy*]. The part of craniology that describes the skull and its parts.

cra·nio·la·cu·nia (kray″nee·o·la·kew′nee·uh) *n.* [*cranio-* + *lacuna* + *-ia*]. Incomplete ossification of the inner table of the vault of the skull in infants, giving the appearance of dense bony ridges separated by radiolucent areas; often associated with spina bifida, meningoceles, meningoencephaloceles, and increased intracranial pressure. Syn. *lacuna skull, Lückenschädel.*

cra·ni·ol·o·gy (kray″nee·ol′uh·jee) *n.* [*cranio-* + *-logy*]. The scientific study of the cranium, comprising craniography and craniometry.

cra·nio·meg·a·ly (kray″nee·o·meg′uh·lee) *n.* Enlargement of the head.

cranio·me·taph·y·se·al (kray″nee·o·me·taf″i·see′ul, ·met″uh·fiz′ee·ul) *adj.* Pertaining to the cranium and the metaphyses.

craniometaphyseal dysplasia. Leontiasis ossea in combination with metaphyseal dysplasia.

cra·ni·om·e·ter (kray″nee·om′e·tur) *n.* [*cranio-* + *-meter*]. A caliper used for measuring the dimensions of the skull.

cra·nio·met·ric (kray″nee·o·met′rick) *adj.* Of or pertaining to craniometry or to a craniometer.

craniometric diameter. A line connecting two corresponding points on opposite surfaces of the cranium.

craniometric point. Any one of the points on the skull used in craniometry. For the main craniometric points, see *acanthion, alveolar point, antinion, apex, asterion, auriculare, basion, Bolton point, bregma, clition, condylion, coronion, crotaphion, dacryon, entomion, frontotemporale, genion, glabella, gnathion, gonion, hormion, infratemporale, inion, jugal point, lacrimale, lambda, maxillofrontale, metopion, nasion, nasospinale, obelion, ophryon, opisthion, opisthocranion, orale, orbitale, porion, prosthion, pterion, rhinion, sphenion, staphylion, staurion, stephanion, symphysion, tylion, vertex, zygion, zygomaxillare.*

cra·ni·om·e·try (kray″nee·om′e·tree) *n.* [*cranio-* + *-metry*]. The science and technique of measuring the skull in order to establish exact, comparable, metric records for use in the comparative study of physical types, variation, and individual peculiarities in the skulls of man and other primates.

cra·ni·op·a·gus (kray″nee·op′uh·gus) *n.*, pl. **craniopa·gi** (·guy, ·jye) [*cranio-* + *-pagus*]. Conjoined twins united by their heads. Syn. *cephalopagus, craniodidymus.* —**craniopagous,** *adj;* **craniopa·gy** (·jee, ·ghee) *n.*

craniopagus fron·ta·lis (fron·tay′lis). Conjoined twins united at the foreheads.

craniopagus oc·ci·pi·ta·lis (ock·sip″i·tay′lis). Conjoined twins united by their occiputs.

craniopagus para·sit·i·cus (păr″uh·sit′i·kus). A parasitic individual or its parts attached cranially.

craniopagus pa·ri·e·ta·lis (pa·rye″e·tay′lis). Conjoined twins united in the parietal region.

cra·ni·op·a·thy (kray″nee·op′uth·ee) *n.* [*cranio-* + *-pathy*]. Any disease of the head, especially of the skull bones.

cra·nio·pha·ryn·ge·al (kray″nee·o·fa·rin′jee·ul, ·făr″in·jee′ul) *adj.* Of or pertaining to the cranium and the pharynx.

craniopharyngeal canal. A fetal canal in the sphenoid bone formed by the growth of the bone about the stalk of the craniobuccal pouch.

cra·nio·pha·ryn·gi·o·ma (kray″nee·o·fa·rin″jee·o′muh) *n.*, pl. **craniopharyngiomas, craniopharyngioma·ta** (·tuh) [*cranio-* + *pharyng-* + *-oma*]. A benign, but infiltrative tumor, usually occurring in children, derived from the epithelium of the embryonal craniopharyngeal canal. The intrasellar type arises from cells dispersed in the adenohypophysis; the suprasellar type, from cells in the infundibulum above the sella turcica. See also *Rathke's pouch cyst.*

cra·nio·plas·ty (kray′nee·o·plas″tee) *n.* [*cranio-* + *-plasty*]. *In surgery,* correction of defects in the cranial bones, usually by implants of metal, plastic material, or bone.

cra·nio·ra·chis·chi·sis, cra·ni·or·rha·chis·chi·sis (kray″nee·o·ra·kis′ki·sis) *n.* [*cranio-* + *rachischisis*]. Congenital fissure of the cranium and vertebral column.

craniorachischisis to·ta·lis (to·tal′is, to·tay′lis). Congenital fissure of the cranium and vertebral column with meningoencephalocele and meningomyelocele.

craniorrhachischisis. CRANIORACHISCHISIS.

cra·nio·sa·cral (kray″nee·o·say′krul) *adj.* Pertaining to the cranium and the sacrum.

craniosacral autonomic nervous system. PARASYMPATHETIC NERVOUS SYSTEM.

craniosacral system. PARASYMPATHETIC NERVOUS SYSTEM.

cra·ni·os·chi·sis (kray″nee·os′ki·sis) *n.*, pl. **cranioschi·ses** (·seez) [*cranio-* + *-schisis*]. Congenital fissure of the cranium.

cra·nio·spi·nal (kray″nee·o·spye′nul) *adj.* [*cranio-* + *spinal*]. Of or pertaining to the cranium and the vertebral column.

cra·nio·stat (kray'nee·o·stat'') *n.* [*cranio-* + *-stat*]. A device for holding the skull during craniometric study.

cra·nio·ste·no·sis (kray''nee·o·ste·no'sis) *n.*, pl. **craniosteno·ses** (·seez) [*cranio-* + *stenosis*]. CRANIOSYNOSTOSIS.

cra·ni·os·to·sis (kray''nee·os·to'sis, ·os'tuh·sis) *n.*, pl. **craniosto·ses** (·seez) [*crani-* + *ostosis*]. CRANIOSYNOSTOSIS.

cra·nio·syn·os·to·sis (kray''nee·o·sin''os·to'sis) *n.*, pl. **cranio·synosto·ses** (·seez) [*cranio-* + *synostosis*]. Premature closure of the sutures of cranial bones, usually present at or shortly after birth, or due to idiopathic hypercalcemia. The resulting head shape and absence or presence of symptoms depend on the sutures involved. See also *oxycephaly, scaphocephaly.*

cra·nio·ta·bes (kray''nee·o·tay'beez) *n.* [*cranio-* + *tabes*]. An acquired change of the cranial bones occurring in infancy, with the formation of small, shallow, conical pits in the bone substance, as seen in rickets and other disease states, and in some newborn infants as localized softening of the parietal bones at the vertex of the skull. —**cranio·ta·bet·ic** (·ta·bet'ick) *adj.*

cra·nio·tome (kray'nee·o·tome) *n.* [*cranio-* + *-tome*]. An instrument used in craniotomy.

cra·ni·ot·o·my (kray''nee·ot'uh·mee) *n.* [*cranio-* + *-tomy*]. 1. Any operation on the skull. 2. An operation reducing the size of the fetal head by cutting or breaking when delivery is otherwise impossible.

craniotomy scissors. A strong S-shaped instrument used in craniotomy for perforating the fetal skull and cutting away portions of bone.

cra·nio·trac·tor (kray''nee·o·track'tur) *n.* [*cranio-* + *tractor*]. A cranioclast designed to be used as a tractor.

cra·nio·tym·pan·ic (kray''nee·o·tim·pan'ick) *adj.* [*cranio-* + *tympanic*]. Of or pertaining to the skull and the tympanum.

cra·nio·ver·te·bral (kray''nee·o·vur'te·brul) *adj.* Of or pertaining to the cranium and the vertebrae.

craniovertebral canal. VERTEBRAL CANAL.

cra·ni·um (kray'nee·um) *n.*, genit. **cra·nii** (·nee·eye), L. pl. **cra·nia** (·nee·uh) [Gk. *kranion*] [NA]. 1. The skull exclusive of the mandible. 2. SKULL. 3. BRAINCASE.

cranium bi·fi·dum (bif'i·dum). A congenital fissure of the cranium, usually midline, often associated with a meningocele or meningoencephalocele.

cranium ce·re·bra·le (serr·e·bray'lee) [BNA]. NEUROCRANIUM.

cranium vis·ce·ra·le (vis·e·ray'lee) [BNA]. VISCERAL CRANIUM.

crap·u·lent (krap'yoo·lunt) *adj.* [L. *crapulentus*, very much intoxicated]. Marked by excess in eating and drinking.

cra·que·lé (krack·lay') *adj.* [F., cracked]. *In dermatology*, scaling, with cracks such as appear in old china or ceramic tile.

-crasia [Gk. *krasis*, mixing, combination, constitution, temperament, + *-ia*]. A combining form designating (results of) *mixing of different humors or substances in the body.*

cra·ter, *n.* A saucer-shaped defect in the interdental soft tissues or interdental bone resulting from periodontal disease. See also *bony crater.*

cra·ter·i·form (kray·terr'i·form) *adj.* [*crater* + *-iform*]. 1. Shaped like a crater or bowl. 2. Conical.

crateriform ulcer. A basal-cell carcinoma, of conical form, resembling a furuncle with fibrotic border.

cra·ter·iza·tion (kray''tur·i·zay'shun) *n.* The removal of part of a bone, leaving a crater, as in operations for osteomyelitis. See also *saucerize.*

crater nipple. RETRACTED NIPPLE.

cra·vat (kruh·vat') *n.* [F. *cravate*]. A triangular bandage folded to form a band, used as a temporary dressing for a wound or fracture.

cre-, creo-, kreo- [Gk. *kreas*]. A combining form meaning *flesh.*

C-reactive protein. A globulin capable of precipitating the C carbohydrate in pneumococcal bodies; found in the serum of patients with inflammation and necrosis, and tests for this protein are used in the diagnosis of rheumatic fever.

cream, *n.* 1. The part of milk rich in butterfat. 2. A solid emulsion for external application, which may contain solutions or suspensions of medicinal agents.

cream of tartar. Potassium bitartrate, $KHC_4H_4O_4$, used as a saline cathartic.

creat-, creato- [Gk. *kreas*]. A combining form meaning (a) *meat, flesh;* (b) *creatine.*

cre·at·ic (kree·at'ick) *adj.* [*creat-* + *-ic*]. Pertaining to or caused by flesh or meat.

creatic nausea. An abnormal aversion to eating meat.

cre·a·tine (kree'uh·teen, ·tin) *n.* [Gk. *kreas*, flesh, + *-ine*]. (α-Methylguanido)acetic acid or *N*-methyl-*N*-guanylglycine, $C_4H_9N_3O_2$, an amino acid present in animal tissues, particularly muscle. Creatine reversibly combines with phosphate to form phosphocreatine, an important compound in the anaerobic phase of muscular contraction. See also Table of Chemical Constituents of Blood in the Appendix.

creatine index or **tolerance.** The ability of the body to retain ingested creatine, as measured under standard conditions. The percentage retained is low in hyperthyroidism and high in hypothyroidism and so may be used as an index of the level of thyroid function or of potency of administered thyroid substance.

creatine kinase. An enzyme found in vertebrate skeletal muscle and myocardium that converts phosphocreatine and ADP to creatine and ATP; used in the diagnosis of myocardial infarction, muscular disorders, and certain other diseases.

cre·a·ti·ne·mia, cre·a·ti·nae·mia (kree''uh·ti·nee'mee·uh) *n.* [*creatine* + *-emia*]. An excess of creatine in the blood.

creatine phosphate. PHOSPHOCREATINE.

creatine phosphokinase. CREATINE KINASE.

cre·a·tine·phos·pho·ric acid (kree''uh·tin·fos·for'ick). PHOSPHOCREATINE.

cre·at·i·nine (kree·at'i·neen, ·nin) *n.* [*creatine* + *-ine*]. 1-Methylhydantoin-2-imide or 1-methylglycocyamidine, $C_4H_7N_3O$, end product of creatine metabolism, excreted in the urine at a constant rate. See also Table of Chemical Constituents of Blood in the Appendix.

creatinine clearance. An index of the glomerular filtration rate, calculated by multiplying the concentration of creatinine in a timed volume of excreted urine by the milliliters of urine produced per minute and dividing the product by the plasma creatinine value. Normal values, when corrected to 1.73 sq m, are greater than 110 ml per minute for males and 100 ml per minute for females.

creatinine coefficient. The value obtained when the number of milligrams of creatinine in the 24-hour urine output is divided by the body weight expressed in kilograms.

cre·a·tin·uria (kree''uh·ti·new'ree·uh) *n.* 1. The occurrence of creatine in the urine. 2. An increase in the amount of creatine in the urine.

creative tension. The state of mind existing under conditions of intellectual challenge and conflict, and self-confidence and stability, which is considered most advantageous to scientists, artists, and other inventive persons to promote achievement.

creato-. See *creat-.*

cre·a·tor·rhe·a, cre·a·tor·rhoea (kree''uh·to·ree'uh) *n.* [*creato-* + *-rrhea*]. Increased amounts of nitrogen in the stool.

Cre·dé's method (kreʸ·deʸ') [K. *Credé*, German gynecologist, 1819–1892]. The prophylactic use of topical 1% silver nitrate in the eyes of newborns; shown to be effective in preventing gonococcal opthalmia neonatorum.

creep·ing eruption. LARVA MIGRANS.

creeping pneumonia. MIGRATORY PNEUMONIA.

creeping ulcer. SERPIGINOUS ULCER.

cre·mas·ter (kre·mas'tur) *n.* [Gk. *kremastēr*, suspender]. CREMASTER MUSCLE. —**crem·as·ter·ic** (krem''as·terr'ick) *adj.*

cremasteric artery. The artery of the cremasteric muscle or spermatic cord. NA *arteria cremasterica.* See also Table of Arteries in the Appendix.

cremasteric fascia. Connective tissue surrounding the cremaster muscle; the middle spermatic fascia covering the spermatic cord and testis. NA *fascia cremasterica.*

cremasteric reflex. Retraction of the testis on the same side induced by stimulation of the skin on the front and inner surface of one thigh.

cremaster muscle. An extension of the internal oblique abdominal muscle over the spermatic cord and testis. There is a similar muscle in the female which is very poorly developed. NA *musculus cremaster.* See also Table of Muscles in the Appendix.

cre·ma·tion (kree·may'shun) *n.* [L. *crematio,* from *cremare,* to burn]. Destruction of a dead body by burning. —**cre·mate** (kree'mate) *v.*

cre·ma·to·ri·um (kree''muh·to'ree·um) *n.*, pl. **cremato·ria** (·ree·uh), **crematoriums.** CREMATORY.

cre·ma·to·ry (kree'muh·tor''ee) *n.* 1. An establishment for burning the bodies of the dead. 2. An incinerator.

crem·no·pho·bia (krem''no·fo'bee·uh) *n.* [Gk. *krēmnos,* crag, + *phobia*]. An abnormal fear of precipices or steep places.

cre·na (kree'nuh) *n.*, pl. **cre·nae** (·nee) [L.]. A notch, especially as seen on the sutural margins of the cranial bones.

crena ani (ay'nigh) [NA]. GLUTEAL FURROW.

crena clu·ni·um (kloo'nee·um). GLUTEAL FURROW.

cre·nate (kree'nate) *adj.* 1. Notched or scalloped. 2. *In botany,* having rounded scalloped edges, as certain leaves. —**cre·nat·ed** (·nay·tid) *adj.*

cre·na·tion (kre·nay'shun) *n.* 1. A notched or cogwheel-like appearance of shrunken erythrocytes; seen when they are exposed to hypertonic solutions. 2. The indentation markings on the tongue caused by a tooth.

cren·el·la·tion method (kren''e·lay'shun). A method of doing differential white blood cell counts in which the blood film is scanned from one narrow margin to the other, then back across the film, and so on. The path thus traced resembles the crenels of castles.

Cren·o·thrix (kren'o·thricks, kree'no·) *n.* [Gk. *krēnē,* spring, + *thrix,* hair]. A genus of bacteria of the family Crenotrichaceae.

Crenothrix po·lys·po·ra (pol·is'por·uh). A species of iron bacteria found growing in the conduits of public water supplies; causes stoppage.

creo-. See *cre-.*

cre·o·sol (kree'o·sol) *n.* 2-Methoxy-4-methylphenol, $C_8H_{10}O_2$, one of the principal phenols contained in creosote.

Creosotal. A trademark for creosote carbonate.

cre·o·sote (kree'o·sote) *n.* [*creo-* + Gk. *sōtēr,* preserver]. A mixture of phenols obtained by the distillation of wood tar, preferably that from the beech, *Fagus sylvatica;* a flammable, oily liquid. Creosote is antiseptic, astringent, styptic, anesthetic, and escharotic. Has been used in the treatment of pulmonary tuberculosis.

creosote carbonate. A mixture of the carbonates of various constituents of creosote. Has been used as an expectorant and antiseptic.

creotoxin. KREOTOXIN.

creotoxism. KREOTOXISM.

crep·i·tant (krep'i·tunt) *adj.* Producing or having a crackling or rattling sound. —**crepi·tance** (·tunce) *n.*

crepitant rale. A fine, dry, crackling rale simulated by the rubbing together of hairs, produced by fluid in the terminal bronchioles; transiently heard at the normal lung base during initial forced inspiration.

crep·i·tate (krep'i·tate) *v.* [L. *crepitare*]. To make sharp repeated crackling sounds, as heard in crepitation.

crep·i·ta·tio (krep''i·tay'shee·o) *n.* [L.]. CREPITATION.

crep·i·ta·tion (krep''i·tay'shun) *n.* 1. The grating of fractured bones. 2. The crackling of the joints. 3. The noise produced by pressure upon tissues containing an abnormal amount of air or gas, as in cellular emphysema. 4. The sound heard at the end of inspiration in the first stage of croupous pneumonia. It closely resembles the sound produced by rubbing the hair between the fingers held close to the ear.

crep·i·tus (krep'i·tus) *n.* [L.]. 1. CREPITATION. 2. Discharge of intestinal flatus.

Cresatin. Trademark for *m*-cresyl acetate, an antiseptic and analgesic useful in treating affections of the nose, throat, and ears.

cres·cent (kres'unt) *n.* [L. *crescens,* growing]. 1. Anything shaped like, or suggestive of, a new moon or a sickle. 2. The curved gametocyte of *Plasmodium falciparum,* infectious for *Anopheles* mosquitoes and the most characteristic diagnostic form of the falciparum malarial parasite. —**cres·cen·tic** (kre·sen'tick) *adj.*

crescent of Gian·nuz·zi (jahⁿn·noot'tsee) [G. *Giannuzzi*]. DEMILUNE.

crescent operation. An operation for lacerated perineum, involving the vaginal entrance only; a crescent-shaped denudation is made from the vulvovaginal entrance, the angles of which extend into the vulvovaginal sulci.

crescents of the spinal cord. The lateral gray bands of the spinal cord as seen in transverse section.

cre·sol (kree'sol) *n.* A mixture of *o-*, *m-*, and *p*-cresol, $CH_3C_6H_4OH$, obtained from coal tar. A colorless, brownish, or pinkish liquid of phenol-like odor; soluble in 50 volumes of water. Used chiefly as a surgical disinfectant, usually in the form of saponated cresol solution which contains 50% cresol. It is superior to phenol both as an antiseptic and as a germicide.

cre·sot·ic acid (kre·sot'ick, ·so'tick). Homosalicylic acid, *o-*, *m-*, and *p-*, $CH_3C_6H_3(OH)COOH$, the sodium salts of which have been used medicinally like the salicylates.

cres·o·tin·ic acid (kres''o·tin'ick). CRESOTIC ACID.

crest, *n.* [L. *crista*]. A ridge or linear prominence, especially of bone. See also *crista.*

crest of the head of a rib. A ridge separating the articular surface of the head of a rib into two parts. NA *crista capitis costae.*

crest of the neck of a rib. A ridge on the superior border of the neck of a rib. NA *crista colli costae.*

cres·yl (kres'il) *n.* TOLYL.

***m*-cres·yl acetate** (met'uh·kres''il). The acetic acid ester of *m*-cresol, $C_9H_{10}O_2$, an oily liquid, practically insoluble in water. An antiseptic and analgesic useful in treating certain affections of the nose, throat, and ears.

cres·yl·ate (kres'il·ate) *n.* Any compound of cresol with a metallic radical.

cre·syl·ic acid (kre·sil'ick). In commerce, a mixture of phenols from coal tar.

cresyl blue. BRILLIANT CRESYL BLUE.

cre·ta (kree'tuh) *n.* [L.]. Chalk; native calcium carbonate. —**cre·ta·ceous** (kre·tay'shus) *adj.*

cre·tin (kree'tin) *n.* [F. *crétin*]. An individual afflicted with cretinism.

cre·tin·ism (kree'tin·iz·um) *n.* [*cretin* + *-ism*]. The congenital and most common form of infantile hypothyroidism with severe deficiency of thyroid hormone; may be due to aplasia, hypoplasia or failure of the thyroid to descend to its normal adult site or locus in the neck resulting from an embryonic developmental defect, the administration of radioiodine to the mother during pregnancy, an autoimmune disease, defective synthesis of thyroid hormone (nonendemic goitrous cretinism), maternal ingestion of medications suppressing thyroid activity, or iodide deficiency (endemic cretinism). Clinically, the infant is characterized, before treatment, by a large protruding tongue, thickened subcutaneous tissues, dry skin, protruding abdomen, mental retardation, and dwarfed stature. Poor muscle tone, depressed tendon reflexes, constipation, and hoarse cry are also common. See also *goitrous cretinism, Pendred's syndrome.* —**cretin·ous** (·us) *adj.;* **cretin·oid** (·oid) *adj. & n.*

Cré·tin method (kreʸ·tæⁿ'). A histochemical method for minerals using gallic acid to obtain blue color for calcium, bright green for barium, blue-green for strontium and cadmium, yellowish-rose for magnesium, violet-brown for iron, dull yellow for zinc and lead, and pure yellow for silicon.

Crétin-Pou·yanne method (poo·yan'). A histochemical method for nickel based on the precipitation of nickel as lilac or blue nickel ammonium phosphate.

Creutz·feldt-Ja·kob disease (kroits'felt, yah'kohp) [H. G. *Creutzfeldt,* German neurologist, b. 1883; and A. M. *Jakob,* German neuropsychiatrist, 1884–1931]. 1. A chronic degenerative disorder of the nervous system described by H. G. Creutzfeldt and identified by W. Spielmeyer with one described by A. M. Jakob. The clinical descriptions included a slowly progressive dementia and signs of corticospinal and extrapyramidal disease; a diffuse loss of neurons in the cerebral cortex, basal ganglia, brainstem nuclei, and sometimes the anterior horns of the spinal cord, was observed pathologically. Identification of this disorder with subacute spongiform encephalopathy is extremely doubtful. Syn. *corticostriatospinal degeneration.* 2. SUBACUTE SPONGIFORM ENCEPHALOPATHY.

crev·ice (krev'is) *n.* [OF. *crevace,* from *crever,* to break, split]. A narrow opening caused by a fissure or crack.

cre·vic·u·lar (kre·vick'yoo·lur) *adj.* Pertaining to or having a crevice, especially of the gingiva.

crevicular epithelium. The epithelium lining the gingival sulcus.

crib·bing, *n.* 1. Air swallowing; AEROPHAGIA. 2. The repeated biting of the crib or manger by horses, resulting in a peculiar wearing of the incisor teeth.

crib death. See sudden infant death syndrome.

crib·rate (krib'rate) *adj.* CRIBRIFORM.

crib·ri·form (krib'ri·form) *adj.* [L. *cribrum,* sieve, + *-iform*]. Perforated like a sieve.

cribriform compress. A compress with holes for drainage or a hole for observation of the skin beneath.

cribriform fascia. The sievelike covering of the fossa ovalis of the thigh. NA *fascia cribrosa.*

cribriform lamina. CRIBRIFORM PLATE.

cribriform plate. 1. The horizontal plate of the ethmoid bone, part of the floor of the anterior cranial fossa, perforated for the passage of the fila olfactoria of the olfactory nerves. NA *lamina cribrosa ossis ethmoidalis.* 2. ALVEOLAR BONE (2).

cribriform spots. MACULAE CRIBROSAE.

crib·rose (krib'roce) *adj. In biology,* sievelike.

Cri·ce·tus (kri·see'tus) *n.* [NL., from Slavic]. A genus of hamsters including the European variety, *Cricetus cricetus* and the golden hamster, *C. auratus.*

Crich·ton-Browne's sign (krye'tun braown') [J. *Crichton-Browne,* British physician, 1840–1938]. Twitching of the outer corners of the eyes and lips, an early sign in general paresis.

crick, *n. Colloq.* Any painful spasmodic affection, as of the back or neck.

crico- [Gk. *krikos,* ring]. A combining form meaning *cricoid.*

cri·co·ar·y·te·noid (krye''ko·ăr''i·tee'noid, ·a·rit'e·noid) *adj. & n.* 1. Pertaining to the cricoid and arytenoid cartilages. 2. One of two muscles attached to the cricoid and arytenoid cartilages, the posterior and lateral cricoarytenoid muscles. NA *musculus cricoarytenoideus lateralis, musculus cricoarytenoideus posterior.* See also Table of Muscles in the Appendix.

cri·co·esoph·a·ge·al (krye''ko·e·sof''uh·jee'ul) *adj.* Of or pertaining to the cricoid cartilage and the esophagus.

cricoesophageal tendon. The tendon of origin of the longitudinal and part of the circular striated musculature of the esophagus, attached to the posterior medial surface of the cricoid cartilage. NA *tendo cricoesophageus.*

cri·coid (krye'koid) *adj. & n.* [Gk. *krikoeidēs,* from *krikos,* ring]. 1. Ring-shaped. 2. CRICOID CARTILAGE.

cricoid cartilage. The ring-shaped cartilage of the larynx. NA *cartilago cricoidea.*

cri·coi·dec·to·my (krye''koy·deck'tuh·mee) *n.* [*cricoid* + *-ectomy*]. The excision of the cricoid cartilage.

cri·co·pha·ryn·ge·al (krye''ko·fa·rin'jee·ul, ·rin·jee'ul) *adj.* Of or pertaining to the cricoid cartilage and the pharynx.

cricopharyngeal ligament. A fibrous band between the posterior aspect of the cricoid cartilage and the pharynx. NA *ligamentum cricopharyngeum.*

cri·co·pha·ryn·ge·us (krye''ko·fa·rin'jee·us) *n.* The portion of the inferior constrictor muscle of the pharynx that arises from the cricoid cartilage. NA *pars cricopharyngea musculi constrictoris pharyngis inferioris.*

cri·co·thy·re·ot·o·my (krye''ko·thigh·ree·ot'uh·mee) *n.* CRICOTHYROTOMY.

cri·co·thy·roid (krye''ko·thigh'roid) *adj. & n.* 1. Pertaining to the cricoid and thyroid cartilages. 2. The muscle, attached to the cricoid and thyroid cartilages, which tenses the vocal folds. NA *musculus cricothyroideus.* See also Table of Muscles in the Appendix.

cricothyroid ligament. The sheet of fibroelastic connective tissue which is attached below to the upper margin of the cricoid cartilage. The central portion (the median cricothyroid ligament) of the upper margin is attached to the lower margin of the thyroid cartilage. The lateral portions of the upper margin of the connective-tissue sheet constitute the vocal ligaments. Syn. *elastic cone, cricovocal membrane.* NA *ligamentum cricothyroideum.*

cricothyroid membrane. CRICOTHYROID LIGAMENT.

cri·co·thy·rot·o·my (krye''ko·thigh·rot'uh·mee) *n.* [*crico-* + *thyro-* + *-tomy*]. Incision of the larynx through the cricothyroid ligament.

cri·cot·o·my (krye·kot'uh·mee) *n.* [*crico-* + *-tomy*]. *In surgery,* the cutting of the cricoid cartilage.

cri·co·tra·che·al (krye''ko·tray'kee·ul) *adj.* Of or pertaining to the cricoid cartilage and the trachea.

cricotracheal ligament. The ligament between the cricoid and the first tracheal cartilage. NA *ligamentum cricotracheale.*

cri·co·tra·che·ot·o·my (krye''ko·tray''kee·ot'uh·mee) *n.* Tracheotomy through the cricoid cartilage.

cri·co·vo·cal (krye''ko·vo'kul) *adj.* Pertaining to the cricoid cartilage and the vocal folds.

cricovocal membrane. CRICOTHYROID LIGAMENT.

cri-du-chat syndrome (kree·due·shah) [F., cat's cry]. A syndrome of congenital defects, including a laryngeal anomaly which is associated with a catlike cry in infants, hypertelorism, epicanthus, brachycephaly, moonface micrognathia, hypotonia, strabismus, and severe mental retardation. The somatic cells of affected individuals display a deletion of the short arm of one of the two number 5 chromosomes. Syn. *deletion-5 syndrome.*

Crig·ler-Naj·jar syndrome [J. F. *Crigler,* U.S. pediatrician, b. 1919; and V. A. *Najjar,* U.S. pediatrician, b. 1914]. A recessively inherited defect in bilirubin conjugation by glucuronide associated with chronic icterus.

crim·i·nal abortion. Interruption of a pregnancy, or the attempt to do so, for reasons and under conditions not authorized by law; an illegal abortion.

criminal anthropology. The study of man in relation to the habitual criminal, utilizing all the measurements and identification data of anthropology; BERTILLON SYSTEM.

criminal degeneracy. *In criminology,* a tendency to commit criminal acts, especially sexual crimes. See also *sociopathic personality disturbance.*

crim·i·nal·is·tics (krim''i·nul·is'ticks) *n.* The solving of crimes by scientific methods, including those associated with many branches of medicine as well as psychology.

criminally insane. *In law,* pertaining to an individual who is committed to a mental hospital by a court or courts after being found not guilty of a crime by reason of insanity.

criminal responsibility. *In forensic medicine,* the concept that a person is responsible for his crime if at the time of committing the act he knew what he was doing and knew it to be wrong. See also *M'Naghten rule.*

crim·i·nol·o·gy (krim″i-nol′uh-jee) *n.* 1. The study of crime and of criminals. 2. CRIMINAL ANTHROPOLOGY.

-crine [Gk. *krinein,* to separate]. A suffix meaning *secretion* or *secreting* (as of a gland).

crines pubis [L.]. The pubic hair(s).

cri·nis (krye′nis) *n.*, pl. **cri·nes** (·neez) [L.]. Hair. —**cri·nos·i·ty** (krye-nos′i-tee, kri·) *n.*; **cri·nous** (krye′nus) *adj.*

crino·gen·ic (krin″o-jen′ick) *adj.* [Gk. *krin*ein, to separate, + *-genic*]. Stimulating the production of secretions.

crise de dé·glo·bu·li·sa·tion (kreez duh de^{y}-gloh^{h}-bu^{e}-lee-za^{h}-syoh^{n}′) [F.]. DEGLOBULINIZATION CRISIS.

cri·sis (krye′sis) *n.*, pl. **cri·ses** (·seez) [Gk. *krisis,* decision, event, turning point]. 1. A turning point for better or worse, as that of a disease or fever; especially, the sudden favorable termination of the acute symptoms of an infectious disease. Contr. *lysis (2).* 2. Paroxysmal disturbance of function accompanied with pain. 3. Paroxysmal intensification of symptoms. 4. The psychological events associated with a specific stage of life. See also *developmental crisis, identity crisis, situational crisis.*

crisis consultation. *In psychiatry,* the optimum use of mental-health consultations through a comprehensive community program in the resolution of personal crisis.

crisis intervention. *In psychiatry,* immediate brief treatment of a patient at a time of personal crisis by a therapist or a therapeutic team, utilizing medications, hospitalization, changes in environmental circumstances, referrals to community agencies, and other means.

cris·pa·tion (kris-pay′shun) *n.* [L. *crispare,* to curl or wave]. 1. A puckering. 2. An annoying involuntary quivering of the muscles.

cris·pa·tu·ra (kris″puh-tew′ruh) *n.* [L.]. CRISPATION.

crispatura ten·di·num (ten′di-num). DUPUYTREN'S CONTRACTURE.

Crisp's aneurysm. Aneurysm of the splenic artery.

cris·ta (kris′tuh) *n.*, pl. & genit. sing. **cris·tae** (·tee) [L.]. A crest or ridge. Adj. *cristal, cristate.*

crista acus·ti·ca (uh-koos′ti-kuh). CRISTA AMPULLARIS.

crista am·pul·la·ris (am″puh-lair′is) [NA]. An elevation projecting into the lumen of an ampulla of the ear containing its sensory end organ. Syn. *crista acustica.*

crista anterior fi·bu·lae (fib′yoo-lee) [BNA]. MARGO ANTERIOR FIBULAE.

crista anterior ti·bi·ae (tib′ee-ee) [BNA]. MARGO ANTERIOR TIBIAE.

crista ar·cu·a·ta (ahr″kew-ay′tuh) [NA]. A ridge on the dorsal surface of the arytenoid cartilage.

crista ba·si·la·ris (bas″i-lair′is) [NA]. The ridge on the spiral ligament to which the basilar membrane of the cochlear duct is attached.

crista buc·ci·na·to·ria (buck″si-na-to′ree-uh) [BNA]. BUCCINATOR CREST.

crista ca·pi·tis cos·tae (kap′i-tis kos′tee) [NA]. CREST OF THE HEAD OF A RIB.

crista ca·pi·tu·li cos·tae (ka-pit′yoo-lye kos′tee) [BNA]. Crista capitis costae (= CREST OF THE HEAD OF A RIB).

crista col·li cos·tae (kol′eye kos′tee) [NA]. CREST OF THE NECK OF A RIB.

crista con·cha·lis max·il·lae (kong-kay′lis mack-sil′ee) [NA]. CONCHAL CREST.

crista conchalis os·sis pa·la·ti·ni (os′is pal-uh-tye′nigh) [NA]. A sharp ridge near the posterior margin of the nasal surface of the perpendicular plate of the palatine bone for articulation with the inferior nasal concha.

crista di·vi·dens (dye′vi-denz, div′i·). The upper margin of the fetal foramen ovale that separates the inferior caval stream of blood into two portions.

cristae. 1. Plural and genitive singular of *crista.* 2. *In electron microscopy,* inward extensions of the inner membrane of the external double membrane system of mitochondria.

cristae cu·tis (kew′tis) [NA]. Ridges of the skin of the palm and sole, which are the basis for identification of fingerprints or toe prints.

cristae ma·tri·cis un·guis (may-trye′sis ung′gwis, may′tri-sis) [NA]. Longitudinal ridges in the matrix of the nail.

cristae sa·cra·les ar·ti·cu·la·res (sa-kray′leez ahr-tick″yoo-lair′eez) [BNA]. Cristae sacrales intermediae, plural of *crista sacralis intermedia.*

cristae sacrales la·te·ra·les (lat″e-ray′leez) [BNA]. Plural of *crista sacralis lateralis.*

crista eth·moi·da·lis max·il·lae (eth″moy-day′lis mack-sil′ee) [NA]. ETHMOID CREST (1).

crista ethmodalis os·sis pa·la·ti·ni (os′is pal-uh-tye′nigh) [NA]. ETHMOID CREST (2).

crista fal·ci·for·mis (fal″si-for′mis). A crest dividing the macula cribrosa into a smaller superior one and a larger inferior one.

crista fe·nes·trae coch·le·ae (fe-nes′tree cock′lee-ee) [NA]. The ridge of bone lying above the cochlear window of the middle ear.

crista fron·ta·lis (fron-tay′lis) [NA]. FRONTAL CREST.

crista gal·li (gal′eye) [NA]. The superior triangular process of the ethmoid bone, so called because it is shaped like a cock's comb.

crista ili·a·ca (il-eye′uh-kuh) [NA]. ILIAC CREST.

crista in·fra·tem·po·ra·lis (in″fruh-tem-po-ray′lis) [NA]. INFRATEMPORAL CREST.

crista in·ter·os·sea fi·bu·lae (in-tur-os′ee-uh fib′yoo-lee) [BNA]. MARGO INTEROSSEUS FIBULAE.

crista interossea ra·dii (ray′dee-eye) [BNA]. MARGO INTEROSSEUS RADII.

crista interossea ti·bi·ae (tib′ee-ee) [BNA]. MARGO INTEROSSEUS TIBIAE.

crista interossea ul·nae (ul′nee) [BNA]. MARGO INTEROSSEUS ULNAE.

crista in·ter·tro·chan·te·ri·ca (in″tur-tro-kan-terr′i-kuh) [NA]. INTERTROCHANTERIC CREST.

cris·tal (kris′tul) *adj.* [L. *crist*a + *-al*]. Of or pertaining to a ridge or crest.

crista la·cri·ma·lis anterior (lack-ri-may′lis) [NA]. A vertical ridge on the lateral surface of the frontal process of the maxillary bone.

crista lacrimalis posterior [NA]. A vertical ridge on the orbital surface of the lacrimal bone.

crista la·te·ra·lis fi·bu·lae (lat-e-ray′lis fib′yoo-lee) [BNA]. MARGO POSTERIOR FIBULAE.

crista mar·gi·na·lis den·tis (mahr-ji-nay′lis den′tis) [NA]. A ridge of a tooth.

crista me·di·a·lis fi·bu·lae (mee-dee-ay′lis fib′yoo-lee) [NA]. The posteromedial border of the fibula, beginning at the medial side of the head and continuing downward into the interosseous crest.

crista mus·cu·li su·pi·na·to·ris (mus′kew-lye sue″pi-na-to′ris) [NA]. SUPINATOR CREST.

crista na·sa·lis max·il·lae (nay-say′lis mack-sil′ee) [NA]. NASAL CREST (1).

crista nasalis os·sis pa·la·ti·ni (os′is pal-uh-tye′nigh) [NA]. NASAL CREST (2).

crista ob·tu·ra·to·ria (ob″tew-ruh-tor′ee-uh) [NA]. OBTURATOR CREST.

crista oc·ci·pi·ta·lis ex·ter·na (ock-sip″i-tay′lis ecks-tur′nuh) [NA]. EXTERNAL OCCIPITAL CREST.

crista occipitalis in·ter·na (in-tur′nuh) [NA]. INTERNAL OCCIPITAL CREST.

crista pa·la·ti·na (pal-uh-tye′nuh) [NA]. A transverse ridge on the inferior surface of the horizontal plate of the palatine bone near the posterior border.

crista pu·bi·ca (pew′bi-kuh) [NA]. PUBIC CREST.

crista sa·cra·lis in·ter·me·dia (sa-kray′lis in-tur-mee′dee-uh) [NA]. An irregular vertical ridge on the posterior surface of the sacrum due to the fusion of the articular processes of the sacral vertebrae. See also *sacral crest.*

crista sacralis la·te·ra·lis (lat-e-ray′lis) [NA]. An irregular vertical ridge on the posterior surface of the sacrum due to the fusion of the transverse processes of the sacral vertebrae.

crista sacralis me·dia (mee'dee·uh) [BNA]. CRISTA SACRALIS MEDIANA.

crista sacralis me·di·a·na (mee·dee·ay'nuh) [NA]. An irregular vertical ridge in the midline of the posterior surface of the sacrum due to the fusion of the spinous processes of the sacral vertebrae. See also *sacral crest.*

crista sep·ti mar·gi·na·lis (sep'tye mahr·ji·nay'lis). The moderator band of the heart when it appears as a prominent ridge.

crista sphe·noi·da·lis (sfee''noy·day'lis) [NA]. SPHENOID CREST.

crista su·pra·ven·tri·cu·la·ris (sue''pruh·ven·trick·yoo·lair'is) [NA]. SUPRAVENTRICULAR CREST.

cris·tate (kris'tate) *adj.* [L. *cristatus,* from *crista,* crest]. Crested; having a crest or ridge.

crista ter·mi·na·lis atrii dex·tri (tur·mi·nay'lis ay'tree·eye decks'trye) [NA]. A crest on the wall of the right atrium derived from the cephalic part of the right valve of the sinus venosus; a point of attachment for the pectinate muscles of the right atrium.

crista trans·ver·sa (trans·vur'suh) [NA]. A transverse ridge at the lateral termination of the internal acoustic meatus.

crista tu·ber·cu·li ma·jo·ris (tew·bur'kew·lye ma·jo'ris) [NA]. The sharp anterior margin of the lateral surface of the greater tubercle of the humerus.

crista tuberculi mi·no·ris (mi·no'ris) [NA]. The sharp posterior margin of the lateral surface of the lesser tubercle of the humerus.

crista ure·thra·lis ure·thrae fe·mi·ni·nae (yoo·re·thray'lis yoo·ree'three fem·i·nigh'nee) [NA]. A longitudinal fold in the posterior wall of the female urethra.

crista urethralis urethrae mas·cu·li·nae (mas·kew·lye'nee) [NA]. A prominent longitudinal ridge in the posterior wall of the prostatic urethra.

crista urethralis urethrae mu·li·e·bris (mew·lee·ee'bris) [BNA]. CRISTA URETHRALIS URETHRAE FEMININAE.

crista urethralis urethrae vi·ri·lis (vir'i·lis, vi·rye'lis) [BNA]. CRISTA URETHRALIS URETHRAE MASCULINAE.

crista ves·ti·bu·li (ves·tib'yoo·lye) [NA]. An oblique ridge on the medial wall of the vestibule of the inner ear.

crit, *n.* 1. In nuclear technology, the mass of a fissionable material which, under a given set of conditions, is critical. 2. HEMATOCRIT.

Cri·thid·ia (kri·thid'ee·uh) *n.* [Gk. *krithidion,* dim. of *krithē,* barleycorn]. A genus of protozoan parasites of the Trypanosomatidae; they occur only in invertebrate hosts.

crit·i·cal (krit'i·kul) *adj.* 1. Pertaining to or characterized by a crisis. 2. Characterized by sharp discernment, severe assessment, or skillful judgement. 3. Of decisive importance as regards outcome; crucial. 4. Involving grave uncertainty or risk; perilous. 5. *In nuclear technology,* of or pertaining to the state of a fissionable material in which it is capable of sustaining, at constant level, a chain reaction.

critical angle. *In optics,* the least angle of incidence at which there is total reflection. It exists when light, traveling in one medium, is incident upon another medium which is less refracting.

critical fusion frequency. FLICKER-FUSION THRESHOLD.

critical illumination. Illumination in which the image of a small source of light is focused exactly at the object on the stage of the microscope.

critical period. *In psychology,* the time period in the development of an organism during which it must be exposed to certain experiences in order to acquire certain behavioral patterns; failure to be so exposed within this period may result in inability to learn not only the particular activity but others.

critical point. The temperature above which a gas cannot be liquefied by pressure.

critical potential. The point at which the electrokinetic or zeta potential between the immobile and mobile ionic layers is lowered by addition of electrolytes so that the double layers of colloidal particles collapse, and the particles aggregate and precipitate.

critical pressure. The pressure on a gas or vapor which will, at the critical temperature, convert it into a liquid.

critical ratio. A statistical term denoting the ratio of the difference between the mean of a series of observations and the true or hypothetical value to the standard deviation of the series.

critical temperature. The temperature at which a gas can, by pressure, be reduced to a liquid.

CR lead. *In electrocardiography,* a precordial exploring electrode paired with an electrode on the right arm.

CRM Abbreviation for *cross-reacting material.*

CRO Abbreviation for *cathode-ray oscillograph.*

Crock·er tumor 180. A poorly differentiated transmissible tumor of mice which originally arose spontaneously in the axilla of a male white mouse.

croc·o·dile tears syndrome. A profuse, paroxysmal flow of tears observed in certain patients with peripheral facial paralysis, when they taste strongly flavored food.

Crocq's disease [J. B. *Crocq,* Belgian physician, 1868–1925]. ACROCYANOSIS.

cro·cus (kro'kus) *n.* [Gk. *krokos,* saffron]. The stigma of the flowers of *Crocus sativus.* Has been used as an aromatic stimulant, emmenagogue, and antispasmodic. Syn. *saffron.*

cro·fil·con A (kro·fil'kon) *n.* A copolymer of methyl methacrylate and 2,3-dihydroxypropyl methacrylate employed as a contact lens material.

Crohn's disease [B. B. *Crohn,* U.S. physician, b. 1884]. REGIONAL ENTERITIS.

Crohn's disease of the colon [B. B. *Crohn*]. GRANULOMATOUS COLITIS.

cro·mo·lyn sodium (kro'mo·lin). The disodium salt of 1,3-bis(2-carboxychroman-5-yloxy)-2-hydroxypropane, $C_{23}H_{14}Na_2O_{11}$, used for the treatment of allergic airway obstruction. Syn. *disodium cromoglycate.*

Cronk·hite-Can·a·da syndrome [B. B. *Cronkhite;* and W. J. *Canada*]. A rare syndrome of diffuse gastrointestinal polyposis, skin pigmentation, alopecia, and atrophy of the nails, with onset in late middle to old age.

Cronolone. Trademark for flurogestone, a progestational steroid used as the acetate ester.

Crooke's cells [A. C. *Crooke,* English endocrinologist, b. 1905]. Beta cells of the adenohypophysis exhibiting Crooke's change.

Crooke's change [A. C. *Crooke*]. Hyalinization and vacuolization of the cytoplasm of pituitary basophils; seen in Cushing's syndrome and other conditions.

Crookes tube [W. *Crookes,* English physicist, 1832–1919]. A highly evacuated tube used to demonstrate the properties of cathode rays (electrons).

crop, *n.* A dilatation of the esophagus of certain kinds of birds, in which relatively large quantities of food are stored, moistened, and released in small portions to the stomach.

cross birth *Obsol.* TRANSVERSE PRESENTATION.

cross·bite, cross bite, *n.* The abnormal occlusal relationship, in a facial or lingual version, of teeth in one arch to those in the opposite arch.

cross·breed·ing, *n.* Production of offspring from the mating of individuals of different breeds, varieties, or strains, or sometimes, different species. —**crossbreed,** *n. & v.*

cross-classification table. CONTINGENCY TABLE.

cross-cultural psychiatry. The comparative study of mental health and disease in different social groups, nations, and cultures.

crossed akinesia. Loss of motor activity on the side opposite that in which a lesion exists in the central nervous system.

crossed anesthesia. Loss or impairment of pain and thermal sense on one side of the body and a cranial nerve palsy on the other, the result of a brainstem lesion that involves a cranial nerve nucleus or its intramedullary fibers and the spinothalamic tract on the same side.

crossed aphasia. Aphasia occurring in a clearly left-handed individual due to a lesion in the left cerebral hemisphere.

crossed cylinders. Two cylindrical lenses placed in apposition to each other with their axes at right angles; used by oculists to determine the strength and the axis of astigmatism.

crossed diplopia. Diplopia in which the false image of the right eye appears upon the left side, and that of the left eye upon the right side; a result of divergent strabismus.

crossed embolus. PARADOXICAL EMBOLUS.

crossed extension reflex. Extension of one leg with plantar flexion when an extensor plantar response is elicited in the passively extended other limb; normally present in the first weeks of life.

crossed hemianesthesia. CROSSED ANESTHESIA.

crossed hemiplegia. CROSSED PARALYSIS.

crossed parallax. Parallax in which the object moves away from the uncovered eye. Syn. *heteronymous parallax.*

crossed paralysis. Paralysis of the arm and leg on one side, associated with contralateral cranial nerve palsies due to a brainstem lesion involving cranial nerve nuclei and the ipsilateral pyramidal tract.

crossed reflex. A response on one side of the body induced by stimulation of the other side.

crossed rubrospinal tract. RUBROBULBAR TRACT.

cross-eye, *n.* ESOTROPIA. —**cross-eyed,** *adj.*

cross-fertilization. *In biology,* the fertilization of the ovules of one species by the seed germs of another.

cross-fire treatment. A method of arranging beams in radiation therapy in such a manner that they overcross in the depth of the body at the site of the tumor, sparing the skin.

cross infection. Any infection which a patient contracts from another patient.

cross·ing-over, *n. In genetics,* an exchange of blocks of genes between homologous chromosomes during synapsis.

cross-legged progression. SCISSORS GAIT.

cross-link, *v.* To unite neighboring long-chain molecules by a chemical bond to form a complex molecule.

cross matching. A test to establish blood compatibility before transfusion by (a) mixing the prospective recipient's serum with the donor's cells (major cross match) or (b) mixing the donor's serum with the recipient's cells (minor cross match). If agglutination, or hemolysis, does not occur in either test when carried out by several acceptable techniques, the bloods are considered compatible, and the donor's blood may be used.

cross-match test. CROSS MATCHING.

cross·over experiment. An experiment or clinical investigation in which subjects are divided randomly into at least as many groups as there are kinds of treatment to be given, and then the groups are interchanged until every subject has received each treatment. Thus it is possible to use each subject as his own control while compensating for any spontaneous time trends, and also to study how long effects persist after treatment is discontinued. See also *double-blind experiment.*

cross-reacting material. The material (protein), formed by a mutant structural gene, which is functionally defective but still able to react as an antigen with an antibody which also reacts with the normally functioning protein. Abbreviated, CRM.

cross reaction. A reaction between an antibody and an antigen which is closely related to, but not identical with, the specific antigen.

cross section. 1. A slice of or a cut through an object made in a plane perpendicular to its longest axis. Syn. *transverse section.* 2. *In nuclear physics,* a measure, commonly expressed in barns, of the probability that a nuclear reaction will occur.

cross-striation. Lines running across the fibers of skeletal muscle in histologic preparations. See also *A band, I band.*

cross suck·ling. Reciprocal foster nursing; a technique now used primarily in animal experimentation, as in viral studies.

cross·way, *n.* [*cross* + path*way*]. The crossing of two nerve paths. See also *chiasma.*

Cro·tal·i·dae (kro·tal'i·dee) *n. pl.* [NL., from *Crotalus,* type genus]. A family of venomous snakes, the pit vipers, differing from Viperidae (true vipers) in possessing a sensory pit situated between the eye and nostril. Found commonly in North and South America, southeastern Asia, and the East Indies.

crot·a·line (krot'uh·leen, ·lin) *adj. & n.* [*Crotal*us + *-ine*]. 1. Of or pertaining to the Crotalidae or, in particular, to the genus *Crotalus.* 2. A protein found in the venom of rattlesnakes. 3. A preparation of venom from the rattlesnakes *Crotalus horridus* and *C. adamanteus* which has been used subcutaneously for immunization against snake bites.

Crot·a·lus (krot'uh·lus) *n.* [L. *crotalum,* rattle]. A genus of the Crotalidae possessing neurotoxic venom; the rattlesnakes. Thirteen species are found in the United States, including *Crotalus adamanteus,* the Florida diamondback found along the Gulf coastal regions; *C. atrox,* the Texas rattler or western diamondback; *C. confluentus,* the prairie rattlesnake; *C. exsul,* the red rattler; *C. horridus,* the timber rattler; *C. oreganus,* the Pacific rattler; *C. durissus durissus* is found in Central America and *C. durissus terrificus* in South America.

***Crotalus* antivenin.** Polyvalent serum for the venom of rattlesnakes.

cro·tam·i·ton (kro·tam'i·ton) *n.* *N*-Ethyl-*o*-crotonotoluidide, $C_{13}H_{17}NO$, used as a scabicide and antipruritic.

cro·taph·i·on (kro·taf'ee·on) *n.* [Gk. *krotaphion,* from *krotaphos,* temple]. *In craniometry,* the point at the posterior extremity of the sphenoparietal suture.

crotch, *n.* The angle formed by the junction of the inner sides of the thighs and the trunk.

crotch·et (krotch'it) *n.* A hook used in extracting the fetus after craniotomy.

-crotic [Gk. *krotos,* beat, clapping, + *-ic*]. A combining form meaning *pulse, heartbeat.*

cro·tin (kro'tin) *n.* [*Cro*ton + *-in*]. A mixture of toxic albuminoids in croton seeds; a protoplasmic poison.

-crotism. A combining form designating *condition of having a* (specified type of) *pulse or heartbeat.*

Cro·ton (kro'ton, ·tun) *n.* [Gk. *krotōn,* castor oil tree]. A genus of plants of the Euphorbiaceae. *Croton eluteria* yields cascarilla, and *C. tiglium* is the source of croton oil.

cro·ton·al·de·hyde (kro''tun·al'de·hide) *n.* *trans*-2-Butenal, C_4H_6O, a pungent liquid; used as a component of tear gas and as an intermediate in chemical syntheses.

Cro·ton bug (kro'tun) [after *Croton* Aqueduct, New York]. A cockroach of the species *Blatella germanica.*

cro·ton·ism (kro'tun·iz·um) *n.* Poisoning by croton oil, characterized by hemorrhagic gastroenteritis.

croton oil. A fixed oil from the seed of *Croton tiglium;* a drastic purgative. Causes pustular eruptions when applied to the skin.

cro·tox·in (kro·tock'sin) *n.* [*Cro*talus + *toxin*]. A neurotoxin from the venom of the rattlesnake *Crotalus durissus terrificus.*

croup (kroop) *n.* Any condition of upper respiratory pathway obstruction, especially acute inflammation of the pharynx, larynx, and trachea of children, characterized by a hoarse, brassy, and stridulent cough and difficulties in breathing, and in some conditions (as in diphtheria), deposition of a localized membrane. See also *spasmodic croup.* —**croup·ous** (kroo'pus), **croupy** (kroo'pee) *adj.*

croup·ine (kroo'peen) *n.* SPASMODIC CROUP.

croup kettle. A kettle for the production of steam or medicated vapor, used for humidification. See also *vaporizer.*

croupous bronchitis. Bronchitis characterized by expectoration of casts of the bronchial tubes, containing Charcot-Leyden crystals and eosinophil cells, after a paroxysm of dyspnea and violent coughing.

croupous membrane. The yellowish white membrane forming in the larynx in laryngotracheobronchitis.

croupous pharyngitis. DIPHTHERITIC PHARYNGITIS.

Crou·zon-Apert disease (kroo·zohⁿ′, a·pehr′) [O. *Crouzon*, French neurologist, 1874–1938; and E. *Apert*]. A syndrome in which there are features of acrocephalosyndactyly and craniofacial dysostosis combined.

Crouzon's disease [O. *Crouzon*]. CRANIOFACIAL DYSOSTOSIS.

Crowe's sign [S. J. *Crowe*, U.S. physician, b. 1883]. The engorgement of the retinal blood vessels when the internal jugular vein is compressed on the normal side; seen in patients with lateral sinus thrombosis.

crown, *n.* [L. *corona*, crown]. Corona; the top part of anything; any structure like a crown.

crown gall. A form of gall found at the root crown near the base of the stem in fruit trees, sugar beets, and other broad-leaved plants, caused by *Agrobacterium tumefaciens;* consists in a tumorlike mass of abnormal cells which continue to multiply independently of the original causative agent, thus resembling cancer in animals. Syn. *plant cancer.*

crown glass. A very hard glass; a silicate of sodium and calcium.

crown of a tooth. The part of the tooth covered with enamel. NA *corona dentis.*

crown of Venus [*Venus*, Roman goddess of love]. A syphilitic lesion about the brow or the hair line with associated patchy alopecia of the area.

crown saw. TREPHINE.

CRST syndrome. A syndrome of calcinosis, Raynaud's phenomenon, sclerodactylia, telangiectasis.

CRT Cathode-ray tube.

cruces. Plural of *crux.*

cruces pi·lo·rum (pi·lo′rum), sing. **crux pilorum** [NA]. Points on the skin or scalp at which hairs oriented toward each other meet and are deflected outward or upward.

cru·cial (kroo′shul) *adj.* [F., from L. *crux*, cross]. 1. Resembling or pertaining to a cross. 2. Critical; decisive.

crucial incision. Two cuts at right angles, made deep into the tissues, usually to ensure free drainage.

cru·ci·ate (kroo′shee·ut, ·ate) *adj.* Resembling a cross; cross-shaped.

cruciate anastomosis. An arterial anastomosis in the upper thigh, formed by the inferior gluteal, medial circumflex femoral, lateral circumflex femoral, and first perforating arteries. It is important in the formation of collateral circulation after ligation of the femoral artery.

cruciate eminence. The intersection of ridges in the form of a cross on the internal surface of the squamous portion of the occipital bone. NA *eminentia cruciformis.*

cruciate ligament. 1. (of the atlas:) The ligament formed by the transverse ligament of the atlas and two vertical bands of fibers, the superior and inferior limbs, passing from the transverse ligament to the occipital bone and to the body of the atlas, respectively. NA *ligamentum cruciforme atlantis.* 2. (of the knee:) Either of two crossing ligaments (NA (pl.) *ligamenta cruciata genus*) connecting the tibia and the femur in the middle of the knee joint and designated as anterior and posterior according to their place of attachment to the tibia, with the anterior cruciate ligament (NA *ligamentum cruciatum anterius*) passing posteriorly and laterally and the posterior cruciate ligament (NA *ligamentum cruciatum posterius*) passing anteriorly and medially. 3. (of the ankle:) INFERIOR EXTENSOR RETINACULUM.

cruciate paralysis. CROSSED PARALYSIS.

cruciate sulcus. One of the two grooves at right angles to each other on the dorsal surface of the mesencephalon between the colliculi of the corpora quadrigemina.

cru·ci·ble (kroo′si·bul) *n.* [ML. *crucibulum*, earthen pot]. A vessel of clay or other refractory material used in melting or igniting substances that require a high degree of heat.

crucifixion attitude. A form of hysterical neurosis characterized by a rigid state of the body with the arms stretched out at right angles, in imitation of the crucifixion position.

cru·ci·form (kroo′si·form) *adj.* Cruciate; shaped like a cross.

crude birth rate. The number of live births in a given year per 1,000 total population at midyear. Contr. *specific birth rate.*

crude death rate. The number of deaths in a given year per 1,000 total population at midyear. Contr. *specific death rate.*

crude drug. 1. A plant or animal drug, fresh or dried, containing all principles characteristic of the drug. 2. More commonly, the dried leaves, bark, or rhizome of a plant containing therapeutically active principles.

cru·fo·mate (kru′fo·mate) *n.* 4-*tert*-Butyl-2-chlorophenyl methyl methylphosphoramidate, $C_{12}H_{19}ClNO_3P$; a veterinary antiparasitic agent.

crup·per (krup′ur) *n.* [OF. *cropiere*]. 1. The buttocks of a horse. 2. The sacrococcygeal region in horses. 3. The base of the tail in mammals.

crura. Plural of *crus.*

crura am·pul·la·ria (am″puh·lair′ee·uh) [BNA]. CRURA OSSEA.

crura ant·hel·i·cis (ant·hel′i·sis) [NA]. CRURA OF THE ANTHELIX.

cru·ral (kroo′rul) *adj.* 1. Pertaining to any of the crura of the body. 2. Pertaining to the lower leg. 3. Loosely, pertaining to the leg including the thigh.

crural arcade. *Obsol.* INGUINAL LIGAMENT.

crural canal. FEMORAL CANAL.

crural cistern. A lateral extension of the interpeduncular cistern.

crural fascia. The deep fascia of the leg, extending from knee to ankle. NA *fascia cruris.*

crural hernia. FEMORAL HERNIA.

crural paralysis. Paralysis involving chiefly the thigh.

crural plexus. FEMORAL PLEXUS.

crural ring. FEMORAL RING.

crural sheath. FEMORAL SHEATH.

crura mem·bra·na·cea (mem·bruh·nay′see·uh) [NA]. The ends of the membranous semicircular canals.

crura membranacea am·pul·la·ria duc·tus se·mi·cir·cu·la·ris (am·puh·lair′ee·uh duck′toos sem″i·sur·kew·lair′is) [NA]. The dilated (ampullary) ends of the membranous semicircular ducts.

crura of the anthelix. The two limbs of the bifurcation of the anthelix. NA *crura anthelicis.*

crura of the incus. The two main processes of the incus. See *long crus of the incus, short crus of the incus.*

crura of the stapes. The two processes that connect the base and head of the stapes: the anterior process (NA *crus anterius stapedis*) and the posterior process (NA *crus posterius stapedis*).

crura os·sea (os′ee·uh) [NA]. The crura of the osseous semicircular canals, including the crura ossea ampullaria, crus osseum commune, and crus osseum simplex.

crura ossea am·pul·la·ria (am·puh·lair′ee·uh) [NA]. The portions of the osseous semicircular canals which house the ampullary crura of the membranous semicircular canals.

cru·re·us (kroo′ree·us) *n.* [L.]. The vastus intermedius muscle. See Table of Muscles in the Appendix.

cru·ro·scro·tal (kroo″ro·skro′tul) *adj.* [*crural* + *scrotal*]. Pertaining to the thighs and scrotum.

cru·ro·ves·i·cal (kroo″ro·ves′i·kul) *adj.* [*crural* + *vesical*]. Pertaining to the thighs and urinary bladder.

crurovesical-gluteal dystrophy. A developmental anomaly of the sacrum and coccyx as well as of the lower spinal cord, resulting in weakness and atrophy of the gluteal muscles and of the muscles innervated by the sacral roots, incontinence of feces and urine, and sensory loss in the sacrococcygeal distribution.

crus (krooce) *n.*, genit. **cru·ris** (kroo′ris), pl. **cru·ra** (kroo′ruh) [L., leg, shin]. 1. [NA] LEG (1). 2. Any of various parts of the body or of an organ suggestive of a leg. Adj. *crural.*

crus an·te·ri·us cap·su·lae in·ter·nae (an·teer′ee·us kap′sue·lee in·tur′nee) [NA]. The portion of the internal capsule lying between the caudate and lentiform nuclei.

crus anterius sta·pe·dis (sta·pee'dis) [NA]. The anterior process of the stapes. See *crura of the stapes.*

crus bre·ve in·cu·dis (brev'ee ing·kew'dis) [NA]. SHORT CRUS OF THE INCUS.

crus ce·re·bri (serr'e·brye) [NA]. CRUS OF THE CEREBRUM.

crus cli·to·ri·dis (kli·tor'i·dis) [NA]. CRUS OF THE CLITORIS.

crus com·mu·ne (kom·yoo'nee) [BNA]. CRUS OSSEUM COMMUNE.

crus dex·trum dia·phrag·ma·tis (decks'trum dye"uh·frag'muh·tis) [NA]. The right crus of the diaphragm. See *crus of the diaphragm.*

crus fas·ci·cu·li atrio·ven·tri·cu·la·ris dex·trum et si·nis·trum (fa·sick'yoo·lye ay"tree·o·ven·trick"yoo·lair'is deck'strum et si·nis'trum) [NA]. Either branch (right or left) of the atrioventricular bundle.

crus for·ni·cis (for'ni·sis) [NA]. CRUS OF THE FORNIX.

crus he·li·cis (hel'i·sis) [NA]. CRUS OF THE HELIX.

crush·ing forceps. A forceps, usually in the form of a clamp, for crushing heavy tissues or pedicles prior to ligation.

crush kidney. ACUTE TUBULAR NECROSIS.

crush syndrome. A severe, often fatal condition that follows a severe crushing injury, particularly involving large muscle masses; characterized by extensive fluid and blood loss in the injured part, hypovolemic shock, hematuria, myoglobinuria, renal tubular necrosis, and renal failure. Syn. *compression syndrome, Bywaters' syndrome.*

crus in·fe·ri·us an·nu·li in·gui·na·lis sub·cu·ta·nei (in·feer'ee·us an'yoo·lye ing·gwi·nay'lis sub"kew·tay'nee·eye) [BNA]. CRUS LATERALE ANULI INGUINALIS SUPERFICIALIS.

crus in·ter·me·di·um dia·phrag·ma·tis (in·tur·mee'dee·um dye"uh·frag'muh·tis) [BNA]. The lateral portion of each right and left crus of the diaphragm.

crus la·te·ra·le anu·li in·gui·na·lis su·per·fi·ci·a·lis (lat·e·ray'lee an'yoo·lye ing·gwi·nay'lis sue"pur·fish·ee·ay'lis) [NA]. The portion of the inguinal ligament on the lateral side of the superficial inguinal ring which attaches to the pubic tubercle.

crus laterale car·ti·la·gi·nis ala·ris ma·jo·ris (kahr·ti·laj'i·nis ay·lair'is ma·jo'ris) [NA]. The lateral portion of the greater alar cartilage of the nose.

crus laterale dia·phrag·ma·tis (dye"uh·frag'muh·tis) [BNA]. The portion of each lateral half of the diaphragm arising from the medial and lateral arcuate ligaments; the lumbar portion of the diaphragm exclusive of the crus proper (crus mediale diaphragmatis).

crus lon·gum in·cu·dis (long'gum ing·kew'dis) [NA]. LONG CRUS OF THE INCUS.

crus me·di·a·le anu·li in·gui·na·lis su·per·fi·ci·a·lis (mee·dee·ay'lee an'yoo·lye ing"gwi·nay'lis sue"pur·fish·ee·ay'lis) [NA]. The portion of the inguinal ligament on the medial side of the superficial inguinal ring which attaches to the symphysis of the pubis.

crus mediale car·ti·la·gi·nis ala·ris ma·jo·ris (kahr·ti·laj'i·nis ay·lair'is ma·jo'ris) [NA]. The medial portion of the greater alar cartilage of the nose.

crus mediale dia·phrag·ma·tis (dye"uh·frag'muh·tis) [BNA]. CRUS OF THE DIAPHRAGM.

crus mem·bra·na·ce·um com·mu·ne (mem·bruh·nay'see·um kom·yoo'nee) [NA]. The combined portion of the anterior and posterior membranous semicircular canals which empties into the utricle.

crus membranaceum sim·plex (sim'plecks) [NA]. The end of the lateral membranous semicircular canal emptying into the utricle.

crus of the cerebellum. CEREBELLAR PEDUNCLE.

crus of the cerebrum. Either of the two peduncles connecting the cerebrum with the pons. NA *crus cerebri.*

crus of the clitoris. The posterior part of either corpus cavernosum clitoridis, attached to the pubic arch. NA *crus clitoridis.*

crus of the diaphragm. Either of the two fibromuscular bands arising from the bodies of the lumbar vertebrae and inserted into the central tendon of the diaphragm: the right crus (NA *crus dextrum diaphragmatis*) and the left crus (NA *crus sinistrum diaphragmatis*).

crus of the fornix. Either one of the two bands of nerve fibers which pass from the hippocampus to the individual posterior portions of the fornix cerebri. NA *crus fornicis.*

crus of the helix. The curved root of the helix above the external acoustic meatus. NA *crus helicis.*

crus of the penis. The posterior part of either corpus cavernosum penis, attached to the pubic arch. NA *crus penis.*

crus os·se·um com·mu·ne (os'ee·um kom·yoo'nee) [NA]. The portion of the osseous lateral semicircular canal which houses the common crus of the anterior and posterior membranous semicircular canals.

crus osseum sim·plex (sim'plecks) [NA]. The portion of the lateral osseous semicircular canal which houses the crus of the lateral membranous semicircular canal emptying into the utricle.

crus·ot·o·my (kroos·ot'uh·mee) *n.* [*crus* + *-tomy*]. PEDUNCULOTOMY.

crus pe·dun·cu·li (pe·dunk'yoo·lye). CRUS OF THE CEREBRUM.

crus pe·nis (pee'nis) [NA]. CRUS OF THE PENIS.

crus phenomenon or **syndrome.** Hemiparetic symptoms homolateral with a cerebral lesion, and thus a false localizing sign, usually found when a chronic subdural hematoma, brain tumor, or brain abscess has caused herniation of the temporal lobe through the incisure of the tentorium with dislocation of the brainstem so as to force the contralateral cerebral peduncle against the tentorium. Syn. *Kernohan-Woltman syndrome.*

crus pos·te·ri·us cap·su·lae in·ter·nae (pos·teer'ee·us kap'sue·lee in·tur'nee) [NA]. The portion of the internal capsule lying between the thalamus and lentiform nucleus.

crus posterius sta·pe·dis (sta·pee'dis) [NA]. The posterior process of the stapes. See *crura of the stapes.*

crus sim·plex (sim'plecks) [BNA]. CRUS OSSEUM SIMPLEX.

crus si·nis·trum dia·phrag·ma·tis (si·nis'trum dye"uh·frag'muh·tis) [NA]. The left crus of the diaphragm. See *crus of the diaphragm.*

crus su·pe·ri·us an·nu·li in·gui·na·lis sub·cu·ta·nei (sue·peer'ee·us an'yoo·lye ing·gwi·nay'lis sub"kew·tay'nee·eye) [BNA]. CRUS MEDIALE ANULI INGUINALIS SUPERFICIALIS.

crust, *n.* [L. *crusta*]. A barklike, hard covering; especially, a dried exudate on the skin.

crus·ta (krus'tuh) *n.*, pl. & genit. sing. **crus·tae** (·tee) [L.]. CRUST.

Crus·ta·cea (krus·tay'shee·uh) *n. pl.* A class of arthropods including the lobsters, crabs, shrimps, barnacles, and sow bugs. —**crus·ta·cean** (krus·tay'shun) *n. & adj.*

crusta lac·tea (lack'tee·uh). [L., lit., milk crust]. CRADLE CAP.

crutch, *n.* A special staff used as a support in walking. The common form has a concave, padded crosspiece to fit the axilla, and a guiding and supporting grip for the hand.

Crutch·field tongs [W. G. *Crutchfield,* U.S. neurosurgeon, b. 1900]. Hinged tongs whose points engage the skull; used to provide traction in the treatment of fracture dislocations of the cervical spine.

crutch paralysis or **palsy.** Weakness or paralysis of the muscles of the upper extremity, due to compression of the brachial plexus and especially of the radial nerve from pressure of the crutch head.

Cru·veil·hier-Baum·gar·ten syndrome or **cirrhosis** (kru^e·veh·ye^y') [J. *Cruveilhier,* French pathologist, 1791–1874; and W. *Baumgarten*]. Distention of the periumbilical veins, associated with a bruit and thrill, due to a large patent umbilical vein, occurring either as a developmental anomaly or as a response to portal hypertension.

Cruveilhier's disease [J. *Cruveilhier*]. PROGRESSIVE SPINAL MUSCULAR ATROPHY.

Cruveilhier's sign [J. *Cruveilhier*]. A sign for saphenous varix in which a tremor or impulse can be palpated over the saphenous vein when the patient coughs.

crux (krucks) *n.*, genit. **cru·cis** (kroo'sis), pl. **cru·ces** (·seez) [L.]. A cross, or a crosslike structure.

Cruz's disease (krooce) [O. G. *Cruz*, Brazilian physician, 1872–1917]. CHAGAS' DISEASE.

cry-, cryo- [Gk. *kryos*]. A combining form meaning *cold, freezing*.

cryaesthesia. CRYESTHESIA.

cry·al·ge·sia (krye″al·jee′zee·uh) *n.* [*cry-* + *algesia*]. Pain from the application of cold.

cry·anes·the·sia, cry·an·aes·the·sia (krye″an·es·theezh′uh, ·theez′ee·uh) *n.* [*cry-* + *anesthesia*].1. Loss of sensation or perception of cold by the skin. 2. Localized anesthesia of a part obtained by the application of cold. See also *refrigeration anesthesia.*

cry·es·the·sia, cry·aes·the·sia (krye″es·theezh′uh, ·theez′ee·uh) *n.* [*cry-* + *esthesia*]. 1. Temperature sense for cold. 2. Extreme sensitivity to cold.

crym-, crymo-, krymo- [Gk. *krymos*, icy cold]. A combining form meaning *cold, frost.*

crymo-. See *crym-.*

cry·mo·dyn·ia (krye″mo·din′ee·uh) *n.* [*crym-* + *-odynia*]. CRYALGESIA; pain coming on in cold or damp weather.

cry·mo·phil·ic (krye″mo·fil′ick) *adj.* [*crymo-* + *-philic*]. PSYCHROPHILIC.

cry·mo·ther·a·py (krye′mo·therr′uh·pee) *n.* [*crymo-* + *therapy*]. CRYOTHERAPY.

cryo-. See *cry-.*

cryo·bi·ol·o·gy (krye″o·bye·ol′uh·jee) *n.* [*cryo-* + *biology*]. The study of frozen or low-temperature life.

cryo·cau·tery (krye″o·kaw′tur·ee) *n.* [*cryo-* + *cautery*]. The destruction of tissues by application of extreme cold which causes an obliterative thrombosis; used especially in removing moles.

cry·o·chem (krye′o·kem) *n.* A desiccation procedure involving rapid freezing of the material to be dried followed by evaporation of the moisture from the frozen state with the aid of a regenerable desiccant.

cryo·ex·trac·tor (krye″o·eck·strack′tur) *n.* [*cryo-* + *extractor*]. *In ophthalmology,* an instrument the tip of which can be cooled to extremely low temperatures by means of Freon, liquid carbon dioxide or nitrogen, or other agents; used in the extraction of cataracts.

cryo·fi·brin·o·gen (krye″o·figh·brin′o·jen) *n.* [*cryo-* + *fibrinogen*]. Any fibrinogen complex that precipitates from the blood at 4°C.

cryo·fi·brin·o·gen·emia (krye″o·figh·brin″o·je·nee′mee·uh) *n.* The presence of cryofibrinogens in the blood.

cryo·glob·u·lin (krye″o·glob′yoo·lin) *n.* [*cryo-* + *globulin*]. An abnormal protein which precipitates from plasma between 4° and 21°C (40 and 70°F).

cryo·glob·u·li·ne·mia, cryo·glob·u·li·nae·mia (krye″o·glob″yoo·li·nee′mee·uh) *n.* [*cryoglobulin* + *-emia*]. A disease state characterized by the presence of cryoglobulin in the blood, associated with malignant plasmacytoma (multiple myeloma) and certain other diseases.

cryo·hy·poph·y·sec·to·my (krye″o·high·pof″i·seck′tuh·mee) *n.* [*cryo-* + *hypophysectomy*]. The partial or total destruction of the hypophysis by means of a freezing lesion.

cryo·im·mu·ni·za·tion (krye″o·im″yoo·ni·zay′shun) *n.* [*cryo-* + *immunization*]. The production or stimulation of immune mechanisms by freezing of tissues with release of antigens from the cells thus disrupted.

cry·om·e·ter (krye·om′e·tur) *n.* [*cryo-* + *meter*]. An instrument for measuring low temperatures.

cryo·phake (krye′o·fake) *n.* [*cryo-* + Gk. *phakos*, lens]. A device for freezing the crystalline lens of the eye to aid in its removal during cataract surgery.

cryo·pre·cip·i·tate (krye″o·pre·sip′·i·tate) *n.* [*cryo-* + *precipitate*]. A slow-melting precipitate rich in factor VIII used in the treatment of hemophilia, prepared from fresh human plasma by freezing and controlled thawing.

cryo·pro·tec·tant (krye″o·pro·teck′tunt) *n.* [*cryo-* + *protectant*]. A substance used to protect against the pathologic changes induced by cold.

cryo·pro·tein (krye″o·pro′tee·in) *n.* [*cryo-* + *protein*]. CRYOGLOBULIN.

cryo·scope (krye′o·skope) *n.* [*cryo-* + *-scope*]. An apparatus for determining the freezing point of a liquid.

cryo·stat (krye′o·stat) *n.* [*cryo-* + *-stat*]. 1. A device consisting of a freezing chamber containing a microtome, so arranged as to allow operation from outside at normal temperature; used to make rapid sections of fresh tissue for microscopic study. 2. Any device for maintaining very low temperatures; as one that operates by compressing, regeneratively cooling, and then expanding helium gas until part of the gas becomes liquid; it can cool contents to −43°C (−45°F).

cryo·sur·gery (krye″o·sur′juh·ree) *n.* [*cryo-* + *surgery*]. Surgery performed with aid of special instruments for local freezing of diseased tissues without significant harm to normal adjacent structures.

cryo·thal·a·mot·o·my (krye″o·thal·uh·mot′uh·mee) *n.* [*cryo-* + *thalamotomy*]. The stereotactical placement of a freezing lesion in the thalamus, primarily in the neurosurgical therapy of movement disorders, particularly parkinsonism, but sometimes to alleviate intractable pain.

cryo·ther·a·py (krye″o·therr′uh·pee) *n.* [*cryo-* + *therapy*]. A form of therapy which consists of local or general use of cold.

cryo·tome (krye′o·tome) *n.* [*cryo-* + *-tome*]. FREEZING MICROTOME.

crypt, *n.* [Gk. *kryptē*, from *kryptos*, hidden]. 1. A small sac or follicle. 2. A glandular cavity.

crypt-, crypto-, krypto- [Gk. *kryptos*]. A combining form meaning (a) *hidden, covered, occult;* (b) *latent;* (c) *crypt.*

cryp·ta (krip′tuh) *n.*, pl. & genit. sing. **cryp·tae** (·tee) [L., from Gk. *kryptē*]. CRYPT.

cryptae ton·sil·la·res (ton·sil·air′eez) [NA]. TONSILLAR CRYPTS.

crypt·am·ne·sia (krip″tam·nee′zhuh, ·zee·uh) *n.* [*crypt-* + *amnesia*]. CRYPTOMNESIA.

crypt·an·am·ne·sia (kript″an·am·nee′zhuh, ·zee·uh) *n.* [*crypt-* + *anamnesis* + *-ia*]. CRYPTOMNESIA.

cryp·ten·a·mine (krip·ten′uh·meen) *n.* A mixture of structurally unidentified alkaloids derived from an extract of *Veratrum viride;* used as an antihypertensive, in the form of the acetate or tannate salts.

cryp·tic depression. *In psychiatry,* a concealed or hidden depression.

cryp·ti·tis (krip·tye′tis) *n.* [*crypt-* + *-itis*]. Inflammation of a crypt, or of crypts.

crypto-. See *crypt-.*

cryp·to·ceph·a·lus (krip″to·sef′uh·lus) *n.*, pl. **cryptocepha·li** (·lye) [*crypto-* + *-cephalus*]. A parasitic conjoined twin with an imperfectly formed and concealed head.

cryp·to·coc·co·sis (krip″to·kock·o′sis) *n.*, pl. **cryptococco·ses** (·seez) [*Cryptococcus* + *-osis*]. A subacute or chronic infection caused by the yeast *Cryptococcus neoformans.* The infection may involve the lungs, bones, or skin, but has a predilection for the central nervous system, causing primarily meningitis. Syn. *torulosis, European blastomycosis.*

Cryp·to·coc·cus (krip″to·kock′us) *n.* [*crypto-* + *coccus*]. A genus of true yeast whose species include the pathogen *Cryptococcus neoformans.*

Cryptococcus neo·for·mans (nee″o·for′manz). The causative organism of cryptococcosis.

cryp·to·did·y·mus (krip″to·did′i·mus) *n.*, pl. **cryptodidy·mi** (·mye) [*crypto-* + *-didymus*]. A form of duplicity in which a fetus or fetal part is included within the body of an individual.

cryp·to·gam (krip′to·gam) *n.* *In botany,* one of the Cryptogamia, a division of the vegetable kingdom comprising all plants without flowers or seeds, as the algae, fungi, mosses, and ferns. Contr. *phanerogam.* —**cryp·tog·a·mous** (krip·tog′uh·mus) *adj.*

cryp·to·gen·ic (krip″to·jen′ick) *adj.* [*crypto-* + *-genic*]. Of unknown or obscure cause. Compare *idiopathic.* Contr. *phanerogenic.* See also *agnogenic.*

cryptogenic anemia. 1. Anemia of undetermined origin. 2. PRIMARY REFRACTORY ANEMIA.

cryptogenic epilepsy. IDIOPATHIC EPILEPSY.

cryptogenic pyemia. A condition in which the primary suppuration occurs in a portion of the body where it is difficult to detect.

cryp·to·in·fec·tion (krip″to·in·feck′shun) *n.* [*crypto-* + *infection*]. A nonapparent, latent, or hidden infection.

cryp·to·lith (krip′to·lith) *n.* [*crypto-* + *-lith*]. A concretion or calculus formed within a crypt, as in the tonsil.

cryp·to·men·or·rhea, cryp·to·men·or·rhoea (krip″to·men″o·ree′uh) *n.* [*crypto-* + *menorrhea*]. A condition in which there is menstrual flow from the uterus, the external escape of which is prevented by an obstruction in the lower genital canal, usually an imperforate hymen.

cryp·to·mero·ra·chis·chi·sis, cryp·to·mer·or·rha·chis·chi·sis (krip″to·merr″o·ra·kis′ki·sis) *n.* [*crypto-* + *mero-* + *rachischisis*]. SPINA BIFIDA OCCULTA.

cryp·tom·ne·sia (krip″tom·nee′zhuh, ·zee·uh) *n.* [*crypto-* + *-mnesia*]. The recall to mind of a forgotten episode which seems entirely new to the patient, and not a part of his experiences. Syn. *subconscious memory.*

cryp·toph·thal·mia (krip″tof·thal′mee·uh) *n.* CRYPTOPHTHALMOS (1).

cryptophthalmia-syndactyly syndrome. Extension of the skin of the forehead to cover one or both eyes, total or partial syndactyly of fingers and toes, coloboma of the alae nasi, abnormal hairline, and urogenital anomalies.

cryp·toph·thal·mos (krip″tof·thal′mos) *n.* [*crypt-* + *ophthalmos*]. 1. Congenital union of the eyelids, usually over imperfect eyes. 2. An individual with this condition.

cryptophthalmos-syndactyly syndrome. CRYPTOPHTHALMIA-SYNDACTYLY SYNDROME.

cryp·toph·thal·mus (krip″tof·thal′mus) *n.* CRYPTOPHTHALMOS.

cryp·to·pine (krip′to·peen, ·pin) *n.* A minor alkaloid, $C_{21}H_{23}NO_5$, in opium.

cryp·top·or·ous (krip·top′or·us) *adj.* [*crypto-* + *porous*]. Having hidden or obscure pores.

cryp·tor·chi·dec·to·my (krip″tor·kid·eck′tuh·mee) *n.* [*crypt-* + *orchidectomy*]. Removal of an undescended testis.

cryp·tor·chid·ism (krip·tor′kid·iz·um) *n.* CRYPTORCHISM.

cryp·tor·chid·o·pexy (krip″tor·kid′o·peck·see, krip·tor′ki·do·) *n.* [*crypt-* + *orchidopexy*]. Fixation, within the scrotum, of an undescended testis.

cryp·tor·chism (krip·tor′kiz·um) *n.* [*crypt* + *orch-* + *-ism*]. A developmental defect in which the testes fail to descend, and remain within the abdomen or inguinal canal. —**cryp·tor·chid** (·kid) *n.* & *adj.*; **cryptor·chis** (·kis) *n.*

cryp·to·xan·thin (krip″to·zan′thin) *n.* [*crypto-* + *xanthine*]. Hydroxy- β-carotene, $C_{40}H_{56}O$, a carotenoid pigment widely distributed in natural sources; possesses vitamin A activity.

cryp·to·zo·ite (krip″to·zo′ite) *n.* [*crypto-* + *zo-* + *-ite*]. The exoerythrocytic stage of malarial parasites which are found in the cells of the liver before gaining access to the erythrocytes.

cryp·to·zy·gous (krip·toz′i·gus, krip″to·zye′gus) *adj.* [*crypto-* + *-zygous*]. Having a wide skull and a narrow face, so that the zygomatic arches are not visible when the skull is viewed from above.

crypts of Lie·ber·kühn (lee′bur·kuᵉn″) [J. L. *Lieberkühn*]. INTESTINAL GLANDS.

crypts of the tongue. Pits in the mucous membrane of the pharyngeal part of the tongue, surrounded by the lymphatic tissue of the lingual tonsils. They often serve also as excretory ducts of the mucous glands of this region.

crys·tal (kris′tul) *n.* [Gk. *krystallos,* ice, crystal]. *In chemistry,* a substance that assumes a definite three-dimensional geometric form.

crys·tal·bu·min (kris″tal·bew′min) *n.* 1. Any crystallized albumin, such as bovine serum albumin. 2. A protein found in the crystalline lens.

crys·tal·fi·brin (kris″tul·figh′brin) *n.* A protein obtained by treating the crystalline lens with hydrochloric acid.

crystall-, crystallo- [Gk. *krystallos*]. A combining form meaning *crystal.*

crys·tal·lin (kris′tul·in) *n.* Either of two globulins of the crystalline lens, separately designated by the prefixes α-, β-.

crys·tal·line (kris′tuh·lin, ·line) *adj.* Like a crystal.

crystalline capsule. CAPSULE OF THE LENS.

crystalline cataract. A cataract in which fine crystalline opacities are found in the axial region of the lens; may be congenital, or acquired from lipid deposition.

crystalline insulin. The crystalline product obtained when insulin is precipitated in the presence of added zinc ion. The rapidity and duration of action are probably no different from that of amorphous insulin.

crystalline lens. The lens of the eye, a refractive organ of accommodation; a biconvex, transparent, elastic body lying in its capsule immediately behind the pupil of the eye, suspended from the ciliary body by the ciliary zonule. NA *lens.*

crys·tal·li·za·tion (kris″tul·i·zay′shun) *n.* The process by which the molecules, atoms, or ions of a substance arrange themselves in geometric forms when passing from a gaseous or a liquid state to a solid state. —**crys·tal·lize** (kris′tul·ize) *v.*

crystallized digitalin. DIGITOXIN.

crystallo-. See *crystall-.*

crys·tal·log·ra·phy (kris″tuh·log′ruh·fee) *n.* [*crystallo-* + *-graphy*]. The science of crystals, their formation, structure, and classification.

crys·tal·loid (kris′tuh·loid) *adj.* [*crystall-* + *-oid*]. Having a crystal-like nature, as distinguished from colloid.

crys·tal·lo·mag·net·ism (kris″tuh·lo·mag′ne·tiz·um) *n.* The property common to certain crystals of orienting themselves in a magnetic field.

crys·tal·lo·pho·bia (kris″tuh·lo·fo′bee·uh) *n.* [*crystallo-* + *-phobia*]. An abnormal fear of glass or things made of glass.

Crystallose. A trademark for sodium saccharine.

crys·tal·lu·ria (kris″tuh·lew′ree·uh) *n.* [*crystall-* + *-uria*]. The presence of crystals in the urine; usually a normal condition.

crystal violet. METHYLROSANILINE CHLORIDE.

Crysticillin. A trademark for procaine penicillin G.

Crystodigin. A trademark for digitoxin, a cardiotonic.

CS Abbreviation for *conditioned stimulus.*

Cs Symbol for cesium.

c/s Cycle(s) per second (= HERTZ).

CSF Abbreviation for *cerebrospinal fluid.*

C-substance. Among the hemolytic streptococci, antigenic group-specific complex polysaccharides of the cell wall which distinguish Group A, B, C, E, G, and probably others.

CT Abbreviation for *computed* or *computerized tomography.*

Cteno·ce·phal·i·des (ten″o·se·fal′i·deez, tee″no·) *n.* [NL., from Gk. *kteis, ktenos,* comb, + *kephalē*]. A genus of fleas which are cosmopolitan in distribution. The species *Ctenocephalides canis,* the dog flea, and *C. felis,* the cat flea, while they infest primarily dogs and cats, may attack man and other mammals. Members of this genus also serve as intermediate hosts of the dog tapeworm, *Dipylidium caninum.*

cten·oids (tee′noidz, ten′oidz) *n.pl.* [Gk. *ktenoeidēs,* comblike]. *In electroencephalography,* 14- and 6-per-second positive spikes.

Cten·o·psyl·lus seg·nis (ten″o·psil′us seg′nis). A species of rodent flea.

Cu Symbol for copper.

cub-, cubi-, cubo-. A combining form meaning (a) *cube;* (b) *cubital;* (c) *cuboid.*

cu·beb (kew′beb) *n.* [Ar. *kabābah*]. The dried, unripe, nearly full-grown fruit of *Piper cubeba,* cultivated in Java and the

West Indies; contains a volatile oil. Has been used as a diuretic, urinary antiseptic, and expectorant.

cu·beb·ism (kew'beb·iz·um) *n.* Poisoning by cubeb, characterized by acute gastroenteritis.

cubic centimeter. A unit of volume represented by a cube one centimeter on edge; for all practical purposes it is equivalent in liquid measure to a milliliter. Abbreviated, c^3, cc.

cu·bi·form (kew'bi·form) *adj.* [*cub-* + *-iform*]. CUBOID.

cubital fossa. ANTECUBITAL FOSSA.

cu·bi·tus (kew'bi·tus) *n.*, pl. & genit. sing. **cubi·ti** (·tye) [LL., from L. *cubitum*]. 1. FOREARM. 2. [NA] ELBOW. 3. *Obsol.* ULNA. —**cubi·tal** (·tul) *adj.*

cubitus val·gus (val'gus). A decrease in the normal carrying angle of the arm.

cubitus va·rus (vair'us). An increase in the normal carrying angle of the arm.

cu·boid (kew'boid) *adj. & n.* [Gk. *kyboeidēs*]. 1. Resembling a cube. 2. The bone of the tarsus between the calcaneus and the fourth and fifth metatarsals. NA *os cuboideum.* See also Table of Bones in the Appendix.

cu·boi·dal (kew·boy'dul) *adj.* Cuboid; cubelike.

cuboidal cell. An epithelial cell in which height and width are nearly equal.

cu·boi·deo·meta·tar·sal (kew·boy"dee·o·met·uh·tahr'sul) *adj.* Pertaining to the cuboid and the metatarsal bones.

cuboideometatarsal articulation. The articulation between the anterior surface of the cuboid and the bases of the fourth and fifth metatarsals. Syn. *lateral tarsometatarsal articulation.*

cu·boi·deo·na·vic·u·lar (kew·boy"dee·o·na·vick'yoo·lur) *adj.* Pertaining to the cuboid and the navicular bones.

cuboideonavicular articulation. The articulation between the cuboid and navicular bones.

cuboideonavicular ligament. Any of the ligaments connecting the cuboid and navicular bones: the dorsal cuboideonavicular ligament (NA *ligamentum cuboideonaviculare dorsale*), the plantar cuboideonavicular ligament (NA *ligamentum cuboideonaviculare plantare*), or the interosseous cuboideonavicular ligament.

cu·boi·do·dig·i·tal (kew·boy"do·dij'i·tul) *adj.* Pertaining to the cuboid bone and the digits.

cuboidodigital reflex. BEKHTEREV-MENDEL REFLEX.

cu·cum·ber shin (kew'kum·bur). Curvature of the tibia with the convexity forward.

Cu·cu·mis (kew'kuh·mis) *n.* [L., cucumber]. A genus of plants of the Cucurbitaceae that includes cucumbers and muskmelons, certain of which have been used medicinally.

Cu·cur·bi·ta (kew·kur'bi·tuh) *n.* [L., gourd]. A genus of plants of the Cucurbitaceae. Several species, such as *Cucurbita pepo,* the pumpkin, yield seeds that have been used as anthelmintics.

cud·bear, *n.* [Dr. *Cuthbert* Gordon, Scottish chemist, 18th century]. A powder prepared from species of *Roccella, Lecanora,* or other lichens; used as a red coloring agent for pharmaceutical preparations.

Cuemid. A trademark for cholestyramine resin.

cuff, *n.* 1. Any bandlike structure that encircles a part. 2. A collection of cells, usually exudative, encircling a blood vessel, especially in the central nervous system.

cuff·ing, *n.* Formation of cuffs (2).

cuff manometry. A variation of the Queckenstedt test in which, to achieve jugular compression, the cuff of a sphygmomanometer is wrapped around the patient's neck and inflated and deflated in a standardized manner; useful in determining the presence of a subarachnoid block.

cui·rass (kwee·ras', kwee'ras) *n.* [F. *cuirasse,* from L. *coriaceus,* made of leather]. A close-fitting or immovable bandage or plate for the front of the chest.

cuirass cancer. CANCER EN CUIRASSE.

cuirass respirator. An apparatus which, by means of an airtight chest piece of plastic and rubber, exerts intermittent negative pressure on the patient's thorax and thus aids breathing. Employed when the patient has some ability to breathe on his own.

cul-de-sac (kul"de·sack') *n.* [F.]. 1. A closed or blind pouch or sac. 2. RECTOUTERINE EXCAVATION.

cul-de-sac of Doug·las [J. *Douglas*]. RECTOUTERINE EXCAVATION.

culdo- [*cul*-de-sac of *Do*uglas]. A combining form meaning *rectouterine excavation.*

cul·do·cen·te·sis (kul"do·sen·tee'sis) *n.*, pl. **culdocente·ses** (·seez) [*culdo-* + *centesis*]. Removal, by aspiration or incision, of intraperitoneal fluid material (transudate, exudate, or blood) through the vagina and the rectouterine excavation.

cul·do·plas·ty (kul'do·plas"tee) *n.* [*culdo-* + *-plasty*]. Plastic surgical repair of the rectouterine excavation.

cul·do·scope (kul'do·skope) *n.* [*culdo-* + *-scope*]. An instrument for the visualization of the female internal genitalia and pelvic tissues, entering through the vagina and a perforation into the rectouterine excavation. —**cul·dos·co·py** (kul·dos'kuh·pee) *n.*

cul·dot·o·my (kul"dot'uh·mee) *n.* [*culdo-* + *-tomy*]. *In surgery,* an incision through the rectouterine excavation.

Cu·lex (kew'lecks) *n.* [L., midge, gnat]. A genus of mosquitoes which are vectors of disease.

Culex fat·i·gans (fat'i·ganz). *CULEX PIPIENS QUINQUEFASCIATUS.*

Culex pi·pi·ens (pye'pee·enz). The species of *Culex* known as the common house mosquito, found in temperate regions; a vector of filariasis.

Culex pipiens quin·que·fas·ci·a·tus (kwin"kwee·fash·ee·ay'tus). A mosquito which is the most common vector of *Wuchereria bancrofti.*

culic-, culici- [L. *culex, culicis,* gnat, midge]. A combining form meaning *gnat, mosquito.*

culici-. See *culic-.*

Cu·lic·i·dae (kew·lis'i·dee) *n.pl.* [from *Culex,* type genus]. A family of the Diptera comprising the mosquitoes.

cu·li·cide (kew'li·side) *n.* [*culic-* + *-cide*]. Any agent that destroys mosquitoes.

cu·lic·i·fuge (kew·lis'i·fewj) *n.* [*culici-* + *-fuge*]. An agent to drive away mosquitoes.

Cu·li·ci·nae (kew"li·sigh'nee) *n.pl.* A subfamily of the Culicidae; contains all species of mosquitoes of medical significance.

Cu·li·coi·des (kew"li·koy'deez) *n.* A genus of ceratopogonid gnats, several species of which serve as intermediate hosts of filarial parasites. *Culicoides austeni* and *C. grahami* are species that transmit the filarial worm, *Acanthocheilonema perstans; C. furens* has been found to transmit *Mansonella ozzardi.*

Cul·len's sign [T. S. *Cullen,* U.S. surgeon, 1868–1953]. A sign for ruptured ectopic pregnancy in which a blue-red discoloration is seen about the umbilicus.

cul·men (kul'min) *n.*, genit. **cul·mi·nis** (kul'mi·nis), pl. **cul·mi·na** (·mi·nuh) [NA]. The superior portion of the monticulus of the vermis of the cerebellum.

cul·ti·va·tion (kul"ti·vay'shun) *n.* Successive transferring of microorganisms to different media favorable to growth. See also *culture.* —**cul·ti·vate** (kul'ti·vate) *v.*

cul·tu·ral anthropology. The study of prehistoric and contemporary human beings with respect to customs, technologies, social, political, and economic life, religions, languages, folklores, and arts, and adaptation to specific settings. See also *sociology.*

cultural deprivation. SOCIAL DEPRIVATION.

cultural-familial mental retardation. Mental retardation, usually mild, of unclear etiology but associated with a family history of borderline or mild retardation and a home environment which was either depriving or was inconsistent with the general culture.

cultural psychiatry. The branch of social psychiatry that deals with mental illness in relation to the cultural setting, as symptoms or behavior regarded as pathological in one society that may be acceptable or approved in another. See also *cross-cultural psychiatry.*

cul·ture (kul'chur) *n. & v.* [L. *cultura,* from *colere,* to till]. 1. The growth of microorganisms or tissue cells in artificial media. 2. A group of microorganisms or cells grown in an artificial medium. 3. *In cultural anthropology,* the total learned way of life of a society. 4. *In archeology,* the material evidence of a particular tradition or complex of traditions. 5. To grow or cultivate (microorganisms, cells) in an artificial medium.

culture medium. Any liquid, solid, or semisolid substance for the cultivation of microorganisms.

culture plate. A culture of bacteria within a petri dish.

cumarin. COUMARIN.

cu·mene (kew'meen) *n.* Isopropylbenzene, C_9H_{12}, a hydrocarbon occurring in pine tar, petroleum, and some volatile oils.

Cumertilin. A trademark for the mercurial diuretic mercumatilin.

cum·in (kum'in, kew'min) *n.* [Gk. *kyminon*]. An umbelliferous plant, *Cuminum cyminum,* native in Egypt and Syria. The fruit has been used as a flavoring agent and carminative. —**cu·mic** (kew'mick) *adj.*

cu·mol (kew''mol) *n.* CUMENE.

Cumopyran. Trademark for cyclocumarol, an anticoagulant.

cu·mu·la·tive action. Sudden and marked action of a drug after administration of a number of ineffectual or slightly effective doses.

cumulative dose. *In radiology,* a total dose delivered in fractions over a period of time.

cu·mu·lus (kew'mew·lus) *n.,* pl. & genit. sing. **cumu·li** (·lye) [L.]. A heap or mound.

cumulus oo·pho·rus (o·off'o·rus) [NA]. The mass of follicular cells surrounding the ovum and protruding into the liquid-filled cavity of a graafian follicle.

cumulus ovi·ge·rus (o·vij'e·rus). CUMULUS OOPHORUS.

cumulus pro·li·ge·rus (pro·lij'e·rus). CUMULUS OOPHORUS.

cune-, cuneo- [L. *cuneus,* wedge]. A combining form meaning *cuneiform.*

cu·ne·ate (kew'nee·ate) *adj.* [L. *cuneatus,* from *cuneus,* wedge]. Wedge-shaped.

cuneate fasciculus. A fiber tract in the lateral part of the dorsal funiculus of the spinal cord. NA *fasciculus cuneatus medullae spinalis.*

cuneate lobule. CUNEUS.

cuneate nucleus. The collection of nerve cells lying in the dorsal aspect of the medulla oblongata in which the fibers of the fasciculus cuneatus terminate and which give origin to part of the fibers of the medial lemniscus. NA *nucleus cuneatus.*

cuneate tubercle. One of the two bilateral ovoid eminences in the caudal end of the fourth ventricle, representing continuations of the fasciculus cuneatus; subjacent to each is a cuneate nucleus. NA *tuberculum nuclei cuneati.*

cunei. Plural and genitive singular of *cuneus.*

cu·ne·i·form (kew·nee'i·form, kew'nee·) *adj. & n.* [*cune-* + *-iform*]. 1. Wedge-shaped; cuneate. 2. Any of three tarsal bones. See Table of Bones in the Appendix. 3. TRIQUETRUM (1).

cuneiform bone of the carpus. TRIQUETRUM (1).

cuneiform cartilage. Either of two small, rod-shaped cartilages of the larynx, located in the aryepiglottic folds anterior to the corniculate cartilages. Syn. *Wrisberg's cartilages.* NA *cartilago cuneiformis.*

cuneiform osteotomy. An ostectomy in which a wedge of bone is removed.

cuneiform tubercle. A rounded eminence on each side of the entrance to the laryngeal cavity lying over the cuneiform cartilage. NA *tuberculum cuneiforme.*

cuneo-. See *cune-.*

cu·neo·cu·boid (kew''nee·o·kew'boid) *adj.* Pertaining to the cuneiform and cuboid bones.

cuneocuboid articulation. The articulation between the cuboid and lateral cuneiform bones.

cuneocuboid ligament. Any of the ligaments connecting the lateral cuneiform and cuboid bones: the dorsal cuneocuboid ligament (NA *ligamentum cuneocuboideum dorsale*), the interosseous cuneocuboid ligament (NA *ligamentum cuneocuboideum interosseum*), or the plantar cuneocuboid ligament (NA *ligamentum cuneocuboideum plantare*).

cu·neo·meta·tar·sal (kew''nee·o·met·uh·tahr'sul) *adj.* Pertaining to the cuneiform and metatarsal bones.

cuneometatarsal articulation. The articulation between the intermediate and lateral cuneiform bones and the second, third, and fourth metatarsals. Syn. *intermediate tarsometatarsal articulation.*

cu·neo·na·vic·u·lar (kew''nee·o·na·vick'yoo·lur) *adj.* Pertaining to the cuneiform and the navicular bones.

cuneonavicular articulation. The gliding joint between the navicular and the three cuneiform bones. NA *articulatio cuneonavicularis.*

cuneonavicular ligament. Any of the ligaments connecting the navicular to the three cuneiform bones, including the dorsal cuneonavicular ligaments (NA *ligamenta cuneonavicularia dorsalia*) and the plantar cuneonavicular ligaments (NA *ligamenta cuneonavicularia plantaria*).

cu·neo·scaph·oid (kew''nee·o·skaf'oid) *adj.* [*cuneo-* + *scaphoid*]. CUNEONAVICULAR.

cu·ne·us (kew'nee·us) *n.,* pl. & genit. sing. **cu·nei** (·nee·eye) [L., wedge] [NA]. A wedge-shaped convolution on the medial aspect of the occipital lobe between the parieto-occipital and calcarine fissures.

cu·nic·u·lar (kew·nick'yoo·lur) *adj.* Furrowed.

cu·nic·u·lus (kew·nick'yoo·lus) *n.,* pl. **cunicu·li** (·lye) [L., rabbit]. A burrow made in the skin by an itch mite.

cun·ni·linc·tus (kun''i·link'tus) *n.* CUNNILINGUS.

cun·ni·lin·guist (kun''i·ling'gwist) *n.* A person who consistently practices cunnilingus.

cun·ni·lin·gus (kun''i·lin'gus) *n.* [*cunn*us + *lingu*ere, to lick]. The sexual practice in which the mouth and tongue are used to lick or stimulate the vulva.

cun·nus (kun'us) *n.,* pl. & genit. sing. **cun·ni** (·eye) [L.]. VULVA.

cu·o·rin (kew'o·rin) *n.* A phospholipid isolated from heart muscle.

cup, *v.* To bleed by means of suction cups or cupping glasses.

cu·po·la (kew'po·luh) *n.* [It., dim. of L. *cupa,* cask, tub]. A dome-shaped structure.

cupped, *adj.* Having the upper surface depressed; applied to the coagulum of blood after phlebotomy.

cupped disk. Excavation of the optic disk, normally present in slight degree, but pathologic if excessive.

cup pessary. A type of pessary for uterine prolapse in which the cervix rests in a cup held in by a belt and straps.

cup·ping, *n.* 1. A method of bloodletting by means of the application of cupping glasses to the surface of the body. 2. Formation of a cuplike depression.

cupping glass. A small bell-shaped glass capable of holding 3 to 4 ounces, in which the air is rarefied by heat or by exhaustion; the glass is applied to the skin, either with or without scarification of the latter. See also *cupping.*

cupr-, cupro-. A combining form meaning (a) *copper;* (b) *cupric.*

cu·pram·mo·nia (kew''pruh·mo'nee·uh) *n.* [*cupr-* + *ammonia*]. A solution of cupric hydroxide in ammonia water used as a solvent for cellulose.

cu·prea bark (kew'pree·uh). The bark of certain species of *Remijia,* containing homoquinine and certain related alkaloids; once used as a substitute for cinchona bark.

cu·pre·ine (kew'pree·een, ·in) *n.* [*curpea* + *-ine*]. Hydroxycinchonine, $C_{19}H_{22}N_2O_2$, an alkaloid in cuprea bark.

cupri-. A combining form meaning (a) *copper;* (b) *cuprous.*

cu·pric (kew'prik) *adj.* Pertaining to or containing copper in the bivalent state.

Cuprimine. Trademark for penicillamine, a metal-chelating degradation product of penicillin used to promote excretion of copper in hepatolenticular degeneration.

cu·pri·myx·in (koo·pri·mick'sin) *n.* Bis(6-methoxy-1-phenazinol 5,10-dioxidato)copper, $C_{26}H_{18}CuN_4O_8$, a veterinary antibacterial agent.

cupro-. See *cupr-.*

cu·prous (kew'prus) *adj.* Pertaining to or containing copper in the univalent state.

cu·prum (kew'prum) [L.]. COPPER.

cu·pu·la (kew'pew·luh) *n.*, pl. & genit. sing. **cupu·lae** (·lee). [NL., from It. *cupola,* dim. of L. *cupa,* cask, tub]. 1. A domelike structure. 2. A body of colorless substance on the crista ampullaris that coagulates and becomes visible upon applying fixing fluids. NA *cupula cristae ampullaris.*

cupula coch·le·ae (kock'lee·ee) [NA]. CUPULA OF THE COCHLEA.

cupula cris·tae am·pul·la·ris (kris'tee am·puh·lair'is) [NA]. CUPULA (2).

cupula of the cochlea. The apex of the osseous cochlea. NA *cupula cochleae.*

cupula of the diaphragm. The right or left dome of the diaphragm.

cupula of the pleura. The part of the pleura covering the apex of the lung in the root of the neck. NA *cupula pleurae.*

cupula op·ti·ca (op'ti·kuh). VESICULA OPTICA INVERSA.

cupula pleu·rae (plew'ree) [NA]. CUPULA OF THE PLEURA.

cu·pu·lar (kew'pew·lur) *adj.* Of or pertaining to a cupula.

cupular cecum. The blind sac which is the termination of the cochlear duct at the apex of the spiral lamina of the internal ear. NA *cecum cupulare.*

cu·pu·lo·gram (kew'pew·lo·gram) *n.* The record, consisting of two lines each for the tracing of the patient's postrotational vertigo and nystagmus during cupulometry.

cu·pu·lom·e·try (kew''pew·lom'e·tree) *n.* [*cupula* + *-metry*]. A test for vestibular function, with the patient in a rotating chair, in which the duration of vertigo and nystagmus after deceleration is recorded for various angular velocities.

Cu·ra·çao aloe (kew''ruh·saow', kew'ruh·so). Aloe obtained from *Aloe barbadensis.*

cu·rage (kewr'ij, kew·rahzh') *n.* [F., from *curer,* to cleanse]. 1. Cleansing of the eye or of an ulcerated or carious surface. 2. Clearing the uterine cavity by means of the finger, as distinguished from the use of the curet. Compare *curettage.*

cu·ran·gin (kew·ran'jin) *n.* A glycoside, $C_{48}H_{76}O_{20}$, obtained from *Curanga amara* (Scrophulariaceae); has been used as a febrifuge and vermifuge in India.

cu·ra·re (kew·rahr'ee) *n.* [Carib]. A drug of uncertain and variable composition prepared from several species of *Strychnos* and *Chondodendron* plants. Curare from *Chondodendron tomentosum* owes its characteristic action to the quaternary base *d*-tubocurarine, which paralyzes the skeletal muscles by a selective blocking of the neuromuscular junction and prevents response to nerve impulses and acetylcholine. Standardized preparations are used to control muscular spasms, particularly in the treatment of certain neurologic disorders; also to relax the skeletal muscles during anesthesia. In South America and elsewhere it is used as an arrow poison.

cu·ra·ri·mi·met·ic (kew·rahr''i·migh·met'ick) *adj.* [*curare* + *mimetic*]. Referring, or pertaining to, the action, similar to that of curare, of an agent that inhibits, at the neuromuscular junction, transmission of an impulse from a nerve to the skeletal muscle fibers that it innervates.

cu·ra·rine (kew·rah'reen, ·rin, kewr'uh·) *n.* [*curare* + *-ine*]. 1. Any of several alkaloids obtained from curare species and identified by use of a preceding letter and a following numeral, as C-curarine I and C-curarine III, obtained from the calabash variety of curare. 2. *Obsol.* TUBOCURARINE CHLORIDE.

cu·ra·ri·za·tion (kew''rahr·i·zay'shun) *n.* Administration of curare or one of its principles or derivatives to produce muscle relaxation or paralysis by blocking impulses at the myoneural junction. —**cu·ra·rize** (kew'ruh·rize) *v.*

Curatin. Trademark for doxepin, an antipruritic agent used as the hydrochloride salt.

cu·ra·tive (kew'ruh·tiv) *adj.* [MF. *curatif,* from *curer,* to heal]. Having a healing tendency; pertaining to the cure of a disease.

cur·cu·ma (kur'kyoo·muh) *n.* [Ar. *kurkum,* saffron, crocus]. The rhizome of *Curcuma longa,* of India, a plant of the Zingiberaceae, with properties similar to ginger; used as a condiment. It contains curcumin, and is occasionally employed as a yellow dye, to color ointments and other preparations.

cur·cu·min (kur'kyoo·min) *n.* Turmeric yellow, $C_{21}H_{20}O_6$, the coloring matter of curcuma. Used as an indicator; gives a brownish-red color with alkalies and a light yellow color with acids.

curd, *n.* The coagulum that separates from milk on the addition of rennin or acids.

curd soap. A soap usually made from sodium hydroxide and animal fats and oils. It is used largely for domestic purposes.

cure, *n.* & *v.* [L. *cura,* care, attention; *curare,* to take care of, attend to]. 1. Recovery from an illness, or correction of a defect, as a result of therapeutic measures. 2. *Colloq.* A course of therapeutic measures. 3. *Colloq.* A remedy. 4. To restore (a patient) to health; to bring about recovery from (an illness); to correct (a defect). 5. To process (a material) from a plastic or raw state to a hard state or finish, usually by means of heat or by a chemical treatment, such as vulcanization or polymerization.

cu·ret, cu·rette (kew·ret') *n.* & *v.* [F., from *curer,* to cleanse]. 1. An instrument, shaped like a spoon or scoop, for scraping away tissue. 2. To scape away tissue with such an instrument.

cu·ret·tage (kewr''e·tahzh') *n.* [F.]. *In surgery,* scraping of the interior of a cavity with a curet. Compare *curage.*

cu·rette·ment (kew·ret'munt) *n.* CURETTAGE.

cu·rie (kewr'ee, kew·ree') *n.* [Marie S. *Curie,* Polish-French chemist, 1867–1934; and Pierre *Curie,* French chemist, 1859–1906]. 1. Formerly, the amount of radon in equilibrium with one gram of radium. 2. That quantity of any radioactive species (radioisotope) undergoing exactly 3.700×10^{10} disintegrations per second. Abbreviated, Ci.

cu·rie·gram (kewr'ee·gram, koor'ee·gram) *n.* [*Curie* + *-gram*]. A photographic print made by radium rays, similar to a radiograph.

cu·rie·ther·a·py (kew''ree·therr'uh·pee) *n.* [Marie S. and P. *Curie*]. Treatment with ionizing radiation from a radium source.

cu·rine (kewr'een, ·in) *n.* [*curare* + *-ine*]. *l*-Bebeerine, $C_{36}H_{38}N_2O_6$, an alkaloid obtained from a kind of curare.

cu·ri·um (kew'ree·um) *n.* [Marie S. and P. *Curie*]. A metallic, artificially produced radioactive element, No. 96. Symbol, Cm.

curled, *adj.* Occurring in parallel chains of wavy strands, as the colonies of anthrax bacillus.

curled-toe paralysis. The characteristic sign of riboflavin deficiency in chickens.

Cur·ling's ulcer [T. B. *Curling,* English surgeon, 1811–1888]. Acute peptic ulcer of the upper gastrointestinal tract, associated with skin burns.

cur·rant-jelly clot or **thrombus.** A red, gelatinous blood clot formed quickly after death, which contains all of the elements of blood.

Cur·rens formula. A ruling, applied only in certain federal courts of the United States, which holds a person not responsible for a crime if, as a consequence of a mental disorder, he did not have "adequate capacity to conform his conduct to the requirements of the law." See also *Durham decision, M'Naghten rule.*

cur·rent, *n.* [OF. *curant,* from L. *currere,* to run]. 1. The flow of electricity (electrons) through a circuit; also, the rate of this flow. See also *Ohm's law.* 2. The movement or flow of a liquid or gas, as of blood in vessels, or of air through the respiratory passages.

current of injury. DEMARCATION CURRENT.

Cursch·mann's spirals (koorsh'mahnn) [H. *Curschmann,* German physician, 1846–1910]. The spiral threads of mucin contained in the small pellets expectorated in asthmatic paroxysm.

cur·sive epilepsy. A form of psychomotor epilepsy manifested by uncontrollable forward running of the patient who appears oblivious to any obstacles in his course; the running phase may be followed by a generalized seizure.

cur·va·tor coc·cy·ge·us (kur·vay'tur cock·sij'ee·us). SACROCOCCYGEUS VENTRALIS.

cur·va·tu·ra (kur"vuh·tew'ruh) *n.,* pl. & genit. sing. **curvatu·rae** (·ree) [L.]. CURVATURE.

curvatura ven·tri·cu·li major (ven·trick'yoo·lye) [NA]. GREATER CURVATURE OF THE STOMACH.

curvatura ventriculi minor [NA]. LESSER CURVATURE OF THE STOMACH.

cur·va·ture (kur'vuh·choor) *n.* [L. *curvatura,* from *curvare,* to bend]. A bending or curving; a curve.

curvature hyperopia. Hyperopia combined with astigmatism; due to changes in curvature of the cornea or lens.

curvature of the microscopic field. An aberration of the optical system which causes the image of a plane object to be curved.

curvature of the spine. Any of various kinds of persistent abnormal curvature of the vertebral column, such as kyphosis, kyphoscoliosis, lordosis, or scoliosis.

curved needle. A needle with a curve of any degree up to a full semicircle.

curve fitting. *In biometry,* the process of determining the graph line that best expresses the relationship between two variables. See also *fit.*

curve of occlusion. A curved surface that makes simultaneous contact with the major portion of the incisal and occlusal prominences of the existing teeth.

curve of Spee (shpey) [F. von *Spee,* German embryologist, 1855–1937]. The anatomic curvature of the occlusal alignment of teeth beginning at the tip of the lower cuspid and following the buccal cusps of the posterior teeth, continuing to the anterior border of the ramus of the mandible.

cur·vi·lin·ear correlation. A nonlinear relationship between two variables; a correlation in which the regression equation cannot be expressed by a straight line.

cus·co bark. The bark of *Cinchona pelletierana* (Rubiaceae), yielding several minor alkaloids of the quinoline group.

cush·ing·oid (koosh'ing·oid) *adj.* 1. Having the appearance of a patient with Cushing's syndrome as the result of therapeutic administration of corticosteroid drugs. 2. Having the habitus of a patient with Cushing's syndrome, but without other features of that disorder.

Cush·ing's incision [Harvey W. *Cushing*]. An incision shaped like a crossbow, used in subtentorial craniotomy.

Cushing's law [Harvey W. *Cushing*]. An increase of intracranial tension causes an increase in blood pressure; the blood pressure remains higher than the intracranial pressure, thus ensuring continuous cerebral circulation.

Cushing's syndrome or **disease** [Harvey W. *Cushing,* U.S. neurosurgeon, 1869–1939]. 1. A clinical condition characterized by truncal and facial adiposity, hypertension, fatigability and weakness, polycythemia, amenorrhea or impotence, hirsutism, purplish striae, purpura-like ecchymoses, edema, glycosuria, osteoporosis, and increased susceptibility to infection, due to excess of the adrenocortical hormone cortisol from adrenal cortical tumor or hyperplasia, basophilic adenoma of the pituitary, certain tumors of nonendocrine origin, or administration of adrenal cortical hormones. Compare *adrenogenital syndrome, hyperaldosteronism.* 2. The symptoms of cerebellopontine angle tumors, usually acoustic neuromas, beginning with subjective noises, followed by hearing loss, ipsilateral paralysis of the abducens and facial nerves, vertigo, nystagmus, and later other cerebellar dysfunctions.

Cushing suture [Hayward W. *Cushing,* U.S. surgeon 1854–1934]. A form of continuous Lembert suture.

Cushing ulcer. An acute ulcer or erosion of the stomach or duodenum occurring in association with central nervous system disease.

cush·ion (koosh'un) *n.* [OF. *coissin*]. *In anatomy,* an aggregate of adipose and fibrous tissue relieving pressure upon tissues lying beneath.

cushion of the epiglottis. EPIGLOTTIC TUBERCLE; a median elevation within the vestibule of the larynx.

cusp, *n.* [L. *cuspis,* point]. 1. A pointed or rounded eminence on or near the masticating surface of a tooth; designed to occlude in the sulcus of a tooth or between two teeth of the opposite dental arch. NA *tuberculum coronae dentis.* 2. One of the flaps or leaflets of a valve in the heart or a vessel. —**cus·pate** (kus'pate), **cuspat·ed** (·id) *adj.*

cus·pid (kus'pid) *adj. & n.* 1. Unicuspid; having one cusp. 2. In the human dentition, CANINE TOOTH. Contr. *bicuspid.* —**cus·pi·dal** (kus'pi·dul) *adj.*

cus·pi·date (kus'pi·date) *adj.* 1. Pertaining to or having one or more cusps. 2. Pointed; coming to a point.

cuspidate fetus. SYMPUS.

cus·pis (kus'pis) *L. n.,* genit. **cus·pidis** (kus'pi'·dis), pl. **cus·pi·des** (kus'pi·deez). CUSP.

cuspis anterior val·vae atrio·ven·tri·cu·la·ris dex·trae (val'vee ay"tree·o·ven·trick·yoo·lair'is decks'tree) [NA]. The anterior cusp of the right atrioventricular valve.

cuspis anterior valvae atrioventricularis si·nis·trae (si·nis'tree) [NA]. The anterior cusp of the left atrioventricular valve.

cuspis anterior val·vu·lae bi·cus·pi·da·lis (val'vew·lee bye·kus"pi·day'lis) [BNA]. CUSPIS ANTERIOR VALVAE ATRIOVENTRICULARIS SINISTRAE.

cuspis anterior valvulae tri·cus·pi·da·lis (trye·kus"pi·day'lis) [BNA]. CUSPIS ANTERIOR VALVAE ATRIOVENTRICULARIS DEXTRAE.

cuspis co·ro·nae den·tis (ko·ro'nee den'tis) [NA]. A small eminence or cusp on the masticating surface of a tooth.

cuspis me·di·a·lis val·vu·lae tri·cus·pi·da·lis (mee·dee·ay'lis val'vew·lee trye·kus"pi·day'lis) [BNA]. CUSPIS SEPTALIS VALVAE ATRIOVENTRICULARIS DEXTRAE.

cuspis posterior val·vae atrio·ven·tri·cu·la·ris dex·trae (val'vee ay"tree·o·ven·trick·yoo·lair'is decks'tree) [NA]. The posterior cusp of the right atrioventricular valve.

cuspis posterior valvae atrioventricularis si·nis·trae (si·nis'tree) [NA]. The posterior cusp of the left atrioventricular valve.

cuspis posterior val·vu·lae bi·cus·pi·da·lis (val'vew·lee bye·kus"pi·day'lis) [BNA]. CUSPIS POSTERIOR VALVAE ATRIOVENTRICULARIS SINISTRAE.

cuspis posterior valvulae tri·cus·pi·da·lis (trye·kus"pi·day'lis) [BNA]. CUSPIS POSTERIOR VALVAE ATRIOVENTRICULARIS DEXTRAE.

cuspis sep·ta·lis val·vae atrio·ven·tri·cu·la·ris dex·trae (sep·tay'lis val'vee ay"tree·o·ven·trick·yoo·lair'is decks'tree) [NA]. The septal cusp of the right atrioventricular valve.

cusp of Carabelli. CARABELLI'S CUSP.

cus·so (koos'o, kus') *n.* [Amharic]. BRAYERA.

cu·ta·neo·gas·tro·in·tes·ti·nal (kew·tay'nee·o·gas"tro·in·tes'ti·nul) *adj.* Involving the skin and the gastrointestinal tract.

cutaneogastrointestinal arteriolar thrombosis. DEGOS' DISEASE.

cu·ta·neo·in·tes·ti·nal (kew·tay"nee·o·in·tes'ti·nul) *adj.* Pertaining to or involving the skin and the intestine.

cutaneointestinal syndrome. DEGOS' DISEASE.

cu·ta·neo·mu·co·sal (kew"tay·nee·o·mew·ko'sul) *adj.* MUCOCUTANEOUS.

cu·ta·ne·ous (kew·tay'nee·us) *adj.* Pertaining to or involving the skin.

cutaneous anaphylaxis. An immunological response occurring 2 or 3 minutes after antigen is injected into the skin of a sensitive person; itching at the injected site is followed within a few minutes by a pale, elevated irregular wheal followed by a zone of erythema, with a complete return to normal appearance in 30 minutes.

cutaneous appendages. Organs and structures of ectodermal origin, attached to or embedded in the skin: the nails, hair, sebaceous glands, sweat glands, and mammary glands.

cutaneous calcinosis. CALCINOSIS CUTIS.

cutaneous calculus. MILIUM.

cutaneous diphtheria. Infection of the skin by *Corynebacterium diphtheriae,* usually manifested by an ulcer with a rolled edge, dirty base, and tending to bulla formation at the periphery; rarely associated with systemic manifestations.

cutaneous emphysema. SUBCUTANEOUS EMPHYSEMA.

cutaneous gland. Any gland of the skin.

cutaneous glomus. GLOMUS BODY.

cutaneous horn. An excrescence, varying in size and more or less in the shape of a miniature horn, seated upon a process that may be precancerous or an already established squamous cell carcinoma. The face, scalp, and chest are common sites for the development.

cutaneous leishmaniasis. An infection characterized by localized cutaneous granulomas with a tendency to ulceration and chronicity; caused by *Leishmania tropica,* transmitted by the bite of the sandfly *Phlebotomus.*

cutaneous muscle. A muscle having an insertion into the skin or both origin and insertion in the skin. NA *musculus cutaneus.*

cutaneous nerve. See Table of Nerves in the Appendix.

cutaneous pupillary reflex. CILIOSPINAL REFLEX.

cutaneous reaction. 1. Any change manifested in the outer layers of the skin, as in sunburn or the rash in measles. 2. The immediate reaction in the skin resulting from antigen-antibody union, such as follows the intracutaneous inoculation of foreign serum in a sensitized individual. 3. A delayed reaction at the site of introduction of the test material, such as tuberculin, based on the phenomenon of delayed hypersensitivity or specific cell mediated immunity. 4. Any reaction resulting from the directly injurious effect of inoculated material, such as diphtheria toxin in the Schick test.

cutaneous reflex. 1. Wrinkling or gooseflesh in response to irritation of the skin. 2. Any reflex, receptors for which are in the skin. See also *superficial reflex.*

cutaneous sensation. Superficial or exteroceptive sensation, comprising the modalities of light touch, pain, and temperature.

cutaneous tag. FIBROMA PENDULUM.

cutaneous test. SKIN TEST.

cutaneous tuberculosis. TUBERCULOSIS CUTIS.

cut·down, *n.* An incision through skin, superficial fascia, or other tissues, permitting access to a cavity or vessel (usually a vein) for insertion of a cannula or other instrumentation.

Cu·te·re·bra (kew″te-ree′bruh) *n.* [*cutis* + L. *terebra,* borer]. A genus of botflies, which attack especially rabbits and other rodents.

Cu·te·re·bri·dae (kew″te-ree′bri-dee) *n. pl.* A family of the Diptera, related to the botfly group. The important genera are *Cuterebra* and *Dermatobia.*

cuti- [L. *cutis*]. A combining form meaning *skin.*

cu·ti·cle (kew′ti-kul) *n.* [L. *cuticula,* dim. of *cutis*]. 1. EPONYCHIUM. 2. EPIDERMIS. 3. Any fine covering. **—cu·tic·u·lar** (kew-tick′yoo-lur) *adj.*

cu·ti·col·or (kew′ti-kul″ur) *adj.* [*cuti-* + *color*]. Simulating the color of skin; said of various ointments and powders used in the treatment of skin diseases.

cu·tic·u·la (kew-tick′yoo-luh) *n.,* pl. & genit. sing. **cuticu·lae** (-lee) [L.]. CUTICLE.

cuticula den·tis (den′tis) [NA]. ENAMEL CUTICLE (2).

cuticular plate. An oar-shaped plate associated with the supporting cells of the spiral organ (of Corti).

cuticular sulci. The many little furrows on the skin which intersect so that they bound polygonal areas. NA *sulci cutis.*

cu·tig·er·al (kew-tij′ur-ul) *adj.* [*cuti-* + L. *gerere,* to bear, + *-al*]. Made up of skin.

cutigeral cavity. The gutterlike cavity situated at the upper and inner portion of the wall of a horse's hoof.

cu·tin (kew′tin) *n.* A waxlike substance found over most of the aerial parts of vascular plants. It serves to protect the underlying cells from too rapid loss of moisture.

cu·ti·re·ac·tion (kew′tee-ree-ack″shun) *n.* CUTANEOUS REACTION.

cu·tis (kew′tis) *n.,* L. pl. **cu·tes** (-teez) [L. (rel. to Gmc. **hudiz* → E. *hide*)] [NA]. SKIN.

cutis an·se·ri·na (an-se-rye′nuh). GOOSE FLESH.

cu·ti·sec·tor (kew′ti-seck″tur) *n.* [*cuti-* + L. *sector,* cutter]. An instrument for taking small sections of skin from the living subject. Syn. *biopsy punch.*

cutis hy·per·elas·ti·ca (high″pur-e-las′ti-kuh). EHLERS-DANLOS SYNDROME.

cutis laxa (lack′suh). 1. DERMATOLYSIS. 2. DERMATOCHALASIS.

cutis mar·mo·ra·ta (mahr″mo-ray′tuh). Blue or purple mottling of the skin; seen in certain young persons as a constant phenomenon or upon exposure of the skin to cold air. Syn. *livedo reticularis, marble skin.*

cutis pen·du·la (pen′dew-luh). DERMATOLYSIS.

cutis plate. DERMATOME; the lateral part of an embryonic somite.

cutis rhom·boi·da·lis nu·chae (rom″boy-day′lis new′kee). The furrowed, leathery skin of the back of the neck caused by exposure to the sun and elements or by degenerative processes of aging. See also *sailor's skin.*

cutis ve·ra (veer′uh, vehr′uh) [L., true]. DERMIS.

cutis ver·ti·cis gy·ra·ta (vur′ti-sis jye-ray′tuh). Hypertrophy and looseness of the skin, particularly of the scalp, with a tendency to hang in folds, resulting in an appearance suggestive of the convolutions of the cerebrum or the wrinkled pate of a bulldog.

cu·ti·za·tion (kew″ti-zay′shun) *n.* Transformation of an exposed mucous membrane into corium at the mucocutaneous margins.

Cut·ler-Pow·er-Wil·der test [H. H. *Cutler,* U.S. physician, 20th century; M. H. *Power,* U.S. physician, 20th century; and R. M. *Wilder,* U.S. physician, 20th century]. A test of adrenal insufficiency (Addison's disease). A patient with adrenal insufficiency, given a diet with supplementary potassium and restricted sodium chloride, continues to excrete greater than normal amounts of sodium chloride in the urine.

cut·ting needle. A needle with a sharp edge, either curved or straight.

Cutting's colloidal mastic test. MASTIC TEST.

cu·vette, cu·vet (kew-vet′) *n.* [F., dim. of *cuve,* a tub]. 1. The absorption cell for spectrophotometry. 2. A small transparent tube or vessel, used in colorimetric determinations.

Cu·vier's canals (kuᵉv-yeʸ′) [G. L. C. *Cuvier,* French scientist, 1769–1832]. Two short vessels opening into the common trunk of the omphalomesenteric veins in the embryo, the right one later becoming the superior vena cava.

Cuvier's ducts [G. L. C. *Cuvier*]. The two common cardinal veins.

CV Abbreviation for *cardiovascular.*

C virus. A group of mosquito-borne viruses of the Bunyamwera supergroup which are found in the tropical and subtropical Western Hemisphere and produce mild disease in humans, with headache and fever.

CVP Abbreviation for *central venous pressure.*

c wave. The positive pressure wave in the atrial and venous pulse produced by bulging of the atrioventricular valves at the onset of ventricular systole, and probably in the jugular venous pulse, by an impulse transmitted from the adjacent carotid artery.

cyan-, cyano- [Gk. *kyanos*]. A combining form meaning (a) *dark blue;* (b) in chemistry, *the presence of the cyanogen group.*

cy·an·a·mide (sigh·an'uh·mide, ·mid) *n.* [*cyan-* + *amide*]. 1. Colorless deliquescent crystals, $H_2N.CN$. 2. CALCIUM CYANAMIDE.

cy·a·nate (sigh'uh·nate) *n.* The univalent radical CNO.

cy·an·eph·i·dro·sis (sigh"an·ef"i·dro'sis) *n.* [*cyan-* + *ephidrosis*]. The excretion of sweat with a blue tint.

cy·an·hem·a·tin, cy·an·haem·a·tin (sigh"an·hem'uh·tin, hee'muh·tin) *n.* [*cyan-* + *hematin*]. A pigment used in hemoglobinometry, produced by the action of acid and cyanide on hemoglobin or the heme pigments.

cy·an·he·mo·glo·bin, cy·an·hae·mo·glo·bin (sigh"an·hee'muh·glo"bin) *n.* [*cyan-* + *hemoglobin*]. A compound of hydrocyanic acid with hemoglobin formed in cases of poisoning with this acid. It gives the blood a bright red color.

cy·an·hi·dro·sis (sigh"an·hi·dro'sis) *n.* CYANEPHIDROSIS.

cy·an·ic acid (sigh·an'ick). A poisonous liquid, HCNO, stable only at low temperatures.

cy·a·nide (sigh'uh·nide) *n.* [*cyan-* + *-ide*]. 1. The univalent radical —CN. 2. Any compound containing this radical, as potassium cyanide, KCN.

cyanide goiter. A goiter produced experimentally by the administration of cyanide; associated with deficient use of the thyroid hormone by the tissues.

cy·an·met·he·mo·glo·bin, cy·an·met·hae·mo·glo·bin (sigh"an·met·hee'muh·glo"bin) *n.* [*cyan-* + *methemoglobin*]. A relatively nontoxic compound formed by the combination of cyanide and methemoglobin.

cyanmethemoglobin method. The determination of blood hemoglobin levels by conversion to the cyanmethemoglobin compound followed by measurement of the light absorption of the solution in a photoelectric colorimeter or spectrophotometer.

cyano-. See *cyan-.*

cy·a·no·chroia (sigh"uh·no·kroy'uh) *n.* [*cyano-* + *-chroia*]. Blueness of the skin. See also *cyanosis.*

cy·a·no·co·bal·a·min (sigh"uh·no·ko·bawl'uh·min, sigh·an") *n.* [*cyano-* + *cobalamin*]. Crystalline vitamin B_{12}, $C_{63}H_{88}CoN_{14}O_{14}P$, a cobalt-containing substance usually produced by the growth of suitable microbial substances, or obtained from liver; dark-red crystals or powder sparingly soluble in water. Appears to be identical with the antianemia factor of liver.

cyanocobalamin Co 57. Cyanocobalamin tagged with radioactive cobalt 57 (Co 57), which has a half-life of 270 days; used for diagnosis of pernicious anemia.

cyanocobalamin Co 60. Cyanocobalamin tagged with radioactive cobalt 60 (Co 60), which has a half-life of 5.27 years; used for diagnosis of pernicious anemia.

cy·a·no·der·ma (sigh"uh·no·dur'muh) *n.* [*cyano-* + *derma*]. Blueness of the skin. See also *cyanosis.*

cy·ano·gen (sigh·an'o·jen) *n.* [*cyano-* + *-gen*]. 1. A colorless toxic gas, NCCN, having the odor of bitter almonds. 2. The radical —CN; cyanide (1).

cy·a·no·ge·net·ic (sigh"uh·no·je·net'ick) *adj.* Capable of producing hydrocyanic acid or a cyanide.

cy·a·nol (sigh'uh·nol) *n.* ANILINE.

cy·a·no·met·he·mo·glo·bin (sigh"uh·no·met·hee'muh·glo"bin) *n.* CYANMETHEMOGLOBIN.

cy·an·o·phil (sigh·an'o·fil, sigh'uh·no·fil") *n.* [*cyano-* + *-phil*]. The blue-staining nuclear substance of cells of plants and animals.—**cy·a·no·phil·ic** (sigh"uh·no·fil'ick), **cy·a·noph·i·lous** (sigh"uh·nof'i·lus) *adj.*

cy·a·no·phose (sigh·an"o·foze, sigh'uh·no·foze") *n.* [*cyano-* + *phose*]. A blue phose.

cy·a·no·pia (sigh"uh·no'pee·uh) *n.* [*cyan-* + *-opia*]. A condition of the vision rendering all objects blue.

cy·a·nop·sia (sigh"uh·nop'see·uh) *n.* [*cyan-* + *-opsia*]. CYANOPIA.

cy·a·nop·sin (sigh"uh·nop'sin) *n.* A compound found in retinal cones, consisting of retinene$_2$ combined with opsin.

cy·a·nosed (sigh'uh·noze'd) *adj.* Affected with cyanosis.

cy·a·no·sis (sigh"uh·no'sis) *n.*, pl. **cyano·ses** (·seez) [Gk. *kyanōsis*, dark blue color]. A bluish-purple discoloration of the mucous membranes and skin, due to the presence of excessive amounts of reduced hemoglobin in capillaries, or less frequently to the presence of methemoglobin. —**cy·a·not·ic** (sigh"uh·not'ick) *adj.*

cyanotic atrophy. Atrophy, especially of the liver, accompanying prolonged passive hyperemia.

cyanotic congenital heart disease. Heart disease present at birth, producing cyanosis by virtue of a significant right-to-left shunt.

cyanotic kidney. A chronically hyperemic kidney, with resultant dilated veins, pigmentation, and some fibrosis.

Cyantin. A trademark for nitrofurantoin, a urinary antibacterial.

cy·as·ma (sigh·az'muh) *n.*, [Gk. *kyein*, to be pregnant]. *Obsol.* The peculiar pigmentation of the skin sometimes seen in pregnant women. Compare *chloasma.*

Cyasorb UV 24. A trademark for dioxybenzone, an ultraviolet screening agent.

cy·ber·net·ics (sigh"bur·net'icks) *n.* [Gk. *kybernetēs*, helmsman, + *-ics*]. The science dealing with communication and control in living and nonliving systems, including control by means of feedback mechanisms, i.e., servomechanisms. —**cybernet·ic** (·ick) *adj.*

cycl-, cyclo- [Gk. *kyklos*]. A combining form meaning (a) *circle, circular, ring, cycle;* (b) *cyclic compound;* (c) *ciliary body;* (d) *fusion.*

cy·cla·cil·lin (sigh·kluh·sil'in) *n.* A 1-aminocyclohexyl derivative of penicillin, $C_{15}H_{23}N_3O_4S$, an antibacterial agent.

Cyclaine. Trademark for hexylcaine, a local anesthetic used as the hydrochloride salt.

cy·cla·mate (sigh'kluh·mate, sick'luh·) *n.* A salt of cyclamic acid.

cy·clam·ic acid (sigh·klam'ick). Cyclohexanesulfamic acid, $C_6H_{11}NHSO_3H$, a nonnutritive sweetening agent; usually used in the form of the calcium or sodium salt.

Cyclamycin. A trademark for troleandomycin, an antibiotic substance.

cy·clan·de·late (sigh·klan'de·late) *n.* 3,3,5-Trimethylcyclohexyl mandelate, $C_{17}H_{24}O_3$, a peripheral vasodilative drug.

cy·claz·o·cine (sigh·klaz'o·seen) *n.* 3-(Cyclopropylmethyl)-1,2,3,4,5,6-hexahydro-6,11-dimethyl-2,6-methano-3-benzazocin-8-ol, $C_{18}H_{25}NO$, an analgesic drug.

cy·cle, *n.* [Gk. *kyklos*, circle]. A regular series of changes which involve a return to the original state or condition, and repetition; a succession of events or symptoms, regularly recurring in an interval of time.

cy·clec·to·my (sigh·kleck'tuh·mee, sick·leck') *n.* [*cycl-* + *-ectomy*]. Excision of part of the ciliary body.

cy·clen·ceph·a·lus (sigh"klen·sef'uh·lus, sick"len·) *n.*, pl. **cyclencepha·li** (·lye) [*cycl-* + *-encephalus*]. A monster showing cyclencephaly.

cy·clen·ceph·a·ly (sigh"klen·sef'uh·lee) *n.* [*cycl-* + *-encephaly*]. The fusion or failure of formation of the cerebral hemispheres.

cycle of generation. Haeckel's term for the successive changes through which an individual passes from its birth to the period when it is capable of reproducing its kind.

cycle of Golgi [C. *Golgi*]. ENDOGENOUS CYCLE.

cycle of Ross [R. R. *Ross*, English parasitologist, 1857–1932]. EXOGENOUS CYCLE.

cy·clic (sigh'klick, sick'lick) *adj.* [Gk. *kyklikos*, circular]. 1. Having cycles or periods of exacerbation or change; intermittent. 2. Having a self-limited course, as certain diseases. 3. Of chemical compounds: having a closed-chain or ring structure of atoms.

cyclic adenosine monophosphate. Adenosine 3′, 5′-monophosphate, a cyclic form of adenosine 5′-monophosphate, found in most animal cells and produced by the action of the enzyme adenyl cyclase on adenosine triphosphate. It mediates many of the actions of a great variety of hormones, performing the functions of the hormones at the intracellular level; it may also have an important role in brain function. A phosphodiesterase enzyme inactivates it by conversion to adenosine 5′-monophosphate. Abbreviated, cyclic AMP.

cyclic albuminuria. CYCLIC PROTEINURIA.

cyclic AMP. Abbreviation for *cyclic adenosine monophosphate.*

cyclic compound. *In chemistry,* an organic compound belonging to the closed-chain series.

cyclic fever. 1. A convulsive equivalent in which recurrent paroxysms of fever not associated with any specific cause are the most prominent symptom. 2. Any fever with a sequential pattern of appearance and disappearance.

cyclic GMP Abbreviation for *cyclic guanosine monophosphate.*

cyclic guanosine monophosphate. The cyclic form of guanosine monophosphate (= ADENYLIC ACID), analogous to cyclic adenosine monophosphate. It appears to act in antagonism to cyclic adenosine monophosphate in many cells. Abbreviated, cyclic GMP.

cyclic headache. Any periodically occurring headache, as a vascular headache or headache associated with menstruation, or as a convulsive equivalent.

cyclic hemorrhage. 1. MENORRHAGIA. 2. Menstrual bleeding of ectopic endometrial implants, as in endometriosis.

cyclic insanity. MANIC-DEPRESSIVE ILLNESS of the circular type.

cyclic neutropenia. An inherited condition which occurs in some gray or silver collies, characterized by severe periodic neutropenia and extreme susceptibility to infections. Syn. *gray collie syndrome.*

cy·cli·cot·o·my (sigh″kli·kot′uh·mee, sick″li·) *n.* CYCLOTOMY.

cyclic proteinuria. Proteinuria in which a small quantity of protein appears in the urine at particular times of the day.

cyclic vomiting. 1. Vomiting recurring at regular intervals. 2. A convulsive equivalent in which recurrent vomiting is the most prominent symptom.

cy·clir·a·mine (sigh·klirr′uh·meen) *n.* 4-[*p*-Chloro-α-(2-pyridyl)benzylidene]-1-methylpiperidine, $C_{18}H_{19}ClN_2$, an antihistaminic drug; used as the maleate salt.

cy·clit·ic (si·klit′ick) *adj.* [*cycl-* + *-itic*]. 1. Pertaining to cyclitis. 2. Pertaining to the ciliary body.

cyclitic membrane. *In ophthalmology,* an inflammatory membrane forming along the plane of the anterior vitreous face anchored on each side at the pars plana.

cy·cli·tis (sigh·klye′tis, si·) *n.* [*cycl-* + *-itis*]. Inflammation of the ciliary body, manifested by a zone of hyperemia in the sclerotic coat surrounding the cornea. It may be serous, plastic, or suppurative.

cy·cli·za·tion (sigh″kli·zay′shun, sick″li·) *n.* *In chemistry,* the formation of closed-chain or ring structures, as of atoms. —**cy·clize** (sigh′klize) *v.*

cy·cli·zine (sigh′kli·zeen) *n.* 1-(Diphenylmethyl)-4-methylpiperazine, $C_{18}H_{22}N_2$, an antinauseant; used as the hydrochloride and lactate salts.

cyclo-. See *cycl-.*

cy·clo·bar·bi·tal (sigh″klo·bahr′bi·tol, ·tal) *n.* 5-(1-Cyclohexenyl)-5-ethylbarbituric acid, $C_{12}H_{16}N_2O_3$, a hypnotic and sedative of short duration of action.

cy·clo·ben·da·zole (sigh″klo·ben′duh·zole) *n.* Methyl 5-(cyclopropylcarbonyl)-2-benzimidazolecarbamate, $C_{13}H_{13}N_3O_3$, an anthelmintic.

cy·clo·ceph·a·lus (sigh″klo·sef′uh·lus) *n.*, pl. **cyclocepha·li** (·lye) [*cyclo-* + *-cephalus*]. A congenital monster showing cyclocephaly.

cy·clo·ceph·a·ly (sigh″klo·sef′uh·lee) *n.* [*cyclo-* + *-cephaly*]. A type of cyclopia in which there is more or less complete absence of the olfactory organs, and intimate union of rudimentary eyes, situated in a single orbit.

cy·clo·cu·ma·rol (sigh″klo·koo′muh·rol) *n.* 3,4-(2′-Methyl-2′-methoxy-4′-phenyl)dihydropyranocoumarin, $C_{20}H_{18}O_4$, an anticoagulant.

cy·clo·di·al·y·sis (sigh″klo·dye·al′i·sis) *n.*, pl. **cyclodialy·ses** (·seez) [*cyclo-* + *dialysis*]. Detaching the ciliary body from the sclera in order to effect reduction of intraocular tension in certain cases of glaucoma, especially in aphakia.

cy·clo·di·a·ther·my (sigh″klo·dye′uh·thur·mee) *n.* [*cyclo-* + *diathermy*]. Destruction, by diathermy, of the ciliary body.

cy·clog·e·ny (sigh·kloj′e·nee) *n.* [*cyclo-* + *-geny*]. The life cycle or development of a microorganism, from its lowest stage to its highest and back to its basal state.

cy·clo·guan·il (sigh″klo·gwah′nil) *n.* 4,6-Diamino-1-(*p*-chlorophenyl)-1,2-dihydro-2,2-dimethyl-*s*-triazine, $C_{11}H_4ClN_5$, an antimalarial drug; used as the pamoate salt.

Cyclogyl. Trademark for cyclopentolate, a cycloplegic and mydriatic drug used as the hydrochloride salt.

cy·clo·hex·ane (sigh″klo·heck′sane) *n.* Hexahydrobenzene, C_6H_{12}, a saturated, cyclic, liquid hydrocarbon, representing a closed chain of six methylene (CH_2) groups; it occurs in some petroleums. Used as a solvent.

cy·clo·hex·a·nol (sigh″klo·heck′suh·nol) *n.* Hexahydrophenol, $C_6H_{12}O$, a widely used solvent with narcotic-like action.

cy·clo·hex·i·mide (sigh″klo·heck′si·mide) *n.* 3-[2-(3,5-Dimethyl-2-oxocyclohexyl)-2-hydroxyethyl]glutarimide, $C_{15}H_{23}NO_4$, an antibiotic produced by some strains of *Streptomyces griseus;* effective against certain yeasts and fungi.

cy·cloid (sigh′kloid) *adj.* [Gk. *kykloeidēs,* circular]. CYCLOTHYMIC.

cycloid personality. CYCLOTHYMIC PERSONALITY.

cy·clol (sigh′klol) *n.* [*cycl*ization + en*ol*ization]. A hypothetical protein structure resulting when an open polypeptide chain undergoes cyclization and enolization at the peptide linkage.

cy·clo·mas·top·a·thy (sigh′klo·mas·top′uth·ee) *n.* [*cyclo-* + *masto-* + *-pathy*]. MAMMARY DYSPLASIA.

cy·clo·meth·y·caine (sigh″klo·meth′i·kane) *n.* 3-(2-Methylpiperidino)propyl *p*-cyclohexyloxybenzoate, $C_{22}H_{33}NO_3$, a topical anesthetic agent; used as the sulfate salt.

Cyclopal. Trademark for 5-allyl-5-(2-cyclopenten-1-yl)barbituric acid, $C_{12}H_{14}N_2O_3$, a sedative and hypnotic of short duration of action.

Cyclopar. A trademark for tetracycline hydrochloride.

cy·clo·par·af·fin (sigh″klo·păr′uh·fin) *n.* A saturated cyclic hydrocarbon of the composition C_nH_{2n}.

cy·clo·pen·ta·mine (sigh″klo·pen′tuh·meen) *n.* *N*,α-Dimethylcyclopentaneëthylamine, $C_9H_{19}N$, a sympathomimetic amine used for systemic pressor and local vasoconstrictor effects; employed as the hydrochloride salt.

cy·clo·pen·tane (sigh″klo·pen′tane) *n.* The cyclic hydrocarbon C_5H_{10}, derivatives of which are moieties of many natural and synthetic compounds.

cy·clo·pen·ta·no·phen·an·threne (sigh″klo·pen·tay″no·fen·an′threen) *n.* $C_{17}H_{24}$. A hydrocarbon representing the fusion of three benzene rings and one cyclopentane ring which is the basic structure of sterols and steroids.

cy·clo·pen·thi·a·zide (sigh″klo·pen·thigh′uh·zide) *n.* 6-Chloro-3-(cyclopentylmethyl)-3,4-dihydro-2*H*-1,2,4-benzothiadiazine-7-sulfonamide 1,1-dioxide, $C_{13}H_{18}ClN_3O_4S_2$, an orally effective diuretic and antihypertensive drug.

cy·clo·pen·to·late (sigh″klo·pen′to·late) *n.* 2-Dimethylaminoethyl 1-hydroxy-α-phenylcyclopentaneacetate, $C_{17}H_{25}NO_3$, a spasmolytic agent that produces cycloplegia and mydriasis and is used for these purposes in ophthalmology; employed as the hydrochloride salt.

cyclopes. Plural of *cyclops.*

cy·clo·phen·a·zine (sigh″klo·fen′uh·zeen) *n.* 10-[3-(4-Cyclopropyl-1-piperazinyl)propyl]-2-(trifluoromethyl)phenothiazine, $C_{23}H_{26}F_3N_3S$, a tranquilizer; used as the dihydrochloride salt.

cy·clo·pho·rase (sigh″klo·fo′race, ·raze). *n.* The group of mitochondria-associated enzymes that catalyze oxidations (as in the tricarboxylic acid cycle), oxidative phosphorylation, and certain reactions of synthesis.

cy·clo·pho·ria (sigh″klo·for′ee·uh) *n.* [*cyclo-* + *-phoria*]. A tendency for the eyes to rotate around their vertical axes held in check by fusion. See also *essential cyclophoria, excyclophoria, incyclophoria, optical cyclophoria.*

cy·clo·phos·pha·mide (sigh″klo·fos′fuh·mide) *n.* *N,N*-Bis(2-chloroethyl)-*N′*-3-(hydroxypropyl)phosphordiamidic acid cyclic ester, $C_7H_{15}Cl_2N_2O_2P$, a cyclic phosphamide of nitrogen mustard; used as an alkylating type of antineoplastic agent.

cy·clo·phre·nia (sigh″klo·free′nee·uh) *n.* [*cyclo-* + *-phrenia*]. CYCLOTHYMIA. —**cyclo·phren·ic** (·fren′ick) *adj.*

cy·clo·pia (sigh·klo′pee·uh) *n.* [*cycl-* + *-opia*]. A large group of terata; characterized externally by fusion of the orbits and various degrees of fusion of the eyes; internally by severe defects of the facial skeleton and brain. A proboscis may or may not be present.

cy·clo·ple·gia (sigh″klo·plee′jee·uh) *n.* [*cyclo-* + *-plegia*]. Paralysis of ciliary muscles of the eyes.

cy·clo·ple·gic (sigh″klo·plee′jick) *adj.* & *n.* 1. Causing temporary paralysis of the ciliary muscle. 2. Any agent that causes temporary paralysis of the ciliary muscle and the muscles of accommodation, such as atropine, homatropine, and other parasympatholytic compounds, used to facilitate ophthalmoscopic examination and refraction. See also *mydriatic.*

cy·clo·pro·pane (sigh″klo·pro′pane) *n.* [*cyclo-* + *propane*]. Trimethylene, C_3H_6, a saturated cyclic hydrocarbon gas having an odor of petroleum benzin; a potent and explosive, but relatively nonirritating and nontoxic inhalation anesthetic which can be administered with a high concentration of oxygen.

cy·clops (sigh′klops) *n.*, pl. **cy·clo·pes** (sigh·klo′peez) [Gk. *Kyklōps,* a one-eyed monster]. An individual with a single eye or congenital fusion of the two eyes into one (synophthalmus).

Cyclops, *n.* A genus of minute crustaceans having a large, median eye; widely distributed throughout fresh and salt waters, but found most commonly in still water. Species have been found to be intermediate hosts of *Dracunculus medinesis, Diphyllobothrium latum, Drepanidotaenia lanceolata,* and *Gnathostoma spinigerum.*

cy·clo·scope (sigh′klo·skope) *n.* [*cyclo-* + *-scope*]. 1. An instrument for determining the width of the field of vision. 2. A device for measuring velocity of rotation.

cy·clo·ser·ine (sigh″klo·serr′een, ·seer′een) *n.* D-4-Amino-3-isoxazolidinone, $C_3H_6N_2O_2$, an antibiotic formed in cultures of several *Streptomyces* species. Used mainly in the treatment of tuberculosis and also in some cases of urinary tract infections.

cy·clo·sis (sigh·klo′sis) *n.*, pl. **cyclo·ses** (·seez) [Gk. *kyklōsis,* surrounding, encirclement]. Streaming of protoplasm; occurs in certain plant cells.

Cyclospasmol. Trademark for cyclandelate, a peripheral vasodilator.

cy·clo·stage (sigh′klo·staij) *n.* [*cyclo-* + *stage*]. A stage in the development of bacteria characterized by coccal and coccoid elements; it represents gonidial forms. If favorable growth conditions continue, these bodies may, by division, return to the higher, or original, stage.

cy·clo·stome (sigh′klo·stome) *n.* [NL. *Cyclostomi,* from *cyclo-* + Gk. *stoma,* mouth]. Any member of the Cyclostomi, comprising lampreys and hagfishes, the most primitive living vertebrates; distinguished from all others in having no jaws.

cy·clo·thi·a·zide (sigh″klo·thigh′uh·zide) *n.* 6-Chloro-3,4-dihydro-3-(5-norbornen-2-yl)-2*H*-1,2,4-benzothiadiazine-7-sulfonamide 1,1-dioxide, $C_{14}H_{16}ClNO_4S_2$, an orally effective diuretic and antihypertensive drug.

cy·clo·thyme (sigh′klo·thime) *n.* An individual with a cyclothymic personality.

cy·clo·thy·mia (sigh″klo·thigh′mee·uh) *n.* [*cyclo-* + *-thymia*]. A condition marked by alternating periods of elation and depression. See also *manic-depressive illness.*

cy·clo·thy·mi·ac (sigh″klo·thigh′mee·ack) *n.* CYCLOTHYME.

cy·clo·thy·mic (sigh″klo·thigh′mick) *adj.* & *n.* 1. Pertaining to or characterized by cyclothymia. 2. CYCLOTHYME.

cyclothymic personality. *In psychiatry,* a disposition marked by alternations of mood between elation and depression out of proportion to apparent external events and rather stimulated by internal factors; it may be hypomanic, depressed, or alternating.

cy·clo·tia (sigh·klo′shuh, ·shee·uh) *n.* [*cycl-* + *ot-* + *-ia*]. Cyclopia associated with more or less complete absence of the lower jaw (agnathia) and approximation or fusion of the ears (synotia).

cy·clo·tome (sigh′klo·tome) *n.* [*cyclo-* + *-tome*]. A knife used in cyclotomy.

cy·clot·o·my (sigh·klot′uh·mee, si·) *n.* [*cyclo-* + *-tomy*]. An operation for the relief of glaucoma, consisting of an incision through the ciliary body.

cy·clo·tron (sigh′klo·tron) *n.* [*cyclo-* + *-tron*]. A device for imparting high speeds to protons or deuterons by a combination of a constant powerful magnet and an alternating high-frequency charge. These high-speed particles can be directed to a target in order to produce neutrons, or they can be made to bombard various substances in order to make them artificially radioactive.

cyclotron cataract. A type of irradiation cataract.

cy·clo·tro·pia (sigh″klo·tro′pee·uh) *n.* [*cyclo-* + *-tropia*]. ESSENTIAL CYCLOPHORIA.

cy·clo·tus (sigh·klo′tus) *n.* An individual with cyclotia.

Cyclural. A trademark for hexobarbital.

cy·cri·mine (sigh′kri·meen) *n.* α-Cyclopentyl-α-phenyl-1-piperidinepropanol, $C_{19}H_{29}NO$, an antiparkinsonian drug; used as the hydrochloride salt.

cy·do·ni·um (sigh·do″nee·um) *n.* [L. *cydonia,* quince]. The seeds of the quince, *Cydonia oblonga;* employed mainly for the bland demulcent mucilage contained in the covering.

cyesio- [Gk. *kyēsis*]. A combining form meaning *pregnancy.*

cy·e·si·og·no·sis (sigh·ee″see·og·no′sis) *n.*, pl. **cyesiogno·ses** (·seez) [*cyesio-* + *-gnosis*]. Diagnosis of pregnancy.

cy·esi·ol·o·gy (sigh·ee″see·ol′uh·jee) *n.* [*cyesio-* + *-logy*]. The science of gestation in its medical aspects.

cy·e·sis (sigh·ee′sis) *n.*, pl. **cye·ses** (·seez) [Gk. *kyēsis*]. PREGNANCY.

cy·hep·ta·mide (sigh·hep′tuh·mide) *n.* 10,11-Dihydro-5*H*-dibenzo[*a,d*]cycloheptene-5-carboxamide, $C_{16}H_{15}NO$, an anticonvulsant drug.

Cyl. An abbreviation for (a) *cylinder;* (b) *cylindrical lens.*

Cylert. A trademark for pemoline.

cyl·in·der (sil′in·dur) *n.* [Gk. *kylindros,* cylinder, roller]. 1. An elongated body of the same transverse diameter throughout and circular on transverse section. 2. A cylindrical cast. 3. CYLINDRICAL LENS. Abbreviated, C., Cyl. —**cy·lin·dric** (si·lin′drick), **cylin·dri·cal** (·dri·kul) *adj.*

cylindr-, cylindro- [Gk. *kylindros*]. A combining form meaning *cylinder, cylindrical.*

cylindrical aneurysm. An aneurysm having a cylindrical shape, commonly seen in dissecting aneurysm.

cylindrical bougie. A bougie that is circular in cross section.

cylindrical bronchiectasis. Uniform dilatation of bronchi.

cylindrical cell. COLUMNAR CELL.

cylindrical-cell carcinoma. ADENOCARCINOMA.

cylindrical epithelium. COLUMNAR EPITHELIUM.

cylindrical lens. A minus or plus lens, with a plane surface in one axis and a concave or convex surface in the axis at right angles to the first. Abbreviated, C., Cyl.

cylindrical syphiloma. A rare growth in a segment of the urethra attributed to syphilis, occurring as a regular, cylindrical mass composed mainly of sclerotic tissue.

cylindric aneurysm. CYLINDRICAL ANEURYSM.

cy·lin·dri·form (si·lin′dri·form) *adj.* [*cylindr-* + *-iform*]. Shaped like a cylinder.

cyl·in·droid (sil′in·droid) *adj.* & *n.* [*cylindr-* + *-oid*]. 1. Resembling a cylinder or tube, i.e., resembling a cylinder with elliptic right sections. 2. One of the bodies sometimes seen on microscopical examination of urine, which resemble hyaline casts but differ by tapering to a slender tail; they have the same significance as casts.

cyl·in·dro·ma (sil″in·dro′muh) *n.*, pl. **cylindromas, cylindroma·ta** (·tuh) [*cylindr-* + *-oma*]. A tumor composed of groups of polygonal epithelial cells surrounded by bands of hyalinized stroma, forming cylinders of cells which give the tumor its name. In the skin, cylindromas are benign hamartomatous masses; in the respiratory tract and salivary glands, they are locally aggressive tumors which occasionally metastasize.

cyl·in·dro·sis (sil″in·dro′sis) *n.*, pl. **cylindro·ses** (·seez) [*cylindr-* + *-osis*]. A type of articulation produced by the approximation of bones on the sides of a cleft or groove in such a manner as to form a tube or canal which contains blood vessels, nerves, or a duct, as the inferior orbital fissure.

cyl·in·dru·ria (sil″in·droo′ree·uh) *n.* [*cylindr-* + *-uria*]. The presence of casts or cylindroids in the urine.

cyl·lo·so·ma (sil″o·so′muh) *n.*, pl. **cyllosomas, cyllosoma·ta** (·tuh) [Gk. *kyllos*, deformed, + *soma*]. A variety of abdominal fissure (gastroschisis) in which a lateral eventration occupies principally the lower portion of the abdomen, with absence or imperfect development of the lower extremity on that side.

cyl·lo·so·mus (sil″o·so′mus) *n.*, pl. **cylloso·mi** (·mye). An individual with cyllosoma.

cy·mar·in (sigh·mahr′in, si·) *n.* A glycoside, $C_{30}H_{44}O_9$, from apocynum, which on hydrolysis yields cymarose and strophanthidin. It has been used as a cardiac tonic and diuretic.

cy·mar·ose (sigh·mahr′oce) *n.* 3-Methyldigitoxose, $C_7H_{14}O_4$; the sugar resulting when certain cardioactive glycosides, as cymarin, undergo hydrolysis.

cym·ba (sim′buh) *n.* [Gk. *kymbē*, boat]. *In biology*, a boat-shaped sponge spicule.

cymba con·chae (kong′kee) [NA]. The upper part of the concha of the ear, above the root of the helix.

cym·bi·form (sim′bi·form) *adj. In biology*, boat-shaped.

cymbo- [Gk. *kymbē*, boat]. A combining form meaning *boat-shaped.*

cym·bo·ceph·a·ly (sim″bo·sef′uh·lee) *n.* [*cymbo-* + *-cephaly*]. SCAPHOCEPHALY. —**cymbo·ce·phal·ic** (·se·fal′ick), **cymbo·ceph·a·lous** (·sef′uh·lus) *adj.*

cy·mene (sigh′meen) *n.* 1-Methyl-4-isopropylbenzene, $C_{10}H_{14}$, a hydrocarbon that occurs in species of caraway, thyme, and other volatile oils. —**cy·mic** (·mick) *adj.*

cy·me·nyl (sigh′me·nil) *n.* The radical $C_{10}H_{13}$—, derived from cymene.

cy·mol (sigh′mol) *n.* CYMENE.

cy·myl (sigh′mil) *n.* CYMENYL.

cyn-, cyno- [Gk. *kyōn, kynos*]. A combining form meaning *dog.*

cy·nan·che (si·nang′kee, sigh·) *n.* [Gk. *kynanchē*, dog-quinsy]. *Obsol.* Severe sore throat, with choking; often due to diphtheria. Syn. *synanche.*

cyn·an·thro·pia (sin″an·thro′pee·uh) *n.* CYNANTHROPY.

cy·nan·thro·py (si·nan′thro·pee, sigh·) *n.* [Gk. *kynanthrōpos*, from *kyn-*, dog, + *anthrōpos*, man.]. A psychotic disorder in which the patient believes himself to be a dog and imitates the actions of one.

cyn·ic (sin′ick) *adj.* [Gk. *kynikos*, doglike]. Like a snarling or grinning dog, as spasm of the facial muscles seen in risus sardonicus.

cyno-. See *cyn-.*

cyno·ceph·a·lous (sin″o·sef′uh·lus, sigh″no·) *adj.* [Gk. *kynokephalos*]. Having a head shaped like a dog's.

cyn·o·dont (sin′o·dont, sigh′no·) *adj.* [Gk. *kynodous, kynodontos*, fang, canine tooth]. 1. Characterized by teeth with small pulp chambers. 2. One of a group of prehistoric reptiles having skulls and teeth relatively similar to those of mammals; considered possibly ancestral to mammals.

Cyn·o·glos·sum (sin″o·glos′um, sigh″no·) *n.* [L., from Gk. *kynoglōsson*, hound's-tongue]. A genus of plants of the Boraginaceae. The powdered herb, *Cynoglossum officinale*, common hound's-tongue, has been used as a demulcent and sedative.

cyn·o·lys·sa (sin″o·lis′uh) *n.* [Gk. *kynolyssos*, from *kyno-*, dog, + *lyssa*, madness]. RABIES.

cyno·pho·bia (sin″of·fo′bee·uh, sigh″no·) *n.* [*cyno-* + *phobia*]. 1. An abnormal fear of dogs. 2. A neurosis, usually hysterical in nature, reproducing the symptoms of rabies, sometimes precipitated by the bite of a dog.

Cy̆no·pi·the·cus (sin″o·pith·ee′kus, ·pith′e·kus, sigh′no·) *n.* [*cyno-* + *Gk. pithēkos*, monkey, ape]. A monotypic genus of Cercopithecidae comprising the so-called black apes.

cyn·o·rex·ia (sin″o·reck′see·uh) *n.* [*cyn-* + *-orexia*]. BULIMIA.

cyn·u·ren·ic acid (sin″yoo·ren′ick). A crystalline acid found in dog's urine. It is a decomposition product of proteins.

cyn·u·rin (sin′yoo·rin) *n.* A base derived from cynurenic acid.

cy·o·pho·ria (sigh″o·fo′ree·uh) *n.* [Gk. *kyophoria*, from *kyos*, fetus]. PREGNANCY.

cy·oph·o·rin (sigh·off′o·rin) *n.* KYESTEIN.

cy·ot·ro·phy (sigh·ot′ruh·fee) *n.* [Gk. *kyos*, fetus, + *-trophy*]. Nutrition of the fetus.

cy·pen·a·mine (sigh·pen′uh·meen) *n.* 2-Phenylcyclopentylamine, $C_{11}H_{15}N$, an antidepressant drug; used as the hydrochloride salt.

Cy·pe·rus (sigh·peer′us, sigh′pur·us) *n.* [Gk. *kypeiron*]. A genus of sedges, species of which have been used medicinally.

cy·pi·o·nate (sigh′pee·o·nate, sigh·pee′o·nate) *n.* Any salt or ester of cyclopentanepropionic acid, $C_5H_9CH_2$-CH_2COOH; a cyclopentanepropionate.

cy·praz·e·pam (sigh·praz′e·pam) *n.* 7-Chloro-2-[(cyclopropylmethyl)amino]-5-phenyl-3H-1,4-benzodiazepine 4-oxide, $C_{19}H_{18}ClN_3O$, a tranquilizer.

cy·pri·do·pho·bia (sigh″pri·do·fo′bee·uh, si·prid″o·) *n.* [Gk. *Kypris, Kypridos*, Venus, + *phobia*]. An abnormal fear of acquiring a venereal disease or of coitus for that reason.

cyp·ri·pe·di·um (sip″ri·pee′dee·um) *n.* The dried rhizome and roots of lady's slipper, *Cypripedium pubescens*, containing a volatile oil, resins, and tannin. Has been used as an antispasmodic and stimulant tonic.

cy·pro·hep·ta·dine (sigh″pro·hep′tuh·deen, sip″ro·) *n.* 1-Methyl-4-(5-dibenzo[*a,e*]cycloheptatrienylidene)piperidine, $C_{21}H_{21}N$, an antagonist of histamine and serotonin; used, as the hydrochloride salt, to relieve pruritus.

cy·pro·li·dol (sigh·pro′li·dol) *n.* Diphenyl[2-(4-pyridyl)cyclopropyl]methanol, $C_{21}H_{19}NO$, an antidepressant drug; used as the hydrochloride salt.

cy·pro·quin·ate (sigh″pro·kwin′ate) *n.* Ethyl 6,7-bis(cyclopropylmethoxy)-4-hydroxy-3-quinolinecarboxylate, $C_{20}H_{23}NO_5$, a coccidiostatic agent.

cy·pro·ter·one (sigh·pro′tur·ohn) *n.* 6-Chloro-17-hydroxy-1α,2α-methylenepregna-4,6-diene-3,20-dione, $C_{22}H_{27}$-ClO_3, a steroid with antiandrogen activity; used as the acetate ester.

cy·prox·im·ide (sigh·prock′si·mide) *n.* 1-(*p*-Chlorophenyl)-1,2-cyclopropanedicarboximide, $C_{11}H_8ClNO_2$, a tranquilizer and antidepressant drug.

Cyprus fever. BRUCELLOSIS.

Cyredin. A trademark for cyanocobalamin.

cy·ren A (sigh′ren). DIETHYLSTILBESTROL.

cyrt-, cyrto- [Gk. *kyrtos*, bulging, convex]. A combining form meaning *bent, curved.*

cyrto-. See *cyrt-.*

cyr·to·ceph·a·lus (sur″to·sef′uh·lus) *n.*, pl. **cyrtocepha·li** (·lye) [*cyrto-* + *-cephalus*]. An individual having a skull that is deformed or distorted in some manner.

cyr·to·cor·y·phus (sur″to·kor′i·fus) *n.* [*cyrto-* + *Gk. koryphē*, crown of the head, + *-us*]. A person having a skull with parietal bones markedly convex in the midsagittal plane. The absolute convexity is measured by the parietal angle of 122 to 131°.

cyr·to·graph (sur'to·graf) *n.* [*cyrto-* + *-graph*]. An instrument used to measure and record the curves of the chest and head.

cyr·toid (sur''toid) *adj.* [*cyrt-* + *-oid*]. Resembling a hump or swelling.

cyr·tom·e·ter (sur·tom'e·tur) *n.* [*cyrto-* + *-meter*]. An instrument for measuring or delineating the curves of parts of the body. Used to demonstrate the dilation and deformation of the chest in certain diseases, or to measure the shape and size of the head. —**cyrtome·try** (·tree) *n.*

cyr·to·me·to·pus (sur''to·met'o·pus) *n.* [*cyrto-* + Gk. *metōpon*, forehead, + *-us*]. A skull with a highly convex frontal bone, or a frontal angle of 120 to 130°.

cyr·to·pis·tho·cra·ni·us (surt''o·pis''tho·kray'nee·us) *n.* [*cyrt-* + *Gk. opisthokranion*, the back part of the skull, + *-us*]. A skull with a very convex occipital bone, or with an occipital angle of 117 to 139.9°.

cyr·to·sis (sur·to'sis) *n.*, pl. **cyrto·ses** (·seez) [Gk. *kyrtōsis*]. KYPHOSIS.

cyr·tu·ran·us (surt''yoo·ran'us, ·ray'nus) *n.* [*cyrt-* + *Gk. ouranos*, roof of the mouth]. A skull with a palate highly arched longitudinally, or with a uranal angle of 132 to 147°.

-cyst [Gk. *kystis*]. A combining form meaning *bladder.*

cyst-, cysti-, cysto- [Gk. *kystis*]. A combining form meaning (a) *gallbladder;* (b) *urinary bladder;* (c) *pouch;* (d) *cyst.*

cyst, *n.* [Gk. *kystis,* bladder]. An enclosed space within a tissue or organ, lined by epithelium and usually filled with fluid or other material.

cyst·ad·e·no·car·ci·no·ma (sist·ad''e·no·kahr·si·no'muh) *n.* An adenocarcinoma in which there is prominent cyst formation.

cyst·ad·e·no·fi·bro·ma (sist·ad''e·no·figh·bro'muh) *n.* [*cyst-* + *adenofibroma*]. A fibroadenoma containing one or more cysts.

cyst·ad·e·no·ma (sist''ad·e·no'muh) *n.* An adenoma containing one or more cysts.

cystadenoma ada·man·ti·num (ad''uh·man'ti·num, ·man·tye'). CYSTIC ADAMANTINOMA.

cystadenoma cy·lin·dro·cel·lu·la·re cel·loi·des ova·rii (si·lin''dro·sel·yoo·lair'ee sel·oy'deez o·vair'ee·eye). PSEUDOMUCINOUS CYSTADENOMA.

cystadenoma pa·pil·lif·er·um (pap''i·lif'ur·um). An adenoma containing cysts with papillae on the inner aspect of the cyst walls.

cyst·ad·e·no·sar·co·ma (sist·ad''e·no·sahr·ko'muh) *n.* [*cyst-* + *adenosarcoma*]. A cystic malignant mixed mesodermal tumor, including both glandular and supportive tissue elements.

cys·tal·gia (sis·tal'jee·uh) *n.* [*cyst-*, bladder, + *-algia,* pain]. Pain in the urinary bladder.

Cystamin. A trademark for methenamine, a urinary antiseptic.

cys·ta·thi·o·nine (sis''tuh·thigh'o·neen) *n.* A mixed thio ether, formed from homocysteine and serine as an intermediate in the conversion of methionine to cysteine.

cys·ta·thi·o·nin·uria (sis''tuh·thigh''o·nin·yoo'ree·uh) *n.* [*cystathionine* + *-uria*]. An inborn error of metabolism in which there is a deficiency of the cystathionine cleavage enzyme, resulting in large amounts of cystathionine in the urine and occasionally slight elevation in blood; manifested clinically by mental retardation, thrombocytopenia, acidosis, and sometimes acromegaly; probably transmitted as a homozygous recessive trait.

cyst·ec·ta·sia (sis''teck·tay'zhuh, ·zee·uh) *n.* [*cyst-* + *ectasia*]. Dilatation of the neck of the bladder.

cys·tec·ta·sy (sis·teck'tuh·see) *n.* CYSTECTASIA.

cys·tec·to·my (sis·teck'tuh·mee) *n.* [*cyst-* + *-ectomy*]. 1. Excision of the gallbladder, or part or all of the urinary bladder. 2. Removal of a cyst. 3. Removal of a piece of the anterior capsule of the lens for the extraction of a cataract.

cys·te·ine (sis'tee·een, ·in, sis·tee'in) *n.* 2-Amino-3-mercaptopropanoic acid, $HSCH_2CH(NH_2)COOH$, obtained by reduction of cystine and important as a constituent of many proteins.

cysteine desulfurase. An enzyme that catalyzes the hydrolysis of cysteine to pyruvic acid, ammonia, and hydrogen sulfide.

cys·te·in·yl (sis''tee·in'il) *n.* The univalent radical, $HSCH_2CH(NH_2)CO$, of the amino acid cysteine.

cysti-. See *cyst-.*

cys·tic (sis'tick) *adj.* [*cyst-* + *-ic*]. 1. Pertaining to or resembling a cyst. 2. Of or pertaining to the urinary bladder or to the gallbladder.

cystic acne. Acne distinguished by the formation of cysts containing purulent or gelatinous material.

cystic adamantinoma. An ameloblastoma containing one or more cysts.

cystic adenoma. An adenoma with one or more foci of cystic change.

cystic artery. The artery supplying the gallbladder; originates in the right branch of the proper hepatic artery. NA *arteria cystica.*

cystic bile. Bile stored in the gallbladder for some time; may be up to 10 times more concentrated than C bile.

cystic calculus. A calculus in the urinary bladder or in the gallbladder.

cystic cataract. MORGAGNIAN CATARACT.

cystic degeneration. Any form of degeneration with cyst formation.

cystic disease. 1. CYSTIC DISEASE OF THE BREAST. 2. CYSTIC FIBROSIS OF THE PANCREAS.

cystic disease of the breast. A condition affecting women, usually in their thirties or forties, characterized by the rapid development in the involuting breast of one or more fairly large cysts which can sometimes be transilluminated. At operation the cysts often show a thin blue dome and contain serous fluid. Syn. *chronic cystic mastitis, cystic mastopathy, fibrocystic disease.*

cystic duct or **canal.** The duct of the gallbladder. NA *ductus cysticus.* See also Plate 13.

cystic endometriosis. A focus of endometriosis which has undergone cavitation.

cysticerci. Plural of *cysticercus.*

cys·ti·cer·coid (sis''ti·sur'koid) *n.* [*cysticercus* + *-oid*]. A larval tapeworm that has a slightly developed bladder and a solid posterior; a stage in the life cycle of *Hymenolepis nana.* Compare *cysticercus.*

cys·ti·cer·co·sis (sis''ti·sur·ko'sis) *n.*, pl. **cysticerco·ses** (·seez) [*cysticercus* + *-osis*]. Infection of man with *Taenia solium* in the larval stages, resulting in invasion of striated muscle, brain, and many other tissues; manifested by fever, myalgia, and neurologic disturbances.

cys·ti·cer·cus (sis''ti·sur'kus) *n.*, pl. **cysticer·ci** (·sigh) [*cysti-* + *Gk. kerkos,* tail]. The larval tapeworm; develops in man after ingestion of the ova of *Taenia solium* or *T. saginata.* Compare *cysticercoid.*

Cysticercus, *n. Obsol.* A genus to which bladder worms were assigned before it was discovered that they were larval tapeworms. *Cysticercus cellulosae,* for example, is the larva of *Taenia solium* and *C. bovis* is that of *T. saginata.*

cystic fibrosis. CYSTIC FIBROSIS OF THE PANCREAS.

cystic fibrosis of the pancreas. A generalized heritable disease of unknown etiology, associated with dysfunction of exocrine and eccrine glands, including mucus-producing glands; observed chiefly in infants, children, and adolescents; manifested mainly by elevated sweat electrolyte concentration, absence of pancreatic enzymes with the clinical appearance of the celiac syndrome, and evidence of chronic lung disease; transmitted as a Mendelian recessive trait. Syn. *mucoviscidosis.*

cystic fossa. A depression on the lower surface of the right lobe of the liver, in which the gallbladder is situated. NA *fossa vesicae felleae.*

cystic goiter. Any thyroid disease accompanied by cysts or cavities; usually represents retrogressive cavity formation in nodular hyperplasia (nodular goiter).

cystic hernia. BLADDER HERNIA.

cystic hygroma. HYGROMA.

cystic kidney. A kidney containing one to several cysts, usually unilateral.

cystic lymphangioma. HYGROMA.

cystic mastitis. CYSTIC DISEASE OF THE BREAST.

cystic mastopathy. CYSTIC DISEASE OF THE BREAST.

cystic mole. HYDATIDIFORM MOLE.

cystic plexus. A nerve plexus near the gallbladder.

cystic teratoma. A teratoma containing one or more cysts, such as a hairy cyst of the ovary.

cystic triangle. TRIANGLE OF CALOT.

cystic tumor of a tendon sheath. GANGLION (2).

cys·ti·form (sis'ti·form) *adj.* [*cyst-* + *-iform*]. Having the form of a cyst or bladder; CYSTOMORPHOUS.

cystinaemia. CYSTINEMIA.

cys·tine (sis'teen, ·tin) *n.* Dicysteine, $(—SCH_2CHNH_2\text{-}COOH)_2$, an amino acid component of many proteins, especially keratin. It may be reduced to cysteine.

cys·tine-ly·sin·uria (sis''teen·lye''sin·yoo'ree·uh) *n.* [*cystine* + *lysine* + *-uria*]. An inborn defect in renal tubular reabsorption, with the presence of excess amounts of cystine and dibasic amino acids in the urine; manifested clinically by the presence of renal calculi. Three types have been described: type I in which cystine and dibasic amino acids are poorly absorbed by the intestine; type II in which only the dibasic amino acids are poorly absorbed; and type III in which there is normal intestinal absorption of amino acids.

cys·ti·ne·mia, cys·ti·nae·mia (sis''ti·nee'mee·uh) *n.* [*cystine* + *-emia*]. The occurrence of cystine in the blood.

cystine storage disease. CYSTINOSIS.

cys·ti·no·sis (sis''ti·no'sis) *n.*, pl. **cystino·ses** (·seez). The form of the Fanconi syndrome in which cystinuria and storage of cystine crystals in the internal organs are prominent features. See also *cystinuria.*

cys·ti·nu·ria (sis''ti·new'ree·uh) *n.* [*cystine* + *-uria*]. A congenital and hereditary anomaly of renal tubular function, in which there is impaired reabsorption of cystine, lysine, arginine, and ornithine, which may result clinically in the formation of urinary calculi composed of almost pure cystine but no other disability; transmitted as a recessive or incompletely recessive trait. See also *cystinosis.*

cys·ti·tis (sis·tye'tis) *n.*, pl. **cys·tit·i·des** (sis·tit'i·deez) [*cyst-* + *-itis*]. Inflammation of the urinary bladder.

cystitis cys·ti·ca (sis'ti·kuh). Chronic inflammation of the urinary bladder characterized by the presence of minute translucent mucus-containing submucosal cysts.

cystitis em·phy·se·ma·to·sa (em''fi·sem·uh·to'suh, ·seem·uh·to'suh). Cystitis in which cystic spaces in the urinary bladder wall are filled with gas; this may result from bacterial fermentation of sugar in the urine, as in diabetes or after glucose infusion.

cystitis fol·lic·u·la·ris (fol·ick''yoo·lair'is). Cystitis in which there are lymphoid nodules or masses of lymphoid cells beneath the epithelium.

cystitis glan·du·la·ris (glan''dew·lair'is). A type of chronic cystitis in which there is metaplastic transformation of nests of transitional epithelium into columnar mucus-secreting epithelium.

cys·ti·tome (sis'ti·tome) *n.* CYSTOTOME.

cys·tit·o·my (sis·tit'uh·mee) *n.* CYSTOTOMY.

cysto-. See *cyst-.*

cys·to·bu·bono·cele (sis''to·bew·bon'o·seel) *n.* [*cysto-* + *bubonocele*]. Hernia of the urinary bladder through the inguinal ring.

cys·to·car·ci·no·ma (sis''to·kahr''si·no'muh) *n.* [*cysto-* + *carcinoma*]. CYSTADENOCARCINOMA.

cys·to·cele (sis'to·seel) *n.* [*cysto-* + *-cele*]. Herniation of the urinary bladder into the vagina.

cys·to·co·los·to·my (sis''to·ko·los'tuh·mee) *n.* [*cysto-* + *colostomy*]. CHOLECYSTOCOLOSTOMY.

cys·to·dyn·ia (sis''to·din'ee·uh) *n.* [*cyst-* + *-odynia*]. CYSTALGIA.

cys·to·en·tero·cele (sis''to·en'tur·o·seel) *n.* [*cysto-* + *entero-* + *-cele*]. Herniation of the urinary bladder and intestine, usually into the vagina.

cyst of a joint capsule. GANGLION (2).

cyst of a semilunar cartilage. GANGLION (2).

cys·to·fi·bro·ma (sis''to·figh·bro'muh) *n.* A fibroma containing cysts.

cystofibroma pap·il·la·re (pap''i·lair'ee). CYSTOSARCOMA PHYLLODES.

Cystogen. A trademark for methenamine, a urinary antiseptic.

cys·to·gen·e·sis (sis''to·jen'e·sis) *n.*, pl. **cystogene·ses** (·seez). The formation or genesis of cysts.

cys·to·gen·ia (sis''to·jen'ee·uh) *n.* CYSTOGENESIS.

Cystografin. A trademark for diatrizoate meglumine, a radiologic contrast agent.

cys·to·gram (sis'to·gram) *n.* [*cysto-* + *-gram*]. 1. A radiograph of the urinary bladder made after the injection of a contrast medium. 2. A radiograph for demonstration of cysts.

cys·tog·ra·phy (sis·tog'ruh·fee) *n.* [*cysto-* + *-graphy*]. Radiography of the urinary bladder after the injection of a contrast medium or contrast media. —**cys·to·graph·ic** (·graf'ick) *adj.*

cys·toid (sis'toid) *adj. & n.* [*cyst-* + *-oid*]. 1. Having the form or appearance of a bladder or cyst. 2. Composed of a collection of cysts. 3. PSEUDOCYST.

cystoid degeneration of the retina. A condition in which cystic spaces are found in the retina. See also *Blessig-Ivanov cystoid degeneration of the retina.*

Cystokon. A trademark for acetrizoate sodium, a radiologic contrast agent.

cys·to·li·thec·to·my (sis''to·li·theck'tuh·mee) *n.* [*cysto-* + *lithectomy*]. CYSTOLITHOTOMY.

cys·to·li·thi·a·sis (sis''to·li·thigh'uh·sis) *n.*, pl. **cystolithia·ses** (·seez) [*cysto-* + *lithiasis*]. Calculi, or a calculus, in the urinary bladder.

cys·to·li·thot·o·my (sis''to·li·thot'uh·mee) *n.* [*cysto-* + *lithotomy*]. Surgical removal of a calculus from the urinary bladder.

cys·to·ma (sis·to'muh) *n.*, pl. **cystomas, cystoma·ta** (·tuh) [*cyst-* + *-oma*]. A cystic mass, especially in or near the ovary; may be neoplastic or inflammatory, or due to retention.

cystoma ova·rii pseu·do·mu·ci·no·sum (o·vair'ee·eye sue''do·mew·si·no'sum). MUCINOUS CYSTADENOMA.

cys·tom·e·ter (sis·tom'e·tur) *n.* [*cysto-* + *-meter*]. An instrument used to determine pressure and capacity in the urinary bladder under standard conditions. —**cystome·try** (·tree) *n.*

cys·to·met·ro·gram (sis''to·met'ro·gram) *n.* [*cysto-* + *metro-* + *-gram*]. Graphic demonstration of the pressure within the urinary bladder with gradual filling, as determined by cystometry.

cys·to·mor·phous (sis''to·mor'fus) *adj.* [*cysto-* + *-morphous*]. Having the structure of, or resembling, a cyst or a bladder.

cys·to·pexy (sis'to·peck''see) *n.* [*cysto-* + *-pexy*]. Surgical fixation of the urinary bladder, or a portion of it, in a new location; vesicofixation.

cys·to·pho·tog·ra·phy (sis''to·fo·tog'ruh·fee) *n.* [*cysto-* + *photography*]. Photography of the interior of the urinary bladder for diagnostic purposes.

cys·to·plas·ty (sis'to·plas''tee) *n.* [*cysto-* + *-plasty*]. A plastic operation upon the urinary bladder; used mainly to increase bladder capacity.

cys·to·pros·ta·tec·to·my (sis''to·pros''tuh·teck'tuh·mee) *n.* [*cysto-* + *prostatectomy*]. *In surgery,* excision of the urinary bladder and the prostate.

cys·to·py·eli·tis (sis''to·pye''e·lye'tis) *n.* [*cysto-* + *pyelitis*]. Inflammation of the urinary bladder and the pelvis of the kidney.

cys·to·py·elo·ne·phri·tis (sis″to·pye″e·lo·nef·rye′tis) *n.* [*cysto-* + *pyelonephritis*]. Inflammation of the urinary bladder, renal pelvis, and renal parenchyma.

cys·to·rec·to·cele (sis″to·reck′to·seel) *n.* [*cysto-* + *recto-* + *-cele*]. Herniation of the urinary bladder and rectum into the vagina.

cys·tor·rha·phy (sis·tor′uh·fee) *n.* [*cysto-* + *-rrhaphy*]. Suture of the urinary bladder.

cys·to·sar·co·ma (sis″to·sahr·ko′muh) *n.* [*cysto-* + *sarcoma*]. Formerly, a fleshy mass containing cysts.

cystosarcoma phyl·lo·des (fi·lo′deez) [Gr. *phyllōdēs*, leafy]. A benign tumor of the mammary gland, which grows slowly but may attain great size, with nodular proliferation of connective tissue and lesser adenomatous proliferation.

cystosarcoma phyl·loi·des (fi·loy′deez). CYSTOSARCOMA PHYLLODES.

cys·to·scope (sis′tuh·skope) *n.* [*cysto-* + *-scope*]. An instrument used in diagnosis and treatment of lesions of the urinary bladder, ureter, and kidney. It consists of an outer sheath bearing the lighting system, a well-fitted obturator, space for the visual system, and room for the passage of ureteral catheters and operative devices to be used under visual control. —**cys·to·scop·ic** (sis″to·skop′ick) *adj.*

cystoscopic lithotrite. A lithotrite which operates under visual control by means of a cystoscopic attachment.

cys·tos·co·py (sis·tos′kuh·pee) *n.* [*cysto-* + *-scopy*]. The procedure of using the cystoscope.

cys·to·sphinc·ter·om·e·try (sis″to·sfink″tur·om′e·tree) *n.* [cysto- + *sphincter* + *-metry*]. Simultaneous measurement of the pressure in the urinary bladder and in the urethra.

cys·to·ste·a·to·ma (sis″to·stee″uh·to′muh, sis·tos″tee·uh·to′muh) *n.* [*cysto-* + *steatoma*]. SEBACEOUS CYST.

cys·tos·to·my (sis·tos′tuh·mee) *n.* [*cysto-* + *-tomy*]. *In surgery*, the formation of a fistulous opening in the urinary bladder wall.

cys·to·tome (sis′tuh·tome) *n.* [*cysto-* + *-tome*]. 1. An instrument for incising the urinary bladder or gallbladder. 2. An instrument for incising the capsule of the lens.

cys·tot·o·my (sis·tot′uh·mee) *n.* [*cysto-* + *-tomy*]. 1. Incision into the urinary bladder or gallbladder. 2. Incision into the anterior capsule of the lens for the extraction of a cataract. Compare *cystectomy*.

cys·to·ure·tero·cele (sis″to·yoo·ree′tur·o·seel) *n.* [*cysto-* + *uretero-* + *-cele*]. Herniation of the urinary bladder and one or both ureters into the vagina.

cys·to·ure·thri·tis (sis″to·yoo″re·thrigh′tis) *n.* [*cysto-* + *urethritis*]. Inflammation of the urinary bladder and the urethra.

cys·to·ure·thro·cele (sis″to·yoo·ree′thro·seel) *n.* [*cysto-* + *urethro-* + *-cele*]. Herniation of the urinary bladder and urethra into the vagina.

cys·to·ure·thro·gram (sis″to·yoo·ree′thro·gram) *n.* [*cysto-* + *urethrogram*]. A radiograph of the urinary bladder and urethra, made after opacification of these structures.

cys·to·ure·throg·ra·phy (sis″to·yoo″re·throg′ruh·fee) *n.* [*cysto-* + *urethrography*]. Radiography of the urinary bladder and urethra. —**cystoure·thro·graph·ic** (·thro·graf′ick) *adj.*

cys·to·ure·thro·scope (sis″to·yoo·ree′thro·skope) *n.* [*cysto-* + *urethroscope*]. An instrument for inspecting the urinary bladder and posterior urethra.

cys·tyl (sis′til) *n.* The divalent radical,— $COCH(NH_2)CH_2SSCH_2CH(NH_2)CO$—, of the amino acid cystine.

cyt-, cyto- [Gk. *kytos*, hollow, vessel]. A combining form meaning (a) *cell, cellular;* (b) *cytoplasm, cytoplasmic.*

cyt·ar·a·bine (sit′ăr·uh·been) *n.* 1-Arabinofuranosylcytosine, $C_9H_{13}N_3O_5$, an inhibitor of deoxyribonucleic acid synthesis and of the proliferation of viruses containing this acid; used as the hydrochloride salt. Syn. *cytosine arabinoside, ara-C, arabinosyl cutosine.*

cy·tase (sigh′tace, ·taze) *n.* [*cyt-* + *-ase*]. 1. Metchnikoff's name for complement, considered as an enzyme. 2. Any enzyme in the seeds of plants that causes solubilization of cell wall components.

cy·tas·ter (sigh·tas′tur, sigh′tas·tur) *n.* [*cyt-* + *aster*]. 1. ASTER. 2. Especially, an accessory aster, not associated with chromosomes, appearing under certain experimental treatment.

-cyte [Gk. *kytos*, vessel, container, hollow]. A combining form meaning *a cell.*

Cytellin. Trademark for a preparation of sitosterols that reduces blood cholesterol levels.

cyth·e·mol·y·sis, cyth·ae·mol·y·sis (sith″e·mol′i·sis, ·mo·lye′sis, sight″he·) *n.* [*cyt-* + *hemolysis*]. Dissolution of erythrocytes and leukocytes.

cyth·er·e·an shield (sith″ur·ee′un) [Gk. *Kythereia*, a name of Aphrodite or Venus]. CONDOM.

cyth·ero·ma·nia (sith″ur·o·may′nee·uh) *n.* [Gk. *Kythereia*, a name of Venus or Aphrodite, + *mania*]. NYMPHOMANIA.

cyt·i·dine (sit′i·deen, ·din) *n.* Cytosine riboside, $C_9H_{13}N_3O_5$, a nucleoside composed of one molecule each of cytosine and D-ribose. One of the four main riboside components of ribonucleic acid.

cytidine monophosphate. CYTIDYLIC ACID.

cyt·i·dyl·ic acid (sit″i·dil′ick). A mononucleotide component, $C_9H_{14}N_3O_8P$, of ribonucleic acid which yields cytosine, D-ribose, and phosphoric acid on complete hydrolysis. Syn. *cytidine monophosphate.*

cyt·i·sine (sit′i·seen, ·sin) *n.* A poisonous alkaloid, $C_{11}H_{14}N_2O$, from *Laburnum anagyroides*, goldenchain laburnum, and from baptisia and other plants. It stimulates, then paralyzes, autonomic ganglions.

cyto-. See *cyt-.*

cy·to·al·bu·mi·no·log·ic (sigh″to·al·bew″mi·no·loj′ick) *adj.* ALBUMINOCYTOLOGIC.

cy·to·ar·chi·tec·ton·ic (sigh″to·ahr″ki·teck·ton′ick) *adj.* [*cyto-* + *architectonic*]. Pertaining to the cellular arrangement of a region, tissue, or organ.

cy·to·ar·chi·tec·ture (sigh″to·ahr′ki·teck″chur) *n.* [*cyto-* + *architecture*]. The cell pattern typical of a region, as of an area of the cerebral cortex.

cy·to·blast (sigh′to·blast) *n.* [*cyto-* + *-blast*]. The nucleus of a cell.

cy·to·blas·te·ma (sigh″to·blas·tee′muh) *n.* [*cyto-* + *blastema*]. The hypothetical formative material from which cells arise. See also *blastema.*

cy·to·cen·trum (sigh″to·sen′trum) *n.* [*cyto-* + *centrum*]. CENTROSOME.

cy·to·cha·la·sin B (sigh″to·ka·lay′sin) [*cyto-* + Gk. *chalasis*, relaxation, + *-in*]. A metabolite obtained from the mold *Helminthosporium dematoiderum* which appears to disrupt microfilaments of cells; used experimentally to inhibit phagocytosis by cells.

cy·to·chem·ism (sigh″to·kem′iz·um) *n.* [*cyto-* + *chem-* + *-ism*]. The reaction of the living cell to chemical agents.

cy·to·chem·is·try (sigh″to·kem′is·tree) *n.* [*cyto-* + *chemistry*]. The science dealing with the chemical constitution of cells and cell constituents, especially as demonstrated in histologic section by specific staining reactions.

cy·to·chrome (sigh′to·krome) *n.* [*cyto-* + *-chrome*]. One of several iron-protoporphyrin cellular pigments (cytochrome a_1, a_2, a_3, b_1, b_2, b_3, etc.) which function in cellular respiration (electron transport) by being alternately oxidized and reduced. Most cytochromes are bound to the protein-lipid complex of the mitochondria. Some 30 such compounds are now known.

cytochrome oxidase. An iron-porphyrin respiratory enzyme in mitochondria in which the prosthetic group undergoes reversible oxidation-reduction, accepting electrons which are transferred subsequently to oxygen. It is identical with indophenol oxidase.

cytochrome reductase. An iron-porphyrin enzyme that serves as a hydrogen acceptor in electron transport.

cy·to·chy·le·ma (sigh″to·kigh·lee′muh) *n.* [NL, from *cyto-* + *Gk. chylos*, juice]. The interreticular portion of protoplasm; cell juice.

cy·to·cide (sigh'to·side) *n.* [*cyto-* + *-cide*]. An agent that is destructive to cells. —**cy·to·ci·dal** (sigh"to·sigh'dul) *adj.*

cy·toc·la·sis (sigh·tock'luh·sis, sigh"to·klay'sis) *n.* [*cyto-* + *-clasis*]. Cell necrosis. —**cy·to·clas·tic** (sigh"to·klas'tick) *adj.*

cy·to·crine theory (sigh'to·krin). The postulated transfer of pigment granules from melanocytes directly into epidermal cells.

cy·to·crin·ia (sigh"to·krin'ee·uh) *n.* [*cyto-* + Gk. *krinein*, to separate, + *-ia*]. The transfer of pigment from melanoblasts to other cells, melanin from basal to intermediate cells of the epidermis in sunburn.

cy·tode (sigh'tode) *n.* [*cyt-* + Gk. *-ōdēs*, -like]. The simplest form of cell, without nucleus or nucleolus.

cy·to·den·drite (sigh"to·den'drite) *n.* [*cyto-* + *dendrite*]. DENDRITE.

cy·to·derm (sigh'to·durm) *n.* [*cyto-* + *-derm*]. *In botany*, CELL WALL.

cy·to·di·ag·no·sis (sigh"to·dye"ug·no'sis) *n.*, pl. **cytodiagno·ses** (·seez) [*cyto-* + *diagnosis*]. The determination of the nature of an abnormal liquid by the study of the cells it contains.

cy·to·di·er·e·sis (sigh"to·dye·err'i·sis) *n.* [*cyto-* + Gk. *diairesis*, dissection, dividing]. CYTOKINESIS.

cy·to·dis·tal (sigh"to·dis'tul) *adj.* [*cyto-* + *distal*]. 1. Of or pertaining to that portion of a nerve fiber farthest removed from the perikaryon. 2. Of or pertaining to a metastatic neoplasm formed at a distance from its cells or origin.

cy·to·gene (sigh'to·jeen) *n.* [*cyto-* + *gene*]. A self-reproducing cytoplasmic particle capable of determining a hereditary characteristic.

cy·to·gen·e·sis (sigh"to·jen'e·sis) *n.*, pl. **cytogene·ses** (·seez) [*cyto-* + *-genesis*]. The genesis and differentiation of a cell. —**cyto·ge·net·ic** (·je·net'ick) *adj.*

cy·to·ge·net·ics (sigh"to·je·net'icks) *n.* [*cyto-* + *genetics*]. The hybrid science in which the methods of cytology are employed to study the chromosomes.

cytogenic gland. A gland producing living cells, as the testis or ovary.

cy·tog·e·ny (sigh·toj'e·nee) *n.* CYTOGENESIS. —**cytoge·nous** (·nus), **cy·to·gen·ic** (sigh"to·jen'ick) *adj.*

cy·to·glob·u·lin (sigh"to·glob'yoo·lin) *n.* [*cyto-* + *globulin*]. A protein obtained from leukocytes and lymph nodes in the form of a white soluble powder.

cy·to·glu·co·pe·nia (sigh"to·gloo"ko·pee'nee·uh) *n.* CYTOGLYCOPENIA.

cy·to·gly·co·pe·nia (sigh"to·glye'ko·pee'nee·uh) *n.* [*cyto-* + *glyco-* + *-penia*]. Deficiency of glucose within cells.

cy·toid (sigh'toid) *adj.* [*cyt-* + *-oid*]. Resembling a cell.

cytoid bodies. Globular bodies located in the nerve fiber layer of the retina and which may represent terminal nerve fiber swellings. A collection of these cytoid bodies gives rise to the cotton-wool exudate.

cy·to·ki·ne·sis (sigh"to·ki·nee'sis, ·kigh·nee'sis) *n.* [*cyto-* + *kinesis*]. The changes in the cytoplasm during cell division. —**cytoki·net·ic** (·net'ick) *adj.*

cy·tol·er·gy (sigh·tol'ur·jee) *n.* [*cytologic* + *-ergy*]. Cell activity.

cy·to·lipo·chrome (sigh"to·lip'o·krome) *n.* [*cyto-* + *lipochrome*]. HEMOFUSCIN.

cytological cancer techniques. Procedures in which cells are obtained by aspirations, washings, smears, or scrapings; and after fixation and staining are studied for anaplasia on the basis of nuclear and cytoplasmic changes, and changes of the cell as a whole.

cytologic mapping. Chromosome mapping in which changes in genetic recombination are correlated with changes in chromosomal structure.

cy·tol·o·gy (sigh·tol'uh·jee) *n.* [*cyto-* + *-logy*]. 1. The subdivision of biology which deals with cells. 2. EXFOLIATIVE CYTOLOGY. —**cy·to·log·ic** (sigh"to·loj'ick), **cytolog·i·cal** (·i·kul) *adj.*; **cy·tol·o·gist** (sigh·tol'uh·jist) *n.*

cy·tol·y·sin (sigh·tol'i·sin, sigh"to·lye'sin) *n.* [*cyto-* + *lysin*]. A specific protein or antibody of blood plasma which brings about the hemolysis of red cells (hemolysin), or the cytolysis of other tissue cells.

cy·tol·y·sis (sigh·tol'i·sis) *n.*, pl. **cytoly·ses** (·seez) [*cyto-* + *lysis*]. The disintegration or dissolution of cells. —**cy·to·lyt·ic** (sigh"to·lit'ick) *adj.*

cy·to·ly·so·some (sigh"to·lye'so·sohm) *n.* An enlarged lysosome containing recognizable organelles such as mitochondria.

-cytoma [*cyt-* + *-oma*]. A combining form meaning *a neoplasm made up of a* (specified) *kind of cell.*

cy·to·me·gal·ic (sigh"to·me·gal'lick) *adj.* [*cyto-* + *megal-* + *-ic*]. Of, pertaining to, or characterizing the greatly enlarged cells, measuring 25 to 40 microns, with enlarged nuclei containing prominent inclusion bodies and sometimes also cytoplasmic inclusions; found in various tissues in cytomegalic inclusion disease.

cytomegalic inclusion disease. Infection with the cytomegaloviruses of man, monkeys, and other animals, characterized by a striking enlargement of epithelial cells of the salivary glands and other organs, and by prominent intranuclear inclusion bodies. In the neonatal period associated with hepatosplenomegaly, thrombocytopenic purpura, hepatitis, jaundice, microcephaly, and subsequent mental retardation; postnatally, may be asymptomatic or associated with pneumonitis and hepatitis. Abbreviated, CID. Syn. *salivary gland virus disease.*

cy·to·meg·a·lo·vi·rus (sigh"to·meg"uh·lo·vye'rus) *n.* [*cyto-* + *megalo-* + *virus*]. A member of a group of DNA viruses closely related to the herpesviruses; the cause of cytomegalic inclusion disease.

cytomegalovirus syndrome. CYTOMEGALIC INCLUSION DISEASE.

Cytomel. Trademark for sodium liothyronine, a thyroid hormone.

cy·tom·e·ter (sigh·tom'e·tur) *n.* [*cyto-* + *meter*]. A device for counting cells, especially blood cells. See also *hemocytometer.* —**cytom·e·try** (sigh·tom'e·tree) *n.*; **cy·to·met·ric** (sigh"to·met'rick) *adj.*

cy·to·mi·cro·some (sigh"to·migh'kro·sohm) *n.* [*cyto-* + *microsome*]. *Obsol.* MICROSOME.

cy·to·mi·tome (sigh"to·migh'tome, sigh·tom'i·tome) *n.* [*cyto-* + *mitome*]. The fibrillar part of cytoplasm. Syn. *cytoreticulum.* See also *mitome.*

cy·to·mor·pho·sis (sigh"to·mor·fo'sis, ·mor'fuh·sis) *n.*, pl. **cytomopho·ses** (·seez) [*cyto-* + *-morphosis*]. All the structural alterations which cells or successive generations of cells undergo from the earliest undifferentiated stage to their final destruction.

cy·to·my·co·sis (sigh"to·migh·ko'sis) *n.*, pl. **cytomyco·ses** (·seez) [*cyto-* + *mycosis*]. 1. Fungal infection in which the organisms primarily grow within cells. 2. HISTOPLASMOSIS.

cy·ton (sigh'ton) *n.* [*cyt-* + *-on*]. CELL BODY.

cy·to·patho·gen·ic (sigh"to·path"o·jen'ick) *adj.* [*cyto-* + *pathogenic*]. Pertaining to the destruction of cells (in tissue culture) by a transmissible agent, such as a virus.

cy·to·pa·thol·o·gy (sigh"to·pa·thol'uh·jee) *n.* [*cyto-* + *pathology*]. The branch of pathology concerned with alterations within cells, especially as demonstrated by techniques such as those of exfoliative cytology.

cy·top·a·thy (sigh·top'uth·ee) *n.* [*cyto-* + *-pathy*]. Disease of the living cell. —**cy·to·path·ic** (sigh"to·path'ick) *adj.*

cy·to·pemp·sis (sigh"to·pemp'sis) *n.* [*cyto-* + Gk. *pempsis*, sending, mission]. Transport of particulate matter or large molecules across an endothelial cell membrane by means of vesicles; of doubtful significance in vivo. Compare *pinocytosis.*

cy·to·pe·nia (sigh"to·pee'nee·uh) *n.* [*cyto-* + *-penia*]. A cell count less than normal. See also *leukopenia, anemia, thrombocytopenia, pancytopenia.*

cy·toph·a·gy (sigh·tof'uh·jee) *n.* [*cyto-* + *-phagy*]. The engulfing of cells by other cells; PHAGOCYTOSIS. —**cytoph·a·gous** (·uh·gus) *adj.*

cy·to·phe·re·sis (sigh"to·fe·ree'sis) *n.* [*cyto-* + *pheresis*]. The removal of cells, especially leukocytes, from whole blood, with return of the remaining blood to the donor.

cy·to·phil (sigh'to·fil) *adj.* [*cyto-* + *-phil*]. Having an affinity for cells; attracted by cells.

cy·to·phil·ic (sigh''to·fil'ick) *adj.* CYTOPHIL.

cy·to·pho·tom·e·ter (sigh''to·fo·tom'e·tur) *n.* [*cyto-* + *photometer*]. A photometer for measuring the intensity of monochromatic light transmitted through individual stained areas of cellular material in a microscopic field. —**cytophotome·try** (·tree) *n.*

cy·to·phys·i·ol·o·gy (sigh''to·fiz''ee·ol'uh·jee) *n.* [*cyto-* + *physiology*]. CELLULAR PHYSIOLOGY.

cy·to·plasm (sigh'to·plaz·um) *n.* [*cyto-* + *-plasm*]. The protoplasm of a cell other than that of the nucleus. Contr. *nucleoplasm.* —**cy·to·plas·mic** (sigh''to·plaz'mick) *adj.*

cytoplasmic inheritance. The acquisition of any trait that is causally dependent upon self-reproducing cytoplasmic bodies, such as chloroplasts, mitochondria, or certain viruses.

cytoplasmic membrane. 1. PLASMA MEMBRANE. 2. Any membrane that bounds cytoplasm, either enclosing a cell or within a cell.

cy·to·plas·tin (sigh'to·plas''tin) *n.* The plastin of cytoplasm.

cy·to·poi·e·sis (sigh''to·poy·ee'sis) *n.* [*cyto-* + *-poiesis*]. The formation and development of a cell.

cy·to·prox·i·mal (sigh''to·prock'si·mul) *adj.* [*cyto-* + *proximal*]. Pertaining to the portion of a nerve fiber near its perikaryon.

cy·to·re·tic·u·lum (sigh''to·re·tick'yoo·lum) *n.* [*cyto-* + *reticulum*]. 1. The network of cells in reticular tissue. 2. CYTOMITOME.

cy·to·ryc·tes, cy·tor·rhyc·tes (sigh''to·rick'teez) *n.* [*cyt-* + Gk. *oryktēs*, digger]. An inclusion body, used originally as the genus name for inclusion bodies in virus diseases under the false assumption that these bodies were protozoan parasites.

Cytosar. A trademark for cytarabine, an antineoplastic.

cy·tos·co·py (sigh·tos'kuh·pee) *n.* [*cyto-* + *-scopy*]. CYTODIAGNOSIS. —**cy·to·scop·ic** (sigh''to·skop'ick) *adj.*

cy·to·se·gre·go·some (sigh''to·se·greg'o·sohm, ·seg're·go·) *n.* A membrane-delineated cytoplasmic organelle, formed within a cell by segregation of a portion of cytoplasm; capable of fusing with a lysosome, it constitutes a mechnanism for removing nonviable parts of a cell.

cy·to·sid·er·in (sigh''to·sid'ur·in) *n.* [*cyto-* + *sider-* + *-in*]. Any of a group of iron-containing lipid pigments found in various tissues.

cy·to·sine (sigh'to·seen, ·sin) *n.* [*cyt-* + *-ose* + *-ine*]. 4-Amino-2(1*H*)-pyrimidone, $C_4H_5N_3O$, a pyrimidine base important mainly as a component of ribonucleic and deoxyribonucleic acids.

cytosine ar·a·bi·no·side (ăr''uh·bin'o·side, a·rab'i·no·side). CYTARABINE.

cy·to·skel·e·ton (sigh''to·skel'e·tun) *n.* [*cyto-* + *skeleton*]. The structural framework of a cell, probably consisting of proteins.

cy·to·smear (sigh'to·smeer) *n.* A smear of some cell-containing material, such as cervical scrapings, for the purpose of cytologic study.

cy·to·sol (sigh'to·sol) *n.* [*cyto-* + *sol*]. The fluid cytoplasmic fraction from which organelles and insoluble cellular components have been removed, as by fractional ultracentrifugation following disruption of the cell membranes.

cy·to·some (sigh'tuh·sohm) *n.* [*cyto-* + *-some*]. A cell body exclusive of the nucleus.

cy·to·spon·gi·um (sigh''to·spon'jee·um) *n.*, pl. **cytospon·gia** (·jee·uh) [*cyto-* + *-spongium*]. The fibrillar protein network of the cytoplasm.

cy·tost (sigh'tost) *n.* A substance, not a histamine, secreted by injured cells and capable of modifying cellular activity.

cy·to·stat·ic (sigh''to·stat'ick) *adj.* [*cyto-* + *static*]. Preventing the multiplication and growth of cells.

cy·to·ste·a·to·ne·cro·sis (sigh''to·stee''uh·to·ne·kro'sis) *n.* [*cyto-* + *steato-* + *necrosis*]. ADIPONECROSIS NEONATORUM.

cy·to·stome (sigh'to·stome) *n.* [*cyto-* + *-stome*]. The oral aperture of a unicellular organism.

cy·to·tax·is (sigh''to·tack'sis) *n.* [*cyto-* + *-taxis*]. The movement of cells toward or away from a stimulus. See also *chemotaxis.* —**cyto·tac·tic** (·tack'tick) *adj.*

cy·to·tech·nol·o·gist (sigh''to·teck·nol'uh·jist) *n.* [*cyto-* + *technologist*]. A person trained and skilled in the preparation and examination of exfoliated cells who conducts a preliminary study of such cells, referring abnormal smears to a specialized physician for final classification.

cy·toth·e·sis (sigh·toth'e·sis, sigh''to·thees'is) *n.* [*cyto-* + Gk. *thesis*, placing, arrangement]. Cell repair.

cy·to·tox·in (sigh''to·tock'sin) *n.* [*cyto-* + *toxin*]. 1. A serum, natural or immune, capable of injuring certain cells without lysis. 2. Any chemical agent which kills cells. —**cyto·tox·ic** (·sick) *adj.*

cy·to·tropho·blast (sigh''to·trof'o·blast) *n.* [*cyto-* + *trophoblast*]. The innermost cellular layer of the trophoblast of embryonic placental mammals, which gives rise to the syntrophoblast layer which ultimately covers the placental villi. Syn. *Langhans' layer.*

cy·tot·ro·phy (sigh·tot'ruh·fee) *n.* [*cyto-* + *-trophy*]. Growth of the cell and sustentation of cell life.

cy·tot·ro·pism (sigh·tot'ruh·piz·um) *n.* [*cyto-* + *tropism*]. 1. The tendency of cells to move toward or away from a stimulus. 2. The tendency of certain chemicals, viruses, and bacteria to be attracted to certain kinds of cells. —**cy·to·tro·pic** (sigh''to·tro'pick, ·trop'ick) *adj.*

Cytoxan. Trademark for cyclophosphamide, an alkylating type of antineoplastic agent.

cy·to·zo·on (sigh''to·zo'on) *n.*, pl. **cyto·zoa** (·zo'uh) [*cyto-* + *-zoon*]. A protozoan intracellular parasite.

cy·to·zyme (sigh'to·zime) *n.* [*cyto-* + *-zyme*]. A substance in various tissues, capable of activating thrombin, the fibrin ferment. See also *thromboplastin.*

Czer·ny's suture (chehr'nee) [V. *Czerny*, German surgeon, 1842–1916]. A type of intestinal suture. 2. A method of repairing ruptured tendons.

D

D Symbol for deuterium.

D *In microbiology,* an abbreviation for *dwarf colony.*

D., d. Abbreviation for (a) *da* (L., give); (b) day, days; (c) dead; (d) *density;* (e) *detur* (L., let it be given); (f) *dexter;* (g) died; (h) *diopter;* (i) *distal;* (j) *dorsal;* (k) *dose;* (l) duration.

2,4-D Abbreviation for *2,4-dichlorophenoxyacetic acid.*

D- *In chemistry,* a configurational descriptor placed before the stereoparent names of amino acids and carbohydrates. With amino acids it relates the configuration of the carbon bearing the amino acid group to serine and for carbohydrates the highest member asymmetric carbon atom to the reference compound, D-glyceraldehyde. Although the symbol D bears no relationship to the rotation of plane polarized light by the compound, the combined symbolic prefix DL always indicates an optically inactive form or a racemic mixture. Compare *R.*

d Abbreviation for *deuteron.*

d- 1. *In chemistry,* a symbol formerly used for dextrorotatory, referring to the direction in which plane polarized light is rotated by a substance; this usage is superseded by the symbol (+). 2. *In chemistry,* a symbol formerly used to indicate the structural configuration of a particular asymmetric carbon atom in a compound, in the manner that the small capital letter D- is now used. Compare D-. See also Table of Medical Signs and Symbols in the Appendix. 3. *In chemistry,* a chemical name followed by the symbol *d* indicates substitution of appropriate hydrogen atoms by deuterium and, if subscripted, also indicates the number of deuterium atoms inserted.

DA Abbreviation for *developmental age.*

da·boia, da·boya (da·boy'uh) *n.* [Hindi *daboyā,* lurker]. RUSSELL'S VIPER.

da·car·ba·zine (day·kahr'buh·zeen) *n.* 5-(3,3-Dimethyl-1-triazeno)imidazole-4-carboxylic acid, $C_6H_{10}N_6O$, an antineoplastic.

Da Cos·ta's syndrome [J. M. *Da Costa,* U.S. surgeon, 1833–1900]. NEUROCIRCULATORY ASTHENIA.

dacry-, dacryo- [Gk. *dakryon,* tear]. A combining form meaning (a) *tears;* (b) *lacrimal apparatus.*

dac·ry·ad·e·ni·tis (dack″ree·ad″e·nigh'tis) *n.* DACRYOADENITIS.

dac·ry·ad·e·no·scir·rhus (dack″ree·ad″e·no·skirr'us) *n.* [*dacry-* + *adeno-* + *scirrhus*]. An indurated tumor of the lacrimal gland.

dac·ry·ag·o·ga·tre·sia (dack″ree·ag″o·ga·tree'zhuh, ·zee·uh, dack″ree·uh·gog″uh·) *n.* [*dacryagogue* + *atresia*]. Obstruction of a lacrimal canaliculus.

dac·ry·a·gog·ic (dack″ree·uh·goj'ick) *adj.* Pertaining to or having the character of a dacryagogue.

dac·ry·a·gogue (dack'ree·uh·gog) *n. & adj.* [*dacry-* + *-agogue*]. 1. An agent causing a flow of tears. 2. Causing a flow of tears; DACRYAGOGIC. See also *lacrimator.*

dacryo-. See *dacry-.*

dac·ryo·ad·e·nal·gia (dack″ree·o·ad″e·nal'jee·uh) *n.* [*dacryo-* + *adenalgia*]. Pain in a lacrimal gland.

dac·ryo·ad·e·nec·to·my (dack″ree·o·ad″e·neck'tuh·mee) *n.* [*dacryo-* + *adenectomy*]. Excision of a lacrimal gland.

dac·ryo·ad·e·ni·tis (dack″ree·o·ad″e·nigh'tis) *n.* [*dacryo-* + *adenitis*]. Inflammation of a lacrimal gland.

dac·ryo·ag·o·ga·tre·sia (dack″ree·o·ag″o·ga·tree'zhuh) *n.* DACRYAGOGATRESIA.

dac·ryo·blen·nor·rhea, dac·ryo·blen·nor·rhoea (dack″ree·o·blen″o·ree'uh) *n.* [*dacryo-* + *blennorrhea*]. Chronic inflammation of and discharge of mucus from the lacrimal sac.

dac·ryo·cele (dack'ree·o·seel) *n.* DACRYOCYSTOCELE.

dac·ryo·cyst (dack'ree·o·sist) *n.* [*dacryo-* + *-cyst*]. LACRIMAL SAC.

dac·ryo·cys·tec·to·my (dack″ree·o·sis·teck'tuh·mee) *n.* [*dacryocyst* + *-ectomy*]. Excision of all or a part of the lacrimal sac.

dac·ryo·cys·ti·tis (dack″ree·o·sis·tye'tis) *n.* [*dacryocyst* + *-itis*]. Inflammation of the lacrimal sac.

dac·ryo·cys·to·blen·nor·rhea, dac·ryo·cys·to·blen·nor·rhoea (dack″ree·o·sis″to·blen·o·ree'uh) *n.* [*dacryocyst* + *blennorrhea*]. DACRYOCYSTITIS.

dac·ryo·cys·to·cele (dack″ree·o·sis'to·seel) *n.* [*dacryocyst* + *-cele*]. Distention of a lacrimal sac.

dac·ryo·cys·top·to·sis (dack″ree·o·sis″top·to'sis) *n.* [*dacryocyst* + *-ptosis*]. Prolapse or downward displacement of a lacrimal sac.

dac·ryo·cys·to·rhi·nos·to·my (dack″ree·o·sis″to·rye·nos'tuh·mee) *n.* [*dacryocyst* + *rhino-* + *-stomy*]. An operation to restore drainage into the nose from the lacrimal sac when the nasolacrimal duct is obliterated or obstructed.

dac·ryo·cys·tos·to·my (dack″ree·o·sis·tos'tuh·mee) *n.* [*dacryocyst* + *-stomy*]. Incision into the lacrimal sac, particularly to promote drainage.

dac·ryo·cys·tot·o·my (dack″ree·o·sis·tot'uh·mee) *n.* [*dacryocyst* + *-tomy*]. Incision of the lacrimal sac.

dac·ry·o·lin (dack'ree·o·lin) *n.* A protein present in tears.

dac·ryo·lith (dack'ree·o·lith) *n.* [*dacryo-* + *-lith*]. A firm, laminated, stonelike structure that develops in the lacrimal sac with obstruction of the nasolacrimal duct.

dac·ryo·li·thi·a·sis (dack″ree·o·li·thigh'uh·sis) *n.* [*dacryolith* + *-iasis*]. The formation and presence of dacryoliths.

dac·ry·o·ma (dack″ree·o'muh) *n.*, pl. **dacryomas, dacryoma·ta** (·tuh) [*dacry-* + *-oma*]. 1. A lacrimal tumor. 2. Obstruction of the lacrimal puncta, causing epiphora.

dac·ry·on (dack'ree·on) *n.*, pl. **dac·rya** (·ree·uh) [*dacry-* (= lacrimal) + *-ion*]. *In craniometry,* the point where the frontomaxillary, the maxillolacrimal, and frontolacrimal sutures meet.

dac·ry·ops, dak·ry·ops (dack'ree·ops) *n.* [*dacry-* + *-ops*]. 1. EPIPHORA. 2. A cyst of an excretory duct of a lacrimal gland.

dac·ry·op·to·sis (dack"ree·op·to'sis) *n.* [*dacryo-* + *-ptosis*]. DACRYOCYSTOPTOSIS.

dac·ry·or·rhea, dac·ry·or·rhoea (dack"ree·o·ree'uh) *n.* [*dacryo-* + *-rrhea*]. An excessive flow of tears.

dac·ryo·so·le·ni·tis (dack"ree·o·so"le·nigh'tis) *n.* [*dacryo-* + Gk. *sōlēn*, pipe, + *-itis*]. Inflammation of the lacrimal drainage system.

dac·ryo·ste·no·sis (dack"ree·o·ste·no'sis) *n.* [*dacryo-* + *stenosis*]. Stenosis or stricture of the lacrimal drainage system.

dac·ryo·syr·inx (dack"ree·o·sirr'inks) *n.*, pl. **dacryo·sy·rin·ges** (·si·rin'jeez), **dacryosyrinxes** [*dacryo-* + *syrinx*]. 1. LACRIMAL FISTULA. 2. A syringe for use in the lacrimal ducts.

Dactil. Trademark for piperidolate, an anticholinergic drug used as the hydrochloride salt.

dac·ti·no·my·cin (dack"ti·no·migh'sin) *n.* An actinomycin antibiotic, produced by *Streptomyces parvullus,* useful in the treatment of various tumors; also useful in the study of genetic transcription because it interferes with the synthesis of messenger RNA. Syn. *actinomycin D.*

dactyl-, dactylo- [Gk. *daktylos*]. A combining form meaning *digit, finger, toe.*

dac·tyl (dack'til) *n.* [Gk. *daktylos*]. *In zoology,* a digit; a finger or toe. —**dacty·lar** (·lur), **dacty·late** (·late) *adj.*

dactyli. Plural of *dactylus.*

-dactylia [*dactyl-* + *-ia*]. A combining form designating *a condition or characteristic involving the digits.*

dac·ty·lif·er·ous (dack"ti·lif'uh·rus) *adj.* [*dactyl-* + *-iferous*]. Having finger or fingerlike parts, organs, or appendages.

dac·tyl·i·on (dack·til'ee·on) *n.* [*dactyl-* + *-ion*]. SYNDACTYLY.

-dactylism. See *-dactylia.*

dac·ty·li·tis (dack"ti·lye'tis) *n.* [*dactyl-* + *-itis*]. Inflammation of a finger or a toe.

dactylitis syph·i·lit·i·ca (sif·i·lit'i·kuh). Gummatous infiltration of the subcutaneous connective tissue and of the joints and bones of the fingers and toes in tertiary syphilis.

dactylo-. See *dactyl-.*

dac·ty·lo·gram (dack·til'o·gram, dack'ti·lo·) *n.* [*dactylo-* + *-gram*]. A fingerprint, generally used for purposes of identification and in genetic studies. See also *dermatoglyphics.*

dac·ty·lol·y·sis (dack"ti·lol'i·sis) *n.* [*dactylo-* + *-lysis*]. Loss or amputation of a digit.

dactylolysis spon·ta·nea (spon·tay'nee·uh). Spontaneous disappearance of fingers or toes, as in ainhum or leprosy.

dac·ty·lo·meg·a·ly (dack"ti·lo·meg'uh·lee) *n.* [*dactylo-* + *-megaly*]. A condition in which one or more of the fingers or toes is abnormally large; MACRODACTYLY.

dac·ty·lo·sym·phy·sis (dack"ti·lo·sim'fi·sis) *n.* [*dactylo-* + *symphysis*]. SYNDACTYLY.

dac·ty·lus (dack'ti·lus) *n.*, pl. **dacty·li** (·lye) [NL., from Gk. *daktylos,* digit]. TOE. Compare *digitus.*

-dactyly [*dactyl-* + *y*]. A combining form designating *a specified condition or number of fingers or toes.*

Da·gni·ni extension-adduction reflex (dahⁿ·nʸee'nee). Percussion of the radial aspect of the back of the hand is followed by extension and slight adduction of the wrist where there is reflex hyperactivity or in pyramidal tract involvement.

Dahl·ia (dahl'yuh, dal'yuh, dayl'yuh) *n.* [A. *Dahl,* Swedish botanist]. A genus of plants of the Compositae whose tuberous roots yield inulin.

dahl·lite (dahl'ite) *n.* [T. and J. *Dahll,* Norwegian geologists, 19th century]. The mineral $CaCO_3.2Ca_3(PO_4)_2$, once said to be structurally close to the chief inorganic constituent of teeth.

daily dose. The total amount of a medicinal to be administered in 24 hours.

Da·kin's solution [H. D. *Dakin,* English chemist in the U.S., 1880–1952]. A 0.4 to 0.5% solution of sodium hypochlorite, buffered with sodium bicarbonate; formerly used extensively as an antiseptic in the treatment of septic wounds.

dakryon. DACRYON.

dakryops. DACRYOPS.

Dalacin C. Trademark for the antibiotic substance clindamycin.

da·le·da·lin (da·lee'duh·lin) *n.* 3-Methyl-3-[3-(methylamino)-propyl]-1-phenylindoline, $C_{19}H_{24}N_2$, an antidepressant usually employed as the tosylate (*p*-toluenesulfonate) salt.

Dal·i·bour water (dal'i·boor, Fr. dahʰ·lee·boor') [*Dalibour,* French dermatologist]. Any of several lotions, especially one containing copper sulfate, zinc sulfate, camphor, and water; used topically for the treatment of certain dermatoses.

Dall·dorf test [G. J. *Dalldorf,* U.S. pathologist, b. 1900]. A test for capillary fragility in which a suction cup is applied to the skin for a measured interval of time and the number of petechiae which result are counted. Syn. *suction test.*

Dalmane. Trademark for flurazepam, a hypnotic agent used as the dihydrochloride salt.

Dalnate. A trademark for tolindate, an antifungal.

dal·ton·ism (dawl'tun·iz·um, dal'tun·) *n.* [J. *Dalton* + *-ism*]. COLOR BLINDNESS.

Dal·ton's law [J. *Dalton,* English chemist and physicist, 1766–1844]. 1. The pressure of a mixture of gases equals the sum of the partial pressures of the constituent gases. 2. So long as no chemical change occurs, each gas in a mixture of gases is absorbed by a given volume of solvent in proportion not to the total pressure of the mixture but to the partial pressure of that gas.

dam, *n.* 1. A thin sheet of rubber used to isolate a tooth during dental operations. 2. A piece of dam used as a drain.

dam·i·ana (dam"ee·an'uh, ·ay'nuh) *n.* The dried leaves of *Turnera diffusa,* found in Mexico and Lower California, containing volatile oil, resins, tannin, and an amaroid; formerly used as a stimulant and laxative, and as an aphrodisiac.

dam·mar, dam·ar (dam'ur) *n.* [Malay *damar*]. A natural resin derived from various East Indian trees of the genus *Shorea,* used in xylene and toluene solutions as a histologic mounting medium.

Da·moi·seau's curve (da·mwa·zo') [L. H. C. *Damoiseau,* French physician, 1815–1891]. ELLIS' CURVE.

Da·na-Put·nam syndrome (day'nuh) [C. L. *Dana,* U.S. neurologist, 1852–1935; and J. J. *Putnam*]. SUBACUTE COMBINED DEGENERATION OF THE SPINAL CORD.

Dana's operation [C. L. *Dana*]. Posterior rhizotomy for the relief of spastic paralysis.

da·na·zol (day'nuh·zole) *n.* 17α-Pregna-2,4-dien-20-yno[2,3-*d*]isoxazol-17-ol, $C_{22}H_{27}NO_2$, an anterior pituitary suppressant.

Dan·bolt-Closs syndrome [N. C. *Danbolt* and K. *Closs*]. ACRODERMATITIS ENTEROPATHICA.

Dance's sign (dahⁿss) [J. B. H. *Dance,* French physician, 1797–1832]. A sign for intussusception consisting of a depression in the right iliac fossa.

dancing chorea. SYDENHAM'S CHOREA.

dancing eye–dancing feet syndrome. Opsoclonus, incoordination, and myoclonic jerks in children, sometimes associated with neuroblastoma, but frequently of unknown cause.

dancing spasm. SALTATORY SPASM.

D and C [*d*ilatation *and c*urettage]. Dilation of the cervix and curettage of the lining of the uterus; a diagnostic and therapeutic procedure in obstetrics and gynecology.

dan·de·li·on root [F. *dent de lion,* lion's tooth]. TARAXACUM.

dan·der (dan'dur) *n.* Scales of animal skin, hair, or feathers; may act as an allergen.

dan·druff, *n.* Scales of greasy keratotic material shed from the scalp.

dan·dy fever (dan'dee). DENGUE.

Dan·dy-Walk·er syndrome [W. E. *Dandy,* U.S. neurosurgeon, 1886–1946; and A. E. *Walker,* U.S. neurosurgeon, b. 1907]. Distension of the fourth ventricle and hydrocephalus, generally attributed to congenital atresia or obstruction of the foramens of Luschka and Magendie.

Dane particle [D. S. *Dane,* English physician, 20th century]. A round particle, about 42 nm in diameter, found in the serum of some patients with serum hepatitis, possibly viral in nature.

Dan·iell cell [J. F. *Daniell,* English physicist and chemist, 1790–1845]. A galvanic cell utilizing zinc and copper electrodes.

Da·niels·sen-Boeck disease [D. C. *Danielssen,* Norwegian physician, 1815–1894; and C. W. *Boeck*]. LEPROSY.

Danlos syndrome [H. A. *Danlos,* French dermatologist, 1844–1912]. EHLERS-DANLOS SYNDROME.

dan·thron (dan'thron) *n.* 1,8-Dihydroxyanthraquinone, $C_{14}H_8O_4$, an orange-colored powder, practically insoluble in water; a laxative and cathartic.

D'An·to·ni stain (It. dahn·toh'nee). A solution containing iodine and potassium iodide used to stain amebic cysts.

Dantrium. A trademark for sodium dantrolene, a skeletal muscle relaxant.

dan·tro·lene (dan'tro·leen) *n.* 1-[[5-(*p*-Nitrophenyl)furfurylidene]amino]hydantoin, $C_{14}H_{10}N_4O_5$, a skeletal muscle relaxant.

Da·nysz phenomenon (dahn'ish) [J. *Danysz,* Polish pathologist in Paris, 1860–1928]. A diminution in the neutralizing power of antitoxin when toxin is added to it in increments instead of all at once, suggesting combination in multiple proportions.

Dan·zer and Hook·er's method. A method for determining capillary blood pressure in which the observer measures the external pressure necessary to obliterate the flow of blood through capillaries while they are being observed microscopically.

Daph·ne (daf'nee) *n.* [Gk., *daphnē,* laurel]. A genus of shrubs, some species of which have been used medicinally.

dap·sone (dap'sone) *n.* 4,4'-Sulfonyldianiline or diaminodiphenylsulfone, $C_{12}H_{12}N_2O_2S$, a leprostatic drug and a suppressant for dermatitis herpetiformis; also used in prophylaxis of falciparum malaria.

DAPT [. . . *di*amino . . . *p*henyl*t*hiazole . . .]. AMIPHENAZOLE; 2,4-diamino-5-phenylthiazole, $C_9H_9N_3S$, a narcotic antagonist.

Daptazole. Trademark for amiphenazole, a narcotic antagonist.

Daranide. Trademark for dichlorphenamide, a carbonic anhydrase inhibitor used for the treatment of glaucoma.

Daraprim. Trademark for pyrimethamine, an antimalarial drug.

Darbid. Trademark for isopropamide iodide, an anticholinergic drug used for treatment of gastrointestinal ailments.

Dare colorimeter. An instrument used in hemoglobinometry. A film of whole blood is arranged between two glass plates and compared with a tinted wedge.

Darenthin. A trademark for bretylium tosylate, a hypotensive agent.

Daricon. A trademark for oxyphencyclimine, an anticholinergic drug used as the hydrochloride salt.

Da·rier's abscess (dăr·yey') [J. F. *Darier,* French dermatologist, 1856–1938]. PAUTRIER'S MICROABSCESS.

Darier's disease [J. F. *Darier*]. A genodermatosis transmitted as a dominant characteristic, consisting of keratotic papules which coalesce to form warty, crusted patches. Syn. *keratosis follicularis.*

Darier's sign [J. F. *Darier*]. A sign of urticaria pigmentosa in which urticaria develops where a macular skin lesion has been stroked with a blunt instrument.

dark adaptation. Adjustment of the iris and retina for vision in dim light or darkness.

dark-field microscopy or **illumination.** A system using a special condenser that transmits only light entering its periphery, so that particles in the object plane are obliquely illuminated and glow against a dark background. Submicroscopic particles and nearly transparent living organisms such as *Treponema* are thus visualized. Contr. *bright-field microscopy.*

Dark·sche·witsch's nucleus (dark·shey'vich) [L. O. *Darkschewitsch,* Russian neurologist, 1858–1925]. An accessory oculomotor nucleus lying dorsal and lateral to the oculomotor complex; its fibers project to the posterior commissure. Syn. *nucleus of the medial longitudinal fasciculus.*

Darkshevic, Darkshevich. See *Darkschewitsch.*

Dar·ling's disease [S. T. *Darling,* U.S. physician, 1872–1925]. HISTOPLASMOSIS.

darm·brand (dahrm'brahnt) *n.* [Ger. *Darm,* bowel, + *Brand,* burning]. ENTERITIS NECROTICANS.

Dar·row's solution [D. C. *Darrow,* U.S. pediatrician, 1895–1965]. A solution of the electrolytes of plasma, containing added amounts of potassium, used in fluid therapy. It contains 122 mEq/liter sodium, 104 mEq/liter chloride, 35 mEq/liter potassium, and 53 mEq/liter lactate.

d'Ar·son·val current (dar·sohn·val') [J. A. *d'Arsonval,* French physiologist, 1851–1940]. A high-frequency alternating flow of electricity of low voltage and high amperage, used in electrotherapy.

d'ar·son·val·iza·tion (dahr"sun·val"i·zay'shun) *n.* [J. A. *d'Arsonval*]. The therapeutic application of high-frequency electric currents. Three types are used: desiccating, coagulating, and cutting. Syn. *arsonvalization.*

Dartal. Trademark for thiopropazate, a tranquilizing drug used as the dihydrochloride salt.

dar·tos (dahr'tos) *n.* [Gk., flayed]. The thin layer of smooth muscle in the deeper part of the corium and the subcutaneous tissue of the scrotum. NA *tunica dartos.* See also Table of Muscles in the Appendix.

dartos muscle reflex. SCROTAL REFLEX.

dar·trous (dahr'trus) *adj.* [F. *dartreux,* from *dartre,* herpes]. 1. Resembling the dartos. 2. HERPETIC.

Darvon. Trademark for propoxyphene, an analgesic drug.

Dar·win·ism (dahr'win·iz·um) *n.* [C. R. *Darwin,* English naturalist, 1809–1882]. The theory of evolution by natural selection.

Dar·win's tubercle [C. R. *Darwin*]. AURICULAR TUBERCLE (1).

da·ta (day'tuh, dah'tuh) *n.,* sing. **da·tum** (·tum) [L. *datum,* something given, from *dare,* to give]. Items of information, especially as collected or processed for some particular kind or kinds of use.

date sore. LEISHMANIASIS.

da·tive bond (day'tiv). COORDINATE COVALENT BOND.

da·tum (day'tum, dah'tum) *n.* 1. Singular of *data.* 2. A point with reference to which positions are measured.

datum plane. Any one of a number of horizontal planes, determined by certain craniometric points, used in craniometry.

Da·tu·ra (dah·tew'ruh) *n.* [Skr. *dhattūra*]. A genus of Solanaceae. Stramonium is produced by the *Datura stramonium.* Alkaloids of the solanaceous group, chiefly scopolamine, hyoscyamine, and atropine, are yielded by several species of *Datura.*

da·tu·rism (da·tew'riz·um, dat'yoo·riz·um) *n.* [*Datura* + *-ism*]. Poisoning by stramonium.

Dau·cus (daw'kus) *n.* [Gk. *daukos,* carrot]. A genus of plants of the Umbelliferae. The seeds of *Daucus carota,* the wild carrot, have been used as a diuretic and anthelmintic.

daugh·ter, *n.* 1. *In radiochemistry,* a radioactive or stable nuclide resulting from the disintegration of a radioactive nuclide, or parent. 2. (*Attributive use*) Resulting from cell division, as daughter nucleus, daughter chromosome.

daughter cell. A cell resulting from the division of a mother cell.

daughter cyst. A satellite cyst in or near larger cysts.

Daunoblastina. Italian trademark for daunorubicin, an antibiotic.

dau·no·my·cin (daw″no·migh′sin) *n.* DAUNORUBICIN.

dau·no·ru·bi·cin (daw″no·roo′bi·sin) *n.* An antibiotic, $C_{27}H_{29}NO_{10}$, produced by *Streptomyces peucetius* or *S. coeruleorubidus*; has been used experimentally in treatment of acute lymphoblastic leukemia and neuroblastoma.

Dauterine. A trademark for hyoscamine, an antimuscarinic agent.

Da·vai·nea (da·vay′nee·uh) *n.* [C. J. *Davaine*, French physician, d. 1882]. A genus of cestode worms, parasitic for fowls.

Davainea for·mo·sa·na (for·mo·say′nuh). *RAILLIETINA CELEBENSIS.*

Davainea ma·da·gas·ca·ri·en·sis (mad″uh·gas·kăr″ee·en′sis). 1. *RAILLIETINA MADAGASCARIENSIS.* 2. *RAILLIETINA DEMERARIENSIS.*

Davainea pro·glot·ti·na (pro″glot·ee′nuh). A common pathogenic cestode found in the small intestine of the domestic chicken and other fowl.

Dav·en·port's alcoholic silver nitrate method. A variation of Cajal's silver methods.

Da·vid·sohn differential test. A test for infectious mononucleosis in which it is shown that the heterophil antibodies produced in infectious mononucleosis are not absorbed by guinea pig kidney whereas those produced in serum disease are readily absorbed.

Davidsohn presumptive test. A sheep cell agglutination test for the presence of heterophil agglutinin which is characteristically produced in the serum of patients with infectious mononucleosis.

Da·vis graft [J. S. *Davis*, U.S. plastic surgeon, 1872–1946]. Small circular pieces of full-thickness skin, cut with minimal trauma, transplanted to raw wound surfaces. Compare *Reverdin graft.*

Daw·son's encephalitis or **disease** [J. R. *Dawson*, U.S. pathologist, b. 1908]. SUBACUTE SCLEROSING PANENCEPHALITIS.

Dawson's subacute inclusion-body encephalitis [J. R. *Dawson*]. SUBACUTE SCLEROSING PANENCEPHALITIS.

day blindness. Low visual acuity in good light; may be congenital, familial, or due to a lesion involving the cones of the fovea. Also considered to be a form of monochromatism or a frequently incomplete form of total color blindness. Syn. *hemeralopia.* Contr. *night blindness.*

day·dream, *n. & v.* 1. An unrealistic, usually wishful reverie experienced while awake. 2. To experience a daydream.

day hospital. A special facility within a hospital setting which enables the patient to come to the hospital for treatment during the day and to return home at night. Contr. *night hospital.*

day sight. NIGHT BLINDNESS.

da·za·drol (day′zuh·drole) *n.* α-(*p*-Chlorophenyl)-α-(2-imidazolin-2-yl)-2-pyridinemethanol, $C_{15}H_{14}ClN_3O$, an antidepressant usually employed as the maleate salt.

daz·zle reflex of Pei·per (pye′pur) [A. *Peiper*, German pediatrician, 20th century]. In infants, the shining of a bright light on the eyes causes an immediate closing of the lids which lasts as long as the stimulus. There may also be slight extension of the head.

db Abbreviation for *decibel.*

DBS Abbreviation for *despeciated bovine serum.*

DC, dc Abbreviation for *direct current.*

D.C. 1. Doctor of Chiropractic. 2. Dental Corps.

DCI Abbreviation for *dichloroisoproterenol.*

D colony. An abbreviation for *dwarf colony.*

d component. DYSPLASIA (2).

DDD Dichlorodiphenyldichloroethane, more specifically 1,1-dichloro-2,2-bis(*p*-chlorophenyl)ethane; an insecticide similar to DDT.

D.D.S. Doctor of Dental Surgery.

DDST Abbreviation for *Denver Developmental Screening Test.*

DDT 1,1,1,-Trichloro-2,2-bis(*p*-chlorophenyl) ethane, an insecticide the medicinal grade of which is chlorophenothane.

de- [L. *de*, from, off, away, down]. A prefix meaning (a) *undoing, reversal;* (b) *removal, loss.*

de·ac·ti·vate (dee·ack′ti·vate) *v.* To become or render inactive. —**de·ac·ti·va·tion** (dee·ack″ti·vay′shun) *n.*

dead, *adj.* No longer living.

dead·ly night·shade. BELLADONNA.

dead space. A cavity left after the closure of a wound. See also *anatomical dead space, physiological dead space.*

dead time. *In radiochemistry,* the time interval, after recording a count, during which a Geiger counter tube and its circuit are completely insensitive and thus incapable of detecting other ionizing events.

deaf, *adj.* Unable to hear because of a defect, disease, or dysfunction of the ear, the vestibulocochlear nerve, or the brain. —**deaf·ness,** *n.*

deaf·ened, *adj.* Rendered deaf after having had normal hearing, especially after having learned to comprehend and produce speech. —**deaf·en,** *v.*

de·af·fer·en·ta·tion (dee·af″ur·en·tay′shun) *n.* The process of interrupting afferent nerve (sensory) fibers.

deaf field or **point.** One of the small areas near the external auditory meatus in which the vibrating tuning fork is not heard.

deaf-mute, *n.* A person who lacks the sense of hearing and the ability to speak.

deaf-mutism, *n.* The condition of being both deaf and mute. See also *congenital deaf-mutism.*

de·al·bate (dee·al′bate) *adj.* [L. *dealbare, dealbatus,* to whitewash, from *albus,* white]. *In biology,* coated with a fine white down or powder.

de·al·co·hol·iza·tion (dee·al″kuh·hol″i·zay′shun) *n. In microscopy,* the removal of alcohol from an object or compound.

de·am·i·dase (dee·am′i·dace, ·daze) *n.* [*de-* + *amid-* + *-ase*]. An enzyme that catalyzes the hydrolysis of an amido compound. —**de·am·i·di·za·tion** (dee·am″i·di·zay′shun) *n.*

de·am·i·nase (dee·am′i·nace, ·naze) *n.* [*de* + *amin-* + *-ase*]. An enzyme that catalyzes the splitting off of an amino group from an organic compound.

de·am·i·nate (dee·am′i·nate) *v.* To remove an amino (NH_2) group from an organic compound, particularly from an amino acid. —**de·am·i·na·tion** (dee·am″i·nay′shun) *n.*

deaminating enzyme. DEAMINIZING ENZYME.

de·am·i·nize (dee·am′i·nize) *v.* DEAMINATE. —**de·am·i·ni·za·tion** (dee·am″i·ni·zay′shun) *n.*

deaminizing enzyme. An enzyme, such as guanase or adenase, that splits off —NH_2 groups; usually followed by a secondary oxidative reaction.

Deaner. A trademark for deanol acetamidobenzoate, an antidepressant.

de·an·es·the·si·ant (dee·an″esth·ee′zhunt, ·zee·unt) *n.* Any agent or means of arousing a patient from a state of anesthesia.

dean·ol acet·am·i·do·ben·zo·ate (deen′ol as″it·am″i·do·ben′zo·ate). $C_{13}H_{20}N_2O_4$, the *p*-acetamidobenzoic acid salt of 2-dimethylaminoethanol, an antidepressant drug.

de·aqua·tion (dee″a·kway′shun) *n.* [*de-* + L. *aqua,* water]. The act or process of removing water from a substance; dehydration.

death, *n.* The cessation of life, beyond the possibility of resuscitation. See also *brain death.*

death adder. *ACANTHOPHIS ANTARCTICUS.*

death certificate. A form, usually required by law, for recording the event of death, its time, place, cause, the name and age of the decedent, and other pertinent data.

death instinct. *In psychoanalytic theory,* the unconscious drive which leads the individual toward dissolution and death, and which coexists with the life instinct.

death mask. A mold of a dead person's face, taken soon after death.

death rate. The proportion of deaths in a given year and area to the mid-year population of that area, usually expressed as the number of deaths per thousand of population. See also *crude death rate, specific death rate.*

death rattle. A gurgling sound heard in dying persons, due to the passage of air through fluid in the trachea.

death struggle. The semiconvulsive twitches often occurring before death.

Dea·ver's incision [J. B. *Deaver,* U.S. surgeon, 1855–1931]. An incision through the sheath of the right rectus abdominis muscle, extending from the costal margin to a point below the level of the umbilicus.

De·bar·y·o·my·ces neoformans (de·băr″ee·o·migh′seez). CRYPTOCOCCUS NEOFORMANS.

de Beur·mann-Gou·ge·rot disease (duh·bœr·mahnn′, goozh·ro′) [C. L. *de Beurmann,* French dermatologist, 1851–1923; and H. *Gougerot*]. SPOROTRICHOSIS.

de·bil·i·tant (de·bil′i·tunt) *adj. & n.* 1. Debilitating, weakening. 2. Any debilitating agent.

de·bil·i·tate (de·bil′i·tate) *v.* [L. *debilitare,* from *debilis,* weak]. To weaken; to make feeble.

de·bil·i·ty (de·bil′i·tee) *n.* [L. *debilitas,* from *debilis,* weak]. Weakness; lack of strength; ASTHENIA.

De·bove's disease (duh·bohv′) [M. G. *Debove,* French physician, 1845–1920]. SPLENOMEGALY.

de·branch·er deficiency (de·branch′ur). LIMIT DEXTRINOSIS.

debrancher deficiency limit dextrinosis. LIMIT DEXTRINOSIS.

debrancher enzyme. Amylo-1,6-glucosidase, an enzyme which acts to free glucose residues from glycogen.

debrancher glycogen storage disease. LIMIT DEXTRINOSIS.

De·bré–de Toni–Fanconi syndrome (duh·brey′) [R. *Debré,* French pediatrician, 20th century; G. *de Toni;* and G. *Fanconi*]. FANCONI SYNDROME.

Debré-Se·me·laigne syndrome (sehm·lehny′) [R. *Debré,* and G. *Semelaigne*]. A symptom complex observed in cretinous children, characterized by enlarged muscles, reduced strength, easy fatigability, and slowness of movements.

de·bride·ment (de·breed″mahn′, de·breed′munt) *n.* [F.]. Removal of foreign material and devitalized tissue from a wound, usually by sharp dissection, sometimes by means of enzymes or other chemical agents. —**de·bride** (de·breed′, day·breed′) *v.*

de·bris (de·bree′, day·bree′) *n.* [F., from OF. *debrisier,* to break]. 1. Foreign material or devitalized tissue. 2. *In dentistry,* soft foreign material loosely attached to the surface of a tooth, as the refuse from the drilling of a cavity.

de·bri·so·quin (de·brye′zo·kwin) *n.* 3,4-Dihydro-2(1*H*)-isoquinolinecarboxamidine, $C_{10}H_{13}N_3$, an antihypertensive drug; used as the sulfate salt.

debt, *n.* [MF. *dette*]. DEFICIT.

dec-, deca- [Gk. *deka*]. A prefix meaning (a) *ten;* (b) *multiplied by ten.*

de·ca·dence (deck′uh·dunce, de·kay′dunce) *n.* [ML. *decadentia,* from *cadere,* to fall]. Decay, decline, deterioration, as in the aging process.

Decadron. A trademark for dexamethasone, an anti-inflammatory glucocorticoid.

Deca-Durabolin. Trademark for nandrolone decanoate, an androgenic steroid ester.

deca·gram (deck′uh·gram) *n.* A metric measure of weight equal to 10 grams. See also Tables of Weights and Measures in the Appendix.

de·cal·ci·fi·ca·tion (dee·kal″si·fi·kay′shun) *n.* Withdrawal or removal of the mineral salts of bone or other calcified substance. See also *demineralization.* —**de·cal·ci·fy** (dee·kal′si·fye) *v.*

deca·li·ter (deck′uh·lee″tur) *n.* A metric measure of volume equal to 10 liters. See also Tables of Weights and Measures in the Appendix.

de·cal·vant (de·kal′vunt) *adj.* [L. *decalvare,* to make bald]. Destroying or removing hair.

deca·me·ter (deck′uh·mee″tur) *n.* A metric measure of length equal to 10 meters. See also Tables of Weights and Measures in the Appendix.

dec·a·me·tho·ni·um (deck″uh·me·tho′nee·um) *n.* One of a homologous series of polymethylene bis(trimethylammonium) ions, of the general formula $(CH_3)_3N^+(CH_2)_nN^+(CH_3)_3$, in which *n* is 10, possessing powerful skeletal muscle relaxant action through blocking of motor impulses at the myoneural junction; used clinically in the form of one of its salts, usually the bromide.

de·can·cel·la·tion (dee·kan″se·lay′shun) *n.* The removal of cancellous bone either for use as bone chips in grafting operations or for correcting deformity.

dec·ane (deck′ane) *n.* [*dec-* + *-ane*]. Any of the isomeric hydrocarbons, $C_{10}H_{22}$, of the paraffin series.

dec·a·no·ate (deck″uh·no′ate) *n.* CAPRATE; a salt or ester of decanoic (capric) acid.

dec·a·no·ic acid (deck″uh·no′ick). CAPRIC ACID.

deca·nor·mal (deck′uh·nor″mul) *adj.* Having 10 times the strength of the normal; said of solutions.

de·cant (dee·kant′) *v.* [ML. *decanthare,* from *canthus,* rim, lip of a vessel, from Gk. *kanthos,* rim, canthus]. To pour off a liquor or solution without disturbing the sediment. —**de·can·ta·tion** (dee·kan·tay′shun) *n.*

deca·pep·tide (deck″uh·pep′tide) *n.* A polypeptide composed of ten amino acid groups.

de·cap·i·tate (dee·kap′i·tate) *v.* To behead; to remove the head of a person, a fetus, an animal, or a bone. —**de·cap·i·ta·tion** (dee·kap″i·tay′shun) *n.*

de·cap·i·ta·tor (dee·kap′i·tay″tur) *n.* An instrument used in performing decapitation in embryotomy.

Decapryn. Trademark for doxylamine, an antihistaminic drug used as the succinate salt.

de·cap·su·la·tion (dee·kap″sue·lay′shun) *n.* The removal of a capsule or enveloping membrane, as the capsule of a kidney.

de·car·bon·ize (dee·kahr′bun·ize) *v.* To remove carbon. —**de·car·bon·iza·tion** (dee·kahr″bun·i·zay′shun, ·eye·zay′shun) *n.*

de·car·box·yl·ase (dee″kahr·bock′sil·ace, ·aze) *n.* An enzyme that removes carbon dioxide without oxidation from various carboxylic acids.

de·car·box·yl·ate (dee″kahr·bock′si·late) *v.* To split off one or more molecules of carbon dioxide from organic acids, especially amino acids. —**decar·box·yl·a·tion** (·bock″si·lay′shun) *n.*

decarboxylating enzyme. An enzyme, such as carboxylase, that cleaves carbon dioxide from organic acids.

de·ca·thec·tion (dee″ka·theck′shun) *n.* [*de-* + *cathect*]. DECATHEXIS.

de·ca·thex·is (dee″ka·theck′sis) *n.* [*de-* + *cathexis*]. *In psychiatry,* the process of dissolving or removing the investment of psychic energy in the form of libidinal or aggressive drives toward one's mental representation of a person or a thing. —**de·ca·thect** (dee″ka·theckt) *v.*

deca·vi·ta·min (deck″uh·vye′tuh·min) *n.* A U.S.P. formulation of vitamin A, vitamin D, ascorbic acid, calcium pantothenate, cyanocobalamin, folic acid, niacinamide, pyridoxine hydrochloride, riboflavin, thiamine, and a suitable form of alpha tocopherol. One capsule or tablet supplies the recommended daily requirement of the vitamins contained therein.

de·cay (de·kay′) *n. & v.* [OF. *decair,* from L. *de-* + *cadere,* to fall]. 1. The progressive chemical decomposition of organic matter in the presence of atmospheric oxygen; due generally to aerobic bacteria and to fungi; rot. 2. A decline in health or strength. 3. SENILITY. 4. DENTAL CARIES. 5. *In physics,* the process or processes of nuclear disintegration by which an unstable, i.e., radioactive, atom is spontaneously converted to a stable one. 6. To undergo decay.

decay constant. The proportion of atoms of any radioactive substance that will disintegrate per unit of time. Radioactive disintegration (decay) is measured by the equation $N = N_0 e^{-kt}$, where N is the number of atoms unchanged at time t, N_0 is the number present initially, e is the base of natural logarithms, and k is the decay constant.

decay curve. *In radiobiology,* a curve showing the percentage of radioactive substance remaining as a function of time.

decay rate. *In radiobiology,* the rate of decay of a radioactive substance, usually expressed as disintegrations per unit time.

Deccox. A trademark for decoquinate, a poultry coccidiostat.

de·ce·dent (de·see'dunt) *n.* [L. *decedere,* to depart, to die]. A deceased person.

decem- [L.]. A combining form meaning *ten.*

de·cen·tered (dee·sen'turd) *adj.* Out of common center; said of a lens when the visual axis and the axis of the lens do not coincide. —**de·cen·tra·tion** (dee"sen·tray'shun) *n.*

de·cer·e·bel·la·tion (dee·serr"e·be·lay'shun) *n.* The experimental removal of the cerebellum for the study of cerebellar functions.

[1]**de·cer·e·brate** (dee·serr'e·brate) *v.* [*de-* + *cerebrum*]. To perform decerebration upon.

[2]**de·cer·e·brate** (dee·serr'e·brut) *adj.* Of, pertaining to, or having undergone interruption of the neuraxis between the inferior and superior colliculi, rendering the cerebrum and higher centers nonfunctional.

decerebrate posture or **position.** The posture assumed by a patient in a state of decerebrate rigidity. The limbs are stiffly extended, the head retracted, and these postures become exaggerated in response to painful stimuli. Compare *decorticate posture.*

decerebrate rigidity. Markedly increased tone in the antigravity muscles resulting from interruption of the neuraxis at a point between the inferior and superior colliculi, with release of the facilitatory pathways of the reticular formation and the vestibulospinal tract.

de·cer·e·bra·tion (dee·serr"e·bray'shun) *n.* [*de-* + *cerebrum*]. Experimental rendering of an animal's cerebrum and higher centers nonfunctional by interruption, usually transection, of the neuraxis at a point between the inferior and superior colliculi.

de·cer·e·brize (dee·serr'e·brize) *v.* To perform decerebration; to decerebrate.

Deceresol OT. Trademark for dioctyl sodium sulfosuccinate, used as a wetting agent.

de·chlo·ri·da·tion (dee·klor"i·day'shun) *n.* Reduction of the quantity of chloride or salt present in tissues.

de·chlo·ri·na·tion (dee·klor"i·nay'shun) *n.* Removal of chlorine, as from water.

de·chlor·u·ra·tion (dee·klor"yoo·ray'shun, ·oo·ray'shun) *n.* Reduction of the amount of chlorides excreted in the urine.

Decholin. A trademark for dehydrocholic acid, a choleretic drug.

deci- [L. *decimus*]. A combining form meaning (a) *tenth;* (b) in the metric system, *a measure one-tenth as large as the unit.*

dec·i·bel (des'i·bel). *n.* One-tenth of a bel. Abbreviated, db.

Decicain. A trademark for tetracaine, a local anesthetic.

de·cid·ua (de·sid'yoo·uh) *n.*, pl. **decid·u·ae** (·yoo·ee) [L., fem. of *deciduus,* falling off]. The endometrium of pregnancy, which is cast off at parturition. —**decid·u·al** (·yoo·ul) *adj.*

decidua ba·sa·lis (ba·say'lis) [NA]. The part of the endometrium of pregnancy between the chorionic vesicle and the myometrium which forms the maternal part of the placenta.

decidua cap·su·la·ris (kap·sue·lair'is) [NA]. The part of the endometrium of pregnancy between the chorionic vesicle and the uterine lumen; the outer investing envelope of the fetus. NA *decidua reflexa.*

decidual cast. The entire decidua expelled from the uterus in a single piece, as with extrauterine gestation.

decidual cell. One of the large, rounded, modified, connective-tissue cells characteristic of the deciduae in pregnancy and responsible for their hypertrophy.

decidual endometritis. DECIDUITIS.

decidual fissure. One of the fissured spaces developing in the decidua basalis, parallel with the uterine wall, in the later months of pregnancy.

decidual membranes. The membranes formed by the superficial part of the endometrium during pregnancy. NA *membranae deciduae.* See also *decidua basalis, decidua capsularis, decidua parietalis.*

decidual reaction. The reaction of tissues, especially the endometrium, to pregnancy; marked by the development of characteristic decidual cells from fibroblasts.

decidua mar·gi·na·lis (mahr"ji·nay'lis). The part of the endometrium of pregnancy at the junction of the decidua basalis, decidua parietalis, and decidua capsularis.

decidua men·stru·a·lis (men"stroo·ay'lis). The outer layer of the uterine mucosa which is shed during menstruation. Syn. *pseudodecidua.*

decidua pa·ri·e·ta·lis (pa·rye"e·tay'lis) [NA]. The endometrium of pregnancy exclusive of the region occupied by the embryo.

decidua re·flexa (re·fleck'suh). DECIDUA CAPSULARIS.

decidua se·ro·ti·na (se·rot'i·nuh). DECIDUA BASALIS.

decidua sub·cho·ri·a·lis (sub·ko·ree·ay'lis). SUBCHORIAL CLOSING RING.

de·cid·u·ate (de·sid'yoo·ut) *adj.* 1. Having, or characterized by, a decidua. 2. Formed in part from a decidua.

de·cid·u·a·tion (de·sid"yoo·ay'shun) *n.* The act or process of dropping off or shedding.

decidua ve·ra (veer'uh) [BNA]. DECIDUA PARIETALIS.

de·cid·u·itis (de·sid"yoo·eye'tis) *n.* [*decidua* + *-itis*]. An acute inflammation of the decidua, frequently the result of attempts to induce abortion.

de·cid·u·o·ma (de·sid"yoo·o'muh) *n.* [*decidua* + *-oma*]. 1. Decidual tissue produced in the uterus by mechanical or other methods in the absence of an embryo. 2. An intrauterine tumor containing decidual remnants believed to arise from hyperplasia of a retained portion of the decidua.

deciduoma ma·lig·num (ma·lig'num). CHORIOADENOMA.

de·cid·u·o·sis (de·sid"yoo·o'sis) *n.* [*decidua* + *-osis*]. A condition in which the decidual tissue develops in an ectopic site, such as the vagina or the cervix of the uterus.

de·cid·u·ous (de·sid'yoo·us) *adj.* [L. *deciduus,* from *de-* + *cadere,* to fall]. Falling off or shed periodically or at a particular stage, as at maturity.

deciduous dentition. PRIMARY DENTITION.

deciduous skin. KERATOLYSIS.

deciduous teeth. The 20 teeth of the primary dentition; those which erupt first and are replaced by succedaneous permanent teeth; there are 8 incisors, 4 canines, and 8 molars. Syn. *primary teeth.* NA *dentes decidui.* Contr. *permanent teeth.* See also Plate 21.

deci·gram (des'i·gram) *n.* One-tenth of a gram. Abbreviated, dg. See also Tables of Weights and Measures in the Appendix.

deci·li·ter (des'i·lee"tur) *n.* One-tenth of a liter. Abbreviated, dl. See also Tables of Weights and Measures in the Appendix.

deci·me·ter (des'i·mee"tur) *n.* One-tenth of a meter. Abbreviated, dm. See also Tables of Weights and Measures in the Appendix.

deci·nor·mal (des'i·nor"mul) *adj.* Having one-tenth the strength of the normal.

de·cip·a·ra (de·sip'uh·ruh) *n.* [*deci-* + *-para*]. A woman who has given birth 10 times.

Declinax. Trademark for debrisoquin, an antihypertensive drug used as the sulfate salt.

de·clive (de·klive') *n.* [L. *declives,* sloping]. A lower or descending part.

declive of the cerebellum. The first portion of the vermis behind the primary fissure, which with the culmen makes the monticulus.

declive of the monticulus. DECLIVE OF THE CEREBELLUM.

Declomycin. Trademark for the antibiotic demeclocycline.

de·coc·tion (de·cock'shun) *n.* [L. *decoctio,* a boiling down]. *In pharmacy,* a liquid dosage form obtained by boiling a medicinal vegetable substance in water.

de·col·la·tion (dee"kol·ay'shun) *n.* [L. *decollatio,* from *collum,* neck]. DECAPITATION.

de·col·la·tor (de·kol'ay·tur, dee'kuh·lay"tur) *n.* An instrument used for fetal decapitation.

de·col·or·ant (dee·kul'ur·unt) *adj. & n.* 1. Employed or having the capacity to alter or remove color. 2. Any of a variety of decolorant chemical agents.

de·col·or·ize (dee·kul'ur·ize) *v.* To remove color. —**de·col·or·iza·tion** (·kul"ur·i·zay'shun) *n.*

de·com·pen·sa·tion (dee·kom"pun·say'shun) *n.* [*de-* + *compensation*]. Failure of compensation, as of the circulation or heart, or of the ego to stress. —**decompensate,** *v.,* **decompensational,** *adj.*

decompensated ileus, decompensational ileus. A late phase in ileus in which the gut is so distended that the smooth muscle has lost its contractile properties.

de·com·po·si·tion (dee"kom·po·zi'shun, dee·kom") *n.* [*de-* + *composition*]. 1. The separation of the component principles of a body. 2. PUTREFACTION. —**de·com·pose** (dee"kum·poze') *v.*

de·com·pres·sion (dee"kum·presh'un) *n.* The removal of compression or pressure; particularly, various techniques for reducing intracranial pressure, or for preventing decompression sickness in divers and caisson workers.

decompression chamber. 1. *In aerospace medicine,* an apparatus for the reduction of barometric pressure, used to study the biologic effects of high-altitude flying and to evaluate the endurance of flight personnel. 2. A compressed-air chamber for the gradual reduction of barometric pressure for deep-sea divers or caisson workers, designed to prevent or treat decompression sickness.

decompression sickness. A condition caused by the formation of nitrogen bubbles in the blood or body tissues due to an abrupt reduction in atmospheric pressure; occurring with rapid return from compressed-air chambers to normal atmospheric pressure or with rapid ascent either from depths in diving apparatus or to high altitudes in open airplanes; symptoms include severe pain in the joints and chest, itching of the skin, pulmonary edema, urticaria, paralysis, convulsions, and sometimes coma. Compare *aeroembolism, aeroemphysema, bends, chokes, dysbarism.*

de·con·di·tion·ing (dee"kun·dish'un·ing) *n.* The breaking-up or extinction of a conditioned response. —**decondition,** *v.*

de·con·ges·tant (dee"kun·jes'tunt) *n. & adj.* 1. Any decongestive agent. 2. Any agent that reduces hyperemia. 3. DECONGESTIVE.

de·con·ges·tive (dee"kun·jes'tiv) *adj.* Relieving or reducing congestion.

de·con·tam·i·nate (dee"kun·tam'i·nate) *v.* [*de-* + *contaminate*]. To make an object or area safe for unprotected personnel by rendering chemical or biological agents harmless, or by removing or blanketing radiological agents. —**decon·tam·i·na·tion** (·tam"i·nay'shun) *n.*

dec·o·quin·ate (deck"o·kwin'ate) *n.* 6-Decycloxy-7-ethoxy-4-hydroxy-3-quinolinecarboxylic acid, ethyl ester, $C_{24}H_{35}NO_5$, a coccidiostat for poultry.

de·cor·ti·cate (dee·kor'ti·kate) *v.* [L. *decorticare,* from *cortex,* bark, husk, shell]. 1. To strip off the bark or husk of a plant. 2. To remove the cortex or external covering from any organ or structure; decapsulation. 3. Specifically, to remove part or all of the cerebral cortex. —**decorti·cate** (·kate, ·kut) *adj.,* **de·cor·ti·ca·tion** (dee·kor"ti·kay'shun) *n.*

decorticate posture or **position.** The posture assumed by a patient with a lesion at the level of the upper brainstem or above, i.e., whose cerebral cortex is essentially nonfunctioning, in which he lies rigidly motionless unless noxious stimuli are applied, with the arms tightly flexed and the fists clenched, and the legs and feet stiffly extended; the trunk may be opisthotonic. Compare *decerebrate posture.*

dec·re·ment (deck're·munt) *n.* [L. *decrementum,* from *decrescere,* to decrease]. 1. Lessening or subtraction. 2. The amount of loss. 3. The stage in which the effects of a disease are decreasing. —**dec·re·men·tal** (deck"re·men'tul) *adj.*

decremental conduction. Conduction in which the intensity of the impulse decreases progressively.

de·cre·scen·do (dee"kre·shen'do) *n.* [*de-* + It. *crescendo,* from *crescere,* to grow]. A gradual decrease in intensity or loudness; applied to cardiac murmurs.

de·cres·cent (de·kres'unt) *adj.* [L. *decrescere,* to decrease]. 1. Gradually becoming less; decreasing; waning. 2. INVOLUTIONAL; SENILE.

decrescent arteriosclerosis. *Obsol.* MEDIAL ARTERIOSCLEROSIS.

dec·ta·flur (deck'tuh·floor) *n.* 9-Octadecenylamine hydrofluoride, $C_{18}H_{37}N{\cdot}HF$, a dental caries prophylactic.

de·cu·ba·tion (dee"kew·bay'shun) *n.* [*de-* + L. *cubare,* to recline]. The period in the course of an infectious disease beginning with the disappearance of the symptoms and lasting until recovery and the absence of infectious organisms. Contr. *incubation (2).*

decubital ulcer. DECUBITUS ULCER.

de·cu·bi·tus (de·kew'bi·tus) *n.,* pl. **decubi·ti** (·tye) [L., from *decumbere,* to lie down]. 1. The recumbent or horizontal posture. 2. DECUBITUS ULCER. —**decubi·tal** (·tul) *adj.*

decubitus ulcer. Ulceration of the skin and subcutaneous tissues, due to protein deficiency and prolonged unrelieved pressure on bony prominences; seen commonly in aged, cachectic, or paralytic bedridden persons. Syn. *bedsore, pressure sore, pressure ulcer.*

de·cur·tate (de·kur'tate) *adj.* [L. *decurtatus,* from *curtare,* to shorten]. Shortened.

decurtate pulse. A pulse characterized by progressive diminution of strength of the beats.

Decurvon. Trademark for a repository form of insulin containing pectin.

de·cus·sate (de·kus'ate) *v.* [L. *decussare,* to divide crosswise in the form of an X]. To intersect; to cross.

de·cus·sa·tio (deck"uh·say'shee·o, dee"kuh·) *n.,* pl. **decus·sa·ti·o·nes** (·say"shee·o'neez) [L.]. DECUSSATION.

decussatio bra·chii con·junc·ti·vi (bray'kee·eye kon·junk·tye'vye) [BNA]. Decussatio pedunculorum cerebellarium superiorum (= DECUSSATION OF THE SUPERIOR CEREBELLAR PEDUNCLES).

decussatio lem·nis·co·rum (lem·nis·ko'rum) [NA]. DECUSSATION OF THE LEMNISCI.

de·cus·sa·tion (dee"kuh·say'shun, deck"uh·) *n.* [L. *decussatio,* from *decussare,* to divide crosswise, from *decussis,* the figure X]. A chiasma or X-shaped crossing, especially of symmetrical parts, as of nerve fibers uniting unlike structures in the two sides of the brain or spinal cord.

decussatio ner·vo·rum tro·chle·a·ri·um (nur·vo'rum trock·lee·air'ee·um) [NA]. TROCHLEAR DECUSSATION.

decussationes. Plural of *decussatio.*

decussationes teg·men·ti (teg·men'tye) [NA]. The dorsal and ventral tegmental decussations.

decussationes teg·men·to·rum (teg·men·to'rum) [BNA]. DECUSSATIONES TEGMENTI.

decussation of Fo·rel (foh·rel') [A. H. *Forel*]. VENTRAL TEGMENTAL DECUSSATION.

decussation of the bra·chia con·junc·ti·va (bray'kee·uh kon·junk·tye'vuh). DECUSSATION OF THE SUPERIOR CEREBELLAR PEDUNCLES.

decussation of the lemnisci. The decussation of the medial lemnisci and associated fiber tracts. NA *decussatio lemniscorum.*

decussation of the optic nerve. OPTIC CHIASMA.

decussation of the superior cerebellar peduncles. Crossing of fibers from the dentate nucleus of each side of the brain to the opposite red nucleus. NA *decussatio pedunculorum cerebellarium superiorum.*

decussatio pe·dun·cu·lo·rum ce·re·bel·la·ri·um su·pe·ri·o·rum (pe·dunk·yoo·lo′rum serr″e·bel·air′ee·um sue·peer·ee·o′rum) [NA]. DECUSSATION OF THE SUPERIOR CEREBELLAR PEDUNCLES.

decussatio py·ra·mi·dum (pi·ram′i·dum) [NA]. PYRAMIDAL DECUSSATION.

de·dif·fer·en·ti·a·tion (dee″dif·ur·en″shee·ay′shun) *n.* [*de-* + *differentiation*]. The process of giving up or losing specific characters and reverting to a more generalized or primitive morphologic state. —**dediffer·en·ti·ate** (·en′shee·ate) *v.*

de-ef·fer·ent·ed state (dee″ef′ur·en·tid). *Informal.* PSEUDOCOMA.

deep, *adj.* Not superficial.

deep cervical fascia. The fascia that invests the muscles of the neck and encloses the vessels and nerves; consists of three fascial planes, one surrounding the trapezius and sternocleidomastoid muscles, a second surrounding the larynx, pharynx, and thyroid gland, and a third, the prevertebral fascia. NA *fascia cervicalis.*

deep fascia. The fibrous tissue between muscles and forming the sheaths of muscles, or investing other deep, definitive structures, as nerves and blood vessels.

deep femoral arch. A band of fibers originating apparently in the transversalis fascia, arching across the femoral sheath and attached to the middle of the inguinal ligament and the pectineal line.

deep folliculitis. SYCOSIS VULGARIS.

deep gland. A gland which has its secreting portion deep to a mucous membrane, usually in the tela submucosa.

deep inguinal ring. The abdominal opening of the inguinal canal. NA *anulus inguinalis profundus.*

deep keratitis. INTERSTITIAL KERATITIS.

deep palmar arch. The anastomosis between the terminal part of the radial artery and the deep palmar branch of the ulnar artery. Syn. *deep volar arch.* NA *arcus palmaris profundus.* See also Table of Arteries in the Appendix.

deep process of the submandibular gland. A tongue-like extension of the submandibular gland which passes around the posterior border of the mylohyoid muscle and then extends forward along with the submandibular duct.

deep reflex. Any stretch or myotatic reflex of the phasic or jerk type. See also *tendon reflex.*

deep reflex of Bekhterev [V. M. *Bekhterev*]. BEKHTEREV'S DEEP REFLEX.

deep sensation. Perception of pressure, tension, and pain in the muscles, joints, tendons, and deep layers of the skin, as contrasted with sensations derived from the superficial layers of the skin.

deep tendon reflex. TENDON REFLEX.

deep transverse metacarpal ligament. A narrow fibrous transverse band connecting the palmar surfaces of the heads of the second, third, fourth, and fifth metacarpals. NA *ligamentum metacarpeum transversum profundum.*

deep transverse metatarsal ligament. The transverse ligament connecting the plantar surfaces of the heads of the metatarsal bones. NA *ligamentum metatarseum transversum profundum.*

deep volar arch. DEEP PALMAR ARCH.

deep water. Water obtained from a porous layer beneath the first impervious stratum of the ground.

deer fly. *Chrysops discalis,* a vector of tularemia; most common in western United States.

deer fly fever. TULAREMIA.

Dees's operation [J. E. *Dees,* U.S. urologist, b. 1910]. A pyelolithotomy in which the stones are enmeshed in an artificial fibrin coagulum and are withdrawn from the kidney as the clot is removed.

Deet·jen's bodies (dey′tyun) [H. *Deetjen,* German physician, 1867–1915]. BLOOD PLATELETS.

def *Decayed, extracted, and filled teeth;* used in the quantitative estimate of dental caries in deciduous teeth.

de·fat·ting (dee·fat′ing) *n.* 1. The removal of lipids from tissue by extraction with fat solvents. 2. The removal of adipose tissue by surgical means, especially from grafts of skin.

def·e·cate, def·ae·cate (def′e·kate) *v.* [L. *defaecare,* to cleanse from dregs, from *faex, faecis,* dregs]. 1. To evacuate the bowels. 2. To purify or refine. —**def·e·ca·tion, def·ae·ca·tion** (def″e·kay′shun), *n.*

defecation reflex. RECTUM REFLEX.

defecation reflex centers. Regions in the lower lumbar and the upper sacral segments of the spinal cord and in the ganglionic plexus of the gut, concerned with controlling the rectum reflex.

de·fect, *n.* [L. *defectus*]. 1. A lack, failure, or deficiency, as of a normal function. 2. Absence of a part or organ.

de·fec·tive, *adj.* & *n.* 1. Falling below an established standard of quality, composition, structure, or behavior. 2. A person lacking a physical or mental quality, especially the latter.

de·fem·i·na·tion (de·fem″i·nay′shun) *n.* DEFEMINIZATION.

de·fem·i·ni·za·tion (de·fem″i·ni·zay′shun) *n.* 1. *In medicine,* the loss or diminution of female sex characteristics, usually as a result of ovarian dysfunction or removal. 2. *In psychiatry,* in cases of antipathic sexual instinct the psychic process in which there is a deep and permanent change of character in a woman, resulting in a giving up of feminine feelings, and the assumption of masculine qualities. Contr. *eviration.* —**de·fem·i·nize** (dee·fem′i·nize) *v.*

defense mechanism or **reaction.** Any psychic device for guarding oneself against blame, guilt, anxiety, and unpleasant or disagreeable memories or experiences, or for concealing unacceptable desires, feelings, and beliefs; an unconscious attempt at self-justification and the maintenance of self-esteem. Specific defense mechanisms are conversion, denial, dissociation, rationalization, repression, and sublimation.

defense reflex. PROTECTIVE REFLEX.

def·er·ent (def′ur·unt) *adj.* [L. *deferens, deferentis,* from *deferre,* to carry away]. 1. Carrying away or down; EFFERENT. 2. Pertaining to the ductus deferens.

deferent canal or **duct.** DUCTUS DEFERENS.

def·er·en·tial (def″ur·en′shul) *adj.* Pertaining to the ductus deferens.

deferential artery. A small branch of the internal iliac artery, supplying the seminal vesicle, ductus deferens, and epididymis; the homologue in the male of the uterine artery. NA *arteria ductus deferentis.*

deferential plexus. A nerve plexus surrounding the ductus deferens and seminal vesicle. NA *plexus deferentialis.*

def·er·en·tio·ves·i·cal (def″ur·en″shee·o·ves′i·kul) *adj.* [*deferential* + *vesical*]. Pertaining to both the ductus deferens and the urinary bladder.

def·er·en·ti·tis (def″ur·en·tye′tis) *n.* [*deferent* + *-itis*]. Inflammation of the ductus deferens.

de·fer·ox·a·mine (dee″ferr·ock′suh·meen) *n.* A complex amine, $C_{25}H_{48}N_6O_8$, of microbial origin, used as an iron-chelating compound in the treatment of hemochromatosis. Syn. *desferrioxamine.*

de·fer·ves·cence (dee″fur·ves′unce, ·def′ur·) *n.* [L. *defervescere,* to cease boiling]. Disappearance of fever.

de·fer·ves·cent (dee″fur·ves′unt, def″ur·) *adj.* & *n.* [L. *defervescens,* ceasing to boil]. 1. Of a fever: diminishing or disappearing. 2. Having the effect of allaying or reducing a fever. 3. A fever-reducing agent.

defervescent stage. The stage in which fever declines.

de·fi·bril·la·tion (dee·fib″ri·lay′shun, ·figh″bri·) *n.* 1. The arrest of fibrillation of the cardiac atria or ventricles. See also *cardioversion.* 2. Blunt dissection of tissue fibers along planes of cleavage. —**de·fi·bril·late** (dee·fib′ri·late, ·figh′bri·) *v.*

de·fi·bril·la·tor (dee·fib′ri·lay″tur, ·figh′bri·) *n.* An apparatus for defibrillating the heart, by the application of electric current.

de·fi·bri·nate (dee·figh′bri·nate) *v.* To remove fibrin from blood or lymph. —**de·fi·bri·na·tion** (dee·figh″bri·nay′shun) *n.*

defibrination syndrome. DISSEMINATED INTRAVASCULAR COAGULATION.

de·fi·cien·cy, *n.* [L. *deficientia,* from *deficere,* to be lacking]. 1. The state or condition of lacking a substance, quality, or characteristic essential for completeness. 2. The amount or extent of lack of an essential substance, quality, or characteristic. 3. *In genetics,* the abnormal lack of a segment of a chromosome; DELETION.

deficiency anemia. HYPOCHROMIC MICROCYTIC ANEMIA.

deficiency disease. A disease resulting from the lack of a necessary dietary constituent, as minerals, vitamins, fatty acids, or essential food elements.

de·fi·cient (de·fish′unt) *adj.* [L. *deficiens,* from *deficere,* to be lacking]. Lacking a substance, quality, or characteristic essential for completeness; below standard.

def·i·cit (def′i·sit) *n.* [L., it fails or is lacking]. 1. A deficiency or lack. 2. An impairment in a particular function. 3. The amount by which something is short of a specified standard. Syn. *debt.*

def·i·ni·tion, *n.* [L. *definitio,* from *definire,* to bound by limits]. 1. The quality of an image with respect to sharpness or clarity of outlines. 2. The quality of a lens with respect to sharpness or clarity of outlines in the images it forms.

de·fin·i·tive, *adj.* [L. *definitivus,* from *definire,* to determine]. 1. Complete; fully developed. 2. Pertaining to the mature or fully developed stage of something. 3. Serving to define.

definitive callus. The permanent callus which is formed between fractured or divided ends of bone and in time is changed into true bone.

definitive host. A host in which the sexual stages of the parasite develop. Contr. *intermediate host.*

definitive kidney. METANEPHROS.

definitive percussion. Percussion whose purpose is to outline the borders of a viscus.

definitive treatment. Any treatment, including surgical and other generally accepted procedures, necessary to produce ultimate recovery of the patient.

definitive urogenital sinus. The distal part of the primitive urogenital sinus forming a common chamber for the openings of the primary urethra and the mesonephric and paramesonephric ducts. NA *sinus urogenitalis.*

def·la·gra·tion (def″luh·gray′shun) *n.* [L. *deflagrare,* to burn up]. A sudden, violent combustion.

de·fla·tion receptors. Vagal nerve fibers that are stimulated by deflation of the lung and reflexly induce inspiration.

de·flec·tion, *n.* [L. *deflectere,* to turn aside]. A turning, or state of being turned, aside.

def·lo·ra·tion (def″lo·ray′shun) *n.* [L. *defloratio,* a plucking of flowers]. Natural loss of the external sexual characteristics which in women indicate virginity, usually typified by rupture of the hymen at the first sexual intercourse.

de·flo·res·cence (dee″flo·res′unce) *n.* [L. *deflorescere,* to drop its blossoms, fade]. Disappearance of the eruption of an exanthematous disease.

de·flu·vi·um (dee·floo′vee·um) *n.* [L., from *defluere,* to flow down]. DEFLUXIO.

defluvium cap·il·lo·rum (kap·i·lo′rum) [L., of the hair]. ALOPECIA.

defluvium un·gui·um (ung′gwee·um). Complete loss of nails.

de·flux·io (dee·fluck′see·o) *n.* [L., from *defluere,* to flow down]. 1. Loss, disappearance. 2. A flowing down.

deforming spondylitis. ANKYLOSING SPONDYLITIS.

de·for·mi·ty, *n.* [L. *deformitas,* from *deformis,* misshapen]. 1. The state of being misshapen. 2. Marked deviation from the normal in size or shape of the body or of a part. —**deform,** *v.*

de·froth·i·cant (de·froth′ick·unt, ·froth′) *n.* A chemical agent that reduces frothing.

de·func·tion·al·iza·tion (de·funk″shun·ul·i·zay′shun) *n.* Loss of function.

de·fu·sion (dee·few′zhun) *n.* [*de-* + *fusion*]. *In psychoanalysis,* the separation of the two primal, or life and death, instincts.

Degalol. A trademark for deoxycholic acid, a choleretic drug.

de·gan·gli·on·ate (dee·gang′glee·un·ate) *v.* To remove a ganglion or ganglia.

de·gas (dee·gas′) *v.* To free an area from toxic gas.

de·gen·er·a·cy (de·jen′ur·uh·see) *n.* 1. A state marked by the deterioration of the mind and body. 2. Sexual perversion as defined by existing social and legal codes; specifically, the committing of or the attempt to commit a sexual offense, such as rape, pederasty, or exhibitionism. 3. The existence in the genetic code of more than one codon for each amino acid.

de·gen·er·ate (de·jen′ur·ate) *v.* [L. *degenerare*]. 1. To undergo the retrogressive changes of degeneration. 2. To deteriorate in physical, mental, or psychic characters.

de·gen·er·ate (de·jen′ur·ut) *adj. & n.* 1. Having undergone degeneration. 2. A person who has changed markedly for the worse in his moral, social, or biological, usually sexual, conduct, or who falls far short of the behavior expected of him in a particular society at a particular time; usually, an individual with markedly deviant sexual behavior.

de·gen·er·a·tion (de·jen″ur·ay′shun) *n.* 1. A retrogressive change in cells characterized by initial cytoplasmic deterioration, then nuclear death in some instances, all with little or no signs of a response to injury. 2. A retrogressive process including even the death of nerves, axons, or tracts of the central nervous system. 3. A sinking to a lower state; progressive deterioration of a physical, mental, or moral state. —**de·gen·er·a·tive** (de·jen′ur·uh·tiv) *adj.*

degeneration of cerebral gray matter in childhood. PROGRESSIVE CEREBRAL POLIODYSTROPHY.

degenerative arthritis. DEGENERATIVE JOINT DISEASE.

degenerative atrophy. A form of atrophy in which cellular degeneration is conspicuous.

degenerative chorea. HUNTINGTON'S CHOREA.

degenerative disease. Disease characterized by the progressive impairment of the function of an organ or organs and not attributable to some cause such as infection or a metabolic defect; for example, Alzheimer's disease or Parkinson's disease. See also *abiotrophy, heredodegenerative.*

degenerative joint disease. A chronic joint disease characterized pathologically by degeneration of articular cartilage and hypertrophy of bone, clinically by pain on activity which subsides with rest; it occurs more commonly in older people, affecting the weight-bearing joints and the distal interphalangeal joints of the fingers; there are no systemic symptoms. Syn. *degenerative arthritis, hypertrophic arthritis, osteoarthritis, senescent arthritis.*

degenerative psychosis. Any psychotic disorder in which the individual regresses to some earlier stage of development or exhibits childish behavior.

de·gen·i·tal·i·ty (dee·jen″i·tal′i·tee) *n.* *In psychoanalysis,* a condition wherein genital instincts are expressed through activities of a nongenital character. —**de·gen·i·tal·ize** (dee·jen′i·tul·ize) *v.*

de·germ (dee·jurm′) *v.* To reduce the normal or abnormal bacterial flora of skin, mucosal surfaces, or open wounds by mechanical cleansing or antiseptic action. —**de·germ·a·tion** (dee″jur·may′shun) *n.*

de·glob·u·li·za·tion crisis (dee·glob″yoo·li·zay′shun). An acute episode in hereditary spherocytosis, characterized by fever, lassitude, palpitation, shortness of breath, violent abdominal pain, vomiting, and anorexia; and associated with anemia resulting from sudden temporary cessation of blood formation. Syn. *crise de deglobulization.*

de·glu·ti·tion (dee″gloo·tish′un, deg″loo·) *n.* [L. *deglutire,* to swallow down]. The act of swallowing. —**de·glu·ti·tive** (de·gloo′ti·tiv), **degluti·to·ry** (·to″ree) *adj.*

deglutition reflex. SWALLOWING REFLEX.

De·gos-De·lort-Tri·cot syndrome (duh·go′, duh·lor′, tree·ko′). DEGOS' DISEASE.

Degos' disease [R. *Degos,* French dermatologist, 20th century]. A combination of slowly evolving painless skin papules, that eventually develop an atrophic center, and multiple infarcts of the viscera, with angiitis common to both. Syn. *malignant papulosis, papulosis atrophicans maligna.*

deg·ra·da·tion (deg″ruh·day′shun) *n.* [L *degradatio,* from *gradus,* step]. The conversion of one organic compound to another containing a smaller number of carbon atoms. —**de·grade** (de·grade′) *v.*

de·grease (dee·greece′) *v.* [*de-* + *grease*]. To remove fat, as from bones in the preparation of skeletons.

de·gree, *n.* [OF. *degré,* from *de-* + L. *gradus,* step]. 1. A position in a graded series. 2. One of the units or intervals of a thermometric or other scale. 3. The unit for measuring arcs or angles. One degree is 1/360 of a circle. A right angle is 90° or one-quarter of a circle. 4. A rank or title conferred by a college or university in recognition of attainment. 5. *In law,* the relative amount of guilt. 6. One remove in the direct line of descent; one remove in the chain of relationship, as a cousin of fourth degree.

degree of freedom. 1. In mechanics, any of the ways in which a point, body, or system may change or move. 2. *In physical chemistry,* a system's capacity for variation due to the variability of one of its factors. 3. *In biometry,* the number of independent values in a statistical table.

de·gus·ta·tion (dee″gus·tay′shun) *n.* [L. *degustare,* to taste, from *gustus,* taste]. The act of tasting.

De·hio's test (d^ye^·^k^hee′uh, d^ye^·gee′uh, Ger. de^y^·hee′o) [K. K. *Dehio,* Russian physician, 1851–1927]. A test to determine the cause of bradycardia; bradycardia abolished by atropine injection is of vagus nerve origin; if not, it is presumed to be due to myocardial factors.

de·his·cence (dee·his′unce) *n.* [L. *dehiscere,* to gape]. 1. The act of splitting open. 2. A defect in the boundary of a bony canal or cavity.

dehydr-, dehydro-. A combining form meaning (a) *dehydrated;* (b) *dehydrogenated.*

de·hy·drase (dee·high′drace) *n.* One of a group of pyridoxal phosphate-dependent enzymes which form ammonia and an α-keto acid from certain amino acids (serine, cysteine, homoserine, and threonine).

de·hy·drate (dee·high′drate) *v.* To remove water from (any source, including the body and its tissues). —**dehydrat·ed,** adj., **de·hy·dra·tion** (dee″high·dray′shun) *n.*

dehydrated alcohol. Ethyl alcohol containing not less than 99.5% by volume of C_2H_5OH. Syn. *absolute alcohol.*

dehydrated creatine. CREATININE.

de·hy·dro·ascor·bic acid (dee·high″dro·uh·skor′bick). The relatively inactive acid resulting from elimination of two hydrogen atoms from ascorbic acid when the latter is oxidized by air or other agents.

de·hy·dro·cho·late (dee·high″dro·ko′late) *n.* A salt of dehydrocholic acid.

7-de·hy·dro·cho·les·ter·ol (dee·high″dro·ko·les′tur·ole, ·ol) *n.* A provitamin of animal origin in the skin of man, in milk, and elsewhere, which upon irradiation with ultraviolet rays becomes vitamin D_3.

de·hy·dro·cho·lic acid (dee·high″dro·ko′lick, ·kol′ick). 3,7,12-Triketocholanic acid, $C_{24}H_{34}O_5$, resulting when the three hydroxyl groups of cholic acid are oxidized to keto groups. Both the acid and its sodium salt are used for their hydrocholeretic and choleretic effects.

de·hy·dro·cor·ti·cos·ter·one (dee-high″dro·kor″ti·kos′tur·ohn) *n.* 11-Dehydrocorticosterone or 21-hydroxypregn-4-ene-3,11,20-trione, $C_{21}H_{28}O_4$, a steroid occurring in the adrenal cortex and possessing biologic activity similar to that of corticosterone.

de·hy·dro·epi·an·dros·ter·one (dee·high″dro·ep″ee·an·dros′tur·ohn) *n.* DEHYDROISOANDROSTERONE.

de·hy·dro·gen·ase (dee·high′druh·je·nace, ·naze, dee″high·droj′e·) *n.* An enzyme that catalyzes the oxidation of a specific substrate by removal of hydrogen; a hydrogen acceptor may or may not be required.

de·hy·dro·gen·ate (dee·high′druh·je·nate, dee″high·droj′e·) *v.* To remove hydrogen from. —**de·hy·dro·gen·a·tion** (dee·high″druh·je·nay′shun) *n.*

de·hy·dro·gen·ize (dee·high′druh·je·nize) *v.* DEHYDROGENATE. —**de·hy·dro·gen·iza·tion** (de·high″druh·je·ni·zay′shun) *n.*

de·hy·dro·iso·an·dros·ter·one (dee·high″dro·eye″so·an·dros′tur·ohn) *n.* Androst-5(6)-en-3-ol-17-one, $C_{19}H_{28}O_2$, an androgenic steroid found in the urine of men and women. Syn. *dehydroepiandrosterone.*

de·ion·ize (dee·eye′un·ize) *v.* To remove ionic constituents from (a liquid, especially water).

deionized water. Water purified by passage through substances which remove contaminating cations and anions and leave finally a water equivalent to distilled water in purity.

de·ion·iz·er (dee·eye′un·eye·zur) *n.* An apparatus, charged with suitable ion-exchanging and ion-removing substances, which effects removal of ionic constituents from liquids, notably from water.

Dei·ters' cells (dye′turss) [O. F. K. *Deiters,* German physician, 1834–1863]. CELLS OF DEITERS (1).

Deiters' nucleus [O. F. K. *Deiters*]. LATERAL VESTIBULAR NUCLEUS.

dé·jà pen·sé (de^y^·zhah pah^n^·se^y^′) [F., already thought]. A feeling of familiarity of some thought, as if one had experienced it previously; may be a symptom of psychomotor epilepsy. Compare *deajas vu.*

dé·jà vu (de^y^·zhah vu^e^′) [F., already seen]. A feeling of familiarity; an illusionary or dream state in which experiences seem to have occurred before, as of a new scene or face that looks familiar; a symptom found in tumors or other lesions of the temporal lobe of the brain. Compare *deajas pensea, jamais vu.*

de·jec·ta (de·jeck′tuh) *n. pl.* [L., from *dejicere,* to throw down, let fall]. EXCREMENT.

de·jec·tion (de·jeck′shun) *n.* [L. *dejectio,* a throwing down]. 1. Depression, lowness of spirits. 2. The discharge of fecal matter; defecation. 3. Feces; excrement.

Dé·je·rine-Klump·ke's syndrome or **paralysis** (de^y^zh·reen′ klump′ke^h^) [Augusta *Déjerine-Klumpke,* French neurologist, 1859–1927]. LOWER BRACHIAL PLEXUS PARALYSIS.

Déjerine-Rous·sy syndrome (roo·see′) [J. J. *Déjerine;* and G. *Roussy,* French pathologist, 1874–1948]. THALAMIC SYNDROME.

Déjerine's anterior bulbar syndrome [J. J. *Déjerine*]. Ipsilateral paralysis of the tongue, contralateral hemiplegia and occasionally contralateral loss of proprioceptive and tactile senses, due to occlusion of the anterior spinal artery.

Déjerine's cortical sensory syndrome [J. J. *Déjerine*]. Loss of proprioception, stereognosis, and other highly integrated sensory functions, but essentially normal appreciation of touch, pain, temperature, and vibration; seen in parietal lobe lesions.

Déjerine-Sot·tas disease or **neuropathy** [J. J. *Déjerine;* and J. *Sottas,* French neurologist, 1866-1943]. HYPERTROPHIC INTERSTITIAL NEUROPATHY (1).

Déjerine-Tho·mas atrophy (toʰ·mah') [J. J. *Déjerine*]. OLIVOPONTOCEREBELLAR ATROPHY.

de·lac·ta·tion (dee"lack·tay'shun) *n.* 1. WEANING. 2. Cessation of lactation.

Del·a·field's hematoxylin [F. *Delafield,* U.S. pathologist, 1841-1915]. A solution of an aluminum complex of hematoxylin, used as a stain for nuclei in histologic sections.

De·la·goa sore (de·lahʰ·go'uh) [*Delagoa* Bay, Mozambique]. CUTANEOUS LEISHMANIASIS.

Delalutin. Trademark for hydroxyprogesterone caproate, an esterified derivative of progesterone that elicits responses similar to those with progesterone.

de·lam·i·na·tion (dee·lam"i·nay'shun) *n.* [*de-* + *lamination*]. Separation or splitting into layers, as in the dividing of cells to form new layers.

de Lange's syndrome. CORNELIA DE LANGE'S SYNDROME.

Delanil. A trademark for propenzolate hydrochloride, an anticholinergic.

Delatestryl. Trademark for testosterone enanthate, an androgenic hormone.

de·layed *adj.* Occurring later than normal, or expected.

delayed hypersensitivity. A specific state of sensitivity induced by infectious agents, chemicals, or foreign animal cells in which the onset of the reaction to the inducer is delayed, and which can be transferred passively by cells but not the serum of sensitive animals. See also *tuberculin reaction.*

delayed menarche. Late onset of first menstruation.

delayed menstruation. Menstruation occurring later than expected from previous cyclic timing.

delayed reaction. An inflammatory lesion of the skin or other phenomenon occurring hours or days after contact between allergen or atopen and hypersensitive tissue cells. Such a reaction may be either local at the site of contact or systemic or constitutional.

delayed reflex. A reflex occurring an abnormally long while after the stimulus.

delayed suture. SECONDARY SUTURE.

delayed tetanus. Tetanus occurring after a prolonged incubation period.

delayed-type hypersensitivity. DELAYED HYPERSENSITIVITY.

Del Cas·ti·llo's syndrome (del kas·tee'yo) [E. B. *Del Castillo,* 20th century]. An endocrinologic syndrome of small testes and sterility in otherwise normal-appearing males. On testicular biopsy, the germinal epithelium is absent, although the Sertoli and Leydig cells are normal. Syn. *testicular dysgenesis syndrome.*

Delestrec. A trademark for estradiol undecylate, an estrogen.

Delestrogen. A trademark for estradiol valerate, an estrogen.

del·e·te·ri·ous (del"e·teer'ee·us) *adj.* [Gk. *dēlētērios,* from *dēleisthai,* to hurt]. Harmful, injurious.

de·le·tion (de·lee'shun) *n.* [L. *deletio,* from *delere,* to wipe out, destroy]. *In genetics,* the abnormal lack of a segment of a chromosome; DEFICIENCY (3).

deletion mapping. A method of chromosome mapping which employs chromosomal deletions to locate the region in which a gene occurs.

deletion-5 syndrome. CRI-DU-CHAT SYNDROME.

Del·hi boil (del'ee) [after *Delhi,* India]. CUTANEOUS LEISHMANIASIS.

De Li·ma's operation. TRANSMAXILLARY ETHMOIDECTOMY.

de·lim·it, *v.* To fix limits or boundaries. **—de·lim·i·ta·tion,** *n.*

de·lim·it·ed, *adj.* Marked by bounds; having a line or lines of demarcation.

delimiting keratotomy. Incision into the cornea at points outside the area of a serpiginous or Mooren's ulcer. Syn. *Gifford's operation.*

de·lin·quen·cy, *n.* [L. *delinquere,* to do wrong]. 1. An offense or violation, especially when committed by a minor, as truancy, vandalism, stealing, or overt sex practices. The term implies a psychologic and therapeutic rather than a punitive attitude toward the offender. 2. The tendency to commit delinquencies; the committing of such offenses.

de·lin·quent, *adj.* & *n.* [from L. *delinquere,* to fail, offend]. 1. Committing or constituting a delinquency. 2. A person who commits a delinquency.

de·lip·i·da·tion (dee·lip"i·day'shun) *n.* Removal of lipids by fat solvents from a tissue or microscopic sections.

del·i·quesce (del"i·kwes') *v.* [L. *deliquescere,* to melt away]. To become liquid by absorption of water from the atmosphere. **—del·i·ques·cence** (·kwes'unce) *n.;* **deliques·cent** (·unt) *adj.*

de·liq·ui·um (de·lick'wee·um) *n.* [L., from *delinquere,* to fail]. 1. Faint or syncope. 2. Mental impairment.

deliquium an·i·mi (an'i·migh). SYNCOPE.

de·lir·i·ant (de·lirr'ee·unt) *adj.* DELIRIFACIENT.

de·lir·i·fa·cient (de·lirr"i·fay'shunt, ·shee·unt) *adj.* [*delirium* + L. *facere,* to cause]. Producing or capable of producing delirium.

de·lir·i·um (de·lirr'ee·um) *n.,* pl. **delir·ia** (·ee·uh) [L., from *delirare,* lit., to deviate from the *lira,* furrow]. A disordered mental state of acute onset and transient nature, characterized by confusion, disorientation, disorders of perception (hallucinations and illusions), delusions, vigilance, and overactivity of psychomotor autonomic nervous system functions. Associated with febrile states, exogenous intoxications, and withdrawal states, occasionally with trauma and other encephalopathies. **—deliri·ous** (·us) *adj.*

delirium cor·dis (kor'dis). Fibrillation of the heart, usually atrial.

delirium gran·di·o·sum (gran·dee·o'sum). MEGALOMANIA.

delirium mi·te (migh'tee, mit'ee). QUIET DELIRIUM.

delirium mus·si·tans (muss'i·tanz). QUIET DELIRIUM.

delirium tre·mens (tree'munz). A special and sometimes lethal form of delirium induced by the withdrawal of alcohol, following a prolonged period of alcoholic intoxication. Wakefulness, tremor, hallucinations, delusions, and signs of autonomic overactivity (fever, dilated pupils, sweating, tachycardia) are particularly prominent. An identical clinical state may follow withdrawal of barbiturates and other sedative-hypnotic drugs, and rarely may be associated with cerebral trauma and infections.

de·liv·ery, *n. In obstetrics,* the expulsion or extraction of a fetus and its membranes; parturition. **—deliver,** *v.*

del·le (del'eh) *n.,* pl. **del·len** (·un) [Ger. *Delle,* a dent]. 1. *In ophthalmology,* a small, saucerlike excavation at the margin of the cornea, occurring most often in processes that produce a localized break in the precorneal oily film layer of tears, which in turn causes the corneal dehydration and thinning. 2. *In hematology,* the central, discoid, usually more lightly colored portion of erythrocytes, as seen in a stained peripheral blood smear.

del·mad·i·none (del·mad'i·nohn) *n.* 6-Chloro-17-hydroxypregna-1,4,6-triene-3,20-dione acetate, $C_{23}H_{27}ClO_4$, a progestin.

de·lo·mor·phous (dee"lo·mor'fus) *adj.* [Gk. *dēlos,* conspicuous, + *-morphous*]. Having a conspicuous form, as a parietal cell of the fundic glands.

delomorphous cell. PARIETAL CELL.

de·louse (dee·lowce', ·lowze') *v.* [*de-* + *louse*]. To free from lice; to destroy lice. **—delous·ing** (·ing) *n.*

Del·phin·i·um (del·fin'ee·um) *n.* [Gk. *delphinion,* larkspur]. A genus of plants of the Ranunculaceae; the larkspurs. *Delphinium ajacis,* larkspur, and *D. staphisagria,* staphisagria or stavesacre, have been used to prepare pediculicide formulations.

del Río Hor·te·ga's silver method (del rree'o or·tehʰ'gahʰ) [P. *del Río Hortega*]. HORTEGA'S SILVER METHOD.

del·ta (del'tuh) *n.* [name of the letter Δ, δ, fourth letter of the Greek alphabet]. 1. The fourth of a series, or any particular member or subset of an arbitrarily ordered set; as in chemistry, the fourth carbon atom starting with the one adjacent to the characteristic functional group. Symbol, δ. 2. *In chemistry,* double bond. Symbol, Δ. 3. *In chemistry,* coefficient of diffusion. Symbol, Δ. 4. *In mathematics,* INCREMENT. Symbol, Δ.

delta cell. 1. A possible third type of cell in the islets of the pancreas. 2. A second type of beta cell of the adenohypophysis.

delta chain, δ chain. The heavy chain of the IgD immunoglobulin molecule.

Delta Cortef. A trademark for prednisolone, an anti-inflammatory adrenocortical steroid.

delta granules. The granules of the delta cells of the islets of the pancreas.

delta hemolysin, δ-hemolysin. A hemolysin of *Staphylococcus aureus,* hemolytic for all species of red blood cells tested, cytotoxic for a variety of other cells, but which is well tolerated by laboratory animals upon injection.

Deltalin. A trademark for vitamin D_2.

delta rhythm. *In electroencephalography,* a succession of slow waves with a frequency of 4 or less per second. Predominate during deep sleep, but also seen in brain damage, especially that involving midline structures.

Deltasone. A trademark for prednisone, an anti-inflammatory adrenocortical steroid.

delta wave. See *delta rhythm.*

del·toid (del'toid) *adj. & n.* [Gk. *deltoeidēs*]. 1. Shaped like a Δ (capital delta). 2. DELTOID MUSCLE. 3. Pertaining to the deltoid muscle.

deltoid ligament. MEDIAL LIGAMENT.

deltoid muscle. The large, thick, delta-shaped muscle covering the shoulder joint. NA *musculus deltoideus.* See also Table of Muscles in the Appendix.

deltoid reflex. Contraction of the deltoid muscle with consequent abduction of the upper arm, resulting from tapping over the insertion of the muscle.

deltoid region. The proximal part of the lateral aspect of the upper arm. NA *regio deltoidea.*

deltoid tuberosity or **tubercle.** A rough elevation about the middle of the anterolateral surface of the humerus for the insertion of the deltoid muscle. NA *tuberositas deltoidea.*

Deltoin. Trademark for methetoin, an anticonvulsant drug.

del·to·pec·to·ral (del''to·peck'tuh·rul) *adj.* Pertaining to the deltoid and pectoral muscles.

Deltra. A trademark for prednisone, an anti-inflammatory adrenocortical steroid.

de·lu·sion (de·lew'zhun) *n.* [L. *delusio,* from *deludere,* to deceive]. A belief maintained in the face of incontrovertible evidence to the contrary, and not in line with the individual's level of knowledge and his cultural group. It results from unconscious needs and may therefore take on various forms.

de·lu·sion·al (de·lew'zhun·ul) *adj.* 1. Characterized by delusions. 2. Pertaining to, or of the nature of, a delusion.

delusional speech. Speech extensively contaminated by delusions of grandeur or persecution or by ideas of reference. See also *paranoia, paranoid state.*

delusion of grandeur. MEGALOMANIA.

delusion of persecution. The false belief that one has been singled out deliberately and without reason for persecution. See also *paranoia, paranoid state, paranoid type of schizophrenia.*

delusions of observation. IDEAS OF REFERENCE.

delusions of reference. IDEAS OF REFERENCE.

de·lu·sive (de·lew'siv) *adj.* Pertaining to a delusion.

de·lu·so·ry (de·lew'suh·ree, ·zuh·ree) *adj.* Pertaining to information or data that appear to support a conclusion, but actually do not, or to alleged facts produced by delusions.

Delvex. A trademark for dithiazanine iodide, an anthelmintic.

dem-, demo- [Gk. *dēmos*]. A combining form meaning *people, population.*

de·mar·ca·tion (dee''mahr·kay'shun) *n.* [Sp. *demarcación,* from *marcar,* to mark]. Separation, establishing of limits. **—de·mar·cate** (de·mahr'kate) *v.*

demarcation current. An electric current that flows toward the depolarized surface of injured tissue from the polarized surface of adjacent intact tissue.

demarcation line. A line forming at the edge of a gangrenous area and marking the limit of the process.

demarcation potential. INJURY POTENTIAL.

de·mas·cu·lin·iza·tion (dee''mas''kew·li·nye·zay'shun) *n.* Loss or diminution of male sex characteristics. **—de·mas·cu·lin·ize** (dee''mas'kew·li·nize) *v.*

De·ma·ti·um (de·may'shee·um) *n.* PULLULARIA.

dem·e·car·i·um bromide (dem''e·kair'ee·um). Diester of (*m*-hydroxyphenyl)trimethylammonium bromide with decamethylenebis(methylcarbamic acid), $C_{32}H_{52}Br_2N_4O_4$, a potent cholinesterase inhibitor used in management of glaucoma and accommodative convergent strabismus.

dem·e·clo·cy·cline (dem''e·klo·sigh'kleen) *n.* 7-Chloro-6-demethyltetracycline, $C_{21}H_{21}ClN_2O_8$, an antibiotic produced by a mutant strain of *Streptomyces aureofaciens;* used, as the hydrochloride salt, for the same purposes as other tetracycline antibiotics. Syn. *demethylchlortetracycline.*

dem·e·cy·cline (dem''e·sigh'kleen) *n.* 4-(Dimethylamino)-1,4,4*a*,5,5*a*,6,11,12*a*-octahydro-3,6,10,12,12*a*-pentahydroxy-1,11-dioxo-2-naphthacenecarboxamide, $C_{21}H_{22}N_2O_8$, an antibiotic.

de·ment·ed (de·men'tid) *adj.* [L. *demens,* out of one's mind]. Deprived of reason. **—dement,** *n. & v.*

de·men·tia (de·men'shuh) *n.*, pl. **dementias, demen·ti·ae** (·shee·ee) [L., from *demens,* out of one's mind, from *mens,* mind]. 1. Deterioration or loss of intellectual faculties, reasoning power, memory, and will due to organic brain disease; characterized by confusion, disorientation, apathy, and stupor of varying degrees. 2. Formerly, madness or insanity.

dementia ag·i·ta·ta (aj''i·tay'tuh). AGITATED DEMENTIA.

dementia par·a·lyt·i·ca (păr''uh·lit'i·kuh). GENERAL PARALYSIS.

dementia par·a·noi·des (păr·uh·noy'deez). PARANOID TYPE OF SCHIZOPHRENIA.

dementia prae·cox or **pre·cox** (pree'kocks), pl. **dementiae prae·co·ces** (pree·ko'seez). Any of a group of psychotic disorders, beginning in adolescence or early adulthood, formerly thought to be a single entity, then categorized by Kraepelin as four, and now classified as simple, hebephrenic, paranoid, and catatonic types of schizophrenia.

dementia pu·gi·lis·ti·ca (pew''ji·lis'ti·kuh) [NL., boxer's dementia, from L. *pugil,* boxer]. PUNCH-DRUNK STATE.

Demerol. Trademark for meperidine, a narcotic analgesic used as the hydrochloride salt.

de·meth·yl·ate (dee·meth'i·late) *v.* To remove one or more methyl (—CH_3) groups from a compound. **—de·meth·yl·a·tion** (dee·meth''i·lay'shun) *n.*

de·meth·yl·chlor·tet·ra·cy·cline (dee·meth''il·klor·tet''ruh·sigh'kleen) *n.* DEMECLOCYCLINE.

demi- [F., from L. *dimidius*]. A prefix signifying *half.*

demi·fac·et (dem''ee·fas'it) *n.* [*demi-* + *facet*]. One-half of an articulation surface adapted to articulate with two bones.

demi·gaunt·let bandage (dem''ee·gawnt'lit). A bandage covering the wrist and hand but not the fingers.

demi·lune (dem'i·lewn) *n.* [F. *demi-lune,* half-moon]. A crescent-shaped aggregation of serous cells capping mucous acini in mixed glands. Syn. *serous crescent.*

demilune cells. The serous cells forming a demilune.

demilune of Gian·nuz·zi (jahⁿ-noot'tsee) [G. *Giannuzzi*]. DEMILUNE.

demilune of Hei·den·hain (high'dᵉn·hine) [R. P. *Heidenhain*]. DEMILUNE.

demi·mon·stros·i·ty (dem''ee·mon·stros'i·tee) *n.* [*demi-* + *monstrosity*]. A variety of congenital deformity that does not give rise to appreciable disorder of function. See also *hemiterata.*

de·min·er·al·iza·tion (dee·min″ur·ul·i·zay′shun) *n.* Loss of mineral salts from the body, as from the bones. See also *decalcification.* —**de·min·er·al·ize** (dee·min′ur·ul·ize) *v.*

demi·pen·ni·form (dem″ee·pen′i·form) *adj.* [*demi-* + *penniform*]. UNIPENNATE.

demo-. See *dem-.*

dem·o·dec·tic (dem″o·deck′tick) *adj.* Of, pertaining to, or caused by mites of the genus *Demodex.*

Dem·o·dex (dem′o·decks, dee′mo·) *n.* [Gk. *dēmos*, fat, + *dēx*, worm]. A genus of parasitic mites. See also *follicular mange.*

Demodex fol·li·cu·lo·rum (fol·ick″yoo·lo′rum). A species of mite which is a parasite of the sebaceous glands and hair follicles. These parasites rarely cause discomfort, but when unusually numerous may cause chronic erythema, with scaling of the epidermis, accompanied by burning sensations.

de·mog·ra·phy (dee·mog′ruh·fee) *n.* [*demo-* + *-graphy*]. The science of populations; specifically, the statistical description of populations according to such characteristics of their members as age, sex, marital status, family structure, geographical distribution, and various other cultural, political, and socioeconomic factors, and of the determinants and consequences of population change. —**de·mo·graph·ic** (dem″uh·graf′ick, dee″muh·) *adj.*

demon-, demono- [Gk. *daimōn*]. A combining form meaning *demon.*

de·mon·mia (dee·mon′mee·uh) *n.* DEMONOMANIA.

demono-. See *demon-.*

de·mon·ol·a·try (dee″mun·ol′uh·tree) *n.* [*demono-* + Gk. *latreia*, service]. Worship of a demon or spirit.

de·mon·o·ma·nia (dee″mun·o·may′nee·uh) *n.* [*demono-* + *mania*]. 1. A state in which one is oppressed by morbid dreams of demons. 2. The delusion of being possessed by evil spirits or a demon. —**demonoma·niac** (·nee·ack) *n.*

de·mon·op·a·thy (dee″mun·op′uth·ee) *n.* [*demono-* + *-pathy*]. DEMONOMANIA.

de·mon·o·pho·bia (dee″mun·o·fo′bee·uh) *n.* [*demono-* + *-phobia*]. Abnormal fear of devils and demons.

de·mo·pho·bia (dee″mo·fo′bee·uh) *n.* [*demo-* + *-phobia*]. OCHLOPHOBIA.

De Mor·gan's spot [C. G. *De Morgan*, English physician, 1811–1876]. PAPILLARY VARIX.

de·mor·phin·iza·tion (dee·mor″fin·i·zay′shun, ·eye·zay′shun) *n.* Treatment of morphinism by gradual withdrawal of the drug.

de·mox·e·pam (de·mock′se·pam) *n.* 7-Chloro-1,3-dihydro-5-phenyl-2*H*-1,4-benzodiazepin-2-one-4-oxide, $C_{15}H_{11}ClN_2O_2$, a minor tranquilizer.

de·mul·cent (de·mul′sunt) *adj.* & *n.* [L. *demulcere*, to stroke down, caress]. 1. Soothing; allaying irritation of surfaces, especially mucous membranes. 2. A soothing substance, particularly a slippery, mucilaginous liquid.

de Mus·sy's point (duh mu^e·see′) [N. F. O. Guéneau *de Mussy*, French physician, 1813–1885]. In diaphragmatic pleurisy, a point of tenderness and referred pain in the epigastrium at the intersection of lines drawn along the left sternal border and along the tenth rib.

de·my·e·lin·at·ed (dee·migh′uh·li·nay·tid) *adj.* Of a nerve or nerve tract: having had its myelin sheath removed or destroyed. Compare *unmyelinated.* —**demyelin·ate** (·nate) *v.*, **demyelin·at·ing** (·nay·ting), **demyelin·at·ive** (·nay·tiv) *adj.*

demyelinating disease. Any one of a large group of diseases of the nervous system which possesses the following pathologic features: (a) destruction of the myelin sheaths with relative sparing of axis cylinders, nerve cells, and supporting structures; (b) an infiltration of inflammatory cells in the adventitial sheaths of blood vessels; (c) a particular distribution of lesions (often perivenous), either in multiple, small, disseminated foci or in large foci, spreading from one or more centers.

de·my·e·lin·a·tion (dee·migh″e·li·nay′shun) *n.* Destruction of myelin; loss of myelin from nerve sheaths or nerve tracts.

de·my·e·lin·iza·tion (dee·migh″e·lin·i·zay′shun) *n.* DEMYELINATION.

de·my·e·lin·ize (dee·migh′e·lin·ize) *v.* DEMYELINATE.

de·nar·co·tize (dee·nahr′kuh·tize) *v.* To deprive of narcotizing qualities. —**denarco·tized** (·tize′d) *adj.*

de·na·to·ni·um benzoate (dee″nay·to′nee·um). Benzyldiethyl[(2,6-xylylcarbamoyl)methyl]ammonium benzoate, $C_{28}H_{34}N_2O_3$, a denaturant for ethanol.

de·na·tur·ant (dee·nay′chur·unt) *n.* 1. A substance added to another to make the latter unfit for certain uses, as when methyl alcohol is added to ethyl alcohol for the purpose of preventing beverage use of the ethyl alcohol. 2. *In nuclear science,* a nonfissionable isotope, which, when added to fissionable material, makes the latter unsuited for use in atomic weapons without considerable processing.

de·na·ture (dee·nay′chur) *v.* [*de-* + *nature*]. To modify, by physical or chemical action, the biological (secondary and tertiary) structure of an organic substance, especially a protein, in order to alter some properties of the substance, such as solubility. —**de·na·tur·a·tion** (de·nay″chur·ay′shun) *n.*

de·na·tured (dee·nay′churd) *adj.* Changed, made different from normal.

denatured alcohol. Alcohol into which some other substance has been introduced, rendering it unfit for drinking but still useful for other purposes.

denatured protein. A protein whose biological (secondary and tertiary) structure and properties have been altered, mainly by the action of chemical or physical agents.

de·na·tur·iza·tion (dee·nay″chur·i·zay′shun) *n.* DENATURATION.

dendr-, dendro- [Gk. *dendron*, tree]. A combining form meaning (a) *tree, arboreal;* (b) *dendritic, arborescent;* (c) *branching process.*

dendra. A plural of *dendron.*

Den·dras·pis (den″dras′pis) *n.* [*dendr-* + L. *aspis*, asp]. A genus of venomous snakes of the Elapidae found in Africa south of the Sahara; the mambas.

Dendrid. A trademark for idoxuridine, a topical antiviral agent used for treatment of dendritic keratitis.

den·drite (den′drite) *n.* [Gk. *dendritēs*, pertaining to a tree, from *dendron*, tree]. The process of a neuron which carries the nerve impulse to the cell body. It is usually branched, like a tree. Syn. *dendron.*

den·drit·ic (den·drit′ick) *adj.* [Gk. *dendritēs*, pertaining to a tree, + *-ic*]. 1. Branching in treelike or rootlike fashion; arborescent. 2. Pertaining to a dendrite.

dendritic calculus. CORAL CALCULUS; STAGHORN CALCULUS.

dendritic keratitis. A superficial form of keratitis attributed to the virus of herpes simplex, also rarely seen with herpes zoster; characterized by a line of infiltration of the corneal tissue near the surface, developing later into an arborescent ulcer. Syn. *furrow keratitis, herpetic keratitis, keratitis arborescens.*

dendritic membrane. POSTSYNAPTIC MEMBRANE.

dendritic ulcer. Benign branching superficial fissures of the cornea caused by infection with herpes simplex virus and rarely with herpes zoster.

dendritic zone. The extensive branching of the dendrite or receptive pole of a neuron.

dendro-. See *dendr-.*

Den·dro·as·pis (den″dro·as′pis) *n.* *DENDRASPIS.*

den·droid (den′droid) *adj.* [Gk. *dendroeidēs*, treelike]. DENDRITIC.

den·dron (den′dron) *n.*, pl. **dendrons, den·dra** (·druh) [Gk., tree]. DENDRITE.

den·dro·phil·ia (den″dro·fil′ee·uh) *n.* [*dendro-* + *-philia*]. *In* *psychiatry,* love of trees; a sexual attraction to trees which are symbolic for the phallus.

de·ner·vate (dee·nur'vate) *v.* To interfere with or cut off the nerve supply to a body part, or to remove a nerve; may occur by excision, drugs, or a disease process.

de·ner·va·tion (dee″nur·vay'shun) *n.* 1. The interruption of the nerve supply to a part by excision, drugs, or disease. 2. The cutting off of the nerve supply to the lower leg and foot to relieve certain types of lameness in a horse.

denervation potential. FIBRILLATION POTENTIAL.

den·gue (deng'gay, ·ghee) *n.* [Sp., of African origin]. An acute febrile, usually epidemic infectious disease caused by a group B togavirus and borne by the *Aëdes* mosquito; characterized by abrupt onset, diphasic course, prostration, muscle and joint pain, exanthems, lymphadenopathy, and leukopenia, with severe residual debility and weakness lasting for about a week.

de·ni·al, *n.* [OF. *denier,* to deny, from L. *denegare*]. *In psychiatry,* the unconscious psychic mechanism or process whereby an observation is denied or refused recognition in order to avoid anxiety or pain; the simplest and commonest form of the ego defense mechanisms, and a part of many normal phenomena, as in the fantasies of children who deny the realities of their own lives to enjoy play.

den·i·da·tion (den″i·day'shun, dee″nigh·) *n.* [*de-* + *nidation*]. Disintegration and ejection of the superficial part of the uterine mucosa.

den·i·grate (den'i·grate) *v.* [L. *denigrare,* to blacken]. 1. To render or become black. 2. To defame. **—den·i·gra·tion** (den″i·gray'shun, dee″nigh·) *n.*

Den·is' method [W. G. *Denis,* U. S. biochemist, b. 1879]. A method for determining serum magnesium in which calcium is removed as oxalate and magnesium is precipitated as magnesium ammonium phosphate which is estimated colorimetrically.

de·ni·tri·fy (dee·nigh'tri·figh) *v.* To remove nitrogen.

de·ni·tro·gen·ate (dee·nigh'tro·je·nate, dee″nigh·troj'e·) *v.* To remove dissolved nitrogen from one's body by breathing nitrogen-free gas. **—de·ni·tro·gen·a·tion** (dee·nigh″tro·je·nay'shun, dee″nigh·troj″e·) *n.*

Den·nie-Mar·fan syndrome [C. C. *Dennie,* U.S. dermatologist, 1883–1971; and A. B. J. *Marfan*]. Spastic paraplegia, usually beginning in early childhood, associated with mental retardation in children with congenital syphilis.

de·no·fun·gin (dee″no·fun'jin) *n.* An antibiotic with antifungal properties, produced by a variant of *Streptomyces hygroscopicus.*

De·non·vil·liers' fascia (duh·nohⁿ·veel·yeʸ') [C. P. *Denonvilliers,* French surgeon, 1808–1872]. The portion of the pelvic fascia between the anterior surface of the rectum and the seminal vesicles and prostate gland.

dens (denz) *n.*, genit. **den·tis** (den'tis), pl. **den·tes** (·teez), genit. pl. **den·ti·um** (den'tee·um, ·shee·um) [L.] [NA]. 1. TOOTH. 2. A toothlike process; specifically, the dens of the axis.

dens ax·is (ack'sis) [NA]. DENS OF THE AXIS.

dense, *adj.* [L. *densus*]. 1. Compact; crowded. 2. Relatively opaque.

dens epi·stro·phei (ep″i·stro'fee·eye) [BNA]. Dens axis (= DENS OF THE AXIS).

den·sim·e·ter (den·sim'e·tur) *n.* [*density* + *-meter*]. An instrument for determining density or specific gravity. See also *hydrometer.* **—den·si·met·ric** (den″si·met'rick) *adj.*

densimetric analysis. Analysis for a substance by determining the density of its solution, thus estimating the amount of dissolved matter.

dens in den·te (denz' in den'tee) [L., a tooth in a tooth]. An abnormality of development in which the enamel organ has invaginated within the dental papilla, producing a deposition of enamel within the tooth.

Densite. Tradename for alpha calcium sulfate hemihydrate of the class II, improved, or modified type; used for making dies. See also *artificial stone.*

den·si·tom·e·ter (den″si·tom'e·tur) *n.* [*density* + *-meter*]. 1. An instrument utilizing the photoelectric principle for measuring the opacity of exposed and processed photographic film. 2. DENSIMETER.

den·si·ty, *n.* 1. Closeness of any space distribution, as for example electron density, the number of electrons per unit volume, or population density, the number of inhabitants per unit area. 2. Any measure of the compactness of substances based on the ratio of weight or mass to volume. Abbreviated, d. See also *specific gravity.* 3. *In radiography and photography,* degree of opacity. See also *absolute density, photographic density.*

dens of the axis. The toothlike process on the body of the axis, going through the front part of the ring of the atlas. Syn. *odontoid process.* NA *dens axis.*

den·sog·ra·phy (den·sog'ruh·fee) *n.* [*dense* + *-graphy*]. The measurement of varying densities of a roentgenogram by a photoelectric cell.

dens se·ro·ti·nus (se·rot'i·nus) [L., late-blooming, late developing] [NA]. WISDOM TOOTH.

dent-, denti-, dento- [L. *dens, dentis*]. A combining form meaning *tooth, dental.*

den·tal (den'tul) *adj.* [*dent-* + *-al*]. Pertaining to the teeth.

dental abscess. ALVEOLAR ABSCESS.

dental alloy. Filings or shavings of an alloy that are triturated with mercury to form amalgam fillings or dies.

dental amalgam. An alloy of silver, tin, zinc, and copper with mercury, used as a tooth-filling material and in the making of dies. See also *silver amalgam.*

dental anesthesia. Anesthesia of the teeth for dental operations.

dental arch. The parabolic curve formed by the cutting edges and masticating surfaces of the upper or lower teeth: the inferior dental arch (NA *arcus dentalis inferior*) or the superior dental arch (NA *arcus dentalis superior*).

dental artery. 1. ALVEOLAR ARTERY. 2. A branch of an alveolar artery supplying a root of a tooth.

dental auxiliary. A dental assistant, dental hygienist, or dental laboratory technician who assists the dentist in the performance of his duties.

dental calculus. A calcareous deposit on the teeth, consisting of organic and mineral matter; formerly divided into salivary calculus and serumal or sanguinary calculus. Syn. *tartar.*

dental canals. ALVEOLAR CANALS (2).

dental caries. A localized, progressive, and molecular disintegration of the teeth believed to begin with the solution of tooth structure by lactic and pyruvic acids, which are the product of enzymic action of oral bacteria upon carbohydrates, followed by bacterial invasion of the dentinal tubules.

dental cavity. 1. CAVITY (2). 2. PULP CAVITY.

dental cone. A medicated conical insert used to prevent infection in the empty socket following extraction of a tooth.

dental crypt. The space filled by a dental sac and a developing tooth.

dental decay. DENTAL CARIES.

dental deposit. Mineralized or nonmineralized material adherent to the surface of a tooth.

dental dysplasia. Abnormal development or growth of the teeth.

dental engine. The motor that provides the power to operate dental rotary cutting or polishing devices such as burs, abrasive disks or wheels, and brushes; it is an integral part of the dental unit.

dental epithelium. The layers of cells that form the boundaries of the enamel organ; divided into the inner and outer dental epithelium.

dental erosion. 1. Loss of tooth substance due to a chemical process of uncertain nature and not associated with bacterial activity, generally occurring in the gingival third of the facial tooth surfaces. 2. Loss of tooth substance due to obvious causes, such as gastric acid from chronic vomiting and habitual ingestion of highly acidic fruits, juices, or beverages. Compare *abrasion* (2), *attrition* (2).

dental excavation. 1. The cavity prepared in a tooth, prior to filling or the insertion of an inlay. 2. The preparation of such a cavity.

dental floss. A string or thread used to clean interdental spaces and tooth surfaces, in the placement of rubber dam, and in the examination of proximal tooth surfaces.

dental fluorosis. CHRONIC DENTAL FLUOROSIS.

dental follicle. DENTAL SAC.

dental forceps. Any one of a variety of forceps adapted for the extraction of teeth.

dental formula. A formula showing the number and arrangement of teeth.

dental germ. TOOTH GERM.

dental granuloma. 1. PERIAPICAL GRANULOMA. 2. ALVEOLAR ABSCESS.

dental hygienist. A person trained and licensed in the technique of removing calcareous deposits and stains from the teeth.

dental identification record. In U.S. military medicine, an official form for recording every characteristic of the condition of a soldier's teeth; used as a means of identification if injuries causing death result in the destruction of other features of the soldier.

dental index. The dental length multiplied by 100 divided by the craniobasal length.

dental lamina. The epithelial ingrowth into the jaw which gives rise to the enamel organs of the developing teeth.

dental organ. ENAMEL ORGAN.

dental papilla. The mass of connective tissue over which fits the enamel organ of a developing tooth and which forms the dentin and dental pulp.

dental plaque. A thin, transparent film on the surfaces of a tooth made up of mucin and colloidal material secreted by the salivary glands. Depending on the predominant component, mucinous and bacterial plaques are recognized.

dental plate. 1. ARTIFICIAL DENTURE. 2. The part of an artificial denture that fits the denture foundation and supports the artificial teeth.

dental plexus. See *inferior dental plexus, superior dental plexus.*

dental prophylaxis. The prevention of dental and oral diseases by preventive measures, such as fluoridation of water and, especially, the mechanical cleansing of the teeth.

dental prosthesis. An appliance to replace missing teeth, as a denture, crown, or bridgework.

dental pulp. The soft vascular tissue which fills the pulp chamber and the root canals of a tooth and is responsible for its vitality, consisting of connective tissue, blood vessels, and nerves with a superficial layer of cells, the odontoblasts, producing and maintaining dentin and supplying branching processes which occupy tubules in the dentin. NA *pulpa dentis.*

dental ridge. An elevation that forms a cusp or margin of a tooth.

dental sac. The connective tissue that encloses the developing tooth. Syn. *dental follicle.*

dental stone. ARTIFICIAL STONE.

dental surgeon. DENTIST.

dental surgery. Surgery pertaining to the teeth.

dental tubercle. CUSP (1).

dental unit. 1. One tooth. 2. A piece of equipment that variously combines the bracket table, cuspidor, dental engine, operating light, saliva ejector, miscellaneous instruments, and outlets for compressed air, gas, and water.

den·ta·phone (den'tuh·fone) *n.* DENTIPHONE.

den·ta·ry (den'tuh·ree) *n.* A bone found chiefly in fishes, regarded as a phylogenetic component of the mammalian mandible.

den·tate (den'tate) *adj.* [L. *dentatus,* toothed]. 1. SERRATED; jagged. 2. Having a concavely scalloped edge or surface. 3. Pertaining to the dentate nucleus.

dentate cerebellar ataxia. DYSSYNERGIA CEREBELLARIS PROGRESSIVA.

den·tat·ec·to·my (den"tait·eck'tuh·mee) *n.* [*dentate* + *-ectomy*]. The ablation of the dentate nucleus in the treatment of a movement disorder, particularly when due to erythroblastosis fetalis.

dentate fissure. HIPPOCAMPAL SULCUS.

dentate fracture. A fracture in which the ends of the fragments are toothed and interlocked.

dentate gyrus. A narrow band of gray matter extending downward and forward above the gyrus parahippocampalis but separated from it by the hippocampal sulcus; anteriorly it is continued into the uncus. NA *gyrus dentatus.*

dentate ligament. A narrow fibrous band separating the dorsal and ventral roots of the spinal cord throughout its entire length. Along its lateral border, triangular toothlike processes are fixed at intervals to the dura mater. NA *ligamentum denticulatum.*

dentate line. The jagged line that indicates the division between the area of columnar epithelium and that of stratified squamous epithelium along the level of the anal valves. Syn. *pectinate line.*

dentate nucleus. An ovoid mass of nerve cells located in the center of each cerebellar hemisphere; the cells give rise to fibers which are found in the superior cerebellar peduncle. NA *nucleus dentatus cerebelli.*

dentate suture. SUTURA SERRATA.

den·ta·tion (den·tay'shun) *n.* 1. The quality or condition of being dentate. 2. A toothlike projection.

dentato- [L. *dentatus*]. A combining form meaning *dentate.*

den·ta·to·re·tic·u·lar (den·tay"to·re·tick'yoo·lur) *adj.* Pertaining to the dentate nucleus and the reticular formation.

dentatoreticular tract. Nerve fibers that arise from the dentate nucleus, separate from the superior cerebellar peduncle just before and beyond its decussation, and descend as crossed and uncrossed fibers in the reticular formation.

den·ta·to·ru·bral (den·tay"to·roo'brul) *adj.* [*dentato-* + *rubr-* + *-al*]. Pertaining to the dentate nucleus and the red nucleus.

dentatorubral tract. Part of the superior cerebellar peduncle; nerve fibers that arise in the dentate nucleus and terminate in the contralateral red nucleus. NA *tractus cerebellorubralis.*

den·ta·to·tha·lam·ic (den·tay"to·thuh·lam'ick) *adj.* Pertaining to the dentate nucleus and the thalamic nucleus.

dentatothalamic tract. The largest component of the superior cerebellar peduncle; nerve fibers that arise in the ventrolateral part of the dentate nucleus and end in the lateral ventral thalamic nucleus. NA *tractus cerebellothalamicus.*

den·ta·to-thal·a·mo-cor·ti·cal (den·tay"to·thal"uh·mo·kor'ti·kul) *adj.* Pertaining to or comprising the dentatothalamic and thalamocortical pathways.

den·ta·tum (den·tay'tum, ·tah'tum) *n.* [L., toothed]. DENTATE NUCLEUS.

den·te·la·tion (den"te·lay'shun) *n.* The state of having toothlike processes.

dentes [NA]. Plural of *dens.*

dentes acu·sti·ci (a·koos'ti·sigh) [NA]. AUDITORY TEETH.

dentes ca·ni·ni (ka·nigh'nigh) [NA]. CANINE TEETH.

dentes de·ci·dui (de·sid'yoo·eye) [NA]. DECIDUOUS TEETH.

dentes in·ci·si·vi (in·si·sigh'vye) [NA]. INCISORS.

dentes mo·la·res (mo·lair'eez) [NA]. MOLAR TEETH.

dentes per·ma·nen·tes (pur·muh·nen'teez) [NA]. PERMANENT TEETH.

dentes prae·mo·la·res (pree″mo·lair′eez) [BNA]. Dentes pre-molares (= PREMOLARS).

dentes pre·mo·la·res (pree″mo·lair′eez) [NA]. PREMOLARS.

denti-. See *dent-*.

den·tia pre·cox (den′shuh pree′kocks) [L.]. The presence of erupted teeth at birth, or shortly thereafter.

dentia tar·da (tahr′duh). Eruption of the teeth delayed beyond the normal expectancy.

den·ti·cle (den′ti·kul) *n.* [L. *denticulus,* a small tooth]. 1. A small tooth or projecting point. 2. A deposit of dentin-like or calcareous material within the pulp of the tooth, associated with degenerative or retrogressive changes of the pulp.

den·tic·u·late (den·tick′yoo·late) *adj.* Having minute dentations; furnished with small teeth or notches.

denticulate ligament. DENTATE LIGAMENT.

den·ti·fi·ca·tion (den″ti·fi·kay′shun) *n.* Formation of teeth.

den·ti·form (den′ti·form) *adj.* [*denti-* + *-form*]. Tooth-shaped; ODONTOID (1).

den·ti·frice (den′ti·fris) *n.* [L. *dentifricium,* from *denti-* + *fricare,* to rub]. A substance or preparation used to aid the mechanical cleaning of the teeth.

den·tig·er·ous (den·tij′ur·us) *adj.* [*denti-* + L. *gerere,* to bear]. Bearing, arising from, or containing teeth.

dentigerous cyst. A cyst originating in the enamel organ of a developing tooth.

den·tin (den′tin) *n.* [*dent-* + *-in*]. The calcified tissue which forms the major part of a tooth. Dentin is related to bone but differs from it in the absence of included cells. It is covered by the enamel over the crown of the tooth, by the cementum over the roots, and itself surrounds the pulp chamber and root canals which contain the dental pulp. **—den·tin·al** (·ti·nul) *adj.*

dentinal canals. DENTINAL TUBULES.

dentinal cell. ODONTOBLAST.

dentinal fiber. ODONTOBLASTIC PROCESS.

dentinal fibril. One of the fibrils of the dentinal matrix.

dentinal sheath. The dentinal matrix immediately adjacent to a dentinal tubule.

dentinal tubules. Canals in the matrix of dentin occupied by odontoblastic processes. NA *canaliculi dentales.*

den·tine (den′teen) *n.* DENTIN.

den·tin·i·fi·ca·tion (den·tin″i·fi·kay′shun) *n.* DENTINOGENESIS.

den·ti·no·blas·to·ma (den″ti·no·blas·to′muh) *n.* [*dentin* + *blastoma*]. A benign odontogenic tumor made up of poorly developed dentin.

den·ti·no·ce·men·tal (den″ti·no·se·men′tul) *adj.* Pertaining to the dentin and cementum of a tooth.

dentinocemental junction. The interface between the dentin and the cementum in the root of a tooth.

den·ti·no·enam·el (den″ti·no·e·nam′ul) *adj.* Pertaining to the dentin and the enamel of a tooth.

dentinoenamel junction. The interface between the enamel and dentin in the crown of a tooth.

den·ti·no·gen·e·sis (den″ti·no·jen′e·sis) *n.* [*dentin* + *genesis*]. The formation of dentin.

dentinogenesis im·per·fec·ta (im·pur·feck′tuh). A hereditary condition of the teeth characterized by a marked reduction in size or obliteration of the pulpal space and a rapid wearing away of the crowns; normal enamel which is weakly attached to the dentin and lost early; and ranging in color from opalescent to bluish to brown. Syn. *hereditary opalescent dentin, odontogenesis imperfecta.*

den·ti·no·gen·ic (den″ti·no·jen′ick) *adj.* [*dentin* + *-genic*]. Pertaining to the formation of dentin.

dentinogenic fibers. The precollagenous fibers that pass between the odontoblasts into the dentin to form the fibrillar component of the dentinal matrix.

den·ti·noid (den′ti·noid) *n.* [*dentin* + *-oid*]. A calcified structure having some but not all of the characteristics of dentin.

den·ti·no·ma (den″ti·no′muh) *n.*, pl. **dentinomas, dentinoma·ta** (·tuh) [*dentin* + *-oma*]. A benign odontogenic tumor made up of dentin.

den·ti·nos·te·oid (den″ti·nos′tee·oid) *n.* [*dentin* + *oste-* + *-oid*]. A hard, calcified structure having some of the histologic appearance of both dentin and bone.

den·ti·num (den·tye′num) *n.* [NA]. DENTIN.

den·tip·a·rous (den·tip′uh·rus) *adj.* [*denti-* + *-parous*]. Producing or bearing teeth.

den·ti·phone (den′ti·fone) *n.* [*denti-* + *-phone*]. A device in which a vibrating disk is attached to or held in contact with the teeth, thus carrying vibration through the bony structures to the vestibulocochlear nerves; used in certain types of deafness.

den·tist (den′tist) *n.* [F. *dentiste,* from *dent,* tooth]. One who practices dentistry.

den·tis·try (den′tis·tree) *n.* 1. The art and science of the prevention, diagnosis, and treatment of diseases of the teeth and adjacent tissues, and the restoration of missing dental and oral structures. 2. The practice of such art and science. 3. The dental profession collectively. 4. RESTORATION (3).

den·ti·tion (den·tish′un) *n.* [L. *dentitio,* from *dentire,* to teethe]. 1. The teeth considered collectively and in place in the dental arch. 2. The character and arrangement of the teeth of an individual or species. 3. The eruption of the teeth. See also *primary dentition, secondary dentition.*

dento-. See *dent-*.

den·to·al·ve·o·lar (den″to·al·vee′o·lur) *adj.* [*dento-* + *alveolar*]. Pertaining to the alveolus of a tooth.

dentoalveolar abscess. ALVEOLAR ABSCESS.

den·to·fa·cial (den″to·fay′shul) *adj.* [*dento-* + *facial*]. Pertaining to the teeth and the face.

dentofacial area. DENTOFACIAL ZONE.

dentofacial relation. The relation which the teeth and alveoli bear to the face.

dentofacial zone. The facial area that includes the teeth and their supporting alveolar processes.

den·toid (den′toid) *adj.* [*dent-* + *-oid*]. Toothlike.

den·tu·lous (den′chuh·lus) *adj.* Having natural teeth. Contr. *edentulous.*

den·ture (den′chur) *n.* [F.]. The natural or artificial teeth of an individual, considered as a unit.

denture flange. The part of an artificial denture that extends from the cervical margins of the teeth to its border; the facial extension of an upper or lower denture and the lingual extension of a lower denture.

denture flask. A sectional housing used to support molds for processing dental materials.

denture foundation. The portion of the oral structures that is available for the support of artificial dentures.

de·nu·cle·at·ed (dee·new′klee·ay″tid) *adj.* Deprived of a nucleus.

de·nude (de·newd′) *v.* [L. *denudare*]. To deprive of covering; to strip, lay bare, as the root of a tooth. **—de·nu·da·tion** (dee″new·day′shun, den″yoo·) *n.*

Denver Developmental Screening Test. A widely used and highly reliable test for evaluating developmental adequacy and identifying developmental delays in personal-social, fine motor-adaptive, language, and gross motor behavior of children from one month to six years of age. Abbreviated, DDST.

de·ob·stru·ent (dee·ob′stroo·unt) *n.* [*de-* + *obstruent*]. Any agent or drug which removes an obstruction or obstructive material, as in the alimentary canal.

de·odor·ant (dee·o′dur·unt) *n. & adj.* 1. A substance that removes or conceals offensive odors. 2. Having the action of a deodorant. **—deodor·ize** (·ize) *v.*

de·oral·i·ty (dee″o·ral′i·tee) *n.* [*de-* + *oral*]. *In psychoanalysis,* the shifting of instinctual activity away from gratification through oral expression.

de·or·sum·duc·tion (dee·or″sum·duck′shun) *n.* [L. *deorsum,* downward, *ducere,* to lead]. A turning downward of a part.

de·or·sum·ver·gence (dee·or″sum·vur′junce) *n.* [L. *deorsum*, downward, + *vergere*, to turn, incline]. A downward inclination, as of the eyes.

de·os·si·fi·ca·tion (dee·os″i·fi·kay′shun) *n.* [*de-* + *ossification*]. 1. The absorption of bony material. 2. The deprivation of the bony character of any part.

deoxy-, desoxy-. A combining form designating (a) *loss of oxygen from a compound;* or specifically (b) *replacement of a hydroxyl group by a hydrogen atom.*

de·oxy·aden·o·sine (dee·ock″see·a·den′o·seen) *n.* One of the principal nucleosides of DNA, composed of adenine and deoxyribose.

de·oxy·cho·late (dee·ock″see·ko′late) *n.* A salt or ester of deoxycholic acid.

deoxycholate-citrate agar. A selective medium for the culture of *Salmonella* and *Shigella.*

de·oxy·cho·lic acid (dee·ock″see·ko′lick, ·kol′ick). 3α,12α-Dihydroxycholanic acid, $C_{24}H_{40}O_4$, one of the unconjugated bile acids; in bile it is largely conjugated with glycine or taurine. Used as a choleretic.

de·oxy·cor·ti·cos·ter·one (dee·ock′see·kor″ti·kos′tur·ohn) *n.* [*deoxy-* + *corticosterone*]. 4-Pregnene-3,20-dione-21-ol, $C_{21}H_{30}O_3$, an adrenocortical hormone. In man it causes an increase in retention of sodium ion and water, and an increase in excretion of potassium ion; it has no demonstrable effect on protein or carbohydrate metabolism. It is used, commonly as the acetate ester, in the management of adrenal insufficiency. Syn. *compound Q (Reichstein's), deoxycortone, deoxycostone.*

de·oxy·cor·tone (dee·ock″see·kor′tone) *n.* British term for DEOXYCORTICOSTERONE.

de·oxy·cos·tone (dee·ock″see·kos′tone) *n.* DEOXYCORTICOSTERONE.

de·oxy·cy·ti·dine (dee·ock″see·sigh′ti·deen) *n.* One of the principal nucleosides of deoxyribonucleic acid, composed of cytosine and deoxyribose.

de·oxy·ephed·rine (dee·ock″see·eh·fed′rin) *n.* [*deoxy-* + *ephedrine*]. METHAMPHETAMINE.

de·ox·y·gen·a·tion (dee·ock″si·je·nay′shun) *n.* [*de-* + *oxygenation*]. The process of removing oxygen from a compound.

de·oxy·gua·nine (dee·ock″see·gwah′neen) *n.* One of the principal nucleosides of deoxyribonucleic acid, composed of guanine and deoxyribose.

de·oxy·pen·tose (dee·ock″see·pen′toce) *n.* Any pentose which contains less oxygen, commonly one atom, than its parent sugar. Biochemically the most important deoxypentose is deoxyribose, in consequence of which the two terms are sometimes used synonymously.

de·oxy·pen·tose·nu·cle·ic acid (dee·ock″see·pen″toce·new·klee′ick). A nucleic acid containing a deoxypentose as the sugar component. The deoxypentose is mostly, if not exclusively, deoxyribose.

de·oxy·pyr·i·dox·ine (dee·ock″see·pirr″i·dock′seen) *n.* 2,4-Dimethyl-3-hydroxy-5-hydroxymethylpyridine, $C_8H_{11}NO_2$, a synthetic antimetabolite which antagonizes the action of pyridoxine in animals and bacteria.

de·oxy·ri·bo·nu·cle·ase (dee·ock″see·rye″bo·new′klee·ace, ·aze) *n.* An enzyme, acting in the presence of magnesium ions, that causes depolymerization of deoxyribonucleic acids.

de·oxy·ri·bo·nu·cle·ic acid (dee·ock″see·rye″bo·new·klee′ick). Any of the high molecular weight polymers of deoxyribonucleotides, found principally in the chromosomes of the nucleus and varying in composition with the source, able to reproduce in the presence of the appropriate enzyme and substrates, and bearing coded genetic information. Abbreviated, DNA.

de·oxy·ri·bo·nu·cleo·pro·tein (dee·ock″see·rye″bo·new″klee·o·pro′tee·in, ·teen). *n.* Any nucleoprotein that yields a deoxyribonucleic acid as a hydrolysis product.

de·oxy·ri·bo·nu·cleo·tide (dee·ock″see·rye″bo·new′klee·o·tide). *n.* A nucleotide in which the sugar component is deoxyribose (2).

de·oxy·ri·bose (dee·ock″see·rye′boce, ·boze) *n.* 1. Any derivative of ribose in which an alcoholic hydroxyl group is replaced by hydrogen. 2. D-2-Deoxyribose, $CHOCH_2$-$HCOHHCOHCH_2OH$, the sugar component of deoxyribonucleic acid and deoxyribonucleotides.

de·oxy·sug·ar (dee·ock″see·shoog′ur) *n.* A sugar derived from or related to another sugar by replacement of a hydroxyl in the latter by hydrogen.

de·oxy·uri·dine (dee·ock″see·yoor′i·deen) *n.* A nucleoside composed of uracil and deoxyribose, intermediate in the synthesis of thymidine.

dep. Abbreviation for *depuratus,* purified.

Depakene. A trademark for valproate, an anticonvulsant.

de·par·af·fin·ize (dee·păr′uh·fin·ize) *v.* To remove the paraffin from something, as a tissue section.

de·pend, *v.* [L. *dependere*, from *pendere*, to hang]. 1. To be contingent. 2. To rely, as for support or maintenance. 3. To hang, hang down.

de·pen·dence, *n.* [MF. *dependance*]. 1. The quality or condition of being contingent upon, requiring the assistance of, being influenced by, or being subject or subservient to someone or something. 2. The causal relationship between two phenomena, as the degree to which one influences the other.

de·pen·den·cy, *n.* 1. DEPENDENCE (1). 2. The quality or condition of lacking independence, and particularly self-reliance, characterized by the need for mothering and the tendency to seek help in making decisions or in carrying out complex and demanding tasks. 3. The state of being dependent (3). See also *dependency needs.*

dependency needs. *In psychiatry,* the vital, originally infantile needs for mothering, love, affection, shelter, protection, security, food, and warmth, which are also present in some degree even in adult life.

de·pen·dent, *adj.* [MF. *dependant*, from L. *dependere*, to hang, to depend]. 1. Determined or controlled by another factor. 2. Relying for support on another person. 3. Hanging down.

dependent differentiation. The differentiation of a tissue partly as a response to an inductor or factor external to itself. Syn. *correlative differentiation.*

de·per·son·al·iza·tion (dee·pur″sun·ul·i·zay′shun, ·eye·zay′shun) *n.* 1. Loss of the sense of one's own reality or identity. 2. *In psychopathology,* a subjective feeling of estrangement or unreality within the personality, often manifested by symptoms of derealization and déjà vu. In mild form, the condition is common; in severe forms, it is a finding in various neuroses, depressive states, and beginning schizophrenias. It is considered to be a pathological defense mechanism.

de·phos·pho·gly·co·gen synthase (dee·fos″fo·glye′ko·jin). The active form of glycogen synthase which catalyzes net formation of glycogen from UDP-glucose. It is converted to inactive form by reaction with ATP and protein kinase in response to increased cyclic AMP levels. Contr. *phospho-glycogen synthase.*

de·phos·pho·phos·pho·ryl·ase kinase (dee·fos″fo·fos′for·i·lace, ·fos·for′i·). The inactive form of phosphorylase kinase which is converted to the active form by reaction with ATP and protein kinase. Activation occurs in response to increased cyclic AMP levels. Contr. *phospho-phosphorylase kinase.*

de·pig·ment (dee·pig′ment) *v.* To remove pigment, cause loss of pigment. —**depigment·ing** (·ing) *adj.*

de·pig·men·ta·tion (dee·pig″men·tay′shun) *n.* Loss of pigment, as from the skin.

dep·i·late (dep′i·late) *v.* [L. *depilare*, from *pilus*, a hair]. To remove hair. —**de·pil·a·to·ry** (de·pil′uh·to·ree) *adj. & n.*

dep·i·lous (dep′i·lus) *adj.* [L. *depilis*, from *pilus*, hair]. Hairless.

Depinar. A trademark for cyanocobalamin.

de·ple·tion (de·plee'shun) *n.* [L. *deplere,* to empty]. 1. The act of diminishing the quantity of fluid or stored materials in the body or in a part, especially by bleeding. 2. The condition of the system produced by the excessive loss of blood or other body constituents; reduction of strength; exhaustion. —**de·plete** (de·pleet') *v.*

de·plu·ma·tion (dee"ploo·may'shun) *n.* [ML. *deplumare,* to pluck, from L. *pluma,* feather, down]. Loss of the eyelashes.

Depo-Cer-O-Cillin. Trademark for chloroprocaine penicillin O, a long-acting penicillin preparation especially useful for patients sensitive to penicillin G.

Depo-Estradiol. A trademark for estradiol cypionate, an estrogenic steroid.

Depo-heparin sodium. Trademark for an injectable preparation of heparin sodium, characterized by prolonged effect of the latter, achieved through combination with gelatin and dextrose.

de·po·lar·iza·tion (dee·po"lur·i·zay'shun) *n.* [*de-* + *polarization*]. The neutralization of polarity; the reduction of differentials of ion distributions across polarized semipermeable membranes, as in nerve or muscle cells in the conduction of impulses. —**de·po·lar·ize** (dee·po'lur·ize) *v.*

de·po·lar·iz·ing electrode (dee·po'lur·eye·zing). An electrode with a resistance greater than that of the part of the body enclosed in the circuit.

de·po·lym·er·ase (dee"po·lim'ur·ace, dee·pol'i·mur·ace) *n.* [*depolymerize* + *-ase*]. One of a group of enzymes which depolymerize high molecular weight plant and animal substances, as nucleic acids.

de·po·lym·er·iza·tion (dee"po·lim"ur·i·zay'shun, dee·pol"i·mur·) *n.* The cleavage, by various means, of a polymer of high molecular weight into simpler units of the same composition. —**de·po·lym·er·ize** (dee"po·lim'ur·ize, dee·pol'i·mur·ize) *v.*

Depo-Medrol. A trademark for methylprednisolone acetate, a glucocorticoid.

Depo-Provera. A trademark for medroxyprogesterone acetate, a progestin.

de·pos·it, *n.* & *v.* [L. *depositum,* from *deponere,* to set down]. 1. An accumulation of material that has settled, precipitated, or formed on surfaces or in hollow or permeable spaces. 2. To cause or allow to accumulate in such a way.

de·pot (dep'o, dee'po) *n.* [F. *dépôt,* from L. *depositum,* deposit]. *In physiology,* the site of accumulation, deposit, or storage of body products not immediately or actively involved in metabolic processes, such as a fat depot.

depot fat. Fat occurring in certain regions such as the abdominal wall or the buttocks, which are called fat depots.

de·pres·sant (de·pres'unt) *n.* & *adj.* [*depress* + *-ant*]. 1. Any agent that diminishes functional activity. 2. Having the action of a depressant.

depressed fracture. A fracture of the skull in which the fractured part is depressed below the normal level.

de·pres·sion, *n.* [ML. *depressio,* from L. *deprimere,* to press down]. 1. A hollow or fossa. 2. An inward displacement of a part. 3. A lowering or reduction of function. 4. *In psychiatry,* extreme sadness, melancholy, or dejection which, unlike grief, is unrealistic and out of proportion to any claimed cause; may be a symptom of any psychiatric disorder or the prime manifestation of a psychotic depressive reaction or of a neurosis. See also *depressive neurosis, manic-depressive illness.* —**de·pressed, de·pres·sive,** *adj.*

depressive insanity. 1. PSYCHOTIC DEPRESSIVE REACTION. 2. INVOLUTIONAL MELANCHOLIA.

depressive neurosis or **reaction.** A psychoneurotic disorder in which the anxiety due to an internal conflict is partially relieved by depression and self-depreciation, frequently precipitated by an identifiable event, such as the loss of a cherished person or object, and associated with guilt feelings. Syn. *reactive depression.*

depressive personality. *In psychiatry,* a type of personality in which there is a pattern of several kinds of character defenses, such as overseriousness, lowered spirits, increased vulnerability to letdown or disappointment, and excessive conscientiousness, dependability, compliance, subservience, and deliberateness; when sufficiently marked to cause interference with normal living or satisfactions, constitutes the depressive neurosis.

depressive states. Certain mental disorders characterized by extreme depression. See also *adolescent depression, agitated depression, depressive neurosis, involutional melancholia, manic-depressive illness, retarded depression.*

de·pres·sor (de·pres'ur) *n.* 1. A muscle, instrument, or apparatus that depresses or lowers. 2. DEPRESSOR NERVE.

depressor alae na·si (ay'lee nay'zye). The alar part of the nasalis muscle.

depressor an·gu·li oris (ang'gew·lye o'ris). A muscle of facial expression which draws down the angle of the mouth. NA *musculus depressor anguli oris.* See also Table of Muscles in the Appendix.

depressor area. The region of the vasomotor center, stimulation of which causes a drop in blood pressure, usually with slowing of the heart rate.

depressor epi·glot·ti·dis (ep·i·glot'i·dis). Certain fibers of the thyroepiglottic muscle.

depressor la·bii in·fe·ri·o·ris (lay'bee·eye in·feer"ee·o'ris). A muscle of facial expression which draws down and everts the lower lip. NA *musculus depressor labii inferioris.* See also Table of Muscles in the Appendix.

depressor nerve. A nerve which, upon stimulation, lowers the blood pressure either in a local part or throughout the body.

depressor reflex. A reflex fall in blood pressure or vasodilatation, which may be evoked by a variety of stimuli, such as increased pressure in the carotid sinus.

depressor sep·ti na·si (sep'tye nay'zye). A muscle of facial expression which draws down the nasal septum. NA *musculus depressor septi nasi.* See also Table of Muscles in the Appendix.

depressor substance. A substance whose pharmacodynamic action results in a lowering of arterial pressure.

depressor su·per·ci·lii (sue·pur·sil'ee·eye). The portion of the orbicularis oculi muscle that draws the eyebrows down. NA *musculus depressor supercilii.* See also Table of Muscles in the Appendix.

dep·ri·va·tion (dep"ri·vay'shun) *n.* [ML. *deprivare,* to deprive, from L. *privare*]. A condition of being in want of anything considered essential for physical or mental well-being; it may be due to a lack, denial, or loss of certain factors, powers, or stimuli.—**de·prive** (de·prive') *v.*

deprivation dwarfism. A syndrome in childhood of short stature, voracious appetite, and delayed bone age secondary to emotional deprivation.

de·pros·til (dee·pros'til) *n.* 15-Hydroxy-15-methyl-9-oxo-prostan-1-oic acid, $C_{21}H_{38}O_4$, a gastric antisecretory.

dep·side (dep'side) *n.* [Gk. *depsein,* to knead, + *-ide*]. Any of a class of compounds characterized by an ester type of union of two or more molecules of phenolic acids, in which the phenolic hydroxyl of one molecule interacts with the carboxyl of another molecule in a manner similar to the combination of amino acids to form peptides. Certain tannins are naturally occurring depsides.

depth, *n.* 1. Distance from top to bottom, from front to back, or inward from a surface. 2. An inner or relatively inaccessible aspect of something.

depth dose. The number of rads within the body at a specified depth below the surface field of roentgen irradiation.

depth perception. The ability to estimate depth or distance between points in the field of vision.

depth psychology. 1. The psychology of unconscious mental activity. 2. Any system of psychology in which the study of unconscious mental processes plays a major role, as in psychoanalysis.

de·pu·li·za·tion (dee·pew″li·zay′shun) *n.* [*de-* + L. *pulex,* flea]. The destruction or removal of fleas, as from infested animals or premises.

de Quer·vain's disease (duh·kehr·væn′) [F. *de Quervain,* Swiss surgeon, 1868–1940]. 1. Subacute or stenosing fibrous tendovaginitis at the styloid process of the radius. 2. Chronic thyroiditis, a granulomatous inflammation of unknown etiology.

der-, dero- [Gk. *derē*]. A combining form meaning *neck.*

der·a·del·phus (derr″uh·del′fus) *n.* [*der-* + *-adelphus*]. CEPHALOTHORACOPAGUS.

de·range·ment (de·rainj′munt) *n.* [F.]. 1. Disturbance of the regular arrangement or function of parts or a system. 2. Disorder of intellect; insanity.

Der·cum's disease [F. X. *Dercum,* U.S. neurologist, 1856–1931]. ADIPOSIS DOLOROSA.

de·re·al·iza·tion (de·ree″ul·i·zay′shun) *n. In psychiatry,* a subjective feeling that other people or objects are unreal, changed or changing, or strange in their particular characteristics and configuration; often accompanies depersonalization.

de·re·ism (dee″ree′iz·um) *n.* [L. *de,* away from, + *re* (*res, rei*), thing, matter, concern, + *-ism*]. *In psychiatry,* a mental state in which the subject is lost in fantasy, showing no interest in external experiences or reality; AUTISM. —**de·re·is·tic** (dee″ree·is′tick) *adj.*

der·en·ceph·a·lus (derr″en·sef′uh·lus) *n.*, pl. **derencepha·li** (·lye). An individual showing derencephaly.

der·en·ceph·a·ly (derr″en·sef′uh·lee) *n.* [*der-* + *-encephaly*]. Cervical rachischisis combined with anencephaly. —**der·encepha·lous** (·lus) *adj.*

de·re·pres·sion (dee″re·presh′un) *n.* [*de-* + *repression*]. *In psychiatry,* the coming back of ideas or impulses into conscious awareness which were earlier pushed from such awareness into the unconscious because they were personally intolerable; occurring when the repressed material becomes too strong or when the repressing forces prove inadequate, and resulting in a strengthening of existing character defenses or in the development of new ones.

der·ic (derr′ick) *adj.* [Gk. *deros,* skin, + *-ic*]. ECTODERMAL.

de·rism (dee′riz·um) *n.* DEREISM.

der·i·va·tion (derr″i·vay′shun) *n.* [L. *derivatio,* from *derivare,* to draw off, divert, from *de-* + *rivus,* stream]. 1. The deflection of blood from one part of the body to another, as by counterirritation; formerly thought to relieve inflammatory hyperemia. 2. *In electrocardiography,* LEAD. 3. Synthesis of a chemical compound from another related to it. 4. The relationship of a substance to its source.

de·riv·a·tive (de·riv′uh·tiv) *adj. & n.* 1. Producing derivation. 2. Derived from another substance. 3. A derivative agent or substance.

de·rived, *adj.* Formed or developed from something else.

derived albumin. A modified albumin resulting from the action of certain reagents upon native albumin.

derived protein. A synthetic protein, a polypeptide, or any product obtained from proteins by the action of acids, alkalies, enzymes, or heat.

-derm [Gk. *derma,* skin, hide]. A combining form meaning (a) *integument;* (b) *germ layer.*

derm-, derma-, dermo-. A combining form meaning (a) *dermis, dermal;* (b) *skin, cutaneous.*

der·ma (dur′muh) *n.* [Gk., hide, skin, from *derein,* to skin, flay]. DERMIS.

-derma [Gk., skin, hide]. A combining form meaning (a) *a* (specified) *kind of skin or integument;* (b) *an abnormal condition of the skin.*

der·ma·bra·sion (dur″muh·bray′zhun) *n.* [*derm-* + *abrasion*]. The removal of skin in variable amounts or to variable depths by such mechanical means as revolving wire brushes or sandpaper, for the purpose of correcting scars.

Der·ma·cen·tor (dur″muh·sen′tur) *n.* [*derma-* + Gk. *kentōr,* goader]. A genus of ticks some species of which are vectors of disease.

Dermacentor an·der·so·ni (an·dur·so′nye). Medically, the most important North American species of tick, transmitting Rocky Mountain spotted fever and tularemia as well as producing tick paralysis. Syn. *wood tick.*

Dermacentor var·i·a·bi·lis (văr·ee·ay′bi·lis). A species of tick widely distributed in North America which has as its principal host the dog and sometimes man and other mammals; transmits Rocky Mountain spotted fever.

Der·ma·cen·trox·e·nus (dur″muh·sen·trock′se·nus) *n.* [*Dermacentor* + Gk. *xenos,* guest]. *RICKETTSIA.*

Dermacentroxenus akari. *RICKETTSIA AKARI.*

Dermacentroxenus pe·dic·u·li (pe·dick′yoo·lye). *ROCHALIMAEA QUINTANA.*

Dermacentroxenus rick·ett·si (ri·ket′sigh). *RICKETTSIA RICKETTSII.*

Dermacentroxenus rickettsi co·no·ri (kon·o′rye). *RICKETTSIA CONORII.*

der·ma·drome (dur′muh·drome) *n.* Any skin manifestation of an internal disorder; the cutaneous aspects of a syndrome.

der·ma·fat (dur′muh·fat) *n.* [*derma-* + *fat*]. The adipose tissue of the skin.

dermafat-fascia graft. A tissue graft employing full-thickness skin, fat, and fascia.

der·ma·he·mia, der·ma·hae·mia (dur″muh·hee′mee·uh) *n.* DERMATHEMIA.

der·mal (dur′mul) *adj.* 1. Pertaining to the dermis. 2. CUTANEOUS.

dermal graft. A skin graft using split or full-thickness dermis.

dermal muscle. CUTANEOUS MUSCLE.

dermal papilla. An elevation of the dermis into a corresponding depression in the overlying epidermis.

dermal sense. The faculty of perceiving heat, cold, pain, or pressure mediated through receptors in the skin.

dermal skeleton. EXOSKELETON (2).

dermal suture. A fine, pliable, comparatively inert skin suture used when a fine scar is desired.

der·ma·my·ia·sis (dur″muh·migh·eye′uh·sis) *n.*, pl. **dermamy·ia·ses** (·seez). Dermal myiasis; any skin disease caused by fly larvae.

dermamyiasis lin·e·ar·is mi·grans oes·tro·sa (lin·ee·air′is migh′granz e·stro′suh). LARVA MIGRANS; properly, that caused by fly larvae such as *Gasterophilus intestinalis.*

der·man·a·plas·ty (dur·man′a·plas″tee) *n.* [*derm-* + *anaplasty*]. SKIN GRAFTING.

der·man sulfate (dur′man). DERMATAN SULFATE.

Der·ma·nys·sus (dur″muh·nis′us) *n.* [NL., from *derma-* + Gk. *nyssein,* to prick]. A genus of itch mites.

Dermanyssus avi·um (ay′vee·um). A mite that is a serious pest of poultry and sometimes of man.

Dermanyssus gal·li·nae (gal·eye′nee). *DERMANYSSUS AVIUM.*

Dermastatin. A trademark for viridofulvin, an antifungal.

dermat-, dermato- [Gk. *derma, dermatos*]. A combining form meaning *skin, cutaneous.*

der·ma·tag·ra (dur″muh·tag′ruh) *n.* 1. PELLAGRA. 2. DERMATALGIA.

der·ma·tal·gia (dur″muh·tal′jee·uh) *n.* [*dermat-* + *-algia*]. Pain, burning, and other sensations of the skin, unaccompanied by any structural change.

der·ma·ta·neu·ria (dur″muh·tuh·new′ree·uh) *n.* [*dermat-* + *a-* + *neur-* + *-ia*]. Derangement of the nerve supply of the skin.

der·ma·tan sulfate (dur′muh·tan). A mucopolysaccharide that is a structural component of certain tissues. Syn. *derman sulfate, chondroitin sulfate B.*

der·mat·he·mia, der·mat·hae·mia (dur″mat·hee′mee·uh, dur″muh·tee′mee·uh) *n.* [*dermat-* + *-hemia*]. Cutaneous hyperemia. Syn. *dermahemia, dermohemia.*

der·ma·therm (dur′muh·thurm) *n.* [*derma-* + *-therm*]. An instrument made up of differential thermocouples, used to measure skin temperature. The apparatus consists of two sensitive thermopiles in parallel with a millivoltmeter, with one thermopile maintained at a constant known temperature and the other applied to the skin. The reading in degrees on the millivoltmeter added to or subtracted from the constant gives the skin temperature.

der·mat·ic (dur·mat′ick) *adj. & n.* [Gk. *dermatikos*]. 1. DERMAL; pertaining to the dermis. 2. CUTANEOUS. 3. A preparation for treating diseases of the skin.

der·ma·ti·tis (dur″muh·tye′tis) *n.*, pl. **derma·tit·i·des** (·tit′i·deez) [*dermat-* + *-itis*]. Inflammation of the skin. Compare *dermatosis.*

dermatitis ac·tin·i·ca (ack·tin′i·kuh). Dermatitis due to the action of actinic rays, from sunlight or artificial ultraviolet radiation.

dermatitis au·to·fac·ti·tia (aw″to·fack·tish′ee·uh). DERMATITIS FACTITIA.

dermatitis ca·lor·i·ca (ka·lor′i·kuh). Dermatitis due to burns and scalds.

dermatitis coc·cid·i·oi·des (kock·sid·ee·oy′deez). COCCIDIOIDOMYCOSIS.

dermatitis con·ge·la·ti·o·nis (kon·je·lay·shee·o′nis). FROSTBITE.

dermatitis con·ti·nu·ée (kon·ti·new·ay′). DERMATITIS REPENS.

dermatitis con·tu·si·for·mis (kon·tew″si·for′mis). ERYTHEMA NODOSUM.

dermatitis dys·men·or·rhe·i·ca (dis·men″o·ree′i·kuh). Wheals, vesicles, or erythematous areas seen during the menstrual period in women having dysmenorrhea.

dermatitis es·cha·rot·i·ca (es·ka·rot′i·kuh). A severe ulcerative dermatitis from exposure to escharotic agents.

dermatitis ex·fo·li·a·ti·va ne·o·na·to·rum (ecks·fo″lee·uh·tye′vuh nee·o·nay·to′rum). An acute dermatitis in infants, in which the epidermis is shed more or less freely in large or small scales; considered to be a consequence of staphylococcal impetigo. Syn. *Ritter's disease.*

dermatitis ex·sic·cans pal·ma·ris (eck·sick′anz pal·mair′is). A scarring tylotic eruption of the hands which may lead to contracture of the fingers, most frequent in women in Formosa.

dermatitis fac·ti·tia (fack·tish′ee·uh). An eruption induced by the patient; varies from simple erythema to gangrene. Syn. *dermatitis autofactitia.* See also *hysterical dermatoneurosis.*

dermatitis gan·gre·no·sa (gang″gre·no′suh). Gangrenous inflammation of the skin; SPHACELODERMA.

dermatitis gangrenosa in·fan·tum (in·fan′tum). A form of ecthyma due to *Pseudomonas,* marked by brown discolorations of the skin, usually surrounded by a halo; the center of these efflorescences rapidly becomes necrotic.

dermatitis her·pet·i·for·mis (hur·pet″i·for′mis, hur″pe·ti·). An inflammatory, recurring skin disease of a herpetic character, the various lesions showing a tendency to group. It is protean, appearing as erythema, vesicles, blebs, and pustules; associated with intense itching and burning. Syn. *Duhring's disease.*

dermatitis hi·e·ma·lis (high·e·may′lis) [L., of winter]. A recurrent inflammation of the skin, associated with cold weather.

dermatitis hy·po·stat·i·ca (high″po·stat′i·kuh). Dermatitis occurring in an area of poor blood supply, usually the lower legs.

dermatitis med·i·ca·men·to·sa (med″i·kuh·men·to′suh). A skin eruption due to the action of certain drugs.

dermatitis nod·u·la·ris ne·crot·i·ca (nod·yoo·lair′is ne·krot′i·kuh). A polymorphous skin eruption of vesicles, pustules, hemorrhagic papules, nodules, ulcers, plaques and their sequels, scars and hyperpigmentation, of unknown cause.

dermatitis pap·il·la·ris cap·il·li·tii (pap″i·lair′is kap″i·lish′ee·eye). KELOID ACNE.

dermatitis pap·u·lo·squa·mo·sa atroph·i·cans (pap″yoo·lo·skway·mo′suh a·trof′i·kanz). DEGOS' DISEASE.

dermatitis re·pens (ree′penz) [L., creeping]. A subacute peripherally spreading dermatitis due to *Staphylococcus aureus* (staphyloderma) usually following minor injuries, and commencing almost exclusively on the distal part of the upper extremity, marked by vesicles or pustules which dry and crust.

dermatitis rhus. Contact dermatitis due to toxic substances from such *Toxicodendron* plants as poison ivy or poison oak, formerly included in the genus *Rhus.*

dermatitis se·bor·rhe·i·ca (seb·o·ree′i·kuh, see·bo·). SEBORRHEIC DERMATITIS.

dermatitis trau·mat·i·ca (trow·mat′i·kuh). Dermatitis resulting from traumatism.

dermatitis veg·e·tans (vej′e·tanz). Elevated, vegetating lesions covered with crusts; very prone to bleeding and believed to be due to infection.

dermatitis ve·ne·na·ta (ven·e·nay′tuh). CONTACT DERMATITIS.

dermatitis ver·ru·co·sa (verr·oo·ko′suh). CHROMOBLASTOMYCOSIS.

dermato-. See *dermat-.*

Der·ma·to·bia (dur″muh·to′bee·uh) *n.* [NL., from *dermato-* + Gk. *bios,* life]. A genus of botflies whose larvae are obligatory sarcobionts, producing cutaneous myiasis in many animals.

Dermatobia hom·i·nis (hom′i·nis). A species of botfly found in tropical America, causing dermal myiasis in man. The eggs are deposited by the adult female on the skin of the host. Upon emergence, the larva burrows into the skin, producing a swelling similar to an ordinary boil.

der·ma·to·bi·a·sis (dur″muh·to·bye′uh·sis) *n.*, pl. **dermatobia·ses** (·seez) [*Dermatobia* + *-iasis*]. Infection with *Dermatobia.*

der·ma·to·cel·lu·li·tis (dur″muh·to·sel″yoo·lye′tis) *n.* [*dermato-* + *cellulitis*]. Acute inflammation of the skin and subcutaneous tissue.

der·ma·to·cha·la·sis (dur″muh·to·kuh·lay′sis) *n.* [*dermato-* + Gk. *chalasis,* slackening]. Diffuse relaxation and abnormal looseness of the skin. Syn. *cutis laxa.*

der·ma·to·co·ni·o·sis, der·ma·to·ko·ni·o·sis (dur″muh·to·ko″nee·o′sis) *n.* [*dermato-* + *coni-* + *-osis*]. Any skin disease due to dust.

der·ma·to·cyst (dur′muh·to·sist″) *n.* [*dermato-* + *cyst*]. Any cyst of the skin.

der·ma·to·dyn·ia (dur″muh·to·din′ee·uh) *n.* [*dermat-* + *-odynia*]. DERMATALGIA.

der·ma·to·fi·bro·ma (dur″muh·to·figh·bro′muh) *n.* [*dermato-* + *fibroma*]. Firm, single, or multiple slowly growing nodules, red, yellow, or bluish-black, found most commonly on the extremities in adults. Histologically, the nodules are composed chiefly of fibroblasts. See also *histiocytoma.*

dermatofibroma len·tic·u·la·re (len·tick·yoo·lair′ee). DERMATOFIBROMA.

der·ma·to·fi·bro·sar·co·ma (dur″muh·to·figh″bro·sahr·ko′muh) *n.* [*dermato-* + *fibrosarcoma*]. A fibrosarcoma arising in the skin.

dermatofibrosarcoma pro·tu·ber·ans (pro·tew′bur·anz). A tumor of dermal fibroblasts forming multinodular red protruding masses; it tends to recur but does not usually metastasize.

der·ma·to·glyph·ics (dur″muh·to·glif′icks) *n.* [*dermato-* + Gk. *glyphē,* carved work]. The skin-pattern lines and whorls of the fingertips, palms, and soles, systematically classified for identification purposes and used in medicine as ancillary findings in chromosomal abnormalities and in individuals with intrauterine exposure to viral infections, such as rubella, during the first trimester of pregnancy. These patterns are individually characteristic and never change.

der·ma·to·graph·ia (dur″muh·to·graf′ee·uh) *n.* DERMOGRAPHIA.

der·ma·tog·ra·phism (dur″muh·tog′ruh·fiz·um, ·to·graf′iz·um) *n.* DERMOGRAPHIA.

der·ma·tog·ra·phy (dur″muh·tog′ruh·fee) *n.* 1. A description of the skin. 2. DERMOGRAPHIA.

der·ma·to·het·ero·plas·ty (dur″muh·to·het′ur·o·plas″tee) *n.* [*dermato-* + *heteroplasty*]. The grafting of heterogenous skin.

dermatokoniosis. DERMATOCONIOSIS.

der·ma·tol (dur′muh·tol) *n.* BISMUTH SUBGALLATE.

der·ma·tol·o·gist (dur″muh·tol′uh·jist) *n.* [*dermatology* + *-ist*]. A skin specialist; a physician who makes a special study of diseases of the skin.

der·ma·tol·o·gy (dur″muh·tol′uh·jee) *n.* [*dermato-* + *-logy*]. The medical specialty dealing with the skin, its structure, functions, diseases, and their treatment. —**derma·to·log·ic** (·to·loj′ick), **dermatolog·i·cal** (·i·kul) *adj.*

der·ma·tol·y·sis (dur″muh·tol′i·sis) *n.* [*dermato-* + *-lysis*]. Fibromas of the skin with masses of pendulous skin. Syn. *cutis laxa, cutis pendula.*

der·ma·tome (dur′muh·tome) *n.* [*derma-* + *-tome*]. 1. The areas of the skin supplied with sensory fibers from a single spinal nerve. 2. An instrument for cutting skin, as in grafting. 3. The lateral part of an embryonic somite; CUTIS PLATE. —**der·ma·tom·ic** (dur″muh·tom′ick) *adj.*

der·ma·to·meg·a·ly (dur″muh·to·meg′uh·lee) *n.* [*dermato-* + *-megaly*]. An excessive amount of skin, producing pendulous folds; may be congenital or acquired.

dermatomic area. The ringlike band of the integument innervated by a segmental spinal nerve.

der·ma·to·mu·co·so·myo·si·tis (dur″muh·to·mew·ko″so·migh″o·sigh′tis) *n.* [*dermato-* + *mucosa-* + *myositis*]. Inflammation of the skin, mucosa of the nose, mouth, and throat, and of the muscles.

der·ma·to·my·ces (dur″muh·to·migh′seez) *n.* [*dermato-* + *myces*]. DERMATOPHYTE.

der·ma·to·my·cete (dur″muh·to·migh′seet) *n.* DERMATOPHYTE.

der·ma·to·my·co·sis (dur″muh·to·migh·ko′sis) *n.* [*dermato-* + *mycosis*]. Any fungous infection of the skin.

der·ma·to·my·o·ma (dur″muh·to·migh·o′muh) *n.* [*dermato-* + *myoma*]. A leiomyoma located in the skin.

der·ma·to·my·o·si·tis (dur″muh·to·migh″o·sigh′tis) *n.* [*dermato-* + *myositis*]. An inflammatory disorder involving skin and muscles, including the muscles of swallowing, often associated with visceral cancer in persons over 40 years old, or occurring as a manifestation of collagen disease.

der·ma·to·neu·rol·o·gy (dur″muh·to·new·rol′uh·jee) *n.* [*dermato-* + *neurology*]. The study of the nerves of the skin.

der·ma·to·neu·ro·sis (dur″muh·to·new·ro′sis) *n.* [*dermato-* + *neurosis*]. A skin disease of nervous origin.

der·ma·to·path·ia (dur″muh·to·path′ee·uh) *n.* [NL.]. DERMATOPATHY.

dermatopathic lymphadenitis. LIPOMELANOTIC RETICULOSIS.

dermatopathic lymphadenopathy. LIPOMELANOTIC RETICULOSIS.

der·ma·to·pa·thol·o·gy (dur″muh·to·pa·thol′uh·jee) *n.* [*dermato-* + *pathology*]. A subspecialty of pathology concerning itself with diseases of the skin.

der·ma·to·patho·pho·bia (dur″muh·to·path″o·fo′bee·uh) *n.* [*dermatopathy* + *-phobia*]. An abnormal fear of having a skin disease.

der·ma·top·a·thy (dur″muh·top′uth·ee) *n.* [*dermato-* + *-pathy*]. Any skin disease. —**derma·to·path·ic** (·to·path′ick) *adj.*

der·ma·to·phi·li·a·sis (dur″muh·to·fil·eye′uh·sis) *n.* [*Dermatophilus* + *-iasis*]. Infection with the impregnated female flea, *Tunga penetrans,* which bores beneath the skin or nail, becomes distended with eggs, and appears as a pea-sized papule.

der·ma·to·phi·lo·sis (dur″muh·to·fil·o′sis) *n.* [*Dermatophilus* + *-osis*]. DERMATOPHILIASIS.

Der·ma·toph·i·lus penetrans (dur″muh·tof′i·lus). TUNGA PENETRANS.

der·ma·to·phyte (dur′muh·to·fite, dur·mat′o·) *n.* [*dermato-* + *-phyte*]. One of a group of keratinophilic fungi which invade the superficial keratinized areas of the body of man and animals, such as the skin, hair, and nails. The dermatophytes include four genera: *Microsporum, Trichophyton, Epidermophyton,* and *Keratomyces.*

der·ma·to·phy·tid (dur″muh·to·figh′tid, ·tof′i·did) *n.* [*dermatophyte* + *-id*]. A skin eruption associated with a skin disease caused by a fungus; fungi are not found in the dermatophytids themselves.

der·ma·to·phy·to·sis (dur″muh·to·figh·to′sis) *n.* [*dermatophyte* + *-osis*]. A skin eruption characterized by the formation of small vesicles on the hands and feet, especially between the toes, with cracking and scaling. There is sometimes secondary infection. The cause may be any one of the dermatophytes. See also *tinea pedis.*

der·ma·to·plas·ty (dur′muh·to·plas″tee) *n.* [*dermato-* + *-plasty*]. A plastic operation on the skin whereby skin losses or defects are replaced by skin flaps or grafts.

der·ma·to·poly·neu·ri·tis (dur″muh·to·pol″ee·new·rye′tis) *n.* [*dermato-* + *polyneuritis*]. ACRODYNIA.

der·ma·tor·rha·gia (dur″muh·to·ray′jee·uh) *n.* [*dermato-* + *-rrhagia*]. Bleeding from the skin.

der·ma·tor·rhex·is (dur″muh·to·reck′sis) *n.* [*dermato-* + *-rrhexis*]. 1. Disruption of skin capillaries. 2. EHLERS-DANLOS SYNDROME.

der·ma·to·scle·ro·sis (dur″muh·to·skle·ro′sis) *n.* [*dermato-* + *sclerosis*]. SCLERODERMA.

der·ma·tos·co·py (dur″muh·tos′kuh·pee) *n.* [*dermato-* + *-scopy*]. Examination of the skin; particularly, microscopical examination of the superficial capillaries of the skin.

dermatoses. Plural of *dermatosis.*

der·ma·to·sio·pho·bia (dur″muh·to″see·o·fo′bee·uh) *n.* [*dermatosis* + *-phobia*]. DERMATOPATHOPHOBIA.

der·ma·to·sis (dur″muh·to′sis) *n.*, pl. **dermato·ses** (·seez) [*dermat-* + *-osis*]. Any disease of the skin. Compare *dermatitis.*

dermatosis pap·u·lo·sa ni·gra (pap·yoo·lo′suh nigh′gruh). A condition commonly seen in Negroes, usually on the face, consisting of many tiny papules on the skin; probably nevoid in origin.

der·ma·to·sto·ma·ti·tis (dur″muh·to·sto″muh·tye′tis) *n.* [*dermato-* + *stomatitis*]. A severe form of erythema multiforme. See also *Stevens-Johnson syndrome.*

der·ma·to·ther·a·py (dur″muh·to·therr′uh·pee) *n.* [*dermato-* + *therapy*]. Treatment of cutaneous disease.

der·ma·to·thla·sia (dur″muh·to·thlay′zhuh, ·zee·uh) *n.* [*dermato-* + Gk. *thlasis*, bruising, + *-ia*]. An abnormal state marked by an uncontrollable impulse to pinch or rub the skin.

der·ma·tot·o·my (dur″muh·tot′uh·mee) *n.* [*dermato-* + *-tomy*]. Anatomy or dissection of the skin.

der·ma·to·zo·on (dur″muh·to·zo′on) *n.*, pl. **dermato·zoa** (·zo′uh) [*dermato-* + Gk. *zōon*, animal]. Any animal parasite of the skin.

der·ma·to·zoo·no·sis (dur″muh·to·zo″uh·no′sis) *n.* [*dermatozoon* + *-osis* (by re-formation of *dermatozoonosus*)]. Any pathologic condition due to a dermatozoon.

der·ma·to·zoo·no·sus (dur″muh·to·zo″uh·no′sus) *n.* [NL., from *dermato-* + *zoo-* + Gr. *nosos*, disease]. DERMATOZOONOSIS.

der·ma·tro·phia (dur″muh·tro′fee·uh) *n.* [*derm-* + *atrophia*]. Atrophy of the skin.

-dermia [*derm-* + *-ia*]. A combining form designating a *condition of the skin.*

der·mic (dur′mick) *adj.* [*derm-* + *-ic*]. DERMAL.

dermic layer. The middle layer of the tympanic membrane.

der·mis (dur′mis) *n.* [ML., from Gk. *derma*, skin, hide] [NA alt.]. The layer of the skin below the epidermis, composed of collagen bundles, elastic fibers, and sparsely arranged fibroblasts, and bearing the appendages (as the hair apparatus, sebaceous glands, and sweat glands), the nerves, and the blood vessels. Syn. *corium [NA], cutis vera, true skin.*

der·mi·tis (dur·migh'tis) *n.* DERMATITIS.

dermo-. See *derm-.*

der·mo·blast (dur'mo·blast) *n.* [*dermo-* + *-blast*]. The part of the mesoderm which develops into the dermis.

der·mo·cy·ma (dur''mo·sigh'muh) *n.* [*dermo-* + Gk. *kyma,* fetus]. A type of cryptodidymus in which the parasitic twin is in the body wall of the host.

der·mo·cy·mus (dur''mo·sigh'mus) *n.* DERMOCYMA.

der·mo·epi·der·mal (dur''mo·ep''i·dur'mul) *adj.* [*dermo-* + *epidermal*]. Pertaining to both the superficial and the deeper layers of the skin; said of skin grafts.

dermoepidermal junction. The area of separation between the basal cell layer of the epidermis and the stratum papillare of the dermis.

der·mo·graph·ia (dur''mo·graf'ee·uh) *n.* [*dermo-* + Gk. *graphein,* to mark, draw, write, + *-ia*]. A condition in which the skin is peculiarly susceptible to irritation; characterized by elevations or wheals with surrounding erythematous axon reflex flare, caused by tracing the fingernail or a blunt instrument over the skin. May or may not be accompanied by urticaria. Syn. *dermatographia, dermographism, autographism.* —**dermograph·ic** (·ick) *adj.*

dermographia al·ba (al'buh). A white line which briefly precedes the development of the initial reddening along the line of scratch as observed in the triple response.

dermographia ru·bra (roo'bruh). The red line of the triple response.

der·mog·ra·phism (dur·mog'ruh·fiz·um) *n.* DERMOGRAPHIA.

der·mog·ra·phy (dur·mog'ruh·fee) *n.* DERMOGRAPHIA.

der·mo·he·mia, der·mo·hae·mia (dur''mo·hee'mee·uh) *n.* DERMATHEMIA.

der·moid (dur'moid) *adj. & n.* [*derm-* + *-oid*]. 1. Resembling skin. 2. DERMOID CYST.

dermoid cyst. A benign cystic teratoma with skin, skin appendages, and their products as the most prominent components, usually involving the ovary or the skin.

der·moid·ec·to·my (dur''moy·deck'tuh·mee) *n.* [*dermoid* + *-ectomy*]. Excision of a dermoid cyst.

der·mo·la·bi·al (dur''mo·lay'bee·ul) *adj.* [*dermo-* + *labial*]. Having relation or pertaining to both the skin and the lips.

der·mo·lath·y·rism (dur''mo·lath'i·riz·um) *n.* [*dermo-* + *lathyrism*]. Collagenous alterations in the skin resulting from experimental penicillamine administration.

der·mo·li·po·ma (dur''mo·li·po'muh) *n.* [*dermo-* + *lip-* + *-oma*]. A congenital increase in adipose tissue beneath the bulbar conjunctiva between the superior and external rectus muscles, appearing as a yellow mass.

der·mom·e·ter (dur·mom'e·tur) *n.* Any instrument used in dermometry.

der·mom·e·try (dur·mom'e·tree) *n.* [*dermo-* + *-metry*]. The measurement of the resistance of the skin to the passage of an electric current; skin areas deprived of their autonomic innervation, where sweat glands are inactive, show increased resistance, and where sweat glands are active, resistance is low.

der·mo·ne·cro·sis (dur''mo·ne·kro'sis) *n.* [*dermo-* + *necrosis*]. Necrosis of the skin.

der·mo·ne·crot·ic (dur''mo·ne·krot'ick) *adj.* [*dermo-* + *necrotic*]. Causing necrosis of the skin.

dermonecrotic toxin. An exotoxin of *Staphylococcus aureus* which produces necrosis of the skin on intradermal injection; ALPHA HEMOLYSIN.

der·mop·a·thy (dur·mop'uth·ee) *n.* DERMATOPATHY.

der·mo·phle·bi·tis (dur''mo·fle·bye'tis) *n.* [*dermo-* + *phlebitis*]. Inflammation of the cutaneous veins.

der·mo·phyte (dur'mo·fite) *n.* DERMATOPHYTE.

der·mo·skel·e·ton (dur''mo·skel'e·tun) *n.* [*dermo-* + *skeleton*]. EXOSKELETON (2).

der·mo·ste·no·sis (dur''mo·ste·no'sis) *n.* [*dermo-* + *stenosis*]. A tightening of the skin, due to swelling or to disease.

dur·mos·to·sis (der''mos·to'sis) *n.* [*derm-* + *oste-* + *-osis*]. OSTEOMA CUTIS.

der·mo·syn·o·vi·tis (dur''mo·sin''o·vye'tis) *n.* [*dermo-* + *synovitis*]. Inflammation of a subcutaneous bursa or tendon sheath and the adjacent skin.

der·mo·syph·i·lop·a·thy (dur''mo·sif''i·lop'uth·ee) *n.* [*dermo-* + *syphilo-* + *-pathy*]. A syphilitic skin disease.

dero-. See *der-.*

dero·did·y·mus (derr''o·did'i·mus) *n.* [*dero-* + *-didymus*]. DICEPHALUS DIAUCHENOS.

de·rom·e·lus (de·rom'e·lus) *n.* [*dero-* + *-melus*]. An individual having an accessory limb attached to the neck or lower jaw.

Deronil. A trademark for dexamethasone, an anti-inflammatory adrenocortical steroid.

der·rid (dur'id, derr'id) *n.* A highly toxic resin from the leguminous plant of Malaya, *Derris elliptica,* used in Borneo as an arrow poison.

de·rrien·gue (derr·yeng'geʰ) *n.* A modified form of rabies transmitted to cattle in parts of Mexico by vampire bats.

DES An abbreviation for *diethylstilbestrol,* a synthetic estrogen.

des- [F. *dés-*]. A prefix designating (a) *reversing or undoing* (of an action); (b) *depriving, ridding of, or freeing from.* See also *de-.*

Desacetyl-Lanatoside C. Trademark for deslanoside, a cardiotonic.

des·am·i·dase (des''am'i·dace, ·daze) *n.* AMIDASE.

des·an·i·ma·nia (des·an''i·may'nee·uh) *n.* [*des-* + *anima* + *-mania*]. Any psychotic disorder with mental deficiency.

de·sat·u·ra·tion (dee·satch''uh·ray'shun) *n.* Conversion of a saturated compound, such as stearin, into an unsaturated compound, such as olein, by the removal of hydrogen.

des·ce·me·ti·tis (des''e·me·tye'tis) *n.* [J. *Descemet,* French anatomist, 1732–1810, + *-itis*]. KERATITIS PUNCTATA.

des·ce·met·o·cele (des''e·met'o·seel) *n.* [J. *Descemet* + *-cele*]. A forward bulging of Descemet's membrane when the overlying cornea is destroyed.

Des·ce·met's membrane (des·meʰ', deh·se·meʰ') [J. *Descemet*]. The posterior elastic lamina of the cornea which covers the posterior surface of the substantia propria; the thickened basement membrane of the corneal epithelium.

de·scen·dens (de·sen'denz) *L. adj.* DESCENDING.

descendens cer·vi·cis (sur'vi·sis). INFERIOR ROOT OF THE ANSA CERVICALIS.

descendens hy·po·glos·si (high·po·glos'eye). SUPERIOR ROOT OF THE ANSA CERVICALIS.

de·scend·ing (de·sen'ding) *adj.* 1. Extending or directed downward or caudally. 2. In the nervous system, EFFERENT; conducting impulses or progressing down the spinal cord or from central to peripheral.

descending aorta. That portion of the aorta between the distal end of the arch, in the thorax, and the bifurcation of the vessel into the iliac arteries in the abdomen. NA *aorta descendens.* See also Plates 5, 7, 8, 14.

descending colon. The portion of the colon that extends from the splenic flexure to the sigmoid colon. NA *colon descendens.*

descending degeneration. Deterioration of myelin sheath and axons of descending tracts progressing caudally from the point of injury.

descending limb. 1. The portion of a renal tubule which extends from the proximal convoluted portion to the bend in the loop of Henle. 2. A downward slope in a graphic wave, representing decrease, as of pressure, volume, or velocity.

descending mesocolon. The descending portion of the mesentery connecting the colon with the posterior abdominal wall. NA *mesocolon descendens.*

descending neuritis. Weakness or paralysis, caused by an inflammatory polyneuritis, of the cranial muscles or proximal muscles of the limbs, followed by involvement of the distal muscles.

descending process. A downward prolongation of the inferior border of the lacrimal bone which articulates with the lacrimal process of the inferior nasal concha, and assists in forming the canal for the nasolacrimal duct.

descending tetanus. A form of tetanus in which the muscle spasms are first noted about the face and throat, later spreading throughout the rest of the patient's body.

descending tract. A collection of nerve fibers conducting impulses down the spinal cord. Syn. *efferent tract.*

descending vestibular nucleus. SPINAL VESTIBULAR NUCLEUS.

descending vestibular root or **tract.** VESTIBULOSPINAL TRACT.

de·scen·sus (de·sen'sus) *n.*, pl. **descensus** [L.]. Descent; fall, prolapse.

descensus tes·tis (tes'tis) [NA]. The descent of the fetal testis from the abdominal cavity through the inguinal canal to the scrotum during the third trimester of gestation.

descensus ute·ri (yoo'tur·eye). PROLAPSE OF THE UTERUS.

descensus ven·tri·cu·li (ven·trick'yoo·lye). GASTROPTOSIS.

de·scent (de·sent') *n.* [L. *descendere,* to descend]. 1. Movement or migration downward. 2. Derivation from an ancestor, especially in regard to evolutionary origin.

des·cin·o·lone acet·o·nide (de·sin'o·lone a·set'o·nide). 9-Fluoro-11β,16α,17-trihydroxypregna-1,4-diene-3,20-dione cyclic 16,17-acetal with acetone, $C_{24}H_{31}FO_5$, a glucocorticoid.

Descotone. A trademark for deoxycorticosterone acetate, an adrenocortical steroid.

descriptive anatomy. Study of the separate and individual portions of the body.

descriptive embryology. A study of the separate and individual portions of the embryo.

descriptive psychiatry. A system of psychiatry based upon the study of readily observable external factors, as in Kraepelin's classification. Contr. *dynamic psychiatry.*

Desenex. Trademark for a fungicidal ointment or powder that contains undecylenic acid and zinc undecylenate.

de·sen·si·tize (dee·sen'si·tize) *v.* 1. To render a person or experimental animal insensitive to an antigen or hapten by the appropriate administration of these agents. 2. *In psychiatry,* to alleviate or remove a mental complex, especially a phobia or an obsessive-compulsive neurosis, by repeated discussion of the stressful experience. See also *abreaction.* —**de·sen·si·ti·za·tion** (dee·sen''si·ti·zay'shun) *n.*

de·ser·pi·dine (dee·sur'pi·deen) *n.* 11-Desmethoxyreserpine, $C_{32}H_{38}N_2O_8$, an alkaloid from *Rauwolfia canescens;* the pharmacologic actions are essentially the same as those of other active *Rauwolfia* alkaloids, including reserpine. Syn. *canescine.*

desert fever or **rheumatism.** PRIMARY COCCIDIOIDOMYCOSIS.

desert sore. VELDT SORE.

de·sex·u·al·iza·tion (dee·seck''shoo·ul·i·zay'shun, ·eye·zay'shun) *n.* 1. Depriving an individual of sexual powers; castration. 2. *In psychiatry,* the act of detaching or neutralizing sexual energy from an object or activity, or removing from an activity any apparent connection with the sexual drive, so that the energy released becomes available to the ego for its wishes and tasks.

Desferal. Trademark for deferoxamine, an iron-chelating compound used in the treatment of hemochromatosis.

des·fer·ri·ox·a·mine (des·ferr''ee·ock'suh·meen) *n.* DEFEROXAMINE.

Desh·ler's salve. Compound rosin cerate; a formulation of rosin, turpentine, yellow wax, prepared suet, and linseed oil, formerly a popular protective and stimulant application.

des·ic·cant (des'ick·unt) *adj. & n.* [L. *desicans,* drying, from *desiccare,* to dry]. 1. Drying; rendering dry. 2. A drying medicine or application.

des·ic·cate (des'i·kate) *v.* [L. *desiccare,* from *siccus,* dry]. To deprive a substance of moisture. —**desic·cat·ed** (·kay·tid) *adj.*, **des·ic·ca·tion** (des''i·kay'shun) *n.*

desiccated ovary or **ovarian substance.** The dried, undefatted, and powdered ovarian substance of domestic animals, usually cattle, swine, or sheep; has been used as a therapeutic agent in the past.

des·ic·ca·tor (des'i·kay''tur) *n.* A vessel containing some strongly hygroscopic substance, such as calcium chloride or sulfuric acid, used to absorb the moisture from any substance placed therein or to maintain it in a moisture-free state.

des·ic·cyte (des'ick·site) *n.* [*desiccate* + *-cyte*]. An erythrocyte with decreased water content, resulting from excessive membrane permeability to potassium as compared with sodium. Contr. *hydrocyte.*

des·ic·cy·to·sis (des''ick·sigh·to'sis) *n.* The presence of an excessive number of desiccytes.

de·sid·er·ize (dee·sid'ur·ize) *v.* [*de-* + Gk. *sidēros,* iron]. To deprive a pigment of its iron.

des·ip·ra·mine (dez·ip'ruh·meen) *n.* 10,11-Dihydro-5-(3-methylaminopropyl)-5*H*-dibenz[*b,f*]azepine, $C_{18}H_{22}N_2$, an antidepressant drug; used as the hydrochloride salt. Syn. *desmethylimipramine.*

-desis [Gk., from *dein,* to bind]. A combining form meaning *binding, fusing.*

Desivac. A process of drying substances which involves quick freezing followed by dehydration under vacuum while in the frozen state. See also *lyophilization.*

des·lan·o·side (des·lan'o·side, dez·) *n.* $C_{47}H_{74}O_{19}$, a cardiotonic glycoside.

desm-, desmo- [Gk. *desmos,* band, bond, from *dein,* to bind]. A combining form meaning (a) *bond, bound;* (b) *connective tissue;* (c) *ligament.*

des·meth·yl·im·ip·ra·mine (dez·meth''il·im·ip'ruh·meen) *n.* DESIPRAMINE.

des·mio·gnath·us (dez''mee·o·nath'us, des'') *n.* [Gk. *desmios,* binding, + *-gnathus*]. DICEPHALUS PARASITICUS.

des·mi·tis (dez·migh'tis, des·) *n.* [*desm-* + *-itis*]. Inflammation of a ligament.

desmo-. See *desm-.*

des·mo·cra·ni·um (dez''mo·kray'nee·um, des'') *n.* [*desmo-* + *cranium*]. The mesenchymal or membranous anlage of the neurocranium from which the chondrocranium develops.

des·mo·cyte (dez'mo·site, des') *n.* [*desmo-* + *-cyte*]. Any kind of supporting-tissue cell.

des·mo·gly·co·gen (dez''mo·glye'ko·jin) *n.* [*desmo-* + *glycogen*]. The bound glycogen of tissues, representing a combination of glycogen with protein; heating the tissue with a solution of alkali releases the glycogen.

des·moid (dez'moid) *adj.* [*desm-* + *-oid*]. Like a ligament; fibrous.

desmoid tumor. A benign tumorlike lesion of subcutaneous tissues or of muscle, as of the rectus abdominis, probably a form of fibroma.

des·mo·lase (dez'mo·lace, ·laze) *n.* Any of a group of enzymes which catalyze rupture of atomic linkages that are not cleaved through hydrolysis, such as the bonds in the carbon chain of D-glucose.

des·mone (dez'mone) *n.* A growth-promoting substance, theoretically present in all cells.

des·mo·pla·sia (dez''mo·play'zhuh, ·zee·uh) *n.* [*desmo-* + *-plasia*]. 1. The formation and proliferation of connective tissue, especially fibrous connective tissue; frequently, prominent proliferation of connective tissue in the growth of tumors. 2. The formation of adhesions. —**desmo·plas·tic** (·plas'tick) *adj.*

des·mo·some (dez'mo·sohm, des') *n.* [*desmo-* + *-some*]. A very strong type of intercellular junction seen on intercellular bridges between epidermal and other epithelial cells and consisting of apposed dense plates (attachment plaques) separated by a narrow space filled with an extracellular substance which is presumed to act as a glue; in each half of the desmosome, delicate fibrils (tonofibrils) extend back from the plaque to the cytoplasm, perhaps to transmit mechanical tension away from the apposing cell membranes. See also *intercellular bridge.*

des·mos·ter·ol (dez·mos'tur·ol, ·ole) *n.* 24-Dehydrocholesterol, the immediate precursor of cholesterol in the biosynthetic pathway.

des·mot·o·my (dez·mot'uh·mee) *n.* [*desmo-* + *-tomy*]. Incision of a ligament.

Des·nos' pneumonia (dess·no^h^ss', ·noce) [L. J. *Desnos,* French physician, 1828–1893]. Splenopneumonia or the hepatization stage of pneumonia.

deso·mor·phine (dez''o·mor'feen) *n.* Dihydrodesoxymorphine-D, $C_{17}H_{21}NO_2$, a morphine derivative reported to be powerfully analgesic but to have greater addiction liability than morphine.

des·o·nide (des'o·nide) *n.* $11\beta,16\alpha,17,21$-Tetrahydroxypregna-1,4-diene-3,20-dione cyclic 16,17-acetal with acetone, $C_{24}H_{32}O_6$, an anti-inflammatory steroid derivative.

de·sorp·tion (dee·sorp'shun) *n.* The process of removing adsorbed matter from an adsorbent; the reverse of the process of adsorption.

des·ox·i·met·a·sone (des·ock''see·met'uh·sone) *n.* 9-Fluoro-11β,21-dihydroxy-16α-methylpregna-1,4-diene-3,20-dione, $C_{22}H_{29}FO_4$, an anti-inflammatory.

desoxy-. See *deoxy-.*

des·oxy·cho·late (des·ock''see·ko'late) *n.* DEOXYCHOLATE.

des·oxy·cho·lic acid (des·ock''si·ko'lick, ·kol'ick). DEOXYCHOLIC ACID.

des·oxy·cor·ti·cos·ter·one (des·ock'see·kor''ti·kos'tur·ohn) *n.* DEOXYCORTICOSTERONE.

des·oxy·ephed·rine (des·ock''see·e·fed'rin) *n.* METHAMPHETAMINE.

Desoxyn. A trademark for methamphetamine, a central stimulant drug used as the hydrochloride salt.

des·oxy·pen·tose (des·ock''see·pen'toce) *n.* DEOXYPENTOSE.

des·oxy·pen·tose·nu·cle·ic acid (des·ock''see·pen''toce·new·klee'ick). DEOXYPENTOSENUCLEIC ACID.

des·oxy·pyr·i·dox·ine (des·ock''see·pirr''i·dock'seen) *n.* DEOXYPYRIDOXINE.

des·oxy·ri·bo·nu·cle·ic acid (des·ock''see·rye''bo·new·klee'ick). DEOXYRIBONUCLEIC ACID.

des·oxy·ri·bose (des·ock''see·rye'boce) *n.* DEOXYRIBOSE.

des·oxy·sug·ar (des·ock''see·shoog'ur) *n.* DEOXYSUGAR.

despeciated bovine serum. A bovine serum altered in such a manner that its species specificity is reduced. Abbreviated, DBS.

de·spe·ci·a·tion (dee·spee''shee·ay'shun) *n.* Change in properties characteristic of the species, as alteration of antigenic properties by digestion with taka-diastase. **—de·spe·ci·at·ed** (dee·spee'shee·ay·tid) *adj.*

d'Es·pine's sign (des·peen') [J. H. A. *d'Espine,* French physician, 1844–1931]. A sign for tracheobronchial adenitis or mediastinal tumor in which whispered voice sounds are heard over the upper thoracic vertebrae.

des·qua·ma·tio in·sen·sib·i·lis (des·kwa·may'shee·o in·sen·sib'i·lis). Peeling of the skin in various-sized flakes and scales, seen in some diseases.

des·qua·ma·tion (des''kwuh·may'shun) *n.* [L. *desquamare,* to scale off, from *squama,* scale]. Shedding; a peeling and casting off of superficial epithelium, such as that of mucous membranes, renal tubules, or skin. **—des·qua·ma·tive** (de·skwam'uh·tiv, des'kwuh·may''tiv) *adj.;* **des·qua·mate** (des'kwuh·mate) *v.*

desquamatio neo·na·to·rum (nee·o·nay·to'rum). Peeling of the superficial epithelium of newborn infants during the first week of life.

desquamative gingivitis. CHRONIC DESQUAMATIVE GINGIVITIS.

des·sert·spoon (de·zurt'spoon) *n.* A spoon of medium size, equal to approximately 2 fluidrachms or 8 ml.

destructive aggression. Aggressiveness which may be physical, verbal, or symbolic, and which is not essential for self-protection or preservation.

destructive distillation. Decomposition of complex organic substances by heat and distillation of the products.

destructive lesion. 1. Any disturbance leading to tissue or organ death. 2. An abnormality of the nervous system caused by destruction of tissue and accompanied by an appropriate tissue reaction, in distinction to a developmental disorder of the nervous system, in which the signs of tissue reaction are absent. Contr. *discharging lesion.*

destructive mole. CHORIOADENOMA.

de·stru·do (de·stroo'do) *n.* [NL., from L. *destruere,* to destroy]. *In psychiatry,* the basic energy associated with the death instinct; the counterpart of libido.

de·sul·fi·nase (dee·sul'fi·nace, ·naze) *n.* An enzyme catalyzing desulfination.

de·sul·fi·na·tion (dee·sul''fi·nay'shun) *n.* The removal of sulfur dioxide from an organic compound such as β-sulfinylpyruvic acid, and its conversion by hydrolysis and ionization to sulfite.

de·sul·fu·rase (dee·sul'few·race) *n.* An enzyme that catalyzes removal of sulfur, commonly as hydrogen sulfide, from organic compounds.

det. Abbreviation for *detur,* let it be given.

de·tach·ment of the retina. Separation of the neural portion of the retina from its pigment layer.

detachment phosphene. A subjective sensation of light or seeing stars due to the movements of a detached retina.

de·ter·e·nol (de·terr'e·nole) *n.* (±)-*p*-Hydroxy-α-[(isopropylamino)methylbenzyl] alcohol, $C_{11}H_{17}NO_2$, an ophthalmic adrenergic, usually used as the hydrochloride salt.

de·ter·gent (de·tur'junt) *adj. & n.* [L. *detergere,* to rub or wipe off]. 1. Cleansing. 2. A cleansing agent or a preparation containing a cleansing agent, which may be useful for medical purposes and may also possess antibacterial activity. 3. A substance that enhances the cleansing action of water or other solvents. See also *anionic detergent, cationic detergent.*

de·te·ri·o·rate (de·teer'ee·uh·rate) *v.* [L. *deteriorare,* from *deterior,* worse]. To become impaired in functioning, quality, or condition from a previously better state; to grow worse; to degenerate. See also *emotional deterioration.* **—de·te·ri·o·ra·tion** (de·teer''ee·uh·ray'shun) *n.*

de·ter·mi·nant (de·tur'mi·nunt) *n.* [L. *determinans,* limiting, determining]. 1. A fact, circumstance, influence, or factor that determines the nature of an entity or an event. 2. *In biology,* a hypothetical unit of the germ plasm which, according to Weismann's theory of heredity, determines the final fate of the cell or the part which receives it during development.

de·ter·mi·nate cleavage (de·tur'mi·nut). Cleavage producing blastomeres, each of which is destined to form some particular part or structure.

determinate reflex. A reflex in which the response occurs at the site of stimulation.

de·ter·mi·na·tion (de·tur''mi·nay'shun) *n.* [L. *determinatio,* boundary, end]. 1. Tendency of the blood to collect in a part. 2. Fixation of the embryologic fate of a tissue or a part of an embryo by an evocator or other agent. 3. The performance of any measurement, as of length, mass, or the quantitative composition of a substance.

de·ter·mi·nism (de·tur'mi·niz·um) *n.* The doctrine that no event, whether in the outer world or within a person, results from chance, but that each is the fixed result of antecedent conditions or forces, known or unknown, physical or emotional.

de To·ni-Fanconi-Debré syndrome (de^y^·toh^h^'nee) [G. *de Toni,* Italian pediatrician, 20th century; G. *Fanconi;* and R. *Debré*]. FANCONI SYNDROME.

de Toni-Fanconi syndrome [G. *de Toni* and G. *Fanconi*]. FANCONI SYNDROME.

de·tor·sion (dee·tor'shun) *n.* The correction of a torsion, as the twisting of a spermatic cord or ureter.

de·tox·i·ca·tion (dee·tock"si·kay'shun) *n.* The process, usually consisting of a series of reactions, by which a toxic substance in the body is changed to a compound or compounds more easily excretable; the latter are not necessarily nontoxic. Syn. *detoxification.* —**de·tox·i·cant** (dee·tock'si·kunt) *n. & adj.;* **detoxi·cate** (·kate) *v.*

de·tox·i·fy (dee·tock'si·figh) *v.* To subject to detoxication. —**de·tox·i·fi·ca·tion** (dee·tock"si·fi·kay'shun) *n.*

Detre's reaction [L. *Detre,* Hungarian pathologist, 1875–1939]. A skin test to differentiate between infection with human and bovine tuberculosis.

de·tri·tion (de·trish'un) *n.* [ML. *detritio,* from L. *deterere,* to wear away]. Wearing away by abrasion.

de·tri·tus (de·trye'tus) *n.*, pl. **detritus** [L., worn away]. 1. Waste matter from disintegration. 2. Waste material adherent to a tooth, or disintegrated tooth substance.

de·trun·cate (dee·trung'kate) *v.* [L. *detruncare,* to cut off, behead]. To decapitate, especially a fetus. —**de·trun·ca·tion** (dee"trung·kay'shun) *n.*

de·tru·sion (de·troo'zhun) *n.* [L. *detrusio,* from *detrudere,* to thrust down]. An ejection or expulsion; thrusting down or out. —**de·trude** (de·trood') *v.*

de·tru·sor (de·troo'zur) *n.* Any muscle that detrudes or thrusts down or out.

detrusor dyssynergia or **irritability.** A condition marked by an unstable urinary bladder which exhibits uninhibited contractions often producing urinary incontinence.

detrusor uri·nae (yoo·rye'nee). 1. The external layer of the muscular coat of the urinary bladder, consisting for the most part of longitudinal fibers. 2. The bulbospongiosus in the male.

detrusor ve·si·cae (ve·sigh'kee, ·see). The smooth muscle in the wall of the urinary bladder which contracts the bladder and expels the urine; applied to all the muscle layers, since all are involved in the contraction.

de·tu·mes·cence (dee"tew·mes'unce) *n.* [L. *detumescere,* to cease swelling]. 1. Subsidence of any swelling. 2. Subsidence of the erectile sexual organs following orgasm.

deut-, deuto- [Gk. *deuteros*]. A combining form meaning (a) *second, secondary;* (b) *second in a regular series of chemical compounds.*

deuter-, deutero- [Gk. *deuteros*]. A combining form meaning (a) *second;* (b) *secondary.*

deu·ter·anom·a·ly (dew"tur·uh·nom'uh·lee) *n.* [*deuter-* + *anomaly*]. A form of partial color blindness in which, of the three basic colors (red, blue, and green), the green spectrum is seen only in part. Compare *deuteranopia.*

deu·ter·an·ope (dew'tur·uh·nope) *n.* An individual with deuteranopia.

deu·ter·an·o·pia (dew"tur·uh·no'pee·uh) *n.* [*deuter-* + *anopia*]. A form of color blindness in which only two of the three basic colors, blue and red, are perceived; green is seen inadequately and shades of red, green, and yellow are confused. Syn. *green blindness.* Compare *deuteranomaly.* —**deuteran·op·ic** (·nop'ick, ·no'pick) *adj.*

deu·ter·anop·sia (dew"tur·uh·nop'see·uh) *n.* [*deuter-* + *anopsia*]. DEUTERANOPIA.

deu·ter·a·tion (dew"tur·ay'shun) *n.* The process of introducing into a chemical compound one or more atoms of deuterium in place of a like number of atoms of ordinary hydrogen (protium) commonly existing in the compound.

deu·te·ri·um (dew·teer'ee·um) *n.* [NL., from Gk. *deuteros,* second]. The isotope of hydrogen of atomic weight approximately 2.0. It constitutes approximately 1 part in 6000 of ordinary hydrogen. Symbol, ^2H, D. Syn. *heavy hydrogen.* See also *heavy water.*

deuterium oxide. Water of composition D_2O, or ^2H_2O; HEAVY WATER.

deutero-. See *deuter-.*

deu·tero·gen·ic (dew"tur·o·jen'ick) *adj.* [*deutero-* + *-genic*]. Of secondary origin.

deu·ter·on (dew'tur·on) *n.* [*deuter*ium + *-on*]. The nucleus of a deuterium atom.

deu·ter·op·a·thy (dew"tur·op'uth·ee) *n.* [*deutero-* + *-pathy*]. A disease occurring secondary to another disease. —**deu·tero·path·ic** (dew"tur·o·path'ick) *adj.*

deu·tero·plasm (dew'tur·o·plaz·um) *n.* [*deutero-* + *-plasm*]. 1. The passive or lifeless components of cytoplasm, especially reserve foodstuffs such as yolk. 2. The store of nutrient material in the ovum. Syn. *deutoplasm.*

deu·tero·plas·mol·y·sis (dew"tur·o·plaz·mol'i·sis) *n.* [*deuteroplasm* + *-lysis*]. In cleavage, the elimination of the yolk from the blastomeres of mammals, especially marsupials.

deu·tero·pro·te·ose (dew"tur·o·pro'tee·oce) *n.* [*deutero-* + *proteose*]. A secondary proteose; a soluble product of proteolysis.

deu·ter·os·to·ma (dew"tur·os'to·muh) *n.*, pl. **deuterostomas, deuter·os·to·ma·ta** (·os·to'muh·tuh) [*deutero-* + *-stoma*]. A second mouth not formed from the blastopore; found in certain worms.

deuto-. See *deut-.*

deu·tom·er·ite (dew·tom'ur·ite) *n.* [*deuto-* + Gk. *meros,* part, + *-ite*]. The second (posterior) cell of a cephaline gregarine.

deu·ton (dew'ton) *n.* DEUTERON.

deu·to·plasm (dew'to·plaz·um) *n.* DEUTEROPLASM.

deu·to·sco·lex (dew"to·sko'lecks) *n.* [*deuto-* + *scolex*]. *In biology,* a secondary or daughter cyst or bladder worm derived from a scolex or primary bladder worm.

Deutsch·län·der's disease (doich'len·dur) [C. E. W. *Deutschländer,* German surgeon, 1872–1942]. MARCH FRACTURE.

de·vas·a·tion (dee"vas·ay'shun) *n.* [L. *de-* + *vas,* vessel]. DEVASCULARIZATION.

de·vas·cu·lar·iza·tion (de·vas"kew·lăr·i·zay'shun) *n.* [*de-* + *vascularization*]. Removal of the blood supply to a given area by vascular destruction or obstruction.

de·vel·op·ment, *n.* [F. *développer,* to unfold, develop, from OF. *des-,* un-, + *voloper,* to wrap]. 1. Change or growth with increase in complexity. 2. *In biology,* the series of events occurring in an organism during the change from the fertilized egg to the adult stage. —**de·vel·op·men·tal,** *adj.*

developmental age. Any index of development stated in age equivalent as determined by specified standardized measurements and observations; especially motor and mental tests, but also body measurements (height, weight), bone age (as measured by serial roentgenograms of the knee or wrist), or social or emotional development. Abbreviated, DA. See also *developmental quotient.*

developmental agraphia. Marked deficiency in learning to write, not based on any obvious skeletal or neuromuscular defect, and out of line with the individual's mental age, accomplishment quotient in other subjects, and general manual dexterity. See also *minimal brain dysfunction syndrome.*

developmental alexia. Marked deficiency in learning to read, not based on obvious visual disturbance and out of line with the individual's mental age and accomplishment quotients in other subjects; may be familial and is seen more frequently in males. See also *minimal brain dysfunction syndrome.*

developmental aneurysm. CONGENITAL ANEURYSM.

developmental aphasia. A deficiency in learning to speak which is not commensurate with the individual's (child's) mental age or development and accomplishment quotients along other lines. See also *minimal brain dysfunction syndrome.*

developmental crisis. *In psychiatry,* any brief, presumably transient period of stress in a child's life related to his attempts to complete successfully such psychosocial tasks as the establishment of trust, autonomy, initiative, and identity; internal forces predominate, as compared to a situational crisis.

developmental dyslexia. Greater than normal difficulties on the part of a school-age child in learning to read, or in reading ability and comprehension; may be hereditary or congenital. See also *minimal brain dysfunction syndrome, strephosymbolia.*

developmental Gerstmann's syndrome [J. *Gerstmann*]. A symptom complex chiefly characterized by difficulties in learning to read, write, do arithmetic, and in left-right disorientation; seen in children with minimal brain dysfunction syndrome. Compare *Gerstmann's syndrome.*

developmental groove. A fine line in the enamel of a tooth which marks the union of two lobes. See also *sulcus.*

developmental horizons. A series of 25 stages proposed by Streeter to express accurately the increasing degrees of morphologic and physiologic complexity of the human embryo from the one-cell stage to the end of 7 weeks of development.

developmental lobe. One of the portions of a tooth germ which initiate formation of dentin and enamel.

developmental milestone. The achievement by an infant or young child of one of a series of sequentially acquired skills in the areas of motor and manipulative ability, general understanding and social behavior, language, and self-feeding, dressing, and toilet training, normally within a given time period. See also *psychomotor development.*

developmental quotient. The score, obtained on the Gesell Developmental Schedules, derived by dividing the child's mental age (measured by the test) by his chronological age and multiplying by 100. Abbreviated DQ, D.Q.

de·vi·a·tion (dee″vee·ay′shun) *n.* [L. *deviare,* to turn from the straight path, from *de-* + *via,* way, road]. 1. Variation from a given or accepted norm or standard. See also *sexual deviation.* 2. Turning from a regular course, standard, or position; deflection. 3. *In ophthalmology,* the inability of the two eyes to focus upon an object at the same time; squint; strabismus. When the unaffected eye is fixed upon the object, the squinting eye is unable to fix and consequently deviates; this is known as primary deviation. When the squinting eye is the one fixed, there is a corresponding deviation of the unaffected eye, known as secondary deviation. —**de·vi·ate** (dee′vee·ate) *v.;* **de·vi·ate** (dee′vee·ut) *adj. & n.*

De·vic's disease or **syndrome** (duh·veek′) [E. *Devic,* French physician, d. 1930]. NEUROMYELITIS OPTICA.

devil's club. FATSIA.

devil's grip. EPIDEMIC PLEURODYNIA.

devil's pinches. Mild skin bruises of obscure origin, usually occurring in women; PURPURA SIMPLEX.

de·vi·om·e·ter (dee″vee·om′e·tur) *n.* [*deviation* + *-meter*]. A variety of strabometer.

de·vi·tal·ize (dee·vye′tul·ize) *v.* To destroy vitality. —**de·vi·tal·iza·tion** (dee·vye″tul·i·zay′shun) *n.*

dev·o·lu·tion (dev″o·lew′shun) *n.* [ML. *devolutio,* from L. *devolvere,* to roll down]. 1. The reverse of evolution; INVOLUTION. 2. CATABOLISM. 3. DEGENERATION.

dew·claw (dew′klaw) *n.* The vestigial first digit located on the medial surface of the feet of some animals, especially dogs and cattle.

dew·lap (dew′lap) *n.* A pendulous fold of skin extending downward from the neck of some animals.

dew point. The temperature at which the atmospheric moisture is deposited as dew.

Dexacaine. A trademark for dexivacaine, an anesthetic.

Dexacillin. A trademark for epicillin, an antibiotic.

Dexameth. A trademark for dexamethasone, an anti-inflammatory adrenocortical steroid.

dex·a·meth·a·sone (deck″suh·meth′uh·sone) *n.* 9α-Fluoro-16α-methylprednisolone, $C_{22}H_{29}FO_5$, a potent anti-inflammatory adrenocortical steroid.

dex·am·i·sole (deck·sam′i·sole) *n.* (*R*)-2,3,5,6-Tetrahydro-6-phenylimidazo[2,1-*b*]thiazole, $C_{11}H_{12}N_2S$, an antidepressant.

dex·am·phet·a·mine (decks″am·fet′uh·min, ·meen) *n.* DEXTROAMPHETAMINE.

Dexawin. A trademark for racephenicol, an antibacterial.

dex·brom·phen·ir·a·mine (decks·brome″fen·irr′uh·meen) *n.* The dextro (+) isomer of brompheniramine having greater antihistaminic activity than the racemic substance, usually used as the maleate salt.

dex·chlor·phen·ir·a·mine (decks·klor″fen·irr′uh·meen) *n.* The dextro (+) isomer of chlorpheniramine having greater antihistaminic activity than the racemic substance, usually used as the maleate salt.

dex·cla·mol (decks′kluh·mole) *n.* (+)-2,3,4,4a*β*,8,9,13b*α*,14-Octahydro-3*α*-isopropyl-1*H*-benzo[6,7]cyclohepta[1,2,3-*de*]pyrido[2,1-*a*]isoquinolin-3-ol, $C_{24}H_{29}NO$, a sedative normally used as the hydrochloride.

Dexedrine. A trademark for dextroamphetamine, the dextrorotatory isomer of amphetamine, a central stimulant drug commonly used as the sulfate salt.

dex·et·i·mide (deck·set′i·mide) *n.* (*S*)-3-Phenyl-1′-(phenylmethyl)-[3,4′-bipiperidine]-2,6-dione, an anticholinergic, also used as the hydrochloride.

dex·im·a·fen (deck·sim′uh·fen, deck·si·may′fen) *n.* (+)-2,3,5,-6-tetrahydro-5-phenyl-1*H*-imidazo[1,2-*a*]imidazole, an antidepressant, also used as the hydrochloride.

dex·io·car·dia (deck″see·o·kahr′dee·uh) *n.* [Gk. *dexios,* right, + *-cardia*]. DEXTROCARDIA.

dex·iv·a·caine (deck·siv′uh·kane) *n.* (+)-1-Methyl-2′,6′-pipecoloxylidide, $C_{15}H_{22}N_2O$, a local anesthetic agent.

Dexon. A trademark for polyglycolic acid, a surgical suture material.

Dexoval. A trademark for methamphetamine, a central stimulant drug used as the hydrochloride salt.

dex·ox·a·drol (deck·sock′suh·drol) *n.* *d*-2-(2,2-Diphenyl-1,3-dioxolan-4-yl)piperidine, $C_{20}H_{23}NO_2$, a central stimulant drug; used as the hydrochloride salt.

dex·pan·the·nol (decks·pan′the·nol) *n.* The D- form of panthenol; possesses pantothenic acid activity said to increase peristalsis and intestinal tone.

dex·pro·pran·o·lol (decks·pro·pran′o·lol) *n.* (*R*)-1-(Isopropylamino)-3-(1-naphthyloxy)-2-propanol, $C_{16}H_{21}NO_2$, an antiarrhythmic cardiac depressant, usually used as the hydrochloride salt.

dex·ter (decks′tur) *n.* [L.]. Right; upon the right side. Abbreviated, d.

dextr-, dextro- [L. *dexter*]. A combining form meaning (a) *toward, of, or pertaining to the right;* (b) *dextrorotatory.*

dex·trad (decks′trad) *adv.* [*dextr-* + *-ad*]. Toward the right side.

dex·tral (decks′trul) *adj.* [*dextr-* + *-al*]. Pertaining to the right side; right-handed.

dex·tral·i·ty (decks·tral′i·tee) *n.* 1. The condition, common to most persons, in which, when there is a choice, the right side of the body is more efficient and hence used more than the left. 2. Specifically, RIGHT-HANDEDNESS.

dex·tral·iza·tion (decks″trul·i·zay′shun) *n.* Development of the control of sensorimotor skill from a dominant area on the left side of the cerebral cortex in right-handed individuals. Contr. *sinistration* (2).

dex·tran (decks′tran) *n.* [*dextr-* + *-an*]. A water-soluble, high molecular weight polymer of glucose produced by the action of *Leuconostoc mesenteroides* on sucrose. Purified forms are usually used to expand plasma volume and maintain blood pressure in emergency treatment of shock. Polymers of lower molecular weight may be useful in preventing intravascular thrombosis and in improving blood circulation in certain conditions. Often written with a number indicating average molecular weight in thousands, as dextran 40, dextran 70, dextran 75.

dex·trates (decks′trates) *n.* A mixture of approximately 92 percent dextrose and other sugars from the enzymatic hydrolysis of starch, used as a tablet binder and diluent.

dex·trau·ral (decks·traw'rul) *adj.* [*dextr-* + *aural*]. 1. Right-eared; characterizing an individual who prefers to listen with the right ear, as with a telephone receiver, or who depends more on the right ear in binaural hearing. 2. Pertaining to the right ear.

dex·tri·ferr·on (decks·tri·ferr'on) *n.* A colloidal solution of ferric hydroxide in complex with partially hydrolyzed dextrin; a hematinic agent used intravenously in the treatment of iron-deficiency anemia.

dex·trin (decks'trin) *n.* [*dextr-* + *-in*]. A white or yellow amorphous powder, $(C_6H_{10}O_5)_n \cdot xH_2O$, produced by incomplete hydrolysis of starch; used as an emulsifying, protective, and thickening agent.

dex·tri·no·sis (deck"stri·no'sis) *n.* [*dextrin* + *-osis*]. Accumulation within the body of abnormal polysaccharides.

dex·trin·uria (decks"tri·new'ree·uh) *n.* The presence of dextrin in the urine.

dextro-. See *dextr-*.

dex·tro·am·phet·a·mine (decks"tro·am·fet'uh·min, ·meen) *n.* The dextrorotatory form of amphetamine, much more active as a central stimulant than the levorotatory form and hence also more active than the racemic mixture; used as the phosphate and sulfate salts.

dex·tro·car·dia (decks"tro·kahr'dee·uh) *n.* [*dextro-* + *-cardia*]. The presence of the heart in the right hemithorax, with the cardiac apex directed to the right. —**dextrocar·di·al** (·dee·ul) *adj.*

dex·tro·car·dio·gram (decks"tro·kahr'dee·o·gram") *n.* [*dextro-* + *cardiogram*]. 1. The component of the normal electrocardiogram or bicardiogram contributed by right ventricular forces. 2. The electrocardiographic complex derived from a unipolar lead facing the right ventricle.

dextro compound. *In chemistry,* a compound which has the property of causing polarized light to rotate to the right; a dextrorotatory compound.

dex·tro·con·dyl·ism (decks"tro·kon'dil·iz·um) *n.* [*dextro-* + *condyl-* + *-ism*]. Deviation of the mandibular condyles toward the right.

dex·troc·u·lar (deck·strock'yoo·lur) *adj.* [*dextr-* + *ocular*]. RIGHT-EYED. —**dex·troc·u·lar·i·ty** (deck·strock"yoo·lăr'i·tee) *n.*

dex·tro·cy·clo·ver·sion (decks"tro·sigh"klo·vur'zhun) *n.* [*dextro-* + *cyclo-* + *version*]. Clockwise torsional movement of both eyes to the right.

dex·tro·duc·tion (deck"stro·duck'shun) *n.* [*dextro-* + L. *ducere,* to lead]. Movement of the visual axis toward the right.

dex·tro·gram (decks'tro·gram) *n.* DEXTROCARDIOGRAM.

dex·tro·gy·rate (decks"tro·jye'rate) *adj.* [*dextro-* + *gyrate*]. DEXTROROTATORY.

dex·tro·man·u·al (decks"tro·man'yoo·ul) *adj.* [*dextro-* + *manus* + *-al*]. RIGHT-HANDED. —**dextro·man·u·al·i·ty** (·man"yoo·al'i·tee) *n.*

dex·tro·meth·or·phan (decks"tro·meth·or'fan) *n.* *d*-3-Methoxy-*N*-methylmorphinan, $C_{18}H_{25}NO$, a nonaddicting antitussive; used as the hydrobromide salt.

dex·tro·mor·am·ide (decks"tro·mor·am'ide) *n.* 4-[2-Methyl-4-oxo-3,3-diphenyl-4-(1-pyrrolidinyl)butyl]morpholine, $C_{25}H_{32}N_2O_2$, an analgesic drug; used as the tartrate salt.

dex·tro·pe·dal (decks"tro·pee'dul, ·trop'e·dul) *adj.* [*dextro-* + *ped-* + *-al*]. RIGHT-FOOTED.

dex·tro·pho·bia (decks"tro·fo'bee·uh) *n.* [*dextro-* + *-phobia*]. Morbid fear of objects on the right side of the body.

dex·tro·po·si·tion (decks"tro·puh·zish'un) *n.* [*dextro-* + *position*]. Displacement to the right.

dextroposition of the heart. Displacement of the heart toward the right or into the right half of the thorax.

dex·tro·ro·ta·to·ry (decks"tro·ro'tuh·tor"ee) *adj.* [*dextro-* + *rotatory*]. Rotating the rays of plane polarized light to the right. See also *d-*.

dex·trose (decks'troce, ·troze) *n.* [*dextr-* + *-ose*]. A dextrorotatory monosaccharide, $C_6H_{12}O_6 \cdot H_2O$, occurring as a white, crystalline powder; odorless and sweet, soluble in about one part of water, it is often prepared by the hydrolysis of starch. An important intermediate in carbohydrate metabolism. Used for nutritional purposes, for temporary increase of blood volume, as a diuretic, and for other purposes. Syn. *grape sugar, starch sugar, bread sugar, d-glucose.* See also *glucose.*

dextrose-nitrogen ratio. D:N RATIO.

dex·tro·sin·is·tral (decks"tro·sin'is·trul) *adj.* [*dextro-* + *sinistral*]. Extending from right to left.

dex·tros·uria (decks"tro·sue'ree·uh) *n.* The presence of dextrose in the urine.

dex·tro·tar·tar·ic acid (deck"stro·tahr·tăr'ick). The ordinary, dextrorotatory, form of tartaric acid. See *tartaric acid.*

dex·tro·thy·rox·ine sodium (decks"tro·thigh·rock'seen, ·sin). Sodium D-3,3',5,5'-tetraiodothyronine, the sodium salt of D-thyroxine, $C_{15}H_{10}I_4NNaO_4$; an anticholesteremic agent.

dex·tro·tor·sion (decks"tro·tor'shun) *n.* [*dextro-* + *torsion*]. A twisting to the right.

dex·trous (decks'trus) *adj.* [*dextr-* + *-ous*]. Skilled; expert. Contr. *sinistrous.*

dex·tro·ver·sion (deck"tro·vur'zhun) *n.* [*dextro-* + *version*]. The act of turning to, or looking toward, the right.

D-form. DWARF COLONY.

DFP Abbreviation for *diisopropyl fluorophosphate.*

dg Abbreviation for *decigram.*

DHE-45. Trademark for dihydroergotamine mesylate.

D hemoglobin. A rare type of hemoglobin, resembling sickle cell hemoglobin (S) in its electrophoretic mobility, but being more soluble.

dho·bie itch (do'bee) [Hindi *dhobī,* laundryman]. TINEA CRURIS.

dhobie mark itch. Dermatitis caused by a laundry-marking ink made from the anacardium or cashew nut.

di-, dis- [Gk. *dis,* twice, doubly]. A prefix meaning *two, twice, double.* Compare *dis-, di-,* and *dia-, di-.*

dia-, di- [Gk. *dia,* through, across]. A prefix meaning (a) *through, by way of, across, between;* (b) *apart, asunder.* Compare *dis-, di-.*

Diabeta. A trademark for glyburide, an antidiabetic.

di·a·be·tes (dye"uh·bee'teez, ·bee'tis) *n.* [Gk. *diabētēs,* siphon]. 1. A disease characterized by the habitual discharge of an excessive quantity of urine and by excessive thirst. 2. Specifically, DIABETES MELLITUS.

diabetes de·cip·i·ens (de·sip'ee·enz) [L., deceiving]. Diabetic glycosuria, without other evidence of diabetes.

diabetes in·si·pi·dus (in·sip'i·dus). A disorder resulting from a deficiency of antidiuretic hormone, characterized by the excretion of large volumes of dilute but otherwise normal urine, associated with compensatory polydipsia; relieved by replacement therapy with vasopressin.

diabetes mel·li·tus (mel·eye'tus) [L., honeyed, from *mel,* honey]. A chronic disorder of carbohydrate metabolism due to a disturbance of the normal insulin mechanism, characterized by hyperglycemia, glycosuria, and alterations of protein and fat metabolism, producing polyuria, polydipsia, weight loss, ketosis, acidosis, and coma; a hereditary predisposition is present in most if not all cases.

di·a·bet·ic (dye"uh·bet'ick) *adj. & n.* 1. Pertaining or relating to diabetes. 2. A person suffering from diabetes.

diabetic acidosis. The metabolic acidosis of uncontrolled diabetes mellitus, due to an excess of ketone bodies; characterized by weakness, headache, thirst, air hunger, and coma.

diabetic amyotrophy. A painful, asymmetric, predominantly motor and proximal neuropathy that tends to occur in older patients with mild or unrecognized diabetes.

diabetic cataract. A form of cataract associated with diabetes.

diabetic diet. A diet used in the treatment of diabetes mellitus, containing calculated amounts of carbohydrate, protein, and fat, with restriction of free sugar.

diabetic dwarf. An individual with growth retardation due to diabetes mellitus.

diabetic gangrene. Moist or dry gangrene occurring in the course of diabetes mellitus, often as a consequence of slight injuries.

diabetic glomerulosclerosis. Renal glomerular abnormalities seen in some cases of diabetes mellitus. The nodular lesion consists of eosinophilic material within lobules of the tuft; the diffuse form of the lesion consists of eosinophilic material within the glomerular mesangium; the fibrin cap or exudative lesion consists of eosinophilic material within a capillary at the periphery of a lobule; and the capsular-drop lesion consists of eosinophilic material within Bowman's capsule.

diabetic glycosuria. Glycosuria resulting from diabetes mellitus.

diabetic milk. Milk that contains only a small amount of lactose.

diabetic mononeuropathy. Acute affection of a single cranial or spinal nerve, particularly the oculomotor, femoral or sciatic, in association with diabetes mellitus and presumably caused by ischemic infarction of the nerve.

diabetic neuropathy or **polyneuropathy**. 1. A distal, symmetric, primary sensory polyneuropathy affecting feet and legs more than hands, in a chronic, slowly progressive manner, and occurring usually in patients with long-established diabetes mellitus. 2. Any affection of peripheral spinal or cranial nerves in association with diabetes mellitus.

diabetic ophthalmoplegia. An acute cranial mononeuropathy, usually of the oculomotor nerve and sometimes of the abducens nerve, in association with diabetes mellitus.

diabetic polyneuritis or **neuritis**. A slowly progressive polyneuritis associated with diabetes.

diabetic pseudotabes. A symptom complex characterized by absent deep tendon reflexes in the lower extremities, lightning pains, delayed appreciation of pain and position sensations, Argyll Robertson pupils, and Charcot's joints, seen in diabetic patients in whom there is no history or serologic evidence of syphilis.

diabetic puncture. Puncture of the floor of the fourth ventricle, which produces glycosuria.

diabetic retinitis. DIABETIC RETINOPATHY.

diabetic retinopathy. Retinal manifestations of diabetes mellitus characterized by capillary microaneurysms, small punctate hemorrhages, yellowish exudates, and neovascularization; saccular dilatations of the retinal veins may also occur and massive hemorrhages into the vitreous may result in blindness.

diabetic tabes. DIABETIC PSEUDOTABES.

di·a·be·to·gen·ic (dye″uh·bee″to·jen′ick, ·bet″o·) *adj.* [*diabetes* + *-genic*]. Causing diabetes.

diabetogenic factor. Originally, the factor in crude anterior pituitary extract which was diabetogenic in dogs. Growth hormone is now known to be the major diabetogenic agent in crude pituitary extract.

diabetogenic hormone. DIABETOGENIC FACTOR; GROWTH HORMONE.

di·a·be·tog·e·nous (dye″uh·be·toj′e·nus) *adj.* [*diabetes* + *-genous*]. Produced by diabetes.

di·a·be·to·pho·bia (dye″uh·bee″to·fo′bee·uh, ·bet″o·) *n.* [*diabetes* + *-phobia*]. Morbid fear of becoming a diabetic.

Diabinese. Trademark for chlorpropamide, an orally effective hypoglycemic agent.

di·ab·o·lep·sy (dye·ab′o·lep″see) *n.* [Gk. *diabolos*, devil, + *-lepsy*]. Diabolical seizure or possession; delusion of supernatural possession. —**di·a·bo·lep·tic** (dye″uh·bo·lep′tick) *adj. & n.*

dia·caus·tic (dye″uh·kaws′tick) *n.* [*dia-* + *caustic*]. *In optics*, a curve formed by the refraction of rays of light.

di·ac·e·te·mia, di·ac·e·tae·mia (dye″as″e·tee′mee·uh) *n.* [*diacetic* + *-emia*]. The presence of diacetic acid (acetoacetic acid) in the blood.

di·ace·tic acid (dye″uh·see′tick, ·set′ick). ACETOACETIC ACID.

di·ac·e·tin (dye·as′i·tin, dye″uh·see′tin) *n.* [*di-* + *acetin*]. Glyceryl diacetate, $C_7H_{12}O_5$, a water-soluble ester of glycerin; sometimes used as a solvent for certain fat-soluble stains.

diacetone alcohol. 4-Hydroxy-4-methyl-2-pentanone, $C_6H_{12}O_2$, used as a reagent and solvent for fats in certain histochemical procedures.

di·ac·e·to·nu·ria (dye·as″e·to·new′ree·uh) *n.* DIACETURIA.

di·ac·e·tu·ria (dye·as″e·tew′ree·uh) *n.* [*diacetic* + *-uria*]. The presence of diacetic acid (acetoacetic acid) in the urine.

di·ac·e·tyl·mor·phine (dye·as″e·til·mor′feen, ·fin) *n.* HEROIN.

Di·ack control. A sterilization detector consisting of a tablet of chemical materials contained in a hermetically sealed glass tube; when placed with a load in a steam sterilizer, the detector indicates adequate conditions for sterilization by melting, fusing, and changing its shape or color.

di·a·cla·sia (dye″uh·klay′zhuh, ·zee·uh) *n.* DIACLASIS.

di·ac·la·sis (dye·ack′luh·sis, dye″uh·klay′sis) *n.*, pl. **diacla·ses** (·seez) [Gk. *diaklasis*, a breaking up]. A fracture produced intentionally. —**di·a·clas·tic** (dye″uh·klas′tick) *adj.*

di·a·clast (dye′uh·klast) *n.* [*dia-* + *-clast*]. An instrument for breaking the fetal head.

di·ac·o·la·tion (dye·ack″o·lay′shun) *n.* [*dia-* + *colation*]. A method of drug extraction involving percolation of a suitable solvent through long narrow columns packed with the drug.

di·ac·ri·sis (dye·ack′ri·sis) *n.* [Gk. *diakrisis*, from *diakrinein*, to distinguish]. DIAGNOSIS.

di·a·crit·ic (dye″uh·krit′ick) *adj.* [Gk. *diakritikos*, from *diakrinein*, to distinguish]. DIAGNOSTIC; distinctive.

dia·crit·i·cal (dye″uh·krit′i·kul) *adj.* Diacritic (= DIAGNOSTIC).

di·ac·tin·ic (dye″ack·tin′ick) *adj.* [*di-*, through, across, + *actinic*]. Capable of transmitting actinic rays.

diad. DYAD.

dia·derm (dye′uh·durm) *n.* [*dia-* + *-derm*]. A two-layered blastoderm composed of ectoderm and entoderm.

diadic. DYADIC.

di·ad·o·cho·ki·ne·sia, di·ad·o·ko·ki·ne·sia (dye·ad″uh·ko·ki·nee′zhuh, ·zee·uh) *n.* [Gk. *diadochos*, succeeding, successive, + *-kinēsis*, motion, + *-ia*]. The normal power of performing alternating movements in rapid succession, such as flipping a hand back and forth.

di·ad·o·cho·ki·ne·sis, di·ad·o·ko·ki·ne·sis (dye·ad″uh·ko·ki·nee′sis) *n.* DIADOCHOKINESIA.

Diafen. Trademark for diphenylpyraline hydrochloride, an antihistaminic.

Diagnex Blue. Trademark for azuresin, a tubeless gastric secretion diagnostic aid, now seldom used.

di·ag·nos·able (dye″ug·no′zuh·bul, ·no′suh·bul) *adj.* Capable of being diagnosed.

di·ag·no·sis (dye″ug·no′sis) *n.*, pl. **diagno·ses** (·seez) [Gk. *diagnōsis*, from *diagignōskein*, to discern]. 1. The art or the act of determining the nature of a patient's disease. 2. A conclusion reached in the identification of a patient's disease. —**diag·nose** (noce′) *v.*

diagnosis by exclusion. The recognition of a disease by excluding all other known conditions.

di·ag·nos·tic (dye″ug·nos′tick) *adj.* [Gk. *diagnōstikos*, able to distinguish]. Pertaining to or serving as evidence in diagnosis; indicating the nature of a disease.

di·ag·nos·ti·cian (dye″ug·nos·tish′un) *n.* One skilled in making diagnoses.

di·ag·o·nal (dye·ag′uh·nul) *adj.* [Gk. *diagōnios*, from angle to angle]. Pertaining to any plane or straight line that is not vertical, perpendicular, or horizontal.

diagonal band of Broca [P. P. *Broca*]. A band of nerve fibers passing from the anterior perforated substance to the region of the amygdaloid nucleus.

diagonal conjugate diameter. The diameter of the pelvis connecting the sacrovertebral angle and the subpubic ligament.

diagonal gyrus. DIAGONAL BAND OF BROCA.

diagonal sulcus. A short, oblique furrow traversing the opercular portion of the inferior frontal gyrus.

dia·ki·ne·sis (dye″uh·kigh·nee′sis) *n.*, pl. **diakine·ses** (·seez) [*dia-* + *kinesis*]. The final stage of the first meiotic prophase, during which the tetrads show terminalization of chiasmata preparatory to separation and formation of dyads.

Dia·kio·gian·nis sign (thyah·kyoh·yah′nis) [*Diakiogiannis*, Greek physician, 20th century]. A sign for pyramidal tract lesions at the spinal cord level, in which light scratching of the skin along the outer border of the tibia and down the dorsum of the foot toward the big toe results in slow extension of the big toe; not seen in pyramidal tract lesions of cortical origin, but a transient positive response may occasionally be seen following status epilepticus.

Dial. A trademark for allobarbital, a sedative and hypnotic of intermediate duration of action.

Di·a·lis·ter (dye″uh·lis′tur) *n.* [*dia-* + Gk. hy*listēr*, filter]. A genus of the family Bacteroidaceae, by some not differentiated from the genus *Bacteroides*, consisting of minute, filtrable, anaerobic nonsporulating gram-negative rods, originally isolated from filtrates of respiratory tract washings in influenza.

Dialister pneu·mo·sin·tes (new″mo·sin′teez). A minute, anaerobic gram-negative rod, which passes through Berkefeld filters V and N and has been recovered from nasopharyngeal washings of man.

di·al·kyl·a·mine (dye·al″kil·uh·meen′) *n.* Secondary alkylamine. See *alkylamine*.

di·al·lyl·bar·bi·tu·ric acid (dye·al″il·bahr″bi·tew′rick). ALLOBARBITAL.

di·al·y·sance (dye·al′i·sunce) *n.* A measure of the rate of exchange between blood and bath fluid used in connection with peritoneal dialysis or hemodialysis; it is the functional equivalent of physiologic renal clearance measurements, being expressed as the net exchange of a substance between blood and bath fluid, per minute.

di·al·y·sate (dye·al′i·sate) *n.* The portion of the liquid which passes through the membrane in dialysis, and contains the substances of greater diffusibility in solution.

di·al·y·sis (dye·al′i·sis) *n.*, pl. **dialy·ses** (·seez) [Gk. a separating]. Separation of substances from one another in solution by taking advantage of their differing diffusibility through porous membranes. See also *hemodialysis*. —**di·a·lyt·ic** (dye·uh·lit′ick) *adj.*

di·al·y·zate (dye·al′i·zate) *n.* DIALYSATE.

di·a·lyze (dye′uh·lize) *v.* To subject to or undergo dialysis. —**di·a·lyz·able** (dye″uh·lye′zuh·bul) *adj.*

di·a·lyz·er (dye′uh·lye·zur) *n.* 1. An apparatus for effecting dialysis. 2. The porous septum or diaphragm of such an apparatus.

dia·mag·net·ic (dye″uh·mag·net′ick) *adj.* [*dia-* + *magnetic*]. Of, pertaining to, or referring to a weakly magnetic substance, having a magnetic permeability less than unity, which is repelled by a magnet. —**dia·mag·net·ism** (dye″uh·mag′ne·tiz·um) *n.*

dia·mer·sul·fon·a·mides (dye″uh·mur·sul·fon′uh·mide′z) *n.* A mixture of equal weights of sulfadiazine and sulfamerazine.

di·am·e·ter (dye·am′e·tur) *n.* [Gk. *diametros*, from *diametrein*, to measure through]. A straight line joining opposite points on the periphery of a body or figure and passing through its center. —**di·a·met·ric** (dye″uh·met′rick), **dia·metric·al** (·ul) *adj.*

diameter obli·qua pel·vis (o·blye′kwuh pel′vis) [NA]. Any oblique diameter of the pelvis, specifically the oblique diameter of the pelvic inlet.

diameter trans·ver·sa pel·vis (trans·vur′suh pel′vis) [NA]. Any transverse diameter of the pelvis, as the transverse diameter of the pelvic inlet or the transverse diameter of the pelvic outlet.

di·am·i·dine (dye·am′i·deen, ·din) *n.* Any compound consisting of two amidine groups, $NH{=}C(NH_2){-}$, linked together by a hydrocarbon chain. Certain ones, of related chemical structure, have been found to possess, in varying degrees, trypanocidal and antibacterial activity. See also *pentamidine*.

di·a·mine (dye′uh·meen, ·min, dye·am′in) *n.* [*di-* + *amine*]. An amine formed by replacing hydrogen in two molecules of ammonia by a hydrocarbon radical.

diamine oxidase. HISTAMINASE.

di·ami·no·di·phen·yl·sul·fone (dye″uh·meen″o·dye·fen″il·sul′fone, ·dye·fee″nil·sul′fone) *n.* DAPSONE.

di·ami·no·pu·rine (dye″uh·meen″o·pew′reen) *n.* 2,6-Diaminopurine or 2-aminoadenine, $C_5H_6N_6$, a compound selectively injurious to certain neoplastic cells in animals, and investigated as a possible chemotherapeutic agent in human neoplastic diseases.

di·a·min·uria (dye″uh·mi·new′ree·uh) *n.* The presence of diamine compounds in the urine.

di·am·mo·ni·um hydrogen phosphate (dye″uh·mo′nee·um). AMMONIUM PHOSPHATE, DIBASIC.

di·am·o·caine cyclamate (dye·am′o·kane) 1-(2-Anilinoethyl)-4-[2-(diethylamino)ethoxy]-4-phenylpiperidine, compound with cyclohexylsulfamic acid, $C_{37}H_{63}N_5O_7S_2$, a local anesthetic.

Dia·mond-Black·fan syndrome or **anemia.** CONGENITAL HYPOPLASTIC ANEMIA.

diamond green. MALACHITE GREEN.

Diamond's method. WALLACE-DIAMOND METHOD.

dia·mor·phine (dye″uh·mor′feen, ·fin) *n.* British term for HEROIN.

Diamox. Trademark for acetazolamide, a carbonic anhydrase inhibitor used as an oral diuretic, in the treatment of hypercapnia, in chronic lung disease, in epilepsy, and in glaucoma.

di·am·tha·zole (dye·am′thuh·zole) *n.* 6-(β-Diethylaminoethoxy)-2-dimethylaminobenzothiazole, $C_{15}H_{23}N_3OS$, a topically applied antifungal agent.

Dianabol. Trademark for methandrostenolone, an anabolic-androgenic steroid.

di·ap·a·mide (dye·ap′uh·mide) *n.* 4-Chloro-*N*-methyl-3-(methylsulfamoyl)benzamide, $C_9H_{11}ClN_2O_3S$, a diuretic and antihypertensive drug.

Diaparene. A trademark for methylbenzethonium chloride, a quaternary ammonium salt used for bacteriostasis of urea-splitting organisms involved in ammonia dermatitis.

di·a·pa·son (dye″uh·pay′zun, ·sun) *n.* [Gk. *diapasōn*, concord of the first and last notes, octave]. A tuning fork, used in the diagnosis of diseases of the ear, especially in determining the presence and extent of deafness.

di·a·pe·de·sis (dye″uh·pe·dee′sis) *n.*, pl. **diapede·ses** (·seez) [Gk. *diapēdēsis*, oozing through]. The passage of blood cells through the unruptured vessel walls into the tissues. —**diape·det·ic** (·det′ick) *adj.*

Diaperene. A trademark for methylbenzethonium chloride, a topical anti-infective.

diaper rash. Maculopapular eruptions which tend to become confluent and may go on to excoriation, seen in the diaper area of infants, due to irritation from moisture, feces, the ammonia formed from decomposed urea, and often monilial infection.

di·a·phane (dye′uh·fane) *n.* [Gk. *diaphanēs*, transparent]. 1. The transparent investing membrane of an organ or cell. 2. A small electric lamp used in transillumination.

di·aph·a·nom·e·ter (dye·af″uh·nom′e·tur) *n.* [*diaphanous* + *-meter*]. An instrument for measuring the transparency of gases, liquids, or solids.

di·aph·a·no·scope (dye·af′uh·nuh·skope) *n.* [*diaphanous* + *-scope*]. A device for lighting an interior body cavity so as to render it visible from the exterior. **—di·aph·a·nos·co·py** (dye·af″uh·nos′kuh·pee) *n.*

di·aph·e·met·ric (dye·af″e·met′rick) *adj.* [*dia-* + Gk. *haphē,* touch, + *-metric*]. Pertaining to measurements of tactile sensibility.

di·aph·o·rase (dye·af′o·race) *n.* Mitochondrial flavoprotein enzymes which catalyze the reduction of dyes, such as methylene blue, by reduced pyridine nucleotides such as NADH.

di·a·pho·re·sis (dye″uh·fo·ree′sis) *n.,* pl. **diaphore·ses** (·seez) [Gk. *diaphorēsis,* from *diaphorein,* to carry through]. Perspiration, especially perceptible perspiration that is artificially induced. Contr. *anaphoresis.*

di·a·pho·ret·ic (dye″uh·fo·ret′ick) *adj. & n.* [Gk. *diaphorētikos*]. 1. Causing an increase of perspiration. 2. A medicinal that induces diaphoresis.

di·a·phragm (dye′uh·fram) *n.* [Gk. *diaphragma*]. 1. *In anatomy,* a musculotendinous partition, especially that partition muscular at the circumference and tendinous at the center, which separates the thorax and abdomen and is the chief muscle of respiration and expulsion. NA *diaphragma.* See also Table of Muscles in the Appendix and Plates 13, 14. 2. A thin septum such as is used in dialysis. 3. *In optics,* an aperture so placed as to control the amount of light passing through an optical system. 4. A device worn during copulation over the ostium uteri for preventing conception or infection; it is usually dome-shaped and of thin rubber or plastic material. 5. *In radiography,* a metal barrier plate with a central aperture designed to limit the beam of radiation to its smallest practical diameter.

dia·phrag·ma (dye·uh·frag′muh) *n.,* pl. **diaphragma·ta** (·tuh) [Gk.] [NA]. DIAPHRAGM (1).

diaphragma pel·vis (pel′vis) [NA]. PELVIC DIAPHRAGM.

diaphragma sel·lae (sel′ee) [NA]. DIAPHRAGM OF THE SELLA.

di·a·phrag·mat·ic (dye″uh·frag·mat′ick) *adj.* Of or pertaining to a diaphragm, especially in the anatomic sense.

diaphragmatic flutter. DIAPHRAGMATIC TIC.

diaphragmatic hernia. A hernia that passes through the diaphragm into the thoracic cavity; may be congenital, acquired, or traumatic, and may contain the stomach, small intestine, and colon; usually a false hernia.

diaphragmatic ligament. The bandlike part of the urogenital fold formed by the degeneration of the cranial mesonephric tubules, extending from the diaphragm to the persisting part of the mesonephros and forming a portion of the suspensory ligament of the ovary.

diaphragmatic myocardial infarction. A myocardial infarction involving the diaphragmatic or inferior portion of the heart.

diaphragmatic pleura. The reflection of the parietal pleura upon the upper surface of the diaphragm. NA *pleura diaphragmatica.*

diaphragmatic plexus. A nerve plexus near the inferior phrenic artery.

diaphragmatic respiration. Respiration effected primarily by movement of the diaphragm, changing the intrathoracic pressure. Contr. *costal respiration.*

diaphragmatic sign. The movement of the diaphragm during respiratory excursions, causing an altered contour of the chest wall. If the patient is observed by means of oblique illumination, a shadow is seen moving up or down the side of the chest. Syn. *Litten's sign.*

diaphragmatic tic. Rapid rhythmic contractions of the diaphragm; may simulate cardiac pain or cardiac arrhythmia.

di·a·phrag·ma·ti·tis (dye″uh·frag″muh·tye′tis) *n.* DIAPHRAGMITIS.

di·a·phrag·mato·cele (dye″uh·frag·mat′o·seel) *n.* [*diaphragm* + *-cele*]. A hernia through the diaphragm.

diaphragma uro·gen·i·ta·le (yoo″ro·jen·i·tay′lee) [NA]. UROGENITAL DIAPHRAGM.

di·a·phrag·mi·tis (dye″uh·frag·migh′tis) *n.* [*diaphragm* + *-itis*]. Inflammation of the diaphragm.

diaphragm of the sella. The circular layer of dura mater which forms the roof of the hypophyseal fossa; its center is pierced by the stalk of the hypophysis. NA *diaphragma sellae.*

diaphragm opening. The opening in the optical system of a microscope through which the rays of light pass.

diaphragm pessary. An occlusive diaphragm for contraception.

diaphragm phenomenon. DIAPHRAGMATIC SIGN.

di·aph·y·se·al (dye·af″i·see′ul, dye″uh·fiz′ee·ul) *adj.* Pertaining to or involving a diaphysis.

diaphyseal aclasis. MULTIPLE HEREDITARY EXOSTOSES.

diaphyseal sclerosis. PROGRESSIVE DIAPHYSEAL DYSPLASIA.

di·aph·y·sec·to·my (dye·af″i·seck′tuh·mee, dye″uh·fi·) *n.* [*diaphysis* + *-ectomy*]. Excision of a portion of the shaft of a long bone.

di·a·phys·i·al (dye″uh·fiz′ee·ul) *adj.* DIAPHYSEAL.

di·aph·y·sis (dye·af′i·sis) *n.,* pl. **diaphy·ses** (·seez) [Gk., ridge on the shaft of the tibia] [NA]. The shaft of a long bone.

Diapid. A trademark for lypressin, a vasoconstrictor.

di·ap·la·sis (dye·ap′luh·sis) *n.,* pl. **diapla·ses** (·seez) [Gk., a putting into shape]. Reduction of a dislocation or of a fracture.

di·apoph·y·sis (dye″uh·pof′i·sis) *n.,* pl. **diapophy·ses** (·seez) [*di-,* across, + *apophysis*]. The articular facet on the transverse process of a thoracic vertebra for articulation with the tubercle of the corresponding rib. Syn. *tubercular process.* **—di·apo·phys·i·al** (dye″uh·po·fiz′ee·ul) *adj.*

diarhemia. SANGUINEOUS ASCITES.

di·ar·rhea, di·ar·rhoea (dye″uh·ree′uh) *n.* [Gk. *diarrhoia,* a flowing through]. A common symptom of gastrointestinal disease; characterized by increased frequency and water content of the stools. See also *dysentery.* **—diar·rhe·al** (·ree′ul), **diarrhe·ic** (·ick) *adj.*

diarrheaogenic. Misformation of DIARRHEOGENIC.

di·ar·rhe·mia, di·ar·rhae·mia (dye″uh·ree′mee·uh) *n.* [*diarrhea* + *-emia*]. SANGUINEOUS ASCITES.

di·ar·rhe·o·gen·ic, di·ar·rhoe·o·gen·ic (dye″uh·ree″o·jen′ick) *adj.* Producing diarrhea.

diarrhoea. DIARRHEA.

diarrhoeogenic. DIARRHEOGENIC.

di·ar·thric (dye·ahr′thrick) *adj.* [*di-* + *arthr-* + *-ic*]. Pertaining to two joints; DIARTICULAR.

di·ar·thro·di·al (dye″ahr·thro′dee·ul) *adj.* Pertaining to or exhibiting diarthrosis.

diarthrodial cartilage. ARTICULAR CARTILAGE.

diarthrodial joint. SYNOVIAL JOINT.

di·ar·thro·sis (dye″ahr·thro′sis) *n.,* pl. **diarthro·ses** (·seez) [Gk. *diarthrōsis,* articulation]. 1. Freely movable articulation. 2. A freely movable joint; SYNOVIAL JOINT. Adj. *diarthrodial.*

di·ar·tic·u·lar (dye″ahr·tick′yoo·lur) *adj.* [*di-* + *articular*]. DIARTHRIC; pertaining to two different joints.

di·as·chi·sis (dye·as′ki·sis) *n.,* pl. **diaschi·ses** (·seez) [Gk., division]. An inhibition or loss of function in a region of the nervous system, due to a localized injury in another region with which it is connected by fiber tracts, such as loss of reflexes following a brain lesion comparable to spinal shock.

dia·schis·tic (dye″uh·skis′tick, ·shis′tick) *adj.* [*dia-* + Gk. *schizein,* to cleave]. Splitting transversely, applied to bivalent or tetrad elements. Contr. *anaschistic.*

dia·scope (dye′uh·skope) *n.* [*dia-* + *-scope*]. A device consisting of a thin piece of glass, used to press against the skin so that superficial lesions may be observed. **—di·as·co·py** (dye·as′kuh·pee) *n.*

Diasone Sodium. Trademark for sulfoxone sodium, now used as a leprostatic drug.

di·a·stal·sis (dye″uh·stal′sis, ·stahl′sis) *n.* [*dia-* + Gk. *stalsis,* a checking]. The downward moving wave of contraction, occurring in the small intestine during digestion, in addition to peristalsis. —**diastal·tic** (·tick) *adj.*

di·a·stase (dye'uh·stace, ·staze) *n.* An enzyme preparation from malt that contains amylases and converts starch to dextrins and maltose by hydrolysis. Syn. *vegetable diastase.*

di·a·sta·sic (dye"uh·stay'zik) *adj.* DIASTATIC.

di·as·ta·sis (dye·as'tuh·sis) *n.*, pl. **diasta·ses** (·seez) [Gk., a separation]. 1. Any simple separation of parts normally joined together, as the separation of an epiphysis from the body of a bone without true fracture, or the dislocation of an amphiarthrosis. 2. The final phase of diastole, the phase of slow ventricular filling.

diastasis rec·ti ab·do·mi·nis (reck'tye ab·dom'i·nis). Separation in the median line of the two rectus abdominis muscles, usually from repeated childbirth.

di·a·stat·ic (dye"uh·stat'ick) *adj.* 1. Pertaining to diastasis. 2. Pertaining to a diastase.

diastatic enzyme. AMYLOLYTIC ENZYME.

diastatic fermentation. Fermentation resulting in the conversion of starch into glucose, as by the action of ptyalin.

di·a·ste·ma (dye"uh·stee'muh) *n.*, pl. **diastema·ta** (·tuh) [Gk. *diastēma,* interval, separation]. 1. A cleft or fissure, especially if congenital. 2. A space between teeth that are normally in approximal contact.

di·a·ste·ma·to·my·e·lia (dye"uh·stee"muh·to·migh·ee'lee·uh) *n.* [*dyastema* + *-myelia*]. A congenital, more or less complete doubling of the spinal cord associated with the formation of a bony or cartilaginous septum from the posterior wall of the vertebral canal, usually in spina bifida.

di·as·ter (dye"as'tur) *n.* [*di-* + *aster*]. AMPHIASTER.

dia·ster·eo·iso·mer (dye"uh·sterr"ee·o·eye'so·mur) *n.* [*dia-* + *stereoisomer*]. A stereoisomer with two or more asymmetric carbon atoms that have identical substituents but is not a mirror image of its reference stereoisomer. In contrast to enantiomers, diastereoisomers need not have the same or similar physical properties. —**diastereo·iso·mer·ic** (·eye"so·merr'ick) *adj.*; **diastereo·isom·er·ism** (·eye·som'ur·iz·um) *n.*

di·as·to·le (dye·as'tuh·lee) *n.* [Gk., dilatation]. 1. The rhythmic period of relaxation and dilatation of a chamber of the heart during which it fills with blood. 2. Specifically, diastole of a cardiac ventricle. —**di·a·stol·ic** (dye"us·tol'ick) *adj.*

diastolic blood pressure. Minimum arterial blood pressure during ventricular diastole.

diastolic murmur. A murmur occurring during ventricular diastole.

diastolic thrill. A vibratory sensation felt on precordial palpation during ventricular diastole.

di·a·stroph·ic dwarfism (dye"uh·strof'ick). A form of osteochondrodysplasia characterized by extremely short stature, abnormal spinal curvature, clubfoot, micromelia, hand deformities, multiple joint contractures or subluxations, deformed ears, and cleft palate; probably inherited as an autosomal recessive trait.

di·atax·ia (dye"uh·tack'see·uh) *n.* [*di-* + *ataxia*]. Ataxia involving both sides of the body.

di·a·ther·mal (dye"uh·thur'mul) *adj.* DIATHERMIC.

di·a·ther·ma·nous (dye"uh·thur'muh·nus) *adj.* [F. *dithermane,* from Gk. *diathermainein,* to warm through]. Allowing passage of heat rays.

di·a·ther·mia (dye"uh·thur'mee·uh) *n.* DIATHERMY.

di·a·ther·mic (dye"uh·thur'mick) *adj.* [*dia-* + *thermic*]. 1. Permitting passage of heat rays. 2. Of or pertaining to diathermy.

di·a·ther·mo·co·ag·u·la·tion (dye"uh·thur"mo·ko·ag"yoo·lay'shun) *n.* [*diathermic* + *coagulation*]. Coagulation secured by the use of a high-frequency electrosurgical knife.

dia·ther·mom·e·ter (dye"uh·thur·mom'e·tur) *n.* [*diathermic* + *-meter*]. *In physics,* an instrument for measuring the heat-conducting capacity of substances.

di·a·ther·my (dye'uh·thur"mee) *n.* [*dia-* + *-thermy*]. 1. The therapeutic use of an oscillating electric current of high frequency to produce local heat in the body tissues below the surface. 2. The electric current so used. 3. The machine producing the electric current. See also *conventional diathermy, medical diathermy, short-wave diathermy.* —**di·a·ther·mize** (dye"uh·thur'mize) *v.*

di·ath·e·sis (dye·ath'e·sis) *n.*, pl. **diathe·ses** (·seez) [Gk., arrangement]. A condition or tendency of the body or a combination of attributes in one individual causing a susceptibility to some abnormality or disease. —**di·a·thet·ic** (dye"uh·thet'ick) *adj.*

di·a·tom (dye'uh·tom, ·tome) *n.* [Gk. *diatomos,* cut in two]. Any of the Diatomaceae, a small family of microscopic, unicellular algae having a cell wall of silica, the skeleton persisting after death of the organism.

di·a·to·ma·ceous (dye"uh·to·may'shus) *adj.* Consisting of diatoms or their siliceous remnants.

diatomaceous earth. A sedimentary rock composed of the empty shells of diatoms and other Protophyta; used as an absorbent, a filtration aid, and an insulating material. Syn. *purified kieselguhr, purified siliceous earth.*

diatomaceous-earth pneumoconiosis. A distinctive type of pneumoconiosis characterized mainly by dyspnea; occurring in workers engaged in the mining and processing of diatomaceous earth; disabling and nondisabling forms have been described.

di·atom·ic (dye"uh·tom'ick) *adj.* 1. Consisting of two atoms; commonly referring to a molecule. 2. Containing two replaceable univalent atoms or radicals.

dia·tri·zo·ate (dye"uh·trye·zo'ate, ·tri·zo'ate) *n.* A salt of diatrizoic acid.

diatrizoate sodium I 125 or **I 131.** The sodium salt of diatrizoic acid labelled with radioactive iodine in the 2, 4 and 6 positions, used as a radiodiagnostic agent.

dia·tri·zo·ic acid (dye"uh·tri·zo'ick, ·trye·zo'ick). 3,5-Diacetamido-2,4,6-triiodobenzoic acid, $C_{11}H_9I_3N_2O_4$, a roentgenographic contrast medium; used as the methylglucamine (meglumine) and sodium salts.

dia·ver·i·dine (dye"uh·verr'i·deen) *n.* 2,4-Diamino-5-veratrylpyrimidine, $C_{13}H_{16}N_4O_2$, an antibacterial agent.

diaz-, diazo- [*di-* + *az-*]. A combining form signifying the *presence* (in an organic compound) *of two nitrogen atoms* as the —N=N— or $(RN{\equiv}N)^+$ group, where R is an organic radical. Compare *disazo-.*

di·az·e·pam (dye·az'e·pam) *n.* 7-Chloro-1,3-dihydro-1-methyl-5-phenyl-2*H*-1,4-benzodiazepin-2-one, $C_{16}H_{13}ClN_2O$, a tranquilizer.

di·a·zine (dye'uh·zeen) *n.* [*diaz-* + *-ine*]. 1. A heterocyclic compound having the formula $C_4H_4N_2$, containing two nitrogen and four carbon atoms in the ring. Three isomers are possible, distinguished as 1,2-diazine (pyridazine), 1,3-diazine (pyrimidine), and 1,4-diazine (pyrazine). 2. Any derivative of any such compound.

di·azo (dye·az'o, dye·ay'zo) *adj.* Of or pertaining to an organic compound containing two nitrogen atoms in the form of the —N=N— group.

diazo-. See *diaz-.*

di·a·zo·ni·um (dye"uh·zo'nee·um) *adj.* Pertaining to or characterizing a compound containing two nitrogen atoms in the form of the $(RN{\equiv}N)^+$ group, where R is an organic radical, the compound being analogous to ammonium compounds in having saltlike properties.

diazo reaction. Any color test using Ehrlich's diazo reagent.

di·azo·res·or·cin·ol (dye·az"o·re·zor'si·nol, ·nole) *n.* RESAZURIN.

di·az·o·tiz·able (dye·az"o·tye'zuh·bul) *adj.* Capable of being diazotized.

di·az·o·ti·za·tion (dye·az"o·ti·zay'shun) *n.* The process of converting certain compounds, notably primary aromatic amines, to their respective diazonium derivatives, commonly by reaction with nitrous acid.

di·az·o·tize (dye·az'o·tize) *v.* To treat a primary aromatic amine with nitrous acid under conditions that produce a diazonium compound.

di·az·ox·ide (dye″az·ock′side) *n.* 7-Chloro-3-methyl-2*H*-1,2,4-benzothiadiazine 1,1-dioxide, $C_8H_7ClN_2O_2S$, an antihypertensive drug devoid of diuretic effect.

di·ba·sic (dye·bay′sick) *adj.* [*di-* + *basic*]. 1. Of a salt, containing two atoms of a monobasic element or radical. 2. Of an acid, having two replaceable hydrogen atoms.

dibasic calcium phosphate. Calcium hydrogen phosphate, $CaHPO_4$.

dibasic potassium phosphate. Dipotassium hydrogen phosphate, K_2HPO_4, sometimes used as a source of potassium ion, and as a purgative.

dibasic sodium phosphate. SODIUM PHOSPHATE.

Dibenamine. Trademark for *N*-(2-chloroethyl)dibenzylamine, employed experimentally as a sympatholytic and adrenolytic agent, in the form of the hydrochloride salt.

di·benz·an·thra·cene (dye″benz·an′thruh·seen) *n.* Dibenz-[*a,h*]anthracene, $C_{22}H_{14}$, a polycyclic hydrocarbon; a carcinogen, said to be the first pure chemical found experimentally to produce cancer in an animal.

di·ben·ze·pin (dye·ben′ze·pin) *n.* 10-[2-(Dimethylamino)ethyl]-5,10-dihydro-5-methyl-11*H*-dibenzo[*b,e*][1,4]diazepin-11-one, $C_{18}H_{21}N_3O$, an antidepressant drug; used as the hydrochloride salt.

Dibenzyline. Trademark for phenoxybenzamine hydrochloride, an adrenergic blocking agent useful in the treatment of peripheral vascular diseases and in certain types of hypertension.

di·both·rio·ceph·a·li·a·sis (dye·both″ree·o·sef″uh·lye′uh·sis) *n.* [*Dibothriocephal*us + *-iasis*]. DIPHYLLOBOTHRIASIS.

Di·both·rio·ceph·a·lus (dye·both″ree·o·sef′uh·lus) *n.* [*di-* + *bothrio-* + *-cephalus*]. *DIPHYLLOBOTHRIUM.*

di·bro·mo·dul·ci·tol (dye·bro″mo·dul′si·tol) *n.* 1,6-Dibromo-1,6-dideoxygalactitol, a halogenated sugar alcohol that acts biologically as an alkylating agent; used in the treatment of cancer.

di·brom·sa·lan (dye·brome′suh·lan) *n.* 4′,5-Dibromosalicylanilide, $C_{13}H_9Br_2NO_2$, a disinfectant.

di·bu·caine (dye·bew′kain) *n.* 2-*n*-Butoxy-*N*-(2-diethylaminoethyl) cinchoninamide, $C_{20}H_{29}N_3O_2$, a local anesthetic; used both as the base and the hydrochloride salt. Syn. *cinchocaine.*

Dibuline Sulfate. Trademark for dibutoline sulfate, a parasympatholytic drug.

di·bu·to·line sulfate (dye·bew′to·leen). Bis[(dibutylcarbamate) of ethyl (2-hydroxyethyl)dimethylammonium] sulfate, $C_{30}H_{66}N_4O_8S$, a parasympatholytic drug useful in the treatment of peptic ulcer and spastic disorders of the biliary and genitourinary tracts.

di·bu·tyl phthal·ate (di·bew′til thal′ate) *n.* *o*-$C_6H_4(COOC_4H_9)_2$ a miticide effective against *Trombicula akamushi,* the insect vector of tsutsugamushi disease.

DIC Abbreviation for *disseminated* (or *diffuse*) *intravascular coagulation.*

di·cal·ci·um (dye·kal′see·um) *adj.* Containing two atoms of calcium in each molecule.

di·car·box·yl·ic acid (dye·kahr″bock·sil′ick). An organic compound with two —COOH groups.

di·cen·tric (dye·sen′trick) *adj.* [*di-* + *centr-* + *-ic*]. Pertaining to a chromosome with two centromeres.

di·ce·pha·lia (dye″se·fay′lee·uh) *n.* DICEPHALISM.

di·ceph·a·lism (dye·sef′uh·liz·um) *n.* [*di-* + *cephal-* + *-ism*]. The condition of having two heads.

di·ceph·a·lous (dye·sef′uh·lus) *adj.* [Gk. *dikephalos*]. Having two heads.

di·ceph·a·lus (dye·sef′uh·lus) *n.*, pl. **dicepha·li** (·lye) [NL., from Gk. *dikephalos,* two-headed]. An individual with two heads.

dicephalus di·auch·e·nos (dye·awk′e·nos) [*di-* + Gk. *auchēn,* neck]. An individual with two heads and two more or less separate necks.

dicephalus mon·auch·e·nos (mon·awk′e·nos) [*mon-* + Gk. *auchēn,* neck]. An individual with two heads on a single neck.

dicephalus monosomus. An individual with two heads and only one body.

dicephalus par·a·sit·i·cus (păr″uh·sit′i·kus). An individual having a more or less incomplete parasitic head attached to the normal head or neck.

dicephalus tet·ra·bra·chi·us (tet″ruh·bray′kee·us) [*tetra-* + *brachi-* + *-us*]. Conjoined twins single below the umbilicus, with two more or less separate thoraces, four arms, two heads, and two necks.

dicephalus tri·bra·chi·us (trye·bray′kee·us) [*tri-* + *brachi-* + *-us*]. Conjoined twins single below the umbilicus; thoraces more or less double, with three arms, two necks, and two heads.

di·ceph·a·ly (dye·sef′uh·lee) *n.* DICEPHALISM.

di·chei·lus, di·chi·lus (dye·kigh′lus) *n.* [*di-* + *cheil-* + *-us*]. Double lip; due to a fold of mucous membrane giving the appearance of duplicity.

di·chei·rus, di·chi·rus (dye·kigh′rus) *n.* [*di-* + *cheir-* + *-us*]. Partial or complete duplication of the hand.

dichilus. DICHEILUS.

di·chlor·a·mine (dye·klor′uh·meen) *n.* DICHLORAMINE-T.

dichloramine-T. *p*-Toluenesulfondichloramide, $CH_3C_6H_4SO_2NCl_2$, a pale-yellow, crystalline powder with the odor of chlorine, almost insoluble in water. It gradually decomposes on exposure to air, releasing chlorine. Has been used as a surgical antiseptic in oil solution. See also *chloramine-T.*

Dichlorman. A trademark for dichlorvos, an anthelmintic.

Dichlor-mapharsen. A trademark for dichlorophenarsine hydrochloride.

di·chlo·ro·ace·tic acid (dye·klor″o·uh·see′tick). $CHCl_2COOH$. A colorless liquid at ordinary temperatures, crystallizing at lower temperatures; soluble in water. Has been used as an escharotic.

di·chlo·ro·ben·zene (dye·klor″o·ben′zeen) *n.* *p*-$C_6H_4Cl_2$, commonly used to preserve fabrics from moths; toxic to moths and their larvae.

di·chlo·ro·di·eth·yl·sul·fide (dye·klor″o·dye·eth″il·sul′fide, ·fid) *n.* MUSTARD GAS.

di·chlo·ro·di·flu·o·ro·meth·ane (dye·klor″o·dye·floo″uh·ro·meth′ane) *n.* CCl_2F_2. A nonflammable gas of low toxicity, used as a refrigerant and as a propellant. See also *propellant 12.*

di·chlo·ro·di·phen·yl·tri·chlo·ro·eth·ane (dye·klor″o·dye·fen″il·trye″klor·o·eth′ane, ·dye·fee″nil·) *n.* DDT.

di·chlo·ro·iso·pro·ter·e·nol (dye·klor″o·eye″so·pro·terr′e·nol) *n.* 3,4-Dichloro-α-(isopropylaminomethyl)benzyl alcohol, $C_{11}H_{15}Cl_2NO$, a beta-adrenergic blocking agent employed experimentally for the treatment of certain cardiovascular diseases. Abbreviated, DCI.

di·chlo·ro·phen·ar·sine hydrochloride (dye·klor″o·fen′ahr·seen, ·sin, ·fen·ahr′sin) 3-Amino-4-hydroxyphenyldichloroarsine hydrochloride, $C_6H_6AsCl_2NO.HCl$, formerly used as an antisyphilitic.

di·chlo·ro·phe·nol·in·do·phe·nol sodium (dye·klo″ro·fee″nol·in″do·fee′nol). Sodium 2,6-dichlorophenolindophenol, $C_{12}H_6Cl_2NNaO_2$, formerly used in the determination of ascorbic acid and commonly used in oxidation-reduction studies where it is employed as an electron acceptor.

di·chlo·ro·phen·oxy·ace·tic acid (dye·klo″ro·fen·ock″see·a·see′tick). 2,4-Dichlorophenoxyacetic acid, $C_8H_6Cl_2O_3$, a substance regulating plant growth and an effective herbicide. Abbreviated, 2,4-D.

di·chlor·phen·a·mide (dye″klor·fen′uh·mide) *n.* 4,5-Dichloro-*m*-benzenedisulfonamide, $C_6H_6Cl_2N_2O_4S_2$, a carbonic anhydrase inhibitor used for the treatment of glaucoma.

di·chlor·vos (dye·klor′voss) *n.* 2,2-Dichlorovinyl dimethyl phosphate, $C_4H_7Cl_2O_4P$, an anthelmintic.

di·cho·ri·al (dye·kor′ee·ul) *adj.* DICHORIONIC.

di·cho·ri·on·ic (dye″ko·ree·on′ick) *adj.* [*di-* + *chorionic*]. Having two chorions.

dichorionic twins. Twins having separate chorions.

di·chot·o·mize (dye·kot′uh·mize) *v.* To make a dichotomy; to divide a distribution, variable, or series into two parts according to a specified classification, as persons with or without a known disease or characteristic.

di·chot·o·my (dye·kot′uh·mee) *n.* [Gk. *dichotomia,* from *dicha,* in two, + *temnein,* to cut]. 1. Division into two equal branches; BIFURCATION. 2. Division of a group into two classes on the basis of the presence or absence of a certain characteristic or characteristics. 3. The type of branching of plants in which there are repeated equal divisions of the stem.

di·chro·ic (dye·kro′ick) *adj.* [Gk. *dichroos,* two-colored]. Having or showing two colors; applied to doubly refracting crystals that show different colors when viewed from different directions, or to solutions that show different colors in varying degrees of concentration.

di·chro·ine (dye·kro′een) *n.* Any of three isomeric alkaloids, designated α-dichroine, β-dichroine, and γ-dichroine, isolated from the herb *Dichroa febrifuga,* which is the probable source of the Chinese antimalarial drug ch'ang shan. α-Dichroine is probably identical with isofebrifugine, while β-dichroine and γ-dichroine appear to be crystalline modifications of febrifugine.

di·chro·ism (dye′kro·iz·um) *n.* The state or condition of being dichroic.

di·chro·ma·sia (dye″kro·may′zhuh, ·zee·uh) *n.* DICHROMATOPSIA.

di·chro·ma·sy (dye·kro′muh·see) *n.* DICHROMATOPSIA.

di·chro·mat (dye′kro·mat) *n.* A person affected with dichromatopsia.

[1]di·chro·mate (dye′kro·mate) *n.* DICHROMAT.

[2]di·chro·mate (dye·kro′mate) *n.* Any salt characterized by the presence of the $Cr_2O_7^{=}$ anion. Syn. *bichromate.*

di·chro·mat·ic (dye″kro·mat′ick) *adj.* [*di-* + *chromatic*]. 1. *In biology,* exhibiting two colors, regardless of sex or age. 2. *In psychology,* pertaining to that form of color blindness in which only two of the four fundamental colors can be seen, usually yellow and blue. 3. *In hematology,* pertaining to an immature nonnucleated erythrocyte.

dichromatic theory of color vision. According to K. E. K. Hering, when two of the four basic-color sensations are missing, most frequently the red-green, wavelength is discriminated along the visible spectrum in terms of two-color processes.

di·chro·ma·tism (dye·kro′muh·tiz·um) *n.* DICHROMATOPSIA.

di·chro·ma·top·sia (dye·kro″muh·top′see·uh) *n.* [*di-* + *chromat-* + *-opsia*]. A condition in which an individual can perceive only two of the three basic hues (red, green, and blue). See also *deuteranopia, protanopia, tritanopia.*

di·chro·mic (dye·kro′mick) *adj.* 1. Marked by two colors. 2. Containing two atoms of chromium.

di·chro·mism (dye′kro·miz·um, dye·kro′miz·um) *n.* DICHROISM.

di·chro·mo·phil (dye·kro′mo·fil) *adj.* [*di-* + *chromophil*]. Characterizing a tissue or cell which takes both an acidic and a basic stain.

di·chro·moph·i·lism (dye″kro·mof′i·liz·um) *n.* [*dichromophil* + *-ism*]. The capacity for double staining.

Dick test [G. F. *Dick* U.S. physician, 1881-1967; and Gladys R. H. *Dick,* U.S. physician 1881-1947]. A test for susceptibility or immunity to scarlet fever in which an intracutaneous inoculation of streptococcal erythrogenic toxin results in a red flush in susceptible individuals lacking the circulating antitoxin, and in no local reaction in individuals immune to scarlet fever.

Dick toxin [G. F. *Dick* and Gladys R. H. *Dick*]. ERYTHROGENIC TOXIN.

di·cli·dot·o·my (dye″kli·dot′uh·mee) *n.* [Gk. *diklis, diklidos,* double door, + *-tomy*]. VALVOTOMY.

di·clo·fen·ac (dye·klo′fe·nack) *n.* [*o*-(2,6-Dichloroanilino)-phenyl]acetic acid, an anti-inflammatory usually used as the sodium salt.

di·clor·al·urea (dye·klor″al·yoo·ree′uh) *n.* *N,N′*-bis(2,2,2-trichloro-1-hydroxyethyl)urea, $C_5H_6Cl_6N_2O_3$, a veterinary food additive.

di·clox·a·cil·lin (dye·klock″suh·sil′in) *n.* 3-(2,6-Dichlorophenyl)-5-methyl-4-isoxazolyl penicillin, $C_{19}H_{17}Cl_2N_3O_5S$, a semisynthetic penicillin antibiotic; used as the sodium salt.

Dicodid. Trademark for hydrocodone (dihydrocodeinone), an antitussive drug used as the bitartrate salt.

di·co·phane (dye′ko·fane) *n.* A medicinal grade of DDT. See also *chlorophenothane.*

di·co·ria (dye·ko′ree·uh) *n.* [di- + *cor-* + *-ia*]. Polycoria in which there are two pupils. Syn. *double pupil.*

di·cot·y·le·do·nous (dye″kot·i·lee′duh·nus) *adj.* [*di-* + *cotyledon* + *-ous*]. Pertaining to the plant subclass Dicotyledoneae; having two cotyledons. Contr. *monocotyledonous.*

di·cou·ma·rin (dye·koo′muh·rin) *n.* DICUMAROL.

di·cou·ma·rol (dye·koo′muh·rol) *n.* DICUMAROL.

Di·cro·coe·li·um (dye″kro·see′lee·um, dick″ro·) *n.* [Gk. *dikroos,* forked, + *koilia,* belly]. A genus of trematodes.

Dicrocoelium den·drit·i·cum (den·drit′i·kum). A species of fluke which has as its definitive host sheep and other herbivorous animals; some cases of human infection have been reported.

di·crot·ic (dye·krot′ick) *adj.* [Gk. *dikrotos,* double-beating, from *krotos,* beat]. Pertaining to a secondary pressure wave on the descending limb of a main wave.

dicrotic notch. A notch on the descending limb of the normal arterial pulse tracing, corresponding to aortic valve closure.

dicrotic pulse. A double-beating arterial pulse, with the second beat occurring during ventricular diastole, due to accentuation of the dicrotic wave; occurs commonly with low diastolic blood pressure.

dicrotic wave. The positive wave following the dicrotic notch of the normal arterial pulse tracing, due to reflected waves from the periphery.

di·cro·tism (dye′kro·tiz·um) *n.* A condition of having a dicrotic pulse.

di·cro·tous (dye′kruh·tus) *adj.* DICROTIC.

dicty-, dictyo- [Gk. *diktyon,* net]. A combining form meaning *network, net-like, reticular.*

dic·tyo·ki·ne·sis (dick″tee·o·ki·nee′sis) *n.* [*dictyo-* + *kinesis*]. Division of the Golgi apparatus in karyokinesis.

dictyoma. DIKTYOMA.

dic·tyo·some (dick′tee·o·sohm) *n.* [*dictyo-* + *-some*]. GOLGI APPARATUS.

dic·tyo·tene (dick′tee·o·teen) *n.* [*dictyo-* + *-tene*]. A resting stage in the first meiotic prophase of the germ cells of female animals, between diplotene and diakinesis; in humans, primary oocytes stay in this stage from fetal life until ovulation.

di·cu·ma·rol (dye·koo′muh·rol, ·kew′) *n.* 3,3′-Methylene-bis(4-hydroxycoumarin), $C_{19}H_{12}O_6$, originally isolated from spoiled sweet clover, eating of which caused hemorrhagic disease in cattle; occurs as a white crystalline powder, practically insoluble in water; used as an anticoagulant. Syn. *bishydroxycoumarin, dicoumarin, dicoumarol, melitoxin.*

Dicurin Procaine. Trademark for merethoxylline procaine, a mercurial diuretic.

di·cy·clo·mine (dye·sigh′klo·meen) *n.* 2-Diethylaminoethyl bicyclohexyl-1-carboxylate, $C_{19}H_{35}NO_2$, an anticholinergic drug with atropine-like effects on the gastrointestinal tract; used as the hydrochloride salt.

Dicynene. Trademark for ethamsylate, a hemostatic agent.

di·cys·te·ine (dye·sis′tee·een, ·in, ·sis·tee′in) *n.* CYSTINE.

di·dac·tic (dye·dack′tick, di·dack′tick) *adj.* [Gk. *didaktos,* from *didaskein,* to teach]. *In medicine,* pertaining to teaching by lectures and textbooks, as opposed to instruction by the clinical method.

di·dac·tyl·ism (dye·dack'til·izm) *n.* [*di-* + *dactyl-* + *-ism*]. BIDACTYLY.

di·del·phia (dye·del'fee·uh) *n.* [*di-* + Gk. *delphys*, womb, + *-ia*]. The condition of having a double uterus. —**didel·phic** (·fick) *adj.*

Di·dot's operation (dee·do') [A. *Didot*, Belgian surgeon, 19th century]. A standard operation for webbed fingers, in which a dorsal flap is moved from one finger and a palmar flap from the other.

Didrex. Trademark for benzphetamine, an anorexigenic drug used as the hydrochloride salt.

didym-, didymo- [Gk, *didymos*]. A combining form meaning (a) *twin;* (b) *testis.*

did·y·mi·tis (did''i·migh'tis) *n.* [*didym-* + *-itis*]. ORCHITIS.

did·y·mous (did'i·mus) *adj.* [*didym-* + *-ous*]. Growing in pairs; arranged in a pair, or in pairs.

-didymus [Gk. *didymos*, twin]. A combining form meaning (a) *a double monstrosity;* (b) *testis.*

[1]die, *v.* To cease to live; to expire. See also *death.*

[2]die, *n.* An exact reproduction in metal, or other substance of suitable hardness, of a tooth, part, object, or cast; used in dentistry for forming an individual tooth restoration or dental appliance. See also *counterdie.*

Die·go blood group. An erythrocyte antigen recognized by its reaction with an antibody, initially detected in a Venezuelan case of erythroblastosis fetalis.

di·el·drin (dye·el'drin) *n.* Generally, an insecticide containing not less than 85% of 1,2,3,4,10,10-hexachloro-6,7-epoxy-1,4,4a,5,6,7,8,8a-octahydro-1,4,5,8-dimethanonaphthalene, a crystalline solid, soluble in many organic solvents but insoluble in water.

di·elec·tric (dye''e·leck'trick) *n.* & *adj.* [*di-*, through, + *electric*]. 1. A nonconductor of direct-current electricity. 2. A medium in which a moderate electric field once established may be maintained with minimum loss of energy. 3. Pertaining to or having the characteristics of a dielectric.

dielectric constant. A measure of the capacity of a material to store electrical potential energy in an electric field; it is the ratio of the capacitance of a condenser filled with the material to the capacitance of the condenser when a vacuum exists between its plates. Syn. *relative permittivity.*

di·em·bry·o·ny (dye·em'bree·o·nee) *n.* [*di-* + *embryon* + *-y*]. The formation or production of two embryos from a single ovum; TWINNING.

di·en·ce·phal·ic (dye''en·se·fal'ick) *adj.* Of, pertaining to, or involving the diencephalon.

diencephalic autonomic epilepsy. An episodic illness characterized by flushing, shivering, hiccups, hyperventilation, tachycardia, hypertension, sweating, and pupillary dilatation presumably due to a discharging seizure focus in the diencephalon.

diencephalic syndrome. 1. A syndrome of early childhood, characterized by progressive emaciation in spite of high caloric intake, a euphoric appearance, and occasionally vertical nystagmus, tremor, and ataxia, due to a tumor in the diencephalon. 2. CONVULSIVE EQUIVALENT.

di·en·ceph·a·lon (dye''en·sef'uh·lon) *n.* [*di-*, through, between, + *encephalon*] [NA]. The part of the brain between the telencephalon and the mesencephalon, including the thalami and most of the third ventricle. Syn. *betweenbrain, interbrain.*

di·en·es·trol, di·en·oes·trol (dye''en·es'trol) *n.* 4,4'- (Diethylidineethylene)diphenol, $C_{18}H_{18}O_2$, a white, crystalline powder, practically insoluble in water; a nonsteroid estrogen.

Di·ent·amoe·ba (dye·en''tuh·mee'buh) *n.* [*di-* + *Entamoeba*]. A genus of parasitic protozoa having two nuclei.

Dientamoeba frag·i·lis (fraj'i·lis). A minute species of intestinal ameba found in the colon of man, lacking a cystic stage, and rarely associated with mild pathogenicity.

di·es·ter·ase (dye·es'tur·ace, ·aze) *n.* An enzyme, such as a nuclease, which splits the linkages binding individual nucleotides of a nucleic acid.

di·es·trum, di·oes·trum (dye·es'trum) *n.* DIESTRUS.

di·es·trus, di·oes·trus (dye·es'trus) *n.* [*di-* + *estrus*]. The period of quiescence or sexual rest of a polyestrous animal; the longest stage of the estrous cycle in which there is a gradual reconstitution of the uterine mucosa or endometrium in preparation for the reception of a fertilized ovum. Compare *anestrus.* —**dies·trous, dioes·trous** (·trus) *adj.*

di·et, *n.* & *v.* [Gk. *diaita*, manner of living, regimen]. 1. Food and drink regularly consumed. 2. Food prescribed, regulated, or restricted as to kind and amount, for therapeutic or other purposes. 3. To take food according to a regimen. 4. To cause to take food according to a regimen.

di·e·tary (dye'e·terr·ee) *adj.* & *n.* 1. Of or pertaining to diet. 2. A rule of diet. 3. A treatise describing such a rule or rules. 4. A fixed allowance of food.

dietary cirrhosis. LAENNEC'S CIRRHOSIS.

di·e·tet·ic (dye''e·tet'ick) *adj.* [Gk. *diaitētikos*]. Pertaining to diet or to dietetics.

dietetic albuminuria. Proteinuria attributed to the ingestion of certain forms of food.

di·e·tet·ics (dye''e·tet'icks) *n.* The science of the systematic regulation of the diet for hygienic or therapeutic purposes.

di·eth·a·nol·amine (dye·eth''uh·nol'uh·meen) *n.* [*di-* + *ethanolamine*]. DIOLAMINE.

di·eth·a·zine (dye·eth'uh·zeen) *n.* 10-(-2-Diethylaminoethyl)-phenothiazine, a drug possessing atropine-like actions and used in the treatment of parkinsonism.

Diet·helm's method (Ger. deet'helm). A method for determining the presence of bromide in the blood, using gold chloride solution to produce a color which is measured colorimetrically.

di·eth·yl·a·mine (dye·eth''il·uh·meen', ·am'in) *n.* $(C_2H_5)_2NH$, a strongly alkaline liquid having many uses in the pharmaceutical and other industries.

di·eth·yl·bar·bi·tu·rate (dye·eth''il·bahr·bitch'oo·rate, ·bahr·bi·tewr'ate) *n.* A salt of diethylbarbituric acid.

di·eth·yl·bar·bi·tu·ric acid (dye·eth''il·bahr''bi·tew'rick). BARBITAL.

di·eth·yl·car·bam·a·zine (dye·eth''il·kahr·bam'uh·zeen) *n.* *N,N*-Diethyl-4-methyl-1-piperazinecarboxamide, $C_{10}H_{21}N_3O$, an antifilarial drug; used as the citrate (dihydrogen citrate) salt.

di·eth·yl·ene·di·a·mine (dye·eth''il·een·dye'uh·meen, ·dye·am'in) *n.* PIPERAZINE.

di·eth·yl·ene glycol (dye·eth'il·een). β,β'-Dihydroxy-diethyl ether, $HOCH_2CH_2OCH_2CH_2OH$, used in histology as a solvent for dyes and as a component of storage fixatives to prevent drying of tissues.

diethylene glycol monoethyl ether. $C_6H_{14}O_3$, used principally as a solvent.

diethylene oxide. DIOXANE.

di·eth·yl ether (dye·eth'il). ETHER (3).

di·eth·yl·mal·o·nyl·urea (dye·eth''il·mal''o·nil·yoo·ree'uh) *n.* BARBITAL.

diethyl oxide. ETHER (3).

di·eth·yl·pro·pion (dye·eth''il·pro'pee·on) *n.* 2-Diethylaminopropiophenone, $C_{13}H_{19}NO$, an anorexic, usually used as the hydrochloride.

di·eth·yl·stil·bes·trol (dye·eth''il·stil·bes'trol) *n.* $(E)\alpha,\alpha'$-Diethyl-4,4'-stilbenediol, $C_{18}H_{20}O_2$, a white, crystalline powder, almost insoluble in water. A nonsteroid estrogen used as a substitute for the natural estrogenic hormones, more readily absorbed from the alimentary canal than most of the natural hormones and hence suitable for oral use. It is marketed under various trademarks. Abbreviated, DES. Syn. *stilbestrol.*

diethylstilbestrol dipropionate. Diethylstilbestrol in which both phenolic groups are esterified with propionic acid. When administered intramuscularly in oil, reactions such as nausea and vomiting are less frequent than with free diethylstilbestrol. The dipropionate is relatively slowly absorbed.

di·eth·yl·to·lu·a·mide (dye·eth″il·to·lew′uh·mide) *n.* *N,N*-Diethyltoluamide, $C_{12}H_{17}NO$, an arthropod repellant.

dietician. DIETITIAN.

di·e·tist (dye′e·tist) *n.* DIETITIAN.

di·e·ti·tian (dye″e·tish′un) *n.* A person trained in dietetics or the scientific management of the meals of individuals or groups; in institutions, one who arranges diet programs for purposes of adequate nutrition of the well and therapeutic nutrition of the sick.

Dietl's crisis (dee′tul) [J. *Dietl,* Polish physician, 1804–1878]. Recurrent attacks of radiating pain in the costovertebral angle, accompanied by nausea, vomiting, tachycardia, and hypotension, due to kinking or twisting of the ureter or renal vasculature; associated with ptosis of the kidney.

di·e·to·ther·a·py (dye″e·to·therr′uh·pee) *n.* The branch of dietetics that has to do with the use of food for therapeutic purposes.

Dieu·la·foy's disease (dyœ·la·fwa′) [G. *Dieulafoy,* French physician, 1839–1911]. Gastric ulceration or erosion complicating pneumonia.

di·fen·ox·i·mide (dye·fen·ock′si·mide) *n.* 4-[[(2,5-dioxo-1-pyrrolidinyl)oxy]carbonyl]-α,α,4-triphenyl-1-piperidinebutanenitrile, $C_{32}H_{31}N_3O_4$, an antiperistaltic, usually used as the hydrochloride salt.

di·fen·ox·in (dye·fen·ock′sin) *n.* 1-(3-Cyano-3,3-diphenylpropyl)-4-phenyl-4-piperidinecarboxylic acid, $C_{28}H_{28}N_2O_2$, an antiperistaltic.

dif·fer·en·tial (dif″ur·en′shul) *adj.* Pertaining to or creating a difference.

differential absorption ratio. *In radiobiology,* the ratio of the concentration of a radioactive substance in a given organ or tissue to the concentration that would be obtained if the same amount of radioactive material were administered and uniformly distributed throughout the body.

differential blood count. DIFFERENTIAL LEUKOCYTE COUNT.

differential bronchospirometry. Bronchospirometry performed on both lungs simultaneously, for comparison.

differential diagnosis. The distinguishing between diseases of similar character by comparing their signs and symptoms.

differential leukocyte count. The percentage of each variety of leukocyte, usually based on counting 100 leukocytes.

differential stain. A stain, as Gram's stain, used to differentiate bacteria or tissue elements.

differential threshold. The lowest limit at which two stimuli can be discriminated.

dif·fer·en·ti·ate (dif″ur·en′shee·ate) *v.* 1. To distinguish or make different. 2. To increase in complexity and organization during development; said of cells and tissues. **—differ·en·ti·a·tion** (·en″shee′ay′shun) *n.*

dif·flu·ence (dif′loo·unce) *n.* [L. *diffluere,* to flow in different directions]. Fluidity.

dif·frac·tion (di·frak′shun) *n.* [NL. *diffractio,* from L. *diffringere,* to break in pieces]. The separation of light into component parts by means of prisms, parallel bars in a grating, or layers of atoms in a crystal, thus producing interference phenomena such as lines, bands, or spot patterns.

diffraction area. A clear area seen in the microscopic image around all bodies of greater or less refractive power.

diffraction method. The determination of mean erythrocyte diameter by optical diffraction.

dif·fu·sate (di·few′zate, dif′yoo·sate) *n.* DIALYSATE.

¹dif·fuse (di·fewce′) *adj.* [L. *diffusus,* from *diffundere,* to spread by pouring]. Scattered; not limited to one tissue or spot. Contr. *localized.*

²diffuse (di·fewz′) *v.* [L. *diffundere, diffusus,* from *dis-,* apart, + *fundere,* to pour, to spread]. To spread, disperse.

diffuse angiokeratosis. ANGIOKERATOMA CORPORIS DIFFUSUM UNIVERSALE.

diffuse arterial ectasia. CIRSOID ANEURYSM (2).

diffuse arteriolar sclerosis. GENERALIZED ARTERIOLAR SCLEROSIS.

diffuse calcinosis. CALCINOSIS UNIVERSALIS.

diffuse choroiditis. Choroiditis characterized by numerous round or irregular spots scattered over the fundus.

diffused aneurysm. CONSECUTIVE ANEURYSM.

diffused light. 1. Light reflected simultaneously from an infinite number of surfaces. 2. Light that has been scattered by means of a concave mirror or lens.

diffuse endothelioma. EWING'S SARCOMA.

diffuse fibromatosis. FIBROMATOSIS GINGIVAE.

diffuse goiter. Thyroid gland enlargement produced by the increased size of all the follicles, or by the increased number of follicles, without the nodule formation characteristic of nodular goiter.

diffuse hypergammaglobulinemia. The general increase in serum concentration of all or many different immunoglobulins, characterized electrophoretically by a diffuse broad band and clinically by hyperplasia of plasma cells throughout the reticuloendothelial system. Main causes include infection, hepatic disease, the so-called collagen diseases, and advanced sarcoidosis.

diffuse hyperplastic sclerosis. Generalized degenerative disease of the arterioles characterized by internal and medial proliferation.

diffuse idiopathic atrophoderma. ACRODERMATITIS CHRONICA ATROPHICANS.

diffuse idiopathic atrophy of the skin. ACRODERMATITIS CHRONICA ATROPHICANS.

diffuse interstitial pulmonary fibrosis. HAMMAN-RICH SYNDROME.

diffuse intravascular coagulation. DISSEMINATED INTRAVASCULAR COAGULATION.

diffuse lung carcinoma. BRONCHIOLAR CARCINOMA.

diffuse lymphoma. A variety of malignant lymphoma, not seen in Hodgkin's disease, in which cellular proliferation is diffuse and without nodular structure; composed of well-differentiated lymphocytes, poorly differentiated lymphocytes, reticulum cells, or a mixture of the last two; prognosis is generally poorer than that of nodular lymphoma.

diffuse nodular cirrhosis. LAENNEC'S CIRRHOSIS.

diffuse scleroderma. Scleroderma in which the cutaneous changes are accompanied by involvement of skeletal muscle and viscera.

diffuse sclerosis. 1. Any diffuse increase of fibrous tissue, glial or collagenous. 2. In the nervous system, a diffuse fibrous glial reaction. 3. SCHILDER'S DISEASE.

diffuse syncytial reticulosarcoma. RETICULUM CELL SARCOMA.

diffuse trachoma. Trachoma in which large growths cover the palpebral conjunctiva.

dif·fus·ible (di·few′zi·bul) *adj.* Capable of being diffused. **—diffus·ibil·i·ty** (·few″zi·bil′i·tee) *n.*

Diffusin. A trademark for lyophilized hyaluronidase.

dif·fu·si·om·e·ter (di·few″zee·om′e·tur) *n.* [*diffusion* + *-meter*]. A device for estimating the diffusion of gases or liquids.

dif·fu·sion (di·few′zhun) *n.* 1. A spreading-out. 2. DIALYSIS. 3. *In optics,* the diversion of an appreciable fraction of energy of any one incident light ray into more than a few directions. See also *immunodiffusion.*

diffusion stasis. Stasis in which there occurs diffusion of serum or lymph.

diffusion vacuole. In the in vitro method of examining living cells, a minute droplet of the surrounding colored liquid which has been absorbed by the cell.

di·flor·a·sone diacetate (dye·flor′uh·sone). 6α,9-Difluoro-11β,17,21-trihydroxy-16β-methylpregna-1,4-diene-3,20-

dione, 17,21-diacetate, $C_{26}H_{32}F_2O_7$, a topical anti-inflammatory.

di·flu·a·nine (dye·floo'uh·neen) *n.* 1-(2-Anilinoethyl)-4-[4,4-bis(*p*-fluorophenyl)butyl]piperazine, $C_{28}H_{33}F_2N_3$, a central nervous system stimulant; used as the trihydrochloride salt.

di·flu·cor·to·lone (dye"floo·kor'tuh·lone) *n.* 6α,9-Difluoro-11β,21-dihydroxy-16α-methylpregna-1,4-diene-3,20-dione, $C_{22}H_{28}F_2O_4$; a glucocorticoid.

di·flu·mi·done (dye·floo'mi·dohn) *n.* 3'-Benzoyl-1,1-difluoromethanesulfonanilide, $C_{14}H_{11}F_2NO_3S$, an anti-inflammatory drug; used as the sodium salt.

di·flu·ni·sal (dye·floo'ni·sal) *n.* 2',4'-Difluoro-4-hydroxy-[1,1'-biphenyl]-3-carboxylic acid, $C_{13}H_8F_2O_3$, an anti-inflammatory.

di·flu·pred·nate (dye"floo·pred'nate) *n.* 21-(Acetyloxy)-6α,9-difluoro-11β-hydroxy-17-(1-oxobutoxy)pregna-1,4-diene-3,20-dione, $C_{27}H_{34}F_2O_7$, an anti-inflammatory.

dif·ta·lone (dif'tuh·lone) *n.* Phthalazino[2,3-*b*]phthalazine-5,12(7*H*,14*H*)-dione, $C_{16}H_{12}N_2O_2$, an anti-inflammatory.

Digalanid. A trademark for lanatoside, a cardiotonic.

di·gal·lic acid (dye·gal'ick). TANNIC ACID.

di·gal·lo·yl tri·o·le·ate (dye·gal'o·il tri·o'lee·ate) *n.* A mixed ester of gallic and oleic acids used as a sun screening agent.

di·gas·tric (dye·gas'trick) *adj.* [*di-* + Gk. *gastēr*, belly, + *-ic*]. 1. Of a muscle, having a fleshy part at each end and a tendinous portion in the middle. 2. Of or pertaining to the digastric muscle.

digastric fossa. 1. A depression on the inside of the mandible for the attachment of the anterior belly of the digastric muscle. NA *fossa digastrica.* 2. MASTOID NOTCH.

digastric groove. MASTOID NOTCH.

digastric muscle. A muscle of the neck having a posterior belly attached to the mastoid process and an anterior belly attached to the mandible with an intermediate tendon attached to the hyoid bone. NA *musculus digastricus.* See also Table of Muscles in the Appendix.

digastric triangle. SUBMANDIBULAR TRIANGLE.

Di·ge·nea (dye·jee'nee·uh, dye"je·nee'uh) *n. pl.* [*di-* + Gk. *genea*, descent, generation]. A subclass of the Trematoda, which in their life cycle exhibit alternation of generations and alternation of hosts. It includes all the species of flatworms parasitic in man, such as the liver flukes. —**di·ge·ne·ous** (dye·jee'nee·us) *adj.*

di·gen·e·sis (dye·jen'e·sis) *n.* [*di-* + *genesis*]. ALTERNATION OF GENERATIONS.

di·ge·net·ic (dye"je·net'ick) *adj.* [*di-* + *genetic*]. 1. Characterized by or pertaining to alternation of generations. 2. Pertaining to the Digenea.

Di·ge·net·i·ca (dye"je·net'ick·uh) *n. pl.* DIGENEA.

di·gen·ic (dye·jen'ick) *adj.* [*di-* + *-genic*]. 1. Characterizing a genetic constitution of nondiploid organisms containing two different genes for any given locus. 2. Of hereditary characters, determined by two different genes.

Di George's syndrome [A. M. *Di George*, U.S. pediatrician, b. 1921]. THYMIC APLASIA.

di·ges·ta (dye·jes'tuh, di·) *n. pl.* [NL., pl. of *digestum*, pass. part. of L. *digerere*, to separate, distribute]. Stomach or intestinal contents in the process of being digested. Compare *chyme.*

di·ges·tant (di·jes'tunt, dye·) *adj.* & *n.* 1. Pertaining to or promoting digestion. 2. An agent that promotes digestion.

di·gest·er (di·jes'tur, dye·) *n.* An apparatus used to subject substances to the action of enzymes or of high temperature and pressure in order to decompose, soften, or cook them.

di·ges·tion (di·jes'chun, dye·jes'chun) *n.* [L. *digestio*, from *digerere*, to separate]. 1. The act or process of converting food into assimilable form, principally through the action of various enzymes in the alimentary canal. 2. The softening of substances by moisture and heat. 3. The disintegration of materials by strong chemical agents. —**di·gest·ible** (di·jest'i·bul) *adj.*; **di·gest·ibil·i·ty** (di·jest"i·bil'i·tee) *n.*; **di·gest** (dye·jest', di·jest') *v.*

di·ges·tive (di·jes'tiv) *adj.* Pertaining to digestion.

digestive canal. ALIMENTARY CANAL.

digestive enzyme. An enzyme concerned with digestion in the alimentary tract.

digestive system. The alimentary canal with its associated glands. NA *apparatus digestorius, systema digestorium.*

digestive tract. ALIMENTARY CANAL.

digestive tube. 1. The portion of the digestive system which includes the esophagus, stomach, intestines, and rectum. 2. The entire alimentary canal from mouth to anus.

digestive vacuole. PHAGOSOME.

Digh·ton syndrome [C. A. A. *Dighton*, English otologist, b. 1885]. VAN DER HOEVE'S SYNDROME.

digi-. A combining form meaning *digitalis.*

Digifortis. A trademark for digitalis, a cardiotonic.

Digiglusin. Trademark for a preparation of digitalis glycosides.

Digilanid. Trademark for a mixture of the cardioactive glycosides from the leaves of *Digitalis lanata* in the approximate proportion in which they occur in the crude drug. The respective glycosides are lanatoside A, B, and C.

Digisidin. A trademark for digitoxin.

dig·it (dij'it) *n.* [L. *digitus*]. 1. A finger or toe. NA *digitus.* 2. One of a set of elementary discrete symbols used for counting and calculating, such as the Arabic numerals (0–9).

dig·i·tal (dij'i·tul) *adj.* 1. Of or pertaining to the digits. 2. Executed or performed by a finger, as a maneuver or an examination. 3. Fingerlike. 4. Functioning, or manipulating data, in terms of digits or discrete units or pulses, as: digital clock, digital computer. Contr. *analogue (4).*

digital compression. Compression of an artery by the fingers.

digital dilatation. Dilatation or stretching of a body cavity or orifice by means of one or more fingers.

digital fossa. 1. TROCHANTERIC FOSSA. 2. A cul-de-sac in the serous membrane which separates the body of the epididymis from the testis. Syn. *epididymal sinus.* NA *sinus epididymidis.* 3. A depression on the posterior inferior end of the fibula. NA *fossa malleoli lateralis.*

digital furrow. One of the transverse lines or furrows on the palmar surface of the fingers.

dig·i·tal·gia (dij"i·tal'jee·uh) *n.* [*digit* + *-algia*]. Pain in a digit.

digitalgia par·es·thet·i·ca (păr"es·thet'i·kuh). Pain and numbness in one of the fingers due to an isolated neuritis of its dorsal digital nerve.

digital impressions or **markings.** CONVOLUTIONAL IMPRESSIONS or MARKINGS.

dig·i·tal·in (dij"i·tal'in, dij'i·tuh·lin) *n.* [*digitalis* + *-in*]. The *Digitalinum verum* of Schmiedeberg and Kiliani, $C_{36}H_{56}O_{14}$, a glycosidal preparation obtained from the seeds of *Digitalis purpurea.*

Digitaline Nativelle. Early name for DIGITOXIN.

Dig·i·tal·is (dij"i·tal'is, ·tay'lis) *n.* [L., pertaining to or resembling fingers]. A genus of herbs whose dried leaves and seeds are cardioactive, including *Digitalis purpurea*, the common foxglove, from which the drug digitalis is derived, and *D. lanata*, from which digoxin and other glycosides are derived.

digitalis, *n.* The dried leaf of *Digitalis purpurea*, the common foxglove, which is a powerful cardiac stimulant that increases contractility of heart muscle, but is frequently followed by a lengthened refractory period and diminished heart size, and that also acts indirectly as a diuretic. Employed mainly in diseases of the heart where compensation is lost. A standardized preparation, powdered digitalis, should be employed medicinally.

digitalis unit. The activity of 100 mg of U.S.P. Digitalis Reference Standard, as determined by biologic assay on the pigeon.

dig·i·tal·i·za·tion (dij"i·tal"i·zay'shun, ·dij"i·tul·eye·zay'shun) *n.* Administration of a variety of digitalis preparations in a dosage schedule producing a therapeutic concentration of digitalis glycosides; maintenance dosage is continued subsequently. —**dig·i·tal·ize** (dij'i·tul·ize, dij''i·tal'ize) *v.*

digital markings. CONVOLUTIONAL IMPRESSIONS or MARKINGS.

dig·i·tal·ose (dij''i·tal'oce, ·tay'loce) *n.* 3-Methyl-D-fucose, $C_7H_{14}O_5$; one of the sugars obtained in the hydrolysis of certain digitalis glycosides.

digital pelvimetry. Measurement of the pelvis by means of the hand.

digital pulp. The sensitive, elastic, convex prominence on the palmar or plantar surface of the terminal phalanx of a finger or toe.

digital reflex. 1. Sudden flexion of the terminal phalanx of the thumb and of the second and third phalanges of some other finger, elicited by snapping the terminal phalanx or tapping the nail of the patient's middle or index finger, usually seen when the tendon reflexes are hyperactive, as in spastic hemiparesis. 2. Reflex finger flexion occurring upon tapping the palmar aspect of the terminal phalanges of the slightly flexed fingers.

digital tonometry. The estimation of intraocular pressure by the palpation of the eyeballs through the upper lids; pathologically high or low tension is readily perceived by the skilled examiner.

dig·i·tate (dij'i·tate) *adj.* Having digits or digitlike processes.

dig·i·ta·tion (dij''i·tay'shun) *n.* A fingerlike process, or a succession of such processes, especially that of a muscle attachment.

digiti. Plural and genitive singular of *digitus.*

dig·i·ti·form (dij'i·ti·form) *adj.* [*digit* + *-iform*]. Finger-shaped.

digiti ma·nus (man'us) [NA]. The digits of the hand.

digiti pe·dis (ped'is) [NA]. The digits of the foot.

dig·i·to·gen·in (dij''i·to·jen'in, ·toj'uh·nin) *n.* The steroid aglycone, $C_{27}H_{44}O_5$, of digitonin.

dig·i·to·nide (dij''i·to'nide) *n.* A sparingly soluble complex formed by the interaction of digitonin with cholesterol and certain other sterols.

dig·i·to·nin (dij''i·to'nin) *n.* A steroid glycoside, $C_{56}H_{92}O_{29}$, from digitalis, lacking in typical digitalis action and reputedly irritant.

dig·i·to·plan·tar (dij''i·to·plan'tur, ·tahr) *adj.* [*digito-* + *plantar*]. Pertaining to the toes and the sole of the foot.

dig·i·tox·i·gen·in (dij''i·tock''si·jen'in) *n.* The steroid aglycone, $C_{23}H_{34}O_4$, formed by removal of three molecules of the sugar digitoxose from digitoxin; also obtained as the aglycone on hydrolysis of lanatoside A.

dig·i·tox·in (dij''i·tock'sin) *n.* [*digitalis* + *toxin*]. The principal active glycoside, $C_{41}H_{64}O_{13}$, of digitalis, introduced as Digitaline Nativelle; it occurs in crystals which are practically insoluble in water. The action is like that of digitalis. Syn. *digitoxoside.*

dig·i·tox·ose (dij''i·tock'soce) *n.* 2-Deoxy-D-altromethylose, $C_6H_{12}O_4$, the sugar resulting when certain digitalis glycosides, notably digitoxin, gitoxin, and gitalin, are hydrolyzed.

dig·i·tox·o·side (dij''i·tock'so·side) *n.* DIGITOXIN.

di·gi·tus (dij'i·tus) *n.*, pl. & genit. sing. **digi·ti** (·tye), genit. pl. **digi·to·rum** (to'rum) [L., lit., pointer] [NA]. A finger or toe; DIGIT.

digitus I [NA alt.]. 1. THUMB. NA alt. *pollex.* 2. GREAT TOE. NA alt. *hallux.*

digitus II. 1. [NA alt.] INDEX FINGER. NA alt. *index.* 2. [NA] The second toe.

digitus III. 1. [NA alt.]. DIGITUS MEDIUS; the middle finger. 2. [NA] The third toe.

digitus IV. 1. [NA]. RING FINGER. NA alt. *digitus anularis.* 2. [NA] The fourth toe.

digitus V [NA alt.]. 1. LITTLE FINGER. NA alt. *digitus minimus.* 2. LITTLE TOE. NA alt. *digitus minimus.*

digitus anu·la·ris (an·yoo·lair'is) [NA]. RING FINGER. NA alt. *digitus IV.*

digitus me·di·us (mee'dee·us) [NA]. The middle finger. NA alt. *digitus III.*

digitus mi·ni·mus (min'i·mus) [NA]. 1. LITTLE FINGER. NA alt. *digitus V.* 2. LITTLE TOE. NA alt. *digitus V.*

digitus pri·mus (prye'mus). DIGITUS I.

digitus quar·tus (kwahr'tus). DIGITUS IV.

digitus quin·tus (kwin'tus). DIGITUS V.

digitus se·cun·dus (se·kun'dus). DIGITUS II.

digitus ter·ti·us (tur'shee·us). DIGITUS III.

di·glos·sia (dye·glos'ee·uh) *n.* [*di-* + *-glossia*]. A form of schistoglossia in which the lateral lingual swellings fail to fuse, producing a bifid tongue.

di·glos·sus (dye·glos'us) *n.* An individual showing diglossia.

di·glu·ta·thi·one (dye·gloo''tuh·thigh'ohn) *n.* The known oxidized form of glutathione in which two molecules of the reduced form are united by loss of two hydrogen atoms.

di·glyc·er·ide (dye·glis'ur·ide) *n.* [*di-* + *glyceride*]. A lipid composed of two molecules of fatty acid esterified with glycerol.

di·gnath·us (dye·nath'us) *n.* [*di-* + *-gnathus*]. An individual with two lower jaws.

dig·ox·i·gen·in (dij·ock''si·jen'in) *n.* The steroid aglycone, $C_{23}H_{34}O_5$, of digoxin and of lanatoside C.

dig·ox·in (dij·ock'sin) *n.* A cardiotonic secondary glycoside, $C_{41}H_{64}O_{14}$, derived from lanatoside C, one of the glycosides of *Digitalis lanata.* On hydrolysis it yields the aglycone digoxigenin and three molecules of digitoxose. The actions and uses of digoxin are similar to those of digitalis.

di Gu·gliel·mo's syndrome or **disease** (dee·goo·lʸel'mo)[G. *di Guglielmo,* Italian hematologist, b. 1886]. ERYTHREMIC MYELOSIS.

di·hex·y·ver·ine (dye·heck''see·verr'een) *n.* 2-Piperidinoethyl ester of bicyclohexyl-1-carboxylic acid, $C_{20}H_{35}NO_2$, an anticholinergic agent; used as the hydrochloride salt.

di·hy·brid (dye·high'brid) *n.* [*di-* + *hybrid*]. The offspring of parents differing in two characters.

dihydr-, dihydro-. A combining form meaning *combined with two atoms of hydrogen.*

di·hy·drate (dye·high'drate) *n.* [*di-* + *hydrate*]. A compound containing two molecules of water.

di·hy·dric (dye·high'drick) *adj.* Containing two hydroxyl groups in the molecule.

dihydro-. See *dihydr-.*

di·hy·dro·cho·les·ter·ol (dye·high''dro·ko·les'tur·ol) *n.* CHOLESTANOL (1).

di·hy·dro·cin·chon·i·dine (dye·high''dro·sing·kon'i·deen) *n.* HYDROCINCHONIDINE.

di·hy·dro·co·de·inone (dye·high''dro·ko·dee'i·nohn) *n.* HYDROCODONE.

di·hy·dro·co·en·zyme I (dye·high''dro·ko·en'zyme). A name given to the reduced form of diphosphopyridine nucleotide (coenzyme I), symbolized as DPNH, but now more often called the reduced form of nicotinamide-adenine dinucleotide and symbolized NADH.

dihydrocoenzyme II. A name given to the reduced form of triphosphopyridine nucleotide (coenzyme II), symbolized as TPNH, but now more often called the reduced form of nicotinamide-adenine dinucleotide phosphate and symbolized as NADPH.

di·hy·dro·er·got·a·mine (dye·high''dro·ur·got'uh·meen, ·ur''guh·tam'een) *n.* A hydrogenated derivative, $C_{33}H_{37}N_5O_5$, of ergotamine, employed parenterally, as the methanesulfonate salt, in the treatment of migraine. It is less toxic than ergotamine and has no uterine effect.

di·hy·dro·mor·phi·none (dye·high''dro·mor'fi·nohn) *n.* HYDROMORPHONE.

di·hy·dro·quin·ine (dye·high''dro·kwin'een, ·kwye'neen) *n.* HYDROQUININE.

di·hy·dro·strep·to·my·cin (dye·high''dro·strep''to·migh'sin) *n.* A hydrogenated derivative, $C_{21}H_{41}N_7O_{12}$, of streptomycin having the antibacterial action of, and used clinically like, streptomycin. It is available as the sulfate for intramuscular injection. Used in patients who cannot tolerate streptomycin, but is toxic to the eighth cranial nerve.

di·hy·dro·ta·chys·ter·ol (dye·high″dro·ta·kis′tuh·role, ·rol, ·tack″i·steer′) *n.* [*dihydro-* + *tachysterol*]. A synthetic steroid, $C_{28}H_{46}O$, derived from ergosterol; possesses some of the biologic properties of vitamin D and of the parathyroid hormone. It produces hypercalcemia and increased urinary excretion of phosphorus. Used in treating hypoparathyroidism.

di·hy·dro·thee·lin (dye·high″dro·thee′lin) *n.* ESTRADIOL.

di·hy·droxy·ace·tic acid (dye″high·drock″see·a·see′tick, ·a·set′ick). GLYOXYLIC ACID.

di·hy·droxy·ac·e·tone (dye″high·drock″see·as′e·tone) *n.* $CH_2OHCOCH_2OH$; a simple ketose derivable from glycerin or dextrose, important in metabolism of carbohydrates; also acts as a sunscreen and reacts with keratin in the stratum corneum to form a dark pigmentation which gives the appearance of a suntan.

dihydroxyacetone phosphate. DIHYDROXYACETONEPHOSPHORIC ACID.

di·hy·droxy·ac·e·tone·phos·phor·ic acid (dye″high·drock″see·as″e·tone·fos·for′ick). $CH_2OHCOCH_2OPO(OH)_2$; a phosphoric acid ester of dihydroxyacetone, produced as an intermediate substance in glycolysis.

di·hy·droxy·alu·mi·num ami·no·ac·e·tate (dye″high·drock″see·uh·lew′mi·num a·mee″no·as′e·tate). A basic aluminum salt of aminoacetic acid, principally $NH_2CH_2COOAl(OH)_2$, a white powder, insoluble in water. It acts as a gastric antacid and is useful for control of hyperacidity in the management of peptic ulcer. It is available under various trademarked names.

di·hy·droxy·an·thra·nol (dye″high·drock″see·an′thruh·nol) *n.* Either of two isomeric substances: (a) 3,4-dihydroxyanthranol or anthrarobin; (b) 1,8-dihydroxyanthranol or anthralin.

***m*-di·hy·droxy·ben·zene** (met′uh dye″high·drock″see·ben′zeen) *n.* RESORCINOL.

di·hy·droxy·es·trin (dye″high·drock″see·es′trin) *n.* ESTRADIOL.

di·hy·droxy·phen·yl·al·a·nine (dye″high·drock″see·fen·il·al′uh·neen) *n.* 3-(3,4-Dihydroxyphenyl)-L-alanine, $C_9H_{11}NO_4$, an amino acid that can be formed by oxidation of tyrosine; it is converted by a series of biochemical transformations, utilizing the enzyme dopa oxidase, to black, pigments known as melanins, and is also the precursor of epinephrine and norepinephrine. Syn. *dopa.* See also *levodopa.*

di·hy·droxy·pro·pane (di″high·drock″see·pro′pane) *n.* PROPYLENE GLYCOL.

di·io·do·hy·droxy·quin (dye″eye·o″do·high·drock′see·kwin) *n.* 5,7-Diiodo-8-quinolinol, $C_9H_5I_2NO$, a light yellowish to tan microcrystalline powder, almost insoluble in water. It is used as an antiprotozoan agent in intestinal amebiasis and in the treatment of *Trichomonas hominis* infections.

di·io·do·hy·droxy·quin·o·line (dye″eye·o″do·high·drock″see·kwin′o·leen, ·lin) *n.* DIIODOHYDROXYQUIN.

di·io·do·thy·ro·nine (dye″eye·o″do·thigh′ro·neen, ·nin) *n.* 3,5-Diiodothyronine, $C_{15}H_{13}I_2NO_4$, a substance obtained as an intermediate product in the manufacture of synthetic thyroxine. It has been used like the latter.

di·io·do·ty·ro·sine (dye″eye·o″do·tye′ro·seen, ·sin) *n.* 3,5-Diiodotyrosine, $C_9H_9I_2NO_3$, a constituent of thyroglobulin; thyroxine may be formed from two molecules of diiodotyrosine by oxidative condensation. Abbreviated, DIT. Syn. *iodogorgoic acid.*

di·iso·pro·pyl flu·o·ro·phos·phate (dye″eye·so·pro′pil floo″uh·ro·fos′fate). Diisopropyl phosphorofluoridate, $[(CH_3)_2CHO]_2PFO$, a colorless, oily liquid. It is a powerful inhibitor of cholinesterase, produces marked and prolonged miosis, and is used topically in the treatment of a variety of ophthalmic afflictions; ISOFLUROPHATE.

diisopropyl phos·pho·ro·flu·o·ri·date (fos″fuh·ro·floo′ur·i·date, ·floo·or′i·date). DIISOPROPYL FLUOROPHOSPHATE; ISOFLUROPHATE.

di·kar·y·on (dye·kăr′ee·on) *n.* [*di-* + *karyon*]. A phase or stage in the growth of the mycelium of many fungi in which the cells each have two haploid nuclei.

di·ke·to·pi·per·a·zine (dye·kee″to·pi·perr′uh·zeen, ·pip′ur·uh·zeen) *n.* Any of a class of heterocyclic compounds formed from two molecules of the same or different amino acids by condensation of the carboxyl group of each with the amino group of the other; the compounds may be considered to be derivatives of piperazine.

dikty-, diktyo-. See *dicty-, dictyo-.*

dik·ty·o·ma, dic·ty·o·ma (dick″tee·o′muh) *n.*, pl. **diktyomas, dictyomas, diktyoma·ta, dictyoma·ta** (·tuh) [*dikty-* + *-oma*]. A tumor derived from the nonpigmented layer of the ciliary epithelium and structurally resembling the embryonic retina. Syn. *medulloepithelioma.*

dik·wa·kwa·di (dick″wah·kwah′dee) *n.* [of Bantu origin]. WITKOP.

Dilabron. Trademark for isoetharine, a bronchodilator drug.

di·lac·er·a·tion (dye·las″uh·ray′shun) *n.* [L. *dilaceratio*, from *dilacerare*, to tear apart]. 1. The act of tearing apart; being torn in pieces. 2. *In dentistry,* a partial alteration of the position of the formative organ during development, resulting in teeth with sharp angulation of the root and crown.

Dilantin. A trademark for phenytoin, an anticonvulsant in the treatment of epilepsy; the compound is also used as the sodium derivative.

Dilantin sodium hyperplasia. Gingival hyperplasia as a side effect of the use of the anticonvulsant drug phenytoin sodium.

di·lat·able (dye·lay′tuh·bul, di·) *adj.* Expandable.

dilatable bougie. A bougie that can be increased in diameter for dilating a stricture.

di·la·tan·cy (dye·lay′tun·see) *n.* A form of thixotropy in which a viscous suspension changes to a solid under the influence of pressure.

dil·a·ta·tion (dil″uh·tay′shun, dye″luh·) *n.* [L. *dilatatio*, from *dilatare*, to spread out]. 1. The state of being stretched. 2. Enlargement, as of a hollow part or organ. Compare *dilation.*

dilatation of the stomach. Increase in size of the stomach from relaxation of the walls and expansion with gas or liquid.

dilatation thrombosis. Thrombosis within a dilated vessel or chamber, due to circulatory slowing or turbulence.

di·late (dye·late′) *v.* [L. *dilatare*, to enlarge, to spread out]. To enlarge or expand. —**di·lat·ing** (dye·lay′ting) *adj.*

dilating bougie. DILATABLE BOUGIE.

dilating pain. Pain accompanying the stretching of the cervix in the first stage of labor.

dilating urethrotome. A combined urethrotome and urethral dilator.

di·la·tion (dye·lay′shun, di·) *n.* The act or process of stretching or dilating. Compare *dilatation.*

dil·a·tom·e·ter (dil″uh·tom′e·tur, dye″luh·) *n.* [*dilate* + *-meter*]. An instrument for measuring volume changes accompanying a chemical reaction or temperature change.

dil·a·to·met·ric (dil″uh·to·met′rick) *adj.* Of or pertaining to a dilatometer.

di·la·tor (dye′lay·tur, dye·lay′tur) *n.* 1. An instrument for stretching or enlarging a cavity or opening. 2. A dilating muscle.

dilator iri·dis (eye′ri·dis, irr′i·dis). DILATOR PUPILLAE.

dilator na·ris (nair′is). A dilating muscle of the nostril; the alar part of the nasalis muscle. NA *pars alaris musculi nasalis.*

dilator pu·pil·lae (pew·pil′ee). The set of radiating smooth involuntary muscle fibers in the iris, dilating the pupil. NA *musculus dilator pupillae.* See also Table of Muscles in the Appendix.

dilator tu·bae (tew'bee). TENSOR VELI PALATINI.

Dilaudid. Trademark for hydromorphone (dihydromorphinone), a respiratory sedative and analgesic used as the hydrochloride salt.

dil·do, *n.* [unkn. orig.]. 1. *Obsol.* Any artifact shaped like or representing a phallus. 2. In current usage, specifically, an artificial penis made of plastic or other appropriate material, used for sexual stimulation.

di·lec·a·nus (dye·leck'uh·nus) *n.* [*di-* + Gk. *lekanē,* basin, "pelvis," + *-us*]. DIPYGUS.

dill, *n.* ANETHUM.

Dil·ling's rule [W. *Dilling,* English, 20th century]. A rule to determine dosage of medicine for children; specifically, dose = age of child in years, multiplied by adult dose, divided by 20.

dill oil. The volatile oil from *Anethum graveolens;* contains carvone. Has been used as a carminative.

dil·u·ent (dil'yoo·unt) *n.* An agent that dilutes the strength of a solution or mixture.

di·lute (di·lewt', dye·) *v. & adj.* [L. *diluere,* to wash away]. 1. To make less concentrated, weaker, or thinner, as by addition of water to an aqueous solution. 2. Diluted.

di·lut·ed acetic acid. An aqueous solution of acetic acid containing about 6% CH_3COOH.

diluted alcohol. A mixture of alcohol and water containing 41 to 42% by weight, or 48.4 to 49.5% by volume at 15.56°C, of C_2H_5OH.

diluted ammonia solution. A 10% solution of ammonia in water; has been used as local irritant, stimulant, and antacid.

diluted hydrochloric acid. An aqueous solution containing 10 g HCl in 100 ml water; used in hydrochloric acid deficiency states.

di·lu·tion (di·lew'shun, dye·) *n.* 1. The process of diluting, as a solution with its solvent or a powder containing an active ingredient with an inactive diluent. 2. A diluted substance; the result of a diluting process. —**dilution·al** (·ul) *adj.*

dilution test. The administration of a water load to test the ability of the kidney to excrete a dilute urine; this ability is lost with renal failure.

Di·mas·tig·a·moe·ba (dye·mas"tig·uh·mee'buh) *n.* [*di-* + Gk. *mastix,* whip, + *amoeba*]. A genus of free-living, coprozoic amebas. The species *Dimastigamoeba gruberi* has been found in decaying feces.

di·mef·a·dane (dye·mef'uh·dane) *n.* *N,N*-Dimethyl-3-phenyl-1-indanamine, $C_{17}H_{19}N$, an analgesic drug.

di·me·fil·con A (dye"me·fil'kon) *n.* A polymer of 2-hydroxyethyl methacrylate, methyl methacrylate and ethylene bis(oxyethylene)dimethacrylate, a hydrophilic contact lens material.

di·me·fline (dye'me·fleen) *n.* 8-[(Dimethylamino)methyl]-7-methoxy-3-methylflavone, $C_{20}H_{21}NO_3$, a respiratory stimulant; used as the hydrochloride salt.

di·meg·a·ly (dye·meg'uh·lee) *n.* [*di-* + *-megaly*]. The condition of having two sizes; applied to spermatozoa.

Dimenformon. A trademark for the estrogen estradiol.

di·men·hy·dri·nate (dye"men·high'dri·nate) *n.* 2-(Benzhydryloxy)-*N,N*-dimethylethylamine 8-chlorotheophyllinate, $C_{17}H_{21}NO.C_7H_7ClN_4O_2$, a white, crystalline powder, slightly soluble in water; an antihistaminic and antinauseant.

di·men·sion (di·men'shun, dye·) *n.* [L. *dimensio*]. A measurable extent.

di·mer (dye'mur) *n.* [*di-* + *-mer*]. The compound resulting from combination of two molecules of the same substance and having twice the molecular weight of the single molecule or monomer.

di·mer·cap·rol (dye"mur·cap'rol) *n.* 2,3-Dimercaptopropanol, $HSCH_2CHSHCH_2OH$, a colorless liquid with a mercaptan-like odor, soluble in water; an antidote for arsenic, gold, and mercury poisoning. Originally developed to counteract the effects of the chemical warfare agent lewisite. Syn. *British anti-lewisite.*

dim·er·ous (dim'ur·us) *adj.* [Gk. *dimerēs,* from *di-* + *meros,* part]. Consisting of two parts; used especially to describe two-parted tarsi of certain insects.

Dimetane. Trademark for brompheniramine, an antihistaminic drug used as the maleate salt.

di·meth·a·di·one (dye·meth"uh·dye'ohn) *n.* 5,5-Dimethyloxazolidine-2,4-dione, $C_5H_7NO_3$, an anticonvulsant drug.

di·meth·i·cone (dye·meth'i·kone) *n.* A silicone oil, with skin-adherent and water-repellent properties, used as a skin-protective agent in petrolatum bases.

di·meth·in·dene (dye"meth·in'deen) *n.* 2-{1-[2-(2-Dimethylaminoethyl)inden-3-yl]ethyl}pyridine, $C_{20}H_{24}N_2$, an antihistaminic drug; used as the maleate salt.

di·meth·iso·quin (dye"meth·eye'so·kwin) *n.* 3-Butyl-1-(2-dimethylaminoethoxy)isoquinoline, $C_{17}H_{24}N_2O$, a surface anesthetic; used as the hydrochloride salt.

di·meth·ox·an·ate (dye"meth·ock'suh·nate) *n.* 2-Dimethylaminoethoxyethyl phenothiazine-10-carboxylate, $C_{19}H_{22}N_2O_3S$, an antitussive with local anesthetic and mild antispasmodic properties; used as the hydrochloride salt.

dimethyl-. A combining form indicating *the presence of two methyl groups.*

di·meth·yl acetal (dye·meth'il). 1. $CH_3CH(OCH_3)_2$. A colorless liquid that has been used as an anesthetic alone or combined with chloroform. 2. The group $—CH(OCH_3)_2$ formed from an aldehyde.

di·meth·yl·ami·no·azo·ben·zene (dye·meth"il·uh·mee"no·az"o·ben'zeen, ·ay"zo·ben'zeen, dye·meth"il·am"i·no·) *n.* $C_{14}H_{15}N_3$; used as yellow leaflets for coloring fats and butter and as an indicator for acid-base titrations. Syn. *methyl yellow.*

di·meth·yl·ami·no·benz·al·de·hyde (dye·meth"il·uh·mee"no·benz·al'de·hide) *n.* *p*-Dimethylaminobenzaldehyde, $CHOC_6H_4N(CH_3)_2$, variously used as a reagent in histochemistry, clinical laboratory diagnosis, and drug analysis. Syn. *Ehrlich's reagent.*

di·meth·yl·ar·sin·ic acid (dye·meth"il·ahr·sin'ick). Cacodylic acid, $(CH_3)_2AsOOH$, a deliquescent, crystalline solid; soluble in water. Has been used, usually in the form of sodium cacodylate, for arsenical therapy, particularly in skin diseases.

di·meth·yl·ben·zene (dye·meth"il·ben'zeen) *n.* XYLENE.

dimethyl carbinol. ISOPROPYL ALCOHOL.

di·meth·yl·gly·ox·ime (dye·meth"il·glye·ock'seem) *n.* Diacetyldioxime, $C_4H_8N_2O_2$, a white crystalline powder, used as a reagent for the detection and determination of nickel.

di·meth·yl·ke·tone (dye·meth"il·kee'tone) *n.* ACETONE.

di·meth·yl·poly·sil·ox·ane (dye·meth"il·pol"ee·sil·ock'sane) *n.* A water-repellant silicone polymer widely used in protective creams and lotions.

dimethyl sulfate. $(CH_3)_2SO_4$, a colorless liquid used as a methylating agent in chemical syntheses. It is a strong caustic, and its vapor is powerfully irritant to the respiratory tract.

dimethyl sulfoxide. CH_3SOCH_3, a colorless liquid, practically odorless when pure, miscible with water. Rapidly absorbed through intact skin, it has local analgesic and anti-inflammatory activity; its use is dangerous. Abbreviated, DMSO.

di·meth·yl·tryp·ta·mine (dye·meth"il·trip'tuh·meen, ·min) *n.* 3-[2-(Dimethylamino)ethyl]indole, $C_{12}H_{10}N_2$, a naturally occurring hallucinogenic agent extracted from the seeds of *Piptadenia peregrina.* Abbreviated, DMT. See also *cohoba snuff.*

dimethyl tubocurarine chloride. Dimethyl ether of *d*-tubocurarine chloride, $C_{40}H_{48}Cl_2N_2O_6$; has the actions and uses of dimethyl tubocurarine iodide.

dimethyl tubocurarine iodide. METOCURINE.

di·meth·yl·xan·thine (dye·meth″il·zan′theen, ·thin) *n.* Either of two isomeric substances: (a) theobromine (3,7-dimethylxanthine); (b) theophylline (1,3-dimethylxanthine).

di·me·tria (dye·mee′tree·uh) *n.* [*di-* + *metr-* + *-ia*]. UTERUS DUPLEX.

Di·mi·tri's disease (dee·mee′tree) [V. *Dimitri,* Argentinian neurologist, 20th century]. STURGE-WEBER DISEASE.

Dimocillin. A trademark for the sodium salt of methicillin, a semisynthetic penicillin antibiotic.

di·mor·phism (dye·mor′fiz·um) *n.* [*di-* + *morph-* + *-ism*]. The property of existing in two distinct structural forms. —**di·mor·phous** (·fus) *adj.*

dimorphous leprosy. A form of leprosy in which cutaneous lesions that are clinically and histologically of both the lepromatous and tuberculoid types are simultaneously present.

dim·ple, *n.* 1. A slight depression. 2. A depression of the skin due to fixation to deep structures or to muscular insertion.

dimp·ling, *n.* An abnormal skin depression from retraction occurring in subcutaneous carcinomas; most commonly seen in breast cancer.

di·neu·ric (dye·new′rick) *adj.* [*di-* + *neur-* + *-ic*]. Provided with two axons; said of a nerve cell.

di·neu·tron (dye·new′tron) *n.* An atomic nuclear particle of neutral electric charge and twice the weight of the ordinary neutron.

di·ni·tro·chlo·ro·ben·zene (dye″nigh″tro·klo″ro·ben′zeen, ·ben·zeen′) *n.* A mixture of 2,4- and 2,6-dinitrochlorobenzenes, but mainly the 2,4 isomer, $C_6H_3ClN_2O_4$; used to evaluate cellular immunity and as a reagent for the detection of nicotinic acid and nicotinamide.

di·ni·tro·phe·nol (dye·nigh″tro·fee′nol) *n.* 2,4-Dinitrophenol, $C_6H_4N_2O_5$; a highly toxic substance, formerly used as a metabolic stimulant to lose weight.

di·ni·tro·phen·yl·hy·dra·zine (dye·nigh″tro·fen″il·high′druh·zeen, ·zin, dye·nigh″tro·fee″nil·) *n.* 2,4-Dinitrophenylhydrazine, $C_6H_3(NO_2)_2NHNH_2$, a red crystalline powder soluble in dilute acids; used in identification and analysis of aldehydes and ketones.

din·ner pad. A removable pad of felt, cotton, or other material placed over the abdomen prior to the application of a plaster jacket, to allow for normal distention after eating.

di·no·prost (dye′no·prost) *n.* (5*Z*,9α,11α,13*E*,15*S*)-9,11,15-Trihydroxyprosta-5,13-dien-1-oic acid, $C_{20}H_{34}O_5$, a prostaglandin oxytocic agent usually used as the tromethamine (trimethanolamine) salt.

di·no·pros·tone (dye·no·pros′tone) *n.* (5*Z*,11α,13*E*,15*S*)-11,15-dihydroxy-9-oxoprosta-5,13-dien-1-oic acid, $C_{20}H_{32}O_5$, an oxytocic prostaglandin, prostaglandin E_2.

di·nu·cle·o·tide (dye·new′klee·o·tide) *n.* A molecule composed of two mononucleotides linked by a phosphodiester bond.

di·o·coele (dye′o·seel) *n.* [*dia-* + *-coele*]. The lumen of the diencephalon, especially in the embryo; it forms part of the third ventricle in the adult.

Di·oc·to·phy·ma (dye·ock″to·figh′muh) *n.* [Gk. *dionk*oun, to distend, + *phyma,* growth, tubercle]. A genus of large nematodes of the superfamily Dioctophymoidea.

Dioctophyma re·na·le (re·nay′lee). A species of kidney worm which occasionally infects man, but principally a parasite of carnivorous and other animals.

di·oc·tyl so·di·um sul·fo·suc·ci·nate (dye·ock′til so′dee·um sul″fo·suck′sin·ate). Sodium bis(2-ethylhexyl) sulfosuccinate, $C_{20}H_{37}NaO_7S$, a white, waxlike, plastic solid, soluble in 70 parts of water; employed as a wetting agent in the formulation of lotions, creams, ointments, and shampoos.

di·o·done (dye′o·dohn) *n.* IODOPYRACET.

Diodoquin. A trademark for diiodohydroxyquin, an antiprotozoan drug.

Diodrast. Trademark for iodopyracet, a radiopaque medium.

Diodrast clearance test. The rate of renal excretion of Diodrast in relation to the blood level is used as a test of renal function and as an approximate measure of renal blood flow.

di·oe·cious (dye·ee′shus) *adj.* [*di-* + Gk. *oikeios,* domestic]. Having separate sexes; used particularly for organisms belonging to larger groups in which hermaphroditism is also common.

dioestrum. DIESTRUS.

dioestrus. DIESTRUS.

Diogyn. A trademark for estradiol, an estrogen.

di·ol·a·mine (dye·ol′uh·meen) *n.* Diethanolamine, $HN(CH_2CH_2OH)_2$, an emulsifier and dispersing agent.

Dioloxol. A trademark for mephenesin, a skeletal muscle relaxant.

Dionin. A trademark for ethylmorphine, a lymphagogue, analgesic, and antitussive; used as the hydrochloride salt.

di·o·nism (dye′o·niz·um) *n.* [after *Dione,* in Greek mythology, the mother of Venus Pandemos]. HETEROSEXUALITY. Contr. *uranism.*

Dionosil. Trademark for propyliodone, a radiopaque contrast medium used in bronchography.

di·op·ter, di·op·tre (dye·op′tur) *n.* [Gk. *dioptra,* an optical instrument for measuring altitudes]. A unit of measurement of the refractive power of an optic lens. It is the refractive power of a lens having a focal distance of one meter. Abbreviated, d. —**di·op·tral** (dye·op′trul) *adj.*

Diopterin. A trademark for pteroyldiglutamic acid, a derivative of folic acid which has been proposed as an adjunct in the treatment of neoplastic diseases.

di·op·tom·e·ter (dye″op·tom′e·tur) *n.* [*diopt*er + *-meter*]. An instrument for determining ocular refraction. —**dioptometry** (·tree) *n.*

dioptre. DIOPTER.

di·op·tric (dye·op′trick) *adj.* [Gk. *dioptrikos,* from *dioptra,* an optical instrument]. Pertaining to transmitted and refracted light.

dioptric aberration. SPHERICAL ABERRATION.

dioptric anamorphosis. The correction of a distorted optical image by means of a pyramidal glass.

di·op·trics (dye·op′tricks) *n.* [*dioptric* + *-s*]. The branch of optics that treats of the refraction of light, especially by the transparent medium of the eye, and by lenses.

di·op·trom·e·ter (dye″op·trom′e·tur) *n.* DIOPTOMETER.

di·or·tho·sis (dye″or·tho′sis) *n.*, pl. **diortho·ses** (·seez) [Gk., *diorthōsis,* making straight]. Surgical correction of a deformity or repair of an injury done to a limb, as diaplasis. —**dior·thot·ic** (·thot′ick) *adj.*

di·os·co·rea (dye″os·ko′ree·uh) *n.* [*Dioscorides,* Greek physician]. The dried rhizome of *Dioscorea villosa,* the wild yam root, indigenous to the eastern United States. It yields an acrid resin and a saponin-like principle; has been used as an expectorant, diuretic, and antispasmodic.

di·os·co·rine (dye·os′ko·reen, ·rin) *n.* An alkaloid, $C_{13}H_{19}NO_2$, obtained from the tubers of *Dioscorea hirsuta.* A bitter and toxic alkaloid resembling picrotoxin; it produces paralysis of the central nervous system.

di·ose (dye′oce, ·oze) *n.* [*di-* + *-ose*]. A monosaccharide containing only two carbon atoms; it is the simplest form of sugar.

di·os·gen·in (dye″os·jen′in, dye″oz·) *n.* A steroid aglycone, $C_{27}H_{42}O_3$, obtained from a saponin in *Dioscorea tokoro* and other sources; it is a starting compound in the synthesis of certain steroid hormones.

di·os·min (dye·oz′min, ·os′min) *n.* BAROSMIN (1).

Di·os·py·ros (dye·os′pi·ros) *n.* [Gk., gromwell, an herbaceous plant]. A genus of trees of the Styraceae. The bark of *Diospyros virginiana,* the persimmon tree of the United States, is astringent and bitter and has been used in diarrhea, intermittent fever, and uterine hemorrhage.

Diothane. Trademark for diperodon, a surface anesthetic and analgesic used as the hydrochloride salt.

di·otic (dye·o'tick, ·ot'ick) *adj.* [*di-* + *otic*]. Pertaining to both ears; BINAURAL.

di·ovu·lar (dye·o'vyoo·lur) *adj.* BIOVULAR.

di·ox·a·drol (dye·ock'suh·drole) *n.* 2-(2,2-Diphenyl-1,3-dioxolan-4-yl)piperidine, $C_{20}H_{23}NO_2$, an antidepressant usually used as the hydrochloride.

di·ox·an (dye·ock'san) *n.* DIOXANE.

di·ox·ane (dye·ock'sane) *n.* [*di-* + *ox-* + *-ane*]. 1,4-Diethylene dioxide, $C_4H_8O_2$, a colorless liquid miscible with water and many organic solvents. Employed as a solvent, and as a dehydrating agent in the process of paraffin embedding in histologic technique.

di·ox·ide (dye·ock'side, ·sid) *n.* [*di-* + *oxide*]. A molecule containing two atoms of oxygen which was formed (or presumably formed) by oxidation of the basic molecule.

Dioxogen. Trademark for a solution of hydrogen peroxide.

di·oxy·an·thra·nol (dye·ock"see·an'thruh·nol, ·nole) *n.* ANTHRALIN.

di·oxy·ben·zone (dye·ock"see·ben'zone) *n.* 2,2′-Dihydroxy-4-methoxybenzophenone, $C_{14}H_{12}O_4$, an ultraviolet screening compound.

di·ox·y·gen·ase (dy"ock'si·je·nace, ·naze) *n.* Any of a group of enzymes that catalyze the insertion of both atoms of an oxygen molecule into an organic substrate.

di·ox·y·line (dye·ock'si·leen) *n.* 1-(4-Ethoxy-3-methoxybenzyl)-6,7-dimethoxy-3-methylisoquinoline, $C_{22}H_{25}NO_4$, a synthetic analogue of papaverine with vasodilative action useful in coronary and other vascular spasms; used as the phosphate salt.

dip, *n.* 1. A bath containing a medicinal agent or agents, of sufficient quantity to allow total immersion, used in veterinary medicine in the treatment and prevention of disease caused by biologic agents active on the external surface of the body. 2. The medicinal substance or substances so used.

Di-Paralene. A trademark for chlorcyclizine, an antihistaminic drug used as the hydrochloride salt.

Diparcol. A trademark for diethazine, a drug used in parkinsonism; employed as the hydrochloride salt.

Dipaxin. Trademark for diphenadione, an orally effective anticoagulant drug.

di·pep·ti·dase (dye·pep'ti·dace, ·daze) *n.* An enzyme that splits dipeptides to amino acids.

di·pep·tide (dye·pep'tide) *n.* A chemical union of two molecules of amino acids obtained by condensation of the acids or by hydrolysis of proteins.

di·per·o·don (dye·perr'o·don) *n.* 3-(1-Piperidyl)-1,2-propanediol dicarbanilate, $C_{22}H_{27}N_3O_4$, a surface anesthetic and analgesic; used as the hydrochloride salt.

Di·pet·a·lo·ne·ma (dye·pet"uh·lo·nee'muh) *n.* A genus of filarial worms.

Dipetalonema per·stans (pur'stanz). A species of filarial worm found extensively in tropical regions, with man the definitive host.

di·pet·a·lo·ne·mi·a·sis (dye·pet"uh·lo·ne·migh'uh·sis) *n.* [*Dipetalonema* + *-iasis*]. Infection with *Dipetalonema perstans,* usually asymptomatic in man but sometimes causing cutaneous edema or elephantiasis.

di·phal·lus (dye·fal'us) *n.* [*di-* + *phallus*]. 1. Partial or complete doubling of the penis or clitoris. 2. An individual with such a condition. —**diphal·lic** (·ick) *adj.*

di·pha·sic (dye·fay'zick) *adj.* [*di-* + *phase* + *-ic*]. Having two phases.

diphasic antigens. Antigens such as those found in *Salmonella,* which exist in two phases, a specific phase and a group phase.

diphasic curve. Any curve consisting of two phases that are opposite in sign.

di·phem·a·nil methylsulfate (dye·fem'uh·nil). 4-Diphenylmethylene-1,1-dimethylpiperidinium methylsulfate, $C_{20}H_{24}N.CH_3SO_4$, a quaternary parasympatholytic agent used to inhibit gastric secretion and motility, relieve pylorospasm, and reduce sweating.

di·phen·a·di·one (dye·fen"uh·dye'ohn) *n.* Diphenylacetylindandione, $C_{23}H_{16}O_3$, an orally effective anticoagulant.

di·phen·an (dye·fen'an) *n.* *p*-Benzylphenyl carbamate, $C_{14}H_{13}NO_2$, a white powder, almost insoluble in water; employed in the treatment of oxyuriasis.

di·phen·hy·dra·mine (dye"fen·high'druh·meen, ·min) *n.* 2-(Benzhydryloxy)-*N,N*-dimethylethylamine, $C_{17}H_{21}NO$, an antihistaminic drug; used as the hydrochloride salt.

di·phen·i·cil·lin (dye·fen"i·sil'in) *n.* 2-Biphenylylpenicillin, $C_{21}H_{20}N_2O_4S$, a semisynthetic penicillin that is acid-resistant; administered as the sodium salt.

di·phen·i·dol (dye·fen'i·dol) *n.* α,α-Diphenyl-1-piperidinebutanol, $C_{21}H_{27}NO$, an antiemetic drug.

di·phen·ox·yl·ate (dye"fen·ock'sil·ate) *n.* 1-(3-Cyano-3,3-diphenylpropyl)-4-phenylpiperidine-4-carboxylic acid ethyl ester, $C_{30}H_{32}N_2O_2$, an antidiarrheal drug; used as the hydrochloride salt.

di·phen·yl·amine (dye·fen"il·uh·meen', ·am'een) *n.* $C_6H_5NHC_6H_5$. A reagent for nitrates, chlorates, and other oxidizing substances with which, in the presence of sulfuric acid, it gives a blue color.

di·phen·yl·chlo·ro·ar·sine (dye·fen"il·klor"o·ahr'seen) *n.* $(C_6H_5)_2AsCl$. A solid used as a sternutator in World War I.

di·phen·yl·hy·dan·to·in (dye·fen"il·high·dan'to·in, ·dan'toin, dye·fee"nil·) *n.* PHENYTOIN.

diphenyl ketone. BENZOPHENONE.

di·phen·yl·pyr·a·line (dye·fen"il·pirr'uh·leen) *n.* 4-(Diphenylmethoxy)-1-methylpiperidine, $C_{19}H_{23}NO$, an antihistaminic drug; used as the hydrochloride salt.

di·pho·nia (dye·fo'nee·uh) *n.* [*di-* + *-phonia*]. The production of two distinct tones during vocal utterance.

di·phos·pha·ti·dyl glycerol (dye"fos·fuh·tye'dil). CARDIOLIPIN.

di·phos·pho·gly·cer·ic acid (dye·fos"fo·gli·serr'ick). $C_3H_8O_9P_2$, an ester of glyceric acid with two molecules of phosphoric acid characterized by a high-energy phosphate bond. 1,3-Diphosphoglyceric acid is a normal glycolytic intermediate found in all cells. 2,3-Diphosphoglyceric acid, an isomer, is found in high concentration in the erythrocytes and is essential for the normal function of hemoglobin.

di·phos·pho·pyr·i·dine nucleotide (dye·fos"fo·pirr'i·deen, ·din). NICOTINAMIDE ADENINE DINUCLEOTIDE; NADIDE.

di·phos·pho·thi·amine (dye·fos"fo·thigh'uh·min) *n.* COCARBOXYLASE. Abbreviated, DPT.

diph·the·ria (dif·theer'ee·uh) *n.* [Gk. *diphthera*, piece of leather, + *-ia*]. An acute infectious disease caused by *Corynebacterium diphtheriae,* characterized by local inflammation and the formation of a false membrane primarily in the pharyngeal area; absorption of toxin may affect the heart and peripheral nerves. —**diphtherial** (·ree·ul), **diph·ther·ic** (·therr'ick, ·theer'ick) *adj.*

diphtheria antitoxin. Any crude or purified serum containing antibodies that specifically neutralize diphtheria toxin.

diphtheria bacillus. *CORYNEBACTERIUM DIPHTHERIAE.*

diphtheria toxin. The crystallized protein purified from culture filtrates of *Corynebacterium diphtheriae* which has deleterious effects on the heart, peripheral nerves, and other tissues, as evidenced in the disease diphtheria.

diphtheria toxin-antitoxin. A mixture of toxin and antitoxin used to produce active immunity against diphtheria; now superseded by diphtheria toxoid.

diphtheria toxoid. A detoxified diphtheria toxin used to produce active immunity against diphtheria, having the advantage over toxin-antitoxin of not producing sensitivity to serum. See also *absorbed diphtheria toxoid.*

diph·the·rit·ic (dif"the·rit'ick) *adj.* Pertaining to, caused by, or like diphtheria.

diphtheritic ataxia. A sequel of diphtheria preceding diphtheritic polyneuritis, in which ataxia is a prominent symptom.

diphtheritic conjunctivitis. A specific purulent inflammation of the conjunctiva due to *Corynebacterium diphtheriae.*

diphtheritic inflammation. A pseudomembranous fibrinous exudate due to infection with *Corynebacterium diphtheriae.*

diphtheritic laryngitis. Inflammation of the larynx with formation of a false membrane, occurring with diphtheria.

diphtheritic membrane. FALSE MEMBRANE.

diphtheritic necrosis. A special type of necrosis of a mucous membrane; characterized by the formation of a tough, leathery membrane composed of coagulated cells and fibrin.

diphtheritic neuritis. A complication of infection with *Corynebacterium diphtheriae,* presumably due to the action of diphtheritic toxin on peripheral nerves and nerve roots, resulting in a polyneuritis.

diphtheritic pharyngitis. Pharyngitis characterized by the presence of a false membrane, the product of the action of *Corynebacterium diphtheriae.*

diphtheritic ulcer. 1. Any ulcer caused by *Corynebacterium diphtheriae,* as in the throat or of the skin. 2. Loosely, any ulcer covered by a fibrinous exudate simulating diphtheria.

diph·the·roid (dif'the·roid) *adj. & n.* [*diphtheria* + *-oid*]. 1. Resembling diphtheria or the bacillus *Corynebacterium diphtheriae.* 2. Any of various unclassified bacteria morphologically resembling *Corynebacterium diphtheriae.* 3. PSEUDODIPHTHERIA.

diph·the·ro·tox·in (dif"the·ro·tock'sin) *n.* DIPHTHERIA TOXIN.

diph·thon·gia (dif·thon'jee·uh) *n.* [*di-* + Gk. *phthongos,* sound, tone, + *-ia*]. DIPHONIA.

diph·y·gen·ic (dif"i·jen'ick) *adj.* [Gk. *diphyēs,* of double form, + *-genic*]. *In zoology,* characterized by or having two types of development.

di·phyl·lo·both·ri·a·sis (dye·fil"o·both·rye'uh·sis) *n.* [*Diphyllobothrium* + *-iasis*]. Infection with *Diphyllobothrium latum.*

Di·phyl·lo·both·ri·um (dye·fil"o·both'ree·um) *n.* [*di-* + *phyllo-* + *bothrium*]. A genus of tapeworms. Formerly called *Dibothriocephalus.*

Diphyllobothrium er·i·na·cei (err·i·nay'see·eye). A species of tapeworm of which only the larval stage is found in man, the adult worm being found only in dogs and cats.

Diphyllobothrium la·tum (lay'tum). The fish tapeworm, a large tapeworm found in the intestine. The head has two suckers or bothria. The adult worm ranges from 3 to 10 meters in length, and may have over 4,000 proglottids. The definitive hosts are man, dog, and cat. The first intermediate hosts are freshwater copepods, and the secondary intermediate hosts are various freshwater fishes. Infection in man may cause disorders of the nervous and digestive systems, malnutrition, and anemia.

di·phy·o·dont (dye·fee'o·dont", dif'ee·o·) *adj.* [Gk. *diphyēs,* of double form, + *-odont*]. Having two sets of teeth, as the deciduous teeth and the permanent teeth.

dipl-, diplo- [Gk. *diploos*]. A combining form meaning *twofold, double, twin.*

dip·la·cu·sis (dip"luh·kew'sis) *n.* [*dipl-* + Gk. *akousis,* hearing]. The hearing of the same sound differently by one ear than by the other.

diplacusis bin·au·ra·lis (bin"aw·ray'lis). Perception of a single tone as having a higher fundamental pitch in one ear than in the other.

diplacusis uni·au·ra·lis (yoo"nee·aw·ray'lis). Hearing of two tones by one ear when only one tone is produced.

di·plas·mat·ic (dye"plaz·mat'ick) *adj.* Containing matter other than protoplasm, said of cells.

di·ple·gia (dye·plee'jee·uh) *n.* [*di-* + *-plegia*]. Paralysis of similar parts on the two sides of the body. See also *spastic diplegia, cerebral palsy.* —**diple·gic** (·jick) *adj.*

diplegia fa·ci·a·lis (fay·shee·ay'lis). Bilateral weakness or paralysis of the facial muscles, referring usually to paralysis of lower motor neuron type.

diplo-. See *dipl-.*

dip·lo·al·bu·min·uria (dip"lo·al·bew"mi·new'ree·uh) *n.* [*diplo-* + *albuminuria*]. The coexistence or alternation of physiologic and pathologic proteinuria in the same individual.

dip·lo·ba·cil·lus (dip"lo·ba·sil'us) *n.* [*diplo-* + *bacillus*]. A pair of bacilli, joined end to end, as the result of incomplete fission.

dip·lo·blas·tic (dip"lo·blas'tick) *adj.* [*diplo-* + *blast-* + *-ic*]. Having two germ layers, ectoderm and entoderm.

dip·lo·car·di·ac (dip"lo·kahr'dee·ack) *adj.* [*diplo-* + *cardiac*]. Having a double heart, or one in which the two sides are more or less separate, as in birds and mammals.

dip·lo·ce·pha·lia (dip"lo·se·fay'lee·uh) *n.* [*diplo-* + *-cephalia*]. *Obsol.* DICEPHALISM.

dip·lo·ceph·a·lus (dip"lo·sef'uh·lus) *n.* [*diplo-* + *-cephalus*]. DICEPHALUS. —**diplocephalous,** *adj.*

dip·lo·ceph·a·ly (dip"lo·sef'uh·lee) *n.* [*diplo-* + *-cephaly*]. *Obsol.* DICEPHALISM.

dip·lo·coc·coid (dip"lo·kock'oid) *adj.* [*diplo-* + *coccoid*]. Resembling a diplococcus.

dip·lo·coc·cus (dip"lo·kock'us) *n.*, pl. **diplococ·ci** (·sigh) [*diplo-* + *coccus*]. A micrococcus that occurs in groups of two, such as the pneumococcus.

Diplococcus, *n.* A genus of bacteria of the family Lactobacteriaceae of the tribe Streptococceae.

Diplococcus go·nor·rhoe·ae (gon"o·ree'ee). *NEISSERIA GONORRHOEAE.*

Diplococcus in·tra·cel·lu·la·ris men·in·git·i·dis (in·truh·sel·yoo·lair'is men·in·jit'i·dis) *NEISSERIA MENINGITIDIS.*

Diplococcus pneu·mo·ni·ae (new·mo'nee·ee). *STREPTOCOCCUS PNEUMONIAE.*

dip·lo·co·ria (dip"lo·ko'ree·uh) *n.* [*diplo-* + *cor-* + *-ia*]. Polycoria in which there are two pupils. Syn. *double pupil.*

dip·loë (dip'lo·ee) *n.* [Gk. *diploē,* fold] [NA]. The cancellous bone between the outer and inner tables of the bones of the skull. —**dip·lo·et·ic** (dip"lo·et'ick) *adj.*

dip·lo·gen·e·sis (dip"lo·jen'e·sis) *n.* [*diplo-* + *genesis*]. Development of a double or twin monstrosity.

Dip·lo·go·nop·o·rus (dip"lo·go·nop'uh·rus) *n.* [*diplo-* + *gono-* + Gk. *poros,* pore]. A genus of cestodes or tapeworms.

Diplogonoporus gran·dis (gran'dis). A species of tapeworm normally infecting whales and seals, with man accidentally infected by the ingestion of saltwater fishes, the second intermediate hosts.

di·plo·ic (di·plo'ick) *adj.* Of or pertaining to the diploë.

di·plo·i·cin (di·plo'i·sin) *n.* An antibiotic substance produced by the lichen *Buellia canescens.*

diploic mastoid. A mastoid process with some marrow within the bone.

diploic veins. The large, thin-walled veins occupying bony channels in the diploë of cranial bones, and communicating with each other, with meningeal veins and sinuses of the dura mater, and, through emissary veins, with the veins of the pericranium. NA *venae diploicae.* See also Table of Veins in the Appendix.

dip·loid (dip'loid) *adj.* [*di-* + *-ploid*]. Having double the haploid or gametic number of chromosomes.

dip·lo·kar·y·on (dip"lo·kăr'ee·on) *n.* [*diplo-* + *karyon*]. A nucleus with twice the diploid number of chromosomes.

dip·lo·mate (dip'lo·mate) *n.* An individual who has received a diploma or certificate; specifically, one who is certified by an American specialty board as having satisfied all its requirements and passed its examinations, and as being qualified to practice that specialty.

dip·lo·mel·li·tu·ria (dip"lo·mel"i·tew'ree·uh) *n.* [*diplo-* + *melituria*]. Coexistence or alternation of diabetic and nondiabetic glycosuria in the same individual.

dip·lo·my·e·lia (dip"lo·migh·ee'lee·uh) *n.* [*diplo-* + *-myelia*]. DIASTEMATOMYELIA.

dip·lo·ne·ma (dip"lo·nee'muh) *n.*, pl. **diplonema·ta** (·tuh),

diplonemas [*diplo-* + *-nema*]. The chromosomes in the diplotene stage.

dip·lo·neu·ral (dip″lo·new′rul) *adj.* [*diplo-* + *neural*]. Pertaining to a muscle supplied by two nerves from different sources.

di·plop·a·gus (di·plop′uh·gus) *n.*, pl. **diplopa·gi** (·guy, ·jye) [*diplo-* + *-pagus*]. Equally developed conjoined twins.

dip·lo·pho·nia (dip″lo·fo′nee·uh) *n.* DIPHONIA.

di·plo·pia (di·plo′pee·uh) *n.* [*dipl-* + *-opia*]. A disorder of sight in which one object is perceived as two. Syn. *double vision.* See also *binocular, crossed, homonymous, monocular, and physiologic diplopia.*

di·plo·pi·om·e·ter (di·plo″pee·om′e·tur) *n.* [*diplopia* + *-meter*]. An instrument for measuring the degree of diplopia.

dip·lo·scope (dip′lo·skope) *n.* [*diplo-* + *-scope*]. An instrument for the investigation of binocular vision.

di·plo·sis (di·plo′sis) *n.*, pl. **diplo·ses** (·seez) [Gk. *diplōsis*, doubling]. The establishment of the full double number of chromosomes by fusion of two haploid sets in fertilization.

dip·lo·tene (dip′lo·teen) *n.* [*diplo-* + *-tene*]. The stage in the first meiotic prophase in which the tetrads exhibit chiasmata. See also *leptotene, pachytene, zygotene.*

Diplovax. A trademark for live oral polio virus vaccine.

di·po·lar (dye·po′lur) *adj.* [*di-* + *polar*]. BIPOLAR.

dipolar ion. ZWITTERION.

di·pole (dye′pole) *n.* [*di-* + *pole*]. 1. A particle or object bearing opposite charges. 2. A pair of electric charges, positive and negative, situated near each other in a conducting medium.

dipole moment. The measure of the electric asymmetry of a molecule. It is equal to the product of the ionic charges and their spatial separation.

di·po·tas·si·um phosphate (dye″po·tas′ee·um). DIBASIC POTASSIUM PHOSPHATE.

Dip·pel's oil [J. C. *Dippel*, German alchemist, 1673–1734]. BONE OIL.

dip·ping, *n.* 1. Palpation of an abdominal organ, particularly the liver, by quick depression of the abdomen. 2. *In veterinary medicine,* the act of submerging an animal for the application of a dip.

dip·pol·dism (dip′ol·diz·um) *n.* [*Dippold*, German schoolteacher tried and convicted of manslaughter]. Flogging of children, especially school children.

di·pro·so·pia (dye″pro·so′pee·uh, dip″ro·) *n.* [*di-* + *prosop-* + *-ia*]. *In teratology,* duplication of the face.

di·pro·so·pus (dye·pro′so·pus, dye″pro·so′pus) *n.* An individual with doubling of the face.

diprosopus dir·rhi·nus (di·rye′nus). An individual with partial or complete doubling of the nose.

diprosopus par·a·sit·i·cus (păr·uh·sit′i·kus). An individual with doubling of the face, one face being markedly smaller or less well formed.

diprosopus tet·roph·thal·mus (tet″rof·thal′mus). An individual exhibiting duplicity of the face with four eyes, two noses, two mouths, and two, three, or four ears.

diprosopus tetrophthalmus te·tro·tus (te·tro′tus). An individual with two complete faces with four eyes and four ears.

di·pros·o·py (dye·pros′uh·pee) *n.* DIPROSOPIA.

dip·set·ic (dip·set′ick) *adj.* [Gk. *dipsētikos*, from *dipsa*, thirst]. Causing or characterized by thirst.

dip·so·ma·nia (dip″so·may′nee·uh) *n.* [Gk. *dipsa*, thirst, + *-mania*]. Recurrent periodic compulsion to excessive drinking of alcoholic beverages. —**dipsoma·ni·ac** (·nee·ack) *n.*

dip·so·pho·bia (dip″so·fo′bee·uh) *n.* [Gk. *dipsa*, thirst, + *-phobia*]. An abnormal fear of drinking, especially of alcoholic beverages.

dip·so·rex·ia, dip·sor·rhex·ia (dip″so·reck′see·uh) *n.* [Gk. *dipsa*, thirst, + *-orexia*]. The early stage of chronic alcoholism before the appearance of neurologic or systemic deficits.

dip·so·ther·a·py (dip″so·therr′uh·pee) *n.* [Gk. *dipsa*, thirst, + *therapy*]. Treatment of certain diseases by reducing the amount of fluid allowed the patient.

Dip·tera (dip′tur·uh) *n. pl.* [Gk. neuter pl. of *dipteros*, two-winged]. An order of two-winged insects; includes mosquitoes, flies, midges.

dip·ter·an (dip′tur·un) *adj. & n.* 1. Of or pertaining to insects of the order Diptera. 2. Any insect of the order Diptera.

Dip·tero·car·pus (dip″tur·o·kahr′pus) *n.* [Gk. *dipteros*, two-winged, + Gk. *karpos*, fruit]. A genus of trees, chiefly found in southern Asia, some of which furnish gurjun balsam.

dip·ter·ous (dip′tur·us) *adj.* [Gk. *dipteros*, from *di-* + Gk. *pteron*, wing]. *In biology,* having two wings or wing-like processes.

di·pus (dye′pus) *adj.* [Gk. *dipous*, from *di-* + *pous*, foot]. Having two feet.

di·py·gus (di·pye′gus, dip′i·gus) *n.* [*di-* + *pyg-* + *-us*]. A monster with more or less duplication of the pelvis, lower parts of the back, and inferior extremities.

dipygus par·a·sit·i·cus (păr″uh·sit′i·kus). A monster having attached to its abdomen a more or less complete parasitic body.

dipygus tet·ra·pus (tet′ruh·pus). A dipygus with four legs.

dipygus tri·pus (trye′pus). A dipygus with three legs.

dip·y·li·di·a·sis (dip″i·li·dye′uh·sis) *n.* [*Dipylidium* + *-iasis*]. Infection with *Dipylidium caninum,* the common tapeworm of dogs.

Di·py·lid·i·um (dye″pye·lid′ee·um) *n.* A genus of tapeworms.

Dipylidium ca·ni·num (ka·nigh′num). A species of tapeworm, 20 to 40 cm in length, of which the dog and cat are definitive hosts, and man is an occasional host; fleas and lice harbor the larval stage, thus acting as vectors.

di·pyr·id·a·mole (dye·pirr′i·duh·mole, ·pi·rid′uh·) *n.* 2,6-Bis-(diethanolamino)-4,8-dipiperidinopyrimidino[5,4-δ-]pyrimidine, $C_{24}H_{40}N_8O_4$, a vasodilator used for relief of anginal pain.

di·pyr·i·thi·one (dye·pirr″i·thigh′ohn) *n.* 2,2′-Dithiobispyridine-1,1-dioxide, $C_{10}H_8N_2O_2S_2$, an antifungal, antibacterial agent.

di·py·rone (dye·pye′rone) *n.* Sodium (antipyrinylmethylamino) methanesulfonate, $C_{13}H_{16}N_3NaO_4S$, an analgesic and antipyretic; may cause agranulocytosis.

direct calorimetry. Actual measurement of the heat produced by an animal enclosed in a box or suitable enclosure; generally used experimentally.

direct cerebellar tract. POSTERIOR SPINOCEREBELLAR TRACT.

direct Coombs test [R. R. A. *Coombs*]. ANTIGLOBULIN TEST.

direct current. An electric current that flows continuously in one direction. Abbreviated, dc, DC. Contr. *alternating current.*

direct developing test. ANTIGLOBULIN TEST.

direct diplopia. HOMONYMOUS DIPLOPIA.

direct emetic. An emetic acting directly on the stomach.

direct emmenagogue. An emmenagogue acting directly on the generative organs.

direct excitation. The stimulation of an electrically excitable tissue by placing an electrode on the tissue itself.

direct hernia. An inguinal hernia in which the sac does not leave the abdominal cavity through the abdominal inguinal ring but through a defect in the floor of the inguinal triangle, between the inferior epigastric artery and the outer edge of the rectus abdominis muscle.

direct illumination. VERTICAL ILLUMINATION.

direct image. An image formed by rays that have not yet come to a focus. Contr. *inverted image.*

directive therapy. *In psychiatry,* a method of treatment which implies that the therapist understands the patient's needs and problems better than the patient, and makes deliberate efforts to change the patient's attitudes, behavior, or mode of living. See also *suppressive psychotherapy, prestige-suggestion.*

direct laryngoscopy. Examination of the interior of the

larynx by direct vision with the aid of a laryngoscope.

direct light reflex. Contraction of the sphincter pupillae induced by a ray of light thrown upon the retina.

direct murmur. A murmur produced by organic obstruction to the flow of blood.

direct ophthalmoscopy. Examination of the ocular fundus using an ophthalmoscope the optics of which gives an erect or upright image.

direct percussion. Percussion performed by striking the skin directly with the pads of one or two fingers without the interposition of a pleximeter.

direct platelet count. A count of suitably diluted platelets in a hemocytometer in contrast to the indirect platelet count, a computation based on the proportion of platelets to erythrocytes in a smear.

direct pupillary reflex. DIRECT LIGHT REFLEX.

direct red C, R, or **Y.** CONGO RED.

direct reflex. A reflex response on the same side as that of the stimulus.

direct respiration. Respiration in which the living substance of an organism, as an ameba, takes oxygen directly from the surrounding medium, and returns carbon dioxide directly to it, no blood being present.

direct symptom. A symptom depending directly upon the disease.

direct transfusion. The transfusion of blood immediately from one person to another without an intermediate container or exposure of the blood to the air.

direct vision. CENTRAL VISION.

dirhinus, dirhynus. DIRRHINUS.

Di·ro·fi·lar·ia (dye″ro·fi·lăr′ee·uh, ·fi·lair′ee·uh) *n.* [L. *dirus*, ominous, + *filaria*]. A genus of filarial worms. Members of the species *Dirofilaria immitis, D. magalhaesi,* and *D. repens* are parasites of dogs.

Dirofilaria con·junc·ti·vae (kon″junk·tye′vee). A species of filarial worm reported in many areas of the Mediterranean basin and found in such diverse sites as the eyelids, conjunctiva, lips, and gastrosplenic ligament.

Dirofilaria im·mi·tis (i·migh′tis). The heartworm, an important filarial parasite of dogs and other Canidae, occurring primarily in tropical and subtropical regions, including the southern and southeastern coastal regions of the United States. The larvae are transmitted by the bite of mosquitoes and fleas, and the adult worms are found in the right ventricle and pulmonary artery of the canine host. Affected animals exhibit weakness, dyspnea, and cardiac hypertrophy, and may die from right heart failure or pulmonary embolism. Rare infections have been reported in man.

di·ro·fil·a·ri·a·sis (dye″ro·fil″uh·rye′uh·sis) *n.* Infection with worms of the genus *Dirofilaria.*

dir·rhi·nus, dir·rhy·nus (di·rye′nus) *n.* [*di-* + *-rrhinus*]. Partial or complete doubling of the nose; a mild degree of diprosopia.

dirt eating. GEOPHAGY.

dis-, di- [L., apart, asunder]. A prefix meaning (a) *separation;* (b) *reversal;* (c) *apart from.* Compare *di-, dis-.*

dis·abil·i·ty, *n.* A persistent physical or mental defect, weakness, or handicap which prevents a person from engaging in ordinary activities or normal life, or from performing a specific job.

di·sac·cha·ri·dase (dye·sack′uh·ri·dace) *n.* An enzyme that causes hydrolysis of disaccharide, producing two monosaccharides.

di·sac·cha·ride (dye·sack′uh·ride, ·rid) *n.* [*di-* + *saccharide*]. A carbohydrate formed by the condensation of two monosaccharide molecules.

dis·ag·gre·ga·tion (dis·ag″re·gay′shun) *n.* [*dis-* + *aggregation*]. 1. A state of perpetual distraction which prevents an individual from entertaining any idea other than the one which dominates or occupies his mind, as in the obsessive compulsive neurosis. 2. In hysteria, an inability to coordinate various new sensations and to connect them with visual impressions.

dis·ar·tic·u·la·tion (dis″ahr·tick″yoo·lay′shun) *n.* [*dis-* + *articulation*]. 1. Amputation at a joint. 2. Separation at a joint. **—disar·tic·u·late** (·tick′yoo·late) *v.*

dis·as·sim·i·la·tion (dis″uh·sim″i·lay′shun) *n.* CATABOLISM.

dis·as·so·ci·a·tion (dis″uh·so″see·ay′shun) *n.* [*dis-* + *association*]. The separation of a substance, initially present in a more complex state of organization, into its simpler parts, as when water in the form of $(H_2O)_2$ or $(H_2O)_3$ disassociates to single molecules of H_2O.

dis·as·sort·a·tive (dis″uh·sor′tuh·tiv) *adj.* [*dis-* + *assortative*]. Pertaining to selection on the basis of dissimilarity.

disassortative mating. Preferential, nonrandom mating based upon phenotypic dissimilarity. Contr. *assortative mating.*

disazo-. A combining form indicating *the presence* (in a compound) *of two azo* (—N=N—) *groups.* Compare *diaz-.*

disc. DISK.

disc-, disco-. A combining form meaning *disk.*

[1]dis·charge (dis·chahrj′) *v.* [MF. *descharger*]. 1. To emit, unload. 2. To release, dismiss.

[2]dis·charge (dis′chahrj) *n.* 1. An emission, unloading, evacuation, or secretion. 2. That which is emitted. 3. *In electricity,* a setting free or escape of stored-up energy; the equalization of differences of potential between the poles of a condenser or other sources of electricity by connecting or nearly connecting them with a conductor. 4. The generation and transmission of impulses by a neuron.

discharging lesion. A brain lesion that may be accompanied by irregular discharges of electrical activity as recorded by the electroencephalogram or as seen clinically in focal seizures. Contr. *destructive lesion (2).*

disci. Plural and genitive singular of *discus.*

dis·ci·form (dis′ki·form, dis′i·form) *adj.* [*disc* + *-iform*]. Disk-shaped; DISCOID.

disciform keratitis. A localized, subacute, nonsuppurative inflammation of the corneal stroma characterized by a discoid opacity, most commonly resulting from herpes simplex infection. Syn. *keratitis disciformis.* Compare *dendritic keratitis.*

disciform macular degeneration. Degeneration of the basal membrane of the choroid in the region of the macula lutea with the deposition of connective tissue under this membrane. Syn. *Kuhnt-Junius disease.*

disci in·ter·ver·te·bra·les (in″tur·vur″te·bray′leez) [NA]. INTERVERTEBRAL DISKS.

dis·cis·sion (di·sish′un, ·sizh′un) *n.* [L. *discissio,* from *discindere,* to tear apart, from *di-* + *scindere,* to tear]. 1. A tearing or being torn apart. 2. *In eye surgery,* an operation for soft cataract in which the capsule is lacerated a number of times to allow the lens substance to be absorbed.

discission needle. An instrument used for cutting the capsule of the lens or for cutting an inflammatory membrane in certain types of cataracts or aftercataract.

dis·ci·tis, dis·ki·tis (disk·eye′tis) *n.* [*disc-* + *-itis*]. Inflammation of a disk, especially of an intervertebral or articular disk.

disc kidney. DISK KIDNEY.

dis·clos·ing material. Wax or a silicone paste applied to the tissue surface of a removable dental prosthesis which, after seating of the denture in function, reveals areas of undesirable pressure.

disclosing solution. A liquid agent used to stain and render more observable deposits on the teeth.

disco-. See *disc-.*

dis·co·blas·tu·la (dis″ko·blas′tew·luh) *n.* A blastula produced by meroblastic, discoidal cleavage.

dis·cob·o·lus attitude (dis·kob′uh·lus) [Gk. *diskobolos,* quoit-thrower]. A position of the body, like that of a discus thrower, assumed as a result of stimulation of one labyrinth. The trunk, head, and arms are turned toward the side stimulated in order to counteract the false sensation of falling in the opposite direction.

dis·co·gas·tru·la (dis″ko·gas′troo·luh) *n.* The modified type of gastrula produced by meroblastic, discoidal cleavage of telolecithal ova.

discogram. DISKOGRAM.

dis·coid (dis′koid) *adj.* & *n.* [Gk. *diskoeidēs*]. 1. Shaped like a disk. 2. Of or pertaining to a disk. 3. A dental carving instrument having a blade in the form of a disk.

dis·coi·dal (dis·koy′dul) *adj.* DISCOID.

discoidal cleavage. Meroblastic cleavage limited to the germinal disk, as in telolecithal avian ova.

discoid lupus erythematosus. CHRONIC DISCOID LUPUS ERYTHEMATOSUS.

discoid placenta. A placenta shaped like a disk.

dis·col·or·a·tion (dis·kul″ur·ay′shun) *n.* Change in color, as of a tissue, part, or fluid. —**dis·col·or** (dis·kul′ur) *v.*

dis·com·po·si·tion (dis″kom·puh·zish′un) *n.* [*dis-* + *composition*]. A process by which an atom is dislodged from its position in a crystal lattice by direct nuclear collision.

dis·con·nec·tion or **dis·con·nex·ion syndrome.** The effects of lesions of cerebral association pathways, either those which lie exclusively within a single hemisphere or those which join the two halves of the brain, as manifested by various types of agnosia, apraxia, and aphasia.

dis·con·tin·u·ous phase. The particles, droplets, or bubbles of an insoluble or immiscible substance that are distributed through the dispersion medium in a colloidal system.

dis·cop·a·thy (dis·kop′uh·thee) *n.* [*disc* + *-pathy*]. Any disease process involving an intervertebral disk.

dis·coph·o·rous (dis·kof′uh·rus) *adj.* [*disco-* + *-phorous*]. Furnished with a disklike organ or part.

dis·co·pla·cen·ta (dis″ko·pluh·sen′tuh) *n.* DISCOID PLACENTA.

dis·cor·dance (dis·kor′dunce) *n.* A state of difference between twins with respect to a particular trait or disease. Contr. *concordance.*

discoria. DYSCORIA.

dis·crete, *adj.* [*discretus,* from L. *discernere,* to separate]. Not running together; separate. Contr. *confluent.*

discrete smallpox. A form of smallpox in which the pustules preserve their distinct form.

disc-shaped cataract. A rare total congenital cataract in which there is a depressed opaque central core surrounded by a clear lens of normal size and thickness, forming a ring resembling a life preserver; usually due to the absence of the embryonic nucleus and inherited as an autosomal dominant, and occasionally the result of discission or a perforating corneal ulcer.

dis·cus (dis′kus) *n.*, pl. & genit. sing. **dis·ci** (·kye, ·eye) [L.]. DISK.

discus ar·ti·cu·la·ris (ahr·tick·yoo·lair′is) [NA]. ARTICULAR DISK.

discus articularis ar·ti·cu·la·ti·o·nis acro·mio·cla·vi·cu·la·ris (ahr·tick″yoo·lay·shee·o′nis a·kro″mee·o·kla·vick″yoo·lair′is) [NA]. The articular disk of the acromioclavicular joint.

discus articularis articulationis man·di·bu·la·ris (man·dib″yoo·lair′is) [BNA]. DISCUS ARTICULARIS ARTICULATIONIS TEMPOROMANDIBULARIS.

discus articularis articulationis ra·dio·ul·na·ris di·sta·lis (ray″dee·o·ul·nair′is dis·tay′lis) [NA]. The articular disk of the distal radioulnar joint.

discus articularis articulationis ster·no·cla·vi·cu·la·ris (stur″no·kla·vick″yoo·lair′is) [NA]. The articular disk of the sternoclavicular joint.

discus articularis articulationis tem·po·ro·man·di·bu·la·ris (tem″puh·ro·man·dib″yoo·lair′is) [NA]. The articular disk of either temporomandibular joint.

discus in·ter·pu·bi·cus (in·tur·pew′bi·kus) [NA]. The fibrocartilage of the pubic symphysis.

discus ner·vi op·ti·ci (nur′vye op′ti·sigh) [NA]. OPTIC DISK.

discus pro·li·ge·rus (pro·lij′e·rus). CUMULUS OOPHORUS.

dis·cu·tient (dis·kew′shee·unt) *adj.* & *n.* [L. *discutere,* to disperse]. 1. Causing dispersion or disappearance, as of a swelling. 2. A discutient remedy.

dis·ease, *n.* [*dis-* + F. *aise,* ease]. 1. The failure of the adaptive mechanisms of an organism to counteract adequately the stimuli or stresses to which it is subject, resulting in a disturbance in function or structure of any part, organ, or system of the body. A response to injury; sickness or illness. 2. A specific entity which is the sum total of the numerous expressions of one or more pathological processes. The cause of a disease entity is represented by the cause of the basic pathological process in combination with important secondary causative factors.

disease potential. The sum of adverse health factors present in a population, which have a bearing upon the incidence of disease to be anticipated.

dis·en·gage·ment (dis″in·gaij′munt) *n.* [F. *désengager*]. 1. Emergence from a confined state; especially the emergence of the head of the fetus from the vagina during parturition. 2. The release from personal ties, obligations, occupation, or other constraints on one's life. —**disengage,** *v.*

dis·equi·lib·ri·um (dis·ee″kwi·lib′ree·um) *n.* [*dis-* + *equilibrium*]. Lack or loss of balance, as of bodily or mental balance, or as between the intellectual and moral faculties.

disgerminoma. DYSGERMINOMA.

dis·gre·ga·tion (dis″gre·gay′shun) *n.* [L. *disgregare,* to separate, from *grex, gregis,* flock]. Dispersion; separation, as of molecules or cells. —**dis·gre·gate** (dis′gre·gate) *v.*

dish-face. SCAPHOID FACE.

dis·im·pact (dis″im·pakt′) *v.* To remove an impaction.

dis·in·fect (dis″in·fekt′) *v.* To kill pathogenic agents by direct application of chemical or physical means, especially in the cleansing of inanimate objects. Compare *antisepsis.* —**disin·fec·tion** (·feck′shun) *n.*

dis·in·fec·tant (dis″in·feck′tunt) *n.* & *adj.* 1. An agent that destroys or inhibits the microorganisms causing disease. 2. Used as or having the action of a disinfectant.

dis·in·fes·ta·tion (dis·in″fes·tay′shun) *n.* [*dis-* + *infestation*]. Extermination of insects, rodents, or animal parasites present on an individual or in his surroundings.

dis·in·hi·bi·tion (dis·in″hi·bish′un) *n.* [*dis-* + *inhibition*]. Revival of an extinguished conditioned response by an unconditioned stimulus.

dis·in·ser·tion (dis″in·sur′shun) *n.* [*dis-* + *insertion*]. 1. Rupture of a tendon at its point of insertion into bone. 2. A circumferentially oriented tear in the extreme periphery of the retina where it terminates at the pars plana; common in juvenile retinal detachment and may occur following trauma. Syn. *retinodialysis.*

dis·in·te·grate (dis·in′te·grate) *v.* [*dis-* + *integrate*]. To break up or decompose. —**dis·in·te·gra·tion** (dis·in″te·gray′shun) *n.*

disintegration constant. DECAY CONSTANT.

disintegration rate. DECAY RATE.

dis·in·te·gra·tor (dis·in′te·gray·tur) *n.* A substance included in the formulation of a tablet to effect its disintegration in the presence of water and release its active ingredient for prompt medicinal action.

dis·in·vag·i·na·tion (dis″in·vaj″i·nay′shun) *n.* The reduction or relief of an invagination.

Disipal. A trademark for orphenadrine, an antispasmodic and antitremor drug used as the hydrochloride salt.

dis·joint, *adj.* [MF. *desjoint,* from *desjoindre*]. Disarticulate; separate, as bones from their natural relations.

dis·junc·tion (dis·junk′shun) *n.* [L. *disjunctio,* from *disjungere,* to disjoin]. 1. Moving apart, divergence. 2. Segregation of homologous chromosomes in first meiotic division or of products of chromosomal duplication in second meiotic division or in mitosis. —**disjunc·tive** (·tiv) *adj.*

disjunctive absorption. Separation of a slough or necrotic part by the absorption of a thin layer of the healthy tissue immediately adjacent to and surrounding it.

disk, disc, *n.* [L. *discus,* quoit, disk, dish, from Gk. *diskos*]. A circular, platelike organ or structure.

diskitis. DISCITIS.

disk kidney. A congenital defect in which both kidneys are fused into one mass, usually on one side of the midline. Compare *cake kidney.*

dis·ko·gram, dis·co·gram (dis'ko·gram) *n.* [*disco-* + *-gram*]. A roentgenogram produced in radiographic examination of intervertebral disks employing the direct injection of radiopaque medium.

dis·lo·ca·tion (dis''lo·kay'shun) *n.* [*dis-* + L. *locare,* to place]. The displacement of one or more bones of a joint or of any organ from the original position. See also *diastasis, displacement, subluxation.* **—dis·lo·cate** (dis'lo·kate, dis·lo'kate) *v.*

dislocation of the lens. A displacement of the crystalline lens of the eye.

dis·mem·bered pyeloplasty. Plastic repair of the uteropelvic junction to overcome obstruction in which the ureter is completely severed from the renal pelvis, then reanastomosed.

dis·mu·ta·tion (dis''mew·tay'shun) *n.* [*dis-* + *mutation*]. *In chemistry,* a reaction in which two molecules of the same compound interact to yield one oxidized and one reduced product.

dis·oc·clude (dis''uh·klude') *v.* [*dis-* + *occlude*]. To grind or level a tooth surface so that it will fail to touch the opposing tooth in the other jaw during mastication.

di·so·di·um cro·mo·gly·cate (dye·so'dee·um kro''mo·glye'sate). CROMOLYN SODIUM.

disodium edathamil. DISODIUM EDETATE.

disodium ed·e·tate (ed'e·tate). Disodium ethylenediaminetetraacetate dihydrate, $C_{10}H_{14}N_2Na_2O_8.2H_2O$, a white, crystalline powder, freely soluble in water. It has an affinity for calcium ions (and metal ions generally) and is used for treatment of diseases in which there is hypercalcemia or pathologic calcification, and in lead poisoning.

disodium EDTA. DISODIUM EDETATE.

disodium hydrogen citrate. $C_6H_6O_7Na_2$, a systemic alkalizer.

disodium hydrogen phosphate. SODIUM PHOSPHATE.

di·so·ma (dye·so'muh) *n.,* pl. **disomas, disoma·ta** (·tuh) [*di-* + *soma*]. A monster having two trunks. In some classifications the term is used to cover all monochorionic twinning.

Disomer. A trademark for dexbrompheniramine maleate, an antihistaminic.

di·so·mus (dye·so'mus) *n.,* pl. **diso·mi** (·migh), **disomuses** [Gk. *disōmos,* double-bodied]. DISOMA.

di·so·pyr·a·mide (dye''so·pirr'uh·mide) *n.* α-[2-(Diisopropylamino)ethyl]-α-phenyl-2-pyridineacetamide, $C_{21}H_{29}N_3O$, an antiarrhythmic cardiac depressant.

dis·or·der, *n.* [*dis-* + *order*]. A disturbance or derangement of regular or normal physical or mental health or function.

dis·ori·en·ta·tion (dis·or''ee·en·tay'shun) *n.* [*dis-* + *orientation*]. Loss of normal relationship to one's surroundings; particularly the ability to comprehend time, place, and people, such as occurs in organic brain syndromes.

Disotate. A trademark for edetate disodium, a calcium chelating agent.

dis·pa·rate (dis'pur·ut) *adj.* [L. *disparatus,* separated; assimilated in meaning to L. *dispar,* unlike]. Not alike; unequal or unmated.

disparate point. One of the points on the retina from which images are projected, not to the same, but to different points in space.

dispareunia. DYSPAREUNIA.

dis·par·i·ty (dis·păr'i·tee) *n.* [F. *disparité,* from *dis-* + L. *paritas,* parity]. Difference; inequality.

dis·pen·sa·ry (dis·pen'suh·ree) *n.* [ML. *dispensaria*]. 1. A place where medicine or medical aid is given free or at low cost to ambulatory patients. 2. In a place of business, a medical office provided by the owner to serve sick or injured employees. 3. *In military medicine,* a medical treatment facility primarily intended to provide examination and treatment for ambulatory patients, to make necessary arrangements for the transfer of patients requiring bed care, and to provide first aid for emergency cases. 4. Any place where drugs or medications are dispensed.

dis·pen·sa·to·ry (dis·pen'suh·to''ree) *n.* A book containing a systematic discussion of medicinal agents, including origin, preparation, description, use, and mode of action.

dis·pense, *v.* [L. *dispensare,* to distribute]. To prepare and distribute (medicines).

di·sper·mine (dye·spur'meen, ·min) *n.* PIPERAZINE.

di·sper·my (dye'spur·mee) *n.* [*di-* + *sperm* + *-y*]. Entrance of two spermatozoa into an ovum.

dispersed or **disperse phase.** DISCONTINUOUS PHASE.

dispersing lens. BICONCAVE LENS.

dis·per·sion (dis·pur'zhun) *n.* [L. *dispersio,* from *dispergere,* to scatter]. 1. The act of scattering; any scattering of light, as that passed through ground glass. 2. A system consisting of an insoluble or immiscible substance dispersed throughout a continuous medium. **—dis·perse** (·purce') *v. & adj.;* **disper·sive** (·siv) *adj.*

dispersion medium. The homogeneous gas, liquid, or solid in which particles, droplets, or bubbles of an insoluble or immiscible substance are dispersed. Syn. *continuous medium.*

dis·per·soid (dis·pur'soid) *n.* [*disperse* + *-oid*]. A colloid or finely divided substance.

displaced testis. A testis in an abnormal situation, as in the pelvic cavity.

dis·place·ment, *n.* 1. Removal from the normal position; dislocation, luxation; dystopia. 2. *In pharmacy,* a process of percolation. 3. *In chemistry,* a change in which one element is replaced by another element. 4. *In psychiatry,* a defense mechanism in which an emotion is unconsciously transferred or displaced from its original object, as a person or situation that is disturbing to the ego, to a more acceptable, less disturbing substitute. **—dis·place,** *v.*

displacement method. A method of treating sinus disease by utilizing negative pressure to displace contents of the sinus.

displacement threshold acuity. In visual acuity, such as vernier or stereoscopic acuity, the minimal displacement of one part of the test object, such as a line, with respect to another part, which can be appreciated.

dis·po·si·tion, *n.* [L. *dispositio,* arrangement, from *disponere,* to arrange]. 1. PREDISPOSITION. 2. TEMPERAMENT.

dis·pro·por·tion, *n.* [*dis-* + *proportion*]. An abnormal size relationship between two elements.

dis·rup·tive, *adj.* [L. *disrumpere,* to burst asunder]. Bursting; rending.

dis·sect (di·sekt', dye·) *v.* [L. *dissecare,* to cut apart, from *secare,* to cut]. 1. To divide or separate along natural lines of cleavage. 2. To cut or separate carefully and methodically, as in anatomical study or surgical operation.

dissecting aneurysm or **hematoma.** An aneurysm produced by blood forcing its way through a tear in the intima and between the layers of an arterial wall, usually that of the aorta.

dissecting forceps. Any of a variety of forceps used for dissection. They may have sharp, smooth, or notched points, may be curved or straight, or self-closing, and come in various sizes.

dissecting microscope. A microscope with a long working distance, allowing adequate space for placement of large unmounted specimens on its stage so as to use magnification during dissection of the specimen.

dis·sec·tion (di·seck'shun, dye·) *n.* [from *dissect*]. 1. Division or separation along natural lines of cleavage. 2. The cutting of structures of the body for purposes of study or operative treatment.

dissection tubercle. TUBERCULOSIS VERRUCOSA.

dis·sec·tor (di·seck'tur) *n.* 1. One who makes a dissection. 2. A handbook or manual of anatomy and instructions for use in dissection.

dis·sem·i·nate (di·sem'i·nate) *v.* [L. *disseminare,* from *seminare,* to sow]. To scatter or disperse. —**dissemi·nat·ed** (·nay·tid) *adj.*

disseminated choroiditis. DIFFUSE CHOROIDITIS.

disseminated coccidioidomycosis. A progressive, often fatal, disease with widespread involvement of the lungs, bones, central nervous system, skin, and subcutaneous tissue; associated with a loss of reactivity to coccidioidin. See also *coccidioidomycosis, primary coccidioidomycosis.*

disseminated follicular lupus. A variety of lupus vulgaris confined to the face, especially in the situations usually occupied by acne. The papules vary from a large pinhead to a pea in size, conical and deep red.

disseminated intravascular coagulation or **clotting.** A complex disorder of the clotting mechanisms, in which coagulation factors are consumed at an accelerated rate, with generalized fibrin deposition and thrombosis, hemorrhages, and further depletion of the coagulation factors. The process may be acute or chronic, and is usually triggered by the entry of large amounts of thromboplastic substances into the circulation, resulting from any of a wide variety of severe diseases and traumas. Abbreviated, DIC. Syn. *consumption coagulopathy, defibrination syndrome, diffuse intravascular coagulation.*

disseminated lipogranulomatosis. An inborn error of lipid metabolism, characterized by the diffuse development of granulomas in many tissues in infancy, resulting in feeding difficulties and hoarse cry due to laryngeal obstruction, periarticular changes suggestive of rheumatoid arthritis, and deposition of abnormal lipids in many other tissues, leading to motor and mental retardation and early death. Syn. *Farber's disease.*

disseminated lupus erythematosus. SYSTEMIC LUPUS ERYTHEMATOSUS.

disseminated myelitis. Diffuse, irregular, patchy inflammatory lesions of the spinal cord.

disseminated necrotizing periarteritis. POLYARTERITIS NODOSA.

disseminated neuritis. POLYNEURITIS.

disseminated sclerosis. MULTIPLE SCLEROSIS.

disseminated trophoneurosis. SCLERODERMA.

disseminate nucleus. The nucleus proprius of the anterior horn.

dis·sem·i·na·tion (di·sem''i·nay'shun) *n.* [L. *disseminatio*]. The scattering or dispersion of disease or disease germs.

dissimilar twins. FRATERNAL TWINS.

dis·sim·i·late (di·sim'i·late) *v.* CATABOLIZE.

dis·sim·u·la·tion (di·sim''yoo·lay'shun) *n.* [L. *dissimulare,* to dissemble]. The act of feigning, disguising, or malingering.

dissociated anesthesia. Loss of pain and temperature sensations, with preservation of touch and proprioception, as seen in syringomyelia.

dissociated jaundice. Selective retention of either bile pigment or bile salts; most frequently acholuric.

dissociated nystagmus. Oscillatory movements of the eyeballs, which are dissimilar both in amount and direction.

dissociated personality. SPLIT PERSONALITY.

dis·so·ci·a·tion (di·so''see·ay'shun, ·shee·) *n.* [L. *dissociare,* to separate from fellowship]. 1. Separation; especially of a chemical compound into ions. 2. *In cardiology,* independent action of atria and ventricles; a form of heart block. 3. *In psychology,* the segregation from consciousness of certain components of mental processes, which then function independently as if they belonged to another person; the separation of ideas from their natural and appropriate affects or feelings. 4. *In bacteriology,* variations due to mutation in colony form and associated properties, including smooth, rough, mucoid, dwarf, gonidial, and L or pleuropneumonia-like colonial forms. —**dis·so·ci·ant** (·so'shee·unt) *adj. & n.;* **dis·so·ci·ate** (·so'shee·ate) *v.;* **dis·so·ci·a·tive** (·so'shee·uh·tiv) *adj.*

dissociation anesthesia or **symptom.** DISSOCIATED ANESTHESIA.

dissociation constant. The equilibrium constant pertaining to a reversible reaction in which a molecule breaks up into two or more products. Symbol, K.

dissociative reaction. DISSOCIATIVE TYPE OF HYSTERICAL NEUROSIS.

dissociative type of hysterical neurosis. The form of hysterical neurosis, leading to alterations in the person's identity or his state of consciousness, that may take the form of depersonalization, dissociation, multiple personality, amnesia, somnambulism, fugue, dream state, or of aimless running or freezing.

dis·sog·e·ny (di·soj'e·nee) *adj.* [Gk. *dissos,* double, + *-geny*]. *In zoology,* having two periods of sexual maturity, one as a larva and one as an adult.

dis·so·lu·tion (dis''uh·lew'shun) *n.* [L. *dissolutio,* from *dissolvere,* to separate]. 1. Separation of a body or compound into its parts. 2. Death; decomposition. 3. SOLUTION.

dis·solve, *v.* [L. *dissolvere,* from *solvere,* to loosen, unbind]. 1. To make a solution of. 2. To become a solution; to pass into solution. —**dis·sol·vent** (di·zol'vunt) *adj. & n.*

dis·sor·ta·tive mating (di·sor'tuh·tiv). Nonrandom mating based on phenotypic dissimilarity.

dist-, disto-. A combining form meaning *distal.*

dis·tad (dis'tad) *adv.* [*dist-* + *-ad*]. Toward the periphery; in a distal direction.

dis·tal (dis'tul) *adj.* 1. Farther or farthest from the point of origin along the course of any asymmetrical structure; nearest the end. Contr. *proximal.* 2. In any symmetrical structure, farther or farthest from the center or midline or median plane. 3. *In dentistry,* away from the sagittal plane along the curve of a dental arch. Contr. *mesial.*

distal angle. The angle formed by the junction of the distal surface with any one of the other surfaces of the crown of a tooth.

distal closed space. The fascial space overlying the palmar surface of a distal phalanx, covered by fascia attached to the tip, lateral margins, and base of the distal phalanx.

distal muscular dystrophy. A rare form of muscular dystrophy of unknown cause, possibly hereditary, involving initially the muscles of the hands or feet, or both, and progressing slowly to affect eventually also the more proximal muscles.

distal myopathy. DISTAL MUSCULAR DYSTROPHY.

distal occlusion. Occlusion occurring when a tooth is situated posterior to its normal position.

dis·tance, *n.* [L. *distantia*]. The measure of space between two objects. —**dis·tant, dis·tan·tial** (dis·tan'shul) *adj.*

distantial aberration. Indistinct vision due to distance.

distant memory. REMOTE MEMORY.

dis·tem·per (dis·tem'pur) *n.* [early mod. E., derangement or imbalance of the humors, from *dis-* + L. *temperare,* to mingle properly]. Any of several infectious, or sometimes contagious, diseases of animals, as: canine distemper, feline distemper (= FELINE PANLEUKOPENIA), equine distemper (= STRANGLES).

dis·ten·si·bil·i·ty (dis·ten''si·bil'i·tee) *n.* The property of being distensible.

dis·ten·si·ble (dis·ten'si·bul) *adj.* Capable of distention.

distension. DISTENTION.

dis·ten·tion (dis·ten'shun) *n.* [L. *distentio,* from *distendere,* to stretch]. A state of dilatation.

distention cyst. A collection of fluid in a cavity.

dis·tich·ia (dis·tick'ee·uh) *n.* [Gk., from *stichos,* row]. A congenital anomaly in which there is an accessory row of eyelashes at the inner lid border, which turn in and rub on the cornea. This row is additional to the two or three rows normally arising at the outer lid border; may be seen in Milroy's disease.

dis·ti·chi·a·sis (dis″ti·kigh′uh·sis) *n.* DISTICHIA.

dis·til·land (dis′ti·land) *n.* The substance being distilled.

dis·til·late (dis′ti·late) *n.* The condensate obtained by distillation.

dis·til·la·tion (dis″ti·lay′shun) *n.* [L. *distillatio,* from *distillare,* to distill, drip, from *stilla,* a drop]. Vaporization and subsequent condensation, used principally to separate liquids from nonvolatile substances. —**dis·till** (dis·til′) *v.*

dis·tilled water. Water purified by distillation.

disto-. See *dist-.*

dis·to·an·gu·lar (dis″to·ang′gew·lur) *adj.* Characterized by angulation in a distal direction; leaning or tipping away from a point of reference.

distoangular impaction. Impaction of a tooth, usually a third molar, with the coronal aspect posterior to the apex.

dis·to·buc·cal (dis″to·buck′ul) *adj.* Pertaining to the distal and buccal surfaces of the premolar and molar teeth.

dis·to·buc·co·oc·clu·sal (dis″to·buck″o·uh·klew′zul) *adj.* Pertaining to the distal, buccal, and occlusal surfaces of a tooth.

dis·to·clu·sion (dis″to·klew′zhun) *n.* [*disto-* + *occlusion*]. Malocclusion of the teeth in which those of the lower jaw are in distal relation to the upper teeth.

dis·to·in·ci·sal (dis″to·in·sigh′zul) *adj.* Pertaining to the distal and incisal surfaces of a tooth.

distoincisal angle. The angle formed by the distal surface and the incisive edge of an incisor.

dis·to·la·bi·al (dis″to·lay′bee·ul) *adj.* Pertaining to the distal and labial surfaces of incisors and canines.

dis·to·lin·gual (dis″to·ling′gwul) *adj.* Pertaining to the distal and lingual surfaces of all teeth.

dis·to·lin·guo·oc·clu·sal (dis″to·ling″gwo·uh·klew′zul) *adj.* Pertaining to the distal, lingual, and occlusal surfaces of a tooth.

Dis·to·ma hae·ma·to·bi·um (dis′to·muh hee·muh·to′bee·um). SCHISTOSOMA HAEMATOBIUM.

Distoma he·pat·i·cum (he·pat′i·kum). FASCIOLA HEPATICA.

Di·sto·ma·ta (di·sto′muh·tuh) *n. pl.* [pl. of *Distoma*]. A suborder of the Trematoda or flukes.

di·sto·mia (dye·sto′mee·uh) *n.* [*di-* + *-stomia*]. Congenital duplication of the mouth.

dis·to·mi·a·sis (dis″to·migh′uh·sis) *n.*, pl. **distomia·ses** (·seez) [*Distoma* + *-iasis*]. Infection with flukes or trematodes.

dis·to·mo·lar (dis″to·mo′lur) *n.* A supernumerary tooth distal to a third molar, hence in the position of a fourth molar.

di·sto·mus (dye·sto′mus, di·sto′mus) *n.* [*di-* + *stom-* + *-us*]. An individual with partial or complete duplicity of the mouth.

dis·to·oc·clu·sal (dis″to·uh·klew′zul) *adj.* Pertaining to the distal and occlusal surfaces of premolar and molar teeth.

distoocclusal angle. The angle of a premolar or molar formed by the junction of its distal and occlusal surfaces. It forms the distal marginal ridge of the occlusal surfaces of these teeth.

dis·tor·tion (dis·tor′shun) *n.* [L. *distortio,* from *distorquere,* to distort, from *torquere,* to twist]. 1. A twisted or bent shape; deformity or malformation, acquired or congenital. 2. A writhing or twisting motion, as of the face. 3. *In optics,* a form of aberration in which objects viewed through certain lenses appear changed in shape but not broken in continuity. 4. *In psychiatry,* the adaptive alteration of an idea or memory to conform with the subject's wishes or prejudices.

dis·to·ver·sion (dis″to·vur′zhun) *n.* [*disto-* + *version*]. Tilting of a tooth so that the crown is directed distally.

distributing artery. Any of the arteries intermediate between the conducting arteries and arterioles, in which a well developed muscular coat of the arterial wall controls the size of the lumen and thereby also the volume of distributed blood.

dis·tri·bu·tion (dis″tri·bew′shun) *n.* [L. *distributio,* from *distribuere,* to distribute]. *In anatomy,* the branching of a nerve or artery, and the arrangement of its branches within those parts that it supplies. —**dis·trib·u·tive** (dis·trib′yoo·tiv) *adj.*

distributive analysis and synthesis. The form of psychotherapy employed in psychobiology which entails extensive but controlled investigation of the patient's entire past experience, and endeavors by better utilization of the individual's assets and diminution of his liabilities to effect a constructive synthesis.

dis·tri·chi·a·sis (dis″tri·kye′uh·sis) *n.* [Gk. *dis,* twice, double, + *trich-* + *-iasis*]. Two hairs growing from a single follicle.

district nurse. A community health nurse working in a designated district for a public health agency.

dis·trix (dis′tricks) *n.* [*dis-* + Gk. *thrix,* hair]. Splitting of the distal ends of the hair.

dis·turbed, *adj.* Troubled, malfunctioning, maladjusted; especially, evincing an emotional disorder.

di·sul·fide (dye·sul′fide, ·fid) *n.* BISULFIDE.

di·sul·fi·ram (dye·sul′fi·ram) *n.* Bis(diethylthiocarbamoyl)disulfide, $C_{10}H_{20}N_2S_4$, an antioxidant that interferes with normal metabolic degradation of alcohol so that acetaldehyde is produced in high concentration; used in the treatment of alcoholism.

disuse arteriosclerosis. Intimal fibrosis of an artery proximal to an occlusion, or in an organ or part that is atrophic, as in an atrophic ovary or leg. Syn. *involutional arteriosclerosis.*

disuse atrophy. Atrophy resulting from inactivity, usually affecting glandular or muscular structures.

DIT Abbreviation for *diiodotyrosine.*

di·ta bark (dee′tuh) [Tagalog]. The bark of *Alstonia scholaris,* native to the Philippine Islands; has been employed as a bitter tonic, antiperiodic, and antimalarial.

di·ter·pene (dye·tur′peen, di·) *n.* Any of the terpene hydrocarbons having the formula $C_{20}H_{32}$, or $(C_5H_8)_4$.

di·thi·az·a·nine iodide (dye″thigh·az′uh·neen). 3-Ethyl-2-[5-(3-ethyl-2-benzothiazolinylidene)-1,3-pentadienyl]benzothiazolium iodide, $C_{23}H_{23}IN_2S_2$, a toxic anthelmintic drug.

di·thi·zone (dye·thigh′zone) *n.* Diphenylthiocarbazone, $C_{13}H_{12}N_4S$, a reagent used as a sensitive test for heavy metals, particularly lead.

dith·ra·nol (dith′ruh·nol) *n.* British name for ANTHRALIN.

di·thy·mol diiodide (dye·thigh′mol). THYMOL IODIDE.

dit·o·kous, dit·o·cous (dit′o·kus) *adj.* [Gk. *ditokos,* from *tokos,* childbirth]. 1. Producing two young at a birth. 2. Producing young of two kinds, as some worms.

Ditt·rich's stenosis (dit′rikh) [F. *Dittrich,* German pathologist, 1815–1859]. Stenosis of the conus arteriosus.

Ditubin. A trademark for isoniazid.

Diucardin. A trademark for hydroflumethiazide, a diuretic.

di·ure·ide (dye·yoo′ree·ide) *n.* 1. A derivative of urea in which a hydrogen of both NH_2 groups is replaced by an acyl radical. 2. An acyl derivative of urea containing residues of two urea molecules.

di·urese (dye″yoo·reece′) *v.* To effect diuresis in (someone).

di·ure·sis (dye″yoo·ree′sis) *n.*, pl. **diure·ses** (·seez) [Gk. *diourein,* to pass urine]. Increased excretion of urine.

di·uret·ic (dye″yoo·ret′ick) *adj.* & *n.* [Gk. *diourētikos*]. 1. Increasing the flow of urine. 2. Any diuretic agent.

Diuril. Trademark for chlorothiazide, an orally effective diuretic and antihypertensive drug.

di·ur·nal (dye·ur′nul) *adj.* [L. *diurnalis,* from *diurnus,* daily]. Occurring in the daytime.

diurnal enuresis. Involuntary urination during the daytime at an age when bladder control is usually established; less common than nocturnal enuresis.

di·ur·nule (dye·urn′yool) *n.* A medicinal product that contains the full quantity of a drug to be administered in 24 hours.

di·va·ga·tion (dye″vuh·gay′shun) *n.* [L. *divagari,* to wander about]. Rambling, incoherent speech and thought.

di·va·lent (dye·vay'lunt) *adj.* 1. BIVALENT. 2. Having the ability to exist in two valence states.
di·var·i·ca·tion (dye·văr"uh·kay'shun) *n.* [L. *divaricare,* to spread asunder]. Separation; divergence.
di·ver·gence (dye·vur'junce, di·) *n.* [ML. *divergere,* to diverge, from *di-,* apart, + *vergere,* to bend]. *In ophthalmology,* the abduction of both eyes simultaneously, or of one eye when the other is fixed. **—diver·gent** (·junt) *adj.*
divergent strabismus. EXOTROPIA.
diverging dislocation. A dislocation of the radius and ulna at the elbow, involving rupture of the annular ligament.
diver's conjunctivitis. INCLUSION CONJUNCTIVITIS.
diver's ear. An inflammation of the middle ear and auditory tube; caused by sudden changes in atmospheric pressure that may occur during a diver's ascent or descent; seen in decompression sickness; similar to barotitis media.
diver's palsy or **paralysis.** Permanent central nervous system damage as a result of decompression sickness.
diverticula. Plural of *diverticulum.*
diverticula am·pul·lae duc·tus de·fe·ren·tis (am·pul'ee duck' tus def·e·ren'tis) [NA]. Small sacs in the wall of the ampulla of the ductus deferens.
di·ver·tic·u·lar (dye"vur·tick'yoo·lur) *adj.* Pertaining to or arising from a diverticulum.
diverticular disease. DIVERTICULITIS.
di·ver·tic·u·lec·to·my (dye"vur·tick"yoo·leck'tuh·mee) *n.* [*diverticul*um + *-ectomy*]. *In surgery,* removal of a diverticulum.
di·ver·tic·u·li·tis (dye"vur·tick"yoo·lye'tis) *n.* [*diverticul*um + *-itis*]. Inflammation of a diverticulum; the clinical condition of inflammation of diverticula. Syn. *diverticular disease.*
di·ver·tic·u·lo·sis (dye"vur·tick"yoo·lo'sis) *n.* [*diverticul*um + *-osis*]. The presence of diverticula of the intestine, with or without clinical symptoms.
diverticulosis co·li (ko'lye). Diverticulosis of the colon.
di·ver·tic·u·lum (dye"vur·tick'yoo·lum) *n.,* pl. **diverticu·la** (·luh) [L. *deverticulum,* byway, from *devertere,* to turn aside]. An outpouching or sac arising from a hollow organ or structure; may be congenital or acquired. In the acquired form, it usually represents a herniation of the mucous membrane through the muscular wall of the organ.
diverticulum hernia. 1. A type of sliding hernia that contains a diverticulum of the urinary bladder. 2. A hernia of an intestinal diverticulum.
diverticulum il·ei (il'ee·eye). A blind tube arising from the antimesenteric border of the terminal ileum at a variable distance from the ileocecal valve. It represents the persistent proximal end of the yolk stalk. Syn. *Meckel's diverticulum.*
di·vide, *v.* 1. To separate into parts. 2. *In surgery,* to sever.
divi-divi (div"ee·div'ee) *n.* [Sp., from Carib]. *Caesalpinia coriaria,* a tree of South America whose seed pods yield tannic and gallic acids; used as an astringent and in tanning.
divine healing. FAITH CURE.
di·vi·nyl ether (dye·vye'nil). VINYL ETHER.
divinyl oxide. VINYL ETHER.
Di·vry–van Bo·gaert disease (dee·vree', vahn bo'ghärt) [P. *Divry,* Belgian neurologist, 20th century; and L. *van Bogaert,* Belgian neuropathologist, 20th century]. A rare heredofamilial disorder characterized clinically by dementia, seizures, pyramidal and extrapyramidal disturbances, defects in the fields of vision, and a progressive course, and characterized pathologically by angiomatosis of the skin and the cerebral meninges and progressive demyelinization.
di·vul·sion (dye·vul'shun, di·) *n.* [L. *divulsio,* from *divellere,* to tear asunder]. A tearing apart. **—di·vulse** (dye·vulce', di·) *v.*
di·vul·sor (dye·vul'sur, di·) *n.* An instrument for the forcible dilatation of a part or of stricture in any organ.
di·xen·ic (dye·zen'ick) *adj.* [*di-* + Gk. *xenos,* guest, stranger, + *-ic*]. Of laboratory animals, deliberately contaminated with two species of microorganisms but otherwise germ-free (axenic). Contr. *monoxenic.*
di·zy·got·ic (dye"zye·got'ick) *adj.* [*di-* + *zygotic*]. Developed from two fertilized ova at a single birth.
dizygotic twins. FRATERNAL TWINS.
di·zy·gous (dye·zye'gus) *adj.* [by false analogy to such words as *heterozygous*]. DIZYGOTIC.
diz·zi·ness, *n.* A sensation of disturbed relations to surrounding objects in space with feelings of rotation or whirling characteristic of vertigo as well as nonrotatory swaying, weakness, faintness, and unsteadiness characteristic of giddiness. **—diz·zy,** *adj.*
DJD Abbreviation for *degenerative joint disease.*
dl Abbreviation for *deciliter.*
dl- *In organic chemistry,* a former symbol indicating a racemic mixture containing both dextrorotatory and levorotatory forms of an organic compound; now replaced by the symbol (±).
dm Abbreviation for *decimeter.*
DMCT DEMECLOCYCLINE HYDROCHLORIDE.
D.M.D. Doctor of Dental Medicine.
DMF *Decayed, missing, and filled teeth;* applied to the quantitative estimate of dental caries in permanent teeth.
DMFS DMF used with the tooth surface as the unit of measurement.
DMFT DMF used with the tooth as the unit of measurement.
DMSO Abbreviation for *dimethyl sulfoxide.*
DMT Abbreviation for *dimethyltryptamine.*
DNA Abbreviation for *deoxyribonucleic acid,* any of the high molecular weight polymers of deoxyribonucleotides, found principally in the chromosomes of the nucleus and varying in composition with the source, able to reproduce in the presence of the appropriate enzyme and substrates, and bearing coded genetic information.
DNA-directed RNA polymerase. RNA POLYMERASE.
DNA ligase. An enzyme which joins the ends of two DNA chains by catalyzing the synthesis of a phosphodiester bond between a 3′-hydroxyl group at the end of one chain and a 5′-phosphate at the end of the other.
DNA polymerase I. An enzyme which catalyzes the addition of deoxyribonucleotide residues to the end of a DNA strand. Originally thought to be responsible for DNA synthesis, but now generally considered to function in the repair of damaged DNA.
DNA polymerase II. An enzyme of unknown biological function similar in action to DNA polymerase I, but with lower activity.
DNA polymerase III. A complex enzyme thought to be the primary enzyme involved in DNA replication in vivo. It utilizes a short priming strand of RNA and sequentially adds deoxyribonucleotides complementary to the template strand of DNA.
DNase Abbreviation for *deoxyribonuclease.*
DNA viruses. Viruses, such as adenoviruses, papovaviruses, herpesviruses, poxviruses, and most bacteriophages, in which the nucleic acid core consists of deoxyribonucleic acid.
D/N quotient. D:N RATIO.
D:N ratio. The ratio of the dextrose to the nitrogen in the urine. In the totally diabetic animal, the average value is 3.65, which is approached in severe human diabetes. It is considered as a measure of the conversion of protein to carbohydrate in the absence of carbohydrate intake.
D.O. Doctor of Osteopathy.
Do·bell's solution (do·bel') [H. B. *Dobell,* English physician, 1828–1917]. Compound sodium borate solution, containing sodium borate, sodium bicarbonate, phenol, glycerin, and water; has been used as an antibacterial, mainly as a gargle and mouthwash.
do·bu·ta·mine (do·bew'tuh·meen) *n.* (±)-4-[2-[[3-(*p*-Hy-

droxyphenyl)-1-methylpropyl]amino]ethyl]pyrocatechol, $C_{18}H_{23}NO_3$, a cardiotonic, also used as the hydrochloride.

Dobutrex. A trademark for dobutamine hydrochloride, a cardiotonic.

Doca. A trademark for deoxycorticosterone (acetate), a salt-regulating adrenocortical hormone.

Do·chez's serum (do·shay') [A. R. *Dochez,* U.S. physician, 1882–1965]. SCARLET FEVER STREPTOCOCCUS ANTITOXIN.

doc·tor, *n. & v.* [L., from *docere,* to teach]. 1. One licensed, usually after special study, and qualifying by examination, to practice medicine, dentistry, or veterinary medicine. 2. The recipient of an academic title signifying competence in a special branch of learning. 3. To treat as a physician; to practice medicine. 4. To tamper with or falsify.

doctrine of Ra·so·ri. RASORIANISM.

doctrine of signatures. A theory that the medicinal uses of a plant can be determined from its fancied physical resemblance to normal or diseased organs (liverwort, lungwort, orchis).

dodec-, dodeca- [Gk. *dōdeka*]. A combining form meaning *twelve.*

do·dec·a·no·ic acid (do·deck"uh·no'ick). LAURIC ACID.

do·dec·yl (do·des'il) *n.* The organic chemical radical $CH_3(CH_2)_{10}CH_2$—.

Dö·der·lein's bacillus (dœh'dur·line) [A. *Döderlein,* German obstetrician, 1860–1941]. Any of various species of *Lactobacillus* found in the vagina.

Doeh·le bodies (dœh'leh) [K. G. P. *Doehle,* German pathologist, 1855–1928]. Irregular peroxidase-negative clumps of ribonucleic acid, 1 to 2 microns in greatest dimension, occurring in the cytoplasm of granulocytes in persons with severe infections and in the May-Hegglin anomaly.

Doerfler-Stewart test. A test for psychogenic deafness employing speech mixed in with a background noise. In individuals with normal hearing or with conduction or perception deafness, the speech sound is not inhibited until the background noise is at least 10 to 25 decibels louder than the speech. In psychogenic hearing loss, the background noise makes the patient forget the level of deafness voluntarily fixed by him when the background noise reaches that level or even when it is well below it.

dog flea. *CTENOCEPHALIDES CANIS.*

Dog·ger Bank itch [After *Dogger Bank* in the North Sea, where the plant is found]. A maculopapular eruption of the skin of the hands, face, and flexor aspects of the forearms resulting from exposure to alcyonidium, a seaweed-like plant.

Do·giel's corpuscle (doh'gyely) [A. S. *Dogiel,* Russian neurophysiologist, 1862–1922]. GENITAL CORPUSCLE.

dog tapeworm. *DIPYLIDIUM CANINUM.*

doigts en lor·gnette (dwah ahn lor·nyet') [F.]. OPERA-GLASS HAND.

doi·sy·nol·ic acid (doy"si·nol'ick) [E. A. *Doisy*]. 1-Ethyl-7-hydroxy-2-methyl-1,2,3,4,4a,9,10,10a-octahydrophenanthrene-2-carboxylic acid, $C_{18}H_{24}O_3$, obtained from estrone by rupture of its cyclopentane ring with alkali; it possesses high estrogenic activity.

Dolantin. A trademark for meperidine, a narcotic analgesic used as the hydrochloride salt.

Dolene. A trademark for propoxyphene hydrochloride, an analgesic.

dolich-, dolicho- [Gk. *dolichos*]. A combining form meaning (a) *long;* (b) *narrow.*

dol·i·cho·ceph·a·lus (dol"i·ko·sef'uh·lus) *n.,* pl. **dolichocepha·li** (·lye) [*dolicho-* + *-cephalus*]. A dolichocephalic or long-headed person.

dol·i·cho·ceph·a·ly (dol"i·ko·sef'uh·lee) *n.* [*dolicho-* + *-cephaly*]. The condition in which the length-breadth index of the head is 75.9 or less, indicating that the head is much longer than it is broad. —**dolicho·ce·phal·ic** (·se·fal'ick), **dolicho·ceph·a·lous** (·sef'uh·lus) *adj.*

dol·i·cho·cham·ae·cra·ni·al (dol"i·ko·kam"i·kray'nee·ul) *adj.* [*dolicho-* + *chamae-* + *cranial*]. *In craniometry,* designating a condition in which a long skull is also markedly low-vaulted, i.e., having a length-breadth index of 74.9 or less and a length-height index of 69.9 or less.

dol·i·cho·cne·mic (dol"i·ko·nee'mick, ·ko·k'nee'mick) *adj.* [*dolicho-* + *cnemic*]. Designating a tibia with a tibiofemoral index of 83 or more, indicating that it is relatively long as compared with the femur.

dol·i·cho·co·lon (dol"i·ko·ko'lun) *n.* [*dolicho-* + *colon*]. An abnormally long colon.

dol·i·cho·cra·ni·al (dol"i·ko·kray'nee·ul) *adj.* [*dolicho-* + *cranial*]. Having a cranial index between 70.0 and 74.9.

dol·i·cho·de·rus (dol"i·ko·deer'us) *n.* [*dolicho-* + Gk. *derē,* neck]. A person having a disproportionately long neck.

dol·i·cho·eu·ro·meso·ceph·a·lus (dol"i·ko·yoor"o·mez"o·sef'uh·lus) *n.* [*dolicho-* + *eury-* + *meso-* + *-cephalus*]. A person having a long skull that is markedly broad in the temporal region.

dol·i·cho·eu·ro·opis·tho·ceph·a·lus (dol"i·ko·yoor"o·o·pis"tho·sef'uh·lus) *n.* [*dolicho-* + *eury-* + *opistho-* + *-cephalus*]. A person having a long skull that is very broad in the occipital region.

dol·i·cho·eu·ro·pro·ceph·a·lus (dol"i·ko·yoor"o·pro·sef'uh·lus) *n.* [*dolicho-* + *eury-* + *pro-* + *-cephalus*]. A person having a long skull that is very broad in the frontal region.

dol·i·cho·fa·cial (dol"i·ko·fay'shul) *adj.* [*dolicho-* + *facial*]. Having an unusually long face.

dol·i·cho·hi·er·ic (dol"i·ko·high·err'ick) *adj.* [*dolicho-* + *hieric*]. Designating a sacrum with a length-breadth index of 99.9 or less, indicating that it is relatively long and narrow.

dol·i·cho·ker·kic (dol"i·ko·kur'kick) *adj.* [*dolicho-* + Gk. *kerkis,* shuttle, radius, tibia, + *-ic*]. Designating a radius with a humeroradial index of 80 or more, indicating that it is relatively long as compared with the humerus.

dol·i·chol (dol'i·kol) *n.* [*dolich-* + alcohol]. Any of various long-chain unsaturated isoprenoid alcohols containing up to 84 carbon atoms, found either free or phosphorylated in membranes of the endoplasmic reticulum and Golgi apparatus, but not in mitochondrial or plasma membranes.

dol·i·cho·lep·to·ceph·a·lus (dol"i·ko·lep"to·sef'uh·lus) *n.* [*dolicho-* + *lepto-* + *-cephalus*]. A person whose skull, in addition to being long, is also high and narrow.

dol·i·cho·mor·phic (dol"i·ko·mor'fick) *adj.* [*dolicho-* + *-morphic*]. Marked by a long or narrow form or build.

dol·i·cho·pel·lic (dol"i·ko·pel'ick) *adj.* [*dolicho-* + *-pellic*]. Designating a pelvis the pelvic index of which is 95.0 or more.

dol·i·cho·pel·vic (dol"i·ko·pel'vick) *adj.* [*dolicho-* + *pelvic*]. DOLICHOPELLIC.

dol·i·cho·platy·ceph·a·lus (dol"i·ko·plat"ee·sef'uh·lus) *n.* [*dolicho-* + *platy-* + *-cephalus*]. A person having a long skull that is also unusually broad.

dol·i·chor·rhine (dol'i·ko·rine, ·reen) *adj.* [*dolicho-* + *-rrhine*]. Having a long nose.

Dol·i·chos (dol'i·kos) *n.* A genus of tropical herbs and woody vines of the pea family (Fabaceae), bearing seed pods covered with stinging hairs.

dol·i·cho·steno·me·lia (dol"i·ko·sten"o·mee'lee·uh) *n.* [*dolicho-* + *steno-* + *-melia*]. Abnormally long, thin extremities, as seen in Marfan's syndrome and in homocystinuria. See also *arachnodactyly.*

dol·i·cho·uran·ic (dol"i·ko·yoo·ran'ick) *adj.* [*dolicho-* + *uran-* + *-ic*]. Having a long palatal alveolar arch, with a palatomaxillary index of 109.9 or less.

doll's-head phenomenon or **eye movements.** Involuntary turning of the eyes upward and downward on passive flexion and extension of the head, an action that has been likened to that of a mechanical doll's eyes. The presence of these movements indicates that the vestibulo-ocular connections are intact.

Dolman test. HOWARD-DOLMAN DEPTH PERCEPTION TEST.

Dolophine. A trademark for methadone hydrochloride, a narcotic analgesic.

do·lor (do'lor) *n.*, pl. **do·lo·res** (do·lo'reez) [L.]. Pain.

dolores prae·sa·gi·en·tes (pree·say''jee·en'teez). Fleeting, false pains occurring a few days before the onset of labor.

do·lo·rim·e·ter (do''luh·rim'e·tur) *n.* [*dolor* + *-meter*]. A device for measuring sensitivity to pain, or pain intensity, utilizing a variety of stimuli such as thermal radiation or a prick and some standard response of the conscious individual as the index of pain threshold.

do·lo·ro·gen·ic (do''luh·ro·jen'ick) *adj.* [*dolor* + *-genic*]. Possessing the quality of pain; causing or arousing pain.

do·lo·rol·o·gy (do''luh·rol'uh·jee) *n.* [*dolor* + *-logy*]. The systematic study of the mechanisms and management of pain.

Doloxene. A trademark for propoxyphene napsylate, an analgesic.

DOM 2,5-Dimethoxy-4-methylamphetamine, $C_{12}H_{20}NO_2$, a psychedelic agent, often abused and known colloquially as STP.

do·ma·to·pho·bia (do''muh·to·fo'bee·uh) *n.* [Gk. *dōma, dōmatos*, house, + *-phobia*]. Abnormal fear of being in a house; a variety of claustrophobia.

do·ma·zo·line (do''muh·zo'leen) *n.* 2-(3,6-Dimethoxy-2,4-dimethylbenzyl)-2-imidazoline, $C_{14}H_{20}N_2O_2$, an anticholinergic usually used as the fumarate salt.

dom·i·nance, *n.* 1. The state of being dominant. See also *cerebral dominance*. 2. *In biology*, the capacity of an allele of a gene for expression in the presence of a different allele which is not expressed. 3. *In psychiatry and psychology*, the disposition of one individual to play a prominent and controlling role in his relationship with another or other individuals.

dom·i·nant, *adj.* & *n.* [L. *dominans*, from *dominare*, to rule, govern]. 1. In any pattern or complex, the quality of being more important or prominent or of taking precedence. 2. DOMINANT CHARACTER.

dominant allele. The member of a pair of contrasted genic alleles which is manifest phenotypically in the heterozygote.

dominant character. The member of a pair of contrasted traits which manifests itself in the heterozygote. Contr. *recessive character*.

dominant eye. The eye that is unconsciously and preferentially chosen to guide decision and action, as leading in reading and writing, or in sighting through a telescope.

dominant hemisphere. The cerebral hemisphere which controls certain motor activities, such as movements of speech; usually the left hemisphere in right-handed individuals. Syn. *categorical hemisphere*. See also *cerebral dominance*.

dominant wavelength. The wavelength of a beam of light which determines its hue.

dom·i·na·tor, *n.* [L., from *dominare*, to rule]. The receptive sense organ in light-adapted eyes representing the preponderant type, occurring in broad spectral response curves or absorption bands, having their maximum in the region of 5600 angstroms; it is regarded as responsible for the sensation of luminosity. Contr. *modulator*.

do·mi·phen bromide (do'mi·fen). Dodecyldimethyl(2-phenoxyethyl)ammonium bromide, $C_{22}H_{40}BrNO$, an antiseptic.

Don·a·hue's syndrome [W. L. *Donahue*, Canadian pathologist, b. 1906]. LEPRECHAUNISM.

Do·nath-Land·stein·er test or **phenomenon** (do'naht) [J. *Donath*, German physician, 1870–1950; and K. *Landsteiner*]. A test for paroxysmal hemoglobinuria based upon a thermolabile isohemolysin occurring in the blood of patients with paroxysmal hemoglobinuria. The cold hemolysin unites with the red cells at low temperatures and causes hemolysis after the cells are warmed to 37°C.

don·a·tism (don'uh·tiz·um) *n.* [*Donato*, professional name of Alfred d'Hont, Belgian "magnetizer," 1845–1900]. A form of hypnosis based on imitation.

Don·ders' law [F. C. *Donders*, Dutch physician and ophthalmologist, 1818–1889]. *In ophthalmology*, when the position of the line of fixation is given with respect to the head, there is correspondingly a definite angle of torsion, independent of the observer's volition and the manner in which the line of fixation arrived in the position in question.

do·nee (do·nee') *n.* A patient who receives transfused blood or other tissues, as skin, bone, or cartilage, from a donor.

Don Juan [*Don Juan*, the legendary Spanish noble, who was a great lover and seducer]. *In psychiatry*, a man who is sexually overactive because of compulsion and anxiety.

Don·nan equilibrium [F. G. *Donnan*, English physical chemist, 1870–1956]. In a system in which a semipermeable membrane separates a solution of an electrolyte with diffusible ions, as sodium chloride, from one containing a salt NaR with a nondiffusible ion R^-, as proteinate, the product of the concentrations of diffusible ions on one side of the membrane is equal to the product of the concentrations of such ions on the other side of the membrane. Syn. *Gibbs-Donnan equilibrium*.

Don·né's corpuscles (dohn·ney') [A. *Donné*, French physician, 1801–1878]. Cells with fatty cytoplasmic vacuoles found in colostrum.

do·nor, *n.* [OF. *doneur*, from L. *donator*, giver]. A person who gives blood or other tissues and organs for use by another person.

donor area. An area, as of skin, from which a graft is taken.

Don·o·van bodies [C. *Donovan*, British physician, 1863–1951]. Chromatin masses at the ends of *Calymmatobacterium granulomatis* bacteria which give them the appearance of a closed safety pin.

Don·o·va·nia gran·u·lo·ma·tis (don·o·vay'nee·uh gran·yoo·lo'muh·tis) [C. *Donovan*]. *CALYMMATOBACTERIUM GRANULOMATIS*.

don·o·va·ni·o·sis (don''o·vay''nee·o'sis, ·van''ee·o'sis) *n.* [*Donovania* + *-osis*]. GRANULOMA INGUINALE.

don·o·van·osis (don''o·vuh·no'sis) *n.* [*Donovan* bodies + *-osis*]. GRANULOMA INGUINALE.

Donovan's solution [E. *Donovan*, Irish chemist, 1798–1837]. A solution of arsenic and mercuric iodides formerly used in chronic diseases of the skin and joints.

do·pa (do'puh) *n.* DIHYDROXYPHENYLALANINE.

L-dopa. LEVODOPA.

dopa decarboxylase. An enzyme which forms dopamine from dopa in the postganglionic sympathetic adrenergic neuron.

do·pa·man·tine (do''puh·man'teen) *n.* *N*-(3,4-Dihydroxyphenethyl)-1-adamantanecarboxamide, $C_{19}H_{25}NO_3$, an antiparkinsonian agent.

do·pa·mine (do'puh·meen) *n.* Hydroxytyramine, $C_8H_{11}NO_2$, the decarboxylation product of dopa; an intermediate in the biosynthesis of epinephrine and norepinephrine.

do·pa·min·er·gic (do''puh·mi·nur'jick) *adj.* Pertaining to the type of activity characteristic of dopamine and dopamine-like substances.

dopa oxidase. An enzyme of the skin that catalyzes the oxidation of dihydroxyphenylalanine to melanin in the melanocytes of the epidermis, thus playing an important role in skin pigmentation.

Dopar. A trademark for levodopa, an antiparkinsonian agent.

dopa reaction. Black coloration induced in melanoblasts by 3,4-dihydroxyphenylalanine.

do·pase (do'pace, ·aze) *n.* DOPA OXIDASE.

dope, *n.* & *v.* [D. *doop*, sauce, from *dopen*, to dip]. 1. Any drug administered to stimulate or to stupefy, temporarily, or taken habitually. 2. To administer a narcotic, stimulant, or habit-forming drug.

dope addict. A person who has become psychologically and physiologically dependent on a narcotic or drug through habitual use.

Dopp·ler principle, phenomenon, or **effect** [C. J. *Doppler,* Austrian physicist and mathematician, 1803–1853]. When a source of light or sound is moving rapidly, the wavelength appears to decrease as the object approaches the observer, or to increase as the object recedes; the pitch of sound becomes higher or lower.

Dopram. A trademark for doxapram hydrochloride, a respiratory stimulant.

do·ra·pho·bia (do″ruh·fo′bee·uh) *n.* [Gk. *dora,* skin, hide, + *-phobia*]. Abnormal fear of touching the skin or fur of animals.

dor·as·tine (dor′us·teen) *n.* 8-Chloro-2,3,4,5-tetrahydro-2-methyl-5-[2-(6-methyl-3-pyridinyl)ethyl]-1*H*-pyrido[4,3-*b*]indole, $C_{20}H_{22}ClN_3$, an antihistaminic.

Dorbane. A trademark for danthron, a cathartic.

Do·rel·lo's canal (do·rel′lo) [P. *Dorello,* Italian anatomist, b. 1872]. A small canal between the apex of the petrous process of the temporal bone, the posterior clinoid, and the petrosphenoid ligament of the dura mater. The abducent nerve passes through it.

Doriden. Trademark for glutethimide, a hypnotic and sedative.

dor·mant (dor′munt) *adj.* [F., sleeping]. Concealed; quiescent; inactive; potential.

Dormate. A trademark for mebutamate, an antihypertensive.

Dormethan. A trademark for dextromethorphan hydrochloride, an antitussive.

Dormison. A trademark for methylparafynol, a hypnotic drug.

Dornavac. Trademark for a preparation of pancreatic dornase used to reduce tenacity of pulmonary secretions and facilitate expectoration in bronchopulmonary infections.

Dor·ner's spore stain. A solution containing nigrosine, formalin, and water; used in staining bacteria.

do·ro·ma·nia (do″ro·may′nee·uh) *n.* [Gk. *dōron,* gift, + *-mania*]. An abnormal wish to give presents.

Dor·o·thy Reed cell [*Dorothy Reed*]. REED-STERNBERG CELL.

Dor·rance's operation [G. M. *Dorrance,* U.S. surgeon, 1877–1949]. A method of surgically repairing the soft palate.

dors-, dorsi-, dorso-. [L. *dorsum*]. A combining form meaning (a) *of* or *on the back;* (b) *dorsal.*

dorsa. Plural of *dorsum.*

Dorsacaine. Trademark for benoxinate, a surface anesthetic agent used as the hydrochloride salt.

dor·sad (dor′sad) *adv.* [*dors-* + *-ad*]. In a ventral-to-dorsal direction. Compare *posteriad.* Contr. *ventrad.*

dor·sal (dor′sul) *adj.* [ML. *dorsalis,* from *dorsum,* back]. 1. Pertaining to, situated at, or relatively near the back, that is, the "backbone side" of the trunk or the body as a whole; in human anatomy: POSTERIOR. Contr. *ventral.* 2. Pertaining to, situated at, or relatively near the back or dorsum of some part, such as a hand or foot. Contr. *volar, palmar, plantar.* —**dorsal·ly** (·lee) *adv.*

dorsal accessory olivary nucleus. A small mass of gray matter lying dorsal to the olivary nucleus. NA *nucleus olivaris accessorius dorsalis.*

dorsal aorta. 1. PRIMITIVE AORTA. 2. THORACIC AORTA.

dorsal calcaneocuboid ligament. A broad, thickened portion of the articular capsule of the calcaneocuboid joint, attached to the dorsal surfaces of the calcaneus and cuboid at some distance from their contiguous margins.

dorsal carpal ligament. EXTENSOR RETINACULUM OF THE WRIST.

dorsal carpal rete. An arterial network on the back of the wrist formed by branches of the dorsal interosseous and the palmar interosseous arteries and terminal branches of the ulnar and radial palmar arteries. NA *rete carpi dorsale.*

dorsal cornu. The posterior column of gray matter of the spinal cord.

dor·sal·gia (dor·sal′jee·uh) *n.* [*dors-* + *-algia*]. Pain in the back.

dorsal horn. The posterior column of gray matter in the spinal cord.

dor·sa·lis (dor·say′lis) *adj.* [L.]. DORSAL.

dorsalis pe·dis (ped′is) [L.]. DORSAL PEDAL ARTERY.

dorsal lateral nucleus of the thalamus. This and the posterior lateral nuclei are in the dorsal division of the lateral nuclei of thalamus. They are continuous with the pulvinar, receive fibers from other thalamic nuclei, and connect with the cortex of the parietal lobe. NA *nucleus lateralis dorsalis thalami.*

dorsal longitudinal fasciculus. PERIVENTRICULAR TRACT.

dorsal longitudinal tract of Schütz (shuets) [H. *Schütz,* German neurologist, 20th century]. PERIVENTRICULAR TRACT.

dorsal median septum. A glial partition continuous with the dorsal median sulcus and extending into the gray matter of the spinal cord.

dorsal mesentery. The mesentery of the digestive tube attached to the dorsal abdominal wall. NA *mesenterium dorsale commune.*

dorsal mesocardium. The dorsal mesentery of the heart.

dorsal mesogaster. The dorsal mesentery of the stomach. The greater omentum is derived from it.

dorsal motor nucleus of the vagus. The column of cells in the medulla oblongata in the floor of the fourth ventricle which gives origin to preganglionic parasympathetic fibers of the vagus nerve. NA *nucleus dorsalis nervi vagi.*

dorsal nucleus. THORACIC NUCLEUS.

dorsal nucleus of Clarke [J. A. L. *Clarke*]. THORACIC NUCLEUS.

dorsal pancreas. DORSAL PANCREATIC BUD.

dorsal pancreatic artery. A large branch of either the splenic or celiac artery which descends dorsal to the pancreas and supplies branches to it at its inferior margin. NA *arteria pancreatica dorsalis.*

dorsal pancreatic bud. An embryonic diverticulum from the roof of the primitive duodenum which forms the dorsal portion of the head and all of the body and tail of the adult pancreas.

dorsal pancreatic duct. The duct of the embryonic dorsal pancreatic bud. In the adult, the distal portion persists as the main duct of the body and tail of the pancreas. The proximal part may persist as the accessory pancreatic duct.

dorsal paramedian nucleus. A band of small cells in the dorsal aspect of the reticular formation of the medulla oblongata on either side of the midline just beneath the ependyma extending the entire length of the fourth ventricle.

dorsal pedal artery. The main artery of the dorsum of the foot. NA *arteria dorsalis pedis.*

dorsal plate. One of the two longitudinal ridges on the dorsal surface of the embryo which subsequently fuse dorsally to form the neural canal.

dorsal position. The posture of a person lying on his back.

dorsal reflex. Contraction of the muscles of the back caused by stimulation of the skin over the sacrospinalis muscle.

dorsal root. A bundle of afferent fibers emerging from a dorsal root ganglion and entering the posterior part of the spinal cord. NA *radix dorsalis nervorum spinalium.*

dorsal root ganglion. SPINAL GANGLION.

dorsal sacroiliac ligament. Any of the several thick, strong bands passing from the lateral sacral crest on the dorsal surface of the sacrum to the tuberosity of the ilium. NA (pl.) *ligamenta sacroiliaca dorsalia.*

dorsal sclerosis. Degeneration of the posterior white columns of the spinal cord, or sclerosis involving the thoracic (dorsal) levels of the spinal cord.

dorsal sensory nucleus of the vagus. A column of nerve cells in the medulla oblongata lateral to the dorsal motor nucleus of the vagus in which part of the fibers of the solitary tract terminate.

dorsal spinocerebellar tract. A nerve tract which arises from the cells of the thoracic nucleus, ascends the spinal cord in the lateral funiculus, and reaches the cerebellum by way of the inferior cerebellar peduncle; it conveys subconscious proprioceptive impulses. NA *tractus spinocerebellaris posterior.*

dorsal supraoptic decussation or **commissure.** The more dorsal of the two decussations lying along the dorsal aspect of the optic chiasma. See also *commissurae supraopticae.*

dorsal talonavicular ligament. TALONAVICULAR LIGAMENT.

dorsal tegmental decussation (of Meynert). The decussation of the tectospinal tracts; it is situated in the midbrain between the red nuclei and dorsal to them.

dorsal tract of Schütz (shu^e^ts) [H. *Schütz,* German neurologist, 20th century]. PERIVENTRICULAR TRACT.

Dorsaphyllin. A trademark for theophylline sodium glycinate, a diuretic and coronary vasodilator.

Dor·set's egg medium. A medium of fresh egg yolk used, with or without diluent, for culture of *Mycobacterium tuberculosis* and other microorganisms.

dorsi-. See *dors-.*

dor·si·flex·ion (dor″si·fleck′shun) *n.* [*dorsi-* + *flexion*]. Bending the foot toward the dorsum, or upper surface of the foot; opposed to plantar flexion. If used with reference to the toes, same as extension or straightening. **—dor·si·flex** (dor′si·flecks) *v.*

dorsiflexion sign. HOMANS' SIGN.

dor·si·flex·or (dor″si·fleck′sur) *n.* [*dorsi-* + *flexor*]. A muscle producing dorsiflexion.

dorso-. See *dors-.*

dor·so·an·te·ri·or (dor″so·an·teer′ee·ur) *adj.* [*dorso-* + *anterior*]. Characterizing the position of a fetus having its back toward the ventral aspect of the mother.

dor·so·ceph·a·lad (dor″so·sef′ul·ad) *adv.* [*dorso-* + *cephalad*]. Toward the dorsal aspect of the head.

dor·so·cu·boi·dal (dor″so·kew·boy′dul) *adj.* Pertaining to or situated on the dorsal aspect of the cuboid bone.

dorsocuboidal reflex or **sign.** BEKHTEREV-MENDEL REFLEX (1).

dor·so·epi·tro·chle·a·ris (dor″so·ep″i·trock·lee·air′is) *n.* [*dorso-* + *epitrochlearis*]. A rare muscle found in the posterior part of the axilla, extending from the tendon of the latissimus dorsi muscle to neighboring structures.

dor·so·lat·er·al (dor″so·lat′ur·ul) *adj.* [*dorso-* + *lateral*]. Pertaining to or toward the back and the side.

dorsolateral placode. One of a series of ectodermal thickenings from which nerves and sense organs of the acoustic and lateral-line systems develop.

dorsolateral sclerosis. Any disorder characterized by degeneration and replacement gliosis in the posterior and lateral columns of the spinal cord.

dorsolateral sulcus. POSTEROLATERAL SPINAL SULCUS.

dorsolateral tract. The narrow bridge of white substance between the apex of the dorsal horn and the periphery of the spinal cord; it is traversed by some of the root fibers. NA *tractus dorsolateralis, fasciculus dorsolateralis.*

dor·so·lum·bar (dor″so·lum′bur, ·bahr) *adj.* LUMBODORSAL.

dor·so·me·di·ad (dor″so·mee′dee·ad) *adv.* Toward the medial part of a dorsal surface of an area.

dor·so·me·di·al (dor″so·mee′dee·ul) *adj.* [*dorso-* + *medial*]. Pertaining to the back and toward the midline.

dorsomedial hypothalamic nucleus. A mass of cells in the dorsal, medial portion of the middle region of the hypothalamus. NA *nucleus dorsomedialis hypothalami.*

dorsomedial nucleus of the thalamus. One of the medial nuclei of the thalamus, located between the internal medullary lamina and the wall of the third ventricle, consisting of a medial part which receives fibers from the midline nuclei and sends fibers to the hypothalamus, and a lateral part which receives fibers from the thalamic nuclei and sends fibers to the frontal lobe. NA *nucleus medialis dorsalis.*

dor·so·me·di·an (dor″so·mee′dee·un) *adj.* [*dorso-* + *median*]. Situated in or pertaining to the midline region of the back.

dor·so·na·sal (dor″so·nay′zul) *adj.* [*dorso-* + *nasal*]. Pertaining to the bridge of the nose.

dor·so·pos·te·ri·or (dor″so·pos·teer′ee·ur) *adj.* [*dorso-* + *posterior*]. Characterizing the position of a fetus having its back toward the dorsal aspect of the mother.

dor·so·ra·di·al (dor″so·ray′dee·ul) *adj.* Pertaining to or situated upon the dorsal aspect and radial border of the hand, finger, or forearm.

dor·so·sa·cral (dor″so·say′krul) *adj.* Pertaining to the dorsal and sacral regions.

dorsosacral position. The posture of a patient lying on the back with the legs flexed on the thighs and the thighs flexed on the abdomen and abducted.

dor·so·ul·nar (dor″so·ul′nur) *adj.* Pertaining to or situated upon the dorsal aspect and ulnar border of the arm, hand, or finger.

dor·so·ven·tral (dor″so·ven′trul) *adj.* Pertaining to the dorsal and ventral regions; extending in a direction from the dorsal surface toward the ventral. See also *posteroanterior.*

dor·sum (dor′sum) *n.*, genit. **dor·si** (dor′sigh), pl. **dor·sa** (·suh) [L.]. 1. [NA] The back. 2. Any part analogous to the back, as the dorsum of the foot or hand.

dorsum lin·guae (ling′gwee) [NA]. The upper surface of the tongue.

dorsum ma·nus (man′us) [NA]. The dorsal surface of the hand, or the back of the hand.

dorsum na·si (nay′zye) [NA]. The anterior border of the external nose, from the root to the apex.

dorsum pe·dis (ped′is) [NA]. The upper surface of the foot.

dorsum pe·nis (pee′nis) [NA]. The upper surface of the erect penis.

dorsum sel·lae (sel′ee) [NA]. A quadrilateral plate of bone forming the posterior boundary of the sella turcica.

dos·age (do′sij) *n.* The proper amount of a medicine or other agent for a given patient or condition.

dosage compensation. *In genetics,* the phenomenon whereby the difference between sexes in doses of X-linked genes is compensated; in mammals this is accomplished by activation of only one X chromosome in each cell, whether male or female in constitution.

dosage rate. DOSE RATE.

dose (doce) *n.* [L. *dosis,* from Gk., gift, portion]. 1. A single prescribed, administered, or received portion or quantity of a therapeutic agent, as medicine or radiation. 2. *In radiology,* an administered quantity of radiation measured at a specific point, as: air dose, depth dose, exit dose, skin dose, and, especially, absorbed dose.

dose-effect curve. *In radiology,* a curve relating the radiation dosage to the biologic effects produced.

dose·me·ter (doce′mee·tur) *n.* DOSIMETER.

dose rate. *In radiology,* the amount of radiation administered per unit time.

dose-rate meter. *In radiology,* an instrument for measuring the radiation dose rate.

do·sim·e·ter (do·sim′e·tur) *n.* [L. *dosis,* dose, + *-meter*]. *In radiology,* an instrument for measuring exposure to x-rays or to radioactive emanations.

do·sim·e·try (do·sim′e·tree) *n.* [L. *dosis,* dose, + *-metry*]. 1. The accurate determination of medicinal doses. 2. The measurement of exposures or doses of x-rays, or of radioactive emanations. **—do·si·met·ric** (do″si·met′rick) *adj.*

dot scan. A rectilinear recording made with a mechanical device (solenoid) of the distribution of radioactivity over a body part.

double aorta. The persistence of both right and left fourth aortic arches and dorsal aortas.

double aortic arch. Failure of the right fourth visceral arch to disappear during normal embryologic development, resulting in two aortic arches or an aortic ring.

double athetosis. A congenital extrapyramidal syndrome, characterized clinically by widespread choreoathetosis and dystonia and pathologically by status marmoratus.

double bind. A type of personal interaction, observed frequently in families with schizophrenic members, in which one person—often the mother—makes mutually contradictory demands of another member—such as the schizophrenic son—who finds it impossible to comply or even to discriminate properly or to escape from the situation because questioning or noncompliance poses a threat to the needed relationship; for example, a mother encourages her son to act independently, but when he does, scolds him for being unloving and disloyal.

double-blind experiment or **test.** An experiment or clinical investigation in which neither the subjects nor the investigator knows which kind of treatment is being given to each individual in order to obviate suggestion and bias of observation. See also *crossover experiment.*

double breech presentation. COMPLETE BREECH PRESENTATION.

double cervix. A congenital malformation usually associated with two uterine cavities.

double consciousness. See *multiple personality.*

double contrast examination. AIR-CONTRAST EXAMINATION.

double decomposition. The mutual interaction of two substances with formation of new substances; METATHESIS.

double diffusion. IMMUNODIFFUSION.

double dislocation. A dislocation in which there are two similar joint dislocations, on opposite sides of the body.

double-flap amputation. An amputation in which there are two opposing skin and muscle flaps.

double fracture. The presence of two fractures in the same bone. Syn. *segmental fracture.*

double gestation. 1. TWIN PREGNANCY. 2. The coexistence of uterine and extrauterine pregnancy.

double harelip. A harelip in which there is a cleft on both sides of the upper lip. Syn. *bilateral harelip.*

double-headed roller bandage. A strip of material rolled from both ends to the middle.

double hearing. DIPLACUSIS.

double image. The two images, known as true and false, which occur when one eye deviates, when the visual lines of the two eyes are not directed toward the same object.

double insanity. FOLIE À DEUX.

double intussusception. A condition in which another area of bowel invaginates into an existing intussusception.

double kidney. A developmental condition in which one of the kidneys is subdivided into two.

double knot. A knot in which the ends of the cord or suture are twisted twice around each other before tying. Syn. *friction knot, surgeon's knot.*

double ligature. The ligation of a vessel at two points, the vessel being divided distal to both.

double pain phenomenon. The phenomenon of feeling two successive sensations of pain following a single pain stimulus, e.g., a pinprick. A brief sensationless inverval, whose duration is directly proportional to the distance between the site of stimulus and site of interpretation (cerebral cortex), separates the two sensations, which are thus considered to be due to the presence of two sets of nerve fibers (delta and C fibers) with different conduction rates.

double pneumonia. Pneumonia involving both lungs.

double point threshold. The smallest distance apart at which two points can be felt as two.

double promontory. An anomaly in which the body of the first sacral vertebra is displaced farther forward than those below it, so that its lower margin projects beyond the general surface.

double pupil. Polycoria in which there are two pupils. Syn. *dicoria, diplocoria.*

double quartan. A form of malaria with a 3-day cycle; characterized by a chill on 2 consecutive days, with an intervening day of normal temperature.

double quotidian fever. A fever having two paroxysms or attacks a day, usually applied to malaria.

double refraction. The property of having more than one refractive index, according to the direction of the traversing light. It is possessed by all except isometric crystals, by transparent substances that have undergone internal strains (e.g., glass), and by substances that have different structures in different directions (e.g., fibers). Syn. *birefringence.* See also *flow birefringence.*

double refraction of flow. FLOW BIREFRINGENCE.

double rhythm. INTERFERENCE DISSOCIATION.

double stain. A mixture of two dyes of contrasting colors, usually an acid stain and a basic stain, or a method involving the successive use of contrasting stains. See also *contrast stain.*

doub·let (dub'lit) *n.* [OF.]. 1. *In optics,* a combination of two lenses of different focal length. 2. *In electricity,* DIPOLE. 3. A spectral line that is actually composed of two narrowly spaced lines.

double tachycardia. INTERFERENCE DISSOCIATION.

double tertian fever. Daily fever paroxysms (quotidian) due to alternation of two generations of tertian malaria parasites.

double touch. Combined vaginal and abdominal or vaginal and rectal palpation.

double variation. The biphasic change in electrical potential produced in a muscle by a single induction shock.

double vision. DIPLOPIA.

double voice. DIPHONIA.

doubling dose. The amount of radiation or other agent that will double the spontaneous mutation rate of a population.

doubting insanity. FOLIE DU DOUTE.

douche (doosh) *n.* [F., shower, spout, from It. *doccia,* conduit, from L. *ducere,* to conduct]. 1. A stream of water or air directed against the body or into a body cavity, commonly used on the body surface for its stimulating effect; may be hot, cold, or alternating. 2. *In gynecology,* lavage of the vagina; used for cleansing or for the application of heat or medication to the parts.

dough·nut pessary. A ring pessary for uterine prolapse.

Doug·las bag [C. G. *Douglas,* English physiologist, 1882–1963]. A collecting bag for expired air, used in determining basal metabolic rate.

Douglas' septum [J. *Douglas,* Scottish anatomist, 1675–1742]. URORECTAL SEPTUM.

Dounce homogenizer. An apparatus consisting of a glass tube with a tight-fitting glass pestle used manually to disrupt tissue suspensions to obtain single cells or subcellular fractions.

Dounce-Lan method. A method for isolation of nuclei of avian erythrocytes, based on hemolysis of cells by saponin and isolation of nuclei by differential centrifugation.

dou·rine (doo·reen', doo'reen) *n.* [F., perhaps from Ar. *darin,* to be filthy]. A contagious venereal disease of horses, characterized by inflammation of the genital organs and lymph nodes, and by paralysis of the hind legs; caused by *Trypanosoma equiperdum.*

dou·rou·cou·li (doo''roo·koo'lee) *n.* A small, nocturnal, South and Central American monkey, *Aotus trivirgatus;* has been used as a model in malaria and oncogenic virus research. Syn. *night monkey, owl monkey.*

Do·ver's powder [T. *Dover,* English physician, 1660–1743]. A powder containing 10% each of ipecac and opium; formerly used as a diaphoretic and sedative. Syn. *ipecac and opium powder.*

dow·el (dow'ul) *n.* A metallic pin inserted into a treated root canal of a tooth in order to attach an artificial crown or other restoration.

down-beat nystagmus. Nystagmus in which the fast component is downward, usually most marked on downward gaze; suggestive of a lesion in the lower brainstem or cerebellum.

Dow·ney cells [H. *Downey,* U.S. hematologist, 1877–1959]. Atypical lymphocytes of the type usually seen in infectious mononucleosis and certain other viral diseases.

Down's syndrome [J. L. H. *Down,* English physician, 1828–1896]. A syndrome of congenital defects, especially mental retardation, typical facies responsible for the older descriptive term *mongoloid idiocy,* or *mongolism,* and cytogenetic abnormality consisting of trisomy 21 or its equivalent in the form of an unbalanced translocation.

dox·a·pram (dock'suh·pram) *n.* 1-Ethyl-4-(2-morpholinoethyl)-3,3-diphenyl-2-pyrrolidinone, $C_{24}H_{30}N_2O_2$, a respiratory and central stimulant; used as the hydrochloride salt.

dox·a·prost (dock'suh·prost) *n.* (13*E*)-15-Hydroxy-15-methyl-9-oxoprost-13-en-1-oic acid, $C_{21}H_{36}O_4$, a prostaglandin bronchodilator.

dox·e·pin (dock'se·pin) *n.* *N,N*-Dimethyldibenz[*b,e*]oxepin-*trans*-$\delta^{11(6H)}$,δ-propylamine, $C_{19}H_{21}NO$, an antidepressant used as the hydrochloride salt.

Doxinate. A trademark for dioctyl sodium sulfosuccinate, a fecal softener.

dox·o·ru·bi·cin (dock''so·roo'bi·sin) *n.* (8*S*-cis)-10-[(3-Amino-2,3,6-trideoxy-α-*L*-*lyxo*-hexapyranosyl)oxy]-7,8,9,10-tetrahydro-6,8,11-trihydroxy-8-(hydroxyacetyl)-1-methoxy-5,12-naphthacenedione, $C_{27}H_{29}NO_{11}$, an antineoplastic.

Doxy II. A trademark for doxycycline, an antibacterial.

Doxychel. A trademark for doxycycline, an antibiotic.

doxy·cy·cline (dock''see·sigh'kleen) *n.* α-6-Deoxy-5-hydroxytetracycline, $C_{22}H_{24}N_2O_8 \cdot H_2O$, a tetracycline antibiotic.

doxycycline hyclate. Doxycycline hydrochloride containing water and ethanol of crystallization, $(C_{22}H_{24}N_2O_8 \cdot HCl)_2C_2H_6O \cdot H_2O$.

dox·yl·a·mine (dock·sil'uh·meen) *n.* 2-[α-(2-Dimethylaminoethoxy)-α-methylbenzyl] pyridine, $C_{17}H_{22}N_2O$, an antihistaminic drug; used as the bisuccinate salt.

Doyne's choroiditis [R. W. *Doyne,* British ophthalmologist, 1857–1916]. A familial disease affecting the macular areas bilaterally, characterized by yellow-white discrete drusen deposits on Bruch's membrane in a mosaic, "honeycomb" pattern, and associated with secondary retinal degeneration in the involved areas.

Doyne's familial colloid degeneration DOYNE'S CHOROIDITIS.

Doyne's honeycomb degeneration DOYNE'S CHOROIDITIS.

D.P.M. Doctor of Podiatric Medicine.

DPN Abbreviation for *diphosphopyridine nucleotide,* now called nicotinamide-adenine dinucleotide and abbreviated NAD.

DPNH Symbol for the reduced form of diphosphopyridine nucleotide, now described as the reduced form of nicotinamide-adenine dinucleotide and symbolized NADH.

DPT 1. Abbreviation for *diphosphothiamine* (= COCARBOXYLASE). 2. Diphtheria-pertussis-tetanus.

DQ, D.Q. Abbreviation for *developmental quotient.*

dr Abbreviation for *dram* or *drachm.*

drachm. DRAM.

drac·on·ti·a·sis (drack''on·tye'uh·sis) *n.* [Gk. *drakontiasis,* from *drakontion,* Guinea worm]. DRACUNCULIASIS.

dra·cun·cu·li·a·sis (dra·kunk''yoo·lye'uh·sis) *n.* [*Dracunculus* + *-iasis*]. Infection with the nematode *Dracunculus medinensis;* characterized by ulcers of the feet and legs produced by the gravid female worm; found in Africa, the Middle East, India, and Brazil. Syn. *guinea worm infection.*

dra·cun·cu·lo·sis (dra·kunk''yoo·lo'sis) *n.* [*Dracunculus* + *-osis*]. DRACUNCULIASIS.

Dra·cun·cu·lus (dra·kunk'yoo·lus) *n.* [NL., dim. of L. *draco,* dragon]. A genus of threadworms belonging to the superfamily Dracunculoidea.

Dracunculus me·di·nen·sis (med·i·nen'sis). A species of filarial worm of which certain species of *Cyclops* are the intermediate hosts and man is a definitive host. Human infection is caused by drinking raw water containing infested *Cyclops.* Syn. *guinea worm.*

draft, draught (draft) *n.* 1. A current of air. 2. A quantity of liquid, usually medicine, taken at one swallow.

dra·gee (drah·zhay') *n.* [F.]. A sugar-coated pill.

drag·on's blood (drag'unz). Any of several resinous secretions, characterized by a dark-red color, obtained from the scale of the fruits of various species of *Daemonorops;* has been used as a coloring agent.

dragon worm. *DRACUNCULUS MEDINENSIS.*

Drag·stedt's operation [L. R. *Dragstedt,* U.S. surgeon, 1893–1975]. Complete vagotomy at the diaphragmatic level combined with gastrojejunostomy for relief of duodenal ulcer.

drain, *n. & v.* 1. A material, such as gauze, rubber tubing, rubber tissue, or twisted suture material, which affords a channel of exit for the discharge from a wound or cavity. 2. *In surgery,* to procure the discharge or evacuation of fluid from a cavity by operation, tapping, or otherwise.

drain·age, *n.* The method of draining; also, the fluid drained off.

drainage headache. LUMBAR PUNCTURE HEADACHE.

drainage tube. A hollow tube of glass, rubber, or other material inserted into a wound or cavity to allow the escape of fluids.

dram, drachm (dram) *n.* [Gk. *drachmē,* as much as one can hold in the hand]. 1. One-eighth of an apothecary ounce. Symbol, ʒ. See also *fluidram* and Table of Medical Signs and Symbols in the Appendix. 2. One-sixteenth of an avoirdupois ounce. Abbreviated, dr. See also Tables of Weights and Measures in the Appendix.

Dramamine. Trademark for dimenhydrinate, an antihistaminic and antinauseant drug.

dram·a·tism (dram'uh·tiz·um) *n.* [*drama* + *-ism*]. Stilted and lofty speech or behavior, observed in some psychoses and neuroses.

dram·a·ti·za·tion, *n. In psychoanalysis,* the transformation of repressed desires into some symbolic form, usually into personifications.

Dramcillin-S. A trademark for the potassium salt of the antibiotic phenethicillin.

drape, *v. & n.* [F. *draper,* from *drap,* cloth]. 1. To cover a part with sterile sheets, so arranged as to leave exposed but protected the particular area to be examined or operated upon. 2. (plural) The sterile sheets or towels used to drape a part for examination or operation.

drap·e·to·ma·nia (drap''e·to·may'nee·uh) *n.* [Gk. *drapetēs,* runaway, + *-mania*]. DROMOMANIA.

dras·tic, *adj. & n.* 1. Extreme, radical; characterizing measures taken as a last resort. 2. A cathartic of the most potent category. Contr. *purgative, laxative.*

draught. DRAFT.

draw, *v. & n.* 1. To cause to soften and discharge; to cause to localize, said of a poultice. 2. The divergence of the walls of a dental cavity preparation that permits the seating and withdrawal of a wax pattern or an inlay.

draw-a-man or **draw-a-person test.** A test based on the subject's drawing of a human figure; employed against children's standardized drawings as a simple and satisfactory estimate of a child's intelligence (Goodenough), as a projective test for personality analysis (Machover), or as a test for the integrity or disturbance of a person's body image.

drawer sign. A sign diagnostic of rupture of a cruciate ligament of the knee; with the knee flexed to a right angle, there is increased anterior or posterior glide of the tibia in rupture of the anterior or posterior ligaments, respectively.

draw·sheet, *n.* A narrow cloth sheet over a waterproof sheet, stretched across the center of the bed, which if soiled can be changed with minimal disturbance to the patient.

dream, *n. & v.* 1. An involuntary series of visual, auditory, or kinesthetic imagery, emotions, and thoughts occurring in the mind during sleep or a sleeplike state, which take the form of a sequence of events or of a story, have a feeling of reality, but totally lack a feeling of free will; believed by Freud to be a mental mechanism whereby impulses are conveyed from the unconscious to the conscious levels of mind. 2. To experience images and trains of thought during sleep, or as if asleep; to have a dream. See also *REM SLEEP.*

dream content. See *latent content, manifest content.*

dreaming sleep. REM SLEEP.

dreamy state. The hallucinations, illusions, and dyscognitive states that accompany temporal lobe epilepsy, and are suggested by hysterical fugues.

dreamy state epilepsy. Psychomotor epilepsy characterized by déjà vu.

drench, *n.* 1. *In veterinary medicine,* the oral administration of a liquid medicinal agent to an animal. 2. The medicinal agent administered in that way.

Dre·pan·i·do·tae·nia (dre·pan″i·do·tee′nee·uh). *n.* A genus of tapeworms of the family Hymenolepididae; *Drepanidotaenia lanceolata* is a parasite of waterfowl.

drep·a·no·cyte (drep′uh·no·site, dre·pan′o·site) *n.* [Gk. *drepanē,* sickle, + *-cyte*]. SICKLE CELL. —**drep·a·no·cyt·ic** (drep″uh·no·sit′ick) *adj.*

drep·a·no·cy·the·mia, drep·a·no·cy·thae·mia (drep″uh·no·sigh·theem′ee·uh, dre·pan″o·) *n.* [*drepanocyte* + *-emia*]. SICKLE CELL ANEMIA.

drepanocytic anemia. SICKLE CELL ANEMIA.

drep·a·no·cy·to·sis (drep″uh·no·sigh·to′sis, dre·pan″o·) *n.* [*drepanocyte* + *-osis*]. The presence of sickle cells in blood. See also *sickle cell anemia.*

Dres·bach's syndrome [M. *Dresbach,* U.S. physician, 1874–1946]. 1. ELLIPTOCYTOSIS. 2. SICKLE CELL ANEMIA.

dress·er, *n.* An attendant in British hospitals, usually a medical student, whose special duty is to dress and bandage wounds.

dress·ing, *n.* Material and medication applied to a wound or infection, and fastened in place to provide protection and to promote healing.

dressing combine. An incision or wound dressing consisting of an unwoven fabric cover which encloses absorbent material and a nonabsorbent layer of cotton or plastic to prevent fluid from passing through; designed to provide warmth and protection and absorb large quantities of fluid.

dressing forceps. A two-limbed, slender-bladed instrument or spring forceps, with blunt or serrated teeth; for use in surgical dressings.

Dress·ler beat [W. *Dressler,* U.S. physician, 1890–1969]. FUSION BEAT.

Dressler's syndrome [W. *Dressler*]. POST-MYOCARDIAL INFARCTION SYNDROME.

drib·ble, *v.* 1. To drool. 2. To void in drops, as urine from a distended or paralyzed bladder.

dried alum. ALUM (3).

dried aluminum hydroxide gel. See *aluminum hydroxide gel.*

dried yeast. BREWER'S YEAST.

Drierite. A trademark for anhydrous calcium sulfate, a dehydrating agent.

Driesch's law of constant volume (dreesh). The differences in the total mass of the organ are due to the number and not to the volume of the cells; e.g., the renal or hepatic cells of a bull, man, or mouse have approximately equal size.

drift, *n.* 1. Movement of teeth from their normal position in the dental arch due to the loss of contiguous teeth. 2. GENETIC DRIFT.

drift·wood cortex. DYSTOPIC CORTICAL MYELINOGENESIS.

drill, *n.* [D. *drillen,* to bore]. A cutting instrument for excavating a tooth or bone by rotary motion.

Drink·er-Col·lins resuscitation [P. *Drinker,* U.S. public health engineer, 1894–1972]. Resuscitation by use of the Drinker respirator.

Drinker respirator [P. *Drinker*]. An iron lung, usually power driven, but also operated manually.

Drinker's method [P. *Drinker*]. Artificial respiration similar to the Schafer method, but with a second operator who kneels at the patient's head and raises the arms to assist in inspiration.

drinking test. WATER-DRINKING TEST.

drip, *n. & v.* 1. The continuous slow introduction of fluid, usually containing nutrients or drugs. 2. To introduce fluid slowly.

drip treatment. The continuous infusion of fluid into the blood or a body cavity so slowly that the rate is measured in drops.

Drisdol. A trademark for vitamin D_2 or calciferol.

drive, *n.* 1. Instinct; basic urge; motivation. 2. *In psychology and psychiatry,* psychic phenomena such as the sexual or aggressive drives in contrast to the more purely biological and physical instincts. 3. *In psychology,* a hypothetical state of an organism necessary before a given stimulus will elicit a certain kind of response, as hunger must be present before the presence of food will elicit eating.

drive conversion. *In psychology,* the turning of a basic or primary drive toward a new goal, converting it into an acquired drive.

driv·ing, *n. In electroencephalography,* the appearance of a certain frequency (hertz) in the electroencephalogram as a result of sensory stimulation at that frequency. See also *photic driving.*

dro·car·bil (dro·kahr′bil) *n.* $C_{16}H_{23}AsN_2O_7$; the acetarsone salt of arecoline, a nearly white or slightly yellow powder, freely soluble in water; used as a veterinary anthelmintic.

dro·cin·o·nide (dro·sin′o·nide) *n.* 9-Fluoro-11β,16α,17,21-tetrahydroxy-5α-pregnane-3,20-dione, cyclic 16,17-acetal with acetone, $C_{24}H_{35}FO_6$, an anti-inflammatory.

Drolban. Trademark for dromostanolone, an antineoplastic drug used as the propionate ester.

drom-, dromo- [Gk. *dromos,* course, race]. A combining form meaning (a) *course*; (b) *running*; (c) *speed.*

dromo·graph (drom′o·graf) *n.* [*dromo-* + *-graph*]. A recording blood flowmeter.

dromo·ma·nia (drom″o·may′nee·uh) *n.* [*dromo-* + *-mania*]. An uncontrollable desire to wander from home.

dromo·pho·bia (drom″o·fo′bee·uh) *n.* [*dromo-* + *-phobia*]. Morbid fear of walking or roaming about.

dro·mos·tan·o·lone (dro·mos′tan·o·lone, dro″mo·stan′o·lone) *n.* 17β-Hydroxy-2α-methylandrostan-3-one, $C_{20}H_{32}O_2$, an antineoplastic agent; used as the propionate ester.

dromo·trop·ic (dro″mo·trop′ick, dromo″o·) *adj.* [*dromo-* + *-tropic*]. Affecting the speed and conduction of nerve fibers.

dromotropic regulation. The regulation of the rate of conduction and duration of the refractory period of the heart, by sympathetic and parasympathetic influences.

drone fly. *ERISTALIS.*

drool, *v.* 1. To let saliva flow out of the mouth, as seen normally in infants. 2. To secrete saliva profusely.

drop, *n.* 1. A minute mass of liquid which in falling or in hanging from a surface forms a spheroid. 2. Commonly, a volume of liquid equal to about 0.05 ml (approximately 1 minim). 3. A lozenge, as a cough drop. 4. *In neurology,* the falling of a part from paralysis, as a foot drop. 5. AKINETIC SEIZURE.

drop attack. Sudden loss of erect posture, with or without loss of consciousness, and due to syncope, brainstem ischemia, akinetic epilepsy, or vertigo, among many other causes.

dro·per·i·dol (dro·perr'i·dol) *n.* 1-[1-[3-(*p*-Fluorobenzoyl)-propyl]-1,2,3,6-tetrahydro-4-pyridyl]-2-benzimidazolinone, $C_{22}H_{22}FN_3O_2$, a tranquilizer and sedative.

drop hand. WRIST-DROP.

drop heart. CARDIOPTOSIS.

drop·let, *n.* A minute particle of moisture, such as that expelled by talking, sneezing, or coughing, which may carry infectious microorganisms from one individual to another.

droplet infection. AIR-BORNE INFECTION.

dropped beat. In second-degree heart block, an atrial deflection (P wave) not followed by a ventricular deflection (QRS complex).

dropped foot. A drop or plantar flexion of the foot, generally due to paralysis of the dorsiflexor muscles of the foot and toes.

drop·per, *n.* A bottle, tube, or pipet, fitted for the emission of a liquid drop by drop.

dropping-mercury electrode. An electrode providing for a steady release of droplets of mercury falling through an electrolyte into a pool of mercury; used in polarography.

drop seizure. AKINETIC SEIZURE.

dropsical ovum. An ovum in which the embryo has entirely disappeared or is represented by only a nodule of deteriorated and nonviable tissue. The amniotic vesicle is distended by an amount of fluid far out of proportion to the duration of pregnancy.

drop·sy (drop'see) *n.* [OF. *ydropesie*, from Gk. *hydrōps*, from *hydōr*, water]. The abnormal accumulation of serous fluid in body tissues and cavities; ANASARCA. —**drop·si·cal** (·si·kul) *adj.*

dropsy of the brain. HYDROCEPHALUS.

Droptainer. A trademark for a plastic container which dispenses one drop of liquid when inverted and squeezed.

Dro·soph·i·la (dro·sof'i·luh) *n.* [Gk. *drosos*, dew, + L. *-phila*, from Gk. *philos*, loving]. A genus of Diptera including common fruit flies.

Drosophila mel·a·no·gas·ter (mel'uh·no·gas"tur) [*melano-* + *-gaster*]. The best known species of fruit fly because of its extensive use in genetic analysis.

Droxone. A trademark for algestone acetophenide, an anti-inflammatory.

Dr. P.H. Doctor of Public Health.

drug, *n.* & *v.* [MF. *drogue*, perhaps from MD. *droge*, dry (as applied to dried herbs and the like)]. 1. Any substance other than food or water that is intended to be taken or administered (ingested, injected, applied, implanted, inhaled, etc.) for the purpose of altering, sustaining, or controlling the recipient's physical, mental, or emotional state. 2. In United States law, any article, other than a food or a device, that is intended for use in the diagnosis, cure, mitigation, treatment, or prevention of disease, or is intended to affect the structure or any function of the body of man or other animals, or is recognized in one or more of the official compendia which provide standards for the evaluation of such articles. 3. To administer a drug to; especially, to NARCOTIZE.

drug-fast, *adj.* Of microorganisms: resistant to antimicrobial drugs. —**drug-fast·ness,** *n.*

drug fever. Fever resulting from the administration of a drug.

drug·gist (drug'ist) *n.* A dealer in medicines.

drum, *n.* [D. *trom*]. TYMPANIC MEMBRANE.

drum·mer's palsy. Paralysis of the extensor of the distal phalanx of the thumb occurring in drummers.

drum·stick, *n.* A small nuclear projection found in 3 to 5 percent of neutrophil leukocytes of females, but not in males.

drum·stick finger. CLUBBED FINGER.

drunk·ard's arm paralysis. Paralysis due to compression of the radial nerve against the humerus during sleep, or when the arm is hung over the edge of a chair or bench during alcoholic stupor.

drunk·en gait. STAGGERING GAIT.

drunk·en·ness, *n.* INTOXICATION (2); especially as produced by drinking alcoholic liquor.

drunk·om·e·ter (drunk·om'e·tur) *n.* [*drunk* + *-meter*]. An instrument used to determine whether or not a person is intoxicated. See also *breath alcohol method.*

drupe (droop) *n.* [Gk. *dryppa*, olive]. A fruit which has a thin epicarp, a fleshy mesocarp, and a stony endocarp which encloses a seed, as the plum or peach.

dru·sen (droo'zun) *n. pl.* [Ger.]. 1. Colloid excrescences on the basal membrane. 2. Granules found in tissues in actinomycosis.

dry, *adj.* 1. Not wet; free from moisture or excess moisture; as dry heat sterilization, dry sponge. 2. Not accompanied by obvious bleeding; as dry operative wound. 3. Not accompanied by mucus or phlegm; as dry rales. 4. Marked by scantiness of effusions or secretions. 5. Dehydrated; as dry tissues.

dry amputation. BLOODLESS AMPUTATION.

dry brain. The paucity of cerebrospinal fluid noted in cases of severe generalized cerebral edema or large space-occupying lesions.

dry-bulb temperature. The actual air temperature, with the exclusion of variations due to radiation or conduction. Contr. *wet-bulb temperature.*

dry cholera. CHOLERA SICCA.

dry cough. A cough unaccompanied by mucus or phlegm.

dry cup. A cup for drawing the blood to the surface.

dry cupping. A form of counterirritation in which the blood is drawn to the surface by means of a cup. This was used mainly in inflammatory affections of the lung.

dry gangrene. Local death of a part due to arterial obstruction without infection. Syn. *mummification.*

dry ice. Carbon dioxide in its solid state; used for cryotherapy.

dry labor. Labor in which there is a deficiency of the liquor amnii, or in which there has been a premature rupture of the amniotic sac.

dry laryngitis. A form of laryngitis characterized by sensations of heat and hoarseness in the throat, persistent cough, and sometimes aphonia.

dry nurse. A nurse who cares for but does not suckle the baby.

Dry·op·ter·is (dry·op'·tur·is) *n.* [Gk. *drys*, *dryos*, oak, + *pteris*, fern]. A large genus of medium-sized ferns of the Polypodiaceae. Syn. *woodfern.*

Dryopteris fil·ix-mas (fil'icks mas'). European aspidium or male fern, the rhizome and stipes of which are a source of aspidium oleoresin.

Dryopteris mar·gi·na·lis (mahr·ji·nay'lis). American aspidium or marginal fern, the rhizome and stipes of which are a source of aspidium oleoresin.

dry socket. Alveolitis following a dental extraction.

dry synovitis. Synovitis with little if any exudate.

dry tap. A tap in which no fluid can be obtained.

Dryvax. A trademark for smallpox vaccine.

dry vomiting. Persistent nausea with attempts at vomiting, but with ejection of nothing but gas.

D. Sc., D. S. Doctor of Science.

DSCG Abbreviation for *disodium chromoglycate* (= CROMOLYN SODIUM).

D-state. REM SLEEP.

DTPA In 111 (or **DTPA In 113m**) The diethylenetetraminepentaacetic acid chelate of indium 111 (or indium 113m), employed as a diagnostic agent in cisternography.

DTPA Tc 99m The diethylenetetraminepentaacetic acid chelate of technetium 99m, employed as a diagnostic agent for brain or kidney visualization and for vascular dynamic studies.

D.T.R. Abbreviation for *deep tendon reflex.*

D trisomy. TRISOMY 13 SYNDROME.

du·al, *adj.* [L. *dualis*]. Consisting of two parts.

Dualar. Trademark for benzodepa, an antineoplastic compound.

du·al·is·tic theory. The theory that the cells of the blood are derived from blast cells of two basically different types.

D^u allele or **factor** (dew) *n.* A clinically important variant of the Rh_0 factor; individuals possessing this variation are considered Rh positive.

dual personality. See *multiple personality.*

Du·ane's retraction syndrome [A. *Duane,* U.S. ophthalmologist, 1858–1926]. A congenital anomaly of the eye, usually involving one only, caused by abnormal fibrous bands attached to the medial rectus muscle or an aplastic and fibrous lateral rectus muscle, in which attempted duction movements often result in retraction of the eyeball with narrowing of the palpebral fissure, poor abduction and limited adduction, and secondary convergence insufficiency.

du·azo·my·cin (dew·az″o·migh′sin) *n.* An antibiotic, produced by *Streptomyces ambofaciens,* that has antineoplastic activity.

Du·bi·ni's chorea or **disease** (doo·bee′nee) [A. *Dubini,* Italian physician, 1813–1902]. An acute febrile disease of unknown nature, accompanied by lancinating pains and myoclonus, sometimes becoming generalized, and progressing rapidly to death in almost all cases.

Du·bin-John·son syndrome [I. N. *Dubin* and F. B. *Johnson,* U.S. physicians, 20th century]. A dominantly inherited defect in liver function in which icterus and hepatic pigmentation are associated with retention of conjugated bilirubin.

Dubin-Sprinz syndrome. DUBIN-JOHNSON SYNDROME.

Du·bois cyst or **abscess** (dueᵉ·bwah′)[P. *Dubois,* French obstetrician, 1795–1871]. A cyst of the thymic corpuscles associated with congenital syphilis.

Du·boi·sia (dew·boy′zee·uh) *n.* [F. N. *Dubois,* French botanist, d. 1824]. A genus of Far Eastern tropical plants, certain members of which contain scopolamine, hyoscyamine, and related alkaloids, while others contain nicotine and associated alkaloids.

Du Bois standards. AUB-DU BOIS STANDARDS.

Du·bos-Bra·chet method (dueᵉ·bo′, bra·sheyʸ′)[R. J. *Dubos,* French microbiologist in America, b. 1901]. A histochemical method for ribonucleic acid using ribonuclease to break down ribonucleic acid and remove its basophilic staining properties.

Du·boscq colorimeter (dueᵉ·boʰsk′) [J. *Duboscq,* French optician, 1817–1886]. An instrument for comparing and matching colors of solutions.

Du·bo·witz method [V. *Dubowitz,* English pediatrician, 20th century, and L. *Dubowitz,* 20th century]. A method, based on neurological function and maturity of skin, ears, genitalia, and other aspects of appearance, for estimating the gestational age of the newborn.

Dubowitz' syndrome. A congenital disorder of unknown cause characterized by shortness of stature; peculiar facies with hypoplasia of the supraorbital ridges, zygoma, malar eminence, and mandible; short palpebral fissures simulating hypertelorism; prominent ears; thick skin with an eczematoid eruption; and sometimes mental retardation.

Du·chenne-Aran disease (dueᵉ·shen′, a·rahⁿ′) [G. B. A. *Duchenne,* French neurologist, 1807–1875; and F. A. *Aran,* French physician, 1817–1861]. PROGRESSIVE SPINAL MUSCULAR ATROPHY.

Duchenne-Erb palsy, paralysis, or **syndrome** [G. B. A. *Duchenne* and W. H. *Erb*]. UPPER BRACHIAL PLEXUS PARALYSIS.

Duchenne-Griesinger disease [G. B. A. *Duchenne* and W. *Griesinger*]. PSEUDOHYPERTROPHIC INFANTILE MUSCULAR DYSTROPHY.

Duchenne's disease [G. B. A. *Duchenne*]. 1. TABES DORSALIS. 2. PROGRESSIVE BULBAR PARALYSIS.

Duchenne's muscular dystrophy [G. B. A. *Duchenne*]. PSEUDOHYPERTROPHIC INFANTILE MUSCULAR DYSTROPHY.

Duchenne's paralysis [G. B. A. *Duchenne*]. PROGRESSIVE BULBAR PARALYSIS.

duck·bill speculum. A bivalve vaginal speculum with flat, broad blades.

duck embryo vaccine. Vaccine prepared in duck embryos for use as active immunization following exposure to rabies.

duck·er·ing (duck′ur·ing) *n.* [G. F. *Duckering*]. A method of disinfecting hair and wool, employed against the *Bacillus anthracis.*

duck virus hepatitis. A usually fatal virus disease of young ducklings, associated with opisthotonus clinically and hemorrhagic lesions of the liver pathologically.

Du·crey's bacillus [A. *Ducrey,* Italian dermatologist, 1860–1940]. *HAEMOPHILUS DUCREYI.*

duct, *n.* [L. *ductus,* from *ducere,* to lead]. 1. A tube or channel, especially one for conveying the secretions of a gland. 2. A small enclosed channel conducting any fluid, as the cochlear duct. —**duc·tal** (duck′tul) *adj.*

ductal carcinoma or **tumor.** Generally, a malignant tumor of the mammary gland, arising from cells lining the ducts.

ductal papillary carcinoma. A papillary carcinoma of the mammary ducts.

ductal papilloma. 1. A benign tumor of the breast limited to the mammary duct system, characterized by atypical papillary structures. 2. Any papilloma growing in a duct.

duc·tile (duck′til, ·tile) *adj.* [L. *ductilis*]. Capable of being reshaped or drawn out without breaking.

duc·tion (duck′shun) *n.* [L. *ductio,* from *ducere,* to lead]. The rotation of the eye around the horizontal axis or the vertical axis.

duct·less, *adj.* Having no excretory duct.

ductless glands. Glands without ducts, such as the endocrine glands, secreting directly into the bloodstream.

duct of Aran·tius (a·ran′chee·us) [G. C. *Aranzi* (*Arantius*), Italian anatomist, 1538–1589]. DUCTUS VENOSUS.

duct of Bel·li·ni (bel·lee′nee) [L. *Bellini,* Italian anatomist, 1643–1704]. PAPILLARY DUCT.

duct of Cu·vier (kueᵉv·yeʸ′) [G. L. C. F. *Cuvier*]. Either of the two common cardinal veins.

duct of San·to·ri·ni (saʰn·to·ree′nee) [G. D. *Santorini*]. ACCESSORY PANCREATIC DUCT.

duct of Ste·no (stee′no, stay′no) [N. *Stensen* (*Steno*)]. PAROTID DUCT.

duct of Sten·sen [N. *Stensen*]. PAROTID DUCT.

duct of the epididymis. EPIDIDYMAL DUCT.

duct of the testis. A duct made up of the epididymal duct, the ductus deferens, and the ejaculatory duct.

duct of Wir·sung (virr′zŏŏng) [J. G. *Wirsung,* German anatomist, 1600–1643]. PANCREATIC DUCT.

duc·tu·lar (duck′tew·lur) *adj.* Pertaining to a ductule.

duc·tule (duck′tewl) *n.* [dim. from *ductus*]. A small duct.

ductuli. Plural of *ductulus.*

ductuli aber·ran·tes (ab″err·an′teez) [NA]. Vestigial remains of caudal mesonephric tubules related to the epididymis. There are superior and inferior ones.

ductuli al·ve·o·la·res (al″vee·o·lair′eez) [NA]. ALVEOLAR DUCTS.

ductuli bi·li·fe·ri (bi·lif′e·rye) [NA]. The small channels that connect the interlobular ductules of the liver with the right and left hepatic ducts.

ductuli ef·fe·ren·tes tes·tis (ef·ur·en′teez tes′tis) [NA]. EFFERENT DUCTULES OF THE TESTIS.

ductuli ex·cre·to·rii glan·du·lae la·cri·ma·lis (ecks·kre·to′ree·eye glan′dew·lee lack·ri·may′lis) [NA]. The numerous small channels that leave the lacrimal gland and open at the fornix of the conjunctiva.

ductuli in·ter·lo·bu·la·res (in″tur·lob·yoo·lair′eez) [NA].

Small channels between the hepatic lobules which drain bile into the ductuli biliferi.

ductuli pro·sta·ti·ci (pro·stat'i·sigh) [NA]. The channels that drain the secretion of the prostate into the prostatic urethra.

ductuli trans·ver·si epo·o·pho·ri (trans·vur'sigh ep"o·of'o·rye) [NA]. Vestigial remains of mesonephric tubules which empty into the ductus epoophori longitudinalis.

duc·tu·lus (duck'tew·lus) *n.*, pl. **ductu·li** (·lye) [NA]. DUCTULE.

ductulus aber·rans superior (ab·err'anz) [NA]. Vestigial remains of a caudal mesonephric tubule attached to the superior portion of the epididymis.

duc·tus (duck'tus) *n.*, pl. & genit. sing. **ductus** (duck'tooss, duck'tus) [L.] [NA]. DUCT.

ductus ar·te·ri·o·sus (ahr·teer"ee·o'sus) [NA]. The distal half of the left sixth aortic arch forming a fetal blood shunt between the left pulmonary artery and the aorta. Syn. *Botallo's duct.*

ductus arteriosus bi·la·te·ra·lis (bye·lat"e·ray'lis). A developmental anomaly in which the right sixth aortic arch persists entirely or in part.

ductus bi·li·fe·ri (bi·lif'e·rye) [BNA]. DUCTULI BILIFERI.

ductus ca·ro·ti·cus (ka·rot'i·kus). The part of the bilateral embryonic dorsal aortae between the third and fourth aortic arches which normally disappears early in development.

ductus cho·le·do·chus (ko·led'o·kus) [NA]. COMMON BILE DUCT.

ductus co·chle·a·ris (kock·lee·air'is) [NA]. COCHLEAR DUCT.

ductus cys·ti·cus (sis'ti·kus) [NA]. CYSTIC DUCT.

ductus de·fe·rens (def'uh·renz), *pl.* **ductus de·fe·ren·tes** (def·e·ren'teez) [NA]. The portion of the excretory duct system of the testis which runs from the epididymal duct to the ejaculatory duct. Syn. *deferent duct, vas deferens.* See also Plate 25.

ductus eja·cu·la·to·ri·us (e·jack"yoo·la·to'ree·us) [NA]. EJACULATORY DUCT.

ductus en·do·lym·pha·ti·cus (en·do·lim·fat'i·kus) [NA]. ENDOLYMPHATIC DUCT (1).

ductus epi·di·dy·mi·dis (ep"ee·di·dim'i·dis) [NA]. EPIDIDYMAL DUCT.

ductus epo·o·pho·ri lon·gi·tu·di·na·lis (ep"o·of'o·rye lon"ji·tew·di·nay'lis) [NA]. The vestigial remnant of the mesonephric duct.

ductus ex·cre·to·ri·us glan·du·lae bul·bo·ure·thra·lis (ecks·kree·to'ree·us glan'dew·lee bul"bo·yoo·re·thray'lis) [BNA]. DUCTUS GLANDULAE BULBOURETHRALIS.

ductus excretorius ve·si·cu·lae se·mi·na·lis (ve·sick'yoo·lee sem·i·nay'lis) [NA]. The duct of the seminal vesicle which unites with the ductus deferens to form the ejaculatory duct.

ductus glan·du·lae bul·bo·ure·thra·lis (glan'dew·lee bul"bo·yoo"re·thray'lis) [NA]. The duct of the bulbourethral gland.

ductus he·pa·ti·cus com·mu·nis (he·pat'i·kus kom·yoo'nis) [NA]. COMMON HEPATIC DUCT.

ductus hepaticus dex·ter (decks'tur) [NA]. The right hepatic duct which unites with the left to form the common hepatic duct.

ductus hepaticus si·nis·ter (sin·is'tur) [NA]. The left hepatic duct which unites with the right to form the common hepatic duct.

ductus in·ci·si·vus (in"si·sigh'vus, in·sigh'si·vus) [NA]. An inconstant channel in the incisive canal connecting the nasal and oral cavities.

ductus in·ter·lo·bu·la·res (in"tur·lob·yoo·lair'eez) [BNA]. DUCTULI INTERLOBULARES.

ductus la·cri·ma·les (lack"ri·may'leez) [BNA]. Canaliculi lacrimales (= LACRIMAL CANALICULI).

ductus lac·ti·fe·ri (lack·tif'ur·eye) [NA]. LACTIFEROUS DUCTS.

ductus lin·gua·lis (ling·gway'lis) [BNA]. The proximal remnant of the thyroglossal duct which may persist and open into the foramen cecum of the tongue.

ductus lo·bi cau·da·ti dex·ter (lo'bye kaw·day'tye decks'tur) [NA]. The right duct of the caudate lobe of the liver.

ductus lobi caudati si·nis·ter (si·nis'tur) [NA]. The left duct of the caudate lobe of the liver.

ductus lym·pha·ti·cus dex·ter (lim·fat'i·kus decks'tur) [NA]. RIGHT LYMPHATIC DUCT. NA alt. *ductus thoracicus dexter.*

ductus me·so·neph·ri·cus (mes'o·nef'ri·kus) [NA]. MESONEPHRIC DUCT.

ductus Muel·leri (mew'lur·eye) [BNA]. Ductus paramesonephricus (= PARAMESONEPHRIC DUCT).

ductus na·so·la·cri·ma·lis (nay"zo·lack·ri·may'lis) [NA]. NASOLACRIMAL DUCT.

ductus pan·cre·a·ti·cus (pan"kree·at'i·kus) [NA]. PANCREATIC DUCT.

ductus pancreaticus ac·ces·so·ri·us (ack"se·so'ree·us) [NA]. ACCESSORY PANCREATIC DUCT.

ductus pa·ra·me·so·neph·ri·cus (păr"uh·mes"o·nef'ri·kus) [NA]. PARAMESONEPHRIC DUCT.

ductus pa·ra·ure·thra·les (păr"uh·yoo·re·thray'leez) [NA]. PARAURETHRAL DUCTS.

ductus pa·ro·ti·de·us (păr"o·ti·dee'us, ·tid'ee·us) [NA]. PAROTID DUCT.

ductus pe·ri·lym·pha·ti·ci (perr·i·lim·fat'i·sigh) [BNA]. Plural of *ductus perilymphaticus.*

ductus pe·ri·lym·pha·ti·cus (perr·i·lim·fat'i·kus) [NA]. AQUEDUCT OF THE COCHLEA. NA alt. *aqueductus cochleae.*

ductus pro·sta·ti·ci (pro·stat'i·sigh) [BNA]. DUCTULI PROSTATICI.

ductus re·u·ni·ens (re·yoo'nee·enz) [NA]. A membranous tube in the inner ear uniting the saccule with the cochlear duct; it contains endolymph. Syn. *Hensen's canal.*

ductus semi·cir·cu·la·res (sem"ee·sur·kew·lair'eez) [NA]. The semicircular ducts (= MEMBRANOUS SEMICIRCULAR CANALS) collectively.

ductus semi·cir·cu·la·ris anterior (sem"ee·sur·kew·lair'is) [NA]. The anterior semicircular duct of the inner ear. See also *membranous semicircular canals.*

ductus semicircularis la·te·ra·lis (lat·e·ray'lis) [NA]. The lateral semicircular duct of the inner ear. See also *membranous semicircular canals.*

ductus semicircularis posterior [NA]. The posterior semicircular duct of the inner ear. See also *membranous semicircular canals.*

ductus semicircularis superior [BNA]. DUCTUS SEMICIRCULARIS ANTERIOR.

ductus sub·lin·gua·les mi·no·res (sub"ling·gway'leez mi·no'reez) [NA]. The minor sublingual ducts. See *sublingual ducts.*

ductus sub·lin·gua·lis major (sub"ling·gway'lis) [NA]. The major sublingual duct. See *sublingual ducts.*

ductus sub·man·di·bu·la·ris (sub"man·dib·yoo·lair'is) [NA]. SUBMANDIBULAR DUCT.

ductus sub·ma·xil·la·ris (sub·mack"si·lair'is) [BNA]. Ductus submandibularis. (= SUBMANDIBULAR DUCT).

ductus su·do·ri·fe·rus (sue"do·rif'uh·rus) [NA]. The duct of any sweat gland.

ductus tho·ra·ci·cus (tho·ras'i·kus) [NA]. THORACIC DUCT.

ductus thoracicus dex·ter (decks'tur). [NA alt.] RIGHT LYMPHATIC DUCT. NA alt. *ductus lymphaticus dexter.*

ductus thy·re·o·glos·sus (thigh"ree·o·glos'us) [BNA]. Ductus thyroglossus. (= THYROGLOSSAL DUCT).

ductus thy·ro·glos·sus (thigh"ro·glos'us) [NA]. THYROGLOSSAL DUCT.

ductus utri·cu·lo·sac·cu·la·ris (yoo·trick"yoo·lo·sack·yoo·lair'is) [NA]. UTRICULOSACCULAR DUCT.

ductus ve·no·sus (ve·no'sus) [NA]. A venous channel of the embryonic liver shunting blood from the left umbilical vein to the enlarging right sinus venosus of the heart. Syn. *duct of Arantius.*

ductus Wolf·fi (wol'fye) [K. F. *Wolff*] [BNA]. Ductus mesonephricus (= MESONEPHRIC DUCT).

Duf·fy blood group. The erythrocyte antigens defined by their reaction with anti-Fy[a] serum, originally found in a multiply transfused patient named Duffy.

Du·gas' test [L. A. *Dugas*, U.S. surgeon, 1806–1884]. A test for dislocation of the shoulder; the elbow cannot be made to touch the side of the chest when the hand of the affected side is placed on the opposite shoulder.

Duh·ring's disease [L. A. *Duhring*, U.S. dermatologist, 1845–1913]. DERMATITIS HERPETIFORMIS.

du·ip·a·ra (dew·ip'uh·ruh) *n.* [L. *duo*, two, + *-para*]. A woman who has given birth twice.

Dukes' disease [C. *Dukes*, English physician, 1845–1925]. EXANTHEM SUBITUM.

Duke test or **method** [W. W. *Duke*, U.S. pathologist, 1883–1945]. A test for bleeding time, performed by puncturing the lobe of the ear and determining the time which elapses until bleeding stops.

dul·ca·ma·ra (dul''kuh·măr'uh, ·mahr'uh) *n.* [L. *dulcis*, sweet, + *amara*, bitter]. The dried stems of *Solanum dulcamara*, bitter nightshade, containing an alkaloid, solanine. Overdoses cause nausea, emesis, and convulsive muscular movements; has been employed in psoriasis and other skin diseases.

dul·cin (dul'sin) *n.* *p*-Phenetolcarbamide or 4-ethoxyphenylurea, $C_9H_{12}N_2O_2$, a crystalline substance, very sweet, that has been employed as a noncaloric sweetening agent but may be toxic on prolonged use.

dul·cite (dul'site, ·sit) *n.* DULCITOL.

dul·ci·tol (dul'si·tol) *n.* A sugar, $C_6H_{14}O_6$, found in a variety of plants.

Dulcolax. Trademark for bisacodyl, a laxative drug.

dull, *adj.* 1. Slow of perception; not clear of mind. 2. Not resonant on percussion; muffled. 3. Not bright in appearance. 4. Not sharp; blunt. —**dull·ness,** *n.*

Du·long and Pe·tit law (dueˡlohn', puh·tee') [P. L. *Dulong*, French physicist and chemist, 1785–1838; and A. T. *Petit*, French physician, 1791–1820]. LAW OF DULONG AND PETIT.

dumb, *adj.* 1. MUTE. 2. *Colloq.* Stupid; lacking in intelligence. —**dumb·ness** *n.*

dumb·bell, *n.* 1. A weight consisting of two identical spheres connected by a short rod. 2. Something shaped like a dumbbell.

dumbbell crystals. Crystals of calcium oxalate or uric acid occurring in acid urine or those of calcium carbonate, in alkaline urine.

dumbbell tumor. A ganglioneuroma or neurofibroma composed of a mass in both the spinal canal and thorax connected by a narrow band of tumor tissue in the intervertebral foramen.

dumb rabies or **madness.** PARALYTIC RABIES.

dum·dum fever (dum'dum) [after *Dum Dum*, W. Bengal, India]. KALA-AZAR.

dum·my, *n.* 1. PONTIC. 2. British term for PLACEBO.

dump·ing, *n.* A sudden, rapid emptying.

dumping syndrome or **stomach.** Disagreeable or painful epigastric fullness, nausea, weakness, giddiness, sweating, palpitations, and diarrhea occurring after meals in patients who have had gastric surgery which interferes with the function of the pylorus.

duo- [L.]. A combining form meaning *two*.

duo·chrome test (dew'o·krohm). A method for determining spherical refraction under complete cycloplegia, based on the fact that the human eye is slightly myopic for the blue end of the color spectrum and slightly hyperopic for the red end.

du·o·crin·in (dew''o·krin'in, dew·ock'rin·in) *n.* An extract from the intestinal mucosa which stimulates duodenal glands. Its hormonal status is uncertain.

duoden-, duodeno-. A combining form meaning *duodenum, duodenal.*

du·o·de·nal (dew''o·dee'nul, dew·od'e·nul) *adj.* Of or pertaining to the duodenum.

duodenal antrum. The normal dilatation presented by the duodenum near its origin.

duodenal bulb or **cap.** *In radiology,* the first part of the duodenum, immediately beyond the pylorus.

duodenal glands. The deep mixed glands of the first part of the duodenum. NA *glandulae duodenales.*

duodenal papilla. See *major duodenal papilla, minor duodenal papilla.*

duodenal regurgitation. The return of chyme from the duodenum into the stomach.

duodenal ulcer. A peptic ulcer situated in the duodenum.

du·o·de·nec·ta·sis (dew''o·de·neck'tuh·sis) *n.*, pl. **duodenecta·ses** (·seez) [*duoden-* + *ectasis*]. Chronic dilatation of the duodenum.

du·o·de·nec·to·my (dew''o·de·neck'tuh·mee) *n.* [*duoden-* + *-ectomy*]. Excision of part of the duodenum.

du·o·de·ni·tis (dew''o·de·nigh'tis) *n.* [*duoden-* + *-itis*]. Inflammation of the duodenum.

duodeno-. See *duoden-*.

du·o·de·no·chol·an·gi·tis (dew''o·dee''no·kol''an·jye'tis) *n.* [*duodeno-* + *cholangitis*]. Inflammation of the duodenum and the common bile duct.

du·o·de·no·chol·e·cys·tos·to·my (dew''o·dee''no·kol''e·sis·tos'tuh·mee) *n.* [*duodeno-* + *cholecystostomy*]. The formation of an anastomosis between the duodenum and gallbladder.

du·o·de·no·cho·led·o·chot·o·my (dew''o·dee''no·ko·led''o·kot'uh·mee) *n.* A modification of choledochotomy by incising the duodenum in order to approach the common duct.

du·o·de·no·co·lic (dew''o·dee''no·kol'ick, ·ko'lick) *adj.* Pertaining to the duodenum and the colon, as: duodenocolic fistula.

du·o·de·no·cys·tos·to·my (dew''o·dee''no·sis·tos'tuh·mee) *n.* [*duodeno-* + *cystostomy*]. DUODENOCHOLECYSTOSTOMY.

du·o·de·no·en·ter·os·to·my (dew''o·dee''no·en''tur·os'tuh·mee) *n.* [*duodeno-* + *enterostomy*]. *In surgery,* the formation of a passage between the duodenum and another part of the intestine.

du·o·de·no·gram (dew''o·dee'no·gram, dew·od'e·) *n.* A radiograph of the duodenum using contrast material.

du·o·de·nog·ra·phy (dew''o·de·nog'ruh·fee) *n.* Radiographic depiction of the duodenum using contrast material.

du·o·de·no·he·pat·ic (dew''o·dee''no·he·pat'ick) *adj.* [*duodeno-* + *hepatic*]. Pertaining to the duodenum and the liver.

du·o·de·no·il·e·os·to·my (dew''o·dee''no·il''ee·os'tuh·mee) *n.* [*duodeno-* + *ileo-* + *-stomy*]. The formation of a passage between the duodenum and the ileum.

du·o·de·no·je·ju·nal (dew''o·dee''no·je·joo'nul) *adj.* Pertaining to the duodenum and the jejunum.

duodenojejunal flexure. The abrupt bend at the junction of the duodenum and jejunum. NA *flexura duodenojejunalis.*

duodenojejunal fold. DUODENOJEJUNAL PLICA.

duodenojejunal fossa. Any one of a variety of pouches or recesses formed by folds of peritoneum from the terminal portion of the duodenum blending with parietal peritoneum. NA *recessus duodenalis superior.*

duodenojejunal hernia. A retroperitoneal hernia into the paraduodenal recess.

duodenojejunal plica. An inconstant fold of peritoneum extending to the left from the duodenojejunal flexure to the posterior abdominal wall; it may contain the main stem of the inferior mesenteric vein. NA *plica duodenalis superior.*

duodenojejunal recess. DUODENOJEJUNAL FOSSA.

du·o·de·no·je·ju·nos·to·my (dew''o·dee''no·jej''oo·nos'tuh·mee) *n.* [*duodeno-* + *jejunostomy*]. *In surgery,* an anastomosis of the duodenum to the jejunum.

du·o·de·no·meso·co·lic (dew''o·dee''no·mez''o·co·lic, ·ko'lick) *adj.* Pertaining to the duodenum and the mesocolon.

duodenomesocolic plica or **fold**. An inconstant fold of peritoneum extending from the ascending part of the duodenum to the posterior abdominal wall. NA *plica duodenalis inferior.*

du·o·de·no·pan·cre·a·tec·to·my (dew″o·dee″no·pan″kree·uh·teck′tuh·mee) *n.* [*duodeno-* + *pancreatectomy*]. *In surgery,* excision of a portion of the duodenum together with the head of the pancreas.

du·o·de·no·plas·ty (dew″o·dee′no·plas″tee) *n.* [*duodeno-* + *-plasty*]. A reparative operation upon some portion of the duodenum. See also *pyloroplasty.*

du·o·de·no·py·lo·rec·to·my (dew″o·dee″no·pye″lo·reck′tuh·mee) *n.* [*duodeno-* + *pylorectomy*]. Resection of a portion of the duodenum and the pylorus.

du·o·de·nor·rha·phy (dew″o·de·nor′uh·fee) *n.* [*duodeno-* + *-rrhaphy*]. The suture and repair of the duodenum after incision, as for the closure of a ruptured duodenal ulcer.

du·o·de·nos·co·py (dew″o·de·nos′kuh·pee) *n.* [*duodeno-* + *-scopy*]. Inspection and visual examination of the duodenum by instrumental means, as by a fiberoptic endoscope.

du·o·de·nos·to·my (dew″o·de·nos′tuh·mee) *n.* [*duodeno-* + *-stomy*]. *In surgery,* the formation, temporarily, of a duodenal fistula.

du·o·de·not·o·my (dew″o·de·not′uh·mee) *n.* [*duodeno-* + *-tomy*]. *In surgery,* incision of the duodenum.

du·o·de·num (dew″o·dee′num, dew·od′e·num) *n.*, pl. **duodena** (·nuh), **duodenums** [ML. *duodenum digitorum,* of 12 finger's breadths][NA]. The first part of the small intestine, beginning at the pylorus. It is 8 to 10 inches long and is the most fixed part of the small intestine; consists of superior, descending, and inferior portions, and contains the openings of the pancreatic duct or ducts and the common bile duct. See also Plates 10, 13.

Duotal. A trademark for guaiacol carbonate, an expectorant.

Duphaston. Trademark for dydrogesterone, a synthetic progestogen.

Du·play's operation (dueᵉ·plehⁿ) [E. S. *Duplay,* French surgeon, 1836–1924]. A reconstructive and corrective operation for epispadias and hypospadias.

du·plex (dew′plecks) *adj.* [L.]. Having two parts.

du·plex·i·ty (dew·pleck′si·tee) *n.* DUPLICITY.

duplex placenta. A placenta with two or more parts separated by membranes, whose vessels do not communicate but unite just before entering the umbilical cord.

du·pli·ca·ta cru·ci·a·ta (dew″pli·kay′tuh kroo″shee·ay′tuh) [L.]. Experimentally produced double monsters obtained by grafting or inversion of the two-celled stage in amphibia.

du·pli·ca·tion, *n.* [L. *duplicatio,* from *duplicare,* to double]. 1. The doubling of any structure which normally occurs singly. 2. *In genetics,* the occurrence of a segment of a chromosome in duplicate.

du·pli·ca·ture (dew′pli·kuh·chur, ·kay″chur) *n.* [L. *duplicare,* to double.]. A fold, as a membrane folding upon itself.

du·plic·i·tas (dew·plis′i·tus, ·tahs) *n.* [L., doubling, duplication]. *In teratology,* an individual with duplication of either the cephalic or pelvic end, or both.

duplicitas cru·ci·a·ta (kroo″shee·ay′tuh). A rare form of conjoined twins in which there is superior and inferior duplicity, the long axes of the bodies forming a cross.

du·plic·i·ty (dew·plis′i·tee) *n.* *In teratology,* the condition of being double. Syn. *duplexity.*

duplicity theory. A theory of vision which states that vision is mediated by two classes of receptors, the rods and cones, whose respective activities are reflected in many visual functions.

Duponol C. Trademark for a pharmaceutical grade of sodium lauryl sulfate.

Du·puys-Du·temps' phenomenon (dueᵉ·pwʸee′ dueᵉ·tahⁿ′) [L. *Dupuys-Dutemps,* French ophthalmologist, b. 1871]. A paradoxical lid retraction present in Bell's palsy.

Du·puy·tren's contracture (dueᵉ·pwʸee·træⁿ′) [G. *Dupuytren,* French surgeon, 1777–1835]. A painless, chronic contracture of the hand, marked by thickening of the digital processes and of the palmar fascia and inability fully to extend the fingers, especially the third and fourth fingers. The disease is of uncertain etiology, and affects chiefly adult males.

Dupuytren's operation [G. *Dupuytren*]. A method of shoulder amputation.

du·ra (dew′ruh) *n.* [L., hard]. DURA MATER.

Durabolin. Trademark for nandrolone phenpropionate, an anabolic steroid.

Duracillin. A trademark for procaine penicillin G.

dura clip. A thin wire suture applied by a special forceps to check hemorrhage in brain operations.

Duraflex. Trademark for flumetramide, a skeletal muscle relaxant.

du·ral (dew′rul) *adj.* Pertaining to or involving the dura mater.

dural endothelioma. MENINGIOMA.

dural sheath. A strong fibrous membrane forming the external investment of the optic nerve. See also *dura mater.*

dural sinus. SINUS OF THE DURA MATER.

Duralumin. Trademark for a noncorroding alloy of aluminum and copper, used in surgical splints and appliances.

dura ma·ter (dew′ruh may′tur, mah′tur) [L., lit., hard mother]. The fibrous membrane forming the outermost covering of the brain and spinal cord.

dura mater en·ce·pha·li (en·sef′uh·lye) [NA]. The dura mater of the brain.

dura mater spi·na·lis (spye·nay′lis) [NA]. The dura mater of the spinal cord.

Du·rand-Ni·co·las-Fa·vre disease (dueᵉ·rahⁿ′, nee·koʰ·lah′, fav′r) [J. *Durand,* French physician, b. 1876; J. *Nicolas;* and M. *Favre*]. LYMPHOGRANULOMA VENEREUM.

Durand's disease [P. *Durand,* French physician, 20th century]. A febrile, presumably viral disease of North Africa, affecting humans and animals and characterized by prominent meningeal and pulmonary symptoms.

Duranest. A trademark for etidocaine, a local anesthetic.

Du·ran-Rey·nals factor [F. *Duran-Reynals,* U.S. physician, 1899–1958]. A substance which can increase connective-tissue permeability. See also *hyaluronidase.*

du·ra·plas·ty (dew′ruh·plas″tee) *n.* [*dura* + *-plasty*]. Repair of defects in the dura mater.

duration tetanus. TETANUS (2).

durch·wan·der·ungs·per·i·to·ni·tis (doorkh″vahn′dur·oongs·perr·i·to·nigh″tis) *n.* [Ger., wandering through]. Peritonitis thought to be due to bacteria escaping through the intestinal wall to the peritoneum even though the mucosa is not ulcerated.

Dürck's nodes (dueᵉrk) [H. *Dürck,* German pathologist, 1869–1941]. Foci of cerebral necrosis occurring in malaria.

Du·ret hemorrhages (dueᵉ·rehⁿ′) [H. *Duret,* French physician, 1849–1921]. 1. Small hemorrhages in the floor of the fourth ventricle which H. Duret produced in animals by blows to the head and attributed to brain concussion. 2. Frequently, secondary brainstem hemorrhages, particularly in the pons and floor of the fourth ventricle, seen after transtentorial herniation or brainstem distortion from other causes such as head trauma.

Dur·ham decision. *In forensic medicine,* the decision by the United States Court of Appeals for the District Court of Columbia in 1954 which states "that an accused is not criminally responsible if his unlawful act was the product of mental disease or mental defect." Objections have centered about the difficulties in defining "mental disease," "mental defect," and "product."

du·ri·tis (dew·rye′tis) *n.* [*dura* + *-itis*]. PACHYMENINGITIS.

du·ro·ar·ach·ni·tis (dew″ro·ăr″ack·nigh′tis) *n.* [*dura* + *arachnitis*]. Inflammation of the dura mater and arachnoid membrane.

du·ro·sar·co·ma (dew″ro·sahr·ko′muh) *n.* [*dura* + *sarcoma*]. MENINGIOMA.

Du·ro·ziez's disease (due·ro·zyey′) [P. L. *Duroziez,* French physician, 1826–1897]. Congenital mitral stenosis.

Duroziez's murmur or **sign** [P. L. *Duroziez*]. A systolic and diastolic murmur (double murmur) heard over the femoral or other large artery when the vessel is compressed in patients with aortic regurgitation or other disease with a wide pulse pressure.

dust, *n.* Fine, dry particles of earth or other material.

dust cell. ALVEOLAR MACROPHAGE; especially, one containing carbon or dust particles.

dust count. The number of particles of dust in a given atmosphere, usually expressed as the number of particles less than 10 microns in diameter per cubic foot of air when counted by the light field method. Used chiefly in evaluation of silicosis hazards in industry.

dust disease. PNEUMOCONIOSIS.

dusting powder. Any fine powder used to dust on the skin to absorb or diminish its secretions or allay irritation.

dust of Mül·ler (muel′ur) [J. *Müller*]. HEMOCONIA.

Dutch cap. A contraceptive device to cover the cervix.

Du·temps' sign (due·tahn′). LEVATOR SIGN.

Dut·ton's disease [J. E. *Dutton,* English physician, 1877–1905]. GAMBIAN TRYPANOSOMIASIS.

Du·val's bacillus [C. W. *Duval,* U.S. pathologist, 1876–1961]. *SHIGELLA SONNEI.*

D.V.M. Doctor of Veterinary Medicine.

D.V.M.S. Doctor of Veterinary Medicine and Surgery.

D.V.S. 1. Doctor of Veterinary Science. 2. Doctor of Veterinary Surgery.

dwale, *n.* [ME., prob. from ON.]. BELLADONNA.

dwarf, *n., adj., & v.* 1. An abnormally small individual; especially, one whose bodily proportions are altered, as in achondroplasia. 2. Being an atypically small form or variety of something. 3. To prevent normal growth.

dwarf bladder. Hypoplasia of the urinary bladder.

dwarf colony. A bacterial colony whose organisms have poorly developed enzyme systems, grow slowly, have little or no virulence, and revert slowly to the original type; frequently isolated from bacterial populations exposed to antibiotics.

dwarf·ism, *n.* Abnormal underdevelopment of the body; the condition of being dwarfed.

dwarf pelvis. Reduction or deformity of the pelvis seen in true hypoplastic, chondrodystrophic, cretin, and rachitic dwarfs.

dwarf pine needle oil. The volatile oil from the leaves of *Pinus mugo;* contains bornyl acetate, *levo*-pinene, sylvestrene, and other principles. An inhalant in bronchitis; has been used as an expectorant and antirheumatic.

dwarf tapeworm. *HYMENOLEPIS NANA.*

dwt Symbol for pennyweight.

Dx Symbol for diagnosis.

Dy Symbol for dysprosium.

dy·ad (dye′ad) *n.* [Gk. *dyas, dyados*]. 1. A pair or a couple. 2. One of the groups of paired chromosomes formed by the division of a tetrad during the first meiotic division. 3. *In chemistry,* a divalent element or radical.

dy·ad·ic, di·ad·ic (dye·ad′ick) *adj.* [*dyad* + *-ic*]. 1. Pertaining to the relationship between a pair. 2. *In psychiatry,* pertaining to the therapeutic relationship between physician and patient, as in dyadic therapy.

Dyclone. Trademark for dyclonine, a topical anesthetic used as the hydrochloride salt.

dy·clo·nine (dye·klo′neen) *n.* 4′-Butoxy-3-piperidinopropiophenone, $C_{18}H_{27}NO_2$, a topical anesthetic; used as the hydrochloride salt.

dy·dro·ges·ter·one (dye″dro·jes′tur·ohn) *n.* 9β-10α-Pregna-4,6-diene-3,20-dione, $C_{21}H_{28}O_2$, a synthetic progestogen.

dye, *n. & v.* 1. A coloring matter, generally used in solution. Certain dyes are used medicinally as antiseptics, as chemotherapeutic or diagnostic agents, or for special effects on tissue cells. 2. To color by means of a dye.

dye inhibition test. DYE TEST.

Dyemelor. A trademark for acetohexamide, an oral hypoglycemic.

dye·stuff, *n.* DYE.

dye test. A test for *Toxoplasma* antibodies which, in the presence of a complement-like accessory factor, prevent the staining of *Toxoplasma* by alkaline methylene blue.

dye-workers' cancer. A carcinoma of the urinary bladder found among aniline-dye workers.

Dylate. Trademark for clonitrate, a coronary vasodilator.

dy·man·thine (dye·man′theen) *n.* *N,N*-Dimethyloctadecylamine, $C_{20}H_{43}N$, an anthelmintic drug; used as the hydrochloride salt.

Dymelor. Trademark for acetohexamide, an oral hypoglycemic.

-dymia [-di*dym*us + *-ia*]. A combining form meaning *conjoined duplicity.*

-dymus [Gk. di*dymos,* twin]. A combining form meaning *superior duplicity in conjoined twins.*

dynam-, dynamo- [Gk. *dynamis*]. A combining form meaning *power, energy, or motion.*

dy·nam·e·ter (dye·nam′e·tur) *n.* DYNAMOMETER.

-dynamia [*dynam-* + *-ia*]. A combining form meaning (a) *strength;* (b) *a condition of having strength.*

dy·nam·ic (dye·nam′ick, di·nam′ick) *adj.* [Gk. *dynamikos,* powerful]. 1. Characterized by energy or great force. 2. Moving; changing; pertaining to motion or process.

dynamic demography. A study of the activities of human communities, their rise, progress, and fall.

dynamic ileus. SPASTIC ILEUS.

dynamic occlusion. The functional application of teeth to their natural purpose, the act of biting or chewing.

dynamic psychiatry. The study of emotional processes, their origins and mental mechanisms, which seeks to analyze the active, energy-filled, and constantly changing factors in human behavior and motivation, and thus convey the concepts of progression or regression. Contr. *descriptive psychiatry.* See also *Kraepelin's classification.*

dynamic psychology. An approach that emphasizes the cause-and-effect relations between conscious and unconscious phenomena and stresses the process nature of personality.

dynamic psychotherapy. INTENSIVE PSYCHOTHERAPY.

dynamic refraction. The static refraction of the eye, plus that secured by the action of the accommodative apparatus.

dy·nam·ics, *n.* The science that treats of matter in motion.

dynamic skiametry. Refraction in which retinoscopy is performed with the accommodation active but controlled.

dynamo-. See *dynam-.*

dy·na·mo, *n.* [*dynamo*electric machine]. A machine for converting mechanical energy into electric energy by means of coils of insulated wire revolving through magnetic fields of force.

dy·na·mo·gen·e·sis (dye″nuh·mo·jen′e·sis) *n.* [*dynamo-* + *-genesis*]. The generation of power, force, or energy.

dy·namo·graph (dye·nam′o·graf) *n.* [*dynamo-* + *-graph*]. An instrument designed to measure and graphically record muscular strength. —**dy·na·mog·ra·phy** (dye″nuh·mog′ruh·fee) *n.*

dy·na·mom·e·ter (dye″nuh·mom′e·tur) *n.* [*dynamo-* + *-meter*]. An instrument for measuring muscular strength, particularly of the hand.

dy·nam·o·neure (dye·nam′o·newr, di·nam′) *n.* [*dynamo-* + *neur*on]. *Obsol.* A spinal motor neuron.

dy·na·moph·a·ny (dye″nuh·mof′uh·nee) *n.* [*dynamo-* + Gk. *phainein,* to show]. The expression or discharge of psychic force.

dy·nam·o·scope (dye·nam′o·scope, di·nam′) *n.* [*dynamo-* + *-scope*]. An apparatus for observing the functioning of an organ or part, as muscular contraction or renal function. —**dy·na·mos·co·py** (dye″nuh·mos′kuh·pee) *n.*

Dynapen. A trademark for dicloxacillin, an antibiotic.

dy·na·therm (dye′nuh·thurm) *n.* [Gk. *dyna*mis, power, + *-therm*]. The apparatus used in diathermy.

dyne (dine) *n.* [F.]. The amount of force which, when acting continuously on a mass of one gram for one second, will accelerate the mass one centimeter per second.

dy·phyl·line (dye·fil′een) *n.* 7-(2,3-Dihydroxypropyl)theophylline, $C_{10}H_{14}N_4O_4$, a drug having the diuretic, myocardial stimulating, vasodilator, and bronchodilator actions of theophylline.

Dyrenium. Trademark for triamterene, a diuretic drug.

dys- [Gk.]. A prefix meaning (a) *abnormal, diseased;* (b) *difficult, painful;* (c) *faulty, impaired;* (d) in biology, *unlike.*

dys·acou·sia, dys·acu·sia (dis″uh·koo′zhuh, ·zee·uh) *n.* [*dys-* + *-acousia*]. 1. A condition in which pain or discomfort is caused by loud or even moderately loud noises. 2. The condition of being hard-of-hearing.

dys·acou·sis (dis″uh·koo′sis) *n.* DYSACOUSIA.

dys·acous·ma (dis″uh·kooz′muh) *n.* [*dys-* + *acousma*]. DYSACOUSIA.

dysacusia. DYSACOUSIA.

dys·ad·ap·ta·tion (dis·ad″ap·tay′shun) *n.* [*dys-* + *adaptation*]. *In ophthalmology,* inability of the iris and retina to accommodate to variable intensities of light.

dysaemia. DYSEMIA.

dysaesthesia. DYSESTHESIA.

dys·an·ag·no·sia (dis·an″ag·no′zhuh, ·zee·uh) *n.* [*dys-* + Gk. *anagnōs*is, reading, + *-ia*]. DYSLEXIA.

dys·an·ti·graph·ia (dis·an″tee·graf′ee·uh) *n.* [*dys-* + *anti-* + *-graphia*]. A form of agraphia in which there is inability to copy writing or print.

dys·aphea (dis·ay′fee·uh, ·af′ee·uh) *n.* [*dys-* + Gk. h*aphē*, touch, + *-ia*]. Disordered sense of touch.

dys·ap·ta·tion (dis″ap·tay′shun) *n.* DYSADAPTATION.

dys·ar·te·ri·ot·o·ny (dis″ahr·teer″ee·ot′uh·nee) *n.* [*dys-* + *arterio-* + Gk. *tonos,* tension]. Abnormal blood pressure.

dys·ar·thria (dis·ahr′three·uh) *n.* [*dys-* + *arthr-* + *-ia*]. Impairment of articulation caused by any disorder or lesion affecting the tongue or speech muscles. —**dysar·thric** (·thrick) *adj.*

dys·ar·thro·sis (dis″ahr·thro′sis) *n.,* pl. **disarthro·ses** (seez) [*dys-* + *arthrosis*]. 1. Deformity, dislocation, or disease of a joint. 2. PSEUDARTHROSIS. 3. DYSARTHRIA.

dys·au·to·no·mia (dis·aw″to·no′mee·uh) *n.* 1. Any dysfunction of the autonomic nervous system. 2. FAMILIAL DYSAUTONOMIA.

dys·bar·ism (dis·băr′iz·um) *n.* [*dys-* + *bar-* + *-ism*]. 1. Any disorder caused by excessive pressure differences between a tissue or part of the body and its surroundings. 2. Specifically, DECOMPRESSION SICKNESS.

dys·ba·sia (dis·bay′zhuh, ·zee·uh) *n.* [*dys-* + Gk. *bas*is, step, + *-ia*]. Difficulty in walking; particularly when due to a nervous system disorder.

dysbasia in·ter·mit·tens an·gio·scle·rot·i·ca (in·tur·mit′enz an″jee·o·skle·rot′i·kuh). INTERMITTENT CLAUDICATION.

dys·bu·lia, dys·bou·lia (dis·boo′lee·uh) *n.* [*dys-* + Gk. *boulē*, will, + *-ia*]. Impairment of will power.

dys·ce·pha·lia man·di·bu·lo·ocu·lo·fa·ci·a·lis (dis″se·fay′lee·uh man·dib″yoo·lo·ock″yoo·lo·fay″shee·ay′lis). HALLERMAN-STREIFF-FRANÇOIS SYNDROME.

dys·chei·ria, dys·chi·ria (dis·kigh′ree·uh) *n.* [*dys-* + Gk. *cheir,* hand, + *-ia*]. Inability to tell which side of the body has been touched, though sensation of touch is not lost; partial allocheiria.

dys·che·zia (dis·kee′zee·uh) *n.* [*dys-* + Gk. *chez*ein, to defecate, + *-ia*]. Painful or difficult defecation.

dys·chi·zia (dis·kigh′zee·uh, dis·kiz′ee·uh) *n.* DYSCHEZIA.

dys·chon·dro·pla·sia (dis·kon″dro·play′zhuh, ·zee·uh) *n.* [*dys-* + *chondro-* + *-plasia*]. ENCHONDROMATOSIS.

dys·chroa (dis′kro·uh) *n.* [*dys-* + Gk. *chroa* (*chroia*), complexion]. DYSCHROIA.

dys·chroia (dis·kroy′uh) *n.* [Gk., from *dys-* + *chroia,* complexion]. Discoloration of the skin; a bad complexion.

dys·chro·ma·to·der·mia (dis·kro″muh·to·dur′mee·uh) *n.* [*dys-* + *chromato-* + *-dermia*]. DYSCHROIA.

dys·chro·ma·top·sia (dis·kro″muh·top′see·uh) *n.* [*dys-* + *chromat-* + *-opsia*]. PARTIAL COLOR BLINDNESS. —**dys·chro·ma·tope** (dis·kro′muh·tope) *n.*

dys·chro·mia (dis·kro′mee·uh) *n.* [*dys-* + *chrom-* + *-ia*]. Discoloration, especially of the skin.

dys·chro·mo·der·mia (dis·kro″mo·dur′mee·uh, dis″kro·mo·) *n.* [*dys-* + *chromo-* + *-dermia*]. DYSCHROIA.

dys·chro·nous (dis′kruh·nus) *adj.* [*dys-* + *chron-* + *-ous*]. Not agreeing as to time. —**dys·chro·na·tion** (dis″kro·nay′shun) *n.*

dys·co·ria (dis·ko′ree·uh) *n.* [*dys-* + *cor-* + *-ia*]. Abnormality of the form of the pupil.

dys·cra·sia (dis·kray′zhuh, ·zee·uh) *n.* [*dys-* + *-crasia*]. 1. An abnormal state or disorder of the body. 2. Formerly, an abnormal mixture of the four humors of the body. —**dys·cra·sic** (·kray′zick), **dys·crat·ic** (krat′ick) *adj.*

dys·cri·nism (dis·krye′niz·um) *n.* [*dys-* + *-crine* + *-ism*]. DYSENDOCRINISM.

dys·di·ad·o·cho·ki·ne·sia, dys·di·ad·o·ko·ki·ne·sia (dis″dye·ad″o·ko·ki·nee′zhuh, ·zee·uh) *n.* [*dys-* + *diadochokinesia*]. Impairment of the power to perform alternating movements in rapid, smooth, and rhythmic succession, such as pronation and supination; a sign of cerebellar disease, but also seen in the so-called clumsy child with minimal brain damage.

dys·eco·ia (dis″e·koy′uh) *n.* [Gk. *dysēkoia,* deafness.]. DYSACOUSIA (2).

dys·em·bry·o·ma (dis·em″bree·o′muh) *n.* [*dys-* + *embryoma*]. TERATOMA.

dys·em·bry·o·pla·sia (dis·em″bree·o·play′zhuh, ·zee·uh) *n.* [*dys-* + *embryo* + *-plasia*]. A malformation that develops during embryonic life.

dys·eme·sia (dis″e·mee′zhuh, ·zee·uh) *n.* [*dys-* + Gk. *emes*is, vomiting, + *-ia*]. Painful vomiting; retching.

dys·em·e·sis (dis·em′e·sis) *n.* [*dys-* + *emesis*]. DYSEMESIA.

dys·emia, dys·ae·mia (dis·ee′mee·uh) *n.* [*dys-* + *-emia*]. Any disease of the blood.

dys·en·ce·pha·lia splanch·no·cys·ti·ca (dis·en″se·fay′lee·uh splank″no·sis′ti·kuh). MECKEL SYNDROME.

dys·en·do·cri·ni·a·sis (dis″en·do·kri·nigh′uh·sis) *n.* [*dys-* + *endocrine* + *-iasis*]. DYSENDOCRINISM.

dys·en·doc·rin·ism (dis″en·dock′rin·iz·um, dis·en′do·krin·iz·um) *n.* [*dys-* + *endocrine* + *-ism*]. Any abnormality in the function of the endocrine glands. —**dys·en·do·crine** (dis·en′do·krin) *adj.*

dys·en·do·cri·si·a·sis (dis″en·do·kri·sigh′uh·sis) *n.* DYSENDOCRINISM.

dys·en·te·ria (dis″en·teer′ee·uh) *n.* [L.]. DYSENTERY.

dys·en·tery (dis′un·terr″ee) *n.* [L. *dysenteria,* from Gk. *dys-* + *enteron,* intestine]. Inflammation of the intestine, particularly the colon, of varied causation, associated with abdominal pain, tenesmus, and diarrhea with blood and mucus. See also *amebic dysentery, bacillary dysentery.* —**dys·en·ter·ic** (dis″un·terr′ick) *adj.*

dys·er·ga·sia (dis″ur·gay′zhuh, ·zee·uh) *n.* [*dys-* + *ergasia*]. *In psychobiology,* a mental disturbance due to toxic factors which are capable of producing delirium, such as uremia or alcohol. See also *toxic encephalopathy.*

dys·er·ga·sy (dis′ur·gay″zee) *n.* DYSERGASIA.

dys·es·the·sia, dys·aes·the·sia (dis″esth·ee′zhuh, ·zee·uh) *n.* [*dys-* + *esthesia*]. 1. Impairment but not absence of the senses, especially of the sense of touch. 2. Painfulness or disagreeableness of any sensation not normally painful.

dys·flu·en·cy (dis·floo′un·see) *n.* Impairment of speech fluency, such as slow, halting delivery, difficulties in enunciation, or disordered rhythm, as seen in certain types of aphasia. —**dysflu·ent,** *adj.*

dys·func·tion (dis·funk'shun) *n.* [*dys-* + *function*]. Any abnormality or impairment of function, as of an organ.

dys·ga·lac·tia (dis"ga·lack'tee·uh, ·shee·uh) *n.* [*dys-* + *galact-* + *-ia*]. Loss or impairment of milk secretion.

dys·gam·ma·glob·u·li·ne·mia (dis"gam·muh·glob"yoo·li·nee'mee·uh) *n.* [*dys-* + *gamma globulin* + *-emia*]. Any abnormality, quantitative or qualitative, of serum gamma globulins.

dys·gen·e·sia (dis"je·nee'zee·uh) *n.* DYSGENESIS.

dys·gen·e·sis (dis·jen'e·sis) *n.*, pl. **dysgene·ses** (·seez) [*dys-* + *-genesis*]. 1. Abnormal development of anything, usually of an organ or individual. 2. Impairment or loss of the ability to procreate.

dys·gen·ic (dis·jen'ick) *adj.* [*dys-* + *-genic*]. Detrimental to the hereditary constitution of a population. Contr. *eugenic.*

dys·ger·mi·no·ma (dis·jur"mi·no'nuh) *n.* [*dys-* + *germin*al + *-oma*]. An ovarian tumor composed of large polygonal cells of germ-cell origin, resembling seminoma of the testis, but less malignant. Syn. *embryoma of the ovary.*

dys·geu·sia (dis·joo'zee·uh, ·see·uh) *n.* [*dys-* + *-geusia*]. Abnormality, impairment, or perversion of the sense of taste.

dys·glan·du·lar (dis·glan'dew·lur) *adj.* [*dys-* + *glandular*]. Pertaining to any abnormality in the function of glands, particularly the glands of internal secretion.

dys·glob·u·li·ne·mia, dys·glob·u·li·nae·mia (dis·glob"yoo·li·nee'mee·uh) *n.* [*dys-* + *globulin* + *-emia*]. Any qualitative or quantitative abnormality of blood globulins.

dys·gnath·ic (dis·nath'ick, ·nay'thick) *adj.* [*dys-* + *gnath-* + *-ic*]. Pertaining to jaws with improper development and in poor relation to each other.

dys·gno·sia (dis·no'zhuh, ·zee·uh) *n.* [*dys-* + *-gnosia*]. Disorder or distortion of intellectual function.

dys·gon·ic (dis·gon'ick) *adj.* [*dys-* + *gonic*]. Growing poorly; said of bacterial cultures.

dys·gram·ma·tism (dis·gram'uh·tiz·um) *n.* AGRAMMATISM.

dys·graph·ia (dis·graf'ee·uh) *n.* [*dys-* + *-graphia*]. Impairment of the power of writing as a result of a brain lesion.

dys·hem·a·to·poi·et·ic, dys·haem·a·to·poi·et·ic (dis·hee"muh·to·poy·et'ick, dis·hem"uh·to·) *n.* [*dys-* + *hematopoietic*]. DYSHEMOPOIETIC.

dys·he·mo·poi·et·ic, dys·hae·mo·poi·et·ic (dis·he"mo·poy·et'ick) *adj.* [*dys-* + *hemopoietic*]. Pertaining to a disturbed formation of blood cells. —**dyshemopoi·e·sis** (·ee'sis) *n.*

dys·hid·ria (dis·hid'ree·uh) *n.* [*dys-* + *hidr-* + *-ia*]. DYSHIDROSIS.

dys·hi·dro·sis (dis·hi·dro'sis) *n.*, pl. **dishidro·ses** (·seez) [*dys-* + *hidrosis*]. 1. Any disturbance in sweat production or excretion. 2. CHEIROPOMPHOLYX. —**dyshi·dros·i·form** (·dros'i·form) *adj.*

dys·hor·ia (dis·hor'ee·uh) *n.* [*dys-* + Gk. *oros,* serum]. Any abnormality of vascular permeability. —**dyshor·ic** (·ick) *adj.*

dys·idro·sis (dis"i·dro'sis) *n.* DYSHIDROSIS.

dys·in·su·lin·ism (dis·in'sue·lin·iz·um) *n.* [*dys-* + *insulin* + *-ism*]. Any condition caused by a disorder of insulin secretion or utilization.

dys·kar·y·o·sis (dis·kăr"ee·o'sis) *n.* [*dys-* + *kary-* + *-osis*]. *In exfoliative cytology,* nuclear abnormalities, especially enlargement, hyperchromatism, irregularity in nuclear shape, and increased number of nuclei per cell without significant change in the cytoplasm or outline of the cell. —**dyskar·y·ot·ic** (·ee·ot'ick) *adj.*

dys·ker·a·to·sis (dis·kerr"uh·to'sis) *n.*, pl. **dyskerato·ses** (·seez) [*dys-* + *kerat-* + *-osis*]. 1. Imperfect keratinization of individual epidermal cells. 2. Keratinization of corneal epithelium. —**dyskera·tot·ic** (tot'ick) *adj.*

dyskeratosis con·gen·i·ta (kon·jen'i·tuh). A familial disorder characterized by telangiectatic erythema of the face, neck, upper chest and hands; atrophy of the manual skin; ungual, dental and eccrine dysplasia; progressive refractory pancytopenia, mental and growth retardation; cutaneous dyschromia; obliteration of puncta lacrimalia; general frailty; atretic external auditory canals and a tendency to develop squamous cell carcinoma of the vulva, anus, oral and esophageal mucosa, as well as a propensity for leukemia in the family.

dys·ki·ne·sia (dis"ki·nee'zhuh, ·zee·uh, dis"kigh·nee') *n.* [*dys-* + *-kinesia*]. 1. Any abnormal or disordered movement, particularly those seen in disorders affecting the extrapyramidal system as in parkinsonism or phenothiazine intoxication. 2. Impairment of the power of voluntary motion, resulting in partial movements. —**dyski·net·ic** (·net'ick) *adj.*

dys·la·lia (dis·lay'lee·uh, dis·lal'ee·uh) *n.* [*dys-* + *-lalia*]. Impairment of the power of speaking, due to a defect of the organs of speech, especially the tongue.

dys·lex·ia (dis·leck'see·uh) *n.* [*dys-* + *-lexia*]. Impairment of the ability to read, particularly in an individual who once knew how or is normally expected to know how to read. See also *developmental dyslexia.* —**dys·lex·ic** (dis·leck'sick) *adj. & n.*

dys·lo·gia (dis·lo'jee·uh) *n.* [*dys-* + *-logia*]. 1. Difficulty in the expression of ideas by speech. 2. Impairment of reasoning or of the faculty to think logically.

dys·ma·se·sia (dis"ma·see'zee·uh) *n.* DYSMASESIS.

dys·ma·se·sis (dis"ma·see'sis) *n.* [*dys-* + Gk. *masēsis,* chewing]. Difficulty in chewing.

dys·ma·tur·i·ty (dis"muh·tewr'i·tee) *n.* [*dys-* + *maturity*]. A disparity in the degree of maturation of various fetal structures.

dys·me·lia (dis·mee'lee·uh) *n.* [*dys-* + *-melia*]. Congenital malformation or absence of a limb or limbs.

dys·men·or·rhea, dys·men·or·rhoea (dis·men"o·ree'uh) *n.* [*dys-* + *menorrhea*]. Difficult or painful menstruation.

dysmenorrhea in·ter·men·stru·a·lis (in"tur·men·stroo·ay'lis). Uterine pain between the menses.

dys·mero·gen·e·sis (dis·merr"o·jen'e·sis) *n.* [*dys-* + *merogenesis*]. Cleavage resulting in unlike parts. —**dysmero·ge·net·ic** (·je·net'ick) *adj.*

dys·met·ria (dis·met'ree·uh) *n.* [*dys-* + Gk. *metr*on, measure, + *-ia*]. Inability to control accurately the range of movement in muscular acts, as observed in cerebellar lesions, with resultant overshooting of a mark; said particularly of hand movements.

dys·mim·ia (dis·mim'ee·uh) *n.* [*dys-* + Gk. *mim*os, mimic, + *ia*]. Impairment of the power to use signs and gestures as a means of expression; inability to imitate.

dys·mne·sia (dis·nee'zhuh, ·zee·uh) *n.* [*dys-* + *-mnesia*]. An impaired or defective memory.

dys·mor·phia (dis·mor'fee·uh) *n.* [Gk., from *dys-* + *morphē,* form]. Deformity; abnormal shape.

dys·mor·phic (dis·mor'fick) *adj.* [*dys-* + *-morphic*]. 1. Ill-shaped, malformed. 2. In the somatotype, of low primary t component.

dys·mor·phol·o·gy (dis"mor·fol'uh·jee) *n.* [*dys-* + morphology]. 1. Abnormal structure, especially as seen in congenital malformations. 2. The study and treatment of such abnormalities.

dys·mor·pho·pho·bia (dis·mor"fo·fo'bee·uh) *n.* [*dysmorph*ia + *-phobia*]. Morbid fear of being deformed.

dys·my·e·lino·gen·ic (dis·migh"e·lin·o·jen'ick) *adj.* [*dys-* + *myelin* + *-genic*]. Characterizing or pertaining to any process that interferes with myelinization.

dysmyelinogenic leukodystrophy. ALEXANDER'S DISEASE.

dys·no·mia (dis·no'mee·uh) *n.* ANOMIA.

dys·odon·ti·a·sis (dis"o·don·tye'uh·sis, ·tee'uh·sis) *n.* [*dys-* + *odontiasis*]. *Obsol.* Difficult or painful dentition.

dys·on·to·gen·e·sis (dis·on"to·jen'e·sis) *n.* [*dys-* + *ontogenesis*]. Defective embryonic development of any tissue or organ. —**dys·on·to·ge·net·ic** (dis·on"to·je·net'ick) *adj.*

dysontogenetic tumor. Any tumor resulting from defective embryologic development.

dys·orex·ia (dis″o·reck′see·uh) *n.* [*dys-* + *-orexia*]. A disordered, diminished, or unnatural appetite.

dys·os·mia (dis·oz′mee·uh) *n.* [*dys-* + *osm-* + *-ia*]. Impairment of the sense of smell.

dys·os·teo·gen·e·sis (dis·os″tee·o·jen′e·sis) *n.* [*dys-* + *osteogenesis*]. DYSOSTOSIS.

dys·os·to·sis (dis″os·to′sis) *n.*, pl. **dysosto·ses** (·seez) [*dys-* + *ostosis*]. Defective formation of bone.

dysostosis clei·do·cra·ni·a·lis (klye″do·kray·nee·ay′lis). CLEIDOCRANIAL DYSOSTOSIS.

dysostosis mul·ti·plex (mul′ti·plecks). MUCOPOLYSACCHARIDOSIS.

dys·para·thy·roid·ism (dis·păr″uh·thigh′roid·iz·um) *n.* [*dys-* + *parathyroid* + *-ism*]. Any disorder of parathyroid gland function.

dys·pa·reu·nia (dis″puh·roo′nee·uh) *n.* [*dys-* + *pareunia*]. Painful or difficult sexual intercourse.

dys·pep·sia (dis·pep′see·uh, ·shuh) *n.* [Gk., from *dys-* + *pepsis*, digestion, + *ia*]. Disturbed digestion.

dys·pep·tic (dis·pep′tick) *adj.* Pertaining to or affected with dyspepsia.

dys·per·i·stal·sis (dis″perr·i·stal′sis, ·stahl′sis) *n.* [*dys-* + *peristalsis*]. Violent or abnormal peristalsis.

dys·pha·gia (dis·fay′jee·uh) *n.* [*dys-* + *-phagia*]. Difficulty in swallowing, or inability to swallow.

dysphagia con·stric·ta (kun·strick′tuh). Difficulty in swallowing due to stenosis of the pharynx or esophagus.

dysphagia glo·bo·sa (glo·bo′suh). GLOBUS HYSTERICUS.

dysphagia lu·so·ria (lew·so′ree·uh) Difficulty in swallowing due to compression of the esophagus by a persistent right aortic arch, a double aortic arch, or an anomalous right subclavian artery.

dys·phag·ic (dis·faj′ick) *adj.* Pertaining to or characterized by dysphagia.

dys·pha·sia (dis·fay′zhuh, ·zee·uh) *n.* [*dys-* + *-phasia*]. Any aphasia which does not produce complete abolition of the facility to use language. See also *aphasia.*

dys·phe·mia (dis·fee′mee·uh) *n.* [*dys-* + *-phemia*]. STAMMERING.

dys·phoi·te·sis (dis″foy·tee′sis) *n.* [*dys-* + Gk. *phoitēsis*, going to school, attendance at school]. Any learning disorder primarily neurophysiologic in character, and not due to mental retardation or to emotional and personality disturbances; often used in a specific sense, such as reading, calculation, graphic, or direction-sense dysphoitesis. See also *developmental dyslexia.*

dys·pho·nia (dis·fo′nee·uh) *n.* [*dys-* + *-phonia*]. An impairment of the voice.

dysphonia spas·ti·ca (spas′ti·kuh). PHONIC SPASM.

dys·pho·ria (dis·fo′ree·uh) *n.* [Gk.]. 1. The condition of not feeling well or of being ill at ease. 2. Morbid impatience and restlessness; anxiety; fidgetiness. 3. Physical discomfort. —**dys·phor·ic** (·for′ick) *adj.*

dys·pho·tia (dis·fo′shuh, ·shee·uh) *n.* [*dys-* + *phot-* + *-ia*]. MYOPIA.

dys·phra·sia (dis·fray′zhuh, ·zee·uh) *n.* [*dys-* + Gk. *phrasis*, expression, phrase, + *-ia*]. DYSPHASIA.

dys·pi·tu·i·ta·rism (dis″pi·tew′i·tuh·riz·um) *n.* [*dys-* + *pituitary* + *-ism*]. A condition due to abnormal function of the pituitary gland.

dys·pla·sia (dis·play′zhuh, ·zee·uh) *n.* [*dys-* + *-plasia*]. 1. Abnormal development or growth, especially of cells. 2. The extent to which an individual presents different components (somatotypes) in different bodily regions, expressed quantitatively by regarding the body as made up of a specific number of regions and somatotyping each. They may be endomorphic, mesomorphic, or ectomorphic. Syn. *d component.*

dysplasia epi·phys·i·a·lis mul·ti·plex (ep″i·fiz·ee·ay′lis mul′ti·plecks). A rare congenital developmental disorder characterized by irregular ossification of several of the developing epiphyses, resulting in dwarfism, joint deformities, and short thick digits.

dysplasia epiphysialis punc·ta·ta (punk·tay′tuh). CHONDRODYSTROPHIA CALCIFICANS CONGENITA.

dysplasia epiphysialis punc·tic·u·la·ris (punk·tick″yoo·lair′is). CHONDRODYSTROPHIA CALCIFICANS CONGENITA.

dys·plas·tic (dis·plas′tick) *adj.* Pertaining to or affected with dysplasia.

dysplastic type. A physique varying greatly from the normal or from such recognized types as the asthenic or athletic.

dys·pnea, dys·pnoea (disp·nee′uh, dis·nee′uh) *n.* [Gk. *dyspnoia*, shortness of breath]. Difficult or labored breathing. —**dys·pne·al** (·nee′ul), **dyspne·ic** (·ick) *adj.*

dys·po·ne·sis (dis″po·nee′sis) *n.* [*dys-* + Gk. *ponos*, work, toil]. A physiopathologic state made up of errors in energy expenditure within the nervous system. —**dyspo·net·ic** (·net′ick) *adj.*

dys·pra·gia (dis·pray′jee·uh) *n.* DYSPRAXIA.

dys·prax·ia (dis·prack′see·uh) *n.* [*dys-* + *-praxia*]. Disturbance in the ability to carry out skilled voluntary movements. See also *apraxia.* —**dys·prac·tic** (dis·prack′tick) *adj.*

dys·pro·si·um (dis·pro′zee·um, ·see·um) *n.* [NL., from Gk. *dysprositos*, difficult of access]. Dy = 162.50. A rare-earth metal. See also Table of Elements in the Appendix.

dys·pros·o·dy (dis·pros′uh·dee) *n.* [*dys-* + *prosody*]. Distortion or obliteration of the normal rhythm and melody of speech, as seen in certain types of aphasia.

dys·ra·phism (dis′ra·fiz·um) *n.* [*dys-* + *raphe* + *-ism*]. Defective raphe formation; defective fusion.

dys·rhyth·mia (dis·rith′mee·uh) *n.* [*dys-* + *rhythm* + *-ia*]. Disordered rhythm, especially of brainwaves or of speech.

dys·se·ba·cia (dis″se·bay′shee·uh) *n.* [*dys-* + *sebaceous* + *-ia*]. Plugging of the sebaceous glands, especially around the nose, mouth, and forehead, with a dry, yellowish material. It occurs in pellagra and other deficiencies of the vitamin-B complex. Syn. *shark skin.*

dys·se·cre·to·sis (dis″see·kre·to′sis) *n.* [*dys-* + *secretion* + *-osis*]. A condition in which there is faulty secretory activity of glands.

dys·so·cial (dis·so′shul) *adj.* [*dys-* + *social*]. *In psychiatry*, pertaining to behavior which is in manifest disregard of existing social codes and patterns, and often in conflict with them, but which is not due to a psychiatric disorder.

dyssocial behavior. *In psychiatry*, a behavioral pattern characteristic of individuals who are not classifiable as antisocial personalities but who manifest disregard for the usual social codes and often come in conflict with them. They tend to be predatory and follow pursuits such as racketeering, gambling, and selling drugs, which they know to be illegal. However, they often exhibit strong loyalties and adherence to the values of the social group to which they belong.

dys·som·nia (dis·som′nee·uh) *n.* [*dys-* + *somn-* + *-ia*]. Any disorder of sleep mechanisms.

dys·sper·ma·tism (dis·spur′muh·tiz·um) *n.* [*dys-* + *spermat-* + *-ism*]. 1. Occurrence of pain or discomfort in discharge of seminal fluid. 2. Any disturbance in the formation of normal spermatozoa.

dys·sper·mia (dis·spur′mee·uh) *n.* [*dys-* + *-spermia*]. DYSSPERMATISM.

dys·splen·ism (dis·splen′iz·um) *n.* [*dys-* + *splen-* + *-ism*]. HYPERSPLENISM.

dys·sta·sia (dis·stay′see·uh, ·zee·uh) *n.* [*dys-* + Gk. *stasis*, standing, + *ia*]. Difficulty in standing. —**dys·stat·ic** (·stat′ick) *adj.*

dys·syn·chro·nous (dis·sin′kruh·nus) *adj.* [*dys-* + *synchronous*]. Characterized by a lack of synchronism; pertaining especially to children with the minimal brain dysfunction syndrome.

dyssynchronous child syndrome. MINIMAL BRAIN DYSFUNCTION SYNDROME.

dys·syn·er·gia (dis″sin·ur′jee·uh) *n.* [*dys-* + *synergia*]. Faulty coordination of groups of organs or muscles normally acting in unison; particularly, the abnormal state of muscle antagonism in cerebellar disease.

dyssynergia ce·re·bel·la·ris my·o·clo·ni·ca (serr″e·bel·air′is migh″o·klon′i·kuh). A frequently familial cerebellar syndrome of childhood described by Ramsay Hunt, the pathologic basis of which was never determined; characterized clinically by progressive ataxia, tremor, and diffuse myoclonus.

dyssynergia cerebellaris pro·gres·si·va (pro″gre·sigh′vuh, pro·gres′i·vuh). A frequently familial cerebellar syndrome of childhood described by Ramsay Hunt, the pathologic basis of which was never determined; characterized clinically by progressive ataxia and tremor.

dys·syn·er·gy (dis·sin′ur·jee) *n.* [*dys-* + *synergy*]. DYSSYNERGIA.

dys·tax·ia (dis·tack′see·uh) *n.* Complete or partial ataxia.

dys·tec·tic (dis·teck′tick) *adj.* [*dys-* + Gk. *tēktikos,* fusible]. *In physical chemistry,* characterizing the specific mixture of two or more substances which has the highest melting point of any mixture of the substances. Contr. *eutectic.*

dys·tha·na·sia (dis″thuh·nay′zhuh, ·zee·uh) *n.* [Gk. *dysthanēs,* unhappy in death, + *-ia*]. A slow and painful death.

dys·the·sia (dis·theezh′uh, ·theez′ee·uh) *n.* [Gk.]. Impatience; fretfulness; ill temper in the sick. —**dys·thet·ic** (·thet′ick) *adj.*

dys·thy·mia (dis·thigh′mee·uh, ·thim′ee·uh) *n.* [*dys-* + *-thymia*]. 1. Any condition due to malfunction of the thymus during childhood. 2. *In psychiatry,* any despondent mood or depressive tendency, often associated with hypochondriasis. 3. Any abnormality of mentation. See also *neurasthenia, cyclothymia.*

dys·thy·mic (dis·thigh′mick) *adj.* 1. Characterizing an individual exhibiting dysthymia. 2. Pertaining to certain reactions that have the appearance of neurasthenia.

dys·thy·roi·dal (dis″thigh·roy′dul) *adj.* Pertaining to imperfect development or function of the thyroid gland.

dysthyroidal infantilism. Physical and mental underdevelopment resulting from hypothyroidism.

dys·tith·ia (dis·tith′ee·uh) *n.* [*dys-* + Gk. *tittheia,* nursing, from *titthos,* breast]. Difficulty of nursing or inability to nurse at the breast.

dys·to·cia (dis·to′shuh, ·see·uh) *n.* [Gk. *dystokia,* from *tokos,* childbirth]. Difficult labor. —**dysto·cic** (·sick) *adj.*

dys·to·nia (dis·to′nee·uh) *n.* [*dys-* + *-tonia*]. Disorder or lack of muscle tonicity. —**dys·ton·ic** (·ton′ick) *adj.*

dystonia mus·cu·lo·rum de·for·mans (mus·kew·lo′rum de·for′manz). A rare disorder characterized by progressive involuntary movements of the trunk and limbs and taking two forms: (a) a primary hereditary disease with a preference for Jews of Russian and Polish descent; (b) a symptomatic form that is associated with other extrapyramidal motor diseases, such as encephalitis lethargica and Wilson's disease.

dys·to·pia (dis·to′pee·uh) *n.* [*dis-* + *top-* + *-ia*]. Displacement or malposition of any organ. —**dys·top·ic** (·top′ick) *adj.*

dystopic cortical myelinogenesis. A type of cortical dysgenesis, consisting of (a) a failure of migration of nerve cells, which persist in the molecular layer of the cortex; (b) presence of myelinated fiber bundles, haphazardly arranged in the outer cortical layers; and (c) an overall disarray of the architecture of the superficial cortical layers. These abnormalities give the cortex the appearance of driftwood.

dys·tro·phia (dis·tro′fee·uh) *n.* DYSTROPHY.

dystrophia ad·i·po·so·ge·ni·ta·lis (ad·i·po″so·jen·i·tay′lis). ADIPOSOGENITAL DYSTROPHY.

dystrophia me·di·a·na ca·nal·i·for·mis (mee·dee·ay′nuh ka·nal·i·for′mis). A rare form of dystrophy characterized by longitudinal grooves occupying the center of the nail from the lunula to the free edge; usually involves the thumb.

dystrophia myo·ton·i·ca (migh″o·ton′i·kuh). MYOTONIC DYSTROPHY.

dystrophia peri·os·ta·lis hy·per·plas·ti·ca fa·mil·i·a·ris (perr″ee·os·tay′lis high″pur·plas′ti·kuh fa·mil″ee·air′is). FAMILIAL HYPERPLASTIC PERIOSTEAL DYSTROPHY.

dystrophia un·gui·um (ung′gwee·um). An abnormality of the finger or toe nails; of any degree, from simple longitudinal fissuring to complete absence.

dys·troph·ic (dis·trof′ick) *adj.* Pertaining to or characterized by dystrophy.

dystrophic gait. WADDLING GAIT.

dys·tro·phy (dis′truh·fee) *n.* [*dys-* + *-trophy*]. 1. Defective nutrition. 2. Defective or abnormal development; degeneration. 3. Specifically, MUSCULAR DYSTROPHY.

dys·uria (dis·yoo′ree·uh) *n.* [*dys-* + *-uria*]. Pain or burning on urination.

E

E 1. [Ger. *e*ntgegen, opposite] *In chemistry,* a stereo descriptor for geometric isomers indicating a configuration of atoms or groups on opposite sides of a theoretical plane intersecting the atoms causing the achiral center. Compare *trans-*. Contr. Z. 2. Symbol for electromotive force.

E. Abbreviation for (a) *eye*; (b) *emmetropia*; (c) *einstein.*

E_0 Symbol for electroaffinity.

e Symbol for electron.

e-. See *ex-*.

EA Abbreviation for *educational age.*

EAE Abbreviation for *experimental allergic encephalomyelitis.*

Ea·gle's media [H. *Eagle,* U.S. pathologist, b. 1905]. A variety of tissue culture media containing various vitamins, amino acids, inorganic salts and serous enrichments, and dextrose.

Eagle test [H. *Eagle*]. 1. A complement-fixation test for syphilis. 2. A flocculation test for syphilis.

Eales' disease [H. *Eales,* English physician, 1852-1913]. Repeated retinal and vitreous hemorrhages or bouts of perivasculitis of uncertain cause and unaccompanied by uveal inflammation, occurring chiefly in young adults, mostly males, manifesting itself by sudden visual impairment, usually in one eye, on awakening, in stress situations, or following trauma. Syn. *retinal periphlebitis, retinal vasculitis.*

ear, *n.* [Gmc. *auz-* (rel. to L. *aur-*, *aus-*, and to Gk. *ous, ōt-*)]. The organ of hearing, consisting of the external ear, the middle ear, and the internal ear or labyrinth. NA *auris.*

ear·ache, *n.* Pain in the ear; otalgia.

ear block. Trauma, inflammation, and pain of the middle ear due to a blocked auditory tube, observed in individuals subjected to sudden and extreme variations in barometric pressure.

ear drops. Liquid medication instilled by drops into the external acoustic meatus.

ear·drum, *n.* 1. TYMPANIC MEMBRANE. 2. MIDDLE EAR.

ear dust. OTOCONIA.

Earle L fibrosarcoma. A transplantable fibrosarcoma, originally developed in an explant of the subcutaneous tissue of a specially bred experimental mouse, grown in tissue culture medium to which 20-methylcholanthrene had been added.

ear·lobe, *n.* The pendulous, fleshy lower portion of the auricle or external ear.

early erythroblast (of Sabin) [F. R. *Sabin,* U.S. anatomist, 1871-1953]. BASOPHILIC NORMOBLAST.

early infantile autism. INFANTILE AUTISM.

early normoblast. BASOPHILIC NORMOBLAST.

early syphilis. Primary, secondary, or latent acquired syphilitic infection of less than four years' duration.

ear·piece, *n.* The part of an apparatus, such as a stethoscope, which fits into each ear.

ear·plug, *n.* A device made of rubber, cotton, or other pliable material, for insertion into the outer ear for protection against water or loud noises.

earth eating. PICA (2).

earth wax. CERESIN.

ear tubercle. AURICULAR TUBERCLE.

ear·wax, *n.* CERUMEN.

East African sleeping sickness. RHODESIAN TRYPANOSOMIASIS.

East Coast fever. A febrile disease of cattle occurring in eastern and southern Africa, caused by the haemosporidium *Theileria parva* and transmitted by several species of tick. See also *theileriasis.*

east·ern equine encephalitis. EASTERN EQUINE ENCEPHALOMYELITIS.

eastern equine encephalomyelitis. A severe, febrile encephalomyelitis with constant polymorphonuclear leukocytosis caused by an arbovirus.

Ea·ton agent or **virus.** *MYCOPLASMA PNEUMONIAE.*

Eaton agent pneumonia. PRIMARY ATYPICAL PNEUMONIA (1).

Eaton-Lam·bert syndrome [L. M. *Eaton,* U.S. neurologist, 1905-1958; and E. H. *Lambert,* U.S. neurologist, b. 1915]. MYASTHENIC SYNDROME.

Ebers papyrus (ey'burss) [G. M. *Ebers,* German Egyptologist, 1837-1898]. An Egyptian papyrus dealing with many fields of medicine, dating from the XVIIIth dynasty (16th century B.C.).

Eber·thel·la (ee"bur·thel'uh, ay"bur·) *n.* [K. J. *Eberth,* German pathologist, 1835-1926]. *SALMONELLA.*

Eberthella typhosa. *SALMONELLA TYPHOSA.*

Eb·ner's glands [V. von *Ebner,* Austrian histologist, 1842-1925]. The serous glands opening into the trenches of the vallate papillae of the tongue.

ébran·le·ment (ay·brahn·luh·mahn', F. eʸ·brahⁿl·mahⁿ') *n.* [F., shaking, shock, loosening]. The removal of a polyp by twisting it until its pedicle ruptures.

ebri·e·ty (e·brye'e·tee) *n.* [L. *ebrietas,* from *ebrius,* drunk]. Inebriety; habitual drunkenness.

ebri·ose (ee'bree·oce) *adj.* [L. *ebriosus*]. Drunk.

ebri·ous (ee'bree·us) *adj.* Drunk.

Eb·stein's anomaly or **malformation** (ep'shtine) [W. *Ebstein,* German physician, 1836-1912]. A symptomatic congenital anomaly of the tricuspid valve in which the septal and posterior leaflets are attached to the right ventricular wall, thus atrializing part of the right ventricle, producing a large right atrium and small ventricle, and sometimes causing obstruction to right ventricular outflow or filling;

arrhythmias, cyanosis, and heart failure are common manifestations.

Ebstein's disease [W. *Ebstein*]. 1. ARMANNI-EBSTEIN LESION. 2. EBSTEIN'S ANOMALY.

ebur (ee'bur) *n.* [L., ivory]. A tissue similar to ivory in appearance or structure.

eb·ur·na·tion (ee"bur·nay'shun, eb"ur·) *n.* [L. *eburneus,* of ivory]. An increase in the density of tooth or bone following some pathologic change. —**eb·ur·nat·ed** (ee'bur·nay·tid, eb'ur·) *adj.*

EBV Abbreviation for *Epstein-Barr virus.*

EB virus. EPSTEIN-BARR VIRUS.

ec- [Gk. *ek*]. A prefix meaning (a) *out;* (b) *outside of.*

Ec·bal·li·um (eck·bal'ee·um) *n.* [NL., from Gk. *ekballein,* to throw out]. A genus of plants of the Cucurbitaceae. See also *elaterium.*

ec·bol·ic (eck·bol'ick) *adj. & n.* [Gk. *ekbolē,* expulsion, + *-ic*]. 1. Producing abortion or accelerating labor. 2. A drug that produces abortion or accelerates labor.

ec·cen·tric (eck·sen'trick) *adj. & n.* [ML. *eccentricus,* from Gk. *ekkentros,* nongeocentric]. 1. Proceeding or situated away from the center or median line. 2. Deviating from the usual, normal, or generally expected behavior or reaction. 3. An individual whose behavioral patterns are generally unconventional or odd, but not necessarily symptomatic of a mental disorder. —**eccentri·cal·ly** (·trick·lee) *adv.*

eccentric atrophy. Atrophy that proceeds from within outward, as atrophy of bone beginning next to the marrow cavity.

eccentric fixation. Fixation of an eye with an area of the retina other than the fovea.

eccentric movement. Any movement of the mandible away from centric occlusion.

eccentric occlusion. The relation of the inclined planes of the teeth when the jaws are closed in any of the excursive movements of the mandible.

eccentric pain. REFERRED PAIN.

eccentric relation. Any relation of the jaws other than centric relation.

ec·cen·tro·chon·dro·os·teo·dys·tro·phy (eck·sen"tro·kon"dro·os"tee·o·dis'truh·fee) *n.* MORQUIO'S SYNDROME.

ec·cen·tro·cyte (eck·sen'tro·site) *n.* [*eccentric* + *-cyte*]. An erythrocyte with hemoglobin concentrated at the periphery.

ec·cen·tro-os·teo·chon·dro·dys·pla·sia (eck·sen"tro·os"tee·o·kon"dro·dis·play'zhuh, ·zee·uh) *n.* MORQUIO'S SYNDROME.

ec·ceph·a·lo·sis (eck·sef"uh·lo'sis) *n.*, pl. **eccephalo·ses** (·seez) [*ec-* + *cephal-* + *-osis*]. CEPHALOTOMY.

ec·chon·dro·ma (eck"on·dro'muh) *n.* [*ec-* + *chondroma*]. A nodular outgrowth from cartilage at the junction of cartilage and bone.

ec·chon·dro·sis (eck"on·dro'sis) *n.*, pl. **ecchondro·ses** (·seez) [*ec-* + *chondr-* + *-osis*]. A cartilaginous outgrowth. See also *exostosis cartilaginea.*

ecchondrosis phy·sa·liph·o·ra (figh·suh·lif'uh·ruh). CHORDOMA.

ec·chon·dro·tome (e·kon'dro·tome) *n.* [*ecchondrosis* + *-tome*]. An instrument for the surgical removal of cartilaginous growths.

ec·chy·mo·sis (eck"i·mo'sis) *n.*, pl. **ecchymo·ses** (·seez) [Gk. *ekchymōsis,* from *ek,* out, + *chyma,* fluid]. 1. Extravasation of blood into the subcutaneous tissues, discoloring the skin. 2. Any extravasation of blood into soft tissue. —**ec·chy·mot·ic** (·mot'ick) *adj.*

ecchymotic mask. The cyanotic facies of traumatic asphyxia.

ec·crine (eck'rin, ·rine, ·reen) *adj.* [*ec-* + *-crine*]. 1. Of sweat glands: MEROCRINE. 2. Of or pertaining to the eccrine glands or their secretion.

eccrine glands. The small sweat glands distributed all over the human body surface. Histologically, they are tubular coiled merocrine glands that secrete the clear aqueous sweat important for heat regulation and hydrating the skin and chemically different from apocrine sweat.

eccrine poroma. A benign skin tumor, usually on a sole and solitary, composed of bands of cuboidal cells suggesting origin from an eccrine sweat gland.

ec·cy·e·sis (eck"sigh·ee'sis) *n.*, pl. **eccye·ses** (·seez) [*ec-* + *cyesis*]. EXTRAUTERINE GESTATION.

ec·dem·ic (eck·dem'ick) *adj.* [Gk. *ekdēmos,* away from home]. Of diseases: brought into a region from without; not endemic or epidemic.

ec·demo·ma·nia (eck·dem"o·may'nee·uh) *n.* [Gk. *ekdēmos,* away from home, + *mania*]. DROMOMANIA.

ec·der·on (eck'dur·on) *n.* [*ec-* + Gk. *deros,* skin]. *Obsol.* The outermost or epithelial layer of the skin and mucous membranes. —**ec·der·on·ic** (eck"dur·on'ick) *adj.*

ec·dy·sis (eck'di·sis) *n.*, pl. **ecdy·ses** (·seez) [Gk. *ekdysis,* stripping]. Sloughing or casting off of the outer integument; molting, as of a crustacean, insect, or reptile.

ECG Abbreviation for *electrocardiogram.*

ec·go·nine (eck'go·neen, ·nin) *n.* 3-Hydroxy-2-tropanecarboxylic acid, $C_9H_{15}NO_3$, the principal part of the cocaine molecule (which is benzoylmethylecgonine); may be obtained from cocaine by hydrolysis.

echid·nase (e·kid'nace) *n.* [Gk. *echidna,* viper, + *-ase*]. A phlogogenic principle found in snake venom.

echid·nin (e·kid'nin) *n.* [Gk. *echidna,* viper, + *-in*]. 1. Snake poison; the poison or venom of the viper and other similar snakes. 2. A nitrogenous and venomous principle found in poisonous secretion of various snakes.

Echid·noph·a·ga (eck"id·nof'uh·guh) *n.* [NL., from Gk. *echidna,* viper, + *phagos,* glutton]. A genus of fleas.

Echidnophaga gal·li·na·cea (gal"i·nay'see·uh). The species of flea which attacks chickens in many parts of the world; may also become a human pest.

echid·no·tox·in (e·kid"no·tock'sin) *n.* [Gk. *echidna,* viper, + *toxin*]. A principle of snake venom which produces a general reaction in the human body and has a powerful effect on the nervous system.

echin-, echino- [Gk. *echinos,* hedgehog, sea urchin]. A combining form meaning (a) *spiny;* (b) *echinoderm.*

ech·i·na·cea (eck"i·nay'shuh) *n.* The dried rhizome and roots of *Echinacea pallida* and *E. angustifolia;* formerly used to treat ulcers and septicemia.

echino-. See *echin-.*

echi·no·chrome (e·kigh'no·krome, eck'i·no·krome) *n.* [*echino-* + *-chrome*]. A respiratory pigment found in the Echinodermata.

echi·no·coc·co·sis (e·kigh"no·kock·o'sis) *n.* Infection of man with *Echinococcus granulosus* in its larval or hydatid stage. Most important site of infection is the liver, and secondly, the lungs.

Echi·no·coc·cus (eh·kigh"no·kock'us) *n.* [NL., from *echino-* + Gk. *kokkos,* grain, berry]. A genus of tapeworms. —**echinoccus,** pl. **echinococ·ci** (·sigh), *com. n.*

echinococcus cyst. A cyst formed by growth of the larval form of *Echinococcus granulosus,* usually in the liver.

echinococcus fremitus. The vibration felt on palpation over an echinococcus cyst.

Echinococcus gran·u·lo·sus (gran·yoo·lo'sus). The species of tapeworm whose ova, when ingested by man or other intermediate hosts, develop into echinococcus cysts.

echinococcus test. CASONI'S TEST.

echi·no·cyte (e·kigh'no·site) *n.* [*echino-* + *-cyte*]. BURR CELL.

echi·no·derm (e·kigh'no·durm) *n.* One of the Echinodermata.

Echi·no·der·ma·ta (e·kigh"no·dur'muh·tuh) *n. pl.* [NL., from *echino-* + Gk. *derma, dermatos,* skin]. A phylum of marine animals including starfish and sea urchins.

ech·i·nop·sine (eck"i·nop'seen, ·sin) *n.* 1-Methyl-4(1)-guinolone, $C_{10}H_9NO$, an alkaloid isolated from the fruits of the herb *Echinops ritro* and other species of *Echinops.*

Echi·no·rhyn·chus (e·kigh"no·ring'kus) *n.* [*echino-* + Gk. *rhynchos,* snout]. A genus of acanthocephalan worms.

Echinorhynchus gi·gas (jye'gas). MACRACANTHORHYNCHUS HIRUDINACEUS.

Echinorhynchus moniliformis. MONILIFORMIS MONILIFORMIS.

ech·i·no·sis (eck''i·no'sis) *n.*, pl. **echino·ses** (·seez) [*echin-* + *-osis*]. CRENATION (1).

Echi·no·sto·ma (e·kigh''no·sto'muh, eck''i·nos'to·muh) *n.* [*echino-* + *-stoma*]. A genus of flukes parasitic in man, but of little pathologic importance.

echi·no·sto·mi·a·sis (e·kigh''no·sto·migh'uh·sis, eck''i·no·) *n.*, pl. **echinostomia·ses** (·seez) [*Echinostoma* + *-iasis*]. Infection by flukes of the genus *Echinostoma* acquired by the ingestion of infected snails in the Far East, and causing diarrhea and abdominal pain.

Ech·is (eck'is) *n.* [Gk., viper]. A genus of vipers found in Africa, Arabia, and India.

Echis car·i·na·tus (kăr''i·nay'tus). The saw-scaled viper, attaining 1½ feet in length, possessing a hemotoxic venom.

echo (eck'o) *n.* [Gk. *ēchō*]. A reverberated sound.

echo$_{10}$. REOVIRUS.

echo·acou·sia (eck''o·a·koo'zhuh, ·zee·uh) *n.* [*echo* + *-acousia*]. A subjective disturbance of hearing in which there appears to be a repetition of a sound just heard.

echo·aor·tog·ra·phy (eck''o·ay''or·tog'ruh·fee) *n.* Echocardiography applied to the aorta.

echo·car·dio·gram (eck''o·kahr'dee·o·gram) *n.* [*echo* + *cardiogram*]. A pictorial representation of the heart, using pulse-echo (ultrasound) techniques.

echo·car·di·og·ra·phy (eck''o·kahr''dee·og'ruh·fee) *n.* The use of ultrasound to delineate structure and motion of the heart and great vessels by means of a reflected acoustic wave, or echo.

echo·en·ceph·a·lo·gram (eck''o·en·sef'uh·lo·gram) *n.* The pictorial representation of intracranial structures, obtained by echoencephalography.

echo·en·ceph·a·lo·graph (eck''o·en·sef'uh·lo·graph) *n.* The instrument employed in echoencephalography.

echo·en·ceph·a·log·ra·phy (eck''o·en·sef''uh·log'ruh·fee) *n.* [*echo* + *encephalo-* + *graphy*]. The study of intracranial structures and disease, employing pulse-echo techniques.

echo·gram (eck'o·gram) *n.* [*echo* + *-gram*]. The pictorial display of anatomic structures, using pulse-echo techniques. Syn. *echosonogram, sonogram.* See also *ultrasound.*

echo·graph·ia (eck''o·graf'ee·uh) *n.* [*echo* + *-graphia*]. A form of aphasia in which the patient copies material presented to him without apparent comprehension.

echo·ki·ne·sis (eck''o·ki·nee'sis, ·kigh·nee'sis) *n.*, pl. **echokine·ses** (·seez). ECHOPRAXIA.

echo·la·lia (eck''o·lay'lee·uh) *n.* [*echo* + *-lalia*]. The purposeless, often seemingly involuntary repetition of words spoken by another person; a disorder seen in certain psychotic states, as in the catatonic type of schizophrenia, in minimal brain dysfunction, and as the only form of speech in so-called isolation of the speech area. Syn. *echophrasia.* —**echo·lal·ic** (·lal'ick) *adj.*

echo·la·lus (eck''o·lay'lus) *n.* [NL., from *echo* + Gk. *lalos,* talkative]. A hypnotized person who repeats words heard without comprehending their meaning.

echo·ma·tism (e·ko'muh·tiz·um, e·kom'uh·tiz·um) *n.* ECHOPRAXIA.

echo·mim·ia (eck''o·mim'ee·uh) *n.* [*echo* + Gk. *mimos*, mime, + *-ia*]. ECHOPRAXIA.

echo·mo·tism (eck''o·mo'tiz·um) *n.* ECHOPRAXIA.

echop·a·thy (eck·op'uth·ee) *n.* [*echo* + *-pathy*]. *In psychiatry,* a morbid condition marked by the automatic and purposeless repetition of a word or sound heard or of an act seen by the patient. See also *echolalia, echopraxia.*

echoph·o·ny (eck·off'uh·nee) *n.* [*echo* + *-phony*]. An echo of a vocal sound heard in auscultation of the chest.

echo·phot·o·ny (eck''o·fot'uh·nee) *n.* [*echo* + *phot-* + Gk. *tonos,* tone]. The mental evocation or association of particular colors by sound waves or tones. See also *phonism, photism.*

echo·phra·sia (eck''o·fray'zhuh, ·zee·uh) *n.* ECHOLALIA.

echo·prax·ia (eck''o·prack'see·uh) *n.* [*echo* + *-praxia*]. Automatic imitation by the patient of another person's movements or mannerisms; seen in various psychoses, as in the catatonic type of schizophrenia.

echo·prax·is (eck''o·prack'sis) *n.* ECHOPRAXIA.

echo·praxy (eck'o·prack''see) *n.* ECHOPRAXIA.

echo·reno·gram (eck''o·ren'o·gram, ·ree'no·) *n.* [*echo* + *reno-* + *-gram*]. The pictorial representation of the kidneys, using pulse-echo (ultrasound) techniques. Syn. *nephrosonogram.*

echo sign. The involuntary repetition of the last syllable, word, or clause of a sentence.

echo·sono·en·ceph·a·lo·gram (eck''o·son''o·en·sef'uh·lo·gram) *n.* [*echo* + *sono-* + *encephalo-* + *-gram*]. ECHOENCEPHALOGRAM.

echo·sono·gram (eck''o·son'o·gram) *n.* [*echo* + *sono-* + *-gram*]. ECHOGRAM.

echo speech. ECHOLALIA.

echo·thi·o·phate iodide (eck''o·thigh'o·fate). (2-Mercaptoethyl)trimethyammonium iodide *O,O*-diethyl phosphorothioate, $C_9H_{23}INO_3PS$, a long-acting cholinesterase inhibitor employed in the treatment of glaucoma.

echo·utero·gram (eck''o·yoo'tur·o·gram) *n.* [*echo* + *utero-* + *-gram*]. The pictorial representation of the uterus, using pulse-echo techniques.

echo·vi·rus or **ECHO virus** [*e*nteric *c*ytopathogenic *h*uman *o*rphan]. A member of a large group of viruses of the picornavirus group which are small, contain RNA, and are ether-resistant. The cause of asymptomatic infection of man as well as a wide variety of syndromes, including aseptic meningitis, exanthems, and diarrhea.

ec·io·ma·nia (eck''ee·o·may'nee·uh) *n.* ECOMANIA.

Eck·er's diluting fluid [E. E. *Ecker,* U.S. bacteriologist, 1887–1966]. REES AND ECKER'S DILUTING FLUID.

Eck's fistula [N. V. *Eck,* Russian physiologist, 1847–1908]. Anastomosis of the portal vein to the inferior vena cava, so that the portal blood bypasses the liver; performed in experimental animals.

ec·la·bi·um (eck·lay'bee·um) *n.* [*ec-* + *labium*]. Eversion of the lip.

eclamp·sia (e·klamp'see·uh) *n.* [NL., fit, convulsion; orig., scintillating visual sensations in neurologic affections, from Gk. *eklampsis,* flash, shining, from *ek-*, out, + *lampein,* to shine]. 1. A disease occurring in the latter half of pregnancy and sometimes in the puerperium, characterized by an acute elevation of blood pressure, proteinuria, edema, sodium retention, convulsions, and sometimes coma. See also *preeclampsia, toxemia of pregnancy.* 2. *Obsol.* Any of various conditions characterized by convulsions. —**eclamp·tic,** *adj.*

eclampsia gra·vi·da·rum (grav·i·dair'um). ECLAMPSIA (1).

eclampsia nu·tans (new'tanz) [L., nodding]. *Obsol.* INFANTILE SPASM.

eclampsia ro·tans (ro'tanz). *Obsol.* SPASMUS NUTANS.

eclamp·sism (e·klamp'siz·um) *n.* [*eclampsia* + *-ism*]. The preeclamptic toxemia of pregnancy which may lead to convulsions and coma; includes the preconvulsive prodromes, nephritis, and vascular disease.

eclamp·to·gen·ic (e·klamp''to·gen'ick) *adj.* [*eclampsia* + *-genic*]. Causing eclampsia.

eclamptogenic toxemia. TOXEMIA OF PREGNANCY.

ec·lec·ti·cism (e·kleck'ti·siz·um) *n.* [Gk. *eklektikos,* selective]. 1. The system of medicine involving the selection of doctrines or elements of various schools of therapeutics according to their utility and combining them into a set of practices. 2. A system of medicine depending primarily on indigenous plant remedies. —**eclec·tic** (·tick) *n. & adj.*

eclipse blindness. Blindness after looking directly at an eclipse of the sun, caused by a thermal lesion in the retina.

ec·ly·sis (eck'li·sis) *n.* [Gk. *eklysis,* release]. *Obsol.* 1. Any loosening, as of the bowels. 2. Faintness; a tendency to faint.

ec·mne·sia (eck·nee'zhuh, ·zee·uh, eck·mnee') *n.* [*ec-* + *-mnesia*]. *Obsol.* ANTEROGRADE AMNESIA.

E. coli Abbreviation for *Escherichia coli.*

Ecolid Chloride. Trademark for chlorisondamine chloride, an antihypertensive drug.

ecol·o·gy (e·kol'uh·jee) *n.* [Gk. *oikos*, house, household, dwelling, + *-logy*]. The study of the environmental relations of organisms.

eco·ma·nia (ee''ko·may'nee·uh) *n.* [Gk. *oikos*, house, + *mania*]. A symptom complex characterized by a domineering, haughty, and irritable attitude toward members of one's own family, but an attitude of humility toward those in authority. See also *authoritarian character.*

eco·na·zole (e·ko'nuh·zole) *n.* 1-[2,4-Dichloro-β-[(*p*-chlorobenzyl)oxy]phenethyl]imidazole, $C_{18}H_{15}Cl_3N_2O$, an antifungal.

Eco·no·mo's disease (eʸ·ko·no'mo) [K. von *Economo*, Austrian neurologist, 1876–1931]. ENCEPHALITIS LETHARGICA.

economy quotient. The ratio of total gain of intake of water over total output of water at any one load. It measures the relative role of gain and of loss during attempts at recovery of water balance.

ecos·tate (ee·kos'tate) *adj.* [*e-* + *costate*]. Without ribs. —**ecos·ta·tion** (ee''kos·tay'shun) *n.*

ecos·ta·tism (ee·kos'tuh·tiz·um) *n.* [*ecostate* + *-ism*]. The condition of being without ribs.

eco·sys·tem (ee''ko·sis''tum, eck''o·) *n.* A system comprised of the abiotic physicochemical environment and the biotic assemblage of plants, animals, and microbes in which an ecological kinship exists. A field, a forest, a pond, or an ocean may constitute such a system.

eco·thio·phate iodide (eck''o·thigh'o·fate) *n.* 2-(Mercaptoethyl)trimethylammonium iodide, *S*-ester with *O,O*-diethyl phosphorothioate, $C_9H_{23}INO_3PS$, an ophthalmic anticholinergic.

ec·pho·ria (eck·for'ee·uh) *n.* [*ec-* + *-phoria*]. *In psychology,* the revival of a memory trace or engram, as by repetition of the original stimuli.

écra·seur (ay·kra·zur') *n.* [F., from *écraser*, to crush]. A surgical instrument armed with a metal loop which can be tightened. Used in veterinary surgery, in castration of stallions, for example; infrequently in human surgery for the control of expected severe hemorrhage, as in excision of large pedicled tumors.

ECS Abbreviation for *electroconvulsive shock.*

ec·sta·sy (eck'stuh·see) *n.* [Gk. *ekstasis*, displacement, trance]. 1. A trancelike state with mental and physical exaltation and often oblivion of environment. 2. *Obsol.* CATALEPSY. —**ec·stat·ic** (eck·stat'ick) *adj.*

ecstatic trance. CATALEPSY.

ECT Abbreviation for *electroconvulsive therapy.*

ect-, ecto- [Gk. *ektos*]. A combining form meaning (a) *outside, outer;* (b) *out of place.*

ec·tad (eck'tad) *adv.* [Gk. *ektos*, outside, + *-ad*]. Outward.

ec·tal (eck'tul) *adj.* [Gk. *ektos*, outside, + *-al*]. External; superficial.

ec·ta·sia (eck·tay'zhuh, ·zee·uh) *n.* [Gk. *ektasis*, a stretching out, + *-ia*]. Dilatation or distention, usually of a hollow structure. —**ec·tat·ic** (·tat'ick) *adj.*

ectasia ven·tric·u·li par·a·doxa (ven·trick'yoo·lye păr''uh·dock'suh). HOURGLASS STOMACH.

ec·ta·sis (eck'tuh·sis) *n.*, pl. **ecta·ses** (·seez). ECTASIA.

ectatic aneurysm. An expansion of a portion of an artery due to distention of all the coats.

ectatic emphysema. COMPENSATORY EMPHYSEMA.

ec·ten·tal (eck·ten'tul) *adj.* [*ect-* + *ent-* + *-al*]. Pertaining to the line of union between the ectoderm and the entoderm.

ect·eth·moid (ekt·eth'moid) *n.* [*ect-* + *ethmoid*]. Either one of the lateral cellular masses of the ethmoid bone.

ectethmoid cartilage. PARANASAL CARTILAGE.

ec·thy·ma (eck·thigh'muh) *n.* [Gk. *ekthyma*, pustule, from *ekthyein* to break out]. An inflammatory skin disease characterized by large, flat pustules that ulcerate and become crusted, and are surrounded by a distinct inflammatory areola. The lesions as a rule appear on the legs and thighs, and occur in crops which persist for an indefinite period.

ecthyma con·ta·gi·o·sum (kon·tay''jee·o'sum). ORF.

ecthyma gan·gre·no·sum (gang''gre·no'sum). DERMATITIS GANGRENOSA INFANTUM.

ecto-. See *ect-.*

ec·to·bat·ic (eck''to·bat'ick) *adj.* [*ecto-* + Gk. *bainein*, to go]. Efferent; centrifugal; moving ectad or distad.

ec·to·blast (eck'to·blast) *n.* [*ecto-* + *-blast*]. 1. ECTODERM. 2. PRIMITIVE ECTODERM. 3. ECTOPLASM.

ec·to·car·dia (eck''to·kahr'dee·uh) *n.* [*ecto-* + *-cardia*]. An abnormal position of the heart. It may be outside the thoracic cavity (ectopia cordis) or misplaced within the thorax.

ec·to·cer·vix (eck''to·sur'vicks) *n.* [*ecto-* + *cervix*]. The portio vaginalis of the uterine cervix; the portion of the cervix bearing stratified squamous epithelium.

ec·to·cho·roi·dea (eck''to·ko·roy'dee·uh) *n.* [*ecto-* + *choroidea*]. The outer layer of the choroid.

ec·to·cor·nea (eck''to·kor'nee·uh) *n.* [*ecto-* + *cornea*]. The outer layer of the cornea.

ec·to·cra·ni·al (eck''to·kray'nee·ul) *adj.* [*ecto-* + *cranial*]. Pertaining to the outside of the skull.

ec·to·derm (eck'to·durm) *n.* [*ecto-* + *-derm*]. The outermost of the three primary germ layers of the embryo. From it arise the epidermis, epithelial lining of stomodeum and proctodeum, and the neural tube, with all derivatives of these. Contr. *entoderm, mesoderm.* —**ec·to·der·mal** (eck''to·dur'mul) *adj.*

ectodermal cloaca. The part of the cloaca derived from the proctodeal invagination after rupture of the cloacal membrane.

ectodermal dysplasia. Abnormal development or growth of tissues and structures arising from the ectoderm.

ec·to·der·mo·sis (eck''to·dur·mo'sis) *n.*, pl. **ectodermo·ses** (·seez) [*ectoderm* + *-osis*]. Any disease entity of the ectoderm.

ectodermosis ero·si·va plu·ri·ori·fi·ci·a·lis (eer·o·sigh'vuh ploor''ee·or·i·fish·ee·ay'lis). STEVENS-JOHNSON SYNDROME.

ec·to·en·zyme (eck''to·en'zime, ·zim) *n.* [*ecto-* + *enzyme*]. 1. An enzyme so situated on the outer surface of a cell membrane that its active site is in contact with the exterior environment of the cell. 2. EXTRACELLULAR ENZYME.

ec·to·gen·e·sis (eck''to·jen'e·sis) *n.* [*ecto-* + *genesis*]. Development of an embryo or of embryonic tissue outside the natural environment. —**ecto·ge·net·ic** (·je·net'ick) *adj.*

ec·to·gen·ic (eck''to·jen'ick) *adj.* [*ecto-* + *-genic*]. ECTOGENOUS.

ec·tog·e·nous (eck·toj'e·nus) *adj.* [*ecto-* + *-genous*]. 1. Capable of growth outside the body of its host; applied to bacteria and other parasites. 2. Due to an external cause; not arising within the organism; exogenous.

ec·tog·o·ny (eck·tog'uh·nee) *n.* [*ecto-* + *-gony*]. The influence of the developing zygote on the mother.

-ectome [*ec-* + *-tome*]. A combining form meaning *an instrument for excising.*

ec·to·me·ninx (eck''to·mee'ninks, ·men'inks) *n.*, pl. **ecto·me·nin·ges** (·me·nin'jeez) [*ecto-* + *meninx*]. The external part of the meninx primitiva, differentiating into dura mater and a more superficial part concerned with the formation of the chondrocranium and osteocranium.

ec·to·mere (eck'to·meer) *n.* A blastomere destined to take part in forming the ectoderm.

ec·to·meso·derm (eck''to·mez'o·durm, ·mes'o·durm) *n.* Mesoderm derived from the primary ectoderm of a bilaminar blastodisk or gastrula. Contr. *endomesoderm.*

ec·to·morph (eck'to·morf) *n.* In the somatotype, an individual exhibiting relative predominance of ectomorphy.

ec·to·mor·phy (eck'to·mor"fee) *n.* [*ecto-* + *-morphy*]. Component III of the somatotype, representing relative predominance of linear and fragile body features; the skin or surface area, derived from ectoderm, is relatively great with respect to body mass. Ectomorphs appear to be more sensitive to their external environment. The counterpart on the behavioral level is cerebrotonia. Contr. *endomorphy, mesomorphy.* —**ec·to·mor·phic** (eck"to·morf'ick) *adj.*

-ectomy [Gk. *ektomē*, excision, from *ek*, out, + *tomē*, cutting]. A combining form meaning *surgical removal.*

ec·to·pa·gia (eck"to·pay'jee·uh) *n.* The condition of being an ectopagus; an ectopagous monstrosity.

ec·top·a·gus (eck·top'uh·gus) *n.*, pl. **ectopa·gi** (·guy, ·jye) [*ecto-* + *-pagus*]. An individual consisting of conjoined twins united laterally at the thorax. —**ectopagous,** *adj.*

ec·top·a·gy (eck·top'uh·jee) *n.* ECTOPAGIA.

ec·to·par·a·site (eck"to·păr'uh·site) *n.* [*ecto-* + *parasite*]. A parasite that lives on the exterior of its host. Contr. *endoparasite.* —**ecto·par·a·sit·ic** (·păr·uh·sit'ick) *adj.*

ec·to·phyte (eck'to·fite) *n.* [*ecto-* + *-phyte*]. 1. An external parasitic plant growth. 2. *In dermatology,* a fungus that infects superficially.

ec·to·phyt·ic (eck"to·fit'ick) *adj.* 1. Of or pertaining to an ectophyte. 2. Characterizing a cutaneous tumor that enlarges outward.

ec·to·pia (eck·to'pee·uh) *n.* [Gk. *ektopos*, away from a place, + *-ia*]. An abnormality of position of an organ or a part of the body; usually congenital.

ectopia cor·dis (kor'dis). A congenital anomaly in which the heart lies outside the thoracic cavity.

ectopia len·tis (len'tis). A subluxated lens, generally seen in Marfan's syndrome and homocystinuria.

ectopia pu·pil·lae (pew·pil'ee). CORECTOPIA.

ectopia re·nis (ree'nis). ECTOPIC KIDNEY.

ectopia tes·tis (tes'tis). A congenital anomaly in which the testis descends into an abnormal location, generally in the perineum or near the pubic bone.

ec·top·ic (eck·top'ick) *adj.* [Gk. *ektopos*, away from a place, foreign, strange, from *ek*, out, + *topos*, place]. 1. Out of place, in an abnormal position. 2. Occurring at an abnormal time.

ectopic ACTH syndrome. Electrolyte abnormalities, edema of the lower limbs, muscle weakness often worsened by diuretics, hyporeflexia, thirst, polyuria, and hyperpigmentation secondary to increased circulating adrenocorticotropin in patients with tumors not involving the pituitary or adrenals. There may be an increased amount of an ACTH-like substance in the primary tumor or its metastases.

ectopic beat. PREMATURE BEAT.

ectopic cardiac rhythm. ECTOPIC RHYTHM.

ectopic eruption. A congenital anomaly in which a permanent tooth erupts in an abnormal position, as at a transposed or an extraoral site.

ectopic gestation. EXTRAUTERINE GESTATION.

ectopic impulse. 1. PREMATURE BEAT. 2. A precordial pulsation, palpable or visible in an abnormal location.

ectopic kidney. A congenital anomaly in which the kidney is held in abnormal position on its own or on the opposite side, where fusion with the other kidney may occur.

ectopic myelopoiesis. EXTRAMEDULLARY HEMOPOIESIS.

ectopic pacemaker. An abnormal focus of impulse initiation in the heart, i.e., not in the sinoatrial node.

ectopic pregnancy. EXTRAUTERINE PREGNANCY.

ectopic rhythm. An abnormal cardiac rhythm originating in a focus other than the sinoatrial node, i.e., from an ectopic pacemaker.

ectopic teratism. A form of teratism in which there is displacement of one or more parts.

ectopic testicle. A testis that has descended through the inguinal canal but does not reside in the scrotum.

ectopic ureter. A ureter emptying at some point other than the trigone of the bladder. Syn. *aberrant ureter.*

ectopic zone. An area in the prosencephalon surrounding the optic vesicle on its dorsal, cephalic, and ventral aspects. From this zone several parts of the telencephalon and diencephalon take origin. Syn. *ectopic zone of Schulte.*

ectopic zone of Schulte. ECTOPIC ZONE.

ec·to·pla·cen·ta (eck"to·pluh·sen'tuh) *n.* [*ecto-* + *placenta*]. TROPHODERM (2). —**ecto·placen·tal** (·tul) *adj.*

ectoplacental amnion. FALSE AMNION.

ectoplacental cavity. FALSE AMNION.

ectoplacental cone. The thickened trophoblast of the early blastocyst of rodents, which forms the fetal placenta.

ec·to·plasm (eck'to·plaz·um) *n.* [*ecto-* + *-plasm*]. The outer denser layer of cytoplasm of a cell or unicellular organism. —**ec·to·plas·mic** (eck"to·plaz'mick) *adj.*

ec·to·plast (eck'to·plast) *n.* [*ecto-* + *-plast*]. ECTOPLASM.

ec·to·pot·o·my (eck"to·pot'uh·mee) *n.* [*ectopic* + *-tomy*]. Laparotomy for the removal of the contents of an extrauterine gestation sac.

ec·to·py (eck'to·pee) *n.* ECTOPIA.

ec·to·sarc (eck'to·sahrk) *n.* [*ecto-* + *-sarc*]. The outer layer of a protozoan.

ec·to·thrix (eck'to·thricks) *n.* [*ecto-* + *-thrix*]. A fungal parasite forming spores on the outside of hair shafts, as certain species of *Microsporum* and *Trichophyton.*

ec·to·zo·on (eck"to·zo'on) *n.*, pl. **ecto·zoa** (·zo'uh) [*ecto-* + *-zoon*]. An external animal parasite; ECTOPARASITE.

ectro- [Gk. *ektrōsis*, miscarriage]. A combining form meaning *congenital absence.*

ec·tro·dac·tyl·ia (eck"tro·dack·til'ee·uh) *n.* [*ectro-* + *-dactylia*]. Congenital absence of any of the fingers or toes or parts of them.

ec·tro·dac·ty·lism (eck"tro·dack'ti·liz·um) *n.* ECTRODACTYLIA.

ec·tro·dac·ty·ly (eck"tro·dack'ti·lee) *n.* ECTRODACTYLIA.

ec·trog·e·ny (eck·troj'e·nee) *n.* [*ectro-* + *-geny*]. Loss or congenital absence of any part or organ. —**ec·tro·gen·ic** (eck"tro·jen'ick) *adj.*

ec·tro·me·lia (eck"tro·mee'lee·uh) *n.* [*ectro-* + *-melia*]. Congenital absence or marked imperfection of one or more of the limbs.

ec·trom·e·lus (eck·trom'e·lus) *n.*, pl. **ectrome·li** (·lye) [*ectro-* + *-melus*]. An individual with one or more congenitally absent or imperfect limbs.

ec·trom·e·ly (eck·trom'e·lee) *n.* ECTROMELIA.

ec·tro·pi·on (eck·tro'pee·on) *n.* [Gk. *ektropion*, from *ek*, out, + *tropē*, turning]. Eversion of a part, especially of an eyelid. —**ectropi·on·ize** (·un·ize) *v.*; **ectropion·iza·tion** (·i·zay'shun) *n.*

ectropion iri·dis (eye'ri·dis). Eversion of a part of the iris.

ec·trop·o·dism (eck·trop'o·diz·um) *n.* [*ectro-* + *pod-* + *-ism*]. Congenital absence of a foot or feet.

ec·tro·syn·dac·ty·ly (eck"tro·sin·dack'ti·lee) *n.* [*ectro-* + *syndactyly*]. A developmental defect in which some of the digits are missing while others are fused.

ec·trot·ic (eck·trot'ick) *adj.* [Gk. *ektrōtikos*, abortive, from *ektrōsis*, abortion]. 1. Tending to cut short; preventing the development of disease. 2. Abortive; abortifacient.

ec·ty·lot·ic (eck"ti·lot'ick) *adj.* & *n.* [Gk. *ektylōtikos*, from *tylos*, callus]. 1. Removing warts or indurations. 2. An agent that removes warts or indurations.

ec·tyl·urea (eck"til·yoo·ree'uh) *n.* 2-Ethyl-*cis*-crotonylurea, $C_7H_{12}N_2O_2$, a tranquilizing drug.

ec·ze·ma (eck'se·muh, eg·zee'muh) *n.* [Gk. *ekzema*, from *ekzein*, to boil over, break out]. An acute or chronic, noncontagious, itching, inflammatory disease of the skin; usually characterized by irregular and varying combinations of edematous, vesicular, papular, pustular, scaling, thickened, or exudative lesions. The skin is reddened, the redness shading off into the surrounding unaffected parts. The cause is unknown. Eruptions of similar appearance due to such known causes as ingested drugs or local irritants are properly referred to as dermatitis medicamentosa, contact dermatitis, or dermatitis venenata.

eczema er·y·the·ma·to·sum (err″i·theem″uh·to′sum, ·themm″). The mildest form of eczema, in which the skin is reddened and slightly swollen.

eczema fis·sum. A form of eczema affecting the hands and skin over the articulations; characterized by deep, painful cracks or fissures.

eczema her·pet·i·cum (hur·pet′i·kum). A rare manifestation of primary herpes simplex infection occurring in patients with eczema or neurodermatitis, with grouped, varicella-like vesicles over large areas of the eczematous skin. See also *eczema vaccinatum.*

eczema hy·per·troph·icum (high″pur·trof′i·kum). A form of eczema characterized by permanent hypertrophy of the papillae of the skin, giving rise to general or limited warty outgrowths.

eczema mad·i·dans (mad′i·danz) [L., from *madidus,* moist]. A form of eczema characterized by large, raw, weeping surfaces studded with red points. It follows eczema vesiculosum. Syn. *eczema rubrum.*

eczema mar·gi·na·tum (mahr·ji·nay′tum). TINEA CRURIS.

eczema num·mu·la·ris (num″yoo·lair′is). NUMMULAR DERMATITIS.

eczema pap·u·lo·sum (pap″yoo·lo′sum). A variety of eczema showing minute papules of deep-red color and firm consistency; accompanied by intense itching.

eczema pus·tu·lo·sum (pus″tew·lo′sum). A stage of eczema characterized by the formation of pustules.

eczema ru·brum (roo′brum). ECZEMA MADIDANS.

eczema se·bor·rhe·i·cum (seb″o·ree′i·kum, see″bo·). SEBORRHEIC DERMATITIS.

eczema so·la·re (so·lair′ee). Eczema due to irritation from the sun's rays. See also *polymorphous light eruption.*

eczema squa·mo·sum (skway·mo′sum). A variety of eczema characterized by the formation of adherent scales of shed epithelium.

eczema strep·to·coc·cum (strep″to·kock′um) Secondary infection with hemolytic streptococci, particularly in infants with weeping eczematoid lesions.

eczema sy·co·ma·to·sum (sigh·ko″muh·to′sum). A pustular form of eczema occurring on the hairy parts and affecting the hair follicles.

eczema sy·co·si·for·me (sigh·ko″si·for′mee). ECZEMA SYCOMATOSUM.

ec·zem·a·tid (eg·zem′uh·tid, eg·zeem′, eck·seem′) *n.* [*eczema* + *-id*]. An exudative dermatitis presumably caused by a circulating allergen.

ec·ze·ma·ti·za·tion (eg·zem″uh·ti·zay′shun, eck·seem′) *n.* The formation or presence of eczema or eczema-like lesions, as from continued physical or chemical irritation or from allergic or autoimmune reactions.

ec·ze·ma·toid (eck·sem′uh·toid, eck·seem′, eg·zem′, eg·zeem′) *adj.* Resembling eczema.

eczematoid dermatitis. ECZEMATOID REACTION.

eczematoid reaction. A dermal and epidermal inflammatory response characterized by erythema, edema, vesiculation, and exudation in the acute stage, and in the chronic stage by erythema, edema, thickening (or lichenification) of the epidermis, and scaling.

ec·ze·ma·to·sis (eg·zem″uh·to′sis, eg·zee″muh·, eck″se·muh·) *n.* Any eczematous skin disease.

ec·ze·ma·tous (eck·sem′uh·tus, eck·seem′, eg·zem′, ·zeem′) *adj.* Of or pertaining to eczema.

eczematous conjunctivitis. PHLYCTENULAR KERATOCONJUNCTIVITIS.

eczema ty·lot·i·cum (tye·lot′i·kum). A form of eczema occurring on the palms; attended with callosity.

eczema vac·ci·na·tum (vack″si·nay′tum). The accidental inoculation of vaccinia virus on lesions of eczema, producing umbilicated vesicles and pustules on eczematous and normal skin, chiefly the former.

eczema ve·sic·u·lo·sum (ve·sick″yoo·lo′sum). An eczema characterized by the presence of vesicles.

Ed·dowes' disease or **syndrome** [A. *Eddowes,* British physician, 1850–1946]. OSTEOGENESIS IMPERFECTA.

Ed·dy·ism (ed′ee·iz·um) *n.* [Mary Baker G. P. *Eddy,* American religious leader, 1821–1910]. CHRISTIAN SCIENCE.

ede-, edeo-, edo- [Gk. *aidoia,* genitals]. A combining form meaning *pertaining to the external genitals.* Most words from this stem are now obsolete.

Ede·bohls' operation [G. M. *Edebohls,* U.S. surgeon, 1853–1908]. A renal decortication procedure formerly used for the relief of chronic nephritis.

Edebohls' position [G. M. *Edebohls*]. An exaggerated lithotomy position for vaginal operations, similar to Simon's position.

Edecrin. Trademark for the diuretic drug ethacrynic acid.

Edel·mann's great toe phenomenon or **sign.** Flexion of the thigh at the hip with the leg remaining extended at the knee results in dorsiflexion of the great toe in meningeal irritation and also in increased intracranial pressure.

ede·ma, oe·de·ma (e·dee′muh) *n.,* pl. **edemas, edema·ta** (·tuh) [Gk. *oidēma,* swelling, from *oidein,* to swell]. Excessive accumulation of fluid in the tissue spaces, due to increased transudation of the fluid from the capillaries; dropsy. **—edem·a·tous** (e·dem′uh·tus, ·deem′) *adj.*

edema neonatorum. SCLEREMA NEONATORUM.

edema of the newborn. SCLEREMA NEONATORUM.

Eden·ta·ta (ee″den·tay′tuh) *n. pl.* [NL., edentate]. An order of mammals in which were formerly grouped certain animals with degenerate or absent dentitions, as tree sloths, South American anteaters, and armadillos.

eden·tate (e·den′tate) *adj. & n.* [L. *edentatus,* from *edentare,* to knock out the teeth, from *dens,* tooth]. 1. Without teeth. Contr. *dentulous.* 2. Pertaining to the order of mammals Edentata. 3. A member of the Edentata.

eden·tia (e·den′shuh) *n.* [*edentate* + *-ia*]. ANODONTIA.

eden·tu·lous (e·den′chuh·lus) *adj.* [L. *edentulus*]. Without teeth. Contr. *dentulous.*

edeo-. See *ede-.*

ede·ol·o·gy, ae·doe·ol·o·gy (ee″dee·ol′uh·jee) *n.* [*edeo-* + *-logy*]. *Obsol.* The science of the organs of generation.

edes·tin (e·des′tin, ee′des·tin) *n.* [Gk. *edestos,* edible]. A globulin type of simple protein; obtained from the seeds of hemp.

ed·e·tate (ed′e·tate) *n.* Any salt of edetic acid; an ethylenediaminetetraacetate.

edet·ic acid (e·det′ick). (Ethylenedinitrilo)tetraacetic acid or ethylenediaminetetraacetic acid, $(HOOC\text{-}CH_2)_2NCH_2\text{-}CH_2N(CH_2COOH)_2$, salts of which, called edetates, are powerful chelating and sequestering agents that form water-soluble complexes with many cations, preventing these from exhibiting their characteristic properties.

edge-to-edge bite. The meeting of the cutting edges of the upper and lower anterior teeth.

ed·i·ble (ed′i·bul) *adj.* [L. *edibilis,* from *edere,* to eat]. Fit to eat.

EDIM Abbreviation for *epidemic diarrhea of infant mice.*

Eding·er-West·phal nucleus (eʸ′ding·ur, vest′fahl) [L. *Edinger,* German neurologist, 1855–1918; and C. F. O. *Westphal*]. AUTONOMIC NUCLEUS OF THE OCULOMOTOR NERVE.

edipal. OEDIPAL.

edipism. OEDIPISM.

edis·yl·ate (e·dis′il·ate) *n.* Any salt or ester of 1,2-ethanedisulfonic acid, $(CH_2SO_3H)_2$; a 1,2-ethanedisulfonate.

edo-. See *ede-.*

edo·ceph·al·us (ee″do·sef′uh·lus) *n.,* pl. **edocepha·li** (·lye) [*edo-* + *-cephalus*]. A type of otocephalus characterized by partially fused eyes in a single orbit (cyclopia), a proboscis above the fused orbit, no mouth, a defective lower jaw, and synotia. **—edocepha·ly** (·lee) *n.*

ed·ro·phon·i·um chloride (ed″ro·fon′ee·um). Dimethylethyl(3-hydroxyphenyl)ammonium chloride, $C_{10}H_{16}ClNO$, a curare antagonist.

EDTA Abbreviation for *ethylenediaminetetraacetic acid* (= EDETIC ACID).

ed·u·ca·ble (ej'oo·kuh·bul) *adj.* 1. Capable of being educated. 2. Specifically, categorizing a mentally retarded individual who can, within limits, profit from educative efforts and become socially and economically self-maintaining or even independent as an adult.

ed·u·ca·tion·al age. The average achievement of a pupil or student in school subjects based on average performances for a given chronological age as measured by standard educational tests; achievement age for a person in school.

educational quotient. The educational age of a pupil divided by his chronological age, multiplied by 100: EQ = EA/CA × 100.

Ed·wards' syndrome [J. H. *Edwards,* British physician, 20th century]. TRISOMY 18 SYNDROME.

Ed·win Smith papyrus [*Edwin Smith,* U.S. Egyptologist, 1822–1906]. An Egyptian papyrus dealing largely with wound surgery, dating from the XVIIIth dynasty (16th century B.C.)

EEC syndrome. A syndrome of ectrodactylia, ectodermal dysplasia, and cleft lip and palate.

EEG Abbreviation for *electroencephalography, electroencephalogram,* or *electroencephalograph.*

E electroretinogram. The type of electroretinogram in which excitatory phenomena are predominant, associated with activity of the rods. Contr. *I electroretinogram.*

EFE Abbreviation for *endocardial fibroelastosis.*

ef·face·ment (e·face'munt) *n.* Loss of form or features; especially, the gradual flattening and obliteration of the uterine cervix during labor.

ef·fec·tive half-life. HALF-LIFE (3).

ef·fec·tor (e·feck'tur) *n.* A motor or secretory nerve ending in an organ, gland, or muscle. Contr. *receptor.*

effector nerve. EFFERENT NERVE.

effector organ. EFFECTOR.

ef·fer·ent (ef'ur·unt) *adj.* [L. *efferens,* from *ex-,* away, + *ferre,* to carry]. Carrying or conducting away. Contr. *afferent.*

efferent duct. A duct that drains the secretion from an exocrine gland.

efferent ductules of the testis. The 8 to 15 coiled ducts that connect the rete testis with the duct of the epididymis and form the head of the epididymis; derived from paragenital mesonephric tubules. NA *ductuli efferentes testis.*

efferent lymphatic. A vessel conveying lymph away from a lymph node.

efferent motor aphasia. A form of motor aphasia characterized by marked disturbance of the serial organization of speech, resulting in perseveration of sounds or syllables and difficulties in transition from pronunciation of separate sounds to a whole phrase; due to a lesion in Broca's area.

efferent nerve. A nerve conducting impulses from the central nervous system to the periphery, as to a muscle.

efferent neuron. 1. A neuron conducting impulses away from a nerve center. 2. In the peripheral nervous system, a neuron conducting impulses away from the central nervous system.

efferent tract. DESCENDING TRACT.

ef·fer·ves·cence (ef"ur·ves'unce) *n.* [L. *effervescere,* to foam up, from *fervere,* to boil, seethe]. 1. The escape of a gas from a liquid; a bubbling. 2. In infectious diseases, the period following the prodrome; the onset or invasion of the disease.

ef·fer·ves·cent (ef"ur·ves'unt) *adj.* Capable of producing effervescence.

effervescent bath. Immersion of the patient in water in which carbon dioxide bubbles are released.

effervescent salt. A mixture of one or more active chemical salts with an effervescent base. The base usually consists of sodium bicarbonate, citric and tartaric acids. The salts formed are usually in the form of coarse granules or powder.

ef·fleu·rage (ef"loo·rahzh', ef"lur·ahzh') *n.* [F.]. The stroking movement used in massage.

ef·flo·res·cence (ef"lo·res'unce) *n.* [L. *efflorescere,* to bloom, from *flos, floris,* flower]. 1. The spontaneous conversion of a crystalline substance into powder by a loss of its water of crystallization. 2. The eruption of an exanthematous disease.

ef·flu·ent (ef'lew·unt) *n.* [L. *effluens,* flowing out]. 1. An outflow. 2. A fluid discharged from a basin or chamber for the treatment of sewage.

ef·flu·vi·um (e·floo'vee·um) *n.,* pl. **efflu·via** (·vee·uh) [L., outflow, outlet]. 1. An efflux, outflow. 2. An exhalation or emanation, especially when unpleasant or noxious.

ef·fort syndrome. NEUROCIRCULATORY ASTHENIA.

effort thrombosis. PAGET-SCHROETTER SYNDROME.

¹ef·fuse (e·fewce') *adj.* [L. *effusus,* from *effundere,* to pour out]. Of growth produced by bacteria on solid media: not projecting above the surface, in contrast with the raised type of growth.

²ef·fuse (e·fewz') *v.* [*effundere, effusus,* to pour out]. Of a fluid: to pour or spread out, as into a body cavity or tissue. —**ef·fu·sion** (e·few'zhun) *n.*

Efroxine. A trademark for methamphetamine, a central stimulant drug used as the hydrochloride salt.

Efudex. A trademark for fluorouracil cream, used in the treatment of solar keratoses.

ega·grop·i·lus (ee"guh·grop'i·lus) *n.* [Gk. *aigagros,* wild goat, + *pilos,* hair wrought into felt]. TRICHOBEZOAR.

eger·sis (e·jur'sis, e·gur'sis) *n.* [Gk., awakening]. *Obsol.* Extreme wakefulness and alertness. —**eger·tic** (·tick) *adj.*

eges·ta (e·jes'tuh) *n.pl.* [L., from *egerere,* to discharge]. Waste material discharged from the intestines or other excretory organs; excrement.

egg, *n.* OVUM.

egg albumin. The form of albumin found in egg white.

egg membrane. Any one of several membranes surrounding an ovum. The primary egg membrane is one formed by the ovum itself, such as the vitelline membrane; the secondary egg membrane is formed by the follicular cells of the ovary, as the zona pellucida; the tertiary egg membrane is one formed by secretions of the oviduct or uterus, as in sauropsids and monotremes.

egg·shell nail. A thin nail which curves upward at its free border and is translucent and blue-white.

egg-white injury or **syndrome.** A syndrome developed in experimental rats fed on raw white of egg; characterized by dermatitis and emaciation resulting in death; caused by the presence of avidin in the white of egg which renders unavailable the biotin of the diet.

eglan·du·lar (e·glan'dew·lur) *adj.* [*e-* + *glandular*]. Without glands; aglandular.

eglan·du·lose (e·glan'dew·loce) *adj.* EGLANDULAR.

ego (ee'go) *n.* [L., I]. 1. *In psychology,* the self, regarded as a succession of mental states, or as the consciousness of the existence of the self as distinct from other selves. 2. *In psychoanalytic theory,* the part of the personality in conscious contact with reality, representing the sum of such mental mechanisms as perception, memory, and specific defense mechanisms, and serving to mediate between the demands of the instinctual drive (id), the superego, and reality.

ego analysis. 1. *In psychoanalysis,* the intensive study of the ego ideal, ego proper, and the superego, seeking to determine how the ego resolves or attempts to resolve intrapsychic conflicts. 2. The study of ego strengths and weaknesses in order to make therapeutic use of these integrative and defensive forces.

ego·bron·choph·o·ny (ee"go·brong·kof'uh·nee) *n.* A combination of egophony and bronchophony.

ego·cen·tric (ee″go·sen′trick) *adj.* [*ego* + *-centric*]. Self-centered. —**ego·cen·tric·i·ty** (·sen·tris′i·tee), **ego·cen·trism** (·sen′ triz·um) *n.*

ego-dys·to·nia (ee″go·dis·to′nee·uh) *n.* A state of mind in which a person's ideas, impulses, and behavior are not acceptable to his ideals or conception of himself; a subjective value judgment. Contr. *ego-syntonia.* —**ego-dys·ton·ic** (·ton′ick) *adj.*

ego erotism. NARCISSISM.

ego ideal. *In psychoanalysis,* the standard of perfection of the ego; usually the idealized significant figures with whom an individual has identified and whom he seeks consciously or unconsciously to emulate. See also *superego.*

ego-identity, *n.* IDENTITY (2).

ego instinct. *In psychoanalysis,* any drive, as for power, prestige, or wealth, which primarily serves the need for self-preservation or self-love.

ego·ism (ee′go·iz·um, eg′o·) *n.* The attitude or philosophical point of view that self-interest is or should be the basis of all human action. Compare *egotism.* —**ego·ist** (·ist) *n.;* **ego·is·tic** (ee″go·is′tick, eg″o·) *adj.*

ego·ma·nia (ee″go·may′nee·uh) *n.* [*ego* + *-mania*]. Pathological self-esteem.

egoph·o·ny (e·gof′uh·nee) *n.* [Gk. *aix, aigos,* goat, + *-phony*]. A modification of bronchophony, in which the voice has a bleating character, like that of a goat; heard over areas of pleural effusion or lung consolidation.

ego restriction. Conscious restriction on behavior, as opposed to repression of instinctual drives.

ego-strength, *n.* The overall ability of a person to maintain himself and to make adjustments between his id, superego, and reality; the effectiveness with which the ego discharges its functions.

ego-syn·to·nia (ee″go·sin·to′nee·uh) *n.* A state of mind in which a person's impulses, ideas, or behavior are consistent with his consciously held ego ideal or conception of himself; i.e., a condition in which ego and superego are in agreement. Contr. *ego-dystonia.* —**ego-syn·ton·ic** (·ton′ick) *adj.*

ego·tism (ee′guh·tiz·um, eg′uh·) *n.* A high degree of self-centeredness and conceit. Compare *egoism.* —**ego·tist** (·tist) *n.;* **ego·tis·tic** (ee″guh·tis′tick, eg″uh·), **egotis·ti·cal** (·ti·kul) *adj.*

Egyp·tian chlorosis. ANCYLOSTOMIASIS.

Egyptian conjunctivitis or **ophthalmia.** TRACHOMA.

Egyptian splenomegaly. Visceral schistosomiasis caused by *Schistosoma mansoni,* common in Egypt, and characterized by splenic enlargement, hepatic cirrhosis, portal hypertension, and ascites.

Eh·lers-Dan·los syndrome (eʸ′lurss, dahⁿ·loce′) [E. *Ehlers,* German dermatologist, 1863–1927; and H. A. *Danlos*]. An autosomal-dominantly inherited systemic connective tissue disorder manifested by skin fragility and hyperelasticity, easy bruising, atrophic scars and soft pseudotumors, subcutaneous ossifications, joint hyperextensibility with frequent luxation, bleeding tendency, and visceral anomalies. Syn. *cutis hyperelastica, dermatorrhexis.*

Eh·ren·rit·ter's ganglion (eʸ′rᵉn·rit·ur) [J. *Ehrenritter,* Austrian anatomist, d. 1790]. SUPERIOR GANGLION (1).

Ehr·lich-Heinz granules (eʸr′likh) [P. *Ehrlich,* German bacteriologist, 1854–1915; and R. *Heinz*]. HEINZ BODIES.

Ehrlich's 606 [P. *Ehrlich*]. ARSPHENAMINE.

Ehrlich's acid hematoxylin [P. *Ehrlich*]. A solution used for staining sections and in the mass; one of the most frequently used hematoxylin stains.

Ehrlich's aniline crystal violet [P. *Ehrlich*]. A solution of 1.2 g gentian violet, 12 ml 95% alcohol, and 100 ml freshly prepared aniline water.

Ehrlich's diazo reagent [P. *Ehrlich*]. A highly acid solution of sodium nitrite and sulfanilic acid used to detect and measure certain aromatic compounds.

Ehrlich's reagent [P. *Ehrlich*]. DIMETHYLAMINOBENZALDEHYDE.

Ehrlich's side-chain theory [P. *Ehrlich*]. SIDE-CHAIN THEORY.

Ehrlich's test [P. *Ehrlich*]. A test for urobilinogen in which bilirubin-free, undiluted urine is added to a solution of *p*-dimethylaminobenzaldehyde in hydrochloric acid. A deep cherry-red color indicates urobilinogen.

Ehrlich tumor [P. *Ehrlich*]. A poorly differentiated transplantable malignant tumor which was originally seen as a spontaneous breast carcinoma in a stock mouse; it grows in both solid and ascitic form.

ei·co·nom·e·ter (eye″ko·nom′e·tur) *n.* ANISEIKOMETER.

ei·co·sane (eye′ko·sane) *n.* 1. Any saturated hydrocarbon having a composition represented by $C_{20}H_{42}$. 2. The normal saturated hydrocarbon having a chain length of 20 carbon atoms; it occurs in paraffin.

eid-, eido- [Gk. *eidos,* form, shape]. A combining form meaning (a) *image;* (b) *form.*

ei·det·ic (eye·det′ick) *adj.* [Gk. *eidētikos,* specific, from *eidos,* form, kind]. Pertaining to forms or images, especially those voluntarily reproducible.

eidetic image. An image (usually visual) so clear as to seem like an external or perceptual experience, but usually recognized as subjective. May be a fantasy, dream, or memory.

eido-. See *eid-.*

ei·do·gen (eye′do·jin) *n.* [*eido-* + *-gen*]. A chemical substance having the power of modifying the form of an embryonic organ after induction has occurred; a second-grade inductor involved in regional differentiation about the neural axis. Compare *organizer.*

ei·dop·tom·e·try (eye″dop·tom′e·tree) *n.* [*eid-* + *optometry*]. The estimation of the acuity of vision.

eighth (VIIIth) cranial nerve. VESTIBULOCOCHLEAR NERVE.

eighth-month anxiety. STRANGER ANXIETY.

eighth-nerve deafness. Deafness due to a lesion of the cochlear portion of the vestibulocochlear nerve.

eighth-nerve tumor. ACOUSTIC NEURILEMMOMA.

eikon-, eikono-. See *icon-.*

ei·ko·nom·e·ter (eye″ko·nom′e·tur) *n.* ANISEIKOMETER.

Ei·me·ria (eye·meer′ee·uh) *n.* [T. *Eimer,* German zoologist, 1843–1898]. A genus of protozoa of the order Coccidia which lives in the body fluids or tissues of vertebrates and invertebrates and has a life cycle characterized by alternation of generations; causes coccidiosis in cattle, sheep, rabbits, and chickens.

Ein·horn's method [M. *Einhorn,* U.S. physician, 1862–1953]. Chemical analysis of duodenal contents to evaluate protein, fat, and carbohydrate digestion.

ein·stein (ine′stine) *n.* [A. *Einstein,* U.S. theoretical physicist, 1879–1955]. A unit of energy (6.06 × 10^{23} quanta) analogous to the faraday (6.06 × 10^{23} electrons); the amount of radiation absorbed by a system to activate one gram molecule of matter. Abbreviated, E.

ein·stein·ium (ine·stye′nee·um) *n.* [A. *Einstein*]. Es = 254. A radioactive element, atomic No. 99, produced artificially, as by bombardment of plutonium with neutrons.

Eint·ho·ven's law, equation, or **formula** (æynt′ho·vun, ·ho·vuh) [W. *Einthoven,* Dutch physiologist, 1860–1927]. *In electrocardiography,* the potential difference in lead II is equal to the algebraic sum of the potential differences of lead I and lead III.

Einthoven's triangle [W. *Einthoven*]. *In electrocardiography,* an equilateral triangle with apices at the right shoulder, left shoulder, and left hip; these apices are assumed to be equidistant from the center of the triangle, the heart. This hypothetical triangle is the basis of Einthoven's law.

ei·san·the·ma (eye″san·theem′uh, eye·san′thi·muh) *n.* [Gk. *eis,* into, + *anthema*]. ENANTHEM.

Ei·sen·meng·er physiology or **reaction** (eye′zun·meng·ur) [V. *Eisenmenger,* Austrian physician, 1864–1932]. A predominant right-to-left shunt, which may originally have been left-to-right, caused by pulmonary vascular disease and producing cyanosis.

Eisenmenger's complex or **tetralogy** [V. *Eisenmenger*]. A congenital cardiac anomaly, characterized by cyanosis, and consisting of a ventricular septal defect, dextroposition of the aorta, pulmonary artery dilatation, and right ventricular hypertrophy.

Eisenmenger syndrome. 1. EISENMENGER'S COMPLEX. 2. EISENMENGER PHYSIOLOGY.

ei·sen·zuck·er (eye'zun·zuck"ur, Ger. ·tsoo͝k"ur) *n.* [Ger.]. Saccharated iron oxide, a hematinic.

ejac·u·la·tion (e·jack'yoo·lay'shun) *n.* [L. *ejaculare,* to throw out]. 1. A sudden expulsion. 2. Ejection of the semen during orgasm. Compare *emission.* —**ejac·u·late** (e·jack'yoo·late, ee·) *v.;* **ejac·u·la·to·ry** (e·jack'yoo·luh·to"ree) *adj.*

ejaculation reflex. GENITAL REFLEX.

ejac·u·la·tio prae·cox (e·jack"yoo·lay'shee·o pree'kocks). PREMATURE EJACULATION.

ejaculatio re·tar·da·ta (ree·tahr·day'tuh, ·dah'tuh). RETARDED EJACULATION.

ejaculator uri·nae (yoo·rye'nee). The bulbospongiosus muscle in the male.

ejaculatory duct. The terminal part of the ductus deferens after junction with the duct of a seminal vesicle, embedded in the prostate gland and opening into the urethra on the colliculus seminalis. NA *ductus ejaculatorius.* See also Plate 25.

ejaculatory reflex. GENITAL REFLEX.

ejec·ta (e·jeck'tuh) *n.pl.* [L.]. Material cast out; excretions or excrementitious matter; dejecta.

ejec·tion (e·jeck'shun) *n.* [L. *ejectio,* from *e-,* out, + *jacere,* to throw, cast]. 1. The act of casting out, as of secretions, excretions, or excrementitious matter. 2. That which is cast out. —**eject** (e·jekt') *v.*

ejection click. A single early systolic extra sound arising from an abnormal great vessel or aortic or pulmonary valve.

ejection phase. The phase of ventricular systole during which blood is pumped out of the heart.

ejec·tor (e·jeck'tur, ·ee) *n.* One who, or that which, casts out or expels.

eka- [Skr., one, first, next]. A combining form which, when prefixed to the name of a recognized chemical element, designates provisionally *a predicted but as yet undiscovered element which should adjoin the former in the same group of the periodic system.*

eka·io·dine (ee"kuh·eye'o·deen, ·din, eck"uh·) *n.* The provisional name of the element of atomic No. 85, adjoining iodine in the halogen group of the periodic table. Now called *astatine.*

EKG [Ger. *E*lektro*k*ardio*g*ramm]. An abbreviation for *electrocardiogram.*

ekis·tics (ee·kis'ticks, e·kis') *n.* [Gk. *oikistikos,* pertaining to settlers, from *oikizein,* to settle, from *oikos,* dwelling]. The science of human settlements or habitations.

elab·o·ra·tion (e·lab"uh·ray'shun) *n.* [L. *elaboratio,* from *elaborare,* to produce, elaborate, from *e-,* out, + *laborare,* to work]. 1. *In physiology,* any anabolic process, such as the production or synthesis of complex substances from simpler precursors or the formation of secretory products in gland cells. 2. *In psychiatry,* an unconscious psychologic process of enlargement and embellishment of detail, especially of a symbol or representation in a dream; this process is also seen in certain psychoses.

el·a·cin (el'uh·sin) *n.* The product of degeneration of elastin.

elaeo-. See *elaio-.*

elaeomyenchysis. ELEOMYENCHYSIS.

elae·o·pho·ro·sis (ee"lee·o·fo·ro'sis) *n.* Infection with the filaria *Elaeophora schneideri.* See also *sorehead* (2).

elaeoptene. ELEOPTENE.

ela·ic acid (e·lay'ick). OLEIC ACID.

el·a·id·ic acid (el"ay·id'ick). *trans*-9-Octadecenoic acid, $CH_3(CH_2)_7CH{=}CH(CH_2)_7COOH$; a solid, unsaturated fatty acid, the trans- stereoisomer of oleic acid.

ela·i·din (e·lay'i·din) *n.* Any glyceryl ester of elaidic acid.

elaio-, elaeo-, eleo- [Gk. *elaion,* olive oil]. A combining form meaning *oil.*

elan·trine (e·lan'treen) *n.* 11-[3-(Dimethylamino)propylidene]-5,6-dihydro-5-methylmorphanthridine, $C_{20}H_{24}N_2$, an anticholinergic.

Elap·i·dae (e·lap'i·dee) *n. pl.* [Gk. *elops,* serpent]. A family of venomous snakes possessing short, erect, immovable front fangs; includes cobras, mambas, kraits, coral snakes, the death adder, and the tiger snake. —**el·a·pid** (el'uh·pid) *adj. & n.*

Elase. A trademark for a mixture of fibrinolysin, obtained from cattle, and deoxyribonuclease from beef pancreas, used topically to lyse fibrin and liquefy pus, facilitating removal of necrotic material.

elast-, elasto-. A combining form meaning *elastic, elasticity.*

elas·tase (e·las'tace, ·taze) *n.* An enzyme that acts on elastin to render it soluble; has been isolated in crystalline form from pancreas.

elas·tic, *adj.* [Gk. *elastos,* ductile, beaten, from *elaunein,* to drive]. Capable of returning to the original form after being stretched or compressed. —**elas·tic·i·ty** (e·las"tis'i·tee) *n.*

elas·ti·ca (e·las'ti·kuh) *n.* [short for *tunica elastica*]. The tunica intima of a blood vessel.

elastic bandage. A bandage of rubber or woven elastic material; used to exert continuous pressure on swollen extremities or joints, fractured ribs, the chest, or varicose veins.

elastic bougie. A bougie made of rubber or other elastic material; used to negotiate angulated or tortuous channels.

elastic cartilage. Cartilage in which a feltwork of elastic fibers pervades the matrix.

elastic cone. CRICOTHYROID LIGAMENT.

elastic fibers. The nonfibrillar, branching, highly elastic fibers of fibroelastic connective tissue, which also form the fenestrated membranes of large arteries. Syn. *yellow fibers.*

elastic ligature. A ligature of live rubber, used for strangulation of tissue and the gradual cutting through of certain areas by constant pressure.

elastic membrane. A thin layer (or layers) of fibers or sheets of elastin, as in the walls of arteries.

elastic membrane of the larynx. The quadrangular membrane and the cricothyroid ligament. NA *membrana fibroelastica laryngis.*

elastic tension. Stretching by means of an elastic material.

elastic tissue. Connective tissue which is composed predominantly of yellow elastic fibers.

elastic traction. Traction exerted by means of rubber bands, usually employed in phalangeal fractures treated with some form of wire frame or plaster splint, or in connection with certain dental splints.

elas·tin (e·las'tin) *n.* The protein base of yellow elastic tissue.

elasto-. See *elast-.*

elas·to·fi·bro·ma (e·las"to·figh·bro'muh) *n.* [*elasto-* + *fibroma*]. A benign soft-tissue tumor, observed in elderly patients in the subscapular area, characterized by large bands of poorly cellular elastic and connective tissue, separated by fat lobules.

elastofibroma dor·si (dor'sigh). ELASTOFIBROMA.

elas·to·ma (e·las·to'muh) *n.,* pl. **elastomas, elastoma·ta** (·tuh) [*elast-* + *-oma*]. A nevoid condition in which there is a localized thickening of the dermis due to increased elastin.

elas·to·mer (e·las'to·mur) *n.* Any substance having the properties of natural or synthetic rubber. —**elas·to·mer·ic** (e·las"to·merr'ick) *adj.*

elas·tom·e·ter (e·las"tom'e·tur) *n.* [*elasto-* + *-meter*]. An instrument which measures the indentation of skin under graded pressure and its return to normal on removal of weights.

elas·tose (e·las′toce) *n.* A proteose obtained from elastin.

elas·to·sis (e·las″to′sis) *n.* [*elast-* + *-osis*]. 1. Retrogressive changes in elastic tissue. 2. Retrogressive changes in cutaneous connective tissue resulting in excessive amounts of material giving the usual staining reactions for elastin.

elastosis se·ni·lis (se·nigh′lis). Degeneration of the elastic connective tissue of the skin in old age.

elat·er·in (e·lat′ur·in) *n.* A neutral principle from juice of the fruit of *Ecballium elaterium;* a powerful hydragogue cathartic.

el·a·te·ri·um (el″uh·teer′ee·um) *n.* [L. from Gk. *elatērion*, from *elatērios*, purgative, driving away]. The dried sediment from the juice of the squirting cucumber, *Ecballium elaterium;* a powerful hydragogue cathartic.

Elavil. Trademark for amitriptyline, an antidepressant and mild tranquilizing drug used as the hydrochloride salt.

el·bow, *n.* [OE. *elnboga*, from *eln*, forearm, ←Gmc. *alinō* (rel. to Gk. *ōlenē* and L. *ulna*)]. The junction of the arm and forearm; the bend of the arm. NA *cubitus.* See also Table of Synovial Joints and Ligaments in the Appendix.

elbow catheter. A catheter of metal or stiff, rubberized material with one or two 45° bends at or near the proximal end.

elbow lameness. Lameness in a horse, due to disease of the elbow joint.

elbow reflex. TRICEPS REFLEX.

el·der, *n.* SAMBUCUS.

Eldopaque. A trademark for hydroquinone used as a skin depigmenting agent.

el·drin (el′drin) *n.* RUTIN.

el·e·cam·pane (el″e·kam·pane′, ·kam′pane) *n.* INULA.

elec·tive mutism. A neurotic symptom complex characterized by a refusal to speak, except occasionally to intimate friends and relatives, which has no neurologic basis and is often precipitated by an emotional crisis.

elective operation. An operation which is not urgent or mandatory, and which may be scheduled well in advance at a time of convenience.

Elec·tra complex [*Electra*, who in Greek mythology urged her brother to kill their mother]. The female analogue of the Oedipus complex.

elec·tric, *adj.* [Gk. *ēlektr*on, amber, + *-ic*]. 1. Of, pertaining to, or caused by electricity. 2. Produced by or as if by electricity.

elec·tri·cal, *adj.* ELECTRIC.

electrical al·ter·nans (awl′tur·nanz). ELECTRICAL ALTERNATION.

electrical alternation. An electrocardiographic pattern characterized by alternating amplitude or configuration of the QRS complex and/or the T wave, indicative of severe myocardial disease or abnormality of the innervation of the heart.

electrical axis. The single resultant vector of the electric activity of all myofibrils of the heart at any particular moment during the electric cycle of cardiac activity. Syn. *QRS axis.*

electrical chorea. 1. BERGERON'S CHOREA. 2. DUBINI'S CHOREA.

electrical systole. The Q-T interval of the electrocardiogram.

electric anesthesia. Transient anesthesia caused by the passage of an electric current through a part.

electric breeze. STATIC BREEZE.

electric burn. A burn due to electric current.

electric cataract. A form of cataract, usually bilateral and developing rapidly peripherally and progressing centrally in the posterior and anterior cortex of the lens; seen in persons shocked by high-voltage current or struck by lightning.

electric-light blindness. A condition similar to snow blindness, caused by exposure of the eyes to intense and prolonged electric illumination.

electric light treatment. The therapeutic application of electric light by means of cabinets in which the patient sits with the light directed upon the affected part. Its therapeutic effect depends on heat.

electric ophthalmia. Actinic keratoconjunctivitis following undue exposure to such bright lights as the electric arc used in welding and the arc lights used in motion-picture studios.

electric shock. The sudden violent effect of the passage of an electric current through the body.

electric shock therapy or **treatment.** ELECTROSHOCK THERAPY.

electric skin response. GALVANIC SKIN RESPONSE.

electric thermometer. A clinical thermometer utilizing measurement of electrical resistance or the voltage of a thermocouple with a calibrated indicating or recording meter to determine temperature.

electric unit. A unit for measuring the strength of an electric current. Three different systems of electric units are used: the electromagnetic, the electrostatic, and the ordinary or practical units. The commonly used practical units are the ampere or unit of current, the volt or unit of electromotive force, the ohm or unit of resistance, the coulomb or unit of quantity, the farad or unit of capacitance, and the watt or unit of power.

elec·tri·fy, *v.* To charge or equip with electricity.

elec·tri·za·tion (e·leck″tri·zay′shun) *n.* The application of electricity to the body.

electro-. A combining form meaning (a) *electric, electricity;* (b) *electron.*

elec·tro·af·fin·ity (e·leck″tro·uh·fin′i·tee) *n.* [*electro-* + *affinity*]. The force by which ions hold their electric charges. Symbol, E_0.

elec·tro·an·es·the·sia, elec·tro·an·aes·the·sia (e·leck″tro·an″es·theezh′uh, ·theez′ee·uh) *n.* Local anesthesia induced by an electric current; electric anesthesia.

elec·tro·bi·ol·o·gy (e·leck″tro·bye·ol′uh·jee) *n.* [*electro-* + *biology*]. The science of electric phenomena in the living organism, either those produced by the organism itself or by outside sources. —**electro·bio·log·ic** (·bye·uh·loj′ick) *adj.*

elec·tro·bi·os·co·py (e·leck″tro·bye·os′kuh·pee) *n.* [*electro-* + *bio-* + *-scopy*]. The use of a galvanic current to determine whether or not a tissue is living.

elec·tro·cap·il·lar·i·ty (e·leck″tro·kap″i·lăr′i·tee) *n.* The effect of an electric current upon the interface between two liquids in a capillary; due to changes in the surface tension. —**electro·cap·il·lary** (·kap′i·lăr″ee) *adj.*

electrocapillary action. The electric phenomena resulting from the chemical reaction between dissimilar fluids connected by a capillary medium.

elec·tro·car·dio·gram (e·leck″tro·kahr′dee·o·gram) *n.* [*electro-* + *cardiogram*]. A graphic record, made by an electrocardiograph, of the electrical forces that produce the contraction of the heart. A typical normal record shows P, Q, R, S, T, and U waves. Abbreviated, ECG, EKG.

elec·tro·car·dio·graph (e·leck″tro·kahr′de·o·graf) *n.* [*electro-* + *cardiograph*]. An instrument that receives electrical impulses as they vary during the cardiac cycle and transforms them into a graphic record; an instrument for recording electrocardiograms. Abbreviated, ECG, EKG. —**electro·car·dio·graph·ic** (·kahr″dee·o·graf′ick) *adj.*

electrocardiographic-auscultatory syndrome. BARLOW'S SYNDROME.

electrocardiographic interval. 1. The intervals (P-R, Q-T, R-R, T-Q) of an electrocardiogram. 2. The duration of the waves (P, QRS, T, U) of an electrocardiogram.

electrocardiographic waves. The various phases of the spread of depolarization and repolarization of the heart, recorded as deflections on the electrocardiogram; indicated by the symbols P, Q, R, S, T, U.

elec·tro·car·di·og·ra·phy (e·leck″tro·kahr″dee·og′ruh·fee) *n.* [*electro-* + *cardiography*]. The specialty or science of recording and interpreting the electrical activity of the heart, i.e., electrocardiograms. Abbreviated, ECG, EKG.

elec·tro·car·dio·pho·nog·ra·phy (e·leck″tro·kahr″dee·o·fo·nog′ruh·fee) *n.* Phonocardiography and electrocardiography performed simultaneously.

elec·tro·car·dio·scope (e·leck″tro·kahr′dee·o·skope) *n.* [*electro-* + *cardioscope*]. CARDIOSCOPE.

elec·tro·ca·tal·y·sis (e·leck″tro·ka·tal′i·sis) *n.*, pl. **electrocatalyses** (·seez). Catalysis or chemical changes produced by the action of electricity.

elec·tro·cau·tery (e·leck″tro·kaw′tur·ee) *n.* [*electro-* + *cautery*]. Cauterization by means of a wire loop or needle heated by a direct galvanic current. Syn. *galvanocautery.*

elec·tro·chem·is·try (e·leck″tro·kem′is·tree) *n.* The science treating of chemical changes produced by electricity and of interconversion of electrical and chemical energy.

elec·tro·chro·ma·tog·ra·phy (e·leck″tro·kro″muh·tog′ruh·fee) *n.* [*electro-* + *chromatography*]. The resolution of mixtures by differential electrical migration from a narrow zone; it applies to such migration of all solutes and suspensoids, ions, and colloids.

elec·tro·co·ag·u·la·tion (e·leck″tro·ko·ag″yoo·lay′shun) *n.* [*electro-* + *coagulation*]. The destruction or hardening of tissues by coagulation induced by the passage of high-frequency currents; surgical diathermy.

elec·tro·co·ma (e·leck″tro·ko′muh) *n.* [*electro-* + *coma*]. The coma induced by electroshock therapy.

elec·tro·con·duc·tiv·i·ty (e·leck″tro·kon″duck·tiv′i·tee) *n.* [*electro-* + *conductivity*]. Facility for transmitting electricity.

elec·tro·con·trac·til·i·ty (e·leck″tro·kon″track·til′i·tee) *n.* [*electro-* + *contractility*]. The capacity of muscular tissue for contraction in response to electric stimulation.

elec·tro·con·vul·sive (e·leck″tro·kun·vul′siv) *adj.* Pertaining to a convulsive response to electrical stimulation.

electroconvulsive therapy or **treatment.** ELECTROSHOCK THERAPY. Abbreviated, ECT.

elec·tro·cor·ti·cal (e·leck″tro·kor′ti·kul) *adj.* [*electro-* + *cortical*]. Pertaining to the electrical activity of the cerebral cortex.

electrocortical potential. Potential electrical differences observed from leads applied to the surface of the cerebral cortex.

elec·tro·cor·ti·cog·ra·phy (e·leck″tro·kor·ti·kog′ruh·fee) *n.* [*electro-* + *cortico-* + *-graphy*]. The process of recording the electric activity of the brain by electrodes placed directly on the cerebral cortex, providing a much higher voltage, greater accuracy, and more exact localization than electroencephalography. —**electro·cor·ti·co·gram** (·kor′ti·ko·gram) *n.*

elec·tro·cor·tin (e·leck″tro·kor′tin) *n.* [*electro-* + *cortin*]. ALDOSTERONE.

elec·tro·cu·tion (e·leck″truh·kew′shun) *n.* [*electro-* + *execution*]. 1. Execution by electricity. 2. Loosely, any electric shock causing death. —**elec·tro·cute** (e·leck′truh·kewt) *v.*

elec·trode (e·leck′trode) *n.* [*electr-* + Gk. *hodos,* way]. 1. A surface of contact between a metallic and a nonmetallic conductor. 2. One of the terminals of metal, salts, or electrolytes through which electricity is applied to, or taken from, the body or an electric device or instrument.

electrode jelly. A jelly for improving the contact between skin and electrode in electrocardiography and electroencephalography.

elec·tro·dep·o·si·tion (e·leck″tro·dep″uh·zish′un) *n.* The process of depositing something, such as a metal, by electrical action.

elec·tro·der·mal response (e·leck″tro·dur′mul). GALVANIC SKIN RESPONSE.

elec·tro·der·ma·tome (e·leck″tro·dur′muh·tome) *n.* [*electro-* + *dermatome*]. An electrically driven cutting instrument used for obtaining split skin grafts.

elec·tro·des·ic·ca·tion (e·leck″tro·des″i·kay′shun) *n.* [*electro-* + *desiccation*]. The diathermic destruction of small growths such as of the urinary bladder, skin, or cervix by means of a single terminal electrode with a small sparking distance.

elec·tro·di·ag·no·sis (e·leck″tro·dye″ug·no′sis) *n.* Diagnosis of disease or aspects of a disease process by recording the spontaneous tissue or organ electrical activity, or by the response to stimulation of electrically excitable tissue.

elec·tro·di·al·y·sis (e·leck″tro·dye·al′i·sis) *n.* A method for rapidly removing electrolytes from colloids by dialysis of the colloidal sol while an electric current is being passed through it.

elec·tro·di·a·phane (e·leck″tro·dye′uh·fane) *n.* [*electro-* + *diaphane*]. An apparatus for illumination of body cavities; DIAPHANOSCOPE. —**electro·di·aph·a·ny** (·dye·af′uh·nee) *n.*

elec·tro·dy·nam·ics (e·leck″tro·dye·nam′icks) *n.* [*electro-* + *dynamics*]. The science of energy transformations as related to electric currents and their magnetic fields.

elec·tro·dy·na·mom·e·ter (e·leck″tro·dye″nuh·mom′e·tur) *n.* [*electro-* + *dynamo-* + *-meter*]. An instrument for measuring the magnitude of electric currents.

elec·tro·en·ceph·a·lo·gram (e·leck″tro·en·sef′uh·lo·gram) *n.* [*electro-* + *encephalo-* + *-gram*]. A graphic record of the minute changes in electric potential associated with the activity of the cerebral cortex, as detected by electrodes applied to the surface of the scalp. Abbreviated, EEG.

elec·tro·en·ceph·a·lo·graph (e·leck″tro·en·sef′ul·lo·graf) *n.* [*electro-* + *encephalo-* + *-graph*]. An instrument for recording the electric activity of the brain. Abbreviated, EEG. —**electro·en·ceph·a·lo·graph·ic** (·en·sef″uh·lo·graf′ick) *adj.*

electroencephalographic lead. A pair of terminals which measures the potential differences resulting from cerebral activity between two points on the skull.

elec·tro·en·ceph·a·log·ra·phy (e·leck″tro·en·sef″uh·log′ruh·fee) *n.* [*electro-* + *encephalo-* + *-graphy*]. A method of recording graphically the electric activity of the brain, particularly the cerebral cortex, by means of electrodes attached to the scalp; used in the diagnosis of epilepsy, trauma, tumors, and degenerations of the brain, as well as in the study of the effect of drugs on the central nervous system and certain psychological and physiological phenomena. Abbreviated, EEG. Compare *electrocorticography.* See also *brain wave.*

elec·tro·end·os·mo·sis (e·leck″tro·en″doz·mo′sis) *n.* [*electro-* + *endosmosis*]. ELECTROOSMOSIS.

elec·tro·fit (e·leck″tro·fit′) *n.* [*electro-* + *fit*]. The convulsion induced by electroshock therapy.

elec·tro·fo·cus·ing (e·leck″tro·fo′kus·ing). ISOELECTRIC FOCUSING.

elec·tro·form (e·leck′tro·form) *v.* To form by the electrodeposition of metal in finished or semifinished form, as sheets or tubes or electrotypes.

elec·tro·gas·tro·graph (e·leck″tro·gas′tro·graf) *n.* [*electro-* + *gastro-* + *-graph*]. A graphic recording of change in electrical potential of the stomach. —**electrogastro·gram,** *n.*

elec·tro·gen·e·sis (e·leck″tro·jen′e·sis) *n.* [*electro-* + *-genesis*]. Production of electricity.

elec·tro·gram (e·leck′tro·gram) *n.* [*electro-* + *-gram*]. The graphic representation of electric events in living tissues; most commonly, an electrocardiogram or electroencephalogram. See also *electromyogram, electroretinogram.* —**elec·trog·ra·phy** (e·leck″trog′ruh·fee) *n.*

elec·tro·he·mos·ta·sis, elec·tro·hae·mos·ta·sis (e·leck″tro·hee·mos′tuh·sis) *n.* [*electro-* + *hemostasis*]. The arrest of hemorrhage by means of a high-frequency current, as in the reduction or prevention of bleeding in operations through use of an electrosurgical knife.

elec·tro·hy·drau·lic lithotrite (e·leck″tro·high·draw′lick). A lithotrite whose action is powered by an electrical pulse generator.

elec·tro·hys·ter·og·ra·phy (e·leck″tro·his″tur·og′ruh·fee) *n.* [*electro-* + *hysterography*]. The recording of electric action potentials of the uterus.

elec·tro·im·mu·no·dif·fu·sion (e·leck″tro·im″yoo·no·di·few′zhun) *n.* Immunodiffusion in which the antigens are separated according to their migration in an electric field. See also *immunoelectrophoresis, rocket electrophoresis.*

elec·tro·ki·net·ic potential. The potential developed across any interface separating two phases as a result of accumulation of electrons in one phase and loss of electrons in the other. Syn. *zeta potential.* See also *bioelectric potential.*

elec·tro·ky·mo·graph (e·leck″tro·kigh′mo·graf) *n.* [*electro-* + *kymograph*]. An apparatus that combines a photoelectric recording system with a fluoroscope so as to make possible the continuous recording of the movements of a shadow within the fluoroscopic field or of changes in density in that shadow; formerly often employed in studying the heart.

elec·tro·ky·mog·ra·phy (e·leck″tro·kigh·mog′ruh·fee) *n.* [*electro-* + *kymography*]. The technique of recording the motions of an organ by means of an electrokymograph.

elec·tro·li·thot·ri·ty (e·leck″tro·lith·ot′ri·tee) *n.* [*electro-* + *lithotrity*]. Disintegration of a vesical calculus by means of electricity.

elec·trol·y·sis (e·leck″trol′i·sis) *n.* [*electro-* + *-lysis*]. The decomposition of a chemical compound by a direct electric current. —**elec·tro·lyze** (e·leck′tro·lize) *v.*

elec·tro·lyte (e·leck′tro·lite) *n.* [*electro-* + *-lyte*]. A substance which, in solution, is dissociated into ions and is capable of conducting an electric current, as the circulating ions of plasma and other body fluids. —**electro·lyt·ic** (e·leck″tro·lit′ick) *adj.*

elec·tro·ly·zer (e·leck′tro·lye″zur) *n.* An instrument for removing or relieving urethral strictures by electrolysis.

elec·tro·mag·net (e·leck″tro·mag′nit) *n.* [*electro-* + *magnet*]. A core of soft iron surrounded by a coil of wire. A current passing through the wire will make the iron temporarily magnetic.

elec·tro·mag·net·ic (e·leck″tro·mag·net′ick) *adj.* Of or pertaining to electromagnetism.

electromagnetic balance. An apparatus for measuring electromagnetic forces by balancing them against gravity.

electromagnetic flowmeter. A flowmeter in which changes in the flow of blood are measured through impedance to electromagnetic lines of force introduced across a stream. It has the great advantage that an intact blood vessel can be used.

electromagnetic radiation. Radiation that is propagated through space or matter in the form of electromagnetic waves.

elec·tro·mag·net·ics (e·leck″tro·mag·net′icks) *n.* ELECTROMAGNETISM (2).

electromagnetic spectrum. The entire continuous range of electromagnetic waves from gamma rays of shortest wavelength to radio waves of longest wavelength.

electromagnetic units. A system of electrical units, based on the centimeter, gram, and second, in which a unit magnetic pole is by definition such that two units of the same sign placed one centimeter apart in free space will repel each other with a force of one dyne. Units in the system are usually characterized by the prefix ab-, as abampere, abvolt.

electromagnetic waves. Any of a continuous spectrum of waves propagated by simultaneous oscillation of electric and magnetic fields perpendicularly to each other and both perpendicularly to the direction of propagation of the waves. Included in the spectrum, in order of increasing frequency (or decreasing wavelength) are the following types of waves: radio, microwave, infrared, visible light, ultraviolet, x-rays, and gamma rays.

elec·tro·mag·net·ism (e·leck″tro·mag′ne·tiz·um) *n.* 1. Magnetism produced by a current of electricity. 2. The science dealing with the relations between electricity and magnetism.

elec·tro·mas·sage (e·leck″tro·muh·sahzh′) *n.* [*electro-* + *massage*]. The transmission of an alternating electric current through body tissues accompanied by manual kneading.

elec·trom·e·ter (e·leck″trom′e·tur) *n.* [*electro-* + *-meter*]. A device for measuring differences in electric potential. —**elec·tro·met·ric** (e·leck″tro·met′rick) *adj.*

electrometric titration. A method of titration in which the end point is detected by measuring the change in potential across suitable electrodes or the change of electric conductance or other electric property during titration.

elec·tro·mo·tive (e·leck″tro·mo′tiv) *n.* [*electro-* + L. *motus,* motion, from *movere,* to move]. Pertaining to or producing electric action.

electromotive force. The force that tends to alter the motion of electricity, measured in volts. Abbreviated, E, emf, EMF.

elec·tro·mus·cu·lar sensibility (e·leck″tro·mus′kew·lur). Responsiveness of muscles to electric stimulus.

elec·tro·myo·gram (e·leck″tro·migh′o·gram) *n.* [*electro-* + *myo-* + *-gram*]. 1. A graphic record of the electric activity of a muscle either spontaneous or in response to artificial electric stimulation. 2. A record of eye movements during reading, obtained by measuring the potential difference between an electrode placed at the center of the forehead and one placed at the temple. Abbreviated, EMG.

elec·tro·my·og·ra·phy (e·leck″tro·migh·og′ruh·fee) *n.* [*electro-* + *myo-* + *-graphy*]. Production and study of the electromyogram. Abbreviated, EMG. —**elec·tro·myo·graph·ic** (e·leck″tro·migh″o·graf′ick) *adj.*

elec·tron (e·leck′tron) *n.* [*electr-* + *-on*]. Commonly the smallest particle of negative electricity, sometimes called negatron. The mass of an electron at rest is 9.109×10^{-28} gram or 1/1845 that of a hydrogen atom. Its electric charge is 4.77×10^{-10} electrostatic unit. Symbol, e. Contr. *proton, positron.*

elec·tro·nar·co·sis (e·leck″tro·nahr·ko′sis) *n.* Narcosis produced by the application of electric currents to the body for therapeutic purposes. See also *electric anesthesia.*

elec·tro·neg·a·tive (e·leck″tro·neg′uh·tiv) *adj.* Pertaining to or charged with negative electricity; tending to attract electrons.

elec·tro·neg·a·tiv·i·ty (e·leck″tro·neg″uh·tiv′i·tee) *n.* The power of an atom in a molecule to attract electrons to itself.

elec·tron·ic (e·leck″tron′ick) *adj.* 1. Of or pertaining to electrons. 2. Pertaining to the emission and transmission of electrons in a vacuum and in gases and semiconductors.

electronic spread. PASSIVE SPREAD.

electron lens. An electric field used to focus a stream of electrons on a target.

electron micrograph. A photograph or other reproduction of the image produced by an electron microscope.

electron microscope. A device for directing streams of electrons by means of electric and magnetic fields in a manner similar to the direction of visible light rays by means of glass lenses in an ordinary microscope. Since electrons carry waves of much smaller wavelengths than light waves, correspondingly greater magnifications are obtainable. The electron microscope will resolve detail 1,000 to 10,000 times finer than the optical microscope. Images can be studied on a fluorescent screen or recorded photographically. See also *scanning electron microscope.*

electron optics. The science of the emission and propagation of electrons and of the factors controlling and modifying their flow, especially when applied to electron microscopy.

electron transport. A process of biological oxidation in which electrons are transferred from a reduced substrate through a series of compounds to oxygen, the energy of the process being conserved by the formation of high-energy bonds in the form of adenosine triphosphate.

electron volt. A unit of energy equivalent to the kinetic energy which an electron acquires in falling through a potential of one volt, equivalent to 1.60×10^{-12} erg. Abbreviated, eV.

elec·tro·nys·tag·mog·ra·phy (e·leck″tro·nis·tag·mog′ruh·fee) *n.* Electroencephalographic recording of eye movements used in qualitative and quantitative assessment of nystagmus.

elec·tro·oc·u·lo·gram (e·leck″tro·ock′yoo·lo·gram) *n.* [*electro-* + *oculo-* + *-gram*]. A record taken of the changes in electric potential with eye movements between two fixed points. Abbreviated, EOG.

elec·tro·os·mo·sis (e·leck″tro·oz·mo′sis) *n.* [*electro-* + *osmosis*]. The movement of a conducting liquid through a permeable membrane under the influence of a potential gradient; it is thought to be caused by the opposite electrification of the membrane and the liquid.

elec·tro·ox·i·da·tion (e·leck″tro·ock·si·day′shun) *n.* Oxidation occurring at the anode of an electrolytic cell. —**electrooxi·diz·able** (·dye′zuh·bul) *adj.*

elec·tro·pa·thol·o·gy (e·leck″tro·pa·thol′uh·jee) *n.* [*electro-* + *pathology*]. The study of morbid conditions produced by the passage of electric current through living tissues.

elec·tro·phil·ic (e·leck″tro·fil′ick) *adj.* [*electro-* + *-philic*]. Having an affinity for electrons whereby a bond is formed when an ion or molecule (the electrophilic agent) accepts a pair of electrons from a nucleophilic ion or molecule.

elec·tro·pho·bia (e·leck″tro·fo′bee·uh) *n.* [*electro-* + *phobia*]. A morbid fear of electricity or anything electrical.

elec·tro·pho·re·sis (e·leck″tro·fo·ree′sis) *n.* [*electro-* + *-phoresis*]. The migration of charged particles through the medium in which they are dispersed, when placed under the influence of an applied electric potential. Syn. *cataphoresis.* See also *microscopic electrophoresis, moving-boundary electrophoresis.* —**elec·tro·pho·ret·ic** (e·leck″tro·fo·ret′ick) *adj.*

elec·troph·o·rus (e·leck″trof′ur·us) *n.*, pl. **electropho·ri** (·eye) [*electro-* + Gk. *phoros,* bearing]. An instrument used to produce small quantities of static electricity by induction.

elec·tro·pho·to·ther·a·py (e·leck″tro·fo″to·therr′uh·pee) *n.* [*electro-* + *photo-* + *therapy*]. Treatment of disease by means of electric light.

elec·tro·phys·i·ol·o·gy (e·leck″tro·fiz′ee·ol′uh·jee) *n.* 1. The branch of physiology dealing with the relations of the body to electricity. 2. The physiologic production of electric phenomena in the normal human body.

elec·tro·pos·i·tive (e·leck″tro·poz′i·tiv) *adj.* Pertaining to or charged with positive electricity; tending to release electrons.

elec·tro·punc·ture (e·leck″tro·punk′chur) *n.* [*electro-* + *puncture*]. *In surgery,* the use of needles as electrodes.

elec·tro·py·rex·ia (e·leck″tro·pye·reck′see·uh) *n.* [*electro-* + *pyrexia*]. The production of high body temperatures by means of an electric current; fever therapy.

elec·tro·re·duc·tion (e·leck″tro·re·duck′shun) *n.* Reduction occurring at the cathode of an electrolytic cell. —**electrore·duc·ible** (·dew′si·bul) *adj.*

elec·tro·re·sec·tion (e·leck″tro·ree·seck′shun) *n.* [*electro-* + *resection*]. Excision by means of electrocautery.

elec·tro·ret·i·no·gram (e·leck″tro·ret′i·no·gram) *n.* [*electro-* + *retino-* + *-gram*]. A record of the electric variations of the retina upon stimulation by lights; made by placing one electrode over the cornea, the other over some indifferent region.

elec·tro·scis·sion (e·leck″tro·sizh′un, ·sish′un) *n.* [*electro-* + *scission*]. Cutting of tissues by an electrocautery knife.

elec·tro·scope (e·leck′truh·skope) *n.* [*electro-* + *-scope*]. An instrument for detecting the presence of static electricity and its relative amount, and for determining whether it is positive or negative.

elec·tro·sec·tion (e·leck″tro·seck′shun) *n.* [*electro-* + *section*]. Tissue division by a knifelike electrode operated by a high-frequency machine.

elec·tro·shock (e·leck″tro·shock′) *n.* Shock produced by electricity.

electroshock therapy or **treatment.** The use of electric current to produce unconsciousness or convulsions in the treatment of psychotic, particularly depressive, disorders. Abbreviated, EST.

elec·tros·mo·sis (e·leck″troz·mo′sis) *n.* ELECTROOSMOSIS.

elec·tro·sol (e·leck′tro·sol) *n.* [*electro-* + *sol*]. A colloidal dispersion of a metal, electrically obtained.

elec·tro·some (e·leck′tro·sohm) *n.* A chondriosome in the cytoplasm which is responsible for chemical action.

electrosome theory. Regaud's theory that the mitochondria are the centers of specific chemical action in cells, capable of synthesizing certain substances from materials selected from the cytoplasm.

elec·tro·stat·ic (e·leck″tro·stat′ick) *adj.* Of or pertaining to static electricity.

electrostatic accelerator. Any device making use of electrostatic forces to establish a large potential difference that can be used to accelerate positive or negative charges; condenser-rectifier circuits or a Van de Graaff generator can accomplish this.

electrostatic attraction. The tendency of bodies to draw together when carrying opposite charges of electricity.

electrostatic generator. An apparatus for producing up to several million volts of electrostatic energy by successive accumulation of small static charges on an insulated high-voltage metal collector.

elec·tro·stat·ics (e·leck″tro·stat′icks) *n.* The science of static electricity.

electrostatic unit of charge. The quantity of electrical charge that repels an equal charge at a point in a vacuum at a distance of one centimeter with a force of one dyne.

electrostatic units. A system of electrical units, based on the centimeter, gram, and second, in which a unit electric charge is by definition such that two units of the same sign placed one centimeter apart in vacuo will repel each other with a force of one dyne. Units in the system are usually characterized by the prefix stat-, as statampere, statvolt.

electrostatic voltmeter. An instrument for measurement of high voltages; built on the principle that like electric charges repel and unlike charges attract each other.

elec·tro·stetho·phone (e·leck″tro·steth′uh·fone) *n.* [*electro-* + *stethophone*]. An electrically amplified stethoscope.

elec·tro·stim·u·la·tion (e·leck″tro·stim·yoo·lay′shun) *n.* Experimental or therapeutic stimulation of a tissue by electrical means.

elec·tro·stric·tion (e·leck″tro·strick′shun) *n.* [*electro-* + *-striction,* narrowing, drawing together, from L. *stringere,* to draw together]. The contraction of a solvent resulting from the development of an electrostatic field by a dissolved electrolyte.

elec·tro·sur·gery (e·leck″tro·sur′jur·ee) *n.* The use of electricity in surgery; surgical diathermy. —**electrosur·gi·cal** (·ji·kul) *adj.*

electrosurgical knife. An instrument, provided with tips of various shapes, which operates on a high-frequency electric current that divides tissues and provides a degree of hemostasis. Used properly, it causes some desiccation but minimal charring.

electrosurgical needle. A needle with high-frequency electric current, capable of coagulating or cutting tissue; an acusector.

elec·tro·syn·the·sis (e·leck″tro·sin′thuh·sis) *n.* [*electro-* + *synthesis*]. Chemical combination caused by electricity.

elec·tro·tax·is (e·leck″tro·tack′sis) *n.* [*electro-* + *taxis*]. The manner of movement of organisms or cells when subjected to an electric current.

elec·tro·thal·a·mo·gram (e·leck"tro·thal'uh·mo·gram) *n.* [*electro-* + *thalamo-* + *-gram*]. A record of the electrical activity of the thalamus, obtained by inserting small electrodes stereotactically.

elec·tro·tha·na·sia (e·leck"tro·thuh·nay'zhuh, ·zee·uh) *n.* [NL., from *electro-* + Gk. *thanatos,* death]. Death due to electricity other than legal electrocution.

elec·tro·ther·a·peu·tics (e·leck"tro·therr·uh·pew'ticks) *n.* ELECTROTHERAPY.

elec·tro·ther·a·py (e·leck"tro·therr'uh·pee) *n.* [*electro-* + *therapy*]. The use of electricity to treat disease.

elec·tro·therm (e·leck'tro·thurm) *n.* [*electro-* + *-therm*]. An apparatus that generates heat electrically for application to the body surface to relieve pain. —**elec·tro·ther·mal** (e·leck"tro·thur'mul), **electrother·mic** (·mick) *adj.;* **elec·tro·ther·my** (e·leck'tro·thur"mee) *n.*

elec·tro·tome (e·leck'tro·tome) *n.* [*electro-* + *-tome*]. A surgical electrocautery device using low current, high voltage, and high frequency, which has a loop for engaging the part to be excised. No macroscopic coagulation of tissues is produced.

elec·tro·ton·ic (e·leck"tro·ton'ick) *adj.* Pertaining to or induced by electrotonus.

electrotonic effect. An altered condition of excitability of a nerve or muscle, produced when in the electrotonic state.

electrotonic potential. 1. The potential led off by electrometers on either side of bipolar electrodes when a nerve is being stimulated by direct current. 2. The potential developed by cells as a result of metabolic activity and circuited through surrounding tissue.

elec·trot·o·nus (e·leck"trot'o·nus, e·leck"tro·to'nus) *n.* [*electro-* + Gk. *tonos,* a stretching]. The transient change of irritability in a nerve or a muscle during the passage of a current of electricity. See also *anelectrotonus, catelectrotonus.*

elec·tro·tro·pism (e·leck"tro·tro'piz·um) *n.* [*electro-* + *-tropism*]. A turning toward or a turning away from a source of electrical energy.

elec·tro·tur·bi·nom·e·ter (e·leck"tro·tur·bi·nom'e·tur) *n.* A small electric turbine placed into the arterial bloodstream for the purpose of measuring blood flow; a flowmeter.

elec·tro·va·go·gram (e·leck"tro·vay'go·gram) *n.* [*electro-* + *vago-* + *-gram*]. A record of the electric changes occurring in the vagus nerve. Syn. *vagogram.*

elec·tro·va·lence (e·leck"tro·vay'lunce) *n.* [*electro-* + *valence*]. The number of electrons that an atom tends to lose or accept by transfer in a chemical reaction.

elec·tro·vi·bra·to·ry massage. Massage performed by means of an electric vibrator.

elec·tro·win (e·leck"tro·win') *v.* To recover, as metals from their ores, by electrodeposition.

elec·tu·ary (e·leck'choo·err"ee) *n.* [L. *electuarium,* from Gk. *ekleigma,* a medicine that melts in the mouth]. CONFECTION.

ele·i·din (e·lee'i·din) *n.* [Gk. *elaioeidēs,* oily, oil-like, + *-in*]. The semifluid, acidophil material in the stratum lucidum of the epidermis.

el·e·ment, *n.* [L. *elementum*]. 1. Any one of the ultimate parts of which anything is composed, as the cellular elements of a tissue. 2. *In chemistry,* any one of the more than 100 ultimate chemical entities of which matter is believed to be composed. Each element is composed wholly of atoms of the same atomic number (having the same charge on their nuclei), although their atomic weights may differ due to differences in nuclear weight. See also *isotope.* For a list of elements see Table of Elements in the Appendix.

el·e·men·tal (el"e·men'tul) *adj.* 1. Of or pertaining to ultimate entities. 2. Not chemically combined; composed of a single element.

el·e·men·ta·ry (el"e·men'tuh·ree) *adj.* 1. Primary or first. 2. Rudimentary; introductory.

elementary body. 1. A cellular inclusion body of a viral disease. 2. BLOOD PLATELET.

elementary cell. EMBRYONIC CELL.

elementary particle. 1. Any of the ultimate components of atoms, such as neutrons, protons, or electrons. 2. A knoblike repeating body, revealed by high-resolution electron microscopy and negative staining techniques, located on the luminal surfaces of mitochondrial cristae.

el·e·mi (el'e·mee) *n.* [Ar. *al-lāmi*]. A resinous exudation frequently derived from *Canarium commune,* as well as from other plants of the Burseraceae. Its action is similar to that of the turpentines, and it has been used in plasters and ointments.

eleo-. See *elaio-.*

el·e·o·ma, el·ae·o·ma (el"ee·o'muh) *n.,* pl. **eleomas, eleoma·ta** (·tuh) [*eleo-* + *-oma*]. A pathologic swelling caused by the injection of an oil into the tissues.

el·e·om·e·ter, el·ae·om·e·ter (el"ee·om'e·tur) *n.* [*eleo-* + *-meter*]. An apparatus for ascertaining the specific gravity of oil.

el·eo·my·en·chy·sis, el·aeo·my·en·chy·sis (el"ee·o·migh·eng'ki·sis, ee"lee·o·) *n.* [*eleo-* + *my-* + Gk. *enchysis,* a pouring in]. *Obsol.* The intramuscular injection of oils in treatment of localized clonic spasm or other disorder.

el·e·op·tene, el·ae·op·tene (el"ee·op'teen) *n.* [*eleo-* + Gk. *ptēnos,* flying]. The permanent liquid portion of volatile oils. Contr. *stearoptene.*

el·eo·ther·a·py (el"ee·o·therr'uh·pee) *n.* [*eleo-* + *therapy*]. OLEOTHERAPY.

el·e·phan·ti·a·sis (el"e·fan·tye'uh·sis) *n.,* pl. **elephantia·ses** (·seez) [Gk., from *elephas, elephantou,* elephant, + *-iasis*]. A chronic enlargement and thickening of the subcutaneous and cutaneous tissues as a result of lymphatic obstruction and lymphatic edema. In the form commonest in the tropics, the recurrent lymphangitis is caused by the filaria *Wuchereria bancrofti.* The legs and scrotum are most commonly affected. —**ele·phan·ti·ac** (·fan'tee·ack) *adj. & n.;* **ele·phan·ti·as·ic** (·fan·tee·az'ick) *adj.*

elephantiasis ar·a·bum (ăr'uh·bum). Elephantiasis, presumably filarial, occurring in the Middle East.

elephantiasis du·ra (dew'ruh). A variety of elephantiasis marked by density and sclerosis of the subcutaneous connective tissues.

elephantiasis fi·lar·i·en·sis (fi·lăr"ee·en'sis). Elephantiasis due to infection with filaria, most commonly *Wuchereria bancrofti.*

elephantiasis ner·vo·rum (nur·vo'rum). PACHYDERMATOCELE.

elephantiasis neu·ro·fi·bro·ma·to·sa (new"ro·figh·bro"muh·to'suh). PACHYDERMATOCELE.

elephantiasis neu·ro·ma·to·sa (new·ro"muh·to'suh). PACHYDERMATOCELE.

elephantiasis nos·tras (nos'tras). Enlargement, especially of the legs, which complicates chronic diseases such as recurrent erysipelas, resulting in lymphatic obstruction.

elephantiasis scir·rho·sa (si·ro'suh, ski·ro'suh). ELEPHANTIASIS DURA.

elephantiasis scle·ro·sa (skle·ro'suh). SCLERODERMA.

el·e·phan·toid (el"e·fan'toid, el'e·fun·toid") *adj.* Pertaining to or resembling elephantiasis.

elephantoid fever. Recurring fever in patients with filariasis, generally attributed to allergy to filarial products, but may represent superimposed streptococcal or fungal infection.

eleu·thera bark (e·lew'thur·uh) [after *Eleuthera* Island, Bahamas]. CASCARILLA.

el·e·va·tor, *n.* An instrument for elevating or lifting a part, or for extracting the roots of teeth.

elev·enth (XIth) cranial nerve. ACCESSORY NERVE.

El·ford membrane. Graded collodion membrane filters employed for the determination of the relative size of different filtrable viruses.

Elft·man-Elft·man method. A histochemical method for the determination of gold using hydrogen peroxide to obtain rose to blue colloidal gold.

elim·i·nant (e·lim′i·nunt) *adj. & n.* 1. Promoting elimination. 2. An agent causing elimination of waste products.

elim·i·na·tion (e·lim″i·nay′shun) *n.* [L. *eliminare,* to put outdoors, from *e-,* out, + *limen,* threshold]. The process of expelling or casting out; especially, the expelling of the waste products of the body. —**elim·i·nate** (e·lim′i·nate) *v.*

elin·gua·tion (ee·ling·gway′shun) *n.* [L. *elinguare,* to deprive of the tongue]. Surgical removal of the tongue.

eli·sion (e·lizh′un) *n.* [L. *elisio,* from *elidere,* to elide]. The omission of one or more sounds or syllables from words when speaking.

elix·ir (e·lik′sur) *n.* [L., from Ar. *al-iksīr*]. A sweetened, aromatic solution, usually hydroalcoholic, commonly containing soluble medicants, but sometimes not containing any medication; intended for use only as a flavor or vehicle, or both.

Elixophyllin. A trademark for theophylline.

El·kin's operation [D. C. *Elkin,* U.S. surgeon, 1893–1958]. A method of suturing a wounded heart by means of a suture passed widely and deeply into the cardiac muscle. This controls bleeding until the edges of the wound are approximated, when the deep suture is removed.

El·liot's operation [E. H. *Elliot,* English ophthalmologist, 1864–1936]. Sclerocorneal trephining for the relief of glaucoma.

Elliot's position [J. W. *Elliot,* U.S. surgeon, 1852–1925]. A position in which the patient is supine, with the upper abdomen raised by a support under the back, facilitating surgical access to the gallbladder and bile ducts.

Elliott treatment [C. H. *Elliott,* U.S. gynecologist, b. 1879]. A former treatment of pelvic infections by an apparatus which delivers circulating heated water to a thin rubber bag inserted in the vagina.

el·lip·sin (e·lip′sin) *n.* The protein constituents of the cell responsible for maintaining its form and structure.

el·lip·soid (e·lip′soid) *adj. & n.* [Gk. *elleipsis,* ellipsis, + *-oid*]. 1. Ellipse-like or oval. 2. A solid figure of which all plane sections are ellipses, or of which some are ellipses and the rest circles. 3. The spindle-shaped sheathed arterial capillary (the second division of the penicillus) in the red pulp of the spleen, consisting of phagocytic cells and reticular fibers. Syn. *Schweigger-Seidel sheath.* —**el·lip·soi·dal** (e·lip″soy′dul) *adj.*

ellipsoid articulation. CONDYLAR JOINT.

el·lip·tic (e·lip′tick) *adj.* [Gk. *elleiptikos,* defective]. Shaped like an ellipse, or an elongated circle.

el·lip·ti·cal (e·lip′ti·kul) *adj.* ELLIPTIC.

elliptical recess. An oval depression in the roof and medial wall of the vestibule lodging the utricle. It contains small foramens for the passage of branches of the acoustic nerve to the utricle and to the ampulla of the superior and lateral semicircular ducts. Syn. *utricular recess.* NA *recessus ellipticus vestibuli.*

elliptic amputation. An amputation similar in performance to the circular amputation, but in which the incision is elliptic.

el·lip·to·cyte (e·lip′to·site) *n.* An elliptic erythrocyte.

el·lip·to·cy·to·sis (e·lip″to·sigh·to′sis) *n.* [*elliptocyte* + *-osis*]. An autosomal dominant anomaly of erythrocytes characterized by an oval shape in 90% or more of peripheral blood erythrocytes, occasionally resulting in hemolysis but usually asymptomatic.

El·lis' curve [C. *Ellis,* U.S. physician, 1826–1883]. The S-shaped curved line on percussion showing the upper limit of dullness of a pleural effusion.

Ellis–van Cre·veld syndrome. CHONDROECTODERMAL DYSPLASIA.

Ells·worth-How·ard test. A test to distinguish pseudohypoparathyroidism from hypoparathyroidism. Failure of injected parathyroid extract to produce a phosphate diuresis indicates pseudohypoparathyroidism.

elm, *n.* ULMUS.

elon·ga·tion factor. Any of the proteins required for the elongation of a growing polypeptide chain during the process of protein synthesis.

elope·ment (e·lope′munt) *n. In psychiatry,* the departure of a patient from a mental hospital without permission. See also *escape, parole.* —**elope,** *v.*

Elorine. Trademark for tricyclamol, an anticholinergic drug used as the methochloride salt.

Elsch·nig's pearls [A. *Elschnig,* German ophthalmologist, 1863–1939]. Nodules of proliferating ocular lens epithelium sometimes developing after trauma or cataract operations, and growing to visible size in the pupillary space.

el·u·ant, el·u·ent (el′yoo·unt) *n.* The solvent used in elution in chromatography.

el·u·ate (el′yoo·ate) *n.* The extract obtained from elution in chromatography; it represents a solution of the formerly adsorbed substance in the eluant.

elu·caine (e·lew′kane) *n.* α-[(Diethylamino)methyl]benzyl alcohol benzoate (ester), $C_{19}H_{23}NO_2$, a gastric anticholinergic, also used as the hydrochloride salt.

elu·sive ulcer. HUNNER'S ULCER.

elu·tion (e·lew′shun) *n.* [L. *elutio,* from *eluere,* to wash out]. 1. The process of extracting by means of a solvent the adsorbed substance from the solid adsorbing medium in chromatography. 2. The removal of antibody from the antigen to which it is attached. —**elute** (e·lewt′) *v.*

elu·tri·a·tion (e·lew″tree·ay′shun) *n.* [L. *elutriare,* to decant, wash out]. A process whereby the coarser particles of an insoluble powder are separated from the finer by mixing the substance with a liquid and decanting the upper layer after the heavier particles have settled. A form of water sifting.

El·ve·hjem and Ken·ne·dy's method. A method for the determination of iron in which urine is ashed, the ash dissolved, and the iron present determined colorimetrically as thiocyanate.

Ely's sign [L. W. *Ely,* U.S. orthopedic surgeon, 1868–1944]. A sign of irritation of the psoas muscle or of hip-joint disease, elicited by having the patient lie prone with feet hanging over the edge of the table. The heel is approximated to the buttock and the thigh is hyperextended. Inability to complete the movement is a positive response.

Ely's table. A table giving approximate dates for expected parturition, based on counting 280 days from date of last menstruation. See Ely's Table of the Duration of Pregnancy in the Appendix.

elytr-, elytro- [Gk. *elytron,* sheath]. A combining form meaning *vagina, vaginal.*

em-. See *en-.*

ema·ci·a·tion (e·may″shee·ay′shun, e·may′see·) *n.* [L. *emaciare,* to make thin, from *macer,* thin]. The process of losing flesh so as to become extremely lean, or the resultant state; a wasted condition. —**ema·ci·ate** (e·may′shee·ate, e·may′see·ate) *v.*

emac·u·la·tion (e·mack″yoo·lay′shun) *n.* [*e-* + *macule*]. The removal of freckles or other skin lesions, especially skin tumors.

em·a·na·tion (em″uh·nay′shun) *n.* [L. *emanatio,* from *emanare,* to spring out of]. 1. That which flows or is emitted from a substance; effluvium. 2. Gaseous, radioactive products formed by the loss of alpha particles from radium (radon), thorium X (thoron), and actinium X (actinon). —**em·a·nate** (em′uh·nate) *v.*

em·a·na·to·ri·um (em″uh·na·to′ree·um) *n.* An institution where patients are treated by radioactive waters and radioactive emanations.

eman·ci·pa·tion (e·man″si·pay′shun) *n.* [L. *emancipatio,* from *emancipare,* to emancipate]. *In embryology,* the process whereby organ districts acquire a definite boundary when forming from the primitive individuation field. —**eman·ci·pate** (e·man'si·pate) *v.*

em·a·no·ther·a·py (em''uh·no·therr'uh·pee) *n.* [*emanation* + *therapy*]. Treatment by radioactive emanations.

eman·sio (e·man'see·o, ·shee·o) *n.* [L.]. A failing.

emansio men·si·um (men'see·um). Delay in the first appearance of the menses.

emas·cu·late (e·mas'kew·late) *v.* [L. *emasculare*]. To castrate; to remove the testes, or the testes and penis. —**emas·cu·la·tion** (e·mas''kew·lay'shun) *n.*

Em·ba·do·mo·nas (em''buh·do·mo'nus, ·dom'o·nus) *n.* [Gk. *embas, embados*, slipper, + *monas*, unit]. A genus of protozoan flagellates, principally found in the gut of arthropods.

Embadomonas in·tes·ti·na·lis (in·tes·ti·nay'lis). A nonpathogenic protozoan found in the intestine of man.

em·balm (em·bahm') *v.* [OF. *embaumer*, from *basme*, balm]. To treat a cadaver with antiseptic and preservative substances for burial or for dissection.

em·bar·rass·ment, *n.* Functional impairment; interference; difficulty.

Emb·den-Mey·er·hof scheme [C. G. *Embden*, German chemist, 1874–1933; and D. *Meyerhof*.]. MEYERHOF PATHWAY.

em·bed (em·bed') *v.* [*em-* + *bed*]. *In histology*, to infiltrate a specimen with a substance, as paraffin or celloidin, to give support during the process of cutting it into sections for microscopical examination.

Em·be·lia (em·bee'lee·uh, em·beel'yuh) *n.* A genus of shrubs of the Myrsinaceae. The berries of *Embelia ribes*, an Asiatic species, have been used as an anthelmintic.

em·bel·ic acid (em·bel'ick). EMBELIN.

em·be·lin (em'be·lin) *n.* 2,5-Dihydroxy-3-undecyl-*p*-benzoquinone, $C_{17}H_{26}O_4$, the anthelmintic principle of *Embelia ribes.*

embol-, embolo-. A combining form meaning *embolus, embolic.*

em·bo·la·lia (em''bo·lay'lee·uh) *n.* EMBOLOLALIA.

em·bo·lec·to·my (em''bo·leck'tuh·mee) *n.* [*embol-* + *-ectomy*]. Surgical removal of an embolus.

em·bo·le·mia, em·bo·lae·mia (em''bo·lee'mee·uh) *n.* [*embol-* + *-emia*]. The presence of emboli in the blood.

emboli. Plural of *embolus.*

em·bol·ic (em·bol'ick) *adj.* Pertaining to an embolus or an embolism.

embolic abscess. An abscess formed at the seat of a septic embolus.

embolic aneurysm. An aneurysm caused by embolism.

embolic glomerulonephritis. FOCAL EMBOLIC GLOMERULONEPHRITIS.

embolic necrosis. Coagulation necrosis in an anemic infarct following embolism.

embolic nephritis. FOCAL EMBOLIC GLOMERULONEPHRITIS.

em·bol·i·form (em·bol'i·form) *adj.* [*embol-* + *-iform*]. Shaped like or resembling an embolus.

emboliform nucleus. A nucleus in the medullary portion of the cerebellum located mediad to the upper part of the dentate nucleus. It receives afferent fibers from the paleocerebellum and sends efferent fibers into the superior cerebellar peduncle. NA *nucleus emboliformis cerebelli.*

em·bo·lism (em'bo·liz·um) *n.* [L. *embolismus*, from Gk. *embolimos*, intercalated, from *emballein*, to throw in]. The occlusion of a blood vessel by an embolus, causing various syndromes depending on the size of the vessel occluded, the part supplied, and the character of the embolus. —**embo·lize** (·lize) *v.*

em·bo·lo·la·lia (em''buh·lo·lay'lee·uh) *n.* [Gk. *embolē*, insertion, + *-lalia*] 1. The insertion of meaningless words into speech, occurring in some aphasic and schizophrenic states. 2. A form of speech disorder, often seen in stutterers, in which short sounds or words are interpolated into the spoken sentence to cover hesitancy.

em·bo·lo·phra·sia (em''buh·lo·fray'zhuh, ·zee·uh) *n.* EMBOLOLALIA.

em·bo·lus (em'buh·lus) *n.*, pl. **embo·li** (·lye) [L., from Gk. *embolos*, stopper]. A bit of matter foreign to the bloodstream, such as blood clot, air, tumor or other tissue cells, fat, cardiac vegetations, clumps of bacteria, or a foreign body (as a needle or bullet) which is carried by the bloodstream until it lodges in a blood vessel and obstructs it. —**embo·loid** (·loid) *adj.*

em·bo·ly (em'buh·lee) *n.* [Gk. *embolē*, insertion]. The process of invagination by which a two-layered gastrula develops from a blastula.

embrace reflex. MORO REFLEX.

em·bra·sure (em·bray'zhur) *n.* [F., from *embraser*, to widen an opening]. The space formed by the sloping or curved proximal surfaces adjacent to the contact area of two teeth in the same arch; it may be facial, or buccal, or labial, lingual, gingival, incisal, or occlusal in accordance with the direction toward which it opens. See also *spillway.*

em·bro·ca·tion (em''bro·kay'shun) *n.* [Gk. *embrochē*, from *embrechein*, to wet]. 1. The application, especially by rubbing, of a liquid to a part of the body. 2. The liquid so applied; liniment.

embry-, embryo-. A combining form meaning *embryo, fetus, embryonic, fetal.*

em·bry·ec·to·my (em''bree·eck'tuh·mee) *n.* [*embry-* + *-ectomy*]. The surgical removal of an extrauterine embryo.

em·bryo (em'bree·o) *n.* [ML., from Gk. *embryon*, from *em-* + *bryein*, to swell, grow]. A young organism in the early stages of development; in human embryology, the product of conception from the moment of fertilization until about the end of the eighth week after fertilization. Compare *fetus.*

embryo-. See *embry-.*

em·bryo·blast (em'bree·o·blast) *n.* [*embryo-* + *-blast*]. The part of the germ disk or inner cell mass from which the embryo proper develops.

em·bryo·car·dia (em''bree·o·kahr'dee·uh) *n.* [*embryo-* + *-cardia*]. A condition in which the heart sounds resemble those of a fetus, the first and second sounds being almost identical in intensity and duration.

em·bryo·chem·i·cal (em''bree·o·kem'i·kul) *adj.* Pertaining to the changes in the chemistry of the ovum or embryo.

em·bryo·ci·dal (em''bree·o·sigh'dul) *adj.* [*embryo-* + *-cidal*]. Capable of killing an embryo.

em·bry·oc·to·ny (em''bree·ock'tuh·nee) *n.* [*embryo-* + Gk. *ktonos*, killing]. The killing of a fetus. —**embry·oc·ton·ic** (·ock·ton'ick) *adj.*

em·bryo·gen·e·sis (em''bree·o·jen'e·sis) *n.* [*embryo-* + *-genesis*]. EMBRYOGENY. —**embryo·ge·net·ic** (·je·net'ick) *adj.*

em·bry·og·e·ny (em''bree·oj'e·nee) *n.* [*embryo-* + *-geny*]. The development of the embryo. —**embry·o·gen·ic** (·o·jen'ick), *adj.*

em·bry·oid (em'bree·oid) *adj.* [*embry-* + *-oid*]. Resembling an embryo.

em·bryo·lem·ma (em''bree·o·lem'uh) *n.*, pl. **embryolemmas, embryolemma·ta** (·tuh) [*embryo-* + *-lemma*]. Any one of the fetal or extraembryonic membranes.

em·bry·ol·o·gist (em''bree·ol'uh·jist) *n.* One skilled in embryology.

em·bry·ol·o·gy (em''bree·ol'uh·jee) *n.* [*embryo-* + *-logy*]. The science dealing with the embryo and its development. —**embry·o·log·ic** (·o·loj'ick), **embryolog·i·cal** (·i·kul) *adj.*

em·bry·o·ma (em''bree·o'muh) *n.*, pl. **embryomas, embryoma·ta** (·tuh) [*embry-* + *-oma*]. 1. MALIGNANT MIXED MESODERMAL TUMOR. 2. TERATOMA.

embryoma of the kidney. WILMS'S TUMOR.

embryoma of the ovary. DYSGERMINOMA.

em·bryo·mor·phous (em''bree·o·mor'fus) *adj.* [*embryo-* + *-morphous*]. Like an embryo; of embryonic origin.

em·bry·on (em'bree·on) *n.* [Gk.]. *Obsol.* EMBRYO.

em·bry·o·nal (em'bree·uh·nul) *adj.* EMBRYONIC.

embryonal adenomyosarcoma. A malignant mixed mesodermal tumor containing glandular and muscular elements.

embryonal cartilage. Developing or young cartilage with a high ratio of cells to matrix and absence of isogenous cell groups.

embryonal-cell lipoma. LIPOSARCOMA.

embryonal leukemia. STEM CELL LEUKEMIA.

embryonal lipomatosis. LIPOSARCOMA.

embryonal medulloepithelioma. DIKTYOMA.

embryonal mixed tumor of the kidney. WILMS'S TUMOR.

embryonal nuclear cataract. A usually nonprogressive cataract most often occurring bilaterally, limited to the embryonic nucleus of the eye and due to some disturbance in the first 3 months of development; vision is rarely affected. Syn. *central pulverulent cataract.*

embryonal rhabdomyoblastoma. A poorly differentiated rhabdomyosarcoma.

embryonal theory. COHNHEIM'S THEORY.

em·bry·o·nate (em'bree·o·nate) *adj.* [*embryon* + *-ate*]. 1. Fecundated. 2. Containing an embryo.

em·bry·on·ic (em″bree·on'ick) *adj.* [*embryon* + *-ic*]. 1. Pertaining to an embryo. 2. Rudimentary; undifferentiated.

embryonic anlage. EMBRYONIC DISK.

embryonic area. EMBRYONIC DISK.

embryonic axis. An imaginary line passing through the future anteroposterior regions of an egg or embryo.

embryonic blastoderm. The part of a blastoderm forming the embryo proper. See also *embryonic disk.*

embryonic carcinoma. A malignant teratoma.

embryonic cell. An undifferentiated developmental cell. See also *blastema.*

embryonic connective tissue. MUCOID TISSUE.

embryonic digestive tube. The digestive tube of the embryo. Sometimes used to include the portion of the alimentary canal between the stomodeum and the proctodeum; includes the foregut, midgut, and hindgut.

embryonic disk. In mammals, the central, circular, or oval area of the bilaminar blastodisk in which the primitive streak arises and from which the embryo proper develops. Syn. *area embryonalis, area germinativa.*

embryonic hormone. EVOCATOR.

embryonic kidney. MESONEPHROS.

embryonic knob. In many mammals, the part of the inner cell mass consisting of primary ectoderm and entoderm after the migration of the endodermal cells forming the yolk sac.

embryonic shield. EMBRYONIC DISK.

embryonic spot. The nucleolus of the ovum.

em·bry·on·i·form (em″bree·on'i·form) *adj.* Like an embryo in form.

em·bry·o·ni·za·tion (em″bree·on·i·zay'shun) *n.* The change of a cell or tissue to an embryonic form of structure.

em·bry·o·noid (em'bree·o·noid) *adj.* EMBRYOID.

em·bry·o·ny (em'bree·uh·nee) *n.* [*embryon* + *-y*]. The condition of constituting an embryo.

em·bry·op·a·thy (em″bree·op'uh·thee) *n.* [*embryo-* + *-pathy*]. Any type of embryonic or congenital defect resulting from faulty development, especially one caused by infection or toxicity from the mother or other damage in utero.

em·bryo·plas·tic (em″bree·o·plas'tick) *adj.* [*embryo-* + *-plastic*]. Participating in the formation of the embryo.

em·bryo·to·cia (em″bree·o·to'shee·uh, ·see·uh) *n.* [*embryo-* + Gk. *tokos*, birth, + *-ia*]. *Obsol.* ABORTION.

em·bryo·tome (em'bree·o·tome) *n.* [Gk. *embryotomos*]. An instrument for performing embryotomy.

em·bry·ot·o·my (em″bree·ot'uh·mee) *n.* [Gk. *embryotomia*, from *embryon* + *tomē*, cutting, section]. Any mutilation of the fetus in the uterus to aid in its removal when natural delivery is impossible.

em·bryo·tox·ic·i·ty (em″bree·o·tock·sis'i·tee) *n.* The state of possessing qualities toxic to embryos.

em·bry·o·tox·on (em″bree·o·tocks'on) *n.* [*embryo* + Gk. *toxon*, bow]. 1. A congenital opaque marginal ring in the cornea. See also *anterior embryotoxon, posterior embryotoxon.* 2. Specifically, ANTERIOR EMBRYOTOXON.

em·bryo·trophe, em·bryo·troph (em'bree·o·trof, ·trofe) *n.* [*embryo-* + *-troph*]. The total nutriment, both histotrophe and hemotrophe, supplied to the embryo during pregnancy. —**em·bryo·troph·ic** (em″bree·o·trof'ick) *adj.*

em·bry·ot·ro·phy (em″bree·ot'ruh·fee) *n.* [*embryo-* + *-trophy*]. The nutrition of the fetus.

em·bry·ul·cia (em″bree·ul'see·uh) *n.* [Gk. *embryoulkia*, from *embryon* + *helkein*, to draw]. Extraction of the fetus from the uterus by means of instruments.

em·bry·ul·cus (em″bree·ul'kus) *n.* [Gk. *embryoulkos*]. A blunt hook, or obstetric forceps, used in performing embryulcia.

Embutal. A trademark for pentobarbital sodium, a barbiturate.

emer·gen·cy, *n.* [ML. *emergentia*, from *emergere*, to emerge]. 1. A suddenly developing pathologic condition in a patient, due to accident or disease, which requires urgent medical or surgical therapeutic attention. 2. A sudden threatening situation, as in warfare, disasters, or epidemics, which calls for immediate correction or defensive measures.

emergency operation. An operation that must be done at once to save the patient from a dangerous extension of the disease or from death.

emergency room. A hospital area with personnel and equipment for the care of acute illness, trauma, or other conditions requiring immediate medical attention.

emergency theory. A concept that the major function of the adrenal medulla is to liberate epinephrine in states of emergency to increase heart rate, raise blood pressure, reduce blood flow to viscera, and mobilize blood glucose, thereby creating optimal conditions for function of skeletal muscles.

emergent stage 1. REM SLEEP.

em·e·sis (em'e·sis) *n.*, pl. **eme·ses** (·seez) [Gk.]. Vomiting; the act of vomiting.

emet-, emeto-. A combining form meaning (a) *emesis, vomiting;* (b) *emetic.*

em·e·ta·mine (em″e·tuh·meen', e·met'uh·meen, ·min) *n.* An alkaloid, $C_{29}H_{36}N_2O_4$, occurring in small amounts in ipecac and obtainable from emetine by dehydrogenation.

emet·a·tro·phia (e·met″uh·tro'fee·uh) *n.* [*emet-* + Gk. *atrophia*, atrophy]. Atrophy or wasting away due to persistent vomiting.

emet·ic (e·met'ick) *adj.* & *n.* [Gk. *emetikos*]. 1. Inducing emesis. 2. An agent that induces emesis.

Emeticon. A trademark for benzquinamide, a tranquilizer.

em·e·tine (em'e·teen, ·tin) *n.* [*emet-* + *-ine*]. Cephaeline methyl ether, $C_{29}H_{40}N_2O_4$, the principal alkaloid of ipecac; a white powder, sparingly soluble in water; an emetic, diaphoretic, and expectorant, but used chiefly as an amebicide, in the form of emetine hydrochloride and emetine bismuth iodide.

emetine bismuth iodide. A complex iodide of emetine and of bismuth; a reddish-orange powder, insoluble in water; used orally in the treatment of amebic dysentery.

emeto-. See *emet-.*

em·e·to·ca·thar·sis (em″e·to·kuh·thahr'sis) *n.*, pl. **emetocathar·ses** (·seez) [*emeto-* + *catharsis*]. Vomiting and purgation at the same time, or produced by a common agent.

em·e·to·ma·nia (em″e·to·may'nee·uh) *n.* [*emeto-* + *-mania*]. An abnormal desire to vomit.

em·e·to·mor·phine (em″e·to·mor'feen, ·fin) *n.* [*emeto-* + *morphine*]. APOMORPHINE.

em·e·to·pho·bia (em″e·to·fo'bee·uh) *n.* [*emeto-* + *phobia*]. A morbid fear of vomiting.

emf, EMF An abbreviation for *electromotive force.*

EMG Abbreviation for *electromyography, electromyogram.*

-emia, -aemia [Gk. *haima*, blood, + *-ia*]. A combining form designating *a* (specified) *condition of the blood or presence in the blood of a* (specified) *substance.*

emic·tion (e·mick'shun) *n.* [L. *emingere,* to urinate, from *e-* + *mingere*]. URINATION.

emic·to·ry (e·mick'tuh·ree) *adj. & n.* DIURETIC.

em·i·gra·tion (em"i·gray'shun) *n.* [L. *emigratio,* from *emigrare,* to depart]. The outward passage of wandering cells or leukocytes through the walls of a small blood vessel; DIAPEDESIS. —**em·i·grate** (em'i·grate) *v.*

em·i·nence (em'i·nunce) *n.* [L. *eminentia,* from *eminere,* to stand out, project]. A projecting, prominent part of an organ, especially a bone.

eminence of the concha. The posterior projection on the pinna corresponding to the concha. NA *eminentia conchae.*

eminence of the scapha. The elevation on the medial side of the auricle corresponding to the scapha on the lateral side. NA *eminentia scaphae.*

eminence of the triangular fossa. The elevation on the medial side of the auricle corresponding to the triangular fossa on the lateral side. NA *eminentia fossae triangularis.*

emi·nen·tia (em"i·nen'shee·uh) *n.* [L.]. EMINENCE.

eminentia ar·cu·a·ta (ahr·kew·ay'tuh) [NA]. ARCUATE EMINENCE.

eminentia car·pi ra·di·a·lis (kahr'pye ray·dee·ay'lis) [BNA]. The prominence on the lateral side of the palmar surface of the articulated carpal bones produced by the tubercles of the scaphoid and trapezium.

eminentia carpi ul·na·ris (ul·nair'is) [BNA]. The prominence on the medial side of the palmar surface of the articulated carpal bones produced by the pisiform and hamulus of the hamate.

eminentia cla·vae (klay'vee). CLAVA.

eminentia col·la·te·ra·lis (ko·lat"e·ray'lis) [NA]. COLLATERAL EMINENCE.

eminentia con·chae (kong'kee) [NA]. EMINENCE OF THE CONCHA.

eminentia cru·ci·a·ta (kroo·shee·ay'tuh) [BNA]. Eminentia cruciformis (= CRUCIATE EMINENCE).

eminentia cru·ci·for·mis (kroo·si·for'mis) [NA]. CRUCIATE EMINENCE.

eminentia fa·ci·a·lis (fay·shee·ay'lis). FACIAL COLLICULUS.

eminentia fos·sae tri·an·gu·la·ris (fos'ee trye·ang"gew·lair'is) [NA]. EMINENCE OF THE TRIANGULAR FOSSA.

eminentia ilio·pec·ti·nea (il"ee·o·peck·tin'ee·uh) [BNA]. Eminentia iliopubica (= ILIOPUBIC EMINENCE).

eminentia ilio·pu·bi·ca (il"ee·o·pew'bi·kuh) [NA]. ILIOPUBIC EMINENCE.

eminentia in·ter·con·dy·la·ris (in"tur·kon·di·lair'is) [NA]. INTERCONDYLAR EMINENCE.

eminentia in·ter·con·dy·loi·dea (in"tur·kon·di·loy'dee·uh) [BNA]. Eminentia intercondylaris (= INTERCONDYLAR EMINENCE).

eminentia me·di·a·lis (mee·dee·ay'lis) [NA]. MEDIAL EMINENCE.

eminentia py·ra·mi·da·lis (pi·ram"i·day'lis) [NA]. PYRAMIDAL EMINENCE.

eminentia sca·phae (skaf'ee, skay'fee) [NA]. EMINENCE OF THE SCAPHA.

eminentia te·res (tee'reez, terr'eez). FACIAL COLLICULUS.

em·io·cy·to·sis (em"ee·o·sigh·to'sis) *n.* [*emet-* + *cyt-* + *-osis*]. Fusion of intracellular granules with the cell membrane, followed by discharge of the granules into the surroundings; applied chiefly to insulin secretion by the islets of Langerhans. Syn. *reverse pinocytosis.*

emis·sa·ri·um (em"i·sair'ee·um) *n.,* pl. **emissa·ria** (·ee·uh) [BNA]. Vena emissaria (= EMISSARY VEIN).

emissarium con·dy·loi·de·um (kon·di·loy'dee·um) [BNA]. Vena emissaria condylaris (= CONDYLOID EMISSARY VEIN).

emissarium ma·stoi·de·um (mas·toy'dee·um) [BNA]. Vena emissaria mastoidea (= MASTOID EMISSARY VEIN).

emissarium oc·ci·pi·ta·le (ock·sip"i·tay'lee) [BNA]. Vena emissaria occipitalis (= OCCIPITAL EMMISSARY VEIN).

emissarium pa·ri·e·ta·le (pa·rye"e·tay'lee) [BNA]. Vena emissaria parietalis (= PARIETAL EMISSARY VEIN).

em·is·sary (vein) (em'i·serr"ee) *n.* [L. *emissarius,* from *emittere,* to send forth]. Any venous channel through the skull, connecting the venous sinuses with the diploic veins and veins of the scalp. NA *vena emissaria.* See also Table of Veins in the Appendix.

emis·sion (e·mish'un) *n.* [L. *emissio,* from *e-,* out, away, + *mittere,* to send, release]. 1. The action or process of emitting. 2. A seminal discharge or ejaculation.

emission histospectroscopy. The identification of certain elements in tissues by means of emission spectra, which are obtained by consuming in a high-frequency spark a chosen region of a tissue section.

emission spectrum. The spectrum of the radiation which a substance emits. Contr. *absorption spectrum.*

Emivan. Trademark for ethamivan, a respiratory stimulant.

em·men·a·gogue (e·men'uh·gog, e·mee'nuh·) *n.* [Gk. *emmēna,* menses, + *-agogue*]. An agent that stimulates the menstrual flow. —**em·men·a·gog·ic** (e·men"uh·goj'ick) *adj.*

em·men·ia (e·men'ee·uh, e·mee'nee·uh) *n.* [Gk. *emmēnia*]. MENSES.

em·men·i·op·a·thy (e·men"ee·op'uth·ee, e·mee"nee·) *n.* [*emmenia* + *-pathy*]. Any menstrual disorder.

em·me·nol·o·gy (em"e·nol'uh·jee) *n.* [Gk. *emmēna,* menses, + *-logy*]. The branch of medicine that treats of menstruation.

em·me·tro·pia (em"e·tro'pee·uh) *n.* [Gk. *emmetros,* in measure, + *-opia*]. Normal or perfect vision. The condition in which parallel rays are focused exactly on the retina without effort of accommodation. Abbreviated, E. —**em·me·trope** (em'e·trope) *n.;* **em·me·trop·ic** (em"e·trop'ick) *adj.*

Em·mon·sia par·va (e·mon'see·uh pahr'vuh). A white mold, bearing conidia, which is a cause of pulmonary haplomycosis in wild rodents and other small mammals.

em·o·din (em'o·din) *n.* 1,3,8-Trihydroxy-6-methylanthraquinone, $C_{15}H_{10}O_5$, a product of hydrolysis or oxidation of glycosidal compounds found in rhubarb, cascara, and other plants; it has also been synthesized. It is an irritant cathartic, acting mainly on the large intestine.

emodin-L-rhamnoside. FRANGULIN.

emol·lient (ee·mol'ee·unt, ·yunt) *adj. & n.* [L. *emolliens,* softening, from *mollis,* soft]. 1. Softening or soothing. 2. A substance used externally to soften the skin; or, internally, to soothe an irritated or inflamed surface.

emo·tio·mo·tor (e·mo"shee·o·mo'tur) *adj.* [*emotion* + *motor*]. Of, pertaining to, or inducing some activity as a result of emotion.

emo·tio·mus·cu·lar (e·mo"shee·o·mus'kew·lur) *adj.* Pertaining to muscular activity which is due to emotion.

emo·tion, *n.* [F., from L. *emovere,* to shake, excite]. 1. Affect, feeling, or sentiment. 2. Strong feeling, often of an agitated nature, accompanied frequently by physical and psychic reactions, as changes in heart action or gastrointestinal and vasomotor disturbances. —**emotion·al,** *adj.*

emotional amenorrhea. Pathological lack of menstruation due to sympathetic vasomotor disturbances caused by fright, emotional disturbances, or hysteria.

emotional castration. 1. CASTRATION ANXIETY. 2. CASTRATION COMPLEX.

emotional deprivation. A lack of adequate and appropriate experience in interpersonal relationships or environmental stimulation or both, usually in the early formative years; may cause pseudoretardation.

emotional deterioration. The clinical picture in which a psychotic patient becomes apathetic and shows a loss of interest in his appearance, environment, and social adjustment.

emotional facial palsy or **paralysis.** A form of supranuclear facial palsy in which weakness, predominantly of the lower face, is more evident with smiling and crying than with voluntary activity.

emotional fatigue. Tiredness or weariness that is out of proportion to the actual amount of physical or mental activity performed, usually traceable to emotional origins.

emotional health. MENTAL HEALTH.

emotional illness. MENTAL DISORDER.

emotional insanity. AFFECTIVE DISORDER.

emotional investment. 1. *In psychiatry,* the investing of an object with emotional meaning or significance. 2. Attachment to an object because of past emotions directed toward the object.

emotionally disturbed. Characterized by inappropriate or disproportionate emotional responses to various life situations; emotionally unstable or labile; neurotic.

emotionally unstable personality. HYSTERICAL PERSONALITY.

emo·tio·vas·cu·lar (e·mo″shee·o·vas′kew·lur) *adj.* Pertaining to any vascular change brought about by emotion.

em·pasm (em′paz·um) *n.* [Gk. *empasma,* dusting powder, from *empassein,* to sprinkle on]. A perfumed dusting powder.

em·pas·ma (em·paz′muh) *n.* [Gk.]. EMPASM.

em·pa·thy (em′puth·ee) *n.* [*em-* + *-pathy*]. 1. The vicarious experience of another person's situation and psychological state, which may facilitate intuitive understanding of that person's feelings, thoughts, and actions. Compare *sympathy.* 2. Attribution of feelings or attitudes to a physical object or an animal.

em·per·io·po·le·sis (em·perr″ee·o·po·lee′sis) *n.* EMPERIPOLESIS.

em·per·i·po·le·sis (em·perr″ee·po·lee′sis) *n.* [Gk. *emperi-,* around, about, + *polēsis,* movement]. Penetration of other cells and wandering about in their cytoplasm, as by lymphocytes and neutrophilic granulocytes.

em·phly·sis (em′fli·sis) *n.* [*em-* + Gk. *phlysis,* eruption]. Any vesicular or exanthematous eruption terminating in scales.

em·phrac·tic (em·frack′tick) *n.* [Gk. *emphraktikos,* obstructive]. Any agent that obstructs the function of an organ, especially the excretory function of the skin.

em·phrax·is (em·frack′sis) *n.,* pl. **emphrax·es** (·eez) [Gk.]. An obstruction, infarction, or congestion.

em·phy·se·ma (em′fi·see′muh) *n.* [Gk. *emphysēma,* inflation, swelling, from *emphysan,* to inflate, from *physan,* to blow]. 1. An anatomic alteration of the lungs characterized by abnormal enlargement of the air spaces distal to the terminal respiratory bronchiole, often accompanied by destructive changes of the alveolar walls. 2. Abnormal presence of air or gas in the body tissues. —**emphy·se·ma·tous** (·sem′uh·tus, ·see′muh·tus) *adj.*

emphysematous anthrax. SYMPTOMATIC ANTHRAX.

emphysematous chest. The altered contour of the chest seen in pulmonary emphysema, with increased anteroposterior diameter, flaring of the lower rib margins, low position of the diaphragm, and minimal respiratory motion. See also *barrel chest.*

emphysematous cystitis. Infection of the urinary bladder by a gas-forming bacterium, usually *Escherichia coli,* causing intraluminal and submucosal gas pockets.

emphysematous gangrene. 1. BLACKLEG. 2. GAS GANGRENE.

emphysematous pyelonephritis. Infection of the kidney by a gas-forming bacterium, characterized by gas in the renal collecting system.

emphysematous vaginitis or **colpitis.** Vaginitis characterized by vesicles that contain a gaseous material.

em·pir·ic (em·pirr′ick) *adj.* & *n.* [Gk. *empeirikos,* experienced; a member of the Empiric school of physicians]. 1. EMPIRICAL. 2. One who in practicing medicine relies solely on actual experience and experimentation.

em·pir·i·cal (em·pirr′i·kul) *adj.* [*empiric* + *-al*]. Based on observation rather than on reasoning, assumption, or speculation.

empirical formula. A formula that indicates only the constituents and their proportions in a molecule, as $C_6H_{12}O_6$, dextrose.

em·pir·i·cism (em·pirr′i·siz·um) *n.* [*empiric* + *-ism*]. 1. Methodological preference for or tendency toward reliance on the directly observable rather than the theoretical, as, in psychology, partiality to behavioral data rather than unobservable mental entities and processes. 2. The philosophical view that all genuine knowledge is empirical.

empiric risk. The probability that a relative of an individual affected by a hereditary disease will also be affected, derived from the pooled data of similar cases without any consideration of the genetic mechanism.

em·plas·trum (em·plas′trum) *n.,* pl. **emplas·tra** (·truh) [L.]. PLASTER (1).

em·pros·thot·o·nos, em·pros·thot·o·nus (em″pros·thot′uh·nus) *n.* [Gk., from *emprosth*en, in front, + *tonos,* stretching]. A tetanic muscular spasm in which the head and feet are flexed forward, tensing the back in a curve with concavity forward. Contr. *opisthotonos.*

em·pros·tho·zy·go·sis (em″pros·tho·zye·go′sis) *n.* [Gk. *emprosth*en, in front, + *zyg-* + *-osis*]. The condition of conjoined twins in which the fusion is anterior.

em·py·e·ma (em″pye·ee′muh, em″pee·ee′muh) *n.,* pl. **empy·ema·ta** (·tuh), **empyemas** [Gk. *empyēma,* gathering, abscess, from *pyon,* pus]. The presence of pus in a cavity, hollow organ, or body space. —**empy·em·a·tous** (·em′uh·tus), **empye·mic** (·mick) *adj.*

empyema ne·ces·si·ta·tis (ne·ses″i·tay′tis). Empyema in which pus from the pleural cavity burrows to the outside, appearing as a swelling in an intercostal space or at the costal border.

empyema of necessity. EMPYEMA NECESSITATIS.

em·py·e·sis (em″pye·ee′sis) *n.,* pl. **empye·ses** (·seez) [Gk. *empyēsis,* suppuration, from *pyon,* pus]. 1. A pustular eruption. 2. Any disease characterized by phlegmonous vesicles filling with purulent fluid. 3. An accumulation of pus.

em·py·reu·mat·ic (em·pye″roo·mat′ick, em″pi·) *adj.* [Gk. *empyreuma, empyreumatos,* ember, coal]. Pertaining to any odorous substance produced by destructive distillation of organic material.

emul·si·fi·er (e·mul′si·figh″ur) *n.* An agent used to assist in the production of an emulsion.

emul·si·fy (e·mul′si·figh) *v.* To make into an emulsion. —**emul·si·fi·ca·tion** (e·mul″si·fi·kay′shun) *n.*

emul·sin (e·mul′sin) *n.* An enzyme, found in bitter almonds and other seeds, which selectively catalyzes hydrolysis of β-glucoside linkages; thus, it effects hydrolysis of amygdalin to benzaldehyde, hydrocyanic acid, and glucose. Syn. *amygdalase, glucosidase.*

emul·sion (e·mul′shun) *n.* [NL. *emulsio,* from L. *emulgere,* to milk out]. A product consisting of minute globules of one liquid dispersed throughout the body of a second liquid. The portion that exists as globules is known as the internal, dispersed, or discontinuous phase; the other liquid is the external or continuous phase or the dispersion medium, for example, a suspension of silver halide salts in gelatin as a component of photographic and x-ray films.

emulsion albuminuria. Proteinuria in which the urine has a milky turbidity which does not clear on heating, filtration, or acidification.

emul·soid (e·mul′soid) *n.* [*emuls*ion + *-oid*]. A colloid system whose internal phase is liquid; a lyophilic colloid.

emunc·to·ry (e·munk′tuh·ree) *adj.* & *n.* [ML. *emunctorius,* from L. *emungere,* to wipe the nose]. 1. EXCRETORY. 2. Any body organ that excretes waste products.

em·yl·cam·ate (em″il·kam′ate) *n.* 1-Ethyl-1-methylpropyl carbamate, $C_7H_{15}NO_2$, a mild tranquilizer.

en-, em- [Gk.]. A prefix meaning *in, inside, into.*

enam·el (e·nam′ul) *n.* [OF. *esmail*]. The hard, calcified substance that covers the crown of a tooth.

enamel cap. The enamel covering the top of a growing dental papilla.

enamel column. ENAMEL PRISM.

enamel cord. In developing enamel organs, a transitory, centrally placed column of cells extending from inner to outer enamel epithelium; it later becomes part of the stellate reticulum.

enamel crypt. ENAMEL NICHE.

enamel cuticle. 1. The primary enamel cuticle which is the transitory remnants of the enamel organ and oral epithelium covering the enamel of a tooth after eruption. Syn. *Nasmyth's membrane.* 2. The secondary enamel cuticle which is a keratinized pellicle found between the gingival epithelium and the surface of a tooth. Syn. *Gottlieb's cuticle.* NA *cuticula dentis.*

enamel drop. ENAMELOMA.

enamel fiber. ENAMEL PRISM.

enamel fissure. FISSURE (3).

enamel knot. A group of cells in the enamel pulp in early stages of the enamel organ which have not yet differentiated into stellate reticulum. Syn. *enamel node.*

enamel lamella. A thin organic sheet extending from the surface of the enamel toward and sometimes into the dentin of a tooth. It may be due to local developmental disturbance or a crack filled with organic matter.

enamel navel. In developing enamel organs, a transitory slight depression in the outer enamel epithelium where it is joined by the enamel cord.

enamel niche. A depression between the lateral dental lamina, the dental lamina itself, and the enamel organ.

enamel node. ENAMEL KNOT.

enam·e·lo·blas·to·ma (e·nam″e·lo·blas·to′muh) *n.* [*enamel* + *blastoma*]. AMELOBLASTOMA.

enam·e·lo·ma (e·nam″e·lo′muh) *n.* [*enamel* + *-oma*]. A benign dysontogenetic tumor composed of enamel-producing connective tissue. It commonly appears as a nodule attached to the root of a tooth, but may lie free in the periodontal ligament.

enam·e·lo·plas·ty (e·nam′e·lo·plas″tee) *n.* [*enamel* + *-plasty*]. The act of grinding away a shallow developmental enamel fault or groove to create a smooth saucer-shaped surface which will be a self-cleansing or easily cleaned area; a prophylactic or preventive measure.

enamel organ. The epithelial ingrowth from the dental lamina which covers the dental papilla, furnishes a mold for the shape of a developing tooth, and forms the dental enamel.

enamel pearl. ENAMELOMA.

enamel prisms. Prismatic columns of four to six sides composing the enamel of the teeth, closely packed together and generally vertical to the surface of the underlying dentin. Syn. *enamel rods.* NA *prismata adamantina.*

enamel pulp. The cells between the outer and inner enamel epithelium of the enamel organ. They include the stellate reticulum and the stratum intermedium.

enamel rods. ENAMEL PRISMS.

enamel spindle. An extension of an odontoblastic process across the dentinoenamel junction into the enamel; it occurs prior to calcification, and the process is thickened at its end.

enam·e·lum (e·nam′e·lum) *n.* [NA]. ENAMEL.

enan·thal·de·hide (ee″nan·thal′de·hide) *n.* HEPTALDEHYDE.

enan·thate (ee·nan′thate) *n.* Any salt or ester of enanthic (heptanoic) acid; a heptanoate.

en·an·them (e·nan′thum) *n.* [NL. *enanthema,* from *en-* + *anthema*]. An eruption on a mucous membrane, or within the body. Contr. *exanthem.* —**en·an·them·a·tous** (en″an·them′uh·tus) *adj.*

en·an·the·ma (en″an·theem′uh) *n.,* pl. **enan·the·ma·ta** (·theem′uh·tuh, ·themm′uh·tuh). ENANTHEM.

enan·thic acid (ee·nan′thick). Heptanoic acid, $C_6H_{13}COOH$, an oily liquid.

enantio- [Gk *enantios,* opposite, contrary]. A combining form meaning (a) *opposite;* (b) *antagonistic.*

en·an·tio·dro·mia (en·an″tee·o·dro′mee·uh) *n.* [*enantio-* + *drom-* + *-ia*]. *In analytical psychology,* the concept that everything is eventually transformed into its opposite, as death from life, and vice versa.

en·an·tio·la·lia (en·an″tee·o·lay′lee·uh) *n.* [*enantio-* + *-lalia*]. Talking contrariwise; a disturbance in mental and speech function which prompts ideas and words opposite to those presented as a stimulus.

en·an·tio·mer (en·an′tee·o·mur) *n.* [*enantio-* + *-mer*]. ENANTIOMORPH (1).

en·an·tio·morph (en·an′tee·o·morf) *n.* [*enantio-* + *-morph*]. 1. *In chemistry,* one of a pair of isomeric substances with asymmetric structures that are mirror images of each other. In general, enantiomorphs possess identical chemical and physical properties, but usually differ in their reactions with other asymmetric molecules or in reactions catalyzed by asymmetric molecules, including enzymes. Under identical conditions, they rotate the plane of polarized light to the same extent but in opposite directions. Syn. *enantiomer, optical antipode.* 2. Either of two forms of a crystal which possesses neither a plane nor a center of symmetry but which has a mirror-image resemblance to the other form; under identical conditions the two forms rotate the plane of polarized light to the same extent but in opposite directions. Compare *antipode.* —**en·an·tio·mor·phic** (e·nan″tee·o·mor′fick), **enantiomor·phous** (·fus) *adj.*

en·ar·thro·sis (en″ahr·thro′sis) *n.,* pl. **enarthro·ses** (·seez) [Gk. *enarthrōsis*]. A ball-and-socket joint, such as that of the hip. —**enarthro·di·al** (·dee·ul) *adj.*

en·can·this (en·kanth′is) *n.,* pl. **encan·thi·des** (·i·deez) [Gk. *enkanthis*]. A neoplasm in the inner canthus of the eye.

en·cap·su·la·tion (en·kap″sue·lay′shun) *n.* The process of surrounding a part with a capsule. —**en·cap·su·late** (en·kap′sue·late) *v.*

en·cap·suled (en·kap′sue′ld) *adj.* Enclosed in a capsule or sheath.

encephal-, encephalo-. A combining form meaning *encephalon, brain.*

en·ceph·a·lal·gia (en·sef″uh·lal′jee·uh) *n.* [*encephal-* + *-algia*]. HEADACHE.

en·ceph·al·at·ro·phy (en·sef″uh·lat′ruh·fee) *n.* [*encephal-* + *atrophy*]. Atrophy of the brain.

-encephalia. See *-encephaly.*

en·ce·phal·ic (en″se·fal′ick) *adj.* Pertaining to or involving the brain or encephalon.

encephalitic meningitis. MENINGOENCEPHALITIS.

encephalitic poliomyelitis. Poliomyelitis in which, in addition to bulbar and spinal lesions, there is involvement of the motor cortex.

en·ceph·a·li·tis (en·sef″uh·lye′tis) *n.,* pl. **encepha·lit·i·des** (·lit′i·deez) [*encephal-* + *-itis*]. Inflammation of the brain. —**en·cepha·lit·ic** (·lit′ick) *adj.*

encephalitis le·thar·gi·ca (le·thahr′ji·kuh). Epidemic encephalitis reported in the first quarter of the 20th century, probably of viral etiology, characterized by lethargy, ophthalmoplegia, hyperkinesia, and at times residual neurologic disability, particularly parkinsonism with oculogyric crisis. Syn. *epidemic encephalitis, sleeping sickness, von Economo's disease.*

encephalitis peri·ax·i·a·lis con·cen·tri·ca (perr″ee·ack·see·ay′lis kon·sen′tri·kuh). CONCENTRIC SCLEROSIS.

encephalitis peri·ax·i·a·lis dif·fu·sa (perr″ee·ack″see·ay′lis di·few′suh). SCHILDER'S DISEASE.

en·ceph·a·li·to·gen·ic (en·sef″uh·li·to·jen′ick) *adj.* [*encephalitis* + *-genic*]. Producing, or capable of producing, encephalitis.

En·ce·phal·i·to·zo·on cu·nic·u·li (en″se·fal″i·to·zo′on kew·nick·yoo·lye) [*encephalitis* + *-zoon;* L. *cuniculi,* of the rabbit]. An intracellular protozoan parasite commonly found in the kidneys and brain of rabbits and less frequently in mice, rats, guinea pigs, and hamsters. Syn. *Nosema cuniculi.* See also *encephalitozoonosis.*

en·ce·phal·i·to·zo·o·no·sis (en″se·fal″i·to·zo″o·no′sis, ·zo·on′o·sis) *n.* Infection by the protozoan parasite *Encephalitozoon cuniculi;* usually asymptomatic, but may be responsible for tremors, paresis, and convulsions in rabbits. Syn. *nosematosis.*

encephalo-. See *encephal-.*

en·ceph·a·lo·cele (en·sef′uh·lo·seel) *n.* [*encephalo-* + *-cele*]. Hernia of the brain through a congenital or traumatic opening in the cranium.

en·ceph·a·lo·clas·tic (en·sef″uh·lo·klas′tick) *adj.* [*encephalo-* + *clastic*]. Destructive of brain tissue.

encephaloclastic porencephaly. A cavity in the cerebrum which connects with one of the lateral ventricles due to destruction of brain tissue; usually congenital, it may be acquired under certain conditions.

en·ceph·a·lo·cra·nio·cu·ta·ne·ous (en·sef″uh·lo·kray″nee·o·kew·tay′nee·us) *adj.* [*encephalo-* + *cranio-* + *cutaneous*]. Pertaining to the brain, the skull, and the skin.

en·ceph·a·lo·cys·to·cele (en·sef″uh·lo·sis′to·seel) *n.* [*encephalo-* + *cysto-* + *-cele*]. HYDRENCEPHALOCELE.

en·ceph·a·lo·cys·to·me·nin·go·cele (en·sef″uh·lo·sis″to·me·ning′go·seel) *n.* [*encephalo-* + *cysto-* + *meningocele*]. HYDRENCEPHALOMENINGOCELE.

en·ceph·a·lo·dys·pla·sia (en·sef″uh·lo·dis·play′zhuh, ·zee·uh) *n.* [*encephalo-* + *dysplasia*]. Maldevelopment of the brain.

en·ceph·a·lo·fa·cial (en·sef″uh·lo·fay′shul) *adj.* [*encephalo-* + *facial*]. Pertaining to the brain and face.

encephalofacial angiomatosis. STURGE-WEBER DISEASE.

en·ceph·a·lo·gram (en·sef′uh·lo·gram) *n.* A roentgenogram of the brain made in encephalography.

en·ceph·a·log·ra·phy (en·sef″uh·log′ruh·fee) *n.* [*encephalo-* + *-graphy*]. Radiography of the brain following removal of cerebrospinal fluid, by lumbar or cisternal puncture, and its replacement by air, other gas, or contrast material.

en·ceph·a·loid (en·sef′uh·loid) *adj.* [*encephal-* + *-oid*]. 1. Resembling the brain or brain tissue. 2. Of soft, brainlike consistency.

encephaloid carcinoma. MEDULLARY CARCINOMA.

en·ceph·a·lo·lith (en·sef′uh·lo·lith) *n.* [*encephalo-* + *-lith*]. A calculus of the brain.

en·ceph·a·lol·o·gy (en·sef″uh·lol′uh·jee) *n.* [*encephalo-* + *-logy*]. The study of the brain; the sum of the knowledge regarding the brain.

en·ceph·a·lo·ma (en·sef″uh·lo′muh) *n.*, pl. **encephalomas, encephaloma·ta** (·tuh) [*encephal-* + *-oma*]. 1. A tumor of the brain. 2. MEDULLARY CARCINOMA.

en·ceph·a·lo·ma·la·cia (en·sef″uh·lo·ma·lay′shuh, shee·uh) *n.* [*encephalo-* + *malacia*]. Softening of the brain due to infarction.

en·ceph·a·lo·men·in·gi·tis (en·sef″uh·lo·men″in·jye′tis) *n.* MENINGOENCEPHALITIS.

en·ceph·a·lo·me·nin·go·cele (en·sef″uh·lo·me·ning′go·seel) *n.* [*encephalo-* + *meningo-* + *-cele*]. Hernia of the membranes and brain substance through an opening in the cranium.

en·ceph·a·lo·men·in·gop·a·thy (en·sef″uh·lo·men″ing·gop′uth·ee) *n.* [*encephalo-* + *meningo-* + *-pathy*]. MENINGOENCEPHALOPATHY.

en·ceph·a·lo·mere (en·sef′uh·lo·meer) *n.* [*encephalo-* + *-mere*]. Any one of the succession of segments of the embryonic brain; a neuromere of the brain. —**en·ceph·a·lo·mer·ic** (en·sef″uh·lo·merr′ick) *adj.*

en·ceph·a·lom·e·ter (en·sef″uh·lom′e·tur) *n.* [*encephalo-* + *-meter*]. An instrument for measuring the cranium, and locating certain regions of the brain. See also *stereoencephalotome.*

en·ceph·a·lo·my·e·li·tis (en·sef″uh·lo·migh″e·lye′tis) *n.* [*encephalo-* + *myel-* + *-itis*]. Inflammation of the brain and spinal cord.

encephalomyelitis of swine. TESCHEN DISEASE.

en·ceph·a·lo·my·e·lo·neu·rop·a·thy (en·sef″uh·lo·migh″e·lo·new·rop′uth·ee) *n.* [*encephalo-* + *myelo-* + *neuro-* + *-pathy*]. Disease of the brain, spinal cord, and peripheral nervous system.

en·ceph·a·lo·my·e·lon·ic (en·sef″uh·lo·migh″e·lon′ick) *adj.* [*encephalo-* + *myelon* + *-ic*]. Pertaining to the brain and spinal cord.

encephalomyelonic axis. CENTRAL NERVOUS SYSTEM.

en·ceph·a·lo·my·e·lop·a·thy (en·sef″uh·lo·migh″e·lop′uth·ee) *n.* [*encephalo-* + *myelo-* + *-pathy*]. Any disease affecting both brain and spinal cord.

en·ceph·a·lo·my·e·lo·sis (en·sef″uh·lo·migh·e·lo′sis) *n.* [*encephalo-* + *myel-* + *-osis*]. ENCEPHALOMYELOPATHY.

en·ceph·a·lo·myo·car·di·tis (en·sef″uh·lo·migh″o·kahr·dye′tis) *n.* [*encephalo-* + *myocarditis*]. An acute febrile illness, usually of infants and children, characterized by encephalitis and myocarditis; caused by a variety of viruses, including the encephalomyocarditis virus (named for this disease), and Columbia-SK, Mengo, and Coxsackie viruses.

en·ceph·a·lon (en·sef′uh·lon) *n.*, genit. **encepha·li** (lye), pl. **encepha·la** (·luh) [Gk. *enkephalos,* from *kephalē,* head] [NA]. BRAIN.

en·ceph·a·lo·nar·co·sis (en·sef″uh·lo·nahr·ko′sis) *n.* [*encephalo-* + *narcosis*]. Stupor from a brain lesion.

en·ceph·a·lop·a·thy (en·sef″uh·lop′uth·ee) *n.* [*encephalo-* + *-pathy*]. Any disease of the brain.

encephalopathy and fatty degeneration of viscera. REYE'S SYNDROME.

en·ceph·a·lo·punc·ture (en·sef′uh·lo·punk″chur) *n.* [*encephalo-* + *puncture*]. Puncture of the substance of the brain, as from trauma or surgical procedure.

en·ceph·a·lo·py·o·sis (en·sef″uh·lo·pye·o′sis) *n.* [*encephalo-* + *pyosis*]. Suppuration or abscess of the brain.

en·ceph·a·lo·ra·chid·i·an (en·sef″uh·lo·ra·kid′ee·un) *adj.* [*encephalo-* + *rachidian*]. CEREBROSPINAL.

en·ceph·a·lor·rha·gia (en·sef″uh·lo·ray′jee·uh) *n.* [*encephalo-* + *-rrhagia*]. A cerebral hemorrhage. See also *pericapillary encephalorrhagia.*

en·ceph·a·lo·scle·ro·sis (en·sef″uh·lo·skle·ro′sis) *n.* [*encephalo-* + *sclerosis*]. Sclerosis of the brain.

en·ceph·a·lo·scope (en·sef′uh·lo·skope) *n.* [*encephalo-* + *-scope*]. An instrument, similar to a cystoscope, for the visualization of a cavity, particularly the ventricles in the brain. —**en·ceph·a·los·co·py** (en·sef″uh·los′kuh·pee) *n.*

en·ceph·a·lo·sep·sis (en·sef″uh·lo·sep′sis) *n.* [*encephalo-* + *sepsis*]. Septic inflammation of brain tissue.

en·ceph·a·lo·sis (en·sef″uh·lo′sis) *n.*, pl. **encephalo·ses** (·seez) [*encephal-* + *-osis*]. ENCEPHALOPATHY.

en·ceph·a·lo·spi·nal (en·sef″uh·lo·spye′nul) *adj.* [*encephalo-* + *spinal*]. Pertaining to the brain and the spinal cord.

encephalospinal axis. CENTRAL NERVOUS SYSTEM.

en·ceph·a·lo·tome (en·sef′uh·lo·tome) *n.* [*encephalo-* + *-tome*]. 1. An instrument for dissecting the brain. 2. A surgical instrument for incising the brain. 3. A surgical instrument for destroying the cranium of a fetus to facilitate delivery.

en·ceph·a·lot·o·my (en·sef″uh·lot′uh·mee) *n.* [*encephalo-* + *-tomy*]. 1. Surgical incision of the brain. 2. Operative destruction of the fetal cranium to facilitate delivery. 3. Dissection of the brain.

en·ceph·a·lo·tri·gem·i·nal (en·sef″uh·lo·trye·jem′i·nul) *adj.* [*encephalo-* + *trigeminal*]. Pertaining to the brain and the trigeminal nerve.

encephalotrigeminal angiomatosis. STURGE-WEBER DISEASE.

-encephalus [Gk. *enkephalos,* brain]. A combining form meaning (a) *individual with a* (specified type of) *brain;* (b) *the condition of having such a brain.*

-encephaly [*encephal-* + *-y*]. A combining form meaning *the condition of having a* (specified type or condition of) *brain.*

en·chon·dral (en·kon′drul) *adj.* [*en-* + *chondral*]. ENDOCHONDRAL.

en·chon·dro·ma (en″kon·dro′muh) *n.*, pl. **enchondroma·ta**

(·tuh), **enchondromas** [*en-* + *chondroma*]. A benign tumor composed of dysplastic cartilage cells, occurring in the metaphysis of cylindric bones, especially of the hands and feet. —**enchon·drom·a·tous** (·dro'muh·tus, ·drom'uh·tus) *adj.*

en·chon·dro·ma·to·sis (en·kon"dro·muh·to'sis, en"kon·dro") *n.* [*enchondroma* + *-osis*]. A rare disorder principally involving tubular bones, especially those of the hands and feet, characterized by hamartomatous proliferation of cartilage in the metaphysis, indistinguishable in single lesions from enchondromas. Chondrosarcomas may appear in the involved areas in later life. Syn. *Ollier's disease.* See also *Maffucci's syndrome.*

en·chon·dro·sar·co·ma (en·kon"dro·sahr·ko'muh) *n.* CHONDROSARCOMA.

en·chon·dro·sis (en"kon·dro'sis) *n.* ENCHONDROMATOSIS.

en·chy·le·ma (en"kigh·lee'muh, eng"ki·) *n.* [*en-* + *chyle* + *-ēma* (noun-formative ending)]. HYALOPLASM.

en·clit·ic (en·klit'ick) *adj.* [Gk. *enklitikos,* from *enklisis,* inclination]. Presenting obliquely; not synclitic; designating the inclination of the pelvic planes to those of the fetal head.

en·clo·mi·phene (en·klo'mi·feen) *n.* (*E*)-2-[*p*-(2-Chloro-1,2-diphenylvinyl)phenoxy]triethylamine, $C_{26}H_{28}ClNO$, the *cis-* form of clomiphene, a gonad-stimulating agent.

en·cod·ing, *n.* The process whereby a message or code is transformed into signals or symbols in a communication system, or converted from one system of communication into another, as the translation of chemical into electrical data.

en·col·pi·tis (en"kol·pye'tis) *n.* Endocolpitis (= MUCOUS VAGINITIS.

en·cop·re·sis (en"kop·ree'sis) *n.* [Gk. *enkopros,* full of manure, + *-esis*]. Psychically caused incontinence of feces; soiling. Compare *enuresis.*

en·cra·ni·us (en·kray'nee·us) *n.* [*en-* + *cranium* + *-us*]. An episphenoid teratoid parasite that lies within the cranium of the autosite.

en·crust, in·crust (in·krust') *v.* To form a crust or hard coating on. —**encrust·ed, incrust·ed,** *adj.*

en·crus·ta·tion (en"krus·tay'shun) *n.* INCRUSTATION.

en·cy·e·sis (en"sigh·ee'sis) *n.* [Gk. *enkyēsis,* germination, from *kyēsis,* pregnancy]. *Obsol.* PREGNANCY.

en·cy·prate (en·sigh'prate) *n.* Ethyl *N*-benzylcyclopropanecarbamate, $C_{13}H_{17}NO_2$, a monoamine oxidase inhibitor used as an antidepressant.

en·cys·ta·tion (en"sis·tay'shun) *n.* 1. Enclosure in a cyst or sac. 2. The process of forming a cyst. —**en·cyst** (en·sist') *v.*

en·cyst·ed (en·sis'tid) *adj.* Enclosed in a cyst or capsule.

encysted bladder. A urinary bladder with communicating cysts.

encysted calculus. A calculus confined in a localized dilatation or diverticulum of the urinary bladder or gallbladder.

encysted hydrocele. A hydrocele that occupies a portion of the tunica vaginalis with closure of the abdominal and scrotal ends.

en·cyst·ment (en·sist'munt) *n.* ENCYSTATION.

end-, endo- [Gk. *endon,* inside]. A combining form meaning (a) *within;* (b) *inner, internal;* (c) *taking in, absorbing, requiring.*

end·adel·phus (end"uh·del'fus) *n.* [*end-* + *-adelphus*]. CRYPTODIDYMUS.

end·am·e·bi·a·sis, end·am·oe·bi·a·sis (end"am·ee·bye'uh·sis) *n.* [*Endamoeba* + *-iasis*]. AMEBIASIS.

End·amoe·ba (end"uh·mee'buh) *n.* ENTAMOEBA.

end·an·gi·i·tis, end·an·ge·i·tis (end"an·jee·eye'tis) *n.* [*end-* + *angiitis*]. Inflammation of the intima of a blood vessel; endarteritis or endophlebitis. Syn. *intimitis.*

end·aor·ti·tis (end"ay·or·tye'tis) *n.* [*end-* + *aortitis*]. Inflammation of the intima of the aorta.

end arborization. One of the small nonmyelinated branches at the end of an axon. Syn. *end branch.*

end·ar·ter·ec·to·my (end"ahr·tur·eck'tuh·mee) *n.* [*end-* + *arterectomy*]. The surgical removal of an organized thrombus and the attached endothelium or an atheromatous intima from a segment of an artery which has become thrombosed or narrowed.

end·ar·te·ri·al (end"ahr·teer'ee·ul) *adj.* 1. Within an artery. 2. Pertaining to the intima of an artery.

end·ar·te·ri·ec·to·my (end"ahr·teer"ee·eck'tuh·mee) *n.* ENDARTERECTOMY.

end·ar·te·ri·tis (end"arh·te·rye'tis) *n.* [*end-* + *arteritis*]. Inflammation of the inner coat or intima of an artery. Contr. *periarteritis.*

endarteritis de·for·mans (de·for'manz). Endarteritis obliterans with calcification.

endarteritis obli·te·rans (ob·lit'e·ranz). A degenerative arterial disease, chiefly of the small arteries of the extremities, in which muscular and fibrous hyperplasia of the media and intima lead to luminal stenosis and, sometimes, occlusion. See also *arteriosclerosis obliterans.*

end artery. An artery without branches or anastomoses.

end·au·ral (end·aw'rul) *adj.* [*end-* + *aural*]. Pertaining to the inner surface or part of the external acoustic meatus.

end·axo·neu·ron (end"ack·so·new'ron) *n.* [*end-* + *axo-* + *neuron*]. *Obsol.* A neuron whose nerve process does not leave the spinal cord.

end·brain, *n.* TELENCEPHALON.

end branch. END ARBORIZATION.

end bud. A mass of indifferent cells produced by the remnant of Hensen's node; it develops into the caudal part of the trunk without forming distinctive germ layers.

end bulb. 1. An end foot, particularly one of the larger end feet. 2. KRAUSE'S CORPUSCLE.

en·dem·ic (en·dem'ick) *adj.* [Gk. *endēmos,* native]. Peculiar to a certain region or people; said of a disease that occurs more or less constantly in any particular locality. Compare *epidemic, ecdemic, sporadic.*

endemic cretinism. Cretinism due to maternal iodide deficiency occurring in regions where little iodide is naturally available in foods; now relatively uncommon as a result of the availability of iodinated salt and other foods.

endemic goiter. Goiter occurring commonly in mountainous or other geographic areas where the diet is deficient in iodine.

endemic influenza. Influenza occurring sporadically, usually less severe than pandemic influenza.

endemic neuritis. BERIBERI.

endemic syphilis. BEJEL.

endemic typhus. MURINE TYPHUS.

Endep. A trademark for amitriptyline hydrochloride, an antidepressant.

end·ep·i·der·mis (end·ep"i·dur'mis) *n.* [*end-* + *epidermis*]. The inner layer of the epidermis.

end·er·gon·ic (end"ur·gon'ick) *adj.* [*end-* + Gk. *ergon,* work, + *-ic*]. Of or pertaining to a chemical reaction in which the final products possess more free energy than the starting materials; usually associated with anabolism. This energy may be drawn from concomitant catabolism or from an external source. Contr. *exergonic.*

en·der·mic (en·dur'mick) *adj.* [*en-* + *derm-* + *-ic*]. Acting through the skin by absorption, as medication applied to the skin.

en·der·mo·sis (en"dur·mo'sis) *n.* [*en-* + *derm-* + *-osis*]. 1. Administration of medicines through the skin, by rubbing. 2. Any herpetic affection of a mucosa.

end feet. Small terminal enlargements of nerve fibers which are in contact with the dendrites or cell bodies of other nerve cells; the synaptic endings of nerve fibers. Syn. *boutons terminaux, end bulbs.*

end gain. PRIMARY GAIN.

endo-. See *end-.*

en·do·ab·dom·i·nal (en"do·ab·dom'i·nul) *adj.* Within the abdomen; intraabdominal.

en·do·an·eu·rys·mor·rha·phy (en″do·an″yoo·riz·mor′uh·fee) *n.* [*endo-* + *aneurysmorrhaphy*]. An operation for aneurysm consisting of opening the sac, suturing the orifices of the communicating arteries, and folding and suturing the walls of the aneurysm, thus leaving a lumen of approximately normal size.

en·do·an·gi·i·tis (en″do·an″jee·eye′tis) *n.* ENDANGIITIS.

en·do·aor·ti·tis (en″do·ay″or·tye′tis) *n.* ENDAORTITIS.

en·do·ar·te·ri·tis (en″do·ahr″te·rye′tis) *n.* ENDARTERITIS.

en·do·bi·ot·ic (en″do·bye·ot′ick) *adj.* [*endo-* + *biotic*]. Of a parasite: living in the tissues of the host.

en·do·bron·chi·al (en″do·bronk′ee·ul) *adj.* [*endo-* + *bronchial*]. 1. Within a bronchus. 2. Within the bronchial tree.

Endocaine. Trademark for pyrrocaine, a local anesthetic.

en·do·car·di·al (en″do·kahr′dee·ul) *adj.* 1. Pertaining to the endocardium. 2. Occurring or situated in the heart.

endocardial blood cyst. Any of the small, circumscribed, nodular, dark-red cystlike lesions usually seen on the atrial surface of the mitral and tricuspid valves, occurring frequently in newborn infants, occasionally in children, and rarely in adults.

endocardial cushion. In the embryonic heart, either of two masses of embryonic connective tissue concerned with the development of the atrioventricular canals and valves.

endocardial fibroelastosis. Fibrous or fibroelastic thickening of the endocardium of unknown cause, but which may be congenital, hereditary, or secondary to other systemic or cardiac disease, usually associated with congestive heart failure and cardiac enlargement.

endocardial fibrosis. ENDOCARDIAL FIBROELASTOSIS.

endocardial murmur. A murmur resulting from endocardial, usually valvular, disease.

endocardial ridge. One of a pair of internal spiral ridges in the embryonic bulbus cordis whose fusion initiates the division of the bulbus into aortic and pulmonary trunks as well as forming part of the septum membranaceum.

endocardial sclerosis. ENDOCARDIAL FIBROELASTOSIS.

en·do·car·di·tis (en″do·kahr·dye′tis) *n.* [*endocardium* + *-itis*]. Inflammation of the endocardium or lining membrane of the heart cavities and its valves. See also *acute bacterial endocarditis, bacterial endocarditis.* —**endocar·dit·ic** (·dit′ick) *adj.*

endocarditis len·ta (len′tuh) [L., slow]. BACTERIAL ENDOCARDITIS.

en·do·car·di·um (en″do·kahr′dee·um) *n.*, pl. **endocar·dia** (·dee·uh) [*endo-* + *-cardium*] [NA]. The membrane lining the interior of the heart, consisting of endothelium and the subjacent connective tissue. See also Plate 5.

en·do·carp (en′do·kahrp) *n.* [*endo-* + *-carp*]. The inner coat of a pericarp.

en·do·ce·li·ac, en·do·coe·li·ac (en″do·see′lee·ack) *adj.* [*endo-* + *celiac*]. Within one of the body cavities, particularly the abdominal cavity.

en·do·cel·lu·lar (en″do·sel′yoo·lur) *adj.* [*endo-* + *cellular*]. INTRACELLULAR.

en·do·cer·vi·cal (en″do·sur′vi·kul) *adj.* [*endo-* + *cervical*]. Pertaining to the inside of the uterine cervix.

endocervical canal. The portion of the uterine cavity situated in the cervix, extending from the isthmus to the ostium of the uterus. Syn. *canal of the cervix of the uterus.* NA *canalis cervicis uteri.*

en·do·cer·vi·ci·tis (en″do·sur″vi·sigh′tis) *n.* [*endocervix* + *-itis*]. Inflammation of the mucous membrane of the uterine cervix.

en·do·cer·vix (en″do·sur′vicks) *n.*, pl. **endocer·vi·ces** (·vi·seez) [*endo-* + *cervix*]. The glandular mucous membrane of the uterine cervix.

en·do·cho·le·doch·al (en″do·ko″le·dock′ul, ·ko·led′uh·kul) *adj.* [*endo-* + *choledochal*]. Within the common bile duct.

en·do·chon·dral (en″do·kon′drul) *adj.* [*endo-* + *chondral*]. Situated within cartilage.

endochondral bone formation. ENDOCHONDRAL OSTEOGENESIS.

endochondral osteogenesis. A type of bone formation in which the osseous tissue produced largely replaces a preexisting mass of cartilage.

en·do·chon·dro·ma (en″do·kon·dro′muh) *n.* [*endo-* + *chondroma*]. ENCHONDROMA.

endocoeliac. ENDOCELIAC.

en·do·col·pi·tis (en″do·kol·pye′tis) *n.* [*endo-* + *colpitis*]. MUCOUS VAGINITIS.

en·do·cra·ni·tis (en″do·kruh·nigh′tis, ·kray·nigh′tis) *n.* [*endo-* + *cranium* + *-itis*]. An epidural abscess of the cranium.

en·do·cra·ni·um (en″do·kray′nee·um) *n.*, pl. **endocra·nia** (·nee·uh) [*endo-* + *cranium*]. The inner lining of the skull; DURA MATER. —**endocrani·al** (·ul) *adj.*

en·do·crine (en′do·krin, ·krine) *adj.* [*endo-* + *-crine*]. 1. Secreting directly into the bloodstream, as a ductless gland. 2. Of or pertaining to the endocrine glands or their secretions. Contr. *exocrine.* —**en·do·crin·ic** (en″do·krin′ick) *adj.*

endocrine gland. Any gland that secretes hormonal substances directly into the bloodstream, as the hypophysis, the islets of the pancreas, the thyroid and parathyroid glands, the adrenal glands, the pineal body, the ovaries and testes. See also Plate 26.

endocrine obesity. Obesity due to dysfunction of the endocrine glands.

endocrine therapy. ENDOCRINOTHERAPY.

en·do·cri·nol·o·gy (en″do·kri·nol′uh·jee) *n.* [*endocrine* + *-logy*]. The study of the endocrine glands and their function.

endocrinopathic amenorrhea. Abnormal amenorrhea due to unphysiologic function or dysfunction of one or more of the endocrine glands. It does not include such cessation of function as normal menopause or lactation amenorrhea.

en·do·cri·nop·a·thy (en″do·kri·nop′uth·ee) *n.* [*endocrine* + *-pathy*]. A disorder resulting from abnormality in one or more of the endocrine glands or their secretions. —**endo·crino·path·ic** (·krin″o·path′ick) *adj.*

en·do·crino·ther·a·py (en″do·krin″o·therr′uh·pee) *n.* [*endocrine* + *therapy*]. Treatment of disease by the administration of endocrine substances.

en·doc·ri·nous (en·dock′ri·nus) *adj.* ENDOCRINE.

en·do·cy·ma (en″do·sigh′muh) *n.* [*endo-* + Gk. *kyma*, fetus]. A type of cryptodidymus in which the parasitic twin is visceral in location.

en·do·cyst (en′do·sist) *n.* [*endo-* + *cyst*]. BROOD MEMBRANE.

en·do·cys·ti·tis (en″do·sis·tye′tis) *n.* [*endo-* + *cystitis*]. Inflammation of the mucous membrane lining the bladder.

en·do·cyte (en′do·site) *n.* [*endo-* + *-cyte*]. A cell inclusion of any type.

en·do·cy·to·sis (en″do·sigh·to′sis) *n.* [*endocyte* + *-osis*]. The engulfment by a cell of a substance or object. Contr. *exocytosis.* See also *phagocytosis, pinocytosis.*

en·do·derm (en′do·durm) *n.* [*endo-* + *-derm*]. The innermost of the three primary germ layers, which forms the lining of the gut, from pharynx to rectum, and its derivatives. Syn. *entoderm.* Contr. *ectoderm, mesoderm.* —**en·do·der·mal** (en″do·dur′mul) *adj.*

en·do·der·ma·to·zoo·no·sis (en″do·dur″muh·to·zo″uh·no′sis) *n.* [*endo-* + *dermatozoonosis*]. A skin disease in which a parasite burrows deeply into and remains embedded within the skin, as certain ascarid and some oestrid larvae.

en·do·der·mo·phy·to·sis (en″do·dur″mo·figh·to′sis) *n.* [*endo-* + *dermophyte* + *-osis*]. TINEA IMBRICATA.

en·do·don·tia (en″do·don′chee·uh) *n.* [*end-* + *-odontia*]. ENDODONTOLOGY.

en·do·don·tics (en″do·don′ticks) *n.* The branch of dental practice that applies the science of endodontology. —**endodontic,** *adj.*

en·do·don·tist (en″do·don′tist) *n.* A dentist who specializes in endodontics.

en·do·don·tol·ogy (en″do·don·tol′uh·jee) *n.* [*end-* + *odontol-*

ogy]. The body of knowledge or science of disease of the dental pulp and associated processes; it deals with etiology, prevention, diagnosis, and treatment. Syn. *endodontia.*

en·do·en·ter·i·tis (en″do·en″tur·eye′tis) *n.* [*endo-* + *enteritis*]. Inflammation of the mucous membrane lining the intestine.

en·do·en·zyme (en″do·en′zime, ·zim) *n.* [*endo-* + *enzyme*]. An intracellular enzyme that is not excreted but is retained in the originating cell.

en·do·er·gic (en″do·ur′jick) *adj.* [*endo-* + *erg-* + *-ic*]. ENDOTHERMIC.

en·dog·a·my (en·dog′uh·mee) *n.* [*endo-* + *-gamy*]. 1. Conjugation between gametes having the same chromatin ancestry. 2. *In anthropology,* marriage between members of the same tribe, community, or other social group, as established by law or custom. Contr. *exogamy.* —**endoga·mous** (·mus) *adj.*

en·do·ge·net·ic (en″do·je·net′ick) *adj.* [*endo-* + *genetic*]. ENDOGENOUS.

en·do·gen·ic (en″do·jen′ick) *adj.* ENDOGENOUS.

endogenic toxicosis. Toxicosis due to toxic substances produced within the body; AUTOINTOXICATION.

en·dog·e·nous (en·doj′e·nus) *adj.* [*endo-* + *-genous*]. 1. Produced within; due to internal causes; applied to the formation of cells or of spores within the parent cell. 2. Pertaining to the metabolism of the nitrogenous elements of tissues. 3. *In psychology,* pertaining to forms of mental disorders and deficiency based on hereditary or constitutional factors; originating within the body and directly affecting the nervous system. Contr. *exogenous.*

endogenous aneurysm. An aneurysm formed by disease of the vessel walls.

endogenous cycle. The phase of development of the *Plasmodium malariae* or other parasite which occurs in the vertebrate host, man.

endogenous lipid pneumonia. LIPID PNEUMONIA (2).

endogenous tuberculosis. Tuberculosis arising from a primary source within the body, even after it has been considered quiescent or healed.

en·dog·e·ny (en·doj′e·nee) *n.* [*endo-* + *-geny*]. *In biology,* growth from within; endogenous formation.

en·do·gna·thi·on (en″do·nay′thee·on, ·nath′ee·on) *n.* [NL., from *endo-* + Gk. *gnathos,* jaw]. A hypothetical medial portion of the premaxilla (incisive bone). Contr. *mesognathion.*

en·do·go·ni·um (en″do·go′nee·um) *n.* [*endo-* + *gonium*]. A gonidium formed inside a receptacle or parent cell.

en·do·la·ryn·ge·al (en″do·la·rin′jee·ul, ·lăr″in·jee′ul) *adj.* [*endo-* + *laryngeal*]. Within the larynx.

En·do·li·max (en″do·lye′macks) *n.* [*endo-* + Gk. *leimax,* slug]. A genus of protozoans of the family Amoebidae, parasitic in man, but nonpathogenic.

Endolimax na·na (nay′nuh). An intestinal commensal ameba of man and other animals in which the nucleus contains a large karyosome; occurs as a trophozoite or as a cyst containing up to four nuclei.

en·do·lymph (en′do·limf) *n.* [*endo-* + *lymph*]. The fluid of the membranous labyrinth of the ear. —**en·do·lym·phat·ic** (en″do·lim·fat′ick), **endo·lym·phic** (·lim′fick) *adj.*

en·do·lym·pha (en″do·lim′fuh) *n.* [NA]. ENDOLYMPH.

en·do·lym·phan·gi·al, en·do·lym·phan·ge·al (en″do·lim·fan′jee·ul) *adj.* [*endo-* + *lymph-* + *-angi-* + *-al*]. Situated or belonging within a lymph vessel.

endolymphatic duct. 1. The duct which unites the endolymphatic sac with the utriculosaccular duct. Syn. *otic duct.* NA *ductus endolymphaticus, aqueductus vestibuli.* 2. *In embryology,* a dorsomedian diverticulum of the otocyst, the anlage of the endolymphatic sac.

endolymphatic hydrops. MÉNIÈRE'S SYNDROME.

endolymphatic sac. The bulblike terminal enlargement of the endolymphatic duct. NA *saccus endolymphaticus.*

endolymphatic shunt. An operation devised to decrease pressure in the endolymphatic system, especially in Ménière's disease.

endolymphatic space. The space containing the endolymphatic sac, situated behind the petrous portion of the temporal bone and communicating with the aqueduct of the vestibule.

endolymphatic stromal myosis. STROMATOSIS.

en·do·ly·sin (en″do·lye′sin, en·dol′i·sin) *n.* [*endo-* + *-lysin*]. A heat-stable endocellular bactericidal substances especially abundant in leukocytes. Syn. *leukin.*

en·do·me·ninx (en″do·mee′ninks, men′inks) *n.,* pl. **endo·me·nin·ges** (·me·nin′jeez) [*endo-* + *meninx*]. The internal part of the meninx primitiva that differentiates into the pia mater and arachnoid membrane.

en·do·meso·derm (en″do·mes′o·durm, ·mez′o·) *n.* [*endo-* + *mesoderm*]. Mesoderm derived from the primary entoderm of a bilaminar blastodisk or gastrula.

en·do·meso·vas·cu·li·tis (en″do·mez″o·vas·kew·lye′tis) *n.* [*endo-* + *meso-* + *vasculitis*]. Abnormal thickening of the intima and media of spinal cord blood vessels, especially veins; noted in subacute necrotic myelopathy.

en·do·me·tri·al (en″do·mee′tree·ul) *adj.* Pertaining to or consisting of endometrium.

endometrial cycle. The periodically recurring series of changes in the uterine mucosa associated with menstruation and the intermenstrual interval in primates, e.g., menstruating endometrium to interval endometrium to secretory endometrium to premenstrual endometrium.

endometrial implantation cyst. CYSTIC ENDOMETRIOSIS.

en·do·me·tri·oid (en″do·mee′tree·oid) *adj.* [*endometri*um + *-oid*]. Resembling endometrium.

endometrioid adenofibrosis. ADENOMYOSIS.

en·do·me·tri·o·ma (en″do·mee″tree·o′muh) *n.,* pl. **endometriomas, endometrioma·ta** (·tuh) [*endometri*um + *-oma*]. Endometriosis in which there is a discrete tumor mass.

en·do·me·tri·o·sis (en″do·mee″tree·o′sis) *n.,* pl. **endometrio·ses** (·seez) [*endometri*um + *-osis*]. The presence of endometrial tissue in abnormal locations, including the uterine wall, ovaries, or extragenital sites. —**endometri·ot·ic** (·ot′ick) *adj.*

en·do·me·tri·tis (en″do·me·trye′tis) *n.* [*endometri*um + *-itis*]. Inflammation of the endometrium.

endometritis ex·fo·li·a·ti·va (ecks·fo″lee·uh·tye′vuh). MEMBRANOUS DYSMENORRHEA.

en·do·me·tri·um (en″do·mee′tree·um) *n.,* pl. **endome·tria** (·tree·uh) [NL., from *endo-* + Gk. *mētra,* womb]. The mucous membrane lining the uterus. NA *tunica mucosa uteri.*

en·dom·e·try (en·dom′e·tree) *n.* [*endo-* + *-metry*]. The measurement of the interior of an organ or cavity.

en·do·mi·to·sis (en″do·migh·to′sis) *n.* [*endo-* + *mitosis*]. The duplication of chromosomes without any accompanying spindle formation or cytokinesis.

en·do·morph (en′do·morf) *n.* [*endo-* + *-morph*]. In the somatotype, an individual exhibiting relative predominance of endomorphy.

en·do·mor·phy (en′do·mor″fee) *n.* [*endo-* + *-morphy*]. Component I of the somatotype, representing relative predominance of soft and round body features. In normal nutritional status, the abdominal viscera, whose functional elements are derived from entoderm, are prominent. Endomorphs tend to be fat. Contr. *ectomorphy, mesomorphy.* See also *viscerotonia.* —**endomor·phic** (·fick) *adj.*

en·do·myo·car·di·tis (en″do·migh″o·kahr·dye′tis) *n.* [*endo-* + *myo-* + *carditis*]. Inflammation of the endocardium and myocardium.

en·do·mys·i·um (en″do·mis′ee·um, ·miz′ee·um) *n.,* pl. **endo·my·sia** (·ee·uh) [NL., from *endo-* + Gk. *mys,* muscle]. The connective tissue between the fibers of a muscle bundle, or fasciculus. —**endomysi·al** (·ul) *adj.*

en·do·na·sal (en″do·nay′zul) *n.* [*endo-* + *nasal*]. Within the nasal cavity.

en·do·neu·ral (en″do·new′rul) *adj.* [*endo-* + *neural*]. Pertaining to or situated in the interior of a nerve.

endoneural fibroma. NEUROFIBROMA.

en·do·neu·ri·um (en″do·new′ree·um) *n.*, pl. **endoneu·ria** (·ree·uh) [NL., from *endo-* + *neuron*, nerve]. The delicate connective tissue surrounding individual nerve fibers and forming intrafascicular partitions. —**endoneuri·al** (·ul) *adj.*

en·do·nu·cle·ase (en″do·new′klee·ace, ·aze) *n.* [*endo-* + *nuclease*]. An enzyme that can degrade DNA or RNA molecules by attacking nucleotide linkages within the polynucleotide chain. Contr. *exonuclease.*

en·do·nu·cle·o·lus (en″do·new·klee′uh·lus) *n.* [*endo-* + *nucleolus*]. A nonstaining area within a nucleolus.

en·do·par·a·site (en″do·păr′uh·site) *n.* [*endo-* + *parasite*]. A parasite living within its host. Contr. *ectoparasite.* —**endo·par·a·sit·ic** (·păr·uh·sit′ick) *adj.*

en·do·pel·vic (en″do·pel′vick) *adj.* [*endo-* + *pelvic*]. Within the pelvis.

endopelvic fascia. The visceral portion of the pelvic fascia.

en·do·pep·ti·dase (en″do·pep′ti·dace, ·daze) *n.* [*endo-* + *peptidase*]. Any of a group of enzymes, including pepsin and trypsin, capable of attacking centrally located peptide bonds; a proteinase. Contr. *exopeptidase.*

en·do·peri·car·di·tis (en″do·perr″i·kahr·dye′tis) *n.* [*endo-* + *peri-* + *carditis*]. Inflammation of the endocardium and pericardium.

en·do·peri·myo·car·di·tis (en″do·perr″ee·migh″o·kahr·dye′tis) *n.* [*endo-* + *peri-* + *myo-* + *carditis*]. PANCARDITIS.

en·do·pha·ryn·ge·al (en″do·fa·rin′jee·ul) *adj.* [*endo-* + *pharyngeal*]. Within the pharynx.

endopharyngeal insufflation. A method of inducing anesthesia through a tube introduced through the mouth or nose to the back of the pharynx.

en·do·phle·bi·tis (en″do·fle·bye′tis) *n.* [*endo-* + *phlebitis*]. Inflammation of the intima of a vein.

en·doph·thal·mi·tis (en·dof″thal·migh′tis) *n.* [*end-* + *ophthalmitis.*]. Inflammation of the internal tissues of the eyeball.

endophthalmitis pha·co·ana·phy·lac·ti·ca (fay″ko·an″uh·fi·lack′ti·kuh). PHACOANAPHYLACTIC ENDOPHTHALMITIS.

en·do·phyte (en′do·fite) *n.* [*endo-* + *-phyte*]. *In dermatology,* a fungus that infects deeply.

en·do·phyt·ic (en″do·fit′ick) *adj.* [*endo-* + *-phyte* + *-ic*]. Tending to grow inward, as certain cutaneous tumors.

en·do·plasm (en′do·plaz·um) *n.* [*endo-* + *-plasm*]. The inner cytoplasm of a protozoon or of certain cells. —**en·do·plas·mic** (en″do·plaz′mick) *adj.*

endoplasmic reticulum. An intracytoplasmic membrane system as seen by electron microscopy. See also *rough-surfaced endoplasmic reticulum, smooth-surfaced endoplasmic reticulum.*

en·do·re·du·pli·ca·tion (en″do·re·dew″pli·kay′shun) *n.* [*endo-* + *reduplication*]. The process in which the chromosomes replicate without cell division.

end organ. The termination of a nerve fiber in muscle, skin, mucous membrane, or other structure.

end·or·phin (en·dor′fin) *n.* [*end-* + m*orphine*]. Any of a group of neurotransmitter peptides with morphine-like action, secreted by the central periaqueductal gray matter of the brain.

end·or·phine (en·dor′feen) *n.* ENDORPHIN.

en·do·sal·pin·gi·o·ma (en″do·sal·pin″jee·o′muh) *n.*, pl. **endosalpingiomas, endosalpingioma·ta** (·tuh) [*endo-* + *salping-* + *-oma*]. A serous cystadenoma of the uterine tube.

en·do·sal·pin·gi·o·sis (en″do·sal·pin″jee·o′sis) *n.* [*endo-* + *salping-* + *-osis*]. ISTHMIC NODULAR SALPINGITIS.

en·do·scope (en″duh·skope) *n.* [*endo-* + *-scope*]. An instrument used for the visual examination of the interior of a body cavity or viscus. —**endo·scop·ic** (·skop′ick) *adj.*; **en·dos·co·py** (·dos′kuh·pee) *n.*

en·do·skel·e·ton (en″do·skel′e·tun) *n.* [*endo-* + *skeleton*]. The internal supporting structure of an animal; the vertebrate skeleton.

end·os·mom·e·ter (en″dos·mom′e·tur, en″doz·) *n.* An instrument for measuring endosmosis.

end·os·mose (en′dos·moce, en′doz·moze) *n.* *Obsol.* ENDOSMOSIS.

end·os·mo·sis (en″dos·mo′sis, en″doz·) *n.* [*end-* + *osmosis*]. The passage of a liquid through a porous septum or membrane into a cavity containing liquid of a different density. —**endosmo·sic** (·sick), **endos·mot·ic** (·mot′ick) *adj.*

endosmotic equivalent. The amount of water that crosses a membrane in the same time interval that a unit volume of water passes out of the cell.

en·do·sperm (en′do·spurm) *n.* [*endo-* + *sperm*]. *In biology,* the nutritional part of a seed, notable for its triploid state in normally diploid plants.

en·do·spore (en′do·spore) *n.* [*endo-* + *spore*]. 1. A spore formed within the parent cell. 2. The inner coat of a spore. —**en·do·spor·u·late** (en″do·spor′yoo·late) *v.*

end·os·te·i·tis (en·dos″tee·eye′tis) *n.* ENDOSTITIS.

end·os·te·o·ma (en·dos″tee·o′muh) *n.* [*end-* + *oste-* + *-oma*]. A tumor within a bone.

end·os·te·um (en·dos′tee·um) *n.*, pl. **endos·tea** (·tee·uh) [NL., from *end-* + Gk. *osteon,* bone]. The membranous layer of connective tissue lining the medullary cavity of a bone. —**endoste·al** (·ul) *adj.*

end·os·ti·tis (en·dos·tye′tis) *n.* [*endost*eum + *-itis*]. Inflammation of endosteum.

end·os·to·ma (en″dos·to′muh) *n.* ENDOSTEOMA.

en·do·sto·mus (en″do·sto′mus) *n.*, pl. **endosto·mi** (·migh) [*endo-* + *stom-* + *-us*]. EPIGNATHUS.

end·os·to·sis (en″dos·to′sis) *n.*, pl. **endosto·ses** (·seez) [*end-* + *ostosis*]. Ossification of a cartilage.

en·do·ten·din·e·um (en″do·ten·din′ee·um) *n.* [NL., from *endo-* + *tendon*]. The delicate connective tissue between the fibers of a tendon bundle or fasciculus.

en·do·ten·on (en″do·ten′on) *n.* [*endo-* + Gk. *tenōn,* tendon]. ENDOTENDINEUM.

endotheli-, endothelio-. A combining form meaning *endothelium, endothelial.*

endothelia. Plural of *endothelium.*

en·do·the·li·al (en″do·theel′ee·ul) *adj.* Pertaining to or involving endothelium.

endothelial cell. One of the thin, flat cells forming the lining (endothelium) of the heart and blood and lymph vessels.

endothelial dystrophy. CORNEA GUTTATA.

endothelial leukocyte. HISTIOCYTE.

endothelial myeloma. EWING'S SARCOMA.

endothelial sarcoma. 1. HEMANGIOENDOTHELIOMA. 2. EWING'S SARCOMA.

endothelio-. See *endotheli-.*

en·do·the·lio·an·gi·i·tis (en″do·theel″ee·o·an″jee·eye′tis) *n.* [*endothelio-* + *angiitis*]. An inflammatory process involving the endothelium of the blood vessels in many organs; used especially in reference to lupus erythematosus.

en·do·the·lio·cho·ri·al (en″do·theel″ee·o·ko′ree·ul) *adj.* Pertaining to maternal endothelium and chorionic ectoderm.

endotheliochorial placenta. A type of placenta in which syncytial chorionic epithelium is in direct contact with the endothelium of uterine blood vessels; found in carnivores.

en·do·the·lio·cyte (en″do·theel′ee·o·site) *n.* [*endothelio-* + *-cyte*]. MACROPHAGE.

en·do·the·li·oid (en″do·theel′ee·oid) *adj.* [*endotheli-* + *-oid*]. Resembling endothelium.

endothelioid cell. 1. A cell resembling an endothelial cell. 2. *Erron.* EPITHELIOID CELL.

en·do·the·li·o·ly·sin (en″do·theel″ee·o·lye′sin, ·theel″ee·ol′i·sin) *n.* [*endotheli*um + *lysin*]. HEMORRHAGIN.

en·do·the·li·o·ma (en″do·theel″ee·o′muh) *n.*, pl. **endotheliomas, endothelioma·ta** (·tuh) [*endotheli-* + *-oma*]. Any tumor arising from, or resembling, endothelium; usually a benign growth, but occasionally, a malignant tumor.

endothelioma an·gi·o·ma·to·sum (an″jee·o·muh·to′sum). A

meningioma with a prominent vascular element; ANGIOBLASTIC MENINGIOMA.

endothelioma cap·i·tis (kap'i·tis). A cylindroma of the scalp.

endothelioma of lymph node. RETICULUM-CELL SARCOMA.

en·do·the·li·o·ma·to·sis (en"do·theel"ee·o·muh·to'sis) *n.* [*endothelioma* + *-osis*]. The presence of multiple endotheliomas.

en·do·the·li·o·sis (en"do·theel"ee·o'sis) *n.* [*endotheli-* + *-osis*]. Overgrowth of endothelium from unknown cause.

en·do·the·lio·tox·in (en"do·thee"lee·o·tock'sin) *n.* [*endothelium* + *toxin*]. HEMORRHAGIN.

en·do·the·li·um (en"do·theel'ee·um) *n.*, pl. **endothe·lia** (ee·uh) [*endo-* + epi*thelium*]. 1. The simple squamous epithelium lining the heart, blood vessels, and lymph vessels; vascular endothelium. 2. *Obsol.* The mesodermally derived simple squamous epithelium lining any closed cavity in the body.

endothelium ca·me·rae an·te·ri·o·ris cor·ne·ae (kam'e·ree an·teer"ee·o"ris kor'nee·ee) [NA]. The endothelium of the anterior chamber of the eye which covers the posterior surface of the cornea.

endothelium camerae anterioris iri·dis (eye'ri·dis) [NA]. The endothelium of the anterior chamber of the eye which covers the iris.

endothelium camerae anterioris ocu·li (ock'yoo·lye) [BNA]. The endothelium of the anterior chamber of the eye.

en·do·ther·mic (en"do·thur'mick) *adj.* [*endo-* + *thermic*]. 1. Pertaining to the absorption of heat. Contr. *exothermic.* 2. Pertaining to diathermy.

en·do·ther·my (en'do·thur"mee) *n.* [*endo-* + *-thermy*]. DIATHERMY.

en·do·thrix (en'do·thricks) *n.* [*endo-* + *-thrix*]. A fungal parasite forming spores inside the hair shaft. Compare *ectothrix.* See also *Trichophyton.*

en·do·tox·i·co·sis (en"do·tock"si·ko'sis) *n.* [*endo-* + *toxic* + *-osis*]. Poisoning by an endotoxin.

en·do·tox·in (en"do·tock'sin) *n.* [*endo-* + *toxin*]. A substance containing lipopolysaccharide complexes found in the cell walls of microorganisms, principally gram-negative bacteria, associated with a wide variety of biological effects, such as fever, shock, transient leukopenia, and thrombocytopenia. Syn. *Boivin antigen.*

en·do·tra·che·al (en"do·tray'kee·ul) *adj.* [*endo-* + *tracheal*]. Within the trachea.

endotracheal anesthesia. General anesthesia in which the anesthetic is administered by means of a tube which conducts the vapor directly into the trachea.

endotracheal tube. A large, specially constructed catheter which is passed through the glottis into the trachea to facilitate controlled, positive-pressure respiration, especially valuable in intrathoracic surgery, in operations on the head or neck, and in respiratory assistance.

en·do·vas·cu·li·tis (en"do·vas"kew·lye'tis) *n.* [*endo-* + *vasculitis*]. Inflammation of the intima of a blood vessel.

en·do·ven·tric·u·lar (en"do·ven·trick'yoo·lur) *adj.* [*endo-* + *ventricular*]. Within a ventricle, as of the heart or brain.

end plate. 1. The structure in which motor nerves terminate in skeletal muscle, involved in the transmission of nerve impulses to muscle. 2. The achromatic mass at the poles of the mitotic spindle of Protozoa.

end·pleas·ure, *n.* The pleasure accompanying sexual discharge or detumescence, brought about by a relief of the tension built up during the forepleasure.

end-point nystagmus. A physiologic, jerky type of nystagmus occurring on extreme lateral gaze after a short latency period, of small amplitude with the fast component in the direction of gaze, and generally exaggerated in fatigue states.

end-positional nystagmus. END-POINT NYSTAGMUS.

end product. The final product formed by a series of reactions.

Endrate. A trademark for sodium ethylenediamenetetracetic acid, a metal-chelating agent.

en·dry·sone (en'dri·sone) *n.* 11β-Hydroxy-6α-methylpregna-1,4-diene-3,20-dione, $C_{22}H_{30}O_3$, a topical anti-inflammatory.

end-stage kidney. A scarred, shrunken kidney resulting from any of several chronic renal diseases, making an etiologic diagnosis difficult or impossible.

end-to-side gastroduodenostomy. Anastomosis of the pyloric end of the stomach to the anterior side of the second portion of the duodenum.

Enduron. Trademark for methyclothiazide, a diuretic.

-ene. *In chemistry,* a suffix used in the naming of certain hydrocarbons; specifically, indicates *the presence of one double bond.*

en·e·ma (en'e·muh) *n.*, pl. **enemas, enem·a·ta** (e·nem'uh·tuh) [Gk., injection]. A rectal infusion for therapeutic, diagnostic, or nutritive purposes.

en·er·get·ics (en"ur·jet'icks) *n.* The branch of physics dealing with energy and the laws and conditions governing its manifestations.

en·er·gom·e·ter (en"ur·gom'e·tur) *n.* [*energy* + *-meter*]. An apparatus for studying energy characteristics of the pulse.

en·er·gy (en'ur·jee) *n.* [Gk. *energeia,* activity, from *energos,* active, from *ergon,* action, work]. The capacity for doing work. All forms of energy are mutually convertible one into the other. The quantity of work done in the process of transfer is a measure of energy. Therefore, work units are commonly used as energy units.

energy balance. The relation of the amount of utilizable energy taken into the body to that which is employed for internal work, external work, and the growth and repair of tissues.

energy metabolism. Physiologic activities concerned with the intake, interchange, and output of energy.

energy-rich phosphate bond. A phosphate bond, as in adenosine triphosphate and phosphocreatine, which on cleavage by hydrolysis releases about 11,000 calories per gram-molecule, as compared with the release of about 3000 calories from ordinary phosphate ester bonds. The bond provides a means of storing chemical energy for subsequent use in muscular activity or biosynthesis. Symbol, ~.

en·er·va·tion (en"ur·vay'shun) *n.* [L. *enervatio,* from *enervare,* to make weak]. 1. Weakness, lassitude, neurasthenia; reduction of strength. 2. Removal of a nerve.

en·flu·rane (en'floo·rane) *n.* 2-Chloro-1-(difluoromethoxy)-1,1,2-trifluoroethane, $C_3H_2ClF_5O$, an inhalation anesthetic.

en·gage·ment, *n. In obstetrics,* the entrance of the presenting part of the fetus into the superior pelvic strait.

en·gas·tri·us (en·gas'tree·us) *n.* [Gk. *engastrios,* in the womb, from *gastēr,* belly, womb]. A form of duplicity in which a parasitic fetus (or fetal parts) is included within the peritoneal cavity of its autosite.

Eng·el·mann's disease (eng'^{e}l·mah^{h}n) [T. W. *Engelmann,* German physiologist, 1843–1909]. PROGRESSIVE DIAPHYSEAL DYSPLASIA.

Eng·el-Reck·ling·hau·sen disease (eng'^{e}l, reck'ling·haow"z^{e}n) [G. *Engel,* German, 19th century; and F. D. von *Recklinghausen*]. OSTEITIS FIBROSA CYSTICA.

En·glish sweating fever. A contagious malignant fever, characterized by black or dark-colored sweat; of historical significance.

en·globe·ment (en·globe'munt) *n.* [F. *englober,* to take in]. PHAGOCYTOSIS. —**englob·ing** (·ing) *adj.*

engorged papilla. PAPILLEDEMA.

en·gorge·ment (en·gorj'munt) *n.* [F.]. 1. HYPEREMIA. 2. The state of being completely filled, or overfilled, as a breast with milk. —**en·gorge,** *v.*

en·gram, en·gramme (en'gram) *n.* [*en-* + *-gram*]. A memory imprint; the alteration that has occurred in nervous tissue as a result of an excitation from a stimulus, which hypothetically accounts for retention of that experience.

en grappes (ahn grap') [F.]. In grapelike clusters; said of fungus spores.

Eng·ström technique (eng'strœm''). ROENTGEN ABSORPTION HISTOSPECTROSCOPY.

en·he·ma·to·spore, en·hae·ma·to·spore (en·hee'muh·to·spore, en·hem'uh·to·) *n.* [*en-* + *hemato-* + *spore*]. A spore of the malarial parasite produced within the human body; MEROZOITE.

en·he·mo·spore, en·hae·mo·spore (en·hee'mo·spore, en·hem'o·) *n.* [*en-* + *hemo-* + *spore*]. ENHEMATOSPORE.

enol (ee'nol, ·nole) *n. In chemistry,* of or designating the form of a compound when it contains the —C=C(OH)— group, as distinguished from that in which it contains the tautomeric $—CH_2CO—$ group, designated *keto.* The enol form is produced from the keto form by migration of a hydrogen atom from the carbon atom adjoining the carbonyl group of the keto form. **—eno·lize** (ee'no·lize) *v.;* **eno·li·za·tion** (ee''no·lye·zay'shun) *n.*

eno·lase (ee'no·lace, ·laze) *n.* The enzyme that converts 2-phosphoglyceric acid to phosphoenolpyruvic acid.

enol·py·ru·vic acid (ee''nol·pye·roo'vick). The enol form of pyruvic acid, $CH_2=C(OH)COOH$; presumably formed in certain metabolic reactions involving pyruvic acid.

eno·ma·nia (ee''no·may'nee·uh) *n.* OINOMANIA.

en·oph·thal·mos (en''off·thal'mus) *n.* [*en-* + *ophthalmos*]. Recession of the eyeball into the orbit.

en·o·si·ma·nia (en''o·si·may'nee·uh) *n.* [Gk. *enosis*, a shaking, + *mania*]. 1. Extreme and irrational terror as a psychotic symptom. 2. The obsessional symptom of having perpetrated an unpardonable act or sin.

en·os·to·sis (en''os·to'sis) *n.,* pl. **enosto·ses** (·seez) [*en-* + *ostosis*]. A bony ingrowth within the medullary canal of a bone, or the cranium. Syn. *entostosis.*

enostosis of calvaria. HYPEROSTOSIS FRONTALIS INTERNA.

Enovid. Trademark for a formulation of norethynodrel, a progestogen, and mestranol, an estrogen, used to inhibit ovulation and control fertility.

en·pro·mate (en'pro·mate) *n.* 1,1-Diphenyl-2-propynyl cyclohexylcarbamate, $C_{22}H_{23}NO_2$, an antineoplastic.

En·roth's sign. Puffy, edematous swelling of the eyelid, often found in thyrotropic exophthalmos.

en·sheathed (en·sheethd', en·sheetht') *adj.* Enclosed, as within a sheath; invaginated; encysted.

Ensidon. Trademark for opipramol, a tranquilizer and antidepressant drug used as the dihydrochloride salt.

en·si·form (en'si·form) *adj.* [L. *ensis*, sword, + *form*]. Shaped like a sword.

ensiform cartilage or **process.** XIPHOID PROCESS.

en·som·pha·lus (en·som'fuh·lus) *n.,* pl. **ensompha·li** (·lye) [Gk. *en-* + *sōma*, body, + *omphalos*]. Conjoined twins (diplopagi) united by a band in the epigastric and lower sternal regions; Siamese twins. Compare *xiphophagus.* **—en·som·phal·ic** (en'som·fal'ick) *adj.*

en·stro·phe (en'stro·fee) *n.* [Gk. *enstrophē*, from *enstrephein*, to turn in]. Inversion, as of the margin of an eyelid.

ent-, ento- [Gk *entos*, within, inside]. A combining form meaning (a) *within;* (b) *inner.*

en·tad (en'tad) *adv.* [*ent-* + *-ad*]. Inward; toward the center.

en·tal (en'tul) *adj.* [*ent-* + *-al*]. Internal.

ent·ame·bi·a·sis, ent·amoe·bi·a·sis (en''tuh·mee·bye'uh·sis) *n.* [*Entamoeba* + *-iasis*]. AMEBIASIS.

Ent·amoe·ba (en''tuh·mee'buh) *n.* [*ent-* + *amoeba*]. A genus of protozoan parasites which includes species parasitic in man.

Entamoeba buc·ca·lis (buh·kay'lis). *ENTAMOEBA GINGIVALIS.*

Entamoeba co·li (ko'lye). A nonpathogenic species of parasite inhabiting the intestinal tract.

Entamoeba gin·gi·va·lis (jin·ji·vay'lis). A species of parasite found in the mouth, about the gums, and in dental plaque.

Entamoeba his·to·lyt·i·ca (his·to·lit'i·kuh). The etiologic agent of amebiasis.

Entamoeba nana. *ENDOLIMAX NANA.*

entamoebiasis. Entamebiasis (= AMEBIASIS).

en·ta·sia (en·tay'zhuh, ·zee·uh) *n.* [Gk. *entasis*, tension, + *-ia*]. *Obsol.* Spasmodic muscular action; TONIC SPASM. **—en·tat·ic** (en·tat'ick) *adj.*

en·ta·sis (en'tuh·sis) *n.* [Gk., tension, straining]. *Obsol.* ENTASIA.

en·tel·e·chy (en·tel'e·kee) *n.* [Gk. *entelecheia*, complete reality, from *entelēs*, complete, + *echein*, to have]. 1. The complete realization or expression of some principle. 2. A vital influence that is supposed to guide living organisms in the right direction.

enter-, entero- [Gk. *enteron*]. A combining form meaning *intestine, intestinal.*

en·ter·al (en'tur·ul) *adj.* [*enter-* + *-al*]. INTESTINAL.

en·ter·al·gia (en''tur·al'jee·uh) *n.* [*enter-* + *-algia*]. Pain in the intestine. **—enteral·gic** (·jick) *adj.*

enteralgic crisis. A paroxysm of pain in the lower part of the abdomen occurring in tabes dorsalis.

en·ter·amine (en''tur·am'een, en'tur·uh·meen) *n.* SEROTONIN.

en·ter·ec·ta·sis (en''tur·eck'tuh·sis) *n.,* pl. **enterecta·ses** (·seez) [*enter-* + *ectasis*]. Dilatation of some part of the small intestine.

en·ter·ec·to·my (en''tur·eck'tuh·mee) *n.* [*enter-* + *-ectomy*]. Excision of a part of the intestine.

en·ter·epip·lo·cele (en''tur·e·pip'lo·seel) *n.* [*enter-* + *epiplocele*]. Hernia in which both the intestine and the greater omentum are involved.

en·ter·ic (en·terr'ick) *adj.* [Gk. *enterikos*]. Pertaining to the intestine.

enteric coating. A coating for pills or tablets or capsules, intended as a protection against solutions found in the stomach, but disintegrating or dissolving in the intestines.

enteric cyst. A congenital cyst formed from a duplicated segment of bowel. See also *neurenteric cyst.*

enteric fever. 1. TYPHOID FEVER. 2. PARATYPHOID FEVER.

enteric ganglions. Small nerve ganglions of the myenteric and submucous plexuses of the intestine.

enteric intussusception. An intussusception involving the small intestine only. Syn. *ileal intussusception.*

en·ter·i·coid (en·terr'i·koid) *adj.* [*enteric* fever + *-oid*]. Resembling typhoid fever.

enteric plexus. The myenteric and submucous plexuses considered together. NA *plexus entericus.*

en·ter·i·tis (en''tur·eye'tis) *n.,* pl. **enter·it·i·des** (·it'i·deez) [*enter-* + *-itis*]. Any inflammation of the intestinal tract, especially of the mucosa.

enteritis ne·crot·i·cans (ne·krot'i·kanz). A form of fulminant gangrenous inflammation of the small intestine, usually due to infection by *Clostridium perfringens.*

entero-. See *enter-.*

en·tero·anas·to·mo·sis (en''tur·o·a·nas''tuh·mo'sis) *n.* [*entero-* + *anastomosis*]. An intestinal anastomosis.

en·tero·an·the·lone (en·tur''o·anth'e·lone) *n.* Urogastrone derived from the mucosa of the small intestine.

En·tero·bac·ter (en''tur·o·back'tur) *n.* [*entero-* + *bacterium*]. A genus of the family Enterobacteriaceae, widely distributed in nature, composed of gram-negative motile or nonmotile rods which ferment glucose and lactose with the production of acid and gas. Reaction to the methyl red test is negative and to the Voges-Proskauer test, positive. **—enterobacter,** *com. n.*

Enterobacter aer·og·e·nes (air·oj'e·neez). A species of *Enterobacter* widely distributed in nature, found in soil, plants, water, milk, and intestinal canals of humans and animals; sometimes a secondary or opportunistic pathogen. Formerly called *Aerobacter aerogenes.*

En·tero·bac·te·ri·a·ce·ae (en''tur·o·back·teer''ee·ay'see·ee) *n. pl.* [*entero-* + *Bacteriaceae*]. A large family of gram-negative bacteria (rods), motile or nonmotile, attacking glucose with the production of acid or acid and gas, forming nitrites from nitrates, of complex antigenic composition with many cross-reactions, and including many animal parasites and saprophytes. They do not possess cytochrome oxidase, and fail to liquefy sodium pectinate. Included are the following principal groups and genera: the *Klebsiella-Enterobacter-Serratia* group, *Salmonella, Shigella, Escherichia coli,* the Arizona group, *Citrobacter, Proteus,* and the Providence group.

en·ter·o·bi·a·sis (en″tur·o·bye′uh·sis) *n.* [*Enterobius* + *-iasis*]. Infection of the intestinal tract with *Enterobius vermicularis,* characterized primarily by perianal pruritus. Syn. *oxyuriasis, pinworm infection.*

En·ter·o·bi·us (en″tur·o′bee·us) *n.* [*entero-* + Gk. *bios,* life]. A genus of nematode parasites of man.

Enterobius ver·mic·u·la·ris (vur·mick·yoo·lair′is). The pinworm or seatworm; the etiologic agent of enterobiasis in man.

en·tero·cele (en′tur·o·seel) *n.* [*entero-* + *-cele*]. A hernia containing a loop of intestine.

en·tero·cen·te·sis (en″tur·o·sen·tee′sis) *n.,* pl. **enterocente·ses** (·seez) [*entero-* + *centesis*]. Surgical puncture of the intestine.

en·tero·cep·tive impulses (en″tur·o·sep′tiv). Afferent nerve impulses that derive their stimulation from internal organs.

en·tero·chro·maf·fin (en″tur·o·kro′muh·fin) *n.* [*entero-* + *chromaffin*]. An intestinal element having an affinity for chromium salts.

enterochromaffin cell. An epithelial cell appearing in solitary fashion among the glandular cells of the crypts of Lieberkühn, with an affinity for silver and chromium salts; analogous to other argentaffin cells of the digestive tube.

en·ter·oc·ly·sis (en″tur·ock′li·sis) *n.,* pl. **enterocly·ses** (·seez) [*entero-* + *clysis*]. Injection of a fluid preparation into the rectum or intestine for nutrient, medicinal, or cleansing purposes.

en·tero·coc·cus (en″tur·o·cock′us) *n.,* pl. **enterococ·ci** (·sigh) [*entero-* + *coccus*]. A streptococcus normally found in the intestinal tract of man and other species, but pathogenic when found elsewhere, as in urinary and respiratory tracts, and the cause of subacute bacterial endocarditis.

en·tero·coele (en′tur·o·seel) *n.* [*entero-* + *-coele*]. A coelom formed by evagination of the wall of the primitive gut. —**en·tero·coe·lic** (en″tur·o·see′lick) *adj.*

en·tero·col·ec·to·my (en″tur·o·ko·leck′tuh·mee, ·kol·eck′) *n.* [*entero-* + *col-* + *-ectomy*]. Resection of parts of both small intestine and colon.

en·tero·co·lic (en″tur·o·ko′lick, ·kol′ick) *adj.* [*entero-* + *colic*]. Pertaining to the small intestine and the colon.

enterocolic intussusception. Invagination of the ileum into the colon. See also *ileocecal intussusception, ileocolic intussusception.*

en·tero·co·li·tis (en″tur·o·ko·lye′tis) *n.* [*entero-* + *colitis*]. Inflammation of small intestine and colon.

en·tero·co·los·to·my (en″tur·o·ko·los′tuh·mee) *n.* [*entero-* + *colostomy*]. *In surgery,* the formation of a communication between the small intestine and colon; enterocolic anastomosis.

en·tero·cri·nin (en″tur·o·krin′in, ·krye′nin, en″tur·ock′rin·in) *n.* [*entero-* + Gk. *krinein,* to secrete, + *-in*]. A hormonal extract from the intestinal mucosa which stimulates the glands of the small intestine.

en·tero·cyst (en′tur·o·sist) *n.* [*entero-* + *cyst*]. An intestinal cyst.

en·tero·cys·to·cele (en″tur·o·sis′tuh·seel) *n.* [*entero-* + *cysto-* + *-cele*]. A hernia involving the urinary bladder and intestine.

en·tero·cys·to·ma (en″tur·o·sis·to′muh) *n.* [*entero-* + *cystoma*]. ENTERIC CYST.

en·tero·cys·to·plas·ty (en″tur·o·sis′to·plas″tee) *n.* [*entero-* + *cystoplasty*]. Surgical anastomosis of a segment of small bowel to the urinary bladder to increase the capacity of the bladder.

en·tero·en·ter·ic (en″tur·o·en·terr′ick) *adj.* [*entero-* + *enteric*]. Involving two separate portions of the intestine.

en·tero·en·ter·os·to·my (en″tur·o·en″tur·os′tuh·mee) *n.* [*entero-* + *enterostomy*]. *In surgery,* the formation of a passage between two parts of the intestine.

en·tero·gas·tri·tis (en″tur·o·gas·trye′tis) *n.* GASTROENTERITIS.

en·tero·gas·tro·cele (en″tur·o·gas′tro·seel) *n.* [*entero-* + *gastro-* + *-cele*]. A hernia containing the stomach and intestine or portions of them; VENTRAL HERNIA.

en·tero·gas·trone (en″tur·o·gas′trone) *n.* [*entero-* + *gastr-* + hormone]. A hormonal extract from the upper intestinal mucosa which inhibits gastric motility and secretion.

en·ter·og·e·nous (en″tur·oj′e·nus) *adj.* [*entero-* + *-genous*]. Originating in the intestine.

enterogenous cyanosis. 1. METHEMOGLOBINEMIA. 2. SULFHEMOGLOBINEMIA.

enterogenous cyst. ENTERIC CYST.

enterogenous peptonuria. Peptonuria due to disease of the intestine.

en·tero·graph (en′tur·o·graf″) *n.* [*entero-* + *-graph*]. An apparatus which records graphically the movements of the intestine.

en·tero·hep·a·ti·tis (en″tur·o·hep·uh·tye′tus) *n.* [*entero-* + *hepat-* + *-itis*]. HISTOMONIASIS.

en·tero·in·su·lar (en″tur·o·in′sue·lur) *adj.* [*entero-* + *insular*]. Pertaining to the intestines and islets of the pancreas.

enteroinsular axis. A regulatory system proposed to account for the stimulation of insulin by substances such as glucose, amino acids, and gastrointestinal hormones in the intestinal tract.

en·tero·ki·nase (en″tur·o·kigh′nace, ·naze, ·kin′ace, ·aze) *n.* [*entero-* + *kinase*]. An enzyme present in the succus entericus which converts inactive trypsinogen into active trypsin.

en·tero·lith (en′tur·o·lith) *n.* [*entero-* + *-lith*]. A concretion formed in the intestine.

en·tero·li·thi·a·sis (en″tur·o·li·thigh′uh·sis) *n.* [*entero-* + *lithiasis*]. The presence of calculi in the intestine.

en·ter·ol·o·gist (en″tur·ol′uh·jist) *n.* GASTROENTEROLOGIST.

en·ter·ol·o·gy (en″tur·ol′uh·jee) *n.* [*entero-* + *-logy*]. GASTROENTEROLOGY.

en·ter·ol·y·sis (en″tur·ol′i·sis) *n.,* pl. **enteroly·ses** (·seez) [*entero-* + *-lysis*]. Removal of adhesions binding the intestine.

en·tero·meg·a·ly (en″tur·o·meg′uh·lee) *n.* [*entero-* + *-megaly*]. Intestinal enlargement. See also *megacolon.*

en·tero·me·ro·cele (en″tur·o·meer′o·seel) *n.* [*entero-* + *mēros,* thigh, + *-cele*]. *Obsol.* A femoral hernia involving intestine.

En·tero·mo·nas (en″tur·o·mo′nas, ·om′o·nas) *n.* [*entero-* + Gk. *monas,* unit]. A genus of the order of Polymastigida possessing four flagella, transmitted from one host to another in the encysted stage. *Enteromonas hominis* is commonly found in diarrheic stools of man.

en·tero·my·co·sis (en″tur·o·migh·ko′sis) *n.,* pl. **enteromyco·ses** (·seez) [*entero-* + *mycosis*]. Any intestinal fungus disease.

en·tero·my·ia·sis (en″tur·o·migh·eye′uh·sis) *n.,* pl. **enteromy·ia·ses** (·seez) [*entero-* + *myiasis*]. Disease due to the presence of the larvae of flies in the intestine.

en·ter·on (en′tur·on) *n.* [Gk.]. 1. INTESTINE. 2. ALIMENTARY CANAL.

en·tero·pa·ral·y·sis (en″tur·o·puh·ral′i·sis) *n.* [*entero-* + *paralysis*]. Paralysis of the intestine.

en·tero·patho·gen·ic (en″tur·o·path·o·jen′ick) *adj.* [*entero-* + *pathogenic*]. Causing intestinal disease.

en·ter·op·a·thy (en″tur·op·uth·ee) *n.* [*entero-* + *-pathy*]. Any disease of the intestine.

en·tero·pexy (en′tur·o·peck″see) *n.* [*entero-* + *-pexy*]. *In surgery,* the fixation of a portion of the intestine to the abdominal wall, for the relief of a condition such as visceroptosis.

en·tero·plas·ty (en′tur·o·plas″tee) *n.* [*entero-* + *-plasty*]. A plastic operation upon the intestine. —**en·tero·plas·tic** (en″tur·o·plas′tick) *adj.*

en·tero·ple·gia (en″tur·o·plee′jee·uh) *n.* [*entero-* + *-plegia*]. ENTEROPARALYSIS.

en·tero·proc·tia (en″tur·o·prock′shee·uh) *n.* [*entero-* + *proct-* + *-ia*]. The existence of an artificial anus.

en·ter·op·to·sis (en″tur·op·to′sis) *n.*, pl. **enteropto·ses** (·seez) [*entero-* + *-ptosis*]. VISCEROPTOSIS. —**enterop·tot·ic** (·tot′ick) *adj.*

en·ter·or·rha·gia (en″tur·o·ray′jee·uh) *n.* [*entero-* + *-rrhagia*]. Intestinal hemorrhage.

en·ter·or·rha·phy (en″tur·or′uh·fee) *n.* [*entero-* + *-rrhaphy*]. Suture of the intestine.

en·ter·or·rhea, en·ter·or·rhoea (en·″tur·o·ree′uh) *n.* [*entero-* + *-rrhea*]. Excessive flow of fluid through the intestine.

en·ter·or·rhex·is (en″tur·o·reck′sis) *n.*, pl. **enterorrhex·es** (·seez) [*entero-* + *-rrhexis*]. Rupture of the intestine.

en·tero·scope (en′tur·o·skope) *n.* [*entero-* + *-scope*]. An endoscope for examining the inside of the intestine.

en·tero·sep·sis (en″tur·o·sep′sis) *n.*, pl. **enterosep·ses** (·seez) [*entero-* + *sepsis*]. Intestinal toxemia or sepsis.

en·tero·sid·er·in (en″tur·o·sid′ur·in) *n.* A glycolipoprotein pigment with iron-positive and iron-negative phases, found in large histiocytoid round cells of the villous and colonic mucosa of man and various mammals. Melanosis coli and pseudomelanosis coli pigments are regarded as phases of enterosiderin.

en·tero·spasm (en′tur·o·spaz″um) *n.* Excessive muscular contraction of the intestine. See also *colic.*

en·tero·sta·sis (en″tur·o·stay′sis) *n.*, pl. **enterosta·ses** (·seez) [*entero-* + *stasis*]. INTESTINAL STASIS.

en·tero·ste·no·sis (en″tur·o·ste·no′sis) *n.*, pl. **enterosteno·ses** (·seez) [*entero-* + *stenosis*]. Stricture or narrowing of the intestinal lumen.

en·ter·os·to·my (en″tur·os′tuh·mee) *n.* [*entero-* + *-stomy*]. 1. The formation of an artificial opening into the intestine through the abdominal wall. 2. An opening, temporary or permanent, in the small intestine for anastomosis or drainage. —**en·tero·sto·mal** (en″tur·o·sto′mul) *adj.*

en·tero·tome (en′tur·o·tome) *n.* [*entero-* + *-tome*]. An instrument for cutting open the intestine.

en·ter·ot·o·my (en″tur·ot′uh·mee) *n.* [*entero-* + *-tomy*]. Incision of the intestine.

en·tero·tox·e·mia, en·tero·tox·ae·mia (en″tur·o·tock·see′mee·uh) *n.* [*entero-* + *toxemia*]. The presence in the bloodstream of toxins produced in the intestine.

en·tero·tox·i·gen·ic (en″tur·o·tock·si·jen′ick) *adj.* [*enterotoxin* + *-genic*]. Producing enterotoxin.

en·tero·tox·in (en″tur·o·tock′sin) *n.* [*entero-* + *toxin*]. A toxin that is specific for intestinal mucosa, such as the thermostable, trypsin-resistant toxin produced by some strains of *Staphylococcus aureus,* and which causes acute food poisoning.

en·tero·ves·i·cal (en″tur·o·ves′i·kul) *adj.* [*entero-* + *vesical*]. Pertaining to the intestine and the urinary bladder.

en·tero·vi·rus (en″tur·o·vye′rus) *n.* [*entero-* + *virus*]. Any of a group of related viruses of human origin, including poliomyelitis, Coxsackie, and ECHO, which are members of the picornaviruses characterized by very small size and the RNA composition of the nucleic acid.

en·tero·zo·on (en″tur·o·zo′on) *n.*, pl. **entero·zoa** (·zo′uh) [*entero-* + *-zoon*]. An animal parasite of the intestine.

en·theo·ma·nia (enth″ee·o·may′nee·uh) *n.* [Gk. *entheos,* inspired (from *theos,* god) + *mania*]. A psychotic symptom in which the patient believes himself to be inspired or especially selected by God for his work.

en·the·sis (en′thuh·sis) *n.*, pl. **enthe·ses** (·seez) [Gk., insertion, graft]. The employment of metallic or other inorganic material to replace lost tissue.

en·thet·ic (en·thet′ick) *adj.* [Gk. *enthetikos,* fit for implanting]. 1. Pertaining to enthesis. 2. EXOGENOUS.

Enthrane. A trademark for enflurane, an inhalation anesthetic.

ent·iris (ent·eye′ris) *n.* [*ent-* + *iris*]. The uvea of the iris, forming its inner and pigmentary layer.

ento-. See *ent-.*

en·to·blast (en′to·blast) *n.* [*ento-* + *-blast*]. ENTODERM.

en·to·cele (en′to·seel) *n.* [*ento-* + *-cele*]. INTERNAL HERNIA.

en·to·cone (en′to·kone) *n.* [*ento-* + *cone*]. The posterior lingual cusp of a maxillary molar tooth.

en·to·co·nid (en″to·ko′nid) *n.* [*ento-* + *cone* + *-id*]. The posterior lingual cusp of a mandibular molar tooth.

en·to·derm (en′to·durm) *n.* [*ento-* + *-derm*]. The innermost of the three primary germ layers, which forms the lining of the gut, from pharynx to rectum, and its derivatives. Syn. *endoderm.* Contr. *ectoderm, mesoderm.* —**en·to·der·mal** (en″to·dur′mul) *adj.*

entodermal cloaca. The part of the cloaca derived from the caudal end of the hindgut.

entom-, entomo- [Gk. *entoma,* insects, from *entomos,* cut up, segmented]. A combining form meaning *insect.*

en·to·mere (en′to·meer) *n.* A blastomere capable of forming entoderm.

en·to·mi·on (en·to′mee·on) *n.*, pl. **ento·mia** (·mee·uh) [Gk. *entomē,* notch, + *-ion*]. *In craniometry,* the point where the tip of the mastoid angle of the parietal bone fits into the parietal notch of the temporal bone.

entomo-. See *entom-.*

en·to·mog·e·nous (en·to·moj′e·nus) *adj.* [*entomo-* + *-genous*]. 1. Originating with insects, their bites, or products. 2. Originating, or growing, within an insect.

en·to·mol·o·gist (en″tuh·mol′uh·jist) *n.* A specialist in that branch of zoology dealing with insects and other arthropods.

en·to·mol·o·gy (en″tuh·mol′uh·jee) *n.* [*entomo-* + *-logy*]. The study of insects and other arthropods.

en·to·mo·pho·bia (en″tuh·mo·fo′bee·uh) *n.* [*entomo-* + *-phobia*]. A morbid fear of insects.

en·to·pe·dun·cu·lar (en″to·pe·dunk′yoo·lur) *adj.* [*ento-* + *peduncular*]. Pertaining to an area situated inside the (thalamic) peduncles.

entopeduncular nucleus. Cells located along the fibers of the ansa lenticularis, which apparently receive fibers from the globus pallidus and project to the reticular substance in the tegmentum of the midbrain.

ent·op·tic (ent·op′tick) *adj.* [*ent-* + *optic*]. Pertaining to the internal parts of the eye.

entoptic image. An image perceived by the retina of objects within the eye, as when one visualizes one's own vascular pattern on rubbing the illuminated bulb of a pocket flashlight against the lower lid while looking upward.

entoptic phenomena. Alterations in normal light perception resulting from intraoptic phenomena, as subjective perception of light resulting from mechanical compression of the eyeball.

entoptic pulse. The subjective illumination of a dark visual field with each heart beat; a condition sometimes noted after violent exercise, and due to the mechanical irritation of the rods by the pulsating retinal arteries.

ent·op·tos·co·py (ent″op·tos′kuh·pee) *n.* [*entoptic* + *-scopy*]. Examination of the interior of the eye, or of the shadows within the eye. —**entop·to·scop·ic** (·tuh·skop′ick) *adj.*

ent·os·te·o·sis (ent·os″tee·o′sis) *n.* ENTOSTOSIS.

ent·os·to·sis (ent″os·to′sis) *n.*, pl. **entosto·ses** (·seez) [*ent-* + *ostosis*]. A benign growth of bone extending from the endosteal cortex into a medullary cavity. Syn. *enostosis.*

ent·otic (ent·o′tick, ·ot′ick) *adj.* [*ent-* + *otic*]. Pertaining to the internal ear.

en·to·zo·on (en″to·zo′on) *n.* [*ento-* + *-zoon*]. An animal parasite living within another animal. —**entozo·al** (·ul) *adj.*

en·train·ment (en·train′munt) *n.* [F. *entraîner,* to draw along]. The act or process of carrying along or over, as when a liquid boils at such a rapid rate as to carry droplets of liquid in the vapor.

entrance heart block. *In electrocardiography,* a variety of unidirectional block which prevents the sinus impulse from discharging an ectopic pacemaker, usually a parasystolic focus, but does not prevent the latter from sending out impulses. Syn. *protection heart block.*

en·trap·ment neuropathy (en·trap'munt). COMPRESSION NEURITIS.

en·tro·pi·on (en·tro'pee·on) *n.* [NL., from Gk. *entropē*, noun from *entrepein*, to turn inward]. Inversion of the eyelid, so that the lashes rub against the globe of the eye. —**entropi·on·ize** (·un·ize) *v.*

en·tro·py (en'truh·pee) *n.* [*en-* (as in energy) + Gk. *tropē*, turn, change]. 1. The portion of the energy of a system, per degree of absolute temperature, that cannot be converted to work. All spontaneous changes—that is, those occurring in nature—are accompanied by an increase in the entropy of the system. 2. *In medicine*, diminished capacity for change such as occurs with aging.

entry zone. ROOT ENTRANCE ZONE.

en·ty·py (en'ti·pee) *n.* [Gk. *entypē*, impression, flattening]. A condition in which the trophoblastic layer remains uninterrupted over the inner cell mass of the blastocyst.

enu·cle·ate (ee·new'klee·ate) *v.* [L. *enucleare*, to take out the kernels]. To remove an organ or a tumor in its entirety, as an eye from its socket. —**enu·cle·a·tion** (ee·new"klee·ay'shun) *n.*, **enuclea·tor** (·tur) *n.*

en·u·re·sis (en"yoo·ree'sis) *n.*, pl. **enure·ses** (·seez) [Gk. *enourein*, to make water in, + *-esis*]. Urinary incontinence at an age when urethral sphincter control may normally be expected, usually a habit disturbance; bed-wetting. Compare *encopresis.* —**enu·ret·ic** (·ret'ick) *adj.* & *n.*

Envacar. Trademark for guanoxan, an antihypertensive drug used as the sulfate salt.

en·ven·om (en·ven'um) *v.* To inject or contaminate with venom, as from a poisonous insect or reptile. —**en·ven·om·ation** (en·ven"um·ay'shun) *n.*

en·vi·ron·ment, *n.* [F. *environ*, about]. The external conditions which surround, act upon, and influence an organism or its parts.

environmental deprivation. Lack of adequate stimulation in early life as a result of severe sensory deprivation in a very limited environment or less often an atypical cultural milieu, even where there may be fairly rich personal interplay, resulting in inadequate opportunities for learning and thus marginal or pseudoretardation. Compare *emotional deprivation.*

en Y anastomosis (en wye, F. ahⁿ·nee·greck') [F., in (the form of) Y]. A Y-shaped enteroenterostomy of small intestine used to drain organs or cavities into the intestinal stream via a defunctionalized side loop.

Enzactin. A trademark for triacetin, an antifungal.

en·zo·ot·ic (en"zo·ot'ick) *adj.* [*en* + *zoo-* + *-ic*]. Pertaining to a disease afflicting animals in a limited district. Contr. *epizootic.*

enzootic ataxia. A syndrome affecting sheep and sometimes cattle grazing on copper-deficient soils, characterized by spastic paralysis and sometimes blindness.

en·zy·got·ic twins (en"zye·got'ick). IDENTICAL TWINS.

enzymatic hydrolysis. ZYMOHYDROLYSIS.

en·zyme (en'zime, ·zim) *n.* [Medieval Gk. *enzymos*, leavened, from Gk. *zymē*, leaven]. A catalytic substance, protein in nature, formed by living cells and having a specific action in promoting a chemical change. Enzymes are classified on the basis of types of reaction catalyzed as oxido-reductases, transferases, hydrolases, lyases, isomerases, and ligases. See also *apoenzyme, ferment.* —**en·zy·mat·ic** (en·zi·mat'ick), **en·zy·mic** (en·zye'mick) *adj.*

en·zy·mol·o·gy (en"zye·mol'o·jee, en"zi·) *n.* [*enzyme* + *-logy*]. The science and study of enzymes and the chemical reactions they catalyze.

en·zy·mol·y·sis (en"zye·mol'i·sis, en"zi·) *n.* [*enzyme* + *-lysis*]. A chemical change produced by enzymic action. —**en·zy·mo·lyt·ic** (en·zye"mo·lit'ick, en"zi·) *adj.*

en·zy·mo·pe·nia (en"zi·mo·pee'nee·uh) *n.* [*enzyme* + *-penia*]. Deficiency or absence of an enzyme in the blood.

en·zy·mo·sis (en"zye·mo'sis, en"zi·) *n.* [*enzyme* + *-osis*]. ENZYMOLYSIS.

en·zym·uria (en"zye·mew'ree·uh, en"zi·) *n.* [*enzyme* + *-uria*]. The presence of enzymes in the urine.

EOG Abbreviation for *electrooculogram.*

eon·ism (ee'on·iz·um) *n.* [Chevalier d'*Eon* de Beaumont, French diplomatic agent, 1728-1810]. The adoption of feminine habits, manners, and costume by a male. Compare *sexoesthetic inversion, transvestism.*

eo·sin, eo·sine (ee'uh·sin, ee'o·seen) *n.* [Gk. *ēōs*, dawn, + *-in*]. A class of red acid dyes of the xanthene group, usually halogenated derivatives of fluorescein. They share the fluorescence of the parent substance to a greater or less extent. Usually eosin Y, $C_{20}H_6Br_4Na_2O_5$, the disodium salt of 2,4,5,7-tetrabromofluorescein, is meant, since it is the most used, but the class includes also ethyl and methyl eosin, eosin B, erythrosin, erythrosin B, phloxine, phloxine B, and rose Bengal. The eosins are variously used as histologic and clinical laboratory stains, and as dyes.

eosin J. ERYTHROSIN B.

eosin-methylene blue stain. MALLORY'S PHLOXINE-METHYLENE BLUE STAIN.

eo·sin·o·pe·nia (ee"o·sin"o·pee'nee·uh) *n.* [*eosin* + *-penia*]. A reduction below normal of the number of eosinophils per unit volume of peripheral blood. —**eosinope·nic** (·nick) *adj.*

eo·sin·o·phil (ee"o·sin'uh·fil) *adj.* & *n.* [*eosin* + *-phil*]. 1. Having an affinity for eosin or any acid stain. 2. EOSINOPHIL LEUKOCYTE. —**eo·sin·o·phil·ic** (ee"o·sin"uh·fil'ick) *adj.*

eo·sin·o·phile (ee"o·sin'uh·file) *adj.* & *n.* EOSINOPHIL.

eo·sin·o·phil·ia (ee"o·sin"uh·fil'ee·uh) *n.* [*eosinophil* + *-ia*]. 1. An increase above normal in the number of eosinophils per unit volume of peripheral blood. 2. The occurrence of increased numbers of eosinophilic granulocytes in certain tissues and organs. 3. The assumption of a deeper shade of red by any cell or tissue in conventional hematoxylin- and eosin-stained material.

eosinophilic adenoma. An adenoma whose cells have moderate to abundant eosinophilic cytoplasm or eosinophilic granules; usually occurs in the pituitary or sweat glands.

eosinophilic erythroblast. NORMOBLAST (1).

eosinophilic granules. Granules staining selectively with eosin, erythrosin, and similar dyes.

eosinophilic granuloma. A benign, chronic, localized, proliferative disorder of reticuloendothelial cells, accompanied by eosinophilic granulocytes and producing one or more bone lesions. Syn. *eosinophilic xanthomatous granuloma.*

eosinophilic leukemia. A rare form of leukemia in which the predominant cells are eosinophilic granulocytes.

eosinophilic leukocyte. EOSINOPHIL LEUKOCYTE.

eosinophilic pneumonitis. LOEFFLER'S SYNDROME.

eosinophilic tumor of the pituitary. EOSINOPHILIC ADENOMA.

eosinophilic xanthomatous granuloma. EOSINOPHILIC GRANULOMA.

eosinophil leukocyte. A leukocyte containing coarse round granules which stain pink to bright red (acid dye) with Wright's stain and usually having a bilobed nucleus.

eo·sin·o·philo·cyt·ic (ee"o·sin·uh·fil"o·sit'ick) *adj. Obsol.* EOSINOPHILIC.

eosin S. ETHYL EOSIN.

eosin Y. $C_{20}H_6Br_4Na_2O_5$, the disodium salt of 2,4,5,7-tetrabromofluorescein. See also *eosin.*

ep-, epi- [Gk. *epi*, on, upon]. A prefix meaning (a) *upon, beside, among, above, anterior, over, on the outside;* (b) in chemistry, *relation of some kind to a* (specified) *compound.*

ep·ac·mas·tic (ep"ack·mas'tick) *adj.* [Gk. *epakmastikos*]. EPACMIC.

ep·ac·mic (ep·ack'mick) *adj.* [*ep-* + *acmic*]. Designating the period of progression of a disease. Contr. *acmic, paracmic.*

epac·tal (e·pack'tul) *adj.* & *n.* [Gk. *epaktos*, brought in]. 1. INTERCALATED. 2. SUPERNUMERARY. 3. An epactal bone, as the interparietal bone, or one of the sutural or wormian bones.

epactal cartilages. Small cartilaginous nodules on the upper edge of the alar cartilages of the nose. NA *cartilagines nasales accessoriae.*

Epanutin. A trademark for phenytoin sodium, an antiepileptic.

ep·ar·te·ri·al (ep″ahr·teer′ee·ul) *adj.* [*ep-* + *arterial*]. Situated upon or above an artery.

eparterial bronchus. The first branch of the right primary bronchus, situated above the right pulmonary artery.

ep·ax·i·al (ep·ack′see·ul) *adj.* [*ep-* + *axial*]. Situated above an axis.

ep·en·dy·ma (ep·en′di·muh) *n.* [Gk., upper garment] [NA]. The nonnervous epithelial cells which abut on all cavities of the brain and spinal cord. —**ependy·mal** (·mul) *adj.*

ependymal cell. 1. A cell of the ependymal zone in the developing neural tube. 2. A type of neuroglia cell lining the central canal of the spinal cord and brain.

ependymal layer or **zone.** 1. In the embryonic neural tube, the innermost cells next to the central canal. 2. EPENDYMA.

ep·en·dy·mi·tis (ep·en″di·migh′tis) *n.* [*ependyma* + *-itis*]. Inflammation of the ependyma.

ep·en·dy·mo·blas·to·ma (ep·en″di·mo·blas·to′muh) *n.* [*ependyma* + *blastoma*]. A poorly differentiated ependymoma.

ep·en·dy·mo·cyte (ep·en′di·mo·site) *n.* [*ependyma* + *-cyte*]. EPENDYMAL CELL.

ep·en·dy·mo·ma (ep·en″di·mo′muh) *n.*, pl. **ependymomas, ependymoma·ta** (·tuh) [*ependyma* + *-oma*]. A central nervous system tumor whose parenchyma consists of cells resembling, and derived from, the ependymal cells. Syn. *blastoma ependymale.*

ep·en·dy·mop·a·thy (ep·en″di·mop′uth·ee) *n.* [*ependyma* + *-pathy*]. Disease of the ependyma.

eph·apse (ef′aps) *n.* [Gk. *ephapsis,* contact, act of touching]. A functional contact in which impulses jump from a nerve or muscle fiber made hyperexcitable to a contiguous inactive fiber. Contr. *synapse.* —**eph·ap·tic** (e·fap′tick) *adj.*

ephaptic conduction, excitation, or **transmission.** The spread of a current from an electrically active nerve not at the synapse, but across the membrane, into a closely contiguous inactive nerve; a mechanism possibly involved in the propagation of an epileptic discharge because of the density of neurons and their processes in the brain.

ephe·bi·a·tri·cian (e·fee″bee·uh·trish′un) *n.* A practitioner of ephebiatrics (adolescent medicine).

ephe·bi·at·rics (e·fee″bee·at′ricks) *n.* [Gr. *ephēbos*, an adolescent, + *-iatrics*]. The practice of adolescent medicine.

ephe·bic (e·fee′bick) *adj.* [Gk. *ephēbikos*]. Adolescent; pubertal.

eph·e·bo·gen·e·sis (ef″e·bo·jen′e·sis) *n.* The spontaneous development of a male germ cell thought to cause chorionic carcinoma or teratoma of the testis.

Ephed·ra (e·fed′rah, ef′e·druh) *n.* [Gk. *ephedra,* horsetail]. A genus of shrubs of the Gnetaceae, from some species of which is obtained the alkaloid ephedrine. Under the name *ma-huang,* species of *Ephedra* have been used in China for many years.

ephed·rine (e·fed′rin, ef′e·dreen, ·drin) *n.* [*Ephedra* + *-ine*]. *l*-α-(1-Methylaminoethyl)benzyl alcohol, $C_{10}H_{15}NO$, an alkaloid present in several *Ephedra* species and produced synthetically; white crystals, soluble in water. A sympathomimetic amine used in the form of the hydrochloride and sulfate salts for its action on the bronchi, blood pressure, blood vessels, and central nervous system.

***dl*-ephedrine.** RACEPHEDRINE.

ephe·lis (e·fee′lis) *n.*, pl. **ephe·li·des** (·li·deez) [Gk. *ephēlis*]. FRECKLE.

ephem·era (e·fem′ur·uh) *n.* An ephemeral fever.

ephem·er·al (e·fem′ur·ul) *adj.* [Gk. *ephēmeros,* short-lived, lasting a day, from *ep-* + *hēmera,* day]. Temporary; transient; applied to fevers that are of short duration.

ephemera ma·lig·na (ma·lig′nuh). ENGLISH SWEATING FEVER.

eph·i·dro·sis (ef″i·dro′sis) *n.* [Gk. *ephidrōsis*]. HYPERHIDROSIS.

ephidrosis cru·en·ta (kroo·en′tuh). HEMATHIDROSIS.

ephidrosis tinc·ta (tink′tuh). CHROMHIDROSIS.

Ephynal. A trademark for alpha tocopherol, a substance having vitamin E activity.

epi-. See *ep-.*

epi·ag·na·thus (ep″ee·ag′nuth·us, ·ag·nay′thus) *n.* [*epi-* + *agnathus*]. An individual with a deficient upper jaw.

epi·an·dros·ter·one (ep″i·an·dros′tur·ohn) *n.* 3β-Hydroxy-17-androstanone, $C_{19}H_{30}O_2$, an androgenic ketosteroid of low activity present in normal human urine as a minor constituent. Syn. *isoandrosterone.* Compare *androsterone.*

epi·blast (ep′i·blast) *n.* [*epi-* + *-blast*]. 1. The epidermal ectoderm after segregation of the neuroblast. 2. The primitive ectoderm of the blastula.

epi·blas·to·trop·ic (ep″i·blas″to·trop′ick) *adj.* [*epi-* + *blasto-* + *-tropic*]. Pertaining to changes in the ectoderm or in ectodermal derivatives.

epiblastotropic reaction. 1. A reaction affecting the ectoderm. 2. The reaction in yaws which produces lesions in the epidermis. Compare *panblastotropic reaction.*

epi·bleph·a·ron (ep″i·blef′uh·ron) *n.* [*epi-* + *blepharon*]. A congenital fold of skin on the lower eyelid, causing lashes to turn inward.

epib·o·ly (e·pib′o·lee) *n.* [Gk. *epibolē,* a throwing on]. A process of overgrowth in gastrulation in telolecithal eggs, in which the blastoporal lips spread over the vegetal hemisphere of the gastrula. —**ep·i·bol·ic** (ep″i·bol′ick) *adj.*

epi·bran·chi·al (ep″ee·brang′kee·ul) *adj.* [*epi-* + *branchial*]. Situated above or dorsal to the branchial grooves.

epibranchial placode. One of a series of ectodermal thickenings at the dorsal ends of the visceral grooves that, in some vertebrates, contributes to the adjacent cranial ganglion.

epi·bul·bar (ep″ee·bul′bur) *adj.* [*epi-* + *bulbar*]. Situated upon the globe of the eye.

epicanthic fold. EPICANTHUS.

epi·can·thus (ep″i·kanth′us) *n.* [*epi-* + *canthus*]. 1. A medial and downward fold of skin from the upper eyelid that hides the inner canthus and caruncle; a normal feature in some Asiatic races of man. Syn. *epicanthic fold.* NA *plica palpebronasalis.* 2. Any similar feature occurring as a congenital anomaly, as, for example, in Down's syndrome. —**epican·thic** (·ick), **epican·thal** (·ul) *adj.*

epi·car·dia (ep″i·kahr′dee·uh) *n.* [*epi-* + *cardia*]. 1. The lower end of the esophagus, between the diaphragm and the stomach. 2. Plural of *epicardium.*

epi·car·di·al (ep″i·kahr′dee·ul) *adj.* 1. Of or pertaining to the epicardium. 2. Of or pertaining to the epicardia.

epi·car·di·um (ep″i·kahr′dee·um) *n.*, pl. **epicar·dia** (·dee·uh) [*epi-* + *-cardium*] [NA]. The visceral layer of serous pericardium. NA *lamina visceralis pericardii.* See also Plate 5.

epi·carp (ep′i·kahrp) *n.* [*epi-* + *-carp*]. The outermost layer of the pericarp of a fruit.

epi·chor·dal (ep″ee·kor′dul) *adj.* [*epi-* + *chordal*]. Located above or dorsad of the notochord; applied especially to cerebral structures.

epi·cho·ri·al (ep″i·kor′ee·ul) *adj.* [*epi-* + *chorial*]. Located on the chorion.

epi·cho·ri·on (ep″i·ko′ree·on) *n.* [*epi-* + *chorion*]. DECIDUA CAPSULARIS.

epi·cil·lin (ep″i·sil′in) *n.* 6-[D-2-Amino-2-(1,4-cyclohexadien-1-yl)acetamido]-3,3-dimethyl-7-oxo-4-thia-1-azabicyclo[3.2.0]heptane-2-carboxylic acid, $C_{16}H_{21}N_3O_4S$, a penicillin-type antibiotic.

Epi-Clear. A trademark for benzoyl peroxide, a keratolytic agent.

epi·co·lic (ep″i·ko′lick, ·kol′ick) *adj.* [*epi-* + *colic*]. Situated over the colon.

epi·co·mus (ep″i·ko′mus) *n.* [*epi-* + Gk. *komē*, hair, + *-us*]. An individual (autosite) with a parasitic accessory head attached to its vertex.

epi·con·dyl·al·gia (ep″i·kon″dil·al′jee·uh) *n.* [*epicondyle* + *-algia*]. Pain, usually muscular, in the vicinity of an epicondyle.

epicondylar fracture. A fracture involving an epicondyle of one of the long bones.

epi·con·dyle (ep″i·kon′dile, ep″ee·) *n.* [*epi-* + *condyle*]. An eminence on a bone upon its condyle. —**epicon·dy·lar** (·di·lur), **epi·con·dyl·i·an** (·kon·dil′ee·un), **epi·con·dyl·ic** (·kon·dil′ick) *adj.*

epicondyli. Plural of *epicondylus.*

epi·con·dy·li·tis (ep″i·kon″di·lye′tis) *n.* [*epicondyle* + *-itis*]. 1. Inflammation of an epicondyle, or of tissues near an epicondyle. 2. Synovitis of the radiohumeral articulation. Syn. *radiohumeral bursitis, tennis elbow.*

ep·i·con·dy·lus (ep″i·kon′di·lus, ep″ee·) *n.*, pl. **epicondy·li** (·lye) [NL.]. EPICONDYLE.

epicondylus la·te·ra·lis fe·mo·ris (lat·e·ray′lis fem′o·ris) [NA]. The lateral epicondyle of the femur.

epicondylus lateralis hu·me·ri (hew′mur·eye) [NA]. The lateral epicondyle of the humerus.

epicondylus me·di·a·lis fe·mo·ris (mee·dee·ay′lis fem′o·ris) [NA]. The medial epicondyle of the femur.

epicondylus medialis hu·me·ri (hew′mur·eye) [NA]. The medial epicondyle of the humerus.

epi·cra·ni·al (ep″i·kray′nee·ul) *adj.* [*epi-* + *cranial*]. Pertaining to or located on the epicranium.

epicranial aponeurosis. GALEA APONEUROTICA.

ep·i·cra·nio·tem·po·ra·lis (ep·i·kray″nee·o·tem·po·ray′lis) *n.* A portion of the anterior auricular muscle.

epi·cra·ni·um (ep″i·kray′nee·um) *n.* [*epi-* + *cranium*]. The structures covering the cranium.

ep·i·cra·ni·us (ep″i·kray′nee·us) *n.* [NL., from *epi-* + Gk. *kranion*, skull]. The muscle of the scalp, consisting of a frontal and an occipital portion with the galea aponeurotica between. NA *musculus epicranius.*

[1]**epi·cri·sis** (ep′ee·krye″sis, ep″i·krye′sis) *n.* [*epi-* + *crisis*]. A secondary crisis in the course of a disease.

[2]**epic·ri·sis** (e·pick′ri·sis) *n.* [Gk. *epikrisis*, determination, judgment]. A critical summary or analysis of the record of a case or of a scientific article.

ep·i·crit·ic (ep″i·krit′ick) *adj.* [Gk. *epikritikos*, determinative]. Characterized by or pertaining to fine sensory discriminations, especially of touch and temperature. See also *epicritic sensibility.*

epicritic sensibility. The peripheral sensory mechanism which, according to the theory of Head and Rivers, subserves light touch, intermediate grades of temperature, and the ability to localize single and simultaneous two-point tactile stimuli.

epi·cys·ti·tis (ep″i·sis·tye′tis) *n.* [*epi-* + *cyst-* + *-itis*]. PERICYSTITIS (2).

epi·cys·tot·o·my (ep″i·sis·tot′uh·mee) *n.* [*epi-* + *cystotomy*]. Suprapubic incision of the urinary bladder.

epi·cyte (ep′i·site) *n.* [*epi-* + *-cyte*]. 1. CELL WALL. 2. A cell of epithelial tissue.

ep·i·dem·ic (ep″i·dem′ick) *adj.* & *n.* [Gk. *epidēmios*, sojourning among the people, from *dēmos*, populace, country]. 1. Of diseases, occurring or tending to occur in extensive outbreaks, or in unusually high incidence at certain times and places. Contr. *endemic, ecdemic, epizootic, sporadic.* 2. An extensive outbreak or period of unusually high incidence of a disease in a community or area. 3. Of or pertaining to epidemics.

epidemic arthritic erythema. HAVERHILL FEVER.

epidemic catalepsy. The occurrence of catalepsy in several individuals at the same time as a result of imitation.

epidemic catarrhal fever. INFLUENZA.

epidemic cerebrospinal meningitis. Meningococcal meningitis of endemic and epidemic incidence.

epidemic diarrhea of infant mice. A viral enteric disease of mice between 7 and 17 days old. Abbreviated, EDIM.

epidemic diarrhea of the newborn. Contagious fulminating diarrhea with high mortality, seen in newborns in hospital nurseries, and caused by enteropathogenic strains of *Escherichia coli*, certain strains of *Staphylococcus*, other bacteria, and possibly viruses.

epidemic dropsy. A disease, epidemic among natives of India, characterized by fever, diarrhea, skin rash, and edema; probably related to the ingestion of contaminated mustard oil.

epidemic encephalitis. 1. ENCEPHALITIS LETHARGICA. 2. Loosely, any of various other encephalitides that occur epidemically, such as Japanese B encephalitis, eastern or western equine encephalomyelitis, Murray Valley encephalitis, St. Louis encephalitis, and others.

epidemic hemoglobinuria. WINCKEL'S DISEASE.

epidemic hemorrhagic fever. An acute febrile epidemic disease of northeast Asia, thought to be due to a virus transmitted by mites; characterized by widespread vascular damage, prostration, vomiting, proteinuria, hemorrhagic manifestations, shock, and renal failure. Syn. *hemorrhagic fever, Far Eastern hemorrhagic fever, hemorrhagic nephrosonephritis.*

epidemic hepatitis or **jaundice.** INFECTIOUS HEPATITIS.

ep·i·de·mic·i·ty (ep″i·de·mis′i·tee) *n.* The state or quality of being epidemic.

epidemic keratoconjunctivitis. An infection caused by adenovirus types 6, 7, and 8, characterized by redness and chemosis of the conjunctiva, edema of periorbital tissues, preauricular lymphadenopathy, and mild constitutional symptoms. Superficial opacities of the cornea sometimes may result in persisting impairment of vision.

epidemic myalgia. EPIDEMIC PLEURODYNIA.

epidemic nausea. EPIDEMIC VOMITING.

epidemic neuromyasthenia. BENIGN MYALGIC ENCEPHALOMYELITIS.

epidemic paralysis. PARALYTIC SPINAL POLIOMYELITIS.

epidemic paralytic vertigo. PARALYTIC VERTIGO.

epidemic parotitis. MUMPS.

epidemic pleurodynia. An acute epidemic disease caused chiefly by Coxsackie B virus, characterized by severe paroxysmal pain in the lower thorax and upper abdomen increased by respiration, and associated with fever, headache, anorexia, and malaise. Syn. *Bornholm disease.*

epidemic roseola. 1. MEASLES. 2. RUBELLA.

epidemic serous meningitis. ASEPTIC MENINGITIS.

epidemic stomatitis. FOOT-AND-MOUTH DISEASE.

epidemic tremor. AVIAN ENCEPHALOMYELITIS.

epidemic tropical acute polyarthritis. A self-limited syndrome of unknown cause, first described among Australian soldiers (1942), characterized by acute polyarthritis, mild fever, lymphadenopathy, and transient rash.

epidemic typhus. An acute infectious louse-borne disease caused by *Rickettsia prowazekii*, characterized by severe headache, high fever, skin rash, and vascular and neurologic disturbances. Syn. *classic epidemic typhus, European typhus, louse-borne typhus.*

epidemic typhus vaccine. 1. COX VACCINE. 2. CASTAÑEDA VACCINE.

epidemic vertigo. PARALYTIC VERTIGO.

epidemic vomiting. Epidemic acute gastroenteritis occurring predominantly in children; may be bacterial or viral in origin.

ep·i·de·mi·ol·o·gist (ep″i·dee″mee·ol′uh·jist, ep″i·dem″ee·) *n.* One who has made a special study of epidemiology.

ep·i·de·mi·ol·o·gy (ep″i·dee″mee·ol′uh·jee, ep″i·dem″ee·) *n.* [*epidemic* + *-logy*]. 1. The study of occurrence and distribution of disease; usually restricted to epidemic and endemic, but sometimes broadened to include all types of disease. 2. The sum of all factors controlling the presence or absence of a disease. —**epidemi·o·log·ic** (·o·loj′ick) *adj.*

ep·i·derm (ep′i·durm) *n.* EPIDERMIS.

epiderm-, epidermo-. A combining form meaning *epidermis.*

epi·der·mal (ep″i·dur′mul) *adj.* Of, pertaining to, or involving the epidermis. Syn. *epidermic.*

epidermal ectoderm. That part of the ectoderm destined to form the epidermis. Syn. *epiblast.*

epidermal nevus. NEVUS VERRUCOSUS.

epi·der·mat·ic (ep″i·dur·mat′ick) *adj.* EPIDERMAL.

epi·der·ma·to·plas·ty (ep″i·dur′muh·to·plas″tee, ·dur·mat′o·) *n.* [*epi-* + *dermato-* + *-plasty*]. Skin grafting by transplanting small pieces to denuded areas.

epi·der·ma·to·zoo·no·sis (ep″i·dur″muh·to·zo″uh·no′sis) *n.* EPIZOONOSIS.

epi·der·mic (ep″i·dur′mick) *adj.* Of or pertaining to the epidermis; EPIDERMAL.

epi·der·mi·dal·iza·tion (ep″i·dur″mi·dul·i·zay′shun) *n.* The conversion of columnar into stratified squamous epithelium.

epi·der·mi·do·sis (ep″i·dur″mi·do′sis) *n.* EPIDERMOSIS.

epi·der·mis (ep″i·dur′mis) *n.* [Gk., from *epi-* + *derma,* skin] [NA]. The superficial portion of the skin, composed of a horny layer (stratum corneum) and a living, cellular part in layers named from outside inward: the stratum lucidum (when present), the stratum granulosum, the stratum spinosum, and the stratum germinativum.

epi·der·mi·tis (ep″i·dur·migh′tis) *n.* [*epiderm-* + *-itis*]. Inflammation of the outer layer of the skin.

epi·der·mi·za·tion (ep″i·dur″mi·zay′shun) *n.* 1. The formation of epidermis as a covering. 2. SKIN GRAFTING.

epidermo-. See *epiderm-.*

epi·der·mo·dys·pla·sia (ep″i·dur″mo·dis·play′zhuh, ·zee·uh) *n.* [*epidermo-* + *dysplasia*]. Abnormal development of the epidermis.

epidermodysplasia ver·ru·ci·for·mis (verr·oo″si·for′mis). A congenital defect in which verrucous lesions caused by a virus occur on the hands, feet, face, or neck.

epi·der·moid (ep″i·dur′moid) *adj.* & *n.* [*epiderm-* + *-oid*]. 1. Resembling epidermis. 2. Any tumor containing or resembling skin with its appendages.

epidermoid carcinoma. SQUAMOUS CELL CARCINOMA.

epidermoid cyst. A cyst lined by stratified squamous epithelium without associated cutaneous glands.

epi·der·moid·oma (ep″i·dur″moid·o′muh) *n.* [*epidermoid* + *-oma*]. An epidermal cyst involving the scalp, the bones of the calvaria, or the extradural space.

epi·der·mol·y·sis (ep″i·dur·mol′i·sis) *n.* [*epidermo-* + *-lysis*]. The easy separation of various layers of skin, primarily of the epidermis from the dermis. See also *Nikolsky's sign.*

epidermolysis bul·lo·sa (buh·lo′suh, bŏŏl·o′suh). A genodermatosis characterized by the development of vesicles and bullae on slight, or even without, trauma.

epidermolysis bullosa dys·troph·i·ca (dis·trof′i·kuh). A condition in which bullae of skin form on slight trauma or without it, followed by scarring and atrophy. Nails become dystrophic and are sometimes destroyed. Oral mucosa may show bullae, infiltration, or patches of leukoplakia. There may be alopecia and electroencephalographic changes.

epidermolysis bullosa he·red·i·tar·ia le·ta·lis (he·red·i·tăr′ee·uh lee·tay′lis). A rare form of epidermolysis bullosa, frequently familial, in which the bullae may appear at birth or shortly thereafter, and may contain lymph or blood. The nails are loosely attached and may be shed, and there are oral lesions. Syn. *Herlitz's disease.*

epidermolysis bullosa sim·plex (sim′plecks). A mild type of epidermolysis bullosa in which bullae form at birth or in early childhood in response to even mild trauma. There is complete healing, tendency to remission at puberty, with none of the other symptoms which occur in the dystrophic type.

epi·der·mo·lyt·ic (ep″i·dur″mo·lit′ick) *adj.* Pertaining to or causing epidermolysis.

epi·der·mo·ma (ep″i·dur·mo′muh) *n.* [*epiderm-* + *-oma*]. A skin mass of any sort, such as verruca vulgaris.

epi·der·mo·my·co·sis (ep″i·dur″mo·migh·ko′sis) *n.* [*epidermo-* + *mycosis*]. Any dermatitis caused by a fungus.

epi·der·moph·y·tid (ep″i·dur·mof′i·tid) *n.* [*Epidermophyton* + *-id*]. A secondary allergic skin eruption thought to occur when the fungus *Epidermophyton floccosum,* or its products, is carried through the blood stream to sensitized areas of the skin.

Epi·der·moph·y·ton (ep″i·dur·mof′i·ton) *n.* [*epidermo-* + Gk. *phyton,* plant]. A genus of fungi of the dermatophyte group; contains but one recognized species.

Epidermophyton floc·co·sum (flock·o′sum). The single species of this genus, found in infections of the skin and nails, and especially of the groin.

Epidermophyton in·gui·na·le (ing·gwi·nay′lee). *EPIDERMOPHYTON FLOCCOSUM.*

epi·der·mo·phy·to·sis (ep″i·dur″mo·figh·to′sis). Infection by *Epidermophyton floccosum.* It has been commonly used to include any fungus infection of the feet producing scaliness and vesicles with pruritus.

epi·der·mo·sis (ep″i·dur·mo′sis) *n.* [*epiderm-* + *-osis*]. A general name for anomalous growths of the skin of epithelial origin and type.

epi·der·mo·tro·pic (ep″i·dur″mo·tro′pick, ·trop′ick) *adj.* Having an affinity for epidermis.

epidermotropic reticulosis. WORINGER-KOLOPP DISEASE.

epi·dia·scope (ep·i·dye′uh·skope) *n.* [*epi-* + *dia-* + *-scope*]. An instrument for projecting either opaque or translucent pictures onto a screen.

epididym-, epididymo-. A combining form meaning *epididymis, epididymal.*

epi·did·y·mal (ep″i·did′i·mul) *adj.* Of or pertaining to the epididymis.

epididymal duct. The highly convoluted part of the duct of the testis which forms the main mass of the epididymis. NA *ductus epididymidis.*

epididymal sinus. DIGITAL FOSSA (2).

epi·did·y·mec·to·my (ep″i·did″i·meck′tuh·mee) *n.* [*epididym-* + *-ectomy*]. Surgical removal of the epididymis.

epi·did·y·mis (ep″i·did′i·mis) *n.,* genit. **epi·di·dy·mi·dis** (ep″i·di·dim′i·dis), pl. **epi·di·dy·mi·des** (·did′i·mi·deez, ·di·dim′i·deez) [Gk.] [NA]. The portion of the seminal duct lying posterior to the testis and connected to it by the efferent ductules of the testis. See also Plate 25.

epi·did·y·mi·tis (ep″i·did″i·migh′tis) *n.* [*epididym-* + *-itis*]. Inflammation of the epididymis.

epididymo-. See *epididym-.*

epi·did·y·mo·or·chi·dec·to·my (ep″i·did″i·mo·or″ki·deck′tuh·mee) *n.* [*epididymo-* + *orchidectomy*]. Surgical removal of a testis and epididymis.

epi·did·y·mo·or·chi·tis (ep″i·did″i·mo·or·kigh′tis) *n.* [*epididymo-* + *orchitis*]. Inflammation of both the epididymis and testis.

epi·did·y·mot·o·my (ep″i·did″i·mot′uh·mee) *n.* [*epididymo-* + *-tomy*]. Incision into the epididymis.

epi·did·y·mo·vas·os·to·my (ep″i·did″i·mo·vas·os′tuh·mee) *n.* [*epididymo-* + *vaso-* + *-stomy*]. *In surgery,* anastomosis of the ductus deferens with the epididymis.

epi·du·ral (ep″i·dew′rul) *adj.* [*epi-* + *dural*]. Situated upon or over the dura mater.

epidural abscess. An abscess located outside the dura mater but within the cranium or spinal canal. Syn. *epidural pachymeningitis, extradural abscess, pachymeningitis externa.*

epidural aerocele. An intracranial extradural accumulation of air or gas, usually resulting from a fracture of the skull.

epidural anesthesia. PERIDURAL ANESTHESIA.

epidural hematoma. The localized accumulation of blood between the dura mater and the skull, usually as a result of rupture of the middle meningeal artery and skull fracture, characterized usually by a brief loss of consciousness, then a lucid interval, and later progressive neurologic involvement with depression of consciousness, hemiparesis, and seizures due to compression of the brain by blood clot.

epidural pachymeningitis. EPIDURAL ABSCESS.

epidural space or **cavity.** The space between the spinal dura mater and the periosteum lining the canal. NA *cavum epidurale.*

epidural spinal hematoma or **hemorrhage.** Bleeding into the epidural space as a result of trauma, vascular abnormality, or bleeding tendency, as with anticoagulant therapy; manifested by signs and symptoms of rapidly progressive spinal cord compression.

epi·fas·cial (ep″ee·fash′ee·uh, ·fash′ul) *adj.* [*epi-* + *fascial*]. Of, pertaining to, or on a fascia.

epi·fol·lic·u·li·tis (ep″i·fol·ick″yoo·lye′tis) *n.* [*epi-* + *folliculitis*]. Inflammation of the hair follicles of the scalp.

epigastraeum. Epigastrium (= EPIGASTRIC REGION).

epi·gas·tral·gia (ep″i·gas·tral′jee·uh) *n.* [*epigastr*ium + *-algia*]. Pain in the epigastric region.

epi·gas·tric (ep″i·gas′trick) *adj.* Of or pertaining to the epigastric region.

epigastric angle. COSTAL ANGLE.

epigastric artery. See Table of Arteries in the Appendix.

epigastric aura. A midline sensation over the gastric area which may ascend to the throat; may precede a major generalized or psychomotor seizure or represent a convulsive equivalent.

epigastric fold. A ridge of peritoneum covering the inferior epigastric vessels.

epigastric fossa. The midline infrasternal depression. NA *fossa epigastrica.*

epigastric hernia. A hernia in the linea alba, between the umbilicus and the xiphoid process, generally found in young adult males; the contents of the sac are usually extraperitoneal fat, lipomas, and, only rarely, bowel.

epigastric plexus. CELIAC PLEXUS.

epigastric region. The upper and middle part of the abdominal surface between the two hypochondriac regions. Syn. *epigastrium.* NA *regio epigastrica.* See also *abdominal regions.*

epi·gas·trio·cele (ep″i·gas′tree·o·seel) *n.* EPIGASTROCELE.

epi·gas·tri·um, epi·gas·trae·um (ep″i·gas′tree·um) *n.*, pl. **epi·gas·tria** (·tree·uh) [NL., from Gk. *epigastrion,* from *epi-* + *gastēr,* belly, stomach]. EPIGASTRIC REGION.

epi·gas·tri·us (ep″i·gas′tree·us) *n.* [*epigastr*ium + *-us*]. A form of unequal conjoined twins in which the parasitic twin or part is attached to the epigastric region of the other.

epigastrius par·a·sit·i·cus (păr·uh·sit′i·kus). A thoracopagus parasiticus in which the parasitic twin is attached in the epigastric region.

epi·gas·tro·cele (ep″i·gas′tro·seel) *n.* [*epigastr*ium + *-cele*]. A hernia in the epigastric region.

epi·gen·e·sis (ep″i·jen′e·sis) *n.* [*epi-* + *-genesis*]. The theory that the fertilized egg gives rise to the organism by the progressive production of new parts, previously nonexistent as such in the egg's original structure. Contr. *preformation.* —**epi·ge·net·ic** (·je·net′ick) *adj.*

epi·gen·i·tal (ep″ee·jen′i·tul) *adj.* [*epi-* + *genital*]. Above a gonad (testis).

epigenital tubule. A mesonephric tubule that becomes one of the ductuli aberrantes.

epi·glot·tal (ep″i·glot′ul) *adj.* Of or pertaining to the epiglottis; EPIGLOTTIC.

epi·glot·tic (ep″i·glot′ick) *adj.* Of or pertaining to the epiglottis; EPIGLOTTAL.

epiglottic cartilage. The cartilage of the epiglottis. NA *cartilago epiglottica.*

epiglottic tubercle. A slight convexity on the dorsal surface of the epiglottis. NA *tuberculum epiglotticum.*

epi·glot·ti·dec·to·my (ep″i·glot″i·deck′tuh·mee) *n.* [*epiglottis* + *-ectomy*]. Excision of the epiglottis or a part of it.

epi·glot·tis (ep″i·glot′is) *n.* [Gk. *epiglōttis*] [NA]. An elastic cartilage covered by mucous membrane, forming the superior part of the larynx which guards the glottis during swallowing. See also Plate 12.

epi·glot·ti·tis (ep″i·glot·eye′tis) *n.* [*epiglott*is + *-itis*]. Inflammation of the epiglottis, frequently caused by *Haemophilus influenzae.*

epig·na·thus (e·pig′nuth·us, ep″i·nath′us) *n.* [*epi-* + *gnath-* + *-us*]. A condition in which a mixed tumor, teratoma, or parasitic twin fetus (or part of a fetus) is attached to the base of the skull or to the jaws, usually to the hard palate.

epig·o·nal (e·pig′uh·nul, ep″i·go′nul) *adj.* [*epi-* + *gon*ad + *-al*]. Located on an embryonic gonad.

epigonal fold. The caudal part of the genital ridge, in which the ovarian ligament or the upper part of the gubernaculum testis develops.

epi·gua·nine, epi·gua·nin (ep″i·gwah′neen, ·nin) *n.* Methylguanine, $C_6H_7N_5O$, a purine base found in human urine.

epi·hy·al (ep″ee·high′ul) *n.* [*epi-* + *hy*oid + *-al*]. One of a series of bones forming the hyoid arch. See also *ceratohyal.*

epi·hy·oid (ep″ee·high′oid) *adj.* [*epi-* + *hyoid*]. Situated upon the hyoid bone.

epi·la·mel·lar (ep″ee·luh·mel′ur, ·lam′e·lur) *adj.* [*epi-* + *lamellar*]. Situated upon a basement membrane.

epilating forceps. Special forceps used for removing the hairs of the lashes, eyebrows, or other areas where hair is not desired.

ep·i·la·tion (ep″i·lay′shun) *n.* [F. *épilation,* from *e-* + L. *pilus,* a hair]. Removal of the hair roots, as by the use of forceps, chemical means, or roentgenotherapy. —**ep·i·late** (ep′i·late) *v.*

ep·i·lem·ma (ep″i·lem′uh) *n.* [*epi-* + *-lemma*]. The perineurium of very small nerves.

ep·i·lep·sia (ep″i·lep′see·uh) *n.* [L.]. EPILEPSY.

epilepsia ar·ith·met·i·ca (ăr″ith·met′i·kuh). A form of reflex epilepsy in which seizures are precipitated by viewing geometric forms, certain line patterns, or solving mathematical problems.

epilepsia mi·tis (migh′tis). ABSENCE ATTACK.

epilepsia par·ti·a·lis con·tin·ua (pahr·shee·ay′lis kon·tin′yoo·uh). STATUS EPILEPTICUS.

epilepsia ver·tig·i·no·sa (vur·tij″i·no′suh). ABSENCE ATTACK.

ep·i·lep·sy (ep′i·lep″see) *n.* [Gk. *epilēpsia,* a seizure, from *epilambanein,* to seize, attack]. A disorder of the brain characterized by a recurring excessive neuronal discharge, manifested by transient episodes of motor, sensory, or psychic dysfunction, with or without unconsciousness or convulsive movements. The seizure is associated with marked changes in recorded electrical brain activity.

epilept-, epilepti-, epilepto-. A combining form meaning *epilepsy, epileptic.*

ep·i·lep·tic (ep″i·lep′tick) *adj.* & *n.* [Gk. *epilēptikos*]. 1. Pertaining to or characterized by epilepsy. 2. An individual who suffers from epilepsy.

epileptic automatism. A complex semipurposeful act performed during a seizure, which the patient later cannot remember. Contr. *postictal automatism, psychomotor seizure.*

epileptic dementia. Severe mental deterioration as a consequence of brain damage, usually anoxic, suffered during prolonged, repeated convulsions.

epileptic equivalent. CONVULSIVE EQUIVALENT.

epileptic stupor. The stupor following an epileptic convulsion.

epileptic vertigo. Vertigo associated with or preceding an attack of epilepsy.

ep·i·lep·ti·form (ep″i·lep′ti·form) *adj.* [*epilept-* + *-iform*]. 1. Resembling epilepsy; specifically, resembling a generalized convulsion. 2. Having the electroencephalographic patterns characteristic of epilepsy, such as 3 per second spikes and waves, generalized paroxysmal activity, and spike or sharp wave discharges.

epilepto-. See *epilept-.*

ep·i·lep·to·gen·ic (ep″i·lep″to·jen′ick) *adj.* [*epilepto-* + *-genic*]. Producing epilepsy.

epileptogenic focus. The exact location in the brain from which an epileptic discharge originates, sometimes identifiable by means of an electroencephalogram or electrocorticogram.

ep·i·lep·tog·e·nous (ep″i·lep·toj′e·nus) *adj.* EPILEPTOGENIC.

ep·i·lep·toid (ep″i·lep′toid) *adj.* [*epilept-* + *-oid*]. Resembling epilepsy.

epileptoid personality disorder. EXPLOSIVE PERSONALITY.

ep·i·lep·tol·o·gist (ep″i·lep·tol′uh·jist) *n.* An individual, usually a physician, who specializes in epileptology.

ep·i·lep·tol·o·gy (ep″i·lep·tol′uh·jee) *n.* [*epilepto-* + *-logy*]. The study and science of the nature, causes, diagnosis, and treatment of epilepsy.

ep·i·loia (ep″i·loy′uh) *n.* [*epi*lepsy + an*oia*]. TUBEROUS SCLEROSIS.

epi·mem·bra·nous nephropathy (ep″ee·mem′bruh·nus). MEMBRANOUS GLOMERULONEPHRITIS.

epi·mer (ep′i·mur) *n.* [*epi-* + *-mer*]. Either of a pair of diastereoisomers with more than one chiral center, the configurations of which are identical, except for the position of groups about one atom, as D-glucose and D-mannose. —**ep·i·mer·ic** (ep·i·merr′ick) *adj.*

epi·mere (ep′i·meer) *n.* [*epi-* + *-mere*]. The dorsal portion of the trunk mesoderm of chordates, forming skeletal musculature and contributing to derma and axial skeleton.

epi·mes·trol (ep″i·mes′trole) *n.* 3-Methoxyestra-1,3,5(10)-triene-16α,17α-diol, $C_{19}H_{26}O_3$, an anterior pituitary activator.

epi·myo·car·di·um (ep″ee·migh″o·kahr′dee·um) *n.* [*epi-* + *myocardium*]. The external part of the embryonic heart that develops into the epicardium and myocardium.

epi·my·si·um (ep″i·miz′ee·um, ·mis′ee·um) *n.*, pl. **epimy·sia** (·ee·uh) [NL., from *epi-* + Gk. *mys*, muscle]. The sheath of connective tissue surrounding a muscle. —**epimysi·al** (·ul) *adj.*

Epinal. A trademark for epinephryl borate, an ophthalmic adrenergic.

epi·neph·rin (ep″i·nef′rin) *n.* EPINEPHRINE.

epinephrinaemia. EPINEPHRINEMIA.

epi·neph·rine (ep″i·nef′rin, ·reen) *n.* [*epi-* + *nephr-* + *-ine*]. *l*-α-3,4-Dihydroxyphenyl-β-methylaminoethanol, $C_9H_{13}NO_3$, the chief catecholamine hormone of the adrenal medulla, occurring as colorless crystals that gradually darken on exposure to light and air; sparingly soluble in water. Increased levels cause a rise in blood glucose levels, elevation of blood pressure, acceleration of the heart, vasoconstriction in such organs as the skin and intestinal tract, but dilation of coronary and skeletal muscle vessels with increased alertness as a response to emergency. Obtained by extraction from the gland or prepared synthetically. In general, the effects of administration are those following stimulation of the sympathetic nervous system. The chief uses medically are as a vasoconstrictor to prolong the action of local anesthetics and as a source of symptomatic relief in allergic states. Its action is fleeting. Syn. *adrenaline*.

epinephrine headache. A pressor headache due to the sudden rise in blood pressure following an injection of epinephrine.

epinephrine hypersensitiveness test. GOETSCH TEST.

epi·neph·ri·ne·mia, epi·neph·ri·nae·mia (ep″i·nef″ri·nee′mee·uh) *n.* [*epinephrin*e + *-emia*]. The presence of epinephrine in the blood.

epinephrine test. 1. BENDA'S TEST. 2. Lowering of blood pressure or elevation of body temperature in a patient with hyperthyroidism after epinephrine injection.

epi·ne·phri·tis (ep″i·ne·frye′tis) *n.* [*epinephros* + *-itis*]. ADRENALITIS.

epi·neph·ros (ep″i·nef′ros) *n.*, pl. **epineph·roi** (·roy) [*epi-* + *nephros*]. ADRENAL GLAND.

epi·neph·ryl borate (ep″i·nef′ril). The cyclic borate ester incorporating the two phenolic hydroxyl groups of epinephrine, $C_9H_{12}BNO_4$; an adrenergic.

epi·neu·ral (ep″ee·new′rul) *adj.* [*epi-* + *neural*]. Attached to a neural arch.

epi·neu·ri·um (ep″i·new′ree·um) *n.* [NL., from *epi-* + Gk. *neuron*, nerve]. The connective-tissue sheath of a nerve trunk. —**epineuri·al** (·ul) *adj.*

epi·otic (ep″ee·ot′ick, ·o′tick) *adj.* [*epi-* + *otic*]. Situated above or on the cartilage of the ear.

epi·pal·a·tum (ep″i·pal′uh·tum, ·pa·lay′tum) *n.* [*epi-* + *palatum*]. The variety of epignathus in which the parasitic fetus or fetal remnant is attached to the palate.

ep·i·pas·tic (ep″i·pas′tick) *adj.* & *n.* [Gk. *epipassein*, to sprinkle over]. 1. Having the qualities of a dusting powder. 2. A powder for use on the surface of the body, as talc.

epi·pa·tel·lar (ep″ee·puh·tel′ur) *adj.* [*epi-* + *patellar*]. Situated above the patella; SUPRAPATELLAR.

epipatellar reflex. SUPRAPATELLAR REFLEX.

epi·peri·car·di·al (ep″ee·perr″i·kahr′dee·ul) *adj.* [*epi-* + *pericardial*]. Situated on or about the pericardium.

epipericardial ridges. Paired areas of loose pharyngeal mesenchyme above the embryonic pericardial cavity; said to form the pathway for migration of occipital premuscle masses and the hypoglossal nerve to the tongue.

epi·pha·ryn·ge·al (ep″ee·fa·rin′jee·ul) *adj.* [*epi-* + *pharyngeal*]. NASOPHARYNGEAL.

epi·phar·ynx (ep″ee·făr′inks) *n.* [*epi-* + *pharynx*]. NASOPHARYNX.

epi·phe·nom·e·non (ep″i·fe·nom′e·nun, ·non) *n.*, pl. **epiphenome·na** (·nuh) [*epi-* + *phenomenon*]. An unusual, accidental, or accessory event or process in the course of a disease, not necessarily related to the disease.

epiph·o·ra (e·pif′o·ruh) *n.* [Gk., from *epipherein*, to bring upon]. A persistent overflow of tears, due to excessive secretion or to impeded outflow.

epi·phre·nal (ep″i·free′nul) *adj.* [*epi-* + *phren-* + *-al*]. EPIPHRENIC.

epi·phren·ic (ep″i·fren′ick) *adj.* [*epi-* + *phrenic*]. Originating or situated above the diaphragm.

epiphrenic diverticulum. A diverticulum originating from the stomach in the region of the cardioesophageal junction.

epi·phy·lax·is (ep″i·fi·lack′sis) *n.*, pl. **epiphylax·es** (·seez) [*epi-* + *phylaxis*]. The reinforcing or increase of the natural defenses of the body, usually by specific therapy.

epi·phy·se·al (e·pif″i·see′ul, ep″i·fiz′ee·ul) *adj.* 1. Pertaining to or involving an epiphysis. 2. Of or pertaining to the pineal body (epiphysis cerebri).

epiphyseal cartilage. EPIPHYSEAL PLATE (2).

epiphyseal chondromatous giant-cell tumor. CHONDROBLASTOMA.

epiphyseal disk. EPIPHYSEAL PLATE (1).

epiphyseal dysplasia. 1. DYSPLASIA EPIPHYSIALIS MULTIPLEX. 2. CHONDRODYSTROPHIA CALCIFICANS CONGENITA.

epiphyseal eye. PINEAL EYE.

epiphyseal fracture. A fracture occurring along the epiphyseal line.

epiphyseal line. 1. The area left at the site of the epiphyseal plate after fusion of an epiphysis with the diaphysis of a long bone. The site is commonly marked by a cribriform bony plate more or less easily demonstrable in sections. NA *linea epiphysialis*. 2. *In radiology*, a strip of decreased density between the metaphysis and the ossified portion of the epiphysis.

epiphyseal plate. 1. The broad, articular surface with slightly elevated rim on each end of the centrum of a vertebra. Syn. *epiphyseal disk*. 2. The thin cartilage mass between an epiphysis and the shaft of a bone; the site of growth in length. It is obliterated by epiphyseal union. NA *cartilago epiphysialis*.

epiphyseal syndrome. PINEAL SYNDROME.

epiphyseolysis. EPIPHYSIOLYSIS.

ep·i·phys·eo·ne·cro·sis, ep·i·phys·io·ne·cro·sis (ep″i·fiz″ee·o·ne·kro′sis) *n.* Aseptic necrosis involving the epiphysis of a long bone.

ep·i·phys·e·op·a·thy (ep″i·fiz″ee·op′uth·ee) *n.* [*epiphysis* + *-pathy*]. 1. Any disorder of an epiphysis of a bone. 2. Any disorder of the pineal body (epiphysis cerebri).

ep·i·phys·i·al (ep″i·fiz′ee·ul) *adj.* EPIPHYSEAL.

ep·i·phys·i·o·de·sis (ep″i·fiz″ee·o·dee′sis, ·od′e·sis) *n.*, pl. **epi-physiode·ses** (·seez) [*epiphysis* + *-desis*]. The surgical production of permanent or temporary arrest of epiphyseal growth.

ep·i·phys·i·o·lis·the·sis (ep″i·fiz″ee·o·lis′thi·sis) *n.*, pl. **epiphys-iolisthe·ses** (·seez) [*epiphysis* + Gk. *olisthēsis*, slipping, dislocation]. The slipping of an epiphysis.

ep·i·phys·i·ol·y·sis, ep·i·phys·e·ol·y·sis (ep″i·fiz″ee·ol′i·sis) *n.*, pl. **epiphysioly·ses** (·seez) [*epiphysis* + *-lysis*]. The separation of an epiphysis from the shaft of a bone.

epiphysionecrosis. EPIPHYSEONECROSIS.

epiph·y·sis (e·pif′i·sis) *n.*, pl. **epiphy·ses** (·seez) [Gk.] [NA]. A portion of bone attached for a time to a bone by cartilage, but subsequently becoming consolidated with the principal bone.

epiphysis ce·re·bri (serr′e·brye). PINEAL BODY.

epiph·y·si·tis (e·pif″i·sigh′tis) *n.* [*epiphysis* + *-itis*]. Inflammation of an epiphysis.

epi·phyte (ep′i·fite) n. [*epi-* + *-phyte*]. 1. A parasitic plant, such as a fungus, growing on the exterior of the body. 2. A plant growing upon another plant, but deriving the moisture required for its development from the air.

epi·pi·al (ep″i·pee′ul, ·pye′ul) *adj.* [*epi-* + *pial*]. Upon or above the pia mater.

epi·pleu·ral (ep″i·ploor′ul) *adj.* [*epi-* + *pleural*]. 1. Pertaining to a pleurapophysis. 2. Located on the side of the thorax.

epiplo-. A combining form meaning *epiploon* or *omentum.*

epiploa. Plural of *epiploon.*

epip·lo·cele (e·pip′lo·seel) *n.* [*epiplo-* + *-cele*]. A hernia containing omentum only.

ep·i·plo·ec·to·my (ep″i·plo·eck′tuh·mee) *n.* [*epiplo-* + *-ectomy*]. Excision of the greater omentum or part of it.

epip·lo·en·tero·cele (e·pip″lo·en′tur·o·seel) *n.* [*epiplo-* + *entero-* + *-cele*]. A hernia containing both omentum and intestine.

ep·i·plo·ic (ep″i·plo′ick) *adj.* Of or pertaining to the epiploon.

epiploic appendages. APPENDICES EPIPLOICAE.

epiploic foramen. An aperture of the peritoneal cavity situated between the liver and the stomach, bounded in front by the portal vein, hepatic artery, and common bile duct, behind by the inferior vena cava, below by the duodenum, and above by the liver. Formed by folds of the peritoneum, it establishes communication between the greater and lesser cavities of the peritoneum. NA *foramen epiploicum.*

epip·lom·phalo·cele (e·pip″lom·fal′o·seel) *n.* [*epiplo-* + *omphalocele*]. An omphalocele containing omentum only.

epip·lo·on (e·pip′lo·on) *n.*, pl. **epip·loa** (·lo·uh) [Gk.]. OMENTUM; specifically, GREATER OMENTUM.

epip·lo·pexy (e·pip′lo·peck″see) *n.* [*epiplo-* + *-pexy*]. Suturing the greater omentum to the anterior abdominal wall for the purpose of establishing a collateral venous circulation in cirrhosis of the liver.

ep·i·plor·rha·phy (ep″i·plor′uh·fee) *n.* [*epiplo-* + *-rrhaphy*]. Suturing of the omentum.

ep·i·pro·pi·dine (ep″i·pro′pi·deen) *n.* 1,1′-Bis(2,3-epoxypropyl)-4,4′-bipiperidine, $C_{16}H_{28}N_2O_2$, an antineoplastic drug.

ep·ip·ter·ic (ep″ip·terr′ick) *adj.* [*epi-* + *pter-* + *-ic*]. Near the pterion, as the wormian bones.

ep·i·py·gus (ep″i·pye′gus, e·pip′i·gus) *n.* [*epi-* + Gk., *pygē*, rump, + *-us*]. PYGOMELUS.

epi·scle·ra (ep″i·skleer′uh) *n.* [*epi-* + *sclera*]. The loose connective tissue lying between the conjunctiva and the sclera.

epi·scle·ral (ep″i·skleer′ul) *adj.* [*epi-* + *scleral*]. 1. Situated on the outside of the sclerotic coat. 2. Pertaining to the episclera.

episcleral space. The interval between the sclera of the eyeball and the investing fascia.

epi·scle·ri·tis (ep″i·skle·rye′tis) *n.* [*episclera* + *-itis*]. Inflammation of the episcleral tissue; can occur as a diffuse form in toxic, allergic, and infectious conditions or as a nodular episcleritis in diffuse connective-tissue diseases.

episio- [Gk. *epision*, pubic region]. A combining form meaning *vulva.*

epis·io·cli·sia (e·piz″ee·o·klye′see·uh, e·pee″see·o·, ep″i·sigh″o·) *n.* [*episio-* + Gk. *kleisis*, closure, + *-ia*]. Surgical closure of the vulva.

epis·io·ely·tror·rha·phy (e·piz″ee·o·el″i·tror′uh·fee) *n.* [*episio-* + *elytro-* + *-rrhaphy*]. Suturing a relaxed or lacerated perineum and narrowing the vagina.

epis·io·per·i·neo·plas·ty (e·piz″ee·o·perr″i·nee′o·plas″tee) *n.* [*episio-* + *perineoplasty*]. Repair of the perineum and vestibule in the female.

epis·io·per·i·ne·or·rha·phy (e·piz″ee·o·perr″i·nee·or′ruh·fee) *n.* [*episio-* + *perineo-* + *-rrhaphy*]. Surgical repair of lacerated vulva and perineum.

epis·io·plas·ty (e·piz′ee·o·plas″tee) *n.* [*episio-* + *-plasty*]. A plastic operation upon the pubic region or the vulva.

epis·i·or·rha·gia (e·piz″ee·o·ray′jee·uh) *n.* [*episio-* + *-rrhagia*]. Hemorrhage from the vulva.

epis·i·or·rha·phy (e·piz″ee·or′uh·fee, e·pee″see·, ep″i·sigh·) *n.* [*episio-* + *-rrhaphy*]. Surgical repair of lacerations about the vulva.

epis·io·ste·no·sis (e·piz″ee·o·ste·no′sis) *n.*, pl. **episiosteno·ses** (·seez) [*episio-* + *stenosis*]. Contraction or narrowing of the vulva.

epis·i·ot·o·my (e·piz″ee·ot′uh·mee, e·pee″see·, ep″i·sigh·) *n.* [*episio-* + *-tomy*]. Medial or lateral incision of the vulva during childbirth, to avoid undue laceration.

ep·i·sode, *n.* [Gk. *epeisodion*, addition, interlude]. 1. An event having a distinct effect on a person's life, or on the course of a disease. 2. SEIZURE. 3. CEREBROVASCULAR ACCIDENT. —**ep·i·sod·ic** (ep·i·sod′ick) *adj.*

epi·some (ep′i·sohm) *n.* [*epi-* + *-some*]. A genetic particle, such as a bacteriophage or the fertility (F) factor of some bacteria, which may exist either in an independent state or in an integrated state as part of a chromosome of a host cell.

epi·spa·dia (ep″i·spay′dee·uh) *n.* EPISPADIAS.

epi·spa·di·as (ep″i·spay′dee·us) *n.* [NL., from *epi-* + *-spadias* as in hypospadias]. A congenital defect of the anterior urethra in which the canal terminates on the dorsum of the penis and posterior to its normal opening or, rarely, above the clitoris. —**epispadi·ac** (·ack) *adj. & n.;* **epispadi·al** (·ul) *adj.*

ep·i·spas·tic (ep″i·spas′tick) *adj. & n.* [Gk. *epispastikos*, drawing in]. 1. Causing blisters. 2. A blistering agent.

epi·sphe·noid (ep″i·sfee′noid) *n.* [*epi-* + *sphenoid*]. A parasitic fetus or fetal parts attached in the sphenoid region; one of the varieties of epignathus.

epi·spi·nal (ep″i·spye′nul) *adj.* [*epi-* + *spinal*]. 1. Upon the spinal column. 2. Upon the spinal cord. 3. Upon any spinelike structure.

epis·ta·sis (e·pis′tuh·sis) *n.*, pl. **epista·ses** (·seez) [Gk., stoppage]. 1. A scum or film of substance floating on the surface of urine. 2. A checking or stoppage of a hemorrhage or other discharge. 3. The suppression of the effect of one gene by another, as in the suppression of genetically determined pigment variation in albinos. —**ep·i·stat·ic** (ep·i·stat′ick) *adj.*

epis·ta·sy (e·pis′tuh·see) *n.* EPISTASIS.

ep·i·stax·is (ep″i·stack′sis) *n.* [Gk., a dripping]. NOSEBLEED.

epi·ster·nal (ep″i·stur′nul) *adj.* [*epi-* + *sternal*]. 1. Situated on or above the sternum. 2. Of or pertaining to the episternum.

episternal bar. EPISTERNAL CARTILAGE.

episternal cartilage. One of a pair of small embryonic cartilages articulating with the clavicle and forming part of the manubrium sterni. Syn. *episternal bar.*

ep·i·stern·um (ep″i·stur′num) *n.* [*epi-* + *sternum*]. A dermal bone or pair of bones ventral to the sternum of certain fishes and reptiles. Compare *prosternum.*

ep·i·stro·phe·us (ep″i·stro′fee·us) *n.* [Gk., from *epistrephein,* to turn about] [BNA]. AXIS (2); the second cervical vertebra. See also Table of Bones in the Appendix.

ep·i·stroph·ic (ep″i·strof′ick) *adj.* Pertaining to the epistropheus or axis.

ep·i·sym·pus di·pus (ep″i·sim′pus dye′pus). An individual in which the legs are rotated as in sympodia, but are united by a membrane only.

epi·tar·sus (ep″i·tahr′sus) *n.* [*epi-* + *tarsus*]. An anomalous fold of conjunctiva passing from the fornix to near the lid border. Syn. *congenital pterygium.*

ep·i·ten·din·e·um (ep″i·ten·din′ee·um) *n.* [NL., from *epi-* + *tendin*ous]. The fibrous sheath surrounding a tendon.

ep·i·ten·on (ep″i·ten′on) *n.* [*epi-* + *Gk. tenōn,* tendon]. EPITENDINEUM.

epi·thal·a·mus (ep″i·thal′uh·mus) *n.*, pl. **epithala·mi** (·migh) [*epi-* + *thalamus*] [NA]. The region of the diencephalon including the habenula, the pineal body, and the posterior commissure.

ep·i·tha·lax·ia (ep″i·tha·lack′see·uh) *n.* [*epith*elium + Gk. *allax*is, a shedding, + *-ia*]. Shedding of epithelial cells, especially in the lining of the intestine.

epitheli-, epithelio-. A combining form meaning *epithelium, epithelial.*

epithelia. A plural of *epithelium.*

ep·i·the·li·al (ep″i·theel′ee·ul) *adj.* Pertaining to or involving epithelium.

epithelial attachment. The union of the gingival epithelium with the tooth.

epithelial body. *Obsol.* PARATHYROID GLAND.

epithelial cord. EPITHELIAL RESTS OF MALASSEZ.

epithelial debris. ²REST (2).

epithelial debris of Malassez. EPITHELIAL RESTS OF MALASSEZ.

epithelial dystrophy. FUCH'S DYSTROPHY.

epithelial gland. A group of glandular cells within an epithelial layer.

epithelial hyalin. The hyalin produced by epithelial cells or resulting from degenerative change, usually in the form of intracytoplasmic droplets and seen in certain tumor cells, plasmacytes, and in various diseases of the liver and kidney.

epithelial ingrowth or **downgrowth.** A complication of faulty wound closure or any form of penetrating trauma of the cornea in which epithelium grows into or down through the wound, preventing its proper healing and eventually producing secondary glaucoma, rarely responsive to treatment.

epi·the·li·al·iza·tion (ep·i·theel″ee·ul·eye·zay′shun) *n.* EPITHELIAZATION.

ep·i·the·li·al·ize (ep·i·theel′ee·uh·lize) *v.* EPITHELIZE.

epithelial mass. The internal mass of cells derived from and covered by the germinal epithelium of the indifferent gonad.

epithelial nevus. A nevoid proliferation, either present at birth or developing later in life, in which hyperplasia of epithelial cells occurs without the presence of melanocytes.

epithelial pearl. PEARL (1).

epithelial plug. A temporary mass of epithelial cells closing the embryonic external naris.

epithelial remnant. EPITHELIAL RESTS OF MALASSEZ.

epithelial rests of Ma·las·sez (ma·la·sey′) [L. C. *Malassez,* French physiologist, 1842–1909]. Remnants of Hertwig's epithelial root sheath which persist in the periodontal ligament. Syn. *epithelial debris of Malassez.*

epithelial sheath of Hertwig [R. *Hertwig*]. HERTWIG'S EPITHELIAL ROOT SHEATH.

epithelial tag. A mass of epithelial cells projecting from the urethral groove on the glans of the embryonic phallus.

epithelial tissue. EPITHELIUM.

epithelial tubercle. EPITHELIAL TAG.

ep·i·the·li·i·tis (ep″i·theel″ee·eye′tis) *n.*, pl. **epitheliitis·es** (·iz), **epitheli·it·i·des** (·it′i·deez) [*epitheli-* + *-itis*]. Infiltration of an epithelial surface by inflammatory cells without ulceration or abscess formation.

epithelio-. See *epitheli-.*

ep·i·the·lio·cho·ri·al (ep″i·theel″ee·o·ko′ree·ul) *adj.* [*epithelio-* + *chorial*]. Pertaining to the relationship of the uterine epithelium and the chorionic membrane in the epitheliochorial placenta.

epitheliochorial placenta. A placenta, especially of mares and sows, in which the endothelial, connective-tissue, and epithelial layers are present in both the uterus and the chorion. The fetal circulation must pass through all of them.

ep·i·the·lio·ge·net·ic (ep″i·theel″ee·o·je·net′ick) *adj.* [*epithelio-* + *-genetic*]. Pertaining to, or caused by, epithelial proliferation.

ep·i·the·li·oid (ep″i·theel′ee·oid) *adj.* [*epitheli-* + *-oid*]. Resembling epithelium.

epithelioid cell. A cell evolved from macrophage and having abundant cytoplasm, which causes it to resemble an epithelial cell; found in granulomas such as those of tuberculosis. Syn. *alveolated cell.* Compare *endothelioid cell.*

ep·i·the·li·o·ma (ep″i·theel″ee·o′muh) *n.*, pl. **epitheliomas, epithelioma·ta** (·tuh) [*epitheli-* + *-oma*]. A tumor derived from epithelium; usually a skin cancer, occasionally cancer of a mucous membrane. —**epithelioma·tous** (·tus) *adj.*

epithelioma ad·e·noi·des cys·ti·cum (ad″e·noy′deez sis′ti·kum). TRICHOEPITHELIOMA.

epithelioma ba·so·cel·lu·la·re (bay″so·sel·yoo·lair′ee). BASAL CELL CARCINOMA.

epithelioma cho·rio·epi·der·ma·le (ko″ree·o·ep″i·dur·may′lee). CHORIOCARCINOMA.

epithelioma con·ta·gi·o·sum (kon·tay″jee·o′sum). FOWL POX.

epi·the·li·o·ma·to·sis (ep″i·theel·ee·o″muh·to′sis) *n.* [*epithelioma* + *-osis*]. The occurrence of multiple squamous-cell carcinomas.

ep·i·the·lio·my·o·sis (ep″i·theel″ee·o·migh·o′sis) *n.*, pl. **epitheliomyo·ses** (·seez) [*epithelio-* + *my-* + *-osis*]. ISTHMIC NODULAR SALPINGITIS.

ep·i·the·li·tis (ep″i·thee·lye′tis) *n.* Inflammation and overgrowth of epithelium of a mucous membrane.

ep·i·the·li·um (ep″i·theel′ee·um) *n.*, pl. **epithe·lia** (·ee·uh) [NL., from *epi-* + Gk. *thēlē,* nipple] [NA]. A tissue composed of contiguous cells with a minimum of intercellular substance. It forms the epidermis and lines hollow organs and all passages of the respiratory, digestive, and genitourinary systems. Epithelium is divided, according to the shape and arrangement of the cells, into columnar, cuboidal, and squamous; simple, pseudostratified, and stratified epithelium; according to function, into protective, sensory, and glandular or secreting. See also *endothelium, mesothelium.*

epithelium an·te·ri·us cor·ne·ae (an·teer′ee·us kor′nee·ee) [NA]. The epithelium covering the surface of the cornea.

epithelium cor·ne·ae (kor′nee·ee) [BNA]. EPITHELIUM ANTERIUS CORNEAE.

epithelium duc·tus se·mi·cir·cu·la·ris (duck′tus sem″ee·sur·kew·lair′is) [NA]. The epithelium lining a semicircular duct.

epithelium len·tis (len′tis) [NA]. The epithelium on the anterior surface of the lens of the eye.

ep·i·the·li·za·tion (ep″i·theel″i·zay′shun) *n.* The growth of epithelium over a raw surface.

ep·i·the·lize (ep″i·theel′ize) *v.* To cover or to become covered with epithelium. Syn. *epithelialize.*

ep·i·them (ep′i·them) *n.* [Gk. *epithēma*, something put on]. Any local application, as a compress, fomentation, lotion, or poultice.

ep·i·thi·a·zide (ep″i·thigh′uh·zide) *n.* 6-Chloro-3,4-dihydro-3-{[(2,2,2-trifluoroethyl)thio]methyl}-2*H*-1,2,4-benzothiadiazine-7-sulfonamide 1,1-dioxide, $C_{10}H_{11}ClF_3N_3O_4S_3$, a diuretic and antihypertensive drug.

ep·i·to·nos (ep″i·to′nos) *n.* [Gk., strained, intense]. 1. The state of exhibiting abnormal tension or muscular tone, or of being overstretched from one point to another. 2. The state of being abnormally tense or overstrained. —**epi·ton·ic** (·ton′ick) *adj.*

ep·i·to·nus (ep″i·to′nus) *n.* EPITONOS.

ep·i·tope (ep′i·tope) *n.* [*epi-* + Gk. *topos*, place, site]. Any structural component of an antigen molecule which is known to function as an antigenic determinant by allowing the attachment of certain antibody molecules. Contr. *paratope.*

Epitrate. A trademark for epinephrine bitartrate, an adrenergic.

ep·i·trich·i·um (ep″i·trick′ee·um) *n.* [NL., from *epi-* + Gk. *trichion*, hair]. 1. PERIDERM. 2. The superficial layers of squamous cells overlying a hair shaft in its canal before it breaks through the epidermis. —**epitrichi·al** (·ul) *adj.*

epi·troch·lea (ep″i·trock′lee·uh) *n.* [*epi-* + *trochlea*]. The medial epicondyle of the humerus.

epi·troch·le·ar (ep″i·trock′lee·ur) *adj.* [*epi-* + *trochlear*]. 1. Of or pertaining to the epitrochlea. 2. Of or pertaining to a lymph node that lies above the trochlea of the elbow joint.

epi·troch·le·a·ris (ep″i·trock″lee·air′is) *n.* CHONDROHUMERALIS MUSCLE.

epi·troch·leo-olec·ra·no·nis (ep″i·trock″lee·o·o·leck″ruh·no′nis) *n.* An occasional bundle of muscle running from the medial epicondyle of the humerus to the olecranon.

epi·tu·ber·cu·lo·sis (ep″i·tew·bur″kew·lo′sis) *n.*, pl. **epitubercu·lo·ses** (·seez) [*epi-* + *tuberculosis*]. A prominent pulmonary shadow (lobar or lobular) seen in x-ray films in active juvenile tuberculosis, probably due to atelectasis secondary to bronchial obstruction; formerly thought to represent pneumonia or allergic reaction to tuberculosis.

epitympanic recess. The attic of the tympanic cavity. NA *recessus epitympanicus.*

epitympanic space. EPITYMPANIC RECESS.

epi·tym·pa·num (ep″i·tim′puh·num) *n.* [*epi-* + *tympanum*]. The attic of the middle ear, or tympanic cavity. —**epi·tym·pan·ic** (·tim·pan′ick) *adj.*

epizoa. Plural of *epizoon.*

epi·zo·ic (ep″i·zo′ick) *adj.* [*epi-* + *-zoic*]. Parasitic on the surface of the body.

epi·zo·i·cide (ep″i·zo′i·side) *n.* [*epizoic* + *-cide*]. A drug or preparation that destroys external parasites.

epi·zo·on (ep″i·zo′on) *n.*, pl. **epi·zoa** (·zo′uh) [*epi-* + *-zoon*]. An animal parasite living upon the exterior of its host; ECTOZOON.

epi·zo·on·o·sis (ep″i·zo·on·o′sis) *n.*, pl. **epizoono·ses** (·seez) [*epizoon* + *-osis*]. A skin disease caused by an epizoon.

epi·zo·ot·ic (ep″i·zo·ot′ick) *adj. & n.* [*epi-* + *zoo-* + *-ic*]. 1. Affecting many animals of one kind in any region simultaneously; widely diffused and rapidly spreading. Contr. *enzootic.* 2. An extensive outbreak of an epizootic disease; a disease of animals which is widely prevalent in contiguous areas. See also *epidemic.*

epizootic equine encephalomyelitis. EQUINE ENCEPHALOMYELITIS.

epizootic lymphangitis. A mycotic disease of the skin and superficial lymphatics of horses, caused by *Histoplasma farciminosum.*

epizootic stomatitis. Foot-and-mouth disease in animals.

epi·zo·ot·i·ol·o·gy (ep″i·zo·ot″ee·ol′uh·jee) *n.* 1. The study of occurrence and distribution of animal diseases, especially those which are epizootic or enzootic. 2. The sum of factors controlling the presence or absence of an animal disease. Compare *epidemiology* (2).

E point. The point of the apex cardiogram at the maximum outward deflection of the cardiac apex impulse, occurring at the onset of ventricular ejection.

Epon. Trademark for a synthetic embedding medium used in electron microscopy.

Eponate. Trademark for epipropidine, an antineoplastic drug.

ep·o·nych·i·um (ep″o·nick′ee·um) *n.* [NL., from *ep-* + Gk. *onyx*, nail]. 1. A horny condition of the epidermis from the second to the eighth month of fetal life, indicating the position of the future nail. 2. [NA] The horny layer (stratum corneum) of the nail fold attached to the nail plate at its margin, representing the remnant of the fetal eponychium.

ep·o·nym (ep′o·nim) *n.* [Gk. *epōnymos*, from *onyma*, name]. A term formed or derived from the name of a person known or assumed to be the first, or one of the first, to discover or describe a disease, symptom complex, or theory. Eponyms often honor persons who are proponents of systems and procedures, methods, or surgical operations, even though these are not original with the person so honored. —**ep·o·nym·ic** (ep″o·nim′ick), **epon·y·mous** (e·pon′i·mus) *adj.*

epoophoral cyst. A congenital cyst derived from mesonephric remnants in the vicinity of the ovary or broad ligament.

ep·o·oph·o·ron (ep″o·off′uh·ron) *n.* [*ep-* + *oophoron*] [NA]. A blind longitudinal duct (Gartner's) and 10 to 15 transverse ductules in the mesosalpinx near the ovary which represent remnants of the reproductive part of the mesonephros in the female; homologue of the head of the epididymis in the male. Syn. *parovarium, Rosenmueller's organ.* —**epo·opho·ral** (·rul) *adj.*

epoxy- [*ep-* + *oxy-*]. A prefix indicating that *two different atoms in a molecule, already otherwise linked, are joined by an atom of oxygen.*

Eppy. A trademark for epinephryl borate, an ophthalmic adrenergic.

Eprolin. A trademark for alpha tocopherol, a substance having vitamin E activity.

EPS Abbreviation for *exophthalmos-producing substance.*

ep·si·lon (ep′si·lon, ·lun) *n.* [name of the letter E, ε, fifth letter of the Greek alphabet]. A designation for the fifth in a series, or any particular member or subset of an arbitrarily ordered set in which other members or subjects are designated α (alpha), β (beta), γ (gamma), and δ (delta); or as a correlate of the letter E, e, in the Roman alphabet. Symbol, E, ϵ (or ε).

epsilon chain, ϵ chain. The heavy chain of the IgE immunoglobulin molecule.

Ep·som salt [after *Epsom*, England]. MAGNESIUM SULFATE.

Ep·stein-Barr virus. Herpes-like virus particles first noted in cultured human lymphoblasts from Burkitt's malignant lymphoma, and of uncertain significance as etiologic agents of such tumors. These viruses may be the cause of, or related to, infectious mononucleosis. Abbreviated, EBV.

Epstein's pearls [A. *Epstein*, Prague pediatrician, 1849–1918]. The small, slightly elevated, yellowish white masses seen on each side of the hard palate in many newborn infants.

Epstein's syndrome [A. A. *Epstein*, U.S. physician, 1880–1965]. NEPHROTIC SYNDROME.

Eptoin. A trademark for phenytoin sodium, an antiepileptic.

epu·lis (e·pew′lis) *n.*, pl. **epu·li·des** (·li·deez) [Gk. *epoulis*, from *oulon*, gum]. Any benign solitary tumorlike lesion of the gingiva. —**ep·u·loid** (ep′yoo·loid) *adj.*

epulis of the newborn. GRANULAR-CELL MYOBLASTOMA.

ep·u·lo·fi·bro·ma (ep″yoo·lo·figh·bro′muh) *n.* [*epulis* + *fibroma*]. A fibroma of the gums.

ep·u·lo·sis (ep″yoo·lo′sis) *n.* [Gk. *epoulōsis*, from *oulē*, scar]. Scarring.

EQ Abbreviation for *educational quotient.*

equal cleavage. Cleavage producing blastomeres of equal size.

equal stereoblastula. A stereoblastula having cells of the same size derived from equal cleavage.

Equanil. A trademark for meprobamate, a tranquilizer drug.

equa·tion (e·kway'zhun) *n.* [L. *aequatio,* from *aequare,* to make equal]. A statement of equality between two parts, as mathematical expressions. **—equation·al** (·ul) *adj.*

equational division. A nuclear division in which daughter chromosomes separate from each other, as in ordinary somatic cell division; applied especially to the second meiotic division in contrast with the reduction division in which maternal and paternal homologous chromosomes disjoin.

equa·tor, ae·qua·tor (e·kway'tur) *n.* [L. *aequator,* equalizer]. 1. Any imaginary circle that divides a body into two equal and symmetrical parts in the manner of the equator of a sphere. 2. Of a cell, the boundary of the plane in which division takes place. 3. (of the eye:) A line joining the four extremities of the transverse and the vertical axis of the eye. NA *equator bulbi oculi.* 4. (of the lens:) The margin of the crystalline lens. NA *equator lentis.* **—equa·to·ri·al** (ee''kwuh·to'ree·ul, ek''wuh·) *adj.*

equator bul·bi ocu·li (bul'bye ock'yoo·lye) [NA]. The equator of the eye. See *equator.*

equatorial cleavage. Cleavage at right angles to the ovum axis, frequently the third cleavage plane.

equatorial plate or **disk.** The compressed mass of chromosomes aggregated at the equator of the nuclear spindle during karyokinesis.

equatorial staphyloma. Staphyloma of the sclera in the equatorial region.

equator len·tis (len'tis) [NA]. The equator of the lens. See *equator.*

equi-. A combining form meaning *equal, equally.*

equi·ax·i·al (ee''kwee·ack'see·ul) *adj.* [*equi-* + *axial*]. Having equal axes.

Eq·ui·dae (eck'wi·dee) *n. pl.* A family of mammals having a single extant genus, *Equus,* which includes the horse, ass, and zebra.

equi·dom·i·nant (ee''kwi·dom'i·nunt, eck''wi·) *adj.* Having equal dominance.

equidominant eyes. Eyes having equal or divided dominance.

eq·ui·len·in (eck''wi·len'in, ee''kwi·len'in) *n.* 3-Hydroxyestra-1,3,5(10),6,8-pentaen-17-one, $C_{18}H_{18}O_2$, an estrogenic steroid hormone, occuring in the urine of pregnant mares; structurally it differs from estrone in containing two additional double bonds.

equil·i·bra·tion (e·kwil''i·bray'shun, ee''kwi·li·) *n.* Development or maintenance of equilibrium. See also *occlusal equilibration.* **—equil·i·brate** (e·kwil'i·brate) *v.*

equil·i·bra·to·ry (ee''kwi·lib'ruh·to·ree, e·kwil'i·bruh·to''ree) *adj.* Maintaining or designed to maintain equilibrium.

equilibratory ataxia. Disturbance of equilibratory coordination, with marked abnormality of station and gait, seen with lesions of the vermis, frontopontocerebellar pathways, and labyrinthine-vestibular apparatus.

equi·lib·ri·um (ee''kwi·lib'ree·um) *n.,* pl. **equilibriums, equilibria** (·ree·uh) [L. *aequilibrium*]. 1. A state of balance; a condition in which opposing forces equalize one another so that no movement occurs. 2. A sense of being well balanced, whether pertaining to posture, or a condition of mind or feeling.

equilibrium constant. The constant pertaining to a reversible chemical reaction; the product of the concentrations or activities of the reaction products divided by the product of the concentrations or activities of the reactants, each concentration or activity term being raised to the power of the number of molecules (or ions) involved in the reaction, determined at the instant the rate of the forward and reverse reactions are equal. Symbol, K.

eq·ui·lin (ee'kwi·lin, eck'wi·lin) *n.* 3-Hydroxy-17-keto-1,3,5,-7-estratetraene, $C_{18}H_{20}O_2$, an estrogenic steroid hormone, occurring in the urine of pregnant mares; structurally it differs from estrone in containing one additional double bond.

equi·mo·lec·u·lar (ee''kwi·mo·leck'yoo·lur) *adj.* [*equi-* + *molecular*]. 1. Containing or representing quantities of substances in the proportion of their molecular weights. 2. Containing or representing an equal number of molecules.

equine (ee'kwine, eck'wine) *adj.* [L. *equinus* from *equus,* horse]. Pertaining to, resembling, or derived from a horse.

equine biliary fever. A form of babesiasis in horses, mules, and donkeys; caused by *Babesia equi* and transmitted by ticks.

equine distemper. STRANGLES.

equine encephalomyelitis or **encephalitis.** An epidemic viral disease of horses and mules, in which birds and reptiles are the main reservoirs and mosquitos the principal vectors of the virus; the disease mitted by mosquitoes; may be communicated to man, in whom it may result in severe illness with paralysis and a wide variety of other neurologic manifestations. Three causative viral strains are known: eastern, western, and Venezuelan.

equine gait. STEPPAGE GAIT.

equine infectious anemia. INFECTIOUS EQUINE ANEMIA.

equine influenza. An acute pantropic virus disease of horses, characterized by inflammation of mucous membranes of the air passages and eyelids, and frequently by inflammation of the tendons and subcutaneous tissues.

equine malaria. INFECTIOUS EQUINE ANEMIA.

equine piroplasmosis. EQUINE BILIARY FEVER.

equine smallpox. HORSEPOX.

equin·ia (e·kwin'ee·uh) *n.* [*equine* + *-ia*]. GLANDERS.

eq·ui·no·ca·vus (eck''wi·no·kay'vus, e·kwye''no·) *n.* TALIPES EQUINOCAVUS.

eq·ui·no·val·gus (eck''wi·no·val'gus, e·kwye''no·) *n.* TALIPES EQUINOVALGUS.

eq·ui·no·va·rus (eck''wi·no·vair'us, e·kwye''no·) *n.* TALIPES EQUINOVARUS.

equi·nus (e·kwye'nus) *n.* [L. *equinus,* equine]. TALIPES EQUINUS.

equi·po·ten·tial (ee''kwi·po·ten'chul, eck''wi·) *adj.* [*equi-* + *potential*]. 1. Having equal capabilities or capacity for development. 2. Having the same electrical potential.

equipotential line. ISOELECTRIC LINE.

equipotential surface. In an electric field, a surface at every point of which the potential energy is equal, and having a contour everywhere normal to the force or flow lines of the field.

eq·ui·se·to·sis (eck''wi·se·to'sis, ee''kwi·) *n.* [*Equisetum* + *-osis*]. Poisoning of horses due to ingestion of plants of the genus *Equisetum.*

Eq·ui·se·tum (eck''wi·see'tum, ee''kwi·) *n.* [L. *equisaetum,* horsetail]. A genus of cryptogamous plants, some of which have a diuretic effect.

equiv·a·lent (e·kwiv'uh·lunt) *adj.* & *n.* [L. *aequivalens*]. 1. Having an equal value. 2. That which is equal in value, size, weight, or in any other respect, to something else. 3. *In chemistry,* the weight of a substance, usually in grams, which combines or otherwise reacts with a standard weight of a reference element or compound, as 8 weight units of oxygen; the weights of the substance and the reference element or compound are related to the respective atomic or molecular weights and the numerical proportions in which the atoms or molecules react.

equivalent weight. EQUIVALENT (3).

Er Symbol for erbium.

era·sion (e·ray'zhun) *n.* [L. *eradere,* to scrape off]. 1. Surgical removal of tissue by scraping. 2. Excision of a joint; ARTHRECTOMY.

Er·a·ty·rus (err″uh·tye′rus) *n.* A genus of bugs of the Reduviidae.

Eratyrus cus·pi·da·tus (kus·pi·day′tus). A South American vector of Chagas' disease.

Erb-Char·cot disease (e^h^rp, shar·ko′) [W. H. *Erb,* German neurologist, 1840–1921; and J. M. *Charcot*]. SPINAL MENINGOVASCULAR SYPHILIS.

Erb-Du·chenne paralysis (du^e^·shen′) [W. H. *Erb* and G. B. A. *Duchenne*]. UPPER BRACHIAL PLEXUS PARALYSIS.

Er·ben's phenomenon, reflex, or **sign** (e^h^r′b^e^n) [S. *Erben,* Austrian neurologist, b. 1863]. Slowing of the pulse, presumed to be due to vagus irritability, when the head and trunk are bent strongly forward.

Erb-Gold·flam symptom complex [W. H. *Erb;* and S. V. *Goldflam,* Polish neurologist, 1852–1932]. MYASTHENIA GRAVIS.

er·bi·um (ur′bee·um) *n.* [after Ytt*erby,* Sweden]. Er = 167.26. A rare-earth metal. See also Table of Elements in the Appendix.

Erb's palsy or **paralysis** [W. H. *Erb*]. UPPER BRACHIAL PLEXUS PARALYSIS.

Erb's point [W. H. *Erb*]. A point 2 to 3 cm above the clavicle and in front of the transverse process of the sixth cervical vertebra. Electric stimulation at this point produces contraction of the various muscles involved in upper brachial plexus paralysis.

Erb's scapulohumeral or **juvenile atrophic muscular dystrophy** [W. H. *Erb*]. SCAPULOHUMERAL MUSCULAR DYSTROPHY (OF ERB).

Erb's sign [W. H. *Erb*]. 1. Loss of the pattellar reflex as an early sign of tabes dorsalis. 2. A sign of tetany in which hyperexcitability can be determined by the use of a galvanic current.

Erb's spastic spinal paraplegia [W. H. *Erb*]. A form of spastic paraplegia attributed by Erb to spinal meningovascular syphilis.

Erb's syphilitic paralysis [W. H. *Erb*]. ERB'S SPASTIC SPINAL PARAPLEGIA.

Erb-Zim·mer·lin type (tsim′ur·lin) [W. H. *Erb* and F. *Zimmerlin*]. SCAPULOHUMERAL MUSCULAR DYSTROPHY.

Erd·mann's reagent (e^y^rt′ma^h^n) [H. *Erdmann,* German chemist, 1862–1910]. A mixture of dilute nitric acid and concentrated sulfuric acid; used in identification of alkaloids.

erect film. A roentgenogram obtained with the subject in the erect position.

erec·tile (e·reck′til) *adj.* Capable of erection.

erectile tissue. A spongelike arrangement of irregular vascular spaces as seen in the corpus cavernosum of the penis or clitoris.

erect image. DIRECT IMAGE.

erec·tion (e·reck′shun) *n.* [L. *erectio,* from *erigere,* to erect, from *regere,* to guide, direct]. The enlarged state of erectile tissue when engorged with blood, as of the penis or clitoris. —**erect** (e·rekt′) *adj. & v.*

erec·tor (e·reck′tur) *n.*, L. pl. **erec·to·res** (e·reck″to′reez). A muscle that produces erection of a part. See also Table of Muscles in the Appendix.

erector cli·to·ri·dis (kli·tor′i·dis). The ischiocavernosus muscle in the female.

erector pe·nis (pee′nis). The ischiocavernosus muscle in the male.

erector pi·li (pye′lye), pl. **erectores pi·lo·rum** (pi·lo′rum). ARRECTOR PILI.

erector spi·nae (spye′nee). A large, complex, deep muscle of the back, having three parts, iliocostalis, longissimus, and spinalis, each with subdivisions. NA *musculus erector spinae.* See also Table of Muscles in the Appendix.

erector spinae reflex. DORSAL REFLEX.

ere·mio·pho·bia (e·ree″mee·o·fo′bee·uh, err″e·migh″o·) *n.* [Gk. *ēremia,* rest, quietude, + *-phobia*]. An abnormal fear of quietude or stillness.

er·e·mo·pho·bia (err″e·mo·fo′bee·uh) *n.* [Gk. *erēmos,* lonely, deserted, + *-phobia*]. 1. An abnormal fear of being lonely. 2. An abnormal fear of large, desolate places; AGORAPHOBIA.

erep·sin (e·rep′sin) *n.* An enzyme mixture produced by the intestinal mucosa, consisting of various peptidases which split peptones and proteoses into simpler products; it has no effect on native proteins.

er·e·thism (err′e·thiz·um) *n.* [Gk. *erethismos,* irritation]. 1. An abnormal increase of nervous irritability. 2. Quick response to stimulus. Contr. *apathism.* —**er·e·this·mic** (err″e·thiz′mick), **ere·this·tic** (·thiss′tick), **ere·thit·ic** (·thit′ick) *adj.*

erethistic ulcer. An exceedingly tender ulcer, such as may occur in the anus or around the fingernails.

ereu·tho·pho·bia (e·rooth″o·fo′bee·uh, err″yoo·tho·) *n.* [Gk. *ereuthos,* redness, + *-phobia*]. ERYTHROPHOBIA.

erg (urg) *n.* [Gk. *ergon,* work]. A unit of work, representing the work done in moving a body against the force of 1 dyne through a distance of 1 cm.

erg-, ergo- [Gk. *ergon*]. A combining form meaning (a) *work;* (b) *activity.*

er·ga·sia (ur·gay′zhuh, ·zee·uh) *n.* [Gk., work, business, function]. 1. *In psychobiology,* the sum total of the functions and reactions of an individual; the actions or responses that spring from the whole organism or personality. 2. A tendency toward work.

er·ga·si·a·try (ur·gay′see·uh·tree, ur″guh·sigh′uh·tree) *n.* [*ergasia* + *-iatry*]. Adolph Meyer's term for psychiatry. See also *psychobiology.*

er·ga·sio·ma·nia (ur·gay″see·o·may′nee·uh) *n.* [*ergasia* + *-mania*]. An exaggerated or obsessive desire for work of any kind; seen in certain neuroses and psychoses.

er·ga·sio·pho·bia (ur·gay″see·o·fo′bee·uh) *n.* [*ergasia* + *-phobia*]. An abnormal fear of work.

er·gas·the·nia (ur″gas·theen′ee·uh) *n.* [*erg-* + *asthenia*]. Weakness or debility due to overwork.

er·gas·tic (ur·gas′tick) *adj.* [Gk. *ergastikos,* working, productive]. 1. Of or pertaining to ergasia. 2. Possessing potential energy; said of certain materials stored in cells, such as lipid.

er·gas·to·plasm (ur·gas′to·plaz·um) *n.* [*ergastic* + *plasm*]. 1. An indefinite collective term for basophil cytoplasmic substances; the expression of the presence of ribonucleic acid in cytoplasm. 2. ROUGH-SURFACED ENDOPLASMIC RETICULUM.

ergo-. See *erg-.*

er·go·ba·sine (ur″go·bay′seen, ·sin) *n.* ERGONOVINE.

er·go·ba·si·nine (ur″go·bay′si·neen, ·nin) *n.* ERGOMETRININE.

er·go·cal·cif·er·ol (ur″go·kal·sif′ur·ol) *n.* Vitamin D_2, prepared from ergosterol; CALCIFEROL.

er·go·cor·nine (ur″go·kor′neen, ·nin) *n.* A levorotatory alkaloid, $C_{31}H_{39}N_5O_5$, from ergot, isomeric with ergocorninine.

er·go·cor·ni·nine (ur″go·kor′ni·neen, ·nin) *n.* The dextrorotatory isomer of ergocornine, occurring in ergot; physiologically, it is relatively inactive.

er·go·cris·tine (ur″go·kris′teen, ·tin) *n.* A levorotatory alkaloid, $C_{35}H_{39}N_5O_5$, from ergot, isomeric with ergocristinine.

er·go·cris·ti·nine (ur″go·kris′ti·neen, ·nin) *n.* The dextrorotatory isomer of ergocristine, occurring in ergot; physiologically, it is relatively inactive.

er·go·cryp·tine (ur″go·krip′teen, ·tin) *n.* A levorotatory alkaloid, $C_{32}H_{41}N_5O_5$, from ergot, isomeric with ergocryptinine.

er·go·cryp·ti·nine (ur″go·krip′ti·neen, ·nin) *n.* The dextrorotatory isomer of ergocryptine, occurring in ergot; physiologically, it is relatively inactive.

er·go·graph (ur′go·graf) *n.* [*ergo-* + *-graph*]. An instrument which, by means of a weight or spring against which a muscle can be contracted, records the extent of movement of that muscle or the amount of work it is capable of doing.

er·gom·e·ter (ur·gom′e·tur) *n.* [*ergo-* + *-meter*]. An instrument that permits a calculation of the work performed (weight multiplied by shortening) by a muscle or muscles over a period of time.

ergometer bicycle. A stationary bicycle on which a person pedals against a measurable load.

er·go·met·rine (ur″go·met′reen, ·rin) *n.* ERGONOVINE.

er·go·met·ri·nine (ur″go·met′ri·neen, ·nin) *n.* The dextrorotatory, relatively inactive isomer of ergonovine. Syn. *ergobasinine.*

er·go·no·vine (ur″go·no′veen, ·vin) *n.* *N*-[α-(Hydroxymethyl)ethyl]-D-lysergamide, $C_{19}H_{23}N_3O_2$, an alkaloid obtained from ergot which causes sustained uterine contractions and is more prompt but less persistent in its action than other ergot alkaloids. Used in the form of its maleate and tartrate salts.

er·go·pho·bia (ur″go·fo′bee·uh) *n.* ERGASIOPHOBIA.

er·go·phore (ur″go·fore) *n.* [*ergo-* + *-phore*]. The chemical group in a molecule, especially of a toxin or agglutinin, which is responsible for the specific activity of the molecule.

er·go·plasm (ur′go·plaz·um) *n.* [*ergo-* + *-plasm*]. ARCHOPLASM.

er·go·sine (ur′go·seen, ·sin) *n.* An alkaloid, $C_{30}H_{37}N_5O_5$, of ergot, having physiologic activity similar to that of ergotoxine.

er·go·si·nine (ur·go′si·neen, ·nin) *n.* The dextrorotatory isomer of ergosine, occurring in ergot; it is nearly devoid of physiologic activity.

er·go·some (ur″go·sohm) *n.* [*ergo-* + *-some*]. POLYRIBOSOME.

er·gos·ta·nol (ur·gos′tay·nol) *n.* A sterol, $C_{28}H_{50}O$, having the structure of ergosterol but with all three double bonds of the latter saturated.

er·gos·te·nol (ur·gos′tee·nol) *n.* Any of a group of sterols of the composition $C_{28}H_{48}O$, differing from ergostanol in having one double bond, the position of which varies and thus characterizes the individual ergostenols.

er·gos·ter·in (ur·gos′tur·in) *n.* ERGOSTEROL.

er·gos·ter·ol (ur·gos′tur·ol) *n.* [*ergot* + *sterol*]. Ergosta-5(6),7(8),22(23)-triene-3-ol, $C_{28}H_{44}O$, an unsaturated sterol found in ergot, yeast, and other fungi; it occurs as crystals, insoluble in water. It is provitamin D_2; on irradiation with ultraviolet light or activation with electrons, it may be converted to vitamin D_2 (ergocalciferol). Syn. *ergosterin.*

er·go·stet·rine (ur″go·stet′reen, ·rin) *n.* ERGONOVINE.

er·got (ur′got) *n.* [F., cock's spur]. The dried sclerotium of *Claviceps purpurea,* a fungus developed on rye plants. It contains at least five optically isomeric pairs of alkaloids; the levorotatory isomers are physiologically active, the dextrorotatory isomers nearly inactive. Originally ergot was used, and now certain of its alkaloids, for oxytocic action; the alkaloid ergotamine is also used for the treatment of migraine headache.

er·got·a·mine (ur·got′uh·meen, ·min) *n.* [*ergot* + *amine*]. A levorotatory alkaloid, $C_{33}H_{35}N_5O_5$, from ergot; while it has oxytocic activity, its principal use, in the form of the tartrate salt, is to relieve pain in the symptomatic treatment of migraine.

er·go·tam·i·nine (ur″go·tam′i·neen, ·nin) *n.* The dextrorotatory isomer of ergotamine; it is nearly devoid of therapeutic activity.

er·go·ther·a·py (ur″go·therr′uh·pee) *n.* [*ergo-* + *therapy*]. Treatment of disease by physical work.

er·go·thi·o·ne·ine (ur″go·thigh″o·nee′een) *n.* THIONEINE.

er·got·in (ur′guh·tin) *n.* An extract of ergot.

er·got·i·nine (ur·got′i·neen, ·nin) *n.* A mixture, originally believed to be a chemical entity, of the ergot alkaloids ergocorninine, ergocristinine, and ergocryptinine; practically inert physiologically.

er·got·ism (ur′got·iz·um, ur′guh·tiz·um) *n.* [*ergot* + *-ism*]. Acute or chronic intoxication resulting from ingestion of grain infected with ergot fungus, *Claviceps purpurae,* or from the chronic use of drugs containing ergot; characterized by vomiting, colic, convulsions, paresthesias, psychotic behavior, and occasionally ischemic gangrene.

er·got·ized (ur′got·ize′d, ur′guh·tize′d) *adj.* Affected by ergot as a result of treatment or poisoning, as wheat infested with the fungus of ergot.

er·go·to·cin (ur″go·to′sin) *n.* ERGONOVINE.

er·go·tox·ine (ur″go·tock′seen, ·sin) *n.* A crystalline alkaloidal substance, long believed to be a chemical entity, isolated from ergot and having pronounced physiologic activity, now known to be a mixture of ergocristine, ergocornine, and ergocryptine.

Ergotrate. A trademark for ergonovine, an oxytocic agent used as the maleate salt.

-ergy [Gk. *-ergeia,* from *ergon,* work]. A combining form meaning *activity, work, function.*

Er·ich·sen's disease (err′ik·sun) [J. E. *Erichsen,* English surgeon, 1818–1896]. RAILWAY SPINE.

Eridone. A trademark for phenindione, an anticoagulant drug.

er·i·gens (err′i·jenz) *adj.* [L., from *erigere,* to erect, arouse]. Pertaining to the sacral parasympathetic preganglionic nerve fibers.

Erig·er·on (e·rij′ur·on) *n.* [Gk. *ērigerōn,* groundsel, lit., early-old]. A genus of the Compositae, several species of which were formerly used, especially in the form of an oil, in treatment of urinary diseases, diarrhea, and dysentery. Syn. *fleabane.*

erigeron oil. A volatile oil consisting chiefly of α-limonene with some terpineol obtained from species of *Erigeron;* formerly used in treatment of diarrhea and internal hemorrhage.

er·i·o·dic·tin (eer″ee·o·dick′tin, err″ee·o·) *n.* Eriodictyol-L-rhamnoside, $C_{21}H_{22}O_{10}$, a constituent of citrin, isolated from citrus fruits.

er·i·o·dic·ty·ol (eer″ee·o·dick′tee·ol, err″ee·o·) *n.* 3′,4′, 5,7-Tetrahydroxyflavanone, $C_{15}H_{12}O_6$, a constituent of *Eriodictyon californicum* leaves. The L-rhamnoside of eriodictyol is eriodictin.

Er·i·o·dic·ty·on (ee″ree·o·dick′tee·on, err″ee·o·) *n.* [Gk. *erion,* wool, + *dictyon,* net]. A genus of shrubs of the Hydrophyllaceae. The leaves of *Eriodictyon californicum,* California yerba santa, have been used as an expectorant and in fluid formations to mask the taste of bitter drugs.

er·i·om·e·ter (err·ee·om′e·tur) *n.* [Gk. *erion,* wool, + *-meter*]. HALOMETER.

erisiphake. ERYSIPHAKE.

eris·o·phake (e·ris′o·fake) *n.* ERYSIPHAKE.

Eris·ta·lis (e·ris′tuh·lis) *n.* A genus of the Diptera of the Syrphidae; commonly called drone flies. The rat-tailed larvae of several species have been known to cause intestinal myiasis in man.

er·len·mey·er flask (e^h^r′l^e^n·migh″ur) [E. *Erlenmeyer,* German chemist, 1825–1909]. A conical flask with a flat bottom, especially suited for certain chemical procedures.

Ero·di·um (e·ro′dee·um) *n.* [NL., from Gk. *erōdios,* heron]. A genus of herbs of the Geraniaceae. *Erodium cicutarium,* alfilaria, has been used as a substitute for hydrastis.

er·o·gen·ic (err″o·jen′ick) *adj.* EROTOGENIC.

erog·e·nous (e·roj′e·nus) *adj.* [Gk. *erōs,* sexual love, + *-genous*]. EROTOGENIC.

erogenous zone. EROTOGENIC ZONE.

ero·ma·nia (err″o·may′nee·uh) *n.* EROTOMANIA.

eros (ee′ros, err′os) *n.* [Gk. *erōs,* sexual love]. *In psychoanalysis,* all the instinctive tendencies that lead the organism toward self-preservation. Syn. *life instinct.* Contr. *death instinct.* See also *libido.*

erose (e·roce′) *adj.* [L. *erosus,* from *erodere,* to gnaw away]. *In botany,* having a margin or border irregularly toothed.

ero·sio in·ter·dig·i·ta·lis blas·to·my·ce·ti·ca (e·ro′see·o in″tur·dij·i·tay′lis blas″to·migh·see′ti·kuh, e·ro′zhee·o, e·ro′zee·o). A form of candidiasis involving the webs of the fingers and particularly the third or fourth interdigital web; seen in those whose hands are exposed to the macerating effects of water and strong alkalies.

ero·sion (e·ro′zhun) *n.* [L. *erosio,* from *erodere,* to gnaw away]. Superficial destruction of a surface area by inflammation or trauma. See also *dental erosion.* —**erode** (e·rode′) *v.;* **ero·sive** (e·ro′siv) *adj.*

erosion of the cervix uteri. Congenital or acquired replacement of the squamous epithelium of the cervix by columnar cells of the endocervix due to inflammation.

erosive aneurysm. An aneurysm due to extension of inflammation from an infected valve (aortic or pulmonic) breaking down the vessel wall.

erot-, eroto- [Gk. *erōs, erōtos*]. A combining form meaning *sexual desire.*

erot·ic (e·rot′ick) *adj.* [Gk. *erōtikos,* amorous, from *erōs,* sexual love]. 1. Pertaining to the libido or sexual passion. 2. Moved by or arousing sexual desire.

erot·i·ca (e·rot′i·kuh) *n.* [Gk. *erōtika*]. Literature devoted to erotic themes; sexual literature.

erot·i·cism (e·rot′i·siz·um) *n.* [*erotic* + *-ism*]. EROTISM.

erot·i·co·ma·nia (e·rot″i·ko·may′nee·uh) *n.* EROTOMANIA.

erotic zoophilism. The desire or impulse to stroke or pet animals for sexual excitement.

er·o·tism (err′o·tiz·um) *n.* [*erot-* + *-ism*]. 1. Sexual excitement or desire. 2. *In psychoanalysis,* any manifestation of the sexual instinct and specifically, the erotic excitement derived from all mucous membranes and special sensory organs, such as anal erotism, oral erotism, or skin erotism. See also *narcissism, alloerotism.*

eroto-. See *erot-.*

ero·to·gen·ic (e·ro″to·jen′ick, err″o·to·, e·rot″o·) *adj.* [*eroto-* + *-genic*]. Pertaining to, causing, or originating from sexual or libidinal feelings.

erotogenic zone. Any part of the body which, on being touched, causes sexual feelings or which most expresses libidinal impulses.

ero·to·ma·nia (e·ro″to·may′nee·uh, err″o·to·, e·rot″o·) *n.* [*eroto-* + *-mania*]. 1. Exaggerated sexual passion, or exaggerated reaction to sexual stimulation. 2. A condition sometimes seen in schizophrenia (and elsewhere) in which one develops an unrealistic persistent infatuation for or sexual fixation upon a certain person, or a delusional belief that a certain person is in love with oneself. —**erotoma·ni·ac** (·nee·ack) *adj.*

er·o·top·a·thy (err″o·top′uth·ee) *n.* [*eroto-* + *-pathy*]. Any perversion of the sexual instinct. —**ero·to·path·ic** (·to·path′ick) *adj.;* **ero·to·path** (e·ro′to·path, e·rot′o·path) *n.*

ero·to·pho·bia (e·ro″to·fo′bee·uh, err″o·to·, e·rot″o·) *n.* [*eroto-* + *-phobia*]. An abnormal fear of love, especially of sexual feelings and their physical expression.

errors of refraction. Departures from the power of producing a normal or well-defined image upon the retina, because of ametropia.

Ertron. A trademark for vitamin D.

eru·cic acid (e·roo′sick). *cis*-13-Docosenoic acid, $C_{22}H_{42}O_2$, an unsaturated acid found in the glycerides of rape oil, mustard oil, and certain other oils.

eruc·ta·tion (ee″ruck·tay′shun, err″uck·) *n.* [L. *eructatio,* from *eructare,* to belch forth]. BELCHING.

er·u·ga·tion (err·oo·gay′shun, err″yoo·) *n.* [L. *erugare,* to remove wrinkles, from *ruga,* wrinkle]. The procedure of removing wrinkles.

eru·ga·to·ry (e·roo′guh·to″ree, err′oo·guh·) *adj. & n.* 1. Pertaining to the removal of wrinkles. 2. A substance that removes wrinkles.

erup·tion (e·rup′shun) *n.* [L. *eruptio,* from *erupmere,* to break forth]. 1. The sudden appearance of lesions on the skin, especially in exanthematous diseases and sometimes as a result of a drug. 2. The appearance of a tooth through the gums.

erup·tive (e·rup′tiv) *adj.* Attended by or producing an eruption; characterized by sudden appearance or development.

eruptive fever. 1. BOUTONNEUSE FEVER. 2. Any fever associated with an exanthema.

eruptive stage. The stage in which an exanthema makes its appearance.

ERV Abbreviation for *expiratory reserve volume.*

Eryn·gi·um (e·rin′jee·um) *n.* [Gk. *ēryngion,* eryngo]. A genus of plants of the Umbelliferae. *Eryngium aquaticum,* button snakeroot, has been used as a diaphoretic, expectorant, and emetic.

er·y·sip·e·las (err″i·sip′e·lus) *n.* [Gk. (rel. to *erythros,* red, and *pella,* skin)]. A form of acute streptococcal cellulitis involving the skin, with a well-demarcated, slightly raised red area having advancing borders, usually accompanied by constitutional symptoms. —**er·y·si·pel·a·tous** (err″i·si·pel′uh·tus) *adj.*

erysipelas am·bu·lans (am′bew·lanz). WANDERING ERYSIPELAS.

erysipelas bul·lo·sum (buh·lo′sum, bo͝ol·o′sum). Erysipelas attended with formation of bullae.

erysipelas chron·i·cum (kron′i·kum). A chronic or relapsing erysipelas leading to elephantiasis of the affected part.

erysipelas dif·fu·sum (di·few′sum). Erysipelas in which the affected area is not sharply defined, the redness merging gradually with the color of the surrounding skin.

erysipelas glab·rum (glab′rum). Erysipelas in which the skin is tightly stretched and has a smooth, shining appearance.

erysipelas med·i·ca·men·to·sum (med″i·kuh·men·to′sum). A rash resembling erysipelas, but marked by rapid development, the absence of well-defined areas, and tenderness on pressure; produced by ingested drugs.

erysipelas mi·grans (migh′granz). WANDERING ERYSIPELAS.

erysipelas per·stans (pur′stanz). A chronic, erysipelas-like condition of the face.

er·y·sip·e·loid (err″i·sip′e·loid) *n. & adj.* [*erysipelas* + *-oid*]. 1. An infection caused by *Erysipelothrix rhusiopathiae,* occurring on the hands of those who handle infected meat or fish and characterized by circumscribed, multiple red lesions with erythema present in some cases. 2. Resembling erysipelas.

erysipeloid cancer. INFLAMMATORY CARCINOMA.

Er·y·sip·e·lo·thrix (err″i·sip′e·lo·thricks) *n.* [*erysipelas* + *-thrix*]. A genus of thin, gram-positive rod-shaped organisms, with a tendency to form long filaments, non-spore-forming and microaerophilic, and with pathogenicity for a wide range of animals, including man.

Erysipelothrix in·sid·i·o·sa (in·sid″ee·o′suh). *Obsol.* *ERYSIPELOTHRIX RHUSIOPATHIAE.*

Erysipelothrix rhu·si·o·path·i·ae (roo″see·o·path′ee·ee). The causative organism of erysipelas, acute septicemia, and chronic arthritis of swine, and of erysipeloid in man.

erys·i·phake, eris·i·phake (e·ris′i·fake) *n.* [Gk. *erysis,* a drawing, pulling, + *phakos,* lens]. A disk-shaped instrument with an opening on one side, capable of producing slight negative pressure and used in cataract extraction.

er·y·the·ma (err″i·thee′muh) *n.* [Gk. *erythēma,* redness, flush]. A redness of the skin occurring in patches of variable size and shape. It can have a variety of causes, such as heat, certain drugs, ultraviolet rays, and ionizing radiation.

erythema ab ig·ne (ab ig′nee) [L., from fire]. An eruption of varying form and color, often with pigmentation; due to prolonged exposure to artificial heat; seen typically on the extremities of stokers or people who sit in front of fires.

erythema an·nu·la·re cen·trif·u·gum (an″yoo·lair′ee sen·trif′yoo·gum). A skin disease characterized by gyrate, annular red macules, with hard cordlike edges and peripheral enlargement.

erythema ar·thrit·i·cum ep·i·dem·i·cum (ahr·thrit′i·kum ep″i·dem′i·kum). HAVERHILL FEVER.

erythema bru·cel·lum (broo·sel′um). Erythema and skin lesions occurring in sensitized individuals coming in contact with cows affected with infectious abortion.

erythema bul·lo·sum (buh·lo'sum, bŏŏl·o'sum). The bullous type of erythema multiforme.

erythema ca·lo·ri·cum (ka·lo'ri·kum). Transitory redness of the skin induced by heat.

erythema chron·i·cum mi·grans (kron'i·kum migh'granz). An afebrile erythema; appears as a single elevated ring, progressive at the border and healing at the center.

erythema chronicum migrans Af·ze·li·us (af·zee'lee·us). A form of annular, peripherally extending erythema progressing from the site of a bite, usually that of a tick.

erythema cir·ci·na·tum (sur''si·nay'tum). A form of erythema multiforme showing lesions with depressed centers and erythematous borders.

erythema el·e·va·tum di·u·ti·num (el·e·vay'tum dye·oo'ti·num) [L., raised, long-lasting]. A dermatosis characterized by firm, painless nodules, which, discrete at first, later coalesce to form flat, raised plaques or nodular tissues.

erythema en·dem·i·cum (en·dem'i·kum). PELLAGRA.

erythema ep·i·dem·i·cum (ep''i·dem'i·kum). ACRODYNIA.

erythema fi·gu·ra·tum per·stans (fig·yoo·ray'tum pur'stanz). ERYTHEMA ANNULARE CENTRIFUGUM.

erythema fu·gax (few'gacks). Transitory redness of the skin, possibly urticarial in nature.

erythema gan·gre·no·sum (gang''gre·no'sum). Dermatitis factitia resulting in gangrene.

erythema glu·te·a·le (gloo·tee·ay'lee). DIAPER RASH.

erythema gy·ra·tum mi·grans (jye·ray'tum migh'granz). A form of erythema annulare centrifugum associated with breast cancer.

erythema hy·per·emi·cum (high''pur·ee'mi·kum). ERYTHEMA SIMPLEX.

erythema in·du·ra·ti·vum (in·dew''ruh·tye'vum). ERYTHEMA INDURATUM.

erythema in·du·ra·tum (in·dew·ray'tum). A chronic recurrent disorder characterized by deep-seated nodosities and subsequent ulcerations; usually involves the skin of the legs of younger women; occasionally tuberculous. Syn. *Bazin's disease.*

erythema in·fec·ti·o·sum (in·feck''shee·o'sum). A benign epidemic infectious disease of early childhood, probably viral in origin, characterized by a rose-red macular rash on the face which may spread to the limbs and the trunk. Syn. *acute infectious erythema, fifth disease, megalerythema.*

erythema intertrigo. INTERTRIGO.

erythema iris [Gk., rainbow, halo]. A variety of erythema multiforme in which the skin lesions appear in variously colored, concentric rings.

erythema mar·gi·na·tum (mahr''ji·nay'tum). A type of erythema multiforme in which an elevated, well-defined band remains as a sequela of an erythematous patch; seen in rheumatic fever.

erythema mi·grans (migh'granz). BENIGN MIGRATORY GLOSSITIS.

erythema mul·ti·for·me (mul''ti·for'mee). An acute, inflammatory skin disease; characterized by red macules, papules, or tubercles; the lesions, varying in appearance, occur usually on neck, face, legs, and dorsal surfaces of hands, forearms, and feet; initial symptoms are often gastric distress and rheumatic pains. Ectodermosis erosiva pluriorificialis and Stevens-Johnson syndrome are clinical variants of erythema multiforme.

erythema no·do·sum (no·do'sum). An eruption, usually on the anterior surfaces of the legs below the knees, of pink to blue, tender nodules appearing in crops; more frequently seen in women; often associated with joint pains.

erythema nu·chae (new'kee). Redness on the back of the neck seen in early infancy, lasting for a variable time, and probably due to pressure.

erythema of ninth day. A morbilliform or scarlatiniform eruption associated with constitutional disturbances; occurs about the ninth day following the administration of arsphenamine or other toxic drugs. Syn. *Milian's ninth-day erythema.*

erythema pal·ma·re he·red·i·ta·ri·um (pal·mair'ee he·red·i·tair'ee·um). Bright red palms resulting from a hereditary disturbance of the local circulation.

erythema pap·u·la·tum (pap''yoo·lay'tum). A type of erythema multiforme in which the lesions are nodular or papular; seen with rheumatic fever.

erythema par·a·lyt·i·cum (păr''uh·lit'i·kum). The early stage of acrodermatitis chronica atrophicans.

erythema pernio. CHILBLAIN.

erythema per·stans (pur'stanz). Persisting, recurring erythema; a group including erythema annulare centrifugum, erythema simplex gyratum, and erythema chronicum migrans.

erythema punc·ta·tum (punk·tay'tum). ERYTHEMA SCARLATINIFORME.

erythema scar·la·ti·ni·for·me (skahr''luh·tee·ni·for'mee, ·tin·i·). An eruption from different causes but simulating the rash of scarlet fever. Syn. *erythema punctatum, scarlatinoid erythema.*

erythema sim·plex (sim'plecks). A hyperemia showing various shades of redness, either diffuse or circumscribed. The symptomatic erythemas may be precursors of systemic disturbances or febrile disorders. Syn. *erythema hyperemicum.*

erythema simplex gy·ra·tum (jye·ray'tum). An eruption of circinate and gyrate lesions disappearing after a few days only to be succeeded by fresh outbursts.

erythema so·la·re (so·lair'ee). SUNBURN.

er·y·the·ma·toid (err''i·theem'uh·toid) *adj.* Resembling erythema.

er·y·the·ma·tous (err''i·theem'uh·tus, ·themm'uh·tus) *adj.* Pertaining to or characterized by erythema.

erythematous stomatitis. Simple inflammation of the oral mucous membrane.

erythema tox·i·cum ne·o·na·to·rum (tock'si·kum nee''o·nay·to'rum). A transient, blotchy erythematous rash occurring usually in the first days of life, of uncertain cause, but attributed to contact dermatitis or to hypersensitivity to human or cow's milk or other allergens.

erythema trau·mat·i·cum (traw·mat'i·kum). Redness of the skin produced by trauma.

erythema tu·ber·cu·la·tum (tew·bur''kew·lay'tum). A type of erythema multiforme in which the lesions are nodular in character.

erythema ur·ti·cans (ur'ti·kanz). A type of erythema multiforme in which the lesions are urticarial in appearance.

erythema ven·e·na·tum (ven''e·nay'tum) [L., from *venenum,* poison]. Redness of the skin produced by external irritants.

erythema ve·sic·u·lo·sum (ve·sick·yoo·lo'sum). A type of erythema multiforme characterized by vesicles.

er·y·the·moid (err''i·theem'oid) *adj.* Resembling erythema.

er·y·ther·mal·gia (err''i·thur·mal'jee·uh) *n.* [*erythr-* + *therm-* + *-algia*]. ERYTHROMELALGIA.

erythr-, erythro- [Gk. *erythros*]. A combining form meaning (a) *red;* (b) *erythrocyte.*

erythraemia. ERYTHREMIA.

er·y·thral·gia (err''i·thral'juh) *n.* [*erythr-* + *-algia*]. ERYTHROMELALGIA.

er·y·thras·ma (err''i·thraz'muh) *n.* [NL., from Gk. *erythros,* red]. A skin disease seen in the axillas or the inguinal or pubic regions. It forms red or brown, sharply defined, slightly raised, desquamating patches which cause little or no inconvenience.

eryth·re·de·ma, eryth·roe·de·ma (e·rith''re·dee'muh) *n.* [*erythr-* + *edema*]. ACRODYNIA.

erythredema polyneuropathy. ACRODYNIA.

er·y·thre·mia, er·y·thrae·mia (err''i·three'mee·uh) *n.* [*erythr-* + *-emia*]. 1. POLYCYTHEMIA VERA. 2. ERYTHROCYTOSIS. **—erythre·mic** (·mick) *adj.*

erythremic myelosis or **disease**. A hemopoietic disease of uncertain nature, characterized by proliferation of atypical primitive red cells, often accompanied by anaplastic granulocytes, and often terminating in granulocytic leukemia. Syn. *DiGuglielmo's disease, erythroleukemia.*

Er·y·thri·na (err″i·three′nuh) *n.* A genus of tropical and subtropical trees and shrubs, various species of which have long been used in folk medicine. The seeds of some species contain one or more alkaloids having curare-like action, including β-erythroidine and its derivative dihydro-β-erythroidine.

er·y·thrite (err′i·thrite, e·rith′rite) *n.* ERYTHRITOL.

eryth·ri·tol (e·rith′ri·tol) *n.* Butanetetrol, $C_4H_{10}O_4$, a polyhydric alcohol existing as several different optical isomers. The meso-isomer occurs in algae and fungi and is also obtained by synthesis; it is very soluble in water, and is about twice as sweet as sucrose.

erythritol tetranitrate. ERYTHRITYL TETRANITRATE.

eryth·ri·tyl tetranitrate (e·rith′ri·til). The tetranitrate of erythritol, $C_4H_6N_4O_{12}$, a coronary vasodilator.

erythro-. See *erythr-*.

eryth·ro·blast (e·rith′ro·blast) *n.* [*erythro-* + *-blast*]. *In hematology,* generally a nucleated precursor of the erythrocyte in which cytoplasmic basophilia is retained. According to size and nuclear characteristics, these cells can be divided into early and late forms. —**eryth·ro·blas·tic** (e·rith″ro·blas′tick) *adj.*

eryth·ro·blas·te·mia, eryth·ro·blas·tae·mia (e·rith″ro·blas·tee′mee·uh) *n.* [*erythroblast* + *-emia*]. The abnormal presence of nucleated erythrocytes in the peripheral blood.

eryth·ro·blas·to·ma (e·rith″ro·blas·to′muh) *n.* [*erythroblast* + *-oma*]. A tumor of bone marrow composed of cells that resemble large erythroblasts; probably a variety of malignant plasmacytoma.

eryth·ro·blas·to·pe·nia (e·rith″ro·blas″to·pee′nee·uh) *n.* [*erythroblast* + *-penia*]. A decrease in number of the erythroblasts in the bone marrow.

eryth·ro·blas·to·sis (e·rith″ro·blas·to′sis) *n.*, pl. **erythroblasto·ses** (·seez) [*erythroblast* + *-osis*]. 1. The presence of erythroblasts in the peripheral blood. 2. ERYTHROBLASTOSIS FETALIS. 3. A proliferative disorder of fowl hematopoiesis caused by a virus and characterized by atypical erythroblasts in the peripheral blood and tissues. —**erythroblas·tot·ic** (·tot′ick) *adj.*

erythroblastosis fe·ta·lis (fee·tay′lis). A hemolytic anemia of the fetus and newborn, occurring when the blood of the infant contains an antigen lacking in the mother's blood, stimulating maternal antibody formation against the infant's erythrocytes. See also *ABO blood group, Rh factor.*

erythroblastosis neonatorum. ERYTHROBLASTOSIS FETALIS.

eryth·ro·chlo·ro·pia (e·rith″ro·klor·o′pee·uh) *n.* [*erythro-* + *chlor-* + *-opia*]. A form of subnormal color perception in which green and red are the only colors correctly distinguished.

eryth·ro·chlo·rop·sia (e·rith″ro·klor·op′see·uh) *n.* ERYTHROCHLOROPIA.

eryth·ro·chlor·o·py (e·rith″ro·klor′o·pee) *n.* ERYTHROCHLOROPIA.

Erythrocin. A trademark for the antibiotic substance erythromycin.

er·y·throc·la·sis (err″i·throck′luh·sis) *n.* [*erythro-* + *-clasis*]. The fragmentation or breaking down of erythrocytes. —**eryth·ro·clas·tic** (e·rith″ro·klas′tick) *adj.*

eryth·ro·conte (e·rith′ro·kont) *n.* [*erythro-* + Gk. *kontos,* pole]. One of the many fine azurophilic rods found in erythrocytes, and especially in stippled cells.

eryth·ro·cru·o·rin (e·rith″ro·kroo′uh·rin, ·kroo·or′in) *n.* Any of the respiratory pigments found in the blood and tissue fluids of some invertebrates; it is an iron-porphyrin protein corresponding to hemoglobin in vertebrates.

eryth·ro·cu·prein (e·rith″ro·kew′preen, ·pree·in) *n.* A copper-containing protein of unknown function, occurring in human erythrocytes.

eryth·ro·cy·a·no·sis (e·rith″ro·sigh·uh·no′sis) *n.* [*erythro-* + *cyan-* + *-osis*]. Irregular red-blue markings on the skin, usually reticular in arrangement; due to a circulatory disturbance of the skin.

eryth·ro·cyte (e·rith′ro·site) *n.* [*erythro-* + *-cyte*]. The nonnucleated and agranular mature cell of vertebrate blood, whose oxygen-carrying pigment, hemoglobin, is responsible for the red color of fresh blood. In man, the cells are generally disk-shaped and biconcave, normally 5 to 9 μm in diameter (mean 7.2 to 7.8) and 1 to 2 μm thick. They number around 5 million /mm³ in the adult, ranging somewhat higher in men and lower in women. Syn. *red blood cell, red cell.* See also *erythrocytic series.* For abnormal forms, see *elliptocyte, macrocyte, microcyte, poikilocyte, sickle cell, spherocyte, target cell.* See also *anisocytosis.*

erythrocyte fragility test. A measure of the resistance of red blood cells to osmotic hemolysis in hypotonic salt solutions of graded dilutions.

erythrocyte-maturing factor. VITAMIN B_{12}.

erythrocyte sedimentation test. The settling rate of erythrocytes in a column of blood kept fluid by anticoagulants, as measured by any of several methods; it is related to content of various blood proteins, and may vary in health and disease.

eryth·ro·cy·the·mia, eryth·ro·cy·thae·mia (eh·rith″ro·sigh·theem′ee·uh) *n.* [*erythrocyte* + *-hemia*]. 1. ERYTHROCYTOSIS. 2. POLYCYTHEMIA VERA.

eryth·ro·cyt·ic (e·rith″ro·sit′ick) *adj.* Of or pertaining to erythrocytes.

erythrocytic series. In hemopoiesis, the cells at progressive stages of development from a primitive cell to the mature erythrocyte. See also *proerythroblast, erythroblast, normoblast, reticulocyte, erythrocyte.*

erythrocyto-. A combining form meaning *erythrocyte.*

eryth·ro·cy·to·blast (e·rith″ro·sigh′to·blast) *n.* [*erythrocyto-* + *-blast*]. ERYTHROBLAST.

eryth·ro·cy·tol·y·sin (e·rith″ro·sigh·tol′i·sin, ·sigh·to·lye′sin) *n.* An agent capable of producing erythrocytolysis; HEMOLYSIN.

eryth·ro·cy·tol·y·sis (e·rith″ro·sigh·tol′i·sis) *n.* [*erythrocyto-* + *lysis*]. Disruption of erythrocytes with discharge of their contents; HEMOLYSIS.

eryth·ro·cy·tom·e·ter (e·rith″ro·sigh·tom′e·tur) *n.* [*erythrocyto-* + *meter*]. HEMOCYTOMETER. —**erythrocytome·try** (·tree) *n.*

eryth·ro·cy·to·op·so·nin (e·rith″ro·sigh″to·op′so·nin) *n.* [*erythrocyto-* + *opsonin*]. A substance that renders erythrocytes liable to phagocytosis, as an opsonin renders bacteria more liable to phagocytosis.

eryth·ro·cy·to·poi·e·sis (e·rith″ro·sigh″to·poy·ee′sis) *n.* [*erythrocyto-* + *-poiesis*]. ERYTHROPOIESIS. —**erythrocytopoi·et·ic** (·et·ick) *adj.*

eryth·ro·cy·tor·rhex·is (e·rith″ro·sigh″to·reck′sis) *n.* [*erythrocyto-* + *-rrhexis*]. The breaking up or fragmentation of erythrocytes. Syn. *erythrorrhexis.*

eryth·ro·cy·tos·chi·sis (e·rith″ro·sigh·tos′ki·sis) *n.* [*erythrocyto-* + *-schisis*]. The fragmentation or splitting up of erythrocytes, the parts retaining hemoglobin.

eryth·ro·cy·to·sis (e·rith″ro·sigh·to′sis) *n.*, pl. **erythrocyto·ses** (·seez) [*erythrocyte* + *-osis*]. Elevation above normal of the numbers of peripheral blood erythrocytes accompanied by an increase in total red cell volume; usually secondary to hypoxia. Compare *polycythemia vera.*

erythrocytosis me·ga·lo·splen·i·ca (meg″uh·lo·splen′i·kuh). POLYCYTHEMIA VERA.

eryth·ro·de·gen·er·a·tive (e·rith″ro·de·jen′ur·uh·tiv) *adj.* Involving degenerative changes in the erythrocytes with increase in polychromatic basophilic stippling.

eryth·ro·der·ma (e·rith″ro·dur′muh) *n.* [*erythro-* + *-derma*]. A dermatosis characterized by an abnormal redness of the skin; ERYTHEMA.

erythroderma des·qua·ma·ti·vum (de·skwam″uh·tye′vum, de·skway″muh·). A generalized redness and scaly eruption seen in children. The nails, scalp, and intestinal tract are usually involved and the outcome is sometimes fatal. Differentiated from dermatitis exfoliativa. Syn. *Leiner's disease, erythrodermia desquamativa.*

erythroderma ich·thy·o·si·for·me con·gen·i·tum (ikth″ee·o″si·for′mee kon·jen′i·tum). A type of congenital dermatosis in which there is a thickening and reddening of the skin, and a tendency to resemble lichen.

erythroderma mac·u·lo·sa per·stans (mack·yoo·lo′suh pur′stanz). A plaque-like variety of psoriasis in which the areas involved are about one-half inch in diameter and without marked desquamation.

erythroderma pso·ri·at·i·cum (so·ree·at′i·kum). Generalized psoriasis, with an increase in the inflammatory changes.

eryth·ro·der·mia (e·rith″ro·dur′mee·uh) *n.* ERYTHRODERMA.

erythrodermia des·qua·ma·ti·va (de·skwam″uh·tye′vuh, de·skway″muh·). ERYTHRODERMA DESQUAMATIVUM.

eryth·ro·dex·trin (e·rith″ro·decks′trin) *n.* A dextrin formed by the partial hydrolysis of starch with acid or amylase. It yields a red color with iodine.

eryth·ro·don·tia (e·rith″ro·don′chee·uh) *n.* [*erythr-* + *-odontia*]. Red discoloration of the teeth.

erythroedema. Erythredema (= ACRODYNIA).

eryth·ro·gen·e·sis (e·rith″ro·jen′e·sis) *n.* [*erythro-* + *-genesis*]. The formation of erythrocytes; ERYTHROPOIESIS.

eryth·ro·gen·ic (e·rith″ro·jen′ick) *adj.* [*erythro-* + *-genic*]. 1. Inducing a rash or redness of the skin. 2. ERYTHROPOIETIC. 3. Producing a color sensation of redness.

erythrogenic toxin. A toxin produced by certain hemolytic streptococci, which is responsible for the rash of scarlet fever. Syn. *Dick toxin.*

eryth·ro·gone (e·rith′ro·gohn) *n.* [*erythro-* + Gk. *gonē*, seed]. A basophilic euchromatic precursor of an erythroblast or a megaloblast; a stem cell.

eryth·ro·go·ni·um (e·rith″ro·go′nee·um) *n.* ERYTHROGONE.

er·y·throid (err′i·throid) *adj.* [*erythr-* + *-oid*]. Reddish; of a red color; used of cells of the erythrocytic series.

er·y·thro·i·dine (err″i·thro′i·deen, ·din) *n.* An alkaloid, $C_{16}H_{19}NO_3$, obtained from species of *Erythrina;* it occurs in α- and β- varieties. β-Erythroidine and its derivative dihydro-β-erythroidine have curare-like activity.

erythroid myeloma. A malignant plasmacytoma.

eryth·ro·ker·a·to·der·mia (e·rith″ro·kerr″uh·to·dur′mee·uh) *n.* [*erythro-* + *kerato-* + *-dermia*]. Papulosquamous erythematous plaques on the skin.

er·y·throl (err′i·throl) *n.* 1. ERYTHRITOL. 2. 3-Butene-1,2-diol; $CH_2OHCHOHCH{=}CH_2$.

eryth·ro·labe (e·rith′ro·labe) *n.* [*erythro-* + *-labe*]. One of the two cone pigments of the normal eye, absorbing light most actively in the red portion of the spectrum. Contr. *chlorolabe.*

eryth·ro·leu·ke·mia (e·rith″ro·lew·kee′mee·uh) *n.* [*erythro-* + *leukemia*]. ERYTHREMIC MYELOSIS.

eryth·ro·leu·ko·blas·to·sis (e·rith″ro·lew″ko·blas·to′sis) *n.* LEUKOERYTHROBLASTOSIS.

eryth·ro·leu·ko·sis (e·rith″ro·lew·ko′sis) *n.*, pl. **erythroleuko·ses** (·seez) [*erythro-* + *leuk-* + *-osis*]. ERYTHROBLASTOSIS (3).

erythrol tetranitrate. ERYTHRITYL TETRANITRATE.

er·y·throl·y·sin (err″i·throl′i·sin, e·rith″ro·lye′sin) *n.* ERYTHROCYTOLYSIN; HEMOLYSIN.

er·y·throl·y·sis (err″i·throl′i·sis) *n.*, pl. **erythroly·ses** (·seez) [*erythro-* + *lysis*]. ERYTHROCYTOLYSIS.

eryth·ro·me·lal·gia (e·rith″ro·me·lal′jee·uh) *n.* [*erythro-* + *melalgia*]. A cutaneous vasodilatation of the feet or, more rarely, of the hands; characterized by redness, mottling, changes in skin temperature, and neuralgic pains. Syn. *acromelalgia, Mitchell's disease.*

erythromelalgia of the head. CLUSTER HEADACHE.

eryth·ro·me·lia (e·rith″·ro·mee′lee·uh) *n.* [*erythro-* + *mel-*, limb, + *-ia*]. A condition of the extensor surfaces of the arms and legs; characterized by painless progressive redness of the skin; distinct from erythromelalgia.

er·y·throm·e·ter (err″i·throm′e·tur) *n.* [*erythro-* + *-meter*]. Apparatus for measuring degree of redness.

eryth·ro·my·cin (e·rith″ro·migh′sin) *n.* [*erythro-* + *-mycin*]. An antibiotic substance, $C_{37}H_{67}NO_{13}$, isolated from cultures of the red-pigment-producing organism *Streptomyces erythreus.* Erythromycin is effective orally against many gram-positive and some gram-negative pathogens. It is used in the form of various salts and esters, as the estolate (propionate lauryl sulfate), ethylcarbonate, ethyl succinate, gluceptate (glucoheptonate), lactobionate, and stearate.

eryth·ro·my·e·lo·sis (e·rith″ro·migh″e·lo′sis) *n.* [*erythro-* + *myel-* + *-osis*]. Proliferation both of erythrocytic and granulocytic bone marrow elements without known cause.

er·y·thron (err′i·thron) *n. In hematology,* the peripheral blood erythrocytes, the erythropoietic bone marrow, and erythroclastic tissues as in the spleen, conceived as one functional organ unit.

eryth·ro·neo·cy·to·sis (e·rith″ro·nee″o·sigh·to′sis) *n.* [*erythro-* + *neo-* + *cyt-* + *-osis*]. The presence of regenerative forms of erythrocytes in the circulating blood.

Er·y·thro·ni·um (err″i·thro′nee·um) *n.* A genus of plants of the Liliaceae.

eryth·ro·no·cla·sia (e·rith″ro·no·klay′zhuh) *n.* [*erythron* + *-clasia*]. Destruction of erythrocytes, not only in circulating blood, but also in the hemopoietic tissues.

eryth·ro·pe·nia (e·rith″ro·pee′nee·uh, err″i·thro·) *n.* [*erythro-* + *-penia*]. Deficiency in the number of erythrocytes.

eryth·ro·phage (e·rith′ro·faje) *n.* [*erythro-* + *-phage*]. A phagocytic cell, as a macrophage, containing ingested erythrocytes.

eryth·ro·pha·gia (e·rith″ro·fay′jee·uh) *n.* [*erythro-* + *-phagia*]. ERYTHROPHAGOCYTOSIS.

eryth·ro·phago·cy·to·sis (e·rith″ro·fag″o·sigh·to′sis) *n.* [*erythro-* + *phagocytosis*]. The ingestion of an erythrocyte by a phagocytic cell, such as a blood monocyte or a tissue macrophage.

eryth·ro·phil (e·rith′ro·fil) *adj.* [*erythro-* + *-phil*]. Having an affinity for a red dye. **—eryth·roph·i·lous** (err″i·throf′i·lus) *adj.*

eryth·ro·phle·ine (e·rith″ro·flee′een, ·in) *n.* An alkaloid, $C_{24}H_{39}NO_5$, from casca bark, having digitalis-like action.

eryth·ro·pho·bia (e·rith″ro·fo′bee·uh) *n.* [*erythro-* + *-phobia*]. 1. An abnormal fear of red colors; may be associated with a fear of blood. 2. Fear of blushing.

eryth·ro·phose (e·rith′ro·foze) *n.* [*erythro-* + *phose*]. A red phose.

er·y·thro·pia (err″i·thro′pee·uh) *n.* [*erythr-* + *-opia*]. ERYTHROPSIA.

eryth·ro·pla·sia of Queyrat (e·rith″ro·play′zhuh, ·zee·uh). QUEYRAT'S ERYTHROPLASIA.

eryth·ro·plas·tid (e·rith″ro·plas′tid) *n.* [*erythro-* + *plastid*]. ERYTHROCYTE.

eryth·ro·poi·e·sis (e·rith″ro·poy·ee′sis) *n.*, pl. **erythropoie·ses** (·seez) [*erythro-* + *-poiesis*]. The formation and development of erythrocytes. See also *erythrocytic series.* **—erythro·poi·et·ic** (·et′ick) *adj.*

erythropoietic porphyria. A rare inborn error of porphyrin metabolism, probably transmitted as a recessive trait, appearing in infancy or early childhood; characterized clinically by photosensitivity with development of blisters, pigmentation and hypertrichosis of the skin exposed to light, redness of the teeth at the gingival margins, splenomegaly, hemolytic anemia, and chemically by the presence of uroporphyrin I and coproporphyrin I in bone marrow, erythrocytes, and urine, and absence of porphobilinogen. Syn. *congenital porphyria, photosensitive porphyria.* Compare *erythropoietic protoporphyria.*

erythropoietic protoporphyria. A congenital and probably inherited form of erythropoietic porphyria in which exposure to sunlight results in intense pruritus, erythema, and edema of the uncovered areas of the body, usually subsiding within one day, and marked increase in the concentration of a free form of protoporphyrin in circulating erythrocytes, and its excretion in stools.

eryth·ro·poi·e·tin (e·rith″ro·poy′e·tin) *n.* [*erythropoietic* + *-in*]. A humoral substance concerned in the regulation of erythrocyte production, found in a variety of animals including man, and characterized as a glycoprotein migrating in blood plasma with alpha-2 globulins.

eryth·ro·pros·o·pal·gia (e·rith″ro·pros″o·pal′jee·uh) *n.* [*erythro-* + *prosopalgia*]. CLUSTER HEADACHE.

er·y·throp·sia (err″i·throp′see·uh) *n.* [*erythr-* + *-opsia*]. An abnormality of vision in which all objects appear red. Syn. *red vision.*

er·y·throp·sin (err″i·throp′sin) *n.* [*erythr-* + *opsin*]. RHODOPSIN.

eryth·ror·rhex·is (e·rith″ro·reck′sis) *n.* [*erythro-* + *-rrhexis*]. ERYTHROCYTORRHEXIS.

eryth·rose (e·rith′roce) *n.* The tetrose sugar CHOCHOHCHOHCH$_2$OH, existing in D- and L- forms, variously obtained.

eryth·ro·sed·i·men·ta·tion (e·rith″ro·sed·i·men·tay′shun) *n.* The settling of erythrocytes. See also *erythrocyte sedimentation test.*

eryth·ro·sin B (e·rith′ro·sin). 2,4,5,7-Tetraiodofluorescein disodium salt, a bluish-red, water-soluble acid dye of the eosin class; used generally as a plasma stain.

erythrosin BB. PHLOXINE.

eryth·ro·sin·o·phil (e·rith″ro·sin′o·fil) *adj.* [*erythrosin* + *-phil*]. Easily stainable with erythrosin.

erythrosin Y. 4,5-Diiodofluorescein disodium salt, a yellowish-red, water-soluble acid dye of the eosin class; used generally as a plasma stain.

er·y·thro·sis (err″i·thro′sis) *n.*, pl. **erythro·ses** (·seez) [*erythr-* + *-osis*]. 1. Overproliferation of erythrocytopoietic tissue as found in polycythemia. 2. The unusual red skin color of individuals with polycythemia.

eryth·ro·sta·sis (e·rith″ro·stay′sis) *n.* [*erythro-* + *stasis*]. The processes to which erythrocytes are subjected when denied free access to fresh plasma, resulting from stasis of the blood.

er·y·throx·y·lon (err″i·throck′si·lon) *n.* COCA.

eryth·ru·lose (e·rith′roo·loce) *n.* The tetrose sugar HOCH$_2$COCHOHCH$_2$OH, existing in D- and L- forms, variously obtained; the sugars are isomeric with the corresponding erythrose form.

er·y·thru·ria (err″i·throo′ree·uh) *n.* [*erythr-* + *-uria*]. Passage of red urine.

Es Symbol for einsteinium.

Es·bach's method (ess·bah^h^k′) [G. H. *Esbach,* French physician, 1843–1890]. A method for detecting protein in urine in which picric acid is added to urine to precipitate protein which settles to the bottom of a graduated tube.

Esbach's reagent [G. H. *Esbach*]. A picric acid–citric acid–water solution used for quantitative protein testing of urine.

es·cape, *n.* 1. *In medicine,* leakage or outflow, as of nervous impulses; release from control. 2. *In psychiatry,* the departure of a patient confined to the maximum security unit of a mental hospital without permission. Compare *elopement, parole.* —**es·cap·ee** (es·kay·pee′) *n.*

escape mechanism. *In psychiatry,* a mode of adjustment to difficult or unpleasant situations by utilizing a means easier or pleasanter than that required for a permanent solution of the difficulty, often resulting in an evasion of responsibility.

-escence [from *-escent*]. A suffix indicating (a) *an incipient state, a process of becoming;* (b) *likeness, similarity.*

-escent [L. *-esc-*, inchoative verb element, + *-ens, -entis,* participial suffix]. A suffix meaning (a) *becoming;* (b) *-like, somewhat.*

es·char (es′kahr, es′kur) *n.* [OF. *eschare,* scar, scab, from L. *eschara,* from Gk., fireplace; burn, scab]. A dry slough, especially that produced by heat or a corrosive or caustic substance.

es·cha·rot·ic (es″kuh·rot′ick) *adj.* & *n.* [Gk. *escharōtikos*]. 1. Caustic; producing a slough. 2. A substance that produces an eschar; a caustic or corrosive. —**escha·ro·sis** (·ro′sis) *n.*

Eschatin. Trademark for an adrenal cortex injection, a preparation of mixed natural adrenocortical hormones.

Esch·e·rich·ia (esh″e·rick′ee·uh) *n.* [T. *Escherich,* German physician, 1857–1911]. A genus of non-spore-forming gram-negative bacteria, widely distributed in nature, belonging to the family Enterobacteriaceae.

Escherichia co·li (ko′lye). A group of normal bacterial inhabitants of the intestine of man and all vertebrates. Toxic strains may cause enteritis, peritonitis, and infections of the urinary tract. Abbreviated, *E. coli.* Syn. *colon bacillus.*

es·chro·la·lia (es″kro·lay′lee·uh) *n.* [Gk. *aischros,* shameful, disgraceful, + *-lalia*]. COPROLALIA.

es·cor·cin (es·kor′sin) *n.* Escorcinol, $C_9H_8O_4$, prepared by the action of sodium amalgam on esculetin; has been used to diagnose corneal and conjunctival lesions.

Escorpal. Trademark for phencarbamide, an anticholinergic drug.

es·cu·le·tin, aes·cu·le·tin (es″kew·lee′tin) *n.* 6,7-Dihydroxycoumarin, $C_9H_6O_4$, a hydrolysis product of esculin.

es·cu·lin, aes·cu·lin (es′kew·lin) *n.* 6,7-Dihydrocoumarin 6-glucoside, $C_{15}H_{16}O_9$, a constituent of the leaves and bark of the horse chestnut, *Aesculus hippocastanum.* Being fluorescent, it absorbs ultraviolet rays and has been used as a sunburn protective.

es·cutch·eon (e·skutch′un) *n.* [OF. *escuchon,* shield, from L. *scutum*]. The pattern of pubic hair growth, which differs in men and women.

es·er·a·mine (e·serr′uh·meen, ·min, es′ur·) *n.* An alkaloid, $C_{16}H_{25}N_4O_3$, from Calabar beans.

es·er·i·dine (e·serr′i·deen, ·din, es′ur·) *n.* An alkaloid, $C_{15}H_{21}N_3O_3$, found in Calabar beans.

es·er·ine (es′ur·een, ·in, ez′) *n.* PHYSOSTIGMINE.

Esidrix. A trademark for hydrochlorothiazide, a diuretic and antihypertensive drug.

-esis [Gk. *-ēsis*]. A suffix meaning (a) *action;* (b) *process.*

Eskadiazine. A trademark for an aqueous suspension of sulfadiazine.

Eskalith. A trademark for lithium carbonate, used in the treatment of manic-depressive psychoses.

Es·march's bandage (ess′mar^k^h) [J. F. A. von *Esmarch,* German surgeon, 1823–1908]. A rubber compression bandage with tourniquet, used to render a limb bloodless during operation.

Esmarch's mask [J. F. A. von *Esmarch*]. A metal frame over which gauze is stretched; used for administration of ether or chloroform by inhalation.

Esmarch's operation [J. F. A. von *Esmarch*]. A method of amputation at the hip joint.

eso- [Gk., from *esō,* within]. A prefix meaning *inner* or *inward.*

esophag-, esophago-, oesophag-, oesophago-. A combining form meaning *esophagus, esophageal.*

esoph·a·gal·gia, oe·soph·a·gal·gia (e·sof″uh·gal′jee·uh) *n.* [*esophag-* + *-algia*]. Pain in the esophagus.

esoph·a·ge·al, oe·soph·a·ge·al (e·sof″uh·jee′ul, ee″so·faj′ee·ul) *adj.* Of or pertaining to the esophagus.

esophageal diverticulum. 1. A herniation through the posterior pharyngeal wall, pulsion in type, presenting most frequently on the left side of the neck. 2. A traction diverticulum of small size and no clinical significance, usually noted only at autopsy.

esophageal fistula. An abnormal tract of congenital origin, communicating between the esophagus and some portion of the skin through an external opening, or between esophagus and some viscus or organ through an internal opening. A similar fistula may result from trauma or disease.

esophageal foramen. ESOPHAGEAL HIATUS.

esophageal forceps. A special forceps for removing foreign bodies from the esophagus.

esophageal hiatus. The opening in the diaphragm for the esophagus. NA *hiatus esophageus.*

esophageal lead. *In electrocardiography,* an exploring electrode placed in the esophagus adjacent to the heart and paired with an indifferent electrode; used to study atrial waves or posterior myocardial infarction.

esophageal plexus. A nerve plexus surrounding the esophagus. NA *plexus esophageus.*

esophageal sound. A long flexible probe for examination of the esophagus.

esophageal speech or **voice.** Speech produced after laryngectomy by swallowing air into the esophagus and expelling it with an eructation past the pharyngeal opening to produce a sound that is then modulated by the lips, tongue, and palate.

esophageal varices. Dilated anastomosing veins of the esophageal plexus, resulting from persistent portal hypertension.

esoph·a·gec·ta·sia, oe·soph·a·gec·ta·sia (e·sof″uh·jeck·tay′zhuh, ·zee·uh) *n.* [*esophag-* + *ectasia*]. Idiopathic dilatation of the esophagus.

esoph·a·gec·ta·sis, oe·soph·a·gec·ta·sis (e·sof″uh·jeck′tuh·sis) *n.* ESOPHAGECTASIA.

esoph·a·gec·to·my, oe·soph·a·gec·to·my (e·sof″uh·jeck′tuh·mee) *n.* [*esophag-* + *-ectomy*]. Surgical resection of part of the esophagus.

esoph·a·gec·to·py, oe·soph·a·gec·to·py (e·sof″uh·jeck′tuh·pee) *n.* [*esophag-* + *ectopy*]. Displacement of the esophagus.

esophagi. Plural and genitive singular of *esophagus.*

esoph·a·gism (e·sof′uh·jiz·um) *n.* ESOPHAGOSPASM.

esoph·a·gis·mus (e·sof″uh·jiz′mus) *n.* ESOPHAGOSPASM.

esoph·a·gi·tis, oe·soph·a·gi·tis (e·sof″uh·jye′tis) *n.* [*esophag-* + *-itis*]. Inflammation of the esophagus.

esophago-. See *esophag-.*

esoph·a·go·bron·chi·al, oe·soph·a·go·bron·chi·al (e·sof″uh·go·brong′kee·ul) *adj.* [*esophago-* + *bronchial*]. Pertaining to the esophagus and a bronchus or the bronchi.

esoph·a·go·cele, oe·soph·a·go·cele (e·sof′uh·go·seel) *n.* [*esophago-* + *-cele*]. 1. An esophageal hernia. 2. An acquired hernia of the inner coats of the esophagus through the tunica muscularis. 3. Abnormal distention of the esophagus.

esoph·a·go·du·o·de·nos·to·my, oe·soph·a·go·du·o·de·nos·to·my (e·sof″uh·go·dew″o·de·nos′tuh·mee) *n.* [*esophago-* + *duodeno-* + *-stomy*]. *In surgery,* an anastomosis between the esophagus and the jejunum.

esoph·a·go·en·ter·os·to·my, oe·soph·a·go·en·ter·os·to·my (e·sof″uh·go·en″tur·os′tuh·mee) *n.* [*esophago-* + *entero-* + *-stomy*]. *In surgery,* anastomosis of the cardiac end of the esophagus to the intestine, following total gastrectomy.

esoph·a·go·esoph·a·gos·to·my, oe·soph·a·gooe·soph·a·gos·to·my (e·sof″uh·go·e·sof″uh·gos′tuh·mee) *n.* [*esophago-* + *esophago-* + *-stomy*]. *In surgery,* reunion of the esophagus after removal of an intervening portion.

esoph·a·go·gas·trec·to·my, oe·soph·a·go·gas·trec·to·my (e·sof″uh·go·gas·treck′tuh·mee) *n.* [*esophago-* + *gastr-* + *-ectomy*]. Excision of parts of the stomach and esophagus.

esoph·a·go·gas·tric, oe·soph·a·go·gas·tric (e·sof″uh·go·gas′trick) *adj.* [*esophago-* + *gastric*]. Pertaining to the esophagus and the stomach.

esophagogastric sphincter. CARDIAC SPHINCTER.

esoph·a·go·gas·tro·du·o·de·no·scope (e·sof″uh·go·gas″tro·dew″o·dee′no·skope) *n.* An instrument for examining the interior of the esophagus, stomach, and duodenum.

esoph·a·go·gas·tro·plas·ty, oe·soph·a·go·gas·tro·plas·ty (e·sof″uh·go·gas′tro·plas″tee) *n.* [*esophago-* + *gastro-* + *-plasty*]. *In surgery,* repair of the stomach and esophagus.

esoph·a·go·gas·tro·scope, oe·soph·a·go·gas·tro·scope (e·sof″uh·go·gas′tro·skope) *n.* [*esophago-* + *gastro-* + *-scope*]. An instrument for examining the interior of the esophagus and the stomach. —**esophago·gas·tros·co·py** (·gas·tros′kuh·pee) *n.*

esoph·a·go·gas·tros·to·my, oe·soph·a·go·gas·tros·to·my (e·sof″uh·go·gas·tros′tuh·mee) *n.* [*esophago-* + *gastro-* + *-stomy*]. *In surgery,* establishment of an anastomosis between the esophagus and the stomach; may be performed by the abdominal route or by transpleural operation.

esoph·a·go·gram, oe·soph·a·go·gram (e·sof′uh·go·gram) *n.* [*esophago-* + *-gram*]. A radiographic image of the esophagus.

esoph·a·go·hi·a·tal, oe·soph·a·go·hi·a·tal (e·sof″uh·go·high·ay′tul) *adj.* [*esophago-* + *hiatal*]. Pertaining to the esophagus and the opening in the diaphragm through which that organ passes.

esoph·a·go·je·ju·nos·to·my, oe·soph·a·go·je·ju·nos·to·my (e·sof″uh·go·je·joo″nos′tuh·mee) *n.* [*esophago-* + *jejuno-* + *-stomy*]. *In surgery,* an anastomosis between the esophagus and the jejunum.

esoph·a·gom·e·ter, oe·soph·a·gom·e·ter (e·sof″uh·gom′e·tur) *n.* [*esophago-* + *-meter*]. An instrument for measuring the esophagus.

esoph·a·gop·a·thy, oe·soph·a·gop·a·thy (e·sof″uh·gop″uhth·ee) *n.* [*esophago-* + *-pathy*]. Any disease of the esophagus.

esoph·a·go·pha·ryn·geal (e·sof″uh·go·fa·rin′jee·ul) *adj.* Pertaining to the esophagus and pharynx.

esoph·a·go·plas·ty, oe·soph·a·go·plas·ty (e·sof′uh·go·plas″tee) *n.* [*esophago-* + *-plasty*]. Plastic surgery of the esophagus.

esoph·a·gop·to·sis, oe·soph·a·gop·to·sis (e·sof″uh·gop·to′sis) *n.* [*esophago-* + *ptosis*]. Prolapse of the esophagus.

esoph·a·go·sal·i·vary reflex (e·sof″uh·go·sal′i·verr·ee). SALIVARY REFLEX.

esoph·a·go·scope, oe·soph·a·go·scope (e·sof′uh·go·skope″) *n.* [*esophago-* + *-scope*]. An endoscopic instrument for examination of the interior of the esophagus. —**esoph·a·gos·co·py** (e·sof″uh·gos′kuh·pee) *n.*

esoph·a·go·spasm, oe·soph·a·go·spasm (e·sof′uh·go·spaz·um) *n.* [*esophago-* + *spasm*]. Spasmodic contraction of the esophagus. See also *dysphagia spastica.*

esoph·a·go·ste·no·sis, oe·soph·a·go·ste·no·sis (e·sof″uh·go·ste·no′sis) *n.* [*esophago-* + *stenosis*]. Constriction of the lumen of the esophagus.

esoph·a·gos·to·ma, oe·soph·a·gos·to·ma (e·sof″uh·gos′tuh·muh) *n.* [*esophago-* + *-stoma*]. An abnormal aperture or passage into the esophagus.

esophagostomiasis. OESOPHAGOSTOMIASIS.

esoph·a·gos·to·my, oe·soph·a·gos·to·my (e·sof″uh·gos′tuh·mee) *n.* [*esophago-* + *-stomy*]. The formation of an artificial opening in the esophagus.

esophagostomy ex·ter·na (ecks·tur′nuh). *In surgery,* the opening of the esophagus from the surface of the neck; for the removal of foreign bodies.

esophagostomy in·ter·na (in·tur′nuh). Incision of the esophagus from the inside by means of the esophagotome; for relief of stricture.

esoph·a·go·tome, oe·soph·a·go·tome (e·sof′uh·go·tome, ee″so·fag′o·tome) *n.* [*esophago-* + *-tome*]. An instrument devised for cutting into the esophagus.

esoph·a·got·o·my, oe·soph·a·got·o·my (e·sof″uh·got′uh·mee) *n.* [*esophago-* + *-tomy*]. Opening of the esophagus by an incision.

esoph·a·gus, oe·soph·a·gus (e·sof′uh·gus) *n.*, pl. & genit. sing. **esopha·gi** (·guy, ·jye) [Gk. *oisophagos* (rel. to *phagein,* to eat)] [NA]. The musculomembranous canal, about nine inches in length, extending from the pharynx to the stomach; the gullet. See also Plate 12.

esoph·o·gram, oe·soph·o·gram (e·sof'o·gram) *n.* ESOPHAGOGRAM.

eso·pho·ria (es"o·fo'ree·uh, ee"so·) *n.* [*eso-* + *-phoria*]. A form of heterophoria in which the visual lines tend inward.

eso·tro·pia (es"o·tro'pee·uh) *n.* [*eso-* + *-tropia*]. Convergent strabismus, occurring when one eye fixes upon an object and the other deviates inward. Contr. *exotropia.*

ESP Abbreviation for *extrasensory perception.*

es·pro·quin (es'pro·kwin) *n.* 2-[3-(Ethylsulfinyl)propyl]-1,2,-3,4-tetrahydroisoquinoline, $C_{14}H_{21}NOS$, an adrenergic agent, usually used as the hydrochloride salt.

es·pun·dia (es·pun'dee·uh, Sp. es·po͞on'dya) *n.* [Sp., orig., a granulomatous ulcer of horses; pseudolatinization from *esponja,* sponge]. A form of American mucocutaneous leishmaniasis caused by *Leishmania brasiliensis,* characterized by erosions of the mucosal surfaces of the nose and mouth and respiratory obstruction, accompanied by fever, anemia, and weight loss, often leading to death, but treatable in the early stages with pentavalent antimonials.

ESR Abbreviation for *erythrocyte sedimentation rate.*

es·sence, *n.* [L. *essentia,* from *esse,* to be]. 1. That which gives to anything its character or peculiar quality. 2. A solution of an essential oil in alcohol.

es·sen·tial, *adj.* 1. Pertaining to the essence of a substance. 2. Of a disease or condition, idiopathic; occurring without a known cause. 3. Necessary in the life of an organism but not producible by it, as an essential amino acid or an essential fatty acid, which cannot be synthesized in the body and must be obtained from the diet.

essential amino acid. An amino acid which must be supplied in the diet because of the inability of an organism to synthesize it; the essential amino acids in humans and other animals are histidine, isoleucine, leucine, lysine, methionine, phenylalanine, threonine, trypotophan, valine, and, on some criteria, arginine.

essential anemia. 1. *Obsol.* PERNICIOUS ANEMIA. 2. IDIOPATHIC ANEMIA.

essential cause. PRIMARY CAUSE.

essential cyclophoria. A form of cyclophoria due to an anatomic or innervational abnormality.

essential dysmenorrhea. PRIMARY DYSMENORRHEA.

essential emphysema. EMPHYSEMA (1).

essential familial hypercholesterolemia. FAMILIAL HYPERBETALIPOPROTEINEMIA.

essential familial hyperlipemia. FAMILIAL HYPERLIPOPROTEINEMIA.

essential fatty acid. Any of the polyunsaturated fatty acids that are required in the diet of mammals; probably needed as precursors of the prostoglandins.

essential fever. A fever of unknown cause.

essential hypercalcinuria. IDIOPATHIC HYPERCALCINURIA.

essential hypercholesterolemia. FAMILIAL HYPERBETALIPOPROTEINEMIA.

essential hyperkinesia. Excessive, often purposeless, muscular activity seen in children with the minimal brain dysfunction syndrome or as a result of anxiety or other emotional disturbance.

essential hypertension. A familial and possibly a genetic form of elevation of blood pressure of unknown origin, which may result in anatomic and physiologic abnormalities of the heart, blood vessels, kidneys, and nervous system. Syn. *primary hypertension.*

essential metabolite. A substance necessary for proper metabolism, such as a vitamin.

essential myoclonia. Myoclonus of unknown cause.

essential oil. VOLATILE OIL.

essential purpura. IDIOPATHIC THROMBOCYTOPENIC PURPURA.

essential tachycardia. Tachycardia occurring in paroxysms, and due to functional disturbance of the cardiac nerves.

essential thrombophilia. Diffuse thrombosis of the arteries and veins not accounted for by infection, stasis, or local inflammatory lesions.

essential tremor. An action tremor of variable frequency, most prominent in the arms and head, exaggerated by activity and emotion, and lessened by alcohol and sedatives.

Es·ser inlay graft [J. F. S. *Esser,* Dutch plastic surgeon, 1877–1946]. A molded, specially prepared epithelial graft used in reconstructive plastic surgery.

Es·sick's cell band [C. *Essick,* U.S. anatomist, 20th century]. CORPUS PONTOBULBARE.

EST Abbreviation for *electroshock therapy.*

es·ter (es'tur) *n.* [Ger., from *Essig,* vinegar, + *Äther,* ether]. A compound formed from an alcohol and an acid by elimination of water, as ethyl acetate, $CH_3COOC_2H_5$.

es·ter·ase (es'tur·ace, ·aze) *n.* [*ester* + *-ase*]. Any enzyme that catalyzes the hydrolysis of an ester into an alcohol and an acid.

ester gum. Any of a group of resinous esters made by esterifying natural acids with a glycol or glycerin; used as a mounting medium in microscopy and in preparing varnishes and lacquers.

es·ter·i·fi·ca·tion (es·terr'i·fi·kay'shun) *n.* The process of converting an alcohol or an acid to an ester. —**es·ter·i·fy** (es·terr'i·figh) *v.*

es·te·trol (es'te·trol, ·trole) *n.* 15 α-hydroxyestriol, an estrogen formed from fetal precursors and dependent upon 15 α-hydroxylation activity in the fetal liver. Synthesis declines during infancy and is absent, or at least undetectable, in adults.

es·the·sia, aes·the·sia (es·theezh'uh, ·theez'ee·uh) *n.* [NL., from Gk. *aisthēsis,* sensation, perception]. Capacity for perception, feeling, or sensation. Contr. *anesthesia.*

-esthesia [Gk. *aisthēsis,* sensation, perception, + *-ia*]. A combining form designating *a condition involving sensation or sense perception.*

esthesio-, aesthesio- [Gk. *aisthēsis*]. A combining form meaning *sense, sensory, sensation.*

es·the·si·ol·o·gy, aes·the·si·ol·o·gy (es·theez"ee·ol'uh·jee) *n.* [*esthesio-* + *-logy*]. The science of the senses and sensations.

es·the·si·om·e·ter, aes·the·si·om·e·ter (es·theez"ee·om'e·tur) *n.* [*esthesio-* + *-meter*]. A two-pronged instrument for measuring tactile sensibility by finding the least distance between two pressure points on the skin which can be perceived as distinct.

es·the·sio·neu·ro·blas·to·ma, aes·the·sio·neu·ro·blas·to·ma (es·theez"ee·o·new"ro·blas·to'muh) *n.* [*esthesio-* + *neuro-* + *blastoma*]. *Obsol.* A neuroblastoma arising in the olfactory apparatus.

es·the·sio·neu·ro·ep·i·the·li·o·ma, aes·the·sio·neu·ro·ep·i·the·li·o·ma (es·theez"ee·o·new"ro·ep"i·theel·ee·o'muh) *n.* [*esthesio-* + *neuroepithelioma*]. *Obsol.* A neuroblastoma arising in the olfactory apparatus.

es·the·sio·neu·ro·ma (es·theez"ee·o·new·ro'muh) *n.* [*enthesio-* + *neuroma*]. A locally invasive tumor of the nasal cavity composed of neural and epithelial elements; metastasis is infrequent.

es·the·sio·phys·i·ol·o·gy, aes·the·sio·phys·i·ol·o·gy (es·theez"ee·o·fiz"ee·ol'uh·jee) *n.* [*esthesio-* + *physiology*]. The physiology of sensation and the sense organs.

es·thet·ic, aes·thet·ic (es·thet'ick) *adj.* [Gk. *aisthētikos,* from *aisthēsis,* sensation, perception]. Pertaining to the senses.

es·thi·om·e·ne (es"thee·om'e·nee) *n.* [F. *esthiomène,* from Gk. *esthiomenos,* decayed]. The chronic ulcerative lesion of the vulva in lymphogranuloma venereum.

Estinyl. A trademark for ethinyl estradiol, an estrogen.

es·ti·val, aes·ti·val (es'ti·vul, es·tye'vul) *adj.* [L. *aestivus,* from *aestas,* summer]. Of or pertaining to the summer.

es·ti·va·tion, aes·ti·va·tion (es"ti·vay'shun) *n.* [L. *aestivare,* to pass the summer]. 1. The adaptation of certain animals to the conditions of summer, or the taking on of certain modifications, which enables them to survive a hot dry summer. 2. The dormant condition of an organism during the summer. Contr. *hibernation.*

es·ti·vo-au·tum·nal, aes·ti·vo-au·tum·nal (es″ti·vo·aw·tum′nul) *adj.* Pertaining to the summer and fall seasons.

estivo-autumnal malaria. FALCIPARUM MALARIA.

Est·lan·der's operation [J. A. *Estlander,* Finnish surgeon, 1831–1881]. 1. Resection of portions of several ribs to produce obliteration of the cavity in the treatment of chronic empyema. 2. Rotation of a flap of lip to fill a defect in the opposing lip.

es·to·late (es′to·late) *n.* Any lauryl sulfate salt of the propionic acid ester of a substance capable of forming such a derivative, as erythromycin.

es·tra·di·ol, oes·tra·di·ol (es·truh·dye′ol) *n.* Estra-1,3,5(10)-triene-3,17-diol, $C_{18}H_{24}O_2$, an estrogenic hormone secreted by the ovary and by the placenta. Two isomers exist: the active isomer 17β-estradiol (once designated α-estradiol) and the inactive isomer 17α-estradiol (once designated β-estradiol). The former is used as an estrogen, commonly as one of its esters: the benzoate, cyclopentylpropionate, dipropionate, undecylate, or valerate. Syn. *dihydrotheelin.*

Estradurin. A trademark for polyestradiol phosphate, a repository form of estradiol.

es·trane (es′trane) *n.* The saturated parent hydrocarbon, $C_{18}H_{30}$, of estrone, estradiol, estratriol, and related estrogenic steroids.

es·tra·zi·nol (es′truh·zi·nol″) *n.* DL-*trans*-3-Methoxy-8-aza-19-nor-17α-pregna-1,3,5-trien-20-yn-17-ol, $C_{20}H_{25}NO_2$, a nitrogen-containing steroidal estrogen; used as the hydrobromide salt.

estriasis. OESTRIASIS.

es·trin (es′trin) *n.* ESTROGEN.

es·tri·ol, oes·tri·ol (es′tree·ole, ·ol, es·trye′ol) *n.* An estrogenic hormone, estra-1,3,5(10)-triene-3,16,17-triol, $C_{18}H_{24}O_3$, which comprises about 90 percent of the estrogen excreted in maternal urine during pregnancy. Since its synthesis then is regulated by enzymes of the placenta and the fetal adrenal gland, the amounts excreted serve as a measure of placental and fetal status, a decline suggesting abnormal function.

Estrobene. A trademark for diethylstilbestrol, an estrogen.

es·tro·fu·rate (es·tro·few′rate) *n.* 21,23-Epoxy-19,24-dinor-17α-chola-1,3,5(10)7,20,22-hexaene-3,17-diol acetate, $C_{24}H_{26}O_4$, an estrogen.

es·tro·gen, oes·tro·gen (es′tro·jin) *n.* [*estrus* + *-gen*]. Any substance possessing the biologic activity of estrus-producing hormones, either occurring naturally or prepared synthetically. —**es·tro·gen·ic, oes·tro·gen·ic** (es″tro·jen′ick) *adj.*

estrogenic hormone. A hormone, found principally in ovaries and also in the placenta, which stimulates the accessory sex structures and the secondary sex characteristics in the female.

es·tro·gen·iza·tion, oes·tro·gen·iza·tion (es″tro·jin·i·zay′shun) *n.* The administration of estrogenic substances.

es·trone, oes·trone (es′trone) *n.* 3-Hydroxyestra-1,3,5(10)-trien-17-one, $C_{18}H_{22}O_2$, an estrogenic hormone present in the ovary, adrenal glands, placenta, and urine. Syn. *theelin, folliculin.*

estrone sulfate. A naturally occurring conjugated form of estrone, in which the hydroxyl group of the latter is esterified with sulfuric acid. The sodium salt of estrone sulfate is soluble in water, and is the principal estrogen in certain commercial products.

estrous cycle. The periodically recurring series of changes in uterus, ovaries, and accessory sexual structures associated with estrus and diestrus in lower mammals.

es·tru·a·tion, oes·tru·a·tion (es″troo·ay′shun) *n.* ESTRUS.

es·trum, oes·trum (es′trum) *n.* ESTRUS.

es·trus, oes·trus (es′trus) *n.* [L. *oestrus,* gadfly, frenzy, from Gk. *oistros*]. 1. Sexual desire in the lower animals; the mating period of animals, especially of the female. Compare *heat, rut.* 2. The whole sequence of changes in the uterine mucosa of mammals, corresponding to the various phases of ovarian activity. —**estrous, oestrous, es·tru·al, oes·tru·al** (es′troo·ul) *adj.*

es·tu·ar·i·um (es″tew·err′ee·um) *n.* [L. *aestuarium,* from *aestus,* swell of the sea, boiling, heat]. VAPOR BATH.

es·y·late (es′i·late) *n.* Any salt or ester of ethanesulfonic acid, $CH_3CH_2SO_3H$; an ethanesulfonate.

et·a·fed·rine (et″uh·fed′reen, ·rin) *n.* *N*-Ethylephedrine, $C_{12}H_{19}NO$, a sympathomimetic amine resembling ephedrine; used as the hydrochloride salt.

état cri·blé (ay·tah′ kree·blay′) [F.]. STATUS CRIBOSUS.

état fi·breux (fee·brœh′) [F.]. STATUS FIBROSUS.

état la·cu·naire (la·kew·nair′) [F.]. LACUNAR STATE.

état ma·me·lon·né (mam″e·lon·ay′) [F., mammilated state]. MÉNÉTRIER'S DISEASE.

état mar·bré (mahr·bray′) [F.]. STATUS MARMORATUS.

eta·zo·late (e·tay′zo·late) *n.* Ethyl 1-ethyl-4-(isopropylidenehydrazino)-1*H*-pyrazolo[3,4-*b*]pyridine-5-carboxylate, $C_{14}H_{19}N_5O_2$, a tranquilizer usually used as the hydrochloride salt.

ete·ro·barb (e·teer′o·bahrb) *n.* 5-Ethyl-1,3-bis(methoxymethyl)-5-phenylbarbituric acid, $C_{16}H_{20}N_2O_5$, an anticonvulsant.

eth·a·cry·nic acid (eth″uh·krye′nick, ·krin′ick). [2,3-Dichloro-4-(2-methylenebutyryl)phenoxy]acetic acid, $C_{13}H_{12}Cl_2O_4$, a diuretic drug.

etham·bu·tol (e·tham′bew·tol) *n.* *d*-2,2′-(Ethylenediimino)di(1-butanol), $C_{10}H_{24}N_2O_2$, a tuberculostatic drug; used as the dihydrochloride salt.

Ethamide. A trademark for ethoxzolamide, a diuretic.

etham·i·van (e·tham′i·van) *n.* *N,N*-Diethylvanillamide, $C_{12}H_{17}NO_3$, a respiratory stimulant.

etham·syl·ate (e·tham′zil·ate) *n.* 2,5-Dihydroxybenzenesulfonic acid compound with diethylamine, $C_6H_6O_5S.C_4H_{11}N$, a hemostatic agent.

eth·a·nal (eth′uh·nal) *n.* ACETALDEHYDE.

eth·ane (eth′ane) *n.* A saturated, gaseous hydrocarbon, C_2H_6, a constituent of natural gas. Syn. *methylmethane.*

eth·a·no·ic acid (eth″uh·no′ick). ACETIC ACID.

eth·a·nol (eth′uh·nol) *n.* ETHYL ALCOHOL.

eth·a·nol·amine (eth″uh·nol′uh·meen) *n.* 2-Aminoethanol, $HOCH_2CH_2NH_2$, a colorless liquid, miscible with water. In animals it may be formed by reduction of glycine or decarboxylation of serine; when methylated by methionine it forms choline. It is the basic component of certain cephalins. Syn. *cholamine, monoethanolamine.*

eth·chlor·vy·nol (eth″klor·vye′nol) *n.* 1-Chloro-3-ethyl-1-penten-4-yn-3-ol, C_7H_9ClO, a sedative-hypnotic with short duration of action.

eth·ene (eth′een) *n.* ETHYLENE.

ether, ae·ther (ee′thur) *n.* [Gk. *aithēr*]. 1. An all-pervading and permeating medium, formerly believed to exist and to transmit light and similar energy. 2. A compound of the general formula ROR, formed hypothetically from H_2O by the substitution of two hydrocarbon radicals for the H. 3. Ethyl ether, $(C_2H_5)_2O$; a thin, colorless, volatile, and highly inflammable liquid. The ether of the U.S.P. contains 96 to 98% by weight of $(C_2H_5)_2O$, the remainder consisting of alcohol and water. Its chief use is as an anesthetic. Syn. *ethyl oxide, sulfuric ether, diethyl ether, diethyl oxide.* —**ethe·re·al, ae·the·re·al** (ee·theer′ee·ul) *adj.*

ether cone. A simple cone-shaped frame, covered with gauze or cloth, once used widely in the administration of ether anesthesia.

ether drunkenness. Inebriation from drinking ether.

ethereal oil. A volatile liquid consisting of equal volumes of ether and a so-called heavy oil of wine made up of ethyl esters of sulfuric acid; has been used for a supposed carminative effect.

ether·ide (ee'thur·ide) *n.* An acid halide representing an organic acid in which the carboxyl OH group is replaced by halogen.

ether·i·fi·ca·tion (ee·therr''i·fi·kay'shun) *n.* The formation of an ether from an alcohol. —**ether·i·fy** (ee·therr'i·figh) *v.*

ether·iza·tion (ee''thur·i·zay'shun) *n.* The administration of ether to produce anesthesia. —**ether·ize** (ee'thur·ize) *v.*

ether spirit. A solution containing 32.5% by volume of ethyl oxide in alcohol; once popular as a carminative. Syn. *Hoffmann's drops.*

eth·ics (eth'icks) *n.* [Gk. *ethikos,* from *ethos,* custom, habit]. A system of moral principles. See also *medical ethics.*

eth·i·nam·ate (eth''i·nam'ate) *n.* 1-Ethynylcyclohexyl carbamate, $C_9H_{13}NO_2$, a central depressant drug of short duration of action; used as a hypnotic.

eth·ine (eth'ine) *n.* ACETYLENE.

ethinyl. ETHYNYL.

ethinyl estradiol. 17-Ethynylestradiol, $C_{20}H_{24}O_2$, an orally effective estrogen.

eth·io·dized oil (eth·eye'uh·dize'd). The iodinated ethyl ester of the fatty acids from poppyseed oil, containing about 37% organically combined iodine; used as a contrast medium.

ethiodized oil I 131. A radioactive iodine addition product of the ethyl ester of the fatty acids of poppyseed oil; used as an antineoplastic agent.

Ethiodol. A trademark for ethiodized oil.

ethi·on·a·mide (e·thigh'on·uh·mide) *n.* 2-Ethylthioisonicotinamide, $C_8H_{10}N_2S$, a tuberculostatic drug.

ethi·o·nine (e·thigh'o·neen, ·nin) *n.* 2-Amino-4-(ethylthio)butyric acid, $C_6H_{13}NO_2S$, the ethyl homologue of methionine; it inhibits growth of experimental animals, presumably by interfering with the metabolism of methionine.

ethis·ter·one (e·thiss'tur·ohn) *n.* 17α-Ethynyltestosterone or anhydrohydroxyprogesterone, $C_{21}H_{28}O_2$, a synthetic progestational steroid.

ethmo-. A combining form meaning *ethmoid, ethmoidal.*

eth·mo·ceph·a·lus (eth''mo·sef'uh·lus) *n.,* pl. **ethmocepha·li** (·lye) [*ethmo-* + *-cephalus*]. A variety of cebocephalus with a rudimentary nose similar to a proboscis, which terminates anteriorly in two imperfect nostrils or in a single opening.

eth·mo·fron·tal (eth''mo·frun'tul) *adj.* Pertaining to the ethmoid and frontal bones.

ethmofrontal suture. The union between the ethmoid and frontal bones.

eth·moid (eth'moid) *n. & adj.* [Gk. *ēthmoeidēs,* perforated, from *ēthmos,* strainer, sieve]. 1. ETHMOID BONE. 2. Pertaining to the ethmoid bone or related structures. —**eth·moi·dal** (eth·moy'dul) *adj.*

ethmoidal or **ethmoid air cells.** ETHMOIDAL CELLS. NA *cellulae ethmoidales.* See also Plate 12.

ethmoidal cells. The small air spaces, lined with mucous membrane and separated by thin bony partitions, which honeycomb the lateral portions of the ethmoid bone, forming the two ethmoid labyrinths, with the anterior cells (NA *cellulae anteriores*) and middle cells (NA *cellulae mediae*) communicating with the middle nasal meatus and the posterior cells (NA *cellulae posteriores*) with the superior nasal meatus. NA *cellulae ethmoidales.* See also *ethmoid sinus* and Plate 12.

ethmoid anfractuosity. *Obsol.* ETHMOIDAL CELL.

ethmoid antrum. ETHMOID SINUS.

ethmoid bone. A delicate bone in the anterior portion of the base of the skull, forming the medial wall of each orbit and part of the lateral wall of each nasal cavity. NA *os ethmoidale.* See also *ethmoidal cells,* Plate 1, and Table of Bones in the Appendix.

ethmoid canal. Ethmoid foramen. See *anterior ethmoid foramen, posterior ethmoid foramen.*

ethmoid cells. ETHMOIDAL CELLS.

ethmoid crest. 1. An oblique ridge on the medial surface of the frontal process of the maxilla. Its posterior end articulates with the middle nasal concha; its anterior part is known as the agger nasi. NA *crista ethmoidalis maxillae.* 2. The superior ridge of the medial surface of the palatine bone, articulating with the middle nasal concha. NA *crista ethmoidalis ossis palatini.*

eth·moid·ec·to·my (eth''moy·deck'tuh·mee) *n.* [*ethmoid* + *-ectomy*]. Removal of the ethmoid sinuses or part of the ethmoid bone.

ethmoid foramen. See *anterior ethmoid foramen, posterior ethmoid foramen.* NA *foramina ethmoidalia.*

ethmoid infundibulum. A crescentic groove connecting the anterior ethmoid cells with the middle nasal meatus. NA *infundibulum ethmoidale.*

eth·moid·itis (eth''moy·dye'tis) *n.* [*ethmoid* + *-itis*]. Inflammation of the ethmoid bone or of the ethmoid sinuses.

ethmoid labyrinth. A labyrinth formed by the air cells in the lateral portions of the ethmoid bone. NA *labyrinthus ethmoidalis.* See also *ethmoidal cells.*

ethmoid notch. The gap between the two orbital plates of the frontal bone, filled in the articulated skull by the cribriform plate of the ethmoid. NA *incisura ethmoidalis.*

eth·moid·ot·o·my (eth''moy·dot'uh·mee) *n.* [*ethmoid* + *-tomy*]. Incision of an ethmoid sinus.

ethmoid process. One of the projections from the superior border of the inferior nasal concha. NA *processus ethmoidalis.*

ethmoid sinus. Either of the paranasal sinuses in the ethmoid bone, each occupying one of the two lateral portions of the bone and consisting of several small air-filled spaces, the ethmoidal cells. NA *sinus ethmoidalis.*

ethmoid spine. The upper end of the sphenoid crest; it articulates with the posterior margin of the cribriform plate of the ethmoid.

eth·mo·lac·ri·mal (eth''mo·lack'ri·mul) *adj.* Pertaining to the ethmoid and lacrimal bones.

ethmoid spine. The upper end of the sphenoid crest; it articulates with the posterior margin of the cribriform plate of the ethmoid.

ethmolacrimal suture. The union between the lacrimal and ethmoid bones.

eth·mo·max·il·lary (eth''mo·mack'si·lerr''ee) *adj.* Pertaining to the ethmoid and the maxillary bone.

eth·mo·na·sal (eth''mo·nay'zul) *adj.* Pertaining to the ethmoid and the nasal bones.

eth·mo·sphe·noid (eth''mo·sfee'noid) *adj.* Pertaining to the ethmoid and the sphenoid bones.

ethmosphenoid suture. SPHENOETHMOID SUTURE.

eth·mo·tur·bi·nal (eth''mo·tur'bi·nul) *adj.* Pertaining to the turbinal portions of the ethmoid bone, forming what are known as the superior and middle turbinates.

eth·nic (eth'nick) *adj.* [Gk. *ethnikos,* national]. Pertaining to races and peoples, and to their traits and customs.

eth·nog·ra·phy (eth·nog'ruh·fee) *n.* [Gk. *ethnos,* nation, people, + *-graphy*]. 1. Descriptive ethnology; the anthropological description of peoples and societies. 2. An anthropological description of a particular community or society. —**eth·no·graph·ic** (eth''no·graf'ick), **ethnograph·i·cal** (·i·kul) *adj.*

eth·nol·o·gy (eth·nol'uh·jee) *n.* [Gk. *ethnos,* nation, people, + *-logy*]. The anthropological study of peoples and societies. —**eth·no·log·ic** (eth''nuh·loj'ick), **ethnolog·i·cal** (·i·kul) *adj.*

etho·caine (eth'o·kane) *n. British.* PROCAINE.

Ethocel. Trademark for ethyl cellulose.

eth·o·hep·ta·zine (eth''o·hep'tuh·zeen) *n.* Ethyl hexahydro-1-methyl-4-phenyl-1*H*-azepine-4-carboxylate, $C_{16}H_{23}NO_2$, an analgesic drug used as the citrate salt.

etho·hexa·di·ol (eth''o·heck''suh·dye'ol) *n.* 2-Ethyl-1,3-hexanediol, $C_8H_{18}O_2$, a colorless, oily liquid; used as an insect repellent and toxicant. Syn. *Rutgers 612.*

ethol·o·gy (e·thol'uh·jee) *n.* [Gk. *ēthologia,* art of depicting character]. 1. *In psychology* and *zoology,* the study of innate behavior patterns; particularly, the study of animal behavior. 2. The empirical study of human character. 3. The study of social behavior, as manners and mores. 4. The study of ethics.

eth·o·nam (eth'o·nam) *n.* Ethyl 1-(1,2,3,4-tetrahydro-1-naphthyl)imidazole-5-carboxylate, $C_{16}H_{18}N_2O_2$, a fungicide; used as the nitrate salt.

etho·pro·pa·zine (eth"o·pro'puh·zeen) *n.* 10-(2-Diethylaminopropyl)phenothiazine, $C_{19}H_{24}N_2S$, used for the treatment of parkinsonism; administered as the hydrochloride salt. Syn. *profenamine.*

etho·sux·i·mide (eth"o·suck'si·mide) *n.* 2-Ethyl-2-methylsuccinimide, $C_7H_{11}NO_2$, an anticonvulsant drug.

eth·o·to·in (eth"o·to'in, eth'o·toin) *n.* 3-Ethyl-5-phenylhydantoin, $C_{11}H_{12}N_2O_2$, an anticonvulsant used in the management of generalized epilepsy.

eth·ox·a·zene (e·thock'suh·zeen) *n.* 4-(*p*-Ethoxyphenylazo)-*m*-phenylenediamine, $C_{14}H_{16}N_4O$, an azo dye having local anesthetic action on urinary tract mucosa and used to relieve pain in chronic infections of the tract; administered as the hydrochloride salt.

eth·oxy (eth·ock'see) *n.* The univalent radical $C_2H_5O—$.

eth·ox·zol·a·mide (eth"ocks·zo'luh·mide) *n.* 6-Ethoxy-2-benzothiazolesulfonamide, $C_9H_{10}N_2O_3S_2$, a diuretic chemically related to acetazolamide but about twice as active.

ethy·benz·tro·pine (eth"i·benz·tro'peen) *n.* 3-(Diphenylmethoxy)-8-ethylnortropane, $C_{22}H_{27}NO$, an anticholinergic compound.

eth·yl (eth'il) *n.* [*eth*er + *-yl*]. The univalent radical $C_2H_5—$.

ethyl acetate. A colorless, pleasantly odorous liquid, $CH_3COOC_2H_5$, used chiefly as a solvent and in artificial fruit essences. Syn. *acetic ether.*

ethyl acetoacetate. ACETOACETIC ESTER.

ethyl alcohol. C_2H_5OH, a colorless, volatile liquid which, as the basis of alcoholic beverages, acts as a central nervous system depressant valued for its euphoric effect but which in immoderate or prolonged use leads to acute or chronic alcoholism. It is used as a pharmaceutical solvent and in medicine as a sedative, for its calorific value in the debilitated, and for its cutaneous vasodilative effect. On the skin, it is antiseptic and astringent. Syn. *ethanol.*

ethyl aminobenzoate. Ethyl *p*-aminobenzoate, $H_2NC_6H_4COOC_2H_5$, a white crystalline powder, slightly soluble in water; a local anesthetic. Syn. *benzocaine.*

eth·yl·ate (eth'i·late) *n.* A compound of ethyl alcohol in which the H of the hydroxyl is replaced by a base.

eth·yl·a·tion (eth"i·lay'shun) *n.* The introduction of an ethyl group into a compound.

ethyl biscoumacetate. 3,3'-Carboxymethylene bis(4-hydroxycoumarin) ethyl ester, $C_{22}H_{16}O_8$, a white, crystalline powder practically insoluble in water; an anticoagulant.

ethyl bromide. A rapid and transient anesthetic, C_2H_5Br, more dangerous than ethyl chloride.

ethyl carbamate. URETHAN (1).

ethyl cellulose. The ethyl ether of cellulose; has been used as a dispersing agent and to increase viscosity in aqueous systems.

ethyl chaulmoograte. The ethyl esters of the mixed acids of chaulmoogra oil, chiefly chaulmoogric and hydnocarpic; has been used in leprosy.

ethyl chloride. A colorless, mobile, very volatile liquid, CH_3CH_2Cl. It acts as a local anesthetic of short duration through the superficial freezing produced by rapid vaporization from the skin. Occasionally used by inhalation as a rapid and fleeting general anesthetic, comparable to nitrous oxide but somewhat more dangerous.

ethyl diacetate. ACETOACETIC ESTER.

ethyl di·bu·nate (dye·bew'nate). Ethyl 3,6-di-*tert*-butyl-1-naphthalenesulfonate, $C_{20}H_{28}O_3S$, an antitussive compound.

eth·yl·ene (eth'i·leen) *n.* A colorless gas, $CH_2{=}CH_2$, used as an inhalation anesthetic. Syn. *ethene, olefiant gas.*

eth·yl·ene·di·amine (eth"i·leen·dye'uh·meen, ·min) *n.* 1,2-Diaminoethane, $H_2NCH_2CH_2NH_2$, a colorless strongly alkaline liquid of ammoniacal odor; used as a solvent and to increase the solubility of certain medicinal substances. See also *aminophylline.*

ethylenediamine dihydrochloride. A urine acidifier.

eth·yl·ene·di·amine·tet·ra·ace·tic acid (eth"il·een·dye"uh·meen·tet"ruh·uh·see'tick). EDETIC ACID.

ethylene glycol. 1,2-Ethanediol, $HOCH_2CH_2OH$, a slightly viscous liquid, miscible with water. It has many industrial uses, and is used as a solvent and humectant.

ethylene oxide. $(CH_2)_2O$. A colorless gas used as a fumigant, insecticide, and sterilizing agent.

ethylene series. A group of hydrocarbons of the general formula, C_nH_{2n}, having one double bond. Syn. *ethene series, alkene series.*

eth·yl·e·nic (eth"i·lee'nick) *adj.* Pertaining to, derived from, or like ethylene, especially in having a double bond.

ethyl eosin. The potassium or sodium salt of the ethyl ester of tetrabromofluorescein; the ethyl ester of eosin Y; a moderately coarse, red powder, used as a histologic stain. Syn. *eosin S.*

eth·yl·ephed·rine (eth"il·e·fed'rin) *n.* *l-N*-Ethylephedrine or *l*-1-phenyl-2-methylethylaminopropan-1-ol, $C_{12}H_{19}NO$, a compound having pharmacologic action similar to *l*-ephedrine, except that its stimulating effect on the central nervous system is slight; used as the hydrochloride salt.

eth·yl·es·tren·ol (eth"il·es'tre·nol) *n.* 19-Nor-17α-pregn-4-en-17-ol, $C_{20}H_{32}O$, an anabolic steroid.

ethyl ether. ETHER (3).

ethyl formate. $HCOOC_2H_5$. A colorless liquid of aromatic odor used as a flavor, fumigant, larvicide, and in organic syntheses.

eth·yl·hy·dro·cu·pre·ine (eth"il·high"dro·kew'pree·een, ·in) *n.* A synthetic derivative, $C_{21}H_{28}N_2O_2$, of cupreine; it is also chemically related to quinine. Has been used internally, as the base, in the treatment of pneumonia and locally, as the hydrochloride, in the treatment of pneumococcal infections of the eye.

eth·yl·i·dene (eth'il·i·deen) *n.* The bivalent hydrocarbon radical $CH_3CH{=}$.

ethyl iodide. CH_3CH_2I. A colorless liquid of ethereal odor; has been used by inhalation in bronchial asthma.

ethyl iodophenylundecylate. IOPHENDYLATE INJECTION.

eth·yl·mor·phine (eth"il·mor'feen, ·fin) *n.* An ethyl ether of morphine; $C_{19}H_{23}NO_3$. The hydrochloride is used topically as a lymphagogue in inflammatory disease of the eye, in rhinitis, and in otitis media, and internally as a narcotic analgesic and antitussive.

ethyl nitrite. C_2H_5ONO. A colorless or pale yellow, exceedingly volatile, liquid of pleasant ethereal odor; slightly soluble in water, miscible with alcohol. Syn. *nitrous ether.*

ethyl nitrite spirit. An alcoholic solution containing 3.5 to 4.5% ethyl nitrite. A popular diaphoretic in mild fevers. Syn. *spirit of nitrous ether, sweet spirit of niter.*

eth·yl·nor·adren·a·line (eth"il·nor"uh·dren'uh·lin) *n.* ETHYLNOREPINEPHRINE.

eth·yl·nor·epi·neph·rine (eth"il·nor·ep"i·nef'reen) *n.* 2-Amino-1-(3,4-dihydroxyphenyl)butan-1-ol, $C_{10}H_{15}NO_3$, a bronchodilator usually used as the hydrochloride salt.

ethyl oxide. ETHER (3).

eth·yl·para·ben (eth"il·păr'uh·ben) *n.* Ethyl *p*-hydroxybenzoate, $C_9H_{10}O_3$, an antimicrobial used to preserve many pharmaceutical dosage forms.

eth·yl·stib·a·mine (eth"il·stib'uh·meen, ·min) *n.* A pentavalent antimony complex consisting principally of the tetramer of *p*-aminobenzenestibonic acid, the dimer of *p*-acetylaminobenzenestibonic acid, antimony pentoxide (Sb_2O_5), and diethylamine; a light yellow to yellow-brown powder, soluble in water; formerly used in the treatment of kala-azar and other forms of leishmaniasis, and also filariasis.

ethyl vanillate. Ethyl 4-hydroxy-3-methoxybenzoate, $CH_3OC_6H_3(OH)COOC_2H_5$, the ethyl ester of vanillic acid. It is a fungicide and has been found useful in the treatment of histoplasmosis, being administered in 40% solution in olive oil by gavage. Compare *ethyl vanillin.*

ethyl vanillin. 3-Ethoxy-4-hydroxybenzaldehyde, $CHOC_6H_3(OC_2H_5)OH$, occurring as white or slightly yellowish crystals, sparingly soluble in water. It has a finer and more intense vanilla odor and taste than has vanillin, and is used as a flavor. Compare *ethyl vanillate.*

ethyl violet. A basic triarylmethane dye, hexaethylpararosaniline hydrochloride, used as a basic dye and in Bowie's neutral stain.

eth·yne (eth'ine) *n.* ACETYLENE.

ethy·ner·one (e·thigh'nur·ohn) *n.* 21-Chloro-17-hydroxy-19-nor-17α-pregna-4,9-dien-20-yn-3-one, $C_{20}H_{23}ClO_2$, a progestational steroid.

ethy·no·di·ol (e·thigh'no·dye''ol) *n.* 19-Nor-17α-pregn-4-en-20-yne-3β,17-diol, $C_{20}H_{28}O_2$, a progestin; used as the diacetate ester.

ethy·nyl, ethi·nyl (e·thigh'nil) *n.* The radical HC≡C—.

ethy·nyl·es·tra·di·ol (e·thigh''nil·es·truh·dye'ol) *n.* ETHINYL ESTRADIOL.

etid·o·caine (e·tid'o·kane) *n.* (±)-2-(Ethylpropylamino)-2',6'-butyroxylidide, $C_{17}H_{28}N_2O$, a local anesthetic also used as the hydrochloride salt.

et·i·dro·nic acid (et''i·dro'nick). (1-Hydroxyethylidene)bi-phosphonic acid, $C_2H_8O_7P_2$, a bone calcium regulator.

étin·ce·lage (ay·tan·se·lahzh') *n.* [F., from *étincelle,* spark, from L. *scintilla*]. FULGURATION.

etio-, aetio- [Gk. *aitia,* cause, responsibility]. A combining form meaning (a) *cause;* (b) *formed by chemical degradation of a compound.*

etio·cho·lan·o·lone (ee''tee·o·ko·lan'o·lone) *n.* Etiocholane-3(α)-ol-17-one, $C_{19}H_{30}O_2$, an isomer of androsterone found in urine.

etiocholanolone fever. Recurrent fever, abdominal pain, arthralgia, and leukocytosis, associated with the presence of unconjugated etiocholanolone in the plasma and elevated urinary etiocholanolone levels. It may be associated with a variety of underlying disease states, including a condition resembling the adrenogenital syndrome, familial Mediterranean fever, and such conditions as malignant lymphoma.

eti·o·la·tion (ee''tee·o·lay'shun) *n.* [F. *étioler,* to etiolate, from *éteule,* stubble]. Pallor caused by the exclusion of light.

eti·ol·o·gy, ae·ti·ol·o·gy (ee''tee·ol'uh·jee) *n.* [Gk. *aitiologia,* investigating causes]. 1. The science or study of the causes of disease, both direct and predisposing, and the mode of their operation. 2. PATHOGENESIS. **—eti·o·log·ic** (·o·loj'ick) *adj.*

etio·patho·gen·e·sis, aetio·patho·gen·e·sis (ee''tee·o·path''o·jen'e·sis) *n.* [*etio-* + *pathogenesis*]. The cause and course of development of a disease or lesion.

etio·por·phy·rin, ae·tio·por·phy·rin (ee''tee·o·por'fi·rin) *n.* [*etio-* + *porphyrin*]. Any of the four isomeric, metal-free porphyrins containing four methyl and four ethyl groups, in different positions, distinguished as etioporphyrins I, II, III, and IV. The particular spatial arrangements of the etioporphyrins provide the basis for classification of naturally occurring porphyrins.

"e" to "a" sign. A sign of pulmonary consolidation or pleural effusion, in which all spoken vowels, including "e", are heard through the stethoscope as "ah." Syn. *Shibley's sign.* See also *egophony.*

eto·do·lic acid (ee''to·do'lick). 1,8-Diethyl-1,3,4,9-tetrahydropyrano[3,4-*b*]indole-1-acetic acid, $C_{17}H_{21}NO_3$, an anti-inflammatory.

eto·for·min (et''o·for'min) *n.* 1-Butyl-2-ethylbiguanide, $C_8H_{19}N_5$, an antidiabetic, used as the hydrochloride salt.

etom·i·date (e·tom'i·date) *n.* (+)-Ethyl 1-(α-methylbenyl)imidazole-5-carboxylate, $C_{14}H_{16}N_2O_2$, a hypnotic.

etox·a·drol (e·tock'suh·drole) *n.* (+)-2-(2-Ethyl-2-phenyl-1,3-dioxolan-4-yl)piperidine, $C_{16}H_{23}NO_2$, an anesthetic used as the hydrochloride salt.

et·o·zo·lin (et''o·zo'lin) *n.* Ethyl [3-methyl-4-oxo-5-(1-piperidinyl)-2-thiazolidinylidene]acetic acid, $C_{13}H_{20}N_2O_3S$, a diuretic.

Etrenol. A trademark for hycanthone mesylate, an antischistosomal.

etryp·ta·mine (e·trip'tuh·meen) *n.* Ethyltryptamine or (2-aminobutyl)indole, $C_{12}H_{16}N_2$, a monoamine oxidase inhibitor that has been used as a central stimulant drug, but is no longer available since cases of agranulocytosis following its administration have been reported.

Eu Symbol for europium.

eu- [Gk. *eus,* good]. A combining form meaning (a) *good, well, easily;* (b) *normal, true, typical;* (c) *improved derivative of a substance.*

euaesthesia. EUESTHESIA.

Eu·bac·te·ri·a·les (yoo''back·teer''ee·ay'leez) *n. pl.* An order of bacteria, class Schizomycetes, including forms least differentiated and least specialized; the true bacteria.

eu·bac·te·ri·um (yoo''back·teer'ee·um) *n.,* pl. **eubacte·ria** (·ee·uh) [*eu-* + *bacterium*]. A member of the order Eubacteriales.

eu·caine (yoo'kane) *n.* α-4-Benzoyloxy-2,2,6-trimethylpiperidine, $C_{15}H_{21}NO_2$, a local anesthetic introduced early as a substitute for cocaine but rarely used today. Syn. *betaeucaine.*

eu·ca·lyp·tene (yoo''kuh·lip'teen) *n.* A terpene, $C_{10}H_{16}$, derived from eucalyptol.

eu·ca·lyp·tol (yoo''kuh·lip'tol) *n.* Cineol, $C_{10}H_{18}O$, the chief constituent of the volatile oils of eucalyptus and cajeput; a mild local irritant; used in bronchitis and coryza, and formerly as a vermifuge and antimalarial.

eu·ca·lyp·tus (yoo''kuh·lip'tus) *n.* [*eu-* + Gk. *kalyptos,* covered]. The leaf of *Eucalyptus globulus,* formerly used medicinally.

eucalyptus gum. The dried gummy exudate from *Eucalyptus camaldulensis* containing kinotannic acid; formerly used as an astringent.

eucalyptus oil. The volatile oil from the leaves of *Eucalyptus globulus* or other species; contains over 70% eucalyptol. Has been used as a local antiseptic and stimulating expectorant.

eucaryote. EUKARYOTE.

euc·at·ro·pine (yook·at'ro·peen, ·pin) *n.* 4-Hydroxy-1,2,2,6-tetramethylpiperidine mandelate, $C_{17}H_{25}NO_3$, used as the hydrochloride salt as a mydriatic.

eu·chlor·hy·dria (yoo''klor·high'dree·uh) *n.* [*eu-* + *chlorhydria*]. The presence of a normal amount of hydrochloric acid in the gastric juice.

eu·chol·ia (yoo·kol'ee·uh, ·ko'lee·uh) *n.* [*eu-* + *chol-* + *-ia*]. Normal condition of the bile.

eu·chro·ma·tin (yoo·kro'muh·tin) *n.* [*eu-* + *chromatin*]. 1. The part of the chromatin which in interphase is dispersed and not readily stainable, and is thought to be genetically and metabolically active. Contr. *basichromatin.* 2. The substance of the autosomes (euchromosomes) in contrast to the substance of heterochromosomes. Contr. *heterochromatin.* **—eu·chro·mat·ic** (yoo''kro·mat'ick) *adj.*

eu·chro·ma·top·sia (yoo·kro''muh·top'see·uh) *n.* [*eu-* + *chromat-* + *-opsia*]. Ability to recognize colors correctly; normal color vision.

eu·chro·mo·some (yoo·kro'muh·sohm) *n.* [*eu-* + *chromosome*]. AUTOSOME.

eu·co·dal (yoo'ko·dal) *n.* A trade name for oxycodone hydrochloride, a narcotic analgesic.

eu·cor·ti·cal·ism (yoo·kor'ti·kul·iz·um) *n.* EUCORTISM.

eu·cor·tism (yoo·kor'tiz·um) *n.* [*eu-* + *cortex* + *-ism*]. Normal adrenal cortical function.

Eucupin. Trademark for euprocin, a local anesthetic used as the dihydrochloride salt.

eu·di·om·e·ter (yoo″dee·om′e·tur) *n.* [Gk. *eudia*, fair weather, + *-meter*]. An instrument for the analysis and volumetric measure of gases. —**eudi·o·met·ric** (·o·met′rick) *adj.*; **eudi·ome·try** (·tree) *n.*

eudiometric analysis. GASOMETRIC ANALYSIS.

eu·es·the·sia, eu·aes·the·sia (yoo″es·theez′ee·uh) *n.* [Gk. *euaisthēsia*]. The sense of well-being; vigor and normal condition of the senses.

Euflavine. A trademark for acriflavine, a local antiseptic.

Eu·ge·nia (yoo·jeen′yuh) *n.* [Prince *Eugene* of Savoy, 1663-1736]. A genus of trees and shrubs of the Myrtaceae, mostly tropical. The species *Eugenia caryophyllata* yields cloves.

eu·gen·ic (yoo·jen′ick) *adj.* 1. Of or pertaining to eugenics. 2. Beneficial to the hereditary constitution of a population. Contr. *dysgenic.*

eu·gen·ics (yoo·jen′icks) *n.* [Gk. *eugenēs*, wellborn]. The applied science concerned with improving the genetic constitution of populations, and specifically, of human populations. Positive eugenics involves selection for desirable types; negative eugenics involves selection against undesirable types.

eugenic sterilization law. Legislation providing for the sterilization of persons with certain inheritable mental disorders and deficiencies, who have been committed to mental institutions, and of certain criminals.

eu·ge·nol (yoo′je·nol) *n.* 4-Allyl-2-methoxyphenol, $C_{10}H_{12}O_2$, a colorless or pale yellow liquid having a clove odor and spicy, pungent taste; obtained from clove oil and other sources. Used in dentistry as a local anesthetic and disinfectant in root canals; in ointments, as an anesthetic and antiseptic.

eu·glob·u·lin (yoo·glob′yoo·lin) *n.* [*eu-* + *globulin*]. True globulin. A globulin fraction soluble in distilled water and dilute salt solutions.

eu·gnath·ic (yoo·nath′ick, ·nay′thick) *adj.* [*eu-* + *gnathic*]. Pertaining to jaws that are well developed and in proper relation to each other.

eu·gon·ic (yoo·gon′ick) *adj.* [Gk. *eugonos*, productive, from *gonos*, seed, procreation]. Growing luxuriantly; used to describe bacterial cultures.

eu·kary·ote, eu·cary·ote (yoo·kăr′ee·ote) *n.* [*eu-* + Gk. *karyon*, nut, kernel]. An organism with a true nucleus, in contrast to bacteria and viruses. Contr. *prokaryote.* —**eu·kary·otic** (yoo″kăr″ee·ot′ick) *adj.*

eu·ker·a·tin (yoo·kerr′uh·tin) *n.* [*eu-* + *keratin*]. One of the two main groups of keratins. Eukeratins are insoluble in water, dilute alkali, and acids; are not digested by common proteolytic enzymes; and contain histidine, lysine, and arginine in the ratio of approximately 1:4:12.

eu·ki·ne·sia (yoo″ki·nee′shuh, ·zee·uh) *n.* [*eu-* + *-kinesia*]. Normal power of movement.

eu·lam·i·nate (yoo·lam′i·nate) *adj.* [*eu-* + *laminate*]. Having the typical number and kinds of layers.

eulaminate cortex. HOMOTYPICAL CORTEX.

Eu·len·burg's disease (oy′l^e^n·boork) [A. *Eulenburg*, German physician, 1840-1917]. PARAMYOTONIA CONGENITA.

eu·mor·phic (yoo·mor′fick) *adj.* [*eu-* + *-morphic*]. Well and normally formed; not misshapen.

Eu·my·ce·tes (yoo″migh·see′teez) *n. pl.* [*eu-* + *mycetes*]. A class of thallophytes containing all the true fungi.

Eumydrin. Trademark for atropine methylnitrate.

eu·noia (yoo·noy′uh) *n.* [Gk., goodwill, from *eu-* + *noos*, mind]. Soundness of mind and will.

eu·nuch (yoo′nuck) *n.* [Gk. *eunouchos*, eunuch, harem attendent; lit. bed watcher, from *eunē*, bed]. A man who has undergone complete loss of testicular function from castration, inflammation, or mechanical injury. If this occurs before puberty, it is associated with failure of development of secondary sex characters and typical changes in skeletal maturation, with increased height and span and disproportionate length of the lower extremities to trunk. —**eu·nuch·ism** (·iz·um) *n.*

eu·nuch·oid (yoo′nuh·koid) *adj.* [Gk. *eunouchoeidēs*]. Characteristic of, or manifesting, eunuchoidism.

eu·nuch·oid·ism (yoo′nuh·koy·diz·um) *n.* [*eunuchoid* + *-ism*]. Deficiency or absence of testicular secretion causing deficient sexual development with persistence of prepuberal characteristics. Compare *agonadism.*

eu·on·y·mus (yoo·on′i·mus) *n.* [Gk. *euōnymos*, of good name]. The dried bark of *Euonymus atropurpureus;* formerly used as a cathartic.

eu·pa·ral (yoo′pa·ral) *n.* A mixture of gum sandarac, eucalyptol, paraldehyde, phenyl salicylate, and camphor; used as a mounting medium for stained sections.

Eu·pa·to·ri·um (yoo″puh·to′ree·um) *n.* [Gk. *eupatorion*, agrimony]. A genus of composite-flowered plants. The leaves and flowering tops of *Eupatorium perfoliatum*, the thoroughwort or boneset, have been used commonly as a bitter tonic, diaphoretic, and feeble emetic.

eu·phen·ics (yoo·fen′icks) *n.* The science of producing a satisfactory phenotype through induction or repression of DNA-RNA synthesis.

eu·pho·nia (yoo·fo′nee·uh) *n.* [Gk. *euphōnia*, from *eu-* + *phōnē*, voice]. A normal, harmonious sound of the voice.

Eu·phor·bia (yoo·for′bee·yuh) *n.* [L. *euphorbea*, from *Euphorbus*, 1st century physician]. A genus of plants of the Euphorbiaceae. *Euphorbia corollata* and *E. ipecacuanhae*, the American species, were formerly employed in medicine because of their emetic and cathartic properties. *E. pilulifera* of South America and Australia is used in asthma and bronchitis. *E. resinifera* of Africa produces euphorbium.

Eu·phor·bi·a·ce·ae (yoo·for″bee·ay′see·ee) *n. pl.* A plant family of herbs, shrubs, or trees.

eu·phor·bi·um (yoo·for′bee·um) *n.* The dried resinous latex obtained from *Euphorbia resinifera.* It is strongly purgative and vesicant; sometimes employed in veterinary medicine.

eu·pho·ria (yoo·fo′ree·uh) *n.* [Gk., sense of well-being]. 1. Elation. 2. *In psychiatry*, an exaggerated sense of physical and emotional well-being, especially when not in keeping with real events; may be of psychogenic origin or due to neurologic or toxic disorders, or as a result of drugs. —**eu·phor·ic** (yoo·for′ick) *adj.*

eu·pho·ri·ant (yoo·fo′ree·unt) *adj.* & *n.* 1. Tending to bring on euphoria. 2. A substance that induces euphoria.

Euphthalmine. Trademark for eucatropine, a mydriatic used as the hydrochloride salt.

eu·phys·io·log·ic (yoo·fiz″ee·o·loj′ick) *adj.* [*eu-* + *physiologic*]. Pertaining to or characterizing the normal range of functions of an organism or part.

eu·ploid (yoo′ploid) *n.* [*eu-* + *-ploid*]. *In biology*, having an exact multiple of the basic haploid number of chromosomes. Contr. *aneuploid.* —**eu·ploidy** (yoo′ploy·dee) *n.*

eup·nea, eup·noea (yoop·nee′uh) *n.* [Gk. *eupnoia*, from *pnoē*, breath]. Normal or easy respiration.

Eupractone. Trademark for dimethadione, an anticonvulsant drug.

eu·prax·ia (yoo·prack′see·uh) *n.* [*eu-* + *-praxia*]. Normal and controlled performance of coordinated movements.

eu·pro·cin (yoo′pro·sin) *n.* (8α,9*R*)-10,11-Dihydro-6′-(3-methylbutoxy)cinchonan-9-ol (also known as isoamylhydrocupreine), $C_{24}H_{34}N_2O_2$, a topical anesthetic; used as the dihydrochloride salt.

Eu·proc·tis chrys·or·rhea (yoo·prock′tis kris″o·ree′uh). The brown-tail moth which causes brown-tail rash.

eu·py·rene (yoo·pye′reen) *adj.* [*eu-* + Gk. *pyrēn*, stone of a fruit]. Of sperm cells, being of the normal functional mature type. Contr. *apyrene, oligopyrene.*

Eurax. Trademark for crotamiton, a scabicide and antipruritic.

Euresol. Trademark for resorcinol monoacetate, a drug used in the treatment of certain skin diseases.

Eu·ro·pe·an blastomycosis. CRYPTOCOCCOSIS.

European noma. NOMA.

European typhus. EPIDEMIC TYPHUS.

eur·o·piso·ceph·a·lus (yoor″o·pis″o·sef′uh·lus) *n.*, pl. **europisocepha·li** (·lye) [*eury-* + Gk. *opisō-*, back, behind, + *-cephalus*]. An individual whose head is unusually broad in the occipital region.

eu·ro·pi·um (yoo·ro′pee·um) *n.* Eu = 151.96. A rare-earth metal found in cerium minerals. See also Table of Elements in the Appendix.

eu·ro·pro·ceph·a·lus (yoo″ro·pro·sef′uh·lus) *n.*, pl. **europrocepha·li** (·lye) [*eury-* + *pro-* + *-cephalus*]. An individual whose head is unusually broad in the frontal region.

eury- [Gk. *eurys*]. A combining form meaning *broad, wide.*

eu·ry·ce·phal·ic (yoo″ree·se·fal′ick) *adj.* [*eury-* + *-cephalic*]. 1. Having or characterizing a head that is unusually broad. 2. Sometimes, designating a brachycephalic head with a cephalic index of 81 to 85.4.

eu·ry·ceph·a·lous (yoo″ree·sef′uh·lus) *adj.* EURYCEPHALIC.

eu·ry·chas·mus (yoo″ree·kaz′mus) *n.* [NL., from *eury-* + Gk. *chasma,* chasm]. An individual with an unusually wide nasopharynx, with corresponding skull differences.

eu·ry·cne·mic (yoo″rick·nee′mick, yoo″ree·nee′mick) *adj.* [*eury-* + *cnemic*]. Characterizing a cnemic index of 70 or above.

eu·ryg·na·thism (yoo·rig′nuh·thiz·um, yoo″ree·nath′iz·um) *n.* [*eury-* + *gnath-* + *-ism*]. A condition in which the jaws are unusually broad. —**eu·ryg·nath·ic** (yoo″rig·nath′ick, yoo″ree·), **eu·ryg·na·thous** (yoo·rig′nuth·us) *adj.*

eu·ry·mer·ic (yoo″ree·merr′ick, yoo″ri·) *adj.* [*eury-* + Gk. *mēros*, thigh, + *-ic*]. *In osteometry,* designating a femur that is nearly circular in cross section in the proximal portion of the shaft; having a platymeric index of 85.0 to 99.9.

eu·ry·on (yoo′ree·on) *n.* [*eury-* + *-ion*]. The point on either lateral surface of the skull which is located at the extremities of the greatest width of the skull.

eu·ry·ther·mal (yoo″ree·thur′mul) *adj.* [*eury-* + *thermal*]. Capable of tolerating a wide range of temperature, as certain organisms.

eu·ry·ther·mic (yoo″ree·thur′mick) *adj.* EURYTHERMAL.

Eu·scor·pi·us (yoo·skor′pee·us) *n.* [NL., from *eu-* + Gk. *skorpios,* scorpion]. A genus of scorpions.

eu·sol (yoo′sol) *n.* [*E*dinburgh *U*niversity *sol*ution]. A solution formerly used as a wound antiseptic, prepared by the interaction of chlorinated lime and boric acid in water.

eu·sta·chian (yoo·stay′kee·un, ·stay′shun) *adj.* 1. Described by or named for Bartolomeo Eustachio, Italian anatomist, 1520–1574. 2. Pertaining to the auditory (eustachian) tube.

eustachian cartilage. TUBAL CARTILAGE.

eustachian catheter. A small catheter with a bend at the leading end, used to relieve obstruction of the auditory tube.

eustachian cushion. TORUS TUBARIUS.

eustachian diverticulum. A small abnormal pouching of the lower portion of the auditory tube.

eustachian salpingitis. Inflammation of the auditory tube.

eustachian tube. AUDITORY TUBE.

eustachian valve. CAVAL VALVE.

Eu·stron·gy·lus gi·gas (yoo·stron′ji·lus jye′gas). *DIOCTOPHYMA RENALE.*

eu·sys·to·le (yoo·sis′tuh·lee) *n.* [*eu-* + *systole*]. Normal systole.

eu·tec·tic (yoo·teck′tick) *adj.* [Gk. *eutēktos,* easily melted, from *tēkein,* to melt]. *In physical chemistry,* of, pertaining to, or designating the specific mixture of two or more substances which has the lowest melting point of any mixture of the substances. Contr. *dystectic.*

eutectic mixture. Through common usage, any mixture which has a lower melting point than the individual constituents; more usually a mixture that softens or melts at room temperature.

eu·tha·na·sia (yoo″thuh·nay′zhuh, ·zee·uh) *n.* [Gk., an easy or happy death, from *eu-* + *thanatos,* death]. The intentional bringing about of an easy and painless death to a person suffering from an incurable or painful disease.

eu·then·ics (yoo·thenn′icks) *n.* [Gk. *euthenein,* to thrive, flourish]. The science of rendering the environment optimal for the particular phenotype, as by the administration of specific diets or drugs. —**euthenic,** *adj.*

Eu·the·ria (yoo·theer′ee·uh) *n.pl.* [NL., from *eu-* + Gk. *thēria,* wild animals]. The true placental mammals. —**eu·the·ri·an** (·ee·un) *adj.*

eu·the·sia (yoo·theez′ee·uh) *n.* EUESTHESIA.

Euthroid. A trademark for liotrix, a mixture of thyroid hormone salts.

eu·thy·roid (yoo·thigh′roid) *adj.* [*eu-* + *thyroid*]. Characterized by or pertaining to normal thyroid function. —**euthyroid·ism,** *n.*

eu·to·cia (yoo·to′shee·uh, ·see·uh) *n.* [Gk. *eutokia,* from *tokos,* childbirth]. Natural or easy childbirth; normal labor.

Eutonyl. Trademark for pargyline, an antihypertensive drug used as the hydrochloride salt.

eu·trep·is·ty (yoo·trep′is·tee, yoo′tre·pis″tee) *n.* [Gk. *eutrepēs,* well-prepared]. Preoperative administration of anti-infection medications.

Eu·tri·at·o·ma (yoo″trye·at′o·muh) *n.* A genus of bugs, some members of which transmit Chagas' disease.

Eu·trom·bic·u·la (yoo″trom·bick′yoo·luh) *n.* [*eu-* + *Trombicula*]. The genus of mites of the Trombiculidae to which chiggers belong.

Eutrombicula al·fred·du·ge·si (al″fred·dew·jee′sigh). The mite species that causes a common type of dermatitis; widely distributed in North and South America; a chigger.

eV Abbreviation for *electron volt.*

evac·u·ant (e·vack′yoo·unt) *adj.* & *n.* 1. Causing evacuation; purgative. 2. Medicine which empties an organ, especially the bowels; a purgative.

evac·u·ate (e·vack′yoo·ate) *v.* [L. *evacuare,* to empty, from *vacuus,* empty].To empty or remove.

evac·u·a·tion (e·vack″yoo·ay′shun) *n.* [L. *evacuatio,* from *evacuare,* to empty]. 1. The voiding of any matter either by the natural passages of the body or by an artificial opening; specifically, defecation. 2. *In military medicine,* the withdrawal of sick and wounded personnel, or material, or both, as from a battle area.

evacuation hospital. *In military medicine,* a mobile hospital or semimobile unit designed to provide facilities, as near the front as possible, for major medical and surgical procedures and for the preparation and sorting of casualties for extended evacuation to the rear.

evac·u·a·tor (e·vack′yoo·ay″tur) *n.* An instrument for the removal of fluid or particles from the urinary bladder or intestine.

evag·i·na·tion (e·vaj″i·nay′shun) *n.* [L. *evaginare,* to unsheathe, from *vagina,* sheath]. 1. The turning inside out of an organ or part. 2. The protrusion of an organ or part by eversion of its inner surface or from its covering. Syn. *outpouching.* Contr. *invagination.* —**evag·i·nate** (e·vaj′i·nate) *v.*

ev·a·nes·cent (ev″uh·nes′unt) *adj.* [L. *evanescens*]. Unstable; tending to vanish quickly.

Ev·ans blue [H. M. *Evans,* U.S. anatomist, 1882–1971]. Tetrasodium salt of 4,4′-bis[7-(1-amino-8-hydroxy-2,4-disulfo)-naphthylazo]-3,3′-bitolyl, $C_{34}H_{24}N_6Na_4O_{14}S_4$, a diazo dye, occurring as a bluish-green or brown iridescent powder, very soluble in water; it is used as an intravenous diagnostic agent for colorimetric determination of blood volume, cardiac output, and residual blood volume in the heart; when injected into the bloodstream it combines with plasma albumin and leaves the circulation slowly. Syn. *T 1824.*

Evans blue method [H. M. *Evans*]. A dye-dilution method using Evans blue (T 1824) for the determination of blood volume, cardiac output, and residual blood volume in the heart.

even·tra·tion (ee″ven·tray′shun) *n.* [F. *éventration,* from *ventre,* belly]. Protrusion of the abdominal viscera through the abdominal wall, as in ventral hernia. Compare *evisceration.*

eventration of the diaphragm. A condition where there is defective muscular action of the diaphragm, the left leaf being abnormally high, not moving through the normal excursion.

Evers·busch's operation (ey′vurs·boosh) [O. *Eversbusch,* German ophthalmologist, 1855–1912]. An operation to relieve ptosis.

ever·sion (e·vur′zhun) *n.* [L. *eversio,* from *evertere,* to turn out]. A turning outward. —**evert** (e·vurt′) *v.*

eversion of the cervix. A turning outward of the cervix of the uterus so that an excessive amount of endocervical tissue, which normally lies inside the os, is visible; it usually follows unrepaired lacerations of the cervix at childbirth.

eversion of the eyelid. 1. A method of folding the lid upon itself for the purpose of exposing the conjunctival surface or sulcus. 2. ECTROPION.

Eve's method [F. C. *Eve,* English physician, 1871–1952]. Artificial respiration by tipping the patient alternately head up and head down on a stretcher, inspiration and expiration occurring as the diaphragm moves up and down from shifting of the abdominal viscera.

ev·i·dence, *n.* [L. *evidentia,* clarity, from *evidens,* clear]. *In legal medicine,* any type of proof or material, as testimony of witnesses, records, or x-ray films, presented at a trial for the purpose of convincing the court or jury as to the truth and accuracy of an alleged fact.

evil eye. The ability to cause misfortune, disease, or death indirectly, or by a glance, believed in many parts of the world to be possessed by certain individuals. The delusion of being a victim of or threatened by the evil eye is frequent among individuals with the paranoid type of schizophrenia. Compare *fascinum.*

Evipal. Trademark for hexobarbital, a sedative and hypnotic of short duration of action.

ev·i·ra·tion (ev″i·ray′shun) *n.* [L. *evirare,* to emasculate, from *e-* + *vir,* man]. 1. Castration; emasculation. 2. Loss of potency. 3. A psychic process in which there is a deep and permanent assumption of feminine qualities, with corresponding loss of manly qualities. Contr. *defeminization.*

evis·cer·a·tion (e·vis″ur·ay′shun) *n.* [L. *eviscerare,* to disembowel]. 1. Removal of the abdominal or thoracic viscera. 2. Protrusion of viscera postoperatively through a disrupted abdominal incision. 3. Removal of the contents of an organ, such as the eyeball.

evo·ca·tion (ev″o·kay′shun, ee″vo·) *n.* [L. *evocatio,* from *evocare,* to call forth]. The part of the morphogenic effect of an organizer which can be referred to the action of a single chemical substance, the evocator.

evo·ca·tor (ev′o·kay″tur, ee′vo·) *n.* [L., one who calls forth]. The chemical substance emitted by an organizer, which acts as all or part of a morphogenic stimulus in an embryonic tissue. Syn. *morphogenic hormone.*

evoked cortical potential. EVOKED POTENTIAL.

evoked potential. The electric response recorded from the cerebral cortex after stimulation of a peripheral sense organ. It may be primary, specific in location, and observed only where the pathway from a particular sense organ ends; or it may be secondary or diffuse, appearing over most of the cortex and other parts of the brain via the nonspecific thalamic nuclei.

evo·lu·tion, *n.* [L. *evolutio,* from *evolvere,* to unroll]. 1. A gradual, usually developmental or directional change in kind or type. 2. *In biology,* specifically, phylogenetic evolution, which is believed to result mainly from natural selection of variants produced by genetic mutations (some few of which are not deleterious and may allow adaptation to new conditions or environments); especially, the totality of those changes whereby the more complex life forms have generally developed from simpler forms. —**evolution·ary,** *adj.*

evul·sion (e·vul′shun) *n.* [L. *evulsio,* from *evellere,* to pull out]. AVULSION.

Ewald's node. SIGNAL NODE.

Ewald tube (ey′vahlt) [C. A. *Ewald,* German physician, 1845–1915]. A large-bore flexible rubber tube designed for aspiration of gastric contents.

Ew·art's sign (yoo′urt) [W. *Ewart,* English physician, 1848–1929]. Dullness to percussion, increased fremitus, and bronchial breathing beneath the angle of the left scapula in pericardial effusion.

E wave. The positive wave of the apex cardiogram occurring late in systole.

Ew·ing's sarcoma or **tumor** (yoo′ing) [J. *Ewing,* U.S. pathologist, 1866–1943]. A malignant tumor of bone whose parenchyma consists of cells resembling endothelial or reticulum cells. Compare *angioendothelioma.*

[1]ex-, e-, ef- [L.]. A prefix meaning (a) *out, away, off;* (b) *without, -less.*

[2]ex-. See *exo-.*

ex·ac·er·ba·tion (eg·zas″ur·bay′shun, eck·sas″ur·) *n.* [L. *exacerbare,* to irritate, from *acerbus,* angry, morose]. Increase in the manifestations or severity of a disease or symptom. —**ex·ac·er·bate** (eg·zas′ur·bait) *v.*

ex·al·ta·tion (eg″zawl·tay′shun) *n.* [L. *exaltatio,* from *exaltare,* to exalt]. A mental state characterized by self-satisfaction, ecstatic joy, abnormal cheerfulness, optimism, or delusions of grandeur.

ex·am·i·na·tion (eg·zam″i·nay′shun) *n.* [L. *examinatio,* from *examinare,* to examine]. 1. Investigation or inspection for the purpose of diagnosis. 2. A formal test of the proficiency or competence of an individual in a given area of learning or training, as for a licensure or certification. —**ex·am·ine** (eg·zam′in) *v.*

ex·am·in·ee (eg·zam″i·nee′) *n.* A patient undergoing examination or any person taking an examination.

ex·an·them (eck·san′thum, eg·zan′thum) *n.* [Gk. *exanthēma,* from *exanthein,* to break out, from *anthein,* to bloom, from *anthos,* flower]. 1. An eruption upon the skin. 2. Any eruptive fever or disease. Contr. *enanthema.* —**exan·them·a·tous** (·themm′uh·tus), **exan·the·mat·ic** (·thi·mat′ick) *adj.*

ex·an·the·ma (eck″san·theem′uh) *n.,* pl. **exanthema·ta** (·tuh), **exanthemas.** EXANTHEM.

exanthematous fever. 1. BOUTONNEUSE FEVER. 2. Any fever associated with an exanthem.

exanthematous lupus erythematosus. SYSTEMIC LUPUS ERYTHEMATOSUS.

exanthematous synovitis. Synovitis secondary to an exanthema.

exanthem su·bi·tum (sue′bi·tum) [L., sudden]. An acute illness of infants, probably of viral origin, characterized by 3 to 4 days of high fever which terminates abruptly and is followed by a transient rubella-like rash. Neurologic complications, particularly convulsions, may occur.

ex·ar·te·ri·tis (ecks·ahr″te·rye′tis) *n.* [*ex-* + *arteritis*]. Inflammation of the outer coat or adventitia of an artery.

ex·ca·va·tio (ecks″ka·vay′shee·o) *n.,* pl. **exca·va·ti·o·nes** (·vay″shee·o′neez) [L.]. EXCAVATION (1).

excavatio dis·ci (dis′kye) [NA]. EXCAVATION OF THE OPTIC DISK.

ex·ca·va·tion (ecks″kuh·vay′shun) *n.* [L. *excavatio,* from *excavare,* to hollow out]. 1. A hollow or cavity, especially one with sharply defined edges. 2. The act or process of making hollow. 3. Removal of carious material from a tooth.

excavation of the optic disk. The depression or cupping in the center of the optic disk. NA *excavatio disci.*

excavatio pa·pil·lae ner·vi op·ti·ci (pap·il′ee nur′vye op′ti·sigh) [BNA]. Excavatio disci (= EXCAVATION OF THE OPTIC DISK).

excavatio rec·to·ute·ri·na (reck″to·yoo·tur·eye′nuh) [NA]. RECTOUTERINE EXCAVATION.

excavatio rec·to·ve·si·ca·lis (reck″to·ves·i·kay′lis) [NA]. RECTOVESICAL EXCAVATION.

excavatio ve·si·co·ute·ri·na (ves″i·ko·yoo·tur·eye′nuh) [NA]. VESICOUTERINE EXCAVATION.

ex·ca·va·tor (ecks′kuh·vay″tur) *n.* 1. An instrument like a gouge or scoop used to scrape away tissue. 2. A dental instrument for removing decayed matter from a tooth cavity.

excentric. ECCENTRIC (1).

ex·cer·e·bra·tion (eck·serr″e·bray′shun) *n.* [*ex-* + *cerebr*um]. CEPHALOTOMY.

exchange transfusion. The replacement of most or all of the recipient's blood in small amounts at a time by blood from a donor, a technique used particularly in cases of erythroblastosis fetalis, in certain types of poisoning such as salicylism, and occasionally in liver failure. Syn. *replacement transfusion.*

ex·cip·i·ent (eck·sip′ee·unt) *n.* [L. *excipere,* to take a thing to one's self]. Any substance combined with an active drug to make of the latter an agreeable or convenient dosage form.

ex·ci·sion (eck·sizh′un) *n.* [L. *excisio,* from *excidere,* to cut out]. 1. The cutting out of a part. 2. Removal of a foreign body, growth, or devitalized or infected tissue from a part, organ, or wound. —**ex·cise** (eck·size′) *v.*

ex·cit·abil·i·ty (eck·sight″uh·bil′i·tee) *n.* Readiness of response to a stimulus; IRRITABILITY. —**ex·cit·able** (eck·sight′uh·bul) *adj.*

excitable membrane. A cell membrane having the property of a regenerative interaction between depolarization and permeability to sodium.

ex·ci·tant (eck·sigh′tunt, eck′si·tunt) *adj.* & *n.* [L. *excitans,* from *excitare,* to arouse]. 1. Stimulating the activity of an organ. 2. An agent that stimulates the activity of an organ.

ex·ci·ta·tion (eck″sigh·tay′shun) *n.* [L. *excitare,* to call forth, summon, from *ciere,* to shake, arouse]. 1. Stimulation or irritation of an organ or tissue. 2. *In physics and chemistry,* the addition of energy to a system, thereby transferring it from its ground state to an excited state. Excitation of a nucleus, atom, or molecule can result from absorption of photons or from inelastic collisions with various atomic or nuclear particles. —**ex·cit·ing** (eck·sigh′ting) *adj.;* **ex·cite** (eck·sight′) *v.*

excitation wave. The progressive wavelike activation of successive muscle fibers in the excitatory process.

ex·cit·ato·ry (eck·sight′uh·to″ree) *adj.* 1. Tending to stimulate or excite. 2. Tending to facilitate or catalyze.

exciting cause. The immediately preceding and conditioning factor associated with a specific event.

exciting eye. The originally injured or diseased eye in sympathetic ophthalmia.

ex·clu·sion (ecks·kloo′zhun) *n.* [L. *exclusio,* from *excludere,* to shut out]. 1. The process of extruding or shutting out. 2. *In surgery,* an operation by which part of an organ is disconnected from the rest, but not excised.

ex·coch·le·a·tion (ecks·kock″lee·ay′shun) *n.* [*ex-* + L. *cochlea,* snail, snail shell]. Removal by scraping.

ex·con·ju·gant (ecks·kon′joo·gunt) *n.* A protozoon or bacterium immediately after the separation following conjugation.

ex·co·ri·a·tion (ecks·ko″ree·ay′shun) *n.* [L. *excoriare,* to skin, from *ex-* + *corium,* skin, hide]. Abrasion of a portion of the skin or other epithelial surface. —**ex·co·ri·ate** (ecks·ko′ree·ate) *v.*

ex·cre·ment (ecks′kre·munt) *n.* [L. *excrementum,* from *excernere,* to sift out]. An excreted substance; specifically, feces. —**ex·cre·men·ti·tious** (ecks″kre·men·tish′us) *adj.*

ex·cres·cence (ecks·kres′unce) *n.* [L. *excrescentia,* from *excrescere,* to grow out]. Abnormal outgrowth upon the body.

ex·cres·cent (ecks·kres′unt) *adj.* Possessing the characteristics of an excrescence.

ex·cre·ta (eck·skree′tuh) *n. pl.* [L., neuter pl. of *excretus,* from *excernere,* to sift out]. The waste material cast out or separated from an organism.

ex·cre·tion (eck·skree′shun) *n.* [L. *excretio,* sifting, sorting out, from *excernere,* to sift out, sort out]. 1. The expulsion of waste-containing substances from cells, tissues, organ systems, or the whole organism. 2. EXCRETA. —**ex·cre·to·ry** (eck′skre·tor″ee) *adj.* & *n.;* **ex·crete** (eck·skreet′) *v.*

excretion threshold. The critical concentration of a substance in the blood, above which the substance is excreted by the kidneys.

excretory duct. A duct, lined by nonsecretory epithelium, which is solely conductive.

excretory urography. The radiographic visualization of the urinary tract, including the renal parenchyma and renal collecting system, ureters, urinary bladder, and sometimes the urethra, following intravenous injection of a contrast medium.

ex·cur·sion (eck·skur′zhun) *n.* [L. *excursio,* from *excurrere,* to run out]. 1. A wandering from the usual course. 2. The extent of movement, as of the eyes from a central position, or of the chest during respiration. —**ex·cur·sive** (eck·skur′siv) *adj.*

ex·cur·va·tion (ecks″kur·vay′shun) *n.* EXCURVATURE.

ex·cur·va·ture (ecks·kur′vuh·chur) *n.* An outward curvature.

ex·cy·clo·pho·ria (eck·sigh″klo·fo′ree·uh) *n.* [*ex-* + *cyclophoria*]. A form of cyclophoria in which the eyes rotate outward.

ex·cy·clo·tro·pia (eck·sigh″klo·tro′pee·uh) *n.* [*ex-* + *cyclotropia*]. Cyclotropia outward.

ex·cys·ta·tion (ecks″sis·tay′shun) *n.* The escape from a cyst by the bursting of the surrounding envelope; a stage in the life of an intestinal parasite which occurs after the parasite has been swallowed by the host.

ex·ec·u·tant ego function (eg·zeck′yoo·tunt). *In psychiatry,* the ego's management of psychologic or mental mechanisms in order to meet the demands of the organism.

ex·e·dens (eck′se·denz) *adj.* [L., consuming, corrosive, from *ex-* + *edere,* to eat]. *In dermatology,* progressively ulcerative.

ex·en·ce·pha·lia (ecks″en·se·fay′lee·uh) *n.* [*ex-* + *-encephalia*]. Cranioschisis and partial anencephalia, with encephalocele, or hydrencephalocele. —**exence·phal·ic** (·fal′ick) *adj.*

ex·en·ceph·a·lus (ecks″en·sef′uh·lus) *n.*, pl. **exencepha·li** (·lye) [*ex-* + *-encephalus*]. An individual showing exencephalia.

ex·en·ceph·a·ly (ecks″en·sef′uh·lee) *n.* EXENCEPHALIA.

ex·en·ter·a·tion (eck·sen″tur·ay′shun) *n.* [L. *exenterare,* to disembowel, from Gk. *exenterizein,* from *ex-* + *enteron,* bowel]. EVISCERATION (1, 3). —**ex·en·ter·ate** (eck·sen′tur·ate) *v.*

ex·er·cise (eck′sur·size) *n.* [L. *exercitium,* from *exercere,* to work at]. Muscular exertion for the purpose of preservation or restoration of health, or development of physical prowess or athletic skill.

exercise gloves. Soft leather gloves used in graduated resistance exercises for patients who lack strength in the upper extremities. They eliminate hazards involved in using the bare hands.

exercise tolerance test. Any of several standardized exercise tests in which the development of chest pain and electrocardiographic abnormalities are interpreted as indicating myocardial ischemia, supporting the diagnosis of angina pectoris.

ex·er·e·sis (eck·serr′e·sis) *n.*, pl. **exere·ses** (·seez) [Gk. *exairesis,* removal]. Surgical excision or extraction.

ex·er·gon·ic (eck″sur·gon′ick) *adj.* [*ex-* + Gk. *ergon,* work, + *-ic*]. Of or pertaining to a chemical reaction in which the end products possess less free energy than the starting materials; usually associated with catabolism. Contr. *endergonic.*

ex·fe·ta·tion (ecks″fe·tay′shun) *n.* Ectopic or extrauterine fetation.

ex·flag·el·la·tion (ecks·flaj″e·lay′shun) *n.* [*ex-* + *flagella* + *-tion*]. The formation of actively motile flagella in the microgametocyte, the male malarial parasite.

ex·fo·li·a·tion (ecks·fo″lee·ay′shun) *n.* [L. *exfoliare,* to strip of leaves, from *folium,* leaf]. 1. The separation of bone or other tissue in thin layers; a superficial sequestrum. 2. A peeling and shedding of the horny layer of the skin, a normal process that may be exaggerated after an inflammation or as part of a skin disease. **—ex·fo·li·ate** (ecks·fo′lee·ate) *v.;* **ex·fo·li·a·tive** (ecks·fo′lee·uh·tiv) *adj.*

exfoliative cytology. The study of desquamated cells.

exfoliative dermatitis. Any dermatitis in which there is extensive involvement of the skin with denudation of large areas, involving hair loss.

exfoliative erythroderma. A dermatosis having a scarlatiniform eruption lasting from 6 to 8 weeks, with free desquamation. Syn. *pityriasis rubra.*

exfoliative vaginitis. Vaginitis characterized by a peeling away or shedding of large fragments of the surface epithelium.

ex·ha·la·tion (ecks″ha·lay′shun) *n.* [L. *exhalatio,* from *exhalare,* to breathe out]. 1. The giving off or sending forth in the form of vapor; expiration. 2. That which is given forth as vapor; emanation. **—ex·hale** (ecks·hail′, ecks′) *v.*

ex·haus·tion (eg·zaws′chun) *n.* [L. *exhaustio,* from *exhaurire,* to exhaust]. 1. The act of using up or consuming all possibilities or resources. 2. Loss of physical and mental power from fatigue, protracted disease, psychogenic causes, or excessive heat or cold. 3. The pharmaceutical process of dissolving out one or more of the constituents of a crude drug by percolation or maceration.

exhaustion atrophy. Atrophy of an endocrine gland, presumably due to prolonged excessive stimulation.

exhaustion delirium. Acute, confusional, delirious reactions brought about by extreme fatigue, long wasting illness, prolonged insomnia, inanition, and marked lowering of psychologic tension; continuing for days to weeks, with recovery usually complete.

ex·haus·tive (eg·zaws′tiv) *adj.* 1. Examining every possibility. 2. Bringing to the point of exhaustion.

exhaustive psychosis. EXHAUSTION DELIRIUM.

ex·hi·bi·tion (eck″si·bish′un) *n.* [L. *exhibitio,* from *exhibere,* to present]. The administration of a remedy. **—ex·hib·it** (eg·zib′it) *v. & n.*

ex·hi·bi·tion·ism (eck″si·bish′un·iz·um) *n.* 1. A sexual perversion in which pleasure is obtained by exposing the genitalia. 2. *In psychoanalysis,* gratification of early sexual impulses in young children by physical activity, such as dancing. **—exhibition·ist** (·ist) *n.*

ex·hil·a·rant (eg·zil′uh·runt) *adj. & n.* [L. *exhilarare,* to make merry]. 1. Exhilarating; causing a rise in spirits. 2. An agent that enlivens or elates. **—ex·hil·a·rate** (eg·zil′uh·rate) *v.;* **ex·hil·a·ra·tion** (eg·zil″uh·ray′shun) *n.*

ex·hu·ma·tion (ecks″hew·may′shun) *n.* [F., from L. *ex-* + *humus,* ground]. Removal from the ground after burial; disinterment. **—ex·hume** (·hewm′) *v.*

ex·is·ten·tial (eg″zis·ten′shul) *adj.* 1. Pertaining to or grounded in existence; readily perceived, experienced, or implied from actuality as opposed to ideal or metaphysical. 2. Specifically, pertaining to human existence. See also *existentialism.*

ex·is·ten·tial·ism (eg″zis·ten′shul·iz·um) *n.* [*existential* + *-ism*]. A school of philosophy which sees the universe as purposeless and hostile and life as absurd unless man, by an act of will, gives it meaning and takes responsibility for his acts.

existential psychiatry. A school of psychiatry based on existentialism.

existential psychology. 1. A school of psychology which sees its task as the observation and description of existent data or of the contents of experience by analysis of the constituent elements, largely through introspection aided by experiment. Syn. *structural psychology.* 2. The psychological theories and doctrines based on existentialism.

exit dose. The amount of radiation which is not absorbed or scattered, but passes through a structure being irradiated.

exit heart block. *In electrocardiography,* a local region of unidirectional block which prevents some of the impulses generated by an ectopic pacemaker (parasystolic focus) from being transmitted to the rest of the heart.

ex·i·tus (eck′si·tus) *n.* [L.]. 1. Exit; outlet. 2. Death.

Exna. Trademark for benzthiazide, a diuretic and antihypertensive agent.

exo-, ex- [Gk.]. A combining form meaning (a) *outside;* (b) *outer layer;* (c) *out of.*

exo·bi·ol·o·gy (eck″so·bye·ol′uh·jee) *n.* [*exo-* + *biology*]. The science that is concerned with life forms occurring outside the earth and its atmosphere.

exo·car·dia (eck″so·kahr′dee·uh) *n.* [*exo-* + *-cardia*]. ECTOCARDIA.

exo·car·di·ac (eck″so·kahr′dee·ack) *adj.* [*exo-* + *cardiac*]. Originating, occurring, or situated outside the heart.

exo·car·di·al (eck″so·kahr′dee·ul) *adj.* EXOCARDIAC.

exocardial murmur. A murmur related to the heart, but produced outside its cavities.

exo·cat·a·pho·ria (eck″so·kat″uh·for′ee·uh) *n.* [*exo-* + *cataphoria*]. The condition in which the visual axis turns outward and downward.

ex·oc·cip·i·tal (ecks″ock·sip′i·tul) *adj.* [*ex-* + *occipital*]. Lying to the side of the foramen magnum, as the exoccipital bone.

exoccipital bone. Either of the two lateral portions of the occipital bone which ossify from separate centers of ossification and fuse to form the adult bone.

exo·cer·vix (eck″so·sur′vicks) *n.* [*exo-* + *cervix*]. ECTOCERVIX.

exo·cho·ri·on (eck″so·kor′ee·on) *n.,* pl. **exocho·ria** (·ee·uh) [*exo-* + *chorion*]. The external layer of the chorion.

exo·coe·lom (eck″so·see′lum) *n.* [*exo-* + *coelum*]. The part of the coelom outside the embryo proper. Originally extensive, it becomes restricted to the proximal umbilical cord by the growth of the amnion. **—exo·coe·lom·ic** (·see·lom′ick) *adj.*

exocoelomic membrane. A delicate, mesothelium-like membrane bounding the exocoelom of the blastocyst; continuous with the extraembryonic mesoderm and with the primary endoderm. It may be derived from either or both.

exo·crine (eck′so·krin, ·krine) *adj.* [*exo-* + *-crine*]. Secreting externally; of or pertaining to glands that deliver their secretion to an epithelial surface, either directly or by ducts. Contr. *endocrine.*

exo·cy·to·sis (eck·so·sigh·to′sis) *n.* [*exo-* + *cyt-* + *-osis*]. The extrusion of material from a cell. Contr. *endocytosis.* **—exocy·tot·ic** (·tot′ick) *adj.*

ex·odon·tia (eck″so·don′chee·uh) *n.* [*ex-* + *-odontia*]. The art and science of the extraction of teeth.

ex·odon·tics (eck″so·don′ticks) *n.* EXODONTIA.

ex·odon·tist (eck″so·don′tist) *n.* Formerly, one who specialized in tooth extraction.

exo·er·gic (eck″so·ur′jick) *adj.* [*exo-* + *erg-* + *-ic*]. EXOTHERMIC.

exo·eryth·ro·cyt·ic (eck″so·e·rith″ro·sit′ick) *adj.* [*exo-* + *erythrocytic*]. Outside of erythrocytes; said of the development of some of the malaria plasmodia in the cells of the lymphatic system of birds, and of human malarial parasites in parenchymal cells of the liver.

ex·og·a·my (ecks·og′uh·mee) *n.* [*exo-* + *-gamy*]. 1. Union of gametes of different ancestry; outbreeding; cross-fertilization. 2. *In anthropology,* marriage between members of different clans, communities, or other social groups, as established by law or custom. Contr. *endogamy.* **—exoga·mous** (·mus) *adj.*

exo·gas·tru·la (eck″so·gas′troo·luh) *n.* [*exo-* + *gastrula*]. An abnormal embryo with evagination of the primitive gut and absence of further development. —**exo·gas·tru·la·tion** (·gas″troo·lay′shun) *n.*

exo·ge·net·ic (eck″so·je·net′ick) *adj.* [*exo-* + *genetic*]. EXOGENOUS.

exo·gen·ic (eck″so·jen′ick) *adj.* [*exo-* + *-genic*]. EXOGENOUS.

exogenic toxicosis. Poisoning induced by toxins taken into the system, as in botulism.

ex·og·e·nous (eck·soj′e·nus) *adj.* [*exo-* + *-genous*]. 1. Due to an external cause; not arising within the organism. 2. *In physiology,* pertaining to those factors in the metabolism of nitrogenous substances obtained from food. 3. Growing by addition to the outer surfaces.

exogenous aneurysm. An aneurysm due to trauma.

exogenous cycle. The phase of development of *Plasmodium malariae* or other parasite which occurs in the invertebrate host, the mosquito.

exogenous tuberculosis. Tuberculosis arising from a source outside the body; may be a primary infection, true reinfection, or superinfection.

exo·hys·tero·pexy (eck″so·his′tur·o·peck″see) *n.* [*exo-* + *hysteropexy*]. Fixation of the uterus in the abdominal wall outside the peritoneum.

exo·me·tri·tis (eck″so·me·trye′tis) *n.* [*exo-* + *metritis*]. PARAMETRITIS.

ex·om·pha·los (ecks·om′fuh·lus) *n.* [*ex-* + *omphalos*]. A prominence of the navel due to umbilical hernia; a congenital hernia into the umbilical cord.

exo·nu·cle·ase (eck·so·new′klee·ace, ·aze) *n.* [*exo-* + *nuclease*]. An enzyme that catalyzes hydrolysis of single nucleotide residues from the end of the DNA chain. Contr. *endonuclease.*

exo·pep·ti·dase (eck″so·pep′ti·dace, ·daze) *n.* [*exo-* + *peptidase*]. Any of a group of enzymes, including aminopeptidases and carboxypeptidases, capable of acting only upon terminal peptide bonds.

exo·pho·ria (eck″so·fo′ree·uh) *n.* [*exo-* + *-phoria*]. A type of heterophoria in which the visual lines tend outward.

ex·oph·thal·mic (eck″sof·thal′mick) *adj.* Characterized by or pertaining to exophthalmos.

exophthalmic goiter. Hyperthyroidism with exophthalmos.

exophthalmic ophthalmoplegia. Extraocular muscle weakness causing strabismus usually accompanied by diplopia, seen with exophthalmos.

exophthalmic syndrome. HYPEROPHTHALMOPATHIC GRAVES' DISEASE.

ex·oph·thal·mom·e·ter (eck″sof·thal·mom′e·tur) *n.* An instrument that measures the degree of exophthalmos.

ex·oph·thal·mom·e·try (eck″sof·thal·mom′e·tree) *n.* [*exophthalmos* + *-metry*]. The mean measurement of the anterior plane of the cornea from the external orbital rim.

ex·oph·thal·mos, ex·oph·thal·mus (eck″sof·thal′mus) *n.* [Gk., having prominent eyes]. Abnormal prominence or protrusion of the eyeball.

exophthalmos-producing substance. A substance, considered to be distinct from thyroid-stimulating hormone, obtained from extracts of the anterior pituitary, which, in experimental animals, produces exophthalmos. Abbreviated, EPS.

exo·phyt·ic (eck′so·fit′ick) *adj.* [*exo-* + *phyte* + *-ic*]. ECTOPHYTIC.

exo·skel·e·ton (eck″so·skel′e·tun) *n.* 1. The usually chitinous external skeleton of invertebrates. 2. The bony or horny supporting structures in the skin of many vertebrates, such as fish scales or the carapace of a turtle.

ex·os·mom·e·ter (eck″soz·mom′e·tur) *n.* [*exosmosis* + *-meter*]. An instrument for measuring the degree of exosmosis.

ex·os·mose (eck′soz·moce, ·moze) *n.* [F.]. EXOSMOSIS.

ex·os·mo·sis (eck″sos·mo′sis, eck″soz·) *n.* [*ex-* + *osmosis*]. Passage of a liquid outward through a porous membrane. —**exos·mot·ic** (·mot′ick) *adj.*

exo·som·es·the·sia, exo·som·aes·the·sia (eck″so·sohm″es·theezh′uh, ·theez′ee·uh) *n.* [*exo-* + *somesthesia*]. A process of disordered perception in which the patient, upon being touched on some part of the body, indicates that some nearby object has been touched.

ex·os·to·sec·to·my (eck·sos″to·seck′tuh·mee) *n.* [*exostosis* + *-ectomy*]. Excision of an exostosis.

ex·os·to·sis (eck″sos·to′sis) *n.*, pl. **exosto·ses** (·seez) [Gk. *exostōsis,* from *ex-* + *ost-* + *-osis*]. A benign cartilage-capped protuberance from the surface of long bones but also seen on flat bones; due to chronic irritation as from infection, trauma, or osteoarthritis. See also *exostosis cartilaginea, multiple hereditary exostoses.* —**exos·tot·ic** (·tot′ick), **ex·os·tosed** (eck·sos′toze′d, eg·zos′) *adj.*

exostosis car·ti·la·gin·ea (kahr″ti·la·jin′ee·uh). A limited or abortive form of multiple hereditary exostosis in which a benign protruding bony lesion capped by growing cartilage appears usually by the end of the second decade of life. Compare *osteochondroma.*

exo·ther·mal (eck″so·thur′mul) *adj.* EXOTHERMIC.

exo·ther·mic (eck″so·thur′mick) *adj.* [*exo-* + *thermic*]. Pertaining to the giving out of energy, especially heat energy. Contr. *endothermic.*

exo·tox·in (eck″so·tock′sin) *n.* [*exo-* + *toxin*]. A toxin which is excreted by a living microorganism and which can afterward be obtained in bacteria-free filtrates without death or disintegration of the microorganisms. —**exotox·ic** (·sick) *adj.*

exo·tro·pia (eck″so·tro′pee·uh) *n.* [*exo-* + *-tropia*]. Divergent strabismus, occurring when one eye fixes upon an object and the other deviates outward. Contr. *esotropia.*

exo·tro·pic (eck″so·tro′pick, ·trop′ick) *adj.* [*exo-* + *-tropic*]. 1. Turning outward. 2. Pertaining to exotropia.

expanded function dental auxiliary. A dental auxiliary who has been trained and certified to perform certain intraoral dental procedures.

Expandex. A trademark for dextran, the plasma-expanding and blood-pressure-maintaining substance.

ex·pan·sile (eck·span′sil, ·sile) *adj.* Prone to or capable of expansion.

ex·pan·sive, *adj.* [L. *expansio,* from *expandere,* to expand]. 1. Comprehensive; extensive. 2. *In psychiatry,* characterized by megalomania, euphoria, talkativeness, overgenerosity, grandiosity. —**expansive·ness,** *n.*

expansive delusion. Megalomania, usually associated with euphoria.

ex·pect·ant, *adj.* [L. *expectare,* to look out for, from *specere,* to look]. 1. In expectation or anticipation of an outcome, as expectant mother. 2. Characterized by expectations, but also uncertainty as to result, as expectant treatment.

ex·pec·ta·tion of life. 1. *In biometry,* the average number of years lived by a group of individuals after reaching a given age, as determined by the mortality experience of a specific time and geographic area. 2. Commonly, the probable number of years of survival for an individual of a given age.

ex·pec·to·rant (eck·speck′to·runt) *adj.* & *n.* [L. *expectorare,* to drive from the chest, from *pectus,* chest, breast]. 1. Promoting expectoration. 2. A medicinal that promotes or modifies expectoration.

expectorant mixture. A nauseating expectorant prepared from fluidextracts of senega and squill, paregoric, ammonium carbonate, and tolu balsam syrup. Syn. *Stokes's expectorant.*

ex·pec·to·ra·tion (eck·speck″tuh·ray′shun) *n.* 1. Ejection of material from the mouth. 2. The fluid or semifluid matter from the lungs and air passages expelled by coughing and spitting; sputum.

ex·pel, *v.* [L. *expellere,* to drive out]. To drive or force out, as the fetus, by means of muscular contractions.

ex·pe·ri·en·tial (eck·speer″ee·en′shul) *adj.* Pertaining to or derived from experience.

ex·per·i·ment, *n.* [L. *experimentum,* from *experiri,* to try]. 1. A trial or test. 2. A procedure undertaken to discover some unknown principle or effect, to test a hypothesis, or to illustrate a known principle or fact. —**ex·per·i·men·tal,** *adj.;* **ex·per·i·men·ta·tion,** *n.*

experimental allergic encephalomyelitis. A demyelinating encephalomyelitis arising from hypersensitivity to neural tissues, induced in experimental animals by injection of brain, spinal cord, or peripheral nerve tissue and important as a laboratory model of acute disseminated encephalomyelitis and similar diseases. Abbreviated, EAE.

experimental animal. An animal which is the subject of experimentation.

experimental diabetes. Diabetes mellitus produced in animals by various methods, such as pancreatectomy or injection of extracts of the anterior pituitary or of alloxan.

experimental embryology. The branch of embryology that uses experimental methods to investigate the development of an embryo.

experimental medicine. Medicine based upon experiments on man or animals by the observation of pathologic changes in disease induced in them and the effect of drugs administered.

experimental oncology. The laboratory study of tumors, either animal or human, naturally occurring or induced, in an attempt to extend knowledge of tumors generally. Contr. *clinical oncology.*

experimental pathology. The branch of pathology that uses experimental methods for the study of disease in animals and in man.

experimental physiology. Experiments carried on in a physiologic laboratory with experimental animals or man.

experimental psychology. The study of psychologic phenomena by experimental methods.

experimental renal hypertension. Hypertension produced in animals by constricting the main renal arteries, simulating the manifestations of human essential hypertension. See also *Goldblatt kidney.*

ex·pert testimony or **evidence.** The testimony given before a court of law by an expert witness. See also *medical expert.*

expert witness. An individual skilled in a profession, science, art, or occupation, who testifies before a court or jury to facts within his own sphere of competence, or who gives an opinion on assumed facts. See also *medical expert.*

ex·pi·ra·tion (eck″spi·ray′shun) *n.* [L. *exspirare,* to breathe out]. The act of breathing forth or expelling air from the lungs; exhalation. —**ex·pi·ra·to·ry** (eck·spye′ruh·tor·ee) *adj.*

expiratory emphysema. EMPHYSEMA (1).

expiratory reserve volume. The maximal volume of air that can be expired after involuntary exhalation, as from the end expiratory level. Abbreviated, ERV.

expiratory standstill. Suspension of action at the end of expiration.

ex·pire (eck·spire′) *v.* [L. *exspirare,* from *spirare,* to breathe]. 1. To breathe out; exhale. 2. To die.

expired air. The air that is exhaled from the lungs by expiration.

¹ex·plant (ecks·plant′) *v.* [L. *explantare,* to pull up (a plant)]. To remove (living tissue) from an organism for tissue culture. —**ex·plan·ta·tion** (ecks″plan·tay′shun) *n.*

²ex·plant (ecks′plant) *n.* Tissue that has been explanted for tissue culture.

ex·plode, *v.* [L. *explodere,* to drive out by clapping]. 1. To burst violently and noisily because of sudden release of energy. 2. To cause to burst violently. 3. To discredit and reject, as a theory. 4. To break out suddenly, as an epidemic. —**ex·plo·sive,** *adj.;* **ex·plo·sion,** *n.*

ex·plo·ra·tion, *n.* [L. *explorare,* to explore]. The act of exploring for diagnostic purposes, through investigation of a part hidden from sight, by means of operation, by touch, by artificial light, or by instruments. —**ex·plor·ato·ry,** *adj.*

exploratory incision. An incision made for the purpose of diagnosis.

exploratory operation. An operation performed for the purpose of diagnosis, often an abdominal operation.

exploratory puncture. The puncture of a cyst or cavity for removal of a portion of the contents for examination.

ex·plor·er, *n.* A probe; an instrument for use in exploration.

exploring electrode. *In electrocardiography,* an electrode designed to determine the potential at single points, paired with an indifferent electrode which registers near-zero potential.

exploring needle. A hollow needle or a trocar with a grooved side, which allows the passage of fluid along it after it is plunged into a part where fluid is suspected.

explosive decompression. *In aerospace medicine,* a reduction of barometric pressure which is so rapid as to cause expansion of the involved gases in an explosive manner.

explosive personality. An individual whose behavior pattern, while often excitable and overresponsive to pressures, is marked periodically by strikingly different outbursts of rage and aggression which he apparently cannot control and for which he is usually sorry afterwards. The lack of amnesia and the presence of serial normal electroencephalograms usually distinguish this from an epileptic disorder.

explosive speech. CEREBELLAR SPEECH.

ex·po·sure, *n.* 1. The act of exposing or laying open. 2. Subjection to some condition or influence that may affect detrimentally, as excessive heat, cold, radiation, or infectious agents. 3. *In radiology,* the dose delivered.

exposure keratitis. Inflammation of the cornea from inability of the eyelid to close over it.

exposure of person. *In legal medicine,* the public display of sexual organs before persons of the opposite sex for gratification or erotic purposes. Syn. *indecent exposure.* See also *exhibitionism* (1).

ex·press, *v.* [L. *exprimere, expressus*]. 1. To press or squeeze out. 2. To show, bring out, manifest, as thoughts or feelings.

expressed almond oil. ALMOND OIL.

expressed nutmeg oil. Mace oil or nutmeg butter; a solid oil obtained by hot expression of bruised nutmegs.

ex·pres·sion, *n.* [L. *expressio,* from *exprimere,* to express, from *premere,* to press]. 1. The act of pressing or squeezing out. 2. The means or the results of expressing something.

expression of fetus. Pressure exerted upon the uterus through the abdominal walls to aid in the expulsion of the fetus.

expressive aphasia. BROCA'S APHASIA.

ex·pres·siv·i·ty (eck″spres·iv′i·tee) *n.* The extent to which a given gene manifests itself in the hereditary characteristic which it governs. See also *penetrance.*

ex·pul·sive pain. A bearing-down sensation accompanying the last two stages of labor.

expulsive stage. The stage of labor which begins when dilatation of the cervix uteri is complete and during which the child is expelled from the uterus.

ex·san·gui·nate (eck·sang′gwi·nate) *v.* To drain of blood. —**exsangui·nat·ed** (·nay·tid) *adj.;* **ex·san·gui·na·tion** (eck·sang″gwi·nay′shun) *n.*

exsanguinate, *adj.* [L. *exsanguinatus,* drained of blood]. EXSANGUINE.

ex·san·guine (eck·sang′gwin) *adj.* [L. *exsanguis,* from *sanguis,* blood]. Bloodless; anemic. —**ex·san·guin·i·ty** (eck″sang·gwin′i·tee) *n.*

ex·sec·tion (eck·seck′shun) *n.* [*ex-* + *section*]. EXCISION.

ex·sic·cant (eck·sick′unt) *adj. & n.* 1. Drying or absorbing moisture. 2. DUSTING POWDER.

exsiccated alum. A form of alum deprived of most of its water of crystallization; used as an astringent.

ex·sic·ca·tion (eck″si·kay′shun) *n.* [L. *exsiccatio,* from *exsiccare,* to dry up]. The act of drying; especially, depriving a crystalline body of its water of crystallization. —**ex·sic·cate** (eck′si·kate) *v.;* **ex·sic·ca·tive** (eck·sick′uh·tiv) *adj.*

ex·sic·ca·tor (eck'si·kay"tur) *n.* DESICCATOR.

ex·stro·phy (eck'stro·fee) *n.* [*ex-* + Gk. *strephein,* to turn]. Eversion; the turning inside out of a part.

exstrophy of the bladder. A rare congenital malformation due to failure of the cloaca to close anteriorly, in which the lower anterior part of the abdominal wall, the anterior wall of the urinary bladder, and usually the symphysis pubis are wanting, and the posterior wall of the bladder presents through the opening; associated with epispadias.

ex·suf·fla·tion (eck"suf·lay'shun) *n.* [L. *exsufflare,* to blow away]. Forcible expiration; forcible expulsion of air from the lungs by a mechanical apparatus. See also *exsufflator.*

ex·suf·fla·tor (eck'suf·lay"tur, eck·suf'lay·tur) *n.* An apparatus that can mimic the effect on the bronchial tree of a vigorous cough, by the sudden production of negative pressure.

ext. Abbreviation for *extract.*

ex·ten·sion, *n.* [L. *extensio,* from *extendere,* to stretch out]. 1. A straightening out, especially the muscular movement by which a flexed part is made straight. 2. Traction upon a fractured or dislocated limb. See also *counterextension.* 3. *In psychiatry,* a mental mechanism operating outside and beyond conscious awareness in which an emotional process comes to include areas associated by physical or psychologic contiguity or by continuity, as for example the progression of a phobia to include related objects and areas. 4. Growth (of a neoplasm) into adjacent structures.

extension for prevention. The principle employed in dental-cavity preparation whereby the outline form is extended to areas that are self-cleansing, easily cleaned, or lie under the free gingival margin.

ex·ten·sor (eck·sten'sur) *n.* [L., from *extendere,* to extend]. A muscle which extends or stretches a limb or part. Contr. *flexor.*

extensor car·pi ra·di·a·lis ac·ces·so·ri·us (kahr'pye ray·dee·ay'lis ack"se·so'ree·us). A variant part of the extensor carpi radialis brevis muscle which is inserted into the base of the first metacarpal, the base of the first phalanx of the thumb, or into the short abductor of the thumb.

extensor carpi radialis bre·vi·or (brev'ee·or). EXTENSOR CARPI RADIALIS BREVIS.

extensor carpi radialis bre·vis (brev'is). The short radial extensor of the wrist. NA *musculus extensor carpi radialis brevis.* See Table of Muscles in the Appendix.

extensor carpi radialis in·ter·me·di·us (in"tur·mee'dee·us). A variant part of the extensor carpi radialis brevis muscle inserted into the base of the second or third metacarpal or both.

extensor carpi radialis lon·gi·or (long'gee·or, lon'jee·or). EXTENSOR CARPI RADIALIS LONGUS.

extensor carpi radialis lon·gus (long'gus). The long radial extensor of the wrist. NA *musculus extensor carpi radialis longus.* See Table of Muscles in the Appendix.

extensor carpi ul·na·ris (ul·nair'is). The ulnar extensor of the wrist. NA *musculus extensor carpi ulnaris.* See Table of Muscles in the Appendix.

extensor carpi ulnaris di·gi·ti mi·ni·mi (dij'i·tye min'i·migh). A rare variant part of the extensor carpi ulnaris muscle inserted into the base of the proximal phalanx of the little finger.

extensor coccygeus. SACROCOCCYGEUS DORSALIS.

extensor com·mu·nis pol·li·cis et in·di·cis (kom·yoo'nis pol'i·sis et in'di·sis). An occasional extra extensor arising from the dorsal surface of the ulna and the interosseous membrane and inserted into both thumb and index finger.

extensor di·gi·ti an·nu·la·ris (dij'i·tye an"yoo·lair'is). A rare anomalous muscle arising from the dorsal surface of the distal end of the ulna and inserted into the ring finger; a variant of the extensor indicis muscle.

extensor digiti me·dii (mee'dee·eye). A rare anomalous muscle arising from the dorsal surface of the distal end of the ulna and inserted into the middle finger; a variant of the extensor indicis muscle.

extensor digiti mi·ni·mi (min'i·migh). The extensor of the little finger. NA *musculus extensor digiti minimi.* See Table of Muscles in the Appendix.

extensor digiti quin·ti pro·pri·us (kwin'tye pro'pree·us). EXTENSOR DIGITI MINIMI.

extensor di·gi·to·rum (dij"i·to'rum). The extensor of the fingers. NA *musculus extensor digitorum.* See Table of Muscles in the Appendix.

extensor digitorum bre·vis (brev'is). The short extensor of the toes. NA *musculus extensor digitorum brevis.* See Table of Muscles in the Appendix.

extensor digitorum brevis ma·nus (man'oos, man'us). Any of various rare anomalous muscle bands arising from the dorsal surface of the ulnar carpal bones and inserted into the usual extensor tendons of the fingers or into the metacarpals.

extensor digitorum com·mu·nis (kom·yoo'nis). EXTENSOR DIGITORUM.

extensor digitorum lon·gus (long'gus). The long extensor of the toes. NA *musculus extensor digitorum longus.* See Table of Muscles in the Appendix.

extensor hal·lu·cis bre·vis (hal'yoo·sis brev'is). The part of the extensor digitorum brevis muscle for the great toe. NA *musculus extensor hallucis brevis.* See Table of Muscles in the Appendix.

extensor hallucis lon·gus (long'gus). The long extensor of the great toe. NA *musculus extensor hallucis longus.* See Table of Muscles in the Appendix.

extensor hallucis pro·pri·us (pro'pree·us). EXTENSOR HALLUCIS LONGUS.

extensor in·di·cis (in'di·sis). The extensor of the index finger. NA *musculus extensor indicis.* See Table of Muscles in the Appendix.

extensor indicis pro·pri·us (pro'pree·us). EXTENSOR INDICIS.

extensor os·sis me·ta·car·pi pol·li·cis (oss'is met"uh·kahr'pye pol'i·sis). ABDUCTOR POLLICIS LONGUS.

extensor ossis me·ta·tar·si hal·lu·cis (met"uh·tahr'sigh hal'yoo·sis). An occasional part of the extensor hallucis longus muscle inserted into the first metatarsal.

extensor plantar reflex or **response.** BABINSKI SIGN (1).

extensor pol·li·cis bre·vis (pol'i·sis brev'is). The short extensor of the thumb. NA *musculus extensor pollicis brevis.* See Table of Muscles in the Appendix.

extensor pollicis lon·gus (long'gus). The long extensor of the thumb. NA *musculus extensor pollicis longus.* See Table of Muscles in the Appendix.

extensor pri·mi in·ter·no·dii lon·gus hal·lu·cis (prye'migh in"tur·no'dee·eye long'gus hal'yoo·sis). An occasional part of the extensor hallucis longus muscle inserted into the proximal phalanx of the great toe.

extensor primi internodii pol·li·cis (pol'i·sis). EXTENSOR POLLICIS BREVIS.

extensor retinaculum. A thickening of deep fascia overlying tendons of extensor muscles. See also *extensor retinaculum of the wrist, inferior extensor retinaculum, superior extensor retinaculum.*

extensor retinaculum of the wrist. A thickened band of deep fascia attached to the radius laterally and the ulna, carpus, and medial ligaments of the wrist medially. It overlies the extensor tendons of the wrist and fingers. Syn. *dorsal carpal ligament.* NA *retinaculum extensorum manus.*

extensor se·cun·di in·ter·no·dii pol·li·cis (se·kun'dye in"tur·no'dee·eye pol'i·sis). EXTENSOR POLLICIS LONGUS.

extensor thrust reflex. Rapid reflex contraction of extensor muscles; occurs in the leg of a spinal animal when the bottom of the foot makes firm contact with a solid surface.

ex·te·ri·or·iza·tion (ecks·teer"ee·ur·i·zay'shun) *n.* 1. *In psychiatry,* the turning of one's interests outward. 2. *In surgery,* an operation that brings an internal organ or part to the surface or exterior of the body, and fixes it in that position.

ex·tern, ex·terne (ecks'turn) *n.* [F. *externe,* from L. *externus,* external]. A medical school student who helps with the care of hospitalized patients.

ex·ter·nal (ecks·tur'nul) *adj.* 1. Exterior; acting from without. 2. *In anatomy,* on or near the outside of the body; away from the center or middle line of the body. 3. Not essential; superficial. —**exter·nad** (·nad) *adv.*

external abdominal ring. SUPERFICIAL INGUINAL RING.

external acoustic meatus. The passage in the external ear from the auricle or pinna to the tympanic membrane. NA *meatus acusticus externus.*

external anal sphincter. Bundles of striate muscle fibers surrounding the anus. NA *musculus sphincter ani externus.* See also Table of Muscles in the Appendix.

external aneurysm. 1. An aneurysm remote from the great body cavities. 2. An aneurysm in which the cavity is entirely or chiefly outside the inner coat of the artery.

external arcuate fibers. Arching fibers running over the surface of the medulla oblongata to the inferior cerebellar peduncle. NA *fibrae arcuatae externae.*

external auditory meatus or **canal.** EXTERNAL ACOUSTIC MEATUS.

external auditory meatus reflex. AURICULOPALPEBRAL REFLEX.

external ballottement. *In obstetrics,* the rebound of the fetal head against the examiner's hand, felt on pressure of the abdominal wall.

external capsule. A layer of white nerve fibers forming part of the external boundary of the lenticular nucleus. Syn. *capsula externa.*

external carotid artery. An artery which originates at the common carotid and has superior thyroid, ascending pharyngeal, lingual, facial, sternocleidomastoid (occasionally), occipital, posterior auricular, superficial temporal, and maxillary branches. It distributes blood to the anterior portion of the neck, face, scalp, side of the head, ear, and dura mater. NA *arteria carotis externa.*

external carotid nerves. Sympathetic nerves which form plexuses on the external carotid artery and its branches. NA *nervi carotici externi.* See also *carotid in Table of Nerves in the Appendix.*

external carotid plexus. A network of sympathetic nerve fibers surrounding the external carotid artery, formed by the external carotid nerves and providing fibers which form networks along the branches of the artery. NA *plexus caroticus externus.*

external cloaca. ECTODERMAL CLOACA.

external conjugate diameter. The distance from the depression above the spine of the first sacral vertebra to the middle of the upper border of the symphysis pubis. Syn. *Baudeloque's diameter.*

external cuneate nucleus. ACCESSORY CUNEATE NUCLEUS.

external ear. The part of the ear that is external to the tympanic membrane, consisting of the external acoustic meatus and the pinna. NA *auris externa.*

external elastic membrane or **lamina.** The membrane of the wall of some arteries forming the boundary between the tunica media and tunica adventitia. See also Plate 6.

external factor. An external component of the environment of an organism, such as heat, gravity.

external fistula. A fistula opening from some body cavity to the skin.

external genitalia. In the male, the penis and testes; in the female, the vulva, vagina, and clitoris. See also *sex organs.*

external genu of the facial nerve. The sharp bend of the facial nerve around the outer border of the vestibule of the inner ear. The geniculate ganglion is located at this bend. NA *geniculum nervi facialis.* Compare *internal genu of the facial nerve.*

external granular layer. 1. (of the cerebellum:) A granular layer in fetal and neonatal cerebellar cortex. 2. (of the cerebrum:) The second layer of the cerebral cortex, containing a large number of small pyramidal and granule cells. Syn. *layer of small pyramidal cells.*

external hamstring reflex. A muscle stretch reflex elicited by tapping the tendon of the biceps femoris muscle just above its insertion on the lateral side of the head of the fibula and the lateral condyle of the tibia. The response is flexion of the leg on the thigh and moderate external rotation of the leg. Syn. *biceps femoris reflex, posterior peroneofemoral reflex.*

external hemorrhoid or **pile.** A hemorrhoid protruding below the anal sphincter.

external hirudiniasis. The form of hirudiniasis produced by leeches of the genus *Haemadipsa,* which attach themselves to and puncture the skin of humans. The leeches suck the blood and secrete an anticoagulating principle, hirudin.

external hordeolum. A circumscribed, acute inflammation on the edge of the lid, produced by staphylococcal infection of one of the ciliary glands or of Zeis' glands.

external hydrocephalus or **hydrocephaly.** *Obsol.* An increased accumulation of fluid in the subarachnoid or the subdural space.

external inguinal ring. SUPERFICIAL INGUINAL RING.

ex·ter·nal·ize (ecks·tur'nul·ize) *v.* 1. *In psychology,* to transform an idea or impression which is on the percipient's mind into an external phantasm. 2. To refer to some outside source, as the voices heard by the subject of hallucinations.

external limiting membrane. 1. In the eye, the thin layer between the outer nuclear layer of the retina and that of the rods and cones; not actually a membrane but a series of junctional complexes between Müller's fibers and the rods and cones. 2. *In embryology,* the membrane investing the outer surface of the neural tube.

external malleolar sign or **reflex.** CHADDOCK'S REFLEX (1).

external malleolus. LATERAL MALLEOLUS.

external maxillary artery. FACIAL ARTERY.

external medullary lamina. Fibers lying along the outer border of the thalamus and separating it from the internal capsule.

external meniscus. LATERAL MENISCUS.

external migration. The passage of the ovum from an ovary to the adjacent oviduct.

external nose. The portion of the nose that protrudes on the face and consists of a framework of bone and cartilage with investing integument and mucous membrane. NA *nasus externus.*

external occipital crest. A vertical ridge on the outer surface of the occipital bone, extending from the occipital protuberance to the foramen magnum. NA *crista occipitalis externa.*

external occipital protuberance. The central prominence on the outer surface of the flat portion of the occipital bone. NA *protuberantia occipitalis externa.*

external ophthalmopathy. An affection of the eyelids, cornea, conjunctiva, or muscles of the eye.

external ophthalmoplegia. Paralysis of the extrinsic ocular muscles, sparing the pupillary muscles.

external os. OSTIUM UTERI.

external os uteri. OSTIUM UTERI.

external pelvimetry. Measurement of the external diameters of the pelvis, to estimate the dimensions of the internal parts.

external pericarditis. Pericarditis chiefly affecting the outer layer of the parietal pericardium.

external phase. DISPERSION MEDIUM.

external pyramidal layer. LAYER OF PYRAMIDAL CELLS.

external ramus of the accessory nerve. The spinal portion of the accessory nerve which innervates the trapezius and sternocleidomastoid muscles. NA *ramus externus nervi accessorii.*

external rectus. Rectus lateralis bulbi. See Table of Muscles in the Appendix.

external respiration. The interchange of gases between the atmosphere and the air in the lungs and between the air in the lungs and the pulmonary capillaries. Contr. *internal respiration.*

external secretion. A secretion thrown out upon any epithelial surface of the body. See also *exocrine.*

external semilunar cartilage or **fibrocartilage**. LATERAL MENISCUS.

external sensation. A sensation transmitted from a peripheral sense organ.

external skeletal fixation. *In dentistry and surgery,* a method of immobilizing bony fragments of fractures by the use of metal pin or screw devices applied externally; adapted especially to edentulous mouths.

external spermatic fascia. The outer covering of the spermatic cord and testis, continuous with the aponeurosis of the external oblique muscle at the subcutaneous inguinal ring. NA *fascia spermatica externa.*

external spermatic nerve. The genital branch of the genitofemoral nerve. See also Table of Nerves in the Appendix.

external strabismus. EXOTROPIA.

external transmigration. The passage of an ovum from one ovary to the opposite oviduct without traversing the uterus.

external urethrotomy. *In surgery,* division of a urethral stricture by an incision from without.

external uterine os. OSTIUM UTERI.

external ventriculostomy. Ventriculostomy accomplished by a communication between a lateral ventricle and an external closed drainage system.

external version. ABDOMINAL VERSION.

externe. EXTERN.

ex·tero·cep·tive (eck″stur·o·sep′tiv) *adj.* [L. *exter,* outward, + *receptive*]. Activated by or pertaining to stimuli impinging on an organism from outside.

exteroceptive impulses. Afferent nerve impulses that derive their stimulation from external sources.

exteroceptive reflex. Any reflex elicited by stimulation of an exteroceptor. The reflex arc is a multineuron arc.

ex·tero·cep·tor (eck″stur·o·sep′tur) *n.* An end organ, in or near the skin or a mucous membrane, which receives stimuli from the external world.

ex·tero·fec·tive (eck″stur·o·feck′tiv) *adj.* [L. *exter,* outward, + ef*fective*]. *Obsol.* Pertaining to the voluntary nervous system (the central nervous system and the somatic nerves).

exterofective system. *Obsol.* The part of the nervous system that is concerned with adapting the body to changes in its external environment.

ex·tinc·tion (eck·stink′shun) *n.* [L. *extinctio,* from *extinguere,* to extinguish]. 1. The act of putting out or extinguishing; destruction. 2. *In neurophysiology,* the disappearance of excitability of a nerve, synapse, or nervous tissue to a previously adequate stimulus. 3. *In clinical neurology,* the failure to recognize one of two simultaneously presented stimuli. 4. *In psychology,* the disappearance of a conditioned reflex when excited repeatedly without reinforcement. Compare *inhibition.*

ex·tir·pa·tion (eck″stur·pay′shun) *n.* [L. *exstirpare,* to pluck out by the stem or root]. Complete removal of a part or surgical destruction of a part.

Ex·ton and Rose's test [W. G. *Exton,* U.S. physician, 1876–1943]. A type of glucose tolerance test.

Exton's method [W. G. *Exton*]. A method for determining the specific gravity of small amounts of fluid by suspending it in an immiscible medium of the same specific gravity as the specimen.

Exton's reagent [W. G. *Exton*]. Either of two slightly different watery solutions of sulfosalicylic acid and sodium sulfate; used in a qualitative and a quantitative urine protein test.

Exton's test [W. G. *Exton*]. A test for urine protein in which equal volumes of clear urine and Exton's qualitative reagent are mixed in a test tube. Cloudiness appearing upon heating indicates protein.

ex·tor·sion (ecks·tor′shun) *n.* [L. *extorsio,* from *extorquere,* to twist out]. 1. Outward rotation of a part. 2. *In ophthalmology,* a turning outward of the vertical meridians.

extra- [L.]. A prefix meaning (a) *outside of;* (b) *beyond the scope of.*

ex·tra·ar·tic·u·lar (ecks″truh·ahr·tick′yoo·lur) *adj.* [*extra-* + *articular*]. Outside a joint.

ex·tra·buc·cal (ecks″truh·buck′ul) *adj.* [*extra-* + *buccal*]. Outside the mouth. Syn. *extraoral.*

extrabuccal feeding. The introduction of food into the system by channels other than the mouth; especially, feeding by nutritive enema, by intravascular injection, or by gastric tubes.

ex·tra·bul·bar (ecks″truh·bul′bur) *adj.* [*extra-* + *bulbar*]. Exterior to a bulb; specifically, exterior to the medulla oblongata.

ex·tra·cam·pine (ecks″truh·kam′pine) *adj.* [*extra* + L. *campus,* field, + *-ine*]. Outside a field of perception, usually the visual field.

extracampine hallucination. A hallucination that occurs outside the normal field of perception of the sense organ involved, as seeing someone behind one's head.

ex·tra·cap·su·lar (ecks″truh·kap′sue·lur) *adj.* [*extra-* + *capsular*]. Outside a capsule; outside the capsular ligament of a joint.

extracapsular ankylosis. Ankylosis due to rigidity of the parts external to the joint, as interference resulting from bony block, adhesions of tendons and tendon sheaths, contractures due to muscles, scars, or thickening of skin in scleroderma, or from heterotopic periarticular bone formation following injury or operation. Syn. *false ankylosis, spurious ankylosis.*

extracapsular fracture. A fracture near a joint but not entering within the joint capsule.

ex·tra·car·di·ac (eck″struh·kahr′dee·ack) *adj.* [*extra-* + *cardiac*]. Outside the heart.

ex·tra·car·di·al (eck″struh·kahr′dee·ul) *adj.* EXTRACARDIAC.

ex·tra·car·pal (ecks″truh·kahr′pul) *adj.* [*extra-* + *carpal*]. Exterior to the wrist bones.

ex·tra·cel·lu·lar (ecks″truh·sel′yoo·lur) *adj.* [*extra-* + *cellular*]. External to the cells of an organism.

extracellular cholesterosis. A disturbance of lipid metabolism, in which reddish-blue nodules appear on the hands and other areas of the body; a variant of erythema elevatum diutinum.

extracellular enzyme. An enzyme which retains its activity when removed from the cell in which it is formed, or which normally exerts its activity at a site removed from the place of formation. Syn. *lyoenzyme.*

ex·tra·cer·e·bral (ecks″truh·serr′e·brul) *adj.* [*extra-* + *cerebral*]. Outside the brain, but within the cranial cavity.

ex·tra·chro·mo·som·al (ecks″truh·kro″muh·so′mul) *adj.* [*extra-* + *chromosomal*]. Outside a chromosome; not involving chromosomes.

extrachromosomal inheritance. Hereditary transmission via a factor not located on a chromosome.

ex·tra·cor·po·ral (eck″struh·kor′puh·rul) *adj.* EXTRACORPOREAL.

ex·tra·cor·po·re·al (ecks″truh·kor·po′ree·ul) *adj.* [*extra-* + *corporeal*]. Outside the body.

ex·tra·cor·pus·cu·lar (ecks″truh·kor·pus′kew·lur) *adj.* [*extra-* + *corpuscular*]. Outside a corpuscle; especially, outside a blood cell.

ex·tra·cra·ni·al (ecks″truh·kray′nee·ul) *adj.* [*extra-* + *cranial*]. Outside the cranial cavity.

ex·tract (eck′strakt) *n.* [L. *extractum,* from *extrahere,* to draw out]. 1. A pharmaceutical preparation obtained by dissolving the active constituents of a drug with a suitable solvent, evaporating the solvent, and adjusting to prescribed standards, often so that one part of the extract represents four to six parts of the drug. Abbreviated, ext. 2. A preparation, usually in a concentrated form, obtained by treating plant or animal tissue with a solvent to remove desired odoriferous, flavorful, or nutritive components of the tissue.

ex·trac·tion (eck·strack'shun) *n.* 1. The act of drawing out. 2. The process of making an extract. 3. The surgical removal of a tooth. —**ex·tract** (eck·strakt') *v.*

extraction of cataract. The surgical removal of a cataractous lens.

ex·trac·tive (eck·strack'tiv) *n.* 1. That which is extracted. 2. An unidentified substance extracted in chemical analyses; as ether extractive, that material which is extracted with ether.

ex·trac·tor (eck·strack'tur) *n.* 1. An instrument or forceps for extracting bullets, sequestra, or foreign bodies. 2. *In dentistry,* an instrument for extracting the root of a tooth.

ex·tra·cyst·ic (ecks"truh·sist'ick) *adj.* [*extra-* + *cystic*]. Outside a cyst, the urinary bladder, or the gallbladder.

ex·tra·du·ral (ecks"truh·dew'rul) *adj.* [*extra-* + *dural*]. EPIDURAL.

extradural abscess. EPIDURAL ABSCESS.

extradural anesthesia. PERIDURAL ANESTHESIA.

extradural cavity. EPIDURAL SPACE.

extradural empyema. EPIDURAL ABSCESS.

extradural hemorrhage. EPIDURAL HEMATOMA.

extradural sacral anesthesia. CAUDAL ANESTHESIA.

ex·tra·em·bry·on·ic (ecks"truh·em"bree·on'ick) *adj.* [*extra-* + *embryonic*]. Situated outside, or not forming a part of, the embryo.

extraembryonic blastoderm. The part of a blastoderm forming the extraembryonic membranes.

extraembryonic coelom. The cavity in the extraembryonic mesoderm; between sheets of chorionic mesoderm and between the mesoderm of the amnion and yolk sac. It is continuous with the embryonic coelom in the region of the umbilicus, and is obliterated by the growth of the amnion.

extraembryonic membrane. Any of the membranes surrounding the embryo or fetus, shed at birth. See also *allantois, amnion, chorion, yolk sac.*

extraembryonic mesoderm. The earliest mesoderm of the embryo, derived from the trophoblast, that forms a part of the amnion, chorion and yolk sac, and the body stalk.

ex·tra·epiph·y·se·al (ecks"truh·ep"i·fiz'ee·ul, ·e·pif"i·see'ul) *adj.* [*extra-* + *epiphyseal*]. Outside, or away from, an epiphysis.

ex·tra·ep·i·phys·i·al (ecks"truh·ep"i·fiz'ee·ul) *adj.* EXTRAEPIPHYSEAL.

ex·tra·eryth·ro·cyt·ic (ecks"truh·e·rith"ro·sit'ick) *adj.* [*extra-* + *erythrocytic*]. EXOERYTHROCYTIC.

ex·tra·esoph·a·ge·al (ecks"truh·e·sof"uh·jee'ul, ·ee"so·faj'ee·ul) *adj.* [*extra-* + *esophageal*]. Immediately surrounding the esophagus, as the extraesophageal region of the mediastinum.

ex·tra·fas·ci·al (eck"struh·fash'ee·ul) *adj.* [*extra-* + *fascial*]. Outside a fascia.

ex·tra·gen·i·tal (ecks"truh·jen'i·tul) *adj.* [*extra-* + *genital*]. Situated outside of, or unrelated to, the genitals.

extragenital syphilis. Syphilis in which the primary lesion is situated elsewhere than on the genital organs.

ex·tra·gin·gi·val (ecks"truh·jin'ji·vul) *adj.* [*extra-* + *gingival*]. Situated outside or above the gingiva.

extragingival calculus. SUPRAGINGIVAL CALCULUS.

ex·tra·he·pat·ic (ecks"truh·he·pat'ick) *adj.* [*extra-* + *hepatic*]. Outside, or not connected with, the liver; especially, referring to disease affecting the liver, in which the primary lesion is external to the organ, as an extrahepatic biliary obstruction.

ex·tra·lig·a·men·tous (ecks"truh·lig"uh·men'tus) *adj.* [*extra-* + *ligamentous*]. External to a ligament.

Extralin. Trademark for a liver-stomach concentrate used orally in the treatment of pernicious anemia.

ex·tra·mam·ma·ry (eck"struh·mam'uh·ree) *adj.* [*extra-* + *mammary*]. Outside the mammary gland; usually referring to a condition associated with the breast but occurring in another location.

extramammary Paget's carcinoma [J. *Paget*]. APOCRINE CARCINOMA.

ex·tra·med·ul·lary (ecks"truh·med'yoo·lerr"ee) *adj.* [*extra-* + *medullary*]. 1. Situated or occurring outside the spinal cord or brainstem. 2. Situated or occurring outside the bone marrow.

extramedullary glioma. A glioma arising in heterotopic glial tissue.

extramedullary hemopoiesis. Formation of blood outside the bone marrow.

extramedullary myelopoiesis. EXTRAMEDULLARY HEMOPOIESIS.

ex·tra·mu·ral (ecks"truh·mew'rul) *adj.* [*extra-* + *mural*]. Outside the wall of an organ.

ex·tra·nu·cle·ar (ecks"truh·new'klee·ur) *adj.* [*extra-* + *nuclear*]. Outside the nucleus of a cell.

ex·tra·oc·u·lar (eck"struh·ock'yoo·lur) *adj.* [*extra-* + *ocular*]. Extrinsic to the eyeball.

extraocular paralysis or **palsy.** Paralysis of the extrinsic muscles of the eye.

ex·tra·oral (ecks"truh·or'ul) *adj.* [*extra-* + *oral*]. Outside the mouth. Syn. *extrabuccal.*

ex·tra·os·se·ous (eck"struh·os'ee·us) *adj.* [*extra-* + *osseous*]. Outside a bone or bones.

ex·tra·pa·ren·chy·mal (ecks"truh·pa·reng'ki·mul) *adj.* [*extra-* + *parenchymal*]. Outside of or unrelated to the parenchyma.

ex·tra·pel·vic (ecks"truh·pel'vick) *adj.* [*extra-* + *pelvic*]. Situated or occurring outside the pelvis.

ex·tra·per·i·ne·al (ecks"truh·perr"i·nee'ul) *adj.* [*extra-* + *perineal*]. Outside or away from the perineum.

ex·tra·peri·to·ne·al (ecks"truh·perr"i·tuh·nee'ul) *adj.* External to the peritoneal cavity.

ex·tra·pla·cen·tal (ecks"truh·pluh·sen'tul) *adj.* [*extra-* + *placental*]. Not connected with the placenta.

ex·tra·pleu·ral (ecks"truh·ploo'rul) *adj.* [*extra-* + *pleural*]. Outside the pleura or the pleural cavity, or both.

extrapleural pneumonolysis. The separation of an area of parietal pleura from the chest wall. See also *apicolysis.*

extrapleural pneumothorax. Pneumothorax in which the parietal pleura is stripped from the thoracic wall, and the air or gas introduced within the space so formed, as in apicolysis.

ex·trap·o·late (ecks·trap'uh·late) *v.* 1. *In statistics,* to estimate a quantity which depends on one or more variables not known by projecting, extending, or expanding such data as are known. 2. To interpret or explain any phenomenon, whether physical or mental, of which the causative factors are secondary or circumstantial. —**ex·trap·o·la·tion** (ecks·trap"uh·lay'shun) *n.*

extrapolation chamber. An ionization chamber for the measurement of roentgen-ray intensities arranged so that the enclosed volume of air may be altered and reduced almost to zero.

ex·tra·pros·tat·ic (ecks"truh·pros·tat'ick) *adj.* [*extra-* + *prostatic*]. Outside or away from the prostate.

ex·tra·psy·chic (ecks"truh·sigh'kick) *adj.* [*extra-* + *psychic*]. Occurring outside the mind or psyche.

extrapsychic conflict. *In psychiatry,* conflict between the self and the outside world.

ex·tra·pul·mo·nary (ecks"truh·pul'muh·nerr"ee) *adj.* [*extra-* + *pulmonary*]. Outside or independent of the lungs.

extrapulmonary bronchus. PRIMARY BRONCHUS.

extrapulmonary tuberculosis. Tuberculous disease in organs or structures other than the lungs.

ex·tra·py·ram·i·dal (ecks"truh·pi·ram'i·dul) *adj.* [*extra-* + *py-*

ramidal]. 1. Outside the pyramidal tracts, applied to other descending motor pathways. 2. Pertaining to or involving the extrapyramidal system.

extrapyramidal disorder or **syndrome.** Any manifestation or complex of symptoms due to a disorder or disease of the extrapyramidal system; manifestations include tremors, muscular rigidity, and dyskinesias, as in hepatolenticular degeneration, Parkinson's disease, or phenothiazine intoxication.

extrapyramidal epilepsy. *Obsol.* STRIATAL EPILEPSY.

extrapyramidal motor areas. Extensive areas of the frontal cerebral cortex other than those which give rise to corticospinal tract fibers, i.e., other than Brodmann's areas 4 and 6a.

extrapyramidal system. A widespread and complicated system of descending fiber tracts arising in the cortex and subcortical motor centers; in the widest sense it includes all nonpyramidal motor tracts; in the usual clinical sense it includes the striatopallidonigral and cerebellar motor systems.

ex·tra·re·nal (ecks"truh·ree'nul) *adj.* [*extra-* + *renal*]. Outside of or not involving a kidney or kidneys.

extrarenal uremia. PRERENAL UREMIA.

ex·tra·sen·so·ry (eck"struh·sen'suh·ree) *adj.* [*extra-* + *sensory*]. 1. Of or pertaining to phenomena outside the realm normally perceived through the senses; not sensory. 2. Of or pertaining to certain capacities of perception unexplainable in relation to the senses. See also *psi phenomena, extrasensory perception.*

extrasensory perception. Direct awareness without the use of the senses; telepathy; clairvoyance; precognition. Abbreviated, ESP. See also *psi phenomena.*

ex·tra·sphinc·ter·ic (ecks"truh·sfink·terr'ick) *adj.* [*extra-* + *sphincteric*]. Outside a sphincter.

extrasphincteric fistula. A rectal or anal fistula external to the sphincter.

ex·tra·spi·nal (ecks"truh·spye'nul) *adj.* [*extra-* + *spinal*]. Outside the spinal or vertebral column.

extraspinal plexus. A large venous plexus extending the length of the vertebral column and lying between it and the multifidus muscle.

ex·tra·sys·to·le (ecks"truh·sis'tuh·lee) *n.* [*extra-* + *systole*]. PREMATURE BEAT.

ex·tra·thy·roi·dal (eck"struh·thigh·roy'dul) *adj.* [*extra-* + *thyroid* + *-al*]. Outside the thyroid gland.

ex·tra·tu·bal (ecks"truh·tew'bul) *adj.* [*extra-* + *tubal*]. Outside a tube, as the uterine tube.

ex·tra·uter·ine (ecks"truh·yoo'tur·in, ·ine) *adj.* [*extra-* + *uterine*]. Outside the uterus.

extrauterine pregnancy or **gestation.** Development of the fertilized ovum outside the uterine cavity.

ex·tra·va·gi·nal (ecks"truh·vaj'i·nul, ·va·jye'nul) *adj.* [*extra-* + *vaginal*]. Outside the vagina or any sheath.

ex·trav·a·sa·tion (ecks·trav"uh·say'shun) *n.* [*extra-* + L. *vas,* vessel]. 1. The passing of a body fluid out of its proper place, as blood into surrounding tissues after rupture of a vessel. 2. Material so discharged. —**ex·trav·a·sate** (ecks·trav'uh·sate) *v. & n.*

extravasation cyst. A cavity formed by encapsulation of extravasated fluid, usually blood, as a hematoma.

ex·tra·vas·cu·lar (ecks"truh·vas'kew·lur) *adj.* [*extra-* + *vascular*]. Outside a vessel.

extravascular theory of erythrocyte formation. A theory that erythrocytes are formed in the reticular mesh of bone marrow outside of the circulatory system and enter it through sinusoids.

ex·tra·ven·tric·u·lar (ecks"truh·ven·trick'yoo·lur) *adj.* [*extra-* + *ventricular*]. Occurring or situated external to a ventricle.

ex·tra·ver·sion (ecks"truh·vur'zhun) *n.* EXTROVERSION.

ex·tra·vert (ecks'truh·vurt) *n. & v.* EXTROVERT.

ex·tra·vis·u·al (ecks"truh·vizh'yoo·ul) *adj.* [*extra-* + *visual*]. Outside the limits of vision.

extreme capsule. A layer of white matter separating the claustrum from the insula.

ex·tre·mi·tas (eck·strem'i·tas) *n.*, genit. **ex·tre·mi·ta·tis** (eck·strem"i·tay'tis), pl. **extremita·tes** (·teez) [L.]. 1. [BNA] The upper or lower extremity or member. 2. [NA] The end of an elongated or pointed structure.

extremitas acro·mi·a·lis cla·vi·cu·lae (a·kro"mee·ay'lis cla·vick'yoo·lee) [NA]. The acromial (lateral) end of the clavicle.

extremitas anterior li·e·nis (lye·ee'nis) [NA]. The lower pole of the spleen.

extremitas inferior [BNA]. Membrum inferius (= LOWER EXTREMITY).

extremitas inferior li·e·nis (lye·ee'nis) [BNA]. EXTREMITAS ANTERIOR LIENIS.

extremitas inferior re·nis (ree'nis) [NA]. The lower pole of the kidney.

extremitas inferior tes·tis (tes'tis) [NA]. The lower end of the testis.

extremitas posterior li·e·nis (lye·ee'nis) [NA]. The upper pole of the spleen.

extremitas ster·na·lis cla·vi·cu·lae (stur·nay'lis kla·vick'yoo·lee) [NA]. The sternal (medial) end of the clavicle.

extremitas superior [BNA]. Membrum superius (= UPPER EXTREMITY).

extremitas superior li·e·nis (lye·ee'nis) [BNA]. EXTREMITAS POSTERIOR LIENIS.

extremitas superior re·nis (ree'nis) [NA]. The superior pole of the kidney.

extremitas superior tes·tis (tes'tis) [NA]. The upper end of the testis.

extremitas tu·ba·ria ova·rii (tew·bair'ee·uh o·vair'ee·eye) [NA]. The end of the ovary related to the free end of the uterine tube.

extremitas ute·ri·na ova·rii (yoo·tur·eye'nuh o·vair'ee·eye) [NA]. The end of the ovary directed toward the uterus.

ex·trem·i·ty, *n.* [L. *extremitas*]. 1. The distal, or terminal, end of any part. 2. An upper or lower limb.

ex·trin·sic (eck·strin'zick, ·sick) *adj.* [L. *extrinsecus,* on the outside]. Originating outside.

extrinsic allergic dermatitis. Allergic dermatitis caused by any external substance capable of penetrating the epidermis, such as that caused by contact with poison ivy.

extrinsic allergy. An allergic reaction caused by an allergen that originates outside the body.

extrinsic asthma. Asthma caused by inhalants, foods, or drugs. Contr. *intrinsic asthma.*

extrinsic factor. VITAMIN B_{12}.

extrinsic muscle. A muscle which has its origin outside, and its insertion into, an organ, as a rectus muscle of the eye. Contr. *intrinsic muscle.*

extrinsic nerve supply. The nerves of an organ or structure that connect it with the central nervous system. Contr. *intrinsic nerve supply.*

extrinsic thromboplastin. Any of several lipid-rich clot accelerators not normally present in blood.

extro-. A prefix meaning (a) *outside;* (b) *outward.*

ex·tro·gas·tru·la·tion (ecks"tro·gas"troo·lay'shun) *n.* [*extro-* + *gastrulation*]. EXOGASTRULATION.

ex·tro·phia (eck·stro'fee·uh) *n.* EXSTROPHY.

ex·tro·phy (ecks'tro·fee) *n.* 1. Malformation of an organ. 2. EXSTROPHY.

ex·tro·ver·sion (ecks"tro·vur'zhun) *n.* [from *extrovert* (verb)]. 1. A turning outward. 2. *In psychoanalytic theory,* the turning of the libido outward, as to a love object. 3. *In psychiatry,* a turning to things and persons outside oneself rather than to one's own thoughts and feelings. Contr. *introversion.* 4. Unusual widening of the dental arch.

ex·tro·vert (ecks'tro·vurt) *v. & n.* [*extro-* + L. *vertere,* to turn]. 1. To turn one's interests to external things rather than to oneself. 2. A person whose interests center in the outside world rather than in subjective activity.

ex·tru·sion (eck·stroo'zhun) *n.* [ML. *extrusio,* from *extrudere,* to drive out]. 1. A forcing out; expulsion. 2. *In dentistry,* movement of a tooth beyond the occlusal plane. —**ex·trude** (eck·strood') *v.*

ex·tu·ba·tion (ecks''tew·bay'shun) *n.* The removal of a tube used for intubation.

ex·u·ber·ant (eg·zew'bur·unt) *adj.* [L. *exuberare,* to be abundant, from *uber,* rich, copious]]. 1. Unrestrained; uninhibited; abundant. 2. Pertaining to or characterized by excessive proliferation or growth of a tissue, as a granulation tissue. —**exuber·ance,** *n.*

exuberant granulation. An excess of granulation tissue in the base of an ulcer or in a healing wound. Syn. *fungous granulation, proud flesh.*

exuberant ulcer. An ulcer which has an excess of granulation tissue growing from the base.

ex·u·date (ecks'yoo·date) *n.* [L. *exudatus, exsudatus,* exuded]. 1. A material, with a high content of protein and cells, that has passed through the walls of vessels into adjacent tissues or spaces, especially in inflammation. 2. Any exuded substance. Compare *transudate.*

ex·u·da·tion (ecks''yoo·day'shun) *n.* [L. *exudare, exsudare,* to sweat out, from *sudare,* to sweat]. The passage of various constituents of the blood through the walls of vessels into adjacent tissues or spaces, especially in inflammation. —**ex·u·da·tive** (ecks·yoo'duh·tiv, ecks'yoo·day''tiv) *adj.;* **ex·ude** (eck·sue'd') *v.*

exudative angina. CROUP.

exudative choroiditis. Choroiditis in which there is production of marked inflammatory exudate thickening the choroid and producing a secondary detachment of the retinal pigment epithelium or of the retina itself.

exudative eczema. An acute eczematous dermatitis with exudation of serum. Syn. *weeping eczema.*

ex·u·vi·a·tion (eg·zew''vee·ay'shun) *n.* [L. *exuviae,* shed skin, from *exuere,* to take off, shed]. The shedding of the primary teeth, or of epidermal structures.

ex vi·vo (ecks vee'vo) [L.]. Outside the living organism; characterizing an operation or other procedure performed on a living organ or tissue that has been removed from the body. Contr. *in vivo.*

ex vivo surgery. BENCH SURGERY.

eye, *n.* [OE. *ēage*←Gmc. *aug-* (rel. to L. *oculus* and to Gk. *op-*)]. The organ of vision which occupies the anterior part of the orbit and which is nearly spherical. It is composed of three concentric coats: the sclera and cornea; the choroid, ciliary body, and iris; and the retina. Abbreviated, E. NA *oculus.* See also Plate 19.

eye·ball, *n.* The globe of the eye. NA *bulbus oculi.* See also Plate 19.

eyeball compression reflex. OCULOCARDIAC REFLEX.

eye·brow, *n.* 1. The arch above the eye. NA *supercilium.* 2. The hair covering the arch. NA *supercilia.*

eye closure reflex. 1. Closure of the eyelids on tapping the cranium in the vicinity of the eye or threatening to do so. 2. AURICULOPALPEBRAL REFLEX.

eye·cup, *n.* 1. OPTIC VESICLE. 2. A small cup that fits over the eye; used for bathing the conjunctiva.

eye dominance. The almost universal condition in which one eye is unconsciously relied on and used more than the other. Syn. *ocular dominance.* See also *dominant eye.*

eye fly or **gnat.** Any of various small dipterans of the family Oscinidae that feed on conjunctival exudates.

eye ground. The fundus of the eye; the internal aspect of the eye as seen through an ophthalmoscope.

eye·lash, *n.* One of the stiff hairs growing on the margin of the eyelid. NA *cilium.*

eye lens. EYEPIECE.

eye·let wiring. SINGLE-LOOP WIRING.

eye·lid, *n.* One of the two protective coverings of the eyeball; a curtain of movable skin lined with conjunctiva, having the tarsus, glands, and cilia in the distal part, muscle in the proximal part. NA *palpebra.* See also Plate 19.

eyelid lag. VON GRAEFE'S SIGN.

eye·piece, *n.* The lens or combination of lenses of an optical instrument, as a microscope or telescope, nearest the eye.

eyepiece micrometer. A micrometer to be used with the eyepiece of a microscope.

eye·point, *n.* The point above an ocular or simple microscope where the greatest number of emerging rays cross.

eye speculum. An instrument for retracting the eyelids.

eye·spot, *n.* A pigmented spot in invertebrates, thought to stimulate reactions in response to light.

eye·strain, *n.* ASTHENOPIA.

eye·tooth, *n.* A canine tooth of the upper jaw. Contr. *stomach tooth.*

eye·wash, *n.* A medicated solution for the eye; a collyrium.

eye worm. *LOA LOA.*

F

F Symbol for fluorine.

F Abbreviation for (a) *Fahrenheit*; (b) fellow; (c) *field of vision*; (d) *formula*.

F Symbol for luminous flux.

F_1 Symbol for first filial generation, offspring of a given mating.

F_2 Symbol for second filial generation, grandchildren of a given mating.

F-12. Abbreviation for *Freon 12*.

fa·bel·la (fa·bel'uh) *n.*, pl. **fabel·lae** (-ee) [dim. of L. *faba*, bean]. A sesamoid fibrocartilage or small bone occasionally developed in the lateral head of the gastrocnemius muscle.

Fa·ber's anemia (fah''bur) [K. H. *Faber*, Danish physician, 1862–1956]. Iron-deficiency anemia associated with achlorhydria.

Fab fragment. The antigen-binding fraction of an immunoglobulin molecule. See also *immunoglobulin fragments*.

fa·bism (fay'biz·um) *n.* FAVISM.

fa·bis·mus (fay·biz'mus) *n.* FAVISM.

fab·ri·ca·tion (fab''ri·kay'shun) *n.* CONFABULATION.

Fa·bri·cus-Mol·ler test. Amylase activity determined by incubating urine with graded dilutions of starch solution, measuring digestion with iodine.

Fa·bry's disease (fah'bree) [J. *Fabry*, German dermatologist, 1860–1930]. ANGIOKERATOMA CORPORIS DIFFUSUM UNIVERSALE.

fab·u·la·tion (fab''yoo·lay'shun) *n.* CONFABULATION.

F.A.C.A. Fellow of the American College of Anesthesiologists.

F.A.C.D. Fellow of the American College of Dentists.

face, *n.* [OF., from L. *facies*, form, face]. The anterior part of the head including forehead and jaws, but not the ears. See also Table of Bones in the Appendix.

face·bow, *n.* A device used to record the spatial relationship between the jaws and the temporomandibular joints and to aid in mounting the dental casts to an articulator.

face gri·pée (fahs gree·pay) [F.]. FACIES ABDOMINALIS.

face-lift, *n.* RHYTIDOPLASTY.

face phenomenon. CHVOSTEK'S SIGN.

face presentation. The fetal presentation of the face at the cervix, where the chin is used as the point of reference.

fac·et (fas'it) *n.* [F. *facette*]. 1. A small plane surface, especially on a bone or a hard body. 2. A worn spot on a surface, as of a tooth.

facet syndrome. A form of traumatic arthritis involving the articular facets of the spinal column, usually in the lumbar region; manifested by sudden onset, with low back pain relieved in certain postures and exaggerated in others, the pain being described as of the locking type.

fac·ial (fay'shul) *adj.* 1. Of, pertaining to, or involving the face. 2. BUCCAL. 3. LABIAL.

facial angle. The angle formed by the union of a line connecting nasion and gnathion with the Frankfort horizontal plane of the head; measured with a craniostat or with the aid of a lateral radiograph.

facial arch. The second visceral arch from which facial structures develop; HYOID ARCH.

facial artery. One of the main branches of the external carotid artery; the principal blood supply of the face. NA *arteria facialis*. See also Table of Arteries in the Appendix.

facial axis. BASIFACIAL AXIS.

facial canal. A channel in the temporal bone for the passage of the facial nerve. NA *canalis facialis*.

facial cleft. 1. An embryonic fissure between facial processes. 2. The facial anomaly produced by failure of the facial processes to fuse.

facial colliculus. One of a pair of rounded eminences in the floor of the fourth ventricle, where the genu of the facial nerve passes around the nucleus of the abducent nerve. NA *colliculus facialis*.

facial coloboma. FACIAL CLEFT (2).

facial eminence. FACIAL COLLICULUS.

facial hemiatrophy. Congenital underdevelopment of the muscles, subcutaneous tissues, and bone on one side of the face. See also *progressive facial hemiatrophy*.

facial hemihypertrophy. Congenital overgrowth of one side of the face and its bony structure.

facial hemispasm. Recurrent irregular clonic muscular twitchings of the facial muscles, on one side only, following Bell's palsy or of unknown cause.

facial hiatus. HIATUS OF THE CANAL FOR THE GREATER PETROSAL NERVE.

facial index. The ratio of the height × 100 to the breadth of the facial part of the skull.

fa·ci·a·lis phenomenon (fay·shee·ay'lis). CHVOSTEK'S SIGN.

facial line. A straight line tangential to the glabella and some point at the lower portion of the face.

facial myokymia. The most common form of myokymia, involving the palpebral (lid) portion of the orbicularis oculi muscle, often occurring in normal but fatigued individuals, and also in debilitated persons or after exposure to cold.

facial myospasm. FACIAL HEMISPASM.

facial nerve. The seventh cranial nerve, which is attached to the brainstem at the inferior border of the pons and innervates the stapedius, stylohyoid, posterior belly of the digastric, and the muscles of facial expression. It also has parasympathetic and sensory components, running by way of the nervus intermedius. NA *nervus facialis.* See also Table of Nerves in the Appendix.

facial neuralgia. TRIGEMINAL NEURALGIA.

facial nucleus. An ovoid collection of nerve cells in the lateral portion of the reticular formation of the pons, giving origin to motor fibers of the facial nerve. NA *nucleus nervi facialis.*

facial palsy or **paralysis.** Partial or total weakness of the muscles of the face. There are two types: the central, or supranuclear, type; and the peripheral, nuclear, or infranuclear, type.

facial plexus. A nerve plexus enveloping part of the facial artery.

facial process of the parotid. A triangular portion of the parotid gland which extends forward, overlapping the masseter muscle.

facial spasm. FACIAL HEMISPASM.

facial triangle. An area bounded by lines between the alveolar point, the basion, and the nasion.

facial trophoneurosis. PROGRESSIVE FACIAL HEMIATROPHY.

-facient [L. *faciens,* from *facere,* to make, do]. A combining form meaning (a) *making;* (b) *causing.*

fa·ci·es (fay'shee·eez) *n.,* genit. **fa·ci·ei** (fay"shee·ee'eye), pl. **facies** [L., face]. 1. The appearance of the face. 2. A surface. 3. [NA] FACE.

facies ab·do·min·a·lis (ab·dom"i·nay'lis). The pinched, dehydrated facial mien of a person with severe abdominal disease, such as peritonitis. Syn. *face gripée.*

facies anterior an·te·bra·chii (an·te·bray'kee·eye) [NA]. The anterior surface of the forearm.

facies anterior bra·chii (bray'kee·eye) [NA]. The anterior surface of the arm.

facies anterior cor·ne·ae (kor'nee·ee) [NA]. The anterior surface of the cornea.

facies anterior cru·ris (kroo'ris) [NA]. The anterior surface of the leg.

facies anterior den·ti·um prae·mo·la·ri·um et mo·la·ri·um (den'shee·um pree·mo·lair'ee·um et mo·lair'ee·um) [BNA]. The mesial aspect of any premolar or molar tooth; the surface that faces the midline.

facies anterior fe·mo·ris (fem'o·ris) [NA]. The anterior surface of the thigh.

facies anterior glan·du·lae su·pra·re·na·lis (glan'dew·lee sue" pruh·re·nay'lis) [NA]. The anterior or ventral surface of an adrenal gland.

facies anterior iri·dis (eye'ri·dis) [NA]. The anterior surface of the iris.

facies anterior la·te·ra·lis hu·me·ri (lat·e·ray'lis hew'mur·eye) [NA]. The anterolateral surface of the shaft of the humerus.

facies anterior len·tis (len'tis) [NA]. The anterior surface of the lens.

facies anterior max·il·lae (mack·sil'ee) [NA]. The anterolateral surface of the body of the maxilla.

facies anterior me·di·a·lis hu·me·ri (mee·dee·ay'lis hew'mur·eye) [NA]. The anteromedial surface of the shaft of the humerus.

facies anterior pal·pe·bra·rum (pal"pe·brair'um) [NA]. The anterior or outer surface of the eyelids.

facies anterior pan·cre·a·tis (pan·kree'uh·tis) [NA]. The anterior or ventral surface of the pancreas.

facies anterior par·tis pe·tro·sae os·sis tem·po·ra·lis (pahr'tis pe·tro'see os'is tem·po·ray'lis) [NA]. The anterior surface of the petrous part of the temporal bone; it helps to form the floor of the middle cranial fossa.

facies anterior pa·tel·lae (pa·tel'ee) [NA]. The anterior surface of the patella.

facies anterior pro·sta·tae (pros'ta·tee) [NA]. The anterior surface of the prostate; the surface directed toward the pubic symphysis.

facies anterior py·ra·mi·dis os·sis tem·po·ra·lis (pi·ram'i·dis os'is tem·po·ray'lis) [BNA]. FACIES ANTERIOR PARTIS PETROSAE OSSIS TEMPORALIS.

facies anterior ra·dii (ray'dee·eye) [NA]. The anterior or palmar surface of the radius.

facies anterior re·nis (ree'nis) [NA]. The anterior or ventral surface of the kidney.

facies anterior ul·nae (ul'nee) [NA]. The anterior or palmar surface of the ulna.

facies an·te·ro·la·te·ra·lis car·ti·la·gi·nis ary·te·noi·de·ae (an" tur·o·lat·e·ray'lis kahr·ti·laj'i·nis ăr"i·te·noy'dee·ee) [NA]. The anterolateral or external surface of the arytenoid cartilage.

facies ar·ti·cu·la·res in·fe·ri·o·res at·lan·tis (ahr·tick·yoo·lair' eez in·feer·ee·o'reez at·lan'tis) [BNA]. FOVEAE ARTICULARES INFERIORES ATLANTIS.

facies articulares inferiores ver·te·brae (vur'te·bree) [BNA]. The articular surfaces on the inferior articular processes of the vertebrae.

facies articulares su·pe·ri·o·res ver·te·brae (sue·peer·ee·o'reez vur'te·bree) [BNA]. The articular facets on the superior articular processes of the vertebrae.

facies ar·ti·cu·la·ris (ahr·tick"yoo·lair'is) [NA]. Articular surface of a bone.

facies articularis acro·mi·a·lis cla·vi·cu·lae (a·kro"mee·ay'lis kla·vick'yoo·lee) [NA]. The articular facet on the lateral end of the clavicle which articulates with the acromion.

facies articularis acro·mii (a·kro'mee·eye) [NA]. The articular facet on the acromion for the lateral end of the clavicle.

facies articularis anterior ax·is (ack'sis) [NA]. The articular facet on the anterior aspect of the dens of the axis which articulates with the atlas.

facies articularis anterior cal·ca·nei (kal·kay'nee·eye) [BNA]. FACIES ARTICULARIS TALARIS ANTERIOR CALCANEI.

facies articularis anterior epi·stro·phei (ep·i·stro'fee·eye) [BNA]. FACIES ARTICULARIS ANTERIOR AXIS.

facies articularis ary·te·noi·dea car·ti·la·gi·nis cri·coi·de·ae (ăr"i·te·noy'dee·uh kahr·ti·laj'i·nis krye·koy'dee·ee) [NA]. The surface of the cricoid cartilage which articulates with an arytenoid cartilage.

facies articularis cal·ca·nea an·te·ri·or ta·li (kal·kay'nee·uh an·teer'ee·or tay'lye) [NA]. The small facet on the head of the talus which articulates with the calcaneus.

facies articularis calcanea me·dia ta·li (mee'dee·uh tay'lye) [NA]. The middle facet on the undersurface of the talus which articulates with the calcaneus.

facies articularis calcanea posterior tali [NA]. The facet on the posterior portion of the undersurface of the talus which articulates with the calcaneus.

facies articularis ca·pi·tis cos·tae (kap'i·tis kos'tee) [NA]. The articular surface on the head of a rib.

facies articularis capitis fi·bu·lae (fib'yoo·lee) [NA]. The facet on the head of the fibula which articulates with the lateral condyle of the tibia.

facies articularis ca·pi·tu·li cos·tae (ka·pit'yoo·lye kos'tee) [BNA]. FACIES ARTICULARIS CAPITIS COSTAE.

facies articularis capituli fi·bu·lae (fib'yoo·lee) [BNA]. FACIES ARTICULARIS CAPITIS FIBULAE.

facies articularis car·pea ra·dii (kahr'pee·uh ray'dee·eye) [NA]. The distal end of the radius.

facies articularis car·ti·la·gi·nis ary·te·noi·de·ae (kahr"ti·laj'i·nis ăr"i·te·noy·dee·ee) [NA]. The facet of an arytenoid cartilage which articulates with the cricoid cartilage.

facies articularis cu·boi·dea cal·ca·nei (kew·boy'dee·uh kal·kay'nee·eye) [NA]. The facet on the anterior surface of the calcaneus which articulates with the cuboid.

facies articularis fi·bu·la·ris ti·bi·ae (fib·yoo·lair'is tib'ee·ee) [NA]. The facet on the lateral condyle of the tibia which articulates with the head of the fibula.

facies articularis inferior tibiae [NA]. The facet on the distal end of the tibia which articulates with the talus.

facies articularis mal·le·o·la·ris fi·bu·lae (mal"ee·o·lair'is fib' yoo·lee) [NA]. The facet on the medial aspect of the lateral malleolus which articulates with the talus.

facies articularis malleolaris ti·bi·ae (tib'ee·ee) [NA]. The facet on the lateral surface of the medial malleolus which articulates with the talus.

facies articularis me·dia cal·ca·nei (mee'dee·uh kal·kay'nee·eye) [BNA]. FACIES ARTICULARIS TALARIS MEDIA CALCANEI.

facies articularis na·vi·cu·la·ris ta·li (na·vick·yoo·lair'is tay'lye) [NA]. The surface of the head of the talus which articulates with the navicular.

facies articularis os·sis tem·po·ra·lis (os'is tem·po·ray'lis) [NA]. The facet in the mandibular fossa of the temporal bone which articulates with the head of the mandible.

facies articularis os·si·um (os'ee·um) [NA]. The articular surface of a bone.

facies articularis pa·tel·lae (pa·tel'ee) [NA]. The posterior surface of the patella which articulates with the femur.

facies articularis posterior ax·is (ack'sis) [NA]. The smooth surface on the posterior aspect of the dens of the axis.

facies articularis posterior cal·ca·nei (kal·kay'nee·eye) [BNA]. FACIES ARTICULARIS TALARIS POSTERIOR CALCANEI.

facies articularis posterior epis·tro·phei (ep·i·stro'fee·eye) [BNA]. FACIES ARTICULARIS POSTERIOR AXIS.

facies articularis ster·na·lis cla·vi·cu·lae (stur·nay'lis kla·vick''yoo·lee) [NA]. The facet on the medial end of the clavicle which articulates with the sternum.

facies articularis superior ti·bi·ae (tib'ee·ee) [NA]. The proximal surface of the tibia which articulates with the femur.

facies articularis ta·la·ris an·te·ri·or cal·ca·nei (tay·lair'is an·teer'ee·or kal·kay'nee·eye) [NA]. The anterior facet on the upper surface of the calcaneus which articulates with the talus.

facies articularis talaris me·dia cal·ca·nei (mee'dee·uh kal·kay'nee·eye) [NA]. The middle facet on the upper surface of the calcaneus which articulates with the talus.

facies articularis talaris posterior calcanei [NA]. The posterior facet on the upper surface of the calcaneus which articulates with the talus.

facies articularis thy·roi·dea car·ti·la·gi·nis cri·coi·de·ae (thigh·roy'dee·uh kahr·ti·laj'i·nis krye·koy'dee·ee) [NA]. The facet on the cricoid cartilage which articulates with the thyroid cartilage.

facies articularis tu·ber·cu·li cos·tae (tew·bur'kew·lye kos'tee) [NA]. The facet on the tubercle of a rib for articulation with the transverse process of the corresponding vertebra.

facies au·ri·cu·la·ris (aw·rick''yoo·lair'is). AURICULAR SURFACE.

facies auricularis os·sis ilii (os'is il'ee·eye) [NA]. The ear-shaped area on the ilium for articulation with the sacrum.

facies auricularis ossis ili·um (il'ee·um) [BNA]. FACIES AURICULARIS OSSIS ILII.

facies auricularis ossis sa·cri (sack'rye, say'krye) [NA]. The ear-shaped area on the sacrum which articulates with the ilium.

facies bo·vi·na (bo·vye'nuh) [L., bovine face]. The characteristic facies of ocular hypertelorism.

facies buc·ca·lis den·tis (buh·kay'lis den'tis). The surface of a tooth that is directed toward the mucous membrane of the cheek.

facies cerebralis alae mag·nae (ay'lee mag'nee) [BNA]. FACIES CEREBRALIS ALAE MAJORIS.

facies cerebralis alae ma·jo·ris (ma·jo'ris) [NA]. The surface of the great wing of the sphenoid bone which forms the anterior part of the floor of the middle cranial fossa.

facies cerebralis os·sis fron·ta·lis (os'is fron·tay'lis) [BNA]. FACIES INTERNA OSSIS FRONTALIS.

facies cerebralis ossis pa·ri·e·ta·lis (pa·rye·e·tay'lis) [BNA]. FACIES INTERNA OSSIS PARIETALIS.

facies cerebralis par·tis squa·mo·sae os·sis tem·po·ra·lis (pahr'tis skway·mo'see os'is tem·po·ray'lis) [NA]. The inner surface of the squamous part of the temporal bone.

facies cerebralis squa·mae tem·po·ra·lis (skway'mee tem·po·ray'lis) [BNA]. FACIES CEREBRALIS PARTIS SQUAMOSAE OSSIS TEMPORALIS.

facies co·li·ca li·e·nis (ko'li·kuh lye·ee'nis) [NA]. The area of the spleen which is in contact with the colon.

facies con·tac·tus den·tis (kon·tack'tus den'tis) [NA]. The surface of a tooth which is in contact with the surface of an adjacent tooth in the same jaw.

facies con·ve·xa ce·re·bri (kon·veck'suh serr'e·brye) [BNA]. FACIES SUPEROLATERALIS CEREBRI.

facies costalis pul·mo·nis (pul·mo'nis) [NA]. The surface of a lung which faces the rib cage.

facies costalis sca·pu·lae (skap'yoo·lee) [NA]. The concave surface of the scapula which faces the rib cage.

facies diaphragmatica cor·dis (kor'dis) [NA]. The surface of the heart which rests upon the diaphragm.

facies diaphragmatica he·pa·tis (hep'uh·tis) [NA]. The surface of the liver which is in contact with the diaphragm.

facies diaphragmatica li·e·nis (lye·ee'nis) [NA]. The surface of the spleen which faces the diaphragm.

facies diaphragmatica pul·mo·nis (pul·mo'nis) [NA]. The surface of a lung which rests on the diaphragm; the base.

facies dis·ta·lis den·tis (dis·tay'lis den'tis) [NA]. The distal surface of a tooth; the surface that is directed away from the midline.

facies dor·sa·les di·gi·to·rum ma·nus (dor·say'leez dij·i·to'rum man'us) [NA]. The dorsal surfaces of the fingers.

facies dorsales digitorum pe·dis (ped'is) [NA]. The dorsal or upper surfaces of the toes.

facies dor·sa·lis an·ti·bra·chii (dor·say'lis an''tee·bray'kee·eye) [BNA]. FACIES POSTERIOR ANTEBRACHII.

facies dorsalis os·sis sa·cri (os'is sack'rye, say'krye) [NA]. The posterior or dorsal surface of the sacrum.

facies dorsalis ra·dii (ray'dee·eye) [BNA]. FACIES POSTERIOR RADII.

facies dorsalis sca·pu·lae (skap'yoo·lee) [NA]. The posterior surface of the scapula.

facies dorsalis ul·nae (ul'nee) [BNA]. FACIES POSTERIOR ULNAE.

facies ex·ter·na os·sis fron·ta·lis (ecks·tur'nuh os'is fron·tay'lis) [NA]. The outer surface of the squamous part of the frontal bone.

facies externa ossis pa·ri·e·ta·lis (pa·rye·e·tay'lis) [NA]. The outer surface of the parietal bone.

facies fa·ci·a·lis den·tis (fay·shee·ay'lis den'tis) [NA alt.]. FACIES VESTIBULARIS DENTIS.

facies fi·bu·la·ris cru·ris (fib·yoo·lair'is kroo'ris) [NA alt.]. FACIES LATERALIS CRURIS.

facies frontalis os·sis fron·ta·lis (os'is fron·tay'lis) [BNA]. FACIES EXTERNA OSSIS FRONTALIS.

facies gastrica li·e·nis (lye·ee'nis) [NA]. The surface of the spleen which is in contact with the stomach.

facies glu·tea os·sis ilii (gloo'tee·uh os'is il'ee·eye) [NA]. The lateral or outer surface of the ala of the ilium.

facies hip·po·crat·i·ca (hip·o·krat'i·kuh). An appearance of the face indicative of the rapid approach of death: the nose is pinched, the temples are hollow, the eyes sunken, the ears leaden and cold, the lips relaxed, the skin livid.

facies inferior ce·re·bri (serr'e·brye) [NA]. The lower surface of the cerebrum.

facies inferior he·mi·sphe·rii ce·re·bel·li (hem·i·sfeer'ee·eye serr·e·bel'eye) [NA]. The inferior surface of the cerebellar hemisphere.

facies inferior hemispherii ce·re·bri (serr'e·brye) [NA]. The inferior surface of the cerebral hemisphere.

facies inferior he·pa·tis (hep'uh·tis) [BNA]. FACIES VISCERALIS HEPATIS.

facies inferior lin·guae (ling'gwee) [NA]. The lower surface of the tongue.

facies inferior me·sen·ce·pha·li (mes·en·sef'uh·lye) [BNA]. The inferior surface of the mesencephalon.

facies inferior pan·cre·a·tis (pan·kree'uh·tis) [NA]. The inferior surface of the pancreas.

facies inferior par·tis pe·tro·sae os·sis tem·po·ra·lis (pahr'tis pe·tro'see os'is tem·po·ray'lis) [NA]. The inferior surface of the petrous part of the temporal bone; the portion which is visible on the lower surface of the base of the skull.

facies inferior py·ra·mi·dis os·sis tem·po·ra·lis (pi·ram'i·dis os'is tem·po·ray'lis) [BNA]. FACIES INFERIOR PARTIS PETROSAE OSSIS TEMPORALIS.

facies in·fe·ro·la·te·ra·lis pro·sta·tae (in"fur·o·lat·e·ray'lis pros'ta·tee) [NA]. The inferolateral surface of the prostate; the portion lying on the pelvic diaphragm.

facies in·fra·tem·po·ra·lis max·il·lae (in"fruh·tem·po·ray'lis mack·sil'ee) [NA]. The posterior convex surface of the maxilla.

facies in·ter·lo·ba·res pul·mo·nis (in"tur·lo·bair'eez pul·mo'nis) [NA]. The interlobar surfaces of the lung; as the surface of any lobe which is in contact with the surface of another lobe.

facies in·ter·na os·sis fron·ta·lis (in·tur'nuh os'is fron·tay'lis) [NA]. The inner surface of the frontal bone.

facies interna ossis pa·ri·e·ta·lis (pa·rye·e·tay'lis) [NA]. The inner surface of the parietal bone.

facies intestinalis ute·ri (yoo'tur·eye) [NA]. The surface of the uterus which is in contact with the intestines.

facies la·bi·a·lis den·tis (lay·bee·ay'lis den'tis) [BNA]. The surface of a tooth which is directed toward a lip.

facies la·te·ra·les di·gi·to·rum ma·nus (lat·e·ray'leez dij·i·to'rum man'us) [NA]. The lateral surfaces of the fingers; the surfaces on the radial sides of the fingers. NA alt. *facies radiales digitorum manus.*

facies laterales digitorum pe·dis (ped'is) [NA]. The lateral surfaces of the toes.

facies lateralis bra·chii (bray'kee·eye) [NA]. The lateral surface of the arm.

facies lateralis cru·ris (kroo'ris) [NA]. The lateral surface of the leg. NA alt. *facies fibularis cruris.*

facies lateralis den·ti·um in·ci·si·vo·rum et ca·ni·no·rum (den'shee·um in"si·sigh·vo'rum et kan·i·no'rum) [BNA]. The distal surface of an incisor or canine tooth; the surface that is directed away from the midline.

facies lateralis fe·mo·ris (fem'o·ris) [NA]. The lateral surface of the thigh.

facies lateralis fi·bu·lae (fib'yoo·lee) [NA]. The lateral surface of the fibula.

facies lateralis os·sis zy·go·ma·ti·ci (os'is zye·go·mat'i·sigh) [NA]. The lateral convex surface of the zygomatic bone.

facies lateralis ova·rii (o·vair'ee·eye) [NA]. The surface of the ovary directed toward the lateral pelvic wall.

facies lateralis ra·dii (ray'dee·eye) [NA]. The lateral surface of the radius.

facies lateralis tes·tis (tes'tis) [NA]. The lateral surface of the testis.

facies lateralis ti·bi·ae (tib'ee·ee) [NA]. The lateral surface of the shaft of the tibia.

facies le·on·ti·na (lee·on·tye'nuh). The "lionlike" face seen in some patients with leprosy.

facies lingualis den·tis (den'tis) [NA]. The surface of a tooth which is directed toward the tongue.

facies lu·na·ta ace·ta·bu·li (lew·nay'tuh as"e·tab'yoo·lye) [NA]. The articular facet of the acetabulum.

facies malaris os·sis zy·go·ma·ti·ci (os'is zye·go·mat'i·sigh) [BNA]. FACIES LATERALIS OSSIS ZYGOMATICI.

facies malleolaris la·te·ra·lis ta·li (lat·e·ray'lis tay'lye) [NA]. The facet on the talus which articulates with the lateral malleolus.

facies malleolaris me·di·a·lis ta·li (mee·dee·ay'lis tay'lye) [NA]. The facet on the talus which articulates with the medial malleolus.

facies mas·ti·ca·to·ria den·tis (mas"ti·ka·to'ree·uh den'tis) [BNA]. The surface of a tooth which is directed toward the surface of its fellow in the other jaw.

facies maxillaris alae ma·jo·ris (ay'lee ma·jo'ris) [NA]. The area of the lower surface of the great wing of the sphenoid bone which contains the foramen rotundum.

facies maxillaris la·mi·nae per·pen·di·cu·la·ris os·sis pa·la·ti·ni (lam'i·nee pur"pen·dick·yoo·lair'is os'is pal·uh·tye'nigh) [NA]. The lateral surface of the perpendicular plate of the palatine bone which is related to the maxilla.

facies maxillaris par·tis per·pen·di·cu·la·ris os·sis pa·la·ti·ni (pahr'tis pur"pen·dick·yoo·lair'is os'is pal·uh·tye'nigh) [BNA]. FACIES MAXILLARIS LAMINAE PERPENDICULARIS OSSIS PALATINI.

facies me·di·a·les di·gi·to·rum ma·nus (mee·dee·ay'leez dij·i·to'rum man'us) [NA]. The medial surfaces of the fingers; the surfaces on the ulnar sides of the fingers. NA alt. *facies ulnares digitorum manus.*

facies mediales digitorum pe·dis (ped'is) [NA]. The medial surfaces of the toes.

facies medialis bra·chii (bray'kee·eye) [NA]. The medial surface of the arm.

facies medialis car·ti·la·gi·nis ary·te·noi·de·ae (kahr·ti·laj'i·nis ăr"i·te·noy'dee·ee) [NA]. The medial surface of the arytenoid cartilage.

facies medialis ce·re·bri (serr'e·brye) [NA]. The medial surface of each cerebral hemisphere; the portion directed toward the midline.

facies medialis cru·ris (kroo'ris) [NA]. The medial surface of the leg. NA alt. *facies tibialis cruris.*

facies medialis den·ti·um in·ci·si·vo·rum et ca·ni·no·rum (den'shee·um in"si·sigh·vo'rum et kan·i·no'rum) [BNA]. The mesial surface of an incisor or a canine tooth; the surface which is directed toward the midline.

facies medialis fe·mo·ris (fem'o·ris) [NA]. The medial surface of the thigh.

facies medialis fi·bu·lae (fib'yoo·lee) [NA]. The medial surface of the shaft of the fibula.

facies medialis he·mi·sphe·rii ce·re·bri (hem·i·sfeer'ee·eye serr'e·brye) [NA]. The medial surface of the cerebral hemisphere; the portion directed toward its fellow on the opposite side.

facies medialis ova·rii (o·vair'ee·eye) [NA]. The surface of the ovary directed toward the fimbriated end of the oviduct.

facies medialis pul·mo·nis (pul·mo'nis) [NA]. The medial surface of the lung.

facies medialis tes·tis (tes'tis) [NA]. The medial surface of the testis.

facies medialis ti·bi·ae (tib'ee·ee) [NA]. The medial surface of the shaft of the tibia.

facies medialis ul·nae (ul'nee) [NA]. The medial surface of the ulna.

facies mediastinalis pul·mo·nis (pul·mo'nis) [BNA]. FACIES MEDIALIS PULMONIS.

facies me·si·a·lis den·tis (mee·see·ay'lis den'tis) [NA]. The mesial surface of a tooth; the surface that is directed toward the midline.

facies my·o·path·i·ca (migh·o·path'i·kuh). MYOPATHIC FACIES.

facies na·sa·lis la·mi·nae ho·ri·zon·ta·lis os·sis pa·la·ti·ni (nay·say'lis lam'i·nee hor"i·zon·tay'lis os'is pal·uh·tye'nigh) [NA]. The upper or nasal surface of the horizontal part of the palatine bone.

facies nasalis laminae per·pen·di·cu·la·ris os·sis pa·la·ti·ni (pur"pen·dick·yoo·lair'is os'is pal·uh·tye'nigh) [NA]. The medial or nasal surface of the perpendicular part of the palatine bone.

facies nasalis max·il·lae (mack·sil'ee) [NA]. The surface of the maxilla which enters into the formation of the lateral wall of the nasal cavity.

facies nasalis par·tis ho·ri·zon·ta·lis os·sis pa·la·ti·ni (pahr'tis hor"i·zon·tay'lis os'is pal·uh·tye'nigh) [BNA]. FACIES NASALIS LAMINAE HORIZONTALIS OSSIS PALATINI.

facies nasalis partis per·pen·di·cu·la·ris os·sis pa·la·ti·ni (pur″pen·dick·yoo·lair′is os′is pal·uh·tye′nigh) [BNA]. FACIES NASALIS LAMINAE PERPENDICULARIS OSSIS PALATINI.

facies oc·clu·sa·lis den·tis (ock·loo·say′lis den′tis) [NA]. The occlusal surface of a tooth.

facies or·bi·ta·lis alae mag·nae (or·bi·tay′lis ay′lee mag′nee) [BNA]. FACIES ORBITALIS ALAE MAJORIS.

facies orbitalis alae ma·jo·ris (ma·jo′ris) [NA]. The surface of the great wing of the sphenoid bone which is part of the lateral wall of the orbit.

facies orbitalis max·il·lae (mack·sil′ee) [NA]. The surface of the maxilla which forms the floor of the orbit.

facies orbitalis os·sis fron·ta·lis (os′is fron·tay′lis) [NA]. The surface of the frontal bone which forms the roof of the orbit.

facies orbitalis ossis zy·go·ma·ti·ci (zye·go·mat′i·sigh) [NA]. The surface of the zygomatic bone which forms part of the lateral wall of the orbit.

facies os·sea (os′ee·uh). The bony portion of the face.

facies (ossea) cra·nii (kray′nee·eye) [BNA]. The portion of the cranium which forms the skeleton of the face.

facies palatina la·mi·nae ho·ri·zon·ta·lis os·sis pa·la·ti·ni (lam′i·nee hor″i·zon·tay′lis os′is pal·uh·tye′nigh) [NA]. The lower surface of the horizontal part of the palatine bone.

facies palatina par·tis ho·ri·zon·ta·lis os·sis pa·la·ti·ni (pahr′tis hor″i·zon·tay′lis os′is pal·uh·tye′nigh) [BNA]. FACIES PALATINA LAMINAE HORIZONTALIS OSSIS PALATINI.

facies pal·ma·res di·gi·to·rum ma·nus (pal·mair′eez dij·i·to′rum man′us) [NA]. The palmar surfaces of the fingers.

facies parietalis os·sis pa·ri·e·ta·lis (os′is pa·rye·e·tay′lis) [BNA]. FACIES EXTERNA OSSIS PARIETALIS.

facies patellaris fe·mo·ris (fem′o·ris) [NA]. The facet on the lower end of the femur for articulation with the patella.

facies pelvina os·sis sa·cri (os′is say′krye, sack′rye) [NA]. The anterior or ventral surface of the sacrum.

facies plan·ta·res di·gi·to·rum pe·dis (plan·tair′eez dij·i·to′rum ped′is) [NA]. The plantar surfaces of the toes.

facies po·pli·tea (pop·lit′ee·uh) [NA]. POPLITEAL PLANE.

facies posterior an·te·bra·chii (an″te·bray′kee·eye) [NA]. The posterior or dorsal surface of the forearm.

facies posterior bra·chii (bray′kee·eye) [NA]. The posterior surface of the arm.

facies posterior car·ti·la·gi·nis ary·te·noi·de·ae (kahr·ti·laj′i·nis ar″i·te·noy′dee·ee) [NA]. The posterior or dorsal surface of the arytenoid cartilage.

facies posterior cor·ne·ae (kor′nee·ee) [NA]. The posterior surface of the cornea.

facies posterior cru·ris (kroo′ris) [NA]. The posterior surface of the leg.

facies posterior den·ti·um prae·mo·la·ri·um et mo·la·ri·um (den′shee·um pree″mo·lair′ee·um et mo·lair′ee·um) [BNA]. The distal surface of the premolar and molar teeth; the surface that is directed away from the midline.

facies posterior fe·mo·ris (fem′o·ris) [NA]. The posterior surface of the thigh.

facies posterior fi·bu·lae (fib′yoo·lee) [NA]. The posterior surface of the fibula.

facies posterior glan·du·lae su·pra·re·na·lis (glan′dew·lee sue″pruh·re·nay′lis) [NA]. The surface of the adrenal gland contacting the posterior body wall.

facies posterior he·pa·tis (hep′uh·tis) [BNA]. PARS POSTERIOR HEPATIS.

facies posterior hu·me·ri (hew′mur·eye) [NA]. The posterior surface of the humerus.

facies posterior iri·dis (eye′ri·dis) [NA]. The posterior surface of the iris.

facies posterior len·tis (len′tis) [NA]. The posterior surface of the lens.

facies posterior pal·pe·bra·rum (pal·pe·bray′rum) [NA]. The inner surface of the eyelids.

facies posterior pan·cre·a·tis (pan·kree′uh·tis) [NA]. The posterior or dorsal surface of the pancreas; the portion in contact with the posterior abdominal wall.

facies posterior par·tis pe·tro·sae os·sis tem·po·ra·lis (pahr′tis pe·tro′see os′is tem·po·ray′lis) [NA]. The posterior surface of the petrous part of the temporal bone; the portion forming part of the posterior cranial fossa.

facies posterior pro·sta·tae (pros′ta·tee) [NA]. The posterior or dorsal surface of the prostate; the portion in contact with the rectum.

facies posterior py·ra·mi·dis os·sis tem·po·ra·lis (pi·ram′i·dis os′is tem·po·ray′lis) [BNA]. FACIES POSTERIOR PARTIS PETROSAE OSSIS TEMPORALIS.

facies posterior ra·dii (ray′dee·eye) [NA]. The posterior or dorsal surface of the radius.

facies posterior re·nis (ree′nis) [NA]. The posterior or dorsal surface of the kidney; the portion in contact with the posterior abdominal wall.

facies posterior ti·bi·ae (tib′ee·ee) [NA]. The posterior surface of the shaft of the tibia.

facies posterior ul·nae (ul′nee) [NA]. The posterior or dorsal surface of the ulna.

facies pul·mo·na·lis cor·dis (pul·mo·nay′lis kor′dis) [NA]. The portion of the surface of the heart directed toward the left lung.

facies ra·di·a·les di·gi·to·rum ma·nus (ray·dee·ay′leez dij·i·to′rum man′us) [NA alt.]. FACIES LATERALES DIGITORUM MANUS.

facies re·na·lis glan·du·lae su·pra·re·na·lis (ree·nay′lis glan′dew·lee sue″pruh·re·nay′lis) [NA]. The surface of the suprarenal gland directed toward the kidney.

facies renalis li·e·nis (lye·ee′nis) [NA]. The surface of the spleen directed toward the left kidney.

facies sa·cro·pel·vi·na os·sis ilii (say·kro·pel·vye′nuh os′is il′ee·eye) [NA]. The irregular posterior portion of the medial surface of the ilium.

facies sphenomaxillaris alae mag·nae (ay′lee mag′nee) [BNA]. FACIES MAXILLARIS ALAE MAJORIS.

facies ster·no·cos·ta·lis cor·dis (stur″no·kos·tay′lis kor′dis) [NA]. The anterior or ventral surface of the heart.

facies superior he·mi·sphe·rii ce·re·bel·li (hem·i·sfeer′ee·eye serr·e·bel′eye) [NA]. The superior surface of the cerebellar hemisphere.

facies superior he·pa·tis (hep′uh·tis) [BNA]. FACIES DIAPHRAGMATICA HEPATIS.

facies superior tro·chle·ae ta·li (trock′lee·ee tay′lye) [NA]. The superior surface of the talus which articulates with the tibia.

facies su·pe·ro·la·te·ra·lis ce·re·bri (sue″pur·o·lat·e·ray′lis serr′e·brye) [NA]. The convex superficial surface of the cerebrum.

facies sym·phy·se·os os·sis pu·bis (sim·fis′ee·os os′is pew′bis) [BNA]. FACIES SYMPHYSIALIS.

facies sym·phy·si·a·lis (sim·fis·ee·ay′lis) [NA]. The surface of a pubic bone which articulates with its fellow of the opposite side.

facies tem·po·ra·lis alae mag·nae (tem·po·ray′lis ay′lee mag′nee) [BNA]. FACIES TEMPORALIS ALAE MAJORIS.

facies temporalis alae ma·jo·ris (ma·jo′ris) [NA]. The outer (inferolateral) lateral surface of the great wing of the sphenoid bone.

facies temporalis os·sis fron·ta·lis (os′is fron·tay′lis) [NA]. The outer or lateral surface of the temporal bone.

facies temporalis ossis zy·go·ma·ti·ci (zye·go·mat′i·sigh) [NA]. The inner, concave surface of the zygomatic bone.

facies temporalis par·tis squa·mo·sae (pahr′tis skway·mo′see) [NA]. The outer surface of the squamous part of the temporal bone.

facies temporalis squa·mae tem·po·ra·lis (skway′mee tem·po·ray′lis) [BNA]. FACIES TEMPORALIS PARTIS SQUAMOSAE.

facies ti·bi·a·lis cru·ris (tib·ee·ay′lis kroo′ris) [NA alt.]. FACIES MEDIALIS CRURIS.

facies ul·na·res di·gi·to·rum ma·nus (ul·nair′eez dij·i·to′rum man'us) [NA alt.]. FACIES MEDIALES DIGITORUM MANUS.

facies ure·thra·lis pe·nis (yoo·re·thray'lis pee'nis) [NA]. The surface of the penis overlying the urethra.

facies ve·si·ca·lis ute·ri (ves·i·kay'lis yoo'tur·eye) [NA]. The surface of the uterus in contact with the bladder.

facies ves·ti·bu·la·ris den·tis (ves·tib·yoo·lay'ris den'tis) [NA]. The surface of a tooth facing the vestibule of the mouth; the surface facing the cheeks and lips. NA alt. *facies facialis dentis.*

facies vis·ce·ra·lis he·pa·tis (vis·ur·ay'lis hep'uh·tis) [NA]. The visceral surface of the liver; the surface making contact with various abdominal viscera.

facies visceralis li·e·nis (lye·ee'nis) [NA]. The visceral surface of the spleen; the surface coming in contact with various abdominal viscera.

facies vo·la·res di·gi·to·rum ma·nus (vo·lair'eez dij·i·to'rum man'us) [BNA]. FACIES PALMARES DIGITORUM MANUS.

facies volaris an·ti·bra·chii (an''tee·bray'kee·eye) [BNA]. FACIES ANTERIOR ANTEBRACHII.

facies volaris ra·dii (ray'dee·eye) [BNA]. FACIES ANTERIOR RADII.

facies volaris ul·nae (ul'nee) [BNA]. FACIES ANTERIOR ULNAE.

fa·cil·i·ta·tion (fa·sil''i·tay'shun) *n.* 1. Increased ease in carrying out an action or function. 2. Enhanced or reinforced reflex or other neural activity by impulses arising other than from a reflex center. 3. An increase in excitatory postsynaptic potential by a slight added quantity of neurotransmitter which enables excitation of the postsynaptic cell.

fa·cil·i·ty (fa·sil'i·tee) *n.* [L. *facilitas,* from *facilis,* easy]. 1. Anything that makes it possible for some particular function to be performed, or which serves toward some specific end. 2. Ease in performance, as the facility to run; freedom from some impediment. 3. Any specific structure, building, establishment, or installation, or part thereof, designed to promote some particular end or purpose, as a hospital or a center for learning or recreation.

fac·ing, *n.* A veneer of porcelain or resin cemented or processed to an artificial tooth crown or pontic to achieve a greater esthetic effect.

facio-. A combining form meaning *face, facial.*

fa·cio·ple·gic (fay''shee·o·plee'jick) *adj.* [*facio-* + *-plegic*]. Pertaining to weakness or paralysis of the facial muscles. See also *Bell's palsy.*

facioplegic migraine. Transient paralysis of facial muscles sometimes accompanying migraine.

fa·cio·scap·u·lo·hu·mer·al (fay''shee·o·skap''yoo·lo·hew'mur·ul) *adj.* [*facio-* + *scapulo-* + *humeral*]. Pertaining to the muscles involving the face, scapula, and humerus.

facioscapulohumeral muscular dystrophy. A hereditary slowly progressive muscular dystrophy affecting both sexes usually beginning in late childhood or early adult life, and involving first the muscles of the face, shoulder girdle, and arm, and eventually those of the pelvis. Syn. *Landouzy-Déjerine muscular dystrophy.*

F.A.C.O.G. Fellow of the American College of Obstetricians and Gynecologists.

F.A.C.P. Fellow of the American College of Physicians.

F.A.C.R. Fellow of the American College of Radiologists.

F.A.C.S. Fellow of the American College of Surgeons.

F-actin. The fibrous form of actin.

fac·ti·tious (fack·tish'us) *adj.* [L. *facticius,* from *facere,* to make]. Pertaining to a state or substance brought about or produced by means other than natural.

factitious urticaria. DERMOGRAPHIA.

fac·tor, *n.* [L., a maker]. 1. A circumstance, fact, or influence which tends to produce a result; a constituent or component. 2. *In biology,* GENE. 3. An essential or desirable element in diet. 4. A substance promoting or functioning in a particular physiologic process, as a coagulation factor.

factor I. FIBRINOGEN.

factor II. PROTHROMBIN.

factor III. *Obsol.* THROMBOPLASTIN.

factor IV. Calcium when it participates in the coagulation of blood.

factor V. A labile procoagulant in normal plasma but deficient in the blood of patients with parahemophilia; essential for rapid conversion of prothrombin to thrombin. It is suggested that during clotting this factor is transformed from an inactive precursor into an active accelerator of prothrombin conversion. Syn. *proaccelerin.*

factor VI. A hypothetical substance believed to be derived from factor V during coagulation.

factor VII. A stable procoagulant in normal plasma but deficient in the blood of patients with a hereditary bleeding disorder; formed in the liver by action of vitamin K. Syn. *proconvertin.*

factor VIII. A procoagulant present in normal plasma but deficient in the blood of patients with hemophilia A.

factor IX. A procoagulant in normal plasma but deficient in the blood of patients with hemophilia B. Syn. *Christmas factor.*

factor X. A procoagulant present in normal plasma but deficient in the blood of patients with a hereditary bleeding disorder. May be closely related to prothrombin since both are formed in the liver by action of vitamin K. Syn. *Stuart-Prower factor.*

factor XI. A procoagulant present in normal plasma but deficient in the blood of patients with a hereditary bleeding disorder.

factor XII. A factor necessary for rapid coagulation in vitro, but apparently not required for hemostasis, present in the normal plasma but deficient in the blood of patients with a hereditary bleeding disorder. Syn. *Hageman factor.*

factor XIII. A factor present in normal plasma which, in the presence of calcium, causes the formation of a highly insoluble fibrin clot resistant to urea and weak acid. Syn. *fibrinase, fibrin stabilizing factor.*

Factorate. A trademark for human antihemophilic factor.

fac·ul·ta·tive (fack'ul·tay''tiv) *adj.* [F. *facultatif,* from L. *facultas,* capability, opportunity]. 1. Voluntary; optional; having the power to do or not to do a thing. 2. *In biology,* capable of existing under differing conditions, as a microorganism that can grow aerobically or anaerobically. Contr. *obligate.*

facultative aerobe. An organism which is normally or usually anaerobic but which, under certain circumstances, may grow aerobically.

facultative anaerobe. An organism which usually grows aerobically, but which can also grow in the absence of molecular oxygen.

facultative hyperopia. Manifest hyperopia that can be concealed by accommodation.

facultative parasite. An organism capable of being free-living as well as parasitic.

facultative sterility. Sterility caused by the prevention of conception.

fac·ul·ty (fack'ul·tee) *n.* [F. *faculté,* from L. *facultas,* ability, power]. 1. A function, power, or capability inherent in a living organism, often in the sense of exceptional development of the function, power, or capability. 2. The teaching staff of an educational institution or one of its divisions. 3. An area of learning or teaching in an institution of higher education.

FAD Abbreviation for *flavin adenine dinucleotide.*

faecal. FECAL.

faeces. FECES.

faeculent. FECULENT.

faex (fecks) *n.* [L.]. The dregs or sediment of any liquid; FECULA.

faex me·dic·i·na·lis (me·dis''i·nay'lis). YEAST.

fa·ga·rine (fay'gur·een, ·in, fag'ur·) *n.* The name applied to the three alkaloids of *Fagara coco,* a tree of Argentina; differentiated by the prefixes α-, β-, and γ-.

fag·o·py·rism (fag″o·pye′riz·um) *n.* [*Fagopyrum,* the genus of buckwheat, + *-ism*]. Photosensitization of the skin and mucous membranes, accompanied by convulsions; produced in white and piebald animals by feeding with the flowers or seed husks of the buckwheat plant (*Fagopyrum sagittatum*) or clovers and grasses containing flavin or carotin and xanthophyll.

Fahr. An abbreviation for *Fahrenheit.*

Fåh·rae·us sedimentation test (fo·rey′o͞os) [R. *Fåhraeus,* Swedish pathologist, b. 1888]. The speed of settling of erythrocytes in an 8-ml sample of blood added directly to 2 ml of 2% sodium citrate in a 17 by 0.9 cm test tube, then measured in the same tube.

Fahr·en·heit (făr′un·hite, ferr′) *adj.* [G. D. *Fahrenheit,* German physicist, 1686–1736]. Pertaining to or designating the Fahrenheit temperature scale in which the interval between the freezing point of water (32°) and its boiling point (212°) is divided into 180 degrees. Abbreviated F, Fahr. Contr. *Celsius.* See also Table of Thermometric Equivalents in the Appendix.

fail·ure, *n. In medicine,* profound inability of an organ to carry out its physiologic functions or the demands upon it, usually resulting in severe impairment of the individual's health.

faint, *adj., n. & v.* 1. Weak or lacking strength or consciousness. 2. Barely perceptible. 3. A sudden, transient loss of consciousness; swoon; syncope. 4. To swoon; lose strength and/or consciousness suddenly.

faint·ness, *n.* A sudden lack of strength with a sensation of impending faint.

Fairley's pigment. METHEMALBUMIN.

fairy cap. DIGITALIS.

faith cure. A system or practice of treating disease by religious faith and prayer, in which results are often obtained by suggestion.

fal·cate (fal′kate) *adj.* [L. *falcatus,* from *falx,* sickle]. Sickle-shaped.

falces. Plural of *falx.*

fal·cial (fal′shul) *adj.* Of or pertaining to a falx.

fal·ci·form (fal′si·form) *adj.* [*falx* + *-iform*]. Having the shape of a sickle.

falciform ligament of the liver. The ventral mesentery of the liver. Its peripheral attachment extends from the diaphragm to the umbilicus and contains the round ligament of the liver. NA *ligamentum falciforme hepatis.* See also Plate 13.

falciform margin. The sharp, crescentic, lateral boundary of the fossa ovalis of the femoral triangle.

falciform process. A thin extension of the sacrotuberous ligament to the ramus of the ischium. NA *processus falciformis ligamenti sacrotuberosi.*

fal·cip·a·rum malaria (fal·sip′ur·um, fawl·). A form of malaria caused by *Plasmodium falciparum* characterized by paroxysms of fever occurring at irregular intervals and often by the localization of the organism in a specific organ, causing capillary blockage in the brain, lungs, intestinal mucosa, spleen, and kidney. Syn. *estivo-autumnal malaria, malignant tertian malaria, subtertian malaria.* See also *algid malaria, blackwater fever.*

fal·cu·la (fal′kew·luh) *n.* [L., small sickle]. FALX CEREBELLI.

fal·cu·lar (fal′kew·lur) *adj.* 1. Sickle-shaped. 2. Pertaining to the falx cerebelli.

fall·ing-drop method. A method of determining the specific gravity of a solution by determining the time taken for a drop of known size to fall a given distance in a nonmiscible fluid of known density.

falling sickness. EPILEPSY.

fal·lo·pi·an (fa·lo′pee·un) *adj.* Pertaining to or designating anatomic structures associated with Gabriele Fallopio (Fallopius), Italian anatomist, 1523–1562.

fallopian aqueduct. FACIAL CANAL.

fallopian tube. UTERINE TUBE.

fall·out, *n.* The radioactive products of nuclear and thermonuclear explosions which originally contaminate the atmosphere, and subsequently are deposited on land or water.

Falls's test [F. H. *Falls,* U.S. obstetrician, b. 1885]. COLOSTRUM TEST.

Falmonox. Trademark for teclozan, an antiamebic drug.

false albuminuria. FALSE PROTEINURIA.

false amnion. A temporary cavity in the trophoblastic knob, resembling the early true amnion.

false amniotic cavity. FALSE AMNION.

false aneurysm. 1. An aneurysm due to a rupture of all the coats of an artery, the effused blood being retained by the surrounding tissues. 2. A swelling in the course of an artery, usually caused by a hematoma, which mimics the appearance of an aneurysm, but does not involve the wall of the artery.

false angina. *Obsol.* ANGINA PECTORIS VASOMOTORIA.

false ankylosis. EXTRACAPSULAR ANKYLOSIS.

false apophysis. PINEAL BODY.

false articulation. PSEUDARTHROSIS.

false associated fixation. ABNORMAL RETINAL CORRESPONDENCE.

false croup. SPASMODIC CROUP.

false diverticulum. PSEUDODIVERTICULUM.

false hematuria. The passage of red urine due to the ingestion of food or drugs containing red pigments.

false hernia. A hernia that has no sac covering the hernial contents.

false hypertrophy. An increase in size of an organ due to an increase in amount of tissue not associated with functional activity, such as connective tissue.

false image. In diplopia, the image of the deviating eye; it is not on the macula, but is projected to a peripheral part of the retina.

false joint. PSEUDARTHROSIS.

false knot. 1. GRANNY KNOT. 2. An external knotlike bulge of the umbilical cord caused by loops in the umbilical blood vessels.

false labor. Painful uterine contractions which simulate labor but are not associated with progressive dilation or effacement of the cervix or descent of the presenting part.

false ligament. Any peritoneal fold which is not a true supporting ligament.

false macula. The point on the retina of a squinting eye which receives the same impression as the macula of the fixing eye.

false membrane. A fibrinous layer formed on a mucous membrane or cutaneous surface and extending downward for a variable depth. It is the result of coagulation necrosis, generally seen in croup and diphtheria. Syn. *pseudomembrane.*

false mole. A mole not containing any tissues derived from a fetus or fetal membranes.

false-negative reaction. An erroneous or deceptive negative reaction. Contr. *false-positive reaction.*

false nucleolus. KARYOSOME (1).

false pains. Mild, recurring lower abdominal cramps, occurring late in pregnancy, but not followed by labor.

false pareira. The root of the species *Cissampelos pareira.*

false passage. A false channel, especially one made by the unskillful introduction of an instrument into the urethra.

false pelvis. The part of the pelvis above the iliopectineal line.

false-positive reaction. An erroneous or deceptive positive reaction, such as a positive serological test for syphilis in the presence of infectious mononucleosis, leprosy, or malaria. Contr. *false-negative reaction.*

false pregnancy. PSEUDOCYESIS.

false projection. The erroneous placement of an object in space in response to the image received by an eye in which one or more of the extraocular muscles are paralyzed. The object is falsely placed in the direction of the normal action of the weak or paralyzed muscle.

false promontory. DOUBLE PROMONTORY.

false proteinuria. Proteinuria from sources other than the usual pathologic states (such as bleeding into the lower urinary tract) associated with this condition. Syn. *accidental proteinuria, false albuminuria.*

false ribs. The five lower ribs on each side not attached to the sternum directly. NA *costae spuriae.*

false spermatorrhea. Involuntary excessive ejaculation of fluid containing no spermatozoa. See also *prostatorrhea.*

false suture. The form of articulation in which the contiguous surfaces are merely roughened, not having dentate or serrate interlocking projections.

false tympanites. PSEUDOTYMPANITES.

false vertebra. One of the sacral or coccygeal vertebrae.

false vocal cord. VESTIBULAR FOLD.

fal·si·fi·ca·tion, *n.* [ML. *falsificatio*]. The act of distorting or altering a fact or object. See also *confabulation, retrospective falsification.* —**fal·si·fy,** *v.*

falx (falks, fawlks) *n.*, genit. **fal·cis** (fal'sis), pl. **fal·ces** (fal'seez) [L.]. A sickle-shaped structure.

falx apo·neu·ro·ti·ca (ap''o·new·rot'i·kuh). FALX INGUINALIS.

falx ce·re·bel·li (serr·e·bel'eye) [NA]. A sickle-like process of dura mater between the lobes of the cerebellum.

falx ce·re·bri (serr'e·brye) [NA]. The process of the dura mater separating the hemispheres of the cerebrum. See also Plate 18.

falx in·gui·na·lis (ing·gwi·nay'lis) [NA]. The combined insertion of the internal oblique abdominal and transverse abdominal muscles into the pubis lateral to the pubic tubercle. Syn. *falx aponeurotica.* NA alt. *tendo conjunctivus.*

falx sep·ti (sep'tye) [NA alt.]. VALVULA FORAMINIS OVALIS.

fa·mes (fay'meez) *n.* [L.]. Hunger.

fa·mil·ial (fa·mil'ee·ul, ·mil'yul) *adj.* Occurring among or pertaining to the members of a family, as a familial disease. Compare *hereditary.*

familial acholuric jaundice. HEREDITARY SPHEROCYTOSIS.

familial aldosterone deficiency. A heritable error of metabolism that occurs in two forms: one due to 18-hydroxylase deficiency, in which affected patients are severely ill with hyperkalemia, sodium depletion, and intermittent fever; the other due to a deficiency of 18-hydroxy dehydrogenase, manifested by mild growth retardation and transient electrolyte disturbances. Both forms show autosomal recessive inheritance.

familial alphalipoprotein deficiency. TANGIER DISEASE.

familial benign pemphigus. A dominantly inherited vesicular and bullous dermatitis localized to the sides of the neck, the axillary spaces, and other flexor surfaces. It is possibly a variant of Darier's disease. Syn. *Hailey-Hailey disease.*

familial broad-beta hyperlipoproteinemia. FAMILIAL HYPERBETALIPOPROTEINEMIA AND HYPERPREBETALIPOPROTEINEMIA.

familial centrolobar sclerosis. PELIZAEUS-MERZBACHER DISEASE.

familial chondrodystrophy. MULTIPLE HEREDITARY EXOSTOSES.

familial combined hyperlipoproteinemia. Familial hyperlipoproteinemia, type IIB, characterized by an increase in total serum cholesterol and triglycerides, with hyperbeta-plus hyperprebetalipoproteinemia. Affected family members may have type IIB, IIA, or IV phenotypes; patients themselves may present these several phenotypes at different times, in response to therapy or varying environmental conditions. Skin xanthomas may be present. There is increased propensity to ischemic heart disease.

familial corneal dystrophy. LATTICE CORNEAL DYSTROPHY.

familial cutaneous col·la·gen·o·ma (kol·aj''e·no'muh). A heritable disorder characterized by multiple asymptomatic, cutaneous nodules limited to the trunk and proximal portions of the upper extremities, which histologically show localized thickening of the dermis due to increased collagen; may be associated with myocarditis, vasculitis, iris atrophy, and sensory-neural hearing loss.

familial disease. Any disorder occurring in several members of the same family; sometimes restricted to mean several members of the same generation. Compare *congenital disease, hereditary disease.*

familial dysautonomia. A hereditary disease, transmitted as an autosomal recessive trait, most common in Jewish children, characterized from infancy by feeding difficulties, absence of overflow tears, indifference to pain, absent or hypoactive deep tendon reflexes, absent corneal reflexes, absence of fungiform papillae on tongue, postural hypotension, emotional lability, abnormal intradermal histidine response, and frequently abnormal temperature control with excessive sweating, abnormal esophageal motility, abnormal pupillary response to methacholine, and excess urinary homovanillic acid, as well as other evidence of autonomic nervous system dysfunctions.

familial eosinophilia. The occurrence within a family of several members whose blood eosinophils are increased per unit volume of blood, without any known cause.

familial erythroblastic anemia. THALASSEMIA.

familial fat-induced hyperlipemia. Familial hyperlipoproteinemia, type I, due to a defect in removal of chylomicrons and other lipoproteins rich in triglycerides, probably as a result of a genetically determined low lipoprotein lipase activity; characterized by an excess of chylomicrons in serum with an ordinary diet and their disappearance with a fat-free diet. Clinically there may be paroxysms of abdominal pain, hepatosplenomegaly, pancreatitis, and xanthomas of various tissues. Syn. *familial lipoprotein lipase deficiency.*

familial fibromatosis. FIBROMATOSIS GINGIVAE.

familial hemolytic anemia. HEREDITARY SPHEROCYTOSIS.

familial hemolytic icterus. HEREDITARY SPHEROCYTOSIS.

familial hemopathy. Any hereditary disease of blood.

familial hemorrhagic nephritis. ALPORT'S SYNDROME.

familial hyperbetalipoproteinemia. The most common form of familial hyperlipoproteinemia, type IIA, characterized by an increase in total serum cholesterol and phospholipids and normal glycerides with an ordinary diet; associated with the formation of xanthelasmas, tendon and tuberous xanthomas, frequently early atheromatosis, and generally a positive family history.

familial hyperbetalipoproteinemia and hyperprebetalipoproteinemia. Familial hyperlipoproteinemia, type III, similar to familial hyperbetalipoproteinemia, but with an increase in total serum cholesterol accompanied by an increase in glycerides which is endogenous and induced by carbohydrates. The plasma very-low-density lipoproteins have unusual electrophoretic mobility, extending from the β to the α_2 zone on paper electrophoresis. Generally, there is an abnormal glucose tolerance curve, as well as tuberous and planar xanthomas, and early ischemic heart disease. Peripheral arteriosclerosis obliterans is often present. Syn. *familial broad-beta hyperlipoproteinemia.*

familial hypercholesterolemia. FAMILIAL HYPERBETALIPOPROTEINEMIA.

familial hypercholesterolemic xanthomatosis. FAMILIAL HYPERBETALIPOPROTEINEMIA.

familial hyperchylomicronemia with hyperprebetalipoproteinemia. Familial hyperlipoproteinemia, type V, characterized by the increase in total serum chylomicrons and prebetalipoproteins which appears to be a combination of fat- and carbohydrate-induced hyperlipemia. There is usually associated moderate diabetes mellitus or other metabolic disorder. Bouts of abdominal pain, eruptive xanthomas of various tissues, and other clinical features similar to those seen in familial fat-induced hyperlipemia may occur.

familial hyperlipoproteinemia. One of several inherited disorders of lipoprotein metabolism, separated on clinical and chemical basis thus far into six types. See also *familial broad-beta lipoproteinemia, familial combined hyperlipoproteinemia, familial fat-induced hyperlipemia, familial hyperbetalipoproteinemia, familial hyperprebetalipoproteinemia, familial hyperchylomicronemia with hyperprebetalipoproteinemia.*

familial hyperplastic periosteal dystrophy. A hereditary disorder in which there is hypertrophy of the subperiosteal bone, characterized by early closure of cranial sutures and thickening of the clavicles and phalanges.

familial hyperprebetalipoproteinemia. Familial hyperlipoproteinemia, type IV, clinically similar to types II and III, characterized by elevated levels of plasma very-low-density lipoproteins, which migrate into the pre-beta region on electrophoresis. Plasma triglyceride levels are elevated with normal diet but there is little or no elevation of total cholesterol. Abdominal pain similar to that seen in other hypertriglyceridemic states is seen clinically.

familial hyperprolinemia. A hereditary disorder in amino acid metabolism probably transmitted as an autosomal recessive trait, occurring in two types, Type I being clinically manifested by renal disease and Type II by mental retardation, generalized seizures, and terminal status epilepticus, patients with both types demonstrating excess urinary excretion of proline, hydroxyproline, and glycine. Syn. *Joseph's syndrome.*

familial hypophosphatemia. An inborn error of metabolism in which hypophosphatemia is the most consistent and often the only anomaly, and where there are various degrees of vitamin D–refractory rickets or osteomalacia, diminished tubular reabsorption of calcium, and at times unusual histologic changes in bone; transmitted as a sex-linked dominant trait.

familial juvenile nephronophthisis. MEDULLARY CYSTIC DISEASE OF THE KIDNEY.

familial Mediterranean fever. An inherited disorder occurring mainly in people of Sephardic Jewish, Armenian, and Arabic ancestry, of unknown etiology characterized by recurrent episodes of fever, abdominal and chest pain, arthralgia, and rash, terminating in some cases in chronic renal failure due to amyloidosis. Abbreviated, FMF. Syn. *familial recurring polyserositis, periodic disease, periodic peritonitis.* See also *etiocholanolone fever.*

familial metaphyseal dysplasia. An exceedingly rare condition marked by symmetrical enlargement of one or both ends of the shafts of long bones.

familial microcytic anemia. THALASSEMIA.

familial neurovisceral lipidosis. G_{M1} GANGLIOSIDOSIS. Deficiency of beta-galactosidase; characterized by peculiar facies, radiologically characteristic bone deformities, visceral enlargement, and vacuolated renal glomerular epithelial cells. Foamy histiocytes and swollen ganglion cells have been observed in most cases, increased ganglioside in liver, spleen, and brain in one. Clinically, there is progressive coarsening of facies, repeated infections, and failure of brain maturation. See also *fucosidosis.*

familial nonhemolytic jaundice. GILBERT'S SYNDROME.

familial osseous dystrophy. MORQUIO'S SYNDROME.

familial osteochondrodystrophy. MORQUIO'S SYNDROME.

familial paroxysmal choreoathetosis. PAROXYSMAL CHOREOATHETOSIS.

familial paroxysmal peritonitis. FAMILIAL MEDITERRANEAN FEVER.

familial periodic paralysis. PERIODIC PARALYSIS.

familial polyposis. An autosomal dominant disease characterized by the appearance before age 30 to 40 of multiple discrete adenomas of the colon; in Type I malignant transformation is common; in Type II (Peutz-Jeghers syndrome) mucocutaneous pigmentation occurs, but malignant transformation is rare; and in Type III (Gardner syndrome) there are sebaceous and inclusion cysts, osteomata of the face, jaw, and calvarium; and the polyps are predisposed to malignancy.

familial recurring polyserositis. FAMILIAL MEDITERRANEAN FEVER.

familial spastic paraplegia or **diplegia.** A heredofamilial disease, usually inherited as a dominant trait, characterized by degeneration of the corticospinal tracts and the development in early life of progressive spasticity and weakness in the lower extremities, eventually often involving the upper extremities, muscles of the trunk, and optic atrophy. There are no cerebellar or sensory defects. Sporadic forms and onset in adult life may occur.

familial splenic anemia. GAUCHER'S DISEASE.

familial steatorrhea. CYSTIC FIBROSIS.

familial tremor. A variety of postural or action tremor, inherited as a dominant trait, which begins in childhood and grows more marked with age and which may be limited to the hands and arms, but often involves the head.

familial xanthoma. FAMILIAL HYPERBETALIPOPROTEINEMIA.

fam·i·ly, *n.* [L. *familia,* household, from *famulus,* servant]. 1. A group of closely related persons; parents and children; those descended from a common ancestor. 2. *In biology,* a classification group higher than a genus; the principal division of an order.

family medicine. General practice; the practice of a family physician.

family nurse practitioner. A nurse practitioner whose primary focus of practice is on the family in ambulatory health care.

family physician. A general physician regularly called by a family in times of illness; one who does not limit his practice to a specialty.

family therapy. *In psychiatry,* the treatment of more than one member in a family during the same session on the assumption that the mental disorder in the patient is a manifestation of disturbed interaction with another member of the family or with the family as a group.

fam·ine dropsy. A form of edema occurring in individuals suffering from protein deprivation, either as the result of disease, or from inadequate intake.

famine edema. NUTRITIONAL EDEMA.

famine fever. 1. RELAPSING FEVER. 2. EPIDEMIC TYPHUS.

fam·o·tine (fam'o·teen) *n.* 1-[(*p*-Chlorophenoxy)methyl]-3,4-dihydroisoquinoline, $C_{16}H_{14}ClNO$, an antiviral.

fa·nat·i·cism (fa·nat'i·siz·um) *n.* [L. *fanaticus,* frantic, inspired by a deity]. Perversion and excess of the religious sentiment; unreasoning zeal in regard to any subject. Sometimes a manifestation of mental disease.

fan·cier's lung. BIRD-BREEDER'S LUNG.

Fan·co·ni's anemia or **disease** (fa^h^ng·ko'nee) [G. *Fanconi,* Swiss pediatrician, b. 1882]. CONGENITAL APLASTIC ANEMIA.

Fanconi syndrome [G. *Fanconi*]. A heritable recessive or sometimes acquired disorder of renal tubular function seen most commonly in children, in which there is rickets or osteomalacia resistant to vitamin D in usual doses, as well as renal glycosuria, generalized aminoaciduria, and hyperphosphaturia in spite of normal or decreased plasma levels of these constituents, and, usually, chronic acidosis and hypokalemia, and sometimes marked growth retardation. (The names of de Toni and Debré are often linked to designate this form of the syndrome.) In many childhood cases, cystinosis, characterized by an excess of cystine in the urine and the deposition of cystine crystals in internal organs and the eyes, is a prominent feature. (The names of Abderhalden, Kaufmann, and Lignac are often associated with this form.) See also *adult Fanconi syndrome.*

fang, *n.* A sharp or pointed tooth; especially, the tooth of a wild beast or serpent.

fan·go (fang'go) *n.* [It., mud]. Clay from the hot springs of Battaglio, Italy; used as a local application.

fan·go·ther·a·py (fang″go·therr'uh·pee) *n.* [*fango* + *therapy*]. Treatment with fango or other mud; used in arthritis or gout.

Fan·nia (fan'ee·uh) *n.* A genus of flies of the family Anthomyiidae. The species *Fannia canicularis,* the lesser house fly, and *F. scalaris,* the latrine fly, breed under unsanitary conditions; occasionally their larvae cause intestinal myiasis in man.

fan·ning, *n. In neurology,* the spreading apart of the fingers or toes like the ribs of an open fan; seen as a normal or abnormal reflex sign, as in the Babinski sign.

fan·ta·sy, *n.* [Gk. *phantasia,* appearance, imagination]. 1. Imagination; the ability to form mental pictures of scenes, occurrences, or objects not actually present; fanciful or dreamlike image making. 2. An image or series of images which may be an expression of unconscious conflicts or a gratification of unconscious wishes.

fan·tri·done (fan'tri·dohn) *n.* 5-[3-(Dimethylamino)propyl]-6(5*H*)-phenanthridinone, $C_{18}H_{20}N_2O$, an antidepressant drug; used as the hydrochloride salt.

Fanzil. Trademark for sulfadoxine, an antibacterial sulfonamide.

Fa·ra·beuf's triangle (fa·ra·bœf') [L. H. *Farabeuf,* French anatomist and surgeon, 1841–1910]. A triangle formed in the upper part of the neck by the internal jugular vein, the common facial vein, and the hypoglossal nerve.

far·ad (făr'ad) *n.* [M. *Farad*ay, English chemist and physicist, 1791–1867]. The unit of electric capacitance; the capacitance of a capacitor that is charged to a potential of 1 volt by 1 coulomb of electricity.

far·a·day (făr'uh·day) *n.* [M. *Faraday*]. The quantity of electricity which will liberate one gram equivalent of an element, specifically 107.88 g of silver, on electrolysis. It equals 96,494 ± 10 international coulombs.

fa·rad·ic (fa·rad'ick) *adj.* [M. *Faraday*]. Pertaining to induced rapidly alternating currents of electricity.

faradic battery. A device that produces induced electricity.

faradic contractility. Ability of muscle to contract in response to a rapidly alternating current.

faradic current. A current produced by an induction coil.

faradic electricity. Electricity produced by induction.

far·a·dim·e·ter (făr″uh·dim'e·tur) *n.* [*faradic* + *meter*]. An instrument for measuring the strength of an induced rapidly alternating electric current.

fa·radi·punc·ture (fa·rad″i·punk'chur) *n.* [*faradic* + *puncture*]. The application of faradic current by means of needle electrodes thrust into the tissues.

far·a·dism (făr'uh·diz·um) *n.* [*faradic* + *-ism*]. The application of a rapidly alternating current of electricity; FARADIZATION.

far·a·di·za·tion (făr″uh·di·zay'shun) *n.* The therapeutic application of induced rapidly alternating current to a diseased part; FARADISM. —**far·a·dize** (făr'uh·dize) *v.*

farado-. A combining form meaning *faradic.*

far·a·do·con·trac·til·i·ty (făr″uh·do·kon″track·til'i·tee) *n.* Contractility in response to faradic stimulus.

far·a·do·mus·cu·lar (făr″uh·do·mus'kew·lur) *adj.* [*farado-* + *muscular*]. Pertaining to the reaction of a muscle when a faradic current is applied.

far·a·do·ther·a·py (făr″uh·do·therr'uh·pee) *n.* Therapeutic use of faradism; FARADIZATION.

far-advanced tuberculosis. Tuberculosis in which there are lesions more extensive than in moderately advanced. Contr. *moderately advanced tuberculosis.*

Far·ber's disease [S. *Farber,* U.S. pathologist, 1903–1973]. DISSEMINATED LIPOGRANULOMATOSIS.

far·cy (fahr'see) *n.* [L. *farcimen,* sausage, from *farcire,* to stuff]. The cutaneous form of glanders, characterized by skin ulcers and thickening of superficial lymphatics.

far·del (fahr'dul) *n.* [OF., parcel, bundle]. *Obsol.* OMASUM.

fardel-bound, *n. & adj.* 1. A condition of cattle or sheep in which the omasum becomes static and the food dry and impacted. 2. Affected with this condition.

Far Eastern hemorrhagic fever. EPIDEMIC HEMORRHAGIC FEVER.

Far Eastern spring-summer encephalitis. A tick-borne encephalitis due to infection with a group B arbovirus, seen in the U.S.S.R., Korea, China, and Malaysia.

fa·ri·na (fa·ree'nuh) *n.* [L.]. 1. Flour or meal, of any origin. 2. A starchy corn-based cereal food. 3. Any powdery substance, such as pollen.

far·i·na·ceous (făr″i·nay'shus) *adj.* [L. *farinaceus,* from *farina,* flour]. Having the nature of or yielding flour; starchy; containing starch.

Far·ley, St. Clair, and Rei·sing·er's method. A method of classifying neutrophils into filament and nonfilament types according to the shape of the nucleus.

farm·er's lung. An acute or chronic inflammatory reaction in the lungs caused by hypersensitivity to thermophilic actinomycetes in moldy hay or grain, characterized by dyspnea, fever, cough, cyanosis, and patchy infiltrates in the lung; may also be caused by other organic dusts.

farmer's skin. SAILOR'S SKIN.

far·ne·sol (fahr'ne·sol) *n.* 3,7,11-Trimethyl-2,6,10-dodecatrien-1-ol, $C_{15}H_{26}O$, an acyclic terpene alcohol in various essential oils, also in Peruvian balsam and tolu balsam. It is used in perfumery to emphasize the odor of certain floral perfumes.

far·ne·syl pyrophosphate (fahr'ne·sil). The pyrophosphate of farnesol, $C_{15}H_{28}O_7P_2$, an intermediate in the synthesis of cholesterol in animal tissues.

far point. The most distant point at which an eye can see distinctly when accommodation is completely relaxed.

Farre's white line [A. *Farre,* British gynecologist, 1811–1877]. The boundary line at the hilus of the ovary.

far·ri·ery (făr'ee·ur·ee) *n.* [*farrier,* blacksmith (from L. *ferrarius*), + *-y*]. 1. The practice of horseshoeing. 2. *Obsol.* The treatment of diseases of horses.

far sight. HYPEROPIA.

far·sight·ed·ness, *n.* HYPEROPIA.

fas·cia (fash'uh, ·ee·uh) *n.*, L. pl. & genit. sing. **fasci·ae** (·shee·ee) [L., band]. 1. The areolar tissue layers under the skin (superficial fascia). 2. The fibrous tissue between muscles and forming the sheaths of muscles, or investing other deep, definitive structures, as nerves and blood vessels (deep fascia). Adj. *fascial.*

fascia an·te·bra·chii (an″te·bray'kee·eye) [NA]. The deep fascia of the forearm.

fascia an·ti·bra·chii (an″tee·bray'kee·eye) [BNA]. FASCIA ANTEBRACHII.

fascia axil·la·ris (ack·si·lair'is) [NA]. The deep fascia of the axilla or armpit.

fascia bra·chii (bray'kee·eye) [NA]. The deep fascia of the arm.

fascia buc·co·pha·ryn·gea (buck″o·fa·rin'jee·uh) [NA]. The deep fascia of the neck covering the constrictor muscles of the pharynx.

fascia bul·bi [Tenoni] (bul'bye) [BNA]. VAGINA BULBI.

fascia cer·vi·ca·lis (sur·vi·kay'lis) [NA]. DEEP CERVICAL FASCIA.

fascia cla·vi·pec·to·ra·lis (klav'i·peck·to·ray'lis) [NA]. CLAVIPECTORAL FASCIA.

fascia cli·to·ri·dis (kli·tor'i·dis) [NA]. The deep fascia of the clitoris.

fascia col·li (kol'eye) [BNA]. Fascia cervicalis (= DEEP CERVICAL FASCIA).

fascia co·ra·co·cla·vi·cu·la·ris (kor″uh·ko·kla·vick″yoo·lair'is) [BNA]. Fascia clavipectoralis (= CLAVIPECTORAL FASCIA).

fascia cre·mas·te·ri·ca (kree·mas·terr'i·kuh) [NA]. CREMASTERIC FASCIA.
fascia cri·bro·sa (kri·bro'suh) [NA]. CRIBRIFORM FASCIA.
fascia cru·ris (kroo'ris) [NA]. CRURAL FASCIA.
fascia den·ta·ta hip·po·cam·pi (den·tay'tuh hip·o·kam'pye) [BNA]. Gyrus dentatus (= DENTATE GYRUS).
fascia di·a·phrag·ma·tis pel·vis inferior (dye·uh·frag'muh·tis pel'vis) [NA]. The deep fascia covering the inferior surface of the pelvic diaphragm.
fascia diaphragmatis pelvis superior [NA]. The deep fascia covering the upper surface of the pelvic diaphragm.
fascia diaphragmatis uro·ge·ni·ta·lis inferior (yoor"o·jen·i·tay'lis) [NA]. PERINEAL MEMBRANE. NA alt. *membrana perinei.*
fascia diaphragmatis urogenitalis superior [NA]. The deep fascia covering the superior surface of the urogenital diaphragm.
fascia dor·sa·lis ma·nus (dor·say'lis man'us) [NA]. The deep fascia of the back of the hand.
fascia dorsalis pe·dis (ped'is) [NA]. The deep fascia of the dorsum of the foot.
fasciae. Plural and genitive singular of *fascia.*
fasciae mus·cu·la·res bul·bi (mus·kew·lair'eez bul'bye) [NA]. The deep fasciae that invest the extrinsic muscles of the eyeball.
fasciae musculares ocu·li (ock'yoo·lye) [BNA]. FASCIAE MUSCULARES BULBI.
fascia en·do·tho·ra·ci·ca (en·do·tho·ras'i·kuh, ·tho·ray'si·kuh) [NA]. The fascia outside the parietal thoracic serous mesothelium.
fasciae or·bi·ta·les (or·bi·tay'leez) [NA]. The deep fasciae within the orbit.
fascia ili·a·ca (i·lye'uh·kuh) [NA]. ILIAC FASCIA.
fascia ilio·pec·ti·nea (il"ee·o·peck·tin'ee·uh) [BNA]. ARCUS ILIOPECTINEUS.
fascia in·fra·spi·na·ta (in"fruh·spye·nay'tuh) [BNA]. The deep fascia over the infraspinatus muscle.
fas·cial (fash'ee·ul) *adj.* Pertaining to or involving a fascia.
fascia la·ta (lay'tuh) [NA]. The deep fascia surrounding the muscles of the thigh.
fascial graft. A strip of fascia lata or aponeurosis; used either for the repair of a defect in muscle or fascia, or for suturing.
fascial plane. Any plane in the body which is oriented along a layer of fascia. It usually represents a cleavage plane, and is used for exposure in surgery; it may limit or direct the spread of infection.
fascial reflex. A deep muscle stretch reflex elicited by a sudden tap over a fascia.
fascial spaces. Potential spaces between layers of fascia, as fascial spaces of the foot.
fascia lum·bo·dor·sa·lis (lum"bo·dor·say'lis) [BNA]. Fascia thoracolumbalis (= THORACOLUMBAR FASCIA).
fascia lu·na·ta (lew·nay'tuh). The deep fascia of the ischiorectal fossa.
fascia mas·se·te·ri·ca (mas"e·terr'i·kuh) [NA]. The deep fascia over the masseter muscle.
fascia nu·chae (new'kee) [NA]. The deep fascia investing the muscles of the back of the neck.
fascia ob·tu·ra·to·ria (ob"tew·ruh·to'ree·uh) [NA]. OBTURATOR FASCIA.
fascia pa·ro·ti·dea (păr"o·tid'ee·uh) [NA]. The deep fascia investing the parotid gland.
fascia pa·ro·ti·deo·mas·se·te·ri·ca (păr·o·tid"ee·o·mas·e·terr'i·kuh) [BNA]. The combined deep fascia investing the parotid gland and covering the masseter muscle.
fascia pec·ti·nea (peck·tin'ee·uh) [BNA]. PECTINEAL FASCIA.
fascia pec·to·ra·lis (peck·to·ray'lis) [NA]. PECTORAL FASCIA.
fascia pel·vis (pel'vis) [NA]. PELVIC FASCIA.
fascia pelvis pa·ri·e·ta·lis (pa·rye"e·tay'lis) [NA]. The deep fascia of the wall of the pelvic cavity.
fascia pelvis vis·ce·ra·lis (vis·e·ray'lis) [NA]. The deep fascia investing the pelvic organs.
fascia pe·nis (pee'nis) [BNA]. 1. FASCIA PENIS PROFUNDA. 2. FASCIA PENIS SUPERFICIALIS.
fascia penis pro·fun·da [NA]. The deep fascia of the penis. Syn. *Buck's fascia.*
fascia penis su·per·fi·ci·a·lis (sue"pur·fish·ee·ay'lis) [NA]. The superficial fascia of the penis.
fascia pe·ri·nei su·per·fi·ci·a·lis (perr·i·nee'eye sue"pur·fish·ee·ay'lis) [NA]. The superficial fascia of the perineum.
fascia pha·ryn·go·ba·si·la·ris (fa·rin"go·bas·i·lair'is) [NA]. The dense fibrous portion of the wall of the pharynx lying outside the mucous membrane.
fascia phre·ni·co·pleu·ra·lis (fren"i·ko·plew·ray'lis) [NA]. The deep fascia covering the upper surface of the diaphragm.
fascia prae·ver·te·bra·lis (pree·vur"te·bray'lis) [BNA]. Lamina prevertebralis fasciae cervicalis (= PREVERTEBRAL FASCIA).
fascia pro·sta·tae (pros'ta·tee) [NA]. The deep fascia surrounding the prostate.
fascia sper·ma·ti·ca ex·ter·na (spur·mat'i·kuh ecks·tur'nuh) [NA]. EXTERNAL SPERMATIC FASCIA.
fascia spermatica in·ter·na (in·tur'nuh) [NA]. INTERNAL SPERMATIC FASCIA.
fascia sub·pe·ri·to·ne·a·lis (sub·perr"i·to·nee·ay'lis) [NA]. The fascia immediately outside the peritoneum.
fascia sub·sca·pu·la·ris (sub·skap"yoo·lair'is) [BNA]. The deep fascia covering the subscapular muscle.
fascia su·per·fi·ci·a·lis (sue"pur·fish·ee·ay'lis) [BNA]. SUPERFICIAL FASCIA.
fascia superficialis pe·ri·nei (perr·i·nee'eye) [BNA]. FASCIA PERINEI SUPERFICIALIS.
fascia su·pra·spi·na·ta (sue"pruh·spye·nay'tuh) [BNA]. The deep fascia over the supraspinatus muscle.
fascia tem·po·ra·lis (tem·po·ray'lis) [NA]. The deep fascia covering the temporal muscle; it consists of a deeper and a more superficial sheet.
fascia tho·ra·co·lum·ba·lis (tho"ruh·ko·lum·bay'lis) [NA]. THORACOLUMBAR FASCIA.
fascia trans·ver·sa·lis (trans·vur·say'lis) [NA]. TRANSVERSALIS FASCIA.
fas·ci·cle (fas'i·kul) *n.* FASCICULUS.
fas·cic·u·lar (fa·sick'yoo·lur) *adj.* Of or pertaining to a fasciculus or to fasciculi.
fascicular degeneration. Degeneration, usually with necrosis, in fasciculi of muscle supplied by diseased or interrupted motor neurons.
fascicular keratitis. A form of phlyctenular conjunctivitis marked by the formation of a fascicle of blood vessels.
fas·cic·u·lat·ed (fa·sick'yoo·lay"tid) *adj.* United into bundles or fasciculi.
fas·cic·u·la·tion (fa·sick"yoo·lay'shun) *n.* 1. An incoordinate contraction of skeletal muscle in which groups of muscle fibers innervated by the same neuron contract together. 2. The formation of fasciculi.
fasciculation potential. *In electromyography,* the electrical activity that represents the spontaneous discharge of a motor unit (the group of muscle fibers innervated by a single axon); may occur in the absence of disease, or may be associated with anterior horn cell disease or with irritative or compressive lesions of the roots or peripheral nerves.
fasciculi. Plural and genitive singular of *fasciculus.*
fasciculi cor·po·ris res·ti·for·mis (kor'po·ris res·ti·for'mis) [BNA]. PEDUNCULUS CEREBELLARIS INFERIOR.
fasciculi cor·ti·co·tha·la·mi·ci (kor"ti·ko·tha·lam'i·sigh) [NA]. A general term for bundles of nerve fibers which project from the cerebral cortex to the thalamus.
fasciculi in·ter·seg·men·ta·les (in"tur·seg·men·tay'leez). [NA alt.]. FASCICULI PROPRII MEDULLAE SPINALIS.
fasciculi lon·gi·tu·di·na·les li·ga·men·ti cru·ci·for·mis at·lan·tis

(lon″ji·tew·di·nay′leez lig·uh·men′tye krew·si·for′mis at·lan′tis) [NA]. The vertical or longitudinal fibers of the cruciate ligament of the atlas.

fasciculi longitudinales pon·tis (pon′tis) [NA]. Various descending pathways from the cerebral cortex which pass through the pons.

fasciculi ma·mil·lo·teg·men·ta·les (ma·mil″o·teg·men·tay′leez). Plural of *fasciculus mamillotegmentalis.*

fasciculi pe·dun·cu·lo·ma·mil·la·res (pe·dunk″yoo·lo·mam·i·lair′eez) [BNA]. Fasciculi mamillotegmentales. See *mamillotegmental tract.*

fasciculi pro·prii me·dul·lae spi·na·lis (pro′pree·eye me·dul′ee spye·nay′lis) [NA]. Bundles of white matter immediately surrounding the gray matter of the spinal cord; they consist of short ascending and descending correlation fibers. NA alt. *fasciculi intersegmentales.*

fasciculi py·ra·mi·da·les (pi·ram″i·day′leez) [BNA]. Tractus pyramidales (= PYRAMIDAL TRACTS).

fasciculi ru·bro·re·ti·cu·la·res (roo″bro·re·tick″yoo·lair′eez) [NA]. Bundles of nerve fibers from the red nucleus to the reticular formation.

fasciculi tha·la·mo·cor·ti·ca·les (thal″uh·mo·kor″ti·kay′leez) [NA]. Bundles of nerve fibers which project from the thalamus to the cerebral cortex.

fas·cic·u·li·tis (fa·sick″yoo·lye′tis) *n.* [*fascicul*us + *-itis*]. Inflammation of a small bundle of muscle or nerve fibers, usually the latter.

fasciculi trans·ver·si apo·neu·ro·sis pal·ma·ris (trans·vur′sigh ap″o·new·ro′sis pal·mair′is) [NA]. Transverse bundles of dense connective tissue in the palmar aponeurosis.

fasciculi transversi aponeurosis plan·ta·ris (plan·tair′is) [NA]. Transverse bundles of dense connective tissue in the plantar aponeurosis.

fas·cic·u·lus (fa·sick′yoo·lus) *n.*, pl. & genit. sing. **fascicu·li** (·lye) [L., dim. of *fascis,* bundle, packet]. 1. *In histology,* a bundle of nerve, muscle, or tendon fibers separated by connective tissue; as that of muscle fibers, by perimysium. 2. *In neurology,* a bundle or tract of nerve fibers presumably having common connections and functions. See also *tract.*

fasciculus anterior pro·pri·us [Flechsigi] (pro′pree·us) [BNA]. The anterior portion of the fasciculi proprii medullae spinalis.

fasciculus an·te·ro·la·te·ra·lis su·per·fi·ci·a·lis [Gowersi] (an″tur·o·lat·e·ray′lis sue″pur·fish·ee·ay′lis) [BNA]. Tractus spinocerebellaris anterior (= VENTRAL SPINOCEREBELLAR TRACT).

fasciculus atrio·ven·tri·cu·la·ris (ay″tree·o·ven·trick·yoo·lair′is) [NA]. ATRIOVENTRICULAR BUNDLE.

fasciculus ce·re·bel·lo·spi·na·lis (serr·e·bel″o·spye·nay′lis) [BNA]. Tractus spinocerebellaris posterior (= DORSAL SPINOCEREBELLAR TRACT).

fasciculus ce·re·bro·spi·na·lis anterior (serr″e·bro·spye·nay′lis) [BNA]. Tractus corticospinalis anterior (= ANTERIOR CORTICOSPINAL TRACT).

fasciculus cerebrospinalis la·te·ra·lis (lat·e·ray′lis) [BNA]. Tractus corticospinalis lateralis (= LATERAL CORTICOSPINAL TRACT).

fasciculus cu·ne·a·tus [Burdachi] (kew·nee·ay′tus) [BNA]. Fasciculus cuneatus medullae spinalis (= CUNEATE FASCICULUS).

fasciculus cuneatus me·dul·lae ob·lon·ga·tae (me·dul′ee ob·long·gay′tee) [NA]. The continuation of the cuneate fasciculus into the medulla oblongata.

fasciculus cuneatus medullae spi·na·lis (spye·nay′lis) [NA]. CUNEATE FASCICULUS.

fasciculus dor·so·la·te·ra·lis (dor″so·lat·ur·ay′lis) [NA]. DORSOLATERAL TRACT.

fasciculus gra·ci·lis me·dul·lae ob·lon·ga·tae (gras′i·lis me·dul′ee ob·long·gay′tee) [NA]. The continuation of the fasciculus gracilis medullae spinalis into the medulla oblongata.

fasciculus gracilis medullae spi·na·lis (spye·nay′lis) [NA]. The medial part of the dorsal funiculus of the spinal cord carrying proprioceptive impulses from the legs and lower regions of the trunk.

fasciculus in·ter·fas·ci·cu·la·ris (in″tur·fa·sick·yoo·lair′is) [NA alt.]. COMMA TRACT. NA alt. *fasciculus semilunaris.*

fasciculus la·te·ra·lis plex·us bra·chi·a·lis (lat·e·ray′lis pleck′sus bray·kee·ay′lis) [NA]. The lateral cord of the brachial plexus.

fasciculus lateralis pro·pri·us (pro′pree·us) [NA]. The lateral part of the fasciculus proprius.

fasciculus lon·gi·tu·di·na·lis dor·sa·lis (lon″ji·tew·di·nay′lis dor·say′lis) [NA]. PERIVENTRICULAR TRACT.

fasciculus longitudinalis inferior [NA]. INFERIOR LONGITUDINAL FASCICULUS.

fasciculus longitudinalis me·di·a·lis (mee·dee·ay′lis) [NA]. MEDIAL LONGITUDINAL FASCICULUS.

fasciculus longitudinalis superior [NA]. SUPERIOR LONGITUDINAL FASCICULUS.

fasciculus ma·mil·lo·teg·men·ta·lis (ma·mil″o·teg″men·tay′lis) [NA]. MAMILLOTEGMENTAL TRACT.

fasciculus ma·mil·lo·tha·la·mi·cus (ma·mil″o·thuh·lam′i·kus) [NA]. MAMILLOTHALAMIC TRACT.

fasciculus me·di·a·lis plex·us bra·chi·a·lis (mee·dee·ay′lis pleck′sus bray·kee·ay′lis) [NA]. The medial cord of the brachial plexus.

fasciculus ob·li·quus pon·tis (ob·lye′kwus pon′tis) [BNA]. An indistinct band of obliquely placed fibers on the inferior surface of the pons.

fasciculus of Türck (tuᵉrk) [L. *Türck,* Austrian neurologist, 1810–1886]. ANTERIOR CORTICOSPINAL TRACT.

fasciculus posterior plex·us bra·chi·a·lis (pleck′sus bray·kee·ay′lis) [NA]. The posterior cord of the brachial plexus.

fasciculus pro·pri·us (pro′pree·us). Singular of *fasciculi proprii (medullae spinalis);* ground bundle.

fasciculus re·tro·flex·us (ret″ro·fleck′sus) [NA]. A bundle of nerve fibers connecting the habenular nucleus with the interpeduncular nucleus of midbrain. It is concerned with olfactory impulses. Syn. *habenulopeduncular tract.*

fasciculus se·mi·lu·na·ris (sem″i·lew·nair′is) [NA]. COMMA TRACT. NA alt. *fasciculus interfascicularis.*

fasciculus sep·to·mar·gi·na·lis (sep″to·mahr·ji·nay′lis) [NA]. SEPTOMARGINAL FASCICULUS.

fasciculus so·li·ta·ri·us (sol·i·tair′ee·us). SOLITARY FASCICULUS.

fasciculus sub·cal·lo·sus (sub·ka·lo′sus) [NA]. SUBCALLOSAL FASCICULUS.

fasciculus tha·la·mo·ma·mil·la·ris (thal″uh·mo·mam·i·lair′is) [BNA]. Fasciculus mamillothalamicus (= MAMILLOTHALAMIC TRACT).

fasciculus un·ci·na·tus (un·si·nay′tus) [NA]. UNCINATE FASCICULUS OF THE HEMISPHERE.

fas·ci·ec·to·my (fash″ee·eck′tuh·mee, fas″ee·) *n.* [*fasci*a + *-ectomy*]. *In surgery,* excision of fascia; specifically, excision of strips from the lateral part of the fascia lata (iliotibial tract) for use in plastic surgery.

fas·ci·itis (fas″ee·eye′tis, fash″) *n.* [*fasci*a + *-itis*]. 1. Inflammation of fascia. 2. A benign proliferative disorder of fascia of unknown cause, often producing nodules.

fas·ci·num (fas′i·num) *n.* [L.]. 1. Literally, a spell, a bewitching; specifically, a spell cast by the evil eye. 2. The belief that certain individuals can cause injury by casting an evil eye upon a person, frequently expressed by patients suffering from the paranoid type of schizophrenia. 3. Any amulet or charm worn to protect against the evil eye, as, in Roman times, a tiny image of a penis hung around the necks of children as a protection against the evil eye and other forms of witchcraft. See also *evil eye.*

fascio-. A combining form meaning *fascia, fascial.*

fas·ci·od·e·sis (fash″ee·od′e·sis, fas″ee·) *n.*, pl. **fasciode·ses** (·seez) [*fascio-* + *-desis*]. The operation of suturing a fascia to another fascia, to a tendon, or to a skeletal attachment.

Fas·ci·o·la (fa·sigh'o·luh) *n.* [L., small bandage]. A genus of trematodes; hermaphroditic flukes.

fasciola, *n.*, pl. **fascio·lae** (·lee). A small strip or bandlike structure.

fasciola ci·ne·rea (si·neer'ee·uh). GYRUS FASCIOLARIS.

Fasciola gi·gan·ti·ca (jye·gant'i·kuh). A species of liver fluke found in Africa, Asia, and Hawaii, which parasitizes cattle, camels, water buffalo, and other herbivorous animals, and occasionally infects man.

Fasciola he·pat·i·ca (he·pat'i·kuh). A species of liver fluke worldwide in distribution, especially in sheep-raising areas, which lives in the biliary passages of the host, producing fascioliasis. Occurs in many mammals, including sheep, goats, camels, elephants, rabbits, monkeys, and man.

fas·ci·o·lar (fa·sigh'o·lur) *adj.* Of or pertaining to a fasciola.

fasciolar gyrus. GYRUS FASCIOLARIS.

fas·ci·o·li·a·sis (fas''ee·o·lye'uh·sis, fa·sigh''o·) *n.*, pl. **fasciolia·ses** (·seez) [*Fasciola* + *-iasis*]. Infection with liver flukes, especially *Fasciola hepatica,* occurring in sheep and other herbivorous animals; man has served as an accidental host. The liver is usually the site of infection.

Fas·cio·loi·des mag·na (fas''ee·o·loy'deez mag'nuh, fa·sigh''o·). A species of flukes occurring in the liver, rarely the lungs, of cattle and other herbivores in North America.

fas·ci·o·loi·di·a·sis (fas''ee·o·loy·dye'uh·sis) *n.* FASCIOLIASIS.

fas·ci·o·lop·si·a·sis (fas''ee·o·lop·sigh'uh·sis, fa·sigh''o·) *n.* [*Fasciolopsis* + *-iasis*]. An intestinal infection of man and hogs by *Fasciolopsis buski,* characterized by diarrhea, abdominal pain, anasarca, and eosinophilia. Generally acquired by the ingestion of water plants, such as the water chestnut, contaminated by infected snails.

Fas·ci·o·lop·sis (fas''ee·o·lop'sis, fa·sigh'o·) *n.* [*Fasciola* + Gk. *opsis,* appearance]. A genus of flukes parasitic in both man and hogs.

Fasciolopsis bus·ki (bus'kye). The largest intestinal fluke of man; endemic only in the Orient; the causative organism of fasciolopsiasis.

fas·cio·plas·ty (fash''ee·o·plas''tee) *n.* [*fascio-* + *-plasty*]. Plastic surgery upon fascia.

fas·ci·or·rha·phy (fash''ee·or'uh·fee) *n.* [*fascio-* + *-rrhaphy*]. Suture of cut or lacerated fascia.

fas·ci·ot·o·my (fash''ee·ot'uh·mee) *n.* [*fascio-* + *-tomy*]. Incision of a fascia.

fas·ci·tis (fas·eye'tis, fash·eye'tis) *n.* FASCIITIS.

Fasigyn. A trademark for tinidazole, an antiprotozoal.

[1]fast, *adj.* 1. Fixed, usually permanently; unable to leave, as a place or thing; immobile. 2. Resistant to change or destructive action.

[2]fast, *v.* & *n.* 1. To abstain from eating. 2. To restrict one's diet. 3. To deny food to someone. 4. Abstention from food.

-fast. A combining form meaning (a) *securely attached, narrowly confined,* as in bedfast; (b) *resistant to a* (specified) *dye, chemical agent, or microorganism,* as in acid-fast.

fast green FCF. An acid dye of the diaminotriphenylmethane series; used as a counterstain.

fas·tid·i·ous (fas·tid'ee·us) *adj.* [L. *fastidiosus,* from *fastidium,* aversion, fastidiousness]. Having exacting nutritional and other requirements for growth, said of microorganisms.

fas·tig·i·al (fas·tij'ee·ul) *adj.* Of or pertaining to the fastigium.

fastigial nucleus. A nucleus in the cerebellum situated near the midline in the roof of the fourth ventricle, which receives fibers from the cerebellar cortex, inferior olivary and vestibular nuclei and sends efferent fibers into the brain stem. NA *nucleus fastigii.*

fas·tig·io·bul·bar (fas·tij''ee·o·bul'bur) *adj.* [*fastigium* + *bulbar*]. Pertaining to the fastigium and the medulla oblongata.

fastigiobulbar tract. A tract arising in the fastigial nuclei, containing crossed and uncrossed fibers, which descends medial to the inferior cerebellar peduncle and is distributed to the vestibular nuclei and to the dorsomedial parts of the reticular formation of the pons and medulla. Syn. *cerebellobulbar tract.*

fas·tig·i·um (fas·tij'ee·um) *n.* [L., summit, top, extremity]. 1. [BNA] The most rostral part of the roof of the fourth ventricle at the junction of the superior medullary velum of each side with the tela choroidea of the fourth ventricle. 2. The acme of a disease or fever.

fat, *adj.* & *n.* 1. Plump, corpulent. 2. Oily, greasy. 3. Any of a class of neutral organic compounds, mixtures of which form the natural fats. They are glyceryl esters of certain acids (in animal fat chiefly oleic, palmitic, and stearic); are soluble in ether but not in water, are combustible, and on saponification yield glycerin. Fat is an energy-yielding foodstuff, 1 g furnishing 9.3 calories. Fat is the chief component of the cell contents of adipose tissue; occurs also in other animal tissue to a lesser degree, and in plant cells. 4. ADIPOSE TISSUE.

fa·tal, *adj.* [L. *fatalis,* from *fatum,* fate]. 1. Causing death; deadly; disastrous. 2. Of or pertaining to whatever is destined or decreed. **—fatal·ly** (·ee) *adv.*

fa·tal·i·ty (fay·tal'i·tee) *n.* 1. Death resulting from a disease, ingestion of a poisonous substance, or a disaster; a fatal outcome. 2. A victim of a fatal outcome.

fat cell. A connective-tissue cell in which fat is stored; LIPOCYTE.

fat embolism. Occlusion of blood vessels in multiple organs by fat droplet emboli, usually resulting from bone or adipose tissue trauma.

fat graft. A portion of fat, implanted to fill a hollow and improve a contour.

father complex. OEDIPUS COMPLEX.

father figure. The male parent figure.

fat·i·ga·ble (fat'i·guh·bul) *adj.* [L. *fatigabilis,* from *fatigare,* to weary]. Susceptible to fatigue; easily tired. **—fat·i·ga·bil·i·ty** (fat''i·guh·bil'i·tee) *n.*

fa·tigue (fa·teeg') *n.* & *v.* [F., from L. *fatigare,* to tire]. 1. Exhaustion of strength; weariness from exertion. 2. Condition of cells or organs in which, through overactivity, the power or capacity to respond to stimulation is diminished or lost. 3. To tire; make or become exhausted.

fatigue contracture. A form of myostatic contracture.

fatigue fracture. A fracture of bone, or of a bone prosthesis, due to repeated loading by weight bearing or muscle contraction. Syn. *stress fracture.* See also *march fracture.*

fatigue nystagmus. A form of pseudonystagmus observed normally after an individual has looked to one side for one or more minutes when nystagmoid jerks may appear along with a disagreeable feeling of fatigue in the eye.

fatigue-postural paradox. SCAPULOCOSTAL SYNDROME.

fatigue state. NEURASTHENIA.

fatigue toxin. A hypothetical toxic material arising from tissue disintegration in excessive fatigue.

fat-induced familial hypertriglyceridemia. A deficiency of lipoprotein lipase, transmitted as an autosomal recessive, resulting in chylomicron accumulation due to defective clearing of dietary fat; manifested clinically by xanthomas, hepatosplenomegaly, attacks of abdominal pain, and lipemia retinalis.

fat infiltration. 1. Deposit of neutral fats in tissues or cells as the result of transport. 2. FATTY INFILTRATION.

fat-metabolizing hormone. *Obsol.* KETOGENIC HORMONE.

fat necrosis. Necrosis in adipose tissue, commonly accompanied by the production of soaps from the hydrolyzed fat, and seen in association with pancreatitis and in injuries to adipose tissue (traumatic fat necrosis).

fat organs. ADIPOSE ORGANS.

fat pad. *In anatomy,* any mass of fatty tissue.

fat·sia (fat'see·uh) *n.* The bark of the root of *Oplopanax horridus,* believed to contain a hypoglycemic principle. Syn. *devil's club.*

fat-soluble, *adj.* Soluble in fats or fat solvents; specifically used with a letter to designate certain vitamins, as fat-soluble A.

fat·ty, *adj.* 1. Pertaining to or containing fat. 2. ALIPHATIC.

fatty acid. An acid derived from the series of open-chain hydrocarbons, usually obtained from the saponification of fats. See also Table of Chemical Constituents of Blood in the Appendix.

fatty acid peroxidase. An enzyme present in germinating plant seeds which catalyzes the oxidation of the carboxyl carbon of fatty acids to CO_2. The α carbon is oxidized to the aldehyde at the expense of hydrogen peroxide.

fatty acid synthetase. The multienzyme complex found in the nonmitochondrial portion of the cellular fluid, which is capable of carrying out the synthesis of fatty acids.

fatty acyl carnitine. A transport form of fatty acids which allows them to cross the mitochondrial membrane; formed by reaction of fatty acyl-CoA with carnitine employing the emzyme carnitine acyltransferase.

fatty acyl-CoA. An activated form of fatty acids formed by the enzyme acyl CoA synthetase at the expense of adenosine triphosphate.

fatty alcohol. An alcohol obtained from a hydrocarbon of the fatty series.

fatty atrophy. FATTY METAMORPHOSIS.

fatty capsule of the kidney. The fat-containing connective tissue encircling the kidney. NA *capsula adiposa renis.*

fatty cirrhosis. Early Laennec's cirrhosis with prominent fatty metamorphosis of liver cells.

fatty degeneration. Fatty metamorphosis, fatty infiltration, or both together.

fatty heart. 1. Fatty degeneration of the cardiac muscle fibers. 2. An increase in the quantity of subpericardial and intramyocardial adipose tissue.

fatty hernia. EPIGASTRIC HERNIA.

fatty infiltration. Excessive accumulation of fat cells in the interstitial tissue of an organ.

fatty kidney. Fatty degeneration of the renal epithelium.

fatty liver. A liver which is the seat of fatty change, as fat infiltration.

fatty metamorphosis. A retrogressive process characterized by the appearance of visible fat and sometimes by other deteriorative changes within cells that do not ordinarily contain visible fat.

fau·ces (faw'seez) *n.pl.,* genit. pl. **fau·ci·um** (faw'see·um) [L., jaws, gullet, throat] [NA]. The space surrounded by the soft palate, palatoglossal and palatopharyngeal arches, and base of the tongue. —**fau·cial** (faw'shul) *adj.*

faucial reflex. Gagging or vomiting produced by irritation of the fauces.

fau·na (faw'nuh) *n.,* pl. **faunas, fau·nae** (·nee) [L. *Faunus,* Roman god of herds and fields]. The entire animal life peculiar to any area or period.

Faust's method. A method of concentrating cysts of protozoa in the stool by using centrifugal flotation with zinc sulfate of specific gravity 1.180.

fa·vag·i·nous (fa·vaj'i·nus) *adj.* 1. Resembling favus. 2. Honeycombed; faveolate.

fa·ve·o·late (fa·vee'uh·late) *adj.* [*faveo*lus + *-ate*]. Honeycombed; alveolate.

fa·ve·o·lus (fa·vee'uh·lus) *n.,* pl. **faveo·li** (·lye) [NL., dim. of *favus*]. A pit or cell like that of the honeycomb.

fa·vi·des (fay'vi·deez) *n. pl.* Allergic skin reactions to favus.

fa·vism (fay'viz·um) *n.* [It. *fava*, broad bean, + *-ism*]. An acute hemolytic anemia, usually in those of Mediterranean area descent, occurring when a person with glucose 6-phosphate dehydrogenase deficiency of erythrocytes eats the beans of *Vicia faba* or inhales its pollen, presumed to be an antigen-antibody interaction with the red blood cells.

Fa·vre's disease (fav'r) [M. *Favre,* French physician, b. 1876]. LYMPHOGRANULOMA VENEREUM.

fa·vus (fay'vus) *n.* [L., honeycomb]. A fungal infection of the scalp, usually caused by *Trichophyton schoenleini,* characterized by round, yellow cup-shaped crusts (scutula, favus cups) having a peculiar mousy odor, which may form honeycomb-like masses; other body areas may occasionally be affected. Syn. *tinea favosa.*

favus of fowls. A fungal infection of the comb and other parts of the head of chickens, turkeys, and other fowl, caused by *Trichophyton megnini,* occurring commonly in Europe. Syn. *comb disease.*

Fa·zio-Londe atrophy or **disease** (fah^t'tsee·o, loh^nd) [E. *Fazio,* Italian physician, 1849-1902; and P. F. L. *Londe*]. A bulbofacial type of progressive muscular atrophy occurring in childhood; frequently heredofamilial.

F.C.A.P. Fellow of the College of American Pathologists.

F.C.C.P. Fellow of the American College of Chest Physicians.

Fc fragment. The crystallizable fraction of immunoglobulin heavy chains. See also *immunoglobulin fragments.*

Fc fragment disease. HEAVY CHAIN DISEASE.

F-Cortef Acetate. A trademark for fluorocortisone acetate, a synthetic glucocorticoid.

FDA Abbreviation for *Food and Drug Administration.*

F. D. & C. Red No. 2. AMARANTH (2).

F. D. & C. Red No. 3. ERYTHROSINE SODIUM.

F.D.I. *Fédération Dentaire Internationale;* International Dental Federation.

Fe [L. *fe*rrum]. Symbol for iron.

fear, *n.* An emotion marked by dread, apprehension, or alarm, sometimes with the visceral manifestations accompanying anxiety. See also *phobia.*

fear reaction. A neurosis, particularly one developed in combat, in which anxiety is manifested by the conscious fear of a particular object or event.

fea·ture, *n.* [MF. *faiture,* from L. *factura,* a making]. Any single part or lineament of a structure, as of the face.

febri- [L. *febris*]. A combining form meaning *fever.*

feb·ri·cant (feb'ri·kunt) *adj.* FEBRIFACIENT.

feb·ri·fa·cient (feb''ri·fay'shunt) *adj.* Producing fever.

fe·brif·ic (fe·brif'ick) *adj.* Producing fever.

feb·ri·fuge (feb'ri·fewj) *n. & adj.* [*febri-* + *-fuge*]. 1. A substance that mitigates or reduces fever; an antipyretic. 2. Tending to reduce fever.

feb·ri·fu·gine (feb''ri·few'jeen) *n.* An alkaloid, possessing antimalarial activity, isolated from the herb *Dichroa febrifuga,* which is the probable source of the Chinese antimalarial drug ch'ang shan. Febrifugine may be identical with α-dichroine *and* β-dichroine from ch'ang shan.

fe·brile (feb'ril, ·rile, feeb') *adj.* [F., from L. *febrilis*]. Pertaining to or characterized by fever.

febrile albuminuria. Proteinuria associated with fever or acute infectious diseases.

febrile convulsion. A generalized (sometimes focal) convulsive seizure accompanying fever, usually in children; febrile seizures in infants with a familial history of epilepsy or with prenatal and birth difficulties often presage recurrent seizures in later life.

febrile crisis. A sudden drop of temperature at the height of a fever, as in lobar pneumonia.

febrile pulse. A pulse that is full, rapid, and often exhibiting dicrotism; common in fever.

feb·ri·pho·bia (feb''ri·fo'bee·uh) *n.* [*febri-* + *phobia*]. PYREXIOPHOBIA.

fe·cal, fae·cal (fee'kul) *adj.* Pertaining to or containing feces.

fecal abscess. An abscess containing feces and communicating with the lumen of the intestine.

fecal fistula. An opening from an intestine through the abdominal wall to the skin, with discharge of intestinal contents; usually applied to openings from the ileum and colon.

fe·ca·lith (fee'kuh·lith) *n.* [*fecal* + *-lith*]. A concretion formed from intermingled fecal material and calcium salts; coprolith.

fe·cal·oid (fee'kuh·loid) *adj.* [*fecal* + *-oid*]. Resembling feces.

fecal vomiting. The vomiting of fecal matter, usually seen with intestinal obstruction.

fe·ces, fae·ces (fee'seez) *n.pl.* [L. *faex, faecis,* dregs]. The excretions of the bowels; the excretions from the intestine of unabsorbed food, indigestible matter, intestinal secretions, and bacteria. —**fe·cal, fae·cal** (·kul) *adj.*

Fech·ner's law (fek^h'nur) [G. T. *Fechner,* German physicist and psychologist, 1801-1887]. The intensity of a sensation produced by a stimulus varies directly as the logarithm of the numerical value of that stimulus. Syn. *Weber-Fechner law.*

fe·co·lith (fee'ko·lith) *n.* FECALITH.

fec·u·la (feck'yoo·luh) *n.*, pl. **fecu·lae** (·lee) [L. *faecula,* dim of *faex*]. 1. The starchy part of a seed. 2. The sediment subsiding from an infusion.

fec·u·lent, fae·cu·lent (feck'yoo·lunt, fee'kew·) *adj.* [L. *faeculentus,* from *faex,* dregs]. 1. Having sediment. 2. Excrementitious.

fe·cun·da·tion (fee"kun·day'shun) *n.* The act of fertilizing; fertilization. —**fe·cun·date** (fee'kun·date, feck'un·) *v.*

fe·cun·di·ty (fe·kun'di·tee) *n.* [L. *funcunditas,* from *fecundus,* fruitful, prolific]. The innate potential reproductive capacity of the individual organism, as denoted by its ability to produce offspring. —**fe·cund** (fee'kund) *adj.*

Fe·de-Ri·ga disease (fe^y'deh, ree'gah) [F. *Fede,* Italian pediatrician, 1832-1913; and A. *Riga*]. Traumatic ulceration of the frenum of the tongue in children, produced by the lower teeth during sucking.

fee·ble·mind·ed, *adj.* Mentally deficient or retarded. —**fee·bleminded·ness,** *n.*

feed·back, *n.* 1. The return to the input, as of an electric, endocrine, or other system, of a part of its output, which frequently leads to an adjustment in this system. See also *positive feedback, negative feedback.* 2. The partial redistribution of the effects or products of a given process to its source so as to modify it.

feedback inhibition. Inhibition of an initial or early step in a sequence of events by the final product of the sequence.

feed·ing, *n.* The taking or giving of food.

feeding center. The region in the lateral hypothalamus presumed to be concerned with food intake and body weight. Syn. *appetite center.*

feeding cup. A cup with a spout or a lip, used for feeding patients incapable of feeding themselves.

feeding tube. A tube for introducing food into the stomach.

feel·ings of inferiority. Conscious unfavorable self-judgment, whether or not justified by the facts, resulting in feelings of depression and shame. Compare *inferiority complex.*

feeling tone. *In psychiatry,* the affective aspect, as the pleasingness or unpleasingness of a person, object, or act.

feeling-type personality. A personality in which the total attitude or reaction is dictated by feeling or emotional tone; one of Jung's functional types of personality.

Feer's disease (fe^yr) [E. *Feer,* Swiss pediatrician, 1864-1955]. ACRODYNIA.

fee splitting. The practice of dividing fees paid for professional services without informing the patient, as between consultants and referring physicians.

Feh·ling's reagent or **solution** (fe^y'ling) [H. von *Fehling,* German chemist, 1812-1855]. A reagent prepared by mixing an aqueous solution of copper sulfate with an aqueous solution of Rochelle salt and either potassium or sodium hydroxide; used to test for glucose and other reducing substances in urine.

Fehling's test [H. von *Fehling*]. A test for reducing substances in urine in which an equal amount of Fehling's reagent and urine are boiled. In the presence of reducing substances, chiefly glucose, a green, yellow, or red precipitate forms, the color depending on the amount of glucose present.

Feil-Klippel syndrome [A. *Feil,* French neurologist, b. 1884; and M. *Klippel*]. KLIPPEL-FEIL SYNDROME.

fel, *n.* [L.]. BILE.

feld·sher (feld'shur) *n.* [Russian, from Ger. *Feldscher,* from *Feld,* field, + *Scherer,* shearer, barber]. In the Soviet Union and other countries, a trained medical worker without the full training or status of a qualified physician, who delivers initial medical care and performs other tasks according to qualifications under the supervision of a physician or medical team; a physician's assistant. See also *syniatrist.*

fe·line (fee'line) *adj.* & *n.* [L. *felinus,* from *felis,* cat]. 1. Pertaining to or derived from cats (genus *Felis*) or the family (Felidae) which includes cats, tigers, lions, leopards. 2. Catlike. 3. A member of the family Felidae.

feline distemper. FELINE PANLEUKOPENIA.

feline enteritis. FELINE PANLEUKOPENIA.

feline infectious anemia. An anemia of cats caused by the rickettsial agent *Hemobartonella felis* and characterized by anorexia, depression, fever, and hemolytic anemia.

feline infectious peritonitis. An invariably fatal disease of domestic cats, suspected to be caused by a virus and characterized by fever, severe depression, anorexia, weight loss, and ascites.

feline leukemia virus. A virus which is widespread in the cat population and known to cause myeloproliferative disorders and lymphosarcoma; probably also responsible for a variety of disease problems related to immunosuppression; horizontal transmission of the virus from cat to cat is possible.

feline panleukopenia. A highly contagious usually fatal virus disease of cats, wild Felidae and mink, characterized by severe leukopenia of the granulocytic series, enteritis, and fever. Syn. *feline distemper, infectious feline enteritis.*

feline pneumonitis. A chlamydial infection of the upper respiratory tract of domestic cats, characterized by sneezing, nasal discharge, fever, and inappetence.

feline viral rhinotracheitis. A viral infection of the upper respiratory tract of cats.

Felix test. WEIL-FELIX TEST.

fel·la·tio (fe·lay'shee·o) *n.* [NL., from L. *fellare,* to suck]. Sexual stimulation of the penis by oral contact.

fel·la·tor (fel'uh·tor, fel·ay'tur) *n.* A male who takes the penis of another into his mouth in fellatio.

fel·la·trice (fel'uh·treece) *n.* A female who takes the penis into her mouth in fellatio.

Fell-O'Dwy·er method [G. E. *Fell,* U.S. physician, 1850-1918; and J. P. *O'Dwyer,* U.S. otolaryngologist 1841-1898]. Artificial respiration by forcing air into the lungs with a bellows through an intubation tube, expiration occurring spontaneously due to elasticity of the chest or by external pressure.

[1]fel·on (fel'un) *n.* [OF., from ML. *fello, fellonis,* perhaps from L. *fel,* gall, venom]. An infection in the closed space of the terminal phalanx of a finger.

[2]felon, *n.* A person who has committed a felony.

fe·lo·ni·ous (fe·lo'nee·us) *adj.* Pertaining to or constituting a felony.

felonious assault. A malicious attack showing criminal intent upon the person of another.

fel·o·ny (fel'uh·nee) *n.* [OF. *felonie,* villainy, treachery, from *felon,* felon, perhaps from L. *fel,* gall, bitterness]. A grave crime; usually one declared such by statute because of the attendant severe punishment.

felt·work, *n.* A tissue composed of closely interwoven fibers.

Fel·ty's syndrome [A. R. *Felty,* U.S. physician, b. 1895]. Adult rheumatoid arthritis, with splenomegaly resulting in granulocytopenia due to hypersplenism.

fe·ly·pres·sin (fel"eye·pres'in, fel"i.) *n.* 2-(Phenylalanine)-8-lysine vasopressin, $C_{46}H_{65}N_{13}O_{11}S_2$, a vasoconstrictor.

fe·male (fee'male) *adj.* & *n.* [F. *femelle,* from L. *femella,* young woman, girl, from *femina,* a woman, a female]. 1. Belonging or pertaining to the sex that produces the ovum. Symbol, ♀. See also Table of Medical Signs and Symbols in the Appendix. 2. Designating that part of a double-limbed instrument that receives the complementary part. 3. A female organism or individual.

female castration. Removal of the ovaries; oophorectomy; spaying.

female catheter. A short catheter for catheterizing women.

female epispadias. A congenital defect in which the urethra, usually dilated, opens between the divided halves of the clitoris; usually associated with absence of all, or at least the upper portion, of the labia minora and other developmental defects.

female gonad. OVARY.

female pseudohermaphroditism. A condition simulating hermaphroditism in which the external sexual characteristics are in part or wholly of male aspect, but internal female genitalia are present. Syn. *gynandry.*

fem·i·nine (fem′i·nin) *adj.* [L. *femininus,* from *femina,* a woman, a female]. Having the appearance or qualities of a woman; female.

fem·i·nism (fem′i·niz·um) *n.* The presence in a male of secondary characteristics of the female sex. —**fem·i·ni·za·tion** (fem″i·ni·zay′shun) *n.;* **fem·i·nize** (fem′i·nize) *v.*

feminizing adenocarcinoma. A malignant feminizing tumor.

feminizing adenoma. An adenoma associated with feminization.

femora. Plural of *femur.*

fem·o·ral (fem′uh·rul) *adj.* [L. *femoralis,* from *femur,* thigh]. Of or pertaining to the femur or to the thigh.

femoral artery. The chief artery of the thigh; it is a continuation of the external iliac artery, beginning where the vessel passes beneath the inguinal ligament. It becomes the popliteal artery when the vessel passes through the hiatus in the adductor magnus muscle. NA *arteria femoralis.* See also Table of Arteries in the Appendix.

femoral canal. The medial compartment of the femoral sheath behind the inguinal ligament. NA *canalis femoralis.*

femoral hernia. A hernia involving the femoral canal; found most often in women, it is usually small and painless, often remaining unnoticed. The neck lies beneath the inguinal ligament and lateral to the tubercle of the pubic bone. Syn. *crural hernia.* See also Plate 4.

femoral nerve. A motor and somatic sensory nerve which is derived from the second, third, and fourth lumbar segments of the cord (lumbar plexus). The motor portion innervates the pectineus, the quadriceps femoris, the iliacus, the sartorius, and the articularis genus muscles; the sensory portion innervates the skin of the anterior aspect of the thigh, the medial aspect of the leg, and the hip and knee joints. NA *nervus femoralis.* See also Table of Nerves in the Appendix.

femoral plexus. A nerve plexus surrounding the femoral artery. NA *plexus femoralis.*

femoral reflex. Extension of the knee and plantar flexion of the toes induced by irritation of the skin over the upper anterior surface of the thigh.

femoral region. The portion of the lower extremity associated with the thighbone. See also Plate 4.

femoral ring. The abdominal opening of the femoral canal. NA *anulus femoralis.*

femoral septum. The layer of areolar tissue closing the femoral ring. NA *septum femorale.*

femoral sheath. A continuation downward of the fasciae that line the abdomen. It contains the femoral vessels.

femoral testis. A testis that has not descended into the scrotum but remains in the inguinal canal near or over the femoral ring.

femoral triangle. A triangle formed laterally by the medial margin of the sartorius, medially by the lateral margin of the adductor longus, and superiorly by the inguinal ligament. NA *trigonum femorale.* Syn. *Scarpa's triangle.*

femoral trigone. FEMORAL TRIANGLE.

femoral vein. A vein accompanying the femoral artery. NA *vena femoralis.*

femoro-. A combining form meaning *femur, femoral.*

fem·o·ro·pop·lit·e·al (fem″uh·ro·pop·lit′ee·ul) *adj.* 1. Pertaining to the femur and the popliteal space. 2. Pertaining to the femoral and popliteal arteries.

fem·o·ro·tib·i·al (fem″uh·ro·tib′ee·ul) *adj.* [*femoro-* + *tibial*]. Pertaining to the femur and the tibia.

fe·mur (fee′mur) *n.,* genit. **fe·mo·ris** (fem′o·ris), pl. **femurs, fe·mo·ra** (fem′o·ruh) [L., thigh] [NA]. The long bone of the thigh; thighbone. See also Table of Bones in the Appendix and Plates 1, 2. Adj. *femoral.*

fen·al·a·mide (fen·al′uh·mide) *n.* Ethyl *N*-[2-(diethylamino)-ethyl]-2-ethyl-2-phenylmalonamate, $C_{19}H_{30}N_2O_3$, a smooth muscle relaxant.

fen·a·mole (fen′uh·mole) *n.* 5-Amino-1-phenyl-1*H*-tetrazole, $C_7H_7N_5$, an inflammation-counteracting drug.

fen·ben·da·zole (fen·ben′duh·zole) *n.* Methyl 5-(phenylthio)-2-benzimidazolecarbamate, $C_{15}H_{13}N_3O_2S$, an anthelmintic.

fen·bu·fen (fen·bew′fen) *n.* γ-Oxo[1,1′-biphenyl]-4-butanoic acid, $C_{16}H_{14}O_3$, an anti-inflammatory.

fen·chone (fen′chone, ·kone) *n.* *d*-1,3,3-Trimethyl-2-norcamphanone, $C_{10}H_{16}O$, a ketone that provides the characteristic bitter taste of some specimens of fennel oil. A levorotatory isomer occurs in thuja oil.

fen·clo·nine (fen·klo′neen) *n.* DL-3-(*p*-Chlorophenyl)alanine, $C_9H_{10}ClNO_2$, an inhibitor of serotonin biosynthesis.

fen·clor·ac (fen·klor′ack) *n.* Chloro(3-chloro-4-cyclohexyphenyl)acetic acid, $C_{14}H_{16}Cl_2O_2$, an anti-inflammatory.

fe·nes·tra (fe·nes′truh) *n.,* pl. & genit. sing. **fenes·trae** (·tree) [L., window]. 1. A small opening. 2. *In anatomy,* an aperture of the medial wall of the middle ear. 3. An opening in a bandage or plaster splint for examination or drainage. 4. The open space in the blade of a forceps. —**fenes·tral** (·trul) *adj.*

fenestra coch·le·ae (kock′lee·ee) [NA]. COCHLEAR WINDOW (= ROUND WINDOW).

fenestra ova·lis (o·vay′lis). OVAL WINDOW (= VESTIBULAR WINDOW).

fenestra ro·tun·da (ro·tun′duh). ROUND WINDOW (= COCHLEAR WINDOW).

fenestrated membrane. One of the layers of elastic tissue in the tunica media and tunica intima of large arteries.

fenestrated skull. Osteoporosis of the skull, as from osteomyelitis.

fen·es·tra·tion (fen″e·stray′shun) *n.* 1. The creation of an opening or openings; perforation. 2. The presence of fenestrae in a structure. 3. An operation to create a permanently mobile window in the lateral semicircular canal; used in cases of deafness caused by stapedial impediment of sound waves. Syn. *Lempert's operation.* 4. *In dentistry,* an isolated area in which a root is denuded of bone and the root surface is covered only by periosteum and the overlying gingiva; usually occurring in the facial alveolar plate in the anterior region, rarely on the lingual surface. See also *dehiscence.* —**fen·es·trat·ed** (fen′e·stray·tid) *adj.*

fenestration compress. CRIBRIFORM COMPRESS.

fenestra ves·ti·bu·li (ves·tib′yoo·lye) [NA]. VESTIBULAR WINDOW (= OVAL WINDOW).

fen·es·trel (fen·es′trel) *n.* 5-Ethyl-6-methyl-4-phenyl-3-cyclohexene-1-carboxylic acid, $C_{16}H_{20}O_2$, an estrogen.

fen·eth·yl·line (fen·eth′il·een) *n.* 7-[2-[α-Methylphenethyl)amino]ethyl]theophylline, $C_{18}H_{23}N_5O_2$, a central stimulant drug; used as the hydrochloride salt.

fen·flur·a·mine (fen·floor′uh·meen) *n.* *N*-Ethyl-α-methyl-*m*-(trifluoromethyl)phenethylamine, $C_{12}H_{16}F_3N$, an anorexigenic drug; used as the hydrochloride salt.

fen·i·mide (fen′i·mide) *n.* 3-Ethyl-2-methyl-2-phenylsuccinimide, $C_{13}H_{15}NO_2$, a tranquilizing drug.

fen·iso·rex (fen·eye'so·recks) *n. cis*-7-Fluoro-1-phenyl-3-isochromanmethylamine, $C_{16}H_{16}FNO$, an anorexic.

fen·met·o·zole (fen·met'uh·zole) *n.* 2-[(3,4-Dichlorophenoxy)methyl]-2-imidazoline, $C_{10}H_{10}Cl_2N_2O$, an antidepressant and narcotic antagonist.

fen·met·ra·mide (fen·met'ruh·mide) *n.* 5-Methyl-6-phenyl-3-morpholinone, $C_{11}H_{13}NO_2$, an antidepressant drug.

fen·nel (fen'ul) *n.* [L. *feniculum*]. The dried, ripe fruit of cultivated varieties of *Foeniculum vulgare;* contains a volatile oil. It is used as a carminative.

fennel oil. The volatile oil from the fruit of *Foeniculum vulgare,* containing anethol; a carminative and flavoring oil.

fen·o·pro·fen (fen″o·pro'fen) *n.* (±)-*m*-Phenoxyhydratropic acid, $C_{15}H_{14}O_3$, an analgesic anti-inflammatory.

fen·o·ter·ol (fen·o·terr'ole) *n.* 3,5-Dihydroxy-α-[[(*p*-hydroxy-α-methylphenethyl)amino]methyl]benzyl alcohol, $C_{17}H_{21}NO_4$, a bronchodilator.

fen·pip·a·lone (fen·pip'uh·lone) *n.* 5-[2-(3,6-Dihydro-4-phenyl-1(2*H*)-pyridinyl)ethyl]-3-methyl-2-oxazolidinone, $C_{17}H_{22}N_2O_2$, an anti-inflammatory.

fen·spir·ide (fen·spirr'ide) *n.* 8-Phenethyl-1-oxa-3,8-diazaspiro[4,5]decan-2-one, $C_{15}H_{20}N_2O_2$, an anti-adrenergic (α-receptor) bronchodilator.

fen·ta·nyl (fen'tuh·nil) *n. N*-(1-Phenethyl-4-piperidyl)propionanilide, $C_{22}H_{28}N_2O$, an analgesic; used as the citrate salt.

fen·ti·clor (fen'ti·klor) *n.* 2,2′-Thiobis[4-chlorophenol], $C_{12}H_8Cl_2O_2S$, a topical anti-infective.

fen·u·greek, foen·u·greek (fen'yoo·greek) *n.* [L. *fenugraecum,* from *fenum,* hay, + *graecus,* Greek]. The *Trigonella foenum-graecum,* a leguminous plant whose seeds are used as a condiment and in preparing emollient applications.

Fen·wal flask. A flask having a heavy rubber cap with a central outlet fitted with a stainless-steel secondary stopper; used for sterilizing fluids by steam.

Fen·wick's disease [S. *Fenwick,* English physician, 1821–1902]. Primary atrophy of the stomach, associated with pernicious anemia.

fen·yr·i·pol (fen·irr'i·pole) *n.* α-[(2-Pyrimidinylamino)methyl]benzyl alcohol, $C_{12}H_{13}N_3O$, a skeletal muscle relaxant; used as the hydrochloride salt.

Feosol. A trademark for certain preparations of ferrous sulfate.

Ferad. A trademark for certain preparations containing ferrous sulfate.

fe·ral (ferr'ul, feer'ul) *adj.* [L. *fera,* wild animal]. 1. Characteristic of or suggestive of an animal, particularly a ferocious one, in its natural state; wild. 2. Living in or being in a natural state; not domesticated, socialized, or humanized, as a child reared in isolation with few human contacts.

fer-de-lance (fair″ duh lahnce') *n.* [F., lance iron]. A large, venomous pit viper of Central and South America; the *Bothrops atrox.*

Fé·ré·ol's node (feʸ·reʸ·ol') [L. H. F. *Féréol,* French physician, 1825–1891]. A subcutaneous nodule in acute rheumatic fever.

Fergon. A trademark for certain preparations containing ferrous gluconate.

Fer·gu·son's operation [A. H. *Ferguson,* Canadian surgeon, 1853–1911]. A simple type of herniorrhaphy in which the cord is not transplanted; high ligation and amputation of the sac are followed by simple closure of the deep inguinal ring and inguinal canal over the cord.

¹fer·ment (fur'ment) *n.* [L. *fermentum,* yeast, leaven]. A catalytic agent produced by, and associated with, a living organism (organized ferment), as distinguished from an enzyme which may be separated from the living organism (unorganized ferment). See also *enzyme, extracellular enzyme, intracellular enzyme.*

²fer·ment (fur·ment') *v.* To undergo or cause to undergo fermentation.

fer·men·ta·tion (fur″men·tay'shun) *n.* The decomposition of complex molecules under the influence of ferments or enzymes. —**fer·men·ta·tive** (fur·men'tuh·tiv) *adj.*

fermentation chemistry. Study of the reactions produced by enzymes and ferments.

fermentation tube. A glass tube used in the fermentation test for carbohydrates.

fer·mi (ferr'mee) *n.* [E. *Fermi,* Italian physicist, 1901–1954]. A unit of distance, equal to 10^{-13} cm., that is used to describe nuclear dimensions.

fer·mi·on (ferr'mee·on, fur') *n.* [E. *Fermi*]. Any elementary particle or atomic nucleus that satisfies the Fermi-Dirac type of quantum statistics. Such particles include atomic nuclei with odd mass numbers, electrons, protons, and neutrons.

fer·mi·um (ferr'mee·um, fur') *n.* [E. *Fermi*]. Fm = 257.0956. A radioactive metallic element, atomic number 100, produced artificially as by bombarding plutonium with neutrons. See also Table of Elements in the Appendix.

fern·ing, *n.* The formation of a crystallized fern pattern in dried mucus from the uterine cervix before ovulation, resulting from estrogen stimulation. Pregnancy and progestational changes prevent ferning; in pregnancy ferning indicates the presence of amniotic fluid in the vagina following premature rupture of membranes. Syn. *arborization.*

fern oil. Aspidium oleoresin; a vermifuge.

fern test. See *ferning.*

-ferous, -iferous [L. *ferre,* to bear, + *-ous*]. A combining form meaning *bearing, producing.*

fer·rat·ed (ferr'ay·tid) *adj.* [L. *ferratus,* from *ferrum,* iron]. Combined with iron; containing iron.

fer·re·dox·in (ferr″e·dock'sin) *n.* Generic name for certain iron-containing proteins of photosynthetic cells and anaerobic bacteria that have the ability to catalyze photoreduction of nicotinamide adenine dinucleotide phosphate by washed chloroplasts.

ferri-. A combining form meaning *ferric, containing iron as a trivalent element.*

fer·ric (ferr'ick) *adj.* [*ferrum* + *-ic*]. 1. Pertaining to or of the nature of iron. 2. Containing iron as a trivalent element.

ferric alum. FERRIC AMMONIUM SULFATE.

ferric ammonium citrate. A complex salt containing 16.5 to 18.5% iron; it occurs in red scales or granules, or as a brownish-yellow powder. Used as a nonastringent hematinic. Syn. *soluble ferric citrate.*

ferric ammonium sulfate. $FeNH_4(SO_4)_2.12H_2O$. Formerly used for its astringent and styptic effects. Syn. *ferric alum, iron alum.*

ferric ammonium tartrate. A salt of somewhat indefinite composition occurring in reddish-brown scales; formerly much used as a mild chalybeate.

ferric cacodylate. Approximately $Fe[(CH_3)_2AsO_2]_3$, a yellowish, amorphous powder, soluble in water; has been used for treatment of leukemias, also in iron-deficiency states.

ferric chloride. $FeCl_3$ + water. Has been used as an astringent and styptic.

ferric glycerophosphate. $Fe_2[C_3H_5(OH)_2PO_4]_3$. Formerly used for treatment of iron-deficiency anemia.

ferric hydroxide. Hydrated iron oxide, $Fe(OH)_3$, an antidote to arsenic.

ferric hydroxide with magnesium oxide. An antidote to arsenic prepared by adding a suspension of magnesium oxide to a ferric sulfate solution.

ferric hypophosphite. $Fe(H_2PO_2)_3$. Formerly used as a chalybeate.

ferric pyrophosphate. Approximately $Fe_4(P_2O_7)_3.9H_2O$; a yellowish-white powder, insoluble in water, and lacking the astringency characteristic of iron salts. It is used in nutrition and medicinally as a source of iron.

ferric pyrophosphate soluble. Ferric pyrophosphate rendered soluble by the inclusion of sodium citrate; has been used as a hematinic.

ferric sulfate. $Fe_2(SO_4)_3$; a salt occurring as a grayish-white powder, very hygroscopic, slowly soluble in water, and forming an acid solution. It is largely used industrially.

fer·ri·cy·a·nide (ferr″eye·sigh′uh·nide, ferr″i·) *n.* [*ferri-* + *cyanide*]. A salt containing the trivalent $[Fe(CN)_6]$ anion.

fer·ri·heme (ferr′eye·heem, ferr′i·) *n.* [*ferri-* + *heme*]. Heme in which the ferrous iron normally present is in the ferric (oxidized) state; the resulting higher valence imparts a positive charge which in alkaline solution attracts a hydroxyl ion, forming hematin, and in hydrochloric acid solution attracts a chloride ion, forming hemin.

fer·ri·he·mo·glo·bin, fer·ri·hae·mo·glo·bin (ferr″i·hee′muh·glo″bin, ferr″eye·) *n.* [*ferri-* + *hemoglobin*]. Methemoglobin, characterized by containing iron in the ferric state.

fer·ri·pro·to·por·phy·rin (ferr″i·pro″to·por′fi·rin) *n.* HEMIN.

fer·ri·tin (ferr′i·tin) *n.* An iron-protein complex occurring in tissues, probably being a storage form of iron. It is in many characteristics similar to hemosiderin. See also *apoferritin.*

ferro-. A combining form meaning (a) *ferrous;* (b) *containing metallic iron.*

fer·ro·che·la·tase (ferr″o·kee′lay·tace, ·taze) *n.* A mitochondrial enzyme catalyzing the incorporation of iron into the protoporphyrin molecule.

fer·ro·cho·li·nate (ferr″o·ko′li·nate) *n.* A compound of iron chelated with choline citrate, used as a hematinic. Syn. *iron choline citrate.*

fer·ro·cy·a·nide (ferr″o·sigh′uh·nide) *n.* A salt containing the divalent $[Fe(CN)_6]$ anion.

fer·ro·heme (ferr′o·heem) *n.* [*ferro-* + *heme*]. HEME.

fer·ro·he·mo·glo·bin, fer·ro·hae·mo·glo·bin (ferr″o·hee′muh·glo″bin) *n.* [*ferro-* + *hemoglobin*]. Hemoglobin in which the iron is in the normal ferrous state.

fer·ro·ki·net·ics (ferr″o·ki·net′icks) *n.* [*ferro-* + *kinetics*]. The study of iron metabolism, especially in regard to hemoglobin metabolism.

Ferrolip. A trademark for ferrocholinate, a hematinic.

fer·ro·mag·net·ic (ferr″o·mag·net′ick) *adj.* [*ferro-* + *magnetic*]. Pertaining to substances that can be magnetized to a high degree, ultimately reaching a saturation value, and that possess abnormally high magnetic permeability.

fer·ro·pro·to·por·phy·rin 9 (ferr″o·pro″to·por′fi·rin) *n.* HEME.

fer·ro·ther·a·py (ferr″o·therr′uh·pee) *n.* [*ferro-* + *therapy*]. Treatment of disease by the use of iron and iron compounds or chalybeates.

fer·rous (ferr′us) *adj.* [*ferr*um + *-ous*]. Containing iron in divalent form.

ferrous carbonate mass. A dosage form of ferrous carbonate, $FeCO_3$, formerly used as a hematinic. Syn. *Vallet's mass.*

ferrous carbonate pills. A pill dosage form of ferrous carbonate, $FeCO_3$, used as a hematinic. Syn. *Blaud's pills.*

ferrous chloride. $FeCl_2.4H_2O$; pale-green, deliquescent crystals or crystalline powder, soluble in acidulated water; used largely industrially.

ferrous fumarate. $FeC_4H_2O_4$. A reddish-orange to reddish-brown powder, slightly soluble in water; used for treatment of iron-deficiency anemias.

ferrous gluconate. $Fe(C_6H_{11}O_7)_2.2H_2O$. A yellowish-gray or pale, greenish-yellow powder; soluble in water. A hematinic better tolerated than other iron salts.

ferrous iodide. $FeI_2.4H_2O$, occurring as almost black, very deliquescent masses, rapidly decomposing in air with liberation of iodine. It has been used in chronic tuberculosis. Ferrous iodide syrup, containing about 5% of FeI_2 by weight, has been used as a hematinic.

ferrous lactate. $Fe(C_3H_5O_3)_2.3H_2O$. A greenish powder; used as a hematinic.

ferrous sulfate. $FeSO_4.7H_2O$. Pale bluish-green crystals or granules. A widely used and effective hematinic, used also as a deodorant. Syn. *copperas, green vitriol.*

fer·ru·gi·na·tion (fe·roo″ji·nay′shun) *n.* Depositions of iron in tissues.

fer·ru·gi·nous (fe·roo′ji·nus) *adj.* [L. *ferruginus,* from *ferrugo,* iron rust]. 1. Of, containing, or pertaining to iron. 2. Having the color of iron rust.

fer·rum (ferr′um) *n.* [L.]. IRON.

fer·tile (fur′til) *adj.* [L. *fertilis*]. 1. Prolific; fruitful. 2. Of an organism: able to reproduce. 3. Of a gamete: able to bring about or undergo fertilization. 4. Of an ovum: fertilized. Contr. *sterile.* —**fer·til·i·ty** (fur·til′i·tee) *n.*

fertility clinic. A clinic to diagnose the causes of infertility in human beings and to assist reproductive ability. Syn. *sterility clinic.*

fertility factor. A factor which imparts to host bacteria the ability to donate genetic material by conjugation to bacteria lacking it, thereby permitting genetic recombination in the recipient. The factor may be transmitted independently to recipient cells and may under certain conditions become associated with its host deoxyribonucleic acid; this ability to exist in two states qualifies the factor as an episome. Syn. *F factor, sex factor.*

fertility vitamin. VITAMIN E.

fer·til·iza·tion (fur″ti·li·zay′shun) *n.* The act of making fruitful; impregnation; union of male and female gametes. —**fer·til·ize** (fur′ti·lize) *v.*

fertilization age. FETAL AGE.

fer·ti·li·zin (fur′ti·lye·zin, fur·til′i·zin) *n.* A colloidal substance in ripe ova, in certain species, which is capable of agglutinating and binding spermatozoa to the ova.

Fer·u·la (ferr′yoo·luh, ferr′oo·luh) *n.* [L., giant fennel]. A genus of the family Umbelliferae whose genera and species yield asafetida, galbanum, and sumbul.

fe·ru·lic acid (fe·roo′lick). 4-Hydroxy-3-methoxycinnamic acid, $C_{10}H_{10}O_4$; widely distributed in plants.

fes·ter, *v.* [OF. *festre,* ulcer, fistula, from L. *fistula*]. 1. To suppurate superficially; to generate pus. 2. To become inflamed and suppurate.

festinating gait. The gait of patients with Parkinson's syndrome, marked by rigidity, shuffling, and festination.

fes·ti·na·tion (fes″ti·nay′shun) *n.* [L. *festinatio,* from *festinare,* to hasten]. An involuntary increase or hastening in gait, seen in Parkinson's syndrome, both paralysis agitans and postencephalitic parkinsonism. —**fes·ti·nate** (fes′ti·nate) *v.* & *adj.*

fes·toon (fes·toon′) *n.* & *v.* [F. *feston,* a garland]. 1. The scalloped appearance that is the natural arrangement of the marginal gingiva. 2. To recreate or reshape the gingival margin to its ideal physiologic contour. 3. To shape the base material in a dental prosthesis to simulate the form of the natural gingiva.

fe·tal, foe·tal (fee′tul) *adj.* Pertaining to, involving, or characteristic of a fetus.

fetal adenoma. A follicular adenoma of the thyroid made up of numerous small follicles of a primitive or fetal type, containing little or no colloid.

fetal adnexa. FETAL APPENDAGES.

fetal age. The age of a fetus computed from the time of conception to any point in time prior to birth. Compare *gestational age.*

fetal alcohol syndrome. A syndrome of various defects, principally small size for gestational age, microcephaly, and retardation, observed in offspring of mothers with excessive alcohol intake during pregnancy.

fetal appendages. The placenta, amnion, chorion, and umbilical cord.

fetal asphyxia. Asphyxia of the fetus while in the uterus caused by interference with its blood supply, as by cord compression or premature placental separation.

fetal cartilage. TEMPORARY CARTILAGE.

fetal circulation. The circulation of the fetus, including the circulation through the placenta and the umbilical cord. See also Plate 6.

fetal cortex. ANDROGENIC ZONE.

fetal cranial diameters. The biparietal, bitemporal, occipitofrontal, occipitomental, and suboccipitobregmatic diameters.

fetal dystocia. Difficult labor due to abnormalities of position or size and shape of the fetus.

fetal fat-cell lipoma. LIPOSARCOMA.

fetal fibroadenoma. FIBROADENOMA.

fetal fissure. CHOROID FISSURE (1).

fetal heart sounds. The sounds produced by the beating of the fetal heart, best heard near the umbilicus of the mother.

fetal hemoglobin. The dominant type of hemoglobin in the fetus, small amounts being produced throughout life; it differs in many chemical properties from adult hemoglobin. Syn. *hemoglobin F.*

fetal integument. *Obsol.* FETAL MEMBRANES.

fe·tal·ism (fee'tul·iz·um) *n.* [*fetal* + *-ism*]. The presence or persistence of certain prenatal conditions in the body after birth.

fetal membranes. The chorion, amnion, and allantois.

fetal movement. The movement of the fetus in the uterus.

fetal pelvis. INFANTILE PELVIS.

fetal respiration. The interchange of gases between the fetal and the maternal blood through the medium of the placenta.

fetal rest. A portion of embryonic tissue, or cells, which remain in the mature tissue or organ.

fetal rest-cell theory. COHNHEIM'S THEORY.

fetal rickets. ACHONDROPLASIA.

fetal souffle. FUNICULAR SOUFFLE.

fetal uterus. A uterus showing defective development, with the cervical canal longer than the uterine cavity.

fe·ta·tion (fee·tay'shun) *n.* 1. The formation of the fetus. 2. PREGNANCY.

fetich. FETISH.

fe·ti·cide, foe·ti·cide (fee'ti·side) *n.* [*fetus* + *-cide*]. The killing of the fetus in the uterus.

fet·id, foet·id (fet'id, fee'tid) *adj.* [L. *fetidus,* from *fetere,* to stink]. Having a foul odor.

fetid perspiration or **sweat.** BROMHIDROSIS.

fet·ish, fet·ich (fet'ish, fee'tish) *n.* [Pg. *feitiço,* from L. *facticius,* artificial]. 1. Any inanimate object thought to have magical power or to bring supernatural aid. 2. *In psychiatry,* a personalized inanimate object, love object, or any maneuver or body part which, through association, arouses erotic feelings. —**fetish·ism** (·iz·um) *n.;* **fetish·ist** (·ist) *n.*

fet·lock, *n.* The region of a horse's leg that extends from the lower extremity of the metacarpal or metatarsal bone to the pastern joint.

feto-, foeto-. A combining form meaning *fetus, fetal.*

fe·to·am·ni·ot·ic (fee"to·am·nee·ot'ick) *adj.* [*feto-* + *amniotic*]. Pertaining to the fetus and the amnion.

fetoamniotic band. AMNIOTIC BAND.

fe·to·glob·u·lin, foe·to·glob·u·lin (fee"to·glob'yoo·lin) *n.* FETOPROTEIN.

fe·to·gram (fee'to·gram) *n.* A radiographic depiction of a fetus, including skin outline and bowel.

fe·tog·ra·phy (fee·tog'ruh·fee) *n.* A method of demonstrating fetal features by injecting the amniotic sac with contrast media designed to show the skin and the intestinal tract.

fe·tol·o·gy (fee·tol'uh·jee) *n.* [*feto-* + *-logy*]. The study, science, and treatment of the fetus. Compare *neonatology.* —**fetolo·gist,** *n.*

fe·tom·e·try (fee·tom'e·tree) *n.* [*feto-* + *-metry*]. The measurement of the fetus, especially of its cranial diameters.

fe·to·pro·tein (fee"to·pro'tee·in, ·teen) *n.* An immunologically homogeneous α_1-globulin containing 22 percent carbohydrate, found in the fetuses of many animal species and in certain patients with hepatoma. See also *fetuin.*

fe·tor, foe·tor (fee'tur, ·tor) *n.* [L.]. Stench.

fetor ex ore (ecks o'ree) [L., from the mouth]. Bad breath; halitosis.

fetor he·pat·i·cus (he·pat'i·kus). A peculiar musty or sweetish odor of the breath occurring in the terminal stage of hepatocellular liver disease.

fe·tox·y·late (fe·tock'si·late) *n.* 2-Phenoxyethyl 1-(3-cyano-3,3-diphenylpropyl)-4-phenylisonipecotate, $C_{36}H_{36}N_2O_3$, an antidiarrheal drug; used as the hydrochloride salt.

fe·tu·in (fee'tew·in) *n.* A fetoprotein found in fetal calf serum.

fe·tus, foe·tus (fee'tus) *n.,* pl. **fetuses, foetuses** [L., bearing, hatching, offspring]. The unborn offspring of viviparous mammals in the later stages of development; in human beings, from about the beginning of the ninth week after fertilization. Compare *embryo.*

fetus com·pres·sus (kom·pres'us). FETUS PAPYRACEUS.

fetus cy·lin·dri·cus (si·lin'dri·kus). A malformed fetus with little indication of head and extremities, roughly cylindrical in form.

fetus in fe·tu (in fee'tew). CRYPTODIDYMUS.

fetus pa·py·ra·ce·us (pap·i·ray'shee·us). A dead twin fetus which has been compressed by the growth of its living twin.

Feul·gen reaction (foil'g^e^n) [R. *Feulgen,* German physiologic chemist, 1884–1955]. A reaction specific for aldehydes based on formation of a purple-colored compound when aldehydes react with fuchsin-sulfuric acid. Deoxyribonucleic acid, but not ribonucleic acid, gives this reaction after the removal of its purine bases by acid hydrolysis.

fe·ver (fee'vur) *n.* [L. *febris*]. 1. Elevation of the body temperature above the normal; in human beings, above an average value of 37°C (98.6°F) orally. Syn. *pyrexia.* 2. A disease whose distinctive feature is elevation of body temperature. —**fever·ish** (·ish) *adj.*

fever blister. HERPES FACIALIS.

fe·ver·et (fee·vur·et') *n.* 1. Any evanescent fever. 2. Influenza or an influenza-like infection.

fever therapy. Treatment of disease by artificially induced fever.

fever thermometer. CLINICAL THERMOMETER.

fex·ism (feck'siz·um) *n.* [G. Berg*fex,* Austrian alpinist, + *-ism*]. Cretinism, once endemic in certain parts of Austria.

F factor. FERTILITY FACTOR.

F.F.P.S. Fellow of the Faculty of Physicians and Surgeons (Glasgow).

FFT Abbreviation for (a) *flicker fusion test;* (b) *flicker fusion threshold.*

ff wave. FIBRILLATION WAVE.

fiant. Plural of *fiat.*

fi·at (figh'at) *v.,* pl. **fi·ant** (·ant, ·unt) [L., pres. subj. of *fieri,* to be made]. Let there be made; used in the writing of prescriptions. Abbreviated, ft.

fi·ber, fi·bre (figh'bur) *n.* [L. *fibra*]. A filamentary or threadlike structure. —**fi·brous** (·brus) *adj.*

fiber baskets. The delicate fibrils extending from the outer limiting membrane of the retina which invest the base of the rods and cones.

fiber cell. Any cell elongated to a fiberlike appearance; as a muscle cell.

fi·ber·op·tic (figh"bur·op'tick) *adj.* Pertaining to or characterizing fine glass or plastic fibers with optical refraction properties such that light can be conveyed along them and reflected around corners; used especially for illumination in endoscopy. —**fiberoptics,** *n.*

fi·ber·scope (figh'bur·skope) *n.* An instrument that has a flexible shaft of light-conducting fibers and a source of illumination and that is used for viewing certain internal tissues.

fibers of Remak [R. *Remak*]. REMAK'S FIBERS.

fibers of Sharpey [W. *Sharpey*]. PERFORATING FIBERS.

Fi·bi·ger's tumor (fee"bi·gur) [J. A. G. *Fibiger,* Danish pathologist, 1867–1928]. Squamous-cell carcinoma of the rat stomach caused by larvae of the nematode *Gongylonema* (formerly *Spiroptera*) *neoplastica*.

Fibocil. A trademark for aprindine hydrochloride, a cardiac depressant.

fibr-, fibro-. A combining form meaning *fiber, fibrous*.

fi·bra (figh'bruh) *n.*, pl. **fi·brae** (·bree) [L.]. FIBER.

fibrae ar·cu·a·tae ce·re·bri (ahr·kew·ay'tee serr'e·brye) [NA] ASSOCIATION FIBERS of the cerebrum.

fibrae arcuatae ex·ter·nae (ecks·tur'nee) [NA]. EXTERNAL ARCUATE FIBERS.

fibrae arcuatae externae dor·sa·les (dor·say'leez) [NA]. The dorsal external arcuate fibers. See *external arcuate fibers*.

fibrae arcuatae externae ven·tra·les (ven·tray'leez) [NA]. The ventral external arcuate fibers. See *external arcuate fibers*.

fibrae arcuatae in·ter·nae (in·tur'nee) [NA]. INTERNAL ARCUATE FIBERS.

fibrae ce·re·bel·lo·oli·va·res (serr·e·bel"o·ol·i·vair'eez) [BNA]. Tractus olivocerebellaris. (= OLIVOCEREBELLAR TRACT)

fibrae cir·cu·la·res mus·cu·li ci·li·a·ris (sur·kew·lair'eez mus'kew·lye sil·ee·air'is) [NA]. Circular muscle fibers within the ciliary body.

fibrae cor·ti·co·nu·cle·a·res (kor"ti·ko·new"klee·air'eez) [NA]. CORTICOBULBAR TRACTS.

fibrae cor·ti·co·pon·ti·nae (kor"ti·ko·pon·tye'nee) [NA]. CORTICOPONTINE FIBERS.

fibrae cor·ti·co·re·ti·cu·la·res me·sen·ce·pha·li (kor"ti·ko·re·tick"yoo·lair'eez mes·en·sef'uh·lye) [NA]. Nerve fibers from the cerebral cortex to nuclei in the reticular substance of the mesencephalon.

fibrae corticoreticulares pon·tis (pon'tis) [NA]. Nerve fibers from the cerebral cortex to nuclei in the reticular substance of the pons.

fibrae cor·ti·co·spi·na·les (kor"ti·ko·spye·nay'leez) [NA]. CORTICOSPINAL TRACTS.

fibrae in·ter·cru·ra·les (in"tur·kroo·ray'leez) [NA]. Arching fibers in the inguinal ligament running between the medial and lateral crura of the superficial inguinal ring.

fibrae len·tis (len'tis) [NA]. LENS FIBERS.

fibrae me·ri·di·o·na·les mus·cu·li ci·li·a·ris (me·rid"ee·o·nay'leez mus'kew·lye sil·ee·air'is) [NA]. Muscle fibers of the ciliary body which run from the pectinate ligament toward the ciliary processes.

fibrae ob·li·quae ven·tri·cu·li (ob·lye'kwee ven·trick'yoo·lye) [NA]. Oblique muscle fibers in the inner part of the muscular coat of the stomach.

fibrae pe·ri·ven·tri·cu·la·res (perr"i·ven·trick·yoo·lair'eez) [NA]. Fibers passing along the wall of the third ventricle descending from the hypothalamus.

fibrae pon·tis pro·fun·dae (pon'tis pro·fun'dee) [BNA]. FIBRAE PONTIS TRANSVERSAE.

fibrae pontis su·per·fi·ci·a·les (sue"pur·fish·ee·ay'leez) [BNA]. Fibers on the surface of the pons.

fibrae pontis trans·ver·sae (trans·vur'see) [NA]. Fibers arising in pontine nuclei and running transversely to the middle cerebellar peduncle; most of these fibers cross the midline.

fibrae py·ra·mi·da·les me·dul·lae ob·lon·ga·tae (pi·ram"i·day'leez me·dul'ee ob·lon·gay'tee). CORTICOSPINAL TRACT.

fibrae zo·nu·la·res (zon·yoo·lair'eez) [NA]. ZONULAR FIBERS.

fibre. FIBER.

fi·bri·form (figh'bri·form) *adj.* [*fibr-* + *-iform*]. Shaped like a fiber.

fi·bril (figh'bril, fib'ril) *n.* [NL. *fibrilla*, dim. of *fibra*]. A component filament of a fiber, as of a muscle or of a nerve. —**fi·bril·lar** (·bri·lur), **fibril·lary** (·lăr·ee) *adj.*

fi·bril·la (figh·bril'uh) *n.*, pl. **fibril·lae** (·ee). FIBRIL.

fibrillary astrocytoma. An astrocytoma with abundant fibrillated cell processes and neuroglial fibrils.

fibrillary contraction. Incoordinate contraction of individual muscle fibers within a fasciculus.

fibrillary neuroma. PLEXIFORM NEUROMA.

fi·bril·late (figh'bri·late, fib'ri·) *v.* 1. To undergo fibrillation. 2. To cause to undergo fibrillation.

fibrillate, *adj.* FIBRILLATED.

fi·bril·lat·ed (figh'bri·lay·tid, fib'ri·) *adj.* Having fibrils; composed of fibrils.

fi·bril·la·tion (figh"bri·lay'shun, fib"ri·) *n.* 1. A noncoordinated twitching involving individual muscle fibers that have been separated from their nerve supply. 2. Very rapid irregular noncoordinated contractions of the heart.

fibrillation potential. *In electromyography,* a monophasic, biphasic, or triphasic spike usually of 25 to 100 microvolts in amplitude and less than 2 milliseconds in duration, producing a sharp clicking sound in the loudspeaker, due to the spontaneous contraction of an individual muscle fiber in a denervated muscle.

fibrillation waves. Electrocardiographic deflections due to atrial excitation in atrial fibrillation, varying in contour, amplitude, and timing; occurring at a rate of about 350 to 600 per minute. Abbreviated, *f waves, ff waves*. Compare *flutter waves*.

fi·bril·lo·gen·e·sis (figh·bril"o·jen'e·sis, figh"bri·lo·) *n.* [*fibril* + *-genesis*]. The formation and development of fibrils.

fibril sheath. A sheath formed by connective-tissue fibrils and surrounding individual nerve fibers.

fi·brin (figh'brin) *n.* The fibrous insoluble protein formed by the interaction of thrombin and fibrinogen.

fibrin-, fibrino-. A combining form meaning *fibrin, fibrinous*.

fi·brin·ase (figh'brin·ace) *n.* [*fibrin-* + *-ase*]. FACTOR XIII.

fibrin aster. Radiation of fibrin lines from centers of platelets or leukocytes.

fi·brin·a·tion (figh"bri·nay'shun) *n.* Formation of fibrin.

fibrin film. A pliable, elastic, translucent film of fibrin, prepared from human blood plasma; used in neurosurgery for the repair of dural defects and in the prevention of meningocerebral adhesions.

fibrin foam. A spongy material made from human fibrin which, when soaked in human thrombin, is a useful hemostatic agent in neurosurgery, in wounds of parenchymatous organs, and in cases of jaundice and hemophilia. It causes little tissue reaction and is absorbable.

fibrino-. See *fibrin-*.

fi·bri·no·cel·lu·lar (figh"bri·no·sel'yoo·lur) *adj.* [*fibrino-* + *cellular*]. Containing both fibrin and cells; usually refers to an exudate.

fi·brin·o·gen (figh·brin'o·jen) *n.* [*fibrino-* + *-gen*]. A protein, which may be bactericidal, of the globulin class present in blood plasma and serous transudations and increasing in quantity during the acute phase of an inflammatory reaction or trauma. The soluble precursor of fibrin. Syn. *factor I*. See also Table of Chemical Constituents of Blood in the Appendix. —**fi·brin·o·gen·ic** (figh"brin·o·jen'ick), **fi·bri·nog·e·nous** (figh"bri·noj'e·nus) *adj.*

fi·brin·o·geno·pe·nia (figh·brin"o·jen"o·pee'nee·uh) *n.* [*fibrinogen* + *-penia*]. A decrease in the fibrinogen content of the blood plasma. Compare *afibrinogenemia*.

fi·bri·no·hem·or·rhag·ic (figh"bri·no·hem"o·raj'ick) *adj.* [*fibrino-* + *hemorrhagic*]. Containing fibrin and blood; usually describes an exudate.

fi·brin·oid (figh'brin·oid) *adj.* & *n.* [*fibrin* + *-oid*]. 1. Having the appearance and the staining properties of fibrin. 2. A homogeneous, refractile, oxyphilic substance occurring in degenerating connective tissue, in term placentas, in rheumatoid nodules, in Aschoff bodies, and in pulmonary alveoli in some prolonged pneumonitides.

fibrinoid degeneration. A form of degeneration in which the tissue involved is converted to a homogeneous or granular acellular mass with bright acidophilic staining reaction resembling that of fibrin.

fi·bri·no·ki·nase (figh"bri·no·kigh'nase) *n.* [*fibrino-* + *kinase*].

An activator of plasminogen derived from animal tissue.
fi·bri·nol·y·sin (figh″bri·nol′i·sin) *n.* [*fibrino-* + *lysin*]. Any enzyme that digests fibrin; a less specific term than plasmin.
fi·bri·nol·y·sis (figh″bri·nol′i·sis) *n.* [*fibrino-* + *-lysis*]. The digestion or degradation of fibrin; may be applied to the proteolysis of fibrin by plasmin, but applies also to other mechanisms. —**fibri·no·lyt·ic** (·no·lit′ick) *adj.*
fi·bri·no·pe·nia (figh″bri·no·pee′nee·uh) *n.* [*fibrino-* + *-penia*]. FIBRINOGENOPENIA.
fi·brin·ous (figh′bri·nus) *adj.* Of, containing, or resembling fibrin.
fibrinous adhesion. Loose attachment of adjacent serous membranes due to the presence of fibrinous exudate.
fibrinous calculus. A mass of fibrin infiltrated with mineral salts.
fibrinous cataract. A false cataract consisting of an effusion on the capsule during severe iridocyclitis.
fibrinous exudate. An exudate in which fibrin is a prominent constituent.
fibrinous inflammation. Inflammation in which the noncellular portion of the exudate is composed largely of fibrin.
fibrinous polyp. A polyp composed of fibrin or organized fibrin.
fibrinous rhinitis. A rare form of rhinitis characterized by the development of a false membrane in the nose.
fibrinous synovitis. DRY SYNOVITIS.
fibrin-stabilizing factor. FACTOR XIII. Abbreviated, FSF.
fibrin star. FIBRIN ASTER.
fi·bri·nu·cle·ase (figh″bri·new′klee·ace) *n.* A mixture of fibrinolysin, obtained from cattle, and deoxyribonuclease from beef pancreas, used topically to lyse fibrin and liquefy pus, facilitating removal of necrotic material.
fibro-. See *fibr-*.
fi·bro·ad·e·no·ma (figh″bro·ad·e·no′muh) *n.* [*fibro-* + *adenoma*]. A benign tumor containing both fibrous and glandular elements.
fibroadenoma xan·tho·ma·to·des (zan″tho·muh·to′deez). FIBROADENOMA.
fi·bro·ad·i·pose (figh″bro·ad′i·poce) *adj.* [*fibro-* + *adipose*]. Both fibrous and fatty.
fi·bro·am·e·lo·blas·to·ma (figh″bro·am″e·lo·blas·to′muh) *n.* An ameloblastoma with an especially abundant fibrous stroma.
fi·bro·an·gio·li·po·ma (figh″bro·an″jee·o·li·po′muh) *n.* [*fibro-* + *angio-* + *lipoma*]. A benign tumor whose parenchyma contains fibrous, vascular, and adipose tissue components.
fi·bro·an·gi·o·ma (figh″bro·an″jee·o′muh) *n.* [*fibro-* + *angioma*]. A benign tumor composed of blood or lymph vessels, with abundant connective tissue.
fi·bro·are·o·lar (figh″bro·a·ree′o·lur) *adj.* Both fibrous and areolar.
fi·bro·blast (figh′bro·blast) *n.* [*fibro-* + *-blast*]. A large stellate cell (spindle-shaped in edge view) in which the nucleus is large, oval, and pale-staining with one or two nucleoli. Fibroblasts are common in developing or repairing tissues where they are concerned in protein and collagen synthesis. Compare *fibrocyte.*
fi·bro·blas·tic (figh″bro·blas′tick) *adj.* 1. Pertaining to fibroblasts. 2. FIBROPLASTIC.
fibroblastic meningioma. A meningioma in which the meningioma cells are highly elongated, resembling fibroblasts, and form interlacing bundles.
fi·bro·blas·to·ma (figh″bro·blas·to′muh) *n.* [*fibroblast* + *-oma*]. A tumor whose parenchyma consists of fibroblasts, as fibromas and fibrosarcomas.
fi·bro·bron·chi·tis (figh″bro·brong·kye′tis) *n.* Bronchitis with expectoration of fibrinous casts.
fi·bro·cal·car·e·ous (figh″bro·kal·kair′ee·us) *adj.* [*fibro-* + *calcareous*]. FIBROCALCIFIC.
fi·bro·cal·cif·ic (figh″bro·kal·sif′ick) *adj.* Consisting of fibrous and calcific elements, the fibrous element being primary.
fi·bro·car·ci·no·ma (figh″bro·kahr·si·no′muh) *n.* A carcinoma with fibrous elements.
fi·bro·car·ti·lage (figh″bro·kahr′ti·lij) *n.* Dense, white, fibrous connective tissue in which the cells have formed small masses of cartilage between the fibers. —**fibro·car·ti·lag·i·nous** (·kahr″ti·laj′i·nus) *adj.*
fibrocartilagines in·ter·ver·te·bra·les (in″tur·vur·te·bray′leez) [BNA]. DISCI INTERVERTEBRALES.
fi·bro·car·ti·la·go (figh″bro·kahr′ti·lay′go) *n.*, pl. **fibrocarti·la·gi·nes** (·laj′i·neez) [NA]. FIBROCARTILAGE.
fibrocartilago ba·sa·lis (ba·say′lis) [BNA]. The cartilage that fills the foramen lacerum.
fibrocartilago na·vi·cu·la·ris (na·vick″yoo·lair′is) [BNA]. A fibrocartilaginous portion of the medial calcaneonavicular ligament.
fi·bro·ca·se·ous (figh″bro·kay′see·us) *adj.* Containing both fibrous and caseous elements, said of certain forms of pulmonary tuberculosis.
fi·bro·cav·i·tary (figh″bro·kav′i·terr·ee) *adj.* Having both fibrosis and cavity formation; said of certain forms of pulmonary tuberculosis.
fi·bro·cel·lu·lar (figh″bro·sel′yoo·lur) *adj.* Both fibrous and cellular.
fi·bro·ce·men·to·ma (figh″bro·see″men·to′muh) *n.* A type of cementoma in which the fibrous component overshadows the cementum component.
fi·bro·chon·dro·ma (figh″bro·kon·dro′muh) *n.* [*fibro-* + *chondr-* + *-oma*]. A benign tumor containing both fibrous and cartilaginous elements.
fi·bro·chon·dro·os·te·o·ma (figh″bro·kon·dro·os·tee·o′muh) *n.* [*fibro-* + *chondroosteoma*]. A type of osteochondroma with a prominent fibrous element.
fi·bro·col·lag·e·nous (figh″bro·kol·aj′e·nus) *adj.* [*fibro-* + *collagenous*]. Pertaining to fibrous tissue in which there is a great deal of collagen and relatively few cells.
fi·bro·cys·tic (figh″bro·sis′tick) *adj.* Having both fibrous and cystic aspects; usually applied to the development of cysts in a gland which is the seat of chronic retrogressive or inflammatory changes accompanied by fibrosis.
fibrocystic disease. CYSTIC DISEASE OF THE BREAST.
fibrocystic disease of the pancreas. CYSTIC FIBROSIS OF THE PANCREAS.
fi·bro·cys·to·ma (figh″bro·sis·to′muh) *n.* [*fibro-* + *cyst-* + *-oma*]. A benign tumor containing both fibrous and cystic elements.
fi·bro·cyte (figh′bro·site) *n.* [*fibro-* + *-cyte*]. A connective-tissue cell present in fully differentiated or mature tissue in which the cytoplasm is less abundant and less basophilic than that of a fibroblast. Fibrocytes are relatively immobile; however, they regain proliferative capacity following tissue injury.
fi·bro·dys·pla·sia (figh″bro·dis·play′zhuh, ·zee·uh) *n.* FIBROUS DYSPLASIA.
fi·bro·elas·tic (figh″bro·e·las′tick) *adj.* Having interlacing collagenous fibers interspersed by more or less strongly developed networks of elastic fibers; applied to connective tissue.
fi·bro·elas·to·sis (figh″bro·e·las·to′sis) *n.* [*fibro-* + *elastic* + *-osis*]. 1. Proliferation of fibrous and elastic tissues. 2. ENDOCARDIAL FIBROELASTOSIS.
fi·bro·en·chon·dro·ma (figh″bro·en″kon·dro′muh) *n.* An enchondroma containing fibrous elements.
fi·bro·en·do·the·li·o·ma (figh″bro·en″do·theel·ee·o′muh) *n.* [*fibro-* + *endothelioma*]. A tumor containing fibrous and endothelium-like structures, as a synovioma.
fibroendothelioma of a joint. A benign synovioma.
fi·bro·fat·ty (figh″bro·fat′ee) *adj.* Both fibrous and fatty.
Fibrogen. Trademark for a suspension of tissue fibrinogen and cephalin in a sodium chloride solution. Possesses thromboplastic activity, and is employed orally as a hemostatic.

fi·brog·lia (figh·brog'lee·uh, fi·) *n.* [*fibro-* + *-glia*]. The ground substance of connective tissue.

fibroglia fibers. Tonofibrils intimately associated with fibroblasts.

fi·bro·he·mo·tho·rax, fi·bro·hae·mo·tho·rax (figh"bro·hee" mo·tho'racks) *n.* [*fibro-* + *hemo-* + *thorax*]. The presence of blood and fibrin in the pleural space. Compare *fibrothorax.*

fi·broid (figh'broid) *adj.* & *n.* [*fibr-* + *-oid*]. 1. Composed largely of fibrous tissue. 2. LEIOMYOMA UTERI. 3. Any fibrous tumor.

fibroid degeneration. Localized fibrosis.

fi·broid·ec·to·my (figh"broy·deck'tuh·mee) *n.* [*fibroid* + *-ectomy*]. Removal of a uterine fibroid; MYOMECTOMY.

fibroid pneumonia. ORGANIZING PNEUMONIA.

fibroid tuberculosis. Chronic tuberculosis with extensive fibrosis and little caseation or cavitation; usually seen in adults.

fibroid tumor. 1. FIBROMA. 2. LEIOMYOMA UTERI.

fi·bro·lam·i·nar (figh"bro·lam'i·nur) *adj.* [*fibro-* + *laminar*]. Pertaining to a fibrous tissue layer.

fibrolaminar thrombus. STRATIFIED THROMBUS.

fi·bro·leio·my·o·ma (figh"bro·lye"o·migh·o'muh) *n.* A leiomyoma containing a fibrous component.

fi·bro·li·po·ma (figh"bro·li·po'muh) *n.* A lipoma with a considerable amount of fibrous tissue. —**fibroli·po·ma·tous** (·pom'uh·tus, ·po'muh·tus) *adj.*

fi·bro·lipo·sar·co·ma (figh"bro·lip"o·sahr·ko'muh) *n.* [*fibro-* + *lipo-* + *sarcoma*]. A malignant tumor with both fibrosarcomatous and liposarcomatous elements.

fi·brol·y·sis (figh·brol'i·sis) *n.*, pl. **fibroly·ses** (·seez) [*fibro-* + *-lysis*]. Resolution of abnormal fibrous tissue, as in a scar.

fi·bro·ma (figh·bro'muh) *n.*, pl. **fibromas, fibroma·ta** (·tuh) [*fibr-* + *-oma*]. A benign tumor composed principally of fibrous connective tissue.

fibroma du·rum (dew'rum). 1. A hard fibroma, firm because of large quantities of collagenous material in comparison with the number of cells. 2. DERMATOFIBROMA.

fibroma fun·goi·des (fung·goy'deez). MYCOSIS FUNGOIDES.

fibroma li·po·ma·to·des (li·po"muh·to'deez). XANTHOMA.

fibroma mol·le (mol'ee). A soft fibroma, containing many cellular components, as compared with collagenous fibers.

fibroma mol·lus·cum (mol·us'kum). The cutaneous lesion of neurofibromatosis.

fibroma pen·du·lum (pen'juh·lum, pend'yoo·lum). A benign, pendulous fibrous tumor attached to the skin by a narrow neck.

fibroma simplex. DERMATOFIBROMA.

fibromata. A plural of *fibroma.*

fi·bro·ma·to·gen·ic (figh·bro"muh·to·jen'ick) *adj.* [*fibroma* + *-genic*]. Pertaining to any process or agent that promotes fibrous connective-tissue formation or fibroma.

fi·bro·ma·toid (figh·bro'muh·toid) *adj.* [*fibroma* + *-oid*]. Resembling a fibroma.

fi·bro·ma·to·sis (figh·bro"muh·to'sis) *n.*, pl. **fibromato·ses** (·seez) [*fibroma* + *-osis*]. 1. The occurrence of multiple fibromas. 2. Localized proliferation of fibroblasts without apparent cause.

fibromatosis gin·gi·vae (jin·jye'vee). A generalized form of gingival hyperplasia of unknown etiology, but having a strong familial or hereditary background. Syn. *diffuse fibromatosis, familial fibromatosis, hereditary gingival fibromatosis.*

fi·bro·ma·tous (figh·bro'muh·tus, ·brom'uh·tus) *adj.* Of or pertaining to a fibroma.

fi·brome en pas·tille (fee·brome' ahn pas·teel', F. fee·bro^{h}m ah^{n} pas·tee$^{y'}$) [F.]. DERMATOFIBROMA.

fi·bro·mus·cu·lar (figh"bro·mus'kew·lur) *adj.* [*fibro-* + *muscular*]. Made up of connective tissue and muscle.

fi·bro·my·o·ma (figh"bro·migh·o'muh) *n.* [*fibro-* + *myoma*]. A benign tumor, usually of smooth muscle, with a prominent fibrous stroma; commonly a LEIOMYOMA UTERI.

fi·bro·my·o·mec·to·my (figh"bro·migh"o·meck'tuh·mee) *n.* [*fibromyoma* + *-ectomy*]. Excision of a fibromyoma.

fi·bro·my·o·si·tis (figh"bro·migh"o·sigh'tis) *n.* 1. FIBROSITIS. 2. FIBROUS MYOSITIS.

fi·bro·myxo·li·po·ma (figh"bro·mick"so·li·po'muh) *n.* [*fibro-* + *myxo-* + *lip-* + *-oma*]. A benign mixed mesodermal tumor of hamartomatous nature, containing fibrous, myxoid, and fatty components.

fi·bro·myx·o·ma (figh"bro·mick·so'muh) *n.* [*fibro-* + *myx-* + *-oma*]. A benign mixed mesodermal tumor of hamartomatous nature, composed of fibrous and myxoid elements.

fi·bro·myxo·sar·co·ma (figh"bro·mick"so·sahr·ko'muh) *n.* [*fibro-* + *myxo-* + *sarcoma*]. A malignant mixed mesodermal tumor with fibrosarcomatous and myxosarcomatous components.

fi·bro·os·teo·chon·dro·ma (figh"bro·os"tee·o·kon·dro'muh) *n.* An osteochondroma with a prominent fibrous element.

fi·bro·os·te·o·ma (figh"bro·os·tee·o'muh) *n.* An osteoma with a prominent fibrous component.

fi·bro·os·teo·sar·co·ma (figh"bro·os"tee·o·sahr·ko'muh) *n.* An osteosarcoma with a significant fibrosarcomatous element.

fi·bro·pap·il·lo·ma (figh"bro·pap"i·lo'muh) *n.* [*fibro-* + *papilloma*]. FIBROADENOMA.

fi·bro·pla·sia (figh"bro·play'zhuh, ·zee·uh) *n.* [*fibro-* + *-plasia*]. The growth of fibrous connective tissue, as in the second phase of wound healing. —**fibro·plas·tic** (·plas'tick) *adj.*

fi·bro·plate (figh'bro·plate) *n.* [*fibro-* + *plate*]. A disk of interarticular fibrocartilage.

fi·bro·psam·mo·ma (figh"bro·sa·mo'muh) *n.* A benign tumor, chiefly fibrous, containing psammoma bodies.

fi·bro·pu·ru·lent (figh"bro·pewr'yoo·lunt, ·pewr'uh·lunt) *adj.* Pertaining to purulent exudate with a prominent fibrinous element.

fi·bro·sar·co·ma (figh"bro·sahr·ko'muh) *n.* [*fibro-* + *sarcoma*]. A malignant tumor whose parenchyma is composed of anaplastic fibrocytes. —**fibrosarcoma·tous** (·tus) *adj.*

fibrosarcoma myx·o·ma·to·des (mick"so·muh·to'deez). FIBROMYXOSARCOMA.

fibrosarcoma of the nerve sheath. NEUROFIBROSARCOMA.

fibrosarcoma phyl·lo·des (fi·lo'deez). CYSTOSARCOMA PHYLLODES.

fi·brose (figh'broce) *adj.* & *v.* 1. FIBROUS. 2. To form fibrous tissue.

fibrosed cyst. Any nonspecific cyst in which the usual structures have been partially replaced by connective tissue.

fi·bro·se·rous (figh"bro·seer'us) *adj.* Having both fibrous and serous elements.

fi·bros·ing (figh'bro·sing) *adj.* 1. Undergoing fibrosis. 2. Having the property of stimulating fibrous tissue production.

fibrosing adenosis or **adenomatosis.** SCLEROSING ADENOMATOSIS.

fibrosing alveolitis. Fibrosis of pulmonary alveoli of unknown cause.

fi·bro·sis (figh·bro'sis) *n.*, pl. **fibro·ses** (·seez) [*fibr-* + *-osis*]. An increment in fibrous connective tissue. —**fi·brot·ic** (figh·brot'ick) *adj.*

fi·bro·si·tis (figh"bro·sigh'tis) *n.* [*fibrose* + *-itis*]. A clinical disease entity characterized by pain, stiffness, and tenderness associated with muscle sheaths and fascial layers. Syn. *muscular rheumatism.* —**fibro·sit·ic** (·sit'ick) *adj.*

fibrositis os·sif·i·cans pro·gres·si·va (os·if'i·kanz pro"gre·sigh'vuh). The multiple progressive form of myositis ossificans.

fi·bro·tho·rax (figh"bro·tho'racks) *n.* [*fibro-* + *thorax*]. Complete adhesion between the visceral and parietal layers of the pleura of a hemithorax, together with fibrosis of the joined surfaces.

fi·brous (figh'brus) *adj.* Containing fibers; similar to fibers.

fibrous adhesion. Firm attachment of adjacent serous membranes by bands or masses of fibrous connective tissue.

fibrous ankylosis. Ankylosis due to fibrosis in the joint capsule or fibrous adhesions between the joint surfaces.

fibrous astrocytes. Neuroglia in the white matter characterized by long, unbranched processes.

fibrous bar. A bar caused by connective-tissue hyperplasia.

fibrous callus. The connective tissue that precedes formation of cartilage or bone in a callus.

fibrous capsule of the kidney. The fibrous investment of the kidney, lying immediately outside the parenchyma and continuous with the connective tissue of the renal pelvis. NA *capsula fibrosa renis.*

fibrous cavernitis. PEYRONIE'S DISEASE.

fibrous connective tissue. The densest connective tissue of the body, including tendons, ligaments, and fibrous membranes. Collagenous fibers form the main constituent and are arranged in parallel bundles between which are rows of connective-tissue cells.

fibrous dysplasia. 1. Fibrous hyperplasia and osseous metaplasia in one bone (monostotic) or several bones (polyostotic); the latter form is often accompanied by segmental café-au-lait spots with ragged edges and, usually in girls, with precocious puberty (Albright's syndrome). 2. A form of mammary dysplasia characterized by abnormal amounts of fibrous tissue in relation to glandular tissue.

fibrous investment. General term describing an outer sheath of connective tissue found about various organs outside the proper capsule of the organ.

fibrous myositis. Chronic myositis with formation of fibrous tissue.

fibrous osteoma. OSSIFYING FIBROMA.

fibrous pericardium. The outer, dense sheet of connective tissue of the parietal pericardium.

fibrous ring. 1. The dense fibrous peripheral portion of an intervertebral disk. NA *anulus fibrosus disci intervertebralis.* 2. Any of the four rings encircling the openings of the heart (aortic, pulmonary, left atrioventricular, right atrioventricular); ANULI FIBROSI CORDIS. See also *skeleton of the heart.* 3. The fibrous attachment of the tympanic membrane to the tympanic sulcus. NA *anulus fibrocartilagineus membranae tympani.* 4. A fibrous loop holding a tendon in place, as in the case of the digastric muscle.

fibrous trigones of the heart. The two triangular masses of fibrous tissue forming the base of the heart. The right trigone is situated between the right and left atrioventricular openings; the left, between the left side of the opening of the aorta and the left atrioventricular opening. NA *trigona fibrosa cordis.*

fi·bro·vas·cu·lar (figh″bro·vas′kew·lur) *adj.* Having both fibrous and vascular components.

fi·bro·xan·tho·ma (figh″bro·zan·tho′muh) *n.* A xanthoma with a prominent fibrous stroma. —**fibroxanthoma·tous** (·tus) *adj.*

fib·u·la (fib′yoo·luh) *n.*, L. pl. & genit. sing. **fibu·lae** (·lee) [L., clasp] [NA]. The slender bone at the outer part of the leg, articulating above with the tibia and below with the talus and tibia. See also Table of Bones in the Appendix and Plates 1, 2. —**fibu·lar** (·lur) *adj.*

fibular artery. PERONEAL ARTERY.

fibular collateral ligament. A strong, fibrous cord on the lateral side of the knee joint, connecting the lateral condyle of the femur and the lateral surface of the head of the fibula. NA *ligamentum collaterale fibulare.*

fibular retinaculum. PERONEAL RETINACULUM.

fib·u·lo·cal·ca·ne·al (fib″yoo·lo·kal·kay′nee·ul) *adj.* [*fibula* + *calcaneal*]. Pertaining to or connecting the fibula and the calcaneus.

fib·u·lo·cal·ca·ne·us (fib″yoo·lo·kal·kay′nee·us) *n.* An occasional muscle arising from the lower third of the fibula and inserted into the tendon of the quadratus plantae or of the flexor digitorum longus, found as an anterior or a medial variant.

fib·u·lo·tib·i·a·lis (fib″yoo·lo·tib·ee·ay′lis) *adj.* [NL.]. Pertaining to the fibula and the tibia.

fibulotibialis muscle. An occasional small muscle arising from the medial side of the head of the fibula and inserted into the posterior surface of the tibia beneath the popliteus.

F.I.C. Fellowship of the Institute of Chemistry.

F.I.C.D. Fellow of the International College of Dentists.

fi·cin (figh′sin) *n.* [L. *ficus*, fig, + *-in*]. A proteolytic enzyme from the sap of the fig-tree. It is an active *Ascaris* and *Trichuris* vermicide.

Fick principle, method, or **equation** [A. *Fick,* German physiologist, 1829–1901]. A method for determining cardiac output based on the principle that the uptake or release of oxygen by an organ is the product of the organ blood flow and the arteriovenous oxygen concentration difference; cardiac output = (oxygen consumption)/(arteriovenous oxygen difference) × 100.

Fick's axes [A. *Fick*]. The vertical, horizontal, and sagittal axes of the eyeball when it is directed straight forward, all of which run through its hypothetical center of rotation; designated X, Y, and Z, respectively.

Fick's law of diffusion [A. *Fick*]. The rate at which a dissolved substance diffuses through a medium (solvent) will depend upon the concentration of the substance diffusing.

fi·co·sis (fye·ko′sis) *n.* [L. *ficus*, fig, + *-osis*]. SYCOSIS.

F.I.C.S. Fellow of the International College of Surgeons.

Fied·ler's disease (feed′lur) [C. L. A. *Fiedler,* German physician, 1835–1921]. WEIL'S DISEASE.

Fiedler's myocarditis [C. L. A. *Fiedler*]. An acute interstitial myocarditis of unknown etiology, with a predominant mononuclear cell infiltrate and varying muscle necrosis.

field, *n.* 1. A space or area of varying size or boundaries. 2. A concept of development in which the whole and the parts of a structure or organism are dynamically interrelated, reacting to each other and to the environment. 3. A region of the embryo that is the anlage of some organ or part. 4. The area within which objects can be seen through a microscope at one time. 5. *In surgery,* the area exposed to the surgeon's vision. 6. A specialty or special branch of knowledge, as the field of neurology. 7. In diagnostic radiology, the projected image of an anatomic organ or region, as lung field. 8. In therapeutic radiology, the area directly encompassed by an external therapy beam; port.

field block anesthesia. Anesthesia produced by injecting a wall of anesthesia solution about an operative field.

field depth. FOCAL DEPTH.

field emission. COLD EMISSION.

field fever. LEPTOSPIROSIS. See also *harvest fever.*

field hospital. *In military medicine,* a hospital, usually under a tent, designed to function as a station hospital at isolated posts or airfields, but adaptable to support ground troops in combat. It is classified as a fixed hospital, but it can be easily moved and even transported by air.

field of fixation. *In optics,* the region bounded by the utmost limits of distinct or central vision, which the eye has under its direct control throughout its excursions when the head is not moved.

field of vision. The space visible to an individual when the eye is fixed steadily on an object in the direct line of vision. Abbreviated, F.

fields of Fo·rel (foʰ·rel′) [A. H. *Forel*]. TEGMENTAL FIELDS OF FOREL.

fiè·vre bou·ton·neuse (fyev′r boo·ton·uhz′, F. boo·toʰn·œhz′) [F.]. BOUTONNEUSE FEVER.

fifth (Vth) cranial nerve. TRIGEMINAL NERVE.

fifth disease. ERYTHEMA INFECTIOSUM.

fifth ventricle. The cavity of the septum pellucidum.

fig, *n.* [OF. *figue,* from L. *ficus*]. The fruit of *Ficus carica,* having nutritive and laxative qualities.

fight-or-flight reaction. 1. *In physiology,* according to W. B. Cannon, the response of the sympathetic nervous system and the adrenal medulla to stress, which results in adjustments in blood flow and metabolism adapted to the preservation of the organism in an emergency situation. Compare *general adaptation syndrome.* See also *homeostasis.* 2. *In psychiatry,* the manner in which a person responds to stress. In the "fight" reaction he strives for adjustment; if he fails he may adopt a neurosis as a compromise. In the "flight" reaction, the patient may take refuge in a psychosis, permitting him to fancy a situation in which he can control the problem or ignore its reality.

fig·ure, *n.* [OF., from L. *figura*]. 1. The visible form of anything; the outline of an organ or part. 2. A group of impressions derived from a single sense and perceived as a whole or one unit set apart from adjacent impressions. Compare *figure-ground.* 3. A person who represents the essential aspects of a certain role; in particular, a father or mother figure.

figure-ground, *n. In psychology,* a general property of perception or awareness, according to which the perceived is divided into two or more parts, each endowed with a different shape or other attribute, but all influencing each other; the most distinct part being the figure and the least formed one, the ground. Inability to separate figure from ground is seen in certain organic brain syndromes.

figure-of-eight bandage. A bandage in which the successive turns cross like the figure eight.

figure-of-eight suture. TRANSFIXION SUTURE.

fig wart. CONDYLOMA ACUMINATUM.

fig·wort, *n.* Any member of the botanical family Scrophulariaceae; specifically, the herb *Scrophularia nodosa* var. *marilandica,* formerly variously used medicinally.

fila. Plural of *filum.*

fila ana·sto·mo·ti·ca ner·vi acu·sti·ci (a·nas″to·mot′i·kuh nur′vye a·koos′ti·sigh) [BNA]. A small bundle of nerve fibers running from the vestibular to the cochlear part of the vestibulocochlear nerve.

fi·la·ceous (fi·lay′shus) *adj.* [L. *fil*um, thread, + *-aceous*]. Consisting of threads or threadlike fibers or parts.

fila co·ro·na·ria (kor·o·nair′ee·uh). Fibrous bands of the cardiac skeleton extending from the base of the medial cusp of the tricuspid valve to the aortic opening and right trigone.

fila la·te·ra·lia pon·tis (lat·e·ray′lee·uh pon′tis) [BNA]. Plural of *filum lateralis pontis.*

fil·a·ment (fil′uh·munt) *n.* [ML. *filamentum,* from L. *filare,* to spin]. A small, threadlike structure. —**fil·a·men·tous** (fil″uh·men′tus), **fil·a·men·ta·ry** (fil″uh·men′tuh·ree) *adj.*

fil·a·men·ta·tion (fil″uh·men·tay′shun) *n.* THREAD REACTION.

filament transformer. A stepdown transformer to provide current for the cathode filament of an x-ray tube.

fila ol·fac·to·ria (ol·fack·to′ree·uh). The component fasciculi of the olfactory nerve before and during their passage through the cribriform plate of the ethmoid bone.

fi·lar (figh′lur) *adj.* [L. *fil*um, thread, + *-ar*]. Filamentous; having or being threadlike structures.

fila ra·di·cu·la·ria (ra·dick″yoo·lair′ee·uh) [NA]. The numerous filaments by which the dorsal root of a spinal nerve enters the spinal cord.

fila radicularia ner·vo·rum spi·na·li·um (nur·vo′rum spye·nay′lee·um) [NA]. The fine filaments that attach the ventral and dorsal roots of the spinal nerves to the spinal cord.

fi·lar·ia (fi·lăr′ee·uh) *n.,* pl. **filar·i·ae** (·ee·ee) [NL., from L. *filum,* thread]. A worm of the superfamily Filarioidea: long filiform nematodes, the adults of which may live in the circulatory or lymphatic systems, the connective tissues, or serous cavities of a vertebrate host. The larval forms, or microfilariae, are commonly found in the circulating blood or lymph spaces from which they are ingested by some form of bloodsucking arthropod. After a series of metamorphoses in the body of the arthropod, the larvae migrate to the proboscis as infestive forms. —**filari·al** (·ul) *adj.*

filarial fever. A recurrent fever occurring irregularly at intervals of months or years in most forms of filariasis. Syn. *elephantoid fever.*

fil·a·ri·a·sis (fil″uh·rye′uh·sis) *n.,* pl. **filaria·ses** (·seez) [*filar*ia + *-iasis*]. An infection with filariae, with or without the production of manifest disease.

fi·lar·i·cide (fi·lăr′i·side) *n.* [*filar*ia + *-cide*]. A drug that destroys filariae. —**fi·lar·i·ci·dal** (fi·lăr″i·sigh′dul) *adj.*

fi·lar·i·form (fi·lăr′i·form) *adj.* In the form of, or resembling, filariae.

fil·a·rin (fil′uh·rin) *n.* The acidic protein found in neurofilaments.

filar ocular micrometer. EYEPIECE MICROMETER.

Fi·la·tov-Dukes disease (fi·lah′tuf) [N. F. *Filatov,* Russian pediatrician, 1846–1902; and C. *Dukes*]. EXANTHEM SUBITUM.

Filatov's disease [N. F. *Filatov*]. INFECTIOUS MONONUCLEOSIS.

Filatov's spots [N. F. *Filatov*]. KOPLIK'S SPOTS.

fil·ial (fil′ee·ul) *adj.* [L. *filialis,* from *filius,* son]. 1. Pertaining to an offspring. 2. *In genetics,* indicating the sequence of an offspring from the original parents, the first being designated F_1, the second F_2, and so forth.

filial regression. The tendency for the mean phenotypic value of offspring to deviate less from a population mean than do parents who demonstrate large deviations.

fi·lic·ic acid (fi·lis′ick). The term applied to one or more constituents of a mixture of related constituents found in aspidium, certain of which appear to be derivatives of a methyl and a dimethyl phloroglucinol.

fil·i·cin (fil′i·sin) *n.* FILICIC ACID.

fil·i·cin·ic acid (fil″i·sin′ick). 1,1-Dimethylcyclohexane-2,4,6-trione, $C_8H_{10}O_3$, a constituent of aspidium or a product of the decomposition of other constituents.

fili·form (fil′i·form, figh′li·) *adj.* [*fil*um + *-iform*]. Threadlike.

filiform bougie. A bougie of very slender caliber, variously tipped.

filiform catheter. A catheter the leading end of which is molded into an extremely slender or thread-shaped form in order to facilitate passage of the larger, following portion through a constricted or irregular passage. Syn. *whip catheter.*

filiform papilla. Any one of the papillae occurring on the dorsum and margins of the oral part of the tongue, consisting of an elevation of connective tissue covered by a layer of epithelium, giving the tongue a velvety appearance.

fil·i·pin (fil′i·pin) *n.* An antibiotic, $C_{35}H_{58}O_{11}$, produced by *Streptomyces filipinensis;* it has antifungal activity.

Fi·li·po·wicz sign (fi·li·po^h′vich) [C. *Filipowicz,* Polish physician, 20th century]. Yellow discoloration of the palms and soles in typhoid fever.

fili·punc·ture (fil′i·punk″chur) *n.* [*fil*um + *puncture*]. A former method of treating aneurysm by inserting wire threads, hair, or the like to promote coagulation.

fil·let (fil′it) *n.* [F. *filet,* dim. of *fil,* thread]. 1. A loop for the purpose of making traction on the fetus. 2. LEMNISCUS.

fill·ing, *n.* A dental restoration; may be applied to a restoration of a temporary nature or for treatment.

filling gallop or **sound.** VENTRICULAR GALLOP.

film, *n.* 1. Any extremely thin covering, coating, or layer, usually nonrigid and translucent or transparent. 2. A pellicle or thin skin. 3. An opacity, as of the cornea. 4. Plastic material coated with a radiation-sensitive emulsion, used to make negatives or transparencies in radiography or photography.

fil·mat·ed gauze (fil′may·tid). A folded absorbent gauze with a thin layer of cotton or rayon evenly distributed over every layer giving ample dressing volume, rapid absorption and extreme softness.

film badge. A device containing photographic film, worn by personnel exposed to radiation to record dosage received. See also *photographic dosimetry.*

film-coated tablet. A compressed tablet covered with a thin film of a water-soluble substance.

filo·po·di·um (fil″o·po′dee·um, figh″lo·) *n.*, pl. **filopo·dia** (·dee·uh) [*fil*um + *-podium*, from Gk. *podion*, dim. of *pous*, foot]. A branching pseudopodium.

fil·ter, *n. & v.* [F. *filtre*, from ML. *filtrum*, piece of felt for straining]. 1. An apparatus that separates one or more components of a mixture from the others. 2. A special part of a high-frequency circuit which suppresses or admits certain frequencies of electric waves. 3. *In acoustics*, a device that suppresses certain frequencies of sound waves. 4. *In photography*, a colored glass or gelatin plate used in front of the photographic lens to alter the relative intensity of different wavelengths in the light beam. 5. To separate one or more components of a mixture from the others.

fil·ter·able (fil′tur·uh·bul) *adj.* FILTRABLE.

filter aid. A substance added to a liquid to be filtered to assist filtration, generally through formation of a bed of the added material which functions as an auxiliary filter, preventing passage of particles that would otherwise either pass through or clog the primary filter.

filtering operation. A surgical procedure performed for various types of glaucoma to form a new route of egress for the aqueous humor.

filter paper. An unglazed paper used for filtration.

fil·tra·ble (fil′truh·bul) *adj.* Able to pass through a filter; usually applied to living agents of disease smaller than the common pathogenic bacteria.

filtrable virus. VIRUS.

fil·trate (fil′trate) *n.* The liquid that has passed through a filter.

filtrate factor. PANTOTHENIC ACID.

fil·tra·tion (fil·tray′shun) *n.* The operation of straining through a filter.

filtration angle. The angle marking the periphery of the anterior chamber of the eye, formed by the attached margin of the iris and the junction of the sclera and cornea and functioning as a drainage route for aqueous humor. Syn. *anterior chamber angle, iridocorneal angle.* NA *angulus iridocornealis.*

fil·trum (fil′trum) *n.*, pl. **fil·tra** (·truh) [ML.]. A filter or strainer.

filtrum ven·tri·cu·li (ven·trick′yoo·lye). A small vertical groove in the mucosa of the lateral wall of the larynx between the cuneiform and arytenoid cartilages.

fi·lum (figh′lum) *n.*, pl. **fi·la** (·luh) [L., thread]. Any threadlike or filamentous structure.

filum du·rae ma·tris spi·na·lis (dew′ree may′tris spye·nay′lis) [NA]. The caudal tip of the filum terminale invested by the dura mater.

filum la·te·ra·lis pon·tis (lat·e·ray′lis pon′tis). *Obsol.* A fiber bundle running along the rostral border of the pons which may go to the cerebellum or connect the pons to the midbrain.

filum ter·mi·na·le (tur·mi·nay′lee) [NA]. The atrophic slender inferior end of the spinal cord, the caudal part of which is mostly pia mater.

fim·bria (fim′bree·uh) *n.*, pl. **fim·bri·ae** (·bree·ee) [L.]. 1. A fringe. 2. The fringelike process of the outer extremity of the uterine tube. 3. A flattened band of white fibers along the medial margin of the hippocampus, continuous with the crus of the fornix. —**fim·bri·al** (fim′bree·ul) *adj.*

fimbria cornu Ammonis. FIMBRIA (3).

fimbriae tu·bae ute·ri·nae (tew′bee yoo·tur·eye′nee) [NA]. The fringelike processes of the lateral end of the uterine tube.

fimbria hip·po·cam·pi (hip·o·kam′pye) [NA]. FIMBRIA (3).

fimbrial cyst. A cyst attached, or adjacent, to the fimbriae of the uterine tubes.

fimbria ova·ri·ca (o·vair′i·kuh) [NA]. FIMBRIA (2).

fim·bri·ate (fim′bree·ate) *adj.* [L. *fimbriatus*, fringed]. Fringed with slender processes that are larger than filaments; possessing pili; said of bacterial cells and of the ostium of the uterine tube.

fim·bri·at·ed (fim′bree·ay″tid) *adj.* FIMBRIATE.

fimbriated fold. A fold of mucous membrane having a fringed, free edge on either side of the frenulum of the tongue. NA *plica fimbriata.*

fim·bri·ec·to·my (fim″bree·eck′tuh·mee) *n.* [*fimbri*a + *-ectomy*]. Surgical resection of the fimbriated portion of the uterine tube.

fim·brio·den·tate (fim″bree·o·den′tate) *adj.* [*fimbri*a + *dentate*]. Pertaining to the fimbria (3) and to the dentate gyrus.

fimbriodentate sulcus. A groove on the superior medial aspect of the temporal lobe, separating the hippocampal fimbria from the dentate gyrus.

final common pathway. LOWER MOTOR NEURON.

Findlay's operation [F. McR. *Findlay*, U.S. surgeon b. 1898]. A method of closing a gastrojejunal fistula.

fine, *adj.* Involving movement through a narrow range. Said of tremors and other involuntary oscillatory movement of skeletal muscle. Contr. *coarse.*

fine structure. Ultramicroscopic structure.

fin·ger, *n.* [Gmc. *fingwraz*, lit., one of five]. A digit of the hand.

finger agnosia. Inability to recognize, name, and select individual fingers when looking at the hands; frequently a component of the Gerstmann syndrome.

finger anomia. A form of aphasia in which the patient has lost the ability to name his fingers though still able to recognize them.

finger cot. A covering of rubber or other material to protect the finger or to prevent infection.

finger-finger test. A cerebellar function test in which the patient is asked to bring the tips of his index fingers together from a position in which the arms are outstretched, or to place his index finger on the examiner's index finger with eyes open. Normally this is carried out smoothly and accurately.

finger flexor reflex. Flexion of the four fingers and the distal phalanx of the thumb, elicited normally when the examiner places his middle and index fingers on the palmar surfaces of the patient's slightly flexed four fingers and then taps his own fingers lightly but briskly. The Hoffman sign, and other pathologic responses are considered the abnormal variants of the finger flexor reflex in corticospinal tract disorders.

finger fracture operation of the mitral valve. A procedure for the relief of mitral stenosis in which the finger of the operator is inserted through the atrial appendage and atrium into the mitral orifice to increase the size of the stenosed opening.

finger-nose test. A cerebellar function test in which the patient is asked to put the tip of the index finger of each hand on the tip of the nose in rapid succession with eyes open. Abnormalities in the rate, range, and force of movement and an ataxic tremor betray the presence of cerebellar disease.

fin·ger·print, *n.* 1. An impression of the cutaneous ridges of a finger tip. May be a direct pressure print or a rolled print, the latter recording the entire flexor and lateral aspects of the phalanx. See also *dermatoglyphics.* 2. Hydrolization of polypeptides into a pattern on a two-dimensional chromatogram. —**fingerprint·ing** (·ing) *n.*

fingerprint body myopathy. A nonprogressive muscle disease characterized by abnormal bodies in red muscle fibers; in electron micrographs the bodies have concentric lamellae reminiscent of a fingerprint.

finger sign or **phenomenon.** SOUQUES' SIGN (1).

fin·ger·stall (fing′gur·stawl) *n.* FINGER COT.

finger-thumb reflex. Apposition and adduction of the thumb, associated with flexion at the metacarpophalangeal joint on firm passive flexion of the third to the fifth finger at the proximal joints. Syn. *Mayer's reflex.*

Fin·kel·dey cells. (fink′el·dye) [W. *Finkeldey*, German pathologist, 20th century]. WARTHIN-FINKELDEY GIANT CELLS.

Fin·ney's operation [J. M. T. *Finney*, U.S. surgeon 1863–1942]. 1. A type of pyloroplasty in which a U-shaped incision is employed that cuts across the sphincter and results in a greatly enlarged pyloric opening. Syn. *Finney's pyloroplasty.* 2. An end-to-side gastroduodenostomy. Syn. *Finney-von Haberer operation.*

Finney's pyloroplasty. FINNEY'S OPERATION (1).

Finney–von Ha·be·rer operation (fo^h^n hah'bur·ur). FINNEY'S OPERATION (2).

Fi·no·chet·ti's stirrup (fee″no·chet'ee, It. fee″no·ket'tee) [E. *Finochetti*, Argentinian surgeon, 1880–1948]. An apparatus used for skeletal traction in leg fractures.

fire·damp, *n.* An explosive mixture of methane and air.

first aid. Emergency treatment given to a casualty before regular medical or surgical care can be administered by trained individuals. —**first-aid,** *adj.;* **first-aider,** *n.*

first-aid kit. A pouch, bag, or box containing sterilized dressings, antiseptics and simple medications, bandages, an emergency airway, and simple instruments; for use in first aid.

first (Ist) cranial nerve. OLFACTORY NERVE.

first-degree burn. A mild burn, characterized by pain and reddening of the skin.

first-degree heart block. An atrioventricular block producing prolongation of the PR interval, but not completely blocking the conduction of any sinus beats to the ventricle.

first heart sound. The heart sound complex related primarily to closure of the atrioventricular valves and rapid ejection of blood from the ventricles. Symbol, S_1 or SI.

first intention. HEALING BY FIRST INTENTION.

first-order reaction. A reaction in which the rate of reaction is proportional to the first power of the concentration of a reactant. Syn. *unimolecular reaction.*

first-set, *adj.* Pertaining to a graft of a genetic constitution to which the recipient has had no previous exposure.

first stage. The stage of labor in which the molding of the fetal head and the dilatation of the cervix are effected.

Fish·berg's test. A concentration test for kidney function in which urinary specific gravity is determined 12 hours after fluid deprivation.

fish·ber·ry, *n.* COCCULUS.

fish glue. Isinglass prepared from the swim bladders of fishes.

fish·hook displacement. A vertical type of stomach, not an actual displacement; an orthotonic stomach.

fishhook stomach. J STOMACH.

fish skin. ICHTHYOSIS.

fishskin disease. ICHTHYOSIS.

fish tapeworm. *DIPHYLLOBOTHRIUM LATUM.*

fis·sile (fis'il, ·ile) *adj.* FISSIONABLE.

fis·sion (fish'un) *n.* [L. *fissio*, from *findere*, to cleave]. 1. Any splitting or cleaving. 2. *In biology,* asexual reproduction by the division of the body into two or more parts, each of which grows into a complete organism. It is the common method of reproduction among the bacteria and protozoa. 3. *In nuclear physics,* the splitting of an atomic nucleus, by bombardment with elementary particles, with release of energy. Contr. *fusion.* —**fission,** *v.;* **fission·able,** *adj.*

fission fungi. BACTERIA.

fis·su·la (fish'oo·luh, fis'yoo·luh) *n.*, pl. & genit. sing. **fissu·lae** (·lee) [L.]. A small fissure.

fissula an·te fe·nes·tram (an'tee fe·nes'tram). A channel, irregular in size and shape and filled with connective tissue, extending from the vestibule of the inner ear from a point just anterior to the fenestra vestibuli toward the tympanic cavity. There may or may not be an external opening. Syn. *Cozzolino's zone.*

fis·su·ra (fi·shoo'ruh, fi·syoo'ruh) *n.*, pl. & genit. sing. **fissu·rae** (·ree) [L.] [NA]. FISSURE.

fissura an·ti·tra·go·he·li·ci·na (an″tee·tray″go·hel·i·sigh'nuh) [NA]. A groove in the cartilage of the auricle between the tail of the helix and the antitragus.

fissura cal·ca·ri·na (kal·kuh·rye'nuh) [BNA]. Sulcus calcarinus (= CALCARINE SULCUS).

fissura ce·re·bri la·te·ra·lis [Sylvii] (serr'e·brye lat·e·ray'lis) [BNA]. Sulcus lateralis cerebri (= LATERAL CEREBRAL SULCUS).

fissura cho·roi·dea (ko·roy'dee·uh) [NA]. CHOROID FISSURE (2).

fissura col·la·te·ra·lis (ko·lat″e·ray'lis) [BNA]. Sulcus collateralis (= COLLATERAL SULCUS).

fissurae ce·re·bel·li (serr·e·bel'eye) [NA]. The grooves on the surface of the cerebellar cortex.

fissura hip·po·cam·pi (hip·o·kam'pye) [BNA]. Sulcus hippocampi (= HIPPOCAMPAL SULCUS).

fissura ho·ri·zon·ta·lis ce·re·bel·li (hor″i·zon·tay'lis serr·e·bel'eye) [NA]. HORIZONTAL FISSURE OF THE CEREBELLUM.

fissura horizontalis pul·mo·nis dex·tri (pul·mo'nis decks'trye) [NA]. HORIZONTAL FISSURE OF THE RIGHT LUNG.

fis·su·ral (fish'yoo·rul) *adj.* Of or pertaining to a fissure.

fissural angioma. A vascular malformation occurring at the site of embryonal fissures, as on the face or neck.

fissura li·ga·men·ti te·re·tis (lig·uh·men'tye terr'e·tis) [NA]. The fissure on the visceral surface of the liver which contains the round ligament after birth.

fissura ligamenti ve·no·si (ve·no'sigh) [NA]. The fissure on the posterior portion of the diaphragmatic surface of the liver which contains the ligamentum venosum after birth.

fissura lon·gi·tu·di·na·lis ce·re·bri (lon″ji·tew·di·nay'lis serr'e·brye) [NA]. LONGITUDINAL FISSURE OF THE CEREBRUM.

fissura me·di·a·na an·te·ri·or me·dul·lae ob·lon·ga·tae (mee·dee·ay'nuh an·teer'ee·or me·dul'ee ob·long·gay'tee) [NA]. The median anterior fissure of the medulla oblongata.

fissura mediana anterior medullae spi·na·lis (spi·nay'lis) [NA]. The anterior median fissure of the spinal cord.

fissura mediana posterior medullae ob·lon·ga·tae (ob·long·gay'tee) [BNA]. SULCUS MEDIANUS POSTERIOR MEDULLAE OBLONGATAE.

fissura ob·li·qua pul·mo·nis (ob·lye'kwuh pul·mo'nis) [NA]. OBLIQUE FISSURE.

fissura or·bi·ta·lis inferior (or·bi·tay'lis) [NA]. INFERIOR ORBITAL FISSURE.

fissura orbitalis superior [NA]. SUPERIOR ORBITAL FISSURE.

fissura pa·ri·e·to·oc·ci·pi·ta·lis (pa·rye″e·to·ock·sip·i·tay'lis) [BNA]. Sulcus parietooccipitalis (= PARIETOOCCIPITAL SULCUS).

fissura pe·tro·oc·ci·pi·ta·lis (pet″ro·ock·sip·i·tay'lis) [NA]. PETROOCCIPITAL FISSURE.

fissura pe·tro·squa·mo·sa (pet″ro·skway·mo'suh) [NA]. PETROSQUAMOUS FISSURE.

fissura pe·tro·tym·pa·ni·ca (pet″ro·tim·pan'i·kuh) [NA]. PETROTYMPANIC FISSURE.

fissura pos·te·ro·la·te·ra·lis ce·re·bel·li (pos″tur·o·lat·e·ray'lis serr·e·bel'eye) [NA]. The posterolateral fissure of the cerebellum, which separates the flocculus and nodulus from the rest of the cerebellum.

fissura pri·ma (prye'muh) [NA]. PRIMARY FISSURE.

fissura pte·ry·goi·dea (terr″i·goy'dee·uh) [BNA]. PTERYGOID FISSURE.

fissura pte·ry·go·ma·xil·la·ris (terr″i·go·mack·si·lair'is) [NA]. PTERYGOMAXILLARY FISSURE.

fissura pte·ry·go·pa·la·ti·na (terr″i·go·pal″uh·tye'nuh). PTERYGOMAXILLARY FISSURE.

fissura se·cun·da (se·kun'duh) [NA]. Postpyramidal sulcus. A sulcus separating the biventral lobule and the tonsilla of the cerebellum.

fissura sphe·no·oc·ci·pi·ta·lis (sfee″no·ock·sip·i·tay'lis) [BNA]. The sphenooccipital fissure between the basilar part of the occipital bone and the body of the sphenoid.

fissura sphe·no·pe·tro·sa (sfee″no·pe·tro'suh) [NA]. SPHENOPETROSAL FISSURE.

fissura ster·ni (stur'nigh). STERNOSCHISIS.

fissura trans·ver·sa ce·re·bel·li (trans·vur'suh serr·e·bel'eye)

[BNA]. Transverse fissure of the cerebellum between the cerebellar peduncles and the nodulus.

fissura transversa ce·re·bri (serr'e·brye) [NA]. TRANSVERSE CEREBRAL FISSURE.

fissura tym·pa·no·ma·stoi·dea (tim''puh·no·ma·stoy'dee·uh) [NA]. Tympanomastoid fissure between the mastoid process and tympanic portion of the temporal bone.

fissura tym·pa·no·squa·mo·sa (tim''puh·no·skway·mo'suh) [NA]. The tympanosquamous suture between the squamous and tympanic parts of the temporal bone.

fis·sure (fish'ur) *n.* [L. *fissura,* cleft]. 1. Any groove or cleft normally occurring in a part or organ such as the skull, liver, or spinal cord. Compare *sulcus.* 2. A crack in skin or an ulcer in mucous membrane. 3. A lineal developmental fault in the surface of a tooth caused by imperfect union of the enamel of adjoining dental lobes. —**fis·sured** (fish'urd) *adj.;* **fis·su·ra·tion** (fish''uh·ray'shun) *n.*

fissured chest. A rare deformity of congenital origin; exists in two forms, vertical fissure of the thoracic wall along the sternum, and lateral fissure. It may be associated with hernia of the lungs or with ectopia cordis. See also *sternoschisis, thoracoschisis.*

fissured fracture. A fracture in which there is an incomplete break; a crack or fissure extending into, but not through, a bone.

fissured tongue. A condition of the tongue in which there are deep furrows in the mucous membrane.

fissure in ano (in ay'no) [L.]. ANAL FISSURE.

fissure of Rolando [L. *Rolando*]. CENTRAL SULCUS (1).

fissure of the anus. ANAL FISSURE.

fissure of the gallbladder. CYSTIC FOSSA.

fissure of the optic cup. The part of the choroid fissure of the embryonic eye located in the optic cup.

fissure of the optic stalk. The part of the choroid fissure of the embryonic eye located in the optic stalk.

fissure of the urinary bladder. EXSTROPHY OF THE BLADDER.

fis·tu·la (fis'tew·luh) *n.,* pl. **fistulas, fistu·lae** (·lee) [L.]. An abnormal congenital or acquired communication between two surfaces or between a viscus or other hollow structure and the exterior. —**fistu·lar** (·lur), **fistu·late** (·late), **fistu·lous** (·lus) *adj.*

fistula au·ris con·ge·ni·ta (aw'ris kon·jen'i·tuh). A congenital, hereditary, narrow, usually blind pit opening at the crus of the helix.

fistula in ano (in ay'no) [L.]. ANAL FISTULA.

fis·tu·la·tion (fis'tew·lay'shun) *n.* FISTULIZATION.

fis·tu·lec·to·my (fis''tew·leck'tuh·mee) *n.* [*fistula* + *-ectomy*]. *In surgery,* excision of a fistula.

fis·tu·li·za·tion (fis''tew·li·zay'shun) *n.* The development or formation of a fistula or the surgical creation of a fistula.

fis·tu·lize (fis'tew·lize) *v.* To cause the formation of a fistula.

fis·tu·lo·en·ter·os·to·my (fis''tew·lo·en·tur·os'tuh·mee) *n.* [*fistula* + *enterostomy*]. *In surgery,* the establishment of an anastomosis between a biliary fistula and the duodenum.

fis·tu·lo·gram (fis'tew·lo·gram) *n.* [*fistula* + *-gram*]. A radiographic depiction of a fistulous tract using contrast material.

fis·tu·lot·o·my (fis''tew·lot'uh·mee) *n.* [*fistula* + *-tomy*]. Incision of a fistula.

¹fit, *n.* Any sudden paroxysm of a disease, especially a seizure.

²fit, *n. & v.* 1. *In biometry,* the agreement of probable data with actual data; in a graphic representation the way in which a curve of specified type approaches a given set of points in a plane. 2. *In biometry,* to adjust obtained data in such a way that it may be expressed by an equation or that the difference between it and the probable data is reduced. See also *curve fitting.*

Fitz·ger·ald-Gard·ner syndrome. GARDNER'S SYNDROME.

Fitz-Hugh–Cur·tis syndrome [T. *Fitz-Hugh,* Jr., U.S. physician, 1894-1963; and A. H. *Curtis,* U.S. obstetrician, 1881-1955]. Pain in the right upper quadrant of the abdomen in women during gonococcic pelvic inflammatory disease due to gonococcic peritonitis.

five-day fever. 1. TRENCH FEVER. 2. Any fever of five days' duration.

five-day schizophrenia. WAR NEUROSIS.

five-glass test. Collection of a urine sample in five containers, sequentially, to aid in localization of disease.

fix, *v.* [L. *figere, fixus,* to fasten]. 1. To render firm, stable, permanent; to fasten. 2. *In histology,* to treat tissue so that it hardens with preservation of the elements in the same relation and form as in life. See also *fixing.* 3. *In ophthalmology,* to turn the eye so that the image in the field of vision falls on the foveola or other point of fixation. 4. *In genetics,* to establish permanently some character of plants or animals by selective inbreeding.

fix·ate (fick'sate) *v.* 1. To become fixed. 2. To render fixed or stable.

fix·a·tion (fick·say'shun) *n.* 1. The act of fixing, establishing firmly, or making permanent. 2. *In surgery,* the immobilization of a part, as of a floating kidney by operative means or of a fractured bone by the use of a metal nail. 3. The intent focusing of the eyes upon an object. See also *fix (3).* 4. *In psychology,* the strengthening of a learned tendency or habit formation; especially, the establishment of a strong or excessive attachment for a person, object, or way of doing something. See also *compulsion, obsession.* 5. *In psychiatry,* the arrest of personality development or of psychosexual maturation at a certain stage. 6. *In microscopy,* the process of preservation of tissue elements in form, position, and reactivity by means of chemical or physical hardening or coagulating agents.

fixation abscess. An abscess produced by the injection of a chemical irritant, in order to attract and hold bacteria in adjacent inflammatory foci.

fixation muscle. A muscle that holds a part from moving to allow more accurate control of a distal part, as a muscle that holds the wrist steady to allow more precise control of finger movement.

fixation of complement. COMPLEMENT FIXATION.

fixation point. The point of sharpest vision in the retina; the point where the visual axis meets the retina.

fixation reflex. A reflex in response to a light stimulus falling on the periphery of the retina which adjusts the movements of each eye so that the image will fall on either fovea.

fixation surface. A curved surface the points of which occupy, in the two monocular fields, positions which are identical horizontally, regardless of vertical disparity.

fix·a·tive (fick'suh·tiv) *n.* 1. *In microscopy,* any substance used to fasten a section on a slide. 2. Any substance used to preserve tissues for microscopic study.

fixed, *adj.* 1. *In clinical medicine,* characterizing a persistent, nongrowing lesion, or one recurring frequently at the same site. 2. *In dermatology,* characterizing a drug eruption that recurs in the same site over and over again upon reexhibition of the causative drug.

fixed alkali. Any metallic hydroxide.

fixed cell. A reticular cell attached to the reticular fibers in reticuloendothelium.

fixed electrode. INDIRECT LEAD.

fixed idea. 1. A delusional idea which the patient refuses to relinquish even after its disproof. 2. Any compulsive drive or obsessive idea.

fixed macrophage. A scavenger cell with the capacity to ingest particulate matter, as found in loose connective tissue fixed to reticular fibers, or lining the sinuses in the liver, spleen, bone marrow, or lymph nodes.

fixed oil. Oil obtained from a vegetable or animal source, consisting chiefly of glyceryl esters of various fatty acids, and containing a higher proportion of esters of unsaturated acids than do fats.

fixed rabies virus. A rabies virus that is injected into rabbits and passed from one animal to another until it acquires a shorter and more constant incubation period than the naturally occurring virus; used in the Pasteur-type vaccines. See also *rabies vaccine, street rabies virus.*

fixed spasm. Permanent or continuous tetanic rigidity of one or more muscles.

fix·ing, *n.* FIXATION (6).

fixing eye. In strabismus, the eye which is directed toward the visual object.

fixing fluid. FIXATIVE.

F.K.Q.C.P. Fellow of the King and Queen's College of Physicians (of Ireland).

fl. Abbreviation for *fluid.*

flac·cid (flack'sid) *adj.* [L. *flaccus,* flabby]. Soft; flabby; relaxed. —**flac·cid·i·ty** (flack·sid'i·tee) *n.*

flaccid neurogenic bladder. MOTOR PARALYTIC BLADDER.

flaccid paralysis. Paralysis of the bladder due to interruption of peripheral motor or sensory innervation of detrusor muscles. See also *lower motor neuron paralysis, motor paralytic bladder.*

flaccid paraplegia. Paralysis of both legs with muscular hypotonia and diminished or absent tendon reflexes.

flaccid talipes. A foot in which there is a complete flaccid paralysis. See also *foot drop.*

Flack's node [M. W. *Flack,* English physiologist, 1882–1931]. SINOATRIAL NODE.

flag, *n.* Any one of several monocotyledonous plants having long ensiform leaves.

flagella. Plural of *flagellum.*

flag·el·lant (flaj'e·lunt) *n.* A person practicing flagellation.

flag·el·lant·ism (flaj'e·lun·tiz·um) *n.* The masochistic or sadistic need for flagellation.

fla·gel·lar (fla·jel'ur) *adj.* Pertaining to a flagellum.

flagellar agglutinin. An agglutinin active against antigens in the flagella of microorganisms. Syn. *H agglutinin.*

flagellar antigen. The antigenic component or components of flagella.

Flag·el·la·ta (flaj''e·lay'tuh) *n. pl.* MASTIGOPHORA.

[1]**flag·el·late** (flaj'e·late) *v.* To practice or indulge in flagellation.

[2]**flag·el·late** (flaj'e·lut, ·late) *n.* A protozoon with slender, whiplike processes.

flag·el·lat·ed (flaj'e·lay·tid) *adj.* Having a flagellum.

flag·el·la·tion (flaj''e·lay'shun) *n.* [L. *flagellatio,* from *flagellare,* to whip]. 1. Flogging or beating, especially as a means of producing erotic or religiously oriented stimulation or gratification. 2. Massage by strokes or blows. 3. By extension, stabbing or cutting with a knife. 4. Having flagella; the pattern of flagella.

fla·gel·li·form (fla·jel'i·form) *adj.* Having the form of a flagellum or whiplash.

fla·gel·lin (fla·jel'in) *n.* A soluble protein that can aggregate to form flagella of bacteria. Different flagellins exist in different strains or species of bacteria.

flag·el·lo·ma·nia (flaj''e·lo·may'nee·uh) *n.* Erotic excitement from flagellation.

flag·el·lo·sis (flaj''e·lo'sis) *n.,* pl. **flagello·ses** (·seez) [*flagell*ate + *-osis*]. Infection with flagellate protozoa.

fla·gel·lum (fla·jel'um) *n.,* pl. **flagel·la** (·luh) [L., whip]. A whiplike process consisting of an axial filament enclosed in thin cytoplasmic sheath; the organ of locomotion of sperm cells, and of certain bacteria and protozoa.

Flagyl. Trademark for metronidazole, a systemic trichomonacide.

flail, *adj.* Abnormally mobile or active; lacking normal control; flaccid.

flail chest. A condition in which there are multiple rib fractures, with or without fracture of the sternum, allowing the occurrence of paradoxic motion of the chest wall and the attendant physiologic disturbances; "stove-in chest."

flail joint. A condition of excessive mobility often following resection of a joint or paralysis.

Fla·ja·ni's disease (fla·yah'nee) [G. *Flajani,* Italian surgeon, 1741–1808]. HYPERTHYROIDISM.

flame photometer. An instrument for the quantitative determination of sodium, potassium, and sometimes other elements, especially in biological fluids. A sample when sprayed into a flame emits light which is resolved into its spectrum; a photoelectric cell measures the intensity of light of the wavelength corresponding to the particular element for which the analysis is made.

flame photometry. The measurement, for the purpose of quantitative analysis, of the intensity of the emission spectra of a metallic element vaporized in a very hot flame.

flame spectrophotometer. FLAME PHOTOMETER.

flam·ma·ble (flam'uh·bul) *adj.* INFLAMMABLE.

flange (flanj) *n.* DENTURE FLANGE.

flank, *n.* [OF. *flanc*]. The fleshy or muscular part of an animal or a man between the ribs and the hip. NA *latus.*

flap, *n.* A partially detached portion of skin or other tissue, either accidentally formed, or created by a surgeon to be used as a graft to fill a defect or to improve contour. Flaps that are composed of special tissue, such as mucous membrane, conjunctiva, dura, wall of intestinal tract, omentum, or muscle are named after the tissue contained, as muscle flap. They may also be named according to the special purpose for which they are used, as a rhinoplastic flap for repair of the nose. See also *graft.*

flapping tremor. ASTERIXIS.

flaps, *n.* Swelling of the lips in horses.

flare, *n.* 1. A vasomotor reaction manifested by a prolonged, widespreading flush of the skin after a pointed instrument has been drawn heavily across it. 2. An area of redness spreading outward from an infected area or lesion that extends beyond the locus of reaction to the irritating stimulus. 3. A widening or extension of a part, as of a bone.

flash burn. A superficial but often extensive burn produced by intense heat of very brief duration, as that of explosions. Syn. *powder burn.*

flash·eye, *n.* ELECTRIC OPHTHALMIA.

flash method. A method of pasteurizing milk by heating it to 178°F and then chilling it promptly.

flash point. The lowest temperature at which vapor of a combustible liquid may be ignited.

flask, *n.* [OF. *flasque,* from L. *flasco,* bottle]. 1. A glass, plastic, or metal vessel having a narrow neck. 2. A sectional metal case in which a sectional mold is made of plaster of paris or artificial stone for the processing of artificial dentures or other resinous dental restorations.

flat, *adj.* 1. Lying in one plane. 2. Having a smooth or even surface. 3. Of a percussion note or a voice sound, lacking in resonance. —**flat·ness,** *n.*

Fla·tau-Schil·der disease (flah'taow) [E. *Flatau,* Polish neurologist, 1869–1932; and P. F. *Schilder*]. SCHILDER'S DISEASE (1).

Flatau's law [E. *Flatau*]. The greater the length of the nerve tracts of the spinal cord, the nearer they are to the periphery of the cord.

flat bone. A bone more or less in the form of a plate, as the parietal bone. NA *os planum.*

flat ear. A large, prominent ear, characterized by inconspicuous ridges and grooves.

flat film. A plain radiograph of the abdomen made with the patient in the supine position. See also *KUB.*

flat·foot, *n.* A depression of the plantar arch of varying degree, which may be congenital or acquired; PES PLANUS.

flat pelvis. Deformity of the pelvis in which all anteroposterior diameters are shortened but the transverse diameters are practically normal.

flat plate. FLAT FILM.

flat·sedge, *n.* A genus of plants of the family Cyperaceae. The root of the jointed flatsedge, *Cyperus articulatus,* has been used as an anthelmintic, aromatic, and stomachic.

flat·u·lence (flatch′oo·lunce) *n.* [F., from L. *flatus*, blowing]. The presence or sensation of excessive gas in the stomach and intestinal tract. —**flatu·lent** (·lunt) *adj.*

flatulent dyspepsia. Dyspepsia marked by a sensation of abdominal fullness. There may be excessive eructation of gas. Syn. *gaseous dyspepsia.*

fla·tus (flay′tus) *n.* [L., a blowing, from *flare*, to blow]. 1. Gas, especially gas or air in the gastrointestinal tract. 2. Air or gas expelled via any body orifice.

flatus va·gi·na·lis (vaj·i·nay′lis). Expulsion of gas from the vagina.

flat·worm, *n.* Any worm of the phylum Platyhelminthes.

flav-, flavo- [L. *flavus*]. A combining form meaning (a) *yellow;* (b) *a series of complex yellow salts of cobalt.*

fla·va·nol (flay′vuh·nol, flav′uh·) *n.* FLAVONOL.

Flavaxin. A trademark for synthetic riboflavin.

fla·ve·do (fla·vee′do) *n.* [NL., from L. *flavus*, yellow]. Yellowness or sallowness, usually referring to the skin.

fla·vi·an·ic acid (flay″vee·an′ick, flav″ee·). 2,4-Dinitro-1-naphthol-7-sulfonic acid, $C_{10}H_{12}N_2O_{11}S$, light-yellow needles, freely soluble in water; employed as a precipitant for arginine and histidine; its salts are used as dyes.

fla·vin (flay′vin, flav′in) *n.* 1. One of a group of yellow pigments, derived from isoalloxazine, isolated from various plant and animal sources. 2. QUERCITRIN.

flavin adenine dinucleotide. $C_{27}H_{33}N_9O_{15}P_2$; a compound resulting from the condensation of a molecule each of riboflavin 5′-phosphate (flavin mononucleotide) and adenosine 5′-phosphate (adenine nucleotide), linkage being effected through the respective phosphoric acid residues. It is the prosthetic group of a number of flavoproteins, including D-amino acid oxidase. Abbreviated, FAD. Syn. *isoalloxazine adenine dinucleotide, riboflavin adenine dinucleotide.*

fla·vine (flay′veen, flav′een) *n.* 1. FLAVIN. 2. ACRIFLAVINE.

flavin mononucleotide. RIBOFLAVIN 5′-PHOSPHATE. Abbreviated, FMN.

flavin phosphate. RIBOFLAVIN 5′-PHOSPHATE. Abbreviated, FP.

flavo-. See *flav-.*

Fla·vo·bac·te·ri·um (flay″vo·back·teer′ee·um) *n.* [*flavo-* + *bacterium*]. A genus of the Achromobacteriaceae consisting of gram-negative rod-shaped bacteria characteristically producing yellow-orange, red, or yellow-brown pigments on media. Commonly proteolytic, they occur widely in water and soil, and are rarely pathogenic.

fla·vo·ki·nase (flay″vo·kigh′nace, ·kin′ace, ·aze, flav″o·) *n.* An enzyme, obtained from yeast, that catalyzes the phosphorylation of riboflavin to riboflavin 5′-phosphate by adenosine triphosphate.

fla·vone (flay′vone, flav′ohn) *n.* 1. 2-Phenyl-1,4-benzopyrone, $C_{15}H_{10}O_2$. 2. One of the yellow vegetable dye derivatives of flavone (1).

fla·vo·noid (flay′vuh·noid, flav′uh·) *n.* & *adj.* 1. A substance obtained from flavone (1), or one of its derivatives. 2. Any of the flavone derivatives, including citrin, hesperetin, hesperidin, rutin, quercetin, and quercitrin, which may reduce capillary fragility in certain cases. 3. Pertaining to or like a flavonoid.

fla·vo·nol (flay′vo·nol, flav′o·) *n.* 1. 3-Hydroxyflavone, $C_{15}H_{10}O_3$. 2. One of a group of vegetable dyes, including the anthocyanins, derived from flavonol (1).

fla·vo·none (flay′vuh·nohn, flav′uh·) *n.* 2,3-Dihydroflavone, $C_{15}H_{12}O_2$, derivatives of which include hesperetin and citrin.

fla·vo·pro·tein (flay″vo·pro′teen, ·tee·in, flav″o·) *n.* One of a group of conjugated proteins of the chromoprotein type which constitute the yellow enzymes. The prosthetic group in the known enzymes of this type is either a phosphoric acid ester of riboflavin or the latter combined with adenylic acid.

fla·vo·xan·thin (flay″vo·zan′thin, flav″o·) *n.* A carotenoid pigment, $C_{40}H_{56}O_3$, often found in plants in minute amounts; it has no vitamin A activity.

fla·vox·ate (flay·vock′sate) *n.* β-Piperidinoethyl 3-methylflavone-8-carboxylate, $C_{24}H_{25}NO_4$, a urinary antispasmodic; used as the hydrochloride salt.

flax-dresser's phthisis. A pneumoconiosis resulting from inhalation of particles of flax.

Flaxedil Triethiodide. Trademark for gallamine triethiodide, a curarimimetic drug employed as a skeletal muscle relaxant.

flax·seed, *n.* LINSEED.

flaxseed oil. LINSEED OIL.

fla·za·lone (flay′zuh·lone) *n.* *p*-Fluorophenyl 4-(*p*-fluorophenyl)-4-hydroxy-1-methyl-3-piperidyl ketone, $C_{19}H_{19}F_2NO_3$, an anti-inflammatory.

flea, *n.* Any bloodsucking, laterally compressed, wingless insect of the order Siphonaptera. Fleas are of medical importance as hosts and transmitters of disease, and their bites produce a form of dermatitis.

flea·bane, *n.* ERIGERON.

flea-borne typhus. MURINE TYPHUS.

Flech·sig's tract (fleck′sikh) [P. E. *Flechsig*, German neurologist, 1847–1929]. The posterior, or dorsal, spinocerebellar tract.

flecked spleen. A spleen containing multiple areas of nonembolic necrosis.

fleck·fie·ber (fleck′fee″bur) *n.* [Ger., spotted fever]. EPIDEMIC TYPHUS.

fleck·milz of Fei·tis (fleck′milts, figh′tis) [Ger.]. FLECKED SPLEEN.

Fleck's test. LEUKERGY TEST.

fleck typhus. EPIDEMIC TYPHUS.

Fleischer-Kayser ring [R. *Fleischer*, German physician, 1848–1909; and B. *Kayser*]. KAYSER-FLEISCHER RING.

flesh, *n.* The soft tissues of the body, especially the muscles. —**fleshy** (flesh′ee) *adj.*

flesh fly. One of the Sarcophagidae.

fleshy mole. 1. A blood mole that has become more solid and has assumed a fleshy appearance. 2. The more or less amorphous remains of a dead fetus in the uterine cavity.

Fletch·er factor. A coagulation factor found in normal plasma which will correct the clotting defect of patients with Fletcher trait.

Fletcher medium. A nutrient agar and rabbit serum used for the culture of *Leptospira.*

Fletcher trait [*Fletcher*, the family in which the trait was discovered]. A coagulation defect found in four siblings of consanguineous parents, characterized by a prolonged partial thromboplastin time despite apparently normal amounts of the factors thought responsible for fibrin formation.

fleu·rette (flur·et′) *n.* [F., dim. of *fleur*, flower]. An arrangement of cells in a retinoblastoma which resembles a fleur-de-lis; considered to represent an aborted process of differentiation into a photoreceptor.

flex, *v.* [L. *flectere, flexus*]. To bend.

flex·i·bil·i·tas ce·rea (fleck″si·bil′i·tas seer′ee·uh) [L.]. WAXY FLEXIBILITY.

flex·i·ble, *adj.* [L. *flexibilis*]. Capable of being bent, without breaking; pliable. —**flex·i·bil·i·ty** (fleck″si·bil′i·tee) *n.*

flexible collodion. Collodion with the addition of castor oil and camphor.

flex·ile (fleck′sil) *adj.* [L. *flexilis*, pliant]. FLEXIBLE.

flex·im·e·ter (fleck·sim′e·tur) *n.* [*flexion* + *-meter*]. An instrument for measuring the amount of flexion possible in a joint.

flex·ion (fleck′shun) *n.* [L. *flexio*, a bending]. 1. The bending of a joint, or of parts having joints. 2. The condition of being bent.

flexion reflex. Flexion or withdrawal of a limb in response to a noxious stimulus.

flexion vertebrae. All the vertebrae except the first two cervical vertebrae.

Flex·ner-Job·ling carcinosarcoma [S. *Flexner,* U.S. pathologist and bacteriologist, 1863–1946; and J. W. *Jobling,* U.S. physician, b. 1876]. A transplantable malignant tumor that arose spontaneously in an albino stock rat, growing in both carcinomatous and sarcomatous fashion.

Flex·ner report [A. *Flexner,* U.S. educator, 1866–1959]. A 1910 study of the 155 medical institutions then existing, made for the Carnegie Foundation for the Advancement of Teaching, and published under the title *Medical Education in the United States and Canada.* It became a basic document in the reform and standardization of medical education and statutory requirements for physicians in these two countries.

Flexner's bacillus [S. *Flexner*]. *Shigella flexneri.* See *Shigella.*

flex·or (fleck'sur, ·sor) *n.* A muscle that bends or flexes a limb or a part. Compare *extensor.* See also Table of Muscles in the Appendix.

flexor ac·ces·so·ri·us (ack"se·so'ree·us). QUADRATUS PLANTAE MUSCLE.

flexor car·pi ra·di·a·lis (kahr'pye ray"dee·ay'lis). The radial flexor of the wrist. NA *musculus flexor carpi radialis.* See also Table of Muscles in the Appendix.

flexor carpi radialis bre·vis (brev'is). An anomalous muscle arising from the lateral or palmar surface of the distal half of the radius and inserted into the carpus, metacarpus, or proximal phalanx of the index finger.

flexor carpi ul·na·ris (ul·nair'is). The ulnar flexor of the wrist. NA *musculus flexor carpi ulnaris.* See Table of Muscles in the Appendix.

flexor carpi ulnaris bre·vis (brev'is). An anomalous muscle arising from the distal fourth of the palmar surface of the ulna and inserted into the ulnar carpals or proximal end of fifth metacarpal. See also Table of Muscles in the Appendix.

flexor di·gi·ti mi·ni·mi bre·vis (dij'i·tye min'i·migh brev'is). The short flexor of the little finger or of the little toe. NA *musculus flexor digiti minimi brevis.* See Table of Muscles in the Appendix.

flexor digiti quin·ti bre·vis (kwin'tye brev'is). FLEXOR DIGITI MINIMI BREVIS.

flexor di·gi·to·rum ac·ces·so·ri·us (dij·i·to'rum ack"se·so'ree·us). QUADRATUS PLANTAE.

flexor digitorum bre·vis (brev'is). The short flexor of the toes. NA *musculus flexor digitorum brevis.* See Table of Muscles in the Appendix.

flexor digitorum lon·gus (long'gus). The long flexor of the toes. NA *musculus flexor digitorum longus.* See Table of Muscles in the Appendix.

flexor digitorum pro·fun·dus (pro·fun'dus). The deeper long flexor of the fingers. NA *musculus flexor digitorum profundus.* See Table of Muscles in the Appendix.

flexor digitorum sub·li·mis (sub·lye'mis). FLEXOR DIGITORUM SUPERFICIALIS.

flexor digitorum su·per·fi·ci·a·lis (sue"pur·fish·ee·ay'lis). The more superficial long flexor of the fingers. NA *musculus flexor digitorum superficialis.* See Table of Muscles in the Appendix.

flexor hal·lu·cis bre·vis (hal'yoo·sis brev'is). The short flexor of the great toe. NA *musculus flexor hallucis brevis.* See Table of Muscles in the Appendix.

flexor hallucis lon·gus (long'gus). The long flexor of the great toe. NA *musculus flexor hallucis longus.* See Table of Muscles in the Appendix.

flexor os·sis me·ta·car·pi pol·li·cis (os'is met"uh·kahr'pye pol'i·sis). OPPONENS POLLICIS.

flexor pollicis bre·vis (brev'is). The short flexor of the thumb. NA *musculus flexor pollicis brevis.* See Table of Muscles in the Appendix.

flexor pollicis lon·gus (long'gus). The long flexor of the thumb. NA *musculus flexor pollicis longus.* See Table of Muscles in the Appendix.

flexor retinaculum. A thickening of deep fascia overlying tendons of flexor muscles. See also *flexor retinaculum of the ankle, flexor retinaculum of the wrist.*

flexor retinaculum of the ankle. A fibrous band of fascia attached to the medial malleolus and the calcaneus. It binds down the tendons of the tibialis posterior and of the long flexors of the toes. NA *retinaculum musculorum flexorum pedis.*

flexor retinaculum of the wrist. A thickened band of deep fascia attached laterally to the scaphoid and trapezium and medially to the pisiform and hamate bones, binding down the tendons of the long flexor of the thumb and of the long flexors of the fingers and completing the carpal canal. Syn. *transverse carpal ligament, transverse ligament of the wrist.* NA *retinaculum flexorum manus.*

flex·u·ous (fleck'shoo·us, flecks'yoo·us) *adj.* [L. *flexuosus,* full of turns]. Curving in an undulating manner.

flex·u·ra (fleck·shoor'uh, ·syoor'uh) *n.,* pl. & genit. sing. **flexu·rae** (·ree) [L.]. FLEXURE.

flexura co·li dex·tra (ko'lye decks'truh) [NA]. HEPATIC FLEXURE.

flexura coli si·nis·tra (si·nis'truh) [NA]. SPLENIC FLEXURE.

flexura du·o·de·ni inferior (dew·o·dee'nigh) [NA]. The bend in the duodenum at the junction of the descending and horizontal parts.

flexura duodeni superior [NA]. The bend in the first part of the duodenum where the descending part begins.

flexura du·o·de·no·je·ju·na·lis (dew·o·dee"no·jee"joo·nay'lis) [NA]. DUODENOJEJUNAL FLEXURE.

flexural dermatitis. Atopic dermatitis seen primarily in infants and children on the face, anterior neck, antecubital and popliteal spaces, and other flexural areas.

flexura pe·ri·ne·a·lis rec·ti (perr·i·nee·ay'lis reck'tye) [NA]. PERINEAL FLEXURE.

flexura sa·cra·lis rec·ti (sa·kray'lis reck'tye) [NA]. SACRAL FLEXURE.

flex·ure (fleck'shur) *n.* [L. *flexura,* a bending]. A bend or fold. —**flexur·al** (·ul) *adj.*

flick·er, *n.* A sensation of fluctuating vision, caused by a light of such slow intermittence that the visual impressions produced do not fuse.

flicker fusion test. An application of the flicker fusion threshold in a test for fatigue and for tolerance to hypoxia; formerly used in the evaluation of hypertension and angina pectoris.

flicker fusion threshold. The minimal frequency of standard flashes of light that will be seen as steady illumination. See also *flicker fusion test.*

flight of ideas. The rapid skipping from one idea to another, even before the last one is thought through, the ideas bearing only a superficial relation to one another and often associated by chance; seen in the manic phase of manic depressive illness or in schizophrenia.

flight-or-fight reaction. FIGHT-OR-FLIGHT REACTION.

Flindt's spots [N. *Flindt,* Danish physician, 1843–1913]. KOPLIK'S SPOTS.

flint disease. 1. CHALICOSIS. 2. Occasionally, silicosis.

flint glass. Glass composed of lead and potassium silicates.

Flint's murmur. AUSTIN FLINT MURMUR.

floatation method. FLOTATION METHOD.

float·ers, *n.* Floating specks in the field of vision, due to opacities in the media of the eye. Syn. *muscae volitantes, mouches volantes.*

float·ing, *adj.* 1. Free or partly free from firm attachment, as a floating rib. 2. Abnormally movable, as a floating kidney. 3. Buoyed up freely, as in a fluid.

floating beta disorder. *Informal.* FAMILIAL HYPERBETALIPOPROTEINEMIA AND HYPERPREBETAPROTEINEMIA.

floating cartilage. A detached segment of cartilage in a joint cavity.

floating head. A freely movable fetal head above the pelvic brim.

floating kidney. A kidney that is displaced from its bed, becoming more freely movable, sometimes causing symptoms, as by kinking the ureter. Syn. *wandering kidney, ren mobilis.*

floating rib. One of the last two ribs which have the anterior end free.

floating spleen. An abnormally movable and perhaps displaced spleen. Syn. *wandering spleen.*

floc·cil·la·tion (flock″si·lay′shun) *n.* [L. *floccus,* flock, tuft]. CARPHOLOGY.

floc·cu·lar (flock′yoo·lur) *adj.* 1. Of or pertaining to the flocculus. 2. Tuftlike.

floccular lobule. One of the paired, small lobules on the inferior surface of the cerebellar hemisphere forming part of the flocculonodular lobe.

floc·cu·la·tion (flock″yoo·lay′shun) *n.* [L. *floccus,* a flock of wool]. The coagulation or coalescence of finely divided or colloidal particles into larger particles which precipitate. —**floc·cu·late** (flock′yoo·late) *v. & n.*

flocculation test. A test in which the antibody reacts directly with the soluble antigen to produce flocculent, as in toxin-antitoxin reactions.

floc·cu·lent (flock′yoo·lunt) *adj. & n.* [L. *flocculus,* dim. of *floccus,* flock, tuft]. 1. Flaky, downy, or woolly, said of such particles in a liquid medium. 2. Causing flocculation. 3. A substance which causes flocculation.

flocculi. Plural of *flocculus.*

floc·cu·lo·nod·u·lar (flock″yoo·lo·nod′yoo·lur) *adj.* Pertaining to the flocculus and nodulus of the cerebellum.

flocculonodular lobe. The part of the cerebellum consisting of the nodule of the vermis and the paired lateral flocculi.

flocculonodular syndrome. A disturbance of equilibrium of the body with sparing of individual movements of the limbs.

floc·cu·lus (flock′yoo·lus) *n.*, pl. **floccu·li** (·lye) [L., a small tuft] [NA]. FLOCCULAR LOBULE. See also Plates 17, 18.

flocculus se·con·da·rii (seck·un·dair′ee·eye) [BNA]. A small lobe occasionally present near the flocculus.

flood fever. TSUTSUGAMUSHI DISEASE.

floor, *n.* The lower inside surface of a hollow organ or open space.

floor of the pelvis. The united mass of tissue forming the inferior boundary of the pelvis, consisting mainly of the muscles of the pelvic diaphragm.

floor plate. The ventral wall of the embryonic neural tube, ependymal in structure.

floppy-infant syndrome. The constellation in infancy of marked deficiency in tone and muscular activity, and usually also delay in motor development; may be due to any of several systemic, neurologic, muscular, and connective-tissue disorders. Syn. *infantile hypotonia.*

flo·ra (flo′ruh) *n.*, pl. **floras, flo·rae** (·ree) [L. *Flora,* goddess of flowers]. 1. The entire plant life of any geographic area or geologic period. 2. The entire bacterial and fungal life normally inhabiting an area of the body, as: intestinal flora, vaginal flora.

flor·an·ty·rone (flor·an′ti·rone) *n.* γ-Oxo-γ-(8-fluoranthene)-butyric acid, $C_{20}H_{14}O_3$, a hydrocholeretic drug.

Floraquin. Trademark for a preparation of diodoquin (diiodohydroxyquin), lactose, dextrose, and boric acid used in the treatment of vaginal infections.

Flor·ence flask. A balloon-shaped flask with a flat bottom used in distillation and other laboratory procedures.

Flo·rence's test (flohⁿ·rahⁿs′) [A. *Florence,* French pharmacologist, 1851–1927]. A test for the presence of semen in which a substance treated with a strong solution of iodine and potassium iodide yields brown crystals in the shape of needles or plates.

flo·res (flor′eez) *n.pl.* [L., plural of *flos,* flower]. 1. The flowers or blossoms of a plant. 2. A flocculent or pulverulent form of certain substances after sublimation.

Flor·ey unit [H. E. *Florey,* English pathologist, 1898–1968]. OXFORD UNIT.

flor·id (flor′id) *adj.* [L. *floridus,* abounding with flowers]. 1. Bright red. 2. Fully developed; manifesting a completely developed clinical syndrome.

florid phthisis. GALLOPING CONSUMPTION.

flo·ri·form cataract (flor′i·form). A rare congenital cataract in which the opacities are arranged like the petals of a flower, commonly in the axial portions of the lens; inherited usually as a dominant and possibly related to the coralliform cataract.

Florinef Acetate. A trademark for fludrocortisone acetate, a synthetic glucocorticoid.

Florone. A trademark for diflorasone diacetate, an anti-inflammatory.

Floropryl. Trademark for diisopropyl fluorophosphate or isoflurophate, a cholinesterase inhibitor.

flo·ta·tion, *n.* The process of separating the valuable constituents (minerals) of ores from the valueless gangue by agitation with water, a small proportion of an oil, and a foaming agent, the mineral rising with the foam and the gangue sinking.

flotation method. A technique employed for separating ova and larvae from stool specimens. The stool is put into a salt solution where it sinks while the ova and larvae, due to their lower specific gravity, rise to the surface.

flotation unit. SVEDBERG FLOTATION UNIT.

flow, *v. & n.* 1. To move freely like liquid or particulate matter. 2. A quantity that flows within a set amount of time, as liquid through an organ. 3. To menstruate. 4. MENSTRUATION.

flow birefringence. Birefringence exhibited by solutions containing long, thin, assymetrical molecules, which are randomly oriented when the solution is at rest but which orient themselves in the direction of flow when the solution is forced through a capillary tube.

flower basket of Boch·da·lek (boᵏh′da·leck) [V. A. *Bochdalek*]. The tuft of the choroid plexus of the fourth ventricle which appears on the external surface of the brain at the outlets of the foramina of Luschka.

flow·ers, *n.pl.* [OF. *flor,* from L. *flos, floris,* flower]. A sublimed form of a substance.

Flower's index [W. H. *Flower,* British physician and anatomist, 1831–1899]. The number obtained by multiplying the dental length by 100 and then dividing by the length of the basinasal line.

flowers of Benjamin. Benzoin flowers; BENZOIC ACID.

flowers of sulfur. A form of sulfur that has been refined by sublimation; sublimed sulfur.

flow·me·ter, *n.* [*flow* + *-meter*]. 1. A physical device for measuring the rate of flow of a gas or liquid. 2. An apparatus for measuring flow characteristics of various substances.

flox·a·cil·lin (flock″suh·sil′in) *n.* 3-(2-Chloro-6-fluorophenyl)-5-methyl-4-isoxazolylpenicillin, $C_{19}H_{17}ClFN_3O_5S$, an antibacterial.

Floxapen. A trademark for floxacillin.

flox·uri·dine (flock·syoor′i·deen) *n.* 2′-Deoxy-5-fluorouridine, $C_9H_{11}FN_2O_5$, an antineoplastic and antiviral agent.

F.L.S. Fellow of the Linnean Society.

flu (floo) *n. Colloq.* INFLUENZA.

flu·aza·cort (floo·ay′zuh·kort) *n.* 5′*H*-Pregna-1,4-dieno[17,16-*d*]oxazole-3,20-dione, $C_{25}H_{30}FNO_6$, an anti-inflammatory.

flu·ban·il·ate (floo·ban′il·ate) *n.* Ethyl *N*-[2-(dimethylamino)-ethyl]-*m*-(trifluoromethyl)carbanilate, $C_{14}H_{19}F_3N_2O_2$, a central stimulant drug; used as the hydrochloride salt.

flu·ben·da·zole (floo·ben′duh·zole) *n.* Methyl 5-(*p*-fluorobenzoyl)-2-benzimidazolecarbamate, $C_{16}H_{12}FN_3O_3$, an antiprotozoal.

flu·clor·o·nide (floo·klor′o·nide) *n.* 9,11β-Dichloro-6α-fluoro-16α,17,21-trihydroxypregna-1,4-diene-3,20-dione 16,17 cyclic acetal with acetone, $C_{24}H_{29}Cl_2FO_5$, a glucocorticoid.

Flucloxacillin. A trademark for floxacillin.

flu·cry·late (floo'kri·late) *n.* 2,2,2-Trifluoro-1-methylethyl 2-cyanoacrylate, $C_7H_6F_3NO_2$, a tissue adhesive used in surgery.

fluc·tu·ance (fluck'tew·uns) *n.* The quality of fluctuation.

fluc·tu·a·tion (fluck"choo· ay'shun) *n.* [L. *fluctuare,* to wave]. 1. The wavelike motion produced by palpation or percussion of a body cavity when it contains fluid. 2. In an organism, a slight structural variation that is not inherited. 3. A recurrent, and often cyclic, alteration. 4. A variation about a fixed value or quantity.

flu·cy·to·sine (floo·sigh'to·seen) *n.* 5-Fluorocytosine, $C_4H_4FN_3O$, an antifungal.

flu·da·zo·ni·um chloride (floo·duh·zo'nee·um) *n.* 1-[2,4-Dichloro-β-[(2,4-dichlorobenzyl)oxy]-phenethyl]-3-(*p*-fluorophenacyl)imidazolium chloride, $C_{26}H_{20}Cl_5FN_2O_2$, an anti-infective.

flu·do·rex (floo'do·recks) *n.* β-Methoxy-*N*-methyl-*m*-(trifluoromethyl)phenethylamine, $C_{11}H_{14}F_3NO$, an anorexic and antiemetic drug.

flu·dro·cor·ti·sone acetate (floo"dro·kor'ti·sone). 9α-Fluoro-17-hydroxycorticosterone-21-acetate, $C_{23}H_{31}FO_6$, a fluorine derivative of hydrocortisone acetate with potent anti-inflammatory action.

fluent aphasia. Aphasia in which speech is effortless, well articulated with normal rhythm, but in which failure to use correct words results in circumlocution, substitution or paraphrasia, neologisms, and often lack of content; due to a lesion in either the temporal or parietal lobes. This form includes anomic aphasia, central (conduction) aphasia, and Wernicke's aphasia. Compare *nonfluent aphasia.*

flu·fen·am·ic acid (floo"fen·am'ick). *N*-(α,α,α-Trifluoro-*m*-tolyl)anthranilic acid, $C_{14}H_{10}F_3NO_2$, a compound with inflammation-counteracting activity.

flu·fen·i·sal (floo·fen'i·sal) *n.* 4'-Fluoro-4-hydroxy-3-biphenylcarboxylic acid acetate, $C_{15}H_{11}FO_4$, an analgesic.

Fluh·mann's test [C. F. *Fluhmann,* U.S. gynecologist, 1898–1966]. A test for determining blood estrogen level performed by injecting blood serum into spayed mice, and using the degree of histologic change in the vaginal epithelium as a guide.

flu·id, *adj.* & *n.* [L. *fluidus,* from *fluere,* to flow]. 1. Of substances: in a state in which the molecules move freely upon one another; flowing. 2. A fluid substance, such as any liquid secretion of the body. Abbreviated, fl.

fluid balance. A state of dynamic equilibrium in the body between the outgo and intake of water. Optimum water content is maintained by homeostatic physiologic mechanisms.

fluid equilibrium. FLUID BALANCE.

flu·id·ex·tract (floo"id·eck'strakt) *n.* [*fluid* + *extract*]. A hydroalcoholic solution of vegetable principles usually so made that each milliliter contains the therapeutic constituents of 1 g of the standardized drug which it represents. Maceration and percolation with suitable solvent are employed as the means of obtaining solution of the desired constituents. Sometimes spelled *fluid extract.* See also *extract, diacolation.*

fluid level. In *radiology,* the interface between gas and liquid or aqueous liquid and liquid fat shown on radiographs as a line when the x-ray beam parallels the interface; seen on films made with the patient in the erect or decubitus positions and using a horizontal x-ray beam. See also *air-fluid level.*

flu·id·ounce (floo"id·aownce') *n.* [*fluid* + *ounce*]. A liquid measure; 8 fluidrams. Equivalent to approximately 29.57 ml. Symbol, f℥. See also Table of Medical Signs and Symbols and Tables of Weights and Measures in the Appendix.

fluidrachm. FLUIDRAM.

flu·i·dram, flu·i·drachm (floo'i·dram") *n.* [*fluid* + *dram*]. A liquid measure equal to one-eighth fluidounce, roughly equivalent to one teaspoonful. 60 minims = 1 fluidram. Symbol, fʒ. See also *dram* (1). See also Table of Medical Signs and Symbols and Tables of Weights and Measures in the Appendix.

fluke, *n.* A trematode worm of the order Digenia.

flu·men (floo'min) *n.,* pl. **flu·mi·na** (·mi·nuh) [L.]. A stream.

flu·me·quine (floo'me·kwin) *n.* 9-Fluoro-6,7-dihydro-5-methyl-1-oxo-1*H*,5*H*-benzo[*ij*]quinolizine-2-carboxylic acid, $C_{14}H_{12}FNO_3$, an antibacterial.

flu·meth·a·sone (floo·meth'uh·sone) *n.* 6α,9α-Difluoro-11β,17,21-trihydroxy-16α-methylpregna-1,4-diene-3,20-dione, $C_{22}H_{28}F_2O_5$, a glucocorticoid.

flu·met·ra·mide (floo·met'ruh·mide) *n.* 6-(α,α,α-Trifluoro-*p*-tolyl)-3-morpholinone, $C_{11}H_{10}F_3NO_2$, a skeletal muscle relaxant.

flumina. Plural of *flumen.*

flumina pi·lo·rum (pi·lor'um) [NA]. Regional hair tracts. Certain areas of the skin have the hairs so arranged that they point in a common direction.

flu·min·o·rex (floo·min'o·recks) *n.* 2-Amino-5-(α,α,α-trifluoro-*p*-tolyl)-2-oxazoline, $C_{10}H_9F_3N_2O$, an anorexigenic drug.

flu·mi·zole (floo'mi·zole) *n.* 4,5-Bis(*p*-methoxyphenyl)-2-(trifluoromethyl)imidazole, $C_{18}H_{15}F_3N_2O_2$, an anti-inflammatory.

flu·nar·i·zine (floo·năr'i·zeen) *n.* (*E*)-1-[Bis(*p*-fluorophenyl)methyl]-4-cinnamylpiperazine, $C_{26}H_{26}F_2N_2$, a vasodilator used as the dihydrochloride salt.

flu·nid·a·zole (floo·nid'uh·zole) *n.* 2-(*p*-Fluorophenyl)-5-nitroimidazole-1-ethanol, $C_{11}H_{10}FN_3O_3$, an antiprotozoal drug.

flu·nis·o·lide (floo·nis'o·lide) *n.* 6α-Fluoro-11β,16α,17,21-tetrahydroxypregna-1,4-diene-3,20-dione cyclic acetal with acetone, $C_{24}H_{31}FO_6$, a glucocorticoid, also used as 21-acetate ester.

flu·ni·traz·e·pam (floo·nigh·traz'e·pam) *n.* 5-(o-Fluorophenyl)-1,3-dihydro-1-methyl-7-nitro-2*H*-1,4-benzodiazepin-2-one, $C_{16}H_{12}FN_3O_3$, a hypnotic.

flu·nix·in (floo·nick'sin) *n.* 2-[[2-Methyl-3-(trifluoromethyl)phenyl]-amino-3-pyridinecarboxylic acid, $C_{14}H_{11}F_3N_2O$, an analgesic anti-inflammatory; also used as the meglumine salt.

fluo-, fluor-, fluori-, fluoro-. A combining form meaning (a) *fluorine;* (b) *fluorescence, fluorescent.*

flu·o·cin·o·lide (floo"o·sin'o·lide) *n.* Former name for fluocinonide.

flu·o·cin·o·lone acet·o·nide (floo"o·sin'uh·lohn a·set'o·nide). 6α,9α-Difluoro-16α-hydroxyprednisolone-16,17-acetonide, $C_{24}H_{30}F_2O_6$, an anti-inflammatory glucocorticoid.

flu·o·cin·o·nide (floo"o·sin'o·nide) *n.* 6α,9-Difluoro-11β,16α,17,21-tetrahydroxypregna-1,4-diene-3,20-dione cyclic acetal with acetone, 21-acetate, $C_{26}H_{32}F_2O_7$, a glucocorticoid.

flu·o·cor·tin butyl (floo"o·kor'tin) *n.* Butyl 6α-fluoro-11β-hydroxy-16α-methyl-3,20-dioxopregna-1,4-diene-21-oate, $C_{26}H_{35}FO_5$, an anti-inflammatory.

flu·o·cor·to·lone (floo"o·kor'tuh·lone) *n.* 6α-Fluoro-11β,21-dihydroxy-16α-methylpregna-1,4-diene-3,20-dione, $C_{22}H_{29}FO_4$, a glucocorticoid.

Fluogen. A trademark for influenza virus vaccine.

Fluonid. A trademark for fluocinolone acetonide, a glucocorticoid.

fluor-. See *fluo-.*

flu·or·chrome (floo'ur·krome) *n.* A dye that fluoresces when irradiated with ultraviolet radiation.

flu·o·rene (floo'uh·reen) *n.* *o*-Biphenylenemethane, $C_{13}H_{10}$, cyclic hydrocarbon from coal tar, employed in the synthesis of several dyes and medicinals.

flu·o·res·ce·in (floo·uh·res'ee·in) *n.* A fluorescent dye, the simplest of the fluorine dyes and the mother substance of eosin, commonly used intravenously to determine the state and adequacy of circulation in the retina, optic nerve head, and to a lesser degree, the choroid and iris and to detect corneal and conjunctival epithelial lesions. Peak excitation occurs with light at a wavelength between 485 and 500 millimicrons, and peak emission occurs between 520 and 530 millimicrons. From 50 to 84 percent of the dye is bound to albumin in the blood.

fluorescein angioretinography. FLUORESCEIN FUNDUSCOPY AND ANGIOGRAPHY.

fluorescein fundus angiography or **photography.** FLUORESCEIN FUNDUSCOPY AND ANGIOGRAPHY.

fluorescein funduscopy and angiography. Observation, and usually photography, of the vascular pattern of the fundus of the eye by special techniques following the injection into a peripheral vein of fluorescein; used in the diagnosis of vascular and neoplastic lesions of the eye and changes of the optic disk.

flu·o·res·cence (floo″uh·res′unce) *n.* [*fluor-* + *-escence*]. A property possessed by certain substances of radiating, when illuminated, a light of a different, usually greater, wavelength. —**fluores·cent,** *adj.;* **flu·o·resce** (floo″uh·res′) *v.*

fluorescence microscope. A microscope equipped with a source of ultraviolet radiation for detection or examination of fluorescent specimens.

fluorescent radiation. Radiation that is emitted by fluorescent bodies.

fluorescent screen. A screen covered with substances which become fluorescent on exposure to rays, as x-rays, which are normally invisible to the eye.

fluorescent stain method. 1. A staining method using a fluorescent dye, such as the method for demonstrating *Mycobacterium tuberculosis* in smears using auramine O, and a fluorescence microscope. 2. Fluorescein labeling of antibodies for identifying and localizing the antigens.

fluorescent treponemal-antibody absorption test. A serologic test for syphilis utilizing *Treponema pallidum* and fluorescein-tagged antibodies, more sensitive than and as specific as the *T. pallidum* immobilization test.

flu·o·res·cin (floo″uh·res′in) *n.* A reduction product, $C_{20}H_{14}O_5$, of fluorescein which readily oxidizes to the latter, occurring as a bright yellow powder, insoluble in water but soluble in alkaline solutions; used as a reagent.

fluori-. See *fluo-*.

flu·o·ri·date (floo′ur·i·date) *v.* To add a fluoride compound to drinking water in such concentration that the incidence rate of caries will be diminished.

flu·o·ri·da·tion (floo″ur·i·day′shun) *n.* The addition of a fluoride to water, especially to the water supply of a community, as an aid in control of dental caries.

flu·o·ride (floo′ur·ide, ·id) *n.* A salt of hydrofluoric acid.

flu·o·ri·dize (floo′ur·i·dize) *v.* To use a fluoride, especially as a therapeutic measure for the prevention of dental caries. —**flu·o·ri·di·za·tion** (floo″ur·i·di·zay′shun) *n.*

flu·o·rim·e·ter (floo″uh·rim′e·tur) *n.* FLUOROMETER.

flu·o·rine (floo′ur·een, ·in) *n.* [NL. *fluor,* fluorite, from L., flow, flux, + *-ine*]. F = 18.9984. A gaseous element belonging to the halogen group. Certain of its salts, the fluorides, have been used in the treatment of goiter and in rheumatism. Fluorides have been shown to prevent dental caries, but in excessive amounts in drinking water they may cause mottling of tooth enamel. See also Table of Elements in the Appendix.

Fluoristan. A trademark for stannous fluoride, a dental caries prophylactic.

flu·o·rite (floo′ur·ite) *n.* Native calcium fluoride, CaF_2; used as a source of fluorine, as a flux, and in the manufacture of certain lenses.

fluoro-. See *fluo-*.

flu·o·ro·ace·tic acid (floo″ur·o·a·see′tick). FCH_2COOH; a crystalline substance, prepared synthetically but occurring in *Dichapetalum (Chailletia) cymosum,* a poisonous South American plant. It is highly poisonous; the sodium salt is used as a water-soluble rodenticide.

flu·o·ro·car·bon (floo″ur·o·kahr′bun) *n.* Any compound composed only of carbon and fluorine, representing a corresponding hydrocarbon in which the hydrogen atoms have been replaced by fluorine. Fluorocarbons are characterized by extreme resistance to chemical action and stability at high temperatures.

flu·o·ro·car·dio·gram (floo″ur·o·kahr′dee·o·gram) *n.* [*fluoro-* + *cardiogram*]. ORTHODIAGRAM.

flu·o·ro·car·dio·graph (floo″ur·o·kahr′dee·o·graf) *n.* [*fluoro-* + *cardiograph*]. ORTHODIAGRAPH.

flu·o·ro·car·di·og·ra·phy (floo″ur·o·kahr″dee·og′ruh·fee) *n.* [*fluoro-* + *cardiography*]. ORTHODIAGRAPHY.

flu·o·ro·chrome (floo′ur·o·krome) *n.* Any fluorescent substance, which may be a dye or an alkaloid, used in biological staining procedures to impart fluorescence to a tissue specimen.

flu·o·ro·cit·rate (floo″ur·o·sit′rate) *n.* A metabolic inhibitor of respiration which interferes with the aconitase reaction in the acid cycle; may be formed intracellularly from fluoroacetic acid.

flu·o·ro·gen (floo′ur·o·jen, floo·or′uh·jen) *n.* Any of the particular groups or arrangements of atoms the presence of which in a compound is essential for development of fluorescence.

flu·o·rog·ra·phy (floo″ur·og′ruh·fee) *n.* [*fluoro-* + *-graphy*]. A combination of fluoroscopy and photography whereby a photograph of small size is made of the fluoroscopic image; used for making large numbers of chest examinations for tuberculosis surveys. —**fluo·ro·graph·ic** (·o·graf′ick) *adj.*

Fluoromar. Trademark for fluroxene, a general anesthetic.

flu·o·rom·e·ter (floo″uh·rom′e·tur) *n.* [*fluoro-* + *-meter*]. An instrument that measures the intensity of fluorescence of substances in solution for the purpose of identification and/or quantitative analysis or that measures the fluorescence produced by x-rays or other radiations. —**fluo·ro·met·ric** (·ro·met′rick) *adj.;* **fluoromet·ri·cal·ly** (·ri·kuh·lee) *adv.*

flu·o·ro·meth·o·lone (floo″ur·o·meth′uh·lohn) *n.* 9-Fluoro-11β,17-dihydroxy-6α-methylpregna-1,4-diene-3,20-dione, $C_{22}H_{29}FO_4$, an anti-inflammatory glucocorticoid.

flu·o·ro·phos·phate (floo″ur·o·fos′fate) *n.* A salt or ester of a fluorophosphoric acid, especially monofluorophosphoric acid, H_2PO_3F.

flu·o·ro·pho·tom·e·try (floo″ur·o·fo·tom′e·tree) *n.* [*fluoro-* + *photometry*]. The quantitative assay of fluorescent substances in solution. The exciting radiation is concentrated upon the substance under investigation, and the intensity of fluorescence is compared, either visually or photoelectrically, against the fluorescence of a standard solution. —**fluoropho·to·met·ric** (·to·met′rick) *adj.*

flu·o·ro·roent·ge·nog·ra·phy (floo″ur·o·rent″ge·nog′ruh·fee) *n.* [*fluoro-* + *roentgenography*]. PHOTOFLUOROGRAPHY.

flu·o·ro·sal·an (floo″ur·o·sal′an) *n.* 3,5-Dibromo-3′-(trifluoromethyl)salicylanilide, $C_{14}H_8Br_2F_3NO_2$, a disinfectant.

flu·o·ro·scope (floo′ur·uh·skope) *n.* [*fluoro-* + *-scope*]. An instrument used for examining the form and motion of the internal structures of the body by means of roentgen rays. It consists of a fluorescent screen composed of fluorescent crystals and excited by x-rays. —**flu·o·ro·scop·ic** (floo″ur·uh·skop′ick) *adj.*

flu·o·ros·co·py (floo″ur·os′kuh·pee) *n.* [*fluoro-* + *-scopy*]. Examination of internal body structures by means of a fluoroscope.

flu·o·ro·sis (floo″ur·o′sis) *n.*, pl. **fluoro·ses** (·seez) [*fluor-* + *-osis*]. 1. Poisoning by absorption of toxic amounts of fluorine. 2. A condition of generalized increased density of the skeleton, resulting from prolonged ingestion of fluorides. In endemic areas, this may lead to rigidity of the spinal column, increased bone fragility, and other symptoms referable to bone and joint changes. See also *chronic dental fluorosis.*

flu·o·ro·ura·cil (floo″ur·o·yoo′ruh·sil) *n.* 5-Fluorouracil, $C_4H_3FN_2O_2$, an antineoplastic agent believed to function as an antimetabolite. Abbreviated, 5-FU.

Fluothane. Trademark for halothane, a general anesthetic.

flu·ox·e·tine (floo·ock′se·teen) *n.* (±)-*N*-Methyl-3-phenyl-3-[α,α,α-trifluoro-*p*-tolyl)oxypropylamine, $C_{17}H_{18}F_3NO$, an antidepressant.

flu·oxy·mes·ter·one (floo″ock·see·mes′tur·ohn) *n.* 9α-Fluoro-11β-hydroxy-17α-methyltestosterone, $C_{20}H_{29}FO_3$, an anabolic and androgenic steroid.

flu·per·a·mide (floo·perr′uh·mide) *n.* 4-(4-Chloro-α,α,α-trifluoro-*m*-tolyl)-4-hydroxy-*N,N*-dimethyl-α,α-diphenyl-1-piperidinebutyramide, $C_{30}H_{32}ClF_3N_2O_2$, an antiperistaltic.

flu·per·o·lone (floo·perr′uh·lone) *n.* 21-Methyl-9α-fluoroprednisolone, $C_{22}H_{29}FO_5$, an anti-inflammatory glucocorticoid; used as the acetate ester.

flu·phen·a·zine (floo·fen′uh·zeen) *n.* 10-[3-[4-(2-Hydroxyethyl)piperazinyl]propyl]-2-trifluoromethylphenothiazine, $C_{22}H_{26}F_3N_3OS$, a tranquilizing drug; used as the decanoate, enanthate, or hydrochloride salt.

flu·pred·nis·o·lone (floo″pred·nis′uh·lone) *n.* 6α-Fluoroprednisolone, $C_{21}H_{27}FO_5$, an anti-inflammatory glucocorticoid.

flu·pros·te·nol (floo·pros′te·nole) *n.* A prostaglandin derivative, used as the sodium salt, $C_{23}H_{28}F_3NaO_6$.

flur·an·dren·o·lide (floo″ran·dren′o·lide, ·dreen′) *n.* 6α-Fluoro-16α-hydroxyhydrocortisone-16,17-acetonide, $C_{24}H_{33}FO_6$, an anti-inflammatory glucocorticoid.

flur·az·e·pam (floo·raz′e·pam, ·ray′ze·) *n.* 7-Chloro-1-[2-(diethylamino)ethyl]-5-(*o*-fluorophenyl)-1,3-dihydro-2*H*-1,4-benzodiazepin-2-one, $C_{21}H_{23}ClFN_3O$, an hypnotic agent; used as the dihydrochloride salt.

flur·o·ges·tone (floo″ro·jes′tone) *n.* 9-Fluoro-11β,17-dihydroxypregn-4-ene-3,20-dione, $C_{21}H_{29}FO_4$, a progestational steroid; used as the 17-acetate ester.

flur·o·thyl (floo′ro·thil) *n.* Bis(2,2,2-trifluoroethyl) ether, $C_4H_4F_6O$, a colorless, volatile liquid; used as an inhalant convulsant in psychiatric therapy. Syn. *hexafluorodiethyl ether.*

flur·ox·ene (floo·rock′seen) *n.* 2,2,2-Trifluoroethyl vinyl ether, $C_4H_5F_3O$, a highly volatile, flammable liquid; employed as a general anesthetic.

Flury strain. A strain of rabies virus, used in the prophylactic immunization of dogs, that has been modified by prolonged cultivation in chick embryos.

flush, *n. & v.* 1. A sudden suffusion and reddening caused by cutaneous vasodilation, as of the face and neck; a blush. 2. A subjective transitory sensation of extreme heat; a hot flush. 3. A more or less persistent reddening of the face, as seen with fever, hyperthyroidism, certain drugs, or in emotional states. 4. To blush; to become suffused, as the cheeks, due to vasodilation of small arteries and arterioles. 5. To cleanse a wound or cavity by a rapid flow of water.

flu·spi·per·one (floo·spye′pur·ohn) *n.* 8-[3-(*p*-Fluorobenzoyl)-propyl]-1-(*p*-fluorophenyl)-1,3,8-triazaspiro[4.5]decan-4-one, $C_{23}H_{25}F_2N_3O_2$, a tranquilizer.

flu·spir·i·lene (floo·spirr′i·leen) *n.* 8-[4,4-Bis(*p*-fluorophenyl)-butyl]-1-phenyl-1,3,8-triazaspiro[4.5]decane-4-one, $C_{29}H_{31}F_2N_3O$, a tranquilizer.

flu·ti·a·zin (floo·tye′uh·zin) *n.* 8-(Trifluoromethyl)phenothiazine-1-carboxylic acid, $C_{14}H_8F_3NO_2S$, a veterinary anti-inflammatory.

flut·ter, *n.* Quick, irregular motion; agitation; tremulousness.

flutter waves. Regular, uniform electrocardiographic deflections due to atrial excitation in atrial flutter; occurring at a rate of about 300 to 350 per minute. Abbreviated, *F waves.* Compare *fibrillation waves.*

flux, *n.* [L. *fluxus,* from *fluere,* to flow]. 1. An excessive flow of any of the excretions of the body, especially the feces. 2. The rate of flow or transfer of a liquid, particles, or energy across a unit area. 3. *In chemistry,* material added to minerals or metals to promote fusion.

fly, *n.* Any of numerous insects of the order Diptera, especially those that are relatively large or thick-bodied. In compound names, also applied to certain non-dipteran flying insects, as caddis fly, ichneumon fly. Compare *midge, gnat, mosquito.*

fly agaric. A poisonous mushroom, *Amanita muscaria,* containing the alkaloid muscarine.

flying bedbug. ASSASSIN BUG.

flying blister. An application of a vesicant substance sufficient to produce erythema, but not a vesicle.

flying fatigue. A chronic psychosomatic disturbance developed by a flier after relatively long exposure to the stresses associated with flying, especially in combat flying.

Fm Symbol for fermium.

FMF Abbreviation for *familial Mediterranean fever.*

FMN Abbreviation for *flavin mononucleotide* (= RIBOFLAVIN 5′-PHOSPHATE).

Foà cell [P. *Foà,* Italian pathologist, 1848–1923]. FOÀ-KURLOV CELL.

Foà-Kur·lov cell (fo·ah′, koor′luf) [P. *Foà* and M. G. *Kurlov*]. Spheroidal cytoplasmic inclusion bodies in the lymphocytes and monocytes of normal guinea pigs, increased after treatment with estrogen.

foam, *n.* A heterogeneous mixture of a gaseous phase, or finely divided gas bubbles, suspended in a liquid. —**foamy** (fo′mee) *adj.*

foam cell. A cell containing lipids in small vacuoles, as seen in leprosy and xanthoma, often a histiocyte but may be some other cell, for example smooth muscle.

foam tablet. A contraceptive tablet containing a spermatocide and a foaming agent, to be inserted in the vagina.

foamy liver. A liver containing many gas-filled spaces which give the organ a spongy appearance and consistency; due to growth of gas-producing anaerobic bacteria, especially *Clostridium perfringens.*

fo·cal, *adj.* 1. Of, pertaining to, or possessing a focus. 2. Limited to one area or part of an organ or of the body; localized.

focal depth. The power of a lens to give clear images of objects at different distances from it.

focal dermal hypoplasia syndrome. A congenital disorder characterized by widespread, usually linear, areas of underdevelopment of the dermis, leading to the appearance of depressed streaks and outpouchings of subcutaneous fat, and associated with diverse osseous, cardiovascular, ocular, dental, and central nervous system defects; observed predominantly in girls since it may be lethal in the male fetus. Syn. *Goltz syndrome, hypoplasia cutis congenita.*

focal distance. The distance between the center of a lens and its focus.

focal embolic glomerulonephritis. The renal lesion seen in subacute bacterial endocarditis, of unknown cause, although allergic mechanisms, rather than embolization are thought responsible; the glomerular tufts are damaged and the kidney appears "flea-bitten." Infarcts may be present. Glomeruli show a lesion characteristic of focal glomerulonephritis. Deposits of IgG, IgM, and C3 within glomeruli have been described. Renal failure is uncommon.

focal epilepsy. Recurrent focal seizures.

focal glomerular hyalinosis or **sclerosis.** FOCAL SCLEROSING GLOMERULONEPHRITIS.

focal glomerulonephritis. A form of glomerulonephritis in which only some glomeruli, or parts thereof, demonstrate lesions.

focal illumination. Light concentrated upon an object by means of a lens or mirror.

focal infection. Infection in a limited area, such as the tonsils, teeth, sinuses, or prostate, to which remote clinical effects have been attributed, often erroneously.

focal interval. *In optics,* the distance between the anterior and posterior focal points.

fo·cal·ize, *v.* 1. To focus. 2. To limit an infection or disease to a particular area. —**fo·cal·iza·tion** (fo″kul·eye·zay·shun) *n.*

focal length. For a thin lens, the image distance of a point object on the lens axis at an infinite distance from the lens.

focal lesion. 1. A pathologic disturbance, such as a tumor, an infection, or an injury, in a well-defined and restricted area of tissue. 2. A circumscribed focus in the brain manifested by symptoms and signs that lead to a diagnosis of its location.

focal motor seizure. A focal seizure manifested by tonic or clonic movements in one part of the body, as in a hand, arm, face, or leg; may spread (Jacksonian march) to involve the rest of the body.

focal plane. The area perpendicular to the axis of a lens or lens system where an object forms its image.

focal point. FOCUS (2).

focal proliferative glomerulonephritis. A form of focal glomerulonephritis in which the predominant lesion consists of endocapillary proliferation with or without sclerosis.

focal sclerosing glomerulonephritis. A form of focal glomerulonephritis in which the predominant lesion consists of hypocellular, progressive sclerosis and hyalinosis of glomerular tufts; usually associated with persistant nephrotic syndrome which progresses to chronic glomerulonephritis and chronic renal failure.

focal sclerosis. Hardening and overgrowth of connective tissue confined to a particular region of the brain and cord. Compare *diffuse sclerosis, multiple sclerosis.*

focal seizure. An epileptic manifestation of a restricted nature, usually without loss of consciousness, due to irritation of a localized area of the brain, often associated with organic lesions such as scar, inflammation, or tumor. May be manifested by the single motor, sensory, or sensorimotor component (Jacksonian convulsion), or may be psychomotor in type; the seizure may also spread to other regions of the brain and develop into a generalized convulsion with loss of consciousness.

focal spot. The area of an x-ray-tube target against which the main electron beam strikes.

focal status. Continuous focal seizures lasting in the order of an hour or more.

fo·cus (fo′kus) *n.*, pl. **focuses, fo·ci** (·sigh) [L., fireplace]. 1. The principal seat of a disease. 2. The point at which rays of any radiant energy, such as light, heat, or sound converge. 3. Adjustment or the position of adjustment for clear, distinct vision. 4. *In cardiology,* the site or locus of a pacemaker.

foenugreek. FENUGREEK.

Foer·ster-Pen·field operation (fœr′stur) [O. *Foerster,* German neurologist and surgeon, 1873–1941; and W. G. *Penfield*]. PENFIELD'S OPERATION.

Foerster's cutaneous numeral test [O. *Foerster*]. A test for graphesthesia.

Foerster sign [O. *Foerster*]. A sign manifested by the usually floppy infant who, when held suspended under the shoulders by the examiner's hands, displays the legs flexed almost rigidly at the hips and knees.

Foerster's operation [O. *Foerster*]. Resection of the posterior spinal root nerves for relief of spastic paralysis and tabetic incoordination.

foetal. FETAL.

foeticide. FETICIDE.

foetid. FETID.

foeto-. See *feto-.*

foetoglobulin. Fetoglobulin (= FETOPROTEIN).

foetor. FETOR.

foetus. FETUS.

fog·ging, *n.* 1. In repression treatment of esophoria, the reduction of vision to about 20/80 by combining prisms (varying with the muscular imbalance), bases in, with a convex sphere; the patient reads with these glasses for a half hour at night before retiring. 2. A method of refracting the eye by using a convex lens sufficiently strong to cause the eye to become artificially myopic and fog the vision. Astigmatism is then corrected by means of minus cylinders, after which the fog is removed by gradually reducing the convex lens. Generally used in adults or when cycloplegia might precipitate glaucoma. 3. The darkening of a radiograph due to any factor other than the intended radiation, caused by light, processing, or stray or scattered radiation.

fo·go sel·va·gem (fo′goo sel·vah′zhem, Pg. ·zhey^n) [Pg., wild fire]. A severe endemic bullous disease found in certain lowland areas of Brazil, believed to be an attenuated tropical form of pemphigus foliaceus.

foil, *n.* [MF. *foille,* from L. *folium,* leaf]. A thin sheet of metal used in dentistry for restoration.

Foix-Ala·joua·nine syndrome (fwah, a·la·zhwa·neen′) [C. *Foix,* French neurologist, 1882–1927; and T. *Alajouanine,* French neurologist, 20th century]. SUBACUTE NECROTIZING MYELOPATHY.

Foix sign [C. *Foix*]. MARIE-FOIX RETRACTION SIGN.

Foix syndrome [C. *Foix*]. Unilateral paralysis of all muscles innervated by the third, fourth and sixth cranial nerves and sensory defect in the distribution of the ophthalmic division of the fifth nerve; indicative of a lesion in the cavernous sinus and the region of the superior orbital fissure. Syn. *Tolosa-Hunt syndrome.*

fo·la·cin (fo′luh·sin) *n.* FOLIC ACID.

fo·late (fo′late) *n.* A salt of folic acid.

fold, *n.* A plication or doubling, as of various parts of the body.

fold of the urachus. MEDIAN UMBILICAL LIGAMENT.

Foley balloon catheter. FOLEY CATHETER.

Fo·ley catheter [F. E. B. *Foley,* U.S. urologist, 1891–1966]. A balloon-tipped rubber catheter used in the urinary bladder.

Foley Y-plasty [F. E. B. *Foley*]. A plastic operation on the ureteropelvic junction for relief of stricture.

folia. Plural of *folium.*

fo·li·a·ceous (fo″lee·ay′shus) *adj.* [L. *foliaceus,* from *folium,* leaf]. Leaflike.

folia ce·re·bel·li (serr·e·bel′eye) [NA]. The narrow folds of cerebellar cortex.

fo·li·ate (fo′li·ate) *adj.* [L. *foliatus,* leaved]. Shaped like a leaf.

foliate papilla. One of the papillae, similar in structure to the vallate papillae, found on the posterolateral margin of the tongue of many mammals, but vestigial or absent in man.

fo·lic acid (fo′lick). [L. *fol*ium, leaf, + *-ic*]. Pteroylglutamic acid, or *N*-{*p*-{[(2-amino-4-hydroxy-6-pteridinyl)methyl] amino} benzoyl} glutamic acid, $C_{19}H_{19}N_7O_6$, a substance occurring in green leaves, liver, and yeast, and also produced synthetically. It is essential for growth of *Lactobacillus casei.* It is effective in the treatment of various megaloblastic anemias and gastrointestinal malabsorption states. In pernicious anemia, it should be used only as an adjunct to treatment with cyanocobalamin or liver injection as it does not prevent or improve the spinal cord lesions.

fo·lie (foh·lee′) *n.* [F., from *fou, folle,* mad, insane]. A mental disorder or psychosis; insanity.

folie à deux (a^h dœh′) [F., double madness]. A type of communicated delusion involving two persons, one of whom suffers from an essential psychosis, and whose control of and influence over the other person is so potent that the latter will simulate or accept elements of the psychosis without question.

folie du doute (du^e doot′) [F., doubting insanity]. A symptom of anxiety, as seen in anxiety neurosis or obsessive-compulsive neurosis, in which a person checks and rechecks an act, such as locking a door, doubting its having been properly done before, so that he may be unable to proceed beyond the act in question, or even to be able to make a simple decision. See also *abulia.*

Fo·lin and Den·is method [O. *Folin,* U.S. biochemist, 1867–1934; and W. G. *Denis*]. 1. A method for determining the presence of phenols in urine, with a solution of phosphotungstic-phosphomolybdic acid and alkali; phenols yield a blue color proportional to their concentration. 2. A method for determining the presence of Bence Jones protein in urine; the urine is heated to 60°C and centrifuged; the precipitated protein is washed with alcohol, dried, and weighed.

Folin and Sved·berg's method [O. *Folin* and T. *Svedberg*]. A method for determining blood urea concentration, in which urease is added to a blood filtrate to produce ammonium carbonate after which the ammonia is distilled off and determined colorimetrically after nesslerization.

Folin and Young·burg's method [O. *Folin*]. A method for determining urea, in which ammonia is removed from urine by an ion-exchange zeolite. The urea is decomposed with urease and the filtrate is nesslerized.

Folin and Wu's method [O. *Folin;* and H. *Wu,* Chinese biochemist, 20th century]. 1. A method for protein-free blood filtrate in which blood is laked and the proteins removed by precipitation with tungstic acid. 2. A method for nonprotein nitrogen in which the nitrogen in the blood filtrate is estimated by the Kjeldahl method; the ammonia formed is determined colorimetrically after direct nesslerization. 3. A method for reducing substances in blood in which the blood filtrate is heated with a copper solution and phosphomolybdic acid is added to form a blue color which is compared with a standard. 4. A method for total acidity in which 25 ml of a mixed 24-hour urine is titrated with O.1N sodium hydroxide using phenolphthalein for an indicator.

Folin, Can·non, and Denis method [O. *Folin,* W. B. *Cannon,* and W. G. *Denis*]. Epinephrine is extracted from the suprarenals with acid. The amount is then determined by its reducing power on the uric acid reagent of Folin and Denis.

Folin-Cio·cal·teu's reagent [O. *Folin*]. A solution of sodium tungstate, sodium molybdate, and phosphoric acid; used in a method of serum alkaline phosphatase determination.

Folin-Far·mer method [O. *Folin*]. A method for determining total nitrogen in urine by a micro-Kjeldahl procedure in which the ammonia solution is nesslerized and compared colorimetrically.

fo·lin·ic acid (fo·lin'ick). 1. Any of a group of factors occurring in liver extracts and also obtained from pteroylglutamic acid by synthesis; essential for growth of *Leuconostoc citrovorum.* 2. 5-Formyl-5,6,7,8-tetrahydrofolic acid, $C_{20}H_{23}N_7O_7$, the form in which folic acid exists and is active in tissues. It is identical with leucovorin and closely related, if not identical, to citrovorum factor. In the form of calcium leucovorin, it is used to counteract the toxic effects of folic acid antagonists and also in the treatment of megaloblastic anemias. Compare *folic acid.*

Folin-McEll·roy test [O. *Folin*]. A copper reduction test used for reducing substances in the urine.

Folin-Shaf·fer method [O. *Folin*]. A method for uric acid in which phosphates and organic matter are removed with uranium acetate. Uric acid is precipitated as ammonium urate which is titrated with potassium permanganate.

Folin's method [O. *Folin*]. 1. A method for uric acid in which tungstic acid filtrate is mixed with a phosphotungstic acid reagent which produces a blue color that is compared with a standard. 2. A method for amino-acid nitrogen in which the color developed by amino acids with β-naphthoquinonesulfonic acid is compared with a standard. 3. A method for ammonia in which alkali is used to set free the ammonia of the urine. The ammonia is collected in a measured amount of acid which is then titrated. 4. A method for creatinine in urine in which the red color produced following the addition of picric acid in alkaline solution is compared with a standard. 5. A method for protein in which protein precipitated by heat and acetic acid is centrifuged, washed, dried, and weighed.

Folin's reagent [O. *Folin*]. 1. A solution of sodium tungstate and orthophosphoric acid in water, used in blood-sugar determinations. 2. A mixture of saturated picric acid and sodium hydroxide; used in creatinine determination.

Folin theory [O. *Folin*]. The bulk of excreted nitrogen is of exogenous origin and does not arise by the metabolism of tissue protein.

Folin-Wu test [O. *Folin* and H. *Wu*]. A method for the quantitative estimation of urea in the blood utilizing urease.

fo·li·um (fo'lee·um) *n.,* pl. **fo·lia** (·lee·uh) [L., leaf]. Any lamina or leaflet of gray matter, forming a part of the arbor vitae of the cerebellum.

folium ca·cu·mi·nis (ka·kew'mi·nis). FOLIUM VERMIS.

folium ce·re·bel·li (serr·e·bel'eye) [NA]. Any one of the narrow folds of the cortex of the cerebellum.

folium ver·mis (vur'mis) [NA]. The terminal lobule in the superior surface of the vermis between the declive and tuber.

folk medicine. Nonprofessional practice of medicine using procedures and remedies, the latter often of plant origin, based largely on empiricism and tradition.

fol·li·cle (fol'i·kul) *n.* [L. *folliculus,* dim. of *follis,* bag]. 1. A lymph nodule. 2. A small secretory cavity or sac, as an acinus or alveolus. —**fol·lic·u·lar** (fol·ick'yoo·lur) *adj.*

follicle-ripening hormone. FOLLICLE-STIMULATING HORMONE.

follicle-stimulating hormone. An adenohypophyseal hormone which stimulates follicular growth in the ovary and spermatogenesis in the testis. Abbreviated, FSH.

fol·li·clis (fol'i·klis) *n. Obsol.* PAPULONECROTIC TUBERCULID.

follicular abscess. An abscess arising in a lymph nodule.

follicular cell. One of the epithelial cells of the ovarian follicle exclusive of the ovum. See also *granulosa cell.*

follicular conjunctivitis. Conjunctivitis characterized by discrete lymphoid follicles in the superficial conjunctival stroma, which often suggest a viral or chlamydial etiology.

follicular cyst. 1. A cyst due to retention of secretion in a follicular space, as in the ovary. 2. DENTIGEROUS CYST.

follicular fluid. The fluid filling the follicle or space about the developing ovum in the graafian (ovarian) follicle. Syn. *liquor folliculi.*

follicular hormone. Estrogen arising in the ovarian follicle.

follicular hyperkeratosis. That form of hyperkeratosis occurring about the openings of the hair follicles.

follicular hyperkeratotic papular dermatitis. PHRYNODERMA.

follicular lutein cells. Cells of the corpus luteum derived from follicular cells of the ovarian follicle. See also *paralutein cells.*

follicular lymphoma. NODULAR LYMPHOMA.

follicular mange. Infection of the hair follicles or sebaceous glands caused by *Demodex folliculorum* in man and by *D. canis* or *D. equi* in animals.

follicular mite. *DEMODEX FOLLICULORUM.*

follicular mucinosis. Mucinosis affecting hair follicles; ALOPECIA MUCINOSA.

follicular sinusitis. A rare type of pathologic lesion in chronically infected sinuses, characterized by numerous lymph follicles.

follicular stigma. The thin, nonvascular area of an ovary overlying the mature follicle marking the spot at which rupture of the follicle will occur; the point of rupture.

follicular tonsillitis. A form of tonsillitis in which the crypts are involved and their contents project as white or yellow spots from the surface of the tonsil.

follicular trachoma. GRANULAR TRACHOMA.

follicular tumor. SEBACEOUS CYST.

follicular ulcer. 1. An ulcer due to breakdown of a lymph follicle on a mucous membrane. 2. Ulceration of a hair follicle.

folliculi. Plural of *folliculus.*

folliculi glan·du·lae thy·roi·de·ae (glan'dew·lee thigh·roy'dee·ee) [NA]. The secretory units of the thyroid gland each consisting of a sac lined with cuboidal epithelium and filled with a colloid secretion.

folliculi lin·gua·les (ling·gway'leez) [NA]. The lymph nodules of the lingual tonsil.

folliculi lym·pha·ti·ci ag·gre·ga·ti ap·pen·di·cis ver·mi·for·mis (lim·fat'i·sigh ag·re·gay'tye a·pen'di·sis vur·mi·for'mis) [NA]. Aggregate follicles or nodules of the vermiform appendix.

folliculi lymphatici aggregati in·te·sti·ni te·nu·is (in·tes·tye'nigh ten'yoo·is) [NA]. AGGREGATE FOLLICLES.

folliculi lymphatici gas·tri·ci (gas'tri·sigh) [NA]. The lymph nodules of the stomach.

folliculi lymphatici la·ryn·gei (la·rin'jee·eye) [NA]. The lymph nodules of the larynx.

folliculi lymphatici li·e·na·les (lye·e·nay'leez) [NA]. The lymph nodules of the spleen.

folliculi lymphatici rec·ti (reck'tye) [NA]. The lymph nodules of the rectum.

folliculi lymphatici so·li·ta·rii in·te·sti·ni cras·si (sol·i·tair'ee·eye in·tes·tye'nigh kras'eye [NA]. The individual lymph nodules of the colon.

folliculi lymphatici solitarii intestini te·nu·is (ten'yoo·is) [NA]. The individual lymph nodules of the small intestine.

fol·lic·u·lin (fol·ick'yoo·lin) *n.* ESTRONE.

folliculi oo·pho·ri pri·ma·rii (o·off'uh·rye pri·mair'ee·eye) [BNA]. FOLLICULI OVARICI PRIMARII.

folliculi oophori ve·si·cu·lo·si [Graafi] (ve·sick"yoo·lo'sigh) [BNA]. FOLLICULI OVARICI VESICULOSI.

folliculi ova·ri·ci pri·ma·rii (o·vair'i·sigh pri·mair'ee·eye) [NA]. Primary ovarian follicles. See *ovarian follicle.*

folliculi ovarici ve·si·cu·lo·si (ve·sick"yoo·lo'sigh) [NA]. Vesicular ovarian follicles. See *ovarian follicle.*

fol·lic·u·li·tis (fol·ick"yoo·lye'tis) *n.* [*follicul*us + *-itis*]. Inflammation of a follicle or group of follicles, usually hair follicles.

folliculitis ab·sce·dens et suf·fo·di·ens (ab·see'denz et suh·fo'dee·enz). A scalp cellulitis with multiple follicular abscess formation.

folliculitis ag·mi·na·ta (ag·mi·nay'tuh). An inflammation of the hair follicles in one region.

folliculitis barbae. SYCOSIS BARBAE.

folliculitis de·cal·vans (de·kal'vanz). An inflammatory condition of hair follicles of the scalp that results in baldness.

folliculitis ke·loi·da·lis (kee"loy·day'lis). KELOID ACNE.

folliculitis sim·plex (sim'plecks). SUPERFICIAL FOLLICULITIS.

folliculitis uler·y·the·ma·to·sa re·tic·u·la·ta (yoo·lerr"i·theem"uh·to'suh re·tick"yoo·lay'tuh). An eruption over the face, especially the cheeks; characterized by small areas of atrophy separated by narrow ridges, producing a reticulated honeycomb appearance. Syn. *atrophoderma vermicularis, atrophoderma reticulatum.*

fol·lic·u·loid (fol·ick'yoo·loid) *adj.* [*follicul*us + *-oid*]. Resembling a follicle.

fol·lic·u·lo·ma (fol·ick"yoo·lo'muh) *n.*, pl. **folliculomas, folliculoma·ta** (·tuh) [*follicul*us + *-oma*]. A granulosa cell tumor of the ovary.

fol·lic·u·lo·sis (fol·ick"yoo·lo'sis) *n.* [*follicul*us + *-osis*]. An excess of lymph follicles caused by a disease process.

fol·li·cu·lus (fol·ick'yoo·lus) *n.*, pl. **follicu·li** (·lye) [NA]. FOLLICLE.

folliculus lym·pha·ti·cus (lim·fat'i·kus) [NA]. LYMPH NODULE.

folliculus pi·li (pye'lye) [NA]. HAIR FOLLICLE.

Follutein. Trademark for a preparation of chorionic gonadotropin obtained from the urine of pregnant women.

Folvite. A trademark for folic acid, a hematopoietic vitamin.

fo·men·ta·tion (fo"men·tay'shun) *n.* [L. *fomentare,* to foment, from *fovere,* to warm]. 1. The application of heat and moisture to a part to relieve pain or reduce inflammation. 2. The substance applied to a part to convey heat or moisture; a poultice.

fo·mes (fo'meez, fom'eez) *n.*, pl. **fomi·tes** (fom'i·teez, fo'mi·) [L., tinder]. FOMITE.

fo·mite (fo'mite) *n.* [from *fomites,* pl. of *fomes*]. Any inanimate object which may be contaminated with infectious organisms and thus serve to transmit disease.

fo·na·zine (fo'nuh·zeen) *n.* 10-[2-(Dimethylamino)propyl]-*N,N*-dimethylphenothiazine-2-sulfonamide, $C_{19}H_{25}N_3O_2S_2$, a serotonin inhibitor employed as the mesylate (methanesulfonate) salt.

Fong's lesion or **syndrome** [E. E. *Fong,* U.S. radiologist, b. 1912]. NAIL-PATELLA SYNDROME.

Fon·se·caea (fon"se·see'uh) *n.* [O. da *Fonseca,* Brazilian physician, 20th century]. *HORMODENDRUM.*

Fon·se·ca's disease (fohn·seʸ'kuh) [O. da *Fonseca*]. CHROMOBLASTOMYCOSIS.

Fon·ta·na's spaces or **canal** (fohn·tah'na) [F. *Fontana,* Italian physiologist and naturalist, 1730–1805]. Spaces of the iridocorneal angle of some lower animals.

Fontana's stain [A. *Fontana,* Italian dermatologist, 1873–1950]. An ammoniacal silver nitrate solution for staining spirochetes by silver impregnation.

fon·ta·nel, fon·ta·nelle (fon"tuh·nel') *n.* [F., dim. of *fontaine,* fountain]. A membranous space between the cranial bones in fetal life and infancy. NA *fonticulus.*

fontanel sign. Constant bulging and tenseness of the anterior fontanel in infants observed in meningitis and other conditions where intracranial pressure is increased.

fonticuli. Plural of *fonticulus.*

fonticuli cra·nii (kray'nee·eye) [NA]. The fontanels of the skull collectively.

fon·ti·cu·lus (fon·tick'yoo·lus) *n.*, pl. **fonticu·li** (·lye) [L., dim. of *fons, fontis,* fountain, spring]. 1. JUGULAR NOTCH OF THE STERNUM. 2. A small artificial ulcer or issue. 3. [NA] FONTANEL.

fonticulus anterior [NA]. ANTERIOR FONTANEL.

fonticulus fron·ta·lis (fron·tay'lis) [BNA]. Fonticulus anterior (= ANTERIOR FONTANEL).

fonticulus ma·stoi·de·us (mas·toy'dee·us) [NA]. The fontanel at the junction of the lambdoid, parietomastoid, and occipitomastoid sutures.

fonticulus oc·ci·pi·ta·lis (ock·sip·i·tay'lis) [BNA]. Fonticulus posterior (= POSTERIOR FONTANEL).

fonticulus posterior [NA]. POSTERIOR FONTANEL.

fonticulus sphe·noi·da·lis (sfee·noy·day'lis) [NA]. The fontanel at the junction of the sutures of the parietal, frontal, great wing of the sphenoid, and squamous part of the temporal bone.

food, *n.* Any organic substance which, when ingested or taken into the body of an organism through some alternate means and assimilated, may be used either to supply energy or to build tissue; classified in three groups: proteins, carbohydrates, and fats, all of which may occur in animal or vegetable substance.

Food and Drug Administration. An agency of the United States federal government responsible for ensuring that food, drugs, and cosmetics sold in the United States are safe, fulfill their stated functions, and are correctly labeled and packaged. Abbreviated, FDA.

food ball. PHYTOBEZOAR.

food infection. FOOD POISONING.

food poisoning. 1. A type of poisoning due to food contaminated by bacterial toxins or by certain living bacteria, particularly those of the *Salmonella* group. 2. The symptoms due to foods naturally poisonous, such as certain fungi, or foods that contain allergens or toxic chemical residues.

food yolk. DEUTEROPLASM.

foot, *n.* [OE. *fōt* ← Gmc. (rel. to Gk. *pod-* and to L. *ped-*)]. 1. The terminal extremity of the leg. Skeletally, it consists of the tarsus, metatarsus, and phalanges. NA *pes.* 2. A measure of length equal to 12 inches, or 30.479 cm. Abbreviated, ft.

foot-and-mouth disease. A highly infectious and acute febrile viral disease producing a vesicular eruption of the mucous membranes of the nose and mouth and of the skin near the interdigital space of cloven-hoofed animals. It is contagious among domestic animals and is occasionally transmitted to man. Syn. *aphthous fever, epidemic stomatitis, epizootic stomatitis.*

foot-candle, *n.* The illumination received at a surface one foot from a standard source of one candela.

foot cell. One of the branching parenchymatous cells of the pineal body.

foot drop, foot-drop. DROPPED FOOT.

foot-drop gait. STEPPAGE GAIT.

foot·ling presentation. Presentation of the fetus with the feet foremost.

foot pad. A cushionlike mass of connective tissue covered by a heavily keratinized hairless epidermis, found on the flexor surface of the feet of certain animals.

foot plate. The flat part of the stapes.

foot-pound, *n.* The work performed when a constant force of one pound is exerted on a body which moves a distance of one foot in the same direction as the force.

foot-print, *n.* An ink impression of the sole of the foot; used for identification of infants and in the study of dermatoglyphics.

foot process. One of the cytoplasmic processes by which the visceral epithelial cells of a glomerular capsule of the kidney attach to the glomerular basement membrane.

foot process disease. A lesion of the nephrotic syndrome, seen by electron microsopy, consisting of flattening, fusion, and loss of the foot processes of the glomerular epithelial cells.

foot rot. A disease of cattle and sheep marked by a necrosis of the skin around the hoof and usually associated with the anaerobic bacterium *Sphaerophorus necrophorus.*

foots, *n.* The bottom portion, sediment, or residue from certain crude liquids, as fixed animal or vegetable oils, obtained in a process of refining.

fo·ra·men (fo·ray'mun) *n.*, genit. **fo·ra·mi·nis** (fo·ram'i·nis, fo·ray'mi·nis), pl. **forami·na, foramens** [L., an opening]. A perforation or opening, especially in a bone.

foramen api·cis den·tis (ay'pi·sis den'tis) [NA]. APICAL FORAMEN.

foramen cae·cum lin·guae (see'kum ling'gwee) [BNA]. Foramen cecum linguae. See *foramen cecum.*

foramen caecum me·dul·lae ob·lon·ga·tae (me·dul'ee ob·long·gay'tee) [BNA]. Foramen cecum of the medulla oblongata. See *foramen cecum.*

foramen caecum os·sis fron·ta·lis (os'is fron·tay'lis) [BNA]. Foramen cecum ossis frontalis. See *foramen cecum.*

foramen ca·ro·ti·cum ex·ter·num (ka·rot'i·kum ecks·tur'num). The outer or lateral opening of the carotid canal.

foramen caroticum in·ter·num (in·tur'num). The inner or medial opening of the carotid canal.

foramen ce·cum (see'kum). A blind foramen, specifically: 1. (of the frontal bone:) A small pit or channel located between the frontal crest and the crista galli. When it is a channel it may transmit an emissary vein. NA *foramen cecum ossis frontalis.* 2. (of the medulla oblongata:) a small pit at the rostral termination of the anterior median fissure of the medulla oblongata. 3. (of the tongue:) a small pit located in the posterior termination of the median raphe of the tongue; the site of the thyroglossal duct. NA *foramen cecum linguae.*

foramen cecum lin·guae (ling'gwee) [NA]. The foramen cecum of the tongue. See *foramen cecum.*

foramen cecum os·sis fron·ta·lis (os'is fron·tay'lis) [NA]. Foramen cecum of the frontal bone. See *foramen cecum.*

foramen cos·to·trans·ver·sa·ri·um (kos''to·trans·vur·sair'ee·um) [NA]. The narrow gap between the upper surface of the neck of a rib and the lower surface of the transverse process of the corresponding vertebra.

foramen dia·phrag·ma·tis sel·lae (dye·uh·frag'muh·tis sel'ee) [BNA]. The opening in the center of the diaphragm of the sella turcica through which the stalk of the hypophysis passes.

foramen epi·plo·i·cum (ep·i·plo'i·kum) [NA]. EPIPLOIC FORAMEN.

foramen eth·moi·da·le an·te·ri·us (eth·moy·day'lee an·teer'ee·us) [NA]. ANTERIOR ETHMOID FORAMEN.

foramen ethmoidale pos·te·ri·us (pos·teer'ee·us) [NA]. POSTERIOR ETHMOID FORAMEN.

foramen fron·ta·le (fron·tay'lee) [NA]. FRONTAL FORAMEN.

foramen in·ci·si·vum (in·si·sigh'vum) [NA]. Singular of *foramina incisiva.* See *incisive foramina.*

foramen in·fra·or·bi·ta·le (in''fruh·or·bi·tay'lee) [NA]. INFRAORBITAL FORAMEN.

foramen in·fra·pi·ri·for·me (in''fra·pirr·i·for'mee). The passageway through the pelvic wall below the piriformis muscle where the inferior gluteal nerve and vessels leave the pelvic cavity; a subdivision of the greater sciatic foramen.

foramen in·no·mi·na·tum (in·nom''i·nay'tum). INNOMINATE CANALICULUS.

foramen in·ter·ven·tri·cu·la·re (in''tur·ven·trick·yoo·lair'ee) [NA]. INTERVENTRICULAR FORAMEN.

foramen in·ter·ver·te·bra·le (in''tur·vur·te·bray'lee) [NA]. INTERVERTEBRAL FORAMEN.

foramen is·chi·a·di·cum ma·jus (is·kee·ad'i·kum may'jus) [NA]. GREATER SCIATIC FORAMEN.

foramen ischiadicum mi·nus (migh'nus) [NA]. LESSER SCIATIC FORAMEN.

foramen ju·gu·la·re (jug·yoo·lair'ee) [NA]. JUGULAR FORAMEN.

foramen la·ce·rum (las'e·rum) [NA]. An irregular aperture in the cranium between the apex of the petrous portion of the temporal bone and the body and great wing of the sphenoid, and the basilar process of the occipital bone. The internal carotid artery with its venous and sympathetic plexuses ascends through the upper end of the foramen.

foramen mag·num (mag'num) [NA]. A large oval aperture centrally placed in the lower and anterior part of the occipital bone; it gives passage to the spinal cord and its membranes and venous plexuses, the spinal accessory nerves, and the vertebral arteries.

foramen man·di·bu·lae (man·dib'yoo·lee) [NA]. MANDIBULAR FORAMEN.

foramen man·di·bu·la·re (man·dib''yoo·lair'ee) [BNA]. Foramen mandibulae (= MANDIBULAR FORAMEN).

foramen mas·toi·de·um (mas·toy'dee·um) [NA]. MASTOID FORAMEN.

foramen men·ta·le (men·tay'lee) [NA]. MENTAL FORAMEN.

foramen nu·tri·ci·um (new·trish'ee·um) [NA]. NUTRIENT FORAMEN.

foramen ob·tu·ra·tum (ob·tew·ray'tum) [NA]. OBTURATOR FORAMEN.

foramen oc·ci·pi·ta·le mag·num (ock·sip''i·tay'lee mag'num) [BNA]. FORAMEN MAGNUM.

foramen of Boch·da·lek (bo^kh'da·leck) [V. A. *Bochdalek*]. Either of two potentially weak areas of the diaphragm between the dorsal or lumbar portion and each costal portion. Either may be the site of a diaphragmatic hernia, but the condition is more common on the left. Compare *foramen of Morgagni.*

foramen of Husch·ke (hŏŏsh'ke^h) [E. *Huschke*]. An inconstant perforation of the tympanic portion of the temporal bone.

foramen of Key (kay) [E. A. H. *Key,* Swedish physician and anatomist, 1832–1901]. FORAMEN OF LUSCHKA.

foramen of Lusch·ka (lŏŏsh'kah) [H. von *Luschka*]. LATERAL APERTURE OF THE FOURTH VENTRICLE.

foramen of Ma·gen·die (ma·zhahⁿ·dee′) [F. *Magendie*]. MEDIAN APERTURE OF THE FOURTH VENTRICLE.

foramen of Mon·ro [A. *Monro* (Secundus)]. INTERVENTRICULAR FORAMEN.

foramen of Mor·ga·gni (mor·gahnʸ′ee) [G. B. *Morgagni*]. Either of two potentially weak areas of the diaphragm between the sternal portion and each costal portion. Either may be the site of a diaphragmatic hernia. Compare *foramen of Bochdalek.*

foramen of Ret·zi·us [M. G. *Retzius*]. LATERAL APERTURE OF THE FOURTH VENTRICLE.

foramen of Scar·pa [A. *Scarpa*]. A median incisive foramen. See *incisive foramina.*

foramen of Sten·sen [N. *Stensen*]. A lateral incisive foramen. See *incisive foramina.*

foramen of Ve·sa·li·us [A. *Vesalius*]. An inconstant foramen in the great wing of the sphenoid, situated between the foramen ovale and foramen rotundum, which when present transmits an emissary vein from the cavernous sinus.

foramen of Wins·low [J. B. *Winslow*]. EPIPLOIC FORAMEN.

foramen op·ti·cum (op′ti·kum) [BNA]. CANALIS OPTICUS.

foramen ova·le (o·vay′lee). 1. FORAMEN OVALE OF THE HEART. 2. FORAMEN OVALE OF THE SPHENOID.

foramen ovale cor·dis (kor′dis) [NA]. FORAMEN OVALE OF THE HEART.

foramen ovale of the heart. A fetal opening between the two atria of the heart, situated at the lower posterior portion of the septum secundum. Through this opening, blood is shunted from the right atrium to the left atrium. Functional closure usually occurs at birth. NA *foramen ovale cordis.*

foramen ovale of the sphenoid. An oval opening near the posterior margin of the great wing of the sphenoid, giving passage to the mandibular branch of the trigeminal nerve, the accessory meningeal artery, and occasionally the lesser petrosal nerve. NA *foramen ovale ossis sphenoidalis.*

foramen ovale os·sis sphe·noi·da·lis (os′is sfee·noy·day′lis) [NA]. FORAMEN OVALE OF THE SPHENOID.

foramen ovale pri·mum (prye′mum). FORAMEN SECUNDUM.

foramen pa·la·ti·num ma·jus (pal·uh·tye′num may′jus) [NA]. GREATER PALATINE FORAMEN.

foramen pa·ri·e·ta·le (pa·rye″e·tay′lee) [NA]. PARIETAL FORAMEN.

foramen pri·mum (prye′mum). The temporary interatrial opening bounded by the growing margins of the septum primum and the endocardial cushions.

foramen ro·tun·dum (ro·tun′dum) [NA]. A round opening in the great wing of the sphenoid bone of the maxillary division of the trigeminal nerve.

foramen se·cun·dum (se·kun′dum). The secondary opening in the septum primum due to thinning and perforation of its cranial portion.

foramen sin·gu·la·re (sing″gew·lair′ee) [NA]. An opening in the inferior portion of the medial end of the internal acoustic meatus for the passage of nerve fibers to the ampulla of the posterior semicircular duct.

foramen sphe·no·pa·la·ti·num (sfee″no·pal·uh·tye′num) [NA]. SPHENOPALATINE FORAMEN.

foramen spi·no·sum (spye·no′sum) [NA]. A passage in the great wing of the sphenoid bone, near its posterior angle, giving passage to the middle meningeal artery and spinosal nerve.

foramen sty·lo·ma·stoi·de·um (stye″lo·mas·toy′dee·um) [NA]. STYLOMASTOID FORAMEN.

foramen su·pra·or·bi·ta·lis (sue″pruh·or·bi·tay′lis) [NA]. SUPRAORBITAL FORAMEN.

foramen su·pra·pi·ri·for·me (sue″pruh·pirr·i·for′mee). The passageway through the pelvic wall above the piriformis muscle where the superior gluteal nerve and vessels leave the pelvic cavity; a subdivision of the greater sciatic foramen.

foramen thy·re·oi·de·um (thigh·ree·oy′dee·um) [BNA]. Foramen thyroideum (= THYROID FORAMEN (1)).

foramen thy·roi·de·um (thigh·roy′dee·um) [NA]. THYROID FORAMEN (1).

foramen trans·ver·sa·ri·um (trans·vur·sair′ee·um) [NA]. A foramen in the transverse process of each of the upper six cervical vertebrae, which transmits the vertebral artery and vein.

foramen ve·nae ca·vae (vee′nee kay′vee) [NA]. The opening in the diaphragm for the transmission of the vena cava inferior.

foramen ve·no·sum (vee·no′sum). Any small opening, especially on the surface of a bone, for the passage of a vein.

foramen ver·te·bra·le (vur·te·bray′lee) [NA]. VERTEBRAL FORAMEN.

foramen zy·go·ma·ti·co·fa·ci·a·le (zye·go·mat″i·ko·fay·shee·ay′lee) [NA]. An opening on the outer aspect of the zygomatic bone for the passage of the zygomaticofacial nerve and accompanying vessels.

foramen zy·go·ma·ti·co·or·bi·ta·le (zye·go·mat″i·ko·or·bi·tay′lee) [NA]. An opening on the orbital surface of the zygomatic bone for the passage of the zygomatic branch of the maxillary nerve and accompanying vessels.

foramen zy·go·ma·ti·co·tem·po·ra·le (zye·go·mat″i·ko·tem·po·ray′lee) [NA]. An opening on the temporal surface of the zygomatic bone for the passage of the zygomaticotemporal nerve.

foramina. Plural of *foramen.*

foramina al·ve·o·la·ria max·il·lae (al″vee·o·lair′ee·uh mack·sil′ee) [NA]. Openings of the alveolar canals on the posterior surface of the maxilla.

foramina eth·moi·da·lia (eth·moy·day′lee·uh) [NA]. The anterior and posterior ethmoid foramens.

foramina in·ci·si·va (in·si·sigh′vuh) [NA]. INCISIVE FORAMINA.

foramina in·ter·ver·te·bra·lia os·sis sa·cri (in″tur·vur·te·bray′lee·uh os′is say′krye) [NA]. The intervertebral foramina of the sacrum. See *anterior sacral foramina, posterior sacral foramina.*

fo·ram·i·nal (fo·ram′i·nul) *adj.* Of or pertaining to a foramen.

foraminal hernia. A false hernia of a loop of bowel through the epiploic foramen.

foramina na·sa·lia (nay·say′lee·uh) [BNA]. The small openings on the outer (facial) surface of the nasal bone which transmit tributaries to the facial vein.

foramina ner·vo·sa (nur·vo′suh) [NA]. Openings in the limbus of the osseous spiral lamina for cochlear nerve fibers.

foramina nervosa la·mi·nae spi·ra·lis (lam′i·nee spye·ray′lis) [BNA]. FORAMINA NERVOSA.

foramina pa·la·ti·na mi·no·ra (pal·uh·tye′nuh mi·no′ruh) [NA]. LESSER PALATINE FORAMINA.

foramina pa·pil·la·ria re·nis (pap·i·lair′ee·uh ree′nis) [NA]. PAPILLARY FORAMINA.

foramina sa·cra·lia an·te·ri·o·ra (sa·kray′lee·uh an·teer·ee·o′ruh) [BNA]. Foramina sacralia pelvina (= ANTERIOR SACRAL FORAMINA).

foramina sacralia dor·sa·lia (dor·say′lee·uh) [NA]. POSTERIOR SACRAL FORAMINA.

foramina sacralia pel·vi·na (pel·vye′nuh) [NA]. ANTERIOR SACRAL FORAMINA.

foramina sacralia pos·te·ri·o·ra (pos·teer·ee·o′ruh) [BNA]. Foramina sacralia dorsalia (= POSTERIOR SACRAL FORAMINA).

foramina ve·na·rum mi·ni·ma·rum cor·dis (ve·nair′um mi·ni·mair′um kor′dis) [NA]. The openings of small veins into the right atrium of the heart.

fo·ram·i·not·o·my (fo·ram″i·not′uh·mee) *n.* [*foramen* + *-tomy*]. Surgical removal of a portion of an intervertebral foramen.

fo·ra·min·u·lum (for″a·min′yoo·lum) *n.*, pl. **foraminu·la** (·luh) [NL.]. A very small foramen. —**foraminu·late** (·late) *adj.*

Forane. A trademark for isoflurane, an inhalation anesthetic.

Forbes' disease [G. B. *Forbes*, U.S. pediatrician, b. 1915]. LIMIT DEXTRINOSIS.

force, *n.* & *v.* [OF., from L. *fortis*, strong]. 1. That which initiates, changes, or arrests motion or results in acceleration of movement of a body. See also *dyne*. 2. To cause to change or move against resistance.

forced beat. An extrasystole initiated by artificial cardiac stimulation.

forced feeding or **alimentation**. 1. The administration of food to a resistant individual, especially feeding through a nasogastric or gastric tube. 2. The administration of food in excess of the amount required by the patient's appetite.

forced grasp reflex. GRASP REFLEX.

forced movement. 1. PASSIVE MOVEMENT. 2. Involuntary movement as a result of injury or exogenous stimulation of the motor centers or the conducting pathways of the nervous system.

forced respiration. Respiration induced by blowing air into the lungs by means of a pump or respirator, or in some other way, as in physiologic experiments or during artificial respiration.

forced version. ACCOUCHEMENT FORCÉ.

for·ceps (for'seps) *n.* [L., pincers, tongs]. 1. A surgical instrument with two opposing blades or limbs; controlled by handles or by direct pressure on the blades. Used to grasp, compress, and hold tissue, a part of the body, needles, or other surgical material. 2. Fiber bundles in the brain resembling forceps.

forceps hand. 1. A hand which has lost the three middle digits. 2. A hand with bidactyly.

forceps major [NA]. A bundle of nerve fibers radiating from the splenum of the corpus callosum into the occipital lobe of the cerebrum.

forceps minor [NA]. A bundle of nerve fibers curving forward from the genu of the corpus callosum and connecting the lateral and medial surfaces of the two frontal lobes.

Forch·heimer's sign [F. *Forchheimer*, U.S. physician, 1853–1913]. A maculopapular, rose-red eruption on the soft palate, seen in early rubella before the skin rash appears.

for·ci·pate (for'si·pate) *adj.* Shaped like a forceps.

for·cip·i·tal (for·sip'i·tul) *adj.* Of or pertaining to a forceps.

for·ci·pres·sure (for'si·presh"ur) *n.* Pressure exerted on a blood vessel by means of a forceps, to prevent hemorrhage.

fore-. Combining form meaning (a) *before, preceding;* (b) *in front, anterior;* (c) *the front* (as of a part of structure).

fore·arm, *n.* The part of the upper extremity between the wrist and the elbow. NA *antebrachium*.

fore·brain, *n.* PROSENCEPHALON.

fore·con·scious, *n.* & *adj.* 1. The portion of the unconscious containing mental experiences that are not in the focus of immediate attention, but which may be recalled to consciousness. 2. Capable of being recalled into the conscious mind, although not in the realm of consciousness.

fore·fin·ger, *n.* INDEX FINGER.

fore·foot, *n.* 1. The anterior part of the foot; from a clinical standpoint, the portion of the foot that includes the toes and the metatarsal, cuneiform, and cuboid bones. 2. Of a quadruped: the foot of the foreleg.

fore·gut, *n.* The cephalic part of the embryonic digestive tube that develops into pharynx, esophagus, stomach, part of the small intestine, liver, pancreas, and respiratory ducts.

fore·head, *n.* The part of the face above the eyes. NA *frons*.

for·eign, *adj.* [OF. *forein*, from L. *foranus*, on the outside]. 1. Derived from other than self, as in tissue transplantation or antigens. 2. Not belonging in the location where found.

foreign body. A substance occurring in any organ or tissue where it is not normally found, especially a substance of extrinsic origin.

foreign-body giant cell. A large cell derived from macrophages, with multiple nuclei and abundant cytoplasm which may contain foreign material; found in granulomatous inflammation in response to foreign bodies.

foreign-body reaction. An inflammation around a foreign body in a tissue or organ. Syn. *perialienitis, perixenitis*.

foreign protein. A protein that differs from the proteins of the animal or person into whom it is introduced.

fore·kid·ney, *n.* PRONEPHROS.

Fo·rel's decussation (fohⁿ·rel') [A. H. *Forel*, Swiss neurologist, 1848–1931]. VENTRAL TEGMENTAL DECUSSATION.

fore·milk, *n.* 1. The milk first withdrawn at each milking. 2. COLOSTRUM.

fo·ren·sic (fo·ren'sick) *adj.* [L. *forensis*, of the forum]. 1. Pertaining or belonging to a court of law. 2. Pertaining to use in legal proceedings or in public discussions.

forensic chemistry. The application of chemical knowledge in the solution of legal problems, especially in the detection of crime.

forensic graphology. The study of handwriting for legal purposes.

forensic medicine. LEGAL MEDICINE.

forensic psychiatry. The branch of psychiatry concerned with the legal aspects of mental disorders.

fore·play, *n.* The fondling of erotogenic zones which usually precedes sexual intercourse and may lead to orgasm; contrectation.

fore·pleas·ure, *n.* The erotic pleasure, both physical and emotional, accompanied by a rise in tension, which precedes the culmination of the sexual act, or end pleasure.

fore·skin, *n.* PREPUCE.

fore·stom·ach, *n.* RUMEN.

forest yaws. A form of American mucocutaneous leishmaniasis resembling espundia.

fore·wa·ters, *n.* HYDRORRHEA GRAVIDARUM.

Forhistal. Trademark for dimethindene, an antihistaminic drug used as the maleate salt.

-form, -iform. A combining form meaning *having the form of, -shaped, resembling*.

form·al·de·hyde (for·mal'de·hide) *n.* Formic aldehyde or methanal, HCHO, a colorless gas obtained by the oxidation of methyl alcohol. It is a powerful disinfectant, generally used in aqueous solution; employed also as a reagent. See also *formalin*.

formaldehyde solution. An aqueous solution containing not less than 37% by weight of formaldehyde. It is a powerful antiseptic. By means of oxidizing agents or heat, it may be converted into a gas, a procedure that has been used for disinfection of rooms and dwellings previously exposed to contagion.

formalin. 1. FORMALDEHYDE SOLUTION. 2. A 4% aqueous solution of formaldehyde; the most common histologic fixative.

form·am·i·dase (form·am'i·dace, ·daze, for'muh·mi·) *n.* An enzyme involved in tryptophane catabolism which catalyzes conversion of *N*-formylkynurenine to kynurenine and formate.

form·am·ide (form·am'ide, ·am'id, for'muh·mide") *n.* 1. $HCONH_2$, the amide of formic acid. 2. A compound containing the HCONH— radical.

for·mate (for'mate) *n.* A salt of formic acid.

for·ma·tio (for·may'shee·o) *n.*, pl. **for·ma·ti·o·nes** (for·may"shee·o'neez) [L.]. FORMATION (2).

for·ma·tion (for·may'shun) *n.* [L. *formatio*, from *formare*, to form]. 1. The process of developing shape or structure. 2. That which is formed; a structure or arrangement.

formatio re·ti·cu·la·ris (re·tick"yoo·lair'is) [NA]. RETICULAR FORMATION.

formatio re·ti·cu·la·ris me·dul·lae ob·lon·ga·tae (re·tick·yoo·lair'is me·dul'ee ob·long·gay'tee) [NA]. The reticular formation of the medulla oblongata.

formatio reticularis medullae spi·na·lis (spye·nay'lis) [NA]. The reticular formation of the spinal cord.

formatio reticularis mes·en·ce·pha·li (mes·en·sef'uh·lye) [NA]. The reticular formation of the mesencephalon.

formatio reticularis pe·dun·cu·li ce·re·bri (pe·dunk'yoo·lye serr'e·brye) [BNA]. The reticular formation of the midbrain.

formatio reticularis pon·tis (pon'tis) [NA]. The reticular formation of the pons.

for·ma·tive (for'muh·tiv) *adj.* 1. Pertaining to the process of development, as of tissue or of the embryo. 2. Forming, producing, originating.

formative blastomere. A blastomere destined to form a part of the embryo, not its membranes.

formative cell. 1. An embryonic cell. 2. Any cell of the inner cell mass of the blastocyst concerned in the formation of the embryo proper.

form·a·zan (form'uh·zan) *n.* A generic name for a deeply colored pigment obtained by reducing 2,3,5-triphenyltetrazolium chloride or certain other related tetrazolium salts by highly labile enzyme systems. The reaction is utilized in testing the ability of seeds to germinate and the function of granulocytes.

forme fruste (form froost, F. fruᵉst) [F., defaced form]. An incomplete, abortive, or atypical form or manifestation of a syndrome or disease.

for·mic (for'mick) *adj.* [L. *formica,* ant]. 1. Of or pertaining to ants. 2. Pertaining to or derived from formic acid.

formic acid. 1. The anhydrous liquid HCOOH; a strong reducing agent, dangerously caustic to the skin. Syn. *methanoic acid.* 2. An aqueous solution containing about 25% HCOOH; it is counterirritant and astringent.

formic aldehyde. FORMALDEHYDE.

for·mi·cant (for'mi·kunt) *adj.* [L. *formicans,* crawling like ants, from *formica,* ant]. Producing a tactile sensation like the crawling of small insects.

formicant pulse. *Obsol.* A small, feeble pulse likened to the movements of ants.

for·mi·ca·tion (for"mi·kay'shun) *n.* [L. *formicatio,* from *formicare,* to crawl like an ant]. An abnormal sensation as of insects crawling in or upon the skin; a common symptom in diseases of the spinal cord and the peripheral nerves; a form of paresthesia; may be a hallucination.

for·mim·i·no·glu·tam·ic acid (for·mim"i·no·gloo·tam'ick). Glutamic acid in which an amino hydrogen is replaced by a formimino (—CH=NH) group. An intermediate in the metabolic conversion of histidine to glutamic acid, it is also involved in the metabolism of tetrahydrofolic acid.

for·mim·i·no·glu·tam·ic·ac·i·du·ria (for·mim"i·no·gloo·tam"ick·as"i·dew'ree·uh) *n.* [*formiminoglutamic acid* + *-uria*]. An inborn error of amino acid metabolism of which there are two types: type A characterized biochemically by a deficiency of formiminotransferase and increased formiminoglutamic acid excretion in urine after a histidine load, and clinically by physical and mental retardation, obesity, and hypersegmentation of polymorphonuclear cells; and type B characterized biochemically by increased formiminoglutamic acid excretion both before and after histidine load, and probably a defect in folic acid transport, and clinically by mental retardation, ataxia, convulsions, and megaloblastic anemia.

for·mim·i·no·trans·fer·ase (for·mim"i·no·trans'fur·ace) *n.* An enzyme that catalyzes transfer of a formimino (—CH=NH) group, as in the reaction of formiminoglutamic acid with tetrahydrofolic acid to produce glutamic acid and formiminotetrahydrofolic acid.

for·mo·cre·sol (for"mo·kree'sol) *n.* A mixture of equal parts of formaldehyde solution and cresol, used in dentistry for treating putrescent pulp chambers.

for·mol (for'mol) *n.* FORMALIN.

for·mo·ni·trile (for"mo·nigh'tril, ·treel, ·tryle) *n.* HYDROCYANIC ACID.

for·mox·yl (for·mock'sil) *n.* FORMYL.

form sense. *In ophthalmology,* acuteness of vision; the faculty of perceiving the shape or form of objects.

for·mu·la (for'mew·luh) *n.,* pl. **formulas, formu·lae** (·lee) [L., dim. of *forma,* form]. 1. A prescribed method. 2. The representation of a chemical compound by symbols. 3. A recipe or prescription. Abbreviated, F.

for·mu·lary (for'mew·lerr"ee) *n.* [F. *formulaire*]. A collection of formulas for making medicinal preparations.

Formvar. A trademark for plastic film used to coat grids to support tissue sections for examination in electron microscopy.

for·myl (for'mil) *n.* HCO—, the radical of formic acid.

for·myl-am·ide (for'mil am'ide). *n.* FORMAMIDE.

for·myl·ase (for'mil·ace, ·aze) *n.* An enzyme, present in the liver of certain animals, which effects hydrolysis of formylkynurenine to tryptophan.

for·myl·a·tion (for"mi·lay'shun) *n.* The introduction of the formyl (HCO—) radical into the molecular structure of an organic compound.

for·myl·fo·lic acid (for"mil·fo'lick). The formyl derivative (at the nitrogen atom of the *p*-aminobenzoyl component) of folic acid; it may be an intermediate in the biogenesis of folic acid. See also *rhizopterin.*

for·myl·for·mic acid (for"mil·for'mick). GLYOXYLIC ACID.

for·myl·gly·cine (for"mil·glye'seen) *n.* $NH_2CH(CHO)$-COOH; a postulated intermediate in the conversion of serine to glycine; it represents serine in which the CH_2OH group has been converted to CHO.

for·myl·me·thi·o·nine (for"mil·me·thigh'o·neen) *n.* A formylated form of the amino acid methionine which initiates peptide chain synthesis in bacteria. Once the complete protein is formed, the formylmethionine is cleaved as such, or as a part of a larger peptide chain.

for·myl·pte·ro·ic acid (for"mil·te·ro'ick). RHIZOPTERIN.

for·ni·cal (for'ni·kul) *adj.* Of or pertaining to a fornix.

fornical commissure. The transverse part of the fornix, uniting the two crura. NA *commissura fornicis.*

for·ni·cate (for'ni·kut, ·kate) *adj.* [L. *fornicatus,* from *fornix,* arch]. Arched or vaulted.

for·ni·ca·tion (for"ni·kay'shun) *n.* [L. *fornicari,* to fornicate, from *fornix,* vaulted dwelling, brothel]. Legally, coitus between unmarried persons. —**for·ni·cate** (for'ni·kate) *v.*

for·nix (for'nicks) *n.,* genit. **for·ni·cis** (for'ni·sis), pl. **forni·ces** (·seez) [L., arch, vault]. An arched body or surface; a concavity or cul-de-sac. See also Plate 18.

fornix ce·re·bri (serr'e·brye) [NA]. An arched fiber tract lying under the corpus callosum; anteriorly it divides into two columns, projecting mainly to the mamillary bodies; posteriorly it divides into two crura, projecting mainly to the hippocampus on each side.

fornix con·junc·ti·vae inferior (kon"junk·tye'vee) [NA]. The line of reflection of the conjunctiva from the lower eyelid onto the eyeball. Syn. *inferior fornix.*

fornix conjunctivae superior [NA]. The line of reflection of the conjunctiva from the upper eyelid to the eyeball. Syn. *superior fornix.*

fornix of the conjunctiva. The cul-de-sac at the line where the bulbar conjunctiva is reflected upon the lid.

fornix of the stomach. FUNDUS VENTRICULI.

fornix of the vagina. The vault of the vagina; the upper part of the vagina which surrounds the cervix of the uterus. May be divided into anterior, posterior, and lateral in relation to the cervix. NA *fornix vaginae.*

fornix pha·ryn·gis (fa·rin'jis) [NA]. The extreme upper portion of the pharynx.

fornix sac·ci la·cri·ma·lis (sack'eye lack·ri·may'lis, sack'sigh) [NA]. The extreme upper part of the lacrimal sac.

fornix va·gi·nae (va·jye'nee) [NA]. FORNIX OF THE VAGINA.

Foroblique. Trademark for a lens system used in a cystoscope that permits observation of instrument use during certain operations.

Fors·gren method. A histochemical method for bile acids, treating the tissue with barium chloride, acid fuchsin, phosphomolybdic acid, and aniline blue-orange G stain to obtain reddish-blue granules.

Forss·man antigens (fors'mahnn) [W. T. O. *Forssman*, German surgeon, b. 1904]. A widely distributed group of heterophil antigens that are thermostable and carbohydrate lipoprotein complex in structure; found in sheep red blood cells, in the tissue of many animals, in bacteria, and in plant cells, but absent in some species, as the rabbit; and detectable by the induction of antibodies reacting with sheep red blood cells by antigens from genetically unrelated species.

Fort Bragg fever [after *Fort Bragg*, N. Carolina]. PRETIBIAL FEVER.

Forthane. Trademark for methylhexamine, a volatile amine employed for vasoconstrictor action on nasal mucosa.

fortification spectrum. SCINTILLATING SCOTOMA.

for·ward failure. Left heart failure in which symptoms result predominantly from low cardiac output; there is weakness and fatigue.

fos·az·e·pam (fos-az'e-pam) *n.* 7-Chloro-1-[(dimethylphosphinyl)methyl]-1,3-dihydro-5-phenyl-2*H*-1,4-benzodiazepin-2-one, $C_{18}H_{18}ClN_2O_2P$, a hypnotic.

fos·fo·my·cin (fos''fo-migh'sin) *n.* (−)-(1*R*,2*S*)-(1,2-Epoxypropyl)phosphonic acid, $C_3H_7O_4P$, an antibiotic produced by *Streptomyces fradiae.*

fos·fo·net (fos'fo-net) *n.* Phosphonoacetic acid, monohydrate, $C_2H_5O_5 \cdot H_2O$, an antiviral agent used as the disodium salt.

Fo·shay's test [L. *Foshay*, U. S. bacteriologist, 1896–1961]. A delayed skin test for the diagnosis of tularemia made by the intradermal injection of a killed suspension of *Francisella tularensis.* A local erythema is considered a positive reaction.

fos·pi·rate (fos'pi-rate) *n.* Dimethyl 3,5,6-trichloro-2-pyridyl phosphate, $C_7H_7C_3NO_4P$, a veterinary anthelmintic drug.

fos·sa (fos'uh) *n.*, pl. & genit. sing. **fos·sae** (-ee) [L., ditch]. A depression or pit.

fossa ace·ta·bu·li (as-e-tab'yoo-lye) [NA]. ACETABULAR FOSSA.

fossa ant·he·li·cis (ant-hel'i-sis) [NA]. A depression on the medial surface of the auricle overlying the anthelix.

fossa axil·la·ris (ack-si-lair'is) [NA]. Axillary fossa; AXILLA.

fossa cae·ca·lis (see-kay'lis) [BNA]. CECAL FOSSA.

fossa ca·ni·na (ka-nye'nuh) [NA]. CANINE FOSSA.

fossa ca·ro·ti·ca (ka-rot'i-kuh) [BNA]. Trigonum caroticum (= SUPERIOR CAROTID TRIANGLE).

fossa ce·re·bri la·te·ra·lis [Sylvii] (serr'e-brye lat-e-ray'lis) [BNA]. FOSSA LATERALIS CEREBRI.

fossa con·dy·la·ris (kon-di-lair'is) [NA]. CONDYLAR FOSSA.

fossa con·dy·loi·dea (kon-di-loy'dee-uh) [BNA]. Fossa condylaris (= CONDYLAR FOSSA).

fossa co·ro·noi·dea (kor-uh-noy'dee-uh) [NA]. CORONOID FOSSA.

fossa cra·nii anterior (kray'nee-eye) [NA]. ANTERIOR CRANIAL FOSSA.

fossa cranii me·dia (mee'dee-uh) [NA]. MIDDLE CRANIAL FOSSA.

fossa cranii posterior [NA]. POSTERIOR CRANIAL FOSSA.

fossa cu·bi·ta·lis (kew-bi-tay'lis) [NA]. ANTECUBITAL FOSSA.

fossa di·gas·tri·ca (dye-gas'tri-kuh) [NA]. DIGASTRIC FOSSA (1).

fossa duc·tus ve·no·si (duck'tus ve-no'sigh) [NA]. A narrow groove on the posterior surface of the liver between the caudate and left lobes, occupied by the ductus venosus in fetal life and by the ligamentum venosum after birth.

fossa epi·gas·tri·ca (ep-i-gas'tri-kuh) [NA]. EPIGASTRIC FOSSA.

fossae sa·git·ta·les dex·trae he·pa·tis (saj-i-tay'leez decks'tree hep'uh-tis) [BNA]. The longitudinal grooves in the right lobe of the liver.

fossa glan·du·lae la·cri·ma·lis (glan'dew-lee lack-ri-may'lis) [NA]. LACRIMAL FOSSA.

fossa hy·a·loi·dea (high-uh-loy'dee-uh) [NA]. HYALOID FOSSA.

fossa hy·po·phy·se·os (high-po-fiz'ee-os) [BNA]. Fossa hypophysialis (= HYPOPHYSEAL FOSSA).

fossa hy·po·phy·si·a·lis (high''po-fiz-ee-ay'lis) [NA]. HYPOPHYSEAL FOSSA.

fossa ili·a·ca (i-lye'uh-kuh) [NA]. ILIAC FOSSA.

fossa ili·a·co·sub·fas·ci·a·lis (i-lye''uh-ko-sub-fash''ee-ay'lis) [BNA]. A depression of the posterior abdominal wall between the psoas muscle and the iliac crest.

fossa ilio·pec·ti·nea (il''ee-o-peck-tin'ee-uh) [BNA]. A depression in the floor of the femoral triangle between the iliopsoas muscle and the pectineus muscle.

fossa in·ci·si·va (in-si-sigh'vuh) [NA]. INCISIVE FOSSA (1).

fossa in·cu·dis (ing-kew'dis) [NA]. A groove in the posterior wall of the tympanic cavity in which is lodged the short process of the incus.

fossa in·fra·spi·na·ta (in''fruh-spye-nay'tuh) [NA]. INFRASPINOUS FOSSA.

fossa in·fra·tem·po·ra·lis (in''fruh-tem-po-ray'lis) [NA]. INFRATEMPORAL FOSSA.

fossa in·gui·na·lis la·te·ra·lis (ing-gwi-nay'lis lat-e-ray'lis) [NA]. LATERAL INGUINAL FOSSA.

fossa inguinalis me·di·a·lis (mee-dee-ay'lis) [NA]. MEDIAL INGUINAL FOSSA.

fossa in·no·mi·na·ta (i-nom''i-nay'tuh). A shallow depression between the vestibular and the aryepiglottic folds of the larynx.

fossa in·ter·con·dy·la·ris (in''tur-kon-di-lair'is) [NA]. INTERCONDYLAR FOSSA.

fossa in·ter·con·dy·loi·dea an·te·ri·or ti·bi·ae (in''tur-kon-di-loy'dee-uh an-teer'ee-or tib'ee-ee) [BNA]. AREA INTERCONDYLARIS ANTERIOR TIBIAE.

fossa intercondyloidea fe·mo·ris (fem'o-ris) [BNA]. Fossa intercondylaris (= INTERCONDYLAR FOSSA).

fossa intercondyloidea posterior ti·bi·ae (tib'ee-ee) [BNA]. AREA INTERCONDYLARIS POSTERIOR TIBIAE.

fossa in·ter·pe·dun·cu·la·ris (in''tur-pe-dunk-yoo-lair'is) [NA]. INTERPEDUNCULAR FOSSA.

fossa is·chio·rec·ta·lis (is''kee-o-reck-tay'lis) [NA]. ISCHIORECTAL FOSSA.

fossa ju·gu·la·ris (jug-yoo-lair'is) [BNA]. A depression in the midline of the neck above the sternum.

fossa jugularis os·sis tem·po·ra·lis (os'is tem-po-ray'lis) [NA]. JUGULAR FOSSA.

fossa la·te·ra·lis ce·re·bri (lat-e-ray'lis serr'e-brye) [NA]. A depression on the lateral aspect of the cerebral hemisphere of the fetus; in the adult brain a portion remains as the lateral sulcus.

fossa mal·le·o·li la·te·ra·lis (ma-lee'o-lye lat-e-ray'lis) [NA]. DIGITAL FOSSA (3).

fossa man·di·bu·la·ris (man-dib''yoo-lair'is) [NA]. MANDIBULAR FOSSA.

fossa na·vi·cu·la·ris ure·thrae (na-vick''yoo-lair'is yoo-ree'three) [NA]. NAVICULAR FOSSA (2).

fossa navicularis ves·ti·bu·li va·gi·nae (ves-tib'yoo-lye va-jye'nee) [BNA]. Fossa vestibuli vaginae (= VESTIBULAR FOSSA OF THE VAGINA).

fossa oc·ci·pi·ta·lis (ock-sip''i-tay'lis). The portion of the posterior cranial fossa which is bounded by the inner surface of the occipital bone; it may be further subdivided into a superior occipital fossa lying above the groove for the transverse sinus and an inferior occipital fossa lying below the groove.

fossa of the ductus venosus. FOSSA DUCTUS VENOSI.

fossa of the incus. FOSSA INCUDIS.

fossa ole·cra·ni (o-le-kray'nigh) [NA]. OLECRANON FOSSA.

fossa ova·lis (o-vay'lis). 1. An oval depression in the interatrial septum; its floor is derived from the embryonic septum primum, and its rim (limbus) from the septum secundum. NA *fossa ovalis cordis.* 2. An opening in the fascia lata of the thigh which gives passage to the great saphenous vein. NA *hiatus saphenus.*

fossa ovalis cor·dis (kor'dis) [NA]. FOSSA OVALIS (1).

fossa ovalis fas·ci·ae la·tae (fash'ee·ee lay'tee) [BNA]. Hiatus saphenus (= FOSSA OVALIS (2)).

fossa ovalis femoris. FOSSA OVALIS (2).

fossa po·pli·tea (pop·lit'ee·uh) [NA]. POPLITEAL SPACE.

fossa prae·na·sa·lis (pree''na·say'lis) [BNA]. INCISIVE FOSSA (2).

fossa pte·ry·goi·dea (terr''i·goy'dee·uh) [NA]. PTERYGOID FOSSA.

fossa pte·ry·go·pa·la·ti·na (terr''i·go·pal·uh·tye'nuh) [NA]. PTERYGOPALATINE FOSSA.

fossa ra·di·a·lis (ray·dee·ay'lis) [NA]. RADIAL FOSSA.

fossa re·tro·man·di·bu·la·ris (ret''ro·man·dib·yoo·lair'is) [BNA]. The depression in the side of the neck below the auricle and behind the angle of the mandible.

fossa rhom·boi·dea (rom·boy'dee·uh) [NA]. RHOMBOID FOSSA.

fossa sac·ci la·cri·ma·lis (sack'eye lack·ri·may'lis) [NA]. The depression in the medial wall of the orbit in which is lodged the lacrimal sac.

fossa sa·git·ta·lis si·nis·tra he·pa·tis (saj·i·tay'lis si·nis'truh hep'uh·tis) [BNA]. The longitudinal groove in the left lobe of the liver.

fossa sca·phoi·dea (ska·foy'dee·uh) [NA]. SCAPHOID FOSSA (1).

fossa Scar·pae major (skahr'pee). FEMORAL TRIANGLE.

fossa se·mi·lu·na·ris (sem''i·lew·nair'is). TROCHLEAR NOTCH.

fossa sub·ar·cu·a·ta (sub·ahr''kew·ay'tuh) [NA]. SUBARCUATE FOSSA.

fossa sub·in·gui·na·lis (sub·ing''gwi·nay'lis) [BNA]. SUBINGUINAL FOSSA.

fossa sub·sca·pu·la·ris (sub·skap''yoo·lair'is) [NA]. SUBSCAPULAR FOSSA.

fossa su·pra·cla·vi·cu·la·ris major (sue''pruh·kla·vick·yoo·lair'is) [NA alt.]. TRIGONUM OMOCLAVICULARE.

fossa supraclavicularis minor [NA]. An indefinite depression in the base of the neck located above the clavicle between the two tendinous attachments of the sternocleidomastoid muscle.

fossa su·pra·spi·na·ta (sue''pruh·spye·nay'tuh) [NA]. SUPRASPINOUS FOSSA.

fossa su·pra·ton·sil·la·ris (sue''pruh·ton·si·lair'is) [NA]. SUPRATONSILLAR FOSSA.

fossa su·pra·ve·si·ca·lis (sue''pruh·ves·i·kay'lis) [NA]. A depression of the inner surface of the anterior abdominal wall between the median and medial umbilical folds.

fossa tem·po·ra·lis (tem·po·ray'lis) [NA]. TEMPORAL FOSSA.

fossa ton·sil·la·ris (ton·si·lair'is) [NA]. TONSILLAR FOSSA.

fossa tri·an·gu·la·ris au·ri·cu·lae (trye·ang''gew·lair'is aw·rick'yoo·lee) [NA]. TRIANGULAR FOSSA.

fossa tro·chan·te·ri·ca (tro''kan·terr'i·kuh) [NA]. TROCHANTERIC FOSSA.

fossa ve·nae ca·vae (vee'nee kay'vee) [BNA]. SULCUS VENAE CAVAE.

fossa venae um·bi·li·ca·lis (um·bil·i·kay'lis) [BNA]. FISSURA LIGAMENTI TERETIS.

fossa ve·si·cae fel·le·ae (ve·sigh'kee fel'ee·ee, ve·sigh'see) [NA]. CYSTIC FOSSA.

fossa ve·sti·bu·li va·gi·nae (ves·tib'yoo·lye va·jye'nee) [NA]. VESTIBULAR FOSSA OF THE VAGINA.

fos·sette (fos·et') *n.* [F., dim. of *fosse,* canal, ditch]. 1. A dimple; a small depression. 2. A small, deep ulcer of the cornea.

fossil wax. CERESIN.

fos·su·la (fos'yoo·luh) *n.*, pl. **fossu·lae** (·lee) [L., little ditch]. A small fossa.

fossulae ton·sil·la·res ton·sil·lae pa·la·ti·nae (ton·si·lair'eez ton·sil'ee pal·uh·tye'nee) [NA]. The small pits on the surface of the palatine tonsil, which are the openings of the tonsillar crypts.

fossulae tonsillares tonsillae pha·ryn·ge·ae (fa·rin'jee·ee) [NA]. The openings of the crypts of the pharyngeal tonsil.

fossula fe·nes·trae coch·le·ae (fe·nes'tree kock'lee·ee) [NA]. The depression in the medial wall of the tympanic cavity surrounding the round window.

fossula fenestrae ves·ti·bu·li (ves·tib'yoo·lye) [NA]. The depression in the medial wall of the tympanic cavity surrounding the oval window.

fossula pe·tro·sa (pe·tro'suh) [NA]. A small depression on the inferior surface of the petrous part of the temporal bone between the jugular fossa and the external opening of the carotid canal.

fossula post fe·nes·tram (pohst fe·nes'tram). A small inconstant outpouching from the vestibule into the otic capsule just posterior to the fenestra vestibuli.

fossula rotunda. FENESTRA COCHLEAE.

Fos·ter Ken·ne·dy syndrome [*Foster Kennedy,* U. S. neurologist, 1884–1952]. Unilateral blindness and optic atrophy, contralateral papilledema, and sometimes anosmia, usually due to a frontal lobe or sphenoid crest tumor or abscess on the side of the atrophy.

foster nursing. Suckling of the young by an animal not the mother.

Fos·ter's rule [Balthazar *Foster,* 1840–1913]. The dictum that it is possible to predict from the radiation of the murmur of aortic regurgitation which aortic cusp is predominantly damaged.

Foth·er·gill's disease [J. *Fothergill,* English physician, 1712–1780]. TRIGEMINAL NEURALGIA.

Fou·chet's reagent (foo·sheh') [A. *Fouchet,* French physician, b. 1894]. A solution of trichloracetic acid and ferric chloride, used in urine bilirubin testing.

fou·droy·ant (foo·droy'unt) *adj.* [F.]. FULMINANT.

foudroyant gangrene. Infectious, fulminating, or spreading gangrene.

foun·der, *n. & v.* [OF. *fondrer,* to fall in]. 1. An acute gastroenteritis in cattle, horses, and sheep caused by the overeating of foods with a high caloric content. 2. Lameness in horses, especially that caused by laminitis. 3. To be afflicted with such lameness.

found·er principle. The principle that the fewer the founders of a new community are, the less representative they are likely to be of their old community's gene pool, and that therefore a population descended from a small group of ancestors may be expected to differ considerably in some gene frequencies from the population in which the ancestors originated.

found·ling, *n.* An infant found after being abandoned by its parents.

fountain decussation. DORSAL TEGMENTAL DECUSSATION (OF MEYNERT).

four·chette, four·chet (foor·shet') *n.* [F., *fork*]. 1. A fold of skin just inside the posterior commissure of the vulva. NA *frenulum labiorum pudendi.* 2. A fork used in dividing the frenulum of the tongue.

Four·neau 309 (foor·no') [E. F. A. *Fourneau,* French chemist and pharmacologist, 1872–1949]. SURAMIN SODIUM.

four-tailed bandage. A strip of cloth with the ends split, used to cover prominent parts, as the elbow, chin, nose, or knee.

fourth (IVth) cranial nerve. TROCHLEAR NERVE.

fourth disease. EXANTHEM SUBITUM.

fourth heart sound. The heart sound following atrial contraction, immediately preceding the first heart sound, to which it may sometimes contribute. Symbol, S_4, or SIV. Syn. *presystolic extra sound.*

fourth stomach. ABOMASUM.

fourth venereal disease. LYMPHOGRANULOMA VENEREUM.

fourth ventricle. The cavity that overlies the pons and medulla and extends from the central canal of the upper cervical spinal cord to the aqueduct of the midbrain. Its roof is the cerebellum and the superior and inferior medullary vela and its floor is the rhomboid fossa. NA *ventriculus quartus.*

fo·vea (fo'vee·uh) *n.*, pl. **fo·ve·ae** (·vee·ee) [L.]. 1. A small pit or depression. 2. *In ophthalmology,* FOVEA CENTRALIS.

fovea ar·ti·cu·la·ris in·fe·ri·or at·lan·tis (ahr·tick″yoo·lair'is in·feer'ee·or at·lan'tis) [NA]. Either of the inferior articular surfaces of the atlas.

fovea articularis superior atlantis [NA]. Either of the superior articular surfaces of the atlas.

fovea ca·pi·tis fe·mo·ris (kap'i·tis fem'o·ris) [NA]. FOVEA OF THE HEAD OF THE FEMUR.

fovea ca·pi·tu·li ra·dii (ka·pit'yoo·lye ray'dee·eye) [BNA]. FOVEA OF THE HEAD OF THE RADIUS.

fovea cen·tra·lis (sen·tray'lis) [NA]. The small depression, measuring approximately 1.85 mm in diameter with a floor of 0.4 mm in the center of the macula lutea of the retina. Its center is 4.0 mm temporal and 0.8 mm inferior to the center of the optic disk.

fovea cos·ta·lis inferior (kos·tay'lis) [NA]. INFERIOR COSTAL FACET. See also *costal fossae.*

fovea costalis superior [NA]. SUPERIOR COSTAL FACET. See also *costal fossae.*

fovea costalis trans·ver·sa·lis (trans·vur·say'lis) [NA]. The facet on the transverse process of a thoracic vertebra for articulation with the tubercle of the corresponding rib.

fovea den·tis at·lan·tis (den'tis at·lan'tis) [NA]. The facet on the posterior (inner) surface of the anterior arch of the atlas which articulates with the dens of the axis.

foveae ar·ti·cu·la·res in·fe·ri·o·res at·lan·tis (ahr·tick·yoo·lair'eez in·feer·ee·o'reez at·lan'tis). Plural of *fovea articularis inferior atlantis.*

fovea hemi·el·lip·ti·ca (hem″ee·e·lip'ti·kuh). ELLIPTICAL RECESS.

fovea he·mi·sphe·ri·ca (hem″i·sfeer'i·kuh). SPHERICAL RECESS.

fovea inferior [NA]. INFERIOR FOVEA.

fovea in·gui·na·lis la·te·ra·lis (ing″gwi·nay'lis lat·e·ray'lis) [BNA]. Fossa inguinalis lateralis (= LATERAL INGUINAL FOSSA).

fovea inguinalis me·di·a·lis (mee·dee·ay'lis) [BNA]. Fossa inguinalis medialis (= MEDIAL INGUINAL FOSSA).

fo·ve·al (fo'vee·ul) *adj.* [*fovea* + *-al*]. 1. Pertaining to a fovea, especially the fovea centralis. 2. Like a fovea; pitted.

foveal reflex. FOVEOLAR REFLEX.

fovea nu·chae (new'kee) [BNA]. The depression at the back of the neck in the midline.

fovea ob·lon·ga car·ti·la·gi·nis ary·te·noi·de·ae (ob·long'guh kahr·ti·laj'i·nis ăr″i·tee·noy'dee·ee) [NA]. An oblong depression on the lateral surface of the arytenoid cartilage.

fovea of the head of the femur. The depression giving attachment to the ligamentum capitis femoris. NA *fovea capitis femoris.*

fovea of the head of the radius. The depression for articulation with the capitulum of the humerus.

fovea of the pharynx. An anomalous depression in the median line of the pharynx.

fovea pa·la·ti·na (pal·uh·tye'nuh). FOVEOLA PALATINA.

fovea pte·ry·goi·dea man·di·bu·lae (terr·i·goy'dee·uh man·dib'yoo·lee) [NA]. A small depression on the anterior aspect of the neck of the mandible where the lateral pterygoid muscle is inserted.

fovea pterygoidea pro·ces·sus con·dy·loi·dei (pro·ses'us kon·di·loy'dee·eye) [BNA]. FOVEA PTERYGOIDEA MANDIBULAE.

fovea sa·cro·coc·cy·gea (say″kro·kock·sij'ee·uh). COCCYGEAL FOVEOLA.

fovea sub·lin·gua·lis (sub″ling·gway'lis) [NA]. SUBLINGUAL FOSSA.

fovea sub·man·di·bu·la·ris (sub″man·dib·yoo·lair'is) [NA]. SUBMANDIBULAR FOSSA.

fovea sub·max·il·la·ris (sub·mack·si·lair'is) [BNA]. Fovea submandibularis (= SUBMANDIBULAR FOSSA).

fovea superior [NA]. SUPERIOR FOVEA.

fovea su·pra·ve·si·ca·lis pe·ri·to·naei (sue″pruh·ves·i·kay'lis perr·i·to·nee'eye) [BNA]. FOSSA SUPRAVESICALIS.

fo·ve·ate (fo'vee·ut, ·ate) *adj.* FOVEAL.

fovea tri·an·gu·la·ris car·ti·la·gi·nis ary·te·noi·de·ae (trye·ang″gew·lair'is kahr″ti·laj'i·nis ăr″i·tee·noy'dee·ee) [NA]. TRIANGULAR FOVEA; a depression on the lateral surface of the arytenoid cartilage.

fovea tro·chle·a·ris (trock·lee·air'is) [NA]. TROCHLEAR FOVEA.

fo·ve·o·la (fo·vee'o·luh) *n.*, pl. **foveo·lae** (·lee), **foveolas** [dim. of *fovea*]. 1. A small fovea or depression. 2. The basal part of the fovea centralis of the retina, containing closely packed, elongated cones.

foveola coc·cy·gea (kock·sij'ee·uh) [NA]. COCCYGEAL FOVEOLA.

foveolae gas·tri·cae (gas'tri·see) [NA]. GASTRIC FOVEOLAE.

foveolae gra·nu·la·res (gran·yoo·lair'eez) [NA]. GRANULAR FOVEOLAE.

foveola pa·la·ti·na (pal·uh·tye'nuh). One of a pair of small depressions in the mucous membrane at the boundary between hard and soft palate, into which several palatine glands open.

fo·ve·o·lar (fo·vee'uh·lur) *adj.* Of or pertaining to a foveola.

foveolar reflex. The bright reflection of light seen with the ophthalmoscope when it is directed upon the fovea. Syn. *foveal reflex.*

fo·ve·o·late (fo·vee'uh·late, ·lut) *adj.* FOVEOLAR.

Fo·ville's paralysis or **syndrome** (fo^h·veel') [A. L. F. *Foville,* French neurologist, 1799–1878]. Seventh- and often sixth-nerve palsy with contralateral hemiplegia and loss of movement of the other eye in attempting to look toward the side of the lesion.

fowl cholera. An often fatal disease of domestic poultry and wild birds, caused by *Pasteurella multocida,* characterized by enteritis, submucosal hemorrhages and vascular congestion.

Fow·ler's position [G. R. *Fowler,* U. S. surgeon, 1848–1906]. A semireclining or sitting position in bed, formerly used in the treatment of peritonitis.

Fowler's solution [T. *Fowler,* English physician, 1736–1801]. Potassium arsenite solution, containing the equivalent of 1% of As_2O_3; formerly frequently employed as a dosage form of arsenic and more recently employed as an antileukemic drug.

fowl paralysis. NEURAL LYMPHOMATOSIS.

fowl plague or **pest.** An acute septicemic disease of chickens, turkeys, and other avian species caused by one of the highly pathogenic myxoviruses of the avian influenza group and characterized by edema of the head, hemorrhage, and focal necrosis of various organs.

fowl pox. AVIAN POX in chickens and turkeys.

fowl typhoid. An infectious disease of domesticated birds, caused by *Salmonella gallinarum.*

fox·glove, *n.* DIGITALIS.

fox·hole arthritis. EPIDEMIC TROPICAL ACUTE POLYARTHRITIS.

FP Abbreviation for *flavin phosphate* (= RIBOFLAVIN 5′-PHOSPHATE).

Fr Symbol for francium.

frac·tion·al (frack'shun·ul) *adj.* 1. Pertaining to a fraction. 2. *In chemistry,* divided successively; applied to any one of the several processes for separating a mixture into its constituents through differences in solubility, boiling point, or other characteristic.

fractional caudal analgesia or **anesthesia.** CONTINUOUS CAUDAL ANESTHESIA.

fractional cultivation. FRACTIONATION (2).

fractional distillation. Separation of a liquid into its components by means of gradually increasing temperature, the different products being vaporized in the order of their respective boiling points.

fractional pneumoencephalography. A technique of lumbar pneumoencephalography in which small quantities, usually 5 to 10 ml, of air are injected at a time into the subarachnoid space with different radiographic views made after each injection. This technique serves to obtain better visualization of various cerebral structures and to lessen the possible complications of pressure changes following the rapid replacement of large amounts of cerebrospinal fluid by air.

fractional precipitation. The separation of substances by precipitating them in increasing order of solubility.

fractional spinal anesthesia. CONTINUOUS SPINAL ANESTHESIA.

fractional sterilization. Sterilization by the intermittent application of steam, as in an Arnold sterilizer, on 3 successive days to permit heat-resistant spores to develop into heat-susceptible vegetative forms.

fractional ultrafiltration. Separation of colloidal particles or macromolecules into certain magnitude ranges by means of ultrafilters of varied pore size.

fractionate contraction. *Obsol.* Contraction of fractions of heart muscle.

frac·tion·a·tion (frack″shun·ay′shun) *n.* 1. *In chemistry,* the separation of a mixture into its constituents, as in fractional distillation. 2. *In microbiology,* the process of obtaining a pure culture by successive culturing of small portions of a colony. Syn. *fractional cultivation.* 3. *In physiology,* the phenomenon whereby maximal stimulation of a given efferent nerve innervating a limb does not evoke as powerful a muscular contraction as direct stimulation of the muscles themselves. Thus the fractionation phenomenon occurs within the motor neuron pool of the spinal cord. —**frac·tion·ate** (frack′shun·ate) *v. & adj.*

fractionation radiation. A method of administration of roentgen rays or other ionizing radiation in fractions of the total dose spread over a period of days.

frac·ture (frack′chur) *n. & v.* [L. *fractura,* from *frangere,* to break (rel. to Gmc. *brekan* → E. *break*)]. 1. A break in a bone, cartilage, tooth, or solid organ, such as the spleen, usually caused by trauma.

fracture bed. A bed especially devised for patients with broken bones.

fracture box. A wooden case for immobilizing fractures of the leg.

fracture by contrecoup. A fracture of the skull caused by transmitted violence to the cranial vault, causing a break at a point distant from, and usually opposite, the site of trauma.

fracture dislocation. A dislocation accompanied by a fracture.

frad·i·cin (frad′i·sin) *n.* An antibiotic substance isolated from cultures of *Streptomyces fradiae;* it is active against certain fungi.

Fraen·kel's glands (frenk′ul) [B. *Fraenkel,* German laryngologist, 1837–1911]. Minute mixed glands immediately inferior to the vocal folds.

Fraenkel's nodule [C. *Fraenkel,* German bacteriologist, 1861–1915]. TYPHUS NODULE.

Fraent·zel murmur. A diastolic murmur of mitral stenosis, which is louder at the beginning and end of diastole than in mid-diastole.

fraenula. FRENULA.

fraenulum. FRENULUM.

fraenum. FRENUM.

fra·gil·i·tas (fra·jil′i·tas) *n.* [L.]. Brittleness.

fragilitas cri·ni·um (krye′nee·um). Atrophic condition of the hair in which individual hairs split into numerous fibrils or break off.

fragilitas os·si·um (os′ee·um). OSTEOGENESIS IMPERFECTA.

fra·gil·i·ty (fra·jil′i·tee) *n.* The quality of being easily broken or destroyed. —**frag·ile** (fraj′il) *adj.*

fragility test. 1. A test of osmotic fragility of erythrocytes. 2. A test of integrity of blood capillaries.

frag·men·ta·tion (frag″men·tay′shun) *n.* [L. *fragmentum,* a piece, from *frangere,* to break]. 1. Division into small portions. 2. AMITOSIS.

fram·be·sia, fram·boe·sia (fram·bee′zhuh, ·zee·uh) *n.* [NL., from F. *framboise,* raspberry]. YAWS.

fram·be·si·form (fram·bee′si·form) *adj.* Pertaining to or like frambesia; said especially of a cutaneous eruption simulating or identical to that of yaws.

Frame, Rus·sell, and Wil·hel·mi's method. A method for amino-acid nitrogen in which the amino nitrogen groups in a protein-free blood filtrate combine with β-naphthoquinone sulfonate to form highly colored compounds which may be compared colorimetrically with a standard.

frame·shift mutation. A mutation in which nucleotide deletion or addition in DNA is not a multiple of three, thereby causing all subsequently transcribed codons to be misread.

Fran·ces·chet·ti syndrome. MANDIBULOFACIAL DYSOSTOSIS.

Fran·ci·sel·la (fran″si·sel′uh) *n.* [E. *Francis,* U. S. bacteriologist, 1872–1957]. The genus of pleomorphic, nutritionally fastidious, cytotropic gram-negative rods, belonging to the family Brucellaceae, of which the type species is *Francisella tularensis.*

Francisella tu·la·ren·sis (too″luh·ren′sis). The causative organism of tularemia in wild mammals, birds, and insects, transmissible to man. Formerly designated *Pasteurella tularensis.*

Fran·cis test [T. *Francis,* Jr., U. S. pathologist, 1900–1969]. An immunologic skin test for determining the presence or absence of antibody in pneumococcal pneumonia, performed by the intradermal injection of the type specific capsular polysaccharide.

fran·ci·um (fran′see·um) *n.* [after *France*]. Fr = 223. Element number 87. Formerly called *virginium.* See also Table of Elements in the Appendix.

Fran·çois' syndrome (frah^{n}·swah′) [J. *François,* Belgian ophthalmologist, 20th century]. HALLERMANN-STREIFF-FRANÇOIS SYNDROME.

fran·gu·la (frang′gew·luh) *n.* [NL., from L. *frangere,* to break]. The bark of *Rhamnus frangula,* or glossy buckthorn. The fresh bark is strongly irritant and causes violent catharsis; when dried it is laxative.

fran·gu·lin (frang′gew·lin) *n.* 4,5,7-Trihydroxy-2-methylanthraquinone-L-rhamnoside, $C_{21}H_{20}O_9$, a glycoside occurring in *Rhamnus* species. On hydrolysis it yields emodin and L-rhamnose.

fran·gu·lo·side (frang′gew·lo·side) *n.* FRANGULIN.

frank, *adj.* Unmistakable, obvious; applied to an unequivocal diagnosis of a fully developed disease state; clinically evident.

frank breech presentation. A breech presentation of the fetus with the buttocks alone presenting at the cervix with the hips flexed and the knees extended along the body so that the feet are near the head.

Frank·en·häu·ser's ganglion (frah^{h}nk′^{e}n·hoy″zur) [F. *Frankenhäuser,* German gynecologist, d. 1894]. GANGLION OF THE CERVIX UTERI.

Franke's method. BENEDICT AND FRANKE'S METHOD.

Frank·fort horizontal plane [after *Frankfurt*-am-Main, Germany, where it was adopted by the International Congress of Anthropologists in 1884]. An anthropometric plane for orienting heads of the living as well as skulls in a definite position, so that measurements and contours of a series will be comparable. The plane was defined as being determined by four points: the two poria and the two orbitalia. In anthropometric practice, only the two poria and left orbitale are used to determine the plane, since only in perfectly symmetrical heads or skulls would all four points fall in the plane. The plane was adopted because it can be determined easily on the living, making comparison between head and skull possible, and it approximates quite closely the position in which the head is carried during life.

frank·in·cense (frank'in·sence) *n.* [OF. *franc encens,* high quality incense]. An aromatic gum resin.

frank·lin·ic electricity (frank·lin'ick) [B. *Franklin,* U. S. statesman and scientist, 1706–1790]. Frictional or static electricity.

frank prolapse. Complete prolapse of the uterus and inversion of the vagina, with both structures hanging outside the vulva.

Frank's capillary toxicosis (frahnk) [A. E. *Frank,* German physician, b. 1884]. Nonthrombocytopenic purpura.

Frank's operation [R. *Frank,* Austrian surgeon, 1862–1913]. A type of gastrostomy in which a cone of stomach wall is brought through a high rectus incision and tunnel of skin, providing a valve-like function. Syn. *Sabaneev-Frank operation.*

Frank-Star·ling law of the heart (frahnk) [O. *Frank,* 19th century; and E. H. *Starling,* English physiologist, 1866–1927]. The force developed by cardiac contraction is proportional to the length of the myocardial fibers in diastole.

fra·ter·nal (fra·tur'nul) *adj.* [ML. *fraternalis,* from L. *frater,* brother]. 1. Of or pertaining to brothers or siblings. 2. Of twins, not identical.

fraternal twins. Twins resulting from the simultaneous fertilization of two ova. They may be of the same or opposite sex, have a different genetic constitution, and each has a separate chorion. Syn. *biovular twins, dizygotic twins.* Contr. *identical twins.*

frat·ri·cide (frat'ri·side) *n.* [L. *fratricidium* and *fratricida*]. 1. Murder of one's own sibling. 2. One who murders one's own sibling.

Fraun·ho·fer's lines (fraown'ho·fur) [J. von *Fraunhofer,* German optician, 1787–1826]. The dark lines of the sun's spectrum resulting from selective absorption by ions, atoms, and molecules in the outer atmosphere of the sun or in the earth's atmosphere.

frax·in (frack'sin) *n.* A glycoside, $C_{16}H_{18}O_{10}$, from the bark of the European ash, *Fraxinus excelsior;* it is diuretic.

FRC Abbreviation for *functional residual capacity.*

F.R.C.P. Fellow of the Royal College of Physicians.

F.R.C.P.E. Fellow of the Royal College of Physicians of Edinburgh.

F.R.C.P.I. Fellow of the Royal College of Physicians of Ireland.

F.R.C.S. Fellow of the Royal College of Surgeons.

F.R.C.S.E. Fellow of the Royal College of Surgeons of Edinburgh.

F.R.C.S.I. Fellow of the Royal College of Surgeons of Ireland.

freak, *n.* 1. *In medicine,* any organism that varies markedly, especially in its physical aspects, from the organisms of its kind or species; a mutation; a monster. 2. Any odd, startling, or unexpected phenomenon, idea, or event.

freck·le, *n.* A pigmented macule resulting from focal increase of melanin, usually associated with exposure to sunlight, commonly on the face. Syn. *ephelis.* See also *lentigo, melanotic freckle.*

Fre·det-Ram·stedt operation (fruh·deh', rahm'shtet) [P. *Fredet,* French surgeon, 1870–1946; and C. *Ramstedt*]. PYLOROMYOTOMY.

free-air ionization chamber. An ionization chamber in which the beam of radiation passes between the electrodes without striking them or other internal parts; the basic standard instrument for roentgen dosimetry.

free association. Spontaneous consciously unrestricted association of ideas or mental images, used to gain an understanding of the organization of the content of the mind in psychoanalysis.

free cell. A reticular cell detached from the reticular mesh and indistinguishable from a free macrophage.

free energy. The portion of the total potential energy of a natural system available for the performance of work.

free-floating anxiety. *In psychiatry,* severe, generalized, persistent anxiety which often precedes panic.

free gingiva. That portion of the marginal gingiva located on the facial and lingual aspects of the tooth.

free gingival groove. The dividing line between the free and attached gingiva.

free gingival margin. The most coronal edge of the free gingiva.

free graft. A graft of any type of tissue which is cut free and transplanted to another area.

free-living, *adj.* 1. Not parasitic or metabolically dependent on another organism. 2. Able to move from place to place; not sessile or permanently attached in one spot.

free macrophage. An actively ameboid macrophage found in the normal connective tissues and in areas of inflammation.

Free·man rule [Case of United States vs. Charles *Freeman,* 1966]. A standard of legal sanity recommended under the Model Penal Code of The American Law Institute, which holds that "a person is not responsible for criminal conduct if at the time of such conduct as a result of mental disease or defect he lacked substantial capacity either to appreciate the wrongfulness of his conduct or to conform his conduct to the requirements of law." Compare *M'Naghten rule, Durham decision.*

free·mar·tin (free'mahr"tin) *n.* An intersexual, usually sterile female calf twinborn with a male; produced by masculinization by sex hormones of the male twin when the placental circulations are partially fused.

free radical. A nonionic compound, highly reactive and of relatively short life, in which the central element is linked to an abnormal number of atoms or groups of atoms, and characterized by the presence of at least one unpaired electron.

free·way space. The distance between the occluding surfaces of the upper and lower teeth when the mandible is at rest.

freeze, *v.* To convert a liquid or gas to a solid by reduction of temperature.

freezing-drying process. Sudden cooling of tissue to very low temperatures and dehydration of the frozen material in a vacuum. The advantages of this method over use of fixing and dehydrating solutions are minimal chemical changes in tissue, a minimum of shifting of diffusible components, and a greater preservation of cytoplasmic inclusions. The freezing is usually carried out at a temperature below the eutectic point of water. Ice crystal formation is thereby avoided and the tissue protected against tearing up and other damage or displacement. See also *lyophilization.*

freezing microtome. A microtome used for cutting frozen tissue, sometimes equipped with a cooling device for the knife or a cold chamber to encase the microtome. See also *cryostat.*

freezing point. The temperature at which a pure liquid is in equilibrium with its solid form, or at which the solid form of the solvent is in equilibrium with a solution.

Frei·berg's disease [A. H. *Freiberg,* U. S. surgeon, 1868–1940]. KÖHLER'S DISEASE (2).

Frei's disease (frye) [W. S. *Frei,* German dermatologist, 1885–1943]. LYMPHOGRANULOMA VENEREUM.

Frei test [W. S. *Frei*]. An intracutaneous test for immunologic changes resulting from infection with the virus of lymphogranuloma venereum, performed by injecting material processed from bubo pus or from infected mouse brain or chick embryo.

frem·i·tus (frem'i·tus) *n.* [L., murmur, roar]. A palpable vibration or thrill.

frena. A plural of *frenum.*

fre·nal (free'nul) *adj.* Of or pertaining to a frenum.

French digitalin. A glycosidal mixture said to consist of digitalin, digitonin, and digitoxin.

French measles. RUBELLA.

fre·nec·to·my (fre·neck'tuh·mee) *n.* [*fren*um + *-ectomy*]. *In surgery,* removal of a frenum.

fre·not·o·my (fre·not'uh·mee) *n.* [*fren*um + *-tomy*]. The cutting of any frenum, particularly of the frenulum of the tongue for tongue-tie.

Frenquel. Trademark for azocyclonol, a drug used as the hydrochloride salt for control of psychotic symptoms.

frenula. Plural of *frenulum.*

frenula of the lips. The frenulum labii superioris and the frenulum labii inferioris.

fren·u·lum, frae·nu·lum (fren'yoo·lum, freen') *n.*, pl. **frenu·la, fraenu·la** (·luh) [dim. of L., *frenum,* bridle]. A small frenum; any small fold of mucous membrane or tissue that restrains a structure or part.

frenulum cli·to·ri·dis (kli·tor'i·dis) [NA]. FRENULUM OF THE CLITORIS.

frenulum la·bii in·fe·ri·o·ris (lay'bee·eye in·feer·ee·o'ris) [NA]. A fold of mucous membrane on the inside of the median portion of the lower lip attached to the gingiva.

frenulum labii su·pe·ri·o·ris (sue·peer·ee·o'ris) [NA]. A fold of mucous membrane on the inside of the median part of the upper lip attached to the gingiva.

frenulum la·bi·o·rum pu·den·di (lay·bee·o'rum pew·den'dye) [NA]. FOURCHETTE (1).

frenulum lin·guae (ling'gwee) [NA]. FRENULUM OF THE TONGUE.

frenulum of Giacomini [C. *Giacomini*]. BAND OF GIACOMINI.

frenulum of the clitoris. Either of two folds of skin coming from the labia minora and being united under the glans of the clitoris. NA *frenulum clitoridis.*

frenulum of the ileocecal valve. The fold at either extremity of the ileocecal valve formed by the union of the upper and lower lips of the valve. NA *frenulum valvae ileocecalis.*

frenulum of the prepuce. The fold on the lower surface of the glans penis connecting it with the prepuce. NA *frenulum preputii penis.*

frenulum of the pudendum. FOURCHETTE (1).

frenulum of the superior medullary velum. The thickened median portion of the anterior medullary velum. NA *frenulum veli medullaris superioris.*

frenulum of the tongue. The vertical fold of mucous membrane under the tongue. NA *frenulum linguae.*

frenulum of the velum. FRENULUM OF THE SUPERIOR MEDULLARY VELUM.

frenulum pre·pu·tii pe·nis (pree·pew'shee·eye pee'nis) [NA]. FRENULUM OF THE PREPUCE.

frenulum val·vae ileo·ce·ca·lis (val'vee il''ee·o·see·kay'lis) [NA]. FRENULUM OF THE ILEOCECAL VALVE.

frenulum val·vu·lae co·li (val'vu·lee ko'lye) [BNA]. Frenulum valvae ileocecalis (= FRENULUM OF THE ILEOCECAL VALVE).

frenulum ve·li me·dul·la·ris an·te·ri·o·ris (vee'lye med·yoo·lair'is an·teer·ee·o'ris) [BNA]. Frenulum veli medullaris superioris (= FRENULUM OF THE SUPERIOR MEDULLARY VELUM).

frenulum veli medullaris su·pe·ri·o·ris (sue·peer·ee·o'ris) [NA]. FRENULUM OF THE SUPERIOR MEDULLARY VELUM.

fre·num, frae·num (free'num) *n.*, pl. **frenums, fraenums, fre·na, frae·na** (·nuh) [L., bridle]. A fold of integument or mucous membrane that checks or limits the movements of any organ. See also *frenulum.*

fren·zy, *n.* [MF. *frenesie,* from ML. *phrenesia*]. 1. Violent temporary mental derangement; the manic phase of manic-depressive illness. 2. Delirious excitement.

Freon. Trademark for a group of halogenated hydrocarbons containing one or more fluorine atoms; widely used as refrigerants and propellants for the dispersion of insecticidal mists.

Freon 11. A trademark for trichloromonofluoromethane, an aerosol propellant.

Freon 12. Trademark for dichlorodifluoromethane, CCl_2F_2, used as a refrigerant and propellant.

fre·quen·cy, *n.* [L. *frequentia,* crowd, abundance, from *frequens,* crowded, frequent]. 1. The rate of occurrence of a periodic or cyclic process. 2. *In biometry,* the ratio of the number of observations falling within a classification group to the total number of observations made.

frequency coding. *In neurophysiology,* the coding of information in terms of nerve impulse frequency.

frequency distribution. *In biometry,* a statistical table showing the frequency, or number, of observations (as test scores, ages) falling in each of certain classification groups or intervals (as 10–19, 20–29).

Fre·rich's theory (freʸ'rikh) [F. T. von *Frerich,* German physician, 1819–1885]. The concept of the toxic action of ammonium carbamate as the cause of uremia.

Freud·i·an (froy'dee·un) *adj. & n.* [S. *Freud,* Austrian psychiatrist, 1856–1939]. 1. Pertaining to Freud, his psychoanalytic theories and methods. 2. A person, often a psychiatrist, who adheres to the basic tenets of Freud's theories and methods.

Freudian censor. CENSOR.

Freud·i·an·ism (froy'dee·un·iz·um) *n.* The psychoanalytic theories and psychotherapeutic methods developed by Freud and his followers.

Freud·ism (froy'diz·um) *n.* FREUDIANISM.

Freund·lich's adsorption equation or **isotherm** (froint'likh) [H. M. F. *Freundlich,* German chemist, 1880–1941]. An adsorption equation, $x/m = kc^n$, in which x is the amount of solute adsorbed at concentration c by mass m of adsorbent and k and n are constants.

Freund's adjuvant (froind) [J. *Freund,* Hungarian bacteriologist in U.S., 1890–1960]. An immunological adjuvant consisting of an emulsion of water in oil, and described as incomplete or complete depending on whether it is mixed with antigen only or with antigen and a killed microorganism (usually *Mycobacterium tuberculosis*).

Frey's syndrome [Lucie *Frey,* Polish physician, 20th century]. AURICULOTEMPORAL SYNDROME.

F.R.F.P.S. Fellow of the Royal Faculty of Physicians and Surgeons.

F.R.F.P.S.G. Fellow of the Royal Faculty of Physicians and Surgeons of Glasgow.

fri·a·ble (frye'uh·bul) *adj.* [L. *friare,* to break into small pieces]. Easily broken or crumbled.

friar's balsam. COMPOUND BENZOIN TINCTURE.

fric·tion (frick'shun) *n.* [L. *frictio,* from *fricare,* to rub]. 1. The act of rubbing, as the rubbing of the body for stimulation of the skin. 2. The resistance offered to motion between two contacting bodies. —**friction·al** (·ul) *adj.*

frictional coefficient. The coefficient for a particle moving through a medium is an indication of the viscous force opposing the motion of the particle and is mathematically represented as the ratio of the opposing force to the velocity.

frictional electricity. The electricity produced by friction.

friction burn. Superficial mechanical and thermal injury from friction, as rope burn of the hands.

friction fremitus. The vibrations produced by the rubbing together of two dry and often inflamed surfaces.

friction knot. DOUBLE KNOT.

friction rub, murmur, or **sound.** The sounds heard on auscultation produced by the rubbing of two dry or roughened surfaces, such as inflamed serous surfaces, upon each other.

Fri·de·rich·sen syndrome (free~~th~~'rick·sᵉn) [C. *Friderichsen,* Danish pediatrician, b. 1886]. WATERHOUSE-FRIDERICHSEN SYNDROME.

Frie·de·mann and Grae·ser's method. A method for lactic acid in which the glucose of the blood is removed and the lactic acid converted to acetaldehyde which is combined with sodium bisulfite. The bound sulfite is then determined iodometrically.

Frie·den·wald's nomogram. A method for computing the coefficient of scleral rigidity and the coefficient of aqueous outflow from the eye.

Fried·län·der cells (freet'len·dur) [C. *Friedländer*, German pathologist, 1847–1887]. The large clear connective-tissue cells of the uterine decidua.

Friedländer pneumonia [C. *Friedländer*]. Pneumonia caused by *Klebsiella pneumoniae.*

Friedländer's bacillus [C. *Friedländer*]. *KLEBSIELLA PNEUMONIAE.*

Fried·man test [M. *Friedman*, U.S. physiologist, b. 1903]. A pregnancy test in which a female rabbit is given an intravenous injection of urine from the patient. Formation of corpora hemorrhagica and corpora lutea in the ovaries indicates a positive test.

Fried·reich's ataxia (freed'rye'^kh) [N. *Friedreich*, German neurologist, 1825–1882]. A hereditary spinocerebellar degenerative disease beginning in childhood and characterized by ataxia, diminished or absent deep tendon reflexes, Babinski signs, dysarthria, nystagmus, scoliosis, and clubfoot. There is degeneration of lateral and posterior columns of the spinal cord and to a variable extent in the cerebellum and medulla.

Friedreich's change of note [N. *Friedreich*]. FRIEDREICH'S SIGN.

Friedreich's disease or **spasms** [N. *Friedreich*]. PARAMYOCLONUS MULTIPLEX.

Friedreich's sign [N. *Friedreich*]. A sign for cavitation of the lungs in which there is a lowering in pitch of the percussion note during inspiration.

Fried·rich-Brau·er operation (freed'ri^kh, braow'ur) [P. L. *Friedrich*, German surgeon, 1864–1916; and L. *Brauer*]. An extensive extrapleural thoracoplasty for lung collapse.

Fried's rule. SOLOMON'S RULE.

fright neurosis or **reaction.** An intense terror reaction to an external frightful situation, as an earthquake or a dangerous fire.

fri·gid·i·ty (fri·jid'i·tee) *n.* [L. *frigiditas*, from *frigidus*, cold]. Lack of libido or interest in sex, usually of psychic origin.

fri·go·ther·a·py (frig"o·therr'uh·pee, frye"go·) *n.* [L. *frigus*, cold, + *therapy*]. CRYOTHERAPY.

fringe, *n.* [OF., from L. *fimbria*, fringe]. One of a number of bands, light or dark, produced by the interference of light.

fringe-tree bark. CHIONANTHUS.

Frisch's bacillus [A. R. von *Frisch*, Austrian surgeon and bacteriologist, 1849–1917]. *KLEBSIELLA RHINOSCLEROMATIS.*

frit fly. Any of various flies of the *Oscinidae.*

Froeh·lich's syndrome (frœh'li^kh) [A. *Froehlich*, Austrian physician, 1871–1953]. ADIPOSOGENITAL DYSTROPHY.

frog, *n.* 1. Any of various tailless, smooth-skinned, web-footed amphibians, primarily of the family Ranidae. 2. An elastic, horny pad, in the middle of the sole of a horse's hoof; it is triangular in shape and serves to separate the two bars.

frog-belly, *n.* The flaccid abdomen of children suffering from rickets as well as other diseases.

frog face. A facial deformity due to growth of polyps or other tumors in the nasal cavities. A temporary condition of this kind may be due to orbital cellulitis or facial erysipelas.

frog position or **posture.** An attitude frequently assumed by premature infants and infants with various central nervous system diseases, especially those resulting in flaccid paralysis, in which the lower extremities are kept flexed and externally rotated at the hips and flexed at the knees.

frog test. A pregnancy test in which urine containing chorionic gonadotropin is injected into the dorsal lymph sac of the male leopard frog (*Rana pipiens*). If spermatozoa are demonstrable in the frog's urine within 3 hours after injection, the test is positive.

Frohde's reagent. A 0.1% solution of sodium molybdate in concentrated sulfuric acid; used for detection of alkaloids.

Froin's syndrome [G. *Froin*, Austrian physician, b. 1874]. A sign of spinal subarachnoid block in which the cerebrospinal fluid below the lesion shows xanthochromia, few or no cells, hyperglobulinemia, and spontaneous clotting.

frôle·ment (frole"mahn') *n.* [F., from *frôler*, to graze, brush]. 1. A succession of slow, brushing movements in massage, done with the palmar surfaces of the hand. 2. A rustling sound sometimes heard on auscultation in pericardial disease.

Fro·ment's sign (fro^h·mah^n') [J. *Froment*, French physician, 20th century]. In ulnar paralysis, when the patient tries to hold a piece of paper between the thumb and first finger on the affected side, flexion of the thumb is substituted for adduction to compensate for paralysis of the adductor pollicis.

From·mel's disease [R. *Frommel*, German gynecologist, 1854–1912]. Atrophy of the uterus sometimes occurring after prolonged lactation.

Frommel's operation [R. *Frommel*]. Shortening of the uterosacral ligaments for correction of uterine retroversion or retroflexion.

frons (fronz) *n.*, genit. **fron·tis** (fron'tis) [NA]. FOREHEAD.

front·ad (frun'tad) *adv.* Toward the frontal aspect or toward the forehead.

fron·tal (frun'tul) *adj.* [L. *frontalis*, from *frons*, forehead]. 1. In humans, pertaining to the anterior part or aspect of an organ or body. 2. Pertaining to the forehead.

frontal adversive field. A zone in the frontal cortex (intermediate precentral region near the midline or area 6a beta), electrical stimulation of which causes a turning of the head and eyes and sometimes the body to the contralateral side.

frontal angle. The angle determined by connecting the point that lies highest in the sagittal curvature of the frontal bone by straight lines with the nasion and bregma, respectively. This angle is greater in a skull with a low, receding forehead. NA *angulus frontalis ossis parietalis.*

frontal arc. The measurement from the nasion to the bregma.

frontal arch. *In comparative anatomy*, the ring formed by the presphenoid, orbitosphenoid, and frontal bones.

frontal ataxia. BRUNS' ATAXIA.

frontal bone. A large cranial bone including the squama-frontalis, the superciliary arches, the glabella, and part of the roofs of the orbitual and nasal cavities. NA *os frontale.* See also Table of Bones in the Appendix and Plate 1.

frontal bossing. Abnormal or excessive frontal protuberance, as in hydrocephalus.

frontal crest. A vertical ridge along the middle line of the internal surface of the frontal bone. NA *crista frontalis.*

frontal eminence. One of two rounded elevations of the frontal bone above the superciliary ridges.

frontal eye field. A region which in man occupies principally the caudal part of the middle frontal gyrus (parts of Brodmann's area 8) and extends into contiguous portions of the inferior frontal gyrus, stimulation of which causes conjugate deviation of the eyes usually to the opposite side. Unilateral lesions of the frontal lobe involving the frontal eye field usually cause the eyes to be turned toward the side of the lesion. Compare *occipital eye field.*

frontal foramen. A foramen commonly present in the supraorbital margin of the frontal bone. NA *foramen frontale.*

frontal gyrectomy. Surgical excision of a block of cortex, bilaterally, from the frontal lobes of the brain, formerly used as a treatment for certain mental illnesses.

frontal internal hyperostosis. HYPEROSTOSIS FRONTALIS INTERNA.

fron·ta·lis (frun·tah'lis, fron·tay'lis) *n.* The frontal portion of the epicranius.

frontal lobe. The part of the cerebral hemisphere in front of the central sulcus and above the lateral cerebral sulcus. NA *lobus frontalis.* See also Plates 16, 17.

frontal lobotomy. PREFRONTAL LOBOTOMY.

frontal nerve. A somatic sensory nerve, attached to the ophthalmic nerve, which innervates the skin of the upper eyelid, the forehead, and the scalp. NA *nervus frontalis.* See also Table of Nerves in the Appendix.

frontal notch. A notch in the superior orbital margin, medial to the supraorbital notch, which transmits the frontal artery and nerve. NA *incisura frontalis.*

frontal operculum. The portion of the frontal lobe which overlies the insula. NA *operculum frontale.*

frontal plane. 1. Any plane parallel with the long axis of the body and perpendicular to the sagittal plane, dividing the body of bipeds into front and back parts. 2. The plane of the limb leads in electrocardiography. 3. The plane defined by combining the Y, or vertical, lead with the X, or horizontal, lead in vectorcardiography.

frontal plate. In the fetus, a cartilaginous plate interposed between the lateral parts of the ethmoid cartilage and the lesser wings and anterior portion of the sphenoid bone.

frontal pole. The tip of the frontal lobe of the cerebrum. NA *polus frontalis.*

frontal process. 1. A prismatic extension from the body of the maxilla, forming part of the medial margin of the orbit and of the lateral side of the nasal cavity. NA *processus frontalis maxillae.* 2. The frontosphenoid process of the zygomatic bone.

frontal protuberance. The prominence of the frontal bone.

frontal region. The area or surface of the forehead. NA *regio frontalis.*

frontal section. A section dividing the body or the head into dorsal and ventral parts.

frontal sinus. The paranasal sinus situated in the frontal bone. NA *sinus frontalis.* See also Plates 12, 20.

frontal spine. NASAL SPINE.

frontal sulcus. One of the longitudinal grooves separating the superior, middle, and inferior frontal gyri. See also *inferior frontal sulcus, superior frontal sulcus,* and Plate 18.

frontal suture. A suture which at birth joins the two frontal bones from the vertex to the root of the nose, but which afterward becomes obliterated. NA *sutura frontalis.*

frontal thalamic peduncle. See *thalamic peduncles.*

frontal vein. The diploic vein of the frontal bone. NA *vena diploica frontalis.*

fronto-. A combining form meaning (a) *frontal;* (b) *forehead.*

fron·to·eth·moid (frun″to·eth′moid) *adj.* Pertaining to the frontal and ethmoid bones.

frontoethmoid suture. A suture between the frontal and ethmoid bones. NA *sutura frontoethmoidalis.*

fron·to·lac·ri·mal (frun″to·lack′ri·mul) *adj.* Of or pertaining to the frontal bone and lacrimal bones.

frontolacrimal suture. The union between the frontal and lacrimal bones. NA *sutura frontolacrimalis.*

fron·to·ma·lar (frun″to·may′lur) *adj.* [*fronto-* + *malar*]. Pertaining to the frontal and zygomatic bones.

frontomalar suture. FRONTOZYGOMATIC SUTURE.

fron·to·max·il·lary (frun″to·mack′si·lerr″ee) *adj.* Pertaining to the frontal bone and the maxilla.

frontomaxillary suture. The union between the maxillary and the frontal bones. NA *sutura frontomaxillaris.*

fron·to·men·tal (frun″to·men′tul) *adj.* [*fronto-* + *mental*]. 1. Running from the top of the forehead to the point of the chin. 2. Pertaining to the forehead and chin.

fron·to·me·taph·y·se·al (frun″to·me·tuh·fiz′ee·ul, ·me·taf″i·see′ul) *adj.* Pertaining to the frontal bone and to the metaphyses of various bones.

fron·to·na·sal (frun″to·nay′zul) *adj.* Pertaining to the frontal and nasal bones.

frontonasal duct. NASOFRONTAL DUCT.

frontonasal process. The anterior region of the embryonic head that later develops into the frontal, median nasal, and lateral nasal processes. NA *nasofrontal process.*

frontonasal suture. The union between the nasal and frontal bones. NA *sutura frontonasalis.*

fron·to·oc·cip·i·tal (frun′to·ock·sip′i·tul) *adj.* OCCIPITOFRONTAL.

fron·to·pa·ri·e·tal (frun″to·pa·rye′e·tul) *adj.* PARIETOFRONTAL.

frontoparietal operculum. The portion of the cerebral cortex overlying the upper part of the insula. Syn. *operculum proper, parietal operculum.* NA *operculum frontoparietale.*

frontoparietal suture. CORONAL SUTURE.

fron·to·pon·tine (frun″to·pon′tine, ·teen) *adj.* [*fronto-* + *pontine*]. Pertaining to the frontal lobe of the cerebrum and the pons.

frontopontine tract. A tract of nerve fibers which arise in the frontal lobe of the cerebrum, descend from the cortex, pass through the internal capsule, and terminate in the pontine nuclei. NA *tractus frontopontinus.*

fron·to·pon·to·cer·e·bel·lar (frun″to·pon″to·serr″e·bel′ur) *adj.* Pertaining to the frontal lobe, the pons, and the cerebellum.

fron·to·sphe·noid (frun″to·sfee′noid) *adj.* Pertaining to the frontal and sphenoid bones.

frontosphenoid process. The thick, serrated, superior angle of the zygomatic bone which articulates with the zygomatic process of the frontal bone and with the great wing of the sphenoid. NA *processus frontalis ossis zygomatici.*

frontosphenoid suture. SPHENOFRONTAL SUTURE.

fron·to·tem·po·ral (frun″to·tem′pur·ul) *adj.* Pertaining to the frontal and temporal bones.

fron·to·tem·po·ra·le (fron″to·tem″po·ray′lee) *n.*, pl. **fronto·tempora·lia** (·lee·uh). *In craniometry,* the point on the superior temporal line on the zygomatic process of the frontal bone which is located most anteriorly and medially. The two frontotemporalia form the points of departure for measuring the least frontal diameter of the skull.

frontotemporal suture. The union between the temporal and frontal bones.

fron·to·zy·go·mat·ic (frun″to·zye·go·mat′ick) *adj.* Pertaining to the frontal and zygomatic bones.

frontozygomatic suture. The union between the frontal and zygomatic bones. NA *sutura frontozygomatica.*

front tap contraction or **reflex.** Contraction of the calf muscles when the muscles of the front of the extended leg are tapped.

Fro·riep's ganglion (fro′reep) [A. von *Froriep,* German anatomist, 1849–1917]. A fetal structure thought to be a rudimentary or vestigial dorsal root ganglion of the hypoglossal nerve.

Froriep's induration [R. *Froriep,* German surgeon, 1804–1861]. Fibrous myositis, usually secondary to inflammation.

frost·bite, *n.* Injury to skin and subcutaneous tissues, and in severe cases to deeper structures also, from exposure to extreme cold; blood vessel damage and cessation of local circulation lead to edema, vesiculation, and tissue necrosis.

frost itch. PRURITUS HIEMALIS.

froth stabilizer. Any of certain oils and chemicals which produce stable froths in water; they function best in the presence of finely divided solids.

frot·tage (frot·ahzh′) *n.* [F.]. 1. Massage, rubbing. 2. A form of masturbation in which orgasm is induced by rubbing against someone, especially in a crowd.

frot·teur (frot·ur′) *n.* [F.]. One who practices frottage to achieve sexual gratification.

fro·zen, *adj.* 1. Converted to a solid by reduction of temperature. 2. Stiff; not easily moved. 3. Not responsive to feeling; incapable of emotion.

frozen section. 1. A histologic section cut from frozen tissues or organs to permit rapid microscopic study. 2. In the teaching of gross anatomy, one of a series of divisions of the body or part which has been frozen before being sectioned.

frozen shoulder. A chronic tenosynovitis of unknown cause, associated with increased vascularity, degeneration, and fibrosis of collagen fibers in and about the shoulder joint, and characterized by pain and limitation of motion.

F.R.S. Fellow of the Royal Society.

F.R.S.E. Fellow of the Royal Society of Edinburgh.

fruc·to·fu·ran·o·san (fruck″to·few·ran′o·san) *n.* One of the polysaccharides of fructose.

fruc·to·fu·ra·nose (fruck″to·few′ruh·noce) *n.* A fructose with a 2, 5-butylene oxide or furanose ring.

fruc·to·fu·ran·o·side (fruck″to·few·ran′o·side) *n.* A glycoside of fructofuranose.

fruc·to·ki·nase (fruck″to·kigh′nace, ·naze) *n.* An enzyme catalyzing transfer of phosphate from a donor to fructose, forming fructose 1-phosphate.

fruc·to·py·ra·nose (fruck″to·pye′ruh·noce) *n.* A fructose with a 2, 6-pyranose ring.

fruc·to·san (fruck′to·san) *n.* A sugar anhydride which yields fructose on hydrolysis. Syn. *levulosan.*

fruc·tose (fruck′toce, frŏŏk′toce) *n.* L. [*fructus*, fruit, + *-ose*]. A monosaccharide, $C_6H_{12}O_6$, occurring as such in many fruits and obtainable also by hydrolysis of sucrose and inulin; a white, crystalline powder, freely soluble in water, at least as sweet as sucrose; used for parenteral alimentation. Syn. *fruit sugar, levulose.*

D-fructose. FRUCTOSE.

fructose 1,6-diphosphate. D-Fructose 1,6-diphosphoric acid, $C_6H_{14}O_{12}P_2$, an ester formed from fructose 6-phosphate and adenosine triphosphate in the presence of magnesium ion and phosphohexokinase; it is an intermediate in carbohydrate metabolism. Syn. *Harden-Young ester, hexosediphosphate.*

fructose intolerance. A hereditary disease characterized by vomiting, sweating, and aversion to fructose-containing foods.

fructose monophosphate. FRUCTOSE 6-PHOSPHATE.

fructose 1-phosphate. D-Fructose 1-phosphoric acid, $C_6H_{13}O_9P$, formed by the action of liver hexokinase upon fructose; presumably it is then converted to fructose 6-phosphate in the presence of phosphofructomutase.

fructose 6-phosphate. D-Fructose 6-phosphoric acid, $C_6H_{13}O_9P$, present in animal tissues in equilibrium with glucose 6-phosphate, into which it may be reversibly converted in the presence of phosphohexoisomerase; it is an intermediate in carbohydrate metabolism. Syn. *fructose monophosphate, hexose monophosphate, Neuberg ester.*

fruc·to·side (fruck′to·side) *n.* A glycoside that yields fructose on hydrolysis.

fruc·tos·uria (fruck″to·syoo′ree·uh) *n.* The presence of fructose in the urine. Syn. *levulosuria.*

fru·giv·o·rous (froo·jiv′uh·rus) *adj.* [L. *frux, frugis*, fruit, + *-vorous*]. Fruit-eating.

fruit, *n.* [OF., from L. *fructus*, proceeds, produce, fruit]. The developed ovary of a plant, including the succulent, fleshy parts gathered about it.

fruit fly. 1. Any of various small dipteran insects of the family Drosophilidae whose larvae feed on decaying fruit or fermenting sap. Those of the genus *Drosophila*, especially *Drosophila melanogaster*, are of great importance in genetic research. 2. Any of various small dipteran orchard pests of the family Trypetidae.

fruit sugar. FRUCTOSE.

fru·men·ta·ceous (froo″men·tay′shus) *adj.* [L. *frumentum*, grain, + *-aceous*]. Pertaining to or resembling grain.

fru·men·tum (froo·men′tum) *n.* [L.]. Wheat or other grain.

frus·tra·tion (frus·tray′shun) *n.* [L. *frustratio*, from *frustrare*, to disappoint, deceive]. 1. The condition that results when an impulse to act or the completion of an act is blocked or thwarted, preventing the satisfaction of attainment. 2. The blocking or thwarting of an impulse, purpose, or action. —**frus·trate** (frus′trate) *v.*

Frutabs. A trademark for fructose.

FSF Abbreviation for *fibrin-stabilizing factor* (= FACTOR XIII).

FSH Abbreviation for *follicle-stimulating hormone.*

ft Abbreviation for (a) in pharmacy, *fiat* or *fiant;* let there be made; (b) *foot.*

ft-lb Abbreviation for *foot-pound.*

ftor·a·fur (tor′uh·foor) *n.* 1-(Tetrahydrofuran-2-yl)-5-fluorouracil, $C_8H_9FN_2O_3$, a potential antineoplastic agent purported to be as efficaceous as 5-fluorouracil with much lower toxicity.

5-FU FLUOROURACIL.

Fuadin. Trademark for stibophen, an organic antimonial employed in the treatment of granuloma inguinale and of schistosomiasis.

Fuchs' combined dystrophy. FUCHS' DYSTROPHY.

Fuchs' dystrophy (fŏŏks) [E. *Fuchs*, Austrian ophthalmologist, 1851–1930]. A familial degenerative condition of the eye, beginning in late middle life and affecting more women than men, progressing from cornea guttata to edema of the epithelium with clouding of the corneal stroma and impaired corneal sensitivity to subepithelial connective-tissue formation and often complicated by glaucoma or infection.

fuch·sin (fook′sin, fyook′sin) *n.* [*fuchsia* + *-in*]. A red dyestuff which can be prepared in two forms, acid fuchsin and basic fuchsin.

fuchsin bodies. Inclusion bodies of keratohyalin, sometimes seen in the cytoplasm of epithelial tumor cells.

fuch·sin·o·phil (fyook·sin′o·fil, fŏŏk·) *adj.* [*fuchsin* + *phil*]. Stainable with fuchsin.

Fuchs' iridocyclitis [E. *Fuchs*]. HETEROCHROMIC UVEITIS.

Fuchs' phenomenon [E. *Fuchs*]. A paradoxical lid retraction associated with eye movements during the healing stage of oculomotor paralysis, characterized by spasmodic raising of the lid which had suffered from ptosis; attributed to aberrant regeneration of the oculomotor nerve.

Fucidin. Trademark for fusidic acid, a steroid antibiotic used as the salt sodium fusidate.

fu·co·san (few′ko·san) *n.* A polysaccharide yielding L-fucose, an aldohexose, upon hydrolysis. Occurs in the seaweed Japanese nori.

fu·cose (few′koce) *n.* 6-Deoxygalactose, $C_6H_{12}O_5$, an aldose terminating in a methyl group at the number 6 carbon atom, existing in D- and L- forms. D-Fucose is obtained by hydrolysis of convolvulin, jalapin, and other glycosides; L-fucose is a component of certain glycoproteins and occurs also in some seaweeds. Syn. D-*galactomethylose.*

fu·co·si·dase (few·ko′si·dace, ·daze) *n.* An enzyme, occurring in alpha- and beta- forms, that catalyzes normal metabolism of fucose and fucose-containing compounds.

fu·co·si·do·sis (few″ko·si·do′sis) *n.* A familial neurovisceral degenerative disease, due to the absence of the enzyme alpha-fucosidase, characterized by normal early development followed by progressive neurologic deterioration, cardiomegaly with myocarditis, thick skin, hyperhidrosis, and early death, with accumulation of fucose-containing sphingolipids and glycoprotein fragments in all tissues and of abnormal carbohydrates especially in brain and liver; inherited as an autosomal recessive trait.

fu·cus (few′kus) *n.* [L., from Gk. *phykos*, seaweed]. The dried thallus of *Fucus vesiculosus* and other common brown algae of the rockweed group. It contains a small amount of combined iodine, and has been used in the treatment of obesity.

FUDR. A trademark for floxuridine, an antineoplastic.

Fuer·bring·er's law (fu^e^r′bring·ur) [P. *Fuerbringer*, (*Fürbringer*), German physician, 1849–1930]. The embryologic origin of a muscle can be traced by its innervation.

Fuerbringer's sign or **test** [P. *Fuerbringer*]. Respiratory movement is transmitted to a needle inserted into a subphrenic abscess; the inserted needle does not move with respiration in an abscess above the diaphragm.

fu·ga·cious (few·gay′shus) *adj.* [L. *fugax, fugacis*, fleeting, transitory]. *In biology,* falling off, as petals after the full bloom of a flower.

-fugal [L. *fuga,* flight, fleeing]. A combining form meaning *tending or acting in a direction away from.*

-fuge [L. *fugare,* to put to flight]. A combining form meaning *that which causes to flee, or drives away.*

fu·gi·tive (few'ji·tiv) *adj.* [L. *fugitivus,* from *fugere,* to flee]. Wandering or transient; inconstant, as a pain.

fugue (fewg) *n.* [L. *fuga,* flight]. A dissociative reaction in hysterical neurosis characterized by amnesia of considerable duration and frequently flight from familiar surroundings. During the fugue, the patient appears to act in a conscious way and retains his mental faculties, but after recovery has no remembrance of the state.

fu·gu poison (foo'goo) [Japanese, globefish]. A toxic principle in the roe and other parts of certain fish of the *Tetrodon* genus, found in Japanese and other eastern Asiatic waters.

ful·gu·rant (ful'gew·runt) *adj.* FULGURATING.

fulgurant pains. LIGHTNING PAINS.

ful·gu·rate (ful'gew·rate) *v.* [L. *fulgurare,* to flash, lighten, from *fulgur,* lightning]. 1. To produce fulguration. 2. To wax and wane with lightning-like speed.

ful·gu·rat·ing (ful'gew·ray"ting) *adj.* Lightning-like; used to describe sudden, lancinating, excruciating pain.

ful·gu·ra·tion (ful"gew·ray'shun) *n.* Destruction of tissue, usually malignant tumors, by means of electric sparks.

fu·lig·i·nous (few·lij'i·nus) *adj.* [L. *fuliginosus,* sooty, from *fuligo,* soot]. Smokelike; very dark; soot-colored.

Ful·ler Al·bright syndrome. ALBRIGHT'S SYNDROME.

ful·ler's asthma. A pneumoconiosis due to the inhalation of lint and dust in the manufacture of wool cloth.

fuller's earth. A clay related to kaolin, and used similarly, as an adsorbent and protective.

Ful·ler's operation [E. *Fuller,* U.S. surgeon, 1858–1930]. *In surgery,* a procedure for drainage of the seminal vesicles.

full-thickness burn. THIRD-DEGREE BURN.

full-thickness graft. A skin graft including all layers of the skin. Syn. *Krause-Wolfe graft.*

Fulmicoton. A trademark for pyroxylin.

ful·mi·nant (ful'mi·nunt) *n.* [L. *fulminare,* to lighten, flash, from *fulmen,* thunderbolt]. Sudden, severe, intense, and rapid in course.

ful·mi·nat·ing (ful'mi·nay"ting) *adj.* FULMINANT.

fulminating adrenal meningitis. WATERHOUSE-FRIDERICHSEN SYNDROME.

Fulton splint. A splint used in the treatment of dislocation of the radius.

Fulvicin-U/F. A trademark for griseofulvin, an orally effective fungistatic antibiotic.

fu·ma·gil·lin (few"muh·jil'in) *n.* An antibiotic substance, $C_{26}H_{34}O_7$, produced by certain strains of *Asperigillus fumigatus,* occurring in light-yellow crystals, practically insoluble in water. It is highly active against *Entamoeba histolytica,* and is used in treating acute intestinal amebiasis.

fu·ma·rase (few'muh·race, ·raze) *n.* An enzyme occurring in bacteria, molds, yeasts, higher plants, and animals, particularly in liver and muscle. It is a specific catalyst for the conversion of fumaric acid (plus water) to L-malic acid.

fu·ma·rate (few'muh·rate, few·mar'ate) *n.* A salt or ester of fumaric acid.

Fu·mar·i·a·ce·ae (few·măr"ee·ay'see·ee) *n.pl.* A family of plants including the genera *Adlumia, Corydalis, Dicentra,* and *Fumaria;* by some authorities this family is ranked as a subfamily (Fumaroidae) of the Papaveraceae. Many alkaloids are found among the plants of the Fumariaceae.

fu·mar·ic acid (few·măr'ick). *trans*-Ethylenedicarboxylic acid, HOOCCH=CHCOOH, the *trans*-isomer of maleic acid. It occurs in *Fumaria officinalis* and in mammalian tissues as an intermediate in the metabolism of carbohydrate.

fu·mig·a·cin (few·mig'uh·sin) *n.* HELVOLIC ACID.

fu·mi·gate (few'mi·gate) *v.* [L. *fumigare,* to smoke, from *fumus,* smoke, fume]. To expose to the fumes of a vaporized disinfectant. —**fumi·gant** (·gunt) *n.;* **fu·mi·ga·tion** (few"mi·gay'shun) *n.*

fum·ing (few'ming) *adj.* Emitting smoke or vapor, as fuming nitric acid or fuming sulfuric acid.

func·tio (funk'shee·o) *n.* [L.]. FUNCTION.

functio lae·sa (lee'suh). Loss of function.

func·tion (funk'shun) *n.* [L. *functio,* performance, from *fungi,* to perform]. 1. The normal or special action of a part. 2. The chemical character, relationships, and properties of a substance contributed by a particular, atom, group of atoms, or type of bond in the substance. 3. A factor related to or dependent upon other factors.

func·tion·al (funk'shun·ul) *adj.* 1. Of or pertaining to a specific function, process, or activity. 2. Pertaining to the physiology or working of a part or system, but not its structure. 3. Useful; able to carry out appropriate tasks though structurally not intact. 4. Pertaining to a condition or illness in which the normal activities are disturbed or cannot be carried out, though there is no apparent organic explanation. Contr. *organic.*

functional albuminuria. Proteinuria without demonstrable renal disease; cyclic albuminuria.

functional amenorrhea. Amenorrhea lacking definite or known organic, endocrine, or nutritional causes, which often results from a psychologic disturbance.

functional contracture. HYPERTONIC CONTRACTURE.

functional disease. A disease in which no definite organic cause or no demonstrable pathologic lesion can be discovered.

functional dysmenorrhea. Dysmenorrhea without anatomic or pathologic explanation.

functional emphysema. EMPHYSEMA (1).

functional imbalance. The contacting of the teeth in such a manner as to preclude optimal dental arch function or to place excessive stress on the supporting structures of the involved teeth.

functional impotence. Impotence due to a psychologic disturbance, usually depression.

functional lesion. An alteration of function or functional capacity without demonstrable morphologic alteration.

functional menorrhagia. Excessive menstruation due to no demonstrable anatomic or pathologic lesion; usually assumed to be due to endocrine dysfunction. Syn. *primary menorrhagia.*

functional murmur. INNOCENT MURMUR.

functional paralysis. HYSTERICAL PARALYSIS.

functional residual air. FUNCTIONAL RESIDUAL CAPACITY.

functional residual capacity. The resting lung volume or the amount of air remaining in the lungs at the end of a quiet expiration. It includes both the expiratory reserve volume and residual volume. Abbreviated, FRC.

functional scoliosis. Scoliosis due to persistent faulty posture, such as standing on one leg or with one shoulder held lower than the other or with the head tilted. Syn. *habit scoliosis.* Contr. *structural scoliosis.*

functioning cortical tumor. CORTICAL ADENOMA.

fun·dal (fun'dul) *adj.* FUNDIC.

fundal placenta. A placenta attached at the fundus of the uterus.

fun·da·ment, *n.* [L. *fundamentum,* foundation, from *fundare,* to found]. 1. The foundation or base. 2. The buttocks.

fun·da·men·tal, *adj.* 1. Basic; underlying. 2. Of essential nature, property, or quality. 3. Elementary.

fundamental column. FASCICULI PROPRII MEDULLAE SPINALIS.

fundamental rule. *In psychoanalysis,* ANALYTIC RULE.

fun·dec·to·my (fun·deck'tuh·mee) *n.* FUNDUSECTOMY.

fundi. Plural of *fundus.*

fun·dic (fun'dick) *adj.* Pertaining to or involving a fundus.

fundic glands. The glands of the corpus and fundus of the stomach.

fun·di·form (fun′di·form) *adj.* [L. *funda*, sling, + *-iform*]. Shaped like a sling, or loop.

fundiform ligament of the penis. A ligament arising from the front of the sheath of the rectus abdominis muscle and the linea alba, splitting into two bands to encircle the root of the penis. NA *ligamentum fundiforme penis.*

fun·do·plasty (fun′do·plas″tee) *n.* [*fundus* + *-plasty*]. Plastic repair of the fundus of an organ.

fun·do·pli·ca·tion (fun″do·pli·kay′shun) *n.* Plication of the gastric fundus around the esophagus.

fun·dos·co·py (fun·dos′kuh·pee) *n.* Examination of the interior of the eye with the use of an ophthalmoscope or slit lamp (biomicroscope) and contact lens; OPHTHALMOSCOPY. —**fun·do·scop·ic** (fun″duh·skop′ick) *adj.*

fun·dus (fun′dus) *n.*, pl. **fun·di** (·dye) [L., bottom, back, base]. The part farthest removed from the opening (exit) of the organ.

fun·du·scope (fun′duh·skope) *n.* [*fundus* + *-scope*]. OPHTHALMOSCOPE.

fun·dus·co·py (fun·dus′kuh·pee) *n.* [*fundus* + *-scopy*]. FUNDOSCOPY. —**fun·du·scop·ic** (fun″duh·skop′ick) *adj.*

fun·du·sec·to·my (fun″duh·seck′tuh·mee) *n.* [*fundus* + *-ectomy*]. 1. Surgical removal of the fundus of an organ, as of the uterus. 2. Surgical removal of a wedge-shaped portion of the fundus of the stomach, used in the treatment of postoperative jejunal ulcer.

fundus fla·vi·mac·u·la·tus (flay″vi·mack·yoo·lay′tus). An uncommon retinal dystrophy with an autosomal recessive mode of transmission, characterized by bilateral symmetrical yellow-white round and linear (pisciform) lesions at the level of the deep retinal layers or retinal pigment epithelium in the posterior region of the eye. Pure forms may or may not have similar lesions in the foveal region. Forms with associated foveal dystrophy have flat atrophic foveal lesions (which may be indistinguishable from Stargardt's disease) or an elevated foveal lesion.

fundus fol·li·cu·li pi·li (fol·ick′yoo·lye pye′lye) [BNA]. The deepest part of a hair follicle.

fundus me·a·tus acu·sti·ci in·ter·ni (mee·ay′tus a·koos′ti·sigh in·tur′nigh) [NA]. The bottom or lateral end of the internal acoustic meatus.

fundus ocu·li (ock′yoo·lye). The posterior portion of the interior of the eye. See also Plate 19.

fundus of the gallbladder. The wide, anterior end of the gallbladder. NA *fundus vesicae felleae.*

fundus of the urinary bladder. The portion of the urinary bladder adjacent to the rectum. NA *fundus vesicae urinariae.*

fundus of the uterus. The part of the uterus most remote from the cervix. NA *fundus uteri.*

fundus reflex test. RETINOSCOPY.

fundus ute·ri (yoo′tur·eye) [NA]. FUNDUS OF THE UTERUS.

fundus ven·tri·cu·li (ven·trick′yoo·lye) [NA]. The large, rounded cul-de-sac cephalad to the cardia of the stomach, when that organ is dilated. Syn. *fornix of the stomach.*

fundus ve·si·cae fel·le·ae (ve·sigh′kee fel′ee·ee, ve·sigh′see) [NA]. FUNDUS OF THE GALLBLADDER.

fundus vesicae uri·na·ri·ae (yoo·ri·nair′ee·ee) [NA]. FUNDUS OF THE URINARY BLADDER.

fun·gal (fung′gul) *adj.* Of or pertaining to fungi. Compare *fungous.*

fun·gate (fung′gate) *v. & adj.* 1. To grow upward from a surface in a fashion resembling a fungus, as certain tumors. 2. Grown into a funguslike form. —**fungat·ing** (·ing) *adj.*

fungating carcinoma. A centrally necrotic carcinoma growing in a sessile polypoid fashion from a surface or into a lumen, giving a resemblance to a fungus.

fun·ge·mia, fun·gae·mia (fun·jee′mee·uh) *n.* [*fungus* + *-emia*]. The presence of fungi in the blood.

fungi. Plural of *fungus.*

fun·gi·cide (fun′ji·side) *n.* [*fungi* + *-cide*]. An agent that destroys fungi. —**fun·gi·ci·dal** (fun″ji·sigh′dul) *adj.*

fun·gi·form (fun′ji·form) *adj.* [*fungus* + *-iform*]. Having the form of a mushroom.

fungiform papilla. One of the low, broad papillae scattered over the dorsum and margins of the tongue.

Fungi Im·per·fec·ti (im″pur·feck′tye). Fungi which lack a known sexual phase of reproduction in their life history.

fun·gi·sta·sis (fun″ji·stay′sis) *n.* [*fungus* + *stasis*]. The inhibition of fungus growth by a chemical or physical agent; to be distinguished from fungicidal action, which involves the killing of fungi. —**fungi·stat·ic** (·stat′ick) *adj.*

Fungizone. Trademark for amphotericin B, a fungistatic antibiotic substance.

fun·goid (fung′goid) *adj.* [*fungus* + *-oid*]. Resembling a fungus.

fun·gos·i·ty (fung·gos′i·tee) *n.* 1. A fungous excrescence. 2. The quality of being fungous.

fun·gous (fung′gus) *adj.* 1. Of or pertaining to fungi; FUNGAL. 2. Caused by or infected with a fungus. 3. Funguslike; FUNGOID.

fungous arthritis or **synovitis.** Tuberculous disease of the joints; white swelling.

fungous granulation. EXUBERANT GRANULATION.

fungous ulcer. EXUBERANT ULCER.

fun·gu·ria (fung·gew′ree·uh) *n.* The presence of fungi in the urine.

fun·gus (fung′gus) *n.*, pl. **fun·gi** (fun′jye), **funguses** [L.]. 1. A low form of plant life, a division of the Thallophytes without chlorophyll. The chief classes of fungi are the Phycomycetes, Ascomycetes, Basidiomycetes, and Fungi Imperfecti. Most of the pathogenic fungi belong to the last group. 2. A spongy morbid excrescence.

fungus ball. A spheroidal mass of fungal elements, mainly mycelia, occupying a lung cavity and usually, but not exclusively, composed of aspergilli. See also *aspergilloma.*

fu·nic (few′nick) *adj.* [*funis* + *-ic*]. Pertaining to the umbilical cord.

fu·ni·cle (few′ni·kul) *n.* [L. *funiculus,* dim. of *funis,* rope]. A slender cord, a funiculus.

funic presentation. A fetal presentation in which the umbilical cord is the foremost structure at the cervix.

funic pulse. The arterial tide in the umbilical cord.

funic souffle. FUNICULAR SOUFFLE.

fu·nic·u·lar (few·nick′yoo·lur) *adj.* Of or pertaining to a funiculus.

funicular hernia. A variety of congenital, indirect hernia confined to the spermatic cord.

funicular myelitis or **myelosis.** SUBACUTE COMBINED DEGENERATION OF THE SPINAL CORD.

funicular process. The portion of the tunica vaginalis that surrounds the spermatic cord.

funicular souffle. A blowing murmur usually synchronous with the fetal heartbeat, heard over the pregnant uterus; thought to originate in the umbilical cord.

funiculi. Plural of *funiculus.*

funiculi me·dul·lae spi·na·lis (me·dul′ee spye·nay′lis) [NA]. The columns of white matter of the spinal cord. See also *funiculus (1).*

fu·nic·u·li·tis (few·nick″yoo·lye′tis) *n.* [*funiculus* + *-itis*]. 1. Inflammation of a funiculus, specifically of the spermatic cord. 2. Inflammation of a spinal nerve root within the vertebral canal.

fu·nic·u·lus (few·nick′yoo·lus) *n.*, pl. **funicu·li** (·lye) [L., cord, string]. 1. One of the three main divisions of white matter, which are named with reference to the gray matter of the cord as dorsal, lateral, and ventral. 2. *Obsol.* FASCICULUS. 3. *Obsol.* The umbilical or spermatic cord.

funiculus anterior me·dul·lae spi·na·lis (me·dul′ee spye·nay′lis) [NA]. The anterior column of white matter of the spinal cord.

funiculus cu·ne·a·tus me·dul·lae ob·lon·ga·tae (kew·nee·ay′

tus me·dul'ee ob·long·gay'tee) [BNA]. Fasciculus cuneatus medullae spinalis (= CUNEATE FASCICULUS).

funiculus gra·ci·lis me·dul·lae ob·lon·ga·tae (gras'i·lis me·dul'ee ob·long·gay'tee) [BNA]. FASCICULUS GRACILIS MEDULLAE OBLONGATAE.

funiculus la·te·ra·lis me·dul·lae ob·lon·ga·tae (lat·e·ray'lis me·dul'ee ob·long·gay'tee) [NA]. The continuation into the medulla oblongata of the lateral column of white matter of the spinal cord.

funiculus lateralis medullae spi·na·lis (spye·nay'lis) [NA]. The lateral column of white matter of the spinal cord.

funiculus posterior medullae spinalis [NA]. The posterior column of white matter of the spinal cord.

funiculus se·pa·rans (sep'uh·ranz) A white ridge of thickened ependyma, separating the ala cinerea from the area postrema.

funiculus sper·ma·ti·cus (spur·mat'i·kus) [NA]. SPERMATIC CORD.

funiculus um·bi·li·ca·lis (um·bil''i·kay'lis) [NA]. UMBILICAL CORD.

fu·nis (few'nis) *n.* [L., rope, cord]. A cord, particularly the umbilical cord.

fun·nel, *n.* [Provençal *fonilh,* from L. *infundibulum*]. A wide-mouthed conical vessel ending in an open tube; for filling bottles or other containers, and as a support for filter papers.

funnel chest or **breast.** A deformity of the sternum, costal cartilages, and anterior portions of the ribs, producing a depression of the lower portion of the chest; usually associated with development of kyphoscoliosis.

funnel pelvis. A deformity in which the usual external measurements are normal while the outlet is contracted, the transverse diameter of the latter being 8 cm or less.

funny bone. The region at the back of the medial condyle of the humerus, crossed superficially by the ulnar nerve. Compression of the nerve at this point induces a painful tingling sensation to the cutaneous area supplied by the ulnar nerve.

F.U.O. Fever of undetermined or unknown origin.

fur, *n.* 1. A coating of epithelial debris, as on the tongue. 2. The hairy coat of some animals. —**furred,** *adj.*

Furacilin. A trademark for nitrofurazone, a topical anti-infective.

Furacin. Trademark for nitrofurazone, a local antibacterial agent.

Furadantin. Trademark for nitrofurantoin, an antibacterial agent for oral administration in the treatment of bacterial infections of the urinary tract.

fu·ral (few'rul) *n.* FURFURAL.

fu·ran (few'ran) *n.* CH=CH—CH=CH (ring closed through O between the terminal CH groups). A constituent of wood tars; a colorless liquid, insoluble in water.

Furanace. A trademark for nifurpirinol, an antibacterial.

fu·rane (few'rane) *n.* FURAN.

fu·ra·nose (few'ruh·noce) *n.* A sugar having a ring structure resembling that of furan.

fur·a·zol·i·done (fewr''uh·zol'i·dohn) *n.* 3-(5-Nitrofurfurylideneamino)-2-oxazolidinone, $C_8H_7N_3O_5$, an antibacterial agent administered orally for treatment of bacterial diarrheal disorders and enteritis, and used topically as an antiprotozoal drug.

fur·a·zo·li·um chloride (fewr''uh·zo'lee·um). 6,7-Dihydro-3-(5-nitro-2-furyl-5*H*-imidazo[2,1-*b*]thiazolium chloride, an antibacterial compound.

fur·az·o·sin (fewr·az'o·sin) *n.* 1-(4-Amino-6,7-dimethoxy-2-quinazolinyl-4-(2-furoyl)piperazine, $C_{19}H_{21}N_5O_4$, an antihypertensive agent; used as the hydrochloride salt.

fur·ca (fur'kuh) *n.*, pl. **fur·cae** (·see) [L.]. A fork. —**fur·cal** (·kul), **fur·cate** (·kate) *adj.*

furca or·bi·ta·lis (or·bi·tay'lis). The orbital fork; one of the earliest signs of the orbit seen in the embryo; it is a mere trace of bifurcated bony tissue.

fur·cu·la (fur'kew·luh) *n.*, pl. **furcu·lae** (·lee) [L., forked prop]. 1. A crescentic median elevation of the floor of the embryonic pharynx, at the level of the third and fourth visceral arches; differentiates into the epiglottis and aryepiglottic folds. Syn. *hypobranchial eminence.* 2. A forked process, especially the joined clavicles of a bird; wishbone.

fur·fur (fur'fur) *n.* [L., bran, scales]. Dandruff; a branny desquamation of the epidermis. —**fur·fu·ra·ceous** (fur''fur·ay'shus, fur''few·ray'shus) *adj.*

fur·fu·ral (fewr'fuh·ral, fur'few·) *n.* 2-Furaldehyde, $C_5H_4O_2$, a liquid used as a solvent and reagent, and as an insecticide and fungicide.

fur·fur·al·de·hyde (fewr''fur·al'de·hide, fur''fewr·) *n.* FURFURAL.

fur·fu·ran (fewr'fuh·ran, fur'few·) *n.* FURAN.

fur·fu·rane (fewr'fuh·rane, fur'few·) *n.* FURAN.

fur·fu·ryl (fewr'fuh·ril, fur'few·) *n.* The monovalent radical C_5H_5O— derived from furfuryl alcohol.

furfuryl alcohol. 2-Furancarbinol, $C_5H_6O_2$, a poisonous liquid obtained from furfural; used as a solvent and in various syntheses.

fu·ri·bund (few'ri·bund) *adj.* [L. *furibundus,* from *furere,* to rage]. Raging; maniacal.

furious rabies. The commoner form of rabies, in which the cerebral involvement is prominent. Compare *paralytic rabies.* See also *rabies.*

fu·ro·bu·fen (few''ro·bew'fen) *n.* 2-Dibenzofuranbutyric acid, $C_{16}H_{14}O_4$, an anti-inflammatory.

fu·ro·ic acid (few·ro'ick). The acid, $C_5H_4O_3$, resulting when the aldehyde group of furfural is oxidized to carboxyl; it occurs in crystals, soluble in water. Syn. *2-furoic acid, a-furoic acid, pyromucic acid.*

fu·role (few'role) *n.* FURFURAL.

fu·ror (few'ror) *n.* [L.]. 1. Madness. 2. The manic phase of manic depressive illness; maniacal attack.

furor am·a·to·ri·us (am·uh·to'ree·us). Excessive sexual desire.

furor ep·i·lep·ti·cus (ep·i·lep'ti·kus). PAROXYSMAL FUROR.

furor gen·i·ta·lis (jen·i·tay'lis). EROTOMANIA.

fur·o·sem·ide (fewr''o·sem'id, ·ide) *n.* 4-Chloro-*N*-furfuryl-5-sulfamoylanthranilic acid, $C_{12}H_{11}ClN_2O_5S$, a diuretic drug. Formerly called *fursemide.*

Furoxone. Trademark for furazolidone, an antibacterial and antiprotozoal drug.

fu·ro·yl (few'ro·il) *n.* The radical C_4H_3OCO—.

furred tongue. A tongue the papillae of which are coated.

fur·row (fur'o) *n.* A groove.

furrowed tongue. FISSURED TONGUE.

furrow keratitis. Any keratitis with a linear surface concavity.

fur·sa·lan (fur'suh·lan, fewr') *n.* 3,4-Dibromo-*N*-(tetrahydrofurfuryl)salicylamide, $C_{12}H_{13}Br_2NO_3$, a disinfectant.

fur·se·mide (fewr'se·mide) *n.* FUROSEMIDE.

Furth pituitary tumor. A transplantable anterior pituitary tumor induced in a special strain of laboratory mice radiothyroidectomized with I^{131}; one transplant subline is autonomous, growing in untreated hosts, while another will grow only in radiothyroidectomized hosts.

fu·run·cle (few'rung·kul) *n.* [L. *furunculus,* petty thief, from *fur,* thief]. A localized infection, usually staphylococcal, of skin and subcutaneous tissue, which usually originates in or about a hair follicle and develops into a solitary abscess that drains externally through a single suppurating tract; a boil. —**fu·run·cu·lar** (few·runk'yoo·lur) *adj.*

furuncular otitis. The formation of furuncles in the external acoustic meatus.

furunculi. Plural of *furunculus.*

fu·run·cu·lo·sis (few·runk''yoo·lo'sis) *n.*, pl. **furunculo·ses** (·seez) [*furunculus* + *-osis*]. A condition in which multiple furuncles form or in which outbreaks of furuncles rapidly succeed one another.

furunculosis ori·en·ta·lis (or″ee·en·tay′lis). CUTANEOUS LEISHMANIASIS.

fu·run·cu·lus (few·runk′yoo·lus) *n.*, pl. **furuncu·li** (·lye) [L.]. FURUNCLE.

fu·ryl (few′ril) *n.* The radical O—CH=CH—CH=C—, known as α-furyl, or the radical CH=CH—O—CH=CH—, known as β-furyl.

Fu·sar·i·um (few·zar′ee·um) *n.* [NL., from L. *fusus,* spindle]. A genus of fungi, including species that may act as allergens and that are pathogenic for plants. Produces verticillate conidiophores, which give rise to sickle-shaped, multiseptate conidia. The spores are airborne.

fus·cin (fus′in, few′sin) *n.* [L. *fuscus,* dusky, + *-in*]. The melanin pigment of the eye.

fuscocaerulius ophthalmomaxillaris of Ota. NEVUS FUSCOCAERULIUS OPHTHALMOMAXILLARIS OF OTA.

fuse, *v.* [L. *fundere, fusus,* to melt]. 1. To unite, melt, or blend. 2. To become united as one.

fu·seau (few·zo′) *n.*, pl. **fuseaux** [F., spindle]. A fusiform macroconidium or spore of a dermatophyte, as of the genus *Trichophyton* or *Microsporum.*

fused bifocals. Bifocals in which greater refractive power is obtained by fusing an insert of denser glass, as flint glass, into a crown-glass lens.

fused kidney. Connection of the inferior poles of the two kidneys anterior to the aorta by an isthmus of renal parenchyma. The most common anomaly is the horseshoe kidney and the sigmoid kidney. Fusion is also seen in the cake kidney. See also *horseshoe kidney.*

fu·sel oil (few′zul) [Ger. *Fusel,* bad liquor]. A by-product, formed from protein materials, in the production of ethyl alcohol by fermentation; it consists chiefly of isoamyl alcohol with varying quantities of other alcohols.

fusi-, fuso- [L. *fusus,* spindle]. A combining form meaning (a) *spindle;* (b) *fusiform.*

fu·si·ble (few′zi·bul) *adj.* [L. *fundere, fusus,* to pour]. Capable of being melted.

fusible calculus. A urinary calculus composed of phosphates of ammonium, calcium, and magnesium.

fu·sid·ic acid (few·sid′ick). A steroid antibiotic, $C_{31}H_{48}O_6$, obtained from the fermentation broth of *Fusidium coccineum.* It is active primarily against gram-positive organisms; used in the form of the salt sodium fusidate.

fu·si·form (few′zi·form, few′si·) *adj.* [*fusi-* + *-form*]. Spindle-shaped.

fusiform aneurysm. A spindle-shaped dilatation of an artery.

fusiform bacillus. A bacterium of spindle-shaped or cigar-shaped morphology, belonging to the genus *Fusobacterium.*

fusiform bougie. A bougie with a spindle-shaped shaft.

fusiform cell. 1. A spindle-shaped cell. 2. SPINDLE CELL.

fusiform gyrus. A long gyrus situated on the inferior aspect of the occipital and temporal lobes between the collateral sulcus and the inferior temporal sulcus. See also *gyrus occipitotemporalis lateralis, gyrus occipitotemporalis medialis.*

Fu·si·for·mis (few″zi·for′mis, few″si·) *n.* *FUSOBACTERIUM.*

Fusiformis den·ti·um (den′shee·um). *FUSOBACTERIUM FUSIFORME.*

fusiform muscle. A spindle-shaped muscle.

fu·si·mo·tor (few″zi·mo′tur) *adj.* [*fusi-* + *motor*]. *In neurophysiology,* pertaining to the motor or efferent innervation of the intrafusal muscle fibers, derived from the gamma efferent neurons of the anterior gray matter of the spinal cord. See also *muscle spindle.*

fu·sion (few′zhun) *n.* [L. *fusio,* from *fundere,* to pour, to melt]. 1. The process of melting. 2. The act of uniting or cohering. 3. The mechanism whereby both eyes are able to act in a conjugate fashion. 4. *In nuclear science,* the union of atomic nuclei to form heavier nuclei, with release of energy. Contr. *fission.*

fusion beat. A QRS complex intermediate in contour between complexes of supraventricular and ventricular origin, representing concomitant supraventricular and ventricular depolarization.

fusion frequency. The lowest frequency at which flashes of light produce on the retina the impression of a steady light rather than a flicker.

fusion tube. A miniature stereoscope by which the two images formed by a straight and a squinting eye may be fused together and seen simultaneously. See also *heteroscope.*

fuso-. See *fusi-.*

Fu·so·bac·te·ri·um (few″zo·back·teer′ee·um) *n.* [*fuso-* + *bacterium*]. A genus of strictly anaerobic or microaerophilic bacteria, consisting of gram-negative rods which are slender, of various length, and often fusiform in shape. They form part of the indigenous flora of man, are found in the mouth, intestinal and genital tracts; in association with spirochetes; and in necrotizing lesions. —**fusobacterium,** pl. **fusobacte·ria,** *com. n.*

Fusobacterium fu·si·for·me (few·zi·for′mee). An anaerobic organism occurring as part of the indigenous flora of the oral cavity and other tracts, found in association with other organisms, including spirochetes, in gingivitis, Vincent's angina, and abscesses of the lungs and other organs.

Fusobacterium plauti-vincenti [H. K. *Plaut,* German physician, 1858–1928; and J. H. *Vincent*]. *FUSOBACTERIUM FUSIFORME.*

fu·so·cel·lu·lar (few″zo·sel′yoo·lur) *adj.* [*fuso-* + *cellular*]. Consisting of spindle-shaped cells.

fu·so·spi·ro·che·tal, fu·so·spi·ro·chae·tal (few″zo·spye″ro·kee′tul) *adj.* Pertaining to the association of fusiform bacteria and spirochetes.

fusospirochetal bronchitis. An infection of the respiratory tract characterized by foul sputum containing anaerobes including fusiform rods and spirilla, probably representing lung abscess or bronchiectasis rather than bronchitis.

fusospirochetal disease. FUSOSPIROCHETOSIS.

fusospirochetal gangrene. Foul, gangrenous lesions of the oropharynx, genitalia, respiratory tract, and other tissues; characterized by the presence of a mixed, largely anaerobic microbial flora, generally including fusobacteria and spirochetes.

fu·so·spi·ro·che·to·sis, fu·so·spi·ro·chae·to·sis (few″zo·spye″ro·kee·to′sis) *n.* Infection with *Fusobacterium fusiforme* and spirochetes, associated with Vincent's infection, lung abscess, vulvovaginitis, or balanitis.

fuzz, *n.* The filamentous glycoprotein coat covering the microvilli of the proximal renal tubules, intestines and certain other epithelia and cells with a free surface.

f waves. FIBRILLATION WAVES.

F waves. FLUTTER WAVES.

G

G 1. *In molecular biology,* a symbol for guanine. 2. *In microbiology,* abbreviation for *gonidial* (colony). 3. Abbreviation for *gravitational unit.*

G, Ĝ, g, ĝ *In electrocardiography,* a symbol for the ventricular gradient, usually as projected on the frontal plane of the body.

G, g 1. Symbol for gravitation constant or Newtonian constant, a constant in Newton's law of gravitation which gives the attraction f between two particles m_1 and m_2 at a distance r as $f = G\,(m_1\,m_2)/r^2$. G is a constant whose value depends on the units in which f, m_1, m_2, and r are expressed. If f is given in dynes, m_1 and m_2 in grams, and r in centimeters, then G is 6.673×10^{-8} dyne cm^2 / g^2. 2. A unit of force of acceleration, equal to that exerted on a body by gravity at the earth's surface, allowing the expression of force of acceleration as a multiple of earth's gravitation.

G_1 Symbol for the period that follows cell division and precedes DNA replication in the life cycle of a cell.

G_2 Symbol for the period between DNA replication and the onset of mitosis in the life cycle of a cell.

g Abbreviation for *gram.*

Ga Symbol for gallium.

Ga·boon viper (ga·boon') [after *Gabon,* Africa]. *BITIS GABONICA.*

G-actin, *n.* The globular form of actin.

gad·fly, *n.* Any of various flies of the Tabanidae.

gad·o·lin·i·um (gad''o·lin'ee·um) *n.* [J. *Gadolin,* Finnish chemist, 1760–1852]. Gd = 157.25. A rare-earth metal discovered in 1880 by Marignac in gadolinite. See also Table of Elements in the Appendix.

Ga·dus (gay'dus) *n.* [Gk. *gados,* a fish]. A genus of soft-finned fish.

Gadus mor·rhua (mor'oo·uh). The common cod; a fish from the livers of which cod liver oil is obtained.

Gaert·ner's tonometer (gehrt'nur) [G. *Gaertner,* Austrian physician, 1855–1937]. An instrument for measuring digital blood pressure.

Gaff·kya (gaf'kee·uh) *n.* [G. T. A. *Gaffky,* German bacteriologist, 1850–1918]. A genus of the Micrococcaceae.

Gaffkya te·trag·e·na (te·traj'e·nuh). A species of micrococci forming tetrads, found in the mucous membranes of the respiratory tract and occasionally pathogenic in man. Syn. *Micrococcus tetragenus.*

gag, *n. & v.* 1. An instrument placed between the jaws to prevent closure of the mouth. 2. To insert a gag. 3. To retch or heave.

gage. GAUGE.

Ga·gel's granuloma (gah'gul) [O. *Gagel*]. A form of histiocytosis X involving the hypothalamus; more broadly, histiocytosis X involving the neurohypophysis.

gag reflex. Contraction of the constrictor muscles of the pharynx in response to stimulation of the posterior pharyngeal wall or neighboring structures.

Gais·böck's disease or **syndrome** (gice'bœck) [L. F. *Gaisböck,* Austrian physician, b. 1868]. Polycythemia vera and hypertension without splenomegaly. Syn. *polycythemia hypertonica.*

gait, *n.* [ON. *gata,* path, way]. Manner of walking.

galact-, galacto- [Gk. *gala, galaktos*]. A combining form meaning (a) *milk;* (b) *milky fluid.*

ga·lac·ta·cra·sia (ga·lack''tuh·kray'zhuh, ·zee·uh) *n.* [*galact-* + Gk. *akrasia,* bad mixture]. Deficiency of or abnormality in mother's milk.

galactaemia. GALACTEMIA.

ga·lac·ta·gogue (ga·lack'tuh·gog) *n.* [*galact-* + *-agogue*]. An agent that induces or increases the secretion of milk.

ga·lac·tan (ga·lack'tan) *n.* [*galact-* + *-an*]. Any polysaccharide composed of galactose units; on hydrolysis it yields galactose. Syn. *galactosan.*

ga·lac·tase (ga·lack'tace, ·taze) *n.* [*galact-* + *-ase*]. A soluble proteolytic enzyme present normally in milk.

gal·ac·te·mia, gal·ac·tae·mia (gal''ack·tee'mee·uh) *n.* [*galact-* + *-emia*]. A milky state or appearance of the blood.

ga·lact·hi·dro·sis (ga·lakt''hi·dro'sis) *n.* [*galact-* + *hidrosis*]. Sweating of a milklike fluid.

ga·lac·tic (ga·lack'tick) *adj.* [Gk. *galaktikos,* pertaining to milk]. Pertaining to or promoting the flow of milk.

ga·lac·tin (ga·lack'tin) *n.* [*galact-* + *-in*]. PROLACTIN.

gal·ac·tis·chia (gal''ack·tis'kee·uh) *n.* [*galact-* + Gk. *ischein,* check, restrain, + *-ia*]. Suppression of the secretion of milk; GALACTOSCHESIS.

galacto-. See *galact-.*

ga·lac·to·blast (ga·lack'to·blast) *n.* [*galacto-* + *-blast*]. COLOSTRUM CORPUSCLE.

ga·lac·to·cele (ga·lack'to·seel) *n.* [*galacto-* + *-cele*]. 1. A retention cyst caused by obstruction of one or more of the mammary ducts. 2. A hydrocele with milky contents.

ga·lac·to·fla·vin (ga·lack''to·flay'vin, ·flav'in) *n.* An analogue of riboflavin in which D-galactose replaces D-ribose; it is a potent riboflavin antagonist.

ga·lac·to·gen (ga·lack'to·jen) *n.* [*galacto-* + *-gen*]. A polysaccharide, occurring in snails, that yields galactose on hydrolysis.

ga·lac·to·gram (ga·lack'to·gram) *n.* A radiograph of the mammary ductal system.

gal·ac·tog·ra·phy (gal''ack·tog'ruh·fee) *n.* Radiographic depiction of the mammary ductal system.

ga·lac·toid (ga·lack'toid) *adj.* [*galact-* + *-oid*]. Resembling milk.

ga·lac·to·ki·nase (ga·lack''to·kigh'nace) *n.* An enzyme that causes reaction of D-galactose with ATP to give D-galactose-1-phosphate and ADP; the first step in the utilization of galactose by cells.

ga·lac·to·lip·id (ga·lack″to·lip′id) *n.* [*galacto-* + *lipid*]. CEREBROSIDE.

ga·lac·to·lip·in (ga·lack″to·lip′in) *n.* [*galacto-* + *lipin*]. CEREBROSIDE.

gal·ac·to·ma (gal″ack·to′muh) *n.*, pl. **galactomas, galactomata** (·tuh) [*galact-* + *-oma*]. GALACTOCELE (1).

gal·ac·tom·e·ter (gal″ack·tom′e·tur) *n.* [*galacto-* + *-meter*]. 1. A graduated glass funnel for determining the fat in milk. 2. An instrument for determining the specific gravity of milk.

D-ga·lac·to·meth·yl·ose (ga·lack″to·meth′il·oce) *n.* FUCOSE.

gal·ac·ton·ic acid (gal″ack·ton′ick). Pentahydroxyhexoic acid, $C_6H_{12}O_7$, a monobasic acid derived from galactose.

gal·ac·toph·a·gous (gal″ack·tof′uh·gus) *adj.* [*galacto-* + *-phagous*]. Subsisting on milk.

gal·ac·toph·ly·sis (gal″ack·tof′li·sis) *n.* [*galacto-* + Gk. *phlysis*, eruption]. 1. A vesicular eruption containing a milk-like fluid. 2. CRADLE CAP.

ga·lac·to·phore (ga·lack′to·fore) *n.* [*galacto-* + *-phore*]. A lactiferous duct. —**gal·ac·toph·o·rous** (gal″ack·tof′uh·rus) *adj.*

gal·ac·toph·o·ri·tis (gal″ack·tof″uh·rye′tis) *n.* [*galactophore* + *-itis*]. Inflammation of a lactiferous duct.

galactophorous ducts or **canals.** LACTIFEROUS DUCTS.

gal·ac·toph·thi·sis (gal″ack·tof′thi·sis) *n.* [*galacto-* + *phthisis*]. Emaciation and debility thought to be due to excessive secretion of milk.

gal·ac·toph·y·gous (gal″ack·tof′i·gus) *adj.* [*galacto-* + Gk. *phygē*, banishment, + *-ous*]. Arresting the secretion of milk.

ga·lac·to·po·et·ic (ga·lack″to·po·et′ick) *adj.* GALACTOPOIETIC.

ga·lac·to·poi·et·ic (ga·lack″to·poy·et′ick) *adj.* [Gk. *galaktopoiētikos*. milk-producing]. Pertaining to the formation and secretion of milk. —**galactopoi·e·sis** (·ee′sis) *n.*

ga·lac·to·py·ra (ga·lack″to·pye′ruh) *n.* [*galacto-* + Gk. *pyr*, fire]. MILK FEVER. —**galacto·py·ret·ic** (·pye·ret′ick) *adj.*

ga·lac·to·py·ra·nose (ga·lack″to·pye′ruh·noce, ·pirr′uh·noce) *n.* A pyranose-type, closed-chain form of galactose.

ga·lac·tor·rhea, ga·lac·tor·rhoea (ga·lack″to·ree′uh) *n.* [*galacto-* + *-rrhea*]. Excessive or spontaneous flow of milk.

ga·lac·to·sac·char·ic acid (ga·lack″to·sa·kăr′ick). MUCIC ACID.

ga·lac·tos·a·mine (ga·lack″to′suh·meen, ·toce·am′een) *n.* Galactose containing an amine group in 2-position, hence 2-amino-D-galactose. Syn. *chondrosamine.*

ga·lac·to·san (ga·lack′to·san) *n.* GALACTAN.

gal·ac·tos·che·sis (gal″ack·tos′ke·sis) *n.* [*galacto-* + Gk. *schesis*, retention]. Retention or suppression of milk secretion.

ga·lac·tose (ga·lack′toce, ·toze) *n.* [*galact-* + *-ose*]. A D-aldohexose, $C_6H_{12}O_6$, obtained by hydrolysis of lactose, occurring also as a component of cerebrosides and of many oligosaccharides and polysaccharides; it exists in α- and β-forms. On oxidation it yields mucic acid. L-Galactose occurs in small amounts in certain polysaccharides, as the mucilage of agar and flaxseed.

galactose diabetes. GALACTOSEMIA.

ga·lac·tos·emia, ga·lac·tos·ae·mia (ga·lack″to·see′mee·uh) *n.* [*galactose* + *-emia*]. An inborn error of metabolism due to absence of galactose 1-phosphate uridyl transferase resulting in inability to convert galactose into glucose; manifested by failure to thrive in infancy, jaundice, involvement of liver and spleen, cataract formation, and mental retardation.

galactose-1-phosphate. A phosphorylated derivative of galactose formed by action of galactokinase in liver.

galactose-1-phosphate uridyl transferase. An enzyme that catalyzes the reaction of galactose-1-phosphate with UTP to form UDP-galactose plus pyrophosphate.

galactose tolerance test. A test of the glycogenic function of the liver, performed by administering 40 g of galactose to a fasting individual. The elimination of more than 3 g of galactose over a 5-hour period indicates hepatic dysfunction.

ga·lac·to·sid·ase (ga·lack″to·sigh′dace, ·daze) *n.* [*galactoside* + *-ase*]. Any enzyme that catalyzes the hydrolysis of a galactoside. Two varieties are known, α- and β-, which act on α- and β- forms, respectively, of galactosides.

ga·lac·to·side (ga·lack′to·side) *n.* A glycoside which, on hydrolysis, yields the sugar galactose and an aglycone.

gal·ac·to·sis (gal″ack·to′sis) *n.* [Gk. *galaktōsis*, conversion into milk]. The secretion of milk by the mammary glands.

ga·lac·to·sphin·go·side (ga·lack″to·sfing′go·side) *n.* Any cerebroside (glycosphingoside) containing galactose as the sugar component.

ga·lac·to·sta·sia (ga·lack″to·stay′zhuh, ·zee·uh) *n.* GALACTOSTASIS.

gal·ac·tos·ta·sis (gal″ack·tos′tuh·sis) *n.* [*galacto-* + *-stasis*]. 1. Suppression of milk secretion. 2. An abnormal collection of milk in a breast.

ga·lac·tos·uria (ga·lack″to·sue′ree·uh) *n.* [*galactose* + *-uria*]. Passage of urine containing galactose.

ga·lac·to·ther·a·py (ga·lack″to·therr′uh·pee) *n.* [*galacto-* + *therapy*]. 1. Treatment by a milk diet; particularly treatment of newborn infants by feeding breast milk. 2. The treatment of disease in nursing infants by the administration of drugs to the mother which are subsequently secreted in the milk. 3. Hypodermic injection of sterile milk as a form of protein therapy.

ga·lac·to·tox·i·con (ga·lack″to·tock′si·kon) *n.* [*galacto-* + Gk. *toxikon*, poison]. A toxin present in decomposed milk.

ga·lac·to·tox·in (ga·lack″to·tock′sin) *n.* [*galacto-* + *toxin*]. A poisonous substance formed in milk by growth of microorganisms.

ga·lac·to·tox·ism (ga·lack″to·tock′siz·um) *n.* [*galacto-* + *tox-* + *-ism*]. Poisoning resulting from ingestion of contaminated or spoiled milk.

gal·ac·tot·ro·phy (gal″ack·tot′ruh·fee) *n.* [*galacto-* + *-trophy*]. Nourishing with milk only.

ga·lac·to·zy·mase (ga·lack″to·zye′mace, ·maze) *n.* [*galacto-* + *zymase*]. An enzyme found in milk that is capable of hydrolyzing starch.

gal·ac·tu·ria (gal″ack·tew′ree·uh) *n.* [*galact-* + *-uria*]. Milkiness of the urine; CHYLURIA.

ga·lac·tu·ron·ic acid (ga·lack″tew·ron′ick). The monobasic acid resulting from oxidation of the primary alcohol group of D-galactose to carboxyl; it is widely distributed as a constituent of pectins and many plant gums and mucilages.

Ga·la·go (ga·lay′go, gal′uh·go) *n.* A widespread African genus of small, leaping primates of the family Lorisidae.

Galalith. Trademark for an absorbent material made by the action of formaldehyde on casein.

Ga·lant's reflex or **response.** A reflex observed in the normal infant in the first months of life, in which scratching the paravertebral region from the shoulder to the buttock causes the trunk to curve with the concavity on the stimulated side. In a transverse lesion of the spinal cord, there is no response below the level of the lesion.

gal·ba·num (gal′buh·num) *n.* [L., from Gk. *chalbanē*, from Heb. *ḥelbĕnāh*]. A gum resin of *Ferula galbaniflua;* formerly used as a stimulant and expectorant and externally in plasters.

ga·lea (gay′lee·uh, gal′ee·uh) *n.*, pl. **galeas, ga·le·ae** (·lee·ee) [L., helmet]. 1. Any structure resembling a helmet. 2. A form of head bandage.

galea apo·neu·ro·ti·ca (ap″o·new·rot′i·kuh) [NA]. The aponeurotic portion of the occipitofrontal muscle. NA alt. *aponeurosis epicranialis.*

galea ca·pi·tis (kap′i·tis). The thin sheath of cytoplasm covering the nucleus and acrosome of the sperm head.

gal·e·an·thro·py (gal″ee·an′thruh·pee, gay′lee·) *n.* [Gk. *galeē*, weasel, polecat, + *anthrōpos*, man, + *-y*]. A form of zoanthropy in which the patient believes himself to be transformed into a cat.

Ga·le·ga (ga·lee'guh) *n.* A genus of the Leguminosae. *Galega officinalis,* goat's rue, was formerly used for supposed galactagogue effect.

ga·le·na (ga·lee'nuh) *n.* [L., lead ore]. Native lead sulfide, PbS.

ga·len·ic (ga·len'ick, ·lee'nick) *adj.* [C. *Galen,* Greek physician in Rome, 2nd century A.D.]. Pertaining to, or consistent with, the system of medicine and teachings of Galen.

ga·len·i·cal (ga·len'i·kul) *adj. & n.* 1. GALENIC. 2. Any medicine prepared from plants, according to standard formulas, as contrasted with chemical entities.

gal·eo·phil·ia (gal''ee·o·fil'ee·uh) *n.* [Gk. *galeē,* weasel, polecat, + *-philia*]. Excessive love of cats.

gal·eo·pho·bia (gal''ee·o·fo'bee·uh) *n.* An abnormal fear of cats.

gal·e·ro·pia (gal''e·ro'pee·uh) *n.* [Gk. *galeros,* cheerful, + *-opia*]. An abnormally clear and light appearance of objects due to some defect in the visual apparatus.

gal·e·rop·sia (gal''e·rop'see·uh) *n.* GALEROPIA.

¹gall (gawl) *n.* BILE.

²gall, *n.* [L. *galla,* gallnut]. 1. A sore on the skin of a horse, caused by a saddle or harness. 2. A swollen mass of disorganized vegetable cells in plant tissue due to fungi, bacteria, or other agents and capable of causing lethal obstruction of water and nutrient flow within the plant. See also *crown gall.*

gal·la·mine tri·eth·io·dide (gal'uh·meen trye''eth·eye'o·dide). 1,2,3-Tris(2-triethylammonium ethoxy)benzene triiodide, $C_{30}H_{60}I_3N_3O_3$, a curarimimetic drug employed as a skeletal muscle relaxant.

gall·blad·der (gawl'blad·ur) *n.* A hollow, pear-shaped, musculomembranous organ, situated on the undersurface of the right lobe of the liver, for the storage and concentration of bile and the secretion of mucus. NA *vesica fellea.* See also Plate 13.

gal·lery, *n.* The burrow or space in the skin occupied by a metazoan parasite.

gal·lic acid (gal'ick) [F. *gallique,* pertaining to gallnuts]. 3,4,5-Trihydroxybenzoic acid, $C_7H_6O_5$, formerly used internally as an astringent; esters of the acid are used as antioxidants.

Gal·lie–Le Me·su·rier operation (luh muh·zuᵉr·yeyʸ') [W. E. *Gallie,* Canadian surgeon, 1889-1959; and A. B. *Le Mesurier,* Canadian surgeon, b. 1889]. GALLIE'S OPERATION.

Gallie's operation [W. E. *Gallie*]. An operation for the radical cure of inguinal hernia, using long, living autogenous strips of fascia lata which are woven through the aponeurotic layers of the oblique and transverse muscles so as to strengthen the repair. Syn. *Gallie-Le Mesurier operation.*

Gallie's transplants. Strips of fascia lata used in Gallie's operation.

gal·li·um (gal'ee·um) *n.* [L. *Gallia,* Gaul]. Ga = 69.72. A rare gray-white metal, element number 31, that melts at 29.7°C.; has been used in high-temperature thermometry.

gallo-. A combining form meaning *gallic acid.*

gal·lo·cy·a·nin (gal''o·sigh'uh·nin) *n.* A basic oxazine dye; used in an aqueous solution with chrome alum as a stain for Nissl bodies; sometimes used as a nuclear stain.

gal·lon, *n.* [OF. *galon,* a measure of capacity]. A standard unit of volume equivalent in the United States to 3785.3 ml or to 231 cubic inches; 4 quarts. Syn. *congius.* See also *imperial gallon and Tables of Weights and Measures in the Appendix.*

galloping consumption. *Colloq.* A rapidly fatal form of pulmonary tuberculosis. Syn. *florid phthisis.*

gallop rhythm. A three-sound sequence resulting from the intensification of the normal third or fourth heart sounds, occurring usually, but not invariably, with a rapid ventricular rate.

gallop sound. A third or fourth heart sound. See also *atrial gallop, summation gallop, ventricular gallop.*

gal·lo·tan·nic acid (gal''o·tan'ick). TANNIC ACID.

gall·stone, *n.* A concretion formed in the gallbladder or the biliary ducts, composed, in varying amounts, of cholesterol, bilirubin, and other elements found in bile.

gal·siek·te, gal·ziek·te (gahl'seek·tuh) *n.* [Afrikaans, from *gal,* gall, + *siekte,* disease]. ANAPLASMOSIS.

Gal·ton's law of filial regression (gawl'tun) [F. *Galton,* English geneticist, 1822–1911]. LAW OF FILIAL REGRESSION.

Galton system [F. *Galton*]. A system of identification based on fingerprints, in which the printed impressions of the 10 digits are recorded in definite order on a card.

gal·van·ic (gal·van'ick) *adj.* Of, pertaining to, or caused by galvanism.

galvanic battery. A device that produces electricity from chemical energy.

galvanic contractility. The ability to contract in response to galvanic currents.

galvanic current. A direct current from a galvanic battery.

galvanic electricity. Electricity generated by chemical action in a galvanic battery.

galvanic skin response. The electrical reactions of the skin to any stimulus as detected by a sensitive galvanometer; most often used experimentally to measure the resistance of the skin to the passage of a weak electric current.

gal·va·nism (gal'vuh·niz·um) *n.* [L. *Galvani,* Italian physician and physicist, 1737–1798]. Primary direct current electricity produced by chemical action, as opposed to that produced by heat, friction, or induction.

gal·va·nize (gal'vuh·nize) *v.* To apply or stimulate with galvanic current. —**gal·va·ni·za·tion** (gal''vuh·ni·zay'shun) *n.*

galvano-. A combining form meaning *galvanic* or *direct current* of electricity.

gal·vano·cau·tery (gal''vuh·no·kaw'tur·ee) *n.* [*galvano-* + *cautery*]. ELECTROCAUTERY.

gal·vano·con·trac·til·i·ty (gal''vuh·no·kon''track·til'i·tee) *n.* [*galvano-* + *contractility*]. The property of being contractile under stimulation by a galvanic current.

gal·vano·far·a·di·za·tion (gal''vuh·no·făr''uh·di·zay'shun) *n.* The simultaneous use of direct galvanic currents and rapidly alternating faradic currents.

gal·va·nom·e·ter (gal''vuh·nom'e·tur) *n.* [*galvano-* + *-meter*]. An instrument for measuring or detecting the presence of relatively small electric currents.

gal·vano·mus·cu·lar (gal''vuh·no·mus'kew·lur) *adj.* [*galvano-* + *muscular*]. Denoting a reaction produced by the application of a galvanic current to a muscle.

gal·vano·punc·ture (gal'vuh·no·punk''chur, gal·van'o·) *n.* [*galvano-* + *puncture*]. ELECTROPUNCTURE.

gal·vano·scope (gal'vuh·no·skope'', gal·van'o·) *n.* [*galvano-* + *-scope*]. An instrument for detecting the presence and direction of small direct or galvanic currents. —**gal·va·nos·co·py** (gal''vuh·nos'kuh·pee) *n.*

gal·vano·sur·gery (gal''vuh·no·sur'jur·ee) *n.* The surgical use of direct or galvanic currents.

gal·vano·tax·is (gal''vuh·no·tack'sis) *n.* [*galvano-* + *-taxis*]. GALVANOTROPISM.

gal·vano·ther·a·py (gal''vuh·no·therr'uh·pee) *n.* [*galvano-* + *therapy*]. Treatment of disease with direct or galvanic currents.

gal·vano·ther·my (gal'vuh·no·thur''mee, gal·van'o·) *n.* [*galvano-* + *-thermy*]. The production of heat by direct or galvanic currents.

gal·va·not·o·nus (gal''vuh·not'o·nus) *n.* [*galvano-* + Gk. *tonos,* tension]. 1. ELECTROTONUS. 2. The continued tetanus of a muscle between the make and break contraction of direct or galvanic current. —**gal·vano·ton·ic** (gal''vuh·no·ton'ick) *adj.*

gal·va·not·ro·pis·um (gal''vuh·not'ro·piz·um) *n.* [*galvano-* + *-tropism*]. The turning movements of a living organism under the influence of direct current.

gal·vo (gal'vo) *n.* METAL FUME FEVER.

galziekte. Galsiekte (= ANAPLASMOSIS).

gam-, gamo- [Gk. *gamos,* marriage]. A combining form meaning (a) *marriage;* (b) in biology, *sexual union;* (c) in botany, *union* or *fusion of parts.*

gam·a·soi·do·sis (gam″uh·soy·do′sis) *n.*, pl. **gamasoido·ses** (·seez). Infestation by Gamasidae, a large group of parasitic mites.

Gam·bi·an sleeping sickness. GAMBIAN TRYPANOSOMIASIS.

Gambian trypanosomiasis. Infection of man with *Trypanosoma brucei gambiense,* acquired by the bite of the tsetse fly, occurring widely throughout central Africa, and characterized by parasitemia, lymphadenitis, and central nervous system lesions causing a chronic, lethal meningoencephalitis. Syn. *mid-African sleeping sickness.*

gam·bir (gam′beer) *n.* [Malay]. An aqueous extract from the twigs and leaves of *Uncaria gambir;* formerly used as an astringent.

gam·boge (gam·boje′) *n.* [after *Cambodia*]. The gum resin obtained from *Garcinia hanburyi;* a drastic, hydragogue cathartic.

Gam·bu·sia (gam·bew′zee·uh, ·see·uh) *n.* [NL., from Sp. *gambusino*]. A genus of top-feeding minnows, found in the southern United States and other warm climates. Their surface-feeding habits make them valuable in the destruction of mosquito larvae.

gamet-, gameto-. A combining form meaning *gamete.*

gam·e·tan·gi·um (gam″e·tan′jee·um) *n.*, pl. **gametan·gia** (·jee·uh) [*gamet-* + *-angium*]. A gamete-producing organ occurring especially in the lower plants.

gam·ete (gam′eet, ga·meet′) *n.* [Gk. *gametē,* wife, *gametēs,* husband, from *gamein,* to marry]. A male or female reproductive cell capable of entering into union with another in the process of fertilization or of conjugation. In higher animals, these sex cells are the egg and sperm; in higher plants, the male gamete is part of the pollen grain, while the ovum is contained in the ovule. In lower forms, the gametes are frequently similar in appearance. See also *conjugation, fertilization.* —**ga·met·ic** (ga·met′ick) *adj.*

gameto-. See *gamet-.*

ga·me·to·cyte (ga·mee′to·site, gam′e·to·site) *n.* [*gameto-* + *-cyte*]. A cell which by division produces gametes; a spermatocyte or oocyte.

gam·e·to·gen·e·sis (gam″e·to·jen′e·sis) *n.* [*gameto-* + *-genesis*]. The origin and formation of gametes. —**gametogen·ic** (·ick) *adj.*

gametogenic hormone. FOLLICLE-STIMULATING HORMONE.

gam·e·tog·o·ny (gam″e·tog′uh·nee) *n.* [*gameto-* + *-gony*]. A process of reproduction leading to the formation of gametocytes and gametes in the sexual phase of the life cycle in certain protozoa.

ga·me·to·phyte (ga·mee′tuh·fite, gam′e·to·) *n.* [*gameto-* + *-phyte*]. A sexual, gamete-producing individual which alternates in the life history of plants with the asexual sporophyte. The leafy moss plant is a gametophyte, but the leafy fern plant is a sporophyte. In the seed plants, the male and female gametophytes are microscopic and are contained in the pollen grain and ovule, respectively. —**ga·me·to·phyt·ic** (ga·mee″tuh·fit′ick, gam″e·to·) *adj.*

gametophytic apomixis. The formation of a gametophyte by asexual reproduction.

gam·fex·ine (gam·feck′seen) *n.* *N,N*-Dimethyl-γ-phenylcyclohexanepropylamine, $C_{17}H_{27}N$, an antidepressant drug.

gam·ic (gam′ick) *adj.* [Gk. *gamikos,* conjugal, connubial, from *gamos,* marriage]. Sexual; applied especially to the members of the bisexual generation in such animals as aphids, in which there is a parthenogenetic-bisexual cycle.

gam·ma (gam′uh) *n.* [name of the letter Γ, γ, third letter of the Greek alphabet]. 1. The third of a series, or any particular member or subset of an arbitrarily ordered set. For many terms so designated, see under the specific noun. Symbol, γ. 2. *In photography,* the contrast of a negative or print, usually controlled by developing time, and expressed as a relationship between the density of the negative and the time of exposure. 3. One-millionth of a gram; MICROGRAM.

gamma-A globulin. The immunoglobulin which comprises about 10 percent of the antibodies of human serum, where it occurs as a monomer with a sedimentation constant of 7 Svedberg units, and which constitutes the principal immunoglobulin in such secretions as parotid saliva, tears, colostrum, and gastrointestinal fluid, where it occurs as a dimer possessing an additional peptide (the secretory piece) and having a sedimentation constant of 11 Svedberg units. Symbol, IgA, γA.

gamma angle. *In ophthalmology,* the angle formed by the line of fixation and the optic axis.

gamma chain, γ chain. The heavy chain of the IgG immunoglobulin molecule.

gam·ma·cism (gam′uh·siz·um) *n.* [*gamma,* the Greek letter corresponding to g, + *-ism*]. Guttural stammering; difficulty in pronouncing velar consonants, especially hard g and k.

Gammacorten. A trademark for dexamethasone, an anti-inflammatory adrenocortical steroid.

gamma-D globulin. An immunoglobulin found in small amounts in normal human serum and on fetal and umbilical cord lymphocytes, having a light chain similar to that of other immunoglobulins, but possessing a heavy chain of unique properties. Symbol, IgD, γD.

gamma efferent nerve fibers. Small motor nerve fibers, 3 to 7 micrometers in diameter, with a conduction velocity of 15 to 30 meters per second, making up nearly one-third of the efferent ventral root fibers and distributed to the motor end plates of the contractile ends of the intrafusal fibers of a muscle spindle. See also *fusimotor.*

gamma-E globulin. The immunoglobulin associated with reaginic antibodies. Symbol, IgE, γE.

Gammagee. A trademark for immune human serum globulin.

gamma-G globulin. The immunoglobulin comprising about 80% of the serum antibodies of the adult, readily transported across the human placenta, having a sedimentation constant of 6.7 Svedberg units and an estimated molecular weight of 145,000. Symbol, IgG, γG.

gamma globulin, γ-globulin. 1. A broad designation for immunoglobulins of differing molecular weights and for certain proteins related to them by chemical structure, many of which have known antibody activity. 2. Sterile concentrated solutions of globulins obtained from pooled human blood of placental or venous origin, containing protective antibodies, and used clinically in viral hepatitis, measles, German measles, or hypogammaglobulinemia. Syn. *immune serum globulin.* 3. Originally, the fraction of serum proteins migrating most slowly toward the anode upon separation by electrophoresis.

gamma granules. The granules of the chromophobe cells of the hypophysis.

gamma hemolysin, γ-hemolysin. A hemolysin of *Staphylococcus aureus* which resembles alpha hemolysin, but differs from it antigenically.

gamma loop. The neural circuits to and from the spinal cord involving the gamma efferent nerve fibers and the muscle spindle.

gamma-M globulin. The immunoglobulin comprising 5 to 10% of the total serum antibodies, and including heterophile and Wassermann antibodies, cold agglutinins, isohemagglutinins, and antibodies to the endotoxins of gram-negative bacteria; characterized by a sedimentation constant of 19 Svedberg units and a molecular weight of about 900,000. Symbol, IgM, γM. Syn. *macroglobin.*

gamma ray. Electromagnetic radiation of high energy and short wavelength emitted by the nucleus of a radioactive atom when it has excess energy.

gamma-ray roentgen. GAMMA ROENTGEN.

gamma rhythm. *In electroencephalography,* very fast waves whose functional significance is unknown; 40 to 50 per second are recorded from the anterior head regions.

gamma roentgen. A unit of radium dosage such that the same amount of ionization in air is produced as by one roentgen unit of gamma rays. Syn. *gamma-ray roentgen.*

gamma streptococci. A group of streptococci that produce no change on blood agar, including organisms of low pathogenicity and many anaerobic strains, often isolated as secondary invaders.

gamma wave. See *gamma rhythm.*

Gam·mel's syndrome. ERYTHEMA GYRATUM MIGRANS.

Gammexane. Trademark for the insecticide lindane.

gam·mop·a·thy (ga·mop'uth·ee) *n.* [*gamma* globulin + *-pathy*]. A condition in which disturbance of immunoglobulin synthesis is presumed to play a primary role; reflected in significant changes of the immunoglobulin profile in the serum of the host.

Gammostan. A trademark for immune human serum globulin.

Gam·na-Fa·vre bodies (gahm'na, fahv'r) [C. *Gamna,* Italian physician, b. 1896; and M. *Favre*]. Small cytoplasmic inclusions said to be characteristic of lymphogranuloma venereum.

Gamna-Gan·dy bodies (gahn·dee') [C. *Gamna* and C. *Gandy*]. Brown nodules noted in the spleen in chronic passive hyperemia, composed of calcium salts and hemosiderin encrusting fibrous connective and reticular tissues.

Gamna nodules. GAMNA-GANDY BODIES.

Gamna's disease [C. *Gamna*]. SPLENOGRANULOMATOSIS SIDEROTICA.

Gamna spleen [C. *Gamna*]. GANDY-GAMNA SPLEEN.

gamo-. See *gam-.*

gamo·ma·nia (gam"o·may'nee·uh) *n.* [*gamo-* + *mania*]. Excessive desire for marriage.

gam·one (gam'ohn) *n.* Any of various substances released by a sperm or ovum and serving to attract the germ cell or gamete of the opposite sex.

gamo·pet·al·ous (gam"o·pet'uh·lus) *adj.* [*gamo-* + *petal* + *-ous*]. *In botany,* with the petals more or less united.

gamo·pho·bia (gam"o·fo'bee·uh) *n.* [*gamo-* + *phobia*]. An abnormal fear of marriage.

gamo·sep·al·ous (gam"o·sep'ul·us) *adj.* [*gamo-* + *sepal* + *-ous*]. *In botany,* with united sepals.

Gam·per's bowing reflex (gahm'pur) [E. *Gamper,* Austrian neurologist, 1887–1938]. A mass reflex in which the head and then the trunk are brought from either the supine or the lateral position with the sacrum held or supported into the erect and then the forward position, like a bowing movement, elicited with the sacrum held or supported by firm, slow extension of the hips and knees to overcome flexor hypertonia in anencephalics, in infants with severe cerebral damage, usually from hypoxia; and in some healthy premature infants; thought to depend on the release of the pons and structures below from cortical, cerebellar, and striatopallidal influences.

Gamstorp's disease [Ingrid *Gamstorp,* Swedish pediatric neurologist, 20th century]. ADYNAMIA EPISODICA HEREDITARIA.

-gamy [L. *-gamia,* from Gk., from *gamos,* marriage]. A combining form designating *a* (specified) *kind of mating, fertilization, or reproduction.*

Gandy-Gamna nodules [C. *Gandy,* French physician, b. 1872; and C. *Gamna*]. GAMNA-GANDY BODIES.

Gandy-Gamna spleen [C. *Gandy* and C. *Gamna*]. Chronic passive splenic hyperemia with siderotic nodule formation.

gangli-, ganglio-. A combining form meaning *ganglion.*

ganglia. A plural of *ganglion.*

ganglia aor·ti·co·re·na·lia (ay·or"ti·ko·re·nay'lee·uh) [NA]. AORTICORENAL GANGLIA.

ganglia car·di·a·ca (kahr·dye'uh·kuh) [NA]. CARDIAC GANGLIA.

ganglia ce·li·a·ca (see·lye'uh·kuh) [NA]. CELIAC GANGLIA.

ganglia coe·li·a·ca (see·lye'uh·kuh) [BNA]. Ganglia celiaca (= CELIAC GANGLIA).

ganglia in·ter·me·dia (in·tur·mee'dee·uh) [NA]. INTERMEDIATE GANGLIA.

ganglia lum·ba·lia (lum·bay'lee·uh) [NA]. LUMBAR GANGLIA.

ganglia pel·vi·na (pel·vye'nuh) [NA]. PELVIC GANGLIA.

ganglia phre·ni·ca (fren'i·kuh) [NA]. PHRENIC GANGLIA.

ganglia plex·u·um au·to·no·mi·co·rum (pleck'sue·um aw"to·nom·i·ko'rum) [NA]. The ganglia of the autonomic nervous system.

ganglia plexuum sym·pa·thi·co·rum (sim·path"i·ko'rum) [BNA]. GANGLIA PLEXUUM AUTONOMICORUM.

gan·gli·ar (gang'glee·ur) *adj.* GANGLIONIC.

ganglia re·na·lia (re·nay'lee·uh) [NA]. RENAL GANGLIA.

ganglia sa·cra·lia (sa·kray'lee·uh) [NA]. The ganglia of the sympathetic nervous system which are associated with the sacral spinal nerves.

gan·gli·at·ed (gang'glee·ay"tid) *adj.* Supplied with ganglia; GANGLIONATED.

ganglia tho·ra·ca·lia (tho·ruh·kay'lee·uh) [BNA]. Ganglia thoracica (= THORACIC GANGLIA).

ganglia tho·ra·ci·ca (tho·ray'si·kuh, tho·ras'i·kuh) [NA]. THORACIC GANGLIA.

ganglia trun·ci sym·pa·thi·ci (trun'sigh sim·path'i·sigh, trunk'eye) [NA]. The ganglia of the sympathetic nervous system.

gan·gli·ec·to·my (gang"glee·eck'tuh·mee) *n.* [*gangli-* + *-ectomy*]. GANGLIONECTOMY.

gan·gli·form (gang'gli·form) *adj.* Formed like or resembling a ganglion.

gan·gli·itis (gang"glee·eye'tis) *n.* [*gangli-* + *-itis*]. GANGLIONITIS.

ganglio-. See *gangli-.*

gan·glio·blast (gang'glee·o·blast) *n.* [*ganglio-* + *-blast*]. 1. An embryonic ganglion cell. 2. *Obsol.* NEUROBLAST.

gan·glio·cyte (gang'glee·o·site) *n.* [*ganglio-* + *-cyte*]. *Obsol.* GANGLION CELL.

gan·glio·cy·to·ma (gang"glee·o·sigh·to'muh) *n.* [*gangliocyte* + *-oma*]. GANGLIONEUROMA.

gan·glio·cy·to·neu·ro·ma (gang"glee·o·site"o·new·ro'muh) *n.* [*ganglio-* + *cyto-* + *neuroma*]. GANGLIONEUROMA.

gan·glio·form (gang'glee·o·form) *adj.* GANGLIFORM.

ganglioform swellings. CYTOID BODIES.

gan·glio·gli·o·ma (gang"glee·o·glye·o'muh) *n.* [*ganglio-* + *glioma*]. A tumor of the central nervous system composed of nerve cells in various stages of differentiation and glial elements.

gan·gli·oid (gang'glee·oid) *adj.* [*gangli-* + *-oid*]. Resembling a ganglion.

gan·gli·o·ma (gang"glee·o'muh) *n.*, pl. **gangliomas, ganglio·ma·ta** (·tuh) [*gangli-* + *-oma*]. GANGLIOGLIOMA.

gan·gli·on (gang'glee·un) *n.*, pl. **gan·glia** (·glee·uh), **ganglions** [Gk.]. 1. A group of nerve cell bodies, usually located outside the brain and spinal cord, as the dorsal root ganglion of a spinal nerve. 2. A cystic, tumorlike, localized lesion in or about a tendon sheath or joint capsule, especially of the hands, wrists, and feet, but also occasionally within other connective tissues. It is composed of stellate cells in a matrix of mucoid hyaluronic acid and reticular fibers. Syn. *cystic tumor of a tendon sheath, cyst of a joint capsule, cyst of a semilunar cartilage, weeping sinew.*

gan·gli·on·at·ed (gang'glee·un·ay"tid) *adj.* Supplied with ganglions; GANGLIATED.

ganglion car·di·a·cum [Wrisbergi] (kahr·dye'uh·kum) [BNA]. CARDIAC GANGLION.

ganglion cell. 1. A nerve cell in a ganglion. 2. Formerly any neuron of the central nervous system.

ganglion-cell glioma. GANGLIOGLIOMA.

ganglion cer·vi·ca·le in·fe·ri·us (sur·vi·kay'lee in·feer'ee·us) [BNA]. The inferior cervical ganglion. See *cervical ganglion* (1).

ganglion cervicale medium [NA]. The middle cervical ganglion. See *cervical ganglion* (1).
ganglion cervicale su·pe·ri·us (sue·peer'ee·us) [NA]. The superior cervical ganglion. See *cervical ganglion* (1).
ganglion cer·vi·co·tho·ra·ci·cum (sur"vi·ko·tho·ray'si·kum) [NA]. STELLATE GANGLION. NA alt. *ganglion stellatum*.
ganglion ci·li·a·re (sil·ee·air'ee) [NA]. CILIARY GANGLION.
gan·gli·on·ec·to·my (gang"glee·un·eck'tuh·mee) *n.* [*ganglion* + *-ectomy*]. Excision of a ganglion.
Gan·gli·o·ne·ma (gang"glee·o·nee'muh) *n.* A genus of nematodes. See also *Fibiger's tumor.*
gan·glio·neu·ro·blas·to·ma (gang"glee·o·new"ro·blas·to'muh) *n.* A tumor sharing features of ganglioneuroma and neuroblastoma that contains incompletely differentiated nerve cells, ranging from embryonal to anaplastic, and that may metastasize.
ganglioneuroblastoma sym·path·i·cum (sim·path'i·kum). A form of ganglioneuroma containing sympathetic ganglion cells.
gan·glio·neu·ro·cy·to·ma (gang"glee·o·new"ro·sigh·to'muh) *n.* [*ganglio-* + *neurocytoma*]. GANGLIONEUROMA.
gan·glio·neu·ro·ma (gang"glee·o·new·ro'muh) *n.* [*ganglio-* + *neuroma*]. A tumor composed predominantly of mature ganglion cells, often lying in groups within abundant interlacing reticulin fibers and Schwann cells, and commonly showing cystic degeneration and microscopic calcification. There is considerable histological variation, even within the same tumor, depending on the degree of neoplastic evolution and the tumor site, with those located in the cerebral hemispheres and brainstem very different from those in the cerebellum and those along the sympathetic ganglia and adrenal medulla. Transitional forms with neuroblastomas, hamartomatous variants, and metastases may occur. Syn. *gangliocytoma.* See also *neuroastrocytoma.*
ganglioneuroma te·lan·gi·ec·ta·tum cys·ti·cum (tel·an"jee·eck·tay'tum sis'ti·kum). A form of ganglioneuroma with a prominent vascular component.
ganglion ge·ni·cu·li (je·nick'yoo·lye) [NA]. GENICULATE GANGLION.
ganglion ha·be·nu·lae (ha·ben'yoo·lee). HABENULAR NUCLEUS.
gan·gli·on·ic (gang"glee·on'ick) *adj.* Pertaining to or containing ganglions.
ganglionic block. Blockade by local anesthetic of an autonomic or central nervous system ganglion.
ganglionic crest. NEURAL CREST.
ganglionic layer of the optic nerve. The innermost cell layer of the retina, composed of large multipolar ganglion cells of the optic nerve. NA *stratum ganglionare nervi optici.*
ganglionic layer of the retina. The layer of the retina which contains the bipolar cells. NA *stratum ganglionare retinae.*
ganglionic neuroglioma. A glioma containing ganglion cells.
ganglionic neuroma. GANGLIONEUROMA.
ganglionic saliva. Saliva produced by stimulating the submandibular ganglion.
ganglion im·par (im'pahr) [NA]. COCCYGEAL GANGLION.
ganglion in·fe·ri·us (in·feer'ee·us). INFERIOR GANGLION.
ganglion inferius ner·vi glos·so·pha·ryn·gei (nur'vye glos·o·fa·rin'jee·eye) [NA]. The inferior ganglion of the glossopharyngeal nerve. See *inferior ganglion.*
ganglion inferius nervi va·gi (vay'guy, ·jye) [NA]. The inferior ganglion of the vagus nerve. See *inferior ganglion.*
gan·gli·on·itis (gang"glee·un·eye'tis) *n.* [*ganglion* + *-itis*]. Inflammation of a ganglion.
ganglion ju·gu·la·re ner·vi va·gi (jug·yoo·layr'ee nur'vye vay'guy, ·jye) [BNA]. Ganglion superius nervi vagi. See *superior ganglion.*
ganglion me·sen·te·ri·cum in·fe·ri·us (mes"en·terr'i·kum in·feer'ee·us) [NA]. INFERIOR MESENTERIC GANGLION.
ganglion mesentericum su·pe·ri·us (sue·peer'ee·us) [NA]. SUPERIOR MESENTERIC GANGLION.
ganglion mol·le (mol'ee). An enlarged and engorged, but nonindurated, lymph node found in African trypanosomiasis.
ganglion no·do·sum (no·do'sum) [BNA]. Ganglion inferius nervi vagi. See *inferior ganglion.*
ganglion nodosum tumor. A tumor of the inferior ganglion of the vagus nerve, histologically indistinguishable from a carotid-body tumor.
ganglion of the cervix uteri. A ganglion of the craniosacral autonomic system, located at the cervix of the uterus. Syn. *Frankenhafuser's ganglion.*
ganglion of the root. SUPERIOR GANGLION (2).
ganglion of the trunk. INFERIOR GANGLION (2).
ganglion oti·cum (o'ti·kum) [NA]. OTIC GANGLION.
ganglion pe·tro·sum (pe·tro'sum) [BNA]. Ganglion inferius nervi glossopharyngei. See *inferior ganglion.*
ganglion pte·ry·go·pa·la·ti·num (terr"i·go·pal·uh·tye'num) [NA]. PTERYGOPALATINE GANGLION.
ganglion ridge. NEURAL CREST.
ganglion sphe·no·pa·la·ti·num (sfee"no·pal·uh·tye'num). PTERYGOPALATINE GANGLION.
ganglion spi·na·le (spye·nay'lee) [NA]. SPINAL GANGLION.
ganglion spi·ra·le coch·le·ae (spye·ray'lee kock'lee·ee) [NA]. SPIRAL GANGLION OF THE COCHLEA.
ganglion splanch·ni·cum (splank'ni·kum) [NA]. SPLANCHNIC GANGLION.
ganglion stel·la·tum (stel·ay'tum) [NA alt.]. STELLATE GANGLION. NA alt. *ganglion cervicothoracicum.*
ganglion sub·man·di·bu·la·re (sub"man·dib·yoo·lair'ee) [NA]. SUBMANDIBULAR GANGLION.
ganglion sub·max·il·la·re (sub·mack·si·lair'ee) [BNA]. Ganglion submandibulare (= SUBMANDIBULAR GANGLION).
ganglion su·pe·ri·us (sue·peer'ee·us). SUPERIOR GANGLION.
ganglion superius ner·vi glos·so·pha·ryn·gei (nur'vye glos"o·fa·rin'jee·eye) [NA]. The superior ganglion of the glossopharyngeal nerve. See *superior ganglion.*
ganglion superius nervi va·gi (vay'guy, ·jye) [NA]. The superior ganglion of the vagus nerve. See *superior ganglion.*
ganglion ter·mi·na·le (tur·mi·nay'lee) [NA]. TERMINAL GANGLION.
ganglion tri·ge·mi·na·le (trye·jem·i·nay'lee) [NA]. TRIGEMINAL GANGLION.
ganglion tym·pa·ni·cum (tim·pan'i·kum) [NA]. TYMPANIC GANGLION.
ganglion ver·te·bra·le (vur·te·bray'lee) [NA]. A small inconstant ganglion associated with the cervical portion of the sympathetic nervous system.
ganglion ve·sti·bu·la·re (ves·tib"yoo·lair'ee) [NA]. VESTIBULAR GANGLION.
gan·gli·o·side (gang'glee·o·side) *n.* [*gangli-* + *-ose* + *-ide*]. One of a group of glycosphingolipids found in neuronal surface membranes and spleen. They contain an *N*-acyl fatty acid derivative of sphingosine linked to a carbohydrate (galactose or glucose). They also contain *N*-acetylglucosamine or *N*-acetylgalactosamine, and *N*-acetylneuraminic acid.
gan·gli·o·si·do·sis (gang"glee·o·si·do'sis, ·sigh·do'sis) *n.*, pl. **gangliosido·ses** (·seez) [*ganglioside* + *-osis*]. 1. Any disorder of the biosynthesis or breakdown of ganglioside, including (a) the generalized or G_{M1} gangliosidoses, (b) the G_{M2} gangliosidoses, and (c) G_{M3} gangliosidosis. 2. *Especially*, a disorder of the breakdown of ganglioside; that is, any of the G_{M1} or G_{M2} gangliosidoses. See also *G_{M1} gangliosidosis, G_{M2} gangliosidosis, G_{M3} gangliosidosis, infantile amaurotic familial idiocy.*
gan·go·sa (gang·go'suh) *n.* [Sp., from *gangoso*, having the voice resonance characteristic of cleft palate]. Destructive lesions of the nose and hard palate, sometimes more extensive, considered to be a tertiary stage of yaws. Syn. *rhinopharyngitis mutilans.*
gan·grae·na oris (gang·gree'nuh or'is). Noma of the mouth.
gan·grene (gang'green, gang·green') *n.* [Gk. *gangraina*].

1. Necrosis of a part; due to failure of the blood supply, to disease, or to direct injury. 2. The putrefactive changes in dead tissue. —**gan·gre·nous** (·gre·nus) *adj.*

gangrene of the appendix. Necrosis of the vermiform appendix in appendicitis, with sloughing of the organ.

gangrene of the lung. A diffuse, putrefactive necrosis of the lung or of a lobe; due to anaerobic or other bacteria; usually a termination of lung abscess in a patient with low resistance.

gangrenous blepharitis. Carbuncle of the eyelids.

gangrenous cystitis. An acute, severe, diffuse inflammation of the urinary bladder involving principally the mucosa and submucosa, due principally to severe infection, x-ray therapy, injection of chemicals, or impaired blood supply and characterized by gross suppuration, necrosis, and gangrene of the involved tissues.

gangrenous inflammation. Severe inflammation complicated by secondary infection with putrefactive bacteria.

gangrenous stomatitis. Noma of the mouth.

gan·ja, gan·jah (gan'juh, ·zhuh) *n.* [Hindi]. The tops, stems, leaves, and twigs of the female hemp plant as used in India for mixing into cakes and for smoking; a form of cannabis more potent than marijuana. See also *cannabis.*

gan·o·blast (gan'o·blast) *n.* [Gk. *ganos*, brightness, + *-blast*]. AMELOBLAST.

Gan·ser's commissure (gahⁿn'zur) [S. J. M. *Ganser*, German psychiatrist, 1853–1931]. ANTERIOR HYPOTHALAMIC DECUSSATION.

Ganser syndrome [S. J. M. *Ganser*]. A mental disorder characterized by the nonsensical performance of simple acts or the giving of wrong, though relevant, answers to questions the correct response to which is known; usually observed in patients, such as prisoners awaiting trial, whose situation might be looked on more leniently by virtue of their confused state.

Gantanol. Trademark for sulfamethoxazole, an antibacterial sulfonamide.

Gantrisin. Trademark for sulfisoxazole, an antibacterial sulfonamide of high solubility in body fluids.

Gantrisin Acetyl. Trademark for acetyl sulfisoxazole, an antibacterial sulfonamide.

Gant's operation [F. J. *Gant*, English surgeon, 1825–1905]. Subtrochanteric osteotomy of the femur for ankylosis of the hip joint with flexion and adduction.

Gant·zer's muscle (gahⁿn'tsur) [C. F. L. *Gantzer*, German anatomist, 19th century]. MUSCLE OF GANTZER.

gapes, *n.* A disease of young fowl caused by the presence of gapeworms in the trachea.

gape·worm (gaip'wurm) *n.* *SYNGAMUS TRACHEALIS.*

Garamycin. Trademark for gentamicin, an antibiotic.

Gar·cin·ia (gahr·sin'ee·uh) *n.* [L. *Garcin*, French botanist, 1683–1752]. A genus of the Guttiferae. *Garcinia hanburyi*, the gamboge tree, yields the gum oleoresin gamboge. *G. mangostana* yields the palatable fruit called mangosteen.

Gardinol W A A trademark for sodium lauryl sulfate, a surfactant.

Gard·ner's syndrome [E. J. *Gardner*, U.S. physician, 20th century.]. An autosomal dominant trait manifested in childhood by multiple osteomas, fibrous and fatty tumors of the skin and the mesentery, epidermoid inclusion cysts of the skin, and the development of intestinal polyps predisposed to malignancy; other tumors, such as carcinoma of the thyroid, may occur.

gar·get (gahr'ghit) *n.* A progressive inflammation of the udder, usually of cattle.

gar·gle, *v. & n.* [OF. *gargouiller*, to gurgle]. 1. To rinse the oropharynx. 2. A solution for rinsing the oropharynx.

gar·goyl·ism (gahr'goil·iz·um) *n.* MUCOPOLYSACCHARIDOSIS.

Gar·land's triangle [G. M. *Garland*, U.S. physician, 1848–1926]. An area of relative resonance in the low back near the spine, found on the same side as a pleural effusion.

gar·lic, *n.* [OE. *gārlēac*, from *gār*, spear, + *lēac*, leek]. The fresh bulb of *Allium sativum*, containing allyl sulfides; has been used medicinally. —**gar·licky,** *adj.*

Gar·ré's osteomyelitis or **disease** (ga·reʸ') [C. *Garré*, Swiss surgeon, 1857–1928]. Chronic sclerosing osteomyelitis with little suppuration, characterized by small areas of necrosis.

Gar·rod's test [A.E. *Garrod*, English physician, 1857–1936]. A test for urinary porphyrins, based on alkaline precipitation of the substances, with resolution in acid alcohol to produce a typical pink-red color.

gar·rot·ing (ga·ro'ting, ga·rot'ing) *n.* [Sp. *garrote*, cudgel]. *In legal medicine*, forcible compression of a victim's neck from behind with intent to rob or kill.

Gart·ner's cyst [H. T. *Gartner*, Danish surgeon, 1785–1827]. A benign cyst arising in the anterolateral vaginal walls from incompletely obliterated remnants of Gartner's duct.

Gartner's duct [H. T. *Gartner*]. The ductus epoophori longitudinalis. It may persist in the mesosalpinx near the ovary or in the lateral wall of the vagina.

gas, *n. & v.* [NL., coined from Gk. *chaos*, chaos, space]. 1. The vaporous or airlike state of matter. A fluid that distributes itself uniformly throughout any space in which it is placed, regardless of its quantity. 2. Any combustible gas used as a source of light or heat. 3. To drench an area with poisonous gas. 4. To execute or attempt to execute a person by means of toxic gas. —**gas·e·ous** (gas'ee·us, gash' us) *adj.*

gas abscess. An abscess filled with gas; TYMPANITIC ABSCESS.

gas chromatography. Chromatography in which the mixture of substances to be separated is vaporized in a stream of carrier gas that moves over a suitably supported stationary liquid phase (gas-liquid chromatography) or a solid phase (gas-solid chromatography); separation occurs by different interactions of the components of the mixture with the stationary phase.

gas cyst. A cyst containing gas, such as gas from the intestinal canal.

gas embolism. AEROEMBOLISM (2).

gaseous dyspepsia. FLATULENT DYSPEPSIA.

gaseous tension. The tendency of a gas to expand.

gas eye. A disease of the eyes characterized by inflammation, tenderness, and sensitivity to light; prevalent among the employees of the gas pumping stations in natural gas regions.

gas gangrene. A form of gangrene occurring in massive wounds, where there is crushing and devitalization of tissue and contamination with dirt. The specific organisms found are anaerobes, including *Clostridium perfringens, C. novyi, C. septicum,* and *C. histolyticum;* nonspecific aerobic pyogens are commonly present also. The condition is characterized by high fever, an offensive, thin, purulent discharge from the wound, and the presence of gas bubbles in the tissues.

gas gangrene bacillus. *CLOSTRIDIUM PERFRINGENS*, type A.

gas gangrene myositis. Inflammation of a muscle followed by or concomitant with a necrotizing infection by anaerobic gas-producing bacteria.

Gas·kell's law of progress. LAW OF PROGRESS.

gas myelography. Radiographic examination of the spinal cord after injecting gas into the subarachnoid spaces.

gas·om·e·ter (gas·om'e·tur) *n.* [*gas* + *-meter*]. A device for holding and measuring gas. —**gas·o·met·ric** (gas"o·met' rick) *adj.*

gasometric analysis. Analysis of a solid or liquid substance by conversion to a gas, or the determination of the constituents of gaseous compounds. Syn. *eudiometric analysis.*

gas sepsis. Sepsis due to the presence of *Clostridium perfringens* or other gas-forming anaerobes.

gas·se·ri·an ganglion (ga·seer'ee·un) [J. L. *Gasser*, Austrian anatomist, d. 1765]. TRIGEMINAL GANGLION.

gas·ter (gas'tur) *n.* [Gk. *gastēr*] [NA alt.]. STOMACH. NA alt. *ventriculus.*

-gaster [Gk. *gastēr*]. A combining form meaning (a) *belly, abdomen;* (b) *stomach.*

Gas·ter·o·phil·i·dae (gas″tur·o·fil′i·dee) *n. pl.* A family of the Diptera, whose larvae, known as bots, are parasitic in the stomach and intestine of horses and related animals. The principal genus is *Gasterophilus.*

Gas·ter·oph·i·lus (gas″tur·off′i·lus) *n.* [NL., from Gk. *gastēr,* stomach, + *philos,* fond of]. A genus of botflies. The larvae are parasites of horses and occasionally infest the cutaneous and subcutaneous tissues in man.

Gasterophilus hem·or·rhoi·da·lis (hem″uh·roy·day′lis). A species of horse botfly in which the eggs attach to the lips and nose of horses, and the mature larvae ultimately leave the stomach to complete their development in the rectum. May cause gastrointestinal disturbances in the horse.

Gasterophilus in·tes·ti·na·lis (in·tes″ti·nay′lis). A species of horse botfly that lays its eggs on the hairs of the foreparts of the horse, with the larvae excavating tunnels under the mucosa of the mouth, and ultimately migrating to the stomach. Human infection similar to the larva migrans caused by *Ancylostoma braziliense* occurs.

Gasterophilus na·sa·lis (nay·say′lis). A species of horse botfly in which the larvae crawl into the mouth of the horse to form pockets between the molars, followed by further development in the stomach and ultimate discharge of the third larval instars in the feces. Rarely causes larva migrans in man.

gastr-, gastro-. A combining form meaning (a) *stomach, gastric;* (b) *belly, abdominal.*

gas·tral·gia (gas·tral′jee·uh) *n.* [*gastr-* + *-algia*]. Pain in the stomach.

gas·tral·go·ke·no·sis (gas·tral″go·ke·no′sis) *n.* [*gastr-* + *algo-* + *ken-* + *-osis*]. Paroxysmal pain due to emptiness of the stomach; relieved by taking food.

gas·tras·the·nia (gas″tras·theen′ee·uh) *n.* [*gastr-* + *asthenia*]. 1. Weakness or lack of tone of the stomach. 2. Weakness of stomach functions.

gas·tra·tro·phia (gas″tra·tro′fee·uh) *n.* [NL., from *gastr-* + *atrophy*]. Atrophy of the stomach.

gas·trec·ta·sia (gas″treck·tay′zhuh, ·zee·uh) *n.* GASTRECTASIS.

gas·trec·ta·sis (gas·treck′tuh·sis) *n.*, pl. **gastrecta·ses** (·seez) [*gastr-* + *ectasis*]. Dilatation of the stomach.

gas·trec·to·my (gas·treck′tuh·mee) *n.* [*gastr-* + *-ectomy*]. Excision of the whole or a part of the stomach.

-gastria [*gastr-* + *-ia*]. A combining form meaning *kind of* or *condition of the stomach.*

gas·tric (gas′trick) *adj.* [Gk. *gastēr, gastros,* stomach, + *-ic*]. Of or pertaining to the stomach.

gastric angle. ANGULAR NOTCH.

gastric antrum. PYLORIC ANTRUM.

gastric areas. The numerous small elevations of the surface of the mucous membrane of the stomach. NA *areae gastricae.*

gastric canal. A longitudinal groove of the mucous membrane of the stomach near the lesser curvature. NA *canalis ventriculi.*

gastric crises. Attacks of intense, paroxysmal pain in the abdomen, often associated with nausea and vomiting, occurring in tabes dorsalis.

gastric cycle. The progression of a peristaltic wave over the stomach; each lasts about 20 seconds.

gastric digestion. Digestion in the stomach by the action of the gastric juice.

gastric fever. BRUCELLOSIS.

gastric foveolae. The pits or grooves in the mucous membrane of the stomach, which receive the secretions of the gastric glands. NA *foveolae gastricae.*

gastric glands. The glands of the stomach, including the cardiac, fundic, and pyloric glands. NA *glandulae gastricae.*

gastric hormone. GASTRIN.

gastric intussusception. An intussusception in which a jejunal loop may escape through a gastroenterostomy into the stomach.

gastric juice. The secretion of the glands of the stomach; a clear, colorless liquid having an acid pH and a specific gravity of about 1.006 and containing about 0.5% of solid matter; contains hydrochloric acid, pepsin, mucin, and, in infants, rennin.

gastric motility. The movements of the stomach walls, including antral peristalsis and fundic contraction in the smooth muscle walls of the stomach.

gastric mucin. A product made from hog stomach linings and once used in the management of peptic ulcers as a demulcent and absorbent.

gastric notch. ANGULAR NOTCH.

gastric pits. GASTRIC FOVEOLAE.

gastric plexus. Any of the nerve plexuses associated with the stomach. The anterior gastric plexus lies along the anterior surface of the lesser curvature of the stomach; its fibers are derived mainly from the left vagus, a few from the right vagus, and some sympathetic fibers. The posterior gastric plexus lies along the posterior surface of the lesser curvature; its fibers are derived mainly from the right vagus. The inferior gastric plexus accompanies the left gastroepiploic artery; its fibers are derived from the splenic plexus. The superior gastric plexus accompanies the left gastric artery, and receives fibers from the celiac plexus. NA (pl.) *plexus gastrici.*

gastric prolapse. Protrusion of gastric mucosa through the pylorus or a surgical stoma.

gastric pyrosis. HEARTBURN.

gastric secretion. GASTRIC JUICE.

gas·tric·sin (gas·trick′sin) *n.* One of the two principal gastric proteases, the other being pepsin.

gastric ulcer. An ulcer affecting the wall of the stomach.

gastric vertigo. Vertigo associated with dyspepsia.

gas·trin (gas′trin) *n.* A polypeptide hormone, secreted by the mucosa of the gastric antrum in response to eating or alkalinization of the stomach; it causes gastric secretion of pepsin and hydrochloric acid and promotes growth of the gastrointestinal mucosa.

gas·tri·tis (gas·trye′tis) *n.*, pl. **gas·trit·i·des** (gas·trit′i·deez) [*gastr-* + *-itis*]. Inflammation of the stomach. —**gas·trit·ic** (gas·trit′ick) *adj.*

gastro-. See *gastr-*.

gas·tro·aceph·a·lus (gas″tro·ay·sef′uh·lus, ·a·sef′) *n.*, pl. **gastroacepha·li** (·lye) [*gastro-* + *acephalus*]. An individual having an acephalic parasitic twin with abdominal attachment.

gas·tro·amor·phus (gas″tro·a·mor′fus) *n.*, pl. **gastroamor·phi** (·figh) [*gastro-* + *amorphus*]. A form of cryptodidymus in which fetal parts are included within the abdomen of the host.

gas·tro·anas·to·mo·sis (gas″tro·uh·nas″tuh·mo′sis) *n.* [*gastro-* + *anastomosis*]. GASTROGASTROSTOMY.

gas·tro·cam·era (gas″tro·kam′e·ruh) *n.* [*gastro-* + *camera*]. A tiny camera with attached light designed to be introduced through the esophagus into the stomach to obtain pictures from within the lumen.

gas·tro·cele (gas′tro·seel) *n.* [*gastro-* + *-cele*]. A hernia of the stomach.

gas·tro·cne·mi·us (gas″tro·nee′mee·us, ·k′nee′mee·us) *n.*, pl. **gastrocne·mii** (·mee·eye) [NL., from Gk. *gastroknēmē,* calf, from *gastēr,* belly, + *knēmē,* leg, shank]. A muscle on the posterior aspect of the leg, arising by two heads from the posterior surfaces of the lateral and medial condyles of the femur, and inserted with the soleus muscle into the calcaneal tendon, and through this into the back of the calcaneus. NA *musculus gastrocnemius.* See also Table of Muscles in the Appendix.

gastrocnemius bursa. Either of the bursas beneath the tendinous origins of the heads of the gastrocnemius muscle, often communicating with the capsule of the knee joint:

the lateral gastrocnemius bursa (NA *bursa subtendinea musculi gastrocnemii lateralis*), between the tendon of the lateral head and the capsule of the knee joint, or the medial gastrocnemius bursa (NA *bursa subtendinea musculi gastrocnemii medialis*), between the tendon of the medial head and the capsule of the knee joint and medial condyle of the femur.

gas·tro·coel, gas·tro·coele (gas'tro·seel) *n.* [*gastro-* + *-coel*]. ARCHENTERON.

gas·tro·co·lic (gas''tro·kol'ick, ·ko'lick) *adj.* [*gastro-* + *colic*]. Pertaining to the stomach and the colon.

gastrocolic ligament. The mesentery or portion of the omentum between stomach and transverse colon produced by fusion of the embryonic mesocolon with part of the greater omentum. NA *ligamentum gastrocolicum.*

gastrocolic omentum. GREATER OMENTUM.

gastrocolic reflex or **response.** Motility of the colon induced by the entrance of food into the stomach.

gas·tro·co·lot·o·my (gas''tro·ko·lot'uh·mee) *n.* [*gastro-* + *colo-* + *-tomy*]. Incision into the stomach and colon.

gas·tro·col·pot·o·my (gas''tro·kol·pot'uh·mee) *n.* [*gastro-* + *colpo-* + *-tomy*]. Cesarean section in which the opening is made through the linea alba and continued into the upper part of the vagina.

gas·tro·did·y·mus (gas''tro·did'i·mus) *n.*, pl. **gastrodidy·mi** (·migh) [*gastro-* + *didymus*]. OMPHALOPAGUS.

gas·tro·dis·ci·a·sis (gas''tro·dis·kigh'uh·sis, ·di·sigh'uh·sis) *n.* [*Gastrodiscoides* + *-iasis*]. Infection of the cecum by *Gastrodiscoides hominis,* causing inflammation and producing diarrhea.

Gas·tro·dis·coi·des (gas''tro·dis·koy'deez) *n.* [*gastro-* + Gk. *diskoeidēs,* disk-shaped]. A genus of flukes of the family Gastrodiscidae.

Gastrodiscoides hom·i·nis (hom'i·nis). A species of small intestinal fluke which has as its natural host the hog; man serves as an accidental host, the fluke attaching to the cecum and ascending colon; the cause of gastrodisciasis.

Gas·tro·dis·cus hominis (gas''tro·dis'kus). *GASTRODISCOIDES HOMINIS.*

gas·tro·disk (gas'tro·disk) *n.* [*gastro-* + *disk*]. GERMINAL DISK.

gas·tro·du·o·de·nal (gas''tro·dew''o·dee'nul, dew·od'e·nul) *adj.* [*gastro-* + *duodenal*]. Pertaining to the stomach and the duodenum.

gastroduodenal artery. See Table of Arteries in the Appendix.

gastroduodenal plexus. A portion of the celiac plexus distributed to the stomach and duodenum.

gas·tro·du·o·de·ni·tis (gas''tro·dew''o·de·nigh'tis, ·dew·od''e·nigh'tis) *n.* [*gastro-* + *duoden-* + *-itis*]. Inflammation of the stomach and duodenum.

gas·tro·du·o·de·nos·to·my (gas''tro·dew''o·de·nos'tuh·mee) *n.* [*gastro-* + *duodeno-* + *-stomy*]. Establishment of an anastomosis between the stomach and duodenum. Compare *gastroenterostomy.*

gas·tro·en·ter·al·gia (gas''tro·en''tur·al'jee·uh) *n.* [*gastro-* + *enter-* + *-algia*]. Pain in the stomach and intestine.

gas·tro·en·ter·ic (gas''tro·en·terr'ick) *adj.* [*gastro-* + *enteric*]. Pertaining to the stomach and the intestines; GASTROINTESTINAL.

gas·tro·en·ter·i·tis (gas''tro·en·tur·eye'tis) *n.* [*gastro-* + *enteritis*]. Inflammation of the mucosa of the stomach and intestines. —**gastroenter·it·ic** (·it'ick) *adj.*

gas·tro·en·tero·anas·to·mo·sis (gas''tro·en''tur·o·uh·nas''tuh·mo'sis) *n.* [*gastro-* + *entero-* + *anastomosis*]. Anastomosis between the intestine and the stomach. Compare *gastroenterostomy.*

gas·tro·en·ter·ol·o·gist (gas''tro·en·tur·ol'uh·jist) *n.* A physician specializing in gastroenterology.

gas·tro·en·ter·ol·o·gy (gas''tro·en''tur·ol'uh·jee) *n.* [*gastro-* + *entero-* + *-logy*]. The study of the stomach and intestine and their diseases.

gas·tro·en·ter·op·a·thy (gas''tro·en''tur·op'uth·ee) *n.* [*gastro-* + *entero-* + *-pathy*]. Any disease of the stomach and intestines.

gas·tro·en·ter·op·to·sis (gas''tro·en''tur·op·to'sis) *n.* [*gastro-* + *entero-* + *-ptosis*]. Sagging or prolapse of the stomach and intestines.

gas·tro·en·ter·os·to·my (gas''tro·en·tur·os'tuh·mee) *n.* [*gastro-* + *entero-* + *-stomy*]. The formation of a communication between the stomach and the small intestine, usually the jejunum. Compare *gastroduodenostomy, gastrojejunostomy, gastroenteroanastomosis.*

gas·tro·ep·i·plo·ic (gas''tro·ep''i·plo'ick) *adj.* [*gastro-* + *epiploic*]. Pertaining to the stomach and greater omentum.

gastroepiploic artery. See Table of Arteries in the Appendix.

gas·tro·esoph·a·ge·al, gas·tro-oe·soph·a·ge·al (gas''tro·e·sof''uh·jee'ul) *adj.* [*gastro-* + *esophageal*]. Pertaining to or involving the stomach and esophagus.

gastroesophageal sphincter. CARDIAC SPHINCTER.

gas·tro·esoph·a·gi·tis (gas''tro·e·sof''uh·jye'tis) *n.* [*gastro-* + *esophag-* + *-itis*]. Inflammation of the stomach and the esophagus.

gas·tro·esoph·a·go·plas·ty, gas·tro-oe·soph·a·go·plas·ty (gas''tro·e·sof'uh·go·plas''tee) *n.* [*gastro-* + *esophago-* + *-plasty*]. Plastic surgical repair of the stomach and esophagus.

gas·tro·gas·tros·to·my (gas''tro·gas·tros'tuh·mee) *n.* [*gastro-* + *gastro-* + *-stomy*]. *In surgery,* anastomosis of one portion of the stomach with another, as the surgical formation of a communication between the two pouches of an hourglass stomach.

gas·tro·ga·vage (gas''tro·ga·vahzh') *n.* [*gastro-* + *gavage*]. Artificial feeding through an opening in the stomach wall.

gas·tro·gen·ic (gas''tro·jen'ick) *adj.* [*gastro-* + *-genic*]. Originating in the stomach.

Gastrografin. Trademark for meglumine diatrizoate in an oral dosage form used for radiological examination of the gastrointestinal tract.

gas·tro·graph (gas'tro·graf) *n.* [*gastro-* + *-graph*]. An apparatus for recording the peristaltic movements of the stomach.

gas·tro·he·pat·ic (gas''tro·he·pat'ick) *adj.* [*gastro-* + *hepatic*]. Pertaining to the stomach and liver.

gastrohepatic ligament. The portion of the lesser omentum extending between the liver and the stomach. NA *ligamentum hepatogastricum.*

gastrohepatic omentum. LESSER OMENTUM.

gas·tro·hy·per·ton·ic (gas''tro·high''pur·ton'ick) *adj.* [*gastro-* + *hypertonic*]. Pertaining to or characterized by morbid or excessive tonicity or irritability of the stomach.

gas·tro·il·e·ac (gas''tro·il'ee·ack) *adj.* [*gastro-* + *ileac*]. Pertaining to the stomach and the ileum.

gastroileac reflex. Altered, usually increased, motility of the ileum resulting from the presence of food in the stomach.

gas·tro·in·tes·ti·nal (gas''tro·in·tes'ti·nul) *adj.* [*gastro-* + *intestinal*]. Pertaining to the stomach and intestine.

gastrointestinal tract. ALIMENTARY CANAL.

gas·tro·je·ju·nal (gas''tro·je·joo'nul) *adj.* Pertaining to the stomach and the jejunum.

gastrojejunal fistula. A fistula between the stomach and the jejunum; a serious complication that develops in about 10% of patients with anastomotic ulcers, especially those ulcers which follow simple posterior gastroenterostomy for peptic ulcer.

gas·tro·je·ju·ni·tis (gas''tro·jee''joo·nigh'tis, ·jej''oo·) *n.* [*gastro-* + *jejun-* + *-itis*]. Inflammation of both the stomach and jejunum; sometimes occurring after gastrojejunostomy.

gas·tro·je·ju·nos·to·my (gas''tro·jee''joo·nos'tuh·mee) *n.* [*gastro-* + *jejuno-* + *-stomy*]. *In surgery,* anastomosis of the jejunum to the anterior or posterior wall of the stomach. Compare *gastroenterostomy.*

gas·tro·la·vage (gas''tro·la·vahzh') *n.* The washing out of the stomach; gastric lavage.

gas·tro·li·e·nal (gas″tro·lye′e·nul) *adj.* [*gastro-* + *lienal*]. GASTROSPLENIC.

gas·tro·lith (gas′tro·lith) *n.* [*gastro-* + *-lith*]. A calcareous formation in the stomach.

gas·tro·li·thi·a·sis (gas″tro·li·thigh′uh·sis) *n.* [*gastrolith* + *-iasis*]. The formation or presence of gastroliths.

gas·trol·o·gy (gas·trol′uh·jee) *n.* [*gastro-* + *-logy*]. The science of the stomach, its functions and diseases.

gas·trol·y·sis (gas·trol′i·sis) *n.*, pl. **gastroly·ses** (·seez) [*gastro-* + *-lysis*]. The breaking up of adhesions between the stomach and adjacent organs.

gas·tro·ma·la·cia (gas″tro·ma·lay′shee·uh, ·see·uh) *n.* [*gastro-* + *malacia*]. An abnormal softening of the walls of the stomach.

gas·tro·meg·a·ly (gas″tro·meg′uh·lee) *n.* [*gastro-* + *-megaly*]. Abnormal enlargement of the stomach.

gas·trom·e·lus (gas·trom′e·lus) *n.*, pl. **gastrome·li** (·lye) [*gastro-* + *-melus*]. An individual with an accessory limb attached to the abdomen.

gas·tro·mes·en·ter·ic (gas″tro·mes″in·terr′ick) *adj.* [*gastro-* + *mesenteric*]. Pertaining to the stomach and the mesentery.

gastromesenteric ileus. ACUTE DUODENAL ILEUS.

gas·tro·my·co·sis (gas″tro·migh·ko′sis) *n.*, pl. **gastromyco·ses** (·seez) [*gastro-* + *mycosis*]. Gastric disease due to fungi.

gas·tro·my·ot·o·my (gas″tro·migh·ot′uh·mee) *n.* [*gastro-* + *myotomy*]. Incision of the circular muscle fibers of the stomach. See also *cardiomyotomy, pyloromyotomy.*

gastro-oesophageal. GASTROESOPHAGEAL.

gas·trop·a·gus (gas·trop′uh·gus) *n.* [*gastro-* + *-pagus*]. SUPRAOMPHALODYMIA.

gas·tro·pan·cre·at·ic (gas″tro·pan″kree·at′ick) *adj.* [*gastro-* + *pancreatic*]. Pertaining to the stomach and the pancreas.

gastropancreatic plicae. Folds of peritoneum on the posterior wall of the omental bursa, extending from the pancreas to the right side of the cardia of the stomach. They contain the left gastric vessels. NA *plicae gastropancreaticae.*

gas·tro·par·a·si·tus (gas″tro·păr·uh·sigh′tus) *n.* [NL., from *gastro-* + Gk. *parasitos,* parasite]. An individual having a more or less complete parasitic twin attached to its abdomen.

gas·trop·a·thy (gas·trop′uth·ee) *n.* [*gastro-* + *-pathy*]. Any disease or disorder of the stomach.

gas·tro·pexy (gas′tro·peck″see) *n.* [*gastro-* + *-pexy*]. The fixation of a prolapsed stomach in its normal position by suturing it to the abdominal wall or other structure.

gas·tro·phren·ic (gas″tro·fren′ick) *adj.* [*gastro-* + *phrenic*]. Pertaining to the stomach and diaphragm.

gastrophrenic ligament. A fold of peritoneum from the diaphragm to the stomach. NA *ligamentum gastrophrenicum.*

gas·tro·plas·ty (gas′tro·plas″tee) *n.* [*gastro-* + *-plasty*]. Plastic operation on the stomach. See also *gastrorrhaphy.*

gas·tro·pli·ca·tion (gas″tro·pli·kay′shun) *n.* [*gastro-* + *plication*]. An operation for relief of chronic dilatation of the stomach, consisting in suturing a large horizontal fold in the stomach wall; plication of the stomach wall for redundancy due to chronic dilatation. Compare *gastrorrhaphy.* See also *gastroplasty.*

gas·tro·pore (gas′tro·pore) *n.* [*gastro-* + *-pore*]. BLASTOPORE.

gas·trop·to·sis (gas″trop·to′sis) *n.* [*gastro-* + *-ptosis*]. Prolapse or downward displacement of the stomach.

gas·tro·py·lo·rec·to·my (gas″tro·pye″lo·reck′tuh·mee) *n.* [*gastro-* + *pylorectomy*]. Excision of the pyloric portion of the stomach.

gas·tror·rha·gia (gas″tro·ray′jee·uh) *n.* [*gastro-* + *-rrhagia*]. Hemorrhage from the stomach.

gas·tror·rha·phy (gas·tror′uh·fee) *n.* [*gastro-* + *-rrhaphy*]. 1. Repair of a stomach wound. 2. GASTROPLICATION. See also *gastroplasty.*

gas·tror·rhea, gas·tror·rhoea (gas″tro·ree′uh) *n.* [*gastro-* + *-rrhea*]. Excessive secretion of gastric mucus or of gastric juice.

gas·tro·sal·i·vary reflex (gas″tro·sal′i·verr·ee). Salivation following the introduction of food into the stomach.

gas·tros·chi·sis (gas·tros′ki·sis) *n.* [*gastro-* + *-schisis*]. A congenital malformation in which the abdomen remains open to the exterior. See also *celosoma.*

gas·tro·scope (gas′truh·skope) *n.* [*gastro-* + *-scope*]. A fiberoptic endoscope for examining the interior of the stomach. —**gas·tros·co·py** (gas·tros′kuh·pee) *n.*

gas·tro·spasm (gas′tro·spaz·um) *n.* [*gastro-* + *spasm*]. Spasm or contraction of the stomach wall.

gas·tro·splen·ic (gas″tro·splen′ick) *adj.* [*gastro-* + *splenic*]. Pertaining to the stomach and the spleen.

gastrosplenic ligament or **omentum.** The fold of peritoneum passing from the stomach to the spleen. NA *ligamentum gastrolienale.*

gas·tro·stax·is (gas″tro·stack′sis) *n.* [*gastro-* + *staxis*]. The oozing of blood from the mucous membrane of the stomach.

gas·tros·to·my (gas·tros′tuh·mee) *n.* [*gastro-* + *-stomy*]. The establishing of a fistulous opening into the stomach, with an external opening in the skin; usually for artificial feeding.

gas·tro·suc·cor·rhea, gas·tro·suc·cor·rhoea (gas″tro·suck″o·ree′uh) *n.* [*gastro-* + *succorrhea*]. REICHMANN'S DISEASE.

gas·tro·tho·ra·cop·a·gus (gas″tro·thor·uh·kop′uh·gus) *n.*, pl. **gastrothoracopa·gi** (·guy, ·jye) [*gastro-* + *thoracopagus*]. Conjoined twins united at the abdomen and thorax.

gas·trot·o·my (gas·trot′uh·mee) *n.* [*gastro-* + *-tomy*]. Incision into the stomach.

gastrotoxic serum. An immune serum which when injected damages the gastric cells, allowing ulceration of the mucosa by the gastric juice; produced by using gastric cells to immunize an animal.

gas·tro·tox·in (gas″tro·tock′sin) *n.* [*gastro-* + *toxin*]. A cytotoxin which has a specific action on the cells lining the stomach. —**gastrotox·ic** (·sick) *adj.*

gas·tro·tym·pa·ni·tes (gas″tro·tim″puh·nigh′teez) *n.* [*gastro-* + *tympanites*]. Gaseous distention of the stomach.

gas·trox·yn·sis (gas″trock·sin′sis) *n.* [*gastro-* + Gk. *oxynein,* to sharpen, to acidify]. Excessive acid secretion by the stomach; HYPERCHLORHYDRIA.

gas·tru·la (gas′troo·luh) *n.*, pl. **gastrulas, gastru·lae** (·lee) [NL., dim. from *gaster*]. An embryo at that stage of its development when it consists of two cellular layers, the primary ectoderm and entoderm, and a primitive gut or archenteron opening externally through the blastopore. The simplest type is derived by the invagination of the spherical blastula, but this is greatly modified in the various animal groups. —**gas·tru·la·tion** (gas″troo·lay′shun) *n.*

gas tube. Early roentgen-ray tube with a relatively low vacuum.

Gatch bed [W. D. *Gatch,* U.S. surgeon, 1878–1963]. A jointed bed frame that permits a patient to be placed in a sitting or semireclining position.

gato·phil·ia (gat″o·fil′ee·uh) *n.* [Mod. Gk. *gatos,* cat, + *-philia*]. GALEOPHILIA.

gato·pho·bia (gat″o·fo′bee·uh) *n.* [Mod. Gk. *gatos,* cat, + *-phobia*]. GALEOPHOBIA.

Gau·cher lipid (go·shey′) [P. C. E. *Gaucher,* French physician, 1854–1918]. KERASIN.

Gaucher's cells [P. C. E. *Gaucher,* French physician, 1854–1918]. Altered macrophages found in Gaucher's disease, 20 to 80 microns in diameter, with single small spherical nuclei and abundant striated cytoplasm containing the characteristic cerebrosides of the disease.

Gaucher's disease [P. C. E. *Gaucher*]. A rare chronic familial deficiency of a glucocerebroside-cleaving enzyme resulting in abnormal storage of cerebrosides in reticuloendothelial cells and characterized by splenomegaly, hepatomegaly, skin pigmentation, pingueculae of the scleras, and bone lesions. Syn. *cerebroside lipidosis, familial splenic anemia.*

gauge (gaje) *n.* An instrument for measuring the dimensions or extent of a structure, or for testing the status of a process or phenomenon.

gaul·the·ria (gawl·theer'ee·uh) *n.* [J. F. *Gaultier,* Canadian physician and botanist, 1708–1756]. The plant *Gaultheria procumbens,* the leaves of which yield a volatile oil. Syn. *teaberry, wintergreen.*

gaultheria oil. A volatile oil from gaultheria consisting principally of methyl salicylate; used as a local irritant, antiseptic, and flavoring agent.

gaul·ther·in (gawl·theer'in, gawl'thur·in) *n.* A glycoside from the bark of sweet birch, *Betula lenta,* and from wintergreen, *Gaultheria procumbens.* On enzymic hydrolysis it yields methyl salicylate and primeverose; on acid hydrolysis the latter yields D-glucose and D-xylose.

gaul·ther·o·lin (gawl·theer'o·lin) *n.* METHYL SALICYLATE.

Gault's reflex. AUDITORY-PALPEBRAL REFLEX.

gaunt·let (gawnt'lit) *n.* [OF. *gantelet,* dim. of *gant,* glove]. A bandage that covers the hand and fingers like a glove.

gauntlet anesthesia. GLOVE-AND-STOCKING ANESTHESIA.

gauntlet bandage. GAUNTLET.

gauntlet flap. A pedicle flap that is raised and applied to a movable part, as from the abdominal wall to a hand.

gauss (gaowss) *n.* [K. F. *Gauss,* German mathematician and optician, 1777–1855]. A unit of magnetic induction, equal to one line of flux per square centimeter.

Gaus·sel sign (go·sel') [A. *Gaussel,* French physician, 19th century]. GRASSET-GAUSSEL PHENOMENON.

Gauss·i·an points (gaow'see·un) [K. F. *Gauss*]. NODAL POINTS.

gauze (gawz) *n.* [OF. *gaze*]. A thin, open-meshed absorbent cloth of varying degrees of fineness, used in surgical operations and for surgical dressings. When sterilized it is called aseptic gauze.

gauze sponge. A flat folded piece of gauze of varying size, used by a surgical assistant to absorb blood from the wound during an operation.

ga·vage (ga·vahzh') *n.* [F., from *gaver,* to stuff, cram]. The administration of nourishment through a stomach tube.

G colony. GONIDIAL COLONY.

g-component. A measure of the amount of gynandromorphy in the somatotype.

Gd Symbol for gadolinium.

Ge Symbol for germanium.

ge-, geo- [Gk. *gē*]. A combining form meaning (a) *earth, ground, soil;* (b) *geographic.*

Gee-Her·ter disease [S. J. *Gee,* English pediatrician, 1839–1911; and C. A. *Herter*]. INFANTILE CELIAC DISEASE.

Gee-Thay·sen disease (tye'sun) [S. J. *Gee;* and T. E. H. *Thaysen,* Danish physician, 1883–1936]. INFANTILE CELIAC DISEASE.

Ge·gen·baur's muscle (geʸ'gun·baow''ur) [C. *Gegenbaur,* German anatomist, 1826–1903]. AURICULOFRONTALIS.

ge·gen·hal·ten (gay'gun·hahl''tun) *n.* [Ger., from *gegen,* against, + *halten,* hold]. PARATONIA.

Gei·gel's reflex (guy'gul) [R. *Geigel,* German physician, 1859–1930]. INGUINAL REFLEX.

Gei·ger counter (guy'gur) [H. *Geiger,* German physicist, 1882–1945]. GEIGER-MÜLLER COUNTER.

Geiger-Mül·ler counter (muᵉl'ur) [H. *Geiger;* and W. *Müller,* German physicist, 20th century]. An instrument for the detection of individual ionizing particles; entry of a charged particle into the apparatus produces ionization and a momentary flow of current which is relayed to a counting device.

Geiger-Müller counting circuit. An amplifier and accessories that make visible or audible, or in other ways record, the pulses from a Geiger-Müller tube.

Geiger-Müller tube [H. *Geiger* and W. *Müller*]. A tube which, when the proper voltage is imposed, will produce an electric pulse each time an ionizing particle penetrates its walls.

Geiger tube. GEIGER-MÜLLER TUBE.

gei·so·ma (guy·so'muh) *n.* [Gk. *geisōma,* penthouse, annex]. 1. EYEBROWS. 2. SUPRAORBITAL RIDGES.

gei·son (guy'son) *n.* [Gk., cornice]. GEISOMA.

gel (jel) *n.* [from *gelatin*]. A colloidal system comprising a solid and a liquid phase which exists as a solid or semisolid mass.

ge·las·ma (je·laz'muh) *n.* [Gk., smile]. GELASMUS.

ge·las·mus (je·laz'mus) *n.* [NL., from Gk. *gelan,* to laugh]. Insane or hysterical spasmodic laughter.

ge·las·tic (je·las'tick) *adj.* [Gk. *gelastikos,* able to laugh]. Pertaining to laughter, laughing.

gelastic epilepsy. A form of epilepsy characterized by laughing.

gel·ate (jel'ate) *v.* To convert or to be converted into a gel. —**gel·at·ed** (·ay·tid) *adj.*

ge·lat·i·fi·ca·tion (je·lat''i·fi·kay'shun) *n.* The conversion of a substance into a jellylike mass.

gel·a·tin (jel'uh·tin) *n.* [It. *gelatina,* from L. *gelare,* to freeze]. The product obtained by partial hydrolysis of collagen, occurring in sheets, flakes, shreds, or as a coarse or fine powder, insoluble in cold water but soluble in hot water; used in many pharmaceutical preparations, in formulations for histochemical examinations, as an ingredient of bacteriologic culture mediums, as a food, as a plasma extender, and as an absorbable film or sponge in operative procedures.

ge·lat·i·nase (je·lat'i·nace, ·naze) *n.* [*gelatin* + *-ase*]. An enzyme, found in some yeasts and molds, that hydrolyzes and liquefies gelatin.

ge·lat·i·nize (je·lat'i·nize) *v.* To convert into a jellylike mass.

ge·lat·i·noid (je·lat'i·noid) *adj.* GELATINOUS.

ge·lat·i·no·lyt·ic (je·lat''i·no·lit'ick) *adj.* [*gelatin* + *-lytic*]. Dissolving or splitting up gelatin.

ge·lat·i·no·sa (je·lat''i·no'suh) *n.* SUBSTANTIA GELATINOSA.

ge·lat·i·nous (je·lat'i·nus) *adj.* 1. Resembling gelatin; jellylike. 2. Of or pertaining to gelatin.

gelatinous ascites or **peritonitis.** PSEUDOMYXOMA PERITONEI.

gelatinous carcinoma. MUCINOUS CARCINOMA.

gelatinous cystadenoma. MUCINOUS CYSTADENOMA.

gelatinous cystosarcoma. CYSTOSARCOMA PHYLLODES.

gelatinous substance of Rolando [L. *Rolando*]. SUBSTANTIA GELATINOSA.

gelatinous tissue. MUCOID TISSUE.

gelatin sponge. A sheet of gelatin, prepared to check bleeding when applied to a raw surface.

ge·la·tion (je·lay'shun) *n.* 1. The change of a colloid from a sol to a gel. 2. Freezing.

gel·a·tose (jel'uh·toce) *n.* An intermediate product in the hydrolysis of gelatin.

geld (gheld) *v.* [ON. *gelda*]. To castrate, as a horse; EMASCULATE.

geld·ing (ghel'ding) *n.* [ON. *geldingr*]. A castrated male horse.

gel electrophoresis. Electrophoresis employing a gel as the supporting medium.

Gelfilm. A trademark for absorbable gelatin film.

gel filtration chromatography. A type of column chromatography which separates molecules on the basis of size, the substances of higher molecular weight passing through the column first. Syn. *molecular exclusion chromatography, molecular sieve chromatography.*

Gelfoam. Trademark for an absorbable gelatin sponge material used as a local hemostatic.

Gé·li·neau–Red·lich syndrome (zheʸ·lee·no', reʸt'likʰ) [J. B. E. *Gélineau,* French physician, b. 1859; and E. *Redlich,* Austrian neurologist, 1866–1930]. NARCOLEPSY.

Gélineau's disease or **syndrome** [J. B. E. *Gélineau*]. NARCOLEPSY.

Gel·lé's test (zhuh·leʸ') [M. E. *Gellé,* French surgeon, 1834–1923]. A hearing test to detect a conductive hearing loss, performed by increasing pressure in the external auditory canal and observing any change in loudness to a bone conduction stimulus. If no change occurs a conductive loss is present.

ge·lo·ple·gia (jel″o·plee′jee·uh) *n.* [Gk. *gelōs*, laughter, + *-plegia*]. GELOTOLEPSY.

ge·lo·sa (je·lo′suh) *n.* AGAR.

gel·ose (jel′oce, je·loce′) *n.* [*gel-* + *-ose*]. The gelatinizing principle of agar, being the calcium salt of a complex carbohydrate substance composed of galactose units.

gel·o·sin (jel′o·sin, je·lo′sin) *n.* A mucilage from a Japanese alga.

ge·lo·sis (je·lo′sis) *n.* [L. *gel*are, to freeze, + *-osis*]. A hardened mass of tissue resembling frozen tissue, especially in skeletal muscle. See also *myogelosis.*

gel·o·to·lep·sy (jel′uh·to·lep″see) *n.* [*gelōs, gelōtos*, laughter, + *-lepsy*]. A sudden loss of muscle tone (cataplexy) induced by uproarious laughter.

gel·se·mine (jel′se·meen, ·min) *n.* [*gelsem*ium + *-ine*]. An alkaloid, $C_{20}H_{22}N_2O_2$, from gelsemium.

gel·se·mi·um (jel·see′mee·um, ·sem′ee·um) *n.* [NL., from It. *gelsomino,* jasmine]. The dried rhizome and roots of *Gelsemium sempervirens,* formerly used as an antispasmodic and antineuralgic. Syn. *yellow jasmine root.*

ge·mel·lus (je·mel′us) *n.*, pl. **gemel·li** (·eye) [L., twin]. Either of two small paired muscles, inserted in the greater trochanter of the femur, which rotate the femur laterally: the inferior gemellus (NA *musculus gemellus inferior*), or the superior gemellus (NA *musculus gemellus superior*). See also Table of Muscles in the Appendix.

¹gem·i·nate (jem′i·nit, ·nate) *adj.* [L. *geminatus,* doubled]. In pairs, coupled.

²gem·i·nate (jem′i·nate) *v.* [L. *geminare,* from *gemini,* twins]. 1. To double. 2. To become doubled.

gem·i·na·tion (jem″i·nay′shun) *n.* An anomaly that represents the attempt of a tooth germ to divide by invagination; it usually presents a tooth having two completely or incompletely separated crowns and a common root or roots and pulp chamber.

gem·i·nous (jem′i·nus) *adj.* ¹GEMINATE.

ge·mis·to·cyte (je·mis′to·site) *n.* [Ger. *gemäst*et, fattened, + *-cyte*]. A large, round type of astrocyte with pale, acidophilic, homogeneous cytoplasm and eccentrically displaced nucleus, observed in certain neuropathologic conditions. —**ge·mis·to·cyt·ic** (je·mis″to·sit′ick) *adj.*

gemistocytic astrocytoma. An astrocytoma composed of gemistocytes. Syn. *gigantocellular astrocytoma.*

gem·ma (jem′uh) *n.*, pl. **gem·mae** (·ee) [L., a bud]. An asexual budlike body, either unicellular or multicellular.

gem·ma·tion (jem·ay′shun) *n.* [L. *gemmare,* to put forth buds]. BUDDING.

gem·mule (jem′yool) *n.* [L. *gemmula,* little bud]. 1. A small bud or gemma. 2. The short thorny processes of the dendrites of pyramidal nerve cells.

Gemonil. Trademark for metharbital, a barbituric acid derivative useful in treating epilepsy.

-gen, -gene [F. *-gène,* from Gk. *-genēs,* born]. A combining form meaning (a) *substance or organism that produces or generates;* (b) *thing produced or generated.*

gen-, geno-. A combining form meaning (a) *gene, genetic;* (b) *genital, sexual;* (c) *generating;* (d) *race, kind.*

ge·na (jee′nuh) *n.*, pl. **ge·nae** (·nee) [L.]. CHEEK. —**ge·nal** (·nul) *adj.*

genal cleft. TRANSVERSE FACIAL CLEFT.

genal coloboma. *Obsol.* TRANSVERSE FACIAL CLEFT.

genal fissure. TRANSVERSE FACIAL CLEFT.

genal line. A line running down from the region of the zygomatic bone to join the nasal line.

gender identity. The sum of those aspects of personal appearance and behavior culturally attributed to masculinity or femininity. While usually based on the external genitalia and body physique, parental attitudes and expectations as well as those of society determine what is masculine and what is feminine, and may cause conflicts. Compare *gender role, sexual identity.*

gender role. The image or behavior a person presents to society whereby that person is categorized as a boy or man, or girl or woman. While gender identity and gender role are usually congruent, the former represents what society or the parents expect, and the latter, what an individual delivers; the two may be in conflict.

Gen·dre's fixing fluid. A fixative used especially for preserving glycogen in tissue; contains alcohol, picric acid, acetic acid, and formaldehyde.

gene (jeen) *n.* [Ger. *Gen,* from *-gen*]. A hereditary factor; the unit of transmission of hereditary characteristics, capable of self-reproduction, which usually occupies a definite locus on a chromosome, although some genes are nonchromosomal. Genes in general are constituted of DNA, although in some viruses they are RNA.

-gene. See *-gen.*

gene flow. The transfer of one or more genetic alleles from one population of an organism to another population of the same organism.

gene frequency. The relative frequency, usually expressed as a decimal, with which an allele of a gene occurs among all the alleles at a given locus in a population.

gene imbalance. A chemical or morphologic change in the gene complex resulting in a modification of hereditary characteristics.

gene pool. The totality of reproductively available genes in a breeding population, characterized by the alleles that are present and their relative frequency.

genera. Plural of *genus.*

gen·er·al, *adj.* [L. *generalis,* generic, general, from *genus,* kind]. 1. Common to a class. 2. Distributed through many parts, diffuse. —**general·ly,** *adv.*

general adaptation syndrome. According to Hans Selye, the sum of all nonspecific systemic reactions of the body which ensue upon long-continued exposure to systemic stress. It is divided into three stages: (a) alarm reaction (shock and countershock), (b) stage of resistance, and (c) stage of exhaustion. Compare *fight-or-flight reaction.*

general anatomy. The study of anatomy that treats of the structure and physiologic properties of the tissues and their arrangement into systems without regard to the disposition of the organs of which they form a part.

general anesthesia. Loss of sensation with loss of consciousness, produced by administration of anesthetic drugs. See also *stages of general anesthesia.*

general anesthetic. An agent that produces general anesthesia either by injection or by inhalation.

general duty nurse. A nurse assigned to a ward or division of a hospital, who performs many different duties for all the patients.

general hospital. 1. A facility in which patients with many types of conditions are cared for; consists of various departments such as medicine, surgery, pediatrics, and obstetrics, all well-equipped and well-staffed. 2. *In military medicine,* a numbered fixed medical treatment facility especially staffed and equipped for observation, treatment, and disposition of patients requiring relatively long periods of hospitalization or highly specialized treatment; normally used in the communications zone.

gen·er·al·iza·tion (jen″rul·i·zay′shun) *n.* 1. The act or process of generalizing; the making of a general assumption or statement on the basis of one or only a few specifics. 2. *In psychiatry,* a mental mechanism operating outside and beyond conscious awareness by which an emotional process extends to include additional areas, as a fear of bridges may progress to a fear of tall buildings, mountains, or any high place.

gen·er·al·ize (jen′ur·ul·ize, jen′rul·) *v.* 1. To make general. 2. To become diffused or widespread.

generalized arteriolar sclerosis. Sclerosis affecting the arterioles of the kidney, liver, brain, meninges, gastrointestinal tract, skeletal muscle, adrenal glands, pancreas, and other organs.

generalized arteriosclerosis. Widespread arterial degenerative disease.

generalized gangliosidosis. G_{M1} GANGLIOSIDOSIS.

generalized glycogenosis. POMPE'S DISEASE.

generalized seizure. An epileptic seizure characterized by sudden loss of consciousness, tonic convulsion, cyanosis, and dilated pupils, followed by a clonic spasm of all voluntary muscles, with the eyes rotated upward, the head extended, frothing at the mouth, and, frequently, incontinence of urine. After the convulsion subsides, the patient is confused and frequently falls into a deep sleep. Syn. *grand mal seizure, major motor seizure.* Compare *tonic-clonic convulsion.*

generalized Shwartzman phenomenon. SHWARTZMAN PHENOMENON (2).

generally contracted pelvis. A pelvis having all diameters symmetrically shortened; a small normally shaped pelvis.

generally enlarged pelvis. A pelvis having all diameters symmetrically enlarged; a large normally shaped pelvis.

general paralysis or **paresis.** A chronic progressive form of central nervous system syphilis occurring 15 to 20 years after the initial infection, taking the form of a meningoencephalitis and resulting in physical and mental dissolution. Syn. *paretic neurosyphilis, syphilitic meningoencephalitis, dementia paralytica.*

general pathology. A study of disturbances that are common to various tissues and organs of the body, as degenerations, hypertrophy, atrophy, or neoplasms.

general practitioner. FAMILY PHYSICIAN.

general sclerosis. A connective-tissue hyperplasia affecting an entire organ. Compare *diffuse sclerosis, multiple sclerosis.*

general semantics. A study or theory of living which stresses a scientific approach to problems and life and emphasizes the way in which language is used as an important factor in adjustment; used in treating certain psychologic maladjustments.

general sensation. One of the body sensations, such as pain, touch, heat, cold.

general surgeon. A surgeon who does not limit his work to a subspecialty, but deals rather with surgery as a whole.

general surgery. Surgery as a whole, not confined to a particular specialty.

general symptom. CONSTITUTIONAL SYMPTOM.

gen·er·a·tion (jen″ur·ay′shun) *n.* [L. *generatio,* from *generare,* to produce, beget, from *genus,* birth, descent]. 1. Production; REPRODUCTION, procreation. 2. The aggregate of individuals descended in the same number of life cycles from a common ancestor or from ancestors that are in some respect equivalent; also, any aggregate of contemporaneous individuals. 3. An aggregate of cells or individuals in the same stage of development from a precursor. 4. The period spanning one life cycle of an organism, from the conception (or birth) of an individual to the conception (or birth) of his offspring.

generative organs. The gonads and secondary sexual organs that are functional in reproduction.

generative tract. The female genital system which consists of ovaries, tubes, uterus, vagina, and the external genitalia. See also Plate 23.

gen·er·a·tor, *n.* [L., begetter, producer, from *generare,* to beget, produce]. 1. A machine that transforms mechanical power into electric power. 2. *In radiology,* a machine that supplies the roentgen-ray tube with the electric energy necessary for the production of roentgen rays. 3. *In chemistry,* an apparatus for the formation of vapor or gas from a liquid or solid by heat or chemical action.

generator potential. *In neurophysiology,* the depolarization of a receptor by any physical stimulus, including light, heat, or mechanical distortion, which is directly related to its intensity; the generated potential produced is graded and remains stationary unless of sufficient intensity to result in an action potential. Syn. *receptor potential.*

ge·ner·ic (je·nerr′ick) *adj.* 1. Of or pertaining to a genus. 2. Not specific. 3. Nonproprietary, as of a drug not registered or protected by a trademark.

gen·es·er·ine (jen·es′ur·een, ·in) *n.* ESERIDINE.

ge·ne·si·al (je·nee′see·ul, ·zee·ul) *adj.* [*genesis* + *-al*]. Pertaining to generation.

genesial cycle. The period between puberty and the menopause; the period of active sexual maturity.

ge·nes·ic (je·nes′ick, je·nee′zick) *adj.* [*genesis* + *-ic*]. Of or pertaining to generation or the genital organs.

genesic sense. SEXUAL INSTINCT.

ge·ne·si·ol·o·gy (je·nee″see·ol′uh·jee, je·nee″zee·) *n.* [*genesis* + *-logy*]. GENETICS.

gen·e·sis (jen′e·sis) *n.,* pl. **gene·ses** (·seez) [Gk.]. 1. The origin or generation of anything. 2. The developmental evolution of a specific thing or type.

-genesis [Gk.]. A combining form meaning (a) *origination;* (b) *development;* (c) *evolution* of a thing or type.

gene spread. The incorporation of a genetic allele into the genetic constitution of a population of organisms.

ge·net·ic (je·net′ick) *adj.* [*genesis* + *-ic*]. 1. Pertaining to or having reference to origin, mode of production, or development. 2. Pertaining to genetics. 3. Produced by genes.

genetic affinity. Relationship by direct descent.

genetic code. The code of the molecules of heredity; the nucleotide "dictionary" that permits the translation of specific gene DNA and messenger RNA molecules into proteins of specific amino acid sequence. The code is triplet and degenerate; each amino acid found in proteins is coded for by more than one triplet. The code is evidently universal for all species. See also *codon.*

genetic drift. The change in allele frequencies from generation to generation which occurs by chance in small populations.

genetic dwarfism. PRIMORDIAL DWARFISM.

genetic-dynamic psychotherapy. INTENSIVE PSYCHOTHERAPY.

genetic equilibrium. The condition that prevails when the relative frequencies of the alleles of a gene are constant from generation to generation.

ge·net·i·cist (je·net′i·sist) *n.* A specialist in genetics.

genetic load. The accumulated deleterious mutant genes in a population, including those maintained by mutation and selection.

genetic mapping. Chromosome mapping by analysis of genetic recombination to provide knowledge of linear order of genes and relative physical distance.

genetic recombination. The formation of new combinations of the alleles of linked genes, as by crossing-over.

ge·net·ics (je·net′icks) *n.* The branch of biology that deals with the phenomena of heredity and variation. It seeks to understand the causes of the resemblances and differences between parents and progeny, and, by extension, between all organisms related to one another by descent.

ge·net·o·troph·ic (je·net″o·trof′ick) *adj.* [*genetic* + *-trophic*]. 1. Of or pertaining to genetics and nutrition. 2. Of, pertaining to, or descriptive of a disease caused by a high inherited demand for some nutrient that is not included in the consumed foods.

gen·e·tous (jen′e·tus) *adj.* CONGENITAL.

Ge·ne·va convention. An agreement signed by the European powers in Geneva, Switzerland, in 1864, guaranteeing humane treatment of the wounded and those caring for them in time of war. Later revisions were accepted by the majority of nations.

geni-, genio- [Gk. *geneion*]. A combining form meaning *chin.*

ge·ni·al (jee′nee·ul) *adj.* [Gk. *geneion,* chin, + *-al*]. Of or pertaining to the chin. Syn. *mental.*

genial spine. MENTAL SPINE.
genial tubercle. MENTAL TUBERCLE.
gen·ic (jee'nick, jen'ick) *adj.* Of or pertaining to a gene or to genes.
-genic. A combining form meaning (a) *producing, forming;* (b) *produced by, formed from;* (c) *of* or *pertaining to a gene.*
genicula. Plural of *geniculum.*
ge·nic·u·lar (je·nick'yoo·lur) *adj.* [L. *genicul*um, knee, + *-ar*]. Of or pertaining to the knee joint.
genicular artery. See Table of Arteries in the Appendix.
ge·nic·u·late (je·nick'yoo·lut) *adj.* [L. *geniculatus,* from *geniculare,* to bend the knee]. Abruptly bent.
geniculate body. See *medial geniculate body, lateral geniculate body.*
geniculate ganglion. The sensory ganglion of the nervus intermedius, lying in the genu of the facial nerve in the facial canal of the temporal bone. NA *ganglion geniculi.*
geniculate herpes. RAMSEY HUNT SYNDROME.
geniculate neuralgia. Severe pain in the middle ear and auditory canal, facial paralysis, hyperacusia, loss of taste, and diminution of tearing and salivation, following a lesion of the facial nerve at the geniculate ganglion; often associated with herpes zoster in the Ramsay Hunt syndrome.
ge·nic·u·lo·cal·ca·rine (je·nick"yoo·lo·kal'kuh·reen) *adj.* Pertaining to the lateral geniculate body and the calcarine sulcus.
geniculocalcarine tract. OPTIC RADIATION.
ge·nic·u·lo·tem·po·ral (je·nick"yoo·lo·temp'ur·ul) *adj.* Pertaining to the medial geniculate body and the temporal cortex.
geniculotemporal radiation or **tract.** ACOUSTIC RADIATION.
ge·nic·u·lum (je·nick"yoo·lum) *n.,* pl. **genicu·la** (·luh) [L., knee, knot]. A small, kneelike structure; a sharp bend in any small organ.
geniculum ca·na·lis fa·ci·a·lis (ka·nay'lis fay·shee·ay'lis). The bend in the facial canal that contains the external genu facialis.
geniculum ner·vi fa·ci·a·lis (nur'vye fay·shee·ay'lis) [NA]. EXTERNAL GENU OF THE FACIAL NERVE.
gen·in (jen'in) *n.* AGLYCONE.
genio-. See *geni-.*
ge·nio·glos·sus (jee"nee·o·glos'us) *n.,* pl. **genioglos·si** (sigh) [NL., from *genio-* + Gk. *glōssa,* tongue]. An extrinsic muscle of the tongue, arising from the superior mental spine of the mandible. NA *musculus genioglossus.* See also Table of Muscles in the Appendix.
ge·nio·hyo·glos·sus (jee"nee·o·high"o·glos'us) *n.,* pl. **genio-hyoglos·si** (·sigh) [NL., from *genio-* + *hyo-* + Gk. *glōssa,* tongue]. GENIOGLOSSUS.
ge·nio·hy·oid (jee"nee·o·high'oid) *n.* A muscle arising from the inferior mental spine of the mandible and inserted into the body of the hyoid. NA *musculus geniohyoideus.* See also Table of Muscles in the Appendix.
ge·ni·on (je·nigh'on, jee'nee·on) *n.* [Gk. *geneion,* chin]. *In craniometry,* the point at the tip of the mental spine. If several spines are present, the point is located between these in the sagittal plane.
ge·nio·pha·ryn·ge·us (jee"nee·o·fa·rin'jee·us) *n.* A variant part of the genioglossus which blends with the superior constrictor of the pharynx.
ge·nio·plas·ty (jee'nee·o·plas"tee, je·nigh'o·) *n.* [*genio-* + *-plasty*]. Plastic operation on the chin.
gen·i·tal (jen'i·tul) *adj.* [L. *genitalis,* from *gignere,* to produce]. Of or pertaining to the organs of generation or to reproduction.
genital canal. *In comparative anatomy,* any canal designated for copulation or for the discharge of ova or offspring.
genital cord. A mesenchymal shelf bridging the coelom, produced by fusion of the caudal part of the urogential folds. It contains the vertical part of the paramesonephric (Müllerian) and the mesonephric (Wolffian) ducts, fuses with the urinary bladder in the male, and is the primordium of the broad ligament and the uterine walls in the female.
genital corpuscle. A complex form of Krause's corpuscle in the skin of the external genitalia and of the nipple. Syn. *Dogiel's corpuscle.* NA (pl.) *corpuscula genitalia.*
genital eminence. GENITAL TUBERCLE.
genital fold. 1. A lateral swelling on either side of the cloacal membrane; produced by the growth of mesoderm. 2. GENITAL RIDGE. 3. URETHRAL FOLD.
genital fossa. URETHRAL GROOVE.
genital furrow. A groove appearing on the genital tubercle of the fetus at the end of the second month.
genital herpes. HERPES PROGENITALIS.
gen·i·ta·lia (jen"i·tay'lee·uh) *n. pl.* [L., from *genitalis,* generative]. The organs of generation, comprising in the male the two testes or seminal glands, their excretory ducts, the prostate, the penis, and the urethra, and in the female the vulva, the vagina, the ovaries, the uterine tubes, and the uterus. See also Plates 23 and 25.
gen·i·tal·i·ty (jen"i·tal'i·tee) *n.* 1. The genital components of sexuality. 2. *In psychoanalysis,* ideally the mutuality of orgasm with a loved partner of the opposite sex, with whom one is able and willing to share a mutual trust and with whom one is able and willing to share work and recreation and, when desired, procreation to secure to the offspring also a satisfactory development.
genital mesonephros. The part of the mesonephros opposite the gonad, the tubules of which become the ductuli efferentes.
gen·i·tal·oid (jen'i·tul·oid) *adj.* [*genital* + *-oid*]. Pertaining to the primordial germ cells, and indicating potentialities for either sex.
genitaloid cells. Primary germ cells of the embryo.
genital papilla. The primitive penis or clitoris.
genital phase. *In psychoanalysis,* the final culminating stage in an individual's psychosexual development, during which a genuinely affectionate and mature relationship with a sex partner is achieved. Compare *phallic phase.*
genital plica. GENITAL RIDGE.
genital prominence. An accumulation of cells on the ventral aspect of the embryonic cloaca, from which generative organs are developed.
genital reflex. A reflex phenomenon involving the autonomic nervous system in which under certain conditions stimulation from the cerebrum or the periphery produces penile erection, priapism, or ejaculation; it may be seen as part of the mass reflex in spinal cord lesions following stimulation of the penis.
genital ridge. A medial ridge or fold on the ventromedial surface of the mesonephros in the embryo produced by growth of the peritoneum; the primordium of the gonads and their ligaments.
gen·i·tals, *n. pl.* GENITALIA.
genital spot. An area on the nasal mucosa which has a tendency to bleed during menstruation, a form of vicarious menstruation.
genital swelling. LABIOSCROTAL SWELLING.
genital system. REPRODUCTIVE SYSTEM.
genital tubercle. A conical elevation in the midventral line between tail and umbilicus that develops into the embryonic phallus.
genito-. A combining form meaning *genital.*
gen·i·to·cru·ral (jen"i·to·kroo'rul) *adj.* [*genito-* + *crural*]. Pertaining to the genitalia and the lower limb.
gen·i·to·fem·o·ral (jen"i·to·fem'uh·rul) *adj.* [*genito-* + *femoral*]. Pertaining to the genitalia and the thigh; GENITOCRURAL.
genitofemoral nerve. See Table of Nerves in the Appendix.
gen·i·to·rec·tal (jen"i·to·reck'tul) *adj.* [*genito-* + *rectal*]. ANOGENITAL.

gen·i·to·uri·nary (jen″i·to·yoor′i·nerr″ee) *adj.* Pertaining to the genitalia and the urinary organs or functions.

genitourinary slit. UROGENITAL APERTURE.

genitourinary surgeon. UROLOGIST.

genitourinary tract. UROGENITAL SYSTEM.

gen·i·to·ves·i·cal (jen″i·to·ves′i·kul) *adj.* [*genito-* + *vesical*]. Pertaining to the genitalia and the urinary bladder.

genitovesical fissure. A groove, developing about the third month of gestation, between the cranial end of the genital cord and the urinary bladder. It disappears in the male, but deepens in the female to form the vesicouterine excavation.

ge·nius (jee′nee·us, jeen′yus) *n.* [L., guardian spirit acquired at birth, from *genus,* birth, origin]. 1. Distinctive character or inherent nature. 2. Unusual creative ability; mental superiority. 3. An individual with unusual creative ability or mental superiority.

genius ep·i·dem·i·cus (ep″i·dem′i·kus). 1. The totality of conditions, atmospheric, cosmic, supernatural, formerly regarded as most favorable to the prevalence of an endemic or epidemic disease. 2. The prevalent picture of an endemic or epidemic disease.

genius mor·bi (mor′bye). The special or predominant feature of a disease.

Gennari's stria. STRIPE OF GENNARI.

geno-. See *gen-.*

geno·cide (jen′uh·side) *n.* [*geno-* + *-cide*]. The systematic extermination of an entire human group. Compare *homicide.*

geno·der·ma·to·sis (jen″o·dur″muh·to′sis) *n.* [*geno-* + *dermatosis*]. Any hereditary skin disease, as ichthyosis, pachyonychia congenita, or epidermolysis bullosa.

ge·nome, ge·nom (jee′nome) *n.* [*gene* + chromos*ome*]. A complete set of the hereditary factors, such as is contained in a haploid set of chromosomes.

geno·pho·bia (jen″o·fo′bee·uh) *n.* [*geno-* + *-phobia*]. An abnormal fear of sex.

Genoscopolamine. Trademark for scopolamine aminoxide, which has the actions and uses of scopolamine.

ge·no·type (jee′no·tipe, jen′o·) *n.* [*geno-* + *type*]. 1. The hereditary constitution of an organism resulting from its particular combination of genes. 2. A class of individuals having the same genetic constitution. —**ge·no·typ·ic** (jee″no·tip′ick, jen″o·), **genotyp·i·cal** (·i·kul) *adj.*

-genous [*gen-* + *-ous*]. A combining form meaning (a) *producing;* (b) *produced by, arising in.*

gen·ta·mi·cin (jen″tuh·migh′sin) *n.* A mixture of two isomeric antibiotics, gentamicin C_1 and gentamicin C_2, produced by the fungi *Micromonospora purpurea* and *M. echinospora.* It is active against many gram-negative pathogens, especially *Pseudomonas aeruginosa,* and also against many gram-positive bacteria; used medicinally, as the sulfate salt, by parenteral injection.

gen·tian (jen′shun) *n.* [L. *gentiana,* after the Illyrian king *Gentius*]. 1. The common name for species of *Gentiana.* 2. The dried rhizome and roots of *Gentiana lutea,* containing a number of glycosides; has been used as a bitter tonic.

gentian violet. A form of methylrosaniline chloride.

gen·tis·ic acid (jen·tis′ick). 2,5-Dihydroxybenzoic acid, $C_7H_6O_4$; occurs in gentian and in urine after ingestion of salicylates.

Gentran. A trademark for dextran, a plasma-expanding and blood-pressure-maintaining glucose polymer.

ge·nu (jen′yoo) *n.,* genit. **ge·nus** (jen′ooss), pl. **ge·nua** (jen′yoo·uh) [L. (rel. to Gk. *gonia,* angle, and to E. *knee*)]. 1. [NA] KNEE. 2. Any of various angular or curved structures suggestive of a bent knee. 3. (of the corpus callosum:) The sharp curve of the anterior portion of the corpus callosum. NA *genu corporis callosi.* See also Plate 18. 4. (of the internal capsule:) The portion of the internal capsule which, in cross section, appears bent at an angle; it occurs where the capsule approaches the cavity of the lateral ventricle. NA *genu capsulae internae.* 5. (of the facial nerve:) Either of the sharp curves in the facial nerve. See also *external genu of the facial nerve, internal genu of the facial nerve.* —**gen·u·al** (jen′yoo·ul) *adj.*

genu cap·su·lae in·ter·nae (kap′sue·lee in·tur′nee) [NA]. The genu of the internal capsule. See *genu.*

genu cor·po·ris cal·lo·si (kor′po·ris ka·lo′sigh) [NA]. The genu of the corpus callosum. See *genu.*

genu·cu·bi·tal (jen″yoo·kew′bi·tul) *adj.* [*genu* + *cubital*]. Pertaining to or supported by the knees and elbows.

genu·fa·cial (jen″yoo·fay′shul) *adj.* [*genu* + *facial*]. Pertaining to or resting on the knees and face.

genu fa·ci·a·lis (fay·shee·ay′lis). GENU (5).

genu ner·vi fa·ci·a·lis (nur′vye fay·shee·ay′lis) [NA]. INTERNAL GENU OF THE FACIAL NERVE.

genu·pec·to·ral (jen″yoo·peck′tur·ul) *adj.* [*genu* + *pectoral*]. Pertaining to or resting on the knees and the chest.

genu ra·di·cis ner·vi fa·ci·a·lis (rad′i·sis nur′vye fay·shee·ay′lis) [BNA]. Genu nervi facialis (= INTERNAL GENU OF THE FACIAL NERVE).

genu re·cur·va·tum (ree″kur·vay′tum, reck″ur·). The backward curvature of the knee joint.

ge·nus (jee′nus) *n.,* pl. **gen·era** (jen′e·ruh) [L., origin, race, kind]. A taxonomic group next above a species and forming the principal subdivision of a family.

genu val·gum (val′gum). Inward or medial curving of the knee. Syn. *knock-knee.*

genu va·rum (vair′um). BOWLEG.

-geny. A combining form meaning *genesis* or *generation.*

geny-, genyo- [Gk. *genys,* jaw, chin]. A combining form meaning the *under jaw.*

geny·chei·lo·plas·ty (jen″i·kigh′lo·plas″tee) *n.* [*geny-* + *cheilo-* + *-plasty*]. Plastic operation on both cheek and lip.

geny·plas·ty (jen′i·plas″tee) *n.* [*geny-* + *-plasty*]. Plastic operation on the lower jaw.

geo-. See *ge-.*

Geocillin. A trademark for carbenicillin indanyl sodium, an antibacterial.

geo·graph·ic (jee″uh·graf′ick) *adj.* [Gk. *geōgraphikos*]. 1. Pertaining to or characteristic of features and regions of the earth. 2. Resembling land masses on a map.

geographic pathology. A study of disease in relation to environmental conditions, such as climate, region, or altitude.

geographic tongue. BENIGN MIGRATORY GLOSSITIS.

geo·med·i·cine (jee″o·med′i·sin) *n.* [*geo-* + *medicine*]. The study of the effects of climate and other environmental conditions on health and disease. See also *nosogeography.*

geo·met·ri·cal axis (jee″uh·met′ri·kul). *In ophthalmology,* a line joining the anterior and posterior poles of the globe of the eye. Compare *visual axis.*

geo·met·ric isomerism (jee″o·met′rick). Isomerism evidenced when substances have the same constitutional formula but differ in the specific arrangement of the atoms and, consequently, in all of their physical properties and in most of their chemical properties. See also *stereoisomerism.*

geometric mean. The antilogarithm of the arithmetic mean of the logarithms of a series of observations; the *n*th root of the product of *n* observations.

geometric-optic, *adj.* Pertaining to the visual appreciation of space, i.e., of dimension and direction.

geometric-optic agnosia. A form of agnosia in which a person can recognize objects, but has lost appreciation of direction or dimension, or both.

Geopen. A trademark for carbenicillin disodium, an antibacterial.

geo·pha·gia (jee·o·fay′jee·uh) *n.* GEOPHAGY.

ge·oph·a·gism (jee·off′uh·jizm) *n.* GEOPHAGY.

ge·oph·a·gy (jee·off′uh·jee) *n.* [*geo-* + *-phagy*]. The practice of eating earth or clay. See also *pica* (2). —**geopha·gous** (·gus) *adj.;* **geopha·gist** (·jist) *n.*

Ge·or·gi-Sachs test (geʰ·or′gee, zaʰks) [W. *Georgi,* German bacteriologist, 1889–1920; and H. *Sachs,* German immunologist, 1877–1945]. A method for testing anticomplementary serums as part of a serodiagnostic test for syphilis.

ge·ot·ri·cho·sis (jee·ot″ri·ko′sis) *n.*, pl. **geotricho·ses** (·seez) [*Geotrich*um + *-osis*]. An infection possibly caused by one or more species of the fungus *Geotrichum.* Lesions may occur in the mouth, intestinal tract, bronchi, and lungs.

Ge·ot·ri·chum (jee·ot′ri·kum) *n.* [NL., from *geo-* + Gk. *thrix, trichos,* hair]. A genus of Fungi Imperfecti, characterized by abundant development of rectangular and rounded arthrospores; of doubtful pathogenicity, but has been isolated from sputum and bronchi.

ge·ot·ro·pism (jee·ot′ruh·piz·um) *n.* [*geo-* + *tropism*]. *In biology,* the gravitational factor which in plants causes roots to grow downward toward the earth and shoots to grow up, and in some animals causes the climbing, swimming, or right-side-up orientation.

ge·phy·ro·pho·bia (je·figh″ro·fo′bee·uh, jef″i·ro·) *n.* [Gk. *gephyra,* bridge, + *-phobia*]. An abnormal fear of crossing a bridge.

ger-, gera-, gero- [Gk. *gēras, gēros*]. A combining form meaning *old age.*

gera-. See *ger-.*

Ger·agh·ty's operation (gerr′uh·tee) [J. T. *Geraghty,* U.S. urologist, 1876–1924]. A modification of Young's perineal prostatectomy.

ge·ra·ni·al (je·ray′nee·al) *n.* One of the geometric isomers of citral.

ge·ra·ni·ol (je·ray′nee·ol) *n.* 3,7-Dimethyl-2,6-octadien-1-ol, $C_{10}H_{18}O$, a terpene alcohol constituent of many volatile oils.

ge·ra·ni·um (je·ray′nee·um) *n.* [L., from Gk. *geranion,* dim. of *geranos,* crane]. The rhizome of *Geranium maculatum,* cranesbill, formerly used as an astringent.

ge·rat·ic (je·rat′ick) *adj.* [Gk. *gēras,* old age, + *-ic*]. Of or pertaining to old age; GERONTIC.

ger·a·tol·o·gy (jerr″uh·tol′uh·jee) *n.* [Gk. *gēras,* old age, + *-logy*]. The scientific study of senescence and its related phenomena; GERONTOLOGY. Compare *geriatrics.*

Ger·hardt's disease (gehr′hart) [C. A. C. J. *Gerhardt,* German physician, 1833–1902]. ERYTHROMELALGIA.

Gerhardt's sign or **change of note** [C. A. C. J. *Gerhardt*]. A sign once used to diagnose cavitation of the lungs in which there is a change in percussion note with change in the patient's position from upright to recumbent.

ger·i·at·ric (jerr″ee·at′rick) *adj.* [*ger-* + *-iatric*]. Of or pertaining to geriatrics or to the process of aging.

ger·i·a·tri·cian (jerr″ee·uh·trish′un) *n.* A physician who specializes in the treatment of the diseases of aging.

ger·i·at·rics (jerr″ee·at′ricks) *n.* The branch of medical science that is concerned with aging and its diseases. Compare *geratology.*

ger·i·a·trist (jerr′ee·uh·trist) *n.* GERIATRICIAN.

gerio- [Gk. *geraios*]. A combining form meaning *old* or *aged.*

ger·io·psy·cho·sis (jerr″ee·o·sigh·ko′sis) *n.*, pl. **geriopsycho·ses** (·seez) [Gk. *gerio-* + *psychosis*]. SENILE DEMENTIA.

Ger·lach's tubal tonsil (geʰr′laᵏh) [J. von *Gerlach,* German histologist, 1820–1896]. TUBAL TONSIL.

Gerlach's valve [J. von *Gerlach*]. A mucosal fold sometimes surrounding the orifice of the vermiform appendix.

Ger·lier's disease or **syndrome** (zheʰrl·yeʸ′) [F. *Gerlier,* Swiss physician, 1840–1914]. An acute transitory disease of unknown cause, characterized by vertigo, visual disorders, and generalized muscular weakness.

germ, *n.* [L. *germen,* sprout]. 1. A small bit of protoplasm capable of developing into a new individual, especially an egg, spore, or seed; any of the early stages in the development of an organism. 2. Any microorganism.

Germanin. A trademark for suramin sodium, an antiprotozoal agent.

ger·ma·ni·um (jur·may′nee·um) *n.* [NL., after *Germany*]. Ge = 72.59. A brittle, grayish white, metallic element. See also Table of Elements in the Appendix.

Ger·man measles. RUBELLA.

germ cell. A spermatozoon or an ovum, or a formative stage of either. Syn. *gonoblast.*

germ center. GERMINAL CENTER.

germ disk. GERMINAL DISK.

germ epithelium. GERMINAL EPITHELIUM.

ger·mi·cide (jur′mi·side) *n.* [*germ* + *-cide*]. An agent that destroys germs. —**germi·ci·dal** (jur″mi·sigh′dul) *adj.*

ger·mi·nal (jur′mi·nul) *adj.* 1. Of, pertaining to, or within a germ or seed. 2. Pertaining to the early developmental stages of an embryo or organism.

germinal area. GERMINAL DISK.

germinal cell. A cell from which other cells are derived, used specifically for dividing cells in the embryonic neural tube.

germinal center. The actively proliferating region of a lymphatic nodule in which lymphocytes are being formed; the site of the high-level antibody formation characteristic of a secondary immune response. Syn. *germ center.*

germinal disk. 1. The protoplasmic area in the eggs of reptiles, birds, and lower animals which becomes the blastoderm, in the center of which arises the definitive embryo. 2. In placental mammals, the inner cell mass which becomes the embryonic disk while the rest of the blastocyst becomes amnion, yolk sac, and trophoblast.

germinal epithelium. A region of the dorsal coelomic epithelium, lying between the dorsal mesentery and the mesonephros, becoming the covering epithelium of the gonad when it arises from the genital ridge; once falsely believed to give rise to the germ cells. Syn. *germ epithelium.*

germinal inclusion cyst. A cyst located near the surface of an ovary, arising from inclusions of germinal epithelium.

germinal membrane. BLASTODERM.

germinal nucleus. PRONUCLEUS.

germinal pole. ANIMAL POLE.

germinal spot. The nucleolus of the egg nucleus.

germinal vesicle. BLASTULA.

ger·mi·na·tion (jur″mi·nay′shun) *n.* [L. *germinatio,* from *germinare,* to germinate]. The beginning of growth of a spore or seed. —**ger·mi·nate** (jur′mi·nate) *v.*

ger·mi·na·tive (jur′mi·nuh·tiv, ·nay″tiv) *adj.* Having the power to begin growth or to develop.

germinative layer. The deeper, proliferative layers of the epidermis; the prickle cell and basal cell layers. Syn. *stratum germinativum.*

ger·mine (jur′meen) *n.* A highly hydroxylated steroidal alkanolamine base, $C_{27}H_{43}NO_8$, various esters of which constitute certain of the alkaloids of *Veratrum viride* and *V. album;* isomeric with cevine and protoverine, which are parent bases of other alkaloids in the veratrums.

ger·mi·no·ma (jur″mi·no′muh) *n.* [*germin*al + *-oma*]. A tumor whose parenchyma is composed of germ cells; usually a malignant teratoma, a seminoma, or a dysgerminoma.

germ layer. One of the epithelial layers of the blastula or blastocyst from which the various organs of the embryo are derived. See also *germ-layer theory.*

germ-layer theory. The theory that a young embryo establishes three superimposed cellular plates, the primary germ layers, which are called ectoderm, mesoderm, and entoderm. According to this theory, the skin, nervous system, and sense organs are derived from ectoderm; the inner lining of the primitive digestive canal from entoderm; and muscles, blood vessels, connective tissues, and organs of excretion and reproduction from mesoderm.

germ membrane. BLASTODERM.

germ plasm. The material basis of inheritance; it is located in the chromosomes.

germ ridge. GENITAL RIDGE.

germ theory. The theory that contagious and infectious diseases are caused by microorganisms.

germ track. The continuity of sexual cells observed through many generations.

germ vesicle. BLASTULA.

gero-. See *ger-.*

ger·o·co·mia (jerr″o·ko′mee·uh) *n.* [Gk. *gērokomia*]. GEROCOMY.

ge·roc·o·my (je·rock′o·mee) *n.* [Gk. *gērokomia,* care of the aged]. The medical and hygienic care of old people. —**ger·o·com·i·cal** (jerr″o·kom′i·kul) *adj.*

gero·der·ma (jerr″o·dur′muh) *n.* [*gero-* + *-derma*]. The skin of old age, showing atrophy, loss of fat, and loss of elasticity.

ger·o·don·tia (jerr″o·don′chee·uh) *n.* [*ger-* + *-odontia*]. Dentistry for the aged.

gero·ma·ras·mus (jerr″o·ma·raz′mus) *n.* [*gero-* + *marasmus*]. Emaciation characteristic of extreme old age.

gero·mor·phism (jerr″o·mor′fiz·um) *n.* [*gero-* + *-morph* + *-ism*]. The condition of appearing prematurely aged.

geront-, geronto- [Gk., from *gerōn, gerontos,* old man]. A combining form meaning *old age.*

ge·ron·tal (je·ron′tul) *adj.* GERONTIC.

ge·ron·tic (je·ron′tick) *adj.* [Gk. *gerontikos,* pertaining to old men]. Pertaining to old age; GERATIC. —**geron·tism** (·tiz·um) *n.*

geronto-. See *geront-.*

ger·on·tol·o·gy (jerr″on·tol′uh·jee) *n.* [*geronto-* + *-logy*]. Scientific study of the phenomena and problems of aging; GERATOLOGY. Compare *geriatrics.*

ge·ron·to·phil·ia (je·ron″to·fil′ee·uh) *n.* [*geronto-* + *-philia*]. Love for and understanding of old people.

ge·ron·to·pho·bia (je·ron″to·fo′bee·uh) *n.* [*geronto-* + *-phobia*]. Unusual fear or dislike of old people or old age.

ge·ron·to·ther·a·peu·tics (je·ron″to·therr″uh·pew′ticks) *n.* GERONTOTHERAPY.

ge·ron·to·ther·a·py (je·ron″to·therr′uh·pee) *n.* [*geronto-* + *therapy*]. 1. Treatment of the aging process. 2. Therapeutic management of aged persons.

ger·on·tox·on (jerr″on·tock′son) *n.* [*geront-* + Gk. *toxon,* bow]. ARCUS SENILIS.

Gerota's fascia [D. *Gerota,* Rumanian surgeon, 1867–1939]. RENAL FASCIA.

-gerous [L. *ger*ere, to carry, bear, + *-ous*]. A combining form meaning (a) *bearing, holding;* (b) *conveying, conducting.*

Gersh-Ma·cal·lum method. A histochemical method for potassium employing the freezing-drying process; potassium is precipitated as yellow sodium potassium cobaltinitrite.

Gerst·mann's syndrome [J. *Gerstmann,* U.S. neuropsychiatrist, b. 1887]. A disorder of cerebral function due to a lesion in the angular gyrus of the dominant cerebral hemisphere and the adjoining area of the middle occipital gyri, consisting of right-left disorientation, finger agnosia, agraphia and acalculia.

Ge·sell developmental schedule (guh·zel′) [A. *Gesell,* U.S. pediatrician and psychologist, 1880–1961]. A test of the mental growth of the preschool child which includes motor development, adaptive behavior, language development, and personal-social behavior.

ges·ta·clone (jes′tuh·klone) *n.* 6-Chloro-1α,2α:16α,17-bismethylene-4,6-pregnadien-3,20-dione, $C_{23}H_{27}ClO_2$, a progestin.

ge·stalt (guh·shtahlt′) *n.* [Ger., form, shape]. The configuration of separate units, both experiential and behavioral, into a pattern or shape which itself seems to function as a unit. See also *gestalt psychology.*

ge·stalt·ism (guh·shtahl′tiz·um) *n.* GESTALT PSYCHOLOGY.

ge·stalt·ist (guh·shtahl′tist) *n.* A psychologist of the gestalt school. See also *gestalt psychology.*

gestalt psychology. A system or theory of psychology that emphasizes the wholeness and organized structure of every experience, maintaining that psychologic processes and behavior cannot be described adequately by analyzing the elements of experience alone, but rather by their integration into one perceptual configuration, and emphasizing sudden learning by insight rather than by trial and error or association.

ges·ta·tion (jes·tay′shun) *n.* [L. *gestatio,* from *gestare,* to carry, bear]. PREGNANCY. —**ges·tate** (jes′tate) *v.;* **ges·ta·tion·al** (jes·tay′shun·ul) *adj.*

gestational age. The age of a conceptus computed from the first day of the last menstrual period to any point in time thereafter, but usually not calculated beyond the first few months of life after birth. Compare *fetal age.*

gestational psychosis. Any serious mental disorder in association with pregnancy or the postpartum period.

gestation period. The period of pregnancy. The average length of human gestation is taken as 10 lunar months (280 days) from the onset of the last menstrual period with a variation between 250 and 310 days. See also Table of the Duration of Pregnancy (Ely's Table) in the Appendix.

ges·to·nor·one (jes″to·nor′ohn) *n.* 17-Hydroxy-19-norpregn-4-ene-3,20-dione, $C_{20}H_{28}O_3$, a progestational steroid; used as the caproate ester.

ges·to·sis (jes·to′sis) *n.*, pl. **gesto·ses** (·seez) [*gest*ation + *-osis*]. Any toxemic manifestation in pregnancy.

Ge·tso·wa's adenoma. Thyroid adenocarcinoma supposedly arising in lateral aberrant thyroid tissue. Syn. *struma postbranchialis.*

geu·ma·pho·bia (gew″muh·fo′bee·uh) *n.* [Gk. *geuma,* taste, + *-phobia*]. A morbid fear of tastes.

-geusia [Gk. *geu*sis, sense of taste, + *-ia*]. A combining form meaning *condition of the taste sense.*

GFR Glomerular filtration rate.

ghat·ti gum (gat′ee). The gummy exudate from stems of *Anogeissus latifolia,* a tree of India and Ceylon. It forms a viscous mucilage, and is sometimes used in place of acacia.

Ghon complex (gohn) [A. *Ghon,* Austrian pathologist, 1866–1936]. The combination of a focus of subpleural tuberculosis (Ghon tubercle) with associated hilar and mediastinal lymph node tuberculosis, usually in children. Syn. *primary complex, Kufss-Ghon focus.*

Ghon primary focus or **lesion.** GHON TUBERCLE.

Ghon tubercle [A. *Ghon*]. The primary lesion of pulmonary tuberculosis, appearing as a radiographic shadow in the lung.

ghost cells or **corpuscles.** 1. The still visible stromata of hemolyzed erythrocytes. Syn. *phantom cells.* 2. *In exfoliative cytology,* the cells of squamous lung cancer in which the nuclei are compressed or destroyed by large amounts of intracytoplasmic keratin.

GI Abbreviation for *gastrointestinal.*

Gia·co·mi·ni's band or **frenulum** (jaʰ″ko·mee′nee) [C. *Giacomini,* Italian anatomist, 1841–1898]. BAND OF GIACOMINI.

Gian·nuz·zi's cells or **crescent** (jaʰn·noot′tsee) [G. *Giannuzzi,* Italian anatomist, 1839–1876]. DEMILUNE.

gi·ant cell. 1. Any large cell. 2. A multinucleate large cell.

giant-cell arteritis. 1. An arterial inflammatory disease characterized by multinucleated cells (giant cells), affecting the carotid artery branches, particularly the temporal artery, of elderly people, accompanied by fever, headache, and a variety of neurologic disturbances, including blindness. Syn. *cranial arteritis, temporal arteritis.* 2. POLYARTERITIS NODOSA. 3. AORTIC ARCH SYNDROME.

giant-cell glioblastoma. MAGNOCELLULAR GLIOBLASTOMA.

giant-cell leukemia. MEGAKARYOCYTIC LEUKEMIA.

giant-cell sarcoma. 1. A usually benign giant-cell tumor. 2. Epulis in malignant form. 3. A malignant synovioma.

giant-cell tumor. 1. A distinctive tumor of bone, thought to arise from nonosteogenic connective tissue or marrow, composed of a richly vascularized reticulum of stromal cells interspersed with multinuclear giant cells. It generally appears after the second decade of life near the end of long limb bones, and it causes thinning of the compact bone. Syn. *central giant-cell tumor, osteoclastoma, myeloid sarcoma, myeloplaxic tumor, chronic hemorrhagic osteomy-*

elitis. 2. EPULIS. 3. CHONDROBLASTOMA. 4. NONOSSIFYING FIBROMA. 5. XANTHOMATOUS GIANT-CELL TUMOR OF TENDON SHEATH.

giant-cell xanthoma. XANTHOMATOUS GIANT-CELL TUMOR OF TENDON SHEATH.

giant colon. MEGACOLON.

giant edema. ANGIOEDEMA.

giant fingers. MACRODACTYLY.

giant follicular lymphoblastoma. NODULAR LYMPHOMA.

giant follicular lymphoma. NODULAR LYMPHOMA.

giant intracanalicular fibroadenomyxoma. CYSTOSARCOMA PHYLLODES.

gi·ant·ism (jye'un·tiz·um) *n.* GIGANTISM.

giant magnet. A large, powerful, stationary magnet for extracting particles of steel from the eye.

giant mammary myxoma. CYSTOSARCOMA PHYLLODES.

giant stellate cells of Meynert [T. H. *Meynert*]. SOLITARY CELLS OF MEYNERT.

giant urticaria. ANGIOEDEMA.

Gi·ar·dia (jee·ahr'dee·uh) *n.* [A. *Giard,* French biologist, 1846–1908]. A genus of flagellated protozoan parasites.

Giardia lam·blia (lam'blee·uh). A species of parasites found in the small intestine of man. It is not a tissue invader but is the cause of giardiasis.

gi·ar·di·a·sis (jee"ahr·dye'uh·sis) *n.*, pl. **giardia·ses** (·seez) [*Giardia* + *-iasis*]. The presence of the *Giardia lamblia* in the small intestine of man, usually without symptoms, but occasionally producing diarrhea and abdominal discomfort. Syn. *lambliasis.*

Gibbon-Landis test. LANDIS-GIBBON TEST.

gib·bos·i·ty (gi·bos'i·tee) *n.* [F. *gibbosité,* from L. *gibbosus,* gibbous]. KYPHOSIS.

gib·bous (gib'us) *adj.* [*gibbus* + *-ous*]. KYPHOTIC; swollen, convex, or protuberant, especially on one side.

Gibbs adsorption law [J. W. *Gibbs,* U.S. physicist, 1839–1903]. A substance that lowers interfacial or surface tension of a dispersion medium will collect at a surface or interface, whereas a substance that increases surface tension is concentrated within the interior of the liquid.

Gibbs-Donnan equilibrium [J. W. *Gibbs* and F. G. *Donnan*]. DONNAN EQUILIBRIUM.

Gibbs-Helm·holtz equation [J. W. *Gibbs* and H. L. F. von *Helmholtz*]. *In thermodynamics,* an equation relating the rate of change in free energy of a system, as an electrochemical cell, with temperature, to other energy quantities.

gib·bus (gib'us) *n.* [L.]. A hump; usually the dorsal convexity seen in tuberculosis of the spine (Pott's disease) or fracture.

Gi·bral·tar fever. BRUCELLOSIS.

Gib·son's bandage [K. C. *Gibson,* U.S. dentist, 1849–1925]. A bandage designed to hold in position the fragments of a fractured mandible.

Gibson's rule [G. A. *Gibson,* Scottish physician, 1854–1913]. In pneumonia, if the systolic blood pressure (mmHg) does not fall below the pulse rate (beats per minute), the prognosis for recovery is good, and vice versa.

gid, *n.* [from *giddy*]. A chronic brain disease of sheep, less frequently of cattle; characterized by forced movements of circling, rolling. Caused by the larval form of the dog tapeworm *Multiceps multiceps.*

gid·di·ness, *n.* An unpleasant sensation of disturbed relation to surrounding objects in space, differing from vertigo in that there is no experience of the external world, or of the patient, being in motion. See also *dizziness.* —**gid·dy,** *adj.*

Giem·sa's stain (gyem'zah) [G. *Giemsa,* German chemist, 1867–1948]. A stain for hemopoietic tissue and hemoprotozoa consisting of a stock glycerol methanol solution of eosinates of Azure B and methylene blue with some excess of the basic dyes.

Gier·ke's corpuscles (geer'kuh) [H. P. B. *Gierke,* German anatomist, 1847–1886]. THYMIC CORPUSCLES.

Gierke's disease [E. von *Gierke*]. VON GIERKE'S DISEASE.

Gierke's respiratory bundle [H. P. B. *Gierke*]. SOLITARY FASCICULUS.

Gif·ford's operation [H. *Gifford,* U.S. ophthalmologist, 1858–1929]. DELIMITING KERATOTOMY.

Gifford's reflex [H. *Gifford*]. Constriction of the pupil when the orbicularis oculi is contracted, the eyelids being held open.

Gifford's sign [H. *Gifford*]. Inability to evert the upper eyelid, or lid lag, in hyperthyroidism.

gift spots. Spots of whiteness of the nails. See also *leukonychia.*

gigant-, giganto- [Gk. *gigas, gigantos*]. A combining form meaning *giant.*

gi·gan·tism (jye·gan'tiz·um) *n.* [*gigant-* + *-ism*]. In man, excessive growth, with a height greater than 78 to 80 inches. Compare *acromegaly.* See also *cerebral gigantism.*

giganto-. See *gigant-.*

gi·gan·to·blast (jye·gan'to·blast) *n.* [*giganto-* + *-blast*]. A large nucleated erythroblast.

gi·gan·to·cel·lu·lar (jye·gan"to·sel'yoo·lur) *adj.* Characterized by or pertaining to giant cells.

gigantocellular astrocytoma. GEMISTOCYTIC ASTROCYTOMA.

gi·gan·to·chro·mo·blast (jye·gan"to·kro'mo·blast) *n.* [*giganto-* + *chromoblast*]. GIGANTOBLAST.

gi·gan·to·cyte (jye·gan'to·site) *n.* [*giganto-* + *-cyte*]. A large nonnucleated red blood corpuscle.

Gi·gli's operation (jeel'lyee) [L. *Gigli,* Italian surgeon and gynecologist, 1863–1908]. Pubiotomy for contracted pelvis in cases of dystocia.

Gigli's saw [L. *Gigli*]. A flexible wire saw with detachable handles at either end. Adapted to cranial and other bone operations.

Gi·la monster (hee'luh) [after *Gila* River, Arizona]. *HELODERMA SUSPECTUM.*

Gil·bert's sign (zheel·behr') [N. A. *Gilbert,* French physician, 1858–1927]. In cirrhosis of the liver, more urine is excreted during fasting than after a meal (opsiuria).

Gilbert's syndrome or **disease** [N. A. *Gilbert*]. An asymptomatic disorder associated with a hereditary (autosomal dominant) glucuronyl transferase deficiency, a compensated hemolytic process, or a nonhemolytic overproduction of bilirubin; characterized by mild fluctuating indirect hyperbilirubinemia and usually with an impaired hepatic uptake or transport of bilirubin, or both.

Gil·christ's disease [T. C. *Gilchrist,* U. S. dermatologist, 1862–1927]. NORTH AMERICAN BLASTOMYCOSIS.

gild·ing, *n.* Application of gold salts to histologic preparations of nerve tissue after fixation and hardening.

Gil·e·ad balm (gil'ee·ad). An oleoresin from the *Commiphora opobalsamum.*

Gilford-Hutchinson disease [H. *Gilford,* English physician, 1861–1941; and J. *Hutchinson*]. HUTCHINSON-GILFORD SYNDROME.

¹gill (jil) *n.* [OF. *gille*]. One-fourth of a pint.

²gill (gil) *n.* A respiratory organ of water-breathing animals.

gill cleft carcinoma. BRANCHIOGENIC CARCINOMA.

Gil·le·nia (ji·lee'nee·uh) *n.* [A. *Gille,* German botanist, 17th century]. A genus of rosaceous herbs, *Gillenia trifoliata,* or bowman's root, and *Gillenia stipulata,* or Indian physic, having emetic power.

Gilles de la Tou·rette disease or **syndrome** (zheel"duh·la·too·ret') [G. *Gilles de la Tourette,* French neurologist, 1857–1904]. A severe form of habit spasm, beginning in late childhood and adolescence and characterized by multiple tics associated with echolalia, obscene utterances, and other compulsive acts.

Gil·lies' operation (gil'is) [H. D. *Gillies,* English surgeon, 1882–1960]. 1. An operation for ectropion, excising scar tissue and grafting the defect. 2. An operation for plastic repair in which a tubed pedicle flap is formed.

gill slit. TREMA (3).

Gim·ber·nat's ligament (Sp. ^{k}heem·behr·na^{h}t', Cat. zheem·behr·na^{h}t') [A. de *Gimbernat*, Spanish surgeon and anatomist, 1734–1816]. LACUNAR LIGAMENT.

gin-drinker's liver. ALCOHOLIC CIRRHOSIS.

gin fever. BYSSINOSIS.

gin·ger, *n.* [Gk. *zingiberi*, from Skr. *sṛṅgavera*]. The dried rhizome of *Zingiber officinale*, formerly used as a carminative and flavoring agent.

ginger paralysis. TRIORTHOCRESYL PHOSPHATE NEUROPATHY.

gin·gi·li (jin'ji·lee) *n.* [Hindi *jinjalī*, from Ar. *jiljilān*]. SESAME.

gingiv-, gingivo-. A combining form meaning *gingiva, gingival.*

gin·gi·va (jin'ji·vuh, jin·jye'vuh) *n.*, pl. & genit. sing. **gingi·vae** (·vee) [L., gum] [NA]. The mucous membrane and underlying soft tissue that covers the alveolar process and surrounds a tooth. **—gingi·val** (·vul) *adj.*; **gingival·ly** (·ee) *adv.*

gingival crevice. GINGIVAL SULCUS.

gingival curvature. A curve of the line of attachment of the gingival tissue at the cervix of a tooth.

gingival groove or **line.** FREE GINGIVAL GROOVE.

gingival margin. 1. The more or less rounded crest of the gingival tissue. 2. The margin of a dental cavity or restoration nearest the apex.

gingival pocket. An abnormally deep gingival sulcus due to inflammatory gingival enlargement, gingival hyperplasia, or incomplete eruption of a tooth; it does not involve the gingival attachment.

gingival septum. The mucous membrane projecting into the interproximal space between two teeth.

gingival sulcus. The space between the free gingiva and the surface of a tooth.

gin·gi·vec·to·my (jin"ji·veck'tuh·mee) *n.* [*gingiv-* + *-ectomy*]. Excision of a portion of the gingiva.

gin·gi·vi·tis (jin"ji·vye'tis) *n.* [*gingiv-* + *-itis*]. Inflammation of the gingiva.

gingivo-. See *gingiv-*.

gin·gi·vo·buc·cal (jin"ji·vo·buck'ul) *adj.* [*gingivo-* + *buccal*]. Pertaining to the gingivae and the mucous membranes of the lips or cheeks.

gin·gi·vo·glos·sal (jin"ji·vo·glos'ul) *adj.* [*gingivo-* + *glossal*]. Pertaining to the gums and the tongue.

gin·gi·vo·plas·ty (jin'ji·vo·plas"tee) *n.* [*gingivo-* + *-plasty*]. The surgical recontouring or reshaping of the gingiva for the achievement of physiologic form.

gin·gi·vo·sis (jin"ji·vo'sis) *n.* [*gingiv-* + *-osis*]. CHRONIC DESQUAMATIVE GINGIVITIS.

gin·gi·vo·sto·ma·ti·tis (jin"ji·vo·sto"muh·tye'tis) *n.* [*gingivo-* + *stomatitis*]. An inflammation of the gingiva and oral mucosa.

gin·gly·mus (jing'gli·mus, ging') *n.*, pl. **gingly·mi** (·migh) [Gk. *ginglymos*, hinge] [NA]. HINGE ARTICULATION. **—gingly·moid** (·moid) *adj.*

gip·py tummy (jip'ee) [for "Egyptian stomach"]. *Slang.* TRAVELER'S DIARRHEA.

Gi·ral·des' organ (zhee·ra^{h}l'dis, ·dish) [J. A. C. C. *Giraldes*, Portuguese surgeon, 1808–1875]. PARADIDYMIS.

gir·dle, *n.* 1. A band designed to go around the body. 2. A structure resembling a circular belt or band.

girdle anesthesia. A zone of anesthesia encircling the body.

girdle pain. A painful sensation as of a cord tied about the waist, symptomatic of disease of the nerve roots.

Gir·dle·stone's operation [G. R. *Girdlestone*, English surgeon, 1881–1950]. A procedure that provides for radical drainage of a dangerously infected hip joint.

girney. GURNEY.

Gitaligin. A trademark for gitalin, a cardiotonic glycoside.

git·a·lin (jit'uh·lin, ji·tay'lin, ji·tal'in) *n.* 1. A crystalline glycoside, $C_{35}H_{56}O_{12}$, from digitalis leaves. 2. An amorphous mixture of digitalis glycosides.

Git·lin's syndrome [D. *Gitlin*, U.S. pediatrician, b. 1921]. PRIMARY LYMPHOPENIC IMMUNOLOGIC DEFICIENCY.

git·o·gen·in (jit"o·jen'in, ji·toj'e·nin) *n.* The steroid aglycone of gitonin.

git·o·nin (jit'o·nin, ji·to'nin) *n.* A saponin from *Digitalis purpurea.* On acid hydrolysis it yields the steroid aglycone gitogenin, galactose, and L-xylose.

gi·tox·i·gen·in (ji·tock"si·jen'in, ji·tock'si·ji·nin) *n.* The steroid aglycone, $C_{23}H_{34}O_5$, of gitoxin and of lanatoside B.

gi·tox·in (ji·tock'sin) *n.* One of the partially hydrolyzed glycosides, $C_{41}H_{64}O_{14}$, obtained from both *Digitalis purpurea* and *D. lanata;* on complete hydrolysis it yields the steroid aglycone gitoxigenin and three molecules of the sugar digitoxose.

git·ter cell (git'ur) [Ger. *Gitter*, lattice, reticulum]. COMPOUND GRANULE CELL.

git·ter·fa·sern (git'ur·fah"zurn) *n. pl.* [Ger., from *Gitter*, lattice, + *Faser*, fiber]. RETICULAR FIBERS.

giz·zard (giz'urd) *n.* [L. *gigeria*, cooked entrails of poultry]. The muscular portion of the upper digestive system of some birds. Syn. *ventriculus.*

gla·bel·la (gla·bel'uh) *n.*, pl. **glabel·lae** (·ee) [L. *glabellus*, dim. of *glaber*, hairless, smooth] [NA]. 1. The bony prominence on the frontal bone joining the supraorbital ridges. 2. *In craniometry,* a point found in the sagittal plane of the bony prominence joining the supraorbital ridges, usually the most anteriorly projecting portion of this region. **—glabel·lar** (·ur) *adj.*

glabellar reflex. MYERSON'S REFLEX.

gla·brate (glay'brate) *adj.* GLABROUS.

gla·brous (glay'brus) *adj.* [*glabr-*, from L. *glaber*, smooth, hairless, + *-ous*]. Smooth; devoid of hairs.

gla·cial (glay'shul) *adj.* [L. *glacialis*, from *glacies*, ice]. Icy; resembling ice in appearance.

glacial acetic acid. A colorless liquid containing not less than 99.4% CH_3COOH; formerly used as a caustic for removing warts and corns.

glad·i·ol·ic acid (glad"ee·ol'ick). An antibiotic substance, $C_{11}H_{10}O_5$, isolated from cultures of *Penicillium gladioli;* it is active against some bacteria and has marked fungistatic properties.

gladi·o·lus (glad"ee·o'lus, gla·dye'o·lus) *n.*, pl. **gladio·li** (·lye) [L., dim. of *gladius*, sword]. The middle or second piece of the sternum.

glair·in (glair'in) *n.* [OF. *glaire*, white of egg, + *-in*]. An organic gelatinous substance of bacterial origin found on the surface of some thermal waters.

glairy (glair'ee) *adj.* [OF. *glaire*, white of egg]. 1. Slimy; VISCOUS; MUCOID. 2. Resembling the white of an egg.

gland, *n.* [F. *glande*, from OF., glandular or lymph-node swelling, from L. *glans, glandis*, acorn]. 1. A cell, tissue, or organ that elaborates and discharges a substance that is used elsewhere in the body (secretion), or is eliminated (excretion). NA *glandula.* 2. GLANS. 3. *Obsol.* LYMPH NODE. Adj. *glandular.*

glan·ders (glan'durz) *n.* [OF. *glandres*, glands, from L. *glandulae*, tonsils, glandular swellings]. A highly contagious acute or chronic disease of horses, mules, and asses, caused by *Pseudomonas mallei* and communicable to dogs, goats, sheep, and man, but not to bovines; characterized by fever, inflammation of mucous membranes (especially of the nose), enlargement and hardening of the regional lymph nodes, formation of nodules which have a tendency to coalesce and then to degenerate to form deep ulcers. In man, the disease runs an acute febrile or a chronic course with granulomas and abscesses in the skin, lungs and elsewhere. Syn. *equinia.* See also *farcy.*

glanders bacillus. *PSEUDOMONAS MALLEI.*

glandes. Plural of *glans.*

gland of Vir·chow-Troi·sier (virr'^{c}ho, firr'^{c}ho, trwa^{h}z·ye^{y}') [R. L. K. *Virchow* and E. *Troisier*]. SIGNAL NODE.

glands of Sham·baugh. The epithelium along the outer wall of the cochlear duct, modified to resemble a glandular epithelium, which rests upon the stria vascularis.

glands of Zeis. ZEIS'S GLANDS.

glan·du·la (glan'dew·luh) *n.*, pl. **glandu·lae** (·lee) [L.] [NA]. GLAND (1).

glandula bul·bo·ure·thra·lis (bul"bo·yoo·re·thray'lis) [NA]. BULBOURETHRAL GLAND.

glandulae are·o·la·res (ăr"ee·o·lair'eez) [NA]. AREOLAR GLANDS.

glandulae bron·chi·a·les (bronk·ee·ay'leez) [NA]. BRONCHIAL GLANDS (1).

glandulae buc·ca·les (buh·kay'leez) [NA]. BUCCAL GLANDS.

glandulae ce·ru·mi·no·sae (se·roo"mi·no'see) [NA]. CERUMINOUS GLANDS.

glandulae cer·vi·ca·les ute·ri (sur·vi·kay'leez yoo'tur·eye) [NA]. The glands of the cervix of the uterus.

glandulae ci·li·a·res (sil·ee·air'eez) [NA]. CILIARY GLANDS.

glandulae cir·cum·ana·les (sur"kum·ay·nay'leez) [NA]. Glands situated around the anus.

glandulae con·junc·ti·va·les (kon·junk"ti·vay'leez) [NA]. CONJUNCTIVAL GLANDS.

glandulae cu·tis (kew'tis) [NA]. The glands associated with the skin.

glandulae duo·de·na·les (dew·o·de·nay'leez) [NA]. DUODENAL GLANDS.

glandulae eso·pha·ge·ae (ee"so·fay'jee·ee) [NA]. The glands associated with the esophagus.

glandulae gas·tri·cae (gas'tri·see) [NA]. GASTRIC GLANDS. NA alt. *glandulae propriae.*

glandulae glo·mi·for·mes (glom"i·for'meez) [NA]. GLOMUS BODIES.

glandulae in·te·sti·na·les in·te·sti·ni cras·si (in·tes·ti·nay'leez in·tes·tye'nigh kras'eye) [NA]. Glands in the mucous membrane of the large intestine.

glandulae intestinales intestini te·nu·is (ten'yoo·is) [NA]. Glands in the mucous membrane of the small intestine.

glandulae intestinales rec·ti (reck'tye) [NA]. Glands in the mucous membrane of the rectum.

glandulae la·bi·a·les (lay·bee·ay'leez) [NA]. LABIAL GLANDS.

glandulae la·cri·ma·les ac·ces·so·ri·ae (lack·ri·may'leez ack·se·so'ree·ee) [NA]. Accessory lacrimal glands occasionally present.

glandulae la·ryn·ge·ae (la·rin'jee·ee) [NA]. Glands in the mucous membrane of the larynx.

glandulae laryngeae an·te·ri·o·res (an·teer"ee·o'reez) [BNA]. Glands located in the anterior part of the mucous membrane of the larynx.

glandulae laryngeae me·di·ae (mee'dee·ee) [BNA]. Glands located in the mucous membrane of the aryepiglottic fold.

glandulae laryngeae pos·te·ri·o·res (pos·teer"ee·o'reez) [BNA]. Glands located in the posterior portion of the mucous membrane of the larynx.

glandulae lin·gua·les (ling·gway'leez) [NA]. Glands of the mucous membrane of the tongue.

glandulae mo·la·res (mo·lair'eez) [NA]. MOLAR GLANDS.

glandulae mu·co·sae bi·li·o·sae (mew·ko'see bil·ee·o'see) [NA]. Glands of the mucous membrane of the gallbladder and bile ducts.

glandulae mucosae tu·ni·cae con·junc·ti·vae (tew'ni·kee kon·junk·tye'vee, tew'ni·see) [BNA]. Glandulae conjunctivales (= CONJUNCTIVAL GLANDS).

glandulae mu·co·sae ure·te·ris (mew·ko'see yoo·re·teer'is, yoo·ree'tur·is) [BNA]. Glands of the mucous membrane of the ureter.

glandulae na·sa·les (na·say'leez) [NA]. Glands associated with the respiratory epithelium of the nose.

glandulae ol·fac·to·ri·ae (ol·fack·to'ree·ee) [NA]. Glands of the olfactory mucous membrane.

glandulae oris (o'ris) [NA]. Glands of the mouth.

glandulae pa·la·ti·nae (pal·uh·tye'nee) [NA]. Glands of the mucous membrane of the palate.

glandulae pel·vis re·na·lis (pel'vis re·nay'lis) [BNA]. Glands in the mucous membrane of the renal pelvis.

glandulae pha·ryn·ge·ae (fa·rin'jee·ee) [NA]. Glands associated with the mucous membrane of the pharynx.

glandulae prae·pu·ti·a·les (pre·pew"shee·ay'leez) [BNA]. Glandulae preputiales (= PREPUTIAL GLANDS).

glandulae pre·pu·ti·a·les (pre·pew"shee·ay'leez) [NA]. PREPUTIAL GLANDS.

glandulae pro·pri·ae (pro'pree·ee) [NA alt.]. GASTRIC GLANDS. NA alt. *glandulae gastricae.*

glandulae py·lo·ri·cae (pye·lo'ri·see) [NA]. PYLORIC GLANDS.

glandulae se·ba·ce·ae (se·bay'see·ee) [NA]. SEBACEOUS GLANDS.

glandulae sebaceae are·o·lae mam·mae (a·ree'o·lee mam'ee) [BNA]. Sebaceous glands associated with the skin of the areola of the nipple.

glandulae sebaceae la·bi·o·rum pu·den·di (lay·bee·o'rum pew·den'dye) [BNA]. Sebaceous glands of the labia majora.

glandulae si·ne duc·ti·bus (sin'ee duck'ti·bus) [NA]. ENDOCRINE GLANDS.

glandulae su·do·ri·fe·rae (sue"dor·if'ur·ee) [NA]. SWEAT GLANDS.

glandulae su·pra·re·na·les ac·ces·so·ri·ae (sue"pruh·re·nay'leez ack"se·so'ree·ee) [NA]. ACCESSORY SUPRARENAL GLANDS.

glandulae tar·sa·les (tahr·say'leez) [NA]. TARSAL GLANDS.

glandulae thy·re·oi·de·ae ac·ces·so·ri·ae (thigh"ree·oy'dee·ee ack"se·so'ree·ee) [BNA]. Glandulae thyroideae accessoriae (= ACCESSORY THYROID GLANDS).

glandulae thy·roi·de·ae ac·ces·so·ri·ae (thigh·roy'dee·ee ack"se·so'ree·ee) [NA]. ACCESSORY THYROID GLANDS.

glandulae tra·che·a·les (tray·kee·ay'leez) [NA]. Glands associated with the trachea.

glandulae tu·ba·ri·ae (tew·bair'ee·ee) [NA]. Glands associated with the auditory tube.

glandulae ure·thra·les (yoo·re·thray'leez) [NA]. URETHRAL GLANDS.

glandulae urethrales ure·thrae mu·li·e·bris (yoo·ree'three mew·lee·ee'bris) [BNA]. Urethral glands of the female urethra.

glandulae ute·ri·nae (yoo·tur·eye'nee) [NA]. UTERINE GLANDS.

glandulae ve·si·ca·les (ves·i·kay'leez) [BNA]. Vestigial glands occurring in the mucous membrane of the urinary bladder near the urethral opening.

glandulae ve·sti·bu·la·res mi·no·res (ves·tib"yoo·lair'eez mi·no'reez) [NA]. The minor vestibular glands. See *vestibular glands.*

glandula la·cri·ma·lis (lack·ri·may'lis) [NA]. LACRIMAL GLAND.

glandula lacrimalis inferior [BNA]. The smaller lower portion of the lacrimal gland.

glandula lacrimalis superior [BNA]. The larger upper portion of the lacrimal gland.

glandula lin·gua·lis anterior (ling·gway'lis) [NA]. ANTERIOR LINGUAL GLAND.

glandula mam·ma·ria (ma·mair'ee·uh) [NA]. MAMMARY GLAND.

glandula mu·co·sa (mew·ko'suh) [NA]. MUCOUS GLAND.

glandula pa·ra·thy·roi·dea inferior (păr"uh·thigh·roy'dee·uh) [NA]. The inferior parathyroid gland.

glandula parathyroidea superior [NA]. The superior parathyroid gland.

glandula pa·ro·tis (pa·ro'tis) [NA]. PAROTID GLAND.

glandula parotis ac·ces·so·ria (ack"se·so'ree·uh) [NA]. ACCESSORY PAROTID GLAND.

glandula pi·tu·i·ta·ria (pi·tew"i·tair'ee·uh) [NA alt.]. HYPOPHYSIS.

glan·du·lar (glan'dew·lur) *adj.* 1. Of or pertaining to a gland or glands. 2. Of or pertaining to the glans of the penis or of the clitoris; BALANIC.

glandular bar. A median bar caused by prostatic hyperplasia.

glandular carcinoma. ADENOCARCINOMA.
glandular cheilitis. A chronic inflammation of the lower lip; characterized by swelling of the labial mucous glands and their ducts. Syn. *cheilitis glandularis, cheilitis glandularis apostematosa, myxadenitis labialis, Puente's disease.*
glandular epithelium. An epithelium in which the cells are predominantly secretory in function.
glandular fever. INFECTIOUS MONONUCLEOSIS.
glandular hypospadias. BALANIC HYPOSPADIAS.
glandular proliferous cysts. CYSTOSARCOMA PHYLLODES.
glandular sinusitis. An extensive hyperplasia of the seromucinous glands of the nose, which in the advanced stage may become cystic. Syn. *adenomatous sinusitis.*
glandular tissue. A group of epithelial cells that elaborate secretions.
glandular tuberculosis. *Obsol.* Tuberculosis affecting the lymph nodes, especially the cervical, bronchial, and mesenteric.
glandula se·ro·mu·co·sa (seer″o·mew·ko′suh) [NA]. MIXED GLAND.
glandula se·ro·sa (se·ro′suh) [NA]. SEROUS GLAND.
glandula sub·lin·gua·lis (sub″ling·gway′lis) [NA]. SUBLINGUAL GLAND.
glandula sub·man·di·bu·la·ris (sub·man·dib″yoo·lair′is) [NA]. SUBMANDIBULAR GLAND.
glandula sub·max·il·la·ris (sub·mack″si·lair′is) [BNA]. Glandula submandibularis (= SUBMANDIBULAR GLAND).
glandula su·pra·re·na·lis (sue″pruh·re·nay′lis) [NA]. ADRENAL GLAND.
glandula thy·re·oi·dea (thigh″ree·oy′dee·uh) [BNA]. Glandula thyroidea (= THYROID GLAND).
glandula thyreoidea ac·ces·so·ria su·pra·hy·oi·dea (ack″se·so′ree·uh sue″pruh·high·oy′dee·uh) [BNA]. An accessory thyroid gland, occasionally present, which is situated above the hyoid bone.
glandula thy·roi·dea (thigh·roy′dee·uh) [NA]. THYROID GLAND.
glandula tym·pa·ni·ca (tim·pan′i·kuh) [BNA]. A small enlargement of the tympanic nerve; not a gland.
glandula ve·sti·bu·la·ris major (ves·tib″yoo·lair′is) [NA]. A major vestibular gland. See *vestibular glands.*
glans (glanz) *n.*, pl. **glan·des** (glan′deez) [L., acorn] [NA]. The conical body that forms the distal end of the clitoris or of the penis.
glans cli·to·ri·dis (kli·tor′i·dis) [NA]. The erectile body at the distal end of the clitoris.
glans pe·nis (pee′nis) [NA]. The erectile body at the distal end of the penis, an expansion of the corpus spongiosum. See also Plate 25.
Glanz·mann and Ri·ni·ker's lymphocytophthisis (glaʰnts′ maʰn, ree′ni·kur) [E. *Glanzmann,* Swiss, 1887–1959; and P. *Riniker,* Swiss, 20th century]. SEVERE COMBINED IMMUNODEFICIENCY.
Glanzmann's disease [E. *Glanzmann*]. THROMBOASTHENIA.
Gla·se·ri·an fissure (gla·zeer′ee·un) [J. H. *Glaser,* Swiss anatomist, 1629–1675]. PETROTYMPANIC FISSURE.
glass, *n.* A brittle, hard, transparent substance, consisting usually of the fused amorphous silicates of potassium and calcium, or sodium and calcium, with an excess of silica.
glass·blower's cataract. HEAT-RAY CATARACT.
glassblower's disease. Infection of the parotid gland.
glass electrode. An electrode used in determining the hydrogen-ion concentration that operates by virtue of the tendency of hydrogen ions to diffuse through a thin glass membrane in contact with a standard solution of an acid.
Gläs·ser's disease (gless′ur). A polyarthritis and polyserositis of young pigs associated with infection with *Haemophilus suis.*
glass factor. FACTOR XII.
glass·pox (glas′pocks) *n.* VARIOLA MINOR.
glass test. A gross test for localizing infection of the urinary tract, in which the urine is voided in sequential fractions into two or more glass containers.
glass wool. White, silky threads obtained by the action of a powerful blast of air on a falling stream of molten glass.
glassy, *adj.* 1. Having the appearance of glass; VITREOUS; HYALINE. 2. Expressionless; dull; lifeless (as applied to the appearance of the eyes).
glassy membrane. Basement membrane of a clear, highly refractive nature, as in the maturing ovarian follicle or in a hair follicle.
glassy swelling. AMYLOID DEGENERATION.
Glau·ber's salt (glaow′bur) [J. R. *Glauber,* German physician, 1604–1668]. SODIUM SULFATE.
glau·ca·ru·bin (glaw″kuh·roo′bin) *n.* A crystalline compound, $C_{25}H_{36}O_{10}$, isolated from the fruit of *Simarouba glauca,* a tropical plant; an intestinal amebicide.
glau·co·ma (glaw·ko′muh, glaow·ko′muh) *n.* [Gk. *glaukōma,* cataract]. An eye disease, the complete clinical picture of which is characterized by increased intraocular pressure, excavation and degeneration of the optic nerve head, and typical nerve fiber bundle defects which produce characteristic defects in the visual field. May be primary, secondary, or congenital.
glau·co·ma·to·cy·clit·ic (glaw·ko″muh·to·si·klit′ick) *adj.* [*glaucoma* + *cyclitic*]. Pertaining to the combination of increased intraocular tension and inflammation of the ciliary body.
glaucomatocyclitic crisis. A discrete, self-limited form of secondary open-angle glaucoma, usually unilateral and recurrent, characterized by inflammatory signs and usually with no synechias. Inflammation may be confined to the trabecular meshwork.
glau·co·ma·tous (glaw·ko′muh·tus, ·kom′uh·tus) *adj.* Pertaining to or affected with glaucoma.
glaucomatous cup. A depression in the optic disk seen in cases of glaucoma.
gleet, *n.* [MF. *glete,* from L. *glittus,* sticky, viscous]. The slight mucopurulent discharge that characterizes the chronic stage of gonorrheal urethritis. —**gleety,** *adj.*
Glé·nard's disease (gleʸ·nahr′) [F. *Glénard,* French physician, 1848–1920]. *Obsol.* VISCEROPTOSIS.
gleno·hu·mer·al (glen″o·hew′mur·ul, glee″no·) *adj.* [Gk. *glēnē,* socket of a joint, + *humeral*]. Pertaining to the glenoid cavity and the humerus.
glenohumeral ligaments. Three variable fibrous thickenings of the capsule of the shoulder joint. NA *ligamenta glenohumeralia.*
gle·noid (glee′noid, glen′oid) *adj.* [Gk. *glēnoeidēs,* like a socket]. Having a shallow cavity; resembling a shallow cavity or socket.
glenoid cavity. The articular surface on the scapula for articulation with the head of the humerus. NA *cavitas glenoidalis.*
glenoid fossa. MANDIBULAR FOSSA.
glenoid lip. LABRUM GLENOIDALE.
Gley's cells (gleʰ) [M. E. E. *Gley,* French physiologist, 1857–1930]. Interstitial cells of the testis.
Gley's glands [M. E. E. *Gley*]. PARATHYROID GLANDS.
gli-, glio- [Gk. *glia,* glue]. A combining form meaning (a) *gluey, gelatinous;* (b) *glia, glial, neuroglia.*
glia (glye′uh, glee′uh) *n.* [Gk., glue]. NEUROGLIA.
-glia. A combining form meaning *neuroglia* of a specified kind or size.
glia·cyte (glye′uh·site, glee′) *n.* [*glia* + *-cyte*]. *Obsol.* NEUROGLIOCYTE.
gli·a·din (glye′uh·din) *n.* A protein derived from gluten of wheat, rye, oats, and other grains.
gli·al (glye′ul, glee′ul) *adj.* [*gli-* + *-al*]. Of or pertaining to neuroglia.
gli·am·i·lide (glye·am′i·lide) *n. endo*-1-[[4-[2-(2-Methoxynicotinamido)ethyl]piperidino]sulfonyl]-3-(5-norbornen-2-ylmethyl)urea, $C_{23}H_{33}N_5O_5S$, an antidiabetic.

Glibenese. A trademark for glipizide, an antidiabetic.

gli·born·u·ride (glye·born'yoo·ride) *n.* *endo,endo*-1-[(1*R*)-(2-Hydroxy-3-bornyl)]-(*p*-tolylsulfonyl)urea, $C_{18}H_{26}N_2O_4S$, an antidiabetic.

glid·ing joint. A synovial joint that allows only gliding movements; formed by the apposition of plane surfaces, or one slightly convex, the other slightly concave. NA *articulatio plana.*

gliding movement. The simplest movement that can take place in a joint, one surface gliding or moving over another, without any angular or rotatory movement.

gli·flu·mide (gli·floo'mide) *n.* (−)-(*S*)-*N*-(5-Fluoro-2-methoxy-α-methylbenzyl)-2-[*p*-[(5-isobutyl-2-pyrimidinyl-sulfamoyl]phenyl]acetamide, $C_{25}H_{29}FN_4O_4S$, an antidiabetic.

glio-. See *gli-.*

glio·bac·te·ria (glye"o·back·teer'ee·uh) *n.* [*glio-* + *bacteria*]. Bacteria embedded in a gelatinous matrix.

glio·blas·to·ma (glye"o·blas·to'muh, glee") *n.* [*glio-* + *blastoma*]. GLIOBLASTOMA MULTIFORME.

glioblastoma iso·mor·phe (eye"so·mor'fee). MEDULLOBLASTOMA.

glioblastoma mul·ti·for·me (mul"ti·for'mee). A central nervous system tumor whose parenchyma is composed of embryonal astrocytes presenting a pleomorphic appearance, accompanied by necrosis, hemorrhages, and reaction and involvement of connective tissue.

glio·car·ci·no·ma (glye"o·kahr"si·no'muh, glee") *n.* [*glio-* + *carcinoma*]. *Obsol.* GLIOBLASTOMA MULTIFORME.

Gli·o·cla·di·um (glye"o·klay'dee·um) *n.* [NL., from *glio-* + Gk. *kladion,* twig, shoot]. A genus of the Ascomycetes.

glio·coc·cus (glye"o·kock'us) *n.*, pl. **gliococ·ci** (·sigh) [*glio-* + *coccus*]. A micrococcus having a gelatinous envelope.

glio·fi·bro·sar·co·ma (glye"o·figh"bro·sahr·ko'muh, glee") *n.* [*glio-* + *fibro-* + *sarcoma*]. GLIOBLASTOMA MULTIFORME.

gli·og·e·nous (glye·oj'e·nus, glee·) *adj.* Productive of glia.

gli·o·ma (glye·o'muh, glee·) *n.*, pl. **gliomas, glioma·ta** (·tuh) [*gli-* + *-oma*]. A tumor composed of cells and fibers representative of the special supporting tissue of the central nervous system, and derived from neuroglial cells or their antecedents; occurs principally in the central nervous system. **—gli·om·a·tous** (·om'uh·tus, ·o'muh·tus) *adj.*

glioma of the retina. Neuroepithelioma of the retina.

glioma sar·coi·des (sahr·koy'deez). GLIOBLASTOMA MULTIFORME.

glioma sar·co·ma·toi·des (sahr·ko·muh·toy'deez). MEDULLOBLASTOMA.

gli·o·ma·to·sis (glye"o·muh·to'sis, glee·o") *n.*, pl. **gliomato·ses** (·seez) [*glioma* + *-osis*]. 1. Multiple hamartomatous nodules of glial cells in the cerebrum. 2. Multifocal gliomas.

gliomatosis cer·e·bri (serr'e·brye). A rare tumor of the central nervous system in which there is widespread infiltration by polar spongioblasts, some of which may be differentiating into astrocytes.

glio·neu·ro·blas·to·ma (glye"o·new"ro·blas·to'muh, glee") *n.* [*glio-* + *neuro-* + *blastoma*]. GANGLIONEUROMA.

glio·neu·ro·ma (glye"o·new·ro'muh, glee") *n.* [*glio-* + *neuroma*]. GANGLIONEUROMA.

glio·sar·co·ma (glye"o·sahr·ko'muh, glee") *n.* [*glio-* + *sarcoma*]. GLIOBLASTOMA MULTIFORME.

gliosarcoma of meninges. MENINGEAL GLIOMATOSIS.

gli·o·sis (glye·o'sis, glee·) *n.*, pl. **glio·ses** (·seez) [*gli-* + *-osis*]. Proliferation of neuroglia in the brain or spinal cord, as a replacement process or a reaction to low-grade inflammation; may be diffuse or focal.

glio·some (glye'o·sohm, glee') *n.* [*glio-* + *-some*]. One of the small granules in the cytoplasm of neuroglial cells.

glio·tox·in (glye"o·tock'sin) *n.* An antibiotic substance, $C_{13}H_{14}N_2O_4S_2$, obtained from cultures of *Trichoderma, Gliocladium,* and *Aspergillus fumigatus.*

glip·i·zide (glip'i·zide) *n.* 1-Cyclohexyl-3-[[*p*-[2-(5-methylpyrazinecarboxamido)ethyl]phenyl]sulfonyl]urea, $C_{21}H_{27}N_5O_4S$, an antidiabetic.

Glis·son's capsule [F. *Glisson,* English physician, 1597–1667]. CAPSULA FIBROSA PERIVASCULARIS.

Glisson's disease [F. *Glisson*]. RICKETS.

Glisson's sling [F. *Glisson*]. A leather collarlike apparatus used with weights and a pulley to extend the vertebral column in treating spinal disease.

glob·al (glo'bul) *adj.* 1. Spherical; shaped like a sphere. 2. Total; comprehensive. 3. Of or pertaining to the eyeball.

global aphasia. Loss of both expression and perception of language and communicative skills.

globe, *n.* [L. *globus*]. 1. A sphere or ball. 2. The earth or the world. 3. *In ophthalmology,* the eyeball.

globe-cell anemia. SPHEROCYTOSIS.

globe lag. KOCHER'S SIGN.

globi. 1. Plural of globus. 2. Rounded masses of lepra bacilli, as seen in tissue sections.

glo·bid·i·o·sis (glo·bid"ee·o'sis) *n.*, pl. **globidio·ses** (·seez). BESNOITIOSIS.

glo·bin (glo'bin) *n.* One of a class of proteins, histone in nature, obtained from the hemoglobins of various animal species; soluble in water, acids, and alkalies and coagulable by heat.

globin zinc insulin. A preparation of insulin modified by the addition of globin (derived from the hemoglobin of beef blood) and zinc chloride; it has intermediate duration of action.

glo·boid (glo'boid) *adj.* Shaped somewhat like a globe; SPHEROID.

globoid leukodystrophy. A heredodegenerative disease transmitted as an autosomal recessive trait, affecting the nervous system of infants with onset in the first months of life and a rapidly progressive course characterized by fretfulness, blindness, dementia, and rigidity. There is a generalized deficit of myelin, more marked in the central than in the peripheral nervous system. Syn. *Krabbe's disease.*

globoid thrombus. BALL THROMBUS.

glo·bose (glo'boce) *adj.* GLOBULAR.

globose nucleus. A nucleus of the cerebellum located between the fastigial and emboliform nuclei. It receives fibers from the paleocerebellum and sends efferent fibers to the red nucleus. NA *nucleus globosus cerebelli.*

glob·u·lar (glob'yoo·lur) *adj.* 1. Shaped like a ball or globule. 2. Made up of globules.

globular albuminuria. Protein and fat in the urine.

globular process. One of the inferior, bilateral bulbous expansions of the median nasal process that fuse in the midline to form the philtrum of the upper lip and adjacent premaxilla. See also *median nasal process.*

globular protein. A protein that in solution tends to assume a spherical or globelike conformation.

glob·ule (glob'yool) *n.* [L. *globulus,* little ball, globule]. A small spherical droplet of fluid or semifluid material.

glob·u·li·cide (glob'yoo·li·side) *n. & adj.* [*globule,* blood cell, + *-cide*]. 1. An agent that destroys blood cells. 2. Destructive to blood cells. **—glob·u·li·ci·dal** (glob"yoo·li·sigh'dul) *adj.*

glob·u·lin (glob'yoo·lin) *n.* [*globule* + *-in*]. Any of a group of animal and plant proteins, including alpha, beta, and gamma globulins, characterized by solubility in dilute salt solutions and differentiated from albumins by lesser solubility, more alkaline isoelectric points, greater molecular weight, faster sedimentation rates, and slower electrophoretic mobilities. See also *euglobulin, immunoglobulin, pseudoglobulin.*

α-globulin. ALPHA GLOBULIN.

β-globulin. BETA GLOBULIN.

γ-globulin. GAMMA GLOBULIN.

glob·u·lin·uria (glob"yoo·li·new'ree·uh) *n.* [*globulin* + *-uria*]. The presence of globulin in the urine.

globulin X. An intracellular protein found in muscular tissue.

glob·u·lo·max·il·lary (glob″yoo·lo·mack′si·lerr·ee) *adj.* Pertaining to the globular and maxillary processes.

globulomaxillary cyst. A cystic embryonal inclusion in the alveolar process between upper lateral incisor and canine teeth, at the site of fusion of the globular and maxillary processes of the upper jaw.

glo·bus (glo′bus) *n.*, pl. **glo·bi** (·bye) [L.]. A ball or globe.

globus hys·ter·i·cus (hi·sterr′i·kus). The choking sensation, or so-called lump in the throat, occurring in hysteria.

globus major epididymidis. HEAD OF THE EPIDIDYMIS.

globus minor epididymidis. TAIL OF THE EPIDIDYMIS.

globus pal·li·dus (pal′i·dus) [NA]. The inner and lighter part of the lenticular nucleus of the corpus striatum.

gloea (glee′uh) *n.* [Gk. *gloia*, glue]. A mucus-like substance secreted about the spore heads of some fungi.

glo·man·gi·o·ma (glo″man·jee·o′muh) *n.* [*glom*us + *angioma*]. GLOMUS TUMOR.

glome, *n.* [L. *glomus*, ball of yarn]. 1. GLOMERULUS. 2. One of the two rounded prominences which form the posterior prolongations of the frog of a horse's foot.

glomera. Plural of *glomus.*

glomera aor·ti·ca (ay·or′ti·kuh). AORTIC BODIES.

glom·er·ate (glom′ur·ut, ·ate) *adj.* [L. *glomeratus*, from *glomerare*, to wind into a ball]. Rolled together like a ball of thread.

glomerul-, glomerulo-. A combining form meaning *glomerulus, glomerular.*

glo·mer·u·lar (glom·err′yoo·lur) *adj.* Pertaining to, produced by, or involving a glomerulus.

glomerular capsule. The sac surrounding the glomerulus of the kidney; the first part of the uriniferous tubule. Syn. *Bowman's capsule.* NA *capsula glomeruli.*

glomerular nephritis. GLOMERULONEPHRITIS.

glom·er·ule (glom′ur·yool) *n.* GLOMERULUS.

glomerule of the pronephros. A fold of the mesothelium arising near the base of the mesentery in the pronephros, and containing a ball of blood vessels.

glomeruli. Plural of *glomerulus.*

glomeruli ar·te·ri·o·si coch·le·ae (ahr·teer·ee·o′sigh cock′lee·ee) [NA]. Arterial loops arising from the cochlear branch of the internal auditory artery.

glomeruli re·nis (ree′nis) [NA]. Capillary loops projecting into the lumens of renal corpuscles.

glo·mer·u·li·tis (glo·merr″yoo·lye′tis) *n.* [*glomerul*us + *-itis*]. Inflammation of renal glomeruli, one or more than one.

glomerulo-. See *glomerul-.*

glo·mer·u·lo·ne·phri·tis (glom·err″yoo·lo·ne·frye′tis) *n.* [*glomerulo-* + *nephritis*]. An acute, subacute, or chronic, usually bilateral, diffuse nonsuppurative inflammatory kidney disease primarily affecting the glomeruli; characterized by proteinuria, cylindruria, hematuria, and often edema, hypertension, and nitrogen retention.

glomerulosa. ZONA GLOMERULOSA.

glo·mer·u·lo·scle·ro·sis (glom·err″yoo·lo·skle·ro′sis) *n.* [*glomerulo-* + *sclerosis*]. Fibrosis of the renal glomeruli.

glo·mer·u·lose (glom·err′yoo·loce) *adj.* Having glomeruli.

glo·mer·u·lus (glom·err′yoo·lus) *n.*, pl. **glomeru·li** (·lye) [L., dim. of *glomus*, ball]. 1. A small rounded mass. 2. [NA]. The tuft of capillary loops projecting into the lumen of a renal corpuscle.

glomiform glands. GLOMUS BODIES.

glo·mus (glo′mus) *n.*, pl. **glom·era** (glom′ur·uh) [L., ball of thread or yarn]. 1. A small mass of tissue composed of a tuft of small arterioles connected with veins and having an abundant nerve supply. 2. A prominent portion of the choroid plexus of the lateral ventricle located at the beginning of the inferior horn. NA *glomus choroideum.* **—glo·mic** (·mick) *adj.*

glomus aor·ti·cum (ay·or′ti·kum). Singular of *glomera aortica;* AORTIC BODY.

glomus bodies. Arteriovenous anastomoses that have a special arrangement of muscle and nerve tissue; usually present in the cutis and subcutis of fingers and toes. NA *glandulae glomiformes.*

glomus ca·ro·ti·cum (ka·rot′i·kum) [NA]. CAROTID BODY.

glomus cho·ri·oi·de·um (ko·ree·oy′dee·um) [BNA]. Glomus choroideum (= GLOMUS (2)).

glomus cho·roi·de·um (ko·roy′dee·um) [NA]. GLOMUS (2).

glomus coc·cy·ge·um (kock·sij′ee·um) [BNA]. CORPUS COCCYGEUM.

glomus ju·gu·la·re (jug·yoo·lair′ee). Any of a number of tiny masses of epithelioid tissue similar in structure to that of the carotid body, usually situated in the adventitia of the superior bulb of the internal jugular vein.

glomus jugulare tumor. A tumor histologically resembling a carotid body tumor, arising mainly in the dome of the jugular bulb but also in many other sites in and around the temporal bone. The clinical syndrome consists of slowly progressive deafness, facial palsy, dysphagia, and unilateral atrophy of the tongue, combined with a vascular polyp in the external auditory meatus.

glomus tumor. A tumor derived from an arteriovenous glomus of the skin, especially of the digits; usually small, blue, painful, and benign.

glon·o·in (glon′o·in, glo′no·in, glo·no′in) *n.* [*gly*ceryl + *o*xygen + *n*itrogen]. NITROGLYCERIN.

gloss-, glosso- [Gk. *glōssa*]. A combining form meaning (a) *tongue;* (b) *language.*

glos·sa (glos′uh) *n.*, pl. & genit. sing. **glos·sae** (·ee) [NL., from Gk. *glōssa*]. TONGUE. **—glos·sal** (·ul) *adj.*

-glossa [Gk. *glōssa*]. A combining form meaning *tongue.*

glos·sal·gia (glos·al′jee·uh) *n.* [*gloss-* + *-algia*]. Pain in the tongue.

glos·san·thrax (glos·an′thracks) *n.* [*gloss-* + *anthrax*]. Anthrax, or carbuncle, of the tongue.

glos·sec·to·my (glos·eck′tuh·mee) *n.* [*gloss-* + *-ectomy*]. Excision of the tongue.

-glossia [*gloss-* + *-ia*]. A combining form meaning *condition of the tongue.*

Glos·si·na (glos·eye′nuh) *n.* A genus of bloodsucking flies, known as tsetse flies; confined to tropical and subtropical Africa. The species *Glossina fusca, G. palpalis,* and *G. morsitans* transmit the trypanosomes of sleeping sickness in man and of nagana and the souma disease of horses, cattle, and sheep.

glos·si·tis (glos·eye′tis) *n.* [*gloss-* + *-itis*]. Inflammation of the tongue. **—glos·sit·ic** (glos·it′ick) *adj.*

glossitis ar·e·a·ta ex·fo·li·a·ti·va (ăr·ee·ay′tuh ecks·fo″lee·uh·tye′vuh). BENIGN MIGRATORY GLOSSITIS.

glosso-. See *gloss-.*

glos·so·cele (glos′o·seel) *n.* [*glosso-* + *-cele*]. Swelling, or edema, of the tongue, with consequent extrusion of the organ.

glos·so·dy·na·mom·e·ter (glos″o·dye″nuh·mom′e·tur) *n.* [*glosso-* + *dynamometer*]. An apparatus for measuring the capacity of the tongue to resist pressure.

glos·so·dyn·ia (glos″o·din′ee·uh) *n.* [*gloss-* + *-odynia*]. Pain in the tongue.

glossodynia ex·fo·li·a·ti·va (ecks·fo·lee·uh·tye′vuh). MOELLER'S GLOSSITIS.

glos·so·epi·glot·tic (glos″o·ep·i·glot′ick) *adj.* [*glosso-* + *epiglottic*]. Pertaining to the tongue and epiglottis.

glossoepiglottic fossa. The depression between the back of the tongue and the epiglottis; it is divided into a right and left vallecula by the median glossoepiglottic fold.

glos·so·epi·glot·tid·e·an (glos″o·ep″i·glot·id′ee·un) *adj.* GLOSSOEPIGLOTTIC.

glos·so·graph (glos′o·graf) *n.* [*glosso-* + *-graph*]. An instrument for registering the movements of the tongue in speech.

glos·so·hy·al (glos″o·high′ul) *adj.* [*glosso-* + *hy-* + *-al*]. Pertaining to the tongue and the hyoid bone.

glossohyal process. A small vestigial process from the anterior surface of the hyoid bone, prominent in some mammals.

glos·so·hy·oid (glos″o·high′oid) *adj.* [*glosso-* + *hyoid*]. GLOSSOHYAL.

glos·so·kin·es·thet·ic, glos·so·kin·aes·thet·ic (glos″o·kin″es·thet′ick) *adj.* [*glosso-* + *kinesthetic*]. Pertaining to the sensations produced by the motions of the tongue in speech.

glos·so·la·bi·al (glos″o·lay′bee·ul) *adj.* [*glosso-* + *labial*]. Relating to the tongue and lips.

glossolabial paralysis. PROGRESSIVE BULBAR PARALYSIS.

glos·so·la·bio·la·ryn·ge·al (glos″o·lay″bee·o·la·rin′jee·ul) *adj.* [*glosso-* + *labio-* + *laryngeal*]. Pertaining to the tongue, lips, and larynx.

glossolabiolaryngeal paralysis. PROGRESSIVE BULBAR PARALYSIS.

glos·so·la·bio·pha·ryn·ge·al (glos″o·lay″bee·o·fa·rin′jee·ul) *adj.* [*glosso-* + *labio-* + *pharyngeal*]. Pertaining to the tongue, lips, and pharynx.

glossolabiopharyngeal paralysis. PROGRESSIVE BULBAR PARALYSIS.

glos·so·la·lia (glos″o·lay′lee·uh) *n.* [NL., from Gk. *glōssais lalein*, "to speak in tongues" (New Testament)]. Gibberish, jargon; speech simulating an unknown foreign language.

glos·sol·o·gy (glos·ol′uh·jee) *n.* [*glosso-* + *-logy*]. 1. The study of the tongue and its diseases. 2. The definition and explanation of terms; NOMENCLATURE.

glos·so·man·tia (glos″o·man′tee·uh) *n.* [*glosso-* + Gk. *manteia*, divination]. Prognosis of a disease based on the appearance of the tongue.

glos·so·pal·a·tine (glos″o·pal′uh·tine, ·tin) *adj.* [*glosso-* + *palatine*]. PALATOGLOSSAL.

glossopalatine arch. PALATOGLOSSAL ARCH.

glos·so·pal·a·ti·nus (glos″o·pal·uh·tye′nus) *n.* PALATOGLOSSUS.

glos·so·pal·a·to·la·bi·al (glos″o·pal″uh·to·lay′bee·ul) *adj.* [*glosso-* + *palato-* + *labial*]. Pertaining to the tongue, palate, and lips.

glossopalatolabial paralysis. PROGRESSIVE BULBAR PARALYSIS.

glos·sop·a·thy (glos·op′uth·ee) *n.* [*glosso-* + *-pathy*]. Any disease of the tongue.

glos·so·pha·ryn·ge·al (glos″o·fa·rin′jee·ul) *adj.* [*glosso-* + *pharyngeal*]. Pertaining to tongue and pharynx.

glossopharyngeal nerve. The ninth cranial nerve with motor, sensory (special and visceral), and parasympathetic components. Motor fibers pass from the nucleus ambiguus to the stylopharyngeus and muscles of the soft palate and pharynx; sensory fibers supply the posterior third of the tongue and taste buds there, the pharynx, middle ear and mastoid air cells; parasympathetic fibers pass from the inferior salivatory nucleus via the otic ganglion to the parotid gland. NA *nervus glossopharyngeus.* See also Table of Nerves in the Appendix.

glossopharyngeal nuclei. The ambiguous nucleus, the inferior salivatory nucleus, and the nucleus of the tractus solitarius.

glossopharyngeal paralysis. Absence of sensation in the pharynx and over the posterior third of the tongue, and loss of the palatal and pharyngeal reflexes, such as the gag reflex, due to a lesion involving the glossopharyngeal or ninth cranial nerve or its nucleus. Sensory disturbances attributed formerly to this nerve are now known to be the result of lesions to the vagus nerve, with which it is intimately associated. See also *Bonnier's syndrome, Vernet's rideau phenomenon.*

glos·so·pha·ryn·geo·la·bi·al (glos″o·fa·rin″jee·o·lay′bee·ul) *adj.* [*glosso-* + *pharyngeal* + *labial*]. Pertaining to the tongue, pharynx, and lips.

glossopharyngeolabial paralysis. PROGRESSIVE BULBAR PARALYSIS.

glos·so·pha·ryn·ge·us (glos″o·fa·rin′jee·us) *n.* [*glosso-* + *pharyngeus*]. PARS GLOSSOPHARYNGEA MUSCULI CONSTRICTORIS PHARYNGIS SUPERIORIS.

glos·so·plas·ty (glos′o·plas″tee) *n.* [*glosso-* + *-plasty*]. Plastic surgery of the tongue.

glos·so·ple·gia (glos″o·plee′jee·uh) *n.* [*glosso-* + *-plegia*]. Paralysis of the tongue.

glos·sop·to·sis (glos″op·to′sis) *n.* [*glosso-* + *-ptosis*]. Downward displacement or a dropping backward of the tongue, usually secondary to underdevelopment of the mandible as in the Robin syndrome.

glos·so·py·ro·sis (glos″o·pye·ro′sis) *n.* [*glosso-* + Gk. *pyrōsis*, burning]. Burning sensation of the tongue.

glos·sor·rha·phy (glos·or′uh·fee) *n.* [*glosso-* + *-rrhaphy*]. Surgical suturing of the tongue.

glos·sos·co·py (glos·os′kuh·pee) *n.* [*glosso-* + *-scopy*]. Diagnostic inspection of the tongue.

glos·so·spasm (glos′o·spaz·um) *n.* [*glosso-* + *spasm*]. Spasm of the tongue.

glos·sot·o·my (glos·ot′uh·mee) *n.* [*glosso-* + *-tomy*]. 1. The dissection of the tongue. 2. An incision of the tongue.

glos·so·trich·ia (glos″o·trick′ee·uh) *n.* [*glosso-* + *-trichia*]. HAIRY TONGUE.

glossy colony. 1. Originally, a smooth colony of streptococci. 2. A colony of streptococci devoid of M substance.

glossy skin. A peculiar shiny skin seen in conditions in which the nerve supply to the skin is interrupted.

glot·tal (glot′ul) *adj.* Of or pertaining to the glottis.

glot·tic (glot′ick) *adj.* GLOTTAL.

glot·tid·ean (glot·id′ee·un) *adj.* GLOTTAL.

glot·tis (glot′is) *n.*, genit. **glot·ti·dis** (·i·dis), L. pl. **glot·ti·des** (·i·deez) [Gk. *glōttis*] [NA]. The two vocal folds and the space (rima glottidis) between them.

glove-and-stocking anesthesia or **hypalgesia.** Distal, symmetrical loss or diminution of sensation in the hands and feet corresponding more or less to the area covered by gloves and stockings; may accompany inflammatory or degenerative diseases affecting peripheral nerves. Absolute loss of all sensations in such a distribution, unaccompanied by objective neurologic findings, is usually a hysterical phenomenon.

glov·er's stitch (gluv′urz). The continuous suture used especially in wounds of the intestines.

glox·a·zone (glock′suh·zone) *n.* (1-Ethoxyethyl)glyoxal bis(thiosemicarbazone), $C_8H_{16}N_6OS_2$, a veterinary agent used to combat anaplasmosis.

gluc-, gluco-. A combining form meaning *glucose.* See also *glyc-, glyco-.*

glu·ca·gon, glu·ca·gone (gloo′kuh·gon) *n.* A polypeptide hormone composed of 29 amino acid residues, secreted by the alpha cells of the islets of Langerhans. Its primary effect is to elevate blood glucose concentration through an adenyl cyclase-dependent mobilization of hepatic glycogen. Its other effects include inhibition of fatty acid synthesis and stimulation of ketone body production. Syn. *hyperglycemic factor, hyperglycemic-glycogenolytic factor, glycogenolytic hormone.*

glu·ca·gon·o·ma (gloo″kuh·gon·o′muh) *n.* A tumor of pancreatic islet alpha cells which produces glucagon; it frequently metastasizes.

glucagonoma syndrome. Necrolytic migratory erythema and glossitis in a patient with a glucagon-producing tumor, usually of alpha cells of the pancreatic islet.

glu·case (gloo′kace) *n. Obsol.* An enzyme that converts starch into glucose.

glu·cep·tate (gloo′sep·tate, gloo·sep′tate) *n.* Any salt or ester of glucoheptonic acid, $C_7H_{14}O_8$; a glucoheptonate.

glu·cide (gloo′side) *n.* A group term for carbohydrates and glycosides. —**glu·cid·ic** (gloo·sid′ick) *adj.*

gluco-. See *gluc-.*

glu·co·ascor·bic acid (gloo″ko·uh·skor′bick). D-Glucoascorbic acid, $C_7H_{10}O_7$, an inactive homologue of ascorbic acid.

glu·co·chlo·ral (gloo″ko·klor′ul, ·al) *n.* CHLORALOSE.

glu·co·cor·ti·coid (gloo″ko·kor′ti·koid) *n.* [*gluco-* + *corticoid*]. 1. An adrenal cortex hormone, such as cortisol, that affects the metabolism of glucose. 2. Any related natural or synthetic substance that functions similarly.

glu·co·fu·ra·nose (gloo″ko·few′ruh·noce) *n.* A cyclic form of glucose having a furanose structure in which carbon atoms 1 and 4 are bridged by an oxygen atom.

glu·co·he·mia, glu·co·hae·mia (gloo″ko·hee′mee·uh) *n.* [*gluco-* + *-hemia*]. HYPERGLYCEMIA.

glu·co·ki·nase (gloo″ko·kigh′nace, ·naze, ·kin′ace, ·aze) *n.* An enzyme, present in liver, which in the course of glycogenesis catalyzes phosphorylation of D-glucose, by adenosine triphosphate, to glucose 6-phosphate.

glu·co·kin·in (gloo″ko·kin′in) *n.* Any substance of vegetable origin that depresses blood-sugar levels in animals. Syn. *plant insulin, vegetable insulin.*

glu·col·y·sis (gloo·kol′i·sis) *n.*, pl. **glucoly·ses** (·seez) [*gluco-* + *-lysis*]. GLYCOLYSIS.

glu·co·neo·gen·e·sis (gloo″ko·nee″o·jen′e·sis) *n.* [*gluco-* + *neo-* + *-genesis*]. The formation of glucose by the liver from noncarbohydrate sources.

glu·con·ic acid (gloo·kon′ick). D-Gluconic acid, $C_6H_{12}O_7$, resulting from oxidation of dextrose and other sugars. Several of its salts, notably calcium gluconate and ferrous gluconate, are used medicinally.

glu·co·no·ki·nase (gloo″kuh·no·kigh′nace, ·naze, ·kin′ace) *n.* An enzyme, present in microorganisms, in muscle, and in liver, which catalyzes phosphorylation of D-gluconic acid, by adenosine triphosphate, to 6-phospho-D-gluconic acid.

glu·co·no·lac·tone (gloo″kuh·no·lack′tone) *n.* A ring form of D-gluconic acid.

glu·co·pro·tein (gloo″ko·pro′tee·in, ·pro′teen) *n.* GLYCOPROTEIN.

glu·co·py·ra·nose (gloo″ko·pye′ruh·noce) *n.* A cyclic form of glucose having a pyranose structure in which carbon atoms 1 and 5 are bridged by an oxygen atom.

glu·co·sac·char·ic acid (gloo″ko·sa·kăr′ick). D-Glucosaccharic acid, $C_6H_{10}O_8$, a dibasic acid resulting from oxidation of D-glucose; SACCHARIC ACID (2).

glu·co·sa·mine (gloo″ko·suh·meen′, ·sam′in) *n.* An amino sugar, $C_6H_{13}NO_5$, derived from D-glucose; it is a structural component of chitin, chondroitin, and heparin, and occurs also in mucus, fungi, and lichens. Syn. *2-aminoglucose, chitosamine, glycosamine.*

glu·co·san (gloo′ko·san) *n.* A polysaccharide that yields glucose on hydrolysis.

glu·co·sa·zone (gloo·ko′suh·zone) *n.* The osazone from glucose, identical with that from fructose and mannose. See also *phenylglucosazone.*

glu·cose (gloo′koce, ·koze) *n.* [F., from Gk. *gleukos,* sweet wine]. 1. The crystalline monosaccharide dextrose, $C_6H_{12}O_6$, sometimes called dextro-glucose, but properly designated D-glucose. 2. A product obtained by the incomplete hydrolysis of starch, consisting chiefly of dextrose (D-glucose), dextrins, maltose, and water; being liquid, it is more correctly designated liquid glucose; employed for its food value, local dehydrating effect, and diuretic action, and in various pharmaceutical and industrial manufacturing operations.

D-glucose. DEXTROSE.

glucose dehydrogenase. The enzyme that catalyzes dehydrogenation of D-glucose to D-gluconic acid in the presence of a hydrogen acceptor.

glucose 6-phosphatase. An enzyme, found in liver but not in muscle, which catalyzes the hydrolysis of glucose 6-phosphate to free glucose and inorganic phosphate; important in the conversion of glycogen to glucose and in the process of gluconeogenesis.

glucose 1-phosphate. α-Glucose 1-phosphoric acid, $C_6H_{13}O_9P$, an ester intermediate formed in the biochemical interactions of glucose. Syn. *Cori ester.*

glucose 6-phosphate. Glucose 6-phosphoric acid, $C_6H_{13}O_9P$, an ester intermediate formed in the biochemical interactions of glucose. Syn. *Robison ester.*

glucose 6-phosphate dehydrogenase deficiency. An inborn error of metabolism affecting the conversion of glucose 6-phosphate to 6-phosphogluconic acid in the erythrocyte, resulting clinically in hemolytic anemia.

glucose syrup. STARCH SYRUP.

glucose tolerance test. Evaluation of the ability of the body to metabolize glucose by administration of a standard dose of glucose to a fasting individual and measurement of blood and urine glucose at regular intervals thereafter.

glu·co·si·dase (gloo·ko′si·dace, ·daze) *n.* 1. An enzyme that catalyzes the hydrolysis of glucosides. 2. EMULSIN.

α-1,4 glucosidase, alpha-1,4 glucosidase. ACID MALTASE.

glu·co·side (gloo′ko·side) *n.* 1. Any member of a series of compounds, usually of plant origin, that may be hydrolyzed into dextrose (D-glucose) and another principle; the latter is often referred to as an aglycone. 2. Any substance, commonly a plant principle, which on hydrolysis yields a sugar and another principle. See also *glycoside.*

glu·co·sin (gloo′ko·sin) *n.* Any one of a series of bases obtained by the action of ammonia on dextrose.

glu·co·sphin·go·side (gloo″ko·sfing′go·side) *n.* Any cerebroside (glycosphingoside) containing glucose as the sugar component.

glu·co·sul·fone sodium (gloo″ko·sul′fone). SODIUM GLUCOSULFONE.

glu·cos·uria (gloo″ko·syoo′ree·uh) *n.* [*glucose* + *-uria*]. Glucose in the urine.

glu·cu·ro·nate (gloo·kew′ruh·nate) *n.* A salt or ester of glucuronic acid.

glu·cu·ron·ic acid (gloo″kew·ron′ick). D-Glucuronic acid, $C_6H_{10}O_7$, the acid resulting from oxidation of the CH_2OH group of D-glucose to COOH; a component of many polysaccharides, and certain vegetable gums. It is a conjugating compound in the metabolism and excretion of many medicinal substances, forming glucuronides. Syn. *glycuronic acid.*

glu·cu·ron·i·dase (gloo″kew·ron′i·dace, ·daze) *n.* An enzyme that catalyzes hydrolysis of glucuronides. Syn. *glycuronidase.*

glu·cu·ro·nide (gloo·kew′ro·nide) *n.* A compound resulting from the interaction, commonly referred to as conjugation, of glucuronic acid with a phenol, an alcohol, or an acid containing a carboxyl group. In man, many of these substances are excreted in the form of glucuronides. Syn. *conjugated glucuronate, glycuronide.*

glue ear. SEROUS OTITIS MEDIA.

glu·side (gloo′side) *n.* SACCHARIN.

Gluside. A trademark for saccharin.

glutaeus. GLUTEUS.

glu·ta·mate (gloo′tuh·mate) *n.* A salt of glutamic acid.

glu·tam·ic acid (gloo·tam′ick) [*glu*ten + *amine* + *-ic*]. 2-Aminopentanedioic acid or α-aminoglutaric acid, $C_5H_9NO_4$, an amino acid obtained on hydrolysis of various proteins. The sodium salt of the naturally occurring L- form of glutamic acid is used for symptomatic treatment of encephalopathies associated with diseases of the liver and for various other therapeutic purposes; it imparts a meat flavor to foods. Syn. *glutaminic acid.*

glutamic acid dehydrogenase. The enzyme that catalyzes conversion of L-glutamic acid into α-ketoglutaric acid in the presence of nicotinamide adenine dinucleotide or nicotinamide adenine dinucleotide phosphate.

glu·tam·ic·ac·i·de·mia, glu·tam·ic·ac·i·dae·mia (glew·tam·ick·as″i·dee′mee·uh) *n.* [*glutamic acid* + *-emia*]. An inborn error of metabolism in which there is an increased amount of glutamic acid in plasma and a slight generalized increase in total urinary amino nitrogen; characterized clinically by sparse, coarse unpigmented hair, mental retardation, failure to thrive, and various congenital malformations. Compare *kinky hair disease.*

glutamic acid hydrochloride. A water-soluble glutamic acid salt that releases hydrochloric acid in the stomach.

glutamic-alanine transaminase. GLUTAMIC-PYRUVIC TRANSAMINASE.

glutamic-aspartic transaminase. GLUTAMIC-OXALOACETIC TRANSAMINASE.

glutamic-oxaloacetic transaminase. An enzyme that catalyzes transfer of the amino group of glutamic acid to oxaloacetic acid, forming α-ketoglutaric acid and aspartic acid. Measurement of the levels of this enzyme in serum is of importance in the diagnosis of liver disease and myocardial infarction. Abbreviated, GOT. Syn. *glutamic-aspartic transaminase, aspartate aminotransferase, l-aspartate:2-oxoglutarate aminotransferase.*

glutamic-pyruvic transaminase. An enzyme that catalyzes transfer of the amino group of glutamic acid to pyruvic acid, forming α-ketoglutaric acid and L-alanine. Measurement of the levels of this enzyme in serum is of importance in the diagnosis of hepatocellular injury. Abbreviated, GPT. Syn. *glutamic-alanine transaminase, alanine aminotransferase, l-alanine:2-oxoglutarate aminotransferase.*

glu·tam·i·nase (gloo·tam'i·nace, ·naze) *n.* The enzyme that catalyzes the conversion of glutamine to glutamic acid and ammonia.

glu·ta·mine (gloo'tuh·meen, ·min) *n.* [*glut*en + *amine*]. The monamide of glutamic acid, $C_5H_{10}N_2O_3$, found in many plant and animal tissues.

glutamine synthetase. An enzyme catalyzing the formation of glutamine from glutamic acid and ammonia, using ATP as a source of energy.

glu·ta·min·ic acid (gloo''tuh·min'ick). GLUTAMIC ACID.

glu·tam·i·nyl (gloo·tam'i·nil) *n.* The univalent radical, $C_5H_9N_2O_2$—, of glutamine, the monamide of glutamic acid.

glu·tam·o·yl (gloo·tam'o·il) *n.* The divalent radical, $C_5H_7NO_2$=, of glutamic acid, an amino acid having two carboxyl groups.

glu·tam·yl (gloo·tam'il, gloo'tuh·mil) *n.* The univalent radical, $C_5H_8NO_3$—, of glutamic acid, an amino acid having two carboxyl groups.

glu·ta·ral (gloo'tuh·ral) *n.* $C_5H_8O_2$, an effective agent against bacteria and spores; employed for cold sterilization of surgical instruments.

glu·tar·al·de·hyde (gloo''tuh·ral'de·hide) *n.* GLUTARAL.

glu·tar·ic acid (gloo·tăr'ick, ·tahr'ick). Pentanedioic acid or 1,3-propanedicarboxylic acid, $C_5H_8O_4$, a constituent of beets and crude wool; formed from lysine by liver homogenates of certain animals.

glu·ta·thi·one (gloo''tuh·thigh'ohn) *n.* The tripeptide γ-L-glutamyl-L-cysteinylglycine, $C_{10}H_{17}N_3O_6S$, widely distributed in plant and animal tissues. It is important in tissue oxidations, acting through the sulfhydryl group (—SH) with the formation of disulfide (—S—S—) linkages. Syn. *GSH.*

glu·te·al (gloo·tee'ul, gloo'tee·ul) *adj.* [NL. *glute*us + *-al*]. Pertaining to the buttocks.

gluteal artery. See Table of Arteries in the Appendix.

gluteal bursa. Any bursa lying under the gluteus maximus muscle, as the ischial bursa of the gluteus maximus.

gluteal fold. The crease between the buttock and thigh. NA *sulcus gluteus.*

gluteal furrow. The groove between the buttocks. NA *crena ani.*

gluteal reflex. Contraction of the gluteal muscles induced by stimulation of the overlying skin.

gluteal region. The region over the gluteal muscles. NA *regio glutea.*

gluteal ridge. GLUTEAL TUBEROSITY.

gluteal sulcus. GLUTEAL FOLD.

gluteal tuberosity. The lateral and upward extension of the linea aspera, which gives attachment to part of the gluteus maximus muscle. NA *tuberositas glutea.*

glu·te·lin (gloo'te·lin, gloo·tel'in) *n.* [from *gluten*]. A class of simple proteins occurring in seeds of cereals; soluble in dilute acids and alkalies, insoluble in neutral solutions, and coagulated by heat.

glu·ten (gloo'tin) *n.* [L., glue]. A mixture of gliadin and glutelin types of proteins found in the seeds of cereals; imparts cohesiveness to dough.

gluten bread. Bread made from wheat flour from which all the starch has been removed; used as a substitute for ordinary bread in diabetes.

gluten casein. VEGETABLE CASEIN.

glu·te·nin (gloo'te·nin) *n.* A glutelin type of protein in wheat.

gluten-induced or **gluten-sensitive enteropathy.** CELIAC SYNDROME.

gluten sensitivity. Hypersensitivity to the gliadin fraction of gluten, leading to infantile celiac disease and some cases of sprue.

gluteo-. A combining form meaning *gluteus, gluteal.*

glu·teo·fas·cial (gloo''tee·o·fash'ee·ul) *adj.* [*gluteo-* + *fascial*]. Pertaining to the gluteus maximus and the deep fascia of the thigh.

gluteofascial bursa. The trochanteric bursa of the gluteus maximus. See *trochanteric bursa.*

glu·teo·fem·o·ral (gloo''tee·o·fem'o·rul) *adj.* [*gluteo-* + *femoral*]. Pertaining to the gluteal muscles and the femur.

gluteofemoral crease. A crease that bounds the buttock below, corresponding nearly to the lower edge of the gluteus maximus. Syn. *iliofemoral crease.*

glu·teo·tro·chan·ter·ic (gloo''tee·o·tro''kan·terr'ick) *adj.* [*gluteo-* + *trochanteric*]. Pertaining to the gluteal muscles and the greater trochanter of the femur.

gluteotrochanteric bursa. The trochanteric bursa of the gluteus maximus. See *trochanteric bursa.*

glu·teth·i·mide (gloo·teth'i·mide) *n.* 2-Ethyl-2-phenylglutarimide, $C_{13}H_{15}NO_2$, a central nervous system depressant used as a short-acting sedative and hypnotic.

glu·te·us, glu·tae·us (gloo·tee'us, gloo'tee·us) *n. & adj.*, pl. & genit. sing. **glu·tei, glu·taei** (gloo·tee'eye, gloo'tee·eye) [NL., from Gk. *gloutos,* buttock]. Being or pertaining to any of the three large muscles of the buttock.

gluteus max·i·mus (mack'si·mus). The largest and most superficial gluteal muscle. NA *musculus gluteus maximus.* See also Table of Muscles in the Appendix.

gluteus me·di·us (mee'dee·us). The gluteal muscle lying between the gluteus maximus and gluteus minimus. NA *musculus gluteus medius.* See also Table of Muscles in the Appendix.

gluteus min·i·mus (min'i·mus). The smallest and deepest gluteal muscle. NA *musculus gluteus minimus.* See also Table of Muscles in the Appendix.

glu·tin (gloo'tin) *n.* 1. A protein obtained from gelatin. 2. VEGETABLE CASEIN.

glu·ti·nous (gloo'ti·nus) *adj.* VISCID; gluelike.

glut·tony (glut'un·ee) *n.* [OF. *glutonie,* from L. *gluto,* glutton]. Excessive indulgence in eating.

gly·bu·ride (glye·bew'ride) *n.* 1-[[*p*-[2-(5-Chloro-*o*-anisamido)ethyl]phenyl]sulfonyl]-3-cyclohexylurea, $C_{23}H_{28}ClN_3O_5S$, an oral hypoglycemic drug.

glyc-, glyco- [Gk. *glykys,* sweet]. A combining form meaning (a) *sweet;* (b) *sugar;* or sometimes specifically (c) *glucose;* (d) *glycerin;* (e) *glycine.*

Glycamine iron. A trademark for a glycine-iron complex used as a hematinic.

gly·case (glye'kase, ·kaze) *n.* MALTASE.

gly·ce·mia, gly·cae·mia (glye·see'mee·uh) *n.* [*glyc-* + *-emia*]. 1. The presence of glucose in the blood. 2. HYPERGLYCEMIA.

glyc·er·al·de·hyde (glis''ur·al'de·hide) *n.* The simplest aldose exhibiting optical activity, formed by mild oxidation of glycerin. It exists as D-glyceraldehyde, as L-glyceraldehyde, or as a racemic mixture of the two (DL-glyceraldehyde). The D- and L- forms are the configurational reference standards for carbohydrates. Glyceraldehyde and phosphoric acid derivatives of it are intermediates in certain biochemical reactions of carbohydrates. Syn. *glyceric aldehyde.*

gly·cer·ic acid (gli·serr'ick). α, β-Dihydroxypropionic acid, $C_3H_6O_4$, occurring in dextrorotatory and levorotatory forms, variously obtained, as by oxidation of glycerin.

glyceric aciduria. OXALOSIS, type II.

glyceric aldehyde. GLYCERALDEHYDE.

glyc·er·i·dase (glis'ur·i·dace, ·daze) *n.* An enzyme catalyzing hydrolysis of glycerides. See also *lipase.*

glyc·er·ide (glis'ur·ide, ·id) *n.* Any ester of glycerin and an organic acid radical. Fats are glycerides of certain long-chain organic acids.

glyc·er·in, glyc·er·ine (glis'ur·in) *n.* [F. *glycérine,* from Gk. *glykeros,* sweet]. 1. Trihydroxypropane, $C_3H_5(OH)_3$, a clear, colorless, syrupy liquid of sweet taste, miscible with water. Obtained by hydrolysis of fats, and also by synthesis, it is the manufactured form of the natural substance glycerol. Used as a vehicle, emollient, and, rectally, as a laxative, particularly in the form of suppositories. 2. British term for GLYCERITE.

glyc·er·in·at·ed (glis'ur·i·nay"tid) *adj.* Treated with or preserved in glycerin.

glycerinated gelatin. A preparation of gelatin and glycerin, used as a vehicle for suppositories and bougies. Syn. *glycerin jelly.*

glycerinated vaccine virus. SMALLPOX VACCINE.

glycerin jelly. GLYCERINATED GELATIN.

glycerin suppository. A suppository prepared from glycerin, sodium stearate, and water; used as a rectal evacuant.

glyc·er·ite (glis'ur·ite) *n.* A solution of one or more medicinal substances in glycerin.

glyc·ero·gel·a·tin (glis"ur·o·jel'uh·tin) *n.* One of a class of pharmaceutical preparations composed of glycerin, gelatin, water, and one or more medicinal substances; they are soft solids, melting at body temperature, and can be applied to the skin or molded as suppositories.

glyc·er·ol (glis'ur·ole, ·ol) *n.* Trihydroxypropane, $C_3H_5(OH)_3$, an important intermediate component in carbohydrate and lipid metabolism. See also *glycerine.*

glycerol kinase. An enzyme which causes ATP to react with free glycerol to give glycerol-3-phosphate and ADP, the first step in the utilization of free glycerol by cells.

glyc·ero·phos·pha·tase (glis"ur·o·fos'fuh·tace, ·taze) *n.* An enzyme, found in pancreatic juice, and generally in cells, capable of liberating phosphoric acid from glycerophosphoric acid and certain of its derivatives.

glyc·ero·phos·phate (glis"ur·o·fos'fate) *n.* Any salt of glycerophosphoric acid.

glycerophosphate dehydrogenase. An enzyme that catalyzes dehydrogenation of glycerophosphate to 3-phosphoglyceraldehyde.

glyc·ero·phos·phor·ic acid (glis"ur·o·fos·for'ick). CH_2OH-$CHOHCH_2OPO(OH)_2$. A pale-yellow, oily liquid, soluble in water. Its salts, especially calcium and sodium glycerophosphate, have been used in the mistaken belief that their phosphorus was more readily utilized than that of other compounds.

glyc·er·ose (glis'ur·oce) *n.* An equilibrium mixture of the interconvertible isomers, glyceraldehyde and dihydroxyacetone, obtained by mild oxidation of glycerin.

glyc·er·yl (glis'ur·il) *n.* The trivalent radical, $C_3H_5\equiv$, combined with fatty acids in fats and in animal and vegetable oils.

glyceryl diacetate. Diacetin, $C_7H_{12}O_5$, a water-soluble ester of glycerin; sometimes used as a solvent for certain fat-soluble stains.

glyceryl guaiacolate. GUAIFENESIN.

glyceryl monostearate. Monostearin, $C_{21}H_{42}O_4$, a white wax-like solid, insoluble in water; employed as a stabilizing agent in various dermatologic preparations.

glyceryl triacetate. Triacetin, $C_9H_{14}O_6$, a water-soluble ester of glycerin; used as a solvent, as for certain local antiseptics.

glyceryl tributyrate. BUTYRIN.

glyceryl trinitrate. NITROGLYCERIN.

glyceryl trioleate. OLEIN.

glyceryl tripalmitate. PALMITIN.

glyceryl tristearate. STEARIN.

gly·ci·nate (glye'si·nate) *n.* Any salt of glycine.

Glyc·i·ne (glis'i·nee) *n.* A genus of legumes. See also *soybean.*

gly·cine (glye'seen, ·sin) *n.* [*glyc-* + *-ine*]. Aminoethanoic acid, NH_2CH_2COOH, a nonessential amino acid. It is a constituent of many proteins from which it may be obtained by hydrolysis. It has been used for treatment of muscular dystrophy and myasthenia gravis. Syn. *aminoacetic acid.*

glycine oxidase. An enzyme, present in liver and kidney, which catalyzes conversion of glycine to glyoxylic acid and ammonia; its prosthetic group is flavin adenine dinucleotide.

gly·ci·nin (glye'si·nin) *n.* The principal protein, a globulin, of the soybean.

gly·ci·nu·ria (glye"si·new'ree·uh) *n.* [*glycine* + *-uria*]. A defect in renal tubular reabsorption, associated with many disorders resulting in the presence of large amounts of glycine in the urine.

Gly·ciph·a·gus do·mes·ti·cus (glye·sif'uh·gus do·mes'ti·kus). A mite that causes grocer's itch.

Glyciphagus pru·no·rum (proo·no'rum). *GLYCIPHAGUS DOMESTICUS.*

glyco-. See *glyc-.*

gly·co·bi·ar·sol (glye"ko·bye·ahr'sol) *n.* Bismuthyl *N*-glycoloylarsanilate, $C_8H_9AsBiNO_6$, an amebicide employed only for treatment of intestinal amebiasis.

gly·co·ca·lyx (glye"ko·kay'licks) *n.* [*glyco-* + *calyx*]. Any polysaccharide-containing structure on the external surface of a cell, as seen by light or electron microscopy.

gly·co·cho·late (glye"ko·ko'late, ·kol'ate) *n.* Any salt of glycocholic acid.

gly·co·cho·lic acid (glye"ko·kol'ick, ·ko'lick). An acid, $C_{26}H_{43}NO_6$, obtained by the conjugation of cholic acid with glycine; found in bile.

gly·co·coll (glye'ko·kol) *n.* GLYCINE.

gly·co·cy·a·mine (glye"ko·sigh'uh·meen) *n.* Guanidinoacetic acid, $C_3H_7N_3O_2$, a product of interaction of aminoacetic acid (glycine) and arginine, which on transmethylation with methionine is converted to creatine. Syn. *guanidineacetic acid.*

gly·co·gen (glye'kuh·jin) *n.* [*glyco-* + *-gen*]. A polysaccharide, $(C_6H_{10}O_5)_n$, in liver cells, all tissues in the embryo, testes, muscles, leukocytes, fresh pus cells, cartilage, and other tissues. It is formed from carbohydrates and is stored in the liver, where it is converted, as the system requires, into sugar (glucose). Syn. *animal starch.*

gly·co·ge·nase (glye'ko·je·nace, glye·koj'e·nace) *n.* An enzyme found in the liver, which hydrolyzes glycogen to maltose and dextrin.

gly·co·gen·e·sis (glye"ko·jen'e·sis) *n.* [*glyco-* + *-genesis*]. The process of formation of glycogen in the animal body. —**glyco·ge·net·ic** (·je·net'ick), **gly·cog·e·nous** (glye·koj'e·nus) *adj.*

gly·co·gen·ic (glye"ko·jen'ick) *adj.* [*glyco-* + *-genic*]. Pertaining to glycogen or to glycogenesis.

glycogenic degeneration. A form of degenerative change resulting from excess deposition of glycogen within cells.

glycogenic heart. Deposits of glycogen in the heart muscles and consequent hypertrophy.

glycogen infiltration. Deposit of glycogen in cells in excessive amounts or in abnormal situation.

gly·co·gen·ol·y·sis (glye"ko·je·nol'i·sis) *n.*, pl. **glycogenoly·ses** (·seez) [*glycogen* + *-lysis*]. The liberation of glucose from glycogen in the liver or other tissues. —**glyco·gen·o·lyt·ic** (·jen″uh·lit′ick) *adj.*

glycogenolytic hormone. GLUCAGON.

gly·co·gen·o·sis (glye″ko·je·no′sis) *n.*, pl. **glycogeno·ses** (·seez) [*glycogen* + *-osis*]. One of several inborn errors in the metabolism of glycogen, classified on the basis of the enzyme deficiency and clinical findings by the Coris as: type I, von Gierke's disease; type II, Pompe's disease; type III, limit dextrinosis; type IV, amylopectinosis; type V, McArdle's disease; type VI, Hers' disease. See also *late infantile acid maltase deficiency, Lewis' disease, Tarui's disease.*

glycogen storage disease. 1. GLYCOGENOSIS. 2. VON GIERKE'S DISEASE.

glycogen synthetase. UDPG-GLYCOGEN TRANSGLUCOSIDASE.

glycogen synthetase deficiency. LEWIS' DISEASE.

gly·cog·e·ny (glye·koj′e·nee) *n.* GLYCOGENESIS.

gly·co·he·mia, gly·co·hae·mia (glye″ko·hee′mee·uh) *n.* [*glyco-* + *-hemia*]. GLYCEMIA.

gly·co·his·tech·ia (glye″ko·his·teck′ee·uh) *n.* [*glyco-* + *hist-* + Gk. *echein*, to have, + *-ia*]. Excessive tissue sugar content.

gly·col (glye′kol) *n.* 1. Any dihydric aliphatic alcohol. 2. ETHYLENE GLYCOL.

glycol aldehyde. The diose $CHOCH_2OH$, a possible intermediate in carbohydrate and protein metabolism.

gly·col·ic acid (glye·kol′ick). Hydroxyacetic acid, $CH_2OHCOOH$, a possible intermediate in protein metabolism.

glycolic aciduria. OXALOSIS, type I.

glycolic aldehyde. GLYCOL ALDEHYDE.

gly·co·lip·id, gly·co·lip·ide (glye″ko·lip′id) *n.* Any cerebroside or similar lipid.

gly·co·lip·in (glye″ko·lip′in) *n.* GLYCOLIPID.

gly·co·lyl (glye′ko·lil, glye·ko′lil) *n.* 1. Properly, the univalent radical, $HOCH_2CO—$, of glycolic acid. 2. The bivalent radical $—CH_2CO—$.

gly·col·y·sis (glye·kol′i·sis) *n.*, pl. **glycoly·ses** (·seez) [*glyco-* + *-lysis*]. The process of conversion of carbohydrate, in tissues, to pyruvic acid or lactic acid, with release of energy. Commonly it is considered to begin with hydrolysis of glycogen to glucose (glycogenolysis), which subsequently undergoes a series of chemical changes. —**gly·co·lyt·ic** (glye″ko·lit′ick) *adj.*

glycolytic enzyme. An enzyme capable of catalyzing hydrolysis or oxidation of sugars.

gly·co·me·tab·o·lism (glye″ko·me·tab′uh·liz·um) *n.* [*glyco-* + *metabolism*]. The metabolism of sugar in the body. —**glyco·met·a·bol·ic** (·met″uh·bol′ick) *adj.*

gly·co·nin (glye′ko·nin) *n.* Glycerite of egg yolk, prepared by mixing strained egg yolk and glycerin; an emulsifying agent.

gly·co·pe·nia (glye″ko·pee′nee·uh) *n.* [*glyco-* + *-penia*]. HYPOGLYCEMIA.

gly·co·pex·is (glye″ko·peck′sis) *n.* [*glyco-* + *pexis*]. The storing of glucose or glycogen.

gly·co·phil·ia (glye″ko·fil′ee·uh) *n.* [*glyco-* + *-philia*]. Tendency to hyperglycemia, after the ingestion of small amounts of glucose.

gly·co·pro·tein (glye″ko·pro′teen, ·pro′tee·in) *n.* One of a group of conjugated proteins which upon decomposition yield a protein and a carbohydrate, or derivatives of the same. See also *mucoprotein.*

gly·co·pty·a·lism (glye″ko·tye′uh·liz·um) *n.* [*glyco-* + *ptyalism*]. Excretion of glucose in the saliva.

gly·co·pyr·ro·late (glye″ko·pirr′o·late) *n.* 3-Hydroxy-1,1-dimethylpyrrolidinium bromide α-cyclopentylmandelate, $C_{18}H_{25}NO_3 \cdot CH_3Br$, a drug used in the management of gastrointestinal disorders in which anticholinergic action is indicated.

gly·cor·rha·chia (glye″ko·ray′kee·uh, ·rack′ee·uh) *n.* [*glyco-* + Gk. *rhachis*, spine, + *-ia*]. 1. Glucose in the cerebrospinal fluid. 2. HYPERGLYCORRHACHIA.

gly·cor·rhea, gly·cor·rhoea (glye″ko·ree′uh) *n.* [*glyco-* + *-rrhea*]. Discharge of sugar-containing fluid from the body.

gly·co·sa·mine (glye″ko·suh·meen′, ·sam′een, ·in) *n.* GLUCOSAMINE.

gly·co·se·cre·to·ry (glye″ko·see′kre·tor·ee) *adj.* [*glyco-* + *secretory*]. Concerned in the secretion of glycogen.

gly·co·se·mia, gly·co·sae·mia (glye″ko·see′mee·uh) *n.* GLYCEMIA.

gly·co·si·al·ia (gly″ko·sigh·al′ee·uh, ·ay′lee·uh) *n.* [*glyco-* + *sial-* + *-ia*]. The presence of glucose in the saliva.

gly·co·si·al·or·rhea (glye″ko·sigh″uh·lo·ree′uh, ·sigh·al″o·) *n.* [*glyco-* + *sialorrhea*]. Excessive salivary secretion containing glucose.

gly·co·side (glye′ko·side) *n.* [*glyc-* + *-ose* + *-ide*]. Any natural or synthetic compound that yields on hydrolysis a sugar and another substance designated as an aglycone. In order to indicate the specific sugar which is formed, a more descriptive term such as glucoside or galactoside may be used. Many glycosides are therapeutically valuable. See also *glucoside.* —**gly·co·si·dal** (glye″ko·sigh′dul), **glyco·sid·ic** (·sid′ick) *adj.*

gly·co·sphin·go·lip·id (glye″ko·sfing″go·lip′id) *n.* A sphingolipid containing galactose or glucose.

gly·co·sphin·go·side (glye″ko·sfing′go·side) *n.* [*glyco-* + *sphingosine* + *-ide*]. CEREBROSIDE.

gly·cos·uria (glye″ko·syoor′ee·uh) *n.* The presence of sugar in the urine. —**glycos·uric** (·syoor′ick) *adj.*

glycosuric acid. HOMOGENTISIC ACID.

gly·co·tro·pic (glye″ko·tro′pick, ·trop′ick) *adj.* [*glyco-* + *-tropic*]. Having an affinity for sugars.

glycotropic factor. *Obsol.* A factor from the adenohypophysis that is capable of antagonizing the action of insulin; probably represents the effects of what are now recognized as growth hormone and adrenocorticotropic hormone.

glyc·ure·sis (glick″yoo·ree′sis, glye″kew·) *n.*, pl. **glycure·ses** (·seez) [*glyc-* + *uresis*]. Excretion of sugar seen normally in the urine.

gly·cu·ron·ic acid (glye″kew·ron′ick). GLUCURONIC ACID.

gly·cu·ron·i·dase (glye″kew·ron′i·dace, ·daze) *n.* GLUCURONIDASE.

gly·cu·ro·nide (glye·kew′ro·nide) *n.* GLUCURONIDE.

gly·cu·ro·nu·ria (glye″kew·ro·new′ree·uh) *n.* The presence of glucuronic acid in the urine.

gly·cyl (glye′sil) *n.* The univalent radical $H_2NCH_2CO—$, of the amino acid glycine.

glyc·yr·rhe·tic acid (glis″ur·ree′tick). GLYCYRRHETINIC ACID.

glyc·yr·rhe·tin·ic acid (glis″ur·e·tin′ic). A pentacyclic terpene acid, $C_{30}H_{46}O_4$, obtained by hydrolysis of glycyrrhizic acid; possesses certain of the physiologic actions of deoxycorticosterone.

glyc·yr·rhi·za (glis″i·rye′zuh) *n.* [Gk. *glykyrriza*, from *glykys*, sweet, + *rhiza*, root]. The dried rhizome and roots of several varieties of *Glycyrrhiza glabra.* Glycyrrhiza extract is used as a flavor. Glycyrrhiza fluid extract is used as a vehicle. Compound opium and glycyrrhiza mixture, called brown mixture, is an expectorant. Glycyrrhiza elixir is used as a vehicle for disguising the taste of bitter substances. Syn. *licorice.*

glyc·yr·rhi·zic acid (glis″i·rye′zick). A crystalline glycoside, $C_{42}H_{62}O_{16}$, salts of which occur in glycyrrhiza; on hydrolysis it yields two molecules of glucuronic acid and one molecule of glycyrrhetinic acid. It appears to have certain of the physiologic actions of deoxycorticosterone.

glyc·yr·rhi·zin (glis″i·rye′zin) *n.* GLYCYRRHIZIC ACID.

gly·hex·a·mide (glye·heck′suh·mide) *n.* 1-Cyclohexyl-3-(5-indanylsulfonyl)urea, $C_{16}H_{22}N_2O_3S$, an orally active hypoglycemic compound.

Glynazan. A trademark for theophylline sodium glycinate.

glyo·ca·lyx (glye″o·kay′licks) *n.* The extracellular carbohydrate-rich coating of cells.

gly·oc·ta·mide (glye·ock'tuh·mide) *n.* 1-Cyclooctyl-3-(*p*-tolylsulfonyl)urea, $C_{16}H_{24}N_2O_3S$, an oral hypoglycemic drug.

gly·ox·al (glye·ock'sal) *n.* Ethanedial, CHOCHO, a compound obtained by oxidation of acetaldehyde.

gly·ox·a·lase (glye·ock'suh·lace, ·laze) *n.* An enzyme present in various body tissues which catalyzes the conversion of methylglyoxal into lactic acid.

gly·ox·al·ic acid (glye"ock·sal'ick). GLYOXYLIC ACID.

gly·ox·a·line (glye·ock'suh·leen, ·lin) *n.* IMIDAZOLE.

gly·ox·yl·ic acid (glye"ock·sil'ick). Formylformic acid, CHOCOOH, a constituent of various plant and animal tissues; it may be obtained by oxidative deamination of glycine, but it may also serve as a precursor of glycine.

glyoxylic acid test. A protein solution is treated with glyoxylic acid. A violet ring is formed at the zone of contact, owing to the presence of the indole group in tryptophan residues of the protein.

gly·par·a·mide (glye·păr'uh·mide) *n.* [1-(*p*-Chlorophenylsulfonyl)]-3-[*p*-(dimethylamino)phenyl]urea, $C_{15}H_{16}ClN_3O_3S$; an oral hypoglycemic drug.

Glysennid. A trademark for senna, a cathartic.

Glytheonate. A trademark for theophylline sodium glycinate.

Glyvenol. A trademark for tribenoside, a sclerosing agent.

Gm, gm A former abbreviation for *gram.*

Gme·lin's test (gmeʸ'leen) [L. *Gmelin,* German chemist, 1788–1853]. Urine is stratified over concentrated nitric acid. In the presence of bilirubin, various colored rings are seen at the junction of the two fluids.

G_{M1} gangliosidosis. Any disorder of the breakdown of the ganglioside G_{M1}. G_{M1} gangliosidoses are due to deficiency of the enzyme ganglioside G_{M1} β-galactosidase, and have been recognized in both infantile (type 1) and juvenile (type 2) forms. The clinical picture in both includes bony deformities and mental and motor deterioration progressing to decerebrate rigidity and death; pathological findings include neuronal lipidosis, visceral histiocytosis, and renal glomerular cytoplasmic ballooning. See also *gangliosidosis.*

G_{M2} gangliosidosis. Any disorder of the breakdown of the ganglioside G_{M2}. G_{M2} gangliosidoses are due to deficiency of one or both of two enzymes, hexosaminidase A and B. Two infantile forms (type 1, or Tay-Sachs disease, and type 2, or Sandhoff's disease) and a juvenile form (type 3) are recognized. See also *infantile amaurotic familial idiocy, gangliosidosis, Tay-Sachs disease, Sandhoff's disease.*

G_{M3} gangliosidosis. A disorder apparently of ganglioside biosynthesis reported in one case, a Jewish child who died in infancy with rapidly progressive neurologic symptoms, spongy degeneration of subcortical white matter, brainstem, optic nerves, and long tracts being found pathologically. An abnormally high concentration of the ganglioside G_{M3} was found in the brain, along with a deficiency of higher homologues and of an enzyme, G_{M3}-UDP-*N*-acetylgalactosaminyl transferase, necessary for their biosynthesis. See also *gangliosidosis.*

Gm groups. Genetically controlled antigenic specificities associated with the heavy chain of gamma-G globulin (IgG), and probably with the heavy chains of other immunoglobulins as well.

GMP Abbreviation for *guanosine monophosphate* (= GUANYLIC ACID).

gnat, *n.* Any of various small pestiferous dipteran insects such as black flies, biting midges, sand flies, or (in British usage) mosquitos.

gnath-, gnatho- [Gk. *gnathos*]. A combining form meaning *jaw* or *jaws.*

gna·thal·gia (na·thal'jee·uh) *n.* [*gnath-* + *-algia*]. Pain or neuralgia of the jaw.

gnath·ic (nath'ick, nay'thick) *adj.* [*gnath-* + *-ic*]. Pertaining to a jaw, or the jaws.

gnathic index. *In craniometry,* the ratio of the facial length (i.e., the distance between basion and prosthion) × 100, to the length of the cranial base (i.e., the distance between nasion and basion). Values of the index are classified as:

orthognathic	x–97.9
mesognathic	98.0–102.9
prognathic	103.0–x

gnathic replicator. An instrument usually driven by a computer-taped program which reproduces jaw movements precisely.

gna·thi·on (nay'thee·on, nath') *n.* [*gnath-* + *-ion*]. *In craniometry,* the most inferior point on the inferior border of the mandible, in the sagittal plane. Syn. *menton.*

gna·thi·tis (na·thigh'tis) *n.* [*gnath-* + *-itis*]. Inflammation of the jaw or cheek.

gnatho-. See *gnath-.*

gnatho·ceph·a·lus (nath"o·sef'uh·lus, nay"tho·) *n.*, pl. **gnathocepha·li** (·lye) [*gnatho-* + *-cephalus*]. An omphalosite lacking all parts of the head except the jaws.

gnatho·dy·na·mom·e·ter (nath"o·dye"nuh·mom'e·tur) *n.* [*gnatho-* + *dynamometer*]. An instrument for recording the force of the bite by measuring the pressure exerted on two rubber pads. Syn. *occlusometer.*

gnath·o·dyn·ia (nath"o·din'ee·uh) *n.* [*gnath-* + *-odynia*]. Pain in the jaw; GNATHALGIA.

gna·thol·ogy (na·thol'uh·jee) *n.* [*gnatho-* + *-logy*]. The study of the functions of the jaws; specifically, a system of reconstruction of the dental apparatus which involves principles of functioning occlusion.

gna·thop·a·gus par·a·sit·i·cus (na·thop'uh·gus păr"uh·sit'i·kus). EPIGNATHUS.

gnatho·pal·a·tos·chi·sis (nath"o·pal·uh·tos'ki·sis, nay"tho·) *n.* [*gnatho-* + *palato-* + *-schisis*]. URANOSCHISIS (2).

gnatho·plas·ty (nay'tho·plas"tee, nath"o·) *n.* [*gnatho-* + *-plasty*]. Plastic surgery of the cheek or jaw.

gna·thos·chi·sis (na·thos'ki·sis) *n.* [*gnatho-* + *-schisis*]. Cleft alveolar process, or jaw.

Gna·thos·to·ma (na·thos'to·muh) *n.* [*gnatho-* + *-stoma*]. A genus of nematode worms of the family Gnathostomatidae.

Gnathostoma his·pi·dum (hiss'pi·dum). A species of nematode worms infecting the stomach walls of hogs and sometimes of cattle in Europe, Asia, Africa, and Australia. Rarely pathogenic for man, but occasionally causing a subcutaneous or ocular infection.

Gnathostoma spi·nig·e·rum (spye·nij'e·rum). A species of nematode worms infecting the subcutaneous tissues and intestinal walls of such animals as domestic and wild felines, dogs, and hogs, restricted geographically to India, Malaya, China, Japan, and Thailand. Man serves as an accidental host in whom the parasites do not fully develop.

gna·thos·to·mi·a·sis (na·thos"to·mye'uh·sis) *n.* [*Gnathostoma* + *-iasis*]. Infection with *Gnathostoma spinigerum* larvae; deep burrows, boils, and abscesses in the skin are caused by this parasite.

-gnathous [*gnath-* + *-ous*]. A combining form meaning *possessing a* (specified) *kind of jaw.*

GNB A trademark for chlorophenothane, a parasiticide.

gno·sia (no'see·uh, no'zhuh) *n.* GNOSIS.

-gnosia. See *-gnosis.*

gno·sis (no'sis) *n.*, pl. **gno·ses** (·seez) [Gk. *gnōsis,* knowledge]. The faculty of knowing in contradistinction to the function of feeling, in respect to any external stimulus.

-gnosis [Gk. *gnōsis*]. A combining form meaning *knowledge, cognition, perception, recognition.*

gnos·tic (nos'tick) *adj.* [Gk. *gnōstikos,* of knowing, cognitive]. Pertaining to discriminative or epicritic sensations in contradistinction to vital or protopathic sensations.

-gnostic [Gk. *gnōstikos*]. A combining form meaning (a) *sensing;* (b) *knowing.*

gnostic sensibility. *In neurology,* the form of sensation which is based on the memory of previous perceptions and which, aroused by primary visual, auditory, tactile, or olfactory sensations, permits recognition and forms the basis of understanding and knowledge.

-gnosy. See *-gnosis*.

gno·to·bi·ot·ics (no″to·bye·ot′icks) *n.* [Gk. *gnōtos*, known, + *biotics*]. The science of raising germ-free animals into which a defined microflora is introduced. —**gnotobiot·ic** (·ick), *adj.*; **gnoto·bi·ote** (·bye′ote) *n.*

G:N ratio. D:N RATIO.

Goa powder (go′uh) [after *Goa*, India]. ARAROBA.

goat fever. BRUCELLOSIS.

goat·pox, *n.* A cutaneous viral disease of goats in Europe, North Africa, and the Middle East, characterized by vesicular skin lesions.

goat's-milk anemia. A macrocytic and megaloblastic nutritional anemia observed in infants fed goat's milk exclusively.

goat's thorn. TRAGACANTH.

gob·let cell. One of the unicellular mucous glands found in the epithelium of certain mucous membranes, such as those of the respiratory passages and the intestine.

goblet-cell carcinoma. MUCINOUS CARCINOMA.

go·det (go·det′) *n.* [F., drinking cup]. SCUTULUM.

Godt·fred·sen's syndrome [E. *Godtfredsen*, British ophthalmologist, 20th century]. A symptom complex consisting of unilateral ophthalmoplegia, amaurosis, trigeminal neuralgia or hypesthesia due to nasopharyngeal tumors, and symptoms referable to paralysis of the hypoglossal (XIIth cranial) nerve occurring on the same side due to compression by enlarged retropharyngeal lymph nodes. Compare *Jacod's syndrome.*

Goetsch test [E. *Goetsch*, U.S. surgeon, b. 1883]. A former test for hyperthyroidism, based on the potentiation of the cardiovascular effects of epinephrine by thyroid hormone, in which a subcutaneous injection of epinephrine produces an increase of heart rate and blood pressure, associated with palpitations and tremor.

Gof·man test. An ultracentrifugal analysis of the low-density β-lipoproteins of serum, based on the relationship of specific classes of serum cholesterol-bearing lipoproteins and atherosclerosis; used as an index of atherogenic potentialities.

G.O.G. Gynecologic Oncology Group.

go·go (go′go) *n.* TINEA IMBRICATA.

goi·ter, goi·tre (goy′tur) *n.* [F., from L. *guttur*, throat]. Enlargement of the thyroid gland; characterized as aberrant when the gland is supernumerary or ectopic.

goiter heart. A condition characterized by atrial fibrillation, cardiac enlargement, and congestive cardiac failure; due to hyperthyroidism. Syn. *thyroid heart, thyrotoxic heart.*

goitre. GOITER.

goi·tro·gen·ic (goy″tro·jen′ick) *adj.* [*goitre* + *-genic*]. Producing goiter; such as iodine-deficient diets or, experimentally, diets of cabbage and other *Brassica* plants, or administration of sulfonamides or drugs of the thiourea group. —**goi·tro·gen** (goy′tro·gen) *n.*

goi·trous (goy′trus) *adj.* Pertaining to or afflicted with goiter.

goitrous cretinism. A congenital, familial form of cretinism, transmitted as an autosomal recessive, in which the early clinical picture is identical with the sporadic form, but in untreated patients compensatory hypertrophy of the thyroid may produce a goiter after months or years without hypothyroidism.

gold, *n.* Au = 196.967. A yellow metallic element, easily malleable and ductile. Gold salts are used principally for treatment of rheumatoid arthritis. See also Table of Elements in the Appendix.

gold Au 198. The radioactive isotope of gold of mass number 198, with a half-life of 2.70 days, used in colloidal solution, by injection, principally for irradiation of closed serous cavities in palliative treatment of ascites and pleural effusion associated with metastatic malignancies.

goldbeater's skin. A thin tenacious sheet from the cecum of cattle, occasionally used as a surgical dressing.

Gold·ber·ger limb lead. AUGMENTED UNIPOLAR LIMB LEAD.

Gold·blatt hypertension [H. *Goldblatt*, U.S. pathologist, b. 1891]. EXPERIMENTAL RENAL HYPERTENSION.

Goldblatt kidney [H. *Goldblatt*]. A kidney to which blood flow is reduced by various experimental procedures in animals or by vascular disease in man. Such kidneys may be associated with hypertension, attributed either to release of vasoconstrictor substances by the kidney or to failure of the ischemic kidney to oppose the action of endogenous vasoconstrictor substances.

gold bromide. Gold tribromide or auric bromide, $AuBr_3$. It has been used in epilepsy and in whooping cough.

golden gargles. Oral solutions of ferric chloride and potassium chlorate employed as gargles.

Gol·den·har's syndrome (go^h^l·d^e^·nahr′) [M. *Goldenhar*, French, 20th century]. OCULOAURICULOVERTEBRAL DYSPLASIA.

gold·en·rod, *n.* The common name for several species of the genus *Solidago* of the Compositae.

gold·en·seal (goal′dun·seel″) *n.* HYDRASTIS.

Gold·flam's disease or **symptom complex** [S. V. *Goldflam*, Polish neurologist, 1852–1932]. MYASTHENIA GRAVIS.

gold leaf. Pure gold in very thin, transparent blue-green sheets; used in some surgical fistula repairs.

Gold·schei·der's disease (go^h^lt′shye·dur) [J. K. A. E. A. *Goldscheider*, German neurologist, 1858–1935]. EPIDERMOLYSIS BULLOSA.

gold sodium thiomalate. [(1,2-Dicarboxyethyl)thio] gold disodium salt, $C_4H_3AuNa_2O_4S.H_2O$, a white to yellowish-white powder, very soluble in water, used in the treatment of rheumatoid arthritis.

gold sodium thiosulfate. $Na_3Au(S_2O_3)_2.2H_2O$, sodium aurothiosulfate, occurring in white crystals, freely soluble in water; used for treatment of rheumatoid arthritis.

Gold·stein catastrophic reaction [K. *Goldstein*, U.S. neurologist, 1878–1965]. Marked disturbance of behavior, such as extreme agitation, anger, or resistance, observed in patients with acute loss of cognitive functions, such as language or arithmetic skills, particularly when attempting tasks that involve the extinct function; otherwise the patient behaves in his usual composed manner or even shows pleasure in performing tasks of which he is capable.

Goldstein-Scheerer tests [K. *Goldstein*]. A battery of tests that measure the impairment of brain function with respect to abstract and concrete thinking, for studying patients with brain injuries.

gold thioglucose. AUROTHIOGLUCOSE.

gold·thread, *n.* An herb, *Coptis groenlandica*, formerly used as a simple bitter tonic.

Gold·thwait's operation [J. E. *Goldthwait*, U.S. orthopedist, 1866–1961]. An operation for recurrent dislocation of the patella.

Gol·gi apparatus (go^h^l′jee) [C. *Golgi*, Italian histologist, 1844–1926]. An organelle, present in the centrosome of virtually all cells but prominent in secretory cells, which encloses secretory material in membrane and may also add a carbohydrate moiety thereto; can be visualized by light microscopy as a branched or reticular apparatus associated with vesicles; by electron microscopy it commonly appears as an array of parallel crescentic membranes about 60Å in thickness, but also frequently as flattened sacs or vesicles and vacuoles of diverse size.

Golgi body. GOLGI APPARATUS.

Golgi bottle neuron [C. *Golgi*]. A short, plump neuron with a thick axon, interposed between the excitatory endings of afferent dorsal root fibers and an anterior motor neuron, whose discharge results in an inhibitory postsynaptic potential.

Golgi cells [C. *Golgi*]. Nerve cells of two types: type I, those with long axons; and type II, those with short axons that branch repeatedly and terminate near the cell body.

Golgi complex. GOLGI APPARATUS.

Golgi corpuscle or **organ** [C. *Golgi*]. CORPUSCLE OF GOLGI.

Golgi element. GOLGI APPARATUS.

Golgi material. GOLGI APPARATUS.

Golgi-Maz·zo·ni corpuscle (mahⁿt·tso'nee) [C. *Golgi* and V. *Mazzoni*]. A small sensory lamellar corpuscle located in the subcutaneous tissue of the fingers and on the surface of tendons.

Golgi membranes. GOLGI APPARATUS.

Golgi network. GOLGI APPARATUS.

gol·gio·ki·ne·sis (gol"jee·o·ki·nee'sis) *n.* The division of the Golgi apparatus during karyokinesis.

Golgi remnant [C. *Golgi*]. ACROSOME.

Golgi-Rez·zo·ni·co spirals or **threads** (ret·tsoʰ'nee·ko) [C. *Golgi*]. Fibrils wound in a spiral funnel-shaped fashion from the surface of the myelin to the axon at the incisure of Schmidt-Lantermann of a nerve fiber; considered to be a supporting apparatus for the myelin, but may be an artifact.

Golgi's law [C. *Golgi*]. The severity of an attack of malaria is proportional to the number of parasites in the red blood cells.

Golgi substance. GOLGI APPARATUS.

Golgi tendon organ [C. *Golgi*]. CORPUSCLE OF GOLGI.

Goll's column or **tract** [F. *Goll*, Swiss anatomist, 1829–1903]. FASCICULUS GRACILIS MEDULLAE SPINALIS.

Goll's nucleus [F. *Goll*]. GRACILIS NUCLEUS.

Goltz syndrome [R. W. *Goltz*, U.S. dermatologist, b. 1923]. FOCAL DERMAL HYPOPLASIA SYNDROME.

Gom·bault-Phi·lippe triangle (gohⁿ·bo', fee·leep') [F. A. A. *Gombault*, French physician, 1844–1904; and C. *Philippe*, French pathologist, 1866–1903]. TRIANGLE OF GOMBAULT-PHILIPPE.

Gombault's degeneration, demyelination, or **neuritis** [F. A. A. *Gombault*, French neurologist, 1844–1904]. SEGMENTAL DEMYELINATION.

Gom·pertz·i·an growth or **curve** (gom·purt'see·un) [B. *Gompertz*, English mathematician, 1779–1865]. A pattern of growth characteristic of embryos and of many animal tumors: early growth is exponential but as time progresses the rate diminishes markedly.

gom·phi·a·sis (gom·fye'uh·sis) *n.* [Gk. *gomph*ios, molar, + *-iasis*]. *Obsol.* Looseness of the teeth in their sockets; PERIODONTOSIS.

gom·pho·sis (gom·fo'sis) *n.*, pl. **gompho·ses** (·seez) [Gk. *gomphōsis*, bolting together] [NA]. A form of synarthrosis, as a tooth in its alveolus.

gon-, gono- [Gk. *gonos*]. A combining form meaning (a) *sexual, generative;* (b) *seed, semen;* (c) *genitalia.*

gon·a·cra·tia (gon"uh·kray'shuh) *n.* [*gon-* + Gk. *akrateia*, incontinence]. SPERMATORRHEA.

go·nad (go'nad) *n.* [NL. *gonas, gonadis*, from Gk. *gonos*, generation, seed, roe]. 1. A gland or organ producing gametes; a general term for ovary or testis. 2. The embryonic sex gland before morphologic identification as ovary or testis is possible. Syn. *indifferent gonad.* —**go·nad·al** (go·nad'ul) *adj.*

gonadal dysgenesis, aplasia, or **hypoplasia.** A chromosomal disorder resulting in failure of the development of the gonads, characterized clinically by various combinations of short stature, webbed neck, deformities of the chest, spine, and extremities, particularly cubitus valgus; abnormalities of skin, face, ears, eyes, and palate; cardiac anomalies; lymphedema of the hands and feet; sexual infantilism; and elevated excretion of urinary gonadotropin. Usually there is a 45,X chromosome complement or sometimes mosaicism. Syn. *Bonnevie-Ullrich syndrome, Turner's syndrome, XO syndrome.*

gonadal fold. The part of a genital ridge containing the gonad and mesorchium or mesovarium.

gonadal ridge. GENITAL RIDGE.

go·nad·ec·to·my (go"nad·eck'tuh·mee) *n.* [*gonad* + *-ectomy*]. *In surgery,* removal of a gonad.

go·na·do·blas·to·ma (go·nad"o·blas·to'muh, gon"uh·do·) *n.* [*gonad* + *blastoma*]. A complex ovarian neoplasm containing primitive sex cords, germ cells, and mesenchyme; occasionally associated with defeminization.

go·na·do·cen·tric (go·nad"o·sen'trick, gon"uh·do·) *adj.* [*gonad* + *-centric*]. Relating to a focusing of the libido upon the genitalia; a phase of psychosexual development normally occurring in puberty.

go·nad·o·rel·in (go·nad"o·rel'in) *n.* A polypeptide, $C_{55}H_{75}N_{17}O_{13}$, obtained from sheep or swine, used as the acetate or hydrochloride; a gonad-stimulating principle. See also *luteinizing hormone releasing factor.*

go·na·do·ther·a·py (go·nad"o·therr'uh·pee, gon"uh·do·) *n.* [*gonad* + *therapy*]. Treatment with gonadal extracts or hormones.

go·na·do·tro·phin (go·nad"o·tro'fin, gon"uh·do·) *n.* GONADOTROPIN.

gonadotropic hormone. Any gonad-stimulating hormone. See also *gonadotropin.*

gonadotropic substance. GONADOTROPIN.

go·na·do·tro·pin (go·nad"o·tro'pin, gon"uh·do·) *n.* [*gonad* + *-trop*ic + *-in*]. A gonad-stimulating hormone, the principal sources of which are the adenohypophysis of various animal species, the urine of pregnant women (chorionic gonadotropin), and the serum of pregnant mares (serum gonadotropin). —**gonado·trop·ic** (·trop'ick, ·tro'pick) *adj.*

gona·duct, gono·duct (gon'uh·dukt) *n.* The duct of a gonad; oviduct or sperm duct.

go·nag·ra (go·nag'ruh, go·nay'gruh) *n.* [*gony-* + *-agra*]. Gout of the knee joint.

go·nal·gia (go·nal'jee·uh) *n.* [*gony-* + *-algia*]. Pain in the knee joint.

gon·an·gi·ec·to·my (gon"an·jee·eck'tuh·mee) *n.* [*gon-* + *angi-* + *-ectomy*]. Excision of part of the ductus deferens; VASECTOMY.

gon·ar·thri·tis (gon"ahr·thrye'tis) *n.* [*gony-* + *arthritis*]. Inflammation of the knee joint.

gon·ar·throt·o·my (gon"ahr·throt'uh·mee) *n.* [*gony-* + *arthrotomy*]. Incision into the knee joint.

go·nato·cele (go·nat'o·seel) *n.* [Gk. *gony, gonatos*, knee, + *-cele*]. A swelling or tumor of the knee.

Gon·da reflex. Extension of the great toe when the last two toes are snapped between the examiner's fingers; indicative of a pyramidal tract lesion.

gon·e·cyst (gon'e·sist) *n.* [Gk. *gonē*, seed, + *cyst*]. SEMINAL VESICLE. —**gon·e·cys·tic** (gon"e·sis'tick) *adj.*

gon·e·cys·tis (gon"e·sis'tis) *n. Obsol.* Gonecyst (= SEMINAL VESICLE).

gon·e·cys·ti·tis (gon"e·sis·tye'tis) *n.* [*gonecyst* + *-itis*]. *Obsol.* Inflammation of the seminal vesicles.

gon·e·cys·to·lith (gon"e·sis'to·lith) *n.* [*gonecyst* + *-lith*]. *Obsol.* A concretion or calculus in a seminal vesicle.

gon·e·cys·to·py·o·sis (gon"e·sis"to·pye·o'sis) *n.* [*gonecyst* + *pyosis*]. *Obsol.* Suppuration of a seminal vesicle.

gon·e·poi·e·sis (gon"e·poy·ee'sis) *n.* [Gk. *gonē*, seed, + *-poiesis*]. *Obsol.* The formation of semen. —**gonepoi·et·ic** (·et'ick) *adj.*

Gon·gy·lo·ne·ma (gon"ji·lo·nee'muh) *n.* [Gk. *gongylos*, round, + *-nema*]. A genus of nematode parasites of the family Spiruridae. The variously named species are usually grouped under the single species *Gongylonema pulchrum.*

Gongylonema pul·chrum (pul'krum). A phasmid nematode found in the upper digestive tract of sheep, cattle, goats, hogs, and horses. In cases of accidental human infection, the worm invades the buccal mucosa.

gon·gy·lo·ne·mi·a·sis (gon"ji·lo·nee·migh'uh·sis) *n.* [*Gongylonema* + *-iasis*]. Infection with filarial nematodes of the genus *Gongylonema.*

goni-, gonio- [Gk. *gōnia,* angle]. A combining form meaning (a) *corner, angle;* (b) *gonion.*

gonia. 1. A plural of *gonion.* 2. Plural of *gonium.*

go·ni·al (go'nee·ul) *adj.* Of or pertaining to the gonion.

gonial angle. ANGLE OF THE MANDIBLE.

gon·ic (gon'ick) *adj.* [Gk. *gonikos,* from *gonē,* seed]. Pertaining to semen or to generation.

go·nid·i·al (go·nid'ee·ul) *adj.* 1. Of or pertaining to gonidia. 2. Similar or analogous to gonidia or spores, as certain minute, more or less inert forms of various bacteria.

gonidial colony. Dwarf variants of bacteria, such as *Staphylococcus aureus,* induced by lithium, antibiotics, and other agents on nonhypertonic media, capable of reversion to the large parent colony when transferred to media lacking the inducers. Abbreviated, G.

go·nid·i·um (go·nid'ee·um) *n.,* pl. **gonid·ia** (·ee·uh) [NL., dim. of Gk. *gonē,* offspring]. 1. The algal component of lichens. 2. A spore produced in a sporangium.

gonio- See *goni-.*

go·nio·chei·los·chi·sis (go"nee·o·kigh·los'ki·sis) *n.* [*gonio-* + *cheilo-* + *-schisis*]. TRANSVERSE FACIAL CLEFT.

go·nio·cra·ni·om·e·try (go"nee·o·kray"nee·om'e·tree) *n.* [*gonio-* + *craniometry*]. Measurement of the various angles of the skull.

go·ni·om·e·ter (go"nee·om'e·tur) *n.* [*gonio-* + *-meter*]. An instrument for measuring angles, as the angle of the mandible.

goniometer test. VON STEIN'S TEST (2).

go·ni·on (go'nee·on) *n.,* pl. **go·nia** [*goni-* + *-ion*]. *In craniometry,* the tip of the angle of the mandible.

go·nio·punc·ture (go'nee·o·punk"chur) *n.* [*gonio-* + *puncture*]. A filtering operation for congenital glaucoma achieved by puncturing the filtration angle with a goniotomy knife and extending it through the sclera.

go·nio·scope (go'nee·o·skope) *n.* [*gonio-* + *-scope*]. A special optical instrument for studying in detail the angle of the anterior chamber of the eye. **—go·ni·os·co·py** (go"nee·os'kuh·pee) *n.*

go·ni·ot·o·my (go"nee·ot'uh·mee) *n.* [*gonio-* + *-tomy*]. An operation for congenital glaucoma in which a segment of the angle is swept with a goniotomy knife in order to cut through mesodermal remnants, allow the iris to fall back, and enable the drainage angle to function.

go·ni·tis (go·nigh'tis) *n.* [*gony-* + *-itis*]. Inflammation of the knee joint.

go·ni·um (go'nee·um) *n.,* pl. **go·nia** (·nee·uh) [NL., from Gk. *gonē,* seed]. A general term for spermatogonium and oogonium.

gono-. See *gon-.*

gono·blast (gon'o·blast) *n.* [*gono-* + *-blast*]. GERM CELL.

gono·coc·cal (gon"uh·kock'ul) *adj.* Of, pertaining to, or caused by gonococci.

gonococcal salpingitis. Salpingitis due to infection with gonococci.

gonococcal urethritis. Urethritis due to infection with gonococci.

gonococcal vaginitis. Vaginitis due to infection with gonococci.

gono·coc·ce·mia, gono·coc·cae·mia (gon"o·cock·see'mee·uh) *n.* [*gonococci* + *-emia*]. The presence of gonococci in the blood.

gonococci. Plural of *gonococcus.*

gono·coc·cic (gon"uh·kock'sick) *adj.* GONOCOCCAL.

gono·coc·cide (gon"uh·kock'side) *n. & adj.* [*gonococci* + *-cide*]. 1. Any substance or agent that destroys gonococci. 2. Having the properties of a gonococcide.

gono·coc·cus (gon"uh·kock'us) *n.,* pl. **gonococ·ci** (·sigh) [*gono-* + *coccus*]. The common name for *Neisseria gonorrhoeae,* the organism causing gonorrhea.

gono·cyte (gon"o·site) *n.* [*gono-* + *-cyte*]. GERM CELL.

gono·cy·to·ma (gon"o·sigh·to'muh) *n.* [*gonocyte* + *-oma*]. A germ-cell tumor of the testis or ovary.

gonoduct. GONADUCT.

go·nom·ery (go·nom'e·ree) *n.* [*gono-* + *mer-* + *-y*]. *In genetics,* the independence of the pronuclei or their chromosomes in the zygote and the first few cleavage stages.

gon·or·rhea, gon·or·rhoea (gon"uh·ree'uh) *n.* [Gk. *gonorroia,* spermatorrhea]. A venereal disease caused by *Neisseria gonorrhoeae,* characterized by mucopurulent inflammation of the mucosa of the genital tract; may produce septicemia with involvement of synovial tissues and serosal surfaces, causing arthritis, endocarditis, or meningitis. **—gonorrhe·al, gonorrhoe·al** (·ul) *adj.*

gonorrheal ophthalmia or **conjunctivitis.** An acute and severe form of purulent conjunctivitis, caused by infection by the *Neisseria gonorrhoeae.*

gonorrheal salpingitis. GONOCOCCAL SALPINGITIS.

-gony [Gk. *goneia,* from *gonos,* offspring]. A combining form meaning *generation, reproduction.*

gony- [Gk. *gony*]. A combining form meaning *knee.*

gony·al·gia par·es·thet·i·ca (gon"ee·al'jee·uh păr"es·thet'i·kuh). Neuralgia of the infrapatellar branch of the saphenous nerve.

gony·camp·sis (gon"ee·kamp'sis) *n.* [*gony-* + Gk. *kampsis,* a bending]. Deformity of knee due to abnormal bending or curving.

gon·yo·cele (gon'ee·o·seel) *n.* [*gony-* + *-cele*]. GONYONCUS.

gony·on·cus (gon"ee·onk'us) *n.* [*gony-* + Gk. *onkos,* mass]. A tumor or swelling of the knee.

Gon·za·les blood group. A blood group character (antigen Go^a) for which the antibody was reported in 1967 in the mother (Mrs. Gonzales) of a newborn infant with erythroblastosis fetalis; apparently limited to individuals of Negro parentage and distinguishable from previously established blood group systems.

Good·ell's sign (gŏŏ·del') [W. *Goodell,* U. S. gynecologist, 1829–1894]. Softening of the cervix of the uterus, considered to be evidence of pregnancy.

Good·enough test [Florence *Goodenough,* U.S., 20th century]. A draw-a-man test used to estimate intelligence.

goodness of fit. A measure of how accurately a particular mathematical equation fits a series of observations.

Good·pas·ture's stain [E. W. *Goodpasture,* U. S. pathologist, 1886–1960]. CARBOL-ANILINE FUCHSIN STAIN.

Goodpasture's syndrome [E. W. *Goodpasture*]. Rapidly progressive glomerulonephritis associated with pulmonary hemorrhage and hemosiderosis; basement membrane antibodies are present in the blood serum and are linearly deposited along the glomerular basement membrane.

Good·sall's rule. *In proctology,* fistulas with external openings in the posterior half of the perianal area have their primary opening in the posterior half of the anus, usually at or near the posterior commissure; fistulas with external openings in the anterior perineum usually have their primary opening in the anterior quadrant of the anus.

Good's syndrome [R. A. *Good,* U. S. pediatrician, b. 1922]. The association of agammaglobulinemia with thymoma, with resulting deficiency in cellular and humoral immunity; clinically frequently characterized by recurrent infections with pyogenic pathogens, but also low resistance to viral and fungal infections.

goose·flesh, *n.* Skin marked by prominence about the hair follicles, resulting from contraction of the arrectores pilorum muscles. Syn. *cutis anserina.*

goose skin. GOOSEFLESH.

Go·pa·lan's syndrome. BURNING FEET SYNDROME.

Gor·di·a·cea (gor"dee·ay'see·uh) *n.pl.* [*Gordius,* who tied the Gordian knot]. A class (or subclass) of Nematomorpha; the so-called hair snakes or horsehair worms. Generally parasites of arthropods, they have also been found in the intestinal and urinary tracts of man, and even in the external ear and in an inflammatory tumor of the orbit.

Gor·don's finger sign [A. *Gordon,* U. S. neurologist, 1874–1953]. GORDON'S REFLEX (2).

Gordon's leg sign [A. *Gordon*]. GORDON'S REFLEX (1).

Gordon's reflex or **sign** [A. *Gordon*]. 1. A variant of the Babinski sign in corticospinal tract disease, in which there is extension of the great toe or of all the toes on compression of the calf muscles. 2. Flexion of all fingers or of the thumb and index finger on compression of the forearm muscles or the pisiform bone; a sign of corticospinal tract disease.

Gordon's test [M. H. *Gordon*, English bacteriologist, 1872–1953]. A test once proposed for Hodgkin's disease in which the intracerebral inoculation of rabbits with suspensions of the lymph nodes from a patient with Hodgkin's disease produces encephalitis. Eosinophils are considered the responsible agent.

gor·get (gor'jit) *n.* [F. *gorgeret*, from *gorge*, throat, gullet]. A channeled instrument similar to a grooved director, formerly used in lithotomy.

Gor·ham's disease or **syndrome** [L.W. *Gorham*, U.S. physician, b. 1885]. Progressive osteolysis associated with vascular malformation of the affected bone.

Gor·lin's syndrome [R. J. *Gorlin*, U. S. oral pathologist, b. 1923]. BASAL CELL NEVUS SYNDROME.

go·ron·dou (go·ron'doo) *n.* GOUNDOU.

Gos·syp·i·um (gos·ip'ee·um) *n.* [L. *gossypion*, cotton tree]. A genus of plants of the Malvaceae from which cotton and cotton-root bark are obtained.

gos·sy·pol (gos'i·pol) *n.* [*Gossyp*ium + -ol]. A complex phenolic compound, $C_{30}H_{30}O_8$, sometimes found in the oil cake after expression of the oil from cottonseed. It has produced toxic symptoms in cattle fed such oil cake.

GOT Abbreviation for *glutamic-oxaloacetic transaminase.*

goth·ic-arch tracing. A registration of mandibular movement.

Gott·lieb's cuticle (goʰt'leep) [B. *Gottlieb*, Austrian dentist, 1885–1950]. ENAMEL CUTICLE (2).

gouge (gaowj) *n.* [F., from L. *gubia*]. A transversely curved chisel for cutting or removing bone or other hard structures.

Gou·ge·rot-Blum disease (goozh·ro', bloom) [H. *Gougerot*, French physician, 1881–1955; and P. *Blum*]. PIGMENTED PURPURIC LICHENOID DERMATITIS.

Gougerot-Houwer-Sjögren syndrome [H. *Gougerot*, A. W. M. *Houwer*, and H. S. C. *Sjögren*]. SJÖGREN'S SYNDROME.

Gougerot's disease [H. *Gougerot*]. NODULAR DERMAL ALLERGID.

Gougerot-Sjögren syndrome [H. *Gougerot* and H. S. C. *Sjögren*]. SJÖGREN'S SYNDROME.

Gougerot's trisymptomatic disease [H. *Gougerot*]. NODULAR DERMAL ALLERGID.

Gou·lard's extract (goo·lahr') [T. *Goulard*, French surgeon, 1724–1784]. A solution of lead subacetate formerly popular as a local astringent and anti-inflammatory application.

Gou·ley's catheter [J. W. S. *Gouley*, U. S. surgeon, 1832–1920]. A solid, curved steel instrument grooved on its inner aspect for passing over a guide inserted through a stricture into the urinary bladder.

goun·dou (goon'doo) *n.* [F., from a native name in West Africa]. An exostosis of the face; probably a sequela of yaws, involving the nasal and adjacent bones to produce a projecting tumorlike mass. Syn. *anakhre, henpue.*

gout (gaowt) *n.* [OF. *goute*, from L. *gutta*, drop]. 1. Primary gout, an inborn error of uric acid metabolism characterized by hyperuricemia and recurrent attacks of acute arthritis, most often of the great toe, and eventually by tophaceous deposits of urates. 2. Secondary gout, the gouty symptom complex which may be acquired as a complication of polycythemia vera and other myeloproliferative disorders, as well as of diuretic therapy. 3. *In veterinary medicine*, a condition usually found in adult hens characterized by the presence of pathologic accumulations of urates in the viscera or joints. —**gouty**, *adj.*

gout diet. A low-purine diet used in the treatment of gout.

gov·ern·men·tal hospital. A hospital supported and administered by a government subdivision; as a municipal, county, state, federal, army, navy, or Veterans Administration hospital.

Gow·er-Hen·ry reflex. A mechanism proposed, but of questionable existence, whereby release of antidiuretic hormone (ADH) occurs as a reflex response to atrial volume depletion.

Gowers' maneuver or **phenomenon.** The characteristic manner in which the patient with the childhood form of muscular dystrophy (or with other forms of proximal muscle weakness) rises from the recumbent or sitting position: the trunk is flexed on the thighs and hands are placed on the knees, and the trunk is raised by working the hands up the thighs.

Gow·ers' myopathy [W. R. *Gowers*, English neurologist, 1845–1915]. DISTAL MUSCULAR DYSTROPHY.

Gowers' sign [W. R. *Gowers*]. 1. In early tabes dorsalis, an irregular contraction of the pupil in response to light. 2. GOWERS' MANEUVER.

Gowers' solution [W. R. *Gowers*]. A dilution fluid used in the erythrocyte count, made up of sodium sulfate and glacial acetic acid dissolved in distilled water.

Gowers' syndrome [W. R. *Gowers*]. VASOVAGAL ATTACK (OF GOWERS).

Gowers' tract, column, or **fasciculus** [W. R. *Gowers*]. ANTERIOR SPINOCEREBELLAR TRACT.

GPT Abbreviation for *glutamic-pyruvic transaminase.*

gr Abbreviation for *grain* (3).

graaf·i·an follicle (graf'ee·un) [R. de *Graaf*, Dutch anatomist, 1641–1673]. A mature ovarian follicle.

graafian vessels [R. de *Graaf*]. EFFERENT DUCTULES OF THE TESTIS.

grac·ile (gras'il) *adj.* [L. *gracilis*]. Long and slender.

grac·i·lis (gras'i·lis) *L. adj.* Gracile; long and slender.

gracilis muscle. A long and slender muscle on the medial aspect of the thigh. NA *musculus gracilis.* See also Table of Muscles in the Appendix.

gracilis nucleus. A nucleus in the dorsal aspect of the medulla oblongata in which fibers of the fasciculus gracilis terminate and which gives origin to part of the fibers of the medial lemniscus. Syn. *nucleus of Goll.* NA *nucleus gracilis.*

gra·da·tim (gra·day'tim) *adv.* [L., from *gradus*, step]. Gradually.

grad·ed responsiveness. The property of manifesting responses which are proportional to the stimulus.

Gra·de·ni·go's sign or **syndrome** (graʰ'deʰ·nee'go) [G. *Gradenigo*, Italian otolaryngologist, 1859–1926]. Intense pain in the temporoparietal region, with paralysis of the lateral rectus muscle of the eye associated with otitis media and mastoiditis; indicative of extradural abscess or mass involving the apex of the petrous part of the temporal bone.

gra·di·ent (gray'dee·unt) *n.* [L. *gradiens*, walking, influenced in meaning by E. *grade*, slope]. 1. The rate of change in a variable magnitude, such as electrical potential, pressure, or concentration, or the curve that represents it. 2. *In biology*, a system of relations within the organism, or a part of it, which involves progressively increasing or decreasing differences in respect to rate of growth, rate of metabolism, or of any other structural or functional property of the cells.

grad·u·ate (graj'oo·ut) *n.* [L. *graduatus*, graduated, from *gradus*, step]. A vessel, usually of glass or plastic, marked with lines at different levels; used for measuring liquids.

grad·u·at·ed (graj'oo·ay·tid) *adj.* Divided into units by a series of lines, as on a barometer, a graduate, or a thermometer.

graduated bath. A bath in which the temperature is gradually lowered.

graduated compress. A compress with folds of varying size, thick in the center and thinner toward the periphery.

graduated cone. A cone-shaped body used for measuring the size of orifices of vessels, etc., especially in postmortem examinations.

graduated-resistance exercise. PROGRESSIVE-RESISTANCE EXERCISE.

graduated tenotomy. The cutting of a part of the fibers of the tendon of an ocular muscle for heterophoria or slight degrees of strabismus.

graduate nurse. A nurse who has been graduated from a recognized school of nursing.

Graefe's sign. VON GRAEFE'S SIGN.

Graeser's method. FRIEDEMANN AND GRAESER'S METHOD.

Gra·fen·berg's ring (grah'fən·behrk) [E. *Grafenberg*, German gynecologist, 1881–1957]. An early type of intrauterine contraceptive device.

Graff method. A histochemical method for cytochrome oxidase based on conversion of Nadi reagent to indophenol to obtain a blue color.

graft, *n. & v.* [OF. *grafe*, (horticultural) graft, from L. *graphium*, stylus]. 1. A portion of tissue, such as skin, periosteum, bone, fascia, or sometimes an entire organ, used to replace a defect in the body. 2. To replace a defect in the body with a portion of suitable tissue. See also *autograft, flap, heterograft, homograft, implantation, implant, transplant, transplantation, zoograft.*

graft-versus-host reaction. The reaction of transferred immunologically competent allogenic cells against host antigens which may take place when immunologically immature or otherwise immunologically deficient animals or humans are the recipients. In animals, the reaction may include runting, failure to thrive, lymph node atrophy, splenomegaly, hepatomegaly, anemia, and death. In humans, the syndrome includes a diffuse rash, diarrhea, hepatosplenomegaly, and sometimes death.

Gra·ham-Cole test [E. A. *Graham*, U.S. surgeon, 1883–1957; and W. H. *Cole*, U.S. surgeon, b. 1898]. CHOLECYSTOGRAPHY.

gra·ham flour, [S. *Graham*, U.S. dietary reform advocate, 1794–1851]. Whole-wheat flour; one that contains all constituents of wheat kernels.

Graham operation [R. R. *Graham*, Canadian surgeon, 1890–1948]. Closure of a perforated gastric or duodenal ulcer by means of an omental plug sutured in place.

Graham's law [T. *Graham*, Scottish chemist, 1805–1869]. The rates of diffusion of any two gases are inversely proportional to the square roots of their densities.

Graham Steell murmur [*Graham Steell*, English physician, 1851–1942]. The murmur of pulmonary insufficiency, associated with pulmonary hypertension of any cause, but often due to mitral stenosis.

grain, *n.* [OF., from L. *granum*]. 1. The seed or seedlike fruit of the cereal grasses. 2. A minute portion or particle, as of sand, or of starch. 3. A unit of weight of the troy, the avoirdupois, and the apothecaries' systems of weights. Abbreviated, gr. See Tables of Weights and Measures in the Appendix.

grain·age (gray'nij) *n.* Weight expressed in grains or fractions of grains.

grain alcohol. Alcohol (especially ethyl alcohol) prepared by distillation of fermented grain.

grain itch. An eruption due to *Pediculoides ventricosus*, acquired by contact with grain or straw, which harbors the parasite. Syn. *prairie itch.* See also *acarodermatitis urticarioides.*

grain itch mite. *PEDICULOIDES VENTRICOSUS.*

grains of paradise. The seed of *Aframomum melegueta*, a reed-like herb of Western Africa; used as a flavor and as a carminative chiefly in veterinary medicine.

-gram [Gk. *gramma*, letter]. A combining form designating a *drawing, writing,* or *record.*

gram, gramme, *n.* [F. *gramme*, from Gk. *gramma*, a small weight unit]. The basic unit of mass, and of weight, in the metric system, and one of the fundamental units of physical measurement; corresponds almost exactly to the weight of a milliliter, or cubic centimeter, of water at the temperature of maximum density. Abbreviated, g, Gm, gm.

gram calorie. CALORIE.

Gram-Clau·dius stain. A stain for fungi in tissue sections.

gram-equivalent weight. EQUIVALENT (3), expressed in grams.

gram·i·ci·din (gram″i·sigh'din) *n.* [*gram*-positive + *-cide* + *-in*]. One of the components of tyrothricin, an antibacterial substance produced by the growth of *Bacillus brevis;* used topically for treatment of localized bacterial infections of the skin.

gram ion. The weight of an ion, in grams, equivalent to its atomic weight or to the sum of the atomic weights of its constituent atoms.

gramme. GRAM.

gram-meter, gramme-metre, *n.* A unit of work, equal to the energy used in raising one gram to a height of one meter.

gram mole. GRAM MOLECULE.

gram molecule. The weight of any substance, in grams, equivalent to its molecular weight. Syn. *gram mole.* See also *mole.*

gram-negative, *adj.* In Gram's stain, pertaining to microorganisms that do not retain gentian or crystal violet when decolorized by alcohol or acetone-ether, being stained only by the counterstain; they appear pink.

gram-positive, *adj.* In Gram's stain, pertaining to microorganisms that retain the gentian or crystal violet stain; they appear blue.

Gram's iodine. A solution of iodine and potassium iodide in distilled water; used for staining smears for protozoan cysts and as a reagent in Gram's stain.

Gram's stain (grahm') [H. C. J. *Gram*, Danish bacteriologist, 1853–1938]. Bacteria are stained with solutions of crystal violet and iodine, followed by exposure to alcohol and then to a counterstain. If the blue color is retained, the organisms are called gram-positive; if it is removed, the organisms appear pink and are called gram-negative.

gra·na (gray'nuh, grah'nuh) *n.pl.* [L., pl. of *granum*, grain]. Minute disks of chlorophyll in the stroma of plants.

gra·na·tum (gra·nay'tum, ·nah'tum) *n.* [L., having many seeds, pomegranate]. Pomegranate. The bark of the stem and root of *Punica granatum;* contains several alkaloids, notably pelletierine. The chief use of pomegranate and its preparations and constituents has been as a taeniacide.

Gran·cher's pneumonia (grahn·shey') [J. J. *Grancher*, French physician, 1843–1907]. Splenopneumonia or the hepatization stage of pneumonia.

Grancher's system [J. J. *Grancher*]. A system for protecting children of tuberculous households from infection by boarding them out of the home.

gran·di·ose (gran'dee·oce) *adj.* [It. *grandioso*]. *In psychiatry,* characterized by a feeling of being important, wealthy, or influential, when there is no true basis for such feeling.

grand mal seizure (grahn mahl, grahn mahl) [Fr., lit., great illness]. GENERALIZED SEIZURE.

grand mal epilepsy. Epilepsy characterized by generalized seizures.

grand mal status. STATUS EPILEPTICUS.

Grand·ry-Mer·kel corpuscle (grahn·ree', mehr'kul) [M. *Grandry*, Belgian physician, 19th century; and F. S. *Merkel*]. TACTILE DISK.

Gran·ger's line [A. *Granger*, U.S. radiologist, 1879–1939]. In posteroanterior radiographs of the skull, a short, dense, curved line bowing upward between the orbits, produced by the roof of the sphenoid in the region of the tuberculum sellae.

gran·ny knot. A double knot in which, unlike the square knot, the loops are not in the same plane, and so tend to slip; a false knot.

grano·plas·ma (gran″o·plaz′muh) *n.* Granular cytoplasm.

granul-, granuli-, granulo-. A combining form meaning *granule, granular, granulation.*

gran·u·la (gran′yoo·luh) *n.* [NL., dim of L. *granum,* grain]. GRANULE.

granula iri·dis (eye′ri·dis). CORPORA NIGRA.

gran·u·lar (gran′yoo·lur) *adj.* Composed of, containing, or having the appearance of, granules.

granular cell carcinoma. A type of renal cell carcinoma whose cells have a granular cytoplasm.

granular cell layer. GRANULAR LAYER.

granular cell myoblastoma. A tumor, usually benign, composed of large cells with granular cytoplasm; the nature of the cells is unknown. The tongue and skin are common sites, though it may occur in many other places.

granular cell myosarcoma. A malignant granular cell myoblastoma.

granular cell neurofibroma. GRANULAR CELL MYOBLASTOMA.

granular cell tumor. 1. GRANULAR CELL MYOBLASTOMA. 2. (of the adrenal cortex:) CORTICAL ADENOMA.

granular conjunctivitis. TRACHOMA.

granular corneal dystrophy. Bilateral corneal opacities, occurring in the first decade of life and slowly progressive, consisting of discrete stromal lesions in the axial area. The intervening stroma and peripheral cornea are clear and vision is usually unaffected. Inherited as an autosomal dominant trait.

granular degeneration. CLOUDY SWELLING.

granular foveolae. The small pits in the cranial bones produced by the arachnoid granulations. NA *foveolae granulares.*

granular layer. 1. GRANULAR LAYER OF THE CEREBELLUM. 2. GRANULAR LAYER OF THE EPIDERMIS.

granular layer of the cerebellum. The innermost of the three layers of the cerebellar cortex, lying deep to the molecular and Purkinje-cell layers; it contains a large number of granule cells. NA *stratum granulosum cerebelli.*

granular layer of the epidermis. The layer of cells containing keratohyalin granules in the epidermis. NA *stratum granulosum epidermidis.*

granular layer of Tomes [J. *Tomes*]. A thin zone of imperfectly calcified dentin immediately under the cementum in the roots of teeth.

granular leukocyte. A leukocyte containing granules in its cytoplasm. See also *granulocyte.*

granular lids. TRACHOMA.

granular myoblastoma. GRANULAR CELL MYOBLASTOMA.

granular neuroma. GRANULAR CELL MYOBLASTOMA.

granular ophthalmia. TRACHOMA.

granular pneumocyte. GREAT ALVEOLAR CELL.

granular trachoma. Trachoma with papillary hypertrophy of the conjunctiva of the lids.

granulated lids. 1. Chronic blepharitis. 2. TRACHOMA.

gra·nu·la·tio (gran″yoo·lay′shee·o) *n.,* pl. **granu·la·ti·o·nes** (·lay·shee·o′neez) [L.]. GRANULATION.

gran·u·la·tion (gran″yoo·lay′shun) *n.* 1. The tiny red granules that are grossly visible in a wound during healing, as in the base of an ulcer; made up of loops of newly formed capillaries and fibroblasts. 2. The process of forming granulation tissue in or around a focus of inflammation. 3. The formation of granules. —**gran·u·lat·ed** (gran′yoo·lay·tid) *adj.*

granulationes arach·noi·de·a·les (a·rack″noy·dee·ay′leez) [NA]. ARACHNOID GRANULATIONS.

granulation stenosis. Narrowing caused by encroachment or contraction of granulations.

granulation tissues. Newly formed capillaries filled with granulocytes, mixed with proliferating fibrocytes, the spaces between them containing an inflammatory exudate, representing a stage in repair of damage associated with inflammation.

gran·ule (gran′yool) *n.* [L. *granulum,* dim. of L. *granum,* grain]. 1. A minute particle or mass. 2. A small, intracellular particle, usually staining selectively. 3. A small pill.

granule cell. One of the small nerve cells of the cerebellar and cerebral cortex.

granuli-. See *granul-.*

gran·u·li·form (gran′yoo·li·form) *n.* Resembling granules or small grains.

granulo-. See *granul-.*

gran·u·lo·blast (gran′yoo·lo·blast) *n.* [*granulo-* + *-blast*]. MYELOBLAST.

gran·u·lo·blas·to·sis (gran″yoo·lo·blas·to′sis) *n.* [*granuloblast* + *-osis*]. 1. MYELOBLASTOSIS. 2. One of the avian leukosis diseases characterized by neoplastic proliferation of primitive cells of the granulocytic series.

gran·u·lo·cyte (gran′yoo·lo·site) *n.* [*granulo-* + *-cyte*]. A mature granular leukocyte; especially, a polymorphonuclear leukocyte, which may be eosinophilic, basophilic, or neutrophilic. —**gran·u·lo·cyt·ic** (gran″yoo·lo·sit′ick) *adj.*

granulocytic hypoplasia. 1. A decrease in the granulocytic cells of the bone marrow. 2. AGRANULOCYTOSIS (2).

granulocytic leukemia. Leukemia in which the predominant cell types belong to the granulocytic series.

granulocytic sarcoma. A focal tumorous proliferation of granulocytes, with or without the blood findings of granulocytic leukemia; the sectioned surfaces of the mass are often green. Syn. *chloroma.*

granulocytic series. The cells concerned in the development of the granular leukocytes (basophil, eosinophil, or neutrophil) from the primitive myeloblasts to the adult segmented cells. Syn. *myeloid series, myelocytic series, leukocytic series.* See also *myelocyte, promyelocyte, metamyelocyte.*

gran·u·lo·cy·to·pe·nia (gran″yoo·lo·sigh″to·pee′nee·uh) *n.* [*granulocyte* + *-penia*]. A deficiency of granular leukocytes in the blood.

gran·u·lo·cy·to·poi·e·sis (gran″yoo·lo·sigh″to·poy·ee′sis) *n.* [*granulocyte* + *-poiesis*]. The process of development of the granular leukocytes, occurring normally in the bone marrow. —**granulocytopoi·et·ic** (·et′ick) *adj.*

gran·u·lo·fil (gran′yoo·lo·fil) *n.* [*granulo-* + L. *filum,* thread]. *Obsol.* RETICULOCYTE (1).

gran·u·lo·ma (gran″yoo·lo′muh) *n.,* pl. **granulomas, granu·loma·ta** (·tuh) [*granul-* + *-oma*]. 1. The aggregation and proliferation of macrophages to form small nodules or granules. 2. A swelling composed of granulation tissue. Adj. *granulomatous.*

granuloma an·nu·la·re (an·yoo·lair′ee). A chronic, self-limiting disease of the skin, usually on the extremities; characterized by reddish nodules, arranged in a circle.

granuloma con·ta·gi·o·sa (kon·tay·jee·o′suh). GRANULOMA INGUINALE.

granuloma fa·ci·a·le (fay″shee·ay′lee). An idiopathic, asymptomatic skin disorder, usually limited to the face, and characterized by soft, purple-red, slowly enlarging patches which usually show marked eosinophilic infiltration microscopically.

granuloma faciale eo·sin·o·phil·i·cum (ee″o·sin″o·fil′i·kum). GRANULOMA FACIALE.

granuloma fis·su·ra·tum (fis″yoo·ray′tum). A discoid mucous membrane inflammatory mass indented by a deep fissure and located in the groove between the lip and the jaw.

granuloma fun·goi·des (fung·goy′deez). MYCOSIS FUNGOIDES.

granuloma gen·i·to·in·gui·na·le (jen″i·to·ing·gwi·nay′lee). GRANULOMA INGUINALE.

granuloma in·gui·na·le (ing·gwi·nay′lee). A chronic, often serpiginous, destructive ulceration of the external genitalia due to a gram-negative rod, *Calymmatobacterium granulomatis,* and exhibiting encapsulated forms (Donovan bodies) in infected tissue.

granuloma of the intestine. REGIONAL ILEITIS.

granuloma pen·du·lum (pen′dew·lum). A granuloma pyogenicum that hangs by a stalk.

granuloma pu·den·di trop·i·cum (pew·den'dye trop'i·kum). GRANULOMA INGUINALE.

granuloma py·o·ge·ni·cum (pye"o·jen'i·kum). A hemangioma with superimposed inflammation, affecting the skin or other epithelial surfaces.

granulomata. A plural of *granuloma.*

granuloma tel·an·gi·ec·ti·cum (tel·an"jee·eck'ti·kum). GRANULOMA PYOGENICUM.

gran·u·lo·ma·to·sis (gran"yoo·lo"muh·to'sis) *n.* [*granuloma* + *-osis*]. A disease characterized by multiple granulomas.

granulomatosis dis·ci·for·mis chron·i·ca pro·gres·si·va (dis"i·for'mis kron'i·kuh pro"gre·sigh'vuh). A variant of necrobiosis lipoidica in which the granulomatous reaction is especially prominent.

granulomatosis in·fan·ti·sep·ti·ca (in·fan"ti·sep'ti·kuh). Fetal infection with *Listeria monocytogenes.*

gran·u·lom·a·tous (gran"yoo·lom'uh·tus, ·lo'muh·tus) *adj.* 1. Of or pertaining to granulomas. 2. Composed of or characteristic of granulomas or granulation tissue.

granulomatous arteritis or **angiitis.** GIANT-CELL ARTERITIS (1).

granulomatous colitis. An inflammatory disease of the colon, differing from ulcerative colitis by being patchy in distribution and being characterized pathologically by granulomas. Compare *ulcerative colitis.*

granulomatous cystitis. Cystitis in which the urinary bladder has been affected by a granulomatous reaction, commonly tuberculosis.

granulomatous inflammation. Inflammation characterized by proliferation of macrophages, usually forming nodules of various sizes. Contr. *nonspecific inflammation.*

granulomatous lymphoma. HODGKIN'S DISEASE.

granulomatous nocardiosis. A granulomatous reaction to infection with *Nocardia.*

granuloma trop·i·cum (trop'i·kum). The third stage of nodule formation in yaws.

granuloma ve·ne·re·um (ve·neer'ee·um). LYMPHOGRANULOMA VENEREUM.

gran·u·lo·mere (gran'yoo·lo·meer) *n.* [*granulo-* + *-mere*]. The mottled purple central portion of a platelet as seen in a peripheral blood film stained with a Romanovsky-type stain.

gran·u·lo·pe·nia (gran"yoo·lo·pee'nee·uh) *n.* GRANULOCYTOPENIA.

gran·u·lo·pex·is (gran"yoo·lo·peck'sis) *n.* [*granulo-* + *pexis*]. Removal of particulate matter by the cells of the reticuloendothelial system; PHAGOCYTOSIS. —**granulo·pec·tic** (·peck'tick) *adj.*

gran·u·lo·pexy (gran'yoo·lo·peck"see) *n.* GRANULOPEXIS.

gran·u·lo·phil (gran'yoo·lo·fil) *n.* [*granulo-* + *-phil*]. *Obsol.* RETICULOCYTE (1).

gran·u·lo·plasm (gran'yoo·lo·plaz·um) *n.* Granular cytoplasm.

gran·u·lo·plas·tic (gran"yoo·lo·plas'tick) *adj.* [*granulo-* + *-plastic*]. Forming granules.

gran·u·lo·poi·e·sis (gran"yoo·lo·poy·ee'sis) *n.* GRANULOCYTOPOIESIS. —**granulopoi·et·ic** (·et'ick) *adj.*

gran·u·lo·sa (gran"yoo·lo'suh) *adj.* [short for *membrana granulosa*]. Pertaining to the layer of epithelial cells lining the ovarian follicle.

granulosa cell. One of the epithelial cells lining the ovarian follicle and constituting the granulosa membrane. See also *follicular cell.*

granulosa cell carcinoma. A malignant granulosa cell tumor.

granulosa cell tumor. An ovarian neoplasm composed of cells resembling those lining the primordial follicle, associated with clinical signs of feminization.

granulosa lutein cells. FOLLICULAR LUTEIN CELLS.

granulosa membrane. The layer of small polyhedral cells within the theca of the graafian follicle.

granulosa–theca cell tumor. An ovarian neoplasm composed of various elements of the wall of the graafian follicle, associated with clinical signs of feminization.

gran·u·lo·sis (gran"yoo·lo'sis) *n.*, pl. **granulo·ses** (·seez) [*granul-* + *-osis*]. The development of a collection of granules or granulomas.

granulosis ru·bra na·si (roo'bruh nay'zigh). An uncommon condition of unknown cause characterized by an eruption of small, red papules and diffuse redness on the nose, cheeks, and chin and by persistent hyperhidrosis; seen in children with delicate constitutions and tending to disappear at puberty.

gran·u·lo·vac·u·o·lar (gran"yoo·lo·vack"yoo·o'lur, ·vack'yoo·o·lur) *adj.* Both granular and vacuolar; having granules and vacuoles.

gra·num (gray'num, grah'num) *n.*, pl. **gra·na** (·nuh) [L.]. GRAIN.

Gran·ville's hammer [J. M. *Granville,* English physician, 1883–1900]. An instrument for vibratory massage, used in the treatment of neuralgia.

grapelike tumor. SARCOMA BOTRYOIDES.

grape sugar. DEXTROSE.

graph, *n.* [*graph*ic formula]. A representation of statistical data by means of points, lines, surfaces, or solids, their positions being determined by a system of coordinates. —**graph·ic** (·ick) *adj.*

graph-, grapho- [Gk. *graphē*]. A combining form meaning *writing.*

-graph [Gk. *-graphos,* from *graphein,* to write]. A combining form meaning *something written or recorded.*

graph·an·es·the·sia, graph·an·aes·the·sia (graf"an·es·theezh'uh) *n.* [*graph-* + *anesthesia*]. Loss of ability to recognize letters or numbers traced on the skin; in the presence of intact peripheral sensation, a contralateral cortical lesion is implied.

graph·es·the·sia, graph·aes·the·sia (graf"es·theezh'uh, ·theez'ee·uh) *n.* [*graph-* + *esthesia*]. The sense or sensation of recognizing a symbol, such as a number, figure, or letter, traced on the skin.

-graphia [*graph-* + *-ia*]. A combining form designating (a) *writing characteristic of a* (specified) *psychologic disorder;* (b) *a condition characterized by* (a specified kind of) *markings or tracings.*

graphic formula. STRUCTURAL FORMULA.

graph·ite (graf'ite) *n.* [from Gk. *graph*ein, to write, + *-ite*]. Plumbago, or black lead; an impure allotropic form of carbon.

grapho-. See *graph-.*

gra·phol·o·gy (gra·fol'uh·jee) *n.* [*grapho-* + *-logy*]. The study of the handwriting; may be used for personal identification, for the analysis of specific psychologic or neurologic states at the time of writing, or for personality analysis.

grapho·ma·nia (graf"o·may'nee·uh) *n.* [*grapho-* + *mania*]. An excessive impulse to write; frequently observed in the paranoid personality and in paranoia. —**graphoma·ni·ac** (·nee·ack) *n.*

grapho·mo·tor (graf"o·mo'tur) *n.* [*grapho-* + *motor*]. Pertaining to or affecting the movements of writing.

grapho·pho·bia (graf"o·fo'bee·uh) *n.* [*grapho-* + *-phobia*]. An abnormal fear of writing.

graph·or·rhea, graph·or·rhoea (graf"o·ree'uh) *n.* [*grapho-* + *-rrhea*]. *In psychiatry,* an uncontrollable desire to write, in which pages are covered with usually unconnected and meaningless words; an intermittent condition, most often seen in manic patients.

-graphy [Gk. *-graphia,* from *graphē,* writing, drawing, delineation]. A combining form meaning (a) *writing, delineating;* (b) *recording;* (c) *description.*

Gra·ser's diverticulum (grah'zur) [E. *Graser,* German surgeon, 1860–1929]. A pulsion diverticulum of the sigmoid colon.

grasp reflex. A grasping motion of the fingers or toes, induced by tactile and then proprioceptive stimulation of the palm of the hand or the sole of the foot, seen in frontal lobe disease. A grasp reflex is normal in young infants.

Gras·set-Gaus·sel phenomenon or **sign** (grah·seh′, go·sel′) [J. *Grasset,* French physician, 1849–1918; and A. *Gaussel,* French physician, 19th century]. 1. A sign of upper motor neuron involvement in which a patient with hemiparesis when lying on his back can raise either leg separately but cannot raise both together. If the paralyzed leg is raised, it falls back heavily when the unaffected leg is lifted passively. 2. HOOVER'S SIGN.

grass sickness. A disease of horses occurring mainly in Scotland, usually in June when the grass is most luxuriant; thought to be caused by a virus similar to that causing poliomyelitis in man.

grass tetany. A disease of cows caused by magnesium deficiency.

gra·ti·o·la (gra·tigh′o·luh, ·tee′o·luh) *n.* [NL., dim. of L. *gratia,* grace]. Hedge hyssop; an herb formerly used as a diuretic, a cathartic, and an emetic.

Gra·tio·let's optic radiation (grah·syoh·leh′) [L. P. *Gratiolet,* French anatomist and zoologist, 1815–1865]. OPTIC RADIATION.

grat·tage (gra·tahzh′) *n.* [F. brushing, scrubbing, scraping]. A method, sometimes used in treatment of trachoma, in which a hard brush, as a toothbrush, is used to scrub the conjunctival surface of the eyelid in order to remove the granulations.

grave, *adj.* [MF., from L. *gravis,* heavy]. Extremely serious; threatening to life; indicating a poor prognosis or fatal outcome.

grav·el (grav′ul) *n.* [OF. *gravele,* dim of *grave,* sandy shore]. 1. A granular, sandlike material forming the substance of renal or vesical calculi. 2. *Informal.* Small calculi.

Graves' disease [R. J. *Graves,* Irish physician, 1797–1853]. A disease of unknown cause, tending to be familial and most commonly affecting women, characterized typically by hyperthyroidism (with diffuse goiter and exophthalmos) and circumscribed myxedema. Syn. *Basedow's disease.*

grav·id (grav′id) *adj.* [L. *gravidus,* from *gravis,* heavy]. Pregnant; of the uterus, containing a fetus; also, pertaining to other than human females when carrying young or eggs. —**gra·vid·i·ty** (gra·vid′i·tee) *n.*

grav·i·da (grav′i·duh) *n.,* pl. **gravidas, gravi·dae** (·dee) [L.]. A pregnant woman.

gra·vid·ic (gra·vid′ick) *adj.* [*gravid* + *-ic*]. Taking place during pregnancy.

grav·i·din (grav′i·din) *n.* KYESTEIN.

grav·i·do·car·di·ac (grav″i·do·kahr′dee·ack) *adj.* [*gravid* + *cardiac*]. *Obsol.* Pertaining to cardiac disorders associated with pregnancy.

gra·vim·e·ter (gra·vim′e·tur) *n.* [L. *gravis,* heavy, + *-meter*]. An instrument used in determining the specific gravity of a substance, especially a hydrometer, aerometer, or urinometer. —**grav·i·met·ric** (grav″i·met′rick) *adj.;* **gra·vim·e·try** (gra·vim′e·tree) *n.*

gravimetric analysis. A quantitative analysis for an element or constituent involving its conversion to a form that can be weighed.

grav·is neonatorum jaundice (grav′is). Severe jaundice of the newborn. See also *erythroblastosis fetalis.*

grav·i·stat·ic (grav″i·stat′ick) *adj.* [*gravitation* + *static*]. Due to gravitation; HYPOSTATIC (1).

grav·i·ta·tion (grav″i·tay′shun) *n.* [NL. *gravitatio,* from L. *gravitas,* weight]. The force by which bodies are drawn together. —**gravitation·al** (·ul) *adj.;* **grav·i·tate** (grav′i·tate) *v.*

gravitation abscess. An abscess resulting from infectious material carried by gravity to the site from an infectious focus above it.

gravitational unit. A unit in which the weight of a standard body is the basic force unit; thus, a unit in which the ratio of a kilogram of force to the weight of a kilogram of mass is one. Abbreviated, G.

gravitation constant. See *G.*

grav·i·ty (grav′i·tee) *n.* [L. *gravitas,* weight]. 1. Seriousness. 2. The effect of the attraction of the earth upon matter.

Gra·witz's tumor (grah′vits) [P. A. *Grawitz,* German pathologist, 1850–1932]. RENAL CELL CARCINOMA.

gray collie syndrome. CYCLIC NEUTROPENIA.

gray commissure of the spinal cord. The transverse band of gray matter connecting the masses of gray matter of the two halves of the spinal cord. It is divided by the central canal into the anterior gray commissure and the posterior gray commissure.

gray crescent. One lateral half of the gray matter of the spinal cord.

gray hepatization. The gross appearance of the lungs in lobar pneumonia just prior to resolution. Compare *red hepatization.*

gray induration. Diffuse fibrosis of the lung without pigmentation in chronic interstitial pneumonitis.

gray matter. GRAY SUBSTANCE.

gray ramus com·mu·ni·cans (kuh·mew′ni·kanz). A communicating branch of a sympathetic ganglion, consisting of unmyelinated postganglionic fibers and connecting it with a peripheral nerve. NA *postganglionic ramus.*

Gray's stain. A stain for flagella in which carbolfuchsin is used to stain the smears which have been treated with a special mordant composed of solution A (potassium alum, saturated aqueous solution; tannic acid and mercuric chloride) and solution B (saturated alcoholic solution of basic fuchsin).

gray substance or **matter.** The part of the central nervous system composed of nerve cell bodies, their dendrites, and the proximal and terminal unmyelinated portions of axons. NA *substantia grisea.* Contr. *white substance.*

gray syndrome. Vasomotor collapse as a manifestation of chloramphenicol toxicity, seen in infants usually under 4 months of age and especially in the premature.

grease (greece) *n.* GREASE HEEL.

grease heel. An infection of the fetlock joint of a horse; characterized by cracking of the skin and an oily exudate.

great alveolar cell. An epithelial cell of the pulmonary alveolus, thought to secrete the surfactant found on the alveolar surface; characterized by a roughly cuboidal shape and the presence in the cytoplasm of multilamellar bodies. Contr. *squamous alveolar cell.*

great ape. Any anthropoid ape of the three large kinds: chimpanzee, gorilla, or orangutan, as distinct from the lesser apes or gibbons.

great calorie. KILOCALORIE.

greater alar cartilage. Major alar cartilage. See *alar cartilages.*

greater arterial circle of the iris. An arterial ring around the circumference of the iris. NA *circulus arteriosus iridis major.*

greater circulation. SYSTEMIC CIRCULATION.

greater curvature of the stomach. The left border of the stomach, to which the greater omentum is attached. NA *curvatura ventriculi major.*

greater omentum. A fold of peritoneum attached to the greater curvature of the stomach above and, after dipping down over the intestine, returning to fuse with the transverse mesocolon. Between the ascending and descending folds is the variable cavity of the greater omentum. NA *omentum majus.* See also Plate 8.

greater palatine foramen. The lower opening of the greater palatine canal; it is formed on the medial side by a notch in the horizontal part of the palatine bone and on the lateral side by the adjacent part of the maxilla. Syn. *major palatine foramen.* NA *foramen palatinum majus.*

greater pelvis. FALSE PELVIS.

greater ring of the iris. The outer of two concentric zones separated by the lesser arterial circle of the iris. NA *anulus iridis major.*

greater sac. The peritoneum forming the main peritoneal cavity.

greater sciatic foramen. The oval space between the sacrotuberous ligament and the hipbone, conveying the piriformis muscle, and the gluteal, sciatic, and pudendal vessels and nerves. NA *foramen ischiadicum majus.*

greater sciatic notch. A notch between the spine of the ischium and the posterior inferior iliac spine; it is converted into a foramen by the sacrospinous and sacrotuberous ligaments. NA *incisura ischiadica major.*

greater splanchnic nerve. A nerve that arises from the fifth to ninth or tenth thoracic ganglions and supplies visceral nerve plexuses in the thorax and to the celiac plexus. NA *nervus splanchnicus major.* See also Table of Nerves in the Appendix.

greater trochanter. A process situated on the outer side of the upper extremity of the femur. NA *trochanter major.*

greater tubercle of the humerus. A prominence on the upper lateral end of the shaft of the humerus into which are inserted the supraspinatus, infraspinatus, and teres minor muscles. NA *tuberculum majus humeri.*

greater tuberosity of the femur. GREATER TROCHANTER.

great fontanel. ANTERIOR FONTANEL.

great pastern bone. The first phalanx of a horse's foot.

great toe. The first or inner digit of the foot. NA *hallux, digitus I.*

great-toe reflex or **phenomenon.** Dorsal extension of the great toe following certain stimuli, seen in the Babinski sign and the Chaddock, Gordon, and Oppenheim reflexes; a sign of corticospinal tract disease.

Green·berg's method. A procedure for determining serum proteins in which proteins are separated with sodium sulfate and determined colorimetrically after treatment with a phenol reagent.

green blindness. DEUTERANOPIA.

green·bot·tle fly. A fly of the family Calliphoridae.

green diarrhea. Infantile diarrhea, characterized by the passage of green stools.

green ferric ammonium citrate. A complex salt of iron, with a higher proportion of citric acid than in ferric ammonium citrate; a hematinic formerly preferred for intramuscular injection.

Green·field's disease [J. G. *Greenfield,* English neuropathologist, 1884–1958]. METACHROMATIC LEUKODYSTROPHY.

green hellebore. VERATRUM VIRIDE.

green jaundice. Obstructive severe jaundice of long duration in which the discoloration of the skin is green or olive-colored.

green monkey. 1. Any monkey of the species (or species group) *Cercopithecus aethiops.* Kidneys of this species are used as a source of tissue cell cultures. 2. More narrowly, a monkey of the West African subspecies, *C. aethiops sabaeus.*

green monkey fever. Infection of man with the Marburg virus, resulting in encephalitis, viremia, and widespread visceral involvement, including the liver and the kidneys.

Gree·nough binocular microscope (gree'no). A binocular compound microscope equipped with erecting prisms; it has an objective for each tube and so is truly stereoscopic.

green sickness. CHLOROSIS.

green soap. Medicinal soft soap prepared by saponification of suitable vegetable oils with potassium hydroxide; a soft, yellowish-white to brownish- or greenish-yellow mass. Used topically as a detergent, commonly in the form of green soap tincture, also called soft soap liniment, which contains 65 g green soap in 100 ml lavender-scented alcohol solution.

green softening. A purulent softening of nervous matter.

green·stick fracture. An incomplete fracture of a long bone, seen in children; the bone is bent but splintered only on the convex side.

green streptococci. ALPHA STREPTOCOCCI.

green sweat. Sweat having a bluish or greenish color, seen mainly in copper workers.

green vitriol. FERROUS SULFATE.

greg·a·rine (greg'uh·rine, ·rin) *adj. & n.* 1. Of or pertaining to the Gregarinida, an order of Sporozoa that are parasitic in invertebrates. 2. Any member of the sporozoan order Gregarinida. See also *Acephalina, Cephalina.*

Gregersen's test. A modification of the benzidine test used for testing for the presence of occult blood in feces.

Greg·o·ry's powder [J. *Gregory,* Scottish physician, 1753–1821]. A powder containing rhubarb, ginger, and magnesium oxide; formerly popular as a laxative antacid.

Greig's syndrome (greg) [D. M. *Greig,* Scottish physician, 1864–1936]. Ocular hypertelorism, often associated with mental retardation and various congenital defects.

grenz rays (grents) [Ger. *Grenzstrahlen,* from *Grenze,* border, limit]. Electromagnetic radiations of about two angstroms, used in x-ray therapy of the skin because of their limited power of penetration.

grenz-ray tube. A roentgen-ray tube for production of soft roentgen rays operated at low potentials, about 10 kilovolts.

Grey Turner's sign. TURNER'S SIGN.

grief, *n.* [OF., from *grever,* to grieve]. The appropriate, self-limited emotional response to an external and consciously recognized loss. Compare *depression (4).*

grief reaction. *In psychiatry,* an overintense and prolonged reaction to a loss, particularly the death of someone close.

Grie·sing·er's disease (gree'zing·ur) [W. *Griesinger,* German neurologist, 1817–1868]. 1. PSEUDOHYPERTROPHIC INFANTILE MUSCULAR DYSTROPHY. 2. ANCYLOSTOMIASIS.

Griesinger's sign [W. *Griesinger*]. Swelling behind the mastoid process, seen in patients with transverse sinus thrombosis.

grif·fin claw. CLAW HAND.

Grif·fith's method. Hippuric acid is extracted with ether. The residue from the ether distillation is treated with bromine and sodium hypobromite. Hippuric acid nitrogen is then determined by the Kjeldahl method.

Grifulvin. A trademark for griseofulvin, an orally effective fungistatic antibiotic.

GRIH Abbreviation for *growth-hormone-release-inhibiting hormone* (= SOMATOSTATIN).

grin·de·lia (grin·dee'lee·uh) *n.* [D. H. *Grindel,* German botanist in Latvia, 1776–1836]. The leaves and flowering tops of *Grindelia camporum, G. humilis,* or *G. squarrosa,* formerly used in bronchitis and asthma as a stimulating expectorant and antispasmodic.

grind·er's asthma or **rot.** An interstitial pneumonitis due to the inhalation of fine particles set free in grinding such materials as steel. See also *silicosis.*

grip. Grippe (= INFLUENZA).

gripe, *n.* A spasmodic intestinal or abdominal pain. —**grip·ing,** *adj.*

grippe, *n.* [F. *grippe,* from *gripper,* to seize]. INFLUENZA.

grip sign. In a patient with hemiparesis, his grip around the examiner's fingers is relaxed when his hand is passively flexed on the forearm, but is increased when his hand is extended.

Grisactin. A trademark for griseofulvin, an orally effective fungistatic antibiotic.

gris·eo·ful·vin (griz''ee·o·ful'vin) *n.* 7-Chloro-2',4,6-trimethoxy-6'-methylspiro[benzofuran-2(3*H*),1'-[2]-cyclohexene]-3,4'-dione, $C_{17}H_{17}ClO_6$, an antibiotic elaborated by *Penicillium griseofulvum* and other *Penicillium* species; an orally administered fungistatic antibiotic.

Gri·solle's sign (gree·zo^hl') [A. *Grisolle,* French physician, 1811–1869]. The persistent palpable nature of an early smallpox papule, even with stretching of the skin, which distinguishes it from the eruption of other exanthems, especially measles.

Grit·ti-Stokes amputation (greet'tee) [R. *Gritti,* Italian surgeon, 1828–1920; and W. *Stokes,* Irish surgeon, 1839–1900]. A supracondylar osteoplastic operation in which the patella is retained in the flap and is attached to the cut end of the femur.

Groc·co's sign (gro^h^k'ko) [P. *Grocco,* Italian physician, 1857–1916]. A sign for pleural effusion in which there is a triangular area of paravertebral dullness on the opposite side.

Grocco's triangle [P. *Grocco*]. PARAVERTEBRAL TRIANGLE. See also *Grocco's sign.*

gro·cer's itch. Acarodermatitis urticarioides caused by *Glyciphagus domesticus* and other food mites.

Groen·blad-Strand·berg syndrome (grœn'blahd, stra^h^nd'bærʸ) [Esther E. *Groenblad* (*Grönblad*), Swedish ophthalmologist, 20th century; and J. *Strandberg,* Swedish dermatologist, 20th century]. Pseudoxanthoma elasticum with angioid streaks.

Groe·nouw's corneal dystrophy (ᵍhroo'noʰw) [A. *Groenouw,* 1862–1945]. 1. MACULAR CORNEAL DYSTROPHY. 2. GRANULAR CORNEAL DYSTROPHY.

groin, *n.* [ME. *grynde,* of uncertain origin]. The depression between the abdomen and thigh. See also *inguinal region* and Plate 4.

Grönblad. See *Groenblad.*

groove, *n.* An elongated depression. See also *sulcus.* —**grooved,** *adj.*

grooved director. An instrument grooved to guide the knife in surgical operations.

gross (groce) *adj.* [MF. *gros,* thick, coarse, from L. *grossus*]. 1. Large enough to be seen without magnification. 2. Pertaining to or describing general aspects or distinctions; not concerned with minute details. 3. Growing or spreading excessively.

gross anatomy. Anatomy that deals with the naked-eye appearance of tissues and organs. Contr. *microscopic anatomy.*

gross pathology. 1. The description of grossly visible changes in the tissues and organs of the body resulting from disease. 2. Grossly visible pathologic changes.

gross stress reaction. *In psychiatry,* an adjustment reaction of adult life in which, under conditions of great or unusual physical or emotional stress (as occurs in combat or civilian catastrophe), a normal personality utilizes neurotic mechanisms to deal with overwhelming danger; differing from neurosis and psychosis with respect to clinical history, reversibility of reaction, and transient character.

ground bundles. FASCICULI PROPRII MEDULLAE SPINALIS.

ground itch. Local irritation of the skin resulting from the entrance of the larvae of any variety of *Ancylostoma* into the skin.

ground lamella. INTERSTITIAL LAMELLA.

ground·nut oil. PEANUT OIL.

ground potential. The electric potential of the earth, arbitrarily used as a standard reference point for all electric measurements.

ground sections. Sections of bones and teeth prepared without demineralization by grinding and polishing until thin enough to transmit light and permit microscopic study of structure.

ground substance. The fluid, semifluid, or solid material, in the connective tissues, cartilage, and bone, which fills in part or all of the space between the cells and fibers. Syn. *matrix, interstitial substance.*

ground water. Water that has penetrated the soil and openings in rocks and is found immediately above the first impervious stratum. It is the water that supplies wells and springs.

group agglutinin. An agglutinating antibody reacting not only with the homologous organisms or antigen, but also with heterologous organisms or antigen. Syn. *minor agglutinin.*

group analysis. *In psychiatry,* a method of intensive therapeutic study and analysis as applied to groups. See also *group psychotherapy.*

group medicine. 1. The practice of medicine by a number of physicians working in systematic association, with joint use of equipment and technical personnel, and with centralized administrative and financial organization. Its objectives are increased professional efficiency, improved medical care of the patient, and increased economic efficiency. 2. The practice of medicine carried on under a legal agreement in a community, by a body of registered physicians and surgeons, for the purpose of caring for a group of persons who have subscribed to such service by the payment of a definite sum for a specified time, which entitles each subscriber to medical care and hospitalization under definite rules and regulations.

group phase. *In immunology,* the group characterized by antigens shared by only a few other species or types.

group psychotherapy. *In psychiatry,* the therapy given to a group of patients by a professional therapist, and based on the effect of the group upon the individual and his interaction with the group.

group reagent. A reagent that reacts in the same manner with each of a group of substances of similar chemical structure.

group-specific substances. Substances derived from a source other than blood which reduce the amount of naturally occurring anti-A or anti-B agglutinins in bloods of the appropriate ABO blood groups. Syn. *Witebsky's substances.*

group therapy. GROUP PSYCHOTHERAPY.

growing follicle. Any stage in the maturation of an ovarian follicle between the primary follicle and the graafian follicle.

growing pains. Soreness of variable degree, duration, and kind in muscles and occasionally in joints in children and adolescents, sometimes during systemic infections.

growth, *n.* 1. The increase in the amount of actively metabolic protoplasm, accompanied by an increase in cell number, or cell size, or both. 2. The increase in the size of the organism or its parts, measured as an increase in weight, volume, or linear dimensions. 3. Any abnormal, localized increase in cells, such as a neoplasm.

growth cartilage. EPIPHYSEAL PLATE (2).

growth factor. 1. GROWTH HORMONE. 2. Any substance, either genetic or extrinsic, which affects growth.

growth hormone. An adenohypophyseal hormone that promotes growth and also has direct influence on the metabolism of carbohydrates, fats, and proteins. Syn. *somatotropin.*

growth-hormone-release-inhibiting hormone. SOMATOSTATIN.

Gru·ber's ligament. PETROSPHENOID LIGAMENT.

Gruber's muscle [W. L. *Gruber,* Bohemian anatomist in Russia, 1814–1890]. PERONEOCALCANEUS EXTERNUS.

Gruber's speculum [J. *Gruber,* Austrian otolaryngologist, 1827–1900]. An aural speculum; no longer in general use.

Gruber's test [J. *Gruber*]. A test for hearing, no longer in general use, in which a tuning fork is held near the ear until it becomes inaudible; the sound should again become audible to the subject when a finger is inserted in the ear and the tuning fork is placed in contact with the finger.

Gruber syndrome [G. B. *Gruber,* German, 20th century]. A complex of central nervous system, somatic, and splanchnic malformations, including occipital encephalocele, microcephaly, abnormal facies with cleft lip and palate, polydactyly, and polycystic kidneys; inherited as an autosomal recessive trait. Syn. *dysencephalia splanchnocystica, Meckel syndrome.*

Grü·bler stain (grue'blur). PANCHROME STAIN.

grume, *n.* [L. *grumus*, a little heap]. A clot, as of blood; a thick and viscid fluid. —**gru·mose** (groo'moce), **gru·mous** (·mus) *adj.*

grumous saccule. A small sac, clump, or bulb of fatty material, representing a degenerated nerve cell; seen particularly in the substantia nigra and locus ceruleus in certain forms of parkinsonism.

Grün·wald stain (gruen'vahlt) [L. *Grünwald*, German otolaryngologist, b. 1863]. MAY-GRÜNWALD STAIN.

Gryn·feltt's triangle (green·felt') [J. C. *Grynfeltt*, French surgeon, 1840–1913]. A triangular space through which lumbar hernia may occur. It is bounded above by the twelfth rib and lower border of the serratus posterior inferior, behind by the quadratus lumborum, and anteriorly by the posterior border of the internal oblique.

gry·o·chrome (grye'o·krome) *n.* [Gk. *gry*, a bit, a little, + *-chrome*]. A nerve cell in which the Nissl substance is in ring arrangement.

gry·po·sis (grye·po'sis, gri·) *n.* [Gk. *grypōsis*, from *grypos*, curved]. Abnormal curvature, especially of the nails.

GSH [*g*lutamyl + *s*ulf*h*ydryl]. GLUTATHIONE.

GSSG [two *g*lutathiones linked by two *s*ulfides]. DIGLUTATHIONE.

g stress. Structural and functional stress on the body from positive or negative acceleratory forces, caused by rapid changes in velocity and direction of motion, as may be experienced in air or space craft.

G-strophanthin. OUABAIN.

g suit. ANTI-G SUIT.

gt. Abbreviation for *gutta*, drop.

gtt. Abbreviation for *guttae*, drops.

GU Abbreviation for *genitourinary*.

gua·co (gwah'ko) *n.* [Sp.]. The plants *Mikania guaco* and other species of *Mikania* and *Aristolochia;* used in South America for snakebites; formerly also used as an antirheumatic, antisyphilitic, and anthelmintic.

guai·ac (gwye'ack) *n.* [NL. *guaiacum*, from Taino *guayacan*]. The resin of the wood of *Guajacum officinale* or of *G. sanctum*, formerly used in treatment of syphilis, chronic rheumatism, and gout; now used in testing for occult blood.

guai·a·col (gwye'uh·kol) *n. o*-Methoxyphenol, $C_7H_8O_2$, a constituent of guaiac and wood creosote, also prepared synthetically; has been used internally as an expectorant, and externally as an antiseptic and anesthetic.

guaiacol benzoate. Benzoylguaiacol, $C_{14}H_{12}O_3$, formerly used for treatment of pulmonary tuberculosis, cystitis, and as an intestinal antiseptic.

guaiacol carbonate. A crystalline derivative, $C_{15}H_{14}O_5$, of guaiacol; formerly used as an expectorant.

guaiacol glyceryl ether. GUAIFENESIN.

guaiac test. A test for blood in which an acetic acid or alcoholic solution of guaiac resin and hydrogen peroxide is mixed with the unknown. The development of a blue color is a positive test.

guai·fen·e·sin (gwye·fen'e·sin) *n.* 3-(*o*-Methoxyphenoxy)-1,2-propanediol, $C_{10}H_{14}O_4$, an expectorant. Syn. *guaiacol glyceryl ether.*

guai·thyl·line (gwye'thi·lin) *n.* A compound of theophylline with guaiafenesin, $C_7H_8N_4O_2 \cdot C_{10}H_{14}O_4$, a bronchodilator; used as an expectorant.

gua·na·benz (gwah'nuh·benz) *n.* [(2,6-Dichlorobenzylidene)-amino]guanidine, $C_8H_8Cl_2N_4$, an antihypertensive.

gua·na·cline (gwah'nuh·kleen) *n.* [2-(3,6-Dihydro-4-methyl-1(2*H*)-pyridyl)ethyl]guanidine, $C_9H_{18}N_4$, an antihypertensive agent; used as the sulfate salt.

gua·na·drel (gwah'nuh·drel) *n.* (1,4-Dioxaspiro[4.5]dec-2-ylmethyl)guanidine, $C_{10}H_{19}N_3O_2$, an antihypertensive agent; used as the sulfate salt.

gua·nase (gwah'nace, ·naze) *n.* A deaminizing enzyme, widely distributed in animal tissues, that catalyzes conversion of guanine into xanthine, with release of ammonia.

Guanatol. A trademark for chloroguanide, an antimalarial drug used as the hydrochloride salt.

gua·na·zo·lo (gwah''nuh·zo'lo) *n.* 8-Azaguanine, $C_4H_4N_6O$, a purine antimetabolite investigated in the therapy of neoplastic diseases.

guan·cy·dine (gwahn'sigh·deen, gwahn·sigh') *n.* 1-Cyano-3-*tert*-pentylguanidine, $C_7H_{14}N_4$, a hypotensive agent.

Guaneran. Trademark for thiamiprine, an antineoplastic agent.

guan·eth·i·dine (gwahn·eth'i·deen) *n.* {2-[Hexahydro-1(2*H*)-azocinyl]ethyl}guanidine, $C_{10}H_{22}N_4$, a potent hypotensive drug used as the sulfate salt.

gua·ni·dine (gwah'ni·deen, ·din, gwan'i·) *n.* Aminomethanamidine, $NH{=}C(NH_2)_2$, a normal product of protein metabolism found in the urine. The hydrochloride has been used for the treatment of myasthenia gravis. Syn. *carbamidine, iminourea.*

guanidine-acetic acid. GLYCOCYAMINE.

gua·ni·di·no·ace·tic acid (gwah·ni·dee''no·a·see'tick, gwah''ni·di·no·). GLYCOCYAMINE.

gua·nine (gwah'neen, ·nin, gwan'een, ·in) *n.* 2-Aminohypoxanthine, $C_5H_5N_5O$, a purine base important mainly as a component of ribonucleic and deoxyribonucleic acids; occurs also in guano.

guanine deaminase. GUANASE.

guan·iso·quin (gwahn''eye'so·kwin) *n.* 7-Bromo-3,4-dihydro-2(1*H*)-isoquinolinecarboxamidine, $C_{10}H_{12}BrN_3$, an antihypertensive compound.

gua·no (gwah'no) *n.* [Sp., from Quechua *huanu*, dung]. The excrement of seafowl found on certain islands in the Pacific Ocean. Contains guanine and various other nitrogen bases; formerly used externally for treatment of certain skin diseases.

gua·no·clor (gwah'no·klor) *n.* {[2-(2,6-Dichlorophenoxy)ethyl]amino}guanidine, $C_9H_{12}Cl_2N_4O$, an antihypertensive compound used as the sulfate salt.

guan·oc·tine (gwahn·ock'teen) *n.* (1,1,3,3-Tetramethylbutyl)-guanidine, $C_9H_{21}N_3$, an antihypertensive drug; used as the hydrochloride salt.

gua·no·sine (gwah'no·seen, ·sin) *n.* Guanine riboside, $C_{10}H_{13}N_5O_5$, a nucleoside composed of one molecule each of guanine and D-ribose. One of the four main riboside components of ribonucleic acid. Syn. *vernine.*

guanosine monophosphate. GUANYLIC ACID. Abbreviated, GMP.

guan·ox·a·benz (gwah·nock'suh·benz) *n.* 1-[(2,6-Dichlorobenzylidene)amino]-3-hydroxyguanidine, $C_8H_8Cl_2N_4O$, an antihypertensive.

guan·ox·an (gwahn'ock·san) *n.* (1,4-Benzodioxan-2-ylmethyl)guanidine, $C_{10}H_{13}N_3O_2$, an antihypertensive drug used as the sulfate salt.

guan·ox·y·fen (gwahn·ock'si·fen) *n.* 3-(Phenoxypropyl)guanidine, $C_{10}H_{15}N_3O$, an antihypertensive drug; used as the sulfate salt.

gua·nyl·ic acid (gwah·nil'ick). A mononucleotide component, $C_{10}H_{14}N_5O_8P$, of ribonucleic acid which yields guanine, D-ribose, and phosphoric acid on complete hydrolysis. Syn. *guanosine monophosphate.* See also *cyclic guanosine monophosphate.*

gua·ra·na (gwah''rah·nah', gwah·rah'nuh) *n.* [Sp. and Pg., from Tupi]. A dried paste prepared from the seeds of *Paullinia cupana*, a Brazilian tree; contains caffeine. Used as an astringent and stimulant.

gua·ra·nine (gwah·rah'neen, ·nin, gwah'ruh·) *n.* An alkaloid from guarana; shown to be identical with caffeine.

guard, *n.* An appliance placed on a knife to prevent too deep an incision.

guar gum (gwahr) [Hindi *guār*]. The ground endosperms of *Cyanopsis tetragonolaba*, cultured in India as a livestock feed; a light-gray powder, about 85% of which is soluble in water and consists of galactose and mannose. The gum is used, like starch, as a tablet-disintegrating material and to prepare mucilages.

Guar·nie·ri bodies (gwar·nyeh'ree) [G. *Guarnieri,* Italian pathologist, 1856–1918]. Eosinophilic cytoplasmic inclusion bodies found in the epidermal cells of patients with smallpox or vaccinia.

gua·za (gwah'zuh, gwaz'uh) *n.* GANJA.

gubernacular fold. A fold of peritoneum containing the lower part of the gubernaculum testis.

gu·ber·nac·u·lum (gew"bur·nack'yoo·lum) *n.*, pl. **gubernacu·la** (·luh) [L., helm, rudder]. A guiding structure. —**gubernacu·lar** (·lur) *adj.*

gubernaculum den·tis (den'tis). A bundle of fibrous tissue connecting the tooth sac of a permanent tooth with the gum.

gubernaculum tes·tis (tes'tis) [NA]. A fibrous cord extending from the fetal testis to the scrotal swellings; it occupies the potential inguinal canal and guides the testis in its descent. See also *chorda gubernaculum.*

Gu·bler's paralysis (gu^e·blehr') [A. *Gubler,* French physician, 1821–1879]. MILLARD-GUBLER SYNDROME.

Gud·den's commissure (gŏŏd'un) [B. A. von *Gudden,* German neurologist, 1824–1886]. The ventral supraoptic decussation. See *commissurae supraopticae.*

Gu·der·natsch's test. A test for thyroid activity, in which if active thyroid is fed to young frogs, metamorphosis is accelerated, resulting in dwarf frogs.

Gué·neau de Mus·sy's point (ge^y·no' duh mu^e·see') DE MUSSY'S POINT.

gue·non (ge·non', ·nohn') *n.* [F.]. Any of various monkeys of the widespread African genus *Cercopithecus,* as for example diana monkeys, green monkeys, mona monkeys, spot-nosed guenons, and many others.

Gué·rin's fold or **valve** (ge^y·ræ^n') [A. F. M. *Guérin,* French surgeon, 1816–1895]. A fold of mucous membrane sometimes found in the roof of the navicular fossa of the urethra. NA *valvula fossae navicularis.*

Guérin's sinus [A. F. M. *Guérin*]. *Obsol.* A diverticulum behind Guérin's fold.

guerney. GURNEY.

Guil·lain-Bar·ré disease or **syndrome** (ghee·læ^n', ba·re^y') [G. *Guillain,* French neurologist, 1876–1961; and J. A. *Barré*]. An acute, more or less symmetrical lower motor neuron paralysis of unknown cause, with areflexia and variable sensory involvement. Proximal as well as distal muscles of the limbs are involved, and, in advanced cases, trunk and cranial muscles as well, with progression to respiratory failure and death within several days. The protein level of the spinal fluid rises after several days, usually without an increase in cells. Syn. *acute idiopathic polyneuritis, acute inflammatory polyradiculoneuropathy, Landry-Guillain-Barrea syndrome.*

Guillain-Barré-Strohl syndrome [G. *Guillain,* J. A. *Barré,* and A. *Strohl*]. GUILLAIN-BARRÉ SYNDROME.

Guillain's sign [G. *Guillain*]. In a patient with meningeal irritation, pinching the skin over the quadriceps femoris muscle on one side, or squeezing the muscle, may result in flexion of the contralateral hip and knee.

guil·lo·tine amputation (gil'uh·teen, gee'o·teen). CIRCULAR AMPUTATION.

guillotine costotome. A specially designed costotome for removal of the first rib in thoracic surgery. Syn. *Lilienthal's costotome.*

guin·ea pig. A prolific rodent of the genus *Cavia,* of South American origin; widely domesticated and used in biological experimentation.

guinea worm. *DRACUNCULUS MEDINENSIS.*

guinea worm infection. DRACUNCULIASIS.

Guld·berg-Waa·ge law (gu^eh l'bærg, vo'guh) [C. *Guldberg,* Norwegian chemist, 1862–1902; and P. *Waage,* Norwegian chemist, 1833–1900]. LAW OF MASS ACTION.

Gull and Sut·ton's disease [W. W. *Gull,* English physician, 1816–1890; and H. G. *Sutton,* English physician, 1837–1891]. GENERALIZED ARTERIOSCLEROSIS.

gul·let, *n.* [OF. *goulet,* dim. of *goule,* throat]. ESOPHAGUS.

Gull's disease [W. W. *Gull*]. Atrophy of the thyroid gland with myxedema. See also *athyreosis.*

gu·lose (gew'loce, ·loze) *n.* An aldohexose, $C_6H_{12}O_6$, synthetically produced; it occurs in D- and L- forms.

¹gum, *n.* [OE. *gōma,* palate]. GINGIVA.

²gum, *n.* [L. *gummi,* from Gk. *kommi,* gum, from Egyptian]. A concrete vegetable juice exuded from many plants, insoluble in alcohol or ether, but swelling or dissolving in water into a viscid mass. Gums consist of glycosidal hexose-uronic acids, partly or wholly combined with calcium, potassium, or magnesium.

gum arabic. ACACIA.

gum benjamin or **benzoin.** BENZOIN.

gum·boil, *n.* The aspect of a periodontal abscess that has extended through the periodontal tissues and involved the gingiva.

gum elemi. ELEMI.

gum ghatti. GHATTI GUM.

gum itch. TINEA CRURIS.

gum·ma (gum'uh) *n.*, pl. **gummas, gumma·ta** (·tuh) [NL., from L. *gummi,* gum]. A mass of rubberlike necrotic tissue found in any of various organs and tissues in tertiary syphilis. —**gumma·tous** (·tus) *adj.*

gum mastic. MASTIC.

gum mastic test. MASTIC TEST.

gummatous meningitis. A granulomatous infection of the meninges occurring in tertiary syphilis.

Gum·precht's shadows (gŏŏm'pre^kht) [F. *Gumprecht,* German physician, b. 1864]. A degenerated nucleus and its contained nucleolus from the abnormal cells of chronic lymphocytic leukemia, where they are commonly seen in peripheral blood films.

gum resin. A solidified plant juice, containing a mixture of gum and resin.

gum sugar. ARABINOSE.

gum thus. TURPENTINE.

gum tragacanth. TRAGACANTH.

gum turpentine. TURPENTINE.

gun-barrel vision. TUBULAR VISION.

gun·cot·ton, *n.* PYROXYLIN.

gun·ja, gun·jah (gun'juh) *n.* GANJA.

Gun·ning's splint [T. B. *Gunning,* U.S. dentist, 1813–1889]. A splint resembling a double dental plate, with a frontal aperture for feeding purposes; used in the treatment of fractured jaw.

gun·stock deformity. A deformity following fracture of either condyle of the humerus in which the long axis of the fully extended forearm deviates outwardly from the arm.

Gün·ther's disease (gu^e nt'ur) [H. *Günther,* German physician, 20th century]. ERYTHROPOIETIC PORPHYRIA.

gur·jun balsam or **oil** (gur'jun). An oleoresin from the East Indian tree, *Dipterocarpus turbinatus,* and other species: formerly used in gonorrhea and coughs.

gur·ney, guer·ney (gur'nee) *n.* A stretcher with wheels for transporting a recumbent patient.

Gur·vich radiation (goor'vich) [A. G. *Gurvich,* Russian pathologist, b. 1874]. MITOGENETIC RADIATION.

gus·ta·tion (gus·tay'shun) *n.* [L. *gustatio,* from *gustare,* to taste]. The sense of taste; the act of tasting.

gus·ta·to·ry (gus'tuh·to"ree) *adj.* Pertaining to or involving the sense of taste.

gustatory audition. A form of synesthesia in which certain sounds are believed to cause a sensation of taste.

gustatory aura. An aura of peculiar taste. See also *gustatory fit.*

gustatory bud or **bulb.** TASTE BUD.

gustatory center. The center for taste; of unknown location. See also *gustatory nucleus.*

gustatory fit or **seizure.** A form of psychomotor or temporal lobe seizure announced by an aura of peculiar taste; frequently followed by disturbance of consciousness and automatisms, such as smacking movements of the tongue and lips; usually indicative of an irritation of the infratemporal cortex. Compare *uncinate fit.*

gustatory hyperhidrosis. The phenomenon of sweating over facial areas, particularly about the mouth and nose, accompanied by flushing of the involved areas, upon smelling or ingestion of spicy or acid foods, or some foods such as chocolate. May be caused even by the thought of these foods, and is found to varying degrees in most people. See also *auriculotemporal syndrome.*

gustatory-lacrimal reflex. CROCODILE TEARS SYNDROME.

gustatory nucleus. The rostral part of the nucleus solitarius in which terminate the gustatory fibers of the chorda tympani and the glossopharyngeal and vagus nerves.

gustatory organ. The organ of taste, comprising the taste buds. NA *organum gustus.*

gustatory papilla. A papilla of the tongue which is furnished with taste buds.

gustatory pore. TASTE PORE.

gustatory region. The tip, margins, and root of the tongue in the neighborhood of the vallate papillae; also the lateral parts of the soft palate and the anterior surface of the palatoglossal arches.

gus·tin (gus'tin) *n.* [L. *gust*are, to taste, + *-in*]. A protein actively secreted into the saliva which acts to cause growth and differentiation of taste buds.

gus·to·lac·ri·mal reflex (gus"to·lack'ri·mul). CROCODILE TEARS SYNDROME.

gut, *n.* 1. INTESTINE. 2. The embryonic digestive tube, consisting of foregut, midgut, and hindgut. 3. Catgut or other suturing material.

Guthrie inhibition assay test. GUTHRIE TEST.

Guth·rie-Smith apparatus [Mrs. O. *Guthrie-Smith,* British physiotherapist, 20th century]. An apparatus in which parts of the body or the entire body is supported by slings and springs; used in physical medicine.

Guthrie test [R. Guthrie, U.S. pediatrician, b. 1916]. A screening test for the detection of phenylketonuria in which the inhibition of growth of a strain of *Bacillus subtilis* by a phenylalanine analogue is reversed by L-phenylalanine, as found in elevated concentration in the plasma of patients with phenylketonuria. Syn. *Guthrie inhibition assay test.*

Gut·stein's stain. An aqueous solution of 1% methyl violet and 2% sodium bicarbonate, used to stain smears of the material from skin lesions of smallpox.

gut·ta (gut'uh) *n.,* pl. **gut·tae** (-ee) [L.]. A drop. Abbreviated, gt.

guttae. Plural of *gutta.* Abbreviated, gtt.

gut·ta-per·cha (gut'uh pur'chuh) *n.* [Malay, from *gĕtah,* sap, + *percha,* cloth]. The latex of various trees of the family Sapotaceae; essentially a polymerized hydrocarbon of the general formula $(C_5H_8)_n$ with other resinous substances. Used to make splints, as a wound dressing, or as an insulator.

gut·tate (gut'ate) *adj.* [L. *guttatus,* from *gutta,* drop]. *In biology,* spotted as if by drops of something colored; resembling a drop.

gut·ta·tim (guh·tay'tim) *adv.* [L.]. Drop by drop.

gut·ter, *n. & v.* [OF. *goutiere,* from L. *gutta,* drop]. 1. A shallow groove. 2. To form a shallow groove; specifically, SAUCERIZE.

gutter fracture. A form of depressed fracture of the skull with an elliptic depression; often caused by a missile.

gut·ti·form (gut'i·form) *adj.* [*gutta* + *-iform*]. Drop-shaped.

Gutt·mann's sign (gŏot'mahn) [P. *Guttmann,* German physician, 1834–1893]. In hyperthyroidism, a bruit heard over the thyroid gland.

gut·tur·al (gut'ur·ul) *adj.* [L. *guttur,* throat, + *-al*]. 1. Pertaining to the throat. 2. Throaty, as certain voice sounds. 3. *Erron.* Of consonant sounds: VELAR; or loosely: velar, uvular, pharyngeal, or laryngeal.

guttural pouch. One of a pair of mucomembranous sacs which are ventral diverticula of the auditory tube in Equidae, located between the base of the cranium and the atlas dorsally and the pharynx ventrally.

guttural pulse. A pulse felt in the throat.

gut·turo·pho·nia (gut"ur·o·fo'nee·uh) *n.* GUTTUROPHONY.

gut·tur·oph·ony (gut"ur·off'uh·nee) *n.* [L. *guttur,* throat, + *-phony*]. A form of dysphonia characterized by a throaty quality of the voice sounds.

gut·turo·tet·a·ny (gut"ur·o·tet'uh·nee) *n.* [L. *guttur,* throat, + *tetany*]. A stammering with difficulties in pronouncing "guttural" sounds due to spasm of the laryngeal muscles.

Gut·zeit's test (goot'tsite) [M. A. *Gutzeit,* German chemist, 1847–1915]. A test for arsenic in which zinc, stannous chloride, and sulfuric acid are added to the sample in a container. If arsenic is present, it is reduced to arsine and evolved as a gas that imparts a characteristic stain to paper previously impregnated with silver nitrate or mercuric chloride.

Gwath·mey's method (gwahth'mee) [J. T. *Gwathmey,* U.S. surgeon, 1863–1944]. A method formerly used for producing general anesthesia by a rectal injection of liquid ether with olive oil or liquid petrolatum.

gym·no·pho·bia (jim"no·fo'bee·uh) *n.* [Gk. *gymnos,* naked, + *-phobia*]. An abnormal fear of nudity.

gym·no·spore (jim'no·spore) *n.* [Gk. *gymnos,* naked, + *spore*]. *In biology,* a naked spore.

gyn-, gyno- [Gk. *gynē,* woman]. A combining form meaning (a) *woman, female;* (b) *female reproductive organ.*

gynaec-, gynaeco- [Gk. *gynē, gynaikos,* woman]. See *gyn-.*

gynaecic. GYNECIC.

gynaecography. GYNECOGRAPHY.

gynaecoid. GYNECOID.

gynaecologist. GYNECOLOGIST.

gynaecology. GYNECOLOGY.

gynaecomania. Gynecomania (= SATYRIASIS).

gynaecomastia. GYNECOMASTIA.

gynaecopathy. GYNECOPATHY.

gynaephobia. GYNEPHOBIA.

gyn·an·der (ji·nan'dur) *n.* [Gk. *gynandros,* of doubtful sex, from *gynē,* woman, + *anēr, andros,* man]. PSEUDOHERMAPHRODITE.

gyn·an·dria (ji·nan'dree·uh) *n.* [NL., from Gk. *gynandr*os, of doubtful sex, + *-ia*]. 1. FEMALE PSEUDOHERMAPHRODITISM. 2. A condition involving secondary characteristics of the opposite sex.

gyn·an·drism (ji·nan'driz·um) *n.* [*gynandr*ia + *-ism*]. 1. FEMALE PSEUDOHERMAPHRODITISM. 2. A condition involving secondary characteristics of the opposite sex.

gynandrism syndrome. SIMPSON'S SYNDROME in boys.

gyn·an·dro·blas·to·ma (ji·nan"dro·blas·to'muh) *n.* [*gyn-* + *andro-* + *blastoma*]. An ovarian tumor, histologically characterized by elements resembling arrhenoblastoma and granulosa cell tumor, associated with hyperestrogenism and masculinization.

gyn·an·dro·morph (ji·nan'dro·morf) *n.* [*gyn-* + *andro-* + *-morph*]. A sex mosaic in which certain areas of the organism have male characters and others female characters due to genetic differences in the cells. —**gyn·an·dro·mor·phic** (ji·nan"dro·mor'fick) *adj.*

gyn·an·dro·mor·phism (ji·nan"dro·mor'fiz·um) *n.* [*gynandromorph* + *-ism*]. An abnormality in which the individual contains both genetically male and genetically female tissue.

gyn·an·dro·mor·phy (ji·nan'dro·mor"fee) *n.* [*gyn-* + *andro-* + *-morphy*]. 1. GYNANDROMORPHISM. 2. In the somatotype, the degree or prominence of feminine characteristics in a male physique, or vice versa, expressed numerically as the g-component.

gyn·an·drous (ji·nan'drus) *adj.* [*gyn-* + *andr-* + *-ous*]. *In bot-*

any, having the stamens and pistils more or less united.

gyn·an·dry (ji·nan′dree) *n.* [NL. *gynandria*]. FEMALE PSEUDOHERMAPHRODITISM. —**gynan·droid** (·droid) *adj. & n.*

gyn·an·thro·pus (ji·nan′thruh·pus) *n.* Gynander (= PSEUDOHERMAPHRODITE).

gyn·atre·sia (jin″uh·tree′zhuh, ·zee·uh) *n.* [*gyn-* + *atresia*]. 1. An imperforate condition of the vagina or of other areas of the female genital system. 2. Occlusion of any portion of the female genital system.

-gyne [Gk. *gynē,* woman]. A combining form meaning *woman* or *female.*

gynec-, gyneco- [Gk. *gynē, gynaikos,* woman]. See *gyn-.*

gy·ne·cic, gy·nae·cic (ji·nee′sick) *adj.* [*gynec-* + *-ic*]. Pertaining to women or the female sex.

gyneco-. See *gyn-.*

gy·ne·co·gen·ic (jin″e·ko·jen′ick, guy″ne·ko·) *adj.* [*gyneco-* + *-genic*]. Causing or producing female characteristics.

gy·ne·cog·ra·phy, gy·nae·cog·ra·phy (jin″e·kog′ruh·fee, guy″ne·) *n.* [*gyneco-* + *-graphy*]. A roentgenologic method of visualization of the female pelvic organs by means of the injection of air or carbon dioxide intraperitoneally.

gy·ne·coid, gy·nae·coid (jin′e·koid, guy′ne·) *adj.* [Gk. *gynaikoeidēs,* womanish]. 1. Pertaining to or like a woman. 2. Specifically, of a pelvis: having a shape typical of that of the female, with a round or nearly round inlet. Contr. *android, anthropoid, platypellic.*

gynecologic pathology. The pathology of the female sexual organs and associated structures.

gy·ne·col·o·gist, gy·nae·col·o·gist (jin″e·kol′uh·jist, guy″ne·, jye″ne·) *n.* A physician who practices gynecology.

gy·ne·col·o·gy, gy·nae·col·o·gy (jin″e·kol′uh·jee, guy″ne·, jye″ne·) *n.* [*gyneco-* + *-logy*]. The science of the diseases of women, especially those affecting the sexual organs. —**gyne·co·log·ic, gynae·co·log·ic** (·ko·loj′ick), **gynecolog·i·cal, gynaecolog·i·cal** (·i·kul) *adj.*

gy·ne·co·ma·nia, gy·nae·co·ma·nia (jin″e·ko·may′nee·uh, guy″ne·) *n.* [Gk. *gynaikomania,* madness for women]. SATYRIASIS.

gy·ne·co·mas·tia, gy·nae·co·mas·tia (jin″e·ko·mas′tee·uh, guy″ne·) *n.* [*gyneco-* + *-mastia*]. Mammary glandular hyperplasia in the male. See also *anisogynecomastia, pseudogynecomastia.*

gynecomastia-and-small-testes syndrome. KLINEFELTER'S SYNDROME.

gynecomastia-aspermatogenesis syndrome. KLINEFELTER'S SYNDROME.

gy·ne·co·mas·ty (jin′e·ko·mas″tee, guy′ne·) *n.* GYNECOMASTIA.

gy·ne·co·ma·zia (jin″e·ko·may′zee·uh, guy″ne·) *n.* [*gyneco-* + *maz-,* breast, + *-ia*]. GYNECOMASTIA.

gy·ne·cop·a·thy, gy·nae·cop·a·thy (jin″e·kop′uth·ee, guy″ne·, jye″ne·) *n.* [*gyneco-* + *-pathy*]. Any disease of, or peculiar to, women.

gy·ne·co·pho·bia (jin″e·ko·fo′bee·uh, guy″ne·, jye″ne·) *n.* GYNEPHOBIA.

gy·ne·co·phor·ic canal (jin″e·ko·for′ick, guy″ne·, jye″ne·). A canal located on the ventral surface of the male of certain species of *Schistosoma* in which the female lies during copulation.

gy·ne·pho·bia, gy·nae·pho·bia (jin″e·fo′bee·uh, jye″ne·, guy″ne·) *n.* [Gk. *gynē,* woman, + *-phobia*]. An abnormal fear of the society of women.

gy·ne·phor·ic (jin″e·for′ick, guy″ne·) *adj.* [*gyn-* + *-phoric*]. Pertaining to inheritance sex-linked to the X chromosome.

Gynergen. A trademark for ergotamine used as the tartrate salt principally to relieve migraine pain.

gy·ni·a·tri·cian (jin″ee·uh·trish′un, jye·, guy·) *n.* A physician who specializes in gyniatrics.

gy·ni·at·rics (jin″ee·at′ricks, jye″nee·, guy″nee·) *n.* [*gyn-* + *-iatrics*]. Treatment of the diseases of women.

gy·nism syndrome (jye′niz·um, guy′). SIMPSON'S SYNDROME in girls.

gyno-. See *gyn-.*

gyno·gam·one (jin″o·gam′ohn) *n.* [*gyno-* + *gamone*]. A gamone present in an ovum.

gy·no·gen·e·sis (jin″o·jen′e·sis, jye″no·, guy″no·) *n.* [*gyno-* + *-genesis*]. Development of the egg without the participation of the sperm nucleus, but after penetration of the egg by the sperm.

gy·nog·ra·phy (jin·og′ruh·fee, jye·nog′, guy·nog′) *n.* [*gyno-* + *-graphy*]. GYNECOGRAPHY.

gy·no·plas·ty (jin′o·plas·tee, jye′no·, guy′no·) *n.* [*gyno-* + *-plasty*]. Plastic surgery of the female genitalia. —**gy·no·plas·tic** (jin″o·plas′tick, guy″no·) *adj.*

Gynorest. A trademark for dydrogesterone, a progestin.

gyp·sum (jip′sum) *n.* [L., from Gk. *gypsos*]. Native calcium sulfate, $CaSO_4.2H_2O$. Deprived of the major portion of its water of crystallization, it constitutes plaster of paris.

gyr-, gyro- [Gk. *gyros*]. A combining form meaning (a) *ring, circle;* (b) *gyral, gyrus.*

gy·ral (jye′rul) *adj.* Of, pertaining to, or involving a gyrus.

gyral fasciculus. ASSOCIATION FIBERS.

gyral isthmus. A narrow gyrus connecting two adjoining gyri; an annectent convolution.

gy·rate (jye′rate) *adj.* [L. *gyratus*]. Coiled; in rings; convoluted.

gyrate atrophy of the choroid and retina. Progressive atrophy of the choroid and pigment epithelium of the retina, beginning with irregular linear patches of destruction around the nerve head which eventually enlarge and coalesce; night blindness and scotomas are common. Cause is unknown, but the disorder is frequently familial.

gy·ra·tion (jye·ray′shun) *n.* [L. *gyratio,* from *gyrare,* to gyrate, from Gk. *gyros,* circle]. 1. A turning in a circle. 2. *Obsol.* The arrangement of gyri in the cerebral hemisphere.

Gy·rau·lus (jye·raw′lus) *n.* [Gk. *gyros,* circular, + *aulos,* tube, pipe]. A genus of freshwater snails.

Gyraulus sai·go·nen·sis (sigh″go·nen′sis). A species of freshwater snails found in China and Formosa which serves as the intermediate host of the oriental fluke, *Fasciolopsis buski.*

gyre, *n. Obsol.* GYRUS.

gy·rec·to·my (jye·reck′tuh·mee) *n.* [*gyr-* + *-ectomy*]. Excision of any gyrus of the brain.

gyr·en·ceph·a·late (jye″ren·sef′uh·late, jirr″en·) *adj.* [*gyr-* + *encephal-* + *-ate*]. Having the surface of the brain convoluted.

gyr·en·ce·phal·ic (jye″ren·se·fal′ick, jirr″en·) *adj.* GYRENCEPHALATE.

gyr·en·ceph·a·lous (jye″ren·sef′uh·lus, jirr″en·) *adj.* GYRENCEPHALATE.

gyri. Plural and genitive singular of *gyrus.*

gyri An·dre·ae Ret·zii (an′dree·ee ret′see·eye) [*Anders* A. *Retzius*]. Two or three inconstant, small, rudimentary gyri, which occupy the angle between the gyrus dentatus and the gyrus parahippocampalis immediately beneath the splenium of the corpus callosum.

gyri an·nec·ten·tes (an″eck·ten′teez). ANNECTENT GYRI.

gyri bre·ves in·su·lae (brev′eez in′sue·lee) [NA]. SHORT GYRI OF THE INSULA.

gyri ce·re·bel·li (serr·e·bel′eye) [BNA]. FOLIA CEREBELLI.

gyri ce·re·bri (serr′e·brye) [NA]. The gyri of the cerebrum.

gyri in·su·lae (in′sue·lee) [NA]. The gyri of the insula. See *long gyrus of the insula, short gyri of the insula.*

gyri oc·ci·pi·ta·les la·te·ra·les (ock·sip″i·tay′leez lat·e·ray′leez) [BNA]. LATERAL OCCIPITAL GYRI.

gyri occipitales su·pe·ri·o·res (sue·peer″ee·o′reez) [BNA]. SUPERIOR OCCIPITAL GYRI.

gyri of Heschl (hesh′[e]l) [R.L. *Heschl*]. TRANSVERSE TEMPORAL GYRI.

gyri oper·ti (o·pur′tye). SHORT GYRI OF THE INSULA.

gyri or·bi·ta·les (or·bi·tay′leez) [NA]. ORBITAL GYRI.

gyri pro·fun·di ce·re·bri (pro·fun'dye serr'e·brye) [BNA]. Annectent gyri that connect two neighboring gyri across the bottom of the intervening fissure or sulcus.

gyri tem·po·ra·les trans·ver·si (tem·po·ray'leez trans·vur'sigh) [NA]. TRANSVERSE TEMPORAL GYRI.

gyri tran·si·ti·vi ce·re·bri (tran·si·tye'vye serr'e·brye) [BNA]. Annectent gyri which are located superficially on the surface of the brain.

gyro-. See *gyr-*.

gy·rose (jye'roce) *adj.* [NL. *gyrosus*, from Gk. *gyros*, ring, circle]. Marked with curved or undulating lines.

gy·ro·spasm (jye'ro·spaz·um) *n.* SPASMUS NUTANS.

gy·rus (jye'rus) *n.*, pl. & genit. sing. **gy·ri** (·rye) [L., circle, circuit, from Gk. *gyros*, circle, ring] [NA]. A convolution on the surface of the cerebral hemisphere. See also Plate 18.

gyrus am·bi·ens (am'bee·enz). A lateral elevation of the upper concealed surface of the uncus of the temporal lobe.

gyrus an·gu·la·ris (ang"gew·lair'is) [NA]. ANGULAR GYRUS.

gyrus cal·lo·sus (ka·lo'sus). CINGULATE GYRUS.

gyrus cen·tra·lis anterior (sen·tray'lis) [BNA]. Gyrus precentralis (= PRECENTRAL GYRUS).

gyrus centralis posterior [BNA]. Gyrus postcentralis (= POSTCENTRAL GYRUS).

gyrus cin·gu·li (sing'gew·lye) [NA]. CINGULATE GYRUS.

gyrus cuneus. CUNEUS.

gyrus den·ta·tus (den·tay'tus) [NA]. DENTATE GYRUS.

gyrus epi·cal·lo·sus (ep·i·ka·lo'sus). INDUSIUM GRISEUM.

gyrus fas·ci·o·la·ris (fash"ee·o·lair'is, fas") [NA]. A small cylindrical strand of cortical substance situated between the dentate gyrus and fimbria in the fimbriodentate sulcus. Syn. *fasciola cinerea.*

gyrus for·ni·ca·tus (for·ni·kay'tus) [BNA]. LIMBIC LOBE.

gyrus fron·ta·lis inferior (fron·tay'lis) [NA]. INFERIOR FRONTAL GYRUS.

gyrus frontalis me·di·us (mee'dee·us) [NA]. MIDDLE FRONTAL GYRUS.

gyrus frontalis superior [NA]. SUPERIOR FRONTAL GYRUS.

gyrus fu·si·for·mis (few·si·for'mis) [BNA]. FUSIFORM GYRUS.

gyrus hip·po·cam·pi (hip·o·kam'pye) [BNA]. Gyrus parahippocampalis (= PARAHIPPOCAMPAL GYRUS).

gyrus in·fra·cal·ca·ri·nus (in"fruh·kal·ka·rye'nus). LINGUAL GYRUS.

gyrus in·tra·lim·bi·cus (in·truh·lim'bi·kus). The posterior tip of the uncus.

gyrus lim·bi·cus (lim'bi·kus). LIMBIC LOBE.

gyrus lin·gua·lis (ling·gway'lis) [NA]. LINGUAL GYRUS.

gyrus lon·gus in·su·lae (long'gus in'sue·lee) [NA]. LONG GYRUS OF THE INSULA.

gyrus mar·gi·na·lis (mahr·ji·nay'lis). PARAHIPPOCAMPAL GYRUS.

gyrus oc·ci·pi·to·tem·po·ra·lis la·te·ra·lis (ock·sip"i·to·tem·po·ray'lis lat·e·ray'lis) [NA]. The lateral portion of a convolution on the inferior surface of the temporal and occipital lobes between the parahippocampal gyrus and the inferior temporal gyrus. The lateral part of the fusiform gyrus.

gyrus occipitotemporalis me·di·a·lis (mee·dee·ay'lis) [NA]. The medial portion of a convolution on the inferior surface of the temporal and occipital lobes between the parahippocampal gyrus and the inferior temporal gyrus; the medial part of the fusiform gyrus.

gyrus of Broca. BROCA'S AREA.

gyrus ol·fac·to·ri·us (ol·fack·to'ree·us). Either of the small gyri on the undersurface of the frontal lobe; there is a medial and a lateral one.

gyrus pa·ra·hip·po·cam·pa·lis (păr"uh·hip·o·kam·pay'lis) [NA]. PARAHIPPOCAMPAL GYRUS.

gyrus pa·ra·ter·mi·na·lis (păr"uh·tur·mi·nay'lis) [NA]. A convolution at the rostrum of the corpus callosum limited anteriorly by the parolfactory sulcus.

gyrus post·cen·tra·lis (pohst"sen·tray'lis) [NA]. POSTCENTRAL GYRUS.

gyrus pre·cen·tra·lis (pree"sen·tray'lis) [NA]. PRECENTRAL GYRUS.

gyrus rec·tus (reck'tus) [NA]. A narrow strip of cortex medial to the olfactory sulcus on the inferior surface of the frontal lobe and continuous with the superior frontal gyrus on the medial surface. Syn. *straight gyrus.*

gyrus ro·lan·di·cus (ro·lan'di·kus) [L. *Rolando*]. A rare anomalous gyrus found in the presence of two central sulci in the brain.

gyrus se·mi·lu·na·ris (sem"ee·lew·nair'is). A median elevation of the upper concealed surface of the uncus of the temporal lobe.

gyrus sub·cal·lo·sus (sub·ka·lo'sus) [BNA]. GYRUS PARATERMINALIS.

gyrus su·pra·cal·lo·sus (sue"pruh·ka·lo'sus). INDUSIUM GRISEUM.

gyrus su·pra·mar·gi·na·lis (sue"pruh·mahr·ji·nay'lis) [NA]. SUPRAMARGINAL GYRUS.

gyrus tem·po·ra·lis inferior (tem·po·ray'lis) [NA]. INFERIOR TEMPORAL GYRUS.

gyrus temporalis me·di·us (mee'dee·us) [NA]. MIDDLE TEMPORAL GYRUS.

gyrus temporalis superior [NA]. SUPERIOR TEMPORAL GYRUS.

gyrus un·ci·na·tus (un·si·nay'tus). PARAHIPPOCAMPAL GYRUS.

H

H Symbol for hydrogen.

H. Abbreviation for *hyperopia.*

H, H *In electrocardiography,* symbol for the longitudinal anatomic axis of the heart as projected on the frontal plane.

H, h Abbreviation for *henry.*

^{1}H Symbol for protium.

^{2}H Symbol for deuterium.

^{3}H Symbol for tritium.

H^+ Symbol for hydrogen ion.

h Abbreviation for (a) height; (b) *hora,* hour; (c) hundred.

h Symbol for Planck's constant.

HAA Abbreviation for *hepatitis-associated antigen.*

Haab's reflex (hahp) [O. *Haab,* Swiss ophthalmologist, 1850–1931]. CEREBRAL CORTEX REFLEX.

Haa·se's rule. A clinical rule for the approximation of crown-heel length of the fetus in centimeters by the use of the lunar month of gestation, and vice versa. Calculated by squaring the lunar month through 5 months (e.g., $5 \times 5 =$ 25 cm) or taking the square root of length up to 25 cm ($\sqrt{25} = 5$ lunar months), and thereafter multiplying the lunar month by 5 (e.g., $7 \times 5 = 35$ cm) or dividing length by 5 (35 cm $\div 5 = 7$ lunar months).

ha·be·na (ha·bee'nuh) *n.* [L., rein, thong, strap]. 1. FRENUM. 2. A bandage. —**habe·nar** (·nur) *adj.*

ha·ben·u·la (ha·ben'yoo·luh) *n.*, pl. & genit. sing. **habenu·lae** (·lee), genit. pl. **ha·be·nu·la·rum** (ha·ben''yoo·lair'um) [L., dim. of *habena*] [NA]. 1. The stalk of the pineal body, attaching it to the thalamus. 2. A ribbonlike structure. —**habenu·lar** (·lur) *adj.*

habenula per·fo·ra·ta (pur·fo·ray'tuh). The upper surface of the tympanic lip of the spiral lamina, having a regular row of holes and giving passage to the cochlear nerves.

habenular calcification. *In radiology,* a commalike calcification seen just anterior to the pineal body and located in the habenular commissure.

habenular commissure. Fibers joining the habenular nuclei on one side to those on the other. NA *commissura habenularum.*

habenular nuclei. Paired groups of nerve cells, medial and lateral, in each habenula, sending fibers to the interpeduncular nucleus by way of the fasciculus retroflexus. NA *nuclei habenulae medialis et lateralis.*

habenular trigone. A small, medial, triangular area on the dorsal aspect of the thalamus between the stalk of the epiphysis and the superior colliculi, and overlying the habenular nucleus; part of the epithalamus. NA *trigonum habenulae.*

ha·ben·u·lo·pe·dun·cu·lar (ha·ben''yoo·lo·pe·dunk'yoo·lur) *adj.* Pertaining to the habenular and the interpeduncular nuclei.

habenulopeduncular tract. FASCICULUS RETROFLEXUS.

ha·bil·i·ta·tion, *n.* [ML. *habilitare,* to capacitate, make fit, from *habilis,* fit, able]. Capacitation, bringing to a state of fitness, as by treatment or training to overcome congenital or early-acquired handicaps. Compare *rehabilitation.*

hab·it, *n.* [L. *habitus,* condition, appearance, disposition]. 1. A behavior pattern fixed by repetition. 2. HABITUS. —**ha·bit·u·al,** *adj.*

hab·i·tat (hab'i·tat) *n.* [L., it inhabits, from *habitare,* to dwell]. The natural place or environment of an organism.

habit scoliosis. FUNCTIONAL SCOLIOSIS.

habit spasm. TIC.

habitual abortion. Spontaneous abortion recurring in three or more successive pregnancies, thought to be due to an endocrinopathic factor or an anatomic defect of the uterus.

habitual dislocation. A dislocation that recurs frequently in a joint, as the shoulder.

ha·bit·u·a·tion, *n.* [L. *habituare,* to bring into a condition]. 1. The gradual adaptation to environment, accompanied by the feeling of certainty that a particular situation will produce a particular response. 2. The gradual increase in efficiency by the elimination of unnecessary motions as a result of repeated reaction to a given stimulus. 3. A condition of tolerance to the effects of a drug or a poison, acquired by its continued use; marked by a craving for the drug when it is withdrawn. 4. Drug addiction, especially a mild form in which withdrawal does not result in severe abstinence symptoms.

hab·i·tus (hab'i·tus) *n.* [L.]. The general appearance of the body, especially as associated with a disease or a predisposition thereto. See also *somatotype.*

Hab·ro·ne·ma (hab''ro·nee'muh) *n.* [Gk. *habros,* graceful, + *-nema*]. A genus of nematodes parasitic in the stomach of horses and mules, and whose larvae may produce dermatitis and conjunctival infection in horses and also in man.

hab·ro·ne·mi·a·sis (hab''ro·ne·migh'uh·sis) *n.*, pl. **habronemia·ses** (·seez) [*Habronema* + *-iasis*]. Infection of horses by nematodes of the genus *Habronema.*

hab·ro·ne·mic (hab''ro·nee'mick) *adj.* Pertaining to or caused by nematodes of the genus *Habronema.*

habronemic ophthalmomyiasis. A granulomatous disease of the eyelids of the horse, caused by any of three species of the nematode *Habronema.* See also *bung-eye.*

ha·bu (hah'boo) *n. Trimeresurus flavoviridis,* a large pit viper found on the Ryukyu Islands.

hache·ment (ahsh·mahn') *n.* [F.]. HACKING (2).

hack·ing, *adj. & n.* 1. Harsh, racking, as hacking cough. 2. A form of massage consisting of a succession of chopping strokes with the edge of the extended fingers or the whole hand, or with firm patting strokes with the extended finger and the whole hand. Syn. *hachement.*

hacking cough. A short, dry cough.

Ha·den-Haus·ser method [R. L. *Haden,* U.S. physician, 1888–1952]. An acid hematin method for hemoglobin using blood diluted in a white cell pipet, in which the color is compared with a glass standard scale through a microscope in a special hemoglobinometer having a wedge-shaped dilution channel.

ha·de·pho·bia (hay″de·fo′bee·uh) *n.* [*Hades* + *-phobia*]. A morbid fear of hell.

HAE Abbreviation for *hereditary angioedema.*

haem. HEME.

haem-, haema-, haemo-. See *hem-.*

Hae·ma·cha·tes (hee″muh·kay′teez) *n.* [*haema-* + Gk. *-chatēs,* craving]. A genus of South African snakes, the ringhalses, of the Elapidae.

Haemachates hae·ma·cha·tus (hee″muh·kay′tus). A species of snake capable of ejecting or spitting its venom at its enemies. The venom is directed toward the eyes and causes intense pain and temporary blindness.

For words beginning HAEM... not found here, see HEM... .

Hae·ma·dip·sa (hee″muh·dip′suh, hem″uh·) *n.* [*haema-* + Gk. *dipsa,* thirst]. A genus of terrestrial leeches species of which produce external hirudiniasis. The most commonly encountered species is the *Haemadipsa zelanica.*

Hae·ma·gog·us (hee″muh·gog′us, ·go′gus, hem′uh·) *n.* [NL., from Gk. *haimagōgos,* drawing blood]. A genus of mosquitoes, one species of which, *Haemagogus capricorni,* has been incriminated in the transmission of jungle yellow fever.

Hae·ma·phy·sa·lis (hee″muh·figh′suh·lis, hem″uh·) *n.* [*haema-* + Gk. *physallis,* bladder]. A genus of ticks which includes the dog tick and the rabbit tick.

Haemaphysalis lep·o·ris pa·lus·tris (lep′o·ris pa·lus′tris). A species of ticks limited to rabbits as hosts, and known to be a natural reservoir of Rocky Mountain spotted fever rickettsia.

Hae·ma·to·bia (hem″uh·to′bee·uh, hee″muh·) *n.* [NL., from *haemato-* + Gk. *bios,* life]. A genus of small flies of the family Muscidae, similar to the common stable fly but more slender.

Haematobia ir·ri·tans (irr′i·tanz). A species known as the horn fly; a great pest of cattle; annoys people but seldom bites them.

Hae·ma·to·si·phon (hee″muh·to·sigh′fon, hem″uh·to·) *n.* [*haemato-* + *siphon*]. A genus of bugs of the family Cimicidae. *Haematosiphon inodora,* a poultry chinch of Central and North America, attacks man as well as fowl. See also *hematosiphoniasis.*

Haem·a·to·ther·ma (hem″uh·to·thur′muh, hee″muh·to·) *n.pl.* [NL., from *haemato-* + Gk. *thermos,* hot]. The warm-blooded vertebrates; birds and mammals.

haem·a·to·ther·mal (hem″uh·to·thur′mul, hee″muh·to·) *adj.* [*haemato-* + *thermal*]. 1. Of or pertaining to the Haematotherma. 2. HEMATOTHERMAL.

-haemia. See *-emia.*

Hae·mo·bar·to·nel·la (hee″mo·bahr″tuh·nel′uh) *n.* [*hemo-* + *Bartonella*]. A genus of gram-negative pleomorphic microorganisms of the family Bartonellaceae which parasitize erythrocytes of several species of wild and domestic animals.

Haemobartonella fe·lis (fee′lis). The agent thought to produce feline infectious anemia.

Haemobartonella mu·ris (mew′ris). A microorganism occasionally found as a latent infection in laboratory rats and mice; following splenectomy, it multiplies rapidly and produces anemia.

Hae·mon·chus (hee·mong′kus) *n.* [NL., from *haem-* + Gk. *onkos,* barb of an arrow]. A genus of nematode worms infecting sheep and cattle.

Haemonchus con·tor·tus (kon·tor′tus). A species of nematode worm parasitic to sheep and other herbivores throughout the world; occasionally infects man.

For words beginning HAEM... not found here, see HEM... .

Hae·moph·i·lus, He·moph·i·lus (hee·mof′i·lus) *n.* [NL., from *hemo-,* blood, + Gk. *philos,* lover of]. A genus of bacteria consisting of parasitic and often pathogenic pleomorphic, gram-negative, nonmotile rods; generally requiring for growth either hemin (X factor) or nicotinamide adenine dinucleotide (V factor), or both.

Haemophilus ae·gyp·ti·us (e·jip′shee·us). A causative agent of catarrhal conjunctivitis. Syn. *Koch-Weeks bacillus.*

Haemophilus bronchiseptica. *BORDETELLA BRONCHISEPTICA.*

Haemophilus con·junc·ti·vi·ti·dis (kun·junk″ti·vye′ti·dis). *HAEMOPHILUS AEGYPTIUS.*

Haemophilus du·creyi (dew·kray′eye). A species of small, gram-negative bacilli tending to grow in short chains; the cause of chancroid.

Haemophilus gal·li·na·rum (gal″i·nair′um). The causative agent of infectious coryza in chickens.

Haemophilus in·flu·en·zae (in″flew·en′zee). A causatic agent of serious pyogenic infection, especially in children, including meningitis, epiglottitis, bacteremia, pneumonia, arthritis, otitis media, and sinusitis.

Haemophilus influenzae suis. *HAEMOPHILUS SUIS.*

Haemophilus parapertussis. *BORDETELLA PARAPERTUSSIS.*

Haemophilus pertussis. *BORDETELLA PERTUSSIS.*

Haemophilus su·is (sue′is). A species of bacteria which together with a virus produces swine influenza. See also *Glafsser's disease.*

Hae·mo·pro·teus (hee″mo·pro′tee·us) *n.* [*haemo-* + Gk. *Prōteus,* sea god who could change his shape readily]. A genus of intracellular parasites found in the red blood cells of birds.

Hae·mo·spo·rid·ia (hee″mo·spo·rid′ee·uh, hem″o·) *n.pl.* [NL., from *haemo-* + Gk. *spora,* seed]. An order of sporozoa that live for a part of their life cycle within the red blood cells of their hosts. **—haemosporidia,** *com. n. pl.,* sing. **haemosporid·i·um; haemosporid·i·an,** *adj. & n.*

Hae·nel's sign (he^y′nul) [H. *Haenel,* German neurologist, b. 1874]. Analgesia to pressure on the eyeball in tabes dorsalis.

Haenel's variant [H. *Haenel*]. Progressive muscular atrophy affecting only the upper extremities.

Hae·ser's formula or **coefficient** (he^y′zur) [H. *Haeser,* German physician, 1811–1884]. If the last two digits expressing specific gravity of urine are multiplied by 2.33 (Haeser's coefficient), the weight of the urine solids in grains is closely approximated. See also *Trapp's formula.*

Haff disease (ha^hff) [after Königsberg *Haff,* an arm of the Baltic Sea, where the first cases were reported]. A disease characterized by muscular weakness, pain in the limbs, and myoglobinuria; caused by ingestion of fish poisoned by industrial wastes from cellulose factories.

Haff·kine vaccine (^kha^hf′kin) [W. M. W. *Haffkine* (*Khavkin*), Russian bacteriologist in India, 1860–1930]. A vaccine for bubonic plague composed of a 6-week-old culture of *Yersinia pestis,* which is killed by heat and phenol.

haf·ni·um (haf′nee·um) *n.* [*Hafnia,* L. name for Copenhagen]. Hf = 178.49. A lanthanide. See also Table of Elements in the Appendix.

Ha·ge·dorn and Jen·sen's method (hah′ge·dorn, yen′s^en) [H. C. *Hagedorn,* Danish physician, b. 1888; and B. N. *Jensen,* Danish biochemist, 20th century]. A method for determining blood sugar in which protein is precipitated with zinc hydroxide, filtered, and the filtrate used to reduce potassium ferricyanide, the excess of which is determined by adding iodide and titrating the liberated iodine with sodium thiosulfate.

Hagedorn needle [W. *Hagedorn,* German surgeon, 1831–1894]. A curved surgical cutting needle with flat sides.

Hageman factor [after *Hageman,* the person in whom the deficiency was first observed]. FACTOR XII. Abbreviated, HF.

Hageman trait. A recessively inherited trait in which there is an in vitro clotting defect attributable to absence of the Hageman factor (factor XII) but in which there is no clinical hemorrhagic disorder.

H agglutinin. FLAGELLAR AGGLUTININ.

Hag·ner bag [F. R. *Hagner,* U.S. surgeon, 1873–1940]. A water-filled bag attached to a rubber tube, used to control bleeding following suprapubic prostatectomy.

Hahn·e·mann·ism (hah'ne·man·iz·um) *n.* [S. *Hahnemann,* German physician, 1755–1843]. HOMEOPATHY.

Hai·ding·er's brushes (high'ding·ur) [W. K. von *Haidinger,* Austrian mineralogist, 1795–1871]. An entoptic phenomenon in which that portion of a beam of polarized light falling on the macula is perceived as a series of brushes or spokes fanning out in opposite directions from a center, due to the double refracting effect of the nerve fibers radially arranged about the macula. Produced by throwing a blue polarized light on the eye which is looking at a sheet of white paper and in other ways; spinning of the polarized filter between the light source and the eye causes the brushes to wheel around like a revolving propeller, with the hub accurately locating the fovea, thus providing a test for foveal vision.

Hai·ley-Hailey disease [W. H. *Hailey,* U.S. dermatologist, b. 1898; and H. E. *Hailey,* U.S. dermatologist, b. 1909]. FAMILIAL BENIGN PEMPHIGUS.

Haines's test [W. S. *Haines,* U.S. chemist, 1850–1923]. A qualitative test for glucose and other reducing sugars in which a yellow or red precipitate is produced in an alkaline solution of cupric sulfate.

hair, *n.* 1. A keratinized filament growing from the skin of mammals; a modified epidermal structure consisting of a shaft, which is the hair itself, exclusive of its sheaths and papilla, and a root. 2. Collectively, the hairs covering the skin. NA *pili.*

hair ball. TRICHOBEZOAR.

hair bulb. The part of the hair apparatus from which the hair shaft develops.

hair canal. The space in the hair follicle occupied by the hair root.

hair cell. An epithelial cell with delicate, hairlike processes, as that of the spiral organ of Corti, which responds to the stimuli of sound waves, and those of the crista ampullaris, macula utriculi, and macula sacculi, which are concerned with equilibrium.

hairdresser's dermatitis. Contact dermatitis due to the irritating effects of substances used in hair dressing.

hair follicle. An epithelial ingrowth of the dermis that surrounds a hair.

hair germ or **column.** The solid epithelial invagination of the germinal layer of the fetal epidermis that forms the primordium of the hair.

hair glands. The sebaceous glands of hair follicles.

hair matrix tumor. PILOMATRICOMA.

hair papilla. The portion of dermis which projects upward into the center of a hair bulb.

hair root. The portion of a hair found within the hair follicle.

hair shaft. A hair, particularly the portion of it that emerges from the hair follicle. NA *scapus pili.*

hairy cell. A circulating mononuclear cell with many cytoplasmic projections. See also *leukemic reticuloendotheliosis.*

hairy-cell leukemia. LEUKEMIC RETICULOENDOTHELIOSIS.

hairy cyst. A cystic teratoma, especially of the ovary, that contains hair.

hairy heart. COR VILLOSUM.

hairy nevus or **mole.** A pigmented nevus covered with downy or stiff hairs.

hairy tongue. A condition in which the filiform papillae of the tongue hypertrophy and are stained from bacteria and food pigments.

Ha·jek's operation (high'eck) [M. *Hajek,* Austrian otolaryngologist, 1861–1941]. An operation for the relief of frontal sinus disease, in which the anterior wall of the sinus is removed and the frontonasal canal enlarged, with removal of diseased tissue.

hal-, halo- [Gk. *hals, halos,* salt]. A combining form meaning (a) *salt;* (b) *halogen.*

ha·la·tion (hay·lay'shun) *n.* [*halo* + *-ation*]. Blurring of the visual image under a powerful direct light coming from a direction different from the line of vision.

hal·az·e·pam (hal·az'e·pam) *n.* 7-Chloro-1,3-dihydro-5-phenyl-1-(2,2,2-trifluoroethyl)-2*H*-1,4-benzodiazepin-2-one, $C_{17}H_{12}ClF_3N_2O$, a tranquilizer.

hal·a·zone (hal'uh·zone) *n.* *p*-Dichlorosulfamoylbenzoic acid, $C_7H_5Cl_2NO_4S$, a disinfectant for drinking water.

Hal·ber·staedt·er bodies (hal'bur·shtet"ur) [L. *Halberstaedter,* German physician, 1876–1949]. PROWAZEK-HALBERSTAEDTER BODIES.

hal·cin·o·nide (hal·sin'o·nide) *n.* 21-Chloro-9-fluoro-11β, 16α,17-trihydroxypregn-4-ene-3,20-dione cyclic acetal with actone, $C_{24}H_{32}ClFO_5$, an anti-inflammatory.

Halcion. A trademark for triazolam, a sedative-hypnotic.

Hal·dane chamber [J. S. *Haldane,* Scottish physiologist, 1860–1936]. An airtight chamber in which the metabolism of animals may be studied.

Haldane scale [J. S. *Haldane*]. A standard for establishing hemoglobin levels in which 13.8 g in 100 ml of blood equals 100 percent.

Haldol. Trademark for haloperidol, a tranquilizer.

Haldrone. Trademark for paramethasone, an anti-inflammatory adrenocortical steroid used as the 21-acetate ester.

Hale method. A histochemical method for hyaluronic acid based on the combination of hyaluronic acid with iron and the development of a blue color by ferrocyanide.

half-life, *n.* 1. The time required for half of any amount of a substance or property to disappear from a mathematically or physically defined space. 2. *In radiology,* the time in which half of any given amount of a radioactive substance will have undergone transmutation; a constant for any given radioactive isotope. Symbol, $t\frac{1}{2}$. 3. *In pharmacology,* the time required for half the amount of a radioactive or nonradioactive substance or drug introduced into an organism to undergo radioactive decay or to be metabolized or excreted.

half-sib·ling, *n.* An individual who shares one parent with another person but has a different father or mother; a half-brother or half-sister.

half-value layer or **thickness.** *In roentgenology,* the thickness of an absorber which reduces the intensity of a given x-ray or gamma-ray beam to half its initial value.

half·way house. *In psychiatry,* a residence specially structured for mental patients who no longer require full hospitalization but who need some protection and support while adjusting to their return to the community and independent living.

hal·i·but-liver oil. The vitamin A-rich fixed oil from the livers of *Hippoglossus hippoglossus;* has been used for prophylaxis and treatment of vitamin A-deficiency states.

hal·ide (hal'ide, hay'lide) *n.* A binary salt in which a halogen serves as anion.

Halinone. Trademark for bromindione, an anticoagulant drug.

hal·i·ste·re·sis (hal"i·ste·ree'sis) *n.*, pl. **halistere·ses** (·seez) [*hal-* + Gk. *sterēsis,* deprivation]. The loss of lime salts from previously well-calcified bone. —**haliste·ret·ic** (·ret'ick) *adj.*

hal·ite (hal'ite, hay'lite) *n.* [*hal-* + *-ite*]. Rock salt; a native sodium chloride occurring in extensive deposits.

hal·i·to·sis (hal"i·to'sis) *n.*, pl. **halito·ses** (·seez) [L. *halitus,* breath, + *-osis*]. The state of having offensive breath. Syn. *bromopnea, fetor ex ore.*

hal·i·tus (hal'i·tus) *n.* [L.]. An exhalation or vapor, as that expired from the lung.

hal·la·chrome (hal'uh·krome) *n.* 5,6-Dihydro-5,6-dioxo-2-indolinecarboxylic acid, $C_9H_7NO_4$, an intermediate compound in the series of transformations by which tyrosine is converted, through the action of tyrosinase, to the black pigment melanin.

Hal·ler·mann-Streiff-Fran·çois syndrome [W. *Hallermann,* German ophthalmologist, 20th century; E. B. *Streiff;* and J. *François*]. A congenital oculocutaneous disorder characterized by relatively short stature, malformation of the skull, hypoplasia of the mandible, a birdlike profile with beak nose, thin scanty hair of the scalp, eyebrows, and eyelashes, atrophy of the skin, dental anomalies, and ocular abnormalities, including congenital cataracts and microphthalmia; other skeletal defects and moderate mental retardation are frequently associated. Compare *oculodentodigital syndrome.*

Hal·ler's habenula [A. von *Haller,* Swiss physiologist and anatomist, 1708–1777]. The solid cord of cells formed when the canal of the vaginal process of the peritoneum closes; it persists for some time after birth.

Haller's isthmus [A. von *Haller*]. The constriction separating the ventricle from the arterial bulb in the fetal heart.

Hal·ler·vor·den-Spatz disease or **syndrome** (ha^h^l'ur·for''dun, shpa^h^ts) [J. *Hallervorden,* German neurologist, 1882–1965; and H. *Spatz,* German neurologist, 1888–1969]. An inherited (autosomal recessive) disease beginning in late childhood or early adolescence and characterized clinically by a slowly progressive pyramidal and extrapyramidal motor syndrome and dementia. There is intense brown pigmentation of the globus pallidus, substantia nigra, and red nucleus. Microscopically, in these parts, there is a loss of neurons and medullated fibers, swollen axon fragments, and deposits of iron mixed with calcium. Syn. *progressive pallidal degeneration syndrome.*

Hal·lé's point (a^h^l·e^y'^) [A. J. M. N. *Hallé,* French physician, 1859–1947]. *Obsol.* The point on the abdomen where a line connecting the anterior superior iliac spines is intersected by a vertical line from the pubic tubercle; this was supposed to correspond to the point where the ureter crosses the pelvic brim.

hal·lex (hal'ecks) *n.* HALLUX.

Hal·lion's law (a^h^l·yoh^n'^) [L. *Hallion,* French physiologist, 1862–1940]. A principle, no longer accepted, that extracts of an organ have a stimulating effect on that organ.

Hal·lo·peau's disease (a^h^·lo^h^·po') [F. H. *Hallopeau,* French dermatologist, 1842–1919]. ACRODERMATITIS CONTINUA.

Hall's muscle. ISCHIOBULBOSUS.

hal·lu·cal (hal'yoo·kul) *adj.* Pertaining to the hallux, or great toe.

halluces. Plural of *hallux.*

hal·lu·ci·na·tion (ha·lew'si·nay'shun) *n.* [L. *hallucinatio,* from *hallucinari, alucinari,* to wander in mind]. A sensory experience of an object not actually existing in the external world or an alteration in perception, which may be in the auditory, visual, tactile (haptic), olfactory, or gustatory fields or any combination; usually occurring in psychosis, in response to certain drugs and toxic substances, following withdrawal of alcohol and barbiturates, and with diseases of and trauma to the brain, particularly in the temporal lobes and diencephalon and in febrile conditions. Syn. *phantasm, socordia, waking dream.* —**hal·lu·ci·nate** (ha·lew'si·nate) *v.;* **hal·lu·ci·na·tive** (ha·lew'si·nuh·tiv), **hallucina·to·ry** (·to''ree) *adj.*

hal·lu·cino·gen (ha·lew'sin·o·jen, hal''yoo·sin'o·jen) *n.* [*hallucination* + *-gen*]. A drug or substance that produces hallucinations.

hal·lu·ci·no·gen·ic (ha·lew''si·no·jen'ick, hal''yoo·sin''o·jen'ick) *adj.* 1. Pertaining to hallucinogens. 2. Pertaining to any stimuli, such as rapidly revolving and changing colored lights, which create the impression of experiencing a hallucination.

hal·lu·ci·no·sis (ha·lew''si·no'sis) *n.,* pl. **hallucino·ses** (·seez) [*hallucination* + *-osis*]. *In psychiatry,* the condition of experiencing persistent hallucinations, especially while fully conscious.

hal·lux (hal'ucks) *n.,* genit. **hal·lu·cis** (hal'yoo·sis), pl. **hallu·ces** (·seez) [L.] [NA]. GREAT TOE. NA alt. *digitus I.*

hallux flex·us (fleck'sus). A condition allied to and perhaps identical with hammertoe, or flexion of the first phalanx of the great toe. The second phalanx is usually extended upon the first, and there is more or less rigidity of the metatarsophalangeal joint.

hallux rig·i·dus (rij'i·dus). A condition in which there is restriction in the range of motion in the first metatarsophalangeal joint; it is frequently secondary to degenerative joint disease.

hallux val·gus (val'gus). A deformity of the great toe, in which the head of the first metatarsal deviates away from the second metatarsal and the phalanges are deviated toward the second toe, causing undue prominence of the metatarsophalangeal joint. See also *bunion.*

hallux va·rus (vair'us). A deformity of the great toe, in which the head of the first metatarsal deviates toward the second metatarsal and the phalanges are deviated away from the second toe.

hal·ma·to·gen·e·sis (hal''muh·to·jen'e·sis) *n.,* pl. **halmatogene·ses** (·seez) [Gk. *halma,* jump, + *-genesis*]. A sudden change of type from one generation to another.

ha·lo (hay'lo) *n.* [Gk. *halōs,* threshing floor, circle]. 1. *In cytology,* a clear area surrounding the nucleus under certain abnormal conditions, especially in cervical cell smears. 2. A luminous circle seen around lights resulting from edema of the cornea or lens; a symptom of glaucoma. 3. The imprint made on the vitreous humor by the ciliary body of the eye. 4. A ring observed ophthalmoscopically around the macula lutea.

halo-. See *hal-.*

halo·chro·mism (hal''o·kro'miz·um) *n.* [*halo-* + *chrom-* + *-ism*]. The phenomenon of the development of color when certain colorless organic compounds, notably those containing a carbonyl group, are dissolved in acids.

hal·o·fen·ate (hal''o·fen'ate) *n.* (*p*-Chlorophenyl)[(α,α,α-trifluoro-*m*-tolyl)oxy]acetic acid ester with *N*-(2-hydroxyethyl)acetamide, $C_{19}H_{17}ClF_3NO_4$, a uricosuric and antihyperlipidemic.

halo·gen (hal'o·jin) *n.* [*halo-* + *-gen*]. Any one of the nonmetallic elements chlorine, iodine, bromine, and fluorine.

hal·o·gen·ate (hal'o·je·nate) *v.* To combine or treat with a halogen. —**halogen·at·ed** (·nay·tid) *adj.*

hal·oid (hal'oid, hay'loid) *adj.* [*hal-* + *-oid*]. Resembling or derived from a halogen.

ha·lom·e·ter (hay·lom'e·tur) *n.* [Gk. *halōs,* disk, halo, + *-meter*]. An instrument for measuring the mean diameter of erythrocytes by the diffraction areas produced. Syn. *eriometer.*

halo nevus. A pigmented nevus surrounded by a depigmented zone, usually occurring as a part of self-involution of the nevus.

hal·o·per·i·dol (hal''o·perr'i·dol) *n.* 4-[4-(*p*-Chlorophenyl)-4-hydroxypiperidino-4'-fluorobutyrophenone, $C_{21}H_{23}ClFNO_2$, a tranquilizer.

halo·pro·ges·ter·one (hal''o·pro·jes'tur·ohn) *n.* 6α-Fluoro-17α-bromoprogesterone, $C_{21}H_{28}BrFO_2$, a progestational drug.

hal·o·pro·gin (hal''o·pro'jin) *n.* 3-Iodo-2-propynyl 2,4,5-trichlorophenyl ether, $C_9H_4Cl_3IO$, an antimicrobial agent.

halo symptom. The colored circles seen around lights in glaucoma.

Halotestin. A trademark for fluoxymesterone, an anabolic and androgenic steroid.

hal·o·thane (hal'o·thane) *n.* 2-Bromo-2-chloro-1,1,1-trifluoroethane, $C_2HBrClF_3$, a colorless, nonflammable liquid; employed as a general anesthetic, by inhalation.

halothane hepatitis. Acute, idiopathic hepatic central lobular necrosis, often fatal, occurring in the post-anesthetic period after use of halothane or other inhalation anesthetics; prodromal symptoms are low-grade fever and malaise.

hal·quin·ols (hal'kwi·nolz, ·nole'z) *n.* A mixture of 5,7-dichloro-8-quinolinol, 5-chloro-8-quinolinol, and 7-chloro-8-quinolinol obtained by chlorination of 8-quinolinol; a topical anti-infective composition.

Hal·stead tests [W. C. *Halstead,* U.S. psychologist, 20th century]. A series of tests requiring psychologic processes fundamental to practical intelligence, used chiefly to assess the effects of cerebral lesions.

Hal·sted school of surgery [W. S. *Halsted,* U.S. surgeon, 1852–1922]. The body of followers of Halsted's teachings, principles, and practice of operative surgery; exact control of hemorrhage, gentle handling of tissues, use of fine silk in sutures and ligatures, avoidance of tension on sutures, careful and unhurried surgery without shock or wound complications.

Halsted's forceps [W. S. *Halsted*]. 1. A delicate, sharp-pointed hemostat. Syn. *mosquito forceps.* 2. A standard-sized artery forceps with relatively narrow jaws designed to catch blood vessels with precision and with minimal crushing of tissues.

Halsted's inguinal herniorrhaphy [W. S. *Halsted*]. 1. An operation in which the spermatic cord is brought directly through the abdominal wall muscle and placed external to the external oblique aponeurosis. 2. A simple type of inguinal herniorrhaphy in which the spermatic cord is left in place.

Halsted's radical mastectomy [W. S. *Halsted*]. Radical removal of the breast for cancer, together with a wide zone of skin, subcutaneous fat, pectoral muscles, and axillary lymph nodes, en masse; and skin grafting if necessary to avoid tension on the skin flaps in closing the wound.

hal·zoun (hal·zoon) *n.* [Ar. *ḥalazūn,* snail, slug]. Pharyngitis due to parasitization by flukes, leeches, or pentastomes; seen especially in Lebanon, usually as a result of eating raw sheep or goat livers infected with *Fasciola hepatica.* See also *fascioliasis.*

HAM Human albumin microspheres (= HUMAN SERUM ALBUMIN MICROSPHERES).

ham, *n.* [OE., from Gmc. **hamma* (rel. to Gk. *knēmē,* leg, shank)]. 1. The posterior portion of the thigh above the popliteal space and below the buttock. 2. POPLITEAL SPACE. 3. The buttock, hip, and thigh.

Ham·a·dry·as hannah (ham''uh·drye'us). OPHIOPHAGUS HANNAH.

Ham·a·me·lis (ham''uh·mee'lis) *n.* [Gk. *hamamēlis,* medlar]. A genus of small trees or shrubs. *Hamamelis virginiana,* witch hazel, is the source of hamamelis water, or witch hazel water, used as an astringent embrocation.

ha·mar·tia (ha·mahr'shee·uh) *n.* [Gk., fault, from *hamartanein,* to err]. A nodular or localized defect of embryonal development; cells and structures natural to the part are not in normal orderly arrangement, giving rise to a hamartoma.

ha·mar·to·blas·to·ma (ha·mahr''to·blas·to'muh) *n.* [*hamartoma* + *blastoma*]. A neoplasm arising from a hamartoma.

hamartoblastoma of the kidney. WILMS'S TUMOR.

ham·ar·to·ma (ham''ahr·to'muh) *n.*, pl. **hamartomas, hamartoma·ta** (·tuh) [*hamartia* + *-oma*]. A developmental anomaly resulting in the formation of a mass composed of tissues normally present in the locality of the mass, but of improper proportion and distribution with dominance of one type of tissue. **—hamar·tom·a·tous** (·tom'uh·tus, ·to'muh·tus) *adj.*

ha·mar·to·pho·bia (ha·mahr''to·fo'bee·uh, ham''ur·to·) *n.* [Gk. *hamartia*, fault, sin, + *-phobia*]. A morbid fear of error or sin.

ha·mate (hay'mate) *adj. & n.* [L. *hamatus,* from *hamus,* hook]. 1. Hook-shaped. 2. HAMATUM.

hamate bone. HAMATUM.

hamate process. UNCINATE PROCESS OF THE ETHMOID BONE.

ha·ma·tum (ha·may'tum) *n.*, pl. **hama·ta** (·tuh) [L. *hamatus,* hooked]. The most ulnar of the distal row of carpal bones. Syn. *hamate bone.* NA *os hamatum.* See also Table of Bones in the Appendix.

Ha·ma·za·ki-We·sen·berg bodies (hah''mah·zah'kee, vey'zen·behrk) [Y. *Hamazaki,* Japanese physician, 20th century; and W. *Wesenberg,*, German physician, 20th century]. Round, ovoid, or angular acid-fast ceroid particles, 1 to 15 μm in their greatest dimension, found in the peripheral sinuses and macrophages of lymph nodes in some patients with sarcoidosis.

Ham·bur·ger's rule. A rule to determine dosage of medicine for children; specifically, dose = weight of child in kilograms, multiplied by adult dose, divided by 70.

Ha·mil·ton's sign. Long hairs growing on the antitragus of the ear, typical of males with normal androgenic function after the age of 25 or 30.

Ham·man-Rich syndrome [L. V. *Hamman,* U.S. physician, 1877–1946; and A. R. *Rich,* U.S. pathologist, 1893–1968]. Progressive idiopathic diffuse interstitial pulmonary fibrosis, with progressive hypoxia, dyspnea, and right ventricular failure.

Hamman's disease [L. V. *Hamman*]. Spontaneous mediastinal emphysema.

Hamman's sign [L. V. *Hamman*]. A crunching sound, synchronous with cardiac systole, heard on auscultation over the precordium in mediastinal emphysema.

Ham·mar·sten's test (hahm'ar·steyn'') [O. *Hammarsten,* Swedish physiologist, 1841–1932]. A test for globulin in which to a neutral solution magnesium sulfate is added to saturation; if globulin is present, it will be precipitated.

ham·mer, *n.* 1. *In anatomy,* MALLEUS. 2. An instrument for striking.

hammer finger. A flexion deformity of the distal interphalangeal joint of a finger due to avulsion or disruption of the extensor tendon. Compare *mallet finger.*

hammer nose. RHINOPHYMA.

Ham·mer·schlag method (hahm'ur·shlahk) [A. *Hammerschlag,* Austrian physician, 1863–1935]. A test for specific gravity of blood in which the amounts of benzene and chloroform are adjusted until an added drop of blood remains suspended; the specific gravity of the mixture is then determined with a hydrometer.

ham·mer·toe, *n.* A condition of the toe, usually the second, in which the proximal phalanx is extremely extended while the two distal phalanges are flexed.

ham·mock bandage. A bandage that retains scalp dressings. The dressings are covered by a broad strip of gauze brought down over the ears and anchored by a circular bandage around the head. The ends of the broad strip are then turned up over the circular bandage and secured by more turns.

hammock ligament. In embryological tooth development, a layer derived from the dental sac related to the growing end of the root of a tooth; constitutes the primitive periodontal ligament.

Ham·mond's syndrome [W. A. *Hammond,* U.S. neurologist, 1828–1900]. ATHETOSIS.

Hamp·ton technique or **maneuver.** A roentgenologic technique for the detection of a peptic ulcer or other gastroduodenal lesion in the presence of recent bleeding, which involves air-contrast films of the stomach and duodenum with the patient in the left posterior oblique position.

ham·ster, *n.* [Ger.]. A short-tailed rodent with large cheek pouches, belonging to the family Cricetidae. Found in Europe, western Asia, and Africa. It is susceptible to a variety of microorganisms, and is used for laboratory purposes.

ham·string, *n.* & *v.* 1. One of the tendons bounding the ham on the outer and inner side. See also Table of Muscles in the Appendix. 2. To cripple by cutting the hamstring tendons.

hamstring muscles. The biceps femoris, semitendinosus, and semimembranosus collectively.

hamstring reflex. See *external hamstring reflex, internal hamstring reflex.*

hamular process. 1. A hooklike process of bone on the lower extremity of the medial pterygoid plate, around which the tendon of the tensor veli palatini muscle bends. 2. The hooklike termination of the lacrimal crest.

ham·u·lus (ham'yoo·lus) *n.* [L., small hook]. A hook-shaped process, as of the hamatum, of the medial plate of the pterygoid process of the sphenoid bone, and of the osseous cochlea at the cupula (hamulus laminae spiralis). —**hamu·lar** (·lur), **hamu·late** (·late) *adj.*

hamulus la·cri·ma·lis (lack·ri·may'lis) [NA]. The inferior hooklike process of the lacrimal bone.

hamulus la·mi·nae spi·ra·lis (lam'i·nee spye·ray'lis) [NA]. The hooklike upper end of the spiral lamina of the inner ear.

hamulus os·sis ha·ma·ti (os'is ha·may'tye) [NA]. The hooklike process on the palmar aspect of the hamate bone.

hamulus pte·ry·goi·de·us (terr·i·goy'dee·us) [NA]. PTERYGOID HAMULUS.

ha·my·cin (hay·migh'sin) *n.* An antibiotic, produced by *Streptomyces pimprina,* that has antifungal activity.

hand, *n.* The organ of prehension, the part of the upper limb at the end of the forearm, composed of the carpus, metacarpus, and phalanges. NA *manus.*

hand crutch. A crutchlike support in which the weight of the body is partially borne by the hand and arm instead of by the axilla, used mainly in training the individual to use an artificial leg or legs after the usual crutch stage of training is ended. See also *Canadian crutch.*

hand·ed·ness, *n.* 1. The favoring of either the right or the left hand for intricate, complex acts, according to cerebral dominance. 2. CHIRALITY.

hand flexor reflex. WRIST FLEXION REFLEX.

hand-foot-and-mouth disease. A highly infectious illness characterized by a maculopapular and vesicular exanthem of the hands and feet, and enanthem of the oropharynx due to infection with any of several Coxsackie A viruses.

hand·i·cap, *n.* 1. A condition that imposes difficulties on functioning and achievement. 2. A mental or physical disability.

hand·i·craft spasms. OCCUPATION SPASMS.

Hand·ley's method [W. S. *Handley,* English surgeon, 1872–1962]. Drainage of elephantiasis by insertion of long pieces of silk or cotton into the affected parts.

hand·piece, *n.* A device used in connection with the dental engine for engaging such instruments as burs and mandrels during operative procedures; held in the hand of the operator.

hand·print, *n.* The dermatoglyphics of the hand.

Hand-Schül·ler-Chris·tian disease or **syndrome** [A. *Hand,* U.S. pediatrician, 1868–1949; A. *Schüller;* and H. A. *Christian*]. A syndrome of childhood, of unknown cause, insidious in onset and progressive, characterized by exophthalmos, diabetes insipidus, and softened or punched-out areas in the bones, particularly in the femurs and those of the skull, shoulder, and pelvic girdle, and with foci of reticuloendothelial proliferation which may be found in every part of the body. Compare *eosinophilic granuloma, Letterer-Siwe disease.*

hand-shoulder syndrome. SHOULDER-HAND SYNDROME.

hand sign of Brun (brœⁿ) [L. *Brun*]. *Obsol.* Genital grasping by patients (especially children) with vesical stones or foreign bodies to prevent involuntary escape of urine. The hands may become macerated and have a strong ammoniacal odor.

Hanf·mann-Ka·sa·nin concept-formation test. A test providing an opportunity to observe the process of concept formation in a problem-solving situation in which there are 22 blocks in 5 different colors, 6 different shapes, and 2 different widths and heights. The testee must sort these into four groups based on a single sorting principle: tall-wide, tall-narrow, low-wide, and low-narrow.

Hang·er's test [F. M. *Hanger,* Jr., U.S. physician, 1894–1971]. CEPHALIN-CHOLESTEROL FLOCCULATION TEST.

hanging-drop culture. A culture in which the microorganism is inoculated into a drop of fluid on a cover glass and the latter is inverted over a glass slide having a central concavity.

hanging-drop preparation. A preparation using a special slide containing a circular concavity, or a regular slide with a petroleum jelly ring, in which a drop of solution to be examined microscopically can be suspended without spreading over the slide.

hanging septum. A broad alar cartilage abnormally overlying the anterior nasal septum.

hang·nail, *n.* [OE. *angnaegl,* from *ang-,* painful, + *-naegl,* nail, spike]. A partly detached piece of skin of the nail fold, friction against which has caused inflammation.

hang·over, *n.* The disagreeable aftereffects following use of alcohol or of certain drugs, such as barbiturates, in large or excessive doses.

Ha·not's cirrhosis or **disease** (aʰ·no') [V. C. *Hanot,* French physician, 1844–1896]. BILIARY CIRRHOSIS.

han·sen·id (han'se·nid) *n.* [G. H. A. *Hansen,* Norwegian physician, 1841–1912]. TUBERCULOID LEPROSY.

Han·sen's bacillus [G. H. A. *Hansen*]. *MYCOBACTERIUM LEPRAE.*

Hansen's disease [G. H. A. *Hansen*]. LEPROSY.

H antigen. A thermolabile, flagellar antigen that confers type specificity like the capsular polysaccharides.

hap·a·lo·nych·ia (hap"uh·lo·nick'ee·uh) *n.* [Gk. *hapalos,* soft, + *onych-* + *-ia*]. A condition in which the nails are soft, may fold, and split easily. They become atrophied due to defective nail production.

Hapamine. Trademark for a histamine-protein complex used subcutaneously for histamine desensitization.

haph·al·ge·sia (haf"al·jee'zee·uh) *n.* [Gk. *haphē,* touch, + *algesia*]. A sensation of pain experienced upon the mere touching of an object.

haph·e·pho·bia (haf"e·fo'bee·uh) *n.* [Gk. *haphē,* touch, + *-phobia*]. A morbid fear of being touched or having to touch objects. Syn. *haptephobia.*

hapl-, haplo- [Gk. *haploos*]. A combining form meaning (a) *single;* (b) *simple.*

hap·lo·dont (hap'lo·dont) *adj.* [*hapl-* + *-odont*]. *In biology,* having or pertaining to molar teeth having simple or single crowns.

hap·loid (hap'loid) *adj.* [Gk. *haploeidēs,* single, simple]. Having the reduced number of chromosomes, as in mature germ cells, as distinguished from the diploid or full number of chromosomes in normal somatic cells.

hap·lo·my·co·sis (hap"lo·migh·ko'sis) *n.* A mycotic infection of wild animals caused by the fungus *Emmonsia parva* (*Haplosporangium parvum*).

ha·plo·pia (ha·plo'pee·uh) *n.* [*hapl-* + *-opia*]. Single vision. Contr. *diplopia.*

hap·lo·scope (hap'lo·skope) *n.* [*haplo-* + *-scope*]. An instrument for measuring the visual axes.

Hap·lo·spo·ran·gi·um parvum (hap"lo·spo·ran'jee·um pahr'vum). *Obsol.* *EMMONSIA PARVA.*

happy-puppet syndrome. A congenital syndrome of unknown cause characterized by severe retardation of psychomotor development, prognathism, brachycephaly, a horizontal occipital depression, certain ocular features, easily provoked and prolonged paroxysms of laughter, ataxic jerky movements like those of a puppet, and seizures, especially infantile spasms associated with slow wave-and-spike activity in the electroencephalogram but not hypsarrhythmia.

hapt-, hapto- [Gk. *haptein,* to fasten, bind, grasp, feel]. A combining form meaning (a) *contact, touch;* (b) *binding, attaching.*

hap·ten (hap'ten) *n.* [Ger., from Gk. *haptein,* to bind, grasp]. A low-molecular-weight substance which reacts with a specific antibody but which by itself is unable to elicit the formation of that antibody. It is antigenic (immunogenic) if coupled to an antigenic carrier. —**hap·ten·ic** (hap·ten'ick) *adj.*

hap·tene (hap'teen) *n.* HAPTEN.

hap·te·pho·bia (hap"te·fo'bee·uh) *n.* [Gk. *haptein,* to grasp, to touch, + *-phobia*]. HAPHEPHOBIA.

hap·tic (hap'tick) *adj.* [Gk. *haptikos*]. Pertaining to the sense of touch; tactile.

hap·tics (hap'ticks) *n.* The branch of psychology dealing with the sense of touch.

hapto-. See *hapt-.*

hap·to·dys·pho·ria (hap"to·dis·fo'ree·uh) *n.* [*hapto-* + *dysphoria*]. The disagreeable sensation sometimes aroused by touching certain objects, such as nylon or fine sandpaper.

hap·to·glo·bin (hap'to·glo"bin) *n.* [*hapto-* + *globin*]. A hemoglobin-binding α_2-globulin of serum, which occurs in at least three different antigenic types.

hap·to·phore (hap'to·fore) *n.* [*hapto-* + *-phore*]. Ehrlich's term for the specific molecular group by which antibodies become attached to the corresponding group of the antigen.

Ha·ra·da's syndrome [E. *Harada,* Japanese, 20th century]. UVEOMENINGOENCEPHALITIS.

hard chancre. The primary lesion of syphilis, a painless papule, usually indurated, which becomes eroded and, histologically, demonstrates mononuclear and histiocytic infiltrates with obliterative endarteritis and periarteritis of small vessels. Syn. *primary sore.*

Har·den-Young ester. FRUCTOSE 1,6-DIPHOSPHATE.

Har·de·ri·an gland (hahr·deer'ee·un) [J. J. *Harder,* Swiss anatomist, 1656–1711]. A racemose gland at the inner canthus of the eye in vertebrates, especially in those having a well-developed nictitating membrane.

Har·der's gland. HARDERIAN GLAND.

Har·ding-Pas·sey melanoma. A transmissible malignant melanoma that arose spontaneously in a noninbred mouse.

hard·ness, *n. In radiology,* a quality of roentgen rays; increased hardness is associated with increased penetrating power, greater energy, and shorter wavelength.

hard-of-hearing, *adj.* Partially deaf.

hard pad. A disease of dogs, probably associated with the canine distemper virus; often characterized by encephalitis and hardening of the foot pads.

hard palate. The anterior part of the palate which is formed by the palatal processes of the maxillary bones and the palatine bones with their covering mucous membranes. NA *palatum durum.*

hard radiation. Radiation with hard rays.

hard rays. Roentgen rays of short wavelength, and with high energy and ability to penetrate deeply, emitted from a tube operated at a high voltage. Contr. *soft rays.*

hard soap. A soap made with sodium hydroxide; a white solid in the form of bars, or a white or yellowish white fine powder.

hard sore. HARD CHANCRE.

hard·ware disease. Traumatic results of the ingestion of hardware or other metal objects in cattle.

hard water. Water containing soluble calcium or magnesium salts and not readily forming a lather with soap.

Har·dy-Wein·berg equilibrium. The condition in which allele frequencies do not change from generation to generation in the absence of mutation, selection, nonrandom mating, and small population size.

hare·lip, *n.* A congenital cleft, or clefts, in the upper lip, resulting from a failure of the union of the maxillary and median nasal processes which may be bilateral and sometimes involves the maxilla and palate. Syn. *cheiloschisis.*

harelip suture. TRANSFIXION SUTURE.

hare's eye. LAGOPHTHALMOS.

Hare's syndrome [E. S. *Hare,* English surgeon, 1812–1838]. PANCOAST SYNDROME.

Har·kins' method [H. N. *Harkins,* U.S. surgeon, b. 1905]. In burn shock, the administration of 100 ml plasma for every point by which the hematocrit exceeds 45.

har·le·quin color-change syndrome (hahr'le·kwin, ·kin). HARLEQUIN SIGN.

harlequin fetus. ICHTHYOSIS CONGENITA.

harlequin sign. A sign of transient vasomotor disturbance in young infants; there is flushing of the body on the dependent side and pallor of the upward side.

harlequin snake. CORAL SNAKE.

Har·ley's disease [G. *Harley,* English physician, 1829–1896]. PAROXYSMAL HEMOGLOBINURIA.

har·mine (hahr'meen, ·min) *n.* An alkaloid, $C_{13}H_{12}N_2O$, from wild rue; chemically identical with banisterine from *Banisteria caapi.* Has been used for treatment of encephalitis lethargica.

Harmonyl. Trademark for deserpidine, a tranquilizing and hypotensive alkaloid from *Rauwolfia canescens.*

har·paxo·pho·bia (hahr"pack·so·fo'bee·uh) *n.* [Gk. *harpax,* robber, + *-phobia*]. An abnormal fear of robbers.

Har·ring·ton's operation [S. W. *Harrington,* U.S. surgeon, b. 1889]. Temporary left phrenic nerve interruption by crushing; used in repair of diaphragmatic hernia.

Har·ris and Ben·edict standards. Multiple prediction equations and tables based on a statistical study of the available data for the basal metabolism of normal men and women.

Har·ri·son Narcotic Act [F. B. *Harrison,* U.S. Representative from New York, 1873–1957]. The federal law regulating the possession, sale, purchase, and prescription of habit-forming drugs.

Harrison's groove [E. *Harrison,* English physician, 1766–1838]. A groove or sulcus extending from the xiphoid process laterally and corresponding to the attachment of the diaphragm; seen in rickets.

Harrison spot test. A test for bilirubin in urine in which urine and barium chloride are mixed and dried on filter paper, and a drop of Fouchet's reagent is added. A green color indicates the presence of bilirubin, which is oxidized to biliverdin.

Har·ris's hematoxylin [D. L. *Harris,* U.S. pathologist, 1875–1956]. A nuclear staining fluid prepared by mixing an alcoholic solution of hematoxylin with an aqueous solution of ammonium alum and ripening by boiling with mercuric oxide.

Har·row·er-Erick·son test [Mollie R. *Harrower-Erickson,* U.S. psychologist, b. 1906]. A modification of the Rorschach test, utilizing a checklist upon which are printed three groups of 10 possible responses to each of the 10 cards.

Hart·ley-Krau·se operation (kraow'zuh) [F. *Hartley,* U.S. surgeon, 1856–1913; and F. *Krause,* German surgeon, 1857–1937]. Intracranial fifth nerve neurectomy for relief of trigeminal neuralgia.

Hart·man·nel·la (hahrt'mun·el"uh) *n.* A genus of nonparasitic, free-living amebas, commonly found in soil and water. Some varieties are pathogenic for the central nervous system of mammals. This organism was formerly incriminated in human meningoencephalitis on the basis of the morphological appearance of the trophozoites, but on culture these cases have proved to be due to an ameboflagellate, *Naegleria fowleri.*

Hartmannella cas·tel·lan·ii (kas"te·lan'ee·eye). A nonparasitic soil ameba that is associated with central nervous system infections.

Hartmannella hy·a·li·na (high·uh·lye′nuh). A species of ameba found in the feces of man.

Hart·mann's fossa (art·mahn′) [H. *Hartmann,* French surgeon, 1860–1952]. A small infundibular fossa of the peritoneum near the mesoappendix.

Hart·mann's pouch (hart′mahn) [R. *Hartmann,* German anatomist, 1831–1893]. A dilatation of the neck of the gallbladder.

Hartmann's solution [A. F. *Hartmann,* U.S. pediatrician, 1898–1964]. LACTATED RINGER'S INJECTION.

Hart·nup disease [*Hartnup,* the first reported family so affected]. A hereditary metabolic disorder in which there is defective intestinal absorption and renal tubular reabsorption of monoamino-monocarboxylic acids, with indicanuria resulting from the bacterial conversion to indole of tryptophan reaching the colon in large amounts; usually manifested by short stature, and clinically by a pellagra-like dermatitis on exposure to sunlight, episodic and reversible ataxia, nystagmus and sometimes pyramidal tract signs, transient psychiatric disorders, and often mild mental retardation; thought to be transmitted as a homozygous autosomal recessive trait. Syn. *H disease.*

harts·horn, *n.* 1. Cornu cervi, the horn of a stag; formerly a source of ammonia, or hartshorn spirit. 2. Popularly, ammonia water. 3. AMMONIUM CARBONATE.

har·vest fever. Leptospirosis affecting field workers.

harvest mite. *EUTROMBICULA ALFREDDUGESI.*

Häser. See *Haeser.*

Ha·shi·mo·to's disease [H. *Hashimoto,* Japanese surgeon, 1881–1934]. STRUMA LYMPHOMATOSA.

hash·ish, hash·eesh (hash′eesh, ha·sheesh′) *n.* [Ar. *ḥashīsh,* grass, hashish]. The pure resinous exudate of the female hemp plant, *Cannabis sativa,* prepared as a tincture and formerly used in medicine, or prepared as a hardened resin and smoked or eaten as an intoxicant and mild hallucinogen. See also *cannabis.*

Has·kins test. OSGOOD-HASKINS TEST.

Has·ner's valve (hahs′nur) [J. R. von *Hasner,* Bohemian ophthalmologist, 1819–1902]. LACRIMAL FOLD.

Has·sall-Hen·le warts [A. H. *Hassall,* English physician, 1817–1894; and F. G. J. *Henle*]. Nodular hyalin thickenings at the periphery of Descemet's membrane, found increasingly after the age of twenty years.

Hassall's body or **corpuscle** [A. H. *Hassall*]. THYMIC CORPUSCLE.

hatch·et face. MYOPATHIC FACIES.

Hau·dek's niche (haow′deck) [M. *Haudek,* Austrian roentgenologist, 1880–1931]. A sign for gastric ulcer, where contrast material fills the ulcer crater and protrudes from the stomach contour on roentgenologic examination.

haunch, *n.* [OF. *hanche*]. The part of the body which includes the hip and the buttock of one side.

Haus·ser method. HADEN-HAUSSER METHOD.

haustra co·li (ko′lye) [NA]. The sacculation of the colon caused by colonic muscle contraction.

haus·tra·tion (haw·stray′shun) *n.* 1. HAUSTRUM. 2. The formation of a haustrum.

haus·trum (haw′strum) *n.*, pl. **haus·tra** (·truh) [L., bucket, scoop]. One of the pouches or sacculations of the colon. —**haus·tral** (·trul) *adj.*

haut mal (o′ mahl′) [F., lit., high illness]. GENERALIZED SEIZURE.

Ha·ver·hill fever [after *Haverhill,* Mass., where in 1926 the disease occurred in epidemic form and was attributed to contaminated milk]. An acute infection due to *Streptobacillus moniliformis,* usually acquired by rat bite, and characterized by acute onset, intermittent fever, erythematous rash, and polyarthritis. Syn. *erythema arthriticum epidemicum, streptobacillary fever.*

Ha·vers' glands [C. *Havers,* English anatomist, 1650–1702]. Aggregates of fat sometimes seen in the synovial fringes of joints.

ha·ver·sian (ha·vur′zhun, hay·) *adj.* Described by or associated with Clopton Havers, English anatomist, 1650–1702.

haversian canal. Any one of the canals penetrating the compact substance of bone in a longitudinal direction and anastomosing with one another by transverse or oblique branches. They contain blood vessels and connective tissue. NA *canalis nutricius.*

haversian glands. HAVERS' GLANDS.

haversian lamella. One of the thin concentric layers of bone surrounding a haversian canal.

haversian system. The concentric layers of bone about a haversian canal; concentric lamellar system. See also *osteon.*

hawk, *v.* To clear the throat by a forcible expiration.

Haw·ley appliance. An orthodontic device used to effect minor movements of teeth or to retain teeth in a stable position following orthodontic treatment.

Haxt·hau·sen's disease (hahkst′haow·zen) [H. *Haxthausen,* German, 1892–1958]. KERATODERMA CLIMACTERICUM.

hay bacillus. *BACILLUS SUBTILIS.*

Ha·yem's corpuscle (a·yem′) [G. *Hayem,* French physician, 1841–1933]. ACHROMACYTE.

Hayem's solution [G. *Hayem*]. A solution of mercuric chloride, anhydrous sodium sulfate, and sodium chloride in water; used as a diluent for erythrocyte counting.

Hayem-Wi·dal syndrome (vee·dahl′) [G. *Hayem* and G. F. I. *Widal*]. ACQUIRED HEMOLYTIC ANEMIA.

hay fever. A seasonal form of allergic rhinitis characterized by sneezing, rhinorrhea, itching of the eyes, and lacrimation; attributed to pollen antigens in the air.

Hay·garth's nodes [J. *Haygarth,* English physician, 1740–1827]. Joint swellings or nodules in rheumatoid arthritis.

Haynes' operation [I. S. *Haynes,* U.S. surgeon, 1861–1946]. Drainage of the cisterna magna for acute suppurative meningitis.

Hb 1. An abbreviation for *hemoglobin.* 2. A symbol for reduced hemoglobin.

HBD Abbreviation for *α-hydroxybutyric dehydrogenase.*

HbO_2 Symbol for oxyhemoglobin.

Hb SC disease. Hemoglobin SC disease: SICKLE CELL–HEMOGLOBIN C DISEASE.

Hb SS disease. Homozygous hemoglobin S disease: SICKLE CELL ANEMIA.

HCG Human chorionic gonadotropin.

H chain. HEAVY CHAIN.

h. d. Abbreviation for *hora decubitus,* at the hour of going to bed.

H disease. HARTNUP DISEASE.

H disk. HENSEN'S DISK.

He Symbol for helium.

head, *n.* [OE. *hēafod*←Gmc. **haubud-* (rel. to L. *caput*)]. 1. The uppermost part of the body, containing the brain, organs of sight, smell, taste, hearing, and part of the organs of speech. NA *caput.* See also Plates 3, 8, 10, 11. 2. The top, beginning, or most prominent part of anything.

head·ache, *n.* Pain in the head. Syn. *cephalalgia.* See also *migraine.*

headache crystals. MENTHOL.

head-bending test. A test for irritation of the meninges or the nerve roots. The test is positive if the patient feels pain or resists flexion when the head is bent forward. The location of the pain indicates grossly the area affected.

head cap. The collapsed acrosomal vesicle that forms a double-layered cap over the anterior two-thirds of the nucleus of developing spermatids.

head cavity. One of three specialized somites in the head region of lower vertebrate embryos that give rise to the somatic eye muscles; in man, represented only by a mesenchymal blastema.

head circumference. OCCIPITOFRONTAL CIRCUMFERENCE.

head-dropping test. With the patient supine and relaxed, the examiner lifts the head suddenly and allows it to drop. In the normal person, the head falls quickly; in a patient with parkinsonism the rigidity affecting the flexor muscles of the neck cause the head to drop slowly; with meningeal irritation, there is resistance to and pain on flexion of the neck.

head fold. A ventral fold formed by rapid growth of the head of the embryo over the embryonic disk, resulting in the formation of the foregut accompanied by anteroposterior reversal of the anterior part of the embryonic disk.

head gut. FOREGUT.

head kidney. PRONEPHROS.

head locking. The entanglement of the heads of twins at the time of birth.

head louse. The louse *Pediculus humanus capitis,* a vector of disease and the cause of pediculosis capitis.

head myotome. One of the specialized head somites present in many vertebrate embryos that give rise to the extrinsic muscles of the eyeball.

head nurse. A nurse who is in charge of a ward or division of a hospital.

head of the epididymus. The superior extremity of the epididymus.

head process. The notochord or notochordal plate formed as an axial outgrowth of the primitive node.

head retraction reflex. A test for bilateral corticospinal tract lesions above the cervical cord. The patient relaxes with the head slightly forward. The test is positive if the head is quickly retracted when the middle part of the upper lip is tapped with the reflex hammer.

Head's areas or **zones** [H. *Head,* English neurologist, 1861–1940]. The segments of skin exhibiting reflex hyperesthesia and hyperalgesia due to disease of the viscera. See also *viscerosensory reflex.*

head traction. Traction exerted upon the head, usually employed in the treatment of injuries of the cervical spine.

heal·er, *n.* 1. One who effects cures. 2. A Christian Science practitioner. 3. A person without formal medical education who claims to cure by some form of suggestion.

heal·ing, *n.* The process or act of getting well or of making whole; the restoration of diseased parts; curing. —**heal,** *v.*

healing by first intention. The primary union of a wound when the incised skin edges are approximated and so held and union takes place without the process of granulation.

healing by second intention. The process of wound closure where the edges remain separated; the wound becomes closed after granulation tissue has filled the cavity to the skin level so that epithelium can grow over the unhealed area.

health, *n.* 1. The state of dynamic equilibrium between the organism and its environment which maintains the structural and functional integrity of the organism within the normal limits for the particular form of life (race, genus, species) and the particular phase of its life cycle. 2. The state of being sound in body and mind; well-being. —**health·ful, healthy** *adj.*

health consumer. A recipient of health services.

health maintenance organization. A public or private organization which provides health services, including minimum emergency treatment, inpatient hospital and physician care, ambulatory physician care, and outpatient preventive medicine, to subscribers for a prepaid fee. Abbreviated, HMO

health physics. The study and practice of various methods of protection from the undesirable effects of ionizing radiation.

health provider. An individual who performs health services.

hear·ing, *n.* 1. The special sense by which sounds are perceived. 2. The process of perceiving sounds.

hearing aid. An instrument that amplifies the intensity of sound waves, used by persons with impaired hearing.

hearing loss. Impairment of ability to hear, sometimes only within certain frequency ranges.

hearing test. Any method of assessing auditory function, as by audiometry or tuning fork testing.

heart, *n.* [Gmc. **hert-* (rel. to Gk. *kard-* and to L. *cord-*)]. A hollow muscular organ in the thorax which functions as a pump to maintain the circulation of the blood. NA *cor.* See also Plate 5.

heart·beat, *n.* The throb or pulsation of the heart with each ventricular systole.

heart block. Any partial or complete interruption in the transmission of the activation process from the sinoatrial node to the ventricular myocardium; especially, ATRIOVENTRICULAR BLOCK. See also *bundle branch block, intra-atrial block.*

heart·burn, *n.* A burning sensation over the precordium or beneath the sternum, usually from the esophagus; gastric pyrosis.

heart catheter. CARDIAC CATHETER.

heart failure. 1. The condition in which the heart is no longer able to pump an adequate supply of blood in relation to venous return and to meet the metabolic needs of body tissues. See also *backward failure, forward failure.* 2. CONGESTIVE HEART FAILURE. 3. CIRCULATORY FAILURE.

heart-failure cell. A macrophage containing hemosiderin granules found in the pulmonary alveoli and stroma of the lung in certain cardiac diseases.

heart-lung preparation. An experimental preparation in which the right atrium of an animal is perfused by a reservoir to which the flow of the ascending aorta is returned, thus isolating the circulation of the heart and lungs.

heart murmur. CARDIAC MURMUR.

heart rate. The number of ventricular contractions per minute.

heart sac. PERICARDIUM.

heart sounds. The sounds produced by normal hemodynamic events heard on auscultation over the heart; the first and second heart sounds are related to closure of the atrioventricular and semilunar valves, respectively, as well as to ventricular systole; the third and fourth are softer, often inaudible, and are related to the early rapid (passive) phase of ventricular filling, and the late (presystolic) active phase produced by atrial contraction, respectively.

heart tamponade. CARDIAC TAMPONADE.

heart·wa·ter disease. A tick-borne disease of ruminants seen in South Africa; due to *Cowdria ruminantium* and characterized by serous exudate in the pericardium.

heart·worm, *n.* *DIROFILARIA IMMITIS.*

heat, *n.* 1. A form of kinetic energy communicable from one body to another by conduction, convection, or radiation; it is that form of molecular motion which is appreciated by a special thermal sense. 2. The periodic sexual excitement in animals. Compare *estrus, rut.*

heat and acid test. A test for protein in urine in which urine is boiled in a test tube for 1 or 2 minutes and then 3 to 5 drops of 5% acetic acid are added. A white precipitate indicates protein.

heat balance. The relation of the amount of heat produced in the body to that which is lost.

heat capacity. The amount of heat necessary to raise the temperature of a body from 15° to 16°C.

heat cramps. Painful voluntary-muscle spasm and cramps following strenuous exercise, usually in persons in good physical condition, due to sodium chloride and water loss from excessive sweating.

heat-curing resin. Resin whose polymerization requires the use of external heat. Contr. *activated resin.*

heat exhaustion, collapse, or **prostration.** A heat-exposure syndrome characterized by weakness, vertigo, headache, nausea, and peripheral vascular collapse, usually precipitated by physical exertion in a hot environment.

heat pyrexia. HEATSTROKE.

heat rash. MILIARIA.

heat-ray cataract. A slowly progressing posterior cortical lens opacity due to prolonged exposure to high temperatures, sometimes seen in persons engaged in the glass-blowing or iron-puddling industries.

heat-regulating centers. Centers in the hypothalamus for the control of heat production and heat elimination and for regulating the relation of these.

heat·stroke, *n.* A heat-exposure syndrome characterized by hyperpyrexia and prostration due to diminution or cessation of sweating, occurring most commonly in persons with underlying disease. See also *sunstroke.*

heat therapy. The treatment of disease with heat by means of hot baths, shortwave electric fields, heat lamps, hot-air cabinets.

heaves, *n.* 1. Chronic diffuse alveolar emphysema of the horse, characterized by difficult and laborious respiration. Syn. *broken wind.* 2. Retching or vomiting.

heavy, *adj.* 1. Of substances: high in density or specific gravity. 2. Of elements: high in atomic weight. 3. Of isotopes: higher in atomic weight than the most common or stable isotope.

heavy chain. Any of the polypeptide subunits (molecular weight 50,000 to 70,000) of immunoglobulin molecules which determine the distinctive properties of each immunoglobulin class and which are classified, depending on the immunoglobulin molecule in which they occur, as alpha chains (IgA), gamma chains (IgG), delta chains (IgD), epsilon chains (IgE), or mu chains (IgM). Contr. *light chain.*

heavy chain disease. Any of several lymphocyte dyscrasias in which globulins composed of heavy polypeptide chains are found in serum and urine; clinically the symptoms mimic malignant lymphoma. Syn. *Fc fragment disease.*

heavy hydrogen. DEUTERIUM. See also *heavy water.*

heavy magnesia. A high-density magnesium oxide, prepared by ignition of heavy magnesium carbonate.

heavy meromyosin. The larger of the two fragments obtained from the muscle protein myosin following limited proteolysis by trypsin or chymotrypsin. Contr. *light meromyosin.*

heavy water. Water that contains double-weight atoms of hydrogen (deuterium) instead of ordinary (lightweight) hydrogen atoms. Syn. *deuterium oxide.*

he·be·phre·nia (hee″be·free′nee·uh) *n.* [Gk. *hēbē,* youth, + *-phrenia*]. HEBEPHRENIC TYPE OF SCHIZOPHRENIA. —**hebe·phren·ic** (·fren′ick) *adj.*

hebephrenic type of schizophrenia. A form of schizophrenia marked by disorganized thinking, mannerisms, and regressive behavior caricaturing that seen in some adolescents, such as silliness, unpredictable giggling, and posturing; delusions and hallucinations, if present, are not well organized and are transient. Syn. *pubescent insanity.*

Heb·er·den-Ro·sen·bach node [W. *Heberden,* Sr., English physician, 1710–1801; and O. *Rosenbach*]. HEBERDEN'S NODE.

Heberden's arthritis [W. *Heberden*]. Degenerative joint disease of the terminal joints of the fingers, producing enlargement (Heberden's nodes) and flexion deformities. Most common in older women; prominent hereditary pattern.

Heberden's disease. 1. HEBERDEN'S ARTHRITIS. 2. ANGINA PECTORIS.

Heberden's node [W. *Heberden*]. Nodose deformity of the fingers in degenerative joint disease. Syn. *Heberden-Rosenbach node.*

he·bet·ic (he·bet′ick) *adj.* [Gk. *hēbētikos,* from *hēbē,* youth]. Relating to, or occurring at, puberty or adolescence.

heb·e·tude (heb′e·tewd) *n.* [L. *hebetudo,* from *hebes, hebetis,* blunt, dull]. Dullness of the special senses and intellect. —**heb·e·tu·di·nous** (heb″e·tew′di·nus) *adj.*

he·bos·te·ot·o·my (he·bos″tee·ot′uh·mee) *n.* [Gk. *hēbē,* pubes, + *osteotomy*]. PUBIOTOMY.

he·bot·o·my (he·bot′uh·mee) *n.* [Gk. *hēbē,* pubes, + *-tomy*]. PUBIOTOMY.

He·bra's pityriasis (heʸ′brah) [F. von *Hebra,* Austrian dermatologist, 1816–1880]. EXFOLIATIVE DERMATITIS.

hec·a·ter·om·er·al (heck″uh·tur·om′ur·ul) *adj.* HECATEROMERIC.

hec·a·ter·o·mer·ic (heck″uh·tur·o·merr′ick) *adj.* [Gk. *hekateros,* each of two, + *mer-* + *-ic*]. Having processes that divide into two parts; as a neuron, with one process going to each side of the spinal cord.

hec·a·to·mer·ic (heck″uh·to·merr′ick) *adj.* HECATEROMERIC.

Hecht-Schlaer adaptometer. A low-brightness adaptometer for measuring the dark-adaptation process of the eyes and indicating both cone and rod function under controlled conditions.

hect-, hecto- [Gk. *hekaton*]. A combining form meaning *one hundred.*

hec·tic (heck′tick) *adj.* [Gk. *hektikos,* habitual; consumptive]. 1. Of a fever: recurring daily and tending to rise in the afternoon, as in tuberculosis or septicemia. 2. Consumptive, tuberculous.

hecto-. See *hect-.*

hec·to·gram (heck′to·gram) *n.* [*hecto-* + *gram*]. One hundred grams, or 1,543.2349 grains. Abbreviated, hg. See also Tables of Weights and Measures in the Appendix.

hec·to·li·ter (heck′to·lee″tur) *n.* [*hecto-* + *liter*]. One hundred liters; equal to 22 imperial or 26.4 United States gallons. Abbreviated, hl. See also Tables of Weights and Measures in the Appendix.

hec·to·me·ter (heck′to·mee″tur) *n.* [*hecto-* + *meter*]. One hundred meters, or 328 feet 1 inch. Abbreviated, hm. See also Tables of Weights and Measures in the Appendix.

Hed·blom's syndrome [C. A. *Hedblom,* U.S. surgeon, 20th century]. Acute primary diaphragmitis.

he·de·o·ma (hee″dee·o′muh, hed″ee·) *n.* [NL., perhaps from Gk. *hēdys,* sweet, + *osmē,* odor]. The leaves and tops of *Hedeoma pulegioides,* the American pennyroyal, which contains a volatile oil; has been used as a carminative.

hedge hyssop. GRATIOLA.

he·do·nia (he·do′nee·uh) *n.* [Gk. *hēdonē,* pleasure, + *-ia*]. Abnormal cheerfulness; AMENOMANIA (2).

he·don·ism (hee′dun·iz·um) *n.* [Gk. *hēdonē,* pleasure, + *-ism*]. 1. The philosophy in which the attainment of pleasure and happiness is the supreme good. 2. *In psychology and psychiatry,* the doctrine that every act is motivated by the desire for pleasure or the aversion from pain and unpleasantness.

he·do·no·pho·bia (hee″duh·no·fo′bee·uh) *n.* [Gk. *hēdonē,* pleasure, + *-phobia*]. An abnormal fear of pleasure.

Hedulin. A trademark for phenindione, an anticoagulant drug.

heel, *n.* The hinder part of the human foot below the ankle.

heel cord. CALCANEAL TENDON.

heel fly. A warble fly of the genus *Hypoderma.*

heel-knee test. HEEL-TO-KNEE-TO-TOE TEST.

heel spur. CALCANEAL SPUR.

heel-to-knee-to-toe test. A test for nonequilibratory coordination in which the patient is asked to place the heel of one foot on the opposite knee, then push the heel along the shin to the big toe. Normally, this is done smoothly and accurately.

Heer·fordt's di·sease or **syndrome** [C. F. *Heerfordt,* Danish ophthalmologist, b. 1871]. UVEOPAROTID FEVER.

Hef·ke-Tur·ner sign [H. W. *Hefke,* U. S. radiologist, b. 1871; and V. C. *Turner,* U. S. surgeon, 20th century]. OBTURATOR SIGN.

He·gar's sign (heʸ′gar) [Alfred *Hegar,* German gynecologist, 1830–1914]. Softening of the isthmic portion of the uterus which occurs at about six weeks of gestation in pregnancy.

he·gem·o·ny (he·jem′uh·nee) *n.* [Gk. *hēgemonia,* from *hēgem-*

on, guide, leader]. Leadership, domination; as the supremacy of one function over a number of others.

Heg·glin anomaly. MAY-HEGGLIN ANOMALY.

Hei·den·hain cells (high'dᵉn·hine) [R. P. H. *Heidenhain,* German physiologist, 1834–1897]. The enterochromaffin cells of the gastric mucosa.

Heidenhain pouch [R. P. H. *Heidenhain*]. A vagally denervated gastric pouch, separated from the remainder of the stomach, having an external fistula; used for experimental study of gastric secretion.

Heidenhain's iron hematoxylin [H. *Heidenhain,* German histologist, 1864–1949]. Mordanting in iron alum solution followed by staining in fresh or ripened hematoxylin solution and differentiation to the desired point with microscopic control in iron alum solutions.

height-breadth index of the nose. *In somatometry,* the ratio of the width of the nose, taken between the two alaria, or the points of farthest lateral projection of the nose, to the height of the nose, taken between nasion and subnasal point, X 100. Its values are classified as:

hyperleptorrhine	x–54.9
leptorrhine	55.0–69.9
mesorrhine	70.0–84.9
chamaerrhine	85.0–99.9
hyperchamaerrhine	100.0–x

height index. LENGTH-HEIGHT INDEX.

height of contour. An imaginary line encircling the crown of a tooth which passes the surface points of greatest radius.

Heim-Krey·sig sign (hime, krye'zikh) [E. L. *Heim,* German physician, 1747–1834; and F. L. *Kreysig,* German physician, 1770–1839]. Intercostal retraction with each cardiac systole; a sign of adherent pericarditis.

Heim·lich maneuver [Henry J. *Heimlich,* U.S. surgeon, 20th century]. The abrupt application of upward pressure to the upper abdomen, used as a technique for explusion of a choking object from the windpipe.

Hei·ne·ke-Mi·ku·licz operation (high'ne·keʰ, mee'koo·litch) [W. H. *Heineke,* German surgeon, 1834–1901; and J. von *Mikulicz*-Radecki, German surgeon, 1850–1905]. An operation to enlarge the pyloric lumen. The pylorus is opened by a short longitudinal incision which is then closed transversely. A type of pylorotomy.

Hei·ne-Me·din disease (high'neʰ, muh·deen') [J. von *Heine,* German orthopedist, 1800–1879; and K. O. *Medin,* Swedish physician, 1847–1927]. PARALYTIC SPINAL POLIOMYELITIS.

Hei·ner's syndrome [D. C. *Heiner,* U. S. pediatrician, b. 1925]. A syndrome of early infancy, characterized by chronic pulmonary disease, iron-deficiency anemia, recurrent diarrhea, and failure to thrive in the presence of precipitating serum antibodies against cow's milk.

Heinz bodies [R. *Heinz,* German physician, 1865–1924]. Refractile areas in red cells, probably representing denatured globin or methemoglobin; seen in hemolytic anemia due to toxic agents.

Heinz-Ehrlich bodies [R. *Heinz* and P. *Ehrlich*]. HEINZ BODIES.

Heis·ter's valve (high'stur) [L. *Heister,* German anatomist, 1683–1758]. The spiral valve of the cystic duct.

Hek·to·en's phenomenon [L. *Hektoen,* U.S. pathologist, 1863–1951]. Nonspecific stimulation of antibodies concerned with remote infections by antigens injected in allergic states.

HeLa cells (hee'luh) [acronym for the name of the patient involved]. A strain of cells derived from a human carcinoma of the cervix uteri. The first carcinoma cells maintained in continuous culture, they are used for culturing viruses and in various cellular biologic studies.

helc-, helco- [Gk. *helkos*]. A combining form meaning *ulcer.*

hel·coid (hel'koid) *adj.* [*helc-* + *-oid*]. Resembling an ulcer; ulcerative.

hel·co·ma (hel·ko'muh) *n.* [Gk. *helkōma*]. ULCER.

hel·cot·ic (hel·kot'ick) *adj.* HELCOID.

Held's stria [H. *Held,* German neuroanatomist, 1866–1942]. Striae of Held (= STRIAE MEDULLARES VENTRICULI QUARTI).

hel·fil·con A (hel·fil'kon). A polymer of 2-hydroxyethyl methacrylate, $(C_6H_{10}O_3)_n$, employed as a contact lens material.

heli-, helio- [Gk. *hēlios*]. A combining form meaning (a) *the sun;* (b) *sunlight.*

he·li·an·thin (hee″lee·an'thin) *n.* [*Helianth*us, genus of the sunflower, + *-in*]. METHYL ORANGE.

he·li·an·thine (hee″lee·an'theen, ·thin) *n.* METHYL ORANGE.

helic-, helico-. A combining form meaning (a) *helix, helical;* (b) *spiral;* (c) *snail.*

hel·i·cal (hel'i·kul) *adj.* 1. Pertaining to a helix. 2. Having the form of a helix.

helical fossa. A furrow between the helix and anthelix.

helical spine. An anterior projection of the cartilage of the auricle of the ear in the region of the helix. NA *spina helicis.*

he·lic·i·form (he·lis'i·form, hel'i·si·) *adj.* [*helic-* + *-iform*]. Spiral; shaped like a snail shell.

hel·i·cin (hel'i·sin) *n.* Salicylaldehyde D-glucoside, $C_{13}H_{16}O_7$, obtained by oxidation of salicin; on hydrolysis it yields D-glucose and salicylaldehyde.

hel·i·cine (hel'i·seen, ·sine, ·sin) *adj.* 1. Spiral, coiled. 2. Pertaining to a helix.

helicine artery. A spiral vessel that empties into the cavernous sinuses of erectile tissue.

hel·i·cis (hel'i·sis) *n.* [L., of the helix]. A vestigial muscle associated with the helix of the external ear; a helicis major and helicis minor have been described. NA *musculus helicis major, musculus helicis minor.* See also Table of Muscles in the Appendix.

helico-. See *helic-.*

hel·i·coid (hel'i·koid) *adj.* [Gk. *helikoeidēs*]. Spiral; coiled like a snail shell.

hel·i·con (hel'i·kon) *n.* ASPIRIN.

hel·i·co·po·dia (hel″i·ko·po'dee·uh) *n.* [*helico-* + *-podia*]. CIRCUMDUCTION. —**hel·i·co·pod** (hel'i·ko·pod″) *adj.*

hel·i·co·ru·bin (hel″i·ko·roo'bin) *n.* [*helico-* + L. *rub*er, red, + *-in*]. A respiratory pigment found in the gut and liver of the snail.

hel·i·co·tre·ma (hel″i·ko·tree'muh) *n.* [*helico-* + Gk. *trēma,* hole] [NA]. The opening connecting the scalae tympani and vestibuli of the spiral canal of the perilymphatic space of the cochlea.

he·li·en·ceph·a·li·tis (hee″lee·en·sef″uh·lye'tis) *n.* [*heli-* + *encephalitis*]. HEATSTROKE.

helio-. See *heli-.*

he·lio·phage (hee'lee·o·faij, ·fahzh) *n.* [*helio-* + *-phage*]. CHROMATOPHORE.

he·lio·phobe (hee'lee·o·fobe) *n.* [*helio-* + *-phobe*]. One who is abnormally sensitive to the effects of the sun's rays, or afraid of them.

he·lio·pho·bia (hee″lee·o·fo'bee·uh) *n.* [*helio-* + *-phobia*]. An abnormal fear of exposure to the sun's rays.

he·lio·stat (hee'lee·o·stat″) *n.* [*helio-* + *-stat*]. A mirror moved by clockwork in such a manner as to reflect continuously the sun's rays on a given spot. —**helio·stat·ic** (·stat'ick) *adj.*

he·lio·tax·is (hee″lee·o·tack'sis) *n.* [*helio-* + *taxis*]. A form of taxis in which there is attraction toward (positive heliotaxis) or repulsion from (negative heliotaxis) the sun or sunlight.

he·lio·ther·a·py (hee″lee·o·therr'uh·pee) *n.* [*helio-* + *therapy*]. SOLAR THERAPY.

he·lio·tro·pin (hee″lee·o·tro'pin, ·ot'ro·pin) *n.* [*heliotrop*e, a flower whose odor it recalls, + *-in*]. PIPERONAL.

he·li·ot·ro·pism (hee″lee·ot'ro·piz·um) *n.* [*helio-* + *tropism*]. *In biology,* property of a plant or plant organ by virtue of which it bends toward or away from the sunlight. Compare *heliotaxis.* —**he·lio·trop·ic** (hee″lee·o·trop'ick) *adj.*

he·li·um (hee'lee·um) *n.* [NL., from Gk. *hēlios,* sun]. He = 4.0026. A chemically inert, colorless, odorless, nonflammable, gaseous element, occurring in certain natural gases and in small amount in the atmosphere; next to the lightest element known. A mixture with oxygen, being less dense than ordinary air, is useful in various types of dyspnea and in cases involving respiratory obstruction. See also Table of Elements in the Appendix.

he·lix (hee'licks) *n.*, genit. **he·li·cis** (hee'li·sis, hel'i·), L. pl. **heli·ces** (hel'i·seez, hee'li·) [Gk.]. 1. [NA] The rounded convex margin of the pinna of the ear. 2. An object or other entity spiral in form, as a coil of wire, the native structure of deoxyribonucleic acid, or a three-dimensional curve with one or more turns about an axis.

α-helix. ALPHA HELIX.

Hel·ke·si·mas·tix (hel"ke·si·mas'ticks) *n.* [Gk. *helkēsi-*, dragging, from *helkein,* to drag, + *mastix,* whip]. A genus of coprozoic flagellates.

Helkesimastix fae·cic·o·la (fe·sick'o·luh). A species of free-living flagellates found in the feces of man.

hel·le·bore (hel'e·bore) *n.* [Gk. *helleboros*]. A plant of the genus *Helleborus,* particularly *Helleborus niger,* black hellebore, which has been used as a purgative.

hel·le·bo·rism (hel'e·bor·iz·um) *n.* [*hellebore* + *-ism*]. 1. The treatment of disease with hellebore. 2. Poisoning due to hellebore.

Hel·ler's test [J. F. *Heller,* Austrian pathologist, 1813–1871]. A test for protein in which clear urine is stratified over concentrated nitric acid in a test tube. A white zone at the junction of the fluids indicates protein.

Hel·lige method. A colorimetric method for determination of hemoglobin by comparing acid hematin (prepared by diluting blood 1 to 100 with hydrochloric acid) with a revolving disk of 18 known glass standards.

Hel·lin's law [D. *Hellin,* Polish pathologist, 1867–1935]. The proposition, stated by Hellin in 1895, that the ratio of twin births to all human births is 1 to 89, and of triplet births to all births is 1 to 89^2, and of quadruplets, 1 to 89^3. Since the ratio of twinning actually varies widely in different populations and at different times, the number 89 has no validity as a constant and the law is better generalized: If the ratio of twin births to all births in a human population is 1:N, then the ratio of triplet births is roughly $1:N^2$, and of quadruplets, $1:N^3$, and so on, the exponent of N being one less than the number of infants in the sets. Thus, in a population with a twinning incidence of 1 in 100 births, the incidence of triplet births will approach 1 in 10,000, and of quadruplets, 1 in 1,000,000.

Hel·ly's fixing fluid. A mixture of potassium bichromate, sodium sulfate, mercuric chloride, distilled water, and formaldehyde.

Helm·holtz's theory of accommodation [H. L. F. von *Helmholtz,* German physiologist and physicist, 1821–1894]. The increased convexity of the lens is produced by a relaxation of the suspensory ligament, thus removing the influence that tends to flatten the lens and permitting the latter, by its elasticity, to become more convex.

hel·minth (hel'minth) *n.* [Gk. *helmins, helminthos,* worm]. Originally any parasitic worm; now includes those worm-like animals, either parasitic or free-living, of the phyla Platyhelminthes and Nemathelminthes as well as members of the phylum Annelida.

helminth-, helmintho-. A combining form meaning *helminth, worm.*

hel·min·tha·gogue (hel·min'thuh·gog) *n.* [*helminth-* + *-agogue*]. ANTHELMINTIC.

hel·min·them·e·sis (hel"min·them'e·sis) *n.* [*helminth-* + *emesis*]. The vomiting of worms.

hel·min·thi·a·sis (hel"min·thigh'uh·sis) *n.*, pl. **helminthia·ses** (·seez) [*helminth-* + *-iasis*]. A disease caused by parasitic worms in the body.

helminthiasis elas·ti·ca (e·las'ti·kuh). Elastic tumors of the axilla and groin due to filarial worms.

hel·min·thic (hel·min'thick) *adj.* Pertaining to or caused by a worm.

helminthic abscess. An abscess initiated by worms, such as filaria.

hel·minth·ism (hel'minth·iz·um) *n.* HELMINTHIASIS.

helmintho-. See *helminth-.*

hel·min·thoid (hel·min'thoid, hel'min·) *adj.* Like a helminth.

hel·min·thol·o·gist (hel"min·thol'uh·jist) *n.* A specialist in the studies of worms, especially parasitic worms.

hel·min·thol·o·gy (hel"min·thol'uh·jee) *n.* [*helmintho-* + *-logy*]. The study of parasitic worms. —**helmin·tho·log·ic** (·tho·loj'ick) *adj.*

hel·min·tho·ma (hel"min·tho'muh) *n.*, pl. **helminthomas, helminthoma·ta** (·tuh) [*helminth-* + *-oma*]. A mass caused by the presence of a parasitic worm.

hel·min·tho·pho·bia (hel·min"tho·fo'bee·uh) *n.* [*helmintho-* + *-phobia*]. An abnormal fear of worms or of becoming infected with worms.

hel·min·thous (hel·minth'us) *adj.* Pertaining to, caused by, or infected with helminths.

Helmitol. A trademark for citramin, a urinary antiseptic.

helo- [Gk. *hēlos,* nailhead, stud]. A combining form meaning (a) *horny, studded;* (b) *corn, callosity.*

He·lo·der·ma (hee"lo·dur'muh) *n.* [*helo-* + *-derma*]. A genus of lizards composed of two species, said to be the only known species of venomous lizards.

Heloderma hor·ri·dum (hor'i·dum). A venomous lizard found in Mexico; the beaded lizard.

Heloderma sus·pec·tum (sus·peck'tum). A species of venomous lizard found in Arizona and New Mexico; the Gila monster.

he·lo·ma (he·lo'muh) *n.*, pl. **helomas, heloma·ta** (·tuh) [*helo-* + *-oma*]. CALLOSITY.

he·lo·ni·as (he·lo'nee·us) *n.* [NL., from Gk. *helos,* marsh]. The dried rhizome and roots of *Chamaelirium luteum,* a plant of the Liliaceae; has been used as a tonic and diuretic.

he·lot·o·my (he·lot'uh·mee) *n.* [*helo-* + *-tomy*]. The cutting of a corn; surgery upon a corn.

hel·vol·ic acid (hel·vol'ick). An antibiotic substance, $C_{33}H_{44}O_8$, produced by *Aspergillus fumigatus;* identical with fumigacin.

Hel·weg's bundle or **tract** [H. K. S. *Helweg,* Danish psychiatrist, 1847–1901]. OLIVOSPINAL TRACT.

hem-, hema-, hemo-, haem-, haema-, haemo- [Gk. *haima*]. A combining form meaning *blood, of or pertaining to blood.*

he·ma·chro·ma·to·sis, hae·ma·chro·ma·to·sis (hee"muh·kro"muh·to'sis) *n.* HEMOCHROMATOSIS.

he·ma·chrome, hae·ma·chrome (hee'muh·krome, hem'uh·) *n.* HEMOCHROME.

he·ma·cy·tom·e·ter, hae·ma·cy·tom·e·ter (hee"muh·sigh·tom'e·tur, hem"uh·) *n.* HEMOCYTOMETER.

he·ma·cy·to·zo·on, hae·ma·cy·to·zo·on (hee"muh·sigh"to·zo'on, hem"uh·) *n.* HEMOCYTOZOON.

he·ma·dromo·graph, hae·ma·dromo·graph (hee"muh·drom'o·graf) *n.* HEMODROMOGRAPH.

he·ma·dro·mom·e·ter, hae·ma·dro·mom·e·ter (hee"muh·dro·mom'e·tur) *n.* HEMODROMOMETER.

he·ma·dy·nam·ics, hae·ma·dy·nam·ics (hee"muh·dye·nam'icks) *n.* HEMODYNAMICS.

he·ma·dy·na·mom·e·ter, hae·ma·dy·na·mom·e·ter (hee"muh·dye"nuh·mom'e·tur) *n.* HEMODYNAMOMETER.

he·mag·glu·ti·na·tion, hae·mag·glu·ti·na·tion (hee"muh·gloo"ti·nay'shun, hem"uh·) *n.* [*hem-* + *agglutination*]. The clumping of red blood cells, as by specific antibodies or by hemagglutinating viruses.

hemagglutination test. Any test in which hemagglutination is used as an indicator.

hem·ag·glu·ti·nin, haem·ag·glu·ti·nin (hee"muh·gloo'ti·nin, hem"uh·) *n.* [*hem-* + *agglutinin*]. 1. An antibody which agglutinates red blood cells. 2. The protein antigen of some viruses, such as the myxoviruses, thought to be the enzyme neuraminidase which reacts with the neuraminic acid of red blood cells to lead to agglutination. 3. Any agent which agglutinates red blood cells.

he·mal, hae·mal (hee'mul) *adj.* [*hem-* + *-al*]. 1. Pertaining to the blood or the vascular system. 2. Pertaining to the part of the body containing the heart and major blood vessels.

hemal arch. *In comparative anatomy,* especially in the caudal vertebrae of lower vertebrates, the inferior loop attached to the vertebral body and enclosing the caudal artery and vein. Syn. *inferior arch.*

hemal axis. AORTA.

hemal node or **gland.** A node of lymphatic tissue, situated in the course of blood vessels, and containing large numbers of erythrocytes; frequently found in ruminants.

hemal spine. The part of the spine that closes in the hemal arch of an ideal vertebra, as in a fish's tail.

he·mal·um, hae·mal·um (he·mal'um) *n.* An alum hematoxylin formula in which hematoxylin is oxidized to hematein by sodium iodate, or prepared hematein is substituted for hematoxylin; generally, a ripened alum hematoxylin.

hem·anal·y·sis, haem·anal·y·sis (hee"muh·nal'i·sis, hem"uh·) *n.*, pl. **hemanaly·ses, haemanaly·ses** (·seez) [*hem-* + *analysis*]. Analysis of the blood.

hemangi-, hemangio- [*hem-* + *angi-, angio-*]. A combining form meaning *blood vessel.*

he·man·gi·ec·ta·sia, hae·man·gi·ec·ta·sia (he·man"jee·eck·tay'zhuh, ·zee·uh) *n.* HEMANGIECTASIS.

he·man·gi·ec·ta·sis, hae·man·gi·ec·ta·sis (he·man"jee·eck'tuh·sis) *n.*, pl. **hemangiecta·ses, haemangiecta·ses** (·seez) [*hemangi-* + *ectasis*]. Dilatation of blood vessels. —**hemangi·ec·tat·ic, haemangi·ec·tat·ic** (·eck·tat'ick) *adj.*

hemangio-. See *hemangi-.*

he·man·gio·am·e·lo·blas·to·ma, hae·man·gio·am·e·lo·blas·to·ma (he·man"jee·o·am"e·lo·blas·to'muh) *n.* [*hemangio-* + *ameloblastoma*]. An ameloblastoma with a prominent vascular stroma.

he·man·gio·blas·to·ma, hae·man·gio·blas·to·ma (he·man"jee·o·blas·to'muh) *n.* [*hemangio-* + *blastoma*]. A variety of hemangioma whose vascular spaces are lined by prominent endothelial cells, found especially in the cerebellum.

he·man·gio·blas·to·ma·to·sis, hae·man·gio·blas·to·ma·to·sis (he·man"jee·o·blas"to·muh·to'sis) *n.* [*hemangioblastoma* + *-osis*]. Widespread occurrence of hemangioblastomas.

he·man·gio·elas·to·myx·o·ma, hae·man·gio·elas·to·myx·o·ma (he·man"jee·o·e·las"to·mick·so'muh) *n.* [*hemangio-* + *elasto-* + *myxoma*]. A type of benign mixed mesodermal tumor, probably hamartomatous, composed of blood vessels and mucinous and elastic connective tissue.

he·man·gio·en·do·the·lio·blas·to·ma, hae·man·gio·en·do·the·lio·blas·to·ma (he·man"jee·o·en"do·theel"ee·o·blas·to'muh) *n.* [*hemangio-* + *endothelio-* + *blastoma*]. HEMANGIOENDOTHELIOMA.

he·man·gio·en·do·the·li·o·ma, hae·man·gio·en·do·the·li·o·ma (he·man"jee·o·en"do·theel·ee·o'muh) *n.* [*hemangio-* + *endothelioma*]. 1. A highly cellular benign hemangioma seen in children. Syn. *benign hemangioendothelioma.* 2. A malignant tumor composed of anaplastic endothelial cells forming vascular spaces in some instances. Syn. *angiosarcoma, malignant hemangioendothelioma.*

he·man·gio·en·do·the·lio·sar·co·ma, hae·man·gio·en·do·the·lio·sar·co·ma (he·man"jee·o·en"do·theel"ee·o·sahr·ko'muh) *n.* [*hemangio-* + *endothelio-* + *sarcoma*]. HEMANGIOENDOTHELIOMA (2).

he·man·gio·li·po·ma, hae·man·gio·li·po·ma (he·man"jee·o·li·po'muh) *n.* [*hemangio-* + *lipoma*]. A hamartomatous mass having hemangiomatous and lipomatous elements.

he·man·gi·o·ma, hae·man·gi·o·ma (he·man"jee·o'muh) *n.* [*hem-* + *angioma*]. An angioma made up of blood vessels. —**hemangioma·tous, haemangioma·tous** (·tus) *adj.*

hemangioma-thrombocytopenia syndrome. Thrombocytopenia associated with large hemangiomas, usually seen in infants. Altered coagulation parameters characteristic of disseminated intravascular coagulation are usually found; KASABACH-MERRITT SYNDROME.

he·man·gi·o·ma·to·sis, hae·man·gi·o·ma·to·sis (he·man"jee·o"muh·to'sis) *n.*, pl. **hemangiomato·ses, haemangiomato·ses** (·seez) [*hemangioma* + *-osis*]. The occurrence of multiple hemangiomas.

hemangiomatosis ret·i·nae (ret'i·nee). VON HIPPEL'S DISEASE.

he·man·gio·myo·li·po·ma, hae·man·gio·myo·li·po·ma (he·man"jee·o·migh"o·li·po'muh) *n.* [*hemangio-* + *myo-* + *lipoma*]. A hamartomatous mass containing hemangiomatous, muscular, and lipomatous elements.

he·man·gio·peri·cy·to·ma, hae·man·gio·peri·cy·to·ma (he·man"jee·o·perr·i·sigh·to'muh) *n.* [*hemangio-* + *pericyte* + *-oma*]. A tumor composed of endothelium-lined tubes or cords of cells, surrounded by spherical cells with supporting reticulin network; the parenchymal cells are presumed to be related to pericytes.

he·man·gio·sar·co·ma, hae·man·gio·sar·co·ma (he·man"jee·o·sahr·ko'muh) *n.* [*hemangio-* + *sarcoma*]. HEMANGIOENDOTHELIOMA (2).

hem·apoph·y·sis, haem·apoph·y·sis (hee"muh·pof'i·sis, hem"uh·) *n.*, pl. **hemapophy·ses, haemapophy·ses** (·seez) [*hem*al + *apophysis*]. The part of an ideal vertebra which forms the ventrolateral part of the hemal arch. In man, all the hemapophyses are detached; represented by the ribs.

hem·ar·thro·sis, haem·ar·thro·sis (hee"mahr·thro'sis, hem"ahr·) *n.*, pl. **hemarthro·ses, haemarthro·ses** (·seez) [*hem-* + *arthrosis*]. Extravasation of blood into a joint.

hemat-, hemato-, haemat-, haemato- [Gk. *haima, haimatos*]. A combining form meaning *blood, of or pertaining to the blood.*

he·ma·te·in, hae·ma·te·in (hee"muh·tee'in, hem"uh·) *n.* A reddish brown substance, $C_{16}H_{12}O_6$, obtained by oxidation of hematoxylin; used as a stain and indicator.

he·ma·tem·e·sis, hae·ma·tem·e·sis (hee"muh·tem'e·sis, hem"uh·) *n.* [*hemat-* + *emesis*]. The vomiting of blood.

he·ma·ther·mous, hae·ma·ther·mous (hee"muh·thur'mus, hem"uh·) *adj.* WARM-BLOODED.

he·mat·hi·dro·sis, hae·mat·hi·dro·sis (hee"mat·hi·dro'sis, hem"at·) *n.* [*hemat-* + *hidrosis*]. The appearance of blood or blood products in sweat gland secretions.

he·mat·ic, hae·mat·ic (hee·mat'ick) *adj.* [Gk. *haimatikos*]. Pertaining to, full of, or having the color of, blood.

hematic abscess. An abscess resulting from blood-borne infectious agents; a hematogenous abscess.

he·ma·ti·dro·sis, hae·ma·ti·dro·sis (hee"ma·ti·dro'sis, hem"uh·) *n.* [*hemat-* + *idrosis*]. HEMATHIDROSIS.

he·ma·tim·e·ter, hae·ma·tim·e·ter (hee"muh·tim'e·tur, hem"uh·) *n.* [*hemat-* + *-meter*]. HEMOCYTOMETER. —**hematime·try, haematime·try** (·tree) *n.*

he·ma·tin, hae·ma·tin (hee'muh·tin, hem'uh·tin) *n.* Ferriheme hydroxide, $C_{34}H_{32}N_4O_4{\cdot}FeOH$, formed from hemin by treatment with alkali; contains iron in the ferric state.

he·ma·ti·ne·mia, haem·a·ti·nae·mia (hem"uh·ti·nee'mee·uh, hee"muh·) *n.* [*hematin* + *-emia*]. The presence of heme in the blood.

he·ma·tin·ic, hae·ma·tin·ic (hee"muh·tin'ick, hem"uh·tin'ick) *n. & adj.* [*hematin* + *-ic*]. 1. An agent that tends to increase the hemoglobin content of the blood. 2. Pertaining to or containing hematin. 3. Pertaining to or acting like a hematinic.

he·ma·tin·om·e·ter, haem·a·tin·om·e·ter (hee"muh·tin·om'e·tur, hem"uh·) *n.* [*hematin* + *-meter*]. HEMOGLOBINOMETER.

he·ma·tin·uria, hae·ma·tin·uria (hee"muh·ti·new'ree·uh, hem"uh·) *n.* [*hematin* + *-uria*]. Hematin in the urine.

he·ma·tite, hae·ma·tite (hem'uh·tite, hee'muh·tite) *n.* [Gk. *lithos haimatitēs,* lit., bloodlike stone]. Ferric oxide, Fe_2O_3, containing little water of hydration; a red powder. See also *iron oxide.*

hemato-. See *hemat-.*

he·ma·to·aer·om·e·ter, hae·ma·to·aer·om·e·ter (hee"muh·to·

ay·ur·om′e·tur, hem″uh·) *n.* [*hemato-* + *aerometer*]. A device for recording the pressure of gases in the blood.

he·ma·to·bil·ia (hee″muh·to·bil′ee·uh, hem″uh·) *n.* [*hemato-* + *bili-* + *-ia*]. A condition in which there is blood in the bile ducts. Syn. *hemobilia.*

he·ma·to·blast, hae·ma·to·blast (hee′muh·to·blast, hem′uh·, he·mat′o·) *n.* [*hemato-* + *-blast*]. An immature form of hematopoietic cell.

he·ma·to·cele, hae·ma·to·cele (hee′muh·to·seel, hem′uh·, he·mat′o·) *n.* [*hemato-* + *-cele*]. The extravasation and collection of blood in a part, especially in the cavity of the tunica vaginalis testis.

he·ma·to·che·zia, hae·ma·to·che·zia (hee″muh·to·kee′zee·uh, hem″uh·) *n.* HEMOCHEZIA.

he·ma·to·chro·ma·to·sis, hae·ma·to·chro·ma·to·sis (hee″muh·to·kro″muh·to′sis, hem″uh·) *n.* HEMOCHROMATOSIS.

he·ma·to·chy·lo·cele, hae·ma·to·chy·lo·cele (hee″muh·to·kigh′lo·seel, hem″uh·to·) *n.* [*hemato-* + *chylo-* + *-cele*]. The extravasation and collection of chyle and blood in a part, especially in the tunica vaginalis testis, complicating filariasis.

he·ma·to·chy·lu·ria, hae·ma·to·chy·lu·ria (hee″muh·to·kigh·lew′ree·uh, hem″uh·to·) *n.* [*hemato-* + *chyl-* + *-uria*]. The presence of blood and chyle in the urine.

he·ma·to·col·pos, hae·ma·to·col·pos (hee″muh·to·kol′pus, hem″uh·to·) *n.* [*hemato-* + *-colpos*]. A retained collection of blood within the vagina, resulting from an imperforate hymen or other obstruction.

he·ma·to·crit, hae·ma·to·crit (he·mat′o·krit, hee′muh·to·krit) *n.* [*hemato-* + Gk. *krit-*, from *krinein,* to separate]. 1. Hematocrit reading. 2. A small centrifuge used to separate blood cells in clinical analysis. 3. The centrifuge tube in which the blood cells are separated.

hematocrit reading. The percentage of the whole blood volume occupied by the red cells after centrifugation.

he·ma·to·crys·tal·lin, hae·ma·to·crys·tal·lin (hee″muh·to·kris′tuh·lin, hem″uh·to·) *n.* [*hemato-* + *crystallin*]. HEMOGLOBIN.

he·ma·to·cyst, hae·ma·to·cyst (he·mat′o·sist, hee′muh·to·) *n.* [*hemato-* + *cyst*]. A cyst containing blood.

he·ma·to·cyte, hae·ma·to·cyte (he·mat′o·site, hee′muh·to·) *n.* HEMOCYTE.

he·ma·to·cy·tol·y·sis, hae·ma·to·cy·tol·y·sis (hee″muh·to·sigh·tol′i·sis, hem″uh·to·) *n.* [*hematocyte* + *-lysis*]. HEMOLYSIS.

he·ma·to·cy·tom·e·ter, hae·ma·to·cy·tom·e·ter (hee″muh·to·sigh·tom′e·tur, hem″uh·to·) *n.* HEMOCYTOMETER.

he·ma·to·cy·to·zo·on, hae·ma·to·cy·to·zo·on (hee″muh·to·sigh″to·zo′on, hem″uh·to·) *n.* HEMOCYTOZOON.

he·ma·to·dy·nam·ics, hae·ma·to·dy·nam·ics (hee″muh·to·dye·nam′icks, hem″uh·to·) *n.* HEMODYNAMICS.

he·ma·to·dy·na·mom·e·ter, hae·ma·to·dy·na·mom·e·ter (hee″muh·to·dye″nuh·mom′e·tur, hem″uh·to·) *n.* HEMODYNAMOMETER.

he·ma·to·dys·cra·sia, hae·ma·to·dys·cra·sia (hee″muh·to·dis·kray′zhuh, ·zee·uh, hem″uh·to·) *n.* [*hemato-* + *dyscrasia*]. A diseased state of the blood.

he·ma·to·en·ce·phal·ic, hae·ma·to·en·ce·phal·ic (hee″muh·to·en″se·fal′ick, hem″uh·to·) *adj.* [*hemato-* + *encephalic*]. Pertaining to the blood and the brain.

hematoencephalic barrier. BLOOD-BRAIN BARRIER.

he·ma·to·gen·e·sis, hae·ma·to·gen·e·sis (hee″muh·to·jen′e·sis, hem″uh·to·) *n.* HEMOGENESIS.

he·ma·to·gen·ic, hae·ma·to·gen·ic (hee″muh·to·jen′ick, hem″uh·to·) *adj.* HEMOGENIC.

hematogenic shock. HYPOVOLEMIC SHOCK.

he·ma·tog·e·nous, hae·ma·tog·e·nous (hee″muh·toj′e·nus, hem″uh·) *adj.* [*hemato-* + *-genous*]. 1. Pertaining to the production of blood or its constituents. 2. Disseminated via the circulation or transported by the bloodstream. 3. Derived from the blood.

hematogenous albuminuria. Proteinuria associated with hematuria.

hematogenous pigment. Any pigment derived from hemoglobin including heme, hemosiderin, methemoglobin, and bile pigments.

hematogenous pyelonephritis. Pyelonephritis which results from a bacterial invasion from the bloodstream.

hematogenous tuberculosis. Any manifestation of tuberculosis resulting from the transmission of tubercle bacilli through the bloodstream.

he·ma·to·glo·bin, hae·ma·to·glo·bin (hee″muh·to·glo′bin, hem″uh·to·) *n.* [*hemato-* + *globin*]. HEMOGLOBIN.

he·ma·to·gone, hae·ma·to·gone (hee′muh·to·gohn, hem′uh·, he·mat′o·) *n.* [*hemato-* + Gk. *gonē,* generation, offspring]. STEM CELL (1).

he·ma·to·hi·dro·sis, hae·ma·to·hi·dro·sis (hee″muh·to·hi·dro′sis, hem″uh·to·) *n.* HEMATHIDROSIS.

he·ma·to·his·tone, hae·ma·to·his·tone (hee″muh·to·his′tone, hem″uh·to·) *n.* [*hemato-* + *histone*]. GLOBIN.

he·ma·toid, hae·ma·toid (hee′muh·toid, hem′uh·) *adj.* [Gk. *haimatoeidēs*]. Bloodlike; resembling blood.

he·ma·toi·din, hae·ma·toi·din (hee″muh·toy′din) *n.* [*hematoid* + *-in*]. A golden yellow, orange, or reddish-brown amorphous or crystalline iron-negative pigment found free or sometimes in macrophages in areas of hemorrhagic infarction.

hematoidin crystals. Yellowish or brown, needlelike or rhombic crystals that may occur in the feces after hemorrhage in the gastrointestinal tract. Syn. *Virchow's crystals.*

hematokrit. HEMATOCRIT.

he·ma·to·lith, hae·ma·to·lith (hee′muh·to·lith, hem′uh·, he·mat′o·) *n.* HEMOLITH.

he·ma·tol·o·gist, hae·ma·tol·o·gist (hee″muh·tol′uh·jist, hem″uh·) *n.* A person who specializes in the study of blood.

he·ma·tol·o·gy, hae·ma·tol·o·gy (hee″muh·tol′uh·jee, hem″uh·) *n.* [*hemato-* + *-logy*]. The science of the blood, its nature, functions, and diseases. —**hema·to·log·ic, haema·to·log·ic** (·to·loj′ick) *adj.*

he·ma·to·lymph·an·gi·o·ma, hae·ma·to·lymph·an·gi·o·ma (hee″muh·to·lim·fan″jee·o′muh, hem″uh·to·) *n.* [*hemato-* + *lymph-* + *angioma*]. A benign tumor composed of blood vessels and lymph vessels.

he·ma·to·lymph·uria, hae·ma·to·lymph·uria (hee″muh·to·lim·few′ree·uh, hem″uh·to·) *n.* [*hemato-* + *lymph-* + *uria*]. The discharge of urine containing lymph and blood.

he·ma·tol·y·sis, hae·ma·tol·y·sis (hee″muh·tol′i·sis, hem″uh·) *n.*, pl. **hematoly·ses, haematoly·ses** (·seez). HEMOLYSIS.

he·ma·to·lyt·o·poi·et·ic, hae·ma·to·lyt·o·poi·et·ic (hee″muh·to·lit″o·poy·et′ick, hem″uh·to·) *adj.* HEMOLYTOPOIETIC.

he·ma·to·ma, hae·ma·to·ma (hee″muh·to′muh, hem″uh·) *n.*, pl. **hematomas, hematoma·ta** (·tuh) [*hemat-* + *-oma*]. A circumscribed extravascular collection of blood, usually clotted, which forms a mass.

hematoma mole. BREUS'S MOLE.

he·ma·to·me·di·as·ti·num, hae·ma·to·me·di·as·ti·num (hee″muh·to·mee″dee·uh·stye′num, hem″uh·to·) *n.* HEMOMEDIASTINUM.

he·ma·tom·e·ter, hae·ma·tom·e·ter (hee″muh·tom′e·tur, hem″uh·) *n.* HEMOMETER. —**hematome·try, haematome·try** (·tree) *n.*

he·ma·to·me·tra, hae·ma·to·me·tra (hee″muh·to·mee′truh, hem″uh·to·) *n.* [*hemato-* + Gk. *mētra,* womb]. An accumulation of blood or menstrual fluid in the uterus.

he·ma·to·mole, hae·ma·to·mole (hee′muh·to·mole) *n.* [*hemato-* + *mole*]. BREUS'S MOLE.

he·ma·to·my·e·lia, hae·ma·to·my·e·lia (hee″muh·to·migh·ee″lee·uh, hem″uh·to·) *n.* [*hemato-* + *myel-* + *-ia*]. Hemorrhage into the spinal cord.

he·ma·to·my·e·li·tis, hae·ma·to·my·e·li·tis (hee″muh·to·migh″e·lye′tis, hem″uh·to·) *n.* [*hemato-* + *myelitis*]. An acute myelitis together with an effusion of blood into the spinal cord.

he·ma·ton·ic, hae·ma·ton·ic (hee″muh·ton′ick, hem″uh·) *n.* [*hema-* + *tonic*]. HEMATINIC.

he·ma·to·pa·thol·o·gy, hae·ma·to·pa·thol·o·gy (hee″muh·to·pa·thol′uh·jee, hem″uh·to·) *n.* HEMOPATHOLOGY.

he·ma·top·a·thy, hae·ma·top·a·thy (hee″muh·top′uth·ee, hem″uh·) *n.* [*hemato-* + *-pathy*]. HEMOPATHY.

he·ma·to·peri·car·di·um, hae·ma·to·peri·car·di·um (hee″muh·to·perr″i·kahr′dee·um, hem″uh·to·) *n.* HEMOPERICARDIUM.

he·ma·to·peri·to·ne·um, hae·ma·to·peri·to·ne·um (hee″muh·to·perr″i·to·nee′um, hem″uh·to·) *n.* HEMOPERITONEUM.

he·ma·to·phage, hae·ma·to·phage (hee′muh·to·faje, he·mat′o·, hem′uh·to·) *n.* HEMOPHAGE.

he·ma·to·pha·gia, hae·ma·to·pha·gia (hee″muh·to·fay′jee·uh, hem″uh·to·) *n.* HEMOPHAGIA.

he·ma·toph·a·gous, hae·ma·toph·a·gous (hee″muh·tof′uh·gus, hem″uh·) *adj.* [*hemato-* + *-phagous*]. Bloodsucking, subsisting on blood.

he·ma·toph·a·gus, hae·ma·toph·a·gus (hee″muh·tof′uh·gus, hem″uh·) *n.* [NL., from *hemato-* + Gk. *phag*ein, to eat]. A bloodsucking insect.

he·ma·to·phil·ia, hae·ma·to·phil·ia (hee″muh·to·fil′ee·uh, hem″uh·to·) *n.* HEMOPHILIA.

he·ma·to·pho·bia, hae·ma·to·pho·bia (hee″muh·to·fo′bee·uh, hem″uh·to·) *n.* HEMOPHOBIA.

he·ma·to·phyte, hae·ma·to·phyte (hee′muh·to·fite, he·mat′o·) *n.* [*hemato-* + *-phyte*]. A plant organism, such as a bacterium or fungus, living in the blood.

he·ma·to·plas·tic, hae·ma·to·plas·tic (hee″muh·to·plas′tick, hem″uh·to·) *adj.* HEMOPLASTIC.

he·ma·to·poi·e·sis, hae·ma·to·poi·e·sis (hee″muh·to·poy·ee′sis, he·mat″o·, hem″uh·to·) *n.* [*hemato-* + *-poiesis*]. The formation and maturation of blood cells and their derivatives. Syn. *hemopoiesis.*

he·ma·to·poi·et·ic, hae·ma·to·poi·et·ic (hee″muh·to·poy·et′ick, he·mat″o·, hem″uh·to·) *adj.* [Gk. *haimatopoiētikos,* from *haima, haimatos*, blood, + *poiētikos,* producing, creative]. Blood-forming; of or pertaining to hematopoiesis. Syn. *hemopoietic.*

he·ma·to·por·phyr·ia, hae·ma·to·por·phyr·ia (hee″muh·to·por·firr′ee·uh, hem″uh·to·) *n.* [*hemato-* + *porphyria*]. PORPHYRIA (1).

he·ma·to·por·phy·rin, hae·ma·to·por·phy·rin (hee″muh·to·por′fi·rin, hem″uh·to·) *n.* HEMOPORPHYRIN.

he·ma·to·por·phy·rin·emia, hae·ma·to·por·phy·rin·ae·mia (hee″muh·to·por″fi·ri·nee′mee·uh, hem″uh·to·) *n.* [*hematoporphyrin* + *-emia*]. The presence of hemoporphyrin in the blood.

he·ma·to·por·phy·rin·uria, hae·ma·to·por·phy·rin·uria (hee″muh·to·por″fi·ri·new′ree·uh, hem″uh·to·) *n.* [*hematoporphyrin* + *-uria*]. The presence of hemoporphyrin in the urine.

he·ma·to·pre·cip·i·tin, hae·ma·to·pre·cip·i·tin (hee″muh·to·pre·sip′i·tin, hem″uh·to·) *n.* HEMOPRECIPITIN.

he·ma·tor·rha·chis, hae·ma·tor·rha·chis (hee″muh·to·ray′kis, hee″muh·tor′uh·kis) *n.* [*hemato-* + *-rrhachis*]. Hemorrhage into the spinal canal.

he·ma·tor·rhea, hae·ma·tor·rhoea (hee″muh·to·ree′uh, hem″uh·to·, he·mat′o·) *n.* [*hemato-* + *-rrhea*]. Copious or profuse hemorrhage.

he·ma·to·sal·pinx, hae·ma·to·sal·pinx (hee″muh·to·sal′pinks, hem″uh·to·) *n.* [*hemato-* + *salpinx*]. A collection of blood in a uterine tube.

he·ma·to·scope, hae·ma·to·scope (hee″muh·to·skope, hem″uh·to·, he·mat′o·) *n.* [*hemato-* + *-scope*]. An instrument used in the spectroscopic or optical examination of the blood.

he·ma·tose, hae·ma·tose (hee′muh·toce) *adj.* [*hemat-* + *-ose*]. Full of blood; bloody.

Hematosiphon. HAEMATOSIPHON.

he·ma·to·si·pho·ni·a·sis (hee″muh·to·sigh″fo·nigh′uh·sis, hem″uh·to·) *n.* [*Hematosiphon* (*Haematosiphon*) + *-iasis*]. The polymorphous dermatitis caused by the bite of *Haematosiphon inodora,* generally localized on the extremities and exposed parts of the body and accompanied by intense itching and systemic manifestations following secondary infection.

he·ma·to·sis, hae·ma·to·sis (hee″muh·to′sis, hem″uh·) *n.* [Gk. *haimatōsis,* conversion into blood]. *Obsol.* 1. HEMATOPOIESIS. 2. Oxygenation of the blood, especially in the lungs.

he·ma·to·spec·tro·scope, hae·ma·to·spec·tro·scope (hee″muh·to·speck′truh·skope, hem″uh·to·) *n.* [*hemato-* + *spectroscope*]. A spectroscope adapted to the study of the blood. —**hemato·spec·tros·co·py, haemato·spec·tros·co·py** (·speck·tros′kuh·pee) *n.*

he·ma·to·sper·ma·to·cele, hae·ma·to·sper·ma·to·cele (hee″muh·to·spur′muh·to·seel, ·spur·mat′o·seel, hem″uh·to·) *n.* [*hemato-* + *spermatocele*]. A spermatocele containing blood.

he·ma·to·sper·mia, hae·ma·to·sper·mia (hee″muh·to·spur′mee·uh, hem″uh·to·) *n.* [*hemato-* + *-spermia*]. The discharge of bloody semen. Syn. *hemospermia.*

he·ma·to·stat·ic, hae·ma·to·stat·ic (hee″muh·to·stat′ick, hem″uh·to·) *adj.* HEMOSTATIC.

he·ma·to·ther·a·py, hae·ma·to·ther·a·py (hee″muh·to·therr′uh·pee, hem″uh·to·) *n.* HEMOTHERAPY.

he·ma·to·ther·mal, hae·ma·to·ther·mal (hee″muh·to·thur′mul, hem″uh·to·) *adj.* [*hemato-* + *thermal*]. WARM-BLOODED.

he·ma·to·ther·mous, hae·ma·to·ther·mous (hee″muh·to·thur′mus, hem″uh·to·) *adj.* Hematothermal (= WARM-BLOODED).

he·ma·to·tho·rax, hae·ma·to·tho·rax (hee″muh·to·tho′racks, hem″uh·to·) *n.* HEMOTHORAX.

he·ma·to·tox·ic, hae·ma·to·tox·ic (hee″muh·to·tock′sick, hem″uh·to·) *adj.* Poisonous to the hematopoietic tissues. —**hemato·tox·ic·i·ty** (·tock·sis′i·tee) *n.*

he·ma·to·tox·i·co·sis, hae·ma·to·tox·i·co·sis (hee″muh·to·tock″si·ko′sis, hem″uh·to·) *n.* [*hemato-* + *toxicosis*]. A state of toxic damage to the hematopoietic system.

he·ma·to·tym·pa·num, hae·ma·to·tym·pa·num (hee″muh·to·tim′puh·num, hem″uh·to·) *n.* HEMOTYMPANUM.

he·ma·tox·y·lin, hae·ma·tox·y·lin (hee″muh·tock′si·lin, hem″uh·) *n.* 1. A colorless crystalline compound, $C_{16}H_{14}O_6$, occurring in hematoxylon. Upon oxidation, it is converted to hematein which forms deeply colored lakes with various metals. Used as a stain in microscopy. 2. ALUM HEMATOXYLIN.

hematoxylin-eosin stain. The most widely used stain for general histologic and histopathologic work; an aqueous solution of blue-purple hematoxylin dye and an alcoholic solution of red eosin dye are used.

he·ma·tox·y·lino·phil·ic, hae·ma·tox·y·lino·phil·ic (hee″muh·tock″so·lin·o·fil′ick) *adj.* [*hematoxylin* + *-philic*]. Having an affinity for hematoxylin.

he·ma·tox·y·lon, hae·ma·tox·y·lon (hee″muh·tock′si·lon, hem′uh·) *n.* [*hemato-* + Gk. *xylon,* wood]. The heartwood of *Haematoxylon campechianum;* contains tannic acid and hematoxylin. Has been used as a mild astringent. Syn. *logwood.*

he·ma·to·zo·on, hae·ma·to·zo·on (hee″muh·to·zo′on, hem″uh·to·) *n.*, pl. **hemato·zoa, haemato·zoa** (·zo′uh) [*hemato-* + *-zoon*]. Any animal parasite living in the blood. —**hemato·zo·al, haematozo·al** (·ul), **hematozo·ic, haematozo·ic** (·ick) *adj.*

he·ma·tu·ria, hae·ma·tu·ria (hee″muh·tew′ree·uh, hem″uh·) *n.* [*hemat-* + *-uria*]. The discharge of urine containing blood.

heme, haem (heem) *n.* $C_{34}H_{32}N_4O_4Fe$; the ferrous complex of protoporphyrin 9, constituting the prosthetic component of hemoglobin. Syn. *ferroheme, reduced heme, ferroprotoporphyrin 9.* See also *hematin, hemin.*

hem·er·a·lo·pia (hem″ur·uh·lo′pee·uh) *n.* [Gk. *hēmer*a, day, + *al*aos, blind, + *-opia*]. 1. DAY BLINDNESS. 2. *Erron.* NIGHT BLINDNESS.

hem·er·a·pho·nia (hem″ur·a·fo′nee·uh) *n.* [Gk. *hēmera*, day, + *aphonia*]. Loss of voice during the day, and recovery of it at night; occurs in hysteria.
he·me·ryth·rin (hee″me·rith′rin, hem″e·) *n.* HEMOERYTHRIN.
heme synthetase. An enzyme which combines protoporphyrin IX, ferrous iron, and globin to form the intact hemoglobin molecule.
hemi- [Gk. *hēmi-*, half]. A prefix meaning (a) *half, partial;* (b) in biology and medicine, either *the right or the left half of the body;* (c) in chemistry, *a combining ratio of one-half.*
-hemia, -haemia. See *-emia.*
hemi·ablep·sia (hem″ee·a·blep′see·uh) *n.* [*hemi-* + *ablepsia*]. HEMIANOPSIA.
hemi·acar·di·us (hem″ee·a·kahr′dee·us) *n.* [*hemi-* + *acardius*]. A placental parasitic twin (omphalosite) in which the principal parts of a fetus are recognizable, with a more or less well-formed, rudimentary heart.
hemi·aceph·a·lus (hem″ee·a·sef′uh·lus) *n.* [*hemi-* + *acephalus*]. ANENCEPHALUS.
hemi·achro·ma·top·sia (hem″ee·a·kro″muh·top′see·uh) *n.* [*hemi-* + *achromatopsia*]. A loss of color vision in corresponding halves of each visual field due to a lesion of one occipital lobe.
hemi·agen·e·sis (hem″ee·ay·jen′e·sis) *n.* [*hemi-* + *agenesis*]. Failure of development of one half or one side of a part, usually one consisting of two nearly symmetrical halves, as the cerebellum.
hemi·ageu·sia (hem″ee·a·gew′zee·uh, ·a·joo′see·uh) *n.* [*hemi-* + *ageusia*]. Loss of the sense of taste on one side of the tongue.
hemi·al·bu·mose (hem″ee·al′bew·moce) *n.* [*hemi-* + *albumose*]. A product of the digestion of certain kinds of proteins. It is a normal constituent of bone marrow, and is found also in the urine of patients with osteomalacia. Syn. *propeptone, pseudopeptone.*
hemi·al·bu·mo·su·ria (hem″ee·al″bew·mo·sue′ree·uh) *n.* [*hemialbumose* + *-uria*]. The presence of hemialbumose in the urine. Syn. *propeptonuria.*
hemi·al·lo·ge·ne·ic (hem″ee·al″o·je·nee′ick) *n.* SEMIALLOGENEIC.
hemi·am·bly·o·pia (hem″ee·am″blee·o′pee·uh) *n.* [*hemi-* + *amblyopia*]. HEMIANOPSIA.
hemi·an·a·cu·sia (hem″ee·an″uh·kew′zhuh, ·zee·uh) *n.* [*hemi-* + *anacusia*]. Deafness in one ear.
hemianaesthesia. HEMIANESTHESIA.
hemi·an·al·ge·sia (hem″ee·an″al·jee′zee·uh) *n.* [*hemi-* + *analgesia*]. Insensibility to pain on one side of the body.
hemi·an·en·ceph·a·ly (hem″ee·an″en·sef′uh·lee) *n.* [*hemi-* + *anencephaly*]. Anencephaly on one side only.
hemi·an·es·the·sia, hemi·an·aes·the·sia (hem″ee·an″es·theezh′uh, ·theez′ee·uh) *n.* [*hemi-* + *anesthesia*]. Loss of sensation on one side of the body; unilateral anesthesia.
hemi·an·o·pia (hem″ee·an·o′pee·uh) *n.* HEMIANOPSIA. —**hemiano·pic** (·pick) *adj. & n.*
hemi·an·op·sia (hem″ee·an·op′see·uh) *n.* [*hemi-* + *anopsia*]. Blindness in one half of the visual field; may be bilateral or unilateral.
hemi·atax·ia (hem″ee·uh·tack′see·uh) *n.* [*hemi-* + *ataxia*]. Ataxia affecting one side of the body.
hemi·ath·e·to·sis (hem″ee·ath″e·to′sis) *n.*, pl. **hemiatheto·ses** (·seez) [*hemi-* + *athetosis*]. Athetosis of one side of the body.
hemi·at·ro·phy (hem″ee·at′ruh·fee) *n.* [*hemi-* + *atrophy*]. Atrophy confined to one side of an organ or region of the body.
hemi·azy·gos, hemi·azy·gous (hem″ee·az′i·gus, uh·zye′gus) *adj.* [*hemi-* + *azygos*]. Partially paired.
hemiazygos vein. The left branch of the ascending lumbar vein. NA *vena hemiazygos.* See also Table of Veins in the Appendix.
hemi·bal·lism (hem″ee·bal′iz·um) *n.* HEMIBALLISMUS.
hemi·bal·lis·mus (hem″ee·ba·liz′mus) *n.* [*hemi-* + *ballismus*]. Sudden, violent, flinging movements involving particularly the proximal portions of the extremities of one side of the body; caused by a destructive lesion of the contralateral subthalamic nucleus or its neighboring structures or pathways; HEMICHOREA.
he·mic, hae·mic (hee′mick) *adj.* [*hem-* + *-ic*]. Pertaining to or developed by the blood.
hemi·car·dia (hem″ee·kahr′dee·uh) *n.* [*hemi-* + *-cardia*]. The presence of only a lateral half of the usual four-chambered heart.
hemi·cel·lu·lose (hem″ee·sel′yoo·loce) *n.* [*hemi-* + *cellulose*]. A group of high-molecular-weight carbohydrates resembling cellulose but less complex.
hemi·cen·trum (hem″ee·sen′trum) *n.* PLEUROCENTRUM.
hemi·ce·phal·ic (hem′ee·se·fal′ick) *adj.* [*hemi-* + *cephalic*]. Pertaining to or involving one side of the head.
hemicephalic vasodilation. CLUSTER HEADACHE.
hemi·ceph·a·lus (hem″ee·sef′uh·lus) *n.*, pl. **hemicepha·li** (·lye) [*hemi-* + *-cephalus*]. An individual exhibiting hemicephaly (HEMIANENCEPHALY).
hemi·ceph·a·ly (hem″ee·sef′uh·lee) *n.* [*hemi-* + *-cephaly*]. HEMIANENCEPHALY; anencephaly on one side only.
hemi·cho·rea (hem″ee·ko·ree′uh) *n.* [*hemi-* + *chorea*]. Chorea in which the involuntary movements are largely confined to one side of the body.
hemi·chro·ma·top·sia (hem″ee·kro″muh·top′see·uh) *n.* HEMIACHROMATOPSIA.
hemic murmur. A cardiac or vascular murmur, usually systolic, heard with anemia or other high cardiac output state; due to increased velocity of blood flow.
hemic myeloma. A malignant plasmacytoma.
hemi·co·lec·to·my (hem″ee·ko·leck′tuh·mee) *n.* [*hemi-* + *colectomy*]. Excision of one side of the colon.
hemi·col·lin (hem″ee·kol′in) *n.* An intermediate product, of indefinite composition, obtained on hydrolysis of gelatin.
hemi·con·vul·sion (hem″ee·kun·vul′shun) *n.* [*hemi-* + *convulsion*]. A form of epilepsy characterized by tonic-clonic movements of one side of the body. See also *H.H.E. syndrome.*
hemiconvulsion-hemiplegia syndrome. ACUTE INFANTILE HEMIPLEGIA.
hemi·cra·nia (hem″i·kray′nee·uh) *n.* [Gk. *hēmikrania*]. 1. MIGRAINE. 2. Pain or headache on one side of the head only.
hemi·cra·ni·o·sis (hem″i·kray″nee·o′sis) *n.* [*hemi-* + *crani-* + *-osis*]. Enlargement of one half of the cranium or face.
hemi·cys·tec·to·my (hem″ee·sis·teck′tuh·mee) *n.* [*hemi-* + *cystectomy*]. Removal of half of the urinary bladder.
hemi·de·cor·ti·ca·tion (hem″ee·dee·kor″ti·kay′shun) *n.* [*hemi-* + *decortication*]. Removal of the cortex from one cerebral hemisphere.
hemi·des·mus (hem″i·dez′mus) *n.* [NL., from *hemi-* + Gk. *desmos*, band]. The dried root of *Hemidesmus indicus;* contains coumarin and a volatile oil. An infusion has been used as a diuretic. Syn. *Indian sarsaparilla.*
hemi·di·a·phragm (hem″ee·dye′uh·fram) *n.* [*hemi-* + *diaphragm*]. 1. A lateral half of the diaphragm. 2. A diaphragm in which the muscle development is deficient on one side.
hem·i·dro·sis, haem·i·dro·sis (hem″i·dro′sis, heem″) *n.* [*hem-* + *idrosis*]. HEMATHIDROSIS.
hemi·dys·es·the·sia, hemi·dys·aes·the·sia (hem″ee·dis″es·theezh′uh, ·theez′ee·uh) *n.* [*hemi-* + *dys-* + *esthesia*]. Impairment of the cutaneous senses, especially of touch, and paresthesias on one side of the body.
hemi·el·lip·tic (hem″ee·e·lip′tick) *adj.* Half elliptical or oval.
hemielliptic fovea. ELLIPTICAL RECESS.
hemi·fa·cial (hem″ee·fay′shul) *adj.* [*hemi-* + *facial*]. Pertaining to one side of the face.
hemifacial spasm. FACIAL HEMISPASM.
hemi·glos·sec·to·my (hem″ee·glos·eck′tuh·mee) *n.* [*hemi-* + *glossectomy*]. Removal of one side of the tongue.
hemi·glos·so·ple·gia (hem″ee·glos″o·plee′jee·uh) *n.* [*hemi-* +

glossoplegia]. Unilateral paralysis of the tongue with relatively minor disturbances of motility; the tongue deviates toward the palsied side upon protrusion.

hemi·gna·thia (hem″i·nay′thee·uh, ·nath′ee·uh) *n.* [*hemi-* + *gnath-* + *-ia*]. Partial or complete absence of the lower jaw on one side. —**hemi·gnath·us** (·nath′us, ·nayth′us) *n.*

hemihypaesthesia. HEMIHYPESTHESIA.

hemi·hyp·al·ge·sia (hem″ee·high″pal·jee′zee·uh) *n.* [*hemi-* + *hypalgesia*]. Decreased sensitivity to pain on one side of the body.

hemi·hy·per·es·the·sia, hemi·hy·per·aes·the·sia (hem″ee·high″pur·es·theezh′uh, ·theez′ee·uh) *n.* [*hemi-* + *hyperesthesia*]. Increased sensitivity to tactile stimulation on one side of the body.

hemi·hy·per·hi·dro·sis (hem″ee·high″pur·hi·dro′sis) *n.* [*hemi-* + *hyperhidrosis*]. Excessive sweating on one side of the body.

hemi·hy·per·i·dro·sis (hem″ee·high″pur·i·dro′sis) *n.* [*hemi-* + *hyperidrosis*]. HEMIHYPERHIDROSIS.

hemi·hy·per·to·nia (hem″ee·high″pur·to′nee·uh) *n.* [*hemi-* + *hypertonia*]. Increased muscular tone confined to one side of the body.

hemi·hy·per·tro·phy (hem″ee·high·pur′truh·fee) *n.* [*hemi-* + *hypertrophy*]. Hypertrophy of one side of the body or unilateral hypertrophy of one or more bodily regions (e.g., the head, an arm).

hemi·hyp·es·the·sia, hemi·hyp·aes·the·sia (hem″ee·high″pes·theezh′uh, theez′ee·uh) *n.* [*hemi-* + *hypesthesia*]. Decreased cutaneous sensitivity in one side of the body.

hemi·hy·po·to·nia (hem″ee·high″po·to′nee·uh) *n.* [*hemi-* + *hypotonia*]. Decreased muscular tone of one side of the body.

hemi·lab·y·rin·thec·to·my (hem″ee·lab″i·rin·theck′tuh·mee) *n.* [*hemi-* + *labyrinthectomy*]. Removal of one or more of the membranous semicircular canals while leaving the ampullated ends and the saccule.

hemi·lam·i·nec·to·my (hem″ee·lam″i·neck′tuh·mee) *n.* [*hemi-* + *laminectomy*]. Laminectomy in which laminae of only one side are removed.

hemi·lar·yn·gec·to·my (hem″ee·lăr″in·jeck′tuh·mee) *n.* [*hemi-* + *laryngectomy*]. Extirpation of one side of the larynx.

hemi·lar·ynx (hem″ee·lăr′inks) *n.* [*hemi-* + *larynx*]. Half of the larynx.

hemi·mac·ro·ceph·a·ly (hem″ee·mack″ro·sef′uh·lee) *n.* [*hemi-* + *macrocephaly*]. Congenital enlargement of one side of the brain.

hemi·man·dib·u·lec·to·my (hem″ee·man″dib·yoo·leck′tuh·mee) *n.* [*hemi-* + *mandibulectomy*]. The surgical removal of one side of the mandible.

hemi·man·di·bu·lo·glos·sec·to·my (hem″ee·man·dib″yoo·lo·glos·eck′tuh·mee) *n.* [*hemi-* + *mandibula* + *gloss-* + *-ectomy*]. Surgical removal of half of the mandible and of the tongue.

hemi·max·il·lec·to·my (hem″ee·mack″si·leck′tuh·mee) *n.* [*hemi-* + *maxilla* + *-ectomy*]. Excision of half of the maxilla.

hemi·me·lia (hem″i·mee′lee·uh) *n.* [*hemi-* + *-melia*]. Congenital absence of all or part of the distal portion of an extremity.

hemi·me·lus (hem″i·mee′lus) *n.*, pl. **hemime·li** (·lye) [*hemi-* + *-melus*]. An individual with incomplete or stunted arms or legs.

hemi·me·tab·o·lous (hem″ee·me·tab′o·lus) *adj.* [*hemi-* + *metabolous*]. Characterizing a type of insect metamorphosis in which the immature stage, known as a nymph, transforms into the adult without an intervening, quiescent, pupal stage; as in grasshoppers, crickets, cockroaches, the true bugs, mayflies, stone flies, and dragonflies. Contr. *holometabolous.*

he·min, hae·min (hee′min) *n.* $C_{34}H_{32}N_4O_4$.FeCl; the chloride of ferriprotoporphyrin, containing iron in the ferric state.

hemin crystals. Reddish-brown, microscopic, prismatic crystals of hemin obtained by heating blood with glacial acetic acid and salt. Syn. *Teichmann's crystals.*

hemi·ne·phrec·to·my (hem″ee·ne·freck′tuh·mee) *n.* [*hemi-* + *nephrectomy*]. Removal of part of a kidney; partial nephrectomy.

hemi·o·pia (hem″ee·o′pee·uh) *n.* [*hemi-* + *-opia*]. HEMIANOPSIA. —**hemi·op·ic** (·op′ick, ·o′pick) *adj.*

he·mip·a·gus (he·mip′uh·gus) *n.* [*hemi-* + *-pagus*]. PROSOPOTHORACOPAGUS.

hemi·pal·at·ec·to·my (hem″ee·pal″uh·teck′tuh·mee) *n.* [*hemi-* + *palate* + *-ectomy*]. Excision of half of the palate.

hemi·pal·a·to·la·ryn·go·ple·gia (hem″ee·pal″uh·to·la·ring″go·plee′jee·uh) *n.* [*hemi-* + *palato-* + *laryngo-* + *-plegia*]. Paralysis of the muscles of the soft palate and larynx on one side.

hemi·pa·ral·y·sis (hem″ee·pa·ral′i·sis) *n.* [*hemi-* + *paralysis*]. HEMIPLEGIA.

hemi·pa·re·sis (hem″ee·pa·ree′sis) *n.*, pl. **hemipare·ses** (·seez) [*hemi-* + *paresis*]. Muscle weakness of one side of the body. —**hemipa·ret·ic** (·ret′ick) *adj.*

hemi-par·kin·son·ism (hem″ee·pahr′kin·sun·iz·um) *n.* [*hemi-* + *parkinsonism*]. Disease of the extrapyramidal system of the brain, manifested by tremor and rigidity of the extremities confined to or predominantly on one side.

hemi·pel·vec·to·my (hem″ee·pel·veck′tuh·mee) *n.* [*hemi-* + *pelv-* + *-ectomy*]. The surgical removal of an entire posterior extremity including the hipbone.

hemi·pel·vis (hem″ee·pel′vis) *n.* [*hemi-* + *pelvis*]. Half of a pelvis.

hemi·pin·to (hem″ee·pin′to) *n.* [*hemi-* + *pinta*]. A unilateral distribution of the cutaneous eruption of pinta.

hemi·ple·gia (hem″i·plee′jee·uh) *n.* [Gk. *hēmiplēgia*, paralysis]. Paralysis of one side of the body. —**hemiple·gic** (·jick) *adj.*

hemiplegia cru·ci·a·ta (kroo·shee·ay′tuh). CROSSED PARALYSIS.

hemiplegic gait. The gait characteristic of a person with hemiplegia, in which the leg on the affected side is stiff and circumducted, the foot scuffing the ground and the arm being held in a stiff, semiflexed position.

He·mip·tera (he·mip′te·ruh) *n.pl.* [*hemi-* + Gk. *ptera*, wings]. 1. An order of insects; the true bugs. 2. Formerly the suborder Heteroptera of the order Hemiptera which also included the suborder Homoptera.

hemi·ra·chis·chi·sis (hem″ee·ra·kis′ki·sis) *n.* [*hemi-* + *rachischisis*]. SPINA BIFIDA OCCULTA.

hemi·sco·to·sis (hem″ee·sko·to′sis) *n.* [*hemi-* + *scotosis*]. HEMIANOPSIA.

hemi·sec·tion (hem″ee·seck′shun) *n.* [*hemi-* + *section*]. 1. The act of division into two lateral halves; bisection. 2. The division of the crown and separation of the roots of a tooth for the removal of the diseased or affected part to accomplish endodontic therapy. —**hemi·sect** (·sekt′) *v.*

hemisection of the spinal cord. Division of one side of the spinal cord. See also *Brown-Séquard's syndrome.*

hemi·sep·tum (hem′i·sep″tum) *n.* The remaining portion of an interdental septum after the mesial or distal portion has been destroyed in periodontal disease.

hemi·so·mus (hem″i·so′mus) *n.* [*hemi-* + *-somus*]. An individual with one side of the body imperfectly developed.

hemi·spasm (hem′ee·spaz·um) *n.* [*hemi-* + *spasm*]. A spasm affecting only one side of the body or part of the body, as in facial hemispasm.

he·mi·sphae·ria bul·bi ure·thrae (hem″i·sfeer′ee·uh bul′bye yoo·ree′three) [BNA]. The lateral halves of the bulb of the urethra.

he·mi·sphae·ri·um ce·re·bel·li (hem″i·sfeer′ee·um serr·e·bel′eye) [BNA]. HEMISPHERIUM CEREBELLI.

hemisphaerium te·len·ce·pha·li (tel″en·sef′uh·lye) [BNA]. HEMISPHERIUM.

hemi·sphere (hem′i·sfeer) *n.* [Gk. *hēmisphairion*]. *In neuroanatomy,* one half of the cerebrum or of the cerebellum.

NA *hemispherium.* —**hemi·sphe·ric** (hem″i·sfeer′ick, ·sferr′ick) *adj.*

hemi·spher·ec·to·my (hem″i·sfeer·eck′tuh·mee) *n.* [*hemisphere* + *-ectomy*]. Surgical excision of one cerebral hemisphere.

hemisphere syndrome. The clinical picture seen in patients with lesions involving one of the cerebral or cerebellar hemispheres.

hemispheric dominance. CEREBRAL DOMINANCE.

hemispheric sulcus. A shallow, circular groove separating the embryonal telencephalon from the diencephalon.

hemispheric syndrome. HEMISPHERE SYNDROME.

he·mi·sphe·ri·um (hem·i·sfeer′ee·um) *n.* [NA]. Either cerebral hemisphere.

hemispherium ce·re·bel·li (serr·e·bel′eye) [NA]. A cerebellar hemisphere; the right or left portion of the cerebellum lateral to the vermis.

hemispherium ce·re·bri (serr′e·brye) [NA]. A cerebral hemisphere; either lateral half of the cerebrum.

hemi·spo·ro·sis (hem″ee·spo·ro′sis) *n.* [*Hemispora*, a fungus, + *-osis*]. Infection with the fungus *Hemispora stellata.*

hemi·syn·er·gia (hem″ee·sin·ur′jee·uh) *n.* [*hemi-* + *synergia*]. Synergia on one side of the body with asynergia on the opposite side.

hemi·sys·to·le (hem″ee·sis′tuh·lee) *n.* [*hemi-* + *systole*]. Contraction of the ventricle after every second atrial contraction so that for each two beats of the atrium only one pulse beat is felt.

hemi·ter·as (hem″ee·terr′us) *n.*, pl. **hemi·ter·a·ta** (·terr′uh·tuh) [*hemi-* + *teras*]. An individual with a malformation not grave enough to be classified as monstrous. —**hemi·te·rat·ic** (·te·rat′ick) *adj.*

hemi·ter·pene (hem″ee·tur′peen) *n.* Any of a group of hydrocarbons of the general formula C_5H_8, as isoprene, related to terpenes.

hemi·tho·rax (hem″ee·tho′racks) *n.* [*hemi-* + *thorax*]. One side of the thorax.

hemi·thy·roid·ec·to·my (hem″ee·thigh″roy·deck′tuh·mee) *n.* [*hemi-* + *thyroidectomy*]. Removal of one lateral lobe of the thyroid gland.

hemi·tri·gone (hem″i·trye′gohn) *n.* One half of the trigone of the urinary bladder, congenital absence of which may denote absence of an ipsilateral kidney.

hemi·ver·te·bra (hem″ee·vur′te·bruh) *n.* [*hemi-* + *vertebra*]. A congenital anomaly of the spine in which one half of a vertebra fails to develop.

hemi·zy·gote (hem″ee·zye′gote) *n.* [*hemi-* + *zygote*]. An individual with only one of a given pair of genes, as in the case of the sex-linked genes in the human male; or with only one of each of all the pairs of genes, as the male bee. —**hemizy·gous** (·gus) *adj.*

hem·lock, *n.* 1. An evergreen tree, genus *Tsuga,* of North America and Asia. 2. A large herb, *Conium maculata,* of the carrot family which yields coniine. See also *conium.*

Hem·me·ler's thrombopathy. A familial anomaly characterized by poor granulation of megakaryocytes, large platelets, normal platelet count, and a bleeding tendency.

hemo-, haemo-. See *hem-.*

he·mo·al·ka·lim·e·ter, hae·mo·al·ka·lim·e·ter (hee″mo·al″kuh·lim′e·tur) *n.* [*hemo-* + *alkalimeter*]. An apparatus for estimating the degree of alkalinity of the blood.

Hemobartonella. *HAEMOBARTONELLA.*

he·mo·bil·ia (hee″mo·bil′ee·uh) *n.* HEMATOBILIA.

he·mo·bil·i·ru·bin, hae·mo·bil·i·ru·bin (hee″mo·bil·i·roo′bin) *n.* [*hemo-* + *bilirubin*]. 1. Bilirubin as it occurs normally in serum before passing through the hepatic cells. 2. A form of bilirubin present normally in blood serum, which is increased in amount in hemolytic jaundice. It gives a negative direct van den Bergh's test. See also *cholebilirubin.*

he·mo·blast, hae·mo·blast (hee′mo·blast) *n.* [*hemo-* + *-blast*]. A primitive blood cell. —**he·mo·blas·tic, hae·mo·blas·tic** (hee″mo·blas′tick) *adj.*

hemoblastic leukemia. STEM CELL LEUKEMIA.

he·mo·che·zia, hae·mo·che·zia (hee″mo·kee′zee·uh) *n.* [*hemo-* + Gk. *chezein*, to defecate, + *-ia*]. The passage of blood, especially bright red blood, in the feces. Sometimes used to distinguish this type of blood from the dark blood characteristic of melena.

he·mo·cho·ri·al, hae·mo·cho·ri·al (hee″mo·kor′ee·ul) *adj.* [*hemo-* + *chorial*]. Pertaining to maternal blood and chorionic ectoderm (trophoblast), especially in their intimate contact in the hemochorial placenta.

hemochorial placenta. A type of placenta in which the chorionic ectoderm is in direct contact with maternal blood; found in insectivores, bats, and anthropoids.

he·mo·chro·ma·to·sis, hae·mo·chro·ma·to·sis (hee″mo·kro″muh·to′sis) *n.* [*hemo-* + *chromatosis*]. A chronic disease characterized pathologically by excessive deposits of iron in the body and clinically by hepatomegaly with cirrhosis, skin pigmentation, diabetes mellitus, and frequently cardiac failure; it may be idiopathic, erythropoietic, dietary, or due to blood transfusion. The idiopathic form is heritable, but the mechanism of its inheritance has not been elucidated. Syn. *bronze diabetes.* —**hemochroma·tot·ic, haemochroma·tot·ic** (·tot′ick) *adj.*

he·mo·chrome, hae·mo·chrome (hee′muh·krome) *n.* [*hemo-* + *-chrome*]. The coloring matter of the blood; HEME.

he·mo·chro·mo·gen, hae·mo·chro·mo·gen (hee″mo·kro′muh·jen) *n.* [*hemochrome* + *-gen*]. The class of substances formed by the union of heme with a nitrogen-containing substance, as a protein or base.

he·mo·chro·mom·e·ter, hae·mo·chro·mom·e·ter (hee″mo·kro·mom′e·tur) *n.* [*hemochrome* + *-meter*]. A colorimeter; an instrument for estimating the amount of hemoglobin in the blood, by comparing a solution of the blood with a standard, such as a solution of ammonium picrocarminate.

he·mo·cla·sia, hae·mo·cla·sia (hee″mo·klay′zhuh, ·zee·uh) *n.* [*hemo-* + *-clasia*]. HEMOLYSIS. —**hemo·clas·tic, haemo·clas·tic** (·klas′tick) *adj.*

he·moc·la·sis, hae·moc·la·sis (he·mock′luh·sis) *n.* [*hemo-* + *-clasis*]. HEMOLYSIS.

he·mo·co·ag·u·la·tion, hae·mo·co·ag·u·la·tion (hee″mo·ko·ag″yoo·lay′shun) *n.* [*hemo-* + *coagulation*]. Blood coagulation.

he·mo·co·ag·u·lin, hae·mo·co·ag·u·lin (hee″mo·ko·ag′yoo·lin) *n.* A compound of certain snake venoms which is associated with intravascular blood clotting.

he·mo·coe·lom, hae·mo·coe·lom (hee″mo·see′lum) *n.* [*hemal-* + *coelom*]. The body cavity of the embryo which contains the heart.

he·mo·con·cen·tra·tion, hae·mo·con·cen·tra·tion (hee″mo·kon″sin·tray′shun) *n.* [*hemo-* + *concentration*]. An increase in the concentration of blood cells resulting from the loss of plasma or water from the bloodstream without a concomitant loss of formed elements, as in extensive burns; ANHYDREMIA.

he·mo·co·nia, hae·mo·co·nia (hee″mo·ko′nee·uh) *n.pl.* [*hemo-* + Gk. *konia*, dust]. Round or dumbbell-shaped refractile, colorless particles found in blood plasma.

he·mo·co·ni·o·sis, hae·mo·co·ni·o·sis (hee″mo·ko″nee·o′sis) *n.* [*hemoconia* + *-osis*]. The condition of having an abnormal amount of hemoconia in the blood.

he·mo·cry·os·co·py, hae·mo·cry·os·co·py (hee″mo·krye·os′kuh·pee) *n.* [*hemo-* + *cryo-* + *-scopy*]. Determination of the freezing point of the blood.

he·mo·cu·pre·in, hae·mo·cu·pre·in (hee″mo·kew′pree·in) *n.* A copper protein, having a molecular weight of about 35,000 and containing two atoms of copper per molecule, obtained from erythrocytes of several animals.

he·mo·cy·a·nin, hae·mo·cy·a·nin (hee″mo·sigh′uh·nin) *n.* A blue respiratory pigment that contains copper, found in the blood of arthropods and mollusks.

he·mo·cyte, hae·mo·cyte (hee'mo·site) *n.* [*hemo-* + *-cyte*]. BLOOD CELL.

he·mo·cy·to·blast, hae·mo·cy·to·blast (hee''mo·sigh'to·blast) *n.* [*hemocyte* + *-blast*]. The cell considered by some to be the primitive stem cell, giving rise to all blood cells. —**hemo·cy·to·blas·tic, haemo·cy·to·blas·tic** (·sigh''to·blas'tick) *adj.*

hemocytoblastic leukemia. STEM CELL LEUKEMIA.

he·mo·cy·to·blas·to·ma, hae·mo·cy·to·blas·to·ma (hee''mo·sigh''to·blas·to'muh) *n.* [*hemocytoblast* + *-oma*]. 1. STEM CELL LEUKEMIA. 2. A tumor that is composed of the most primitive bone marrow cells.

he·mo·cy·to·gen·e·sis, hae·mo·cy·to·gen·e·sis (hee''mo·sigh''to·jen'e·sis) *n.* [*hemocyte* + *-genesis*]. HEMATOPOIESIS.

he·mo·cy·tol·y·sis, hae·mo·cy·tol·y·sis (hee''mo·sigh·tol'i·sis) *n.*, pl. **hemocytoly·ses, haemocytoly·ses** (·seez) [*hemocyte* + *-lysis*]. The dissolution of blood cells.

he·mo·cy·tom·e·ter, hae·mo·cy·tom·e·ter (hee''mo·sigh·tom'e·tur) *n.* [*hemocyte* + *-meter*]. An instrument for counting the number of blood cells. —**hemocytome·try, haemocytome·try** (·tree) *n.*

he·mo·cy·to·poi·e·sis, hae·mo·cy·to·poi·e·sis (hee''mo·sigh''to·poy·ee'sis) *n.* HEMATOPOIESIS.

he·mo·cy·to·zo·on, hae·mo·cy·to·zo·on (hee''mo·sigh''to·zo'on) *n.*, pl. **hemocyto·zoa, haemocyto·zoa** (·zo'uh) [*hemocyte* + *-zoon*]. A protozoan parasite inhabiting the red blood cells.

he·mo·di·ag·no·sis, hae·mo·di·ag·no·sis (hee''mo·dye·ug·no'sis) *n.*, pl. **hemodiagno·ses, haemodiagno·ses** (·seez) [*hemo-* + *diagnosis*]. Diagnosis by examination of the blood.

he·mo·di·al·y·sis, hae·mo·di·al·y·sis (hee''mo·dye·al'i·sis) *n.* [*hemo-* + *dialysis*]. The process of exposing blood to a semipermeable membrane, thereby removing from it or adding to it diffusible materials, rate and direction being a function of the concentration gradient across that membrane.

he·mo·di·a·stase, hae·mo·di·a·stase (hee''mo·dye'uh·stace) *n.* [*hemo-* + *diastase*]. The amylolytic enzyme of blood.

he·mo·di·lu·tion, hae·mo·di·lu·tion (hee''mo·di·lew'shun) *n.* [*hemo-* + *dilution*]. A condition of the blood in which the ratio of blood cells to plasma is reduced.

he·mo·dromo·graph, hae·mo·dromo·graph (hee''mo·drom'o·graf) *n.* [*hemo-* + *dromo-* + *-graph*]. An instrument for recording the velocity of the blood flow.

he·mo·dro·mom·e·ter, hae·mo·dro·mom·e·ter (hee''mo·dro·mom'e·tur) *n.* [*hemo-* + *dromo-* + *-meter*]. An instrument for measuring the velocity of the blood flow. —**hemodro·mome·try, haemodromome·try** (·tree) *n.*

he·mo·dy·nam·ics, hae·mo·dy·nam·ics (hee''mo·dye·nam'icks) *n.* [*hemo-* + *dynamics*]. The study of the interrelationship of blood pressure, blood flow, vascular volumes, physical properties of the blood, heart rate, and ventricular function. —**hemodynamic,** *adj.*

he·mo·dy·na·mom·e·ter, hae·mo·dy·na·mom·e·ter (hee''mo·dye''nuh·mom'e·tur) *n.* [*hemo-* + *dynamo-* + *-meter*]. An instrument for measuring the pressure of the blood within the arteries. —**hemodynamome·try** (·tree) *adj.*

he·mo·en·do·the·li·al, hae·mo·en·do·the·li·al (hee''mo·en''do·theel'ee·ul) *adj.* [*hemo-* + *endothelial*]. Pertaining to maternal blood and to the endothelium of the chorionic villi.

hemoendothelial placenta. A type of placenta in which the endothelium of vessels of chorionic villi is in direct contact with maternal blood; found in the rat and guinea pig.

he·mo·eryth·rin, hae·mo·eryth·rin (hee''mo·e·rith'rin, hee''mo·err'i·thrin) *n.* [*hemo-* + Gk. *erythros*, red, + *-in*]. A red pigment found in the blood of worms and other invertebrates.

he·mo·flag·el·late, hae·mo·flag·el·late (hee''mo·flaj'e·late) *n.* [*hemo-* + *flagellate*]. Any protozoan flagellate living in the blood of its host.

he·mo·fus·cin, hae·mo·fus·cin (hee''mo·fus'in) *n.* [*hemo-* + *fuscin*]. An insoluble lipid pigment found in liver cells.

he·mo·gen·e·sis, hae·mo·gen·e·sis (hee''mo·jen'e·sis) *n.* [*hemo-* + *-genesis*]. Formation of blood or blood cells; HEMATOPOIESIS.

he·mo·gen·ic, hae·mo·gen·ic (hee''mo·jen'ick) *adj.* 1. Of or pertaining to hemogenesis; HEMATOPOIETIC. 2. Derived from blood or caused by a condition of the blood.

hemogenic-hemolytic balance. The balance in the body between the production of normal erythrocytes and their destruction, which maintains the count and the hemoglobin at the optimum level by physiologic processes.

hemogenic shock. HYPOVOLEMIC SHOCK.

he·mo·glo·bin, hae·mo·glo·bin (hee'muh·glo''bin) *n.* [*hemo-* + *globulin*]. The respiratory pigment of erythrocytes, having the reversible property of taking up oxygen (oxyhemoglobin, HbO_2) or of releasing it (reduced hemoglobin, Hb), depending primarily on the oxygen tension of the medium surrounding it. At tensions of 100 mmHg or more, hemoglobin is fully saturated with oxygen; at 50 mmHg, oxygen is progressively more rapidly dissociated. Other factors affecting dissociation of oxyhemoglobin are temperature, electrolytes, and carbon dioxide tension (Bohr effect). Human hemoglobin consists of four heme molecules (iron-protoporphyrin) linked to the protein globin, which is composed of complexly folded polypeptide chains. Globin may vary in its essential properties, resulting in definite normal and genetically determined abnormal types, which may be differentiated on biochemical, pathophysiological, and genetic bases; it may differ in the fetus and in the adult, and also in different animal species. The average molecular weight of hemoglobin is about 67,000. Hemoglobin combines with carbon monoxide to form the stable compound carboxyhemoglobin. Oxidation of the ferrous iron of hemoglobin to the ferric state produces methemoglobin. Abbreviated, Hb. See also Table of Chemical Constituents of Blood in the Appendix.

hemoglobin A. The type of hemoglobin found in normal adults, which moves as a single component in an electrophoretic field, is rapidly denatured by highly alkaline solutions, and contains two titratable sulfhydryl groups per molecule. It forms orthorhombic crystals. Specific hemoglobin A antibodies have been obtained.

hemoglobin C. A slow-moving abnormal hemoglobin associated with intraerythrocytic crystal formation, target cells, and chronic hemolytic anemia; it may occur together with sickle-cell hemoglobin.

hemoglobin carbamate. CARBAMINOHEMOGLOBIN.

hemoglobin C disease. A disease largely of blacks, characterized by anemia, splenomegaly, target erythrocytes, intraerythrocytic hemoglobin crystals, and presence of hemoglobin C.

hemoglobin E. An abnormal hemoglobin found in Southeast Asia, migrating slightly faster than hemoglobin C; in the homozygous form it causes a mild hemolytic anemia with normochromic target cells.

he·mo·glo·bi·ne·mia, hae·mo·glo·bi·nae·mia (hee''muh·glo''bi·nee'mee·uh) *n.* [*hemoglobin* + *-emia*]. The presence in the blood plasma of hemoglobin.

hemoglobin F. FETAL HEMOGLOBIN.

hemoglobin H. An abnormal hemoglobin migrating more rapidly than normal hemoglobin on electrophoresis, and usually associated with thalassemia.

he·mo·glo·bin·if·er·ous, hae·mo·glo·bin·if·er·ous (hee''muh·glo''bi·nif'ur·us) *adj.* [*hemoglobin* + *-iferous*]. Yielding or carrying hemoglobin.

hemoglobin M. An abnormal hemoglobin associated with hereditary methemoglobinemia, which can be differentiated from normal hemoglobin in its electrophoretic mobility by the starch-block method.

he·mo·glo·bi·nom·e·ter, hae·mo·glo·bi·nom·e·ter (hee''muh·glo''bi·nom'e·tur) *n.* [*hemoglobin* + *-meter*]. An instrument for determining the hemoglobin concentration of the blood. —**hemoglobinome·try, haemoglobinome·try** (·tree) *n.;* **hemoglobi·no·met·ric, haemoglobi·no·met·ric** (·no·met′rick) *adj.*

he·mo·glo·bin·op·a·thy (hee″muh·glo·bi·nop′uh·thee) *n.* Any disease caused by abnormal hemoglobin.

he·mo·glo·bi·no·phil·ic, hae·mo·glo·bi·no·phil·ic (hee″muh·glo″bi·no·fil′ick) *adj.* [*hemoglobin* + *-philic*]. HEMOPHILIC (1).

hemoglobin S. SICKLE CELL HEMOGLOBIN.

he·mo·glo·bin·uria, hae·mo·glo·bin·uria (hee″muh·glo″bi·new′ree·uh) *n.* The presence of hemoglobin in the urine. —**hemoglobin·uric, haemoglobin·uric** (·new′rick) *adj.*

hemoglobinuric fever. BLACKWATER FEVER.

hemoglobinuric nephrosis. ACUTE TUBULAR NECROSIS.

he·mo·gram, hae·mo·gram (hee′mo·gram) *n.* [*hemo-* + *-gram*]. 1. The number of erythrocytes and leukocytes per cubic millimeter of blood plus the differential leukocyte count and hemoglobin level in grams per 100 ml blood. 2. The differential leukocyte count.

he·mo·his·tio·blast, hae·mo·his·tio·blast (hee″mo·his′tee·o·blast) *n.* [*hemo-* + *histioblast*]. The hypothetical reticuloendothelial cell from which all the cells of the blood are eventually differentiated; a stem cell.

he·mo·hy·dro·sal·pinx, hae·mo·hy·dro·sal·pinx (hee″mo·high″dro·sal′pinks) *n.* [*hemo-* + *hydro-* + *salpinx*]. A state in which blood and watery fluid distend a uterine tube.

hemokonia, haemokonia. HEMOCONIA.

hemokoniosis, haemokoniosis. HEMOCONIOSIS.

he·mo·lith, hae·mo·lith (hee′mo·lith) *n.* [*hemo-* + *-lith*]. A stone or concretion within the lumen of a blood vessel, or incorporated in the wall of a blood vessel.

he·mo·lymph, hae·mo·lymph (hee′mo·limf) *n.* [*hemo-* + *lymph*]. The circulating nutritive fluid of certain invertebrates.

hemolymph gland or **node.** HEMAL NODE.

he·mol·y·sate (he·mol′i·sate) *n.* The product obtained when blood or a material containing blood undergoes hemolysis.

he·mol·y·sin, hae·mol·y·sin (he·mol′i·sin, hee″mo·lye′sin) *n.* [*hemo-* + *lysin*]. A substance that frees hemoglobin from the red cells.

α-hemolysin. ALPHA HEMOLYSIN.

β-hemolysin. BETA HEMOLYSIN.

δ-hemolysin. DELTA HEMOLYSIN.

γ-hemolysin. GAMMA HEMOLYSIN.

he·mol·y·sis, hae·mol·y·sis (he·mol′i·sis) *n.*, pl. **hemoly·ses, haemoly·ses** (·seez) [*hemo-* + *-lysis*]. The destruction of red blood cells and the resultant escape of hemoglobin. —**he·mo·lyt·ic, hae·mo·lyt·ic** (hee″mo·lit′ick, hem″o·) *adj.*

α-hemolysis. ALPHA HEMOLYSIS.

β-hemolysis. BETA HEMOLYSIS.

α-hemolytic. ALPHA-HEMOLYTIC.

β-hemolytic. BETA-HEMOLYTIC.

hemolytic anemia. Anemia resulting from excessive destruction of erythrocytes.

hemolytic anemia of pregnancy. Any anemia of pregnancy which results in excessive destruction of erythrocytes; may be due to extrinsic causes, as drugs, or intrinsic causes, as congenital ones, or to immunologic reactions.

hemolytic crisis. Sudden rapid erythrocyte destruction or cessation of blood formation, usually referring to a hemolytic anemia.

hemolytic disease of the newborn. ERYTHROBLASTOSIS FETALIS.

hemolytic index. The ratio of urobilinogen excretion to total circulating hemoglobin. The normal ratio is 11 to 21 mg per 100 g hemoglobin.

hemolytic jaundice. 1. Jaundice due to excessive red blood cell destruction. 2. HEREDITARY SPHEROCYTOSIS.

hemolytic splenomegaly. HEREDITARY SPHEROCYTOSIS.

hemolytic streptococci. A group of β-hemolytic streptococci, especially varieties of *Streptococcus pyogenes,* that produce complete hemolysis on blood agar. It includes Lancefield groups A, B, C, E, F, G, H, K, L, M, O. Occasionally strains not producing complete hemolysis elaborate C-substance identical with the above Lancefield groups, and are therefore classified in this group. Group A and less commonly groups C and G are pathogenic for man. Group A is subdivided into 40 or more types on the basis of a type-specific protein (M-substance) produced by matt colonies; especially, types 12 and 4 are thought to be associated with acute glomerulonephritis. Members of this group also cause scarlet fever, erysipelas, sore throat, and other infections.

hemolytic-uremic syndrome. An acute illness of unknown cause, principally of infants and sometimes of older children and adults, that may follow a nonspecific respiratory infection; characterized clinically by bloody diarrhea, hemolytic anemia with abnormally shaped erythrocytes, thrombocytopenia, and azotemia, and pathologically by findings similar to those seen in the Shwartzman phenomenon, as well as by fibrin deposits, endothelial proliferation, and hyalin necrosis of the walls of blood vessels.

he·mo·lyto·poi·et·ic, hae·mo·lyto·poi·et·ic (hee″mo·lit″o·poy·et′ick, hem″o·) *adj.* [*hemolytic* + *hemopoietic*]. Pertaining to the processes of blood destruction and blood formation.

he·mo·lyze, hae·mo·lyze (hee′mo·lize, hem′o·) *v.* To produce hemolysis. —**he·mo·ly·za·tion, hae·mo·ly·za·tion** (hee″mo·li·zay′shun, hem″o·) *n.*

he·mo·ma·nom·e·ter, hae·mo·ma·nom·e·ter (hee″mo·ma·nom′e·tur) *n.* [*hemo-* + *manometer*]. A manometer for determining blood pressure.

he·mo·me·di·as·ti·num, hae·mo·me·di·as·ti·num (hee″mo·mee″dee·uh·stye′num) *n.* [*hemo-* + *mediastinum*]. The presence of blood in the mediastinal space.

he·mo·meta·ki·ne·sia, hae·mo·meta·ki·ne·sia (hee″mo·met″uh·kigh·nee′zee·uh, ·ki·nee′zhuh) *n.* HEMOMETAKINESIS.

he·mo·meta·ki·ne·sis, hae·mo·meta·ki·ne·sis (hee″mo·met″uh·kigh·nee′sis, ·ki·nee′sis) *n.* [*hemo-* + Gk. *metakinēsis,* shifting, dislocation]. The borrowing-lending hemodynamic phenomena consisting of proper temperature control and adequate variation of blood flow to satisfy local demands by the normal uninterrupted flow of sympathetic nervous impulses.

he·mom·e·ter, hae·mom·e·ter (he·mom′e·tur) *n.* [*hemo-* + *-meter*]. 1. HEMOGLOBINOMETER. 2. HEMODYNAMOMETER. —**hemome·try, haemome·try** (·tree) *n.*

he·mo·me·tra, hae·mo·me·tra (hee″mo·mee′truh) *n.* HEMATOMETRA.

he·mo·my·e·lo·gram, hae·mo·my·e·lo·gram (hee″mo·migh′e·lo·gram) *n.* [*hemo-* + *myelo-* + *-gram*]. A differential count of the leukocytes.

he·mo·pa·thol·o·gy, hae·mo·pa·thol·o·gy (hee″mo·pa·thol′uh·jee) *n.* [*hemo-* + *pathology*]. The science of the diseases of the blood.

he·mop·a·thy, hae·mop·a·thy (hee·mop′uth·ee) *n.* [*hemo-* + *-pathy*]. Any disease of the blood.

he·mo·peri·car·di·um, hae·mo·peri·car·di·um (hee″mo·perr″i·kahr′dee·um) *n.* [*hemo-* + *pericardium*]. The presence of blood or bloody effusion in the pericardial sac.

he·mo·peri·to·ne·um, hae·mo·peri·to·ne·um (hee″mo·perr″i·tuh·nee′um) *n.* [*hemo-* + *peritoneum*]. An effusion of blood into the peritoneal cavity.

he·mo·pex·in, hae·mo·pex·in (hee·mo·peck′sin) *n.* [*hemo-* + Gk. *pexis,* fixation, + *-in*]. A heme-binding protein in human plasma that may be a regulator of heme and drug metabolism, and a distributor of heme. Measurement of its levels in serum and amniotic fluid may aid in assessing the severity of porphyria and certain hemolytic conditions.

he·mo·phage, hae·mo·phage (hee′mo·faij) *n.* [*hemo-* + *-phage*]. A phagocytic cell that destroys red blood cells. —**he·mo·phag·ic, hae·mo·phag·ic** (hee″mo·faj′ick, hem″o·), **he·moph·a·gous, hae·moph·a·gous** (he·mof′uh·gus) *adj.*

he·mo·pha·gia, hae·mo·pha·gia (hee″mo·fay′jee·uh, hem″o·) *n.* [*hemo-* + *-phagia*]. 1. Ingestion of blood as a therapeutic agent. 2. Feeding on the blood of another organism. 3. Phagocytosis of the red blood cells.

he·mo·phil, hae·mo·phil (hee′mo·fil) *adj.* [*hemo-* + *-phil*]. Characterizing an organism that grows preferably on blood media.

he·mo·phil·ia, hae·mo·phil·ia (hee″mo·fil′ee·uh) *n.* [*hemo-* + *-philia*]. 1. An X-linked recessive hereditary bleeding disorder caused by factor VIII or factor IX deficiency and characterized clinically by hemarthrosis, hematomas, ecchymoses, gastrointestinal and genitourinary bleeding, and excessive traumatic bleeding. See also *hemophilia A, hemophilia B.* 2. Broadly, any of various other hereditary procoagulant deficiencies clinically similar to hemophilia A or B.

hemophilia A. Hemophilia resulting from deficiency of factor VIII; the typical and most common hemophilia.

hemophilia B. CHRISTMAS DISEASE; hemophilia resulting from deficiency of factor IX.

he·mo·phil·i·ac, hae·mo·phil·i·ac (hee″mo·fil′ee·ack) *n.* An individual who is affected with hemophilia.

hemophilia neonatorum. HEMORRHAGIC DISEASE OF THE NEWBORN.

he·mo·phil·ic, hae·mo·phil·ic (hee″mo·fil′ick, hem″o·) *adj.* [*hemophil* + *-ic*]. 1. *In biology,* pertaining to bacteria growing well in culture media containing hemoglobin. 2. Pertaining to hemophilia or to a hemophiliac.

hemophilic arthritis. Arthritis that is the result of repeated bleeding into the joints in a hemophilic patient.

hemophilic factor A. FACTOR VIII.

hemophilic factor B. FACTOR IX.

hemophilic factor C. FACTOR XI.

he·mo·phil·i·oid, hae·mo·phil·i·oid (hee″mo·fil′ee·oid) *adj.* [*hemophilia* + *-oid*]. Designating any coagulation disorder that resembles hemophilia, but that is the result of a genetic defect different from that in hemophilia.

Hemophilus. *HAEMOPHILUS.*

he·mo·pho·bia, hae·mo·pho·bia (hee″mo·fo′bee·uh) *n.* [*hemo-* + *-phobia*]. An abnormal fear of the sight of blood or of bleeding.

he·moph·thal·mia, hae·moph·thal·mia (hee″mof·thal′mee·uh) *n.* [*hem-* + *ophthalm-* + *-ia*]. Hemorrhage into the vitreous.

he·moph·thal·mos, hae·moph·thal·mos (hee″mof·thal′mus) *n.* [*hem-* + *ophthalmos*]. HEMOPHTHALMIA.

he·moph·thi·sis, hae·moph·thi·sis (he·mof″thi·sis, hee″mof·thigh′sis) *n.* [*hemo-* + Gk. *phthisis,* a wasting away]. Anemia caused by degeneration or inadequate formation of red blood cells.

he·mo·plas·tic, hae·mo·plas·tic (hee″mo·plas′tick) *adj.* [*hemo-* + *-plastic*]. Blood-forming.

he·mo·pleu·ra, hae·mo·pleu·ra (hee″mo·plew′ruh) *n.* [*hemo-* + *pleura*]. HEMOTHORAX.

he·mo·pneu·mo·tho·rax, hae·mo·pneu·mo·tho·rax (hee″mo·new″mo·thor′acks) *n.* [*hemo-* + *pneumo-* + *thorax*]. A collection of blood and air within the pleural cavity.

he·mo·poi·e·sis, hae·mo·poi·e·sis (hee″mo·poy·ee′sis, hem″o·) *n.*, pl. **hemopoie·ses, haemopoie·ses** (·seez) [*hemo-* + *-poiesis*]. HEMATOPOIESIS. —**hemo·poi·et·ic, haemo·poi·et·ic** (·poy·et′ick) *adj.*

he·mo·poi·e·tin, hae·mo·poi·e·tin (hee″mo·poy′e·tin) *n.* INTRINSIC FACTOR.

he·mo·por·phy·rin, hae·mo·por·phy·rin (hee″mo·por′fi·rin) *n.* Iron-free heme, $C_{34}H_{38}N_4O_6$; a porphyrin obtained in vitro by treating hemoglobin with sulfuric acid. It is closely related to the naturally occurring porphyrins.

he·mo·pre·cip·i·tin, hae·mo·pre·cip·i·tin (hee″mo·pre·sip′i·tin) *n.* A precipitin specific for blood.

he·mo·pro·to·zoa (hee″mo·pro·tuh·zo′uh) *n.pl.* [*hemo-* + *protozoa*]. Protozoan parasites that circulate in the host's blood stream during some particular stage in their life cycle, as for example trypanosomes and plasmodia.

he·mop·ty·sis, hae·mop·ty·sis (hee·mop′ti·sis) *n.* [*hemo-* + *ptysis*]. The spitting of blood or blood-stained sputum from the lungs, trachea, or bronchi.

he·mo·pyr·role, he·mo·pyr·rol, hae·mo·pyr·role (hee″mo·pi·role′, ·pirr′ole) *n.* Any of several pyrrole derivatives formed by reduction of heme.

hem·or·rhage, haem·or·rhage (hem′uh·rij) *n.* [Gk. *haimorrhagia,* from *haima,* blood, + *rēgnynai,* to burst forth]. An escape of blood from the vessels, either by diapedesis through intact capillary walls or by flow through ruptured walls; bleeding. —**hem·or·rhag·ic, haem·or·rhag·ic** (hem″uh·raj′ick) *adj.*

hemorrhagic abscess. An abscess with a prominent admixture of blood.

hemorrhagic anemia. Anemia following gross hemorrhage.

hemorrhagic cyst. 1. A circumscribed collection of blood, representing a focus of hemorrhage into a solid tissue or organ. 2. A cyst in which hemorrhage into the lumen has occurred.

hemorrhagic diathesis. An abnormal bleeding tendency as in hemophilia, purpura, scurvy, or vitamin K deficiency.

hemorrhagic disease of the newborn. A bleeding tendency occurring in the neonatal period as a result of vitamin K deficiency.

hemorrhagic encephalitis. ACUTE NECROTIZING HEMORRHAGIC ENCEPHALOMYELITIS.

hemorrhagic exudate. SANGUINEOUS EXUDATE.

hemorrhagic fever. EPIDEMIC HEMORRHAGIC FEVER.

hemorrhagic infarct. RED INFARCT.

hemorrhagic infarction. RED SOFTENING.

hemorrhagic inflammation or **mucositis.** Inflammation in which the exudate contains blood, usually as the result of vascular damage by the inflammatory process.

hemorrhagic measles. A grave variety of measles with a hemorrhagic eruption and severe constitutional symptoms. Syn. *black measles.*

hemorrhagic mucositis. Hemorrhagic inflammation invading a mucous membrane.

hemorrhagic nephrosonephritis. EPIDEMIC HEMORRHAGIC FEVER.

hemorrhagic pachymeningitis. *Obsol.* Chronic subdural hematoma.

hemorrhagic polioencephalitis. POLIOENCEPHALITIS HEMORRHAGICA.

hemorrhagic purpura. IDIOPATHIC THROMBOCYTOPENIC PURPURA.

hemorrhagic salpingitis. HEMATOSALPINX.

hemorrhagic scarlet fever. A toxic form of scarlet fever with hemorrhagic erythema.

hemorrhagic septicemia. SHIPPING FEVER.

hemorrhagic softening. The softening of parts involved in a hemorrhage.

hem·or·rhag·in, haem·or·rhag·in (hem″o·raj′in, ·ray′jin) *n.* [*hemorrhage* + *-in*]. A cytolysin found in venoms of snakes and other animals which can destroy blood vessels and endothelial cells.

he·mor·rhe·ol·o·gy (hee″mo·ree·ol′uh·jee, hem″o·) *n.* [*hemo-* + *rheology*]. A branch of medical science which seeks to ascertain physical laws obeyed by circulating blood.

hem·or·rhoid, haem·or·rhoid (hem′uh·roid) *n.* [Gk. *haimorrhois, haimorrhoidos,* from *haima,* blood, + *-rrhoos,* flowing]. A varix in the lower rectal or anal wall; a pile.

hem·or·rhoi·dal, haem·or·rhoi·dal (hem″uh·roy′dul) *adj.* 1. Pertaining to or affected with hemorrhoids. 2. Of or pertaining to blood vessels or nerves of the anus.

hemorrhoidal anthrax. A contagious type of anthrax affecting the rectum of animals and marked by dark bloody feces.

hemorrhoidal plexus. RECTAL PLEXUS (1).

hemorrhoidal ring. A circular swelling of the wall of the anal canal at the level of the external sphincter muscle; it contains the rectal venous plexus. When enlarged, it forms hemorrhoids. NA *zona hemorrhoidalis.*

hem·or·rhoid·ec·to·my, haem·or·rhoid·ec·to·my (hem″o·roy·deck′tuh·mee) *n.* [*hemorrhoid* + *-ectomy*]. Surgical removal of hemorrhoids.

hem·or·rhoids, haem·or·rhoids (hem′uh·roidz) *n.pl.* [Gk. *haimorrhoides*]. A plexus or multiple plexuses of varicose veins in the lower rectum or anus. Syn. *piles.*

he·mo·sal·pinx, hae·mo·sal·pinx (hee″mo·sal′pinks) *n.* [*hemo-* + *salpinx*]. HEMATOSALPINX.

he·mo·sid·er·in, hae·mo·sid·er·in (hee″mo·sid′ur·in) *n.* [*hemo-* + *sider-* + *-in*]. An iron-containing glycoprotein pigment found in liver and in most tissues, representing colloidal iron in the form of granules much larger than ferritin molecules. It is insoluble in water and differs from ferritin in electrophoretic mobility. Pathologic accumulations are known to occur in a number of disease states.

he·mo·sid·er·ino·pe·nia, hae·mo·sid·er·ino·pe·nia (hee″mo·sid″ur·in·o·pee′nee·uh) *n.* HEMOSIDEROPENIA.

he·mo·sid·er·in·uria, hae·mo·sid·er·in·uria (hee″mo·sid″ur·i·new′ree·uh) *n.* The presence of hemosiderin in the urine.

he·mo·sid·ero·pe·nia, hae·mo·sid·ero·pe·nia (hee″mo·sid″ur·o·pee′nee·uh) *n.* [*hemosiderin* + *-penia*]. Hemosiderin deficiency in the bone marrow and other storage sites.

he·mo·sid·er·o·sis, hae·mo·sid·er·o·sis (hee″mo·sid″ur·o′sis) *n.*, pl. **hemosider·ses, haemosidero·ses** (·seez) [*hemosiderin* + *-osis*]. Deposition of hemosiderin in body tissues without tissue damage, reflecting an increase in body iron stores. See also *hemochromatosis.*

he·mo·sper·mia, hae·mo·sper·mia (hee″mo·spur′mee·uh) *n.* The discharge of bloody semen; HEMATOSPERMIA.

he·mo·sta·sia, hae·mo·sta·sia (hee″mo·stay′zhuh, ·zee·uh) *n.* HEMOSTASIS.

he·mo·sta·sis, hae·mo·sta·sis (hee″mo·stay′sis, hee·mos′tuh·sis) *n.*, pl. **hemosta·ses, haemosta·ses** (·seez) [Gk. *haimostasis,* styptic]. 1. The arrest of a flow of blood or hemorrhage either physiologically via vasoconstriction and clotting or by surgical intervention. 2. The stopping or slowing of the circulation through a vessel or area of the body.

he·mo·stat, hae·mo·stat (hee′mo·stat) *n.* [*hemo-* + *-stat*]. An agent or instrument that arrests the flow of blood.

he·mo·stat·ic, hae·mo·stat·ic (hee″mo·stat′ick) *n.* [*hemo-* + *-static*]. An agent that arrests hemorrhage. Syn. *hemostyptic.*

hemostatic forceps. ARTERY FORCEPS.

he·mo·styp·tic, hae·mo·styp·tic (hee″mo·stip′tick) *n.* [*hemo-* + *styptic*]. HEMOSTATIC.

he·mo·ta·chom·e·ter, hae·mo·ta·chom·e·ter (hee″mo·ta·kom′e·tur) *n.* [*hemo-* + *tacho-* + *-meter*]. An instrument for measuring the rate of blood flow. **—hemotachome·try, haemotachome·try** (·tree) *n.*

he·mo·ther·a·peu·tics, hae·mo·ther·a·peu·tics (hee″mo·therr″uh·pew′ticks) *n.* HEMOTHERAPY.

he·mo·ther·a·py, hae·mo·ther·a·py (hee″mo·therr′uh·pee) *n.* [*hemo-* + *therapy*]. The treatment of disease by means of blood or blood derivatives.

he·mo·tho·rax, hae·mo·tho·rax (he″mo·tho′racks) *n.* [*hemo-* + *thorax*]. An accumulation of blood in the pleural cavity. Syn. *hemopleura.*

he·mo·tox·ic·i·ty, hae·mo·tox·ic·i·ty (hee″mo·tock·sis′i·tee) *n.* [*hemo-* + *toxicity*]. The property of being injurious to blood or blood-forming organs.

he·mo·tox·in, hae·mo·tox·in (hee″mo·tock′sin) *n.* [*hemo-* + *toxin*]. A cytotoxin capable of destroying red blood cells. **—hemotox·ic, haemotox·ic** (·sick) *adj.*

he·mot·ro·phe, hae·mot·ro·phe (hee′mo·trofe, ·trof, he·mot′ro·fee) *n.* [*hemo-* + Gk. *trophē,* nourishment]. All the nutritive substances supplied to the embryo from the maternal bloodstream in viviparous animals having a deciduate placenta. See also *embryotrophe.* **—he·mo·troph·ic, hae·mo·troph·ic** (hee″mo·trof′ick) *adj.*

he·mo·tym·pa·num, hae·mo·tym·pa·num (hee″mo·tim′puh·num) *n.* [*hemo-* + *tympanum*]. The presence of blood in the tympanic cavity.

he·mo·zo·in, hae·mo·zo·in (hee″mo·zo′in) *n.* [*hemozoon* + *-in*]. A dark-brown or red-brown pigment, seen within plasmodia; formed from the disintegrated hemoglobin.

he·mo·zo·on, hae·mo·zo·on (hee″mo·zo′on) *n.* [*hemo-* + *-zoon*]. HEMATOZOON.

hemp, *n.* [OE. *haenep* ← Gmc. **hanipiz* (rel. to Gk. *kannabis*)]. *Cannabis sativa,* the bast fiber of which is used for textile purposes. See also *cannabis.*

hemp-worker's disease. BYSSINOSIS.

hen·bane, *n.* HYOSCYAMUS.

Hench and Al·drich's test [P. S. *Hench,* U.S. physician, 1896–1965; and Martha *Aldrich,* U.S. biochemist, b. 1897]. A test for retention of urea in the blood by measuring the amount of urea in the saliva.

hen·dec·yl (hen·des′il) *n.* UNDECYL.

Hen·der·son-Has·sel·balch equation [L. J. *Henderson,* U.S. biochemist, 1879-1942; and K. *Hasselbalch,* Danish biochemist and physician, b. 1874]. An equation expressing the pH of a buffer solution as a function of the concentrations of weak acid (or weak base) and salt components of the buffer. For a weak acid-salt buffer system, the equation is $pH = pK_a + \log(\text{salt}/\text{acid})$, where pK_a is the negative logarithm of the ionization constant of the acid.

Henderson's operation [M. S. *Henderson,* U.S. orthopedist, 1883-1954]. An operation for habitual dislocation of the shoulder, a section of peroneus longus tendon being used to anchor the head of the humerus in place.

Hen·le's ampulla (hen′leh) [F. G. J. *Henle,* German anatomist, 1809–1885]. AMPULLA OF THE DUCTUS DEFERENS.

Henle's fenestrated membrane [F. G. J. *Henle*]. FENESTRATED MEMBRANE.

Henle's layer [F. G. J. *Henle*]. LAYER OF HENLE.

Henle's ligament [F. G. J. *Henle*]. The lateral expansion of the tendinous insertion of the rectus abdominis muscle situated posterior to the falx inguinalis.

Henle's loop [F. G. J. *Henle*]. LOOP OF HENLE.

Henle's muscle [F. G. J. *Henle*]. The anterior auricular muscle. See Table of Muscles in the Appendix.

Henle's sheath [F. G. J. *Henle*]. ENDONEURIUM.

Henle's spine [F. G. J. *Henle*]. SUPRAMEATAL SPINE.

Henle's warts [F. G. J. *Henle*]. HASSALL-HENLE WARTS.

Henneberg's disease [R. *Henneberg*]. METACHROMATIC LEUKODYSTROPHY.

He·noch-Schön·lein purpura (heʸ′nokh, shœhn′line) [E. H. *Henoch,* German pediatrician, 1820–1910; and J. L. *Schönlein*]. Purpura having features of both Henoch's purpura and Schönlein's purpura, such as abdominal pain, gastrointestinal bleeding, joint pain, and nephritis.

Henoch's purpura [E. H. *Henoch*]. A type of allergic, nonthrombocytopenic purpura associated with attacks of gastrointestinal pain and bleeding and with erythematous or urticarial exanthema. See also *Henoch-Schofnlein purpura.*

hen·pue (hen′poo·ee) *n.* [West African]. GOUNDOU.

Hen·ri·ques-Sør·en·sen method (sœr″n·sun) [V. *Henriques,* Danish biochemist, 1864–1936; and S. P. L. *Sørensen,* Danish chemist, 1868–1939]. A method for determining the presence of amino acid nitrogen. If formaldehyde is added to a solution of amino acids, interaction with amino groups destroys their basic property so that the carboxyl groups may be titrated with alkali.

hen·ry (hen′ree) *n.*, pl. **hen·rys, hen·ries** (·reez) [J. *Henry,* U.S. physicist, 1797–1878]. The unit of electric inductance; the inductance in a circuit such that an electromotive force of 1 volt is induced in the circuit by variation of an inducing current at the rate of 1 ampere per second. Abbreviated, h.

Hen·ry's law [W. *Henry,* English chemist, 1774–1836]. The amount of gas dissolved in a liquid is proportional to the pressure of the gas; hence, if the temperature is constant, the ratio of the concentrations of the gas in gaseous form and in solution is constant.

Hen·ry's melano-flocculation test [A. F. G. *Henry*, Turkish pathologist, b. 1894]. A test for malaria which depends upon changes in the serum proteins; gives a high percentage of positive reactions in malaria, but sometimes is positive in syphilis and other diseases.

Hen·sen's canal or **duct** (hen'z^{e}n) [V. *Hensen*, German pathologist, 1835–1924]. DUCTUS REUNIENS.

Hensen's disk [V. *Hensen*]. The low-density region bisecting A disk of a striated myofibril, occupied by myosin filaments only. Syn. *H zone.*

Hensen's node or **knot** [V. *Hensen*]. In the embryo, an accumulation of cells at the anterior end of the primitive streak, through which the neurenteric canal passes from the outside into the blastodermic vesicle. Syn. *primitive node or knot.*

hep·ap·to·sis (hep"ap·to'sis) *n.* [*hepar* + *ptosis*]. HEPATOPTOSIS.

he·par (hee'pahr) *n.* [Gk *hēpar, hēpatos* (rel. to L. *iecur*)]. 1. [NA] LIVER. 2. *Obsol.* A substance having the color of liver, generally a compound of sulfur, as hepar sulfuris.

hep·a·ran sulfate (hep'uh·ran). HEPARITIN SULFATE.

hep·a·rin (hep'uh·rin) *n.* [L. *hepar*, liver, + *-in*]. An acid mucopolysaccharide acting as an antithrombin, antithromboplastin, and antiplatelet factor to prolong the clotting time of whole blood; it occurs in a variety of tissues, most abundantly in the liver. Employed parenterally as an anticoagulant, in the form of the sodium salt. —**heparin·ize** (·ize) *v.*; **heparin·oid** (·oid) *adj.*

hep·a·ri·ne·mia, hep·a·ri·nae·mia (hep"uh·ri·nee'mee·uh) *n.* [*heparin* + *-emia*]. The presence of heparin in the circulating blood.

hep·a·rino·cyte (hep"uh·rin'o·site) *n.* [*heparin* + *-cyte*]. A cell that produces heparin; a mast cell.

hep·a·ri·tin sulfate (hep'uh·ri·tin). A sulfate ester of an acetylated heparin.

hep·a·ri·tin·uria (hep"uh·ri·ti·new'ree·uh) *n.* [*heparitin* sulfate + *-uria*]. Heparitin sulfate in the urine; characteristic of the mucopolysaccharidoses, particularly of Sanfillipo's syndrome.

hepar lo·ba·tum (lo·bay'tum). The nodular lobulated liver of syphilitic cirrhosis; gummatous pseudolobation.

hepar sul·fu·ris (sul'few·ris). SULFURATED POTASH.

hepat-, hepato- [Gk. *hēpar, hēpatos*]. A combining form meaning *liver, hepatic.*

hep·a·tal·gia (hep"uh·tal'jee·uh) *n.* [*hepat-* + *-algia*]. Pain in the liver. —**hepatal·gic** (·jick) *adj.*

hep·a·tec·to·my (hep"uh·teck'tuh·mee) *n.* [*hepat-* + *-ectomy*]. Excision of the liver or of a part of it.

he·pat·ic (he·pat'ick) *adj.* [Gk. *hēpatikos*, from *hēpar*, liver]. Of, pertaining to, or involving the liver.

He·pat·i·ca (he·pat'i·kuh) *n.* Liverwort; a genus of ranunculaceous plants. *Hepatica triloba* and *H. acutiloba* formerly were employed in the treatment of hepatic, renal, and pulmonary complaints.

hepatic artery. One of the three branches of the celiac trunk. The common hepatic artery (arteria hepatica communis) gives off the right gastric and gastroduodenal arteries and continues as the proper hepatic artery (arteria hepatica propria) to the liver.

hepatic calculus. A biliary calculus situated in the intrahepatic biliary passages.

hepatic coma. 1. A state of unconsciousness seen in patients severely ill with liver disease. 2. The precomatose state of hepatic encephalopathy.

hepatic cords. The anastomosing columns of liver cells separated by the hepatic sinusoids.

hepatic diverticulum. The primordium of the liver, gallbladder, and their ducts.

hepatic duct. The common hepatic duct or any of its branches.

hepatic duct system. The biliary tract including the hepatic ducts, gallbladder, cystic duct, and common bile duct.

hepatic encephalopathy. Disturbance of central nervous function involving the changes in consciousness, mentation, behavior, and neurologic status occurring in advanced liver disease. See also *hepatic coma.*

hepatic facies. The sharp, pinched features, sunken eyes, and yellowish skin seen in patients with chronic liver disorders.

hepatic failure. LIVER FAILURE.

hepatic fetor. FETOR HEPATICUS.

hepatic fever. VIRAL HEPATITIS.

hepatic flexure. An abrupt bend where the ascending colon becomes the transverse colon. NA *flexura coli dextra.*

hepatic glycogenosis. VON GIERKE'S DISEASE.

hepatic gutter. HEPATIC DIVERTICULUM.

hepatic infantilism. Failure to grow associated with liver disease.

hepatico-. A combining form meaning *hepatic.*

he·pat·i·co·du·o·de·nos·to·my (he·pat"i·ko·dew"o·de·nos'tuh·mee) *n.* [*hepatico-* + *duodeno-* + *-stomy*]. Establishment of an anastomosis between the hepatic duct and the duodenum.

he·pat·i·co·en·ter·os·to·my (he·pat"i·ko·en"tur·os'tuh·mee) *n.* [*hepatico-* + *entero-* + *-stomy*]. Establishment of an anastomosis between the hepatic duct and the intestine.

he·pat·i·co·gas·tros·to·my (he·pat"i·ko·gas·tros'tuh·mee) *n.* [*hepatico-* + *gastro-* + *-stomy*]. Establishment of an anastomosis between the hepatic duct and the stomach.

he·pat·i·co·je·ju·nos·to·my (he·pat"i·ko·jej"oo·nos'tuh·mee) *n.* [*hepatico-* + *jejuno-* + *-stomy*]. Surgical connection of the hepatic duct and the jejunum.

he·pat·i·co·li·thot·o·my (he·pat"i·ko·li·thot'uh·mee) *n.* [*hepatico-* + *lithotomy*]. Removal of a biliary calculus from the liver or any of its ducts.

he·pat·i·co·pan·cre·at·ic (he·pat"i·ko·pan"kree·at'ick) *adj.* [*hepatico-* + *pancreatic*]. Pertaining to the liver and the pancreas.

hepaticopancreatic ampulla. The dilation of the common bile duct and pancreatic duct where they join the duodenum. NA *ampulla hepatopancreatica.*

he·pat·i·co·re·nal (he·pat"i·ko·ree'nul) *adj.* HEPATORENAL.

hepaticorenal syndrome. HEPATORENAL SYNDROME.

he·pat·i·cos·to·my (he·pat"i·kos'tuh·mee) *n.* [*hepatico-* + *-stomy*]. The formation of a fistula in the hepatic duct for the purpose of drainage.

he·pat·i·cot·o·my (he·pat"i·kot'uh·mee) *n.* [*hepatico-* + *-tomy*]. Incision into the hepatic duct.

hepatic plexus. A visceral nerve network accompanying the hepatic artery to the liver. NA *plexus hepaticus.*

hepatic porphyria. ACUTE INTERMITTENT PORPHYRIA.

hepatic tubules. HEPATIC CORDS.

hepatic vein occlusion. BUDD-CHIARI SYNDROME.

hepatic veins. The veins which drain blood from the liver into the inferior vena cava. NA *venae hepaticae.* See also Table of Veins in the Appendix.

hepatic zones. The central, midzonal, and peripheral parts of the liver lobule.

hepatitides. Plural of *hepatitis;* inflammatory diseases of the liver.

hep·a·ti·tis (hep"uh·tye'tis) *n.*, pl. **hepa·tit·i·des** (·tit'i·deez) [Gk. *hēpatitis*]. Inflammation of the liver. See also *infectious hepatitis, serum hepatitis, halothane hepatitis.*

hepatitis A. INFECTIOUS HEPATITIS.

hepatitis-associated antigen. An antigen associated with a spherical lipid-containing particle 200 to 250 Å in diameter and virus-like in appearance, found in the blood of most individuals with serum hepatitis. Abbreviated, HAA. Syn. *Australia antigen.*

hepatitis B. SERUM HEPATITIS.

hepatitis virus A. The virus of infectious hepatitis.

hepatitis virus B. The virus of serum hepatitis.

hep·a·ti·za·tion (hep″uh·ti·zay′shun) *n.* The conversion of tissue, as of the lungs during the exudative stage of pneumonia, into a liverlike substance. See also *gray hepatization, red hepatization, yellow hepatization.* —**hep·a·tized** (hep′uh·tize′d) *adj.*

hepato-. See *hepat-.*

hep·a·to·can·a·lic·u·lar (hep″uh·to·kan″uh·lick′yoo·lur) *adj.* [*hepato-* + *canalicular*]. Pertaining to the intrahepatic bile duct tributaries, especially the very small ones.

hepatocanalicular jaundice. CHOLESTATIC HEPATITIS.

hep·a·to·cel·lu·lar (hep″uh·to·sel′yoo·lur) *adj.* [*hepato-* + *cellular*]. Of or pertaining to the liver cells.

hepatocellular jaundice. Jaundice due to destruction or functional impairment of the liver cells.

hep·a·to·chol·an·gio·du·o·de·nos·to·my (hep″uh·to·ko·lan″jee·o·dew″o·de·nos′tuh·mee) *n.* [*hepato-* + *cholangio-* + *duodenostomy*]. Establishment of a communication between the hepatic duct and the duodenum.

hep·a·to·chol·an·gio·en·ter·os·to·my (hep″uh·to·ko·lan″jee·o·en″tur·os′tuh·mee) *n.* [*hepato-* + *cholangio-* + *entero-* + *-stomy*]. Establishment of an anastomosis between the hepatic duct and some portion of the small intestine.

hep·a·to·chol·an·gio·gas·tros·to·my (hep″uh·to·ko·lan″jee·o·gas·tros′tuh·mee) *n.* [*hepato-* + *cholangio-* + *gastro-* + *-stomy*]. Establishment of an anastomosis between the hepatic duct and the stomach.

hep·a·to·chol·an·gio·je·ju·nos·to·my (hep″uh·to·ko·lan″jee·o·jej·oo·nos′tuh·mee) *n.* [*hepato-* + *cholangio-* + *jejuno-* + *-stomy*]. Establishment of a communication between the hepatic duct and the jejunum.

hep·a·to·co·lic (hep″uh·to·ko′lick, ·kol′ick) *adj.* [*hepato-* + *colic*]. Pertaining to the liver and the colon.

hepatocolic ligament. A prolongation of the hepatoduodenal ligament downward to the transverse colon. NA *ligamentum hepatocolicum.*

hep·a·to·cu·pre·in (hep″uh·to·kew′pree·in) *n.* A copper-containing protein, similar to hemocuprein, but isolated from liver.

hep·a·to·cys·tic (hep″uh·to·sist′ick) *adj.* [*hepato-* + *cystic*]. Pertaining to the liver and the gallbladder.

hepatocystic duct. A bile duct connected directly with the gallbladder.

he·pa·to·cyte (he·pat′o·site, hep′uh·to·) *n.* [*hepato-* + *-cyte*]. An epithelial cell constituting the major cell type in the liver.

hep·a·to·du·o·de·nal (hep″uh·to·dew″o·dee′nul, ·dew·od′e·nul) *adj.* [*hepato-* + *duodenal*]. Pertaining to the liver and the duodenum.

hepatoduodenal ligament. The portion of the lesser omentum extending between the liver and the duodenum. NA *ligamentum hepatoduodenale.*

hep·a·to·du·o·de·nos·to·my (hep″uh·to·dew″o·de·nos′tuh·mee) *n.* HEPATICODUODENOSTOMY.

hep·a·to·fla·vin (hep″uh·to·flay′vin) *n.* Riboflavin isolated from liver.

hep·a·to·gen·ic (hep″uh·to·jen′ick) *adj.* [*hepato-* + *-genic*]. HEPATOGENOUS.

hep·a·tog·e·nous (hep″uh·toj′e·nus) *adj.* [*hepato-* + *-genous*]. Produced by or originating in the liver.

hepatogenous jaundice. Jaundice due to liver disease.

hepatogenous peptonuria. Peptonuria accompanying certain liver diseases.

hepatogenous pigment. BILE PIGMENT.

hep·a·to·gram (hep′uh·to·gram) *n.* [*hepato-* + *-gram*]. 1. A graphic record of the liver pulse. 2. A radiograph of the liver, usually a phase of hepatic angiography.

hep·a·to·je·ju·nal (hep″uh·to·je·joo′nul) *adj.* [*hepato-* + *jejunal*]. Pertaining to the liver and jejunum.

hep·a·to·jug·u·lar reflux (hep″uh·to·jug′yoo·lur). Compression of the abdomen, especially, but not necessarily, over the liver with marked jugular venous distention and pulsation when right-sided heart failure is present.

hep·a·to·len·tic·u·lar (hep″uh·to·len·tick′yoo·lur) *adj.* [*hepato-* + *lenticular*]. Pertaining to the liver and the lentiform nucleus.

hepatolenticular degeneration. A recessive autosomal disorder associated with abnormalities of copper metabolism, characterized by decreased serum ceruloplasmin and copper values and increased urinary copper excretion. Untreated patients develop tissue copper deposits associated with hepatic cirrhosis, deep marginal pigmentation of the cornea (Kayser-Fleischer rings), and extensive degenerative changes in the central nervous system, particularly the basal ganglions. Syn. *Wilson's disease.*

hep·a·to·li·enal (hep″uh·to·lye·ee′nul, ·lye′e·nul) *adj.* [*hepato-* + *lienal*]. Pertaining to the liver and the spleen.

hep·a·to·li·en·og·ra·phy (hep″uh·to·lye″e·nog′ruh·fee) *n.* [*hepato-* + *lieno-* + *-graphy*]. Radiographic examination of the liver and the spleen.

hep·a·to·lith (hep′uh·to·lith) *n.* [*hepato-* + *-lith*]. A calculus in the biliary passages of the liver.

hep·a·to·li·thec·to·my (hep″uh·to·li·theck′tuh·mee) *n.* [*hepatolith* + *-ectomy*]. HEPATICOLITHOTOMY.

hep·a·to·li·thi·a·sis (hep″uh·to·li·thigh′uh·sis) *n.* [*hepatolith* + *-iasis*]. The presence or formation of calculi in the biliary passages of the liver.

hep·a·tol·o·gy (hep″uh·tol′uh·jee) *n.* [*hepato-* + *-logy*]. The medical study and treatment of the liver. —**hepatolo·gist,** *n.*

hep·a·to·ma (hep″uh·to′muh) *n.*, pl. **hepatomas, hepatoma·ta** (·tuh) [*hepat-* + *-oma*]. 1. A malignant tumor whose parenchymal cells resemble those of the liver. 2. Any tumor of the liver.

hep·a·to·me·ga·lia (hep″uh·to·me·gay′lee·uh) *n.* HEPATOMEGALY.

hep·a·to·meg·a·ly (hep″uh·to·meg′uh·lee) *n.* [*hepato-* + *-megaly*]. Enlargement of the liver.

hep·a·tom·pha·lo·cele (hep″uh·tom·fal′o·seel, ·tom′fuh·lo·) *n.* [*hepat-* + *omphalocele*]. An umbilical hernia containing liver.

hep·a·to·pan·cre·at·ic (hep″uh·to·pan″kree·at′ick) *adj.* [*hepato-* + *pancreatic*]. HEPATICOPANCREATIC.

hepatopancreatic duct. The terminal part of the embryonic common bile duct which also drains the ventral pancreas.

hep·a·to·pexy (hep′uh·to·peck″see) *n.* [*hepato-* + *-pexy*]. Surgical fixation of a movable, or ptosed, liver; usually by utilizing additional supportive power of the round and the falciform ligaments.

hep·a·top·to·sia (hep″uh·top·to′zee·uh, ·zhuh, hep″uh·to·to′zee·uh) *n.* HEPATOPTOSIS.

hep·a·top·to·sis (hep″uh·top·to′sis, hep″uh·to·to′sis) *n.* [*hepato-* + *-ptosis*]. Abnormally low position of the liver in the abdomen.

hep·a·to·re·nal (hep″uh·to·ree′nul) *adj.* [*hepato-* + *renal*]. Pertaining to both the liver and the kidney.

hepatorenal glycogenosis. VON GIERKE'S DISEASE.

hepatorenal ligament. A fold of peritoneum extending from the inferior surface of the liver to the right kidney. NA *ligamentum hepatorenale.*

hepatorenal pouch. The portion of the peritoneal cavity situated behind the right lobe of the liver and in front of the right kidney and right portion of the transverse mesocolon. Syn. *pouch of Morison.* NA *recessus hepatorenalis.*

hepatorenal recess. HEPATORENAL POUCH.

hepatorenal syndrome. 1. Hyperpyrexia, oliguria, azotemia, and coma; the renal failure once thought to be of toxic origin, related to hepatic decompensation, now is generally agreed to be concomitant hepatic and renal failure, due to infection, dehydration, hemorrhage, or shock. Syn. *Heyd's syndrome.* 2. Renal failure occurring in any severe chronic hepatic disease, probably related to change in renal blood flow.

hep·a·tor·rha·phy (hep″uh·tor′uh·fee) *n.* [*hepato-* + *-rrhaphy*]. Suturing of the liver following an injury or an operation.

hep·a·tor·rhex·is (hep″uh·to·reck′sis) *n.*, pl. **hepatorrhex·es** (·seez) [*hepato-* + *-rrhexis*]. Rupture of the liver.

hep·a·tos·co·py (hep″uh·tos′kuh·pee) *n.* [*hepato-* + *-scopy*] Inspection of the liver, as by laparotomy or peritoneoscopy.

hep·a·to·sis (hep″uh·to′sis) *n.*, pl. **hepato·ses** (·seez) [*hepat-* + *-osis*]. Any noninflammatory disorder of the liver.

hep·a·to·sple·no·meg·a·ly (hep″uh·to·splee″no·meg′uh·lee) *n.* [*hepato-* + *spleno-* + *-megaly*]. Enlargement of the liver and spleen.

hep·a·to·sple·nop·a·thy (hep″uh·to·splee·nop′uth·ee) *n.* [*hepato-* + *spleno-* + *-pathy*]. Any combination of disorders of the liver and spleen.

hep·a·to·ther·a·py (hep″uh·to·therr′uh·pee) *n.* [*hepato-* + *therapy*]. Therapeutic use of liver or liver extract.

hep·a·tot·o·my (hep″uh·tot′uh·mee) *n.* [*hepato-* + *-tomy*]. Incision into the liver.

hep·a·to·tox·in (hep″uh·to·tock′sin) *n.* [*hepato-* + *toxin*]. 1. Any substance that produces injury or death of parenchymal liver cells. 2. A poisonous or deleterious product elaborated in the liver. —**hepatotox·ic** (·sick) *adj.*

hep·a·to·uro·log·ic (hep″uh·to·yoor·uh·loj′ick) *adj.* [*hepato-* + *urologic*]. HEPATORENAL.

hepatourologic syndrome. HEPATORENAL SYNDROME.

hept-, hepta- [Gk. *hepta*]. A combining form meaning *seven, seventh.*

hepta-. See *hept-.*

hep·ta·bar·bi·tal (hep″tuh·bahr′bi·tol, ·tal) *n.* 5-(1-Cyclohepten-1-yl)-5-ethylbarbituric acid, $C_{13}H_{18}N_2O_3$, a sedative and hypnotic having short duration of action.

hept·al·de·hyde (hep·tal′de·hide) *n.* Heptyl aldehyde, $C_7H_{14}O$, a colorless liquid of aromatic odor. Has been used experimentally to induce certain retrogressive changes in tumors of animals. Syn. *enanthaldehyde.*

hep·tane (hep′tane) *n. n*-Heptane, C_7H_{16}, liquid hydrocarbon of the paraffin series, present in petroleum; used as a solvent.

hep·tose (hep′toce, ·toze) *n.* Any member of the group of the monosaccharides containing seven carbon atoms.

hep·tyl (hep′til) *n.* The univalent radical $CH_3(CH_2)_6$—.

heptyl aldehyde. HEPTALDEHYDE.

her·a·path·ite (herr′uh·pa·thite, herr·ap′uh·thite) *n.* [W. *Herapath,* English chemist, 1796–1868]. Quinine iodosulfate; plate-like crystals of a pale olive green by transmitted light, and a golden green by reflected light. Has strong polarizing ability.

herb, *n.* [L. *herba,* grass, herb]. 1. A plant without a woody stem. 2. A plant used for medicinal purposes or for its odor or flavor.

her·ba·ceous (hur·bay′shus) *adj.* [L. *herbaceus,* grassy]. 1. Of plants: having stems or other organs that have a tender, juicy consistency and perish at the close of the growing season. 2. Of the nature of herbs.

herb·al, *adj.* & *n.* 1. Of or pertaining to herbs. 2. A book on the medicinal virtues of herbs.

her·bi·cide (hur′bi·side) *n.* [*herb* + *-cide*]. A substance used to destroy herbaceous plants; weed killer.

her·biv·o·rous (hur·biv′ur·us) *adj.* [*herb* + L. *vor*are, to devour, + *-ous*]. Living on vegetable food; applied mainly to grazing and browsing mammals. —**her·bi·vore** (hur′bi·vore) *n.*

Herbst's bodies or **corpuscles** (hehrpst) [E. F. G. *Herbst,* German anatomist, 1803–1893]. A type of sensory end organs, resembling Pacinian corpuscles, found in the mucous membrane of the tongue of the duck.

herd immunity. Resistance of a large group of animals or humans to one or more specific infections, as a result of individual immunities in large enough proportion to make spread of infection within the group uncommon; may be due to both specific and nonspecific factors.

herd instinct. The fundamental psychic urge to identify oneself with a group and to function in the same manner as the group; group feeling. Syn. *gregariousness.*

he·red·i·tary (he·red′i·terr·ee) *adj.* 1. Of or pertaining to heredity. 2. Of or pertaining to inheritance; inborn; inherited. Compare *congenital, familial.*

hereditary angioedema. A hereditary disorder, transmitted as an autosomal dominant trait, characterized by recurrent rapid attacks of edema, particularly around the glottis, caused by failure to produce the inhibitor of the first component of complement, or by production of a nonfunctional form of that protein. Abbreviated, HAE.

hereditary anhidrosis. HEREDITARY ANHIDROTIC ECTODERMAL DYSPLASIA.

hereditary anhidrotic ectodermal dysplasia. One of a very large group of primarily cutaneous congenital abnormalities, marked chiefly by deficient or absent sweat-gland function (anhidrosis), deficient development of the teeth (hypodontia) or their absence (anodontia), and by congenital alopecia. Transmitted in a mild form as a dominant trait, and in a severe form as an X-linked recessive trait. Syn. *Siemen's syndrome.*

hereditary cerebellar ataxia. 1. FRIEDREICH'S ATAXIA. 2. MARIE'S ATAXIA.

hereditary cerebellar sclerosis. MARIE'S ATAXIA.

hereditary chorea. HUNTINGTON'S CHOREA.

hereditary deforming chondrodysplasia. MULTIPLE HEREDITARY EXOSTOSES.

hereditary disease. A disorder transmitted from parent to offspring through the genes; may be dominant or recessive, sex-linked or autosomal. Compare *congenital disease, familial disease.*

hereditary dystrophic lipidosis. ANGIOKERATOMA CORPORIS DIFFUSUM UNIVERSALE.

hereditary edema. MILROY'S DISEASE.

hereditary gingival fibromatosis. FIBROMATOSIS GINGIVAE.

hereditary hemorrhagic telangiectasia. A hereditary disease characterized by multiple telangiectases and a tendency to habitual hemorrhages, most commonly epistaxis. Syn. *Osler-Rendu-Weber disease.*

hereditary kinesthetic reflex epilepsy. PAROXYSMAL CHOREOATHETOSIS.

hereditary leptocytosis. THALASSEMIA.

hereditary multiple cartilaginous exostoses. MULTIPLE HEREDITARY EXOSTOSES.

hereditary multiple neurofibromatosis. NEUROFIBROMATOSIS.

hereditary multiple polyposis. Any of various hereditary polypoid conditions of the gastrointestinal tract, such as Peutz-Jeghers syndrome and familial polyposis.

hereditary nephritis. ALPORT'S SYNDROME.

hereditary nonhemolytic hyperbilirubinemia. GILBERT'S DISEASE.

hereditary opalescent dentin. DENTINOGENESIS IMPERFECTA.

hereditary osteoonychodystrophia. NAIL-PATELLA SYNDROME.

hereditary perforating ulcer of the foot. HEREDITARY SENSORY NEUROPATHY.

hereditary progressive ar·thro·oph·thal·mop·a·thy (ahr″thro·off″thal·mop′uth·ee). A dominantly inherited disease, manifesting abnormal epiphyseal development, degenerative joint changes beginning in childhood, progressive myopia with retinal detachment and blindness, and sensorineural loss.

hereditary pseudohemophilia. VASCULAR HEMOPHILIA.

hereditary sensory neuropathy. Any of a group of inherited neuropathies which have their basis in a chronic and selective degeneration of sensory neurons, often associated with areflexia, painless infections of the feet and toes, perforating ulcers over the pressure points of the soles, and mutilation of the extremities, and sometimes with sensorineural hearing loss.

hereditary spherocytosis. A chronic dominantly inherited disorder characterized by spherocytosis, increased osmotic fragility of the red corpuscles, splenomegaly, and a variable degree of hemolytic anemia. Syn. *chronic acholuric jaundice, chronic familial jaundice, congenital hemolytic anemia, hemolytic splenomegaly, spherocytic anemia.*

hereditary spinal ataxia or **sclerosis.** FRIEDREICH'S ATAXIA.

he·red·i·ty, *n.* [L. *hereditas,* inheritance]. The inborn capacity of the organism to develop ancestral characteristics; it is dependent upon the constitution and organization of the cell or cells that form the starting point of the new individual. In biparental reproduction, this starting point is the fertilized egg.

heredo- [L. *heres, heredis,* heir]. A combining form meaning *hereditary.*

her·e·do·de·gen·er·a·tion (herr″e·do·de·jen″uh·ray′shun) *n.* A degenerative process or state which results from a hereditary defect. —**heredode·gen·er·a·tive** (·jen′ur·uh·tiv) *adj.*

her·e·do·fa·mil·i·al (herr″e·do·fa·mil′ee·ul) *adj.* [*heredo-* + *familial*]. Characterizing a disease or condition that occurs in more than one member of a family and is suspected of being inherited.

heredofamilial tremor. FAMILIAL TREMOR.

her·e·do·mac·u·lar (herr″e·do·mack′yoo·lur) *adj.* Of hereditary diseases, involving the macular part of the retina.

heredomacular degeneration. Genetically transmitted macular degeneration.

her·e·do·path·ia atac·ti·ca poly·neu·ri·ti·for·mis (herr″e·do·path′ee·uh a·tack′ti·kuh pol″ee·new·rye″ti·for′mis). REFSUM'S SYNDROME.

He·ring-Breu·er reflex (heʸr′ing, broy′ur) [H. E. *Hering,* German physiologist, 1866–1948; and J. *Breuer,* Austrian psychiatrist, 1842–1925]. The neural mechanism that controls respiration automatically by impulses transmitted via the pulmonary fibers of the vagus nerves.

Hering's canal [K. E. K. *Hering,* German physiologist, 1834–1918]. Any one of the passages from the bile canaliculi to the smallest radicles of the bile ducts.

Hering's theory of color vision [K. E. K. *Hering*]. DICHROMATIC THEORY OF COLOR VISION.

her·i·ta·bil·i·ty, *n.* The ratio of the variance due to genetic effects to the total variance, used as an index of the extent to which the phenotype is genetically determined and responsive to selection.

her·i·ta·ble, *adj.* [MF.]. Able to be inherited.

her·i·tage, *n.* [OF., from *heriter,* to inherit]. *In genetics,* the sum total of the genes of characteristics transmitted from parents to their children.

Her·litz's disease or **syndrome** [G. *Herlitz,* 20th century]. EPIDERMOLYSIS BULLOSA HEREDITARIA LETALIS.

Her·man·sky-Pud·lak syndrome (herr′maʰn·skiʰ, pood′laʰk) [F. *Hermansky* and P. *Pudlak,* Czech physicians, 20th century]. The triad of tyrosinase-positive oculocutaneous albinism, hemorrhagic diathesis due to storage pool-deficient platelets that do not aggregate normally, and an accumulation of a ceroid-like material in the reticuloendothelial system, oral mucosa, and urine.

her·maph·ro·dism (hur·maf′ro·diz·um) *n.* HERMAPHRODITISM.

her·maph·ro·dite (hur·maf′ro·dite) *n.* [Gk. *hermaphroditos,* a person partaking of the primary attributes of both sexes, from *Hermaphroditos,* son of Hermes and Aphrodite]. An individual showing hermaphroditism. Compare *pseudohermaphrodite.* —**her·maph·ro·dit·ic** (hur·maf″ro·dit′ick) *adj.*

her·maph·ro·dit·ism (hur·maf′ro·dye·tiz·um) *n.* [*hermaphrodite* + *-ism*]. A condition characterized by the coexistence in an individual of ovarian and testicular tissue.

Her·me·tia (hur·mee′shee·uh) *n.* A genus of the soldier fly family, Stratiomyiidae. The species *Hermetia illucens* is an occasional cause of intestinal myiasis.

her·met·ic (hur·met′ick) *adj.* [NL. *hermeticus,* after *Hermes* Trismegistus, the Egyptian god Thoth, said to have invented an airtight seal]. Protected from exposure to air; airtight. —**hermet·i·cal·ly** (·ick·uh·lee) *adv.*

her·nia (hur′nee·uh) *n.,* pl. **hernias, her·ni·ae** (·nee·ee) [L.]. The abnormal protrusion of an organ or a part through the containing wall of its cavity, usually the abdominal cavity, beyond its normal confines. Syn. *rupture.* Compare *prolapse.* —**her·nial** (·nee·ul) *adj.*

hernial aneurysm. An aneurysm in which the internal coat of the artery, with or without the middle coat, forms the aneurysmal sac that has forced its way through an opening in the outer coat.

hernial canal. A canal giving passage to a hernia.

hernial sac. The pouch or protrusion of peritoneum containing a herniated organ or part, formed gradually by pressure against a defect in the containing wall or present at birth.

hernia of the brain. Protrusion of a portion of the brain through a defect in the skull.

hernia of the lungs. A rare, congenital anomaly associated with fissured chest, in which a portion of the lung protrudes through the opening, the swelling enlarging with each expiration.

her·ni·ate (hur′nee·ate) *v.* To form a hernia. —**herni·at·ed** (·ay·tid) *adj.;* **her·ni·a·tion** (hur″nee·ay′shun) *n.*

herniated disk. An intervertebral disk in which the nucleus pulposus has protruded through the surrounding fibrocartilage, occurring most frequently in the lower lumbar region, less commonly in the cervical region. Mild to severe symptoms may result from pressure on spinal nerves. Syn. *ruptured intervertebral disk, slipped disk.* See also *sciatica.*

herniation of the nucleus pulposus. HERNIATED DISK.

hernio-. A combining form meaning *hernia.*

her·nio·gram (hur′nee·o·gram) *n.* A depiction of a hernia made by herniography.

her·ni·og·ra·phy (hur″nee·og′ruh·fee) *n.* The radiographic depiction of a hernia aided by injection of contrast medium into the sac.

her·nio·plas·ty (hur′nee·o·plas″tee) *n.* [*hernio-* + *-plasty*]. Plastic operation for the radical cure of hernia.

her·ni·or·rha·phy (hur″nee·or′uh·fee) *n.* [*hernio-* + *-rrhaphy*]. Any operation which includes suturing for the repair of hernia.

her·nio·tome (hur′nee·o·tome) *n.* [*hernio-* + *-tome*]. A special knife or curved bistoury, with a blunt end, sometimes used in operations for hernia.

her·ni·ot·o·my (hur″nee·ot′uh·mee) *n.* [*hernio-* + *-tomy*]. 1. An operation for the relief of irreducible hernia, by cutting through the neck of the sac. 2. HERNIOPLASTY.

her·o·in (herr′o·in) *n.* [Ger. *Heroin,* a trademark]. Diacetylmorphine, $C_{21}H_{23}NO_5$, a morphine derivative, a white, crystalline, odorless powder, formerly used as an analgesic, a sedative, and to relieve coughs, but since 1956 banned from use or manufacture because of its addictive properties.

her·o·in·ism (herr′o·in·iz·um) *n.* [*heroin* + *-ism*]. Addiction to heroin.

her·pan·gi·na (hur″pan·jye′nuh, hur·pan′ji·nuh) *n.* [*herpes* + *angina*]. A mild disease caused by any of various Coxsackie group A viruses and characterized by fever, anorexia, dysphagia, and grayish-white papules or vesicles surrounded by a red areola on the pharynx, uvula, palate, and tonsils, or tongue.

Herperal. A trademark for stallimycin hydrochloride, an antibacterial.

her·pes (hur′peez) *n.* [Gk. *herpēs,* a spreading cutaneous affection, from *herpein,* to creep]. HERPES SIMPLEX.

herpes cir·ci·na·tus (sur″si·nay′tus). DERMATITIS HERPETIFORMIS.

herpes des·qua·mans (de·skway′manz, des′kwuh·manz). TINEA IMBRICATA.

herpes fa·ci·a·lis (fay·shee·ay′lis). A type of herpes simplex occurring on the face, usually about the lips. May also occur in the mouth and pharynx. Syn. *cold sore, herpes febrilis.*

herpes fe·bri·lis (fe·brye'lis). Fever blister (= HERPES FACIALIS).

herpes gen·i·ta·lis (jen''i·tay'lis). HERPES PROGENITALIS.

herpes ges·ta·ti·o·nis (jes·tay''shee·o'nis). A vesicular or bullous skin eruption occurring during pregnancy; probably related to erythema multiforme.

herpes glad·i·a·to·rum (glad''ee·a·to'rum). A herpesvirus infection contracted from persons or contaminated material by close contact, especially in conjunction with skin trauma; seen frequently in athletes, especially wrestlers.

herpes iris (eye'ris). A form of erythema multiforme, characterized by vesicles growing in a ring. It is usually seen on the backs of the hands and feet.

herpes la·bi·a·lis (lay''bee·ay'lis). Herpes facialis on the lip.

herpes oph·thal·mi·cus (off·thal'mi·kus). HERPES ZOSTER OPHTHALMICUS.

herpes prae·pu·ti·a·lis (pree·pew''shee·ay'lis). HERPES PROGENITALIS.

herpes pro·gen·i·ta·lis (pro·jen''i·tay'lis). Vesicles on the genitalia caused by herpes simplex virus, type 2. Syn. *herpes praeputialis, herpes genitalis.*

herpes sim·plex (sim'plecks). A viral disorder, characterized by groups of vesicles on an erythematous base. Commonly recurrent, and at times seen in the same place.

herpes simplex virus. A herpesvirus that causes a variety of human diseases notable for their persistence in a latent state and tendency to recur at irregular intervals. The virus usually enters the body through breaks in mucous membranes or skin. Of the two principal strains, type 1 usually causes oral, ocular, cutaneous, and encephalitic infections and type 2, genital (and various congenital) infections. Syn. *Herpesvirus hominis.* See also *herpetic encephalitis.*

herpes ton·su·rans (ton·sue'ranz, ton'sue·ranz). TINEA CAPITIS.

herpes ton·su·rans mac·u·lo·sus (ton'sue·ranz mack''yoo·lo'sus). PITYRIASIS ROSEA.

Her·pes·vi·rus (hur''peez·vye'rus) *n.* A group of ether-sensitive, large DNA viruses that form eosinophilic intranuclear inclusion bodies, and include among others the viruses of herpes simplex, varicella, herpes zoster, pseudorabies, infectious bovine rhinotracheitis, and equine abortion. —**herpesvirus,** *com. n.*

Herpesvirus hom·i·nis (hom'i·nis). HERPES SIMPLEX VIRUS.

Herpesvirus sim·i·ae (sim'ee·ee). A virus that causes a usually mild disease similar to herpes simplex in Old World monkeys, but which may cause fatal myelitis or encephalomyelitis in man. Syn. *B virus.*

herpes zos·ter (zos'tur). An acute viral infectious disease of man, characterized by unilateral segmental inflammation of the posterior root ganglia and roots (and sometimes of anterior roots and posterior horn), or sensory ganglia of cranial nerves and by a painful vesicular eruption of the skin or mucous membranes in the peripheral distribution of the individual nerve or nerves. Syn. *shingles.*

herpes zoster au·ric·u·la·ris (aw·rick''yoo·lair'is). RAMSAY HUNT SYNDROME (1).

herpes zoster oph·thal·mi·cus (off·thal'mi·kus). A virus infection of the trigeminal ganglion, sometimes giving rise to a vesicular skin eruption in the distribution of the ophthalmic division of the trigeminal nerve. Corneal and intraocular involvement may sometimes occur.

herpes zoster oti·cus (o'ti·kus). RAMSAY HUNT SYNDROME (1).

her·pet·ic (hur·pet'ick) *adj.* Of or pertaining to herpes.

herpetic encephalitis. An acute encephalitis, frequently lethal, which occurs sporadically throughout the year in all age groups and throughout the world, usually caused by type 1 herpes simplex virus. Type 2 virus causes acute encephalitis rarely and only in the neonate, in relation to maternal genital herpetic infection.

herpetic fever. A herpetic eruption on the face associated with chills, fever, and sore throat.

herpetic keratitis. Keratitis due to either herpes simplex or zoster.

herpetic neuralgia. The severe pain associated with some cases of herpes zoster; it follows the course of the affected nerve or nerves.

herpetic stomatitis. Stomatitis characterized by fever blisters or cold sores.

herpetic tonsillitis. Tonsillitis characterized by an eruption of herpetic vesicles, leaving small circular ulcers that coalesce and become covered with a fibrinous exudation. The disease has an acute onset, a continuous fever, and a critical decline, affects individuals subject to herpes elsewhere, and tends to recur.

her·pet·i·form (hur·pet'i·form) *adj.* [*herpetic* + *-form*]. Resembling herpes; having groups of vesicles.

her·pe·tol·o·gy (hur''pe·tol'uh·jee) *n.* [Gk. *herpeton*, creeping thing, reptile, + *-logy*]. The branch of zoology concerned with the study of reptiles.

Her·pe·tom·o·nas (hur''pe·tom'uh·nas) *n.* [Gk. *herpetos*, crawling, + *monas*, single unit]. A genus of flagellates of the family Trypanosomatidae; parasitic only in invertebrate hosts. —**herpetomo·nad** (·nad) *adj. & n.*

Herplex. A trademark for idoxuridine, a topical antiviral agent used for treatment of dendritic keratitis.

Her·rick's anemia [J. B. *Herrick*, U. S. physician, 1861-1954]. SICKLE CELL ANEMIA.

Her·ring bodies [P. T. *Herring*, British physiologist, b. 1872]. Granular masses, apparent with special stains, seen in the nerve endings of fibers of the hypothalamo-hypophyseal tract; thought to be aggregates of neurosecretory material.

herring-worm disease. ANISAKIASIS.

Hers' disease [H. G. *Hers*, 20th century]. Glycogenosis caused by a deficiency of the enzyme liver phosphorylase, with abnormal storage of glycogen in liver, and clinically similar to von Gierke's disease with marked hepatomegaly and varying degrees of hypoglycemia and its manifestations. Syn. *type VI of Cori.*

Her·tel apparatus. EXOPHTHALMOMETER.

Her·ter-Fos·ter method [C. A. *Herter*, U. S. physician, 1865–1910]. A test for indole employing an alkaline solution of β-naphthoquinone sodium monosulfonate. A red color indicates the presence of indole.

Herter's infantilism [C. A. *Herter*]. PANCREATIC INFANTILISM.

Hert·wig's epithelial root sheath (hehrt'vikh) [W. A. O. *Hertwig*, German embryologist, 1849–1922]. An epithelial sheath, derived from the enamel organ, which molds the shape of tooth roots and initiates dentin formation; remnants persist as epithelial rests of Malassez in the periodontal ligament.

hertz (hurtz) *n.* [H. R. *Hertz*, German physicist, 1857–1894]. *In physics*, a unit of frequency of a periodic process, equal to one cycle per second.

Hertz·ian waves (hurt'see·un, hehrt'see·un) [H. R. *Hertz*]. Electromagnetic waves, used for radio transmission, having wavelengths between the arbitrary limits of 1 millimeter to several kilometers.

Herx·hei·mer-Mans·feld phenomenon (hehrks'high·mur, mahns'felt) [K. *Herxheimer*, German dermatologist, 1861–1944]. Hypoglycemia associated with pancreatic secretory obstruction.

He·ryng's sign (hehr'ink) [T. *Heryng*, Polish otolaryngologist, 1847–1925]. An infraorbital shadow, indicating empyema of the maxillary sinus; seen when an electric light is placed in the mouth.

herz·stoss (hairts'shtoce) *n.* [Ger., heartbeat]. The widespread impact of the heart during systole against a large part of the entire precordium, seen especially in thin patients with cardiac hypertrophy, in contradistinction to the circumscribed apex impulse seen normally.

Heschl's gyri (hesh'^{e}l) [R. L. *Heschl,* Austrian pathologist, 1824–1881]. TRANSVERSE TEMPORAL GYRI.

hes·per·e·tin (hes·perr'e·tin) *n.* 3′,5,7-Trihydroxy-4′-methoxyflavanone, $C_{16}H_{14}O_6$, the aglycone of hesperidin, obtained by hydrolysis of the latter or by synthesis. Certain derivatives were claimed to have a favorable effect in certain types of capillary fragility. See also *citrin.*

hes·per·i·din (hes·perr'i·din) *n.* [*hesperidium,* the form characteristic of citrus fruits, + *-in*]. Hesperetin-1-rhamnosido-D-glucoside, $C_{28}H_{34}O_{15}$, occurring in the rind of many citrus fruits; on hydrolysis it yields hesperetin, rhamnose, and D-glucose. Certain water-soluble derivatives were claimed to provide protection against capillary fragility. See also *citrin.*

Hes·sel·bach's ligament (hess'^{e}l·bak^{h}h) [F. C. *Hesselbach,* German anatomist, 1759–1816]. INTERFOVEOLAR LIGAMENT.

Hesselbach's triangle [F. C. *Hesselbach*]. INGUINAL TRIANGLE.

het·a·cil·lin (het''uh·sil'in) *n.* 6-(2,2-Dimethyl-5-oxo-4-phenyl-1-imidazolidinyl)penicillanic acid, $C_{19}H_{23}N_3O_4S$, a semisynthetic penicillin antibiotic.

het·a·flur (het'uh·flure) *n.* Hexadecylamine hydrofluoride, $C_{16}H_{35}N{\cdot}HF$, a dental caries prophylactic.

heta·starch [het'uh·stahrch] *n.* A starch which is primarily amylopectin partially etherified with ethylene oxide, used as a plasma volume extender.

heter-, hetero- [Gk. *heteros*]. A combining form meaning (a) *other, another;* (b) *different, unlike;* (c) *various, diverse;* (d) *irregular, abnormal.*

het·er·a·del·phus (het''ur·uh·del'fus) *n.* [*heter-* + *-adelphus*]. THORACOACEPHALUS. —**heteradel·phia** (fee·uh) *n.* —**heteradelphous,** *adj.*

het·er·ade·nia (het''ur·a·dee'nee·uh) *n.* [*heter-* + *aden-* + *-ia*]. Any abnormality in the formation or location of gland tissue. —**heter·aden·ic** (·a·den'ick) *adj.*

het·er·a·li·us (het''ur·ay'lee·us) *n.* [*heter-* + Gk. *halios,* useless]. Asymmetric uniovular twins in which the parasite is only rudimentary, and with no direct connection with the umbilical cord of its host.

het·er·aux·e·sis (het''ur·awk·see'sis) *n.* [*heter-* + *auxesis*]. Allometric change during the course of an organism's growth and development. Contr. *allomorphosis.*

het·er·e·cious, het·er·oe·cious (het''ur·ee'shus) *adj.* [*heter-* + Gk. *oikos,* house, + *-ous*]. Parasitic upon different hosts at different stages of growth. —**hetere·cism, heteroe·cism** (·siz·um) *n.*

het·er·er·gic (het''ur·ur'jick) *adj.* [*heter-* + *erg-* + *-ic*]. Of or pertaining to drugs that elicit different qualities of effect. Contr. *homergic.*

het·er·es·the·sia, het·er·aes·the·sia (het''ur·es·theez'ee·uh) *n.* [*heter-* + *esthesia*]. Variations in the degree of response to a cutaneous stimulus from one point to another on the body.

hetero-. See *heter-.*

heteroaesthesia. Heteroesthesia (= HETERESTHESIA).

het·ero·ag·glu·ti·nin (het''ur·o·uh·gloo'ti·nin) *n.* [*hetero-* + *agglutinin*]. An agglutinin in normal blood having the property of agglutinating foreign cells, including the blood corpuscles of other species of animals.

het·ero·al·bu·mose (het''ur·o·al'bew·moce, ·moze) *n.* A variety of albumose soluble in salt solutions, insoluble in water, and precipitated by saturation with sodium chloride or magnesium sulfate.

het·ero·al·bu·mo·su·ria (het''ur·o·al''bew·mo·sue'ree·uh) *n.* [*heteroalbumose* + *-uria*]. The presence of heteroalbumose in the urine.

het·ero·al·lele (het''ur·o·a·leel') *n.* [*hetero-* + *allele*]. One of a set of alleles which differ at more than one intragenic site. Contr. *homoallele.* See also *pseudoallele.*

het·ero·at·om (het''ur·o·at'um) *n.* [*hetero-* + *atom*]. Any atom, linked in the ring of a heterocyclic compound, other than a carbon atom, as the nitrogen atom of pyridine, C_5H_5N.

het·ero·aux·in (het''ur·o·awk'sin) *n.* Indole-3-acetic acid, $C_{10}H_9NO_2$, an activator of growth substance (auxin); used as a plant growth stimulant.

het·ero·aux·one (het''ur·o·awk'sone) *n.* A growth-promoting substance. See also *heteroauxin.*

het·ero·blas·tic (het''ur·o·blas'tick) *adj.* [*hetero-* + *-blastic*]. Arising from tissue of a different kind.

heterocaryon. HETEROKARYON.

heterocaryosis. HETEROKARYOSIS.

het·ero·cel·lu·lar (het''ur·o·sel'yoo·lur) *adj.* [*hetero-* + *cellular*]. Formed of cells of different kinds.

het·ero·ceph·a·lus (het''ur·o·sef'uh·lus) *n.,* pl. **heterocepha·li** (·lye) [*hetero-* + *-cephalus*]. A dicephalus with heads of unequal size.

het·ero·chro·ma·tin (het''ur·o·kro'muh·tin) *n.* [*hetero-* + *chromatin*]. 1. BASICHROMATIN. 2. Originally, the substance of heterochromosomes (allosomes), as of the Y chromosome. —**hetero·chro·mat·ic** (·kro·mat'ick) *adj.*

het·ero·chro·mia (iri·dis) (het''ur·o·kro'mee·uh eye'ri·dis) *n.* [*hetero-* + *-chromia*]. A condition in which the two irises are of different colors, or a portion of an iris is a different color from the remainder. Syn. *anisochromia, chromheterotropia.* —**heterochro·mous** (·mus), **heterochro·mic** (·mick) *adj.*

heterochromic uveitis. Chronic uveitis which causes loss of iris pigments resulting in a disparity of color in the two eyes. Syn. *Fuchs' iridocyclitis.*

het·ero·chro·mo·some (het''ur·o·kro'muh·sohm) *n.* [*hetero-* + *chromosome*]. ALLOSOME (1).

het·ero·chro·nia (het''ur·o·kro'nee·uh) *n.* [*hetero-* + *chron-* + *-ia*]. 1. Variation in time relationships. 2. Departure from the typical sequence in the time of formation of organs or parts. 3. Difference in chronaxies of tissue elements functionally related, as a difference of 100 percent or more between the chronaxie of a muscle and the nerve that innervates it. —**hetero·chron·ic** (·kron'ick), **het·er·och·ro·nous** (het''ur·ock'ruh·nus) *adj.*

het·ero·cy·clic (het''ur·o·sigh'click, ·sick'lick) *adj.* [*hetero-* + *cyclic*]. *In chemistry,* pertaining to compounds of the closed-chain or ring type in which the ring atoms are of two or more dissimilar elements. Contr. *homocyclic.*

het·ero·cy·to·tro·pic (het''ur·o·sigh·to·tro'pick) *adj.* [*hetero-* + *cytotropic*]. Of an antibody; having an affinity for cells of a species of animal different from the one in which it originated. Contr. *homocytotropic.*

Het·er·od·era (het''ur·od'e·ruh) *n.* [NL., from *hetero-* + Gk. *derē,* neck]. A genus of minute nematodes of the superfamily Tylenchicae.

Heterodera ra·di·cic·o·la (rad''i·sick'o·luh). A species of minute nematodes parasitic on the roots and stems of many edible plants. The ova are sometimes found in human feces and may be mistaken for hookworm eggs.

het·ero·did·y·mus (het''ur·o·did'i·mus) *n.* [*hetero-* + *-didymus*]. HETERODYMUS.

het·er·o·dont (het'ur·o·dont) *adj.* [*heter-* + *-odont*]. *In biology,* having teeth of more than one shape, as does man. Contr. *homodont.*

het·er·od·y·mus (het''ur·od'i·mus) *n.,* pl. **heterody·mi** (·mye) [*hetero-* + *-dymus*]. A type of thoracopagus parasiticus in which the parasitic twin is represented by a head, neck, and thorax implanted in the thoracic or the epigastric wall of the host.

heteroecious. HETERECIOUS.

het·ero·er·o·tism (het''ur·o·err'o·tiz·um) *n.* [*hetero-* + *erotism*]. The direction of the sexual desire toward another person or toward any object other than oneself. Contr. *autoerotism.* —**hetero·erot·ic** (·e·rot'ick) *adj.*

het·ero·es·the·sia, het·ero·aes·the·sia (het''ur·o·es·thee'zee·uh) *n.* [*hetero-* + *esthesia*]. HETERESTHESIA.

het·ero·fer·men·ta·tive (het''ur·o·fur·men'tuh·tiv) *adj.* [*hetero-* + *fermentative*]. Pertaining to the ability of certain bacteria, such as *Lactobacillus brevis, L. buchneri,* and *Leuconos-*

toc dextranicum, to form lactic acid, ethyl alcohol, acetic acid, carbon dioxide, and glycerol from glucose, as well as mannitol from levulose. Contr. *homofermentative*.

het·ero·ga·met·ic (het″ur·o·ga·met′ick) *adj.* [*hetero-* + *gametic*]. Referring to the production of two types of germ cells in regard to the sex chromosomes. The male, being XY in constitution, is the heterogametic sex.

het·er·og·a·my (het″ur·og′uh·mee) *n.* [*hetero-* + *-gamy*]. The conjugation of gametes of unlike size and structure, as in higher plants and animals.

het·ero·ge·ne·ic (het″ur·o·je·nee′ick) *adj.* XENOGENEIC.

het·er·o·ge·ne·ous (het″ur·o·jee′nee·us) *adj.* [Gk. *heterogenēs*, from *hetero-* + *genos*, kind]. 1. Differing in kind or nature; composed of different substances or constituents. 2. Not uniform in composition or structure. Contr. *homogeneous*. —**hetero·ge·ne·i·ty** (·je·nee′i·tee) *n.*

heterogeneous radiation. Radiation of more than one wavelength.

het·ero·gen·e·sis (het″ur·o·jen′e·sis) *n.* [*hetero-* + *-genesis*]. Alternation of generations in the complete life cycle, especially the alternation of a dioecious generation with one or more parthenogenetic generations and sometimes with an alternation of hosts, as in many trematode parasites. —**het·ero·ge·net·ic** (·je·net′ick) *adj.*

heterogenetic cortex. ALLOCORTEX.

heterogenetic rhythm. ECTOPIC RHYTHM.

het·ero·gen·ic (het″ur·o·jen′ick) *adj.* [*hetero-* + *-genic*]. Pertaining to polysomic or polyploid organisms which contain different alleles for any given locus. Compare *heterozygous*.

het·er·og·e·nous (het″ur·oj′e·nus) *adj.* [*hetero-* + *-genous*]. 1. Of, relating to, or derived from a different species. Contr. *homogenous*. 2. Not originating within the same body. Contr. *autogenous*.

heterogenous vaccine. A vaccine prepared from organisms derived from some source other than the patient in whose treatment they are to be used; the source is usually a stock culture.

het·ero·geu·sia (het″ur·o·gew′see·uh, ·joo′see·uh) *n.* [*hetero-* + *-geusia*]. A sensation of taste which is inappropriate for the food or drink stimulating it.

het·er·og·o·ny (het″ur·og′uh·nee) *n.* [*hetero-* + *-gony*]. An alternation of generations in which a generation of males and females is followed by a hermaphroditic generation.

het·ero·graft (het′ur·o·graft) *n.* [*hetero-* + *graft*]. A graft of tissue obtained from an animal of one species and transferred to the body of another animal of a different species. Syn. *xenograft*. Contr. *homograft*.

heterograft rejection. The immunologic process by which an animal causes the destruction or sloughing of tissue transplanted to it from an animal of another species.

het·ero·hem·ag·glu·ti·nin, het·ero·haem·ag·glu·ti·nin (het″ur·o·hee″muh·gloo′ti·nin) *n.* [*hetero-* + *hemagglutinin*]. HETEROAGGLUTININ.

het·ero·he·mol·y·sin, het·ero·hae·mol·y·sin (het″ur·o·he·mol′i·sin) *n.* [*hetero-* + *hemolysin*]. A hemolytic amboceptor, natural or developed by immunization, against the red cells of a species different from that used to obtain the amboceptor.

het·ero·hyp·no·sis (het″ur·o·hip·no′sis) *n.* [*hetero-* + *hypnosis*]. Hypnosis induced by another. Contr. *autohypnosis*.

het·er·oid (het′ur·oid) *adj.* [Gk. *heteroeidēs*]. Formed diversely, as enclosed structures that differ from their investment.

het·ero·in·tox·i·ca·ti·on (het″ur·o·in·tock″si·kay′shun) *n.* [*hetero-* + *intoxication*]. Intoxication by a poison not produced within the body.

het·ero·ion (het″ur·o·eye′on) *n.* [*hetero-* + *ion*]. A complex ion resulting from absorption of a simple ion by a relatively large molecule, as by a protein.

het·ero·kar·y·on, het·ero·car·y·on (het″ur·o·kăr′ee·on) *n.* [*hetero-* + *karyon*]. A cell with two or more nuclei of unlike genetic constitution.

het·ero·kary·o·sis, het·ero·cary·o·sis (het″ur·o·kăr″ee·o′sis) *n.* [*heterokaryon* + *-osis*]. Differing genetic constitution among the nuclei of multinuclear cells. —**heterokar·y·ot·ic, heterocar·y·ot·ic** (·ee·ot′ick) *adj.*

het·ero·ki·ne·sis (het″ur·o·ki·nee′sis) *n.* [*hetero-* + *kinesis*]. Differential distribution of sex chromosomes during meiosis.

het·ero·lac·tic (het″ur·o·lack′tick) *adj.* [*hetero-* + *lactic*]. Pertaining to a type of sugar fermentation in which lactic acid and several other products, as carbon dioxide and alcohol, are produced; ordinarily indicating fermentation by microorganisms.

het·ero·la·lia (het″ur·o·lay′lee·uh) *n.* [*hetero-* + *-lalia*]. *Obsol.* 1. The unconscious saying of one thing when something else is intended. 2. A form of motor aphasia in which the patient habitually says one thing but means something else. 3. ECHOLALIA; the echoing of someone else's words. Contr. *autoecholalia*.

het·ero·lat·er·al (het″ur·o·lat′ur·ul) *adj.* [*hetero-* + *lateral*]. Pertaining to or situated on the opposite side.

het·er·ol·o·gous (het″ur·ol′uh·gus) *adj.* 1. Characterized by heterology. 2. Derived from an organism of a different species. Contr. *homologous*.

heterologous graft. HETEROGRAFT.

heterologous stimulus. A form of energy capable of exciting any sensory receptor or form of nervous tissue. Contr. *homologous stimulus*.

heterologous tumor. A tumor composed of tissues different from those in which it grows.

het·er·ol·o·gy (het″ur·ol′uh·jee) *n.* [Gk. *heterologia*, unorthodox speech]. Deviation from the normal in structure, organization, or time or manner of formation.

het·ero·ly·sin (het″ur·o·lye′sin, het″ur·ol′i·sin) *n.* [*hetero-* + *lysin*]. HETEROHEMOLYSIN.

het·er·om·e·ral (het″ur·om′e·rul) *adj.* HETEROMERIC.

het·ero·mer·ic (het″ur·o·merr′ick) *adj.* [Gk. *heteromerēs*, one-sided]. Of neurons, originating in one side of the spinal cord and sending processes to the other side.

heteromeric cell. COMMISSURAL CELL.

het·er·om·er·ous (het″ur·om′ur·us) *adj.* [*hetero-* + *mer-* + *-ous*]. Characterizing substances unlike in chemical composition.

het·ero·meta·pla·sia (het″ur·o·met·uh·play′zhuh, ·zee·uh) *n.* [*hetero-* + *metaplasia*]. The change in the character of a tissue after transplantation to another part of the body.

het·ero·met·ric (het″ur·o·met′rick) *adj.* [*hetero-* + *metric*]. Involving changes in length.

heterometric autoregulation. Intrinsic self-regulation of the heart which varies with different initial myocardial fiber lengths; the family of ventricular function curves depicts the relationship between change in initial myocardial fiber length and change in myocardial contractility. Contr. *homeometric autoregulation*. See also *Frank-Starling law of the heart*.

het·ero·me·tro·pia (het″ur·o·me·tro′pee·uh) *n.* [*hetero-* + Gk. *metron*, measure, + *-opia*]. The condition in which the refraction in the two eyes is dissimilar.

het·ero·mor·phic (het″ur·o·mor′fick) *adj.* [*hetero-* + *-morphic*]. 1. Differing in size or form as compared with the normal. 2. *In chemistry*, crystallizing in different forms. 3. *In zoology*, having different forms at different stages of the life history. 4. *In cytology*, unlike in form or size; applied to either chromosome of a synaptic pair of unlike chromosomes, as an X and a Y chromosome. —**heteromor·phism** (·fiz·um) *n.*

heteromorphic gliosis. HETEROMORPHOUS GLIOSIS.

het·ero·mor·pho·sis (het″ur·o·mor′fuh·sis, ·mor·fo′sis) *n.* [*hetero-* + *-morphosis*]. *In biology*, the regeneration of an organ or part different from that normal to the site, as the production in certain Crustacea of an antenna-like structure after the removal of an eye and its ganglion. Compare *homeosis.*

het·ero·mor·phous (het″ur·o·mor′fus) *adj.* [Gk. *heteromorphos*]. 1. Differing from the normal in form. 2. Of varied or irregular form.

heteromorphous gliosis. A form of astrocytic proliferation in which the glial fibers are arranged in an irregular meshwork.

het·er·o·ni·um bromide (het″ur·o′nee·um). 3-Hydroxy-1,1-dimethylpyrrolidinium bromide α-phenyl-2-thiopheneglycolate, $C_{18}H_{22}BrNO_3S$, an anticholinergic drug.

het·er·on·o·mous (het″ur·on′uh·mus) *adj.* [*hetero-* + Gk. *nomos*, law, + *-ous*]. *In biology,* pertaining to the condition in which the metameres of a segmented animal are dissimilar.

het·er·on·y·mous (het″ur·on′i·mus) *adj.* [Gk. *heterōnymos,* having a different denominator]. *In optics,* pertaining to crossed images of an object seen double.

heteronymous diplopia. CROSSED DIPLOPIA.

heteronymous hemianopsia. Loss of vision affecting either the inner halves or the outer halves of both visual fields. Contr. *homonymous hemianopsia.* See also *binasal hemianopsia, bitemporal hemianopsia.*

heteronymous parallax. CROSSED PARALLAX.

het·ero·os·teo·plas·ty (het″ur·o·os′tee·o·plas″tee) *n.* [*hetero-* + *osteoplasty*]. The grafting, by operation, of bone taken from an animal. See also *bone graft.*

het·er·op·a·gus (het″ur·op′uh·gus) *n.,* pl. **heteropa·gi** (·jye, ·guy) [*hetero-* + *-pagus*]. A type of thoracopagus parasiticus in which the parasite, although imperfectly developed, has a head and extremities.

het·er·op·a·thy (het″ur·op′uth·ee) *n.* [*hetero-* + *-pathy*]. 1. The condition of being abnormally sensitive to stimuli; hypersensitivity. 2. ALLOPATHY. —**het·ero·path·ic** (het″ur·o·path′ick) *adj.*

het·ero·pha·sia (het″ur·o·fay′zhuh, ·zee·uh) *n.* [*hetero-* + *-phasia*]. HETEROLALIA (2).

het·ero·phe·mia (het″ur·o·fee′mee·uh) *n.* [*hetero-* + Gk. *phēmē,* voice, speech, + *-ia*]. *Obsol.* HETEROLALIA (1).

het·er·o·phe·my (het′ur·o·fee″mee, het″ur·off′e·mee) *n.* [*hetero-* + Gk. *phēmē,* voice, speech]. HETEROLALIA (1).

het·ero·phil (het′ur·o·fil) *adj.* [*hetero-* + *-phil*]. Of or pertaining to antigens occurring in apparently unrelated animals and microorganisms that are closely related immunologically so that antibodies produced against one antigen cross-react with the others.

heterophil antibody. An antibody that is produced in response to a heterophil antigen, as exemplified in the Paul-Bunnell test for infectious mononucleosis.

heterophil antibody test. Any test of human serum for the detection of heterophil antibodies.

het·ero·phile (het′ur·o·file, ·fil) *adj.* HETEROPHIL.

heterophil leukocyte. A neutrophil leukocyte, especially of vertebrates other than man.

het·ero·pho·nia (het″ur·o·fo′nee·uh) *n.* [Gk. *heterophōnia,* diversity of note]. Abnormal quality or change of voice.

het·ero·pho·ral·gia (het″ur·o·fo·ral′jee·uh) *n.* [*heterophoria* + *-algia*]. Pain caused by heterophoria.

het·ero·pho·ria (het″ur·o·fo′ree·uh) *n.* [*hetero-* + *-phoria*]. Any tendency of the eyes to turn away from the position correct for binocular vision; latent squint or deviation. See also *esophoria, exophoria, hyperesophoria, hyperexophoria, hyperphoria.*

het·er·o·phy·di·a·sis (het″ur·o·figh·dye′uh·sis) *n.* HETEROPHYIDIASIS.

Het·er·oph·y·es (het″ur·off′ee·eez) *n.* [Gk. *heterophyēs,* of different form or nature]. A genus of trematode worms, found in Egypt and the Far East, which produces heterophyidiasis in humans.

Heterophyes heterophyes. A trematode species that has as definitive hosts man, cats, dogs, foxes, hogs, and other fish-eating animals; as first intermediate hosts, the snails; and as second intermediate hosts, mullet fish.

het·er·o·phy·i·a·sis (het″ur·o·figh·eye′uh·sis) *n.* [*Heterophyes* + *-iasis*]. HETEROPHYIDIASIS.

het·er·o·phy·id·i·a·sis (het″ur·o·figh″id·eye′uh·sis) *n.* [*Heterophyidae* + *-iasis*]. Infection by any fluke of the family Heterophyidae, of which the species *Heterophyes heterophyes* and *Metagonimus yokogawai* are the most important and most common in humans. The flukes inhabit the small intestine but may also pass into the muscles of the heart through the lymphatics.

het·ero·pla·sia (het″ur·o·play′zhuh, ·zee·uh) *n.* [*hetero-* + *-plasia*]. 1. The presence of a tissue in an abnormal location. 2. A process whereby tissues are displaced to or developed in locations foreign to their normal habitats. —**hetero·plas·tic** (·plas′tick) *adj.*

het·ero·plas·ty (het′ur·o·plas″tee) *n.* [*hetero-* + *-plasty*]. The operation of grafting parts taken from another species. Compare *alloplasty.* Contr. *homoplasty.*—**het·ero·plas·tic** (het″ur·o·plas′tick) *adj.*

het·ero·ploid (het′ur·o·ploid) *adj.* [*hetero-* + *-ploid*]. Having a chromosome number that is not an exact multiple of the haploid number characteristic for the species. —**hetero·ploi·dy** (·ploy·dee) *n.*

het·ero·poly·ac·id (het″ur·o·pol″ee·as′id) *n.* Any of a large group of complex oxygen-containing acids, formed by condensation of at least two different types of acid anhydrides, such as the phosphomolybdic acids of the formulas $P_2O_5.24MoO_3.xH_2O$ and $P_2O_5.18MoO_3.xH_2O$, or the silicotungstic acids of the formulas $SiO_2.12WO_3.xH_2O$ and $SiO_2.10WO_3.xH_2O$.

het·ero·poly·sac·cha·ride (het″ur·o·pol·ee·sack′uh·ride, ·rid) *n.* Any polysaccharide that yields on hydrolysis a mixture of monosaccharides and derived products. Contr. *homopolysaccharide.*

het·ero·pro·so·pus (het′ur·o·pro′suh·pus, ·pro·so′pus) *n.* [NL., from *hetero-* + Gk. *prosōpon,* face]. A diprosopus with three or four eyes and two ears.

het·ero·pro·te·ose (het″ur·o·pro′tee·oce) *n.* [*hetero-* + *proteose*]. One of a group of hydrolytic products, intermediate in the conversion of proteins to peptones; formed during gastric digestion or by autolysis of tissue protein.

het·er·op·sia (het″ur·op′see·uh) *n.* [*heter-* + *-opsia*]. Inequality of vision in the two eyes.

Het·er·op·tera (het″ur·op′tur·uh) *n.pl.* [*hetero-* + Gk. *ptera,* wings]. An order of insects including the true bugs. Formerly classified as a suborder of the Hemiptera.

het·er·op·tics (het″ur·op′ticks) *n.* [*heter-* + *optics*]. Perverted vision.

heteropycnosis. HETEROPYKNOSIS.

het·ero·pyk·no·sis (het″er·o·pick·no′sis) *n.* [*hetero-* + Gk. *pyknōsis,* condensation]. 1. A staining property of nuclei characterized by areas of heavier staining (positive heteropyknosis) and areas of lighter staining (negative heteropyknosis). 2. The state of differing in degree of condensation, said of chromosomes, such as one of the X chromosomes in somatic cells of human females. —**hetero·pyk·not·ic** (·not′ick) *adj.*

het·ero·sac·cha·ride (het″ur·o·sack′uh·ride) *n.* A polysaccharide that yields, on hydrolysis, both sugars and nonsugars.

het·ero·scope (het′ur·o·skope) *n.* [*hetero-* + *-scope*]. An instrument for determining the range of vision in strabismus. —**het·er·os·co·py** (het″ur·os′kuh·pee) *n.*

het·ero·sex·u·al·i·ty (het″ur·o·seck″shoo·al′i·tee) *n.* [*hetero-* + *sexuality*]. Sexual orientation toward the opposite sex. Contr. *homosexuality.*

het·ero·side (het′ur·o·side) *n.* [*hetero-* + glyco*side*]. A glycoside that yields, on hydrolysis, a noncarbohydrate as well as a sugar. Contr. *holoside.*

het·er·o·sis (het″ur·o′sis) *n.,* pl. **hetero·ses** (·seez) [Gk. *heteroiōsis,* alteration]. HYBRID VIGOR.

het·er·os·mia (het″ur·oz′mee·uh) *n.* [*heter-* + *osm-* + *-ia*]. An odor which is inappropriate for the substance producing it.

het·ero·sug·ges·ti·bil·i·ty (het″ur·o·sug·jes″ti·bil′i·tee) *n.* SUGGESTIBILITY.

het·ero·sug·ges·tion (het″ur·o·sug·jes′chun) *n.* [*hetero-* + *suggestion*]. Suggestion originating from a source outside the individual's mind; suggestion by another. Contr. *autosuggestion.*

het·ero·tax·ia (het″ur·o·tack′see·uh) *n.* HETEROTAXIS.

het·ero·tax·is (het″ur·o·tack′sis) *n.*, pl. **heterotax·es** (·seez) [*hetero-* + *taxis*]. Anomalous position or transposition of organs. Compare *dextrocardia, situs inversus.*

het·ero·taxy (het′ur·o·tack″see) *n.* HETEROTAXIS.

het·ero·to·nia (het″ur·o·to′nee·uh) *n.* [*hetero-* + *-tonia*]. Variability in tension or tone.

het·ero·to·pia (het″ur·o·to′pee·uh) *n.* [*hetero-* + Gk. *topos*, place, + *-ia*]. Displacement or deviation from natural position, as of an organ or a part.

het·ero·top·ic (het″ur·o·top′ick) *adj.* [*hetero-* + Gk. *topos*, place, + *-ic*]. 1. Occurring in an abnormal location, as intestinal epithelial cells occurring in the gastric epithelium. 2. Of or pertaining to a graft transplanted to an abnormal anatomic location in the host, as bone of the donor to muscle of the recipient. Contr. *orthotopic.*

heterotopic epithelium. Epithelium found in a part of the digestive tract for which it is not typical, as intestinal epithelial cells, including goblet cells, found in the stomach.

heterotopic glioma. A benign tumor of glial tissue outside the bony confines of the central nervous system.

heterotopic pain. REFERRED PAIN.

heterotopic pregnancy. Double gestation, with one fetus inside and the other outside the uterine cavity.

heterotopic transplantation. A graft transplanted to a different location in the host than it had in the donor. Contr. *orthotopic transplantation.*

het·ero·tox·in (het″ur·o·tock′sin) *n.* [*hetero-* + *toxin*]. A toxin introduced into, but formed outside of, the body.

het·ero·trans·plan·ta·tion (het″ur·o·trans·plan·tay′shun) *n.* [*hetero-* + *transplantation*]. Transplantation of a tissue or part from one species to another. —**hetero·trans·plant** (·trans′plant) *n.*

het·ero·troph (het′ur·o·trof, ·trofe) *n.* [*hetero-* + Gk. *trophē*, nourishment]. Any of those bacteria, including all those pathogenic for man, which require for growth a source of carbon more complex than carbon dioxide. Wide variation exists in respect to utilizable organic carbon sources and requirements for accessory growth factors. Contr. *autotroph.*

het·ero·troph·ic (het″ur·o·trof′ick, ·tro′fick) *adj.* [*hetero-* + *-trophic*]. Pertaining to heterotrophs. Contr. *autotrophic.*

het·ero·tro·pia (het″ur·o·tro′pee·uh) *n.* [*hetero-* + *tropia*]. STRABISMUS.

het·ero·tro·pic enzyme (het″ur·o·tro′pick). A type of allosteric enzyme in which a small molecule other than the substrate serves as the allosteric effector. Contr. *homotropic enzyme.*

het·ero·typ·ic (het″ur·o·tip′ick) *adj.* [*hetero-* + Gk. *typos*, pattern, + *-ic*]. Pertaining to the first division in meiosis, as distinguished from the second, or regular, cell division.

het·ero·typ·i·cal (het″ur·o·tip′i·kul) *adj.* HETEROTYPIC.

heterotypical cortex. ALLOCORTEX.

heterotypic mitosis. The first meiotic division in the maturation of the germ cells; the reduction division.

het·ero·ty·pus (het″ur·o·tye′pus) *n.* [*hetero-* + Gk. *typos*, form, replica]. PARACEPHALUS.

het·er·ox·e·nous (het″ur·ock′se·nus) *adj.* [*hetero-* + *-xenous*]. Infecting more than one kind of host during the life cycle. —**heteroxe·ny** (·nee) *n.*

het·ero·zy·go·sis (het″ur·o·zye·go′sis) *n.* [*heterozygous* + *-osis*]. In the genotype, the presence of one or many pairs of genes in the heterozygous phase, which results from crossbreeding. Contr. *homozygosis.*

het·er·o·zy·gote (het″ur·o·zye′gote) *n.* [*hetero-* + *zygote*]. A heterozygous individual.

het·ero·zy·gous (het″ur·o·zye′gus) *adj.* [Gk. *heterozygos*, unevenly yoked, not matched]. Having the two members of one or more pairs of genes dissimilar. Contr. *homozygous.* —**hetero·zy·gos·i·ty** (·zye·gos′i·tee) *n.*

Heth·er·ing·ton's stain [D. C. *Hetherington*, U.S. anatomist, b. 1895]. A supravital technique for the demonstration of mitochondria.

Hetrazan. Trademark for diethylcarbamazine, an antifilarial drug used as the citrate salt.

Hetrum Bromide. Trademark for heteronium bromide, an anticholinergic drug.

Heub·ner-Her·ter disease (huᵉb′nur) [O. J. L. *Heubner*, German pediatrician, 1843–1926; and C. A. *Herter*]. INFANTILE CELIAC DISEASE.

Heubner's disease or **endarteritis** [O. J. L. *Heubner*]. Syphilitic endarteritis of cerebral vessels.

Heu·ser's membrane. EXOCOELOMIC MEMBRANE.

HEW Department of Health, Education and Welfare, a United States federal agency.

hex-, hexa- [Gk. *hex*]. A combining form meaning *six.*

Hexa-Betalin. A trademark for pyridoxine hydrochloride.

hex·a·canth (heck′suh·kanth) *n.* [*hex-* + Gk. *akantha*, thorn]. A six-hooked larva of a tapeworm.

Hexachlorane. A trademark for gamma benzene hexachloride, a pediculicide.

hexa·chlo·ro·phene (heck″suh·klor′uh·feen) *n.* 2,2′-Methylenebis(3,4,6-trichlorophenol), $C_{13}H_6Cl_6O_2$, a germicide active in the presence of soap. Syn. *compound G-11.*

hexa·chro·mic (heck″suh·kro′mick) *adj.* [*hexa-* + *chrom-* + *-ic*]. Capable of distinguishing only six of the seven spectrum colors, indigo not being distinguished.

hex·ad (heck′sad) *n.* [*hex-* + *-ad*]. An element which has a valence of six.

hexa·dac·ty·lism (heck″suh·dack′ti·liz·um) *n.* [Gk. *hexadaktylia*, from *hexa-* + *daktilos*, finger]. The state of having six fingers or toes.

hex·a·dec·yl (heck″suh·des′il) *n.* CETYL.

hexa·di·meth·rine bromide (heck″suh·dye·meth′reen). Poly[(1,5-dimethyl)-1,5-diazaundecamethylene dimethobromide], $(C_{13}H_{30}Br_2N_2)_x$, a heparin-neutralizing agent.

Hexadrol. A trademark for dexamethasone, an anti-inflammatory adrenocortical steroid.

hexa·eth·yl tet·ra·phos·phate (heck″suh·eth′il tet″ruh·fos′fate). $(C_2H_5O)_6P_4O_7$. A liquid, probably a mixture of compounds, of which tetraethylpyrophosphate is the predominant constituent. It inhibits cholinesterase and is used as an insecticide.

hexa·flu·o·ren·i·um bromide (heck″suh·floo″uh·reen′ee·um, ·ren′ee·um). Hexamethylenebis(fluoren-9-yl)dimethylammonium bromide, $C_{36}H_{42}Br_2N_2$, used in conjunction with succinylcholine to reduce the dose of the latter and prolong its action as a skeletal-muscle relaxant.

hexa·flu·o·ro·di·eth·yl ether (heck″suh·floo″uh·ro·dye·eth′il). FLUROTHYL.

hexa·gen·ic (heck″suh·jen′ick) *adj.* [*hexa-* + *-genic*]. Referring to genotypes of polysomic or polyploid organisms that contain six different alleles for any given locus.

hexa·hy·dric (heck″suh·high′drick) *adj.* [*hexa-* + *hydr-* + *-ic*]. Containing six atoms of replaceable hydrogen.

hexa·hy·dro·hem·a·to·por·phy·rin, hexa·hy·dro·haem·a·to·por·phy·rin (heck″suh·high″dro·hee″muh·to·por′fi·rin) *n.* A reduction product of hematin.

hexa·hy·dro·phe·nol (heck″suh·high·dro·fee′nol) *n.* CYCLOHEXANOL.

hexa·hy·droxy·cy·clo·hex·ane (heck″suh·high·drock″see·sigh″klo·heck′sane) *n.* INOSITOL.

hex·al·de·hyde (heck·sal′de·hide) *n.* HEXANAL.

hexa·me·tho·ni·um chloride (heck″suh·me·tho′nee·um). One of a homologous series of polymethylene bis(trimethylammonium) ions, of the general formula $(CH_3)_3N^+(CH_2)_nN^+(CH_3)_3$, in which n is 6. It possesses potent ganglion-blocking action, effecting reduction in blood pressure. It is used clinically in the form of one of its salts, commonly the bromide or iodide.

hexa·meth·yl·en·a·mine (heck″suh·meth″il·en′uh·meen) *n.* METHENAMINE.

hexa·meth·yl·ene·tet·ra·mine (heck″suh·meth″il·een·tet′ruh·meen) *n.* METHENAMINE.

Hexamic acid. A trademark for cyclamic acid, a sweetening agent.

hex·a·mine (heck′suh·meen) *n.* A former British name for methenamine.

hex·a·nal (heck′suh·nal) *n.* *n*-Hexaldehyde, $C_5H_{11}CHO$, a pleasantly odorous liquid; used in the preparation of dyes, perfumes, and other synthetics.

hex·ane (heck′sane) *n.* Any one of the isomeric liquid hydrocarbons, C_6H_{14}, of the paraffin series.

hex·ane·di·o·ic acid (heck″sane·dye·o′ick). ADIPIC ACID.

hex·a·no·ic acid (heck″suh·no′ick). CAPROIC ACID.

hexa·pep·tide (heck″suh·pep′tide) *n.* A polypeptide composed of six amino acid groups.

hexa·va·lent (heck″suh·vay′lunt) *adj.* Having a valence of six.

Hexavibex. A trademark for pyridoxine hydrochloride (vitamin B_6).

hexa·vi·ta·min (heck″suh·vye′tuh·min) *n.* [*hexa-* + *vitamin*]. A capsule or tablet formulation of vitamin A, vitamin D, ascorbic acid, niacinamide, riboflavin, and thiamine.

hex·ax·i·al (hecks·ack′see·ul) *adj.* [*hex-* + *axial*]. Having six axes.

hexaxial reference system. *In electrocardiography,* a diagram of six bisecting lines produced by the superimposition of unipolar limb lead axes on the triaxial reference system used to plot the frontal plane electrical axis of various electrocardiographic deflections or of portions of such deflections.

hex·es·trol (heck′ses·trol) *n.* 4,4′-(1,2-Diethylene)diphenol, $C_{18}H_{22}O_2$, a synthetic estrogen.

hex·e·thal (heck′se·thal) *n.* 5-Ethyl-5-*n*-hexylbarbituric acid, $C_{12}H_{20}N_2O_3$, a sedative and hypnotic of short duration of action; used as the sodium derivative.

hex·et·i·dine (heck·set′i·deen) *n.* 5-Amino-1,3-bis(β-ethylhexyl)-5-methylhexahydropyrimidine, $C_{21}H_{45}N_3$, a local antibacterial, antifungal, and antitrichomonal agent.

hexo·bar·bi·tal (heck″so·bahr′bi·tol, ·tal) *n.* 5-(1-Cyclohexen-1-yl)-1,5-dimethylbarbituric acid, $C_{12}H_{16}N_2O_3$, a sedative and hypnotic of short duration of action; used also, as the sodium derivative, to induce surgical anesthesia.

hexo·bar·bi·tone (heck″so·bahr′bi·tone) *n.* British name for hexobarbital.

hexo·ben·dine (heck″so·ben′deen) *n.* 3,3′-[Ethylenebis(methylimino)]di-1-propyl ester of 3,4,5-trimethoxybenzoic acid, $C_{30}H_{44}N_2O_{10}$, a vasodilator.

hex·o·cy·cli·um methylsulfate (heck″so·sigh′klee·um). *N*-(β-Cyclohexyl-β-hydroxy-β-phenylethyl)-*N*′-methylpiperazine dimethylsulfate, $C_{21}H_{36}N_2O_5S$, a parasympatholytic agent used for its gastrointestinal antisecretory and antispasmodic effects.

hexo·ki·nase (heck″so·kigh′nace, ·naze) *n.* An enzyme that catalyzes the transfer of phosphate from adenosine triphosphate to glucose or fructose, forming glucose 6-phosphate or fructose 6-phosphate and adenosine diphosphate.

hex·one base (heck′sohn). One of the diaminomonocarboxylic acids (arginine, lysine, and histidine) each containing six carbon atoms, basic in reaction.

hex·os·a·mine (heck″so·suh·meen′, heck·so′suh·meen″) *n.* A primary amine derivative of a hexose resulting from replacement of hydroxyl in the latter by an amine group. Glucosamine is an important hexosamine.

hex·os·a·min·i·dase A (heck″so·suh·min′i·dace). An enzyme which catalyzes the hydrolysis of the *N*-acetylgalactosamine residue from certain gangliosides. This enzyme is defective in Tay-Sachs disease.

hex·o·san (heck′so·san) *n.* Any complex carbohydrate yielding a hexose on hydrolysis. Cellulose, starch, and glycogen are important hexosans.

hex·ose (heck′soce) *n.* Any monosaccharide that contains six carbon atoms in the molecule.

hexose diphosphate. A diester of phosphoric acid and a hexose; usually in reference to fructose 1,6-diphosphate, a product of anaerobic glycolysis.

hexose monophosphate. A monoester of phosphoric acid and a hexose; usually in reference either to glucose 1-phosphate or glucose 6-phosphate, products of anaerobic glycolysis.

hexose monophosphate shunt. A pathway of glucose metabolism in virtually all tissues by which five-carbon sugars are formed. NADP is a required cofactor for the first two enzymes which provide an important source of NADPH within the cell. Syn. *pentose phosphate pathway, phosphogluconate pathway.*

hexose phosphate. Any one of the phosphoric acid esters of a hexose, notably glucose, formed during the metabolism of carbohydrates by living organisms.

hex·u·ron·ic acid (heck″syoo·ron′ick) *n.* 1. An acid formed by oxidation of the primary alcohol group of a hexose sugar, as glucuronic acid from glucose. 2. *Obsol.* ASCORBIC ACID.

hex·yl (heck′sil) *n.* The univalent radical, C_6H_{13} —.

hex·yl·caine (heck′sil·kane) *n.* 1-Cyclohexylamino-2-propyl benzoate, $C_{16}H_{23}NO_2$, a local anesthetic suitable for infiltration, spinal anesthesia, surface anesthesia, and nerve block; used as the hydrochloride salt, primarily for surface anesthesia.

hex·yl·res·or·cin·ol (heck″sil·re·zor′sin·ole, ·ol) *n.* 4-Hexylresorcinol, $C_{12}H_{18}O_2$; an anthelmintic active against intestinal roundworms and trematodes and also employed as an antiseptic and germicide.

Heyd's syndrome [C. G. *Heyd,* U. S. surgeon, 1884–1970]. HEPATORENAL SYNDROME (1).

Hey's amputation [W. *Hey,* English surgeon, 1736–1819]. The same as Lisfranc's amputation except that the medial cuneiform bone is sawed through in a line with the articulation of the second metatarsal bone, instead of being disarticulated.

Hey's saw [W. *Hey*]. A serrated disk affixed to a handle, and used for enlarging an opening in a bone.

HF Abbreviation for *Hageman factor* (= FACTOR XII).

Hf Symbol for hafnium.

H fields. FIELDS of FOREL.

Hg [NL. *hydrargyrum*]. Symbol for mercury.

hg Abbreviation for (a) *hectogram;* (b) *hyperglycemic factor.*

hgb An abbreviation for *hemoglobin.*

HGF Abbreviation for *hyperglycemic factor* (*hyperglycemic-glycogenolytic factor*).

HGPTase Abbreviation for *hypoxanthine-guanine phosphoribosyl transferase.*

H.H.E. syndrome [*h*emiplegia + *h*emiconvulsions + *e*pilepsy]. Acute hemiplegia in infancy or early childhood, usually following a febrile illness, hemiconvulsions, and subsequently, epilepsy.

hi·a·tus (high·ay′tus) *n.* [L., from *hiare,* to stand open]. A space or opening. —**hia·tal** (·tul) *adj.*

hiatus ad·duc·to·ri·us (ad″uck·to′ree·us). [NA alt.]. ADDUCTOR HIATUS. NA alt. *hiatus tendineus.*

hiatus aor·ti·cus (ay·or′ti·kus) [NA]. AORTIC HIATUS.

hiatus ca·na·lis fa·ci·a·lis (ka·nay′lis fay·shee·ay′lis) [BNA]. Hiatus canalis nervi petrosi majoris (= HIATUS OF THE CANAL FOR THE GREATER PETROSAL NERVE).

hiatus canalis ner·vi pe·tro·si ma·jo·ris (ner′vye pe·tro′sigh ma·jo′ris) [NA]. HIATUS OF THE CANAL FOR THE GREATER PETROSAL NERVE.

hiatus canalis nervi petrosi mi·no·ris (mi·no'ris) [NA]. HIATUS OF THE CANAL FOR THE LESSER PETROSAL NERVE.

hiatus eso·pha·ge·us (ee"so·faj'ee·us) [NA]. ESOPHAGEAL HIATUS.

hiatus eth·moi·da·lis (eth·moy·day'lis) [BNA]. Hiatus semilunaris (= SEMILUNAR HIATUS (1)).

hiatus hernia. A form of hernia through the esophageal hiatus; usually a small, intermittent hernia of a part of the stomach.

hiatus max·il·la·ris (mack·si·lair'is) [NA]. The opening of the maxillary air sinus into the middle nasal meatus.

hiatus oe·so·pha·ge·us (ee"so·faj'ee·us) [BNA]. Hiatus esophageus (= ESOPHAGEAL HIATUS).

hiatus of Fal·lo·pi·us [G. *Fallopius*]. HIATUS OF THE CANAL FOR THE GREATER PETROSAL NERVE.

hiatus of Schwal·be (shvahl'beh) [G. A. *Schwalbe*]. A gap occasionally found in the pelvic fascia due to improper fusion of the obturator fascia with the tendinous arch.

hiatus of the canal for the greater petrosal nerve. The opening in the petrous portion of the temporal bone which transmits the greater petrosal nerve as it leaves the geniculate ganglion. NA *hiatus canalis nervi petrosi majoris.*

hiatus of the canal for the lesser petrosal nerve. A small lateral opening in the petrous portion of the temporal bone which transmits the lesser petrosal nerve. NA *hiatus canalis nervi petrosi minoris.*

hiatus of the facial canal. HIATUS OF THE CANAL FOR THE GREATER PETROSAL NERVE.

hiatus pleu·ro·pe·ri·to·ne·a·lis (plew'ro·perr"i·to·nee·ay'lis). A fetal opening in the posterior part of the diaphragm. If it fails to close, it may be the site of hernia. See also *foramen of Bochdalek.*

hiatus sa·cra·lis (sa·kray'lis) [NA]. SACRAL HIATUS.

hiatus sa·phe·nus (sa·fee'nus) [NA]. FOSSA OVALIS (2).

hiatus se·mi·lu·na·ris (sem"i·lew·nair'is) [NA]. SEMILUNAR HIATUS (1).

hiatus ten·di·ne·us (ten·din'ee·us) [NA]. ADDUCTOR HIATUS. NA alt. *hiatus adductorius.*

Hibbs' operation [R. A. *Hibbs*, U. S. orthopedist, 1869–1932]. A method of spinal fusion formerly used in the treatment of Pott's disease. The spinous processes of several vertebrae are fractured, and each is bent down to rest on the fractured surface of the next spine below.

hibernating gland. The brown fat of hibernating animals. See also *brown fat.*

hi·ber·na·tion (high"bur·nay'shun) *n.* [L. *hibernare*, to spend the winter, from *hibernus*, of winter]. The dormant condition of certain animals in the winter, characterized by twilight sleep, muscle relaxation, a fall in metabolic rate, and, hence, lowered body temperature. —**hi·ber·nate** (high'bur·nate) *v.*

hi·ber·no·ma (high"bur·no'muh) *n.* A benign tumor composed of adipose tissue cells with a high lipochrome content, giving it the appearance of the brown fat organs of hibernating animals.

Hibitane. Trademark for chlorhexidine hydrochloride, an anti-infective.

hic·cough (hick'up, ·off) *n.* HICCUP.

hic·cup (hick'up) *n.* A sudden contraction of the diaphragm causing inspiration, followed by a sudden closure of the glottis.

Hicks sign [J. Braxton *Hicks*]. BRAXTON HICKS SIGN.

Hicks version [J. Braxton *Hicks*]. BRAXTON HICKS VERSION.

hide·bound skin. DIFFUSE SCLERODERMA.

hidr-, hidro- [Gk. *hidrōs*]. A combining form meaning *sweat, perspiration.*

hi·drad·e·ni·tis, hy·drad·e·ni·tis (hi·drad"e·nigh'tis, high·) *n.* [*hidr-* + *adenitis*]. Inflammation of the sweat glands.

hidradenitis ax·il·la·ris (ack"si·lair'is). Inflammation of the apocrine glands of the axillae. See also *hidradenitis suppurativa.*

hidradenitis sup·pu·ra·ti·va (sup"yoo·ruh·tye'vuh). Suppurative inflammation of apocrine glands, usually of the axillae. A characteristic condition marked by abscesses, sinus formation, and great chronicity.

hi·drad·e·no·car·ci·no·ma (hi·drad"e·no·kahr"si·no'muh, high·) *n.* [*hidr-* + *adeno-* + *carcinoma*]. SWEAT GLAND CARCINOMA.

hi·drad·e·no·cyte (hi·drad'e·no·site, high·drad') *n.* [*hidr-* + *adeno-* + *-cyte*]. A metaplastic cell, occurring in the cystic disease form of mammary dysplasia, which resembles the epithelium of apocrine sweat glands. —**hi·drad·e·no·cyt·ic** (hi·drad"e·no·sit'ick) *adj.*

hidradenocytic cyst. A benign cyst, sometimes occurring in the breast, lined by hidradenocytes and derived from a sweat or apocrine gland.

hi·drad·e·noid (hi·drad'e·noid, high·) *adj.* [*hidr-* + *aden-* + *-oid*]. Resembling or having the form or appearance of a sweat gland.

hidradenoid carcinoma. SWEAT GLAND CARCINOMA.

hi·drad·e·no·ma, hy·drad·e·no·ma (hi·drad"e·no'muh, high·) *n.* [*hidr-* + *adenoma*]. 1. Any benign sweat-gland tumor. 2. HIDRADENOMA PAPILLIFERUM. 3. SYRINGOMA. 4. CYLINDROMA.

hidradenoma pap·il·lif·e·rum (pap·i·lif'e·rum). A benign sweat-gland tumor whose parenchymal cells are arranged into papillary processes extending into a cystic space, usually occurring on the vulva or perineum.

hidro-. See *hidr-.*

hi·droa (hi·dro'uh, high·dro'uh) *n.* [Gk. *hidrōa*, heat spots, pustules, from *hidrōs*, sweat]. 1. Any skin lesion associated with, or caused by, profuse sweating. 2. HYDROA.

hid·ro·cyst·ad·e·no·ma (hid"ro·sist"ad·e·no'muh, high"dro·) *n.* [*hidro-* + *cyst* + *adenoma*]. HIDROCYSTOMA.

hid·ro·cys·to·ma (hid"ro·sis·to'muh, high"dro·) *n.*, pl. **hidrocystomas, hidrocystoma·ta** (·tuh) [*hidro-* + *cyst* + *-oma*]. A retention cyst of a sweat gland.

hid·ro·poi·e·sis (hid"ro·poy·ee'sis, high"dro·) *n.* [*hidro-* + *-poeisis*]. The formation and secretion of sweat. —**hidropoi·et·ic** (·et'ick) *adj.*

hid·ror·rhea, hid·ror·rhoea (hid"ro·ree'uh, high"dro·) *n.* [*hidro-* + *-rrhea*]. Excessive flow of sweat.

hi·dros·ad·e·ni·tis, hy·dros·ad·e·ni·tis (high"dro·sad·i·nigh'tis, hid"ro·) *n.* [Gk. *hidrōs*, sweat, + *adenitis*]. HIDRADENITIS.

hi·dros·che·sis (hi·dros'ke·sis, high·dros') *n.* [*hidro-* + Gk. *schesis*, retention]. Retention or suppression of sweat; ANHIDROSIS.

hi·dro·sis (hi·dro'sis, high·) *n.*, pl. **hidro·ses** (·seez) [Gk. *hidrōsis*, from *hidrōs*, sweat]. 1. The formation and excretion of sweat. 2. Abnormally profuse sweating. —**hi·drose** (high'droce) *adj.*

hi·drot·ic (hi·drot'ick, high·) *adj. & n.* [Gk. *hidrōtikos*, from *hidrōs*, sweat] 1. Diaphoretic or sudorific. 2. A medicine that causes sweating.

hidrotic, *n.* A medicine that causes sweating.

hier-, hiero- [Gk. *hieros*]. A combining form meaning (a) *sacred;* (b) *sacral, hieric.*

hi·er·ic (high·err'ick) *adj.* [*hier-* + *-ic*]. SACRAL.

hieric index. The ratio of the width of the sacrum, taken between the tips of the greatest anterolateral extension of the facies auriculares, to the length, taken in the sagittal plane from the sacral promontory to the ventral edge of the apex, × 100. Values of the index are classified as:

dolichohieric (narrow sacrum)	x–99.9
subplatyhieric (moderately broad)	100.0–105.9
platyhieric (broad sacrum)	106.0–x

hi·er·on·o·sus (high"ur·on'o·sus) *n.* [*hiero-* + Gk. *nosos*, disease]. *Obsol.* EPILEPSY.

hi·ero·pho·bia (high"ur·o·fo'bee·uh) *n.* [*hiero-* + *-phobia*]. Morbid fear of religious objects or rituals, clergymen, or places of religious worship.

high-alcoholic elixir. A vehicle for various medicaments consisting of orange spirit, saccharin, and glycerin, containing about 80% alcohol.

high-altitude erythremia. The increased erythrocyte count, or physiologic polycythemia, seen in persons living at high altitudes.

high-altitude pulmonary edema. Pulmonary edema occurring in certain predisposed individuals after a rapid change from low to high altitude, usually over 3,000 m.

high-bush cranberry bark. VIBURNUM OPULUS.

high-caloric diet. A diet containing a large number (3000 to 5000) of calories per day.

high enema. An enema injected into the colon.

higher center. An aggregate of neuronal elements usually located in the cerebrum; associated with consciousness, language, and intellectual function and the regulation of intricate and complex movements.

high-explosive injury. Damage to tissues from the action of high explosives, as shells, dynamite, or TNT; may be of all degrees of severity.

high forceps. An obstetric forceps applied to the fetal head which has descended into the pelvic canal, when its greatest diameter is still above the superior strait.

high-frequency current. A rapidly alternating short-wave flow of electricity, used to produce warmth or heat. See also *d'Arsonval current, Tesla current.*

high hyperopia. Manifest hyperopia, especially the absolute form.

high incidence factors. PUBLIC ANTIGENS.

high-mountain disease. BRISKET DISEASE.

high myopia. A degree of myopia greater than 6.5 diopters.

high operation. The application of forceps to the fetal head at the superior strait.

high pelvic position. TRENDELENBURG POSITION.

high-performance liquid chromatography. A separation process similar to gas chromatography in which the mobile phase is a liquid.

high takeoff. *In electrocardiography,* elevation of the RST segment at its junction with QRS complex, seen in conditions such as early repolarization, epicardial injury (pericarditis, trauma, ischemia, neoplasm), and ventricular aneurysm.

high-tension pulse. A pulse that is gradual in its impulse, long in duration, slow in subsiding, and with difficulty compressible; the artery between the beats feels like a firm round cord. Syn. *cordy pulse.*

high-vitamin diet. A diet rich in vitamins, used in such conditions as vitamin-deficiency diseases, anemia, hyperthyroidism, and tuberculosis. It is often combined with a high-caloric diet.

hila. Plural of *hilum.*

hi·lar (high'lur) *adj.* Pertaining to or located near a hilus.

hilar cyst. A bronchogenic cyst attached to one of the main or lobar bronchi.

hilar dance. Increased amplitude of pulsation of the pulmonary arteries on fluoroscopic examination.

hili. Plural and genitive singular of *hilus.*

hill diarrhea. A sprue-like diarrhea occurring at high altitudes in hot climates, particularly in the hill country of India.

Hill-Flack sign [L. *Hill,* English physician, 20th century; and M. W. *Flack,* English physiologist, 1882–1931]. HILL'S SIGN.

Hil·liard's lupus [named after a patient of J. Hutchinson]. A form of lupus vulgaris affecting the hands and arms.

hill·ock, *n.* A slight prominence or elevation; COLLICULUS.

Hill's sign [L. *Hill*]. An increase in femoral artery pressure over brachial artery pressure of more than the normal difference of 20 mmHg; a sign of severe aortic regurgitation.

Hil·ton's law [J. *Hilton,* English surgeon and anatomist, 1804–1878]. The nerve trunk supplying a joint also supplies the overlying skin and the muscles that move the joint.

hi·lum (high'lum) *n.*, pl. **hi·la** (·luh) [L., a little thing]. 1. *In botany,* the scar on a seed marking its point of attachment. 2. *In anatomy,* HILUS.

hi·lus (high'lus) *n.*, pl. & genit. sing. **hi·li** (·lye) [NL., from *hilum*]. A pit, recess, or opening in an organ, usually for the entrance and exit of vessels or ducts.

hilus cells. Cells in the hilus of the ovary, which may be functional, hormone-producing cells, analogous to the interstitial (Leydig) cells of the testis.

hilus-cell tumor. ADRENOCORTICOID ADENOMA OF THE OVARY.

hilus glan·du·lae su·pra·re·na·lis (glan'dew·lee sue"pruh·re·nay'lis) [NA]. The small groove on the ventromedial surface of the suprarenal gland where the suprarenal vein leaves.

hilus li·e·nis (lye·ee'nis) [NA]. The deep groove on the gastric surface of the spleen where the splenic vessels reach the spleen.

hilus lym·pho·glan·du·lae (lim·fo·glan'dew·lee) [BNA]. HILUS NODI LYMPHATICI.

hilus no·di lym·pha·ti·ci (no'dye lim·fat'i·sigh) [NA]. The groove on the surface of a lymph node where the arteries enter and the veins and efferent lymphatic vessels leave the node.

hilus nu·clei den·ta·ti (new'klee·eye den·tay'tye) [NA]. The cup-shaped opening on the medial side of the dentate nucleus. It is filled with white matter.

hilus nuclei oli·va·ris (ol·i·vair'is) [NA]. The area on the medial side of the olive filled with white matter.

hilus ova·rii (o·vair'ee·eye) [NA]. The border of the ovary to which is attached the mesovarium. Here the vessels and nerves reach the ovary.

hilus pul·mo·nis (pul·mo'nis) [NA]. The area on the medial aspect of each lung where the pulmonary artery and bronchus enter the lung and the pulmonary veins leave.

hilus re·na·lis (re·nay'lis) [NA]. The fissure on the medial margin of the kidney to which is attached the renal pelvis. The renal vessels reach the kidney here. Syn. *renal hilus.*

hind·brain, *n.* RHOMBENCEPHALON.

hindbrain sleep. REM SLEEP.

hind·gut, *n.* The caudal part of the embryonic digestive tube formed by the development of the tail fold.

Hines and Brown test [E. A. *Hines,* U. S. physician, b. 1906; and G. E. *Brown,* U. S. physician, 1885–1935]. COLD PRESSOR TEST.

hinge articulation or **joint.** A synovial joint in which a convex cylindrical surface is grooved at right angles to the axis of the cylinder, or trochlea, and meets a concave cylindrical surface that is ridged to fit the trochlea in such a manner as to permit motion in only one plane. NA *ginglymus.*

hinge axis. An imaginary line between the two mandibular condyles around which the mandible can rotate without translatory movement.

Hink·le's pill. A laxative pill containing aloin, belladonna, cascara, and podophyllum as active ingredients.

Hin·ton test [W. A. *Hinton,* U. S. *bacteriologist,* 1883–1959]. A macroscopic flocculation test for syphilis.

hip, *n.* 1. The upper part of the thigh at its junction with the buttocks. NA *coxa.* See also *hip joint.* 2. The lateral prominence of the body at the level of the hip joint.

hip·bone, *n.* The irregular bone forming one side and the anterior wall of the pelvic cavity, and composed of the ilium, ischium, and pubis. Syn. *innominate bone.* NA *os coxae.* See also Table of Bones in the Appendix.

hip displacement. Congenital acetabular dysplasia with or without subluxation or dislocation of the femoral head.

hip joint. The articulation of the head of the femur with the acetabulum of the hip bone. NA *articulatio coxae.* See also Table of Synovial Joints and Ligaments in the Appendix and Plate 2.

hip lift-prone pressure method. Artificial respiration in which the Schafer method is combined with lifting the hips in expiration; the hips also may be rolled to one side, an action that is less effective but less exhausting for the operator.

hipp-, hippo- [Gk. *hippos*]. A combining form meaning *horse, equine.*

Hip·pe·la·tes (hip″e·lay′teez) *n.* [Gk. *hippelatēs,* horse driver]. A genus of minute flies of the family Oscinidae.

Hippelates col·lu·sor (col·yoo′sor). HIPPELATES FLAVIPES.

Hippelates fla·vi·pes (flay′vi·peez). A species of eye fly found in southeastern United States, Mexico, Central and South America. Syn. *H.* collusor.

Hippelates pal·li·pes (pal′i·peez). The Egyptian eye fly; feeds on conjunctival exudates. Syn. *Oscinis pallipes.*

Hippelates pu·sio (pew′see·o). The American eye fly; a pest of both man and animals which feeds on drops of blood on the skin, open wounds, and mucous membranes; a factor in spreading pinkeye.

Hip·pel-Lin·dau disease [E. von *Hippel,* German ophthalmologist, 1867–1939; and A. *Lindau,* Swedish pathologist, b. 1892]. Angiomatosis of the retina (von Hippel's disease) associated with cerebellar angioma (Lindau's disease) and angioma of other viscera.

hippo-. See *hipp-.*

Hip·po·bos·ci·dae (hip″o·bos′i·dee) *n.pl.* [*hippo-* + Gk. *boskein,* to feed]. A family of the Diptera which includes the louse flies, bloodsucking ectoparasites of birds and mammals.

hip·po·cam·pal (hip″o·kam′pul) *adj.* Of or pertaining to the hippocampus.

hippocampal commissure. COMMISSURE OF THE FORNIX.

hippocampal fissure. HIPPOCAMPAL SULCUS.

hippocampal gyrus. PARAHIPPOCAMPAL GYRUS.

hippocampal sulcus. A fissure situated between the parahippocampal gyrus and the fimbria hippocampi. NA *sulcus hippocampi.*

hip·po·cam·pus (hip″o·kam′pus) *n.,* pl. & genit. sing. **hippo·cam·pi** (·pye) [Gk. *hippokampos,* sea monster, sea horse] [NA]. A curved elevation consisting largely of gray matter, in the floor of the inferior horn of the lateral ventricle.

Hip·po·crat·ic (hip″o·krat′ick) *adj.* Originated by or associated with Hippocrates, Greek physician, 460–377 B.C.

Hippocratic face. FACIES HIPPOCRATICA.

Hippocratic finger. CLUBBED FINGER.

Hippocratic nail. The nail of a clubbed finger.

Hippocratic oath. [*Hippocrates.* Greek physician, 460–377 B. C.]. An oath setting forth the duties of the physician to his patients, as follows: I swear by Apollo the physician, and Asklepios, and health, and All-heal, and all the gods and goddesses, that, according to my ability and judgment. I will keep this Oath and this stipulation—to reckon him who taught me this Art equally dear to me as my parents, to share my substance with him, and relieve his necessities if required; to look upon his offspring in the same footing as my own brothers, and to teach them this art, if they shall wish to learn it, without fee or stipulation; and that by precept, lecture, and every other mode of instruction, I will impart a knowledge of the Art to my own sons, and those of my teachers, and to disciples bound by a stipulation and oath according to the law of medicine, but to none others.

I will follow that system of regimen which, according to my ability and judgment, I consider for the benefit of my patients, and abstain from whatever is deleterious and mischievous, I will give no deadly medicine to any one if asked, nor suggest any such counsel; and in like manner I will not give to a woman a pessary to produce abortion. With purity and holiness I will pass my life and practice my Art.

I will not cut persons labouring under the stone, but will leave this to be done by men who are practitioners of this work. Into whatever houses I enter, I will go into them for the benefit of the sick, and will abstain from every voluntary act of mischief and corruption; and, further, from the seduction of females or males, of freemen and slaves. Whatever, in connection with my professional practice, or not in connection with it, I see or hear, in the life of men, which ought not to be spoken of abroad, I will not divulge, as reckoning that all such should be kept secret. While I continue to keep this Oath unviolated, may it be granted to me to enjoy life and the practice of the art, respected by all men, in all times! But should I trespass and violate this Oath, may the reverse be my lot!

hip·po·lith (hip′o·lith) *n.* [*hippo-* + *-lith*]. A calculus or bezoar found in the stomach of the horse.

hip·po·myx·o·ma (hip″o·mick·so′muh) *n.* [*hippo-* + *myxoma*]. The swelling attending glanders.

hip·pu·rase (hip′yoo·race) *n.* HIPPURICASE.

hip·pu·ria (hi·pew′ree·uh) *n.* Excess of hippuric acid in the urine.

hip·pu·ric acid (hi·pew′rick) [*hipp-* + *uric*]. Benzoylaminoacetic acid, $C_9H_9NO_3$, an acid found in high concentration in the urine of herbivorous animals and to a lesser extent in the urine of man; it is a metabolic product of benzoic acid. Syn. *urobenzoic acid.*

hippuric acid test. A test for liver function based upon the ability of the liver to synthesize glycine and to conjugate it with benzoic acid to form hippuric acid. Given 6 g of sodium benzoate, in 4 hours a normal person will eliminate 3 g or more of hippuric acid in the urine, whereas a person with liver dysfunction will eliminate less than 3 g.

hip·pu·ri·case (hi·purr′ri·kace, ·kaze, hi·pew′ri·) *n.* An enzyme found in kidney, liver, muscle, and pancreas which catalyzes the hydrolysis of hippuric acid to benzoic acid and glycine. The hippuricase occurring in liver and kidney probably exerts a synthetic, rather than a hydrolytic, action, metabolizing benzoic acid by the formation of hippuric acid. Syn. *hippurase, histozyme.*

hip·pus (hip′us) *n.* [Gk. *hippos,* horse; name of an eye condition involving blinking]. Spasmodic pupillary movement, independent of the action of light.

Hiprex. A trademark for methenamine hippurate, a urinary antibacterial.

hip roll–prone pressure method. HIP LIFT–PRONE PRESSURE METHOD.

hir·ci (hur′sigh) *n.,* sing. **hir·cus** (·kus) [L., he-goats] [NA]. The hair in the axilla.

hir·cis·mus (hur·siz′mus, hear·sis′mus) *n.* [NL., from L. *hircus,* he-goat]. The peculiar odor of axillary apocrine secretion.

Hirsch·berg's reflex or **sign** [L. K. *Hirschberg,* U. S. neurologist, b. 1877]. ADDUCTOR REFLEX OF THE FOOT.

Hirsch·berg's test for strabismus (hirrsh′behrk) [J. *Hirschberg,* German ophthalmologist, 1843–1925]. A rough estimate of the degree of strabismus.

Hirsch·feld's nerve (hirrsh′feld) [L. M. *Hirschfeld,* Polish anatomist, 1816–1876]. An inconstant lingual branch of the facial nerve.

Hirsch·sprung's disease [H. *Hirschsprung,* Danish physician, 1830–1916]. A congenital, often familial disorder manifested by inability to defecate due to absence of ganglion cells in the submucosal or myenteric plexuses in a given segment of the colon or proximal rectum, which is unable to relax to permit passage of the stool. The normal colon proximal to the aganglionic segment is narrow, with dilatation above. Treatment is surgical, and if untreated, the disease results in growth retardation.

hir·sute (hur′sewt) *adj.* [L. *hirsutus*]. Shaggy; hairy.

hir·su·tic acid (hur·sue′tick). Generic term for a series of substances, derived from the fungus *Stereum hirsutum,* certain of which have antibiotic activity.

hir·su·ti·es (hur·sue′shee·eez) *n.* [L., from *hirsutus,* hairy]. Excessive growth of hair; HYPERTRICHOSIS.

hir·sut·ism (hur′sewt·iz·um) *n.* [*hirsute* + *-ism*]. A condition characterized by growth of hair in unusual places and in unusual amounts.

Hirtz's rale. A moist, metallic sound accompanying tuberculous softening.

hiru·din (hirr'yoo·din) *n.* [L. *hirudo*, leech, + *-in*]. The active principle of a secretion derived from the buccal glands of leeches. It prevents the coagulation of blood.

Hir·u·din·ea (hirr''yoo·din'nee·uh) *n.pl.* [NL., from *Hirudo*]. A class of predatory or parasitic annelids; the leeches.

hir·u·di·ni·a·sis (hirr''yoo·di·nigh'uh·sis) *n.*, pl. **huridinia·ses** (·seez) [L. *hirudo, hirudinis*, leech, + *-iasis*]. Infestation by leeches.

hi·ru·di·ni·cul·ture (hi·roo'di·ni·kul''chur, hirr·yoo'di·ni·) *n.* [L. *hirudo, hirudinis*, leech, + *culture*]. The artificial breeding of leeches.

Hi·ru·do (hi·roo'do) *n.* [L., leech]. A genus of leeches.

Hirudo me·dic·i·na·lis (me·dis''i·nay'lis). The medicinal leech; formerly extensively used for bloodletting.

His bundle (hiss) [W. *His*, Jr.]. Bundle of His (= ATRIOVENTRICULAR BUNDLE).

His-Held spaces (hiss, helt) [W. *His*, Swiss anatomist and embryologist, 1831-1904; and H. *Held*]. PERIVASCULAR SPACES OF VIRCHOW-ROBIN.

his operon. A sequence of nine genes in many bacteria which code for all the enzymes involved in histidine biosynthesis.

His's spaces [W. *His*]. PERIVASCULAR SPACES OF VIRCHOW-ROBIN.

Hiss's serum water [P. H. *Hiss*, U. S. bacteriologist, 1868-1913]. Serum diluted with two or three times its volume of distilled water; used in bacteriology to aid the growth of fastidious organisms.

Hiss's serum water medium [P. H. *Hiss*]. A medium used for determining fermentative capacities of bacteria, containing water, serum, carbohydrate, phenol red, or other indicator.

hist-, histo- [Gk. *histos*, web, web-beam of loom, orig. upright beam, mast, from *histanai*, to set upright, stand]. A combining form meaning *tissue*.

Histadur. A trademark for chlorpheniramine maleate, an antihistaminic.

Histadyl. A trademark for methapyrilene, an antihistaminic drug used as the hydrochloride salt.

Histalog. Trademark for betazole, a gastric secretion diagnostic agent used as the dihydrochloride salt.

his·tam·i·nase (his·tam'i·nace, ·naze, his''tuh·mi·naze') *n.* An enzyme, obtainable from extracts of kidney and intestinal mucosa, capable of inactivating histamine and other diamines; has been used in the treatment of anaphylactic shock, asthma, hay fever, serum sickness, and other allergic conditions which may be due to, or accompanied by, liberation of histamine in the body. Syn. *diamine oxidase*.

his·ta·mine (his'tuh·meen, ·min) *n.* 4-(2-Aminoethyl)imidazole, $C_5H_9N_3$, an amine occurring as a decomposition product of histidine and prepared synthetically from that substance. It stimulates visceral muscles, dilates capillaries, and stimulates salivary, pancreatic, and gastric secretions. Used as the hydrochloride or phosphate salt as a diagnostic agent in testing gastric secretion. —**his·ta·min·ic** (his''tuh·min'ick) *adj.*

histamine cephalalgia or **headache**. CLUSTER HEADACHE.

histamine test. 1. The subcutaneous injection of histamine stimulating the gastric secretion of hydrochloric acid. 2. The precipitation of an attack of cephalalgia (vasomotor headache) by the injection of histamine done for purposes of diagnosis. 3. The intradermal injections of histamine at various points along a limb, resulting normally in the appearance within 5 minutes of a wheal with an erythematous areola. Absence of these phenomena indicates insufficient pressure in skin vessels, arterial spasm, or nonfunctioning sensory nerves of the skin.

histaminic headache. CLUSTER HEADACHE.

his·ta·min·o·lyt·ic (his''tuh·min·o·lit'ick) *adj.* [*histamine* + *-lytic*]. Breaking down histamine.

Histan. A trademark for pyrilamine maleate, an antihistaminic.

his·ta·nox·ia (his''tuh·nock'see·uh) *n.* [*hist-* + *anoxia*]. Decreased tissue oxygenation due to diminution of the blood supply.

Histaspan. A trademark for chlorpheniramine maleate, an antihistaminic.

His-Ta·wa·ra node (hiss, tah'wa·rah) [W. *His*, Jr., German physician, 1863-1934; and S. *Tawara*, Japanese pathologist, 1873-1952]. ATRIOVENTRICULAR NODE.

His-Tawara system [W. *His*, Jr., and S. *Tawara*]. The conduction system of the heart, composed of the atrioventricular node and the atrioventricular bundle.

histi-, histio- [Gk. *histion*, web]. A combining form meaning (a) *web, weblike;* (b) *tissue*.

his·tic (his'tick) *adj.* [*hist-* + *-ic*]. *Obsol.* Pertaining to tissue.

his·ti·dase (his''ti·dace, ·daze) *n.* An enzyme, found in the liver of higher animals, acting on L-histidine, but not on D-histidine or other imidazole compounds, to open the imidazole ring with formation of urocanic acid.

histidinaemia. HISTIDINEMIA.

his·ti·dine (his'ti·deen, ·din) *n.* [*hist-* + *-id* + *-ine*]. β-Imidazole-α-alanine, $C_6H_9N_3O_2$, an amino acid resulting from hydrolysis of many proteins. By elimination of a molecule of carbon dioxide, it is converted to histamine. The hydrochloride has been used for the treatment of peptic ulcers.

histidine decarboxylase. The enzyme that catalyzes decarboxylation of histidine to histamine.

his·ti·di·ne·mia, his·ti·di·nae·mia (his''ti·di·nee'mee·uh) *n.* [*histidine* + *-emia*]. A rare hereditary (probably autosomal recessive) metabolic disorder in which there is a deficiency of histidase (L-hystidine ammonia lysase) with a high blood level of histidine and often alanine, increased urinary excretion of imidazolepyruvate, imidazoleacetate, and imidazolelactate, as well as absence of urocanic acid in sweat and urine after an oral histidine load; manifested clinically by speech disorders and often mild mental retardation, as well as lowered growth rates and heightened susceptibility to infection.

histidine test. A pregnancy test based on the quantity of histidine excreted in the urine during pregnancy.

his·ti·di·nu·ria (his''ti·di·new'ree·uh) *n.* [*histidine* + *-uria*]. The presence of histidine in the urine.

his·ti·dyl (his'ti·dil) *n.* The univalent radical, $C_6H_8N_3O_2$—, of the amino acid histidine.

his·tio·cyte (his'tee·o·site) *n.* [*histio-* + *-cyte*]. A fixed macrophage of the loose connective tissue, usually one which has not ingested material and which, in common with other cells belonging to the reticuloendothelial system, stores electively certain dyes such as trypan blue or lithium carmine. —**his·tio·cyt·ic** (his''tee·o·sit'ick) *adj.*

histiocytic leukemia. SCHILLING TYPE LEUKEMIA.

histiocytic sarcoma. RETICULUM-CELL SARCOMA.

his·tio·cy·toid (his'tee·o·sigh''toid) *adj.* Like a histiocyte.

his·tio·cy·to·ma (his''tee·o·sigh·to'muh) *n.*, pl. **histiocytomas, histiocytoma·ta** (·tuh) [*histiocyte* + *-oma*]. 1. A benign tumor composed of histiocytes. 2. DERMATOFIBROMA.

his·tio·cy·to·sar·co·ma (his''tee·o·sigh''to·sahr·ko'muh) *n.* A sarcoma whose parenchyma is composed of anaplastic histiocytes.

his·tio·cy·to·sis (his''tee·o·sigh·to'sis) *n.*, pl. **histiocyto·ses** (·seez) [*histiocyte* + *-osis*]. An excessive number of histiocytes, usually generalized.

histiocytosis X. Any of a group of proliferative disorders of the reticuloendothelial system of unknown cause, characterized by local or general proliferation of histiocytes which often show phagocytosis. Among the subtypes are Letterer-Siwe disease, Hand-Schüller-Christian disease, and eosinophilic granuloma of bone. Syn. *reticuloendotheliosis*.

his·ti·oid (his'tee·oid) *adj.* HISTOID.

histioid tumor. A tumor made up almost entirely of a single type of cell.

his·ti·o·ma (his·tee·o'muh) *n.* HISTOMA.

his·tio·troph·ic (his''tee·o·trof'ick) *adj.* [*histio-* + *trophic*]. Having a protective or anabolic influence on the energy of cells, as the histiotrophic functions of the autonomic nervous system.

histo-. See *hist-*.

his·to·blast (his'to·blast) *n.* [*histo-* + *-blast*]. *Obsol.* A cell engaged in the formation of tissue.

his·to·chem·is·try (his''to·kem'is·tree) *n.* [*histo-* + *chemistry*]. 1. The chemistry of the tissues of the body. 2. The study of microscopic localization and analysis of substances in cells and tissues. —**histochem·i·cal** (·i·kul) *adj.*

his·to·com·pat·i·bil·i·ty (his''to·kum·pat''i·bil'i·tee) *n.* [*histo-* + *compatibility*]. Sufficient compatibility between different tissues for a graft to be accepted and remain functional without rejection. —**histocom·pat·i·ble** (·pat'i·bul) *adj.*

his·to·cyte (his'to·site) *n.* HISTIOCYTE.

his·to·di·al·y·sis (his''to·dye·al'i·sis) *n.* [*histo-* + *dialysis*]. The dissolution of organic tissue.

his·to·dif·fe·ren·ti·a·tion (his''to·dif''ur·en·shee·ay'shun) *n.* The differentiation of cell groups into tissues having characteristic cytologic and histologic appearances.

his·to·flu·o·res·cence (his''to·floo''uh·res'unce) *n.* [*histo-* + *fluorescence*]. Fluorescence of the tissues during x-ray treatment, produced by the prior administration of fluorescing drugs.

his·to·gen·e·sis (his''to·jen'e·sis) *n.* [*histo-* + *-genesis*]. Differentiation of cells and cell products from their earliest appearance to the completion of mature tissues. —**histo·ge·net·ic** (·je·net'ick) *adj.*

his·tog·e·ny (his·toj'e·nee) *n.* [*histo-* + *-geny*]. HISTOGENESIS.

his·to·gram (his'to·gram) *n.* [*history* + *-gram*]. A type of chart used in descriptive statistics to show the frequency distribution of a set of data.

his·tog·ra·phy (his·tog'ruh·fee) *n.* [*histo-* + *-graphy*]. Description of tissues.

his·to·he·ma·tin, his·to·hae·ma·tin (his''to·hee'muh·tin, ·hem'uh·tin) *n.* [*histo-* + *hematin*]. CYTOCHROME.

his·toid (his''toid) *adj.* [*hist-* + *-oid*]. 1. Resembling tissue. 2. Composed of only one kind of tissue.

his·to·in·com·pat·i·bil·i·ty (his''to·in''kum·pat·i·bil'i·tee) *n.* Lack of histocompatibility; incompatibility of tissues. —**histoincom·pat·i·ble** (·pat'i·bul) *adj.*

his·to·ki·ne·sis (his''to·ki·nee'sis, ·kigh·nee'sis) *n.* [*histo-* + *kinesis*]. Movement that takes place in the minute structural elements of the body.

his·to·log·ic (his''tuh·loj'ick) *adj.* 1. Of or pertaining to tissues. 2. Of or pertaining to histology. —**histolog·i·cal** (·i·kul) *adj.*; **histologi·cal·ly** (·kuh·lee) *adv.*

histologic accommodation. Microscopic changes in the form, structure, and function of cells and tissues after adapting to new conditions.

histologic chemistry. HISTOCHEMISTRY.

his·tol·o·gy (his·tol'uh·jee) *n.* [*histo-* + *-logy*]. The branch of biology that deals with the minute structure of tissues, including the study of cells and of organs. —**histolo·gist**, *n.*

his·tol·y·sis (his·tol'i·sis) *n.* [*histo-* + *-lysis*]. Disintegration and dissolution of organic tissue. —**his·to·lyt·ic** (his''to·lit'ick) *adj.*

his·to·ma (his·to'muh) *n.* [*hist-* + *-oma*]. A tumor whose cells are typical of a tissue, such as a fibroma. Syn. *histioma*.

his·to·meta·plas·tic (his''to·met''uh·plas'tick) *adj.* [*histo-* + *metaplastic*]. Causing the transformation of one tissue into another type. See also *metaplasia*.

His·tom·o·nas (his·tom'o·nas) *n.* [*histo-* + Gk. *monas*, unit, single]. A genus of flagellate protozoans. *Histomonas meleagridis* is an endoparasite of fowl, and the causative agent of histomoniasis.

his·tom·o·ni·a·sis (his·tom''o·nigh'uh·sis, his''to·mo·) *n.* [*Histomonas* + *-iasis*]. A disease of the ceca and liver of poultry, and wild gallinaceous birds caused by the protozoan *Histomonas meleagridis*. Syn. *blackhead enterohepatitis*.

his·to·mor·phol·o·gy (his''to·mor·fol'uh·jee) *n.* [*histo-* + *morphology*]. The morphology of the tissues of the body; histology.

his·to·my·co·sis (his''to·migh·ko'sis) *n.* [*histo-* + *mycosis*]. Fungal infection of the deep tissues, as opposed to surface growth.

his·tone (his'tone) *n.* Any one of a group of strongly basic proteins found in cell nuclei, such as thymus histone; soluble in water but insoluble in, or precipitated by, ammonium hydroxide, and coagulable by heat.

histone insulin. A preparation containing insulin and thymus histone which precipitates the insulin, the resulting suspension producing a prolonged hypoglycemic effect, as compared to amorphous or crystalline insulin solutions, and combined with zinc as histone zinc insulin, it is comparable in action to protamine zinc insulin.

his·to·neu·rol·o·gy (his''to·new·rol'uh·jee) *n.* NEUROHISTOLOGY.

his·ton·o·my (his·ton'uh·mee) *n.* [*histo-* + Gk. *nomos*, law, + *-y*]. The laws of the development and arrangement of organic tissue.

his·to·nu·ria (his''to·new'ree·uh) *n.* The presence of histone in the urine.

his·to·pa·thol·o·gy (his''to·puh·thol'uh·jee) *n.* [*histo-* + *pathology*]. The study of microscopically visible changes in diseased tissue. —**histo·patho·log·ic** (·path''uh·loj'ick) *adj.*

his·to·phys·i·ol·o·gy (his''to·fiz''ee·ol'uh·jee) *n.* [*histo-* + *physiology*]. The science of tissue functions.

His·to·plas·ma (his''to·plaz'muh) *n.* [NL., from *histo-* + *plasm*]. A genus of parasitic fungi.

Histoplasma cap·su·la·tum (kap·sue·lay'tum). The species of parasitic fungi that is the causative agent of histoplasmosis.

Histoplasma far·ci·mi·no·sum (fahr''si·mi·no'sum). The causative agent of epizootic lymphangitis.

his·to·plas·min (his''to·plaz'min) *n.* A standardized liquid concentrate of soluble growth factors developed by the fungus *Histoplasma capsulatum*; used as a dermal reactivity indicator in the diagnosis of histoplasmosis.

histoplasmin test. A skin test for delayed hypersensitivity to products of *Histoplasma capsulatum*, as an indicator of past or present infection with *H. capsulatum*. Cross-reactions occur with coccidioidomycosis and blastomycosis, and anergy may occur with disseminated histoplasmosis.

his·to·plas·mo·ma (his''to·plaz·mo'muh) *n.* [*histoplasma* + *-oma*]. A tumorlike swelling produced by an inflammatory reaction to *Histoplasma capsulatum*.

his·to·plas·mo·sis (his''to·plaz·mo'sis) *n.*, pl. **histoplasmo·ses** (·seez) [*Histoplasma* + *-osis*]. A reticuloendothelial cell infection with the fungus *Histoplasma capsulatum*, varying from a mild respiratory infection to severe disseminated disease, usually characterized by fever, anemia, hepatomegaly, splenomegaly, leukopenia, pulmonary lesions, gastrointestinal ulcerations, and suprarenal necrosis. Syn. *cytomycosis, Darling's histoplasmosis*.

his·to·ra·di·og·ra·phy (his''to·ray·dee·og'ruh·fee) *n.* [*histo-* + *radiography*]. MICRORADIOGRAPHY.

his·tor·ic typhus. EPIDEMIC TYPHUS.

his·to·ry (his'tur·ee) *n.* [Gk. *historia*, inquiry, information, narrative]. MEDICAL HISTORY.

his·to·spec·tros·co·py (his''to·speck·tros'ko·pee) *n.* The application of spectroscopy to histochemistry.

Histostat-50. A trademark for nitarsone, an antiprotozoal.

his·to·ther·a·py (his''to·therr'uh·pee) *n.* [*histo-* + *therapy*]. The remedial use of animal tissues.

his·to·throm·bin (his''to·throm'bin) *n.* [*histo-* + *thrombin*]. A thrombin supposedly formed from connective tissues.

his·to·tome (his'tuh·tome) *n.* [*histo-* + *-tome*]. An instrument for cutting tissue in preparation for microscopic study; MICROTOME.

his·tot·o·my (his·tot'uh·mee) *n.* [*histo-* + *-tomy*]. 1. The dissection of tissues. 2. The cutting of thin sections of tissues; microtomy.

his·to·tox·ic (his''to·tock'sick) *adj.* [*histo-* + *toxic*]. Deleterious or poisonous to the tissues, wholly or in part.

histotoxic hypoxia. Reduction in oxygen utilization due to interference in cellular metabolism by agents such as cyanide which poison the respiratory enzymes, or through deficiency of a respiratory enzyme, as in certain infections or deficiency diseases.

his·to·trip·sy (his'to·trip''see) *n.* [*histo-* + *-tripsy*]. The crushing of tissue by an écraseur.

his·to·trophe, his·to·troph (his'to·trof, ·trofe) *n.* [*histo-* + *-troph*]. 1. In deciduate placentation, the temporary nutritive substances supplied from sources other than the circulating blood, such as glandular secretion, extravasated blood. See also *embryotrophe.* 2. In nondeciduate placentation, the uterine secretion and transudates bathing the chorion and furnishing nutritive materials throughout gestation. —**his·to·troph·ic** (·trof'ick) *adj.*

his·to·zo·ic (his''to·zo'ick) *adj.* [*histo-* + *-zoic*]. Living on or within the tissues; denoting certain protozoan parasites.

his·to·zyme (his'to·zime) *n.* [*histo-* + *-zyme*]. HIPPURICASE.

his·tri·on·ic (his''tree·on'ick) *adj.* [L. *histrionicus,* from *histrio, histrionis,* actor]. 1. Characterized by exaggerated, dramatic gestures, attitudes, speech, and facial expressions, as are used by some actors. 2. Pertaining to the muscles producing facial expression.

histrionic personality. HYSTERICAL PERSONALITY.

histrionic spasm. A condition in which facial tics, acquired in childhood, persist during adult life, and are increased by emotional causes.

his·tri·o·nism (his'tree·o·niz·um) *n.* [*histrion*ic + *-ism*]. Dramatic action or attitude, as seen in some mental disorders.

His-Werner disease [W. *His,* Jr., and H. *Werner*]. TRENCH FEVER.

Hitch·cock's reagent. BENEDICT AND HITCHCOCK'S REAGENT.

hitch·hik·er's thumb deformity. Malformation of the first metatarsal occurring as part of diastrophic dwarfism, and producing the abducted thumb appearance used as a signal by hitchhikers.

Hit·zig's center (hits'i^{k}h)[E. *Hitzig,* German neurologist and psychiatrist, 1838-1907]. *Obsol.* The cortical motor area, especially that in dogs and monkeys.

hives, *n.pl.* URTICARIA.

Hjär·re's disease (yehr'e^{h})[A. *Hjärre,* German pathologist, 20th century]. A disease of chickens characterized by granulomatous lesions of the ceca, liver, duodenum, and mesentery. Syn. *coligranuloma.*

hl Abbreviation for *hectoliter.*

Hl. Symbol for latent hyperopia.

HLA [*h*uman *l*eukocyte, locus *A*]. The complex of antigens controlled by the major histocompatibility complex of gene loci for leukocyte antigens in man. Also written *HL-A.*

HLP Abbreviation for *hyperlipoproteinemia.*

Hm. Symbol for manifest hyperopia.

hm Abbreviation for *hectometer.*

HMO Abbreviation for *Health Maintenance Organization.*

HMS-Liquifilm. A trademark for medrysone, an ophthalmologic anti-inflammatory.

HN2 A trademark for mechlorethamine hydrochloride, a nitrogen mustard cytotoxic agent.

Ho Symbol for holmium.

hoarse, *adj.* 1. Of the voice: harsh, grating. 2. Having a harsh, discordant voice, caused by an abnormal condition of the larynx or throat. —**hoarse·ness,** *n.*

hoary, *adj.* Gray or white with age; said of the hair. —**hoar·i·ness,** *n.*

hob·ble, *v.* & *n.* 1. To have an uneven gait; to limp. 2. *In veterinary medicine,* a bond or shackle used to confine the foot of an animal. 3. Anything that restrains motion.

hob·nail liver. The liver as seen in Laennec's cirrhosis, in which masses of regenerated liver cells among weblike fibrous septa form a nodular or "hobnail" surface.

Hoch·sing·er's sign (hohk^{h}'zing·ur) [K. *Hochsinger,* Austrian pediatrician, b. 1860]. A sign suggestive of hypoparathyroidism; when the inner side of the biceps muscle of the arm is pressed, the fist closes. Compare *Trousseau's phenomenon.*

hock, *n.* The joint on the hind leg of a quadruped between the knee and the fetlock, corresponding to the ankle joint in man.

hock disease. *In veterinary medicine,* a deficiency disease of unknown etiology, characterized by the occurrence of deformed legs. Syn. *slipped tendon.*

hod-carrier's palsy. Paralysis of the muscles innervated by the long thoracic nerve, usually from carrying heavy objects on the shoulder, characterized by unilateral "winging" of the scapula.

Hodg·en splint [J. T. *Hodgen,* U.S. surgeon, 1826-1882]. A metal frame with supporting muslin straps, formerly used in the treatment of fractures of the shaft of the femur.

Hodg·kin's disease or **lymphoreticuloma** [T. *Hodgkin,* English physician, 1798-1866]. A malignant lymphoma composed of anaplastic reticuloendothelial cells of a distinctive type (Reed-Sternberg cells) and varying numbers of stromal cells including fibrocytes, lymphocytes, and eosinophils, with or without foci of necrosis.

Hodgkin's granuloma [T. *Hodgkin*]. A form of Hodgkin's disease in which anaplastic reticulum cells are associated with necrosis, eosinophils, and lymphocytes, producing lesions resembling those of infectious granulomas.

Hodgkin's sarcoma [T. *Hodgkin*]. A form of Hodgkin's disease in which the anaplastic reticuloendothelial cells are very prominent and stromal cells inconspicuous.

Hodg·son's disease [J. *Hodgson,* English physician, 1788-1869]. Nonsaccular aneurysmal dilatation of the aortic arch.

ho·do·pho·bia (ho''do·fo'bee·uh) *n.* [Gk. *hodos,* way, road, + *-phobia*]. An abnormal fear of travel.

hoe, *n.* 1. A scraping instrument used in operations for cleft palate. 2. A type of instrument used in the preparation of a dental cavity for restoration. 3. A periodontal instrument with a single blade, usually at a right angle to the shank, used for removing deposits of calculus from the tooth surface.

Hoeh·ne's sign (hœh'ne^{h}) [O. *Hoehne,* German gynecologist, 1871-1932]. Disappearance of uterine contractions during delivery, indicating that rupture of the uterus may have occurred.

hof (hofe) *n.* [Ger., courtyard, halo, areola]. 1. An open area. 2. *In hematology,* a space without granules in a granulocyte, or the lighter staining area adjacent to the nucleus of a plasma cell.

Hof·bau·er cell [J. I. I. *Hofbauer,* U.S. gynecologist, 1878-1961]. A large, sometimes binucleate, apparently phagocytic cell found in chorionic villi.

Hof·fa's disease (ho^{h}f'ah) [A. *Hoffa,* German orthopedist, 1859-1908]. Traumatic solitary lipoma of the knee joint.

Hoff·mann's anodyne (ho^{h}f'ma^{h}n) [F. *Hoffmann,* German physician, 1660-1742]. COMPOUND ETHER SPIRIT.

Hoffmann's atrophy [J. *Hoffmann,* German neurologist, 1857-1919]. INFANTILE SPINAL MUSCULAR ATROPHY.

Hoffmann's drops [F. *Hoffmann*]. ETHER SPIRIT.

Hoffmann's duct [M. *Hoffmann,* German anatomist, 1622-1698]. PANCREATIC DUCT.

Hoffmann's finger reflex or **sign** [J. *Hoffmann*]. DIGITAL REFLEX (1).

Hoffmann's phenomenon [J. *Hoffmann*]. The increased sensitivity of the sensory nerves to electrical stimuli in tetany.

Hoffmann's syndrome [J. *Hoffmann*]. Muscle enlargement, weakness, and fatigue, accompanied by slow, clumsy movements, associated with myxedema in adults.

Hoffmann-Werdnig disease or **syndrome** [J. *Hoffmann* and G. *Werdnig*]. INFANTILE SPINAL MUSCULAR ATROPHY.

Hof·mann's bacillus (hofe'mahn) [G. von *Hofmann*-Wellenhof, Austrian bacteriologist, 19th century]. *CORYNEBACTERIUM PSEUDODIPHTHERITICUM.*

Hof·meis·ter-Fin·ster·er operation (hofe'migh·stur, fin'stur·ur) [F. von *Hofmeister,* German surgeon, 1867–1926; and H. *Finsterer,* Austrian surgeon, 1877–1955]. A modification of Polya's operation of subtotal gastrectomy with posterior gastrojejunostomy.

Hofmeister series [F. *Hofmeister,* Czechoslovakian chemist, 1850–1922]. LYOTROPIC SERIES.

hog cholera. An epizootic infectious disease of swine caused by a filtrable virus. *Salmonella choleraesuis* is a common secondary invader. The disease is characterized by fever, diarrhea, emaciation, patchy redness of the skin with inflammation and ulceration of the intestines. Syn. *swine fever.*

hog cholera bacillus. *SALMONELLA CHOLERAESUIS.*

hog gum. TRAGACANTH.

Hö·gyes' treatment (hœ'dyesh) [E. *Högyes,* Hungarian physician, 1847–1906]. A prophylactic treatment for rabies with diluted rabies virus.

Hoke's operation [N. *Hoke,* U.S. orthopedist, 1874–1944]. An operation for flatfoot, with removal of the navicular and cuneiform bones, fusion of the joints, and lengthening of the calcaneal tendon.

hol-, holo- [Gk. *holos,* whole]. A combining form meaning (a) *complete, entire;* (b) *homogeneous, like.*

hol·an·dric (hol·an'drick, ho·lan') *adj.* [*hol-* + *andr-* + *-ic*]. Pertaining to genes carried by the Y chromosomes; inherited only through the paternal line. Contr. *hologynic.* —**hol·an·dry** (hol'an·dree) *n.*

holding back. The deliberate avoidance of orgasm by a woman in the erroneous belief that this will prevent conception.

hol·er·ga·sia (hol''ur·gay'zhuh, ·zee·uh, ho''lur·) *n.* [*hol-* + *ergasia*]. A mental disorder, or major psychosis, that disrupts the entire structure of the personality, such as schizophrenia.

Hol·ger Niel·sen method [*Holger Nielsen,* Danish army officer, 20th century]. A method for artificial respiration in which the patient lies prone and the operator extends the patient's arms in inspiration and presses on the scapulae in expiration.

ho·lism (ho'liz·um) *n.* [*hol-* + *-ism*]. A concept in modern biological and psychological thinking which states that for complex systems such as a cell, an organism, or a personality the whole is greater than the sum of its parts from a functional point of view. Syn. *organicism.* —**ho·lis·tic** (ho·lis'tick) *adj.*

Hol·la disease [after *Holla,* Norway]. Epidemic hemolytic jaundice, with recurrent episodes of anemic crisis.

Hol·lan·der test [F. *Hollander,* U.S. physiologist, b. 1899]. A test for the presence of intact vagus nerves based on the rise in gastric acidity after the production of hypoglycemia by giving insulin.

Hol·len·horst bodies [R. W. *Hollenhorst,* U.S. ophthalmologist, b. 1913]. Pieces of atheromatous plaques that have broken off and lodged at a retinal bifurcation; seen as shiny irregular yellow patches on funduscopic examination.

hol·low back. Excessive lumbar lordosis.

hollow foot. TALIPES CAVUS.

hollow respiration. AMPHORIC RESPIRATION.

Holmes phenomenon or **sign** [G. M. *Holmes,* English neurologist, 1876–1966]. If the patient flexes an arm against a resistance that is suddenly released, the patient may be unable to check the flexion movement, to the point of striking the face, because of a delay in contraction of the triceps muscle, which would ordinarily arrest overflexion of the arm.

Holm·gren-Gol·gi canals (hohlm'greyn, gohl'jee) [E. A. *Holmgren,* Swedish histologist, 1866–1922; and C. *Golgi,* Italian histologist, 1844–1926]. Clear canals present in the cytoplasm of many cells which are similar to those of the Golgi apparatus.

Holmgren's wool-skein test. HOLMGREN TEST.

Holmgren test [A. F. *Holmgren,* Swedish physiologist, 1831–1897]. A test for color vision in which the subject is required to choose from a large number of pieces (100 or more) of colored wool yarn those that match a sample, such as red, green, or rose, momentarily exposed.

hol·mi·um (hole'mee·um, hol'mee·um) *n.* [*Holmia,* L. name for Stockholm]. Ho = 164.930. A lanthanide.

holo-. See *hol-.*

ho·lo·acar·di·us (hol''o·a·kahr'dee·us, ho''lo·) *n.* [*holo-* + *acardius*]. 1. ACARDIACUS. 2. ACARDIUS.

holoacardius acephalus. A placental parasitic twin (omphalosite) that is headless, but has a rudimentary heart.

holoacardius acormus. A placental parasitic twin (omphalosite) in which there is little more than a head.

holoacardius amorphus. ANIDEUS.

ho·lo·acra·nia (hol''o·a·kray'nee·uh, ho''lo·) *n.* [*holo-* + *acrania*]. Complete absence of the cranial vault, with partial or complete anencephalia.

ho·lo·blas·tic (hol''o·blas'tick, ho''lo·) *adj.* [*holo-* + *-blastic*]. Dividing completely into cells during cleavage. Contr. *meroblastic.*

holoblastic cleavage. Total cleavage of the ovum.

holoblastic ovum. An ovum having total or complete cleavage.

Holocaine. Trademark for phenacaine, a local anesthetic used as the hydrochloride salt.

ho·lo·ce·phal·ic (hol''o·se·fal'ick, ho''lo·) *adj.* [*holo-* + *-cephalic*]. Pertaining to a form of teratism with deficiency of certain parts, but with the head complete.

ho·lo·crine (hol'o·krin, ho'lo·) *adj.* [*holo-* + *-crine*]. Of or pertaining to glands in which the secretion is formed by degeneration of the glandular cells. Contr. *merocrine.* —**ho·loc·ri·nous** (ho·lock'ri·nus) *adj.*

ho·lo·di·as·tol·ic (hol''o·dye''as·tol'ick, ho''lo·) *adj.* [*holo-* + *diastolic*]. Lasting throughout diastole, especially as the murmurs of major aortic or pulmonic valve insufficiency or the diastolic portion of a continuous murmur.

ho·lo·en·zyme (hol''o·en'zyme, ho''lo·) *n.* [*holo-* + *enzyme*]. A complete enzyme formed from the purely protein part, or apoenzyme, combined with the coenzyme.

ho·lo·gas·tros·chi·sis (hol''o·gas·tros'ki·sis, ho''lo·) *n.* [*holo-* + *gastroschisis*]. A congenital fissure involving the entire length of the abdominal wall, exposing the abdominal organs.

ho·lo·gram (hol'o·gram, ho'lo·) *n.* [*holo-* + *-gram*]. The record of the diffraction pattern of the image of an object obtained by holography.

ho·log·ra·phy (ho·log'ruh·fee) *n.* [*holo-* + *-graphy*]. A lensless type of photography in which monochromatic light, as from a laser, is split into two beams, one of which enters the lensless camera directly, while the other enters after passing through a transparent image of the object; the two beams combine to form a diffraction pattern of the image which is recorded on film, this record being the hologram. To reconstruct the image, a beam of laser light is transmitted through the hologram to generate a second diffraction pattern, a component of which reproduces the original image on a screen.

ho·lo·gyn·ic (hol''o·jin'ick, ·jye'nick, ho''lo·) *adj.* [*holo-* + *gyn-* + *-ic*]. Pertaining to genes transmitted only in the female line from mother to daughter generation after generation, as in the case of attached X chromosomes. Contr. *holandric.*

ho·lo·met·a·bol·ic (hol''o·met''uh·bol'ick, ho''lo·) *adj.* HOLOMETABOLOUS.

ho·lo·me·tab·o·lous (hol''o·me·tab'uh·lus, ho''lo·) *adj.* [*holo-*

+ *-metabolous*]. Characterizing a mode of insect metamorphosis in which there is a quiescent pupal stage between the larva and the adult, as in beetles, moths, butterflies, midges, flies, ants, bees, and wasps. Contr. *hemimetabolous.*

ho·lo·mi·crog·ra·phy (hol″o·migh·krog′ruh·fee, ho″lo·) *n.* [*holo-* + *micrography*]. The technique of photographing reconstructed images.

ho·lo·phyt·ic (ho″lo·fit′ick) *adj.* [*holo-* + *phyt-* + *-ic*]. Not requiring the ingestion of exogenous complex organic substances for nutrition; characteristic of green plants. Contr. *holozoic.*

ho·lo·pros·en·ceph·a·ly (ho″lo·pros″en·sef′uh·lee) *n.* [*holoprosencephal*on + *-y*]. ARRHINENCEPHALIA.

ho·lo·ra·chis·chi·sis (hol″o·ra·kis′ki·sis, ho″lo·) *n.* [*holo-* + *rachischisis*]. The type of spina bifida in which the entire spinal canal is open.

ho·lo·sac·cha·ride (hol″o·sack′uh·ride, ho″lo·) *n.* [*holo-* + *saccharide*]. A polysaccharide that yields, on hydrolysis, only sugars. Compare *heterosaccharide.*

hol·o·side (hol′o·side) *n.* [*holo-* + glyco*side*]. A glycoside that yields, on hydrolysis, only sugars. Contr. *heteroside.*

ho·lo·so·ma·tic (hol″o·so·mat′ick, ho″lo·) *adj.* [*holo-* + *somatic*]. Pertaining to the whole body, in contrast to a local lesion.

ho·lo·sys·tol·ic (hol″o·sis·tol′ick, ho″lo·) *adj.* [*holo-* + *systolic*]. Lasting throughout systole, as the murmurs of major mitral or tricuspid valve insufficiency or ventricular septal defect.

ho·lo·zo·ic (hol″o·zo′ick, ho″lo·) *adj.* [*holo-* + *-zoic*]. Requiring the ingestion of complex organic materials for nutrition. Contr. *holophytic.*

Hol·ter-Doyle method. A titrimetric method for catalase based on the oxidation of iodide to iodine, by oxygen liberated from hydrogen peroxide, and titration of iodine with thiosulfate.

Holt-Oram syndrome. Atrial septal defect and associated bony abnormalities of the upper extremity, especially loss of opposition of the thumb.

Holtz machine [W. *Holtz*, German physicist, 1836–1913]. An early form of electrostatic generator for the production of high potentials.

hom-, homo- [Gk. *homos*, same]. A combining form meaning (a) *common, like, same;* (b) in chemistry and biology, *homologous.*

homal-, homalo- [Gk. *homalos*]. A combining form meaning (a) *level, even;* (b) *equal.*

hom·a·lo·ceph·a·lus (hom″uh·lo·sef′uh·lus) *n.*, pl. **homalocepha·li** (·lye) [*homalo-* + *-cephalus*]. An individual with a flat head.

hom·a·lo·cor·y·phus (hom″uh·lo·kor′i·fus) *n.* [*homalo-* + Gk. *koryphē*, head, + *-us*]. *In craniometry*, a skull with a parietal angle of 132 to 141°, indicating a moderate degree of convexity of the parietal bone in the sagittal plane. The angle is formed by locating the point in the arch of the parietal bone that lies highest above the straight line which connects the points bregma and lambda, and then connecting this point with bregma and lambda, respectively. The angle included between these two lines is the parietal angle.

hom·a·lo·me·to·pus (hom″uh·lo·me·to′pus) *n.* [*homalo-* + Gk. *metōpon*, forehead, + *-us*]. *In craniometry*, a skull having a frontal angle between 130.5 and 141°.

hom·al·o·pis·tho·cra·ni·us (hom″uh·lo·pis″tho·kray′nee·us) *n.* [*homal-* + *opistho-* + Gk. *kranion*, skull, + *-us*]. *In craniometry*, a skull in which the angle formed by lines joining the external occipital protuberance and the occipital point with the highest point of the skull is 140 to 154°.

hom·al·u·ra·nus (hom″uh·lew·ray′nus) *n.* [*homal-* + Gk. *ouranos*, vault]. *In craniometry*, a skull with an angle of the palatal arch of 147.5 to 164°, indicating a moderately flattened arching of the palate in the sagittal plane. The angle is formed by locating the point in the palatal arch that lies highest above the straight line which connects the inferior point of the premaxilla with the tip of the posterior nasal spine, and then connecting this point with the inferior point of the premaxilla and the tip of the posterior nasal spine, respectively. The angle included between these two lines is the angle of the palatal arch.

Ho·mans' sign [J. *Homans*, U. S. surgeon, 1877–1954]. Pain in the calf and popliteal area on passive dorsiflexion of the foot, indicating deep venous thrombosis of calf. Syn. *dorsiflexion sign.*

hom·a·rine (ho′muh·rine, ·rin, hom′uh·) *n.* A methylated picolinic acid, isomeric with trigonelline, isolated from mammalian urine.

hom·at·ro·pine (ho·mat′ro·peen, ·pin) *n.* An alkaloid, $C_{16}H_{21}NO_3$, prepared from atropine and mandelic acid. It causes dilatation of the pupil and paralysis of accommodation, as does atropine, but its effects pass off more quickly, usually in two or three days. Variously used, in the form of its hydrobromide, hydrochloride, or methylbromide salt, as a parasympatholytic drug.

hom·ax·i·al (ho·mack′see·ul) *adj.* [*hom-* + *axial*]. Having all axes equal.

hom·ax·o·ni·al (ho″mack·so′nee·ul) *adj.* HOMAXIAL.

homeo-, homoeo-, homoio- [Gk. *homoios*]. A combining form meaning *like, similar.*

ho·meo·chrome (ho′mee·o·krome) *adj.* [*homeo-* + *-chrome*]. Characterizing those special serous cells of salivary glands staining with mucin stains after fixation in a Formalin-bichromate mixture. Contr. *tropochrome.*

ho·meo·ki·ne·sis (ho″mee·o·ki·nee′sis) *n.*, pl. **homeokine·ses** (·seez) [*homeo-* + *-kinesis*]. A mitosis in which equal amounts of chromatin go to each daughter nucleus.

ho·meo·met·ric (ho″mee·o·met′rick) *adj.* [*homeo-* + *metric*]. Maintaining equal lengths.

homeometric autoregulation. An increase in the metabolic rate of the myocardium that develops gradually when the heart is distended by augmented filling pressures; the elevated metabolic rate is maintained as long as the increased filling pressure continues. Contr. *heterometric autoregulation.*

ho·meo·mor·phous, ho·moeo·mor·phous (ho″mee·o·mor′fus) *adj.* [Gk. *homoiomorphos*]. Like or similar in form and structure.

ho·meo·path·ic, ho·moeo·path·ic (ho″mee·o·path′ick) *adj.* Of or pertaining to homeopathy, and to its practice and principles.

homeopathic principle. ISOPATHIC PRINCIPLE.

ho·me·op·a·thy, ho·moe·op·a·thy (ho″mee·op′uth·ee) *n.* [*homeo-* + *-pathy*]. A system of medicine expounded by Samuel Hahnemann based on the simile phenomenon (*similia similibus curantur*). Cure of disease is effected by minute doses of drugs which produce the same signs and symptoms in a healthy person as are present in the disease for which they are administered. Syn. *Hahnemannism.* —**ho·meo·path, ho·moeo·path** (ho′mee·o·path), **ho·me·op·a·thist, ho·moe·op·a·thist** (ho″mee·op′uh·thist) *n.*

ho·meo·pla·sia, ho·moeo·pla·sia (ho″mee·o·play′zhuh, ·zee·uh) *n.* [*homeo-* + *-plasia*]. 1. The growth of tissue resembling the normal tissue, or matrix, in its form and properties. 2. The tissue so formed. —**homeo·plas·tic, homoeo·plas·tic** (·plas′tick) *adj.*

ho·me·o·sis, ho·moe·o·sis (ho″mee·o′sis) *n.*, pl. **homeo·ses, homoeo·ses** (·seez) [Gk. *homoiōsis*, resemblance, assimilation]. The appearance of an organ or appendage not normal to its location, as a leg in place of a proboscis in a fly. —**home·ot·ic, homoe·ot·ic** (·ot′ick) *adj.*

ho·meo·sta·sis (ho″mee·os′tuh·sis, ho″mee·o·stay′sis) *n.*, pl. **homeosta·ses** (·seez) [*homeo-* + *-stasis*]. The maintenance of steady states in the organism by coordinated physiologic processes or feedback mechanisms. Thus all organ systems are integrated by automatic adjustments to keep within narrow limits disturbances excited by, or directly resulting from, changes in the organism or in the surroundings of the organism. See also *milieu intearieur.* —**ho·meo·stat·ic** (ho″mee·o·stat′ick) *adj.*

ho·meo·therm (ho′mee·o·thurm) *n.* A homeothermic organism.

ho·meo·ther·mal (ho″mee·o·thur′mul) *adj.* HOMEOTHERMIC.

ho·meo·ther·mic (ho″mee·o·thur′mick) *adj.* [*homeo-* + *thermic*]. Of an organism: able to regulate physiologically the rate of heat production and heat loss so as to maintain itself at constant temperature independently of the environmental temperature; WARM-BLOODED. Contr. *poikilothermic.* —**ho·meo·ther·my** (ho′mee·o·thur″mee) *n.*

ho·meo·typ·ic (ho″mee·o·tip′ick) *adj.* [*homeo-* + Gk. *typos*, image, type, + *-ic*]. Resembling the normal type or the usual type.

homeotypic mitosis. The second meiotic division in the maturation of the germ cells; an equational division.

hom·er·gic (hom·ur′jick, ho·mur′jick) *adj.* [*hom-* + *erg-* + *-ic*]. Of or pertaining to drugs that elicit the same quality of effect irrespective of the manner in which the effect originates. Contr. *heterergic.*

Home's gland or **lobe** [E. *Home*, British surgeon, 1756–1832]. SUBTRIGONAL GLAND.

home·sick·ness, *n.* An urgent desire to return to one's home, which may be accompanied by a morbid sluggishness of the functions of the various organs of the body, and may develop into depression and morbid anxiety.

home visit. PAROLE.

ho·mi·chlo·pho·bia (ho·mick″lo·fo′bee·uh, hom″i·klo·) *n.* [Gk. *homichlē*, mist, fog, + *-phobia*]. An abnormal fear of fog.

hom·i·cide (hom′i·side) *n.* [L. *homicidium*, from *homo*, man, + *caedere*, to kill]. 1. The killing of a fellow human being. 2. A person who takes the life of another. —**hom·i·ci·dal** (hom″i·sigh′dul) *adj.*

Ho·min·i·dae (ho·min′i·dee) *n.pl.* A family of the Hominoidea that includes the genus *Homo*, and, in recent classifications, also genera of extinct "ape-men" or "man-apes" such as *Australopithecus.* —**hom·i·nid** (hom′i·nid) *adj. & n.*

Hom·i·noi·dea (hom″i·noy′dee·uh) *n.pl.* A superfamily of Primates that includes men and apes. Contr. *Cercopithecoidea, Ceboidea.* —**hom·i·noid** (hom′i·noid) *adj.*

Ho·mo (ho′mo) *n.* [L., man, human being]. The hominid genus that includes *Homo sapiens*, modern man, together with extinct species known from fossil remains such as *H. erectus* (formerly assigned to another genus, *Pithecanthropus*) and *H. neanderthalensis* (regarded by some as *H. sapiens neanderthalensis*, conspecific with modern man).

homo-. See *hom-*.

ho·mo·al·lele (ho′mo·a·leel′) *n.* [*homo-* + *allele*]. One of a set of alleles that differ at the same intragenic site. Contr. *heteroallele.* See also *pseudoallele.*

ho·mo·bi·o·tin (ho″mo·bye′o·tin) *n.* A homologue of biotin containing an additional CH_2 group in the side chain; it is a potent antagonist of biotin toward some bacteria but is capable of replacing biotin in certain of its functions toward other organisms.

ho·mo·cen·tric (ho″me·sen′trick, hom″o·) *adj.* [*homo-* + *-centric*]. Concentric; having the same center. —**homocen·tri·cal·ly** (·tri·kul·lee) *adv.*

ho·mo·cen·tri·cal (ho″mo·sen′tri·kul) *adj.* HOMOCENTRIC.

homocentric rays. Light rays that have a common focus or are parallel.

ho·mo·chrome (ho′muh·krome) *adj.* [*homo-* + *-chrome*]. Pertaining to one of two types of serous cells of the salivary glands, which takes the same color as the stain.

ho·mo·chro·mo·isom·er·ism (ho″mo·kro″mo·eye·som′ur·iz·um) *n.* [*homo-* + *chromo-* + *isomerism*]. The phenomenon of two or more organic substances of different structure exhibiting similar absorption spectra in solution.

ho·mo·clad·ic (ho″mo·klad′ick) *adj.* [*homo-* + Gk. *klados*, branch, + *-ic*]. Referring to an anastomosis between twigs of the same artery.

ho·mo·cy·clic (ho″mo·sigh′click, ·sick′lick) *adj.* [*homo-* + *cyclic*]. *In chemistry,* pertaining to compounds of the closed-chain or ring type in which all the ring atoms are of the same element, usually carbon. Contr. *heterocyclic.* See also *carbocyclic.*

ho·mo·cys·te·ine (ho″mo·sis′tee·een, ·in) *n.* 2-Amino-4-mercaptobutyric acid, $C_4H_9NO_2S$, a demethylated product of methionine. Capable of conversion to methionine in the animal body by a transmethylation reaction with choline, betaine, etc.

ho·mo·cys·tine (ho″mo·sis′teen, ·tin) *n.* 4,4′-Dithiobis-[2-aminobutyric acid], $C_8H_{16}N_2O_4S_2$, the oxidized, disulfide form of homocysteine; capable of replacing methionine in the diet provided choline is present.

ho·mo·cys·ti·nu·ria (ho″mo·sis·ti·new′ree·uh) *n.* [*homocystine* + *-uria*]. A recessively inherited disorder clinically resembling Marfan's syndrome; manifested by subluxated lenses regularly developing after the age of 10, frequently thromboembolic phenomena, and usually mental retardation. Homocystine is excreted in the urine as a result of absence of cystathionine synthetase activity.

ho·mo·cy·to·tro·pic (ho″mo·sigh″to·tro′pick) *adj.* [*homo-* + *cytotropic*]. Of an antibody; having an affinity for cells of the species of animal in which it originated. Contr. *heterocytotropic.*

homo·dont (ho′mo·dont) *adj.* [*hom-* + *-odont*]. *In biology,* having all the teeth alike, as the porpoises. Contr. *heterodont.*

ho·mo·dy·nam·ic (ho″mo·dye·nam′ick) *adj.* [*homo-* + *dynamic*]. Of or pertaining to homergic drugs that are agonists of the same receptor and thus have the same response system.

ho·mo·dy·na·my (ho″mo·dye′nuh·mee) *n.* [*homo-* + Gk. *dynamis*, force, value, + *-y*]. Serial homology; the correspondence of parts arranged in series along the main axis of the body. —**homo·dy·nam·ic** (·dye·nam′ick) *adj.*

homoeo-. See *homeo-.*

homoeomorphous. HOMEOMORPHOUS.

homoeopathic. HOMEOPATHIC.

homoeopathy. HOMEOPATHY.

homoeoplasia. HOMEOPLASIA.

homoeosis. HOMEOSIS.

homoeostasis. HOMEOSTASIS.

ho·mo·erot·i·cism (ho″mo·e·rot′i·siz·um) *n.* [*homo-* + *eroticism*]. HOMOEROTISM.

ho·mo·er·o·tism (ho″mo·err′o·tiz·um) *n.* [*homo-* + *erotism*]. 1. The direction of the libido toward a member of the same sex; HOMOSEXUALITY. 2. Specifically, homosexual orientation in which the erotic feeling is well sublimated, not requiring genital expression. Contr. *homogenitality.* —**homo·erot·ic** (·e·rot′ick) *adj. & n.*

ho·mo·fer·men·ta·tive (ho″mo·fur·men′tuh·tiv) *adj.* [*homo-* + *fermentative*]. Pertaining to the ability of certain bacteria to produce only lactic acid from glucose and other sugars. Contr. *heterofermentative.*

ho·mo·ga·met·ic (ho″mo·ga·met′ick) *adj.* [*homo-* + *gametic*]. Producing one kind of germ cell in regard to the sex chromosomes. The female, being XX in constitution, is the homogametic sex.

ho·mog·a·my (ho·mog′uh·mee) *n.* [*homo-* + *-gamy*]. INBREEDING.

ho·mog·e·nate (ho·moj′e·nate) *n.* The substance produced by homogenization.

ho·mo·ge·ne·ous (ho″mo·jee′nee·us, hom″o·) *adj.* [ML. *homogeneus*, from Gk. *homogenēs*, from *homo-*, same, + *genos*, race, kind]. Having the same nature or qualities; of uniform character in all parts. —**homo·ge·ne·i·ty** (·je·nee′i·tee) *n.*

homogeneous immersion. A fluid between the objective or condenser of a microscope, and the cover glass or slide, having about the same refractive and dispersive power as the glass.

homogeneous radiation. Radiation of uniform wavelength.

ho·mo·ge·net·ic (ho″mo·je·net′ick) *adj.* HOMOGENOUS.

homogenetic cortex. ISOCORTEX.

homogenetic rhythm. Cardiac rhythm caused by an impulse arising normally in the specialized tissues of the heart.

ho·mo·gen·ic (ho″mo·jen′ick) *adj.* [*homo-* + *-genic*]. Pertaining to genotypes of polysomic or polyploid organisms that contain the same allele for any given locus; similar to the term homozygous, used for diploid organisms.

ho·mo·gen·i·tal·i·ty (ho″mo·jen″i·tal′i·tee) *n.* Homoerotism in which the sexual impulses are given genital expression; HOMOSEXUALITY (1). —**ho·mo·gen·i·tal** (·jen′i·tul) *adj.*

ho·mog·e·ni·za·tion (ho·moj″e·ni·zay′shun) *n.* 1. The process of becoming homogeneous. 2. The production of a uniform dispersion, suspension, or emulsion from two or more normally immiscible substances. —**ho·mog·e·nize** (huh·moj′e·nize) *v.*

homogenized milk. Milk especially processed so that fat globules are minute and emulsification so complete that cream does not separate from the rest of the milk.

ho·mog·e·niz·er (huh·moj′e·nigh″zur) *n.* An apparatus for effecting a dispersion of a solid or liquid substance uniformly in a continuous medium, commonly water or one containing a considerable proportion of water.

ho·mog·e·nous (ho·moj′e·nus) *adj.* [Gk. *homogenēs*, of the same race or family]. 1. Of or derived from an individual of a closely related or similar strain of the same species. 2. Of two or more individuals, genetically or otherwise identical in certain characteristics.

ho·mo·gen·tis·ic acid (ho″mo·jen·tiz′ick, ·jen·tis′ick, hom″o·) [*homo-* + *gentisic*]. 2,5-Dihydroxyphenylacetic acid, $C_8H_8O_4$, found in urine in alkaptonuria; it is an intermediate in the oxidation of tyrosine and phenylalanine. Formerly called *glycosuric acid.*

ho·mo·glan·du·lar (ho″mo·glan′dew·lur) *adj.* [*homo-* + *glandular*]. Pertaining to the same gland.

ho·mo·graft (ho′mo·graft) *n.* [*homo-* + *graft*]. A tissue graft taken from a genetically nonidentical donor of the same species as the recipient. Syn. *allograft, homologous graft.* Compare *autograft.* Contr. *heterograft.*

homograft rejection. The immunologic process by which an animal causes the destruction or sloughing of tissue transplanted to it from an animal of the same species. See also *graft-versus-host reaction.*

homoio-. See *homeo-.*

ho·moio·ther·mic (ho·moy″o·thur′mick) *adj.* HOMEOTHERMIC.

ho·moio·top·ic transplantation (ho·moy″o·top′ick). ORTHOTOPIC TRANSPLANTATION.

ho·mo·lac·tic (ho″mo·lack′tick) *adj.* [*homo-* + *lactic*]. Pertaining to a type of sugar fermentation in which the only product is lactic acid; usually said of fermentation by microorganisms.

ho·mo·lat·er·al (ho″mo·lat′ur·ul) *adj.* [*homo-* + *lateral*]. IPSILATERAL.

homolog. HOMOLOGUE.

ho·mo·log·ic (ho″mo·loj′ick) *adj.* Of or pertaining to homology.

homologic anatomy. Study of the correlations of the several parts of the body with those of other groups of animals.

ho·mol·o·gous (ho·mol′uh·gus) *adj.* [Gk. *homologos*, in agreement]. 1. Corresponding in structure, either directly or as referred to a fundamental type. 2. Derived from a different organism of the same species. Compare *autologous.* Contr. *heterologous.* 3. *In chemistry*, being of the same type or series; differing by a multiple, such as CH_2, or by an arithmetic ratio in certain constituents.

homologous analogue. ANALOGUE (1).

homologous chromosomes. Chromosomes that have like gene loci in the same sequence; in man there are 23 pairs of homologous chromosomes; one member of each pair is derived from the mother and one from the father.

homologous graft. HOMOGRAFT.

homologous series. A group of compounds differing from one another by a definite radical or group, as CH_2.

homologous serum hepatitis or **jaundice.** SERUM HEPATITIS.

homologous stimulus. A form of energy to which a specific sensory receptor is most sensitive. Contr. *heterologous stimulus.*

homologous tissues. Tissues that are identical in type of structure.

homologous tumor. A tumor consisting of tissue identical with that of the organ from which it springs.

homologous vaccine. AUTOGENOUS VACCINE.

ho·mo·logue (ho′muh·log, hom′uh·log) *n.* Something homologous.

ho·mol·o·gy (ho·mol′uh·jee) *n.* [Gk. *homologia*, agreement, conformity]. Structural correspondence; especially, that attributable to common origin.

ho·mo·mor·phic (ho″mo·mor′fick) *adj.* [*homo-* + *-morphic*]. Having similar structure without definite relation to bodily axes.

ho·mon·y·mous (ho·mon′i·mus) *adj.* [Gk. *homōnymos*, from *homos*, same, + *onyma*, name]. 1. Having the same name; of words, having the same form. 2. *In ophthalmology*, pertaining to the same sides of the field of vision. —**homonymy** (·mee) *n.*

homonymous diplopia. The reverse of crossed diplopia; found in convergent strabismus. Syn. *direct diplopia.*

homonymous hemianopsia. Loss of vision affecting the inner half of one and the outer half of the other visual field; generally caused by lesions involving the optic radiations posterior to the optic chiasm; the more congruous the defect, the closer the lesion to the occipital cortex. Contr. *heteronymous hemianopsia.*

homonymous parallax. Parallax in which the object moves toward the uncovered eye.

ho·mo·plast (ho′mo·plast, hom′o·) *n.* [*homo-* + *-plast*]. *In biology*, a formative compound of one tissue. Contr. *alloplast.*

ho·mo·plas·ty (ho′mo·plas″tee) *n.* [*homo-* + *-plasty*]. Surgery using grafts from another individual of the same species. Compare *autoplasty.* Contr. *heteroplasty.* —**ho·mo·plas·tic** (ho″mo·plas′tick) *adj.*

ho·mo·po·lar (ho″mo·po′lur) *adj.* [*homo-* + *polar*]. Covalent; exhibiting covalence.

ho·mo·poly·sac·cha·ride (ho″mo·pol·ee·sack′uh·ride, hom″o·, ·rid) *n.* Any polysaccharide that yields on hydrolysis a single monosaccharide. Contr. *heteropolysaccharide.*

Ho·mop·ter·a (ho·mop′tur·uh) *n.pl.* [*homo-* + Gk. *ptera*, wings]. An order of insects; includes cicadas, plant lice, and scale insects. Formerly a suborder of the old order Hemiptera.

ho·mo·qui·nine (ho″mo·kwye′nine, ·kwi·neen′) *n.* A molecular compound of quinine and cupreine obtained from cuprea bark.

ho·mo·sal·ate (ho″mo·sal′ate) *n.* 3,3,5-Trimethylcyclohexyl salicylate, $C_{16}H_{22}O_3$, an ultraviolet screening agent used mainly to promote tanning.

Homo sa·pi·ens (say′pee·unz, sap′ee·enz) [L., wise, sensible, from *sapere*, to taste, discern]. The human species; the species of *Homo* that includes all extant races of man.

ho·mo·ser·ine (ho″mo·serr′een, ·seer′een) *n.* 2-Amino-4-hydroxybutyric acid, $C_4H_9NO_3$, an amino acid formed in the breakdown of cystathionine to cysteine in animal tissues.

ho·mo·sex·u·al·i·ty (ho″mo·seck″shoo·al′i·tee) *n.* [*homo-* + *sexuality*]. 1. The practice of sexual relations with members of one's own sex. 2. The disposition to be sexually attracted to, or to fall in love with, members of one's own sex. Compare *homoerotism.* 3. *Colloq.* Male homosexuality. Contr. *lesbianism.* —**homo·sex·u·al** (·seck′shoo·ul) *adj.* & *n.*

homosexual panic. An acute undifferentiated syndrome that comes as the climax of prolonged tension from unconscious homosexual conflicts or sometimes bisexual tendencies. The attack is characterized by a high degree of fear, paranoid ideas, great excitement, and a tendency toward disorganization. It may mark the onset of schizophrenia.

ho·mo·ther·mal (ho″mo·thur′mul) *adj.* HOMEOTHERMIC.

ho·mo·ther·mic (ho″mo·thur′mick) *adj.* HOMEOTHERMIC.

ho·mo·tope (hom′o·tope, ho′mo·) *n.* [*homo-* + Gk. *topos,* place]. Any member of a particular group of elements in the periodic table, thus, sodium is a homotope of lithium, potassium, rubidium, cesium, and francium.

ho·mo·top·ic (ho·mo·top′ick) *adj.* [*homo-* + *topic*]. Pertaining to the same or corresponding places or parts.

homotopic transplantation. ORTHOTOPIC TRANSPLANTATION.

ho·mo·trans·plan·ta·tion (ho″mo·trans″plan·tay′shun) *n.* [*homo-* + *transplantation*]. Transplantation of tissue from one to another genetically different individual of the same species. —**homo·trans·plant** (·trans′plant) *n.*

ho·mo·tro·pic enzyme (ho″mo·tro′pick) [*homo-* + *-tropic*]. A type of allosteric enzyme in which the substrate serves as the allosteric effector. Contr. *heterotropic enzyme.*

ho·mo·type (ho′mo·tipe, hom′o·) *n.* [*homo-* + *type*]. A part corresponding to a part on the lateral half of the body. —**ho·mo·typ·ic** (ho·mo·tip′ick) *adj.*

ho·mo·typ·i·cal (ho″mo·tip′i·kul) *adj.* [*homo-* + *typical*]. Pertaining to a common structure.

homotypical cortex. The typical six-layered cerebral cortex, distinguished from other areas of the isocortex, such as the agranular cortex of the primary motor area, which lacks a definite fourth layer, and the koniocortex of the primary sensory areas, which has a dense inner granular layer as well as small granular cells throughout. Within this cortex three association areas—the prefrontal, the anterior temporal, and the parietotemporopreoccipital—are recognized.

ho·mo·zy·go·sis (ho″mo·zye·go′sis) *n.* [*homozyg*ous + *-osis*]. In the genotype, presence of one or many pairs of genes in the homozygous phase, which results from inbreeding. Contr. *heterozygosis.*

ho·mo·zy·gote (ho″mo·zye′gote) *n.* [*homo-* + *zygote*]. A homozygous individual.

ho·mo·zy·gous (ho″mo·zye′gus) *adj.* [Gk. *homozygos,* yoked together, corresponding, matching]. Having both members of a given pair of genes alike. Contr. *heterozygous.* —**homo·zy·gos·i·ty** (·zye·gos′i·tee) *n.*

ho·mun·cu·lus (ho·munk′yoo·lus) *n.,* pl. **homuncu·li** (·lye) [L., dim. of *homo,* man]. 1. A midget. 2. A manikin or a small-scale model of the human form. 3. A miniature human body, as was once believed to exist preformed in the sperm or in the ovum; hence also a human embryo or fetus. 4. An analogic representation of the human body, as sometimes used to show the functional topography of the cerebral cortex.

hon·ey, *n.* 1. The saccharine secretion deposited in the honeycomb by the bee, *Apis mellifera;* the principal constituents are fructose and dextrose; it is used as a food and pharmaceutical excipient. 2. A preparation of honey with some medicinal substance.

hon·ey·comb lung. An emphysematous lung, or occasionally a lung containing numerous small pus-filled cavities.

honey sugar. DEXTROSE.

Hong Kong influenza [after the British crown colony of *Hong Kong,* where the virus responsible was first isolated]. An acute respiratory illness which first appeared in a moderate pandemic in 1968; due to certain strains of influenza A virus.

hoof, *n.* The horny covering of the distal end of a digit in the ungulates. —**hoofed,** *adj.*

hoof-and-mouth disease. FOOT-AND-MOUTH DISEASE.

hook, *n.* & *v.* 1. An elongate structure with a bend or curve at one end which serves to exert traction or to perform functions based on traction. 2. To exert traction in the manner of a hook; a function of the hand with fingers flexed but without participation of the opposed thumb. Contr. *grasp, pinch.*

hook bundle. UNCINATE FASCICULUS OF THE HEMISPHERE.

Hooker's method. DANZER AND HOOKER'S METHOD.

hook·worm, *n.* Any nematode belonging to the superfamily Strongyloidea, particularly the species *Ancylostoma duodenale* and *Necator americanus.*

hookworm disease. ANCYLOSTOMIASIS.

hoove, *n.* BLOAT (2).

hoo·ven (hoo′vun) *n.* BLOAT (2).

Hoo·ver's sign [C. F. *Hoover,* U.S. physician, 1865–1927]. 1. A sign of organic hemiplegia. The examiner places his palms under the heels of the recumbent patient and asks him to press down as hard as he can; pressure will be felt only from the nonparalyzed leg. The examiner then places his hand on top of the nonparalyzed foot and asks the patient to raise that leg. In true hemiplegia, no added pressure will be felt by the hand which had remained beneath the heel of the paralyzed leg, whereas in hemiplegia of hysterical origin the heel of the supposedly paralyzed leg presses down on the palm as an attempt is made to raise the well leg. 2. A test for hemiplegia in which the examiner places his hand under the sound heel while the recumbent patient attempts to raise the paralyzed leg; the pressure on the examiner's hand by the sound leg is then much greater than that observed in a normal or hysterical individual. Syn. *Grasset-Gaussel sign.*

hop, *n.* HUMULUS.

hop dermatitis. A contact dermatitis due to fresh hop oil, seen in hop pickers.

Hope's murmur [J. *Hope,* English physician, 1801–1841]. The apical systolic murmur of mitral regurgitation.

Hopf's disease (ho^{h}pf) [G. *Hopf,* German dermatologist, b. 1931]. ACROKERATOSIS VERRUCIFORMIS.

Hop·kins-Cole reaction [F. G. *Hopkins,* English biochemist, 1861–1947; and S. W. *Cole,* English biochemist, b. 1877]. GLYOXYLIC ACID TEST.

Hop·mann's polyp (ho^{h}p′ma^{h}n) [C. M. *Hopmann,* German otolaryngologist, 1844–1925]. Polypoid hyperplasia of the nasal mucous membrane.

Hop·pe-Gold·flam disease or **symptom complex** [H. H. *Hoppe,* U.S. neurologist, 1867–1929; and S. V. *Goldflam*]. MYASTHENIA GRAVIS.

ho·qui·zil (ho′kwi·zil) *n.* 2-Hydroxy-2-methylpropyl 4-(6,7-dimethoxy-4-quinazolinyl)-1-piperazinecarboxylate, $C_{19}H_{26}N_4O_5$, a bronchodilator drug; used as the hydrochloride salt.

ho·ra (ho′ruh) *n.* [L.]. Hour; at the hour. Abbreviated, h.

hora de·cu·bi·tus (de·kew′bi·tus) [L., lit., at the hour of lying down]. At bedtime. Abbreviated, h. d.

hora som·ni (som′nigh) [L., lit., at the hour of sleep]. At bedtime. Abbreviated, h. s.

hor·de·in (hor′dee·in) *n.* A protein found in barley, the seed of *Hordeum sativum.*

hor·de·nine (hor′di·neen, ·nin) *n.* *p*-(2-Dimethylaminoethyl)phenol, $C_{10}H_{15}NO$, an alkaloid from germinating barley. Has been used in diarrhea and dysentery, and as a cardiac tonic.

hor·de·o·lum (hor·dee′o·lum) *n.,* pl. **hordeo·la** (·luh) [L., sty, dim. of *hordeum*]. A suppurative infection of the tarsal glands or the ciliary glands of the eyelid; a sty.

Hor·de·um (hor′dee·um) *n.* [L.]. The genus of barley.

ho·ris·ma·scope (ho·riz′muh·skope) *n.* [Gk. *horisma,* boundary, + *-scope*]. An instrument intended to facilitate the making of "ring" tests such as Heller's. If care is taken, there is no possibility of mixing the two solutions, and a definitely defined ring is easily obtained at the zone of contact. Syn. *albumoscope.*

hor·i·zon·tal, *adj.* In a plane parallel to the ground or a base line.

horizontal cells. Neurons of the inner nuclear layer of the retina, the axons of which run parallel to the retina.

horizontal fissure of the cerebellum. A deep groove encircling the cerebellum and separating the superior and inferior surfaces. NA *fissura horizontalis cerebelli.*

horizontal fissure of the right lung. The fissure between the upper and middle lobes of the right lung. NA *fissura horizontalis pulmonis dextri.*

horizontal hemianopsia. Loss of the upper (superior) or lower (inferior) field of vision, due to lesions affecting, respectively, the lower or upper visual cortex bilaterally.

horizontal nystagmus. LATERAL NYSTAGMUS.

horizontal plane. 1. Any transverse plane at right angles to the long axis of the body dividing it into upper and lower parts. 2. A plane at right angles with the long axis of a tooth. 3. *In electrocardiography and vectorcardiography,* the plane established by combining a transverse (X) lead with an anteroposterior (Z) lead.

horizontal raphe of the eye. The portion of the meridian of the eye at which the arcs of nerve fibers from the upper and lower temporal quadrants meet; functionally a sharp line in certain optic nerve fiber lesions. Syn. *median raphe.*

horizontal transmission. Transmission (of a disease) to victims postnatally. Contr. *vertical transmission.*

hor·me·pho·bia (hor″me·fo′bee·uh) *n.* [Gk. *hormē,* assault, shock, + *-phobia*]. Morbid fear of shock.

hor·mi·on (hor′mee·on) *n.* [Gk. *hormē,* start, onset, + *-ion*]. *In craniometry,* the point in the sagittal plane, between the alae of the vomer, where the vomer is attached to the body of the sphenoid bone.

Hor·mo·den·drum (hor″mo·den′drum) *n.* [Gk. *hormos,* chain, + *dendron,* tree]. A genus of saprophytic fungi whose species act as common allergens. *Hormodendrum compactum* and *H. pedrosoi* are pathogenic to man, and have been isolated from chromoblastomycosis.

hor·mone (hor′mone) *n.* [Gk. *hormōn,* present participle of *horman,* to set in motion, excite]. A specific chemical product of an organ or of certain cells of an organ, transported by the blood or other body fluids, and having a specific regulatory effect upon cells remote from its origin. Compare *autacoid.* —**hor·mo·nal** (hor·mo′nul), **hor·mon·ic** (hor·mon′ick) *adj.*

hor·mo·no·poi·e·sis (hor·mo″no·poy·ee′sis) *n.* [*hormone* + *-poiesis*]. The production of hormones. —**hormonopoi·et·ic** (·et′ick) *adj.*

horn, *n.* [Gmc. *khurnaz* (rel. to L. *cornu* and to Gk. *keras*)]. 1. A substance composed chiefly of keratin. 2. CORNU. —**horny,** *adj.*

horned viper. *Cerastes cornutus,* a viper of the African deserts, characterized by a scaly projection above each eye.

Horner-Bernard syndrome. HORNER'S SYNDROME.

Hor·ner's muscle [W. E. *Horner,* U.S. anatomist, 1793–1853]. The lacrimal part of the orbicularis oculi muscle.

Horner's oculopupillary syndrome [J. H. *Horner,* Swiss ophthalmologist, 1831–1886]. HORNER'S SYNDROME.

Horner's syndrome [J. H. *Horner*]. Unilateral ptosis, miosis, enophthalmos, diminished sweating on the same side of the face and neck, and redness of the conjunctiva due to interruption of the sympathetic nerve fibers on the affected side.

horn fly. *HAEMATOBIA IRRITANS.*

horn·i·fi·ca·tion (hor″ni·fi·kay′shun) *n.* CORNIFICATION.

horny layer. STRATUM CORNEUM.

ho·rop·ter (ho·rop′tur) *n.* [Gk. *horos,* limit, + *optēr,* observer]. The sum of all the points seen singly by the two retinas while the fixation point remains stationary. —**ho·rop·ter·ic** (hor″op·terr′ick) *adj.*

hor·rip·i·la·tion (ho·rip″i·lay′shun) *n.* [L. *horripilatio,* from *horrere,* to bristle, + *pilus,* hair]. PILOERECTION.

horse·fly, *n.* A large fly of the family Tabanidae.

horse·foot, *n.* TALIPES EQUINUS.

horse·hair probang. BRISTLE PROBANG.

horsehair suture. A fine-gauge, flexible suture obtained from the tail and mane of the horse; causes minimal tissue reaction and leaves inconspicuous scars.

horse·pox, *n.* A virus disease of horses characterized by fever, mucopurulent discharge, and pox lesions on the mouth, vulva, leg, and occasionally over the entire body.

horse serum. Serum obtained from the blood of horses. Some therapeutically useful serums are obtained from horses immunized against a specific organism or its toxin.

horse·shoe, *n.* 1. A metal bow for the attachment of Steinmann pins and threaded (Kirschner) wires. 2. Something shaped like a horseshoe.

horseshoe fistula. A semicircular fistulous tract in the perineum near the anus.

horseshoe kidney. Greater or lesser degree of congenital fusion of the two kidneys, usually at the lower poles.

horseshoe magnet. An iron magnet having the shape of a horseshoe.

horseshoe placenta. In twin pregnancy, a condition in which two placentas are joined.

Hors·ley's operation [J. S. *Horsley,* U.S. surgeon, 1870–1946]. A type of gastrojejunostomy following subtotal gastric resection.

Hors·ley's sign [V. A. H. *Horsley,* English neurosurgeon, 1857–1916]. A sign for middle meningeal hemorrhage in which the axillary temperature is higher on the paralyzed side.

Hor·te·ga cell (or·te^y′ga^h) [P. del Río *Hortega,* Argentinian neuroanatomist, 1882–1945]. A microglial cell.

Hortega's silver stain or **method** [P. del Río *Hortega*]. An ammoniacal silver carbonate method for staining oligodendroglia.

Hor·ton's headache or **syndrome** [B. T. *Horton,* U. S. physician, b. 1895]. CLUSTER HEADACHE.

hos·pice (hos′pis) *n.* [OF., from L. *hospitium,* orig., hospitality]. 1. A shelter or lodging for paupers, destitute travelers, or abandoned children, usually maintained by a charitable institution. 2. An institution for the care and comfort of the terminally ill.

hos·pi·tal, *n.* [OF. *hospice,* from L. *hospitalis,* pertaining to guests]. A medical treatment facility intended, staffed, and equipped to provide diagnostic and therapeutic service in general medicine and surgery or in some circumscribed field or fields of restorative medical care, together with bed care, nursing, and dietetic service to patients requiring such care and treatment.

hospital center. *In military medicine,* an aggregation of one or more general hospitals, often including schools, central laboratories, and utilities, all administered under the central authority of a commanding officer, generally an officer of the Medical Department of the army or navy.

hospital fever. EPIDEMIC TYPHUS.

hospital gangrene. A type of gangrene associated with severe, contagious, often fatal infections, involving especially amputation stumps and extensive war wounds; once commonly seen in crowded hospitals, but now infrequently encountered in modern countries.

hos·pi·tal·ism, *n.* [*hospital* + *-ism*]. The anaclitic depression observed in young children who are separated for several months from their mother figures for reasons of hospitalization.

hos·pi·tal·i·za·tion, *n.* Placement of patients in a hospital for diagnostic study or treatment.

hospitalization unit. *In military medicine,* a complete self-contained hospital unit able to function independently; one of three identical units that make up a field hospital.

hospital nurse. A nurse who works for a hospital rather than for one special patient or physician.

hospital plant. *In military medicine,* a permanent physical facility operated by a medical treatment facility in a theater of operations.

host, *n.* [OF. *hoste,* from L. *hospes,* host]. 1. An organism on or in which another organism, known as a parasite, lives and from which the parasite obtains nourishment during all or part of its existence. 2. *In teratology,* a relatively normal fetus to which a less complete fetus or fetal part is attached. 3. The recipient of a transplanted organ or tissue. 4. The tissue invaded by a tumor.

hos·tile, *adj.* [L. *hostilis,* from *hostis,* enemy]. Marked by hostility.

hostile identification. *In psychiatry,* the assumption by an individual, particularly a child, of socially undesirable characteristics of a parent or other important person so as to gain some special strength or merit.

hos·til·i·ty, *n.* Antagonism, animosity, anger, or resistance toward an individual or group.

hot, *adj. Slang.* Highly radioactive.

hot air treatment. The local application of superheated dry air, the affected part being introduced into a cylinder or chamber.

hot atom. An atom that has high internal energy or high kinetic energy as a result of a nuclear process, such as neutron capture or beta decay.

hot cathode tube. A modern highly evacuated roentgen-ray tube with a heated filament cathode for the production of an abundant and controllable stream of cathode rays.

Hotch·kiss method. PERIODIC ACID SCHIFF REACTION.

Hotchkiss operation [L. W. *Hotchkiss,* U. S. surgeon, 1859–1926]. An operation for resection of carcinoma involving the jaw, followed by plastic repair of the cheek defect.

hot flash. A sudden transitory sensation of heat, often involving the whole body, due to cessation of ovarian function; a symptom of menopause.

hot flush. A vasomotor symptom of menopause; sudden vasodilatation and sensation of heat involving the upper portion of the body, often accompanied by sweating. Syn. *menopausal flush.*

hot laboratory. A laboratory designed for research with radioactive materials where the quantities of radioactive sources employed require special facilities and precautions in handling.

hot pack. A blanket wrung out of hot water and wrapped about the body.

hot spot. 1. A site in a gene peculiarly susceptible to mutation. 2. An area on the surface of the skin overlying a group of sense organs that are stimulated by heat.

hot stage. The febrile stage of a malarial paroxysm.

Hot·ten·tot apron (hot'un·tot). An overgrowth of the labia minora, seen in Hottentots.

Hottentot bustle. STEATOPYGIA.

hot·ten·tot·ism (hot'un·tot·iz·um) *n.* An extreme form of stammering.

hour·glass bladder. A urinary bladder in which there is a horizontal midvesical constriction.

hourglass contraction. A contraction of an organ, as the stomach or uterus, at the middle.

hourglass stomach. A stomach divided more or less completely into two compartments by an equatorial constriction, usually resulting from chronic gastric ulcer. Syn. *bilocular stomach, ectasia ventricula paradoxa.*

hourglass tumor or **ganglioneuroma.** DUMBBELL TUMOR.

house·fly, *n.* A fly of the genus *Musca.*

house·maid's knee. Inflammation of the bursa in front of the patella.

house physician. A physician employed by, and constantly available at, a particular place, as an intern at a hospital or a physician at a hotel.

house staff. The group of physicians and surgeons employed by a hospital, and receiving postgraduate training there; those having the status of intern or resident.

house surgeon. A surgeon employed by a hospital and constantly available.

Hous·say animal (oo·sigh') [B. A. *Houssay,* Argentinian physiologist, 1887–1971]. An animal in which the pancreas and hypophysis both have been excised.

Houssay phenomenon [B. A. *Houssay*]. Occasional abrupt amelioration of preexisting diabetes mellitus, with sudden lowering of insulin requirement, after pituitary destruction.

Hous·ton's muscle (hoos'tun) [J. *Houston,* Irish surgeon, 1802–1845]. COMPRESSOR VENAE DORSALIS.

Houston's valves [J. *Houston*]. TRANSVERSE RECTAL FOLDS.

hove, *n.* BLOAT (2).

How·ard-Dol·man depth perception test. A test of the average error in setting a moving rod equidistant to a fixed rod at a distance of 20 feet. All clues to depth perception other than those furnished by binocular vision are eliminated.

Howard's method [B. D. *Howard,* U. S. physician, 1840–1900]. A formerly used method for artificial respiration, in which the patient is supine, head low, and pressure is applied rhythmically over the lower ribs.

Howard test. A renal function test using bilateral ureteral catheterization to identify a kidney producing renovascular hypertension.

How·ell-Jol·ly bodies [W. H. *Howell,* U. S. physiologist, 1860–1945; and J. *Jolly*]. Dot-shaped basophilic inclusions of nuclear material occurring in the peripheral blood erythrocytes of splenectomized persons.

Howe's ammoniacal silver nitrate. A solution of silver diammino nitrate, used by dentists to deposit silver in exposed dentin.

How·ship-Rom·berg syndrome or **sign** [J. *Howship,* British surgeon, 1781–1841; and M. H. *Romberg*]. Pain or paresthesia on the medial aspect of the thigh down to and usually most marked at the knee, as a result of pressure on the obturator nerve by an obturator hernia.

Howship's lacunas [J. *Howship*]. Minute depressions in the surface of bone undergoing resorption; usually contain osteoclasts.

HPLC Abbreviation for *high-performance liquid chromatography.*

H_1-receptors. Pharmacological receptor sites involved in histamine responses sensitive to pyrilamine or any typical antihistamine.

H_2-receptors. Pharmacological receptor sites involved in histamine-induced gastric acid secretion.

H reflex [P. *H*offmann, German neurophysiologist, 20th century]. A monosynaptic reflex, evoked by stimulating a nerve, particulary the tibial nerve, with a single electrical shock.

HRIG Trademark for rabies immune human globulin.

h.s. Abbreviation for *hora somni,* bedtime.

H-substance, *n.* A substance similar to, if not identical with, histamine; believed to play a prominent role in the response of local blood vessels to tissue damage.

HSV Abbreviation for *herpes simplex virus.*

Hub·bard tank [L. W. *Hubbard,* U.S. surgeon, 1857–1938]. A large, specially designed tank in which a patient may be immersed for various therapeutic underwater exercises.

Hu·chard's disease (ue·shahr') [H. *Huchard,* French physician, 1844–1910]. ARTERIAL HYPERTENSION.

Huchard's sign [H. *Huchard*]. A less than normal diminution of the heart rate in changing from the standing to the recumbent position, seen in hypertension.

Hud·dle·son's test [I. F. *Huddleson,* U. S. bacteriologist, b. 1893]. An agglutination test for brucellosis in humans or cattle, using *Brucella abortus* as an antigen.

Hud·son's bone drill [W. H. *Hudson,* U. S. physician, 1862–1915]. A drill designed to open the skull without injuring the dura mater.

Hudson's line [A. C. *Hudson,* British ophthalmologist, 20th century]. STAEHLI'S PIGMENT LINE.

Hudson-Staehli line. STAEHLI'S PIGMENT LINE.

hue, *n.* [OE. *hīw,* appearance, color]. The quality of visual sensation which permits the observer to distinguish different wavelengths of light.

Huggins-Miller-Jensen test. IODOACETATE INDEX.

Hug·gins test [C. B. *Huggins,* U. S. urologist, b. 1901]. IODOACETATE INDEX.

Hugh·lings Jack·son syndrome [J. *Hughlings Jackson*]. JACKSON'S SYNDROME.

Hu·guier's canal (ueg·yey') [P. C. *Huguier,* French surgeon, 1804–1874]. ITER CHORDAE ANTERIUS.

Huguier's disease [P. C. *Huguier*]. LEIOMYOMA.

Huh·ner's test [M. *Huhner,* U. S. urologist, 1873–1947]. An examination of seminal fluid obtained from the vaginal fornix and cervical canal after a specified interval following coitus; used in fertility studies to evaluate spermatozoal survival and activity in the lower female genital tract.

hum, *n.* A low murmuring sound.

hu·man, *adj. & n.* [L. *humanus*]. 1. Belonging or pertaining to the species *Homo sapiens.* 2. A human being; a member of the species *Homo sapiens.*

human blood ratio. In malarial investigations, the percentage of freshly fed mosquitoes that contain human blood.

human flea. *PULEX IRRITANS.*

human immune serum. A sterile serum obtained from the blood of a healthy person who has survived an attack of a disease, administered during the incubation period to prevent or modify the expected attack of a specific disease; immune sera exist for measles, varicella, vaccinia, diphtheria, etc.

hu·man·ized vaccine. The vaccine obtained from vaccinal vesicles of man.

hu·mano·scope (hew·man'uh·skope) *n.* A series of overlapping anatomic plates so arranged as to allow the examiner to study the relative sizes, shapes, and relationships of various parts of the human body, as the pages are turned.

human runt disease. A form of graft-versus-host reaction occurring in early infancy and characterized chiefly by failure to thrive.

human serum albumin microspheres. Sterile, pyrogen-free spheres radiolabeled with Tc99m, In111, In113m or Pb203 used principally for lung-imaging.

Humatin. Trademark for paromomycin, an antibiotic.

hu·mec·tant (hew·meck'tunt) *adj. & n.* [L. *humectare,* to moisten, from *humere,* to be moist]. 1. Moistening. 2. A substance used to retain moisture.

Humegon. A trademark for menotropins, an extract of postmenopausal urine which contains follicle-stimulating hormone (FSH) and luteinizing hormone (LH), used to stimulate ovulation.

hu·mer·al (hew'mur·ul) *adj.* Of or pertaining to the humerus.

humeri. Plural and genitive singular of *humerus.*

humero-. A combining form meaning *humerus, humeral.*

hu·mero·ra·di·al (hew''mur·o·ray'dee·ul) *adj.* Pertaining to the humerus and the radius; applied to the joint between these two bones and to the ligaments joining them.

humeroradial index. The ratio of (length of humerus × 100) / length of radius.

hu·mero·scap·u·lar (hew''mur·o·skap'yoo·lur) *adj.* Pertaining to both the humerus and the scapula.

hu·mero·ul·nar (hew''mur·o·ul'nur) *adj.* Pertaining to the humerus and the ulna; applied to the joint between these two bones and to the ligaments joining them.

hu·mer·us (hew'mur·us) *n.,* pl. & genit. sing. **hu·meri** (·mur·eye) [L., shoulder] [NA]. The bone of the upper arm, or brachium. See also Table of Bones in the Appendix and Plates 1, 2.

hu·mic acid (hew'mick). Any acid substance derived from humus.

hu·mic·o·lin (hew·mick'o·lin) *n.* A weakly acidic antifungal substance produced by *Aspergillus humicola.*

hu·mid·i·fi·ca·tion (hew·mid''i·fi·kay'shun) *n.* The process of moistening or humidifying air; specifically, in respiration, by moisture from mucous membranes.

hu·mid·i·ty, *n.* [L. *humidus,* moist]. The state or quality of being moist; moisture; dampness. —**hu·mid** (hew'mid) *adj.*

hu·min (hew'min) *n.* 1. Any of several varied substances, including humic acid, obtained from humus; sometimes humus itself. 2. A dark-colored substance or substances formed when proteins undergo acid hydrolysis, probably resulting from condensation of tryptophan with an aldehyde.

humming-top murmur. VENOUS HUM.

hu·mor, hu·mour, *n.* [L., a liquid]. 1. Any fluid or semifluid part of the body. 2. *In old physiology,* one of the four cardinal body fluids of Galen: the choleric, the melancholic, the phlegmatic, and the sanguine, said to determine a person's health and temperament. 3. Disposition, temperament. —**humor·al** (·ul) *adj.*

humoral antibody. Any antibody found in solution in lymph, plasma, or another fluid part of the body, as contrasted with antibody bound to the surface of a cell.

humoral immunity. Immunity which is maintained by antibody molecules secreted by B lymphocytes and plasma cells and circulating freely throughout the plasma, lymph, and other body fluids, as distinguished from cell-mediated immunity, which is maintained by T lymphocytes; seen in immune response to bacterial infections and reinfection by virus.

humoral pathology. A historical theory that disease is caused by alterations in constitution of the blood and various secretions.

humoral reflex. CHEMICAL REFLEX.

humoral transmission. Transmission of impulse over a synapse by means of chemical substances released at the synapse.

humor aquo·sus (a·kwo'sus) [NA]. AQUEOUS HUMOR.

Humorsol. Trademark for demecarium bromide, a cholinesterase inhibitor used for treatment of glaucoma and strabismus.

humor vi·tre·us (vit'ree·us) [NA]. VITREOUS HUMOR.

hump·back, *n.* KYPHOSIS.

Hum·phry's operation [G. M. *Humphry,* English surgeon, 1820–1896]. Excision of the condyle of the lower jaw.

hu·mu·lene (hew'mew·leen) *n.* A sesquiterpene, $C_{15}H_{24}$, contained in the volatile oil from hops.

hu·mu·lin (hew'mew·lin) *n.* LUPULIN.

hu·mu·lus (hew'mew·lus) *n.* [ML.]. Hops. The dried strobile of *Humulus lupulus* bearing the glandular trichomes known as lupulin. Hops have been used as a calmative, stomachic, and tonic.

hu·mus (hew'mus) *n.* [L., earth, ground]. A dark material in soil, consisting of decaying organic matter.

hunch·back, *n.* 1. A person with kyphosis. 2. KYPHOSIS.

hun·ger, *n.* A sensation of longing for food.

hunger contractions. Movements of the stomach formerly thought to be associated with hunger.

hunger disease. HYPERINSULINISM.

hunger edema. NUTRITIONAL EDEMA.

Hun·ner's ulcer [G. L. R. *Hunner,* U.S. surgeon, 1868–1957]. A chronic ulcer of the urinary bladder, of unknown etiology, found frequently near the vertex and in association with interstitial cystitis. Syn. *elusive ulcer.*

Hun·te·ri·an chancre (hun·teer'ee·un) [J. *Hunter,* Scottish surgeon, 1728–1793]. A syphilitic chancre.

Hun·ter's canal [J. *Hunter*]. ADDUCTOR CANAL.

Hunter-Schre·ger bands (shrey'gur) [J. *Hunter* and C. H. T. *Schreger,* German anatomist, 1768–1833]. Alternating dark and light strips of varying widths seen in a longitudinal ground section of dental enamel under oblique reflected light. Whether this phenomenon is due to the more or less regular change in direction of enamel rods, variations in mineralization, zones of varying permeability and organic content, or some combination of these factors, is not clear.

Hunter's glossitis [W. *Hunter,* English physician, 1861–1937]. Glossitis associated with pernicious anemia, characterized by atrophy of the papillae and by redness, burning, and pain. Syn. *atrophic glossitis.*

Hunter's operation [J. *Hunter*]. Proximal ligation of an artery at some distance from the aneurysm.

Hunter's syndrome [C. H. *Hunter,* Canadian physician, 20th century]. Mucopolysaccharidosis II, transmitted as an X-linked recessive, characterized chemically by excessive dermatan sulfate and heparitin sulfate in tissues and urine, and clinically by an appearance similar to that seen in the more common Hurler's syndrome, but a milder course. Mental deterioration progresses more slowly, lumbar gibbus does not occur, and clouding of the cornea of clinically evident degree does not appear.

Hunt·ing·ton's chorea or **disease** [G. *Huntington,* U.S. physician, 1851–1916]. A dominantly heritable disorder of the central nervous system characterized by the onset, usually in adult life, of progressive choreoathetosis, emotional disturbances, and dementia. Compare *senile chorea.*

Hunt's atrophy [J. Ramsay *Hunt,* U.S. neurologist, 1874–1937]. Neurotrophic atrophy of the small muscles of the hand without sensory alteration.

Hunt's neuralgia or **syndrome** [J. Ramsay *Hunt*]. 1. GENICULATE NEURALGIA. 2. RAMSAY HUNT SYNDROME (1).

Hup·pert's test (hoop'urt) [C. H. *Huppert,* Bohemian physician, 1832–1904]. A test for bile pigments based upon their oxidation by concentrated hydrochloric acid to produce a green-colored derivative.

Hur·ler's syndrome (hoor'lur) [Gertrud *Hurler,* German pediatrician, 20th century]. Mucopolysaccharidosis I, transmitted as an autosomal recessive, characterized chemically by excessive dermatan sulfate and heparitin sulfate in tissues and urine, and clinically by a rather grotesque appearance due to a disproportionately large head and coarse facies with flat nose and thick lips, skeletal changes including shortness of stature, gibbus, chest deformities, marked limitation in extensibility of joints, spadelike hands, enlarged tongue and hepatosplenomegaly, skin and cardiac changes, and early progressive clouding of the cornea, mental deficit, and often deafness.

Hürth·le-cell adenoma (huert'leh) [K. W. *Hürthle,* German histologist, 1860–1945]. A thyroid adenoma whose parenchyma is composed of Hürthle cells.

Hürthle cells [K. W. *Hürthle*]. 1. Thyroid follicular epithelial cells that are enlarged and have acidophilic cytoplasm, seen especially in adenomas. 2. Sometimes, cells of similar appearance in the parathyroid.

Husch·ke's cartilage (hoosh'keh) [E. *Huschke,* German anatomist, 1797–1858]. VOMERONASAL CARTILAGE.

Huschke's foramen [E. *Huschke*]. FORAMEN OF HUSCHKE.

Huschke's papilla [E. *Huschke*]. SPIRAL ORGAN (OF CORTI).

Huschke's teeth [E. *Huschke*]. AUDITORY TEETH.

Hutch·in·son-Boeck disease [J. *Hutchinson,* English surgeon, 1828–1913; and C. P. M. *Boeck*]. SARCOIDOSIS.

Hutchinson-Gil·ford syndrome or **disease** [J. *Hutchinson;* and H. *Gilford,* English physician, 1861–1941]. A disorder of unknown cause appearing in early childhood, characterized by cessation of growth, senile-like changes, large skull, "birdlike" features with crowding of teeth, atrophic skin, and loss of subcutaneous fat in the face, chest, and extremities, often with severe mental defects, high levels of serum lipoproteins and consequent atherosclerosis and its complications. Syn. *progeria of children.*

hutch·in·so·ni·an (hutch"in·so'nee·un) *adj.* Described by or associated with Jonathan Hutchinson, English surgeon, 1828–1913.

Hutchinson's disease [J. *Hutchinson*]. ANGIOMA SERPIGINOSUM.

Hutchinson's freckle [J. *Hutchinson*]. LENTIGO MALIGNA.

Hutchinson's prurigo [J. *Hutchinson*]. HYDROA VACCINIFORME.

Hutchinson's pupil [J. *Hutchinson*]. A widely dilated, inactive pupil that demonstrates no reflex activity, seen in lesions or compression of the third cranial nerve.

Hutchinson's teeth [J. *Hutchinson*]. Deformity of permanent incisor teeth associated with congenital syphilis. The crown of such a tooth is wider in the cervical portion than at the incisal edge; the incisal edge has a characteristic crescent-shaped notch.

Hutchinson's triad [J. *Hutchinson*]. Interstitial keratitis, eighth-nerve deafness, and notched permanent teeth signifying congenital syphilis.

Hutch·i·son syndrome [R. G. *Hutchison,* British pediatrician, 1871–1943]. Neuroblastoma with prominent skull metastasis, exophthalmos, and periorbital discoloration.

Huy·ge·ni·an ocular (high·ghee'nee·un, ·ghen'ee·un) [C. *Huygens,* Dutch physicist, 1629–1695]. A lens consisting of two planoconvex lenses, the convexities being directed toward the objective; the lower lens is the field lens, the upper, the eye lens.

h wave. A small positive wave on the venous pulse pressure curve, occasionally occurring prior to the a wave.

hy·al (high'ul) *adj.* HYOID.

hyal-, hyalo- [Gk. *hyalos,* glass]. A combining form meaning (a) *glass;* (b) *glassy, transparent;* (c) *vitreous, hyaloid;* (d) *hyaline.*

hy·a·line, hy·a·lin (high'uh·lin) *n. & adj.* [*hyal-* + *-in*]. 1. A clear, structureless, homogeneous, glassy material occurring normally in matrix of cartilage, vitreous body, colloid of thyroid gland, mucin, glycogen, Wharton's jelly; occurs pathologically in degenerations of connective tissue, epithelial cells, and in the form of mucinous and colloid degenerations and glycogen infiltration. 2. Consisting of or pertaining to hyaline.

hyaline capsulitis. PERISPLENITIS CARTILAGINEA.

hyaline cartilage. Cartilage in which the matrix is clear and homogeneous.

hyaline degeneration. A form of degeneration in which a clear, structureless or homogeneous, translucent change in tissues or cells is produced.

hyaline membrane. 1. A layer of fibrinoid material lying on part or all of the pulmonary alveoli in a variety of disorders that damage alveolar walls, especially the respiratory distress syndrome of the newborn. 2. BASEMENT MEMBRANE. 3. The basement membrane of a graafian follicle; GLASSY MEMBRANE. 4. The membrane between the inner fibrous layer of a hair follicle and its outer root sheath.

hyaline membrane disease. RESPIRATORY DISTRESS SYNDROME OF THE NEWBORN.

hyaline thrombus. A thrombus found in the smaller blood vessel as a glossy fibrinous mass.

hy·a·lin·ize (high'uh·lin·ize) *v.* To undergo, or to cause to undergo, hyaline degeneration. —**hy·a·lin·iza·tion** (high"uh·lin·i·zay'shun) *n.*

hy·a·li·no·sis (high"uh·li·no'sis) *n.,* pl. **hyalino·ses** (·seez) [*hyalin* + *-osis*]. HYALINE DEGENERATION.

hy·a·lin·uria (high"uh·li·new'ree·uh) *n.* [*hyalin* + *-uria*]. The presence of hyalin or of hyalin casts in the urine.

hy·a·li·tis (high"uh·lye'tis) *n.* [*hyal-* + *-itis*]. Inflammation of the vitreous body, or of the hyaloid membrane of the vitreous body.

hyalo-. See *hyal-.*

hy·a·lo·cap·su·li·tis (high"uh·lo·kap"sue·lye'tis) *n.* Hyalinization of a capsule, usually of the liver or spleen.

hy·al·o·gen (high·al'o·jen) *n.* [*hyalo-* + *-gen*]. 1. Any of the insoluble substances resembling mucin found in such areas as the walls of echinococcus cysts and the vitreous body, and yielding hyalin on hydrolysis. 2. An albuminoid found in cartilage.

hy·a·loid (high'uh·loid) *adj.* [Gk. *hyaloeidēs,* glassy]. 1. Transparent; glasslike. 2. Pertaining to the vitreous body.

hyaloid artery. In the embryo, a forward continuation of the central artery of the retina traversing the vitreous body to ramify on the posterior surface of the lens capsule. NA *arteria hyaloidea.*

hyaloid canal. A canal running posteroanteriorly through the vitreous through which, in the fetus, the hyaloid artery passes to ramify on the posterior surface of the crystalline lens. Syn. *Cloquet's canal.* NA *canalis hyaloideus.*

hyaloid capsule. HYALOID MEMBRANE.

hy·a·loi·deo·cap·su·lar (high″uh·loy″dee·o·kap′sue·lur) *adj.* Pertaining to the hyaloid capsule or membrane.

hyaloideocapsular ligament. The circular fibers at the area of contact of the vitreous body and the posterior surface of the capsule of the lens of the eye.

hyaloid fossa. A depression in the anterior surface of the vitreous body for the crystalline lens. NA *fossa hyaloidea.*

hy·a·loid·i·tis (high″uh·loy·dye′tis) *n.* HYALITIS.

hyaloid membrane. The dense layer of fibrils surrounding the vitreous body. NA *membrana vitrea.*

hy·a·lo·mere (high′uh·lo·meer) *n.* [*hyalo-* + *-mere*]. The clear part of a blood platelet after staining with stains of the Romanovsky type.

Hy·a·lom·ma (high″uh·lom′uh) *n.* [*hyal-* + Gk. *omma*, eye]. A genus of ticks the males of which are characterized by submarginal eyes, ventral plates, and two protrusions from the tip of the abdomen which are capped with chitinous points. *Hyalomma aegyptium,* the most important species, is found on cattle and other large mammals in Africa, Asia, and southern Europe.

hy·a·lo·nyx·is (high″uh·lo·nick′sis) *n.* [*hyalo-* + Gk. *nyxis*, a pricking]. Puncture of the vitreous body of the eye.

hy·a·lo·pho·bia (high″uh·lo·fo′bee·uh) *n.* [*hyalo-* + *-phobia*]. A morbid fear of glass.

hy·a·lo·plasm (high′uh·lo·plaz·um) *n.* [*hyalo-* + *-plasm*]. The fluid portion of the protoplasm. Syn. *enchylema, interfilar mass, paraplasm, paramitome.*

hy·a·lo·se·ro·si·tis (high″uh·lo·seer″o·sigh′tis) *n.* [*hyalo-* + *serositis*]. HYALOCAPSULITIS.

hy·al·uron·ic acid (high″uh·lew·ron′ick). A viscous mucopolysaccharide occurring in connective tissues and in bacterial capsules.

hy·a·lu·ron·i·dase (high″uh·lew·ron′i·dace, ·daze) *n.* An enzyme occurring in pathogenic bacteria, snake venoms, and sperm capable of catalyzing depolymerization and hydrolysis of hyaluronic acid in protective polysaccharide barriers, promoting penetration of cells and tissues by an agent in contact with them; it is a spreading factor. Hyaluronidase is used to promote diffusion and absorption of various injected medicaments.

Hyamate. Trademark for buramate, an anticonvulsant and tranquilizer.

Hyamine. A trademark for benzalkonium chloride, an anti-infective.

Hyazyme. A trademark for hyaluronidase for injection.

hy·ben·zate (high·ben′zate) *n.* Any salt or ester of *o*-(4-hydroxybenzoyl)benzoic acid, $C_{14}H_{10}O_4$.

hy·brid, *n. & adj.* [L. *hibrida*, crossbreed]. 1. The offspring of parents belonging to different species, varieties, or genotypes. 2. Being or pertaining to a hybrid. —**hybrid·ism** (·iz·um), **hy·brid·i·ty** (high·brid′i·tee) *n.*

hy·brid·iza·tion (high″brid·i·zay′shun) *n.* 1. CROSSBREEDING. 2. *In chemistry,* a distribution of electrons in different types of orbitals in an atom to give equivalent orbitals and bonds. 3. The pairing of single complementary strands of deoxyribonucleic acid and ribonucleic acid to form a double-stranded molecule.

hybrid vigor. The increased vitality of a hybrid over an inbred organism; especially used in agriculture.

hy·can·thone (high·kan′thone) *n.* 1-[[2-(Diethylamino)ethyl]amino]-4-(hydroxymethyl)thioxanthen-9-one, $C_{20}H_{24}N_2O_2S$, an antischistosomal drug.

hy·clate (high′klate) *n.* A contraction for (mono)hydrochloride hemiethanolate hemihydrate, $2HCl{\cdot}C_2H_5OH{\cdot}H_2O$.

Hycortole. A trademark for hydrocortisone, an anti-inflammatory adrenocortical steroid.

hy·dan·to·ic acid (high″dan·to′ick). An acid, $C_3H_6N_2O_3$, resulting from the union of aminoacetic acid and carbamic acid which is an intermediary in the production of creatine in the body.

hy·dan·to·in (high·dan′to·in, high″dan·to′in) *n.* 2,4-(3*H*,5*H*)-Imidazoledione or glycolylurea, $C_3H_4N_2O_2$, a crystalline substance derived from allantoin and related to urea.

hy·dat·id (high·dat′id) *n.* [Gk. *hydatis, hydatidos,* watery vesicle]. 1. A cyst formed in tissues due to growth of the larval stage of *Echinococcus granulosus* (dog tapeworm). 2. A cystic remnant of an embryonal structure. —**hydat·ic** (·ick), **hy·da·tid·i·form** (high″duh·tid′i·form) *adj.*

hydatid cyst. ECHINOCOCCUS CYST.

hydatid fremitus. ECHINOCOCCUS FREMITUS.

hydatidiform mole. Transformation of all or part of the placenta into grapelike cysts, characterized by poorly vascularized and edematous villi and trophoblastic proliferation. Syn. *hydatid mole.*

hydatid mole. HYDATIDIFORM MOLE.

hy·da·ti·do·cele (high″duh·tid′o·seel) *n.* [*hydatid* + *-cele*]. A scrotal hernia containing echinococcus cysts.

hydatid of Morgagni [G. B. *Morgagni*]. APPENDIX TESTIS.

hy·da·ti·do·sis (high″duh·ti·do′sis) *n.*, pl. **hydatido·ses** (·seez) [*hydatid* + *-osis*]. Multiple echinococcus cysts.

hydatid pregnancy. Gestation in which the chorionic sac develops into a hydatidiform mole.

Hydeltra. Trademark for prednisolone, an anti-inflammatory adrenocortical steroid.

Hydeltrasol. Trademark for prednisolone sodium phosphate, a water-soluble anti-inflammatory adrenocortical steroid.

Hydergine. Trademark for a mixture of the methanesulfonates of dihydroergocornine, dihydroergocristine, and dihydroergocryptine used clinically to produce adrenergic blocking and peripheral vasodilatation.

Hyde's disease [J. N. *Hyde*, U. S. dermatologist, 1840–1910]. PRURIGO NODULARIS.

hyd·no·car·pic acid (hid″no·kahr′pick) [*hydnocarpus* + *-ic*]. An unsaturated acid, $C_{15}H_{27}COOH$, occurring as the glyceride in chaulmoogra oil.

hyd·no·car·pus oil (hid″no·kahr′pus) [Gk. *hydnon*, truffle, + *karpos*, fruit]. A British name for chaulmoogra oil.

Hydoxin. A trademark for pyridoxine hydrochloride (vitamin B_6).

hydr-, hydro- [Gk. *hydōr*, from earlier *wudōr* (rel. to Gmc. *watar-* → E. *water*)]. A combining form meaning (a) *water;* (b) *presence of hydrogen* or *the addition of hydrogen to a compound;* (c) *a disease characterized by an accumulation of water or other fluid in a bodily part.*

hy·dra·bam·ine penicillin V (high″druh·bam′een). HYDRABAMINE PHENOXYMETHYL PENICILLIN.

hydrabamine phenoxymethyl penicillin. A mixture of crystalline phenoxymethyl penicillin salts, chiefly of the salt of *N,N′*-bis(dehydroabietyl)ethylenediamine, with smaller amounts of the salts of the dihydro- and tetrahydro- derivatives; a water-insoluble dosage form of phenoxymethyl penicillin. Syn. *hydrabamine penicillin V.*

hy·drac·id (high·dras′id) *n.* An acid containing no oxygen.

hydradenitis. HIDRADENITIS.

hydradenoma. HIDRADENOMA.

hydraemia. HYDREMIA.

hy·dra·ero·peri·to·ne·um (high·dray″ur·o·perr″i·tuh·nee′um) *n.* [*hydr-* + *aero-* + *peritoneum*]. HYDROPNEUMOPERITONEUM.

hy·dra·gogue, hy·dra·gog (high″druh·gog) *adj. & n.* [Gk. *hydragōgos*]. 1. Causing the discharge of watery fluid, especially from the bowel. 2. A purgative that causes copious watery discharges.

hy·dral·a·zine (high·dral′uh·zeen) *n.* 1-Hydrazinophthalazine, $C_8H_8N_4$, an antihypertensive drug; used as the hydrochloride salt.

hydralazine syndrome. The production of an illness resembling acute lupus erythematosus as a toxic reaction to the prolonged administration of hydralazine.

hy·dram·ni·on (high·dram'nee·on) *n.* [*hydr-* + *amnion*]. POLYHYDRAMNIOS.

hy·dram·ni·os (high·dram'nee·os) *n.* POLYHYDRAMNIOS.

hy·dram·ni·ot·ic (high·dram''nee·ot'ick) *adj.* [from *hydramnios*]. Having a greater than normal amount of amniotic fluid.

hy·dran·en·ceph·a·ly (high''dran·en·sef'uh·lee) *n.* [*hydr-* + *anencephaly*]. A developmental disorder of the nervous system due to a failure of evagination of the greater part of the cerebral hemispheres, resulting in large fluid-filled cavities in communication with the third ventricle. The disorder is characterized clinically by postnatal enlargement and transillumination of the head, retention of brainstem reflexes, and a failure of development of cerebral functions.

hy·dran·gea, *n.* [NL., from *hydr-* + Gk. *angeion,* vessel]. The dried rhizome and roots of *Hydrangea arborescens;* has been used as a diuretic and antilithic.

hy·drar·gyr·ia (high''drahr·jirr'ee·uh, ·jye'ree·uh) *n.* [*hydrargyrum* + *-ia*]. Chronic mercurial poisoning.

hy·drar·gy·ri·a·sis (high''drahr·ji·rye'uh·sis) *n.*, pl. **hydrargyria·ses** (·seez). HYDRARGYRIA.

hy·drar·gy·rism (high·drahr'ji·riz·um) *n.* HYDRARGYRIA.

hy·drar·gy·ro·pho·bia (high·drahr''ji·ro·fo'bee·uh) *n.* [*hydrargyrum* + *-phobia*]. An abnormal fear of mercurial medicines.

hy·drar·gyr·oph·thal·mia (high·drahr''jirr·off·thal'mee·uh) *n.* [*hydrargyrum* + *ophthalmia*]. Ophthalmia due to mercurial poisoning.

hy·drar·gy·rum (high·drahr'ji·rum) *n.* [NL., from Gk. *hydrargyros,* from *hydōr,* water, + *argyros,* silver]. MERCURY.

hy·drar·thro·sis (high''drahr·thro'sis) *n.*, pl. **hydrarthro·ses** (·seez) [*hydr-* + *arthrosis*]. An accumulation of fluid in a joint.

hy·drase (high'drace, ·draze) *n.* An enzyme that catalyzes removal or addition of water to a substrate without hydrolyzing it.

hy·dras·tine (high·dras'teen, ·tin) *n.* An alkaloid, $C_{21}H_{21}NO_6$, from hydrastis; has been used, generally in the form of the hydrochloride, as an astringent, hemostatic, and uterine stimulant.

hy·dras·ti·nine (high·dras'ti·neen, ·nin) *n.* An oxidation product, $C_{11}H_{13}NO_3$, of hydrastine; has been used, in the form of the hydrochloride, in uterine hemorrhage as a stimulant and hemostatic.

hy·dras·tis (high·dras'tis) *n.* The rhizome and roots of *Hydrastis canadensis,* which contain the alkaloids hydrastine, berberine, and canadine. Has been used as a hemostatic and astringent. Syn. *goldenseal, yellowroot.*

hy·drate (high'drate) *n.* 1. A compound containing water in chemical combination; water of crystallization. 2. *Obsol.* HYDROXIDE. —**hydrat·ed** (·id) *adj.*

hy·dra·tion, *n.* 1. Absorption of, or combination with, water. 2. In histologic procedures, successively transferring a specimen from an anhydrous reagent or solvent through mixtures of solvent with an increasing proportion of water and finally to water alone. 3. Fluid replacement.

hy·drau·lics (high·draw'licks) *n.* [Gk. *hydraulikos,* from *hydraulis,* hydraulic organ]. The science that deals with the mechanical properties of liquids. —**hydrau·lic** (·lick) *adj.*

hy·dra·zine (high'druh·zeen, ·zin) *n.* 1. H_2NNH_2. Diamine; a colorless liquid, soluble in water, having a strong alkaline reaction. The sulfate is used as a reducing agent. 2. One of a class of bodies derived from hydrazine by replacing one or more hydrogen atoms by a radical.

Hydrea. Trademark for hydroxyurea, an antineoplastic agent.

hy·dre·lat·ic (high''dre·lat'ick) *adj.* [*hydr-* + Gk. *elatēs,* driver, driving, from *elaunein,* to drive]. Pertaining to the secretory effect of nerves or hormones upon glands, causing them to discharge the watery part of their secretion.

hy·dre·mia, hy·drae·mia (high·dree'mee·uh) *n.* [*hydr-* + *-emia*]. An excessive amount of water in the blood; disproportionate increase in plasma volume as compared with red blood cell volume. —**hydre·mic, hydrae·mic** (·mick) *adj.*

hy·dren·ceph·a·lo·cele (high''dren·sef'uh·lo·seel) *n.* [*hydr-* + *encephalocele*]. Protrusion through a defect in the cranium of a sac and brain substance in which a cystic cavity contains fluid.

hy·dren·ceph·a·lo·me·nin·go·cele (high''dren·sef''uh·lo·me·ning'go·seel) *n.* [*hydr-* + *encephalo-* + *meningo-* + *-cele*]. A hernia through a cranial defect of meninges and brain substance, fluid filling the space between these.

hy·dri·a·try (high·drye'uh·tree) *n.* [*hydr-* + *-iatry*]. HYDROTHERAPY.

hy·dride (high'dride) *n.* A compound containing hydrogen united to a more positive element or to a radical.

hy·dri·od·ic acid (high''dree·od'ick). The gas hydrogen iodide, HI, or an aqueous solution thereof. Diluted hydriodic acid, containing 10% weight by volume HI, and hydriodic acid syrup, containing 1.4% weight by volume HI, are sometimes used medicinally for the effects of iodide ion.

hy·dri·o·dide (high·drye'o·dide, ·did) *n.* An iodide formed by interaction of an organic nitrogenous base with hydriodic acid.

hy·dri·on (high·drye'on, high'dree·on) *n.* Hydrogen in the ionized form.

Hydrionic. A trademark for glutamic acid hydrochloride, a gastric acidifier.

hydro-. See *hydr-.*

hy·droa (high·dro'uh) *n.* [alteration of *hidroa*]. Any skin disease characterized by vesicles or bullae.

hy·dro·ab·do·men (high''dro·ab·do'mun, ·ab'do·mun) *n.* [*hydro-* + *abdomen*]. *Obsol.* ASCITES.

hydroa her·pet·i·for·me (hur·pet''i·for'mee). DERMATITIS HERPETIFORMIS.

hy·dro·al·co·hol·ic (high''dro·al·kuh·hol'ick) *adj.* [*hydro-* + *alcoholic*]. Consisting of or containing water and alcohol.

hydroa vac·ci·ni·for·me (vack·sin''i·for'mee). A dermatosis consisting of delicate blisters that appear on exposed skin during the summer and that heal by scarring. Erythropoietic protoporphyria is the underlying condition.

hy·dro·bil·i·ru·bin (high''dro·bil''i·roo'bin) *n.* A red pigment, a reduction product from bilirubin; probably the same as urobilin.

hy·dro·bro·mate (high''dro·bro'mate) *n.* A hydrobromic acid salt; a hydrobromide.

hy·dro·bro·mic (high''dro·bro'mick) *adj.* Composed of hydrogen and bromine.

hydrobromic acid. 1. Hydrogen bromide, HBr; a heavy, colorless gas with a pungent irritating odor. 2. An aqueous solution of hydrogen bromide.

hy·dro·bro·mide (high''dro·bro'mide) *n.* A bromide formed by interaction of an organic nitrogenous base with hydrobromic acid.

Hydrocal. Trade name for the original alpha calcium sulfate hemihydrate; a class I artificial stone used for making casts or models. See also *artificial stone.*

hydrocalix. HYDROCALYX.

hy·dro·cal·y·co·sis, hy·dro·cal·i·co·sis (high''dro·kal''i·ko'sis, ·kay''li·ko'sis) *n.* [*hydrocalyx* + *-osis*]. CALICEAL DIVERTICULUM.

hy·dro·ca·lyx, hy·dro·ca·lix (high''dro·kay'licks) *n.* [*hydro-* + *calyx*]. Cystic dilatation of a renal calix, usually solitary.

hy·dro·car·bon (high''dro·kahr'bun) *n.* [*hydro-* + *carbon*]. Any compound composed only of hydrogen and carbon.

hy·dro·cele (high'dro·seel) *n.* [Gk. *hydrokēlē,* from *hydōr,* water, + *kēlē,* tumor, hernia]. An accumulation of clear, slightly viscid fluid in the processus vaginalis or sac of the tunica vaginalis of the testis. In communicating hydrocele, a patent processus vaginalis permits peritoneal fluid to distend the tunica vaginalis in the upright position. In hydrocele of the cord, there is loculation of fluid along the incompletely involuted processus vaginalis.

hy·dro·ce·lec·to·my (high″dro·se·leck′tuh·mee) *n.* [*hydrocele* + *-ectomy*]. Surgical removal of part of the tunica vaginalis or drainage of the tunica vaginalis.

hydrocele her·ni·a·lis (hur″nee·ay′lis). An accumulation of peritoneal fluid in a hernial sac, especially when hernia accompanies congenital or infantile hydrocele.

hy·dro·ce·phal·ic (high″dro·se·fal′ick) *adj.* Of or pertaining to hydrocephalus.

hydrocephalic dementia. Progressive intellectual deterioration resulting from hydrocephalus.

hy·dro·ceph·a·lo·cele (high″dro·sef′uh·lo·seel) *n.* [*hydro-* + *cephalocele*]. HYDRENCEPHALOCELE.

hy·dro·ceph·a·lus (high″dro·sef′uh·lus) *n.* [Gk. *hydrokephalon*, from *hydōr*, water, + *kephalē*, head]. 1. Distention of the cerebral ventricles with cerebrospinal fluid due to obstruction of the flow of spinal fluid within the ventricular system or in the subarachnoid space, preventing its absorption. See also *communicating hydrocephalus, external hydrocephalus, obstructive hydrocephalus, occult hydrocephalus.* 2. An individual with hydrocephalus.

hy·dro·ceph·a·ly (high″dro·sef′uh·lee) *n.* HYDROCEPHALUS(1).

hydrocephaly ex vac·uo (ecks vack′yoo·o). EXTERNAL HYDROCEPHALUS.

hy·dro·chin·one (high″dro·kin′ohn) *n.* HYDROQUINONE.

hy·dro·chin·on·uria (high″dro·kin″o·new′ree·uh) *n.* [*hydrochinone* + *-uria*]. The presence in the urine of hydroquinone; due to ingestion of substances such as salol and resorcin.

hy·dro·chlo·rate (high″dro·klor′ate) *n. Obsol.* A misnomer for salts formed by hydrochloric acid with certain organic nitrogenous bases, especially alkaloids.

hy·dro·chlo·ric acid (high″druh·klor′ick). 1. Hydrogen chloride, HCl, a colorless gas of pungent odor which can be liquefied under pressure. 2. An aqueous solution containing 35 to 38% of HCl.

hy·dro·chlo·ride (high″druh·klor′ide) *n.* A chloride formed by interaction of an organic nitrogenous base with hydrochloric acid.

hy·dro·chlo·ro·thi·a·zide (high″druh·klor″o·thigh′uh·zide) *n.* 6-Chloro-3,4-dihydro-2*H*-1,2,4-benzothiadiazine-7-sulfonamide 1,1-dioxide, $C_7H_8ClN_3O_4S_2$, an orally effective diuretic and antihypertensive drug.

hy·dro·chol·e·re·sis (high″dro·kol″ur·ee′sis, ·ko″lur·ee′sis) *n.* [*hydro-* + *choleresis*]. Choleresis characterized by an increase of water output, or of a bile relatively low in specific gravity, viscosity, and content of total solids. —**hydrochol·er·et·ic** (·et′ick) *adj.*

Hydrocholin. A trademark for dehydrocholic acid.

hy·dro·cin·chon·i·dine (high″dro·sing·kon′i·deen, ·din) *n.* An alkaloid, $C_{19}H_{24}N_2O$, from species of *Cinchona.*

hy·dro·co·done (high″dro·ko′dohn) *n.* Dihydrocodeinone, $C_{18}H_{21}NO_3$, a compound isomeric with codeine and prepared from it by catalytic rearrangement. Used mainly as an antitussive, as the bitartrate salt.

hy·dro·col·li·dine (high″dro·kol′i·deen, ·din) *n.* A highly poisonous ptomaine obtained from putrefying mackerel, horseflesh, and oxflesh.

hy·dro·col·loid (high″dro·kol′oid) *n.* A type of dental impression material derived from marine kelp. It is introduced into the mouth as a viscous sol which sets into an elastic, insoluble gel. See also *alginate.*

hy·dro·col·pos (high″dro·kol′pos) *n.* [*hydro-* + *-colpos*]. A vaginal retention cyst containing a watery fluid.

hy·dro·co·ni·on (high″dro·ko′nee·on) *n.* [*hydro-* + Gk. *konion,* dust]. An atomizer; a spraying apparatus.

hy·dro·con·qui·nine (high″dro·kon′kwi·neen, ·nin) *n.* HYDROQUINIDINE.

hy·dro·cor·ta·mate (high″dro·kor′tuh·mate) *n.* Hydrocortisone 21-diethylaminoacetate, $C_{27}H_{41}NO_6$, an adrenocortical steroid used topically, as the hydrochloride salt, for the treatment of dermatoses.

hy·dro·cor·ti·sone (high″dro·kor′ti·sone) *n.* 11β,17,21-Trihydroxypregn-4-ene-3,20-dione or 17-hydroxycorticosterone, $C_{21}H_{30}O_5$, an adrenocortical steroid occurring naturally and prepared synthetically; its metabolic and therapeutic effects are qualitatively similar to those of cortisone, but it is considerably more active. Used therapeutically in the form of free hydrocortisone, hydrocortisone acetate, hydrocortisone cypionate, and hydrocortisone sodium succinate. Syn. *Kendall's compound F, Reichstein's substance M.*

Hydrocortole. A trademark for hydrocortisone, an anti-inflammatory adrenocortical steroid.

Hydrocortone. A trademark for hydrocortisone, an anti-inflammatory adrenocortical steroid.

hy·dro·co·tar·nine (high″dro·ko·tahr′neen, ·nin) *n.* An alkaloid, $C_{12}H_{15}NO_3$, derived from narcotine and occurring in small amount in opium.

Hy·dro·cot·y·le (high″dro·cot′i·lee) *n.* [*hydro-* + Gk. *kotylē*, cup]. A genus of umbelliferous herbs, several species of which have been variously employed in therapeutics. Syn. *pennywort.*

hy·dro·cy·an·ic acid (high″dro·sigh·an′ick, ·see·an′ick). Hydrogen cyanide, HCN, a liquid boiling at 26°C; used as a fumigant to rid vessels, buildings, or orchards of vermin. It is a powerful, rapidly acting blood and nerve poison. Syn. *prussic acid.*

hydrocystoma. HIDROCYSTOMA.

hy·dro·cyte (high′dro·site) *n.* [*hydro-* + *-cyte*]. An erythrocyte containing excess water, resulting from excessive membrane permeability to sodium as compared with potassium. Contr. *desiccyte.*

hy·dro·cy·to·sis (high″dro·sigh·to′sis) *n.* The presence of an excessive number of hydrocytes.

hy·dro·dip·so·ma·nia (high″dro·dip″so·may′nee·uh) *n.* [*hydro-* + *dipsomania*]. Periodic attacks of uncontrollable thirst; psychogenic thirst.

HydroDiuril. A trademark for hydrochlorothiazide, an orally effective diuretic and antihypertensive drug.

hy·dro·dy·nam·ics (high″dro·dye·nam′icks) *n.* [*hydro-* + *dynamics*]. The branch of mechanics that deals with liquids. —**hydrodynam·ic** (·ick) *adj.*

hy·dro·elec·tric bath (high″dro·e·leck′trick). A process of immersing the body, or parts of it, in water through which faradic, galvanic, or sinusoidal currents are running.

hy·dro·er·got·i·nine (high″dro·ur·got′i·neen, ·nin) *n.* A name given to ergotoxine before the latter was found to be a mixture of alkaloids.

hy·dro·flu·me·thi·a·zide (high″dro·floo″me·thigh′uh·zide) *n.* 3,4-Dihydro-6-(trifluoromethyl)-2*H*-1,2,4-benzothiadiazine-7-sulfonamide 1,1-dioxide, $C_8H_8F_3N_3O_4S_2$, an orally effective diuretic and antihypertensive drug.

hy·dro·flu·or·ic acid (high″dro·floo·or′ick). 1. Hydrogen fluoride, HF; a highly corrosive, colorless gas. 2. An aqueous solution containing about 50% of HF; used for etching glass.

hy·dro·gel (high′dro·jel) *n.* [*hydro-* + *gel*]. A colloidal gel in which water is the dispersion medium.

hy·dro·gen (high′druh·jin) *n.* [F. *hydrogène,* from *hydro-* + *-gène,* -gen]. H= 1.0080. A univalent, flammable, gaseous element; the lightest element known. It occurs in water and in practically all organic compounds. It is used in various syntheses, as a reducing agent, for the hydrogenation of vegetable oils to form solid products, and in many other industrial applications. Three isotopes of hydrogen (namely, protium, deuterium, and tritium, having atomic masses of approximately one, two, and three, respectively) have been discovered.

hydrogen acceptor. A substance that, on reduction, accepts hydrogen atoms from another substance (hydrogen donor). See also *coenzyme.*

hydrogen arsenide. ARSINE.

hy·dro·gen·a·tion (high″druh·je·nay′shun) *n.* The process of combining with hydrogen. —**hy·dro·gen·at·ed** (high'druh·je·nay''tid) *adj.;* **hy·dro·gen·ate** (high·droj'e·nate, high'druh·je·nate) *v.*

hydrogen bond or **bridge.** The bond formed between two molecules when the nucleus of a hydrogen atom, originally attached to an electronegative atom of a molecule, is attracted to the highly electronegative fluorine, nitrogen, or oxygen atom of the same or a different substance. Water molecules are joined to each other through hydrogen bond formation.

hydrogen bromide. HBr. A heavy, colorless gas with a pungent irritating odor; HYDROBROMIC ACID (1).

hydrogen chloride. HCl. A colorless gas of pungent odor, liquefied under pressure; HYDROCHLORIC ACID (1).

hydrogen cyanide. HYDROCYANIC ACID.

hydrogen dioxide. HYDROGEN PEROXIDE.

hydrogen donor. A chemical compound capable of transferring hydrogen atoms to another substance (hydrogen acceptor), thereby reducing the latter and oxidizing the donor.

hydrogen electrode. An electrode made of platinum saturated with hydrogen. Used as a standard in the determination of hydrogen-ion concentration.

hydrogen fluoride. HYDROFLUORIC ACID (1).

hydrogen iodide. HYDRIODIC ACID.

hydrogen ion. The positively charged nucleus of the hydrogen atom, a proton. Acids are characterized by their ability to liberate hydrogen ions when in aqueous solution. Symbol, H^+. See also *hydronium.*

hydrogen-ion concentration. The number of gram ions of hydrogen per liter of solution. See also *pH.*

hy·dro·gen·ly·ase (high''dro·jin·lye'ace, ·aze) *n.* An enzyme, present in *Escherichia coli,* which catalyzes reversible decomposition of formic acid to molecular hydrogen and carbon dioxide, a reaction which appears to be associated with the anaerobic decomposition, by extracts of *E. coli,* of pyruvic acid to acetic acid and formic acid.

hydrogen peroxide. H_2O_2, a colorless, caustic liquid, highly explosive in contact with oxidizable material. A 3% solution is used as an antiseptic and germicide.

hydrogen sulfide. H_2S. A colorless, highly toxic gas of unpleasant odor.

hy·dro·glos·sa (high''dro·glos'uh) *n.* [*hydro-* + Gk. *glōssa,* tongue]. RANULA.

hy·dro·gym·nas·tics (high''dro·jim·nas'ticks) *n.* [*hydro-* + *gymnastics*]. Active exercises performed in water; the buoyancy thus obtained enables weakened muscles to move the limbs more easily.

hy·dro·he·ma·to·ne·phro·sis, hy·dro·hae·ma·to·ne·phro·sis (high''dro·hee''muh·to·ne·fro'sis, ·hem''uh·to·) *n.* [*hydro-* + *hemato-* + *nephrosis*]. The presence of blood and urine in a dilated renal pelvis.

hy·dro·he·ma·to·sal·pinx, hy·dro·hae·ma·to·sal·pinx (high''dro·hee''muh·to·sal'pincks) *n.* [*hydro-* + *hemato-* + *salpinx*]. HEMOHYDROSALPINX.

hy·dro·hep·a·to·sis (high''dro·hep''uh·to'sis) *n.* [*hydro-* + *hepatosis*]. An abnormal collection of watery fluid in the liver.

hy·dro·ki·net·ics (high''dro·ki·net'icks) *n.* [*hydro-* + *kinetics*]. The science of the motion of liquids. —**hydrokinetic,** *adj.*

hy·dro·lac·tom·e·ter (high''dro·lack·tom'e·tur) *n.* [*hydro-* + *lacto-* + *-meter*]. An instrument used in estimating the percentage of water in milk.

hy·dro·lase (high'dro·lace, ·laze) *n.* An enzyme catalyzing hydrolysis.

hy·drol·o·gy (high·drol'uh·jee) *n.* [*hydro-* + *-logy*]. The science of the properties of water, as it occurs in the atmosphere and in the environment.

hy·drol·y·sate (high·drol'i·sate) *n.* The product of hydrolysis.

hy·drol·y·sis (high·drol'i·sis) *n.* [*hydro-* + *-lysis*]. Any reaction with water, frequently of the type AB + HOH → AOH + HB, the latter being the reverse reaction of neutralization. —**hy·dro·lyt·ic** (high''dro·lit'ick) *adj.;* **hy·dro·lyze** (high'dro·lize) *v.*

hy·dro·lyte (high'dro·lite) *n.* The substance undergoing hydrolysis.

hydrolytic enzyme. An enzyme capable of catalyzing hydrolytic reactions, as carbohydrase, esterase, or protease.

hy·drol·y·zate (high·drol'i·zate) *n.* HYDROLYSATE.

hy·dro·ma (high·dro'muh) *n.* [*hydr-* + *-oma*]. HYGROMA.

hy·dro·ma·nia (high''dro·may'nee·uh) *n.* [*hydro-* + *-mania*]. 1. Abnormal thirst, especially for water. 2. A severe depressive neurosis with a morbid desire for suicide by drowning.

hy·dro·mas·sage (high''dro·ma·sahzh') *n.* [*hydro-* + *massage*]. Massage by means of moving water.

hy·dro·mel (high'dro·mel) *n.* [Gk. *hydromeli*]. A mixture of honey and water, with or without a medicinal substance.

hy·dro·me·nin·go·cele (high''dro·me·ning'go·seel) *n.* [*hydro-* + *meningocele*]. A meningocele with prominent distention by cerebrospinal fluid.

hy·drom·e·ter (high·drom'e·tur) *n.* [*hydro-* + *-meter*]. An instrument for determining the specific gravity of liquids. —**hy·dro·met·ric** (high''dro·met'rick) *adj.;* **hy·drom·e·try** (high·drom'e·tree) *n.*

hy·dro·me·tra (high''dro·mee'truh) *n.* [*hydro-* + Gk. *mētra,* womb]. Accumulation of watery fluid in the uterus.

hy·dro·me·tro·col·pos (high''dro·mee''tro·kol'pos) *n.* [*hydro-* + *metro-* + *-colpos*]. Accumulation of watery fluid in the uterus and vagina.

hy·dro·mi·cro·ceph·a·ly (high''dro·migh''kro·sef'uh·lee) *n.* [*hydro-* + *microcephaly*]. Microcephaly with increased cerebrospinal fluid.

hy·dro·mor·phone (high''dro·mor'fone) *n.* Dihydromorphinone, $C_{17}H_{19}NO_3$, prepared by hydrogenation of morphine; a respiratory sedative and analgesic considerably more powerful than morphine. Used as the hydrochloride salt.

Hydromox. Trademark for quinethazone, an orally effective diuretic and antihypertensive drug.

hy·dro·my·e·lia (high''dro·migh·ee'lee·uh) *n.* [*hydro-* + *-myelia*]. A dilatation of the central canal of the spinal cord.

hy·dro·my·e·lo·cele (high''dro·migh'e·lo·seel'') *n.* [*hydro-* + *myelo-* + *-cele*]. HYDROMYELIA.

hy·dro·my·rinx (high''dro·migh'rinks) *n.* [*hydro-* + *myrinx*]. HYDROTYMPANUM.

hy·dro·ne·phro·sis (high''dro·ne·fro'sis) *n.* [*hydro-* + *nephrosis*]. Dilatation of the pelvis and calyces of the kidney secondary to urinary tract obstruction; eventually kidney parenchymal atrophy results. —**hydrone·phrot·ic** (·frot'ick) *adj.*

hy·dro·ni·um (high·dro'nee·um) *n.* The solvated hydrogen ion, $H^+(H_2O)$ or H_3O^+, considered to be present in aqueous solutions of all acids.

hy·dro·nol (high'dro·nol) *n.* A postulated form of water in the double molecule form, $(HOH)_2$, in which one of the molecules is resolved into H and OH, with increased chemical activity.

Hydronol. Trademark for isosorbide, a diuretic.

hy·drop·a·thy (high·drop'uth·ee) *n.* [*hydro-* + *-pathy*]. The system of internal and external use of water in attempting to cure disease. —**hy·dro·path·ic** (high''dro·path'ick) *adj.*

hy·dro·pel·vis (high''dro·pel'vis) *n.* [*hydro-* + *pelvis*]. Distention of the renal pelvis by urine, with little or no calyceal distention; PELVIECTASIS.

hy·dro·peri·car·di·tis (high''dro·perr''i·kahr·dye'tis) *n.* [*hydro-* + *pericarditis*]. Pericarditis accompanied by serous effusion into the pericardial cavity.

hy·dro·peri·car·di·um (high''dro·perr''i·kahr'dee·um) *n.* [*hydro-* + *pericardium*]. A collection of a serous effusion in the pericardial cavity.

hy·dro·per·i·on (high''dro·perr'ee·on) *n.* [*hydro-* + *peri-* + Gk. *ōon,* egg]. The liquid existing between the decidua parietalis and the decidua capsularis.

hy·dro·peri·to·ne·um (high″dro·perr″i·to·nee′um) *n.* [*hydro-* + *peritoneum*]. ASCITES.

Hy·droph·i·dae (high·drof′i·dee) *n.pl.* [NL., from *hydr-* + Gk. *ophis*, serpent]. A family of poisonous snakes, the sea snakes, which because of certain modifications are adapted to life in the sea. These snakes occur most abundantly in the seas of northern Australia and southern Asia; although their venom is the most toxic known, bites are relatively rare.

hy·dro·phil (high′dro·fil) *n. & adj.* [*hydro-* + *-phil*]. 1. A substance, usually in the colloidal state, which is capable of combining with, or attracting, water. 2. Capable of combining with, or attracting, water. —**hy·dro·phil·ic** (high″dro·fil′ick) *adj.*

hy·dro·phile (high′dro·fil, ·file) *n. & adj.* HYDROPHIL.

hy·dro·phil·ia (high″dro·fil′ee·uh) *n.* HYDROPHILISM.

hydrophilic colloid. A colloid that has a strong affinity for water and forms stable dispersions in water by virtue of this property.

hydrophilic ointment. An official oil-in-water type of ointment base, containing stearyl alcohol, white petrolatum, propylene glycol, sodium lauryl sulfate, and water, preserved with methylparaben and propylparaben.

hydrophilic petrolatum. A protectant and ointment base, capable of absorbing aqueous solutions, containing 3% cholesterol, 3% stearyl alcohol, 8% white wax, and 86% white petrolatum.

hy·droph·i·lism (high·drof′i·liz·um) *n.* [*hydrophil* + *-ism*]. The property of colloids, cells, and tissues of attracting and holding water.

hy·droph·i·lous (high·drof′i·lus) *adj.* [*hydro-* + *-philous*]. 1. Pertaining to or designating plants that are fertilized through the agency of water. 2. Absorbing water.

hy·dro·phobe (high′druh·fobe) *n.* [Gk. *hydrophobos*, dreading water]. 1. A substance, usually in the colloidal state, which lacks affinity for water. 2. A person who has a fear of water.

hy·dro·pho·bia (high″druh·fo′bee·uh) *n.* [Gk., from *hydōr*, water, + *-phobia*]. 1. Spasticity and paralysis of the muscles of deglutition, with consequent aversion to liquids, as a manifestation of rabies. 2. RABIES. 3. Morbid fear of water.

hy·dro·pho·bic (high″druh·fo′bick) *adj.* [Gk. *hydrophobikos*]. 1. Of or pertaining to a hydrophobe (2). 2. Pertaining to or suffering from rabies.

hydrophobic colloid. A colloid lacking affinity for water and capable of forming dispersions in water only by virtue of adsorption of ions by individual particles of the colloid.

hydrophobic tetanus. Tetanus characterized by violent spasm of the muscles of the throat.

hy·dro·pho·bo·pho·bia (high″druh·fo″bo·fo′bee·uh) *n.* [*hydrophobia* + *-phobia*]. An intense dread of hydrophobia, sometimes producing a state simulating true hydrophobia.

hy·dro·phone (high′druh·fone) *n.* [*hydro-* + *-phone*]. An instrument used in auscultatory percussion, the sound being conveyed to the ear through a liquid column.

hy·droph·thal·mos (high″drof·thal′mus) *n.* [*hydr-* + *ophthalmos*]. CONGENITAL GLAUCOMA.

hy·drop·ic (high·drop′ick) *adj.* [Gk. *hydrōpikos*]. Characterized by swelling or retention of fluid; specifically, characterized by or pertaining to hydrops.

hydropic degeneration. A retrogressive change characterized by the appearance of water droplets in the affected parts of the cell.

hy·dro·plasm (high′dro·plaz·um) *n.* [*hydro-* + *-plasm*]. The fluid constituent of protoplasm.

hy·dro·pleu·ra (high″dro·ploo′ruh) *n.* [*hydro-* + *pleura*]. HYDROTHORAX.

hy·dro·pneu·ma·to·sis (high″dro·new″muh·to′sis) *n.* [*hydro-* + *pneumat-* + *-osis*]. A collection of liquid and gas within the tissues.

hy·dro·pneu·mo·peri·car·di·um (high″dro·new″mo·perr·i·kahr′dee·um) *n.* [*hydro-* + *pneumo-* + *pericardium*]. A collection of fluid and gas in the pericardial sac.

hy·dro·pneu·mo·peri·to·ne·um (high″dro·new″mo·perr·i·tuh·nee′um) *n.* [*hydro-* + *pneumo-* + *peritoneum*]. A collection of fluid and gas within the peritoneal cavity.

hy·dro·pneu·mo·tho·rax (high″dro·new″mo·tho′racks) *n.* [*hydro-* + *pneumo-* + *thorax*]. The presence of fluid and gas in the pleural cavity.

hy·drops (high′drops) *n.* [Gk. *hydrōps*]. The accumulation of fluid in body tissues or cavities; dropsy.

hydrops an·tri (an′trye). Effusion of fluid into the maxillary sinus.

hydrops ar·tic·u·lo·rum (ahr·tick″yoo·lo′rum). HYDRARTHROSIS.

hydrops fe·ta·lis (fee·tay′lis). A severe form of erythroblastosis fetalis characterized by marked anasarca; the fetus is usually dead at delivery.

hydrops grav·i·da·rum (grav·i·dair′rum). Edema in pregnancy.

hydrops of the labyrinth. A condition of the labyrinth caused by increased endolymphatic pressure producing tinnitus, hearing loss, and vertigo. See also *Meaniesre's disease.*

hy·dro·pyo·ne·phro·sis (high″dro·pye″o·ne·fro′sis) *n.* [*hydro-* + *pyo-* + *nephrosis*]. Dilatation of the pelvis of the kidney with urine and pus, usually caused by bacterial infection complicating an obstruction of the urinary tract.

hy·dro·quin·i·dine (high″dro·kwin′i·deen, ·din) *n.* An alkaloid, $C_{20}H_{26}N_2O_2$, in cinchona bark. Syn. *hydroconquinine.*

hy·dro·quin·ine (high″dro·kwin′een, ·in, ·kwye′nine) *n.* An alkaloid, $C_{20}H_{26}N_2O_2$, obtained from cinchona, and frequently contaminating quinine. It is effective against malaria, but more toxic than quinine. Syn. *dihydroquinine.*

hy·dro·quin·ol (high″dro·kwin′ol) *n.* HYDROQUINONE.

hy·dro·qui·none (high″dro·kwi·nohn′, ·kwin′ohn) *n.* *p*-Dihydroxybenzene, $C_6H_6O_2$, an isomer of resorcinol and pyrocatechin. A photographic developer; used as a skin depigmenting agent.

hy·dror·rhea, hy·dror·rhoea (high″dro·ree′uh) *n.* [*hydro-* + *-rrhea*]. A copious flow of a watery fluid.

hydrorrhea grav·i·da·rum (grav·i·dair′rum). A chronic discharge from the vagina, prior to parturition, of watery fluid resembling amniotic fluid, but with no evidence of ruptured membranes. It may be formed by the decidua.

hydrosadenitis. HIDRADENITIS.

hy·dro·sal·pinx (high″dro·sal′pinks) *n.* [*hydro-* + *salpinx*]. A distention of a uterine tube with fluid.

hydrosis. HIDROSIS.

hy·dro·sol (high′dro·sol) *n.* [*hydro-* + *sol*]. A colloid system in which water is the dispersion medium.

hy·dro·sol·u·ble (high″dro·sol′yoo·bul) *adj.* [*hydro-* + *soluble*]. Soluble in water.

hy·dro·sper·ma·to·cele (high″dro·spur′muh·to·seel, ·spur·mat′o·) *n.* [*hydro-* + *spermatocele*]. SPERMATOCELE.

hy·dro·sper·ma·to·cyst (high″dro·spur′muh·to·sist, ·spur·mat′o·) *n.* [*hydro-* + *spermato-* + *cyst*]. A hydrocele whose fluid contains spermatozoa. See also *spermatocele.*

hy·dro·spi·rom·e·ter (high″dro·spye·rom′e·tur) *n.* [*hydro-* + *spirometer*]. A spirometer in which air pressure is indicated by the rise and fall of a column of water.

hy·dro·stat·ic (high″dro·stat′ick) *adj.* [*hydro-* + *static*]. 1. Functioning by means of a liquid in equilibrium. 2. Pertaining to hydrostatics.

hydrostatic bed. A bed with a water mattress.

hydrostatic dilatation. Dilatation of a cavity or part by an introduced elastic bag that is subsequently distended with water.

hydrostatic pressure. A pressure created in a fluid system.

hy·dro·stat·ics (high″dro·stat′icks) *n.* [*hydro-* + *statics*]. The branch of hydraulics that treats of the properties and characteristics of liquids in a state of equilibrium.

hydrostatic test. A test, not regarded as reliable by forensic authorities, in which a live birth is indicated if the lungs of a dead infant float in water.

hy·dro·sul·fu·ric acid (high″dro·sul·few′rick). 1. HYDROGEN SULFIDE. 2. Dithionic acid, $H_2S_2O_6$. 3. Any organic acid of the formula RCSSH.

hy·dro·sy·rin·go·my·e·lia (high″dro·si·ring″go·migh·ee′lee·uh) *n.* [*hydro-* + *syringo-* + *-myelia*]. *Obsol.* Dilatation of the central canal of the spinal cord by cerebrospinal fluid, accompanied by degeneration and the formation of cavities.

hy·dro·tax·is (high″dro·tack′sis) *n.* [*hydro-* + *-taxis*]. The response of organisms to the stimulus of moisture. See also *hydrotropism.*

hy·dro·ther·a·peu·tics (high″dro·therr·uh·pew′ticks) *n.* [*hydro-* + *therapeutics*]. The branch of therapeutics that deals with the curative use of water.

hy·dro·ther·a·py (high″dro·therr′uh·pee) *n.* [*hydro-* + *therapy*]. The treatment of disease by the external use of water.

hy·dro·ther·mal (high″dro·thur′mul) *adj.* [*hydro-* + *thermal*]. Of or pertaining to warm water; said of springs.

hy·dro·thi·o·nu·ria (high″dro·thigh″o·new′ree·uh) *n.* [*hydro-* + *thion-* + *-uria*]. The presence of hydrogen sulfide in the urine.

hy·dro·tho·rax (high″dro·tho′racks) *n.* [*hydro-* + *thorax*]. A collection of fluid in the pleural cavity. —**hydro·tho·rac·ic** (·tho·ras′ick) *adj.*

hydrotic. HIDROTIC.

hy·dro·tis (high·dro′tis) *n.* [NL., from *hydr-* + Gk. *ous, ōtos,* ear]. Watery effusion into the external ear, the middle ear, or the inner ear, seldom in combination.

hy·dro·trop·ic (high″dro·trop′ick) *adj.* 1. Of or pertaining to hydrotropism. 2. Of or pertaining to hydrotropy.

hydrotropic action. An action that confers water solubility on substances ordinarily not soluble in water, such as that of bile salts on fatty acids.

hy·drot·ro·pism (high·drot′ro·piz·um) *n.* [*hydro-* + *-tropism*]. *In botany,* the tendency of a growing plant or organ, as roots, to turn either away from, or toward, moisture.

hy·drot·ro·py (high·drot′ruh·pee) *n.* [*hydro-* + *-tropy*]. The power that certain substances have of making water-insoluble substances dissolve in water without any apparent chemical alteration of the dissolved substances, as the solubilizing action of bile salts on fatty acids.

hy·dro·tym·pa·num (high″dro·tim′puh·num) *n.* [*hydro-* + *tympanum*]. Effusion of fluid into the cavity of the middle ear.

hy·dro·ure·ter (high″dro·yoo·ree′tur, ·yoor′e·tur) *n.* [*hydro-* + *ureter*]. Abnormal distention of the ureter with urine, usually due to partial obstruction.

hy·dro·ure·tero·ne·phro·sis (high″dro·yoo·ree″tur·o·ne·fro′sis) *n.* [*hydro-* + *ureter* + *nephrosis*]. Abnormal unilateral or bilateral distention and dilatation of both kidney and ureter with urine or other watery fluid, from obstructed outflow.

hy·dro·ure·ter·o·sis (high″dro·yoo·ree″tur·o′sis) *n.* [*hydro-* + *ureter* + *osis*]. HYDROURETER.

hy·drous (high′drus) *adj.* [*hydr-* + *-ous*]. Containing water.

hydrous wool fat. LANOLIN.

hy·drox·ide (high·drock′side, ·sid) *n.* Any compound formed by the union of a metal, or of an inorganic or organic radical, with one or more hydroxyl (OH) groups.

hy·droxo·co·bal·a·min (high·drock″so·ko·bawl′uh·min) *n.* Cyanocobalamin in which the cyano group has been replaced by hydroxyl. Hydroxocobalamin, although absorbed more slowly than cyanocobalamin from the site of injection, results in higher and more prolonged levels of cobalamin in blood serum.

hydroxy-. A combining form indicating *the hydroxyl group —OH.*

hy·droxy·ace·tic acid (high·drock″see·uh·seet′ick). GLYCOLIC ACID.

hy·droxy·am·phet·a·mine (high·drock″see·am·fet′uh·min, ·meen) *n.* *p*-(2-Aminopropyl)phenol, $C_9H_{13}NO$, a sympathomimetic amine used as the hydrobromide salt orally as a pressor drug and locally as a mydriatic and nasal decongestant.

***p*-hy·droxy·am·pi·cil·lin** (high·drock″see·am·pi·sil′in) *n.* AMOXICILLIN.

hy·droxy·ap·a·tite (high·drock″see·ap′uh·tite) *n.* $3Ca_3(PO_4)_2.Ca(OH)_2$. The basic inorganic constituent of bone. In bone, the hydroxyl groups are partially substituted by other elements and radicals, such as fluoride or carbonate.

hy·droxy·ben·zene (high·drock″see·ben′zeen) *n.* PHENOL.

hy·droxy·ben·zo·ic acid (high·drock″see·ben·zo′ick). Any of three isomeric acids, HOC_6H_4COOH, differing in the position of the OH and COOH groups, and distinguished by the prefixes ortho-, meta-, and para-. Ortho-hydroxybenzoic acid is salicylic acid; esters of para-hydroxybenzoic acid are used as preservatives against microbial action in various preparations.

β-hy·droxy·bu·tyr·ic acid (high·drock″see·bew·tirr′ick). 3-Hydroxybutanoic acid, $C_4H_8O_3$, an intermediate acid formed in fat metabolism. It is a member of a group of compounds called acetone bodies or ketone bodies. In ketosis, increased amounts of these compounds appear in blood and urine.

α-hydroxybutyric dehydrogenase. Any of a group of isoenzymes of lactic dehydrogenase, largely the isoenzyme chiefly found in cardiac muscle; determination of serum levels is sometimes used in the diagnosis of myocardial infarction.

β-hydroxybutyric dehydrogenase. The enzyme that catalyzes removal of hydrogen from L-β-hydroxybutyric acid to form acetoacetic acid, in the presence of coenzyme I (nicotinamide adenine dinucleotide).

hy·droxy·chlo·ro·quine (high·drock″see·klo′ro·kween) *n.* 7-Chloro-4-{4-[ethyl(2-hydroxyethyl)amino]-1-methylbutylamino}-quinoline, $C_{18}H_{26}ClN_3O$, used as the sulfate salt for the treatment of malaria, lupus erythematosus, and rheumatoid arthritis.

17-hy·droxy·cor·ti·cos·ter·one (high·drock″see·kor″ti·kos′tur·ohn) *n.* HYDROCORTISONE.

17-hydroxy-11-dehydrocorticosterone, *n.* CORTISONE.

hy·droxy·di·one sodium succinate (high·drock″see·dye′ohn). SODIUM HYDROXYDIONE SUCCINATE.

hy·droxy·eth·ane (high·drock″see·eth′ane) *n.* ETHYL ALCOHOL.

5-hy·droxy·in·dole·ace·tic acid (high·drock″see·in″dole·a·see′tick). $C_{10}H_9NO_3$. A metabolite of serotonin present in cerebrospinal fluid and in small amounts in normal urine, and markedly increased in some cases of carcinoid syndrome.

hy·drox·yl (high·drock′sil) *n.* The univalent radical —OH, the combination of which with a basic element or radical forms a hydroxide.

hy·drox·yl·amine (high·drock″sil·uh·meen′) *n.* A basic substance, NH_2OH, known only in solution in water or in combination with acids. The hydrochloride salt is used as a reagent.

hy·drox·yl·ase (high·drock′si·lace, ·laze) *n.* Any enzyme that results in the formation or introduction of a hydroxyl group in a substrate.

hy·drox·yl·ation (high·drock″si·lay′shun) *n.* Introduction or formation, by various chemical procedures, of one or more hydroxyl radicals in a compound. —**hy·drox·yl·at·ed** (high·drock′si·lay·tid) *adj.*

hy·droxy·ly·sine (high·drock″see·lye′seen) *n.* The amino acid 2,6-diamino-3-hydroxycaproic acid, $C_6H_{14}N_2O_3$.

hy·droxy·phen·a·mate (high·drock″see·fen′uh·mate) *n.* 2-Hydroxy-2-phenylbutyl carbamate, $C_{11}H_{15}NO_3$, a tranquilizer drug.

hy·droxy·pro·ges·ter·one (high·drock″see·pro·jes′tur·ohn) *n.* 17α-Hydroxyprogesterone, $C_{21}H_{30}O_3$, used as the caproate (hexanoate) ester for progestational therapy.

hy·droxy·pro·line (high·drock″see·pro′leen, ·lin) *n.* 4-Hydroxy-2-pyrrolidinecarboxylic acid, $C_5H_9NO_3$, a naturally occurring amino acid.

hy·droxy·pro·lin·emia, hy·droxy·pro·lin·ae·mia (high·drock″see·pro·lin·ee′mee·uh) *n.* [*hydroxyproline* + *-emia*]. An inborn error of metabolism in which there is a deficiency of hydroxyproline oxidase with increased blood levels of hydroxyproline; mental retardation is the main clinical manifestation.

hy·droxy·quin·o·line (high·drock″see·kwin′o·leen, ·lin) *n.* 8-Hydroxyquinoline, C_9H_7NO, used as an analytical reagent for metals and for arginine. The base and certain of its salts, especially the citrate and sulfate, have been used as fungicides, antiseptics, and deodorants. Syn. *oxyquinoline.*

hy·droxy·stea·rin sulfate (high·drock″see·stee′uh·rin). A substance prepared by sulfating hydrogenated castor oil; it is a pale yellow-brown, semisoft, unctuous mass, dispersible in water; has been used in the formulation of hydrophilic ointment bases.

hy·droxy·stil·bam·i·dine (high·drock″see·stil·bam′i·deen) *n.* 2-Hydroxy-4,4′-stilbenedicarboxamidine, $C_{16}H_{16}N_4O$, a stilbamidine derivative useful for the treatment of blastomycosis, leishmaniasis, and trypanosomiasis; employed in this treatment as the diisethionate (di-β-hydroxyethanesulfonate) salt.

5-hy·droxy·trypt·amine (high·drock″see·trip′tuh·meen) *n.* SEROTONIN.

hy·droxy·urea (high·drock″see·yoo·ree′uh) *n.* Hydroxycarbamide, $H_2NCONHOH$, an antineoplastic agent.

hy·droxy·zine (high·drock′si·zeen) *n.* 1-(*p*-Chlorobenzhydryl)-4-[2-(2-hydroxyethoxy)ethyl]piperazine, $C_{21}H_{27}ClN_2O_2$, a tranquilizer also possessing antiemetic and antihistaminic effects; used as the hydrochloride or pamoate salt.

Hy·dro·zoa (high″druh·zo′uh) *n.pl.* [*hydro-* + Gk. *zōa,* animals]. A class of coelenterates, most of the sort commonly called jellyfish.

hy·dru·ria (high·droo′ree·uh) *n.* [*hydr-* + *-uria*]. The passage of large amounts of urine of low specific gravity, as in diabetes insipidus; polyuria. —**hydru·ric** (·rick) *adj.*

hy·e·tom·e·try (high″e·tom′e·tree) *n.* [Gk. *hyetos,* rain, + *-metry*]. Measurement of the quantity of rainfall.

Hy·ge·ia (high·jee′uh) *n.* [Gk. *hygieia,* health, from *hygiēs,* healthy]. In Greek mythology, the goddess of health; daughter of Asklepios.

hy·giene (high′jeen) *n.* [Gk. *hygieinos,* healthful]. The science that treats of the laws of health and the methods of their observation. —**hy·gien·ic** (high·jee·en′ick) *adj.*

hy·gien·ist (high′jeen·ist, high·jen′ist) *n.* 1. One trained in the science of health. 2. A dental hygienist.

hygr-, hygro- [Gk. *hygros*]. A combining form meaning *moist, moisture, humidity.*

hy·gre·che·ma (high″gre·kee′muh) *n.* [*hygr-* + Gk. *ēchēma,* sound]. The sound produced by a liquid in a body tissue or cavity as heard by auscultation.

hy·gric (high′grick) *adj.* [*hygr-* + *-ic*]. Of or pertaining to moisture.

hy·grine (high′green, ·grin) *n.* *N*-Methyl-2-acetonylpyrrolidine, $C_8H_{15}NO$, a liquid alkaloid occurring in the leaves of certain species of coca.

hy·gro·ble·phar·ic (high″gro·ble·făr′ick) *adj.* [*hygro-* + *blephar-* + *-ic*]. Serving to moisten the eyelid.

hy·gro·ma (high·gro′muh) *n.*, pl. **hygromas, hygroma·ta** (·tuh) [*hygr-* + *-oma*]. A cystic cavity derived from distended lymphatics and filled with lymph; a congenital malformation, most often seen in young children. Syn. *cavernous lymphangioma, cystic hygroma.* —**hy·grom·a·tous** (high·grom′uh·tus) *adj.*

hygroma cys·ti·cum col·li (sis′ti·kum kol′eye). A hygroma in the neck.

hy·grom·e·ter (high·grom′e·tur) *n.* [*hygro-* + *-meter*]. An instrument for determining quantitatively the amount of moisture in the air. —**hygrome·try** (·tree) *n.*

hy·gro·met·ric (high″gro·met′rick) *adj.* 1. Pertaining to hygrometry. 2. Readily absorbing water; HYGROSCOPIC (2). —**hygromet·ri·cal** (·ri·kul) *adj.;* **hygromet·ri·cal·ly** (·ri·kul·ee) *adv.*

hy·gro·my·cin (high″gro·migh′sin) *n.* A broad-spectrum antibiotic, $C_{23}H_{29}NO_{12}$, obtained from various strains of *Streptomyces hygroscopicus.*

hy·gro·pho·bia (high″gro·fo′bee·uh) *n.* [*hygro-* + *-phobia*]. Morbid fear of liquids or of moisture.

hy·gro·scope (high′gro·skope) *n.* [*hygro-* + *-scope*]. An instrument for indicating the humidity of the atmosphere. —**hy·gros·co·py** (high·gros′kuh·pee) *n.*

hy·gro·scop·ic (high″gro·skop′ick) *adj.* 1. Pertaining to a hygroscope. 2. Sensitive to moisture; readily absorbing moisture.

hy·gro·sto·mia (high″gro·sto′mee·uh) *n.* [*hygro-* + *-stomia*]. Chronic excess salivation.

Hygroton. Trademark for chlorthalidone, an orally effective diuretic and antihypertensive drug.

Hykinone. Trademark for menadione sodium bisulfite, a water-soluble derivative of menadione with the actions and uses of the latter.

hyl-, hylo- [Gk. *hylē*]. A combining form meaning (a) *wood;* (b) *material, substance, matter.*

hy·lic (high′lick) *adj.* [Gk. *hylikos,* from *hylē,* matter]. Of or pertaining to matter; material.

hylo-. See *hyl-.*

Hy·lob·a·tes (high·lob′uh·teez, high″lo·bay′teez) *n.* [Gk. *hylobatēs,* one who haunts the woods, from *hylē,* wood, forest]. A Southeast Asian and Indonesian genus of arboreal apes comprising the gibbons.

Hy·lo·bat·i·dae (high″lo·bat′i·dee) *n. pl.* A family of the Hominoidea that includes the genera *Hylobates* and *Symphalangus;* the lesser apes. Contr. *Pongidae.*

hy·lo·pho·bia (high″lo·fo′bee·uh) *n.* [*hylo-* + *-phobia*]. Morbid fear of forests.

hy·lo·trop·ic (high″lo·trop′ick) *adj.* [*hylo-* + *-tropic*]. Characterizing a substance capable of changing its form without changing its composition, as a solid that can be melted or distilled.

hy·lo·zo·ism (high″lo·zo′iz·um) *n.* [*hylo-* + Gk. *zōē,* life, + *-ism*]. The theory that all matter is endowed with life.

hy·men (high′mun) *n.* [Gk. *hymēn,* membrane] [NA]. A membranous partition partially, or in some cases wholly, blocking the orifice of the vagina. It may be of several forms, such as circular, or crescentic; it may be multiple, entirely lacking, or imperforate. —**hymen·al** (·ul) *adj.*

hymen-, hymeno-. A combining form meaning (a) *hymen;* (b) *membrane.*

hymenal caruncles. The small irregular nodules which are the remains of the hymen. NA *carunculae hymenales.*

hy·men·ec·to·my (high″me·neck′tuh·mee) *n.* [*hymen* + *-ectomy*]. Excision of the hymen.

hy·men·i·tis (high″me·nigh′tis) *n.* [*hymen* + *-itis*]. Inflammation of the hymen.

hymeno-. See *hymen-.*

hy·me·no·le·pi·a·sis (high″me·no·le·pye′uh·sis) *n.*, pl. **hymenolepia·ses** (·seez) [*Hymenolepis* + *-iasis*]. Infection of the intestines by tapeworms of the genus *Hymenolepis,* usually producing only mild abdominal distress.

Hy·me·no·le·pid·i·dae (high″me·no·le·pid′i·dee) *n.pl.* A family of tapeworms (class Cestoda) of the phylum Platyhelminthes.

Hy·me·nol·e·pis (high″me·nol′e·pis) *n.* [*hymeno-* + Gk. *lepis,* scale]. A genus of tapeworms; any dwarf tapeworm.

Hymenolepis dim·i·nu·ta (dim·i·new′tuh). A species of tapeworm found commonly in rats and mice and occasionally in man.

Hymenolepis na·na (nay′nuh). A species of tapeworm, cosmopolitan in distribution, which infects man; the smallest of the dwarf tapeworms.

hy·me·nol·o·gy (high″me·nol′uh·jee) *n.* [*hymeno-* + *-logy*]. The science of the nature, structure, functions, and diseases of membranes.

Hy·me·nop·tera (high″me·nop′tur·uh) *n.pl.* [Gk., from *hymenopteros,* membranous-winged]. An order of insects which includes the bees, ants, wasps, sawflies, and gallflies. They are the most highly specialized group of invertebrates. —**hymenopter·ous** (·us) *adj.*

hy·men·or·rha·phy (high″me·nor′uh·fee) *n.* [*hymeno-* + *-rrhaphy*]. 1. Suture of the hymen to occlude the vagina. 2. Suture of any membrane.

hy·meno·tome (high·men′uh·tohm) *n.* [*hymeno-* + *-tome*]. A surgical instrument used for cutting membranes.

hy·men·ot·o·my (high″me·not′uh·mee) *n.* [*hymeno-* + *-tomy*]. 1. Surgical incision of the hymen. 2. Dissection or anatomy of membranes.

Hymorphan. A trademark for hydromorphone hydrochloride, a narcotic analgesic.

hyo-. A combining form meaning *hyoid.*

hyo·epi·glot·tic (high″o·ep·i·glot′ick) *adj.* Relating to the hyoid bone and the epiglottis.

hyoepiglottic ligament. A band of tissue from the hyoid to the upper anterior surface of the epiglottis. NA *ligamentum hyoepiglotticum.*

hyo·epi·glot·tid·e·an (high″o·ep″i·glot·tid′ee·un) *adj.* HYOEPIGLOTTIC.

hyo·glos·sal (high″o·glos′ul) *adj.* [*hyo-* + *glossal*]. 1. Pertaining to the hyoglossus. 2. Extending from the hyoid bone to the tongue.

hyoglossal membrane. The membrane at the posterior portion of the tongue, uniting the tongue to the hyoid bone and giving attachment to the posterior fibers of the genioglossus muscle.

hyo·glos·sus (high″o·glos′us) *n.,* pl. **hyoglos·si** (·sigh) [NL., from *hyo-* + Gk. *glōssa,* tongue]. An extrinsic muscle of the tongue arising from the hyoid bone. NA *musculus hyoglossus.* See also Table of Muscles in the Appendix.

hy·oid (high′oid) *n. & adj.* [Gk. *hyoeidēs,* shaped like the letter *υ* (upsilon)]. 1. A bone between the root of the tongue and the larynx, supporting the tongue and giving attachment to several muscles. NA *os hyoideum.* See also Plate 15 and Table of Bones in the Appendix. 2. Of or pertaining to the hyoid.

hyoid arch. The second visceral arch.

hyoid bars. The pair of cartilaginous plates forming the ventral ends of the second visceral (hyoid) arch.

hyoid tubercle. One of three auricular tubercles on the anterior surface of the hyoid arch of the embryo.

hyo·man·dib·u·lar (high″o·man·dib′yoo·lur) *adj. & n.* 1. Pertaining to the hyoid and mandibular arches of the embryo or to the groove and pouch between them. 2. The upper cartilaginous or osseous element of the hyoid arch in fishes.

hy·o·scine (high′o·seen, ·sin) *n.* SCOPOLAMINE.

hyo·scy·a·mine (high″o·sigh′uh·meen, ·min) *n.* An alkaloid, $C_{17}H_{23}NO_3$, occurring in many of the Solanaceae, notably belladonna, hyoscyamus, and stramonium. It is the levorotatory component of racemic atropine, the pharmacologic activity of the latter being due largely to hyoscyamine. Used as the hydrobromide and sulfate salts.

hyo·scy·a·mus (high″o·sigh′uh·mus) *n.* [Gk. *hyoskyamos*]. Henbane. The dried leaf, with or without flowering tops, of *Hyoscyamus niger;* contains the alkaloids hyoscyamine and scopolamine. Its therapeutic effects are similar to those of belladonna but it is variable in its action. An extract and tincture were popular dosage forms.

hyo·sta·pe·di·al (high″o·stay·pee′dee·ul) *adj.* [*hyo-* + *stapedial*]. Of or pertaining to the hyoid bar and the stapes, which are continuous in early embryologic development.

hyo·thy·roid (high″o·thigh′roid) *adj.* THYROHYOID.

hyothyroid ligament. THYROHYOID LIGAMENT.

hyothyroid membrane. THYROHYOID MEMBRANE.

hyo·ver·te·brot·o·my (high″o·vur″te·brot′uh·mee) *n.* [*hyo-* + *vertebro-* + *-tomy*]. *In veterinary medicine,* the operation of incising the guttural pouch. Syn. *hypospondylotomy.*

hyp-, hypo- [Gk. *hypo-,* beneath]. A prefix meaning (a) *deficiency, lack;* (b) *below, beneath;* (c) (of acids and salts) *having the least number of atoms of oxygen* (as in a series of compounds of the same elements).

hyp·acid·i·ty (hip″uh·sid′i·tee, hipe″) *n.* HYPOACIDITY.

hyp·acu·sia (hip″a·kew′zhuh, ·zee·uh, high″pa·) *n.* [*hyp-* + *-acusia*]. Impairment of hearing. Syn. *hypoacusia.*

hyp·acu·sis (hip″a·kew′sis, high″pa·) *n.* HYPACUSIA.

hypaesthesia. HYPESTHESIA.

hyp·al·bu·min·emia, hyp·al·bu·min·ae·mia (hip″al·bew″min·ee′mee·uh, hipe″) *n.* HYPOALBUMINEMIA.

hyp·al·bu·mi·no·sis (hip″al·bew″mi·no′sis, hipe″) *n.* [*hyp-* + *albumin* + *-osis*]. HYPOALBUMINEMIA.

hyp·al·ge·sia (hip″al·jee′zee·uh, high″pal·) *n.* [*hyp-* + *algesia*]. Diminished sensitivity to pain. —**hypalge·sic** (·zick) *adj.*

hyp·al·gia (hip·al′jee·uh, high·pal′) *n.* [*hyp-* + *-algia*]. HYPALGESIA.

hyp·am·ni·on (hip·am′nee·on, high·pam′) *n.* [*hyp-* + *amnion*]. A small amount of amniotic fluid; OLIGOHYDRAMNIOS.

hyp·an·i·sog·na·thism (hi·pan″i·sog′nuth·iz·um, high·pan″i·) *n.* [*hyp-* + *aniso-* + *gnath-* + *-ism*]. The condition of having the upper teeth broader than the lower, with a lack of correspondence between the jaws. —**hypanisogna·thous** (·us) *adj.*

hy·paph·o·rine (high·paf′o·reen, ·rin) *n.* $C_{14}H_{18}N_2O_2$; the betaine of tryptophan, occurring in various *Erythrina* species; it is a convulsive poison.

Hypaque. Trademark for sodium diatrizoate, a roentgenographic contrast medium for excretory urography and angiography.

hyp·ar·te·ri·al (high″pahr·teer′ee·ul, hip″ahr·) *adj.* [*hyp-* + *arterial*]. Situated beneath an artery; specifically applied to branches of the stem bronchi.

hyparterial bronchus. Any one of the first collateral branches of the stem bronchi except the eparterial bronchus.

hyp·as·the·nia (high″pas·theen′ee·uh, hip″as·) *n.* [*hyp-* + *asthenia*]. Slight loss of strength.

hyp·ax·i·al (high·pack′see·ul, hip·ack′) *adj.* [*hyp-* + *axial*]. Situated beneath the vertebral column; ventral.

hyp·az·o·tu·ria (hip·az″o·tew′ree·uh, high·paz″) *n.* HYPOAZOTURIA.

hy·pen·gyo·pho·bia (high·pen″jee·o·fo′bee·uh) *n.* [Gk. *hypengyos,* liable, accountable, + *-phobia*]. Morbid fear of responsibility.

hyp·eo·sin·o·phil, hyp·eo·sin·o·phile (high″pee·o·sin′uh·fil) *adj. & n.* [*hyp-* + *eosinophil*]. 1. Not staining completely with eosin. 2. A histologic element that does not stain completely with eosin.

hyper- [Gk. *hyper,* beyond, above, over]. A prefix meaning (a) *excessive, excessively;* (b) *above normal;* (c) in anatomy and zoology, *situated above.*

hy·per·ab·duc·tion (high″pur·ab·duck′shun) *n.* [*hyper-* + *abduction*]. Excessive abduction of a limb or part. Syn. *superabduction.*

hyperabduction syndrome. WRIGHT'S SYNDROME.

hy·per·ac·id (high″pur·as′id) *adj.* [*hyper-* + *acid*]. Containing more than the usual or normal concentration of acid.

hy·per·ac·id·am·i·nu·ria (high″pur·as″id·am·i·new′ree·uh) *n.* HYPERAMINOACIDURIA.

hy·per·acid·i·ty (high″pur·a·sid′i·tee) *n.* [*hyper-* + *acidity*]. Excessive acidity.

hyperactive child syndrome. MINIMAL BRAIN DYSFUNCTION SYNDROME.

hy·per·ac·tiv·i·ty (high″pur·ack·tiv′i·tee) *n.* [*hyper-* + *activity*]. Excessive or abnormal activity. See also *hyperactive child syndrome* (= minimal brain dysfunction syndrome). —**hy·per·ac·tive** (high″pur·ack′tiv) *adj.*

hy·per·acu·i·ty (high″pur·uh·kew′i·tee) *n.* [*hyper-* + *acuity*]. Unusual sensory acuity or sharpness, especially of vision.

hy·per·acu·sia (high″pur·a·kew′zhuh, ·zee·uh) *n.* [*hyper-* + *-acusia*]. Abnormal acuteness of the sense of hearing; painful sensitivity to sounds, as in cases of Bell's palsy, with involvement of the nerve to the stapedius.

hy·per·acu·sis (high″pur·a·kew′sis) *n.* HYPERACUSIA.

hy·per·acute (high″pur·uh·kewt′) *adj.* Of extremely rapid onset or course.

hy·per·ad·e·no·sis (high″pur·ad″e·no′sis) *n.* [*hyper-* + *adenosis*]. Enlargement of the lymph nodes.

hy·per·adre·nal·cor·ti·cal·ism (high″pur·a·dree″nul·kor′ti·kul·iz·um) *n.* HYPERADRENALISM.

hy·per·adre·nal·ism (high″pur·uh·dree′nul·iz·um) *n.* [*hyper-* + *adrenal* + *-ism*]. A condition due either to hyperfunction of the adrenal cortex or prolonged or excessive treatment with adrenal cortical hormones, resulting in several clinical syndromes reflecting excessive glucocorticoid, mineralocorticoid, estrogen, or androgen secretion. Syn. *hyperadrenocorticism.*

hy·per·adre·nia (high″pur·a·dree′nee·uh) *n.* [*hyper-* + *adren-* + *-ia*]. HYPERADRENALISM.

hy·per·adre·no·cor·ti·cism (high″pur·a·dree″no·kor′ti·siz·um) *n.* [*hyper-* + *adreno-* + *-cortico-* + *-ism*]. HYPERADRENALISM.

hyperaemia. HYPEREMIA.

hy·per·aer·a·tion (high″pur·ay·ur·ay′shun) *n.* [*hyper-* + *aeration*]. HYPERVENTILATION (1).

hyperaesthesia. HYPERESTHESIA.

hy·per·af·fec·tiv·i·ty (high″pur·a·feck·tiv′i·tee) *n.* A pathologic increase in reaction to normal or mild sensory stimuli.

hy·per·al·do·ste·ron·ism (high″pur·al″do·sterr′o·niz·um, al″do·ste·ro′niz·um) *n.* [*hyper-* + *aldosterone* + *-ism*]. The clinical syndrome of muscle weakness, polyuria, hypertension, hypokalemia, and alkalosis associated with hypersecretion of the mineralocorticoid aldosterone by the adrenal cortex; described as primary hyperaldosteronism when due to adrenal hyperplasia or tumor and as secondary hyperaldosteronism when due to stimuli external to the adrenal gland. Compare *adrenogenital syndrome, Cushing's syndrome.*

hy·per·al·ge·sia (high″pur·al·jee′zee·uh) *n.* [*hyper-* + *algesia*]. Excessive sensitivity to pain. —**hyperalge·sic** (·zick) *adj.*

hy·per·al·gia (high″pur·al′jee·uh) *n.* [*hyper-* + *-algia*]. HYPERALGESIA.

hy·per·al·i·men·ta·tion (high″pur·al″i·men·tay′shun) *n.* [*hyper-* + *alimentation*]. 1. Overfeeding; superalimentation. 2. Prolonged maintenance of full nutritional requirements by intravenous infusion of carbohydrate, fat, amino acids, electrolytes, and vitamins.

hy·per·al·i·men·to·sis (high″pur·al″i·men·to′sis) *n.* [*hyper-* + *aliment* + *-osis*]. Any disease due to excessive eating.

hy·per·ami·no·ac·id·uria (high″pur·am″in·o·as″i·dew′ree·uh, high″pur·a·mee″no·) *n.* [*hyper-* + *aminoaciduria*]. Abnormally high urinary excretion of amino acids.

hy·per·am·mo·ne·mia, hy·per·am·mo·nae·mia (high″pur·am″o·nee′mee·uh) *n.* [*hyper-* + *ammonia* + *-emia*]. 1. An elevation of ammonia in blood; characteristic of a number of metabolic diseases and hepatic encephalopathy. 2. A rare inborn error of metabolism divided into types I and II according to the location of the metabolic block in the urea cycle. Type I is carbamylphosphate synthetase deficiency. Type II is ornithine carbamyl transferase deficiency. Both are accompanied by elevation of ammonia in blood and cerebrospinal fluid; manifested clinically, especially after a meal rich in proteins, by vomiting, agitation and then lethargy, and later by ataxia, slurred speech, ptosis, and mental retardation. Pneumoencephalography may reveal cortical atrophy.

hy·per·am·ne·sia (high″pur·am·nee′zhuh, ·zee·uh) *n.* HYPERMNESIA.

hy·per·am·y·las·emia, hy·per·am·y·las·ae·mia (high″pur·am″i·lay·see′mee·uh) *n.* [*hyper-* + *amylase* + *-emia*]. The presence of abnormally large amounts of amylase or of a macroamylase in the serum.

hy·per·an·a·ki·ne·sia (high″pur·an″uh·ki·nee′zhuh, zee·uh, ·an″uh·kigh·nee′) *n.* [*hyper-* + Gk. *anakinēsis*, a swinging to and fro, + *-ia*]. Excessive activity of a part; hyperkinesia.

hyperanakinesia ven·tric·u·li (ven·trick′yoo·lye). *Obsol.* Exaggerated motor activity of the stomach.

hy·per·aphia (high″pur·ay′fee·uh, ·af′ee·uh) *n.* [*hyper-* + Gk. *haphē*, touch, + *-ia*]. An abnormally acute sense of touch. —**hyper·aph·ic** (·af′ick) *adj.*

hy·per·az·o·te·mia, hy·per·az·o·tae·mia (high″pur·az″o·tee′mee·uh) *n.* AZOTEMIA.

hy·per·az·o·tu·ria (high″pur·az″o·tew′ree·uh) *n.* AZOTURIA.

hy·per·bar·ic (high″pur·băr′ick) *adj.* [*hyper-* + *bar-* + *-ic*]. 1. Of greater weight, density, or pressure. 2. Of an anesthetic solution: having a specific gravity greater than that of the cerebrospinal fluid.

hyperbaric oxygenation. HYPERBARIC OXYGEN TREATMENT.

hyperbaric oxygen treatment. The administration of oxygen, under greater than atmospheric pressure, usually by placing the patient within a room or chamber especially designed for this purpose.

hy·per·bar·ism (high″pur·băr′iz·um) *n.* [*hyper-* + *bar-* + *-ism*]. A condition resulting from an excess of the ambient gas pressure over that within the body tissues, fluids, and cavities.

hy·per·beta·al·a·ni·ne·mia, hy·per·beta·al·a·ni·nae·mia (high″per·bay″tuh·al″uh·neen·ee′mee·uh) *n.* [*hyper-* + *β-alanine* + *-emia*]. An inborn error of metabolism in which there appears to be a deficiency of beta-alanyl-alpha-ketoglutaric amino transferase, resulting in elevated levels of beta-alanine and gamma-aminobutyric acid in blood and cerebrospinal fluid, and increased excretion of beta-aminoisobutyric acid, gamma-aminobutyric acid, and taurine in the urine; manifested clinically by excessive somnolence and seizures.

hy·per·beta·lipo·pro·tein·emia (high″pur·bay″tuh·lip″o·pro·tee·nee′mee·uh) *n.* [*hyper-* + *β-lipoprotein* + *-emia*]. Abnormally high concentration of low-density lipoproteins in the plasma. See also *familial hyperbetalipoproteinemia.*

hy·per·bil·i·ru·bi·ne·mia, hy·per·bil·i·ru·bi·nae·mia (high″pur·bil″i·roo″bi·nee′mee·uh) *n.* [*hyper-* + *bilirubinemia*]. 1. Excessive amount of bilirubin in the blood. 2. A severe and prolonged physiologic jaundice, sometimes seen in a premature newborn.

hy·per·brachy·ceph·a·ly (high″pur·brack″ee·sef′uh·lee) *n.* [*hyper-* + *brachycephaly*]. Extreme brachycephalia, usually a cephalic index over 85.5.

hy·per·brachy·cra·ni·al (high″pur·brack·ee·kray′nee·ul) *adj.* [*hyper-* + *brachycranial*]. Having a cranial index between 85.0 and 89.9.

hy·per·bu·lia (high″pur·bew′lee·uh) *n.* [*hyper-* + Gk. *boulē*, will, + *-ia*]. Exaggerated willfulness.

hy·per·cal·ce·mia, hy·per·cal·cae·mia (high″pur·kal·see′mee·uh) *n.* [*hyper-* + *calc-* + *-emia*]. Excessive quantity of calcium in the blood. Syn. *calcemia.*

hy·per·cal·ci·nu·ria (high″pur·kal·si·new′ree·uh) *n.* [*hyper-* + *calci-* + *-uria*]. An abnormally high level of calcium in the urine.

hy·per·cal·ci·uria (high″pur·kal·si·yoo′ree·uh) *n.* [*hyper-* + *calciuria*]. HYPERCALCINURIA.

hy·per·cal·cu·ria (high″pur·kal·kew′ree·uh) *n.* [*hyper-* + *calc-* + *-uria*]. HYPERCALCINURIA.

hy·per·cap·nia (high″pur·kap′nee·uh) *n.* [*hyper-* + *-capnia*]. Excessive amount of carbon dioxide in the blood.

hy·per·car·bia (high″pur·kahr′bee·uh) *n.* [*hyper-* + *carb-* + *-ia*]. HYPERCAPNIA.

hy·per·car·o·ten·emia, hy·per·car·o·te·nae·mia (high″pur·kăr″o·te·nee′mee·uh) *n.* CAROTENEMIA.

hy·per·ca·thar·sis (high″pur·ka·thahr′sis) *n.* [*hyper-* + *catharsis*]. Excessive purgation of the bowels. —**hypercathar·tic** (·tick) *adj.*

hy·per·ca·thex·is (high″pur·ka·theck′sis) *n.* [*hyper-* + *cathexis*]. Excessive concentration of the psychic energy upon a particular focus.

hy·per·ce·men·to·sis (high″pur·see″men·to′sis, ·sem″en·to′sis) *n.*, pl. **hypercemento·ses** (·seez) [*hyper-* + *cementum* + *-osis*]. Excessive formation of cementum on the root of a tooth.

hy·per·ce·nes·the·sia, hy·per·coe·naes·the·sia (high″pur·see″nes·theezh′uh, ·theez′ee·uh, ·sen″es·) *n.* [*hyper-* + *cenesthesia*]. EUPHORIA (2).

hy·per·cham·aer·rhine (high″pur·kam′e·rine) *adj.* [*hyper-* + *chamaerrhine*]. 1. *In craniometry,* designating an apertura piriformis that is relatively very broad and short; having a nasal index of 58.0 or more. 2. *In somatometry,* designating a nose that is as broad as, or broader than, it is long; having a height-breadth index of 100.0 or more.

hy·per·chlo·re·mia, hy·per·chlo·rae·mia (high″pur·klo·ree′mee·uh) *n.* [*hyper-* + *chlor-* + *-emia*]. An increase in the chloride content of the blood. —**hyperchlo·re·mic, hyperchlo·rae·mic** (·ree′mick) *adj.*

hyperchloremic acidosis. A metabolic acidosis characterized by low blood pH, low blood carbon dioxide, and elevated blood chloride; most commonly seen with renal disease.

hy·per·chlor·hy·dria (high″pur·klor·high′dree·uh) *n.* [*hyper-* + *chlorhydria*]. Excessive secretion of hydrochloric acid in the stomach.

hy·per·cho·les·ter·emia, hy·per·cho·les·ter·ae·mia (high″pur·ko·les″tur·ee′mee·uh) *n.* [*hyper-* + *cholesteremia*]. HYPERCHOLESTEROLEMIA.

hy·per·cho·les·ter·ol·emia, hy·per·cho·les·ter·ol·aemia (high″pur·ko·les″tur·o·lee′mee·uh) *n.* [*hyper-* + *cholesterolemia*]. An excess of cholesterol in the blood. See also *familial hyperlipoproteinemia.* —**hypercholesterole·mic** (·mick) *adj.*

hy·per·cho·lia (high″pur·ko′lee·uh) *n.* [*hyper-* + *chol-* + *-ia*]. Excessive secretion of bile.

hy·per·chro·mat·ic (high″pur·kro·mat′ick) *adj.* [*hyper-* + *chromatic*]. Pertaining to a cell or a portion of a cell which stains more intensely than is normal. Compare *hyperchromic.* —**hyperchro·ma·sia** (·may′zhuh, ·zee·uh) *n.*

hy·per·chro·ma·tism (high″pur·kro′muh·tiz·um) *n.* [*hyperchromatic* + *-ism*]. 1. Excessive formation of the pigment of the skin. 2. A condition in which cells or parts of cells stain more intensely than is normal.

hy·per·chro·ma·to·sis (high″pur·kro″muh·to′sis) *n.* [*hyper-* + *chromatosis*]. Excessive pigmentation, as of the skin.

hy·per·chro·mia (high″pur·kro′mee·uh) *n.* [*hyper-* + *-chromia*]. HYPERCHROMATISM.

hy·per·chro·mic (high″pur·kro′mick) *adj.* [*hyper-* + *chrom-* + *-ic*]. Pertaining to or describing the microscopic appearance of cells of the erythropoietic series, in which dense staining is due not to increased concentration of hemoglobin, but to increased thickness of the cells. Compare *hyperchromatic.*

hyperchromic anemia. 1. Anemia in which the erythrocytes are more deeply colored than usual as a result of increased thickness. See also *macrocytic anemia.* 2. Anemia associated with a lack of vitamin B_{12} and related substances. 3. Megaloblastic anemia associated with pregnancy.

hy·per·chy·lia (high″pur·kigh′lee·uh) *n.* [*hyper-* + *chyl-* + *-ia*]. Excess secretion or formation of chyle.

hy·per·chy·lo·mi·cro·ne·mia, hy·per·chy·lo·mi·cro·nae·mia (high″pur·kigh″lo·migh″kro·nee′mee·uh) *n.* [*hyper-* + *chylomicron* + *-emia*]. FAT-INDUCED FAMILIAL HYPERTRIGLYCERIDEMIA.

Hypercillin. A trademark for penicillin G procaine, an antibacterial.

hy·per·ci·ne·sis (high″pur·si·nee′sis) *n.* [*hyper-* + Gk. *kinēsis,* motion]. HYPERKINESIA.

hy·per·co·ag·u·la·bil·i·ty (high″pur·ko·ag″yoo·luh·bil′i·tee) *n.* A condition in which the blood coagulates more readily than normally.

hypercoenaesthesia. Hypercenesthesia (= EUPHORIA (2)).

hy·per·cor·ti·cism (high″pur·kor′ti·siz·um) *n.* [*hyper-* + *cortico-* + *-ism*]. HYPERADRENALISM.

hy·per·cor·ti·sol·ism (high″pur·kor′ti·so·liz·um) *n.* [*hyper-* + *cortisol* + *-ism*]. Excessive production of hydrocortisone (cortisol) by the adrenal cortex, as in Cushing's syndrome.

hy·per·cry·al·ge·sia (high″pur·krye″al·jee′zee·uh) *n.* [*hyper-* + *cryalgesia*]. Abnormal sensitivity to cold.

hy·per·cry·es·the·sia, hy·per·cry·aes·the·sia (high″pur·krye″es·theez′ee·uh) *n.* [*hyper-* + *cryesthesia*]. HYPERCRYALGESIA.

hy·per·cu·pri·uria (high″pur·koo″pri·yoo′ree·uh) *n.* [*hyper-* + *cupri-* + *-uria*]. Excessive urinary excretion of copper.

hy·per·cy·a·not·ic (high″pur·sigh″uh·not′ick) *adj.* [*hyper-* + *cyanotic*]. Characterized by an extreme degree of cyanosis.

hypercyanotic angina. Angina pectoris in cyanotic patients with congenital heart disease or chronic pulmonary disease; the pain is associated with increased cyanosis occurring with exertion.

hy·per·dac·tyl·ia (high″pur·dack·til′ee·uh) *n.* [*hyper-* + *-dactylia*]. POLYDACTYLY.

hy·per·di·crot·ic (high″pur·dye·krot′ick) *adj.* [*hyper-* + *dicrotic*]. Pertaining to the dicrotic wave of the peripheral pulse which is increased in amplitude, so that it may be detected by palpation. —**hyper·di·cro·tism** (·dye′kro·tiz·um) *n.*

hy·per·dis·ten·tion (high″pur·dis·ten′shun) *n.* [*hyper-* + *distention*]. Forcible or extreme distention.

hy·per·dol·i·cho·cra·ni·al (high″pur·dol″i·ko·kray′nee·ul) *adj.* [*hyper-* + *dolichocranial*]. Having a cranial index between 65.0 and 69.9.

hy·per·dy·na·mia (high″pur·dye·nay′mee·uh, ·di·nay′mee·uh, ·dye·nam′ee·uh) *n.* [*hyper-* + *-dynamia*]. Excessive strength or exaggeration of function, as of nerves or muscles. —**hyperdy·nam·ic** (·nam′ick) *adj.*

hyperdynamic ileus. SPASTIC ILEUS.

hy·per·e·che·ma (high″pur·e·kee′muh) *n.* [*hyper-* + Gk. *ēchēma,* sound]. A normal sound abnormally exaggerated.

hy·per·elas·tic (high″pur·e·las′tick) *adj.* [*hyper-* + *elastic*]. Possessing excessive elasticity. —**hyper·elas·tic·i·ty** (·e·las″tis′i·tee) *n.*

hy·per·em·e·sis (high″pur·em′e·sis) *n.* [*hyper-* + *emesis*]. Excessive vomiting. —**hyper·emet·ic** (·e·met′ick) *adj.*

hyperemesis gra·vi·da·rum (grav·i·dair′rum). PERNICIOUS VOMITING in pregnancy.

hyperemesis lac·ten·ti·um (lack·ten′tee·um, ·chee·um). Vomiting of nurslings.

hy·per·emia, hy·per·ae·mia (high″pur·ee′mee·uh) *n.* [*hyper-* + *-emia*]. Increased blood in a part, resulting in distention of the blood vessels. Hyperemia may be active, when due to dilatation of blood vessels, or passive, when the drainage is hindered. —**hyper·emic, hyper·ae·mic** (ee′mick) *adj.*

hyperemia test. MOSCHCOWITZ TEST.

hy·per·en·ceph·a·lus (high″pur·en·sef′uh·lus) *n.*, pl. **hyperencepha·li** (·lye) [*hyper-* + *-encephalus*]. A type of anencephalus in which the entire cranial vault above the level of the occipital protuberance is absent.

hy·per·eo·sin·o·phil·ia (high″pur·ee″o·sin″uh·fil′ee·uh) *n.* EOSINOPHILIA.—**hypereosinophil·ic** (·ick) *adj.*

hy·per·ep·i·thy·mia (high″pur·ep″i·thigh′mee·uh) *n.* [*hyper-* + Gk. *epithymia,* desire]. Exaggerated desire.

hy·per·equi·lib·ri·um (high″pur·ee″kwi·lib′ree·um) *n.* [*hyper-* + *equilibrium*]. A tendency to vertigo on even slight rotary movement.

hy·per·er·ga·sia (high″pur·ur·gay′zhuh, ·zee·uh) *n.* [*hyper-* + *ergasia*]. HYPERERGIA.

hy·per·er·gia (high″pur·ur′jee·uh) *n.* [*hyper-* + *erg-* + *-ia*]. 1. HYPERERGY. 2. Increased functional activity.

hy·per·er·gy (high′pur·ur·jee) *n.* [*hyper-* + *-ergy*]. An altered state of reactivity, in which the response is more marked than usual; hypersensitivity. It is one form of allergy or pathergy.

hy·per·eso·pho·ria (high″pur·es″o·fo′ree·uh) *n.* [*hyper-* + *esophoria*]. A form of heterophoria in which the visual axis tends to deviate upward and inward.

hy·per·es·the·sia, hy·per·aes·the·sia (high″pur·es·theezh′uh, ·theez′ee·uh) *n.* [*hyper-* + *-esthesia*]. Increased sensitivity (usually cutaneous) to tactile, painful, thermal, and other stimuli. —**hyperes·thet·ic, hyperaes·thet·ic** (·thet′ick) *adj.*

hyperesthesia un·gui·um (ung′gwee·um). ONYCHALGIA NERVOSA.

hy·per·es·trin·emia, hy·per·oes·trin·ae·mia (high″pur·es″tri·nee′mee·uh) *n.* [*hyper-* + *estrin* + *emia*]. HYPERESTROGENEMIA.

hy·per·es·trin·ism, hy·per·oes·trin·ism (high″pur·es′trin·iz·um) *n.* [*hyper-* + *estrin* + *-ism*]. Excessive or prolonged secretion, or both, of the female estrogenic hormones.

hy·per·es·tro·gen·emia, hy·per·oes·tro·gen·ae·mia (high″pur·es″tro·je·nee′mee·uh) *n.* [*hyper-* + *estrogen* + *-emia*]. An excess of estrogens in the blood.

hy·per·es·tro·gen·ism, hy·per·oes·tro·gen·ism (high″pur·es′tro·je·niz·um) *n.* [*hyper-* + *estrogen* + *-ism*]. HYPERESTRINISM.

hy·per·ex·cit·abil·i·ty (high″pur·eck·sight″uh·bil′i·tee) *n.* [*hyper-* + *excitability*]. 1. Excessive excitability. 2. A lowered threshold to excitation.

hyperexcitability syndrome. MINIMAL BRAIN DYSFUNCTION SYNDROME.

hy·per·exo·pho·ria (high″pur·eck″so·fo′ree·uh) *n.* [*hyper-* + *exophoria*]. A form of heterophoria in which the visual axis has a tendency to deviate upward and outward.

hy·per·ex·ten·si·ble (high″pur·ick·sten′si·bul) *adj.* Able to be extended or flexed to a greater extent than normal. —**hy·per·ex·ten·si·bil·i·ty** (·ick·sten″si·bil′i·tee) *n.*

hy·per·ex·ten·sion (high″pur·ick·sten′shun) *n.* [*hyper-* + *extension*]. Overextension of a limb or part for the correction of deformity or for the retention of fractured bones in proper position and alignment.

hy·per·fer·re·mia, hy·per·fer·rae·mia (high″pur·ferr·ee′mee·uh) *n.* [*hyper-* + *ferr*um + *-emia*]. Excessive amounts of iron in the blood plasma. —**hyperferre·mic** (·mick) *adj.*

hy·per·fer·ri·ce·mia, hy·per·fer·ri·cae·mia (high″pur·ferr″i·see′mee·uh) *n.* [*hyper-* + *ferric* + *-emia*]. HYPERFERREMIA.

hy·per·fi·bri·nol·y·sis (high″pur·fye″bri·nol′i·sis) *n.* [*hyper-* + *fibrinolysis*]. Markedly increased fibrinolysis.

hy·per·flex·ion (high″pur·fleck′shun) *n.* [*hyper-* + *flexion*]. Overflexion of a limb or part of the body.

hy·per·fo·cal distance (high″pur·fo′kul). In photography, the nearest point to a lens at which objects will appear sharp in the image space when the lens is focused for objects at an infinite distance.

hy·per·fo·lic·ac·id·emia, hy·per·fo·lic·ac·id·ae·mia (high″pur·fo″lick·as″i·dee′mee·uh) *n.* [*hyper-* + *folic acid* + *-emia*]. A rare inborn error of metabolism, due to formiminotransferase deficiency, in which there is high serum folic acid level, excessive urinary excretion of formiminoglutamic acid following histidine loading, and, clinically, physical and mental retardation, round facies, and obesity. Pathologically there is hypersegmentation of polymorphonuclear cell nuclei. Syn. *glutamate formiminotransferase deficiency syndrome.*

hy·per·func·tion (high″pur·funk′shun) *n.* [*hyper-* + *function*]. Excessive function; excessive activity.

hy·per·gam·ma·glob·u·li·ne·mia, hy·per·gam·ma·glob·u·li·nae·mia (high″pur·gam″uh·glob″yoo·lin·ee′mee·uh) *n.* [*hyper-* + *gamma globulin* + *-emia*]. The increased concentration of immunoglobulins in the blood seen in a wide variety of clinical disorders. See also *diffuse hypergammaglobulinemia, M-component hypergammaglobulinemia.*

hy·per·gen·e·sis (high″pur·jen′e·sis) *n.* [*hyper-* + *-genesis*]. Excessive development or redundancy of the parts or organs of the body. —**hyper·ge·net·ic** (·je·net′ick) *adj.*

hypergenetic teratism. Teratism in which certain organs are disproportionately large.

hy·per·geu·sia (high″pur·gew′see·uh, ·joo′see·uh) *n.* [*hyper-* + *-geusia*]. Abnormal acuteness of the sense of taste.

hy·per·gi·gan·to·so·ma (high″pur·jye·gan″to·so′muh) *n.* [*hyper-* + *giganto-* + *soma*]. *Obsol.* Extraordinary gigantism.

hy·per·glob·u·li·ne·mia, hy·per·glob·u·li·nae·mia (high″pur·glob″yoo·lin·ee′mee·uh) *n.* [*hyper-* + *globulin* + *-emia*]. Increased amount of globulin in the blood plasma or serum.

hy·per·gly·ce·mia, hy·per·gly·cae·mia (high″pur·glye·see′mee·uh) *n.* [*hyper-* + *glycemia*]. Excess of sugar in the blood. —**hyperglyce·mic, hyperglycae·mic** (·mick) *adj.*

hyperglycemic factor. GLUCAGON.

hyperglycemic-glycogenolytic factor. GLUCAGON. Abbreviated, HGF.

hy·per·gly·cin·emia, hy·per·gly·cin·ae·mia (high″pur·glye″sin·ee′mee·uh) *n.* [*hyper-* + *glycine* + *-emia*]. A hereditary (autosomal recessive) metabolic disorder, resulting in abnormally high glycine levels in the blood and glycinuria. The disorder is manifested clinically by episodes of vomiting, severe dehydration with acidosis and ketosis, hypotonia, repeated infections and neutropenia, osteoporosis, and physical and mental retardation. Death usually occurs in early infancy. Pathologically, there is an abnormality of myelination of the central nervous system, with spongy degeneration and lipid-filled glial cells.

hy·per·gly·co·ge·nol·y·sis (high″pur·glye″ko·je·nol′i·sis) *n.* [*hyper-* + *glycogenolysis*]. Excessive glycogenolysis.

hy·per·gly·cor·rha·chia (high″pur·glye″ko·ray′kee·uh, ·rack′ee·uh) *n.* [*hyper-* + *glycorrhachia*]. An excess of glucose in the cerebrospinal fluid; usually secondary to an elevated concentration of glucose in the blood.

hy·per·gly·cos·uria (high″pur·glye″ko·sue′ree·uh) *n.* [*hyper-* + *glycosuria*]. The presence of excessive amounts of sugar in the urine.

hy·per·gly·ox·a·la·tu·ria (high″pur·glye·ock″suh·lay·tew′ree·uh) *n.* [*hyper-* + *glyoxalate* + *-uria*]. An excess of glyoxalate in the urine.

hy·per·go·nad·ism (high″pur·go′nad·iz·um, ·gon′uh·diz·um) *n.* [*hyper-* + *gonad* + *-ism*]. Excessive internal secretion of the sexual glands (testes or ovaries).

hy·per·go·nia (high″pur·go′nee·uh) *n.* [*hyper-* + Gk. *gōnia*, angle]. Increase in size of the gonial angle.

hy·per·he·do·nia (high″pur·he·do′nee·uh) *n.* [*hyper-* + Gk. *hēdonē*, pleasure, + *-ia*]. 1. An excessive feeling of pleasure in any sensation or the gratification of a desire. 2. Erethism relating to the sexual organs.

hy·per·he·don·ism (high″pur·hee′dun·iz·um) *n.* HYPERHEDONIA.

hy·per·he·mo·lyt·ic, hy·per·hae·mo·lyt·ic (high″pur·hee″mo·lit′ick) *adj.* [*hyper-* + *hemolytic*]. Of, pertaining to, or caused by excessive hemolysis.

hyperhemolytic jaundice. Hemolytic jaundice due to inability of the liver to excrete the quantity of pigment presented to it as the result of excessive hemolysis.

hy·per·hep·a·rin·emia, hy·per·hep·a·rin·ae·mia (high″pur·hep″uh·rin·ee′mee·uh) *n.* [*hyper-* + *heparin* + *-emia*]. Excessive amounts of heparin in the blood.

hy·per·hi·dro·sis (high″pur·hi·dro′sis, ·high·dro′sis) *n.* [*hyper-* + *hidrosis*]. Excessive sweating; may be localized or generalized, chronic or acute; the sweat often accumulates in visible drops on the skin. Syn. *ephidrosis, polyhidrosis, sudatoria.*

hy·per·his·ta·mi·ne·mia, hy·per·his·ta·mi·nae·mia (high″pur·his″tuh·min·ee″mee·uh) *n.* [*hyper-* + *histamine* + *-emia*]. An increase of histamine in the blood.

hy·per·hor·mo·nal (high″pur·hor·mo′nul) *adj.* [*hyper-* + *hormonal*]. Containing, or due to, excess of a hormone.

hy·per·i·dro·sis (high″pur·i·dro′sis) *n.* HYPERHIDROSIS.

hy·per·im·mu·no·glob·u·lin·emia, hy·per·im·mu·no·glob·u·lin·ae·mia (high″pur·im″mew·no·glob″yoo·lin·ee′mee·uh) *n.*

[*hyper-* + *immunoglobulin* + *-emia*]. HYPERGAMMAGLOBULINEMIA.

hy·per·in·fla·tion (high"pur·in·flay'shun) *n.* Overdistention of an inflatable structure.

hy·per·ino·se·mia, hy·per·ino·sae·mia (high"pur·in"o·see' mee·uh, ·eye"no·) *n.* [*hyper-* + *inosemia*]. Excessive formation of fibrin in the blood; hypercoagulability of the blood.

hy·per·ino·sis (high"pur·i·no'sis) *n.* HYPERINOSEMIA.

hy·per·in·su·lin·ism (high"pur·in'sue·lin·iz·um) *n.* [*hyper-* + *insulin* + *-ism*]. The presence of high circulating blood levels of endogenous insulin, seen in a variety of conditions, such as obesity and insulin-producing tumors, and in newborns of diabetic mothers. Symptoms may or may not be present.

hy·per·in·vo·lu·tion (high"pur·in·vuh·lew'shun) *n.* [*hyper-* + *involution*]. A rapid shrinking to less than normal size of an organ that has been enlarged, as of the uterus after delivery.

hy·per·ir·ri·ta·bil·i·ty (high"pur·irr"i·tuh·bil'i·tee) *n.* [*hyper-* + *irritability*]. The pathologically excessive reaction of an individual, organ, or part to a given stimulus.

hy·per·ka·le·mia (high"pur·ka·lee'mee·uh) *n.* [*hyper-* + *kalemia*]. An elevation above normal of potassium in the blood. **—hyperkale·mic** (·mick) *adj.*

hy·per·kal·i·emia, hy·per·kal·i·ae·mia (high"pur·kal·ee·ee' mee·uh) *n.* HYPERKALEMIA.

hy·per·ker·a·tin·iza·tion (high"pur·kerr"uh·tin·i·zay'shun) *n.* [*hyper-* + *keratinization*]. Excessive production of keratin.

hy·per·ker·a·to·sis (high"pur·kerr"uh·to'sis) *n.*, pl. **hyperker·ato·ses** (·seez) [*hyper-* + *keratosis*]. Hypertrophy of the horny layer of the skin, usually associated with hypertrophy of the granular and prickle-cell layers.

hyperkeratosis ex·cen·tri·ca (eck·sen'tri·kuh). POROKERATOSIS.

hyperkeratosis fol·lic·u·la·ris et para·fol·lic·u·la·ris in cu·tem pen·e·trans (fol·ick"yoo·lair'is et păr"uh·fol·ick"yoo·lair'is in kew'tem pen'e·tranz). KYRLE'S DISEASE.

hyperkeratosis lac·u·na·ris pha·ryn·gis (lack"yoo·nair'is fa·rin'jis). A condition characterized by numerous hard white masses sometimes developing into long horny spines, projecting from the nodules of the lymphatic ring about the pharynx.

hyperkeratosis lin·guae (ling'gwee). BLACK, HAIRY TONGUE.

hyperkeratosis sub·un·gua·lis (sub"ung·gway'lis). Hyperkeratosis affecting the nail bed.

hy·per·ker·a·tot·ic (high"pur·kerr"uh·tot'ick) *adj.* Of, pertaining to, or characterized by hyperkeratosis.

hyperkeratotic eczema. The type of eczema in which the stratum corneum is thickened.

hyperkeratotic ulcer. A chronic, nonmalignant, cutaneous ulcer with hyperkeratosis of the margin.

hy·per·ke·to·ne·mia, hy·per·ke·to·nae·mia (high"pur·kee"to·nee'mee·uh) *n.* KETONEMIA.

hy·per·ke·to·nu·ria (high"pur·kee"to·new'ree·uh) *n.* [*hyper-* + *ketonuria*]. The presence of an excess of ketone in the urine.

hy·per·ki·ne·mia, hy·per·ki·nae·mia (high"pur·ki·nee'mee·uh) *n.* [*hyper-* + *kin-* + *-emia*]. A condition marked by an abnormally increased cardiac output at rest and lying supine.

hy·per·ki·ne·sia (high"pur·ki·nee'zhuh, ·zee·uh, ·kigh·nee') *n.* [*hyper-* + *-kinesia*]. Excessive movement; excessive muscular activity. Contr. *hypokinesia.* See also *hyperactivity.* **—hyperki·net·ic** (·net'ick) *adj.*

hy·per·ki·ne·sis (high"pur·ki·nee'sis) *n.* HYPERKINESIA.

hyperkinetic behavior syndrome. MINIMAL BRAIN DYSFUNCTION SYNDROME.

hyperkinetic child syndrome. MINIMAL BRAIN DYSFUNCTION SYNDROME.

hyperkinetic heart syndrome. A syndrome of unknown cause in young adults, characterized by an increased cardiac output at rest, increased rate of ventricular ejection, and in some patients, the development of heart failure.

hyperkinetic impulse disorder. MINIMAL BRAIN DYSFUNCTION SYNDROME.

hyperkinetic syndrome. MINIMAL BRAIN DYSFUNCTION SYNDROME.

hy·per·lac·ta·tion (high"pur·lack·tay'shun) *n.* [*hyper-* + *lactation*]. Excessive or prolonged secretion of milk.

hy·per·lep·tor·rhine (high"pur·lep'to·rine) *adj.* [*hyper-* + *leptorrhine*]. *In somatometry,* designating a nose that is relatively very long and narrow, having a height-breadth index of 54.9 or less.

hy·per·leu·ko·cy·to·sis (high"pur·lew"ko·sigh·to'sis) *n.* [*hyper-* + *leukocytosis*]. An excessive increase in leukocytes per unit volume of blood.

hy·per·lip·ac·i·de·mia (high"pur·lip·as"i·dee'mee·uh) *n.* [*hyper-* + *lip-* + *acid* + *-emia*]. Excessive blood levels of fatty acids.

hy·per·li·pe·mia, hy·per·li·pae·mia (high"pur·li·pee'mee·uh) *n.* An excess of lipemic substances in the blood. See also *familial hyperlipoproteinemia.* **—hyperlipe·mic, hyperlipae·mic** (·mick) *adj.*

hy·per·lip·id·emia, hy·per·lip·id·ae·mia (high"pur·lip"i·dee' mee·uh) *n.* [*hyper-* + *lipid* + *-emia*]. HYPERLIPEMIA.

hy·per·lipo·pro·tein·emia, hy·per·lipo·pro·tein·ae·mia (high" pur·lip"o·pro·tee·nee'mee·uh) *n.* An excess of lipoproteins in the blood. See also *familial hyperlipoproteinemia.*

hy·per·li·thu·ria (high"pur·lith·yoo'ree·uh) *n.* [*hyper-* + *lith*ic acid + *-uria*]. An excess of uric (lithic) acid in the urine.

hy·per·lo·gia (high"pur·lo'jee·uh) *n.* [*hyper-* + *-logia*]. Excessive or manic loquacity.

hy·per·ly·si·ne·mia, hy·per·ly·si·nae·mia (high"pur·lye"si·nee'mee·uh) *n.* [*hyper-* + *lysine* + *-emia*]. A hereditary metabolic disorder of unknown cause, in which there is an abnormally high blood level of lysine and excessive urinary excretion of ornithine, gamma-aminobutyric acid and ethanolamine, and delayed conversion of injected lysine to carbon dioxide; the disorder is manifested clinically by physical and mental retardation, lax ligaments and hypotonia, seizures in early life, and impaired sexual development.

hy·per·mag·ne·se·mia, hy·per·mag·ne·sae·mia (high"pur·mag"ne·see'mee·uh) *n.* [*hyper-* + *magnes*ium + *-emia*]. Abnormally high serum magnesium levels.

hy·per·ma·nia (high"pur·may'nee·uh) *n.* [*hyper-* + *mania*]. An advanced manic type of manic-depressive illness. **—hyper·man·ic** (·man'ick) *adj.*

hy·per·mas·tia (high"pur·mas'tee·uh) *n.* [*hyper-* + *-mastia*]. Overgrowth of the mammary gland.

hy·per·ma·ture (high"pur·muh·tewr') *adj.* [*hyper-* + *mature*]. Overmature; overripe.

hypermature cataract. A cataract which has become liquified with partial escape of lens substance. Contr. *immature cataract, mature cataract.* See also *Morgagnian cataract.*

hy·per·meg·a·so·ma (high"pur·meg"uh·so'muh) *n.* [*hyper-* + *mega-* + *-soma*]. *Obsol.* HYPERGIGANTOSOMA.

hy·per·mel·a·no·sis (high"pur·mel·uh·no'sis) *n.* [*hyper-* + *melan-* + *-osis*]. Increase in melanin pigmentation. **—hyper·mela·not·ic** (·not'ick) *adj.*

hy·per·men·or·rhea, hy·per·men·or·rhoea (high"pur·men"o·ree'uh) *n.* [*hyper-* + *menorrhea*]. MENORRHAGIA.

hy·per·me·tab·o·lism (high"pur·me·tab'uh·liz·um) *n.* [*hyper-* + *metabolism*]. Any state in which there is an abnormal increase in metabolic rate. **—hyper·met·a·bol·ic** (·met"uh·bol'ick) *adj.*

hy·per·me·tro·pia (high"pur·me·tro'pee·uh) *n.* [*hyper-* + *metr-* + *-opia*]. HYPEROPIA. **—hyper·met·rope** (·met'rope) *n.* **—hyperme·tro·pic** (·trop'ick, ·tro'pick) *adj.*

hypermetropic astigmatism. HYPEROPIC ASTIGMATISM.

hy·per·mi·cro·so·ma (high"pur·migh"kro·so'muh) *n.* [*hyper-* + *micro-* + *-soma*]. Extreme dwarfism.

hy·per·mim·ia (high"pur·mim'ee·uh) *n.* [*hyper-* + Gk. *mimos,* actor, mime, + *-ia*]. Excessive emotional expression or mimetic movement.

hy·per·min·er·alo·cor·ti·coid·ism (hy″pur·min″ur·uh·lo·kor′ti·koid·iz·um) *n.* [*hyper-* + *mineral* + *corticoid* + *-ism*]. A pathologic state resulting from the excessive production of adrenal cortical steroids affecting mineral metabolism.

hy·perm·ne·sia (high″purm·nee′zhuh, ·zee·uh) *n.* [*hyper-* + *-mnesia*]. Unusual ability of memory.

hy·perm·ne·sis (high″purm·nee′sis) *n.* HYPERMNESIA.

hy·per·mo·til·i·ty (high″pur·mo·til′i·tee) *n.* [*hyper-* + *motility*]. Increased motility, as of the stomach or intestines.

hy·per·na·tre·mia, hy·per·na·trae·mia (high″pur·na·tree′mee·uh) *n.* [*hyper-* + *natremia*]. Abnormally high sodium level in the blood. **—hypernatre·mic** (·mick) *adj.*

hy·per·nea, hy·per·noea (high″pur·nee′uh) *n.* [NL., variant of *hypernoia*]. HYPERPSYCHOSIS.

hy·per·neph·roid (high″pur·nef′roid) *adj.* [*hyper-* (= *supra*) + *nephr-* (= *renal*) + *-oid*]. Resembling the adrenal gland.

hypernephroid tumor. A tumor whose cells resemble those of the adrenal gland.

hy·per·ne·phro·ma (high″pur·ne·fro′muh) *n.*, pl. **hypernephromas, hypernephroma·ta** (·tuh) [*hyper-* (= *supra-*) + *nephr-* (= *renal*) + *-oma*]. 1. Originally, a variety of tumor of the kidney supposed to be derived from embryonal inclusions of adrenocortical tissue in the kidney. 2. RENAL CELL CARCINOMA.

hy·per·noia (high″pur·noy′uh) *n.* [*hyper-* + Gk. *noos*, mind, + *-ia*]. HYPERPSYCHOSIS.

hy·per·nu·tri·tion (high″pur·new·trish′un) *n.* [*hyper-* + *nutrition*]. SUPERALIMENTATION.

hyperoestrinaemia. Hyperestrinemia (= HYPERESTROGENEMIA).

hyperoestrinism. HYPERESTRINISM.

hyperoestrogenaemia. HYPERESTROGENEMIA.

hyperoestrogenism. Hyperestrogenism (= HYPERESTRINISM).

hy·per·on (high′pur·on) *n.* [*hyper-* + *-on*]. A short-lived elementary nuclear particle with a mass greater than that of the neutron.

hy·per·on·to·morph (high″pur·on′to·morf) *n.* [*hyper-* + *onto-* + *-morph*]. A person of a long, thin body type.

hy·per·onych·ia (high″pur·o·nick′ee·uh) *n.* [*hyper-* + *onych-* + *-ia*]. Hypertrophy of the nails.

hy·per·ope (high′pur·ope) *n.* A person with hyperopia.

hy·per·oph·thal·mo·path·ic Graves' disease (high″pur·off·thal″mo·path′ick). Graves' disease in which ophthalmopathy is the predominant feature, usually characterized pathologically by an inflammatory infiltrate of the orbital contents, whose cellular components are mainly lymphocytes, mast cells, and plasma cells and by degeneration and fibrosis of muscle fibers, which causes the globe to protrude.

hy·per·opia (high″pur·o′pee·uh) *n.* [*hyper-* + *-opia*]. A refractive error in which, with suspended accommodation, the focus of parallel rays of light falls behind the retina; due to an abnormally short anteroposterior diameter of the eye or to subnormal refractive power. Abbreviated, H. Syn. *hypermetropia, farsightedness.*

hy·per·opic (high″pur·o′pick) *adj.* Pertaining to or having hyperopia.

hyperopic astigmatism. Hyperopia with astigmatism; it may be simple, with one principal meridian hyperopic and the other normal; or compound, with both meridians hyperopic but one more so than the other. Symbol, ah.

hy·per·orex·ia (high″pur·o·reck′see·uh) *n.* [*hyper-* + *-orexia*]. BULIMIA.

hy·per·or·ni·thi·ne·mia (high″pur·or″ni·thi·nee′mee·uh) *n.* [*hyper-* + *ornithene* + *-emia*]. A rare inherited metabolic disorder associated with hyperammonemia.

hy·per·or·thog·na·thy (high″pur·or·thog′nuth·ee) *n.* [*hyper-* + *ortho-* + *gnath-* + *-y*]. 1. The condition of having a profile angle of greater than 93°. 2. The condition of having an exceedingly low gnathic (alveolar) index. **—hyperorthog·na·thous** (·nuth·us) *adj.*

hy·per·os·mia (high″pur·oz′mee·uh, ·os′mee·uh) *n.* [*hyper-* + *osm-* + *-ia*]. An abnormally acute sense of smell.

hy·per·os·mo·lar (high″pur·oz″mo′lur) *n.* [*hyper-* + *osmolarity*]. Of solutions: having an osmotic pressure greater than that of normal plasma. Compare *osmolar* **—hyperos·mo·lar·i·ty** (·mo·lăr′i·tee) *n.*

hy·per·os·te·og·e·ny (high″pur·os″tee·oj′e·nee) *n.* [*hyper-* + *osteogeny*]. Excessive development of bone.

hy·per·os·to·sis (high″pur·os·to′sis) *n.*, pl. **hyperosto·ses** (·seez) [*hyper-* + *ostosis*]. Exostosis or hypertrophy of bone tissue. **—hyperos·tot·ic** (·tot′ick) *adj.*

hyperostosis fron·ta·lis in·ter·na (fron·tay′lis in·tur′nuh). An idiopathic condition occurring almost exclusively in women, in which new bone is formed in a symmetrical pattern on the inner aspect of the frontal bone; usually of no clinical significance but historically associated with the Stewart-Morel-Morgagni syndrome.

hy·per·ox·al·uria (high″pur·ock″suh·lew′ree·uh) *n.* [*hyper-* + *oxaluria*]. The excessive excretion of oxalates in the urine. See also *oxalosis.*

hyperoxaluria, type I. OXALOSIS, type I.

hyperoxaluria, type II. OXALOSIS, type II.

hy·per·ox·emia, hy·per·ox·ae·mia (high″pur·ock·see′mee·uh) *n.* [*hyper-* + *ox-* + *-emia*]. Extreme acidity of the blood.

hy·per·ox·ia (high″pur·ock′see·uh) *n.* [*hyper-* + *ox-* + *-ia*]. An excessive amount of oxygen.

hy·per·ox·y·gen·a·tion (high″pur·ock″si·je·nay′shun) *n.* [*hyper-* + *oxygenation*]. An excessive amount of oxygen in the body.

hy·per·par·a·site (high″pur·păr′uh·site) *n.* [*hyper-* + *parasite*]. A secondary parasite interfering with the development of a previously existing parasite. **—hyperpara·sit·ism** (·si·tiz·um) *n.*

hy·per·para·thy·roid·ism (high″pur·păr″uh·thigh′roy·diz·um) *n.* [*hyper-* + *parathyroid* + *-ism*]. A state produced by an increased functioning of the parathyroid glands.

hy·per·path·ia (high″pur·path′ee·uh) *n.* [*hyper-* + *-pathia*]. 1. An exaggerated or excessive perception of or response to any painful stimulus. 2. A condition in which all tactile, painful, and thermal stimuli have a severely painful and unpleasant quality, usually associated with an elevated threshold to these stimuli. Compare *hyperesthesia.*

hy·per·pep·sin·ia (high″pur·pep·sin′ee·uh) *n.* [*hyper-* + *pepsin* + *-ia*]. Excessive secretion of pepsin in the stomach.

hy·per·peri·stal·sis (high″pur·perr″i·stal′sis, ·stahl′sis) *n.* [*hyper-* + *peristalsis*]. An increase in the occurrence, rate, or depth of peristaltic waves.

hy·per·pex·ia (high″pur·peck′see·uh) *n.* [*hyper-* + *-pexia*]. The binding of an excessive amount of a substance by a tissue.

hy·per·pha·gia (high·pur·fay′jee·uh) *n.* [*hyper-* + *-phagia*]. BULIMIA.

hy·per·pha·lan·gia (high″pur·fuh·lan′jee·uh) *n.* HYPERPHALANGISM.

hy·per·pha·lan·gism (high″pur·fuh·lan′jiz·um) *n.* [*hyper-* + *phalang-* + *-ism*]. The presence of supernumerary phalanges. See also *triphalangism.*

hy·per·pha·lan·gy (high″pur·fuh·lan′jee) *n.* HYPERPHALANGISM.

hy·per·phen·yl·al·a·nin·emia, hy·per·phen·yl·al·a·nin·ae·mia (high″per·fen″il·al″uh·ni·nee′mee·uh) *n.* [*hyper-* + *phenylalanine* + *-emia*]. The presence of abnormally high blood levels of phenylalanine, which may or may not be associated with elevated tyrosine levels, observed in premature and also in full-term newborn infants and associated with the heterozygous state of phenylketonuria, maternal phenylketonuria, or transient deficiency of phenylalanine hydroxylase or *p*-hydroxyphenylpyruvic acid oxidase.

hy·per·pho·ne·sis (high″pur·fo·nee′sis) *n.* [*hyper-* + Gk. *phōnēsis*, a sound, call, utterance]. Increased intensity of the percussion note or of the voice sound on auscultation.

hy·per·pho·nia (high″pur·fo′nee·uh) *n.* [*hyper-* + *-phonia*]. Excessive utterance of vocal sounds, especially in stuttering.

hy·per·pho·ria (high″pur·fo′ree·uh) *n.* [*hyper-* + *-phoria*]. A condition of latent strabismus or intermittent hypertropia in which the visual axis of one eye tends to deviate upward as compared with that of the other.

hy·per·phos·pha·te·mia, hy·per·phos·pha·tae·mia (high″pur·fos·fay·tee′mee·uh, ·fos·fuh·tee′mee·uh) *n.* [*hyper-* + *phosphatemia*]. Increased levels of inorganic phosphate in serum.

hy·per·phos·pha·tu·ria (high″pur·fos″fay·tew′ree·uh, ·fos·fuh·tew′) *n.* [*hyper-* + *phosphaturia*]. An excess of phosphates in the urine.

hy·per·pi·e·sia (high″pur·pye·ee′zhuh, ·zee·uh) *n.* [*hyper-* + Gk. *piesis*, pressure, + *-ia*]. Abnormally high blood pressure; especially, essential hypertension. —**hyperpi·et·ic** (·et′ick) *adj.*

hy·per·pi·e·sis (high″pur·pye·ee′sis) *n.* HYPERPIESIA.

hy·per·pig·men·ta·tion (high″pur·pig″men·tay′shun) *n.* [*hyper-* + *pigmentation*]. Excessive or increased pigmentation.

hy·per·pi·tu·i·ta·rism (high″pur·pi·tew′i·tuh·riz·um) *n.* [*hyper-* + *pituitary* + *-ism*]. 1. Increased growth-hormone secretion from the anterior lobe of the hypophysis with resultant gigantism or acromegaly. 2. Increased secretion of any anterior pituitary trophic hormone, particularly ACTH, producing Cushing's syndrome.

hy·per·pla·sia (high″pur·play′zhuh, ·zee·uh) *n.* [*hyper-* + *-plasia*]. Excessive formation of tissue; an increase in the size of a tissue or organ owing to an increase in the number of cells. Compare *hypertrophy.* —**hyper·plas·tic** (·plas′tick) *adj.*

hyperplastic inflammation. PRODUCTIVE INFLAMMATION.

hyperplastic periostosis. INFANTILE CORTICAL HYPEROSTOSIS.

hyperplastic pulpitis. A chronic inflammatory response characterized by protrusion of the pulp of a tooth through an opening in the pulp chamber, usually seen in young individuals with a deep carious lesion that exposes the pulp. Syn. *hypertrophic pulp, pulp polyp.*

hy·per·platy·mer·ic (high″pur·plat″i·merr′ick) *adj.* [*hyper-* + *platymeric*]. *In osteometry,* designating a femur with an exaggerated anteroposterior compression of the proximal portion of the diaphysis; having a platymeric index of 74.9 or less.

hy·per·pnea, hy·per·pnoea (high″pur·nee′uh, ·pnee′uh) *n.* [*hyper-* + *-pnea*]. Increase in depth and rate of respiration.

hy·per·po·lar·iza·tion (high″pur·po″lur·i·zay′shun) *n.* An increase in polarity, as across a cell membrane.

hy·per·po·lar·iza·tion block. An increase of the negative charge on the inside of a nerve membrane, which diminishes depolarization of the nerve membrane and blocks nerve impulse conduction.

hy·per·po·ro·sis (high″pur·po·ro′sis) *n.* [*hyper-* + Gk. *pōros*, callus, + *-osis*]. An excessive formation of callus in the reunion of fractured bones.

hy·per·po·tas·se·mia, hy·per·po·tas·sae·mia (high″pur·po·ta·see′mee·uh) *n.* [*hyper-* + *potassemia*]. HYPERKALEMIA.

hy·per·pra·gia (high″pur·pray′jee·uh) *n.* [*hyper-* + *-pragia*]. An excess of thinking and feeling, commonly observed in the manic type of the manic-depressive illness. —**hyper·prag·ic** (·praj′ick) *adj.*

hy·per·prax·ia (high″pur·prack′see·uh) *n.* [*hyper-* + *-praxia*]. Restlessness of movement; HYPERACTIVITY.

hy·per·pre·beta·lipo·pro·tein·emia (high″pur·pree″bay″tuh·lip″o·pro·tee·nee′mee·uh) *n.* [*hyper-* + *prebetalipoprotein* + *-emia*]. An excessive concentration of very low-density lipoproteins in the plasma. See also *familial hyperprebetalipoproteinemia, familial hyperchylomicronemia.*

hy·per·pres·by·opia (high″pur·prez″bee·o′pee·uh) *n.* [*hyper-* + *presbyopia*]. Excessive presbyopia.

hy·per·pro·cho·re·sis (high″pur·pro″ko·ree′sis) *n.* [*hyper-* + Gk. *prochōrēsis*, progress, progression]. Excessive motor function of the gastrointestinal tract.

hy·per·pro·lin·emia, hy·per·pro·lin·ae·mia (high″pur·pro″li·nee′mee·uh) *n.* [*hyper-* + *proline* + *-emia*]. A hereditary metabolic disorder in which there is an abnormally high blood level of proline, and mental retardation clinically. In type I of this disorder, there is a deficiency of proline oxidase, increased urinary excretion of hydroxyproline and glycine, and an association with renal disease. In type II, there is a deficiency of Δ^1-pyrroline-5-carboxylate dehydrogenase, excessive urinary excretion of Δ^1-pyrroline-5-carboxylate, as well as proline, hydroxyproline, and glycine; clinically there are seizures and mental retardation.

hy·per·pro·sex·ia (high″pur·pro·seck′see·uh) *n.* [*hyper-* + Gk. *prosexis*, application, + *-ia*]. Marked attention to one subject, as to one idea or symptom. Compare *fixed idea.*

hy·per·pro·tein·emia, hy·per·pro·tein·ae·mia (high″pur·pro″tee·in·ee′mee·uh) *n.* [*hyper-* + *protein* + *-emia*]. Abnormally high blood protein level.

hy·per·psy·cho·sis (high″pur·sigh·ko′sis) *n.* [*hyper-* + *psych-* + *-osis*]. Exaggerated mental activity.

hy·per·py·rex·ia (high′pur·pye·reck′see·uh) *n.* [*hyper-* + *pyrexia*]. Excessively high fever. —**hyperpy·ret·ic** (·ret′ick) *adj.*

hy·per·re·flex·ia (high″pur·re·fleck′see·uh) *n.* [*hyper-* + *reflex* + *-ia*]. A condition in which reflexes are increased above normal, due to a variety of causes. —**hyperreflex·ic** (·sick) *adj.*

hy·per·res·o·nance (high″pur·rez′uh·nunce) *n.* [*hyper-* + *resonance*]. Exaggeration of normal resonance on percussion; heard chiefly in pulmonary emphysema and pneumothorax.

hy·per·ru·gos·i·ty (high″pur·roo·gos′i·tee) *n.* [*hyper-* + *rugosity*]. An excessive number of folds or excessively prominent folds.

hy·per·sal·i·va·tion (high″pur·sal″i·vay′shun) *n.* [*hyper-* + *salivation*]. Abnormally increased secretion of saliva.

hy·per·se·cre·tion (high″pur·se·kree′shun) *n.* [*hyper-* + *secretion*]. Excessive secretion. —**hypersecre·to·ry** (·tuh·ree) *adj.*

hy·per·seg·men·ta·tion (high″pur·seg·men·tay′shun) *n.* Division into more than the usual number of segments or lobes.

hy·per·sen·si·tiv·i·ty (high″pur·sen″si·tiv′i·tee) *n.* [*hyper-* + *sensitivity*]. The state of being abnormally sensitive or susceptible, as to the action of allergens. See also *allergy.*

hy·per·sen·si·ti·za·tion (high″pur·sen″si·ti·zay′shun) *n.* The process of producing hypersensitivity.

hy·per·se·ro·to·nin·emia, hy·per·se·ro·to·nin·ae·mia (high″pur·serr″o·to″ni·nee′mee·uh, ·seer″o·) *n.* [*hyper-* + *serotonin* + *-emia*]. 1. Excessive amounts of circulating serotonin. See also *carcinoid syndrome.* 2. A rare inborn error of metabolism of unknown cause in which abnormally high blood levels of serotonin are associated over a long period of time with episodes of flushing, rage attacks, ataxia, seizures, intermittent hypertension, and other manifestations of disturbances of the autonomic and central nervous systems.

hy·per·som·nia (high″pur·som′nee·uh) *n.* [*hyper-* + *somn-* + *-ia*]. Excessive sleepiness.

hypersomnia-bulimia syndrome. KLEINE-LEVIN SYNDROME.

hy·per·splen·ism (high″pur·splen′iz·um, ·spleen′iz·um) *n.* [*hyper-* + *splen-* + *-ism*]. A pattern of reaction in which the peripheral blood lacks one or more formed elements whose precursors in the bone marrow are present in normal or increased numbers; removal of the spleen leads, at least temporarily, to return toward normal levels. The reaction may accompany any recognized splenic disease, or may occur idiopathically. Syn. *dyssplenism.*

Hyperstat. A trademark for diazoxide, an antihypertensive.

hy·per·sthe·nia (high″pur·sthee′nee·uh) *n.* [*hyper-* + Gk.

sthenos, strength, + *-ia*]. A condition of exalted strength or tone of the body. —**hyper·sthen·ic** (·sthen'ick) *adj.*

hy·per·tel·or·ism (high"pur·tel'ur·iz·um) *n.* [*hyper-* + Gk. *tēle*, far off, + *horizein*, to be separated, + *-ism*]. Excessive width between two organs or parts. Contr. *hypotelorism*. See also *ocular hypertelorism*.

Hypertensin. Trademark for the vasoconstrictor and vasopressor drug angiotensin amide.

hy·per·ten·sin (high"pur·ten'sin) *n.* ANGIOTENSIN.

hy·per·ten·sin·o·gen (high"pur·ten·sin'uh·jen) *n.* ANGIOTENSINOGEN. —**hyperten·sin·o·gen·ic** (·sin·o·jen'ick) *adj.*

hy·per·ten·sion (high"pur·ten'shun) *n.* [*hyper-* + *tension*]. 1. Excessive tension or pressure, especially that exerted by bodily fluids such as blood or aqueous humor. 2. Specifically, high blood pressure. Contr. *normotension*. See *essential hypertension, malignant hypertension, portal hypertension.*

hy·per·ten·sive (high"pur·ten'siv) *adj. & n.* 1. Pertaining to, characterized by, or causing hypertension. 2. A person affected with hypertension.

hypertensive meningeal hydrops. PSEUDOTUMOR CEREBRI.

hypertensive retinopathy. A vascular retinopathy associated with arteriolar sclerosis; characterized by cotton-wool exudates, linear hemmorrhages, and AV nicking.

hy·per·ten·sor (high"pur·ten'sur, ·sor) *n.* A substance capable of raising blood pressure.

Hyper-tet. A trademark for tetanus immune human globulin.

hy·per·the·co·sis (high"pur·thee·ko'sis) *n.* [*hyper-* + *theca* + *-osis*]. Hyperplasia of the ovarian theca interna, with increased luteinization of the cells.

hy·per·the·lia (high"pur·theel'ee·uh) *n.* [*hyper-* + *thel-* + *-ia*]. The presence of supernumerary nipples.

hy·per·therm·al·ge·sia (high"pur·thur"mal·jee'zee·uh, ·see·uh) *n.* [*hyper-* + *therm-* + *algesia*]. Abnormal sensitivity to heat.

hy·per·ther·mia (high"pur·thur'mee·uh) *n.* [*hyper-* + *-thermia*]. 1. HYPERPYREXIA. 2. The treatment of disease by the induction of fever, as by inoculation with malaria, by injection of foreign proteins, or by physical means.

hy·per·ther·mo·es·the·sia, hy·per·ther·mo·aes·the·sia (high"pur·thur"mo·es·theezh'uh, ·theez'ee·uh) *n.* [*hyper-* + *thermo-* + *esthesia*]. HYPERTHERMALGESIA.

hy·per·ther·my (high'pur·thur"mee) *n.* HYPERTHERMIA.

hy·per·thy·mia (high"pur·thigh'mee·uh) *n.* [Gk. *hyperthymos*, vehement, angry, + *-ia*]. 1. Excessive sensibility or oversensitiveness. 2. Vehement cruelty or foolhardiness as a symptom of mental disorder. 3. Pathologically labile or unstable emotionality.

hy·per·thy·mism (high"pur·thigh'miz·um) *n.* [*hyper-* + *thymus* + *-ism*]. Excessive activity of the thymus gland.

hy·per·thy·mi·za·tion (high"pur·thigh"mi·zay'shun) *n.* HYPERTHYMISM.

hy·per·thy·roid·ism (high"pur·thigh'roy·diz·um) *n.* [*hyper-* + *thyroid* + *-ism*]. The constellation of signs and symptoms due to excessive thyroid hormone in the blood, either from exaggerated functional activity of the thyroid gland or from excessive administration of thyroid hormone; manifested by thyroid enlargement, emaciation, sweating, tachycardia, exophthalmos, and tremor.

hy·per·thy·ro·tro·pin·ism (high"pur·thigh"ro·tro'pin·iz·um, ·thigh·rot'ro·pin·iz·um) *n.* [*hyper-* + *thyrotropin* + *-ism*]. Excessive secretion of thyrotropic hormone by the adenohypophysis.

hy·per·to·nia (high"pur·to'nee·uh) *n.* [*hyper-* + *-tonia*]. Abnormally great muscular tonicity or contractility. Compare *spasticity*.

hy·per·ton·ic (high"pur·ton'ick) *adj.* [*hyper-* + *tonic*]. 1. Excessive or above normal in tone or tension. 2. Having an osmotic pressure greater than that of physiologic salt solution or of any other solution taken as a standard. —**hyper·to·nic·i·ty** (·to·nis'i·tee) *n.*

hypertonic bladder. A condition of persistently increased muscular activity of the urinary bladder, such as that which appears after recovery from the shock following section of its voluntary innervation.

hypertonic contracture. In spastic paralysis, the contracture that results from chronic overactivity of tonic myotatic reflexes.

hypertonic solution. A solution that produces a change in the tone of a tissue immersed in it through passage of water from the tissue into the solution. With reference to erythrocytes, a hypertonic solution of sodium chloride is one that contains more than 0.9 g of sodium chloride in each 100 ml.

hy·per·to·nus (high"pur·to'nus) *n.* [*hyper-* + *tonus*]. HYPERTONIA.

hy·per·tri·chi·a·sis (high"pur·tri·kigh'uh·sis) *n.* [*hyper-* + *trich-* + *-iasis*]. HYPERTRICHOSIS.

hy·per·tri·cho·sis (high"pur·tri·ko'sis) *n.* [*hyper-* + Gk. *trichōsis*, hairiness, growth of hair, from *thrix, trichos*, hair]. Excessive growth of normal hair; superfluous hair; abnormal hairiness. —**hypertri·chot·ic** (·kot'ick) *adj.*

hy·per·tri·glyc·er·id·emia, hy·per·tri·glyc·er·id·ae·mia (high"pur·trye·glis"ur·i·dee'mee·uh) *n.* [*hyper-* + *triglyceride* + *-emia*]. An excessively high level of serum triglycerides.

hy·per·tro·phic (high"pur·trof'ick) *adj.* Pertaining to or characterized by hypertrophy.

hypertrophic arthritis. DEGENERATIVE JOINT DISEASE.

hypertrophic cervical pachymeningitis. Spinal pachymeningitis attacking the cervical region.

hypertrophic cirrhosis. *Obsol.* BILIARY CIRRHOSIS.

hypertrophic conjunctivitis. Chronic catarrhal conjunctivitis attended with enlargement of the conjunctival papillae.

hypertrophic emphysema. EMPHYSEMA (1).

hypertrophic gastritis. A chronic form of gastritis with increased thickness of mucosa, exaggerated granulation, and larger, more numerous rugae.

hypertrophic interstitial neuropathy or **radiculoneuropathy.** 1. A rare genetically determined syndrome of undetermined etiology, characterized by onset between 10 to 40 years of age, a slowly progressive motor and sensory radiculoneuropathy with palpable thickening of nerve trunks, weakness, atrophy, kyphoscoliosis, impaired coordination, nystagmus, and other neurologic deficits. Microscopically, the nerves show a nonspecific "onion-bulb" formation, which may be the result of successive demyelination and regeneration. Syn. *Dejerine-Sottas disease*. 2. Any condition which may result in thickening of the nerves with the "onion-bulb" microscopic appearance mentioned above.

hypertrophic obstructive cardiomyopathy. IDIOPATHIC HYPERTROPHIC SUBAORTIC STENOSIS.

hypertrophic pharyngitis. Chronic pharyngitis associated with hypertrophy of the mucous membranes.

hypertrophic pulmonary osteoarthropathy. The clubbing of the fingers and toes associated with enlargement of the ends of the long bones, encountered in chronic pulmonary disease. Syn. *osteopulmonary arthropathy, pseudoacromegaly*.

hypertrophic pulp. HYPERPLASTIC PULPITIS.

hypertrophic rhinitis. Rhinitis marked by hypertrophy of the nasal mucous membrane.

hypertrophic secondary osteoarthropathy. HYPERTROPHIC PULMONARY OSTEOARTHROPATHY.

hypertrophic spinal pachymeningitis. A localized or diffuse chronic inflammation of the dura mater, attributed to syphilis, tuberculosis, trauma, and other causes, giving rise to symptoms of irritation of spinal roots and compression of the spinal cord. It attacks any level of the spinal cord or brain but most often the lower cervical region.

hypertrophic subaortic stenosis. IDIOPATHIC HYPERTROPHIC SUBAORTIC STENOSIS.

hypertrophic sycosis. KELOID SYCOSIS.

hy·per·tro·phy (high·pur'truh·fee) *n.* [*hyper-* + *-trophy*]. An increase in size of an organ, independent of natural growth, due to enlargement of its constituent cells; usually with an accompanying increase in functional capacity. Compare *hyperplasia.*

hy·per·tro·pia (high″pur·tro′pee·uh) *n.* [*hyper-* + *-tropia*]. Vertical strabismus in which the visual axis of one eye deviates upward. **—hypertro·pic,** *adj.*

Hypertussis. A trademark for pertussis immune human globulin.

hy·per·ty·ro·sin·emia, hy·per·ty·ro·sin·ae·mia (high″pur·tye″ ro·si·nee′mee·uh) *n.* [*hyper-* + *tyrosine* + *-emia*]. 1. TYROSINOSIS. 2. TYROSINEMIA.

hy·per·ure·sis (high″pur·yoo·ree′sis) *n.* [*hyper-* + *uresis*]. POLYURIA.

hy·per·uric·ac·id·emia, hy·per·u·ric·ac·id·ae·mia (high″pur· yoo″rick·as″id·ee′mee·uh) *n.* [*hyper-* + *uric acid* + *-emia*]. HYPERURICEMIA.

hy·per·uri·ce·mia, hy·per·uri·cae·mia (high″pur·yoo″ri·see′ mee·uh) *n.* [*hyper-* + *uricemia*]. Abnormally high level of uric acid in the blood. See also *gout, Lesch-Nyhan disease.*

hy·per·val·in·emia, hy·per·val·in·ae·mia (high″pur·val″i·nee′ mee·uh, ·vay″li·) *n.* [*hyper-* + *valine* + *-emia*]. A hereditary metabolic disorder in which there is believed to be a deficiency of valine alpha-ketoglutarate transaminase resulting in abnormally high levels of valine in blood and urine; manifested clinically by failure to thrive, vomiting, nystagmus, hypotonia, and mental retardation.

hy·per·vas·cu·lar (high″pur·vas′kew·lur) *adj.* [*hyper-* + *vascular*]. Excessively vascular.

hy·per·veg·e·ta·tive (high″pur·vej′e·tay″tiv) *adj.* [*hyper-* + *vegetative*]. Referring to a constitutional body type in which visceral or nutritional function dominates the somatic or neuromuscular system. Compare *pyknic.*

hy·per·ven·ti·la·tion (high″pur·ven″ti·lay′shun) *n.* [*hyper-* + *ventilation*]. 1. Abnormally rapid, deep breathing. 2. Overbreathing, usually due to anxiety, producing hypocapnia and symptoms of dizziness, paresthesia, and carpopedal spasm caused by the respiratory alkalosis that develops.

hyperventilation syndrome. HYPERVENTILATION (2).

hyperventilation tetany. Tetany due to alkalosis from loss of carbon dioxide from the blood following hyperventilation. See also *respiratory alkalosis.*

hy·per·vis·cos·i·ty (high″pur·vis·kos′i·tee) *n.* Abnormally high viscosity. **—hyper·vis·cous** (·vis′kus) *adj.*

hy·per·vi·ta·min·osis (high″pur·vye″tuh·min·o′sis) *n.*, pl. **hypervitamin·oses** (·o′seez) [*hyper-* + *vitamin* + *-osis*]. A condition due to administration of excessive amounts of a vitamin, as: hypervitaminosis A, hypervitaminosis D.

hy·per·vo·le·mia, hy·per·vo·lae·mia (high″pur·vo·lee′mee· uh) *n.* [*hyper-* + *volume* + *-emia*]. A total circulating blood volume greater than normal. **—hypervole·mic, hypervolae· mic** (·mick) *adj.*

hy·per·vo·lu·mic (high″pur·vol·yoo′mick) *adj.* [*hyper-* + *volume* + *-ic*]. Pertaining to a greater than normal volume or bulk of a body part, such as muscle or brain.

hyp·es·the·sia, hyp·aes·the·sia (hip″es·thee′zhuh, ·theez′ee· uh, high″pes·) *n.* [*hyp-* + *esthesia*]. Impairment of sensation; lessened tactile sensibility. **—hypesthe·sic, hypaesthe· sic** (·zick), **hypes·thet·ic, hypaes·thet·ic** (·thet′ick) *adj.*

hy·pha (high′fuh) *n.*, pl. **hy·phae** (·fee) [NL., from Gk. *hyphē*, web]. A filament that develops from the germ tube of a fungus. The septate hyphae are those divided into a chain of cells by cross walls forming at regular intervals. Those without cross walls, the nonseptate hyphae, are described as being coenocytic. **—hy·phal** (·ful) *adj.*

hyphaema. HYPHEMA.

hyphaemia. Hyphemia (= HYPHEMA or OLIGEMIA).

hyphal cell. A cell of the hypha of a mold.

hyp·he·do·nia (hip″he·do′nee·uh, hype″he·do′nee·uh) *n.* [*hyp-* + Gk. *hēdonē*, pleasure, + *-ia*]. Abnormal diminution of pleasure.

hy·phe·ma, hy·phae·ma (high·fee′muh) *n.* [Gk. *hyphaimos*, bloodshot, from *haima*, blood]. Blood in the anterior chamber of the eye.

hy·phe·mia, hy·phae·mia (high·fee′mee·uh) *n.* [*hyp-* + *-hemia*]. 1. HYPHEMA. 2. OLIGEMIA.

hyp·hi·dro·sis (hip″hi·dro′sis, hipe″hi·) *n.* [*hyp-* + *hidrosis*]. Deficiency of perspiration.

hy·pho·gen·ic sycosis (high″fo·jen′ick). TINEA BARBAE.

Hy·pho·my·ce·tes (high′fo·migh·see′teez) *n.pl.* [Gk. *hyphē*, web, + *mycetes*]. FUNGI IMPERFECTI.

hyp·i·no·sis (hip″i·no′sis) *n.* [*hyp-* + Gk. *is, inos*, fiber, + *-osis*]. A deficiency of fibrin factors in the blood.

hyp·iso·ton·ic (hip″i·so·ton′ick, hip·eye″so·) *adj.* [*hyp-* + *isotonic*]. HYPOTONIC (2).

hypn-, hypno- [Gk. *hypnos*, sleep]. A combining form meaning (a) *sleep;* (b) *hypnotism, hypnosis.*

hyp·na·gog·ic (hip″nuh·goj′ick) *adj.* [*hypn-* + Gk. *agōgos*, leading, + *-ic*]. 1. Pertaining to the inception or the induction of sleep. 2. Occurring at the inception or induction of sleep, before stage 1 is reached. Contr. *hypnopompic.*

hypnagogic hallucination. A mental image or series of images perceived just at the moment of falling asleep or at the beginning of sleep paralysis, but differentiated from a dream in that it does not occur during REM sleep; may be a normal phenomenon or part of the syndrome of narcolepsy and cataplexy. Compare *hypnopompic hallucination.*

hypnagogic paralysis. Paralysis during the period of falling asleep. See also *sleep paralysis.*

hypnagogic state. The state between sleeping and waking.

hyp·na·gogue (hip′nuh·gog) *n.* [*hypn-* + *-agogue*]. A hypnotic drug.

hyp·nal·gia (hip·nal′jee·uh) *n.* [*hypn-* + *-algia*]. Pain occurring during sleep.

hyp·nic (hip′nick) *adj.* & *n.* [Gk. *hypnikos*, producing sleep]. 1. Pertaining to or inducing sleep; hypnotic. 2. An agent that induces sleep.

hypno-. See *hypn-.*

hyp·no·anal·y·sis (hip″no·uh·nal′i·sis) *n.*, pl. **hypnoanaly·ses** (·seez). A form of psychotherapy combining psychoanalytic techniques with hypnosis.

hyp·no·ge·net·ic (hip″no·je·net′ick) *adj.* HYPNOGENIC.

hyp·no·gen·ic (hip″no·jen′ick) *adj.* [*hypno-* + *-genic*]. 1. Producing or inducing sleep. 2. Inducing hypnosis. **—hypno·gen·e·sis** (·e·sis) *n.*

hyp·no·gog·ic (hip″no·goj′ick) *adj.* HYPNAGOGIC.

hyp·noid (hip′noid) *adj.* [*hypn-* + *-oid*]. Resembling sleep or hypnosis.

hyp·noi·dal (hip·noy′dul) *adj.* HYPNOID.

hyp·no·lep·sy (hip′no·lep″see) *n.* [*hypno-* + *-lepsy*]. NARCOLEPSY.

hyp·nol·o·gy (hip·nol′uh·jee) *n.* [*hypno-* + *-logy*]. 1. The science dealing with sleep 2. The scientific study of hypnosis.

hyp·no·nar·co·sis (hip″no·nahr·ko′sis) *n.* [*hypno-* + *narcosis*]. 1. Deep sleep induced through hypnosis. 2. Combined hypnosis and narcosis.

hyp·no·pho·bia (hip″no·fo′bee·uh) *n.* [*hypno-* + *-phobia*]. Morbid dread of sleep or of falling asleep. **—hypnopho·bic** (·bick) *adj.*

hyp·no·pho·by (hip′no·fo″bee) *n.* HYPNOPHOBIA.

hyp·no·phre·no·sis (hip″no·fre·no′sis) *n.*, pl. **hypnophreno·ses** (·seez) [*hypno-* + *phren-* + *-osis*]. Any sleep disorder.

hyp·no·pom·pic (hip″no·pom′pick) *adj.* [*hypno-* + Gk. *pompē*, a sending away, + *-ic*]. Pertaining to or occurring during the process of awakening. Contr. *hypnagogic.*

hypnopompic hallucination. A mental image or series of mental images that occur at the moment of awakening from sleep or prior to complete awakening, observed in otherwise normal persons or in those with the syndrome of narcolepsy and cataplexy. Compare *hypnagogic hallucination.*

hypnopompic paralysis. Paralysis during the period of awakening. See also *sleep paralysis.*

hyp·no·si·gen·e·sis (hip″no·si·jen′e·sis) *n.* [*hypnosis* + *-genesis*]. Induction of hypnosis.

hyp·no·sis (hip·no′sis) *n.*, pl. **hypno·ses** (·seez) [*hypn-* + *-osis*]. A state of altered consciousness, sleep, or trance; induced artificially in a subject by means of verbal suggestion by the hypnotist or by the subject's concentration upon some object; characterized by extreme responsiveness to suggestions made by the hypnotist. The degree of the hypnotic state may vary from mild increased suggestibility to that comparable to surgical anesthesia.

hyp·no·ther·a·py (hip″no·therr′uh·pee) *n.* [*hypno-* + *therapy*]. 1. The treatment of disease by means of hypnotism. 2. The induction of sleep for therapeutic purposes.

hyp·not·ic (hip·not′ick) *adj.* & *n.* [Gk. *hypnōtikos*, sleepy, inducing sleep]. 1. Inducing sleep. 2. Pertaining to hypnosis or to hypnotism. 3. A drug that causes sleep. 4. A person who is susceptible to hypnotism; one who is hypnotized.

hypnotic somnambulism. A condition of hypnosis in which the subject is possessed of his or her senses and often has the appearance of one awake, though his or her consciousness is under the control of the hypnotizer.

hypnotic suggestion. A suggestion made to an individual in the hypnotic state.

hyp·no·tism (hip′nuh·tiz·um) *n.* The practice and principles of inducing hypnosis. —**hypno·tist** (·tist) *n.*

hyp·no·tize (hip′nuh·tize) *v.* 1. To bring into a state of hypnosis. 2. To influence another person, usually by suggestion or strong personal attributes. —**hyp·no·ti·za·tion** (hip″nuh·ti·zay′shun) *n.*

hyp·no·toid (hip′no·toid) *adj.* Resembling hypnosis or hypnotism.

¹hypo, *n.* Short for *hypodermic* syringe or medication.

²hypo, *n.* [from *hypo*sulfite]. SODIUM THIOSULFATE.

hypo-. See *hyp-*.

hy·po·acid·i·ty (high″po·a·sid′i·tee) *n.* [*hypo-* + *acidity*]. Deficiency in acid constituents.

hy·po·ac·tiv·i·ty (high″po·ack·tiv′i·tee) *n.* [*hypo-* + *activity*]. Diminished activity.

hy·po·acu·sia (high″po·a·kew′zhuh, ·zee·uh) *n.* [*hypo-* + *-acusia*]. HYPACUSIA.

hy·po·adren·a·lin·emia (high″po·uh·dren″uh·li·nee′mee·uh) *n.* [*hypo-* + *adrenalin* + *-emia*]. A condition in which the epinephrine content of the blood is insufficient.

hy·po·adre·nal·ism (high″po·uh·dree′nul·iz·um) *n.* [*hypo-* + *adrenal* + *-ism*]. 1. Abnormally diminished adrenal gland function; adrenal insufficiency. 2. HYPOADRENOCORTICISM. —**hypoadrenal,** *adj.*

hy·po·adre·nia (high″po·uh·dree′nee·uh) *n.* HYPOADRENALISM.

hy·po·adre·no·cor·ti·cism (high″po·uh·dree″no·kor′ti·siz·um) *n.* Diminished activity of the adrenal cortex.

hypoaesthesia. HYPESTHESIA.

hy·po·ag·na·thus (high″po·ag′nuth·us) *n.* [*hypo-* + *agnathus*]. An individual with no lower jaw.

hy·po·al·bu·min·emia, hy·po·al·bu·min·ae·mia (high″po·al·bew″min·ee′mee·uh) *n.* [*hypo-* + *albumin* + *-emia*]. Abnormally low blood content of albumin.

hy·po·al·do·ste·ro·nism (high″po·al·do·sterr′o·niz·um) *n.* [*hypo-* + *aldosterone* + *-ism*]. Deficient production or secretion of aldosterone.

hy·po·al·i·men·ta·tion (high″po·al″i·men·tay′shun) *n.* [*hypo-* + *alimentation*]. The state produced by insufficient or inadequate food intake.

hy·po·al·ler·gen·ic (high″po·al″ur·jen′ick) *adj.* [*hypo-* + *allergenic*]. Having a low tendency to induce allergic reactions, especially with reference to dermatologic preparations so formulated and produced as to have this quality to a high degree.

hy·po·az·o·tu·ria (high″po·az″o·tew′ree·uh) *n.* [*hypo-* + *azote* + *-uria*]. A diminished amount of nitrogenous substances in the urine.

hy·po·bar·ic (high″po·băr′ick) *adj.* [*hypo-* + Gk. *baros*, weight, + *-ic*]. 1. Of less weight or pressure. 2. Pertaining to an anesthetic solution of specific gravity lower than the cerebrospinal fluid.

hy·po·bar·ism (high″po·băr′iz·um) *n.* [*hypo-* + *bar-* + *-ism*]. A condition resulting from an excess of gas pressure within the body fluids, tissues, or cavities over the ambient gas pressure.

hy·po·ba·rop·a·thy (high″po·ba·rop′uth·ee) *n.* [*hypo-* + *baro-* + *-pathy*]. ALTITUDE SICKNESS.

hy·po·bil·i·ru·bi·ne·mia, hy·po·bil·i·ru·bi·nae·mia (high″po·bil″i·roo″bi·nee′mee·uh) *n.* [*hypo-* + *bilirubin* + *-emia*]. A reduction below normal of bilirubin in the blood.

hy·po·blast (high′po·blast) *n.* [*hypo-* + *-blast*]. ENTODERM. —**hy·po·blas·tic** (high″po·blas′tick) *adj.*

hy·po·bran·chi·al (high″po·brang′kee·ul) *adj.* & *n.* [*hypo-* + *branchial*]. 1. Located below or under the branchial or visceral arches. 2. A bone or cartilage located under the branchial arches.

hypobranchial eminence. FURCULA (1).

hy·po·bro·mite (high″po·bro′mite) *n.* A salt of hypobromous acid.

hy·po·bro·mous acid (high″po·bro′mus) *n.* HBrO. An unstable acid containing bromine having a positive valence number of one.

hy·po·bu·lia (high″po·bew′lee·uh) *n.* [*hypo-* + Gk. *boulē*, will, + *-ia*]. Deficiency of will power.

hy·po·cal·ce·mia, hy·po·cal·cae·mia (high″po·kal·see′mee·uh) *n.* [*hypo* + *calc-* + *-emia*]. A condition in which there is a diminished amount of calcium in the blood. —**hypocalcemic** (·mick) *adj.*

hy·po·cal·ci·fi·ca·tion (high″po·kal″si·fi·kay′shun) *n.* [*hypo-* + *calcification*]. Reduction of the normal amount of mineral salts in calcified tissues, as bone, dentin, or dental enamel. —**hypo·cal·cif·ic** (·kal·sif′ick) *adj.*; **hypo·cal·ci·fy** (·kal′si·figh) *v.*

hy·po·cal·ci·uria (high″po·kal″see·yoo′ree·uh) *n.* [*hypo-* + *calci-* + *-uria*]. Decreased urinary calcium excretion.

hy·po·cap·nia (high″po·kap′nee·uh) *n.* [*hypo-* + *-capnia*]. Subnormal concentration of carbon dioxide in the blood. Syn. *acapnia.*

hy·po·car·bia (high″po·kahr′bee·uh) *n.* [*hypo-* + *carb-* + *-ia*]. HYPOCAPNIA.

hy·po·ca·thex·is (high″po·ka·theck′sis) *n.* [*hypo-* + *cathexis*]. A lack of concentration of the psychic energy upon a particular object, as a parent or spouse.

hy·po·cel·lu·lar (high″po·sel′yoo·lur) *adj.* [*hypo-* + *cellular*]. Characterized by an abnormally low number or density of cells. —**hypo·cel·lu·lar·i·ty** (·sel″yoo·lăr′i·tee) *n.*

hypocelom. HYPOCOELOM.

hy·po·ce·ru·lo·plas·min·emia, hy·po·ce·ru·lo·plas·min·ae·mia (high″po·se·roo″lo·plaz″mi·nee′mee·uh) *n.* [*hypo-* + *ceruloplasmin* + *-emia*]. Decreased amounts of ceruloplasmin in the blood plasma.

hy·po·chlo·re·mia, hy·po·chlo·rae·mia (high″po·klor·ee′mee·uh) *n.* [*hypo-* + *chlor-* + *-emia*]. Reduction in the amount of blood chlorides.

hy·po·chlor·hy·dria (high″po·klor·high′dree·uh, ·klor·hid′ree·uh) *n.* [*hypo-* + *chlorhydria*]. Diminished hydrochloric acid secretion by the stomach.

hy·po·chlo·rite (high″po·klor′ite) *n.* Any salt of hypochlorous acid, HClO.

hy·po·chlo·ri·za·tion (high″po·klo″ri·zay′shun) *n.* Reduction in the dietary intake of sodium chloride.

hy·po·chlo·rous acid (high″po·klor′us). HClO. An unstable compound, known only in solution. It has disinfectant and bleaching properties and is used mostly in the form of its sodium and calcium salts.

hy·po·chlor·uria (high″po·klor·yoo′ree·uh) *n.* [*hypo-* + *chlor-* + *-uria*]. A diminution in the amount of chlorides excreted in the urine.

hy·po·cho·les·ter·emia, hy·po·cho·les·ter·ae·mia (high″po·ko·

les″tur·ee′mee·uh) *n.* HYPOCHOLESTEROLEMIA. —**hypocholester·emic, hypocholester·ae·mic** (·ee′mick) *adj.*

hy·po·cho·les·ter·ol·emia, hy·po·cho·les·ter·ol·ae·mia (high″po·ko·les″tur·ol·ee′mee·uh) *n.* [*hypo-* + *cholesterol* + *-emia*]. An abnormally low level of serum cholesterol.

hy·po·chon·dria (high″po·kon′dree·uh) *n.* 1. HYPOCHONDRIASIS. 2. Plural of *hypochondrium.*

hy·po·chon·dri·ac (high″po·kon′dree·ack) *adj. & n.* [Gk. *hypochondriakos,* of the hypochondrium]. 1. Pertaining to the hypochondriac region. 2. Affected with or caused by hypochondriasis. 3. A person who is affected with hypochondriasis.

hy·po·chon·dri·a·cal (high″po·kon·drye′uh·kul) *adj.* Of, pertaining to, or characterized by hypochondriasis.

hypochondriacal neurosis. A neurosis characterized by preoccupation with one's own body and obsessive thoughts about presumed illnesses, which, though not delusional, persist despite reassurances.

hypochondriac region. The right or the left upper lateral region of the abdomen below the lower ribs. Syn. *hypochondrium.* NA *regio hypochondriaca (dextra et sinistra).* See also *abdominal regions.*

hy·po·chon·dri·al (high″po·kon′dree·ul) *adj.* Pertaining to or involving the hypochondriac region.

hypochondrial reflex. Sudden inspiration produced by sudden pressure below the costal border.

hy·po·chon·dri·a·sis (high″po·kon·drye′uh·sis) *n.,* pl. **hypochondria·ses** (·seez) [*hypochondr*ium (as the supposed source of melancholy and classic locus of complaints) + *-iasis*]. A chronic condition in which one is morbidly concerned with one's own physical or mental health, and believes himself or herself to be suffering from a grave, usually bodily, disease often focused upon one organ, without demonstrable organic findings; this condition is traceable to some longstanding intrapsychic conflict.

hy·po·chon·dri·um (high″po·kon′dree·um) *n.,* pl. **hypochondria** (·dree·uh) [Gk. *hypochondrion,* from *hypo-* + *chondros,* cartilage, xiphoid cartilage]. HYPOCHONDRIAC REGION.

hy·po·chon·dro·pla·sia (high″po·kon″dro·play′zhuh, ·zee·uh) *n.* [*hypo-* + *chondro-* + *-plasia*]. A type of chondrodystrophy with radiologic changes similar to, but less pronounced than, achondroplasia.

hy·po·chord·al (high″po·kor′dul) *adj.* [*hypo-* + *chordal*]. Located below or ventral to the notochord.

hypochordal bar or **arch.** *In embryology,* a band of mesodermal tissue found in the upper cervical vertebrae connecting the ends of the vertebral arches across the ventral surfaces of the intervertebral cartilages. The bars are transitory, except for the first which is the anlage of the anterior arch of the atlas.

hy·po·chro·ma·sia (high″po·kro·may′zee·uh, ·zhuh) *n.* HYPOCHROMIA.

hy·po·chro·mat·ic (high″po·kro·mat′ick) *adj.* [*hypo-* + *chromatic*]. HYPOCHROMIC.

hy·po·chro·ma·tism (high″po·kro′muh·tiz·um) *n.* [*hypo-* + *chromat-* + *-ism*]. HYPOCHROMIA.

hy·po·chro·mia (high″po·kro′mee·uh) *n.* [*hypo-* + *chrom-* + *-ia*]. 1. A lack of color. 2. A lack of complete saturation of the erythrocytic stroma with hemoglobin, as judged by pallor of the unstained or stained erythrocytes when examined microscopically. —**hypochro·mic** (·mick) *adj.*

hypochromic anemia. Anemia characterized by a reduced average hemoglobin concentration in erythrocytes.

hypochromic anemia of prematurity, infancy, childhood, or **pregnancy.** IRON-DEFICIENCY ANEMIA.

hypochromic microcytic anemia. Anemia characterized by erythrocytes of decreased size and decreased hemoglobin content such as iron-deficiency anemia.

hy·po·chy·lia (high″po·kigh′lee·uh) *n.* [*hypo-* + *chyl-* + *-ia*]. Deficiency of chyle.

hy·po·ci·ne·sia (high″po·si·nee′zee·uh, ·zhuh) *n.* HYPOKINESIA.

hy·po·ci·ne·sis (high″po·si·nee′sis) *n.* HYPOKINESIA.

hy·po·coe·lom, hy·po·ce·lom (high″po·see′lum) *n.* [*hypo-* + *coelom*]. The ventral part of the coelom.

hy·po·com·ple·men·te·mia (high″po·kom″ple·men·tee′mee·uh) *n.* [*hypo-* + *complement* + *-emia*]. Abnormally low blood levels of one or more complement components, most frequently secondary to fixation or activation of complement by antigen-antibody reactions, but sometimes the result of decreased production or excessive loss of complement. —**hypocomplemente·mic** (·mick) *adj.*

hy·po·cone (high′po·kone) *n.* [*hypo-* + *cone*]. The distolingual cusp of an upper molar tooth.

hy·po·con·id (high″po·kon′id) *n.* [*hypocone* + *-id*]. The distobuccal cusp of a lower molar tooth.

hy·po·con·ule (high″po·kon′yool) *n.* [dim. of *hypocone*]. The fifth, or distal, cusp of an upper molar tooth.

hy·po·con·u·lid (high″po·kon′yoo·lid) *n.* [*hypoconule* + *-id*]. The fifth or distal cusp of a lower molar tooth.

hy·po·cu·pre·mia, hy·po·cu·prae·mia (high″po·kew·pree′mee·uh) *n.* [*hypo-* + *cupr-* + *-emia*]. An abnormally low level of copper in the blood plasma.

hy·po·cy·clo·sis (high″po·sigh·klo′sis) *n.,* pl. **hypocyclo·ses** (·seez) [*hypo-* + *cycl-* + *-osis*]. *In ophthalmology,* deficient accommodation.

hy·po·cy·the·mia, hy·po·cy·thae·mia (high″po·sigh·theem′ee·uh) *n.* [*hypo-* + *cyt-* + *-hemia*]. Any deficiency of the formed elements of blood, especially of erythrocytes.

Hy·po·der·ma (high″po·dur′muh) *n.* [*hypo-* + *-derma*]. A genus of warble flies whose larvae are parasitic to cattle and occasionally to humans.

hy·po·der·mat·ic (high″po·dur·mat′ick) *adj.* [*hypo-* + *dermat-* + *-ic*]. HYPODERMIC.

hy·po·der·ma·toc·ly·sis (high″po·dur″muh·tock′li·sis) *n.* [*hypo-* + *dermato-* + *clysis*]. HYPODERMOCLYSIS.

hy·po·der·mi·a·sis (high″po·dur·mye′uh·sis) *n.* [*hypoderma* + *-iasis*] A condition in which warble fly larvae invade the subcutaneous tissue and produce a form of creeping eruption. See also *warbles.*

hy·po·der·mic (high″po·dur′mick) *adj. & n.* [*hypo-* + *dermic*]. 1. Pertaining to the region beneath the skin. 2. Placed or introduced beneath the skin. 3. A substance, as a medicine or drug, introduced or injected beneath the skin. 4. A syringe used for a hypodermic injection.

hypodermic needle. A hollow needle, with a slanted point, used for subcutaneous and intramuscular injections of fluid.

hy·po·der·mis (high″po·dur′mis) *n.* [*hypo-* + *dermis*]. 1. The outermost layer of cells of invertebrates, which corresponds to the epidermis. It secretes the cuticular exoskeleton of arthropods, annelids, mollusks, and other forms. 2. In human anatomy, SUBCUTANEOUS TISSUE.

hy·po·der·moc·ly·sis (high″po·dur·mock′li·sis) *n.,* pl. **hypodermocly·ses** (·seez) [*hypo-* + *dermo-* + *clysis*]. The therapeutic introduction into the subcutaneous tissues of large quantities of fluids.

hy·po·der·mo·li·thi·a·sis (high″po·dur″mo·li·thigh′uh·sis) *n.* [*hypo-* + *dermo-* + *lithiasis*]. CALCINOSIS CUTIS CIRCUMSCRIPTA.

hy·po·don·tia (high″po·don′chee·uh) *n.* [*hyp-* + *-odontia*]. Partial anodontia.

hy·po·er·gy (high′po·ur·jee) *n.* [*hypo-* + *-ergy*]. A state of less than normal reactivity, in which the response is less marked than usual; hyposensitivity; one form of allergy or pathergy.

hy·po·eso·pho·ria (high″po·es″o·fo′ree·uh) *n.* [*hypo-* + *esophoria*]. A type of heterophoria in which the visual lines tend downward and inward.

hy·po·es·the·sia, hy·po·aes·the·sia (high″po·es·theezh′uh, ·theez′ee·uh) *n.* HYPESTHESIA.

hy·po·es·trin·ism, hy·po·oes·trin·ism (high″po·es′trin·iz·um) *n.* [*hypo-* + *estrin* + *-ism*]. The state of deficient production of estrogen by the ovaries.

hy·po·exo·pho·ria (high″po·eck″so·fo′ree·uh) *n.* [*hypo-* + *exophoria*]. A type of heterophoria in which the visual lines tend downward and outward.

hy·po·fer·re·mia, hy·po·fer·rae·mia (high″po·ferr·ee′mee·uh) *n.* [*hypo-* + *ferr*um + *-emia*]. Diminished or abnormally low iron level in the blood.

hy·po·fi·brin·o·gen·emia, hy·po·fi·brin·o·gen·ae·mia (high″po·figh″bri·no·je·nee′mee·uh) *n.* [*hypo-* + *fibrinogen* + *-emia*]. A decrease in plasma fibrinogen level.

hy·po·func·tion (high″po·funk′shun) *n.* [*hypo-* + *function*]. Diminished function. —**hypofunction·al** (·ul) *adj.*

hy·po·ga·lac·tia (high″po·ga·lack′shee·uh) *n.* [*hypo-* + *galact-* + *-ia*]. Decreased milk secretion.

hy·po·gam·ma·glob·u·lin·emia, hy·po·gam·ma·glob·u·lin·ae·mia (high″po·gam″uh·glob″yoo·li·nee′mee·uh) *n.* [*hypo-* + *gamma globulin* + *-emia*]. A decrease in plasma gamma globulin. See also *agammaglobulinemia.*

hy·po·gan·gli·on·o·sis (high″po·gang″glee·uh·no′sis) *n.* [*hypo-* + *ganglion* + *-osis*]. A reduction in the number of ganglia, especially of the ganglia of the myenteric plexus.

hy·po·gas·tric (high″po·gas′trick) *adj.* Of or pertaining to the hypogastrium or pubic region.

hypogastric artery. INTERNAL ILIAC ARTERY.

hypogastric fold. LATERAL UMBILICAL FOLD.

hypogastric nerve. NA *nervus hypogastricus (dexter et sinister).* See Table of Nerves in the Appendix.

hypogastric plexus. See *inferior hypogastric plexus, superior hypogastric plexus.*

hypogastric reflex. Contraction of the muscles of the lower abdomen induced by stroking of the skin of the inner surface of the thigh.

hypogastric region. PUBIC REGION.

hy·po·gas·tri·um (high″po·gas′tree·um) *n.*, pl. **hypogas·tria** (·tree·uh) [Gk. *hypogastrion,* from *hypo-* + *gastēr,* belly]. PUBIC REGION.

hy·po·gas·tro·did·y·mus (high·po·gas″tro·did′i·mus) *n.* [*hypogastr*ium + *didymus*]. HYPOGASTROPAGUS.

hy·po·gas·trop·a·gus (high″po·gas·trop′uh·gus) *n.* [*hypogastr*ium + *-pagus*]. Conjoined twins united at the hypogastric region.

hy·po·gas·tros·chi·sis (high″po·gas·tros′ki·sis) *n.* Abdominal fissure (gastroschisis) limited to the hypogastric region.

hy·po·gen·e·sis (high″po·jen′e·sis) *n.* [*hypo-* + *-genesis*]. Underdevelopment.

hy·po·gen·i·tal·ism (high″po·jen′i·tul·iz·um) *n.* [*hypo-* + *genital* + *-ism*]. Underdevelopment of the genital system. See also *eunuchoidism, hypogonadism.*

hy·po·geu·sia (high″po·gew′see·uh, ·joo′see·uh) *n.* [*hypo-* + *-geusia*]. Diminution in the sense of taste.

hy·po·glos·sal (high″po·glos′ul) *adj.* [*hypo-* + *glossal*]. Situated under the tongue.

hypoglossal canal. The passageway for the hypoglossal nerve in the occipital bone. Syn. *anterior condylar canal.* NA *canalis hypoglossi.*

hypoglossal eminence. TRIGONE OF THE HYPOGLOSSAL NERVE.

hypoglossal nerve. The twelfth cranial nerve; a motor nerve, attached to the medulla oblongata, which innervates the intrinsic and extrinsic muscles of the tongue. NA *nervus hypoglossus.* See also Table of Nerves in the Appendix.

hypoglossal nucleus. A long and cylindrical nucleus located lateral to the midline extending throughout most of the length of the medulla oblongata whose cells give origin to the fibers of the hypoglossal nerve. NA *nucleus nervi hypoglossi.*

hypoglossal trigone. TRIGONE OF THE HYPOGLOSSAL NERVE.

hy·po·glos·sis (high″po·glos′is) *n.* HYPOGLOTTIS.

hy·po·glos·si·tis (high″po·glos·eye′tis) *n.* [*hypogloss*al + *-itis*]. Inflammation of the tissue under the tongue.

hy·po·glos·sus (high″po·glos′us) *n.*, pl. **hypoglos·si** (·eye) [NL., from *hypo-* + Gk. *glōssa,* tongue]. HYPOGLOSSAL NERVE.

hy·po·glot·tis (high″po·glot′is) *n.* [Gk. *hypoglōttis,* from *hypo-* + *glōtta,* tongue]. The underpart of the tongue.

hy·po·gly·ce·mia, hy·po·gly·cae·mia (high″po·glye·see′mee·uh) *n.* [*hypo-* + *glyc-* + *-emia*]. 1. A reduction below normal in blood glucose. 2. The clinical state associated with decrease of blood glucose below a critical level for the individual, characterized by hunger, nervousness, profuse sweating, faintness, and sometimes convulsions.

hy·po·gly·ce·mic, hy·po·gly·cae·mic (high″po·glye·see′mick) *adj.* 1. Of or pertaining to hypoglycemia. 2. Lowering the concentration of glucose in the blood.

hypoglycemic shock therapy or **treatment.** INSULIN SHOCK THERAPY.

hy·po·gly·ce·mo·sis (high″po·glye·se·mo′sis) *n.* [*hypoglycem*ia + *-osis*]. HYPOGLYCEMIA (2).

hy·po·gly·cin (high″po·glye′sin) *n.* A toxin (L-α-amino-β-methylenecyclopropanepropionic acid) found in the unripe fruit of the akee, associated with Jamaican vomiting sickness; it produces marked hypoglycemia by interfering with oxidation of long-chain fatty acids and gluconeogenesis.

hy·po·gly·co·ge·nol·y·sis (high″po·glye″ko·je·nol′i·sis) *n.* [*hypo-* + *glycogenolysis*]. Diminished glycogenolysis.

hy·po·gly·cor·rha·chia (high″po·glye″ko·ray′kee·uh) *n.* [*hypo-* + *glycorrhachia*]. Abnormally low concentration of glucose in the cerebrospinal fluid; usually values below 40 mg per 100 ml or less than two-thirds of the blood sugar value.

hy·po·gnath·ous (high″po·nath′us) *adj.* [*hypo-* + *-gnathous*]. Having the lower jaw abnormally small.

hy·po·gnath·us (high″po·nath′us) *n.* [*hypo-* + *-gnathus*]. *In teratology,* an individual having a parasite attached to the lower jaw.

hy·po·go·nad·ism (high″po·go′nad·iz·um, ·gon′uh·diz·um) *n.* [*hypo-* + *gonad* + *-ism*]. Diminished internal secretion of the testes or ovaries which may be due to a primary defect or secondary to insufficient stimulation by the adenohypophysis.

hy·po·gran·u·lo·cy·to·sis (high″po·gran″yoo·lo·sigh·to′sis) *n.* [*hypo-* + *granulocyte* + *-osis*]. AGRANULOCYTOSIS.

hy·po·hi·dro·sis (high″po·hi·dro′sis) *n.* [*hypo-* + *hidrosis*]. Deficient perspiration.

hy·po·in·su·lin·ism (high″po·in′sue·lin·iz·um) *n.* [*hypo-* + *insulin* + *-ism*]. Diminished secretion of insulin by the pancreas.

hy·po·io·dism (high″po·eye′uh·diz·um) *n.* [*hypo-* + *iod-* + *ism*]. Iodine deficiency.

hy·po·ka·le·mia, hy·po·ka·lae·mia (high″po·ka·lee′mee·uh) *n.* [*hypo-* + *kal*ium + *-emia*]. A deficiency of potassium in the blood. —**hypokale·mic, hypokalae·mic** (·mick) *adj.*

hy·po·kal·i·emia, hy·po·kal·i·ae·mia (high″po·kal″ee·ee′mee·uh) *n.* HYPOKALEMIA.

hy·po·ker·a·to·sis (high″po·kerr″uh·to′sis) *n.* [*hypo-* + *kerat-* + *-osis*]. A deficiency of keratinization.

hy·po·ki·ne·sia (high″po·ki·nee′zhuh, ·zee·uh, ·kigh·nee′) *n.* [*hypo-* + *-kinesia*]. Abnormally decreased muscular movement. Contr. *hyperkinesia.* —**hypoki·net·ic** (·net′ick) *adj.*

hy·po·ki·ne·sis (high″po·ki·nee′sis, ·kigh·nee′) *n.* HYPOKINESIA.

hypokinetic syndrome. A form of the minimal brain dysfunction syndrome in which decreased motor activity is an outstanding feature.

hy·po·lem·mal (high″po·lem′ul) *adj.* [*hypo-* + Gk. *lemma,* rind, husk, + *-al*]. Lying under a sheath, as the motor end plates under the sarcolemma or sheath of a muscle fiber.

hy·po·lep·sio·ma·nia (high″po·lep″see·o·may′nee·uh) *n.* [*hypo-* + Gk. *lēpsis,* seizure, + *-mania*]. Any form of monomania.

hy·po·leu·ko·cyt·ic, hy·po·leu·co·cyt·ic (high″po·lew″ko·sit′ick) *adj.* [*hypo-* + *leukocyte* + *-ic*]. 1. LEUKOPENIC. 2. AGRANULOCYTIC.

hypoleukocytic angina. AGRANULOCYTOSIS (2).

hy·po·ley·dig·ism (high″po·lye′dig·iz·um) *n.* [*hypo-* + *Leydig* cells + *-ism*]. Retarded sexual development, or loss of some male sexual characteristics, as a result of a decrease or absence in the function of the interstitial (Leydig) cells of the testes. Compare *aleydigism.*

hy·po·li·pe·mia, hy·po·li·pae·mia (high″po·li·pee′mee·uh) *n.* [*hypo-* + *lip-* + *-emia*]. Lowered fat concentration in the blood. —**hypolipe·mic, hypolipae·mic** (·mick) *adj.*

hy·po·lo·gia (high″po·lo′jee·uh) *n.* [*hypo-* + *-logia*]. Poverty of speech as a symptom of cerebral disease.

hy·po·mag·ne·se·mia, hy·po·mag·ne·sae·mia (high″po·mag″ne·see′mee·uh) *n.* [*hypo-* + *magnes*ium + *-emia*]. An abnormally low level of magnesium in the blood.

hy·po·ma·nia (high″po·may′nee·uh) *n.* [*hypo-* + *mania*]. A common, mild form of the manic type of manic depressive illness, in which the person generally exhibits rapid fluctuations between elation and irritation, great energy, impatience, euphoria, and occasionally bouts of depression; in an otherwise normal person, this state of stimulation may be very productive. —**hypo·man·ic** (man′ick) *adj.*

hy·po·mas·tia (high″po·mas′tee·uh) *n.* [*hypo-* + *-mastia*]. Abnormal smallness of the mammary glands.

hy·po·ma·ture (high″po·muh·tewr′) *adj.* [*hypo-* + *mature*]. IMMATURE.

hy·po·ma·zia (high″po·may′zee·uh) *n.* [*hypo-* + *maz-* + *-ia*]. HYPOMASTIA.

hy·po·mel·a·no·sis (high″po·mel″uh·no′sis) *n.* [*hypo-* + *melan-* + *-osis*]. Decrease in melanin pigmentation. —**hypo-mela·not·ic** (·not′ick) *adj.*

hy·po·men·or·rhea, hy·po·men·or·rhoea (high″po·men″o·ree′uh) *n.* [*hypo-* + *menorrhea*]. A small amount of menstrual flow over a shortened duration at the regular period. Compare *oligomenorrhea.*

hy·po·mere (high′po·meer) *n.* [*hypo-* + *-mere*]. The ventral portion of the mesothelial lining of the coelom of primitive chordates, forming pleura, pericardium, and peritoneum.

hy·po·me·tab·o·lism (high″po·me·tab′uh·liz·um) *n.* [*hypo-* + *metabolism*]. Metabolism below the normal rate.

hy·po·me·tro·pia (high″po·me·tro′pee·uh) *n.* [*hypo-* + *metr-* + *-opia*]. MYOPIA.

hy·po·mi·cro·gnath·us (high″po·migh″kro·nath′us) *n.* [*hypo-* + *micro-* + *-gnathus*]. An individual having an abnormally small lower jaw.

hy·po·mi·cron (high″po·migh′kron) *n.* [*hypo-* + *micron*]. A particle capable of being recognized by the ultramicroscope, but not be the ordinary microscope; SUBMICRON.

hy·po·mi·cro·so·ma (high″po·migh″kro·so′muh) *n.* [*hypo-* + *micro-* + *-soma*]. The lowest stature that is not dwarfism.

hy·pom·ne·sia (high″pom·nee′zhuh, ·zee·uh) *n.* [*hypo-* + *-mnesia*]. Poor or defective memory.

hy·po·morph (high′po·morf) *n.* [*hypo-* + *-morph*]. A mutation in which the mutant allele acts in the same direction as the normal one, but at a level too low to effect normal development. Compare *amorph.*

hy·po·mo·til·i·ty (high″po·mo·til′i·tee) *n.* [*hypo-* + *motility*]. 1. Decreased movement or motility, especially of the gastrointestinal tract. 2. HYPOKINESIA.

hy·po·na·tre·mia, hy·po·na·trae·mia (high″po·na·tree′mee·uh) *n.* [*hypo-* + *natr-* + *-emia*]. Abnormally low blood sodium level. —**hyponatre·mic** (·mick) *adj.*

hyponatremic syndrome. 1. LOW-SALT SYNDROME. 2. Specifically, a renal salt-wasting disorder usually associated with chronic renal disease, such as renal tubular disorders and chronic pyelonephritis. Hyponatremia, hypochloremia, and various degrees of azotemia are present.

hy·po·ni·trous oxide (high″po·nigh′trus). NITROUS OXIDE.

hy·po·nych·i·um (high″po·nick′ee·um) *n.* [NL., from *hyp-* + Gk. *onyx, onychos,* nail]. The thickened stratum corneum of the epidermis which lies under the free edge of a nail. —**hyponychi·al** (·ul) *adj.*

hy·po·os·to·sis (high″po·os·to′sis) *n.*, pl. **hypoosto·ses** (·seez) [*hypo-* + *ostosis*]. Hypoplasia of bone. —**hypoos·tot·ic** (·tot′ick) *adj.*

hy·po·ovar·i·an·ism (high″po·o·văr′ee·un·iz·um, ·o·vair′) *n.* [*hypo-* + *ovarian* + *-ism*]. Decrease in ovarian endocrine activity.

hy·po·para·thy·roid·ism (high″po·păr″uh·thigh′roy·diz·um) *n.* [*hypo-* + *parathyroid* + *-ism*]. The functional state resulting from insufficiency of parathyroid hormone, characterized by hypocalcemia, hyperphosphatemia, and increased neuromuscular excitability, sometimes progressing to seizures or tetany. —**hypoparathyroid,** *adj.*

hy·po·per·fu·sion (high″po·pur·few′zhun) *n.* [*hypo-* + *perfusion*]. A reduction of blood flow through a part.

hy·po·per·me·abil·i·ty (high″po·pur″mee·uh·bil′i·tee) *n.* [*hypo-* + *permeability*]. A state in which membranes have reduced permeability for electrolytes, and other solutes, or colloids.

hy·po·pha·lan·gism (high″po·fuh·lan′jiz·um) *n.* [*hypo-* + *phalang-* + *-ism*]. Congenital absence of one or more phalanges in a finger or toe.

hy·po·phar·yn·gi·tis (high″po·făr″in·jye′tis) *n.* [*hypopharyn*x + *-itis*]. Inflammation of the laryngopharynx.

hy·po·phar·yn·gos·co·py (high″po·făr″ing·gos′kuh·pee) *n.* [*hypopharyn*x + *-scopy*]. Inspection of the laryngopharynx.

hy·po·phar·ynx (high″po·făr′inks) *n.* [*hypo-* + *pharynx*]. LARYNGOPHARYNX.

hy·po·pho·ria (high″po·fo′ree·uh) *n.* [*hypo-* + *-phoria*]. A tendency of the visual axis of one eye to deviate below that of the other.

hy·po·phos·pha·ta·sia (high″po·fos″fuh·tay′zee·uh) *n.* [*hypo-* + *phosphatas*e + *-ia*]. 1. A deficiency of alkaline phosphatase, as in rickets. 2. An inborn error of metabolism, probably due to an autosomal recessive trait, characterized by a deficiency of tissue alkaline phosphatase; manifested by skeletal abnormalities resembling rickets or osteomalacia, defective development of teeth, and the presence of phosphoethanolamine (ethanolamine phosphate) in the urine.

hy·po·phos·pha·te·mia, hy·po·phos·pha·tae·mia (high″po·fos″fuh·tee′mee·uh, ·fos″fay·) *n.* [*hypo-* + *phosphat*e + *-emia*]. Abnormally low concentration of phosphates in the blood serum. See also *hypophosphatasia, familial hypophosphatemia.*

hy·po·phos·pha·tu·ria (high″po·fos″fuh·tew′ree·uh, ·fos″fay·) *n.* [*hypo-* + *phosphat*e + *-uria*]. Reduced urinary phosphate excretion.

hy·po·phos·phite (high″po·fos′fite) *n.* A salt of hypophosphorous acid.

hy·po·phos·pho·rous acid (high″po·fos′fuh·rus, ·fos·fo′rus). An aqueous solution containing HPH_2O_2. It is easily oxidized and, therefore, may prevent oxidation of other substances.

hy·po·phre·nia (high″po·free′nee·uh) *n.* [*hypo-* + *-phrenia*]. MENTAL RETARDATION. —**hypo·phren·ic** (·fren′ick) *adj.*

hy·poph·y·se·al (high·pof″i·see′ul, high″po·fiz′ee·ul) *adj.* Of or pertaining to the hypophysis.

hypophyseal cachexia. SIMMONDS' DISEASE.

hypophyseal cyst. RATHKE'S POUCH CYST.

hypophyseal-duct tumor. Any of the tumors derived from epithelial remnants of the involuted pouch of Rathke. Usually suprasellar, they include the craniopharyngioma and teratoma, which originate in the residual stalk, and cystic neoplasms, which originate from the residual cleft. More frequent in children than in adults.

hypophyseal fossa. A depression in the sphenoid bone lodging the hypophysis. Syn. *pituitary fossa.* NA *fossa hypophysialis.*

hypophyseal portal system. HYPOPHYSEOPORTAL CIRCULATION.

hypophyseal stalk. The combined infundibulum and pars tuberalis of the hypophysis.

hypophyseal stalk cyst. CRANIOPHARYNGIOMA.

hy·poph·y·sec·to·my (high·pof″i·seck′tuh·mee) *n.* [*hypophys*is

+ *-ectomy*]. Surgical removal of the hypophysis or pituitary gland. —**hypophysecto·mize** (·mize) *v.*

hy·poph·y·seo·por·tal (high·pof″i·see″o·por′tul, high″po·fiz″ee·o·) *adj.* Related to the hypophysis and its portal type of circulation.

hypophyseoportal circulation. The passage of blood from superior hypophyseal arteries through capillary clusters in the median eminence of the hypothalamus and the neural stalk through a second capillary bed in the adenohypophysis.

hy·po·phys·eo·priv·ic, hy·po·phys·io·priv·ic (high″po·fiz″ee·o·priv′ick) *adj.* [*hypophys*is + L. *priv*us, deprived of, + *-ic*]. Lacking in hypophyseal hormones.

hy·po·phys·i·al (high″po·fiz′ee·ul) *adj.* HYPOPHYSEAL.

hy·po·phys·io·por·tal (high″po·fiz″ee·o·por′tul) *adj.* HYPOPHYSEOPORTAL.

hy·poph·y·sis (high·pof′i·sis) *n.*, genit. **hy·po·phy·se·os** (high″po·fiz′ee·os), pl. **hypophy·ses** (·seez) [Gk., outgrowth] [NA]. A small, rounded, bilobate endocrine gland, averaging about 0.5 g in weight, which lies in the sella turcica of the sphenoid bone, is attached by a stalk, the infundibulum, to the floor of the third ventricle of the brain at the hypothalamus, and consists of an anterior lobe, the adenohypophysis, which produces and secretes various important hormones, including several which regulate other endocrine glands, and a less important posterior lobe, the neurohypophysis, which holds and secretes antidiuretic hormone and oxytocin produced in the hypothalamus. Syn. *pituitary gland.* NA alt. *glandula pituitaria.* See also *adenohypophysis, neurohypophysis, and Plates 17, 18, 26.*

hypophysis cer·e·bri (serr′e·brye). HYPOPHYSIS.

hy·po·pi·e·sia (high″po·pye·ee′zhuh, ·zee·uh) *n.* [*hypo-* + Gk. *piesis*, pressure, + *-ia*]. Subnormal arterial blood pressure resulting from an organic or specific cause.

hy·po·pi·e·sis (high″po·pye·ee′sis) *n.* HYPOPIESIA.

hy·po·pi·ne·al·ism (high″po·pin′ee·ul·iz·um, ·pi·nee′ul·iz·um) *n.* [*hypo-* + *pineal* + *-ism*]. Hypothetical lessened secretion of the pineal gland.

hy·po·pi·tu·i·ta·rism (high″po·pi·tew′i·tuh·riz·um) *n.* [*hypo-* + *pituitary* + *-ism*]. The clinical condition resulting from hypofunction of the anterior pituitary gland with secondary atrophy of the gonads, thyroid gland, and/or adrenal cortex; due to tumor or metastasis of neoplastic disease or to postpartum necrosis of the hypophysis. Syn. *adult hypopituitarism, pituitary insufficiency.* Compare *pituitary hypoadrenocorticism, pituitary hypogonadism, pituitary myxedema, Sheehan's syndrome.*

hypopituitary cachexia. SIMMONDS' DISEASE.

hy·po·pla·sia (high″po·play′zhuh, ·zee·uh) *n.* [*hypo-* + *-plasia*]. Underdevelopment of a tissue or organ, usually associated with a decreased number of cells. Compare *aplasia.* Contr. *hyperplasia.*

hypoplasia cu·tis con·ge·ni·ta (kew′tis kon·jen′i·tuh). FOCAL DERMAL HYPOPLASIA SYNDROME.

hy·po·plas·tic (high″po·plas′tick) *adj.* [*hypo-* + *-plastic*]. Pertaining to or characterized by hypoplasia.

hypoplastic anemia. PRIMARY REFRACTORY ANEMIA.

hypoplastic dwarf. An individual with usual proportions of bodily parts, but markedly smaller than normal. Contr. *achondroplastic dwarf.*

hypoplastic left-heart syndrome. Aortic atresia, or severe aortic stenosis, aortic arch atresia, or mitral atresia with hypoplasia of the left ventricle; there is severe cyanosis and heart failure.

hy·po·plas·ty (high′po·plas″tee) *n.* HYPOPLASIA.

hy·po·pnea (high″po·nee′uh) *n.* [*hypo-* + *-pnea*]. Diminution of breathing; abnormally slow or shallow breathing.

hy·po·po·tas·se·mia, hy·po·po·tas·sae·mia (high″po·po·ta·see′mee·uh) *n.* [*hypo-* + *potassemia*]. HYPOKALEMIA.

hy·po·prax·ia (high″po·prack′see·uh) *n.* [*hypo-* + *-praxia*]. 1. Deficient activity; inactivity. 2. Listlessness.

hy·po·pro·sex·ia (high″po·pro·seck′see·uh) *n.* [*hypo-* + Gk. *prosexis*, application, + *-ia*]. Inadequate attention or inability to pay attention.

hy·po·pro·tein·emia, hy·po·pro·tein·ae·mia (high″po·pro″tee·in·ee′mee·uh) *n.* [*hypo-* + *protein* + *-emia*]. Abnormally low concentration of protein in the blood.

hy·po·pro·throm·bin·emia, hy·po·pro·throm·bin·ae·mia (high″po·pro·throm″bin·ee′mee·uh) *n.* [*hypo-* + *prothrombin* + *-emia*]. Deficient supply of prothrombin in the blood.

hy·po·psel·a·phe·sia (high″po·sel″uh·fee′zee·uh, ·zhuh) *n.* [*hypo-* + Gk. *psēlaphēsis*, a touching, + *-ia*]. *Obsol.* Diminution of sensitivity to tactile impressions.

hy·po·psy·cho·sis (high″po·sigh·ko′sis) *n.* [*hypo-* + *psych-* + *-osis*]. Diminution or blunting of thought.

hy·po·py·on (high·po′pee·on, hi·po′) *n.* [Gk., ulcer, from *hypopyos*, suppurative, from *pyon*, pus]. A collection of pus in the anterior chamber of the eye.

hy·po·re·ac·tive (high″po·ree·ack′tiv) *adj.* [*hypo-* + *reactive*]. Characterized by decreased responsiveness to stimuli.

hy·po·re·flex·ia (high″po·re·fleck′see·uh) *n.* [*hypo-* + *reflex* + *-ia*]. Reflexes below normal. —**hyporeflex·ic** (·sick) *adj.*

hy·po·sal·i·va·tion (high″po·sal″i·vay′shun) *n.* [*hypo-* + *salivation*]. Pathologically insufficient secretion of saliva.

hy·po·scle·ral (high″po·skleer′ul, ·sklerr′ul) *adj.* [*hypo-* + *scleral*]. Beneath the sclera.

hy·po·se·cre·tion (high″po·se·kree′shun) *n.* [*hypo-* + *secretion*]. Diminished secretion.

hy·po·sen·si·tiv·i·ty (high″po·sen″si·tiv′i·tee) *n.* [*hypo-* + *sensitivity*]. A state of diminished sensitiveness, especially to appropriate external stimuli. —**hypo·sen·si·tive** (·sen′si·tiv) *adj.*; **hyposensitive·ness** (·nis) *n.*

hy·po·sen·si·ti·za·tion (high″po·sen″si·ti·zay′shun) *n.* 1. The process of producing hyposensitivity. 2. The lowering of the sensitivity of an individual to an antigen or hapten, usually by repeated injections of small amounts of the substance.

hy·pos·mia (high·poz′mee·uh, hi·poz′) *n.* [*hyp-* + *osm-* + *-ia*]. Diminution of the sense of smell.

hy·po·som·nia (high″po·som′nee·uh) *n.* [*hypo-* + L. *somnus*, sleep, + *-ia*]. An insufficient number of hours of sleep.

hy·po·spa·di·ac (high″po·spay′dee·ack) *adj.* & *n.* 1. Pertaining to hypospadias. 2. An individual with hypospadias.

hy·po·spa·di·as (high″po·spay′dee·us) *n.* [Gk., from *hypo-* + *span*, to tear, rend]. 1. A congenital anomaly of the penis and urethra in which the urethra opens upon the ventral surface of the penis or in the perineum. 2. A congenital malformation in which the urethra opens into the vagina.

hy·po·sper·ma·to·gen·e·sis (high″po·spur″muh·to·jen′e·sis, ·spur·mat″o·) *n.* [*hypo-* + *spermato-* + *-genesis*]. A decreased production of male germ cells, caused by such factors as diseased testes or hypoleydigism.

hy·pos·phre·sia (high″pos·free′zhuh, ·zee·uh) *n.* [*hyp-* + Gk. *osphrēsis*, sense of smell, + *-ia*]. HYPOSMIA.

hy·po·spon·dy·lot·o·my (high″po·spon″di·lot′uh·mee) *n.* [*hypo-* + *spondylo-* + *-tomy*]. HYOVERTEBROTOMY.

Hypospray. Trademark for a device for administering jet injections.

Hypospray anesthesia. Loss of sensation produced by administering anesthetic by Hypospray.

hy·pos·ta·sis (high·pos′tuh·sis, hi·) *n.*, pl. **hyposta·ses** (·seez) [Gk., sediment]. 1. A deposit that forms at the bottom of a liquid; a sediment. 2. The formation of a sediment, especially the settling of blood in dependent parts of the body.

hy·po·stat·ic (high″po·stat′ick) *adj.* [Gk. *hypostatikos*, substantial; patient]. 1. Due to, or of the nature of, hypostasis. 2. *In genetics*, subject to being suppressed, as a gene whose effect is suppressed by another gene that affects the same part of the organism.

hypostatic abscess. An abscess that gravitates to a lower position in the body.

hypostatic albuminuria. Proteinuria present in a supine position, but disappearing when standing erect.

hypostatic ectasia. Dilatation of a blood vessel in a dependent part, due to gravitational pooling of blood.

hypostatic pneumonia. Pneumonia in dependent parts of lungs which are hyperemic, seen in patients who remain in one position for long periods of time.

hy·po·sthe·nia (high″po·sthee′nee·uh) *n.* [*hypo-* + *sthenia*]. ASTHENIA. —**hyposthe·ni·ant** (·nee·unt), **hypo·sthen·ic** (·sthen′ick) *adj.*

hy·pos·the·nu·ria (high·pos″thi·new′ree·uh) *n.* [*hypo-* + Gk. *sthenos*, strength, + *-uria*]. The constant secretion of urine of low specific gravity.

hy·po·sto·mia (high″po·sto′mee′uh) *n.* [*hypo-* + *-stomia*]. A form of microstomia in which the mouth is a vertical slit opening into a pharyngeal sac.

hy·po·sul·fite, hy·po·sul·phite (high″po·sul′fite) *n.* A name, which has formerly been applied to salts both of thiosulfuric acid and of hydrosulfurous acid.

hy·po·syn·er·gia (high″po·sin·ur′jee·uh) *n.* [*hypo-* + Gk. *synergia*, cooperation]. DYSSYNERGIA.

hy·po·tax·ia (high″po·tack′see·uh) *n.* [Gk. *hypotaxis*, subjection, submission, + *-ia*]. A condition of emotional rapport existing in the beginning of hypnosis between the subject and the hypnotizer.

hy·po·tax·is (high″po·tack′sis) *n.* [Gk., subjection, submission]. Light hypnotic sleep.

hy·po·tel·or·ism (high″po·tel′ur·iz·um) *n.* [*hypo-* + Gk. *tēle*, far, + *horizein*, to be separated, + *-ism*]. Decrease in distance between two organs or parts. Contr. *hypertelorism.* See also *ocular hypotelorism.*

hy·po·ten·sion (high″po·ten′shun) *n.* [*hypo-* + *tension*]. 1. Diminished or abnormally low tension. 2. Specifically, low blood pressure.

hy·po·ten·sive (high″po·ten′siv) *adj.* 1. Pertaining to or characterized by hypotension. 2. Serving to reduce tension or to lower blood pressure.

hypotensive encephalopathy. HYPOXIC ENCEPHALOPATHY.

hy·po·ten·sor (high″po·ten′sur) *n.* [*hypotension* + *-or*]. Any substance capable of lowering blood pressure. It implies a persistent effect, as opposed to the fleeting effect of a depressor.

hy·po·tha·lam·ic (high″po·thuh·lam′ick) *adj.* Pertaining to or involving the hypothalamus.

hypothalamic amenorrhea. EMOTIONAL AMENORRHEA.

hypothalamic centers. Neuronal aggregates in the hypothalamus concerned with the regulation of autonomic functions, including body temperature, water balance, oxytocin secretion, adenohypophyseal function, food intake, and gastric secretion. See also *hypothalamus.*

hypothalamic epilepsy. DIENCEPHALIC EPILEPSY.

hypothalamic inhibitory factors. Hormonelike substances released from the hypothalamus which inhibit the release of specific hormones from the anterior pituitary gland. Compare *hypothalamic releasing factors.*

hypothalamic nucleus. SUBTHALAMIC NUCLEUS.

hypothalamic obesity. Obesity resulting from a disturbance of function of the appetite-regulating centers of the hypothalamus.

hypothalamic releasing factors. Hormones secreted by the hypothalamus which travel via nerve fibers to the anterior pituitary where they cause selective release of specific pituitary hormones. Compare *hypothalamic inhibitory factors.*

hypothalamic sulcus. A groove on the lower medial surface of each thalamus at the level of the third ventricle. NA *sulcus hypothalamicus.*

hypothalamic-thalamic seizure. The episodes of diencephalic autonomic epilepsy.

hy·po·thal·a·mo·hy·poph·y·se·al tract (high″po·thal″uh·mo·high·pof″i·see′ul, ·high·po·fiz′ee·ul). A tract of nerve fibers, with cells of origin in the supraoptic and paraventricular nuclei of the hypothalamus and also in the tuber cinereum, which runs through the median eminence and infundibular stem to the neurohypophysis and which distributes fibers to these parts. Its component parts are also referred to as supraopticohypophyseal tract, paraventricular fibers, and tuberohypophyseal tract, respectively.

hy·po·thal·a·mus (high″po·thal′uh·mus) *n.* [*hypo-* + *thalamus*] [NA]. The region of the diencephalon forming the floor of the third ventricle, including neighboring, associated nuclei. It is divided into three regions: (a) The anterior region, or pars supraoptica, which is superior to the optic chiasma, and includes the supraoptic and paraventricular nuclei and a less differentiated nucleus that merges with the preoptic area (the anterior hypothalamic nucleus). (b) The middle region, the pars tuberalis or tuber cinereum, including the lateral hypothalamic and tuberal nuclei, lateral to a sagittal plane passing through the anterior column of the fornix, and the dorsomedial, ventromedial, and posterior hypothalamic nuclei, medial to the above plane. (c) The caudal region, pars mamillaris or mamillary bodies, including medial, lateral, and intercalated mamillary nuclei and premamillary and supramamillary nuclei.

hy·po·the·nar (high″po·theen′ur, high·poth′e·nahr) *adj.* [Gk., from *hypo-* + *thenar*, palm]. Designating or pertaining to the fleshy eminence on the ulnar side of the palm of the hand.

hypothenar area. The region of the hypothenar eminence.

hypothenar eminence. An elevation on the ulnar side of the palm corresponding to the muscles of the little finger.

hypothenar reflex. Contraction of the palmaris brevis muscle upon stimulation over the pisiform bone.

hypothenar space. A potential space in the fascia surrounding the muscles of the hypothenar eminence in the hand.

hy·po·therm·es·the·sia, hy·po·therm·aes·the·sia (high″po·thur″mes·theezh′uh) *n.* [*hypo-* + *therm-* + *esthesia*]. Decreased temperature sensibility.

hy·po·ther·mia (high″po·thur′mee·uh) *n.* [*hypo-* + *-thermia*]. 1. Subnormal temperature of the body. 2. The artificial reduction of body temperature to below normal to slow physiologic processes for operative or therapeutic purposes. —**hypother·mal** (·mul), **hypother·mic** (·mick) *adj.*

hy·po·ther·my (high′po·thur″mee) *n.* HYPOTHERMIA.

hy·poth·e·sis (high·poth′e·sis) *n.*, pl. **hypothe·ses** (·seez) [Gk., proposal]. A supposition or conjecture put forth to account for known facts.

hy·po·thy·mia (high″po·thigh′mee·uh) *n.* [*hypo-* + *-thymia*]. 1. Despondency; depression of spirits. 2. A diminution in the intensity of emotions.

hy·po·thy·roid (high″po·thigh′roid) *adj.* Characterized or caused by, or pertaining to, hypothyroidism.

hy·po·thy·roid·ism (high″po·thigh′roid·iz·um) *n.* [*hypo-* + *thyroid* + *ism*]. The functional state resulting from insufficiency of thyroid hormones; the clinical manifestations depend upon the stage of development of the patient and the degree of insufficiency. See also *infantile hypothyroidism, cretinism, myxedema.*

hy·po·thy·ro·sis (high″po·thigh·ro′sis) *n.* [*hypo-* + *thyrosis*]. HYPOTHYROIDISM.

hy·po·to·nia (high″po·to′nee·uh) *n.* [*hypo-* + *-tonia*]. Decrease of normal tonicity or tension; especially diminution of intraocular pressure or of muscle tone.

hy·po·ton·ic (high″po·ton′ick) *adj.* [*hypo-* + *tonic*]. 1. Below the normal strength or tension. 2. Characterizing or pertaining to a solution whose osmotic pressure is less than that of sodium chloride solution, or any other solution taken as standard. —**hypo·to·nic·i·ty** (·to·nis′i·tee) *n.*

hypotonic bladder. ATONIC BLADDER.

hypotonic diplegia. A form of spastic diplegia (2), characterized by atonicity of the muscles of the extremities with retention of postural reflexes, preservation of tendon reflexes, and mental backwardness.

hypotonic infant syndrome. FLOPPY-INFANT SYNDROME.

hypotonic solution. A solution that produces a change in the tone of a tissue immersed in it through passage of water from the solution into the tissue. With reference to erythrocytes, a hypotonic solution of sodium chloride is one that contains less than 0.9 g of sodium chloride in each 100 ml.

hy·pot·o·ny (high·pot'uh·nee) *n.* HYPOTONIA.

hy·po·tri·chi·a·sis (high"po·tri·kigh'uh·sis) *n.* [*hypo-* + *trich-* + *-iasis*]. HYPOTRICHOSIS.

hy·po·tri·cho·sis (high"po·tri·ko'sis) *n.* [*hypo-* + *trich-* + *-osis*]. A condition in which there is less than normal hair.

hy·pot·ro·phy (high·pot'ruh·fee) *n.* [*hypo-* + *-trophy*]. 1. Subnormal growth. 2. Bacterial nutrition dependent on the host nutrition.

hy·po·tro·pia (high"po·tro'pee·uh) *n.* [*hypo-* + *-tropia*]. A form of strabismus in which one eye looks downward.

hy·po·tym·pa·num (high"po·tim'puh·num) *n.* [*hypo-* + *tympanum*]. The part of the tympanum lying below the level of the tympanic membrane. —**hypo·tym·pan·ic** (tim·pan'ick) *adj.*

hy·po·vaso·pres·sin·emia, hy·po·vaso·pres·sin·ae·mia (high"po·vay"zo·pres·in·ee'mee·uh, ·vas"o·) *n.* A decrease in circulating vasopressin leading to diabetes insipidus.

hy·po·veg·e·ta·tive (high"po·vej'e·tay"tiv) *adj.* [*hypo-* + *vegetative*]. Characterizing or pertaining to a human biotype in which purely somatic systems dominate over the visceral or nutritional organs.

hy·po·ven·ti·la·tion (high"po·ven·ti·lay'shun) *n.* [*hypo-* + *ventilation*]. 1. Reduced respiratory effort. 2. Reduced alveolar ventilation.

hy·po·vi·ta·min·osis (high"po·vye"tuh·min·o'sis) *n.*, pl. **hypo·vitamin·oses** (·o'seez) [*hypo-* + *vitamin* + *-osis*]. A condition due to deficiency of one or more vitamins in the diet.

hy·po·vo·le·mia, hy·po·vo·lae·mia (high"po·vo·le'mee·uh) *n.* [*hypo-* + *vol*ume- + *-emia*]. Low, or decreased, blood volume. —**hypovole·mic, hypovolae·mic** (·mick) *adj.*

hypovolemic shock. Shock caused by a reduced circulating blood volume which may be due to loss of blood or plasma as in burns, the crush syndrome, perforating wounds, or other trauma. Syn. *wound shock.*

hy·po·vo·lu·mic (high"po·vol·yoo'mick) *adj.* [*hypo-* + *volum*e + *-ic*]. Pertaining to a decreased volume of a body part, such as muscle or brain.

hy·po·xan·thine (high"po·zan'theen, ·thin) *n.* 6-Oxypurine or 6-ketopurine, $C_5H_4N_4O$, an intermediate product resulting when adenine, an amino purine formed by hydrolysis of nucleic acid, is transformed into uric acid and allantoin.

hypoxanthine-guanine phos·pho·ri·bo·syl transferase (fos"fo·rye'bo·sil). An enzyme which salvages and recycles guanine and hypoxanthine, preventing their further degradation and excretion as uric acid. Partial deficiency causes gout; complete deficiency causes Lesch-Nyhan disease. Abbreviated, HGPTase.

hypoxanthine-guanine phosphoribosyltransferase deficiency. An enzyme deficiency associated with Lesch-Nyhan disease.

hy·po·xan·thyl·ic acid (high"po·zan·thil'ick). INOSINIC ACID.

hyp·ox·emia, hy·pox·ae·mia (high"pock·see'mee·uh) *n.* [*hyp-* + *ox-* + *-emia*]. HYPOXIA. —**hypoxe·mic, hypoxae·mic** (·mick) *adj.*

hypoxemia test. The production of chest pain and electrocardiographic abnormalities by having the patient breathe a low oxygen mixture; formerly used as a diagnostic test for angina pectoris.

hypoxemic hypoxia. HYPOXIC HYPOXIA.

hyp·ox·ia (high·pock'see·uh, hi·pock') *n.* [*hyp-* + *ox-* + *-ia*]. Oxygen want or deficiency; any state wherein a physiologically inadequate amount of oxygen is available to, or utilized by, tissue without respect to cause or degree. Compare *asphyxia.* See also *anoxia.* —**hypox·ic** (·sick) *adj.*

hypoxic emphysema. EMPHYSEMA (1).

hypoxic encephalopathy. Brain damage resulting from oxygen deprivation due to failure of the heart and circulation or of the lungs and respiration; manifested clinically as disturbances of intellect, vision, and motor functioning progressing to recurrent convulsions, coma, the decorticate or decerebrate state, and even death; and manifested pathologically by cerebral edema, with scattered loss of neurons, gliosis, and patchy but widespread destruction of subcortical white matter, depending on the intensity and duration of the arterial oxygen unsaturation.

hypoxic hypoxia. Reduction in availability of oxygen to tissue due to a decrease in the partial pressure of oxygen in the arterial blood, as in low oxygen tension in inspired air, interference with gas exchange in the lungs, and arteriovenous shunts.

hyps-, hypsi-, hypso- [Gk. *hypsos,* height]. A combining form meaning *height, high.*

hyp·sar·rhyth·mia, hyp·sa·rhyth·mia (hip"sa·rith'mee·uh) *n.* [*hyps-* + *arrhythmia*]. An electroencephalographic abnormality consisting of continuous multifocal spikes and slow waves of large amplitude; characteristic of, but not specific for, infantile spasms.

hyp·sar·rhyth·moid, hyp·sa·rhyth·moid (hip"sa·rith'moid) *adj.* Pertaining to or characterized by hypsarrhythmia.

hypsi-. See *hyps-.*

hyp·si·brachy·ce·phal·ic (hip"si·brack"ee·se·fal'ick) *adj.* [*hypsi-* + *brachy-* + *cephalic*]. Having a skull that is high and broad.

hyp·si·ceph·a·ly (hip"si·sef'uh·lee) *n.* [*hypsi-* + *-cephaly*]. The condition of a skull with a cranial index of over 75.1.

hyp·si·conch (hip'si·konk) *adj.* [*hypsi-* + Gk. *konchē,* shell-like cavity]. *In craniometry,* designating an orbit that appears high because of an elongation of the superoinferior diameter; having an orbital index of 85.0 or more.

hyp·si·sta·phyl·ia (hip"si·sta·fil'ee·uh) *n.* [*hypsi-* + *staphyl-* + *-ia*]. The condition in which the palatal arch is high and narrow. —**hypsistaphyl·ic** (·ick), **hypsi·staph·y·line** (·staf'i·line) *adj.*

hypso-. See *hyps-.*

hyp·so·ceph·a·ly (hip"so·sef'uh·lee) *n.* HYPSICEPHALY.

hyp·so·chrome (hip'suh·krome) *n.* [*hypso-* + *-chrome*]. An atom or a group of atoms having the effect when introduced into a molecule or ion of displacing absorption in its spectrum to a higher frequency (shorter wavelength). Contr. *bathochrome.* —**hyp·so·chro·mic** (hip"suh·kro'mick) *adj.*

hyp·so·pho·bia (hip"so·fo'bee·uh) *n.* [*hypso-* + *-phobia*]. Morbid dread of being at a great height.

Hyrtl's loop (hirr'tel) [J. *Hyrtl,* Austrian anatomist, 1810–1894]. An anastomosis sometimes found between the two hypoglossal nerves.

Hyrtl's sphincter [J. *Hyrtl*]. NÉLATON'S SPHINCTER.

hys·sop (hiss'up) *n.* [Gk. *hyssōpos*]. The leaves and tops of *Hyssopus officinalis;* has been used as an aromatic stimulant and carminative.

hyster-, hystero- [Gk. *hystera,* womb]. A combining form meaning (a) *uterus, uterine;* (b) *hysteria, hysterical.*

hys·ter·al·gia (his"tur·al'jee·uh) *n.* [*hyster-* + *-algia*]. Neuralgic pain in the uterus. —**hysteral·gic** (·jick) *adj.*

hys·ter·ec·to·my (his"tur·eck'tuh·mee) *n.* [*hyster-* + *-ectomy*]. Total or partial surgical removal of the uterus.

hys·ter·e·sis (his"tur·ee'sis) *n.*, pl. **hystere·ses** (·seez) [Gk. *hysterēsis,* deficiency]. 1. *In medicine,* a delayed reaction in the formation of gels, as the retraction of a blood clot after coagulation. 2. *In physics,* the retention of a magnetic state of iron in a changing magnetic field. 3. *In chemistry,* the lag of a chemical system in attaining equilibrium.

hys·ter·eu·ryn·ter (his"tur·yoo·rin'tur) *n.* [*hyster-* + Gk. *eurynein,* to make wide]. A metreurynter used for dilating the cervix of the uterus.

hys·te·ria (his·teer'ee·uh, ·terr') *n.* [NL., lit., a uterine condition]. 1. *In psychiatry,* a neurosis resulting from repression of emotional conflicts from the conscious; characterized by immature, impulsive, dependent, and attention-seeking behavior, and conversion and dissociation symptoms. Usually through a process of suggestion or autosuggestion, the symptoms may take any form and involve any mental or bodily function under voluntary control. Compare *hysterical neurosis.* 2. *Loosely,* any excessive emotional response.

hys·te·ri·ac (his·teer'ee·ack) *n.* HYSTERIC.

hysteric, *n. & adj.* 1. An individual in a state of hysteria. 2. An overemotional individual. 3. HYSTERICAL.

hys·ter·i·cal (his·terr'i·kul) *adj.* Pertaining to or characterized by hysteria.

hysterical amblyopia or **blindness.** A unilateral or bilateral functional loss of vision involving great variations in the extent of the visual fields; seen in hysteria. See also *tubular vision.*

hysterical anesthesia. Loss of pain sense in the skin, seen in hysteria, usually taking on geometric configuration or conforming to zones covered by various articles of apparel, but not conforming to any dermatomes. See also *glove-and-stocking anesthesia.*

hysterical aphonia. Inability to speak, seen in the conversion type of hysterical neurosis.

hysterical ataxia. ASTASIA-ABASIA.

hysterical convulsion. HYSTEROEPILEPSY.

hysterical dermatoneurosis. A psychophysiologic disorder involving the skin.

hysterical dysbasia. The apparent difficulty in gait seen in hysterical individuals, often characterized by marked swaying, zigzag steps, superfluous movements, and faked falling by which the person dramatizes the disability.

hysterical epilepsy. HYSTEROEPILEPSY.

hysterical imitation. The complaints or acting out by an individual of the symptoms of an illness or of a behavior disorder known to him from experience, hearsay, or reading; a hysterical phenomenon, as in hysteroepilepsy.

hysterical mutism. ELECTIVE MUTISM.

hysterical neurosis. A form of neurosis in which there is an involuntary disturbance or loss of psychogenic origin of motor, sensory, or mental function. Characteristically, the symptoms begin and end suddenly in situations which are emotionally charged and which are symbolic of underlying, usually repressed conflicts; frequently the symptoms can be modified by suggestion. It can be classified as conversion type or dissociative type.

hysterical paralysis or **paraplegia.** Muscle weakness or paralysis without loss of reflex activity, in which no organic lesion can be demonstrated. See also *hysterical neurosis.*

hysterical personality. An individual whose behavior is characterized by excitability, instability under, and overreaction to, minor stress; self-dramatization; attention-seeking; and often seductiveness. Such individuals tend to be immature, undependable in their judgment, self-centered, vain, and dependent on others. Compare *hysterical neurosis.*

hysterical psychosis. *In psychiatry,* a term sometimes used to describe an acute episode or gross stress reaction in a hysterical personality, usually manifested by sudden, bizarre, histrionic, violent, and volatile behavior. See also *amuck, jumping Frenchman of Maine, lata.*

hysterical seizure. HYSTEROEPILEPSY.

hysterical stigmas. The specific, peculiar phenomena or symptoms of hysteria or hysterical neurosis, as anesthesia, hyperesthesia, hysterogenic zones, reversal of the color field, contraction of the visual field, amblyopia of sudden onset with normal pupillary responses, and impairment of the senses of hearing and of taste and of muscular sense. Syn. *neurasthenic stigmas.*

hysterical torticollis. Spasmodic torticollis due to psychogenic causes.

hys·ter·i·cism (his·terr'i·siz·um) *n.* [*hysteric* + *-ism*]. A tendency to hysteria.

hys·ter·ics (his·terr'icks) *n.* 1. A hysterical attack. 2. Extreme emotional display, as a fit of laughing, crying, or anger.

hys·ter·i·form (his·terr'i·form) *adj.* [*hyster-* + *-form*]. Resembling hysteria.

hys·ter·i·tis (his''tur·eye'tis) *n.* [*hyster-* + *-itis*]. METRITIS.

hystero-. See *hyster-.*

hys·tero·bu·bono·cele (his''tur·o·bew·bon'o·seel) *n.* [*hystero-* + *bubonocele*]. An inguinal hysterocele.

hys·tero·cele (his'tur·o·seel) *n.* [*hystero-* + *-cele*]. A hernia containing all or part of the uterus.

hys·tero·clei·sis (his''tur·o·klye'sis) *n.* [*hystero-* + *-cleisis*]. The closure of the uterus by suturing the edges of the os.

hys·tero·cys·tic (his''tur·o·sis'tick) *adj.* [*hystero-* + *cystic*]. Pertaining to the uterus and the urinary bladder.

hys·tero·cys·to·pexy (his''tur·o·sis'to·peck''see) *n.* [*hystero-* + *cysto-* + *-pexy*]. Suturing of the uterus to the bladder and abdominal wall.

hys·tero·de·mon·op·a·thy (his''tur·o·dee''mun·op'uth·ee) *n.* [*hystero-* + *demono-* + *-pathy*]. Demonomania in hysteria.

hys·ter·o·dyn·ia (his''tur·o·din'ee·uh) *n.* [*hyster-* + *-odynia*]. Pain in the uterus.

hys·tero·ep·i·lep·sy (his''tur·o·ep'i·lep·see) *n.* [*hystero-* + *epilepsy*]. Hysteria in which seizures usually occur only in the presence of others; they are frequently triggered by some emotional situation, are imitative of true epileptic phenomena including disorganized violent muscular movements, and are abruptly terminated without the confusion and lethargy which frequently occur in true epilepsy.

hys·tero·fren·a·to·ry (his''tur·o·fren'uh·tor·ee) *adj.* HYSTEROFRENIC.

hys·tero·fren·ic (his''tur·o·fren'ick) *adj.* [*hystero-* + L. *frenum,* curb, + *-ic*]. Capable of arresting an attack of hysteria, as pressure on a certain point or part of the body.

hys·tero·gen·ic (his''tur·o·jen'ick) *adj.* [*hystero-* + *-genic*]. Producing hysterical phenomena or symptoms.

hysterogenic zone. 1. A painful spot occurring in hysteria, not due to organic disease. 2. An area of the body such as the inguinal and mammary regions which, when pressed, produces hysterical attacks in susceptible individuals.

hys·ter·og·e·nous (his''tur·oj'e·nus) *adj.* HYSTEROGENIC.

hysterogenous point. HYSTEROGENIC ZONE.

hys·ter·og·e·ny (his''tur·oj'e·nee) *n.* [*hystero-* + *-geny*]. The induction of hysteria.

hys·tero·gram (his'tur·o·gram) *n.* [*hystero-* + *-gram*]. A roentgenogram obtained after the injection of the uterine cavity with contrast material.

hys·ter·og·ra·phy (his''tur·og'ruh·fee) *n.* [*hystero-* + *-graphy*]. Roentgenologic examination of the uterus after the introduction of a contrast medium.

hys·ter·oid (his'tur·oid) *adj.* [*hyster-* + *-oid*]. Resembling hysteria.

hys·ter·oi·dal (his''tur·oy'dul) *adj.* HYSTEROID.

hys·tero·lap·a·rot·o·my (his''tur·o·lap''uh·rot'uh·mee) *n.* [*hystero-* + *laparotomy*]. Abdominal hysterectomy or hysterotomy.

hys·tero·lith (his'tur·o·lith) *n.* [*hystero-* + *-lith*]. A calculus in the uterus.

hys·tero·li·thi·a·sis (his''tur·o·li·thigh'uh·sis) *n.,* pl. **hysterolithia·ses** (·seez) [*hysterolith* + *-iasis*]. The formation of a concretion in the uterus.

hys·ter·ol·o·gy (his''tur·ol'uh·jee) *n.* [*hystero-* + *-logy*]. The branch of medical science dealing with the anatomy, physiology, and pathology of the uterus.

hys·ter·ol·y·sis (his''tur·ol'i·sis) *n.,* pl. **hysteroly·ses** (·seez) [*hystero-* + *-lysis*]. Severing the attachments or adhesions of the uterus.

hys·tero·ma·nia (his''tur·o·may'nee·uh) *n.* [*hystero-* + *-mania*]. 1. Psychomotor overactivity seen in hysteria. 2. NYMPHOMANIA.

hys·ter·om·e·ter (his''tur·om'e·tur) *n.* [*hystero-* + *-meter*]. An instrument for measuring the length of the intrauterine cavity. —**hysterome·try** (·tree) *n.*

hys·tero·my·o·ma (his″tur·o·migh·o′muh) *n.* [*hystero-* + *myoma*]. A uterine leiomyoma.

hys·tero·my·o·mec·to·my (his″tur·o·migh″o·meck′tuh·mee) *n.* [*hysteromyoma* + *-ectomy*]. *In surgery,* removal of a fibroid tumor of the uterus.

hys·tero·my·ot·o·my (his″tur·o·migh·ot′uh·mee) *n.* [*hystero-* + *myo-* + *-tomy*]. Incision into the uterus for removal of a solid tumor.

hys·tero-oo·pho·rec·to·my (his″tur·o·o″uh·fo·reck′tuh·mee) *n.* [*hystero-* + *oophor-* + *-ectomy*]. *In surgery,* removal of the uterus and ovaries.

hys·ter·op·a·thy (his″tur·op′uth·ee) *n.* [*hystero-* + *-pathy*]. Any disease or disorder of the uterus. —**hys·tero·path·ic** (his″tur·o·path′ick) *adj.*

hys·tero·pexy (his′tur·o·peck″see) *n.* [*hystero-* + *-pexy*]. Fixation of the uterus by a surgical operation to correct displacement.

hys·tero·phil·ia (his″tur·o·fil′ee·uh) *n.* [*hystero-* + *-philia*]. A tendency to develop symptoms of the conversion type of hysterical neurosis.

hys·tero·plas·ty (his′tur·o·plas″tee) *n.* [*hystero-* + *-plasty*]. A plastic operation on the uterus.

hys·ter·op·to·sis (his″tur·op·to′sis) *n.* [*hystero-* + *-ptosis*]. Falling or inversion of the uterus.

hys·ter·or·rha·phy (his″tur·or′uh·fee) *n.* [*hystero-* + *-rrhaphy*]. The closure of a uterine incision or rent by suture.

hys·ter·or·rhex·is (his″tur·o·reck′sis) *n.*, pl. **hysterorrhex·es** (·seez) [*hystero-* + *-rrhexis*]. Rupture of the uterus.

hys·tero·sal·pin·gec·to·my (his″tur·o·sal″pin·jeck′tuh·mee) *n.* [*hystero-* + *salping-* + *-ectomy*]. Excision of the uterus and oviducts.

hys·tero·sal·pin·gog·ra·phy (his″tur·o·sal″ping·gog′ruh·fee) *n.* [*hystero-* + *salpingo-* + *-graphy*]. Radiographic examination of the uterus and oviducts after injection of a radiopaque substance into their cavities. See also *combined gynecography.*

hys·tero·sal·pin·go-oo·pho·rec·to·my (his″tur·o·sal·ping″go·o″uh·fo·reck′tuh·mee) *n.* [*hystero-* + *salpingo-* + *oophor-* + *-ectomy*]. Excision of the uterus, oviducts, and ovaries.

hys·tero·sal·pin·go-oo·the·cec·to·my (his″tur·o·sal·ping″go·o″o·thi·seck′tuh·mee) *n.* [*hystero-* + *salpingo-* + *oothec-* + *-ectomy*]. *Obsol.* HYSTEROSALPINGO-OOPHORECTOMY.

hys·tero·sal·pin·gos·to·my (his″tur·o·sal″ping·gos′tuh·mee) *n.* [*hystero-* + *salpingo-* + *-stomy*]. The establishment of an anastomosis between an oviduct and the uterus.

hys·tero·scope (his′tur·o·skope) *n.* [*hystero-* + *-scope*]. A uterine speculum with a reflector. —**hys·ter·os·co·py** (his″tur·os′kuh·pee) *n.*

hys·tero·tome (his′tur·o·tome) *n.* [*hystero-* + *-tome*]. An instrument for incising the uterus.

hys·ter·ot·o·my (his″tur·ot′uh·mee) *n.* [*hystero-* + *-tomy*]. 1. Incision of the uterus. 2. CESAREAN SECTION.

hys·tero·trach·e·lec·to·my (his″tur·o·tray″ke·leck′tuh·mee, ·track″e·leck′) *n.* [*hystero-* + *trachel-* + *-ectomy*]. Amputation of the cervix of the uterus.

hys·tero·trach·e·lo·plas·ty (his″tur·o·tray′ke·lo·plas″tee, ·track′e·lo·) *n.* [*hystero-* + *trachelo-* + *plasty*]. Plastic surgery on the cervix of the uterus.

hys·tero·trach·e·lor·rha·phy (his″tur·o·tray″ke·lor′uh·fee, ·track″e·lor′) *n.* [*hystero-* + *trachelo-* + *-rrhaphy*]. A plastic operation for the restoration of a lacerated cervix of the uterus.

hys·tero·trach·e·lot·o·my (his″tur·o·tray″ke·lot′uh·mee, ·track″e·lot′) *n.* [*hystero-* + *trachelo-* + *-tomy*]. Surgical incision of the cervix of the uterus.

hys·tero·trau·mat·ic (his″tur·o·traw·mat′ick, ·trow·) *adj.* [*hystero-* + *traumatic*]. Pertaining to hysterotraumatism.

hys·tero·trau·ma·tism (his″tur·o·traw′muh·tiz·um, ·traow′) *n.* [*hystero-* + *traumatism*]. Hysterical symptoms arising in association with a severe injury.

hys·trix (his′tricks) *n.* [Gk., porcupine]. NEVUS VERRUCOSUS.

Hytakerol. A trademark for dihydrotachysterol, a blood-calcium regulator.

hy·ther (high′thur) *n.* [Gk. *hydōr*, water, + *thermē*, heat]. The combined effect of the atmospheric heat and humidity on an organism.

Hyzyd. A trademark for isoniazid, a tuberculostatic.

H zone. The region of low density bisecting the A disk of a striated myofibril, occupied by myosin filaments only. Syn. *Hensen's disk.*

I

I Symbol for iodine.

^{125}I Symbol for the radioactive isotope of iodine of atomic weight 125. Formerly written I^{125}. See also Table of Common Radioactive Pharmaceuticals in the Appendix.

^{131}I Symbol for the radioactive isotope of iodine of atomic weight 131. Formerly written I^{131}. See also *radioiodine,* and Table of Common Radioactive Pharmaceuticals in the Appendix.

i- *In chemistry,* symbol for is-, iso-.

-ia [L. and Gk. abstract noun suffix]. A suffix indicating a *condition, especially an abnormal or pathologic condition.*

I.A.D.R. International Association for Dental Research.

iam·a·tol·o·gy (eye·am″uh·tol′uh·jee) *n.* [Gk. *iama, iamatos,* remedy, + *-logy*]. The science or study of remedies or therapeutics.

-iasis [Gk. verb-nominalizing suffix]. A suffix indicating *a diseased condition caused by or resembling.*

-iatric [Gk. *iatrikos,* of a physician, medical]. A combining form meaning *pertaining to medical treatment of* (a specified category or aspect of patients).

iatro- [Gk. *iatros,* physician]. A combining form signifying a *relation to medicine or to physicians.*

iat·ro·chem·is·try (eye·at″ro·kem′is·tree) *n.* [*iatro-* + *chemistry*]. 1. The application of chemistry to therapeutics; the treatment of disease by chemical means. 2. A seventeenth century theory that physiology and disease and its treatment are explicable on a chemical basis.

iat·ro·gen·ic (eye·at″ro·jen′ick) *adj.* [*iatro-* + *-genic*]. Induced by a physician or by medical treatment; of or pertaining to the effects of a physician's words, actions, or treatments upon the patient. —**iatro·gen·e·sis** (·jen′e·sis) *n.*

iat·ro·phys·ics (eye·at″ro·fiz′icks) *n.* [*iatro-* + *physics*]. 1. The treatment of disease by physical measures. 2. A seventeenth century school of medicine which used physical principles to explain normal physiology, as well as disease and treatment.

iat·ro·tech·ni·cal (eye·at″ro·teck′ni·kul) *adj.* [*iatro-* + *technical*]. Pertaining to medical techniques.

-iatry [Gk. *iatreia*]. A combining form meaning *medical treatment.*

I band [*i*sotropic band]. The zone of relatively low density and low birefringence between two A bands of a striated muscle fibril; represents a zone occupied by actin filaments only. The I band is transected by the Z line. Contr. *A band.*

ibid (ib′id) [L. *ibidem*]. In the same book, paper, or place.

I blood group. The erythrocyte antigens defined by reactions with anti-I and anti-i antibodies, which occur both in acquired hemolytic anemia and naturally in certain normal persons of the rare phenotype i.

ibo·ga·ine (eye″bo·gay′een, ·in, i·bo′gay·een, ·in) *n.* An alkaloid, $C_{20}H_{26}N_2O$, from the roots of *Tabernanthe iboga,* a plant of the Congo; a stimulant like caffeine, which produces hallucination and paralysis in overdose.

ibu·fen·ac (eye·bew′fe·nack) *n.* (*p*-Isobutylphenyl)acetic acid, $C_{12}H_{16}O_2$, an analgesic and inflammation-counteracting drug.

ibu·pro·fen (eye·bew′pro·fen) *n.* 2-(*p*-Isobutylphenyl)propionic acid, $C_{13}H_{18}O_2$, an anti-inflammatory drug.

-ic [L. *-icus,* from Gk. *-ikos*]. 1. A general adjective-forming suffix meaning *of* or *pertaining to.* 2. *In chemistry,* a suffix designating the higher of two valencies assumed by an element and, incidentally, in many cases, a larger amount of oxygen. Contr. *-ous.*

ice, *n.* Water in its solid state, which at 1 atmosphere it assumes at a temperature of 0°C, or 32°F.

ice bag. A bag, usually of rubber, to hold cracked ice; used to reduce the temperature of a part locally, sometimes in attempts to control acute localized swelling or inflammation.

iced spleen. A spleen with a clear, translucent, pearl-gray or pale-blue hyalinized capsule. Syn. *sugar-coated spleen, zuckerguss spleen.*

Ice·land disease. BENIGN MYALGIC ENCEPHALOMYELITIS.

Iceland moss. A lichen, *Cetraria islandica,* found in Iceland and other northern countries. It contains a starchlike substance, lechenin, that gelatinizes when boiled with water. It has been used as a demulcent and nutrient.

Iceland spar. A crystalline form of calcium carbonate, having doubly refracting properties; used in polariscopes.

ich·no·gram (ick′no·gram) *n.* [Gk. *ichnos,* track, + *-gram*]. *In legal medicine,* the record of a footprint.

ichor (eye′kor, eye′kur) *n.* [Gk. *ichōr,* juice, serous discharge]. A thin discharge from an ulcer or wound. —**ichor·ous** (·us), **ichor·oid** (·oid) *adj.*

ichor·rhea, ichor·rhoea (eye″ko·ree′uh) *n.* [*ichor* + *-rrhea*]. A copious flow of ichor.

ichor·rhe·mia, ichor·rhae·mia (eye″ko·ree′mee·uh) *n.* [*ichor* + *-hemia*]. 1. PYEMIA. 2. SEPTICEMIA.

ich·tham·mol (ick′thuh·mole, ·mol) *n.* [*ichthy-* (from fossil fish in the shale originally used in its production) + *ammonia* + *-ol*]. A reddish-brown to brownish-black, viscid fluid of characteristic odor; obtained by the destructive distillation of certain bituminous schists, followed by sulfonation of the distillate and neutralization with ammonia. It is used as a weak antiseptic and stimulant in skin diseases, usually in ointment form; it has been occasionally used internally as an expectorant.

ichthy-, ichthyo- [Gk. *ichthys*]. A combining form meaning *fish.*

ich·thy·ism (ikth'ee·iz·um) *n.* [*ichthy-* + *-ism*]. Poisoning from eating fish containing toxic substances, as of bacterial origin.

ich·thy·is·mus (ikth"ee·iz'mus) *n.* ICHTHYISM.

Ichthymall. A trademark for ichthammol.

Ichthynat. A trademark for ichthammol.

ichthyo-. See *ichthy-*.

ich·thyo·col·la (ikth"ee·o·kol'uh) *n.* [Gk. *ichthyokolla,* fish glue]. Isinglass; a gelatinous substance prepared from the air bladders of the sturgeon and other fish. Used as a food, adhesive, and clarifying agent.

ich·thy·oid (ikth'ee·oid) *adj.* [Gk. *ichthyoeidēs*]. Resembling or shaped like a fish.

Ichthyol. A trademark for ichthammol.

ich·thy·ol·o·gy (ikth"ee·ol'uh·jee) *n.* [*ichthyo-* + *-logy*]. The study of fishes.

ich·thy·oph·a·gous (ikth"ee·off'uh·gus) *adj.* [Gk. *ichthyophagos,* from *ichthyo-* + *phagein,* to eat]. Eating or subsisting on fish.

ich·thyo·pho·bia (ikth"ee·o·fo'bee·uh) *n.* [*ichthyo-* + *-phobia*]. 1. A morbid fear of fish. 2. An intense dislike for the taste or smell of fish. —**ichthyopho·bic** (·bick) *adj.*

ich·thyo·sar·co·tox·in (ikth"ee·o·sahr"ko·tock'sin) *n.* [*ichthyo-* + *sarco-* + *toxin*]. Toxin found in the flesh of poisonous fishes. —**ichthyosarcotox·ic** (·sick) *adj.*

ich·thyo·sar·co·tox·ism (ikth"ee·o·sahr"ko·tock'siz·um) *n.* Poisoning from ichthyosarcotoxin. Compare *ichthyotoxism.*

ich·thy·o·si·form (ikth"ee·o'si·form) *adj.* [*ichthyosis* + *-iform*]. Resembling ichthyosis.

ich·thy·o·sis (ikth"ee·o'sis) *n.*, pl. **ichthyo·ses** (·seez) [*ichthy-* + *-osis*]. A genodermatosis characterized by a dry harsh skin with adherent scales, most severe on the extensor surfaces of the extremities. —**ichthy·ot·ic** (·ot'ick) *adj.*

ichthyosis con·gen·i·ta (kon·jen'i·tuh). A severe, probably familial form of ichthyosis present at birth; the fetus may be stillborn or live a few days. The skin and mucous membranes are markedly cracked and thickened, producing a bizarre checked appearance. Syn. *harlequin fetus.*

ichthyosis fe·ta·lis (fee·tay'lis). ICHTHYOSIS CONGENITA.

ichthyosis fol·lic·u·la·ris (fol·ick'yoo·lair'is). The genodermatosis with moderate ichthyosis and associated baldness, absence of eyebrows and eyelashes, thickened lens, and conjunctivitis.

ichthyosis hystrix. NEVUS VERRUCOSUS.

ichthyosis le·tha·lis (lee·thay'lis). ICHTHYOSIS CONGENITA.

ichthyosis sim·plex (sim'plecks). The common form of ichthyosis developing in early life; characterized by large, finely corrugated, papery scales with deficient secretions of the sebaceous glands and sometimes of the sweat glands.

ichthyosis vul·ga·ris (vul·gair'is). ICHTHYOSIS SIMPLEX.

ich·thyo·tox·in (ikth"ee·o·tock'sin) *n.* [*ichthyo-* + *toxin*]. The toxic constituent of eel serum.

ich·thyo·tox·ism (ikth"ee·o·tock'siz·um) *n.* [*ichthyo-* + *tox-* + *-ism*]. ICHTHYISM.

ich·thyo·tox·is·mus (ikth"ee·o·tock·siz'mus) *n.* ICHTHYISM.

ic·ing liver. Hyaline thickening of the liver capsule, giving the appearance of white cake icing.

icon (eye'kon) *n.* [Gk. *eikōn*]. An image or model. —**icon·ic** (eye·kon'ick) *adj.*

icon-, icono- [Gk. *eikōn*]. A combining form meaning *image.*

ico·nog·ra·phy (eye"kuh·nog'ruh·fee) *n.* [Gk. *eikonographia,* description, from *eikōn,* image]. 1. Graphic or plastic representation or illustration. 2. History and theory of the techniques and styles of illustration or representation.

icon·o·lag·ny (eye·kon"o·lag'nee, eye·kon'o·lag"nee) *n.* [*icono-* + Gk. *lagneia,* salaciousness]. Sexual stimulation induced by the sight of statues or pictures.

icono·ma·nia (eye·kon"o·may'nee·uh) *n.* [*icono-* + *-mania*]. A morbid interest in images. See also *iconolagny.*

-ics [*-ic* + *-s*]. A suffix meaning *a field of organized knowledge or practice.*

ICSH Abbreviation for *interstitial-cell stimulating hormone* (= LUTEINIZING HORMONE).

ICT Abbreviation for *insulin coma therapy* (= INSULIN SHOCK THERAPY).

ic·tal (ick'tul) *adj.* Pertaining to or caused by ictus.

ictal automatism. EPILEPTIC AUTOMATISM.

ic·ta·sol (ick'tuh·sole) *n.* A material with the tentative formula of $C_{28}H_{36}Na_2O_6S_3$, obtained by the destructive distillation of bituminous schists, followed by sulfonation of the distillate; employed as a disinfectant.

icter-, ictero-. A combining form meaning *icterus, jaundice.*

ic·ter·ic (ick·terr'ick) *adj.* [Gk. *ikterikos,* from *ikteros,* jaundice]. Pertaining to or characterized by jaundice.

ic·tero·gen·ic (ick"tur·o·jen'ick) *adj.* [*ictero-* + *-genic*]. Causing jaundice.

ic·ter·og·e·nous (ick"tur·oj'e·nus) *adj.* ICTEROGENIC.

ic·tero·he·mo·lyt·ic anemia (ick"tur·o·hee·mo·lit'ick). HEMOLYTIC ANEMIA.

ic·tero·hem·or·rhag·ic fever (ick"tur·o·hem·o·raj'ick). WEIL'S DISEASE.

ic·ter·oid (ick'tur·oid) *adj.* [*icter-* + *-oid*]. Resembling the color of, or having the nature of, jaundice.

ic·ter·us (ick'tur·us) *n.* [Gk. *ikteros*]. JAUNDICE.

icterus grav·is (grav'is). ACUTE YELLOW ATROPHY.

icterus gravis neonatorum. ERYTHROBLASTOSIS FETALIS.

icterus index. A measurement of the yellow color of blood serum when compared with standard solutions of potassium dichromate; roughly correlated with serum bilirubin levels.

icterus index test. A colorimetric test for jaundice in which blood serum is compared with a standard solution of sodium dichromate.

icterus neonatorum. JAUNDICE OF THE NEWBORN.

ic·tus (ick'tus) *n.* [L., a blow]. 1. An acute attack, or stroke, as a cerebrovascular accident. 2. Specifically, an epileptic attack, usually a generalized or psychomotor seizure.

ICU Abbreviation for *intensive care unit.*

IC wave. Abbreviation for *isovolumetric contraction wave.*

id, *n.* [L., it]. *In psychoanalysis,* an unconscious part of the personality consisting of those wishes and needs which are the mental representations of the sexual and aggressive instinctual drives as well as of wishes resulting from perceptions and memories of the earlier gratification of basic physiologic needs. Contr. *ego, superego.*

-id [Gk. *-idēs,* descendent of, related to]. A suffix designating (a) *a stage in the maturation of a kind of cell or organism,* as spermatid; (b) *one of a* (specified) *family of animals,* as mustelid, one of the Mustelidae; (c) *a skin lesion related to a* (specified) *agent or cause,* as tuberculid, angiectid; (d) *a mandibular tooth element corresponding to a* (specified) *maxillary element,* as entoconid, corresponding to entocone; (e) in chemistry, *-ide* (b), as lipid.

-idae. *In biology,* a suffix indicating a taxonomic *family.*

-ide [F., from L. *-idus* (adjective suffix)]. A suffix indicating (a) *the nonmetallic element in a binary compound,* as chloride; (b) *a compound derived from another compound,* as ureide; (c) *certain sugar derivatives,* as glycoside, cerebroside; (d) *a member of certain groups of chemical elements,* as actinide, lanthanide.

idea, *n.* [Gk., form]. 1. A mental impression or thought; a belief or object existing in the mind or thought. 2. *In psychology,* an experience or thought not directly due to an external sensory stimulation.

idea chase. FLIGHT OF IDEAS.

ide·al·iza·tion, *n.* 1. Seeing or conceiving a person, situation, or object as ideal, perfect, or far better than it is, with an exaggeration of the virtues and an overlooking of faults. 2. *In psychiatry,* a defense mechanism in which there is a gross overestimation of another person or a situation. 3. *In psychoanalysis,* a sexual overevaluation of the love object.

ideas of influence. *In psychiatry,* a clinical manifestation of certain psychoses in which one may believe that one's thoughts are read, that one's limbs move involuntarily, or that one is under the control of someone else or some external force or influence.

ideas of reference. *In psychopathology,* the symptom complex in which, through the mechanism of projection, every casual remark or incident is believed directed at the individual with hostile intent; observed in various paranoid states, the paranoid type of schizophrenia, and in manic-depressive illness.

ide·a·tion (eye″dee·ay′shun) *n.* The formation of a mental conception; the mental action by which, or in accord with which, an idea is formed. —**ideation·al** (·ul) *adj.*

ideational apraxia. One of the now largely abandoned divisions of the apractic syndromes, including those syndromes thought to be due to affection of a presumed ideation area rather than of motor association cortex or of fibers connecting the ideation area with it. Contr. *ideomotor apraxia, motor apraxia.*

idée fixe (ee·day feeks) [F.]. FIXED IDEA.

idem (eye′dim, id′im) [L.]. The same author as previously mentioned.

-idene. A suffix designating *a radical having two valence bonds at the point of attachment.*

iden·ti·cal points. Corresponding points of the two retinas, upon which the rays from an object must be focused so that it may be seen as one.

identical twins. Twins developed from a single ovum, always of the same sex, the same genetic constitution, and ordinarily the same chorion. Syn. *monozygotic twins.* Contr. *fraternal twins.*

iden·ti·fi·ca·tion, *n.* 1. Verification of identity. 2. Establishment of a specimen's classification or composition. 3. *In psychiatry,* a defense mechanism whereby one unconsciously patterns one's self, on the basis of love or aggression, after the characteristics of another. Identification normally plays a major role in the development of the personality and especially of the superego, but when used to excess, may disturb the development of an integrated and independent ego. See also *hostile identification.*

iden·ti·ty, *n.* [F. *identité,* from L. *identitas,* from *idem,* the same]. 1. Exact sameness; selfsameness. 2. *In psychiatry,* the sense of unity and of continuity of one's own self in the face of changing experiences. Syn. *ego-identity.*

ileal bladder. ILEAL CONDUIT.

ileal conduit. A segment of ileum which is surgically prepared to receive both ureters and to serve as a substitute bladder.

identity crisis. The critical period in emotional maturation and personality development, occurring usually during adolescence, which involves the reworking and abandonment of childhood identifications and the integration of new personal and social identifications.

ideo-. A combining form meaning (a) *idea;* (b) *pertaining to the mind.*

ideo·ge·net·ic (id″ee·o·je·net′ick, eye″dee·o·) *adj.* [*ideo-* + *genetic*]. 1. Pertaining to mental activity in which primary sense impressions are employed in place of completed ideas that are ready for expression. 2. Produced within the mind, as the assumption that judgment or a sense of responsibility is a primary mental activity and not due to experience.

ide·og·e·nous (id″ee·oj′e·nus, eye″dee·) *adj.* IDEOGENETIC.

ideo·glan·du·lar (id″ee·o·glan′dew·lur, eye″dee·o·) *adj.* [*ideo-* + *glandular*]. Pertaining to glandular activity as evoked by a mental concept, as salivating at the thought of a good meal.

ideo·ki·net·ic (id″ee·o·ki·net′ick, eye″dee·o·) *adj.* [*ideo-* + *kinetic*]. IDEOMOTOR.

ideokinetic apraxia. IDEOMOTOR APRAXIA.

ide·ol·o·gy (id″ee·ol′uh·jee, eye″dee·) *n.* [*ideo-* + *-logy*]. 1. The science of ideas and of intellectual operations. 2. A program of ideas or world view.

ideo·me·tab·o·lism (id″ee·o·me·tab′uh·liz·um, eye″dee·o·) *n.* [*ideo-* + *metabolism*]. Metabolic processes induced by mental and emotional causes. —**ideo·met·a·bol·ic** (·met″uh·bol′ick) *adj.*

ideo·mo·tor (id″ee·o·mo′tur) *adj.* [*ideo-* + *motor*]. 1. Pertaining to involuntary movement resulting from or accompanying some mental activity, as moving the lips while reading. 2. Pertaining to both ideation and motor activity.

ideomotor apraxia. One of the now largely abandoned divisions of the apractic syndromes, including those syndromes thought to be due to disconnection of a presumed ideation area in the supramarginal gyrus of the dominant hemisphere from association cortex, either by interruption of long association fibers within the dominant hemisphere (causing an apraxia of both sides of the body) or by disconnection of the motor areas of the two hemispheres by a callosal lesion (causing an apraxia on the non-dominant side only). Contr. *ideational apraxia, motor apraxia.*

ideo·mus·cu·lar (id″ee·o·mus′kew·lur) *adj.* [*ideo-* + *muscular*]. IDEOMOTOR.

ideo·pho·bia (id″ee·o·fo′bee·uh, eye″dee·o·) *n.* [*ideo-* + *-phobia*]. A morbid fear of ideas.

ideo·plas·ty (id′ee·o·plas″tee, eye″dee·o·) *n.* [*ideo-* + *-plasty*]. The process of making the subject's mind receptive to the suggestions of the hypnotizer. —**ideo·plas·tic** (id″ee·o·plas′tick) *adj.*

ideo·syn·chy·sia (id″ee·o·sin·kigh′zee·uh, eye″dee·o·) *n.* [*ideo-synchysis* + *-ia*]. *Obsol.* DELIRIUM.

ideo·syn·chy·sis (id″ee·o·sin′ki·sis, eye″dee·o·) *n.* [*ideo-* + Gk. *synchysis,* confusion]. *Obsol.* DELIRIUM.

ideo·vas·cu·lar (id″ee·o·vas′kew·lur, eye″dee·o·) *adj.* [*ideo-* + *vascular*]. Designating a vascular change resulting from a mental or emotional activity, as blushing in response to an embarrassing memory.

-idin, -idine. A suffix designating *a chemical compound related in origin or structure to another compound.*

idio- [Gk. *idios*]. A combining form meaning (a) *one's own;* (b) *separate, distinct;* (c) *self-produced.*

id·io·blast (id′ee·o·blast) *n.* [*idio-* + *-blast*]. BIOPHORE.

id·io·chro·mo·some (id″ee·o·kro′muh·sohm) *n.* [*idio-* + *chromosome*]. SEX CHROMOSOME.

id·io·cra·sia (id″ee·o·kray′zee·uh, ·zhuh) *n.* [Gk. *idiokrasia,* peculiar temperament]. IDIOSYNCRASY.

id·i·oc·ra·sis (id″ee·ock′ruh·sis) *n.* [*idio-* + Gk. *krasis,* mixing, temperament]. IDIOSYNCRASY.

id·i·oc·ra·sy (id″ee·ock′ruh·see) *n.* [Gk. *idiokrasia*]. IDIOSYNCRASY. —**id·io·crat·ic** (id″ee·o·krat′ick) *adj.*

id·i·oc·to·nia (id″ee·ock·to′nee·uh) *n.* [*idio-* + Gk. *ktonos,* murder, + *-ia*]. SUICIDE.

id·i·o·cy (id′ee·uh·see) *n.* [*idiot* + *-y*]. The lowest grade of mental deficiency, in which the subject's mental age is under 3 years, or if a child, the intelligence quotient is under 20. Custodial or complete protective care is usually required.

id·i·og·a·mist (id″ee·og′uh·mist) *n.* [*idio-* + Gk. *gamos,* marriage, + *-ist*]. A man capable of coitus only with his marital partner or with certain women, but impotent with women in general.

id·io·gen·e·sis (id″ee·o·jen′e·sis) *n.* [*idio-* + *-genesis*]. Idiopathic or spontaneous origin.

id·io·glos·sia (id″ee·o·glos′ee·uh) *n.* [*idio-* + *-glossia*]. Any form of speech invented by an individual and unique, usually incomprehensible to others; in a very young child, a transition stage toward normal speech which may be understood by parents and associates; in one in whom normal speech development may be expected, it represents a neuropathological process, such as congenital auditory aphasia or auditory imperception. —**idio·glot·ic** (·glot′ick) *adj.*

id·io·gram (id'ee·o·gram) *n.* [*idio-* + *-gram*]. Schematic representation of the karyotype.

id·io·hyp·no·tism (id''ee·o·hip'nuh·tiz·um) *n.* [*idio-* + *hypnotism*]. The practice of self-hypnosis.

id·i·ol·o·gism (id''ee·ol'uh·jiz·um) *n.* [*idio-* + *log-* + *-ism*]. A form of utterance peculiar to and constantly employed by a particular person, and incomprehensible to all others, as seen in certain psychoses. Compare *neologism.*

id·io·me·tri·tis (id''ee·o·me·trye'tis) *n.* [*idio-* + *metritis*]. Inflammation of the parenchymatous substance of the uterus.

id·io·mus·cu·lar (id''ee·o·mus'kew·lur) *adj.* [*idio-* + *muscular*]. Characterizing phenomena occurring in a muscle which are independent of outside stimuli.

idiomuscular contractility. Capacity of a muscle fiber to contract independently, despite separation from its nerve supply.

idiomuscular contraction or **contracture.** Persistent local shortening in muscle resulting from a single direct stimulus, as a mechanical blow or extreme fatigue.

id·io·neu·ro·sis (id''ee·o·new·ro'sis) *n.* [*idio-* + *neurosis*]. NEUROSIS.

id·io·pa·thet·ic (id''ee·o·puh·thet'ick) *adj.* IDIOPATHIC.

id·io·path·ic (id''ee·o·path'ick) *adj.* [*idio-* + *-pathic*]. 1. Primary, spontaneous; not resulting from another disease. 2. Of a pathological condition: having an unknown or obscure cause. Compare *cryptogenic.*

idiopathic adult steatorrhea. NONTROPICAL SPRUE.

idiopathic anemia. Anemia of unknown origin.

idiopathic blennorrheal arthritis. REITER'S SYNDROME.

idiopathic epilepsy. Recurrent seizures of unknown cause. Contr. *symptomatic epilepsy.*

idiopathic erysipelas. Erysipelas occurring without any visible wound.

idiopathic eunuchoidism. A type of eunuchoidism without enlargement of the mammary glands, in which the testes are similar in histologic appearance to those of a prepuberal male. There is a normal to low level of urinary 17-ketosteroids.

idiopathic generalized glycogenosis. POMPE'S DISEASE.

idiopathic hypercalcinuria. A high level of calcium in the urine in the absence of acidosis. Syn. *essential hypercalcinuria.*

idiopathic hypertrophic subaortic stenosis. A cardiomyopathy characterized by left ventricular hypertrophy, particularly marked hypertrophy of the interventricular septum. During systole, left ventricular ejection is obstructed. Abbreviated, IHSS.

idiopathic hypochromic anemia. Hypochromic microcytic anemia of unknown cause.

idiopathic infantile steatorrhea. INFANTILE CELIAC DISEASE.

idiopathic leukopenia. AGRANULOCYTOSIS (2).

idiopathic megacolon. Hypertrophy and dilatation of the colon resulting in moderate constipation; sometimes due to a congenital anomaly of the colon, but usually due to psychogenic causes and faulty bowel habits. Compare *Hirschsprung's disease.*

idiopathic parkinsonism. PARKINSON'S DISEASE.

idiopathic peritonitis. PRIMARY PERITONITIS.

idiopathic pulmonary hemosiderosis. An uncommon disease of unknown etiology characterized by widespread recurrent pulmonary capillary hemorrhages; manifested by hemoptysis, progressive dyspnea, anemia, cyanosis, and finally chronic cor pulmonale.

idiopathic respiratory distress of the newborn. RESPIRATORY DISTRESS SYNDROME OF THE NEWBORN.

idiopathic retroperitoneal fibrosis. RETROPERITONEAL FIBROSIS.

idiopathic steatorrhea. CELIAC SYNDROME.

idiopathic thrombocytopenic purpura. Thrombocytopenic purpura of unknown cause but suspected to be immunogenic in character. Abbreviated, ITP.

idiopathic uveoneuraxitis. UVEOMENINGOENCEPHALITIS.

id·i·op·a·thy (id''ee·op'uth·ee) *n.* [Gk. *idiopatheia*]. 1. A primary disease; one not a result of any other disease, but of spontaneous origin. 2. Disease for which no cause is known. Adj. *idiopathic.*

id·io·plasm (id'ee·o·plaz·um) *n.* [*idio-* + *-plasm*]. *In biology,* a hypothetic structural unit of the germ plasm, according to Weismann's theory.

id·io·psy·chol·o·gy (id''ee·o·sigh·kol'uh·jee) *n.* [*idio-* + *psychology*]. The psychological study by a person of his own mental acts and dynamics. Compare *self-analysis.*

id·io·re·flex (id''ee·o·ree'flecks) *n.* [*idio-* + *reflex*]. A reflex arising from a stimulus originating within the organ itself.

id·io·ret·i·nal (id''ee·o·ret'i·nul) *adj.* [*idio-* + *retinal*]. Peculiar or proper to the retina.

id·io·some (id'ee·o·sohm) *n.* [*idio-* + *-some*]. The central apparatus of an auxocyte, especially a spermatocyte, including the surrounding Golgi apparatus and mitochondria.

id·io·spasm (id'ee·o·spaz·um) *n.* [*idio-* + *spasm*]. A spasm confined to one part. —**id·io·spas·tic** (id''ee·o·spas'tick) *adj.*

id·io·syn·cra·sy (id''ee·o·sing'kruh·see) *n.* [Gk. *idiosynkrasia,* from *idios,* personal, peculiar, + *synkrasis,* temperament]. 1. Any special or peculiar characteristic or temperament by which a person differs from other persons. 2. A peculiarity of constitution that makes an individual react differently from most persons to drugs, diet, treatments, or other situations. —**idio·syn·crat·ic** (·sing·krat'ick) *adj.*

id·i·ot, *n.* [Gk. *idiōtēs,* private individual, layman, ignorant person]. A person afflicted with idiocy.

idi·ot sa·vant (ee·dee·o' sa·vahn') [F.]. An individual with general mental retardation as measured by the intelligence quotient, but capable of performing some isolated mental feat, such as calculating or puzzle-solving.

id·io·ven·tric·u·lar (id''ee·o·ven·trick'yoo·lur) *adj.* [*idio-* + *ventricular*]. Pertaining to the cardiac ventricles alone, and not involving the atria.

idioventricular beat. A cardiac impulse originating from an ectopic focus in the ventricle.

idioventricular pacemaker. An ectopic focus of impulse initiation in the ventricle.

idioventricular rhythm. The heart rhythm in which an ectopic focus below the bifurcation of the bundle of His is the pacemaker.

id·io·zome (id'ee·o·zome) *n.* [*idio-* + Gk. *zōma,* girdle, loin cloth]. IDIOSOME.

I disk. The transverse segment of a myofibril (or of a whole muscle fiber) which appears longitudinally as an I band.

id·i·tol (id'i·tol) *n.* L-Iditol, $C_6H_{14}O_6$, a hexahydroxy alcohol formed by reduction of the ketohexose L-sorbose.

ido·lo·ma·nia (eye·duh·lo·may'nee·uh, eye·dol''o·) *n.* Exaggerated idolatry.

id·ose (id'oce, ·oze) *n.* A synthetic hexose sugar, $C_6H_{12}O_6$, isomeric with glucose; occurs in D- and L- forms.

idox·uri·dine (eye''docks·yoor'i·deen) *n.* 2'-Deoxy-5-iodouridine, $C_9H_{11}IN_2O_5$, a topical antiviral agent used for the treatment of dendritic keratitis. Abbreviated, IDU.

id reaction [from the suffix *-id*]. Papulovesicular exanthematic eruptions that appear suddenly after exacerbation of foci of some superficial fungous infections, particularly on the hands from tinea pedis and on the trunk from tinea capitis.

idro·sis (i·dro'sis) *n.* HIDROSIS.

IDU Abbreviation for *idoxuridine.*

id·uron·ic acid (id''yoo·ron'ick). Uronic acid derived from idose; a constituent of the heparin molecule.

I electroretinogram. The type of electroretinogram in which inhibitory phenomena are dominant; associated with activity of the cones. Contr. *E electroretinogram.*

-iferous. See *-ferous.*

-iform. See *-form.*

Ig Abbreviation for *immunoglobulin.*

IgA A symbol for gamma-A globulin.

IgD A symbol for gamma-D globulin.

IgE A symbol for gamma-E globulin.

i gene [*i*nhibitory]. A regulatory gene which is capable of inhibiting the transcription of a given structural gene.

IgG A symbol for gamma-G globulin.

Igle·sias resectoscope. An instrument used with one hand to perform transurethral operations. Recent models are equipped with a continuous two-way fluid irrigation system.

IgM A symbol for gamma-M globulin.

ig·na·tia (ig·nay'shuh) *n.* The seed of *Strychnos ignatii;* contains the alkaloids strychnine and brucine. Its therapeutic effects are similar to those of nux vomica.

ig·ni·punc·ture (ig'ni·punk"chur) *n.* [L. *ignis,* fire, + *puncture*]. Puncture with metal needles heated to either red or white heat.

ig·ni·tion, *n.* The process of heating solids until all volatile matter has been driven off. When performed in the presence of air, oxidizable matter such as carbon is burned.

IHSA Radioactive iodine-tagged human serum albumin.

IHSS Abbreviation for *idiopathic hypertrophic subaortic stenosis.*

IH virus. HEPATITIS VIRUS A.

Il Symbol for illinium.

ile-, ileo-. A combining form meaning *ileum, ileal.*

ilea. Plural of *ileum.*

il·e·ac (il'ee·ack) *adj.* ILEAL.

il·e·al (il'ee·ul) *adj.* Pertaining to, or involving the ileum.

ileal bladder. ILEAL CONDUIT.

ileal conduit. A segment of ileum which is surgically prepared to receive both ureters and to serve as a substitute bladder.

ileal graft. *In urology,* the use of a loop of ileum to replace a part of the genitourinary tract, usually a ureter. See also *ureteroileal neocystostomy.*

ileal intussusception. ENTERIC INTUSSUSCEPTION.

ile·ec·to·my (il"ee·eck'tuh·mee) *n.* [*ile-* + *-ectomy*]. Excision of the ileum.

il·e·itis (il"ee·eye'tis) *n.,* pl. **il·e·it·i·des** (il"ee·it'i·deez) [*ile-* + *-itis*]. Inflammation of the ileum. —**ile·it·ic** (·it'ick) *adj.*

ileo-. See *ile-.*

il·eo·ap·pen·dic·u·lar fold (il"ee·o·ap"en·dick'yoo·lur). ILEOCECAL FOLD.

ileoappendicular hernia. A type of retroperitoneal hernia.

ileocaecostomy. ILEOCECOSTOMY.

ileocaecum. ILEOCECUM.

il·eo·ce·cal, il·eo·cae·cal (il"ee·o·see'kul) *adj.* Pertaining to or involving the ileum and the cecum.

ileocecal fold. A fold of the peritoneum extending from the terminal part of the ileum to the cecum and to the mesentery of the vermiform appendix, or to the appendix itself. Syn. *bloodless fold of Treves, ileoappendicular fold, ileocolic fold.* NA *plica ileocecalis.*

ileocecal fossae. ILEOCECAL RECESSES.

ileocecal intussusception. An intussusception that takes place at the ileocecal valve, the cecum as well as the ileum being invaginated into the colon.

ileocecal recesses. Peritoneal pouches, inferior (NA *recessus ileocecalis inferior*) and superior (NA *recessus ileocecalis superior*), in the region of the ileocecal junction.

ileocecal valve. The valve at the junction of the terminal ileum and the cecum which consists of a superior and inferior lip and partially prevents reflux from the cecum into the ileum. NA *valva ileocecalis.*

il·eo·ce·cos·to·my, il·eo·cae·cos·to·my (il"ee·o·see·kos'tuh·mee) *n.* [*ileo-* + *ceco-* + *-stomy*]. The formation of an anastomosis between the cecum and the ileum.

il·eo·ce·cum, il·eo·cae·cum (il"ee·o·see'kum) *n.* The ileum and the cecum regarded as one organ.

il·eo·co·lic (il"ee·o·ko'lick) *adj.* Pertaining conjointly to the ileum and the colon. See also Table of Arteries in the Appendix.

ileocolic fold. ILEOCECAL FOLD.

ileocolic intussusception. An intussusception of the ileum through the ileocecal valve, without invagination of the cecum.

ileocolic valve. ILEOCECAL VALVE.

il·eo·co·li·tis (il"ee·o·ko·lye'tis) *n.* [*ileo-* + *col-* + *-itis*]. Inflammation of the ileum and the colon.

il·eo·co·lon·ic (il"ee·o·ko·lon'ick) *adj.* [*ileo-* + *colonic*]. ILEOCOLIC.

il·eo·co·los·to·my (il"ee·o·ko·los'tuh·mee) *n.* [*ileo-* + *colo-* + *-stomy*]. The establishment of an anastomosis between the ileum and the colon.

il·eo·cu·ta·ne·ous (il"ee·o·kew·tay'nee·us) *adj.* [*ileo-* + *cutaneous*]. Pertaining to the ileum and the skin, usually to a fistulous connection between the two.

il·eo·cys·to·plas·ty (il"ee·o·sis'to·plas"tee) *n.* [*ileo-* + *cystoplasty*]. An operation in which a segment of ileum is sutured to the urinary bladder, to increase bladder capacity.

il·eo·il·e·al (il"ee·o·il'ee·ul) *adj.* [*ileo-* + *ileal*]. Pertaining to two different portions of the ileum, usually to a communication or other connection between two parts of the ileum.

il·eo·il·e·os·to·my (il"ee·o·il·ee·os'tuh·mee) *n.* [*ileo-* + *ileo-* + *-stomy*]. The establishment of an anastomosis between two different parts of the ileum.

ileopagus. ILIOPAGUS.

il·eo·proc·tos·to·my (il"ee·o·prock·tos'tuh·mee) *n.* [*ileo-* + *procto-* + *-stomy*]. The surgical formation of a connection between the ileum and the rectum.

il·e·or·rha·phy (il"ee·or'uh·fee) *n.* [*ileo-* + *-rrhaphy*]. Suture of the ileum.

il·eo·sig·moid·os·to·my (il"ee·o·sig"moid·os'tuh·mee) *n.* [*ileo-* + *sigmoid* + *-stomy*]. The surgical formation of an anastomosis between the ileum and the sigmoid colon.

il·e·os·to·my (il"ee·os'tuh·mee) *n.* [*ileo-* + *-stomy*]. The surgical formation of a fistula or artificial anus through the abdominal wall into the ileum.

il·e·ot·o·my (il"ee·ot'uh·mee) *n.* [*ileo-* + *-tomy*]. Surgical incision of the ileum.

il·eo·trans·verse (il"ee·o·trans·vurce') *adj.* Pertaining to the ileum and transverse colon.

il·eo·trans·ver·sos·to·my (il"ee·o·trans·vur·sos'tuh·mee) *n.* [*ileo-* + *transverse* + *-stomy*]. *In surgery,* the formation of a connection between the ileum and the transverse colon.

il·eo·typh·li·tis (il"ee·o·tif·lye'tis) *n.* [*ileo-* + *typhl-* + *-itis*]. Inflammation of the cecum and the ileum.

il·eo·ves·i·cal (il"ee·o·ves'i·kul) *adj.* [*ileo-* + *vesical*]. Pertaining to the ileum and the urinary bladder.

Iletin. A trademark for insulin.

il·e·um (il'ee·um) *n.,* genit. **ilei** (il'ee·eye), pl. **il·ea** (·ee·uh) [ML., from Gk. *eileon,* from *eileos,* twisted] [NA]. The lower portion of the small intestine, extending from the jejunum to the large intestine. See also Plate 13.

il·e·us (il'ee·us) *n.* [L., from Gk. *eileos,* from *eilein,* to block, to twist]. Acute intestinal obstruction characterized by diminished or absent intestinal peristalsis, distention, obstipation, abdominal pain, and vomiting.

ili-, ilio-. A combining form meaning *ilium, iliac.*

ilia. Plural of *ilium.*

il·i·ac (il'ee·ack) *adj.* Pertaining to the ilium.

iliac abscess. A wandering abscess of the iliac region.

iliac artery. See Table of Arteries in the Appendix.

iliac bone. ILIUM (2).

iliac crest. The thickened and expanded upper border of the ilium. NA *crista iliaca.* See also Plate 13.

iliac fascia. The fascia covering the pelvic surface of the iliacus muscle. NA *fascia iliaca.*

iliac fossa. A wide depression on the internal surface of the ilium. NA *fossa iliaca.*

iliac horns. Bilateral exostoses arising from the posterior surfaces of the iliac bones. See also *nail-patella syndrome.*

iliac plexus. A nerve plexus surrounding the common iliac artery. NA *plexus iliacus.*

iliac region. 1. The region of the ilium. 2. INGUINAL REGION.

iliac spines. Four spines of the ilium: ANTERIOR INFERIOR ILIAC SPINE, ANTERIOR SUPERIOR ILIAC SPINE, POSTERIOR INFERIOR ILIAC SPINE, POSTERIOR SUPERIOR ILIAC SPINE.

iliac subtendinous bursa. A bursa lying between the tendon of the iliopsoas muscle and the lesser trochanter. NA *bursa subtendinea iliaca.*

iliac tuberosity. A rough, elevated area above the articular surface on the inner aspect of the ala of the ilium, which gives attachment to the posterior sacroiliac ligament, and from which the erector spinae and multifidus muscles take origin. NA *tuberositas iliaca.*

ili·a·cus (i·lye′uh·kus) *n.* The portion of the iliopsoas muscle arising from the iliac fossa and sacrum. NA *musculus iliacus.* See also Table of Muscles in the Appendix.

iliacus minor. A variant of the iliacus muscle inserted into the capsule of the hip joint.

ili·a·del·phus (il″ee·uh·del′fus) *n.* [*ili-* + *-adelphus*]. ILIOPAGUS.

Ilidar. Trademark for azapetine, an adrenergic blocking agent used as the phosphate salt.

ilio-. See *ili-.*

il·io·cap·su·la·ris (il″ee·o·kap″sue·lair′is) *n.* [NL., from *ilio-* + *capsular*]. ILIACUS MINOR.

il·io·cap·su·lo·tro·chan·te·ri·cus (il″ee·o·kap″sue·lo·tro″kan·terr′i·kus) *n.* A variant of the iliacus minor muscle in which some fibers are inserted into the lesser trochanter.

il·io·coc·cyg·e·al (il″ee·o·kock·sij′ee·ul) *adj.* Pertaining to the ilium and the coccyx.

iliococcygeal muscle. ILIOCOCCYGEUS.

il·io·coc·cy·ge·us (il″ee·o·kock·sij′ee·us) *n.* The portion of the levator ani muscle overlying the obturator internus muscle. NA *musculus iliococcygeus.*

il·io·cos·ta·lis (il″ee·o·kos·tay′lis) *n.* [NL., from *ilio-* + *costal*]. The lateral portion of the erector spinae muscle. NA *musculus iliocostalis.* See also Table of Muscles in the Appendix.

iliocostalis cer·vi·cis (sur′vi·sis). The portion of the erector spinae muscle arising from the upper six ribs and inserted into the posterior tubercle of the transverse processes of the middle cervical vertebrae. NA *musculus iliocostalis cervicis.* See also Table of Muscles in the Appendix.

iliocostalis dor·si (dor′sigh). ILIOCOSTALIS THORACIS.

iliocostalis lum·bo·rum (lum·bo′rum). The portion of the erector spinae muscle that arises from the lumbar vertebrae and adjacent area and is inserted into the lower six ribs. NA *musculus iliocostalis lumborum.* See also Table of Muscles in the Appendix.

iliocostalis tho·ra·cis (tho·ray′sis). The portion of the erector spinae muscle arising from the lower six ribs and inserted into the upper six ribs. Syn. *accessorius.* NA *musculus iliocostalis thoracis.* See also Table of Muscles in the Appendix.

il·io·cos·to·cer·vi·ca·lis (il″ee·o·kos″to·sur·vi·kay′lis) *n.* A muscle composed of the iliocostalis cervicis and the iliocostalis thoracis.

il·io·fem·o·ral (il″ee·o·fem′o·rul) *adj.* Pertaining to the ilium and the femur.

iliofemoral crease. GLUTEOFEMORAL CREASE.

iliofemoral ligament. A strong band of dense fibrous tissue extending from the anterior inferior iliac spine to the lesser trochanter and the intertrochanteric line. Syn. *Y ligament.* NA *ligamentum iliofemorale.* See also Plate 2.

iliofemoral triangle. A triangle formed by a line from the anterior superior iliac spine to the top of the greater trochanter, a horizontal line from the anterior superior iliac spine, and a vertical line from the top of the greater trochanter. Syn. *Bryant's triangle.*

il·io·hy·po·gas·tric (il″ee·o·high″po·gas′trick) *adj.* Pertaining to the ilium and the pubic (hypogastric) region.

iliohypogastric nerve. NA *nervus iliohypogastricus.* See Table of Nerves in the Appendix.

il·io·in·gui·nal (il″ee·o·ing′gwi·nul) *adj.* Pertaining to the ilium and the groin.

ilioinguinal nerve. NA *nervus ilioinguinalis.* See Table of Nerves in the Appendix.

il·io·lum·bar (il″ee·o·lum′bur) *adj.* Pertaining to the ilium and the lumbar vertebrae, or to the iliac and lumbar regions.

iliolumbar ligament. A fibrous band radiating laterally from the transverse processes of the fourth and fifth lumbar vertebrae to attach to the pelvis by two main bands. The lower part blends with the anterior sacroiliac ligament and the upper is attached to the ilium and is continuous above with the lumbodorsal fascia. NA *ligamentum iliolumbale.* See also Plate 2.

il·i·op·a·gus (il″ee·op′uh·gus) *n.* [*ilio-* + *-pagus*]. Conjoined twins united in the iliac region. Syn. *iliadelphus.*

il·io·par·a·si·tus (il″ee·o·păr″uh·sigh′tus) *n.* Parasitic, supernumerary limbs attached to one or both ilia.

il·io·pec·tin·e·al (il″ee·o·peck·tin′ee·ul) *adj.* Pertaining jointly to the ilium and the pecten of the pubic bone.

iliopectineal bursa. A bursa separating the tendon of the iliopsoas muscle from the iliopubic eminence and the capsule of the hip joint. NA *bursa iliopectinea.*

iliopectineal eminence. ILIOPUBIC EMINENCE.

iliopectineal line. The bony ridge marking the brim of the true pelvis, the pecten of the pubic bone, plus its lateral extension to the iliopubic eminence. NA *linea terminalis.*

il·io·pso·as (il″ee·o·so′us, il″ee·op′so·us) *n.* The combined iliacus and psoas muscles. NA *musculus iliopsoas.*

il·io·pu·bic (il″ee·o·pew′bick) *adj.* Pertaining to the ilium and the pubis.

iliopubic eminence. A ridge on the hipbone marking the site of union of ilium and pubis. NA *eminentia iliopubica.*

il·io·sa·cra·lis (il″ee·o·sa·kray′lis) *n.* An occasional band of muscle ventral to the coccygeus, extending from the iliopectineal line to the lateral border of the sacrum.

il·io·tho·ra·cop·a·gus (il″ee·o·tho″ruh·kop′uh·gus) *n.* [*ilio-* + *thoraco-* + *-pagus*]. Conjoined twins united laterally at their thoracic and iliac regions.

il·io·tib·i·al (il″ee·o·tib′ee·ul) *adj.* Pertaining to the ilium and the tibia.

iliotibial tract or **band.** A thickened portion of fascia lata extending from the lateral condyle of the tibia to the iliac crest. NA *tractus iliotibialis.*

il·io·xi·phop·a·gus (il″ee·o·zi·fop′uh·gus) *n.* [*ilio-* + *xipho-* + *-pagus*]. Conjoined twins united from the xiphoid to the iliac (inguinal) region.

il·i·um (il′ee·um) *n.*, genit. **ilii** (il′ee·eye), pl. **il·ia** (·ee·uh) [L.]. 1. The flank. 2. The superior broad portion of the hipbone. NA *os ilium.* See also Plates 1, 2, 14 and Table of Bones in the Appendix.

ill, *adj.* & *n.* 1. Not healthy; sick; indisposed. 2. An ailment, illness, disease, or misfortune.

il·laq·ue·a·te (i·lack′wee·ate) *v.* [L. *illaqueare,* to ensnare, from *laqueus,* a snare]. To correct an ingrowing eyelash by drawing it with a loop through an opening in the lid. —**il·laq·ue·a·tion** (i·lack″wee·ay′shun) *n.*

il·le·git·i·mate, *adj.* [L. *illegitimus,* unlawful]. 1. Not in accordance with statutory law. 2. Not recognized by statutory law as a lawful offspring; bastard. —**illegiti·ma·cy,** *n.*

il·lic·i·um (i·lis′ee·um, i·lish′) *n.* [L., that which entices]. The fruit of *Illicium verum,* which yields a volatile oil consisting chiefly of anethole; may be used to prepare anise oil.

il·li·ni·tion (il″i·nish′un) *n.* [L. *illinire,* to smear, spread over, from *linere,* to daub, anoint]. A rubbing in or on; inunction.

il·lin·i·um (i·lin′ee·um) *n.* [after *Illinois,* U.S.]. A rare-earth element, atomic number 61, reported in 1926 by B. S. Hopkins. Other discoverers called the element florentium, cyclonium, and promethium, the last now being the accepted name.

ill·ness, *n.* 1. The state of being ill or sick. 2. A malady; sickness; disease; disorder.

il·lu·mi·nance (i·lew'mi·nunce) *n.* The amount of light incident per unit area of a surface.

il·lu·mi·na·tion, *n.* [L. *illuminatio,* from *lumen,* light]. 1. The lighting up or illuminating, as of a surface or cavity in the examination of a patient or of an object under microscopical examination. 2. The quantity of light thrown upon an object. —**il·lu·mi·nate,** *v.*

il·lu·mi·nism (i·lew'mi·niz·um) *n.* The mental state in which one imagines that one receives messages from or converses with supernatural beings.

il·lu·sion, *n.* [L. *illusio,* from *illudere,* to mock]. A false interpretation of a real sensation; a perception that misinterprets the object perceived. —**illusion·al, illu·so·ry,** *adj.*

illusory visual spread. 1. Perseveration in space of a visual image. 2. Extension of part of a visual image outside its own boundaries.

Ilopan. A trademark for dexpanthenol, the D- form of pantothenyl alcohol.

Ilosone. Trademark for erythromycin estolate, an acid-stable dosage form of the antibiotic erythromycin.

Ilotycin. A trademark for the antibiotic substance erythromycin.

Ilozyme. A trademark for pancrelipase.

I.M., i.m. Abbreviation for *intramuscular.*

im-. See *in-.*

ima (eye'muh) *L. adj.* [fem. of *imus,* superlative of *inferus,* lower, below]. Lowest.

im·age, *n.* [L. *imago*]. 1. A more or less accurate representation of an object. 2. The picture of an object formed by a lens; a collection of foci, each corresponding to a point in the object. 3. A mental picture of an object in the absence of viewing or directly perceiving that object. 4. IMAGO (2). See also *afterimage, imaging.*

image space. The space around an optical system each point of which is an image of a corresponding point in the object space. Properties relating to the image are said to be in the image space, and properties relating to the object are said to be in the object space.

imag·i·nary, *adj.* Produced by the picture-making power of the mind; fictitious; often used in relation to pain or other sensations or ailments for which no objective cause can be demonstrated.

imag·i·na·tion, *n.* [L. *imaginatio,* from *imaginari,* to imagine]. The picture-making power of the mind. The faculty by which one creates new ideas or mental pictures by means of separate data derived from experience, ideally revivified, extended, and combined in new forms.

im·ag·ing, *n.* Production of an image; usually refers to the production of a photographable image by a radionuclide concentrated in an organ or other part of the body.

ima·go (i·may'go) *n.,* pl. **imagoes, imag·i·nes** (i·maj'i·neez) [L., image]. 1. The adult, sexually mature stage of an insect. 2. *In analytic psychology,* an unconscious mental picture, usually idealized, of a parent or loved person important in the early development of an individual and carried into adulthood.

Imap. A trademark for fluspirilene, a tranquilizer.

im·a·pun·ga (im''uh·pung'guh) *n.* A disease occurring to a limited extent among African cattle; closely related pathologically to African horse sickness.

im·bal·ance, *n.* [*im-* + *balance*]. 1. Lack of balance. 2. Lack of muscular balance, especially between the muscles of the eyes. See also *heterophoria.* 3. Absence of biological equilibrium, as between the number of males and females in a population. 4. Lack of physiologic balance between parts or functions of the body. See also *intellectual imbalance.*

im·be·cile (im'bi·sil) *n.* [L. *imbecillus,* weak, feeble]. A person afflicted with imbecility.

im·be·cil·i·ty (im''be·sil'i·tee) *n.* An intermediate grade of mental deficiency, in which the subject's mental age is between 3 and 7 years with an intelligence quotient between 20 and 45.

im·bed, *v.* EMBED.

im·bi·bi·tion, *n.* [L. *imbibere,* to drink in]. The absorption of liquid by a solid or a gel. —**im·bibe,** *v.*

imbibition pressure. Pressure due to the increase in volume of a gel as a result of the imbibition of liquid.

im·bri·ca·tion (im''bri·kay'shun) *n.* [L. *imbricare,* to cover with tiles]. *In surgery,* the closing of wounds or the covering of deficiencies with tissue arranged in layers overlapping one another. —**im·bri·cate** (im'bri·kate) *v.;* **imbri·cat·ed** (·kay·tid) *adj.*

imbrication lines. PERIKYMATA.

imbrication lines of Pickerill [*Pickerill,* New Zealand dental histologist]. PERIKYMATA.

Imferon. Trademark for iron-dextran complex, a preparation for parenteral treatment of iron-deficiency anemias.

im·id (im'id) *n.* IMIDE.

imid-, imido-. A combining form meaning *imide.*

im·id·az·ole (im''id·az'ole, ·ay'zole, im'id·uh·zole'') *n.* 1,3-Diaza-2,4-cyclopentadiene, $C_3H_4N_2$, a compound, readily synthesized, which is of interest because of the importance of a number of its derivatives, such as histamine, histidine, privine. Syn. *glyoxaline.*

im·id·az·o·line (im''id·az'o·leen) *n.* Any of three dihydro derivatives of imidazole, or compounds derived from the former.

im·id·az·o·lyl (im''id·az'o·lil) *n.* One of four univalent, isomeric radicals, $C_3H_3N_2$—, derived from imidazole.

im·ide (im'ide) *n.* Any compound containing the radical NH= united to a divalent acid radical.

imido-. See *imid-.*

im·id·o·carb (i·mid'o·kahrb) *n.* 3,3′-Di-2-imidazolin-2-ylcarbanilide, $C_{19}H_{20}N_6O$, an antiprotozoal employed for the genus *Babesia* and usually used as the hydrochloride salt.

im·id·o·line (im·id'o·leen) *n.* 1-(*m*-Chlorophenyl)-3-[2-(dimethylamino)ethyl]-2-imidazolidinone, a tranquilizer; used as the hydrochloride salt.

imin-, imino-. A combining form designating *the bivalent group NH= when attached to or in nonacid radicals.*

im·in·az·ole (im''in·az'ole, ·ay'zole, ·uh·zole') *n.* IMIDAZOLE.

im·i·no acid (im'i·no). An organic acid that contains the bivalent imino group (=NH). Imino acids are in some instances intermediaries in the metabolism of amino acids.

im·i·no·urea (im''i·no·yoo·ree'uh) *n.* GUANIDINE.

imip·ra·mine (i·mip'ruh·meen) *n.* 5-(3-Dimethylaminopropyl)-10,11-dihydro-5*H*-dibenz[*b,f*]azepine, $C_{19}H_{24}N_2$, a drug useful in the treatment of depression; used as the hydrochloride salt.

im·i·tate, *v.* [L. *imitari*]. To copy an act, a manner of behavior, or a characteristic of another.

im·i·ta·tion, *n.* The assumption of characteristics or behavior of others. Compare *identification* (3), *mimesis.* See also *hysterical imitation.*

im·i·ta·tive, *adj.* Having some of the qualities of or imitating an original model, pattern, or process.

imitative chorea. Choreic movements developed usually in children from association with choreic subjects; a habit spasm.

imitative insanity. A form of folie à deux marked by mimicry of the insane characteristics of another.

imitative tetanus. A conversion symptom simulating tetanus.

im·ma·ture, *adj.* [L. *immaturus,* unripe]. Not yet adult or fully developed; unripe. —**imma·tur·i·ty,** *n.*

immature cataract. A cataract in which only a part of the lens substance is cataractous.

im·me·di·ate, *adj.* Direct; without the intervention of anything.

immediate allergy. IMMEDIATE HYPERSENSITIVITY.

immediate auscultation. The direct application of the examiner's ear to the patient's skin overlying the area to be auscultated in order to listen to the heart and lungs without a stethoscope.

immediate denture. A dental prosthesis that is placed in position immediately following the removal of natural teeth.

immediate hypersensitivity. Hypersensitivity in which reaction commences within seconds or minutes of exposure to antigens; always associated with prior presence of serum antibodies, generally of the IgE class. Contr. *delayed hypersensitivity.*

immediate memory. 1. SHORT-TERM MEMORY. 2. RECENT MEMORY.

immediate percussion. DIRECT PERCUSSION.

immediate transfusion. DIRECT TRANSFUSION.

immediate union. HEALING BY FIRST INTENTION.

im·med·i·ca·ble (i·med'i·kuh·bul) *adj.* Characterizing that which does not yield to medicine or treatment; incurable.

im·mer·sion, *n.* [L. *immersio,* from *immergere,* to plunge into]. The plunging of a body or an object into a liquid so that it is completely covered by the liquid. —**im·merse,** *v.*

immersion blast injury. Blast injury resulting from the transmission of the shock wave of an underwater explosion, as from a depth charge.

immersion foot. Skin, peripheral vessel, nerve, and muscle damage of the foot due to prolonged exposure to low but not freezing temperatures, combined with dampness or actual immersion in water. See also *trench foot.*

immersion lens. A microscope objective lens designed for use with a liquid (usually oil) filling the space between it and the cover glass over the specimen.

immersion microscopy. Microscopy with the lower lens of an objective immersed in a medium of refractive index of glass, thus preventing light losses by reflection and interface refraction and enhancing the resolving power of the lens system. Immersion of the top lens of the substage condenser is less often used for the same purpose.

immersion oil. An oil, such as cedar, used as a medium of contact between the objective of a microscope and the object being examined.

im·mis·ci·ble (i·mis'i·bul) *adj.* [*im-,* not, + *miscible*]. Not capable of being mixed.

im·mo·bi·lize, *v.* [L. *immobilis,* immovable]. To render motionless or to fix in place, as by splints or surgery. —**im·mo·bi·li·za·tion,** *n.*

im·mov·able bandage. A bandage for immobilizing any part.

im·mune, *adj.* [L. *immunis,* exempt]. 1. Safe from attack; protected against a disease by an innate or an acquired immunity. 2. Pertaining to or conferring immunity.

immune-adherence phenomenon. An immunologically specific in vitro reaction involving microorganisms sensitized with antibody, phagocytic cells, and complement resulting in enhanced phagocytosis. Syn. *adhesion phenomenon.*

immune bacteriolysis. Intracellular or extracellular dissolution of bacteria mediated by a specific antibody or complement.

immune body. ANTIBODY.

immune complex. A complex of antigen and antibody molecules bound together, either circulating in the blood or forming a precipitate; often associated with such pathologic lesions as glomerulonephritis, vasculitis, and arthritis.

immune globulin. IMMUNOGLOBULIN.

immune hemolysin. A hemolysin formed in response to the injection of erythrocytes of another species.

immune horse serum. A serum obtained from an immunized horse. See also *horse serum.*

immune opsonin. An opsonin in the serum resulting from infection or inoculation with dead microorganisms of the same species, and active only against the microorganism that created it. See also *bacteriotropin.*

immune protein. ANTIBODY.

immune reaction or **response.** Any reaction involving demonstrated specific antibody response to antigen, or the specifically altered reactivity of host cells following antigenic stimulation.

immune serum. The serum of an immunized animal or person, which carries specific antibodies for the organism or antigen introduced.

immune serum globulin. GAMMA GLOBULIN (2).

im·mu·ni·ty (i·mew'ni·tee) *n.* The condition of a living organism whereby it resists and overcomes infection or disease. Contr. *susceptibility.*

im·mu·ni·za·tion (im"yoo·ni·zay'shun) *n.* The act or process of rendering immune. See also *vaccination.*

immunization register. A form on which are recorded all immunizations or inoculations given to an individual.

immunization therapy. The use of vaccines or antiserums to produce immunity against a specific disease.

im·mu·nize (im'yoo·nize) *v.* To render immune.

immunizing unit. ANTITOXIC UNIT.

immuno-. A combining form meaning *immune, immunity.*

im·mu·no·blast (im'yoo·no·blast") *n.* [*immuno-* + *-blast*]. An immature cell of the plasmacytic series, actively synthesizing antibodies. —**im·mu·no·blas·tic** (im"yoo·no·blas'tick) *adj.*

immunoblastic adenopathy. IMMUNOBLASTIC LYMPHADENOPATHY.

immunoblastic lymphadenopathy. A disorder of the reticuloendothelial system, usually with a progressively worsening course, characterized histologically by proliferation of small blood vessels, prominent immunoblastic proliferation, and amorphous acidophilic interstitial material. Clinically, there is usually generalized lymphadenopathy, fever, night sweats, and weight loss. Syn. *angioimmunoblastic lymphadenopathy, immunoblastic adenopathy.*

im·mu·no·chem·is·try (im"yoo·no·kem'is·tree) *n.* The branch of science that deals with the chemical changes and phenomena of immunity; specifically, the chemistry of antigens, antibodies, and their reactions.

im·mu·no·con·glu·ti·nin (im"yoo·no·kon·gloo'ti·nin) *n.* [*immuno-* + *conglutinin*]. A gamma-M antibody to altered complement, measured by reacting the serum with sensitized erythrocytes coated with complement.

im·mu·no·de·fi·cien·cy (im"yoo·no·de·fish'un·see) *n.* Any deficiency of immune reaction, involving humoral immunity or cell-mediated immunity only, or both, as in severe combined immunodeficiency.

im·mu·no·de·pres·sion (im"yoo·no·de·presh'un) *n.* IMMUNOSUPPRESSION.

im·mu·no·dif·fu·sion (im"yoo·no·di·few'zhun) *n.* Any of a number of techniques favoring the formation of immune precipitates by the diffusion of antigens and antibodies in gels.

im·mu·no·elec·tro·pho·re·sis (im"yoo·no·e·leck"tro·fo·ree'sis) *n.* [*immuno-* + *electrophoresis*]. The technique of first separating antigens according to their migration in an electric field in a supporting medium, such as agar, and then demonstrating their presence by means of precipitation zones with antibody. —**immunoelectropho·ret·ic** (·ret'ick) *adj.*

im·mu·no·flu·o·res·cence (im"yoo·no·floo"ur·es'unce) *n.* Fluorescence as the result of, or identifying, an immune response.

im·mu·no·gen (im'yoo·no·jen) *n.* [*immuno-* + *-gen*]. Any substance capable of stimulating an immune response.

im·mu·no·ge·net·ics (im"yoo·no·je·net'icks) *n.* The discipline encompassing the study of immunoglobulins, including genetic markers and histocompatibility antigens.

im·mu·no·gen·ic (im"yoo·no·jen'ick) *adj.* [*immuno-* + *-genic*]. 1. Producing immunity. 2. Pertaining to an immunogen.

im·mu·no·ge·nic·i·ty (im"yoo·no·je·nis'i·tee) *n.* The capacity to produce an immune response; the state or quality of being an immunogen.

im·mu·no·glob·u·lin (im″yoo·no·glob′yoo·lin) *n.* [*immuno-* + *globulin*]. Any one of the proteins of animal origin having known antibody activity, or a protein related by chemical structure and hence antigenic specificity; may be found in plasma, urine, spinal fluid, and other body tissues and fluids, and includes such proteins as myeloma and Bence Jones protein. Abbreviated, Ig. See also *gamma globulin.*

immunoglobulin chain. Any of the major groups of polypeptide chains found in immunoglobulin molecules. See also *heavy chain, light chain.*

immunoglobulin fragments. Portions of the molecule of immunoglobulins obtained by cleavage of the peptide bonds by proteolytic enzymes, and further subdivided into such fractions as Fab and Fc fragments.

im·mu·no·gran·u·lom·a·tous disease (im″yoo·no·gran″yoo·lom′uh·tus, ·lo′muh·tus). A disease in which an aberration in immune mechanisms is thought to be associated with the development of granulomas in various organs, as in sarcoidosis.

im·mu·no·he·ma·tol·o·gy, im·mu·no·hae·ma·tol·o·gy (im″yoo·no·hee″muh·tol′uh·jee) *n.* The branch of immunology and hematology concerned with immunologic aspects of normal and diseased blood; includes studies of antigen-antibody systems of the formed blood elements, hemolytic anemias, and other autoimmune phenomena.

im·mu·no·he·mo·lyt·ic anemia (im″yoo·no·hee·mo·lit′ick). Hemolytic anemia resulting from abnormal immune responses on the part of the patient.

im·mu·no·log·ic (im″yoo·no·loj′ick) *adj.* Pertaining to immunology.

immunologic paralysis. A state in which immunologic mechanisms for antibody formation are partially or completely inhibited.

immunologic test for pregnancy. A pregnancy test in which urine containing chorionic gonadotropin prevents the agglutination of red blood cells or of latex particles coated by antiserum to human chorionic gonadotropin. Absence of agglutination on a slide preparation indicates a positive test.

immunologic tolerance. 1. A condition, natural or induced, in which a graft will be accepted without the occurrence of homograft rejection. 2. A state of specific unresponsiveness to an antigen or antigens in adult life as a consequence of exposure to the antigen in utero or in the neonatal period, administration of modified antigen, administration of specific blocking antibody, or administration of antigen with immunosuppressive agents.

im·mu·nol·o·gist (im″yoo·nol′uh·jist) *n.* A specialist in immunology.

im·mu·nol·o·gy (im″yoo·nol′uh·jee) *n.* [*immuno-* + *-logy*]. The science dealing with specific mechanisms, including antigen-antibody and cell-mediated reactions, by which living tissues react to foreign or autologous biological material that may result in enhanced resistance or immunity or, as in allergy, in heightened reactivity that may be damaging to the host.

im·mu·no·pa·thol·o·gy (im″yoo·no·pa·thol′uh·jee) *n.* [*immuno-* + *pathology*]. 1. The study of diseases and other changes caused by immunologic reactions in the host. 2. The changes caused by immunologic reactions.

im·mu·nop·a·thy (im″yoo·nop′uth·ee) *n.* [*immuno-* + *-pathy*]. Any disorder of the immune system of the body.

im·mu·no·pho·re·sis (im″yoo·no·fo·ree′sis) *n.* [*immuno-* + *-phoresis*]. IMMUNOELECTROPHORESIS.

im·mu·no·re·ac·tant (im″yoo·no·ree·ack′tunt) *n.* Any of the substances involved in immunologically mediated reactions, including immunoglobulins, complement components, and specific antigens.

im·mu·no·sup·pres·sant (im″yoo·no·suh·press′unt) *n. & adj.* IMMUNOSUPPRESSIVE.

im·mu·no·sup·pres·sion (im″yoo·no·suh·presh′un) *n.* Suppression of immune responses produced primarily by any of a variety of immunosuppressive agents or secondarily during any of a number of diseases.

im·mu·no·sup·pres·sive (im″yoo·no·suh·pres′iv) *adj. & n.* 1. Capable of suppressing an immune response. 2. An agent, such as a chemical, a drug, or x-rays, for suppressing immunologic reactions, as in autoimmune diseases or for enhancing successful foreign tissue grafts.

im·mu·no·ther·a·py (im″yoo·no·therr′uh·pee) *n.* [*immuno-* + *therapy*]. 1. SEROTHERAPY. 2. Therapy utilizing immunosuppressives. 3. Therapy using vaccines or allergenic extracts.

im·mu·no·trans·fu·sion (im″yoo·no·trans·few′zhun) *n.* Transfusion with the blood or plasma of a donor previously rendered immune to a specific infection.

IMP Abbreviation for *inosine monophosphate* (= INOSINIC ACID).

impacted fracture. A fracture in which one fragment has been driven into another fragment.

im·pac·tion, *n.* [L. *impactio,* from *impingere,* to drive against]. 1. The state of being lodged and retained in a part or strait. 2. Confinement of a tooth in the jaw so that its eruption is prevented. 3. A condition in which one fragment of a fractured bone is driven into another and is fixed in that position. 4. A large accumulation of inspissated feces in the rectum or colon, difficult to move. —**im·pact·ed,** *adj.*

im·pal·pa·ble, *adj.* [*im-,* not, + *palpable*]. Not capable of being felt; imperceptible to the touch.

impalpable powder. A powder so fine that its separate particles cannot be felt.

im·par (im′pahr) *adj.* [L., unequal]. Without a fellow; AZYGOUS.

im·pari·dig·i·tate (im·păr″i·dij′i·tate) *adj.* [*im-,* not, + *pari-,* even, + *digitate*]. Having an uneven number of fingers or toes.

im·passe, *n.* [F.]. *In psychoanalysis,* a stalemate in the therapeutic process with a breakdown in controlled emotional communication between patient and therapist.

im·ped·ance (im·peed′unce) *n.* [*impede* + *-ance*]. The apparent resistance of a circuit to the flow of an alternating electric current. Symbol, Z.

im·per·a·tive, *adj.* [L. *imperativus,* from *imperare,* to order]. Peremptory, absolute; compulsory; binding.

imperative conception or **idea.** OBSESSION.

im·per·cep·tion, *n.* Defective or absent perception. See also *visual agnosia.*

imperfect fungus. Any of the Fungi Imperfecti.

im·per·fo·rate (im·pur′fuh·rit, ·rate) *adj.* [*im-,* not, + *perforate*]. Without the normal opening. —**im·per·fo·ra·tion** (im·pur″fuh·ray′shun) *n.*

imperforate anus. Congenital closure of the anal opening, usually by a membranous septum.

im·pe·ri·al gallon. A unit of volume, used in the United Kingdom and other Commonwealth Nations, equal to 4.546 liters and equivalent to approximately 1.201 U.S. gallons.

imperial green. PARIS GREEN.

imperial pint. One-eighth of an imperial gallon or 20 fluidounces.

imperial quart. One-fourth of an imperial gallon or 40 fluidounces; 1.136 liters.

im·per·me·able, *adj.* [*im-,* not, + *permeable*]. Not permitting passage through a substance.

im·per·vi·ous, *adj.* [*im-,* not, + *pervious*]. Not permitting a passage; impermeable.

im·pe·tig·i·ni·za·tion (im″pe·tij″i·ni·zay′shun) *n.* Lesions of impetigo occurring on a previous skin lesion.

im·pe·tig·i·noid (im″pe·tij′i·noid) *adj.* [*impetigo* + *-oid*]. Resembling impetigo.

im·pe·ti·go (im″pe·tye′go, ·tee′go) *n.* [L., an attack]. An acute, inflammatory skin disease caused by streptococci or staphylococci, and characterized by subcorneal vesicles and bullae which rupture and develop distinct yellow crusts. —**impe·tig·i·nous** (·tij'i·nus) *adj.*

impetigo cir·ci·na·ta (sur''si·nay'tuh). A form of impetigo characterized by a circle or a semicircle of small vesicles or pustules; there are usually many such circles.

impetigo cir·cum·pi·la·ris (sur''kum·pi·lair'is). IMPETIGO FOLLICULARIS.

impetigo con·ta·gi·o·sa (kon·tay''jee·o'suh). IMPETIGO.

impetigo fol·lic·u·la·ris (fol·ick''yoo·lair'is). A form of staphylococcal infection of hair follicles characterized by vesicles at the pilosebaceous orifice, which form yellowish crusts. Syn. *Bockhart's impetigo, impetigo circumpilaris.*

impetigo her·pet·i·for·mis (hur·pet''i·for'mis). A variant form of psoriasis resembling pustular psoriasis, but occurring in hypocalcemic patients following parathyroidectomy or during pregnancy, and not associated with pre-existing psoriasis.

impetigo neonatorum. NEONATAL IMPETIGO.

impetigo vul·ga·ris (vul·gair'is). IMPETIGO.

im·pin·ger (im·pin'jur) *n.* An instrument for collecting dust particles in a measured volume of air by impinging them on a plate or dispersing them in water, after which the particles are counted.

[1]im·plant (im·plant') *v.* [F. *implanter,* from *im-,* in, + *planter,* to plant]. To embed, set in.

[2]im·plant (im'plant) *n.* 1. A small tube or needle which contains radioactive material, placed in a tissue or tumor to deliver therapeutic doses of radiation. 2. A tissue graft placed in depth. See also *graft, implantation.*

im·plan·ta·tion, *n.* 1. The act of implanting, as the transplantation of a tissue, tooth, duct, or organ from one place in the body to another, or from the body of one person to that of another, implying the placement of the tissue in depth, as distinguished from the placement of a surface graft. Tissue implants are sometimes used as guides or ladders for the restoration of damaged nerve trunks and tendons. 2. The placement within the body tissues of a substance, such as tantalum, vitallium, or wire filigree, for restoration by mechanical means; as, for example, the closure of a bone defect or the repair of a ventral hernia. 3. The embedding of the embryo into, or on, the endometrium.

implantation graft. [2]IMPLANT (2).

implantation of the bile ducts. The placement of the proximal end of the common or the hepatic duct into the wall of the duodenum, stomach, or jejunum for the cure of biliary fistula or to bypass an obstruction.

implantation of the ureters. The transfer of the distal ends of the ureters into the intestine or the skin after cystectomy for malignant disease and in certain cases of exstrophy.

implant biotelemetry. A technique of biomedical instrumentation for conveying information transmitted by radio frequency waves from within the body of a living organism to a receiver at a remote location. Data can be obtained from a free-ranging animal, for example, concerning its location, body temperature, heart rate, blood pressure, etc.

im·pon·der·a·ble, *adj.* [*im-,* not, + *ponderable*]. Incapable of being weighed, evaluated, or measured.

imposed insanity. Delusional ideas imposed by one person upon another. See also *suggestion.*

im·po·tence (im'puh·tunce) *n.* [L. *impotentia,* from *impotens,* powerless]. 1. Inability in the male to perform the sexual act, most frequently for psychologic reasons. 2. By extension, lack of sexual vigor or of power generally. —**impo·tent** (·tunt) *adj.*

im·po·ten·cy (im'puh·tun·see) *n.* IMPOTENCE.

im·preg·nate (im·preg'nate) *v.* [ML. *impraegnare,* from L. *praegnans,* pregnant]. 1. To inseminate and fertilize; make pregnant. 2. To saturate or mix with another substance. —**im·preg·na·tion** (im''preg·nay'shun) *n.*

impregnated bandage. A wide-meshed bandage impregnated with such substances as plaster of Paris, sodium silicate, starch, or dextrin, put up in rolls and used for stiffening, immobilizing, and making molds of various parts of the body.

im·pres·sio (im·pres'ee·o) *n.*, pl. **im·pres·si·o·nes** (im·pres''ee·o'neez) [L.]. IMPRESSION (1).

impressio car·di·a·ca he·pa·tis (kahr·dye'uh·kuh hep'uh·tis) [NA]. A shallow depression on the diaphragmatic surface of the liver corresponding to the position of the heart.

impressio cardiaca pul·mo·nis (pul·mo'nis) [NA]. A concavity on the medial surface of each lung corresponding to the heart; the one on the left lung is deeper.

impressio co·li·ca (ko'li·kuh) [NA]. A variable indentation on the visceral surface of the right lobe of the liver corresponding to the hepatic flexure of the colon.

impressio du·o·de·na·lis he·pa·tis (dew·o·de·nay'lis hep'uh·tis) [NA]. A faint depression on the visceral surface of the right lobe of the liver corresponding to the descending duodenum.

impressio eso·pha·gea he·pa·tis (ee''so·fay'jee·uh, es''o·faj'ee·uh hep'uh·tis) [NA]. A faint depression on the diaphragmatic surface of the left lobe of the liver corresponding to the distal portion of the esophagus.

impressio gas·tri·ca he·pa·tis (gas'tri·kuh hep'uh·tis) [NA]. A depression on the visceral surface of the left lobe of the liver corresponding to the stomach.

impressio gastrica re·nis (ree'nis) [BNA]. A depression on the anterior surface of the left kidney corresponding to the stomach.

impressio he·pa·ti·ca re·nis (he·pat'i·kuh ree'nis) [BNA]. A depression on the anterior surface of the left kidney corresponding to the left lobe of the liver.

impressio li·ga·men·ti cos·to·cla·vi·cu·la·ris (lig·uh·men'tye kos''to·kla·vick''yoo·lair'is) [NA]. COSTAL TUBEROSITY.

impressio mus·cu·la·ris re·nis (mus·kew·lair'is ree'nis) [BNA]. A variable depression on the posterior surface of the kidney corresponding to the psoas muscle.

im·pres·sion, *n.* [L. *impressio,* from *imprimere,* to press into]. 1. A mark produced upon a surface by pressure. 2. A mold or imprint of a bodily part or parts from which a positive likeness or cast is made, usually from material, as plaster of Paris, wax compounds, or hydrocolloids. 3. The effect or sensation, usually the initial one, produced by a person, situation, or other phenomenon upon an individual's mind or feelings.

impression compound. Any one of many thermoplastic organic materials used for making dental impressions; individual formulas vary but usually contain combinations of shellac, resin, gums, stearic acid, glycerin, talc, or chalk.

impressiones. Plural of *impressio.*

impressiones di·gi·ta·tae (dij·i·tay'tee) [NA]. CONVOLUTIONAL IMPRESSIONS.

impression tonometry. INDENTATION TONOMETRY.

impression tray. A device shaped to cover the dental arch or ridge in which a plastic material is placed for making impressions of the teeth and/or alveolar ridges.

impressio oe·so·pha·gea he·pa·tis (ee''so·fay'jee·uh, ·faj'ee·uh hep'uh·tis) [BNA]. IMPRESSIO ESOPHAGEA HEPATIS.

impressio pe·tro·sa ce·re·bri (pe·tro'suh serr'e·brye) [BNA]. A groove on the base of the brain corresponding to the petrous portion of the temporal bone.

impressio re·na·lis he·pa·tis (re·nay'lis hep'uh·tis) [NA]. A depression on the visceral surface of the right lobe of the liver corresponding to the right kidney.

impressio su·pra·re·na·lis he·pa·tis (sue''pruh·re·nay'lis hep'uh·tis) [NA]. A faint indentation on the visceral surface of the right lobe of the liver corresponding to the right suprarenal gland.

impressio tri·ge·mi·ni os·sis tem·po·ra·lis (trye·jem'i·nigh os'is tem·po·ray'lis) [NA]. A shallow depression in the floor of the middle cranial fossa which lodges the trigeminal ganglion.

im·print·ing, *n.* A particular mode of learning in animals occurring at critical periods in early development, characterized by patterning on adult models, rapid acquisition, and relative resistance to forgetting or extinction. Observed chiefly in animal behavior; the extent to which it applies to human behavior has not been determined. **—imprint,** *v.*

im·pro·cre·ant (im·pro'kree·unt) *adj.* [*im-*, not, + L. *procreare,* to beget]. Incapable of procreating; impotent. **—improcre·ance** (·unce) *n.*

im·pu·ber·al (im·pew'bur·ul) *adj.* [L. *impubes, impuberis*]. 1. Destitute of hair on the pubes. 2. Not of adult age; immature.

im·pu·bic (im·pew'bick) *adj.* IMPUBERAL.

im·pulse, *n.* [L. *impulsus,* from *impellere,* to impel]. 1. A push or communicated force. 2. A mechanical or electrical force or action generally of brief duration. 3. *In neurophysiology,* NERVE IMPULSE. 4. A sudden mental urge to an action. Compare *drive.*

impulse disorder. Any nonpsychotic mental disorder in which control of one's impulses is weak, with the resultant impulsive behavior usually irresistible, pleasurable, and ego-syntonic.

im·pul·sion, *n.* [L. *impulsio,* from *impellere,* to impel]. 1. The act of driving or urging onward, either mentally or physically. 2. The sudden and spontaneous drive to perform a usually forbidden or illegal act. **—impul·sive,** *adj.*

impulsive behavior. 1. IMPULSE DISORDER. 2. Behavior with lack of impulse control commonly seen in children, especially those with the minimal brain dysfunction syndrome.

impulsive insanity. Any mental disorder accompanied by an uncontrollable desire to commit acts of violence.

im·put·abil·i·ty (im·pew''tuh·bil'i·tee) *n.* [L. *imputare,* to bring into the reckoning]. *In legal medicine,* the degree of mental soundness which makes a person responsible for his own acts.

Imuran. Trademark for azathioprine, a drug used in treating leukemia, as a suppressive agent in diseases produced by altered immune mechanisms, in the induction of immune tolerance, and in the prevention of rejection of allografts.

imvic. A mnemonic designating four reactions (*i*ndole, *m*ethyl red, *V*oges-Proskauer, *c*itrate). *Escherichia coli* forms are indole and methyl red positive. They do not produce acetylmethylcarbinol and do not attack sodium citrate. Organisms classified as *Enterobacter aerogenes* are indole and methyl red negative, produce acetylmethylcarbinol, and attack sodium citrate. A symbol for *Escherichia coli* becomes then + + − −, and the symbol for *Enterobacter aerogenes* is − − + +.

In Symbol for indium.

[1]in-, im- [L.]. A prefix meaning *not, non-, un-.*

[2]in-, im- [L.]. A prefix meaning *in, into, on, onto, toward.*

[3]in-. See *ino-.*

-in [L. *-inus*]. 1. A suffix designating (a) *a neutral nitrogenous substance* (as a protein or bitter principle); (b) *an ester* (as palmitin); (c) *the name of a glycoside* or *neutral principle.* See also *-ine.* 2. A suffix designating *the product derived from* a particular organism or substance (as tuberculin or coccidioidin).

in·acid·i·ty (in''a·sid'i·tee) *n.* Lack of acidity; especially deficiency of hydrochloric acid in the gastric juice.

in·ac·ti·vate, *v.* To render inactive, as by heating fresh serum to destroy its complement.

in·ac·tive, *adj.* 1. Of a substance: exhibiting no activity of a given sort, as optical, chemical, or biological. 2. Of a disease: exhibiting no activity or progress; in remission. **—inactiv·i·ty,** *n.*

inactive cavitary tuberculosis. Tuberculosis with persisting pulmonary cavity, but with 18 consecutive months of negative bacteriologic findings.

inactive mandelic acid. MANDELIC ACID.

inactive noncavitary tuberculosis. Tuberculosis with negative bacteriology on monthly examination for at least 6 months, and in which serial chest roentgenograms are stable, without cavities, for 6 months.

inactive paraganglioma. CAROTID-BODY TUMOR.

inactive tuberculosis. The stage of tuberculosis in which bacteriologic tests are negative upon monthly examination for 6 months and serial radiographs for the same period show stability or slight clearing and contraction of the lesions, without cavitation.

inactivity atrophy. DISUSE ATROPHY.

in·ad·e·qua·cy, *n.* Insufficiency of function or capacity. **—inade·quate,** *adj.*

inadequate personality. An individual showing no obvious mental or physical defect, but characterized by inappropriate or inadequate response to intellectual, social, emotional, and physical demands, and whose behavior pattern shows inadaptability, ineptitude, poor judgment, lack of physical and emotional stamina, and social incompatibility.

inadequate stimulus. A stimulus unable to produce a response; a subthreshold stimulus.

in·al·i·men·tal (in·al''i·men'tul) *adj.* [*in-* + *aliment* + *-al*]. Not nourishing; not suitable for food.

in·a·ni·tion (in''a·nish'un) *n.* [L. *inanire,* to empty]. A pathologic state of the body due to the lack of food and water; starvation.

in·ap·pe·tence (in·ap'e·tunce) *n.* [*in-* + L. *appetere,* to strive after]. Loss of appetite or desire.

Inapsine. A trademark for droperidol, a tranquilizer.

in·ar·tic·u·late (in''ahr·tick'yoo·lut) *adj.* Not articulate.

in ar·tic·u·lo mor·tis (in ahr·tick'yoo·lo mor'tis) [L.]. At the moment of death; in the act of dying.

in·as·sim·i·la·ble (in''a·sim'i·luh·bul) *adj.* Incapable of being assimilated.

in·born, *adj.* Of a constitutional characteristic: inherited or implanted during intrauterine life; innate; congenital.

inborn reflex. UNCONDITIONED REFLEX.

in·bred, *adj.* Derived from closely related parents.

in·breed·ing, *n.* Any system of mating which gives a smaller number of ancestors than the maximum possible, the closest inbreeding being self-fertilization, as in plants, or brother-by-sister mating in animals.

inbreeding coefficient. A measure of the probability that the two genes at a locus came from a common ancestor.

In·ca bone (ink'uh). INCARIAL BONE.

in·ca·nous (in·kay'nus) *adj.* [L. *incanus*]. Hoary white.

INCAP Institute of Nutrition of Central America and Panama.

in·cap·a·ri·na (in·kap''uh·rye'nuh, ·ree·nuh) *n.* [*INCAP* + Sp. h*arina,* flour]. A cereal food mixture with added yeast and vitamin A supplied to increase protein intake to combat kwashiorkor in Central America.

in·car·cer·ate (in·kahr'sur·ate) *v.* [*in-* + L. *carcer,* prison]. To imprison, confine, or enclose. **—incarcer·at·ed** (·ay·tid) *adj.*

incarcerated calculus. ENCYSTED CALCULUS.

incarcerated hernia. An irreducible hernia, frequently due to adhesions, particularly of the omentum, to the sac. If bowel is present in the hernia, it may become obstructed.

incarcerated placenta. A placenta retained by contraction of the uterus including the cervix, which traps the placenta.

in·car·cer·a·tion (in·kahr''sur·ay'shun) *n.* The abnormal imprisonment of a part, as in some forms of hernia.

in·ca·ri·al bone (ing·kair'ee·ul). The human interparietal bone as it occurs anomalously separated from the rest of the occipital bone by a suture or sutures; so called because common in the ancient Incas. Syn. *Inca bone.*

in·car·nant (in·kahr'nunt) *adj.* & *n.* [L. *incarnare,* to make flesh]. 1. Flesh-forming; promoting granulation. 2. An agent that promotes granulation.

in·car·na·tive (in·kahr'nuh·tiv) *adj.* & *n.* INCARNANT.

in·cep·tus (in·sep'tus) *n.* [L., a beginning, from *incipere,* to begin]. ANLAGE.

in·cest (in′sest) *n.* [L. *incestus,* unchaste]. Sexual intercourse between persons of such close genetic relationship that their marriage is prohibited by law.

inch, *n.* [OE. *ince,* from L. *uncia,* twelfth part]. The twelfth part of a foot; 2.54 cm.

in·ci·dence, *n.* [MF., from L. *incidere,* to fall upon]. 1. The act or manner of falling upon; the way in which one body strikes another. 2. The rate of occurrence, as of a disease.

incidence rate. The number of new cases of a disease or injury that occur per population at risk in a particular geographic area within a defined time interval such as a year; usually expressed as the number of new cases of a disease or injury per 1,000 or 100,000 population.

in·ci·dent, *adj.* [L. *incidens, incidentis*]. 1. Falling upon, as an incident ray. 2. External. 3. Likely to occur. **—in·ci·den·tal** (in″si·dent′ul) *adj.*

incidental parasite. A parasitic organism as parasite of a host other than its usual one.

incident ray. The ray of light that forms the angle of incidence.

in·cin·er·ate, *v.* [L. *incinerare,* from *cinis, cineris,* ashes]. To heat an organic substance until all the organic matter is driven off and only ash remains; to cremate. **—in·cin·er·a·tion,** *n.;* **in·cin·er·a·tor,** *n.*

in·cip·i·ent, *adj.* [L. *incipiens,* from *incipere,* to begin]. Initial, commencing; coming into being, as a disease. **—incipi·ence, incipi·en·cy,** *n.*

in·ci·sal (in·sigh′zul) *adj.* Of or pertaining to the cutting edge of incisor and canine teeth.

incisal angle. The junction of the incisal edge of an anterior tooth with a proximal surface.

incisal guidance. The effect of the occluding surfaces of the upper and lower anterior teeth on mandibular movements.

in·cise (in·size′) *v.* [L. *incidere, incisus,* to cut into, from *caedere,* to cut]. To cut into a body tissue or organ with a knife or scalpel.

in·ci·sion (in·sizh′un) *n.* [L. *incisio,* from *incidere,* to cut into]. 1. A cut or wound of the body tissue, as an abdominal incision or a vertical or oblique incision. 2. The act of cutting. **—incision·al** (·ul) *adj.*

incisional hernia. A hernia occurring from an operative or accidental incision, the predisposing factors being wound infection, prolonged drainage, or interference with nerve supply.

in·ci·sive (in·sigh′siv, ·ziv) *adj.* 1. Cutting; penetrating. 2. Pertaining to the incisor teeth.

incisive bone. The intermaxillary bone which bears the upper incisor teeth. Fused with the maxilla in man; a separate bone in most mammals. NA *os incisivum.*

incisive canal. The bifurcated bony passage from the floor of the nasal cavity to the incisive fossa. On each side, the branches open by a median and a lateral incisive foramen transmitting, respectively, the nasopalatine nerve and a branch of the greater palatine artery. NA *canalis incisivus.*

incisive foramina. The two to four openings of the incisive canal or canals on the floor of the incisive fossa (1). A pair in the midline, the median incisive foramina (foramina of Scarpa) transmit the nasopalatine nerves from the anterior nasal floor to the anterior hard palate. A pair of lateral incisive foramina (foramina of Stensen) transmit terminal branches of the greater palatine arteries from the palate to the floor of the nasal cavities. NA *foramina incisiva.*

incisive fossa. 1. A bony pit behind the upper incisors into which the incisive canals open. NA *fossa incisiva.* 2. A depression on the maxilla at the origin of the depressor muscle of the nose. 3. A depression on the mandible at the origin of the mentalis muscle.

incisive papilla or **pad.** The oval or pear-shaped thickening of the palatine mucous membrane overlying the incisive fossa and containing vestiges of the nasopalatine ducts. Syn. *palatine papilla.* NA *papilla incisiva.*

incisive recess. A depression on the nasal septum immediately above the incisive canal.

incisive suture. The suture between the premaxilla and maxilla in the embryo and fetus; union usually occurs before birth. It is rarely visible in the adult. NA *sutura incisiva.*

in·ci·si·vus la·bii in·fe·ri·o·ris (in″si·sigh′vus lay′bee·eye in·feer″ee·o′ris). A portion of the orbicularis oris muscle extending from the vicinity of the base of the lower canine tooth to the corner of the mouth.

incisivus labii su·pe·ri·o·ris (sue·peer″ee·o′ris). A portion of the orbicularis oris muscle extending from the vicinity of the base of the upper canine tooth to the corner of the mouth.

in·ci·so·la·bi·al (in·sigh″zo·lay′bee·ul) *adj.* Pertaining to the incisal and labial surfaces of an anterior tooth.

in·ci·so·lin·gual (in·sigh″zo·ling′gwul) *adj.* Pertaining to the incisal and lingual surfaces of an anterior tooth.

in·ci·so·prox·i·mal (in·sigh″zo·prock′si·mul) *adj.* Pertaining to the incisal and proximal surfaces of an anterior tooth.

in·ci·sor (in·sigh′zur) *n.* [L., cutter, from *incidere,* to cut into, cut through]. A cutting tooth; in the human dentition, one of the four front teeth of either jaw. NA *dens incisivus* (pl. *dentes incisivi*).

incisor crest. The forward prolongation of the nasal crest of the maxilla, terminating in the anterior nasal spine; the cartilage of the nasal septum rests upon it.

in·ci·su·ra (in″sigh·zew′ruh, in″si·) *n.,* pl. & genit. sing. **incisu·rae** (·ree) [L.]. INCISURE.

incisura ace·ta·bu·li (as·e·tab′yoo·lye) [NA]. ACETABULAR NOTCH.

incisura an·gu·la·ris (ang″gew·lair′is) [NA]. ANGULAR NOTCH.

incisura anterior au·ris (aw′ris) [NA]. A notch between the tragus and the crus of the helix of the auricle.

incisura api·cis cor·dis (ap′i·sis kor′dis) [NA]. An indefinite notch at the apex of the heart marking the septum between the right and left ventricles.

incisura car·di·a·ca (kahr·dye′uh·kuh) [BNA]. Incisura cardiaca pulmonis sinistri (= CARDIAC INCISURE (2)).

incisura cardiaca pul·mo·nis si·nis·tri (pul·mo′nis si·nis′trye) [NA]. CARDIAC INCISURE (2).

incisura cardiaca ven·tri·cu·li (ven·trick′yoo·lye) [NA]. CARDIAC INCISURE (1).

incisura ce·re·bel·li anterior (serr″e·bel′eye) [BNA]. ANTERIOR CEREBELLAR NOTCH.

incisura cerebelli posterior [BNA]. POSTERIOR CEREBELLAR NOTCH.

incisura cla·vi·cu·la·ris (kla·vick″yoo·lair′is) [NA]. CLAVICULAR NOTCH.

incisura cos·ta·lis (kos·tay′lis) [NA]. COSTAL NOTCH.

incisurae. Plural and genitive singular of *incisura.*

incisurae car·ti·la·gi·nis me·a·tus acu·sti·ci (kahr·ti·laj′i·nis mee·ay′tus a·koos′ti·sigh) [NA]. Two fissures usually present in the anterior wall of the cartilage of the external acoustic meatus.

incisurae cartilaginis meatus acustici ex·ter·ni [San·to·ri·ni] (ecks·tur′nigh san·to·ree′nee) [BNA]. INCISURAE CARTILAGINIS MEATUS ACUSTICI.

incisurae cos·ta·les (kos·tay′leez) [NA]. COSTAL NOTCHES.

incisurae he·li·cis (hel′i·sis). A vestigial band of muscle occasionally associated with the incisura of the helix of the external ear. NA *musculus incisurae helicis.*

incisura eth·moi·da·lis (eth·moy·day′lis) [NA]. ETHMOID NOTCH.

incisura fi·bu·la·ris (fib·yoo·lair′is) [NA]. A notch on the lateral side of the distal end of the shaft of the tibia, which articulates with the lower end of the fibula.

incisura fron·ta·lis (fron·tay′lis) [NA]. FRONTAL NOTCH.

incisura in·ter·ary·te·noi·dea (in″tur·ăr″i·te·noy′dee·uh) [NA]. INTERARYTENOID INCISURE.

incisura in·ter·lo·ba·ris pul·mo·nis (in″tur·lo·bair′is pul·mo′nis) [BNA]. INTERLOBAR FISSURE.

incisura in·ter·tra·gi·ca (in″tur·traj′i·kuh) [NA]. INTERTRAGIC INCISURE.
incisura is·chi·a·di·ca major (is·kee·ad′i·kuh) [NA]. GREATER SCIATIC NOTCH.
incisura ischiadica minor [NA]. LESSER SCIATIC NOTCH.
incisura ju·gu·la·ris os·sis oc·ci·pi·ta·lis (jug·yoo·lair′is os′is ock·sip·i·tay′lis) [NA]. JUGULAR NOTCH OF THE OCCIPITAL BONE.
incisura jugularis ossis tem·po·ra·lis (tem·po·ray′lis) [NA]. JUGULAR NOTCH OF THE TEMPORAL BONE.
incisura jugularis ster·ni (stur′nigh) [NA]. JUGULAR NOTCH OF THE STERNUM.
in·ci·su·ral (in·sigh′zhur·ul, in″sigh·zew′rul) *adj.* Of or pertaining to an incisure.
incisura la·cri·ma·lis (lack·ri·may′lis) [NA]. LACRIMAL NOTCH.
incisura li·ga·men·ti te·re·tis (lig·uh·men′tye teer′e·tis) [NA]. UMBILICAL NOTCH.
incisural sclerosis. MESIAL TEMPORAL SCLEROSIS.
incisura man·di·bu·lae (man·dib′yoo·lee) [NA]. MANDIBULAR NOTCH.
incisura mas·toi·dea (mas·toy′dee·uh) [NA]. MASTOID NOTCH.
incisura na·sa·lis (na·say′lis) [NA]. NASAL NOTCH (1).
incisura pan·cre·a·tis (pan·kree′uh·tis) [NA]. PANCREATIC NOTCH.
incisura pa·ri·e·ta·lis (pa·rye·e·tay′lis) [NA]. PARIETAL NOTCH.
incisura pre·oc·ci·pi·ta·lis (pree″ock·sip·i·tay′lis) [NA]. An inconstant notch on the lower lateral margin of the cerebral hemisphere between the parietal and occipital lobes.
incisura pte·ry·goi·dea (terr″i·goy′dee·uh) [NA]. PTERYGOID FISSURE.
incisura ra·di·a·lis (ray·dee·ay′lis) [NA]. RADIAL NOTCH.
incisura sca·pu·lae (skap′yoo·lee) [NA]. SCAPULAR NOTCH.
incisura se·mi·lu·na·ris (sem″i·lew·nair′is) [BNA]. Incisura trochlearis (= TROCHLEAR NOTCH).
incisura sphe·no·pa·la·ti·na (sfee″no·pal·uh·tye′nuh) [NA]. SPHENOPALATINE NOTCH.
incisura su·pra·or·bi·ta·lis (sue″pruh·or·bi·tay′lis) [NA]. SUPRAORBITAL NOTCH.
incisura ten·to·rii (ten·to′ree·eye) [NA]. INCISURE OF THE TENTORIUM.
incisura ter·mi·na·lis au·ris (tur·mi·nay′lis aw′ris) [NA]. A notch in the auricular cartilage between the tragal portion and the portion forming the external acoustic meatus.
incisura thy·roi·dea inferior (thigh·roy′dee·uh) [NA]. INFERIOR THYROID NOTCH.
incisura thyroidea superior [NA]. SUPERIOR THYROID NOTCH.
incisura tro·chle·a·ris (trock·lee·air′is) [NA]. TROCHLEAR NOTCH.
incisura tym·pa·ni·ca (tim·pan′i·kuh) [NA]. TYMPANIC NOTCH.
incisura ul·na·ris (ul·nair′is) [NA]. ULNAR NOTCH.
incisura um·bi·li·ca·lis (um·bil·i·kay′lis) [BNA]. Incisura ligamenti teretis (= UMBILICAL NOTCH).
incisura ver·te·bra·lis inferior (vur″te·bray′lis) [NA]. INFERIOR VERTEBRAL INCISURE.
incisura vertebralis superior [NA]. SUPERIOR VERTEBRAL INCISURE.
in·ci·sure (in·sigh′zhur) *n.* [L. *incisura*]. A notch, fissure, or groove.
incisure of Ri·vi·nus (ri·vee′nŏŏs, angl. ri·vye′nus) [A. Q. *Rivinus,* German anatomist, 1652–1723]. TYMPANIC NOTCH.
incisure of Schmidt-Lantermann SCHMIDT-LANTERMANN INCISURE.
incisure of the acetabulum. ACETABULAR NOTCH.
incisure of the cerebellum. One of the notches separating the cerebellar hemispheres. See also *anterior cerebellar notch, posterior cerebellar notch.*
incisure of the gallbladder. CYSTIC FOSSA.
incisure of the tentorium. A deep notch in the tentorium of the cerebellum for the midbrain. NA *incisura tentorii.*
in·cli·na·tio (in″kli·nay′shee·o) *n.,* pl. **incli·na·ti·o·nes** (·nay″shee·o′neez) [L.]. INCLINATION.
in·cli·na·tion (in″kli·nay′shun) *n.* [L. *inclinatio,* a leaning]. 1. A propensity; a leaning. 2. The deviation of the long axis of a tooth from the vertical. 3. A slope. —**in·cline** (in·kline′) *v.;* **in·cline** (in′kline) *n.*
inclination of the pelvis. In the erect position, the angle that the plane of the pelvic inlet makes with the horizontal plane, normally 55° to 60°. NA *inclinatio pelvis.*
inclinatio pel·vis (pel′vis) [NA]. INCLINATION OF THE PELVIS.
inclined plane. Any one of the inclined cuspal surfaces of a tooth.
in·cli·nom·e·ter (in″kli·nom′e·tur) *n.* [*incline* + *meter*]. A device for determining the diameter of the eye from the horizontal and vertical lines.
in·clu·sion blennorrhea. INCLUSION CONJUNCTIVITIS.
inclusion body. A minute foreign particle found in cells under special conditions; especially in cells infected by any of various viruses.
inclusion body encephalitis. Encephalitis characterized pathologically by large intranuclear inclusion bodies in astrocytes, oligodendrocytes, and nerve cells; classified as acute (HERPETIC ENCEPHALITIS) and subacute (SUBACUTE SCLEROSING PANENCEPHALITIS).
inclusion conjunctivitis. An acute purulent conjunctivitis, caused by *Chlamidia trachomatis,* and having a different clinical appearance in the neonate than in the adult. In the neonate the organism is transmitted from the mother's genital tract during birth, and the condition is characterized by swelling and redness of the lids, purulent discharge, and chemosis, involving both eyes. In the adult the condition is less severe and often acquired in swimming pools or venereally; it is characterized by a less purulent discharge, but by larger papillae and preauricular adenopathy, frequently involving one eye only. Confirmed clinically in both instances by finding of epithelial-cell inclusion bodies in conjunctival scrapings.
inclusion cyst. A cyst due to embryonal or traumatic implantation of epithelium into another structure, as an epidermal inclusion cyst.
inclusion encephalitis. Inclusion body encephalitis (= SUBACUTE SCLEROSING PANENCEPHALITIS or HERPETIC ENCEPHALITIS).
in·co·ag·u·la·ble (in″ko·ag′yoo·luh·bul) *adj.* Incapable of coagulating or curdling.
in·com·bus·ti·ble (in″kum·bus′ti·bul) *adj.* Incapable of being burned.
in·com·pat·i·ble (in″kum·pat′i·bul) *adj.* Incapable of being used or put together because of resulting chemical change or of antagonistic qualities, as two drugs or two types of blood. —**incom·pat·i·bil·i·ty** (·pat″i·bil′i·tee) *n.*
in·com·pen·sa·tion (in″kom″pen·say′shun) *n.* Lack of compensation.
in·com·pe·tence (in·kom′pe·tunce) *n.* [F. *incompétence*]. 1. Insufficiency; inadequacy in performing natural functions. 2. *In legal medicine,* incapacity; want of legal fitness, as the incompetence of a drunken man to drive a car. —**incompe·tent** (·tunt) *adj.*
in·com·plete abortion. Partial expulsion of the products of conception before 20 weeks gestation, with some of the placenta and/or membranes remaining within the uterus.
incomplete antibody. An antibody that combines with its antigen but is not grossly detectable unless shown to inhibit or block a reaction.
incomplete antigen. HAPTEN.
incomplete bundle branch block. A delay in activation of a portion of the ventricles due to slow conduction through one of the bundle branches, with lengthening of the QRS interval to over 0.10 seconds but not over 0.12 seconds.
incomplete disinfectant. A disinfectant that destroys the vegetative cells but not the spores.
incomplete dislocation. A dislocation in which there has been only a partial separation of the joint surfaces. Syn. *subluxation.*

incomplete fracture. A fracture that does not extend through the entire bone.

incomplete heart block. A first- or second-degree atrioventricular block.

incomplete (inguinal) hernia. An inguinal hernia in which the sac has not passed through the subcutaneous inguinal ring.

in·con·gru·ence (in·kong'groo·unce) *n.* INCONGRUITY. —**in·con·gru·ent** (·groo·unt) *adj.*

incongruent articulation. An articulation in which two or more opposing surfaces may differ in form or present curves of unequal radii resulting in imperfect fitting.

in·con·gru·i·ty (in''kong·groo'i·tee) *n.* [ML. *incongruitas,* from *incongruus,* incongruous]. Absence of agreement, correspondence, or needful harmony.

in·con·stant (in·kon'stunt) *adj.* Not always present.

in·con·ti·nence (in·kon'ti·nunce) *n.* [L. *incontinentia,* lack of restraint]. Inability to control the natural evacuations, as the feces or the urine; specifically, involuntary evacuation due to organic causes.

in·con·ti·nen·tia pig·men·ti (in·kon''ti·nen'shee·uh pig·men'tye). A skin disorder seen almost exclusively in female infants, characterized by widespread pigmented macules of bizarre shape usually located on the sides of the trunk; often associated with defects of the teeth, brain, eyes, and scalp hair. Inherited as a dominant trait, it is usually lethal to the male (fetus). Syn. *Bloch-Sulzberger syndrome.*

in·co·or·di·na·tion (in''ko·or''di·nay'shun) *n.* Inability to bring into common, harmonious movement or action, as inability to produce voluntary muscular movements in proper order or sequence. See also *ataxia.* —**inco·or·di·nate** (·or'di·nut) *adj.*

in·cor·po·ra·tion (in·kor''puh·ray'shun) *n.* [L. *incorporatio,* from *incorporare,* to embody]. 1. The intimate mingling, union, or embodiment of something, as an idea, a feeling, a chemical substance, or an individual, with an existing whole into a new or composite, usually permanent, whole. 2. *In psychiatry,* a defense mechanism, operating unconsciously, in which the psychic representation of another person or part of him has been figuratively ingested into one's body, as the infant's fantasy of having eaten the maternal breast, making it part of his own self. Compare *internalization, introjection.* —**in·cor·po·rate** (in·kor'puh·rate) *v.*

in·co·sta·pe·di·al (ing''ko·stay·pee'dee·ul) *adj.* INCUDOSTAPEDIAL.

in·cre·ment (in'kre·munt) *n.* [L. *incrementum,* increase]. The amount of increase or growth in a given period of time. —**in·cre·men·tal** (in''kre·men'tul) *adj.*

incremental lines. Lines seen in histologic sections that are manifestations of variations in structure and mineralization during the periodic growth of dental enamel, dentin, and cementum. See also *incremental lines of Retzius.*

incremental lines of Ret·zi·us (ret'see·ōōs) [M. G. *Retzius,* Swedish histologist, 1842–1919]. Brownish bands that represent the successive apposition of layers of enamel matrix; seen in ground sections of dental enamel.

in·cre·tion (in·kree'shun) *n.* An internal secretion. —**in·cre·to·ry** (in'kre·to·ree, in·kree'tuh·ree) *adj.*

incretory gland. ENDOCRINE GLAND.

in·crust, en·crust (in·krust') *v.* To form a crust or hard coating on.

in·crus·ta·tion (in''krus·tay'shun) *n.* The formation of a crust or hard coating, as from an exudate; scab, scale.

incrusted cystitis. Chronic severe cystitis characterized by deposits of calcium phosphate or other crystalline material on the bladder wall, with alkaline urine; usually due to infection by *Proteus.* Syn. *alkaline incrusted cystitis.*

in·cu·ba·tion (ing''kew·bay'shun) *n.* [L. *incubatio,* from *incubare,* to lie on, to hatch]. 1. The act or process of hatching or developing, as eggs or bacteria. 2. The phase of an infectious disease from the time of infection to the appearance of symptoms. Contr. *decubation.* 3. The process of culturing bacteria for qualitative or quantitative growth studies, as in microbiologic assays. 4. The process of maintaining mixtures of substances in suspension or solution at definite temperatures for varying periods of time for the study of enzyme action or other chemical reactions. 5. In ancient Greek medicine, sleep within the precincts of the temples of healing gods, for the purpose of curing disease. —**in·cu·bate** (ing'kew·bate) *v.*

incubation period. The period of time required for development, as of symptoms of disease after infection, or of altered reactivity after exposure to an allergen.

in·cu·ba·tor (ing'kew·bay''tur) *n.* 1. A small chamber with controlled oxygen, temperature, and humidity for newborns requiring special care. 2. A laboratory cabinet with controlled temperature for the cultivation of bacteria or for facilitating biologic tests. 3. A device for the artificial hatching of eggs.

incubi. A plural of *incubus.*

in·cu·bus (ing'kew·bus) *n.*, pl. **incu·bi** (·bye), **incubuses** [L.]. 1. A demon supposed to have sexual intercourse with sleeping men or women or to enter their bodies and thus direct and influence their behavior. Compare *succubus.* 2. A stifling or suffocating dream; NIGHTMARE.

incud-, incudo-. A combining form meaning *incus, incudal.*

incudal ligament. See *posterior ligament of the incus, superior ligament of the incus.*

in·cu·dec·to·my (ing''kew·deck'tuh·mee) *n.* [*incud-* + *-ectomy*]. Surgical removal of the incus.

incudes. Plural of *incus.*

in·cu·do·mal·le·al (in''kew·do·mal'ee·ul, ing'') *adj.* [*incudo-* + *malleal*]. Pertaining to the incus and the malleus, as the ligaments joining these two bones.

in·cu·do·sta·pe·di·al (in''kew·do·stay·pee'dee·ul, ing'') *adj.* [*incudo-* + *stapedial*]. Pertaining to the incus and the stapes, as the ligaments joining these two bones.

in·cur·able (in·kewr'uh·bul) *adj. & n.* 1. Not capable of being cured. 2. A person suffering from an incurable disease.

in·cur·va·tion (in·kur·vay'shun) *n.* A state or condition of being turned inward. —**in·cur·vate** (in'kur·vate) *v. & adj.*

incurvation-of-the-trunk response. GALANT'S REFLEX.

in·cus (ing'kus) *n.*, genit. **in·cu·dis** (ing·kew'dis), pl. **in·cu·des** (ing·kew'deez) [L., anvil] [NA]. The middle one of the chain of ossicles in the middle ear, so termed from its resemblance to an anvil. See also Plate 20 and Table of Bones in the Appendix. —**in·cu·dal** (ing'kew·dul, ing·kew'dul) *adj.*

in·cy·clo·pho·ria (in·sigh''klo·fo'ree·uh) *n.* Cyclophoria in which the eyes rotate inward.

in·cy·clo·tro·pia (in·sigh''klo·tro'pee·uh) *n.* Cyclotropia (ESSENTIAL CYCLOPHORIA) in which the eyes rotate inward.

IND Investigational New Drug Application; a document filed with the Federal Food and Drug Administration giving complete details of the manufacture and testing of a new drug.

in d. Abbreviation for *in dies,* daily.

in·da·ga·tion (in''duh·gay'shun) *n.* [L. *indagare,* to trace out]. 1. Close investigation or examination. 2. Digital examination.

Indalone. A trademark for butopyronoxyl, an insect repellent and toxicant.

in·de·cent (in·dee'sunt) *adj.* [L. *indecens,* unseemly]. Characterizing any act or material that is lewd or obscene, or specifically designed to arouse the kind of sexual interest that is outside the accepted mores of the community.

indecent assault. Any overture or bodily gesture, such as pinching or touching another person with indecent intent.

indecent exposure. EXPOSURE OF PERSON.

in·de·ci·sion (in''de·sizh'un) *n.* 1. A state characterized by inability to make up one's mind; want of firmness or of will. 2. Abnormal irresolution, usually a symptom of anxiety and depression.

in·dent, *v.* To notch or dent; to form a depression in a surface. —**in·den·ta·tion,** *n.*

indentation of the tongue. Notching of the borders of the tongue made by the teeth.

indentation tonometry. A method of determining the intraocular pressure by measuring the depth of the impression produced upon the ocular wall by a given force represented by a plunger which has a small bearing area. Compare *applanation tonometry.*

in·de·pen·dent assortment. Independent segregation of two or more gene pairs during sexual reproduction (Mendel's second law).

independent cutaneous glycohistechia. Rise in the skin sugar content without a corresponding increase in the blood sugar.

Inderal. Trademark for propranolol, a β-adrenergic blocking agent for the treatment of hypertension, used as the hydrochloride salt.

in·de·ter·mi·nate cleavage (in″de·tur′mi·nut). Cleavage producing blastomeres having similar developmental potencies, each of which can produce a whole embryo. Syn. *regulative cleavage.*

indeterminate leprosy. A form of leprosy, usually early in the disease, in which an inflammatory process marked by mild erythema and hypopigmentation appears and from which the direction of development to lepromatous or tuberculoid forms cannot yet be predicted by clinical, histopathologic, or immunologic means.

in·dex (in′decks) *n.*, genit. **in·di·cis** (in′di·sis), pl. **in·di·ces** (in′di·seez) [L., indicator; forefinger]. 1. [NA]. INDEX FINGER. NA alt. *digitus II.* 2. The ratio, or the formula expressing the ratio, of one dimension of a thing to another dimension. See also *cranial index.*

index case. A case of a disease or abnormality whose identification leads to the investigation and identification of further cases in other members of the same family; PROBAND; PROPOSITUS.

index finger. The second digit of the hand, next to the thumb. Syn. *forefinger.* NA *index, digitus II.*

index hyperopia. Hyperopia due to deficient refractive power of the lens.

Index Medicus. A citation index of publications pertaining to medicine and related fields, by subject headings and authors, published by the U.S. National Library of Medicine.

index of Flow·er [W. H. *Flower*]. 1. NASOMALAR INDEX. 2. DENTAL INDEX.

index of refraction. REFRACTIVE INDEX.

index of relative refraction. The ratio of the refractive index of a substance to the index of its surrounding medium.

In·dia ink method. The use of wet mounts of India ink to outline unstained microbes, especially useful for the demonstration of such structures as capsules.

India ink nucleus. *In exfoliative cytology,* a staining aberration in the nuclei of small squamous lung cancer cells, consisting of deeply and evenly hyperchromatic nuclei resembling India ink droplets.

In·di·an balsam. PERUVIAN BALSAM.

Indian gum. Any of several different gums, including karaya gum and ghatti gum.

Indian hemp. See *cannabis.*

Indian physic. *GILLENIA STIPULATA.*

Indian sarsaparilla. HEMIDESMUS.

Indian sickness. An epidemic gangrenous proctitis, occurring in parts of South America and some islands of the South Pacific, which begins as a severe spreading inflammation of the rectum and progresses to ulceration and gangrene; seen most frequently in children.

Indian tobacco. LOBELIA.

India rubber. RUBBER.

India rubber skin. The hyperelastic skin characteristic of Ehlers-Danlos syndrome.

in·di·can (in′di·kan) *n.* 1. Indoxyl glucoside, $C_{14}H_{17}NO_6 \cdot 3H_2O$, occurring in indigo plants; upon hydrolysis and subsequent oxidation, it is converted to indigotin, the chief constituent of indigo. 2. Indoxyl sulfuric acid or, more commonly, its potassium salt, $C_8H_6NSO_4K$, a substance occurring in urine and formed from indole.

in·di·cant (in′di·kunt) *adj. & n.* 1. Serving as an index or as an indication. 2. A fact or symptom that indicates a particular diagnosis or treatment. 3. That which serves as an index or an indication.

in·di·can·uria (in″di·kuh·new′ree·uh) *n.* The presence of an excess of indican in the urine.

in·di·ca·tion, *n.* [ML. *indicatio,* from L. *indicare,* to indicate]. Any symptom, sign, or occurrence in a disease which points out its cause, diagnosis, course of treatment, or prognosis.

in·di·ca·tor, *n. In chemistry,* a substance used to show by a color or other change when a reaction has taken place or a chemical affinity has been satisfied.

indicator-dilution techniques or **methods.** The measurement of fluid volume or flow by injection of a known amount of indicator and subsequent sampling of its concentration in the fluid.

indicator paper. Strong white filter paper, saturated with the proper strength indicator solution or other particular substance, and dried; used for testing acidity or alkalinity (pH) or for the presence or absence of a particular substance. Syn. *test paper.*

indicator yellow. An intermediary substance formed in the conversion of rhodopsin to retinene.

indices. Plural of *index.*

in·di·co·phose (in′di·ko·foze) *n.* [L. *indic*um, indigo, + *phose*]. A blue-colored phose.

In·di·el·la (in″dee·el′uh) *n.* A genus of Fungi Imperfecti. It is one of several genera whose species cause mycetoma.

in di·es (in dee′es) [L.]. Daily. Abbreviated, in d.

in·dif·fer·ent (in·dif′runt) *adj.* [L. *indifferens*]. Neutral; undifferentiated or nonspecialized, as indifferent cells.

indifferent electrode. INDIRECT LEAD.

indifferent genitalia. The genitalia of the embryo before sexual differences are recognizable.

indifferent gonad. GONAD (2).

in·dif·fer·ent·ism (in·dif′ur·un·tiz·um) *n.* 1. Nondifferentiation. 2. Indifference, apathy.

indifferent streptococci. GAMMA STREPTOCOCCI.

indifferent tissue. Undifferentiated tissue.

in·dig·e·nous (in·dij′e·nus) *adj.* [L. *indigena,* a native]. 1. Native; originating or belonging to a certain locality or country. 2. INBORN.

indigenous sprue. CELIAC SYNDROME.

in·di·ges·tion (in″di·jesh′chun) *n.* 1. Imperfect or disturbed digestion. 2. Failure to digest.

in·dig·i·ta·tion (in·dij″i·tay′shun) *n.* [*in-* + *digitation*]. 1. INTUSSUSCEPTION. 2. Interlocking of fibers, as between muscle and tendons.

in·di·go (in′di·go) *n.* [L. *indicum,* from Gk. *indikon,* from *Indikos,* Indian]. A blue pigment formed by the hydrolysis and oxidation of the indican contained in various species of the shrub *Indigofera* (*Indigofera tinctoria, I. anil, I. argentea*); the chief constituent of indigo is indigotin, but varying amounts of such dyes as indigo brown, indigo red, and indigo yellow are also present.

indigo blue. INDIGOTIN.

indigo carmine. SODIUM INDIGOTINDISULFONATE.

indigo carmine test. A test of kidney function. Indigo carmine should appear in the urine 5 to 7 minutes after intramuscular or intravenous injection if the kidneys are functioning normally.

in·di·go·tin (in·dig′uh·tin, in″di·go′tin) *n.* The chief constituent, $C_{16}H_{10}N_2O_2$, of indigo. Syn. *indigo blue.* See also *indican.*

in·di·go·uria (in″di·go·yoo′ree·uh) *n.* The presence of indigo in the urine, due to a decomposition of indican.

in·di·rect calorimetry. Indirect measurement of heat production in an individual by calculation from oxygen inspired, carbon dioxide expired, and nitrogen excreted in the urine. See also *respiration calorimeter.*

indirect Coombs test [R. *Coombs,* British pathologist, b. 1921]. A means of detecting certain agglutinins that are not capable of producing agglutination by themselves. Test particles are exposed to the unknown serum, then washed and exposed to antihuman serum (Coombs serum) and examined for agglutination.

indirect developing test. INDIRECT COOMBS TEST.

indirect emetic. An emetic acting through the blood upon the vomiting center. Syn. *systemic emetic.*

indirect emmenagogue. An emmenagogue acting by relieving an underlying condition, such as anemia or constipation.

indirect excitation. The stimulation of a muscle through its nerves. Contr. *direct excitation.*

indirect funduscopy. INDIRECT OPHTHALMOSCOPY.

indirect hernia. An inguinal form of hernia that follows the spermatic cord into the scrotum or, in the female, the round ligament into the labium majus. The hernial sac leaves the abdomen through the deep inguinal ring, traverses the inguinal canal, and passes through the superficial inguinal ring. Syn. *lateral hernia, oblique hernia.*

indirect inhibition. *In neurophysiology,* inhibition of postsynaptic potential excitation due to the effects of previous postsynaptic neuron discharge, as during a refractory period.

indirect laryngoscopy. Examination of the interior of the larynx by means of a laryngeal mirror.

indirect lead. An electrical connection in which all electrodes or the exploring electrodes are not in direct contact with, but are distant from, the current source, such as the heart, brain, muscle, or spinal cord, body tissues or fluids serving as a conducting medium.

indirect ophthalmoscopy. The method of the inverted image; the observer's eye is placed about 16 inches from that of the patient, and a high plus biconvex lens is held about 2 inches in front of the observed eye, thereby forming an aerial inverted image of the fundus.

indirect percussion. Percussion effected by placing a pleximeter against the skin surface to receive the tap. Syn. *mediate percussion.*

indirect platelet count. Enumeration of blood platelets by counting them in a stained blood film, together with a count of the erythrocytes in the same microscopic fields. If the number of erythrocytes per unit volume of blood is known, the number of platelets in the same volume can be calculated.

indirect reflex. CROSSED REFLEX.

indirect transfusion. The introduction of blood that was first drawn from the donor into a container and mixed with an anticoagulant. Syn. *mediate transfusion.*

indirect vision. PERIPHERAL VISION.

in·dis·po·si·tion (in·dis″po·zish′un) *n.* The state of being slightly ill or somewhat unwell. —**in·dis·posed** (in″di·spoze′d′) *adj.*

in·di·um (in′dee·um) *n.* [NL., from *indigo* blue (in spectrum)]. In = 114.82. A rare metal that is very soft, resembles lead in its properties, and is used in many alloys.

in·di·vid·u·al immunity. The particular power of certain individuals to resist or overcome infection. Contr. *herd immunity, racial immunity.*

in·di·vid·u·al·iza·tion (in″di·vij″oo·ul·i·zay′shun) *n.* 1. The process whereby an organism becomes an individual, distinct and independent from others in the same category. 2. The process by which an observer recognizes an organism, in particular a person, as an individual with distinctive qualities. 3. The adaptation of any method, such as a therapeutic or educational process, to the needs of a particular person. —**indi·vid·u·al·ize** (·vij′oo·ul·ize) *v.*

individual psychology. A system developed by Alfred Adler, in which the individual is regarded as an indivisible unit of human society; his individual traits are compared, in terms of a striving for superiority which is assumed to exist in everyone, and then restated to provide a composite picture of a single tendency expressed in many ways. The mechanisms of compensation and overt compensation to deal with feelings of inferiority are stressed.

in·di·vid·u·a·tion (in″di·vij″oo·ay′shun) *n.* 1. The process whereby a part of a whole becomes progressively more independent and distinct. 2. INDIVIDUALIZATION.

individuation field. The ability of an organizer to rearrange the regional structure of both itself and the adjacent tissue, to make the adjacent tissue part of a complete embryo.

Indocin. Trademark for indomethacin, a drug with anti-inflammatory, antipyretic, and analgesic activities used in the management of arthritic disorders.

in·do·cy·a·nine green (in″do·sigh′uh·neen). A green dye, $C_{43}H_{47}N_2NaO_6S_2$, used as a diagnostic to determine cardiac output, hepatic function, and liver blood flow.

Indoklon. Trademark for flurothyl, an inhalant convulsant used in psychiatry for shock therapy.

in·dol·ac·e·tu·ria (in″dol·as·i·tew′ree·uh, in″dole·) *n.* The presence of indoleacetic acid in the urine.

in·dole (in′dole) *n.* 2,3-Benzopyrrole, C_8H_7N, a substance formed from tryptophan during intestinal putrefaction. It is responsible, in part, for the odor of feces. In intestinal obstruction it is converted into indican, which is eliminated in the urine.

in·dole·ace·tic acid (in″dole·a·see′tick). Indole-3-acetic acid, $C_{10}H_9NO_2$, a bacterial decomposition product of tryptophan, found in the urine and feces. It promotes and accelerates rooting of plant clippings.

in·do·lent (in′duh·lunt) *adj.* [*in-*, not, + L. *dolens,* from *dolere,* to hurt, be painful]. 1. Painless. 2. Sluggish; of tumors: slow in developing; of ulcers: slow in healing.

in·dole·pro·pi·on·ic acid (in″dole·pro″pee·on′ick). The acid produced when tryptophan loses its NH_2 group.

in·dole·py·ru·vic acid (in″dole·pye·roo′vick). A product of tryptophan upon oxidative deamination of the α-amino group.

in·do·log·e·nous (in″do·loj′e·nus) *adj.* [*indole* + *-genous*]. Producing indole.

in·do·lu·ria (in″do·lew′ree·uh) *n.* [*indole* + *-uria*]. The excretion of indole in the urine.

in·do·lyl·acrylo·yl·gly·cine (in″do·lil·a·kril″o·il·glye′seen) *n.* A product of colonic fermentation of tryptophan, found in abnormal quantities in the urine of certain mentally retarded patients.

in·do·lyl·acrylo·yl·gly·ci·nu·ria (in″do·lil·a·kril″o·il·glye″si·new′ree·uh) *n.* [*indolylacryloylglycine* + *-uria*]. A rare hereditary metabolic disorder in which indolylacryloylglycine is present in the urine, possibly as a result of defective transport across the intestinal and renal mucosa; associated clinically with mental retardation; seen in Hartnup disease.

in·do·meth·a·cin (in″do·meth′uh·sin) *n.* 1-(*p*-Chlorobenzoyl)-5-methoxy-2-methylindole-3-acetic acid, $C_{19}H_{16}ClNO_4$, a drug with anti-inflammatory, antipyretic, and analgesic activities used in the management of arthritic disorders.

in·do·phe·nol (in″do·fee′nole, ·nol) *n.* Any of a series of dyes, derived from quinone imine, used as electron acceptors in biological oxidation studies.

indophenol oxidase. The oxidizing enzyme, present in animal and plant tissues, that catalyzes formation of indophenol blue from dimethyl-*p*-phenylenediamine and α-naphthol when these are injected into tissue; it is identical with cytochrome oxidase.

in·dor·a·min (in·dor'uh·min) *n.* *N*-[1-(2-Indol-3-ylethyl)-4-piperidyl]benzamide, $C_{22}H_{25}N_3O$, an antihypertensive.

in·dox·ole (in·dock'sole) *n.* 2,3-Bis(*p*-methoxyphenyl)indole, $C_{22}H_{19}NO_2$, an antipyretic and inflammation-counteracting drug.

in·dox·yl (in·dock'sil) *n.* An oxidation product, C_8H_7NO, of indole and skatole found in the urine among the products of intestinal putrefaction.

indoxyl glucoside. INDICAN (1).

in·dox·yl·og·e·nous (in·dock''si·loj'e·nus) *adj.* [*indoxyl* + *-genous*]. Producing indoxyl.

indoxyl potassium sulfate. INDICAN (2).

in·dox·yl·sul·fate (in·dock''sil·sul'fate) *n.* INDICAN (2).

in·dox·yl·sul·fu·ric acid (in·dock''sil·sul·few'rick). INDICAN (2).

in·dox·yl·uria (in·dock''sil·yoo'ree·uh) *n.* The presence of indoxyl in the urine.

in·dri·line (in'dri·leen) *n.* *N,N*-Dimethyl-1-phenylindene-1-ethylamine, $C_{19}H_{21}N$, a central nervous system stimulant; used as the hydrochloride salt.

in·duce, *v.* [L. *inducere,* to lead in]. To bring on, produce, as by application of a stimulus.

induced abortion. Intentional premature termination of pregnancy by medicinal or mechanical means. Syn. *artificial abortion.*

induced association. A form of controlled association in which the person to be tested calls out the first word that comes to mind in response to a specific stimulus word.

induced current. The momentary current produced in a coil of insulated wire, introduced within the field of another coil, when the circuit is made or broken in the latter.

induced electricity. The electricity produced in a body by proximity to an electrified body.

induced insanity. FOLIE À DEUX.

induced labor. Labor brought on by artificial means.

induced mutation. Mutation produced by experimental treatment, as by x-rays.

in·duc·ible enzyme (in·dew'si·bul). An enzyme normally present in extremely minute quantities within a cell but whose concentration increases dramatically in the presence of substrate molecules. Contr. *constitutive enzyme.*

in·duc·tion, *n.* [L. *inductio,* from *inducere,* to lead in]. 1. The act of bringing on or causing. 2. The bringing about of an electric or magnetic state in a body by the proximity (without actual contact) of an electrified or magnetized body. 3. The period from first administration of the anesthetic until consciousness is lost and the patient is stabilized in the desired surgical plane of anesthesia. 4. *In embryology,* the specific morphogenetic effect brought about by the action of one tissue upon another, acting through organizers or evocators. 5. The process whereby a lysogenic bacterium is caused to produce infective bacteriophage. 6. The process of initiating or increasing cellular production of an inducible enzyme. —**in·duct,** *v.;* **in·duc·tor,** *n.*

induction coil. Rolls of wire used to transform a current of low potential into a current of high potential by electric induction.

induction current. Current produced in a coil of insulated wire by a changing magnetic field of force surrounding the coil.

in·duc·to·py·rex·ia (in·duck''to·pye·reck'see·uh) *n.* ELECTROPYREXIA.

in·duc·to·ri·um (in''duck·to'ree·um) *n.* *In physiology,* an instrument for the generation and administration of electric shocks by induction; it consists of a primary and a secondary coil mounted on a stand.

in·duc·to·ther·my (in·duck'to·thur''mee) *n.* [*induction* + *-thermy*]. The application of energy to tissue through the agency of a high-frequency magnetic field; usually applied to local parts, but may be used to produce general artificial fever.

in·du·lin (in'dew·lin) *n.* Any one of a group of aniline dyes, certain of which, notably nigrosine, are sometimes used as biological stains.

in·du·ra·tion (in''dew·ray'shun) *n.* [L. *induratio,* from *indurare,* to harden, from *durus,* hard]. 1. The hardening of a tissue or part, resulting from hyperemia, inflammation, or infiltration by neoplasm. 2. A hardened area of tissue. —**in·du·rate** (in'dew·rate) *v.;* **in·dú·ra·tive** (in'dew·ray''tiv) *adj.*

indurative headache. MUSCLE-CONTRACTION HEADACHE.

in·du·si·um (in·dew'zee·um) *n.,* pl. **indu·sia** (·zee·uh) [L., a kind of tunic]. A membranous covering.

indusium gri·se·um (gris'ee·um) [NA]. A thin layer of gray matter in contact with the upper surface of the corpus callosum and continuous laterally with the gyrus fasciolaris and the dentate gyrus. Syn. *supracallosal gyrus.*

in·dus·tri·al (in·dus'tree·ul) *adj.* 1. Of or pertaining to industry. 2. Caused by certain types of work or by processes used in industry.

industrial chemistry. Chemistry applied to industry; the chemistry of industrial processes.

industrial hygiene. The branch of preventive medicine concerned with the promotion of healthful conditions in industry, the prevention of occupational accidents and sickness, and measures for their emergency treatment.

industrial medicine. OCCUPATIONAL MEDICINE.

industrial photophthalmia. ACTINIC KERATOCONJUNCTIVITIS.

industrial psychology. Psychology applied to problems in industry dealing chiefly with the selection and mental health of personnel and their efficiency.

in·dwell·ing (in'dwel·ing) *adj.* Of a catheter or similar tube: left within an organ, duct or vessel for a time to provide drainage, prevent obstruction, or maintain a passage for administration of food or drugs.

¹-ine [L. *-inus*]. An adjective-forming suffix meaning *pertaining to* or *-like,* as bovine, saccharine.

²-ine. A suffix designating (a) a *basic nitrogenous compound,* as morphine or purine; (b) *a halogen,* as bromine. See also *-in.*

in·ebri·ant (in·ee'bree·unt) *adj.* & *n.* 1. Inebriating; causing inebriation. 2. An agent that causes inebriation; an intoxicant.

in·ebri·ate (in·ee'bree·ate) *v.* [L. *inebriare,* from *ebrius,* drunk]. To make drunk; to intoxicate. —**in·ebri·a·tion** (in·ee''bree·ay'shun) *n.*

in·ebri·e·ty (in''e·brye'e·tee) *n.* Habitual drunkenness.

in·ef·fi·ca·cious (in''ef·i·kay'shus) *adj.* [*in-,* not, + *efficacious*]. Failing to produce the desired effect. —**in·ef·fi·ca·cy** (in·ef'i·kuh·see) *n.*

in·elas·tic (in''e·las'tick) *adj.* Not elastic.

inelastic gel. A gel that loses its property of elasticity and pulverizes when dried, becoming amorphous.

in·ert (in·urt') *adj.* [L. *iners, inertis,* inactive, unskilled, from *in-,* not, + *ars,* art, skill]. Lacking in physical activity, in chemical reactivity, or in an expected biologic or pharmacologic effect.

in·er·tia, *n.* [L., sluggishness, from *iners,* sluggish]. 1. Dynamic opposition to acceleration, common to all forms of matter, including electrons and quanta. 2. Lack of activity; sluggishness. See also *uterine inertia.*

inertia time. The time elapsed between the introduction of a stimulus and the response to it; LATENT PERIOD (2).

in·ev·i·ta·ble abortion. An abortion that has advanced to a stage where termination of the pregnancy no longer can be prevented.

in ex·tre·mis (in ecks·tree'mis) [L.]. At the end; at the last; at the point of death.

in·fant, *n.* [MF. *enfant,* from L. *infans, infantis,* from *in-,* not, + *fans,* speaking]. A baby; often more specifically, a child 12 months old or less or, by some criteria, two years old or less. —**in·fan·cy,** *n.*

in·fan·ti·cide (in·fan'ti·side) *n.* [*infant* + *-cide*]. 1. The murder of an infant. 2. The murderer of an infant.

in·fan·tile (in'fun·tile, ·til) *adj.* [L. *infantilis,* of infants]. 1. Pertaining to or occurring during infancy or early childhood. 2. Like or characteristic of an infant.

infantile acquired hemiplegia. ACUTE INFANTILE HEMIPLEGIA.

infantile amaurotic familial idiocy. Either or both of the infantile forms of G_{M2} gangliosidosis: TAY-SACHS DISEASE and SANDHOFF'S DISEASE.

infantile autism. AUTISM (2).

infantile celiac disease. A form of the celiac syndrome of infants and young children, associated with an intolerance to the gliadin fraction of gluten found in wheat, oats, and rye. The patient presents marked abdominal distention, characteristic bulky, greasy, and foul-smelling stools, malnutrition, and growth retardation. See also *nontropical sprue, celiac syndrome.*

infantile cerebral palsy. CEREBRAL PALSY.

infantile cortical hyperostosis. A self-limited painful swelling of the soft parts of the lower jaw, associated with irritability and fever and characterized by periosteal proliferation of the mandible, occurring in the first 3 months of life. The clavicles, scapulae, and long bones are sometimes affected. Syn. *Caffey's disease.*

infantile diarrhea. An acute form of diarrhea in infants, frequently during the summer, caused by bacterial and viral infection of the intestinal tract or other body systems. The pathogens cannot always be identified, and there may be predisposing factors, such as allergic or nutritional ones.

infantile eczema. Dermatitis seen in young children, often associated with personal or family histories of allergy. Allergies to food or inhalants may be identified.

infantile genitalia. 1. The organs of generation of an infant. 2. Underdevelopment to a marked degree of the chronologically adult organs of generation.

infantile glaucoma. CONGENITAL GLAUCOMA.

infantile hernia. A congenital, indirect, inguinal hernia.

infantile hydrocele. Peritoneal fluid in the tunica vaginalis and the vaginal process, but with the process closed at the deep inguinal ring.

infantile hypothyroidism. Hypothyroidism in infancy or early childhood, frequently congenital but may be acquired. Of the congenital types, cretinism is the most severe, but milder forms, often diagnosed later, exist. The acquired forms may be the result of pituitary dysfunction, ingestion of medications containing iodides or cobalt, deficiency of iodides, surgical excision of the thyroid, or lymphocytic thyroiditis or various chronic infections.

infantile hypotonia. FLOPPY-INFANT SYNDROME.

infantile leishmaniasis. A form of kala azar, observed primarily in small children in the Mediterranean area, clinically identical with that of adults. It is acquired from dogs who act as reservoirs for the parasite *Leishmania infantum.*

infantile macular degeneration. BEST'S DISEASE.

infantile muscular dystrophy. PSEUDOHYPERTROPHIC INFANTILE MUSCULAR DYSTROPHY.

infantile myoclonic spasm or **seizure.** INFANTILE SPASM.

infantile neuroaxonal dystrophy. A hereditary (autosomal recessive) disease of the central nervous system of early onset, characterized by the widespread distribution of eosinophilic spheroids of swollen axoplasm, and manifested clinically by arrest in development and regression, the frequent coexistence of upper and lower motor neuron involvement, nystagmus, and optic atrophy and blindness late in the disease, which may run a course over several years.

infantile nuclear aplasia. MÖBIUS' SYNDROME.

infantile osteomalacia. RICKETS.

infantile paralysis. PARALYTIC SPINAL POLIOMYELITIS.

infantile pelvis. An adult pelvis retaining the infantile shape.

infantile polycystic disease. A form of polycystic disease appearing usually at birth but also later before adolescence and probably inherited as an autosomal recessive trait; hepatic cysts are usually associated, and hypertension and respiratory difficulties are common.

infantile pseudohypertrophic muscular dystrophy. PSEUDOHYPERTROPHIC INFANTILE MUSCULAR DYSTROPHY.

infantile pseudoleukemia. VON JAKSCH'S ANEMIA.

infantile pseudoleukemic anemia. VON JAKSCH'S ANEMIA.

infantile scurvy. An acute form of scurvy in infants and children, characterized especially by subperiosteal hemorrhage, particularly of the long bones, with painful swellings. Syn. *Cheadle's disease, Moeller-Barlow disease.*

infantile sexuality. *In psychoanalysis,* the infant's or young child's capacity for, and pleasure derived from, experiences that are essentially sexual in nature, which may include excitation of erotogenic zones, as well as the sexual coloring of the child's relation to close and significant persons, especially the parents.

infantile spasm. A type of seizure seen in infants and young children, characterized by a sudden, brief, massive myoclonic jerk. The commonest form is the flexion spasm, salaam or jack-knife seizure in which the arms are flung forward and out and the legs flex at the hips, resembling the Moro reflex, or there may be simply a sudden nodding of the head or extension of the legs at the hips. Frequently there is an associated cry. The spasms tend to occur on waking or going to sleep and to run in series, and to be accompanied by hypsarrhythmia and mental regression.

infantile spastic paralysis. CEREBRAL PALSY.

infantile spinal muscular atrophy. The commonest and most rapidly progressive heredofamilial form of progressive spinal muscular atrophy, becoming clinically manifest in the prenatal period or in the three months after birth and characterized by general hypotonia and atrophy of skeletal muscle, with death occurring in infancy or childhood. Syn. *Werdnig-Hoffmann atrophy.* See also *progressive spinal muscular atrophy.*

infantile spongy degeneration. SPONGY DEGENERATION OF INFANCY.

infantile subacute necrotizing encephalopathy. SUBACUTE NECROTIZING ENCEPHALOMYELOPATHY.

infantile uterus. A uterus normally formed, but arrested in development.

in·fan·ti·lism (in·fan'ti·liz·um, in'fun·ti·liz·um) *n.* [*infantile* + *-ism*]. 1. The persistence of infantile or childish physical, sexual, or mental characteristics into adolescent and adult life. 2. Specifically such a condition due to a malfunctioning organ or to a disease state, as in Down's syndrome. See also *pituitary dwarfism.* 3. *In psychiatry,* a behavioral pattern characteristic of the state of infancy prolonged into childhood or adult life, such as temper tantrums.

infant mortality rate. The number of deaths reported among infants under 1 year of age in a calendar year per 1,000 live births reported in the same year and place.

in·fan·tum (in·fan'tum) *L. n.* Genitive plural of *infans,* infant; of infants.

in·farct (in'fahrkt, in·fahrkt') *n.* [L. *infarcire,* to stuff into]. A localized or circumscribed area of ischemic tissue necrosis due to inadequate blood flow.

in·farc·tec·to·my (in·fahrk·teck'tuh·mee) *n.* [*infarct* + *-ectomy*]. Removal by surgery of an infarct.

in·farc·tion (in·fahrk'shun) *n.* 1. The process leading to the formation or development of an infarct. 2. INFARCT.

in·fect, *v.* [L. *inficere,* to poison, to taint]. 1. To contaminate with a disease or a pathogenic organism. 2. To invade a body or organ, as by disease-producing pathogens; to cause an infection. Compare *infest.*

in·fec·tion, *n.* 1. The invasion of a host by organisms such as bacteria, fungi, viruses, protozoa, helminths, or insects, with or without manifest disease. Compare *contagion, infestation.* 2. The pathologic state caused in the host by such organisms.

infection immunity. Immunity due to the persistence of an infection, as in syphilis or a virus disease.

in·fec·tious (in·feck'shus) *adj.* Caused by infection.

infectious abortion. An infectious disease in animals which causes premature termination of gestation. The specific organisms are *Brucella abortus* for cattle, *Salmonella abortivoequina* for horses, and *Salmonella abortusovis* for sheep.

infectious adenitis. INFECTIOUS MONONUCLEOSIS.

infectious allergy. Delayed hypersensitivity induced by an infectious agent.

infectious arthritis. An acute or chronic inflammatory disease of a joint caused by invasion of the articular tissue by microorganisms. Infection is usually hematogenous in origin.

infectious bovine rhinotracheitis. An upper respiratory infection of cattle caused by a herpesvirus.

infectious bronchitis. A highly contagious respiratory viral disease of chickens.

infectious bulbar paralysis. PSEUDORABIES.

infectious chorea. SYDENHAM'S CHOREA.

infectious cirrhosis. 1. Cirrhosis usually of Laennec's type in which bacteria are present; there is no conclusive proof that the bacteria cause the disease. 2. Cirrhosis as a sequel of hepatitis.

infectious conjunctivitis. A conjunctivitis caused by microorganisms that may or may not be contagious.

infectious coryza. A respiratory disease of chickens caused by *Haemophilus gallinarum.*

infectious disease. A disease due to invasion of the body by pathogenic organisms, which subsequently grow and multiply. Compare *contagious disease, communicable disease.*

infectious ectromelia. MOUSEPOX.

infectious eczematoid dermatitis. An acute eczematous dermatitis secondary to an infectious exudate.

infectious enterotoxemia of sheep. A toxemia of sheep occurring in Australia and in scattered parts of the United States, thought to be caused by *Clostridium perfringens,* type D. Syn. *overeating disease.*

infectious equine anemia. A virus disease of solipeds (horse, mule, ass), characterized by fever, progressive anemia, edema, and emaciation. Syn. *swamp fever of horses.*

infectious feline enteritis. FELINE PANLEUKOPENIA.

infectious hepatitis. An acute infectious inflammatory disease of the liver, often epidemic, due to hepatitis A virus, characterized in many cases by fever, hepatomegaly, and jaundice. There is oral transmission of the virus, and the incubation period varies from 2 to 6 weeks. Syn. *hepatitis A, short-incubation hepatitis.* Compare *serum hepatitis.*

infectious jaundice. INFECTIOUS HEPATITIS.

infectious laryngotracheitis. A highly contagious respiratory disease of viral etiology affecting chickens.

infectious lymphocytosis. A self-limited contagious and infectious disease, chiefly of children, with or without such systematic manifestations as fever and diarrhea, and characterized by a marked increase in small lymphocytes in the peripheral blood.

infectious mononucleosis. A usually benign, probably infectious disorder, now associated with the Epstein-Barr virus, characterized by irregular fever, sore throat, lymphadenopathy, splenomegaly, lymphocytosis with abnormal lymphocytes, and the development of an abnormally high serum concentration of a specific type of heterophil antibodies against sheep erythrocytes. Syn. *glandular fever, kissing disease, lymphocytic angina, monocytic angina, Pfeiffer's disease.*

infectious myoclonia. SYDENHAM'S CHOREA.

infectious myxomatosis. An infectious disease in rabbits, transmitted by a virus, with widespread lesions resembling myxomas.

infectious neuritis. GUILLAIN-BARRÉ SYNDROME.

infectious oral papillomatosis of dogs. A viral disease of young dogs, characterized by the formation of multiple pedunculated growths on the oral mucosa. The growths disappear spontaneously and leave the animal with a high degree of immunity.

infectious papillomatosis of cattle. A viral disease of cattle, characterized by the formation of warts on various parts of the body.

infectious parotitis. Any infection of the parotid gland, including the mumps virus and bacterial agents complicating systemic disease, as well as an infection complicating obstruction of the parotid duct.

infectious polyneuritis. GUILLAIN-BARRÉ SYNDROME.

infectious pustular dematitis. ORF.

infectious uro·ar·thri·tis (yoor''o·ahr·thrigh'tis). REITER'S SYNDROME.

in·fec·tive (in·feck'tiv) *adj.* 1. Capable of producing infection. 2. INFECTIOUS.

infective hepatitis. INFECTIOUS HEPATITIS.

infective neuritis or **neuronitis.** GUILLAIN-BARRÉ SYNDROME.

in·fe·cun·di·ty (in''fe·kun'di·tee) *n.* [L. *infecundus,* unfruitful]. Sterility; barrenness.

in·fe·ri·ad (in·feer'ee·ad) *adv.* In anatomy, downward; in a superior-to-inferior direction. Compare *caudad.*

in·fe·ri·or (in·feer'ee·ur) *adj.* [L.]. *In anatomy* (with reference to the human or animal body as poised for its usual manner of locomotion): lower; nearer the ground or surface of locomotion. Compare *caudal.* Contr. *superior.* —**inferior·ly,** *adv.*

inferior alveolar canal. MANDIBULAR CANAL.

inferior angle of the scapula. The angle formed by the junction of the lateral and medial margins of the scapula. NA *angulus inferior scapulae.*

inferior arch. HEMAL ARCH.

inferior articular process. One of a pair of processes projecting downward from a vertebral arch and articulating with a superior articular process of the vertebra next below. NA *processus articularis inferior.*

inferior bulb of the internal jugular vein. An enlargement of the internal jugular vein immediately above its union with the subclavian vein. NA *bulbus venae jugularis inferior.*

inferior carotid triangle. A triangle bounded by the median line of the neck, the sternocleidomastoid muscle, and the superior belly of the omohyoid muscle. Syn. *triangle of necessity, muscular triangle, tracheal triangle.*

inferior central nucleus. NUCLEUS OF THE RAPHE.

inferior cerebellar peduncle. A large bundle of nerve fibers running from the medulla oblongata to the cerebellum. It contains the dorsal spinocerebellar tract from the nucleus dorsalis of the spinal cord, olivocerebellar fibers from the olivary nuclei, dorsal external arcuate fibers from the lateral cuneate nucleus, and ventral external arcuate fibers from the arcuate and lateral reticular nuclei. Syn. *restiform body.* NA *pedunculus cerebellaris inferior.*

inferior colliculus. One of the posterior pair of rounded eminences arising from the dorsal portion of the mesencephalon. It contains centers for reflexes in response to sound. Syn. *inferior quadrigeminal body.* NA *colliculus inferior.*

inferior cornu of the thyroid cartilage. See *cornua of the thyroid cartilage.*

inferior costal facet. The inferior facet on the body of a vertebra for articulation with the head of a rib. NA *fovea costalis inferior.* See also *costal fossae.*

inferior curved line of the ilium. INFERIOR GLUTEAL LINE.

inferior curved line of the occipital bone. INFERIOR NUCHAL LINE.

inferior dental canal. MANDIBULAR CANAL.

inferior dental plexus. A plexus of nerve fibers in the lower jaw derived from the inferior alveolar nerve. NA *plexus dentalis inferior.*

inferior duodenal fossa. A small pocket of peritoneum formed on the left of the terminal portion of the duodenum by a triangular fold of peritoneum and having the opening directed upward.

inferior duplicity. *In teratology,* duplicity involving at least infraumbilical parts, with union chiefly by heads or by heads and thoraces.

inferior extensor retinaculum. A thickened band of deep fascia attached laterally to the calcaneus and medially to the medial malleolus and medial cuneiform. It overlies the tendons of the extensor muscles on the dorsal aspect of the foot. Syn. *cruciate ligament of the ankle.* NA *retinaculum musculorum extensorum inferius.*

inferior fascia of the urogenital diaphragm. PERINEAL MEMBRANE.

inferior fovea. The pit in the inferior part of the floor of the fourth ventricle, marking the end of the sulcus limitans. NA *fovea inferior.*

inferior frontal gyrus. The most inferior of the three frontal convolutions, situated in relation to the horizontal and ascending branches of the lateral sulcus. NA *gyrus frontalis inferior.* See also Plate 18.

inferior frontal sulcus. A longitudinal groove separating the inferior and middle frontal gyri. NA *sulcus frontalis inferior.*

inferior ganglion. 1. (of the glossopharyngeal nerve:) The lower sensory ganglion on the glossopharyngeal nerve located in the lower part of the jugular foramen. NA *ganglion inferius nervi glossopharyngei.* 2. (of the vagus nerve:) The lower sensory ganglion on the vagus nerve located below the jugular foramen and anterior to the upper part of the internal jugular vein. NA *ganglion inferius nervi vagi.*

inferior gluteal line. A line extending from the anterior inferior spine of the ilium to the middle of the greater sciatic notch. NA *linea glutea inferior.*

inferior horn of the thyroid cartilage. The inferior cornu of the thyroid cartilage. See *cornua of the thyroid cartilage.*

inferior hypogastric plexus. A nerve plexus in the pelvic fascia; it contains sympathetic, parasympathetic, and visceral sensory elements. Syn. *pelvic plexus.* NA *plexus hypogastricus inferior.*

in·fe·ri·or·i·ty complex. Repressed unconscious fears and feelings of physical or social inadequacy or both, which may result in excessive anxiety, and inability to function, or actual failure; or because of overcompensation, the individual may exhibit excessive ambition and develop skills, often in the area of the real or imagined handicaps. Compare *feelings of inferiority.*

inferior laryngotomy. CRICOTHYROTOMY.

inferior ligament of the epididymis. The fold of the tunica vaginalis testis connecting the testis and the body or tail of the epididymis; the lower lip of the digital fossa. NA *ligamentum epididymidis inferius.*

inferior longitudinal diameter. SAGITTAL DIAMETER OF THE SKULL.

inferior longitudinal fasciculus. A bundle of long association fibers coursing horizontally in the lateral wall of the inferior and posterior horns of the lateral ventricle, extending from the occipital to the temporal lobe. NA *fasciculus longitudinalis inferior.*

inferior mediastinal syndrome. INFERIOR VENA CAVA SYNDROME.

inferior medullary velum. A thin band of white substance which forms the roof of the inferior part of the fourth ventricle. NA *velum medullare inferius.*

inferior mesenteric ganglion. An outlying or collateral sympathetic ganglion lying in the inferior mesenteric plexus near the aorta at the origin of the inferior mesenteric artery. NA *ganglion mesentericum inferius.* See also Plate 15.

inferior mesenteric plexus. A visceral nerve plexus surrounding the inferior mesenteric artery, derived from the aortic plexus. NA *plexus mesentericus inferior.*

inferior nasal concha. The scroll-like bone covered with mucous membrane situated in the lower part of the lateral nasal wall. NA *concha nasalis inferior.* See also Table of Bones in the Appendix.

inferior nasal meatus. The part of the nasal cavity between the floor of the nose and the inferior nasal concha. NA *meatus nasi inferior.*

inferior nasal turbinate. INFERIOR NASAL CONCHA.

inferior nuchal line. A transverse ridge extending from the median nuchal line across the outer surface of the occipital bone, a short distance below the superior nuchal. NA *linea nuchae inferior.*

inferior occipital fossae. CEREBELLAR FOSSAE.

inferior olivary nucleus. OLIVARY NUCLEUS.

inferior olive. OLIVARY NUCLEUS.

inferior orbital fissure. A fissure of the orbit which gives passage to the infraorbital blood vessels, and ascending branches from the pterygopalatine ganglion. NA *fissura orbitalis inferior.*

inferior pancreatic artery. The left, principal branch of the dorsal pancreatic artery, supplying the body and the tail of the pancreas from its inferior margin. NA *arteria pancreatica inferior.*

inferior parietal lobule. The subdivision of the parietal lobe of the cerebrum that contains the supramarginal gyrus and the angular gyrus. NA *lobulus parietalis inferior.*

inferior pelvic aperture or **strait.** The lower opening of the pelvic canal; OUTLET OF THE PELVIS. Syn. *pelvic outlet.* NA *apertura pelvis inferior.* See also *pelvis.*

inferior peroneal retinaculum. A band of fascia overlying the tendons of the peroneus longus and peroneus brevis muscles at the ankle and attached to the lateral aspect of the calcaneus. NA *retinaculum musculorum peroneorum inferius.*

inferior petrosal sinus. A sinus of the dura mater running posteriorly from the cavernous sinus along the line of the petrooccipital suture to the beginning of the internal jugular vein at the jugular foramen. NA *sinus petrosus inferior.* See also Table of Veins in the Appendix.

inferior polioencephalitis. *Obsol.* A pathologic state of uncertain type as characterized by Strümpell; probably acute necrotizing hemorrhagic encephalitis.

inferior quadrigeminal body. INFERIOR COLLICULUS.

inferior quadrigeminal brachium. BRACHIUM OF THE INFERIOR COLLICULUS.

inferior recess of the omental bursa. The downward extension of the omental bursa for a variable distance into the greater omentum. NA *recessus inferior omentalis.*

inferior rectus. An extrinsic muscle of the eye. See *rectus inferior bulbi* in Table of Muscles in the Appendix.

inferior root of the ansa cervicalis. A nerve, formed of fibers from the second and third cervical nerves, which joins the superior root to form the ansa cervicalis. Syn. *descendens cervicis.* NA *radix inferior ansae cervicalis.*

inferior sagittal sinus. A sinus of the dura mater which extends along the posterior half of the lower border of the falx cerebri and terminates in the straight sinus. NA *sinus sagittalis inferior.* See also Table of Veins in the Appendix and Plates 10, 18.

inferior salivatory nucleus. An ill-defined nucleus anterior to the ambiguous nucleus which sends preganglionic autonomic fibers to the otic ganglion via the lesser petrosal nerve. Concerned in the regulation of secretion of the parotid gland. NA *nucleus salivatorius inferior.*

inferior semilunar lobule. The portion of the posterior lobe of the cerebellum lying just inferior to the horizontal cerebellar fissure. NA *lobulus semilunaris inferior.*

inferior sternal region. The part of the sternal region lying below the margins of the third costal cartilages.

inferior strait of the pelvis. INFERIOR PELVIC APERTURE or STRAIT.

inferior tegmental tympanic process. A narrow plate of bone which proceeds from the anterior margin of the anterior pyramidal surface of the temporal bone and forms part of the petrotympanic fissure.

inferior temporal arcade. ZYGOMATIC ARCH.

inferior temporal gyrus. A convolution of the temporal lobe which lies below the middle temporal sulcus and extends around the inferolateral border onto the inferior surface of the temporal lobe, where it is limited by the inferior sulcus. NA *gyrus temporalis inferior.*

inferior temporal line. A line arching across the side of the cranium, marking the upper limit of the temporal fossa and of the attachment of the temporalis muscle. NA *linea temporalis inferior.*

inferior thyroid notch. The notch in the lower margin of the thyroid cartilage between the two laminas. NA *incisura thyroidea inferior.*

inferior transverse ligament of the scapula. A fibrous band which crosses from the lateral border of the spine of the scapula to the margin of the glenoid cavity and under which the suprascapular vessels and nerve pass to the infraspinous fossa. NA *ligamentum transversum scapulae inferius.*

inferior tympanic canaliculus. TYMPANIC CANALICULUS. Contr. *superior tympanic canaliculus* (= CANAL OF THE LESSER PETROSAL NERVE).

inferior vena cava. A vein formed by the junction of the two common iliac veins and emptying into the right atrium of the heart. It receives the lumbar, right spermatic, renal, right suprarenal, phrenic, and hepatic veins. See also Plates 5, 8, 9, 10, 14.

inferior vena caval valve. CAVAL VALVE.

inferior vena cava syndrome. Venous distention and edema of the legs and abdomen, often with hepatic hyperemia, due to inferior vena cava obstruction by thrombosis, tumor, or aneurysm. Syn. *inferior mediastinal syndrome.*

inferior vermis. The inferior portion of the vermis, which includes the lobules called nodulus, uvula, pyramid, and tuber vermis.

inferior vertebral incisure. A notch on the caudal border of a pedicle of a vertebra. NA *incisura vertebralis inferior.*

inferior vestibular nucleus. One of the four vestibular nuclei that receive fibers from the vestibular nerve. It begins caudally in the medulla, medial to the accessory cuneate nucleus and extends rostrally medial to the inferior cerebellar peduncle to the point near the entrance of the vestibular nerve root. Syn. *spinal vestibular nucleus, descending vestibular nucleus.* NA *nucleus vestibularis inferior.*

infero- [L. *inferus,* below, lower]. A combining form meaning *inferior, below.*

in·fe·ro·lat·er·al (in″fur·o·lat′ur·ul) *adj.* [*infero-* + *lateral*]. Located below and to one side.

in·fe·ro·me·di·al (in″fur·o·mee′dee·ul) *adj.* [*infero-* + *medial*]. Located below and in the middle.

in·fe·ro·pa·ri·etal (in″fur·o·pa·rye′e·tul) *adj.* [*infero-* + *parietal*]. Pertaining to the inferior portion of the parietal bone or parietal lobe of the brain.

in·fe·ro·pos·te·ri·or (in″fur·o·pos·teer′ee·ur) *adj.* [*infero-* + *posterior*]. Located below and behind.

in·fer·til·i·ty (in″fur·til′i·tee) *n.* [L. *infertilitas,* from *infertilis,* unfruitful]. Involuntary reduction in reproductive ability. Compare *sterility.* —**in·fer·tile** (in·fur′til) *adj.*

in·fest, *v.* [L. *infestare,* to harass, from *infestus,* hostile]. To live on or within the skin of the host, as in the case of certain insects and other arthropods in relation to their hosts. Compare *infect.*

in·fes·ta·tion, *n.* The state or condition of being infested. Often used as a synonym for infection in reference to animal parasites but, more properly, restricted to the presence of animal parasites, such as arthropods, on the surface of the host or in his environment.

in·fes·tive, *adj.* Prone to infest.

in·fib·u·la·tion (in·fib″yoo·lay′shun) *n.* [L. *infibulare,* to clasp or buckle together, from *fibula,* clasp, pin]. The act of clasping or fastening a ring, clasp, or frame to the genital organs to prevent copulation.

Infiltrase. A trademark for hyaluronidase.

in·fil·trate (in·fil′trate, in′fil·) *v. & n.* [*in-* + *filtrate,* to filter]. 1. To pass into tissue spaces or cells, as fluids, cells, or other substances. 2. The material that has infiltrated.

infiltrating lipoma. LIPOSARCOMA.

in·fil·tra·tion, *n.* [*in-* + *filtration*]. 1. A process by which cells, fluid, or other substances pass into tissue spaces or into cells. The various substances may be natural to the part or cell, but in excess; or they may be foreign to the part or cell. 2. The material taking part in the process.

infiltration analgesia. Paralyzing the nerve endings at the site of operation by subcutaneous injection of an anesthetic.

infiltration anesthesia. Anesthesia induced by the injection of the anesthetic solution directly into the tissues that are to be anesthetized.

infiltration block anesthesia. Anesthesia produced by injection of an anesthetic solution close to the nerves supplying an operative field.

infinite distance. *In optics,* a distance of 20 feet or more, so established because the rays from an object at that distance to the lens of the eye are practically parallel.

in·fin·i·ty, *n.* [L. *infinitas,* from *infinitus,* endless]. 1. Unlimited extent of space, time, or quantity. 2. *In optics,* a distance so great that light rays from a point source at that distance may be considered parallel. —**in·fi·nite,** *adj.*

in·firm, *adj.* [L. *infirmus,* from *in-,* not, + *firmus,* strong, robust]. In poor health; feeble.

in·fir·ma·ry, *n.* [ML. *infirmaria,* from *infirmus,* infirm]. 1. A medical facility serving a live-in institution providing beds and treatment primarily on a short-term or nonintensive basis. 2. A hospital.

in·fir·mi·ty, *n.* [L. *infirmitas*]. 1. Poor health; feebleness. 2. An illness or disability.

in·flamed, *adj.* Exhibiting or in a state of inflammation.

in·flam·ma·ble, *adj.* Tending to ignite and burn readily.

in·flam·ma·tion, *n.* [L. *inflammatio,* from *inflammare,* to set on fire]. The reaction of the tissues to injury, characterized clinically by heat, swelling, redness, pain, and loss of function; pathologically, by vasoconstriction followed by vasodilatation, stasis, hyperemia, accumulation of leukocytes, exudation of fluid, and deposition of fibrin; and according to some authorities, the processes of repair, the production of new capillaries and fibroblasts, organization, and cicatrization. —**in·flam·ma·to·ry,** *adj.;* **in·flame,** *v.*

inflammatory carcinoma. A fast-spreading carcinoma which may clinically resemble a benign inflammatory process, usually of the breast.

inflammatory cell. Any cell appearing as an integral part of an inflammatory exudate, including the neutrophil, eosinophil, lymphocyte, plasmacyte, and histiocyte.

inflammatory dysmenorrhea. Dysmenorrhea due to inflammation.

inflammatory macrophage. FREE MACROPHAGE.

inflammatory polyps. A structure of polypoid configuration resulting from inflammation rather than epithelial proliferation.

inflammatory pseudotumor of the orbit. A benign inflammatory lesion in the orbit which in its clinical presentation simulates a neoplasm.

inflammatory tissue. Tissue in which there is exudation or proliferation as a result of injury.

in·fla·tion, *n.* [L. *inflatio,* from *inflare,* to blow up]. Distention with air or fluid; or the process of filling with air or fluid to produce distention. —**in·flate,** *v.*

inflation receptor. STRETCH RECEPTOR.

in·flec·tion, in·flex·ion, *n.* [L. *inflexio,* a bending]. 1. A bending inward. 2. Modification of the pitch of the voice in speaking.

in·flo·res·cence (in″flo·res′unce) *n.* [*in-* + L. *florescere,* to begin to bloom, from *flos, floris,* flower, blossom]. The structure and position of the flowering parts of a plant and their relation to each other.

in·flu·en·za (in″floo·en′zuh) *n.* genit. sing. **influen·zae** (·zee) [It., (astral) influence, epidemic]. An acute respiratory infection of specific viral etiology, usually epidemic, characterized by sudden onset of headache, myalgia, fever, and prostration. Three major antigenic types of the causative organism exist: the influenza A, B, and C viruses. Syn. *flu (colloq.).* See also *Asian influenza virus, endemic influenza, swine influenza, Hong Kong influenza.* —**influen·zal** (·zul) *adj.*

influenzal meningitis. Inflammation of the meninges due to infection with *Haemophilus influenzae,* most commonly occurring in infants and young children.

in·fold, *v.* To enclose within folds.

in·foot·ed, *adj.* PIGEON-TOED.

in·formed consent. Consent, preferably in writing, obtained from a patient regarding the use of specific therapy, especially in case of operative intervention, radiation, new or unusual use of drugs, or other unconventional treatment, or participation in a research project, or to allow use of medical or other records for research purposes, after the proposed procedure and risks involved have been explained fully in nontechnical terms. If the patient is a minor, or is incapable of understanding or communicating, such consent may be obtained from a close adult relative or legal guardian.

infra- [L., below, under]. A prefix meaning (a) *below, beneath, inferior;* (b) *within.*

in·fra·al·ve·o·lar (in″fruh·al·vee′uh·lur) *adj.* [*infra-* + *alveolar*]. Below an alveolus, especially of a tooth.

in·fra·au·ric·u·lar (in″fruh·aw·rick′yoo·lur) *adj.* [*infra-* + *auricular*]. Below the external ear.

in·fra·ax·il·lary (in″fruh·ack′si·lerr·ee) *adj.* [*infra-* + *axillary*]. Situated below the axilla.

infraaxillary region. The space between the anterior and posterior axillary lines.

in·fra·bony pocket. Any periodontal pocket that extends apically from the alveolar crest. Contr. *suprabony pocket.*

in·fra·car·di·ac (in″fruh·kahr′dee·ack) *adj.* [*infra-* + *cardiac*]. Situated below or beneath the heart.

infracardiac bursa. The cephalic end of the embryonic mesenteric recess lying in the mesentery between the esophagus and right lung bud, or a small cyst in the right pulmonary ligament derived from it.

in·fra·cla·vic·u·lar (in″fruh·kla·vick′yoo·lur) *adj.* [*infra-* + *clavicular*]. Below the clavicle.

infraclavicular fossa. The triangular area bounded by clavicle, deltoid muscle, and pectoralis major muscle.

in·fra·cla·vic·u·la·ris (in″fruh·kla·vick″yoo·lair′is) *n.* A rare muscle extending from above the clavicular part of the pectoralis major to the fascia over the deltoid muscle.

infraclavicular region. The area bounded superiorly by the lower border of the clavicle, inferiorly by the lower border of the third rib, on one side by a line extending from the acromion to the pubic spine, and on the other side by the edge of the sternum. NA *regio infraclavicularis.*

in·fra·cli·noid (in″fruh·klye′noid) *adj.* [*infra-* + *clinoid*]. Below one or more of the clinoid processes of the sphenoid bone.

in·fra·clu·sion (in″fruh·kloo′zhun) *n.* INFRAOCCLUSION.

in·fra·con·dyl·ism (in″fruh·kon′di·liz·um) *n.* [*infra-* + *condyle* + *-ism*]. Downward deviation of the mandibular condyles.

in·fra·cos·tal (in″fruh·kos′tul) *adj. & n.* [*infra-* + *costal*]. SUBCOSTAL.

infracostal plane. SUBCOSTAL PLANE.

in·frac·tion (in·frack′shun) *n.* [L. *infractio,* from *infringere,* to break]. Incomplete fracture of a bone.

in·fra·den·ta·le (in″fruh·den·tay′lee) *n.* The highest anterior point on the gums between the central incisors of the mandible.

in·fra·di·an (in·fray′dee·un) *adj.* [*infra-* + L. *dies,* day]. Recurring in or manifesting cycles less frequent than once a day. Contr. *circadian, ultradian.*

in·fra·di·a·phrag·mat·ic (in″fruh·dye″uh·frag·mat′ick) *adj.* [*infra-* + *diaphragmatic*]. Situated below the diaphragm.

in·fra·gle·noid (in″fruh·glee′noid, ·glen′oid) *adj.* [*infra-* + *glenoid*]. Located below the glenoid cavity of the scapula.

infraglenoid tubercle. A rough impression below the glenoid cavity, from which the long head of the triceps muscle arises. NA *tuberculum infraglenoidale.*

infraglenoid tuberosity. INFRAGLENOID TUBERCLE.

in·fra·glot·tic (in″fruh·glot′ick) *adj.* [*infra-* + *glottic*]. Below the glottis.

in·fra·gran·u·lar layer (in″fruh·gran′yoo·lur). The ganglionic layer and the layer of fusiform cells of the cerebral cortex collectively.

in·fra·hy·oid (in″fruh·high′oid) *adj.* [*infra-* + *hyoid*]. Situated below the hyoid bone.

infrahyoid muscles. The muscles attached to the lower border of the hyoid. NA *musculi infrahyoidei.*

infrahyoid region. The space below the hyoid bone, between the sternocleidomastoid muscles and the sternum.

in·fra·mam·ma·ry (in″fruh·mam′uh·ree) *adj.* [*infra-* + *mammary*]. Below a breast.

inframammary region. The area immediately below each breast and above the costal margin.

in·fra·na·sal area (in″fruh·nay′zul). The ventral part of the median nasal process between the globular processes; forms the mobile septum of the nose.

in·fra·nu·cle·ar (in″fruh·new′klee·ur) *adj.* [*infra-* + *nuclear*]. In the nervous system, peripheral to a nucleus; below or away from the nucleus of a nerve.

infranuclear paralysis. Paralysis of the motor function of a cranial nerve, due to a lesion of the nerve peripheral to its nucleus.

in·fra·oc·clu·sion (in″fruh·o·klew′zhun) *adj.* [*infra-* + *occlusion*]. Failure of one or more teeth to reach the plane of occlusion.

in·fra·or·bit·al (in″fruh·or′bi·tul) *adj.* [*infra-* + *orbital*]. Beneath or below the floor of the orbit.

infraorbital canal. A channel running obliquely through the bony floor of the orbit; it gives passage to the infraorbital artery and nerve. NA *canalis infraorbitalis.*

infraorbital foramen. In the maxilla, the external aperture of the infraorbital canal; it gives passage to the infraorbital nerve and vessels. NA *foramen infraorbitale.*

infraorbital groove. INFRAORBITAL SULCUS.

infraorbital plexus. A nerve plexus lying under the levator labii superioris muscle and formed by branches of the maxillary and facial nerves. See also Table of Nerves in the Appendix.

infraorbital point. The lowest point on the anterior margin of the orbit.

infraorbital process. The anterior angle of the zygomatic bone, sharp and pointed, which articulates with the maxilla and occasionally forms the superior boundary of the infraorbital foramen.

infraorbital sulcus. A groove in the middle of the floor of the orbit, lodging the infraorbital nerve and vessels. NA *sulcus infraorbitalis.*

in·fra·pa·tel·lar (in″fruh·puh·tel′ur) *adj.* [*infra-* + *patellar*]. Below the patella.

infrapatellar bursa. The bursa situated between the patellar ligament and the tibia. NA *bursa infrapatellaris profunda.*

infrapatellar synovial fold. A fold of synovial membrane in the knee joint which extends from the infrapatellar fatty mass to the anterior part of the intercondylar fossa of the femur. NA *plica synovialis infrapatellaris.*

in·fra·phys·i·o·log·ic (in″fruh·fiz″ee·o·loj′ick) *adj.* [*infra-* + *physiologic*]. Of or having less than normal function; hypofunctional; said of an organ or part.

in·fra·red (in″fruh·red′) *adj. & n.* 1. Beyond the red end of the spectrum of visible light; pertaining specifically to the thermal region of the electromagnetic spectrum with wavelengths longer than those of the red end of the visible spectrum and shorter than those of microwaves. 2. Radiation or waves in the infrared region of the electromagnetic spectrum.

infrared lamp. A source of heat rays, which emanate from a surface heated to a temperature of 300 to 800°C. The spectral emission ranges through infrared from 8000 to 150,000 angstroms. Such rays have poor penetrability for skin.

in·fra·roent·gen rays (in″fruh·rent′gun). GRENZ RAYS.

in·fra·scap·u·lar (in″fruh·skap′yoo·lur) *adj.* [*infra-* + *scapular*]. Below the scapula.

infrascapular region. A region on either side of the vertebral column below a horizontal line drawn through the inferior angle of each scapula. NA *regio infrascapularis.*

in·fra·spi·na·tus (in″fruh·spye·nay′tus) *n.* A muscle arising from the infraspinous fossa of the scapula and inserted into the greater tubercle of the humerus. NA *musculus infraspinatus.* See also Table of Muscles in the Appendix.

infraspinatus reflex. Extension of the elbow and lateral rotation of the arm induced by a sudden sharp tap over the infraspinatus muscle.

in·fra·spi·nous (in″fruh·spye′nus) *adj.* [*infra-* + *spinous*]. Below the spine of the scapula.

infraspinous fossa. The recess on the posterior surface of the scapula occupied by the infraspinatus muscle. NA *fossa infraspinata.*

infraspinous region. The region corresponding to the infraspinous fossa of the scapula.

in·fra·ster·nal (in″fruh·stur′nul) *adj.* [*infra-* + *sternal*]. Below the sternum.

infrasternal angle. COSTAL ANGLE.

infrasternal notch. The depression in the anterior abdominal wall, superficial to the xiphoid cartilage.

in·fra·tem·po·ral (in″fruh·tem′puh·rul) *adj.* [*infra-* + *temporal*]. Situated below the temporal fossa.

infratemporal crest. A crest on the outer aspect of the great wing of the sphenoid and separating the part of the bone which partly forms the temporal fossa from that which aids in forming the zygomatic fossa. NA *crista infratemporalis.*

in·fra·tem·po·ra·le (in″fruh·tem″po·rah′lee, ·ray′lee) *n. In craniometry,* a point on the infratemporal crest of the great wing of the sphenoid bone; used in measuring the least cranial breadth.

infratemporal fossa. An irregular space situated below and medial to the zygomatic arch, behind the maxilla and medial to the upper part of the ramus of the mandible. Syn. *zygomatic fossa.* NA *fossa infratemporalis.*

infratemporal region. The area below the temporal fossa and deep to the ramus of the mandible. NA *regio infratemporalis.*

in·fra·ten·to·ri·al (in″fruh·ten·to′ree·ul) *adj.* [*infra-* + *tentorial*]. Below the tentorium.

in·fra·troch·le·ar (in″fruh·trock′lee·ur) *adj.* Below a trochlea.

infratrochlear nerve. A branch of the nasociliary nerve situated below the trochlea of the superior oblique muscle of the eye and supplying the skin of the eyelid and root of the nose. NA *nervus infratrochlearis.* See also Table of Nerves in the Appendix.

in·fra·um·bil·i·cal (in″fruh·um·bil′i·kul) *adj.* [*infra-* + *umbilical*]. Below the navel; caudal to a transverse plane at the umbilicus.

in·fra·va·gi·nal (in″fruh·vaj′i·nul, ·va·jye′nul) *adj.* [*infra-* + *vaginal*]. Below the vagina.

in·fra·ver·sion (in″fruh·vur′zhun) *n.* [*infra-* + *version*]. 1. Downward turning of an eye. 2. INFRAOCCLUSION.

in·fra·ves·i·cal (in″fruh·ves′i·kul) *adj.* [*infra-* + *vesical*]. Below the urinary bladder.

in·fra·zy·go·mat·ic (in″fruh·zye·go·mat′ick) *adj.* [*infra-* + *zygomatic*]. Below the cheekbone.

infrequent pulse. A pulse that has a slower rate than normal; BRADYCARDIA.

in·fric·tion (in·frick′shun) *n.* [L. *infrictio,* from *infricare,* to rub in]. The rubbing of a body surface with an ointment or liniment.

in·fun·dib·u·lar (in″fun·dib′yoo·lur) *adj.* 1. Resembling a funnel. 2. Pertaining to an infundibulum.

infundibular process. The main body of the neurohypophysis. Syn. *neural lobe.*

infundibular recess. A recess in the anterior part of the floor of the third ventricle extending through the tuber cinereum into the infundibulum (2). NA *recessus infundibuli.* See also Plate 18.

infundibular stem or **stalk.** The lower part of the infundibulum of the neurohypophysis, between the median eminence and the infundibular process.

in·fun·dib·u·li·form (in″fun·dib′yoo·li·form) *adj.* [*infundibulum* + *-iform*]. Funnel-shaped.

infundibuliform anus. A relaxed condition of the anal canal with loss of the natural folds.

infundibuliform fascia. INTERNAL SPERMATIC FASCIA.

in·fun·dib·u·lo·ma (in″fun·dib·yoo·lo′muh) *n.* [*infundibulum* + *-oma*]. A glioma, characteristically a pilocytic astrocytoma, involving the infundibulum (2).

in·fun·dib·u·lo·pel·vic ligament (in″fun·dib″yoo·lo·pel′vick). SUSPENSORY LIGAMENT OF THE OVARY.

in·fun·dib·u·lo·ven·tric·u·lar crest (in·fun·dib″yoo·lo·ven·trick′yoo·lur). SUPRAVENTRICULAR CREST.

in·fun·dib·u·lum (in″fun·dib′yoo·lum) *n.,* genit. **infundibu·li** (·lye), pl. **infundibu·la** (·luh) [L., funnel]. 1. A funnel-shaped passage or part. 2. (of the hypophysis:) The stalk by which the neurohypophysis is attached to the tuber cinereum of the hypothalamus; consists of the medial eminence and infundibular stem. NA *infundibulum hypothalami.* 3. (of the uterine tube:) The wide, funnel-shaped portion of the uterine tube at its fimbriated end. NA *infundibulum tubae uterinae.* 4. (of the frontal sinus:) NASOFRONTAL DUCT. 5. [NA alt.] CONUS ARTERIOSUS.

infundibulum eth·moi·da·le (eth·moy·day′lee) [NA]. ETHMOID INFUNDIBULUM.

infundibulum hy·po·tha·la·mi (high″po·thal′uh·migh) [NA]. The infundibulum of the hypophysis. See *infundibulum.*

infundibulum tu·bae ute·ri·nae (tew′bee yoo·tur·eye′nee) [NA]. The infundibulum of the uterine tube. See *infundibulum.*

in·fu·sion (in·few′zhun) *n.* [L. *infusio,* from *infundere,* to pour into]. 1. The process of extracting the active principles of a substance by means of water, but without boiling. 2. The product of such a process. 3. The slow injection of a solution into a vein or into subcutaneous or other tissue of the body, from which it is absorbed into the bloodstream.

infusion reaction. An acute febrile response to the infusion of pyrogenic agents present as contaminants in parenteral fluids.

In·fu·so·ria (in″few·sor′ee·uh, ·zor′ee·uh) *n.pl.* [NL., from L. *infusio,* infusion]. 1. CILIATA. 2. Originally, a group including diverse kinds of microorganisms, principally protozoans. —**infuso·ri·al** (·ee·ul) *adj.;* **infuso·ri·an** (·ee·un) *n. & adj.*

infusorial earth. DIATOMACEOUS EARTH.

in·ges·ta (in·jes′tuh) *n.pl.* [L. *ingestum,* from *ingerere,* to put in]. Substances taken into the body, especially foods.

in·ges·tion (in·jes′chun) *n.* [L. *ingestio,* from *ingerere,* to put or pour in]. 1. The act of taking substances, especially food, into the body. 2. The process by which a cell takes up nutrients or foreign matter, such as bacilli or smaller cells. See also *endocytosis, phagocytosis, pinocytosis.* —**ingest,** *v.;* **inges·tive,** *adj.*

In·gras·sia's wings (ing″grah^{h}s·see′a^h) [G. F. *Ingrassia,* Italian physician and anatomist, 1510–1580]. The small wings of the sphenoid bone.

in·gra·ves·cent (in″gra·ves′unt) *adj.* [L. *ingravescere,* to become heavy, from *gravis,* heavy, severe]. Increasing in severity.

ingravescent apoplexy. A cerebrovascular accident with slowly evolving neurologic deficits, as from a gradual leakage of blood from a ruptured vessel.

in·gre·di·ent, *n.* [L. *ingredi,* to enter]. Any substance that enters into the formation of a compound or mixture.

in·grown, *adj.* Of a hair or nail, grown inward so that the normally free end is embedded in or under the skin. —**in·grow·ing,** *adj.;* **in·growth,** *n.*

in·guen (ing′gwen) *n.,* genit. **in·gui·nis** (ing′gwi·nis), pl. **in·gui·na** (ing′gwi·nuh) [NA]. GROIN.

inguin-, inguino- [L. *inguen, inguinis*]. A combining form meaning *groin, inguinal.*

in·gui·nal (ing′gwi·nul) *adj.* [L. *inguinalis,* from *inguen,* groin]. Pertaining to or in the vicinity of the groin.

inguinal adenitis. BUBO.

inguinal canal. A canal about 4 cm long, running obliquely downward and medially from the deep to the superficial inguinal ring; the channel through which an inguinal hernia descends; it gives passage to the ilioinguinal nerve and to the spermatic cord in the male and to the round ligament of the uterus in the female. NA *canalis inguinalis.*

inguinal crest. A prominence on the ventrolateral abdominal wall in the embryo within which develops a part of the chorda gubernaculum. Its base marks the site of the internal opening of the inguinal canal.

inguinal fold. A fold, developing on the urogenital ridge, which unites with the inguinal crest at the brim of the embryonic pelvis. The gubernaculum testis develops within these structures. Syn. *inguinal fold of the mesonephros.* NA *plica inguinalis.*

inguinal fold of the mesonephros. INGUINAL FOLD.

inguinal hernia. A hernia through the inguinal canal. This variety constitutes more than four-fifths of all hernias. See also Plate 4.

inguinal ligament. The lower portion of the aponeurosis of the external oblique muscle extending from the anterior superior spine of the ilium to the tubercle of the pubis and the pectineal line. Syn. *Poupart's ligament.* NA *ligamentum inguinale.* See also Plate 2.

inguinal reflex. In the female, contraction of muscle fibers above the inguinal ligament, induced by stimulation of the skin over the upper and inner aspect of the thigh; comparable to the cremasteric reflex in the male.

inguinal region. The right or left lower abdominal region, on either side of the pubic region. The right inguinal region includes the abdominal surface covering the cecum and the vermiform appendix, the ureter, and the spermatic vessels. The left inguinal region includes the abdominal surface covering the sigmoid flexure of the colon, the ureter, and the spermatic vessels. Syn. *iliac region.* NA *regio inguinalis (dextra et sinistra).* See also *abdominal regions* and Plate 4.

inguinal testis. An undescended testis remaining in the inguinal canal.

inguinal triangle. An area bounded laterally by the inferior epigastric artery, medially by the rectus abdominis, and inferiorly by the medial half of the inguinal ligament. NA *trigonum inguinale.*

inguino-. See *inguin-.*

in·gui·no·cru·ral (ing″gwi·no·kroo′rul) *adj.* [*inguino-* + *crural*]. Pertaining to the groin and the thigh.

in·gui·no·dyn·ia (ing″gwi·no·din′ee·uh) *n.* [*inguin-* + *-odynia*]. Pain in the groin.

in·gui·no·la·bi·al (ing″gwi·no·lay′bee·ul) *adj.* [*inguino-* + *labial*]. Pertaining to the groin and the labium.

inguinolabial hernia. An inguinal hernia that has descended into the labium majus.

in·gui·no·scro·tal (ing″gwi·no·skro′tul) *adj.* [*inguino-* + *scrotal*]. Relating to the groin and the scrotum.

INH Abbreviation for *isonicotinic acid hydrazide (isoniazid).*

in·hal·ant (in·hay′lunt) *n. & adj.* 1. That which is inhaled, either from the atmosphere or as a medicine. 2. Occurring as, or used as, an inhalant.

in·ha·la·tion (in″huh·lay′shun) *n.* 1. The process of inhaling. 2. A medicinal substance to be inhaled; an inhalant.

inhalation anesthesia. Anesthesia produced by the inhalation of anesthetic gases or vapors.

in·ha·la·tor (in′huh·lay″tur, in″huh·lay′tur) *n.* A device for facilitating the inhalation of a gas or spray, as for providing oxygen or oxygen-carbon dioxide mixtures for respiration in resuscitation.

in·hale, *v.* [*in-* + L. *halare,* to breathe]. To breathe in, as air or vapor; inspire.

inhalent. INHALANT.

in·hal·er (in·hail′ur) *n.* 1. A device containing a solid medication through which air is drawn into the air passages. 2. An atomizer. 3. An apparatus used to filter or condition air, etc., for inhalation, to protect the lungs against the entry of damp or cold air, dust, smoke, or gases.

in·her·ent, *adj.* [L. *inhaerens,* from *inhaerere,* to stick in, adhere]. Innate; natural to the organism.

inherent filter. The intrinsic filtration of a roentgen-ray tube, consisting of tube wall plus any oil layer or plastic layer in the mounting covering the aperture.

in·her·it, *v.* [MF. *enheriter,* to make heir, from L. *heres, heredis,* heir]. To derive from an ancestor.

in·her·i·tance, *n.* 1. The acquisition of characteristics by transmission of germ plasm from ancestor to descendant. 2. The sum total of characteristics dependent upon the constitution of the fertilized ovum; also, the total set of genes in the fertilized ovum.

inherited response. UNCONDITIONED REFLEX.

in·hib·in (in·hib′in) *n.* 1. A postulated testicular hormone inhibiting the gonadotropic secretion of the adenohypophysis. 2. Generic name for various antibacterial substances occurring in normal saliva, urine, and other body fluids. 3. An antibiotic substance present in honey.

inhibiter. INHIBITOR.

inhibiting antibody. BLOCKING ANTIBODY.

in·hi·bi·tion, *n.* [L. *inhibitio,* from *inhibere,* to restrain]. 1. The act of checking or restraining the action of an organ, cell, or chemical, as the process of rusting, or the action of an enzyme. See also *competitive inhibition.* 2. *In psychiatry,* an unconscious restraining of or interference with an instinctual drive, leading to restricted patterns of behavior. —**in·hib·i·to·ry** (in·hib′i·to·ree) *adj.;* **in·hib·it,** *v.*

inhibition-action balance. *In psychiatry,* the relative balance maintained in every individual between the experiencing of emotional feelings and outward behavior in response to them; may be used as an index in appraising emotional health.

inhibition index. The amount of an antimetabolite that is needed to overcome the biological effect of a unit weight of a metabolite; the index is a measure of the antagonism between metabolite and antimetabolite.

in·hib·i·tor, *n.* 1. A substance that checks or stops a chemical action. 2. A neuron whose stimulation stops, or suppresses, the activity of the part it innervates, or of a neuron on which it synapses. 3. Any substance or structure that prevents, slows, or stops a process.

inhibitory equilibrium potential. *In neurophysiology,* the membrane potential at which activation of an inhibitory synapse causes neither depolarization nor hyperpolarization of the postsynaptic cell.

inhibitory ileus. ADYNAMIC ILEUS.

inhibitory interneuron. RENSHAW CELL.

inhibitory nerve. Any nerve which, upon stimulation, reduces the activity of a nerve center or end organ.

Inhiston. A trademark for pheniramine maleate, an antihistaminic.

in·i·en·ceph·a·lus (in″ee·en·sef′uh·lus) *n.* [*inion* + *-enceph-*

alus]. An individual with occipital fissure of the cranium, with exposure of brain substance, usually combined with rachischisis and retroflexion of the cervical spine. —**inien·cepha·ly** (·lee) *n.*

in·i·od·y·mus (in″ee·od′i·mus) *n.* [*inion* + *-dymus*]. DIPROSOPUS TETROPHTHALMUS.

in·i·on (in′ee·on) *n.* [Gk., occiput] [NA]. *In craniometry,* the external protuberance of the occipital bone.

in·i·op·a·gus (in″ee·op′uh·gus) *n.* [*inion* + *-pagus*]. CRANIOPAGUS OCCIPITALIS.

in·i·ops (in′ee·ops) *n.* [*inion* + Gk. *ōps,* face, eye]. CEPHALOTHORACOPAGUS MONOSYMMETROS.

ini·ti·a·tion codon. A sequence of three bases in messenger RNA which signals for the initiation of synthesis of a protein chain. In certain bacteria, the initiation codon is AUG (adenine-uracil-guanine).

ini·ti·a·tor, *n.* Any substance capable of starting a reaction as peroxide in the polymerization of acrylic resins.

in·ject, *v.* [L. *injicere, injectus,* to throw in]. To introduce into, as a fluid into the skin, subcutaneous tissue, muscle, blood vessels, spinal canal, or any body cavity.

in·ject·able (in·jeck′tuh·bul) *adj. & n.* 1. Suitable for injection into the body. 2. Any drug preparation intended for injection.

in·jec·tion, *n.* [L. *injectio,* from *injicere,* to throw in]. 1. The act of injecting. 2. The substance injected. 3. A state of hyperemia.

in·ju·ry, *n.* [L. *injuria,* injustice, wrong]. 1. Any stress upon an organism that disrupts its structure or function, or both, and results in a pathologic process. 2. The resultant hurt, wound, or damage. See also *trauma.*

injury current. INJURY POTENTIAL.

injury potential. A potential difference, measuring about 30 to 40 millivolts, between injured and uninjured portions of a damaged cell or tissue at rest. Syn. *demarcation potential.* See also *demarcation current.*

ink·blot test. RORSCHACH TEST.

in·lay, *n.* A dental restoration that is formed outside the tooth cavity and subsequently secured in place with a cementing medium; usually made of metal or porcelain.

inlay graft. A graft placed beneath the tissue, as a bone graft placed in the medullary cavity of a bone, or an Esser inlay beneath the skin or mucous membrane.

in·let, *n.* The entrance to a cavity.

inlet of the pelvis. The space within the brim of the pelvis; the superior pelvic strait. See also *pelvis.*

in·ly·ing, *adj.* INDWELLING.

in·nate, *adj.* [L. *innatus,* inborn, from *natus,* born]. Dependent upon the genetic constitution; inherent; natural to the organism.

innate immunity. NATIVE IMMUNITY.

inner cell mass. The mass at the animal pole of the blastocyst, from which the embryo and certain adnexa are derived.

inner dental epithelium. The layer of cells of the enamel organ which lies at the concavity and next to the dental papilla.

inner ear. INTERNAL EAR.

inner germinal layer. BROOD MEMBRANE.

inner hamstrings. The tendons of the semimembranosus and semitendinosus muscles.

inner horizontal cell. AMACRINE CELL.

inner longitudinal arch. NA *pars medialis arcus pedis longitudinalis.* See *longitudinal arch of the foot.*

inner nuclear layer. The layer of the retina made up chiefly of the cell bodies of the bipolar neurons.

inner spiral sulcus. SPIRAL SULCUS.

in·ner·vate, *v.* Of nerves, to supply a part; to stimulate a part by nerve impulses.

in·ner·va·tion, *n.* 1. The distribution of nerves to a part. 2. The amount of nerve stimulation received by a part. —**innervation·al,** *adj.*

innervation ratio. The proportion of skeletal muscle fibers innervated by a nerve fiber in a motor unit.

in·no·cent, *adj.* [MF., from L. *innocens,* from *in-,* not, + *nocens,* harmful]. Benign; not malignant; not apparently harmful.

innocent murmur. A murmur, systolic in time, occurring in the absence of any cardiac abnormality. Syn. *functional murmur, inorganic murmur, physiologic murmur.*

in·noc·u·ous, *adj.* [L. *innocuus*]. Not injurious; harmless.

in·nom·i·nate (i·nom′i·nut) *adj. & n.* [L. *innominatus,* from *in-,* not, + *nominatus,* named, from *nominare,* to name]. 1. Unnamed, nameless; a designation traditionally applied to certain anatomical structures. 2. The innominate bone (= HIPBONE).

innominate artery. BRACHIOCEPHALIC TRUNK.

innominate bone. HIPBONE.

innominate canaliculus. A small inconstant channel in the great wing of the sphenoid bone, which, when present, transmits the lesser petrosal nerve.

innominate cartilage. CRICOID CARTILAGE.

innominate foramen. INNOMINATE CANALICULUS.

innominate veins. The brachiocephalic veins. See Table of Veins in the Appendix.

in·nox·ious (i·nock′shus, in·nock′shus) *adj.* [L. *innoxius,* from *in-,* not, + *noxius,* noxious]. Innocuous; not harmful.

ino-, in- [Gk. *is, inos,* fiber, sinew]. A combining form meaning (a) *fiber, fibrous;* (b) *muscle fiber, muscle.*

ino·blast (in′o·blast) *n.* [*ino-* + *-blast*]. FIBROBLAST.

in·oc·ci·pit·ia (in″ock·si·pit′ee·uh) *n.* [*in-,* lack, + *occipit-* + *-ia*]. Deficiency of the occipital lobe of the brain.

ino·chon·dri·tis (in″o·kon·drye′tis) *n.* [*ino-* + *chrondr-* + *-itis*]. Inflammation of fibrocartilage.

in·oc·u·la·ble (in·ock′yoo·luh·bul) *adj.* 1. Capable of transmission by inoculation. 2. Susceptible to inoculation for a disease. —**in·oc·u·la·bil·i·ty** (in·ock″yoo·luh·bil′i·tee) *n.*

in·oc·u·late (in·ock′yoo·late) *v.* [L. *inoculare,* to ingraft a bud]. 1. To introduce a small amount of a pathogenic substance such as bacteria, viruses, spores, antibodies, or antigens into (an organism), as for therapeutic, prophylactic, or experimental purposes. See also *vaccinate.* 2. *In bacteriology,* to plant microorganisms in or on (a culture medium). —**in·oc·u·la·tion** (in·ock″yoo·lay′shun) *n.*

inoculation jaundice. SERUM HEPATITIS.

in·oc·u·la·tor (in·ock′yoo·lay″tur) *n.* One who or that which inoculates; an instrument used in inoculation.

in·oc·u·lum (in·ock′yoo·lum) *n.,* pl. **inocu·la** (·luh) [NL., from L. *inoculare,* to ingraft a bud]. A substance containing bacteria, spores, viruses, or other material for use in inoculation.

ino·cyte (in′o·site) *n.* [*ino-* + *-cyte*]. FIBROCYTE.

in·o·gen (in′o·jen) *n.* [*ino-* + *-gen*]. A hypothetical complex substance of high energy in muscle whose breakdown was thought to supply the energy for muscular contraction.

inog·lia (in·og′lee·uh, in·o′glee·uh) *n.* [*ino-* + *glia*]. FIBROGLIA.

in·o·kom·ma (in″o·kom′uh) *n.* [Gk. *is, inos,* sinew, muscle fiber, + *komma,* piece, section]. SARCOMERE.

in·op·er·a·ble (in·op′ur·uh·bul) *adj.* Not to be operated upon; of or pertaining to a condition in which the prognosis is unfavorable if an operation is undertaken.

in·or·gan·ic (in″or·gan′ick) *adj.* Not organic.

inorganic acid. Any acid, except H_2CO_3, which does not contain carbon.

inorganic chemistry. The branch of chemistry that treats of substances other than carbon compounds.

inorganic murmur. INNOCENT MURMUR.

inosaemia. INOSEMIA.

in·os·cu·late (in·os′kew·late) *v.* [*in-* + L. *osculare,* to supply with a mouth, from *osculum,* small mouth]. To unite by small openings, as in anastomosis.

in·os·cu·la·tion (in·os″kew·lay′shun) *n.* The joining of blood vessels by direct communication.

in·ose (in′oce, ·oze) *n.* INOSITOL.

in·o·se·mia, in·o·sae·mia (in″o·see′mee·uh) *n.* [Gk. *is, inos,* sinew, fiber, + *-emia*]. 1. An excess of fibrin in the blood. 2. The presence of inositol in the blood.

ino·sine (in′o·seen, ·sin, eye′no·) *n.* Hypoxanthine riboside, $C_{10}H_{12}N_4O_5$, a compound occurring in muscle. It is a hydrolysis product of inosinic acid.

inosine monophosphate. INOSINIC ACID.

ino·sin·ic acid (in″o·sin′ick, eye″no·). Hypoxanthine riboside 5-phosphoric acid, $C_{10}H_{13}N_4O_8P$, a nucleotide constituent of muscle, formed by deamination of adenylic acid; on hydrolysis with acid it yields hypoxanthine and D-ribose 5-phosphoric acid. Syn. *inosine monophosphate.*

in·o·site (in′o·site) *n.* INOSITOL.

ino·si·tol (i·no′si·tole, ·tol) *n.* [Gk. *is, inos,* sinew, muscle, + *-ite* + *-ol*]. Hexahydroxycyclohexane, $C_6H_6(OH)_6$, a sugarlike alcohol widely distributed in plants and animals. It is a growth factor for animals and microorganisms.

ino·si·tol·hexa·phos·phor·ic acid (in·o″si·tol·heck″suh·fos·for′ick). PHYTIC ACID.

in·o·si·tu·ria (in″o·si·tew′ree·uh) *n.* [*inosite* + *-uria*]. The presence of inositol in the urine.

in·o·su·ria (in″o·sue′ree·uh) *n.* INOSITURIA.

ino·trop·ic (in″o·trop′ick) *adj.* [*ino-* + *-tropic*]. Modifying the force of muscular contractions.

in·pa·tient, *n.* A person admitted to a hospital who receives lodging and food as well as treatment. Contr. *outpatient.*

in·put, *n.* 1. Energy or matter entering a structure or system of structures. 2. A stimulus or contribution; may be emotional or physical.

in·quest, *n.* [OF. *enqueste,* from L. *inquirere,* to inquire, investigate]. *In legal medicine,* a judicial inquiry, as a coroner's inquest, for the purpose of determining the cause of death of one who has died by violence or in some unknown way.

in·qui·si·tion, *n.* [L. *inquisitio,* from *inquirere,* to inquire, investigate]. An inquiry, especially one into the sanity or mental incompetence of a person.

in·sal·i·va·tion (in·sal″i·vay′shun) *n.* The mixture of the food with saliva during mastication. —**in·sal·i·vate** (in·sal′i·vate) *v.*

in·sa·lu·bri·ous (in″sa·lew′bree·us) *adj.* [*in-* + L. *salubris,* healthy]. Unhealthful; not wholesome.

in·sa·lu·bri·ty (in″sa·lew′bri·tee) *adj.* Unwholesomeness or unhealthfulness, as of air or climate.

in·san·i·tary, *adj.* Not sanitary; not in a proper condition to preserve health.

in·san·i·ty, *n.* [L. *insanitas,* from *insanus,* insane]. 1. Loosely, any mental disorder or derangement. See also *organic brain syndrome, psychosis.* 2. *In legal medicine,* a mental disorder of such severity that the individual (a) is unable to manage his or her own affairs and fulfill social duties, (b) cannot distinguish "right from wrong," or (c) is dangerous to him- or herself or to others. See also *Briggs law, Durham decision, M'Naghten rule.* —**in·sane,** *adj.*

in·scrip·tio (in·skrip′shee·o, ·tee·o) *n.,* pl. **in·scrip·ti·o·nes** (in·skrip″shee·o′neez) [L.]. Inscription; INTERSECTIO.

in·scrip·tion, *n.* [L. *inscriptio,* from *inscribere,* to write on]. 1. The body or main part of a prescription that specifies the ingredients and amounts to be used. 2. *In anatomy,* INTERSECTIO.

inscriptiones. Plural of *inscriptio.*

inscriptiones ten·di·ne·ae (ten·din′ee·ee), sing. **inscriptio ten·di·nea** (ten·din′ee·uh) [BNA]. INTERSECTIONES TENDINEAE.

in·sect, *n.* [L. *insectum,* cut in pieces, segmented]. A member of the class Insecta of the phylum Arthropoda. In the adult, the body is segmented and is divided into head, thorax, and abdomen; there are three pairs of legs and a single pair of antennae. Usually there are one pair or two pairs of wings, but sometimes none.

in·sec·ti·cide (in·seck′ti·side) *n.* [*insect* + *-cide*]. A substance that is used to kill insects. —**in·sec·ti·ci·dal** (in·seck″ti·sigh′dul) *adj.*

in·sec·ti·fuge (in·seck′ti·fewj) *n.* [*insect* + *-fuge*]. A substance that is used to repel insects.

in·se·cu·ri·ty, *n.* The state, feeling, or quality of being uncertain or unsafe; an attitude of apprehensiveness, as in respect to one's social status, circumstances, or safety.

in·sem·i·na·tion (in·sem″i·nay′shun) *n.* [L. *inseminare,* to implant]. The introduction of semen into the female genital tract. See also *artificial insemination.*

in·sen·si·ble, *adj.* [L. *insensibilis*]. 1. Incapable of sensation or feeling; unconscious. 2. Incapable of being perceived or recognized by the senses. —**in·sen·si·bil·i·ty** (in·sen″si·bil′i·tee) *n.*

insensible perspiration. Perspiration that takes place constantly, the fluid being evaporated as fast as excreted.

insensible water loss. Loss of water from the body by way of the lungs, from the skin apart from sweat gland secretion, and from sweat gland secretion which evaporates so quickly that detectable perspiration does not occur.

in·ser·tion, *n.* [L. *insertio,* from *inserere,* to insert, from *serere,* to connect]. *In anatomy,* the attachment of a muscle that is relatively more movable during contraction of that muscle. Contr. *origin.*

insheathed. ENSHEATHED.

in·sid·i·ous, *adj.* [L. *insidiosus,* deceitful]. Coming on gradually or almost imperceptibly, as a disease whose onset is gradual or inappreciable.

in·sight, *n.* 1. Self-understanding; a person's ability to understand the origin, nature, mechanisms, and meaning of his behavior, feelings, and attitudes. 2. Superficially, the ability of a mentally disturbed person to recognize that he is ill.

in·sip·id (in·sip′id) *adj.* [L. *insipidus,* from *in-,* not, + *sapidus,* tasty]. Tasteless.

in si·tu (in sigh′too, sigh′tew) [L.]. In a given or natural position; undisturbed.

in·so·la·tion (in″so·lay′shun) *n.* [L. *insolatio,* from *insolare,* to place in the sun]. 1. Exposure to the rays of the sun. 2. Treatment of disease by such exposure. 3. HEATSTROKE.

in·sol·u·ble (in·sol′yoo·bul) *adj.* Not soluble; incapable of dissolving in a liquid. —**in·sol·u·bil·i·ty** (in·sol″yoo·bil′i·tee) *n.*

insoluble digitalin. FRENCH DIGITALIN.

in·som·nia (in·som′nee·uh) *n.* [L., from *somnus,* sleep]. Sleeplessness; disturbed sleep; prolonged inability to sleep.

in·som·ni·ac (in·som′nee·ack) *n.* A person who is susceptible to insomnia.

in·spec·tion, *n.* [L. *inspectio,* from *inspicere,* to examine]. *In medicine,* the examination of the body or any part of it by the eye.

in·sper·sion (in·spur′zhun) *n.* [L. *inspergere, inspersus,* to sprinkle]. Sprinkling.

in·spi·ra·tion, *n.* [L. *inspiratio,* from *inspirare,* to breathe into]. The drawing in of the breath; inhalation. —**in·spire,** *v.*

in·spi·ra·tor (in′spi·ray″tur) *n.* 1. INHALATOR. 2. RESPIRATOR.

in·spi·ra·to·ry (in·spye′ruh·to·ree) *adj.* Pertaining to the act of inspiration.

inspiratory capacity. The amount of air that can be inhaled after a normal expiration.

inspiratory emphysema. EMPHYSEMA (1).

inspiratory reserve volume. COMPLEMENTAL AIR.

inspiratory spasm. A spasmodic contraction of nearly all the inspiratory muscles.

inspiratory standstill. A halt in the respiratory cycle at the end of inspiration when the lungs are filled with air. The condition can be produced by stimulating the central end of the cut vagus nerve.

inspired air. The air that is taken in by inspiration.

in·spi·rom·e·ter (in″spi·rom′e·tur) *n.* [*inspire* + *-meter*]. An instrument for measuring the amount of air inspired.

in·spis·sate (in·spis′ate, in′spi·sate) *v.* [L. *inspissare,* from *spissus,* thick]. To make thick by evaporation or by absorption of fluid. —**inspissat·ed,** *adj.;* **in·spis·sa·tion** (in″spi·say′shun) *n.*

in·sta·bil·i·ty, *n.* 1. Lack of stability; insecurity of support or balance. 2. Lack of fixed purpose; inconstancy in opinions or beliefs.

in·stance, *n.* [OF., from L. *instantia,* presence, urgency]. *In psychoanalysis,* the dominance or perseverance of one level of mental function in comparison to others.

in·star (in′stahr) *n.* [L., image, form]. Any one of the larval stages of arthropods.

in·step, *n.* The arch on the medial side of the foot.

in·stil·la·tion (in″sti·lay′shun) *n.* [L. *instillatio,* from *instillare,* to pour in by drops, from *stilla,* a drop]. The introduction of a liquid into a cavity drop by drop.

in·stil·la·tor (in′sti·lay″tur) *n.* An apparatus for introducing, by drops, a liquid into a cavity or space.

in·stinct, *n.* [L. *instinctus,* instigation, incitement, from *instinguere,* to incite]. 1. A precise, inherited pattern of unlearned behavior in which there is an invariable association of a particular series of responses with specific stimuli; an unconditioned complex reflex. 2. *In psychiatry,* a primary tendency or inborn drive, as toward life, sexual reproduction, and death.

in·stinc·tive, *adj.* Prompted or determined by instinct; of the nature of instinct.

instinctive reflex. UNCONDITIONED REFLEX.

in·stinc·tu·al (in·stink′choo·ul, ·tew·ul) *adj.* 1. INSTINCTIVE. 2. *In psychiatry,* pertaining to a psychic process or behavior which is a function of, or motivated by, the id, and which is more or less emotional, impulsive, and unreasoned.

in·stru·ment, *n.* [L. *instrumentum.* from *instruere,* to build]. A mechanical tool or implement; a mechanical device having a specific function. —**in·stru·men·tal,** *adj.*

instrumental amusia. Loss of the ability to play a musical instrument; a form of aphasia.

instrumental conditioning. OPERANT CONDITIONING.

instrumental labor. Labor requiring instrumental means to extract the child.

in·stru·men·ta·tion (in″stroo·men·tay′shun) *n.* The use of instruments in treating a patient.

in·su·date (in′sue·date) *n.* A substance accumulated by insudation.

in·su·da·tion (in″sue·day′shun) *n.* [L. *insudare,* to sweat into]. Accumulation within a tissue or organ of a substance or substances derived from the blood. Compare *exudation, transudation.* —**in·su·date** (in′sue·date) *v.*

in·suf·fi·cien·cy (in″suh·fish′un·see) *n.* The state of being inadequate; incapacity to perform a normal function. —**insuffi·cient** (·unt) *adj.*

in·suf·fla·tion (in″suh·flay′shun) *n.* [L. *insufflatio,* from *insufflare,* to breathe into]. The act of blowing into, as blowing a gas, powder, or vapor into one of the cavities of the body.

insufflation anesthesia. Anesthesia produced by the delivery of anesthetic gases under pressure into the respiratory system, used during bronchoscopy or laryngoscopy.

in·suf·fla·tor (in′suh·flay″tur) *n.* An instrument used in insufflation.

in·su·la (in′sue·luh) *n.,* pl. & genit. sing. **insu·lae** (·lee) [L., island] [NA]. The portion of the cortex overlying the corpus striatum; it lies hidden from view in the adult brain at the bottom of the lateral fissure. See also Plate 17.

in·su·lae·mia (in″sue·lee′mee·uh) *n.* INSULINEMIA.

in·su·lar (in′sue·lur) *adj.* [L. *insularis,* from *insula,* island]. Pertaining to or characterized by islands or islets.

insular cirrhosis. LAENNEC'S CIRRHOSIS.

insular sclerosis. MULTIPLE SCLEROSIS; a mnemonic acronym of its principal symptoms: *i*ntention tremor, *n*ystagmus, *s*canning speech, *u*rogenital disturbances, *l*abile emotions, *a*taxia, and retrobulbar *r*etinitis.

insulated plastic boot. A high boot, consisting of an inner and outer sleeve with a filler of spun glass, used to increase blood flow to the lower extremities by conserving body heat and raising cutaneous temperature.

in·su·lin (in′suh·lin, ·sue·) *n.* [L. *insul*a, island, + *-in*]. The hypoglycemic hormone secreted by the beta cells of the islets of the pancreas; a protein with a molecular weight of about 6000. It participates, together with other biochemical entities, in regulating carbohydrate and fat metabolism. The principal effect of insulin may be to facilitate conversion of extracellular glucose to intracellular glucose 6-phosphate. Deficiency of insulin causes diabetes mellitus, for the treatment of which one or more forms of insulin may be used; these differ in speed and duration of action, mainly because of difference in solubility. Globin zinc insulin, which is insulin modified by addition of globin and zinc, has longer duration of action than regular insulin. Protamine zinc insulin, prepared by adding protamine and zinc to insulin, is a long-acting insulin. Isophane insulin contains crystals of insulin, protamine, and zinc, in such proportion (the isophane ratio) as to produce an intermediate-acting preparation. By using insulin modified by the addition of zinc, it is possible to prepare amorphous or crystalline forms of insulin zinc, which differ in particle size and hence in solubility and duration of action; long-acting, intermediate-acting, and rapid-acting forms are available.

in·su·lin·ase (in′suh·li·nace, ·naze) *n.* An enzyme, present in liver, capable of inactivating insulin.

insulin atrophy. Atrophy of the subcutaneous, chiefly fatty tissues about the site of injection of insulin.

insulin coma therapy. INSULIN SHOCK THERAPY. Abbreviated, ICT.

in·su·lin·emia, in·su·lin·ae·mia (in″sue·li·nee′mee·uh) *n.* [*insulin* + *-emia*]. The presence of insulin in the circulating blood.

insulin hypertrophy. A painless, locally indurated, raised, rubbery area of adipose tissue hypertrophy seen in some patients in an area repeatedly injected with insulin.

insulin hypoglycemia test. HOLLANDER TEST.

in·su·li·no·ma (in″sue·li·no′muh) *n.* [*insulin* + *-oma*]. An islet-cell tumor that produces insulin.

insulin shock. Hypoglycemia with coma as a result of overdosage of insulin in diabetes or in the treatment of psychoses.

insulin shock therapy or **treatment.** The treatment of certain psychoses, especially severe depressive disorders and schizophrenia, by the induction of a series of hypoglycemic comas through the injection of appropriate amounts of insulin, with subsequent termination of the coma by the administration of glucose. Abbreviated, IST.

in·su·li·tis (in″sue·lye′tis) *n.* [L. *insul*a, island, + *-itis*]. Inflammation of the islets of the pancreas.

in·su·lo·ma (in″sue·lo′muh) *n.* [L. *insul*a, island (of Langerhans), + *-oma*]. 1. ISLET-CELL TUMOR. 2. Specifically, INSULINOMA.

in·sult, *n.* Trauma or other harmful stress to tissues or organs.

in·sul·to·ic membrane (in″sul·to′ick) [*insul*ate + allan*toic*]. A protective membrane for denuded surfaces prepared from the allantoic membrane of bovine embryos.

in·sus·cep·ti·bil·i·ty, *n.* Lack of susceptibility.

in·take, *n. In medicine,* the total amount of fluid and other substances entering the body by ingestion or parenterally.

Intal. A trademark for cromolyn sodium used in the treatment of bronchial asthma.

in·te·gral dose. *In radiology,* the total energy absorbed by a patient during an exposure or series of exposures to radiation. See also *volume dose.*

integrating dose meter or **dosimeter.** *In radiology,* a measuring system designed to determine the total radiation administered during a single exposure or series of exposures.

in·te·gra·tion, *n.* [L. *integratio,* restoration, from *integer,* whole, sound]. 1. The process of unifying different elements into a single whole. 2. The combination of bodily activities to cooperate in the welfare of the whole organism. 3. *In neurology,* the impingement of impulses from various centers upon one final, common pathway, resulting in an adaptive response. 4. The useful and harmonious incorporation and organization of old and new information and experiences into the personality, including the amalgamation of functions at different levels of psychosexual development.

in·te·gra·tor gene. A gene in eukaryotic cells which is such that when an adjacent sensor site is activated the gene is transcribed to yield activator RNA.

in·teg·u·ment (in·teg'yoo·munt) *n.* [L. *integumentum,* from *integere,* to cover]. A covering, especially the skin. —**in·teg·u·men·ta·ry** (in·teg"yoo·men'tuh·ree) *adj.*

integumentary system. A system pertaining to the body covering, as the skin, hair, nails.

in·te·gu·men·tum (in·teg"yoo·men'tum) *n.* [L.]. INTEGUMENT.

integumentum com·mu·ne (kom·yoo'nee) [NA]. The skin and its appendages.

in·tel·lect, *n.* [L. *intellectus,* from *intelligere,* to understand]. The mind, the understanding, the reasoning or thinking power. —**in·tel·lec·tu·al,** *adj.*

intellectual imbalance. The state of a person who exhibits special abilities in some areas of mental activity and is more or less deficient in others, so that there are marked discrepancies in performance and he or she appears to be poorly integrated.

in·tel·lec·tu·al·iza·tion, *n.* 1. Analysis of an emotional or social problem in rational, intellectual terms to the exclusion or neglect of feelings or practical considerations. 2. *In psychiatry,* a defense mechanism utilizing reasoning against consciously facing an unconscious conflict and the stress and affect connected with it. Compare *rationalization.*

in·tel·li·gence, *n.* [L. *intelligentia*]. 1. The understanding, intellect, or mind. 2. The ability to perceive qualities and attributes of the objective world, and to employ purposively a means toward the attainment of an end. 3. The general capacity of an organism endowed with a cerebrum to meet a novel situation by improvising a novel adaptive response, that is, to solve a problem and to engage in abstract thought. 4. Mental astuteness, insight, sagacity.

intelligence quotient. A numerical rating used to designate a person's intelligence; a ratio of an individual's performance on some standardized mental test as compared to the normal or average for age and even social situation. The most common such ratio is arrived at by dividing the mental age by the chronologic age (up to 16 years) and multiplying by 10. The most common scale employed in the United States is the Stanford-Binet test. The three grades of mental deficiency are marked by intelligence quotients of 69 or lower. Above 69 the classification is as follows: dull normal, 70 to 90; normal 90 to 110; superior, 110 to 125; very superior, 125 to 140; and genius, 140 and above. Abbreviated, I.Q.

intelligence test. Any task or series of problems presented to an individual to carry out or solve with a view toward determining the level of ability to think, conceive, or reason. Such tests seek to measure innate capacity rather than achievement resulting from formal education and are standardized by finding the average level of performance of individuals who by other, independent criteria are judged to have a certain degree of intelligence. Among the most widely used tests are the Cattell infant intelligence scale, the Stanford-Binet test, and the Wechsler-Bellevue intelligence scale.

in·tem·per·ance, *n.* [L. *intemperantia*]. Lack of moderation; immoderate indulgence, especially in alcoholic beverages. —**intemper·ate,** *adj.* & *n.*

Intensain. Trademark for chromonar, a coronary vasodilator used as the hydrochloride salt.

in·tense, *adj.* [L. *intensus,* stretched]. 1. Extreme in degree; showing to a high degree the characteristic attribute. 2. Feeling deeply.

in·ten·si·fi·ca·tion, *n.* 1. An increase in intensity, concentration, or strength of any kind. 2. The condition occurring in cutaneous sensory disturbances in which certain sensations are abnormally vivid. 3. *In radiology,* the enhancement of the radiographic image produced on film by the use of intensifying screens or in fluoroscopy by means of an electron multiplier tube. —**in·ten·si·fy,** *v.*

intensifying screen. A screen composed of fluorescent material, used in a cassette in close contact with x-ray film to increase the photographic effect of the x-ray beam. It decreases the dose and shortens exposure time.

in·ten·sim·e·ter (in"ten·sim'e·tur, in·ten'si·mee"tur) *n.* An instrument for measuring the intensity or dosage per unit time of radiation.

in·ten·si·ty, *n.* 1. The state or condition of being intense. 2. Amount or degree of strength or power. 3. *In radiology,* the amount of energy per unit time passing through a unit area perpendicular to the line of propagation.

intensity of an electric field. At any point, the force per unit charge upon a charged particle, placed at that point.

intensity of a magnetic field. At any point, the force per unit pole upon a free pole, placed at that point.

intensity of x-rays. The dose of radiation in roentgens divided by the time required to deliver it; dose per unit time.

in·ten·sive, *adj.* Characterized by intensity; occurring or administered in high concentration.

intensive care. 1. The services, such as continuous close medical and nursing attention and the use of complex equipment, offered in a hospital for care of certain critically ill patients, with a view to restoring, when possible, normal life processes. 2. *Informal.* INTENSIVE CARE UNIT.

intensive care unit. An area within a hospital facility for patients whose health conditions require close medical attention, constant nursing care, and the use of complex medical equipment. Abbreviated, ICU.

intensive psychotherapy. Any one of the methods of psychiatric treatment which aims at helping the patient to gain insight into the origin and dynamics of his conflicts and feelings so that the patient can release for useful purposes much ego energy previously spent in defense against his feelings about himself in relation to others. Compare *supportive therapy* (2). See also *psychoanalysis* (1), *psychobiology.*

in·ten·tion, *n.* [L. *intentio*]. 1. Aim, purpose. 2. A process or manner of healing. See also *healing by first intention, healing by second intention.*

intention tremor. A jerky, four-to-six-per-second tremor, which is absent when the limbs are inactive, but becomes more prominent as action continues and fine adjustment of the movement is demanded; indicative of disease of the cerebellum or its connections. Syn. *ataxic tremor.*

inter- [L., between]. A prefix meaning (a) *between, among;* (b) *mutual, reciprocal.*

in·ter·ac·ces·so·ry (in"tur·ack·ses'uh·ree) *adj.* Situated between accessory processes of the vertebrae.

in·ter·ac·i·nar (in"tur·as'i·nur) *adj.* [*inter-* + *acinar*]. Situated between acini.

in·ter·ac·i·nous (in"tur·as'i·nus) *adj.* INTERACINAR.

in·ter·al·ve·o·lar (in"tur·al·vee'uh·lur) *adj.* [*inter-* + *alveolar*]. Between alveoli.

interalveolar septum. 1. INTERDENTAL SEPTUM. 2. One of the septa between alveoli of the lung.

in·ter·an·nu·lar (in"tur·an'yoo·lur) *adj.* [*inter-* + *annular*]. 1. Between two cardiac valve rings. 2. Between nodes of Ranvier.

interannular segment. The portion of a nerve included between two consecutive nodes of Ranvier.

in·ter·ar·tic·u·lar (in"tur·ahr·tick'yoo·lur) *adj.* [*inter-* + *articular*]. Situated between articulating surfaces.

interarticular cartilage or **fibrocartilage.** A flat fibrocartilage situated between the articulating surfaces of some joints. See also *articular disk, meniscus* (1).

in·ter·ar·y·te·noid (in″tur·ăr″i·tee′noid) *adj.* Between arytenoid cartilages or muscles.

interarytenoid cartilage. An inconstant cartilage found between the arytenoid cartilages.

in·ter·ar·y·te·noi·de·us (in″tur·ăr″i·te·noy′dee·us) *n.* A variant name for the combined oblique and transverse arytenoid muscles.

interarytenoid fissure. The narrow cleft between the embryonic arytenoid folds.

interarytenoid incisure. A small vertical notch between the corniculate cartilages and the apexes of the arytenoid cartilages of the two sides. NA *incisura interarytenoidea.*

in·ter·atri·al (in″tur·ay′tree·ul) *adj.* [*inter-* + *atrial*]. Between the atria of the heart.

interatrial groove. INTERATRIAL SULCUS.

interatrial septum. The septum between the right and left atria of the heart. Syn. *atrial septum.* NA *septum interatriale.*

interatrial sulcus. An indefinite furrow on the posterior surface of the heart marking the location of the interatrial septum.

in·ter·ax·o·nal (in″tur·ack′suh·nul) *adj.* [*inter-* + *axonal*]. Occurring between nerve fibers.

interaxonal current. The electric stimulation or modification of excitability produced in one group of nerve fibers by the action potential of a contiguous group. See also *ephapse.*

in·ter·blink interval (in″tur·blink′). The average period between blinks, which is about 2.8 seconds in men and just under 4 seconds in women.

in·ter·body, *n.* [*inter-* + *body*]. AMBOCEPTOR.

in·ter·brain, *n.* [*inter-* + *brain*]. DIENCEPHALON.

in·ter·ca·lary (in·tur′kuh·lerr″ee) *adj.* [L. *intercalarius,* from *intercalare,* to insert]. Situated between; intercalated.

intercalary staphyloma. A staphyloma developing in that region of the sclera which is united with the periphery of the iris.

in·ter·ca·lat·ed (in·tur′kuh·lay″tid) *adj.* [L. *intercalare, intercalatus,* to insert]. Placed or inserted between.

intercalated disk. Transverse thickening, representing an intercellular junction, occurring at the abutting surface of cardiac muscle cells.

intercalated duct. The narrow portion of the intralobular ducts of the pancreas, or of the parotid or submandibular glands.

intercalated mamillary nucleus. A nucleus in the mamillary body, lateral to the medial mamillary nucleus.

intercalated neuron. INTERNEURON.

intercalated nucleus. A nucleus of the medulla oblongata in the central gray matter of the ventricular floor located between the hypoglossal nucleus and the dorsal motor nucleus of the vagus. NA *nucleus intercalatus.*

intercalated vein. SUBLOBULAR VEIN.

in·ter·can·a·lic·u·lar (in″tur·kan″uh·lick′yoo·lur) *adj.* [*inter-* + *canalicular*]. Situated between canaliculi, particularly of the small ducts of the breasts.

in·ter·cap·il·lary (in″tur·kap′i·lerr·ee) *adj.* Between capillaries.

intercapillary glomerulosclerosis. A nodular eosinophilic hyalin deposit at the periphery of the renal glomerular tufts in diabetic patients, usually associated with the clinical syndrome of hypertension, proteinuria, and edema. See also *Kimmelstiel-Wilson syndrome.*

in·ter·ca·rot·id (in″tur·ka·rot′id) *adj.* Situated between the internal and external carotid arteries.

in·ter·car·pal (in″tur·kahr′pul) *adj.* Between carpal bones.

intercarpal articulation. 1. Any articulation between carpal bones, including the mediocarpal and pisiform articulations. 2. Any of the articulations between adjacent bones within either row of carpals. NA (pl.) *articulationes intercarpeae.*

intercarpal ligament. Any of certain ligaments which interconnect the carpal bones on their dorsal, palmar, and adjacent surfaces; described respectively as dorsal intercarpal ligaments (NA *ligamenta intercarpea dorsalia*), palmar intercarpal ligaments (NA *ligamenta intercarpea palmeria*), and interosseous intercarpal ligaments (NA *ligamenta intercarpea interossea*). See also *intercarpal* in Table of Synovial Joints and Ligaments in the Appendix.

in·ter·cav·ern·ous (in″tur·kav′ur·nus) *adj.* Situated between the two cavernous sinuses.

intercavernous sinuses. Sinuses of the dura mater running across the median line of the hypophyseal fossa in front of and behind the hypophysis, connecting the cavernous sinuses of each side. NA *sinus intercavernosi.*

in·ter·cel·lu·lar (in″tur·sel′yoo·lur) *adj.* Between cells.

intercellular bridge. An attachment structure formed by the protrusion of apposing cell membrane processes from adjacent epidermal and other stratified squamous epithelial cells; once thought to constitute a continuous cytoplasmic connection between cells, but now known to include a narrow space separating the apposing processes. See also *desmosome.*

intercellular cement. A material of low density found between the two halves of a desmosome and presumed to act as a glue.

intercellular spaces. Cavities between adjacent cells.

intercellular substance. The part of a tissue that lies between the cells.

in·ter·cep·tive orthodontics (in″tur·sep′tiv). The early treatment of malocclusion wherein growth or eruptive forces may be used to accomplish improved tooth or jaw relationships.

in·ter·chon·dral (in″tur·kon′drul) *adj.* [*inter-* + *chondral*]. Between cartilages.

in·ter·cil·i·um (in″tur·sil′ee·um) *n.* [NL., from *inter-* + *cilia*]. The space between the eyebrows.

in·ter·cla·vic·u·lar (in″tur·kla·vick′yoo·lur) *adj.* Between the clavicles.

interclavicular ligament. A fibrous band connecting the upper surface of the sternal end of one clavicle with that of the other. NA *ligamentum interclaviculare.*

in·ter·cli·noid (in″tur·klye′noid) *adj.* Between the clinoid processes of the sphenoid bone.

in·ter·co·lum·nar (in″tur·kuh·lum′nur) *adj.* [*inter-* + *columnar*]. Between pillars or columns.

intercolumnar fascia. 1. A fascia attached to the crura of the superficial inguinal ring. 2. The superficial inguinal portion of the diaphragmatic fascia located between the two pubococcygeus muscles.

in·ter·con·dy·lar (in″tur·kon′di·lur) *adj.* [*inter-* + *condylar*]. Between condyles.

intercondylar eminence. The spinous process lying between the two articular facets on the superior articular surface of the tibia. NA *eminentia intercondylaris.*

intercondylar fossa. A notch on the back of the femur between the condyles. NA *fossa intercondylaris.*

intercondylar line. A ridge on the posterior surface of the lower end of the femur, forming the upper limit of the intercondylar fossa. NA *linea intercondylaris.*

intercondylar tubercles. The two sharp elongations on the summit of the intercondylar eminence of the tibia, the lateral intercondylar tubercle and the medial intercondylar tubercle.

in·ter·con·dy·loid (in″tur·kon′di·loid) *adj.* INTERCONDYLAR.

intercondyloid notch or **fossa.** INTERCONDYLAR FOSSA.

in·ter·cor·o·nary (in″tur·kor′uh·nerr·ee) *adj.* [*inter-* + *coronary*]. Among or between coronary arteries.

intercoronary reflex. Change in caliber of a coronary artery presumed due to reflexes arising in another coronary artery.

intercortical sensory aphasia of Starr. VISUAL APHASIA.

in·ter·cos·tal (in″tur·kos′tul) *adj.* [*inter-* + *costal*]. Between the ribs.

intercostal artery. See Table of Arteries in the Appendix.

intercostal membrane. Either of the thin membranes passing between adjacent ribs in the intercostal space. Specifically, the external intercostal membrane (NA *membrana intercostalis externa*), which replaces the external intercostal muscle at the anterior, sternal end of the intercostal space, or the internal intercostal membrane (NA *membrana intercostalis interna*), which replaces the internal intercostal muscle at the posterior end of the intercostal space from the angles of the ribs to the vertebrae.

intercostal muscles. Muscles lying between adjacent ribs, divided into external (NA *musculi intercostales externi*), internal (NA *musculi intercostales interni*), and the innermost (NA *musculi intercostales intimi*) as a subdivision of the internal. See also Table of Muscles in the Appendix.

intercostal nerves. The branches of the thoracic nerves in the intercostal spaces. NA *rami ventrales nervorum thoracicorum, nervi intercostales.*

intercostal space. The space between two adjacent ribs. NA *spatium intercostale.*

in·ter·cos·to·bra·chi·al (in″tur·kos″to·bray′kee·ul) *adj.* [*intercostal* + *brachial*]. Associated with an intercostal space and the arm.

intercostobrachial nerves. NA *nervi intercostobrachiales.* See Table of Nerves in the Appendix.

in·ter·coup·ler (in″tur·kup′lur) *n.* An apparatus used during the administration of an inflammable anesthetic to equalize the electric potential among anesthetist, patient, operating table, and anesthetic machine; designed to prevent explosions or fires due to static electricity.

in·ter·course, *n.* [L. *intercursus,* intervention, from *intercurrere,* to run between]. 1. Personal communication or interaction. 2. Specifically, sexual intercourse; coitus.

in·ter·cri·co·thy·rot·o·my (in″tur·krye″ko·thigh·rot′uh·mee) *n.* [*inter-* + *cricothyroid* + *-tomy*]. A cut into the larynx by transverse section of the cricothyroid ligament.

in·ter·cris·tal (in″tur·kris′tul) *adj.* [*inter-* + L. *crista,* crest]. Between the surmounting ridges of a bone, organ, or process.

intercristal diameter. The distance between the middle points of the iliac crests.

in·ter·cru·ral (in″tur·kroo′rul) *adj.* [*inter-* + *crural*]. Situated between the crura, particularly of the superficial inguinal ring.

in·ter·cu·ne·i·form (in″tur·kew·nee′i·form) *adj.* Between cuneiform bones.

intercuneiform articulation. Either of the gliding joints connecting the cuneiform bones.

intercuneiform ligament. Any of the ligaments connecting the cuneiform bones, including the dorsal intercuneiform ligaments (NA *ligamenta intercuneiformia dorsalia*), the interosseous intercuneiform ligaments (NA *ligamenta intercuneiformia interossea*), and the plantar intercuneiform ligaments (NA *ligamenta intercuneiformia plantaria*).

in·ter·cur·rent (in″tur·kur′unt) *adj.* [L. *intercurrens,* running along with, from *currere,* to run]. Partially concurrent; occurring during the course of another condition.

intercurrent disease. COMPLICATING DISEASE.

in·ter·cus·pa·tion (in″tur·kus·pay′shun) *n.* The fitting together of the occlusal surfaces of the maxillary and mandibular teeth in jaw closure.

in·ter·cusp·ing (in″tur·kus′ping) *n.* INTERCUSPATION.

in·ter·den·tal (in″tur·den′tul) *adj.* [*inter-* + *dental*]. Located or placed between teeth in the same arch.

interdental papilla. The portion of the gingiva between two contiguous teeth.

interdental septum. The alveolar process between adjoining teeth.

interdental space. INTERDENTIUM.

interdental splint. A dental apparatus for holding the ends of fractured maxillas or mandibles in place by means of wires passing about the teeth.

in·ter·den·ti·um (in″tur·den′shee·um) *n.* [NL., from L. *inter,* between, + *dentes,* teeth]. The space between any two approximating teeth.

in·ter·dic·tion, *n.* [L. *interdictio,* from *interdicere,* to prohibit]. *In legal medicine,* a judicial or voluntary restraint placed upon a person suffering from, or suspected of suffering from, a mental disorder, preventing that person from managing his or her own affairs or the affairs of others.

in·ter·dig·i·tal (in″tur·dij′i·tul) *adj.* [*inter-* + *digital*]. Between digits.

in·ter·dig·i·ta·tion (in″tur·dij″i·tay′shun) *n.* [*inter-* + L. *digitus,* finger]. 1. The locking or dovetailing of similar parts, as the fingers of one hand with those of the other; or of the ends of the obliquus abdominis externus muscle with those of the serratus anterior. 2. In closure of the jaws, the fitting of the cusps of the teeth of one arch fairly into the occluding sulci of the other arch. —**inter·dig·i·tate** (·dij′i·tate) *v.*

in·ter·duc·tal (in″tur·duck′tul) *adj.* [*inter-* + *duct* + *-al*]. Between ducts.

in·ter·face, *n.* A surface which forms the boundary between two phases or systems. —**in·ter·fa·cial,** *adj.*

interfacial tension. A measure of the work that must be done in increasing the interface between two phases by a given unit of surface. When one of the phases is gas, then the interfacial tension is commonly called surface tension.

in·ter·fas·cic·u·lar (in″tur·fa·sick′yoo·lur) *adj.* [*inter-* + *fascicular*]. Between fasciculi or fascicles.

interfascicular cells. Oligodendroglial cells that often appear in rows between myelinated fibers in the white matter.

in·ter·fere, *v.* [*inter-* + L. *ferire,* to strike]. In horses, to strike one hoof or the shoe of one hoof against the opposite leg or fetlock.

in·ter·fer·ence, *n.* 1. *In physics,* the mutual action of two beams of light, or of two series of sound vibrations, or, in general, of two series of any types of waves when they coincide or cross. 2. The mutual extinction of two excitation waves that meet in any portion of the heart.

interference dissociation. Interruption of the regular cadence of the QRS complex by a conducted supraventricular impulse, in the course of an arrhythmia characterized by independent pacemaker control of the atria and ventricles; the combination of interference beats and atrioventricular dissociation.

interference phenomenon. *In virology,* the inhibition of the simultaneous infection of host cells by certain other viruses; e.g., the neurotropic yellow fever virus protects against the viscerotropic virus. See also *interferon.*

in·ter·fero·gen·e·sis (in″tur·feer″o·jen′e·sis) *n.* The production or stimulation of interferon.

in·ter·fer·om·e·ter (in″tur·fe·rom′e·tur) *n.* [*interfere* + *-meter*]. An apparatus for the production and demonstration of interference fringes between two or more wave trains of light from the same area. It is chiefly used to compare wavelengths with a standard wavelength, by means of interference fringes.

in·ter·fer·om·e·try (in″tur·fe·rom′e·tree) *n.* Use of the interferometer to compare wavelengths with observable displacements of reflectors. —**inter·fer·o·met·ric,** *adj.*

in·ter·fer·on (in″tur·feer′on) *n.* A protein, formed by animal cells in the presence of a virus, or other inducing agent, that prevents viral reproduction and that is capable of inducing in fresh cells of the same animal species resistance to a variety of viruses.

in·ter·fer·on·o·gen (in″tur·feer·on′o·jen) *n.* [*interferon* + *-gen*]. Inactivated virus or synthetic polyribonucleotides used to stimulate interferon production.

in·ter·fi·bril·lar (in″tur·figh′bri·lur, ·fib′ri·lur) *adj.* [*inter-* + *fibrillar*]. Situated between the fibrils of tissues, as interfibrillar substances.

in·ter·fi·lar (in″tur·fye′lur) *adj.* [*inter-* + *filar*]. Between filaments.

interfilar mass. HYALOPLASM.

in·ter·fol·lic·u·lar (in″tur·fol·ick′yoo·lur) *adj.* [*inter-* + *follicular*]. Between follicles.

interfollicular cells. 1. Tangential sections of acini of the thyroid gland simulating solid masses of cells between the acini. 2. PARAFOLLICULAR CELLS.

in·ter·fo·ve·o·lar ligament (in″tur·fo·vee′uh·lur). Tendinous bands of the transversalis fascia curving downward medial to the deep inguinal ring. Syn. *Hesselbach's ligament.* NA *ligamentum interfoveolare.*

in·ter·fur·ca (in″tur·fur′kuh) *n.*, pl. **interfur·cae** (·kee, ·see) [*inter-* + *furca*]. The region between, and at the base of, three or more normally divided tooth roots.

in·ter·gem·mal (in″tur·jem′ul) *adj.* [*inter-* + *gemma* + *-al*]. Situated between the taste buds, or other buds.

in·ter·glob·u·lar (in″tur·glob′yoo·lur) *adj.* Situated between globules.

interglobular dentin. A small region of poorly calcified dentin found along the course of the incremental lines.

interglobular spaces. Small, irregular cavities in the outer surface of the dentin of a tooth, resulting from imperfect calcification. NA *spatia interglobularia.*

in·ter·glu·te·al (in″tur·gloo·tee′ul) *adj.* [*inter-* + *gluteal*]. Between the buttocks.

in·ter·go·ni·al (in″tur·go′nee·ul) *adj.* [*inter-* + *gonial*]. Between the two gonia (angles of the lower jaw).

in·ter·he·mal cartilages (in″tur·hee′mul). Nodules of cartilage which aid in the formation of the hemal arch of a vertebra.

in·ter·hemi·sphe·ric (in″tur·hem·is·ferr′ick, ·feer′ick) *adj.* Situated between the cerebral hemispheres.

interhemispheric fissure. LONGITUDINAL FISSURE OF THE CEREBRUM.

in·ter·ic·tal (in″tur·ick′tul) *adj.* [*inter-* + *ictus* + *-al*]. Between seizures or paroxysms.

in·te·ri·or (in·teer′ee·ur) *adj.* [L., inner]. Situated within, with reference to a cavity, part, or organ.

in·ter·ja·cent (in″tur·jay′sunt) *adj.* [L. *interjacens*]. Being, falling, or lying between or among others.

interjacent child. A child with minimal brain dysfunction syndrome.

in·ter·jec·tion·al speech (in″tur·jeck′shun·ul). The communication of emotions by inarticulate sounds or expletives, as seen in motor aphasia.

in·ter·kin·e·sis (in″tur·ki·nee′sis) *n.* [*inter-* + *kinesis*]. INTERPHASE.

in·ter·la·bi·al (in″tur·lay′bee·ul) *adj.* [*inter-* + *labial*]. Between the lips, or between the labia pudendi.

in·ter·la·mel·lar (in″tur·la·mel′ur) *adj.* [*inter-* + *lamellar*]. Between lamellas.

in·ter·lam·i·nar (in″tur·lam′i·nur) *adj.* [*inter-* + *laminar*]. Situated between laminas.

in·ter·lig·a·men·ta·ry (in″tur·lig″uh·men′tuh·ree) *adj.* INTERLIGAMENTOUS.

in·ter·lig·a·men·tous (in″tur·lig″uh·men′tus) *adj.* [*inter-* + *ligamentous*]. Between ligaments.

in·ter·lo·bar (in″tur·lo′bur) *adj.* [*inter-* + *lobar*]. Situated or occurring between lobes of an organ or structure.

interlobar arteries of the kidney. Branches of a renal artery, running in the renal columns. NA *arteriae interlobares renis.*

interlobar fissure. A fissure separating lobes of the lung. See also *horizontal fissure of the right lung, oblique fissure.*

interlobar veins. In the kidney, the veins running in the renal columns and draining into the renal vein. NA *venae interlobares renis.*

in·ter·lob·u·lar (in″tur·lob′yoo·lur) *adj.* [*inter-* + *lobular*]. Between lobules.

interlobular artery. 1. (of the kidney:) Any of the radial branches of an arcuate artery, running in the radial cortex of the kidney. NA (pl.) *arteriae interlobulares renis.* 2. (of the liver:) Any of the branches of the proper hepatic artery located in the portal canals of the liver. NA (pl.) *arteriae interlobulares hepatis.*

interlobular emphysema. INTERSTITIAL EMPHYSEMA.

interlobular vein. 1. (of the kidney:) Any of the tributaries of an arcuate vein of the kidney that lie in the cortical substance between the medullary rays. NA (pl.) *venae interlobulares renis.* 2. (of the liver:) Any of the branches of the portal vein located in the portal canals of the liver. NA (pl.) *venae interlobulares hepatis.*

interlocking ligature. CHAIN LIGATURE.

interlocking twins. Twins in which the neck of the first child becomes engaged with the head of the second above the superior strait. Such locking is possible when the first is a breech and the second a vertex presentation.

in·ter·mam·ma·ry (in″tur·mam′uh·ree) *adj.* [*inter-* + *mammary*]. Between breasts.

in·ter·mar·riage, *n.* 1. Marriage of blood relations. 2. Marriage between persons of different ethnic groups.

in·ter·max·il·lary (in″tur·mack′si·lerr″ee) *adj.* & *n.* [*inter-* + *maxillary*]. 1. Between the maxillary bones. 2. INCISIVE BONE.

intermaxillary suture. The union between the maxillary bones. NA *sutura intermaxillaris.*

in·ter·me·di·ary, *adj.* & *n.* Intermediate; mediating, mediator.

intermediary carcinoma. INTERMEDIATE-CELL CARCINOMA.

intermediary cartilage. 1. Cartilage bone in the process of transformation into true bone. 2. EPIPHYSEAL PLATE (2).

intermediary metabolism. The intermediate chemical steps in the intracellular transformation of foodstuffs within the body.

in·ter·me·di·ate, *n.* [L. *intermedius*]. 1. A biological substance or type necessary in the change of one form into another. 2. A chemical substance formed as part of a necessary step between one organic compound and another, as an amino acid or dye intermediate.

intermediate body of Flem·ming [W. *Flemming,* German anatomist, 1843–1905]. In mitosis, a small darkly staining, acidophilic body to which the two daughter cells are briefly attached during the telophase.

intermediate-cell carcinoma. A carcinoma derived from surface epithelium, but composed almost entirely of intermediate cells with intercellular bridges, the prickle cells. Syn. *intermediary carcinoma.*

intermediate cell mass. NEPHROTOME.

intermediate cervical septum. The septum formed by the union of the cervical spinal arachnoid and dura mater in the posterior midline. NA *septum cervicale intermedium.*

intermediate colony. A bacterial colony which is intermediate between the typical smooth (S) and rough (R) forms, and designated according to the resemblance to the S or R form, Sr, SR, or sR.

intermediate coronary syndrome. CORONARY INSUFFICIENCY.

intermediate disk. In a muscle fiber, the thin, dark, doubly refractive disk in the middle of the isotropic disk. Not confined to a single myofibril, it passes through the entire diameter of a striated muscle fiber. Syn. *Krause's membrane, Z disk.*

intermediate ganglia. Small variable groups of sympathetic nerve cells found on the communicating rami of spinal nerves. NA *ganglia intermedia.*

intermediate host. A host in which the parasite passes its larval or asexual stage. Contr. *definitive host.*

intermediate leprosy. DIMORPHOUS LEPROSY.

intermediate line. A ridge on the iliac crest between the inner and outer lips. NA *linea intermedia.*

intermediate lobe of the hypophysis. PARS INTERMEDIA (1).

intermediate mamillary nucleus. INTERCALATED MAMILLARY NUCLEUS.

intermediate mesoderm. NEPHROTOME.

intermediate plexus. A nerve plexus found in the embryo between the bulbar and atrial plexuses.

intermediate split graft. A graft consisting of the epidermis, papillary layer, and reticular layer of intermediate thickness. Syn. *Blair-Brown graft.*

intermediate sulcus. A slight groove on the greater curvature of the stomach, opposite the angular incisure, separating the pyloric antrum and vestibule.

intermediate tarsometatarsal articulation. CUNEOMETATARSAL ARTICULATION.

in·ter·me·din (in″tur·mee′din) *n.* A hypophyseal substance influencing pigmentation and found in greatest concentration in the intermediate portion of the hypophysis in certain animal species. A similar or identical principle active in man is now called melanocyte-stimulating hormone (MSH).

in·ter·me·dio·lat·er·al (in″tur·mee″dee·o·lat′ur·ul) *adj.* Both lateral and intermediate.

intermediolateral cell column. A division of the lateral gray column of the spinal cord, extending from the thoracic region to the upper lumbar segments, and composed of small neurons whose axons form preganglionic sympathetic fibers.

in·ter·me·dio·me·di·al (in″tur·mee″dee·o·mee′dee·ul) *adj.* Both intermediate and medial.

intermediomedial nucleus. A group of small and medium-sized cells in the intermediate gray column of the spinal cord (lamina VII). It receives fibers from the dorsal root at all levels, and may serve as an intermediary relay in transmission of impulses to visceral motor neurons. NA *nucleus medialis medullae spinalis, nucleus intermediomedialis.*

in·ter·me·di·us (in″tur·mee′dee·us) *adj. & n.* [L.]. 1. Intermediate, middle. 2. NERVUS INTERMEDIUS.

in·ter·mem·bra·nous (in″tur·mem′bruh·nus) *adj.* [*inter-* + *membranous*]. Lying between membranes.

in·ter·me·nin·ge·al (in″tur·me·nin′jee·ul) *adj.* [*inter-* + *meningeal*]. Between the dura mater and the arachnoid, or between the arachnoid and the pia mater, as intermeningeal hemorrhage.

in·ter·men·stru·al (in″tur·men′stroo·ul) *adj.* Between menstrual periods.

intermenstrual flow. METRORRHAGIA.

intermenstrual pain. MITTELSCHMERZ.

in·ter·ment (in·tur′munt) *n.* [OF. *enterrement,* from *enterrer,* to bury, from L. *terra,* earth]. The burial of a body.

in·ter·meso·blas·tic (in″tur·mez″o·blas′tick) *adj.* Between the layers or between the lateral plates of the mesoderm.

in·ter·meta·car·pal (in″tur·met·uh·kahr′pul) *adj.* Between metacarpal bones.

intermetacarpal articulation. Any of the joints between the bases of the four medial metacarpal bones. NA (pl.) *articulationes intermetacarpeae.* See also Table of Synovial Joints and Ligaments in the Appendix.

in·ter·meta·mer·ic (in″tur·met″uh·merr′ick) *adj.* Between two metameres, as the intermetameric or intersegmental ribs.

in·ter·meta·tar·sal (in″tur·met·uh·tahr′sul) *adj.* Between metatarsal bones.

intermetatarsal articulation. Any of the articulations between the bases of the metatarsal bones. NA (pl.) *articulationes intermetatarseae.* See also Table of Synovial Joints and Ligaments in the Appendix.

intermetatarsal ligament. METATARSAL LIGAMENT.

in·ter·mi·cel·lar fluid (in″ter·mi·sel′ur). *In colloid chemistry,* a liquid medium in which the colloidal particles (micelles) are dispersed.

in·ter·mi·tot·ic (in″tur·migh·tot′ick) *adj.* [*inter-* + *mitotic*]. Pertaining to the interphase stage of mitosis.

in·ter·mit·tent, *adj.* [L. *intermittens,* interrupting, leaving off]. Occurring at intervals; not continuous; recurring periodically.

intermittent biliary fever. CHARCOT'S INTERMITTENT FEVER.

intermittent branched-chain ketonuria. A form of maple syrup urine disease.

intermittent claudication. Cramplike pains and weakness in the legs, particularly the calves; induced by walking and relieved by rest; associated with atherosclerosis and perhaps with vascular spasm. Syn. *angina cruris, dysbasia intermittens angiosclerotica.*

intermittent convergent strabismus. Squint, usually first noted between 1 and 5 years of age, which is not present on casual gaze but only under special circumstances, as when the child is tired, upset, or looking at near objects. See also *accommodative esotropia.*

intermittent fever. 1. MALARIA. 2. Any febrile state interrupted by periods of normal temperature.

intermittent hepatic fever. CHARCOT'S INTERMITTENT FEVER.

intermittent hydrarthrosis. A condition characterized by acute regularly recurring effusions of fluid into a joint cavity.

intermittent insanity. MANIC-DEPRESSIVE ILLNESS.

intermittent ionization. Further ionization of ions at a surface, occurring at the same time as neutralization of electrons at the surface.

intermittent pulse. A pulse in which one or more beats are absent or dropped.

intermittent torticollis. SPASMODIC TORTICOLLIS.

intermittent tremor. The tremor commonly observed in hemiplegics on any attempt at voluntary motion.

in·ter·mu·ral (in″tur·mew′rul) *adj.* [*inter-* + *mural*]. Situated between the walls of an organ.

in·ter·mus·cu·lar (in″tur·mus′kew·lur) *adj.* [*inter-* + *muscular*]. Situated between muscles.

intermuscular hernia. INTERSTITIAL HERNIA.

intermuscular septum. A connective-tissue septum between muscles, particularly one from which the muscles take origin, as the septum between the brachialis and the triceps muscles in the arm.

in·tern, in·terne, *n.* [F. *interne,* from L. *internus,* internal]. A resident physician in a hospital, usually in the first year of service following graduation from medical school.

in·ter·nal, *adj.* [L. *internus*]. Situated within or on the inside. **—inter·nad** (·nad) *adv.*

internal abdominal ring. DEEP INGUINAL RING.

internal absorption. Normal digestive assimilation of a substance, as of foods or water. Syn. *molecular, nutritive,* or *organic absorption.*

internal acoustic meatus. A passage in the petrous portion of the temporal bone which gives passage to the facial and eighth cranial nerves and internal labyrinthine or internal auditory vessels. NA *meatus acusticus internus.*

internal anal sphincter. A thickening of the inner circular (smooth) muscle layer of the anal canal. NA *musculus sphincter ani internus.* Contr. *external anal sphincter.*

internal arcuate fibers. Arching fibers within the substance of the medulla oblongata. NA *fibrae arcuatae internae.*

internal auditory artery. LABYRINTHINE ARTERY.

internal auditory foramen. INTERNAL ACOUSTIC MEATUS.

internal auditory meatus or **canal.** INTERNAL ACOUSTIC MEATUS.

internal ballottement. VAGINAL BALLOTTEMENT.

internal capsule. A layer of nerve fibers on the outer side of the thalamus and caudate nucleus, which it separates from the lenticular nucleus; it is continuous with the cerebral peduncle and the corona radiata and consists of fibers to and from the cerebral cortex. NA *capsula interna.*

internal carotid artery. An artery that originates at the common carotid and has three sets of branches: the petrous portion has a corticotympanic branch and the artery of the pterygoid (Vidian) canal (inconstant); the cavernous portion has cavernous, hypophyseal, semilunar, anterior meningeal, and ophthalmic branches; and the cerebral portion has anterior cerebral, middle cerebral, posterior communicating, and choroid branches. The artery distributes blood to the cerebrum, the eye and its appendages, the forehead, nose, internal ear, trigeminal nerve, dura mater, and hypophysis. NA *arteria carotis interna.*

internal carotid nerve. A sympathetic nerve which forms plexuses on the internal carotid artery and its branches. NA *nervus caroticus internus.* See also Table of Nerves in the Appendix.

internal carotid plexus. A network of sympathetic fibers from the internal carotid nerve, surrounding the internal carotid artery and supplying fibers to its branches as well as to the abducens nerve, the pterygopalatine ganglion, the tympanic plexus, and the cerebral arteries. NA *plexus cardiacus internus.*

internal cervical os. OS UTERI INTERNUM.

internal conjugate diameter. The distance from the middle of the sacral promontory to the posterior surface of the symphysis pubis. Syn. *conjugata vera.*

internal derangement of the knee. A condition of abnormal joint mobility with painful symptoms, usually due to injury to a semilunar cartilage or cruciate ligament.

internal derangement syndrome. INTERNAL DERANGEMENT OF THE KNEE.

internal ear. The labyrinth, containing the essential organs of hearing and equilibrium, the sensory receptors of the vestibulocochlear nerve. The osseous labyrinth, consisting of the vestibule, the osseous semicircular canals, and the cochlea, houses the membranous labyrinth, which consists of the membranous semicircular canals, the cochlear duct, the utricle, saccule, and associated structures. NA *auris interna.*

internal elastic coat. The internal elastic membrane of an artery.

internal elastic membrane. A thin sheet (or fibers) of elastin which forms the boundary between the tunica intima and the tunica media, being prominent in arteries of medium and small caliber. See also Plate 6.

internal endometriosis. ADENOMYOSIS (1).

internal factor. An internal component of the environment of an organism. See also *milieu intérieur.*

internal fistula. A fistula in which all openings are within the body without communication through the skin; often used in reference to fistulous communication between two hollow organs.

internal genitalia. In the female, the uterus, uterine tubes, and ovaries; in the male, the prostate, ductus deferentes, and seminal vesicles. See also *sex organs.*

internal genu of the facial nerve. The C-shaped curve of the intracranial part of the motor nerve root of the facial nerve around the nucleus of the abducens nerve; produced by a shift in the positions of the nuclei of both facial and abducens nerves late in development. NA *genu nervi facialis.* Compare *external genu of the facial nerve.*

internal granular layer. The fourth layer of the cerebral cortex containing many small multipolar cells with short axons, and scattered small pyramidal cells.

internal hamstring reflex. A muscle stretch reflex elicited by tapping the tendons of the semitendinosus and semimembranosus muscles just above their insertions along the medial condyle of the tibia. The response is flexion of the leg on the thigh.

internal hemorrhage. Bleeding that is concealed by escape into a cavity, as the intestine, peritoneal cavity, or within the cranium.

internal hemorrhoids. Hemorrhoids within the anal orifice or sphincter.

internal hernia. A hernia occurring within the abdominal cavity; a sac of peritoneum, containing intraabdominal contents, protrudes through a normal or abnormal opening. It may be retroperitoneal or intraperitoneal.

internal hirudiniasis. A pathologic state caused by the ingestion of aquatic leeches of the genus *Limnatis,* or by their invasion of the genitourinary tract.

internal hordeolum. A suppurative infection of a tarsal (Meibomian) gland.

internal hydrocephalus. OBSTRUCTIVE HYDROCEPHALUS.

internal iliac artery. The medial terminal division of the common iliac artery. Syn. *hypogastric artery.* NA *arteria iliaca interna.* See also Table of Arteries in the Appendix.

internal inguinal ring. DEEP INGUINAL RING.

internal injury. Damage from violence to the organs of the abdominal or thoracic cavity.

in·ter·nal·iza·tion (in·tur″nul·i·zay′shun) *n. In psychiatry,* an unconscious process by which the attributes, attitudes, or standards of the parents and cultural environment are taken within oneself. Compare *incorporation* (2), *introjection.*

internal malleolus. MEDIAL MALLEOLUS.

internal medicine. The branch of medicine which deals with the diagnosis and medical therapy of diseases of the internal organ systems; the nonsurgical management of disease.

internal medullary lamina. A delicate band of fibers which divides the dorsal thalamus into medial and lateral nuclear groups.

internal meniscus. MEDIAL MENISCUS.

internal migration of the ovum. The passage of the ovum through the oviduct into the uterus.

internal naris. CHOANA (2).

internal negativism. PASSIVE NEGATIVISM.

internal occipital crest. The crest on the inner surface of the occipital bone, from the internal occipital protuberance to the foramen magnum. NA *crista occipitalis interna.*

internal occipital protuberance. A slight central prominence on the inner surface of the tabular portion of the occipital bone. NA *protuberantia occipitalis interna.*

internal ophthalmopathy. Any disease affecting the eyeball.

internal ophthalmoplegia. Paralysis of the intrinsic muscles of the eye, specifically those of the iris and the ciliary body.

internal os. OS UTERI INTERNUM.

internal pelvimetry. Measurement of the internal dimensions of the pelvis by hand or by pelvimeter.

internal phase. DISCONTINUOUS PHASE.

internal pyramidal layer. GANGLIONIC LAYER OF THE OPTIC NERVE.

internal ramus of the accessory nerve. The nerve derived from the most caudal cells of the nucleus ambiguus and which runs with the vagus, sending motor fibers to the striate muscles of the larynx and pharynx. NA *ramus internus nervi accessorii.*

internal resorption. Idiopathic resorption of the dentin of a tooth from within.

internal respiration. The exchange of respiratory gases between the systemic blood in the capillaries and tissues.

internal reticular apparatus. GOLGI APPARATUS.

internal secretion. A secretion that is not secreted upon a surface, but is released into and transported by the blood.

internal semilunar cartilage or **fibrocartilage.** MEDIAL MENISCUS.

internal sensation. A sensation from viscera, such as hunger, thirst, satiety; VISCERAL SENSATION.

internal spermatic fascia. The inner covering of the spermatic cord and testis, continuous with the transversalis fascia at the deep inguinal ring. NA *fascia spermatica interna.*

internal standard flame photometry. Flame photometry in which the intensity of the unknown element is simultaneously compared with a fixed or known concentration of another element, usually lithium.

internal strabismus. ESOTROPIA.

internal transmigration. The passage of an ovum through its proper oviduct into the uterus and across to the opposite oviduct.

internal urethral orifice. OSTIUM URETHRAE INTERNUM.
internal urethrotomy. Incision for treatment of a urethral stricture or obstruction from within the urethra.
internal ventriculostomy. Establishment of a communication between the third ventricle and the basal cistern. Syn. *third ventriculostomy.*
internal version. Turning of the fetus by introducing the entire hand within the uterus.
in·ter·nar·i·al (in″tur·năr′ee′ul, ·nair′ee·ul) *adj.* [*inter-* + *narial*]. Situated between the nostrils.
in·ter·na·sal (in″tur·nay′zul) *adj.* Situated between the nasal bones.
internasal suture. The union between the nasal bones. NA *sutura internasalis.*
in·ter·na·tal (in″tur·nay′tul) *adj.* Situated between the nates, or buttocks.
internatal cleft. The cleft of the buttocks, in which is situated the anus.
international angstrom. ANGSTROM (2).
international ohm. OHM (2).
international unit. The amount of a substance, commonly a vitamin, hormone, enzyme, or antibiotic, that produces a specified biological effect and is internationally accepted as a measure of the activity or potency of the substance. Such units are usually used only when the substance is not sufficiently pure to express its activity or potency in units of weight or volume. Abbreviated, I.U.
interne. INTERN.
in·ter·neu·ral cartilages (in″tur·new′rul). Nodules of cartilage which aid in the formation of the neural arch of a vertebra.
in·ter·neu·ron (in″tur·new′ron) *n.* Any neuron that is intermediary in position in a chain of neurons. Syn. *internuncial neuron, intercalated neuron.*
in·ter·neu·ro·nal (in″tur·new′ruh·nul) *adj.* [*inter-* + *neuronal*]. Between neurons.
in·ter·nist (in·tur′nist) *n.* A physician who specializes in internal medicine.
in·ter·no·dal (in″tur·no′dul) *adj.* Between nodes.
internodal segment. INTERNODE.
in·ter·node (in′tur·node) *n.* [*inter-* + *node*]. The space between two nodes of a nerve fiber, as the internode between the nodes of Ranvier. Syn. *internodal segment.*
in·tern·ship, *n.* The period of service of an intern.
in·ter·nu·cle·ar ophthalmoplegia. MEDIAL LONGITUDINAL FASCICULUS SYNDROME.
in·ter·nun·ci·al (in″tur·nun′see·ul, ·shul) *adj.* [L. *internuntius,* go-between, from *nuntius,* messenger]. Serving as a connecting or announcing medium.
internuncial cell or **neuron.** INTERNEURON.
in·ter·nus (in·tur′nus) *adj.* [L.]. INTERNAL.
intero-. A combining form meaning *interior, internal.*
in·ter·oc·clu·sal (in″tur·uh·kloo′zul) *adj.* Situated between the occlusal surfaces of teeth in opposite arches.
interocclusal record. A record of the positional relationship of the teeth of opposite arches made of a plastic material, such as wax, plaster of Paris, or zinc oxide and eugenol paste.
in·tero·cep·tive (in″tur·o·sep′tiv) *adj.* Pertaining to an interoceptor.
in·tero·cep·tor (in″tur·o·sep′tur) *n.* [*intero-* + receptor]. Any sensory receptor situated in the viscera and responding to such stimuli as digestion, excretion, and blood pressure. Syn. *visceroceptor.*
in·tero·fec·tive (in″tur·o·feck′tiv) *adj.* [*intero-* + ef*fective*]. Bringing about internal changes; referring specifically to the nerves of the autonomic nervous system. —**interofec·tion** (·shun) *n.*
interofective system. The part of the nervous system concerned with the regulation of the internal environment of the body; essentially, equivalent to the autonomic nervous system.
in·tero·ges·tate (in″tur·o·jes′tate) *adj.* & *n.* [*intero-* + L. *gestatus,* borne]. 1. Forming in the uterus. 2. During gestation. 3. An intrauterine fetus.
in·ter·ol·i·vary (in″tur·ol′i·verr·ee) *adj.* Between the olivary nuclei.
in·ter·os·sei (in″tur·os′ee·eye) *n.,* sing. **interos·se·us** (·ee·us). Small muscles inserting on the phalanges of the hand and foot. See also Table of Muscles in the Appendix.
in·ter·os·se·ous (in″tur·os′ee·us) *adj.* [*inter-* + *osseus*]. Between bones.
interosseous crest. INTEROSSEOUS MARGIN.
interosseous cuneometatarsal ligament. Any of the interosseous ligaments between the cuneiform and metatarsal bones. NA (pl.) *ligamenta cuneometatarsea interossea.*
interosseous margin. The sharp ridge along the shaft of a bone, such as the ulna or fibula, for the attachment of the interosseous ligament.
interosseous membrane of the forearm. The strong fibrous membrane between the interosseous margins of the radius and ulna. NA *membrana interossea antebrachii.*
interosseous membrane of the leg. The strong fibrous sheet between the interosseous margins of the tibia and fibula, extending distally into the tibiofibular syndesmosis, where it forms an interosseous ligament composed of short, strong fibers. NA *membrana interossea cruris.*
interosseous ridge. INTEROSSEOUS MARGIN.
interosseous sacroiliac ligament. Any of the numerous short, strong fibers passing between the tuberosities of the sacrum and ilium just anterior to the dorsal sacroiliac ligaments. NA (pl.) *ligamenta sacroiliaca interossea.*
interosseous talocalcaneal ligament. The thick, strong ligament occupying the sinus tarsi, consisting of layers of fibrous tissue attached to the talus and calcaneus along the calcaneal and talar sulci. NA *ligamentum talocalcaneum interosseum.*
interosseus. Singular of *interossei.*
in·ter·pal·a·tine (in″tur·pal′uh·tine) *adj.* Between the palatine bones.
interpalatine suture. The junction between the two palatine bones; the posterior segment of the median palatine suture.
in·ter·pal·pe·bral (in″tur·pal′pe·brul) *adj.* [*inter-* + *palpebral*]. Between the palpebrae, or eyelids.
in·ter·pap·il·lary (in″tur·pap′i·lerr·ee) *adj.* [*inter-* + *papillary*]. Between papillae.
in·ter·pa·ri·etal (in″tur·pa·rye′e·tul) *adj.* [*inter-* + *parietal*]. 1. Between walls or layers. 2. Between the parietal bones. 3. Between the parietal lobules.
interparietal bone. The part of the squamous portion of the occipital bone which is intramembranous in development. It forms a separate bone in most mammals and is separate abnormally in the human cranium. NA *os interparietale.* See also *incarial bone.*
interparietal hernia. INTERSTITIAL HERNIA.
interparietal sulcus. INTRAPARIETAL SULCUS.
interparietal suture. SAGITTAL SUTURE.
in·ter·pe·dun·cu·lar (in″tur·pe·dunk′yoo·lur) *adj.* [*inter-* + *peduncular*]. Situated between the cerebral peduncles.
interpeduncular cistern. The subarachnoid space between the cerebral peduncles. NA *cisterna interpeduncularis.*
interpeduncular fossa. A deep groove in the anterior surface of the midbrain. NA *fossa interpeduncularis.*
interpeduncular ganglion. INTERPEDUNCULAR NUCLEUS.
interpeduncular nucleus. A nucleus of the brainstem located between the cerebral peduncles, in which terminate the fibers of the habenulopeduncular tract. NA *nucleus interpeduncularis.*
interpeduncular space. The region between the cerebral peduncles. See also *interpeduncular cistern.*
in·ter·pel·vio·ab·dom·i·nal amputation (in″tur·pel″vee·o·ab·dom′i·nul). Amputation of the thigh with a portion of the adjoining half of the pelvis.

in·ter·pha·lan·ge·al (in″tur-fuh-lan′jee-ul) *adj.* [*inter-* + *phalangeal*]. Between the phalanges of the fingers or toes.

interphalangeal articulation. Any of the joints between the phalanges of the hand (NA (pl.) *articulationes interphalangeae manus*) or the foot (NA (pl.) *articulationes interphalangeae pedis*).

interphalangeal ligament. Any of the ligaments connecting the phalanges of the fingers or toes. See also *collateral ligaments, plantar ligaments, palmar ligaments.*

in·ter·phase (in′tur-faze) *n.* A period in the life of a cell during which there is no mitotic division before and after that interval in the intermitotic period. Syn. *interkinesis.* —**in·ter·pha·sic** (·fay′zick) *adj.*

in·ter·plas·mic reactions (in·tur·plaz′mick). Reactions taking place in interspaces between the protoplasmic micelles or molecules of cytoplasm.

in·ter·pleu·ral (in″tur-ploo′rul) *adj.* [*inter-* + *pleural*]. Between two layers of pleura, particularly of the visceral and parietal pleurae.

interpleural space. MEDIASTINUM.

in·ter·po·late (in·tur′puh·late) *v.* [L. *interpolare,* to alter, furbish]. To estimate values of a variable between two calculated or experimentally determined values of the same variable.

interpolated beat. An ectopic beat, usually ventricular in origin, occurring between two normal beats without disturbing the basic rhythm of the heart.

interpolated extrasystole. INTERPOLATED BEAT.

in·ter·po·si·tion (in″tur·puh·zish′un) *n.* The act of placing in between or in an intermediate position. —**inter·pose** (·poze′) *v.*

interposition operation. An operation occasionally performed in aged women for relief of cystocele and prolapse of the uterus, performed through vaginal incision. The body of the uterus is fastened below the urinary bladder, and the pelvic floor is repaired.

in·ter·pre·ta·tion, *n. In psychiatry,* the process by which the therapist communicates to the patient understanding or insight into some particular aspect of his or her problems or behavior on a deep level.

in·ter·pris·mat·ic (in″tur·priz·mat′ick) *adj.* Situated between prisms.

interprismatic cement. INTERPRISMATIC SUBSTANCE.

interprismatic substance. The cementing substance between enamel prisms.

in·ter·prox·i·mal (in″tur·prock′si·mul) *adj.* [*inter-* + *proximal*]. Between two adjacent teeth.

interproximal gingiva. INTERDENTAL PAPILLA.

interproximal space. The V-shaped space between the proximal surfaces of the teeth and the alveolar septum which is normally occupied by gingival tissue.

in·ter·prox·i·mate (in″tur·prock′si·mut) *adj.* INTERPROXIMAL.

in·ter·pu·pil·lary (in″tur·pew′pi·lerr·ee) *adj.* [*inter-* + *pupillary*]. Between the pupils.

interpupillary distance. The distance between the centers of the pupils of the two eyes.

in·ter·py·ram·i·dal (in″tur·pi·ram′i·dul) *adj.* Between pyramids.

interpyramidal cortex. RENAL COLUMN.

in·ter·ra·dic·u·lar septum (in″tur·ra·dick′yoo·lur). The bony partition between the roots of a tooth.

in·ter·re·tic·u·lar (in″tur·re·tick′yoo·lur) *adj.* [*inter-* + *reticular*]. Between or external to elements of endoplastic reticulum.

in·ter·rupt·ed, *adj.* Not continuous.

interrupted respiration. Respiration in which either inspiration or expiration is not continuous but is divided into two or more sounds. Syn. *jerky respiration, cogwheel respiration.*

interrupted suture. A type of suture in which each stitch is tied and cut individually.

in·ter·sca·lene (in″tur′skay′leen) *adj.* Between scalene muscles.

in·ter·scap·u·lar (in″tur·skap′yoo·lur) *adj.* [*inter-* + *scapular*]. Situated between the scapulae.

interscapular gland. The brown fat between the scapulae of certain rodents. See also *hibernating gland.*

interscapular reflex. SCAPULAR REFLEX.

interscapular region. The space between the scapulae. NA *regio interscapularis.*

in·ter·scap·u·lo·tho·ra·cic (in″tur·skap″yoo·lo·tho·ras′ick) *adj.* Between the scapula and the thorax.

in·ter·sec·tio (in″tur·seck′shee·o) *n.*, pl. **inter·sec·ti·o·nes** (·seck″shee·o′neez) [L.]. A cross line marking the site of union of two structures; intersection.

intersectiones ten·di·ne·ae (ten·din′ee·ee), sing. **intersectio tendi·nea** (·ee·uh) [NA]. The horizontal fibrous bands on the rectus abdominis muscle marking the site of fusion of segments of the muscle.

in·ter·seg·men·tal (in″tur·seg·men′tul) *adj.* Situated between or involving segments.

intersegmental reflex. Any reflex involving more than one segment of the spinal cord for the completion of its arc.

intersegmental septum. The space intervening between two mesodermal somites.

in·ter·sep·to·val·vu·lar (in·tur·sep″to·val′vew·lur) *adj.* Situated between a septum and a valve.

interseptovalvular space. A narrow cleft between the left valve of the sinus venosus and the septum primum after the latter develops.

in·ter·sex (in′tur·secks) *n.* [*inter-* + *sex*]. An individual whose constitution is intermediate between male and female, and who may be a true or a pseudohermaphrodite. —**in·ter·sex·u·al** (in″tur·seck′shoo·ul) *adj.*; **inter·sex·u·al·i·ty** (in″tur·seck″shoo·al′i·tee) *n.*

in·ter·sig·moid (in″tur·sig′moid) *adj.* Between portions of the sigmoid colon.

intersigmoid fossa. INTERSIGMOID RECESS.

intersigmoid hernia. A hernia involving the prolapse of a loop of intestine into a subsigmoid fossa at the root of the sigmoid mesocolon.

intersigmoid recess. A peritoneal diverticulum occasionally found at the apex of the attachment of the sigmoid mesocolon. NA *recessus intersigmoideus.*

in·ter·space, *n.* An interval between the ribs or the fibers or lobules of a tissue or organ.

in·ter·sphe·noid cartilage (in″tur·sfee′noid). The cartilage between the basisphenoid and orbitosphenoid ossification centers in the fetus.

in·ter·spi·nal (in″tur·spye′nul) *adj.* [*inter-* + *spinal*]. Situated between or connecting spinous processes; interspinous.

in·ter·spi·na·les (in″tur·spye·nay′leez) *n.*, sing. **interspina·lis** (·lis) [NL., interspinal]. Variable small muscles running between adjacent spinous processes of the vertebrae. NA *musculi interspinales.* See also Table of Muscles in the Appendix.

interspinal ligament. Any of the thin membranous bands connecting adjacent spinous processes of the vertebrae. NA *ligamentum interspinale.*

in·ter·spi·nous (in″tur·spye′nus) *adj.* Situated between or connecting spines or spinous processes.

interspinous diameter. The distance between the anterior superior iliac spines.

interspinous notch. The notch between the posterior superior and posterior inferior iliac spines.

in·ter·stage (in′tur·staje) *n.* INTERPHASE.

in·ter·sti·ces (in·tur′sti·siz) *n.*, sing. **inter·stice** (·stis) [L. *interstitium,* a place between]. Spaces or intervals.

in·ter·sti·tial (in″tur·stish′ul) *adj.* 1. Situated between parts; occupying the interspaces or interstices of a part. 2. Pertaining to the finest connective tissue of organs.

interstitial absorption. The taking up of metabolites and waste materials by the absorbent system.

interstitial calcinosis. CALCINOSIS UNIVERSALIS.

interstitial cell. A cell that lies between the germ cells or germinal tubules of a gonad, poorly represented in the adult human ovary. In the testis they are the Leydig cells.

interstitial-cell stimulating hormone. LUTEINIZING HORMONE. Abbreviated, ICSH.

interstitial-cell tumor. A usually benign tumor of the testis composed of interstitial cells (Leydig cells), which may be associated with hypersecretion of male sex hormones. Syn. *interstitioma, Leydig-cell tumor.*

interstitial cystitis. Chronic cystitis of unknown etiology with painful inflammation principally in the subepithelial connective tissue, extending in variable degree into the deeper tissues. Ulcers frequently accompany the process and are known as Hunner's ulcer or elusive ulcer.

interstitial emphysema. Escape of air from the alveoli into the interstices of the lung, commonly due to trauma or violent cough.

interstitial endometriosis. STROMATOSIS.

interstitial gestation. Gestation in the uterine part of a uterine tube.

interstitial gland. 1. Cell groups in the testis which secrete androgen; LEYDIG CELLS. 2. Mass of epithelioid cells in the medulla of the ovary of many lower animals. It is questionable whether or not it is present in women. The term has been applied to the hypertrophic theca cells about the periphery of follicles.

interstitial granules. The granules occurring in the sarcoplasm of muscle.

interstitial hepatitis. Associated degeneration or necrosis of hepatic parenchymal cells and infiltration of lymphocytes, plasma cells, large mononuclear cells, and sometimes polymorphonuclear leukocytes in the portal canals. Syn. *acute nonsuppurative hepatitis, nonspecific hepatitis.*

interstitial hernia. An intestinal hernia that lies between the muscular or fascial planes of the abdominal wall, rather than in the subcutaneous area. Syn. *intermuscular hernia, interparietal hernia.*

interstitial inflammation. Inflammation chiefly in the supportive or interstitial tissues of an organ.

interstitial irradiation therapy. Therapy of tumors with various types of implants or seeds containing radioactive material.

interstitial keratitis. An inflammatory process that involves the corneal stroma, characteristically seen in congenital syphilis.

interstitial lamella. One of the layers of bone of the regions between haversian systems.

interstitial mastitis. Inflammation of the connective tissue of the breast.

interstitial myocarditis. 1. Inflammation of the myocardium characterized primarily by cellular infiltration of the interstitial tissues. 2. FIEDLER'S MYOCARDITIS.

interstitial myositis. Inflammation of the stroma of muscle.

interstitial nephritis. 1. Inflammation primarily localized in the renal interstitium and involving the tubules. It may be seen as an acute form in drug-induced reactions, a chronic form in congenital renal diseases, and an accompanying lesion in many cases of chronic glomerulonephritis. It is characterized by various degrees of mononuclear cell infiltrates, tubular atrophy and dilatation, and interstitial fibrosis and edema. 2. PYELONEPHRITIS.

interstitial neuritis. HYPERTROPHIC INTERSTITIAL NEUROPATHY.

interstitial nucleus of Ca·jal (ka·^{k}ha^{h}l') [S. Ramón y *Cajal*]. A small nucleus in the dorsomedial part of the rostral midbrain just anterior to the oculomotor nucleus. It projects fibers contralaterally to the oculomotor nucleus, bilaterally to the trochlear nuclei, and ipsilaterally to the medial vestibular nucleus. NA *nucleus interstitialis.*

interstitial plasma-cell pneumonia. *PNEUMOCYSTIS CARINII* PNEUMONIA.

interstitial pneumonia. Inflammation particularly of the stroma of the lungs including the peribronchial tissues and the septa between alveoli, often viral or rickettsial in origin.

interstitial pneumonitis. PNEUMONITIS (2).

interstitial pregnancy. Gestation in the uterine part of a uterine tube. Syn. *intramural pregnancy.*

interstitial radiation. Radiation delivered by inserting a source or a number of sources of radioactive material (implants) directly into the tissue.

interstitial salpingitis. Salpingitis marked by excessive formation of connective tissue in response to an inflammatory stimulus.

interstitial substance. GROUND SUBSTANCE.

interstitial therapy. INTERSTITIAL IRRADIATION THERAPY.

interstitial tissue. The intercellular connective tissue.

in·ter·sti·ti·o·ma (in″tur·stish·ee·o′muh) *n.* [*interstiti*al + *-oma*]. INTERSTITIAL-CELL TUMOR.

in·ter·sti·tio·spi·nal tract (in″tur·stish″ee·o·spye′nul). Descending nerve fibers that arise in the interstitial nucleus of Cajal and enter the medial longitudinal fasciculus.

in·ter·sti·ti·um (in″tur·stish′ee·um) *n.* [NL.]. The interstitial tissue; intercellular connective tissue.

in·ter·sub·car·di·nal (in″tur·sub·kahr′di·nul) *adj.* Situated between the subcardinal veins.

intersubcardinal anastomosis. A transverse anastomosis between the paired subcardinal veins of the early embryo, ventral to the aorta.

in·ter·sys·tol·ic (in″tur·sis·tol′ick) *adj.* Between atrial and ventricular systole.

in·ter·tar·sal (in″tur·tahr′sul) *adj.* Situated between adjacent tarsal bones.

intertarsal articulation. Any of the various named joints between the tarsal bones. NA (pl.) *articulationes intertarseae.* See also Table of Synovial Joints and Ligaments in the Appendix.

in·ter·ter·ri·to·ri·al matrix (in″tur·terr·i·to′ree·ul). The lighter stained area that separates the areas of territorial matrix from each other in hyalin cartilage.

in·ter·tho·rac·i·co·scap·u·lar (in″tur·tho·ras″i·ko·skap′yoo·lur) *adj.* Between the thorax and the scapula.

interthoracicoscapular amputation. Amputation of the upper extremity at the shoulder girdle with disarticulation of the humerus. It includes removal of the scapula and outer portion of the clavicle.

in·ter·tra·gic (in″tur·tray′jick) *adj.* [*inter-* + *tragus* + *-ic*]. Situated between the tragus and the antitragus.

intertragic incisure or **notch.** The notch between the tragus and antitragus. NA *incisura intertragica.*

in·ter·trans·ver·sa·les (in″tur·tranz·vur·say′leez) *n.pl.* [NL]. INTERTRANSVERSARII.

in·ter·trans·ver·sa·rii (in″tur·tranz·vur·sair′ee·eye) *n.pl.* Short bundles of muscular fibers extending between the transverse processes of contiguous vertebrae. NA *musculi intertransversarii.* See also Table of Muscles in the Appendix.

in·ter·trans·verse (in″tur·tranz·vurce′) *adj.* Connecting the transverse processes of contiguous vertebrae.

intertransverse ligament. Any of the ligaments connecting two adjacent transverse processes in the vertebral column. NA *ligamentum intertransversarium.*

intertriginous vulvitis. Vulvitis secondary to the irritation that follows the rubbing together of adjacent parts.

in·ter·tri·go (in″tur·trye′go) *n.* [L., from *inter-* + *terere,* to rub]. An erythematous eruption of the skin produced by friction of adjacent parts. —**in·ter·trig·i·nous** (·trij′i·nus) *adj.*

in·ter·tro·chan·ter·ic (in″tur·tro″kan·terr′ick) *adj.* [*inter-* + *trochanteric*]. Between the trochanters.

intertrochanteric crest. A ridge between the greater and lesser trochanters of the femur. NA *crista intertrochanterica.*

intertrochanteric fossa. A fossa located medial to the intertrochanteric crest of the femur.

intertrochanteric line. A line upon the anterior surface of the femur, between the neck and shaft, and extending from the tubercle of the greater trochanter to a point below the lesser trochanter. NA *linea intertrochanterica.*

in·ter·tu·ber·al (in″tur·tew′bur·ul) *adj.* [*inter-* + *tuberal*]. Between tubers or tuberosities; specifically, between the ischial tuberosities.

intertuberal diameter. TRANSVERSE DIAMETER OF THE PELVIC OUTLET; the distance between the ischial tuberosities.

in·ter·tu·ber·cu·lar (in″tur·tew·bur′kew·lur) *adj.* [*inter-* + *tubercular*]. Situated between tubercles.

intertubercular groove. INTERTUBERCULAR SULCUS.

intertubercular line. An imaginary transverse line drawn across the abdomen at the level of the tubercles on the iliac crests.

intertubercular plane. A horizontal plane, usually at the level of the fifth lumbar vertebra, passing through the tubercles on the crests of the ilia.

intertubercular sulcus. A deep groove on the anterior surface of the upper end of the humerus, separating the greater and lesser tubercles; it contains the tendon of the long head of the biceps brachii muscle. Syn. *bicipital groove.* NA *sulcus intertubercularis.*

in·ter·tu·bu·lar (in″tur·tew′bew·lur) *adj.* [*inter-* + *tubular*]. Between tubes or tubules.

intertubular substance. The matrix of dentin, containing the dentinal tubules.

in·ter·ure·ter·ic (in″ter·yoo″re·terr′ick) *adj.* [*inter-* + *ureteric*]. Situated between the ureters.

interureteric bar or **ridge.** BAR OF THE BLADDER.

in·ter·vag·i·nal (in″tur·vaj′i·nul) *adj.* [*inter-* + *vaginal*]. Situated between sheaths.

intervaginal spaces. The subdural and subarachnoid spaces of the optic sheaths. NA *spatia intervaginalia.*

in·ter·val, *n.* [L. *intervallum,* from *vallum,* wall, rampart]. 1. The time intervening between two points of time. 2. The lapse of time between two recurrences of the same phenomenon. 3. The space between any two things or parts of the same thing.

interval operation. An operation performed between acute attacks of a disease, as an interval appendectomy.

in·ter·vas·cu·lar (in″tur·vas′kew·lur) *adj.* [*inter-* + *vascular*]. Situated between vessels.

in·ter·ve·nous (in″tur·vee′nus) *adj.* [*inter-* + *venous*]. Between veins; specifically, in the right atrium between the two venae cavae.

intervenous tubercle. A tubercle formed by the superior limbic band of cardiac muscle developing in the posterior wall of the sinus venosus between the superior and inferior caval openings. Syn. *Lower's tubercle.* NA *tuberculum intervenosum.*

in·ter·ven·tric·u·lar (in″tur·ven·trick′yoo·lur) *adj.* [*inter-* + *ventricular*]. Situated between or connecting ventricles.

interventricular foramen. Either one of the two foramina that connect the third ventricle with each lateral ventricle. Syn. *foramen of Monro.* NA *foramen interventriculare.* See also Plate 18.

interventricular furrows. Two longitudinal grooves, the anterior interventricular sulcus and the posterior interventricular sulcus, marking the location of the interventricular septum.

interventricular groove. An external, longitudinal groove indicating the beginning of separation of right and left ventricles in the developing heart.

interventricular septum. The wall between the ventricles of the heart, largely muscular, partly membranaceous. NA *septum interventriculare.*

interventricular sulcus. See *anterior interventricular sulcus, posterior interventricular sulcus.*

in·ter·ver·te·bral (in″tur·vur′te·brul) *adj.* Between vertebrae.

intervertebral cartilages. INTERVERTEBRAL DISKS.

intervertebral disks. The masses of fibrocartilage between adjacent surfaces of most of the vertebrae. NA *disci intervertebrales.*

intervertebral foramen. The aperture formed by the notches opposite to each other in the laminas of the adjacent vertebrae; a passage for the spinal nerves and vessels. NA *foramen intervertebrale.*

in·ter·vil·lous (in″tur·vil′us) *adj.* Between villi.

intervillous circulation. The circulation of maternal blood in the intervillous spaces of the placenta.

intervillous spaces. Spaces within the placenta developed from the trophoblastic lacunas and the dilated maternal veins, with which the maternal vessels communicate.

intervillous thrombosis. Coagulation of blood in the intervillous spaces of the placenta, usually seen near the end of pregnancy. Syn. *placentosis.*

in·ter·zon·al (in″tur·zo′nul) *adj.* [*inter-* + *zonal*]. Between zones, applied to filaments between daughter cells in the telophase of mitosis.

in·tes·ti·nal (in·tes′ti·nul) *adj.* Of or pertaining to the intestine.

intestinal angina. ABDOMINAL ANGINA.

intestinal arteries. The jejunal and ileal arteries. See Table of Arteries in the Appendix.

intestinal calculus. ENTEROLITH.

intestinal canal. The portion of the gastrointestinal tract extending from the pylorus to the anus.

intestinal capillariasis. A chronic wasting disease caused by the nematode worm *Capillaria philippinensis,* characterized clinically by abdominal pain, muscle wasting, and edema, often leading to death within several months; observed in epidemics in the Philippines since 1966.

intestinal decompression. Release of pressure by means of suction through a tube inserted into the intestine, usually by way of the nose.

intestinal digestion. Digestion by the action of the intestinal juices, including the action of the bile and the pancreatic fluid.

intestinal dyspepsia. Indigestion due to impairment of intestinal secretions or lack of tone in intestinal wall.

intestinal flu. Gastroenteritis of viral or bacterial origin. See also *viral gastroenteritis.*

intestinal fluke. A member of the species *Fasciolopsis buski, Heterophyes heterophyes,* or *Metagonimus yokogawai.*

intestinal glands. The simple straight tubular glands of the intestinal mucous membrane, containing goblet cells and Paneth cells which produce lysozyme, believed to have a role in the regulation of intestinal flora. Syn. *Lieberkuḟhn's glands, crypts of Lieberkuḟhn.* NA *glandulae intestinales.*

intestinal hormones. The hormones produced in the intestine: secretin and cholecystokinin.

intestinal infantilism. PANCREATIC INFANTILISM.

intestinal juice. The combined secretions of the various intestinal glands, a pale yellow fluid, alkaline in reaction, having a specific gravity of 1.001, and possessing diastasic and proteolytic properties. It also to a certain extent emulsifies and decomposes fats.

intestinal lipodystrophy. WHIPPLE'S DISEASE.

intestinal obstruction. Any hindrance to the passage of the chyme.

intestinal polyposis–cutaneous pigmentation syndrome. PEUTZ-JEGHERS SYNDROME.

intestinal portal. The opening of the foregut or of the hindgut into the midgut or yolk sac.

intestinal reflex. MYENTERIC REFLEX.

intestinal stasis. An undue delay in the passage of chyme along the intestines usually due to inadequate peristaltic contractions.

intestinal trunks. The collecting lymph trunks receiving lymph from the stomach, intestine, pancreas, spleen, and the lower and anterior part of the liver. They empty into the cisterna chyli. NA *trunci intestinales.*

intestinal villi. The villi of the mucous membrane of the small intestine. Each consists of an epithelially covered, vascular core of connective tissue containing smooth muscle cells and an efferent lacteal end capillary. NA *villi intestinales.*

in·tes·tine (in·tes'tin) *n.* [L. *intestinum,* from *intestinus,* internal, inward, from *intus,* inside]. The part of the digestive tube extending from the pylorus to the anus. It consists of the small and large intestine. The small intestine (NA *intestinum tenue*) extends from the pylorus to the junction with the large intestine at the cecum. Three divisions are described: the duodenum, the jejunum, and the ileum. The large intestine (NA *intestinum crassum*) consists of the cecum (with the vermiform appendix), the colon, the rectum, and the anal canal. See also Plates 13, 14.

in·tes·ti·num (in"tes·tye'num) *n.,* genit. **intesti·ni** (nye), pl. **intesti·na** (·nuh) [L.]. INTESTINE.

intestinum cae·cum (see'kum) [BNA]. CECUM.

intestinum cras·sum (kras'um) [NA]. LARGE INTESTINE.

intestinum ile·um (il'ee·um) [BNA]. ILEUM.

intestinum je·ju·num (je·joo'num) [BNA]. JEJUNUM.

intestinum rec·tum (reck'tum) [BNA]. RECTUM.

intestinum te·nue (ten'yoo·ee) [NA]. SMALL INTESTINE.

intestinum tenue me·sen·te·ri·a·le (mes"en·terr·ee·ay'lee) [BNA]. The portion of the small intestine which has a mesentery, namely, the jejunum and ileum.

in·ti·ma (in'ti·muh) *n.* TUNICA INTIMA; the innermost of the three coats of a blood vessel. See also Plate 6. —**inti·mal** (·mul) *adj.*

intimal arteriosclerosis. ATHEROSCLEROSIS.

intimal bodies. Mineralized hyaline bodies occasionally found in the vascular endothelium of horses.

in·ti·mate, *adj.* [L. *intimatus,* intimated, made known, from *intimus,* inmost]. 1. Pertaining to something which is innermost or of an essential character, as something which is reflective of the deepest part of oneself or someone very close to oneself. 2. Pertaining to highly personal matters, especially to emotions and drives, marriage, coitus. 3. Pertaining to detailed knowledge of a person or subject matter, as from a close and long association.

in·ti·mec·to·my (in"ti·meck'tuh·mee) *n.* [*intima* + *-ectomy*]. Surgical removal of a portion of the intima of an artery, especially to relieve obstruction of blood flow.

in·ti·mi·tis (in"ti·migh'tis) *n.* [*intima* + *-itis*]. Inflammation of the intima of a blood vessel.

in·tine (in'tine, ·teen) *n.* [L. *intus,* within]. The thin, inner coat of an endospore.

in·toe·ing, *adj.* & *n.* Walking pigeon-toed.

in·tol·er·ance, *n.* [L. *intolerantia,* from *intolerans,* intolerant]. 1. Lack of capacity to endure, as intolerance of light or pain. 2. Sensitivity, as to a drug.

in·tor·sion, in·tor·tion (in·tor'shun) *n.* [L. *intortio,* from *intorquere,* to curl]. 1. Inward rotation of a part. 2. *In ophthalmology,* an inward rotation of the vertical meridan, so that the superior point of the cornea turns nasally.

in·tort (in·tort') *v.* [L. *intorquere, intortus,* to twist round, turn]. To tilt the vertical meridian of the eye inward.

in·tort·er (in·tor'tur) *n.* [from *intort*]. The muscle tilting the vertical meridian of the eye inward; the superior rectus muscle.

intortion. INTORSION.

in·tox·i·cant (in·tock'si·kunt) *n.* & *adj.* 1. An agent capable of producing intoxication. 2. Producing intoxication.

in·tox·i·ca·tion (in·tock"si·kay'shun) *n.* [ML. *intoxicatio,* from *intoxicare,* to put poison in]. 1. Poisoning, or the pathological state produced by a drug, a serum, alcohol, or any toxic substance. 2. The state of being intoxicated, especially the acute condition produced by overindulgence in alcohol; drunkenness. 3. A state of mental excitement or emotional frenzy.

intoxication parkinsonism. Parkinsonism symptomatic of a toxic state as from carbon monoxide or manganese poisoning or, usually, certain drugs, as the phenothiazine compounds.

intra- [L.]. A prefix meaning *within, inside, inward, into.*

in·tra·ab·dom·i·nal (in"truh·ab·dom'i·nul) *adj.* [*intra-* + *abdominal*]. Within the cavity of the abdomen.

intraabdominal pressure. The pressure exerted upon the walls of the peritoneal cavity by the abdominal viscera.

in·tra·ac·i·nar (in"truh·as'i·nur) *adj.* [*intra-* + *acinar*]. Situated or occurring within an acinus.

in·tra·al·ve·o·lar (in"truh·al·vee'uh·lur) *adj.* [*intra-* + *alveolar*]. Within an alveolus.

in·tra·am·ni·ot·ic (in"truh·am"nee·ot'ick) *adj.* [*intra-* + *amniotic*]. Within or into the amniotic sac.

intraamniotic injection. Injection of hypertonic saline or glucose solution into amniotic fluid to induce abortion, usually in the second trimester.

in·tra·ar·te·ri·al (in"truh·ahr·teer'ee·ul) *adj.* Within or directly into an artery.

in·tra·ar·tic·u·lar (in"truh·arh·tick'yoo·lur) *adj.* [*intra-* + *articular*]. Within a joint.

intraarticular sternocostal ligament. A fibrocartilage within the joint of the second rib with the sternum. NA *ligamentum sternocostale intraarticulare.*

in·tra·atri·al (in"truh·ay'tree·ul) *adj.* [*intra-* + *atrial*]. Within an atrium, usually of the heart.

intraatrial heart block. Delayed or abnormal conduction within the atria, recognized on the electrocardiogram by a prolonged and often notched P wave.

in·tra·bony pocket (in"truh·bo'nee). INFRABONY POCKET.

in·tra·bron·chi·al (in"truh·bronk'ee·ul) *adj.* [*intra-* + *bronchial*]. Within a bronchus; for use within or by way of a bronchus, as an intrabronchial catheter.

in·tra·bron·chi·o·lar (in"truh·brong·kigh'o·lur, ·brong·kee·o'lur) *adj.* [*intra-* + *bronchiolar*]. Within a bronchiole.

in·tra·cal·i·ce·al, in·tra·cal·y·ce·al (in"truh·kal"i·see'ul) *adj.* [*intra-* + *caliceal*]. Within a calix.

in·tra·can·a·lic·u·lar (in"truh·kan"uh·lick'yoo·lur) *adj.* [*intra-* + *canalicular*]. Located within a canaliculus.

intracanalicular fibroadenoma. A benign breast tumor with proliferation of connective tissue causing distortion of the glands and ducts in the tumor.

intracanalicular myxoma. INTRACANALICULAR FIBROADENOMA.

intracanalicular sarcoma. CYSTOSARCOMA PHYLLODES.

in·tra·cap·su·lar (in"truh·kap'sue·lur) *adj.* [*intra-* + *capsular*]. Within the fibrous capsule of a joint.

intracapsular ankylosis. Ankylosis due to rigidity of structures within a joint.

intracapsular fracture. A fracture within the joint capsule.

in·tra·car·di·ac (in"truh·kahr'dee·ack) *adj.* [*intra-* + *cardiac*]. Within the heart.

in·tra·car·ti·lag·i·nous (in"truh·kahr"ti·laj'i·nus) *adj.* [*intra-* + *cartilaginous*]. Within a cartilage; endochondral.

intracartilaginous bone formation. ENDOCHONDRAL OSTEOGENESIS.

in·tra·cav·ern·ous (in"truh·kav'ur·nus) *adj.* [*intra-* + *cavernous*]. Within a cavernous sinus.

intracavernous aneurysm. A nonfistulous aneurysm of the internal carotid artery within the cavernous sinus. Syn. *subclinoid aneurysm.*

in·tra·cav·i·tary (in"truh·kav'i·terr·ee) *adj.* [*intra-* + *cavitary*]. Within a cavity.

intracavitary irradiation therapy. Therapy by means of radioactive tubes, capsules, or applicators inserted into a cavity of the body.

in·tra·cel·lu·lar (in"truh·sel'yoo·lur) *adj.* [*intra-* + *cellular*]. Within a cell.

intracellular canaliculi. A system of fine canaliculi within certain gland cells which apparently drain their secretion and increase the surface area of the cells, as that of the parietal cells of the gastric glands.

intracellular enzyme. An enzyme which exerts its activity within the cell in which it is formed.

in·tra·cer·e·bel·lar (in"truh·serr"e·bel'ur) *adj.* [*intra-* + *cerebellar*]. Within the cerebellum.

in·tra·cer·e·bral (in"truh·serr'e·brul, ·se·ree'brul) *adj.* Within or into the cerebrum.

in·tra·cho·ri·on·ic (in"truh·ko·ree·on'ick) *adj.* Within the chorion or chorionic cavity.

intrachorionic rudiment. AMNIOEMBRYONIC RUDIMENT.

in·tra·cho·roi·dal membrane (in"truh·ko·roy'dul). An ependymal membrane below the choroidal fissure in the embryo.

in·tra·cis·ter·nal (in"truh·sis·tur'nul) *adj.* [*intra-* + *cisternal*]. In a cistern, usually the cisterna magna.

in·tra·cor·ne·al (in"truh·kor'nee·ul) *adj.* [*intra-* + *corne-* + *-al*]. 1. Within the cornea of the eye. 2. Within the horny layer of the skin.

in·tra·cor·pus·cu·lar (in"truh·kor·pus'kew·lur) *adj.* Within a corpuscle, usually an erythrocyte.

in·tra·cra·ni·al (in"truh·kray'nee·ul) *adj.* [*intra-* + *cranial*]. Within the cranium, as intracranial pressure or calcifications.

intracranial aneurysm. An aneurysm located on any of the cerebral arteries. The most frequent is berry aneurysm.

intracranial angiography. Radiography of the blood vessels within the cranial cavity following the intravascular injection of a radiopaque material.

in·trac·ta·ble (in·track'tuh·bul) *adj.* Not easily managed.

in·tra·cu·ta·ne·ous (in"truh·kew·tay'nee·us) *adj.* [*intra-* + *cutaneous*]. Within the skin.

intracutaneous test. SCRATCH TEST.

in·tra·cu·tic·u·lar (in"truh·kew·tick'yoo·lur) *adj.* [*intra-* + *cuticular*]. Within the epidermis.

in·tra·cys·tic (in"truh·sis'tick) *adj.* [*intra-* + *cystic*]. Situated or occurring within a cyst or bladder.

in·tra·cy·to·plas·mic (in"truh·sigh"to·plaz'mick) *adj.* [*intra-* + *cytoplasmic*]. Within or surrounded by cytoplasm.

in·tra·der·mal (in"truh·dur'mul) *adj.* [*intra-* + *dermal*]. Within the dermis.

intradermal nevus. A skin lesion containing melanocytes located chiefly or entirely in the dermis, with little or no dermoepidermal junctional proliferation.

intradermal vitamin-C test. A test for vitamin-C levels which is based upon the length of time that an intradermal injection of dichlorophenolindophenol takes to decolorize.

in·tra·der·mic (in"truh·dur'mick) *adj.* INTRADERMAL.

in·tra·duc·tal (in"truh·duck'tul) *adj.* [*intra-* + *ductal*]. Within a duct.

intraductal papilloma. DUCTAL PAPILLOMA (1).

in·tra·du·ral (in"truh·dew'rul) *adj.* [*intra-* + *dural*]. Within the dura mater.

in·tra·em·bry·on·ic (in"truh·em·bree·on'ick) *adj.* [*intra-* + *embryonic*]. Within the embryo.

intraembryonic mesoderm. The mesoderm of the embryo formed largely from the primitive streak.

in·tra·epi·der·mal (in"truh·ep·i·dur'mul) *adj.* [*intra-* + *epidermal*]. Within the epidermis.

intraepidermal epithelioma. Carcinoma in situ, of either the squamous cell or basal cell type.

in·tra·epi·the·li·al (in"truh·ep·i·theel'ee·ul) *adj.* [*intra-* + *epithelial*]. Within the epithelial layer.

intraepithelial gland. A small aggregation of mucous cells within an epithelial layer.

in·tra·eryth·ro·cyt·ic (in"truh·e·rith"ro·sit'ick) *adj.* Within erythrocytes.

in·tra·esoph·a·ge·al (in"truh·e·sof"uh·jee'ul) *adj.* [*intra-* + *esophageal*]. Within the esophagus.

intraesophageal pressure. Air pressure within the relaxed esophagus, closely reflecting intrapleural pressure.

in·tra·fa·cial (in"truh·fay'shul) *adj.* Pertaining to interconnections between branches or fibers of the facial nerve on one side, as sometimes formed in reinnervation following an injury.

in·tra·fas·cic·u·lar (in"truh·fa·sick'yoo·lur) *adj.* Within a fasciculus.

in·tra·fu·sal (in"truh·few'zul) *adj.* [*intra-* + L. *fusus*, spindle, + *-al*]. Pertaining to the striated muscular fibers contained in a muscle spindle.

in·tra·gem·mal (in"truh·jem'ul) *adj.* [*intra-* + L. *gemma*, bud, + *-al*]. Within a bud or a bulbous nerve end, as a taste bud of the tongue.

in·tra·ge·ner·ic (in"truh·je·nerr'ick) *adj.* [*intra-* + *generic*]. Within a genus.

in·tra·gen·ic (in"truh·jen'ick, ·jee'nick) *adj.* [*intra-* + *-genic*]. Within a gene.

in·tra·glu·te·al (in"truh·gloo·tee'ul, ·gloo'tee·ul) *adj.* [*intra-* + *gluteal*]. Within a buttock.

in·tra·group (in"truh·groop') *adj.* [*intra-* + *group*]. Within a group.

in·tra·group·al (in"truh·groop'ul) *adj.* INTRAGROUP.

in·tra·he·pat·ic (in"truh·he·pat'ick) *adj.* [*intra-* + *hepatic*]. Within the liver.

in·tra·jug·u·lar process (in"truh·jug'yoo·lur). 1. A small curved process on some occipital bones which partially or completely divides the jugular foramen into lateral and medial parts. NA *processus intrajugularis ossis occipitalis.* 2. A small process on the petrous portion of the temporal bone which completely or partially separates the jugular foramen into medial and lateral parts. NA *processus intrajugularis ossis temporalis.*

in·tra·lam·i·nar nuclei of the thalamus (in"truh·lam'i·nur). Diffusely organized thalamic nuclei located in the internal medullary lamina which separates the medial from the lateral thalamic mass. The lateral central nucleus, paracentral nucleus, parafascicular nucleus, and submedial nucleus belong to this group. NA *nuclei intralaminares thalami.*

in·tra·le·sion·al (in"truh·lee'zhun·ul) *adj.* Within a lesion, either by natural occurrence or introduction.

in·tra·lig·a·men·ta·ry (in"truh·lig·uh·men'tuh·ree) *adj.* INTRALIGAMENTOUS.

intraligamentary pregnancy. Gestation within the broad ligament.

in·tra·lig·a·men·tous (in"truh·lig·uh·men'tus) *adj.* [*intra-* + *ligamentous*]. 1. Within the broad ligament of the uterus. 2. Within a ligament.

intraligamentous cyst. A cyst of the broad ligament.

in·tra·lo·bar (in"truh·lo'bur) *adj.* [*intra-* + *lobar*]. Within a lobe.

in·tra·lob·u·lar (in"truh·lob'yoo·lur) *adj.* [*intra-* + *lobular*]. Within a lobule.

intralobular artery. An artery lying within the lobule of an organ.

intralobular jaundice. HEPATOCELLULAR JAUNDICE.

intralobular veins. CENTRAL VEINS OF THE LIVER.

in·tra·lu·mi·nal (in"truh·lew'mi·nul) *adj.* [*intra-* + *luminal*]. Within the lumen of a hollow or tubelike structure.

in·tra·ma·tri·cal (in"truh·may'tri·kul, ·mat'ri·kul) *adj.* Within a matrix.

in·tra·mam·ma·ry (in"truh·mam'uh·ree) *adj.* [*intra-* + *mammary*]. Within breast tissue.

in·tra·med·ul·lary (in"truh·med'yoo·lerr·ee) *adj.* [*intra-* + *medullary*]. 1. Within the substance of the spinal cord or medulla oblongata. 2. Within the substance of the bone marrow, as an intramedullary nail. 3. Within the substance of the adrenal medulla.

intramedullary fixation. A method of holding a fractured bone in proper alignment by means of a metal pin or nail in the marrow cavity. See also *intramedullary nail.*

intramedullary nail. A metal rod or nail inserted into the medullary canal of a tubular bone to provide internal immobilization of fractures. It is long enough to pass across the fracture site to obtain fixation of both fragments of the bone.

in·tra·mem·bra·nous (in"truh·mem'bruh·nus) *adj.* [*intra-* + *membranous*]. Developed or taking place within a membrane.

intramembranous bone formation. The formation of bone by or within a connective tissue without involvement of a cartilage stage.

in·tra·men·stru·al (in″truh·men′stroo·ul) *adj.* Occurring during a menstrual period.

in·tra·mu·co·sal (in″truh·mew·ko′sul, ·zul) *adj.* Within a mucous membrane.

in·tra·mu·ral (in″truh·mew′rul) *adj.* [*intra-* + *mural*]. Within the substance of the walls of an organ, as intramural fibroid of the uterus.

intramural aneurysm. DISSECTING ANEURYSM.

intramural plexus. A plexus located within the wall of an organ, as the submucous or myenteric plexus.

intramural pregnancy. INTERSTITIAL PREGNANCY.

in·tra·mus·cu·lar (in″truh·mus′kew·lur) *adj.* [*intra-* + *muscular*]. Within or into the substance of a muscle.

intramuscular fibrositis. MYOSITIS.

in·tra·myo·car·di·al (in″truh·migh·o·kahr′dee·ul) *adj.* [*intra-* + *myocardial*]. Within the myocardium.

in·tra·myo·me·tri·al (in″truh·migh″o·mee′tree·ul) *adj.* [*intra-* + *myometrium* + *-al*]. Within the muscular part of the uterine wall.

in·tra·na·sal (in″truh·nay′zul) *adj.* [*intra-* + *nasal*]. Within the cavity of the nose.

in·tra·neu·ral (in″truh·new′rul) *adj.* [*intra-* + *neural*]. Within a nerve.

in·tra·nu·cle·ar (in″truh·new′klee·ur) *adj.* [*intra-* + *nuclear*]. Within a nucleus.

in·tra·oc·u·lar (in″truh·ock′yoo·lur) *adj.* [*intra-* + *ocular*]. Within the globe of the eye.

intraocular pressure or **tension.** The pressure within the eyeball, which in the normal population usually ranges between 14 and 20 mm of mercury; aqueous humor dynamics are mainly responsible for maintaining the intraocular pressure.

in·tra·op·er·a·tive (in″truh·op′ur·uh·tiv) *adj.* [*intra-* + *operative*]. During the time of a surgical operation.

in·tra·op·tic (in″truh·op′tick) *adj.* [*intra-* + *optic*]. Within the eye.

in·tra·oral (in″truh·o′rul) *adj.* [*intra-* + *oral*]. Within the mouth.

in·tra·or·bit·al (in″truh·or′bi·tul) *adj.* [*intra-* + *orbital*]. Within an orbit.

in·tra·pan·cre·at·ic (in″truh·pan″kree·at′ick) *adj.* Within the pancreas.

in·tra·pa·ren·chy·mal (in″truh·pa·renk′i·mul) *adj.* Within the parenchyma of an organ.

in·tra·pa·ri·etal (in″truh·pa·rye′e·tul) *adj.* [*intra-* + *parietal*]. 1. Within the wall of an organ. 2. Within the parietal region of the cerebrum. 3. Within the body wall.

intraparietal sulcus. A well-marked furrow separating the superior and inferior parietal lobules. This furrow has a complex and variable form having the following subdivisions: superior postcentral sulcus, inferior postcentral sulcus, and transverse occipital sulcus. NA *sulcus intraparietalis.* See also Plate 18.

in·tra·par·tum (in″truh·pahr′tum) *adj.* [NL., from *intra,* during, + *partus,* childbirth]. Occurring during parturition.

in·tra·pel·vic (in″truh·pel′vick) *adj.* [*intra-* + *pelvic*]. Within the pelvic cavity.

in·tra·peri·car·di·al (in″truh·perr·i·kahr′dee·ul) *adj.* Within the pericardial sac.

in·tra·peri·to·ne·al (in″truh·perr·i·tuh·nee′ul) *adj.* [*intra-* + *peritoneal*]. Within the peritoneum, or peritoneal cavity.

intraperitoneal hernia. A type of false, internal hernia in which some of the intraabdominal contents pass through an anomalous opening in the mesentery, omentum, or broad ligaments.

in·tra·pha·lan·ge·al (in″truh·fuh·lan′jee·ul) *adj.* Within a phalanx or phalanges.

in·tra·pleu·ral (in″truh·ploo′rul) *adj.* Within the pleura or pleural cavity.

intrapleural pneumonolysis. The severance of adhesion bands between the visceral and parietal layers of pleura. May be closed when performed by the use of a thoracoscope, and open when an incision is made through the chest wall to permit direct vision.

intrapleural pressure. Normally, the negative pressure existing in the potential space between the parietal and visceral pleura of the lungs and wall of the thoracic cavity. It fluctuates rhythmically throughout the respiratory cycle but normally is subatmospheric. In pneumothoraxes, this may be a negative, atmospheric, or positive pressure.

in·tra·psy·chic (in″truh·sigh′kick) *adj.* [*intra-* + *psychic*]. Pertaining to that which takes place within the mind or psyche.

intrapsychic adjustment. MENTAL ADJUSTMENT.

intrapsychic conflict. *In psychiatry,* a conflict between forces within the personality. Contr. *extrapsychic conflict.*

in·tra·pul·mo·nary (in″truh·pool′muh·nerr·ee) *adj.* [*intra-* + *pulmonary*]. Within the parenchyma of a lung.

in·tra·re·nal (in″truh·ree′nul) *adj.* [*intra-* + *renal*]. Within a kidney or kidneys.

in·tra·scap·u·lar (in″truh·skap′yoo·lur) *adj.* Within the scapula.

in·tra·scro·tal (in″truh·skro′tul) *adj.* [*intra-* + *scrotal*]. Within the scrotal sac.

in·tra·seg·men·tal (in″truh·seg·men′tul) *adj.* Within a segment.

intrasegmental reflex. Any reflex involving only one segment of the spinal cord.

in·tra·sel·lar (in″truh·sel′ur) *adj.* [*intra-* + *sellar*]. Within the sella turcica.

in·tra·spi·nal (in″truh·spye′nul) *adj.* Within the spinal canal.

intraspinal block. Spinal anesthesia produced by injection of an anesthetic.

in·tra·spi·nous (in″truh·spye′nus) *adj.* Within a spinous process, usually of a vertebra.

in·tra·splen·ic (in″truh·splen′ick, splee′nick) *adj.* Within the spleen.

in·tra·stro·mal (in″truh·stro′mul) *adj.* [*intra-* + *stromal*]. Within the stroma of an organ, part, or tissue.

in·tra·sy·no·vi·al (in″truh·si·no′vee·ul) *adj.* 1. Within a synovial cavity. 2. Within a synovial membrane.

in·tra·the·cal (in″truh·theek′ul) *adj.* [*intra-* + *thecal*]. In the subarachnoid space.

intrathecal therapy. Introduction into the spinal subarachnoid space of a therapeutic agent, such as an antibiotic or antimetabolite.

in·tra·tho·rac·ic (in″truh·tho·ras′ick) *adj.* [*intra-* + *thoracic*]. Within the thoracic cavity.

intrathoracic kidney. A kidney situated within the thoracic cavity, as in some cases of diaphragmatic hernia.

intrathoracic pressure. The pressure within the thoracic cavity; usually refers also to the pressure within the pleural cavity.

in·tra·ton·sil·lar (in″truh·ton′si·lur) *adj.* [*intra-* + *tonsillar*]. Within a tonsil.

in·tra·tra·che·al (in″truh·tray′kee·ul) *adj.* [*intra-* + *tracheal*]. Within the trachea.

intratracheal insufflation. Insufflation through an endotracheal tube introduced through the larynx into the trachea.

in·tra·tro·chan·ter·ic (in″truh·tro″kan·terr′ick) *adj.* Within a trochanter.

in·tra·tu·bal (in″truh·tew′bul) *adj.* [*intra-* + *tubal*]. Within a tube; specifically, within a uterine tube.

in·tra·tu·bu·lar (in″truh·tew′bew·lur) *adj.* [*intra-* + *tubular*]. Within a tubule.

in·tra·um·bil·i·cal (in″truh·um·bil′i·kul) *adj.* [*intra-* + *umbilical*]. Within the umbilicus.

in·tra·ure·ter·al (in″truh·yoo·ree′tur·ul) *adj.* [*intra-* + *ureteral*]. Within a ureter.

in·tra·ure·thral (in″truh·yoo·ree′thrul) *adj.* [*intra-* + *urethral*]. Within the urethra.

in·tra·uter·ine (in″truh·yoo′tur·in, ·ine) *adj.* [*intra-* + *uterine*]. Within the uterus.

intrauterine amputation. CONGENITAL AMPUTATION.

intrauterine asphyxia. FETAL ASPHYXIA.

intrauterine contraceptive device. Any mechanical device placed in the uterine cavity to prevent implantation or growth of the embryo. Abbreviated, IUD.

intrauterine dwarfism. Growth retardation evident at birth.

intrauterine fracture. A fracture occurring during fetal life, as in osteogenesis imperfecta.

intrauterine respiration. Respiration by the fetus before delivery.

in·tra·vag·i·nal (in″truh·vaj′i·nul) *adj.* [*intra-* + *vagina* + *-al*]. 1. Within the female vagina. 2. Within a tendon sheath.

in·trav·a·sate (in·trav′uh·sate) *n.* [*intra-* + L. *vas,* vessel]. The material accumulated in a tissue or organ by insudation.

in·tra·vas·cu·lar (in″truh·vas′kew·lur) *adj.* [*intra-* + *vascular*]. Within the blood vessels.

intravascular theory of erythrocyte formation. A theory that erythrocytes are formed inside delicate blood vessels in bone marrow from the lining of these vessels.

in·tra·ve·nous (in″truh·vee′nus) *adj.* [*intra-* + *venous*]. Within, or into, the veins.

intravenous anesthesia. The injection of an anesthetic into a vein, as thiopenthal sodium for general anesthesia or a local anesthetic for Bier block.

intravenous cholangiography. Roentgenologic demonstration of the biliary drainage system by the intravenous injection of an appropriate contrast agent.

intravenous pyelogram. A pyelogram in which the contrast material is given intravenously and excreted by the kidneys to permit their radiographic visualization; an intravenous urogram.

intravenous tension. The degree of stretch to which the wall of a vein is subjected by the pressure of the blood.

intravenous urography. EXCRETORY UROGRAPHY.

in·tra·ven·tric·u·lar (in″truh·ven·trick′yoo·lur) *adj.* [*intra-* + *ventricular*]. Located, or occurring, within a ventricle.

intraventricular conduction delay. INTRAVENTRICULAR HEART BLOCK. Abbreviated, IVCD.

intraventricular heart block. A prolongation of the QRS complex of the electrocardiogram, not fitting the criteria for a typical bundle branch block. See also *arborization block, parietal block, periinfarction block.*

in·tra·ver·te·bral (in″truh·vur′te·brul) *adj.* Within a vertebra.

in·tra·ves·i·cal (in″truh·ves′i·kul) *adj.* [*intra-* + *vesical*]. Within the urinary bladder.

in·tra·vi·tal (in″truh·vye′tul) *adj.* [*intra-* + *vital*]. Occurring during life; pertaining to the tissues or cells of living organisms. Compare *supravital.*

intravital stain. A dye, introduced by injection into the body of man or animal, which stains certain tissues or cells selectively; the stain must be minimally toxic so as not to kill cells. Syn. *vital stain.*

in·tra·zole (in′truh·zole) *n.* 1-(*p*-Chlorobenzoyl)-3-(1*H*-tetrazol-5-ylmethyl)indole, $C_{17}H_{12}ClN_5O$, an anti-inflammatory, also used as the sodium salt.

in·trin·sic (in·trin′sick) *adj.* [L. *intrinsecus,* inward]. Inherent; situated within; peculiar to a part; originating or due to causes or factors within a body, organ, or part.

intrinsic albuminuria. Albuminuria associated with renal glomerular disease.

intrinsic allergy. An allergic reaction in which the allergen may possibly originate within the body.

intrinsic asthma. Asthma caused by factors such as bronchial or other infection of the respiratory tract or by unknown factors. Contr. *extrinsic asthma.*

intrinsic deflection. The rapid downward deflection from the peak of maximum positivity to that of greatest negativity, as recorded directly when muscle underlying a surface electrode is depolarized during passage of an action potential.

intrinsic factor. A substance, produced by the stomach, which combines with the extrinsic factor (vitamin B_{12}) in food to yield an antianemic principle; lack of the intrinsic factor is believed to be a cause of pernicious anemia. Syn. *intrinsic factor of Castle.*

intrinsic muscle. A muscle that has both its origin and its insertion within an organ, as the transverse muscle of the tongue. Contr. *extrinsic muscle.*

intrinsic nerve supply. The nerves of an organ or structure which are entirely contained within that organ or structure, as the myenteric and submucous plexuses of the intestine. Contr. *extrinsic nerve supply.*

in·trin·si·coid deflection (in·trin′si·koid). 1. The deflection in precordial leads analogous to the intrinsic deflection in direct leads. 2. In clinical electrocardiography, the line extending from the apex of the R wave to the baseline or to the nadir of the S wave, representing passage of the ventricular activation process under the exploring electrode.

intrinsic thromboplastin. Any of several lipid-rich clot accelerators present in blood, primarily in blood platelets.

in·trip·ty·line (in·trip′ti·leen) *n.* 4-(5*H*-Dibenzo[*a,d*]cyclohepten-5-ylidene)-*N,N*-dimethyl-2-butynylamine, $C_{21}H_{19}N$, an antidepressant, used as the hydrochloride.

intro- [L.]. A prefix meaning *inward, into.*

in·tro·ces·sion (in″tro·sesh′un) *n.* [ML. *introcessio,* from L. *introcedere,* to go into]. A depression, as of a surface.

in·tro·fi·er (in′tro·figh·ur) *n.* [*intro-* + *-fier* as in emulsifier]. A liquid that aids emulsification by lowering the interfacial tension.

in·tro·flex·ion (in″tro·fleck′shun) *n.* [*intro-* + *flexion*]. A bending in; inward flexion.

in·troi·tus (in·tro′i·tus) *n.,* pl. **introitus** [L., entrance, from *introire,* to enter]. An aperture or entrance, particularly the entrance to the vagina. —**introi·tal** (·tul) *adj.*

in·tro·jec·tion (in″tro·jeck′shun) *n.* [*intro-* + *-jection,* from *jacere,* to throw, cast]. *In psychiatry* and *psychoanalysis,* the symbolic absorption into and toward oneself of concepts and feelings generated toward another person or object; an unconscious process which may serve as a defense against conscious recognition of overwhelming or intolerable impulses. Its effect in mental disorders is to motivate irrational behavior toward oneself, such as self-neglect or suicide arising from aggression stimulated by others, then introjected. Compare *incorporation, internalization.*

in·tro·mis·sion (in″tro·mish′un) *n.* [L. *intromittere, intromissus,* to send into]. Insertion, the act of putting in, the introduction of one body into another, as of the penis into the vagina.

in·tro·mit·tent (in″tro·mit′unt) *adj.* Conveying or allowing to pass into or within, as into a cavity; refers usually to the penis, which carries the semen into the vagina.

Intropin. A trademark for dopamine.

in·tro·spec·tion (in″tro·speck′shun) *n.* [L. *introspicere, introspectus,* to look into]. The act of looking inward, as into one's own mind and feelings.

introspective diplopia. PHYSIOLOGIC DIPLOPIA.

in·tro·sus·cep·tion (in″tro·suh·sep′shun) *n.* INTUSSUSCEPTION.

in·tro·ver·sion (in″tro·vur′zhun) *n.* [from *introvert* (verb)]. 1. A turning within, as a sinking within itself of the uterus. 2. *In psychiatry,* the preoccupation with oneself, with concomitant reduction of interest in the outside world. Contr. *extroversion.*

¹in·tro·vert (in″tro·vurt′) *v.* [*intro-* + L. *vertere,* to turn]. To turn one's interests to oneself rather than to external things.

²in·tro·vert (in′tro·vurt) *n.* A person whose interests are directed inwardly upon himself and not toward the outside world. Contr. *extrovert.*

introverted personality. An individual whose instinctual energy is weak and whose inadequate libido is directed inwardly.

in·trude, *v.* [L. *intrudere*, to force in]. To move a tooth apically.

in·tu·ba·tion (in″tew·bay′shun) *n.* The introduction of a tube into a hollow organ to keep it open, especially into the trachea to ensure the passage of air.

intubation tube. A tube for insertion through the larynx into the trachea to maintain an airway, primarily used in anesthesia or cardiopulmonary resuscitation.

in·tu·ba·tor (in′tew·bay″tur) *n.* An instrument used as a guide to facilitate intubation of the trachea.

in·tu·i·tion, *n.* [L. *intuitio*, from *intueri*, to look at, contemplate]. 1. Knowledge of something attained without conscious reasoning. 2. A sudden understanding or insight. —**intuition·al,** *adj.*

intuitional-type personality. An individual largely directed by unconscious indications or by vaguely conscious stimuli; one of Jung's functional types of personality.

in·tu·i·tive, *adj.* Knowing or known by intuition.

in·tu·mes·cence (in″tew·mes′unce) *n.* [L. *intumescere*, to swell up, from *tumere*, to swell or be swollen]. 1. A swelling of any kind, as an increase of the volume of any organ or part of the body. 2. The process of becoming swollen. 3. *Obsol. In neuroanatomy*, the cervical and lumbar enlargements. —**intumes·cent** (·unt) *adj.*

intumescent cataract. A cataract presenting a swollen appearance from breakdown of lens protein with an increase in osmotic pressure, resulting in imbibition of water.

in·tu·mes·cen·tia (in·tew″mee·sen′shee·uh) *n.*, pl. **intumescen·ti·ae** (·shee·ee) [NL.]. A swelling or enlargement; INTUMESCENCE.

intumescentia cer·vi·ca·lis (sur·vi·kay′lis) [NA]. CERVICAL ENLARGEMENT.

intumescentia lum·ba·lis (lum·bay′lis) [NA]. LUMBAR ENLARGEMENT.

intumescentia tym·pa·ni·ca (tim·pan′i·kuh) [BNA]. Ganglion tympanicum (= TYMPANIC GANGLION).

in·tus·sus·cep·tion (in″tuh·suh·sep′shun) *n.* [L. *intus*, within, *suscipere, susceptus*, to receive]. The receiving of one part within another; especially, the invagination, slipping, or passage of one part of the intestine into another, occurring usually in young children. Acute intussusception is characterized by paroxysmal pain, vomiting, the presence of a sausage-shaped tumor in the lower abdomen, and the passage of blood and mucus per rectum.

in·tus·sus·cep·tum (in″tuh·suh·sep′tum) *n.* [NL.]. In intussusception, the invaginated portion of intestine.

in·tus·sus·cip·i·ens (in″tuh·suh·sip′ee·enz) *n.* [NL.]. In intussusception, the segment of the intestine receiving the other segment.

in·u·la (in′yoo·luh) *n.* [L., from Gk. *helenion*]. The root of *Inula helenium*, of the family Compositae; contains inulin, a volatile oil, and certain crystallizable principles. It has been variously used for treatment of diseases. Syn. *elecampane.*

in·u·lase (in′yoo·lace, ·laze) *n.* An enzyme capable of converting inulin into levulose.

in·u·lin (in′yoo·lin) *n.* [*inul*a + *-in*]. A polysaccharide, $(C_6H_{10}O_5)_n$, in Jerusalem artichoke and certain other plants, made up of polymerized fructofuranose units, and yielding fructose on hydrolysis; used to measure glomerular filtration rate (inulin clearance).

in·unc·tion (in·unk′shun) *n.* [L. *inunctio*, from *in-* + *unguere*, to anoint]. 1. The act of rubbing an oily or fatty substance into the skin. 2. The substance thus used.

in ute·ro (in yoo′te·ro) [L.]. Within the uterus; not yet born.

in vac·uo (in vack′yoo·o) [L.]. In a vacuum; in a space from which most of the air has been exhausted.

in·vade, *v.* [L. *invadere*, from *in-* + *vadere*, to go]. To enter or penetrate into an area or sphere of which one is not naturally a part, usually with resultant injury to that part, as a virus invades a cell, or cancer invades healthy tissue. —**in·vad·er,** *n.*

in·vag·i·na·tion (in·vaj″i·nay′shun) *n.* [ML. *invaginare*, from L. *vagina*, sheath]. 1. The act of ensheathing or becoming ensheathed. 2. The process of burrowing or infolding to form a hollow space within a previously solid structure, as the invagination of the nasal mucosa within a bone of the skull to form a paranasal sinus. 3. INTUSSUSCEPTION. 4. *In embryology*, the infolding of a part of the wall of the blastula to form a gastrula. —**in·vag·i·nate** (in·vaj′i·nate) *v.*

¹in·va·lid (in′vuh·lid) *n.* [F. *invalide*, from L. *invalidus*, powerless, feeble, from *validus*, strong, healthy]. A person with a long-term, usually acquired, disability or illness which seriously limits self-sufficiency, as one confined to bed or wheelchair. —**invalid·ism** (·iz·um) *n.*

²in·val·id (in·val′id) *adj.* Not valid; unsound.

invariably lethal dose. The dose of an injurious agent (drug, virus, radiation) given to a population of animals or man, such that 100 percent die within a given time period. Symbol, LD 100. Contr. *median lethal dose.*

in·va·sin (in·vay′zin) *n.* HYALURONIDASE.

in·va·sion, *n.* [L. *invasio*, from *invadere*, to invade]. 1. One period in the course of disease, especially an infectious disease, during which the pathogen multiplies and is distributed preceding prodromal signs and symptoms. 2. The process whereby bacteria or other microorganisms enter the body. Compare *infection.*

in·va·sive (in·vay′siv) *adj.* 1. Tending to invade healthy cells or tissues; said of microorganisms or tumors. 2. Characterized by instrumental penetration of the viscera or nonsuperficial tissues of the body; said especially of diagnostic or therapeutic techniques such as biopsy, catheterization. —**invasive·ness** (·nis) *n.*

invasive mole. CHORIOADENOMA.

in·verse, *adj.* [L. *inversus*, inverted]. Inverted, reversed; reciprocal; opposite.

inverse Marcus Gunn phenomenon. MARÍN AMAT SYNDROME.

inverse temperature. Variations of body temperature through the day, opposite to normal, so that the morning temperature is higher than the evening temperature.

inverse voltage. The voltage between the filament cathode and the anode in a roentgen-ray tube during the part of the cycle that the anode is negatively charged, occurring only in a self-rectifying circuit.

Inversine. Trademark for mecamylamine, a ganglionic blocking agent used, as the hydrochloride salt, for treatment of hypertension.

in·ver·sion (in·vur′zhun) *n.* [L. *inversio*, from *invertere*, to turn upside down]. 1. Reversal in order, form, or structure; specifically, a change in configuration or orientation resulting in a structure that is inside out, upside down, backward, or opposite with respect to a prior or more usual one, as: *in chemistry*, the alteration of configuration about a chiral center to produce the enantiomorphic isomer, or, *in genetics*, the reattachment of a detached chromosome segment in its original place but reversed end for end, so that the order of its genetic material with respect to the rest of the chromosome is the opposite of what it was. 2. A turning inward. Contr. *eversion.* 3. HOMOSEXUALITY.

inversion of the bladder. A condition, occurring only in females, in which the urinary bladder is in part or completely pushed into the dilated urethra.

inversion of the foot. A turning of the sole of the foot inward, so that the medial margin is elevated.

inversion of the uterus. A rare condition in which the fundus of the uterus is forced or pulled through the cervix and comes into close contact with, or protrudes through, the os and even through the vagina.

in·ver·sive (in·vur′siv) *adj.* Characterizing or pertaining to enzymes which convert sucrose into invert sugar.

¹in·vert (in·vurt′) *v.* [*in* + L. *vertere*, to turn]. 1. To turn inside out, outside in, upside down; to reverse in position or relationship, especially from one that is natural to one less usual. 2. To turn inward. See also *inversion.*

²in·vert (in'vurt) *adj. & n.* 1. INVERTED. 2. A homosexual.

in·ver·tase (in·vur'tace, in'vur·taze) *n.* SACCHARASE.

in·ver·te·bral (in·vur'te·brul) *adj.* Without a spinal column; invertebrate.

in·ver·te·brate (in·vur'te·brut) *adj. & n.* [*in-* + *vertebrate*]. 1. Without a vertebral column. 2. Any animal without a vertebral column, including mainly achordates such as coelenterates, flatworms, nematodes, mollusks, annelids, echinoderms, and arthropods, but including also a few primitive chordates such as the lancelet *Amphioxus.*

in·vert·ed, *adj.* Subjected to inversion; reversed in position or orientation.

inverted image. An image that is turned upside down, such as the image produced on the retina by the convergence of rays coming from the object. Contr. *direct image.*

inverted Marcus Gunn phenomenon. MARÍN AMAT SYNDROME.

inverted oculocardiac reflex. Acceleration of the heart rate in response to compression of the eyeballs.

inverted radial reflex. Flexion of the fingers without flexion of the forearm when the lower end of the radius is tapped; presumed to indicate a lesion involving the fifth cervical segment of the spinal cord.

inverted testis. A testis that is so placed in the scrotum that the epididymis is attached to the anterior part of the gland.

in·vert·in (in·vurt'in, in'vur·tin) *n.* SACCHARASE.

in·ver·tose (in'vur·toce, ·toze) *n.* INVERT SUGAR.

invert sugar. A mixture of equal parts of glucose and levulose obtained by hydrolysis of sucrose, the sign of optical rotation having been inverted from (+) for sucrose, to (−) for the mixture.

in·vest, *v.* [ML. *investire,* from *in-* + *vestire,* to clothe]. To envelop, enclose, cover.

investing cartilage. ARTICULAR CARTILAGE.

investing technique. The process of enveloping or covering wholly or in part an object, such as a denture, artificial tooth, wax pattern, crown, band, or bar, with some form of heat-resisting material before curing, soldering, or casting.

in·vest·ment, *n.* A sheath; a covering.

in·vet·er·ate (in·vet'ur·ut) *adj.* [L. *inveteratus,* of long standing, from *vetus, veteris,* old]. Long established, chronic, resisting treatment.

in·vi·ril·i·ty (in"vi·ril'i·tee) *n.* IMPOTENCE.

in·vis·ca·tion (in"vis·kay'shun) *n.* [*in-* + L. *viscare,* to besmear]. 1. The mixing of saliva with food during chewing. 2. Smearing with mucilaginous material.

in·vis·i·ble differentiation. Differentiation that is determined but not yet apparent microscopically; CHEMODIFFERENTIATION.

in vi·tro (in vee'tro) [L.]. In glass; referring to a process or reaction carried out in a culture dish or test tube. Contr. *in vivo.*

in vi·vo (in vee'vo) [L.]. In the living organism. Contr. *ex vivo, in vitro.*

in·vo·lu·crum (in"vo·lew'krum) *n.,* pl. **involu·cra** (·kruh) [L., wrapper, cover]. 1. The covering of a part. 2. New bone laid down by periosteum around a sequestrum in osteomyelitis.

in·vol·un·tary, *adj.* [L. *involunterius*]. 1. Performed or acting independently of the will, as involuntary contractions of visceral muscles. See also *autonomic.* 2. Resulting from an irresistible impulse or accident, rather than from a conscious or purposeful act.

involuntary impulse. An impulse not activated by the will of the person, as the cardiac impulse.

involuntary movements. Unintentional bodily movements; applied particularly to movements that characterize extrapyramidal disorders, such as athetosis, chorea, and ballism.

involuntary muscle. Muscle not under the control of the will; usually consists of smooth muscle fibers and lies within a viscus, or is associated with skin.

involuntary nervous system. AUTONOMIC NERVOUS SYSTEM.

in·vo·lute (in'vo·lewt) *adj.* [L. *involutum,* from *involvere,* to roll up]. *In biology,* rolled up, as the edges of certain leaves in the bud.

in·vo·lu·tion (in"vo·lew'shun) *n.* [L. *involutio,* from *involvere,* to roll in, roll up]. 1. A turning or rolling inward. 2. The retrogressive change to their normal condition that certain organs undergo after fulfilling their functional purposes, as the uterus after pregnancy. 3. The period of regression or the process of decline or decay that occurs in all organ systems of the body after middle life. —**involution·al** (·ul) *adj.*

involutional arteriosclerosis. DISUSE ARTERIOSCLEROSIS.

involutional cyst. Cystic dilatation of glands or ducts during the course of involution of a gland, as in the mammary gland in abnormal involution.

involutional depression. INVOLUTIONAL MELANCHOLIA.

involutional melancholia. A sometimes prolonged severe mental disorder occurring in late middle life, usually characterized by depression and sometimes by paranoid ideas; manifested by excessive worry, narrow mental interests, lack of adaptability, severe insomnia, guilt, anxiety, agitation, delusional and nihilistic ideas, and somatic concerns.

involutional paranoid state. A paranoid psychosis with onset after middle life, characterized chiefly by delusion formation.

involutional paraphrenia. INVOLUTIONAL PARANOID STATE.

involutional psychosis. INVOLUTIONAL MELANCHOLIA.

involution form. A form seen in microorganisms that have undergone degenerative changes as a result of unfavorable environment or age.

involution of the uterus. The return of the uterus to its usual mass and physiologic state after childbirth.

in·ward aggression. Aggression, often destructive, directed toward the self.

io·ben·zam·ic acid (eye"o·ben·zam'ick). *N*-(3-Amino-2,4,6-triiodobenzoyl)-*N*-phenyl-*β*-alanine, $C_{16}H_{13}I_3N_2O_3$, a cholecystographic contrast medium.

io·car·mic acid (eye"o·kahr'mick). 5,5'-(Adipoyldiimino)bis-2,4,6-triiodo-*N*-methylisophthalamic acid, $C_{24}H_{20}I_6N_4O_8$, a radiopaque diagnostic aid.

io·ce·tam·ic acid (eye"o·se·tam'ick). *N*-Acetyl-*N*-(3-amino-2,4,6-triiodophenyl)-2-methyl-*β*-alanine, $C_{12}H_{13}I_3N_2O_3$, a radiopaque agent.

iod-, iodo-. A combining form meaning (a) *iodine;* (b) *violet.*

io·da·mide (eye·o'duh·mide, eye·od'uh·mide) *n.* 3-Acetamido-5-(acetamidomethyl)-2,4,6-triiodobenzoic acid, $C_{12}H_{11}I_3N_2O_4$, a radiopaque diagnostic agent.

Iod·amoe·ba (eye·o"duh·mee'buh, eye·od"uh·) *n.* [*iod-* + *amoeba*]. A genus of amebas.

Iodamoeba bütsch·lii (bootch'lee·eye). A species of small, sluggish ameba that is nonpathogenic but is parasitic in the large intestine of man.

Iodamoeba wil·liam·si (wil·yam'zye). *IODAMOEBA BÜTSCHLII.*

io·date (eye'o·date) *n.* Any salt of iodic acid.

iod·ic acid (eye·od'ick). A crystalline powder, HIO_3, soluble in water. In 1 to 3% solution it has been employed in the treatment of trachoma and indolent corneal ulcers.

io·dide (eye'uh·dide) *n.* Any binary compound, such as a salt or ester, containing iodine having a negative valence of 1.

io·dim·e·try (eye"o·dim'e·tree) *n.* [*iod-* + *-metry*]. Volumetric analysis by titration with an iodine solution.

io·din·at·ed I 125 serum albumin (eye'o·di·nay"tid). A preparation of normal human serum albumin containing radioactive iodine 125, used similarly to iodinated I 131 serum albumin but having the advantages of longer radiological half-life of the isotope and reduced radiation dose because iodine 125 emits no beta radiation and its gamma radiation is relatively soft.

iodinated I 131 serum albumin. A preparation of normal human serum albumin containing radioactive iodine 131 to facilitate quantitative determination of the albumin. Solutions of the preparation are used to determine blood or plasma volume and circulation time or cardiac output; also to aid detection and localization of brain tumors.

io·dine (eye'uh·dine, ·deen, ·din) *n.* [F. *iode,* from Gk. *ioeidēs,* violet-colored, from *ion,* violet]. I = 126.9045. A nonmetallic element occurring as gray-black plates or granules with metallic luster and characteristic odor. Sparingly soluble in water but more soluble in iodide solutions; soluble in 13 parts of alcohol or 80 parts of glycerin. A local irritant and germicide, generally applied for the latter purpose in the form of a 2 or 3% solution. Iodine is a normal constituent of the thyroid gland and essential for its proper functioning. See Table of Chemical Constituents of Blood in the Appendix.

iodine 131. A radioactive isotope of iodine, which emits beta and gamma rays, used in the form of sodium iodide in the diagnosis of thyroid disease and in the treatment of hyperthyroidism. Symbol, ^{131}I.

iodine antiseptic solution. IODINE TINCTURE.

iodine number. A measure of unsaturation of fats and fatty acids usually expressed as the number of grams of iodine capable of absorption by 100 g of the substance in question.

iodine pentoxide. I_2O_5. Iodic anhydride. A white, crystalline powder used in determining carbon monoxide content of gases.

iodine solution. A solution of 20 g iodine and 24 g sodium iodide in purified water to 1,000 ml; a local anti-infective.

iodine test for bile pigments. A test in which tincture of iodine is slowly poured into urine. The development of a green-blue color indicates bile pigments.

iodine test for starch. A test in which a potassium iodide solution of iodine reacts with starch to produce a blue color.

iodine tincture. A solution of iodine and sodium iodide in diluted alcohol; a local anti-infective.

iodine value. IODINE NUMBER.

iod·i·nin (eye·od'i·nin) *n.* A purple-bronze antibiotic pigment, $C_{12}H_8N_2O_4$, produced by *Chromobacterium iodinum;* it inhibits the growth of streptococci.

io·din·o·phil (eye"o·din'uh·fil) *adj.* & *n.* [*iodine* + *-phil*]. 1. Having an affinity for iodine stain. 2. A histologic element staining readily with iodine.

io·din·o·phile (eye"o·din'uh·file, ·fil) *adj.* & *n.* IODINOPHIL.

io·din·o·phil·ia (eye"o·din"uh·fil'ee·uh) *n.* IODOPHILIA.

io·din·o·phil·ic (eye"o·din"uh·fil'ick) *adj.* IODINOPHIL.

io·dip·a·mide (eye"o·dip'uh·mide) *n.* 3,3'-(Adipoyldiimino)-bis[2,4,6-triiodobenzoic acid], $C_{20}H_{14}I_6N_2O_6$, a roentgenographic contrast medium; used as the methylglucamine (meglumine) and sodium salts.

io·dism (eye'uh·diz·um) *n.* [*iod-* + *-ism*]. A condition arising from the excessive or prolonged use of iodine or iodine compounds; marked by frontal headache, coryza, ptyalism, and various skin eruptions, especially acne.

io·dize (eye'uh·dize) *v.* To impregnate with iodine. —**io·dized** (eye'uh·dize'd) *adj.*

iodized oil. An iodine addition product of vegetable oils, containing 38 to 42% of organically combined iodine. Used for the therapeutic effect of iodine and as an x-ray contrast medium.

iodo-. See *iod-*.

io·do·ac·e·tate (eye·o"do·as'e·tate, eye·od"o·) *n.* A salt or ester of iodoacetic acid.

iodoacetate index. The ratio of the smallest amount of iodoacetate that, under constant conditions, prevents heat coagulation of serum to the total protein concentration of the serum. A low index occurs after major surgery, in some cancers, and sometimes in other pathological states. Syn. *Huggins test, Huggins-Miller-Jensen test.*

io·do·ace·tic acid (eye·o"do·uh·see'tick). ICH_2COOH, a compound of importance in experimental biochemistry because it has the ability to interfere with phosphorylating enzyme activity, thereby inhibiting absorption of glucose.

io·do·al·phi·on·ic acid (eye·o"do·al"fee·on'ick). 3-(4-Hydroxy-3,5-diiodophenyl)-2-phenylpropionic acid, $C_{15}H_{12}I_2O_3$, used orally as a contrast medium in cholecystography.

io·do·chlor·hy·droxy·quin (eye·o"do·klor"high·drock'see·kwin) *n.* 5-Chloro-7-iodo-8-quinolinol, C_9H_5ClINO, a brownish-yellow powder; formerly used for treatment of amebiasis, trichomonas vaginitis, and coccogenic infections of the skin; now used mainly for treatment of dermatitides.

19-io·do·cho·les·ter·ol (eye·o"do·ko·les'tur·ol) *n.* $C_{27}H_{45}IO$, labelled with ^{131}I, used as a radiopaque for the adrenal gland to identify specific dysfunctions such as Cushing's disease, adrenal adenoma, and hyperaldosteronism.

io·do·der·ma (eye·o"do·dur"muh) *n.* [*iodo-* + *-derma*]. Skin eruption due to iodine; generally used in reference to a pustular eruption caused by the ingestion of iodine compounds.

io·do·form (eye·o'duh·form, eye·od'uh·) *n.* Triiodomethane, CHI_3, a yellow, crystalline powder, used locally as an antiseptic and anesthetic.

iodoform test for acetone. LIEBEN'S TEST.

io·do·gor·go·ic acid (eye·o"do·gor·go'ick). DIIODOTYROSINE.

io·dom·e·try (eye"o·dom'e·tree) *n.* [*iodo-* + *-metry*]. Usually, volumetric analysis for iodine present in, or liberated by, a compound. —**io·do·met·ric** (eye·o"duh·met'rick) *adj.*

io·do·pa·no·ic acid (eye·o"do·pa·no'ick). IOPANOIC ACID.

io·do·phe·nol (eye·o"do·fee'nole, ·nol, ·fe·nole') *n.* *p*-Iodophenol, C_6H_5IO; has been used as an antiseptic.

io·do·phil (eye·o'duh·fil, eye·od'o·fil) *adj.* & *n.* [*iodo-* + *-phil*]. IODINOPHIL.

io·do·phil·ia (eye·o"duh·fil'ee·uh, eye·od"o·) *n.* [*iodo-* + *-philia*]. A pronounced affinity for iodine; applied to the protoplasm of leukocytes in purulent conditions.

io·do·phor (eye·o'duh·fore, eye·od'o·fore) *n.* [*iodo-* + *-phor*]. A type of antiseptic in which iodine is combined with a detergent, a solubilizing agent, or other carrier in relatively stable form, which produces its effect by slow release of the iodine when in contact with tissues or bacteria.

io·do·phthal·ein (eye·o"do·thal'een) *n.* Tetraiodophenolphthalein, $C_{20}H_{10}I_4O_4$, formerly used as a local antiseptic. The disodium salt has been used as a radiopaque medium for cholecystography. Syn. *tetiothalein.*

io·dop·sin (eye"o·dop'sin) *n.* [*iod-,* violet, + *ops-* + *-in*]. The visual pigment found in the cones, consisting of retinene$_1$ combined with photopsin. Contr. *rhodopsin.*

io·do·pyr·a·cet (eye·o"do·pirr'uh·set) *n.* Diethanolamine 3,5-diiodo-4-pyridone-*N*-acetate, $C_{11}H_{16}I_2N_2O_5$, a radiopaque medium for urography, pyelography, and angiocardiography. Syn. *diodone.*

io·do·ther·a·py (eye·o"do·therr'uh·pee) *n.* [*iodo-* + *therapy*]. The treatment of disease by the use of iodine or iodide compounds.

io·do·thy·mol (eye·o"do·thigh'mol) *n.* THYMOL IODIDE.

io·do·thy·ro·glob·u·lin (eye"o·do·thigh"ro·glob'yoo·lin) *n.* [*iodo-* + *thyro-* + *globulin*]. An iodine-containing globulin found in the thyroid gland.

Iodotope-I 131. A trademark for sodium iodide I 131, a diagnostic and therapeutic radioisotope.

io·dox·am·ic acid (eye"o·dock·sam'ick). 3,3'-[Ethylenebis(oxyethyleneoxyethylenecarbonylimino)]-bis[2,4,6-triiodobenzoic acid], $C_{26}H_{26}I_6N_2O_{10}$, a radiopaque diagnostic aid.

io·dox·yl (eye″o·dock′sil) *n.* British name for sodium iodomethamate, a radiopaque medium.

io·glic·ic acid (eye″o·glis′ick). 5-Acetamido-2,4,6-triiodo-*N*-[(methylcarbamoyl)methyl]isophthalamic acid, $C_{13}H_{12}I_3N_3O_5$, a radiopaque diagnostic aid.

io·gly·cam·ic acid (eye″o·glye·kam′ick). 3,3′-(Diglycoloyldiimino)bis[2,4,6-triiodobenzoic acid], $C_{18}H_{10}I_6N_2O_7$, a radiopaque (cholecystographic) medium; used as the methylglucamine (meglumine) and sodium salts.

iom·e·ter (eye·om′e·tur) *n.* [*ion* + *-meter*]. A special type of monitor ionization chamber for the measurement of roentgen rays.

io·meth·in I 125 (eye″o·meth′in). 4-[[3-(Dimethylamino)propyl]amino]-7-iodo-^{125}I-quinoline, $C_{14}H_{18}$-$^{125}IN_3$, a radiopaque diagnostic agent. Also available with ^{131}I labelling (iomethin I 131).

-ion [Gk. neuter diminutive suffix]. A suffix meaning (a) *small;* (b) *craniometric point.*

ion (eye′on) *n.* [Gk. *iōn,* going (as toward an electrode), from *ienai,* to go]. An atom or group of atoms which, by a suitable application of energy (for example, by collision with alpha or beta particles or gamma rays, or by dissociation of a molecule), has lost or gained one or more orbital electrons and has thereby become capable of conducting electricity.

Ionamin. Trademark for phentermine, an anorexigenic drug prepared as a complex with an ion-exchange resin to provide sustained action.

ion exchange. The reversible exchange of ions in a solution with ions present in an ion exchanger.

ion-exchange chromatography. Separation of charged molecules by differential evolution from a column containing ion-exchange resin.

ion exchanger. A matrix of insoluble material, which may be inorganic or organic, interspersed with cations and anions, certain of which may participate in the exchange process.

ion-exchange resin. A synthetic polymer containing fixed ionizable groups capable of exchanging ions of opposite charge in a solution in contact with the polymer.

ion·ic (eye·on′ick) *adj.* Pertaining to, characterized by, or existing as ions.

ionic bond. A bond formed between two atoms when one or more electrons are transferred from one atom to another, thereby completing a stable electron configuration for each.

ionic strength. A measure of the intensity of the electric field in a solution; half the sum of the activity of each ion in solution, multiplied by the square of its ionic charge.

io·ni·um (eye·o′nee·um) *n.* A radioactive isotope of thorium.

ion·iza·tion (eye″un·i·zay′shun) *n.* The production of ions. —**ion·ize** (eye′un·ize) *v.;* **ion·iz·ing** (·eye·zing) *adj.*

ionization chamber. An instrument for collecting and measuring ions produced in a definite volume of air by a beam of roentgen rays or rays emitted from radioactive substances.

ionization current. A current produced in an ionized gas by an electric field.

ionization potential. The lowest potential capable of removing an electron from an atom.

ionizing event. Any occurrence of a process in which an ion or group of ions is produced, as by passage of alpha or beta particles or gamma rays through a gas.

ionizing radiation. Radiation which directly or indirectly produces ionization.

ion·om·e·ter (eye″on·om′e·tur) *n.* [*ion* + *-meter*]. An instrument for measuring dosages of ionizing radiation based upon the production of ions in air.

io·none (eye′uh·nohn) *n.* A mixture of isomeric ketones, $C_{13}H_{20}O$, used in perfumery.

ion·o·phore (eye·on′o·fore) *n.* [*ion* + *-phore*]. An organic substance, such as the potassium ionophore, valinomycin, which serves to transport either univalent or divalent cations across membranes.

iono·phose (eye·on′o·foze, eye′uh·no·foze) *n.* [Gk. *ion,* violet, + *phose*]. A violet phose.

ion·o·sphere (eye·on′uh·sfeer) *n.* [*ion* + *sphere*]. The part of the earth's atmosphere which is sufficiently ionized by solar ultraviolet radiation for the concentration of free electrons to affect the propagation of radio waves; extends outward an indefinite distance from the upper boundary of the stratosphere at roughly 70 or 80 kilometers from the earth's surface. Contr. *stratosphere, troposphere.*

ionto- [Gk. *iōn, iontos,* going, from *ienai,* to go]. A combining form meaning *ion, ionic.*

ion·to·pho·re·sis (eye·on″to·fo·ree′sis) *n.,* pl. **iontophore·ses** (·seez) [*ionto-* + *-phoresis*]. 1. ELECTROPHORESIS. 2. *In medicine,* a method of introducing therapeutic particles into the skin or other tissues by means of an electric current.

io·pa·no·ic acid (eye″o·pa·no′ick). 3-Amino-α-ethyl-2,4,6-triiodohydrocinnamic acid, $C_{11}H_{12}I_3NO_2$, a radiopaque medium for cholecystography. Syn. *iodopanoic acid.*

io·phen·dyl·ate (eye″o·fen′di·late) *n.* A mixture of isomers of ethyl iodophenylundecanoate, $C_{19}H_{29}IO_2$, a radiopaque medium for myelography, cisternography, and sialography.

io·phen·ox·ic acid (eye″o·fen·ock′sick). α-Ethyl-β-(3-hydroxy-2,4,6-triiodophenyl)propionic acid, $C_{11}H_{11}I_3O_3$, a radiopaque agent for cholecystography. Syn. *triiodoethionic acid.*

io·pho·bia (eye″o·fo′bee·uh) *n.* [Gk. *ios,* poison, + *-phobia*]. A morbid fear of poison or being poisoned.

io·pro·nic acid (eye″o·pro′nick). (±)-2-[[2-(3-Acetamido-2,4,6-triiodophenoxy)ethoxy]methyl]butyric acid, $C_{15}H_{18}I_3NO_5$, a cholecystographic diagnostic aid.

io·py·dol (eye″o·pye′dol) *n.* 1-(2,3-Dihydroxypropyl)-3,5-diiodo-4(1*H*)-pyridone, $C_8H_9I_2NO_3$, a radiopaque (bronchographic) medium.

io·py·done (eye″o·pye′dohn) *n.* 3,5-Diiodo-4(1*H*)-pyridone, $C_5H_3I_2NO$, a radiopaque (bronchographic) medium.

io·se·fam·ic acid (eye″o·se·fam′ick). 5,5′-(Sebacoyldiimino)bis[2,4,6-triiodo-*N*-methylisophthalmic acid], $C_{28}H_{28}I_6N_4O_8$, a radiopaque medium.

io·ser·ic acid (eye″o·serr′ick). *N*-[2-Hydroxy-1-(methylcarbamoyl)ethyl]-2,4,6-triiodo-5-(2-methoxyacetamido)isophthalamic acid, $C_{15}H_{16}I_3N_3O_7$, a radiopaque diagnostic aid.

io·su·met·ic acid (eye″o·soo·met′ick). *N*-Ethyl-2′,4′,6′-triiodo-3′-(methylamino)succinanilic acid, $C_{13}H_{15}I_3N_2O_3$, a radiopaque diagnostic aid.

io·tha·lam·ic acid (eye″o·thuh·lam′ick). 5-Acetamido-2,4,6-triiodo-*N*-methylisophthalamic acid, $C_{11}H_9I_3N_2O_4$, a roentgenographic contrast medium; used as the methylglucamine (meglumine) and sodium salts.

io·thio·ura·cil (eye″o·thigh″o·yoo′ruh·sil) *n.* 5-Iodo-2-thiouracil, $C_4H_3IN_2OS$, an antithyroid drug; used as the sodium derivative.

io·trox·ic acid (eye″o·trock′sick). 3,3′-[Oxybis-(ethyleneoxymethylenecarbonylimino)]-bis[2,4,6-triiodobenzoic acid], $C_{22}H_{18}I_6N_2O_9$, a radiopaque diagnostic aid.

ioxo·tri·zo·ic acid (eye·ock″so·trye·zo′ick). 3-(Acetylamino)-5-[(hydroxyacetyl)amino]-2,4,6-triiodobenzoic acid, $C_{11}H_9I_3N_2O_5$, a radiopaque diagnostic aid.

ip·e·cac (ip′e·kack) *n.* [Pg. *ipecacuanha,* from Tupi]. The dried rhizome and roots of *Cephaëlis ipecacuanha,* known as Rio or Brazilian ipecac, or of *C. acuminata,* known as Cartagena, Nicaragua, or Panama ipecac. It contains emetine, cephaeline, and other alkaloids, Used, in various dosage forms, as an emetic and nauseating expectorant.

ipecac and opium powder. DOVER'S POWDER.

"I"-per·so·na (eye′pur·so″nuh) *n.* The sum of all the cortical or discriminative functions of the human brain which produce sentiment and partitive feeling, as contrasted with the primary instinctual and affective functions which motivate the organism as a whole.

ip·o·mea, ip·o·moea (ip″o·mee′uh, eye″po·) *n.* [Gk. *ips*, woodworm, + h*omoios*, like]. The dried root of *Ipomoea orizabensis*, the resin of which has been used as a cathartic. Syn. *Mexican scammony, Orizaba jalap.*

iprin·dole (i·prin′dole) *n.* 5-[3-(Dimethylamino)propyl]-6,7,8,9,10,11-hexahydro-5*H*-cyclooct[*b*]indole, $C_{19}H_{28}N_2$, an antidepressant drug.

ipro·ni·a·zid (eye″pro·nigh′uh·zid) *n.* Isonicotinic acid 2-isopropylhydrazide, $C_9H_{13}N_3O$, formerly used as an antituberculosis drug and psychic energizer.

ipro·nid·a·zole (eye″pro·nid′uh·zole) *n.* 2-Isopropyl-1-methyl-5-nitroimidazole, $C_7H_{11}N_3O_2$, a drug used for treatment of histomoniasis.

iprox·a·mine (eye·prock′suh·meen) *n.* 5-[2-(Dimethylamino)ethoxy]carvacryl isopropyl carbonate, $C_{18}H_{29}NO_4$, a vasodilator used as the hydrochloride.

ip·sa·tion (ip·say′shun) *n.* [L. *ipse*, self]. MASTURBATION.

ip·si·lat·er·al (ip″si·lat′ur·ul) *adj.* [L. *ipse*, same, self, + *lateral*]. Situated on the same side, as for example paralytic (or similar) symptoms which occur on the same side as the lesion causing them. Contr. *contralateral.*

ip·si·ver·sive seizure (ip″si·vur′siv) [L. *ipse*, same, self, + *vertere, versus*, to turn]. A rare form of seizure in which movements of the eyes, head, neck, and body are toward the side of the epileptogenic focus.

IQ, I.Q. Abbreviation for *intelligence quotient.*

Ir Symbol for iridium.

iral·gia (eye·ral′juh, ·jee·uh) *n.* IRIDALGIA.

iras·ci·bil·i·ty (i·ras″i·bil′i·tee) *n.* [L. *irasci*, to be angry]. The quality of being choleric, irritable, or of hasty temper; frequently a symptom in some mental disorders.

Irgasan DP300. A trademark for triclosan, a disinfectant.

irid-, irido- [Gk. *iris, iridos*]. A combining form meaning *iris.*

iridaemia. IRIDEMIA.

iri·dal (eye′ri·dul, irr′i·dul) *adj.* Pertaining to the iris.

iri·dal·gia (eye″ri·dal′jee·uh, irr″i·) *n.* [*irid-* + *-algia*]. Pain referable to the iris.

irid·aux·e·sis (eye″ri·dawk·see′sis, irr″i·) *n.* [*irid-* + *auxesis*]. Auxesis or tumefaction of the iris.

irid·avul·sion (eye″ri·duh·vul′shun, irr″i·) *n.* [*irid-* + *avulsion*]. Surgical avulsion of the iris; iridoavulsion. See also *iridectomy.*

iri·dec·tome (eye″ri·deck′tome, irr″i·) *n.* A cutting instrument used in iridectomy.

iri·dec·to·mize (eye″ri·deck′tuh·mize, irr″i·) *v.* To excise a part of the iris; to perform iridectomy.

iri·dec·to·my (eye″ri·deck′tuh·mee, irr″i·) *n.* [*irid-* + *-ectomy*]. The cutting out of part of the iris.

iri·dec·tro·pi·um (eye″ri·deck·tro′pee·um, irr″i·) *n.* [NL., from *irid-* + Gk. *ektropion*, eversion]. Eversion of a part of the iris; ECTROPION IRIDIS.

iri·de·mia, iri·dae·mia (eye″ri·dee′mee·uh, irr″i·) *n.* [*irid-* + *-emia*]. Hemorrhage of the iris.

iri·den·clei·sis (eye″ri·den·klye′sis, irr·i·) *n.*, pl. **iridenclei·ses** (·seez) [*irid-* + Gk. *enklein*, to shut in]. An operation, as for glaucoma, in which, in addition to inclusion of iris in the wound, a piece of limbus may be excised to permit better drainage of aqueous humor under the conjunctiva.

iri·den·tro·pi·um (eye″ri·den·tro′pee·um, irr″i·) *n.* [NL., from *irid-* + Gk. *entropē*, turning toward, inward]. Inversion of a part of the iris.

iri·de·re·mia (eye″ri·de·ree′mee·uh, irr·i·) *n.* [*irid-* + Gk. *erēmia*, absence]. Total or partial absence of the iris.

irides. Plural of *iris.*

ir·i·des·cence (irr″i·des′unce) *n.* A rainbow-like display of intermingling and changing colors, as in mother-of-pearl. —**irides·cent** (·unt) *adj.*

irid·e·sis (i·rid′e·sis, eye″ri·dee′sis) *n.* [*irid-* + *-desis*]. IRIDOTASIS.

iri·di·ag·no·sis (eye″ri·dye″ug·no′sis, irr″i·) *n.* IRIDODIAGNOSIS.

irid·i·al (eye·rid′ee·ul, i·rid′) *adj.* IRIDAL.

iridial angle. FILTRATION ANGLE.

irid·i·an (eye·rid′ee·un, i·rid′) *adj.* IRIDAL.

irid·ic (eye·rid′ick, i·rid′ick) *adj.* Pertaining to the iris.

Iriditope. A trademark for cobalt-60 and iridium-192 radioactive gamma sources.

irid·i·um (i·rid′ee·um, eye·rid′ee·um) *n.* Ir = 192.2. An element of the platinum family; alloyed in small proportion with platinum, it confers rigidity upon the latter.

iri·di·za·tion (irr″i·di·zay′shun) *n.* The appearance of an iridescent halo, seen by persons affected with glaucoma.

irido-. See *irid-.*

iri·do·avul·sion (eye″ri·do·a·vul′shun, irr″i·) *n.* [*irido-* + *avulsion*]. Avulsion of the iris.

iri·do·cap·su·li·tis (eye″ri·do·kap·sue·lye′tis, irr″i·) *n.* [*irido-* + *capsule* + *-itis*]. Inflammation involving the iris and the capsule of the lens.

iri·do·cap·su·lot·o·my (eye″ri·do·kap″sue·lot′uh·mee, irr″i·) *n.* [*irido-* + *capsule* + *-tomy*]. An incision through the iris and adherent secondary membrane to create a pupillary opening.

iri·do·cele (i·rid′o·seel, eye·rid′o·, irr″i·do·) *n.* [*irido-* + *-cele*]. Protrusion of part of the iris through a wound or ulcer.

iri·do·cho·roid·itis (eye″ri·do·ko″roy·dye′tis, irr″i·) *n.* [*irido-* + *choroid* + *-itis*]. Inflammation of both the iris and the choroid of the eye.

iri·do·col·o·bo·ma (eye″ri·do·kol″uh·bo′muh, irr″i·) *n.* [*irido-* + *coloboma*]. A coloboma of the iris.

iri·do·cor·ne·al angle (eye″ri·do·kor′nee·ul, irr″i·do·). The angle marking the periphery of the anterior chamber of the eye, formed by the attached margin of the iris and the junction of the sclera and cornea and functioning as a drainage route for aqueous humor. Syn. *anterior chamber angle, filtration angle.* NA *angulus iridocornealis.*

iri·do·cy·clec·to·my (eye″ri·do·si·kleck′tuh·mee, irr″i·) *n.* [*irido-* + *cycl-* + *-ectomy*]. En bloc excision of the iris and of the ciliary body.

iri·do·cy·cli·tis (eye″ri·do·sigh·klye′tis, irr″i·) *n.* [*irido-* + *cycl-* + *-itis*]. Inflammation of the iris and the ciliary body; IRITIS.

iri·do·cy·clo·cho·roid·itis (eye″ri·do·sigh″klo·ko″roy·dye′tis, irr″i·) *n.* [*irido-* + *cyclo-* + *choroid* + *-itis*]. Combined inflammation of the iris, the ciliary body, and the choroid; uveitis.

iri·do·cys·tec·to·my (eye″ri·do·sis·teck′tuh·mee, irr″i·) *n.* [*irido-* + *cyst-* + *-ectomy*]. An operation for making a new pupil; the edge of the iris and the capsule are drawn out through an incision in the cornea and cut off.

iri·do·cyte (irr′i·do·site, eye·rid′o·site) *n.* [*irido-* + *-cyte*]. A special cell in which an insoluble substance, guanine (2-amino-6-oxypurine), is deposited in crystalline form.

iri·dod·e·sis (eye″ri·dod′e·sis, irr″i·) *n.* [*irido-* + *-desis*]. IRIDOTASIS.

iri·do·di·ag·no·sis (eye″ri·do·dye″ug·no′sis, irr″i·) *n.* [*irido-* + *diagnosis*]. Diagnosis of disease from examination of the iris.

iri·do·di·al·y·sis (eye″ri·do·dye·al′i·sis, irr″i·) *n.* [*irido-* + *dialysis*]. A separation of the base of the iris from its normal insertion.

iri·do·di·la·tor (eye″ri·do·dye·lay′tur, irr″i·do·) *n.* [*irido-* + *dilator*]. Anything which dilates the iris.

iri·do·do·ne·sis (eye″ri·do·do·nee′sis, irr″i·) *n.*, pl. **irido·done·ses** (·seez) [*irido-* + Gk. *donein*, to shake]. Quivering movements of the iris with motion of the eye, seen in aphakia or as a sign of subluxation of the lens; HIPPUS.

iri·do·ki·ne·sia (eye″ri·do·kigh·nee′zee·uh, irr″i·) *n.* [*irido-* + *-kinesia*]. Any movement of the iris, normal or otherwise, as in contracting and dilating the pupil.

iri·do·ki·ne·sis (eye″ri·do·ki·nee′sis, ·kigh·nee′sis, irr″i·) *n.* IRIDOKINESIA.

iri·do·ma·la·cia (eye″ri·do·ma·lay′shuh, ·see·uh, irr″i·) *n.* [*irido-* + *malacia*]. Pathologic softening of the iris.

ir·id·on·co·sis (eye″ri·dong·ko′sis, irr″i·) *n.* [*irid-* + *oncosis*]. Thickening of the iris.

iri·do·pa·ral·y·sis (eye″ri·do·puh·ral′i·sis, irr″i·) *n.* [*irido-* + *paralysis*]. IRIDOPLEGIA.

iri·do·pa·re·sis (eye″ri·do·pa·ree′sis, ·păr′e·sis, irr″i·) *n.* [*irido-* + *paresis*]. A slight or partial paralysis of the smooth muscle of the iris.

iri·dop·a·thy (eye″ri·dop′uth·ee, irr″i·) *n.* [*irido-* + *-pathy*]. 1. Any disease of the iris. 2. A degenerative disease of the iris generally localized to the pigment epithelium. Consists of vacuoles forming in the pigment epithelium and can occur in diabetes and in some systemic mucopolysaccharidoses.

iri·do·plat·i·num (irr″i·do·plat′i·num) *n.* An alloy of iridium and platinum; used in making electrodes.

iri·do·ple·gia (eye″ri·do·plee′jee·uh, irr″i·) *n.* [*irido-* + *-plegia*]. Paralysis of the sphincter pupillae of the iris.

iri·dop·to·sis (irr″i·dop·to′sis, eye″ri·) *n.*, pl. **iridopto·ses** (·seez) [*irido-* + *-ptosis*]. Prolapse of the iris.

iri·do·pu·pil·lary (eye″ri·do·pew′pi·lerr·ee, irr″i·) *adj.* [*irido-* + *pupillary*]. Pertaining to the iris and the pupil.

iri·do·rhex·is, iri·dor·rhex·is (eye″ri·do·reck′sis, irr″i·) *n.*, pl. **iridorhex·es, iridorrhex·es** (·seez) [*irido-* + *-rrhexis*]. 1. Rupture of the iris. 2. The tearing away of the iris from its attachment.

iri·dos·chi·sis (eye″ri·dos′ki·sis, irr″i·) *n.*, pl. **iridoschi·ses** (·seez) [*irido-* + *-schisis*]. A pathologic process characterized by separation of the anterior portions of the iris stroma from the deeper portions. Eventually, the inner-layer fibers may break, with free ends floating in the aqueous humor.

iri·do·schis·ma (eye″ri·do·skiz′muh, irr″i·) *n.* [*irido-* + Gk. *schisma*, cleft]. IRIDOCOLOBOMA.

iri·do·scle·rot·o·my (eye″ri·do·skle·rot′uh·mee, irr″i·) *n.* [*irido-* + *sclero-* + *-tomy*]. Puncture of the sclera with division of the iris.

iri·do·ste·re·sis (eye″ri·do·ste·ree′sis, irr″i·) *n.* [*irido-* + Gk. *sterēsis*, loss]. IRIDEREMIA.

iri·dot·a·sis (eye″ri·dot′uh·sis, irr″i·) *n.*, pl. **iridota·ses** (·seez) [*irido-* + Gk. *tasis*, a stretching]. Stretching the iris, as in glaucoma; in place of iridotomy. The stretched iris is left in the wound, under the conjunctiva. See also *iridencleisis.*

iri·do·tome (eye″ti·duh·tome, irr″i·) *n.* [*irido-* + *-tome*]. An instrument for incising the iris. See also *keratome.*

iri·dot·o·my (eye″ri·dot′uh·mee, irr″i·) *n.* [*irido-* + *-tomy*]. A small incision into the iris.

iri·dot·ro·mos (eye″ri·dot′ruh·mus, irr″i·) *n.* [*irido-* + Gk. *tromos*, trembling]. HIPPUS.

iris (eye′ris) *n.*, genit. **iri·dis** (eye′ri·dis), L. pl. **iri·des** (eye′ri·deez) [L., from Gk., rainbow, colored halo; iris] [NA]. The anterior portion of the uvea of the eye, suspended in the aqueous humor from the ciliary body. Its posterior surface rests on the lens, hence it separates the anterior and posterior chambers. It is perforated by the adjustable pupil. It consists of loose stroma with radial vessels and melanocytes, a layer of smooth muscle (sphincter and dilator of the pupil), and pigmented epithelium. The two smooth muscles control the size of the pupil; one, circularly arranged in the pupillary border, forms the sphincter pupillae; the other, radially arranged, is the dilator pupillae. The color is governed by the number of melanocytes in the stroma. See also Plate 19.

Iris, *n.* [L., from Gk.]. A genus of plants of the Iridaceae. The dried rhizome of *Iris versicolor* (blue flag iris) has been used as a cathartic, emetic, and diuretic.

iris block glaucoma. Pupillary block glaucoma, which may be the mechanism of glaucoma in narrow-angle glaucoma.

iris bom·bé (bom·bay′) [F.]. A condition in which the iris bulges forward at the periphery due to an accumulation of the intraocular fluid in the posterior chamber; due to seclusion of the pupil.

iris contraction reflex. PUPILLARY REFLEX (1).

iris diaphragm. A device for changing or regulating the amount of light directed upon an object under the microscope.

iris hernia. Prolapse of the iris after iridectomy or following trauma.

Irish moss. See *Chondrus crispus.*

iris inclusion operation. 1. IRIDENCLEISIS. 2. IRIDOTASIS.

iris pigment. The pigment contained in the melanocytes in the stroma of the iris and the iris pigment epithelium.

iris scissors. Scissors having flat blades bent in such a manner that they may be applied to the eyeball.

iri·tis (eye·rye′tis, irr·eye′tis) *n.* [*iris* + *-itis*]. 1. Inflammation of the iris. 2. Inflammation of the iris and the ciliary body; IRIDOCYCLITIS. —**irit·ic** (eye·rit′ick) *adj.*

iri·to·ec·to·my (eye″ri·to·eck′tuh·mee, irr″i·to·) *n.* [*irito-* (as in *iritomy*) + *-ectomy*]. The removal of a portion of the iris for occlusion of the pupil.

irit·o·my (eye·rit′uh·mee, i·rit′uh·mee) *n.* [*iris* + *-tomy*]. IRIDOTOMY.

iron, *n.* Fe = 55.847. A silver-white or gray, hard, ductile, malleable metal. Iron forms two classes of salts: ferrous, in which it has a valence of 2; and ferric, in which it has a valence of 3. In medicine, iron is used in the form of one of its salts in the treatment of certain anemias, especially of the hypochromic type. See also Table of Chemical Constituents of Blood in the Appendix.

iron alum. FERRIC AMMONIUM SULFATE.

iron and ammonium acetate solution. A solution formerly widely used as a hematinic and diuretic. Syn. *Basham's mixture.*

iron and ammonium citrate. FERRIC AMMONIUM CITRATE.

iron and potassium tartrate. Ferric potassium tartrate, approximately $K(FeO)C_4H_4O_6.xH_2O$; formerly used for treatment of iron-deficiency anemia.

iron arsenate. Ferrous arsenate, $Fe_3(AsO_4)_2.6H_2O$, formerly used for its arsenic content in chronic skin affections.

iron ascorbate. Ferrous ascorbate. A purple powder, soluble in water; has been used for treatment of anemia.

iron by hydrogen. REDUCED IRON.

iron cacodylate. Ferric cacodylate, approximately $Fe[(CH_3)_2AsO_2]_3$; has been used for treatment of chlorosis and other anemias.

iron chloride. FERRIC CHLORIDE.

iron choline citrate. FERROCHOLINATE.

iron-deficiency anemia. Hypochromic microcytic anemia due to excessive loss, deficient intake, or poor absorption of iron.

iron-dextran complex. A colloidal solution of ferric hydroxide in complex with partially hydrolyzed dextran of low molecular weight; used parenterally for treatment of iron-deficiency anemias.

iron enzyme. One of the group of enzymes that contain iron in the prosthetic group.

iron gluconate. FERROUS GLUCONATE.

iron glycerophosphate. FERRIC GLYCEROPHOSPHATE.

iron hydroxide. FERRIC HYDROXIDE.

iron iodide. FERROUS IODIDE.

iron lactate. FERROUS LACTATE.

iron lung. A metal tank respirator which encloses the body up to the neck; alternating negative and positive pressure within the respirator produces expansion and contraction of the patient's chest, inducing artificial breathing. Syn. *artificial lung, Drinker respirator.*

iron oxide. Ferric oxide, Fe_2O_3, the color of which varies from red to yellow depending on the degree of hydration. See also *limonite, hematite.*

iron pheophytin. A chlorophyll derivative in which the

magnesium has been replaced by iron; it has been used in anemias.

iron-porphyrin protein. One of a large group of proteins which contain iron and porphyrin; these include hemoglobin, the cytochromes, cytochrome oxidase, catalase, and peroxidase.

iron-porphyrin-protein enzymes. Iron porphyrin proteins with enzymic function.

iron resorcin fuchsin. WEIGERT'S STAIN.

iron sor·bi·tex (sor'bi·tecks). A sterile, colloidal solution of a complex of trivalent iron, sorbitol, and citric acid, stabilized with dextrin and sorbitol; a hematinic preparation.

iron sulfate. FERROUS SULFATE.

irot·o·my (eye·rot'uh·mee) *n.* IRIDOTOMY.

ir·ra·di·ate (i·ray'dee·ate) *v.* [L. *irradiare,* to shine forth, from *radius,* ray]. To treat with radiation, either roentgen rays or radiation from radioactive isotopes; to expose to radiation.

irradiated ergosterol. ERGOCALCIFEROL. See also *vitamin D.*

ir·ra·di·a·tion (i·ray''dee·ay'shun) *n.* Exposure to radiation such as infrared, ultraviolet, roentgen rays, gamma rays.

irradiation cataract. A slowly developing cataract, beginning peripherally and progressing centrally in the posterior cortex, occurring 6 months to 2 years after prolonged or intense exposure to radium or roentgen rays. Syn. *cyclotron cataract, radiation cataract.*

irradiation cystitis. Inflammation of the urinary bladder, which may follow exposure to any of the modalities of radiation therapy to the pelvic organs.

ir·ra·tio·nal, *adj.* 1. Contrary to reason or logical thinking. 2. Of a personality type, tending to rely on the affective, intuitive domains, rather than on reason and logic.

ir·re·duc·ible (irr''e·dew'si·bul) *adj.* Not reducible; not capable of being replaced in a normal position.

irreducible hernia. A hernia that cannot be returned through the opening by manipulation; usually due to hyperemia, adhesions, and edema, or to blocking by fecal impaction; INCARCERATED HERNIA.

ir·reg·u·lar articulation. A type of synovial joint in which the surfaces are small, irregular, flat, or slightly curved.

irregular astigmatism. Astigmatism in which different parts of the meridian have varying refractive powers.

irregular dentin. SECONDARY DENTIN.

ir·reg·u·lar·i·ty, *n. In medicine,* a deviation from a rhythmic activity or regular interval.

irregular pulse. A pulse in which the interval between beats, or the force of successive beats, or both vary.

ir·re·me·able (i·ree'mee·uh·bul) *adj.* [L. *irremeabilis,* from *in-,* not, + *remeare,* to go back, from *meare,* to go, pass]. IRREVERSIBLE.

ir·re·me·di·a·ble, *adj.* [L. *irremediabilis,* from *remedium,* remedy]. Not capable of correction.

ir·re·sist·ible impulse test. *In forensic medicine,* a test for determining criminal responsibility, which holds that a person cannot be held criminally responsible for an act demonstrably committed as the result of an irresistible impulse. This is based on the assumption that mental disorders produce sudden, spontaneous impulses to commit illegal acts. Compare *Durham decision, M'Naghten rule.*

ir·re·sus·ci·ta·ble (irr''e·sus'si·tuh·bul) *adj.* Not capable of being resuscitated or revived.

ir·re·vers·i·ble, *adj.* Not capable of being reversed; characterizing a state or process from which recovery is impossible. —**irre·ver·si·bil·i·ty,** *n.*

irreversible colloid. A colloid which, on being precipitated or otherwise separated from its dispersion medium, cannot be restored to its original state merely by adding the dispersion medium.

irreversible emphysema. EMPHYSEMA (1).

irreversible gel. A gel transformed from a sol, which cannot be reversed to a sol.

ir·ri·ga·tion *n.* [L. *irrigatio,* from *irrigare,* to irrigate, from *rigare,* to water]. The act of washing out by a stream of water, as irrigation of the urinary bladder or a wound.

ir·ri·ga·tor (irr'i·gay''tur) *n.* An apparatus, or device, for accomplishing the irrigation or washing of a part, surface, or cavity.

ir·ri·ta·bil·i·ty, *n.* 1. A condition or quality of being excitable; the ability to respond to a stimulus. 2. A condition of abnormal excitability of an organism, organ, or part, when it reacts excessively to a slight stimulation.

ir·ri·ta·ble, *adj.* 1. Capable of reacting to appropriate stimuli. 2. Easily excited; susceptible of irritation. 3. Likely to become disturbed, or otherwise mentally distraught.

irritable bladder. A condition in which there is frequent desire to urinate with inability to perform the act perfectly.

irritable colon. Any of a variety of disturbances of colonic function, with accompanying emotional tension, which participate in the general bodily adaptation to nonspecific stress. Syn. *adaptive colitis, mucous colitis, spastic colon, unstable colon.*

irritable heart. NEUROCIRCULATORY ASTHENIA.

ir·ri·tant, *adj. & n.* 1. Causing or giving rise to irritation. 2. An agent that induces irritation.

irritant poison. A poison that causes irritation at the point of entrance or at the point of elimination.

irritant smoke. *Obsol.* VOMITING GAS.

ir·ri·ta·tion, *n.* [L. *irritatio,* from *irritare,* to irritate]. 1. A condition of excitement or irritability. 2. The act of irritating or stimulating. 3. The stimulus necessary to elicit a response.

ir·ru·ma·tion (irr''oo·may'shun) *n.* [L. *irrumatio,* from *irrumare,* to suckle]. FELLATIO.

IR wave. Abbreviation for *isovolumetric relaxation wave.*

is-, iso- [Gk. *isos,* equal, level]. A combining form indicating (a) *equality, similarity, uniformity;* (b) in biology, *for or from different individuals of the same species;* (c) in chemistry, *a compound isomeric with another, or a compound with a straight chain of carbon atoms containing a functional group at one end and an isopropyl group at the opposite end.* Symbol, *i-.*

Isaac's granules [R. *Isaacs,* U.S. physician b.1891]. Small solitary refractile granules seen in normal erythrocytes in unstained and vitally stained moist preparations.

Isacen. Trademark for acetphenolisatin, a laxative.

isa·del·phia (eye''suh·del'fee·uh, iss''uh·) *n.* [*is-* + Gk. *adelphos,* brother, + *-ia*]. Conjoined twins united by unimportant tissues; each body is normal in the development of all essential organs.

Isam·bert's disease (ee·zah^{n}·behr') [E. *Isambert,* French physician, 1827–1876]. Tuberculous ulceration of the larynx and pharynx.

is·aux·e·sis (eye''sawk·see'sis) *n.* [*is-* + *auxesis*]. A type of relative growth in which a part grows at the same rate as the whole organism or other part.

isch-, ischo- [Gk. *ischein,* to check]. A combining form meaning *suppression, checking, stoppage,* or *deficiency.*

isch·emia, isch·ae·mia (is·kee'mee·uh) *n.* [Gk. *ischaimos,* styptic (from *ischein,* to check, + *haima,* blood) + *-ia*]. Local diminution in the blood supply, due to obstruction of inflow of arterial blood or to vasoconstriction; localized tissue anemia. —**isch·emic, isch·ae·mic** (is·kee'mick) *adj.*

ischemic contracture. Shortening of muscle, often with fibrosis, due to interference with the blood supply. See also *Volkmann's contracture.*

ischemic myositis. Inflammatory reaction in muscle due to marked reduction of blood supply, as by prolonged tight bandaging of a fracture.

ischemic necrosis. Death of tissue due to lack of blood flow.

ischemic nephrosis. Acute renal failure presumably due to renal vascular ischemia.

ischemic neuropathy or **neuritis.** Lesions of a nerve or nerves with reflex, sensory, and motor loss of the parts involved, associated with occlusion of the blood vessels to the nerve, as in atherosclerosis, diabetes, thromboangiitis obliterans, polyarteritis nodosa, surgical ligation of an artery, or prolonged use of a tourniquet.

ischemic paralysis. Inability to move a part due to stoppage of the circulation, as in certain cases of embolism or thrombosis.

ischemic tubulorrhexis. Severe necrosis of renal tubular cells, including the renal tubular basement membranes, the etiology of which is thought to be renal vascular ischemia.

is·che·sis (is·kee'sis, is'ki·sis) *n.* [Gk. *ischein*, to check, staunch]. Retention of a discharge or secretion.

ischi-, ischio-. A combining form meaning *ischium, ischial.*

ischia. Plural of *ischium.*

is·chi·ad·ic (is"kee·ad'ick) *adj.* [Gk. *ischiadikos*]. ISCHIAL; SCIATIC.

ischiadic hernia. SCIATIC HERNIA.

ischiadic nerve. SCIATIC NERVE.

is·chi·al (is'kee·ul) *adj.* Of or pertaining to the ischium.

ischial bursa. 1. (of the gluteus maximus muscle:) A small bursa between the gluteus maximus and the ischial tuberosity. NA *bursa ischiadica musculi glutei maximi.* 2. (of the obturator internus muscle:) The bursa between the tendon of the obturator internus and the ischial tuberosity; the obturator bursa. NA *bursa ischiadica musculi obturatorii interni.*

is·chi·al·gia (is"kee·al'jee·uh) *n.* [*ischi-* + *-algia*]. *Obsol.* SCIATICA. —**ischial·gic** (·jick) *adj.*

ischial spine. SPINE OF THE ISCHIUM.

ischial tuber or **tuberosity.** A protuberance on the posterior portion of the superior ramus of the ischium, upon which the body rests in sitting. NA *tuber ischiadicum.*

is·chi·at·ic (is"kee·at'ick) *adj.* ISCHIAL; SCIATIC.

ischiatic artery. SCIATIC ARTERY.

is·chi·a·ti·tis (is"kee·uh·tye'tis) *n.* [*ischiat*ic + *-itis*]. *Obsol.* Inflammation of the sciatic nerve.

is·chi·dro·sis (is"ki·dro'sis) *n.* [*isch-* + h*idrosis*]. Suppression of the secretion of sweat. —**ischi·drot·ic** (·drot'ick) *adj.*

is·chi·ec·to·my (is"kee·eck'tuh·mee) *n.* [*ischi-* + *-ectomy*]. Resection of the ischium.

ischio-. See *ischi-.*

is·chio·bul·bo·sus (is"kee·o·bul·bo'sus) *n.* A variable part of the bulbospongiosus muscle. See also Table of Muscles in the Appendix.

is·chio·cap·su·lar (is"kee·o·kap'sue·lur) *adj.* [*ischio-* + *capsular*]. Pertaining to the ischium and the fibrous capsule of the hip, as in ischiocapsular ligament of the hip joint.

is·chio·ca·ver·no·sus (is"kee·o·kav"ur·no'sus) *n.* A muscle arising from the ischium, encircling each crus of the penis or clitoris. NA *musculus ischiocavernosus.* See also Table of Muscles in the Appendix.

is·chio·cav·ern·ous (is"kee·o·kav'ur·nus) *adj.* [*ischio-* + *cavernous*]. Pertaining to the ischium and one or both of the corpora cavernosa of the penis or clitoris.

is·chio·coc·cyg·e·al (is"kee·o·cock·sij'ee·ul) *adj.* [*ischio-* + *coccygeal*]. Pertaining to the ischium and the coccyx.

is·chio·coc·cyg·e·us (is"kee·o·kock·sij'ee·us) *n.* COCCYGEUS.

is·chio·did·y·mus (is"kee·o·did'i·mus) *n.* [*ischio-* + *-didymus*]. ISCHIOPAGUS.

is·chio·fem·o·ral (is"kee·o·fem'uh·rul) *adj.* Pertaining to the ischium and the femur, as the ischiofemoral ligament of the hip joint.

ischiofemoral ligament. A wide, strong band in the hip joint, attached to the ischium just beneath and behind the margin of the acetabulum and passing to the greater trochanter and the trochanteric fossa. NA *ligamentum ischiofemorale.*

is·chio·fem·o·ra·lis (is"kee·o·fem·o·ray'lis) *n.* An occasional slip of the gluteus maximus muscle, attached to the ischial tuberosity.

is·chi·om·e·lus (is"kee·om'e·lus) *n.* [*ischio-* + *-melus*]. An individual with an accessory limb attached in the ischial region.

is·chio·my·e·li·tis (is"kee·o·migh"e·lye'tis) *n.* [*ischio-* + *myelitis*]. Lumbar myelitis.

is·chio·neu·ral·gia (is"kee·o·new·ral'jee·uh) *n.* [*ischio-* + *neuralgia*]. *Obsol.* SCIATICA.

is·chi·op·a·gus (is"kee·op'uh·gus) *n.* [*ischio-* + *-pagus*]. Conjoined twins united by their sacral or ischial regions.

ischiopagus tet·ra·pus (tet'ruh·pus) [Gk. *tetrapous*, quadruped]. An ischiopagus with four legs.

ischiopagus tri·pus (trye'pus) [Gk. *tripous*, three-footed]. An ischiopagus with three legs.

is·chi·op·a·gy (is"kee·op'uh·jee) *n.* [*ischio-* + *-pagy*]. The condition exhibited by an ischiopagus.

is·chio·pu·bic (is"kee·o·pew'bick) *adj.* [*ischio-* + *pubic*]. Pertaining to the ischial and pubic bones.

is·chio·pu·bi·cus (is"kee·o·pew'bi·kus) *n.* A variable part of the sphincter urethrae muscle.

is·chio·pu·bi·ot·o·my (is"kee·o·pew·bee·ot'uh·mee) *n.* [*ischio-* + *pubio-* + *-tomy*]. *Obsol.* Division of the ischial and pubic rami in otherwise impossible labor.

is·chio·pu·bis (is"kee·o·pew'bis) *n.* 1. The site of junction of the ischium and the pubis. 2. The ischium and pubis considered together. —**ischiopu·bic** (·bick) *adj.*

is·chio·rec·tal (is"kee·o·reck'tul) *adj.* Pertaining to both the ischium and the rectum.

ischiorectal fascia. The fascia covering the perineal aspect of the levator ani muscle and filling the ischiorectal fossa.

ischiorectal fossa. The region on either side of the rectum, bounded laterally by the obturator internus muscle, medially by the levator ani and coccygeus muscles, and posteriorly by the gluteus maximus muscle. NA *fossa ischiorectalis.*

ischiorectal hernia. PERINEAL HERNIA.

ischiorectal region. The region corresponding to the posterior part of the pelvic outlet, between the ischium and the rectum.

ischiorectal space. ISCHIORECTAL FOSSA.

is·chi·um (is'kee·um) *n.*, genit. **is·chii** (is'kee·eye), pl. **is·chia** (·kee·uh) [L., hip joint, from Gk. *ischion*] [NA]. The inferior part of the hipbone; the bone upon which the body rests in sitting. NA *os ischii.* See also Table of Bones in the Appendix and Plate 2.

ischium-pubis index. The ratio (length of pubis × 100/(length of ischium) by which the sex of an adult pelvis may be determined in most cases, the index being greater than 90 in the female, and less than 90 in the male.

isch·no·pho·nia (isk"no·fo'nee·uh) *n.* [Gk. *ischnophōnia*, from *ischnophōnos*, having a speech impediment (from *ischnos*, feeble, + *phōnē*, voice)]. STAMMERING.

ischo-. See *isch-.*

is·cho·ga·lac·tia (is"ko·guh·lack'tee·uh, ·shee·uh) *n.* [*ischo-* + *galact-* + *-ia*]. Suppression of the normal flow of milk.

is·cho·ga·lac·tic (is"ko·guh·lack'tick) *adj.* & *n.* [*ischo-* + *galactic*]. 1. Suppressing the secretion of milk. 2. An agent that suppresses the secretion of milk.

is·cho·gy·ria (is"ko·jye'ree·uh) *n.* [*ischo-* + *gyr-* + *-ia*]. *Obsol.* A jagged appearance of the cerebral convolutions, produced by atrophy.

is·cho·me·nia (is"ko·mee'nee·uh) *n.* [*ischo-* + *men-* + *-ia*]. Suppression of the menstrual flow.

isch·uria (is·kew'ree·uh) *n.* [Gk. *ischouria*, from *ischein*, to hold back, + *ouron*, urine]. Retention or suppression of the urine. See also *anuria.* —**isch·uret·ic** (is"kew·ret'ick) *adj.*

is·ei·ko·nia (eye"sigh·ko'nee·uh) *n.* [*is-* + Gk. *eikōn*, image, + *-ia*]. The condition in which the images are of equal size in the two eyes. Syn. *isoiconia.* Contr. *aniseikonia.*

is·ei·kon·ic lens (eye"sigh·kon'ick) [*is-* + *eikonic*, iconic]. A temporary lens, known as a fitover; may be of two kinds, over-all or meridional.

is·ethi·o·nate (eye″se·thigh′o·nate) *n.* Any salt or ester of isethionic acid.

is·ethi·on·ic acid (eye″se·thigh·on′ick) *n.* 2-Hydroxyethanesulfonic acid, $HOCH_2CH_2SO_3H$, an acid sometimes used to prepare crystallizable salts of organic bases.

Ishi·ha·ra's test [S. *Ishihara,* Japanese ophthalmologist, b.1879]. A color vision test made by using a series of plates upon which are printed round dots of various sizes, colors, and combinations.

isin·glass (eye′zing·glas″, eye′zin·) *n.* [D. *huizenblas* (*obsol.*), lit., sturgeon's bladder]. ICHTHYOCOLLA.

is·land, *n.* 1. An isolated structure; particularly, a group of cells differentiated from the surrounding tissue by staining or arrangement. 2. INSULA.

island of Lang·er·hans (lahng′ur·hahnss) [P. *Langerhans,* German physician and anatomist, 1847–1888]. ISLET OF THE PANCREAS.

island of Reil (rile) [J. C. *Reil,* German anatomist and physician, 1759–1813]. INSULA.

is·let, *n.* [MF. *islette,* dim. of *isle,* island]. A small island.

islet-cell adenoma. ISLET-CELL TUMOR.

islet-cell carcinoma. An islet-cell tumor of aggressive behavior as demonstrated by metastasis.

islet-cell tumor. A benign tumor arising from cells of the islets of the pancreas, clinically classified as functioning, producing insulin or other polypeptide hormones, or as nonfunctioning. Syn. *Langerhansian adenoma, insuloma.*

islet of Lang·er·hans (lahng′ur·hahnss) [P. *Langerhans*]. ISLET OF THE PANCREAS.

islet of the pancreas. One of the small irregular islands of cell cords, found in the pancreas; it has no connection with the functioning duct system, and is delimited from the acini by a reticular membrane. It is of an endocrine nature, as indicated by its great vascularity, and consists mainly of alpha and beta cells, the former secreting a hormone believed to be glucagon, and the latter secreting insulin. The islets also secrete a growth-homone-release-inhibiting factor, somatostatin. Syn. *island of Langerhans.*

-ism [Gk. *-isma, -ismos,* noun-forming suffixes]. A suffix indicating (a) *a condition or disease resulting from or involving,* as embolism, alcoholism; (b) *a doctrine or practice,* as Freudianism, hypnotism; (c) *-ismus.*

Ismelin. Trademark for guanethidine, a potent hypotensive drug used as the sulfate salt.

-ismus [L., from Gk. *-ismos,* noun-of-action suffix]. A suffix meaning *spasm, contraction, displacement.*

iso-. See *is-.*

iso·ag·glu·ti·nin (eye″so·uh·gloo′ti·nin) *n.* [*iso-* + *agglutinin*]. An agglutinin which acts upon the cells of members of the same species.

iso·ag·glu·ti·no·gen (eye″so·a·gloo′ti·no·jen, ·ag″lew·tin′o·jen) *n.* [*iso-* + *agglutinogen*]. An antigen which distinguishes the cells of some individuals from those of other individuals of the same species.

iso·aj·ma·line (eye″so·aj′muh·leen) *n.* An alkaloid from *Rauwolfia serpentina.*

iso-al·co·hol·ic elixir (eye″so·al·kuh·hol′ick). An elixir of the particular alcohol concentration which is most suitable for the intended medicament. It is prepared by combining in suitable proportions a high-alcoholic elixir and a low-alcoholic elixir, the former containing 73 to 78% of alcohol, the latter 8 to 10%. Syn. *iso-elixir.*

iso·al·lox·a·zine (eye″so·a̤·lock′suh·zeen) *n.* The tricyclic compound benzo[*g*]pteridine-2,4(3*H*,10*H*)dione, $C_{10}H_6N_4O_2$; an isomer of alloxazine. Derivatives of the compound are widely distributed in plants and animals and include such substances as riboflavin and the *yellow* enzymes; these substances are sometimes incorrectly named as derivatives of alloxazine. 2. Loosely, any derivative of isoalloxazine.

isoalloxazine adenine dinucleotide. FLAVIN ADENINE DINUCLEOTIDE.

isoalloxazine mononucleotide. RIBOFLAVIN 5′-PHOSPHATE.

iso·am·yl alcohol (eye″so·am′il). 3-Methyl-1-butanol or fermentation amyl alcohol, $(CH_3)_2CHCH_2CH_2OH$, a colorless liquid of disagreeable odor. It constitutes the major portion of fusel oil, which name is commonly applied to technical isoamyl alcohol.

iso·am·yl·a·mine (eye″so·am″il·uh·meen′, ·am″il·am′een, ·in) *n.* A ptomaine, $C_5H_{11}NH_2$, formed by the putrefaction of yeast.

isoamyl nitrite. AMYL NITRITE.

iso·an·dros·ter·one (eye″so·an·dros′tur·ohn) *n.* EPIANDROSTERONE.

iso·an·ti·body (eye″so·an′ti·bod″ee) *n.* [*iso-* + *antibody*]. An antibody in certain members of a species against cells or cell constituents of certain other members of the same species.

iso·an·ti·gen (eye″so·an′ti·jin) *n.* [*iso-* + *antigen*]. An antigen found in an animal, capable of stimulating the production of a specific antibody in some other animal of the same species but not in itself.

iso·bar (eye′so·bahr) *n.* [*iso-* + Gk. *baros,* weight]. 1. Any one of two or more atoms which have the same atomic mass but different atomic numbers. 2. A line drawn through points having equal barometric or manometric pressure. —**iso·bar·ic** (eye″so·băr′ick) *adj.*

iso·bas·tique point (eye″so·bas′tick). ISOBESTIC POINT.

iso·bes·tic point (eye″so·bes′tick). *In applied spectroscopy,* the wavelength at which the absorbance of two substances, one of which can be converted into the other, is the same.

iso·bor·nyl thio·cy·a·no·ac·e·tate (eye″so·bor′nil thigh″o·sigh″un·o·as′e·tate). Terpinyl thiocyanoacetate, $C_{13}H_{19}NO_2S$, a yellow, oily liquid, practically insoluble in water; the technical grade, which contains 82% or more of isobornyl thiocyanoacetate, is used as a pediculicide and insecticide.

iso·bu·caine (eye″so·bew′kain) *n.* 2-Isobutylamino-2-methylpropyl benzoate, $C_{15}H_{23}NO_2$, a local anesthetic used as the hydrochloride salt.

iso·bu·tyl (eye″so·bew′til) *n.* The univalent hydrocarbon radical $(CH_3)_2CHCH_2$—.

isobutyl alcohol. 3-Methyl-1-propanol, $(CH_3)_2CHCH_2OH$, a colorless, flammable liquid, soluble in water; it is produced by fermentation of carbohydrates and is a constituent of fusel oil. Used as a solvent.

iso·car·box·a·zid (eye″so·kahr·bock′suh·zid) *n.* 1-Benzyl-2-(5-methyl-3-isoxazolylcarbonyl)hydrazine, $C_{12}H_{13}N_3O_2$, a monoamine oxidase inhibitor used in treating mental depression and angina pectoris.

iso·cel·lo·bi·ose (eye″so·sel″o·bye′oce) *n.* A disaccharide formed during hydrolysis of cellulose.

iso·cel·lu·lar (eye″so·sel′yoo·lur) *adj.* [*iso-* + *cellular*]. Composed of cells of the same size or character.

iso·cho·les·ter·ol (eye″so·ko·les′tur·ol) *n.* A substance isolated from wool fat; originally considered to be a sterol but now believed to consist of several complex terpene alcohols.

iso·chore (eye′so·kore) *n.* [*iso-* + Gk. *chōra,* space]. A curve showing the variation of pressure with temperature of a substance, the volume of which is maintained constant. —**iso·chor·ic** (eye″so·kor′ick) *adj.*

iso·chro·mat·ic (eye″so·kro·mat′ick) *adj.* [*iso-* + *chromatic*]. Having the same color throughout.

iso·chro·ma·to·phil (eye″so·kro′muh·to·fil, ·kro·mat′o·) *adj.* [*iso-* + *chromato-* + *-phil*]. Of cells and tissues: equally stainable by the same dye.

iso·chro·ma·to·phile (eye″so·kro′muh·to·file, ·fil, ·kro·mat′o·) *adj.* ISOCHROMATOPHIL.

iso·chro·mo·some (eye″so·kro′muh·sohm) *n.* [*iso-* +

chromosome]. An abnormal chromosome with a medial centromere which arises through transverse splitting of the centromere rather than the normal longitudinal splitting between two chromatids so that the arms are identical.

isoch·ro·nal (eye·sock'ruh·nul, eye''so·kro'nul) *adj.* [Gk. *isochronos,* from *isos,* equal, + *chronos,* time]. Occurring at or occupying equal intervals of time. —**isochro·nism** (·niz·um) *n.*

isoch·ro·nous (eye·sock'ruh·nus) *adj.* ISOCHRONAL.

iso·cit·ric acid (eye''so·sit'rick). An intermediate compound, $HOOCCH_2CH(OH)COOH$, in the tricarboxylic acid cycle.

isocitric dehydrogenase. The enzyme that, in the presence of nicotinamide adenine dinucleotide phosphate, converts L-isocitric acid to oxalosuccinic acid.

iso·com·ple·ment (eye''so·kom'ple·munt) *n.* [*iso-* + *complement*]. A complement from an individual of the same species.

iso·co·na·zole (eye''so·ko'nuh·zole) *n.* 1-[2,4-Dichloro-β-[2,6-dichlorobenzyl)oxy]phenethyl]imidazole, $C_{18}H_{14}Cl_4N_2O$, an antifungal, antibacterial agent; also used as the nitrate salt.

iso·co·ria (eye''so·ko'ree·uh) *n.* [*iso-* + *cor-* + *-ia*]. Equality in diameter of the two pupils.

iso·cor·tex (eye''so·kor'tecks) *n.* [*iso-* + *cortex*]. The parts of the cerebral cortex exhibiting the six characteristic layers or strata, each layer having certain predominant cells and histologic features common to all isocortical areas; NEOCORTEX. Syn. *homogenetic cortex.*

iso·cy·a·nide (eye''so·sigh'uh·nide) *n.* Any organic compound of the formula RNC, isomeric with but differing from RCN, which is a cyanide. On hydrolysis a cyanide (RCN) yields RCOOH and NH_3; an isocyanide (RNC) yields RNH_2 and HCOOH (formic acid). Syn. *carbylamine, isonitrile.*

iso·cy·tol·y·sin (eye''so·sigh·tol'i·sin, ·sigh''to·lye'sin) *n.* [*iso-* + *cytolysin*]. A cytolysin capable of acting against the cells of other animals of the same species.

iso·dac·tyl·ism (eye''so·dack'ti·liz·um) *n.* [*iso-* + *-dactylism*]. The condition of having fingers or toes of equal length. —**isodacty·lous** (·lus) *adj.*

iso·di·a·phere (eye''so·dye'uh·feer) *n.* [*iso-* + Gk. *diapherein,* to differ]. One of two or more species of atoms which have the same difference between the numbers of neutrons and protons in their respective nuclei.

iso·dont (eye'so·dont) *adj.* [*is-* + *-odont*]. *In zoology,* having teeth of the same size and shape.

iso·dose (eye''so·doce) *adj.* [*iso-* + *dose*]. Pertaining to surfaces that receive equal radiation intensities.

isodose curve. A graphic presentation of the distribution of radiation dosage about a radiant source usually consisting of lines connecting points of equal doses.

isodose pattern or **plot.** A graphic presentation of the distribution of radiation dosage from one or more radiant sources.

iso·do·ses (eye''so·do'seez) *n.pl.* [*iso-* + Gk. *doses,* pl. of *dosis,* contribution]. Surfaces of equal radiation intensities in irradiated tissue.

iso·dul·ci·tol (eye''so·dul'si·tol) *n.* RHAMNOSE.

iso·dy·nam·ic (eye''so·dye·nam'ick, ·di·nam'ick) *adj.* [Gk. *isodynamos*]. Having or generating equal amounts of force, or energy, as isodynamic foods. —**isody·nam·ia** (·nam'ee·uh) *n.*

isodynamic law. In metabolism, different foods are interchangeable in accordance with their caloric values.

iso·elec·tric (eye''so·e·leck'trick) *adj.* [*iso-* + *electric*]. Having the same electric properties throughout.

isoelectric focusing. A separation technique in which a mixture of protein molecules is resolved into its components by subjecting the mixture to an electric field in a supporting gel in which a pH gradient has been generated. Syn. *electrofocusing.*

isoelectric level or **line.** *In electrocardiography,* the zero position of the string, needle, pen, or heated stylus of a galvanometer when no current from the heart is flowing through it. The base line of the electrocardiogram, from which all deflections are measured.

isoelectric period. A period of the cardiac cycle when there is no potential to be recorded on the electrocardiogram.

isoelectric point. The pH at which the concentration of an amphoteric electrolyte in cation form equals that in anion form; the pH at which the net electric charge on the electrolyte is zero.

iso-elix·ir (eye''so·e·lick'sur) *n.* ISO-ALCOHOLIC ELIXIR.

iso·en·zyme (eye''so·en'zime) *n.* [*iso-* + *enzyme*]. Any of the electrophoretically distinct forms of an enzyme having the same function. Syn. *isozyme.*

iso·er·y·throl·y·sis (eye''so·err·i·throl'i·sis) *n.* Erythrocytolysis caused by an isoimmune mechanism.

iso·eth·a·rine (eye''so·eth'uh·reen) *n.* 3,4-Dihydrox-α-[1-(isopropylamino)propyl]benzyl alcohol, $C_{13}H_{21}NO_3$, a bronchodilator drug.

iso·feb·ri·fu·gine (eye''so·feb''ri·few'jeen) *n.* An alkaloid, possessing some antimalarial activity, isolated from the herb *Dichroa febrifuga,* which is the probable source of Chinese antimalarial drug ch'ang shan. Isofebrifugine may be identical with α-dichroine.

iso·flur·ane (eye''so·floo'rane) *n.* 1-Chloro-2,2,2-trifluoroethyl difluoromethyl ether, $C_3H_2ClF_5O$, an inhalation anesthetic.

iso·flu·ro·phate (eye''so·floo'ro·fate) *n.* Diisopropyl phosphorofluoridate, $[(CH_3)_2CHO]_2PFO$, a colorless, oily liquid. It is a powerful inhibitor of cholinesterase, produces marked and prolonged miosis, and is used topically in the treatment of a variety of ophthalmic afflictions.

iso·gam·ete (eye''so·gam'eet) *n.* [*iso-* + *gamete*]. A reproductive cell, similar in form and size to the cell with which it unites; found in certain protozoans and thallophytes.

isog·a·my (eye·sog'uh·mee) *n.* [*iso-* + *-gamy*]. Sexual union between gametes of similar form and structure. —**isoga·mous** (·mus) *adj.*

iso·gen·e·sis (eye''so·jen'e·sis) *n.* [*iso-* + *-genesis*]. Identity of origin of development.

iso·gen·ic (eye''so·jen'ick) *adj.* [*iso-* + *-genic*]. Having the same genotype. Contr. *allogenic.*

isog·en·ous (eye·soj'e·nus) *adj.* [*iso-* + *-genous*]. 1. ISOGENIC. 2. Characterized by isogenesis.

iso·ger·mine (eye''so·jur'meen) *n.* An isomeric form of germine, obtained from the latter under certain conditions of chemical treatment.

isog·na·thous (eye·sog'nuth·us, eye''so·nath'us) *adj.* [*iso-* + *-gnathous*]. Having jaws of equal size.

iso·graft (eye''so·graft) *n.* [*iso-* + *graft*]. A graft between a genetically identical donor and recipient; transplantation of tissues between identical twins.

iso·hem·ag·glu·ti·nin, iso·haem·ag·glu·ti·nin (eye''so·hee''muh·gloo'ti·nin, eye''so·hem''uh·) *n.* [*iso-* + *hemagglutinin*]. An agglutinin in the serum of an individual which agglutinates the red blood cells of another individual of the same species.

iso·he·mol·y·sin, iso·hae·mol·y·sin (eye''so·he·mol'i·sin) *n.* [*iso-* + *hemolysin*]. A hemolysin produced by injecting red blood cells into an animal of the same species. An isohemolysin will destroy the red blood cells of any animal of the same species except the immunized individual. Syn. *isolysin.* —**iso·he·mo·lyt·ic, iso·hae·mo·lyt·ic** (eye''so·hee''mo·lit'ick, ·hem''o·) *adj.*

iso·he·mol·y·sis, iso·hae·mol·y·sis (eye''so·he·mol'i·sis) *n.* [*iso-* + *hemolysis*]. The hemolytic action of an isohemolysin.

iso·hy·dric (eye''so·high'drick) *adj.* [*iso-* + *hydr-* + *-ic*].

Pertaining to a solution having the same hydrogen-ion concentration as another so that no change in the concentration of this ion takes place when the solutions are mixed.

isohydric shift. The reversible binding and release of protons by the imidazole nitrogen of the histidine residues in hemoglobin, due to the difference in pK_a of reduced hemoglobin and oxyhemoglobin. This process allows the transport of the majority of hydrogen ions formed from carbonic acid, with no change in blood pH.

iso·ico·nia, iso·iko·nia (eye″so·eye·ko′nee·uh) *n.* [*iso-* + *icon* + *-ia*]. ISEIKONIA. —**iso·icon·ic** (·eye·kon′ick) *adj.*

iso·im·mune (eye″so·i·mewn′) *adj.* Pertaining to or characterized by isoimmunization.

isoimmune hemolytic disease of the newborn. ERYTHROBLASTOSIS FETALIS.

iso·im·mu·ni·za·tion (eye″so·im″yoo·ni·zay′shun) *n.* [*iso-* + *immunization*]. Immunization of a species of animal with antigens of the same species; for example, the development of anti-Rh serum may be produced by transfusing Rh-positive blood into an Rh-negative individual or by an Rh-negative woman being pregnant with an Rh-positive fetus.

iso·ion·ic point (eye″so·eye·on′ick). The pH at which the number of protons dissociated from proton donors in a system equals the number of protons combined with proton acceptors. In solutions in which a protein is the only ionic species present, the isoionic point is identical with the isoelectric point.

iso·lac·tose (eye″so·lack′toce, ·toze) *n.* [*iso-* + *lactose*]. A disaccharide synthesized by the action of a lactase on a solution of glucose and galactose.

iso·lat·er·al (eye″so·lat′ur·ul) *adj.* 1. IPSILATERAL. 2. Equilateral.

iso·la·tion, *n.* [It. *isolato,* isolated, from *isola,* island]. 1. *In medicine,* the separation of a patient from the rest of the community or from other patients because of a communicable disease or for other reasons. 2. *In psychoanalysis,* the dissociation of an idea or memory from its emotional content or the feelings attached to it, or from other facts related to it, so as to render it a matter of indifference; a common defense mechanism against anxiety. 3. *In microbiology,* the derivation of a pure culture of an organism. 4. *In chemistry,* the purification or separation of a substance or compound. 5. *In physiology and experimental medicine,* the separation of cells, a body part, organ, tissue, or system from the organism for the purpose of studying its functions. —**iso·late,** *v.*

iso·lec·i·thal (eye″so·les′i·thul) *adj.* [*iso-* + *lecithal*]. Having yolk evenly distributed in the ovum, usually in small amount.

Isolette. Trade name for a self-contained incubator permitting isolation and manipulations of an infant, usually a premature or neonate requiring special care.

iso·leu·cine (eye″so·lew′seen, ·sin) *n.* α-Amino-β-methylvaleric acid, $C_2H_5CH(CH_3)CH(NH_2)COOH$; an essential amino acid.

iso·leu·cyl (eye″so·lew′sil) *n.* The univalent radical, $CH_3CH_2CH(CH_3)CH(NH_2)CO$—, of the amino acid isoleucine.

isol·o·gous (eye·sol′uh·gus) *adj.* [*isologue* + *-ous*]. ISOGENIC.

iso·logue, iso·log (eye′so·log) *n.* One of a series of compounds of similar structure, but having different atoms of the same valency and usually of the same periodic group.

iso·ly·ser·gic acid (eye″so·lye·sur′jick). The parent constituent, $C_{16}H_{16}N_2O_2$, along with lysergic acid, of certain ergot alkaloids; it may be obtained from such alkaloids by hydrolysis.

iso·ly·sin (eye″so·lye′sin, eye·sol′i·sin) *n.* ISOHEMOLYSIN.

iso·mal·tose (eye″so·mahl′toce) *n.* An isomer of maltose claimed to be produced by the action of certain enzymes upon maltose.

iso·mer (eye′suh·mur) *n.* [*iso-* + *-mer*]. 1. One of two or more compounds having the same molecular formula but differing in the relative positions of the atoms within the molecule. See also *isomerism.* 2. *In nuclear science,* one of two or more nuclides with the same numbers of neutrons and protons in the nucleus, but with different energy.

isom·er·ase (eye·som′ur·ace, ·aze) *n.* An enzyme that catalyzes an intramolecular rearrangement with the formation of an isomeric compound, such as the interconversion of aldose and ketose sugars.

iso·mer·ic (eye″so·merr′ick) *adj.* 1. Pertaining to isomerism. 2. Existing as an isomer of another substance.

isom·er·ide (eye·som′ur·ide, ·id) *n.* One of two or more compounds that have similar structural groups but not necessarily the same number of atoms.

isom·er·ism (eye·som′ur·iz·um) *n.* The relationship between two isomers. The phenomenon wherein two or more compounds possess the same molecular formula but differ in the relative position of the atoms within the molecule and may have different properties.

isom·er·iza·tion (eye·som″ur·i·zay′shun) *n.* Conversion of one isomer to another. —**isomer·ize** (·ize) *v.*

iso·meth·a·done (eye″so·meth′uh·dohn) *n.* 1,6-Dimethylamino-4,4-diphenyl-5-methyl-3-hexanone; an oily liquid, $C_{21}H_{27}NO$; the levorotatory isomer has been employed as an analgesic and narcotic, though it is not as active as methadone.

iso·me·thep·tene (eye″so·me·thep′teen) *n.* *N*,1,5-Trimethyl-4-hexenylamine, $C_9H_{19}N$, an antispasmodic and vasoconstrictor drug used as the hydrochloride or mucate salt.

iso·met·ric (eye″so·met′rick) *adj.* [Gk. *isometros,* of equal measure]. 1. Having equal measurements in several dimensions. 2. Characterized by maintenance of equal distance, area, or volume.

isometric contraction. Contraction of muscle characterized by increase in tension without significant shortening of the length of the fibers. 2. Contraction of the cardiac ventricles characterized by increase in tension without volume change as the heart valves are closed. Syn. *isovolumetric contraction.* Contr. *isotonic contraction.*

isometric exercise. Muscular exercise in which contraction, and bodily movement ordinarily produced thereby, is counteracted in equal force by opposing muscles, in the same individual.

isometric interval or **period**. ISOVOLUMETRIC INTERVAL.

iso·me·tro·pia (eye″so·me·tro′pee·uh) *n.* [*iso-* + *metr-* + *-opia*]. Equality of kind and degree in the refraction of the two eyes.

isom·e·try (eye·som′e·tree) *n.* [Gk. *isometria*]. Equality of measurement. See also *Cieszynski's rule of isometry.*

iso·morph (eye′so·morf) *n.* [*iso-* + *-morph*]. 1. *In chemistry,* one of two or more substances of different composition which have the same crystalline form. 2. *In chemistry,* one of a group of elements whose compounds with the same other atoms or radicals have the same crystalline form. 3. *In biology,* an animal or plant having superficial similarity to another which is phylogenetically different.

iso·mor·phic (eye″so·mor′fick) *adj.* [*iso-* + *-morphic*]. 1. Identical or similar in form or structure. 2. *In genetics,* descriptive of genotypes of polysomic or polyploid organisms which, although containing the same number of linked genes in different combinations on homologous chromosomes, yet are similar in the series of gametes which they can produce. 3. *In chemistry,* pertaining to similar crystalline forms. —**isomor·phism** (·fiz·um) *n.*

isomorphic gliosis. ISOMORPHOUS GLIOSIS.

iso·mor·phous (eye″so·mor′fus) *adj.* [*iso-* + *-morphous*]. ISOMORPHIC.

isomorphous gliosis. Gliosis in which the astroglial fibers are parallel to the degenerating nerve fibers.

isomorphous irritation effect. ISOMORPHOUS PROVOCATIVE REACTION.

isomorphous provocative reaction. The appearance of cutaneous lesions at sites of trauma, originally observed in psoriasis, now applied equally to diseases such as lichen planus, atopic dermatitis, necrobiosis lipoidica. Syn. *isomorphous irritation effect, Koebner's phenomenon.*

iso·myl·a·mine (eye''so·mil'uh·meen) *n.* 2-(Diethylamino)ethyl 1-isopentylcyclohexanecarboxylate, $C_{18}H_{35}NO_2$, a smooth muscle relaxant, used as the hydrochloride salt.

iso·ni·a·zid (eye''so·nigh'uh·zid) *n.* Isonicotinic acid hydrazide, $C_6H_7N_3O$, a tuberculostatic drug.

iso·nic·o·tin·ic acid hydrazide (eye''so·nick·o·tin'ick). ISONIAZID.

iso·nip·e·caine (eye''so·nip'e·kane) *n.* MEPERIDINE.

iso·ni·trile (eye·so·nigh'trile, ·tril, ·treel) *n.* ISOCYANIDE.

Isonorin. A trademark for isoproterenol, a sympathomimetic amine used principally as a bronchodilator in the form of the sulfate salt.

iso·os·mot·ic (eye''so·oz·mot'ick) *adj.* [*iso-* + *osmotic*]. Characterizing or pertaining to a solution which has the same osmotic pressure as that of any reference physiological fluid, particularly that enclosed in red blood cells. An isoosmotic solution is also isotonic only when the tissue concerned, by virtue of its lack of permeability to the solutes present or to any interaction with them, maintains its normal state or tone. Syn. *isosmotic.*

isoosmotic solution. ISOSMOTIC SOLUTION.

Isopaque. A trademark for metrizoate sodium.

isopathic principle. The apparently paradoxical rule according to which the cause cures the effect, as a feeling of guilt can be relieved by an expression of the cause of the guilt, namely, expression of hate.

isop·a·thy (eye·sop'uth·ee) *n.* [*iso-* + *-pathy*]. The treatment of a disease by the administration of the causative agent or of its products, as the treatment of smallpox by the administration of variolous matter. Syn. *isotherapy.* —**iso·path·ic** (eye''so·path'ick) *adj.*

iso·phane insulin (eye'so·fane). A preparation of protamine and insulin, commonly zinc-insulin, in which the two substances are present in their combining proportion (isophane ratio); has intermediate duration of action. NPH insulin is an isophane insulin.

isophane ratio. The proportion in which insulin and protamine combine in preparations containing both substances. See also *isophane insulin.*

iso·phen·ic (eye''so·fen'ick) *adj.* Pertaining to or characterizing different genes that produce similar phenotypic effects.

iso·pho·ria (eye''so·fo'ree·uh) *n.* [*iso-* + *-phoria*]. A condition in which the eyes lie in the same horizontal plane, the tension of the vertical muscles being equal in both eyes, and the visual lines lying in the same plane.

iso·pia (eye·so'pee·uh) *n.* [*is-* + *-opia*]. Equal acuteness of vision in the two eyes.

iso·po·ten·tial line (eye''so·po·ten·chul). ISOELECTRIC LINE.

iso·pre·cip·i·tin (eye''so·pre·sip'i·tin) *n.* [*iso-* + *precipitin*]. A precipitin which is active only against the serum of animals of the same species as that from which it is derived.

iso·pren·a·line (eye''so·pren'uh·leen) *n.* British name for isoproterenol.

iso·prene (eye'so·preen) *n.* 2-Methylbutadiene, $CH_2{=}CHC(CH_3){=}CH_2$, a hydrocarbon formed in the dry distillation of rubber.

iso·pro·pa·mide iodide (eye''so·pro'puh·mide). (3-Carbamoyl-3,3-diphenylpropyl)diisopropylmethylammonium iodide, $C_{23}H_{33}IN_2O$, an anticholinergic drug employed for antispasmodic and antisecretory effects on the gastrointestinal tract.

iso·pro·pa·nol (eye''so·pro'puh·nole, ·nol) *n.* ISOPROPYL ALCOHOL.

iso·pro·pyl (eye''so·pro'pil) *n.* The univalent hydrocarbon radical $(CH_3)_2CH—$.

iso·pro·pyl·ace·tic acid (eye''so·pro''pil·a·see'tick). ISOVALERIC ACID.

isopropyl alcohol. 2-Propanol, $CH_3CH(OH)CH_3$, a homologue of ethyl alcohol; used as a solvent and rubefacient. Syn. *isopropanol.*

iso·pro·pyl·ar·ter·e·nol (eye''so·pro''pil·ahr·teer'e·nole, ·ahr·terr'e·nole) *n.* ISOPROTERENOL.

isopropyl my·ris·tate (mi·ris'tate). A pharmaceutic aid, used as an emollient in topical medicinal preparations, which is said to enhance absorption through the skin.

iso·pro·ter·e·nol (eye''so·pro·teer'e·nole, ·terr'e·nole) *n.* 3,4-Dihydroxy-α-[(isopropylamino)methyl]benzyl alcohol, $C_{11}H_{17}NO_3$, a sympathomimetic amine; used principally as a bronchodilator as the hydrochloride and sulfate salts. Syn. *isopropylarterenol.*

isop·ters (eye·sop'turz) *n.pl.* [*is-* + Gk. *optēr,* observer]. The curves of relative visual acuity of the retina, at different distances from the macula, for form and for color.

iso·quin·o·line (eye''so·kwin'o·leen, ·lin) *n.* Benzo[*b*]pyridine, C_9H_7N, a substance important in the synthesis of some antimalarials and other medicinals.

iso·rau·wol·fine (eye''so·raw·wol'feen, ·fin) *n.* An alkaloid isolated from *Rauwolfia serpentina.*

Isordil. A trademark for isosorbide dinitrate, a coronary vasodilator.

iso·ri·bo·fla·vin (eye''so·rye'bo·flay''vin) *n.* 5,6-Dimethyl-9-(D-1'-ribityl)isoalloxazine; an isomer of riboflavin, which is 6,7-dimethyl-9-(D-1'-ribityl)isoalloxazine. Isoriboflavin is an effective metabolite antagonist for riboflavin in the rat, but not in certain bacterial systems.

iso·scope (eye'so·skope) *n.* [*iso-* + *-scope*]. An instrument consisting of two sets of parallel vertical wires, one of which can be superimposed on the other; it is designed to show that the vertical lines of separation of the retina do not correspond exactly to the vertical meridians.

iso·ser·ine (eye''so·serr'een, ·seer'een) *n.* α-Hydroxy-β-aminopropionic acid, $NH_2CH_2CHOHCOOH$, isomeric with serine; it is an analogue of β-alanine and inhibits the growth-promoting action of the latter.

iso·sex·u·al (eye''so·seck'shoo·ul) *adj.* [*iso-* + *sexual*]. Characteristic of or pertaining to the same sex, as: isosexual precocity, precocious sexual development appropriate to the sex of the individual undergoing it.

is·os·mot·ic (eye''soz·mot'ick) *adj.* ISOOSMOTIC.

isosmotic solution. A solution which has the same osmotic pressure as that of a selected reference solution; commonly accepted as synonymous with isotonic solution, but the two are identical only when there is no diffusion of solute across the membrane of a tissue immersed in the solution. Syn. *isoosmotic solution.*

iso·sor·bide (eye''so·sor'bide) *n.* 1,4:3,6-Dianhydro-D-glucitol, $C_6H_{10}O_4$, an osmotic diuretic.

isosorbide di·ni·trate (dye·nigh'trate). 1,4:3,6-Dianhydro-D-glucitol dinitrate, $C_6H_8N_2O_8$, a coronary vasodilator.

Isos·po·ra (eye·sos'puh·ruh) *n.* [*iso-* + Gk. *spora,* seed]. A genus of coccidia.

Isospora hom·i·nis (hom'i·nis). A species of coccidia parasitic in the small intestine of man, but rarely pathogenic.

iso·spo·ro·sis (eye''so·spo·ro'sis) *n.* [*Isospora* + *-osis*]. Human infection by members of the genus *Isospora.*

iso·stere (eye'so·steer, ·stair) *n.* [*iso-* + Gk. *stereos,* solid, three-dimensional]. Generally, any of two or more compounds having essentially identical molecular configurations, including molecular volumes, and similar electrical fields. Criteria for deciding whether two dissimilar compounds are isosteres vary. —**iso·ster·ic** (eye''so·steer'ick) *adj.*

isos·ter·ism (eye·sos'tur·iz·um) *n.* [*isostere* + *-ism*]. The relationship between two or more compounds which are isosteres. In medicinal chemistry, the concept of isosterism involves the possibility that compounds having such a relationship may have the same or quite similar pharmacologic actions.

isos·the·nu·ria (eye″sos·thi·new′ree·uh) *n.* [*iso-* + Gk. *sthenos*, strength, + *-uria*]. Inability of the kidneys to produce either a concentrated or dilute urine.

iso·tel (eye′so·tel) *n.* [Gk. *isotelēs*, bearing equal burdens]. A food factor capable of replacing another in a given diet for a specified species; thus, for the human species, carotene is isotelic with vitamin A; for the cat, it is not, since the cat is incapable of converting carotene into vitamin A. —**iso·tel·ic** (eye″so·tel′ick) *adj.*

iso·ther·a·py (eye″so·therr′uh·pee) *n.* [*iso-* + *therapy*]. ISOPATHY.

iso·therm (eye′so·thurm) *n.* [*iso-* + *-therm*]. A graph or curve representing the dependence of one quantity upon another at constant temperature, such as the dependence of gas pressure upon volume.

iso·ther·mal (eye″so·thur′mul) *adj.* [*iso-* + *thermal*]. Of equal or uniform temperature; without change in temperature.

iso·ther·mic (eye″so·thur′mick) *adj.* ISOTHERMAL.

iso·thio·cy·a·nate (eye″so·thigh″o·sigh′uh·nate) *n.* Any organic compound of the formula RNCS, isomeric with but differing from RCNS, which is a thiocyanate.

iso·tone (eye′so·tone) *n.* One of two or more species of atoms which contain the same number of neutrons.

iso·ton·ic (eye″so·ton′ick) *adj.* [Gk. *isotonos*, even, pulling evenly]. Pertaining to a solution in which cells or a tissue, especially erythrocytes, maintain the normal state without undergoing lysis or crenation. Compare *isoosmotic*. 2. *In physiology*, having uniform tension under pressure.

isotonic coefficient. The lowest concentration of a solution of a salt in which laking of blood does not occur.

isotonic contraction. Muscular contraction characterized by decrease in length of the muscle fibers whereas the tone remains the same as the fibers shorten. Contr. *isometric contraction*.

isotonic sodium chloride injection. SODIUM CHLORIDE INJECTION.

isotonic sodium chloride solution. SODIUM CHLORIDE IRRIGATION.

isotonic solution. A solution that causes no change in the tone of a tissue, such as erythrocytes, immersed in the solution. In the absence of solute diffusing through the tissue membrane, a solution which is isotonic is isoosmotic with the fluid phase of the tissue.

iso·tope (eye′suh·tope) *n.* [*iso-* + Gk. *topos*, place]. An element which has the same atomic number as another but a different atomic weight. Many elements have been shown to consist of several isotopes, the apparent atomic weight of the element actually representing an average of the atomic weights of the isotopes. —**iso·top·ic** (·top′ick) *adj.*

isotope dilution analysis. A method of analysis for a component of a mixture in which a known amount of the same component, commonly labeled with a radioactive isotope of predetermined activity, is added to the mixture. A pure sample of the compound is then isolated, and from the decrease in activity of the tracer substance, the original concentration of the component may be calculated.

isotope effect. The effect of difference of mass between isotopes of the same element on the rate of reaction, position of equilibrium, or both, of chemical reactions involving the isotopes; the effect may be particularly prominent in the case of an element of low atomic weight.

isotope exchange reaction. A chemical reaction in which interchange of the atoms of a given element between two or more chemical forms of the element occurs, the atoms in one form being isotopically labeled so as to distinguish them from atoms in the other form. Study of the course of the reaction is thereby possible.

isotopic abundance. The relative number of atoms of a particular isotope in a particular sample of an element.

isotopic dilution analysis. ISOTOPE DILUTION ANALYSIS.

iso·tro·pic (eye″so·tro′pick, trop′ick) *adj.* [*iso-* + *-tropic*]. 1. Having the same values of a property (as refractive index, tensile strength, elasticity, electrical or heat conductivity, or rate of solution) in different directions, especially in crystal. 2. Having the same shape and appearance from whatever point observed. 3. *In biology*, having equal growth tendency in all directions. 4. In an ovum, lacking a predetermined axis or axes. Contr. *anisotropic*.

isotropic band. I BAND.

isotropic disk. I DISK.

isot·ro·py (eye·sot′ruh·pee) *n.* The property or quality of being isotropic.

iso·va·ler·ic acid (eye″so·va·lerr′ick, ·va·leer′ick) *n.* Isopropylacetic acid, $(CH_3)_2CHCH_2COOH$, the valeric acid of commerce, obtained from valerian root; it has been used medicinally in the form of the ammonium salt. See also *valeric acid*.

isovaleric acidemia. Elevated serum isovaleric acid content associated with recurrent episodes of coma, acidosis, and malodorous sweat.

iso·vol·u·met·ric (eye″so·vol″yoo·met′rick) *adj.* Isometric in volume.

isovolumetric contraction. ISOMETRIC CONTRACTION (2).

isovolumetric contraction wave. The outward deflection of the apex cardiogram corresponding to ventricular isovolumetric contraction. Abbreviated, IC wave.

isovolumetric interval. The first phase of ventricular systole, beginning with the first detectable rise in ventricular pressure after closure of the atrioventricular valves to the beginning of ejection of blood from the ventricles.

isovolumetric relaxation wave. The inward deflection of the apex cardiogram corresponding to ventricular isovolumetric relaxation. Abbreviated, IR wave.

iso·vo·lu·mic (eye″so·vol·yoo′mick) *adj.* ISOVOLUMETRIC.

isox·i·cam (eye·sock′si·kam) *n.* 4-Hydroxy-2-methyl-*N*-(5-methyl-3-isoxozolyl)-2*H*-1,2-benzothiazine-3-carboxamide 1,1-dioxide, $C_{14}H_{13}N_3O_5S$, an anti-inflammatory agent.

isox·su·prine (eye·sock′sue·preen) *n.* *p*-(Hydroxy-α-[1-[(1-methyl-2-phenoxyethyl)amino]ethyl]benzyl alcohol, $C_{18}H_{23}NO_3$, a sympathomimetic with vasodilator activity.

iso·zyme (eye′so·zime) *n.* ISOENZYME.

is·pa·ghul (is′puh·gul, ·gool) *n.* [Persian *ispaghōl*]. The seeds of *Plantago ispaghula*, used as a purgative in India; they contain mucilage and have been used for treatment of bacillary dysentery.

is·sue, *n.* [OF., from L. *exitus*, from *exire*, to go out]. 1. Offspring. 2. A bloody or purulent discharge from a wound or cavity.

-ist [OF. *-iste*, from L. *-ista*, from Gk. *-istēs*]. A suffix meaning *one who does, practices, or deals with*.

IST Abbreviation for *insulin shock therapy*.

isth·mec·to·my (is·meck′tuh·mee, isth·) *n.* [*isthmus* + *-ectomy*]. Excision of an isthmus; specifically, excision of the isthmus of the thyroid gland in goiter.

isthmic endometrium. The portion of the endometrium lining the isthmus uteri, whose tubules are neither racemose nor secretory, and which does not show the cyclic changes characteristic of the rest of the endometrium.

isthmic nodular salpingitis. Follicular inflammation of the small constricted portion (isthmus) of the oviduct, with formation of small nodules of muscular and connective tissue. Syn. *endosalpingiosis*.

isth·mus (is′mus, isth′mus) *n.* [Gk. *isthmos*]. The neck or constricted part of an organ. —**isth·mic** (·mick) *adj.*

isthmus aor·tae (ay·or′tee) [NA]. AORTIC ISTHMUS.

isthmus car·ti·la·gi·nis au·ris (kahr·ti·laj'i·nis aw'ris) [NA]. The portion of the cartilage of the external ear between the portion forming the auricle and that forming the external acoustic meatus.

isthmus fau·ci·um (faw'see·um) [NA]. ISTHMUS OF THE FAUCES.

isthmus glandulae thy·roi·de·ae (thigh·roy'dee·ee) [NA]. ISTHMUS OF THE THYROID GLAND.

isthmus gy·ri cin·gu·li (jye'rye sing'gew·lye) [NA]. ISTHMUS OF THE CINGULATE GYRUS.

isthmus gyri for·ni·ca·ti (for·ni·kay'tye) [BNA]. Isthmus gyri cinguli (= ISTHMUS OF THE CINGULATE GYRUS).

isthmus hip·po·cam·pi (hip·o·kam'pye). ISTHMUS OF THE CINGULATE GYRUS.

isthmus of the cingulate gyrus. The narrow portion of the cingulate gyrus which connects with the parahippocampal gyrus. NA *isthmus gyri cinguli.*

isthmus of the fauces. The passage between the oral cavity and the oral pharynx. NA *isthmus faucium.*

isthmus of the gyrus fornicatus. ISTHMUS OF THE CINGULATE GYRUS.

isthmus of the limbic lobe. ISTHMUS OF THE CINGULATE GYRUS.

isthmus of the thyroid gland. The narrow transverse part connecting the lobes of the thyroid gland. NA *isthmus glandulae thyroideae.* See also Plate 26.

isthmus of the uterine tube. The part of the uterine tube nearest the uterus. NA *isthmus tubae uterinae.*

isthmus pro·sta·tae (pros'tuh·tee) [NA]. The portion of the prostate between the lateral lobes.

isthmus rhom·ben·ce·pha·li (rom''ben·sef'uh·lye) [NA]. The narrow portion of the hindbrain, situated rostral to the cerebellum, which merges with the midbrain.

isthmus tu·bae au·di·ti·vae (tew'bee aw·di·tye'vee) [NA]. The narrowest portion of the auditory tube.

isthmus tubae ute·ri·nae (yoo·tur·eye'nee) [NA]. ISTHMUS OF THE UTERINE TUBE.

isthmus ute·ri (yoo'tur·eye) [NA]. The constricted part of the uterus between the cervix and body. It corresponds to the lower uterine segment.

Istizin. Trademark for danthron, a laxative and cathartic.

Isuprel. A trademark for isoproterenol, a sympathomimetic amine used principally as a bronchodilator in the form of the hydrochloride salt.

isu·ria (eye·sue'ree·uh, i·sue'ree·uh) *n.* [*is-* + *-uria*]. Excretion of equal amounts of urine in equal periods of time.

Ital·ian juice root. GLYCYRRHIZA.

Itard's catheter (ee·tahr') [J. M. G. *Itard,* French otolaryngologist, 1775–1838]. A type of eustachian catheter.

itch, *n.* 1. An irritating sensation in the skin. 2. Any of various skin diseases accompanied by itching, particularly scabies.

itch·ing, *n.* A sensation of tickling and irritation in the skin, producing a desire to scratch; pruritis.

itch mite. *SARCOPTES SCABIEI.*

itch points or **spots.** PAIN SPOTS.

[1]-ite [Gk. *-itēs,* adj. and n. derivational suffix]. A suffix designating (a) *a mineral or rock;* (b) *a division of the body or of a part.*

[2]-ite. A suffix designating *the salt or ester from an acid with the termination -ous.* Compare *-ide, -ate.*

iter (eye'tur, it'ur) *n.* [L., journey, way]. A passageway.

iter ad infundibulum. The passage between the third ventricle of the brain and the infundibulum (2).

it·er·a·tion (it''ur·ay'shun) *n.* [L. *iteratio,* from *iterum,* again]. Repetition.

iter chor·dae an·te·ri·us (kor'dee an·teer'ee·us). The aperture through which the chorda tympani nerve leaves the tympanum. Syn. *Huguier's canal.*

iter chordae pos·te·ri·us (pos·teer'ee·us). The aperture through which the chorda tympani nerve enters the tympanum; POSTERIOR ITER. NA *apertura tympanica canaliculi chordae tympani.*

iter den·ti·um (den'chee·um, den'tee·um). An opening in the alveolar process lingual to or between the roots of a primary tooth, occupied by an extension of the dental sac of the permanent (succedaneous) tooth.

ithy·lor·do·sis (ith''i·lor·do'sis) *n.* [NL., from Gk. *ithys,* straight, + *lordosis*]. Lordosis unaccompanied by lateral curvature.

ithyo·ky·pho·sis (ith''ee·o·kigh·fo'sis) *n.* [NL., from Gk. *ithys,* straight, + *kyphosis*]. Backward bending of the vertebral column.

-itis [Gk.]. A suffix meaning *inflammation of a* (specified) *part.*

Itobarbital. A trademark for butalbital, a sedative-hypnotic.

Ito cells (ee'to) [T. *Ito,* Japanese, 20th century]. Lipid-containing cells of mesenchymal origin found in human liver in certain diseases.

-itol. A suffix designating *a polyhydroxy alcohol, usually related to a sugar.*

Ito-Reen·stier·na test or **reaction.** An allergic skin test of aid in the diagnosis or exclusion of chancroid, performed by the intradermal injection of a vaccine of killed *Haemophilus ducreyi.*

ITP Abbreviation for *idiopathic thrombocytopenic purpura.*

Itrumil. Trademark for iothiouracil, an antithyroid drug used as the sodium derivative.

I.U. Abbreviation for *international unit.*

IUD Abbreviation for *intrauterine contraceptive device.*

-ium [NL.]. A suffix in chemistry designating (a) *a chemical element;* (b) *a chemical radical;* (c) *an ion with a positive charge.*

IUPAC International Union of Pure and Applied Chemistry, an organization which coordinates international acceptance of chemical standards and provides a uniform system of nomenclature.

I.V., i.v. Abbreviation for *intravenous.*

IVCD Abbreviation for *intraventricular conduction delay* (= INTRAVENTRICULAR HEART BLOCK).

Ive·mark syndrome (ee've·mark'') [B. I. *Ivemark,* Swedish physician, 20th century]. A syndrome of unknown etiology, characterized by visceral symmetry, absence, rudimentary development, or situs inversus of the spleen, and complex cardiac malformations leading to early death. Syn. *asplenia syndrome.*

ivo·ry, *n.* [OF. *ivoire,* from L. *ebur*]. The dentin, particularly of commerce, such as that obtained from the tusks of the elephant, walrus, or hippopotamus.

ivory black. ANIMAL CHARCOAL.

ivory bones. Very dense bones, as seen in osteopetroses, osteoblastic metastases, etc.

ivory osteosis. OSTEOMA DURUM.

IVP Abbreviation for *intravenous pyelogram.*

Ivy method or **test.** A test for bleeding time, in which a small puncture wound is made in a relatively avascular part of the forearm and the time which elapses until bleeding stops is recorded.

Iwa·noff's cysts (ee·vah'nuf, ee·vah·noff') [W. P. *Iwanoff* (V. P. Ivanov), Russian ophthalmologist b. 1861]. BLESSIG-IVANOV CYSTIC DEGENERATION OF THE RETINA.

Ix·o·des (ick·so'deez) *n.* [Gk. *ixōdēs,* sticky, from *ixos,* birdlime]. A genus of parasitic ticks, some species of which cause tick paralysis and are important vectors of diseases of cattle, sheep, and dogs, as well as transmitters of encephalomyelitis and tularemia to man.

ix·o·di·a·sis (ick''so·dye'uh·sis) *n.* [*Ixodes* + *-iasis*]. Lesions or disease caused by infestation with ticks.

ix·od·ic (ick·sod'ick, ·so'dick) *adj.* Caused by or pertaining to ticks.

ix·od·id (ick·sod'id, ·so'did) *adj. & n.* 1. Pertaining to ticks as distinguished from mites. 2. A tick of one of the 60 species of the genus *Ixodes,* implicated as vectors of rickettsial and other infectious diseases.

Ix·od·i·dae (ick·sod'i·dee) *n.pl.* A family of hardbodied ticks, which includes the genera *Boöphilus, Amblyomma, Dermacentor, Haemaphysalis, Hyalomma, Ixodes,* and *Rhipicephalus,* all of some pathologic significance to man.

ix·yo·my·e·li·tis (ick''see·o·migh''e·lye'tis) *n.* [Gk. *ixys, ixyos,* waist, + *myelitis*]. *Obsol.* Inflammation of the lumbar portion of the spinal cord.

J

J Symbol for joule.

j Used as a Roman numeral (in prescriptions) as the equivalent of i for one, usually at the end of a number, as j, ij, iij, vj, vij.

jaag·siek·te (yahk'seek''te) *n.* [Afrikaans, from *jag,* hunt, + *siekte,* sickness]. A contagious disease of sheep, sometimes of goats and guinea pigs, resembling the more benign and diffuse forms of bronchiolar carcinoma in man.

jab·o·ran·di (jab''o·ran'dee) *n.* [Pg., from Tupi]. PILOCARPUS.

Ja·bou·lay's operation (zhah·boo·leh') [M. *Jaboulay,* French surgeon, 1860-1913]. An early method of gastroduodenostomy.

Jac·coud's arthritis (zhah·koo') [S. *Jaccoud,* French physician, 1830-1913]. Progressive periarticular fibrosis with later pain or loss of mobility developing after severe recurrent rheumatic fever arthritis.

Jaccoud's dissociated fever [S. *Jaccoud*]. *Obsol.* Febrile meningitis with a slow pulse rate, observed in patients with tuberculous meningitis.

Jaccoud's sign [S. *Jaccoud*]. Prominence of the aorta in the suprasternal notch; originally described as a sign of leukemia, but in fact suggesting aortic dilatation.

jack bean. The seed of *Canavalia,* from which urease is prepared for use in the estimation of urea.

jack·et, *n.* 1. *In medicine,* a supporting, therapeutic, or restraining apparatus covering the upper part or trunk of the body. 2. JACKET CROWN.

jacket crown. An artificial crown of a tooth consisting of a covering of porcelain or resin.

jack·knife convulsion or **seizure.** INFANTILE SPASM.

jackknife position. A position in which the patient reclines on his back with the shoulders elevated, the legs flexed on the thighs, and the thighs at right angles to the abdomen; a position for urethral instrumentation.

jackknife sign. A sign of peritoneal irritation in acute appendicitis, in which sudden pressure over the appendix causes immediate involuntary flexion of the right thigh.

jack·screw, *n.* A threaded screw in a socket, used in various types of appliances to exert orthodontic forces or to position the parts of a fracture.

Jack·son-Bab·cock operation [Chevalier *Jackson,* U.S. laryngologist, 1866-1958; and W. W. *Babcock*]. An operation for radical removal of an esophageal diverticulum.

Jack·so·nian convulsion or **seizure** (jack·so'nee·un) [J. Hughlings *Jackson,* English neurologist, 1835-1911]. A focal seizure originating in one part of the motor or sensorimotor cortex, and manifested usually by spasmodic contractions or paroxysmal paresthesias of part of the fingers, toes, and face, whence it spreads to involve one side of the body with retention of consciousness (Jacksonian march); or it may become generalized with loss of consciousness.

Jacksonian epilepsy [J. Hughlings *Jackson*]. Epilepsy characterized by recurrent focal seizures.

Jacksonian march [J. Hughlings *Jackson*]. A focal motor or sensorimotor seizure of the fingers, toes, or face, spreading to involve the rest of the body.

Jackson-Mackenzie syndrome [S. *Mackenzie*]. JACKSON'S SYNDROME.

Jackson's membrane [J. N. *Jackson,* U.S. surgeon, 1868-1935]. 1. A thin membrane arising from the peritoneum on the right and extending across the colon to the hepatic flexure, sometimes causing intestinal obstruction. 2. Any peritoneal band or adhesion. Syn. *Jackson's veil.*

Jackson's reevolution [J. Hughlings *Jackson*]. REEVOLUTION.

Jackson's sign [Chevalier *Jackson*]. In patients with pulmonary tuberculosis, a prolonged wheezing expiratory sound heard over the affected area.

Jackson's syndrome [J. Hughlings *Jackson*]. Paralysis of half the soft palate, pharynx, and larynx, and flaccid paralysis of the homolateral sternocleidomastoid and part of the trapezius and of the tongue due to a nuclear or radicular lesion of the tenth, eleventh, and twelfth cranial nerves on one side.

Jackson's veil [J. N. *Jackson*]. JACKSON'S MEMBRANE.

Ja·co·be·us operation (yah·koh·bey'ōōs) [H.C. *Jacobeus,* Swedish surgeon, 1879-1937]. An operation for pneumonolysis in which pleural adhesions are divided with a galvanocautery.

Ja·cob·sohn's reflex (yah'kohp·zone). Flexion of the fingers induced by a mild tap on the lower end of the radius or in its neighborhood on the dorsal side of the forearm; a sign of reflex overactivity.

Ja·cob·son's cartilage (yah'kohb·sen) [L. L. *Jacobson,* Danish anatomist, 1783-1843]. VOMERONASAL CARTILAGE.

Jacobson's nerve [L. L. *Jacobson*]. TYMPANIC NERVE.

Jacobson's plexus [L. L. *Jacobson*]. TYMPANIC PLEXUS.

Ja·cob's ulcer [A. *Jacob,* Irish ophthalmologist, 1790-1874]. Basal cell carcinoma of the eyelid.

Ja·cod's syndrome or **triad** (zhah·ko') [M. *Jacod,* 20th century]. Unilateral optic atrophy with blindness, total ophthalmoplegia, and trigeminal neuralgia involving the distribution of the ophthalmic branch, due to tumors or aneurysms in the petrosphenoid space. Compare *Godtfredsen's syndrome.*

Ja·cquet's erythema (zha·keh') [L. M. L. *Jacquet,* French dermatologist, 1860-1914]. DIAPER RASH.

jac·ta·tion (jack·tay'shun) *n.* JACTITATION.

jac·ti·ta·tion (jack''ti·tay'shun) *n.* [L. *jactitare,* frequentative of *jactare,* to throw, to toss about]. A tossing about, great restlessness; seen with acute illness, high fever, and great exhaustion.

jac·u·lif·er·ous (jack″yoo·lif′ur·us) *adj.* [L. *jacul*um, dart, + *-ferous*]. Prickly, bearing spines.

Ja·das·sohn-Le·wan·dow·sky law (yah′dahs·zone, ley·van·dof′skee) [J. *Jadassohn,* German dermatologist, 1863–1936; and F. *Lewandowsky,* German dermatologist, 1879–1921]. A law of doubtful validity stating that tubercles or tuberculoid structures tend to appear wherever microorganisms or their products are neutralized or overcome by the local immunologic reactions. Thus chronic infections other than tuberculosis can produce the tuberculoid structure.

Jadassohn's disease [J. *Jadassohn*]. 1. ANETODERMA. 2. GRANULOSIS RUBRA NASI. 3. EXFOLIATIVE DERMATITIS.

Jadassohn's nevus [J. *Jadassohn*]. NEVUS SEBACEUS.

Jadassohn-Tièche nevus (tyesh) [J. *Jadassohn* and M. *Tièche*]. BLUE NEVUS.

Jae·ger test. SCRATCH-PATCH TEST.

Jaf·fé-Lich·ten·stein disease or **syndrome** [H. L. *Jaffé,* U.S. physician, b. 1907; and L. *Lichtenstein,* U.S. physician, b. 1906]. The monostotic form of fibrous dysplasia.

Jaf·fé's test or **reaction** (yah·fey′) [M. *Jaffé,* German biochemist, 1841–1911]. Creatinine forms a red compound with picric acid in alkaline solution.

jagziekte. JAAGSIEKTE.

jail fever. EPIDEMIC TYPHUS.

jake palsy or **paralysis.** [from *jake,* slang for *extract of Jamaica Ginger,* an alcoholic preparation used as a beverage during prohibition and sometimes contaminated with triorthocresyl phosphate]. TRIORTHOCRESYL PHOSPHATE NEUROPATHY. Polyneuropathy and myelopathy from triorthocresylphosphate poisoning.

Jakob-Creutzfeldt disease or **syndrome.** CREUTZFELDT-JAKOB DISEASE.

jal·ap (jal′up) *n.* [after *Jalapa,* Mexico]. The tuberous root of *Exogonium purga,* a plant of the Convolvulaceae. Its active principle is a resin that contains a glycoside, convolvulin. Jalap is an active hydragogue cathartic.

jal·a·pin (jal′uh·pin) *n.* A name sometimes applied to the resin from jalap.

Ja·mai·ca dogwood. PISCIDIA.

Jamaica ginger paralysis or **polyneuritis.** [from the alcoholic extract of Jamaica Ginger used as a beverage during prohibition and sometimes contaminated with triorthocresyl phosphate]. TRIORTHOCRESYL PHOSPHATE NEUROPATHY.

Jamaican neuropathy. STRACHAN'S SYNDROME.

Jamaican vomiting sickness. AKEE POISONING.

ja·mais vu (zha·meh vue′) [F., never seen]. A psychic phenomenon in which the patient has the sensation of never having seen or being an utter stranger to surroundings which are normally thoroughly familiar to him; observed particularly in lesions of the temporal lobe and in temporal lobe epilepsy. Compare *deajas vu.*

jam·bul (jam′bul) *n. Eugenia jambolana,* the bark and seeds of which have been variously used in medicine.

James's powder [R. *James,* English physician, 1705–1776]. ANTIMONY POWDER.

James·town weed [after *Jamestown,* Va.]. STRAMONIUM.

Jam·shi·di needle. An instrument used to perform percutaneous bone marrow biopsy.

Ja·net's disease (zha·neh′) [P. M. F. *Janet,* French psychiatrist, 1859–1947]. PSYCHASTHENIA.

Jane·way lesions [E. G. *Janeway,* U.S. physician, 1841–1911]. Small painless hemorrhagic macular lesions on the palms of the hand and soles of the feet in bacterial endocarditis.

Janeway nodes or **spots** [E. G. *Janeway*]. JANEWAY LESIONS.

jan·i·ceps (jan′i·seps) *n.* [*Jan*us + *-ceps,* -headed, from L. *caput,* head]. CEPHALOTHORACOPAGUS DISYMMETROS.

janiceps asym·me·tros (a·sim′e·tros). CEPHALOTHORACOPAGUS ASYMMETROS.

janiceps ate·le·us (a·tee′lee·us, a·tel′ee·us) [NL., from Gk. *atelēs,* incomplete, imperfect]. CEPHALOTHORACOPAGUS MONOSYMMETROS.

Jan·sen's operation (yahn′zen) [A. *Jansen,* German otolaryngologist, 1859–1933]. An operation, no longer in use, for disease of the frontal sinus in which the frontal sinus is curetted after removing the lower wall and the inferior portion of the anterior wall.

Jansen's syndrome [M. *Jansen,* 1863–1934]. METAPHYSEAL DYSOSTOSIS.

Jan·ský's classification or **groups** (yahn′skee) [J. *Janský,* Czech physician, 1873–1921]. An early system of classification of the ABO blood groups in which O,A,B, and AB were designated groups I,II,III, and IV, respectively.

ja·nus (jay′nus) *n.* [*Janus,* a two-faced Roman god]. CEPHALOTHORACOPAGUS.

janus asym·me·tros (a·sim′e·tros). CEPHALOTHORACOPAGUS ASYMMETROS.

Janus green B. A basic azo dye, $C_{30}H_{31}ClN_6$, used as a supravital stain for mitochondria, as a nuclear stain in contrast staining for fats, and for other purposes.

Ja·nu·si·an thinking (ja·noo′zee·un) [from *Janus,* a two-faced Roman god (coined erroneously by addition of the adjectival suffix *-ian* directly to the Latin nominative rather than to the stem *Jan-*)]. The process of conceiving two or more opposite or contradictory ideas, concepts or images simultaneously; an important thought process in creativity. Differs from dialectical thinking, conflict, ambivalence, and Jung's formulations about opposition in psychic life.

Japanese B encephalitis. An arbovirus encephalitis, epidemic in Japan, most commonly producing subclinical infection; symptomatic disease is characterized by fever, cortical, cerebellar, motor, and sensory deficits, and coma.

Jap·a·nese macaque or **ape.** *Macaca fuscata,* a large, stub-tailed, pink- or red-faced monkey native to Japan.

Japanese river fever. TSUTSUGAMUSHI DISEASE.

ja·ra·ra·ca (zhah″ruh·rah′kuh) *n.* [Pg.]. A poisonous snake, a member of the genus *Bothrops,* found in Brazil.

jar·gon (jahr′gun) *n.* [MF.]. The production, as a manifestation of aphasia, of linguistic segments whose combinations cannot be recognized as vocabulary items of a language; gibberish. Compare *agrammatism.*

jargon aphasia. Aphasia characterized by the occurrence of jargon; usually central aphasia.

Ja·risch-Herx·hei·mer reaction (yah′rish, hehrks′high·mur) [A. *Jarisch,* Austrian dermatologist, 1850–1902; and K. *Herxheimer*]. An acute systemic reaction following initial dose of a therapeutic agent, characterized by fever, chill, malaise, headache, and myalgia, with exacerbations of the clinical signs of the infection being treated, most commonly seen in the treatment of syphilis; thought to be due to rapid release of large amounts of the antigen.

Jat·ro·pha (jat′ro·fuh) *n.* [NL., from Gk. *iatros,* physician, + *trophē,* nourishment]. A genus of plants of the Euphorbiaceae; different species have been variously used as medicinal agents.

jaun·dice (jawn′dis) *n.* [MF. *jaunisse,* from *jaune,* yellow]. Yellowness of the skin, mucous membranes, and secretions; due to hyperbilirubinemia. Syn. *icterus.*

jaundice of the newborn. Yellowness of skin and hyperbilirubinemia observed in infants during the first few days after birth. The causes are various and range from physiologic jaundice, which has no aftereffects, through that of erythroblastosis fetalis and septic jaundice, to the severe jaundice due to absence of the bile ducts. See also *physiologic jaundice of the newborn.*

jaw, *n.* Either of the two structures that constitute the framework of the mouth; skeletally, the upper jaw is formed by the maxillae, and the lower jaw by the mandible.

jaw·bone, *n.* One of the bones of the jaw; especially, the mandible.

jaw jerk. Contraction of the muscles of mastication and elevation of the mandible, elicited by striking the relaxed and dependent jaw with a percussion hammer, the mouth being open. Absent in nuclear and peripheral lesions of the trigeminal nerve, and exaggerated with supranuclear lesions, when jaw clonus may be elicited.

Ja·wor·ski's corpuscles (yah·vor'skee) [V. *Jaworski,* Polish physician, 1849–1925]. Spiral fragments of mucus occurring in the gastric secretion of patients with marked hyperchlorhydria.

Jaworski's test [V. *Jaworski*]. In hourglass deformity of the stomach, the production of a splashing sound over the pyloric area by percussion after gastric aspiration.

jaw-winking phenomenon or **reflex.** MARCUS GUNN PHENOMENON.

J disk. I DISK.

Jean·selme's nodule (zhahⁿ·selm') [A. E. *Jeanselme,* French dermatologist, 1858–1935]. JUXTA-ARTICULAR NODE.

Jectofer. Trademark for iron sorbitex, a hematinic preparation.

Jed·dah ulcer [after *Jidda,* Arabia]. An ulcer of cutaneous leishmaniasis.

Jeghers-Peutz syndrome. PEUTZ-JEGHERS SYNDROME.

jejun-, jejuno-. A combining form meaning *jejunum.*

jejuna. Plural of *jejunum.*

je·ju·nal (je·joo'nul) *adj.* Of or pertaining to the jejunum.

jejunal ulcer. An ulcer of the jejunum. See also *marginal ulcer.*

je·ju·nec·to·my (jej"oo·neck'tuh·mee) *n.* [*jejun-* + *-ectomy*]. Excision of part or all of the jejunum.

je·ju·ni·tis (jej"oo·nigh'tis) *n.* [*jejun-* + *-itis*]. Inflammation of the jejunum.

je·ju·no·ce·cos·to·my, je·ju·no·cae·cos·to·my (je·joo"no·se·kos'tuh·mee, jej"oo·no·) *n.* [*jejuno-* + *ceco-* + *-stomy*]. *In surgery,* formation of an anastomosis between the jejunum and the cecum.

je·ju·no·co·los·to·my (je·joo"no·ko·los'tuh·mee, jej"oo·no·) *n.* [*jejuno-* + *colo-* + *-stomy*]. *In surgery,* the formation of an anastomosis between the jejunum and the colon.

je·ju·no·gas·tric (je·joo"no·gas'trick, jej"oo·no·) *adj.* [*jejuno-* + *gastric*]. GASTROJEJUNAL.

je·ju·no·il·e·itis (je·joo"no·il"ee·eye'tis, jej"oo·no·) *n.* [*jejuno-* + *ile-* + *-itis*]. Inflammation of the jejunum and the ileum.

je·ju·no·il·e·os·to·my (je·joo"no·il·ee·os'tuh·mee, jej"oo·no·) *n.* [*jejuno-* + *ileo-* + *-stomy*]. *In surgery,* the formation of an anastomosis between the jejunum and the ileum.

je·ju·no·il·e·um (jej"oo·no·il'ee·um, je·joo"no·) *n.* [*jejuno-* + *ileum*]. The part of the small intestine extending from the duodenum to the cecum.

je·ju·no·je·ju·nos·to·my (je·joo"no·jej"oo·nos'tuh·mee) *n.* [*jejuno-* + *jejuno-* + *-stomy*]. Formation of an anastomosis between two parts of the jejunum.

je·ju·nor·rha·phy (jej"oo·nor'uh·fee) *n.* [*jejuno-* + *-rrhaphy*]. Suture of the jejunum.

je·ju·nos·to·my (jej"oo·nos'tuh·mee) *n.* [*jejuno-* + *-stomy*]. The making of an artificial opening (jejunal fistula) through the abdominal wall into the jejunum.

je·ju·not·o·my (jej"oo·not'uh·mee) *n.* [*jejuno-* + *-tomy*]. Incision into the jejunum.

je·ju·num (je·joo'num) *n.*, pl. **jeju·na** (·nuh) [L. *jejunus,* fasting, empty]. The portion of the small intestine extending between the duodenum and the ileum. It is usually considered to be about the proximal two-fifths of the combined jejunum and ileum. See also Plate 13.

Jel·li·nek's sign (yel'i·neck) [S. *Jellinek,* Austrian physician, b. 1871]. Increased pigmentation of the lids and area around the eyes in hyperthyroidism.

jel·ly, *n.* [MF. *gellee,* from L. *gelata,* frozen]. A semisolid colloidal system of a liquid suspended in a solid, as water in gelatin.

jelly boot. UNNA'S PASTE BOOT.

jelly of Wharton. WHARTON'S JELLY.

Je·na Nomina Anatomica (yeʸ'nah). A list of anatomic terms proposed in 1936 at Jena by German anatomists. It has been superseded by the current Nomina Anatomica. Abbreviated, JNA.

Jen·dras·sik's maneuver (yen'drah·sick) [E. *Jendrassik,* Hungarian physician, 1858–1921]. A method used in neurologic examination to facilitate testing of a peripheral reflex, particularly the knee jerk, wherein the patient is asked to interlink his hands and pull them apart at time of testing.

Jen·ne·ri·an vaccination (je·neer'ee·un) [E. *Jenner,* English physician, 1749–1823]. Vaccination for smallpox.

Jennerian vaccine. SMALLPOX VACCINE.

Jen·ner's stain [L. L. *Jenner,* English physician, 1866–1904]. MAY-GRÜNWALD STAIN.

Jen·sen's chorioretinitis (yen'sᵉn) [E. Z. *Jensen,* Danish ophthalmologist, 1861–1950]. JUXTAPAPILLARY CHOROIDITIS.

Jensen's method [O. *Jensen,* Danish bacteriologist, 20th century]. HAGEDORN AND JENSEN'S METHOD.

Jensen's retinopathy or **disease** [E. Z. *Jensen,* Danish ophthalmologist, 1861–1950]. JUXTAPAPILLARY CHOROIDITIS.

Jensen's sarcoma [C. O. *Jensen,* Danish veterinary pathologist, 1864–1934]. A transmissible, poorly differentiated malignant tumor of diverse cellular pattern; it arose originally in a grey rat inoculated with acid-fast bacteria obtained from a cow with pseudotuberculous enteritis.

jerk, *n.* 1. A sudden, spasmodic movement. 2. A muscle stretch reflex, as jaw jerk, knee jerk. —**jerky,** *adj.*

jerky pulse. A pulse in which the artery is suddenly and markedly distended, as in aortic regurgitation.

jerky respiration. INTERRUPTED RESPIRATION.

Jer·vell and Lange-Niel·sen's syndrome [A. *Jervell,* U.S. cardiologist, 20th century; and F. *Lange-Nielsen*]. CARDIOAUDITORY SYNDROME.

jer·vine (jur'veen, ·vin) *n.* A steroidal alkaloid, $C_{27}H_{39}NO_3$, occurring in veratrum species; it is practically inert physiologically.

Je·su·its' balsam. COMPOUND BENZOIN TINCTURE.

Jesuits' bark. CINCHONA.

jet injection. A technique for administering injections intracutaneously and subcutaneously; the fluid is ejected with high velocity through an orifice 75 to 80 μm in diameter and penetrates the unbroken skin without pain.

Jew·ett angle nail [E. L. *Jewett,* U.S. surgeon, b. 1900]. A nail for internal fixation of intertrochanteric fractures; a three-flanged spike is driven into the neck and head of the femur, and an attached flat plate conforms to the side of the shaft.

Jewett operation [H. J. *Jewett,* U.S. urologist, b. 1903]. A two-stage anastomosis between the ureter and the sigmoid.

Jez·ler-Ta·ka·ta test. TAKATA-ARA TEST.

jig·ger, *n.* *TUNGA PENETRANS.*

Jim·son weed [*Jamestown* weed]. STRAMONIUM.

Jirgl's reaction. A test for the presence of abnormal lipoproteins with an excess of phospholipids in the blood.

JNA Abbreviation for *Jena Nomina Anatomica.*

Jo·bert's fossa (zhoʰ·behr') [A. J. *Jobert* de Lamballe, French surgeon, 1799–1867]. A potential hollow in the upper part of the popliteal space.

Job's syndrome (jobe) [*Job,* Old Testament patriarch]. Recurrent cold staphylococcal abscesses; the patient may have diminished local resistance to staphylococcal infection due to defective function of neutrophil leukocytes.

jock itch. TINEA CRURIS.

jock·strap, *n.* [from slang *jock,* penis, + *strap*]. A scrotal supporter.

Jof·froy's reflex (zhoʰ·frwahʰ') [A. *Joffroy,* French neuropsychiatrist, 1844–1908]. Twitching of the gluteal muscles when pressure is made against the buttocks; observed in spastic paralysis.

Joffroy's sign [A. *Joffroy*]. A sign for hyperthyroidism in which the forehead does not wrinkle when the patient looks up with the head bent down.

Joh·ne's bacillus (yo'nuh) [H. A. *Johne,* German bacteriologist, 1839–1910]. MYCOBACTERIUM PARATUBERCULOSIS.

Johne's disease [H. A. *Johne*]. A chronic granulomatous enteritis of cattle, sheep, and deer, caused by *Mycobacterium paratuberculosis* and characterized by intermittent diarrhea and progressive emaciation without fever. Gross thickening of the mucosa of the small intestine and enlargement of the mesenteric lymph nodes without ulceration may occur. Syn. *paratuberculosis.*

joh·nin (yo'nin) *n.* [H. A. *Johne*]. A vaccine prepared from cultures of *Mycobacterium paratuberculosis.* Syn. *paratuberculin.*

johnin reaction. A diagnostic skin test for Johne's disease in cattle.

joint, *n.* [OF. *jointe* from *joindre,* to join, from L. *jungere, junctus,* lit., to yoke]. Any junction of two or more bones or skeletal parts, including the fibrous joints (syndesmoses, sutures, and gomphoses), cartilaginous joints (synchondroses and symphyses), and synovial joints (the movable joints). Syn. *articulation.* NA *articulatio, junctura ossium.* For synovial joints listed by name, see Table of Synovial Joints and Ligaments in the Appendix. See also Plate 2.

joint body. JOINT MOUSE.

joint capsule. The fibrous sheet enclosing a synovial joint. Syn. *capsular ligament.* NA *capsula articularis.* See also Plate 2.

joint cavity. The closed space in a synovial joint, formed by the synovial membrane and containing synovial fluid; the cavity enclosed by the synovial sac. NA *cavum articulare.*

joint·ed, *adj.* Forming a joint.

joint fever. DENGUE.

joint fusion. ARTHRODESIS.

joint-ill, *n.* A pyosepticemia of newborn animals resulting from an infection of the navel, characteristically accompanied by a suppurative arthritis.

joint mouse. A small loose body within a synovial joint, frequently calcified, derived from synovial membrane, organized fibrin fragments of articular cartilage, or arthritic osteophytes. Syn. *joint body.*

Jol·ly bodies (zhoʰ·lee') [J. *Jolly,* French histologist, 1870–1953]. HOWELL-JOLLY BODIES.

Jol·ly's reaction (yoʰl'ee) [F. *Jolly,* German neurologist, 1844–1904]. A reaction, said to occur in certain amyotrophies, in which the contractility of a muscle that has been exhausted by faradism can still be excited by the influence of the will; inversely, when voluntary movements are impossible, the muscle can contract on faradization.

jolt headache. A form of traction headache, usually transient and localized to the frontal or temporal area on one or both sides, due to sudden and vigorous head movements.

Jones criteria [T. D. *Jones,* U.S. physician, 1899–1954]. A listing of findings of major and minor importance for making the diagnosis of acute rheumatic fever.

Jones splint [R. *Jones,* English orthopedist, 1858–1933]. A modification of the Thomas splint, designed for fractures of the humerus.

Jones's position [R. *Jones*]. Hyperflexion of the forearm on the arm, in the treatment of elbow fractures involving the condyles.

Jones test. BOERNER-LUKENS TEST.

Jor·ge Lo·bo's blastomycosis (zhor'zhiʰ lo'boo) [*Jorge Lobo,* Brazilian, 20th century]. A form of South American blastomycosis reported only in Brazil, characterized clinically by pseudokeloid conglomerate cutaneous nodules, variable in number and size, which may become fistulous and suppurative.

Jo·seph's syndrome (zhoʰ·zef') [R. *Joseph,* French pediatrician, 20th century]. A hereditary defect in renal tubular reabsorption resulting in exceedingly high urinary excretion of proline, hydroxyproline, and glycine; manifested clinically by generalized seizures beginning in early life, terminal status epilepticus, and elevated cerebrospinal fluid protein. Syn. *familial hyperprolinemia.* See also *benign prolinuria.*

joule (jool) *n.* [J. P. *Joule,* English physicist, 1818–1889]. 1. The absolute joule: an mks unit of work or energy equivalent to 10^7 ergs. 2. The international joule: a unit equivalent to the work done when a current of 1 international ampere is passed for 1 second through a conductor having a resistance of 1 international ohm; an international joule = 1.00019 absolute joules. Symbol, J.

Joule's equivalent [J. P. *Joule*]. The mechanical or work equivalent of heat, 4.1840 absolute joules being equivalent to 1 calorie.

J point. The junction point of the QRS complex and the S-T segment of the electrocardiogram.

J stomach. A long, longitudinally oriented stomach.

Ju·det prosthesis (zhuᵉ·deʰ') [R. *Judet,* French orthopedic surgeon, 20th century]. A femoral head prosthesis consisting of an acrylic head component attached to an acrylic or metalic stem. See also *Judet's operation.*

Judet's operation [R. *Judet*]. Replacement of the head of the femur by an acrylic prosthesis to relieve arthritis deformans, congenital dislocation in the adult, pseudoarthrosis of the femoral neck.

juga. Plural of *jugum.*

juga al·ve·o·la·ria man·di·bu·lae (al·vee·o·lair'ee·uh man·dib'yoo·lee) [NA]. The ridges on the anterior surface of the alveolar process of the mandible.

juga alveolaria max·il·lae (mack·sil'ee) [NA]. The ridges on the anterior surface of the alveolar process of the maxilla.

juga ce·re·bra·lia os·si·um cra·nii (serr·e·bray'lee·uh os'ee·um kray'nee·eye) [BNA]. The variable ridges on the inner surface of the cranial vault.

ju·gal (joo'gul) *adj.* [L. *jugalis,* from *jugum,* yoke]. 1. Connecting or uniting, as by a yoke. 2. Pertaining to the zygoma.

jugal point. *In craniometry,* the point which is situated at the angle that the posterior border of the frontosphenoid process of the zygoma makes with the superior border of its temporal process.

ju·glans (joo'glanz) *n.* The dried inner bark from the roots of *Juglans cinerea;* formerly used as a laxative. Syn. *butternut bark.*

ju·glone (joo'glone) *n.* 5-Hydroxy-1,4-naphthoquinone, $C_{10}H_6O_3$, obtained from various species of *Juglans* (the walnut trees); antifungal activity has been claimed for it.

jug·u·lar (jug'yoo·lur) *adj. & n.* [L. *jugularis,* from *jugulum,* collarbone; throat, neck]. 1. Pertaining to the neck above the clavicle. 2. Any of the jugular veins. See Table of Veins in the Appendix.

jugular arch. JUGULAR VENOUS ARCH.

jugular bulb. 1. SUPERIOR BULB OF THE INTERNAL JUGULAR VEIN. 2. See *inferior bulb of the internal jugular vein, superior bulb of the internal jugular vein.*

jugular compression. A technique for determining the absence or presence of a spinal subarachnoid block, in which, after the initial spinal fluid pressure has been recorded and before any fluid has been removed, the jugular veins are compressed either manually (Queckenstedt test) or by the use of a sphygmomanometer (cuff manometrics) and then released, and the rise and rate of fall of the spinal fluid pressure noted. Unilateral compression may be useful in diagnosing lateral sinus thrombosis. The test should not be performed in patients with or suspected of having increased intracranial pressure.

jugular eminence. The spinelike extremity of the jugular process of the occipital bone.

jugular foramen. The space formed by the jugular notches of the occipital and temporal bones, divided into two portions, the posterior portion giving passage to an internal jugular vein and the anterior portion giving passage to the ninth, tenth, and eleventh cranial nerves and the inferior petrosal sinus. NA *foramen jugulare.*

jugular foramen syndrome. Paralysis of the ipsilateral glossopharyngeal, vagus, and spinal accessory nerves; caused by a lesion involving the jugular foramen, usually a basilar skull fracture.

jugular fossa. The fossa between the carotid canal and the stylomastoid foramen, containing the superior bulb of the internal jugular vein. NA *fossa jugularis ossis temporalis.*

jugular ganglion. SUPERIOR GANGLION (2).

jugular notch of the occipital bone. A concavity in the inferior border, posterior to the jugular process, which, in the articulated skull, forms the posterior part of the jugular foramen. NA *incisura jugularis ossis occipitalis.*

jugular notch of the sternum. The depression on the upper surface of the manubrium between the two clavicles. NA *incisura jugularis sterni.*

jugular notch of the temporal bone. A small notch in the petrous portion which corresponds to the jugular notch of the occipital bone, with which it forms the jugular foramen. NA *incisura jugularis ossis temporalis.*

jugular process. A rough process external to the condyle of the occipital bone. NA *processus jugularis ossis occipitalis.*

jugular pulse. Pulsation of the jugular veins.

jugular trunk. One of two collecting lymph trunks, right and left, draining the head and neck. The one on the right empties into the right lymphatic duct or into the right subclavian vein at its angle of junction with the right internal jugular vein; the one on the left empties into the thoracic duct. NA *truncus jugularis.*

jugular tubercle. One of a pair of eminences on the basilar portion of the occipital bone between the foramen magnum and the jugular foramen. NA *tuberculum jugulare ossis occipitalis.*

jugular vein. Any of several major veins of the neck. See *anterior jugular, external jugular,* and *internal jugular* in Table of Veins in the Appendix.

jugular venous arch. A communicating vein between the anterior jugular veins situated in the suprasternal space. NA *arcus venosus juguli.*

ju·gum (joo'gum) *n.*, pl. **ju·ga** (·guh) [L., yoke]. A yoke or bridge.

jugum sphe·noi·da·le (sfee·noy·day'lee) [NA]. The bridge of bone between the roots of the lesser wings of the sphenoid.

juice, *n.* [L. *jus,* broth]. 1. The liquid contained in vegetable or animal tissues. 2. Any of the secretions of the body.

ju·jube (joo'joob) *n.* [F., from Gk. *zizyphon*]. The fruit of the jujube tree, *Zizyphus jujuba;* formerly used as a demulcent in the form of a lozenge or syrup.

Jukes. A fictitious name given to the descendants of certain sisters in a study of the occurrence among them of crime, immorality, pauperism, and disease in relation to heredity.

Jukes unit. BOURQUIN-SHERMAN UNIT.

ju·men·tous (joo·men'tus) *adj.* [L. *jumen*tum, beast of burden, + *-ous*]. Similar to that of a horse; applied to the odor of urine.

jump·ers, *n. pl.* JUMPING FRENCHMEN OF MAINE.

jumping disease or **spasm.** JUMPING FRENCHMEN OF MAINE.

jumping Frenchmen of Maine. A bizarre paroxysmal disorder of unknown cause characterized by episodes of a single, violent jump evoked by sound, touch, or a sudden movement, and accompanied by echolalia; usually the disorder begins in childhood, is lifelong, familial, and observed only in males of French-Canadian descent. See also *lata, paroxysmal choreoathetosis, Gilles de la Tourette disease.*

jumping the bite. *In orthodontics,* a procedure used to correct a cross bite by temporarily opening the bite and moving the tooth or dental segment into the desired position.

junc·tion (junk'shun) *n.* [L. *junctio,* from *jungere,* to yoke, join]. The point or line of union of two parts; juncture, interface. —**junction·al** (·ul) *adj.*

junctional capillary. PRECAPILLARY.

junctional rhythm. A regular cardiac rhythm with the dominant pacemaker located in the atrioventricular junctional tissues. The rate is usually between 40 and 70 per minute. The P wave of the electrocardiogram is usually abnormal and may precede, follow, or be hidden in the QRS complex. Syn. *nodal rhythm.*

junctional tachycardia. A cardiac arrhythmia characterized by a heart rate of 140 to 220 per minute, with the impulses originating in the atrioventricular node or adjacent junctional tissue. Syn. *nodal tachycardia.*

junction nevus. A benign skin lesion containing nevus cells at the junction of the epidermis and dermis, but not in the dermis.

junc·tu·ra (junk·tew'ruh) *n.*, pl. & genit. sing. **junctu·rae** (·ree) [L.]. A joint or junction.

junctura car·ti·la·gi·nea (kahr·ti·la·jin'ee·uh) [NA]. A cartilaginous joint.

juncturae. Plural and genitive singular of *junctura.*

juncturae cin·gu·li mem·bri in·fe·ri·o·ris (sing'gew·lye mem'brye in·feer·ee·o'ris) [NA]. The joints of the pelvic girdle.

juncturae cinguli membri su·pe·ri·o·ris (sue·peer·ee·o'ris) [NA]. The joints of the shoulder girdle.

juncturae co·lum·nae ver·te·bra·lis, tho·ra·cis, et cra·nii (ko·lum'nee vur·te·bray'lis, tho·ray'sis et kray'nee·eye) [NA]. The combined joints of the vertebral column, thorax, and cranium.

juncturae mem·bri in·fe·ri·o·ris li·be·ri (mem'brye in·feer·ee·o'ris lye'bur·eye, lib'ur·eye) [NA]. The joints of the lower extremity proper.

juncturae membri su·pe·ri·o·ris li·be·ri (sue·peer·ee·o'ris lye'ber·eye, lib'ur·eye) [NA]. The joints of the upper extremity proper.

juncturae os·si·um (os'ee·um) [NA alt.]. JOINTS. NA alt. *articulationes.*

juncturae ten·di·num (ten'di·num) [BNA]. CONNEXUS INTERTENDINEUS.

juncturae zy·ga·po·phy·se·a·les (zig"uh·pof"i·see·ay'leez) [NA]. The joints between the articular processes of the vertebrae.

junctura fi·bro·sa (figh·bro'suh) [NA]. A fibrous joint.

junctura lum·bo·sa·cra·lis (lum"bo·sa·kray'lis) [NA]. The joint between the sacrum and lumbar vertebrae right or left.

junctura os·si·um (os'ee·um) [NA alt.]. JOINT. NA alt. *articulatio.*

junctura sa·cro·coc·cy·gea (sack"ro·kock·sij'ee·uh) [NA]. The joint between the sacrum and coccyx.

junctura sy·no·vi·a·lis (si·no·vee·ay'lis) [NA]. SYNOVIAL JOINT.

Jung·i·an (yoong'ee·un) *adj.* [C. J. *Jung,* Swiss psychiatrist, 1875–1961]. Pertaining to Jung, his psychoanalytic theories and methods.

Jungian psychology [C. J. *Jung*]. ANALYTIC PSYCHOLOGY.

jungle fever. 1. MALARIA. 2. YELLOW FEVER.

jun·gle yellow fever. A form of yellow fever endemic in South and Central America and Africa; occurs in or near forested areas where the disease is present in monkeys and is transmitted by *Haemagogus* and some *Aëdes* mosquitoes. Syn. *sylvan yellow fever.*

Jüng·ling's disease (yuᵉng'ling) [O. *Jüngling,* German surgeon, b. 1884]. OSTEITIS CYSTICA.

Jung's muscle (yoong) [C. G. *Jung,* German anatomist in Switzerland, 1793–1864]. The pyramidal muscle of the ear. See Table of Muscles in the Appendix.

ju·ni·per (joo'ni·pur) *n.* [L. *juniperus*]. 1. The fruit of *Juniperus communis,* containing a volatile oil, resin, and fixed oil. 2. Any of various evergreen shrubs or trees of the genus *Juniperus.*

juniper oil. The volatile oil from the fruit of *Juniperus communis;* has been used as a diuretic.

juniper tar. The empyreumatic volatile oil from the wood of the prickly juniper, *Juniperus oxycedrus.* A thick, dark-brown liquid, slightly soluble in water; used as a local antieczematic. Syn. *cade oil.*

Ju·nip·er·us (joo·nip'ur·us) *n.* [L., juniper]. A widespread genus of coniferous shrubs and trees comprising the junipers and including the red cedar of eastern North America.

Ju·nius-Kuhnt disease [H. *Kuhnt*]. DISCIFORM MACULAR DEGENERATION.

ju·ry, *n.* [OF. *juree,* oath, from L. *jurare,* to swear]. A body of adult persons chosen according to law to attend a judicial tribunal and sworn to determine upon the evidence to be placed before them the true verdict concerning a matter being tried or inquired into.

jury mast. An iron rod fixed in a plaster jacket; used to support the head in disease or fracture of the cervical spine.

jury of inquest. CORONER'S JURY.

jus·ta·ma·jor (jus"tuh·may'jur) *adj.* JUSTO MAJOR.

jus·ta·mi·nor (jus"tuh·migh'nur) *adj.* JUSTO MINOR.

jus·to major (jus'to) [L., regularly larger]. Greater than normal, larger in all dimensions than normal, applied to a pelvis.

justo minor [L., regularly smaller]. Abnormally small in all dimensions, applied to a pelvis.

jute, *n.* [Bengali *jūṭ*]. The bast fiber of several species of the genus *Corchorus,* grown chiefly in India and Ceylon; has been used in absorbent dressings.

ju·ve·nile (joo've·nil, ·nile) *adj.* [L. *juvenilis,* from *juvenis,* young]. 1. Pertaining to or characteristic of youth or childhood. 2. Young; immature.

juvenile acanthosis. A variety of acanthosis nigricans.

juvenile amaurotic familial idiocy. SPIELMEYER-VOGT DISEASE.

juvenile cell. METAMYELOCYTE.

juvenile histiocytoma. JUVENILE XANTHOGRANULOMA.

juvenile kyphosis. SCHEURMANN'S DISEASE.

juvenile macular degeneration. The most common familial form of macular degeneration, with onset between ages 8 to 20, characterized by slowly progressive loss of foveal reflex, granular appearance of the macula, and eventually pigmentary or atrophic macular changes; resulting in loss of central vision and markedly decreased visual acuity, but with no mental or neurologic dysfunctions. Inherited as either a dominant or recessive trait. Syn. *Stargardt's disease.*

juvenile melanoma. A type of benign compound nevus, principally occurring in young people, whose histologic appearance superficially resembles that of malignant melanoma.

juvenile metagranulocyte. METAMYELOCYTE.

juvenile-onset diabetes. Diabetes mellitus which develops early in life, presenting much more severe symptoms than the more common maturity-onset diabetes.

juvenile osteomalacia. RICKETS.

juvenile paralysis agitans (of J. R. Hunt). Typical Parkinson's disease, sometimes familial, beginning in late childhood and characterized by loss of cells in the putamen, pallidum, and substantia nigra. Syn. *progressive pallidal atrophy.*

juvenile parkinsonism. JUVENILE PARALYSIS AGITANS.

juvenile progressive spinal muscular atrophy. JUVENILE SPINAL MUSCULAR ATROPHY.

juvenile rheumatoid arthritis. Rheumatoid arthritis beginning before puberty, often ushered in by symptoms such as fever, erythematous rash, and weight loss, which often precede the onset of arthritis, and with lymphadenopathy, hepatosplenomegaly, and pericarditis. See also *Still's disease.*

juvenile spinal muscular atrophy. A hereditary, slowly progressive degenerative disorder of the anterior horn cells of the spinal cord, with onset in the first or second decade of life, usually affecting the larger proximal muscles first, especially of the pelvic girdle, and those of the arms and the distal muscles later. Commonly inherited as an autosomal recessive. Syn. *Kugelberg-Welander syndrome.* See also *infantile spinal muscular atrophy.*

juvenile type of progressive muscular dystrophy. LIMB-GIRDLE MUSCULAR DYSTROPHY.

juvenile T-wave pattern. Inverted or diphasic T waves in the right precordial leads of the electrocardiogram in adolescence and early adulthood.

juvenile wave pattern. JUVENILE T-WAVE PATTERN.

juvenile xanthogranuloma. A benign self-limited disorder of unknown cause, often familial and found at birth or early childhood, characterized clinically by yellowish-brown or red nodules on the extensor surfaces of the extremities as well as on the face, scalp, and trunk, and histologically by the presence of many histiocytes, foam cells, and Touton giant cells. The lesions disappear gradually. Lack of bone and other systemic involvement differentiates the disorder from Hand-Schüller-Christian disease, Letterer-Siwe disease, and eosinophilic granuloma. Syn. *nevoxanthoendothelioma, juvenile histiocytoma, juvenile xanthoma.*

juvenile xanthoma. JUVENILE XANTHOGRANULOMA.

juxta- [L.]. A combining form meaning *near, next to.*

jux·ta-ar·tic·u·lar (jucks"tuh·ahr·tick'yoo·lur) *adj.* [*juxta-* + *articular*]. Near a joint.

juxta-articular node or **nodule.** 1. A nodule adjacent to a joint. 2. A very hard, well-outlined tumefaction about a joint, frequently multiple, usually found about the elbows; most often seen in patients with syphilis, yaws, or pinta. Syn. *Jeanselme's nodule, Steiner's tumor.*

jux·ta·cor·ti·cal (jucks"tuh·kor'ti·kul) *adj.* [*juxta-* + *cortical*]. Near the cortex.

jux·ta·glo·mer·u·lar (jucks"tuh·glom·err'yoo·lur) *adj.* [*juxta-* + *glomerular*]. Next to a glomerulus.

juxtaglomerular apparatus. A cuff of epithelioid cells in the muscularis of an afferent arteriole near its entrance into the renal glomerulus and in contact with the distal convoluted tubules; it is concerned with renin production and sodium metabolism.

jux·ta·pap·il·lary (jucks"tuh·pap'i·lerr·ee) *adj.* [*juxta-* + *papillary*]. Situated near the optic disk.

juxtapapillary choroiditis. Choroiditis adjacent to the optic disk, resulting in a visual field defect; may be confused in the active stage with optic neuritis. Syn. *Jensen's chorioretinitis.*

jux·ta·po·si·tion (juck"stuh·po·zish'un) *n.* [*juxta-* + *position*]. Situation adjacent to another; close relationship; apposition. —**juxta·pose** (·poze') *v.*

jux·ta·py·lo·ric (jucks"tuh·pye·lor'ick, ·pi·lor'ick) *adj.* [*juxta-* + *pyloric*]. Near the pylorus.

jux·ta·res·ti·form body (jucks"tuh·res'ti·form). A structure in the medulla oblongata lying just medial to the inferior cerebellar peduncle proper; it contains fibers connecting the cerebellum with vestibular nuclei and other nuclei in the medulla.

K

K [NL. *kalium*]. Symbol for potassium.
K. An abbreviation for *cathode.*
K_a Symbol for the dissociation constant of an acid.
K_b Symbol for the dissociation constant of a base.
K_m Symbol for Michaelis constant.
Ka., ka. Abbreviation for *cathode.*
Ka·der-Senn operation (kah'derr) [B. *Kader,* Polish surgeon, 1863–1937; and N. *Senn,* U.S. surgeon, 1844–1908]. KADER'S OPERATION.
Kader's operation [B. *Kader*]. A gastrostomy with a fold which acts like a valve when the tube is removed.
Kaes-Bekhterev layer, lines, or **stripes** [T. *Kaes,* German neurologist, 1852–1913; and V. M. *Bekhterev*]. KAES'S LAYER.
Kaes's layer, lines, or **stripes** (keʸss) [T. *Kaes*]. A horizontal layer of fibers in the most superficial part of the external pyramidal layer of the cerebral cortex.
Kaf·fir pox (kaf'ur). [Ar. *kāfir,* infidel; an outmoded or derogatory name for the Xhosa and other South African Bantu]. A mild form of smallpox; VARIOLA MINOR.
Kahl·den's tumor. GRANULOSA CELL TUMOR.
Kah·ler's disease (kah'lur) [O. *Kahler,* Austrian physician, 1849–1893]. MULTIPLE MYELOMA.
Kahn's method. LEIBOFF AND KAHN'S METHOD.
Kahn test [R. L. *Kahn,* U.S. bacteriologist, b. 1887]. A precipitin test for syphilis.
kai·no·pho·bia (kigh''no·fo'bee·uh) *n.* [Gk. *kainos,* new, + *-phobia*]. A morbid fear of anything new. **—kai·no·phobe** (kigh'no·fobe) *n.*
Kai·ser·ling's method (kigh'zur·ling) [K. *Kaiserling,* German pathologist, 1869–1942]. A method of preparing museum specimens of human or animal organs to preserve their color.
kak-, kako-. See *cac-.*
kak·er·ga·sia (kack''ur·gay'zhuh) *n.* [*kak-* + *ergasia*]. MERERGASIA.
kak·ke (kahk'eh) *n.* [Jap.]. BERIBERI.
kak·or·rhaph·io·pho·bia (kack''o·raf''ee·o·fo'bee·uh) *n.* [Gk. *kakorraphia,* contrivance of ill, + *-phobia*]. Morbid fear of failure.
ka·la azar, kala-azar (kah'lah ah·zahr', ah'zahr, kal''uh ay'zur, az'ur) [Hindi *kālā,* black, + *āzār,* disease]. Visceral leishmaniasis due to the protozoan *Leishmania donovani,* transmitted by sandflies of the genus *Phlebotomus.* It is characterized by irregular fever of long duration, chronicity, enlargment of the spleen and liver, emaciation, anemia, leukopenia, and hyperglobulinemia.
ka·la·fun·gin (kay''luh·fung'gin, ·fun'jin) *n.* An antibiotic, $C_{15}H_{10}O_7$, produced by *Streptomyces tanashiensis, Kala* strain, that has antifungal activity.
ka·le·mia (ka·lee'mee·uh) *n.* [*kal*ium + *-emia*]. HYPERKALEMIA.
kal·i·emia, kal·i·ae·mia (kal''ee·ee'mee·uh) *n.* [*kal*ium + *-emia*]. HYPERKALEMIA.
kal·io·pe·nia (kal''ee·o·pee'nee·uh) *n.* [*kal*ium + *-penia*]. Low potassium concentration in the blood; HYPOKALEMIA. **—kaliope·nic** (·nick) *adj.*
Ka·lisch·er's disease (kah'li·shur) [O. *Kalischer,* German physician, 1842–1910]. STURGE-WEBER DISEASE.
ka·li·um (kay'lee·um) *n.* [NL., from Ar. *qalī,* ashes of saltwort, from *qala,* to fry]. POTASSIUM.
kal·li·din (kal'i·din) *n.* Either or both of two polypeptide plasma kinins released from the plasma alpha globulin kallidinogen (bradykininogen) by a kallikrein. The individual kallidins are identified as kallidin-9 (identical with bradykinin), which contains nine amino acid residues, and kallidin-10, which contains an additional amino acid residue. Kallidins cause vasodilatation, increase capillary permeability, produce edema, and contract or relax a variety of extravascular smooth muscles.
kal·li·din·o·gen (kal''i·din'o·jen) *n.* [*kallidin* + *-gen*]. An alpha globulin present in blood plasma which serves as the precursor for the kallidins and the substrate for kallikreins. Kallidinogen appears to be identical with bradykininogen.
Kal·li·kak (kal'i·kack) *n.* A fictitious name given to the descendants of a Revolutionary War soldier in a study of the occurrence among them of feeblemindedness and of immorality and the bearing of heredity on intelligence, personality, and behavior.
kal·li·kre·in (kal''i·kree'in) *n.* [Gk. *kallikre*as, pancreas, + *-in*]. A proteolytic enzyme present in pancreatic juice, blood plasma, urine, saliva, and other body fluids that releases a kallidin from the plasma alpha globulin kallidinogen (bradykininogen). Kallikrein from blood plasma releases only kallidin-9, but kallikrein from urine releases kallidin-9 and kallidin-10.
Kall·mann's syndrome. An inherited form of hypogonadotropic hypogonadism associated with infertility and anosmia.
ka·ma·la (kuh·may'luh, kam'uh·luh) *n.* [Skr.]. The glands and hairs from the capsules of *Mallotus philippinensis* (kamala tree); has been used as a purgative and anthelmintic.
ka·me·la (kuh·mee'luh, kam'e·luh) *n.* KAMALA.
Kam·mer·er-Bat·tle incision [F. *Kammerer,* U.S. surgeon, 1856–1928; and W. H. *Battle*]. A vertical abdominal incision through the rectus sheath, with medial retraction of the muscle.
kan·a·my·cin (kan''uh·migh'sin) *n.* An antibiotic substance,

$C_{18}H_{36}N_4O_{11}$, derived from strains of *Streptomyces kanamyceticus;* used as the sulfate salt. Absorbed rapidly from intramuscular sites but only slightly from the gastrointestinal tract. It is active against many bacteria.

Ka·na·vel's operation (ka·nay'vul) [A. B. *Kanavel,* U.S. surgeon, 1874–1938]. An operation in which full-thickness skin grafts, with all fat removed, are used for the relief of Dupuytren's contracture.

Kanavel's sign [A. B. *Kanavel*]. A sign for ulnar bursitis in which there is a point of maximal tenderness in the center of the hypothenar eminence.

Kan·da·har sore (kan″da·hadr′) [after *Kandahar,* Afghanistan]. CUTANEOUS LEISHMANIASIS.

Kan·din·sky complex (kahn·dyin'skee) [V. C. *Kandinsky,* Russian psychiatrist, 1825–1889]. CLÉRAMBAULT-KANDINSKY COMPLEX.

kan·ga·roo tendon. A tendon obtained from the tail of the kangaroo; used for surgical ligatures and sutures.

"kan·gri basket" cancer. (kang'gree, kung'gree). A nonmetastasizing squamous cell carcinoma of the abdominal skin occurring in Kashmir and Tibet where people warm the belly by means of a wicker-covered clay pot (kangri) of hot coals.

kangri burn. "KANGRI BASKET" CANCER.

Kan·ner's syndrome [L. *Kanner,* U.S. psychiatrist, b. 1894]. AUTISM (2).

Kantrex. Trademark for the antibiotic kanamycin.

ka·o·lin (kay'o·lin) *n.* [F., after *Kao Ling,* high hill, the place in China where it was first obtained]. A native, hydrated aluminum silicate, powdered and freed from gritty particles by elutriation. Used externally as a protective and absorbent; internally it is sometimes used as an adsorbent.

kaolin cataplasm. A mixture of kaolin, glycerin, and boric acid, with small amounts of thymol, methyl salicylate, and peppermint oil; has been used as a local counterirritant.

ka·o·li·no·sis (kay″o·li·no'sis) *n.* [*kaolin* + *-osis*]. A pneumoconiosis due to the inhalation of kaolin dust.

Ka·po·si's disease (kah'po·zee) [M. K. *Kaposi,* Austrian dermatologist, 1837–1902]. 1. XERODERMA PIGMENTOSUM. 2. MULTIPLE IDIOPATHIC HEMORRHAGIC SARCOMA. 3. ECZEMA HERPETICUM.

Kaposi's sarcoma or **syndrome** [M. K. *Kaposi*]. MULTIPLE IDIOPATHIC HEMORRHAGIC SARCOMA.

Kaposi's varicelliform eruption [M. *Kaposi*]. ECZEMA HERPETICUM.

kap·pa (kap'uh) *n.* [name of the letter K, κ, tenth letter of the Greek alphabet]. A designation used for various categories and quantities, sometimes as one of a series or set along with other Greek letters, and sometimes as a correlate of the letter K,k in the Roman alphabet. Symbol, K, κ.

kappa angle. The angle formed by the visual and pupillary axes; when the pupillary axis is temporal to the visual axis, the angle is positive.

kappa chain, κ chain. See *light chain.*

Kappadione. A trademark for menadiol sodium diphosphate, a water-soluble prothrombinogenic compound with the actions and uses of menadione.

kappa factor. A cytoplasmic genic factor in paramecia, believed to be a deoxyribonucleoprotein. When this factor is transmitted to a susceptible paramecium through cytoplasmic conjugation, it causes cell death.

kappa toxin. COLLAGENASE.

Kappaxin. A trademark for menadione, a prothrombinogenic compound.

ka·ra·ya gum (ka·rah'yuh, kăr'ay·uh). An exudate from trees of the *Sterculia* or *Cochlospermum* species; with water, it swells to form a bulky mass. Karaya gum is sometimes employed as a mechanical laxative. Syn. *sterculia gum.*

Ka·rell diet [P. J. *Karell,* Russian physician, 1806–1886]. A sodium and fluid-restricted diet consisting only of 800 ml of milk; once used to treat patients with congestive heart failure.

Karr's method [W. G. *Karr,* U.S. biochemist, b. 1892]. A method for the detection of urea in blood, similar to Folin and Svedberg's method except that the ammonium carbonate is nesslerized directly in the presence of gum ghatti as a protective colloid.

Kar·ta·ge·ner's syndrome or **triad** (kar·tah'ge·nur) [M. *Kartagener,* Swiss physician, b. 1897]. A hereditary symptom complex consisting of transposition of the viscera, maldevelopment of the sinuses leading to sinusitis, and bronchiectasis.

kary-, karyo- [Gk. *karyon,* nut, kernel]. *In biology,* a combining form meaning *nucleus, nuclear.*

kary·en·chy·ma (kăr″ee·eng'ki·muh) *n.* [*kary-* + Gk. *enchyma,* liquid contents, from *enchein,* to pour in]. NUCLEAR SAP.

karyo·blast (kăr'ee·o·blast) *n.* [*karyo-* + *-blast*]. *Obsol.* PRONORMOBLAST.

karyo·chrome (kăr'ee·o·krome) *n.* [*karyo-* + *-chrome*]. KARYOCHROME CELL.

karyochrome cell. *Obsol.* 1. A nerve cell which has a high nucleocytoplasmic ratio. 2. A nerve cell in which the nucleus stains intensely.

kary·oc·la·sis (kăr″ee·ock'luh·sis) *n.* [*karyo-* + *-clasis*]. KARYORRHEXIS. —**karyo·clas·tic** (kăr″ee·o·klas'tick) *adj.*

karyo·cyte (kăr'ee·o·site) *n.* [*karyo-* + *-cyte*]. NORMOBLAST (1).

kary·og·a·my (kăr″ee·og'uh·mee) *n.* [*karyo-* + *-gamy*]. A conjugation of cells characterized by a fusion of the nuclei. —**karyo·gam·ic** (kăr″ee·o·gam'ick) *adj.*

karyo·gram (kăr'ee·o·gram) *n.* KARYOTYPE (2).

karyo·ki·ne·sis (kăr″ee·o·ki·nee'sis, ·kigh·nee'sis) *n.* [*karyo-* + *-kinesis*]. Mitosis, especially the nuclear transformations. Syn. *karyomitosis.* Contr. *cytokinesis.* —**karyoki·net·ic** (·net'ick) *adj.*

karyo·lo·bic (kăr″ee·o·lo'bick) *adj.* [*karyo-* + *lobe* + *-ic*]. Having or pertaining to a lobated nucleus.

karyo·lymph (kăr'ee·o·limf) *n.* [*karyo-* + *lymph*]. NUCLEAR SAP.

kary·ol·y·sis (kăr″ee·ol'i·sis) *n.* [*karyo-* + *-lysis*]. The dissolution of the nucleus of the cell. —**karyo·lit·ic** (kăr″ee·o·lit'ick) *adj.*

karyo·meg·a·ly (kăr″ee·o·meg'uh·lee) *n.* [*karyo-* + *-megaly*]. *In exfoliative cytology,* slight but uniform nuclear enlargement in superficial and intermediate squamous cells of the uterine cervical epithelium.

karyo·mere (kăr'ee·o·meer) *n.* [*karyo-* + *-mere*]. A segment of a chromosome. See also *chromomere.*

kary·om·e·try (kăr″ee·om'e·try) *n.* [*karyo-* + *-metry*]. The measurement of the nucleus of a cell.

karyo·mi·cro·so·ma (kăr″ee·o·migh″kro·so'muh) *n.* [*karyo-* + *micro-* + Gk. *sōma,* body]. A chromatin particle of the nucleus.

karyo·mi·tome (kăr″ee·o·migh'tome) *n.* [*karyo-* + *mitome*]. The fibrillar part of nucleoplasm. See also *mitome.*

karyo·mi·to·sis (kăr″ee·o·mi·to'sis, ·migh·to'sis) *n.* [*karyo-* + *mitosis*]. KARYOKINESIS.

kar·y·on (kăr'ee·on) *n.* [Gk., nut, kernel]. The nucleus of a cell.

karyo·phage (kăr'ee·o·faje, ·fahzh) *n.* [*karyo-* + *-phage*]. A cell capable of phagocytizing the nucleus of an infected cell.

karyo·plasm (kăr'ee·o·plaz·um) *n.* [*karyo-* + *-plasm*]. NUCLEOPLASM. —**karyo·plas·mic** (kăr″ee·o·plaz'mick) *adj.*

karyoplasmic ratio. NUCLEOCYTOPLASMIC RATIO.

kary·or·rhex·is (kăr″ee·o·reck'sis) *n.*, pl. **karyorrhex·es** (·seez) [*karyo-* + *-rrhexis*]. Fragmentation or splitting up of a nucleus into a number of pieces which become scattered in the cytoplasm. —**karyor·rhec·tic** (·reck'tick) *adj.*

karyo·some (kăr'ee·o·sohm) *n.* [*karyo-* + *-some*]. 1. An aggregated mass of chromatin in the nucleus, confused with the nucleolus. 2. A large, deeply staining body in the nucleus of many Protista, associated with the chromosomes or other structures.

kary·os·ta·sis (kăr″ee·os′tuh·sis) *n.* [*karyo-* + *-stasis*]. The stage of the nucleus between mitotic divisions.

karyo·the·ca (kăr″ee·o·theek′uh) *n.* [*karyo-* + *theca*]. NUCLEAR MEMBRANE.

karyo·type (kăr′ee·o·tipe) *n.* [*karyo-* + *type*]. 1. The total of characteristics, including number, form, and size, of chromosomes and their grouping in a cell nucleus; it is characteristic of an individual, race, species, genus, or larger grouping. 2. The arrangement of chromosome photomicrographs according to a standard classification.

Kas·a·bach-Mer·ritt syndrome [H. H. *Kasabach*, U.S. pediatrician, 20th century; and K. K. *Merritt*, U.S. pediatrician, b. 1886]. Giant capillary hemangioma, thrombocytopenia, and purpura, occurring principally in childhood; HEMANGIOMA-THROMBOCYTOPENIA SYNDROME.

ka·sai (kah·sigh′) *n.* A syndrome seen in the Democratic Republic of the Congo, characterized by depigmentation of the skin, anemia, edema, and digestive disturbances, attributed to iron deficiency. Syn. *Belgian Congo anemia.*

Ka·shi·da's thermic sign. In tetany, the appearance of hyperesthesias and spasms after the application of cold and warm stimuli.

Ka·shin-Beck disease (kah′shin) [N. I. *Kashin*, Russian physician, 1825–1872; and E. V. *Bek* (*Beck*)]. A chronic degenerative generalized osteoarthrosis occurring chiefly in children in Siberia, northern China, and northern Korea; believed to be a form of mycotoxicosis due to ingestion of cereals infected with the fungus *Fusarium sporotrichiella.* Syn. *Urov disease.*

Kast's syndrome (kahst) [A. *Kast*, German physician, 1856–1903]. Multiple cavernous hemangiomas associated with chondromas or enchondromatosis. Some patients show pigmentary skin changes. It is thought to be a variant of Maffucci's syndrome.

kata-. See *cata-.*

kata·did·y·mus (kat″uh·did′i·mus) *n.* [*kata-* + *-didymus*]. Duplication of the superior pole, as in diprosopia or dicephalism. Has been incorrectly used for inferior duplicity. Syn. *superior duplicity.*

kataplasia. CATAPLASIA.

kata·ther·mom·e·ter, cata·ther·mom·e·ter (kat″uh·thur·mom′e·tur) *n.* [*kata-* + *thermometer*]. An alcohol thermometer, with a dry bulb and a wet bulb, that measures how quickly air is cooling, thus permitting an estimate of evaporation of moisture from the body.

katatonia. CATATONIA.

Ka·ta·ya·ma (kat″uh·yah′muh, kah″tuh·) *n.* [Jap.]. A genus of amphibious snails, usually included in the genus *Oncomelania.*

Katayama formosana. ONCOMELANIA FORMOSANA.

Katayama nosophora. ONCOMELANIA NOSOPHORA.

kathepsin. CATHEPSIN.

kath·i·so·pho·bia (kath″i·so·fo′bee·uh) *n.* [Gk. *kathisis*, sitting, + *-phobia*]. Morbid fear of or anxiety about sitting down; AKATHISIA (2).

kathode. CATHODE.

kation. CATION.

Katz-Wach·tel sign [L. N. *Katz*, U.S. physician, 20th century; and H. *Wachtel*, U.S. physician, 20th century]. High-voltage QRS complexes in the midprecordial leads of the electrocardiogram; a sign of ventricular septal defect.

Kauff·mann's tetrathionate broth medium. TETRATHIONATE BROTH BASE MEDIUM.

kau·ri (kaow′ree) *n.* [Maori]. The fossilized resinous exudate from the Kauri pine; used largely in the arts. A solution in alcohol has been used as a substitute for collodion in treating wounds.

ka·va (kah′vuh, kav′uh) *n.* [Tongan, bitter]. 1. An intoxicating beverage prepared in the Hawaiian Islands from the root of *Piper methysticum.* 2. The root of *Piper methysticum*, containing a resin, kawine, and other constituents; formerly used for treatment of genitourinary tract inflammation.

ka·va-ka·va (kah″vuh·kah′vuh) *n.* KAVA.

Kayexalate. Trademark for sodium polystyrene sulfonate, an ion-exchange resin used for the treatment of hyperkalemia.

Kay-Gra·ham pasteurization test [H. D. *Kay*, Canadian biochemist, b. 1893; and G. S. *Graham*, U.S. pathologist, 1879–1942]. The destructive effect of heat on the natural phosphatase in raw milk is used as a basis for testing the efficiency of pasteurization. Phosphatase activity is measured by the hydrolysis of disodium phenyl phosphate and colorimetric estimation of the released phenol by means of Folin-Ciocalteu's reagent.

kay·ser (kigh′zur) *n.* [J. H. G. *Kayser*, German physicist, 1853–1940]. *In spectroscopy*, a unit for expressing frequency of electromagnetic radiation as the number of wavelengths per centimeter; it is the reciprocal of the wavelength in centimeters.

Kayser-Fleischer ring [B. *Kayser*, German ophthalmologist, 1869–1954; and R. *Fleischer*]. A ring of golden-brown or brownish green pigmentation in the periphery of the cornea due to the deposition of copper in the area of Descemet's membrane and deep corneal stroma; diagnostic of hepatolenticular degeneration. It may be visible only on slit-lamp examination.

kcal Abbreviation for *kilocalorie.*

Kedani fever. TSUTSUGAMUSHI DISEASE.

Kee·ler's lie detector or **polygraph** [L. *Keeler*, U.S. psychologist and criminologist, 1903–1949]. A polygraph adapted for the questioning of a person considered to be or suspected of being guilty of a crime.

Keen's point [W. W. *Keen*, U.S. surgeon, 1837–1932]. A point 3 cm above and 3 cm behind the external auditory meatus from which to needle the lateral ventricle on that side.

keep·er, *n.* The armature of a horseshoe magnet.

kef·ir (kef′ur, ke·feer′) *n.* [Russ., from a Caucasian language]. A beverage prepared, especially in certain European countries, from the milk of cows, sheep, or goats through fermentation by kefir grains, these containing unidentified species of yeast or bacterial organisms.

Keflex. A trademark for cephalexin, an antibacterial agent.

Keflin. Trademark for cephalothin, a bactericidal antibiotic drug.

Kefloridin. A trademark for cephaloridine, an antibacterial agent.

Keforal. A trademark for cephalexin, an antibacterial agent.

Kefzol. A trademark for cefazolin, an antibacterial agent.

Keh·rer's reflex (keyr′ur) [F. A. *Kehrer*, German neurologist, b. 1883]. AURICULOPALPEBRAL REFLEX.

Kehr's operation [H. *Kehr*, German surgeon, 1862–1916]. A form of cholangioenterostomy. A segment of liver is resected so that several moderate-sized bile ducts are opened; this area is then sutured, preferably to an opening in the duodenum.

Kehr's sign [H. *Kehr*]. An inconstant sign for rupture of the spleen in which there is an area of hyperesthesia and pain over the left shoulder.

Keith's node [A. *Keith*, Scottish anatomist and anthropologist, 1866–1955]. SINOATRIAL NODE.

Keith-Wagener-Barker classification. A classification of funduscopic changes observed in hypertensive patients, graded 1 to 4 according to the severity of the changes: group 1, moderate attenuation of the retinal arterioles with focal constrictions at times; group 2, more marked arteriolar constriction and retinal hemorrhages; group 3, cotton-wool exudates regardless of other findings; group 4, papilledema regardless of other findings.

k electron. Either of the two electrons in the first shell or orbit surrounding the nucleus of an atom.

Kelene. A trademark for ethyl chloride.

ke·lis (kee'lis) *n.* [Gk. *kēlis*, stain, spot]. 1. Localized scleroderma. 2. KELOID.

Kell blood group system [after Mrs. *Kell*, in whose serum the antibody was first found]. A family of antigens, first described in 1946, found in erythrocytes designated as K,k, Kp^a, Kp^b, and Ku. Antibodies to the K antigen, which occurs in about 10 percent of the population of England, have been associated with hemolytic transfusion reactions and with hemolytic disease.

Kel·ler-Blake splint. A hinged, half-ring splint of the Thomas type for the lower extremity.

Keller operation [W. L. *Keller*, U.S. surgeon, 1874–1959]. Arthroplasty of the first metatarsophalangeal joint to correct hallux valgus or hallux rigidus; the proximal phalanx of the great toe is partially resected and the toe shortened.

Keller's micromethod. A method for detecting urea in which the solution resulting from incubation of a protein-free blood filtrate with urease and buffer is nesslerized and compared colorimetrically with a similarly treated standard urea solution.

kellin. KHELLIN.

Kel·ling's test [G. *Kelling*, German surgeon, b. 1866]. A test for lactic acid in which ferric chloride added to gastric juice produces a deep yellow color if lactic acid is present.

Kel·ly cystoscope [H. A. *Kelly*, U.S. gynecologist, 1858–1943]. A short, open-air cystoscope through which, with the help of a head mirror, the interior of a female urinary bladder can be visualized. With the patient in a knee-chest posture, the bladder automatically becomes distended with air.

Kelly forceps [H. A. *Kelly*]. A curved surgical clamp which can be used either as a hemostat for large vessels or to grasp bundles of vascular tissues prior to dividing them.

Kelly-Paterson syndrome [A. Brown *Kelly*, British laryngologist, 1865–1941; and D. R. *Paterson*]. PLUMMER-VINSON SYNDROME.

Kelly plication. Surgical plication of the bladder neck and urethra for stress incontinence of urine.

Kelly speculum [H. A. *Kelly*]. A tubular speculum fitted with an obturator designed principally for use in the rectum.

Kelly's sign [H. A. *Kelly*]. During operation, if a ureter is nudged with an instrument, it will contract; this enables one to recognize the structure.

ke·loid, che·loid (kee'loid) *n.* [F. *keloïde, cheloïde*, from Gk. *kēlē*, tumor, + *-oïde*, -oid, -like]. A fibrous hyperplasia usually at the site of a scar, elevated, rounded, firm, and with ill-defined borders. There is predilection for the upper trunk and face, and the condition is observed especially in young female adults and in blacks. —**ke·loid·al** (kee·loy'dul) *adj.*

keloid acne. Follicular infection, resembling acne in papular and pustular form, and resulting in hypertrophic or keloidal scarring. The nape of the neck is the commonest site of such process; blacks are frequently affected. Syn. *folliculitis keloidalis, dermatitis papillaris capillitii.*

keloidal folliculitis. KELOID ACNE.

keloid sycosis. Sycosis in which keloidal change occurs in the cicatrices resulting from the follicular inflammation. NA *ulerythema sycosiforme.*

ke·lo·ma (kee·lo'muh) *n.* [Gk. *kēlis*, blemish, nevus, + *-oma*]. KELOID.

Kelox. Trademark for tetroquinone, a systemic keratolytic drug.

kelp, *n.* 1. A common name for a group of large brown algae growing in the cool ocean waters. 2. Burnt seaweed from which potassium salts and iodine formerly were prepared.

kel·vin, *n.* [W. Thomson, Lord *Kelvin*, British physicist, 1824–1907]. A commercial unit of electricity; 1,000 watt-hours.

Kelvin scale [Lord *Kelvin*]. An absolute scale of temperature which has its zero at −273°C.

Kemadrin. Trademark for the antiparkinsonism drug procyclidine, used as the hydrochloride salt.

Kemp·ner rice diet [W. *Kempner*, U.S. physician, b. 1903]. A rigid diet of rice, fruit, and sugar, providing about 7 mEq per day of sodium and averaging about 2000 calories per day; used in the treatment of hypertension.

ken-, keno- [Gk. *kenos*]. A combining form meaning *empty.*

Kenacort. A trademark for the adrenocortical steroid triamcinolone and its diacetate ester.

Kenalog. A trademark for triamcinolone acetonide.

Ken·dall's compound A [E. C. *Kendall*, U.S. physiologist and biochemist, 1886–1972]. DEHYDROCORTICOSTERONE.

Kendall's compound B [E. C. *Kendall*]. CORTICOSTERONE.

Kendall's compound C [E. C. *Kendall*]. COMPOUND C.

Kendall's compound D [E. C. *Kendall*]. COMPOUND D.

Kendall's compound E [E. C. *Kendall*]. CORTISONE.

Kendall's compound F [E. C. *Kendall*]. HYDROCORTISONE.

ken·es·the·sia (ken"es·theezh'uh) *n.* CENESTHESIA.

Ken·ne·dy syndrome [F. *Kennedy*, U. S. neurologist, 1884–1952]. FOSTER KENNEDY SYNDROME.

Ken·ny treatment [Elizabeth *Kenny*, Australian nurse, 1886–1952]. Treatment of weak or paralyzed muscles in poliomyelitis with hot moist packs, followed by passive and then active exercises with muscle reeducation.

keno-. See *ken-*.

keno·pho·bia (ken"o·fo'bee·uh) *n.* [*keno-* + *-phobia*]. A morbid fear of large, empty spaces.

keno·tox·in (ken"o·tock'sin) *n.* [*keno-* + *toxin*]. A hypothetical poisonous substance developed in the tissues during their activity which has been said to be responsible for their fatigue and for sleep.

Kent mental test [G. H. *Kent*, U.S. psychologist, b. 1875]. An oral test for intelligence consisting of 25 questions for emergency use in clinics.

Ke·nya tick typhus (kee'nyuh, ken'yuh) [after *Kenya*, East Africa]. One of the tick-borne typhus fevers of Africa.

keph·a·lin (kef'uh·lin) *n.* CEPHALIN.

kephir, kephyr. KEFIR.

Ke·ran·del's sign or **symptom** (key·rah^n·del') [J. F. *Kerandel*, French physician, 1873–1934]. Deep hyperesthesia, later possibly followed by pain, resulting from slight trauma over a bony prominence, especially at the elbow; seen in Gambian trypanosomiasis.

ker·a·phyl·lo·cele (kerr"uh·fil'o·seel) *n.* [*keraphyllous* + *-cele*]. A horny tumor on the inner side of the wall of a horse's hoof.

ker·a·phyl·lous (kerr"uh·fil'us, ke·raf'i·lus) *adj.* [Gk. *keras*, horn, + *phyllon*, leaf, + *-ous*]. *In veterinary medicine*, composed of horny layers.

ker·a·sin (kerr'uh·sin) *n.* A cerebroside separated from the brain; contains sphingosine, galactose, and fatty acid.

kerat-, kerato- [Gk. *keras, keratos*, horn]. A combining form meaning (a) *horn, horny;* (b) *cornea, corneal.*

ker·a·tal·gia (kerr"uh·tal'jee·uh) *n.* [*kerat-* + *-algia*]. Pain in the cornea.

ker·a·tec·ta·sia (kerr"uh·teck·tay'zhuh) *n.* [*kerat-* + *ectasia*]. Thinning with protrusion of the cornea as seen following ulceration or with keratoconus. See also *descemetocele.*

ker·a·tec·to·my (kerr"uh·teck'tuh·mee) *n.* [*kerat-* + *-ectomy*]. Surgical excision of a part of the cornea, usually for removal of a localized opacity or for diagnostic purposes.

ke·rat·ic (ke·rat'ick) *adj.* [*kerat-* + *-ic*]. Pertaining to the cornea.

keratic precipitates. Clumps of inflammatory cells deposited upon the endothelial surface of the cornea, occurring with intraocular inflammations such as uveitis. Round-cell precipitates are generally the result of an acute, nongranulomatous infection, while the larger "mutton-fat" precipitates of epithelioid cells indicate a chronic, granulomatous process.

ker·a·tin (kerr'uh·tin) *n.* [*kerat-* + *-in*]. Any of a group of albuminoids or scleroproteins characteristic of horny tissues, hair, nails, feathers, insoluble in protein solvents, and having a high content of sulfur. Two main groups are distinguished: eukeratins, which are not digested by common proteolytic enzymes, and pseudokeratins, which are partly digested. Both contain various amino acids; cystine and arginine generally predominate.

ker·a·tin·iza·tion (kerr″uh·tin·i·zay′shun) *n.* 1. Development of a horny quality in a tissue. 2. The process whereby keratin is formed. 3. The coating of pills with keratin. —**ker·a·tin·ize** (kerr′uh·tin·ize) *v.;* **keratin·ized** (·ize′d) *adj.*

ke·rat·i·no·cyte (ke·rat′i·no·site) *n.* [*keratin* + *-cyte*]. An epidermal cell that synthesizes keratin.

ke·rat·i·no·phil·ic (ke·rat″i·no·fil′ick) *adj.* [*keratin* + *-philic*]. Having an affinity for horny or keratinized tissue, as certain fungi.

ke·rat·i·nous (ke·rat′i·nus) *adj.* 1. Of or pertaining to keratin. 2. HORNY.

keratinous degeneration. The appearance of keratin granules in the cytoplasm of a cell which does not ordinarily undergo keratinization.

ké·ra·tite en ban·de·lette (kerr·a·teet′ ahn bahnd·let′) [F.]. BAND KERATOPATHY.

ker·a·ti·tis (kerr″uh·tye′tis) *n.*, pl. **kera·tit·i·des** (·tit′i·deez) [*kerat-* + *-itis*]. Inflammation of the cornea. —**kera·tit·ic** (·tit′ick) *adj.*

keratitis ar·bo·res·cens (ahr·bo·res′enz). DENDRITIC KERATITIS.

keratitis bul·lo·sa (bo͝ol·o′suh). The formation of large or small blebs upon the cornea in cases of iridocyclitis, glaucoma, interstitial keratitis, or Fuch's dystrophy. Syn. *bullous keratitis.*

keratitis dis·ci·for·mis (dis″i·for′mis, dis″ki·). DISCIFORM KERATITIS.

keratitis hypopyon. Keratitis with accumulation of neutrophils, gravitating inferiorly, in the anterior chamber; seen most commonly with pneumococcal and aspergillus infections.

keratitis neu·ro·par·a·lyt·i·ca (new″ro·păr·uh·lit′i·kuh). NEUROPARALYTIC KERATITIS.

keratitis pa·ren·chy·ma·to·sa (pa·renk″i·muh·to′suh). INTERSTITIAL KERATITIS.

keratitis punc·ta·ta (punk·tay′tuh). The presence of leukocytes on the back of Descemet's membrane. Not a primary inflammation of Descemet's membrane, since the cells derive from the ciliary body as a result of its inflammation. Syn. *descemetitis.*

keratitis punctata le·pro·sa (le·pro′suh). Keratitis punctata of leprous origin.

keratitis punctata pro·fun·da (pro·fun′duh). Keratitis punctata of syphilitic origin.

keratitis pu·ru·len·ta (pewr″yoo·len′tuh). KERATITIS HYPOPYON.

keratitis pus·tu·li·for·mis pro·fun·da (pus″tew·li·form′is pro·fun′duh). KERATITIS PUNCTATA PROFUNDA.

keratitis ro·sa·cea (ro·zay′see·uh, ·shee·uh). The occurrence of small, sterile infiltrates at the periphery of the cornea, which are approached but not invaded by small blood vessels. They are most frequently seen unaccompanied by acne rosacea, but are most severe in this connection.

keratitis sic·ca (sick′uh). XEROSIS INFANTILIS.

kerato-. See *kerat-.*

ker·a·to·ac·an·tho·ma (kerr″uh·to·ack″an·tho′muh) *n.* [*kerato-* + *acanthoma*]. A firm skin nodule with a center of keratotic material, occurring on the hairy parts of the body, especially the exposed sites, developing and regressing over a period usually less than six months; it has a histologic resemblance to squamous cell cancer of the skin, and is usually solitary.

ker·a·to·cele (kerr′uh·to·seel) *n.* [*kerato-* + *-cele*]. A hernia of Descemet's membrane through the cornea; DESCEMETOCELE.

ker·a·to·cen·te·sis (kerr″uh·to·sen·tee′sis) *n.*, pl. **keratocente·ses** (·seez) [*kerato-* + *centesis*]. Corneal puncture.

ker·a·to·chro·ma·to·sis (kerr″uh·to·kro·muh·to′sis) *n.* [*kerato-* + *chromatosis*]. Discoloration of the cornea.

ker·a·to·con·junc·ti·vi·tis (kerr″uh·to·kun·junk·ti·vye′tis) *n.* [*kerato-* + *conjunctivitis*]. Simultaneous inflammation of the cornea and the conjunctiva.

keratoconjunctivitis sic·ca (sick′uh). Keratinization of the cornea and conjunctiva resulting from dryness.

ker·a·to·co·nus (kerr″uh·to·ko′nus) *n.* [*kerato-* + *conus*]. Conical axial ectasia of the cornea. The anterior form is an acquired lesion for adults, may be associated with an allergic diathesis, and is also a component of Down's syndrome; posterior keratoconus is a congenital lesion considered to be the mildest form of Peter's anomaly.

ker·a·to·der·ma (kerr″uh·to·dur′muh) *n.* [*kerato-* + *-derma*]. A horny condition of the skin, especially of the palms and soles.

keratoderma blen·nor·rhag·i·cum (blen″o·raj′i·kum). KERATOSIS BLENNORRHAGICA.

keratoderma cli·mac·ter·i·cum (klye″mack·terr′i·kum). A circumscribed hyperkeratosis of the palms and soles occurring in women during the menopause, and accompanied chiefly by obesity and hypertension. Syn. *Haxthausen's disease.*

keratoderma punc·ta·tum (punk·tay′tum). KERATOSIS PUNCTATA.

ker·a·to·der·ma·to·cele (kerr″uh·to·dur·mat′o·seel, ·dur′muh·to·) *n.* [*kerato-* + *dermato-* + *-cele*]. KERATOCELE.

ker·a·to·der·mia (kerr″uh·to·dur′mee·uh) *n.* [*kerato-* + *-dermia*]. KERATODERMA.

ker·a·to·gen·e·sis (kerr″uh·to·jen′e·sis) *n.* [*kerato-* + *-genesis*]. Development of horny growths.

ker·a·to·glo·bus (kerr″uh·to·glo′bus) *n.* [*kerato-* + L. *globus,* ball]. A globular protrusion of the cornea due to thinning of the entire cornea. May be congenital or acquired as with arrested congenital or juvenile glaucoma.

ker·a·to·hel·co·sis (kerr″uh·to·hel·ko′sis) *n.* [*kerato-* + Gk. *helkōsis,* ulcerations]. Ulceration of the cornea.

ker·a·to·he·mia, ker·a·to·hae·mia (kerr″uh·to·hee′mee·uh) *n.* [*kerato-* + *-hemia*]. The presence of blood or its breakdown products in or staining the cornea.

ker·a·to·hy·a·lin (kerr″uh·to·high′uh·lin) *n.* [*kerato-* + *hyalin*]. The substance of the granules in the stratum granulosum of keratinized stratified squamous epithelium; an early phase in the formation of keratin. —**keratohya·line** (·lin, ·leen) *adj.*

ker·a·toid (kerr′uh·toid) *adj.* [Gk. *keratoeidēs*]. Hornlike.

ker·a·to·iri·tis (kerr″uh·to·eye·rye′tis, ·i·rye′tis) *n.* [*kerato-* + *iritis*]. Combined inflammation of the cornea and the iris, as seen especially in herpetic keratouveitis.

ker·a·to·leu·ko·ma (kerr″uh·to·lew·ko′muh) *n.* [*kerato-* + *leukoma*]. A leukoma or whitish opacity of the cornea.

ker·a·tol·y·sis (kerr″uh·tol′i·sis) *n.* [*kerato-* + *-lysis*]. 1. Exfoliation of the epidermis. 2. A congenital anomaly in which the skin is shed periodically.

keratolysis neonatorum. DERMATITIS EXFOLIATIVA NEONATORUM.

ker·a·to·lyt·ic (kerr″uh·to·lit′ick) *adj.* & *n.* 1. Characterized by or pertaining to keratolysis. 2. An agent which causes exfoliation of the epidermis to a greater degree than that which occurs normally.

ke·ra·to·ma (kerr″uh·to′muh) *n.* [*kerat-* + *-oma*]. CALLOSITY.

ker·a·to·ma·la·cia (kerr″uh·to·ma·lay′shee·uh) *n.* [*kerato-* + *malacia*]. Degeneration of the cornea characterized by keratinization of the epithelium, eventually leading to ulceration and perforation of the cornea; seen in vitamin A deficiency.

keratoma plan·ta·re sul·ca·tum (plan·tair′ee sul·kay′tum). KERATOMA SULCATUM PLANTARUM.

keratoma sul·ca·tum plan·ta·rum (sul·kay′tum plan·tair′um).

An idiopathic pitted thickening of the soles seen in barefooted native adults in the tropics.

ker·a·tome (kerr'uh·tome) *n.* [*kerat-* + *-tome*]. A knife with a trowel-like blade, for incising the cornea.

ker·a·to·meg·a·ly (kerr''uh·to·meg'uh·lee) *n.* [*kerato-* + *-megaly*]. MEGALOCORNEA.

ker·a·tom·e·ter (kerr''uh·tom'e·tur) *n.* [*kerato-* + *-meter*]. An instrument for measuring the curves of the cornea. —**keratome·try** (·tree) *n.*

ker·a·to·my·co·sis (kerr''uh·to·migh·ko'sis) *n.* [*kerato-* + *mycosis*]. A fungus disease of the cornea.

ker·a·top·a·thy (kerr''uh·top'uth·ee) *n.* [*kerato-* + *-pathy*]. A degenerative process of the cornea. See also *band keratopathy.*

ker·a·to·plas·ty (kerr'uh·to·plas''tee) *n.* [*kerato-* + *-plasty*]. A plastic operation upon the cornea, especially the transplantation of a portion of cornea; may be full thickness or partial. —**ker·a·to·plas·tic** (kerr''uh·to·plas'tick) *adj.*

ker·a·tor·rhex·is (kerr''uh·to·reck'sis) *n.*, pl. **keratorrhex·es** (·seez) [*kerato-* + *-rrhexis*]. Rupture of the cornea, due to ulceration or trauma.

ker·a·to·scle·ri·tis (kerr''uh·to·skle·rye'tis) *n.* [*kerato-* + *scleritis*]. Inflammation of the cornea and the sclera.

ker·a·to·scope (kerr'uh·to·skope) *n.* [*kerato-* + *-scope*]. An instrument for examining the cornea and testing the symmetry of its meridians of curvature. Syn. *Placido's disk.*

ker·a·tos·co·py (kerr''uh·tos'kuh·pee) *n.* [*kerato-* + *-scopy*]. Examination of the cornea with the keratoscope.

ker·a·tose (kerr''uh·toce) *adj.* [*kerat-* + *-ose*]. Horny.

ker·a·to·sis (kerr''uh·to'sis) *n.* [*kerat-* + *-osis*]. 1. Any disease of the skin characterized by an overgrowth of the cornified epithelium. 2. ACTINIC KERATOSIS.

keratosis blen·nor·rhag·i·ca (blen''o·raj'i·kuh). A disease characterized by rupial, pustular, and crusted lesions, usually on the palms and soles. Found in association with gonococcal arthritis or with Reiter's disease. Syn. *keratoderma blennorrhagicum.*

keratosis fol·lic·u·la·ris (fol·ick''yoo·lair'is). DARIER'S DISEASE.

keratosis nigricans. ACANTHOSIS NIGRICANS.

keratosis pal·ma·ris et plan·ta·ris (pal·mair'is et plan·tair'is). A marked, congenital thickening of the volar surfaces of the hands and feet, frequently complicated by painful fissures; occurs as a dominant hereditary trait.

keratosis pha·ryn·ge·us (fa·rin'jee·us). A rare affection in which there is an outgrowth composed of horny desquamated epithelium from the crypts of the tonsils.

keratosis pi·la·ris (pi·lair'is). A chronic disorder of the skin marked by hard, conical elevations in the pilosebaceous orifices on the arms and thighs.

keratosis punc·ta·ta (punk·tay'tuh). Keratosis of the palms and soles, characterized by numerous minute, crateriform pits set in patches of thickening of the stratum corneum. Syn. *keratoderma punctatum.*

keratosis seb·or·rhe·i·ca (seb''o·ree'i·kuh). SEBORRHEIC KERATOSIS.

keratosis se·ni·lis (se·nigh'lis). ACTINIC KERATOSIS.

keratosis uni·ver·sa·lis con·gen·i·ta (yoo''ni·vur·say'lis kon·jen'i·tuh). DARIER'S DISEASE.

ker·a·to·sul·fate (kerr''uh·to·sul'fate) *n.* A sulfated mucopolysaccharide in which the uronic acid component is replaced by D-galactose.

ker·a·to·sul·fa·tu·ria (kerr''uh·to·sul''fuh·tew'ree·uh, ·sul''fay·) *n.* [*keratosulfate* + *-uria*]. MORQUIO'S SYNDROME.

ker·a·tot·ic (ker·uh·tot'ick) *adj.* Pertaining to or affected with keratosis.

keratotic nevus. NEVUS VERRUCOSUS.

ker·a·to·tome (kerr'uh·to·tome, ke·rat'o·tome) *n.* [*kerato-* + *-tome*]. KERATOME.

ker·a·tot·o·my (kerr''uh·tot'uh·mee) *n.* [*kerato-* + *-tomy*]. Incision of the cornea.

ke·rau·no·pho·bia (ke·raw''no·fo'bee·uh) *n.* [Gk. *keraunos*, thunderbolt, + *-phobia*]. Abnormal excessive fear of lightning and thunderstorms.

Kerck·ring's f ·lds (kerrk'ring) [T. *Kerckring*, German anatomist, 1640–1693]. CIRCULAR FOLDS.

Kerckring's ossicle [T. *Kerckring*]. An independent ossification center in the occipital bone at the posterior margin of the foramen magnum.

ke·rec·to·my (ke·reck'tuh·mee) *n.* KERATECTOMY.

ke·ri·on (keer'ee·on, kerr'ee·on) *n.* [Gk. *kērion*, honeycomb, from *kēros*, beeswax]. A pustular eruption with boggy abscess on a hair-bearing area of the body.

kerion cel·si (sel'sigh) [L., of Celsus]. A type of dermatophytosis of the scalp or beard, with deep, boggy infiltration.

Ker·ley lines [P. J. *Kerley*, British roentgenologist, b. 1900]. Thickened interlobular septa visible radiographically usually in the region of the costophrenic angles (Kerley B lines) but also in the upper and middle portion of the lungs as longer lines or extending peripherally from the hilum (Kerley A lines). The thickening is due to edema and lymphatic distention in chronic pulmonary venous hypertension, but may be due to cellular infiltrate or fibrous tissue in other conditions.

ker·mes (kur'meez) *n.* [Ar. *qirmiz*]. The dried bodies of an insect found on the oak *Quercus coccifera;* contain a purplish-red coloring matter said to be the oldest dyestuff known; has been used in medicine.

kern·echt·rot (kehrn''ekht'rote) *n.* [Ger.]. NUCLEAR FAST RED.

ker·nic·ter·us (kair·nick'tur·us, kur·) *n.* [Ger., from *Kern*, nucleus, + *icterus*]. Bilirubin pigmentation of gray matter of the central nervous system, especially basal ganglions, accompanied by degeneration of nerve cells; occurring as complication of erythroblastosis fetalis and other causes of severe hyperbilirubinemia of the newborn, and accompanied and followed by a variety of severe neurological deficits or death. Syn. *nuclear icterus.*

Ker·nig's sign (kʸerr'nʸik) [V. M. *Kernig*, Russian physician, 1840–1917]. In meningeal irritation, with the patient supine and the thigh flexed at the hip, an attempt to completely extend the leg at the knee causes pain and spasm of the hamstring muscles.

Ker·no·han's notch [J. W. *Kernohan*, U.S. pathologist, b. 1897]. CRUS PHENOMENON.

Kernohan-Woltman syndrome [J. W. *Kernohan* and H. W. *Woltman*]. CRUS PHENOMENON.

ker·o·sene oil (kerr'uh·seen). A liquid mixture of hydrocarbons distilled from petroleum. Syn. *coal oil.*

ket-, keto-. *In chemistry*, a combining form designating *the presence of the ketone group.*

ke·ta·mine (kee'tuh·meen) *n.* 2-(*o*-Chlorophenyl)-2-(methylamino) cyclohexanone, $C_{13}H_{16}ClNO$, an anesthetic given intravenously or intramuscularly as the hydrochloride salt; may produce vivid and sometimes unpleasant dreams.

ke·ta·zo·cine (kee·tay'zo·seen) *n.* (2*R*,6*S*11*S*)-3-(Cyclopropylmethyl)-3,4,5,6-tetrahydro-8-hydroxy-6,11-dimethyl-2,6-methano-3-benzazocin-1-(2*H*)-one, $C_{18}H_{23}NO_2$, an analgesic.

ke·ta·zo·lam (kee·tay'zo·lam) *n.* 4*H*-[1,3]-Oxazino[3,2-*d*][1,4]benzodiazapene-4,7(6*H*)-dione, $C_{20}H_{17}ClN_2O_3$, a minor tranquilizer.

ke·tene (kee'teen) *n.* Ethenone, $H_2C{=}CO$, a colorless gas that forms acetic acid on hydrolysis; used to effect acetylization of free amino and hydroxyl groups.

ke·tip·ra·mine (kee·tip'ruh·meen) *n.* 5-[3-(Dimethylamino)-propyl]-5,11-dihydro-10*H*-dibenz[*b,f*]azepin-10-one, $C_{19}H_{22}N_2O$, an antidepressant drug; usually used as the fumarate salt.

ke·to (kee'to) *adj.* Characterizing the tautomeric and usually most stable form of certain ketones, which exhibit keto-enol tautomerism. Contr. *enol.*

keto-. See *ket-*.

ke·to acid (kee'to). Any compound containing both a ketone (—CO—) and a carboxyl (—COOH) group.

α-keto acid carboxylase. CARBOXYLASE (1).

α-keto acid decarboxylase. CARBOXYLASE (1).

ke·to·ac·i·do·sis (kee"to·as"i·do'sis) *n.* Acidosis accompanied by an increase in the blood of such ketone bodies as β-hydroxybutyric and acetoacetic acids.

ke·to·ac·i·du·ria (kee"to·as·i·dew'ree·uh) *n.* [*keto-* + *acid* + *-uria*]. The excretion, especially the excessive excretion, in the urine of organic molecules which have both a ketone and an acid group.

ke·to·adip·ic acid (kee"to·uh·dip'ick). α-Ketoadipic acid, $HOOCCOCH_2CH_2COOH$; an intermediate compound in the biochemical conversion of lysine to glutaric acid.

ke·to·bem·i·done (kee"to·bem'i·dohn) *n.* 4-(*m*-Hydroxyphenyl)-1-methyl-4-piperidyl ethyl ketone, $C_{15}H_{21}NO_2$, a narcotic related to morphine and causing true addiction; used experimentally as an analgesic.

Ketochol. Trademark for a combination of the keto forms of the biliary acids in approximately the same proportions as found in normal human bile. The preparation is used in gallbladder disorders.

ke·to·cho·lan·ic acid (kee"to·ko·lan'ick). Cholic acid in which one or more of the secondary alcohol groups have been oxidized to ketone groups.

α-ke·to·de·car·box·yl·ase (al'fuh kee"to·dee·kahr·bock'sil·ace) *n.* CARBOXYLASE (1).

Keto-Diastix. A trademark for a reagent strip containing sodium nitroprusside used to test for glucose and ketones in urine.

ke·to·gen·e·sis (kee"to·jen'e·sis) *n.* [*keto-* + *-genesis*]. The production of ketone bodies.

ke·to·gen·ic (kee"to·jen'ick) *adj.* [*keto-* + *-genic*]. Producing ketone bodies.

ketogenic diet. A diet in which an excessive proportion of the allotted calories is derived from fats, which are reduced to ketones; used in the therapy of epilepsy, especially in children with myoclonic and akinetic seizures and absence attacks refractory to conventional anticonvulsant drugs.

ketogenic hormone. Originally, the factor in crude extract of the anterior hypophysis which stimulated the rate of fatty acid metabolism. The metabolic actions which the term designates are now known to be induced by adrenocorticotropin and the growth hormone. Syn. *fat-metabolizing hormone.*

ketogenic substance. A foodstuff from which ketone bodies are produced.

ke·to·glu·tar·ic acid (kee"to·gloo·tăr'ick, ·tahr'ick). A dibasic keto acid, $HOOC(CH_2)_2COCOOH$, an intermediate product in the metabolism of carbohydrates and proteins.

ke·to·hep·tose (kee"to·hep'toce) *n.* A general term for monosaccharides consisting of a seven-carbon chain and containing a ketone group.

ke·to·hex·ose (kee"to·heck'soce) *n.* A general term for monosaccharides consisting of a six-carbon chain and containing a ketone group.

ke·to·hy·droxy·es·trin (kee"to·high·drock"see·es'trin, ·ees'trin) *n.* ESTRONE.

ke·tol (kee'tole, ·tol) *n.* Any compound containing both a ketone (—CO—) group and an alcohol (—OH) group.

ke·tole (kee'tole) *n.* INDOLE.

ke·tol·y·sis (kee·tol'i·sis) *n.* [*keto-* + *-lysis*]. The dissolution of ketone bodies. —**ke·to·lyt·ic** (kee"to·lit'ic) *adj.*

ke·tone (kee'tone) *n.* [Ger. *Keton*, from *Azeton*, acetone]. An organic compound derived by oxidation from a secondary alcohol; it contains the characterizing group —CO—.

ketone acid. KETO ACID.

ketone body. A group name for any of the compounds, β-hydroxybutyric acid, acetoacetic acid, or acetone, which simultaneously increase in blood and urine in diabetic acidosis, starvation, pregnancy, after ether anesthesia, and in other conditions. See also Table of Chemical Constituents of Blood in the Appendix.

ke·to·ne·mia, ke·to·nae·mia (kee"to·nee'mee·uh) *n.* [*ketone* + *-emia*]. The presence of increased concentrations of ketone bodies in the blood.

ke·to·nu·ria (kee"to·new'ree·uh) *n.* The presence of ketone bodies in the urine.

ke·to·pro·fen (kee"to·pro'fen) *n.* *m*-Benzoylhydratropic acid, $C_{16}H_{14}O_3$, an anti-inflammatory agent.

ke·to·pro·pi·on·ic acid (kee"to·pro"pee·on'ick). α-Ketopropionic acid; PYRUVIC ACID.

ke·to·re·duc·tase (kee"to·re·duck'tace, ·taze) *n.* An enzyme occurring in muscle, liver, and kidney, which converts acetoacetic acid into beta-oxybutyric acid.

ke·tose (kee'toce) *n.* A carbohydrate containing the ketone group.

ke·to·side (kee'to·side) *n.* Any glycoside that yields, on hydrolysis, a ketose.

ke·to·sis (kee·to'sis) *n.*, pl. **keto·ses** (·seez) [*ket-* + *-osis*]. 1. A condition in which ketones are present in the body in excessive amount. 2. The acidosis of diabetes mellitus. —**ke·tot·ic** (kee·tot'ick) *adj.*

ke·to·ste·roid (kee"to·sterr'oid, ·steer'oid, ke·tos'te·roid) *n.* One of a group of neutral steroids possessing ketone substitution, which produces a characteristic red color with *m*-dinitrobenzene in alkaline solution. The ketosteroids are principally metabolites of adrenal cortical and gonadal steroids. Syn. *17-ketosteroid.*

17-ketosteroid. KETOSTEROID.

ke·tox·ime (ke·tock'seem) *n.* An oxime resulting from action of hydroxylamine upon a ketone, having the general formula R(R')C=NOH.

Kety method. A method for determination of cerebral blood flow employing nitrous oxide.

key·way (kee'way) *n.* The receptacle attachment of a precision prosthodontic partial denture.

kg Abbreviation for *kilogram.*

khel·lin (kel'in) *n.* [Ar. *khilla* + *-in*]. 2-Methyl-5,8-dimethoxyfuranochromone, $C_{14}H_{12}O_5$, a constituent of the umbelliferous plant *Ammi visnaga*, the fruits of which have been used in Egypt as an antispasmodic in renal colic and ureteral spasm. Khellin has been used as a coronary vasodilator and bronchodilator. Syn. *kellin, chellin, visammin.*

khel·li·nin (kel'i·nin) *n.* 2-Hydroxymethyl-5-methoxyfuranochrome glucoside, $C_{19}H_{20}O_{10}$, a minor constituent of the umbelliferous plant *Ammi visnaga.* Syn. *khellol-glucoside.*

khel·lol-glu·co·side (kel"ol·gloo'ko·side) *n.* KHELLININ.

Kidd blood group system. The erythrocyte antigens defined by reactions to anti-Jk^a antibodies originally found in the mother (Mrs. Kidd) of an erythroblastotic infant, and to anti-Jk^b.

kid·ney, *n.* [ME., obsc. orig.]. One of the pair of glandular organs of the urinary system which, by filtration and excretory activity of its component units, the nephrons, elaborates the urine. NA *ren.* Comb. form *nephr-, ren-.* See also Plates 7, 8, 14, 26.

kidney basin. A kidney-shaped basin; emesis basin.

kidney failure. A reduction in kidney function, acute or chronic, to a level at which the kidneys are unable to maintain normal biological homeostasis. Syn. *renal failure.*

kidney film. A small flexible cassette containing x-ray film used in intraoperative radiography of the kidney.

kidney stone. A concretion in the kidney. Syn. *renal calculus.*

kidney worm. *DIOCTOPHYMA RENALE.*

kidney worm disease. STEPHANURIASIS.

kidney worm infection. Infection of the dog, mink, and occasionally of man by *Dioctophyma renale.*

Kien·böck's atrophy (keen'bœck) [R. *Kienböck*, Austrian radiologist, 1871-1953]. Acute atrophy of bone seen in inflammatory conditions of the extremities.

Kienböck's disease [R. *Kienböck*]. Osteochondrosis of the lunate bone.

kie·sel·guhr (kee'zul·goor'') *n.* [Ger. *Kieselgur*, from *Kiesel*, flint, silica]. DIATOMACEOUS EARTH.

Kies·sel·bach's area or **triangle** (kee'sul·bakh) [W. *Kiesselbach*, German laryngologist, 1839–1902]. An area of the anterior of the nasal septum which may be the site of epistaxis or of perforation.

Kil·ham rat virus (kil·um). A parvovirus occurring commonly in both laboratory and wild rats which produces disease and mortality in immunodepressed animals.

Kil·lian's operation (kil'yahn) [G. *Killian*, German laryngologist, 1860–1921]. Excision of the anterior wall of the frontal sinus, and formation of a permanent opening into the nose.

kilo- [Gk. *chilioi*]. A prefix meaning *thousand*.

kilo·cal·o·rie, kilo·cal·o·ry (kil'o·kal''o·ree) *n.* [*kilo-* + *calorie*]. Any one of several heat units that represent the quantity of heat required to raise the temperature of one kilogram of water 1 degree centigrade but that differ slightly from each other in the specific 1-degree interval of temperature selected. Kilocalorie units are used in metabolic studies, when they are also called large calories or Calories. Abbreviated, kcal.

kilo·gram (kil'uh·gram) *n.* [*kilo-* + *gram*]. One thousand grams, or about 2.2 pounds avoirdupois. Abbreviated, kg.

kilo·gram-me·ter, kilo·gram-me·tre (kil'uh·gram mee'tur) *n.* A unit of energy; the amount of energy required to raise one kilogram one meter; approximately 7.233 foot-pounds.

kilo·joule (kil'o·jool'') *n.* [*kilo-* + *joule*]. A unit of heat, equivalent to 239.1 small calories.

kilo·li·ter, kilo·li·tre (kil'o·lee''tur) *n.* [*kilo-* + *liter*]. One thousand liters, or 35.31 cubic feet. Abbreviated, kl.

ki·lo·me·ter, ki·lo·me·tre (ki·lom'e·tur, kil'uh·mee''tur) *n.* [*kilo-* + *meter*]. One thousand meters, or 1093.6 yards. Abbreviated, km.

kilo·nem (kil'o·nem) *n.* [*kilo-* + *nem*]. A nutritional unit representing 1000 nems, equivalent to approximately 667 calories.

kilo·volt (kil'o·vohlt) *n.* [*kilo-* + *volt*]. A unit of electric power equal to 1000 volts. Abbreviated, kv.

kilo·watt (kil'uh·wot) *n.* [*kilo-* + *watt*]. A unit of electric power; one thousand watts. Abbreviated, kw.

kilowatt hour. A unit of energy equivalent to the energy supplied by a power of 1000 watts operating for 1 hour.

Kim·mel·stiel-Wil·son syndrome [P. *Kimmelstiel*, U.S. pathologist, 1900–1970; and C. *Wilson*, British physician, b. 1906]. Hypertension, proteinuria, edema, and renal failure in association with diabetic glomerulosclerosis.

kin-, kine-, kino- [Gk. *kinein*, to move]. A combining form meaning *action, motion.*

kinaesthesia. KINESTHESIA.

kinaesthesis. KINESTHESIA.

kinaesthesiometer. KINESTHESIOMETER.

ki·nase (kigh'nace, kin'ace, kin'aze) *n.* [*kin*etic + *-ase*]. An enzyme that catalyzes the transfer of phosphate from adenosine triphosphate to an acceptor.

kind·ling. A progressive intensification of stimulus-induced seizure resulting from periodic administration of initially subconvulsive electrical stimuli. Once developed, the enhanced sensitivity to electrical stimulation is permanent.

kin·dred, *n.* 1. A more or less broad and cohesive kinship group such as an extended family or a clan. 2. Any aggregate of relatives, such as might be studied for genetic purposes, that is broader than an immediate family of parents and offspring.

kine-. See *kin-*.

kin·e·ma·di·ag·ra·phy (kin''e·muh·dye·ag'ruh·fee) *n.* [Gk. *kinēma*, movement, + *dia-* + *-graphy*]. CINEROENTGENOGRAPHY.

ki·ne·mat·ic (kin·e·mat'ick, kigh''ne·) *adj.* [Gk. *kinēma, kinēmatos*, movement, + *-ic*]. 1. Of or pertaining to motion. 2. Of or pertaining to kinematics.

kinematic amputation. An amputation in which a muscular stump is left so as to allow for movement of an artificial limb; KINEPLASTY.

ki·ne·mat·ics (kin''e·mat'icks, kigh''ne·) *n.* The science of motion.

ki·ne·mato·graph (kin''e·mat'o·graf, kigh''ne·) *n.* A device for making and demonstrating a continuous record or pictures of a moving body such as a motion picture camera.

kineplastic amputation. KINEPLASTY.

kin·e·plas·ty (kin'e·plas''tee) *n.* [*kine-* + *-plasty*]. An amputation in which tendons are arranged in the stump to permit their use in moving parts of the prosthetic appliance. Types of kineplastic amputations include the club, the loop, the tendon tunnel, and the muscle tunnel. See also *plastic motor.* —**kin·e·plas·tic** (kin''e·plas'tick) *adj.*

ki·ne·ra·dio·ther·a·py (kin''e·ray''dee·o·therr'uh·pee) *n.* [*kine-* + *radio-* + *therapy*]. X-ray therapy whereby the tube is moved in relation to the patient, or the patient in relation to the stationary tube. The object is the attainment of larger depth doses with sparing of the skin.

kin·e·scope (kin'e·skope) *n.* [*kine-* + *-scope*]. An instrument for testing the refraction of the eye; consists of a moving disk with a slit of variable width, through which the patient observes a fixed object.

kinesi-, kinesio-. A combining form meaning *kinesis, movement.*

ki·ne·sia (ki·nee'zhuh, ·see·uh, kigh·nee') *n.* Motion sickness or other disorder caused by motion. Syn. *kinetosis.*

-kinesia [Gk. *kinēsis*, movement, + *-ia*]. A combining form meaning *a condition involving movements.*

kinesiaesthesiometer. KINESIESTHESIOMETER.

ki·ne·si·at·rics (ki·nee''see·at'ricks) *n.* [*kinesi-* + *-iatric* + *-s*]. The treatment of disease by systematic active or passive movements. Syn. *kinesitherapy, kinetotherapy.*

ki·ne·sic (ki·nee'sick) *adj.* KINETIC.

ki·ne·si·es·the·si·om·e·ter, ki·ne·si·aes·the·si·om·e·ter (ki·nee''see·es·theez''ee·om'e·tur) *n.* [*kinesi-* + *esthesio-* + *-meter*]. 1. An instrument for testing the proprioceptive sense; kinesthesiometer. 2. Specifically: an instrument employed to measure the perception of changes in the angles of joints.

ki·ne·si·gen·ic (ki·nee''si·jen'ick) *adj.* [*kinesi-* + *-genic*]. Brought on or triggered by movements.

ki·ne·sim·e·ter (kin''e·sim'e·tur, kigh''ne·) *n.* [*kinesi-* + *-meter*]. An instrument for determining quantitatively the motions of a part.

kinesio-. See *kinesi-*.

ki·ne·si·ol·o·gy (ki·nee''see·ol'uh·jee) *n.* [*kinesio-* + *-logy*]. The science of the anatomy, physiology, and mechanics of purposeful muscle movement in man.

ki·ne·si·om·e·ter (ki·nee''see·om'e·tur) *n.* KINESIMETER.

ki·ne·sis (ki·nee'sis, kigh·nee'sis) *n.*, pl. **kine·ses** (·seez) [Gk. *kinēsis*, from *kinein*, to move]. The general term for physical movement, including that induced by stimulation, as by light.

kinesis par·a·doxa (păr''uh·dock'suh). SOUQUES' SIGN (3).

ki·ne·si·ther·a·py (ki·nee''si·therr'uh·pee) *n.* KINESIATRICS.

kinesthetic apraxia. In the theories of Luria, disturbance of voluntary movement characterized by a failure to select the required kinesthetic impulses for bringing about a movement.

ki·ne·so·pho·bia (ki·nee''so·fo'bee·uh) *n.* [*kines*is + *-phobia*]. Morbid fear of motion.

kin·es·the·sia, kin·aes·the·sia (kin''es·theezh'uh, ·theez'ee·uh) *n.* [*kin-* + *esthesia*]. The proprioceptive sense; the sense of perception of movement, weight, resistance, and position. —**kines·thet·ic** (·thet'ick) *adj.*

kin·es·the·si·om·e·ter, kin·aes·the·si·om·e·ter (kin''es·theez''ee·om'e·tur) *n.* [*kinesthes*ia + *-meter*]. An instrument for measuring the degree of proprioceptive sense.

kin·es·the·sis (kin″es·thees′is) *n.* KINESTHESIA.

kinesthetic memory. KINESTHESIA.

kinesthetic motor aphasia. AFFERENT MOTOR APHASIA.

kinesthetic sensations. Sensations of weight, resistance, acceleration, velocity, and position of a part of the body in space.

kinet-, kineto-. A combining form meaning *motion, movement, kinesis, kinetic.*

ki·net·ic (ki·net′ick, kigh·net′ick) *adj.* [Gk. *kinētikos,* from *kinein,* to move]. Pertaining to motion; producing motion.

kinetic apraxia. APRAXIA.

kinetic ataxia. MOTOR ATAXIA.

kinetic energy. The part of the total energy of a body in motion which is caused by its motion.

kinetic motor aphasia. EFFERENT MOTOR APHASIA.

kinetic reflex. Any reflex that results in movement.

ki·net·ics (ki·net′icks, kigh·) *n.* [*kinetic* + *-s*]. 1. The science of the effects of forces on the motions of matter. 2. *In chemistry,* the study of the rates of reaction of systems; often referred to as reaction kinetics.

kinetic tremor. ACTION TREMOR.

ki·ne·tism (ki·nee′tiz·um, kin′e·) *n.* [*kinet-* + *-ism*]. The ability to initiate or perform independent movement such as muscular activity.

kineto-. See *kinet-.*

ki·neto·car·dio·gram (ki·net″o·kahr′dee·o·gram) *n.* [*kineto-* + *cardiogram*]. The record of the pulsations and vibrations over the anterior chest, used in the diagnosis of cardiac disease. See also *apex cardiogram, ballistocardiogram.* —**ki·neto·car·di·og·ra·phy** (·kahr·dee·og′ruh·fee) *n.*

ki·neto·chore (ki·nee′to·kore, ki·net′o·, kigh·) *n.* [*kineto-* + Gk. *chōra,* space]. The constriction in the chromosome where the spindle fiber is attached. Syn. *centromere.*

ki·neto·nu·cle·us (ki·nee″to·new′klee·us, ki·net″o·) *n.* PARABASAL BODY.

ki·neto·plast (ki·nee′to·plast, ki·net″o·) *n.* [*kineto-* + *-plast*]. PARABASAL BODY.

kin·e·to·sis (kin″e·to′sis) *n.*, pl. **kineto·ses** (·seez) [*kinet-* + *-osis*]. Motion sickness or any other disorder caused by motion. Syn. *kinesia.*

ki·neto·ther·a·py (ki·nee″to·therr′uh·pee, ki·net″o·, kigh·) *n.* [*kineto-* + *-therapy*]. KINESIATRICS.

Kings·bury's test [F. B. *Kingsbury,* U.S. biochemist, b. 1886]. A test for protein concentration performed by adding 3% sulfosalicylic acid to urine and comparing turbidity with a set of standards.

king's evil. SCROFULA.

Kings·ley's splint [N. W. *Kingsley,* U.S. dentist, 1829–1913]. A splint for fractures of the maxilla; it consists of a curved metal bar passing around the face with its lower edge at the level of the mandible, and a headpiece fixed in a plaster cast. A rubber band suspended from the headpiece may be stretched around the curved bar to exert downward traction.

King's operation. An extralaryngeal arytenoidopexy.

ki·nin (kin′in, kigh′nin) *n.* [Gk. *kin*ein, to move, + *-in*]. Any of a group of polypeptides, as bradykinin, that are hypotensive, contract most isolated smooth muscle preparations, increase capillary permeability, and have certain other pharmacologic properties in common. Certain other polypeptides that are hypertensive, such as angiotensins, may also be included in the group.

kinin hormone. KININ.

kink, *n.* ANGULATION.

kinky hair disease. A sex-linked recessive disorder of unknown cause, with onset in early infancy, characterized clinically by light, kinky hair, developmental failure, death in early childhood, and focal cerebral and cerebellar degeneration. Syn. *Menkes' syndrome.*

Kin·ney's law. In acquired deafness, speech changes develop over a period of time in direct proportion to the length of time during which normal speech had been present.

Kin·nier Wilson sign (ki·neer′) [S. A. *Kinnier Wilson,* English neurologist, 1877–1937]. WILSON'S SIGN.

ki·no (kee′no, kigh′no) *n.* [West African origin]. The dried juice obtained from the trunk of *Pterocarpus marsupium;* a powerful astringent that has been used in the treatment of diarrhea.

kino-. See *kin-.*

ki·no·cen·trum (kigh″no·sen′trum, kin″o·) *n.* [*kino-* + *centrum*]. CENTROSOME.

kino·plasm (kin′o·plaz·um, kigh′no·) *n.* [*kino-* + *-plasm*]. *Obsol.* ARCHOPLASM.

Kinyoun stain. PONDER-KINYOUN STAIN.

ki·ot·o·my (kigh·ot′o·mee) *n.* [Gk. *kiōn,* pillar, uvula, + *-tomy*]. UVULECTOMY.

Kirk-Bent·ley method. A microtitrimetric method for iron based on the reduction of iron by cadmium amalgam, the addition of excess ceric sulfate, and the titration of the excess with ferrous ammonium sulfate.

Kirch·ner's diverticulum (kirr^{k}h′nur) [W. *Kirchner,* German otologist, 1849–1935]. A small diverticulum of the lower portion of the auditory tube.

Kir·mis·sion's operation (kerr·mee·syo^{n}′) [E. *Kirmission,* French surgeon, 1848–1927]. An operation for talipes varus, involving transplantation of the calcaneal tendon.

Kirsch·ner's traction (kirrsh′nur) [M. *Kirschner,* German surgeon, 1879–1942]. A form of skeletal traction used in the treatment of bone fractures. Kirschner's wires, passed through holes drilled in the bones, and attached to stirrups, are used to apply the traction.

Kirschner's wires [M. *Kirschner*]. Metallic wires, usually 9 inches in length, either threaded or smooth, usually supplied in three diameters of .035, .045, and .062 inches, used for the application of percutaneous skeletal traction or internal fixation of small fractures.

Kisch's reflex [B. *Kisch,* German physiologist, b. 1890]. AURICULOPALPEBRAL REFLEX.

kiss·ing bug. 1. ASSASSIN BUG. 2. Specifically, *REDUVIUS PERSONATUS.*

kissing disease. INFECTIOUS MONONUCLEOSIS.

kissing ulcer. An ulcer that appears to be due to transmission from one apposing part to another, or due to pressure of apposing parts.

ki·ta·sa·my·cin (ki·tah″suh·migh′sin) *n.* An antibiotic substance obtained from cultures of *Streptomyces kitasatoensis.*

ki·tol (kee′tol, kit′ol) *n.* [Gk. *kētos,* whale]. A precursor of vitamin A in whale-liver oil, which yields vitamin A on heating under low pressures.

Kjel·dahl method (kel″dahl) [J. G. C. *Kjeldahl,* Danish chemist, 1849–1900]. A method to determine the amount of nitrogen in an organic compound by interaction with sulfuric acid to produce ammonium ion which is converted to ammonia by alkali and distilled into standard acid.

kl Abbreviation for *kiloliter.*

Klatsch preparation. A cover-glass preparation made by pressing the cover glass lightly on a bacterial colony in plate culture.

Klebs' disease (kle^{y}ps) [T. A. E. *Klebs,* German bacteriologist, 1834–1913]. GLOMERULONEPHRITIS.

Kleb·si·el·la (kleb″zee·el′uh) *n.* [T. A. E. *Klebs*]. A genus of bacteria of the family Enterobacteriaceae; frequently associated with infections of the respiratory tract and pathologic conditions of other parts of the body.

Klebsiella gra·nu·lo·ma·tis (gray·yoo·lo′muh·tis). *CALYMMATOBACTERIUM GRANULOMATIS.*

Klebsiella ozae·nae (o·zee′nee). A gram-negative encapsulated rod found in association with ozena and atrophic rhinitis.

Klebsiella pneu·mo·ni·ae (new·mo′nee·ee). A species of short, plump, heavily capsulated, nonmotile, and gram-negative bacteria, responsible for severe pneumonitis in man. Syn.

Bacillus mucosus capsulatum, Friedländer's bacillus, pneumobacillus.

Klebsiella rhi·no·scle·ro·ma·tis (rye''no·skle·ro'muh·tis). Encapsulated gram-negative rod recovered from nasal granulomas of patients with rhinoscleroma. Syn. *Frisch's bacillus.*

Klebs-Loeffler bacillus [T. A. E. *Klebs*, German bacteriologist, 1834–1913; and F. A. J. *Loeffler*]. CORYNEBACTERIUM DIPHTHERIAE.

klee·blatt·schä·del deformity syndrome (klay'blot·shay''dul) [Ger.]. CLOVERLEAF SKULL DEFORMITY SYNDROME.

Klei·ne-Le·vin syndrome (klye'neʰ, le·vin') [W. *Kleine*, German neuropsychiatrist, 20th century; and M. *Levin*, U.S. neurologist, b. 1901]. Periodic attacks of excessive sleepiness and food intake (bulimia) frequently associated with mild mental confusion, irritability, and amnesia for portions of the attacks; of unknown cause.

klein·re·gel (kline'ray''gul) *n.* [Ger. *klein*, small, + *Regel*, menstruation]. Scant uterine bleeding at the midinterval of the menstrual cycle. It may be associated with mittelschmerz.

Klein's muscle [E. E. *Klein*, Hungarian histologist in England, 1844–1925]. COMPRESSOR LABII MUSCLE.

Klem·per·er's tuberculin [G. *Klemperer*, German physician, 1865–1946]. P.T.O.

klept-, klepto- [Gk. from *kleptein*, to steal]. A combining form meaning *stealing, theft.*

klep·to·lag·nia (klep''to·lag'nee·uh) *n.* [*klepto-* + Gk. *lagneia*, salaciousness]. Sexual gratification induced by theft.

klep·to·ma·nia (klep''to·may'nee·uh) *n.* [*klepto-* + *-mania*]. A morbid desire to steal; obsessive stealing; a mental disorder in which the objects stolen are usually of symbolic value only, being petty and useless items.

klep·to·pho·bia (klep''to·fo'bee·uh) *n.* [*klepto-* + *-phobia*]. 1. A morbid dread of thieves or of suffering theft. 2. A morbid dread of becoming a kleptomaniac.

klieg conjunctivitis or **eyes.** A condition caused by ultraviolet rays from klieg lights used in motion-picture studios or the theater.

Kline·fel·ter-Rei·fen·stein-Al·bright syndrome [H. F. *Klinefelter*, E. C. *Reifenstein*, and F. *Albright*]. KLINEFELTER'S SYNDROME.

Klinefelter's syndrome [H. F. *Klinefelter*, Jr., U.S. physician, b. 1912]. The clinical syndrome of hypogonadism including gynecomastia, eunuchoidism, elevated urinary gonadotropins, and decreased testicular size associated with hyalinization of the tubules. The sex chromosome constitution of somatic cells is abnormal in that a Y chromosome is associated with more than one X chromosome.

Kline test [B. S. *Kline*, U.S. pathologist, 1886–1968]. A flocculation test for syphilis.

klino-. See *clin-.*

Klip·pel-Feil syndrome or **deformity** (klee·pel', fel) [M. *Klippel*, French neurologist, 1858–1942; and A. *Feil*]. Congenital fusion of the bodies of two or more cervical vertebrae; the spines are small, deficient, or bifid; atlanto-occipital fusion is common. As a result the neck is short and wide with markedly limited movements. Platybasia and its associated neurologic deficits may occur.

Klippel's disease [M. *Klippel*]. Weakness (psuedoparalysis) due to severe generalized arthritis.

Klippel-Tré·nau·nay-We·ber syndrome (treʸ·no·neʰ', wee'bur) [M. *Klippel;* P. *Trénaunay*, French physician, 20th century; and F. P. *Weber*]. Cutaneous hemangioma of an extremity, often extending to the trunk, followed as the child grows by hypertrophy of the involved limb and, if a leg, by varicose veins. Mild mental retardation is frequently present.

Klippel-Weil sign (vay) [M. *Klippel;* and M. P. *Weil*, French physician, b. 1884]. In corticospinal tract lesions, where there is some degree of flexion contracture of the involved fingers, their passive extension results in involuntary flexion, opposition, and adduction of the thumb on that side.

kliseometer. CLISEOMETER.

klop·e·ma·nia (klop''e·may'nee·uh) *n.* [Gk. *klopē*, theft, + *-mania*]. KLEPTOMANIA.

Klos·si·el·la (klos''ee·el'uh) *n.* A genus of coccidia of low pathogenicity which is sometimes observed upon microscopic examination of the kidneys of mice (*Klossiella muris*), guinea pigs (*K. cobayae*), and horses (*K. equi*).

Klump·ke's paralysis or **palsy** (klump'kee) [Augusta Déjerine-*Klumpke*, French neurologist, 1859–1927]. LOWER BRACHIAL PLEXUS PARALYSIS.

km Abbreviation for *kilometer.*

knee, *n.* [Gmc. *kniwam* (rel. to L. *genu*; also to Gk. *gonia*, angle)]. 1. The part of the leg containing the articulation of the femur, tibia, and patella. NA *genu.* 2. The knee joint (NA *articulatio genus*). See also Table of Synovial Joints and Ligaments in the Appendix and Plate 2. 3. An analogous part or joint in the leg of certain animals, as for example the carpus of ungulates.

knee·cap, *n.* PATELLA.

knee-chest position. A position assumed by a patient resting on the knees and chest as an exercise after childbirth, or for the purposes of examination and treatment.

knee-dropping test. A simple test for the early detection of hemiplegia. The relaxed patient lies supine on a hard surface with legs drawn into a flexed position (slightly more than 45° at the knees); on the side of the pyramidal lesion, the knee drops continuously and evenly, with speed proportionate to severity of lesion, until the leg lies flat. The knee-drop should occur on successive examinations before the test may be considered positive.

knee-elbow position. KNEE-CHEST POSITION.

knee jerk. PATELLAR REFLEX.

knee reflex or **phenomenon.** PATELLAR REFLEX.

knee-sprung, *adj.* Of a horse: having bucked knees, anterior deviation of the carpus resulting in constant partial flexion.

Knies' sign. Unequal dilatation of the pupils, found in thyrotoxicosis and other conditions.

knife, *n.* A cutting instrument of varying shape, size, and design, used in surgery and in dissecting; a scalpel. See also *bistoury.*

knit·ting, *n.* A lay term to indicate the process of union in a fractured bone.

knob, *n.* 1. A rounded prominence or protuberance. 2. An end foot.

knob motor. PLASTIC MOTOR.

knock, *n.* A term used in the jargon of sports medicine to denote a blow to the head which is followed by a severe dazed state.

knock-knee, *n.* GENU VALGUM.

knock·out drops. Chloral hydrate solution; so called because of the rapid action of small doses of the compound, sometimes given in food or drink to render a victim helpless.

Knoop's theory (knope) [F. *Knoop*, German physiologist, b. 1875]. The theory that fats are metabolized by beta oxidation.

Knop test. TRACTION TEST.

Knopf's treatment [S. A. *Knopf*, U.S. physician 1857–1940]. Training of tuberculous patients in diaphragmatic respiration, in an attempt to rest the apices of the lungs.

knop·pie spider (nop'ee) [Afrikaans, dim. of *knop*, knob]. A southern African form of the black widow spider.

knot·ting hair. TRICHONODOSIS.

knuck·le, *n.* 1. An articulation of the phalanges with the metacarpal bones or with each other. 2. The distal convex ends of the metacarpals.

knuck·ling, *n.* A condition in which the hoof of a horse is turned under; due to excessive flexion of the fetlock joint.

Ko·belt's cyst [G. L. *Kobelt*, German anatomist, 1804–1857].

A small cystic remnant of the mesonephric duct in the vicinity of the ovary and broad ligament.

Ko·bert's test [E. R. *Kobert*, German biochemist, 1854–1918]. A test in which hemoglobin is precipitated by powdered zinc or zinc sulfate and turns red when alkali is added.

Koch·er-De·bré-Sé·mé·laigne syndrome (kokh'ur, duh·brey', sey·mey·lehny') [E. T. *Kocher*, Swiss surgeon, 1841–1917; R. *Debré;* and G. *Sémélaigne*, French pediatrician, 20th century]. A rare symptom complex of childhood in which hypothyroidism is associated with muscular enlargement, particularly of the extremities, giving the child an athletic or Herculean appearance.

Kocher forceps [E. T. *Kocher*]. A strong surgical clamp having serrated jaws and sharp interlocking teeth at the tip.

Kocher maneuver [E. T. *Kocher*]. A method of reducing dislocation of the shoulder.

Kocher's reflex [E. T. *Kocher*]. TESTICULAR COMPRESSION REFLEX.

Kocher's sign [E. T. *Kocher*]. A sign of hyperthyroidism in which, as the patient looks up, the eyelid retracts faster than the eyeball is raised, thus exposing the sclera above the cornea. Syn. *globe lag.*

Koch-McMee·kin's method [F. C. *Koch*, U.S. biochemist, 1876–1948; and T. L. *McMeekin*]. A method for nonprotein nitrogen in which the organic matter is digested with sulfuric acid and hydrogen peroxide and the resulting solution is nesslerized. It may also be used for total nitrogen of urine.

Koch phenomenon (kokh) [R. *Koch*, German bacteriologist, 1843–1910]. The altered reactivity of guinea pigs, previously infected with tubercle bacilli, to reinoculation with living or killed tubercle bacilli, or with tuberculin, characterized by an acceleration and intensification of the reaction at the local site. Serves as the basis of the general concept of delayed hypersensitivity.

Koch's law or **postulate** [R. *Koch*]. The four conditions that are required to establish an organism as the causative agent of a disease are: (a) the microorganism must be present in every case of the disease; (b) it must be capable of cultivation in pure culture; (c) it must, when inoculated in pure culture, produce the disease in susceptible animals; (d) it must be recovered and again grown in pure culture. Syn. *law of specificity of bacteria.*

Koch-Weeks bacillus [R. *Koch;* and J. E. *Weeks*, U.S. ophthalmologist, 1853–1949]. *HAEMOPHILUS AEGYPTIUS.*

Koch-Weeks conjunctivitis [R. *Koch* and J. E. *Weeks*]. Catarrhal conjunctivitis due to infection by *Haemophilus aegyptius.*

Koeb·ner's phenomenon (kœb'nur) [H. *Koebner*, German dermatologist, 1838–1904]. ISOMORPHOUS PROVOCATIVE REACTION.

Koer·ber-Sa·lus-El·schnig syndrome (kœr'bur, zah'lōos, el' shnikh). SYLVIAN AQUEDUCT SYNDROME.

Koep·pe's nodules (kœp'eh) [L. *Koeppe*, German ophthalmologist, b. 1884]. Nonspecific gray lumps found on the pupillary margin in a variety of inflammatory diseases of the uvea; most commonly a feature of sarcoid uveitis.

Köh·ler's disease (kœh'lur) [Alban *Köhler*, German physician, 1874–1947]. 1. Osteochondrosis of the navicular bone; a variety of aseptic necrosis of bone. Syn. *Kofhler's tarsal scaphoiditis.* 2. Osteochondrosis of the second metatarsal head. Syn. *Freiberg's disease.*

Köhler's method of illumination [August *Köhler*, German microscopist, 1866–1948]. A method of microscopical illumination in which an image of the source is focused in the lower focal plane of the microscope condenser, and the condenser, in turn, focuses an image of the lamp lens in the object field.

Köhler's tarsal scaphoiditis. KÖHLER'S DISEASE (1).

Köhl·mei·er-Degos disease (kœhl'migh·ur) [W. *Köhlmeier*, German, 20th century; and R. *Degos*]. DEGOS' DISEASE.

koilo- [Gk. *koilos*]. A combining form meaning *hollow, concave.*

koi·lo·cy·to·sis (koy''lo·sigh·to'sis) *n.* [*koilo-* + *cyto-* + *-osis*]. The hollow appearance of a cell due to large perinuclear vacuoles, as seen in certain desquamated cells of the uterine cervix. —**koilocy·tot·ic** (·tot'ick) *adj.*

koilocytotic atypia. A pattern of nuclear abnormalities of the stratified squamous epithelium of the uterine cervix, associated with vacuolization and ballooning of the upper layer of cells.

koil·onych·ia (koy''lo·nick'ee·uh) *n.* [*koilo-* + *onych-* + *-ia*]. A spoon-shaped deformity of the nails; may be familial, or associated with other diseases, such as iron-deficiency anemia and lichen planus. Syn. *spoon nail.*

koi·lo·ster·nia (koy''lo·stur'nee·uh) *n.* [*koilo-* + *stern-* + *-ia*]. FUNNEL CHEST.

koi·not·ro·py (koy·not'ruh·pee) *n.* [Gk. *koinos*, common, + *-tropy*]. *In psychobiology*, the state of being socialized; the condition of being identified with the common interest of the people. —**koi·no·trop·ic** (koy''no·trop'ick) *adj.*

Kojewnikoff. See *Kozhevnikov.*

ko·jic acid (ko'jick). 3-Hydroxy-5-hydroxymethyl-γ-pyrone, $C_6H_6O_4$, formed from glucose by the action of certain molds; it possesses antibiotic activity against various bacterial species.

ko·la (ko'luh) *n.* [West African origin]. The dried cotyledon of *Cola nitida* or of other species of *Cola* (cola nut); the chief constituent is caffeine, with traces of theobromine also present. The effect of kola is the same as that of other sources of caffeine, as coffee and tea.

Kol·mer's test [J. A. *Kolmer*, U.S. pathologist, 1886–1962]. 1. A complement-fixation test for syphilis. 2. A complement-fixation test for bacterial, spirochetal, viral, protozoal, or metazoal diseases.

kolp-, kolpo-. See *colp-.*

Kom·me·rell's diverticulum (kohm'ur·el) [B. *Kommerell*, German radiologist, 20th century]. A large, aneurysm-like swelling on the descending aorta, from which an aberrant right subclavian artery arises and passes posterior to the esophagus; the swelling represents the remnant of a persistent right aortic arch.

Kon·do·lé·on's operation [E. *Kondoléon*, Greek surgeon, 1879–1939]. An operation for elephantiasis, in which extensive strips of skin, subcutaneous tissue, and scarred fascia are excised.

koni-, konio-. See *coni-.*

Kö·nig's disease (kœh'nikh) [F. *König*, German surgeon, 1832–1910]. OSTEOCHONDRITIS DISSECANS.

ko·nim·e·ter (ko·nim'e·tur) *n.* [Gk. *konia*, dust, sand, + *-meter*]. A device for determining the number of dust particles in air.

ko·nio·cor·tex (ko''nee·o·kor'tecks) *n.* [Gk. *konia*, dust, sand, + *cortex*]. Granular cortex characteristic of sensory areas.

koniosis. CONIOSIS.

ko·nom·e·ter (ko·nom'e·tur) *n.* KONIMETER.

Konseal. A trademark for a form of cachet.

ko·phe·mia (ko·fee'mee·uh) *n.* [Gk. *kōphos*, deaf, + *-phemia*]. *Obsol.* AUDITORY VERBAL AGNOSIA.

Kop·lik's spots or **sign** [H. *Koplik*, U.S. pediatrician, 1858–1927]. The characteristic oral enanthem of measles, at the end of the prodromal stage, consisting of tiny gray-white areas on a bright red base, grouped around the orifice of the parotid duct opposite the premolar teeth.

kop·o·pho·bia (kop''o·fo'bee·uh) *n.* [Gk. *kopos*, exertion, + *-phobia*]. Morbid fear of fatigue or exhaustion.

kop·ro·stea·rin (kop''ro·stee'ur·in, ·steer'in) *n.* [Gk. *kopros*, excrement, + *stearin*]. COPROSTEROL.

Korff's fibers. OSTEOGENIC FIBERS.

Kor·ner-Shil·ling·ford method [P. I. *Korner*, English physician, 20th century; and J. P. *Shillingford*, English physician, 20th century]. A method of quantitative estimation of the regurgitant blood flow in cardiac valvular regurgitation by indicator dilution techniques.

ko·ro (ko'ro) *n. In psychiatry,* a hysterical neurosis of the conversion type, observed chiefly in certain Far Eastern countries among males, characterized by the fear that the penis is retracted into the abdomen.

ko·ros·co·py (ko·ros'kuh·pee) *n.* [Gk. *korē*, pupil, + *-scopy*]. RETINOSCOPY.

Korotkoff. See *Korotkov.*

Ko·rot·kov's method (kor'ut·kuf) [N. S. *Korotkov,* Russian physician, b. 1874]. The auscultatory method for determining the blood pressure, by applying a stethoscope to the brachial artery below the pressure cuff of a sphygmomanometer.

Korotkov sounds [N. S. *Korotkov*]. The sounds heard with the stethoscope during the auscultatory determination of the blood pressure.

Korotkov test [N. S. *Korotkov*]. A test for collateral circulation in an aneurysm; with compression of the artery proximal to the aneurysm, if there is adequate pulsation or blood pressure distal to the aneurysm, the collateral circulation is adequate.

Kor·sa·koff's syndrome, psychosis, or **neurosis** (kor'suh·kuf) [S. S. *Korsakoff,* Russian neuropsychiatrist, 1853-1900]. An amnestic-confabulatory syndrome characterized by confusion, retrograde and anteograde amnesia, confabulation, and apathy seen most often in chronic alcoholism and other causes of vitamin B deficiency as well as in other diseases that involve the diencephalon or hippocampal formations bilaterally.

Korsakov. See *Korsakoff.*

Kos·sel's test [A. *Kossel,* German biochemist, 1853-1927]. A test for hypoxanthine in which the unknown solution is treated with hydrochloric acid, zinc, and sodium hydroxide. A ruby-red color indicates the presence of hypoxanthine.

Koss's koilocytotic atypia [L. G. *Koss,* U.S. pathologist, b. 1920]. KOILOCYTOTIC ATYPIA.

kous·so (kŏŏs'o) *n.* [Galla *kosso*]. BRAYERA.

Ko·zhev·ni·kov's epilepsy (kah·zhev'nee·kuf) [A. Y. *Kozhevnikov,* Russian neurologist, 1836-1902]. STATUS EPILEPTICUS.

Kr Symbol for krypton.

Krab·be's disease [K. H. *Krabbe,* Danish neurologist, 1885-1961]. GLOBOID LEUKODYSTROPHY.

Krae·pe·lin-Mo·rel disease (kreh'pe·leen, moh·rel') [E. *Kraepelin,* German psychiatrist, 1856-1926; and B. A. *Morel*]. DEMENTIA PRAECOX.

Kraepelin's classification [E. *Kraepelin*]. An extensive systematic, descriptive classification of mental disorders, which employed the term dementia praecox for schizophrenia and divided it into the simple, hebephrenic, catatonic, and paranoid types. See also *descriptive psychiatry.*

krait (krite) *n.* [Hindi *karait*]. Any snake of the genus *Bungarus.*

kra·me·ria (kra·meer'ee·uh) *n.* [J. G. H. *Kramer,* Austrian physician and botanist, d. 1742]. The dried root of *Krameria triandra,* known in commerce as Peruvian rhatany, or of *Krameria argentea,* known in commerce as Para or Brazilian rhatany; has been used as an astringent.

Kra·mer-Tis·dall method [B. *Kramer,* U.S. physician, b. 1888; and F. F. *Tisdall*]. A method for serum calcium (the Clark-Collip modification) in which calcium is precipitated from serum as oxalate and titrated with potassium permanganate.

Kras·ke's operation (krahs'keh) [P. *Kraske,* German surgeon, 1851-1930]. An operation for rectal carcinoma in which the coccyx and part of the sacrum are removed.

K ration. A complete emergency ration for three meals put up in pocket size for United States Armed Forces personnel.

kra·tom·e·ter (kra·tom'e·tur) *n.* [Gk. *kratos*, power, + *-meter*]. A device consisting of prisms, used for correcting nystagmus or in orthoptic exercises.

krau·ro·sis (kraw·ro'sis) *n.* [NL., from Gk. *krauros*, brittle, + *-osis*]. A progressive, sclerosing, shriveling process of the skin.

kraurosis of the penis. BALANITIS XEROTICA OBLITERANS.

kraurosis of the vulva. A disease of elderly women, characterized by pruritus, atrophy, and dryness of the external genitalia. Stenosis of the vaginal orifice and carcinoma may develop.

Krau·se's corpuscle (kraow'zeh) [W. J. F. *Krause,* German anatomist, 1833-1910]. One of the spheroid nerve end organs resembling lamellar corpuscles, but having a more delicate capsule; found especially in the conjunctiva, the mucosa of the tongue, and in the external genitalia.

Krause's end bulb [W. J. F. *Krause*]. KRAUSE'S CORPUSCLE.

Krause's glands [C. F. T. *Krause,* German anatomist, 1797-1868]. Accessory lacrimal glands in the forniceal areas of the conjunctiva.

Krause's membrane [W. J. F. *Krause*]. INTERMEDIATE DISK.

Krause-Wolfe graft [F. V. *Krause,* German surgeon, 1857-1937; and J. R. *Wolfe*]. FULL-THICKNESS GRAFT.

Kraus's fetal cells [E. J. *Kraus*]. Columnar cells around blood vessels in the anterior hypophysis.

kre·a·tin (kree'uh·tin) *n.* CREATINE.

kreatinine. CREATININE.

Krebs cycle [H. A. *Krebs,* British biochemist, b. 1900]. CITRIC ACID CYCLE.

Krebs-Hen·se·leit cycle (hen'ze·lite) [H. A. *Krebs;* and K. *Henseleit,* German internist, b. 1907]. UREA CYCLE.

Krebs 2 tumor. A transmissible poorly-differentiated malignant tumor of mice which originated spontaneously as a carcinoma, probably of breast origin.

kreo-. See *cre-.*

kreo·tox·in (kree''o·tock'sin) *n.* [Gk. *kreas*, flesh, + *toxin*]. A meat poison that is formed by bacteria.

kreo·tox·ism (kree''o·tock'siz·um) *n.* [*kreo-* + *tox-* + *-ism*]. Poisoning by infected meat.

Kretsch·mer type [E. *Kretschmer,* German psychiatrist, 1888-1964]. The type of physique associated with certain psychic or temperamental traits a person possesses, such as the pyknic, asthenic, athletic, or dysplastic type.

Krey·sig's sign (krye'zikh) [F. L. *Kreysig,* German physician, 1770-1839]. Retraction of the intercostal spaces with cardiac systole; a sign of adherent pericarditis. Syn. *Heim-Kreysig sign.*

Krom·pech·er's tumor [E. *Krompecher,* Hungarian pathologist, 1870-1926]. BASAL CELL CARCINOMA.

Krö·nig's fields (krœh'nikh) [G. *Krönig,* German physician, 1856-1911]. Anterior and posterior areas of resonance over the apices of the lungs.

Krönig's isthmus [G. *Krönig*]. A narrow area of resonance, connecting the anterior and posterior areas of resonance, found on percussion over the apices of the lungs above the clavicles (Krönig's fields).

Kru·ken·berg's spindle (kroo'ken·behrk) [E. F. *Krukenberg,* German pathologist, 1871-1946]. A vertical line or spindle-shaped deposit of melanin on the posterior surface of the cornea.

Krukenberg's tumor [E. F. *Krukenberg*]. Bilateral primary ovarian carcinoma, as originally described, but most widely used to denote metastatic ovarian carcinoma, usually of gastric origin.

krymo-. See *crym-.*

kry·mo·ther·a·py (krye''mo·therr'uh·pee) *n.* [Gk. *krymos*, frost, + *therapy*]. CRYOTHERAPY.

krypto-. See *crypt-.*

kryp·ton (krip'ton) *n.* [Gk. *kryptos*, hidden, + *-on*]. Kr = 83.80; a colorless, inert gaseous element which occurs in the atmosphere.

KUB (kay yoo bee) [*k*idneys, *u*reters, *b*ladder]. A plain film of the abdomen, including the areas of the kidneys, ureters, and the bladder.

ku·bis·a·ga·ri (koo·bis″uh·gah′ree) *n.* [Jap.]. PARALYTIC VERTIGO, endemic in Japan.

ku·bis·ga·ri (koo″bis·gah′ree) *n.* [Jap.]. Kubisagari (= PARALYTIC VERTIGO).

Kufs' disease (koofs) [H. *Kufs,* German neurologist, 1871–1955]. A hereditary disorder of lipid metabolism, usually manifesting itself in adolescence and early adult life, characterized by slowly progressive dementia, seizures, ataxia, increasing rigidity, and occasionally retinal pigmentation. Though the pathologic findings are similar to those of other forms of amaurotic familial idiocy, vision is not lost. Syn. *late juvenile amaurotic familial idiocy.* See also *amaurotic familial idiocy.*

Ku·gel·berg-We·lan·der syndrome (kueʹgel·bæry, veyʹlahn·dur) [E. *Kugelberg,* Swedish neurologist, 20th century, and L. *Welander,* Swedish neurologist, 20th century]. JUVENILE SPINAL MUSCULAR ATROPHY.

Ku·gel's artery. The artery to the atrioventricular node.

Kuhnt-Ju·nius disease (koont, yoon′yo͞os) [H. *Kuhnt,* German ophthalmologist, 1850–1925]. DISCIFORM MACULAR DEGENERATION.

Kulchitsky. See *Kultschitzsky.*

Kul·tschitz·sky cells (ko͝oly·chits′kee) [N. *Kultschitzsky,* Russian histologist, 1856–1925]. CELLS OF KULTSCHITZSKY.

Kultschitzsky's carcinoma [N. *Kultschitzsky*]. CARCINOID.

Kultschitzsky's hematoxylin [N. *Kultschitzsky*]. A valuable myelin-sheath stain. Used in the Smith-Dietrich stain for lipids.

Kum·linge disease (ko͞om′ling·uh). A form of viral meningoencephalitis occurring in the Åland Islands, related to louping ill.

Küm·mell's disease (kuem′el) [H. *Kümmell,* German surgeon, 1852–1937]. A syndrome which follows compression fracture of the vertebrae and traumatic spondylitis.

Kun·drat's lymphosarcoma (ko͞on′draht) [H. *Kundrat,* Austrian physician, 1845–1893]. Lymphosarcoma confined to lymph nodes and sparing viscera, accompanied by anemia and lymphocytopenia.

Kun·kel test [H. G. *Kunkel,* U.S. physician, b. 1916]. A test for gamma globulin in which the turbidity resulting on addition of zinc sulfate solution is compared with suitable standards.

Künt·scher nail (kuench′ur) [G. *Küntscher,* German surgeon, b. 1902]. A stainless-steel rod used for intramedullary fixation of fractures of long bones, especially the femur, tibia, humerus, radius, and ulna. Syn. *Kufntscher intramedullary nail.*

Kupf·fer cells (ko͞op′fur) [K. W. *Kupffer,* German anatomist, 1829–1902]. Fixed macrophages lining the hepatic sinusoids.

kur·chi (ko͞or′chee) *n.* [Skr. *kūrcin,* long-bearded]. An extract of kurchi bark used in amebic dysentery.

Kur·lov bodies (koor′luf) [M. G. *Kurlov,* Russian physician, 1859–1932]. Cytoplasmic inclusion bodies found in peripheral blood mononuclear cells in guinea pigs which are increased in size and number by estrogen stimulation; their significance is unknown.

Kurlov cell [M. G. *Kurlov*]. FOÀ-KURLOV CELL.

ku·ru (koo′roo) *n.* [Fore, trembling]. A subacute degenerative disease of the central nervous system unique to certain groups, especially the Fore tribe of New Guinea, but now disappearing, characterized clinically by cerebellar ataxia, trembling, spasticity and progressive dementia, due to a transmissible agent once acquired by ritual cannibalism.

Kus·ko·kwim disease [after *Kuskokwim,* Alaska]. Arthrogryposis occurring in the Yupik Eskimos of southwestern Alaska.

Küss-Ghon focus (kuess, gohn) [G. *Küss,* French physician, 1867–1936; and A. *Ghon*]. GHON COMPLEX.

Kuss·maul-Mai·er disease (ko͞os′maowl, migh′ur) [A. *Kussmaul,* German physician, 1822–1902; and R. *Maier,* German physician, 1824–1888]. POLYARTERITIS NODOSA.

Kussmaul's disease [A. *Kussmaul*]. POLYARTERITIS NODOSA.

Kussmaul's respiration, breathing, or **sign** [A. *Kussmaul*]. AIR HUNGER.

kus·so (ko͞os′o, kuss′o) *n.* [Galla *kosso*]. BRAYERA.

kv Abbreviation for *kilovolt.*

Kveim antigen [M. A. *Kveim,* Norwegian physician, b. 1892]. Emulsified material from a lymph node proved to be sarcoid, which, on injection into an individual with sarcoidosis, usually results in the formation of sarcoid tubercles. Used in the Kveim test.

Kveim test [M. A. *Kveim*]. A test for the diagnosis of sarcoidosis, in which intradermal administration of Kveim antigen results in the appearance of noncaseating granulomas at the site of injection 4 to 8 weeks later. Syn. *Nickerson-Kveim test.*

K virus. A polyomavirus commonly found in both wild and laboratory mice which may produce interstitial pneumonitis and death in suckling mice less than 10 days old.

kw Abbreviation for *kilowatt.*

kwa·shi·or·kor (kwah″shee·or′kor) *n.* [local name in Ghana]. A disease of infants and young children, mainly in the tropics and subtropics, occurring soon after weaning, due primarily to deficient quality and quantity of dietary protein; characterized by edema, skin and hair changes, impaired growth, fatty liver, severe apathy, and weakness. See also *marasmic kwashiorkor.*

Kwi·lecki's method. A method for protein determination in which a solution of ferric chloride is added to urine before proceeding with Esbach's method.

ky·a·nop·sia (kigh″uh·nop′see·uh) *n.* [Gk. *kyanos,* blue, + *-opsia*]. CYANOPIA.

Kya·sa·nur forest disease. One of the Russian tick-borne encephalitides.

ky·es·te·in (kigh·es′tee·in) *n.* [Gk. *kyein,* to be pregnant]. A filmy deposit upon decomposing urine, once thought to be diagnostic of pregnancy.

ky·mo·gram (kigh′mo·gram) *n.* The record made on a kymograph.

ky·mo·graph (kigh′mo·graf) *n.* [Gk. *kyma,* wave, + *-graph*]. An instrument for recording physiologic cycles or actions in a patient, an experimental animal, or in an isolated muscle or heart; consists of a clock- or motor-driven cylinder, covered with paper on which the record is made. Time intervals can be recorded simultaneously with the phenomena. —**ky·mo·graph·ic** (kigh″mo·graf′ick) *adj.*

ky·mog·ra·phy (kigh·mog′ruh·fee) *n.* [Gk. *kyma,* wave, + *-graphy*]. Any method or technique for recording motions or contractions in an organ, usually by means of a kymograph or electrokymograph.

ky·no·pho·bia (kigh″no·fo′bee·uh) *n.* CYNOPHOBIA.

kyn·uren·ic acid (kin″yoo·ree′nick, ·ren′ick, kigh″new·). γ-Hydroxy-β-quinolinecarboxylic acid, $C_{10}H_7NO_3$, a product of the metabolism of tryptophan occurring in the urine of mammals.

kyn·uren·ine (kigh·new′ri·neen, kin″yoo·ree′nin) *n.* An intermediate product, $C_{10}H_{12}N_2O_3$, of tryptophan metabolism isolated from the urine of mammals.

kyphorachitic pelvis. A deformity of the pelvis associated with rickets in which changes are slight because the effect of kyphosis tends to counterbalance that of rickets.

ky·pho·ra·chi·tis (kigh″fo·ra·kigh′tis) *n.* [Gk. *kyphos,* hump, hunchbacked, + *rachi-* + *-itis*]. Rachitic deformity of the thorax and spine, resulting in an anteroposterior hump. The pelvis is sometimes involved. —**kyphora·chit·ic** (·kit′ick) *adj.*

ky·phos (kye′fos) *n.* [Gk.]. The convex part (the hump) of the deformed back in kyphoscoliosis.

kyphoscoliorachitic pelvis. A deformity of the pelvis resembling the kyphorachitic type because the kyphotic and rachitic effects counterbalance each other. However, a considerable degree of oblique deformity of the superior strait is usually present.

ky·pho·sco·lio·ra·chi·tis (kigh″fo·sko″lee·o·ra·kigh′tis) *n.* [*kyphos* + Gk. *scolios*, curved, + *rachi*- + -*itis*]. A combined kyphosis and scoliosis due to rickets. The pelvis and thorax may be involved in the deformity. —**kyphoscoliora·chit·ic** (·kit′ick) *adj.*

ky·pho·sco·li·o·sis (kigh″fo·sko″lee·o′sis) *n.* [*kyphos* + *scoliosis*]. Lateral curvature of the spine with vertebral rotation, associated with an anteroposterior hump in the spinal column. —**kyphoscoli·ot·ic** (·ot′ick) *adj.*

kyphoscoliotic heart disease. Cardiorespiratory disease or failure due to functional abnormalities imposed by kyphoscoliosis.

kyphoscoliotic pelvis. A deformity of the pelvis varying in character with the predominance of the kyphosis or scoliosis of the vertebral column.

ky·pho·sis (kigh·fo′sis) *n.*, pl. **kypho·ses** (·seez) [Gk. *kyphōsis*, being hunchbacked]. Angular curvature of the spine, the convexity of the curve being posterior, usually situated in the thoracic region, and involving few or many vertebrae; the result of such diseases as tuberculosis, osteochondritis or ankylosing spondylitis of the spine, or an improper posture habit. Syn. *humpback, hunchback.* See also *round shoulders.* —**ky·phot·ic** (kigh·fot′ick) *adj.*

kyphotic pelvis. A pelvis characterized by increase of the conjugata vera, but decrease of the transverse diameter of the outlet, through approximation of the ischial spines and tuberosities. Associated with kyphosis of the vertebral column.

Kyr·le's disease (kirr′leʰ) [J. *Kyrle*, Austrian dermatologist, 1880–1921]. A condition in which excessive horn forms in and around the hair follicles and tends to penetrate the living structure of the skin. Syn. *hyperkeratosis follicularis et parafollicularis in cutem penetrans.*

kyto-. See *cyt-*.

L

l. Abbreviation for (a) left; (b) left eye; (c) *libra*; (d) *lethal*; (e) *liter*.

L_+ Symbol for limes death.

L_0 Symbol for limes zero.

L- *In chemistry*, a configurational descriptor placed before the stereoparent names of amino acids and carbohydrates. For usage, see definition of D. Compare *S*.

***l*-** 1. *In chemistry*, a symbol formerly employed for levorotatory, referring to the direction in which the plane of polarized light is rotated by a substance; this usage is superseded by the symbol (−). 2. *In chemistry*, a symbol formerly used to indicate the structural configuration of a particular asymmetric carbon atom in a compound, in the manner that the small capital letter L- is now used.

La Symbol for lanthanum.

lab. *Obsol.* RENNIN.

Lab·ar·raque's solution (lahʰ·bahʰ·rahʰck') [A. G. *Labarraque*, French chemist, 1777–1850]. A solution of sodium hypochlorite, with an equivalent amount of sodium chloride; used as a disinfectant and antiseptic.

lab·da·cism (lab'duh·siz·um) *n.* LAMBDACISM.

-labe [Gk. *-labos*, from *lambanein*, to take]. A combining form designating *something that takes, removes, takes up, or absorbs.*

la·bel, *v.* To convert a small portion of the atoms of a specific element in a compound or system to a radioactive isotope, or to add a radioactive isotope or an isotope of unusual mass of the element for the purpose of tracing the element through one or more chemical reactions. Syn. *tag.* —**la·beled, la·belled,** *adj.*

la belle indifférence. BELLE INDIFFÉRENCE.

lab ferment. *Obsol.* RENNIN.

labia. Plural of *labium*.

la·bi·al (lay'bee·ul) *adj.* Pertaining to a lip or labium.

labial angle. ANGLE OF THE MOUTH.

labial glands. Glands of the mucous membrane of the lips. NA *glandulae labiales.*

labial groove. A groove, developing in the vestibular lamina by disintegration of its central cells, which deepens to form the vestibule of the oral cavity.

labial hernia. Complete, indirect inguinal hernia into the labium majus.

la·bi·al·ism (lay'bee·ul·iz·um) *n.* 1. The tendency to substitute labial sounds, as *b, p, m,* or *w,* for other speech sounds. 2. The addition of a labial or labiodental quality to any speech sound. 3. The tendency to confuse one labial consonant with any other.

labial lamina. LABIOGINGIVAL LAMINA.

labial ligament. A ligamentous cord located in the labial swellings that forms the distal end of the round ligament of the uterus.

labial occlusion. A situation in which the alignment of a tooth is external to the line of occlusion.

labial swelling. LABIOSCROTAL SWELLING.

labial tubercle. A small, inconstant median tubercle of the philtrum of the upper lip. NA *tuberculum labii superioris.*

labial villi. Minute, conical projections from the inner aspect of the fetal lips, sometimes retained until birth.

labia ma·jo·ra (ma·jo'ruh). Plural of *labium majus.*

labia mi·no·ra (mi·no'ruh). Plural of *labium minus.*

labia oris (o'ris) [NA]. The lips of the mouth, including the upper lip (NA *labium superius*) and the lower lip (NA *labium inferius*).

labia pu·den·di (pew·den'dye). The lips of the vulva, including the labia majora and the labia minora.

La·bi·a·tae (lay''bee·ay'tee) *n.pl.* A family of herbs, mostly aromatic. Syn. *Lamiaceae, Menthaceae.*

la·bile (lay'bil, ·bile) *adj.* [L. *labilis,* from *labi,* to slip, glide]. 1. Unstable, particularly when applied to moods. 2. Readily changed as by heat, oxidation, or other processes, particularly when applied to chemical substances, microorganisms, antibodies, and so on. 3. Moving from place to place. 4. Fluctuating widely.

labile current. An electric current which results when electrodes are moved over the surface of the body.

labile factor. FACTOR V.

la·bil·i·ty (lay·bil'i·tee) *n.* The quality of being labile. Specifically: 1. *In neurology and psychiatry,* very rapid fluctuations in intensity and modality of emotions, without apparent adequate cause and with inadequate control of their expression, seen most dramatically in the affective reactions or in pseudobulbar palsy. 2. *In chemistry,* readily susceptible to change, such as a rearrangement or cleavage of an organic molecule.

labio- [L. *labium*]. A combining form meaning *lip, labial.*

la·bio·al·ve·o·lar (lay''bee·o·al·vee'uh·lur) *adj.* [*labio-* + *alveolar*]. Pertaining to the lip and to the alveolar process of maxilla or mandible.

la·bio·cer·vi·cal (lay''bee·o·sur'vi·kul) *adj.* [*labio-* + *cervical*]. 1. Pertaining to a lip and a neck. 2. Pertaining to the labial surface of the neck of a tooth.

la·bio·den·tal (lay''bee·o·den'tul) *adj.* [*labio-* + *dental*]. Pertaining to the lips and the teeth.

labiodental lamina. The epithelial ingrowth which forms the labiogingival lamina and the dental lamina.

la·bio·gin·gi·val (lay''bee·o·jin'ji·vul, ·jin·jye'vul) *adj.* [*labio-* + *gingival*]. Pertaining to the lips and gums.

labiogingival lamina. The portion of the vestibular lamina opposite the lips. Syn. *labial lamina.*

la·bio·glos·so·la·ryn·ge·al (lay″bee·o·glos″o·la·rin′jee·ul) *adj.* [*labio-* + *glosso-* + *laryngeal*]. Pertaining conjointly to the lips, tongue, and larynx.

labioglossolaryngeal paralysis. A form of bulbar paralysis involving the lips, tongue, and larynx.

la·bio·glos·so·pha·ryn·ge·al (lay″bee·o·glos″o·fa·rin′jee·ul) *adj.* [*labio-* + *glosso-* + *pharyngeal*]. Pertaining to the lips, tongue, and pharynx.

labioglossopharyngeal paralysis. Paralysis of lips, tongue, and pharynx.

la·bio·men·tal (lay″bee·o·men′tul) *adj.* [*labio-* + *mental*]. Pertaining to the lip and chin.

la·bio·pal·a·tine (lay″bee·o·pal′uh·tine, ·tin) *adj.* [*labio-* + *palatine*]. Pertaining to the lip and palate.

la·bio·plas·ty (lay′bee·o·plas″tee) *n.* [*labio-* + *-plasty*]. CHEILOPLASTY.

la·bio·scro·tal swelling (lay″bee·o·skro′tul). The eminence or ridge on either side of the base of the embryonic phallus that is the primordium of half the scrotum in the male or of a labium majus in the female.

la·bi·um (lay′bee·um) *n.*, genit. **la·bii** (·bee·eye), pl. **la·bia** (·bee·uh) [L.]. 1. A lip. 2. *In invertebrate zoology,* the lower lip, as opposed to the labrum, the upper lip.

labium an·te·ri·us os·tii ute·ri (an·teer′ee·us os′tee·eye yoo′tur·eye) [NA]. The anterior lip of the cervix of the uterus.

labium anterius por·ti·o·nis va·gi·na·lis ute·ri (por·shee·o′nis vaj·i·nay′lis yoo′tur·eye) [BNA]. LABIUM ANTERIUS OSTII UTERI.

labium anterius tu·bae au·di·ti·vae (tew′bee aw·di·tye′vee) [BNA]. The anterior lip of the medial opening of the auditory tube.

labium ex·ter·num cris·tae ili·a·cae (ecks·tur′num kris′tee i·lye′uh·see) [NA]. The external lip of the iliac crest.

labium in·fe·ri·us (in·feer′ee·us) [NA]. The lower lip (of the mouth).

labium inferius val·vu·lae co·li (val′vew·lee ko′lye) [BNA]. The lower lip of the ileocecal valve.

labium internum cris·tae ili·a·cae (kris′tee i·lye′uh·see) [NA]. The internal lip of the iliac crest.

labium la·te·ra·le li·ne·ae as·pe·rae fe·mo·ris (lat′e·ray′lee lin′ee·ee as′pe·ree fem′o·ris) [NA]. The lateral lip of the linea aspera of the femur.

labium lep·o·ri·num (lep·o·rye′num) [L., from *lepus,* hare]. HARELIP.

labium lim·bi tym·pa·ni·cum (lim′bye tim·pan′i·kum) [NA]. The lower lip of the osseous spiral lamina.

labium limbi ves·ti·bu·la·re (ves·tib·yoo·lair′ee) [NA]. The upper lip of the osseous spiral lamina.

labium ma·jus (may′jus). One of two folds (labia majora) of the female external genital organs, arising just below the mons pubis, and surrounding the vulval entrance or rima pudendi. Syn. *major lip.* NA *labium majus pudendi.* See also Plate 23.

labium majus pu·den·di (pew·den′dye) [NA]. LABIUM MAJUS.

labium me·di·a·le li·ne·ae as·pe·rae fe·mo·ris (mee·dee·ay′lee lin′ee·ee as′pe·ree fem′o·ris) [NA]. The medial lip of the linea aspera of the femur.

labium mi·nus (migh′nus). One of the two folds (labia minora) at the inner surfaces of the labia majora. Syn. *minor lip.* NA *labium minus pudendi.* See also Plate 23.

labium minus pu·den·di (pew·den′dye) [NA]. LABIUM MINUS.

labium pos·te·ri·us os·tii ute·ri (pos·teer′ee·us os′tee·eye yoo′tur·eye) [NA]. The posterior lip of the cervix of the uterus.

labium posterius por·ti·o·nis va·gi·na·lis ute·ri (por·shee·o′nis vaj·i·nay′lis yoo′tur·eye) [BNA]. LABIUM POSTERIUS OSTII UTERI.

labium posterius tu·bae au·di·ti·vae (tew′bee aw·di·tye′vee) [BNA]. The posterior lip of the medial opening of the auditory tube.

labium su·pe·ri·us (sue·peer′ee·us) [NA]. The upper lip (of the mouth).

labium superius val·vu·lae co·li (val′vew·lee ko′lye) [BNA]. The upper lip of the ileocecal valve.

labium tym·pa·ni·cum (tim·pan′i·kum) [BNA]. LABIUM LIMBI TYMPANICUM.

labium ves·ti·bu·la·re (ves·tib·yoo·lair′ee) [BNA]. LABIUM LIMBI VESTIBULARE.

labium vo·ca·le (vo·kay′lee) [BNA]. VOCAL LIP.

la·bor, la·bour, *n.* [L., work, travail]. The series of processes, especially the coordinated, periodic uterine contractions, whereby the fetus is expelled in parturition.

lab·o·ra·to·ry, *n.* [ML. *laboratorium,* workshop, from L. *laborare,* to work]. 1. A place for experimental work in any branch of science. 2. In the 17th and 18th century, a place where medicines were prepared.

laboratory animal. EXPERIMENTAL ANIMAL.

laboratory diagnosis. A diagnosis arrived at from the results of tests on and examination of various tissues, excretions, and secretions.

La·borde's method (la·bord′) [J. B. V. *Laborde,* French physician, 1830–1903]. A method of artificial respiration in which the respiratory center is stimulated by rhythmic traction of the tongue with the fingers or a specially designed forceps.

la·bored respiration. Respiration performed with difficulty with the use of the accessory muscles of respiration.

labor pains. The pains associated with parturition due to uterine contractions.

labour. LABOR.

lab·ro·cyte (lab′ro·site) *n.* [Gk. *labros,* turbulent, hasty, + *-cyte*]. MAST CELL.

la·brum (lay′brum, lab′rum) *n.* [L., lip]. 1. A liplike structure. 2. *In invertebrate zoology,* the upper lip, as opposed to the labium, the lower lip.

labrum ace·ta·bu·la·re (as″e·tab″yoo·lair′ee) [NA]. ACETABULAR LIP.

labrum gle·noi·da·le (glee·noy·day′lee) [NA]. The fibrocartilaginous ring that surrounds the glenoid cavity of the scapula.

labrum glenoidale ar·ti·cu·la·ti·o·nis cox·ae (ahr·tick″yoo·lay″shee·o′nis kock′see) [BNA]. LABRUM ACETABULARE.

labrum glenoidale articulationis hu·me·ri (hew′mur·eye) [BNA]. LABRUM GLENOIDALE.

Labstix. A trademark for reagent strips employed to test urine for pH, proteins, glucose, ketones, or blood.

lab·y·rinth (lab′i·rinth) *n.* [Gk. *labyrinthos*]. 1. An intricate system of connecting passageways; maze. 2. The system of intercommunicating canals and cavities that makes up the inner ear. —**lab·y·rin·thine** (lab″i·rin′theen) *adj.*

lab·y·rin·thec·to·my (lab″i·rin·theck′tuh·mee) *n.* [*labyrinth* + *-ectomy*]. The complete removal of the membranous labyrinth of the inner ear. See also *hemilabyrinthectomy.*

labyrinthine artery. A branch of the basilar or anterior inferior cerebellar artery which supplies the inner ear. NA *arteria labyrinthi.*

labyrinthine fluid. PERILYMPH.

labyrinthine hydrops or **syndrome.** MÉNIÈRE'S SYNDROME.

labyrinthine nystagmus. Nystagmus occurring when the labyrinths are stimulated or diseased.

labyrinthine recess. A diverticulum of the auditory vesicle which finally becomes the endolymphatic duct and sac.

labyrinthine reflex. A reflex initiated by stimulation of the vestibular apparatus of the inner ear. See also *vestibular reflexes.*

labyrinthine test. Any test to check the function of the vestibular nerve and labyrinth. See also *Bárány's pointing test, caloric test.*

labyrinthine vertigo or **syndrome.** Vertigo that has its origin in labyrinthine structures, as in Ménière's syndrome.

lab·y·rin·thi·tis (lab″i·rin·thigh′tis) *n.* [*labyrinth* + *-itis*]. Inflammation of the labyrinth of the inner ear. Syn. *otitis interna.*

lab·y·rin·thot·o·my (lab″i·rin·thot′uh·mee) *n.* [*labyrinth* +

-tomy]. Incision into the labyrinth, specifically, into that of the inner ear.

la·by·rin·thus (lab″i·rinth′us) *n.*, pl. & genit. sing. **labyrin·thi** (·eye) [L.]. LABYRINTH.

labyrinthus eth·moi·da·lis (eth″moy·day′lis) [NA]. ETHMOID LABYRINTH.

labyrinthus mem·bra·na·ce·us (mem″bruh·nay′see·us) [NA]. MEMBRANOUS LABYRINTH.

labyrinthus os·se·us (os′ee·us) [NA]. OSSEOUS LABYRINTH.

[1]lac (lack) *n.*, pl. **lac·ta** (·tuh) [L.]. MILK (1).

[2]lac, *n.* [Hindi *lākh*]. Any of various natural resins used in preparing shellac.

lac·case (lack′ace) *n.* 1. An oxidizing enzyme present in many plants. 2. A class of oxidases which act on phenols.

lac·er·ate (las′ur·ate) *v.* [L. *lacerare*, from *lacer*, torn, maimed]. To wound by tearing. —**lacer·at·ed** (·ay·tid) *adj.*

lacerated foramen. FORAMEN LACERUM.

lac·er·a·tion (las″ur·ay′shun) *n.* [L. *laceratio*]. 1. A tear, or a wound made by tearing. 2. The act of tearing or lacerating.

laceration of the perineum. A tearing of the wall separating the lower portion of the vagina and anal canal occurring occasionally during parturition.

lac·ero·con·dy·lar (las″ur·o·kon′di·lur) *adj.* Pertaining to the foramen lacerum and the condylus occipitalis.

la·cer·tus (la·sur′tus) *n.*, pl. **lacer·ti** (·tye) [L., muscular part of the arm]. A small bundle of fibers.

lacertus fi·bro·sus (figh·bro′sus) [BNA]. APONEUROSIS MUSCULI BICIPITALIS BRACHII.

lacertus mus·cu·li rec·ti la·te·ra·lis (mus′kew·lye reck′tye lat·e·ray′lis) [NA]. The attachment of the lateral rectus muscle to the lateral palpebral ligament.

lac fe·mi·ni·num (fem″i·nigh′num) [BNA]. Secretion of the mammary gland.

Lach·e·sis (lack′e·sis) *n.* [Gk., one of the three Fates]. A genus of the Crotalidae. See also *bushmaster.*

lachrymal. LACRIMAL.

la·cin·i·ate (la·sin′ee·ate) *adj.* [L. *lacinia*, fringe]. Jagged, fringed; cut into narrow flaps.

laciniate ligament. FLEXOR RETINACULUM OF THE ANKLE.

la·cis cells (la·see′) [F., meshwork]. Mesangial cells of the renal juxtaglomerular apparatus.

lac operon. A section of chromosome involved in lactose metabolism, consisting of three structural genes which are regulated by a single i gene and a single operator; the model system used in developing the operon theory.

lac·ri·ma (lack′ri·muh) *n.*, pl. **lacri·mae** (·mee) [L., from OL. *dacruma* (rel. to Gk. *dakryon* and to Gmc. *ta*[k]*hr-* → E. *tear*)]. Tear.

lac·ri·mal (lack′ri·mul) *adj.* & *n.* [ML. *lacrimalis*, from L. *lacrima*, a tear]. 1. Pertaining to tears, or to the organs secreting and conveying tears. 2. LACRIMAL BONE.

lacrimal adenitis. DACRYOADENITIS.

lacrimal apparatus. The mechanism for secreting tears and draining them into the nasal cavity, consisting of the lacrimal gland, lake, puncta, canaliculi, sac, and the nasolacrimal duct. See also Plate 19.

lacrimal bone. A thin, delicate bone at the anterior part of the medial wall of the orbit; the smallest bone of the face. NA *os lacrimale.* See also Table of Bones in the Appendix.

lacrimal canal. NASOLACRIMAL CANAL.

lacrimal canaliculus. A small tube lined with stratified squamous epithelium which runs vertically a short distance from the punctum of each eyelid and then turns horizontally in the lacrimal part of the lid margin to the lacrimal sac. NA *canaliculus lacrimalis.*

lacrimal caruncle. A small, rounded elevation covered by modified skin lying in the lacrimal lake at each medial palpebral commissure. NA *caruncula lacrimalis.*

lacrimal crest. POSTERIOR LACRIMAL CREST.

lacrimal duct. LACRIMAL CANALICULUS.

lac·ri·ma·le (lack″ri·mah′lee, ·may′lee) *n. In craniometry*, the point where the posterior lacrimal crest meets the frontolacrimal suture. This point may occasionally be coincident with the dacryon, and cannot be located in skulls from which the lacrimal bones have been lost.

lacrimal fistula. A fistula communicating with a lacrimal canaliculus.

lacrimal fold. An inconstant, valvular fold of mucosa at the inferior meatus of the nasolacrimal duct. Syn. *Hasner's valve.* NA *plica lacrimalis.*

lacrimal fossa. The depression in the frontal bone for the reception of the lacrimal gland.

lacrimal gland. The compound tubuloalveolar gland secreting the tears, situated in the orbit in a depression of the frontal bone. NA *glandula lacrimalis.* See also Plate 19.

lacrimal groove. LACRIMAL SULCUS.

lacrimal lake. The space at the inner canthus of the eye, near the lacrimal punctum, in which there is some pooling of tear fluid. NA *lacus lacrimalis.*

lacrimal notch. A notch on the inner margin of the orbital surface of the maxilla which receives the lacrimal bone. NA *incisura lacrimalis.*

lacrimal papilla. One of the small papillary prominences at the margin of the eyelids in the center of which is the lacrimal punctum. NA *papilla lacrimalis.*

lacrimal point. LACRIMAL PUNCTUM.

lacrimal process. A short process of the inferior nasal concha that articulates with the descending process of the lacrimal bone. NA *processus lacrimalis.*

lacrimal punctum. The orifice of either lacrimal canaliculus at the inner canthus of the eye. NA *punctum lacrimale.*

lacrimal reflex. Secretion of tears induced by irritation of the corneal conjunctiva.

lacrimal sac. The dilated upper portion of the nasolacrimal duct. NA *saccus lacrimalis.* See also Plate 19.

lacrimal sound. A fine sound for exploring or dilating a lacrimal canaliculus.

lacrimal sulcus. A groove on the medial aspect of the frontal process of the maxilla which lodges the lacrimal sac. NA *sulcus lacrimalis maxillae.*

lacrimal tubercle. LACRIMAL PAPILLA.

lac·ri·ma·tion (lack″ri·may′shun) *n.* [L. *lacrimare*, to shed tears]. 1. Normal secretion of tears. 2. Excessive secretion, as in weeping.

lac·ri·ma·tor (lack′ri·may″tur) *n.* Any substance, as a tear gas, which irritates the conjunctiva and causes secretion of the tears.

lac·ri·ma·to·ry (lack′ri·muh·to″ree) *adj.* Pertaining to or causing lacrimation.

lacrimatory nucleus. An indefinite group of nerve cells located near the superior salivatory nucleus at the junction of the pons and medulla. Its fibers project to the pterygopalatine ganglion.

lac·ri·mo·max·il·lary suture (lack″ri·mo·mack′si·lerr·ee). MAXILLOLACRIMAL SUTURE.

lac·ri·mo·na·sal (lack″ri·mo·nay′zul) *adj.* [*lacrimal-* + *nasal*]. Pertaining to the lacrimal apparatus and the nose.

lacrimonasal duct. NASOLACRIMAL DUCT.

lac·ri·mot·o·my (lack″ri·mot′uh·mee) *n.* [*lacrimal* + *-tomy*]. Incision of the nasolacrimal duct.

lac sul·fu·ris (sul·few′ris). PRECIPITATED SULFUR.

lact-, lacti-, lacto- [L. *lac, lactis*]. A combining form meaning (a) *milk, lacteal;* (b) *lactic, lactic acid.*

lac·tac·i·de·mia, lac·tac·i·dae·mia (lack·tas″i·dee′mee·uh) *n.* [*lact-* + *acid* + *-emia*]. The presence of lactic acid in the blood.

lac·tac·i·du·ria (lack·tas″i·dew′ree·uh) *n.* [*lact-* + *acid* + *-uria*]. The presence of lactic acid in the urine.

lac·ta·gogue (lack′tuh·gog) *n.* [*lact-* + *-agogue*]. GALACTAGOGUE.

lac·tal·bu·min (lack″tal·bew′min) *n.* [*lact-* + *albumin*]. A simple protein contained in milk which resembles serum albumin and is of high nutritional quality.

lac·tam (lack′tam) *n.* An organic compound, containing a

—NH—CO— group in ring form, produced by the elimination of a molecule of water from certain amino acids. It is the keto form of its isomer, lactim.

lac·tam·ic acid (lack·tam'ick). ALANINE.

lac·tam·ide (lack·tam'id, ·ide, lack'tuh·mide, ·mid) *n.* The amide, $CH_3CHOHCONH_2$, of lactic acid.

lac·ta·mine (lack'tuh·meen) *n.* ALANINE.

lac·tar·o·vi·o·lin (lack·tăr″o·vye'o·lin) *n.* An antibiotic pigment, $C_{15}H_{14}O$, from *Lactarius deliciosus.*

lac·tase (lack'tace, ·taze) *n.* A soluble enzyme found in the animal body which hydrolyzes lactose to dextrose and galactose.

lactase deficiency syndrome. Diarrhea induced by ingestion of a lactose-containing food such as milk, secondary to a congenital or acquired deficiency of the disaccharide-splitting enzyme lactase in the intestinal mucosa.

¹lac·tate (lack'tate) *n.* A salt or ester of lactic acid. —**lac·tat·ed** (·tay·tid) *adj.*

²lactate, *v.* [L. *lactare,* from *lac,* milk]. To secrete milk.

lactate dehydrogenase. LACTIC ACID DEHYDROGENASE.

lactated Ringer's injection [S. *Ringer*]. A sterile solution of 0.6 g sodium chloride, 0.03 g potassium chloride, 0.02 g calcium chloride, and 0.31 g sodium lactate in sufficient water for injection to make 100 ml. Used intravenously as a systemic alkalizer, and as a fluid and electrolyte replenisher. Syn. *Hartmann's solution, Ringer's lactate solution.*

lac·ta·tion (lack·tay'shun) *n.* [L. *lactatio,* from *lactare,* to give milk]. 1. The period during which the child is nourished from the breast. 2. The formation or secretion of milk. —**lactation·al** (·ul) *adj.*

lactation amenorrhea. Postpartum amenorrhea due to lactation and nursing. It is probably a result of pituitary inhibition of the ovaries and indirectly or directly related to prolactin.

lactation hormone. PROLACTIN.

lactation mastitis. PUERPERAL MASTITIS.

lac·te·al (lack'tee·ul) *adj.* & *n.* [L. *lacteus,* from *lac,* milk]. 1. Pertaining to milk. 2. Milky. 3. Any of the lymphatics of the small intestine that take up the chyle.

lacteal calculus. MAMMARY CALCULUS.

lac·tes·cence (lack·tes'unce) *n.* [L. *lactescere,* to turn to milk]. Milkiness; often applied to the chyle.

lacti-. See *lact-.*

lac·tic (lack'tick) *adj.* [*lact-* + *-ic*]. Pertaining to milk or its derivatives.

lactic acid. 2-Hydroxypropanoic acid or α-hydroxypropionic acid, existing in three forms: (a) D(−)-lactic acid, $CH_3HCOHCOOH$, levorotatory, biochemically produced from methylglyoxal under certain conditions; (b) L(+)-lactic acid, $CH_3HOCHCOOH$, dextrorotatory, the product of anaerobic glycolysis in muscle, hence called sarcolactic acid; (c) DL-lactic acid, a racemic mixture of (a) and (b), produced by the action of bacteria on sour milk and other foods, and prepared synthetically by fermentation. The last occurs as a colorless, syrupy liquid, miscible with water. It is used as an ingredient of infant-feeding formulas, and has been variously used for medicinal purposes.

lactic acid dehydrogenase. A polymeric enzyme in mammalian tissues that exists in different forms and that catalyzes dehydrogenation of L(+)-lactic acid to pyruvic acid. Measurement of the levels of this enzyme in serum is useful in the diagnosis of myocardial infarction. Abbreviated, LAD.

lactic acidosis. A condition brought about by the accumulation of lactic acid in the tissues, as in circulatory failure, hypotension, or hypoxemia.

lactic dehydrogenase. LACTIC ACID DEHYDROGENASE.

lactic fermentation. Fermentation resulting in the souring of milk.

lac·tide (lack'tide) *n.* 1. The ring compound produced by interaction of two molecules of an α-hydroxyacid in such a way that the carboxyl group of one molecule is esterified with the hydroxyl group of the other, and vice versa. 2. The ring compound formed, according to the preceding definition, from two molecules of lactic acid.

lac·tif·er·ous (lack·tif'ur·us) *adj.* [*lacti-* + *-ferous*]. Conveying or secreting milk. Syn. *lactigerous.*

lactiferous ducts. The excretory ducts of the mammary gland, opening on the nipple. Syn. *milk ducts.* NA *ductus lactiferi.* See also Plate 24.

lactiferous sinuses. Dilatations of lactiferous ducts where milk may accumulate. NA *sinus lactiferi.* See also Plate 24.

lactiferous tubules. LACTIFEROUS DUCTS.

lac·ti·fuge (lack'ti·fewj) *n.* & *adj.* [*lacti-* + *-fuge*]. 1. A drug or agent that lessens the secretion of milk. 2. Having the action of a lactifuge.

lac·tig·e·nous (lack·tij'e·nus) *adj.* [*lacti-* + *-genous*]. Milk-producing.

lac·tig·er·ous (lack·tij'ur·us) *adj.* [*lacti-* + *-gerous*]. LACTIFEROUS.

lac·tim (lack'tim) *n.* An organic compound, containing a —NCOH— group in ring form, produced by the elimination of a molecule of water from certain amino acids. It is the enol form of its isomer, lactam.

lac·tin (lack'tin) *n.* LACTOSE.

Lactinex. A trademark for a mixture containing *Lactobacillus acidophilus* and *L. bulgaricus* used to restore intestinal flora.

lac·ti·su·gi·um (lack″ti·sue'jee·um) *n.* [NL., from *lacti-* + L. *sugere,* to suck]. BREAST PUMP.

lac·tiv·o·rous (lack·tiv'uh·rus) *adj.* [*lacti-* + L. *vorare,* to devour]. Subsisting on milk.

lacto-. See *lact-.*

lac·to·ba·cil·lic acid (lack″to·ba·sil'ick). 2-Hexylcyclopropanedecanoic acid, $C_{19}H_{36}O_2$, a lipid constituent of various microorganisms.

Lac·to·ba·cil·lus (lack″to·ba·sil'us) *n.* [*lacto-* + *bacillus*]. A genus of bacteria that are capable of producing lactic acid from carbohydrates and carbohydrate-like compounds, and which are able to withstand a degree of acidity usually destructive to nonsporulating bacteria. —**lactobacillus,** pl. **lactobacil·li** (·eye), *com. n.*

Lactobacillus ac·i·doph·i·lus (as″i·dof'i·lus). A gram-positive rod-shaped microorganism found in milk, feces, saliva, and carious teeth, nonpathogenic and unusually resistant to acid. Formerly called *Bacillus acidophilus, B. gastrophilus, Lactobacillus gastrophilus.*

Lactobacillus bi·fi·dus (bye'fi·dus, bif'i·). A nonmotile, anaerobic, gram-positive rod-shaped bacterium; the predominant organism in the intestine and feces of breast-fed infants.

Lactobacillus bul·gar·i·cus (bul·găr'i·kus). A species of bacteria isolated from Bulgarian fermented milk.

***Lactobacillus ca·sei* factor** (kay'see·eye). FOLIC ACID.

lactobacillus count. A count of the number of *Lactobacillus acidophilus* in a sample of saliva; used in testing for dental caries activity.

Lactobacillus gas·troph·i·lus (gas·trof'i·lus). *LACTOBACILLUS ACIDOPHILUS.*

***Lactobacillus lac·tis* Dorner** (lack'tis). A microorganism which is used in qualitative tests for vitamin B_{12} since it requires this vitamin for growth.

***Lactobacillus lactis* Dorner factor.** VITAMIN B_{12}; CYANOCOBALAMIN. Abbreviated, LLD factor.

lactobacillus of Boas-Oppler [I. I. *Boas;* and B. *Oppler,* German physician, 20th century]. A gram-positive rod-shaped microorganism originally found in the gastric juice of patients with carcinoma of the stomach, but bearing no known causative relationship to this; probably *Lactobacillus acidophilus.*

lac·to·cele (lack'to·seel) *n.* [*lacto-* + *-cele*]. GALACTOCELE.

lac·to·crit (lack'to·krit) *n.* [*lacto-* + Gk. *kritēs,* judge]. An apparatus for testing the quantity of fat in milk.

lac·to·fla·vin (lack″to·flay′vin, ·flav′in) *n.* RIBOFLAVIN.

lac·to·gen (lack′to·jen) *n.* [*lacto-* + *-gen*]. Any agent or substance that stimulates the secretion of milk.

lac·to·gen·ic (lack″to·jen′ick) *adj.* [*lacto-* + *-genic*]. Activating or stimulating the mammary glands.

lactogenic hormone. PROLACTIN.

lac·to·glob·u·lin (lack″to·glob′yoo·lin) *n.* [*lacto-* + *globulin*]. One of the proteins of milk.

lac·tom·e·ter (lack·tom′e·tur) *n.* [*lacto-* + *-meter*]. An instrument for determining the specific gravity of milk.

lac·tone (lack′tone) *n.* [*lact-* + *-one*]. An anhydro-ring compound produced by elimination of water from a molecule of an oxyacid.

lac·ton·ic acid (lack·ton′ick). GALACTONIC ACID.

lac·to·per·ox·i·dase (lack″to·pur·ock′si·dace) *n.* A peroxidase present in milk; it has been isolated in crystalline form.

lac·to·phos·phate (lack″to·fos′fate) *n.* A salt composed of a base combined with lactic and phosphoric acids.

lac·to·pro·te·in (lack″to·pro′tee·in, ·pro′teen) *n.* A protein of milk.

lac·tor·rhea, lac·tor·rhoea (lack″to·ree′uh) *n.* [*lacto-* + *-rrhea*]. GALACTORRHEA.

lac·to·sa·zone (lack·to′suh·zone) *n.* The characteristic osazone of lactose.

lac·tose (lack′toce) *n.* 4-(β-D-Galactopyranosido)-D-glucopyranose or 4-D-glucopyranosyl-β-D-galactopyranoside, $C_{12}H_{22}O_{11}$, a disaccharide representing D-glucose and D-galactose joined by a 1,4-glycosidic bond; on hydrolysis it is converted to these sugars. Two forms are known, alpha-lactose and beta-lactose; milk of mammals contains an equilibrium mixture of the two. Lactose is commonly the alpha form; crystallization at higher temperatures yields the beta form, which is more soluble in water. Both are used as nutrients and occasionally as diuretic agents; in pharmacy both are widely used as diluents and tablet excipients. Syn. *lactin, milk sugar.*

lac·tos·uria (lack″to·sue′ree·uh) *n.* [*lactose* + *-uria*]. The presence of lactose in the urine.

lac·to·syl ce·ram·i·do·sis (lack′to·sil serr″uh·mi·do′sis, se·ram″i·). A rare neurovisceral storage disorder due to a galactosyl hydrolase deficiency and characterized by elevation of lactosyl ceramide in erythrocytes, plasma, bone marrow, urine sediment, liver, and brain.

lac·to·ther·a·py (lack″to·therr′uh·pee) *n.* [*lacto-* + *therapy*]. GALACTOTHERAPY.

lac·to·tox·in (lack″to·tock′sin) *n.* [*lacto-* + *toxin*]. Any toxic substance formed in milk by decomposition of one of its proteins.

lac·to·veg·e·tar·i·an (lack″to·vej″e·terr′ee·un) *adj. & n.* [*lacto-* + *vegetarian*]. 1. Subsisting on or pertaining to a diet of milk and vegetables. 2. One who lives on a diet of milk and vegetables.

lac·to·vo·veg·e·tar·i·an (lack·to″vo·vej″e·terr′ee·un) *n.* [*lact-* + *ovo-* + *vegetarian*]. A person who lives on a diet of milk, eggs, and vegetables.

lac·tu·ca·ri·um (lack″tew·kair′ee·um, lack″tuh·) *n.* [NL., from L. *lactuca,* lettuce]. The dried milky juice of *Lactuca virosa,* alleged to have sedative activity; has been used for treatment of coughs and nervous irritability.

lac·tu·lose (lack′tew·loce) *n.* 4-*o*-β-D-Galactopyranosyl-D-frutose, $C_{12}H_{22}O_{11}$, a cathartic carbohydrate.

lac·tyl (lack′til) *n.* The monovalent radical $CH_3CHOHCO$— derived from lactic acid.

la·cu·na (la·kew′nuh) *n.*, pl. **lacunas, lacu·nae** (·nee) [L., from *lacus,* lake, basin]. 1. A little depression or space. 2. The space in the matrix occupied by a cartilage cell or by the body of a bone cell. 3. Gap; lapse; something missing.

lacunae la·te·ra·les (lat·e·ray′leez) [NA]. Venous pockets on either side of the superior sagittal sinus.

lacunae ure·thra·les (yoo·re·thray′leez) [NA]. URETHRAL LACUNAE.

lacuna mag·na (mag′nuh). An inconstant pouch extending upward from the dorsal wall of the navicular fossa of the penis.

lacuna mus·cu·lo·rum (mus·kew·lo′rum) [NA]. The space beneath the inguinal ligament which contains the iliopsoas muscle and femoral nerve.

la·cu·nar (la·kew′nur) *adj.* Pertaining to or characterized by lacunae.

lacunar abscess. An abscess involving a lacuna, usually of the urethra.

lacunar amnesia. Amnesia characterized by gaps or hiatuses in recall of a given stretch of time; spotty memory loss.

lacunar ligament. The part of the aponeurosis of the external oblique muscle which is reflected backward and laterally to be attached to the pecten of the pubic bone. Its base is thin and sharp and forms the medial boundary of the femoral ring. NA *ligamentum lacunare.*

lacunar state. The occurrence of small cerebral infarcts, the result of occlusion of small penetrating branches. There is a high correlation of the lacunar state with a combination of hypertension and atherosclerosis, and to a lesser degree with diabetes. Syn. *état lacunaire.*

lacunar tonsillitis. FOLLICULAR TONSILLITIS.

lacuna skull. CRANIOLACUNIA.

lacunas of Morgagni [G. B. *Morgagni*]. The orifices of the urethral glands.

lacuna va·so·rum (va·so′rum) [NA]. The space beneath the inguinal ligament which contains the femoral artery and vein.

lacuna ve·no·sa du·rae ma·tris (ve·no′suh dew′ree may′tris). Any small venous cleft between the layers of the dura mater, connecting the emissary and diploic veins with the venous sinuses.

la·cune (la·kyoon′) *n.* [F., from L. *lacuna*]. A small cavity left in the brain by the healing of a cerebral infarct. See also *lacunar state.*

la·cu·nu·la (la·kew′new·luh) *n.*, pl. **lacunulas, lacunu·lae** (·lee) [dim. of *lacuna*]. A small or minute lacuna; an air space, as seen in a gray hair when magnified.

la·cu·nule (la·kew′newl) *n.* [dim. of *lacuna*]. LACUNULA.

la·cus (lay′kus, lack′us) *n.* [L.]. [1]LAKE.

lacus la·cri·ma·lis (lack·ri·may′lis) [NA]. LACRIMAL LAKE.

LAD Abbreviation for *lactic acid dehydrogenase.*

lad·der splint. A splint with crossbars resembling a ladder.

Ladd-Frank·lin theory of color vision [Christine *Ladd-Franklin,* U.S. psychologist, 1847–1930]. A theory of the evolution of color vision. From a primitive black-white substance operative in rod vision in retinas without cones, the first stage in the development of color vision is said to have produced yellow and blue substances and cones; in the final stage, red and green substances were produced from the yellow, finishing the series of substances for white, yellow, red, and green vision.

lad·re·rie (lad′re·ree) *n.* [F., from *ladre,* measly]. A chronic cutaneous helminthiasis characterized by multiple painless nodules containing parts of taenias *(Cysticercus cellulosae).*

La·en·nec's cirrhosis (la·eh·neck′) [R. T. H. *Laennec,* French physician, 1781–1826]. Replacement of normal liver structure by abnormal lobules of liver cells, often hyperplastic, delimited by bands of fibrous tissue, giving the gross appearance of a finely nodular surface; alcoholism and malnutrition are chronically associated factors. Syn. *atrophic cirrhosis, diffuse nodular cirrhosis.* See also *alcoholic cirrhosis, portal cirrhosis, fatty cirrhosis.*

Laennec's pearl [R. T. H. *Laennec*]. PEARL (3).

Laennec's thrombus [R. T. H. *Laennec*]. A globular thrombus formed in the heart.

La·e·trile (lay′e·tril) *n.* A British trademark for *l*-mandelnitrile-β-glucuronic acid, $C_{14}H_{15}HO_7$, a product obtained by hydrolysis of amygdalin and oxidation of the resulting glycoside. It has been proposed as a valuable agent in the treatment of cancer, but, to date, this has not been confirmed by scientific studies.

laev-, laevo-. See *levo-.*

La·for·a bodies (lahˑfo'rahˑ) [G. Rodríguez *Lafora,* Spanish physician, b. 1887]. Basophilic, cytoplasmic bodies composed of an unusual polyglucosan and found in the dentate, brainstem, and thalamic neurons in progressive familial myoclonic epilepsy.

Lafora's disease [G. Rodríguez *Lafora*]. PROGRESSIVE FAMILIAL MYOCLONIC EPILEPSY.

lag, *n.* 1. The time between the application of a stimulus and resulting response; LATENT PERIOD. 2. LAG PHASE.

la·ge·na (la·jee'nuh) *n.*, pl. **lagenas, lage·nae** (·nee) [L., flask]. The curved, flasklike organ of hearing in lower vertebrates corresponding to the cochlea of higher forms.

la·ge·ni·form (la·jee'ni·form, la·jen'i·) *adj.* [*lagena* + *-iform*]. Flask-shaped.

lag·neia (lag·nigh'uh) *n.* [Gk., coition; salaciousness]. EROTOMANIA.

lag·neu·o·ma·nia (lag"new·o·may'nee·uh) *n.* [Gk. *lagneu*ein, to have sexual intercourse, + *-mania*]. A mental disorder characterized by lustful, sadistic, lewd, and lecherous actions; particularly, sadism in the male.

Lag·o·mor·pha (lag"o·mor'fuh) *n. pl.* [NL., from Gk. *lagos,* hare]. An order of gnawing placental mammals comprising the rabbits, hares, and pikas; this order is differentiated from the order Rodentia by having six incisor teeth as compared to four found in rodents. **—lag·o·morph** (lag'o·morf) *com. n.*

lag·oph·thal·mia (lag"off·thal'mee·uh) *n.* LAGOPHTHALMOS.

lagophthalmic keratitis. Keratitis due to the failure of the eyelids to close completely; a form of exposure keratitis.

lag·oph·thal·mos (lag"off·thal'mus) *n.* [Gk. *lagōs,* hare, + *ophthalmos*]. A condition in which the eyelids do not entirely close. **—lagophthal·mic** (·mick) *adj.*

Lag·o·thrix (lag'o·thricks) *n.* [NL., from Gk. *lagōs,* hare, + *-thrix*]. A genus of the Cebidae comprising the woolly monkeys.

lag phase or **period.** The early period of slow growth of bacteria when first inoculated in a culture medium.

La·grange's operation (la·grahⁿzh') [P. F. *Lagrange,* French ophthalmologist, 1857–1928]. A combination of iridectomy and sclerectomy for relief of glaucoma.

la grippe (lah greep) [F.]. INFLUENZA.

Laid·law's stain. Silver stain for normal ectodermal cells except basal epidermal cells and Schwann cells. It also stains ectodermal tumors.

Laid·low method for dopa oxidase. An adaptation of Bloch's method for dopa oxidase.

la·i·ty (lay'i·tee) *n.* Lay people; nonprofessional people as opposed to any particular professional group.

[1]lake, *n.* [L. *lacus,* lake, trough, basin]. A small, fluid-filled hollow or cavity.

[2]lake, *n.* [F. *laque,* from Per. *lak,* lac]. A pigment prepared by precipitating a vegetable or animal coloring matter or synthetic dye with a metallic compound.

[3]lake, *v.* To hemolyze.

laked blood. Blood in which the red blood cells are hemolyzed.

laky (lay'kee) *adj.* [from [3]*lake*]. Purplish red; said of blood serum which has a transparent red color after hemolysis.

-lalia [Gk. *lalia,* talk, conversation]. A combining form designating *a condition involving speech.*

lal·io·pho·bia (lal"ee·o·fo'bee·uh) *n.* [Gk. *lali*a, talk, + *-phobia*]. Morbid fear of talking or of stuttering.

lal·la·tion (lal·ay'shun) *n.* [L. *lallare,* to babble, to sing a lullaby]. 1. Any unintelligible stammering of speech, particularly that in which difficult consonants are avoided so that the speech sounds like the prattling of a baby. 2. Pronunciation of *l* sounds in place of *r* sounds.

lall·ing (lal'ing) *n.* LALLATION.

lalo- [Gk. *lalein,* to talk, chat]. A combining form meaning *speech.*

lal·og·no·sis (lal"og·no'sis) *n.* [*lalo-* + *-gnosis*]. Recognition of words.

la·lop·a·thy (la·lop'uth·ee) *n.* [*lalo-* + *-pathy*]. Any disorder of speech or disturbance of language.

lalo·pho·bia (lal"o·fo'bee·uh) *n.* LALIOPHOBIA.

lalo·pho·mi·a·trist (lal"o·fo·migh'uh·trist) *n.* SPEECH PATHOLOGIST.

lalo·ple·gia (lal"o·plee'jee·uh) *n.* [*lalo-* + *-plegia*]. Inability to speak, due to paralysis of the muscles concerned in speech, except those of the tongue.

lal·or·rhea, lal·or·rhoea (lal"o·ree'uh) *n.* [*lalo-* + *-rrhea*]. LOGORRHEA.

La·marck·ism (la·mahrk'iz·um) *n.* [J. R. *Lamarck,* French biologist, 1744–1820]. The theory that organic evolution takes place through the inheritance of modifications caused by the environment, and by the effects of use and disuse of organs.

lamb·da (lam'duh) *n.* [name of the letter Λ, λ, eleventh letter of the Greek alphabet]. 1. A designation used for various categories and quantities, sometimes as one of a series or set along with other Greek letters, and sometimes as a correlate of the Roman letter L, l. Symbol, Λ, λ. 2. *In craniometry,* the point where the sagittal suture meets the lambdoid suture.

lambda chain, λ chain. See *light chain.*

lamb·da·cism (lam'duh·siz·um) *n.* [Gk. *labdakismos,* from *labda,* lambda]. 1. Difficulty in uttering the sound of the letter *l.* 2. Too frequent use of the *l* sound, or its substitution for the *r* sound.

lamb·doid (lam'doid) *adj.* [Gk. *lambdoeidēs*]. Resembling the Greek letter lambda (Λ, λ).

lambdoid suture. The union between the two superior borders of the occipital bone with the parietal bones. NA *sutura lambdoidea.*

lamb dysentery. An acute enteritis occurring among lambs chiefly along the English-Scottish border. The etiological agent is *Clostridium perfringens,* type B. In other geographic locations, conditions known by the same name are caused by other agents.

lam·bert (lam'burt) *n.* [after J. H. *Lambert,* German physicist, 1728–1777]. A photometric unit for describing the brightness of light reflected from a surface. One lambert is the equivalent of one lumen per square centimeter.

Lam·bert's law (lahˑm'behrt) [J. H. *Lambert*]. The fraction of light absorbed on passage through a medium is proportional to the thickness of the medium.

Lam·blia (lam'blee·uh) *n.* [W. D. *Lambl,* Bohemian physician, 1824–1895]. *GIARDIA.*

lam·bli·a·sis (lam·blye'uh·sis) *n.* [*Lambl*ia + *-iasis*]. GIARDIASIS.

Lambl's excrescences. Fine, hairlike proliferations of fibrous connective tissue in the region of the nodules of the aortic valves.

lame, *adj.* Having a weakness or partial loss of function of a leg, so that the gait is abnormal, whether due to acute disease, shortening, atrophy of muscle, pain, or to any other disturbance of the member. **—lame·ness,** *n.*

la·mel·la (la·mel'uh) *n.*, pl. **lamellas, lamel·lae** (·ee) [L., dim. of *lamina*]. 1. A thin scale or plate. 2. Specifically: a thin layer of bone deposited during one period of osteogenic activity. 3. *In ophthalmology,* a medicated disk, usually prepared with gelatin, intended to be inserted under the eyelid.

la·mel·lar (la·mel'ur) *adj.* Resembling a thin plate; composed of lamellas or thin plates.

lamellar body. A cytoplasmic inclusion of unknown function found in human Sertoli cells and composed of concentric rings of fenestrated agranular reticulum.

lamellar bone. Bone which exhibits microscopic laminations (lamellas) of its matrix.

lamellar cataract. ZONULAR CATARACT.

lamellar corpuscle. A large, ellipsoid end organ made up of many concentric lamellas of connective tissue around a core containing the termination of a nerve fiber. Found in the deeper layers of the skin, under mucous membranes, in association with tendons, intermuscular septums, periosteum, and serous membranes. Syn. *pacinian corpuscle, Vater-Pacini corpuscle.* NA *corpuscula lamellosa.*

lamellar keratoplasty. Keratoplasty in which the more superficial stromata or the stromata near Descemet's membrane are excised and replaced by donor corneal tissue.

lamellar sheath. PERINEURIUM.

lames fo·li·a·cées (lam fo·lee·a·say') [F., foliated laminas]. Fibrous tissue in a concentric arrangement, resembling Meissner corpuscles found in the intradermal type of nevus pigmentosus.

La·mi·a·ce·ae (lay''mee·ay'see·ee) *n.pl.* [NL., from the genus *Lamium*]. LABIATAE.

lam·i·na (lam'i·nuh) *n.*, pl. **laminas, lami·nae** (·nee) [L.]. A thin plate or layer.

lamina af·fixa (a·fick'suh) [NA]. A thin strip of fibers covered by ependyma, along the line of union of a cerebral hemisphere with the thalamus.

lamina ala·ris (ay·lair'is) [NA]. ALAR PLATE.

lamina anterior va·gi·nae mus·cu·li rec·ti ab·do·mi·nis (va·jye'nee mus'kew·lye reck'tye ab·dom'i·nis) [NA]. The anterior leaf of the sheath of the rectus abdominis muscle.

lamina ar·cus ver·te·brae (ahr'kus vur'te·bree) [NA]. The portion of a vertebra between the spinous process and the posterior part of a transverse process.

lamina ba·sa·lis (ba·say'lis) [NA]. *In embryology*, the basal plate of the neural tube.

lamina basalis cho·roi·de·ae (ko·roy'dee·ee) [NA]. The basal lamina of the choroid.

lamina basalis cor·po·ris ci·li·a·ris (kor'po·ris sil·ee·air'is) [NA]. The inner layer of the ciliary body.

lamina ba·si·la·ris (bas·i·lair'is) [NA]. BASILAR MEMBRANE.

lamina car·ti·la·gi·nis cri·coi·de·ae (kahr·ti·laj'i·nis kri·koy'dee·ee) [NA]. The posterior part of the cricoid cartilage.

lamina cartilaginis la·te·ra·lis tu·bae au·di·ti·vae (lat·e·ray'lis tew'bee aw·di·tye'vee) [NA]. The lateral plate of the cartilage of the auditory tube.

lamina cartilaginis me·di·a·lis tu·bae au·di·ti·vae (mee·dee·ay'lis tew'bee aw·di·tye'vee) [NA]. The medial plate of the cartilage of the auditory tube.

lamina cho·rio·ca·pil·la·ris (ko''ree·o·kap·i·lair'is) [BNA]. Lamina choroidocapillaris (= CHORIOCAPILLARY LAMINA).

lamina chorioidea epi·the·li·a·lis ven·tri·cu·li la·te·ra·lis (ep''i·theel·ee·ay'lis ven·trick'yoo·lye lat·e·ray'lis) [BNA]. A thin epithelial layer which lines the roof of the lateral ventricle.

lamina chorioidea epithelialis ventriculi quar·ti (kwahr'tye) [BNA]. A thin epithelial layer which lines the roof of the fourth ventricle.

lamina cho·roi·do·ca·pil·la·ris (ko·roy''do·cap·i·lair'is) [NA]. CHORIOCAPILLARY LAMINA.

lamina ci·ne·rea (si·neer'ee·uh). *Obsol.* LAMINA TERMINALIS.

lamina cri·bro·sa (kri·bro'suh). 1. The portion of the sclera which is perforated for the passage of the optic nerve. 2. The fascia covering the saphenous opening. 3. The anterior or posterior perforated space of the brain. 4. The perforated plates of bone through which pass branches of the cochlear part of the vestibulocochlear nerve.

lamina cribrosa os·sis eth·moi·da·lis (os'is eth·moy·day'lis) [NA]. CRIBRIFORM PLATE (1).

lamina cribrosa scle·rae (skleer'ee) [BNA]. LAMINA CRIBROSA (1).

lamina dex·tra car·ti·la·gi·nis thy·roi·de·ae (deck'struh kahr·ti·laj'i·nis thigh·roy'dee·ee) [NA]. The right lamina of the thyroid cartilage.

lamina du·ra (dew'ruh). 1. DURA MATER. 2. The bone lining a dental alveolus which appears more radiopaque than the surrounding spongy bone; ALVEOLAR BONE (2).

laminae al·bae ce·re·bel·li (al'bee serr·e·bel'eye) [NA]. Sheets of white matter as seen in sections of the cerebellum.

laminae car·ti·la·gi·nis thy·roi·de·ae (kahr·ti·laj'i·nis thigh·roy'dee·ee). The laminae of the thyroid cartilage.

lamina elas·ti·ca (e·las'ti·kuh). The layer of interlacing elastic fibers in the mucous membrane of the pharynx, larynx, and respiratory tree.

lamina elastica anterior [BNA]. LAMINA LIMITANS ANTERIOR CORNEAE.

lamina elastica posterior [BNA]. LAMINA LIMITANS POSTERIOR CORNEAE.

laminae me·di·a·sti·na·les (mee·dee·as''ti·nay'leez) [BNA]. The mediastinal layers of the pleura.

laminae me·dul·la·res ce·re·bel·li (med''uh·lair'eez serr·e·bel'eye) [BNA]. LAMINAE ALBAE CEREBELLI.

laminae medullares tha·la·mi (thal'uh·migh) [NA]. Sheets of white matter seen in sections of the thalamus. See also *external medullary lamina, internal medullary lamina.*

lamina epi·scle·ra·lis (ep''i·skle·ray'lis) [NA]. A layer of connective tissue covering the sclera.

lamina epi·the·li·a·lis (ep''i·theel·ee·ay'lis) [NA]. The epithelial layer covering a choroid plexus.

lamina ex·ter·na os·si·um cra·nii (ecks·tur'nuh os'ee·um kray'nee·eye) [NA]. The outer layer of compact bone of the bones of the cranial vault.

lamina fi·bro·car·ti·la·gi·nea in·ter·pu·bi·ca (figh''bro·kahr·ti·la·jin'ee·uh in''tur·pew'bi·kuh) [BNA]. DISCUS INTERPUBICUS.

lamina for·ni·cis (for'ni·sis). FORNIX.

lamina fus·ca scle·rae (fus'kuh skleer'ee) [NA]. The thin pigmented inner layer of the sclera.

lam·i·na·gram (lam'i·nuh·gram) *n.* [*lamina* + *-gram*]. TOMOGRAM.

lam·i·nag·ra·phy (lam''i·nag'ruh·fee) *n.* [*lamina* + *-graphy*]. SECTIONAL RADIOGRAPHY.

lamina ho·ri·zon·ta·lis os·sis pa·la·ti·ni (hor''i·zon·tay'lis os'is pal·uh·tye'nigh) [NA]. The horizontal plate of the palatine bone.

lamina in·ter·na os·si·um cra·nii (in·tur'nuh os'ee·um kray'nee·eye) [NA]. The inner layer of compact bone of the bones of the cranial vault.

lamina la·te·ra·lis pro·ces·sus pte·ry·goi·dei (lat·e·ray'lis pro·ses'us terr·i·goy'dee·eye) [NA]. LATERAL PTERYGOID PLATE.

lamina li·mi·tans an·te·ri·or cor·ne·ae (lim'i·tanz an·teer'ee·or kor'nee·ee) [NA]. The basement membrane of the corneal epithelium.

lamina limitans posterior corneae [NA]. The basement membrane of the epithelium of the anterior chamber of the eye on the inner surface of the cornea.

lamina me·di·a·lis pro·ces·sus pte·ry·goi·dei (mee·dee·ay'lis pro·ses'us terr''i·goy'dee·eye) [NA]. MEDIAL PTERYGOID PLATE.

lamina me·dul·la·ris la·te·ra·lis cor·po·ris stri·a·ti (med·uh·lair'is lat·e·ray'lis kor'po·ris strye·ay'tye) [NA]. In cross sections of the corpus striatum, a sheet of white matter separating putamen from globus pallidus.

lamina medullaris me·di·a·lis cor·po·ris stri·a·ti (mee·dee·ay'lis kor'po·ris strye·ay'tye) [NA]. In cross sections of the corpus striatum, a sheet of white matter separating the medial and lateral parts of the globus pallidus.

lamina mem·bra·na·cea tu·bae au·di·ti·vae (mem·bra·nay'see·uh tew'bee aw·di·tye'vee) [NA]. A sheet of connective tissue forming the lower part of the cartilaginous portion of the auditory tube.

lamina mo·di·o·li (mo·dye'o·lye) [NA]. The upper part of the osseous spiral lamina.

lamina mus·cu·la·ris mu·co·sae (mus·kew·lay'ris mew·ko'see). The layer or layers of smooth muscle at the deep face of the mucous membrane of the digestive tube.

lamina muscularis mucosae co·li (ko'lye) [NA]. A thin layer of smooth muscle in the tunica mucosa of the colon.

lamina muscularis mucosae eso·pha·gi (e·sof'uh·jye) [NA]. A thin layer of muscle in the tunica mucosa of the esophagus.

lamina muscularis mucosae in·tes·ti·ni cras·si (in·tes·tye'nigh kras'eye) [BNA]. A thin layer of smooth muscle in the tunica mucosa of the large intestine.

lamina muscularis mucosae intestini te·nu·is (ten'yoo·is) [NA]. A thin layer of smooth muscle in the tunica mucosa of the small intestine.

lamina muscularis mucosae oe·so·pha·gi (e·sof'uh·jye) [BNA]. LAMINA MUSCULARIS MUCOSAE ESOPHAGI.

lamina muscularis mucosae rec·ti (reck'tye) [NA]. A thin layer of smooth muscle in the tunica mucosa of the rectum.

lamina muscularis mucosae ven·tri·cu·li (ven·trick'yoo·lye) [NA]. A thin layer of smooth muscle in the tunica mucosa of the stomach.

lamina or·bi·ta·lis (or·bi·tay'lis) [NA]. A thin, smooth, oblong plate of bone which closes in the ethmoid cells and forms a large part of the medial wall of the orbit.

lamina pa·py·ra·cea (pap·i·ray'see·uh) [BNA]. LAMINA ORBITALIS.

lamina pa·ri·e·ta·lis pe·ri·car·dii (pa·rye"e·tay'lis perr·i·kahr'dee·eye) [NA]. The parietal layer of serous pericardium.

lamina parietalis tu·ni·cae va·gi·na·lis pro·pri·ae tes·tis (tew'ni·see vaj·i·nay'lis pro'pree·ee tes'tis) [BNA]. LAMINA PARIETALIS TUNICAE VAGINALIS TESTIS.

lamina parietalis tunicae vaginalis testis [NA]. The parietal layer of the tunica vaginalis of the testis.

lamina per·pen·di·cu·la·ris os·sis eth·moi·da·lis (pur"pen·dick"yoo·lair'is os'is eth·moy·day'lis) [NA]. PERPENDICULAR PLATE OF THE ETHMOID BONE.

lamina perpendicularis ossis pa·la·ti·ni (pal·uh·tye'nigh) [NA]. PERPENDICULAR PLATE OF THE PALATINE BONE.

lamina posterior va·gi·nae mus·cu·li rec·ti ab·do·mi·nis (va·jye'nee mus'kew·lye reck'tye ab·dom'i·nis) [NA]. The posterior sheet of the sheath of the rectus abdominis muscle.

lamina pre·tra·che·a·lis fas·ci·ae cer·vi·ca·lis (pree·tray·kee·ay'lis fash'ee·ee sur·vi·kay'lis) [NA]. The layer of deep cervical fascia anterior to the trachea.

lamina pre·ver·te·bra·lis fas·ci·ae cer·vi·ca·lis (pree·vur·te·bray'lis fash'ee·ee sur·vi·kay'lis) [NA]. PREVERTEBRAL FASCIA.

lamina pro·fun·da fas·ci·ae tem·po·ra·lis (pro·fun'duh fash'ee·ee tem·po·ray'lis) [NA]. The deep layer of temporal fascia.

lamina profunda mus·cu·li le·va·to·ris pal·pe·brae su·pe·ri·o·ris (mus'kew·lye lev·uh·to'ris pal·pee'bree sue·peer·ee·o'ris) [NA]. The deep layer of the levator palpebrae superioris muscle.

lamina pro·pria mem·bra·nae tym·pa·ni (pro'pree·uh mem·bray'nee tim'puh·nigh). The middle or fibrous layer of the tympanic membrane.

lamina propria mu·co·sae (mew·ko'see) [NA]. The connective tissue of a mucous membrane. Syn. *tunica propria mucosae.*

lamina qua·dri·ge·mi·na (qwah·dri·jem'i·nuh) [BNA]. LAMINA TECTI.

lam·i·nar (lam'i·nur) *adj.* Of or pertaining to a lamina.

lam·i·nar·ia tent (lam"i·năr'ee·uh). A cone-shaped plug made from *Laminaria digitata,* a seaweed. When wet, the plug dilates; sometimes used in gynecologic procedures.

lamina ros·tra·lis (ros·tray'lis) [BNA]. ROSTRAL LAMINA.

lamina sep·ti pel·lu·ci·di (sep'tye pe·lew'si·dye) [NA]. Either one of the two thin sheets which form the septum pellucidum.

lamina si·nis·tra car·ti·la·gi·nis thy·roi·de·ae (si·nis'truh kahr·ti·laj'i·nis thigh·roy'dee·ee) [NA]. The left lamina of the thyroid cartilage.

lamina spi·ra·lis os·sea (spi·ray'lis os'ee·uh) [NA]. OSSEOUS SPIRAL LAMINA.

lamina spiralis se·cun·da·ria (seck·un·dair'ee·uh) [NA]. SECONDARY SPIRAL LAMINA.

lamina su·per·fi·ci·a·lis fasci·ae cer·vi·ca·lis (sue"pur·fish·ee·ay'lis fash'ee·ee sur·vi·kay'lis) [NA]. The superficial layer of deep cervical fascia.

lamina superficialis fasciae tem·po·ra·lis (tem·po·ray'lis) [NA]. The superficial layer of temporal fascia.

lamina superficialis mus·cu·li le·va·to·ris pal·pe·brae su·pe·ri·o·ris (mus'kew·lye lev·uh·to'ris pal·pee'bree sue·peer·ee·o'ris) [NA]. The superficial layer of the levator palpebrae superioris muscle.

lamina su·pra·cho·roi·dea (sue"pruh·ko·roy'dee·uh) [NA]. The delicate connective-tissue membrane uniting the choroid and sclerotic coats of the eye.

lam·i·nate (lam'i·nut, ·nate) *adj.* Consisting of layers or laminae; laminated.

lamina tec·ti (teck'tye) [NA]. The alar plate of the midbrain containing the superior and inferior colliculi.

laminated calculus. A calculus made up of layers of different materials.

laminated epithelium. STRATIFIED EPITHELIUM.

laminated tubercle. NODULUS (2).

lamina ter·mi·na·lis (tur·mi·nay'lis) [NA]. The connecting layer of gray matter between the optic chiasma and the anterior commissure where it becomes continuous with the rostral lamina.

lam·i·na·tion (lam"i·nay'shun) *n.* 1. Arrangement in plates or layers. 2. An operation in embryotomy consisting in cutting the skull in slices.

lamina tra·gi (tray'jye) [NA]. The portion of the cartilage of the external ear forming the tragus.

lamina vasculosa cho·roi·de·ae (ko·roy'dee·ee) [NA]. The outer, pigmented layer of the choroid, composed of small arteries and veins.

lamina vasculosa tes·tis (tes'tis). The vascular connective tissue deep to the tunica albuginea testis.

lamina vis·ce·ra·lis pe·ri·car·dii (vis·e·ray'lis perr·i·kahr'dee·eye) [NA]. EPICARDIUM.

lamina visceralis tu·ni·cae va·gi·na·lis pro·pri·ae tes·tis (tew'ni·see vaj·i·nay'lis pro'pree·ee tes'tis) [BNA]. LAMINA VISCERALIS TUNICAE VAGINALIS TESTIS.

lamina visceralis tunicae vaginalis testis [NA]. The visceral layer of the tunica vaginalis of the testis.

lamina vi·trea (vit'ree·uh). BASAL MEMBRANE.

lam·i·nec·to·my (lam"i·neck'tuh·mee) *n.* [*lamina* + *-ectomy*]. Surgical removal of one or more laminas of the vertebrae, often including the spinous processes of the vertebrae.

lam·i·ni·tis (lam"i·nigh'tis) *n.* [*lamina* + *-itis*]. An inflammatory disease of the laminae of a horse's hoof which may follow a variety of stressful events including acute gastroenteritis, parturition, overdosing with strong purgatives, temperature extremes, septicemic infections, and trauma. See also *founder.*

lam·i·nog·ra·phy (lam"i·nog'ruh·fee) *n.* [*lamina* + *-graphy*]. SECTIONAL RADIOGRAPHY. —**lam·i·no·gram** (lam'i·no·gram) *n.*

lam·i·not·o·my (lam"i·not'uh·mee) *n.* [*lamina* + *-tomy*]. Division of a lamina of a vertebra.

lam·pas (lam'pus) *n.* [F., from *lamper,* to guzzle]. *In veterinary medicine,* hyperemia of the mucous membrane of the hard palate just posterior to the incisor teeth in horses.

lamp·black, *n.* A fine black substance, almost pure carbon, made by burning oils, tars, fats, or resins in an atmosphere deficient in oxygen. The similar product (sometimes called lampblack), obtained by allowing a gas flame to impinge on a cold surface, is more properly designated gas black or carbon black.

lamp·brush chromosome. An especially large, unique chromosome characterized by many fine lateral projections giving the appearance of a test-tube brush or lamp brush, as seen in newt oocytes. Active ribonucleic acid and protein synthesis is associated with the projections.

lamp-chimney drain. A tubular drain of large-caliber glass or metal, anchored over selected areas within the abdomen and adapted to gastric, colonic, and urinary bladder surgery.

lam·pro·pho·nia (lam″pro·fo′nee·uh) *n.* LAMPROPHONY.

lam·proph·o·ny (lam·prof′uh·nee) *n.* [Gk. *lamprophōnia*, from *lampros*, clear, + *phōnē*, voice]. Clearness of voice. —**lam·pro·phon·ic** (lam″pro·fon′ick) *adj.*

La·mus me·gis·tus (lay′mus me·jis′tus). *PANSTRONGYLUS MEGISTUS.*

lam·ziek·te (lahm′zeek·tuh) *n.* [Afrikaans, lit., lame-sickness]. A bone disease of cattle in South Africa, resulting from the eating of contaminated carrion. The disease is due to *Clostridium botulinum*, type D.

la·na (lay′nuh, lan′uh) *n.* [L.]. Wool. See also *wool fat.*

la·nat·o·side (la·nat′o·side) *n.* A natural glycoside from the leaves of *Digitalis lanata;* three such glycosides have been isolated and are designated lanatoside A, lanatoside B, and lanatoside C, formerly called digilanid A, digilanid B, and digilanid C, respectively. The aglycones are, respectively, digitoxigenin, gitoxigenin, and digoxigenin. All three lanatosides yield, on hydrolysis with acid, one molecule of D-glucose, three molecules of digitoxose, and one molecule of acetic acid. They are cardioactive.

Lan·cas·ter's advancement [W. B. *Lancaster*, U.S. ophthalmologist, 1863–1915]. A modification of advancement (2) in which the shortened muscle, rather than its tendon, is attached anterior to the stump.

lance, *v.* To cut or open, as with a lancet or bistoury.

Lance·field groups [Rebecca C. *Lancefield*, U.S. bacteriologist, b. 1895]. An antigenic classification of streptococci. See also *streptococci, hemolytic streptococci.*

Lan·ce·reaux's diabetes (lahⁿs·ro′) [E. *Lancereaux*, French physician, 1829–1910]. Diabetes mellitus with extreme emaciation.

Lancereaux's law of thrombosis [E. *Lancereaux*]. Marantic thromboses occur at the points where there is the greatest tendency to stasis.

lan·cet (lan′sit) *n.* [F. *lancette*]. A small, pointed, double-edged surgical knife; rarely used nowadays.

lan·ci·nat·ing (lan′si·nay·ting) *adj.* [L. *lancinare*, to tear to pieces]. Tearing; shooting, sharply cutting, as lancinating pain. —**lanci·nate** (·nate) *v.*

Lan·ci·si's sign (lahⁿ·chee′zee) [G. M. *Lancisi*, Italian physician, 1654–1720]. A sign of tricuspid regurgitation; a large positive systolic wave in the jugular venous pulse.

Lancisi's striae or **nerves** [G. M. *Lancisi*]. Medial and lateral longitudinal striae on the superior surface of the corpus callosum.

Lan·dau position, posture, reflex, or **response.** Antigravity movements of an infant held suspended in the air with the examiner's hands around his chest. On being lifted, the baby normally elevates his head and to some degree extends his legs. Passive flexion of the head in this position results in loss of extensor tone of the legs. The response is poor in floppy infants, who remain draped over the examiner's hand like an inverted U, but is exaggerated in hypertonic and opisthotonic babies.

Lan·dis-Gib·bon test [E. M. *Landis*, U.S. physiologist, b. 1901; and J. H. *Gibbon*, U.S. surgeon, b. 1903]. A test for the evaluation of vasospasm in peripheral vascular disease, based on reflex vasodilatation which normally occurs in an unheated extremity when the other extremity is heated. In obliterative vascular disease, little or no rise in skin temperature occurs in the affected extremity when the uninvolved extremity is heated; a normal response occurs in vasospastic disorders.

land·marks, *n.pl.* Superficial marks, as eminences, lines, and depressions, that serve as guides to, or indications of, deeper parts.

Lan·dolt ring (lahⁿ·doʰlt′) [E. *Landolt*, French ophthalmologist, 1846–1926]. *In ophthalmology,* an incomplete ring used as a test object for visual acuity.

Landolt's broken C test [E. *Landolt*]. A test for visual acuity wherein the subject is to determine in which segment the gap in the ring (or letter C) lies, a factor which is determined by the size of the image of the gap on the retina.

Landouzy-Gras·set law (graʰ·seʰ′) [L. T. J. *Landouzy* and J. *Grasset*]. In disease of one cerebral hemisphere, producing hemiplegia, the head is turned toward the side of the cerebral lesion if there is flaccidity and away from the side of the cerebral lesion if there is spasticity; of questionable validity.

Landouzy's disease [L. T. J. *Landouzy*]. LEPTOSPIROSIS.

Landouzy's purpura [L. T. J. *Landouzy*]. Purpura with serious systemic symptoms.

Landouzy's sciatica [L. T. J. *Landouzy*]. Sciatic neuritis with muscle atrophy of the affected leg.

Landromil. A trademark for ticlatone, an antibacterial agent.

Landry-Guillain-Barré disease or **syndrome.** GUILLAIN-BARRÉ DISEASE.

Lan·dry's ascending paralysis (lahⁿ·dree′) [J. B. O. *Landry* de Thézillat, French physician, 1826–1895]. GUILLAIN-BARRÉ DISEASE.

land scurvy. IDIOPATHIC THROMBOCYTOPENIC PURPURA.

Land·stei·ner classification [K. *Landsteiner*, U.S. pathologist, 1868–1943]. Designation of the major blood groups as O, A, B, and AB. See also *blood groups.*

Land·ström's muscle (laʰnd′strœm″) [J. *Landström*, Swedish surgeon, 1869–1910]. MUSCLE OF LANDSTRÖM.

Lane's disease [W. A. *Lane*, English surgeon, 1856–1943]. *Obsol.* INTESTINAL STASIS.

Lane's kink [W. A. *Lane*]. *Obsol.* An obstructive bend or twist of the terminal ileum.

Lane's operation [W. A. *Lane*]. Ileosigmoidostomy for relief of chronic constipation.

Lane's plates [W. A. *Lane*]. Steel plates of various shapes, with holes for screws, for fixing fragments in position in cases of fracture.

Lang·don Down anomaly [J. *Langdon* Haydon *Down*]. DOWN'S SYNDROME.

Lang·en·beck's operation (laʰng′ᵉn·beck) [B. R. K. von *Langenbeck*, German surgeon, 1810–1887]. An operation for cleft palate in which closure is effected by means of periosteal flaps obtained from either side and sutured in the midline.

Lang·en·dorf preparation. An isolated mammalian heart preparation in which the coronary vessels are perfused in warm oxygenated Locke-Ringer's or Tyrode solution.

Lang·er·hans cell (laʰng′ur·haʰnss) [P. *Langerhans*, German anatomist, 1847–1888]. A star-shaped structure of the mammalian epidermis and dermis, revealed by gold impregnation and containing nonmelanized disklike organelles.

Lang·er·hans·ian adenoma (lahng″ur·hahns′ee·un) [P. *Langerhans*]. ISLET-CELL TUMOR.

Lang·er's lines (laʰng′ur) [C. von *Langer*, Austrian anatomist, 1819–1887]. Cleavage lines of the skin.

Lange's test. COLLOIDAL GOLD TEST.

Lang·hans' cell (laʰng′haʰnss) [T. *Langhans*, German pathologist, 1834–1915]. One of the discrete cuboidal cells forming the cytotrophoblast layer of the chorionic villi during the first half of pregnancy.

Langhans' giant cell [T. *Langhans*]. A multinucleated giant cell with peripheral, radially arranged nuclei found in certain granulomatous lesions, as tuberculosis, leprosy, and tularemia.

Langhans' layer [T. *Langhans*]. CYTOTROPHOBLAST.

Langhans' stria [T. *Langhans*]. STRIA OF LANGHANS.

lan·gur (lahng·goor′) *n.* [Hindi, from Skr. *lāṅgūla*, tailed]. Any of various Asian colobine monkeys, mainly those of the genus *Presbytis.*

Lan·ne·longue's operation (lan·lohⁿg') [O. M. *Lannelongue,* French surgeon, 1840–1911]. A craniectomy in which a narrow strip of parietal bone near the sagittal suture is resected, for decompression as in craniosynostosis.

lan·o·lin (lan'uh·lin) *n.* [Ger., from L. *lana,* wool]. Wool fat containing about 30% water; used as an ointment base. Syn. *hydrous wool fat.*

lanolin rosin. A cement for sealing coverslips.

la·nos·ter·ol (la·nos'tur·ol) *n.* 8,24-Lanostadien-3-ol, $C_{30}H_{50}O$, an unsaturated sterol in wool fat.

Lanoxin. Trademark for the cardioactive glycoside digoxin.

Lan·sing virus. Poliomyelitis virus type 2; a strain of virus that can infect human beings. It was adapted to the cotton rat and white mouse in 1937, and is useful in vaccines and in serologic studies of poliomyelitis.

Lan·ter·mann's cleft or **incisure** [A. J. *Lantermann,* Alsatian anatomist, 19th century]. SCHMIDT-LANTERMANN INCISURE.

lan·tha·nic (lan'thuh·nick, lan·than'ick) *adj.* [Gk. *lanthanein,* to escape notice]. Pertaining to patients who are medically diagnosed as having a particular disease but have a symptom or complaint that is not attributable to that disease.

lan·tha·nide (lan'thuh·nide) *n.* Any chemical element of a series beginning with lanthanum, and including cerium, praseodymium, neodymium, promethium, samarium, europium, gadolinium, terbium, dysprosium, holmium, erbium, thulium, ytterbium, and lutetium, the group constituting the lanthanide series of elements, formerly called the rare-earth elements.

lan·tha·non (lan'thuh·non) *n.* Any element belonging to the lanthanide series of elements.

lan·tha·num (lan'thuh·num) *n.* [NL., from Gk. *lanthanein,* to escape notice]. La = 138.9055. A rare metallic element.

lan·thi·o·nine (lan·thigh'o·neen) *n.* 3,3'-Thiodialanine, $C_6H_{12}N_2O_4S$, an amino acid constituent of proteins.

lan·tho·pine (lan'tho·peen) *n.* A minor alkaloid, $C_{23}H_{25}NO_4$, from opium.

la·nu·go (la·new'go) *n.* [L., down, from *lana,* wool]. 1. [NA] The downlike hair that covers the fetus from about the fifth month of gestation. 2. VELLUS. —**lanu·gi·nous** (·ji·nus) *adj.*

lan·u·lous (lan'yoo·lus) *adj.* [L. *lanula,* a small lock of wool]. Covered with short, fine hair.

Lanum. Trade name for hydrous wool fat.

la·pac·tic (la·pack'tick) *n.* [Gk. *lapaktikos,* from *lapassein,* to empty]. 1. An evacuant. 2. Any purgative substance.

lapar-, laparo- [Gk. *lapara*]. A combining form meaning *flank* or, more loosely, *abdomen.*

lap·a·ror·rha·phy (lap''uh·ror'uh·fee) *n.* [*laparo-* + *-rrhaphy*]. Suture of the abdominal wall.

lap·a·ro·scope (lap'uh·ro·skope) *n.* [*laparo-* + *-scope*]. PERITONEOSCOPE.

lap·a·ros·co·py (lap''uh·ros'kuh·pee) *n.* [*laparo-* + *-scopy*]. PERITONEOSCOPY.

lap·a·rot·o·my (lap''uh·rot'uh·mee) *n.* [*laparo-* + *-tomy*]. 1. An incision through the abdominal wall; CELIOTOMY. 2. The operation of cutting into the abdominal cavity through the loin or flank.

lap·a·ro·trach·e·lot·o·my (lap''uh·ro·tray''ke·lot'uh·mee, ·track''e·lot'uh·mee) *n.* [*laparo-* + *trachelo-* + *-tomy*]. A low cervical cesarean section in which the uterine incision is made in the lower uterine segment following entry into the peritoneal cavity.

la·pis (lap'is, lay'pis) *n.* [L.]. A stone; an alchemic term applied to any nonvolatile substance.

lapis cal·a·mi·na·ris (kal''uh·mi·nair'is, ka·lam''i·). CALAMINE.

lapis im·pe·ri·a·lis (im·peer''ee·ay'lis). SILVER NITRATE.

lapis in·fer·na·lis (in''fur·nay'lis). SILVER NITRATE.

Laplace's law. LAW OF LAPLACE.

lap·pa (lap'uh) *n.* [L., bur]. The root of the common burdock, *Arctium lappa,* or of *A. minus;* has been used as an aperient, diuretic, and alterative.

lapping murmur. A murmur that occurs following rupture of the aorta, resembling the sound of a cat lapping milk.

lapse attack. ABSENCE ATTACK.

lap·sus (lap'sus) *n.* [L., from *labi,* to fall]. 1. *In psychiatry,* a slip thought to reveal an unconscious desire. 2. PTOSIS.

lapsus cal·a·mi (kal'uh·migh). Slip of the pen; from the psychoanalytic point of view, it reveals an unconscious desire.

lapsus lin·guae (ling'gwee). Slip of the tongue, considered by psychoanalysts to reveal an unconscious desire.

lapsus pal·pe·brae su·pe·ri·o·ris (pal·pee'bree sue·peer''ee·o'ris). Ptosis of the eyelid.

lapsus pi·lo·rum (pi·lo'rum). ALOPECIA.

lapsus un·gui·um (ung'gwee·um). Falling of the nails.

la·pyr·i·um chloride (la·peer'·ee·um). 1[[(2-Hydroxyethyl)carbamoyl]methyl]pyridinim chloride, laurate ester, $C_{21}H_{35}ClN_2O_3$, a surfactant.

lar·bish (lahr'bish) *n.* A form of larva migrans that is seen in Senegal.

lard, *n.* [OF., from L. *laridum*]. The purified internal fat of the abdomen of the domestic hog. Has been used in pharmacy as an ingredient of ointment and cerate bases.

lar·da·ceous (lahr·day'shus) *adj.* 1. Resembling lard. 2. Containing diffuse amyloid deposits.

lardaceous degeneration. AMYLOID DEGENERATION.

lardaceous spleen. A spleen with diffuse amyloid degeneration. Syn. *waxy spleen.*

Largactil. A trademark for chlorpromazine, a tranquilizer used as the hydrochloride salt.

large alveolar cell. GREAT ALVEOLAR CELL.

large calorie. KILOCALORIE.

large intestine. The distal portion of the intestine, extending from the ileum to the anus, and consisting of the cecum, the colon, and the rectum. NA *intestinum crassum.*

large-lung emphysema. EMPHYSEMA (1).

Largon. Trademark for propiomazine, a sedative used as the hydrochloride salt.

lark·spur, *n.* The dried ripe seed of *Delphinium ajacis;* preparations of the seed have been used as a pediculicide.

Larocin. A trademark for amoxicillin, an antibacterial.

Larodopa. A trademark for levodopa, an anticholinergic.

La Roque's sign. A sign of acute appendicitis in which pressure over the appendix may cause the right testis to be drawn up.

La·ro·yenne's operation (laʰ·rwaʰ·yen') [L. *Laroyenne,* French surgeon, 1832–1902]. An operation for drainage of a pelvic abscess by an incision through the rectouterine excavation.

Lar·rey's sign (la·rehʼ) [D. J. de *Larrey,* French surgeon, 1766–1842]. A sign for sacroiliac disease in which pain in the joint is felt when the patient sits down abruptly on a hard seat.

Lar·sen-Jo·hans·son disease (lahr'sᵉn, yoo'aʰn·soʰnn'') [C. M. F. Sinding-*Larsen;* and S. *Johansson,* Swedish surgeon, b. 1880]. A form of osteochondrosis involving an accessory center of ossification in the apex of the patella. Syn. *Sinding-Larsen disease.*

lar·va (lahr'vuh) *n.,* pl. **lar·vae** (·vee) [L., ghost]. An immature and independent developmental stage in the life cycle of various animals which reach the adult form by undergoing metamorphosis.

lar·val (lahr'vul) *adj.* 1. Pertaining to or in the condition of a larva. 2. LARVATE.

larval seizures. *In electroencephalography,* subliminal seizures which produce no clinical symptoms but which are recognized by abnormal brain-wave discharges.

larva mi·grans (migh'granz). Invasion of the epidermis by various larvae, characterized by bizarre red irregular lines which are broad at one end and fade at the other, produced by burrowing larvae, most commonly in the United States by those of *Ancylostoma braziliense.* Syn. *creeping eruption.* See also *dermamyiasis linearis migrans oestrosa.*

lar·vate (lahr'vate) *adj.* [L. *larvatus,* masked]. Concealed; masked; applied to diseases and conditions that are hidden or atypical.

lar·vi·cide (lahr'vi·side) *n.* [*larva* + *-cide*]. Any agent destroying insect larvae.

laryng-, laryngo-. A combining form meaning *larynx, laryngeal.*

lar·yn·gal·gia (lăr"in·gal'jee·uh) *n.* [*laryng-* + *-algia*]. Pain or neuralgia of the larynx.

la·ryn·ge·al (la·rin'jee·ul, ·jul, lăr"in·jee'ul) *adj.* Of or pertaining to the larynx.

laryngeal cartilages. The cartilages forming the framework of the larynx. NA *cartilagines laryngis.*

laryngeal crisis. An acute laryngeal spasm, sometimes occurring in tabes dorsalis.

laryngeal mirror. 1. A small circular mirror affixed to a long handle, used in laryngoscopy. 2. A similar instrument used by dentists in the examination of the teeth.

laryngeal mirror test. A test for tuberculosis used to replace the usual sputum test where the patient swallows the sputum. A laryngeal mirror is placed in the back of the throat so that the vocal folds may be seen. The patient coughs, and the sputum on the mirror is examined for acid-fast bacilli.

laryngeal nerves. See Table of Nerves in the Appendix.

laryngeal pharynx. LARYNGOPHARYNX.

laryngeal pouch or **saccule.** SACCULE OF THE LARYNX.

laryngeal prominence. The tubercle of the thyroid cartilage and the bulging in the midline of the neck caused by it. Syn. *Adam's apple, laryngeal protuberance.* NA *prominentia laryngea.*

laryngeal protuberance. LARYNGEAL PROMINENCE.

laryngeal reflex. A cough resulting from irritation of the larynx.

laryngeal sinus. LARYNGEAL VENTRICLE.

laryngeal speech. Speech produced by means of an artificial larynx following laryngectomy; less commonly employed than esophageal speech.

laryngeal stridor. Stridor due to laryngeal obstruction.

laryngeal venous plexus. A venous plexus draining blood from the larynx to the anterior and inferior laryngeal veins and communicating with the pharyngeal venous plexus.

laryngeal ventricle. The portion of the cavity of the larynx between the vestibular and the vocal folds. NA *ventriculus laryngis.*

laryngeal-vertigo syndrome. COUGH SYNCOPE.

lar·yn·gec·to·my (lăr"in·jeck'tuh·mee) *n.* [*laryng-* + *-ectomy*]. Extirpation or partial excision of the larynx.

lar·yn·gem·phrax·is (lăr"in·jem·frack'sis) *n.* [*laryng-* + *emphraxis*]. Closure or obstruction of the larynx.

lar·yn·gis·mus (lăr"in·jiz'mus) *n.*, pl. **laryngis·mi** (·migh). A spasm of the larynx. —**laryngis·mal** (·mul) *adj.*

laryngismus stri·du·lus (strye'dew·lus, strid'yoo·lus). 1. SPASMODIC CROUP. 2. The laryngeal spasm sometimes seen in hypocalcemic states.

lar·yn·gi·tis (lăr"in·jye'tis) *n.*, pl. **laryn·git·i·des** (·jit'i·deez) [*laryng-* + *-itis*]. Inflammation of the larynx. It may be acute or chronic, catarrhal, suppurative, croupous (diphtheritic), tuberculous, or syphilitic. —**laryn·git·ic** (·jit'ick) *adj.*

laryngitis sic·ca (sick'uh). DRY LARYNGITIS.

laryngo-. See *laryng-.*

la·ryn·go·cele (la·ring'go·seel) *n.* [*laryngo-* + *-cele*]. An aerocele connected with the larynx.

la·ryn·go·cen·te·sis (la·ring"go·sen·tee'sis) *n.* [*laryngo-* + *centesis*]. Puncture of the larynx.

la·ryn·go·fis·sure (la·ring"go·fish'ur) *n.* [*laryngo-* + *fissure*]. 1. Surgical division of the larynx for the removal of tumors or foreign bodies. 2. The aperture made in the operation of laryngofissure.

la·ryn·go·gram (la·ring'go·gram) *n.* [*laryngo-* + *-gram*]. A representation of the larynx, usually radiographic, after the introduction of contrast material.

la·ryn·go·graph (la·ring'go·graf) *n.* [*laryngo-* + *-graph*]. An instrument for recording laryngeal movements. —**laryn·gog·ra·phy** (la"rin·gog'ruh·fee) *n.*

lar·yn·gol·o·gist (lăr"ing·gol'uh·jist) *n.* A person who specializes in laryngology.

lar·yn·gol·o·gy (lăr"ing·gol'uh·jee) *n.* [*laryngo-* + *-logy*]. The science of the anatomy, physiology, and diseases of the larynx. —**laryn·go·log·ic** (·go·loj'ick) *adj.*

lar·yn·gom·e·try (lăr"ing·gom'e·tree) *n.* [*laryngo-* + *-metry*]. The systematic measurement of the larynx.

la·ryn·go·pa·ral·y·sis (la·ring"go·puh·ral'i·sis) *n.* [*laryngo-* + *paralysis*]. Paralysis of the laryngeal muscles.

lar·yn·gop·a·thy (lăr"ing·gop'uth·ee) *n.* [*laryngo-* + *-pathy*]. Any disease of the larynx.

la·ryn·go·phan·tom (la·ring"go·fan'tum) *n.* [*laryngo-* + *phantom*]. *Obsol.* An artificial larynx designed for illustrative purposes.

la·ryn·go·pha·ryn·ge·al (la·ring"go·fa·rin'jee·ul) *adj.* [*laryngo-* + *pharyngeal*]. Pertaining conjointly to the larynx and pharynx.

laryngopharyngeal recess. The lower pyramidal part of the pharynx from which open the esophagus and the larynx.

la·ryn·go·phar·yn·gec·to·my (la·ring"go·făr"in·jeck'tuh·mee) *n.* [*laryngo-* + *pharyng-* + *-ectomy*]. Surgical removal of the larynx and a portion of the pharynx.

la·ryn·go·pha·ryn·ge·us (la·ring"go·fa·rin'jee·us) *n.* The inferior constrictor of the pharynx. See Table of Muscles in the Appendix.

la·ryn·go·phar·yn·gi·tis (la·ring"go·făr"in·jye'tis) *n.* [*laryngo-* + *pharyng-* + *-itis*]. 1. Inflammation of the laryngopharynx. 2. Inflammation of the larynx and the pharynx.

la·ryn·go·phar·ynx (la·ring"go·făr'inks) *n.* [*laryngo-* + *-pharynx*]. The inferior portion of the pharynx. It extends from the level of the greater cornua of the hyoid bone to that of the inferior border of the cricoid cartilage. Syn. *hypopharynx, laryngeal pharynx.* NA *pars laryngea pharyngis.*

lar·yn·goph·o·ny (lăr"ing·gof'uh·nee) *n.* [*laryngo-* + *-phony*]. The sound of the voice observed in auscultation of the larynx.

la·ryn·go·plas·ty (la·ring'go·plas"tee) *n.* [*laryngo-* + *-plasty*]. Plastic reparative operation upon the larynx.

la·ryn·go·ple·gia (la·ring"go·plee'jee·uh) *n.* [*laryngo-* + *-plegia*]. Paralysis of the laryngeal muscles.

la·ryn·go·pto·sis (la·ring"go·to'sis) *n.* [*laryngo-* + *ptosis*]. Mobility and falling of the larynx; sometimes occurs in old age.

la·ryn·go·rhi·nol·o·gy (la·ring"go·rye·nol'uh·jee) *n.* [*laryngo-* + *rhino-* + *-logy*]. The branch of medicine which treats of diseases of the larynx and the nose.

la·ryn·gor·rha·gia (la·ring"go·ray'jee·uh) *n.* [*laryngo-* + *-rrhagia*]. Hemorrhage from the larynx.

lar·yn·gor·rha·phy (lăr"ing·gor'uh·fee) *n.* [*laryngo-* + *-rrhaphy*]. Suture of the larynx.

la·ryn·gor·rhea, la·ryn·gor·rhoea (la·ring"go·ree'uh) *n.* [*laryngo-* + *-rrhea*]. Excessive secretion of mucus from the larynx, especially when it is used in phonation.

la·ryn·go·scle·ro·ma (la·ring"go·skle·ro'muh) *n.* [*laryngo-* + *scleroma*]. Induration of the larynx.

la·ryn·go·scope (la·ring'go·skope) *n.* [*laryngo-* + *-scope*]. A tubular instrument, combining a light system and a telescopic system, used in the visualization of the interior larynx and adaptable for diagnostic, therapeutic, and surgical procedures. —**la·ryn·go·scop·ic** (la·ring"go·skop'ick) *adj.*

lar·yn·gos·co·pist (lăr"ing·gos'kuh·pist) *n.* An expert in laryngoscopy.

lar·yn·gos·co·py (lăr"ing·gos'kuh·pee) *n.* [*laryngo-* + *-scopy*]. Examination of the interior of the larynx directly with a laryngoscope or indirectly with a laryngeal mirror or telescope.

la·ryn·go·spasm (la·ring'go·spaz·um) *n.* [*laryngo-* + *spasm*]. Spasmodic closure of the glottis; LARYNGISMUS STRIDULUS.

lar·yn·gos·ta·sis (lăr"ing·gos'tuh·sis) *n.* [*laryngo-* + *-stasis*]. CROUP.

la·ryn·go·ste·no·sis (la·ring"go·ste·no'sis) *n.* [*laryngo-* + *stenosis*]. Contraction or stricture of the larynx.

lar·yn·gos·to·my (lăr"ing·gos'tuh·mee) *n.* [*laryngo-* + *-stomy*]. The establishing of a permanent opening into the larynx through the neck.

la·ryn·go·stro·bo·scope (la·ring"go·stro'buh·scope) *n.* [*laryngo-* + *stroboscope*]. A laryngoscope combined with an adjustable intermittent source of illumination, used in the observation of the vocal folds. —**laryngo·stro·bos·copy** (·stro·bos'kuh·pee) *n.*

la·ryn·go·tome (la·ring'go·tome) *n.* [*laryngo-* + *-tome*]. A cutting instrument used in laryngotomy.

lar·yn·got·o·my (lăr"ing·got'uh·mee) *n.* [*laryngo-* + *-tomy*]. The operation of incising the larynx.

la·ryn·go·tra·che·al (la·ring"go·tray'kee·ul) *adj.* [*laryngo-* + *tracheal*]. Pertaining conjointly to the larynx and the trachea.

laryngotracheal groove. A gutterlike groove of the floor of the embryonic pharynx, which is the anlage of the respiratory system.

la·ryn·go·tra·che·i·tis (la·ring"go·tray"kee·eye'tis) *n.* [*laryngo-* + *trachea* + *-itis*]. Inflammation of the larynx and the trachea.

la·ryn·go·tra·cheo·bron·chi·tis (la·ring"go·tray"kee·o·brong·kigh'tis) *n.* [*laryngo-* + *tracheo-* + *bronch-* + *-itis*]. Acute inflammation of the mucosa of the larynx, trachea, and bronchi. See also *croup.*

la·ryn·go·tra·che·os·co·py (la·ring"go·tray"kee·os'kuh·pee) *n.* [*laryngo-* + *tracheo-* + *-scopy*]. Laryngoscopy combined with tracheoscopy.

la·ryn·go·tra·che·ot·o·my (la·ring"go·tray"kee·ot'uh·mee) *n.* [*laryngo-* + *tracheo-* + *-tomy*]. Incision of the larynx and trachea.

la·ryn·go·xe·ro·sis (la·ring"go·ze·ro'sis) *n.* [*laryngo-* + *xerosis*]. Dryness of the larynx or throat.

lar·ynx (lăr'inks) *n.*, genit. **la·rin·gis** (la·rin'jis), pl. **larynxes, la·ryn·ges** (la·rin'jeez) [NL., from Gk.] [NA]. The organ of the voice, situated between the trachea and the base of the tongue. It consists of a series of cartilages: the thyroid, the cricoid, and the epiglottis, and three pairs of cartilages: the arytenoid, corniculate, and cuneiform, all of which are lined by mucous membrane and are moved by the muscles of the larynx. The mucous membrane is, on each side, thrown into two transverse folds that constitute the vocal bands or folds, the upper being the false, the lower the true, vocal folds. See also Plate 12.

la·sal·o·cid (la·sal'·o·sid) *n.* A complex ester of 2,3-cresotic acid, $C_{34}H_{54}O_8$, a coccidiostat used in veterinary medicine.

las·civ·ia (la·siv'ee·uh) *n.* [L., wantonness, from *lascivus*, wanton]. EROTOMANIA.

las·civ·i·ous (la·siv'ee·us) *adj.* [*lascivia* + *-ous*]. Wanton; having an unlawful desire; lustful.

La·sègue's law (lah·seg') [E. C. *Lasègue*, French physician, 1816–1883]. Reflexes are increased in functional illness, decreased in organic disease.

Lasègue's sign [E. C. *Lasègue*]. A sign elicited in patients with low back pain and sciatica. With the patient supine, the entire lower extremity is raised gently keeping the knee in full extension. The sign becomes positive at whatever angle of elevation pain or muscle spasm is produced, resulting in limitation of movement.

la·ser (lay'zur) *n.* [*l*ight *a*mplification by *s*timulated *e*mission of *r*adiation]. An operating assembly for utilizing the property of certain molecules to emit essentially monochromatic radiation when stimulated with radiation of optical frequencies (near ultraviolet, visible, and infrared). The emitted radiation may be produced as a directional beam of great power, which has been used as a surgical tool, and in research. Syn. *optical maser.*

lash, *n.* 1. EYELASH. 2. FLAGELLUM.

Lash·met and New·burgh's test. A concentration test for kidney function based upon the specific gravity of urine voided during the day with the patient on a special diet with no fluids.

Lasix. Trademark for furosemide, a diuretic drug.

Las·kow·ski method. A method for isolation of nuclei of avian erythrocytes, based on hemolysis of cells by lysolecithin and isolation of nuclei by differential centrifugation.

Las·sa fever [after *Lassa*, Nigeria]. A disease caused by Lassa virus, characterized by high fever, headache, myalgia, ulcerative pharyngitis, hemorrhagic signs, and renal and cardiac failure.

Las·saigne test. A test for organic nitrogen in which the organic compound containing nitrogen is fused with sodium to form sodium cyanide. This, when heated with ferrous sulfate in alkaline solution, forms sodium ferrocyanide. The sodium ferrocyanide reacts with ferric iron, to form the blue ferric ferrocyanide.

Lassa virus. A highly infectious, virulent, and pathogenic arenavirus, antigenically related to the virus of lymphocytic choriomeningitis and to some South American hemorrhagic fevers. Believed to be spherical, with a lipid envelope and having ribonucleic acid as its genetic material. See also *Lassa fever.*

Las·sar's paste [O. *Lassar*, German dermatologist, 1849–1907]. A paste containing zinc oxide, starch, and salicylic acid, dispersed in white petrolatum, used in dermatologic practice.

las·si·tude (las'i·tewd) *n.* [L. *lassitudo*, from *lassus*, weary]. A state of exhaustion or weakness; debility.

la·ta, la·tah (lah'tuh) *n.* [Malay]. An abnormal behavior pattern among the Malays and other peoples, more common in females, usually provoked by a startle, fright, or being tickled, characterized by imitative behavior and coprolalia.

late arsphenamine jaundice. SERUM HEPATITIS.

late erythroblast. An erythroblast characterized by a less vesicular and smaller nucleus, absence of nucleoli, and incipient cytoplasmic polychromatophilia indicating beginning hemoglobin synthesis. It is generally smaller than the basophilic normoblast but larger than the normoblast. See also *normoblast.*

late infantile acid maltase deficiency. A form of glycogenosis, caused by deficit of the enzyme α-1,4-glucosidase, clinically manifested later in infancy than Pompe's disease, and like it exhibiting progressive muscle weakness but neither cardiac or visceral symptoms.

late infantile amaurotic familial idiocy. BIELSCHOWSKY-JANSKÝ DISEASE.

late juvenile amaurotic familial idiocy. KUFS' DISEASE.

la·ten·cy (lay'tun·see) *n.* 1. The state or quality of being latent. 2. *In psychoanalytic theory*, the phase between the oedipal period and adolescence, lasting approximately 5 to 7 years, and characterized by an apparent cessation in psychosexual development. 3. LATENT PERIOD (1, 2).

la·tent (lay'tunt) *adj.* [L. *latens*, concealed, hidden]. Not manifest; dormant; potential.

latent content. *In psychiatry*, the hidden unconscious meaning of thoughts or actions, especially in dreams and fantasies, where such meaning appears in condensed, disguised, and symbolic form. Contr. *manifest content.*

latent energy. POTENTIAL ENERGY.

latent gout. Hyperuricemia without gouty symptoms.

latent heat. The quantity of heat necessary to convert a body into another state without changing its temperature.

latent homosexuality. *In psychiatry*, an erotic desire for a member of the same sex, present in the unconscious but not felt or expressed overtly.

latent hyperopia. The part of the total hyperopia which

cannot be overcome by the accommodation, or the difference between the manifest and the total hyperopia, detected only after using a cycloplegic. Symbol, Hl.

la·ten·ti·a·tion (lay·ten″shee·ay′shun) *n.* The chemical modification of an active drug to form a new compound or precursor, which upon enzymatic or other action in vivo will liberate or form the parent compound, for the purpose of delaying the action or prolonging the effect of the parent drug or avoiding any local reaction or unpleasant taste it may produce.

latent jaundice. Hyperbilirubinemia of insufficient degree to show jaundice clinically.

latent microbism. The presence in the body of inactive organisms awaiting favorable conditions to become active.

latent neurosyphilis. ASYMPTOMATIC NEUROSYPHILIS.

latent nystagmus. Nystagmus which appears only or is markedly increased when one eye is covered.

latent period. 1. Any stage of an infectious disease in which there are no clinical signs of symptoms of the infection. 2. *In physiology,* the period of time which elapses between the introduction of a stimulus and the response to it. Syn. *inertia time.* 3. *In radiology,* the elapsed time between the exposure to radiation and the appearance of morphologic or physiologic effects.

latent schizophrenia. A form of mental disorder in which there are definite symptoms of schizophrenia, but because of the absence of a history of a psychotic schizophrenic episode, the disorder is regarded as incipient, prepsychotic, pseudoneurotic, pseudopsychopathic, or borderline.

latent stimulus. *In psychiatry,* the unconscious basis for a symptom or a behavioral manifestation such as the unconscious conflict which underlies the formation of a phobia. Contr. *manifest stimulus.*

latent syphilis. Absence of clinical manifestations in syphilis as after spontaneous healing of primary and secondary lesions; the existence of the disease is recognized only by serologic tests.

latent tuberculosis. Tuberculosis which is quiescent.

latent zone. The part of the cerebral cortex in which a lesion produces no recognized symptoms.

lat·er·ad (lat′ur·ad) *adv.* [L. *latus, lateris,* side, + *-ad,* toward]. Toward the lateral aspect.

lat·er·al (lat′ur·ul) *adj.* [L. *lateralis,* from *latus,* side]. 1. At, belonging to, or pertaining to the side; situated on either side of the median vertical plane. 2. External, as opposed to medial (internal), away from the midline of the body.

lateral aberration. Deviation of a ray in any direction from the axis, measured in the focal plane perpendicularly to the axis.

lateral aneurysm. An aneurysm projecting on one side of a vessel, the rest of the circumference being intact.

lateral angle of the eye. The angle formed at the lateral junction of the eyelids. Syn. *outer canthus.* NA *angulus oculi lateralis.*

lateral angle of the scapula. The angle formed by the junction of the lateral and superior margins of the scapula, including the portion forming the head of the scapula and the glenoid cavity. NA *angulus lateralis scapulae.*

lateral aperture of the fourth ventricle. The aperture at the tip of each of the lateral recesses of the fourth ventricle, through which cerebrospinal fluid passes into the subarachnoid space. Syn. *foramen of Luschka.* NA *apertura lateralis ventriculi quarti.*

lateral arcuate ligament. A thick band of fascia extending from the tip of the transverse process of the second lumbar vertebra to the twelfth rib. NA *ligamentum arcuatum laterale.* See also *lumbocostal arch.*

lateral atlantoaxial joint. Either of the two lateral joints between the atlas and the axis. NA *articulatio atlantoaxialis lateralis.* See also Table of Synovial Joints and Ligaments in the Appendix.

lateral atlantooccipital ligament. A thickened lateral portion of the atlantooccipital joint capsule analogous to an intertransverse ligament in the vertebral column; passes obliquely mediad and upward from the transverse process of the atlas to the jugular process of the occipital bone. NA *ligamentum atlantooccipitalis lateralis.*

lateral central nucleus of the thalamus. One of the intralaminar nuclei of the thalamus, located dorsally in the internal medullary lamina.

lateral cerebellar syndrome. HEMISPHERE SYNDROME.

lateral cerebral peduncular sulcus. A longitudinal furrow on the lateral surface of each cerebral peduncle separating it from the tegmentum dorsally. Syn. *lateral mesencephalic sulcus.*

lateral cerebral sulcus. A deep fissure of the brain, beginning on the outer side of the anterior perforated space, and extending outward to the lateral surface of the hemisphere. It has two branches, a short vertical and a long horizontal, the latter separating the temporal from the frontal and parietal lobes. NA *sulcus lateralis cerebri.* See also Plate 18.

lateral chain ganglion. Any ganglion of the sympathetic trunk.

lateral check ligament. A thickening of the orbital fascia running from the insertion of the lateral rectus muscle to the lateral orbital wall.

lateral column. A division of the longitudinal columns of gray matter in the spinal cord. NA *columna lateralis medullae spinalis.*

lateral cornu. CORNU LATERALE MEDULLAE SPINALIS.

lateral corticospinal tract. The fibers of the corticospinal tract that run in the dorsolateral zone of the spinal cord. Most of these fibers originate in the contralateral motor cortex and decussate in the medulla; a smaller number originate in the ipsilateral motor cortex. NA *tractus corticospinalis lateralis, tractus pyramidalis lateralis.*

lateral costotransverse ligament. A short, strong ligament which connects the nonarticular surface of the tubercle of a rib to the tip of the corresponding transverse process. NA *ligamentum costotransversarium laterale.*

lateral cuneate nucleus. ACCESSORY CUNEATE NUCLEUS.

lateral curvature. SCOLIOSIS.

lateral decubitus. 1. A position employed in radiography, with the patient lying on his side on a table and the x-ray beam directed through the patient parallel to the tabletop and perpendicular to the x-ray film. Described as left lateral decubitus when patient's left side is down, and as right lateral decubitus when patient's right side is down. 2. A position also used in lumbar puncture.

lateral excursion. The sideways movement of the mandible causing the inclined planes of the opposing teeth to glide upon each other.

lateral fillet. LATERAL LEMNISCUS.

lateral fistula of the neck. A congenital fistula opening lateral to the midline, anywhere from the mandible to the sternum, and communicating with the pharynx, a cyst, a fetal rest, or a duct; due to faulty closure of pharyngeal pouches or the thymopharyngeal duct, or to other developmental defects.

lateral fontanels. The anterolateral and posterolateral fontanels.

lateral ganglion. 1. In fishes and certain amphibians, a ganglion associated with cranial nerve VII and another with X, whose postganglionic fibers supply the lateral line organs. 2. *In comparative anatomy,* a ganglion of the sympathetic trunk.

lateral geniculate body. A flattened area in the posterolateral surface of the thalamus containing nerve cells which receive impulses from the retinas and relay them to the occipital cortex via the geniculocalcarine tracts. NA *corpus geniculatum laterale.*

lateral glossoepiglottic fold. A fold of mucous membrane extending from the side of the base of the tongue to the lateral margin of the epiglottis; there is a right and a left one. NA *plica glossoepiglottica lateralis.*

lateral hemianopsia. HOMONYMOUS HEMIANOPSIA.

lateral hermaphroditism. The form of human hermaphroditism in which there is an ovary on one side and a testis on the other. Syn. *alternating hermaphroditism.*

lateral hernia. INDIRECT HERNIA.

lateral horn. The lateral column of gray matter as seen in a cross section of the spinal cord. NA *cornu laterale medullae spinalis.*

lateral hypothalamic nucleus. A group of cells located in the lateral part of the middle region of the hypothalamus.

lateral inguinal fossa. A slight depression of the peritoneum lateral to the lateral umbilical fold.

lateral inguinal fovea. LATERAL INGUINAL FOSSA.

lateral intercondylar tubercle. The spine on the lateral side of the intercondylar eminence of the tibia. NA *tuberculum intercondylare laterale.*

lat·er·al·i·ty (lat″ur·al′i·tee) *n.* Functional predominance of one side of an anatomically bilateral structure, such as greater proficiency in the use of one side of the body or language-related dominance of one cerebral hemisphere. See also *dextrality, sinistrality.*

lat·er·al·iza·tion (lat″ur·ul·i·zay′shun) *n.* Localization on one side of the body, as in one of the cerebral hemispheres. —**lat·er·al·ize** (lat′ur·ul·ize) *v.*

lateral lemniscus. The secondary auditory pathway arising in the cochlear nuclei and terminating in the inferior colliculus and medial geniculate body; it crosses in the trapezoid body. NA *lemniscus lateralis.*

lateral ligament of the malleus. A short, thick band connecting the typanic notch and the neck of the malleus. NA *ligamentum mallei laterale.*

lateral ligament of the temporomandibular joint. A strong ligament on the lateral side of the temporomandibular joint, passing anterosuperiorly from the condylar process of the mandible to the zygomatic process of the temporal bone. NA *ligamentum laterale.*

lateral lingual swelling. One of the paired swellings of the floor of the first visceral arch that form the primordia of the oral part of the tongue.

lateral longitudinal arch. NA *pars lateralis arcus pedis longitudinalis.* See *longitudinal arch of the foot.*

lateral longitudinal stria. The lateral of two long bundles of fibers on the upper surface of the corpus callosum. NA *stria longitudinalis lateralis corporis callosi.*

lateral lumbocostal arch. LATERAL ARCUATE LIGAMENT.

lateral malleolus. The distal end of the fibula. Syn. *external malleolus.* NA *malleolus lateralis.* See also Plate 1.

lateral mamillary nucleus. A nucleus in the mamillary body, ventrolateral to the intercalated mamillary nucleus.

lateral medullary syndrome. WALLENBERG'S SYNDROME.

lateral meniscus. The articular disk in the knee joint between the lateral condyles of the tibia and femur; a crescentic, nearly circular fibrocartilaginous disk attached to the margin of the lateral condyle of the tibia, resting on and serving to deepen the tibia's lateral articular surface. Syn. *external semilunar cartilage.* NA *meniscus lateralis.*

lateral mesencephalic sulcus. LATERAL CEREBRAL PEDUNCULAR SULCUS.

lateral mesoderm. The mesoderm lateral to the intermediate mesoderm. After formation of the coelom, it is separated into the somatic and the splanchnic mesoderm.

lateral midpalmar space. A deep fascial space on the radial side of the palm; thenar space.

lateral nasal cartilage. The upper lateral cartilage of the nose. An extension on either side of the cartilage of the nasal septum. NA *cartilago nasi lateralis.*

lateral nasal process. The embryonic process bounding the lateral margin of the olfactory pit that forms a side and wing of the nose.

lateral nuclei of the thalamus. The nuclei lying between the internal medullary lamina and the internal capsule. NA *nuclei laterales thalami.*

lateral nystagmus. Horizontal nystagmus that appears on right or left lateral gaze.

lateral occipital gyri. Convolutions on the lower lateral surface of the occipital lobe of the cerebrum. Contr. *superior occipital gyri.*

lateral occipital sulcus. The longitudinal groove dividing the lateral surface of the occipital lobe into a superior and an inferior gyrus. See also Plate 18.

lateral palatine process. PALATINE PROCESS (1).

lateral palpebral artery. NA (pl.) *arteriae palpebrales laterales.* See *palpebral artery.*

lateral phallic groove. A groove on either side of the phallus, separating it from the labioscrotal swellings.

lateral pharyngeal fossa. PHARYNGEAL RECESS.

lateral pharyngotomy. An external incision entering one side of the pharynx.

lateral plate. Either of the thickened side walls of the neural tube.

lateral process of the malleus. A slight projection from the root of the manubrium of the malleus, lying in contact with the tympanic membrane. NA *processus lateralis mallei.*

lateral process of the talus. A process passing downward and laterally from the lateral surface of the talar bone. NA *processus lateralis tali.*

lateral pterygoid plate or **lamina.** A broad, thin process whose lateral surface forms part of the medial wall of the infratemporal fossa and gives attachment to the lateral pterygoid muscle, and whose medial surface forms part of the pterygoid fossa and gives attachment to the medial pterygoid muscle. NA *lamina lateralis processus pterygoidei.*

lateral recess. The lateral extension of the fourth ventricle in the angle between the cerebellum and the medulla oblongata. NA *recessus lateralis ventriculi quarti.*

lateral rectus. An extrinsic muscle of the eye. See *rectus lateralis bulbi* in Table of Muscles in the Appendix.

lateral region of the abdomen. The right or left abdominal region on either side of the umbilical region. NA *regio lateralis abdominis [dextra et sinistra].* See also *abdominal regions.*

lateral reticular nucleus. A nucleus, in the ventrolateral part of the reticular formation of the medulla, which receives spinoreticular fibers from the dorsal gray columns of the spinal cord and perhaps also collaterals from the spinothalamic tract. Its axons project to specific portions of the cerebellum via the ipsilateral inferior cerebellar peduncle.

lateral root abscess. An alveolar abscess originating along a lateral surface of the root of the tooth, usually the result of periodontal disease.

lateral sclerosis. See *amyotrophic lateral sclerosis, primary lateral sclerosis.*

lateral sinus. The sinus of the dura mater running from the internal occipital protuberance, following for part of its course the attached margin of the tentorium cerebelli, then over the jugular process of the occipital bone to reach the jugular foramen. Syn. *transverse sinus.* NA *sinus transversus durae matris.*

lateral spinothalamic tract. A tract of nerve fibers which arise from cells of the posterior horn of spinal gray matter, cross in the anterior white commissure, ascend in the lateral funiculus, and terminate in the posterior nuclei of the thalamus; it conducts mainly pain and temperature impulses. NA *tractus spinothalamicus lateralis.*

lateral sympathetic nucleus. Cells of the intermediolateral cell column of the spinal cord, extending from the first thoracic to the second lumbar segment. NA *nucleus intermediolateralis, nucleus lateralis medullae spinalis.*

lateral sympathetic veins. SUPRACARDINAL VEINS.

lateral tarsometatarsal articulation. CUBOIDEOMETATARSAL ARTICULATION.

lateral thrombus. 1. PARIETAL THROMBUS. 2. MURAL THROMBUS.

lateral thyrohyoid ligament. The dorsal margin of the thyrohyoid membrane on either side. NA *ligamentum thyrohyoideum.*

lateral thyroids. ULTIMOBRANCHIAL BODIES.

lateral umbilical fold. A fold of peritoneum covering the inferior epigastric vessels. NA *plica umbilicalis laterale.*

lateral umbilical ligament. MEDIAL UMBILICAL LIGAMENT.

lateral ventral nucleus of the thalamus. One of the nuclei of the ventral division of the lateral nuclei of the thalamus which receives fibers from the pallidum and the superior cerebellar peduncle and sends fibers to the motor cortex and premotor cortex of the frontal lobe.

lateral ventricle. The cavity of either cerebral hemisphere communicating with the third ventricle through the interventricular foramen, and consisting of a triangular central cavity or body and three smaller cavities or cornua. NA *ventriculus lateralis.* See also Plates 10, 17.

lateral vestibular nucleus. One of four vestibular nuclei, consisting of large cells at the caudal border of the pons between the inferior cerebellar peduncle and the spinal tract of the trigeminal nerve. Syn. *Deiter's nucleus.* NA *nucleus vestibularis lateralis.*

lat·er·i·ceous (lat″ur·ish′us) *adj.* LATERITIOUS.

late rickets. OSTEOMALACIA. See also *vitamin D-refractory rickets.*

lat·er·i·tious (lat″ur·ish′us) *adj.* [L. *lateritius,* made of brick, from *later,* brick]. Resembling brick dust, as the lateritious sediment of the urine.

lat·er·i·ver·sion (lat″ur·i·vur′zhun) *n.* LATEROVERSION.

latero-. A combining form meaning *lateral.*

lat·ero·ab·dom·i·nal (lat″ur·o·ab·dom′i·nul) *adj.* Pertaining to either lateral portion of the abdomen.

lateroabdominal position. SIM'S POSITION.

lat·ero·duc·tion (lat″ur·o·duck′shun) *n.* [*latero-* + L. *ducere,* to lead]. Lateral movement, as of the eye.

lat·ero·flex·ion (lat″ur·o·fleck′shun) *n.* Lateral flexion, as the alteration in position of the uterus in which the uterine axis is bent upon itself to one side.

lat·ero·mar·gin·al (lat″ur·o·mahr′ji·nul) *adj.* [*latero-* + *marginal*]. Situated on the lateral edge.

lat·ero·pul·sion (lat″ur·o·pul′shun) *n.* [*latero-* + *pulsion*]. An involuntary tendency to move to one side in forward locomotion.

lat·ero·tor·sion (lat″ur·o·tor′shun) *n.* [*latero-* + *torsion*]. A twisting to one side.

lat·ero·ver·sion (lat″ur·o·vur′zhun) *n.* Lateral version, as the alteration in position of the uterus in which the entire uterine axis is displaced to one side.

late syphilis. Stages of infection occurring after secondary syphilis, and including asymptomatic and symptomatic neurosyphilis, cardiovascular syphilis, and gumma.

la·tex (lay′tecks) *n.,* pl. **lat·i·ces** (lat′i·seez), **latexes** [L., liquid]. The milky juice of certain plants and trees. Rubber and gutta-percha are commercial products of latex.

latex cells. Cells giving rise to latex or milky juice.

lath·y·rism (lath′i·riz·um) *n.* 1. An affection attributed to the ingestion of the peas or meal from varieties of the chickpea, chiefly *Lathyrus sativus* and toxins derived from the common vetch, *Vicia sativa,* characterized by spastic paraplegia with tremor, hyperreflexia, and Babinski responses, but normal sensation. 2. A disease produced by feeding experimental animals extracts of *Lathyrus odoratus* seeds, or more commonly, beta-aminopropionitrile; it is characterized in rats by gross bony deformity of the limb epiphyses and vertebrae, hind limb paresis, aortic medial hemorrhage and, in some cases, hernias.

lath·y·ro·gen·ic (lath″i·ro·jen′ick) *adj.* Producing lathyrism.

la·tis·si·mo·con·dy·la·ris (la·tis″i·mo·kon·di·lair′is) *n.* DORSOEPITROCHLEARIS.

la·tis·si·mus (la·tis′i·mus) *adj.* [L., superlative of *latus,* wide]. Widest.

latissimus dor·si (dor′sigh). The widest muscle of the back. NA *musculus latissimus dorsi.* See also Table of Muscles in the Appendix.

latissimus tho·ra·cis (tho·ray′sis). LATISSIMUS DORSI.

la·trine (la·treen′) *n.* [F., from L. *latrina*]. A water closet or other place for urination or defecation, especially any of a number of types used in military installations, permanent or temporary.

latrine fly. *FANNIA.*

Lat·ro·dec·tus (lat′ro·deck′tus) *n.* A genus of spiders of the family Theridiidae, of which the females are sedentary in webs, have globose abdomens, and a bite poisonous to man. Excepting the more northerly parts of Europe, Asia, and North America, species are found in most parts of the inhabited world, including almost all of the contiguous United States. The most dangerous species is *Latrodectus mactans,* the black widow. See also *black widow.*

LATS Abbreviation for *long-acting thyroid stimulator.*

lat·tice (lat′is) *n.* [OF. *lattis,* from *latte,* lath]. 1. A network or framework, as of fibers or filaments; a reticulum. 2. *In physics,* the structural pattern of ions or molecules in a crystal.

lattice corneal dystrophy. A type of primary localized amyloidosis inherited as an autosomal dominant trait, clinically manifest as progressive corneal opacities which include a filamentous branching network rarely associated with systemic amyloidosis.

lattice fibers. RETICULAR FIBERS.

lattice keratitis. LATTICE CORNEAL DYSTROPHY.

la·tus (lay′tus, lat′us) *n.* [L.] [NA]. FLANK.

Lau·bry-Soulle syndrome (lo·bree′, sool). Abnormal accumulations of gas in the splenic flexure of the colon and in the stomach of patients with three-to-four-day-old myocardial infarcts, accompanied by chest and abdominal pain.

laud·able (law′duh·bul) *adj.* [L. *laudabilis,* from *laudare,* to praise]. Healthy; formerly used to describe thick, copious pus thought to indicate an improved condition of a wound.

lau·dan·i·dine (law·dan′i·deen) *n.* *l*-Laudanine, $C_{20}H_{25}NO_4$, an alkaloid from opium.

lau·da·nine (law′duh·neen, ·nin) *n.* *dl*-Laudanine, $C_{20}H_{25}NO_4$, an alkaloid from opium.

lau·dan·o·sine (law·dan′o·seen, ·sin) *n.* *l-N*-Methyltetrahydropapaverine, $C_{21}H_{27}NO_4$, an alkaloid from opium.

lau·da·num (law′duh·num) *n.* A tincture of opium.

laughing disease. KURU.

laughing epilepsy. GELASTIC EPILEPSY.

laughing gas. NITROUS OXIDE.

Laugh·len test [G. F. *Laughlen,* Canadian pathologist, b. 1888]. A flocculation test for syphilis.

laugh·ter, *n.* A succession of rhythmic, spasmodic expirations with open glottis and vibration of the vocal folds normally expressing mirth, but also a response to tickling, or a manifestation of pseudobulbar palsy or rarely of epilepsy.

laundryman's itch. TINEA CRURIS.

laur-, lauro-. In chemistry, a combining form meaning *lauric acid.*

lau·re·ate (law′ree·ut, lor′ee·ut) *n.* [L. *laureatus,* crowned with laurel]. A recipient of an award or honor; a prizewinner.

Laurence-Moon-Biedl syndrome [J. Z. *Laurence,* English ophthalmological surgeon, 1829–1870; R C. *Moon,* U.S. ophthalmologist, 1844–1914; and A. *Biedl,* Czechoslovakian physician, 1869–1933]. A heredodegenerative disease probably due to recessive mutations of two genes in the same chromosome, and more frequent in males; characterized by girdle-type obesity, hypogenitalism, mental retardation, polydactyly, skull deformations, pigmentary retinal degeneration, and generally a shortened life-span.

lau·reth-9 (law'reth) *n.* A mixture of polyethylene glycol monodecyl ethers of the average formula, $C_{30}H_{62}O_{10}$, a surfactant employed as a spermaticide.

lau·ric acid (law'rick). Dodecanoic acid, $CH_3(CH_2)_{10}COOH$, a fatty acid from the glycerides of laurel oil, coconut oil, and other fats.

lauro-. See *laur-*.

lau·rus (law'rus) *n.* The leaves of *Laurus nobilis* (bay laurel) containing cineole, *l*-linalool, geraniol, eugenol, etc; used as a spice.

lau·ryl (law'ril) *n.* The univalent radical $C_{12}H_{25}$— present in lauric acid.

Lauth's violet [C. *Lauth,* English chemist, 1836–1913]. THIONINE.

la·vage (lah·vahzh, lav'ij) *n.* [F., washing, from *laver,* to wash]. The irrigation or washing out of an organ, such as the stomach, bowel, urinary bladder, or paranasal sinus.

la·va·tion (la·vay'shun) *n.* [L. *lavatio,* from *lavare,* to wash]. LAVAGE; ablution.

lav·en·der, *n.* [ML. *lavendula*]. The flowers of *Lavandula officinalis;* formerly used as an aromatic stimulant.

lavender oil. The volatile oil distilled from the fresh flowering tops of *Lavandula officinalis;* contains linalyl acetate. Used chiefly as a perfume.

La·ve·ran's bodies (lav·rahn') [C. L. A. *Laveran,* French physician, 1845–1922]. Malarial parasites in erythrocytes.

Lavrentiev's phenomenon. MULTIPLICATION PHENOMENON OF LAVRENTIEV.

law, *n.* 1. Statement of a relation or sequence of phenomena invariable under the same conditions. 2. A rule of conduct prescribed by authority.

law of Avogadro [A. *Avogadro*]. Equal volumes of gases at the same pressure contain equal numbers of molecules.

law of Bunsen-Roscoe [R. W. E. von *Bunsen;* and H. E. *Roscoe,* English chemist, 1833–1915]. The time required for a reaction to light is inversely proportional to the intensity of the light.

law of definite proportions. Any chemical compound is formed always by the same elements in the same proportion by weight.

law of Dulong and Petit [P. L. *Dulong* and A. T. *Petit*]. The specific heat of an element varies inversely as its atomic weight.

law of filial regression. Children whose parents deviate from the average of the population likewise deviate from the average in the same direction as the parents, but regress by about one-third of the parental deviation toward the mean. For example, children whose parents are 3 inches above the average stature are themselves on the average about 2 inches above the mean stature of the population. Syn. *Galton's law of filial regression.*

law of independent assortment. The members of different gene-pairs segregate at meiosis independently of one another. See also *Mendel's laws.*

law of inverse squares. For point sources of radiant energy, the intensity of the radiation at any point varies inversely as the square of the distance from the point source.

law of Lambert. LAMBERT'S LAW.

law of Laplace (lah·plahss') [P. S. *Laplace,* French physicist, 1749-1827]. A law of fluid mechanics which, as applied to blood flow, states that the wall tension of a blood vessel is directly proportional to its radius and inversely proportional to its thickness. Syn. *Laplace's law.*

law of mass action. The speed of a chemical reaction is proportional to the active masses of the reacting substances. Syn. *Guldberg-Waage law.*

law of multiple proportions. If more than one compound is formed by two elements, the weight of one of the elements remains constant, that of the other element varies as a multiple of the lowest amount of that element in the series of compounds.

law of parsimony. Economy in the use of a specific means to an end.

law of progress. The nervous system has been the dominant factor in evolution. Syn. *Gaskell's law of progress.*

law of reciprocal proportions. Two elements, which unite with each other, will unite singly with a third element in proportions which are the same as, or multiples of, the proportions in which they unite with each other.

law of refraction. *In optics,* a ray of light passing from a rarer to a denser medium is turned toward a perpendicular to the interface and in passing from a denser to a rarer medium it is turned away from that perpendicular.

law of refreshment. The rate of recovery of muscle from fatigue is proportional to its blood supply.

law of segregation. The two members of any given pair of genes separate at meiosis so that a mature germ cell receives one or the other member of each pair of genes. See also *Mendel's laws.*

law of similars. *In homeopathy,* the rule *similia similibus curantur,* like cures like.

law of small numbers. POISSON DISTRIBUTION.

law of specific energy. MÜLLER'S LAW.

law of specific irritability. Every sensory nerve reacts to one form of stimulus and gives rise to one form of sensation. If under abnormal circumstances it is stimulated by other forms of excitation, the sensation produced is the same.

law of specificity of bacteria. KOCH'S LAW.

law of the eccentric situation of the long tracts. FLATAU'S LAW.

law of the heart. FRANK-STARLING LAW OF THE HEART.

law of the intestines. A stimulus applied to a given point in the intestinal wall initiates a band of constriction on the proximal side and relaxation on the distal side of the stimulated point.

law of universal affect. *In psychology,* the premise that every idea, thought, or object, no matter how apparently minor or neutral, possesses a distinct quantum of affect.

law of wallerian degeneration. WALLERIAN LAW.

Leeu·wen·hoek's disease (ley'wen·hook) *n.* [A. van *Leeuwenhoek,* Dutch scientist, 1632–1723]. DIAPHRAGMATIC TIC.

Law position. LAW'S PROJECTION.

Law's projection [F. M. *Law*]. A radiographic view of the temporal bone with the beam angled 15 degrees anteriorly and 15 degrees caudally to obtain a lateral radiograph of one mastoid without overlap of the other.

lax·a·tion (lack·say'shun) *n.* DEFECATION.

lax·a·tive (lack'suh·tiv) *adj. & n.* [L. *laxare,* to lighten, relieve]. 1. Relieving constipation; causing evacuation of the bowels. 2. An agent employed for its laxative properties; a cathartic of the least potent category. Contr. *purgative.*

lax·i·ty (lack'si·tee) *n.* [L. *laxitas,* roominess]. 1. Absence or loss of tone, tension, or firmness. 2. Lack of strictness or precision. —**lax,** *adj.*

lay, *adj.* [OF. *lai,* from L. *laicus,* from Gk. *laikos*]. Nonprofessional.

lay·er, *n.* A deposited material of uniform or nearly uniform thickness, spread over a comparatively considerable area; cover. Syn. *stratum.*

layer of fusiform cells. The deepest layer of the cerebral cortex, with irregular fusiform and angular cells, whose axons enter the subjacent white matter. Syn. *multiform layer.*

layer of Henle [F. G. H. *Henle*]. The outermost layer of the internal root sheath of hair.

layer of Langhans [T. *Langhans*]. CYTOTROPHOBLAST.

layer of pyramidal cells. The third layer of the cerebral cortex, having a superficial stratum containing chiefly medium-sized pyramidal cells and a deeper stratum containing large pyramidal cells. Syn. *external pyramidal layer.*

layer of rods and cones. The neuroepithelial layer of the retina. NA *stratum neuroepitheliale retinae.* See also *retina.*

layer of small pyramidal cells. The external granular layer of the cerebrum. See *external granular layer.*

lay·ette (lay·et') *n.* [F., from OF. *laie,* box, drawer]. A full outfit of garments and bedding for a newborn child.

lay·man, *n.* A member of the laity; a person not a member of a given professional group, as distinguished from a member of the group.

laz·ar (laz'ur) *n.* [L. *Lazarus,* a beggar mentioned in the Gospel of Luke]. A patient with leprosy, or any person having a repulsive disease.

laz·a·ret, laz·a·rette (laz"uh·ret', laz'uh·ret) *n.* LAZARETTO.

laz·a·ret·to (laz"uh·ret'o) *n.* [It., from *lazzaro,* leper]. 1. A public hospital for the care of persons suffering from contagious diseases, especially lepers; a pesthouse. 2. A building or vessel used for quarantine.

laz·a·rine leprosy (laz'uh·rine, ·reen) [*lazar* + *-ine*]. A form of lepromatous leprosy marked by continuous ulceration and resultant scarring.

Lazarow method. A method for isolation of lipoprotein and glycogen particles from liver cells, based on centrifugation. The resulting red precipitate, containing lipoprotein and glycogen, is treated with diastase to obtain pure lipoprotein.

℔. Abbreviation for *libra,* pound.

£. Symbol for *libra,* pound (usually apothecaries').

L band. PSEUDO H ZONE.

LBBB. Left bundle branch block.

L.C.L. bodies [*L*eventhal, *C*ole, and *L*illie]. Clusters of minute spherical or coccoid elementary inclusion bodies found within reticuloendothelial cells and in body fluids of birds and humans infected with psittacosis (ornithosis).

LD Abbreviation for (a) *lethal dose;* (b) *light difference.*

LD 50, LD_{50} Symbol for median lethal dose.

LD 50 time. Symbol for median lethal time.

LD 100, LD_{100} Symbol for invariably lethal dose.

L.D.A. Abbreviation for *left dorsoanterior* position of the fetus.

L.D.H. Abbreviation for *lactic (acid) dehydrogenase.*

L.D.P. Abbreviation for *left dorsoposterior* position of the fetus.

L.E. Abbreviation for *lupus erythematosus.*

leach, *v.* To wash or extract the soluble constituents from insoluble material.

¹lead (leed) *n.* 1. A pair of terminals or electrodes or electrode arrays situated within or upon the body, each connected either directly or through resistors to a recording instrument for the purpose of measuring the difference in electrical potential between them. 2. The electrocardiogram or other recording obtained from a pair of electrodes.

²lead (led) *n.* Pb = 207.2. A soft, bluish-gray, malleable metal, occurring in nature chiefly as the sulfide, PbS, known as galena. Its soluble salts are violent irritant poisons, formerly used as local astringents. Insoluble lead salts at one time were used as protectives, but because of the danger of absorption, the therapeutic use of lead compounds has been discontinued.

lead IV. A precordial lead, in which the positive electrode placed near the cardiac apex is paired with an extremity or back electrode. Also designated as CR_4, CL_4, CF_4, or CB_4 when the right or left arm, left leg, or back, respectively, is the location of the negative electrode. See also *precordial lead.*

lead acetate. $(CH_3COO)_2Pb.3H_2O$. Occurs as white crystals. Has been used as a local astringent. Syn. *sugar of lead.*

lead anemia. Anemia resulting from lead poisoning.

lead arsenate. Approximately $PbHAsO_4$; a dense, white powder, insoluble in water, used as a constituent of insecticides.

lead arsenite. Approximately $Pb(AsO_2)_2$; a white powder, insoluble in water, used as a constituent of insecticides.

lead axis. An imaginary line through the body between the sites of attachment of the positive and negative electrodes of a lead.

Lead·bet·ter's maneuver or **procedure** [G. W. *Leadbetter,* U.S. orthopedist, 1893–1945]. A method of reduction in fracture of the femoral neck.

lead borosilicate. A mixture of the borate and silicate of lead; a constituent of certain optical glasses.

lead chromate. $PbCrO_4$; a yellow powder; used as a pigment. Syn. *chrome yellow.*

lead encephalopathy. A form of lead poisoning, occurring mainly in children, characterized by swelling of the brain, herniation of the temporal lobes and cerebellum, multiple ischemic foci, and perivascular deposition of proteinaceous material and mononuclear inflammatory cells. The clinical syndrome consists of vomiting, seizures, stupor, and coma.

lead equivalent. The thickness of lead which absorbs a specific radiation which is the same amount as the material in question.

lead·er, *n. Obsol.* 1. A sinew or tendon. 2. An inflamed lymphatic channel.

lead line. The blue line at the dental margin of the gums in chronic lead poisoning.

lead monoxide. PbO; a yellowish or reddish powder, almost insoluble in water. Has been used as an ingredient of external applications for relieving inflammation. Syn. *litharge, yellow lead oxide.*

lead orthoplumbate. Pb_2PbO_4 (or Pb_3O_4); an orange-red powder, almost insoluble in water; formerly used externally as a protective. Syn. *minium, red lead, red lead oxide.*

lead oxide. 1. LEAD MONOXIDE. 2. LEAD ORTHOPLUMBATE.

lead palsy or **paralysis.** LEAD POLYNEUROPATHY.

lead-pencil stools. Fecal discharges of very small caliber.

lead-pipe rigidity. RIGIDITY (2).

lead poisoning. Poisoning caused by prolonged ingestion or absorption of lead or lead-containing materials, manifested by colic, encephalopathy, polyneuropathy, and hemolytic anemia. See also *lead encephalopathy, lead polyneuropathy.*

lead polyneuropathy. A distal symmetrical polyneuropathy, affecting mainly the wrists and hands, seen principally in adults with chronic lead poisoning; characterized by weakness, paresthesias, pain, and less often by sensory loss.

lead subacetate solution. GOULARD'S EXTRACT.

lead tetraethyl. $Pb(C_2H_5)_4$, a colorless, flammable liquid; used as an antiknock ingredient in motor fuels. Acute or chronic poisoning may result from its inhalation.

lead water. Diluted lead subacetate solution; formerly used as a local astringent and sedative.

lead water and laudanum. A mixture of lead subacetate solution with an equal volume of opium tincture: formerly used as an external application to sprains and bruises.

leaf, *n. In anatomy,* a flat leaflike structure, as for example the right and left leaves of the diaphragm.

leak·age headache. LUMBAR PUNCTURE HEADACHE.

Leake and Guy's method. A method for counting platelets which consists of diluting the blood in order to count the platelets in a solution composed of formalin, sodium oxalate, crystal violet, and water.

Leão's spreading depression (lyaʊwⁿ) [A. A. P. *Leão,* Brazilian physiologist, b. 1914]. A marked enduring reduction of the "spontaneous" electrical activity of the cerebral cortex, following repeated local electrical, mechanical, or chemical stimulation of any area, and spreading slowly from the region stimulated to involve successively more distant parts of the cerebral cortex; also manifested by decreased cortical excitability, slow change in steady potential, and vascular dilatation.

leaping mydriasis. ALTERNATING MYDRIASIS.

learning disorder, disturbance, or **defect.** Any specific defect in the ability of a child to learn one of the basic academic disciplines, or a general defect in learning to read or write, or in learning mathematics. It is often complicated by behavior disturbances. See also *minimal brain dysfunction syndrome.*

learning-theory therapy. BEHAVIOR THERAPY.

least splanchnic nerve. A nerve that arises from the lowest thoracic ganglion and goes to the renal plexus. NA *nervus splanchnicus imus.* See also Table of Nerves in the Appendix.

least squares method. The method of finding a statistical constant or the equation of a straight line or curve in such a manner that the sum of the squares of the deviations about the mean, line, or curve is a minimum.

leather bottle stomach. LINITIS PLASTICA.

Le·ber's disease or **optic atrophy** (leʸ'bur) [T. von *Leber,* German ophthalmologist, 1840-1917]. A hereditary form of optic atrophy, characterized by loss of central vision with usually relatively well-preserved peripheral vision, occurring in young males; usually acute in onset, often preceded by transient optic neuritis, and commonly reaching its maximum within a few weeks, it rarely progresses to total blindness; it is transmitted as a sex-linked recessive through the female.

lec·a·nop·a·gus (leck''uh·nop'uh·gus) *n.*, pl. **lecanopa·gi** (·guy, ·jye) [Gk. *lekanē*, dish, basin, + *-pagus*]. Conjoined twins with union of the pelves and lower parts, and separate heads, necks and upper thoraxes.

lec·a·no·so·ma·top·a·gus (leck''uh·no·so''muh·top'uh·gus) *n.*, pl. **lecanosomatopa·gi** (·guy, ·jye) [Gk. *lekanē*, dish, basin, + *somato-* + *-pagus*]. Equal twins conjoined by the pelves and thoraxes, or by the vertebral columns; a form of dicephalism.

Le·cat's gulf (luh·kahʰ') [C. N. *Lecat,* French surgeon and anatomist, 1700-1768]. *Obsol.* A dilatation of the bulbous portion of the urethra.

L.E. cell. Abbreviation for *lupus erythematosus cell.*

L.E. cell test. Any procedure that provides optimum conditions for the formation and detection of lupus erythematosus cells.

le·che de hi·gue·rón (leʰ'chehʰ deʰ ee·geh·roʰn') [Sp.]. The crude sap (lit., milk) of the bastard fig tree, *Ficus glabrata* or *F. doliara;* used in Central and South America as an anthelmintic, especially in trichuriasis.

lech·o·py·ra (leck''o·pye'ruh, leck·op'i·ruh) *n.* [Gk. *lechō*, woman in childbed, + *pyr*, fire, fever]. PUERPERAL FEVER.

lecith-, lecitho- [Gk. *lekithos*]. A combining form meaning *yolk, lecithal.*

lec·i·thal (les'i·thul) *adj.* [*lecith-* + *-al*]. Having a yolk; used especially in combination, as alecithal and telolecithal.

lec·ith·al·bu·min (les''ith·al·bew'min) *n.* A more or less stable compound of albumin and lecithin, found in various organs.

lec·i·thin (les'i·thin) *n.* [*lecith-* + *-in*]. A phospholipid in which phosphatidic acid is esterified to choline. Syn. *phosphatidyl choline.* —**leci·thoid** (·thoid) *adj.*

lec·i·thi·nase (les'i·thi·nace, ·naze) *n.* [*lecithin* + *-ase*]. An enzyme that catalyzes the hydrolysis of a lecithin to its constituents. See also *phospholipase.*

lecithinase A. An enzyme catalyzing the removal of only one fatty acid from lecithin and yielding lysolecithin.

lecithinase B. An enzyme that catalyzes the removal of acyl groups from both the alpha and beta positions of a phospholipid.

lecithinase C. An enzyme found in many plant tissues that catalyzes the removal of the nitrogenous base of lecithin to produce the base and a phosphatidic acid.

lecithinase D. An enzyme found in the toxin of clostridia and in other bacteria, which catalyzes the removal of the phosphorylated base from lecithins, producing an α,β-diglyceride.

lecitho-. See *lecith-.*

lec·i·tho·blast (les'ith·o·blast, le·sith'o·blast) *n.* [*lecitho-* + *-blast*]. The entoblast or primitive entoderm of the bilaminar blastodisk.

lec·i·tho·pro·te·in (les''i·tho·pro'tee·in, ·teen) *n.* A compound of lecithin with a protein molecule.

lec·i·tho·vi·tel·lin (les''i·tho·vi·tel'in) *n.* [*lecitho-* + *vitellin*]. The lecithin-phosphoprotein complex as found in egg yolk.

lec·tin (leck'tin) *n.* [L. *lectus*, selected, + *-in*]. A substance occurring in seeds and other parts of certain plants which displays specific antibody-like activity toward animal cells or their components, as in specific agglutination of mammalian erythrocytes.

Led·der·hose's disease (led'ur·ho'zeʰ) [G. *Ledderhose,* German surgeon, 1855-1925]. Dupuytren's contracture involving the plantar aponeurosis.

Lederer's acute anemia [M. *Lederer,* U.S. pathologist, 1855-1952]. A form of acute acquired hemolytic anemia, occurring mostly in children, characterized by sudden onset, short duration, and spontaneous recovery; the cause may be infectious, and transfusions are required to maintain adequate hemoglobin levels.

Le·duc's current (luh·dueᵏ') [S. A. N. *Leduc,* French physicist, 1853-1939]. An interrupted, direct electric current whose pulses are of constant strength and duration; used to produce electronarcosis as long as the current is applied.

leech, *n.* Any parasitic annelid of the class Hirudinea; some leeches have been detrimental, and some have aided medically. Infestation by leeches (hirudiniasis) may be either internal or external.

leech·es, *n.pl.* Cutaneous granulomatous lesions which occur on the limbs of horses as a result of phycomycosis or cutaneous habronemiasis. So called because early horsemen thought the elongated necrotic masses within the lesions were leeches.

Lee's test. A test for rennin in gastric juice based upon its ability to coagulate the protein of milk.

Lee-White method. A test-tube method for estimating the coagulation time of whole blood.

L.E. factor. A substance occurring in the blood and other body fluids of patients with systemic lupus erythematosus and, occasionally, in other diseases. Syn. *lupus erythematosus factor, L.E.* plasma factor, L.E. serum factor.

Le Fort's operation (luh·fohr') [L. C. *Le Fort,* French surgeon, 1829-1893]. An operation for uterine prolapse; partial colpocleisis.

left anterior oblique. A position assumed by a patient for x-ray examination, with the anterior aspect of his left side closest to the film so that the x-ray beam passes diagonally through his body.

left aorta. The left primitive or dorsal aorta, especially in the aortic arch region where fusion of the aortas does not occur.

left atrioventricular valve. MITRAL VALVE.

left axis deviation or **shift.** Leftward deviation of the mean frontal plane axis of the QRS complex of the electrocardiogram less than O°; usually beyond −15 or −30° for the adult.

left-eyed, *adj.* Tending to use the left eye in preference to the right, as in looking through a monocular telescope.

left-footed, *adj.* Tending to use the left foot in preference to the right, as in hopping or kicking.

left-handed, *adj.* Having the left hand stronger or more expert than the right, or using the left hand in preference to the right.

left heart. The part of the heart which pumps blood to the systemic and coronary vessels; the left atrium and left ventricle.

left hepatic artery. The left branch of the proper hepatic artery. NA *ramus sinister arteriae hepaticae propriae.*

left lateral. A position assumed by a patient for x-ray examination, with his left side closest to the film and the x-ray beam perpendicular to the film.

left posterior oblique. A position assumed by a patient for x-ray examination, with the posterior aspect of his left side closest to the film so that x-ray beam passes diagonally through his body.

left-to-right shunt. A cardiac defect characterized by the return of oxygenated blood from the left side of the heart directly to the right side of the heart or pulmonary artery, without passage through the systemic circulation. See also *cyanotic congenital heart disease.*

left ventricle of the heart. The chamber that forces the blood through the aorta and throughout the body. NA *ventriculus sinister.* See also Plate 5.

left ventricular thrust. APEX IMPULSE.

leg, *n.* 1. *In human anatomy,* the lower extremity between the knee and the foot. NA *crus.* 2. Popularly, the lower extremity including the thigh, but usually excluding the foot.

le·gal medicine. The branch of medicine, involving any and all of its disciplines, employed by the legal authorities for the solution of legal problems. Syn. *forensic medicine.*

Leg·al's disease (ley·gahl') [E. *Legal,* German physician, 1859–1922]. Paroxysmal pain and tenderness of the scalp in the region supplied by the auriculotemporal nerve, associated with pharyngotympanic inflammation.

Legal's test [E. *Legal*]. An alkaline urine distillate containing acetone produces a red color in the presence of sodium nitroferricyanide.

Legg-Calvé-Perthes disease or **syndrome** [A. T. *Legg,* U.S. orthopedist, 1874–1939; J. *Calvé;* and G. C. *Perthes*]. OSTEOCHONDRITIS DEFORMANS JUVENILIS.

Legg-Perthes disease [A. T. *Legg* and G. C. *Perthes*]. OSTEOCHONDRITIS DEFORMANS JUVENILIS.

Le·gion·naires' bacillus (lee''juh·nairz'). A small gram-negative bacillus, the causative organism of Legionnaires' disease.

Legionnaires' disease. An acute lobar pneumonia often producing renal, intestinal, neurologic, and hepatic symptoms, due to the Legionnaires' bacillus; first recognized in an outbreak at a convention of the American Legion in July 1976.

leg scissoring. 1. SCISSORING. 2. SCISSORS GAIT.

leg sign. SOUQUES' SIGN (2).

le·gu·min (le·gew'min, leg'yoo·min) *n.* A globulin found in the seeds of many plants belonging to the Leguminosae.

Le·gu·mi·no·sae (le·gew''mi·no'see) *n.pl.* The family of leguminous plants, such as peas, beans, peanuts, and alfalfa, characteristically bearing pods and harboring nitrogen-fixing bacteria in root nodules.

Lei·boff and Kahn's method. A test for urea in which the urea in a blood filtrate is converted to ammonia by acid hydrolysis under pressure and directly nesslerized.

Leich·ten·stern's phenomenon or **sign** (lye'kh'tᵉn·shterrn) [O. M. *Leichtenstern,* German physician, 1845–1900]. In meningitis, the wincing or violent jerk of a patient with cries of pain when any part of the skeleton is tapped.

Leif·son's method [E. *Leifson,* U.S bacteriologist, b. 1902]. A stain for bacterial flagella, composed of pararosaniline acetate, tannic acid, sodium chloride, ethyl alcohol, and distilled water and applied to a dried smear of the culture for 10 minutes, washed with water, and examined after drying without any counterstain.

Leigh's syndrome or **disease** (lee) [D. *Leigh,* English neuropathologist, 20th century]. SUBACUTE NECROTIZING ENCEPHALOMYELOPATHY.

Lei·ner's disease (lye'nur) [K. *Leiner,* Austrian pediatrician, 1871–1930]. ERYTHRODERMA DESQUAMATIVUM.

leio-, lio- [Gk. *leios*]. A combining form signifying *smooth.*

leio·der·ma·tous (lye''o·dur'muh·tus) *adj.* [*leio-* + *dermat-* + *-ous*]. Smooth-skinned.

leio·der·mia, lio·der·mia (lye''o·dur'mee·uh) *n.* [*leio-* + *-dermia*]. A condition of abnormal smoothness and glossiness of the skin.

leio·myo·fi·bro·ma (lye''o·migh''o·figh·bro'muh) *n.* [*leio-* + *myo-* + *fibroma*]. A benign tumor composed of smooth muscle cells and fibrocytes.

leio·my·o·ma (lye''o·migh·o'muh) *n.,* pl. **leiomyomas, leiomy·oma·ta** (·tuh) [*leio-* + *myoma*]. A benign tumor whose parenchyma is composed of smooth muscle cells; occurs most often in the uterus. See also *leiomyoma uteri.*

leiomyoma ute·ri (yoo'tur·eye). A leiomyoma of the uterus. Syn. *fibroid tumor, uterine fibroid.*

leio·myo·sar·co·ma (lye''o·migh''o·sahr·ko'muh) *n.* [*leio-* + *myo-* + *sarcoma*]. A malignant tumor whose parenchyma is composed of anaplastic smooth muscle cells. Syn. *malignant leiomyosarcoma, metastasizing leiomyosarcoma.*

lei·ot·ri·chous (lye·ot'ri·kus) *adj.* [*leio-* + *trich-* + *-ous*]. Having smooth or straight hair.

lei·po·mer·ia (lye''po·meer'ee·uh, ·merr'ee·uh) *n.* [Gk. *leipein,* to leave, + *mer-* + *-ia*]. Congenital absence of one or more limbs.

Leish·man-Don·o·van bodies (leesh'mun) [W. B. *Leishman,* British Army pathologist, 1865–1926; and C. *Donovan*]. Small, oval protozoa lacking flagellum and undulating membrane, occurring in the vertebrate host intracellularly in macrophages of areas such as the skin, liver, spleen, and common to leishmanial infections such as kala azar, oriental sore, and mucocutaneous leishmaniasis.

Leish·man·ia (leesh·man'ee·uh, ·may'nee·uh) *n.* [W. B. *Leishman*]. A genus of the Trypanosomatidae whose species are morphologically similar but differ in serologic reactions; transmitted to man by the bite of species of *Phlebotomus.* They have a single flagellum when in the invertebrate host, but assume the leishmania (nonflagellated) form in the vertebrate host. —**leishma·ni·al** (·nee·ul) *adj.*

leishmania, *n.,* pl. **leishmania.** 1. An organism of the genus *Leishmania.* 2. The nonflagellated form in the life cycle of any of the Trypanosomatidae.

Leishmania bra·sil·i·en·sis (bra·zil''i·en'sis). A species of *Leishmania* confined largely to Central and South America. This parasite shows a predilection for the mucocutaneous borders of the nose and mouth and produces mucocutaneous leishmaniasis. Syn. *Leishmania peruviana, Leishmania tropica var.* americana.

Leishmania don·o·va·ni (don''o·vay'nigh, ·van'eye). A species of protozoan flagellate which is the etiologic agent of kala azar, the visceral form of leishmaniasis.

Leishmania in·fan·tum (in·fan'tum). A parasite, observed in the Mediterranean area, believed generally to belong to the species *Leishmania donovani;* the causative agent of infantile leishmaniasis.

Leishmania pe·ru·vi·a·na (pe·roo''vee·ay'nuh). LEISHMANIA BRASILIENSIS.

leish·man·i·a·sis (leesh''muh·nigh'uh·sis) *n.,* pl. **leishmania·ses** (·seez) [*Leishmania* + *-iasis*]. A variety of visceral and tegumentary infections caused by protozoan parasites of the genus *Leishmania.* Several species of biting flies of the genus *Phlebotomus* are responsible for transmission. In India, man constitutes the main reservoir, but in the Mediterranean region infected dogs are the reservoirs for the infantile form of the disease.

leishmaniasis amer·i·ca·na (a·merr''i·kay'nuh). AMERICAN MUCOCUTANEOUS LEISHMANIASIS.

Leishmania trop·i·ca (trop'i·kuh). A species of protozoan flagellate that affects primarily the skin and produces oriental sore.

Leishmania tropica* var. *americana. LEISHMANIA BRASILIENSIS.

leish·man·in test (leesh·man'in, leesh'muh·nin). An intradermal test of the delayed-sensitivity type in which formalinized leishmania are used as antigen; it is positive after recovery from infection with *Leishmania* but negative in active kala azar.

leish·man·oid (leesh'mun·oid) *n.* A cutaneous lesion in which leishmania are present.

Leishman's stain [W. B. *Leishman*]. A blood stain of the Romanovsky type, the eosinate of polychrome methylene blue, available as a powder used in 0.15% solution in methanol.

l electron. An electron in the l or second shell surrounding the nucleus of an atom.

le·ma (lee'muh) *n.* [Gk. *lēmē*, a humor in the corner of the eye, rheum]. A collection of dried secretion of the tarsal glands at the inner canthus of the eye.

Lem·bert's suture (lahⁿ·behr') [A. *Lembert*, French surgeon, 1802–1851]. An interrupted suture used to approximate serous surfaces of the intestine.

-lemma [Gk. *lemma*, peel, husk]. A combining form meaning *a sheath or envelope.*

lemmo- [Gk. *lemma*, peel, husk]. A combining form meaning *neurilemma.*

lem·mo·blast (lem'o·blast) *n.* [*lemmo-* + *-blast*]. An immature lemmocyte.

lem·mo·blas·to·ma (lem''o·blas·to'muh) *n.* [*lemmoblast* + *-oma*]. NEURILEMMOMA.

lem·mo·cyte (lem'o·site) *n.* [*lemmo-* + *-cyte*]. A formative cell for the neurilemma.

lem·mo·cy·to·ma (lem''o·sigh·to'muh) *n.* [*lemmocyte* + *-oma*]. NEURILEMMOMA.

lem·nis·cus (lem·nis'kus) *n.*, pl. **lemnis·ci** (·kigh, ·igh) [L., ribbon, from Gk. *lēmniskos*]. A secondary sensory pathway of the central nervous system, which usually decussates and terminates in the thalamus. —**leminis·cal** (·kul) *adj.*

lemniscus acu·sti·cus (a·koos'ti·kus). LATERAL LEMNISCUS.

lemniscus la·te·ra·lis (lat·e·ray'lis) [NA]. LATERAL LEMNISCUS.

lemniscus me·di·a·lis (mee·dee·ay'lis) [NA]. MEDIAL LEMNISCUS.

lemniscus op·ti·cus (op'ti·kus). OPTIC TRACT.

lemniscus sen·si·ti·vus (sen·si·tye'vus). MEDIAL LEMNISCUS.

lemniscus spi·na·lis (spye·nay'lis) [NA]. SPINAL LEMNISCUS.

lemniscus tri·ge·mi·na·lis (trye·jem''i·nay'lis) [NA]. TRIGEMINAL LEMNISCUS.

lem·no·blast (lem'no·blast) *n.* LEMMOBLAST.

lem·no·cyte (lem'no·site) *n.* LEMMOCYTE.

lem·on, *n.* [OF. *limon*, from Ar. *laymūn*, from Per. *līmūn*]. The fruit of *Citrus limon.*

lemon oil. The volatile oil obtained from the fresh peel of the fruit of *Citrus limon;* characteristic odor is due chiefly to citral, an aldehyde. Used as a flavor.

le·mo·pa·ral·y·sis (lee''mo·pa·ral'i·sis) *n.* [Gk. *laimos*, gullet, + *paralysis*]. Paralysis of the esophagus.

le·mo·ste·no·sis (lee''mo·ste·no'sis) *n.* [Gk. *laimos*, gullet, + *stenosis*]. Constriction or narrowing of the pharynx or esophagus.

Lem·pert's operation [J. *Lempert*, U.S. otolaryngologist, 1891–1974]. FENESTRATION (2).

le·mur (lee'mur) *n.* [L. *lemures*, ghosts]. 1. Any of the prosimian primates native to Madagascar. 2. Loosely, any prosimian primate other than tarsiers and tree shrews.

Len·drum's inclusion-body stain [A. C. *Lendrum*, Scottish pathologist, 20th century]. A hematoxylin-phloxine stain which colors certain inclusion bodies red.

length·en·ing reaction. Sudden inhibition of the stretch reflex when extensor muscles are subjected to an excessive degree of stretching by forceful flexion of a limb. See also *stretch reflex.*

length-height index. The ratio of the basion-bregma height of the skull to its greatest length × 100. Syn. *altitudinal index, height index.*

Len·hartz diet (leʸn'harts) [H. A. D. *Lenhartz*, German physician, 1854–1910]. A high protein regimen for the treatment of peptic ulcer, consisting chiefly of milk and eggs.

len·i·ceps (len'i·seps) *n.* [L. *lenis*, mild, gentle, + for*ceps*]. Obstetric forceps with short handles.

len·i·quin·sin (len''i·kwin'sin) *n.* 6,7-Dimethoxy-4-(veratrylideneamino) quinoline, $C_{20}H_{20}N_2O_4$, an antihypertensive agent.

len·i·tive (len'i·tiv) *adj.* & *n.* [ML. *lenitivus*, from *lenire*, to soften]. 1. Soothing, emollient, demulcent. 2. An emollient remedy or application.

Len·nert's lymphoma. A malignant lymphoma characterized by a high content of epithelioid histiocytes; possibly a variant of Hodgkin's disease.

Len·nox-Gas·taut syndrome (gaʰs·to') [W. G. *Lennox*, U.S. neurologist, 20th century; and H. *Gastaut*, French neurologist, b. 1915]. The occurrence, in infants and young children, of akinetic seizures, succeeded by tonic seizures and mental retardation, and associated with slow spike-and-wave complexes in the electroencephalogram.

len·per·one (len'pur·ohn) *n.* 4'-Fluoro-4-[4-(*p*-fluorobenzoyl)piperidino]butyrophenone, a tranquilizer, sometimes used as the hydrochloride salt.

lens (lenz) *n.*, genit. sing. **len·tis** (len'tis), L. pl. **len·tes** (·teez) [L., lentil]. 1. A piece of glass or crystal for the refraction of rays of light. 2. [NA] CRYSTALLINE LENS. See also Plate 19.

lens capsule. CAPSULE OF THE LENS.

lens crys·tal·li·na (kris·tuh·lye'nuh) [BNA]. Lens (2) (= CRYSTALLINE LENS).

lens fibers. The highly modified epithelial cells that form the main mass of the lens of the eye. NA *fibrae lentis.*

lens-induced uveitis. Intraocular inflammation caused by the lens. See also *phacoanaphylactic endophthalmitis, phacotoxic uveitis.*

lens·om·e·ter (len·zom'e·tur) *n.* [*lens* + *-meter*]. An instrument for determining the optical centers and refractive power of spheres and lenses, to locate the axes of cylindrical lenses, and to measure the power and locate the direction of prisms. Syn. *phacometer.*

lens placode. The ectodermal anlage of the lens of the eye; its formation is induced by the presence of the underlying optic vesicle.

lens star. The starlike arrangement of the lens sutures, having three to nine rays, produced by the growth of the lens fibers.

lens vesicle. The ectodermal vesicle that differentiates into the lens of the eye.

lent-, lenti- [L. *lens, lentis*, lentil]. A combining form meaning *lens, lenticular.*

Lente Iletin. Trademark for lente insulin or insulin zinc suspension.

len·te insulin (len'tee). One of a series of protein-free injectable preparations of insulin, with adjustable duration of action, obtained by mixing proper proportions of crystalline, long-acting zinc insulin with amorphous, short-acting zinc insulin, the mixture being suspended in an acetate-buffered medium of pH 7.3. A mixture of approximately 7 parts of the crystalline form and 3 parts of the amorphous variety is known as insulin zinc suspension.

len·ti·co·nus (len''ti·ko'nus) *n.* [*lenti-* + *conus*]. A rare, usually congenital, anomaly of the lens; marked by a conical prominence upon its anterior or, more rarely, upon its posterior surface; may be seen in Alport's syndrome.

len·tic·u·lar (len·tick'yoo·lur) *adj.* [L. *lenticularis*, from *lenticula*, dim. of *lens*, lentil]. 1. Pertaining to or resembling a lens. 2. Pertaining to the crystalline lens. 3. Pertaining to the lentiform nucleus of the brain.

lenticular apophysis. The lenticular process of the incus.

lenticular astigmatism. Astigmatism due to defective curvature or refractive surface of the lens of an eye.

lenticular degeneration. HEPATOLENTICULAR DEGENERATION.

lenticular fasciculus. A bundle of nerve fibers from the globus pallidus which pass through the H_2 field of Forel. Many of the fibers continue into the midbrain.

lenticular loop. ANSA LENTICULARIS.

lenticular nucleus. The globus pallidus and putamen together. Syn. *lentiform nucleus.*

lenticular papilla. One of the irregularly distributed, low folds of mucous membrane in the anterior part of the dorsum of the base of the tongue.

lenticular process. The extremity of the long process of the incus, covered with cartilage and articulating with the stapes. NA *processus lenticularis incudis.*

lenticular progressive degeneration. HEPATOLENTICULAR DEGENERATION.

len·tic·u·late (len·tick′yoo·lut, ·late) *adj.* Lens-shaped.

len·tic·u·lo·stri·ate (len·tick″yoo·lo·strye′ate) *adj.* Pertaining to the lenticular nucleus of the corpus striatum, as lenticulostriate artery.

len·tic·u·lo·tha·lam·ic (len·tick″yoo·lo·tha·lam′ick) *adj.* [*lenticular* + *thalamic*]. Extending from the lentiform nucleus to the thalamus.

lenticulothalamic tract. Fibers from the lentiform nucleus to the thalamus.

len·ti·form (len′ti·form) *adj.* Lens-shaped or lentil-shaped.

lentiform nucleus. The globus pallidus and putamen together. Syn. *lenticular nucleus.* NA *nucleus lentiformis.*

lentigines. Plural of *lentigo.*

lentigines le·pro·sae (le·pro′see). The pigmented macular lesions of leprosy.

len·ti·glo·bus (len″ti·glo′bus) *n.* [*lenti-* + *globus*]. A spherical bulging of the lens of the eye, as in intumescent cataract.

len·ti·go (len·tye′go) *n.*, pl. **len·tig·i·nes** (len·tij′i·neez) [L., from *lens, lentis,* lentil]. A smooth, dark brown spot on the skin, usually of an exposed part, of a person of middle years or older. Histologically there is elongation of rete ridges with increased numbers of melanocytes. See also *freckle.*

lentigo ma·lig·na (muh·lig′nuh). A slowly growing variety of junction nevus characteristically occurring on the face of people over age 50, which may evolve into an invasive malignant melanoma. Syn. *Hutchinson's freckle, malignant freckle, melanosis circumscripta preblastomatosa of Dubreuilh, melanotic freckle, senile freckle.*

lentigo maligna melanoma. Lentigo maligna with dermal invasion by spindle-shaped anaplastic melanocytes.

lentigo se·ni·lis (se·nigh′lis) A flat, uniformly colored spot that appears on exposed areas of skin during middle age and after. Syn. *liver spots.*

le·on·ti·a·sis (lee″on·tye′uh·sis) *n.*, pl. **leontia·ses** (·seez) [Gk., from *leōn, leontos,* lion]. A "lionlike" appearance of the face, seen in lepromatous leprosy.

leontiasis os·sea (os′ee·uh). An overgrowth of the bones of the face and cranium as the result of which the features acquire a "lionlike" appearance.

Leon virus. POLIOMYELITIS VIRUS, type 3.

lep·er (lep′ur) *n.* [ME. *lepre,* leprosy, from OF., from L. *lepra*]. One affected with leprosy.

lepid-, lepido- [Gk. *lepis, lepidos*]. A combining form meaning *a scale, scaly.*

lep·i·do·ma (lep″i·do′muh) *n.* [*lepid-* + *-oma*]. A tumor arising from a lining membrane.

Lep·i·dop·tera (lep″i·dop′te·ruh) *n.pl.* [*lepido-* + Gk. *ptera,* wings]. An order of insects distinguished by featherlike scales and spirally coiled suctorial apparatus. The order includes butterflies, moths, and skippers. The larvae of certain species cause caterpillar dermatitis.

L.E. plasma factor. L.E. FACTOR.

lep·o·thrix (lep′o·thricks) *n.* [Gk. *lepos,* scale, husk, + *-thrix*]. A skin disorder in which masses of reddish, black, and yellow fungous material are found in nodular or diffuse distribution about the axillary or genital hair; usually seen in those who sweat freely. Syn. *trichomycosis nodosa.*

lepr-, lepro-. A combining form meaning *leprous, leprosy.*

lep·ra (lep′ruh) *n.* [L., from Gk., psoriasis, from *lepros,* scaly, scabby]. LEPROSY.

lepra bo·ni·ta (bo·nee′tuh). Infiltrative changes in the face causing a smooth, plump appearance seen in diffuse lepromatous leprosy.

lepra cell. A large mononuclear cell associated with lepromatous lesions, which often contains the acid-fast organisms of leprosy.

lepra major. Tuberculoid leprosy with massive lesions.

lepra minor. Tuberculoid leprosy with small, discrete patches.

lepra reaction. Exacerbation of the inflammatory process in lepromatous leprosy, either spontaneous or provoked by treatment.

lep·re·chaun·ism (lep′re·kawn″iz·um) *n.* [*leprechaun,* Irish elf, + *-ism*]. A congenital disorder, presumably autosomal recessive, in which the infant is small and cachectic, with a small hirsute face but nearly normal-sized ears, eyes, and nasal tip, giving it a gnome-like appearance; there is also premature ovarian follicular maturation, enlargement of the nipples and external genitalia, and various visceral abnormalities. Syn. *Donahue's syndrome.*

lep·rid (lep′rid) *n.* [*lepr-* + *-id*]. 1. Any skin lesion of leprosy. 2. A type of skin lesion seen in tuberculoid leprosy.

lep·ride (lep′ride, ·rid) *n.* LEPRID.

lepro-. See *lepr-.*

lep·ro·lin (lep′ro·lin) *n.* A vaccine prepared from an acid-fast bacillus; used unsatisfactorily in the treatment of leprosy.

leprolin test. An intradermal test with a vaccine used as a diagnostic procedure in leprosy.

lep·rol·o·gist (lep·rol′uh·jist) *n.* An individual who specializes in the study and treatment of leprosy.

lep·rol·o·gy (lep·rol′uh·jee) *n.* [*lepro-* + *-logy*]. The study of leprosy. —**lep·ro·log·ic** (lep″ro·loj′ick) *adj.*

lep·ro·ma (lep·ro′muh) *n.*, pl. **lepromas, leproma·ta** (·tuh) [*lepr-* + *-oma*]. The cutaneous nodular lesion of leprosy. —**lep·rom·a·tous** (lep·rom′uh·tus) *adj.*

lepromatous leprosy. One of the two principal forms of leprosy, characterized by the presence of large numbers of *Mycobacterium leprae* in the lesions, a negative lepromin reaction, and diffuse skin lesions which may be macular or nodular, with later involvement of peripheral nerve trunks. In advanced cases, destructive lesions of the nose, mouth, throat, and larynx and deformities of the extremities are common. Contr. *tuberculoid leprosy.*

lep·ro·min (lep′ro·min) *n.* An emulsion prepared from ground and sterilized tissue containing the leprosy bacillus (*Mycobacterium leprae*); used for intradermal skin tests in leprosy but of little diagnostic utility although of prognostic significance.

lepromin test. The intradermal injection of lepromin as a skin test, useful in the classification and prognosis of leprosy, generally positive in the tuberculoid and negative in the lepromatous form.

lep·ro·pho·bia (lep″ro·fo′bee·uh) *n.* [*lepro-* + *-phobia*]. Morbid dread of leprosy.

lep·ro·sar·i·um (lep″ro·săr′ee·um) *n.*, pl. **leprosariums, lepro·sar·ia** (·ee·uh). An institution for the treatment of persons affected with leprosy.

lep·ro·sery, lep·ro·sary (lep′ro·serr″ee) *n.* [F. *léproserie*]. LEPROSARIUM.

lep·ro·stat·ic (lep″ro·stat′ick) *adj.* [*lepro-* + *-static*]. Having an action inhibiting the growth of *Mycobacterium leprae,* the organism causing leprosy.

lep·ro·sy (lep′ruh·see) *n.* [*leprous* (q.v.) + *-y*]. An infectious disease of low communicability, due to invasion of nerves by acid-fast *Mycobacterium leprae;* followed by progressive local invasion of tissues or hematogenous spread to skin, ciliary bodies, testes, lymph nodes, and nerves.

lep·rot·ic (lep·rot′ick) *adj.* LEPROUS.

lep·rous (lep′rus) *adj.* [OF., from L. *leprosus,* from *lepra,* leprosy, from Gk. *lepra,* psoriasis, from *lepros,* scaly, scabby]. 1. Pertaining to, or characteristic of leprosy. 2. Affected with leprosy.

-lepsis. See *-lepsy.*

-lepsy [Gk. *-lēpsia,* from *lēpsis,* seizure, from *lambanein,* to seize, take]. A combining form meaning *seizure.*

lept-, lepto- [Gk. *leptos*]. A combining form meaning (a) *thin, narrow, fine;* (b) *small;* (c) *slight, mild.*

lep·tan·dra (lep·tan'druh) *n.* The dried rhizome and roots of *Veronicastrum virginicum (Leptandra virginica)*; formerly used as a cathartic.

lep·ta·zol (lep'tuh·zole, ·zol) *n.* British name for pentylenetetrazol.

lep·to·ce·pha·lia (lep"to·se·fay'lee·uh) *n.* [*lepto-* + *-cephalia*]. Abnormal smallness of the skull.

lep·to·ceph·a·lus (lep"to·sef'uh·lus) *n.,* pl. **leptocepha·li** (·lye) [*lepto-* + *-cephalus*]. An individual with an abnormally small head from premature union of the frontal and sphenoid bones.

lep·to·ceph·a·ly (lep"to·sef'uh·lee) *n.* LEPTOCEPHALIA.

lep·to·chro·mat·ic (lep"to·kro·mat'ick) *adj.* [*lepto-* + *chromatic*]. Having chromatin of a thin-stranded or fine appearance.

lep·to·cyte (lep'to·site) *n.* [*lepto-* + *-cyte*]. An abnormally thin erythrocyte, often characterized also by other abnormalities of shape.

lep·to·cyt·ic (lep"to·sit'ick) *adj.* 1. Of or pertaining to leptocytes. 2. Pertaining to or characterizing a condition in which leptocytosis is evident microscopically, and in which the hypochromic microcytic anemia present is not amenable to iron therapy.

lep·to·cy·to·sis (lep"to·sigh·to'sis) *n.* [*leptocyte* + *-osis*]. A preponderance of leptocytes in the blood. See also *thalassemia.*

lep·to·dac·ty·lous (lep"to·dack'ti·lus) *adj.* [*lepto-* + *dactyl-* + *-ous*]. Characterized by slenderness of the fingers or toes, or both.

lep·to·don·tous (lep"to·don'tus) *adj.* [*lept-* + *-odont* + *-ous*]. Having thin or slender teeth.

lep·to·me·nin·ges (lep"to·me·nin'jeez) *n.pl.* [*lepto-* + *meninges*]. The arachnoid and the pia mater considered together.

lep·to·me·nin·gi·o·ma (lep"to·me·nin"jee·o'muh) *n.* [*leptomeninges* + *-oma*]. A tumor of the pia mater or arachnoid.

lep·to·men·in·gi·tis (lep"to·men"in·jye'tis) *n.* [*leptomeninges* + *-itis*]. Inflammation of the pia mater and arachnoid of the brain or the spinal cord or both.

lep·to·men·in·gop·a·thy (lep"to·men"ing·gop'uth·ee) *n.* [*leptomeninges* + *-pathy*]. Disease of the leptomeninges, or pia mater and arachnoid.

lep·to·me·ninx (lep"to·mee'ninks) *n.,* pl. **lepto·me·nin·ges** (·me·nin'jeez) [*lepto-* + *meninx*]. PIA-ARACHNOID.

lep·to·mi·cro·gnath·ia (lep"to·migh"kro·nath'ee·uh, ·naith'ee·uh, ·migh"krog·) *n.* [*lepto-* + *micrognathia*]. A mild degree of micrognathia.

Lep·to·mi·cru·rus (lep"to·migh·kroor'us) *n.* [*lepto-* + *Micrurus*]. A genus of coral snakes found in the Americas, with neurotoxic venom.

Lep·tom·o·nas (lep·tom'o·nas, lep"to·mo'nas) *n.* [*lepto-* + Gk. *monas,* unit]. A genus of the Trypanosomatidae whose members are hemoflagellates of invertebrates.

lep·ton (lep'ton) *n.* [*lept-* + *-on*]. An elementary particle of small mass, as the electron, positron, neutrino, or antineutrino.

lep·to·pel·lic (lep"to·pel'ick) *adj.* [*lepto-* + *-pellic*]. Having a very narrow pelvis.

lep·to·pho·nia (lep"to·fo'nee·uh) *n.* [*lepto-* + *-phonia*]. Delicacy, gentleness, or weakness of the voice. —**lepto·phon·ic** (·fon'ick) *adj.*

lep·to·pro·so·pia (lep"to·pro·so'pee·uh) *n.* [*lepto-* + *prosop-* + *-ia*]. Narrowness of the face. —**leptopro·sop·ic** (·sop'ick, ·so'pick) *adj.*

lep·tor·rhine (lep'to·rine, ·rin) *n.* [*lepto-* + *-rrhine*]. 1. *In craniometry,* designating an apertura piriformis that is relatively long and narrow; having a nasal index of 46.9 or less. 2. *In somatometry,* designating a nose that is long and narrow; having a height-breadth index of 55.0 to 69.9.

lep·to·scope (lep'to·skope) *n.* [*lepto-* + *-scope*]. An optical device for measuring the thickness and composition of the plasma membrane of a cell.

Lep·to·spi·ra (lep"to·spye'ruh) *n.* [*lepto-* + L. *spira,* coil]. A genus of spirochetes able to survive in water; characterized by sharply twisted filaments with one or both extremities hooked or recurved. These organisms are not predominantly blood parasites, but are also found in other tissues. —**leptospira,** pl. **leptospiras, lep·to·spi·rae** (lep"to·spye'ree) *com. n.*

Leptospira au·tum·na·lis (aw·tum·nay'lis). The causative agent of pretibial fever.

Leptospira ca·nic·o·la (ka·nick'o·luh) [NL., from L. *canis,* dog, + *colere,* to inhabit, to cultivate]. The etiologic agent of Stuttgart disease in dogs and of canicola fever in man.

Leptospira grip·po·ty·pho·sa (grip·o·tye·fo'suh). One of the etiological agents of leptospirosis.

Leptospira heb·dom·a·dis (heb·dom'uh·dis) [L., from Gk. *hebdomas, hebdomados,* a week, from *hepta,* seven]. The spirochete which is the causative agent of seven-day fever in eastern Asia.

Leptospira ic·tero·hae·mor·rha·gi·ae (ick"tur·o·hem·o·ray'jee·ee). A species of spirochete which produces leptospirosis in man, in common with other species such as *Leptospira canicola, L. grippotyphosa.*

lep·to·spire (lep'tuh·spire) *n.* A spirochete of the genus *Leptospira.*

lep·to·spi·rol·y·sin (lep"to·spye·rol'i·sin, ·spye"ro·lye'sin) *n.* A lysin that dissolves leptospiras.

lep·to·spi·ro·sis (lep"to·spye·ro'sis) *n.,* pl. **leptospiro·ses** (·seez) [*Leptospira* + *-osis*]. A systemic infection with spirochetal microorganisms of the genus *Leptospira,* usually a short self-limited febrile illness, but at times producing distinctive clinical syndromes of aseptic meningitis, hemorrhagic jaundice, or glomerulonephritis. Syn. *Landouzy's disease.* See also *Weil's disease.*

leptospirosis ic·te·ro·he·mor·rhag·i·ca (ick"tur·o·hem·o·raj"i·kuh). WEIL'S DISEASE.

lep·to·tene (lep'to·teen) *n.* [*lepto-* + *-tene*]. The initial stage in the first meiotic prophase in which the chromosomes are first visualized. See also *diplotene, pachytene, zygotene.*

lep·to·thri·co·sis (lep"to·thri·ko'sis) *n.* LEPTOTRICHOSIS.

Lep·to·thrix (lep'to·thricks) *n.* [Gk., having fine hair, from *lepto-* + *thrix,* hair]. A genus of unbranched filamentous organisms of the Chlamydobacteriaceae.

Leptothrix buc·ca·lis (buh·kay'lis). A species of organism which is a common inhabitant of the oral cavity.

lep·to·tri·chal (lep"to·trye'kul, ·trick'ul) *adj.* Pertaining to or caused by organisms of the genus *Leptothrix.*

leptotrichal conjunctivitis. A syndrome caused by members of the genus *Leptothrix,* characterized by unilateral conjunctivitis, usually follicular, with preauricular lymphadenopathy on the affected side, and low-grade fever for several weeks; diagnosis is confirmed by biopsy and pathologic examination of one of the nodules, which shows the organisms in the pinpoint foci of necrosis. Syn. *Parinaud's conjunctivitis.*

Lep·to·trich·ia (lep"to·trick'ee·uh) *n.* A genus of anaerobic, nonmotile, filamentous microorganisms, gram-positive but easily decolorized, indigenous to the oral cavity, but also found in the genitourinary tract of man.

lep·to·tri·cho·sis (lep"to·tri·ko'sis) *n.,* pl. **leptotricho·ses** (·seez) [*Leptothrix* + *-osis*]. Any disease caused by a species of *Leptothrix.*

leptotrichosis con·junc·ti·vae (kon"junk·tye'vee). LEPTOTRICHAL CONJUNCTIVITIS.

lep·tus (lep'tus) *n.,* pl. **leptuses, lep·ti** (·tye) [NL., from Gk. *leptos,* small]. CHIGGER.

le·re·sis (le·ree'sis) *n.* [Gk. *lērēsis,* silly talk, from *lēros,* silly]. Garrulousness; senile loquacity.

ler·go·trile (lur'go·trile) *n.* 2-Chloro-6-methylergoline-8β-

acetonitrile, $C_{17}H_{18}ClN_3$, a prolactin inhibitor, also used as the methanesulfonate (mesylate) salt.

Le·riche's operation (le·reesh') [R. *Leriche*, French surgeon, 1870–1955]. A periarterial sympathectomy for relief of vasomotor disturbances.

Leriche syndrome [R. *Leriche*]. Thrombotic obliteration or occlusion of the aortic bifurcation producing intermittent claudication of the low back, buttocks, thighs, or calves; symmetrical atrophy and pallor of the legs; impotence; and weakness or absence of the femoral pulses.

Lé·ri's disease (ley·ree') [A. *Léri*, French physician, 1875–1930]. PLEONOSTEOSIS OF LÉRI.

Léri's sign [A. *Léri*]. In spastic hemiplegia, absence of normal flexion at the elbow following the passive folding of the fingers into the hollows of the hand and forcible flexion of the wrist.

Leritine. Trademark for anileridine, an analgesic used as the hydrochloride and phosphate salts.

Léri type of osteopetrosis [A. *Léri*]. MELORHEOSTOSIS.

Ler·man-Means scratch [J. *Lerman*, U.S. physician, b. 1902; and J. H. *Means*, U.S. physician, 1885–1967]. A left sternal border sound or rub, seen in thyrotoxicosis, possibly due to pulmonary conus dilatation and/or increased blood flow.

Ler·moy·ez syndrome (lehr·mwa·yey') [M. *Lermoyez*, French otolaryngologist, 1858–1929]. Attacks or episodes of diminished hearing followed by attacks of vertigo, after which hearing improves or returns to normal. Cause and mechanism are unclear.

LES Abbreviation for *lower esophageal sphincter* (= CARDIAC SPHINCTER).

les·bi·an (lez'bee·un) *adj. & n.* [Gk. *lesbios*, of the island of *Lesbos*, home of the poetess Sappho]. 1. Pertaining to or practicing female homosexuality. 2. One who practices female homosexuality.

les·bi·an·ism (lez'bee·un·iz·um) *n.* [*lesbian* + *-ism*]. Female homosexuality. Syn. *sapphism*.

Lesch·ke method. A histochemical method for urea based on treatment with mercuric nitrate followed by hydrogen sulfide to obtain black mercuric sulfide precipitate at the site of urea in the tissue.

Lesch-Ny·han disease or **syndrome.** [M. *Lesch*, U.S. cardiologist, b. 1939; and W. L. *Nyhan*, U.S. pediatrician, b. 1926]. A disease of male children characterized by hyperuricemia, deficiency of hypoxanthine-guanine phosphoribosyltransferase, mental retardation, spasticity, tremor, choreoathetosis, and self-mutilating biting; transmitted as an X-linked recessive.

L. E. serum factor. L. E. FACTOR.

le·sion (lee'zhun) *n.* [OF., harm, injury, from L. *laesio*, from *laedere*, to injure]. An alteration, structural or functional, due to disease; most commonly applied to morphological alterations.

les·ser alar cartilages. The minor alar cartilages. See *alar cartilages*.

lesser arterial circle of the iris. An arterial circle around the free margin of the iris. NA *circulus arteriosus iridis minor*.

lesser cavity of the peritoneum. OMENTAL BURSA.

lesser circulation. PULMONARY CIRCULATION.

lesser curvature of the stomach. The right border of the stomach, to which the lesser omentum is attached. NA *curvatura ventriculi minor*.

lesser omentum. A fold of peritoneum passing from the lesser curvature of the stomach to the transverse fissure of the liver. On the right its edge is free and encloses all the structures issuing from or entering the transverse fissure of the liver: portal vein, hepatic artery, bile duct, nerves, and lymphatics. Behind the free edge is the epiploic foramen. Syn. *gastrohepatic omentum*. NA *omentum minus*.

lesser palatine foramen. Any of the lower openings of the lesser palatine canals on the lower surface of the palatine bone. Syn. *minor palatine foramen*. NA (pl.) *foramina palatina minora*.

lesser pancreas. A small, partially detached portion of the gland, lying posteriorly to its head, and occasionally having a separate duct that opens into the pancreatic duct proper.

lesser pelvis. TRUE PELVIS.

lesser peritoneal cavity. OMENTAL BURSA.

lesser ring of the iris. The inner of two concentric zones separated by the lesser arterial circle of the iris. NA *anulus iridis minor*.

lesser sac. OMENTAL BURSA.

lesser sciatic foramen. The space included between the sacrotuberous and sacrospinous ligaments and the portion of the hipbone between the spine and ischial tuberosity, giving passage to the internal obturator muscle and the internal pudendal vessels and pudendal nerve. NA *foramen ischiadicum minus*.

lesser sciatic notch. The notch below the spine of the ischium which is converted to a foramen by the sacrotuberous and sacrospinous ligaments; it transmits the tendon of the internal obturator muscle and the internal pudendal vessels and pudendal nerve. NA *incisura ischiadica minor*.

lesser splanchnic nerve. A nerve that arises from the ninth and tenth thoracic ganglions and goes to the celiac plexus. NA *nervus splanchnicus minor*. See also Table of Nerves in the Appendix.

Les·ser's triangle. An area of the neck bounded above by the hypoglossal nerve and below by the anterior and posterior bellies of the digastric muscle.

lesser trochanter. A process situated on the inner side of the upper extremity of the femur below the neck. NA *trochanter minor*.

lesser tubercle of the humerus. A prominence on the upper anterior end of the shaft of the humerus into which is inserted the subscapularis muscle. NA *tuberculum minus humeri*.

lesser tuberosity of the femur. LESSER TROCHANTER.

let·down, *n.* Transport of milk to the ducts from the alveoli where it is formed.

let·down factor. One of the psychosomatic mechanisms influencing the course of lactation by the expulsion of already secreted milk from the breast. Pain, fear, and emotional tension inhibit letdown.

letdown reflex. A neuroendocrine reflex responsible for producing milk letdown.

L. E. test. 1. L. E. CELL TEST. 2. Any test for systemic lupus erythematosus.

le·thal (lee'thul) *adj.* [L. *letalis*, from *letum*, death]. Deadly; pertaining to or producing death. Abbreviated, l.

lethal dose. A dose sufficient to kill. Abbreviated, LD.

lethal gene. An allele that causes the death of the gamete or the zygote before development is completed, or at least before the organism reaches sexual maturity.

lethal intestinal virus of infant mice. A coronavirus that produces epizootics of diarrhea with high mortality in suckling mice; though originally thought to be a distinct syndrome caused by a specific etiological agent, the disease is now believed to be caused by a variant of mouse hepatitis virus studied in genetic research. Abbreviated, LIVIM. See also *mouse hepatitis virus*.

lethal mutation. A mutation causing death of the organism during any stage of its development prior to reproduction.

lethargic encephalitis. ENCEPHALITIS LETHARGICA.

leth·ar·gy (leth'ur·jee) *n.* [Gk. *lēthargia*, from *lēthē*, forgetfulness]. Drowsiness or stupor; mental torpor. —**le·thar·gic** (le·thahr'jick) *adj.*

let·i·mide (let'i·mide) *n.* 3-[2-(Diethylamino)ethyl]-2*H*-1,3-benzoxazine-2,4(3*H*)-dione, $C_{14}H_{18}N_2O_3$, an analgesic, usually employed as the hydrochloride salt.

Letonoff and Rein·hold's method [J. G. *Reinhold*]. A method for determining inorganic sulfate in serum in which, after deproteinization with uranium acetate, the sulfate is precipitated, dissolved, and determined colorimetrically.

Letter. A trademark for levothyroxine sodium, used for thyroid hormone replacement therapy.

Let·ter·er-Si·we disease (let'ur·ur, see'vuh) [E. *Letterer,* German pathologist, b. 1895; and S. A. *Siwe,* Swedish physician, b. 1897]. A usually fatal disease of infancy and childhood, of unknown cause, characterized by hyperplasia of the reticuloendothelial system without lipid storage. Manifestations include enlargement of spleen, liver, and lymph nodes, histiocytic infiltration of the lungs, perivascular white matter of brain and meninges, osseous defects particularly in the skull, and involvement of the bone marrow resulting in secondary anemia. Cutaneous eruptions and purpura are frequently present. Syn. *nonlipid reticuloendotheliosis, nonlipid histiocytosis.*

leuc-, leuco-. See *leuk-.*

leuc·ae·thi·op (lew·seeth'ee·op, lew·keeth'ee·op) *n.* [*leuc-* + Gk. *aithiops,* Ethiopian]. A Negro albino. —**leuc·ae·thi·op·ic** (lew·seeth''ee·op'ick, ·keeth'') *adj.*

leu·ce·mia, leu·cae·mia (lew·see'mee·uh) *n.* LEUKEMIA.

leu·cine (lew'seen, ·sin) *n.* [*leuc-* + *-ine*]. CH_3-$CH(CH_3)CH_2CH(NH_2)COOH$. The α-aminoisocaproic acid, an amino acid obtainable by the hydrolysis of milk and other protein-containing substances, and found in various tissues of the human body. It is essential to the growth of man. —**leu·cic** (lew'sick) *adj.*

leucine aminopeptidase. An enzyme acting on peptides which have a terminal free α-amino group, causing the sequential liberation of free amino acids from the peptide. The enzyme acts most rapidly on terminal leucine residues, and is useful in determining the structure of proteins. Marked increase in the serum level of the enzyme has been observed in pancreatic carcinoma but also in certain other diseases.

leucine intolerance or **sensitivity.** A condition of hypoglycemia primarily in infants caused by the ingestion of proteins rich in leucine. Thought to be genetic in origin, the condition appears to be caused by stimulation of insulin secretion.

leucine tolerance test. A sensitivity test based on the difference in the level of blood sugar in the fasting state and at specified intervals after administering L-leucine or casein; a fall in blood glucose to 50% of control or less in 30-45 minutes occurs in patients with leucine sensitivity.

leu·ci·nu·ria (lew''si·new'ree·uh) *n.* [*leucine* + *-uria*]. The occurrence of leucine in the urine.

leuco-. See *leuk-.*

leucoblast. LEUKOBLAST.

leucoblastosis. LEUKOBLASTOSIS.

leucocidin. LEUKOCIDIN.

leucocyte. LEUKOCYTE.

leucocythaemia. Leukocythemia (= LEUKEMIA).

leucocytoblast. LEUKOCYTOBLAST.

leucocytogenesis. LEUKOCYTOGENESIS.

leucocytolysin. LEUKOCYTOLYSIN.

leucocytolysis. LEUKOCYTOLYSIS.

leucocytoma. LEUKOCYTOMA.

leucocytometer. LEUKOCYTOMETER.

leucocytopenia. Leukocytopenia (= LEUKOPENIA).

leucocytopoiesis. LEUKOCYTOPOIESIS.

leucocytosis. LEUKOCYTOSIS.

leucoderma. LEUKODERMA.

leucodermia. LEUKODERMA.

leucodystrophy. LEUKODYSTROPHY.

leucoencephalitis. LEUKOENCEPHALITIS.

leucoencephalopathy. LEUKOENCEPHALOPATHY.

leucoerythroblastosis. LEUKOERYTHROBLASTOSIS.

leu·co·fla·vin (lew''ko·flay'vin, ·flav'in) *n.* LEUCORIBOFLAVIN.

leucokeratosis. Leukokeratosis (= LEUKOPLAKIA).

leu·co·lac·to·fla·vin (lew''ko·lack·to·flay'vin, ·flav'in) *n.* LEUCORIBOFLAVIN.

leucolymphosarcoma. Leukolymphosarcoma (= LEUKOSARCOMA (1)).

leucolysis. Leukolysis (= LEUKOCYTOLYSIS).

leucoma. LEUKOMA.

leu·co·maine (lew'ko·mane, lew''ko·may'een, ·in) *n.* [*leuco-* + *-maine* (as in *ptomaine*)]. Any one of the nitrogenous bases normally developed by the metabolic activity of living organisms, as distinguished from the bases developed by putrefactive processes, and called ptomaines.

leu·co·main·emia, leuco·main·ae·mia (lew''ko·may·i·nee'mee·uh, ·may·nee') *n.* [*leucomaine* + *-emia*]. An excess of leucomaines in the blood.

leucomyoma. Leukomyoma (= LIPOMYOMA).

Leu·co·nos·toc (lew''ko·nos'tock) *n.* [*leuco-* + *Nostoc,* a genus of algae]. A genus of saprophytic bacteria of the family Lactobacteriaceae. Species of this genus are found in milk, fermenting vegetables, and slimy sugar solutions. Used in the manufacture of dextrans.

leuconychia. LEUKONYCHIA.

leucopathia. Leukopathia (= LEUKOPATHY).

leucopathy. LEUKOPATHY.

leucopedesis. LEUKOPEDESIS.

leucopenia. LEUKOPENIA.

leucopheresis. Leukopheresis (= LEUKAPHERESIS).

leucophlegmasia. LEUKOPHLEGMASIA.

leucophthalmous. LEUKOPHTHALMOUS.

leucoplakia. LEUKOPLAKIA.

leucoplasia. LEUKOPLAKIA.

leucoplastid. LEUKOPLASTID.

leucopoiesis. Leukopoiesis (= LEUKOCYTOPOIESIS).

leucoprotease. LEUKOPROTEASE.

leucopsin. LEUKOPSIN.

leu·co·ri·bo·fla·vin (lew''ko·rye''bo·flay'vin, ·flav'in) *n.* The dihydro compound resulting from reduction of riboflavin. It is colorless and shows no fluorescence. Syn. *leucoflavin.*

leucorrhagia. LEUKORRHAGIA.

leucorrhoea. LEUKORRHEA.

leucosarcoma. LEUKOSARCOMA.

leucosarcomatosis. LEUKOSARCOMATOSIS.

leu·co·sin (lew'ko·sin) *n.* A simple protein of the albumin type found in wheat and other cereals.

leucosis. LEUKOSIS.

leucotaxine. LEUKOTAXINE.

leucotome. LEUKOTOME.

leucotomy. Leukotomy (= LOBOTOMY).

leucotoxic. LEUKOTOXIC.

leucotoxin. LEUKOTOXIN.

leucourobilin. LEUKOUROBILIN.

leucous. LEUKOUS.

leu·co·vor·in (lew''ko·vor'in, lew·kov'uh·rin) *n.* Folinic acid (2); used as the calcium salt to counteract the toxic effects of folic acid antagonists and for treatment of megaloblastic anemias.

leu·cyl (lew'sil) *n.* The univalent radical $(CH_3)_2$-$CHCH_2CH(NH_2)CO$—, of the amino acid leucine.

Leu·det's sign (lœh·de[h]') [T. E. *Leudet,* French physician, 1825-1887]. In catarrhal or nervous diseases of the ear, the patient hears a fine, crackling sound in the ear.

leuk-, leuc-, leuko-, leuco- [Gk. *leukos,* light, white]. A combining form meaning (a) *white, colorless, weakly colored;* (b) *leukocyte, leukocytic.*

leukaemia. LEUKEMIA.

leukaemic. LEUKEMIC.

leukaemoid. LEUKEMOID.

leuk·ane·mia (lew''kuh·nee'mee·uh) *n.* A blood disease having characteristics of granulocytic leukemia and pernicious anemia.

leu·ka·phe·re·sis (lew''kuh·fe·ree'sis) *n.* [*leuk-* + Gk. *aphairesis,* removal]. The removal from a blood donor of a quantity of leukocytes, followed by return to the donor of the remaining portions of the blood.

leu·kas·mus (lew·kaz'mus) *n.* LEUKODERMA; ALBINISM.

leu·ke·mia, leu·kae·mia (lew·kee'mee·uh) *n.* [*leuk-* + *-emia*]. Any disease of the hemolytopoietic system characterized by uncontrolled proliferation of the leukocytes. Anaplastic leukocytes usually are present in the blood, often in large numbers, and characteristically involve various organs. Leukemias are classified on the basis of rapidity of course (acute, subacute, or chronic), the cell count, the cell type, and the degree of differentiation. Syn. *leukosis, leukocythemia.*

leu·ke·mic (lew·kee'mick) *adj.* 1. Of or pertaining to leukemia. 2. Characterized by an increase in leukocytes.

leukemic adenia. Enlargement of lymph nodes associated with a leukemia.

leukemic leukemia. Leukemia in which the leukocyte count in peripheral blood is above 15,000 per mm^3, and the cell types are in accord with the diagnosis of leukemia. Contr. *aleukemic leukemia.*

leukemic reticuloendotheliosis. A rare neoplastic disease of the hematopoietic system characterized by a chronic course, splenomegaly, and pancytopenia, and marked by "hairy cells," circulating mononuclear cells with numerous cytoplasmic projections. Syn. *hairy-cell leukemia.*

leukemic retinitis or **retinopathy.** A form of retinitis characterized by pallor of the retinal vessels and optic disk, the boundary of the latter being indistinct. Hemorrhages appear at various points of the membrane, while numerous white patches and round bodies are visible about the disk in the retina.

leu·ke·mid (lew·kee'mid) *n.* [*leukem*ia + *-id*]. A cutaneous lesion which accompanies leukemia; sometimes restricted to those which do not contain leukemic cells.

leu·ke·moid, leu·kae·moid (lew·kee'moid) *adj.* [*leukem*ia + *-oid*]. Similar to leukemia, but due to other conditions; usually refers to the presence of immature cells in the blood in conditions other than leukemia.

Leukeran. Trademark for chlorambucil, an antineoplastic drug.

leu·ker·gy (lew'kur·jee) *n.* [*leuk-* + *-ergy*]. The tendency of leukocytes in the bloodstream of subjects with various inflammatory states to aggregate in groups of cytologically similar cells.

leukergy test. Increased agglomeration of leukocytes in citrated blood, as a test for rheumatic disease. Syn. *Fleck's test.*

leu·kin (lew'kin) *n.* [*leuk-* + *-in*]. ENDOLYSIN.

leukobasic fuchsin stain. SCHIFF'S REAGENT.

leu·ko·blast, leu·co·blast (lew'ko·blast) *n.* [*leuko-* + *-blast*]. A general term for the parent cell of the leukocytes.

leu·ko·blas·to·sis, leu·co·blas·to·sis (lew"ko·blas·to'sis) *n.* [*leukoblast* + *-osis*]. Excessive proliferation of immature leukocytes.

leu·ko·ci·din, leu·co·ci·din (lew·ko·sigh'din, lew·ko'si·din) *n.* [*leuko-* + *-cide* + *-in*]. A toxic substance capable of killing and destroying neutrophil leukocytes.

leu·ko·cyte, leu·co·cyte (lew'ko·site) *n.* [*leuko-* + *-cyte*]. 1. One of the colorless, more or less ameboid cells of the blood, having a nucleus and cytoplasm. Those found in normal blood are usually divided according to their staining reaction into granular leukocytes, including neutrophils, eosinophils, and basophils, and nongranular leukocytes, including lymphocytes and monocytes. The kinds found in abnormal blood are myeloblasts, promyelocytes, neutrophilic myelocytes, eosinophilic myelocytes, basophilic myelocytes, lymphoblasts, and plasma cells. Syn. *white blood cell, white corpuscle.* Contr. *erythrocyte.* 2. Specifically, NEUTROPHIL LEUKOCYTE.

leukocyte antigens. Transplantation antigens found on leukocytes, used for clinical purposes because easily detectable and roughly representative of the antigenic content of body tissue. See also *transplantation antigen.*

leukocyte series. GRANULOCYTIC SERIES.

leu·ko·cy·the·mia, leu·co·cy·thae·mia (lew"ko·sigh·theem'ee·uh) *n.* [*leukocyte* + *-hemia*]. LEUKEMIA.

leu·ko·cyt·ic (lew"ko·sit'ick) *adj.* Of or pertaining to leukocytes.

leukocytic series. GRANULOCYTIC SERIES.

leu·ko·cy·to·blast, leu·co·cy·to·blast (lew"ko·sigh'to·blast) *n.* [*leukocyte* + *-blast*]. The precursor of a leukocyte.

leu·ko·cy·to·gen·e·sis, leu·co·cy·to·gen·e·sis (lew"ko·sigh"to·jen'e·sis) *n.*, pl. **leukocytogene·ses, leucocytogene·ses** (·seez) [*leukocyte* + *-genesis*]. The formation of leukocytes.

leu·ko·cy·to·ly·sin, leu·co·cy·to·ly·sin (lew"ko·sigh"to·lye'sin, ·sigh·tol'i·sin) *n.* [*leukocyte* + *lysin*]. A lysin which disintegrates leukocytes.

leu·ko·cy·tol·y·sis, leu·co·cy·tol·y·sis (lew"ko·sigh·tol'i·sis) *n.*, pl. **leukocytoly·ses, leucocytoly·ses** (·seez) [*leukocyte* + *-lysis*]. The destruction of leukocytes. —**leukocy·to·lit·ic, leucocy·to·lit·ic** (·to·lit'ick) *adj.*

leu·ko·cy·to·ma, leu·co·cy·to·ma (lew"ko·sigh·to'muh) *n.* [*leukocyte* + *-oma*]. A tumor composed of leukocytes.

leu·ko·cy·tom·e·ter, leu·co·cy·tom·e·ter (lew"ko·sigh·tom'e·tur) *n.* [*leukocyte* + *-meter*]. A graduated capillary tube used for counting leukocytes.

leu·ko·cy·to·pe·nia, leu·co·cy·to·pe·nia (lew"ko·sigh"to·pee'nee·uh) *n.* [*leukocyte* + *-penia*]. LEUKOPENIA.

leu·ko·cy·to·poi·e·sis, leu·co·cy·to·poi·e·sis (lew"ko·sigh"to·poy·ee'sis) *n.*, pl. **leukocytopoie·ses, leucocytopoie·ses** (·seez) [*leukocyte* + *-poiesis*]. The formation of leukocytes. Syn. *leukopoiesis.* —**leukocytopoi·et·ic, leucocytopoi·et·ic** (·et'ick) *adj.*

leu·ko·cy·to·sis, leu·co·cy·to·sis (lew"ko·sigh·to'sis) *n.*, pl. **leukocyto·ses, leucocyto·ses** (·seez) [*leukocyte* + *-osis*]. An increase in the leukocyte count above the upper limits of normal. —**leukocy·tot·ic, leucocy·tot·ic** (·tot'ick) *adj.*

leu·ko·cy·tu·ria (lew"ko·sigh·tew'ree·uh) *n.* The presence of leukocytes in the urine.

leu·ko·der·ma (lew"ko·dur'muh) *n.* [*leuko-* + *-derma*]. Loss of skin melanin secondary to a cause which is known or reasonably certain. —**leukoder·mic** (·mick) *adj.*

leukoderma ac·qui·si·tum cen·trif·u·gum (ak"wi·sigh'tum sen·trif'yoo·gum). HALO NEVUS.

leukoderma col·li (kol'eye). A condition coincident with the appearance of the macular eruption of cutaneous syphilis; characterized by mottled skin on the neck, chin, or rarely on other parts.

leukoderma pso·ri·at·i·cum (so"ree·at'i·kum). Areas of skin hypopigmentation following psoriatic inflammation.

leukoderma punc·ta·tum (punk·tay'tum). An affection of the skin characterized by minute areas of hypopigmentation scattered through the melanosis following prolonged intake of arsenic.

leu·ko·der·mia, leu·co·der·mia (lew"ko·dur'mee·uh) *n.* LEUKODERMA.

leu·ko·dys·tro·phy, leu·co·dys·tro·phy (lew"ko·dis'truh·fee) *n.* [*leuko-* + *dystrophy*]. Any disorder characterized by progressive degeneration of the cerebral white matter, or by defective building up of myelin, and most often due to an inborn error of metabolism.

leu·ko·en·ceph·a·li·tis, leu·co·en·ceph·a·li·tis (lew"ko·en·sef"uh·lye'tis) *n.* [*leuko-* + *encephalitis*]. Any inflammatory disease affecting chiefly the cerebral white matter; may be acute, subacute, or chronic.

leukoencephalitis con·cen·tri·ca (kun·sen'tri·kuh). CONCENTRIC SCLEROSIS.

leu·ko·en·ceph·a·lop·a·thy, leu·co·en·ceph·a·lop·a·thy (lew"ko·en·sef"uh·lop'uth·ee) *n.* [*leuko-* + *encephalopathy*]. Any pathologic condition involving chiefly the white matter; may be inflammatory (leukoencephalitis) or degenerative (leukodystrophy).

leu·ko·eryth·ro·blas·tic anemia (lew"ko·e·rith"ro·blas'tick). Anemia accompanied by immature erythrocytes and leukocytes in the peripheral blood.

leu·ko·eryth·ro·blas·to·sis, leu·co·eryth·ro·blas·to·sis (lew"ko·

e·rith″ro·blas·to′sis) *n.* [*leuko-* + *erythro-* + *-blast* + *-osis*]. Immature erythrocytes and leukocytes simultaneously present in the peripheral blood.

leu·ko·ker·a·to·sis, leu·co·ker·a·to·sis (lew″ko·kerr·uh·to′sis) *n.* [*leuko-* + *kerat-* + *-osis*]. LEUKOPLAKIA.

leu·ko·lym·pho·sar·co·ma, leu·co·lym·pho·sar·co·ma (lew″ko·lim″fo·sahr·ko′muh) *n.* LEUKOSARCOMA (1).

leu·kol·y·sis, leu·col·y·sis (lew·kol′i·sis) *n.*, pl. **leukoly·ses, leucoly·ses** (·seez). LEUKOCYTOLYSIS.

leu·ko·ma, leu·co·ma (lew·ko′muh) *n.*, pl. **leukomas, leucomas, leukoma·ta, leucoma·ta** (·tuh) [Gk. *leukōma*, white spot in the eye]. 1. A dense opacity of the cornea as a result of an ulcer, wound, or inflammation, which presents an appearance of ground glass. 2. LEUKOPLAKIA BUCCALIS. 3. LEUKOSARCOMA. —**leu·kom·a·tous, leu·com·a·tous** (·kom′uh·tus), **leukoma·toid, leucoma·toid** (·toid) *adj.*

leukomaine. LEUCOMAINE.

leu·ko·my·o·ma, leu·co·my·o·ma (lew″ko·migh·o′muh) *n.* [*leuko-* + *myoma*]. LIPOMYOMA.

leuk·onych·ia, leuc·onych·ia (lew″ko·nick′ee·uh) *n.* [*leuk-* + *onych-* + *-ia*]. Whitish discoloration of the nails. —**leuk·ony·chit·ic, leuc·ony·chit·ic** (·ni·kit′ick) *adj.*

leukonychia par·ti·a·lis (pahr″shee·ay′lis). Partial whitening of the nails.

leukonychia stri·a·ta (strye·ay′tuh). Horizontal streaks of whiteness of the nails.

leukonychia stria·ta lon·gi·tu·di·na·lis (strye·ay′tuh lon″ji·tew″di·nay′lis). Persistence of a longitudinal white streak on a finger nail for several years.

leukonychia to·ta·lis (to·tay′lis). Pure white nails; probably congenital.

leu·ko·path·ia, leu·co·path·ia (lew″ko·path′ee·uh) *n.* LEUKOPATHY.

leu·kop·a·thy, leu·cop·a·thy (lew·kop′uth·ee) *n.* [*leuko-* + *-pathy*]. 1. Any deficiency of coloring matter. 2. ALBINISM.

leu·ko·pe·de·sis, leu·co·pe·de·sis (lew″ko·pe·dee′sis) *n.* Diapedesis of leukocytes through the walls of blood vessels, especially the capillaries.

leukopedesis gas·tri·ca (gas′tri·kuh). Leukocytes, particularly in increased numbers, in the gastric secretion.

leu·ko·pe·nia, leu·co·pe·nia (lew″ko·pee′nee·uh) *n.* [*leuko-* + *-penia*]. A decrease below the normal number of leukocytes in the peripheral blood. Syn. *leukocytopenia.* See also *agranulocytosis.* —**leukope·nic, leucope·nic** (·nick) *adj.*

leukopenic index. An index depending on the capacity of certain substances to reduce the leukocytes after ingestion. The total count is made before and after taking the specific substance.

leukopenic leukemia. ALEUKEMIC LEUKEMIA.

leukopenic myelosis. ALEUKEMIC LEUKEMIA.

leu·ko·phe·re·sis (lew″ko·fe·ree′sis) *n.* LEUKAPHERESIS.

leu·ko·phleg·ma·sia, leu·co·phleg·ma·sia (lew″ko·fleg·may′zhuh, ·zee·uh) *n.* [*leuko-* + *phlegmasia*]. 1. A condition due to obstruction (usually venous thrombosis) of the iliac and/or femoral vein and characterized by pallor and edema of the thigh and leg. 2. PHLEGMASIA ALBA DOLENS.

leu·ko·pho·re·sis (lew″ko·fo·ree′sis) *n.* LEUKAPHERESIS.

leu·koph·thal·mous, leu·coph·thal·mous (lew″kof·thal′mus) *n.* [*leuk-* + *ophthalm-* + *-ous*]. Having unusually white eyes.

leu·ko·pla·kia, leu·co·pla·kia (lew″ko·play′kee·uh) *n.* [*leuko-* + Gk. *plax, plakos*, flat surface, slab, + *-ia*]. Abnormal thickening and whitening of the epithelium of a mucous membrane; it is considered to be precancerous in some cases. —**leukopla·ki·al** (·kee·ul) *adj.*

leukoplakia buc·ca·lis (buh·kay′lis). Leukoplakia characterized by pearly-white or bluish-white patches on the surface of the tongue or the mucous membrane of the cheeks.

leukoplakia oris (o′ris). LEUKOPLAKIA BUCCALIS.

leukoplakia vul·vae (vul′vee). Irregular white patches on the mucosa of the vulva. There is thickening of the epithelium, and the papillae may be hypertrophied. Carcinoma may develop. See also *kraurosis of the vulva.*

leu·ko·pla·sia, leu·co·pla·sia (lew″ko·play′zhuh, ·zee·uh) *n.* [*leuko-* + *-plasia*]. LEUKOPLAKIA.

leu·ko·plas·tid, leu·co·plas·tid (lew″ko·plas′tid) *n.* [*leuko-* + *plastid*]. A colorless plastid which under proper stimulus may become a chloroplast, chromoplast, or amyloplast.

leu·ko·poi·e·sis, leu·co·poi·e·sis (lew″ko·poy·ee′sis) *n.*, pl. **leukopoie·ses, leucopoie·ses** (·seez) [*leuko-* + *-poiesis*]. LEUKOCYTOPOIESIS.

leu·ko·pro·te·ase, leu·co·pro·te·ase (lew″ko·pro′tee·ace, ·aze) *n.* [*leuko-* + *protease*]. An enzyme in leukocytes which splits protein. In inflammation, it causes liquefaction of necrotic tissue.

leu·kop·sin, leu·cop·sin (lew·kop′sin) *n.* [*leuk-* + *ops-* + *-in*]. Visual white, produced by reaction of light on rhodopsin (visual purple) derived from vitamin A.

leu·kor·rha·gia, leu·cor·rha·gia (lew″ko·ray′jee·uh) *n.* [*leuko-* + *-rrhagia*]. An excessive leukorrheal flow.

leu·kor·rhea, leu·cor·rhoea (lew″ko·ree′uh) *n.* [*leuko-* + *-rrhea*]. A whitish, mucopurulent discharge from the female genital canal. —**leukor·rhe·al, leucor·rhe·al** (·ree′ul) *adj.*

leu·ko·sar·co·ma, leu·co·sar·co·ma (lew″ko·sahr·ko′muh) *n.* [*leuko-* + *sarcoma*]. 1. Lymphosarcoma accompanied by involvement of the peripheral blood with anaplastic lymphoid cells. Syn. *leukolymphosarcoma, sarcoleukemia.* 2. LYMPHOCYTIC LEUKEMIA.

leu·ko·sar·co·ma·to·sis, leu·co·sar·co·ma·to·sis (lew″ko·sahr·ko″muh·to′sis) *n.* A generalized form of leukosarcoma.

leu·ko·sis, leu·co·sis (lew·ko′sis) *n.*, pl. **leuko·ses, leuco·ses** (·seez) [*leuk-* + *-osis*]. An excess of white blood cells. See also *avian leukosis complex.*

leu·ko·tax·ine, leu·co·tax·ine (lew″ko·tack′seen, ·sin) *n.* [*leuko-* + Gk. *taxis*, arrangement, + *-ine*]. A crystalline, nitrogenous substance present in inflammatory exudates, which exerts positive chemotaxis and appears to increase capillary permeability. It is probably produced by injured cells.

leu·ko·tome, leu·co·tome (lew′ko·tome) *n.* [*leuko-* + *-tome*]. An instrument for dividing nerve fibers of the white matter of the brain in lobotomy.

leu·kot·o·my, leu·cot·o·my (lew·kot′uh·mee) *n.* [*leuko-* + *-tomy*]. LOBOTOMY.

leu·ko·tox·ic, leu·co·tox·ic (lew″ko·tock′sick) *adj.* [*leuko-* + *toxic*]. Destructive to leukocytes.

leu·ko·tox·in, leu·co·tox·in (lew″ko·tock′sin) *n.* [*leuko-* + *toxin*]. A cytotoxin obtained from lymph nodes.

leu·ko·trich·ia (lew″ko·trick′ee·uh) *n.* [*leuko-* + *-trichia*]. Whiteness of the hair; CANITIES. —**leu·kot·ri·chous** (lew·kot′ri·kus) *adj.*

leu·ko·uro·bil·in, leu·co·uro·bil·in (lew″ko·yoor″o·bil′in, ·bye′lin) *n.* [*leuko-* + *urobilin*]. A colorless decomposition product of bilirubin.

leu·kous, leu·cous (lew′kus) *adj.* [*leuk-* + *-ous*]. White.

leu·ro·cris·tine (lew″ro·kris′teen) *n.* VINCRISTINE.

Le·va·di·ti's method [C. *Levaditi*, Rumanian bacteriologist in Paris, 1874–1928]. A method for staining *Treponema pallidum* in sections which is a modification of Cajal's method of staining nerve fibers; a silver nitrate solution is used, which stains the treponema a dense black.

Levaditi spirochete stain [C. *Levaditi*]. A silver nitrate-pyrogallol method which blackens spirochetes in tissue sections.

lev·al·lor·phan (lev″al·or′fan) *n.* 17-Allylmorphinan-3-ol, $C_{19}H_{25}NO$, a narcotic antagonist used as the tartrate salt to counteract narcotic-induced respiratory depression.

lev·am·fet·a·mine (lev″am·fet′uh·meen) *n.* (−)-α-Methylphenethylamine, $C_9H_{13}N$, an anorexigenic drug; used as the succinate and sulfate salts.

lev·am·i·sole (le·vam′i·sole) *n.* (−)2,3,5,6-Tetrahydro-6-

phenylimidazo [2,1-*b*] thiazole, a veterinary anthelmintic usually used as the hydrochloride salt.

levamphetamine. LEVAMFETAMINE.

lev·an (lev'an) *n.* A levulosan polysaccharide, composed of furanose-type D-fructose (D-fructofuranose) units linked by 2,6-β-glycosidic bonds, elaborated from sucrose by certain microorganisms, as *Bacillus subtilis* and *B. pumilus.*

Levanil. A trademark for ectylurea, a tranquilizing drug.

levan sucrase. An enzyme that catalyzes formation of levan from sucrose.

Levant wormseed. SANTONICA.

lev·ar·ter·e·nol (lev"ahr·teer'e·nole, ·ahr·terr'e·nole) *n.* *l*-α-(Aminomethyl)-3,4-dihydroxybenzyl alcohol, $C_8H_{11}NO_3$, the levo isomer of the pressor amine *l*-arterenol (*l*-norepinephrine); used as a vasopressor in the form of the bitartrate salt.

le·va·tor (le·vay'tur) *n.*, pl. **le·va·to·res** (lev"uh·to'reez) [L., from *levare*, to lift up]. 1. Any of various muscles that raise or elevate. 2. An instrument used for raising a depressed portion of the skull.

levator an·gu·li oris (ang'gew·lye o'ris). A muscle of facial expression attached to the skin at the angle of the mouth. NA *musculus levator anguli oris.*

levator anguli sca·pu·lae (skap'yoo·lee). LEVATOR SCAPULAE.

levator ani (ay'nigh). The chief muscle of the pelvic diaphragm. NA *musculus levator ani.* See also Table of Muscles in the Appendix.

levator cla·vi·cu·lae (kla·vick'yoo·lee). An occasional muscle arising from the transverse process of the first or second cervical vertebra and extending to the lateral end of the clavicle.

levator epi·glot·ti·dis (ep"i·glot'i·dis). A variant part of the genioglossus muscle inserted into the epiglottis.

levatores cos·ta·rum (kos·tair'um). Small deep muscles of the back which aid in raising the ribs. They are divided into levatores costarum breves (NA *musculi levatores costarum breves*), and levatores costarum longi (NA *musculi levatores costarum longi*). See also Table of Muscles in the Appendix.

levator glandulae thy·roi·de·ae (thigh·roy'dee·ee). An occasional slip of muscle extending from the body of the hyoid to the isthmus of the thyroid gland. NA *musculus levator glandulae thyroideae.*

levator la·bii su·pe·ri·o·ris (lay'bee·eye sue·peer"ee·o'ris). A muscle of facial expression attached to the skin of the upper lip. NA *musculus levator labii superioris.*

levator labii superioris alae·que na·si (ay·lee'kwee nay'zye). A muscle of facial expression. NA *musculus levator labii superioris alaeque nasi.* See also Table of Muscles in the Appendix.

levator men·ti (men'tye). MENTALIS.

levator pa·la·ti (pa·lay'tye, pa·lah'tye). LEVATOR VELI PALATINI.

levator pal·pe·brae su·pe·ri·o·ris (pal·pee'bree sue·peer·ee·o' ris). The muscle that raises the upper eyelid. NA *musculus levator palpebrae superioris.* See also Table of Muscles in the Appendix.

levator pro·sta·tae (pros'tuh·tee). A few medial fibers of the pubococcygeus part of the levator ani muscle. NA *musculus levator prostatae.*

levator sca·pu·lae (skap'yoo·lee). The muscle that raises the shoulder and rotates the inferior angle of the scapula medially. NA *musculus levator scapulae.* See also Table of Muscles in the Appendix.

levator sign. In paralysis of the facial nerve, when the patient is asked to look down and then close his eyes slowly, the upper lid on the paralyzed side moves upward slightly, being elevated by the levator palpebrae superioris whose action is no longer opposed by the orbicularis. Syn. *Cestan's sign.*

levator ve·li pa·la·ti·ni (vee'lye pal·uh·tye'nigh). The muscle that raises the soft palate. NA *musculus levator veli palatini.* See also Table of Muscles in the Appendix.

le·ver (lee'vur, lev'ur) *n.* [OF. *levier*, from *lever*, to raise]. A vectis or one-armed tractor, used in obstetrics.

le·vid·u·lin·ose (le·vid'yoo·lin·oce) *n.* A trisaccharide occurring in manna; on hydrolysis it yields one molecule of glucose and two molecules of mannose.

lev·i·ga·tion (lev"i·gay'shun) *n.* [L. *levigare*, to make smooth, from *lēvis*, smooth]. The reduction of a substance to a powder by grinding in water, followed by fractional sedimentation, in order to separate the coarser from the finer particles. See also *porphyrization.* —**lev·i·gate** (lev'i·gate) *v.*

Lé·vi-Lo·rain disease or **dwarfism** (leʸ·vee', loʰ·ræⁿ') [L. *Lévi* and P. J. *Lorain*]. PITUITARY DWARFISM.

Le·vine's clenched-fist sign [S. A. *Levine*, U.S. physician, 1891–1966]. A sign of angina pectoris; the clenched fist over the sternum depicts the location and constricting nature of the discomfort.

Lev·in·son test. A test for tuberculous meningitis in which a characteristic ratio is said to be obtained between the alkaloidal precipitate formed by sulfosalicylic acid and the metallic precipitate formed by mercuric chloride in cerebrospinal fluid.

Le·vin tube [A. L. *Levin*, U.S. physician, 1880–1940]. A nasal gastroduodenal catheter, used in connection with gastric and intestinal operations.

Lé·vi's syndrome [L. *Lévi*, French endocrinologist, 1868–1933]. PITUITARY DWARFISM.

lev·i·ta·tion (lev"i·tay'shun) *n.* [L. *lēvitas*, lightness]. 1. The subjective sense of rising into the air or being aloft without support, as in dreams or certain mental disorders. 2. The illusion of the suspension of a body in air; performed by modern magicians.

levo-, laevo- [L. *laevus*]. A combining form meaning (a) *left, on the left;* (b) in chemistry, *levorotatory.*

le·vo·car·dia (lee"vo·kahr'dee·uh) *n.* [*levo-* + *-cardia*]. 1. Normal position of the heart in the left hemithorax. Contr. *dextrocardia.* 2. A form of congenital heart disease associated with situs inversus, in which the heart paradoxically remains in the left chest, usually with intrinsic anomalies of its own.

le·vo·car·dio·gram (lee"vo·kahr'dee·o·gram) *n.* [*levo-* + *cardiogram*]. 1. That component of the normal electrocardiogram contributed by left ventricular forces. 2. The electrocardiographic complex derived from a unipolar lead facing the left ventricle.

le·vo·con·dy·lism (lee"vo·kon'di·liz·um) *n.* [*levo-* + *condyle* + *-ism*]. Deviation of the mandibular condyles toward the left.

le·vo·cy·clo·ver·sion (lee"vo·sigh"klo·vur'zhun, ·sick"lo·) *n.* [*levo-* + *cyclo-* + *version*]. Counterclockwise torsional movement of both eyes to the left.

le·vo·do·pa (lee"vo·do'puh) *n.* (−)-3-(3,4-Dihydroxyphenyl)-L-alanine, $C_9H_{11}NO_4$, an antiparkinson drug.

Levo-Dromoran. Trademark for levorphanol, a synthetic narcotic analgesic used as the bitartrate salt.

le·vo·duc·tion (lee"vo·duck'shun) *n.* [*levo-* + L. *ducere*, to lead]. Movement to the left, said especially of an eye.

le·vo·fur·al·ta·done (lee"vo·few·ral'tuh·dohn) *n.* (−)-5-(Morpholinomethyl)-3-[(5-nitrofurfurylidene)amino)-2-oxazolidinone, $C_{13}H_{16}N_4O_6$, an antibacterial and antiprotozoan drug.

le·vo·gram (lee'vo·gram) *n.* LEVOCARDIOGRAM.

le·vo·gy·rate (lee"vo·jye'rate, lev'o·) *adj.* [*levo-* + *gyrate*]. LEVOROTATORY.

le·vo·gy·rous (lee"vo·jye'rus) *adj.* [*levo-* + *gyr-* + *-ous*]. LEVOROTATORY.

le·vo·me·pro·ma·zine (lee"vo·me·pro'muh·zeen) *n.* METHOTRIMEPRAZINE.

le·vo·meth·a·dyl acetate (lee"vo·meth'uh·dil). (−)-6-(Dimethylamino)-4,4-diphenyl-3-heptanol acetate(ester), $C_{23}H_{31}NO_2$, a narcotic analgesic.

le·vo·nor·de·frin (lee″vo·nor′de·frin) *n.* *l*-α-(1-Aminoethyl)-3,4-dihydroxybenzyl alcohol, $C_9H_{13}NO_3$, a vasoconstrictor used in solutions of local anesthetics for dental practice.

Levophed. Trademark for levarterenol, a pressor amine used as the bitartrate salt.

le·vo·pho·bia (lee″vo·fo′bee·uh) *n.* [*levo-* + *-phobia*]. Morbid fear of objects on the left side of the body.

Levoprome. Trademark for methotrimeprazine, a tranquilizer, nonnarcotic analgesic, and sedative.

le·vo·pro·pox·y·phene (lee″vo·pro·pock′si·feen) *n.* α-(−)-4-(Dimethylamino)-3-methyl-1,2-diphenyl-2-butanol propionate, $C_{22}H_{29}NO_2$, an antitussive drug; used as the 2-naphthalenesulfonate (napsylate) salt.

le·vo·ro·ta·tion (lee″vo·ro·tay′shun) *n.* [*levo-* + *rotation*]. Rotation toward the left, especially of the plane of polarization of light.

le·vo·ro·ta·to·ry (lee″vo·ro′tuh·to″ree, lev″o·) *adj.* [*levo-* + *rotatory*]. Rotating the plane of polarized light from right to left (counterclockwise).

lev·or·phan·ol (lev·or′fuh·nol) *n.* *l*-3-Hydroxy-*N*-methylmorphinan, $C_{17}H_{23}NO$, a synthetic narcotic analgesic; used as the bitartrate salt.

le·vo·tar·tar·ic acid (lee″vo·tahr·tăr′ick, lev″o·). The optical isomer of tartaric acid which rotates polarized light to the left.

le·vo·thy·rox·ine (lee″vo·thigh·rock′seen, ·sin) *n.* L-3-[4-(4-Hydroxy-3,5-diiodophenoxy)-3,5-diiodophenyl]alanine, or L-3,3′,5,5′-tetraiodothyronine, $C_{15}H_{11}I_4NO_4$, the active isomer of thyroxine occurring in the thyroid gland.

levothyroxine sodium. The sodium salt of levothyroxine, used for treatment, by oral or parenteral administration, of hypothyroid states.

le·vo·ver·sion (lee″vo·vur′zhun) *n.* [*levo-* + *version*]. A turning to the left.

le·vox·a·drol (lee·vock′suh·drole) *n.* (−)-2-(2,2-Diphenyl-1,3-dioxolan-4-yl)piperidine $C_{20}H_{23}NO_2$, a local anesthetic and smooth muscle relaxant; used as the hydrochloride salt.

lev·u·lin (lev′yoo·lin) *n.* A substance resembling starch occurring in some tubers; easily converted into levulose.

lev·u·lin·ic acid (lev″yoo·lin′ick). 4-Oxopentanoic acid, $C_5H_8O_3$, an acid obtained by boiling dextrose, sucrose, starch, or similar derivatives with dilute hydrochloric acid.

lev·u·lo·san (lev″yoo·lo′san, lev′yoo·lo·san″) *n.* FRUCTOSAN.

lev·u·lose (lev′yoo·loce) *n.* FRUCTOSE.

lev·u·lo·se·mia, lev·u·lo·sae·mia (lev″yoo·lo·see′mee·uh) *n.* [*levulose* + *-emia*]. The presence of levulose in the blood.

levulose test. SELIWANOFF'S TEST.

levulose tolerance test. A test for liver function based on the observation that the blood sugar level is normally unaffected by the oral administration of levulose, whereas it is supposedly increased in the presence of hepatic disease.

lev·u·lo·su·ria (lev″yoo·lo·sue′ree·uh) *n.* [*levulose* + *-uria*]. Presence of levulose in the urine.

lev·u·rid (lev′yoo·rid) *n.* [F. *levure*, yeast, + *-id*]. CANDIDID.

Levy-Palmer method. A colorimetric method for total nitrogen based on the reaction of ammonia with excess hypobromite and measurement of the excess iodometrically.

Lévy-Roussy syndrome. ROUSSY-LÉVY DISEASE.

Lew·is blood group system. First recognized in a Mrs. Lewis in 1946, an antigen occurring in some 22% of the population, designated Le[a] and detected by anti-Le[a] antibodies. Le[b] and Le[c] antigens and antibodies have since been recognized. The system is unique in being primarily composed of soluble antigens of serum and body fluids like saliva, with secondary adsorption by erythrocytes, in that Le[a] positive individuals are nonsecretors of blood group substances A,B, and H, and in that the frequency of Le[a] positives is highest in infancy up to the age of 18 months.

Lewis' disease. An inborn error of glycogen metabolism, caused by a deficiency of the enzyme glycogen synthetase or UDPG-glycogen transglucosidase, resulting in diminished glycogen storage in liver.

lew·is·ite (lew′is·ite) *n.* [Wilford L. *Lewis*, U.S. chemist, 1879–1943]. Chlorovinyldichloroarsine, $ClCH{=}CHAsCl_2$, an oily substance having vesicant, lacrimatory, and lung irritant effects; it was developed for use as a chemical warfare agent.

Lewy body. A concentric hyaline cytoplasmic inclusion, especially numerous in pigmented neurons of the substantia nigra and locus ceruleus, characteristic of idiopathic Parkinson's disease.

-lexia [Gk. *lexis*, word, speech, + *-ia*; assimilated in meaning to L. *lectio*, reading]. A combining form meaning (a) *impairment of reading;* (b) *impairment of word recognition.*

Leyden battery. A series of Leyden jars connected in parallel. See also *Leyden jar.*

Ley·den crystals (lye′d^en) [E. V. von *Leyden*, German physician, 1832–1910]. CHARCOT-LEYDEN CRYSTALS.

Leyden jar [after *Leiden*, Netherlands]. A glass jar coated within and without, for its lower two-thirds, with metal foil, surmounted by a knobbed conductor in connection with the inner coating. It is designed for the temporary accumulation of electricity. See also *Leyden battery.*

Leyden-Möbius dystrophy [E. V. von *Leyden* and P. J. *Möbius*]. A form of progressive muscular dystrophy seen in children and usually beginning in the pelvic girdle and thighs, but without pseudohypertrophy, with wasting predominantly in the legs, and occasionally facial involvement. Compare *scapulohumeral muscular dystrophy.* See also *limb-girdle muscular dystrophy.*

ley·dig·ar·che (lye″dig·ahr′kee) *n.* [*Leydig* cell + Gk. *archē*, beginning]. The time at which production of androgen by the interstitial cells of the testis begins.

Leydig cell (lye′di^kh) [F. von *Leydig*, German histologist, 1821–1908]. One of the interstitial cells of the testis; it produces the male sex hormone.

Leydig-cell tumor. INTERSTITIAL-CELL TUMOR.

Leydig pause. The hypothetical time of physiologic cessation of the function of the interstitial (Leydig) cells of the testis. See also *male climacteric.*

Lf Abbreviation for *limit of flocculation.*

L.F.A. Abbreviation for *left frontoanterior* position of the fetus.

L.F.P. Abbreviation for *left frontoposterior* position of the fetus.

LGB disease. Abbreviation for *Landry-Guillain-Barré disease* (= GUILLAIN-BARRÉ DISEASE).

LGV Abbreviation for *lymphogranuloma venereum.*

LH Abbreviation for *luteinizing hormone.*

Lher·mitte's sign (lehr·meet′) [J. J. *Lhermitte*, French neurologist, 1877–1959]. Flexion of the neck is accompanied by the sensation of an electric shock shooting into the extremities in multiple sclerosis and other diseases involving the cervical spinal cord.

LHRF Abbreviation for *luteinizing hormone releasing factor.*

LHRH Abbreviation for *luteinizing hormone releasing hormone* (= LUTEINIZING HORMONE RELEASING FACTOR).

Li Symbol for lithium.

lib·er·a·tion of the arms. In breech presentations, a lowering of the arms of the fetus when they have become extended along the sides of the child's head.

li·bid·i·nal (li·bid′i·nul) *adj.* Of or pertaining to the libido.

libidinal development. PSYCHOSEXUAL DEVELOPMENT.

libidinal object. LOVE OBJECT (2).

li·bi·do (li·bee′do, li·bye′do) *n.* [L., desire, lust, from *libere* (*lubere*), to please (rel. to Gmc. *lubō* → E. *love*)].1. Sexual desire. 2. *In psychoanalysis*, psychic energy or drive usually associated with the sexual instinct, that is, for pleasure and the seeking out of a love object. —**li·bid·i·nous** (li·bid′i·nus) *adj.*

Lib·man-Sacks endocarditis, syndrome, or **disease** [E. *Lib-*

man, U.S. physician, 1872–1946; and B. *Sacks*, U.S. physician, 1873–1939]. Verrucous endocarditis complicating systemic lupus erythematosus.

li·bra (lye'bruh, lee'bruh) *n.*, pl. **li·brae** (·bree) [L., a balance]. A pound; a weight of 12 troy ounces. Abbreviated, l. Symbol, ℔.

Librium. Trademark for chlordiazepoxide, a tranquilizer used as the hydrochloride salt.

lice. Plural of *louse*.

li·cense, *n.* [MF., from L. *licentia*, from *licet*, it is allowed]. An official permit or authority conferring on the recipient the right and privilege of practicing his profession.

licensed practical nurse. A nursing assistant who has graduated from a vocational or technical school of nursing and passed requirements of state licensure. Abbreviated, LPN.

li·cen·ti·ate (lye·sen'shee·ut, ·ate) *n.* 1. One who practices a profession by the authority of a license. 2. Specifically, in some countries, a licensed medical practitioner who has no medical degree and whose professional training is less than those who do have such a degree.

li·chen (lye'kin) *n.* [Gk. *leichēn*]. 1. A plant consisting of a symbiotically associated alga and fungus, usually growing as an incrustation on dry rock or wood. 2. Any of various lesions of the skin which consist of solid papules with exaggerated skin markings.

lichen amyloidosis. LICHENOID AMYLOIDOSIS.

lichen chron·i·cus sim·plex (kron'i·kus sim'plecks). The chronic stage of neurodermatitis characterized by lichenification of lesions in various regions. Syn. *neurodermatitis circumscripta*.

lichen cor·ne·us hy·per·troph·i·cus (kor'nee·us high''pur·trof'i·kus). Thickening and induration of the skin, found in lichen chronicus simplex and the plaque type of lichen planus. Syn. *lichenificatio gigantea*.

li·chen·i·fi·ca·tio gi·gan·tea (lye·ken''i·fi·kay'shee·o, ·tee·o jye·gan'tee·uh). LICHEN CORNEUS HYPERTROPHICUS.

li·chen·i·fi·ca·tion (lye·ken''i·fi·kay'shun) *n.* The process whereby the skin becomes leathery and hardened; often the result of chronic pruritis and the irritation produced by scratching or rubbing eruptions.

li·chen·in (lye'ke·nin) *n.* [*lichen* + *-in*]. A carbohydrate obtained from Iceland moss. Does not give the starch reaction with iodine. Insoluble in cold water; forms a jelly with hot water. See also *Cetraria*.

li·chen·iza·tion (lye''ke·ni·zay'shun) *n.* LICHENIFICATION.

lichen myx·ede·ma·to·sus (mick''se·dee''muh·to'sus). A widespread eruption of asymptomatic nodules resulting from focal mucinosis of the upper dermis. Syn. *papular mucinosis*.

lichen nit·i·dus (nit'i·dus). A chronic, inflammatory skin disease characterized by groups of tiny papules which are asymptomatic; found frequently in the genital region and the flexor region of a joint.

lichen ob·tu·sus cor·ne·us (ob·tew'sus kor'nee·us). PRURIGO NODULARIS.

li·chen·oid (lye'ke·noid) *adj.* Resembling lichen.

lichenoid amyloidosis. A primary amyloidosis involving only the skin, usually of the legs, characterized by small subepidermal amyloid deposits producing papules resembling those of lichen planus; they are conical or flat, discrete, brown-red, and may coalesce to form plaques.

lichenoid eczema. Eczema marked by acuminate papules on reddened and infiltrated bases, and accompanied by intense itching.

li·chen·ous (lye'ke·nus) *adj.* 1. Of or pertaining to lichen. 2. Resembling lichen; LICHENOID.

lichen pilaris. KERATOSIS PILARIS.

lichen pla·nus (play'nus). A subacute or chronic idiopathic skin disease characterized by small, flat violaceous papules, often combining to form plaques; it is often pruritic and chiefly affects the flexor surfaces of the wrist, the legs, penis, and buccal mucosa.

lichen ru·ber acu·mi·na·tus (roo'bur a·kew''mi·nay'tus). PITYRIASIS RUBRA PILARIS.

lichen ruber mo·nil·i·for·mis (mo·nil''i·for'mis). A disease of unknown cause, with linear lesions of flat papules which resemble those of lichen planus.

lichen scle·ro·sus et atroph·i·cus (skle·ro'sus et a·trof'i·kus). A chronic skin disease characterized by flat-topped white macules or patches, often with a central hair follicle plugged by keratin; the neck, trunk, vulva, and glans penis are sites of predilection.

lichen scrof·u·lo·sus (skrof''yoo·lo'sus). TUBERCULOSIS LICHENOIDES.

lichen spi·nu·lo·sis (spin''yoo·lo'sus, spye''new·lo'sus). A skin disease of children, occasionally due to a vitamin-A deficiency; characterized by keratotic spines protruding from hair follicles or follicular papules.

lichen stri·a·tus (strye·ay'tus). A rare, sudden, self-limited disorder of the skin, occurring mostly in children, appearing as long strips of small lichenoid papules, usually on the extremities.

lichen trop·i·cus (trop'i·kus). MILIARIA.

lichen ur·ti·ca·tus (ur''ti·kay'tus). URTICARIA PAPULOSA.

Licht·heim's aphasia or **disease** (li^k^ht'hime) [L. *Lichtheim*, German physician, 1845–1928]. An unusual symptom of aphasia in which the patient, though unable to articulate a word, can indicate by signs the number of syllables in it. Now regarded as a historical curiosity, not a disease.

Lichtheim's syndrome [L. *Lichtheim*]. Subacute combined degeneration of the spinal cord associated with pernicious anemia.

lick, *n.* A term used in the jargon of sports medicine to denote a dazed state following a blow to the head.

lic·o·rice, liq·uo·rice (lick'ur·is) *n.* [OF., from L. *liquiritia*, from Gk. *glykyrriza*, lit., sweet-root]. GLYCYRRHIZA.

lid, *n.* EYELID.

lid drop. Ptosis of the upper eyelid.

lid lag. Lagging of the upper lid behind the eyeball when the patient looks downward, seen in thyrotoxic exophthalmos (von Graefe's sign) and other myopathies.

lid·o·caine (lid'o·kane) *n.* 2-(Diethylamino)-2',6'-acetoxylidide, $C_{14}H_{22}N_2O$, a local anesthetic; usually used as the hydrochloride salt. Syn. *lignocaine*. (*Brit.*).

li·do·fla·zine (lye''do·flay'zeen) *n.* 4-[4,4-Bis(*p*-fluorophenyl)-butyl]-1-piperazineaceto-2',6'-xylidide, $C_{30}H_{35}F_2N_3O$, a coronary vasodilator.

lid reflex. CONJUNCTIVAL REFLEX.

lid vibration test. A test for facial paralysis in which diminished vibration of the upper lid of the closed eye against resistance is used as an index of facial paralysis.

Lie·ben's test (lee'b^e^n) [A. *Lieben*, Austrian chemist, 1836–1914]. A test for acetone in urine in which to a urine distillate, sodium hydroxide and Lugol's solution are added. Turbidity changing to a yellow precipitate of iodoform is a positive test.

Lie·ber·kühn's glands (lee'bur·ku^e^n) [J. N. *Lieberkühn*, German anatomist, 1711–1756]. INTESTINAL GLANDS.

Lie·ber·mann-Bur·chard reaction or **test** (lee'bur·mahn) [L. von S. *Liebermann*, Austrian physician, 1852–1926; and H. *Burchard*]. A test for cholesterol, in which a solution of cholesterol in acetic anhydride, when treated with concentrated sulfuric acid, develops a color display going from red to purple to green.

Liebermann reaction [L. von S. *Liebermann*]. Proteins containing tryptophan give a violet or bluish color in the presence of hydrochloric acid after prior treatment of the protein with alcohol and ether.

Lie·big's test (lee'bi^k^h) [J. von *Liebig*, German chemist, 1803–1873]. 1. A test for cyanide in which to a distillate prepared from the suspected material, yellow ammonium sulfide is added and evaporated to dryness. Hydrochloric acid and ferric chloride solution are added to the residue. A deep red color indicates the presence of cyanide. 2. A test for cystine in which the substance is boiled with caustic alkali containing lead oxide. In the presence of cystine, a precipitate of black lead sulfide is formed.

lie detector. An instrument such as a polygraph used to record graphically changes in pulse rate, respiration, blood pressure, and perspiration in a person confronted by questions pertaining to past behavior; sudden marked changes are assumed to be indicative of a repressed sense of guilt or fear of detection when answering a question untruthfully. See also *Keeler's lie detector.*

li·en (lye'en) *n.*, genit. **li·e·nis** (lye·ee'nis) [L.] [NA]. SPLEEN. —**li·enal** (lye·ee'nul, lye'e·nul) *adj.*

lien-, lieno- [L. *lien*]. A combining form meaning *spleen, splenic.*

lien ac·ces·so·ri·us (ack·se·sor'ee·us) [NA]. ACCESSORY SPLEEN.

lienal recess. The extension of the omental bursa to the left toward the hilus of the spleen. NA *recessus lienalis.*

li·en·cu·lus (lye·eng'kew·lus) *n.*, pl. **liencu·li** (·lye) [NL., dim. from *lien,* spleen]. ACCESSORY SPLEEN.

lienic penicilli. PENICILLI LIENIS.

li·en·itis (lye''e·nigh'tis) *n.* [*lien-* + *-itis*]. SPLENITIS.

lieno-. See *lien-.*

li·eno·cele (lye·ee'no·seel, lye''e·no·) *n.* [*lieno-* + *-cele*]. Hernia of the spleen.

li·en·og·ra·phy (lye''e·nog'ruh·fee) *n.* [*lieno-* + *-graphy*]. Radiography of the spleen.

li·eno·ma·la·cia (lye·ee''no·ma·lay'shee·uh, lye''e·no·) *n.* [*lieno-* + *-malacia*]. Abnormal softening of the spleen.

li·eno·my·e·lo·ma·la·cia (lye·ee''no·migh''e·lo·ma·lay'shee·uh) *n.* [*lieno-* + *myelo-* + *malacia*]. Abnormal softening of the spleen and bone marrow.

li·en·op·a·thy (lye''e·nop'uth·ee) *n.* [*lieno-* + *-pathy*]. Disease of the spleen.

li·eno·re·nal (lye·ee''no·ree'nul, lye''e·no·) *adj.* [*lieno-* + *renal*]. Pertaining to the spleen and the kidneys; SPLENORENAL.

lienorenal ligament. PHRENICOLIENAL LIGAMENT.

lienorenal shunt. SPLENORENAL SHUNT.

li·eno·tox·in (lye·ee''no·tock'sin, lye''e·no·) *n.* [*lieno-* + *toxin*]. A cytotoxin with specific action on spleen cells.

lienteric diarrhea. Diarrhea with stools containing undigested food.

li·en·tery (lye'un·terr''ee) *n.* [Gk. *leienteria,* from *leios,* smooth, soft, + *entera,* bowels]. LIENTERIC DIARRHEA. —**lien·ter·ic** (·terr'ick) *adj.*

li·en·un·cu·lus (lye''un·ung'kew·lus) *n.*, pl. **lienuncu·li** (·lye) [NL., dim. from *lien,* spleen]. ACCESSORY SPLEEN.

Liep·mann's apraxia (leep'mahn) [H. C. *Liepmann,* German neurologist, 1863–1925]. APRAXIA.

Lie·se·gang's phenomenon (lee'zᵉ·gahng) [R. E. *Liesegang,* German chemist, 1869–1947]. A rhythmic precipitation of salts in colloids in the form of concentric rings, which may occur in calculus formation.

life, *n.* The sum of properties by which an organism grows, reproduces, maintains its structure, and adapts itself to its environment; the quality by which an organism differs from inorganic or dead organic bodies.

life-buoy cataract. DISC-SHAPED CATARACT.

life cycle. 1. The characteristic sequence of changes beginning with any given stage in the life of a particular kind of organism and ending with the first recurrence of that stage in its descendants. 2. The sequence of biologically significant periods in the lifetime of an individual.

life expectancy. EXPECTATION OF LIFE.

life instinct. EROS.

life insurance method. BENEDICT'S PICRATE METHOD.

life insurance method for protein. Clarified urine is treated with sulfosalicylic acid and the turbidity is compared with artificial standards.

li·fi·brate (li·fye'·brate) *n.* Bis(4-chlorophenoxy)acetic acid, 1-methyl-4-piperdinyl ester, $C_{20}H_{21}Cl_2NO_4$, an antihyperlipidemic.

lig·a·ment (lig'uh·munt) *n.* [L. *ligamentum,* from *ligare,* to tie, bind]. 1. A band of flexible, tough, dense white fibrous connective tissue connecting the articular ends of the bones, and sometimes enveloping them in a capsule. Syn. *ligamentum.* For ligaments listed according to associated joint, see Table of Synovial Joints and Ligaments in the Appendix. See also Plate 2. 2. Certain folds and processes of the peritoneum.

ligamenta. Plural of *ligamentum* (= LIGAMENT).

ligamenta ac·ces·so·ria plan·ta·ria (ack''se·so'ree·uh plan·tair'ee·uh) [BNA]. Ligamenta plantaria articulationum metatarsophalangearum. See *plantar ligaments.*

ligamenta accessoria vo·la·ria (vo·lair'i·uh) [BNA]. Ligamenta palmaria articulationum metacarpophalangearum. See *palmar ligaments.*

ligamenta ala·ria ar·ti·cu·la·tio·nis at·lan·to·ax·i·a·lis me·di·a·nae (ay·lair'ee·uh ahr·tick''yoo·lay·shee·o'nis at·lan''to·ack·see·ay'lis mee·dee·ay'nee) [NA]. ALAR ODONTOID LIGAMENTS.

ligamenta an·nu·la·ria di·gi·to·rum ma·nus (an·yoo·lair'ee·uh dij·i·to'rum man'us) [BNA]. PARS ANULARIS VAGINAE FIBROSAE DIGITORUM MANUS.

ligamenta annularia digitorum pe·dis (ped'is) [BNA]. PARS ANULARIS VAGINAE FIBROSAE DIGITORUM PEDIS.

ligamenta annularia tra·che·a·lia (tray·kee·ay'lee·uh) [BNA]. LIGAMENTA ANULARIA TRACHEALIA.

ligamenta anu·la·ria tra·che·a·lia (an''yoo·lair'ee·uh tray·kee·ay'lee·uh) [NA]. The portions of the membranous wall of the trachea between the tracheal cartilages.

ligamenta au·ri·cu·la·ria (aw·rick''yoo·lair'ee·uh) [NA]. AURICULAR LIGAMENTS.

ligamenta ba·si·um os·si·um me·ta·car·pa·li·um dor·sa·lia (bay'see·um os'ee·um met''uh·kahr·pay'lee·um dor·say'lee·uh) [BNA]. Ligamenta metacarpea dorsalia. See *metacarpal ligament.*

ligamenta basium ossium metacarpalium in·ter·os·sea (in''tur·os'ee·uh) [BNA]. Ligamenta metacarpea interossea. See *metacarpal ligament.*

ligamenta basium ossium metacarpalium vo·la·ria (vo·lair'ee·uh) [BNA]. Ligamenta metacarpea palmaria. See *metacarpal ligament.*

ligamenta basium ossium me·ta·tar·sa·li·um dor·sa·lia (met''uh·tahr·say'lee·um dor·say'lee·uh) [BNA]. LIGAMENTA METATARSEA DORSALIA.

ligamenta basium ossium metatarsalium in·ter·os·sea (in·tur·os'ee·uh) [BNA]. LIGAMENTA METATARSEA INTEROSSEA.

ligamenta basium ossium metatarsalium plan·ta·ria (plan·tair'ee·uh) [BNA]. LIGAMENTA METATARSEA PLANTARIA.

ligamenta ca·pi·tu·li fi·bu·lae (ka·pit'yoo·lye fib'yoo·lee) [BNA]. The ligaments of the head of the fibula. See *ligamentum capitis fibulae anterius, ligamentum capitis fibulae posterius.*

ligamenta ca·pi·tu·lo·rum os·si·um me·ta·car·pa·li·um trans·ver·sa (ka·pit·yoo·lo'rum os'ee·um met''uh·kahr·pay'lee·um trans·vur'suh) [BNA]. The transverse ligaments joining the heads of adjacent metacarpal bones; now described as one continuous band, the deep transverse metacarpal ligament.

ligamenta capitulorum ossium me·ta·tar·sa·li·um trans·ver·sa (met''uh·tahr·say'lee·um trans·vur'suh) [BNA]. The transverse ligaments joining the heads of adjacent metatarsal bones; now described as one continuous band, the deep transverse metatarsal ligament.

ligamenta car·po·me·ta·car·pea dor·sa·lia (kahr''po·met·uh·kahr'pee·uh dor·say'lee·uh), sing. **ligamentum carpometa·car·pe·um dorsa·le** [NA]. The dorsal carpometacarpal ligaments. See *carpometacarpal ligament.*

ligamenta carpometacarpea pal·ma·ria (pal·mair'ee·uh), sing. **ligamentum carpometacarpeum palma·re** [NA]. The palmar carpometacarpal ligaments. See *carpometacarpal ligament.*

ligamenta carpometacarpea vo·la·ria (vo·lair'ee·uh) [BNA]. Ligamenta carpometacarpea palmaria. See *carpometacarpal ligament.*

ligamenta ce·ra·to·cri·coi·dea la·te·ra·lia (serr"uh·to·kri·koy' dee·uh lat·e·ray'lee·uh) [BNA]. Fibrous bands from the tip of the inferior cornu of the thyroid cartilage to the lateral side of the cricoid cartilage.

ligamenta ceratocricoidea pos·te·ri·o·ra (pos·teer"ee·o'ruh) [BNA]. Fibrous bands from the tip of the inferior cornu of the thyroid cartilage to the posterior part of the cricoid cartilage.

ligamenta cin·gu·li ex·tre·mi·ta·tis in·fe·ri·o·ris (sing'gew·lye eck·strem"i·tay'tis in·feer"ee·o'ris) [BNA]. A general term for the ligaments of the lower extremity.

ligamenta cinguli extremitatis su·pe·ri·o·ris (sue·peer"ee·o' ris) [BNA]. A general term for the ligaments of the upper extremity.

ligamenta col·la·te·ra·lia ar·ti·cu·la·tio·num di·gi·to·rum ma·nus (ko·lat"e·ray'lee·uh ahr·tick"yoo·lay·shee·o'num dij·i·to'rum man'us) [BNA]. LIGAMENTA COLLATERALIA ARTICULATIONUM INTERPHALANGEARUM MANUS.

ligamenta collateralia articulationum digitorum pe·dis (ped' is) [BNA]. LIGAMENTA COLLATERALIA ARTICULATIONUM INTERPHALANGEARUM PEDIS.

ligamenta collateralia articulationum in·ter·pha·lan·ge·a·rum ma·nus (in"tur·fa·lan"jee·air'um man'us) [NA]. The collateral ligaments of the interphalangeal joints of the hand. See also *collateral ligament.*

ligamenta collateralia articulationum interphalangearum ped·is (ped'is) [NA]. The collateral ligaments of the interphalangeal joints of the foot. See also *collateral ligament.*

ligamenta collateralia articulationum me·ta·car·po·pha·lan·ge·a·rum (met"uh·kahr"po·fa·lan·jee·air'um) [NA]. The collateral ligaments of the metacarpophalangeal joints. See also *collateral ligament.*

ligamenta collateralia articulationum me·ta·tar·so·pha·lan·ge·a·rum (met"uh·tahr"so·fa·lan·jee·air'um) [NA]. The collateral ligaments of the metatarsophalangeal joints. See also *collateral ligament.*

ligamenta co·lum·nae ver·te·bra·lis et cra·nii (ko·lum'nee vur·te·bray'lis et kray'nee·eye) [BNA]. A general term for the ligaments of the vertebral column and cranium.

ligamenta cos·to·xi·phoi·dea (kos"to·zi·foy'dee·uh) [NA]. COSTOXIPHOID LIGAMENTS.

ligamenta cru·ci·a·ta di·gi·to·rum ma·nus (kroo·shee·ay'tuh dij·i·to'rum man'us) [BNA]. PARS CRUCIFORMIS VAGINAE FIBROSAE DIGITORUM MANUS.

ligamenta cruciata digitorum pe·dis (ped'is) [BNA]. PARS CRUCIFORMIS VAGINAE FIBROSAE DIGITORUM PEDIS.

ligamenta cruciata ge·nu (jen'yoo) [BNA]. Ligamenta cruciata genus. See *cruciate ligament.*

ligamenta cruciata ge·nus (jen'us) [NA]. The cruciate ligaments of the knee. See *cruciate ligament.*

ligamenta cu·neo·me·ta·tar·sea in·ter·os·sea (kew"nee·o·met·uh·tahr'see·uh in"tur·os'ee·uh) [NA]. INTEROSSEOUS CUNEOMETATARSAL LIGAMENTS.

ligamenta cu·neo·na·vi·cu·la·ria dor·sa·lia (kew"nee·o·na·vick"yoo·lair'ee·uh dor·say'lee·uh) [NA]. The dorsal cuneonavicular ligaments, passing from the dorsal surface of the navicular to the dorsal surfaces of the cuneiform bones.

ligamenta cuneonavicularia plan·ta·ria (plan·tair'ee·uh) [NA]. The plantar cuneonavicular ligaments, which pass from the plantar surface of the navicular to the plantar surfaces of the cuneiform bones.

ligamenta ex·tra·cap·su·la·ria (ecks"truh·kap·sue·lair'ee·uh) [NA]. A general term for ligaments which are outside the capsular ligament of a joint.

ligamenta fla·va (flay'vuh) [BNA]. Plural of *ligamentum flavum.*

ligamenta gle·no·hu·me·ra·lia (glen"o·hew·me·ray'lee·uh) [NA]. GLENOHUMERAL LIGAMENTS.

ligamenta in·ter·car·pea dor·sa·lia (in"tur·kahr'pee·uh dor·say'lee·uh) [NA]. The dorsal intercarpal ligaments. See *intercarpal ligament.*

ligamenta intercarpea in·ter·os·sea (in"tur·os'ee·uh) [NA]. The interosseous intercarpal ligaments. See *intercarpal ligament.*

ligamenta intercarpea pal·ma·ria (pal·mair'ee·uh) [NA]. The palmar intercarpal ligaments. See *intercarpal ligament.*

ligamenta intercarpea vo·la·ria (vo·lair'ee·uh) [BNA]. Ligamenta intercarpea palmaria. See *intercarpal ligament.*

ligamenta in·ter·cos·ta·lia (in"tur·kos·tay'lee·uh) [BNA]. Ligaments between the ribs; INTERCOSTAL MEMBRANES.

ligamenta intercostalia ex·ter·na (ecks·tur'nuh) [BNA]. Membrana intercostalis externa. See *intercostal membrane.*

ligamenta intercostalia in·ter·na (in·tur'nuh) [BNA]. Membrana intercostalis interna. See *intercostal membrane.*

ligamenta in·ter·cu·ne·i·for·mia dor·sa·lia (in"tur·kew·nee·i·for'mee·uh dor·say'lee·uh) [NA]. The two dorsal intercuneiform ligaments, which connect the dorsal surfaces of the three cuneiform bones.

ligamenta intercuneiformia in·ter·os·sea (in"tur·os'ee·uh) [NA]. The interosseous intercuneiform ligaments, which connect the facing surfaces of the cuneiform bones.

ligamenta intercuneiformia plan·ta·ria (plan·tair'ee·uh) [NA]. The two plantar intercuneiform ligaments which connect the plantar surfaces of the cuneiform bones.

ligamenta in·ter·spi·na·lia (in"tur·spye·nay'lee·uh) [BNA]. Plural of *ligamentum interspinale.*

ligamenta in·ter·trans·ver·sa·ria (in"tur·trans·vur·sair'ee·uh) [BNA]. Plural of *ligamentum intertransversarium* (= INTERTRANSVERSE LIGAMENT).

ligamenta in·tra·cap·su·la·ria (in"truh·kap"sue·lair'ee·uh) [NA]. Ligaments which are within the joint capsule of a joint.

lig·a·men·tal (lig"uh·men'tul) *adj.* Of or pertaining to a ligament or ligaments.

ligamenta me·ta·car·pea dor·sa·lia (met"uh·kahr'pee·uh dor·say'lee·uh) [NA]. The dorsal metacarpal ligaments. See *metacarpal ligament.*

ligamenta metacarpea in·ter·os·sea (in·tur·os'ee·uh) [NA]. The interosseous metacarpal ligaments. See *metacarpal ligament.*

ligamenta metacarpea pal·ma·ria (pal·mair'ee·uh) [NA]. The palmar metacarpal ligaments. See *metacarpal ligament.*

ligamenta me·ta·tar·sea dor·sa·lia (met"uh·tahr'see·uh dor·say'lee·uh) [NA]. The dorsal metatarsal ligaments, which connect the dorsal surfaces of the bases of the lateral four metatarsal bones.

ligamenta metatarsea in·ter·os·sea (in"tur·os'ee·uh) [NA]. The interosseous metatarsal ligaments, which connect the facing surfaces of the bases of the five metatarsal bones.

ligamenta metatarsea plan·ta·ria (plan·tair'ee·uh) [NA]. The plantar metatarsal ligaments, which connect the plantar surfaces of the bases of the lateral four metatarsal bones.

ligamenta os·si·cu·lo·rum au·di·tus (os·ick·yoo·lo'rum aw·dye'tus, aw'di·tus) [NA]. The ligaments associated with the bones of the middle ear.

ligamenta pal·ma·ria ar·ti·cu·la·ti·o·num in·ter·pha·lan·ge·a·rum ma·nus (pal·mair'ee·uh ahr·tick"yoo·lay·shee·o'num in·tur·fa·lan·jee·air'um man'us) [NA]. The palmar ligaments of the interphalangeal joints of the hand. See *palmar ligaments.*

ligamenta palmaria articulationum me·ta·car·po·pha·lan·ge·a·rum (met"uh·kahr"po·fa·lan·jee·air'um) [NA]. The palmar ligaments of the metacarpophalangeal joints. See *palmar ligaments.*

ligamenta plan·ta·ria ar·ti·cu·la·ti·o·num in·ter·pha·lan·ge·a·rum pe·dis (plan·tair'ee·uh ahr·tick"yoo·lay·shee·o'num in"tur·fa·lan·jee·air'um ped'is) [NA]. The plantar ligaments of the interphalangeal joints of the foot. See *plantar ligaments.*

ligamenta plantaria articulationum me·ta·tar·so·pha·lan·ge·a·rum (met·uh·tahr″so·fa·lan·jee·air′um) [NA]. The plantar ligaments of the metatarsophalangeal joints. See *plantar ligaments.*

ligamenta py·lo·ri (pi·lo′rye) [BNA]. Longitudinal bands of fibromuscular tissue on the anterior and posterior aspects of the pyloric area.

ligamenta sa·cro·ili·a·ca an·te·ri·o·ra (sack·ro·i·lye′uh·kuh an·teer·ee·o′ruh) [BNA]. Ligamenta sacroiliaca ventralia (= VENTRAL SACROILIAC LIGAMENTS).

ligamenta sacroiliaca dor·sa·lia (dor·say′lee·uh) [NA]. DORSAL SACROILIAC LIGAMENTS.

ligamenta sacroiliaca in·ter·os·sea (in″tur·os′ee·uh) [NA]. INTEROSSEOUS SACROILIAC LIGAMENTS.

ligamenta sacroiliaca ven·tra·lia (ven·tray′lee·uh) [NA]. VENTRAL SACROILIAC LIGAMENTS.

ligamenta ster·no·cos·ta·lia ra·di·a·ta (stur″no·kos·tay′lee·uh ray″dee·ay′tuh) [NA]. RADIATE STERNOCOSTAL LIGAMENTS.

ligamenta ster·no·pe·ri·car·di·a·ca (stur″no·perr·i·kahr·dye′uh·kuh) [NA]. STERNOPERICARDIAL LIGAMENTS.

ligamenta sus·pen·so·ria mam·mae (sus·pen·so′ree·uh mam′ee) [NA]. The suspensory ligaments of the breast. See *suspensory ligament.*

ligamenta tar·si dor·sa·lia (tahr′sigh dor·say′lee·uh) [NA]. The dorsal ligaments of the foot; specifically, the talonavicular, bifurcate, and dorsal intercuneiform, cuneocuboid, cuboideonavicular, and cuneonavicular ligaments.

ligamenta tarsi in·ter·os·sea (in·tur·os′ee·uh) [NA]. The interosseous ligaments of the foot; specifically, the interosseous talocalcaneal, cuneocuboid, and intercuneiform ligaments.

ligamenta tarsi plan·ta·ria (plan·tair′ee·uh) [NA]. The plantar ligaments of the foot; specifically, the long plantar and the plantar calcaneocuboid, calcaneonavicular, cuneonavicular, cuboideonavicular, intercuneiform, and cuneocuboid ligaments.

ligamenta tarsi pro·fun·da (pro·fun′duh) [BNA]. The deep ligaments of the tarsal bones.

ligamenta tar·so·me·ta·tar·sea dor·sa·lia (tahr″so·met·uh·tahr′see·uh dor·say′lee·uh) [NA]. The dorsal tarsometatarsal ligaments. See *tarsometatarsal ligament.*

ligamenta tarsometatarsea in·ter·os·sea (in·tur·os′ee·uh) [BNA]. The interosseous tarsometatarsal ligaments. See *tarsometatarsal ligament.*

ligamenta tarsometatarsea plan·ta·ria (plan·tair′ee·uh) [NA]. The plantar tarsometatarsal ligaments. See *tarsometatarsal ligament.*

ligamenta va·gi·na·lia di·gi·to·rum ma·nus (vaj·i·nay′lee·uh dij·i·to′rum man′us) [BNA]. VAGINAE FIBROSAE DIGITORUM MANUS.

ligamenta vaginalia digitorum pe·dis (ped′is) [BNA]. VAGINAE FIBROSAE DIGITORUM PEDIS.

ligament of Cooper [A. P. *Cooper*]. 1. Any of the suspensory ligaments of the breast. See *suspensory ligament.* 2. A band of fibrous connective tissue overlying the pecten of the pubis.

ligament of the left vena cava. A fold of pericardium, between the left pulmonary artery and the left superior pulmonary vein, enclosing the fibrous remnant of part of the left common cardinal vein. NA *plica venae cavae sinistrae.*

ligament of Treitz [W. *Treitz*]. The suspensory ligament of the duodenum. See *suspensory ligament.*

ligament of Zinn [J. G. *Zinn*]. The fibrous ring from which arise the four rectus muscles of the eye and which is attached to the dural sheath of the optic nerve and to the upper and medial margins of the optic canal; it bridges the superior orbital fissure. NA *anulus tendineus communis.*

lig·a·men·to·pexy (lig″uh·men′to·peck″see) *n.* [*ligament* + *-pexy*]. Suspension of the uterus by shortening or fixation of the round ligaments.

lig·a·men·tous (lig″uh·men′tus) *adj.* Of or pertaining to a ligament or ligaments.

ligamentous ankylosis. FIBROUS ANKYLOSIS.

lig·a·men·tum (lig″uh·men′tum) *n.*, pl. **ligamen·ta** (·tuh) [L.]. LIGAMENT.

ligamentum acro·mio·cla·vi·cu·la·re (a·kro″mee·o·kla·vick·yoo·lair′ee) [NA]. ACROMIOCLAVICULAR LIGAMENT.

ligamentum an·nu·la·re ba·se·os sta·pe·dis (an″yoo·lair′ee bay′see·os sta·pee′dis) [BNA]. Ligamentum anulare stapedis. See *annular ligament.*

ligamentum annulare ra·dii (ray′dee·eye) [BNA]. Ligamentum anulare radii. See *annular ligament.*

ligamentum ano·coc·cy·ge·um (ay″no·kock·sij′ee·um) [NA]. ANOCOCCYGEAL LIGAMENT.

ligamentum anu·la·re ra·dii (an·yoo·lair′ee ray′dee·eye) [NA]. The annular ligament of the radius. See *annular ligament.*

ligamentum anulare sta·pe·dis (sta·pee′dis) [NA]. The annular ligament of the stapedial base. See *annular ligament.*

ligamentum api·cis den·tis (ay′pi·sis den·tis) [NA]. APICAL DENTAL LIGAMENT.

ligamentum ar·cu·a·tum la·te·ra·le (ahr·kew·ay′tum lat·e·ray′lee) [NA]. LATERAL ARCUATE LIGAMENT.

ligamentum arcuatum me·di·a·le (mee·dee·ay′lee) [NA]. MEDIAL ARCUATE LIGAMENT.

ligamentum arcuatum me·di·a·num (mee·dee·ay′num) [NA]. MEDIAN ARCUATE LIGAMENT.

ligamentum arcuatum pu·bis (pew′bis) [NA]. ARCUATE PUBIC LIGAMENT.

ligamentum ar·te·ri·o·sum (ahr·teer·ee·o′sum) [NA]. The remains of the fetal ductus arteriosus, extending from the pulmonary trunk to the arch of the aorta.

ligamentum at·lan·to·oc·ci·pi·ta·lis (at·lan″to·ock·sip·i·tay′lis). Membrana atlantooccipitalis anterior (= ANTERIOR ATLANTOOCCIPITAL MEMBRANE).

ligamentum atlantooccipitalis lateralis [NA]. LATERAL ATLANTOOCCIPITAL LIGAMENT.

ligamentum au·ri·cu·la·re an·te·ri·us (aw·rick″yoo·lair′ee an·teer′ee·us) [NA]. The anterior auricular ligament. See *auricular ligament.*

ligamentum auriculare pos·te·ri·us (pos·teer′ee·us) [NA]. The posterior auricular ligament. See *auricular ligament.*

ligamentum auriculare su·pe·ri·us (sue·peer′ee·us) [NA]. The superior auricular ligament. See *auricular ligament.*

ligamentum bi·fur·ca·tum (bye·fur·kay′tum) [NA]. BIFURCATE LIGAMENT.

ligamentum cal·ca·neo·cu·boi·de·um (kal·kay″nee·o·kew·boy′dee·um) [NA]. CALCANEOCUBOID LIGAMENT.

ligamentum calcaneocuboideum plan·ta·re (plan·tair′ee) [NA]. PLANTAR CALCANEOCUBOID LIGAMENT.

ligamentum cal·ca·neo·fi·bu·la·re (kal·kay″nee·o·fib·yoo·lair′ee) [NA]. CALCANEOFIBULAR LIGAMENT.

ligamentum cal·ca·neo·na·vi·cu·la·re (kal·kay″nee·o·na·vick″yoo·lair′ee) [NA]. CALCANEONAVICULAR LIGAMENT.

ligamentum calcaneonaviculare dor·sa·le (dor·say′lee) [BNA]. A ligament between the dorsal surfaces of the navicular and the calcaneus.

ligamentum calcaneonaviculare plan·ta·re (plan·tair′ee) [NA]. PLANTAR CALCANEONAVICULAR LIGAMENT.

ligamentum cal·ca·neo·ti·bi·a·le (kal·kay″nee·o·tib″ee·ay′lee) [BNA]. PARS TIBIOCALCANEA LIGAMENTI MEDIALIS.

ligamentum ca·pi·tis cos·tae in·tra·ar·ti·cu·la·re (kap′i·tis kos′tee in″truh·ahr·tick″yoo·lair′ee) [NA]. The intraarticular ligament of the joint of the head of a rib with a vertebra.

ligamentum capitis costae ra·di·a·tum (ray·dee·ay′tum) [NA]. RADIATE LIGAMENT (1).

ligamentum capitis fe·mo·ris (fem′o·ris) [NA]. The round ligament of the femur. See *round ligament.*

ligamentum capitis fi·bu·lae an·te·ri·us (fib′yoo·lee an·teer′ee·us) [NA]. The anterior ligament of the head of the fibula;

the anterior band or bands connecting the head of the fibula and the lateral condyle of the tibia.

ligamentum capitis fibulae pos·te·ri·us (pos·teer'ee·us) [NA]. The posterior ligament of the head of the fibula; the posterior band connecting the head of the fibula and the lateral condyle of the tibia.

ligamentum ca·pi·tu·li cos·tae in·ter·ar·ti·cu·la·re (ka·pit'yoo·lye kos'tee in"tur·ahr·tick·yoo·lair'ee) [BNA]. LIGAMENTUM CAPITIS COSTAE INTRAARTICULARE.

ligamentum capituli costae ra·di·a·tum (ray·dee·ay'tum) [BNA]. Ligamentum capitis costae radiatum (= RADIATE LIGAMENT (1)).

ligamentum car·pi dor·sa·le (kahr'pye dor·say'lee) [BNA]. Retinaculum extensorum manus (= EXTENSOR RETINACULUM OF THE WRIST).

ligamentum carpi ra·di·a·tum (ray·dee·ay'tum) [NA]. RADIATE CARPAL LIGAMENT.

ligamentum carpi trans·ver·sum (kahr'pye trans·vur'sum) [BNA]. Retinaculum flexorum manus (= FLEXOR RETINACULUM OF THE WRIST).

ligamentum carpi vo·la·re (vo·lair'ee) [BNA]. CARPAL PALMAR LIGAMENT.

ligamentum cau·da·le (kaw·day'lee) [BNA]. RETINACULUM CAUDALE.

ligamentum ce·ra·to·cri·coi·de·um an·te·ri·us (serr"uh·to·kri·koy'dee·um an·teer'ee·us) [BNA]. An anterior ligament between the tip of the inferior cornu of the thyroid cartilage and the cricoid cartilage.

ligamentum col·la·te·ra·le car·pi ra·di·a·le (ko·lat·e·ray'lee kahr'pye ray·di·ay'lee) [NA]. The radial collateral ligament of the wrist. See *radial collateral ligament.*

ligamentum collaterale carpi ul·na·re (ul·nair'ee) [NA]. The ulnar collateral ligament of the wrist. See *ulnar collateral ligament.*

ligamentum collaterale fi·bu·la·re (fib·yoo·lair'ee) [NA]. FIBULAR COLLATERAL LIGAMENT.

ligamentum collaterale ra·di·a·le (ray·dee·ay'lee) [NA]. The radial collateral ligament of the elbow. See *radial collateral ligament.*

ligamentum collaterale ti·bi·a·le (tib·i·ay'lee) [NA]. TIBIAL COLLATERAL LIGAMENT.

ligamentum collaterale ul·na·re (ul·nair'ee) [NA]. The ulnar collateral ligament of the elbow. See *ulnar collateral ligament.*

ligamentum col·li cos·tae (kol'eye kos'tee) [BNA]. Ligamentum costotransversarium (= COSTOTRANSVERSE LIGAMENT).

ligamentum co·noi·de·um (ko·noy'dee·um) [NA]. CONOID LIGAMENT.

ligamentum co·ra·co·acro·mi·a·le (kor"uh·ko·a·kro"mee·ay'lee) [NA]. CORACOACROMIAL LIGAMENT.

ligamentum co·ra·co·cla·vi·cu·la·re (kor"uh·ko·kla·vick"yoo·lair'ee) [NA]. CORACOCLAVICULAR LIGAMENT.

ligamentum co·ra·co·hu·me·ra·le (kor"uh·ko·hew·me·ray'lee) [NA]. CORACOHUMERAL LIGAMENT.

ligamentum co·ro·na·ri·um he·pa·tis (kor"o·nair'ee·um hep'uh·tis) [NA]. The coronary ligament of the liver. See *coronary ligament.*

ligamentum cos·to·cla·vi·cu·la·re (kos"to·kla·vick"yoo·lair'ee) [NA]. COSTOCLAVICULAR LIGAMENT.

ligamentum cos·to·trans·ver·sa·ri·um (kos"to·trans"vur·sair'ee·um) [NA]. COSTOTRANSVERSE LIGAMENT.

ligamentum costotransversarium an·te·ri·us (an·teer'ee·us) [BNA]. Ligamentum costotransversarium superius (= SUPERIOR COSTOTRANSVERSE LIGAMENT).

ligamentum costotransversarium la·te·ra·le (lat·e·ray'lee) [NA]. LATERAL COSTOTRANSVERSE LIGAMENT.

ligamentum costotransversarium pos·te·ri·us (pos·teer'ee·us) [BNA]. Ligamentum costotransversarium laterale (= LATERAL COSTOTRANSVERSE LIGAMENT).

ligamentum costotransversarium su·pe·ri·us (sue·peer'ee·us) [NA]. SUPERIOR COSTOTRANSVERSE LIGAMENT.

ligamentum cri·co·ary·te·noi·de·um pos·te·ri·us (krye"ko·ăr·i·tee·noy'dee·um pos·teer'ee·us) [NA]. POSTERIOR CRICOARYTENOID LIGAMENT.

ligamentum cri·co·pha·ryn·ge·um (krye"ko·fa·rin'jee·um) [NA]. CRICOPHARYNGEAL LIGAMENT.

ligamentum cri·co·thy·re·oi·de·um (krye"ko·thigh·ree·oy'dee·um) [BNA]. Ligamentum cricothyroideum (= CRICOTHYROID LIGAMENT).

ligamentum cri·co·thy·roi·de·um (krye"ko·thigh·roy'dee·um) [NA]. CRICOTHYROID LIGAMENT.

ligamentum cri·co·tra·che·a·le (krye"ko·tray·kee·ay'lee) [NA]. CRICOTRACHEAL LIGAMENT.

ligamentum cru·ci·a·tum an·te·ri·us (krew·see·ay'tum an·teer'ee·us) [NA]. The anterior cruciate ligament of the knee. See *cruciate ligament.*

ligamentum cruciatum at·lan·tis (at·lan'tis) [BNA]. Ligamentum cruciforme atlantis. See *cruciate ligament.*

ligamentum cruciatum cru·ris (kroo'ris) [BNA]. Retinaculum musculorum extensorum pedis inferius (= INFERIOR EXTENSOR RETINACULUM).

ligamentum cruciatum pos·te·ri·us (pos·teer'ee·us) [NA]. The posterior cruciate ligament of the knee. See *cruciate ligament.*

ligamentum cru·ci·for·me at·lan·tis (kroo·si·for'mee at·lan'tis) [NA]. The cruciate ligament of the atlas. See *cruciate ligament.*

ligamentum cu·boi·deo·na·vi·cu·la·re dor·sa·le (kew·boy"dee·o·na·vick"yoo·lair'ee dor·say'lee) [NA]. The dorsal cuboideonavicular ligament, which connects the dorsal surfaces of the cuboid and navicular.

ligamentum cuboideonaviculare plan·ta·re (plan·tair'ee) [NA]. The plantar cuboideonavicular ligament, which connects the plantar surfaces of the navicular and cuboid.

ligamentum cu·neo·cu·boi·de·um dor·sa·le (kew"nee·o·kew·boy'dee·um dor·say'lee) [NA]. The dorsal cuneocuboid ligament, which connects the dorsal surfaces of the cuboid and lateral cuneiform.

ligamentum cuneocuboideum in·ter·os·se·um (in"tur·os'ee·um) [NA]. The interosseous cuneocuboid ligament, which connects the facing surfaces of the cuboid and lateral cuneiform.

ligamentum cuneocuboideum plan·ta·re (plan·tair'ee) [NA]. The plantar cuneocuboid ligament, which connects the plantar surfaces of the cuboid and lateral cuneiform.

ligamentum del·toi·de·um (del·toy'dee·um) [NA alt.]. MEDIAL LIGAMENT. NA alt. *ligamentum mediale.*

ligamentum den·ti·cu·la·tum (den·tick"yoo·lay'tum) [NA]. DENTATE LIGAMENT.

ligamentum du·o·de·no·re·na·le (dew·o·dee"no·re·nay'lee) [BNA]. A fold of peritoneum between the duodenum and the right kidney.

ligamentum epi·di·dy·mi·dis in·fe·ri·us (ep"i·di·dim'i·dis in·feer'ee·us) [NA]. INFERIOR LIGAMENT OF THE EPIDIDYMIS.

ligamentum epididymidis su·pe·ri·us (sue·peer'ee·us) [NA]. SUPERIOR LIGAMENT OF THE EPIDIDYMIS.

ligamentum fal·ci·for·me he·pa·tis (fal·si·for'mee hep'uh·tis) [NA]. FALCIFORM LIGAMENT OF THE LIVER.

ligamentum fla·vum (flay'vum) [NA]. Yellow elastic tissue that connects the laminas of contiguous vertebrae.

ligamentum fun·di·for·me pe·nis (fun·di·for'mee pee'nis) [NA]. FUNDIFORM LIGAMENT OF THE PENIS.

ligamentum gas·tro·co·li·cum (gas·tro·ko'li·kum) [NA]. GASTROCOLIC LIGAMENT.

ligamentum gas·tro·li·e·na·le (gas"tro·lye·e·nay'lee) [NA]. GASTROSPLENIC LIGAMENT.

ligamentum gas·tro·phre·ni·cum (gas"tro·fren'i·kum) [NA]. GASTROPHRENIC LIGAMENT.

ligamentum ge·ni·to·in·gui·na·le (jen"i·to·ing·gwi·nay'lee) [NA]. The precursor of the gubernaculum of the testis.

ligamentum he·pa·to·co·li·cum (hep"uh·to·ko'li·kum) [NA]. HEPATOCOLIC LIGAMENT.

ligamentum he·pa·to·du·o·de·na·le (hep″uh·to·dew″o·de·nay′lee) [NA]. HEPATODUODENAL LIGAMENT.

ligamentum he·pa·to·gas·tri·cum (hep″uh·to·gas′tri·kum) [NA]. GASTROHEPATIC LIGAMENT.

ligamentum he·pa·to·re·na·le (hep″uh·to·re·nay′lee) [NA]. HEPATORENAL LIGAMENT.

ligamentum hyo·epi·glot·ti·cum (high″o·ep·i·glot′i·kum) [NA]. HYOEPIGLOTTIC LIGAMENT.

ligamentum hyo·thy·re·oi·de·um la·te·ra·le (high″o·thigh·ree·oy′dee·um lat·e·ray′lee) [BNA]. Ligamentum thyrohyoideum (= LATERAL THYROHYOID LIGAMENT).

ligamentum hyothyreoideum medium [BNA]. Ligamentum thyrohyoideum medianum (= MEDIAN THYROHYOID LIGAMENT).

ligamentum ilio·fe·mo·ra·le (il″ee·o·fem·o·ray′lee) [NA]. ILIOFEMORAL LIGAMENT.

ligamentum ilio·lum·ba·le (il″ee·o·lum·bay′lee) [NA]. ILIOLUMBAR LIGAMENT.

ligamentum in·cu·dis pos·te·ri·us (ing·kew′dis pos·teer′ee·us) [NA]. POSTERIOR LIGAMENT OF THE INCUS.

ligamentum incudis su·pe·ri·us (sue·peer′ee·us) [NA]. SUPERIOR LIGAMENT OF THE INCUS.

ligamentum in·gui·na·le (ing·gwi·nay′lee) [NA]. INGUINAL LIGAMENT.

ligamentum in·ter·cla·vi·cu·la·re (in″tur·kla·vick·yoo·lair′ee) [NA]. INTERCLAVICULAR LIGAMENT.

ligamentum in·ter·fo·ve·o·la·re (in″tur·fo″vee·o·lair′ee) [NA]. INTERFOVEOLAR LIGAMENT.

ligamentum in·ter·spi·na·le (in″tur·spye·nay′lee) [NA]. INTERSPINAL LIGAMENT.

ligamentum in·ter·trans·ver·sa·ri·um (in″tur·trans″vur·sair′ee·um) [NA]. INTERTRANSVERSE LIGAMENT.

ligamentum is·chio·cap·su·la·re (is″kee·o·kap″sue·lair′ee) [BNA]. Ligamentum ischiofemorale (= ISCHIOFEMORAL LIGAMENT).

ligamentum is·chio·fe·mo·ra·le (is″kee·o·fem·o·ray′lee) [NA]. ISCHIOFEMORAL LIGAMENT.

ligamentum la·ci·ni·a·tum (la·sin·ee·ay′tum) [BNA]. Retinaculum musculorum flexorum pedis (= FLEXOR RETINACULUM OF THE ANKLE).

ligamentum la·cu·na·re (lack·yoo·nair′ee) [NA]. LACUNAR LIGAMENT.

ligamentum la·te·ra·le (lat·e·ray′lee) [NA]. LATERAL LIGAMENT OF THE TEMPOROMANDIBULAR JOINT.

ligamentum la·tum ute·ri (lay′tum yoo′tur·eye) [NA]. BROAD LIGAMENT OF THE UTERUS.

ligamentum li·e·no·re·na·le (lye·ee′no·re·nay′lee) [NA alt.]. PHRENICOLIENAL LIGAMENT. NA alt. *ligamentum phrenicolienale.*

ligamentum lon·gi·tu·di·na·le an·te·ri·us (lon″ji·tew·di·nay′lee an·teer′ee·us) [NA]. ANTERIOR LONGITUDINAL LIGAMENT.

ligamentum longitudinale pos·te·ri·us (pos·teer′ee·us) [NA]. POSTERIOR LONGITUDINAL LIGAMENT.

ligamentum lum·bo·cos·ta·le (lum″bo·kos·tay′lee) [NA]. LUMBOCOSTAL LIGAMENT.

ligamentum mal·lei an·te·ri·us (mal′ee·eye an·teer′ee·us) [NA]. ANTERIOR LIGAMENT OF THE MALLEUS.

ligamentum mallei la·te·ra·le (lat·e·ray′lee) [NA]. LATERAL LIGAMENT OF THE MALLEUS.

ligamentum mallei su·pe·ri·us (sue·peer′ee·us) [NA]. SUPERIOR LIGAMENT OF THE MALLEUS.

ligamentum mal·le·o·li la·te·ra·lis an·te·ri·us (ma·lee′o·lye lat·e·ray′lis an·teer·ee·us) [BNA]. Ligamentum tibiofibulare anterius. See *tibiofibular ligament.*

ligamentum malleoli lateralis pos·te·ri·us (pos·teer′ee·us) [BNA]. Ligamentum tibiofibulare posterius. See *tibiofibular ligament.*

ligamentum me·di·a·le (mee·dee·ay′lee) [NA]. MEDIAL LIGAMENT. NA alt. *ligamentum deltoideum.*

ligamentum me·nis·co·fe·mo·ra·le an·te·ri·us (me·nis″ko·fem·o·ray′lee an·teer′ee·us) [NA]. The anterior meniscofemoral ligament. See *meniscofemoral ligament.*

ligamentum meniscofemorale pos·te·ri·us (pos·teer′ee·us) [NA]. The posterior meniscofemoral ligament. See *meniscofemoral ligament.*

ligamentum me·ta·car·pe·um trans·ver·sum pro·fun·dum (met″uh·kahr′pee·um trans·vur′sum pro·fun′dum) [NA]. DEEP TRANSVERSE METACARPAL LIGAMENT.

ligamentum metacarpeum transversum su·per·fi·ci·a·le (sue·pur·fish·ee·ay′lee) [NA]. SUPERFICIAL TRANSVERSE METACARPAL LIGAMENT.

ligamentum me·ta·tar·se·um trans·ver·sum pro·fun·dum (met″uh·tahr′see·um trans·vur′sum pro·fun′dum) [NA]. DEEP TRANSVERSE METATARSAL LIGAMENT.

ligamentum metatarseum transversum su·per·fi·ci·a·le (sue·pur·fish·ee·ay′lee) [NA]. SUPERFICIAL TRANSVERSE METATARSAL LIGAMENT.

ligamentum nu·chae (new′kee) [NA]. NUCHAL LIGAMENT.

ligamentum ova·rii pro·pri·um (o·vair′ee·eye pro′pree·um) [NA]. OVARIAN LIGAMENT.

ligamentum pal·pe·bra·le la·te·ra·le (pal·pe·bray′lee lat·e·ray′lee) [NA]. The lateral palpebral ligament. See *palpebral ligament.*

ligamentum palpebrale me·di·a·le (mee·dee·ay′lee) [NA]. The medial palpebral ligament. See *palpebral ligament.*

ligamentum pa·tel·lae (pa·tel′ee) [NA]. PATELLAR LIGAMENT.

ligamentum pec·ti·na·tum an·gu·li iri·do·cor·ne·a·lis (peck·ti·nay′tum ang′gew·lye eye″ri·do·kor·nee·ay′lis) [NA]. PECTINATE LIGAMENT.

ligamentum pectinatum iri·dis (eye′ri·dis) [BNA]. Ligamentum pectinatum anguli iridocornealis (= PECTINATE LIGAMENT).

ligamentum pec·ti·ne·a·le (peck·tin·ee·ay′lee) [NA]. PECTINEAL LIGAMENT.

ligamentum phre·ni·co·co·li·cum (fren″i·ko·ko′li·kum) [NA]. PHRENICOCOLIC LIGAMENT.

ligamentum phre·ni·co·li·e·na·le (fren″i·ko·lye·e·nay′lee) [NA]. PHRENICOLIENAL LIGAMENT. NA alt. *ligamentum lienorenale.*

ligamentum pi·so·ha·ma·tum (pye″so·ha·may′tum) [NA]. PISOHAMATE LIGAMENT.

ligamentum pi·so·me·ta·car·pe·um (pye″so·met·uh·kahr′pee·um) [NA]. PISOMETACARPAL LIGAMENT.

ligamentum plan·ta·re lon·gum (plan·tair′ee long′gum) [NA]. LONG PLANTAR LIGAMENT.

ligamentum po·pli·te·um ar·cu·a·tum (pop·lit′ee·um ahr·kew·ay′tum) [NA]. ARCUATE POPLITEAL LIGAMENT.

ligamentum popliteum obli·quum (o·blye′kwum) [NA]. OBLIQUE POPLITEAL LIGAMENT.

ligamentum pte·ry·go·spi·na·le (terr″i·go·spi·nay′lee) [NA]. PTERYGOSPINOUS LIGAMENT.

ligamentum pte·ry·go·spi·no·sum (terr″i·go·spi·no′sum) [BNA]. Ligamentum pterygospinale (= PTERYGOSPINOUS LIGAMENT).

ligamentum pu·bi·cum su·pe·ri·us (pew′bi·kum sue·peer′ee·us) [NA]. SUPERIOR PUBIC LIGAMENT.

ligamentum pu·bo·cap·su·la·re (pew″bo·kap·sue·lair′ee) [BNA]. Ligamentum pubofemorale (= PUBOFEMORAL LIGAMENT).

ligamentum pu·bo·fe·mo·ra·le (pew″bo·fem·o·ray′lee) [NA]. PUBOFEMORAL LIGAMENT.

ligamentum pu·bo·pro·sta·ti·cum (pew″bo·pros·tat′i·kum) [NA]. PUBOPROSTATIC LIGAMENT.

ligamentum puboprostaticum la·te·ra·le (lat·e·ray′lee) [BNA]. The lateral puboprostatic ligament. See *puboprostatic ligament.*

ligamentum puboprostaticum medium [BNA]. The medial puboprostatic ligament. See *puboprostatic ligament.*

ligamentum pu·bo·ve·si·ca·le (pew″bo·ves·i·kay′lee) [NA]. PUBOVESICAL LIGAMENT.

ligamentum pubovesicale la·te·ra·le (lat·e·ray′lee) [BNA]. The lateral pubovesical ligament. See *pubovesical ligament.*

ligamentum pubovesicale medium [BNA]. The medial pubovesical ligament. See *pubovesical ligament.*

ligamentum pul·mo·na·le (pul·mo·nay'lee) [NA]. PULMONARY LIGAMENT.

ligamentum pul·mo·nis (pul·mo'nis). PULMONARY LIGAMENT.

ligamentum qua·dra·tum (kwah·dray'tum) [NA]. QUADRATE LIGAMENT.

ligamentum ra·dio·car·pe·um dor·sa·le (ray·dee·o·kahr'pee·um dor·say'lee) [NA]. The dorsal radiocarpal ligament. See *radiocarpal ligament.*

ligamentum radiocarpeum pal·ma·re (pal·mair'ee) [NA]. The palmar radiocarpal ligament. See *radiocarpal ligament.*

ligamentum radiocarpeum vo·la·re (vo·lair'ee) [BNA]. Ligamentum radiocarpeum palmare. See *radiocarpal ligament.*

ligamentum re·flex·um (re·fleck'sum) [NA]. REFLECTED LIGAMENT.

ligamentum sa·cro·coc·cy·ge·um an·te·ri·us (sack"ro·kock·sij'ee·um an·teer'ee·us) [BNA]. Ligamentum sacrococcygeum ventrale. See *sacrococcygeal ligament.*

ligamentum sacrococcygeum dor·sa·le pro·fun·dum (dor·say'lee pro·fun'dum) [NA]. The deep dorsal sacrococcygeal ligament. See *sacrococcygeal ligament.*

ligamentum sacrococcygeum dorsale su·per·fi·ci·a·le (sue"pur·fish·ee·ay'lee) [NA]. The superficial dorsal sacrococcygeal ligament. See *sacrococcygeal ligament.*

ligamentum sacrococcygeum la·te·ra·le (lat·e·ray'lee) [NA]. The lateral sacrococcygeal ligament. See *sacrococcygeal ligament.*

ligamentum sacrococcygeum pos·te·ri·us pro·fun·dum (pos·teer'ee·us pro·fun'dum) [BNA]. Ligamentum sacrococcygeum dorsale profundum. See *sacrococcygeal ligament.*

ligamentum sacrococcygeum posterius su·per·fi·ci·a·lis (sue·pur·fish·ee·ay'lis) [BNA]. Ligamentum sacrococcygeum dorsale superficiale. See *sacrococcygeal ligament.*

ligamentum sacrococcygeum ven·tra·le (ven·tray'lee) [NA]. The ventral sacrococcygeal ligament. See *sacrococcygeal ligament.*

ligamentum sa·cro·ili·a·cum pos·te·ri·us bre·ve (sack"ro·i·lye'uh·kum pos·teer'ee·us brev'ee) [BNA]. The short posterior sacroiliac ligament; one of the dorsal sacroiliac ligaments.

ligamentum sacroiliacum posterius lon·gum (long'gum) [BNA]. The long posterior sacroiliac ligament; one of the dorsal sacroiliac ligaments.

ligamentum sa·cro·spi·na·le (sack"ro·spi·nay'lee) [NA]. SACROSPINOUS LIGAMENT.

ligamentum sa·cro·spi·no·sum (sack"ro·spi·no'sum) [BNA]. Ligamentum sacrospinale (= SACROSPINOUS LIGAMENT).

ligamentum sa·cro·tu·be·ra·le (sack"ro·tew·be·ray'lee) [NA]. SACROTUBEROUS LIGAMENT.

ligamentum sa·cro·tu·be·ro·sum (sack"ro·tew·be·ro'sum) [BNA]. Ligamentum sacrotuberale (= SACROTUBEROUS LIGAMENT).

ligamentum se·ro·sum (se·ro'sum) [BNA]. A general term for any fold of a serous membrane.

ligamentum sphe·no·man·di·bu·la·re (sfee"no·man·dib·yoo·lair'ee) [NA]. SPHENOMANDIBULAR LIGAMENT.

ligamentum spi·ra·le coch·le·ae (spi·ray'lee kock'lee·ee) [NA]. SPIRAL LIGAMENT.

ligamentum ster·no·cla·vi·cu·la·re (stur"no·kla·vick"yoo·lair"ee) [BNA]. STERNOCLAVICULAR LIGAMENT.

ligamentum sternoclaviculare an·te·ri·us (an·teer'ee·us) [NA]. The anterior sternoclavicular ligament. See *sternoclavicular ligament.*

ligamentum sternoclaviculare pos·te·ri·us (pos·teer'ee·us) [NA]. The posterior sternoclavicular ligament. See *sternoclavicular ligament.*

ligamentum ster·no·cos·ta·le in·ter·ar·ti·cu·la·re (stur"no·kos·tay'lee in"tur·ahr·tick·yoo·lair'ee) [BNA]. Ligamentum sternocostale intraarticulare (= INTRAARTICULAR STERNOCOSTAL LIGAMENT).

ligamentum sternocostale in·tra·ar·ti·cu·la·re (in"truh·ahr·tick·yoo·lair'ee) [NA]. INTRAARTICULAR STERNOCOSTAL LIGAMENT.

ligamentum sty·lo·hy·oi·de·um (stye"lo·high·oy'dee·um) [NA]. STYLOHYOID LIGAMENT.

ligamentum sty·lo·man·di·bu·la·re (stye"lo·man·dib·yoo·lair'ee) [NA]. STYLOMANDIBULAR LIGAMENT.

ligamentum su·pra·spi·na·le (sue"pruh·spi·nay'lee) [NA]. SUPRASPINAL LIGAMENT.

ligamentum sus·pen·so·ri·um cli·to·ri·dis (sus·pen·so'ree·um kli·tor'i·dis) [NA]. The suspensory ligament of the clitoris. See *suspensory ligament.*

ligamentum suspensorium ova·rii (o·vair'ee·eye) [NA]. The suspensory ligament of the ovary. See *suspensory ligament.*

ligamentum suspensorium pe·nis (pee'nis) [NA]. The suspensory ligament of the penis. See *suspensory ligament.*

ligamentum ta·lo·cal·ca·ne·um an·te·ri·us (tay"lo·kal·kay'nee·um an·teer'ee·us) [BNA]. The anterior talocalcaneal ligament. See *talocalcaneal ligament.*

ligamentum talocalcaneum in·ter·os·se·um (in·tur·os'ee·um) [NA]. The interosseous talocalcaneal ligament. See *talocalcaneal ligament.*

ligamentum talocalcaneum la·te·ra·le (lat·e·ray'lee) [NA]. The lateral talocalcaneal ligament. See *talocalcaneal ligament.*

ligamentum talocalcaneum me·di·a·le (mee·dee·ay'lee) [NA]. The medial talocalcaneal ligament. See *talocalcaneal ligament.*

ligamentum talocalcaneum pos·te·ri·us (pos·teer'ee·us) [BNA]. The posterior talocalcaneal ligament. See *talocalcaneal ligament.*

ligamentum ta·lo·fi·bu·la·re an·te·ri·us (tay"lo·fib·yoo·lair'ee an·teer'ee·us) [NA]. The anterior talofibular ligament. See *talofibular ligament.*

ligamentum talofibulare pos·te·ri·us (pos·teer'ee·us) [NA]. The posterior talofibular ligament. See *talofibular ligament.*

ligamentum ta·lo·na·vi·cu·la·re (tay"lo·na·vick·yoo·lair'ee) [NA]. TALONAVICULAR LIGAMENT.

ligamentum ta·lo·ti·bi·a·le an·te·ri·us (tay"lo·tib·ee·ay'lee an·teer'ee·us) [BNA]. PARS TIBIOTALARIS ANTERIOR LIGAMENTI MEDIALIS.

ligamentum talotibiale pos·te·ri·us (pos·teer'ee·us) [BNA]. PARS TIBIOTALARIS POSTERIOR LIGAMENTI MEDIALIS.

ligamentum tem·po·ro·man·di·bu·la·re (tem"pur·o·man·dib·yoo·lair'ee) [BNA]. Ligamentum laterale (= LATERAL LIGAMENT OF THE TEMPOROMANDIBULAR JOINT).

ligamentum te·res fe·mo·ris (tee'reez fem'o·ris) [BNA]. Ligamentum capitis femoris. See *round ligament.*

ligamentum teres he·pa·tis (hep'uh·tis) [NA]. The round ligament of the liver. See *round ligament.*

ligamentum teres ute·ri (yoo'tur·eye) [NA]. The round ligament of the uterus. See *round ligament.*

ligamentum tes·tis (tes'tis). A short embryonic ligament developing in the caudal genital ridge forming the upper part of the gubernaculum testis.

ligamentum thy·reo·epi·glot·ti·cum (thigh"ree·o·ep·i·glot'i·kum) [BNA]. Ligamentum thyroepiglotticum (= THYROEPIGLOTTIC LIGAMENT).

ligamentum thy·ro·epi·glot·ti·cum (thigh"ro·ep·i·glot'i·kum) [NA]. THYROEPIGLOTTIC LIGAMENT.

ligamentum thy·ro·hy·oi·de·um (thigh"ro·high·oy'dee·um) [NA]. LATERAL THYROHYOID LIGAMENT.

ligamentum thyrohyoideum me·di·a·num (mee·dee·ay'num) [NA]. MEDIAN THYROHYOID LIGAMENT.

ligamentum ti·bio·fi·bu·la·re an·te·ri·us (tib"ee·o·fib·yoo·lair'ee an·teer'ee·us) [NA]. The anterior tibiofibular ligament. See *tibiofibular ligament.*

ligamentum tibiofibulare pos·te·ri·us (pos·teer'ee·us) [NA]. The posterior tibiofibular ligament. See *tibiofibular ligament.*

ligamentum ti·bio·na·vi·cu·la·re (tib"ee·o·na·vick·yoo·lair'ee) [BNA]. PARS TIBIONAVICULARIS LIGAMENTI MEDIALIS.

ligamentum trans·ver·sum ace·ta·bu·li (trans·vur'sum as"e·tab'yoo·lye) [NA]. The transverse ligament of the acetabulum (= TRANSVERSE ACETABULAR LIGAMENT).

ligamentum transversum at·lan·tis (at·lan'tis) [NA]. The transverse ligament of the atlas. See *transverse ligament.*

ligamentum transversum cru·ris (kroo'ris) [BNA]. Retinaculum musculorum extensorum pedis superius (= SUPERIOR EXTENSOR RETINACULUM).

ligamentum transversum ge·nu (jen'yoo) [BNA]. Ligamentum transversum genus. See *transverse ligament.*

ligamentum transversum ge·nus (jen'oos, jen'us) [NA]. The transverse ligament of the knee. See *transverse ligament.*

ligamentum transversum pel·vis (pel'vis) [BNA]. Ligamentum transversum perinei (= TRANSVERSE PERINEAL LIGAMENT).

ligamentum transversum pe·ri·nei (perr·i·nee'eye) [NA]. TRANSVERSE PERINEAL LIGAMENT.

ligamentum transversum sca·pu·lae in·fe·ri·us (skap'yoo·lee in·feer'ee·us) [NA]. INFERIOR TRANSVERSE LIGAMENT OF THE SCAPULA.

ligamentum transversum scapulae su·pe·ri·us (sue·peer'i·us) [NA]. SUPERIOR TRANSVERSE LIGAMENT OF THE SCAPULA.

ligamentum tra·pe·zoi·de·um (trap''e·zoy'dee·um) [NA]. TRAPEZOID LIGAMENT.

ligamentum tri·an·gu·la·re dex·trum (trye·ang·gew·lair'ee decks'trum) [NA]. The right triangular ligament. See *triangular ligament.*

ligamentum triangulare si·nis·trum (si·nis'trum) [NA]. The left triangular ligament. See *triangular ligament.*

ligamentum tu·ber·cu·li cos·tae (tew·bur'kew·lye kos'tee) [BNA]. Ligamentum costotransversarium laterale (= LATERAL COSTOTRANSVERSE LIGAMENT).

ligamentum ul·no·car·pe·um pal·ma·re (ul''no·kahr'pee·um pal·mair'ee) [NA]. PALMAR ULNOCARPAL LIGAMENT.

ligamentum um·bi·li·ca·le la·te·ra·le (um·bil''i·kay'lee lat·e·ray'lee). NA predecessor of *ligamentum umbilicale mediale.*

ligamentum umbilicale me·di·a·le (mee·dee·ay'lee) [NA]. MEDIAL UMBILICAL LIGAMENT.

ligamentum umbilicale me·di·a·num (mee·dee·ay'num) [NA]. MEDIAN UMBILICAL LIGAMENT.

ligamentum umbilicale medium [BNA]. Ligamentum umbilicale medianum (= MEDIAN UMBILICAL LIGAMENT).

ligamentum va·gi·na·le (vaj·i·nay'lee) [BNA]. Vestigium processus vaginalis (= VAGINAL LIGAMENT).

ligamentum ve·nae ca·vae si·nis·trae (vee'nee kay'vee si·nis'tree) [BNA]. PLICA VENAE CAVAE SINISTRAE.

ligamentum ve·no·sum (ve·no'sum) [NA]. A ligament of the liver representing the remains of the embryonic ductus venosus.

ligamentum ven·tri·cu·la·re (ven·trick·yoo·lair'ee) [BNA]. Ligamentum vestibulare (= VESTIBULAR LIGAMENT).

ligamentum ve·sti·bu·la·re (ves·tib·yoo·lair'ee) [NA]. VESTIBULAR LIGAMENT.

ligamentum vo·ca·le (vo·kay'lee) [NA]. VOCAL LIGAMENT.

lig·and (lig'and, lye'gand) *n.* [L. *ligandum,* from *ligare,* to bind]. 1. *In biochemistry,* a molecule which is bound by a protein surface. 2. *In inorganic chemistry,* any ion or molecule that by donating one or more pairs of electrons to a central metal ion is coordinated with it to form a complex ion or molecule, as in the compound $[CoCl(NH_3)_5]\ Cl_2$, in which Cl and NH_3 in the bracketed portion are ligands coordinated with Co.

li·gase (lye'gace, ·gaze, lig'ace) *n.* Any enzyme that catalyzes the joining of two molecules and that involves also the participation of a nucleoside triphosphate, such as adenosine triphosphate, which is converted to nucleoside diphosphate or monophosphate. Syn. *synthetase.*

li·ga·tion (lye·gay'shun) *n.* [L. *ligatio,* from *ligare,* to bind]. The operation of tying, especially arteries, veins, or ducts, with some form of knotted ligature. —**li·gate** (lye'gate) *v.*

lig·a·ture (lig'uh·chur, ·choor) *n.* [L. *ligatura,* a bond]. 1. A cord or thread for tying vessels. 2. The act of tying or binding; ligation. 3. A wire or other material used to secure an orthodontic attachment to an arch wire or to bind teeth together temporarily.

ligature carrier. A specially designed forceps for passing or drawing ligatures through tissues.

Liget's sign. A sign of acute appendicitis; the skin in Sherren's triangle is hyperesthetic when it is lifted and pinched gently.

light, *n.* Electromagnetic radiations that give rise to the sensation of vision when the rays impinge upon the retina.

light adaptation. The disappearance of dark adaptation; the chemical processes by which the eyes, after exposure to a dim environment, become accustomed to bright illumination, which initially is perceived as quite intense and uncomfortable.

light chain. Any of the polypeptide subunits of approximate molecular weight 22,000 common to molecules of all classes of immunoglobulins and classified, irrespective of immunoglobulin class, as kappa chains or lambda chains on the basis of distinctive amino acid sequence characteristics. Contr. *heavy chain.*

light chain disease. A variant of multiple myeloma in which the principal paraprotein is an immunoglobulin light chain.

light difference. 1. The difference between the two eyes in respect to their sensitivity to light. 2. The smallest difference in illumination which can be distinguished by the eyes. Abbreviated, L.D.

light·en·ing (lite'un·ing) *n.* The sinking of the fetus into the pelvic inlet with an accompanying descent of the uterus.

light·er·man's bottom (lite'ur·munz). Inflammation of the bursa over the tuberosity of the ischium; due to prolonged sitting. Syn. *weaver's bottom.*

light-head·ed (lite'hed''id) *adj.* Dizzy, delirious, disordered in the head; faint. —**light-head·ed·ness** (lite''hed'id·nis) *n.*

light hydrogen. PROTIUM.

light magnesia. A low-density magnesium oxide, prepared by ignition of light magnesium carbonate.

light meromyosin. The smaller of two fragments obtained from the muscle protein myosin following limited proteolysis by trypsin or chymotrypsin. Contr. *heavy meromyosin.*

light minimum. MINIMUM VISIBLE.

light-negative disease. LIPOID NEPHROSIS.

lightning cataract. ELECTRIC CATARACT.

lightning major convulsion. INFANTILE SPASM.

lightning pains. Lancinating pains coming on and disappearing with lightninglike rapidity and most commonly felt in the legs. They may come in bouts lasting several hours or days. They are characteristic of tabes dorsalis, but occur occasionally in other forms of neuropathy and radiculopathy.

light reflex. 1. A cone of light on the anterior and inferior part of the tympanic membrane, with its apex directed toward the umbo. 2. A circular area of light reflected from the retina during retinoscopic examination or from any light source. 3. The contraction of the pupil in response to light. Syn. *Whytt's reflex.*

light sense. *In ophthalmology,* the faculty of perceiving light and recognizing gradations of its intensity.

light sense tester. Any instrument used to test the sensitivity of the eye to light.

light spot. LIGHT REFLEX (1).

light treatment. Treatment by sunlight or artificial light; PHOTOTHERAPY.

Lig·nac-de Toni-Fan·coni syndrome. FANCONI SYNDROME.

Lignac-Fanconi syndrome. FANCONI SYNDROME.

lig·ne·ous (lig'nee·us) *adj.* [L. *ligneus,* from *lignum,* wood]. Woody, or having a woody texture.

ligneous thyroiditis. RIEDEL'S DISEASE.

lig·ni·fi·ca·tion (lig''ni·fi·kay'shun) *n.* The process by which the cell wall of a plant acquires greater rigidity by deposition of lignin.

lig·nin (lig'nin) *n.* [*lignum* + *-in*]. A modification of cellulose, constituting the greater part of the weight of most dry wood. A substance deposited in the cell walls of plants.

lig·no·caine (lig'no·kane) *n.* British name for lidocaine, a local anesthetic usually used as the hydrochloride salt.

lig·no·cer·ic acid (lig''no·serr'ick, ·seer'ick). A fatty acid, $C_{23}H_{47}COOH$, derived from kerasin.

lig·num (lig'num) *n.* [L.]. WOOD.

lig·ro·in (lig'ro·in) *n.* A liquid fraction obtained from petroleum; used as a solvent.

Lil·ien·thal's costotome [H. *Lilienthal,* U.S. surgeon, 1861–1946]. A guillotine type of costotome for use in removing the first rib. Syn. *guillotine costotome.*

Lilienthal's operation [H. *Lilienthal*]. An esophagogastrostomy through a posterior approach.

Lil·li·pu·tian hallucination (lil''i·pew'shun). A false visual perception in which all objects and persons appear diminutive, often seen in febrile or intoxicated states, psychomotor seizures, and in manic-depressive illness. Syn. *microptic hallucination.*

limb, *n.* 1. One of the extremities attached to the trunk and used for prehension or locomotion. NA *membrum.* 2. An elongated limblike structure, as one of the limbs of the internal capsule.

limb bud. A lateral swelling of the embryonic trunk; the anlage of an appendage.

lim·ber·neck (lim'bur·neck) *n.* An avian type of botulism; a disease caused by *Clostridium botulinum* toxin and characterized by muscular incoordination, weakness, and death.

limb-girdle muscular dystrophy. A form of muscular dystrophy with onset in late childhood or even the second or third decade of life, involving either the pelvic girdle (Leyden-Möbius type) or the shoulder girdle (Erb's type), then spreading to other parts. The face is rarely affected and pseudohypertrophy of calves is uncommon. Course is variable, but usually slower than in pseudohypertrophic muscular dystrophy, and more rapid than in the facioscapulohumeral variety. Inherited as an autosomal recessive trait, it also often occurs sporadically.

limbi. Plural of *limbus.*

lim·bic (lim'bick) *adj.* 1. Pertaining to or of the nature of a limbus or border; circumferential; marginal. 2. Pertaining to the limbic system or lobes of the brain.

limbic cortex, lobe, or **system.** A ring of cerebral cortex, composed of archipallium and paleopallium, which includes the paraterminal gyrus and parolfactory area, the gyrus cinguli, part of the gyrus parahippocampalis, and uncus. It is the oldest portion of the cortex which has its evolutionary rudiment in the reptiles, amphibians, and fish. Now thought to control various emotional and behavioral patterns.

limbi pal·pe·bra·les an·te·ri·o·res (pal''pe·bray'leez an·teer''ee·o'reez) [NA]. Plural of *limbus palpebralis anterior.*

limbi palpebrales pos·te·ri·o·res (pos·teer''ee·o'reez) [NA]. Plural of *limbus palpebralis posterior.*

lim·bus (lim'bus) *n.,* pl. **lim·bi** (·bye) [L., fringe, border]. A border; the circumferential edge of any flat organ or part.

limbus al·ve·o·la·ris man·di·bu·lae (al·ve·o·lair'is man·dib'yoo·lee) [BNA]. ARCUS ALVEOLARIS MANDIBULAE.

limbus alveolaris max·il·lae (mack·sil'ee) [BNA]. ARCUS ALVEOLARIS MAXILLAE.

limbus cor·ne·ae (kor'nee·ee) [NA]. CORNEOSCLERAL LIMBUS.

limbus fos·sae ova·lis (fos'ee o·vay'lis) [NA]. ANNULUS OVALIS.

limbus la·mi·nae spi·ra·lis os·se·ae (lam'i·nee spye·ray'lis os'ee·ee) [NA]. LIMBUS OF THE SPIRAL LAMINA.

limbus mem·bra·nae tym·pa·ni (mem·bray'nee tim'puh·nye) [BNA]. The margin of the tympanic membrane.

limbus of the spiral lamina. A thickening of the periosteum at the border of the osseous spiral lamina of the cochlea; to it is attached the tectorial membrane. NA *limbus laminae spiralis osseae.*

limbus pal·pe·bra·lis anterior (pal·pe·bray'lis). The rounded anterior edge of the margin of the eyelid from which the eyelashes grow.

limbus palpebralis posterior. The sharp posterior edge of the margin of the eyelid that is applied to the eyeball; it is the point of transition of skin to the conjunctival mucous membrane.

limbus sphe·noi·da·lis (sfee''noy·day'lis). The sharp anterior edge of the groove on the sphenoid bone for the optic chiasma.

limbus spi·ra·lis (spye·ray'lis). LIMBUS OF THE SPIRAL LAMINA.

[1]lime, *n.* [OE. *līm,* glue, paste, cement (rel. to *slīm,* slime, and to L. *limus,* mud)]. CALCIUM OXIDE.

[2]lime, *n.* [F., from Ar. *līm*]. The fruit of *Citrus aurantifolia;* its juice is antiscorbutic.

lime chloride. CHLORINATED LIME.

lime liniment. CARRON OIL.

li·men (lye'mun) *n.,* pl. **lim·i·na** (lim'i·nuh) [L., threshold]. 1. A boundary line. 2. THRESHOLD.

limen in·su·lae (in'sue·lee) [NA]. The imaginary line separating the anterior perforated substance from the insula.

limen na·si (nay'zye) [NA]. The boundary line between the osseous and the cartilaginous portions of the nasal cavity.

li·mes (lye'meez) *n.,* pl. **li·mi·tes** (·mi·teez) [L.]. Limit, boundary.

limes death. The least amount of diphtheria toxin which, when mixed with one unit of antitoxin and injected into a guinea pig weighing 250 g, kills within 5 days. Symbol, L_+.

limes zero. The greatest amount of diphtheria toxin which causes no local edema when mixed with one unit of antitoxin and injected into a guinea pig weighing 250 g. Symbol, L_0.

lime water. An aqueous solution containing 0.14% $Ca(OH)_2$ at 25°C. Used as an antacid.

limina. Plural of *limen.*

lim·i·nal (lim'i·nul) *adj.* Pertaining to the limen or threshold, especially pertaining to the lowest limit of perception to a sensory stimulus.

liminal stimulus. THRESHOLD STIMULUS.

limit dextrinosis. Glycogenosis caused by a deficiency of amylo-1,6-glucosidase (debrancher enzyme), with abnormal storage of excessively branched glycogen in liver, heart, and muscle in various combinations depending on which organs are enzyme deficient; manifested clinically by moderate to marked hepatomegaly and varying degrees of skeletal weakness and cardiomegaly. Involvement of erythrocytes results in high levels of blood glycogen. Syn. *type III of Cori, Forbes' disease.*

limites. Plural of *limes.*

limiting angle. CRITICAL ANGLE.

limiting membrane. The membrane surrounding the vitreous body. See also *hyaloid membrane.*

limiting sulcus of Reil [J. C. *Reil*]. CIRCULAR SULCUS.

limit of flocculation. The amount of diphtheria toxin or toxoid which gives the most rapid flocculation with one standard unit of antitoxin. Abbreviated, Lf.

lim·i·troph·ic (lim''i·trof'ick) *adj.* Controlling nutrition.

limitrophic area or **cortex.** LIMITROPHIC ZONE.

limitrophic zone. Any area of the cerebral cortex transitional between two neighboring well-defined areas.

Lim·na·tis (lim·nay'tis) *n.* A genus of aquatic leeches.

Limnatis ni·lo·ti·ca (nye·lot'i·kuh). A widely distributed species of leech which produces internal hirudiniasis in man.

lim·nol·o·gy (lim·nol'o·jee) *n.* [Gk. *limnē,* marsh, + *-logy*]. The study of inland waters; particularly the study of biological, chemical, and physical conditions in ponds, lakes, and streams.

lim·o·nene (lim'o·neen) *n.* A monocyclic terpene hydrocarbon, $C_{10}H_{16}$, existing in optically active and racemic forms, occurring in many volatile oils.

li·mo·nite (lye'mo·nite, lim'o·) *n.* Ferric oxide, of the approximate formula $2Fe_2O_3.3H_2O$; a yellow powder. See also *iron oxide.*

li·moph·thi·sis (li·mof'thi·sis, lye·) *n.* [Gk. *limos*, hunger, + *phthisis*, a wasting away]. Wasting of the body, due to starvation; INANITION.

¹limp, *n.* An abnormal gait resulting from one or a combination of malfunctions of musculoskeletal structures pertinent to locomotion, or pain in a joint or other lower extremity structure.

²limp, *adj.* Floppy, flaccid; HYPOTONIC (1).

***Limulus* assay test.** A method in which minute quantities of endotoxin causes the gelation of an extract from the amebocyte lysate of the king crab, *Limulus polyphemus;* has been used as a means of detecting clinical septicemia due to gram-negative bacteria.

limy bile syndrome. Opacification of the gallbladder or common duct on a plain abdominal x-ray film, due to excessive calcium salts in the bile.

lin·al·o·ol (lin·al'o·ole, ·ol, lin"uh·lool') *n.* 3,7-Dimethyl-1,6-octadien-3-ol, $C_{10}H_{17}OH$, an alcohol in coriander, lavender, and bergamot oils. It exists in both dextrorotatory and levorotatory forms, designated *d*-linalool and *l*-linalool, respectively. *d*-Linalool is the chief constituent of coriander oil.

lin·a·mar·in (lin"uh·măr'in) *n.* The toxic cyanogenetic glycoside, $C_{10}H_{17}NO_6$, of linseed.

Lincocin. Trademark for the antibiotic substance lincomycin.

lin·co·my·cin (lin·ko·migh'sin) *n.* Methyl 6,8-dideoxy-6-(1-methyl-4-propyl-L-2-pyrrolidinecarboxamido)-1-thio-D-*erythro*-α-D-*galacto*-octopyranoside, $C_{18}H_{34}N_2O_6S$, an antibiotic produced by *Streptomyces lincolnensis.* Its spectrum of action is limited to gram-positive bacteria, especially cocci.

linc·tus (link'tus) *n.* [participle of L. *lingere,* to lick]. A syrupy preparation, usually containing sugar, of a medicinal that will alleviate irritation of the mucous membrane of the throat.

lin·dane (lin'dane) *n.* The gamma isomer of 1,2,3,4,5,6-hexachlorocyclohexane, $C_6H_6Cl_6$, known also as benzene hexachloride, of a purity of not less than 99%; a powerful insecticide.

Lin·dau's disease [A. *Lindau,* Swedish pathologist, b. 1892]. Cerebellar angioma sometimes associated with von Hippel's disease. See also *Hippel-Lindau disease.*

Lind·bergh flask [C. A. *Lindbergh,* U.S. aviator, 1902–1974]. A two-chambered vessel, one above the other, for cultivating a large number of tissue fragments in a thin layer of well-oxygenated medium. See also *Carrel-Lindbergh pump.*

Lin·der·strøm-Lang-Duspiva method. A microtitrimetric method for protease based on exposure of peptides to protease and titration of the carboxyl groups of the proteolytic products with tetraethylammonium hydroxide.

Linderstrøm-Lang-Engel method. A titrimetric method for amylase based on the measurement of an increase in reducing sugar after the action of the enzyme on starch.

Linderstrøm-Lang-Glick method. A Cartesian diver method for cholinesterase based upon the fact that when a choline ester is broken down in a bicarbonate buffer, the acid produced causes equivalent liberation of carbon dioxide which is measured by the Warburg apparatus.

Linderstrøm-Lang-Holter method. 1. A titrimetric method for protease based upon the addition of acetone indicator to the products and the titration of their amino groups with hydrochloric acid. 2. A microtitrimetric method for reducing sugars based on reduction of iodine to iodide and titration of the excess of the former with thiosulfate.

Linderstrøm-Lang-Lanz method. A dilatometric method for peptidase using DL-alanylglycine as the substrate for peptidase.

Linderstrøm-Lang method. A microtitrimetric method for combined potassium and sodium based on the conversion of potassium and sodium to chlorides by an ashing reagent, removal of other chlorides, and electrometric titration of the residual chloride with silver nitrate.

Linderstrøm-Lang-Weil-Holter methods. Two methods for detecting arginase: 1. The *urease method:* a titrimetric method based on the action of the enzyme on arginine to liberate urea, the action of urease on urea to release ammonia, and the measurement of ammonia. 2. The *acetone-alcohol method:* a method based on titration of ornithine and urea, formed on the breakdown of arginine by acetone-alcohol mixture.

line, *n.* [L. *linea*]. 1. Extension of dimension having length, but neither breadth nor thickness. 2. *In anatomy,* anything resembling a mathematical line in having length without breadth or thickness; a boundary or guide mark. 3. *In genetics,* lineage; the succession of progenitors and progeny. 4. *Obsol.* The 1/12 part of an inch.

lin·ea (lin'ee·uh) *n.,* pl. **lin·e·ae** (·ee·ee) [L.]. LINE.

linea al·ba (al'buh) [NA]. A tendinous raphe extending in the median line of the abdomen from the pubes to the xiphoid process; it is formed by the blending of the aponeuroses of the oblique and transverse muscles of the abdomen. See also Plate 4.

linea ar·cu·a·ta os·sis il·ii (ahr"kew·ay'tuh os'is il'ee·eye) [NA]. ARCUATE LINE (1).

linea arcuata ossis il·i·um (il'ee·um) [BNA]. Linea arcuata ossis ilii (= ARCUATE LINE (1)).

linea arcuata va·gi·nae mus·cu·li rec·ti ab·do·mi·nis (va·jye'nee mus'kew·lye reck·tye ab·dom'i·nis) [NA]. SEMICIRCULAR LINE.

linea as·pe·ra (as'pe·ruh) [NA]. A rough longitudinal ridge on the posterior surface of the middle third of the femur serving as attachment for muscles.

linea ax·il·la·ris (ack·si·lair'is) [NA]. MIDAXILLARY LINE.

lineae. Plural of *linea* (= LINE).

lineae al·bi·can·tes (al·bi·kan'teez). Glistening white lines seen in the skin, especially that of the anterior abdominal wall, after reduction from extreme distention, as in pregnancy; produced by rupture of the elastic fibers.

lineae gra·vi·da·rum (grav"i·dair'um). LINEAE ALBICANTES.

lineae mus·cu·la·res sca·pu·lae (mus·kew·lair'eez skap'yoo·lee) [BNA]. Several oblique ridges on the costal surface of the scapula.

linea epi·phy·si·a·lis (ep"i·fiz·i·ay'lis) [NA]. EPIPHYSEAL LINE (1).

lineae trans·ver·sae os·sis sa·cri (trans·vur'see os'is say'krye) [NA]. Transverse lines on the pelvic surface of the adult sacrum, marking the positions of the intervertebral disks of the immature bone.

linea glu·taea an·te·ri·or (gloo'tee·uh an·teer'ee·or) [BNA]. Linea glutea anterior (= ANTERIOR GLUTEAL LINE).

linea glutaea inferior [BNA]. Linea glutea inferior (= INFERIOR GLUTEAL LINE).

linea glutaea posterior [BNA]. Linea glutea posterior (= POSTERIOR GLUTEAL LINE).

linea glu·tea an·te·ri·or (gloo'tee·uh an·teer'ee·or) [NA]. ANTERIOR GLUTEAL LINE.

linea glutea inferior [NA]. INFERIOR GLUTEAL LINE.

linea glutea posterior [NA]. POSTERIOR GLUTEAL LINE.

linea in·ter·con·dy·la·ris (in"tur·kon·di·lair'is) [NA]. INTERCONDYLAR LINE.

linea in·ter·con·dy·loi·dea (in"tur·kon·di·loy'dee·uh) [BNA]. Linea intercondylaris (= INTERCONDYLAR LINE).

linea in·ter·me·dia (in"tur·mee'dee·uh) [NA]. INTERMEDIATE LINE.

linea in·ter·tro·chan·te·ri·ca (in"tur·tro·kan·terr'i·kuh) [NA]. INTERTROCHANTERIC LINE.

lin·eal (lin'ee·ul) *adj.* [L. *linealis,* from *linea,* line]. 1. Of or pertaining to a line of descent or lineage. 2. Being in a direct line of descent. 3. Linear.

linea ma·mil·la·ris (mam·i·lair'is) [NA]. MAMILLARY LINE.

linea me·di·a·na anterior (mee·dee·ay'nuh) [NA]. The anterior midline of the body.

linea mediana posterior [NA]. The posterior midline of the body.

linea me·dio·cla·vi·cu·la·ris (mee''dee·o·kla·vick·yoo·lair'is) [NA alt.]. MAMILLARY LINE. NA alt. *linea mamillaris.*

linea men·sa·lis (men·say'lis). Any one of the principal creases of the palm; often designated as proximal, middle, or distal.

linea mus·cu·li so·lei (mus'kew·lye so'lee·eye) [NA]. SOLEAL LINE.

linea my·lo·hy·oi·dea (migh''lo·high·oy'dee·uh) [NA]. MYLOHYOID LINE.

line angle. An angle formed by the meeting of two tooth surfaces.

linea ni·gra (nigh'gruh). A dark pigmented line often present in pregnant women and extending from the pubes upward in the median line.

linea nu·chae inferior (new'kee) [NA]. INFERIOR NUCHAL LINE.

linea nuchae superior [NA]. SUPERIOR NUCHAL LINE.

linea nuchae su·pre·ma (sue·pree'muh) [NA]. An indistinct line arching up and out from the external occipital protuberance.

linea obliqua cartilaginis thy·roi·de·ae (thigh·roy'dee·ee) [NA]. OBLIQUE LINE OF THE THYROID CARTILAGE.

linea obliqua man·di·bu·lae (man·dib'yoo·lee) [NA]. OBLIQUE LINE OF THE MANDIBLE.

linea pa·ra·ster·na·lis (păr''uh·stur·nay'lis) [BNA]. PARASTERNAL LINE.

linea pec·ti·nea (peck·tin'ee·uh) [NA]. PECTINEAL LINE.

linea po·pli·tea (pop·lit'ee·uh) [BNA]. Linea musculi solei (= SOLEAL LINE).

lin·ear (lin'ee·ur) *adj.* [L. *linearis*]. Pertaining to or resembling a line or lines.

linear correlation. A correlation between two variables in which the regression equation is represented by a straight line; a relationship that can be described graphically by a straight line.

linear craniotomy. CRANIECTOMY.

linear nevus. A nevus verrucosus of linear shape.

linear nevus sebaceus syndrome. A neurocutaneous syndrome in which there is an association of a nevus sebaceus on one side of the face and truck with mental retardation, seizures, and sometimes other anomalies.

linear osteotomy. Simple surgical division of a bone.

linear streak cau·tery. A type of cautery used in an everted cervix uteri, in which the cautery strokes radiate like the spokes of a wheel.

linea sca·pu·la·ris (skap''yoo·lair'is) [NA]. SCAPULAR LINE.

linea se·mi·cir·cu·la·ris (Doug·la·si) (sem''i·sur·kew·lair'is dug'luh·sigh) [BNA]. Linea arcuata vaginae musculi recti abdominis (= SEMICIRCULAR LINES).

linea se·mi·lu·na·ris (sem'i·lew·nair'is) [NA]. SEMILUNAR LINE.

linea si·nu·o·sa ana·lis (sin''yoo·o'suh ay·nay'lis). The junction between the rectum and the anal canal. Syn. *anorectal junction.*

linea splen·dens (splen'denz). A longitudinal fibrous band of pia mater along the median line of the anterior surface of the spinal cord.

linea ster·na·lis (stur·nay'lis) [BNA]. STERNAL LINE.

linea tem·po·ra·lis in·fe·ri·or os·sis pa·ri·e·ta·lis (tem·po·ray'lis in·feer'ee·or os'is pa·rye·e·tay'lis) [NA]. INFERIOR TEMPORAL LINE.

linea temporalis ossis fron·ta·lis (fron·tay'lis) [NA]. TEMPORAL LINE.

linea temporalis superior ossis pa·ri·e·ta·lis (pa·rye·e·tay'lis) [NA]. SUPERIOR TEMPORAL LINE.

linea ter·mi·na·lis (tur·mi·nay'lis) [NA]. ILIOPECTINEAL LINE.

linea tra·pe·zoi·dea (trap·e·zoy'dee·uh) [NA]. TRAPEZOID LINE.

line of demarcation. A line of division between healthy and gangrenous tissue.

line of fixation. An imaginary line drawn from the object viewed through the center of rotation of the eye.

line of Gennari [F. *Gennari*]. STRIPE OF GENNARI.

line of incidence. The path of a ray or a projectile.

line of occlusion. An imaginary line formed by the opposing arches of teeth when they are in maximum contact.

line of sight. An imaginary line drawn from the object viewed to the center of the pupil.

line of the soleus muscle. SOLEAL LINE.

lines of Baillarger. STRIPES OF BAILLARGER.

lines of Owen. CONTOUR LINES OF OWEN.

lines of Retzius. INCREMENTAL LINES OF RETZIUS.

lines of Sal·ter [S. J. A. *Salter*]. Incremental lines of the dentin.

lines of Schreger. HUNTER-SCHREGER BANDS.

line test. A test developed to study the progress of rickets in experimental animals. The radius or tibia is split lengthwise, immersed briefly in 2% $AgNO_3$, washed in water, and exposed to bright light. A black deposit of metallic silver appears in the epiphyseal region and is proportional to the degree of calcification. In extreme rickets no silver will appear in the epiphysis, but when healing has begun the calcium deposits are so located that the corresponding silver stain appears along a distinct line.

lingu-, lingua-, lingui-, linguo-. A combining form meaning *tongue, lingual.*

lin·gua (ling'gwuh) *n.* [L., ←OL. *dingua* (rel. to Gmc. *tung-* →E. *tongue*)] [NA]. TONGUE.

lin·gual (ling'gwul) *adj. & n.* [ML. *lingualis,* from L. *lingua,* tongue]. 1. Of or pertaining to the tongue. 2. Toward or nearest the tongue. 3. Either the inferior or superior intrinsic longitudinalis muscle of the tongue.

lingual artery. NA *arteria lingualis.* See Table of Arteries in the Appendix.

lingual bar. A metal bar on the lingual side of the mandibular arch, connecting the two or more parts of a mandibular removable partial denture.

lingual gland. Any one of the glands opening onto the surface of the tongue.

lingual goiter. A mass of thyroid tissue, at the upper end of the original thyroglossal duct, near the foramen cecum of the tongue.

lingual gyrus. A gyrus of the medial surface of the occipital lobe, lying between the calcarine sulcus and the posterior part of the collateral sulcus. NA *gyrus lingualis.*

lingual nerve. NA *nervus lingualis.* See Table of Nerves in the Appendix.

lingual occlusion. An occlusion where the line of a tooth is internal.

lingual papilla. Any one of the papillae on the tongue.

lingual plexus. A nerve plexus surrounding the lingual artery. Syn. *plexus lingualis.*

lingual quinsy. Quinsy originating in the lingual tonsil and involving the tongue.

lingual septum. The vertical median partition of the tongue which divides the muscular tissue into halves. NA *septum linguae.*

lingual spasm. APHTHONGIA.

lingual titubation. Stammering; stuttering.

lingual tonsil. Accumulations of lymphatic tissue more or less closely associated with crypts which serve also as ducts of the mucous glands of the base of the tongue. NA *tonsilla lingualis.*

lingua ni·gra (nigh'gruh). BLACK, HAIRY TONGUE.

lingua pli·ca·ta (pli·kay'tuh). FISSURED TONGUE.

Lin·guat·u·la (ling·gwach'oo·luh) *n.* A genus of the class Pentastomida, degenerate arthropods, endoparasites of vertebrates; commonly known as tongue worms.

Linguatula ser·ra·ta (se·ray'tuh). A tongue worm found in the nose or paranasal sinuses of dogs and other carnivores; rarely infests man.

Linguet. Trademark for a tablet designed to permit absorption of active ingredient through the buccal mucosa into the venous system.

lin·gu·la (ling'gew·luh) *n.*, pl. **lingu·lae** (·lee) [L., dim. from *lingua*, tongue]. 1. LINGULA CEREBELLI. 2. A tonguelike structure. —**lingu·lar** (·lur) *adj.*

lingula ce·re·bel·li (serr·e·bel'eye) [NA]. The portion of the vermis of the cerebellum attached to the superior medullary velum.

lingula man·di·bu·lae (man·dib'yoo·lee) [NA]. LINGULA OF THE MANDIBLE.

lingula of the ear. The cartilaginous projection toward or into the upper portion of the lobe of the ear.

lingula of the mandible. The prominent, thin process of bone partly surrounding the mandibular foramen. NA *lingula mandibulae.*

lingula of the sphenoid. A small, tonguelike process extending backward in the angle formed by the body of the sphenoid and one of its greater wings. NA *lingula sphenoidalis.*

lingula pul·mo·nis si·nis·tri (pul·mo'nis si·nis'trye) [NA]. A projection of the inferior border of the upper lobe of the left lung.

lingula sphe·noi·da·lis (sfee·noy·day'lis) [NA]. LINGULA OF THE SPHENOID.

lin·gu·lec·to·my (ling''gew·leck'tuh·mee) *n.* [*lingula* + *-ectomy*]. Surgical removal of the lingula of the upper lobe of the left lung.

linguo-. See *lingu-.*

lin·guo·dis·tal (ling''gwo·dis'tul) *adj.* [*linguo-* + *distal*]. Distally and toward the tongue, as the inclination of a tooth.

lin·guo·gin·gi·val (ling''gwo·jin'ji·vul, ·jin·jye'vul) *adj.* [*linguo-* + *gingival*]. Pertaining to the tongue and the gingiva.

lin·i·ment (lin'i·munt) *n.* [L. *linimentum*, from *linire*, to smear]. A liquid intended for application to the skin by gentle friction.

li·nin (lye'nin) *n.* 1. A strongly purgative principle obtainable from *Linum catharticum*, or purging flax. 2. *In biology*, the substance of the achromatic network of the nucleus of a cell.

lin·ing cells. The endothelium of vascular sinuses; once thought to be phagocytic.

li·ni·tis (li·nigh'tis, lye·nigh'tis) *n.* [Gk. *linon*, thread, linen, net, + *-itis*]. GASTRITIS.

linitis plas·ti·ca (plas'ti·kuh). Infiltrating, poorly differentiated carcinoma of the stomach involving all coats of the wall. Syn. *leather-bottle stomach.*

link·age (link'ij) *n.* 1. *In chemistry*, the lines used in structural formulas to represent valency connections between the atoms: a single line represents a valency of one, a double line a valency of two. 2. *In genetics*, the association of genes located in the same chromosome.

linkage law. Different gene pairs tend to segregate together if they are located on the same pair of homologous chromosomes. Linked genes may be separated with a frequency which varies from 0 to 50%, depending chiefly upon the relative linear distances between them.

lin·o·le·ic acid (lin''o·lee'ick, li·no'lee·ick). 9,12-Octadecadienoic acid, $C_{17}H_{31}COOH$, an unsaturated acid containing two double bonds, occurring in the glycerides of linseed and other oils. Syn. *linolic acid.*

li·no·le·in (li·no'lee·in) *n.* The glyceride of linoleic acid found in all drying oils.

lin·o·le·nic acid (lin''o·lee'nick, ·len'ick). 9,12-15-Octadecatrienoic acid, $C_{17}H_{29}COOH$, an unsaturated acid containing three double bonds, occurring in the glycerides of linseed and other oils; essential for normal nutrition.

li·no·lic acid (li·nol'ick, li·no'lick). LINOLEIC ACID.

lin·ono·pho·bia (lin''on·o·fo'bee·uh) *n.* [Gk. *linon*, thread, + *-phobia*]. Morbid fear of string.

lin·seed, *n.* The dried ripe seed of *Linum usitatissimum;* it contains 30 to 40% of a fixed oil, together with wax, resin, tannin, gum, and protein. Linseed is demulcent and emollient; infusions of the whole seed have been used in respiratory infections, and the whole seed is sometimes employed as a laxative. Syn. *flaxseed.*

linseed oil. The fixed oil obtained from linseed (oil that has been boiled or treated with a drier must not be used medicinally); used mostly in liniments and cerates, occasionally given for its laxative effect.

lint, *n.* [L. *linteum*, linen cloth]. A loosely woven or partly felted mass of broken linen fibers, made by scraping or picking linen cloth. It was once much used as a dressing for wounds.

lin·tin (lin'tin) *n.* Absorbent cotton rolled or compressed into sheets; used for dressing wounds.

lio-. See *leio-.*

liodermia. LEIODERMIA.

lion-jawed forceps. A bone-holding forceps with large strong teeth.

li·o·thy·ro·nine (lye''o·thigh'ro·neen) *n.* L-3-[3-(4-Hydroxy-3-iodophenoxy)-3,5-diiodophenyl]alanine, or L-3,5,3'-triiodothyronine, $C_{15}H_{12}I_3NO_4$, a thyroid hormone also prepared synthetically; it produces the metabolic and clinical effects of desiccated thyroid and thyroxine but is much more potent and rapid in action.

liothyronine sodium. The sodium salt of liothyronine, used for treatment, by oral administration, of thyroid states.

li·o·trix (lye'o·tricks) *n.* A mixture of liothyronine sodium and levothyroxine sodium, salts of thyroid hormones used for the treatment of hypothyroidism.

lip, *n.* [Gmc. *lep-* (rel. to L. *labium*)]. 1. One of the two fleshy folds surrounding the orifice of the mouth. NA *labia oris.* 2. One of the labia majora or labia minora. 3. A projecting margin; rim.

lip-, lipo- [Gk. *lipos*]. A combining form meaning (a) *fat, fatty;* (b) *lipid.*

li·pa (lye'puh) *n.* [Gk., oil]. FAT (3).

lip·ac·i·de·mia (lip·as''i·dee'mee·uh) *n.* [*lip-* + *acid* + *-emia*]. The presence of fatty acids in the blood.

lip·ac·i·du·ria (lip·as''i·dew'ree·uh) *n.* [*lip-* + *acid* + *uria*]. The presence of fatty acids in the urine.

lipaemia. LIPEMIA.

lip·a·ro·trich·ia (lip''uh·ro·trick'ee·uh) *n.* [Gk. *liparos*, oily, shiny, + *-trichia*]. Abnormal oiliness of the hair.

lip·a·rous (lip'uh·rus) *adj.* [Gk. *liparos*, oily, shiny]. Fat; obese.

li·pase (lye'pace, lip'ace) *n.* [*lip-* + *-ase*]. A fat-splitting enzyme contained in the pancreatic juice, in blood plasma, and in many plants.

li·pa·su·ria (lip'ay·syoo'ree·uh, lye''pay·) *n.* [*lipase* + *-uria*]. The presence of lipase in the urine.

li·pec·to·my (li·peck'tuh·mee) *n.* [*lip-* + *-ectomy*]. Excision of fatty tissue.

li·pe·mia, li·pae·mia (li·pee''mee·uh) *n.* [*lip-* + *-emia*]. The presence of a fine emulsion of fatty substance in the blood. Syn. *lipidemia, lipoidemia.* —**lipe·mic, li·pae·mic** (li·pee'mick) *adj.*

lipemia ret·i·na·lis (ret''i·nay'lis). Fatty infiltration of the retina and its blood vessels in hyperlipemic states.

lipemic nephrosis. *Obsol.* LIPID NEPHROSIS.

lip·fan·o·gen (lip·fan'o·jen) *n.* [*lip-* + Gk. *phaneros*, conspicuous, + *-gen*]. Any lipid substance present in blood serum (for example, long-chain soaps, monoglycerides) which can be taken up by animal cells in tissue culture and converted to visible fat granules.

lip fissure. HARELIP.

lip furrow band. VESTIBULAR LAMINA.

lip herpes. HERPES LABIALIS.

lip·id (lip'id, lye'pid) *n.* [*lip-* + *-id*]. Any one of a group of fats and fatlike substances having in common the property of insolubility in water and solubility in the fat solvents. Included are fats, fatty acids, fatty oils, waxes, sterols, and esters of fatty acids containing other groups such as phosphoric acid (phospholipids) and carbohydrates (glycolipids). Syn. *lipin.*

lipid-cell tumor of the ovary. LUTEOMA.

lip·ide (lip'ide, ·id, lye'pid) *n.* LIPID.

lip·id·emia, lip·i·dae·mia (lip"i·dee'mee·uh) *n.* [*lipid* + *-emia*]. LIPEMIA.

lipid granulomatosis. HAND-SCHÜLLER-CHRISTIAN DISEASE.

lipid histiocytosis. 1. Any collection of lipid-containing histiocytes. 2. NIEMANN-PICK DISEASE.

li·pid·ic (li·pid'ick) *adj.* 1. Of or pertaining to a lipid; having the nature of a lipid.

lipid keratopathy. LIPOIDOSIS CORNEAE.

lipid nephrosis. *Obsol.* A chronic renal disease chiefly of children, characterized clinically by severe proteinuria, edema, hypoalbuminemia, hypercholesterolemia, and normal blood pressure, and associated with glomerular basement membrane thickening.

lip·i·dol·y·sis (lip"i·dol'i·sis) *n.* LIPOLYSIS.

lip·i·do·sis (lip"i·do'sis) *n.*, pl. **lipido·ses** (·seez) [*lipid* + *-osis*]. The generalized deposition of fat or fat-containing substances in cells of the reticuloendothelial system. See also *lipid storage diseases.*

lipid pneumonia. 1. Pneumonia due to aspiration of oily substances, particularly kerosene, mineral oil, or cod-liver oil; more common in children or in adults when the cough reflex is impaired. 2. The deposition of cholesterol and other lipids in chronically inflamed pulmonary tissue.

lipid proteinosis. A hereditary disorder characterized by extracellular deposits of phospholipid-protein conjugate involving various areas of the body including the skin and air passages.

lipid storage disease. Any of a group of rare diseases, including Gaucher's disease, Niemann-Pick disease, and the amaurotic familial idiocies; characterized by an accumulation of large, lipid-containing cells throughout the viscera and nervous system. They occur primarily in childhood. See also *sphingolipidosis.*

lip·i·du·ria (lip"i·dew'ree·uh) *n.* The presence of fats or other lipids in the urine.

lip·in (lip'in, lye'pin) *n.* LIPID.

Lipiodol. The trademark for an iodized poppy seed oil used as a contrast medium for roentgenologic work.

[1]lipo-. See *lip-.*

[2]lipo- [Gk., from *lipein,* to leave]. A combining form meaning *lack, absence.*

Lipo-Adrenal cortex. Trademark for a preparation of adrenal cortical hormones dissolved in cottonseed oil.

lipo·blast (lip'o·blast) *n.* [*lipo-* + *-blast*]. A formative fat cell, small or moderate in size, polyhedral, and having numerous tiny droplets of fat in its cytoplasm. —**lipo·blas·tic** (lip" o·blas'tick) *adj.*

lipoblastic lipoma. LIPOSARCOMA.

lipo·blas·to·ma (lip"o·blas·to'muh) *n.* [*lipoblast* + *-oma*]. LIPOSARCOMA.

lipo·blas·to·sis (lip"o·blas·to'sis) *n.* [*lipoblast* + *-osis*]. Multiple lipomas in subcutaneous and visceral fat deposits. Syn. *systemic multiple lipomas.*

lip·o·ca·ic (lip"o·kay'ick) *n.* [*lipo-* + Gk. *kaiein*, to burn, + *-ic*]. A substance, probably a hormone, found in the pancreas which prevents deposition of lipids in the liver.

lipo·cal·ci·no·gran·u·lo·ma·to·sis (lip"o·kal"si·no·gran·yoo·lo"muh·to'sis) *n.* [*lipo-* + *calci-* + *granuloma* + *-osis*]. Lipidosis characterized by painless symmetric tumors in the bursae, mucosae, and musculature. Syn. *tumoral calcinosis.*

lipo·cele (lip'o·seel) *n.* [*lipo-* + *-cele*]. ADIPOCELE.

lipo·cere (lip'o·seer) *n.* ADIPOCERE.

lipo·chon·dro·dys·tro·phy (lip"o·kon"dro·dis'truh·fee) *n.* [*lipo-* + *chondrodystrophy*]. MUCOPOLYSACCHARIDOSIS.

lipo·chon·dro·ma (lip"o·kon·dro'muh) *n.* [*lipo-* + *chondroma*]. Chondroma containing fat cells.

lipo·chrome (lip'o·krohm) *n.* [*lipo-* + *-chrome*]. 1. A readily soluble carotenoid pigment giving a blue color with sulfuric acid. 2. LIPOFUSCIN.

lipo·cyte (lip'o·site) *n.* [*lipo-* + *-cyte*]. A specialized cell for fat storage. Syn. *adipocyte.*

lipo·di·er·e·sis (lip"o·dye·err'e·sis) *n.* [*lipo-* + Gk. *diairesis,* division, separation]. LIPOLYSIS.

lipo·dys·tro·phia (lip"o·dis·tro'fee·uh) *n.* [*lipo-* + *dystrophia*]. LIPODYSTROPHY.

lipodystrophia pro·gres·si·va (pro·gre·sigh'vuh). PROGRESSIVE LIPODYSTROPHY.

lipo·dys·tro·phy (lip"o·dis'truh·fee) *n.* [*lipo-* + *dystrophy*]. A disturbance of fat metabolism in which the subcutaneous fat disappears over some regions of the body, but is unaffected in others.

lipo·fi·bro·ma (lip"o·figh·bro'muh) *n.* [*lipo-* + *fibr-* + *-oma*]. A benign connective tissue tumor composed of adipose and fibrous tissue.

lipo·fi·bro·myx·o·ma (lip"o·figh"bro·mick·so'muh) *n.* [*lipo-* + *fibro-* + *myx-* + *-oma*]. A benign mesodermal mixed tumor, containing fatty tissue, fibrous tissue, and mucoid or myxomatous tissue.

lipo·fi·bro·sar·co·ma (lip"o·figh"bro·sahr·ko'muh) *n.* [*lipo-* + *fibro-* + *sarcoma*]. A malignant tumor whose parenchyma is composed of anaplastic fibrous and adipose tissue cells.

lip of the cervix of the uterus. One of two lips surrounding the cervical os, usually designated anterior (NA *labium anterius ostii uteri*) and posterior (NA *labium posterius ostii uteri*).

lipo·fus·cin (lip"o·fus'in, ·few'sin) *n.* [*lipo-* + *fuscin*]. One of a group of at least partly insoluble lipid pigments occurring in cardiac and smooth muscle cells, in macrophages and in parenchyma and interstitial cells of various organs; characterized by sudanophilia, Nile blue staining, fatty acid, glycol, and ethylene reactions, slow reduction of diammine silver, osmic acid, and ferric ferricyanide.

lipo·gen·e·sis (lip"o·jen'e·sis) *n.* [*lipo-* + *-genesis*]. The formation or deposit of fat. —**lipogen·ic** (·ick) *adj.*

li·pog·e·nous (li·poj'e·nus) *adj.* [*lipo-* + *-genous*]. Fat-producing.

lipo·gran·u·lo·ma (lip"o·gran·yoo·lo'muh) *n.* [*lipo-* + *granuloma*]. A nodule of fatty tissue, consisting of a center of degenerated and necrotic fat associated with granulomatous inflammation.

lipo·gran·u·lo·ma·to·sis (lip"o·gran·yoo·lo"muh·to'sis) *n.* [*lipogranuloma* + *-osis*]. A condition marked by the presence of one or more lipogranulomas.

lipo·he·mar·thro·sis, lipo·hae·mar·thro·sis (lip"o·hee"mahr·thro'sis) *n.*, pl. **lipohemarthro·ses, lipohaemarthro·ses** (·seez) [*lipo-* + *hem-* + *arthrosis*]. The presence of blood and lipids in the joint cavity following injury.

li·po·ic acid (li·po'ick). 6,8-Dithio-*n*-octanoic acid, $C_8H_{14}O_2S_2$, first isolated from yeast and liver, which participates in the enzymatic oxidative decarboxylation of alpha-keto acids in a stage between thiamine pyrophosphate and coenzyme A, and which is produced by resting cells of *Streptococcus fecalis* and other organisms. See also *protogen, thioctic acid.*

lip·oid (lip'oid, lye'poid) *adj. & n.* [*lip-* + *-oid*]. 1. Resembling fat or oil. 2. Having the character of a lipid; lipidic. 3. Lipid, particularly one of the intracellular lipids which contain nitrogen. The chemists have officially adopted the term lipid, but many histologists still use the term lipoid.

lip·oi·de·mia, lip·oi·dae·mia (lip"oy·dee'mee·uh) *n.* [*lipoid* + *-emia*]. LIPEMIA.

li·poid·ic (li·poy'dick) *adj.* Of or pertaining to a lipoid.

lipoid nephrosis. A disease state characterized by the nephrotic syndrome, with renal glomeruli demonstrating no histopathologic changes by light microscopy but with ultrastructural abnormalities, mainly fusion of epithelial foot processes. Syn. *minimal change glomerular disease.*

lip·oi·do·sis (lip"oy·do'sis) *n.*, pl. **lipoido·ses** (·seez) [*lipoid* + *-osis*]. LIPIDOSIS.

lipoidosis cor·ne·ae (kor'nee·ee). Fatty deposits in the cornea.

lipoidosis cutis et mu·co·sae (mew·ko'see). LIPID PROTEINOSIS.

Lipoiodine. Trademark for ethyl diiodobrassidate, $C_{21}H_{39}I_2$-$COOC_2H_5$, used where iodide therapy is indicated and as a roentgenographic contrast medium.

lipoid pneumonia. LIPID PNEUMONIA.

li·pol·y·sis (li·pol'i·sis) *n.*, pl. **lipoly·ses** (·seez) [*lipo-* + *-lysis*]. The hydrolysis of fat. —**lipo·lyt·ic** (lip"o·lit'ick) *adj.*

lipolytic enzyme. An enzyme that hydrolyzes fats to glycerin and fatty acids, as pancreatic lipase.

li·po·ma (li·po'muh, lye·) *n.*, pl. **lipomas, lipoma·ta** (·tuh) [*lip-* + *-oma*]. A benign tumor whose parenchyma is composed of mature adipose tissue cells. —**li·pom·a·tous** (li·pom'uh·tus), **lipoma·toid** (·toid) *adj.*

lipoma foe·ta·lo·cel·lu·la·re (fee·tay"lo·sel"yoo·lair'ee). HIBERNOMA.

li·po·ma·to·sis (li·po"muh·to'sis, lye·) *n.*, pl. **lipomato·ses** (·seez) [*lipoma* + *-osis*]. 1. Multiple lipomas. 2. A general deposition of fat; obesity.

lipomatous synovitis. Synovitis in which there is fatty degeneration.

lipo·mel·a·not·ic (lip"o·mel·uh·not'ick) *adj.* [*lipo-* + *melanotic*]. Pertaining both to fat and melanin.

lipomelanotic reticular hyperplasia. LIPOMELANOTIC RETICULOSIS.

lipomelanotic reticulosis. A form of lymph-node hyperplasia characterized by preservation of the architectural structure, inflammatory exudate, and hyperplasia of the reticulum cells which show phagocytosis of hemosiderin, melanin, and occasionally fat. It is often secondary to an extensive dermatitis. Syn. *lipomelanotic reticular hyperplasia, dermatopathic lymphadenitis.*

lipo·me·nin·go·cele (lip"o·me·ning'go·seel) *n.* [*lipo-* + *meningocele*]. The association of lobules of adipose tissue with a meningocele.

li·po·me·ria (lye"po·meer'ee·uh, lip"o·) *n.* LEIPOMERIA.

lipo·me·tab·o·lism (lip"o·me·tab'uh·liz·um) *n.* [*lipo-* + *metabolism*]. The absorption and metabolism of fat.

li·pom·pha·lus (li·pom'fuh·lus) *n.* [*lip-* + Gk. *omphalos,* navel]. A fatty umbilical hernia.

lipo·my·e·lo·me·nin·go·cele (lip"o·migh"e·lo·me·ning'go·seel) *n.* [*lipo-* + *myelomeningocele*]. The association of masses of adipose tissue with a myelomeningocele.

lipo·myo·he·man·gi·o·ma, lipo·myo·hae·man·gi·o·ma (lip"o·migh"o·he·man"jee·o'muh) *n.* [*lipo-* + *myo-* + *hemangi-* + *-oma*]. A benign hamartomatous tumor whose parenchyma is composed of adipose tissue, muscle, and blood vessels.

lipo·my·o·ma (lip"o·migh·o'muh) *n.* [*lipo-* + *my-* + *-oma*]. A benign hamartomatous tumor whose parenchyma is composed of adipose tissue and muscle.

lipo·myo·sar·co·ma (lip"o·migh"o·sahr·ko'muh) *n.* [*lipo-* + *myo-* + *sarcoma*]. A malignant tumor whose parenchyma is composed of anaplastic adipose tissue and muscle cells.

lipo·myx·o·ma (lip"o·mick·so'muh) *n.* [*lipo-* + *myx-* + *-oma*]. A benign tumor whose parenchyma is composed of adipose tissue and mucinous connective tissue elements.

lipo·myxo·sar·co·ma (lip"o·mick"so·sahr·ko'muh) *n.* [*lipo-* + *myxo-* + *sarcoma*]. A malignant tumor whose parenchyma is composed of anaplastic adipose tissue and mucinous connective-tissue cells.

Lip·o·nys·sus (lip"o·nis'us) *n.* [*lipo-* + Gk. *nyss*ein, to prick, sting]. *BDELLONYSSUS.*

Liponyssus bacoti. *BDELLONYSSUS BACOTI.*

lipo·pathy (lip'o·path"ee) *n.* Any disease of lipid metabolism.

lipo·pe·nia (lip"o·pee'nee·uh) *n.* [*lipo-* + *-penia*]. Abnormal diminution of fat in tissues.

lipo·pep·tide (lip"o·pep'tide) *n.* AMINOLIPID; a compound belonging to a poorly defined group of fatlike substances containing amino acids.

lipo·phage (lip"o·faje, ·fahzh) *n.* [*lipo-* + *-phage*]. A cell which has taken up fat in its cytoplasm.

lipo·pha·gia (lip"o·fay'jee·uh) *n.* LIPOPHAGY.

lipo·pha·gic (lip"o·fay'jick, ·faj'ick) *adj.* Pertaining to lipophagy.

lipophagic granuloma. A granuloma whose macrophages contain fat derived from the breakdown of adipose tissue in the area.

lipo·pha·gy (lip'o·fay"jee, li·pof'uh·jee) *n.* [*lipo-* + *-phagy*]. The destruction of adipose tissue, associated with cellular elements which ingest products of fat breakdown.

lipo·phil (lip'o·fil) *adj.* [*lipo-* + *-phil*]. Having affinity for lipids; LIPOTROPIC (1).

lipo·phil·ia (lip"o·fil'ee·uh) *n.* [*lipo-* + *-philia*]. Affinity for fat.

li·po·phre·nia (lye"po·free'nee·uh, lip"o·) *n.* [*lipo-*, lack, + *-phrenia*]. *Obsol.* Failure of mental capacity.

lipo·plas·tic (lip'o·plas'tick) *adj.* [*lipo-* + *plastic*]. Producing adipose tissue.

lipoplastic lymphadenopathy. Lymph node enlargement due to an increment in adipose tissue, largely in the hilum.

lipo·poly·sac·cha·ride (lip"o·pol"ee·sack'uh·ride) *n.* A compound of a lipid with a polysaccharide.

lipo·pro·tein (lip"o·pro'tee·in, ·teen) *n.* One of a group of conjugated proteins consisting of a simple protein combined with a lipid. A lipoprotein may be classified according to its physical properties or density as alpha-lipoprotein, containing more protein and having high density; beta-lipoprotein, containing more lipid compared to protein and having low density; or omega-lipoprotein, containing the largest amount of lipids and appearing as chylomicra in the serum.

lipo·rho·din (lip"o·ro'din) *n.* [*lipo-* + *rhod-* + *-in*]. A red lipochrome.

lipo·sar·co·ma (lip"o·sahr·ko'muh) *n.* [*lipo-* + *sarcoma*]. A malignant tumor whose parenchyma is composed of anaplastic adipose tissue cells. —**liposarcoma·tous** (·tus) *adj.*

li·po·sis (li·po'sis) *n.*, pl. **lipo·ses** (·seez) [*lip-* + *-osis*]. LIPOMATOSIS.

li·po·si·tol (li·po'si·tol) *n.* A name proposed by Folch and Woolley for inositol phospholipids.

lipo·sol·u·ble (lip"o·sol'yoo·bul) *adj.* [*lipo-* + *soluble*]. Soluble in fats.

li·pos·to·my (li·pos'tuh·mee, lye·) *n.* [*lipo-*, absence, + *-stomy*]. The congenital absence of a mouth.

li·po·thy·mia (lye"po·thigh'mee·uh) *n.* [Gk., from *lipothymein,* to faint]. *Obsol.* Faintness or giddiness.

lipo·tro·pia (lip"o·tro'pee·uh) *n.* [*lipo-* + *-tropia*]. LIPOTROPIC FACTOR.

lipo·trop·ic (lip"o·trop'ick) *adj.* [*lipo-* + *-tropic*]. 1. Having an affinity for lipids, particularly fats and oils. 2. Having a preventive or curative effect on the deposition of excessive fat in abnormal sites.

lipotropic factor. A substance that reduces the amount of liver fat; more specifically, choline or any compound, or compounds, which metabolically can give rise to choline. Syn. *lipotropia.*

lipo·vac·cine (lip"o·vack'seen, ·vack·seen') *n.* [*lipo-* + *vaccine*]. A vaccine with a fatty or oily menstruum.

lipo·vi·tel·lin (lip"o·vi·tel'in) *n.* [*lipo-* + *vitellin*]. A lipoprotein occurring in egg yolk; a conjugated protein containing approximately 18% of phospholipid.

lipo·xan·thin (lip"o·zan'thin) *n.* [*lipo-* + *xanth-* + *-in*]. A yellow lipochrome.

li·pox·e·nous (li·pock'se·nus, lye·) *adj.* [Gk. *leip*ein, to leave, + *xen-* + *-ous*]. Of or pertaining to a parasite which leaves its host after completing its development. —**lipoxe·ny** (·nee) *n.*

li·pox·i·dase (li·pock'si·dace, ·daze) *n.* An enzyme catalyzing the oxidation of the double bonds of an unsaturated fatty acid.

lip·pa (lip'uh) *n.* MARGINAL BLEPHARITIS.

lip·ping, *n.* The perichondral growth of osteophytes which project beyond the margin of the joint in degenerative joint disease.

lip·pi·tude (lip'i·tewd) *n.* LIPPITUDO.

lip·pi·tu·do (lip"i·tew'do) *n.* [L., blearedness, inflammation of the eyes, from *lippus,* blear-eyed]. A condition of the eyes marked by ulcerative marginal blepharitis; a state of being blear-eyed.

lip reading. Understanding what a person is saying by observing the movements of the lips and other facial muscles; important in instruction of the deaf.

Lip·schütz body (lip'shuᵉts) [B. *Lipschütz,* Austrian dermatologist, 1878–1931]. Eosinophilic nuclear inclusion, granular or amorphous, designated as type A, found in cells infected with such viruses as herpes simplex, herpes zoster, cytomegalovirus, and yellow fever.

Lipschütz cell [B. *Lipschütz*]. CENTROCYTE.

li·pu·ria (li·pew'ree·uh) *n.* [*lip-* + *-uria*]. The presence of fat in the urine; ADIPOSURIA.

Liquaemin. A trademark for a sterile solution of the sodium salt of heparin.

Liquamar. Trademark for phenprocoumon, a synthetic, coumarin-type anticoagulant drug.

liq·ue·fa·cient (lick"we·fay'shunt) *n.* [L. *liquefaciens*]. An agent capable of producing liquefaction.

liq·ue·fac·tion (lick"wi·fack'shun) *n.* [L. *liquefacere,* to make liquid]. 1. The change to a liquid form, usually of a solid tissue to a fluid or semifluid state. 2. Condensation of a gas to a liquid or the conversion of a solid to a liquid.

liquefaction necrosis. Tissue death in which the remains are converted to a liquid state.

liq·ue·fac·tive (lick"wi·fack'tiv) *adj.* Pertaining to, causing, or characterized by liquefaction.

liquefactive degeneration. LIQUEFACTION NECROSIS.

liquefactive necrosis. LIQUEFACTION NECROSIS.

liquefied phenol. Phenol maintained in the liquid state by the presence of 10% of water.

li·ques·cent (li·kwes'unt) *adj.* Becoming liquid.

liq·uid (lick'wid) *n.* [L. *liquidus,* fluid, flowing, from *liquere,* to be liquid]. A fluid or substance that flows readily. A state of matter intermediate between a solid and a gas, shapeless and fluid, taking the shape of the container and seeking the lowest level.

liquid air. Air that has been liquefied by subjecting it to great pressure; extreme cold is produced by its evaporation.

liquid apiol. The liquid oleoresin prepared from parsley fruit, not identical with apiol but formerly used similarly. Syn. *parsley oleoresin.*

liquid paraffin. MINERAL OIL.

liquid petrolatum. MINERAL OIL.

liq·uo·gel (lick'wo·jel) *n.* A gel which, when melted, yields a sol of low viscosity.

li·quor (lye'kwor, lick'wor; in senses 3 and 4, lick'ur) *n.* [L., a liquid]. 1. Any of certain medicinal solutions, usually including aqueous solutions of nonvolatile substances, except those solutions which belong to the class of syrups, infusions, or decoctions. 2. In Latin anatomical terms, a body fluid. 3. Any of various liquids occurring in nature or, more usually, in the preparation of certain man-made products, as dye liquor, mother liquor. 4. A distilled alcoholic drink.

liquor am·nii (am'nee·eye). AMNIOTIC FLUID.

liquor amnii spu·ri·us (spew'ree·us). *Obsol.* Allantoic fluid.

liquor ce·re·bro·spi·na·lis (serr"e·bro·spi·nay'lis) [NA]. CEREBROSPINAL FLUID.

liquor fol·li·cu·li (fol·ick'yoo·lye) [BNA]. FOLLICULAR FLUID.

liquorice. Licorice (= GLYCYRRHIZA).

liquor pe·ri·car·dii (perr"i·kahr'dee·eye) [BNA]. PERICARDIAL FLUID.

liquor san·gui·nis (sang'gwi·nis). BLOOD PLASMA.

liquor se·mi·nis (see'mi·nis). SEMEN (2).

Lis·franc's amputation (lees·frahⁿ') [J. *Lisfranc* de Saint Martin, French surgeon, 1790–1847]. Partial amputation of the foot by disarticulation of the metatarsal bones from the tarsus.

Lisfranc's tubercle [J. *Lisfranc*]. SCALENE TUBERCLE.

lisp, *n.* & *v.* 1. A speech defect consisting in the substitution of interdental spirant sounds (th, t̶h̶) for sibilants (s, z). 2. Any of various other speech defects or affectations, especially those reminiscent of baby talk. 3. To speak with a lisp.

Lis·sau·er's cerebral sclerosis (lis'aow·ur) [H. *Lissauer,* German neurologist, 1861–1891]. LISSAUER'S PARALYSIS.

Lissauer's column, fasciculus, tract, or **zone.** DORSOLATERAL TRACT.

Lissauer's paralysis [H. *Lissauer*]. General paresis of rapid onset and progression with seizures and prominent focal signs of unilateral frontal or temporal lobe disease. Syn. *Lissauer's cerebral sclerosis.*

lis·sen·ce·pha·lia (lis"en·se·fay'lee·uh) *n.* [Gk. *lissos,* smooth, + *-encephalia*]. Smallness of the brain and failure of sulcal formation, resulting in a smooth brain.

lis·sen·ceph·a·lous (lis"en·sef'uh·lus) *adj.* [Gk. *lissos,* smooth, + *encephal-* + *-ous*]. Having a brain with few or no convolutions.

lis·sen·ceph·a·ly (lis"en·sef'uh·lee) *n.* LISSENCEPHALIA.

Lissephen. A trademark for mephenesin, a skeletal muscle relaxant.

lister bag. LYSTER BAG.

Lis·ter·el·la (lis"tur·el'uh) *n.* LISTERIA.

lis·ter·el·lo·sis (lis"tur·el·o'sis) *n.*, pl. **listerello·ses** (·seez) [*Listerella* + *-osis*]. LISTERIOSIS.

Lis·te·ria (lis·teer'ee·uh) *n.* [J. *Lister,* English surgeon, 1827–1912]. A genus of bacteria of the family Corynebacteriaceae. Its members are small, non-spore-forming, gram-positive rods, motile by means of a single terminal flagellum. —**lis·te·ric** (·rick) *adj.*

Listeria mono·cy·tog·e·nes (mon"o·sigh·toj'e·neez). One cause of sporadic cases of purulent meningitis in man, granulomatosis infantasepticum, septicemia, and less commonly, mononucleosis and conjunctivitis.

lis·te·ri·o·sis (lis·teer"ee·o'sis) *n.*, pl. **listerio·ses** (·seez) [*Listeria* + *-osis*]. Infection of animals and man with the gram-positive bacillus *Listeria monocytogenes;* the protean manifestations include meningitis, lymphadenopathy, disseminated granulomas, respiratory symptoms, and ill-defined acute febrile illness; it can produce abortion and fetal or neonatal death.

Lis·ter·ism (lis'tur·iz·um) *n.* A general name for the antiseptic and aseptic treatment of wounds according to the principles of Joseph Lister.

Listica. Trademark for hydroxyphenamate, a tranquilizer.

Lis·ting's law [J. B. *Listing,* German physicist and physiologist, 1808–1882]. When the eyeball moves from the position of rest, its angle of rotation is the same as if it rotated on an axis perpendicular to both the line of vision in its new position and the line of vision in its former position.

Lis·ton forceps [R. *Liston,* Scottish surgeon in England, 1794–1847]. A type of bone-cutting forceps.

Liston's knives [R. *Liston*]. Long-bladed amputation knives of various sizes.

Liston's splint [R. *Liston*]. A straight splint for the side of the leg, or the body.

li·ter, li·tre (lee'tur) *n.* [Gk. *litra,* pound]. The metric unit of volume, representing 0.001 cubic meter or 1000 cubic centimeters. Formerly defined as the volume occupied by 1 kg of pure water at 4°C and 760 mm pressure. It is equal to 1.056 United States quarts. Abbreviated, l.

lith-, litho- [Gk. *lithos*]. A combining form meaning *stone, calculus.*

-lith [Gk. *lithos*]. A combining form meaning *stone, calculus.*

lith·a·gogue (lith'uh·gog) *n.* [*lith-* + *-agogue*]. Any agent that is supposed to expel calculi from the urinary bladder.

lith·arge (lith'ahrj, li·thahrj') *n.* [Gk. *lithargyros,* from *lithos,* stone, + *argyros,* silver]. LEAD MONOXIDE.

li·thec·to·my (li·theck'tuh·mee) *n.* [*lith-* + *-ectomy*]. LITHOTOMY.

li·the·mia, li·thae·mia (li·theem'ee·uh) *n.* [*lith-* + *-emia*]. HYPERURICEMIA.

lith·ia (lith'ee·uh) *n.* [NL., from Gk. *litheios*, of stone]. Li_2O. Lithium oxide. Lithia water is a mineral water containing lithium salts in solution.

li·thi·a·sis (li·thigh'uh·sis) *n.*, pl. **lithia·ses** (·seez) [Gk.]. The formation of calculi in the body. —**lithia·sic** (·sick) *adj.*

lithiasis conjunctivitis. Irritation of the conjunctiva due to deposition of calcareous matter in the tissue of the palpebral conjunctiva.

lith·ic (lith'ick) *adj.* [Gk. *lithikos*, from *lithos*, stone]. 1. Pertaining to calculi. 2. Pertaining to lithium.

lithic acid. URIC ACID.

lith·i·co·sis (lith·i·ko'sis) *n.* [Gk. *lithik*os, of stone, + *-osis*]. Silicosis or other pneumoconiosis occurring in stonecutters.

lith·i·um (lith'ee·um) *n.* [NL., from *lithia*]. Li = 6.941. A soft, silver-white metal belonging to the alkali group. It is the lightest solid element, having a density of 0.534. Salts of lithium have been used like salts of other alkali metals; under certain conditions they are toxic; now widely used in the treatment of hypomanic and manic states. See also Table of Elements in the Appendix.

lithium carbonate. Li_2CO_3, an antidepressant.

lithium carmine (Orth's). Contains 2.5 to 5.0 g of carmine in 100 ml of saturated aqueous lithium carbonate solution; used to stain histologic sections, the nuclei being stained bright red, and as a vital stain.

litho-. See *lith-*.

litho·cho·lic acid (lith''o·ko'lick, ·kol'ick). 3α-Hydroxycholanic acid, $C_{24}H_{40}O_3$, found in human and animal bile, also in gallstones from certain animals.

litho·di·al·y·sis (lith''o·dye·al'i·sis) *n.* [*litho-* + *dialysis*]. 1. The solution of calculi in the urinary bladder. 2. The breaking of a vesical calculus previous to its removal.

litho·fel·lic acid (lith''o·fel'ick). An acid, $C_{20}H_{36}O_4$, occurring in the intestinal concretions of ruminants.

litho·gen·e·sis (lith''o·jen'e·sis) *n.* [*litho-* + *-genesis*]. The formation of calculi or stones. —**litho·ge·net·ic** (·je·net'ick), **li·thog·e·nous** (li·thoj'e·nus) *adj.*

li·thog·e·ny (li·thoj'e·nee) *n.* [*litho-* + *-geny*]. LITHOGENESIS.

lith·oid (lith'oid) *adj.* [Gk. *lithoeidēs*]. Resembling a stone.

li·thoi·dal (li·thoy'dul) *adj.* LITHOID.

litho·kel·y·pho·pe·di·on (lith''o·kel''i·fo·pee'dee·on) *n.* [*litho-kelyphos* + Gk. *paidion*, child]. A calcified fetus (lithopedion) enclosed in calcified fetal membranes.

lith·o·kel·y·phos (lith''o·kel'i·fos) *n.* [*litho-* + Gk. *kelyphos*, sheath, membrane]. Calcified fetal membranes without calcification of the dead fetus. Compare *lithopedion*.

litho·labe (lith'o·labe) *n.* [*litho-* + *-labe*]. An instrument formerly used for grasping and holding a vesical calculus during operation.

li·thol·a·paxy (li·thol'uh·pack''see, lith'o·luh·) *n.* [*litho-* + Gk. *lapax*is, evacuation]. The operation of crushing a urinary calculus in the bladder by means of the lithotrite, and then removing the fragments by irrigation, a procedure now performed by a transurethral approach. Syn. *lithotrity*.

litho·ne·phri·tis (lith''o·ne·frye'tis) *n.* [*litho-* + *nephritis*]. Inflammation of the kidney, associated with the presence of renal calculi.

litho·ne·phrot·o·my (lith''o·ne·frot'uh·mee) *n.* [*litho-* + *nephrotomy*]. Lithotomy performed by means of an incision into the kidney parenchyma or the renal pelvis; renal lithotomy.

lith·o·pe·di·on (lith''o·pee'dee·on) *n.* [*litho-* + Gk. *paidion*, child]. A retained fetus that has become calcified. See also *lithokelyphopedion*.

litho·phone (lith'uh·fone) *n.* [*litho-* + *-phone*]. An instrument formerly used to detect by sound the presence of calculi in the urinary bladder.

litho·scope (lith'uh·skope) *n.* [*litho-* + *-scope*]. An instrument for the visual detection and examination of vesical calculi; CYSTOSCOPE.

li·tho·sis (li·tho'sis) *n.* [*lith-* + *-osis*]. LITHICOSIS.

li·thot·o·mist (li·thot'uh·mist) *n.* 1. A surgeon who performs lithotomies. 2. Formerly, an individual who cut for stone in the urinary bladder.

li·thot·o·my (li·thot'uh·mee) *n.* [Gk. *lithotomia*, from *lithos*, stone, calculus]. The removal of a calculus, usually vesical, through an operative incision.

lithotomy forceps. A special type of forceps for removing a stone from the urinary bladder or ureter.

lithotomy position. DORSOSACRAL POSITION.

litho·trip·sy (lith''o·trip'see) *n.* [*litho-* + *-tripsy*]. The operation of crushing calculi in the urinary bladder.

litho·trip·to·scope (lith''o·trip'tuh·skope) *n.* [*lithotrip*sy + *-scope*]. CYSTOSCOPIC LITHOTRITE.

lith·o·trite (lith'o·trite) *n.* [*litho-* + L. *terere, tritum* to rub, grind]. An instrument for crushing a vesical calculus. See also *electrohydraulic lithotrite*. —**lith·o·trit·ic** (lith''o·trit'ick) *adj.*

li·thot·ri·ty (li·thot'ri·tee) *n.* [*litho-* + L. *terere, tritum*, to rub, grind]. LITHOLAPAXY.

lith·ous (lith'us) *adj.* [*lith-* + *-ous*]. Having the nature of a calculus.

lith·u·re·sis (lith''yoo·ree'sis) *n.* [*lith-* + *uresis*]. Voiding of small calculi with the urine; gravel urine.

li·thu·ria (lith·yoo'ree·uh) *n.* [*lith*ic acid + *-uria*]. A condition marked by excess of uric (lithic) acid or its salts in the urine.

li·ti·gious paranoia (li·tij'us). A paranoid state in which the main symptom is a desire to initiate lawsuits which have no rational basis.

lit·mus (lit'mus) *n.* [ON. *litmosi*, literally, dye-moss]. A blue pigment obtained from *Roccella tinctoria*, a lichen; used as an acid-base indicator.

litmus milk. Milk that contains litmus; used as an indicator in bacteriology.

litre. LITER.

Lit·ten's sign [M. *Litten*, German physician, 1845–1907]. DIAPHRAGMATIC SIGN.

lit·ter (lit'ur) *n.* [OF. *litiere*, from L. *lectus*, bed]. 1. A stretcher, basket, or bed with handles, used for carrying the sick or injured. 2. In animals, the group of young brought forth at one birth.

lit·tle finger. The fifth digit of the hand, on the ulnar side. NA *digitus minimus, digitus V*.

Little's disease [W. J. *Little*, English surgeon, 1810–1894]. Cerebral palsy; especially the spastic diplegic type, considered by Little to be due to perinatal asphyxia and prematurity.

little toe. The fifth or outer digit of the foot. NA *digitus minimus, digitus V*.

little-toe reflex. PUUSSEPP'S REFLEX.

Litt·man ox-gall medium. A selective medium containing bile salts, crystal violet, and streptomycin, used in the primary isolation of fungi from specimens having a mixed bacterial and fungal flora.

lit·to·ral (lit'uh·rul) *adj.* [L. *littoralis*, coastal, from *littus, litus*, seashore, coast]. Pertaining to a lining, as of a sinus; an endothelium.

littoral cells. The cells that line lymph sinuses in lymphatic tissue, or the sinusoids of bone marrow. They form a type of endothelium once thought to be phagocytic.

Lit·tré's glands (lee·trey') [A. *Littré*, French anatomist, 1658–1726]. URETHRAL GLANDS.

lit·tri·tis (li·trye'tis) *n.* [*Littré's* glands + *-itis*]. Inflammation of the urethral glands.

Litz·mann's obliquity [K. K. T. *Litzmann*, German gynecologist, 1815–1890]. POSTERIOR ASYNCLITISM.

live-born, *adj.* Born in such a state that acts of life are manifested after the extrusion of the whole body. Contr. *stillborn*.

li·ve·do (li·vee′do) *n.* [L., from *livere,* to be bluish]. A mottled discoloration of the skin.

livedo re·tic·u·la·ris (re·tick″yoo·lair′is). CUTIS MARMORATA.

livedo vasculitis. A chronic, recurrent hyalinizing vasculitis limited to the lower extremities, manifested by patches of purpura and ulcerations, but without the true findings of cutis marmorata (livedo reticularis).

live flesh. MYOKYMIA.

liv·er, *n.* [Gmc. *librō* (rel. to Gk. *lip-,* fat, and probably also to Gmc. *līb-,* life)]. The largest glandular organ in the body, situated directly beneath the diaphragm mainly on the right side of the abdominal cavity. It is encapsulated and consists of two principal lobes: a larger right and a smaller left. Its specific functions are many and include secretion of bile, storage of glycogen and fat, protein breakdown, and detoxification. It receives nutrients and oxygen for cellular metabolism via the hepatic portal circulatory system. The gall bladder lies within the cystic fossa, a depression on its inferior surface. NA *hepar.* Comb. form *hepat(o)-.*

liver breath. FETOR HEPATICUS.

liver cords. HEPATIC CORDS.

liver failure. Severe inability of the liver to carry out its normal functions or the demands made upon it, as evidenced by such clinical phenomena as severe jaundice, disturbed mental functioning including coma, and abnormal levels of blood ammonia, bilirubin, alkaline phosphatase, glutamic oxaloacetic transaminase, lactic dehydrogenase, and reversal of the albumin/globulin ratio.

liver flap. ASTERIXIS.

liver fluke. A trematode that lodges in the intrahepatic biliary passages, most frequently *Clonorchis sinensis,* rarely *Fasciola hepatica.*

liver injection. A sterile solution in water for injection of the soluble thermostable fraction of mammalian livers which increases the number of red blood cells in the blood of persons affected with pernicious anemia. The potency is expressed in terms of the equivalent of cyanocobalamin.

liver injury. 1. Contusion or laceration of the liver, usually of the right lobe; may be due to crushing injuries, fractured ribs, gunshot wounds, stab wounds, or operations. 2. Necrosis of liver cells from poisoning and infectious disease, as from malaria or jaundice.

liver *Lactobacillus casei* factor. FOLIC ACID.

liver lobules. LOBULES OF THE LIVER.

liver of lime. CALCIUM SULFIDE.

liver of sulfur. SULFURATED POTASH.

liver phosphorylase deficiency. HERS' DISEASE.

liver rot. A severe form of fascioliasis which occurs in sheep and results in anemia and sudden death.

liver spot. LENTIGO SENILIS.

liver sugar. GLYCOGEN.

liv·er·wort (liv′ur·wurt) *n.* HEPATICA.

liv·e·tin (liv′e·tin) *n.* A protein occurring in the yolk of egg.

liv·id (liv′id) *adj.* [L. *lividus,* of a leaden, bluish color]. Of a pale lead color; black and blue; discolored, as flesh from contusion or from hyperemia. —**li·vid·i·ty** (li·vid′i·tee) *n.*

Li·vie·ra·to's sign (leev·yeh·rah′to) [P. *Livierato,* Italian physician, 1860–1936]. 1. Vasoconstriction upon mechanical stimulation of the abdominal sympathetic (aortic) plexus by striking the anterior abdomen on the xiphoumbilical line. This increases venous return to the heart and increases the area of cardiac dullness on the right cardiac border. Syn. *abdominocardiac sign.* 2. Enlargement of the right side of the heart, occurring with change from recumbent to erect posture, with spontaneous regression on resuming the recumbent position. Syn. *orthocardiac sign.*

LIVIM. Abbreviation for *lethal intestinal virus of infant mice.*

li·vor (lye′vor, ·vur) *n.* [L., leaden color]. 1. LIVIDITY. 2. LIVOR MORTIS.

livor mor·tis (mor′tis). Mottled purple-red discoloration of the dependent parts of the body after death, related to pooling of blood in those regions. Syn. *cadaveric lividity.*

lix·iv·i·a·tion (lick·siv″ee·ay′shun) *n.* [L. *lixivius,* of lye, from *lixa,* ashes, lye]. The extraction and separation of a soluble substance from a mixture with insoluble matter, such as the leaching of salts from ashes.

Li·zars' operation (li·zahrz′) [J. *Lizars,* Scottish surgeon, 1783–1860]. An excision of the upper jaw through an incision running from the corner of the mouth to the zygoma.

Lju·bin·sky's stain. A stain for bacterial granules consisting of methyl violet 2B or crystal violet in 5% acetic acid; counterstain, Bismarck brown, 0.1% aqueous solution.

LLD factor. Abbreviation for *Lactobacillus lactis Dorner factor.*

L.M.A. Abbreviation for *left mentoanterior* position of the fetus.

LMD. A trademark for dextran 40, a plasma volume extender.

L.M.P. Abbreviation for *left mentoposterior* position of the fetus.

L.O.A. Abbreviation for *left occipitoanterior* position of the fetus.

Loa (lo′uh) *n.* [Kongo *lowa*]. A genus of filarial worms.

load, *n. & v.* 1. A supported mass, weight, or force. 2. Something given to a patient to test a physiologic process. See also *loading test.* 3. To place a weight or physical stress on something. 4. To stress a process or to weight a test or experimental situation in order to observe or to influence the outcome.

load-assisting exercise. An exercise to increase the power of a weakened muscle in which the load with which the patient performs the exercise serves as a counterbalance, i.e., helps the muscle. See also *progressive-resistance exercise.*

loading test. *In medicine,* the administration of a substance to a patient to test his capacity for handling that substance, as the administration of phenylalanine to carriers of phenylketonuria, or of xylose for the detection of intestinal malabsorption.

load-resisting exercise. An exercise to increase the power of a weakened muscle in which the load with which the patient performs the exercise resists the muscle. See also *progressive-resistance exercise.*

lo·a·i·a·sis (lo″uh·eye′uh·sis) *n.* LOIASIS.

Loa loa. A species of filaria that invades human subcutaneous tissues; the eye worm.

lo·bar (lo′bur, bahr) *adj.* Of or pertaining to a lobe.

lobar atrophy. LOBAR SCLEROSIS.

lobar bronchus. Any bronchus which originates in a primary bronchus and through its branches, the segmental bronchi, ventilates a lobe of a lung; the right superior (NA *bronchus lobaris superior dexter*), right middle (NA *bronchus lobaris medius dexter*), right lower (NA *bronchus lobaris inferior dexter*), left superior (NA *bronchus lobaris superior sinister*), or left lower (NA *bronchus lobaris inferior sinister*) *lobar bronchus.* NA (pl.) *bronchi lobares* (sing. *bronchus lobaris*).

lobar pneumonia. Pneumonia involving one or more lobes of the lung, usually pneumococcal pneumonia; characterized by abrupt onset with chill, fever, pleuritic pain, cough, and dyspnea. The pathologic changes are of hyperemia, hepatization, and finally, resolution.

lobar sclerosis. Gliosis and atrophy of a lobe of the cerebrum, resulting in mental and neurologic deficits; applied particularly to the hardening and shrinkage seen in the brains of infants and children who suffered prolonged intrauterine or neonatal hypoxia. See also *Pick's disease.*

lo·bate (lo′bate) *adj.* Arranged in lobes.

lo·bat·ed (lo′bay·tid) *adj.* LOBATE.

lobated spleen. MULTILOBATE SPLEEN.

lobe, *n.* [L. *lobus,* from Gk. *lobos*]. 1. A more or less rounded part or projection of an organ, separated from neighboring parts by fissures and constrictions. NA *lobus.* 2. A division or part of a tooth formed from a separate point of the beginning of calcification.

lo·bec·to·my (lo·beck'tuh·mee) *n.* [*lobe* + *-ectomy*]. Excision of a lobe of an organ or gland; specifically, the excision of a lobe of the lung or a frontal or temporal lobe of the brain.

lo·be·lia (lo·bee'lee·uh, lo·beel'yuh) *n.* [M. de *Lobel*, Flemish botanist, 1538–1616]. The leaves and tops of *Lobelia inflata;* contains several alkaloids including lobeline. It has been used as an expectorant.

lo·be·line (lo'be·leen, ·lin, lo·bee') *n.* 1. A mixture of alkaloids obtained from lobelia; these have been separated into alpha-, beta-, and gamma- forms. 2. Alpha-lobeline, $C_{22}H_{27}NO_2$, an alkaloid from lobelia having emetic, respiratory, and vasomotor actions similar to those of nicotine.

lo·ben·da·zole (lo·ben'duh·zole) *n.* Ethyl 2-benzimidazolecarbamate, $C_{10}H_{11}N_3O_2$, a veterinary anthelmintic.

lobi. Plural and genitive singular of *lobus* (= LOBE).

lobi ce·re·bri (serr'e·brye) [NA]. The lobes of the cerebrum.

lobi glan·du·lae mam·ma·ri·ae (glan'dew·lee ma·mair'ee·ee) [NA]. The lobes of the mammary gland.

lobi mam·mae (mam'ee) [BNA]. LOBI GLANDULAE MAMMARIAE.

lobi re·na·les (re·nay'leez) [NA]. RENAL LOBES.

lo·bo·cyte (lo'bo·site) *n.* [*lobe* + *-cyte*]. SEGMENTED CELL.

lo·bo·po·di·um (lo''bo·po'dee·um) *n.*, pl. **lobopo·dia** (·dee·uh) [NL., from *lobe* + Gk. *podion*, small foot]. A stout, cylindrical pseudopodium.

lo·bot·o·my (lo·bot'uh·mee) *n.* [*lobe* + *-tomy*]. Surgical sectioning of brain tissue, particularly of the frontal lobe for the relief of mental disorders.

Lob·stein's disease (lohp'shtine) [J. G. C. F. *Lobstein*, Alsatian pathologist, 1777–1835]. OSTEOGENESIS IMPERFECTA.

lobster-claw deformity. BIDACTYLY.

lobular carcinoma. A form of breast cancer.

lobular pneumonia. BRONCHOPNEUMONIA.

lob·ule (lob'yool) *n.* [F., dim. of L. *lobus*, lobe]. A small lobe or a subdivision of a lobe. —**lob·u·lar** (lob'yoo·lur), **lob·u·lat·ed** (lob'yoo·lay·tid) *adj.*

lobules of the epididymis. The series of cones forming the head of the epididymis, each composed of an efferent ductule. Syn. *vascular cones.* NA *lobuli epididymidis.*

lobules of the liver. 1. Polygonal prisms making up the parenchyma of the liver, each with a central vein running longitudinally through the center, and with branches of the portal vein, the interlobular bile ducts, and branches of the hepatic artery and lymph vessels in the periphery. NA *lobuli hepatis.* 2. The physiologic lobules of the liver; portions of liver tissue each of which surrounds and is drained by an interlobular bile duct.

lobules of the testis. The conoid compartments of the testis, each of whose cavities contains the terminal portions of one to three seminiferous tubules. NA *lobuli testis.*

lobuli. Plural of *lobulus.*

lobuli cor·ti·ca·les re·nis (kor·ti·kay'leez ree'nis) [NA]. Lobules of the cortex of the kidney.

lobuli epi·di·dy·mi·dis (ep''i·di·dim'i·dis) [NA]. LOBULES OF THE EPIDIDYMIS.

lobuli glan·du·lae mam·ma·ri·ae (glan'dew·lee ma·mair'ee·ee) [NA]. The lobules of the mammary gland.

lobuli glandulae thy·roi·de·ae (thigh·roy'dee·ee) [NA]. Lobules of the thyroid gland.

lobuli he·pa·tis (hep'uh·tis) [NA]. LOBULES OF THE LIVER.

lobuli mam·mae (mam'ee) [BNA]. LOBULI GLANDULAE MAMMARIAE.

lobuli pul·mo·num (pul·mo'num) [BNA]. PULMONARY LOBULES.

lobuli tes·tis (tes'tis) [NA]. LOBULES OF THE TESTIS.

lobuli thy·mi (thigh'migh) [NA]. Lobules of the thymus.

lob·u·lus (lob'yoo·lus) *n.*, pl. **lobu·li** (·lye) [NA]. LOBULE.

lobulus an·si·for·mis (an''si·for'mis). ANSIFORM LOBULE.

lobulus au·ri·cu·lae (aw·rick'yoo·lee) [NA]. The lobule of the ear; the dependent portion of the auricle.

lobulus bi·ven·ter (bye·ven'tur) [NA]. Biventral lobule (= PARAMEDIAN LOBULE).

lobulus cen·tra·lis (sen·tray'lis) [NA]. CENTRAL LOBULE.

lobulus me·di·us me·di·a·nus (mee'dee·us mee·dee·ay'nus). A small lobule of the cerebellum comprising the folium and tuber of the vermis.

lobulus pa·ra·cen·tra·lis (păr''uh·sen·tray'lis) [NA]. PARACENTRAL LOBULE.

lobulus pa·ri·e·ta·lis inferior (pa·rye''e·tay'lis) [NA]. INFERIOR PARIETAL LOBULE.

lobulus parietalis superior [NA]. SUPERIOR PARIETAL LOBULE.

lobulus qua·dran·gu·la·ris (kwah·drang''gew·lair'is) [NA]. QUADRANGULAR LOBULE.

lobulus se·mi·lu·na·ris inferior (sem''ee·lew·nair'is) [NA]. INFERIOR SEMILUNAR LOBULE.

lobulus semilunaris superior [NA]. SUPERIOR SEMILUNAR LOBULE.

lobulus sim·plex (sim'plecks) [NA]. The most rostral part of the posterior lobe of the cerebellum, forming a broad crescentic band across the superior surface.

lo·bus (lo'bus) *n.*, pl. & genit. sing. **lo·bi** (·bye) [L., from Gk. *lobos*] [NA]. LOBE.

lobus anterior hy·po·phy·se·os (high''po·fis'ee·os) [NA]. The anterior lobe of the hypophysis (= ADENOHYPOPHYSIS).

lobus cau·da·tus (kaw·day'tus) [NA]. CAUDATE LOBE.

lobus fron·ta·lis (fron·tay'lis) [NA]. FRONTAL LOBE.

lobus glandulae thy·roi·de·ae (thigh·roy'dee·ee) [NA]. The lobe of the thyroid gland, right or left.

lobus he·pa·tis dex·ter (hep'uh·tis decks'tur) [NA]. The right lobe of the liver.

lobus hepatis si·nis·ter (si·nis'tur) [NA]. The left lobe of the liver.

lobus inferior pul·mo·nis (pul·mo'nis) [NA]. The inferior lobe of the lung, right or left.

lobus inferior pul·mo·nis dex·tri (pul·mo'nis decks'trye) [NA]. The inferior lobe of the right lung.

lobus inferior pulmonis si·nis·tri (si·nis'trye) [NA]. The inferior lobe of the left lung.

lobus me·di·us pro·sta·tae (mee'dee·us pros'tuh·tee) [NA]. The median lobe of the prostate.

lobus medius pulmonis dex·tri (decks'trye) [NA]. The middle lobe of the right lung.

lobus oc·ci·pi·ta·lis (ock·sip''i·tay'lis) [NA]. OCCIPITAL LOBE.

lobus ol·fac·to·ri·us (ol·fack·to'ree·us) [BNA]. OLFACTORY LOBE.

lobus pa·ri·e·ta·lis (pa·rye·e·tay'lis) [NA]. PARIETAL LOBE.

lobus posterior hy·po·phy·se·os (high''po·fis'ee·os) [NA]. The posterior lobe of the hypophysis (= NEUROHYPOPHYSIS).

lobus pro·sta·tae (pros'tuh·tee) [NA]. The lobe of the prostate, right or left.

lobus py·ra·mi·da·lis (pi·ram''i·day'lis) [NA]. PYRAMIDAL LOBE.

lobus qua·dra·tus (kwah·dray'tus) [NA]. QUADRATE LOBE.

lobus superior pul·mo·nis (pul·mo'nis) [NA]. The superior lobe of the lung, right or left.

lobus superior pulmonis dex·tri (decks'trye) [NA]. The superior lobe of the right lung.

lobus superior pulmonis si·nis·tri (si·nis'trye) [NA]. The superior lobe of the left lung.

lobus tem·po·ra·lis (tem·po·ray'lis) [NA]. TEMPORAL LOBE.

lobus thy·mi (thigh'migh) [NA]. The lobe of the thymus, right or left.

lo·cal (lo'kul) *adj.* [L. *localis*, from *locus*, place]. Limited to a part or place; not general. Contr. *systemic.*

local anaphylaxis. A reaction at the site of injections, dependent upon the union in the tissues of the circulating precipitin and its specific antigen, as edema, induration, and necrosis caused by repeated subcutaneous injections of horse serum into rabbits. See also *Arthus' phenomenon.*

local anemia. A lack of blood in a particular organ or part; ISCHEMIA.

local anesthesia. Anesthesia produced in a local area usually by infiltration technique.

local anesthetic. A drug which, topically applied or injected into the tissues, causes local insensibility to pain by neural blockade. Sympathetic sensory or motor block may be produced.

local asphyxia. Stagnation or diminution of the circulation in a part, as the fingers, hands, toes, or feet; often used in reference to Raynaud's disease.

local catalepsy. Catalepsy affecting an associated group of muscles, such as only one limb.

local convulsion. FOCAL SEIZURE.

local death. Death of one part of the body.

local immunity. Immunity confined to a given tissue or area of the body. Syn. *tissue immunity.*

lo·cal·iza·tion (lo″kul·i·zay′shun) *n.* 1. The determination of the site of a lesion or process. 2. The limitation or restriction of a process to a circumscribed area. —**lo·cal·ize** (lo′kul·ize) *v.*

lo·cal·ized (lo′kul·ize′d) *adj.* Confined to a particular situation or place. Contr. *diffuse.*

localized myxedema. CIRCUMSCRIBED MYXEDEMA.

localized pericarditis. A form of pericarditis characterized by localized white areas, the so-called milk spots.

localized peritonitis. Peritonitis in which only a part of the peritoneum is involved. Syn. *circumscribed peritonitis.*

localized tetanus. A clinical type of tetanus, in which rigidity and spasms are limited to the muscles in the neighborhood of a wound of the arm or hand or of the abdomen, after an operation.

lo·cal·iz·er (lo′kul·eye″zur) *n.* An instrument used in roentgenographic examination of the eye for localizing opaque foreign bodies.

local reaction. The phenomena or lesions occurring at the site of application of an exciting agent.

local Shwartzman phenomenon. SHWARTZMAN PHENOMENON (1).

local stimulant. A stimulant acting directly on the end organs of the sensory nerves of the skin.

lo·chia (lo′kee·uh, lock′ee·uh) *n.* [Gk., from *lochos,* childbirth]. The discharge from the uterus and vagina during the first few weeks after labor. —**lo·chi·al** (lo′kee·ul, lock′ee·ul) *adj.*

lochia al·ba (al′buh). The whitish or yellowish flow that takes place after the seventh day after labor.

lochia cru·en·ta (kroo·en′tuh). The sanguineous flow of the first few days after labor. Syn. *lochia rubra.*

lochia ru·bra (roo′bruh). LOCHIA CRUENTA.

lochia se·ro·sa (se·ro′suh). The serous discharge taking place about the fifth day after labor.

lo·chio·col·pos (lo″kee·o·kol′pos) *n.* [*lochia* + *-colpos*]. Distention of the vagina by retained lochia.

lo·chio·cyte (lo′kee·o·site) *n.* [*lochia* + *-cyte*]. A decidual cell found in the lochia.

lo·chio·me·tra (lo″kee·o·mee′truh) *n.* [*lochia* + *-metra*]. A retention of lochia in the uterus.

lo·chio·me·tri·tis (lo″kee·o·me·trye′tis) *n.* [*lochia* + *metritis*]. PUERPERAL METRITIS.

lo·chi·or·rha·gia (lo″kee·o·ray′jee·uh) *n.* [*lochia* + *-rrhagia*]. LOCHIORRHEA.

lo·chi·or·rhea, lo·chi·or·rhoea (lo″kee·o·ree′uh) *n.* [*lochia* + *-rrhea*]. An abnormal flow of the lochia.

lo·chi·os·che·sis (lo″kee·os′ke·sis) *n.* [*lochia* + Gk. *schesis,* a checking]. Suppression or retention of the lochia.

lo·cho·me·tri·tis (lo″ko·me·trye′tis, lock″o·) *n.* [Gk. *lochos,* childbirth, + *metritis*]. PUERPERAL METRITIS.

lo·cho·per·i·to·ni·tis (lo″ko·perr·i·tuh·nigh′tis, lock″o·) *n.* [Gk. *lochos,* childbirth, + *peritonitis*]. Inflammation of the peritoneum following childbirth.

loci. Plural of *locus.*

lock and key theory. An enzyme to be effective must fit the molecule of the substrate somewhat as a key fits into a lock. Some enzymes appear to be "master keys" in that they fit into a considerable number of substrates. This analogy of enzyme specificity was suggested by Emil Fischer.

locked bite. Interdigitation of the teeth in such a manner that normal excursions of the mandible are restricted or prevented while the teeth are in occlusion.

locked-in syndrome. PSEUDOCOMA.

Locke-Ring·er's solution [F. S. *Locke,* British physiologist, 1871–1949; and S. *Ringer,* English physiologist, 1835–1910]. A solution containing sodium, potassium, calcium, and magnesium chlorides with sodium bicarbonate and dextrose used in experimental physiology and pharmacology.

lock finger. A peculiar affection of the fingers in which they suddenly become fixed in a flexed position, due to the presence of a fibrous constriction of the tendon sheath or a nodular enlargement in the tendon.

lock·jaw, *n.* TRISMUS.

Lock·wood's sign [C. B. *Lockwood,* English surgeon, 1858–1914]. *Obsol.* A sign for appendiceal adhesions in which flatus can be palpated trickling through the ileocecal valve.

lo·co disease (lo′ko) [Sp., crazy]. A poisoning produced in livestock by eating plants which take up selenium from the soil; the symptoms of the disease are loss of flesh, disordered vision, delirium, convulsive movements, and stupor, often terminating fatally.

lo·co·mo·tion (lo″kuh·mo′shun) *n.* [L. *locus,* place, + *motion*]. The act of moving from place to place. —**locomo·tive** (·tiv), **locomo·tor** (·tur) *adj.*

locomotor ataxia. TABES DORSALIS.

locomotor system. The extremities and their parts, as the bones, muscles, and joints concerned with locomotion, or the motor activities of the body.

loco weed. Those species of *Astragalus* which contain selenium. See also *loco disease.*

loc·u·la·tion (lock″yoo·lay′shun) *n.* The formation of loculi in tissue. —**loc·u·lat·ed** (lock′yoo·lay·tid), *adj.*

loculation syndrome. FROIN'S SYNDROME.

loc·u·lus (lock′yoo·lus) *n.,* pl. **locu·li** (·lye) [L.]. A small space or compartment. —**locu·lar** (·lur), **locu·late** (·late) *adj.*

lo·cum te·nens (lo′kum ten′enz) [ML., lit., holding the place]. A physician who temporarily acts as a substitute for another physician.

lo·cus (lo′kus) *n.,* pl. **lo·ci** (·sigh) [L.]. 1. Place, site. 2. *In genetics,* the position on a chromosome occupied by a particular gene.

locus ce·ru·le·us (se·roo′lee·us) [NA]. A bluish-tinted eminence on the floor of the fourth ventricle of the brain, subjacent to which is an aggregation of pigmented cells. Syn. *nucleus pigmentosus pontis.*

locus mi·no·ris re·sis·ten·ti·ae (mi·no′ris rez″is·ten′shee·ee). A site of diminished resistance.

locus per·fo·ra·tus (pur·fo·ray′tus). *Obsol.* The anterior and the posterior perforated substance at the base of the brain through which the blood vessels pass.

Loeb's decidual reaction [L. *Loeb,* U.S. pathologist, 1869–1959]. Nodules of uterine decidual tissue induced in nonpregnant animals by mechanical stimulation.

Loeff·ler's alkaline methylene blue (lœf′lur) [F. A. J. *Loeffler,* German bacteriologist, 1852–1915]. Methylene blue made alkaline by adding a small amount of potassium hydroxide.

Loeffler's disease [W. *Loeffler,* Swiss physician, b.1887]. Fibroplastic parietal endocarditis, characterized by progressive congestive heart failure, eosinophilia, and multiple embolic systemic infarct.

Loeffler's pneumonia or **eosinophilia** [W. *Loeffler*]. LOEFFLER'S SYNDROME.

Loeffler's stain [F. A. J. *Loeffler*]. A stain for flagella.

Loeffler's syndrome [W. *Loeffler*]. Transient pulmonary infiltration by eosinophils associated with peripheral blood eosinophilia and minimal or no symptoms; sometimes associated with parasitic infections in which their lodging in the lungs causes inflammatory reactions. Syn. *eosinophilic pneumonitis.*

Loele method. A histochemical method for alphanaphthol oxidase based on the effect of the enzyme on alphanaphthol dissolved in potassium hydroxide to give violet or black granules.

Loe·wen·thal's tract (lœh'vᵉn·tahl) [N. *Loewenthal,* Swiss histologist, 20th century]. TECTOSPINAL TRACT.

Loewi's sign [O. *Loewi,* U.S. pharmacologist, 1873–1961]. Dilatation of the pupil within 30 to 60 minutes following instillation of a weak (1:1000) solution of epinephrine, demonstrating irritability of the sympathetic nervous system; due to previous denervation.

Löffler. See *Loeffler.*

Lof·strand crutch. A forearm crutch, usually of metal, consisting of a vertical member, handle, and open forearm clip.

log-, logo- [Gk. *logos*]. A combining form meaning (a) *word, speech;* (b) *thought, reason.*

lo·ga·nin (lo'guh·nin) *n.* [*Logani*aceae, the botanical family that includes *Strychnos*]. A glycoside extracted from the seeds and pulp of the fruit of *Strychnos nux-vomica.*

Log Etronic. An electronic device for reproducing radiographs by adding or lowering density or diminishing contrast by compressing a film's gray scale. A reproduction by this method is called a Log Egram.

-logia [*log-* + *-ia*]. A combining form meaning (a) *a condition involving the faculty of speech or of reasoning;* (b) *-logy, a field of study.*

logo-. See *log-.*

logo·clo·nia (log"o·klo'nee·uh) *n.* [*logo-* + Gk. *klon*ein, to agitate]. LOGOSPASM.

logo·ma·nia (log"o·may'nee·uh) *n.* [*logo-* + *mania*]. Logorrhea so excessive as to be a form of a manic state; new words may be invented to keep up the garrulity.

logo·neu·ro·sis (log"o·new·ro'sis) *n.* [*logo-* + *neurosis*]. Any neurosis associated with a speech defect.

log·op·a·thy (log·op'uth·ee) *n.* [*logo-* + *-pathy*]. Any disorder of speech.

logo·pe·dia, logo·pae·dia (log"o·pee'dee·uh) *n.* LOGOPEDICS.

logo·pe·dics, logo·pae·dics (log"o·pee'dicks) *n.* [*logo-* + orthopedics]. The study, knowledge, and treatment of defective speech.

log·or·rhea, log·or·rhoea (log"o·ree'uh) *n.* [*logo-* + *-rrhoea*]. Excessive, uncontrollable, or abnormal talkativeness or loquacity; may be exceedingly rapid and even incoherent. See also *logomania.*

log·wood, *n.* HEMATOXYLON.

-logy [Gk. *-logia,* from *logos,* discourse, explanation]. A combining form meaning (a) *a field of study;* (b) *discourse, treatise.*

Loh·mann reaction (lo'mahn) [K. *Lohmann,* German biochemist, b.1898]. The transference of a phosphate radical from adenosine triphosphate to creatine, or to adenosine diphosphate from phosphocreatine.

lo·i·a·sis (lo·eye'uh·sis) *n.,* pl. **loia·ses** (·seez) [*Loa* + *-iasis*]. A filariasis of tropical Africa, caused by the filaria *Loa,* acquired from bites by *Chrysops dimidiata* and *C. silacea,* and characterized by diurnal periodicity of microfilariae in the blood and transient cutaneous swelling caused by migrating adult worms. The eye may be involved.

loin, *n.* [OF. *loigne,* from L. *lumbus*]. The lateral and posterior region of the body between the false ribs and the iliac crest. NA *lumbus.*

lol·ism (lol'iz·um, lo'liz·um) *n.* Poisoning by the seeds of *Lolium temulentum* (darnel ryegrass).

lo·met·ra·line (lo·met'ruh·leen) *n.* 8-Chloro-1,2,3,4-tetrahydro-5-methoxy-*N,N*-dimethyl-1-naphthylamine, $C_{13}H_{18}ClNO$, a tranquilizer and antiparkinsonian used as the hydrochloride salt.

lo·mo·fun·gin (lo"mo·fun'jin) *n.* An antibiotic substance, produced by *Streptomyces lomondensis* var. *lomondensis,* that has antifungal activity.

Lomotil. Trademark for diphenoxylate hydrochloride with atropine sulfate, an antidiarrheal drug combination.

lo·mus·tine (lo·mus'teen) *n.* 1-(2-Chloroethyl)-3-cyclohexyl-1-nitrosourea, $C_9H_{16}ClN_3O_2$, an antineoplastic. Syn. *CCNU.*

Londe's atrophy (lohⁿd) [P. F. L. *Londe,* French neurologist, 1864–1944]. FAZIO-LONDE DISEASE.

long-acting thyroid stimulator. A circulating gamma globulin whose action resembles that of thyroid-stimulating hormone of the pituitary, found in the serum of some patients with Grave's disease, occasionally in exophthalmos without other evidence of Grave's disease, and in pretibial myxedema. It is probably produced by lymphocytes and may represent an autoantibody to a thyroid antigen. Abbreviated, LATS.

long bone. A bone in which the length markedly exceeds the width. NA *os longum.*

long circuit reflex. A reflex which involves the higher centers in the medulla, midbrain, basal ganglions, or cerebral cortex, as opposed to the segmental reflex.

long-cone technique. PARALLEL TECHNIQUE.

long crus of the incus. A slender process or long limb that descends vertically from the body of the incus and articulates with the head of the stapes. NA *crus longum incudis.*

lon·gev·i·ty (lon·jev'i·tee) *n.* [L. *longaevitas,* from *longaevus,* long-lived, from *aevus,* age]. Long life; length of life.

long gyrus of the insula. The furrowed gyrus occupying the posterior portion of the insula, separated from the short gyri of the anterior portion by the central sulcus of the insula. NA *gyrus longus insulae.*

lon·gi·lin·e·al (lon"ji·lin'ee·ul) *adj.* [L. *long*us, long, + *line*a, line, + *al*]. Referring to a long, lean type of body build.

lon·gi·ma·nous (lon"ji·may'nus, ·man'us, lon·jim'uh·nus) *adj.* [L. *longimanus,* from *manus,* hand]. Long-handed.

long-incubation hepatitis. SERUM HEPATITIS.

lon·gi·ped·ate (lon"ji·ped'ate, ·pee'date) *adj.* [L. *long*us, long, + *pes, ped*is, foot, + *-ate*]. Long-footed.

lon·gis·si·mus (lon·jis'i·mus) *adj. & n.* [L.]. 1. Longest; applied to muscles, as longissimus thoracis. 2. The middle part of the erector spinae muscle. NA *musculus longissimus.* See also Table of Muscles in the Appendix.

lon·gi·tu·di·nal (lon"ji·tew'di·nul) *adj.* [L. *longitudo, longitudinis,* length]. 1. Lengthwise; in the direction of the long axis of a body. 2. Over a protracted period of time, as of a study of population growth.

longitudinal aberration. Deviation of a ray from the focus, measured along the axis above or below the focal plane.

longitudinal arch of the foot. The anteroposterior arch (NA *arcus pedis longitudinalis*) formed by the tarsal and metatarsal bones, consisting of the inner, or medial, longitudinal arch (NA *pars medialis arcus longitudinalis*) formed by the calcaneus, the talus, the navicular, three cuneiform bones, and the first three metatarsals, and the outer, or lateral, longitudinal arch (NA *pars lateralis arcus pedis longitudinalis*) formed by the calcaneus, the cuboid, and the fourth and fifth metatarsals. Contr. *transverse arch of the foot.*

longitudinal duct of the epoophoron. DUCTUS EPOOPHORI LONGITUDINALIS.

longitudinal duodenal plica. A variable fold in the medial wall of the descending portion of the duodenum extending upward from the major duodenal papilla, it marks the opening of the common bile duct. NA *plica longitudinalis duodeni.*

longitudinal fissure of the cerebrum. The deep fissure that divides the cerebrum into two hemispheres. Syn. *interhemispheric fissure.* NA *fissura longitudinalis cerebri.*

longitudinal fissure of the liver. A fissure on the lower border of the liver, through which passes the round ligament.

lon·gi·tu·di·na·lis (lon"ji·tew"di·nay'lis) *n.* Either of the longitudinal intrinsic muscles of the tongue: the inferior (NA *musculus longitudinalis inferior linguae*) or the superior (NA *musculus longitudinalis superior linguae*). See also Table of Muscles in the Appendix.

longitudinal line. A longitudinal ridge on a nail produced by unequal growth.

longitudinal sinus. 1. INFERIOR SAGITTAL SINUS. 2. SUPERIOR SAGITTAL SINUS.

longitudinal suture. SAGITTAL SUTURE.

lon·gi·typ·i·cal (lon″ji·tip′i·kul) *adj.* [L. *longus*, long, + *typical*]. LONGILINEAL.

long plantar ligament. A strong, compact ligament, the longest in the foot, attached posteriorly to the anterior plantar surface of the calcaneus and anteriorly to the plantar surface of the cuboid and the bases of the second through fifth metatarsals. NA *ligamentum plantare longum.* Compare *plantar ligaments.*

long process of the malleus. ANTERIOR PROCESS OF THE MALLEUS.

Long's coefficient [J. H. *Long*, U.S. biochemist, 1856–1918]. The number 2.6 is multiplied by the last two figures of the urine specific gravity, determined at 25°C, to derive the number of grams of solids per liter of urine.

long-term care. Medical care providing symptomatic treatment or maintenance and rehabilitative services for patients of all age groups in a variety of settings. Contr. *intensive care, primary care.*

long-term memory. 1. Memory store in which the rate of loss is relatively low and where information is held without active rehearsal. Syn. *secondary memory.* Contr. *short-term memory.* 2. Generally, anything retained for more than a very brief period of time, from minutes to years, sometimes thought of as a person's total store of knowledge.

lon·gus (long′gus) *adj. & n.* [L.]. 1. Long. 2. A long muscle.

longus ca·pi·tis (kap′i·tis). The long muscle of the head. NA *musculus longus capitis.* See also Table of Muscles in Appendix.

longus cer·vi·cis (sur′vi·sis, sur·vye′sis). LONGUS COLLI.

longus col·li (kol′eye). A deep muscle of the anterior neck region attached to the anterior surfaces of the bodies of the cervical vertebrae. NA *musculus longus colli.* See also Table of Muscles in the Appendix.

Loo·ney and Dy·er method for potassium in blood. Potassium is precipitated from the protein-free, chloride-free serum filtrate as the insoluble potassium silver cobaltinitrite. The washed precipitate is decomposed by alkali to liberate the nitrite, which is then determined colorimetrically.

loop, *n.* 1. A bend in a cord or cordlike structure. 2. A platinum wire, in a handle, with its extremity bent in a circular form; used to transfer bacterial cultures.

loop motor. A type of tissue motor used in kineplastic amputations. See also *plastic motor.*

loop of Henle [F. G. J. *Henle*]. The U-shaped section of a uriniferous tubule which is formed by a descending and an ascending limb.

Looser's lines. LOOSER'S ZONES.

Loo·ser's zones (lo′zur) [E. *Looser*, Swiss surgeon, 1877–1936]. Transverse ribbonlike radiolucent zones usually found in the tibia and other long bones representing deficient calcification, united but uncalcified pseudofractures, or decalcification along nutrient arteries, characteristically seen on radiographs in osteomalacia, including Milkman's syndrome and rickets.

L.O.P. Abbreviation for *left occipitoposterior* position of the fetus in utero.

lo·per·a·mide (lo·perr′·uh·mide) *n.* 4-(*p*-Chlorophenyl)-4-hydroxy-*N*,*N*-dimethyl-α,α-diphenyl-1-piperidinebutyramide, $C_{29}H_{33}ClN_2O_2$, an antiperistaltic.

loph·o·dont (lof′o·dont, lo′fo·) *adj.* [Gk. *lophos*, crest, ridge, + *-odont*]. Having the crowns of the molar teeth formed in crests or ridges. Contr. *bunodont.*

Lo·phoph·o·ra (lo·fof′uh·ruh) *n.* [Gk. *lophēphora*, crested, tufted]. A genus of cacti, formerly called *Anhalonium. Lophophora williamsii* yields mescal (1).

lo·phoph·o·rine (lo·fof′o·reen, ·rin) *n.* [*Lophophora* + *-ine*]. *N*-Methylanhalonine, $C_{13}H_{17}NO_3$, the most active of the alkaloids from mescal buttons. Has been used experimentally as a hypnotic.

lo·phot·ri·chous (lo·fot′ri·kus) *adj.* [Gk. *lophos*, crest, tuft, + *trich-* + *-ous*]. Pertaining to microorganisms characterized by a tuft of cilia or flagella at each pole.

lo·pre·mone (lo′pre·mone) *n.* PROTIRELIN.

lo·quac·i·ty (lo·kwas′i·tee) *n.* [L. *loquacitas*, from *loquax*, talkative, from *loqui*, to talk]. Volubility of speech; talkativeness; a condition frequently excessive in various mental disorders. See also *logorrhea.*

Lo·rain-Lé·vi syndrome (loʰ·ræⁿ′, leʸ·vee′) [P. J. *Lorain*, French physician, 1827–1875; and L. *Lévi*]. PITUITARY DWARFISM.

lor·aj·mine (lor·aj′meen) *n.* Ajmaline 17-(chloroacetate)ester, $C_{22}H_{27}ClN_2O_3$, an antiarrhythmic cardiac depressant used as the hydrochloride salt.

lor·az·e·pam (lor·az′e·pam) *n.* 7-Chloro-5-(2-chlorophenyl)-1,3-dihydro-3-hydroxy-2*H*-1,4-benzodiazepin-2-one, $C_{15}H_{10}Cl_2N_2O_2$, a minor tranquilizer.

lor·bam·ate (lor·bam′ate) *n.* 2-(Hydroxymethyl)-2-methylpentyl cyclopropanecarbamate carbamate ester, $C_{12}H_{22}N_2O_4$, a muscle relaxant.

lor·do·sis (lor·do′sis) *n.*, pl. **lordo·ses** (·seez) [Gk. *lordōsis*, from *lordos*, bent backward, concavely]. Forward curvature of the lumbar spine; spinal curvature in the sagittal plane which is concave to the dorsal aspect. —**lor·dot·ic** (·dot′ick) *adj.*

Lo·renz method (lo′rents) [A. *Lorenz*, Austrian surgeon, 1854–1946]. A method of forcible closed reduction and treatment of congenital dislocation of the hip.

Lorfan. A trademark for levallorphan, a narcotic antagonist.

L organisms. Forms derived from various bacteria which may or may not revert to the parent strains, occurring spontaneously or favored by penicillin and other agents, pleomorphic, lacking cell walls, and growing in minute colonies. Compare *Mycoplasma, pleuropneumonia-like organisms.*

lo·ri·ca (lo·rye′kuh) *n.* [L., cuirass]. A protective external covering or case.

Loridine. Trademark for the antibiotic substance cephaloridine.

Loriga's disease. PNEUMATIC-HAMMER DISEASE.

Lormin. A trademark for chlormadinone acetate, a progestin.

Lor·rain Smith's stain for fatty acids. NILE BLUE A.

Lo·theis·sen's operation (lo′tye·sᵉn) [G. *Lotheissen*, Swiss surgeon in Austria, 1868–1941]. An operation, using the inguinal approach, for the radical cure of femoral hernia.

lo·tio (lo′shee·o, lo′tee·o) *n.* [L., from *lavare*, to wash]. LOTION.

lo·tion (lo′shun) *n.* [L. *lotio*]. Any of a class of liquid medicinal preparations, either suspensions or dispersions, intended for local application.

Lotrimin. A trademark for clotrimazole, an antifungal.

Lotusate. Trademark for talbutal, a barbiturate with intermediate duration of action used as a sedative and hypnotic.

Lou·is-Bar syndrome (lwee baʰr) [Denise *Louis-Bar*, Belgian neuropathologist, 20th century]. ATAXIA-TELANGIECTASIA.

loupe (loop) *n.* [F.]. A magnifying lens.

loup·ing ill (laʊwp′ing, lo′ping) [Scottish *loup*, leap]. An enzootic and sometimes epizootic disease of sheep; a form of encephalomyelitis caused by a group B encephalitis virus and transmitted by the tick *Ixodes ricinus.* The virus is infectious also for monkeys, mice, horses, and cattle. Infected animals display ataxia. Syn. *ovine encephalomyelitis, trembling ill.*

louse (laʊwce) *n.*, pl. **lice.** A small, wingless, dorsoventrally flattened insect which lacks true metamorphosis. An ectoparasite of birds and mammals, it is medically important as a vector of disease and as a producer of irritating dermatitis.

louse-borne typhus. EPIDEMIC TYPHUS.

louse fly. Any of various wingless, parasitic flies of the family Hippoboscidae.

lousy (laowz'ee) *adj.* Infested with lice. See also *pediculosis, phthiriasis.* —**lous·i·ness,** *n.*

lov·age (luv'ij) *n.* [OF. *luvesche,* from L. *Ligusticus,* Ligurian]. The root of *Levisticum officinale;* formerly used as a stimulant, aromatic, carminative, and emmenagogue.

Lo·vén's reflex (loo·veʸn') [O. C. *Lovén,* Swedish physiologist, 1835–1904]. Vasodilatation in an organ in response to stimulation of its afferent nerve.

love object. 1. Any person or object that regularly excites or receives a person's affection or love. 2. *In psychoanalysis,* the person or object with which libido is concerned, and which stimulates the instinctual activity generated by it. Syn. *libidinal object.*

Lovibond unit. One Lovibond unit of vitamin A = 208 international (or U.S.P.) units.

low-caloric diet. A diet containing a small number (600 to 1500) of calories.

low cervical cesarean section. Delivery through an incision made through the lower uterine segment.

Lö·wen·stein-Jen·sen medium (lœh'vᵉn·shtine, yen'zᵉn) [E. *Löwenstein,* Austrian pathologist, b. 1878]. An egg-potato-glycerin medium used for culture of *Mycobacterium tuberculosis.*

lower abdominal reflex. SUPRAPUBIC REFLEX.

lower brachial plexus paralysis. Weakness of the small hand muscles and flexors of the wrist resulting in claw hand, and ulnar-type sensory loss, due to injury to the eighth cervical and first thoracic roots or the lower trunk of the brachial plexus; usually caused by birth injury; the prognosis is favorable. Syn. *Klumpke's paralysis.* Contr. *upper brachial plexus paralysis.*

lower center. A functional nerve center of the brainstem or spinal cord, one concerned with a reflex pathway or one receiving impulses from a higher center.

lower extremity. In human anatomy, the extremity comprising the hip, thigh, leg, ankle, and foot. NA *membrum inferius.* See also Plates 7, 9, 16.

lower horizontal plane. INTERTUBERCULAR PLANE.

lower-leg syndrome. POSTPHLEBITIC SYNDROME.

lower motor neuron. An efferent neuron which has its cell body located in the anterior gray column of the spinal cord or in the brainstem nuclei and its axon passing by way of a peripheral nerve to skeletal muscle. Syn. *final common pathway.* Contr. *upper motor neuron.*

lower motor neuron disease, lesion, or **paralysis.** An injury to the cell bodies or axons of lower motor neurons, characterized by flaccid paralysis of the muscle(s), diminished or absent reflexes, absence of pathological reflexes, reaction of degeneration (about two weeks after injury), and progressive muscle atrophy.

lower nephron nephrosis or **syndrome.** ACUTE TUBULAR NECROSIS.

Low·er's tubercle [R. *Lower,* English physician, 1631–1691]. INTERVENOUS TUBERCLE.

lower urinary tract. The part of the urinary tract concerned with the storage and expulsion of the urine; the bladder and urethra. Contr. *upper urinary tract.*

lower uterine segment. The isthmus of the uterus which expands as pregnancy progresses, and whose muscle fibers are stretched passively during labor, together with the cervix, allowing the upper uterine musculature to retract and thus to expel the fetus. See also *retraction ring.*

Lowe's syndrome [C. U. *Lowe,* U.S. pediatrician, b. 1921]. OCULOCEREBRORENAL SYNDROME.

lowest splanchnic nerve. LEAST SPLANCHNIC NERVE.

low forceps. An obstetric forceps applied to the fetal head when it is well within the lower portion of the pelvic canal.

low myopia. Myopia of less than 2 diopters.

low-pressure hydrocephalus. A form of communicating hydrocephalus in adult life, in which the syndrome of gait disorder, incontinence, and dementia is associated with cerebrospinal fluid pressures of less than 180 mm water, no clinical evidence of increased intracranial pressure, marked ventricular enlargement, and an abnormal isotopic cisternogram. Syn. *normal pressure hydrocephalus.*

Low·ry-Lo·pez-Bes·sey method. A colorimetric method for ascorbic acid based on the conversion of ascorbic acid to dehydroascorbic acid which is treated with 2,4-dinitrophenylhydrazine to give an osazone; the osazone is treated with sulfuric acid to give a colored dehydration product.

low-salt diet. A diet low in its content of sodium salt; used in the treatment of hypertension and edema.

low-salt syndrome. A clinical syndrome characterized by a low serum sodium concentration, occurring acutely in heat exhaustion or water intoxication; and chronically in cardiac or renal disease, especially with prolonged restriction of sodium chloride intake and diuretic therapy. There are postural hypotension, tachycardia, nausea, vomiting, drowsiness, muscle cramps, azotemia, oliguria, convulsions, and coma.

Lowsley's operation [O. S. *Lowsley,* U.S. urologist, 1884–1955]. A three-stage repair of hypospadias.

low-tension pulse. A pulse sudden in its onset, short, and quickly declining. It is easily obliterated by pressure.

loxa bark (lock'suh) [after *Loja,* Ecuador]. Pale cinchona; the bark of *Cinchona officinalis.*

lox·ia (lock'see·uh) *n.* [Gk. *loxos,* oblique, + *-ia*]. TORTICOLLIS.

lox·ic (lock'sick) *adj.* LOXOTIC.

Lox·os·ce·les (lock·sos'e·leez) *n.* [NL., from Gk. *loxos,* slanting, + *skelos,* leg]. A genus of spiders that includes the poisonous brown recluse, *Loxosceles reclusa,* of south central United States, and the larger *L. laeta* of South America, both of which are often found in human dwellings. See also *loxoscelism.*

lox·os·ce·lism (lock·sos'e·liz·um) *n.* [*Loxosceles* + *-ism*]. The clinical state resulting from the bite of the brown recluse spider, which includes pain and vesiculation at the bite site, ischemic changes in the affected area, and systemic complaints.

lox·ot·ic (lock·sot'ick) *adj.* [Gk. *loxos,* slanting, oblique, + *-ic*]. Slanting; twisted.

loz·enge (loz'inj) *n.* [OF. *losenge,* diamond-shaped figure]. A solid dosage form containing one or more medicinal agents and, usually, flavor, sugar, and a demulcent substance, for therapeutic application in the throat and bronchial area.

L-PAM [*L-p*henylalanine *m*ustard]. MELPHALAN.

LPN Abbreviation for *licensed practical nurse.*

L. R. C. S. Licentiate of the Royal College of Surgeons.

L. R. C. S. E. Licentiate of the Royal College of Surgeons of Edinburgh.

L. R. C. S. I. Licentiate of the Royal College of Surgeons of Ireland.

L. R. F. P. S. Licentiate of the Royal Faculty of Physicians and Surgeons.

L. S. A. 1. Abbreviation for *left sacroanterior* position of the fetus. 2. Licentiate of the Society of Apothecaries.

LSD Abbreviation for *lysergic acid diethylamide.*

L-shaped kidney. A form of congenital renal fusion. See *cake kidney.*

L. S. P. Abbreviation for *left sacroposterior* position of the fetus.

LTH Abbreviation for *luteotropic hormone* (= PROLACTIN).

Lu Symbol for *lutetium.*

Lu·barsch-Pick syndrome (loo'barsh) [O. *Lubarsch,* German pathologist, 1860–1933; and L. *Pick,* German pediatrician, 1868–1935]. Atypical amyloidosis frequently associated with a diffuse enlargement of the tongue (amyloid macroglossia), involvement of the skeletal muscles, and scleroderma.

Lubarsch's crystals [O. *Lubarsch*]. Crystals in the Sertoli cells of the testicular tubules.

lu·can·thone (lew·kan'thone) *n.* 1-{[2-(Diethylamino)ethyl]-amino}-4-methylthioxanthen-9-one, $C_{20}H_{24}N_2OS$, an antischistosomal drug; used as the hydrochloride salt. Syn. *miracil D.*

Lu·cas-Cham·pion·nière disease (lue·kah' shahn·pyohn·yehr') [J. M. M. *Lucas-Championnière,* French surgeon, 1843–1913]. CHRONIC PSEUDOMEMBRANOUS BRONCHITIS.

Lu·cas' sign [R. L. *Lucas,* English surgeon, 1846–1915]. Distention of the abdomen early in rickets.

lu·cent (lew'sunt) *adj.* [L. *lucens,* from *lucere,* to shine]. 1. Luminous. 2. Translucent; readily transmitting rays, as x-rays. —**lu·cen·cy** (lew'sun·see) *n.*

Lu·cia·ni's triad (loo·chah'nee) [L. *Luciani,* Italian physiologist, 1840–1919]. Asthenia (weakness), atonia (hypotonia), and ataxia as manifestations of cerebellar disease.

lu·cid (lew'sid) *adj.* [L. *lucidus,* bright, clear]. 1. Clear and enlightening. 2. In a clear state of mind; in full possession of one's senses. —**lu·cid·i·ty** (lew·sid'i·tee) *n.*

lucid interval. *In neurology* and *psychiatry,* a transitory return of the normal state of consciousness following the initial loss of consciousness, sometimes observed in cerebral trauma, particularly in cases of temporal or parietal fracture with rupture of the middle meningeal artery and epidural hematoma.

lu·cif·er·ase (lew·sif'ur·ace, ·aze) *n.* An oxidative enzyme that catalyzes the reaction between oxygen and luciferin to produce luminescence.

lu·cif·er·in (lew·sif'ur·in) *n.* [L. *lucifer,* light-bearing, + *-in*]. An organic substrate found in luminescent organisms which when oxidized in the presence of the enzyme luciferase emits light, as in fireflies and glow-worms.

lu·cif·u·gal (lew·sif'yoo·gul) *adj.* [L. *lux, lucis,* light, + *-fugal*]. Fleeing from, or avoiding, light.

Lu·cil·ia (lew·sil'ee·uh) *n.* A genus of blowflies whose species, *Lucilia caesar, L. sericata,* may cause myiasis in man. Species of this genus have also been found feeding on human wounds and occasionally attacking the adjacent healthy tissue.

Lu·cio leprosy or **phenomenon** (loo'syo) [R. *Lucio,* Mexican physician, 1819–1866]. An unusual form of severe lepromatous leprosy occurring in Mexico and in Central and South America, characterized by diffuse cutaneous infiltration, later with vesiculation, ulceration, and necrosis, and with necrotizing lesions of blood vessels.

Lück·en·schä·del (lick'un·shay"dul, Ger. luek'en·shey·del) *n.* [Ger., from *Lücke,* gap, + *Schädel,* cranium]. CRANIOLACUNIA.

Lucké renal adenocarcinoma. A kidney tumor of leopard frogs, *Rana pipiens*; thought to be etiologically related to a herpesvirus and widely used in the study of viral oncogenesis.

lu·dic (lew'dick) *adj.* [L. *lud*ere, to play, + *-ic*]. Pertaining to the element of play in automatic action.

Ludiomil. A trademark for maprotiline, an antidepressant.

Lud·wig's angina (loot'vikh) [W. F. von *Ludwig,* German surgeon, 1790–1865]. A indurated cellulitis of the submandibular space, often rapidly progressive, and usually caused by hemolytic streptococci.

Ludwig's filtration theory [K. F. W. *Ludwig,* German physiologist, 1816–1895]. The kidney glomeruli filter a protein-free dilute urine which in passing through the tubules becomes concentrated because of the resorption of water.

Ludwig's muscle [W. F. von *Ludwig*]. ARYVOCALIS.

Luer-Lok syringe. LUER SYRINGE.

Luer syringe [*Luer,* German instrument maker in France, 19th century]. A glass syringe for intravenous and hypodermic injections with a mechanism to attach the needle securely.

lu·es (lew'eez) *n.* [L., pestilence]. SYPHILIS. —**lu·et·ic** (lew·et'ick) *adj.*

luetic aneurysm. SYPHILITIC ANEURYSM.

lu·e·tin (lew'e·tin) *n.* An extract of killed cultures of several strains of the *Treponema pallidum;* once used in skin tests for syphilis.

Lu·gol's solution (lue·gohl') [J. G. *Lugol,* French physician, 1786–1851]. STRONG IODINE SOLUTION.

Lukens test. BOERNER-LUKENS TEST.

luke·warm (lewk"wawrm') *adj.* Tepid; about the temperature of the body, approximately 37°C.

lum·ba·go (lum·bay'go) *n.* [L., from *lumbus,* loin]. 1. Backache in the lumbar or lumbosacral region. 2. AZOTURIA (2).

lum·bar (lum'bur, ·bahr) *adj.* [NL. *lumbaris,* from *lumbus,* loin]. Pertaining to the loins.

lumbar abscess. An abscess of the lumbar region.

lumbar arteries. NA *arteriae lumbales.* See Table of Arteries in the Appendix.

lumbar enlargement. Broadening of the spinal cord starting at the level of the ninth and maximal at the level of the twelfth thoracic vertebra. Syn. *lumbar intumescence.* NA *intumescentia lumbalis.*

lumbar ganglia. The ganglia of the lumbar sympathetic trunk. NA *ganglia lumbalia.*

lumbar hernia. A hernia passing out of the abdomen through the lumbar triangle, resulting usually from operation, lumbar abscess, or injury.

lumbar intumescence. LUMBAR ENLARGEMENT.

lum·bar·iza·tion (lum"bur·i·zay'shun) *n.* A condition in which the first segment of the sacrum is partially or completely separate from the remainder of the sacrum.

lumbar nephrectomy. Nephrectomy through an incision in the loin.

lumbar nephrotomy. Nephrotomy through an incision in the loin.

lumbar nerves. NA *nervi lumbales.* See Table of Nerves in the Appendix.

lumbar plexus. A plexus formed by the anterior divisions of the upper four lumbar spinal nerves in the posterior part of the psoas major muscle. NA *plexus lumbalis.*

lumbar puncture. Puncture of the spinal canal, in the subarachnoid space usually between the third and fourth lumbar vertebrae, for the removal of cerebrospinal fluid, especially for diagnostic purposes, or for the introduction of medication. Syn. *spinal tap.*

lumbar puncture headache. A diffuse self-limited headache due to cerebrospinal fluid loss after lumbar puncture, accentuated by sitting or standing and relieved by lying flat.

lumbar reflex. DORSAL REFLEX.

lumbar region. 1. The area of the back lying lateral to the lumbar vertebrae. NA *regio lumbalis.* 2. The lateral region of the abdomen.

lumbar triangle. Lateral abdominal wall triangle bounded by the iliac crest below, the external oblique in front, the latissimus dorsi behind, and floored by the internal oblique. Syn. *Petit's triangle.* NA *trigonum lumbale.*

lumbar trunks. Two collecting lymph trunks, right and left, receiving lymph from the lower limbs, walls of the pelvis and abdomen, pelvic viscera, kidneys, and adrenal glands, and emptying into the cisterna chyli. NA *trunci lumbales (dexter et sinister).*

lumbar vertebrae. The five vertebrae associated with the lower part of the back.

lumbo-. A combining form meaning *lumbar, loin.*

lum·bo·co·los·to·my (lum"bo·ko·los'tuh·mee) *n.* Colostomy in the left lumbar region.

lum·bo·co·lot·o·my (lum"bo·ko·lot'uh·mee) *n.* [*lumbo-* + *colotomy*]. Incision of the colon through the lumbar region.

lum·bo·cos·tal (lum″bo·kos′tul) *adj.* [*lumbo-* + *costal*]. Pertaining to the loins and ribs, as lumbocostal arch.

lumbocostal arch. The lateral arcuate ligament or the medial arcuate ligament.

lumbocostal ligament. A portion of the ventral layer of the thoracolumbar fascia connecting the neck of the twelfth rib to the transverse processes of the first two lumbar vertebrae. NA *ligamentum lumbocostale.*

lumbocostal triangle of Boch·da·lek (boᵏh′daʰ·leck) [Victor *Bochdalek*]. An area of potential weakness in the left half of the diaphragm, bounded medially by the lateral margin of the lumbar part of the diaphragm, laterally by the posterior margin of the costal part, and posteriorly by the lateral arcuate ligament. In the embryo, it is occupied by the left pleuroperitoneal canal. Syn. *vertebrocostal triangle.*

lum·bo·dor·sal (lum″bo·dor′sul) *adj.* [*lumbo-* + *dorsal*]. Pertaining to the lumbar region of the back.

lumbodorsal fascia. THORACOLUMBAR FASCIA.

lumbodorsal splanchnicectomy. SMITHWICK'S OPERATION.

lumbodorsal sympathectomy. Surgical removal of a portion or all of the lumbar and thoracic ganglia of the sympathetic trunk.

lum·bo·in·gui·nal (lum″bo·ing′gwi·nul) *adj.* Pertaining to the lumbar and inguinal regions.

lumboinguinal nerve. A branch of the genitofemoral nerve, distributed to the skin on the front of the thigh. NA *ramus femoralis nervi genitofemoralis.* See also Table of Nerves in the Appendix.

lum·bo·is·chi·al (lum″bo·is′kee·ul) *adj.* [*lumbo-* + *ischial*]. Pertaining to the ischium and the lumbar part of the vertebral column.

lum·bo·sa·cral (lum″bo·say′krul) *adj.* [*lumbo-* + *sacral*]. Pertaining to the lumbar vertebrae and to the sacrum.

lumbosacral plexus. A network formed by the anterior branches of lumbar, sacral, and coccygeal nerves which for descriptive purposes are divided into the lumbar, sacral, and pudendal plexuses. NA *plexus lumbosacralis.* See also Plate 16.

lumbosacral trunk. A trunk formed by the anterior ramus of the fifth lumbar nerve and the smaller part of the anterior ramus of the fourth, and forming the liason between the lumbar and the sacral plexuses. NA *truncus lumbosacralis.*

lum·bo·ver·te·bral (lum″bo·vur′te·brul) *adj.* [*lumbo-* + *vertebral*]. Pertaining to the lumbar region and the vertebrae.

lum·bri·cal (lum′bri·kul) *adj.* & *n.* [L. *lumbricus*, earthworm]. 1. Pertaining to, or resembling, an earthworm or *Lumbricus.* 2. Any of four small muscles in the hand or foot. NA *musculi lumbricales.* See also Table of Muscles in the Appendix.

Lum·bri·cus (lum′bri·kus) *n.* [L.]. A genus of earthworms, formerly erroneously regarded as an intestinal worm.

lum·bus (lum′bus) *n.*, pl. & genit. sing. **lum·bi** (·bye), genit. pl. **lum·bo·rum** (lum·bo′rum) [L.] [NA]. LOIN.

lu·men (lew′min) *n.*, pl. **lu·mi·na** (·mi·nuh), **lumens** [L., light, opening]. 1. The space inside of a tube, as the lumen of a thermometer, blood vessel, or duct. 2. The unit of flux of light; the flux in a unit of solid angle from a source having a uniform luminous intensity of one candela.

lumi-. A combining form designating *irradiation or fluorescence.*

lu·mi·chrome (lew′mi·krome) *n.* [*lumi-* + *-chrome*]. 7,8-Dimethylalloxazine, $C_{12}H_{10}N_4O_2$, an oxidation product of riboflavin.

lu·mi·fla·vin (lew″mi·flay′vin, ·flav′in) *n.* [*lumi-* + *-flavin*]. A derivative of riboflavin; produced by irradiation of riboflavin in alkaline solution.

lumin-. A combining form meaning *luminosity.*

lu·mi·nal, lu·me·nal (lew′mi·nul) *adj.* Of or pertaining to a lumen (1).

Luminal. A trademark for phenobarbital, a sedative and hypnotic.

lu·mi·nance (lew′mi·nunce) *n.* The amount of light emitted from a source and projected on a measuring surface; also called brightness, although, technically, brightness is a subjective quality of light as measured by the eye.

lu·mi·nes·cence (lew″mi·nes′unce) *n.* An emission of light without a production of heat sufficient to cause incandescence. It is encountered in certain animals, as some protozoa and fireflies.

lu·mi·nif·er·ous (lew″mi·nif′ur·us) *adj.* [*lumin-* + *-ferous*]. Conveying or bearing light.

lu·mi·nol (lew′mi·nole, ·nol) *n.* 3-Aminophthalhydrazide, $C_8H_7N_3O_2$, a substance which becomes strongly luminescent as it undergoes oxidation. See also *chemiluminescence.*

lu·mi·nous (lew′mi·nus) *adj.* [L. *luminosus*, from *lumen*, light]. Emitting light. —**lu·mi·nos·i·ty** (lew″mi·nos′i·tee) *n.*

luminous flux. Radiant flux applied to visible light; symbol, *F.*

luminous intensity. From a point source of light, the flux emitted per unit angle in a certain direction.

lu·mi·rho·dop·sin (lew″mi·ro·dop′sin) *n.* The first intermediate product of the bleaching of rhodopsin.

lu·mis·ter·ol (lew·mis′tur·ol) *n.* [*lumi-* + *sterol*]. The first product obtained in the irradiation of ergosterol with ultraviolet light; further irradiation produces calciferol (vitamin D_2).

lump, *n.* 1. A small mass; a protuberant part. 2. Any localized swelling or tumor.

lump·ec·to·my (lum·peck′tuh·mee) *n. Informal.* Surgical removal of a neoplasm or cyst in the breast.

lump kidney. A form of congenital renal fusion. See *cake kidney.*

lumpy jaw. Actinomycosis of cattle and swine. See also *wooden tongue, bighead.*

lu·na·cy (lew′nuh·see) *n.* [from *lunatic*]. *In legal medicine,* mental disorder in which the individual is not legally responsible; insanity. See also *psychosis.*

lu·nar (lew′nur) *adj.* [L. *lunaris*, from *luna*, moon]. 1. Pertaining to the moon. 2. Pertaining to silver (*luna* of the alchemists).

lunar caustic. TOUGHENED SILVER NITRATE.

lu·nate (lew′nate) *n.* [L. *lunatus*, crescent-shaped, from *luna*, moon]. One of the carpal bones. NA *os lunatum.* See also Table of Bones in the Appendix.

lunate sulcus. An inconstant sulcus in the superolateral surface of the occipital lobe of the cerebrum marking the cephalic limit of the visual area. NA *sulcus lunatus.* See also *ape fissure.*

lu·na·tic (lew′nuh·tick) *n.* [L. *lunaticus*, insane, moonstruck, from *luna*, moon]. A psychotic person.

lu·na·to·ma·la·cia (lew″nuh·to·ma·lay′shuh) *n.* [*lunate* + *malacia*]. KIENBÖCK'S DISEASE.

lu·nel·la (lew·nel′uh) *n.* [NL., lit., little moon]. HYPOPYON.

lung, *n.* The organ of respiration, in which venous blood is relieved of carbon dioxide and oxygenated by air drawn through the trachea and bronchi into the alveoli. There are two lungs, a right and a left, the former consisting of three, the latter of two, lobes. The lungs are situated in the thoracic cavity, and are enveloped by the pleura. NA *pulmo.* See also Plates 5, 12, 13, 14.

lung bud. One of the primary outgrowths of the embryonic trachea whose growth and subsequent division produce a primary bronchus and all its branches.

lung fluke. *PARAGONIMUS WESTERMANI.*

lung·mo·tor (lung′mo·tur) *n.* An apparatus for pumping air or air and oxygen into the lungs, as treatment for asphyxia.

lu·nu·la (loo′new·luh) *n.*, pl. **lunu·lae** (·lee) [NA]. 1. The white, semilunar area of a nail near the root. 2. The thin, crescentic area of a semilunar valve of the heart, on either side of the nodule.

lunulae val·vu·la·rum se·mi·lu·na·ri·um aor·tae (val·vew·lair′um sem″ee·lew·nair′ee·um ay·or′tee) [NA]. The thin crescentic areas of the semilunar valves of the aorta.

lunulae valvularum semilunarium trun·ci pul·mo·nis (trunk′

eye, trun'sigh pul·mo'nis) [NA]. The thin crescentic areas of the semilunar valves of the pulmonary trunk.

lu·pa·nine (lew'puh·neen) *n.* An alkaloid, $C_{15}H_{24}N_2O$, from various species of *Lupinus.*

lu·pi·form (lew'pi·form) *adj.* [*lupus* + *-iform*]. LUPOID.

lu·pine (lew'pin, ·pine, ·peen) *n.* [L. *lupinus*]. A plant of the genus *Lupinus.* One or more poisonous alkaloids have been found in various species of the genus. The bruised seeds of *L. albus* have been used as an external application to ulcers.

lu·pi·no·sis (lew''pi·no'sis) *n.* [*lupine* + *-osis*]. LATHYRISM.

lu·poid (lew'poid) *adj.* [*lupus* + *-oid*]. Resembling lupus.

lupoid hepatitis. A form of chronic active hepatitis in which the serologic reactions characteristic of lupus erythematosus are present, although other features of that disease are not present.

lupoid sycosis. KELOID SYCOSIS.

lupoid ulcer. An ulcer of the skin with a resemblance to lupus vulgaris.

lu·pu·lin (lew'pew·lin) *n.* The glandular trichomes separated from the strobiles of *Humulus lupulus;* formerly used as an antispasmodic and sedative.

lu·pu·lus (lew'pew·lus) *n.* [NL., dim. of L. *lupus,* hop plant]. HUMULUS.

lu·pus (lew'pus) *n.* [L., wolf]. 1. LUPUS ERYTHEMATOSUS. 2. Any chronic progressive ulcerative skin lesion. 3. LUPUS VULGARIS.

lupus band test. A test which is positive in most patients with systemic lupus erythematous, in which immunoglobulins are shown to be bound to the basement membrane of the epidermis on a skin biopsy specimen.

lupus crus·to·sus (krus·to'sus). A crusted form of lupus vulgaris.

lupus en·dem·i·cus (en·dem'i·kus). CUTANEOUS LEISHMANIASIS.

lupus er·y·the·ma·to·sus (err''i·theem''uh·to'sus, ·them''). A disease of unknown causation and variable manifestations, ranging from a skin disorder (discoid lupus erythematosus) to a generalized disorder involving the skin and viscera (systemic lupus erythematosus).

lupus erythematosus body. A mass of altered nuclear material found in a lupus erythematosus cell.

lupus erythematosus cell. A polymorphonuclear leukocyte which has ingested nuclear material from another cell which has been denatured in a specific way by the action of a substance occurring in the blood and body fluids of patients with systemic lupus erythematosus and, occasionally, other diseases. Syn. *L.E. cell.*

lupus erythematosus cell test. L.E. CELL TEST.

lupus erythematosus factor. L.E. FACTOR.

lupus erythematosus un·gui·um mu·ti·lans (ung'gwee·um mew'ti·lanz). A type of chronic discoid lupus erythematosus affecting the dorsum of both hands in which the nails become reduced to irregular, discolored, "worm-eaten" strips adherent to the ungual bed, with deformities of the ends of the fingers.

lupus ex·ce·dens (eck·see'denz). The ulcerating type of lupus vulgaris.

lupus hy·per·troph·i·cus (high''pur·trof'i·kus). The variety of lupus vulgaris in which new connective-tissue formation predominates over the destructive process, and markedly raised, thick patches result.

lupus keloid. A scar-tissue overgrowth in an area of lupus vulgaris.

lupus lym·phat·i·cus (lim·fat'i·kus). LYMPHANGIOMA CIRCUMSCRIPTUM CONGENITALE.

lupus mac·u·lo·sus (mack''yoo·lo'sus). A variety of lupus vulgaris characterized by the eruption of very soft, smooth, brownish red, semitranslucent miliary nodules that develop in the connective tissue of otherwise healthy skin without subjective sensations.

lupus mil·i·a·ris dis·sem·i·na·tus fa·ci·ei (mil·ee·air'is di·sem·i·nay'tus fay·shee·ee'eye). A papular dermatosis on the face whose histopathology is tuberculoid, course benign, and cause uncertain.

lupus of the larynx. A condition caused by *Mycobacterium tuberculosis* which usually follows lupus of the nasopharynx or face; rarer and less destructive than tuberculous laryngitis. The nodules occur on the epiglottis or the aryepiglottic folds.

lupus per·nio (pur'nee·o). SARCOIDOSIS.

lupus pernio of Besnier [E. *Besnier*]. A granulomatous process in the nature of sarcoid histologically and clinically resembling frostbite; occurs on the face, particularly on the nose.

lupus se·ba·ce·us (se·bay'see·us). CHRONIC DISCOID LUPUS ERYTHEMATOSUS.

lupus ser·pig·i·no·sus (sur·pij·i·no'sus). A form of lupus vulgaris which spreads peripherally while cicatrizing centrally.

lupus su·per·fi·ci·a·lis (sue''pur·fish·ee·ay'lis). CHRONIC DISCOID LUPUS ERYTHEMATOSUS.

lupus tu·mi·dus (tew'mi·dus). A form of lupus vulgaris with edematous infiltration.

lupus veg·e·tans (vej'e·tanz). A form of lupus vulgaris characterized by warty-looking patches liable to secondary infection.

lupus ver·ru·co·sus (verr''oo·ko'sus). LUPUS VEGETANS.

lupus vul·gar·is (vul·gair'is). True tuberculosis of the skin; a slow-developing, scarring, and deforming disease, often asymptomatic, often involving the face, and occurring in a wide variety of appearances. Syn. *tuberculosis luposa.*

Lusch·ka's bursa (lo͝osh'kah) [H. von *Luschka,* German anatomist, 1820–1875]. PHARYNGEAL BURSA.

Luschka's cartilage [H. von *Luschka*]. An inconstant, small, cartilaginous nodule, enclosed in the front of the true vocal folds.

Luschka's foramen [H. von *Luschka*]. LATERAL APERTURE OF THE FOURTH VENTRICLE.

Luschka's glands or **ducts** [H. von *Luschka*]. Aberrant bile ducts in the wall of the gallbladder.

Luschka's subpharyngeal cartilage [H. von *Luschka*]. A small, inconstant body of hyaline cartilage, situated in the capsule or in a septum of the palatine tonsil.

Luschka's tonsil [H. von *Luschka*]. ADENOID (3).

Luschka's tubercle [H. von *Luschka*]. An osteochondroma located at the superior angle of the scapula.

Lust's phenomenon, reflex, or **sign.** Dorsal flexion and eversion of the foot in response to percussion over the common peroneal nerve as a sign of increased neuromuscular irritability.

lu·sus na·tu·rae (lew'sus na·tew'ree) [L. *lusus,* game, sport, trick]. A freak of nature, a monstrosity.

lute, *n.* [L. *lutum,* mud]. A pasty substance which hardens when dry; used sometimes to make joints waterproof in laboratory apparatus.

lute-, luteo- [L. *luteus,* yellow]. A combining form designating (a) *yellow, yellowish, orange-yellow, brownish yellow;* (b) in chemistry, *a yellow ammoniacal cobaltic salt;* (c) *luteal, corpus luteum.*

lu·te·al (lew'tee·ul) *adj.* Of or pertaining to the corpus luteum or to its principle.

luteal cyst. A cyst of the corpus luteum.

luteal hormone. The hormone secreted by the corpus luteum; PROGESTERONE.

lu·te·ci·um (lew·tee'shee·um) *n.* LUTETIUM.

lu·tein (lew'tee·in) *n.* [L. *lute*us, yellow, + *-in*]. 1. A yellow dihydroxy-α-carotene, $C_{40}H_{56}O_2$, first isolated from egg yolk, but widely distributed in nature. Syn. *xanthophyll.* 2. A dried, powdered preparation of corpus luteum.

lutein cells. Cells of the corpus luteum. See also *follicular lutein cells, paralutein cells.*

lutein cyst. LUTEAL CYST.

lu·tein·iza·tion (lew''tee·in·i·zay'shun) *n.* The acquisition by ovarian follicle cells of the characteristics of lutein cells following release of the ovum they surround.

lu·tein·ize (lew'tee·in·ize) *v.* To form lutein.

luteinized granulosa cell carcinoma. LUTEOMA.

luteinizing hormone. An adenohypophyseal hormone which stimulates both epithelial and interstitial cells in the ovary, where together with the follicle-stimulating hormone it induces follicular maturation and formation of corpora lutea. In the male, where it acts only on the interstitial cells of the testis, it is more appropriately called interstitial cell-stimulating hormone (ICSH). Abbreviated, L.H. Syn. *corpus luteum-stimulating hormone, metakentrin, pituitary B gonadotropin.*

luteinizing hormone releasing factor or **hormone.** A small peptide hormone released from the hypothalamus which acts on the pituitary gland to cause release of luteinizing hormone. Abbreviated, LHRF, LHRH.

lu·tein·o·ma (lew"tee·in·o'muh) *n.* [*lutein* + *-oma*]. LUTEOMA.

Lu·tem·ba·cher's complex or **disease.** (lue·tæn·bah·kehr') [R. *Lutembacher,* French cardiologist, b. 1884]. LUTEMBACHER'S SYNDROME.

Lutembacher's syndrome. An atrial septal defect associated with congenital mitral stenosis.

lu·te·no·ma (lew"tee·no'muh) *n.* LUTEOMA.

luteo-. See *lute-.*

lu·teo·blas·to·ma (lew"tee·o·blas·to'muh) *n.* [*luteo-* + *blastoma*]. LUTEOMA.

lu·te·o·lin (lew'tee·o·lin) *n.* 3',4',5,7-Tetrahydroxyflavone, $C_{15}H_{10}O_6$, occurring in many plants in glycosidic combination.

lu·te·o·ma (lew"tee·o'muh) *n.*, pl. **luteomas, luteoma·ta** (·tuh) [*lute-* + *-oma*]. An ovarian tumor made up of cells resembling those of the corpus luteum. Syn. *luteinized granulosa-cell carcinoma, lutenoma, luteinoma, luteoblastoma, struma ovarii luteinocellulare, lipid-cell tumor of the ovary.*

lu·teo·tro·pic (lew"tee·o·tro'·pick) *adj.* [*luteo-* + *-tropic*]. Having an affinity for or having an effect on the corpus luteum.

luteotropic hormone. PROLACTIN. Abbreviated, LTH.

lu·te·ti·um (lew·tee'shee·um) *n.* [L. *Lutetia,* pre-Roman Paris]. Lu = 174.967. One of the lanthanide series of elements.

Lu·ther·an blood group. The erythrocyte antigens defined by reactions with an antibody designated anti-Lu[a], initially detected in the serum of a multiply transfused patient with lupus erythematosus who developed antibodies against the erythrocytes of a donor named Lutheran, and by anti-Lu[b].

lu·tu·trin (lew'too·trin) *n.* A uterine relaxing factor, a protein or polypeptide, obtained from corpus luteum; used in the treatment of functional dysmenorrhea.

Lutz-Splen·do·re-Al·mei·da disease (loots, splen·do're[h], ahl·me[y]'duh) [A. *Lutz,* Brazilian, 20th century; A. *Splendore,* Italian, 20th century; and F. P. de *Almeida,* Brazilian, 20th century]. SOUTH AMERICAN BLASTOMYCOSIS.

lux (lucks) *n.*, pl. **lux, luxes** [L., light]. A unit of illumination equivalent to one lumen per square meter.

lux·a·tio cox·ae con·gen·i·ta (luck·say'shee·o kock'see kon·jen'i·tuh). CONGENITAL DISLOCATION OF THE HIP.

luxatio erec·ta (e·reck'tuh). Inferior dislocation of the shoulder in which the arm is elevated and unable to be lowered.

lux·a·tion (luck·say'shun) *n.* [L. *luxatio,* from *luxus,* dislocated]. 1. A dislocation, especially a complete dislocation of a joint. 2. The partial or complete separation of a tooth from its socket by mechanical force.

lux·u·ri·ant (lug·zhoor'ee·unt) *adj.* [L. *luxurians,* from *luxuria,* rankness, excess]. Growing to excess, exuberant; specifically referring to the abnormal growth of certain body cells, as in granulation tissue.

lux·us (luck'sus) *n.* [L.]. Excess.

luxus breathing. Voluntary hyperventilation.

luxus consumption. A reserve of protein in the body in excess of the amount required by metabolism.

luxus heart. Dilatation and hypertrophy of the left ventricle.

Luys body lesion (lw[y]ee) [J. B. *Luys,* French neurologist, 1828–1897]. HEMIBALLISMUS.

LVH Left ventricular hypertrophy.

L wave. Large irregular atrial contraction waves seen with high-speed cinematography in atrial fibrillation, occurring at a rate of 400 to 800 per minute.

ly·can·thro·py (lye·kan'thruh·pee) *n.* [Gk. *lykanthrōpia,* from *lykanthrōpos,* werewolf, from *lykos,* wolf, + *anthrōpos,* man]. The delusion of being a wolf or some other wild beast, seen in schizophrenic patients. —**ly·can·throp·ic** (lye"kan·throp'ick) *adj.;* **ly·can·thrope** (lye'kun·thrope) *n.*

ly·cine (lye'seen, ·sin) *n.* BETAINE (1).

ly·co·ma·nia (lye"ko·may'nee·uh) *n.* [Gk. *lykos,* wolf, + *-mania*]. LYCANTHROPY.

ly·co·pene (lye'ko·peen) *n.* [*Lyco*persicon, genus of the tomato plant, + *-ene*]. A red carotenoid pigment, $C_{40}H_{56}$, occurring in ripe fruit, especially tomatoes.

ly·co·pen·emia (lye"ko·pe·nee'mee·uh) *n.* 1. An excess of lycopene in the blood. 2. A clinical disorder characterized by orange-yellow skin pigmentation, with similar discoloration of the liver, resulting from excessive ingestion of tomato juice.

ly·co·per·don·o·sis (lye"ko·pur"dun·o'sis) *n.* [*Lycoperdon* + *-osis*]. A respiratory disease caused by inhalation of large quantities of spores from the mature puffball mushroom, *Lycoperdon.*

ly·co·po·di·um (lye"ko·po'dee·um) *n.* [NL., from Gk. *lykos,* wolf, + *pous,* foot]. The spores of *Lycopodium clavatum,* occurring as a light, fine, yellowish powder. Has been used as a desiccant and absorbent on moist and excoriated surfaces, and as an inert powder in which to embed pills to prevent their adhering to one another. Syn. *club moss, witch meal, wolf's claw.*

Lycopodium, *n.* The large type genus of the evergreen plant family Lycopodiaceae. *Lycopodium saururus* is the source of the alkaloids sauroxine and saururine; the spores of *Lycopodium clavatum* (lycopodium) have various uses.

ly·co·pus (lye'ko·pus) *n.* [NL., from Gk. *lykos,* wolf, + *pous,* foot]. Bugle weed, *Lycopus virginicus;* formerly used as an astringent and hemostatic.

ly·co·rex·ia (lye"ko·reck'see·uh) *n.* [Gk. *lykos,* wolf, + *-orexia*]. A wolfish or ravenous appetite.

ly·di·my·cin (lye·di·migh'sin) *n.* An antibiotic substance, with antifungal activity, derived from *Streptomyces lydicus.*

lye, *n.* [OE. *lēag* ← Gmc. *laugō* (rel. to L. *lavere,* to wash)]. 1. An alkaline solution obtained by leaching wood ashes. 2. A solution of sodium or potassium hydroxide.

Ly·ell's syndrome [A. *Lyell,* British dermatologist, contemporary]. TOXIC EPIDERMAL NECROLYSIS.

ly·go·phil·ia (lye"go·fil'ee·uh) *n.* [Gk. *lygē,* twilight, + *-philia*]. Morbid love of dark places.

Lygranum. Trademark for antigens employed in the complement-fixation test and the Frei test for lymphogranuloma venereum. They are prepared by growing the virus on the chick embryo.

ly·ing-in. 1. PARTURITION. 2. PUERPERIUM (1).

Lym·naea (lim'nee·uh) *n.* [Gk. *limnaios,* of the marsh]. A snail genus which contains species acting as invertebrate hosts for *Fasciola hepatica.*

Lyme arthritis. An acute, transient, epidemic form of arthritis, accompanied by fever and a skin lesion resembling an insect bite; presumably due to a transmissible, possibly arthropod-borne agent which has not been identified. It has been observed near Lyme, Connecticut beginning in 1974.

lymph (limf) *n.* [L. *lympha,* clear water]. 1. Interstitial fluid that has entered and is circulating in the lymphatic system; composed of water, proteins, salts, and other substances derived from the blood plasma and contains lymphocytes and other cells. Concentrations of cells and other ingredients vary in specific regions of the body. 2. EXUDATE. —**lym·phoid** (·oid) *adj.*

lymph-, lympho-. A combining form meaning (a) *lymph, lymphatic;* (b) *lymphocyte.*

lym·pha (lim'fuh) *n.* [NA]. LYMPH (1).

lymphaden-, lymphadeno- [*lymph-* + *aden-*]. A combining form meaning *lymph node.*

lymph·ad·e·nec·to·my (lim·fad''e·neck'tuh·mee) *n.* [*lymphaden-* + *-ectomy*]. Excision of a lymph node.

lymph·ad·e·ni·tis (lim·fad''e·nigh'tis) *n.* [*lymphaden-* + *-itis*]. Inflammation of the lymph nodes.

lymphadeno-. See *lymphaden-.*

lymph·ad·e·noid (lim·fad'e·noid) *adj.* [*lymphaden-* + *-oid*]. Resembling a lymph node.

lymphadenoid goiter. STRUMA LYMPHOMATOSA.

lymph·ad·e·no·ma (lim·fad''e·no'muh) *n.*, pl. **lymphadenomas, lymphadenoma·ta** (·tuh) [*lymphaden-* + *-oma*]. Tumorlike enlargement of a lymph node; it probably exists in two forms, the neoplastic and the hyperplastic.

lymph·ad·e·no·ma·to·sis (lim·fad''e·no''muh·to'sis) *n.* [*lymphadenoma* + *-osis*]. A malignant lymphoma.

lymph·ad·e·nop·a·thy (lim·fad''e·nop'uth·ee) *n.* [*lymphadeno-* + *-pathy*]. 1. Lymph node enlargement in response to any disease. 2. Any disease of the lymph nodes.

lymph·ad·e·no·sis (lim·fad''e·no'sis) *n.*, pl. **lymphadeno·ses** (·seez) [*lymphaden-* + *-osis*]. Hyperplasia or neoplasia affecting the lymph nodes.

lymphadenosis be·nig·na cu·tis (be·nig'nuh kew'tis). LYMPHOCYTOMA CUTIS.

lymph·ad·e·not·o·my (lim·fad''e·not'uh·mee) *n.* [*lymphadeno-* + *-tomy*]. Incision of a lymph node.

lym·pha·gogue (lim'fuh·gog) *n.* [*lymph-* + *-agogue*]. An agent that stimulates the flow of lymph.

lymphangi-, lymphangio- [*lymph-* + *angi-*]. A combining form meaning *lymphatic vessel.*

lym·phan·gi·ec·ta·sia (lim·fan''jee·eck·tay'zhuh, ·zee·uh) *n.* LYMPHANGIECTASIS.

lym·phan·gi·ec·ta·sis (lim·fan''jee·eck'tuh·sis) *n.* [*lymphangi-* + *ectasis*]. Dilatation of the lymphatic vessels. —**lym·phangi·ec·tat·ic** (·eck·tat'ick) *adj.*

lym·phan·gi·ec·to·des (lim·fan''jee·eck·to'deez) *n.* LYMPHANGIOMA CIRCUMSCRIPTUM CONGENITALE.

lym·phan·gi·ec·to·my (lim·fan''jee·eck'tuh·mee) *n.* [*lymphangi-* + *-ectomy*]. Excision of a pathologic lymphatic channel, as in surgery for cancer.

lymphangio-. See *lymphangi-.*

lym·phan·gio·en·do·the·li·al sarcoma (lim·fan''jee·o·en''do·theel'ee·ul). LYMPHANGIOSARCOMA.

lym·phan·gio·en·do·the·li·o·ma (lim·fan''jee·o·en''do·theel·ee·o'muh) *n.* [*lymphangio-* + *endotheli-* + *-oma*]. A tumor composed of a congeries of lymphatic vessels, between which are many large mononuclear cells presumed to be endothelial cells.

lym·phan·gio·fi·bro·ma (lim·fan''jee·o·figh·bro'muh) *n.* A benign tumor whose parenchyma contains both lymphangiomatous and fibromatous elements.

lym·phan·gio·gram (lim·fan'jee·o·gram) *n.* [*lymphangio-* + *-gram*]. A radiographic representation of lymph nodes and lymph vessels produced by lymphangiography.

lym·phan·gi·og·ra·phy (lim·fan''jee·og'ruh·fee) *n.* [*lymphangio-* + *-graphy*]. The process of radiographic visualization of lymph channels and lymph nodes by injection of radiopaque contrast media into afferent lymphatic channels.

lym·phan·gi·o·ma (lim·fan''jee·o'muh) *n.*, pl. **lymphangiomas, lymphangioma·ta** (·tuh) [*lymphangi-* + *-oma*]. A benign, abnormal collection of lymphatic vessels forming a mass. Syn. *simple lymphangioma.* See also *hygroma.*

lymphangioma cir·cum·scrip·tum con·gen·i·ta·le (sur''kum·skrip'tum kon·jen''i·tay'lee). A rare skin disease of unknown cause, occurring in early life. Marked by the formation of straw-yellow vesicles, deeply situated in the skin, with thick and tense walls, and connected with the lymphatics.

lymphangioma tu·be·ro·sum mul·ti·plex (tew''be·ro'sum mul'ti·plecks). A skin disease characterized by the formation of large, brownish-red papules or tubercles, not arranged in groups or clusters, but scattered indiscriminately over the trunk.

lym·phan·gio·plas·ty (lim·fan'jee·o·plas''tee, lim·fan''jee·o·plas'tee) *n.* [*lymphangio-* + *-plasty*]. Replacement of lymphatics by artificial channels.

lym·phan·gio·sar·co·ma (lim·fan''jee·o·sahr·ko'muh) *n.* [*lymphangio-* + *sarcoma*]. A sarcoma whose parenchymal cells form vascular channels resembling lymphatics; often associated with preexisting lymphedema.

lym·phan·gi·ot·o·my (lim·fan''jee·ot'uh·mee) *n.* [*lymphangio-* + *-tomy*]. Cutting or dissection of lymphatic channels.

lym·phan·gi·tis (lim''fan·jye'tis) *n.*, pl. **lymphan·git·i·des** (·jit'i·deez) [*lymphangi-* + *-itis*]. Inflammation of a lymphatic vessel or vessels. —**lymphan·git·ic** (·jit'ick) *adj.*

lym·phat·ic (lim·fat'ick) *adj. & n.* 1. Pertaining to lymph. 2. A vessel conveying lymph. NA *vas lymphaticum.*

lymphatic abscess. An abscess associated with lymphadenitis and/or lymphangitis.

lymphatic anemia. HODGKIN'S DISEASE.

lymphatic blockade. Obstruction of lymphatic drainage.

lymphatic cachexia. Cachexia resulting from malignant lymphoma.

lymphatic leukemia. LYMPHOCYTIC LEUKEMIA.

lym·phat·i·cos·to·my (lim·fat''i·kos'tuh·mee) *n.* [*lymphatic* + *-stomy*]. Formation of an opening into a lymphatic trunk, as the thoracic duct.

lymphatic system. A system of vessels and nodes accessory to the blood vascular system, conveying lymph. Its functions are to return water and proteins from the interstitial fluid to the blood and to produce lymphocytes and other cells in response to the presence of antigens and inflammations. NA *systema lymphaticum.* See also Plate 11.

lymphatic tissue. Tissue consisting of networks of reticular and collagenous fibers and lymphocytes.

lym·pha·tism (lim'fuh·tiz·um) *n.* [*lymphatic* + *-ism*]. STATUS THYMICOLYMPHATICUS.

lymphato-. A combining form meaning *lymphatic.*

lym·phato·cele (lim·fat'o·seel) *n.* [*lymphato-* + *-cele*]. LYMPHANGIOMA.

lym·phato·gogue (lim·fat'uh·gog, lim'fuh·to·) *n.* LYMPHAGOGUE.

lymph channel. A tissue space or lymphatic.

lymph·ede·ma, lymph·oe·de·ma (lim''fe·dee'muh) *n.* [*lymph* + *edema*]. Edema due to obstruction of lymph vessels.

lymph follicle. LYMPH NODULE.

lymph glands. LYMPH NODES.

lymph nodes. Masses of lymphatic tissue 1 to 25 mm long, often bean-shaped, intercalated in the course of lymph vessels, more or less well organized by a connective-tissue capsule and trabeculae into cortical nodules and medullary cords which form lymphocytes, and into lymph sinuses through which lymph filters, permitting phagocytic activity of reticular cells and macrophages. Syn. *lymph glands.* NA *nodi lymphatici.* See also Plate 11.

lymph nodule. A small mass of dense lymphatic tissue in which new lymphocytes are formed. NA *folliculus lymphaticus.*

lympho-. See *lymph-.*

lym·pho·blast (lim'fo·blast) *n.* [*lympho-* + *-blast*]. A blast cell, considered a precursor or early form of a lymphocyte. —**lym·pho·blas·tic** (lim''fo·blas'tick) *adj.*

lymphoblastic leukemia. A form of lymphocytic leukemia in which the cells are poorly differentiated but recognizably of the lymphocytic series; associated with an acute course, if untreated.

lymphoblastic plasma cell. 1. PLASMABLAST. 2. PROPLASMACYTE (1).

lymphoblastic reticulosarcoma. RETICULUM-CELL SARCOMA.

lym·pho·blas·to·ma (lim″fo·blas·to′muh) *n.* [*lymphoblast* + *-oma*]. A type of malignant lymphoma whose parenchyma is composed of lymphoblasts. See also *lymphocytoma, lymphosarcoma.*

lymphoblastoma ma·lig·num (ma·lig′num). HODGKIN'S DISEASE.

lym·pho·blas·to·sis (lim″fo·blas·to′sis) *n.* [*lymphoblast* + *-osis*]. An excessive number of lymphoblasts in peripheral blood; occasionally found also in tissues.

lym·pho·cyte (lim′fo·site) *n.* [*lympho-* + *-cyte*]. A leukocyte found in the lymphoid tissue, blood, and lymph, characterized by a round, centrally located nucleus, cytoplasm showing various degrees of basophilia due to the presence of free ribosomes, and a lack of specific granules. Two major classes, B and T lymphocytes, are active in the immune response. See also *B lymphocyte, T lymphocyte.* —**lym·pho·cyt·ic** (lim″fo·sit′ick) *adj.*

lymphocyte transformation. Growth of a lymphocyte with DNA synthesis, assumption of morphologic characteristics of a blast cell, and finally mitotic division.

lym·pho·cy·the·mia, lym·pho·cy·thae·mia (lim″fo·sigh·theem′ee·uh) *n.* [*lymphocyte* + *-hemia*]. An absolute increase in the number of peripheral blood lymphocytes.

lymphocytic angina. INFECTIOUS MONONUCLEOSIS.

lymphocytic choriomeningitis. An acute viral meningitis due to a specific virus endemic in mice; characterized clinically by the syndrome of aseptic meningitis, and a short, benign course with usual recovery.

lymphocytic leukemia. A form of leukemia, acute or chronic, in which the predominating cell type belongs to the lymphocytic series. Syn. *lymphoid leukemia, lymphogenous leukemia.*

lymphocytic lymphoma. A form of malignant lymphoma in which the predominating cell type belongs to the lymphocytic series.

lymphocytic myeloma. A malignant plasmacytoma.

lymphocytic sarcoma. LYMPHOSARCOMA.

lymphocytic series. In lymphocytopoiesis, the cells at progressive stages of development from a primitive cell (lymphoblast) through an intermediate stage (prolymphocyte) to a mature cell (lymphocyte).

lym·pho·cy·toid (lim″fo·sigh′toid) *adj.* Resembling a lymphocyte.

lym·pho·cy·to·ma (lim″fo·sigh·to′muh) *n.*, pl. **lymphocytomas, lymphocytoma·ta** (·tuh) [*lymphocyte* + *-oma*]. A type of malignant lymphoma in which the predominant cell type closely resembles mature lymphocytes. Syn. *pseudolymphoma.* See also *lymphoblastoma, lymphosarcoma.*

lymphocytoma cu·tis (kew′tis). A benign collection of lymphocytes, with or without germinal centers, in the dermis. Syn. *Spiegler-Fendt sarcoid, lymphadenosis benigna cutis.*

lym·pho·cy·to·pe·nia (lim″fo·sigh″to·pee′nee·uh) *n.* [*lymphocyte* + *-penia*]. Reduction of the absolute number of lymphocytes per unit volume of peripheral blood. Syn. *lymphopenia.*

lym·pho·cy·toph·thi·sis (lim″fo·sigh·tof′thi·sis) *n.* [*lymphocyte* + *phthisis*]. SWISS TYPE AGAMMAGLOBULINEMIA.

lym·pho·cy·to·poi·e·sis (lim″fo·sigh″to·poy·ee′sis) *n.*, pl. **lymphocytopoie·ses** (·seez) [*lymphocyte* + *-poiesis*]. The genesis of lymphocytes.

lym·pho·cy·to·sis (lim″fo·sigh·to′sis) *n.*, pl. **lymphocyto·ses** (·seez) [*lymphocyte* + *-osis*]. An abnormally large number of lymphocytes in peripheral blood.

lym·pho·cy·to·tox·ic (lim″fo·sigh″to·tock′sick) *adj.* Having deleterious effects on lymphocytes. —**lymphocyto·tox·ic·i·ty** (·tock·sis′i·tee) *n.*

lym·pho·cy·tu·ria (lim″fo·sigh·tew′ree·uh) *n.* The presence of abnormal numbers of lymphocytes in the urine; may be associated with renal allograft rejection.

lym·pho·der·mia (lim″fo·dur′mee·uh) *n.* [*lympho-* + *-dermia*]. A disease of the lymphatics of the skin.

lymphodermia per·ni·ci·o·sa (pur·nish·ee·o′suh). Leukemic enlargement of the lymph nodes.

lymphoedema. LYMPHEDEMA.

lym·pho·ep·i·the·li·al (lim″fo·ep·i·theel′ee·ul) *adj.* Pertaining to or characterizing epithelial tissue infiltrated by lymphocytes.

lym·pho·ep·i·the·li·o·ma (lim″fo·ep″i·theel·ee·o′muh) *n.* [*lympho-* + *epitheli-* + *-oma*]. A poorly differentiated squamous cell carcinoma of the nasopharynx whose parenchymal cells resemble elements of the reticuloendothelial system. —**lymphoepithelioma·tous** (·tus) *adj.*

lymphoepitheliomatous blastoma. LYMPHOEPITHELIOMA.

lym·pho·gen·ic (lim·fo·jen′ick) *adj.* LYMPHOGENOUS.

lymphogenic tuberculosis. Tuberculosis spread from any focus to another by way of the lymph channels. Syn. *lymphogenous tuberculosis.*

lym·phog·e·nous (lim·foj′e·nus) *adj.* [*lympho-* + *-genous*]. 1. Producing lymph. 2. Produced or spread in the lymphatic system.

lymphogenous leukemia. LYMPHOCYTIC LEUKEMIA.

lymphogenous tuberculosis. LYMPHOGENIC TUBERCULOSIS.

lym·pho·glan·du·la (lim″fo·glan′dew·luh) *n.*, pl. **lymphoglandu·lae** (·lee) [BNA]. Nodus lymphaticus (= LYMPH NODE).

lym·pho·go·nia (lim″fo·go′nee·uh) *n.pl.* [NL., from *lympho-* + Gk. *gonos*, offspring]. Large lymphocytes having a relatively large nucleus deficient in chromatin and a faintly basophil nongranular cytoplasm.

lym·pho·gran·u·lo·ma (lim″fo·gran″yoo·lo′muh) *n.*, pl. **lymphogranulomas, lymphogranuloma·ta** (·tuh) [*lympho-* + *granul-* + *-oma*]. HODGKIN'S DISEASE.

lymphogranuloma in·gui·na·le (ing·gwi·nay′lee). LYMPHOGRANULOMA VENEREUM.

lym·pho·gran·u·lo·ma·to·sis (lim″fo·gran·yoo·lo″muh·to′sis) *n.*, pl. **lymphogranulomato·ses** (·seez) [*lymphogranuloma* + *-osis*]. HODGKIN'S DISEASE.

lymphogranulomatosis cu·tis (kew′tis). Any form of malignant lymphoma, especially Hodgkin's disease, involving the skin.

lymphogranulomatosis of Schaumann [J. *Schaumann*]. SARCOIDOSIS.

lymphogranuloma ve·ne·re·um (ve·neer′ee·um). A systemic infectious disease, due to a member of the psittacosis-lymphogranuloma group of agents, transmitted by sexual contact and characterized by genital ulceration, regional lymphadenitis, and constitutional symptoms. Abbreviated, LGV.

lym·pho·his·tio·cyt·ic (lim″fo·his″tee·o·sit′ick) *adj.* Involving both lymphocytes and histiocytes.

lym·phoid (lim′foid) *adj.* Resembling or pertaining to lymphocytes, lymph nodes, or lymph.

lymphoid cell. Any mononuclear cell resembling a lymphocyte.

lymphoid hemoblast (of Pap·pen·heim) [A. *Pappenheim*, German pathologist, 1870–1916]. PRONORMOBLAST.

lymphoid leukemia. LYMPHOCYTIC LEUKEMIA.

lymphoid leukocyte. A nongranular leukocyte including lymphocytes and monocytes.

lymphoid megakaryocyte. PROMEGAKARYOCYTE.

lymphoid myeloma. A malignant plasmacytoma.

lym·phoi·do·cyte (lim·foy′do·site) *n.* [*lymphoid* + *-cyte*]. HEMOCYTOBLAST.

lymphoid series. LYMPHOCYTIC SERIES.

lymphoid stem cells. LYMPHOBLASTS; HEMOCYTOBLASTS.

lymphoid tissue. LYMPHATIC TISSUE.

lymphoid wandering cells. Lymphocytes or monocytes in connective tissue.

lym·pho·ken·tric (lim″fo·ken′trick) *adj.* [*lympho-* + Gk. *kentron*, goad, spur, + *-ic*]. Stimulating lymphocyte formation.

lym·pho·kine (lim′fo·kine) *n.* [*lympho-* + Gk *kinein*, to move, alter, arouse]. Any of certain low-molecular-weight factors, produced by activated T lymphocytes, that have various effects including stimulation of mitosis in other lymphocytes, immobilization of macrophages, and lysis of other cells.

lym·pho·ma (lim·fo'muh) *n.*, pl. **lymphomas, lymphoma·ta** (·tuh) [*lymph-* + *-oma*]. Any neoplasm, usually malignant, of the lymphatic tissues. See also *Hodgkin's disease, leukosarcoma, lymphosarcoma, reticulum-cell sarcoma, nodular lymphoma, lymphocytic leukemia.*

lym·pho·ma·toid (lim·fo'muh·toid) *adj.* Resembling a malignant lymphoma.

lym·pho·ma·to·sis (lim"fo·muh·to'sis) *n.*, pl. **lymphomato·ses** (·seez) [*lymphoma* + *-osis*]. 1. Involvement of multiple body sites by malignant lymphoma. 2. A disease of animals, especially chickens, characterized by widespread involvement of the viscera by malignant lymphoma.

lym·pho·mono·cyte (lim"fo·mon'o·site) *n.* A peripheral blood leukocyte having morphologic characteristics of both a monocyte and a lymphocyte.

lym·pho·mono·cy·to·sis (lim"fo·mon"o·sigh·to'sis) *n.*, pl. **lymphomonocyto·ses** (·seez) [*lympho-* + *mono-* + *-cyte* + *-osis*]. An increase in both lymphocytes and monocytes.

lym·pho·no·dus (lim"fo·no'dus) *n.*, pl. **lymphono·di** (·dye) [*lympho-* + *nodus*] [NA alt.]. LYMPH NODE. NA alt. *nodus lymphaticus.*

lym·pho·path·ia ve·ne·re·um (lim"fo·path'ee·uh ve·neer'ee·um). LYMPHOGRANULOMA VENEREUM.

lym·pho·pe·nia (lim"fo·pee'nee·uh) *n.* [*lympho-* + *-penia*]. 1. LYMPHOCYTOPENIA. 2. A reduction in the amount of lymph.

lym·pho·poi·e·sis (lim"fo·poy·ee'sis) *n.*, pl. **lymphopoie·ses** (·seez) [*lympho-* + *-poiesis*]. 1. LYMPHOCYTOPOIESIS. 2. Lymph production. —**lymphopoi·et·ic** (·et'ick) *adj.*

lym·pho·pro·lif·er·a·tive (lim"fo·pro·lif'ur·uh·tiv) *adj.* Characterized by proliferation—benign, malignant, or undetermined—of lymphoid tissues.

lymphoproliferative disease or **syndrome.** Any condition featured by a lymphoproliferative response by host tissues; included are the malignant lymphomas.

lym·pho·pro·te·ase (lim"fo·pro'tee·ace, ·aze) *n.* An enzyme, capable of catalyzing hydrolysis of proteins, occurring in lymphocytes.

lym·pho·re·tic·u·lar system (lim"fo·re·tick'yoo·lur). RETICULOENDOTHELIAL SYSTEM.

lym·pho·re·tic·u·lo·sis (lim"fo·re·tick·yoo·lo'sis) *n.* [*lymphoreticul*ar + *-osis*]. 1. NODULAR LYMPHOMA. 2. Reticuloendothelial hyperplasia in lymphatic organs, especially lymph nodes.

lym·phor·rhage (lim'fuh·rij) *n.* [*lympho-* + *-rrhage* (as in hemorrhage)]. 1. A flow of lymph from a ruptured lymphatic vessel. 2. An aggregation of lymphocytes, usually seen in muscle tissue.

lym·phor·rha·gia (lim"fo·ray'jee·uh) *n.* [*lympho-* + *-rrhagia*]. LYMPHORRHAGE.

lym·phor·rhea, lym·phor·rhoea (lim"fo·ree'uh) *n.* [*lympho-* + *-rrhea*]. LYMPHORRHAGE (1).

lym·pho·sar·co·ma (lim"fo·sahr·ko'muh) *n.* [*lympho-* + *sarcoma*]. A malignant lymphoma composed of anaplastic lymphoid cells resembling lymphocytes or lymphoblasts, according to the degree of differentiation. Syn. *lymphocytic sarcoma.* See also *lymphoblastoma, lymphocytoma, reticulum-cell sarcoma.*

lymphosarcoma-cell leukemia. LEUKOSARCOMA.

lym·pho·sar·co·ma·to·sis (lim"fo·sahr·ko·muh·to'sis) *n.* [*lymphosarcoma* + *-osis*]. Diffuse involvement of various anatomic sites by lymphosarcoma.

lym·pho·tox·in (lim"fo·tock'sin) *n.* A lymphokine having direct cytotoxic or cytostatic action against tissue culture cells derived from human tumors.

lymph scrotum. Elephantiasis of the scrotum.

lymph sinus or **space.** One of the tracts of diffuse lymphatic tissue between the cords and nodules, and the septa and capsule of a lymph node.

lymph·uria (lim·few'ree·uh) *n.* [*lymph* + *-uria*]. The presence of lymph in the urine.

lyn·es·tre·nol (lin·es'tre·nol) *n.* 17α-Ethinyl-17β-hydroxyestr-4-ene, $C_{20}H_{28}O$, a progestational steroid.

lyo- [Gk. *lyein*, to loosen, dissolve]. A combining form meaning *dissolution, dispersion.*

lyo·chrome (lye'o·krome) *n.* [*lyo-* + *-chrome*]. FLAVIN.

lyo·en·zyme (lye"o·en'zime) *n.* [*lyo-* + *enzyme*]. EXTRACELLULAR ENZYME.

lyo·gel (lye'o·jel) *n.* [*lyo-* + *gel*]. A gel rich in liquid.

lyo·gly·co·gen (lye"o·glye'ko·jen) *n.* [*lyo-* + *glycogen*]. The portion of glycogen in tissue readily extractable with water.

Ly·on hypothesis [Mary *Lyon*, English geneticist, 20th century]. The hypothesis that in each somatic cell of the female only one of the two X chromosomes is functional, that inactivation of one occurs randomly in early embryogenesis, and that female somatic cells are consequently mosaic with respect to the X chromosomes. The DNA of the inactive X chromosomes is late replicating in the mitotic cycle and in interphase cells is visualized as the sex chromatin, or Barr body.

lyo·phile (lye'o·file, ·fil) *adj.* [*lyo-* + *-phile*]. Pertaining to the dispersed phase of a colloidal system when there is strong affinity between the dispersion medium and the dispersed phase. Contr. *lyophobe.*

lyophile complement. Complement prepared by freezing guinea pig serum and dehydrating it rapidly under high vacuum.

lyo·phil·ic (lye"o·fil'ick) *adj.* LYOPHILE.

lyophilic colloid. A colloid capable of combining with, or attracting to it, the dispersion medium.

ly·oph·i·li·za·tion (lye·off"i·li·zay'shun) *n.* The process of rapidly freezing a substance (pollen, blood plasma, antitoxin, serum) at an unusually low temperature, and then quickly dehydrating the frozen mass in a high vacuum. —**ly·oph·i·lized** (lye·off'i·lize'd) *adj.*

lyophilized biologicals. Any biologic substance, such as blood plasma, antitoxins, toxins, serums, which has been prepared in dry form by rapid freezing and dehydration, while in the frozen state, under high vacuum. Such a preparation is more stable than the product from which it is derived, does not require refrigeration, and is made ready for use by the addition of sterile distilled water.

lyo·phobe (lye'o·fobe) *adj.* [*lyo-* + *-phobe*]. Pertaining to the dispersed phase of a colloidal system when there is lack of strong affinity between the dispersed phase and the dispersion medium. Contr. *lyophile.*

lyo·pho·bic (lye"o·fo'bick) *adj.* LYOPHOBE.

lyophobic colloid. A colloid incapable of combining with, or attracting to it, the dispersion medium.

ly·o·sol (lye'o·sol) *n.* [*lyo-* + *sol*]. A disperse system wherein a liquid is the dispersing medium for suspended liquid or solid particles.

lyo·sorp·tion (lye"o·sorp'shun) *n.* [*lyo-* + ad*sorption*]. The preferential adsorption of the solvent constituent of a solution or of the dispersing medium of a colloidal system.

lyo·trope (lye'o·trope) *n.* [*lyo-* + *-trope*]. 1. One of a group of ions which, when arranged in a series, influence in the same order different phenomena which involve forces existing between the solvent and one or more other components of a solution. 2. A readily soluble substance. —**lyo·tro·pic** (lye"o·tro'pick, ·trop'ick) *adj.*

lyotropic series. An arrangement of the ions in the order of their behavior, such as their effect in salting-out of proteins or on the viscosity of colloids. Syn. *Hofmeister series.*

ly·pe·ma·nia (lye"pe·may'nee·uh, lip"e·) *n.* [Gk. *lypē*, grief, + *-mania*]. MELANCHOLIA. See also *involutional psychosis.*

ly·po·thy·mia (lye"po·thigh'mee·uh, lip"o·) *n.* [*lypē*, grief, + *-thymia*]. MELANCHOLIA. See also *involutional psychosis.*

ly·pres·sin (lye·pres'in) *n.* 8-Lysine vasopressin, $C_{46}H_{65}N_{13}O_{12}S_2$, the vasopressin obtained from the posterior pituitary of swine; an antidiuretic and vasopressor hormone.

ly·ra Da·vi·dis (lye'ruh day'vi·dis) [L., lyre of David]. COMMISSURE OF THE FORNIX.

lys-, lysi-, lyso-. A combining form meaning *lysis, dissolution, solution.*

ly·sate (lye'sate) *n.* The product of lysis.

lyse (lize) *v.* To cause or undergo lysis (1).

ly·ser·gic acid (lye·sur'jick) [*lys-* + *ergot* + *-ic*]. The tetracyclic moiety, $C_{16}H_{16}N_2O_2$, of many ergot alkaloids and obtained from these on hydrolysis.

lysergic acid di·eth·yl·am·ide (dye·eth"il·am'ide). *N,N*-Diethyl-D-lysergamide, $C_{20}H_{25}N_3O$, a synthetic compound structurally related to ergot alkaloids but differing from these in being a very potent psychotogen. Abbreviated, LSD.

Lys·holm grid (lues'hohlm) [E. *Lysholm*, Swedish radiologist, 1892–1947]. A stationary, thin grid of fine lead strips used to diminish scattered x-rays and improve the quality of roentgenograms.

Lysholm projection [E. *Lysholm*]. *In radiology,* 1. an oblique lateral projection of the vault and adjacent base of the skull; 2. an oblique view of the orbit; 3. an en face view of the posterior face of the petrous portion of the temporal bone.

Lysholm's line [E. *Lysholm*]. In neuroradiology, a line from the clivus through the cerebral aqueduct to the skull vault; the aqueduct normally lies below the junction of the first and middle thirds of this line.

lysi-. See *lys-.*

ly·sig·e·nous (lye·sij'e·nus) *adj.* [*lysi-* + *-genous*]. Formed by the breaking down of adjoining cells; used especially of some intercellular spaces. Contr. *schizogenous.*

ly·sim·eter (lye·sim'e·tur) *n.* [*lysi-* + *-meter*]. An apparatus for determining the solubility of a substance.

ly·sin (lye'sin) *n.* A substance, especially an antibody, capable of causing lysis.

ly·sine (lye'seen, ·sin) *n.* α, ε-Diaminocaproic acid, $NH_2(CH_2)_4CHNH_2COOH$, an amino acid present in many proteins. The hydrochloride salt is used to produce systemic acidosis and increase responsiveness to mercurial diuretics.

ly·sis (lye'sis) *n.*, pl. **ly·ses** (·seez) [Gk., loosing, release, from *lyein,* to unbind, loosen]. 1. Disintegration or dissolution, as of cells, bacteria, or tissue. See also *lysin.* 2. Gradual decline in the manifestations of a disease, especially an infectious disease, or of fever. 3. Loosening of or detachment from adhesions.

-lysis [Gk. *lysis*]. 1. A combining form signifying *dissolving, loosening, dissolution,* or *decomposition.* 2. In medicine, a combining form meaning *reduction or abatement; remission of fever.*

Lysivane. A trademark for ethopropazine, also known as profenamine, used for the treatment of parkinsonism as the hydrochloride salt.

lyso-. See *lys-.*

ly·so·ceph·a·lin (lye"so·sef'uh·lin) *n.* A substance derived from cephalin by the removal of one of the fatty acid components of the molecule, by the action of an enzyme contained in cobra venom. It possesses powerful hemolytic properties.

ly·so·chrome (lye'so·krome) *n.* [*lyso-* + *-chrome*]. An oil-soluble dye employed as a fat stain.

ly·so·gen·e·sis (lye"so·jen'e·sis) *n.* [*lyso-* + *-genesis*]. The production of lysins or lysis. —**lysogen·ic** (·jen'ick) *adj.*

ly·sog·eny (lye"soj'e·nee) *n.* [*lyso-* + *-geny*]. The phenomenon in which a viral genome is integrated into that of its host bacterium.

ly·so·ki·nase (lye"so·kigh'nace, ·naze) *n.* [*lyso-* + *kinase*]. Any substance of the fibrinolytic system which activates the plasma activators.

ly·so·lec·i·thin (lye"so·les'i·thin) *n.* [*lyso-* + *lecithin*]. LYSOPHOSPHATIDYLCHOLINE.

ly·so·phos·pha·ti·dyl·cho·line (lye"so·fos·fuh·tye"dil·ko'leen, ·fos·fat"i·dil·) *n.* A substance having strong hemolytic properties produced from phosphatidylcholine (lecithin) by the action of snake venom, which removes unsaturated fatty acids from the lecithin molecules. Syn. *lysolecithin.*

ly·so·some (lye'so·sohm) *n.* [*lyso-* + *-some*]. A cytoplasmic body bound by a single membrane, present in most types of cells but especially abundant in the liver and kidney, that contains various hydrolytic enzymes whose pH optima are acid. —**ly·so·so·mal** (lye"so·so'mul) *adj.*

ly·so·zyme (lye'so·zime) *n.* [*lyso-* + *-zyme*]. An enzyme present in the tears (as well as in other secretions) which has a hydrolytic action on certain bacterial cell walls (composed of specific polysaccharide units); can induce pinocytosis. It has been isolated in the granules of intestinal Paneth cells and may play a role in the regulation of intestinal flora. Syn. *muramidase.*

ly·so·zy·mu·ria (lye"so·zye·mew'ree·uh) *n.* [*lysozyme* + *-uria*]. The presence of lysozyme in the urine.

lys·sa (lis'uh) *n.* [Gk., rage, madness, rabies]. *Obsol.* RABIES.

lyssa bodies. Structures that appear similar to Negri bodies but lack the inner basophilic core of the latter; they are often found in large numbers in rabid brains and were originally though to be an intracellular phase of the parasite *Encephalitozoon lyssae.* They are now recognized to be nonspecific for rabies, having been found in normal animals of many species, in human senescence, and in some human degenerative diseases.

lys·sic (lis'ick) *adj.* [*lyssa* + *-ic*]. Pertaining to or caused by rabies.

lys·soid (lis'oid) *adj.* [*lyssa* + *-oid*]. Resembling rabies.

lys·so·pho·bia (lis"o·fo'bee·uh) *n.* [*lyssa* + *-phobia*]. 1. CYNOPHOBIA (2). 2. Morbid fear of becoming insane.

Lys·ter bag [W. J. L. *Lyster,* U. S. army surgeon, 1869–1947]. A heavy canvas or rubberized cloth bag used to prepare and dispense chemically disinfected water.

ly·syl (lye'sil) *n.* The univalent radical, $H_2NCH_2CH_2CH_2CH_2CH(NH_2)CO$—, of the amino acid lysine.

lysyl oxidase. An enzyme found in bone and connective tissue which oxidizes terminal amino groups of lysine residues in tropocollagen molecules to aldehyde residues. Such oxidation is necessary for normal cross-linking between tropocollagen molecules.

-lyte [Gk. *lytos,* soluble]. A combining form designating *a substance capable of undergoing lysis.*

ly·te·ri·an (lye·teer'ee·un) *adj.* [Gk. *lytērios,* loosing, healing, from *lyein,* to loosen]. Indicative of a lysis, or of abatement of an attack of disease.

lyt·ic (lit'ick) *adj.* [Gk. *lytikos,* loosening, laxative]. Pertaining to or causing lysis.

-lytic. A combining form meaning *pertaining to lysis or a lysin.*

Lyt·ta ves·i·ca·to·ria (lit'uh ves"i·kuh·to'ree·uh). SPANISH FLY; a species of Meloidae of the order Coleoptera. Characterized by the formation of cantharidin, a toxin which may produce blisters of the skin.

lyxo·fla·vin, lyxo·fla·vine (lick"so·flay'vin) *n.* $C_{17}H_{20}N_4O_6$. The L-lyxose analogue of riboflavin, first isolated from human cardiac muscle. It has no riboflavin activity but possesses growth-promoting activity in rats.

lyx·ose (lick'soze, ·soce) *n.* A synthetic pentose sugar that is isomeric with arabinose, ribose, and xylose.

lyze. LYSE.

L zone. PSEUDO H ZONE.

M

M Roman numeral for one thousand.
M Abbreviation for *mucoid* (colony); (b) *matt* (colony).
M. An abbreviation for (a) *mass*; (b) *molar*; (c) *misce*, mix.
m, m. Abbreviation for *meter*.
***m*-** In chemistry, symbol for *meta-*.
mμ Abbreviation for *millimicron* (= NANOMETER).
MA, M.A. Abbreviation for *mental age*.
M.A. Master of Arts.
ma, mA Abbreviation for *milliampere*.
ma·ba·ta (ma·bah'tuh) *n.* An African name for *Ornithodorus moubata*, a parasitic tick infesting birds, small mammals, domestic animals, and occasionally man; an important vector of relapsing fever. Syn. *tampan*.
Ma·ca·ca (muh·kah'kuh) *n.* [NL., from Pg. *macaco*, monkey]. A widespread, predominantly Asian genus of the Cercopithecidae. Among especially important species are *Macaca mulatta* (rhesus monkey), *M. fascicularis* (crab-eating macaque), *M. nemestrina* (pig-tailed macaque), *M. fuscata* (Japanese macaque), and *M. sylvanus* (Barbary ape).
ma·ca·cus ear (muh·kah'kus, muh·kay'kus). An ear with a prominent auricular (Darwin's) tubercle.
Mac·al·lis·ter's muscle. A medial variant of the fibulocalcaneus muscle.
ma·caque (muh·kack', ·kahk') *n.* [F., from Pg. *macaco*, monkey]. Any of various monkeys of the genus *Macaca*.
***McArdle-Schmid-Pearson disease.** MCARDLE'S SYNDROME.
Mc·Ar·dle's syndrome or **disease** [B. *McArdle*, English neurologist, 20th century]. Glycogenosis caused by a deficiency of the muscle phosphorylase, with abnormal accumulation of glycogen in skeletal muscle, manifested clinically by temporary weakness and cramping of muscles after exercise, and no rise in blood lactic acid during exercise. Muscle fibers are destroyed to a variable degree. Syn. *myophosphorylase deficiency glycogenesis, type V of Cori.*
Mc·Bur·ney's incision [C. *McBurney*, U.S. surgeon, 1845–1913]. A short diagonal incision in the lower right quadrant, used for appendectomy, in which the muscle fibers are separated rather than cut.
McBurney's operation. Appendectomy through a McBurney incision.
McBurney's point [C. *McBurney*]. A point halfway between the umbilicus and the anterior superior iliac spine. A point of extreme tenderness in appendicitis, and usually the approximate location of the base of the appendix.
McBurney's sign. A sign for acute appendicitis in which the area of maximum tenderness is over McBurney's point.

*Names beginning with Mc or M' are alphabetized as if spelled Mac. . . . .

Mc·Call's festoon. A thickening, rolled formation, or piling up of the gingiva along its margin.
Mac·Cal·lum's patch [W. G. *MacCallum*, U.S. pathologist, 1874–1944]. An irregular area of endocardial thickening on the posterior surface of the left atrium, usually representing the effects of rheumatic fever.
MacCallum's stain [W. G. *MacCallum*]. A method of staining for gram-positive and gram-negative bacteria in tissues.
Mc·Car·thy's electrotome. MCCARTHY'S RESECTOSCOPE.
McCarthy's reflex [D. J. *McCarthy*, U.S. neurologist, 1874–1958]. SUPRAORBITAL REFLEX.
McCarthy's resectoscope [J. F. *McCarthy*, U.S. urologist, 1874–1965]. A modification of the cystoscope for use in transurethral surgery. Syn. *McCarthy's electrotome.*
Mac·chia·vel·lo's stain (for Rickettsiae). BASIC FUCHSIN.
Mac·Cor·mac's reflex [W. *MacCormac*, Irish surgeon, 1836–1901]. PATELLOADDUCTOR REFLEX.
Mc·Cune-Al·bright syndrome [D. J. *McCune*, U.S. pediatrician, b.1902; and F. *Albright*]. ALBRIGHT'S SYNDROME.
mace, *n.* [F. *macis*]. A spice derived from the dried covering of the seed of the nutmeg.
Mace, *n.* A lacrimatory agent consisting of a *m*ethylchloroform solution of chloro*ace*tophenone, used in riot control.
Mc·Ell·roy test. FOLIN-MCELLROY TEST.
mac·er·ate (mas'ur·ate) *v.* [L. *macerare*]. To soften a solid or a tissue, or remove therefrom certain constituents, by steeping in a fluid. —**mac·er·a·tive** (mas'ur·ay''tiv) *adj.*
mac·er·a·tion (mas''ur·ay'shun) *n.* 1. The act or process of macerating. 2. *In obstetrics*, the changes undergone by a dead fetus as it is retained in utero, characterized by reddening, loss of skin, and distortion of features.
Mac·ew·en's osteotomes (muh·kew'un) [W. *Macewen*, Scottish surgeon, 1848–1924]. Specially designed bone-cutting instruments in three sizes.
Macewen's osteotomy [W. *Macewen*]. A supracondylar, wedge-shaped osteotomy for correction of genu valgum (knock-knee).
Macewen's sign [W. *Macewen*]. Tympany on percussion of the skull in hydrocephalus, large cystic lesions, and occasionally cerebral abscess. See also *cranial cracked-pot sound.*
Macewen's triangle [W. *Macewen*]. SUPRAMEATAL TRIANGLE.
Mc·Gill's operation [A. F. *McGill*, English surgeon, 1846–1890]. SUPRAPUBIC PROSTATECTOMY.
Mc·Gun·kin method. A histochemical method for catalase based on the oxidation of benzidine by the oxygen liberated from hydrogen peroxide, to give a blue color which changes to brown.
Ma·cha·do-Guer·rei·ro reaction (mah·shah'doo, ge·rrey'roo). An early complement fixation test for Chagas' disease and

visceral leishmaniasis, in which the antigens were prepared from organs of laboratory animals infected with *Trypanosoma cruzi.*

Mache unit (Ger. mah^kh'e^h) [H. *Mache,* Austrian physicist, b.1876]. A unit of radioactive emanation, equivalent to the quantity of radon, free from decay products, which gives rise to a saturation current of 1×10^{-3} electrostatic unit.

machinery murmur. A continuous murmur; usually used to describe the rumbling murmur of patent ductus arteriosus or other arteriovenous communication.

Mach number (mah^k; Ger. mah^kh) [E. *Mach,* Austrian scientist, 1838-1916]. The ratio of the speed of an object to the speed of sound in the same medium.

Machover test [Karen *Machover,* U.S., b.1902]. DRAW-A-MAN TEST.

Mc·In·tosh test. UREA CLEARANCE TEST.

Mac·Kee-Herr·mann-Ba·ker-Sulz·berg·er method. A histochemical method for sulfonamides based on the formation of a yellow to orange precipitate of *p*-dimethylaminobenzylidene derivative when sulfonamides react with *p*-dimethylaminobenzaldehyde.

Mack·en·rodt's ligament (mah^hk'^en·rote) [A. K. *Mackenrodt,* German gynecologist, 1859-1925]. CARDINAL LIGAMENT.

Mac·ken·zie's amputation [Richard James *Mackenzie,* Scottish surgeon, 1821-1854]. A method of amputation at the ankle joint, a modification of Syme's amputation.

Mackenzie's disease [James *Mackenzie,* Scottish physician, 1853-1925]. X-DISEASE (1).

Mackenzie's syndrome [Stephen *Mackenzie,* British physician, 1844-1909]. Associated paralysis of the tongue, soft palate, vocal cord, trapezius and sternocleidomastoid on the same side, due to lesion of the tenth, eleventh, and twelfth cranial nerves, or their nuclei of origin.

Mc·Lean's formula or **index** [F. C. *McLean,* U.S. physiologist, b.1888]. An index of urea secretion, computed by the formula $(D\sqrt{C} \times 8.96)/(Wt. \times Ur^2)$, in which D is the grams of urea excreted in 24 hours, C is the grams of urea per liter of urine, Wt. is the weight of the individual in kilograms, and Ur is the grams of urea per liter of blood.

Mac·Lean's test. A test for lactic acid in which a reagent containing ferric chloride, mercuric chloride, and hydrochloric acid is added to gastric juice. A yellow color indicates lactic acid.

Mac·leod's syndrome (muh·klaowd') [W. M. *Macleod,* British physician, 20th century]. Unilateral translucency of the lung.

Mc·Mee·kin's method [T. L. *McMeekin,* U.S. biochemist, b.1900]. KOCH-MCMEEKIN'S METHOD.

Mc·Mur·ray's sign [T. P. *McMurray,* British surgeon, b.1887]. A sign for posterior tears of the lateral and medial menisci of the knee.

Mc·Naghten (muck·naw'tun). See *M'Naghten.*

M'Naghten rule [Daniel *M'Naghten,* accused English murderer, 1843]. The formula for criminal responsibility still widely in use in the United States that holds a person not responsible for a crime if the accused "was laboring under such a defect of reason from the mind as not to know the nature and quality of the act; or, if he did know it, that he did not know that he was doing what was wrong." See also *Currens formula, Durham decision, irresistible impulse test.*

McNaughten or **McNaughton.** See *M'Naghten.*

Mac·Neal's tetrachrome stain [W. J. *MacNeal,* U.S. pathologist and hematologist, 1881-1946]. A blood stain containing eosin, methylene azure A, methylene blue, and methylene violet in methyl alcohol; it is used like Wright's stain.

M.A.C.P. Master of the American College of Physicians.

macr-, macro- [Gk. *makros*]. A combining form meaning (a) *large, great;* (b) *long, length.*

Mac·ra·can·tho·rhyn·chus (mack"ruh·kan"tho·ring'kus) *n.* [*macr-,* long, + *acantho-,* thorn, + Gk. *rhynchos,* snout]. A genus of acanthocephalan worms.

Macracanthorhynchus hi·ru·di·na·ce·us (hi·roo"di·nay'see·us, hir"yoo·). A species of acanthocephalan worm infecting swine, and formerly man in the Volga valley in Russia.

mac·ren·ceph·a·ly (mack"ren·sef'uh·lee) *n.* [*macr-* + *en-cephal-* + *-y*]. MEGALENCEPHALY. —**macrencepha·lous** (·lus), **macren·ce·phal·ic** (·se·fal'ick) *adj.*

macro-. See *macr-.*

mac·ro·am·y·lase (mack"ro·am'i·lace, ·laze) *n.* An amylase of abnormally large size occurring in the blood serum of patients with macroamylasemia.

mac·ro·am·y·la·se·mia (mack"ro·am"i·lay·see'mee·uh) *n.* [*macroamylase* + *-emia*]. The presence of high-molecular-weight amylase molecules in the serum.

mac·ro·an·gi·op·a·thy (mack"ro·an"jee·op'uth·ee) *n.* [*macro-* + *angiopathy*]. Any disease of the larger blood vessels. Contr. *microangiopathy.*

mac·ro·bac·te·ri·um (mack"ro·back·teer'ee·um) *n.* A large bacterium.

mac·ro·blast (mack'ro·blast) *n.* [*macro-* + *-blast*]. PRONORMOBLAST.

mac·ro·ble·phar·ia (mack"ro·ble·făr'ee·uh) *n.* [*macro-* + *blephar-* + *-ia*]. Abnormal largeness of the eyelid.

mac·ro·bra·chia (mack"ro·bray'kee·uh) *n.* [*macro-* + *brachi-* + *-ia*]. Excessive development of the arms.

mac·ro·car·di·us (mack"ro·kahr'dee·us) *n.* [*macro-* + *cardi-* + *-us*]. A fetus with a greatly enlarged heart.

mac·ro·ce·pha·lia (mack"ro·se·fay'lee·uh) *n.* MACROCEPHALY.

mac·ro·ce·phal·ic (mack"ro·se·fal'ick) *adj.* [*macro-* + *cephalic*]. Having an abnormally large head.

mac·ro·ceph·a·lous (mack"ro·sef'uh·lus) *adj.* MACROCEPHALIC.

mac·ro·ceph·a·lus (mack"ro·sef'uh·lus) *n.* [*macro-* + *cephal-* + *-us*]. An individual with excessive development of the head.

mac·ro·ceph·a·ly (mack"ro·sef'uh·lee) *n.* [*macro-* + *cephal-* + *-y*]. Abnormal largeness of the head; megalocephaly.

mac·ro·chei·lia (mack"ro·kigh'lee·uh) *n.* [*macro-* + *cheil-* + *-ia*]. 1. Relatively large size of the lips as a normal human variation. 2. Enlargement of the lips resulting from disease.

mac·ro·chei·ria (mack"ro·kigh'ree·uh) *n.* [*macro-* + *cheir-* + *-ia*]. Abnormal enlargement of the hands.

mac·ro·co·nid·i·um (mack"ro·ko·nid'ee·um) *n.,* pl. **macroco·nid·ia** (·ee·uh). *In botany,* a large and usually multicelled conidium.

mac·ro·cra·nia (mack"ro·kray'nee·uh) *n.* [*macro-* + *-crania*]. Disproportionately large head size compared with face size.

mac·ro·cyst (mack'ro·sist) *n.* 1. A cyst visible to the naked eye. 2. A very large cyst.

mac·ro·cyte (mack'ro·site) *n.* [*macro-* + *-cyte*]. An erythrocyte having either a diameter or a mean corpuscular volume (MCV), or both, exceeding by more than two standard deviations that of the mean normal, as determined by the same method on the blood of healthy persons of the patient's age and sex group. Syn. *macronormocyte.* See also *macrocytic anemia.* —**mac·ro·cyt·ic** (mack"ro·sit'ick) *adj.*

macrocytic anemia. Any anemia characterized by the presence in the blood of abnormally large erythrocytes (MCV greater than 100 $\mu\mu^3$), with or without megaloblastic bone marrow changes. See also *hyperchromic anemia* (1), *megaloblastic anemia.*

macrocytic anemia of pregnancy. A megaloblastic anemia of pregnancy due to folic acid deficiency.

mac·ro·cy·to·sis (mack"ro·sigh·to'sis) *n.* The presence of macrocytes, or abnormally large erythrocytes, in the blood as determined microscopically or by measurement of cell volume.

mac·ro·dac·tyl·ia (mack"ro·dack·til'ee·uh) *n.* MACRODACTYLY.

mac·ro·dac·ty·lism (mack″ro·dack′til·iz·um) *n.* MACRODACTYLY.

mac·ro·dac·ty·ly (mack″ro·dack′til·ee) *n.* [*macro-* + *dactyl-* + *-y*]. Abnormally large size of the fingers or toes; DACTYLOMEGALY.

Macrodantin. A trademark for nitrofurantoin, a urinary antibacterial.

mac·ro·don·tia (mack″ro·don′chee·uh) *n.* [*macr-* + *-odontia*]. The condition of having abnormally large teeth. Syn. *megalodontia.* —**mac·ro·dont** (mack′ro·dont) *adj.*

mac·ro·en·ceph·a·ly (mack″ro·en·sef′uh·lee) *n.* [*macro-* + *-encephal-* + *-y*]. MEGALENCEPHALY.

mac·ro·fol·lic·u·lar (mack″ro·fol·ick′yoo·lur) *adj.* [*macro-* + *follicular*]. Having large follicles.

macrofollicular adenoma. 1. A thyroid adenoma with large follicles. 2. A variety of malignant lymphoma.

mac·ro·gam·ete (mack″ro·gam′eet) *n.* [*macro-* + *gamete*]. A relatively large, nonmotile reproductive cell of certain protozoans and thallophytes, comparable to an ovum of the metazoans.

mac·ro·ga·me·to·cyte (mack″ro·ga·mee′to·site, ·gam′e·to·) *n.* [*macro-* + *gametocyte*]. The enlarged merozoite before maturation into the female cell, in propagative reproduction in sporozoa.

ma·crog·a·my (ma·krog′uh·mee) *n.* [*macro-* + *-gamy*]. Conjugation of two adult protozoan cells.

mac·ro·gen·i·to·so·mia (mack″ro·jen″i·to·so′mee·uh) *n.* [*macro-* + *genito-* + *-somia*]. Excessive bodily development, especially of the external genitalia.

macrogenitosomia precox. The occurrence, in childhood, of the somatic and genital changes associated with puberty. May be due to a functioning testicular tumor or to altered hypothalamic-pituitary function, due to a tumor in the region of the third ventricle.

mac·rog·lia (ma·krog′lee·uh) *n.* [*macro-* + *glia*]. *Obsol.* ASTROCYTES. Contr. *microglia.*

mac·ro·glob·u·lin (mack″ro·glob′yoo·lin) *n.* GAMMA-M GLOBULIN.

mac·ro·glob·u·li·ne·mia, mac·ro·glob·u·li·nae·mia (mack″ro·glob″yoo·lin·ee′mee·uh) *n.* 1. A disorder of the hemolytopoietic system characterized by proliferation of cells of the lymphocytic and plasmacytic series and the presence of abnormally large amounts of macroglobulin in the blood. 2. A marked increase in blood macroglobulins.

mac·ro·glos·sia (mack″ro·glos′ee·uh) *n.* [*macro-* + *-glossia*]. Enlargement of the tongue.

mac·ro·gnath·ic (mack″ro·nath′ick, ·nay′thick, mack″rog·) *adj.* [*macro-* + *gnathic*]. Having long jaws; prognathous. —**mac·rog·na·thism** (ma·krog′nuh·thiz·um) *n.*

mac·ro·gy·ria (mack″ro·jye′ree·uh) *n.* [*macro-* + Gk. *gyros*, circle, + *-ia*]. A congenital condition of excessively large convolutions of the brain, often associated with retardation.

mac·ro·lym·pho·cyte (mack″ro·lim′fo·site) *n.* A large lymphocyte.

mac·ro·mas·tia (mack″ro·mas′tee·uh) *n.* [*macro-* + *mast-* + *-ia*]. Abnormal enlargement of the breast.

mac·ro·ma·zia (mack″ro·may′zee·uh) *n.* [*macro-* + Gk. *mazos*, breast, + *-ia*]. MACROMASTIA.

mac·ro·me·lia (mack″ro·mee′lee·uh) *n.* [*macro-* + *mel-* + *-ia*]. Abnormally large size of arms or legs.

ma·crom·e·lus (ma·krom′e·lus) *n.* [*macro-* + *mel-* + *-us*]. An individual having excessively large limbs.

ma·crom·e·ly (ma·krom′e·lee) *n.* MACROMELIA.

mac·ro·mero·zo·ite (mack″ro·merr″o·zo′ite) *n.* A large merozoite.

mac·ro·mo·lec·u·lar (mack″ro·mo·leck′yoo·lur) *adj.* Having large molecules.

mac·ro·mol·e·cule (mack″ro·mol′e·kyool) *n.* A very large molecule, as of a protein, polysaccharide, rubber, or synthetic polymer.

mac·ro·mono·cyte (mack″ro·mon′o·site) *n.* An abnormally large monocyte.

mac·ro·my·e·lo·blast (mack″ro·mye′e·lo·blast) *n.* An excessively large myeloblast.

mac·ro·nor·mo·blast (mack″ro·nor′mo·blast) *n.* PRONORMOBLAST.

mac·ro·nor·mo·cyte (mack″ro·nor′mo·site) *n.* MACROCYTE.

mac·ro·nu·cle·us (mack″ro·new′klee·us) *n.* The vegetative or trophic nucleus of protozoa as contrasted with the micronucleus which is reproductive in function.

mac·ro·nych·ia (mack″ro·nick′ee·uh) *n.* [*macr-* + *onych-* + *-ia*]. Excessive size of the nails.

mac·ro·pe·nis (mack′ro·pe″nis) *n.* MACROPHALLUS.

mac·ro·phage (mack′ro·faij) *n.* [*macro-* + *-phage*]. A phagocytic cell belonging to the reticuloendothelial system; important in resistance to infection and in immunological responses. It has the capacity for accumulating certain aniline dyes, as trypan blue or lithium carmine, in its cytoplasm in the form of granules.

ma·croph·a·gy (ma·krof′uh·jee) *n.* The activity of macrophages.

mac·ro·phal·lus (mack′ro·phal″lus) *n.* Large penis or phallus.

mac·ro·po·dia (mack″ro·po′dee·uh) *n.* [*macro-* + *pod-* + *-ia*]. Abnormally large size of the foot or feet. Syn. *pes gigas, sciapody.*

ma·crop·o·dy (ma·krop′uh·dee) *n.* MACROPODIA.

mac·ro·poly·cyte (mack″ro·pol′ee·site) *n.* [*macro-* + *poly-* + *-cyte*]. An unusually large, neutrophilic leukocyte with six or more lobes in the nucleus.

mac·ro·pro·so·pia (mack″ro·pruh·so′pee·uh) *n.* [*macro-* + *prosop-* + *-ia*]. Abnormal enlargement of the face.

mac·ro·pro·so·pus (mack″ro·pro′suh·pus, ·pruh·so′pus) *n.* [Gk. *makroprosōpos*, long-faced, from *prosōpon*, face]. An individual with an abnormally large face.

mac·ro·pro·so·py (mack″ro·pro′suh·pee) *n.* MACROPROSOPIA.

ma·crop·sia (ma·krop′see·uh) *n.* [*macr-* + *-opsia*]. A disturbance of vision in which objects seem larger than they are. Syn. *megalopia.*

mac·rop·sy (mack′rop·see) *n.* MACROPSIA.

mac·ro·scop·ic (mack″ro·skop′ick) *adj.* [*macro-* + Gk. *skopein*, to examine, + *-ic*]. Large enough to be seen by the naked eye; gross; not microscopic.

mac·ros·mat·ic (mack″roz·mat′ick) *adj.* [*macr-* + *osmatic*]. Possessing a highly developed sense of smell.

mac·ro·so·mia (mack″ro·so′mee·uh) *n.* [*macro-* + *-somia*]. GIGANTISM.

mac·ro·spore (mack′ro·spore) *n.* 1. A spore of relatively large size. 2. One of the larger spores arising in the reproduction of certain protozoans. —**mac·ro·spor·ic** (mack″ro·spor′ick) *adj.*

mac·ro·sto·mia (mack″ro·sto′mee·uh) *n.* [*macro-* + Gk. *stoma*, mouth, + *-ia*]. Abnormally large mouth; a mild form of transverse facial cleft.

mac·ro·throm·bo·cy·to·path·ia (mack″ro·throm″bo·sigh″to·path′ee·uh) *n.* [*macro-* + *thrombocyte* + *-pathia*]. A platelet disorder characterized by thrombocytopenia, giant platelets with abnormal structure, prolonged bleeding time, and defective adherence of platelets to glass.

mac·ro·tia (mack·ro′shee·uh, ·shuh) *n.* [*macr-* + *ot-* + *-ia*]. Abnormal largeness of the external ear.

Ma·cruz index [R. *Macruz*, U.S., contemporary]. The ratio of P wave duration to P-R segment duration in the electrocardiogram, used as a criterion of atrial enlargement.

mac·u·la (mack′yoo·luh) *n.*, pl. **macu·lae** (·lee) [L.]. 1. In general, a spot. 2. [NA] MACULA LUTEA. 3. A circumscribed corneal scar or opacity. 4. MACULE.

macula acu·sti·ca sac·cu·li (a·koos′ti·kuh sack′yoo·lye). MACULA SACCULI.

macula acustica utriculi. MACULA UTRICULI.

macula ad·hae·rens or **ad·he·rens** (ad·heer′enz), pl. **maculae ad·hae·ren·tes** (ad·heer·en′teez). *In electron microscopy,* DESMOSOME.

macula ce·ru·lea (se·roo'lee·uh). BLUE SPOT.
macula com·mu·nis (kom·yoo'nis). The thickening in the medial wall of the auditory vesicle, which divides to form the maculae, cristae, and spiral organ (of Corti) of the internal ear.
macula cor·ne·ae (kor'nee·ee). A permanent corneal opacity from an ulcer or keratitis.
macula cri·bro·sa inferior (kri·bro'suh) [NA]. A small area in the wall of the vestibule perforated by nerve filaments to ampulla of the posterior membranous semicircular canal.
macula cribrosa me·dia (mee'dee·uh) [NA]. A small circular depression in the spherical recess of the vestibule of the internal ear, perforated by filaments of the vestibular nerve to the saccule.
macula cribrosa superior [NA]. A small oval depression in the elliptical recess of the vestibule of the inner ear, perforated by filaments of the vestibular nerve to the utricle and the anterior and lateral semicircular canals.
macula den·sa (den'suh). A thickening of the epithelium of the ascending limb of the loop of Henle, at the level of attachment to the vascular pole of the renal corpuscle.
maculae. Plural of *macula.*
maculae acu·sti·cae (a·koos'ti·see) [BNA]. The macula sacculi and macula utriculi.
maculae cri·bro·sae (kri·bro'see) [NA]. Three areas of perforations in the wall of the vestibule for the passage of filaments of the vestibular nerve; the macula cribrosa inferior, macula cribrosa media, and macula cribrosa superior.
macula fla·va (flay'vuh) [BNA]. A yellow spot or nodule.
macula ger·mi·na·ti·va (jur''mi·nuh·tye'vuh). The nucleolus of the ovum.
macula lu·tea (lew'tee·uh) [BNA]. The yellow spot of the retina; the point of clearest vision. See also Plate 19.
mac·u·lar (mack'yoo·lur) *adj.* 1. Of or pertaining to the macula of the retina. 2. Characterized by corneal maculae. 3. Characterized by macules.
macular corneal dystrophy. A heredodegenerative disease of the eye, characterized by irregular gray opacities with a diffuse cloudiness of the corneal stroma between the opacities, as well as involvement of the periphery, resulting usually in severe early impairment of vision; transmitted as a recessive trait.
macular degeneration or **dystrophy.** Pathologic changes of the macula lutea, occurring bilaterally at any age, characterized by spots of pigmentation, a moth-eaten appearance or other alterations, and producing a reduction or loss of central vision; may be hereditary, traumatic, senile, or atherosclerotic. Compare *cerebroretinal degeneration.*
macular dysplasia. A congenital macular defect which may show pigmentation or abnormality of the retinal vessels; rarely, the macula is absent; usually due to intrauterine choroiditis. See also *coloboma.*
macular sparing. Preservation of central vision in homonymous hemianopsia, most commonly seen with lesions near the tip of the occipital lobe; the exact mechanism is still uncertain.
macular vision. CENTRAL VISION.
macula sac·cu·li (sack'yoo·lye) [NA]. An oval thickened area in the anterior portion of the saccule where the saccular nerve filaments attach. Syn. *macula acustica sacculi.*
macula utri·cu·li (yoo·trick'yoo·lye) [NA]. An oval thickened area in the floor and anterior portion of the utricle where the utricular nerve filaments attach. Syn. *macula acustica utriculi.*
mac·ule (mack'yool) *n.* [L. *macula,* spot, blemish]. A small, circumscribed, discolored spot on the skin; especially, one not perceptibly raised above the surrounding level. Compare *papule.*
mac·u·lo·an·es·thet·ic (mack''yoo·lo·an''is·thet'ick) *adj.* Having the appearance of a macule and being insensitive to pain in the affected area; said of certain leprous lesions.
maculoanesthetic leprosy. TUBERCULOID LEPROSY.
mac·u·lo·pap·ule (mack''yoo·lo·pap'yool) *n.* A small, circumscribed, discolored elevation of the skin; a macule and papule combined. —**maculopap·u·lar** (·yoo·lur) *adj.*
mac·u·lop·a·thy (mack''yoo·lop'uth·ee) *n.* Any disease of the macula lutea of the retina.
mad, *adj.* 1. Insane. 2. Affected with rabies; rabid.
mad·a·ro·sis (mad''uh·ro'sis) *n.* [Gk. *madarōsis,* falling hair, eyelashes]. Loss of the eyelashes or eyebrows. —**mada·rot·ic** (·rot'ick), **mad·a·rous** (mad'uh·rus) *adj.*
mad·der, *n.* 1. The Eurasian herb *Rubia tinctorum* and other species. 2. The root of *Rubia tinctorum* and other species, used for dyeing and from which alizarin and purpurin may be obtained; formerly used medicinally.
Mad·dox rod [E. E. *Maddox,* English ophthalmologist, 1860–1933]. An instrument used to demonstrate latent or manifest strabismus, composed of one or several red or green glass rods in the form of a lens. When placed in front of an eye, it changes a spot of light into a colored line, thus breaking up binocular vision by interfering with fusion.
Ma·de·lung's deformity (mah'd^e·lŏŏng) [O. W. *Madelung,* German surgeon, 1846-1926]. A congenital or developmental deformity of the wrist characterized by palmar angulation of the distal end of the radius and dorsal dislocation of the head of the ulna.
mad·i·dans (mad'i·danz, ·dance) *adj.* [L., from *madidus,* wet, moist]. Weeping, oozing.
mad itch. PSEUDORABIES.
mad·ness *n.* Mental disorder.
Madribon. Trademark for sulfadimethoxine, a sulfonamide for general use.
ma·du·ra foot (ma·dew'ruh, mad'yoo·ruh) [after *Madura,* in India]. MYCETOMA.
Mad·u·rel·la (mad''yoo·rel'uh) *n.* [*Madura* + L. *-ella,* diminutive suffix]. A genus of fungi of the Fungi Imperfecti; species of this genus are often isolated in cases of mycetoma.
mad·u·ro·my·co·sis (mad''yoo·ro·migh·ko'sis) *n.* [*Madura* + *mycosis*]. MYCETOMA.
mae·di (mye'dee) *n.* A slow viral infection of sheep causing a chronic interstitial pneumonitis; observed primarily in Iceland.
maelenic. MELENIC.
ma·fe·nide (may'fe·nide) *n.* α-Amino-*p*-toluenesulfonamide, $C_7H_{10}N_2O_2S$, an antibacterial drug. Syn. *sulfbenzamine.*
Maf·fuc·ci's syndrome (maf·fooch'ee) [A. *Maffucci,* Italian physician, 1845-1903]. Cutaneous hemangiomas associated with enchondromatosis. See also *Kast's syndrome.*
mag·al·drate (mag'al·drate) *n.* Tetrakis-(hydroxymagnesium)decahydroxydialuminate dihydrate, $Al_2H_{14}Mg_4O_{14}.2H_2O$, a chemical combination of aluminum hydroxide and magnesium hydroxide; employed as a gastric antacid.
Magcyl. A trademark for poloxalkol, a surface-active compound used in the treatment of chronic constipation.
ma·gen·bla·se (mah'gun·blah''zeh) *n.* [Ger., stomach bubble]. *In radiology,* the bubble of gas in the fundus of the stomach, usually seen in erect films of the chest or abdomen beneath the left hemidiaphragm.
Ma·gen·die's foramen (mah·zhahn·dee') [F. *Magendie,* French physiologist, 1783–1855]. MEDIAN APERTURE OF THE FOURTH VENTRICLE.
Magendie's law [F. *Magendie*]. Anterior spinal roots are motor; posterior roots are sensory. Syn. *Bell's law.*
ma·gen·stras·se (mah'gun·shtrah''seh) *n.* [Ger., from *Magen,* stomach, + *Strasse,* street, way]. GASTRIC CANAL.
ma·gen·ta (muh·jen'tuh) *n.* [after *Magenta,* Italy]. BASIC FUCHSIN.
mag·got, *n.* A fly larva, especially one of the kinds that live on decaying animal matter.
maggot therapy. Implantation of sterile cultivated maggots

of the bluebottle fly into wounds in the treatment of chronic soft tissue infections and chronic osteomyelitis.

magical thinking. *In psychiatry,* a person's confusion of imagining with doing, wish with fulfilment, cause with effect, or symbol with event. So called by analogy to certain magical beliefs and practices, it is commonly observed in dreams and in children's thinking as well as in a variety of mental disorders.

mag·is·tery (maj'i·sterr"ee) *n.* [ML. *magisterium,* philosopher's stone]. Formerly, a preparation considered to have especial virtue as a remedy.

mag·is·tral (maj'i·strul) *adj.* [L. *magistralis,* of the master]. Pertaining to medicines prepared on prescription.

mag·ma (mag'muh) *n.* [Gk., thick unguent]. 1. Any pulpy mass; a paste. 2. *In pharmacy,* a more or less permanent suspension of a precipitate in water.

magma cavity. A cavity in the extraembryonic mesoderm of the blastocyst.

magma re·tic·u·la·re (re·tick"yoo·lair'ee). The jellylike strands of extraembryonic mesoderm bridging the extraembryonic coelom of the young human embryo.

Magnamycin. Trademark for the antibiotic substance carbomycin.

Ma·gnan's sign (mah·nyahn') [V. J. J. *Magnan,* French psychiatrist, 1835–1916]. An illusory sensation of a small foreign body under the skin, as in cocaine addiction.

mag·ne·sia (mag·nee'zhuh, ·shuh, ·zee·uh) *n.* [Gk. *magnēsia,* a name given to several ores and amalgams]. Magnesium oxide, MgO.

magnesia magma. MILK OF MAGNESIA.

mag·ne·site (mag'ne·site) *n.* Native magnesium carbonate; sometimes used as a substitute for plaster of Paris.

mag·ne·sium (mag·nee'zhum, ·zee·um, ·shum) *n.* [NL., from *magnesia*]. Mg = 24.305. A bluish white metal of the group of elements to which calcium and barium belong. Abundantly distributed throughout inorganic and organic nature and essential to life; certain of its salts are used in medicine. See also Table of Chemical Constituents of Blood in the Appendix. —**magne·sic** (·zick, ·sick) *adj.*

magnesium carbonate. Basic or normal hydrated magnesium carbonate, $(MgCO_3)_4.Mg(OH)_2.5H_2O$ or $MgCO_3.H_2O$. Exists in two densities: light and heavy magnesium carbonate. Used as an antacid and laxative.

magnesium hydrate. MAGNESIUM HYDROXIDE.

magnesium hydroxide. $Mg(OH)_2$. A white powder, used as an antacid and cathartic. Syn. *magnesium hydrate.*

magnesium oxide. MgO. Obtained by calcining magnesium carbonate. Exists in two densities: light and heavy. Used as an antacid and laxative and as a dusting powder. See also *light magnesia, heavy magnesia.*

magnesium sulfate. $MgSO_4.7H_2O$. Epsom salt, an active cathartic, especially useful in inflammatory affections; has central depressant action when administered intravenously.

magnesium trisilicate. Approximately $2MgO.3SiO_2$ with varying amounts of water. Almost insoluble in water; reacts slowly with acid. Used as an antacid and absorbent.

mag·net, *n.* [Gk. *Magnētis lithos*]. 1. A variety of iron ore or mineral, as lodestone, that attracts iron. 2. Any body having the power to attract iron. See also *electromagnet.* —**mag·net·ic,** *adj.*

magnetic field. The portion of space around a magnet in which its action can be felt.

mag·ne·tism, *n.* 1. The power possessed by a magnet to attract or repel other masses. 2. ANIMAL MAGNETISM.

mag·ne·tize, *v.* To render magnetic. —**mag·ne·ti·za·tion,** *n.*

mag·ne·to·car·di·og·ra·phy (mag"ne·to·kahr"dee·og'ruh·fee) *n.* [*magneto-* + *cardiography*]. Measurement of the magnetic field of the heart.

mag·ne·to·elec·tric·i·ty (mag·nee"to·e·leck·tris'i·tee, mag"ne·to·, mag·net"o·) *n.* Electricity produced by moving a conductor through a magnetic field.

mag·ne·to·graph (mag·nee"to·graf, mag·net'o·, mag'ne·to·) *n.* An instrument for determining and recording the strength of a magnetic field.

mag·ne·to·in·duc·tion (mag·nee"to·in·duck'shun, mag"ne·to·) *n.* The induction of an electric current by placing a permanent or temporary magnet within a coil of wire.

mag·ne·tom·e·ter (mag"ne·tom'e·tur) *n.* An instrument with a series of magnets suspended to record graphically variations in direction and intensity of magnetic force.

mag·ne·to·op·tic (mag"ne·to·op'tick, mag·nee"to·, mag·net"o·) *adj.* Pertaining to optic phenomena influenced by magnetic fields.

mag·ne·to·stric·tion (mag"ne·to·strick'shun, mag·nee"to·) *n.* [*magnetic* + *-striction* (as in *constriction*)]. A magnetic phenomenon involving the change in length of a rod or tube of ferromagnetic material when it is exposed to a magnetic field parallel to its length.

mag·ne·to·ther·a·py (mag·nee"to·therr'uh·pee, mag"ne·to·) *n.* The treatment of diseases by magnets or magnetism.

magnet reaction or **reflex.** Reflex extension of the leg initiated by pressure of the foot against a surface, seen in the newborn and in early infancy.

mag·ne·tron (mag'ne·tron) *n.* [*magnet* + *-tron*]. A thermionic tube used to generate microwaves using a magnetic field acting transversely to the cathode-anode path.

mag·ni·fi·ca·tion, *n.* [L. *magnificatio,* extolling, glorification, from *magnus,* large]. 1. Apparent enlargement; the production of an image larger than that produced by the naked eye. 2. A ratio, usually expressed in diameters or in degrees of arc subtended, between the dimensions of an image produced by an optical instrument and the dimensions of the object. 3. Exaggeration.

mag·no·cel·lu·lar (mag"no·sel'yoo·lur) *adj.* [L. *magnus,* large, + *cellular*]. Having large cell bodies; said of various nuclei of the central nervous system.

magnocellular glioblastoma. A well-circumscribed tumor, found in all parts of the central nervous system but particularly the temporal lobe and brainstem, composed of very large plump cells usually with one eccentric giant nucleus and a dense network of reticulin fibers; its relationship to glioblastoma or sarcoma remains unclear. Syn. *monstrocellular sarcoma.*

magnocellular nucleus of the dorsal column. ACCESSORY CUNEATE NUCLEUS.

magnocellular nucleus of the hypothalamus. PARAVENTRICULAR NUCLEUS OF THE HYPOTHALAMUS.

magnocellular nucleus of the thalamus. A part of the ventral thalamic nuclei.

magnocellular nucleus of the vestibular nerve. LATERAL VESTIBULAR NUCLEUS.

mag·num (mag'num) *adj.* [L., neuter of *magnus*]. Large, as in foramen magnum.

magnum, *n.* CAPITATE.

Mag·nus-de Kleijn reflexes (mag'noos, duh·klæyn') [R. *Magnus,* German physiologist, 1873–1927]. The postural, especially the tonic neck and tonic labyrinthine, reflexes.

Mag·nu·son splint [U.S. surgeon, 20th century]. An abduction splint used in the treatment of fractures of the humerus.

Ma·haim fibers [I. *Mahaim,* French physician, 20th century]. Connections between the atrioventricular node of the heart and the ventricular septal myocardium; probably constitute an accessory conduction bundle and may be associated with pre-excitation syndromes.

MAHC. Microangiopathic hemolytic aneurysm.

ma-huang (mah hwahng) *n.* [Chinese]. EPHEDRA.

maid·en·head, *n.* HYMEN; the intact hymen of a virgin.

ma·ieu·sio·ma·nia (migh·yoo"see·o·may'nee·uh, may·) *n.* [Gk. *maieusis,* delivery of a woman in childbirth, + *-mania*]. PUERPERAL PSYCHOSIS.

ma·ieu·sio·pho·bia (migh·yoo"see·o·fo'bee·uh, may·) *n.* [Gk.

maieusis, delivery of a woman in childbirth, + *-phobia*]. Morbid fear of childbirth.

ma·ieu·tic (migh·yoo'tick, may·) *adj. & n.* [Gk. *maieutikos*, skilled in or pertaining to midwifery]. 1. Obstetrical. 2. A rubber bag used for dilating the cervix uteri.

ma·ieu·tics (migh·yoo'ticks) *n.* [*maieutic* + *-s*]. OBSTETRICS.

ma·ieu·tol·o·gist (migh"yoo·tol'uh·jist) *n.* A practitioner of maieutics; an obstetrician.

maim, *v.* [OF. *mayner*]. To mutilate or disable; to commit mayhem, especially by destroying or crippling a limb.

main en griffe (man ahn greef; F. mæⁿ ahⁿ) [F.]. CLAW HAND.

main en lor·gnette (man ahn lor·nyet'; F. mæⁿ ahⁿ) [F.]. OPERA-GLASS HAND.

main sensory nucleus of the trigeminal nerve. A large group of nerve cells in the tegmentum of the pons dorsolateral to the entering fibers of the fifth nerve in which most of the afferent fibers terminate. Probably concerned with touch and pressure. NA *nucleus sensorius principalis nervi trigemini.*

Main syndrome [T. F. *Main*, U.S. psychiatrist, 20th century]. *In psychiatry*, a personality disorder in which the patient gains satisfaction from manipulating persons in the environment so that they argue with each other over his management. The patient assumes the role of a helpless, misunderstood, but deserving individual mistreated by his family or the hospital staff, and thus is frequently responsible for causing much turmoil.

Mai·son·neuve's urethrotome (meʰ·zohⁿ·nœv') [J. G. T. *Maisonneuve*, French surgeon, 1809–1897]. A urethrotome with a concealed knife which is retracted until the instrument reaches the stricture.

Mais·sat's band (meʰ·saʰ') [J. H. *Maissat*, French anatomist, 1805–1878]. ILIOTIBIAL TRACT.

maize, *n.* [Sp. *maíz*, from Taino *mahiz*]. The cereal grain *Zea mays*; corn, Indian corn. One of the principal foodstuffs, but deficient in niacin (nicotinic acid) and other vitamins.

maize oil. CORN OIL.

Ma·joc·chi's disease or **purpura** (maʰ·yoʰk'kee) [D. *Majocchi*, Italian physician, 1849–1929]. PURPURA ANNULARIS TELANGIECTODES.

ma·jor (may'jur) *adj.* [L.]. Larger, greater.

major agglutinin. CHIEF AGGLUTININ.

major alar cartilage. NA *cartilago alaris major.* See *alar cartilages.*

major amputation. Any amputation through the long bones of the upper or lower extremities; disarticulation at the hip joint or shoulder girdle.

major calices. The primary divisions of the renal pelvis; derived from the embryonic pole tubules, usually two or three in number. NA *calices renales majores.*

major cross match. See *cross matching.*

major duodenal papilla. A small elevation of the mucosa of the medial wall of the second part of the duodenum where the common bile duct and the main pancreatic duct empty. NA *papilla duodeni major.*

major histocompatibility complex. The human chromosomal segment situated on a pair of autosomes not yet identified, which determines the major leukocyte antigens and certain other characteristics of lymphocytes. Abbreviated, MHC

major lip. LABIUM MAJUS.

major motor epilepsy. Recurrent generalized seizures.

major motor seizure. GENERALIZED SEIZURE.

major operation. An extensive, relatively difficult, potentially dangerous surgical procedure, frequently involving a major cavity of the body, or requiring general anesthesia; one which demands of the surgeon a special degree of experience and skill.

major palatine foramen. GREATER PALATINE FORAMEN.

Ma·jor·ström method. A method of managing the second stage of labor by the use of a vacuum extractor.

major surgery. MAJOR OPERATION.

MAKA Major karyotypic abnormalities.

Makarol. A trademark for diethylstilbestrol, an estrogen.

make, *n.* In electricity, the establishing of the flow of an electric current.

makro-. See *macr-*.

mal- [F., from L. *malus*, bad, *male*, badly]. A prefix meaning *wrong, abnormal, bad, badly.*

mal, *n.* [F., Sp., It.]. Sickness, disease.

ma·la (may'luh) *n.* [L., cheek, cheekbone] [NA alt.]. CHEEK. NA alt. *bucca.*

Mal·a·bar itch [after *Malabar*, west coastal region of southern India]. TINEA IMBRICATA.

mal·ab·sorp·tion (mal"ub·sorp'shun) *n.* [*mal-* + *absorption*]. Defective absorption of nutritive substances from the alimentary canal.

malabsorption syndrome. A syndrome in which intestinal malabsorption of fat results in bulky, loose, foul-smelling stools, high in fatty acid content, as well as failure to gain or loss of weight, weakness, anorexia, and vitamin deficiencies with their accompanying symptoms. This syndrome is common to a number of different diseases, including infantile celiac disease, nontropical and tropical sprue, cystic fibrosis of the pancreas, and other specific enzyme deficiencies, as well as obstruction of digestive and absorptive pathways as in Whipple's disease, Hirschsprung's disease, giardiasis, and tuberculous and lymphomatous infiltration of mesenteric nodes.

mal·a·chite (mal'uh·kite) *n.* [Gk. *molochītis lithos*, a kind of precious stone]. A green mineral containing basic copper carbonate, $Cu_2CO_3(OH)_2$.

malachite green. A weakly basic dye of the triphenylmethane series, commonly used as a counter stain for safranin or carmine. A 1% aqueous solution may be used.

ma·la·cia (ma·lay'shee·uh, ·shuh) *n.* [Gk. *malakia*, softness, from *malakos*, soft]. Abnormal softening of part of an organ or structure. See also *encephalomalacia, osteomalacia.*

malacia cor·dis (kor'dis) [L., of the heart]. Softening of areas of the myocardium after infarction.

mal·a·co·pla·kia, mal·a·ko·pla·kia (mal"uh·ko·play'kee·uh) *n.* [Gk. *malakos*, soft, + *plax*, *plakos*, slab, + *-ia*]. The accumulation of histiocytes containing Michaelis-Gutmann calcospherules to produce soft, pale elevated plaques, usually in the urinary bladder of middle-aged women.

malacoplakia cell. A large, plump histiocytic cell, occasionally multinucleate, often with Michaelis-Gutmann bodies in its cytoplasm, seen in malacoplakia of the urinary tract.

ma·la·die (ma·la·dee') *n.* [F.]. Malady, sickness, disease.

maladie bleu (F. blœh) [F., blue disease]. Cyanosis in congenital heart disease.

maladie de Roger [H. L. *Roger*]. VENTRICULAR SEPTAL DEFECT.

maladie des tics (day teek) [F.]. GILLES DE LA TOURETTE DISEASE.

maladie de tic con·vul·sif (duh teek' kohn·vul·seef; F. kohⁿ·vuᵉl·seef') [F.]. GILLES DE LA TOURETTE DISEASE.

maladie du doute (duᵉ doot) [F., malady of doubt]. Obsessive doubting.

mal·ad·just·ment (mal"uh·just'munt) *n.* A state of faulty or inadequate conformity to one's environment, due to the inability to adjust one's desires, attitudes, or feelings to social requirements. —**maladjust·ed** (·id) *adj.*

mal·a·dy (mal'uh·dee) *n.* [F. *maladie*]. Disease, illness.

mal·aise (mal·aiz') *n.* [F., from *mal-*, dis-, + *aise*, comfort]. A general feeling of illness or discomfort.

malakoplakia. MALACOPLAKIA.

mal·align·ment (mal"uh·line'munt) *n.* Improper alignment, as of fragments of a fractured bone, or of teeth.

ma·lar (may'lur) *adj. & n.* [NL. *malaris*, from L. *mala*, cheek, cheekbone]. 1. Pertaining to the cheek or to the zygoma. 2. ZYGOMATIC BONE.

ma·lar·ia (muh·lăr'ee·uh) *n.* [It., from *mala aria*, bad air (orginally thought to be the cause of the disease)]. An infectious febrile disease produced by several species of the protozoan genus *Plasmodium*, transmitted from host to host by the bite of an infected anopheline mosquito. It is characterized by paroxysms of severe chills, fever, and sweating, splenomegaly, anemia, and a chronic relapsing course. —**malar·i·al** (·ee·ul) adj.

malarial nephropathy. Nephrotic syndrome associated with quartan malaria. Soluble immune-complex injury has been postulated as a cause of the glomerular alterations. Syn. *quartan malarial nephropathy.*

malarial therapy. The artificial induction of vivax malaria for its therapeutic effect, as in central nervous system syphilis. Syn. *malariotherapy.*

malaria pigment. Dark brown amorphous or microcrystalline and birefringent pigment found in parasitized erythrocytes (especially with quartan parasites) and in littoral phagocytes of spleen, liver, and bone marrow. It is apparently related to the acid hematins and must be distinguished from formaldehyde pigment.

ma·lar·i·ol·o·gist (muh·lăr″ee·ol′uh·jist) *n.* An expert in the diagnosis, treatment, and control of malaria.

ma·lar·i·ol·o·gy (muh·lăr″ee·ol′uh·jee) *n.* The study of malaria.

ma·lar·io·ther·a·py (muh·lăr″ee·o·therr′uh·pee) *n.* MALARIAL THERAPY.

malar point. The most prominent point on the outer surface of the zygomatic bone.

mal·ar·tic·u·la·tion (mal″ahr·tick″yoo·lay′shun) *n.* [*mal-* + *articulation*]. 1. Defective production of speech sounds. 2. Defective positioning of joint surfaces.

malar tubercle or **tuberosity.** MARGINAL TUBERCLE OF THE ZYGOMATIC BONE.

Mal·as·se·zia (mal″a·see′zee·uh) *n.* [L. C. *Malassez*, French physiologist, 1842–1909]. A genus of fungi.

Malassezia furfur. *PITYROSPORUM FURFUR.*

mal·as·sim·i·la·tion (mal″uh·sim″i·lay′shun) *n.* Defective assimilation.

mal·ate (mal′ate) *n.* Any salt or ester of malic acid.

malate-aspartute shuttle. A method of transporting NADH from the cytoplasm of the cell to the electron transport chain in the mitochondrion, using both soluble and mitochondrial forms of the enzymes malic acid dehydrogenase and glutamic oxaloacetic transaminase.

malate dehydrogenase. MALIC ENZYME.

Malayan filariasis. Filariasis of man caused by *Brugia malayi*, occurring in southeast Asia, transmitted by mosquitoes of the genera *Mansonia* and *Anopheles*. Lymphadenopathy, lymphadenitis, and elephantiasis, principally of the lower limbs, occur.

Malayan scrub typhus. TSUTSUGAMUSHI DISEASE.

Malayan typhus. TSUTSUGAMUSHI DISEASE.

mal de ca·de·ras (ka·deh′ras) [Sp., haunch disease]. A South American disease affecting domestic animals; characterized by fever, emaciation, and paralysis of the hind legs; caused by *Trypanosoma hippicum.*

mal de Ca·yenne (ka·yen′) [F., after *Cayenne*, French Guiana]. Elephantiasis due to filariasis.

mal de coït (mal duh ko·eet′) [F., disease of coitus]. DOURINE.

mal de la ro·sa (ro′sah) [Sp., lit., disease of the rose]. PELLAGRA.

mal del pin·to (mal del pin′to) [Sp.]. PINTA.

mal del sole (mahl del so′leh) [It., sun disease]. PELLAGRA.

mal de Meleda (mal duh me·lay′duh) [F., after the Yugoslav island of Mljit (It. *Meleda*)]. KERATOSIS PALMARIS ET PLANTARIS.

mal de mer (mal duh mehr) [F.]. SEASICKNESS.

mal des bas·sines (mal day ba·seen′) [F., lit., of the basins]. A dermatitis affecting those in the silkworm industry; due to handling cocoons.

mal·de·vel·op·ment (mal″de·vel′up·munt) *n.* Faulty development.

mal·di·ges·tion, *n.* Disordered or imperfect digestion.

male, *adj. & n.* [OF., from L. *masculus*]. 1. Of or pertaining to the sex that produces small motile gametes, as spermatozoa, which fertilize ova. 2. Of instruments or connecting tubes, having a protuberance which fits into a corresponding (female) part in order to function. 3. An individual of the male sex. Symbol, □, ♂. 4. *In botany*, a plant having stamens only.

ma·le·ate (mal′ee·ate) *n.* Any salt or ester of maleic acid.

male climacteric. A condition presumably due to loss of testicular function, associated with an elevated urinary excretion of gonadotropins and symptoms such as loss of sexual desire and potency, hot flashes, and vasomotor instability: rarely, if ever, seen clinically.

male fern. ASPIDIUM.

male gonad. TESTIS.

ma·le·ic acid (ma·lee′ick, ma·lay′ick). *cis*-Ethylene carboxylic acid, HOOCCH=CHCOOH. A dibasic acid, the cis-isomer of fumaric acid. Does not occur in nature.

male pseudohermaphroditism. Androgyny; a condition simulating hermaphroditism in which the individual has external sexual characteristics of female aspect, but has testes (usually undescended). Syn. *pseudohermaphroditismus masculinus.*

mal·eth·a·mer (mal·eth′uh·mur) *n.* A high molecular weight copolymer of ethylene with maleic anhydride, cross-linked with 1 to 2% of vinyl crotonate; an antiperistaltic agent.

male-toad test. A pregnancy test in which urine containing chorionic gonadotropin is injected into a male toad, *Bufo arenarum Hensel.* If spermatozoa are demonstrable in the toad's urine within 3 hours after injection, the test is positive.

male Turner's syndrome. ULLRICH-TURNER SYNDROME.

mal·for·ma·tion, *n.* An abnormal development or formation of a part of the body; deformity.

mal·func·tion, *n. & v.* [*mal-* + *function*]. 1. Failure to function normally or properly. 2. To function abnormally or improperly.

Mal·gaigne's amputation (mal·gehnʸ′) [J. F. *Malgaigne*, French surgeon, 1806–1865]. A subtalar disarticulation of the foot.

Mal·i·bu disease (mal′i·boo) [after *Malibu* Beach, California]. SURFER'S LUMPS.

mal·ic acid (mal′ick, may′lick). Hydroxysuccinic acid, $HOOCCH_2CHOHCOOH$, a dibasic hydroxy acid found in apples and many other fruits. Exists in two optically active isomers and a racemic form. The acid and various of its salts have been used medicinally.

malic dehydrogenase. An enzyme that catalyzes, in the presence of diphosphopyridine nucleotide as the coenzyme, oxidation of L-malic acid to oxaloacetic acid in the tricarboxylic acid cycle.

malic enzyme. An enzyme that utilizes NADP to catalyze oxidative decarboxylation of malic acid to pyruvic acid and carbon dioxide; the NADP being reduced to NADPH in the process. Syn. *malate dehydrogenase.*

ma·lig·nant (muh·lig′nunt) *adj.* [L. *malignans*, malicious, mischief-working]. 1. Endangering health or life. 2. Specifically, characterizing the progressive growth of certain tumors which if not checked by treatment spread to distant sites, terminating in death. —**malig·nan·cy** (·nun·see) *n.*

malignant acanthosis nigricans. Acanthosis nigricans associated with visceral adenocarcinoma.

malignant adenoma. A tumor with cytologic features of an adenoma which gives rise to local or distant metastases.

malignant angiochondroma. A sarcoma with vascular and cartilaginous differentiation.

malignant anthrax. ANTHRAX (1).

malignant atrophic papulosis. DEGOS' DISEASE.

malignant bone aneurysm. OSTEOGENIC SARCOMA.

malignant bone cyst. OSTEOGENIC SARCOMA.
malignant carbuncle. An anthrax carbuncle; infection of the skin and subcutaneous tissue with *Bacillus anthracis.*
malignant catarrhal fever. BOVINE MALIGNANT CATARRH.
malignant chromaffinoma. PHEOCHROMOCYTOMA.
malignant disease. 1. Any disease in a particularly violent form, threatening to produce death in a short time. 2. CANCER.
malignant edema. 1. An acute toxemic infection of ungulates usually caused by *Clostridium septicum.* 2. An inflammatory edema in humans caused by *Clostridium* species.
malignant exophthalmos. Rapidly progressive severe exophthalmos in hyperthyroidism.
malignant freckle. LENTIGO MALIGNA.
malignant glaucoma. Glaucoma attended with violent pain and rapidly leading to blindness. Generally occurs following ocular surgery for glaucoma.
malignant goiter. A goiter that contains carcinoma or sarcoma.
malignant granuloma. HODGKIN'S DISEASE.
malignant hemangioendothelioma. HEMANGIOENDOTHELIOMA (2).
malignant hemorrhagic bone cyst. OSTEOGENIC SARCOMA.
malignant hydatidiform mole. CHORIOADENOMA.
malignant hyperlipemia of infancy. A severe form of familial fat-induced hyperlipemia occurring in infancy, characterized by an increase in total serum triglycerides, hepatosplenomegaly, pancytopenia possibly due to replacement of bone marrow by lipid and consequently a high degree of susceptibility to infections, and the presence of neutral-fat-containing, granuloma-like cells in various organs.
malignant hypertension. The accelerated phase of essential hypertension, with papilledema, retinal hemorrhages and exudates, higher and less labile blood pressure levels, progressive cardiac, renal and vascular disease, and encephalopathy. Syn. *accelerated hypertension.*
malignant hyperthermia. A condition in which rapid temperature elevation and often hypertonicity results from anesthesia induction; inherited as an autosomal dominant trait.
malignant leiomyosarcoma. LEIOMYOSARCOMA.
malignant leprosy. LEPROMATOUS LEPROSY.
malignant leukopenia. AGRANULOCYTOSIS (2).
malignant malaria. FALCIPARUM MALARIA.
malignant malnutrition. KWASHIORKOR.
malignant mixed mesodermal tumor. A tumor whose parenchyma is composed of anaplastic cells resembling two or more derivatives of the mesoderm.
malignant mole of placenta. CHORIOADENOMA.
malignant myopia. Rapidly progressing myopia.
malignant nephrosclerosis. Specific histologic changes seen in kidneys of patients with malignant hypertension that include a proliferative endarteritis, necrotizing arteriolitis, and necrotizing glomerulitis.
malignant neurilemmoma. NEUROFIBROSARCOMA.
malignant neurinoma. NEUROFIBROSARCOMA.
malignant neurofibroma. NEUROFIBROSARCOMA.
malignant neutropenia. AGRANULOCYTOSIS.
malignant papulosis. DEGOS' DISEASE.
malignant peripheral glioma. NEUROFIBROSARCOMA.
malignant pheochromocytoma. PHEOCHROMOBLASTOMA.
malignant pustule. A localized skin lesion of anthrax.
malignant rhabdomyoma. RHABDOMYOSARCOMA.
malignant schwannoma. NEUROFIBROSARCOMA.
malignant tertian malaria. FALCIPARUM MALARIA.
malignant transformation. A permanent genetic change in a somatic cell, which may be induced by physical, chemical, or viral means, resulting in formation of a cancer cell.
ma·lin·ger (muh·ling'gur) *v.* [F. *malingre*, sickly]. To feign or exaggerate illness or incapacity in order to avoid work or other responsibilities. —**malinger·er** (·ur) *n.*
mal·lea·ble (mal'ee·uh·bul) *adj.* [L. *malleabilis*, from *malleus*, hammer]. Capable of being beaten or rolled into thin sheets. —**mal·le·a·bil·i·ty** (mal''ee·uh·bil'i·tee) *n.*
malleable spinal needle. An especially annealed stainless-steel or German-silver pliable, nonbreakable needle which assumes, through ligamental and bony pressure, the proper curves within the vertebral canal for continued or serial injections without stress; used for continuous spinal, caudal, or peridural anesthesia.
mal·le·al (mal'ee·ul) *adj.* MALLEAR.
malleal ligament. See *anterior, lateral,* and *superior ligament of the malleus.*
mal·le·ar (mal'ee·ur) *adj.* Pertaining to the malleus.
mallear folds or **plicae.** See *anterior mallear fold, posterior mallear fold.*
mallear prominence. The bulge on the medial surface of the tympanic membrane overlying the lateral process of the malleus. NA *prominentia mallearis.*
mal·le·a·tion (mal''ee·ay'shun) *n.* [L. *malleatio*, from *malleare*, to hammer]. A spasmodic ticlike action of the hands, consisting in regularly striking any near object.
mal·lei (mal'ee·eye) [L.] 1. Plural of *malleus.* 2. Genitive singular of *malleus;* of or pertaining to the malleus. 3. Of or pertaining to malleus (glanders).
mal·le·in (mal'ee·in) *n.* A protein concentrate of *Actinobacillus mallei*, used in a skin test for the diagnosis of glanders, analogous to the tuberculin test.
mal·leo·in·cu·dal (mal''ee·o·ing'kew·dul, ·in'kew·dul) *adj.* Pertaining to the malleus and the incus.
mal·le·o·lar (mal·lee'uh·lur) *adj.* 1. Pertaining to a malleolus. 2. MALLEAR.
malleolar folds or **plicae.** MALLEAR FOLDS.
malleolar sulcus. A shallow groove on the posterior border of the medial malleolus for the passage of the tendons of the tibialis posterior and flexor digitorum longus muscles. NA *sulcus malleolaris.*
mal·le·o·lus (ma·lee'o·lus) *n.*, pl. & genit. sing. **malleo·li** (·lye) [L., small hammer]. A part or process of bone having a hammerhead shape.
malleolus la·te·ra·lis (lat·e·ray'lis) [NA]. LATERAL MALLEOLUS.
malleolus me·di·a·lis (mee·dee·ay'lis) [NA]. MEDIAL MALLEOLUS.
Mal·leo·my·ces (mal''ee·o·mye'seez) *n.* [*malle*us, glanders, + *-myces*]. *ACTINOBACILLUS.*
Malleomyces mallei. *Obsol.* *PSEUDOMONAS MALLEI.*
Malleomyces pseudomallei. *PSEUDOMONAS PSEUDOMALLEI.*
mal·leo·my·rin·go·plas·ty (mal''ee·o·mi·ring'go·plas·tee) *n.* [*malleo-* + *myringo-* + *-plasty*]. A method of reestablishing an effective sound-conducting method when the tympanic membrane and the handle of the malleus have been destroyed, by reconstructing the tympanic membrane from adherent fascial layers covering the temporalis muscle and the handle of the malleus, incorporating a shaped bone graft between the layers.
mal·le·ot·o·my (mal''ee·ot'um·ee) *n.* [*malle*us + *-tomy*]. 1. Incision or division of the malleus. 2. Division of the ligaments attached to the malleoli.
mallet finger. A deformity marked by undue flexion of the last phalanx.
mal·le·us (mal'ee·us) *n.*, pl. & genit. sing. **mal·lei** (·ee·eye) [L., hammer]. 1. [NA] One of the ossicles of the internal ear, having the shape of a hammer. See also Table of Bones in the Appendix and Plate 20. 2. *In veterinary medicine,* GLANDERS. Adj. *malleal, mallear.*
Mal·loph·a·ga (ma·lof'uh·guh) *n.pl.* [Gk. *mallos*, tuft of wool, hair, + *-phaga*, eaters]. An order of small, wingless, flat insects which feed on hair, feathers, and epidermal scales, parasitic on birds and occasionally man; the bird lice.
Mallophene. A trademark for phenazopyridine, a urinary analgesic drug that is used as the hydrochloride salt.
Mal·lo·ry bodies [F. B. *Mallory*, U.S. pathologist, 1862–1941]. Oval acidophilic hyalin inclusion bodies of cyto-

plasm of hepatic cells, observed in Laennec's cirrhosis.

Mallory's acid fuchsin stain. A staining method for fibroglia and collagen.

Mallory's connective-tissue stain. MALLORY'S TRIPLE STAIN.

Mallory's phloxine–methylene blue stain [F. B. *Mallory*]. A histologic stain using the named dyes, similar in application to hematoxylin-eosin staining.

Mallory's phosphotungstic acid hematoxylin [F. B. *Mallory*]. A method of differential staining of tissue components used especially for muscle and nerve fibers.

Mallory's triple stain. A stain which differentially colors different tissue components; contains acid fuchsin, orange G, and aniline blue dyes.

Mallory-Weiss syndrome [G. K. *Mallory*, U.S. pathologist, b. 1900; and S. *Weiss*, U.S. internist, 1898–1942]. Painless hematemesis secondary to lacerations of the distal esophagus and esophagogastric junction, involving only the mucosa and submucosa, usually a result of prolonged violent vomiting, coughing, or hiccuping. Compare *Boerhaave syndrome.*

mal·low (mal'o) *n.* [L. *malva*]. Any plant of the genus *Malva*, certain species of which have been used medicinally as demulcents.

Mal·loy-Eve·lyn method. A method for bilirubin in which blood is treated with Ehrlich's reagent and the bilirubin reacts to form a colored compound, azorubin or azobilirubin. The quantity of azorubin formed is determined photometrically.

Mall's formula [F. P. *Mall*, U.S. embryologist and anatomist, 1862–1917]. A formula for estimating the age of human embryos with a vertex-breech length of 100 mm. or less: Age in days $= \sqrt{VB \times 100}$. VB represents vertex-breech length in millimeters. When Mall's formula was introduced, the Peters embryo was thought to be three or four days old. Since the Peters embryo is now known to be about 14 days old, it is necessary to correct the formula as follows: Age in days $= \sqrt{VB \times 100} + 10$.

Mall's technique [F. P. *Mall*]. A vascular injection technique for liver to demonstrate selectively the distribution of finely ground carbon particles in portal and hepatic venules.

mal·nu·tri·tion (mal''new·trish'un) *n.* Defective nutrition. —**mal·nour·ish** (·nur'ish) *v.*

mal·oc·clu·sion (mal''uh·kloo'zhun) *n.* Any deviation from a physiologically normal occlusion of the teeth. See also *Angle's classification.*

mal·o·nate (mal'o·nate, mal'un·ut) *n.* Any salt or ester of malonic acid.

ma·lo·nic acid (ma·lo'nick, ·lon'ick). Propanedioic acid, $HOOCCH_2COOH$, a dibasic acid found in many plants and obtainable from malic acid by oxidation.

mal·o·nyl (mal'o·nil, ·neel) *n.* $—COCH_2CO—$. The bivalent radical of malonic acid.

malonyl-ACP. A molecule formed as a result of esterification of a malonyl group (derived from malonyl CoA) with acyl carrier protein. It is required in the de novo synthesis of fatty acids.

malonyl-CoA. An activated form of malonic acid formed by the enzymatic carboxylation of acetyl coenzyme A. Malonyl-CoA is required in the de novo synthesis of fatty acids.

mal·o·nyl·urea (mal''o·nil·yoo·ree'uh) *n.* [*malonyl* + *urea*]. BARBITURIC ACID.

mal per·fo·rant (perr·fo·rahn', F. pehr·fo^h·rah^n') [F.]. Perforating ulcer of the foot.

mal·pigh·i·an (mal·pig'ee·un) *adj.* Discovered or described by Marcello Malpighi, Italian anatomist, 1628–1691.

malpighian capsule. GLOMERULAR CAPSULE.

malpighian corpuscle or **body.** 1. A lymph nodule of the spleen. 2. RENAL CORPUSCLE.

malpighian epithelium. MUCOUS EPITHELIUM.

malpighian layer. GERMINATIVE LAYER of the epidermis.

malpighian pyramid. RENAL PYRAMID.

mal·po·si·tion (mal''puh·zish'un, mal''po·) *n.* An abnormal position of any part or organ, as of the fetus.

mal·pos·ture (mal·pos'chur) *n.* Faulty posture.

mal·prac·tice (mal·prack'tis) *n.* Improper or injurious medical or surgical treatment, through carelessness, ignorance, or intent.

mal·pre·sen·ta·tion (mal''prez''un·tay'shun, ·pree''zen·tay'shun) *n.* Abnormal position of the child at birth, making delivery difficult or impossible.

mal·re·duc·tion (mal''re·duck'shun) *n.* Faulty or incomplete reduction of a fracture.

malt, *n.* Grain, commonly of one or more varieties of barley, which has been soaked, made to germinate, and dried. The germinated grains contain diastase, dextrin, maltose, and proteins. Malt has been used as a nutrient and digestant.

Mal·ta fever. BRUCELLOSIS.

malt agar. A medium for the culture of fungi.

malt·ase (mawl·tace, ·taze) *n.* An enzyme found in the saliva and pancreatic juice which converts maltose into dextrose.

Mal·thu·sian·ism (mal·thoo'zhun·iz·um, mawl·, ·zee·un·) *n.* [T. R. *Malthus*, English economist, 1766–1834]. The theory that in the absence of such checks as epidemics and war, population tends to increase more rapidly than the food supply. —**Malthusian,** *adj.*

mal·to·bi·ose (mawl''to·bye'oce) *n.* MALTOSE.

malt·ose (mawl'toce) *n.* 4-(α-D-Glucopyranosido)-D-glucopyranose, $C_{12}H_{22}O_{11}.H_2O$, a reducing disaccharide representing 2 molecules of D-glucose joined by α-glycosidic linkage, and yielding 2 molecules of D-glucose on hydrolysis. It does not appear to exist free in nature, being a product of enzymatic hydrolysis of starch by diastase, as in malt. It exists in 2 forms, α-maltose and β-maltose. Syn. *maltobiose, malt sugar.*

malt·os·uria (mawl''to·sue'ree·uh) *n.* [*maltose* + *-uria*]. The presence of maltose in the urine.

malt sugar. MALTOSE.

mal·um (mal'um, mah'lum, may'lum) *n.* [L., harm, evil]. DISEASE.

malum cox·ae (kock'see). Hip joint disease.

malum coxae se·ni·lis (se·nigh'lis). Hypertrophic arthritis of the hip joint in the aged.

malum per·fo·rans ped·is (pur'fo·ranz ped'is). Perforating ulcer of the foot.

malum ve·ne·re·um (ve·neer'ee·um). SYPHILIS.

mal·un·ion (mal·yoon'yun) *n.* Incomplete or faulty union of the fragments of a fractured bone.

ma·man pi·an, ma·man·pi·an (ma·mahn' pee·ahn', F. ma·mah^n' pee·ah^n') *n.* [F. *maman*, mother, + *pian*]. MOTHER YAW.

mam·ba (mahm'buh) *n.* [Xhosa and Zulu *-mamba*]. Any snake of *Dendraspis*, a genus of venomous snakes of Africa south of the Sahara, allied to cobras but without a hood. The common black mamba is *D. angusticeps.*

mam·e·lon (mam'e·lon, ·lun) *n.* [F., diminutive of *mamelle*, teat]. One of the three elevations on the incisal edge of a recently erupted or little-worn incisor tooth.

mamill-, mamillo- [L. *mamilla*]. A combining form meaning (a) *mamilla* or *nipple;* (b) *mamillary.*

ma·mil·la, mam·mil·la (ma·mil'uh) *n.*, pl. **ma·mil·lae, mam·mil·lae** (·ee) [L., nipple]. A small prominence or papilla; nipple.

mam·il·lary, mam·mil·lary (mam'i·lerr''ee) *adj.* 1. Pertaining to a nipple or mamilla. 2. Nipple-shaped; breast-shaped.

mamillary body. Either of the two small, spherical masses of gray matter in the interpeduncular space at the base of the brain. They receive projections from the hippocampus by means of the fornix and relay them to the anterior nucleus of the thalamus via the mamillothalamic tract and to the tegmentum of the pons and medulla oblongata via the mamillotegmental bundle. NA *corpus mamillare.* See also Plate 18.

mamillary line. A vertical line passing through the center of the nipple. NA *linea mamillaris.*

mamillary process. One of the tubercles on the posterior part of the superior articular processes of the lumbar vertebrae. NA *processus mamillaris.*

mam·il·lat·ed, mam·mil·lat·ed (mam'i·lay·tid) *adj.* Covered with nipplelike protuberances.

mam·il·la·tion, mam·mil·la·tion (mam''i·lay'shun) *n.* [from *mamilla*]. Small, dome-shaped elevations of varied causation, mainly seen on mucous surfaces.

ma·mil·li·form, mam·mil·li·form (ma·mil'i·form) *adj.* [*mamill-* + *-iform*]. Nipple-shaped.

ma·mil·li·plas·ty, mam·mil·li·plas·ty (ma·mil'i·plas''tee) *n.* [*mamill-* + *-plasty*]. Plastic surgery of the nipple. Syn. *thelyplasty.*

mam·il·li·tis, mam·mil·li·tis (mam''i·lye'tis) *n.* [*mamill-* + *-itis*]. Inflammation of the mamilla, or nipple. Syn. *thelitis.*

mam·il·lo·teg·men·tal, mam·mil·lo·teg·men·tal (mam''i·lo·teg·men'tul) *adj.* Pertaining to the mamillary bodies and the tegmentum.

mamillotegmental tract. A tract that projects caudally from the mamillary nuclei into the midbrain tegmentum, where fibers of the tract terminate in the dorsal and ventral tegmental nuclei. NA *fasciculus mamillotegmentalis.*

mam·il·lo·tha·lam·ic, mam·mil·lo·tha·lam·ic (mam''i·lo·tha·lam'ick) *adj.* Pertaining to the mamillary bodies and the thalamus.

mamillothalamic tract. A tract of nerve fibers passing from the mamillary body to the anterior nuclei of the thalamus. NA *fasciculus mamillothalamicus.*

mamm-, mammo- [L. *mamma*]. A combining form meaning *mamma* or *breast.*

mam·ma (mam'uh) *n.*, pl. **mam·mae** (·mee) [L.] [NA]. The breast; the milk-secreting gland.

mamma ab·er·rans (a·berr'anz). A supernumerary breast.

mammae ac·ces·so·ri·ae fe·mi·ni·nae et mas·cu·li·nae (fem''i·nigh'nee et mas''kew·lye'nee) [NA]. Accessory mammary glands, occurring in either the male or female.

mammae accessoriae mu·li·e·bres et vi·ri·les (mew''lee·ee'breez et vi·rye'leez) [BNA]. MAMMAE ACCESSORIAE FEMININAE ET MASCULINAE.

mamma er·rat·i·ca (e·rat'i·kuh). MAMMA ABERRANS.

mam·mal (mam'ul) *n.* An individual of the class Mammalia.

mam·mal·gia (ma·mal'jee·uh) *n.* [*mamm-* + *-algia*]. Pain in the mammary gland; mastalgia.

Mam·ma·lia (ma·may'lee·uh) *n.pl.* [NL., from *mammalis,* of the breast]. The class of vertebrates that includes all animals that have hair and suckle their young. **—mamma·li·an** (·lee·un) *adj.*

mamma mas·cu·li·na (mas''kew·lye'nuh) [NA]. The male breast.

mam·ma·plas·ty (mam'uh·plas''tee) *n.* MAMMOPLASTY.

mam·ma·ry (mam'uh·ree) *adj.* Pertaining to the mammae.

mammary calculus. A calcified mass of secretion or exudate in the ducts of the mammary gland.

mammary dysplasia. A group of common pathologic conditions in the breasts of women during sexual maturity. Included are adenosis of breast, cystic disease, and mastodynia. Syn. *chronic cystic mastitis.*

mammary fold. MAMMARY RIDGE.

mammary gland. A gland that secretes milk. NA *glandula mammaria.* See also Plate 24.

mammary line. MAMMARY RIDGE.

mammary lymphatic plexus. A lymphatic plexus originating in the walls of the ducts and between the lobules of the mamma which also drains the overlying skin, areola, and nipple. The efferent vessels empty into the pectoral group of axillary nodes laterally, the sternal group medially, and occasionally the subclavian nodes superiorly. See also Plate 11.

mammary papilla. The nipple of the breast. See also Plate 24.

mammary region. The space on the anterior surface of the chest between a line drawn through the lower border of the third rib, and one drawn through the upper border of the xiphoid cartilage. NA *regio mammaria.*

mammary ridge. A longitudinal elevation of thickened ectoderm between the bases of the limb buds in the embryo from which develop the mammary glands. Syn. *milk ridge.*

mammary-stimulating hormone. 1. PROLACTIN. 2. More appropriately, estrogen and progesterone, which induce proliferation of the ductal and acinous elements of the mammary glands, respectively.

mammary venous plexus. A venous plexus draining blood from the mammary glands to the axillary vein.

mamma vi·ri·lis (vi·rye'lis, vir'i·lis) [BNA]. MAMMA MASCULINA.

mam·mec·to·my (ma·meck'tum·ee) *n.* [*mamm-* + *-ectomy*]. MASTECTOMY.

mam·mi·form (mam'i·form) *adj.* [*mamm-* + *-iform*]. Shaped like a breast or nipple.

mammill-, mammillo-. See *mamill-.*

mammilla. MAMILLA.

Mam·mil·lar·ia (mam''i·lăr'ee·uh) *n.* [NL., from *mamilla*]. A genus of cacti. The mescal or peyote cactus, once assigned to this genus, is now properly designated *Lophophora williamsii.*

mammillary. MAMILLARY.

mammillated. MAMILLATED.

mammilation. MAMILLATION.

mammilliform. MAMILLIFORM.

mammilliplasty. MAMILLIPLASTY.

mammillitis. MAMILLITIS.

mammillotegmental. MAMILLOTEGMENTAL.

mammillothalamic. MAMILLOTHALAMIC.

mam·mi·tis (mam·eye'tis) *n.* [*mamm-* + *-itis*]. MASTITIS.

mam·mo·gen (mam'uh·jin, ·jen'') *n.* [*mammo-* + *-gen*]. PROLACTIN. **—mammogen·ic** (mam''o·jen'ick) *adj.*

mammogenic hormone. 1. PROLACTIN. 2. Loosely, any hormone known to influence the mammary gland.

mam·mo·gram (mam'o·gram) *n.* [*mammo-* + *-gram*]. A radiographic depiction of the breast.

mam·mog·ra·phy (ma·mog'ruh·fee) *n.* [*mammo-* + *-graphy*]. Radiographic examination of the breast, occasionally performed with a contrast medium injected into the ducts of the mammary gland, usually without.

mam·mo·pla·sia (mam''o·play'zhuh, ·zee·uh) *n.* [*mammo-* + *-plasia*]. Development of breast tissue.

mam·mo·plas·ty (mam'o·plas·tee) *n.* [*mammo-* + *-plasty*]. Any plastic surgery operation altering the shape of the breast. See also *augmentation mammoplasty.*

mam·mose (mam'oce, ma·moce') *adj.* [L. *mammosus*]. Having full or abnormally large breasts.

mam·mot·o·my (ma·mot'um·ee) *n.* [*mammo-* + *-tomy*]. MASTOTOMY.

mam·mo·tro·phin (mam''o·tro'fin) *n.* PROLACTIN.

mam·mo·tro·pin (mam''o·tro'pin) *n.* [*mammo-* + *-tropin*]. PROLACTIN.

mam·pir·ra (mam·pirr'uh) *n.* A tiny ceratopogonid gnat of the tropics which causes urticaria and subjective symptoms of burning pruritis. Syn. *merutu.*

man, *n.* 1. *Homo sapiens;* the human race, mankind. 2. An adult male human being.

man·a·ca (man'uh·kuh) *n.* [Brazilian Pg. *manacá*]. The dried root of *Brunfelsia hopeana.* Has been used as an antirheumatic and antisyphilitic.

Manadrin. A trademark for ephedrine, an adrenergic.

man·cha·da (man·chah'duh) *n.* [Sp., blotchy, spotted, stained]. LUCIO LEPROSY.

man·chette (mahn·shet') *n.* [F., cuff]. A cylindrical structure in the developing spermatid, formed by straight filaments that extend caudally from a ringlike structure surrounding the nucleus.

Man·chu·ri·an fever. EPIDEMIC HEMORRHAGIC FEVER.

Mancke-Sommer test. A test for liver function which is a modification of the Takata-Ara test.

Mancke's test. Insulin-glucose-water tolerance test.

Mandelamine. Trademark for methenamine mandelate, a salt of methenamine and mandelic acid used as a urinary antibacterial agent.

man·del·ate (man'de·late) *n.* A salt of mandelic acid.

Man·del·baum's reaction (mahn'del·baowm) [M. *Mandelbaum*, German physician, 1881-1947]. THREAD REACTION.

man·del·ic acid (man·del'ick, ·dee'lick) [Ger. *Mandel*, almond, + *-ic*]. Alpha-hydroxyphenylacetic acid, $C_6H_5CH(OH)COOH$, a urinary antiseptic; usually used in the form of one of its salts.

man·di·ble (man'di·bul) *n.* [L. *mandibula* from *mandere*, to chew (rel. to Gmc. *munthā* → E. *mouth*)]. The lower jawbone. NA *mandibula*. See also Table of Bones in the Appendix and Plate 1.

mandibul-, mandibulo-. A combining form meaning *mandible, mandibular.*

man·di·bu·la (man·dib'yoo·luh) *n.*, pl. & genit. sing. **mandibu·lae** (·lee) [L.] [NA]. MANDIBLE.

man·dib·u·lar (man·dib'yoo·lur) *adj.* Of or pertaining to the mandible. See also Table of Synovial Joints and Ligaments in the Appendix.

mandibular arch. The first visceral arch, including the maxillary process. Syn. *oral arch.*

mandibular canal. The canal in the mandible which transmits the inferior alveolar vessels and nerve. NA *canalis mandibulae.*

mandibular cartilage. The bar of cartilage of the mandibular arch.

mandibular foramen. The aperture of the inferior dental or alveolar canal in the ramus of the mandible; it transmits the inferior dental or alveolar vessels and nerve to the lower jaw. NA *foramen mandibulae.*

mandibular fossa. The fossa in the temporal bone that receives the condyle of the mandible. NA *fossa mandibularis.*

mandibular gland. SUBMANDIBULAR GLAND.

mandibular hinge position. The most posterior position in which one can effect a hinge movement of one's mandible.

mandibular nerve. A motor (masticator nerve) and somatic sensory nerve, attached to the trigeminal nerve, which innervates the tensor tympani, tensor veli palatini, mylohyoid, anterior belly of the digastric, and muscles of mastication, the lower teeth, the mucosa of the anterior two-thirds of the tongue, the floor of the mouth, the cheek and the skin of the lower portion of the face, and the meninges. NA *nervus mandibularis.*

mandibular notch. The deep concavity between the condyle and the coronoid process of the mandible. NA *incisura mandibulae.*

mandibular process. The chief part of the embryonic mandibular arch that forms the lower jaw.

mandibular reflex. JAW JERK.

mandibular torus. Ridge of the mandible situated in the anterior portion of the inner aspect of the bone approximately at the junction between the body and the alveolar process in the region of the incisors, canines, and premolars, rarely in the molar region, due to an overgrowth of the bone.

mandibular tubercle. One of three auricular tubercles on the posterior surface of the embryonic mandibular arch.

man·dib·u·lec·to·my (man·dib"yoo·leck'tum·ee) *n.* [*mandibul-* + *-ectomy*]. Surgical removal of the mandible.

mandibulo-. See *mandibul-.*

man·dib·u·lo·fa·cial dysostosis (man·dib"yoo·lo·fay'shul). Hypoplasia of the facial bones, especially of the zygoma and the mandible. With this are associated a lateral downward sloping of the palpebral fissures, defects of the ear, macrostomia, and a peculiar "fish-face" appearance. It is presumed to be a dominant trait. Syn. *Treacher Collins syndrome.*

man·dib·u·lo·glos·sus (man·dib"yoo·lo·glos'us) *n.* A variant portion of the genioglossus muscle extending from the posterior border of the mandible to the side of the tongue.

man·dib·u·lo·mar·gi·na·lis (man·dib"yoo·lo·mahr"ji·nay'lis, ·nal'is) *n.* A variant part of the platysma muscle extending from the mastoid process forward over the angle of the mandible.

Mand·ler filter. The American modification of the German Berkefeld filter made of diatomaceous earth, and used in the recovery and study of viruses, or to render solutions bacteria-free.

Man·dl's operation (mahn'del) [F. *Mandl*, Austrian surgeon, b. 1892]. Extirpation of parathyroid adenoma for the relief of osteitis fibrosa cystica.

man·drel (man'dril) *n.* A shank or shaft that fits into a dental handpiece and which holds a cup, disk, or stone for polishing or grinding.

man·drin (man'drin) *n.* [F.]. A guide or stylet.

man·du·cate (man'dew·kate) *v.* [L. *manducare*]. *Obsol.* To masticate, chew. —**man·du·ca·tion** (man"dew·kay'shun) *n.*

man·du·ca·to·ry (man'dew·kuh·tor"ee) *adj. Obsol.* Used for or pertaining to manducation, chewing.

ma·neu·ver (muh·new'vur) *n.* [F. *manoeuvre*, from L. *manu operari*, to work by hand]. Skillful procedure or manual method.

man·ga·nese (mang'guh·neece, ·neez, man'guh·) *n.* [It., from ML. *magnesia*]. Mn = 54.9380. A brittle, hard, grayish-white metal resembling iron in its properties. Manganese salts have been used in medicine, but proof of their value is lacking.

man·gan·ic (mang·gan'ick) *adj.* Pertaining to compounds of manganese when it has a valence of three.

man·ga·nous (mang'guh·nus) *adj.* Pertaining to compounds of manganese when it has a valence of two.

mange (mainj) *n.* [OF. *mangeue*, itch, from *mangier*, to eat, to itch]. Infestation of the skin of mammals by mange mites which burrow into the epidermal layer of the skin; characterized by multiple lesions in the skin with vesiculation and papule formation accompanied by intense itching. See also *scabies.*

mange mite. Any species of the Sarcoptoidea.

mango fly. Any of various species of the genus *Chrysops.*

-mania [Gk.]. A combining form designating *obsession, abnormal preoccupation,* or *compulsion.*

ma·nia (may'nee·uh) *n.* [Gk.]. 1. Excessive enthusiasm or excitement; a violent desire or passion. 2. PSYCHOSIS. See also *manic-depressive illness.* —**man·ic** (man'ick) *adj.*

mania a po·tu (ah po'too, ay po'tew) [L., from drink]. PATHOLOGIC INTOXICATION.

ma·ni·ac (may'nee·ack) *n.* [L. *maniacus*, from Gk. *mania*, mania]. 1. A psychotic person with violent or destructive tendencies. 2. A person with a mania for something. —**ma·ni·a·cal** (muh·nigh'uh·kul) *adj.*

maniacal chorea. CHOREA INSANIENS.

manic-depressive illness, reaction, or **psychosis.** One of a group of psychotic reactions, fundamentally marked by severe mood swings from normal to elation or to depression or alternating, and a tendency to remission and recurrence. Illusions, delusions, and hallucinations are often associated with the change of affect, but milder forms are often observed. The manic type is characterized by elation or irritability, overtalkativeness, flight of ideas, and increased motor activity; the depressive type exhibits outstanding depression of mood, mental and motor retardation, and inhibition. Marked mixture of these phases is the mixed type; continuous alternation of phases is the circular type. Compare *psychotic depressive reaction.*

manifest content. *In psychiatry,* any idea, feeling or action considered to be the conscious expression of repressed motives or desires, particularly the remembered content of a dream or fantasy which conceals and distorts its unconscious meaning. Contr. *latent content.*

manifest hyperopia. The amount of hyperopia represented by the strongest convex lens that a person will accept without paralysis of the accommodation; may be facultative or absolute. Symbol, Hm.

manifest stimulus. *In psychiatry,* the obvious or external basis for anxiety, fear, or dread, such as the immediate or apparent cause for a phobic reaction. Contr. *latent stimulus.*

man·i·kin (man'i·kin) *n.* [D. *manneken,* dim. from *man,* man]. 1. A model of the body; made of plaster, papier-mâché, or other material, and showing, by means of movable parts, the relations of the organs. 2. A model of a term fetus; used for the teaching of obstetrics.

man·i·ple (man'i·pul) *n.* [L. *manipulus*]. A handful.

ma·nip·u·la·tion (muh·nip"yoo·lay'shun) *n.* [L. *manipulus,* handful, + *-ation*]. The use of the hands in a skillful manner, as reducing a dislocation, returning a hernia into its cavity, or changing the position of a fetus.

Manite. A trademark for mannitol hexanitrate, a vasodilator.

man·na (man'uh) *n.* [Gk., from Heb. *mān,* manna]. The concrete, saccharine exudation of the flowering ash, *Fraxinus ornus;* contains mannitol, sugar, mucilage, and resin. Has been used as a mild laxative.

man·nan (man'un, ·an) *n.* MANNOSAN.

manna sugar. MANNITOL.

Mann-Boll·man fistula [F. C. *Mann,* U.S. physiologist, 1887–1962; and J. L. *Bollman,* U.S. pathologist, b. 1896]. A fistula of the small intestine produced in animal experimentation by suturing the proximal end of a loop of small intestine to the edges of the opening in the abdominal wall and anastomosing the distal end with the functioning intestine, thus preventing movement of material out through the skin by peristalsis.

man·ni·tan (man'i·tan) *n.* Mannitol anhydride, $C_6H_{12}O_6$, a sweet, syrupy liquid.

man·nite (man'ite) *n.* MANNITOL.

man·ni·tol (man'i·tol) *n.* D-Mannitol, $HOCH_2(CHOH)_4CH_2OH$; a hexahydric alcohol from manna and other plant sources. Hypertonic solutions are administered intravenously to promote diuresis. Sometimes used to measure the rate of glomerular filtration, and as an irrigating fluid in transurethral resection of the prostate; in pharmacy used as a diluent and excipient. Syn. *manna sugar, mannite.*

mannitol hexanitrate. An ester, $C_6H_8(ONO_2)_6$, formed by nitration of mannitol, occurring as explosive, colorless crystals, insoluble in water; supplied only in admixture with carbohydrates to render it nonexplosive. Used as a vasodilator. Syn. *nitromannite, nitromannitol.*

man·non·ic acid (ma·non'ick, ma·no'nick). $HOCH_2(CHOH)_4COOH$. An acid derived by the oxidation of mannitol.

man·no·sac·char·ic acid (man"o·sa·kăr'ick). $HOOC(CHOH)_4COOH$; the saccharic acid produced when both the aldehyde and primary alcohol groups of mannose are oxidized.

man·no·san (man'o·san) *n.* A polysaccharide, occurring in plants, which upon hydrolysis yields mannose. Syn. *mannan.*

man·nose (man'oce) *n.* A fermentable monosaccharide, $C_6H_{12}O_6$, obtained from manna. Occurs in two optically active forms.

man·no·side (man'o·side) *n.* A glycoside of mannose.

man·no·sid·o·sis (man"o·si·do'sis) *n.* A rare hereditary disorder brought about by a deficiency of the enzyme α-mannosidase, occurring in the first two years; characterized by skeletal deformities, Hurler-like facial deformities, mental retardation and some motor disability. Its neuropathology is presently unknown.

Mann's palsy (ma^{h}n) [Ludwig *Mann,* German neurologist, 1866–1936]. WERNICKE-MANN PARALYSIS.

Mann's sign [J. D. *Mann,* English physician, 1840–1912]. 1. Decreased electrical resistance of the skin, thought to be associated with neuroses. 2. An ocular sign of thyrotoxicosis in which the eyes do not appear to be on the same level.

man·nu·ron·ic acid (man"yoo·ron'ick). D-Mannuronic acid, $HOOC(CHOH)_4CHO$, the uronic acid resulting when the primary alcohol group of mannose is oxidized to carboxyl.

Mann-Wil·liam·son ulcer [F. C. *Mann,* U.S. surgeon and physiologist, 1887–1962; and C. A. *Williamson,* U.S. surgeon, 1896–1952]. Experimental peptic ulcer occurring in dogs after gastroenterostomy.

ma·nom·e·ter (ma·nom'e·tur) *n.* [Gk. *manos,* rare, loose, sparse, + *-meter*]. An instrument for measuring the pressure of liquids and gases. —**mano·met·ric** (man"uh·met'rick) *adj.*

manometric block. A partial or complete obstruction to the free flow of cerebrospinal fluid as measured usually by pressure on the abdomen or jugular veins during a lumbar or cisternal puncture or both. See also *Queckenstedt test, cuff manometry.*

manometric flames. Flames of different heights and characters seen in a rotating mirror and due to the reflection of a pulsating gas flame, when the supplying gas is set in motion by sound waves.

manometric test. 1. QUECKENSTEDT TEST. 2. CUFF MANOMETRY.

ma·nom·e·try (ma·nom'e·tree) *n.* Use of manometers. See also *Queckenstedt test, cuff manometry.*

mano·scope (man'uh·skope) *n.* [Gk. *manos,* rare, sparse, + *-scope*]. An instrument for measuring the density of gases.

Man·son·el·la (man"suh·nel'uh) *n.* [P. *Manson,* Scottish physician and parasitologist, 1844–1922]. A genus of filarial worms that are transmitted to man by mosquitoes of the genus *Culicoides.*

Mansonella oz·zar·di (oz·ahr'dee, ·dye). A species of filarial worm found in the Western Hemisphere, living in body cavities and generally producing no symptoms in man.

Man·so·nia (man·so'nee·uh) *n.* [P. *Manson*]. A genus of mosquitoes which are important as vectors of human disease. Species of *Mansonia,* subgenus *Mansonioides,* are the principal carriers of *Wuchereria malayi,* and also are carriers of *Wuchereria bancrofti.*

Man·son's pyosis [P. *Manson*]. PEMPHIGUS CONTAGIOSUS.

man·tle, *n.* [L. *mantellum,* covering, veil]. 1. An enveloping layer. 2. The portion of brain substance that includes the convolutions, corpus callosum, and fornix.

mantle dentin. The thin superficial layer of dentin.

mantle layer. A layer of neuroblasts between the ependymal and marginal layers of the (developing) neural tube.

mantle sclerosis. ULEGYRIA.

Man·toux test (mah^n·too') [Charles *Mantoux,* French physician, 1877–1947]. Any intradermal test for tuberculin hypersensitivity.

manual pelvimetry. DIGITAL PELVIMETRY.

ma·nu·bri·um (ma·new'bree·um) *n.,* pl. **manu·bria** (·bree·uh) [L., handle, haft]. 1. A handlelike process. 2. MANUBRIUM STERNI. —**manubri·al** (·ul) *adj.*

manubrium mal·lei (mal'lee·eye) [NA]. MANUBRIUM OF THE MALLEUS.

manubrium of the malleus. The handle-shaped process of the malleus of the ear.

manubrium ster·ni (stur'nigh) [NA]. The upper segment of the sternum.

man·u·duc·tion (man"yoo·duck'shun) *n.* [L. *manuductio,* from *manu ducere,* to lead by hand]. Operation performed by the hands in surgical and obstetric practice.

manu·dy·na·mom·e·ter (man"yoo·dye·nuh·mom'e·tur) *n.* [L. *manu,* by hand, artificially, + *dynamometer*]. An apparatus that measures the force exerted by the thrust of an instrument.

ma·nus (man'us) *n.,* pl. & genit. sing. **manus** (man'oos, man'us) [L.] [NA]. HAND.

manus ca·va (kay'vuh). Excessive concavity of the palm of the hand.

manus cur·ta (kur'tuh). CLUBHAND.

manus ex·ten·sa (eck·sten'suh). Clubhand with a backward deviation.

manus flexa (fleck'suh). Clubhand with a forward deviation.

manu·stu·pra·tion (man''yoo·stew·pray'shun, ·stuh·pray'shun) *n.* [L. *manu*, by hand, + *stupration*, defilement]. MASTURBATION.

manus val·ga (val'guh) [L., bowed, bent inward]. Clubhand with ulnar deviation.

manus va·ra (vair'uh, vahr'uh) [L., bent outward]. Clubhand with radial deviation.

many·plies (men'ee·plize) *n.* [E. *many* + plural of *ply*, fold]. OMASUM.

many-tailed bandage. An irregular bandage having four or more cut or torn ends which are tied together to hold a dressing. See also *scultetus bandage.*

MAO Abbreviation for *monoamine oxidase.*

MAOI Abbreviation for *monoamine oxidase inhibitor.*

Maolate. Trademark for chlorphenesin carbamate, a skeletal muscle relaxant drug.

maple bark disease. CONIOSPORIOSIS.

maple syrup urine disease. A hereditary metabolic disorder in which there is a deficiency of branched-chain keto acid decarboxylase with abnormally high concentrations of valine, leucine, isoleucine, and the presence of alloisoleucine in blood, urine, and cerebrospinal fluid; manifested clinically by the aromatic maple syruplike odor of urine noted shortly after birth. In the severe infantile form, in which the enzyme deficiency is nearly complete, there is protracted vomiting and hypertonicity and, unless treated by diet, severe mental retardation, seizures, and death. In the intermittent form, the enzyme activity is decreased to about 10 to 20% of normal, and the above symptoms occur usually only with infection or trauma; the patient may die in status epilepticus unless treated by diet. Syn. *branched-chain ketoaciduria.*

ma·pro·ti·line (ma·pro'ti·leen) *n.* *N*-Methyl-9,10-ethanoanthracene-9(10*H*)-propylamine, $C_{20}H_{23}N$, an antidepressant.

Ma·ran·ta (ma·ran'tuh) *n.* [B. *Maranta*, Italian physician and botanist, 16th century]. A genus of tropical American herbs with tuberous roots containing starch. See also *arrowroot.*

ma·ran·tic (muh·ran'tick) *adj.* [Gk. *marantikos*, wasting away]. 1. Pertaining to marasmus. 2. Pertaining to slowed circulation.

marantic endocarditis. Nonbacterial thrombotic endocarditis, usually associated with neoplasm or other debilitating diseases.

marantic thrombosis. Thrombosis, usually of a cerebral sinus, associated with a wasting disease.

marantic thrombus. A thrombus occurring in an area of retarded blood flow, as the atria.

marasmic kwashiorkor. Kwashiorkor in which there is caloric deficiency as well as protein deficiency.

marasmic thrombosis. MARANTIC THROMBOSIS.

ma·ras·mus (muh·raz'mus) *n.* [NL., from Gk. *marasmos*, a wasting, withering]. Chronic severe wasting of the tissues of the body, particularly in children, resulting in loss of subcutaneous fat, inelastic, wrinkled skin, loss of muscle tissue and strength, growth failure, lethargy, and often acidosis and hypoproteinemia; may be due to chronic severe malnutrition or defective absorption or utilization of a good food supply. —**maras·mic** (·mick) *adj.*

marble bone. 1. OSTEOPETROSIS. 2. The osteopetrotic form of lymphomatosis in chickens.

mar·ble·iza·tion (mahr''bul·eye·zay'shun, ·i·zay'shun) *n.* The condition of being marked or veined like marble.

marble skin. CUTIS MARMORATA.

Marboran. Trademark for methisazone, an antiviral agent.

Mar·burg virus [*Marburg*, West Germany]. A large arbovirus transmitted by green monkeys, *Cercopithecus aethiops*, to man; reported in 1968 in Marburg and Frankfurt, West Germany. See also *green monkey fever.*

Marburg virus disease. GREEN MONKEY FEVER.

marc, *n.* [F., from MF. *marchier*, to trample]. The residue remaining after the extraction of the active principles from a vegetable drug, or after the extraction of the juice or oil from fruits.

Marcaine. A trademark for bupivacaine, a local anesthetic.

march albuminuria. Proteinuria associated with long walks or runs.

marche à pe·tit pas (mahrsh ah p'tee pah') [F., gait with a small step]. A slow, shuffling, short-stepped uncertain gait, associated with a slightly flexed posture and a loss of adaptive movements; observed usually in the aged and senile.

Mar·che·sa·ni syndrome (mar''ke·zah'nee) [O. *Marchesani*, German ophthalmologist, 1900–1952]. WEILL-MARCHESANI SYNDROME.

march foot. A foot crippled by march fracture.

march fracture. A fracture usually of the metatarsal bones, without obvious trauma, as a result of marching, running, etc. See also *fatigue fracture.*

march hemoglobinuria. A paroxysmal hemoglobinuria noted sometimes after strenuous marching.

Mar·chia·fa·va-Bi·gna·mi disease (mar''kyah·fah'vah, been·nyah'mee) [E. *Marchiafava*, Italian physician, 1847–1935; and A. *Bignami*, Italian pathologist, 1862–1929]. A disease of unknown cause, observed almost exclusively in alcoholic men and characterized by a degeneration of the middle portion of the corpus callosum and, in advanced cases, of the central portions of the anterior and posterior commissures, the superior cerebellar peduncles and centrum ovale. The clinical manifestations are variable and may include coma, dementia, seizures, focal neurologic signs and a frontal lobe syndrome. Syn. *primary degeneration of the corpus callosum.*

Marchiafava-Micheli syndrome [E. *Marchiafava* and F. *Micheli*]. PAROXYSMAL NOCTURNAL HEMOGLOBINURIA.

Marchiafava's disease. MARCHIAFAVA-BIGNAMI DISEASE.

Mar·chi's globules (mar'kee) [V. *Marchi*, Italian neurohistologist, 1851–1908]. Portions of myelin, stained with osmic acid, found in degenerating myelin sheaths.

Marck·wald's operation (mark'vahlt) [M. *Marckwald*, German surgeon, 1844–1923]. Removal of two wedge-shaped pieces of the cervix for relief of stenosis of the cervical os.

mar·cor (mahr'kor) *n.* [L., decay]. MARASMUS.

Mar·cus Gunn phenomenon [R. *Marcus Gunn*, English ophthalmologist, 1850–1909]. A partial, usually unilateral congenital and sometimes hereditary ptosis, in which opening of the mouth or chewing and lateral movements of the jaw cause an exaggerated reflex elevation of the upper lid. Compare *Marín Amat syndrome.*

mard el bicha (mahrd'' ul bish'ah) [Ar. *mard el-bisha'*, the bad, or ugly, disease]. KALA AZAR.

Maretin. A trademark for naftalofos, an anthelmintic.

Marey reflex. Changes in the heart rate as specified in Marey's law.

Ma·rey's law (mah·reh') [E. J. *Marey*, French physiologist, 1830–1904]. The heart rate is inversely related to the pressure in the aortic arch and the carotid sinus. Increased pressure produces a reflex bradycardia; decreased pressure produces a reflex tachycardia.

Marezine. Trademark for cyclizine, an antinauseant drug used as the hydrochloride and lactate salts.

Mar·fan's syndrome (mar·fahn') [A. B. J. *Marfan*, French pediatrician, 1858–1942]. 1. A heritable disorder of connective tissue, clinically manifested by skeletal changes such as abnormally long, thin extremities (dolichostenomelia), spidery fingers and toes (arachnodactyly), as well as high-arched palate, defects of the spine and chest, redundant ligaments and joint capsules; by ocular changes including subluxation of the lens, cataract, coloboma, enlarged cornea, strabismus and nystagmus; and by congenital heart disease, particularly weakness of the media of the ascending aorta causing diffuse dilatation and dissection. Chemically there may be an altered ratio of chondroitin sulfate to keratosulfate in costal cartilage, decreased serum mucoproteins, and increased urinary excretion of hydroxyproline. Transmitted as a simple Mendelian dominant with a high degree of penetrance. Compare *homocystinuria.* 2. DENNIE-MARFAN SYNDROME.

mar·ga·ri·to·ma (mahr″guh·ri·to′muh) *n.* [Gk. *margaritēs*, pearl, + *-oma*]. A true primary cholesteatoma formation in the auditory canal.

Mar·gar·o·pus annulatus (mahr·găr′o·pus). *BOÖPHILUS ANNULATUS.*

mar·gin (mahr′jin) *n.* [L. *margo, marginis*]. The boundary or edge of a surface. —**margin·al** (·ul) *adj.*

marginal abscess. An abscess situated near the margin of an orifice, specifically, near the anal orifice.

marginal blepharitis. Inflammation of the hair follicles and sebaceous glands along the margins of the lids.

marginal dystrophy (of Bietti). A form of arcus senilis associated with degeneration of the cornea.

marginal gingiva. The unattached gingiva that surrounds a tooth; it lies occlusally or incisally to the floor of the gingival sulcus and forms its soft tissue wall.

marginal gyrus. PARAHIPPOCAMPAL GYRUS.

marginal infarct. Zone of degeneration forming a yellowish-white fibrous ring, found at term about the edge of the placenta.

marginal keratitis. An inflammation around the periphery of the cornea. Syn. *annular keratitis.*

marginal layer. A narrow nonnuclear zone in the external part of the neural tube.

marginal nucleus. POSTEROMARGINAL NUCLEUS.

marginal process. A prominence situated on the lateral margin of the frontosphenoidal process of the zygomatic bone.

marginal rale. CREPITANT RALE.

marginal ridges. The elevations of enamel located on the mesial and distal aspects of the occlusal surfaces of posterior teeth and the lingual surfaces of maxillary incisors and cuspids.

marginal sinus. 1. An enlarged venous sinus incompletely encircling the margin of the placenta. 2. One of the bilateral, small sinuses of the dura mater which skirt the edge of the foramen magnum, usually uniting posteriorly to form the occipital sinus. 3. A venous sinus surrounding a portion of the white pulp of the spleen. 4. TERMINAL SINUS.

marginal sulcus. A continuation of the cingulate sulcus which turns dorsally at the level of the splenium and forms the caudal margin of the paracentral lobule.

marginal tubercle of the zygomatic bone. The blunt, thickened inferior angle of the zygomatic bone. NA *tuberculum marginale ossis zygomatici.*

marginal ulcer. A peptic ulcer of the jejunum on the efferent margin of a gastrojejunostomy, due to action of acid gastric juice upon the jejunum; associated with pain and bleeding and sometimes with perforation.

marginal zone. The band of tissue lying between the white pulp and red pulp of the spleen.

mar·gin·ation (mahr″ji·nay′shun) *n.* 1. Adhesion of leukocytes to the walls of capillaries in the early stage of inflammation. 2. The establishment or finishing of a dental cavity preparation or restoration.

mar·gino·plas·ty (mahr′ji·no·plas″tee) *n.* Plastic surgery of the marginal portion of the eyelid.

mar·go (mahr′go) *n.*, genit. **mar·gi·nis** (mahr′ji·nis), pl. **margi·nes** (·neez) [L.]. MARGIN.

margo acu·tus cor·dis (a·kew′tus kor′dis). *Obsol.* Right border of the heart.

margo anterior fi·bu·lae (fib′yoo·lee) [NA]. The anterior margin of the fibula.

margo anterior he·pa·tis (hep′uh·tis) [BNA]. MARGO INFERIOR HEPATIS.

margo anterior li·e·nis (lye·ee′nis) [BNA]. MARGO SUPERIOR LIENIS.

margo anterior pan·cre·a·tis (pan·kree′uh·tis) [NA]. The anterior margin of the pancreas.

margo anterior pul·mo·nis (pŏŏl·mo′nis, pul·) [NA]. The anterior margin of either lung.

margo anterior ra·dii (ray′dee·eye) [NA]. The anterior or volar margin of the radius.

margo anterior tes·tis (tes′tis) [NA]. The free border of the testis.

margo anterior ti·bi·ae (tib′ee·ee) [NA]. TIBIAL CREST.

margo anterior ul·nae (ul′nee) [NA]. The anterior margin of the ulna.

margo axil·la·ris sca·pu·lae (ack·si·lair′is skap′yoo·lee) [BNA]. MARGO LATERALIS SCAPULAE.

margo ci·li·a·ris (sil·ee·air′is) [NA]. CILIARY MARGIN.

margo dex·ter cor·dis (decks′tur kor′dis) [NA]. The right border of the heart.

margo dor·sa·lis ra·dii (dor·say′lis ray′dee·eye) [BNA]. MARGO POSTERIOR RADII.

margo dorsalis ul·nae (ul′nee) [BNA]. MARGO POSTERIOR ULNAE.

margo fal·ci·for·mis fas·ci·ae la·tae (fal·si·for′mis fash′ee·ee lay′tee) [BNA]. MARGO FALCIFORMIS HIATUS SAPHENI.

margo falciformis hi·a·tus sa·phe·ni (high·ay′tus sa·fee′nigh) [NA]. The lateral side of the saphenous opening in the fascia lata of the thigh.

margo fi·bu·la·ris pe·dis (fib·yoo·lair′is ped′is) [NA alt.]. MARGO LATERALIS PEDIS.

margo fron·ta·lis alae mag·nae (fron·tay′lis ay′lee mag′nee) [BNA]. MARGO FRONTALIS ALAE MAJORIS.

margo frontalis alae ma·jo·ris (ma·jo′ris) [NA]. The upper border of the greater wing of the sphenoid.

margo frontalis os·sis pa·ri·e·ta·lis (os′is pa·rye″e·tay′lis) [NA]. The anterior border of the parietal bone.

margo in·ci·sa·lis (in·sigh·say′lis) [NA]. The occlusal margin of an incisor tooth.

margo inferior ce·re·bri (serr′e·brye) [NA]. The inferior lateral border of the cerebrum. NA alt. *margo inferolateralis cerebri.*

margo inferior he·pa·tis (hep′uh·tis) [NA]. The anteroinferior border of the liver.

margo inferior li·e·nis (lye·ee′nis) [NA]. The border of the spleen between the diaphragmatic and visceral surfaces.

margo inferior pan·cre·a·tis (pan·kree′uh·tis) [NA]. The inferior margin of the pancreas.

margo inferior pul·mo·nis (pŏŏl·mo′nis) [NA]. The inferior border of the lung.

margo in·fe·ro·la·te·ra·lis ce·re·bri (in″fe·ro·lat·e·ray′lis serr′e·brye) [NA alt.]. MARGO INFERIOR CEREBRI.

margo in·fe·ro·me·di·a·lis ce·re·bri (in″fe·ro·mee·dee·ay′lis serr′e·brye) [NA alt.]. MARGO MEDIALIS CEREBRI.

margo in·fra·gle·noi·da·lis (in″fruh·glen·oy·day′lis) [BNA]. The anterior border of the proximal end of the tibia.

margo in·fra·or·bi·ta·lis (in″fruh·or·bi·tay′lis) [NA]. The lower border of the orbit.

margo in·ter·os·se·us fi·bu·lae (in·tur·os′ee·us fib′yoo·lee) [NA]. The ridge on the medial side of the fibula to which is attached the interosseous membrane.

margo interosseus ra·dii (ray′dee·eye) [NA]. The ridge on the medial side of the radius to which is attached the interosseous membrane.

margo interosseus ti·bi·ae (tib′ee·ee) [NA]. The sharp ridge on the lateral aspect of the shaft of the tibia for the attachment of the interosseous membrane.

margo interosseus ul·nae (ul′nee) [NA]. The sharp margin on the lateral aspect of the shaft of the ulna for the attachment of the interosseous membrane.

margo la·cri·ma·lis max·il·lae (lack·ri·may'lis mack·sil'ee) [NA]. The border of the maxilla which articulates with the lacrimal bone.
margo lamb·doi·de·us (lam·doy'dee·us) [NA]. The border of the occipital bone which articulates with the parietal bones.
margo la·te·ra·lis an·te·bra·chii (lat·e·ray'lis an''te·bray'kee·eye) [NA]. The lateral or radial border of the forearm. NA alt. *margo radialis antebrachii.*
margo lateralis hu·me·ri (hew'mur·eye) [NA]. The lateral border of the humerus.
margo lateralis lin·guae (ling'gwee) [BNA]. The lateral border of the tongue.
margo lateralis pe·dis (ped'is) [NA]. The lateral border of the foot. NA alt. *margo fibularis pedis.*
margo lateralis re·nis (ree'nis) [NA]. The convex border of the kidney.
margo lateralis sca·pu·lae (skap'yoo·lee) [NA]. The lateral or axillary border of the scapula.
margo lateralis un·guis (ung'gwis) [NA]. The lateral margin of a nail, the edge on either side.
margo li·ber ova·rii (lye'bur o·vair'ee·eye) [NA]. The distal or free margin of an ovary.
margo liber un·guis (ung'gwis) [NA]. The distal or free edge of a nail.
margo lin·guae (ling'gwee) [NA]. The border of the tongue.
margo ma·stoi·de·us (mas·toy'dee·us) [NA]. The border of the occipital bone which articulates with the mastoid portion of the temporal bone.
margo me·di·a·lis an·te·bra·chii (mee·dee·ay'lis an''te·bray'kee·eye) [NA]. The medial or ulnar border of the forearm. NA alt. *margo ulnaris antebrachii.*
margo medialis ce·re·bri (serr'e·brye) [NA]. The inferior medial border of the cerebrum. NA alt. *margo inferomedialis cerebri.*
margo medialis glan·du·lae su·pra·re·na·lis (glan'dew·lee sue·pruh·re·nay'lis) [NA]. The medial margin of the suprarenal gland.
margo medialis hu·me·ri (hew'mur·eye) [NA]. The medial border of the humerus.
margo medialis pe·dis (ped'is) [NA]. The medial border of the foot. NA alt. *margo tibialis pedis.*
margo medialis re·nis (ree'nis) [NA]. The medial or concave border of the kidney.
margo medialis sca·pu·lae (skap'yoo·lee) [NA]. The medial or vertebral border of the scapula.
margo medialis ti·bi·ae (tib'ee·ee) [NA]. The medial border of the tibia.
margo me·so·va·ri·cus (mes''o·vair'i·kus) [NA]. The border of the ovary to which is attached the mesovarium.
margo na·sa·lis (na·say'lis) [NA]. The border of the frontal bone which articulates with the nasal bones.
margo na·si (nay'zye) [BNA]. MARGO NASALIS.
margo ob·tu·sus cor·dis (ob·tew'sus kor'dis). *Obsol.* The left border of the heart.
margo oc·ci·pi·ta·lis os·sis pa·ri·e·ta·lis (ock·sip·i·tay'lis os'is pa·rye''e·tay'lis) [NA]. The border of the parietal bone which articulates with the occipital bone.
margo occipitalis ossis tem·po·ra·lis (tem·po·ray'lis). The border of the temporal bone which articulates with the occipital bone.
margo oc·cul·tus un·guis (o·kul'tus ung'gwis) [NA]. The buried proximal end of the nail.
margo pa·ri·e·ta·lis alae ma·jo·ris (pa·rye''e·tay'lis ay'lee ma·jo'ris) [NA]. The border of the greater wing of the sphenoid bone which articulates with the parietal bone.
margo parietalis os·sis fron·ta·lis (os'is fron·tay'lis) [NA]. The border of the frontal bone which articulates with the parietal bones.
margo parietalis ossis tem·po·ra·lis (tem·po·ray'lis) [NA]. The border of the temporal bone which articulates with the parietal bone.
margo pe·dis la·te·ra·lis (ped'is lat·e·ray'lis) [BNA]. MARGO LATERALIS PEDIS.
margo pedis me·di·a·lis (mee·dee·ay'lis) [BNA]. MARGO MEDIALIS PEDIS.
margo posterior fi·bu·lae (fib'yoo·lee) [NA]. A vertical ridge on the shaft of the fibula; it is more properly regarded as being on the posterior aspect than on the lateral aspect.
margo posterior li·e·nis (lye·ee'nis) [BNA]. MARGO INFERIOR LIENIS.
margo posterior pan·cre·a·tis (pan·kree'uh·tis) [BNA]. MARGO INFERIOR PANCREATIS.
margo posterior par·tis pe·tro·sae (pahr'tis pe·tro'see) [NA]. The margin on the petrous portion of the temporal bone that separates the posterior and inferior surfaces of that portion.
margo posterior ra·dii (ray'dee·eye) [NA]. The posterior border of the radius.
margo posterior tes·tis (tes'tis) [NA]. The posterior border of the testis to which is attached the epididymis and ductus deferens.
margo posterior ul·nae (ul'nee) [NA]. The posterior border of the ulna.
margo pu·pil·la·ris iri·dis (pew·pi·lair'is eye'ri·dis) [NA]. The inner circular border of the iris surrounding the pupil.
margo ra·di·a·lis an·te·bra·chii (ray·dee·ay'lis an''te·bray'kee·eye) [NA alt.]. MARGO LATERALIS ANTEBRACHII.
margo sa·git·ta·lis (saj·i·tay'lis) [NA]. The border of a parietal bone which articulates with the corresponding border of the other parietal bone.
margo sphe·noi·da·lis (sfee·noy·day'lis) [NA]. The border of the temporal bone which articulates with the greater wing of the sphenoid bone.
margo squa·mo·sus alae mag·nae (skway·mo'sus ay'lee mag'nae) [BNA]. MARGO SQUAMOSUS ALAE MAJORIS.
margo squamosus alae ma·jo·ris (ma·jo'ris) [NA]. The border of the greater wing of the sphenoid bone which articulates with the squamous portion of the temporal bone.
margo squamosus os·sis pa·ri·e·ta·lis (os'is pa·rye·e·tay'lis) [NA]. The border of the parietal bone which articulates with the squamous portion of the temporal bone.
margo superior ce·re·bri (serr'e·brye) [NA]. The superior medial border of the cerebrum. NA alt. *margo superior cerebri.*
margo superior glan·du·lae su·pra·re·na·lis (glan'dew·lee sue''pruh·re·nay'lis) [NA]. The upper border of the suprarenal gland.
margo superior li·e·nis (lye·ee'nis) [NA]. The sharp, serrated border of the spleen.
margo superior pan·cre·a·tis (pan·kree'uh·tis) [NA]. The superior border of the pancreas.
margo superior par·tis pe·tro·sae (pahr'tis pe·tro'see) [NA]. The margin that separates the posterior surface of the petrous portion of the temporal bone from the anterior surface.
margo superior sca·pu·lae (skap'yoo·lee) [NA]. The superior border of the scapula.
margo su·pe·ro·me·di·a·lis ce·re·bri (sue''pur·o·mee·dee·ay'lis serr'e·brye) [NA alt.]. MARGO SUPERIOR CEREBRI.
margo su·pra·or·bi·ta·lis (sue''pruh·or·bi·tay'lis) [NA]. The upper portion of the margin of the orbit.
margo ti·bi·a·lis pe·dis (tib·ee·ay'lis ped'is) [NA alt.]. MARGO MEDIALIS PEDIS.
margo ul·na·ris an·te·bra·chii (ul·nair'is an''te·bray'kee·eye) [NA alt.]. MARGO MEDIALIS ANTEBRACHII.
margo ute·ri (yoo'tur·eye) [NA]. The edge on either side of the uterus to which the broad ligament is attached.
margo ver·te·bra·lis sca·pu·lae (vur·te·bray'lis skap'yoo·lee) [BNA]. MARGO MEDIALIS SCAPULAE.
margo vo·la·ris ra·dii (vo·lair'is ray'dee·eye) [BNA]. MARGO ANTERIOR RADII.
margo volaris ul·nae (ul'nee) [BNA]. MARGO ANTERIOR ULNAE.

margo zy·go·ma·ti·cus alae mag·nae (zye·go·mat'i·kus ay'lee mag'nee) [BNA]. Margo zygomaticus alae majoris. (= ZYGOMATIC MARGIN).

margo zygomaticus alae ma·jo·ris (ma·jo'ris) [NA]. ZYGOMATIC MARGIN.

Ma·rie-Bam·ber·ger disease [P. *Marie*, French neurologist, 1853–1940; and E. *Bamberger*]. HYPERTROPHIC PULMONARY OSTEOARTHROPATHY.

Marie-Foix retraction sign [P. *Marie* and C. *Foix*]. In upper motor neuron paralysis of the legs, squeezing of the toes or forcing the toes or foot downward results in dorsiflexion at the ankle and flexion withdrawal at the hip and knee; a spinal defense mechanism.

Marie's ataxia [P. *Marie*]. MARIE'S HEREDITARY CEREBELLAR ATAXIA.

Marie's disease [P. *Marie*]. Rheumatic spondylitis involving the spine only, or invading the shoulders and hips. See also *Strümpell-Marie disease.*

Marie's hereditary cerebellar ataxia. A category of hereditary ataxia, created by Pierre Marie in 1893, to designate a form of ataxia which he presumed to be related to atrophy of the cerebellum rather than to atrophy of the spinal cord. The distinguishing features of the cerebellar form were said to be a later age of onset, more definite hereditary transmission, persistence of hyperactivity of tendon reflexes, and more frequent occurrence of ophthalmoplegia and optic atrophy.

Marie's syndrome [P. *Marie*]. ACROMEGALY.

Marie-Strümpell arthritis, disease, or **spondylitis** [P. *Marie* and E. *Strümpell*]. ANKYLOSING SPONDYLITIS.

Marie-Strümpell encephalitis [P. *Marie* and E. *Strümpell*]. A focal imflammatory lesion of the brain observed in an infant with acute hemiplegia. In the light of current knowledge, the lesion probably represented acute necrotizing hemorrhagic encephalitis.

Marie-Tooth disease [P. *Marie* and H. *Tooth*]. PERONEAL MUSCULAR ATROPHY.

marihuana. MARIJUANA.

mar·i·jua·na. (măr''i·wah'nuh) *n.* [Mexican Sp. *marihuana*]. A relatively crude preparation of cannabis used most often for smoking; a mood-altering or mildly hallucinogenic drug. Compare *hashish.*

Ma·rín Amat syndrome (ma·reen' ah·maht') [M. *Marín Amat*, Spanish, 19th-20th century]. Automatic closure of one eye on opening the mouth, seen in patients who have had a peripheral facial palsy; considered to be an intrafacial associated movement. Syn. *inverse Marcus Gunn phenomenon.* Compare *Marcus Gunn phenomenon.*

Ma·ri·nes·co's hand or **sign** [G. *Marinesco*, Rumanian physician, 1864–1938]. The cold, livid, edematous hand sometimes seen in patients with syringomyelia or other trophic disturbances.

Marinesco-Sjögren-Garland syndrome [G. *Marinesco*, T. *Sjögren*, and H. *Garland*]. A rare hereditary syndrome, transmitted as an autosomal recessive trait and characterized by congenital cerebellar ataxia, cataracts which form in childhood and are progressive, bone abnormalities, dwarfism, and mental retardation.

Marinesco's succulent hand. MARINESCO'S HAND.

Ma·riotte's blind spot (măr·yoht') [E. *Mariotte*, French physicist, 1620–1684]. BLIND SPOT.

Mar·jo·lin's ulcer (mar·zhoh·læn') [J. N. *Marjolin*, French surgeon, 1780–1850]. An ulcer due to malignant change in an indolent ulcer or in a scar.

mark·er. A gene or gene-associated genetic element which is identifiable in individuals possessing it.

marker rescue. The recovery of a gene present in an individual incapable of independent reproduction by recombination with another related individual.

mar·mo·ri·za·tion (mahr''mo·ri·zay'shun) *n.* [L. *marmor*, marble]. MARBLEIZATION.

mar·mo·set (mahr'muh·set) *n.* [OF., grotesque figure]. Any of various small arboreal primates belonging to the family Callitrichidae, which inhabit tropical rain forests in South America; used in dental research and in studies on viral oncology.

Ma·ro·teaux-La·my syndrome (mah·roh·to', lah·mee') [P. *Maroteaux* and M. *Lamy*]. Mucopolysaccharidosis VI, transmitted as an autosomal recessive, characterized chemically by the excessive excretion of chondroitin sulfate B in the urine, and clinically by an appearance similar to that seen in the more common Hurler's syndrome, including marked skeletal changes and corneal opacities, but normal intellectual development.

Marplan. Trademark for isocarboxazid, a monoamine oxidase inhibitor used as an antidepressant drug.

mar·row (măr'o) *n.* [OE. *mærg* ← Gmc. *mazgā* (rel. to Russ. *mozg*, marrow, brain)]. 1. A fatty or soft substance occupying certain cavities; MEDULLA. 2. Specifically, bone marrow: the soft tissues contained in the medullary canals of long bones and in the interstices of cancellous bone. See also *red marrow, yellow marrow.*

marrow space. A marrow-filled space between the trabeculae of cancellous bone.

Mar·schal·ko's plasma cell. PLASMA CELL.

Mar·seilles fever. One of the tick-borne typhus fevers of Africa.

Mar·shall Hall's method [*Marshall Hall*, English physician, 1790–1857]. A method of artificial respiration, no longer used, in which the patient is alternately rolled from his side or back to his abdomen to expand or compress the lungs, expiration being augmented by pressure on the chest. Compare *Holger Nielsen method.*

Marshall's vein [J. *Marshall*, English surgeon and anatomist, 1818–1891]. OBLIQUE VEIN OF THE LEFT ATRIUM.

marsh fever. 1. LEPTOSPIROSIS. 2. MALARIA.

marsh gas. The gaseous products, chiefly methane, formed from decaying, moist organic matter in marshes and mines.

marsh·mal·low, *n.* ALTHEA.

Marsh's test [J. *Marsh*, English chemist, 1794–1846]. A test for arsenic or antimony in which the metal is dissolved in dilute acid, reduced to arsine or stibine in the presence of zinc, and then deposited as metal on a cold surface. Potassium hypochlorite will dissolve arsenic but leave antimony.

Marsilid. A trademark for iproniazid, a tuberculostatic.

Mar·ston deception test [W. M. *Marston*, U.S. psychologist, 1893–1947]. A lie detector test based on changes in systolic blood pressure.

mar·su·pi·al·iza·tion (mahr·sue''pee·ul·eye·zay'shun) *n.* [from *marsupial*, pouched mammal]. An operation for pancreatic, hydatid, and other cysts when extirpation of the cyst walls and complete closure are not possible. The cyst is evacuated and its walls sutured to the edges of the wound, leaving the packed cavity to close by granulation. The procedure has been used also in cases of extrauterine pregnancy when the placenta cannot be removed. —**marsupial·ize** (mahr·sue'pee·ul·ize) *v.*

Mar·ti·not·ti's cells (mar''tee·noht'tee) [Giovanni *Martinotti*, Italian pathologist, 1857–1928]. Nerve cells in the cerebral cortex with axons running toward the surface and ramifying horizontally.

Mar·to·rell's syndrome (Sp. mar·to·rel', Cat. murr·too·rely') [F. *Martorell* Otzet, Spanish, 20th century]. AORTIC ARCH SYNDROME.

Mar·we·del's operation (mar'vey·del) [G. *Marwedel*, German surgeon, contemporary]. A method of gastrostomy similar to Witzel's.

mas·cu·line (mas'kew·lin) *adj.* [L. *masculinus*, from *masculus*, male]. Having the appearance or qualities of a male. —**mas·cu·lin·i·ty** (mas''kew·lin'i·tee) *n.*

masculine pelvis. A pelvis resembling the normal male pelvis; an android pelvis.

masculine protest. 1. *In individual psychology,* the struggle to dominate, which, in excess, is the core of all neurotic disorders. Characterized by aggressive behavior, masculine habits, and the desire to escape identification with the feminine role, which is presumably a more submissive one. Masculine protest is exhibited primarily by women, but to some extent also by men. 2. By extension, the desire of a female to be like a man and have masculine rights and privileges, or of a male to avoid traits presumed to be typical of the female.

mas·cu·lin·ize (mas'kew·lin·ize) *v.* To induce male secondary sex characteristics in a female or in a sexually immature animal. —**masculin·iza·tion** (mas''kew·lin·eye·zay'shun) *n.*

mas·cu·lin·o·ma (mas''kew·lin·o'muh) *n.* ADRENOCORTICOID ADENOMA OF THE OVARY.

mas·cu·lin·ovo·blas·to·ma (mas''kew·lin·o''vo·blas·to'muh) *n.* ADRENOCORTICOID ADENOMA OF THE OVARY.

ma·ser (may'zur) *n.* [*m*icrowave *a*mplification by *s*timulated *e*mission of *r*adiation]. An operating assembly for utilizing the property of certain molecules to emit essentially monochromatic radiation when stimulated with radiation of microwave frequencies. The emitted radiation may be produced as a directional beam of great power. When the stimulating radiation is in the range of optical frequencies (near ultraviolet, visible, and infrared), the operating assembly is called an optical maser or laser.

mask, *n.* [F. *masque*]. 1. A bandage applied to the face. 2. A gauze shield, fitted with tapes, to enclose the mouth and nose during surgical operations. 3. An apparatus for covering the nose and mouth in giving anesthetics.

masked, *adj.* Disguised; concealed; covert, latent.

masked epilepsy. CONVULSIVE EQUIVALENT.

masked facies. MASK FACE.

masked hernia. A type of ventral hernia in which the hernial sac is situated within the abdominal wall.

mask face. An immobile, expressionless face, with flattened and smoother than usual features, seen in pseudobulbar palsy and in parkinsonism. In the latter disorder there may be near-normal voluntary movements of the face and an exaggerated frozen smile, but blinking, spontaneous smiling, and other associated involuntary movements are infrequent.

mask·ing, *n. In audiometry,* the use of a sound stimulus to interfere with the perception of one ear while testing the other.

masklike face. MASK FACE.

mask of pregnancy. Irregularly shaped, brownish patches of varying size which frequently appear on the face and neck during pregnancy; CHLOASMA (1).

mas·o·chism (maz'uh·kiz·um, mas'o·) *n.* [L. von Sacher-*Masoch,* Austrian novelist, 1836–1895]. Pleasure derived from physical or psychological pain inflicted by oneself or by others, often unconsciously invited but sometimes sought out consciously as in flagellation; a sexual component is always present; and in moral masochism there is an implication of punishment for some feeling of guilt. Masochistic tendencies exist to some extent in many human relationships and to a larger degree in most psychiatric disorders. It is the opposite of sadism but the two conditions tend to coexist in the same individual. —**maso·chist** (·kist) *n.;* **masochis·tic** (maz''uh·kis'tick) *adj.*

Ma·son's incision [J. T. *Mason,* U.S. surgeon, 1882–1936]. A vertical zigzag incision which permits wide exposure of the upper abdominal cavity while preserving the nerve supply of the rectus muscles.

masque bi·liare (bee·lyair') [F., lit., biliary mask]. Excess pigmentation of the eyelids; seen more often in women. Syn. *periocular hyperpigmentation.*

mass, *n.* [L. *massa,* from Gk. *maza,* lump, mass]. 1. That essential property of matter which is responsible for inertia and weight. See also *atomic mass.* 2. A relatively solid or bulky piece of any substance or part of any object. 3. A cohesive medicinal substance that may be formed into pills. 4. (*In attributive use*) Space-occupying (as: mass lesion).

mas·sa (mas'uh) *n.,* pl. & genit. sing. **mas·sae** (·ee) [L.]. MASS (2).

mas·sage (muh·sahzh') *n.* [F., from *masser,* to massage]. The act of rubbing, kneading, or stroking the superficial parts of the body with the hand or with an instrument, for therapeutic purposes such as modifying nutrition, restoring power of movement, breaking up adhesions, or improving the circulation.

massa in·ter·me·dia (in''tur·mee'dee·uh) [BNA]. ADHESIO INTERTHALAMICA.

massa la·te·ra·lis at·lan·tis (lat·e·ray'lis at·lan'tis) [NA]. The strong lateral portion of each side of the atlas with which the occipital condyles articulate.

mass defect. The difference between the mass of an isotope and its mass number expressed in atomic mass units; energy equivalent to the mass defect is considered to be the binding energy of the atom.

mas·se·ter (ma·see'tur) *n.* [Gk. *masētēr,* chewer]. A muscle of mastication, arising from the zygomatic arch, and inserted into the mandible. NA *musculus masseter.* See also Table of Muscles in the Appendix.

mas·se·ter·ic (mas·e·terr'ick) *adj.* Of or pertaining to the masseter.

masseter reflex. JAW JERK.

mas·seur (ma·sur') *n.* [F.]. 1. A man who practices massage. 2. An instrument used for mechanical massage.

mas·seuse (ma·suhz', ·soos') *n.* [F.]. A woman who practices massage.

mas·sive myoclonic jerk. INFANTILE SPASM.

massive spasm. INFANTILE SPASM.

mass lesion. Any space-occupying lesion in the central nervous system, particularly the brain, such as an abscess, hematoma, or tumor.

mass number. The whole number nearest the atomic weight of a given atomic species; the total number of nucleons (protons and neutrons) in the nucleus of the atom described.

Mas·son body (mah·sohn') [Pierre *Masson,* Canadian pathologist, 1880–1959]. Fibrin and macrophages in the pulmonary alveoli in organizing pneumonia of any cause, originally thought to be associated with rheumatic pneumonitis.

Masson's trichrome stain. A method for differentiating tissue components using hematoxylin, acid fuchsin, ponceau, and aniline blue dyes.

mas·so·ther·a·py (mas''o·therr'uh·pee) *n.* Treatment by massage.

mass reflex. Exaggerated withdrawal reflexes accompanied by profuse sweating, piloerection, and automatic emptying of the bladder and occasionally of the rectum; observed in patients with transection of the spinal cord, during the stage of heightened reflex activity. See also *Riddoch's mass reflex.*

mass spectrometer. An instrument which magnetically separates a beam of positively charged ions of different masses into beams of ions of the same mass, and electrically or photographically records the intensity of the beams thus produced.

mast-, masto- [Gk. *mastos,* breast]. A combining form meaning (a) *breast;* (b) *mastoid.*

mast·ad·e·ni·tis (mast''ad·e·nigh'tis) *n.* [*mast-* + *adenitis*]. MASTITIS.

mast·ad·e·no·ma (mast''ad·e·no'muh) *n.* [*mast-* + *adenoma*]. A glandular tumor of the breast.

mas·tal·gia (mas·tal'juh, ·jee·uh) *n.* [*mast-* + *-algia*]. Pain in the breast. Syn. *mastodynia* (1).

mas·ta·tro·phia (mas''ta·tro'fee·uh) *n.* MASTATROPHY.

mast·at·ro·phy (mast·at'ruh·fee) *n.* [*mast-* + *-atrophy*]. Atrophy of the breast.

mas·tauxy (mas·tawk'see) *n.* [*mast-* + Gk. *auxē*, growth, increase]. Increase in size, or excessive size, of the breast.
mast cell [Ger. *Mastzelle*, from *Mast*, forced fattening, + *Zelle*, cell]. A type of connective tissue cell associated with the formation and storage of heparin, histamine, and other pharmacologically active substances. It is characterized by numerous large, basophil, metachromatic granules.
mast-cell disease. MASTOCYTOSIS.
mast-cell leukemia. Leukemia in which the anaplastic cells resemble mast cells.
mast-cell tumor. MASTOCYTOMA.
mast·ec·chy·mo·sis (mas·teck''i·mo'sis) *n.* Ecchymosis of the breast.
mas·tec·to·my (mas·teck'tuh·mee) *n.* [*mast-* + *-ectomy*]. Excision, or amputation, of the breast.
Mas·ter's two-step test [A. M. *Master*, U.S. physician, 1895–1973]. TWO-STEP TEST.
mast·hel·co·sis (mast''hel·ko'sis, mas''thel·) *n.* [*mast-* + Gk. *helkōsis*, ulceration]. Ulceration of the breast.
-mastia [*mast-* + *-ia*]. A combining form meaning *condition of the breast.*
mas·tic (mas'tick) *n.* [Gk. *mastichē*]. The resin flowing from the incised bark of the *Pistacia lentiscus*. Formerly used as a styptic and as a varnish in microscopy.
mas·ti·cate (mas'ti·kate) *v.* [L. *masticare*]. To chew. —**mas·ti·ca·tion** (mas''ti·kay'shun) *n.*
mas·ti·ca·tor (mas'ti·kay''tur) *adj.* Of or pertaining to chewing or mastication.
masticator nerve. The motor portion of the trigeminal nerve. See also Table of Nerves in the Appendix.
masticator nucleus. MOTOR NUCLEUS OF THE TRIGEMINAL NERVE.
mas·ti·ca·to·ry (mas'ti·kuh·to''ree) *adj.* & *n.* 1. For or pertaining to mastication. 2. A medicinal preparation to be chewed but not swallowed; used for its local action in the mouth.
masticatory spasm of the face. TRISMUS.
masticatory surface. The occlusal or biting surface of a tooth.
masticatory system. The functional unit of mastication composed of the teeth, their surrounding and supportive structures, the jaws, the temporomandibular joints, the muscles which are attached to the mandible, lip and tongue muscles, and the vascular and nervous systems for these tissues.
mastic test. A test similar in principle to Lange's colloidal gold test but using a colloidal suspension of gum mastic as the reagent with varying dilutions of cerebrospinal fluid.
Mas·ti·goph·o·ra (mas''ti·gof'ur·uh) *n.pl.* [Gk. *mastix*, *mastigos*, whip, + *phoros*, bearing]. A class of flagellated protozoa which includes both free-living and parasitic species.
mas·ti·tis (mas·tye'tis) *n.* [*mast-* + *-itis*]. Inflammation of the breast.
masto-. See *mast-*.
mas·to·car·ci·no·ma (mas''to·kahr''si·no'muh) *n.* A mammary carcinoma.
mas·to·cyte (mas'to·site) *n.* MAST CELL.
mas·to·cy·to·ma (mas''to·sigh·to'muh) *n.* [*mastocyte* + *-oma*]. A local proliferation of mast cells forming a tumorous nodule, seen most commonly in dogs, less frequently in cats, oxen, and men.
mas·to·cy·to·sis (mas''to·sigh·to'sis) *n.* [*mastocyte* + *-osis*]. Excessive proliferation of mast cells, either local (mastocytoma) or systemic.
mas·to·dyn·ia (mas''to·din'ee·uh) *n.* [*mast-* + *-odynia*]. 1. A pain in the breast. Syn. *mastalgia*. 2. A type of mammary dysplasia in which pain and tenderness are prominent symptoms.
mas·to·de·al·gia (mas''to·dee·al'jee·uh) *n.* MASTOIDALGIA.
mas·toid (mas'toid) *adj.* & *n.* [Gk. *mastoeidēs*, like a breast]. 1. Breast-shaped, as the mastoid process of the temporal bone. 2. The mastoid portion of the temporal bone.
mastoid air cell. MASTOID CELL.
mas·toid·al·gia (mas''toy·dal'jee·uh) *n.* [*mastoid* + *-algia*]. Pain in, or over, the mastoid process.
mastoid angle. The posterior inferior corner of the parietal bone where it articulates with the mastoid part of the temporal bone. NA *angulus mastoideus ossis parietalis.*
mastoid antrum. The pneumatic space between the epitympanic recess and the mastoid cells. NA *antrum mastoideum.*
mastoid canaliculus. A canaliculus opening in the jugular fossa just above the stylomastoid foramen, through which the auricular branch of the vagus nerve enters the temporal bone. NA *canaliculus mastoideus.*
mastoid cell. One of the compartments in the mastoid part of the temporal bone, connected with the mastoid antrum and lined with a thin mucous membrane. Syn. *mastoid air cell.*
mas·toid·ec·to·my (mas''toy·deck'tuh·mee) *n.* [*mastoid* + *-ectomy*]. Exenteration of the mastoid cells.
mastoid emissary vein. A fairly constant venous channel passing through the mastoid process of the temporal bone and connecting the sigmoid sinus with the occipital vein. NA *vena emissaria mastoidea.*
mastoid fontanel. POSTEROLATERAL FONTANEL.
mastoid foramen. A small foramen behind the mastoid process; it transmits a small artery from the dura mater and a vein opening into the lateral sinus. NA *foramen mastoideum.*
mastoid fossa. The fossa on the lateral surface of the temporal bone, behind the suprameatal spine.
mas·toid·itis (mas''toid·eye'tis) *n.*, pl. **mastoid·it·i·des** (·it'i·deez) [*mastoid* + *-itis*]. Inflammation of the mastoid cells.
mastoid notch. A groove on the medial surface of the mastoid process, which serves as the site of origin of the posterior belly of the digastric muscle. Syn. *digastric groove.* NA *incisura mastoidea.*
mas·toid·ot·o·my (mas''toy·dot'uh·mee) *n.* [*mastoid* + *-tomy*]. Incision into mastoid cells or the mastoid antrum.
mastoid process. The blunt inferior projection of the mastoid part of the temporal bone; it may be described as nipple-shaped. NA *processus mastoideus.*
mastoid ridge. The bony ridge on the mastoid process for the attachment of the sternocleidomastoid muscle.
mastoid sinus. MASTOID CELL.
mas·ton·cus (mas·tonk'us) *n.* [*mast-* + Gk. *onkos*, tumor]. Any tumor of the mammary gland or nipple.
mas·to·pa·ri·etal (mas''to·puh·rye'uh·tul) *adj.* [*masto-* + *parietal*]. PARIETOMASTOID.
mas·top·a·thy (mas·top'uth·ee) *n.* [*masto-* + *-pathy*]. Any disease or pain of the mammary gland.
mas·to·pexy (mas'to·peck''see) *n.* [*masto-* + *-pexy*]. Surgical fixation of a pendulous breast.
mas·to·pla·sia (mas''to·play'zhuh, ·zee·uh) *n.* [*masto-* + *-plasia*]. 1. Hyperplasia of breast tissue. 2. MASTODYNIA (2).
mas·to·plas·tia (mas''to·plas'tee·uh) *n.* MASTOPLASIA.
mas·to·plas·ty (mas'to·plas''tee) *n.* [*masto-* + *-plasty*]. Plastic surgery on the breast.
mas·tor·rha·gia (mas''to·ray'jee·uh) *n.* [*masto-* + *-rrhagia*]. Hemorrhage from the breast.
mas·to·scir·rhus (mas''to·skirr'us, ·sirr'us) *n.* Hardening, or scirrhus, of the breast; usually cancer.
mas·tos·to·my (mas·tos'tuh·mee) *n.* [*masto-* + *-stomy*]. Incision into the breast.
mas·tot·o·my (mas·tot'uh·mee) *n.* [*masto-* + *-tomy*]. Incision of the breast.
mas·tous (mas'tus) *adj.* [*mast-* + *-ous*]. Having large breasts.
mas·tur·bate (mas'tur·bate) *v.* [L. *masturbari*]. To manipulate the genitalia, usually producing an orgasm. —**mas·tur·ba·tion** (mas''tur·bay'shun) *n.*
Mat·as' operation (mat'us) [R. *Matas*, U.S. surgeon, 1860–1957]. A method of endoaneurysmorrhaphy.
match, *v.* To supply as nearly exact a counterpart as possible of a desired object, through comparison of the character-

istics of that object with possible sources of counterparts, as the selection of blood donors whose erythrocytes have the same antigens as those of the recipient. See also *cross matching.*

mate, *v.* To pair for breeding; to copulate.

ma·te·ria al·ba (ma·teer'ee·uh al'buh) [L., white material]. A soft, cheeselike, white deposit on the necks of teeth and adjacent gums, made up of epithelial cells, leukocytes, bacteria, and molds.

materia med·i·ca (med'i·kuh) [L.]. 1. The science that treats of the sources, properties, and preparation of medicinal substances. 2. A treatise on these substances.

ma·te·ri·es mor·bi (ma·teer'ee·eez mor'bye, mor'bee) [L.]. The material or principle that is the cause of a disease.

materies pec·cans (peck'anz) [L., the offending matter]. MATERIES MORBI.

ma·ter·nal (muh·tur'nul) *adj.* [L. *maternus*]. Pertaining to a mother.

maternal dystocia. Difficult labor due to deformities within the mother.

maternal impressions. The congenital developmental effects formerly thought to be produced upon the fetus in the uterus by mental impressions of a vivid character received by the mother during pregnancy.

maternal inheritance. The acquisition of any characteristic that is causally dependent upon a peculiarity of the egg cytoplasm, as dextral and sinistral coiling of snail shells.

maternal mortality rate. The number of deaths reported as due to puerperal causes in a calendar year per 100,000 live births reported in the same year and place.

maternal phenylketonuria. Physical and mental retardation, particularly with microcephaly, in non-phenylketonuric offspring of mothers who have phenylketonuria; thought to be due to the effects of elevated phenylalanine levels in the heterozygous fetus whose own phenylalanine hydroxylase may as yet be insufficient.

maternal placenta. The external layer developed from the decidua basalis.

ma·ter·ni·ty (muh·tur'ni·tee) *n.* [L. *maternitas*]. 1. Motherhood. 2. PARTURITION.

maternity hospital. A hospital restricted to the care of women during pregnancy and parturition.

ma·ti·co (ma·tee'ko) *n.* [Sp., dim. from *Mateo,* Matthew]. The leaves of *Piper angustifolium,* of the Piperaceae. Aromatic and stimulant; has been used as a local and general hemostatic and as a stimulant to mucous membranes.

mat·ri·car·ia (mat"ri·kăr'ee·uh) *n.* [L., from *matrix,* womb]. German chamomile; the flower tops of *Matricaria chamomilla,* of the family Compositae. Has been used as an aromatic bitter.

matrices. A plural of *matrix.*

mat·ri·cide (mat'ri·side) *n.* [L. *matricidium* and *matricida*]. 1. The murder of one's own mother. 2. A person who murders his own mother.

ma·trix (may'tricks) *n.,* pl. **mat·ri·ces** (mat'ri·seez), **matrixes** [L.]. 1. A mold; the cavity in which anything is formed. 2. That part of tissue into which any organ or process is set, as the matrix of a nail. 3. GROUND SUBSTANCE. 4. An arrangement of mathematical elements in rows and columns for special algebraic evaluation. Adj. *matrical.*

matrix un·guis (ung'gwis) [NA]. NAIL BED.

Matromycin. A trademark for oleandomycin, an antibacterial.

matt, *adj.* [F. *mat, matte*]. 1. Dull, not glossy; rough. 2. Specifically, of hemolytic streptococci, having a flattened and rough colonial form resulting from the collapse of the capsular hyaluronate gel. Abbreviated, M.

mat·ter, *n.* [F. *matière,* from L. *materia*]. 1. Any material or substance, described as having three states of aggregation, solid, liquid, or gaseous. 2. PUS.

mat·tress suture. A suture in which the needle, after being drawn through both skin edges, is reinserted on the far side and drawn through the original side again. This may be continuous or interrupted.

Matulane. Trademark for procarbazine, an antineoplastic agent used as the hydrochloride salt.

mat·u·rate (mat'yoo·rate) *v.* 1. To bring or come to maturity, to ripen. 2. Of a boil, to bring or come to a head.

mat·u·ra·tion (match"oo·ray'shun, mat"yoo·) *n.* [L. *maturatio,* ripening]. 1. The process of coming to full development. 2. The final series of changes in the growth and formation of the germ cells. It includes two divisions of the cell body but only one division of the chromosomes, with the result that the number of chromosomes in the mature germ cell is reduced to one-half (haploid, n) the original number (diploid, 2n). The term also includes the cytoplasmic changes which occur in the preparation of the germ cell for fertilization. 3. The achievement of emotional and intellectual maturity. Compare *psychomotor development.*

ma·ture (muh·tewr') *adj. & v.* [L. *maturus*]. 1. Fully developed, full grown, ripe. 2. To become ripe, to attain full development.

mature cataract. A cataract in which the whole lens is opaque, of a dull gray or amber color, and in which the opacity has advanced to the anterior capsule and no shadow is thrown by the iris on the lens with focal illumination. Such a cataract is suitable for extraction.

ma·tur·i·ty (muh·tewr'i·tee) *n.* 1. The state of being mature. 2. The period of life when the organs of reproduction become and remain best capable of functioning. 3. The stage between adolescence or youth and old age or senescense.

maturity-onset diabetes. Diabetes mellitus which develops later in life, characterized by more gradual development and less severe symptoms than juvenile-onset diabetes.

ma·tu·ti·nal (muh·tew'ti·nul) *adj.* [L. *matutinalis,* of the morning]. Occurring in the morning, as matutinal nausea.

Mauch·art's ligaments (mαwkh'art) [B. D. *Mauchart,* German anatomist, 1696–1751]. The alar ligaments of the median atlantoaxial articulation.

Mau·noir's hydrocele (mo·nwahr') [J. P. *Maunoir,* Swiss surgeon, 1768–1861]. A congenital lymphatic cyst of the neck.

Maurer's clefts. MAURER'S DOTS.

Mau·rer's dots (mαw'rur) [G. *Maurer,* German physician, 20th century]. Red dots in Leishman-stained erythrocytes infected by *Plasmodium falciparum.*

Mau·riac syndrome (mo·ryahk') [P. *Mauriac,* French physician, b. 1882]. Juvenile diabetes mellitus, growth retardation, obesity, and hepatomegaly, probably related to inadequate control of the diabetic state.

Mau·ri·ceau's method (mo·ree·so') [F. *Mauriceau,* French obstetrician, 1637–1709]. In breech delivery, the fingers of the physician are introduced into the vagina to guide the aftercoming head with the infant resting on the physician's forearm. Gentle pressure is applied above the symphysis pubis by an assistant.

Mauth·ner's sheath (mαwt'nur) [L. *Mauthner,* Austrian ophthalmologist, 1840–1894]. AXOLEMMA.

maw worm. *ASCARIS EQUORUM.*

Maxibolin. Trademark for ethylestrenol, an anabolic steroid.

max·il·la (mack·sil'uh) *n.,* pl. & genit. sing. **maxil·lae** (·ee) [L., jaw] [NA]. The bone of the upper jaw. See also Table of Bones in the Appendix and Plate 1.

max·il·lary (mack"si·lerr·ee) *adj.* Of or pertaining to the maxilla. See also Table of Arteries in the Appendix.

maxillary air sinus. MAXILLARY SINUS.

maxillary antrum. MAXILLARY SINUS.

maxillary arch. PALATOMAXILLARY ARCH.

maxillary artery. NA *arteria maxillaris.* See Table of Arteries in the Appendix.

maxillary bone. MAXILLA.

maxillary canals. The alveolar canals of the maxilla. See *alveolar canals.*

maxillary hiatus. A hiatus on the inner aspect of the body of the maxilla, establishing communication between the nasal cavity and maxillary sinus.

maxillary nerve. A somatic sensory nerve, attached to the trigeminal nerve, which innervates the meninges, the skin of the upper portion of the face, the upper teeth, and the mucosa of the nose, palate, and cheeks. NA *nervus maxillaris.*

maxillary palatal process. MAXILLARY PROCESS (3).

maxillary plexuses. Nerve plexuses found around facial and maxillary arteries, designated the external and internal maxillary plexuses, respectively.

maxillary process. 1. (of the embryo:) An embryonic outgrowth from the dorsal part of the mandibular arch that forms the lateral part of the upper lip, the upper cheek region, and the upper jaw except the premaxilla. 2. (of the inferior nasal concha:) A thin plate of bone descending from the ethmoid process of the inferior nasal concha, and hooking over the lower edge of the maxillary hiatus. NA *processus maxillaris conchae nasalis inferioris.* 3. (of the palatine bone:) A variable projecting lamina of the anterior border of the palatine bone which is directed forward and closes in the lower and back part of the maxillary hiatus. 4. (of the zygomatic bone:) A rough, triangular process from the anterior surface of the zygomatic bone which articulates with the maxilla; usually given as part of the infraorbital process.

maxillary sinus. The paranasal sinus in the maxilla. Syn. *antrum of Highmore.* NA *sinus maxillaris.* See also Plate 12.

maxillary tuber or **tuberosity.** A protuberance on the lower part of the infratemporal surface of the maxillary bone; the medial side articulates with the pyramidal process of the palatine bone. NA *tuber maxillae.*

max·il·lo·fa·cial (mack·sil″o·fay′shul) *adj.* [*maxilla* + *facial*]. Pertaining to the lower half of the face.

maxillofacial prosthesis. A substitute for a jaw, nose, or cheek, when the loss is too extensive for surgical repair alone.

max·il·lo-fron·ta·le (mack·sil″o·fron·tah′lee, ·fron·tay′lee) *n.* [*maxilla* + os *frontale*]. *In craniometry,* the point where the anterior lacrimal crest or its prolongation meets the frontomaxillary suture.

max·il·lo·lac·ri·mal (mack·sil″o·lack′ri·mul) *adj.* Pertaining to the maxilla and the lacrimal bone.

maxillolacrimal suture. The union between the lacrimal and maxillary bones. NA *sutura lacrimomaxillaris.*

max·il·lo·man·dib·u·lar (mack·sil″o·man·dib′yoo·lur) *adj.* Pertaining to the maxillae and the mandible.

max·il·lo·tur·bi·nal (mack·sil″o·tur′bi·nul) *n.* [*maxilla* + *turbinate*]. INFERIOR NASAL CONCHA.

max·i·mal (mack′si·mul) *adj.* Pertaining to the maximum; highest; greatest.

maximal ejection phase. RAPID EJECTION PHASE.

maximal stimulus. A stimulus of such intensity that an increment in stimulus intensity produces no increment of response.

max·i·mum, *n.*, pl. **maxi·ma** (·muh) [L., largest, greatest]. The greatest possible degree or amount of anything; the highest point attained or attainable by anything.

maximum and minimum thermometer. A thermometer that registers the maximum and minimum temperatures to which it has been exposed.

maximum breathing capacity. The greatest amount of air which can be voluntarily breathed during a 10-to-30-second period, and expressed as liters of air per minute. It is a test of many factors, including patient cooperation, his physical state, muscular function and lung compliance. Adequately performed, it is a reliable test of the ventilatory capacity of the thoracic bellows. Abbreviated, MBC.

maximum dose. The largest dose consistent with safety.

maximum occipital point. OPISTHOCRANION.

maximum security unit. *In medicine,* a prisonlike ward or building within a general or mental hospital for confining and treating patients, especially mental ones, whose symptoms are a physical threat to the safety of others or who have committed major crimes.

maximum transverse arc. The measurement across the face from a point on each side just anterior to the external auditory meatus.

Maxipen. A trademark for the potassium salt of the antibiotic phenethicillin.

May apple, may·ap·ple. PODOPHYLLUM.

Maydl's operation (migh′dᵉl) [K. *Maydl,* Bohemian surgeon, 1853–1903]. 1. An operation in which the ureters are transplanted into the rectum, for exstrophy of the bladder. 2. A colostomy in which the unopened colon is held in place by means of a glass rod until adhesions have formed.

Mayer position [E. G. *Mayer*]. A position for obtaining a superior-inferior radiographic view of the temporal bone.

May·er's alum hematoxylin or **hemalum** (migh′ur) [P. *Mayer,* German histologist, 1848–1923]. Several formulas of varying hematoxylin content, containing water, ammonium alum, and sometimes glycerol, and used as a stain for large objects.

Mayer's mucicarmine stain [P. *Mayer*]. A stain composed of carmine and aluminum hydroxide or aluminum chloride which is diluted in water or alcohol for staining epithelial mucins, including gastric mucin, red.

Mayer's reflex [K. *Mayer,* Austrian neurologist, 1862–1932]. When the extended middle finger is flexed against resistance, the thumb goes into a position of extension and opposition; seen in a normal but not a hemiplegic hand. Syn. *finger-thumb reflex.*

May-Grünwald stain. A stain for blood which is a saturated solution of methylene blue eosinate in methyl alcohol. Syn. *Jenner's stain.*

May-Hegg·lin anomaly. Inclusions of basophilic RNA (Doehle bodies) in the cytoplasm of the granulocytes and marked variation in the size and shape of the platelets, inherited as an autosomal dominant trait.

may·hem (may′hem) *n.* [MF.]. *In legal medicine,* the willful, malicious, and usually permanent depriving of a person, by violence, of any limb, member, or organ, or causing any mutilation of the body.

Mayo-Rob·son incision [A. W. *Mayo-Robson,* English surgeon, 1853–1933]. A vertical right rectus incision, extended if necessary toward the xiphoid process, used in biliary surgery.

Mayo-Robson point [A. W. *Mayo-Robson*]. A point of extreme tenderness, above and to the right of the umbilicus, in gallbladder disease.

Mayo-Robson position [A. W. *Mayo-Robson*]. Elevation of the prone patient by a sandbag or other device under the right costolumbar region, to facilitate operations on the gallbladder and bile ducts.

Mayo's operation [W. J. *Mayo,* 1861–1939]. Repair of umbilical hernia with a transverse, elliptical incision and overlap of the fascial layers.

¹maz-, mazo- [Gk. *mazos*]. A combining form meaning *breast.*

²maz-, mazo- [*maza*]. A combining form meaning *placenta, placental.*

maza (maz′uh, may′zuh) *n.* [Gk., barley cake, lump, mass]. PLACENTA. —**maz·ic** (maz′ick, may′zick) *adj.*

ma·zal·gia (may·zal′juh, ·jee·uh) *n.* [*maz-* + *-algia*]. MASTALGIA.

maze, *n.* A network of paths, blind alleys, and compartments; used in intelligence tests and in experimental psychology for developing learning curves.

ma·zin·dol (may′zin·dole) *n.* 5-(*p*-Chlorophenyl)-2,5-dihydro-3*H*-imidazo[2,1-*a*]isoindol-5-ol, $C_{16}H_{13}ClN_2O$, an anorexic.

mazo-. See *maz-.*

ma·zo·ca·coth·e·sis (may″zo·ka·koth′e·sis) *n.* [*mazo-* + *caco-*

+ Gk. *thesis*, placing, position]. Faulty implantation of the placenta.

ma·zo·dyn·ia (may″zo·din′ee·uh) *n.* [*maz-* + *-odynia*]. MASTODYNIA.

ma·zo·i·tis (may″zo·eye′tis) *n.* [*mazo-* + *-itis*]. MASTITIS.

ma·zol·y·sis (may·zol′i·sis) *n.* [*mazo-* + *-lysis*]. Separation of the placenta.

ma·zop·a·thy (may·zop′uth·ee) *n.* [*mazo-* + *-pathy*]. 1. Any disease of the placenta. 2. MASTOPATHY.

ma·zo·pexy (may′zo·peck·see) *n.* [*mazo-* + *-pexy*]. Surgical fixation of a pendulous breast; MASTOPEXY.

ma·zo·pla·sia (may″zo·play′zhuh) *n.* [*mazo-* + *-plasia*]. MASTODYNIA (2).

Maz·za·mar·ra itch. An itch caused by ancylostomiasis.

Maz·zi·ni test [L. Y. *Mazzini*, U.S. serologist, b. 1894]. A rapid cardiolipin slide flocculation test for syphilis.

Maz·zo·ni's corpuscle (maht·tso′nee) [V. *Mazzoni*, Italian physician, 19th century]. CORPUSCLE OF GOLGI.

Maz·zot·ti test. A test for onchoceriasis in which ingestion of 50 mg of diethylcarbamazine, in positive cases, induces a pruritic skin reaction over the subcutaneous nodules.

mb Abbreviation for *millibar.*

M. B. *Medicinae Baccalaureus*, Bachelor of Medicine.

MBC Abbreviation for *maximum breathing capacity.*

M. C., M. Ch. *Magister Chirurgiae*, Master of Surgery.

mcg An abbreviation for *microgram.*

MCH Abbreviation for *mean corpuscular hemoglobin.*

MCHC Abbreviation for *mean corpuscular hemoglobin concentration.*

mCi Abbreviation for *millicurie.*

M-component. A single homogeneous (monoclonal) species of immunoglobulin; may be found in excess in benign or in malignant forms of hypergammaglobulinemia.

M-component hypergammaglobulinemia. A form of hypergammaglobulinemia characterized by a single, prominent, more or less narrow band occurring anywhere from the slow gamma (γ) to the fast alpha$_1$ (α_1) region of the electrophoretic strip; associated clinically with neoplasia of the plasma cell, lymphoid, and reticuloendothelial cell series in such diseases as multiple myeloma, Waldenström syndrome leukemia, lymphoma, and carcinoma, but also found in apparently normal individuals. See also *benign M-component hypergammaglobulinemia, Fc fragment disease.*

MCV Abbreviation for *mean corpuscular volume.*

M.D. *Medicinae Doctor*, Doctor of Medicine.

M disk. The region of projections from thick myosin filaments of a striated myofibril appearing longitudinally as the M line.

M.D.S. Master of Dental Surgery.

MEA Abbreviation for *multiple endocrine adenomatosis.*

mead·ow saffron. COLCHICUM.

mean, *adj. & n.* [OF. *meien*, from L. *medianus*, in the middle]. 1. Midway between extremes. 2. A point or value midway between two extremes, commonly of mathematical forms. See also *arithmetic mean, geometric mean.*

mean afterlifetime. EXPECTATION OF LIFE.

mean blood pressure. The average level of blood pressure as determined by actual blood pressure throughout systole and diastole.

mean cell volume. MEAN CORPUSCULAR VOLUME.

mean corpuscular hemoglobin. An expression, in absolute terms, of the average content of hemoglobin of the individual erythrocyte, calculated from the equation

$$\text{MCH} = \frac{\text{hemoglobin [(g/100 ml)} \times 10]}{\text{erythrocyte count } (10^6/\text{mm}^3)}$$

and stated in picograms (10^{-12} g) per cell. Normal values are 28 to 32 pg. Abbreviated, MCH.

mean corpuscular hemoglobin concentration. An expression, in absolute terms, of the average hemoglobin concentration per unit volume (per 100 ml) of packed erythrocytes, calculated from the equation

$$\text{MCHC} = \frac{\text{hemoglobin [(g/100 ml)} \times 100]}{\text{hematocrit}}$$

and stated in grams per 100 ml of packed red cells, or in percent. Normal values for adults are 32 to 36%. Abbreviated, MCHC.

mean corpuscular volume. An expression, in absolute terms, of the average volume of the individual erythrocyte, calculated from the equation

$$\text{MCV} = \frac{\text{hematocrit (percent)} \times 10}{\text{erythrocyte count } (10^6/\text{mm}^3)}$$

and stated in cubic micrometers per cell. Normal values are 82 to 92 μm^3, or 80 to 96 μm^3, depending on methods used. Abbreviated, MCV.

mean deviation. The arithmetic average of the differences between each observation in a series and the mean of the series, disregarding the sign of the differences.

mean life. AVERAGE LIFE.

mean temperature. The average temperature in a locality for a given period of time.

mea·sle (mee′zul) *n.* CYSTICERCUS.

mea·sles (mee′zulz) *n.* 1. An acute infectious viral disease, characterized by a fine dusty rose-red, maculopapular eruption and by catarrhal inflammation of the conjunctiva and of the air passages. After a period of incubation of nearly two weeks, the disease begins with coryza, cough, conjunctivitis, and the appearance of Koplik spots on the oral mucous membranes; on the third or fourth day chills and fever and dusky rose-red maculopapular eruptions appear, arranged in the form of crescentic groups, at times becoming confluent, usually appearing first on the face or behind the ears. In three or four days, the eruption gradually fades and is followed by a branny desquamation. The symptoms are worse at the height of the eruption. The disease affects principally the young, is exceedingly contagious, and one attack or the vaccine usually confers immunity. Central nervous system involvement may occur. Syn. *rubeola*. Compare *rubella*. 2. Plural of *measle;* CYSTICERCI.

measles convalescent serum. The human immune serum for measles.

measles encephalitis. Acute disseminated encephalomyelitis as a result of measles.

measles immune globulin. A sterile solution of globulins from the blood plasma of human donors; used for passive immunization against measles.

measles virus vaccine. A vaccine prepared from measles virus. Two principal types are available: live attenuated measles virus vaccine, and inactivated measles virus vaccine. Both vaccines produce active immunity against measles, although only the live attenuated vaccine is in current use.

mea·sly (meez′lee) *adj.* 1. Infected with measles; spotted with measles. 2. Containing cysticerci; said of pork.

measured work therapy. METRIC OCCUPATIONAL THERAPY.

meat-, meato-. A combining form meaning *meatus.*

meatal plate. A solid mass of cells seen in a two-month embryo, formed by the ingrowth of ectoderm from the bottom of the branchial groove toward the tympanic cavity.

me·a·ti·tis (mee″ay·tigh′tis, mee″uh·) *n.* [*meat-* + *-itis*]. Inflammation of the wall of a meatus.

me·a·tot·o·my (mee″uh·tot′um·ee) *n.* [*meato-* + *-tomy*]. Incision into and enlargement of a meatus.

meat peptone. PEPTONE.

meat sugar. INOSITOL.

me·a·tus (mee·ay′tus) *n.*, L. pl. & genit. sing. **meatus** [L., from *meare*, to pass]. An opening or passage. —**mea·tal** (·tul) *adj.*

meatus acu·sti·cus ex·ter·nus (a·koos'ti·kus ecks·tur'nus) [NA]. EXTERNAL ACOUSTIC MEATUS.

meatus acusticus externus car·ti·la·gi·ne·us (kahr"ti·la·jin'ee·us) [NA]. The cartilaginous portion of the external acoustic meatus.

meatus acusticus in·ter·nus (in·tur'nus) [NA]. INTERNAL ACOUSTIC MEATUS.

meatus na·si com·mu·nis (nay'zye kom·ew'nis) [BNA]. The portion of each nasal cavity adjacent to the nasal septum.

meatus nasi inferior [NA]. INFERIOR NASAL MEATUS.

meatus nasi me·di·us (mee'dee·us) [NA]. MIDDLE NASAL MEATUS.

meatus nasi superior [NA]. SUPERIOR NASAL MEATUS.

meatus na·so·pha·ryn·ge·us (nay"zo·fa·rin'jee·us) [NA]. The opening between the nose and the pharynx.

meatus ure·thrae (yoo·ree'three). The orifice or external ostium of the urethra.

Mebaral. A trademark for mephobarbital.

me·ben·da·zole (me·ben'·duh·zole) *n.* Methyl 5-benzoyl-2-benzimidazolecarbamate, $C_{16}H_{13}N_3O_3$, an anthelmintic.

me·bev·er·ine (me·bev'ur·een) *n.* 4-[Ethyl(*p*-methoxy-α-methylphenethyl)amino]butyl veratrate, $C_{25}H_{35}NO_5$, a smooth muscle relaxant; used as the hydrochloride salt.

me·bu·ta·mate (me·bew'tuh·mate) *n.* 2-*sec*-Butyl-2-methyl-1,3-propanediol dicarbamate, $C_{10}H_{20}N_2O_4$, a central nervous system depressant, related to meprobamate, with mild antihypertensive action.

mec·a·myl·a·mine (meck"a·mil'uh·meen) *n.* *N*,2,3,3-Tetramethyl-2-norbornanamine, $C_{11}H_{21}N$, a ganglionic blocking agent used, as the hydrochloride salt, for treatment of hypertension.

me·chan·i·cal (me·kan'i·kul) *adj.* [L. *mechanicus*, from Gk. *mēchanikos*]. Caused by or pertaining to gross physical forces as opposed to chemical, electrical, or other forces.

mechanical al·ter·nans (ahl'tur·nanz). Regular variation in the pulse pressure because alternate ventricular contractions are more forceful; demonstrable by sphygmomanometry, palpation of arterial pulse, or direct intravascular manometry.

mechanical ascites. Ascites associated with portal venous obstruction. Syn. *passive ascites.*

mechanical bronchitis. Bronchitis caused by the inhalation of dust or other particulate matter.

mechanical dropsy. Edema due to mechanical obstruction of the veins or lymphatics.

mechanical dysmenorrhea. Dysmenorrhea due to mechanical obstruction to the free escape of the menstrual fluid. Syn. *obstructive dysmenorrhea.*

mechanical equivalent of heat. The mechanical energy which is required to produce a given amount of heat. One calorie is equivalent to 4.1855 × 10^7 ergs of work.

mechanical fragility. The susceptibility to breakage of erythrocytes when mechanically agitated under standard conditions as with glass beads in a flask.

mechanical hearing aid. A hearing device that amplifies the intensity of sound waves by some physical means other than electricity.

mechanical ileus. Obstruction of the intestines by extrinsic pressure or internal blockage, due to a variety of causes.

mechanical purpura. Purpura due to violent muscular contractions or application of a tourniquet, not associated with any blood or vascular defects.

mechanical restraint. Restraining a psychotic or otherwise uncontrollable individual or child by mechanical means.

mechanical stage. A device for moving slides in a precise and controlled manner usually on a microscope stage, either laterally or to and from the observer, to facilitate systematic scanning of smears and sections; often equipped with vernier scales, so that the same field may be again found by duplicating the vernier readings.

mechanical stimulus. A stimulus by physical means, as pinching, striking, or stretching.

mech·a·nism (meck'uh·niz·um) *n.* 1. An aggregation of parts arranged in a mechanical way to perform a specific function. 2. A series or combination of processes by which a given change in the state of matter or energy is brought about.

mechanism of labor. The mechanism by which a fetus and its appendages traverse the birth canal.

mech·a·no·re·cep·tor (meck"uh·no·re·sep'tur) *n.* [*mechano-* + *receptor*]. A specialized structure of sensory nerve terminals which responds to mechanical stimuli such as pressure or touch.

mech·a·no·ther·a·py (meck"uh·no·therr'uh·pee) *n.* Treatment of injury or disease by mechanical means. —**mechanothera·pist** (·pist) *n.*

me·chlor·eth·a·mine hydrochloride (meck"lor·eth'uh·meen). 2,2'-Dichloro-*N*-methyldiethylamine hydrochloride, $C_5H_{11}Cl_2N.HCl$; white, crystalline, hygroscopic powder. A cytotoxic drug used for the treatment of various neoplastic diseases. Syn. *mustine hydrochloride, nitrogen mustard* (1).

me·cism (mee'siz·um) *n.* [Gk. *mēkysmos*, lengthening, from *mēkos*, length]. A condition marked by abnormal lengthening of one or more parts of the body.

Meck·el's cartilage [J. F. *Meckel*, the Younger, German anatomist, 1781–1833]. The bar of cartilage in the mandibular arch of the embryo and fetus.

Meckel's cavity [J. F. *Meckel*, the Elder, German anatomist, 1724–1774]. CAVUM TRIGEMINALE.

Meckel's diverticulum [J. F. *Meckel*, Younger]. DIVERTICULUM ILEI.

Meckel's ganglion [J. F. *Meckel*, Elder]. PTERYGOPALATINE GANGLION.

Meckel's stalk [J. F. *Meckel*, Younger]. VITELLINE STALK.

Meckel syndrome. A complex of central nervous system, somatic, and splanchnic malformations transmitted as an autosomal recessive trait, including occipital encephalocele, microcephaly, abnormal facies with cleft lip and palate, polydactyly, and polycystic kidneys. Syn. *Gruber syndrome.*

mec·li·zine (meck'li·zeen) *n.* 1-(*p*-Chloro-α-phenylbenzyl)-4-(*m*-methylbenzyl)piperazine, $C_{25}H_{27}ClN_2$, an antinauseant drug used as the hydrochloride salt.

mec·lo·cy·cline (meck"lo·sigh'kleen) *n.* A tetracycline-type antibiotic, $C_{22}H_{21}ClN_2O_8$.

mec·lo·fe·nam·ic acid (meck"lo·fe·nam'ick) *n.* *N*-(2,6-Dichloro-*m*-tolyl) anthranilic acid, $C_{14}H_{11}Cl_2NO_2$, an anti-inflammatory.

mec·lo·qua·lone (meck"lo·kway'lone) *n.* 3-(*o*-Chlorophenyl)-2-methyl-4(3*H*)-quinazolinone, $C_{15}H_{11}ClN_2O$, a sedative and hypnotic drug.

me·co·bal·a·min (meck"o·bal'uh·min) *n.* A derivative of cobalamine with ribofuranosylbenzimidazole, $C_{63}H_{91}CoN_{13}O_{14}P$, a hemotopoietic vitamin.

me·com·e·ter (me·kom'e·tur) *n.* [Gk. *mēkos*, length, height, + *-meter*]. An instrument resembling calipers with attached scales used in measuring fetuses or newborn infants.

mecon-, mecono- [Gk. *mēkōn*, poppy]. A combining form meaning *opium.*

me·co·nal·gia (mee"ko·nal'jee·uh, meck"on·al'jee·uh) *n.* [*mecon-* + *-algia*]. Pain or neuralgia when the use of opium is discontinued.

mec·o·nate (meck'o·nate, mee'ko·nate) *n.* A salt of meconic acid.

me·con·ic (me·kon'ick, ·ko'nick) *adj.* 1. Pertaining to or derived from opium. 2. Pertaining to the meconium.

meconic acid. 3-Hydroxy-4-oxo-1,4-pyran-2,6-dicarboxylic acid, $C_7H_4O_7$, a dibasic acid occurring in opium.

meconic membrane. A layer within the rectum of the fetus supposed to invest the meconium.

me·co·ni·or·rhea (me·ko'nee·o·ree'uh, meck"o·nigh"o·) *n.* [*meconium* + *-rrhea*]. An excessive discharge of meconium.

me·co·ni·um (me·ko'nee·um) *n.* [Gk. *mēkōnion*]. The pasty, greenish mass, consisting of mucus, desquamated epithelial cells, bile, lanugo hairs, and vernix caseosa, that collects in the intestine of the fetus. It forms the first fecal discharge of the newborn and is not wholly expelled until the third or fourth day after birth.

meconium ileus. Intestinal obstruction caused by inspissation of the meconium due to deficiency of trypsin production, occurring in the newborn with cystic fibrosis of the pancreas.

mec·ry·late (meck'ri·late) *n.* Methyl 2-cyanoacrylate, $C_5H_5NO_2$, a tissue adhesive used as a surgical aid.

me·cys·ta·sis (me·sis'tuh·sis) *n.* [Gk. *mēky-*, from *mēkos*, length, + *stasis*, state, position]. A process in which a muscle increases in length but maintains its original degree of tension. —**mecy·stat·ic** (mes''i·stat'ick) *adj.*

mecystatic relaxation. MECYSTASIS.

me·daz·e·pam (me·daz'e·pam, me·day'ze·pam) *n.* 7-Chloro-2,3-dihydro-1-methyl-5-phenyl-1*H*-1,4-benzodiazepine, $C_{16}H_{15}ClN_2$, a tranquilizing drug; used as the hydrochloride salt.

medi-, medio-. A combining form meaning *middle, medial, median,* or *intermediate.*

me·dia (mee'dee·uh) *n.* 1. TUNICA MEDIA; the middle coat of a vein, artery, or lymph vessel. See also Plate 6. 2. Plural of *medium.*

me·di·ad (mee'dee·ad) *adv.* [*medi-* + *-ad*]. Toward the median plane or line.

me·di·al (mee'dee·ul) *adj.* [L. *medialis*]. 1. Internal, as opposed to lateral (external); toward the midline of the body. 2. Of or pertaining to the tunica media or middle coat of a blood vessel.

medial accessory olivary nucleus. A small mass of gray matter lying medial to the olivary nucleus. NA *nucleus olivaris accessorius medialis.*

medial angle of the eye. The angle formed at the medial junction of the eyelids. NA *angulus oculi medialis.*

medial angular process of the frontal bone. The medial end of the supraorbital margin.

medial aperture of the fourth ventricle. MEDIAN APERTURE OF THE FOURTH VENTRICLE.

medial arcuate ligament. A thick band of fascia extending from the body of the second lumbar vertebra to the tip of the transverse process of the same vertebra. NA *ligamentum arcuatum mediale.* See also *lumbocostal arch.*

medial arteriosclerosis or **calcinosis.** Calcification of the middle coat of the small- and medium-sized muscular arteries. Syn. *Mönckeberg's arteriosclerosis.*

medial check ligament. A thickening of the orbital fascia running from the insertion of the medial rectus muscle to the medial orbital wall.

me·di·a·lec·i·thal (me''dee·uh·les'i·thul) *adj.* MESOLECITHAL.

medial eminence. A longitudinal ridge in the floor of the fourth ventricle, bounded by the median sulcus medially and the sulcus limitans laterally. It includes the facial colliculus and the trigone of the hypoglossal nerve. NA *eminentia medialis.*

medial eminence of the neurohypophysis. A midline prominence in the floor of the third ventricle which is the upper part of the neurohypophysis.

medial fillet. MEDIAL LEMNISCUS.

medial geniculate body. A nuclear mass just lateral to the posterior thalamic zone which receives auditory impulses from the inferior colliculus and relays them to the superior temporal (Heschl's) gyri via the auditory radiation. NA *corpus geniculatum mediale.*

medial inguinal fossa. A slight depression of the peritoneum between the medial and lateral umbilical folds.

medial inguinal fovea. MEDIAL INGUINAL FOSSA.

medial intercondylar tubercle. The spine on the medial side of the intercondylar eminence of the tibia. NA *tuberculum intercondylare mediale.*

medial lemniscus. A lemniscus arising in the nucleus gracilis and nucleus cuneatus, crossing almost immediately as internal arcuate fibers, and terminating mainly in the posterolateral ventral nucleus of the thalamus. NA *lemniscus medialis.*

medial ligament. The ligament on the medial side of the ankle joint, attached to the tibia at the medial malleolus and consisting of an anterior and posterior tibiotalar part (NA *pars tibiotalaris anterior, pars tibiotalaris posterior*), a tibiocalcaneal part (NA *pars tibiocalcanea*), and a tibionavicular part (NA *pars tibionavicularis*). Syn. *deltoid ligament.* NA *ligamentum mediale, ligamentum deltoideum.*

medial longitudinal arch. NA *pars medialis arcus pedis longitudinalis.* See *longitudinal arch of the foot.*

medial longitudinal fasciculus. One of two heavily medullated bundles close to the midline, just ventral to the central gray matter and extending from the upper spinal cord to the rostral end of the midbrain. NA *fasciculus longitudinalis medialis.*

medial longitudinal fasciculus syndrome. On lateral gaze, paresis of the medial rectus muscle of the adducting eye and horizontal nystagmus of the abducting eye, often with impaired convergence (anterior internuclear ophthalmoplegia) or with sixth nerve palsy and intact convergence (posterior internuclear ophthalmoplegia); when present to one side only, usually associated with a vascular lesion of a medial longitudinal fasciculus in the brainstem; when bilateral, almost always due to demyelinating lesions. Syn. *internuclear ophthalmoplegia.*

medial longitudinal stria. The medial one of the two long bundles of fibers on the upper surface of the corpus callosum. NA *stria longitudinalis medialis corporis callosi.*

medial lumbocostal arch. MEDIAL ARCUATE LIGAMENT.

medial malleolus. A process on the internal surface of the lower extremity of the tibia. Syn. *internal malleolus.* NA *malleolus medialis.* See also Plate 1.

medial mammillary nucleus. The main nucleus of the mammillary body located on its medial aspect.

medial meniscus. The articular disk in the knee joint between the medial condyles of the tibia and femur; a crescentic fibrocartilaginous disk attached to the margin of the medial condyle of the tibia, resting on and serving to deepen the tibia's medial articular surface. Syn. *internal semilunar cartilage.* NA *meniscus medialis.*

medial (muscle) necrosis. The death of cells in the middle coat (media) of the walls of arteries.

medial nasal process. MEDIAN NASAL PROCESS.

medial necrosis of aorta. MEDIONECROSIS AORTAE IDIOPATHICA CYSTICA.

medial nucleus of the thalamus. An aggregate of nuclei located between the midline nuclei of the thalamus and the internal medullary lamina.

medial palmar space. MIDPALMAR SPACE.

medial palpebral artery. NA (pl.) *arteriae palpebrales mediales.* See *palpebral artery.*

medial pterygoid plate or **lamina.** A long, narrow plate whose lateral surface forms part of the pterygoid fossa and whose medial surface constitutes the lateral boundary of the choana. Its lower extremity forms a hook, the pterygoid hamulus, for the tendon of the tensor veli palatini muscle. NA *lamina medialis processus pterygoidei.*

medial rectus. An extrinsic muscle of the eye. See *rectus medialis bulbi* in Table of Muscles in the Appendix.

medial sympathetic veins. Longitudinal venous channels of the embryo medial to the sympathetic ganglions, forming the azygos and hemiazygos veins. Syn. *azygos line veins, supracardinal veins.*

medial tarsometatarsal articulation. The articulation between the medial cuneiform and the first and second metatarsals.

medial umbilical fold. The fold of peritoneum overlying the medial umbilical ligament. NA *plica umbilicalis medialis.*

medial umbilical ligament. A cordlike fold extending from the urinary bladder to the umbilicus representing the fibrosed distal part of the umbilical artery. NA *ligamentum umbilicale mediale.*

medial vestibular nucleus. A nucleus in the floor of the fourth ventricle medial and lateral to the ala cinerea. NA *nucleus vestibularis medialis.*

me·di·an (mee'dee·un) *adj. & n.* [L. *medianus,* middle]. 1. Situated or placed in the middle of the body or in the middle of a part of the body, as the arm. 2. That value on the numerical scale of classification in a frequency distribution below which and above which half the observations fall.

median aperture of the fourth ventricle. An aperture in the posterior central portion of the fourth ventricle through which cerebrospinal fluid passes into the subarachnoid space. Syn. *foramen of Magendie.* NA *apertura mediana ventriculi quarti.*

median arcuate ligament. The fibrous margin interconnecting the two crura of the diaphragm in front of the aorta. NA *ligamentum arcuatum medianum.*

median atlantoaxial joint. The joint between the atlas and the dens of the axis. NA *articulatio atlantoaxialis mediana.* See also Table of Synovial Joints and Ligaments in the Appendix.

median bar. Contracture of the vesical neck, or constriction of the prostatic urethra, caused by prostatic hyperplasia (glandular bar) or by overgrowth of connective tissue across the posterior lip of the vesical orifice or of the vesical trigone (fibrous bar).

median cricothyroid ligament. The central portion of the cricothyroid ligament.

median eminence of the tuber cinereum. MEDIAL EMINENCE OF THE NEUROHYPOPHYSIS.

median facial cleft. An embryonic fissure between the mandibular or the median nasal processes which may involve both mandible and maxilla or only one.

median fistula of the neck. A rare congenital fistula with its opening in the midline, due to imperfect closure of the cervical sinus.

median glossoepiglottic fold. A fold of mucous membrane extending in the midline from the back of the tongue to the epiglottis. NA *plica glossoepiglottica mediana.*

median harelip. A median facial cleft which has failed to fuse in embryonic or fetal life.

median laryngotomy. Incision of the larynx through the thyroid cartilage; THYROTOMY.

median lethal dose. That dose of an injurious agent (drug, virus, radiation) given to a population of animals or man, such that 50 per cent will die within a specific time period. Symbol, LD 50, LD_{50}.

median lethal time. The amount of time required for 50 percent of the organisms in a large group to die following a specific dose of a drug, infective agent, or radiation.

median lingual sulcus. A narrow median longitudinal groove on the dorsum of the tongue. NA *sulcus medianus linguae.*

median maxillary cyst. Cystic dilatation of embryonal inclusions in the incisive fossa or between the roots of the central incisors. Syn. *nasopalatine cyst.*

median nasal process. The entire region between the olfactory sacs and below the frontonasal sulcus of the embryo. It forms the bridge, mobile septum, and anterior portion of the cartilaginous septum of the nose, the philtrum of the lip, and the premaxillary portion of the upper jaw.

median nerve. See Table of Nerves in the Appendix.

median nuchal line. EXTERNAL OCCIPITAL CREST.

median palatine suture. The median suture joining the bones of the palate. Syn. *palatine suture.* NA *sutura palatina mediana.*

median plane. A plane that bisects a structure in the anteroposterior direction, dividing it into right and left halves. See also *sagittal plane.*

median posterior sulcus. A longitudinal groove incompletely dividing the spinal cord posteriorly into two symmetrical parts.

median prostatic notch. A notch in the posterior border of the base of the prostate.

median raphe. HORIZONTAL RAPHE OF THE EYE.

median rhomboidal glossitis. A congenital anomaly of the tongue in which an oval or rhomboidal area, devoid of papillae and sometimes elevated, is found on the dorsal surface anterior to the circumvallate papillae.

median sulcus. The longitudinal groove in the floor of the fourth ventricle of the brain. NA *sulcus medianus ventriculi quarti.*

median thyrohyoid ligament. The median portion of the thyrohyoid membrane. NA *ligamentum thyrohyoideum medianum.*

median umbilical fold. A fold of peritoneum covering the urachus or its remains. NA *plica umbilicalis mediana.*

median umbilical ligament. A cordlike structure extending in the midline from the urinary bladder to the umbilicus representing the fibrosed urachus. NA *ligamentum umbilicale medianum.*

mediastina. Plural of *mediastinum.*

me·di·as·ti·nal (mee"dee·as·tye'nul) *adj.* Of or pertaining to a mediastinum.

mediastinal emphysema. Accumulation of air in the tissues of the mediastinum.

mediastinal pleura. A continuation of the parietal pleura covering the mediastinum. NA *pleura mediastinalis.*

mediastinal septum. MEDIASTINUM.

mediastinal space. MEDIASTINUM (2).

me·di·as·ti·ni·tis (mee"dee·as"ti·nigh'tis) *n.* [*mediastinum* + *-itis*]. Inflammation of the tissues of the mediastinum.

me·di·as·ti·no·peri·car·di·tis (mee·dee·as·tigh"no·perr"i·kahr·dye'tis) *n.* 1. Combined inflammation of the mediastinum and the pericardium. 2. POLYSEROSITIS.

me·di·as·tino·scope (mee"dee·as·tin'o·skope) *n.* [*mediastinum* + *-scope*]. An instrument for examining the mediastinum through a skin incision.

me·di·as·ti·nos·co·py (mee"dee·as"ti·nos'kuh·pee) *n.* Examination of the mediastinum using the mediastinoscope.

me·di·as·ti·not·o·my (mee"dee·as"ti·not'um·ee) *n.* [*mediastinum* + *-tomy*]. Incision into the mediastinum.

me·di·as·ti·num (mee"dee·as·tye'num) *n.,* pl. **mediasti·na** (·nuh) [L.]. 1. A partition separating adjacent parts. 2. [NA] The space left in the middle of the chest between the two pleurae, divided into the anterior, middle, posterior, and superior mediastinum.

mediastinum an·te·ri·us (an·teer'ee·us) [NA]. ANTERIOR MEDIASTINUM.

mediastinum medium [NA]. MIDDLE MEDIASTINUM.

mediastinum pos·te·ri·us (pos·teer'ee·us) [NA]. POSTERIOR MEDIASTINUM.

mediastinum su·pe·ri·us (sue·peer'ee·us) [NA]. SUPERIOR MEDIASTINUM.

mediastinum tes·tis (tes'tis) [NA]. A septum in the posterior portion of the testis, formed by a projection inward of the tunica albuginea. Syn. *body of Highmore.*

¹me·di·ate (mee'dee·ate) *v.* [L. *mediare*]. To function as an interposed action in a chain of actions, as adrenocorticotrophin mediates the hypothalamic regulation of cortisol secretion.

²me·di·ate (mee'dee·ut) *adj.* [L. *mediatus*]. Indirect; performed through something interposed.

mediate auscultation. Listening with the aid of a stethoscope interposed between the ear and the part being examined.

mediate percussion. INDIRECT PERCUSSION.

mediate transfusion. INDIRECT TRANSFUSION.

me·di·a·tor (mee'dee·ay"tur) *n.* [L.]. An agent, such as a hormone, that mediates a chemical reaction or a process of a particular type.

med·i·ca·ble (med'i·kuh·bul) *adj.* [L. *medicabilis*]. 1. Amenable to cure. 2. Specifically, amenable to drug therapy.

med·i·cal (med'i·kul) *adj.* [L. *medicalis,* from *medicus,* healing; physician]. 1. Pertaining to medicine. 2. Pertaining to the nonsurgical treatment of disease.

medical aneurysm. An aneurysm that cannot be treated surgically.

medical center. 1. A medical clinic usually serving a discrete geographical area. 2. A group of medical facilities, incorporating all the medical specialities, and possessing the capacity for medical education, and the diagnosis, care, and treatment of patients.

medical de·pot (dep'o). An installation for concentrating, storing, and issuing medical supplies, usually for the armed forces.

medical diathermy. Diathermy in which the tissues are heated to a point less than destructive temperature.

medical ethics. Principles of proper medical conduct; the set of moral values, as well as professionally endorsed principles and practices, which govern the conduct of a member of the medical profession in its exercise.

medical examiner. 1. A professionally qualified physician duly authorized and charged by a governmental unit, such as a municipality, county, or state, to determine facts concerning causes of death, particularly when not occurring under natural circumstances, and to testify thereto in courts of law. Such a physician now frequently replaces or works with a coroner, who may not be a physician, or a coroner's jury of laymen. 2. An officer of a corporation or bureau, whose duty is to determine facts relating to injuries and deaths alleged to have occurred, to place responsibility on the part of the corporation or other agency, and to make recommendations as to compensation. In certain cases, as in life insurance applications, the examiner is charged with passing upon the state of health.

medical expert or **witness.** *In legal medicine,* any licensed physician found qualified by the court to testify before it as an expert witness, regardless of the special medical subject matter under consideration. The physician is expected to be familiar with and possessed of the skill and care ordinarily exercised by reputable medical practitioners in the community, or similar communities, in cases similar to that before the court.

medical gymnastics. Systematic exercises designed to bring ailing or feeble parts of the body back to normal.

medical history. An account of the past and present medical status of a patient. Compare *anamnesis* (2).

medical in·di·gen·cy (in'di·jun·see). The inability to pay for needed medical and related services without severely curtailing the ability to pay for other necessities of life.

medical jurisprudence. LEGAL MEDICINE.

medical pathology. The study of diseases not of surgical importance.

medical referee. MEDICAL EXAMINER (1).

medical statistics. Statistics relating to facts and data concerning human health.

me·dic·a·ment (me·dick'uh·munt, med'i·kuh·munt) *n.* [L. *medicamentum*]. A medicinal substance used for the treatment of disease.

med·i·ca·men·to·sus (med''i·kuh·men·to'sus) *L. adj.* [L., medicinal]. Pertaining to a drug or a drug eruption.

med·i·cant (med'i·kunt) *n.* MEDICATION (3).

Medicare. Popular designation for 1965 amendments to the U.S. Social Security Act, providing hospitalization and certain other benefits to qualified people, most of them over age 65.

med·i·cate (med'i·kate) *v.* [L. *medicare,* to heal, treat, to medicate]. 1. To impregnate with medicine. 2. To treat with a medicine.

med·i·cat·ed (med'i·kay·tid) *adj.* Containing a medicinal substance.

medicated bougie. A suppository containing a medicinal agent.

med·i·ca·tion (med''i·kay'shun) *n.* [L. *medicatio*]. 1. Impregnation with a medicine. 2. Treatment by medicines; the administration of medicines. 3. A medicine or combination of medicines administered.

med·i·ca·tor (med'i·kay·tur) *n.* 1. A person who gives medicines for the relief of disease. 2. An applicator for medicines.

me·dic·i·nal (me·dis'i·nul) *adj.* [L. *medicinalis*]. Pertaining to, due to, or having the nature of medicine.

medicinal leech. *HIRUDO MEDICINALIS.*

medicinal restraint. The use of narcotics and sedatives in quieting an uncontrollable or psychotic individual.

medicinal soft soap. GREEN SOAP.

med·i·cine (med'i·sin) *n.* [OF., from L. *medicina,* from *medicus,* healing, physician, from *mederi,* to heal, cure]. 1. Any substance used for treating disease. 2. The science of treating disease; the healing art. 3. In a restricted sense, that branch of the healing art dealing with internal diseases, which can be treated by a physician rather than by a surgeon.

med·i·co·chi·rur·gi·cal (med''i·ko·kigh·rur'ji·kul) *adj.* [*medical* + *chirurgical*]. MEDICOSURGICAL.

med·i·co·le·gal (med''i·ko·lee'gul) *adj.* Pertaining both to medicine and law.

med·i·co·psy·chol·o·gy (med''i·ko·sigh·kol'uh·jee) *n.* The study of mental diseases in relation to medicine.

med·i·co·sta·tis·tic (med''i·ko·stuh·tis'tick) *adj.* Pertaining to medical statistics.

med·i·co·sur·gi·cal (med''i·ko·sur'ji·kul) *adj.* Pertaining conjointly to medicine and surgery.

Medinal. A trademark for barbital sodium.

Me·di·na worm (me·dee'nuh) [after *Médine,* (*Medina*), Mali]. *DRACUNCULUS MEDINENSIS.*

Me·din's disease (muh·deen') [K. O. *Medin,* Swedish physician, 1847–1927]. PARALYTIC SPINAL POLIOMYELITIS.

medio-. See *medi-.*

me·dio·car·pal (mee''dee·o·kahr'pul) *adj.* Between the two rows of carpal bones.

mediocarpal articulation. The joint between the proximal row and the distal row of carpal bones. NA *articulatio mediocarpea.*

me·dio·cen·tric (mee''dee·o·sen'trick) *adj.* METACENTRIC.

me·dio·dor·sal (mee''dee·o·dor'sul) *adj.* Both median and dorsal; on the median line of the back.

me·dio·fron·tal (mee''dee·o·frun'tul, ·fron'tul) *adj.* [*medio-* + *frontal*]. Pertaining to the middle of the forehead.

me·dio·lat·er·al (mee''dee·o·lat'ur·al) *adj.* [*medio-* + *lateral*]. Pertaining to the median plane and one side.

me·dio·ne·cro·sis (mee''dee·o·ne·kro'sis) *n.* Necrosis occurring in the tunica media of an artery.

medionecrosis aor·tae id·io·path·i·ca cys·ti·ca (ay·or'tee id''ee·o·path'i·kuh sis'ti·kuh) [L.]. Degeneration of the muscle and elastic fibers of the aorta. Syn. *medial necrosis of aorta.*

me·dio·plan·tar (mee''dee·o·plan'tahr, ·tur) *adj.* [*medio-* + *plantar*]. Pertaining to the midsole.

medioplantar reflex. In corticospinal tract lesions, tapping of the midsole of the involved foot produces plantar flexion with fanning of the toes.

me·dio·su·pe·ri·or (mee''dee·o·sue·peer'ee·ur) *adj.* Toward the middle and above.

me·dio·tar·sal (mee''dee·o·tahr'sul) *adj.* Pertaining to the middle articulations of the tarsal bones.

mediotarsal amputation. Amputation of the distal portion of the foot. Syn. *midtarsal amputation.* See also *Chopart's amputation.*

Med·i·ter·ra·nean anemia or **disease.** THALASSEMIA.

Mediterranean dengue. WEST NILE FEVER.

Mediterranean fever. BRUCELLOSIS.

Mediterranean tick fever. BOUTONNEUSE FEVER.

me·di·um (mee'dee·um) *n.,* pl. **me·dia** (·dee·uh) [L., middle, midst]. 1. That in which anything moves or through which it acts. 2. *In microbiology,* any substrate on which microorganisms are cultivated. See also *culture.*

medium-grade medical worker. MIDDLE MEDICAL PERSONNEL.

me·di·us (mee'dee·us) *adj. & n.* [L.]. 1. Middle. 2. The middle finger.

Med·lar bodies. The spherical, dark brown elements of the causative fungi of chromoblastomycosis.

MEDLARS [*M*edical *L*iterature *A*nalysis and *R*etrieval *S*ystem]. A computerized system to aid in the search and retrieval of articles published in medical and related journals, based on the citations in Index Medicus, and made available through the U.S. National Library of Medicine.

Medomin. Trademark for heptabarbital, a sedative and hypnotic having short duration of action.

Medrocort. A trademark for medrysone, a glucocorticoid steroid.

med·ro·ges·tone (med''ro·jes'tone) *n.* 6,17-Dimethylpregna-4,6-diene-3,20-dione, $C_{23}H_{32}O_2$, a progestational steroid.

Medrol. Trademark for methylprednisolone and certain of its derivatives.

me·droxy·pro·ges·ter·one acetate (me·drock''see·pro·jes'tur·ohn). 17-Hydroxy-6α-methylpregn-4-ene-3,20-dione 17-acetate, $C_{24}H_{34}O_4$, an orally and parenterally active steroid progestogen.

med·ry·sone (med'ri·sone) *n.* 11β-Hydroxy-6α-methylpregn-4-ene-3,20-dione, $C_{22}H_{32}O_3$, an anti-inflammatory adrenocorticoid.

me·dul·la (me·dul'uh) *n.*, pl. & genit. sing. **medul·lae** (·ee) [L.]. 1. A fatty or soft substance occupying certain cavities; MARROW. 2. The central part of certain organs as distinguished from the cortex. 3. MEDULLA OBLONGATA.

medulla glan·du·lae su·pra·re·na·lis (glan'dew·lee sue·pruh·re·nay'lis) [NA]. The soft, inner, reddish-brown portion of the suprarenal gland.

medulla no·di lym·pha·ti·ci (no'dye lim·fat'i·sigh) [NA]. The inner portion of a lymph node, composed of irregular cords of cells.

medulla ob·lon·ga·ta (ob''long·gay'tuh, ·gah'tuh) [NA]. The most caudal part of the brain and extending from the pons to the spinal cord. See also Plates 15, 18.

medulla os·si·um (os'ee·um) [BNA]. Bone marrow; MARROW (2).

medulla ossium fla·va (flay'vuh) [NA]. YELLOW MARROW.

medulla ossium ru·bra (roo'bruh) [NA]. RED MARROW.

medulla re·nis (ree'nis) [NA]. The inner portion of a kidney composed of renal pyramids.

med·ul·lar·in (med''uh·lăr'in) *n.* A hypothetical morphogenetic inductor secreted by the medullary component of a developing embryonic vertebrate gonad which inhibits differentiation of the cortical gonadal component, resulting in development of a testis. See also *corticin.*

med·ul·lary (med'yoo·lerr·ee, med'uh·, me·dul'ur·ee) *adj.* 1. Pertaining to a medulla. 2. Pertaining to or resembling marrow. 3. Pertaining to the spinal cord or medulla oblongata.

medullary canal. The cavity of a long bone, containing the marrow.

medullary carcinoma. A form of poorly differentiated adenocarcinoma, usually of the breast, grossly well circumscribed, gray-pink and firm. Syn. *encephaloid carcinoma.*

medullary center. *Obsol.* CENTRUM OVALE.

medullary chondroma. ENCHONDROMA.

medullary coccygeal vesicle. The enlarged caudal termination of the spinal cord present in embryos of 10 to 17 mm.

medullary cords. 1. The primary invaginations of the germinal epithelium of the embryonic gonad that differentiate into rete testis and seminiferous tubules or into rete ovarii. Syn. *primary cords, testis cords.* 2. The cords of dense, lymphatic tissue separated by sinuses in the medulla of a lymph node.

medullary cystic disease of the kidney. A slowly progressive familial disease characterized by multiple renal medullary cysts, usually located at the corticomedullary junction, in association with interstitial fibrosis; it appears clinically in childhood as a salt-wasting syndrome with anemia and uremia. Syn. *familial juvenile nephronophthisis.*

medullary foramen. NUTRIENT FORAMEN.

medullary groove. NEURAL GROOVE.

medullary membrane. ENDOSTEUM.

medullary necrosis. PAPILLARY NECROSIS.

medullary plate. NEURAL PLATE.

medullary rays. Raylike extensions of medullary substance of the kidney projected from the base of the medullary pyramid into the cortex. Syn. *cortical rays.*

medullary sheath. MYELIN SHEATH.

medullary sinus. A lymph sinus in the medulla of a lymph node.

medullary sponge kidney. A congenital condition characterized by bilateral cystic dilatations of the papillary collecting ducts; occasionally renal calculi or pyelonephritis develop.

medullary streak. NEURAL PLATE.

medullary syndrome. Any clinical complex or disorder resulting from involvement of the motor and sensory pathways and of the cranial nerve nuclei within the medulla oblongata.

medullary tractotomy. Surgical incision of the spinothalamic tract in the medulla or of the descending or spinal root of the trigeminal nerve. Syn. *bulbar tractotomy.*

medulla spi·na·lis (spye·nay'lis) [NA]. SPINAL CORD.

med·ul·lat·ed (med'uh·lay·tid, med'yoo·, me·dul'ay·tid) *adj.* [L. *medullatus,* having marrow]. MYELINATED.

med·ul·la·tion (med''uh·lay'shun, med''yoo·) *n.* MYELINIZATION.

med·ul·li·za·tion (med''uh·lye·zay'shun, med''yoo·li·zay'shun) *n.* Conversion into marrow, as the replacement of bone tissue in the course of osteitis.

med·ul·lo·blast (med'uh·lo·blast, med'yoo·lo·, me·dul'o·) *n.* [*medulla* + *-blast*]. A primitive brain cell of the neural tube.

med·ul·lo·blas·to·ma (med''uh·lo·blas·to'muh, med''yoo·lo·, me·dul''o·) *n.* [*medulloblast* + *-oma*]. A malignant brain tumor with a tendency to spread in the meninges; most common in the cerebellum of children. The cells are small, with scanty cytoplasm, dense spheroid or oval nuclei, many mitoses, and a tendency to form pseudorosettes.

med·ul·lo·ep·i·the·li·o·ma (med''uh·lo·ep''i·theel·ee·o'muh) *n.* [*medulla* + *epithelioma*]. *Obsol.* 1. EPENDYMOMA. 2. A locally invasive tumor of the eye arising from the ciliary epithelium or iris.

Me·du·na's method (med'oo·nahⁿ) [L. von *Meduna,* Hungarian psychiatrist, 20th century]. Shock therapy with convulsions, induced chemically as by Metrazol, in the treatment of manic-depressive illness and schizophrenia.

Meek·rin-Ehlers-Danlos syndrome. EHLERS-DANLOS SYNDROME.

Mees' lines (meʸss) [R. A. *Mees,* Dutch neurologist, b. 1873]. The transverse white streaks seen above the crescents of the nails 30 to 40 days after onset of arsenical poisoning.

mef·e·nam·ic acid (mef''e·nam'ick). *N*-(2,3-Xylyl)anthranilic acid, $C_{15}H_{15}NO_2$, an inflammation-counteracting drug.

me·fen·o·rex (me·fen'o·recks) *n.* *N*-(3-Chloropropyl)-α-methylphenethylamine, $C_{12}H_{18}ClN$, an anorexiant drug used as the hydrochloride salt.

me·fex·a·mide (me·feck'suh·mide) *n.* *N*-[α-(Diethylamino)-ethyl]-2-(*p*-methoxyphenoxy)acetamide, $C_{15}H_{24}N_2O_3$, a central nervous system stimulant.

mef·lo·quine (mef'lo·kwin) *n.* (*R**,*S**)-(±)α-2-Piperidinyl-2,8-bis(trifluoromethyl)-4-quinolinemethanol, $C_{17}H_{16}F_6N_2O$, a central stimulant.

Mefoxin. A trademark for cefoxitin, an antibacterial.

mef·ru·side (mef'ruh·side) *n.* 4-Chloro-N^1-methyl-N^1-(tetrahydro-2-methylfurfuryl)-*m*-benzenedisulfonamide, $C_{13}H_{19}ClN_2O_5S_2$, a diuretic.

meg-, mega- [Gk. *megas*, large]. A combining form meaning (a) *large, extended, enlarged;* (b) *unit one million times as large as a* specified unit of measure.

mega·blad·der (meg'uh·blad''ur) *n.* MEGALOCYSTIS.

mega·cal·y·co·sis, mega·cal·i·co·sis (meg''uh·kal''i·ko'sis, ·kay''li·) *n.* Enlargement of the minor calices of the kidney. See also *congenital megacalycosis.*

mega·car·dia (meg''uh·kahr'dee·uh) *n.* [*mega-* + *-cardia*]. MEGALOCARDIA.

Megace. Trademark for megestrol acetate, a progestational agent used in the treatment of breast cancer.

mega·ce·cum, mega·cae·cum (meg''uh·see'kum) *n.* A cecum with a markedly distended lumen.

mega·ceph·a·ly (meg''uh·sef'uh·lee) *n.* MEGALOCEPHALY.

mega·coc·cus (meg''uh·kock'us) *n.*, pl. **mega·coc·ci** (·kock' sigh). A large coccus.

mega·co·lon (meg'uh·ko''lun) *n.* Hypertrophy and dilatation of the colon, usually first seen in childhood, associated with prolonged constipation and consequent abdominal distention. See also *Hirschsprung's disease, idiopathic megacolon.*

mega·co·ni·al (meg''uh·ko'nee·ul) *adj.* [*mega-* + *coni-* + *-al*]. Pertaining to or characterized by large mitochondria or particles seen in certain cells with the electron microscope.

megaconial myopathy. A rare disorder of muscle, observed in childhood, characterized by the presence of very large mitochondria containing bar-shaped and other inclusions, and associated clinically with proximal, slowly progressive weakness. Similar mitochondrial changes have been found in muscles of patients with a variety of nonmuscular diseases.

mega·cys·tis (meg''uh·sis'tis) *n.* MEGALOCYSTIS.

megacystis syndrome. A large, thin walled urinary bladder with poor muscular development, often associated with ureteral reflux; usually congenital in origin.

mega·dont (meg'uh·dont) *adj.* [*mega-* + Gk. *odous, odontos*, tooth]. Having abnormally large teeth; MACRODONT.

mega·du·o·de·num (meg''uh·dew·o·dee'num, dew·od'e·num) *n.* Idiopathic dilatation of the duodenum.

mega·dyne (meg'uh·dine) *n.* A million dynes.

mega·esoph·a·gus, mega·oe·soph·a·gus (meg''uh·e·sof'uh·gus) *n.* [*mega-* + *esophagus*]. A markedly dilated esophagus.

mega·far·ad (meg'uh·făr''ad) *n.* A million farads.

mega·ga·mete (meg''uh·gam'eet, ·ga·meet') *n.* MACROGAMETE.

mega·gna·thus (meg''uh·naith'us) *n.* [*mega-* + *gnath-* + *-us*]. An individual having an abnormally large jaw.

mega·karyo·blast (meg''uh·kăr'ee·o·blast) *n.* [*mega-* + *karyo-blast*]. An immature, developing megakaryocyte. It is a large cell with nongranular, deeply basophilic cytoplasm, and a nucleus showing a fine chromatin structure and numerous nucleoli.

mega·karyo·blas·to·ma (meg''uh·kăr''ee·o·blas·to'muh) *n.* [*megakaryoblast* + *-oma*]. HODGKIN'S DISEASE.

mega·karyo·cyte (meg''uh·kăr'ee·o·site) *n.* [*mega-* + *karyo-* + *-cyte*]. A giant cell of bone marrow, 30 to 70μm, containing a large, irregularly lobulated nucleus; the progenitor of blood platelets. The cytoplasm contains fine azurophil granules. —**mega·karyo·cyt·ic** (·kăr''ee·o·sit'ick) *adj.*

megakaryocytic leukemia. Leukemia in which proliferation of anaplastic megakaryocytes is a prominent feature; usually a variety of granulocytic leukemia. Syn. *giant-cell leukemia.*

mega·karyo·cy·to·pe·nia (meg''uh·kăr''ee·o·sigh''to·pee'nee·uh) *n.* [*megakaryocyte* + *-penia*]. MEGAKARYOPHTHISIS.

mega·karyo·cy·to·sis (meg''uh·kăr''ee·o·sigh·to'sis) *n.* Excessive numbers of megakaryocytes.

mega·karyo·phthi·sis (meg''uh·kăr·ee·off'thi·sis, ·kăr''ee·o·thigh'sis) *n.* [*megakaryocyte* + *-phthisis*]. A scarcity of megakaryocytes in the bone marrow.

megal-, megalo- [Gk. *megalos*]. A combining form meaning (a) *large, great;* (b) *abnormally large.*

mega·lec·i·thal (meg'uh·les'i·thul) *adj.* [*mega-* + *lecithal*]. Large-yolked.

meg·al·en·ceph·a·ly (meg''uh·len·sef'uh·lee) *n.* [*megal-* + *-encephaly*]. The condition of having an abnormally large brain.

meg·al·er·y·the·ma (meg''ul·err·ith·ee'muh) *n.* [*megal-* + *erythema*]. ERYTHEMA INFECTIOSUM.

me·gal·gia (meg·al'jee·uh) *n.* [*meg-* + *-algia*]. Excessively severe pain.

megalo-. See *megal-.*

meg·a·lo·blast (meg'ul·o·blast) *n.* [*megalo-* + *-blast*]. A large erythroblast with a characteristic nuclear pattern formed in marrow in vitamin B_{12} or folic acid deficiency. —**meg·a·lo·blas·tic** (meg''ul·o·blas'tick) *adj.*

megaloblastic anemia. Any anemia characterized by the presence of megaloblasts in the bone marrow, usually associated with macrocytosis in the peripheral blood.

megaloblast of Sa·bin [Florence R. *Sabin*, U. S. anatomist, 1871–1953]. PRONORMOBLAST.

meg·a·lo·blas·toid (meg''ul·o·blas'toid) *adj.* Resembling a megaloblast.

meg·a·lo·car·dia (meg''ul·o·kahr'dee·uh) *n.* [*megalo-* + *-cardia*]. Enlargement of the heart.

meg·a·lo·ceph·a·ly (meg''ul·o·sef'uh·lee) *n.* [*megalo-* + *-cephaly*]. 1. The condition of having a head whose maximum fronto-occipital circumference is greater than two standard deviations above the mean for age and sex. 2. LEONTIASIS OSSEA. —**megalo·ce·phal·ic** (·se·fal'ick) *adj.*

meg·a·loc·er·us (meg''uh·los'ur·us) *n.* [Gk. *megalokerōs*, large-horned, from *megalo-* + *keras*, horn]. An individual with hornlike projections on the forehead.

meg·a·lo·chei·rous (meg''ul·o·kigh'rus) *adj.* [*megalo-* + *cheir-* + *-ous*]. Abnormally large-handed.

meg·a·lo·cor·nea (meg''ul·o·kor'nee·uh) *n.* An enlarged cornea.

meg·a·lo·cys·tis (meg''uh·lo·sis'tis) *n.* [*megalo-* + Gk. *kystis*, bladder]. Abnormal enlargement of the urinary bladder.

meg·a·lo·cyte (meg'ul·o·site) *n.* [*megalo-* + *-cyte*]. A large, nonnucleated, red blood corpuscle, usually oval, derived from a megaloblast. —**meg·a·lo·cyt·ic** (meg''ul·o·sit'ick) *adj.*

meg·a·lo·cy·to·sis (meg''ul·o·sigh·to'sis) *n.* [*megalocyte* + *-osis*]. The occurrence of megalocytes in the peripheral blood.

meg·a·lo·dac·ty·ly (meg''ul·o·dack'ti·lee) *n.* [*megal-* + *dactyl-* + *-y*]. MACRODACTYLY.

meg·a·lo·don·tia (meg''ul·o·don'chee·uh) *n.* [*megal-* + *-odontia*]. MACRODONTIA.

meg·a·lo·en·ter·on (meg''ul·o·en'tur·on) *n.* [*megalo-* + *enteron*]. An excessively large intestine.

meg·a·lo·gas·tria (meg''ul·o·gas'tree·uh) *n.* [*megalo-* + *gastr-* + *-ia*]. Abnormal enlargement of the stomach.

meg·a·lo·glos·sia (meg''uh·lo·glos'ee·uh) *n.* [*megalo-* + *-glossia*]. MACROGLOSSIA.

meg·a·lo·he·pat·ia (meg''ul·o·he·pat'ee·uh) *n.* [*megalo-* + *hepat-* + *-ia*]. Enlargement of the liver; HEPATOMEGALY.

meg·a·lo·karyo·blast (meg''ul·o·kăr'ee·o·blast) *n.* MEGAKARYOBLAST.

meg·a·lo·karyo·cyte (meg''ul·o·kăr'ee·o·site) *n.* MEGAKARYOCYTE.

meg·a·lo·ma·nia (meg''ul·o·may'nee·uh) *n.* [*megalo-* + *-mania*]. A delusion of personal greatness; the patient is pathologically preoccupied with or expresses in words or actions ideas of exalted attainment, power, or wealth, a symptom common in schizophrenia and other psychoses. See also *paranoia, paranoid state, paranoid type of schizophrenia.* —**megalo·man·ic** (·man'ick) *adj.*; **megalo·ma·ni·ac** (·may'nee·ack) *n.*

meg·a·lo·mas·tia (meg″ul·o·mas′tee·uh) *n.* [*megalo-* + *mast-* + *-ia*]. MACROMASTIA.

meg·a·lo·me·lia (meg″ul·o·mee′lee·uh) *n.* [*megalo-* + *-melia*]. Excessive enlargement of one or more limbs.

meg·al·on·y·cho·sis (meg″uh·lon·i·ko′sis) *n.* [*megal-* + *onychosis*]. Universal, noninflammatory hypertrophy of the nails.

meg·a·lo·po·dia (meg″ul·o·po′dee·uh) *n.* [*megalo-* + *pod-* + *-ia*]. The condition of having abnormally large feet.

meg·a·lo·pe·nis (meg″ul·o·pee′nis) *n.* Abnormally large penis; MACROPHALLUS.

meg·a·loph·thal·mos, meg·a·loph·thal·mus (meg″ul·off·thal′mus) *n.* [*megal-* + *ophthalmos*]. Excessive largeness of the eyes.

meg·a·lo·pia (meg″uh·lo′pee·uh) *n.* [*megal-* + *-opia*]. MACROPSIA.

meg·a·lop·sia (meg″uh·lop′see·uh) *n.* [*megal-* + *-opsia*]. MACROPSIA.

meg·a·lo·splanch·nic (meg″ul·o·splank′nick) *adj.* [*megalo-* + *splanchnic*]. Possessing large viscera, especially a large liver.

meg·a·lo·sple·nia (meg″ul·o·splee′nee·uh) *n.* [*megalo-* + *splen-* + *-ia*]. SPLENOMEGALY.

meg·a·lo·spore (meg′ul·o·spore) *n.* A large spore; MACROSPORE.

meg·a·lo·ure·ter (meg″ul·o·yoo·ree′tur) *n.* A greatly enlarged ureter.

-megaly [*megal-* + *-y*]. A combining form designating *abnormal enlargement.*

mega·mero·zo·ite (meg″uh·merr″o·zo′ite) *n.* A large merozoite.

mega·nu·cle·us (meg″uh·new′klee·us) *n.* MACRONUCLEUS.

megaoesophagus. MEGAESOPHAGUS.

mega·phone (meg′uh·fone) *n.* [*mega-* + *-phone*]. An instrument used for assisting the hearing of the deaf, by means of large reflectors of the sound waves.

mega·pros·o·pous (meg″uh·pros′uh·pus) *adj.* [*mega-* + *prosop-* + *-ous*]. Having an unusually large face.

mega·rec·tum (meg″uh·reck′tum) *n.* A greatly enlarged rectum.

mega·sig·moid (meg″uh·sig′moid) *n.* A greatly enlarged sigmoid colon.

mega·spore (meg′uh·spore) *n.* MACROSPORE.

mega·throm·bo·cyte (meg″uh·throm′bo·site) *n.* [*mega-* + *thrombocyte*]. An abnormally large blood platelet.

mega·ure·ter (meg″uh·yoo′re·tur, ·yoo·ree′tur) *n.* [*mega-* + *ureter*]. MEGALOURETER.

mega·volt (meg′uh·vohlt) *n.* A unit equal to 1 million volts.

Megazyme. A trademark for asperkinase, a proteolytic enzyme.

me·ges·trol (me·jes′trol) *n.* 17-Hydroxy-6-methylpregna-4,6-diene-3,20-dione, $C_{22}H_{30}O_3$, a progestational steroid; used as the acetate ester.

Megimide. Trademark for the analeptic drug bemegride.

me·glu·mine (me·gloo′meen, meg′loo·meen) *n. N*-Methylglucamine, $C_7H_{17}NO_5$, a crystalline base; used to prepare salts of certain acidic radiopaque and therapeutic substances.

meglumine di·a·tri·zo·ate (dye″uh·tri·zo′ate, ·trye·zo′ate). A salt of 3,5-diacetamido-2,4,6-triiodobenzoic acid (diatrizoic acid) with *N*-methylglucamine (meglumine); $C_{18}H_{26}I_3N_3O_9$; a roentgenographic contrast medium.

meglumine io·dip·a·mide (eye″o·dip′uh·mide). A salt of 3,3′-(adipoyldiimino)-bis [2,4,6-triiodobenzoic acid] (iodipamide) and *N*-methylglucamine (meglumine); $C_{34}H_{48}I_6N_4O_{16}$; a roentgenographic contrast medium.

meglumine io·tha·lam·ate (eye″o·thuh·lam′ate, eye″o·thal′uh·mate). A salt of 5-acetamido-2,4,6-triiodo-*N*-methylisophthalamic acid (iothalamic acid) and *N*-methylglucamine (meglumine); $C_{18}H_{26}I_3N_3O_9$; a roentgenographic contrast medium.

meg·ohm (meg′ome) *n.* An electric unit equal to 1 million ohms.

meg·oph·thal·mus (meg″off·thal′mus) *n.* MEGALOPHTHALMOS.

me·grim (mee′grim) *n. Obsol.* MIGRAINE.

Mei·bo·mi·an cyst (migh·bo′mee·un) [H. *Meibom,* German anatomist, 1638–1700]. CHALAZION.

Meibomian glands [H. *Meibom*]. TARSAL GLANDS.

mei·bo·mi·a·ni·tis (migh·bo″mee·uh·nigh′tis) *n.* [*Meibomian* glands + *-itis*]. Inflammation of tarsal glands.

mei·bo·mi·tis (migh″bo·migh′tis) *n.* MEIBOMIANITIS.

Meige's disease (mezh) [Henri *Meige,* French physician, 1866–1940]. Hereditary lymphedema with onset at puberty or later. Compare *Milroy's disease.*

Meigs's syndrome (megz) [J. V. *Meigs,* U.S. gynecologist, 1892–1963]. Ovarian fibroma with ascites and hydrothorax.

Mei·nicke's test (migh′ni·ke^h) [E. *Meinicke,* German physician, b. 1878]. A flocculation test for syphilis.

meio-. See *mio-.*

meio·lec·i·thal, mio·lec·i·thal (migh″o·les′i·thul) *adj.* [*mio-* + *lecithal*]. ALECITHAL.

mei·o·sis (migh·o′sis) *n.*, pl. **meio·ses** (·seez) [Gk. *meiōsis,* diminution]. The nuclear changes which take place in the last two cell divisions in the formation of the germ cells. The chromosomes separate from one another once but the cell body divides twice with the result that the nucleus of the mature egg or sperm contains the reduced (haploid) number of chromosomes. In addition, by mechanisms such as crossing-over, chromosomal segments are exchanged between chromatids and genetic variation is achieved. Syn. *reduction division.* —**mei·ot·ic** (migh·ot′ick) *adj.*

Mei·row·sky phenomenon. The increase in epidermal pigment post mortem or in excised skin from living subjects after incubation at 37°C or exposure to ultraviolet light.

Meiss·ner's corpuscle (mice′nur) [G. *Meissner,* German anatomist and physiologist, 1829–1905]. An ovoid end organ connected with one or more myelinated nerve fibers which lose their sheaths as they enter a surrounding capsule, make several spiral turns, and break up into a complex network of branches. Found in the dermal papillae especially of the volar surfaces of the fingers and toes.

Meissner's plexus [G. *Meissner*]. SUBMUCOUS PLEXUS.

mel [L.]. HONEY.

¹mel-, melo- [Gk. *melos*]. A combining form meaning *limb, extremity.*

²mel-, melo- [Gk. *mēlon,* apple; cheek]. A combining form meaning *cheek.*

melaena. MELENA.

me·lag·ra (me·lag′ruh) *n.* [*mel-,* limb, + *-agra*]. Muscular pains in the extremities.

me·lal·gia (me·lal′jee·uh) *n.* [*mel-,* limb, + *-algia*]. Pain or neuralgia in the extremities.

melan-, melano- [Gk. *melas, melanos,* black, dark]. A combining form meaning (a) *black, dark;* (b) *pertaining to melanin.*

mel·an·cho·lia (mel″un·ko′lee·uh) *n.* [Gk., melancholy]. Severe depression, usually of psychotic proportion. See also *agitated depression, involutional melancholia, manic-depressive illness, retarded depression.* —**melan·chol·ic** (·kol′ick), *adj.;* **melan·cho·li·ac** (·ko′lee·ack) *n.*

melancholia ag·i·ta·ta (aj″i·tay′tuh). 1. The excited phase in catatonia. 2. A form of manic-depressive illness or involutional melancholia associated with excessive motor excitement.

melancholia at·ton·i·ta (a·ton′i·tuh). The immobile stage of catatonia.

melancholia simplex. A simple depression, without delusions.

melancholic insanity. INVOLUTIONAL MELANCHOLIA.

mel·an·choly (mel′un·kol·ee) *n.* [Gk. *melancholia,* from *melas,* black, + *cholē,* bile]. 1. Dejection, gloom, sadness. 2. MELANCHOLIA.

mel·a·ne·mia (mel″uh·nee′mee·uh) *n.* [*melan-* + *-emia*]. The presence of melanin in the blood.

Melanex. A trademark for metahexamide, a hypoglycemic.

Me·la·nia (me·lay′nee·uh) *n.* A genus of freshwater snails whose species serve as important intermediate hosts of the trematodes *Paragonimus westermani* and *Metagonimus yokogawai.*

mel·an·idro·sis (mel″uh·ni·dro′sis, me·lan″i·) *n.* [*melan-* + *idrosis*]. A form of chromhidrosis in which the sweat is dark-colored or black.

mel·a·nif·er·ous (mel″uh·nif′ur·us) *adj.* [*melan-* + *-iferous*]. Containing melanin.

mel·a·nin (mel′uh·nin) *n.* [*melan-* + *-in*]. A group of black or dark-brown pigments produced by many kinds of cells. Occurs naturally in the choroid coat of the eye, the skin, hair, cardiac muscle, pia mater, adrenal medulla, and nervous tissue. Chemically, melanins are polymers of indole-5,6-quinone, which may be derived from 3,4-dihydroxyphenylalanine, from epinephrine, from homogentisic acid, or from *p*-phenylenediamine.

melanin granule. Any melanin-containing particle observable with the light microscope.

mel·a·nism (mel′uh·nizum) *n.* Abnormal deposition of dark pigment (melanin) in tissues, in organs, or in the skin.

mel·a·nize (mel′uh·nize) *v.* To form and deposit melanin in a tissue or organ. —**mel·a·ni·za·tion** (mel″uh·nigh·zay′shun) *n.*

melano-. See *melan-.*

mel·a·no·am·e·lo·blas·to·ma (mel″uh·no·am″e·lo·blas·to′muh) *n.* Ameloblastoma in which melanin is found.

mel·a·no·blast (mel′uh·no·blast) *n.* [*melano-* + *blast*]. 1. The precursor of all melanocytes and melanophores. 2. *In biology,* an immature pigment cell, of neural crest origin, in certain vertebrates. 3. *In medicine,* the mature melanin-elaborating cell.

mel·a·no·blas·to·ma (mel″uh·no·blas·to′muh) *n.* [*melanoblast* + *-oma*]. A malignant melanoma.

mel·a·no·car·ci·no·ma (mel″uh·no·kahr·si·no′muh) *n.* [*melano-* + *carcinoma*]. A malignant melanoma.

mel·a·no·cyte (mel′uh·no·site, me·lan′o·) *n.* [*melano-* + *-cyte*]. A fully differentiated melanin-forming cell; a cell which synthesizes melanosomes.

melanocyte-stimulating hormone. A substance found in the pituitary gland which causes darkening of human skin and nevi, formation of new pigmented nevi, and pigmentary changes in fish and amphibia, where it has been called intermedin. Abbreviated, MSH. Syn. *melanophore hormone, melanophore-dilating principle.*

mel·a·no·cy·to·ma (mel″uh·no·sigh·to′muh) *n.* 1. Any benign tumor of melanocytes. 2. A benign, heavily pigmented tumor of melanocytes arising at the optic disk.

mel·a·no·cy·to·sis (mel″uh·no·sigh·to′sis) *n.* An excessive number of melanocytes.

mel·a·no·der·ma (mel″uh·no·dur′muh) *n.* [*melano-* + *-derma*]. Any abnormal darkening of the skin, either diffuse or in patches, and either by accumulation of melanin or by deposition of other substances as, for example, silver salts in argyria. —**melanoder·mic** (·mick) *adj.*

mel·a·no·der·ma·ti·tis (mel″uh·no·dur″muh·tigh′tis) *n.* [*melano-* + *dermatitis*]. Any inflammatory skin disease accompanied by increased skin pigmentation.

melanodermatitis tox·i·ca (tock′si·kuh). A form of contact dermatitis resulting from combined exposure to tars, oils or greases, and sunlight.

mel·a·no·der·mia (mel″uh·no·dur′mee·uh) *n.* MELANODERMA.

melanodermic leukodystrophy. ADRENOLEUKODYSTROPHY.

mel·a·no·ep·i·the·li·o·ma (mel″uh·no·ep·i·theel·ee·o′muh) *n.* [*melano-* + *epithelioma*]. A malignant melanoma.

me·lano·gen (me·lan′o·jin) *n.* [*melano-* + *-gen*]. A colorless precursor which is transformed into melanin. Patients, especially those with widespread melanomas, may excrete urine containing melanogen; on standing, the urine becomes dark brown or black.

mel·a·no·gen·e·sis (mel″uh·no·jen′e·sis) *n.* [*melano-* + *genesis*]. The formation of melanin.

mel·a·no·glos·sia (mel″uh·no·glos′ee·uh) *n.* [*melano-* + *gloss-* + *-ia*]. BLACKTONGUE.

mel·a·noid (mel′uh·noid) *adj.* Dark-colored; resembling melanin.

mel·a·no·leu·ko·der·ma col·li (mel″uh·no·lew·ko·dur′muh kol′eye). COLLAR OF VENUS.

mel·a·no·ma (mel″uh·no′muh) *n.* [*melan-* + *-oma*]. 1. A malignant tumor whose parenchyma is composed of anaplastic melanocytes. 2. Any tumor, benign or malignant, of melanocytes.

melanoma su·pra·re·na·le (sue″pruh·re·nay′lee). ADDISON'S DISEASE.

mel·a·no·ma·to·sis (mel″uh·no″muh·to′sis) *n.* [*melanoma* + *-osis*]. Widespread distribution of melanoma.

mel·a·no·nych·ia (mel″uh·no·nick′ee·uh) *n.* [*melan-* + *-onychia*]. Blackening of the fingernails or toenails.

mel·a·no·phage (mel′uh·no·faje) *n.* [*melano-* + *-phage*]. A cell, unrelated to the pigment-producing cells, which contains phagocytized melanin.

mel·a·no·phore (mel′uh·no·fore, me·lan′o·) *n.* [*melano-* + *-phore*]. A type of melanocyte which participates with other pigment cells in the rapid color changes of certain animals; rearrangement of melanosomes within the cell is probably responsible.

melanophore-dilating principle. MELANOCYTE-STIMULATING HORMONE.

melanophore hormone. MELANOCYTE-STIMULATING HORMONE.

melanophore-stimulating factor. A hormone or part of a hormone, intermedin, present in lower vertebrates, that effects the dispersion of pigment granules in the melanophores.

mel·a·no·pla·kia (mel″uh·no·play′kee·uh) *n.* [*melano-* + Gk. *plax,* flat surface, + *-ia*]. Pigmentation of the mucous membrane of the mouth, usually in patches and occasionally with leukoplakia superimposed.

mel·a·no·pro·te·in (mel″uh·no·pro′tee·in, ·teen) *n.* A conjugated protein in which melanin is the associated chromogen.

mel·a·nor·rha·gia (mel″uh·no·ray′jee·uh) *n.* [*melano-* + *-rrhagia*]. MELENA.

mel·a·nor·rhea (mel″uh·no·ree′uh) *n.* [*melano-* + *-rrhea*]. MELENA.

mel·a·no·sar·co·ma (mel″uh·no·sahr·ko′muh) *n.* [*melano-* + *sarcoma*]. A malignant melanoma.

mel·a·no·sis (mel″uh·no′sis) *n.* [*melan-* + *-osis*]. Dark-brown or brownish-black pigmentation of surfaces by melanins or, in some instances, by hematogenous pigments. —**mel·a·not·ic** (mel″uh·not′ick) *adj.*

melanosis cir·cum·scrip·ta pre·blas·to·ma·to·sa of Du·breuilh (sur″kum·skrip′tuh pree·blas″to·muh·to′suh) [M. W. *Dubreuilh*]. LENTIGO MALIGNA.

melanosis co·li (ko′lye). Brown-black pigmentation of mucosa of the colon in innumerable, approximated, minute foci.

melanosis iri·dis (irr′i·dis, eye′ri·dis). Abnormal melanotic pigmentation of the iris.

mel·a·no·some (mel′uh·no·sohm) *n.* [*melano-* + *-some*]. A discrete, melanin-containing organelle, ovoid, about 0.2 nm. in diameter; membrane-bound and has longitudinally arranged fibers on which the pigment is located.

melanotic freckle. LENTIGO MALIGNA.

melanotic freckle of Hutchinson [J. *Hutchinson*]. LENTIGO MALIGNA.

melanotic sarcoma. A malignant melanoma.

melanotic whitlow. A malignant melanoma of the nail bed.

mel·a·no·trich·ia lin·guae (mel″uh·no·trick′ee·uh ling′gwee). BLACK, HAIRY TONGUE.

mel·a·not·ri·chous (mel″uh·not′ri·kus) *adj.* [Gk. *melanothrix, melanotrichos,* from *melano-* + *thrix,* hair]. Black-haired.

mel·a·nu·ria (mel″uh·new′ree·uh) *n.* [*melan-* + *-uria*]. The presence of black pigment in the urine, the result of oxidation of melanogens. —**melanu·ric** (·rick) *adj.*

mel·ar·sen (mel·ahr′sin) *n.* Disodium *p*-melaminylphenylarsonate, a pentavalent arsenical which has been used as a trypanocidal agent.

mel·ar·so·prol (mel·ahr′so·prol) *n.* 2-*p*-(4,6-Diamino-1,3,5-triazin-2-ylamino)phenyl-4-hydroxymethyl-1,3,2-dithioarsolan, $C_{12}H_{15}AsN_6OS_2$, a trypanocidal drug. Syn. *Mel B.*

me·las·ma (me·laz′muh) *n.* [Gk., a black spot, from *melas,* black]. MELANODERMA.

mel·a·to·nin (mel″uh·to′nin) *n.* *N*-acetyl-5-methoxytryptamine, $C_{13}H_{16}O_2N_2$, a compound secreted by the pineal gland which has been found to inhibit the estrous cycle.

Mel B. MELARSOPROL.

Melbex. A trademark for mycophenolic acid, an antineoplastic.

m electron. An electron in the m or third shell surrounding the nucleus of an atom.

me·le·na, me·lae·na (me·lee′nuh) *n.* [Gk. *melaina,* from *melas,* black]. The discharge of stools colored black by altered blood.

melena neonatorum. A melena occurring most often in the first few hours after birth.

Me·le·ney's ulcer [F. L. *Meleney,* U.S. surgeon, 1889-1963]. Spreading gangrenous ulceration of the skin due to infection with anaerobic or micro-aerophilic streptococci, mixed with other organisms indigenous to the skin.

mel·en·ges·trol (mel″in·jes′trol) *n.* 17-Hydroxy-6-methyl-16-methylene-pregna-4,6-diene-3,20-dione, $C_{23}H_{30}O_3$, an antineoplastic and progestational steroid; used as the acetate ester.

me·le·nic, me·lae·nic (me·lee′nick) *adj.* [*melena* + *-ic*]. Pertaining to, or marked by, melena.

mel·e·tin (mel′e·tin) *n.* QUERCETIN.

me·lez·i·tose (me·lez′i·toce) *n.* A nonreducing trisaccharide obtained from an exudate of the Douglas fir and the larch.

meli- [Gk. *meli,* honey]. A combining form meaning *sugar.*

-melia [*mel-* + *-ia*]. A combining form designating *a condition of the limbs or extremities.*

meli·bi·ase (mel″i·bye′ace, ·aze) *n.* An enzyme from certain brewer's yeasts catalyzing the hydrolysis of melibiose to dextrose and galactose.

meli·bi·ose (mel″i·bye′oce, ·oze) *n.* A disaccharide, $C_{12}H_{22}O_{11}$, resulting from hydrolysis of raffinose and also occurring naturally; it may be hydrolyzed to glucose and galactose.

mel·i·lo·tox·in (mel″i·lo·tock′sin) *n.* [*Melilotus,* sweet clover, + *toxin*]. BISHYDROXYCOUMARIN.

mel·in (mel′in) *n.* RUTIN.

mel·i·oi·do·sis (mel″ee·oy·do′sis) *n.* [Gk. *mēlis,* glanders, + *-oid,* -like, + *-osis*]. A disease characterized by infectious granulomas similar to glanders; it is primarily a disease of rodents but is occasionally communicable to man. This disease has been observed in Malaysia, Indochina, and Ceylon and is caused by *Pseudomonas pseudomallei.*

me·lis·sic acid (me·lis′ick) [Gk. *melissa,* bee, + *-ic*]. An acid, $CH_3(CH_2)_{28}COOH$, occurring in beeswax.

me·lis·so·pho·bia (me·lis″o·fo′bee·uh) *n.* [Gk. *melissa,* bee, + *-phobia*]. APIOPHOBIA.

me·lis·syl (me·lis′il) *n.* MYRICYL.

me·li·tis (me·lye′tis) *n.* [*mel-,* cheek, + *-itis*]. Inflammation of the cheek.

mel·i·tose (mel′i·toce, ·toze) *n.* RAFFINOSE.

meli·tox·in (mel″i·tock′sin) *n.* BISHYDROXYCOUMARIN.

meli·tra·cen (mel″i·tray′sen) *n.* 9-(3-Dimethylaminopropylidene)-10,10-dimethyl-9,10-dihydroanthracene, $C_{21}H_{25}N$, an antidepressant drug; used as the hydrochloride salt.

meli·tri·ose (mel″i·trye′oce, ·oze) *n.* RAFFINOSE.

mel·i·tu·ria (mel″i·tew′ree·uh) *n.* [Gk. *meli, melitos,* honey, + *-uria*]. The presence of any sugar in urine.

mel·i·zame (mel′·i·zame) *n.* 5-(*m*-Hydroxyphenoxy)-1*H*-tetrazole, $C_7H_6N_4O_2$, a synthetic sweetener.

Mel·kers·son-Ro·sen·thal syndrome [E. *Melkersson,* Swedish physician, 20th century; and C. *Rosenthal*]. A disease of unknown cause, usually beginning in childhood or adolescence characterized by recurrent peripheral facial paralysis, swelling of the face and lips, and deep furrows in the tongue. May be hereditary.

Melkersson syndrome [E. *Melkersson*]. MELKERSSON-ROSENTHAL SYNDROME.

Mellaril. Trademark for thioridazine, a tranquilizer used as the hydrochloride salt in the treatment of various psychotic conditions.

Mellinger magnet. A type of giant magnet, with a magnetized core held in the surgeon's hand, the coil being over the patient's eye, and devised for extracting steel particles from the eyeball.

mel·lit·ic acid (me·lit′ick). Benzenehexacarboxylic acid, $C_6(COOH)_6$, a crystalline substance occurring in certain coal and wood products and synthesized by oxidation of carbon with nitric acid. Has been used medicinally.

mellituria. MELITURIA.

melo-. See *mel-.*

melo·di·dy·mia (mel″o·di·dye′mee·uh, ·di·dim′ee·uh) *n.* [*melo-,* limb, + *didymus* + *-ia*]. The presence of an accessory limb or limbs.

melo·did·y·mus (mel″o·did′i·mus) *n.* [*melo-,* limb, + *didymus*]. An individual with an accessory limb or limbs.

melo·ma·nia (mel″o·may′nee·uh) *n.* [Gk. *melos,* song, tune, + *-mania*]. A psychotic disorder marked by an inordinate devotion to music. —**melomani·ac** (·ack) *n.*

me·lom·e·lus (me·lom′e·lus) *n.* [*melo-,* limb, + Gk. *melos,* limb]. An individual with one or more rudimentary accessory limbs attached to a limb.

mel·on·seed bodies. Loose, ovoid fragments of inflamed synovial tissue found in bursitis.

Me·loph·a·gus (me·lof′uh·gus) *n.* [Gk. *mēlon,* sheep, goat, + *-phagus,* eater, from Gk. *phagein,* to eat]. A genus of the family Hippoboscidae (louse flies) ectoparasitic on mammals and birds.

Melophagus ovi·nus (o·vye′nus). The species of louse fly known as the sheep tick or ked, which transmits *Rickettsia melophagi* and the trypanosomiasis of sheep.

melo·rhe·os·to·sis (mel″o·ree″os·to′sis) *n.* [*melo-,* limb, + *rheostosis*]. A very rare condition of unknown cause in which certain bones, or parts of bones, undergo asymmetrical or local enlargement and sclerotic changes, typically confined to the bones of one extremity, with distortion of affected bone, limitation of movement in the joints between the bones, and marked pain. Syn. *Léri type of osteopetrosis.*

me·los·chi·sis (me·los′ki·sis) *n.* [*melo-,* cheek, + *-schisis*]. A facial cleft, usually a transverse one.

melo·trid·y·mus (mel″o·trid′i·mus) *n.* [*melo-,* limb, + Gk. *tridymos,* triplet]. DIPYGUS TRIPUS.

me·lo·tus (me·lo′tus) *n.* [*mel-,* cheek, + *ot-* + *-us*]. An individual showing congenital displacement of the ear, which lies on the cheek.

Meloxine. Trademark for methoxsalen, a compound that induces formation of melanin pigment in the skin.

mel·pha·lan (mel′fuh·lan) *n.* L-3-*p*-[Bis(2-chloroethyl)amino]-phenylalanine, $C_{13}H_{18}Cl_2N_2O_2$, an antineoplastic drug. Syn. *L-phenylalanine mustard, L-sarcolysin, L-PAM.*

melting point. The temperature at which a fusible solid melts. Abbreviated, m.p.

Melt·zer's method [S. J. *Meltzer,* U.S. physiologist, 1851-1920]. A method of anesthesia by intratracheal insufflation.

-melus [NL., from Gk. *melos*, limb]. A combining form designating *an individual having a* (specified) *abnormality of the limbs.*

mem·ber, *n.* [L. *membrum*]. A part of the body, especially a projecting part, as the upper or lower extremity.

membra. Plural of *membrum* (= MEMBER).

mem·bra·na (mem·bray'nuh) *n.*, pl. & genit. sing. **membra·nae** (·nee) [L.]. MEMBRANE.

membrana at·lan·to·oc·ci·pi·ta·lis anterior (at·lan''to·ock·sip·i·tay'lis) [NA]. ANTERIOR ATLANTOOCCIPITAL MEMBRANE.

membrana atlantooccipitalis posterior [NA]. POSTERIOR ATLANTOOCCIPITAL MEMBRANE.

membrana ba·sa·lis duc·tus se·mi·cir·cu·la·ris (ba·say'lis duck'tus sem''ee·sur·kew·lair'is) [NA]. Basal membrane of a semicircular duct of the inner ear.

membrana de·ci·dua (de·sid'yoo·uh). DECIDUA.

membranae de·ci·du·ae (de·sid'yoo·ee) [NA]. DECIDUAL MEMBRANES.

membrana elas·ti·ca la·ryn·gis (e·las'ti·kuh la·rin'jis) [BNA]. Membrana fibroelastica laryngis (= ELASTIC MEMBRANE OF THE LARYNX).

membrana fi·bro·elas·ti·ca la·ryn·gis (figh''bro·e·las'ti·kuh la·rin'jis) [NA]. ELASTIC MEMBRANE OF THE LARYNX.

membrana fi·bro·sa cap·su·lae ar·ti·cu·la·ris (figh·bro'suh kap'sue·lee ahr·tick·yoo·lair'ris) [NA]. The outer fibrous portion of any articular capsule.

membrana gran·u·lo·sa (gran''yoo·lo'suh). GRANULOSA MEMBRANE.

membrana hy·a·loi·dea (high''uh·loy'dee·uh) [BNA]. Membrana vitrea (= HYALOID MEMBRANE).

membrana hyo·thy·re·oi·dea (high''o·thigh·ree·oy'dee·uh) [BNA]. MEMBRANA THYROHYOIDEA.

membrana in·ter·cos·ta·lis ex·ter·na (in''tur·kos·tay'lis ecks·tur'nuh) [NA]. External intercostal membrane.

membrane intercostalis in·ter·na (in·tur'nuh) [NA]. Internal intercostal membrane.

membrana in·ter·os·sea an·te·bra·chii (in''tur·os'ee·uh an·te·bray'kee·eye) [NA]. INTEROSSEOUS MEMBRANE OF THE FOREARM.

membrana interossea cru·ris (kroo'ris) [NA]. INTEROSSEOUS MEMBRANE OF THE LEG.

membrana mu·co·sa na·si (mew·ko'suh nay'zye) [BNA]. TUNICA MUCOSA NASI.

membrana nic·ti·tans (nick'ti·tanz). NICTITATING MEMBRANE.

membrana ob·tu·ra·to·ria (ob''tew·ruh·to'ree·uh) [NA]. OBTURATOR MEMBRANE (1).

membrana obturatoria sta·pe·dis (sta·pee'dis) [BNA]. Membrana stapedis (= OBTURATOR MEMBRANE (2)).

membrana pe·ri·nei (perr·i·nee'eye) [NA alt.]. PERINEAL MEMBRANE. NA alt. *fascia diaphragmatis urogenitalis inferior.*

membrana pro·pria duc·tus se·mi·cir·cu·la·ris (pro'pree·uh duck'tus sem''i·sur·kew·lair'is) [NA]. The outer connective-tissue layer of a semicircular duct.

membrana pu·pil·la·ris (pew·pi·lair'is) [NA]. PUPILLARY MEMBRANE.

membrana pupillaris per·sis·tens (pur·sis'tenz). ATRETOPSIA.

membrana qua·dran·gu·la·ris (kwah·drang·gew·lair'is) [NA]. QUADRANGULAR MEMBRANE.

membrana re·ti·cu·la·ris (re·tick·yoo·lair'is) [NA]. RETICULAR MEMBRANE.

membrana spi·ra·lis (spi·ray'lis) [NA alt.]. PARIES TYMPANICUS DUCTUS COCHLEARIS.

membrana sta·pe·dis (sta·pee'dis) [NA]. OBTURATOR MEMBRANE (2).

membrana sta·to·co·ni·o·rum ma·cu·la·rum (stat''o·ko·nee·o'rum mack·yoo·lair'um) [NA]. A gelatinous membrane containing otoconia which overlies the maculae of the semicircular canals.

membrana ster·ni (stur'nigh) [NA]. STERNAL MEMBRANE.

membrana su·pra·pleu·ra·lis (sue''pruh·ploo·ray'lis) [NA]. SUPRAPLEURAL MEMBRANE.

membrana sy·no·vi·a·lis (si·no·vee·ay'lis) [NA]. SYNOVIAL MEMBRANE.

membrana tec·to·ria (teck·to'ree·uh) [NA]. TECTORIAL MEMBRANE (2).

membrana tectoria duc·tus coch·le·a·ris (duck'tus kock''lee·air'is) [NA]. TECTORIAL MEMBRANE (1).

membrana thy·ro·hy·oi·dea (thigh''ro·high·oy'dee·uh) [NA]. THYROHYOID MEMBRANE.

membrana tym·pa·ni (tim'puh·nigh) [NA]. TYMPANIC MEMBRANE.

membrana tympani reflex. LIGHT REFLEX (1).

membrana tympani se·cun·da·ria (seck''un·dair'ee·uh) [NA]. SECONDARY TYMPANIC MEMBRANE.

membrana ve·sti·bu·la·ris (ves·tib·yoo·lair'is) [NA alt.]. VESTIBULAR MEMBRANE. NA alt. *paries vestibularis ductus cochlearis.*

membrana vi·trea (vit'ree·uh) [NA]. HYALOID MEMBRANE.

mem·brane (mem'brane) *n.* [L. *membrana*]. A thin layer of tissue surrounding a part, separating adjacent cavities, lining a cavity, or connecting adjacent structures.

membrane bone. Osseous tissue formed by or within a connective tissue, as by a periosteum.

membrane equilibrium. DONNAN EQUILIBRIUM.

membrane potential. Potential difference across the membrane of a living cell usually measured in millivolts. Syn. *transmembrane potential, resting potential.*

mem·bra·no·cra·ni·um (mem''bruh·no·kray'nee·um) *n.* DESMOCRANIUM.

mem·bra·no·pro·lif·er·a·tive (mem''bruh·no·pro·lif'ur·uh·tiv, mem·bray''no·) *adj.* Affecting membranes and associated with proliferative activity on the part of the cells of the area; said especially of the renal glomeruli.

membranoproliferative glomerulonephritis. A renal glomerular disease characterized by lobular accentuation of capillary tufts due to an increase in numbers of mesangial cells and amounts of mesangial matrix and diffuse thickening of capillary walls. Immunologic features include variable C3 hypocomplementemia with mesangial deposits of C3 and properdin and minimal deposits of immunoglobin and C4. Clinically, combined features of a nephritic-nephrotic syndrome are seen. The disease is slowly progressive to chronic renal failure.

mem·bra·nous (mem'bruh·nus) *adj.* Pertaining to or characterized by a membrane or membranes.

membranous ampullae. The ampullae occurring at one end of the membranous semicircular canals near their junction with the utricle, and containing the end organs of the sense of equilibrium. NA *ampullae membranaceae.*

membranous cataract. A cataractous lens, flattened in the anteroposterior direction, consisting of lens capsule, variable amounts of proliferated lens epithelium, and fibrous tissue; may be unilateral or bilateral, and is often due to intrauterine iritis and associated with other anomalies of the eye. Syn. *pseudoaphakia.*

membranous cochlea. COCHLEAR DUCT.

membranous cochlear canal. COCHLEAR DUCT.

membranous dysmenorrhea. Dysmenorrhea characterized by discharge of a cast of uterine mucosa.

membranous enteritis. ACUTE FIBRINOUS ENTERITIS.

membranous glomerulonephritis. A form of glomerulonephritis characterized clinically by proteinuria or nephrotic syndrome which usually follows a benign course. The characteristic lesions of the glomerular basement membrane are seen by the electron microscope and consist of subendothelial or intramembranous electron-dense deposits interspersed by a thickened basement membrane. Proliferation of endocapillary cells is absent. Syn. *epimembranous nephropathy.*

membranous labyrinth. Those membranous canals corresponding to the shape of the osseous labyrinth, suspended in the perilymph, and containing endolymph. NA *labyrinthus membranaceus.*

membranous nephropathy. MEMBRANOUS GLOMERULONEPHRITIS.

membranous pneumocyte. SQUAMOUS ALVEOLAR CELL.

membranous pregnancy. Gestation in which there has been a rupture of the amniotic sac and the fetus is in direct contact with the wall of the uterus.

membranous semicircular canals. Three loop-shaped tubes in the membranous labyrinth of the ear lying at right angles to one another and communicating with the utricle. The superior (frontal) semicircular canal and the posterior (sagittal) semicircular canal lie in the vertical plane, making a right angle which opens laterally. The lateral or horizontal canal lies in the horizontal plane. Syn. *semicircular ducts.* NA *ductus semicirculares.*

membranous semicircular ducts. MEMBRANOUS SEMICIRCULAR CANALS.

membranous stomatitis. Stomatitis with the formation of an adventitious membrane.

membranous urethra. The part of the urethra between the two fascial layers of the urogenital diaphragm.

mem·brum (mem'brum) *n.*, pl. **mem·bra** (·bruh) [L.]. MEMBER.

membrum in·fe·ri·us (in·feer'ee·us) [NA]. LOWER EXTREMITY.

membrum mu·li·e·bre (mew''lee·ee'bree) [L., of woman]. CLITORIS.

membrum su·pe·ri·us (sue·peer'ee·us) [NA]. UPPER EXTREMITY.

membrum vi·ri·le (vi·rye'lee) [L.]. PENIS.

mem·o·ry (mem'uh·ree) *n.* [L. *memoria,* from *memor,* mindful]. 1. That faculty of mind by which ideas and sensations are recalled. 2. The mental process of recalling and reproducing that which has been learned and retained. 3. The capacity of an object to resume its original shape after being deformed, as, for example, a plastic IUD after being stretched during insertion.

memory trace. 1. ENGRAM. 2. *In psychiatry,* an experience intentionally forgotten but not fully repressed, which may result in a neurotic conflict.

mem·o·tine (mem'o·teen) *n.* 3,4-Dihydro-1-(4-methoxyphenoxy)methylisoquinoline, $C_{17}H_{17}NO_2$, an antiviral, used as the hydrochloride salt.

men-, meno- [Gk. *mēn,* month]. A combining form meaning *menses.*

men·ac·me (me·nack'mee) *n.* [*men-* + *acme*]. The period of a woman's life during which menstruation persists.

men·a·di·ol (men''uh·dye'ol) *n.* 2-Methyl-1,4-naphthohydroquinone or 2-methyl-1,4-naphthalenediol, $C_{11}H_{10}O_2$, a prothrombinogenic compound obtained by reduction of the C=O groups of menadione.

menadiol diacetate. ACETOMENAPHTHONE.

menadiol sodium diphosphate. Tetrasodium 2-methyl-1,4-naphthalenediolbis(dihydrogenphosphate), $C_{11}H_8Na_4O_8P_2.6H_2O$, a water-soluble prothrombogenic compound having the actions and uses of menadione. Syn. *sodium menadiol phosphate.*

men·a·di·one (men''uh·dye'ohn) *n.* 2-Methyl-1,4-naphthoquinone, $C_{11}H_8O_2$; practically insoluble in water but soluble in vegetable oils. Has vitamin-K activity in promoting synthesis of prothrombin and possibly other clotting factors in blood; used for the treatment of conditions characterized by hypoprothrombinemia. Syn. *menaphthone, vitamin* K_3.

menadione sodium bisulfite. 2-Methyl-1,4-naphthoquinone sodium bisulfite, $C_{11}H_8O_2.NaHSO_3.H_2O$, a water-soluble derivative of menadione with the actions and uses of the latter.

men·a·gogue (men'uh·gog) *n.* [*men-* + *-agogue*]. EMMENAGOGUE.

me·naph·thone (me·naf'thone) *n.* British Pharmacopoeia name for menadione.

men·ar·che (me·nahr'kee) *n.* [*men-* + Gk. *archē,* beginning]. The time when menstruation starts.

Men·de·lé·ev's law (men·dye·lye'yef) [D. I. *Mendeléev,* Russian chemist, 1834–1907]. PERIODIC LAW.

Mendelian ratio [G. *Mendel*]. The approximate numerical relation between various types of progeny in crosses involving sharply contrasted characters that conform to Mendel's law of heredity; the typical ratios for the F_2 generation are 3:1 for one pair of characters, 9:3:3:1 for two pairs.

Men·del·ism (men'duh·liz·um) *n.* The body of knowledge growing out of the application of Mendel's laws; this knowledge refers to all inheritance through the chromosomes. —**Men·de·lian** (men·dee'lee·un) *adj.*

Men·del reaction or **test** [F. *Mendel,* German physician, 1862–1925]. MANTOUX TEST.

Mendel's dorsal reflex of the foot [K. *Mendel,* German neurologist, 1874–1946]. BEKHTEREV-MENDEL REFLEX (1).

Mendel's laws [G. *Mendel,* Austrian botanist, 1822–1884]. The laws of heredity, concerning the way in which the hereditary units, the genes, pass from one generation to the next by way of the germ cells. In neo-Mendelian terms the principles may be stated as follows: Genes segregate at the time of maturation, with the result that a mature germ cell gets either the maternal or the paternal gene of any pair (first law). Genes of different pairs segregate independently of one another, provided they are located on different pairs of chromosomes (second law). If they are located on the same pair of chromosomes, they are linked and consequently segregate in larger or smaller blocks depending mainly on their relative distances apart on the chromosome, that is, on the percentage of crossing over (a discovery made after Mendel's time).

Men·del·son's syndrome [C. L. *Mendelson,* U.S. obstetrician, 20th century]. Postoperative chemical pneumonitis caused by silent aspiration of gastric contents.

Mendel's test [F. *Mendel*]. MANTOUX TEST.

men·el·lip·sis (men''e·lip'sis) *n.* [*men-* + *ellipsis*]. MENOLIPSIS.

Mé·né·tri·er's disease (mey·ney·tree·ey') [P. *Ménétrier,* French physician, 1859–1935]. Diffuse giant hypertrophic gastritis, benign, of unknown etiology. Symptoms include vomiting, diarrhea, weight loss, excessive mucus secretion, and hypoproteinemia.

Menformon. A trademark for preparations containing estrogens in oil.

Men·go virus. A strain of encephalomyocarditis virus, belonging to the picornavirus group.

men·hi·dro·sis (men''hi·dro'sis) *n.* [*men-* + *hidrosis*]. Replacement of the menstrual flow by bloody sweat.

men·idro·sis (men''i·dro'sis) *n.* MENHIDROSIS.

Mé·niè·re's syndrome or **disease** (mey·nyehr') [P. *Ménière,* French otologist, 1799–1862]. A disease of the internal ear characterized by deafness, vertigo, and tinnitus, frequently accompanied by nausea, vomiting, and nystagmus. An allergic mechanism for some cases has been suggested but not proven. Syn. *endolymphatic hydrops, labyrinthine hydrops* or *syndrome.*

mening-, meningo-. A combining form meaning (a) *meninx, meninges;* (b) *membrane, membranous.*

meninge-, meningeo-. See *mening-.*

me·nin·ge·al (me·nin'jee·ul) *adj.* Pertaining to the meninges.

meningeal arteries. See Table of Arteries in the Appendix.

meningeal carcinomatosis. Diffuse infiltration of the leptomeninges by tumor cells, such as of leukemia, medulloblastoma, or melanoma.

meningeal fibroblastoma. MENINGIOMA.

meningeal gliomatosis. Widespread involvement of the subarachnoid space by cells originating in a glioma. Syn. *gliosarcoma of the meninges, meningeal sarcomatosis.*

meningeal hydrops. PSEUDOTUMOR CEREBRI.

meningeal plexus. A nerve plexus found about the middle meningeal artery.

meningeal sarcoma. A sarcoma arising from dural fibroblasts.

meningeal sarcomatosis. MENINGEAL GLIOMATOSIS.
meningeal spaces. The subdural and subarachnoid spaces.
meningeo-. See *mening-.*
me·nin·ge·or·rha·phy (me·nin″jee·or′uh·fee) *n.* [*meningeo-* + *-rrhaphy*]. 1. Suture of membranes. 2. Suture of the meninges of the brain or spinal cord.
meninges [NA]. Plural of *meninx.*
meningi-, meningio-. See *mening-.*
me·nin·gio·blas·to·ma (me·nin″jee·o·blas·to′muh) *n.* [*meningio-* + *blastoma*]. MENINGIOMA.
me·nin·gio·fi·bro·blas·to·ma (me·nin″jee·o·figh″bro·blas·to′muh) *n.* [*meningio-* + *fibroblastoma*]. MENINGIOMA.
me·nin·gi·o·ma (me·nin″jee·o′muh) *n.* [*meningi-* + *-oma*]. A tumor derived from arachnoidal cells or dural fibroblasts, arranged in various patterns, involving the meninges or other central nervous system structures, and usually confined to local growth. Syn. *arachnothelioma, dural endothelioma, meningeal fibroblastoma, meningioblastoma, meningiothelioma.*
meningioma-en-plaque (ahn″plack′) [F.]. A meningioma forming a thin sheath of tumor tissue along the undersurface of the dura mater.
me·nin·gi·o·ma·to·sis (me·nin″jee·o″muh·to′sis) *n.* [*meningioma* + *-osis*]. Multiple meningiomas.
me·nin·gio·sar·co·ma (me·nin″jee·o·sahr·ko′muh) *n.* [*meningio-* + *sarcoma*]. MENINGEAL SARCOMA.
me·nin·gio·the·li·o·ma (me·nin″jee·o·theel·ee·o′muh) *n.* [*meningio-* + endo*thelioma*]. MENINGIOMA.
me·nin·gism (me·nin′jiz·um, men′in·) *n.* [*mening-* + *-ism*]. A condition in which there are signs and often symptoms of meningeal irritation, particularly nuchal rigidity, suggesting meningitis, but no evidence of this on examination of the cerebrospinal fluid; associated with many acute febrile illnesses in childhood.
men·in·gis·mus (men″in·jiz′mus) *n.* MENINGISM.
meningitic streak. TACHE CÉRÉBRALE.
men·in·gi·tis (men″in·jye′tis) *n.*, pl. **menin·git·i·des** (·jit′i·deez) [*mening-* + *-itis*]. 1. Any inflammation of the membranes of the brain or spinal cord. Meningitides may be classified according to the causative agent, as tuberculous meningitis, pneumococcal meningitis. 2. LEPTOMENINGITIS. See also *pachymeningitis, meningoencephalitis.* —**menin·git·ic** (·jit′ick) *adj.*
meningitis cir·cum·scrip·ta spi·na·lis (sur″kum·skrip′tuh spye·nay′lis). Arachnoiditis of the spinal cord only, with localized symptoms.
meningitis se·ro·sa circumscripta (se·ro′suh, ·zuh). Inflammation of the meninges with adhesions and formation of cystic accumulations of fluid which cause localized symptoms of pressure.
meningitis serosa spinalis. MENINGITIS CIRCUMSCRIPTA SPINALIS.
meningitis serum. ANTIMENINGOCOCCIC SERUM.
men·in·gito·pho·bia (men″in·jit″o·fo′bee·uh) *n.* 1. A morbid fear of meningitis. 2. A pseudomeningitis due to fear of that disease.
meningo-. See *mening-.*
me·nin·go·ar·te·ri·tis (me·ning″go·ahr″tur·eye′tis) *n.* Inflammation of the arteries of the meninges.
me·nin·go·cele (me·ning′go·seel) *n.* [*meningo-* + *-cele*]. A protrusion of the cerebral or spinal meninges through a defect in the skull or vertebral column, forming a cyst filled with cerebrospinal fluid.
me·nin·go·ceph·a·li·tis (me·ning″go·sef″uh·lye′tis) *n.* MENINGOENCEPHALITIS.
me·nin·go·cer·e·bral (me·ning′go·serr″e·brul) *adj.* [*meningo-* + *cerebral*]. Pertaining to the cerebrum and the meninges.
me·nin·go·cer·e·bri·tis (me·ning″go·serr″e·brigh′tis) *n.* [*meningo-* + *cerebr-* + *-itis*]. MENINGOENCEPHALITIS.
meningococcal meningitis. Meningitis caused by *Neisseria meningitidis* (meningococcus).
me·nin·go·coc·ce·mia (me·ning″go·kock·see′mee·uh) *n.* 1. The presence of meningococci in the blood. 2. A clinical disorder consisting of fever, skin hemorrhages, varying degrees of shock and meningococci in the blood. See also *Waterhouse-Friderichsen syndrome.*
meningococcic adrenal syndrome. WATERHOUSE-FRIDERICHSEN SYNDROME.
me·nin·go·coc·cus (me·ning″go·kock′us) *n.*, pl. **meningococ·ci** (·sigh) [*meningo-* + *coccus*]. Common name for *Neisseria meningitidis.* —**meningococ·cal** (·ul), **meningococ·cic** (·sick) *adj.*
meningococcus serum. ANTIMENINGOCOCCIC SERUM.
me·nin·go·cor·ti·cal (me·ning″go·kor′ti·kul) *adj.* [*meningo-* + *cortical*]. Pertaining to the meninges and the cortex of the cerebral hemispheres.
me·nin·go·cyte (me·ning′go·site) *n.* [*meningo-* + *-cyte*]. A flattened epithelioid cell lining a subarachnoid space, which may become phagocytic.
me·nin·go·en·ceph·a·li·tis (me·ning″go·en·sef″uh·lye′tis) *n.* [*meningo-* + *encephalitis*]. Inflammation of the brain and its membranes. —**meningoencepha·lit·ic** (·lit′ick) *adj.*
me·nin·go·en·ceph·a·lo·cele (me·ning″go·en·sef′uh·lo·seel) *n.* [*meningo-* + *encephalo-* + *-cele*]. Hernia of the brain and its meninges through a defect in the skull.
me·nin·go·en·ceph·a·lo·my·e·li·tis (me·ning″go·en·sef″uh·lo·migh″e·lye′tis) *n.* [*meningo-* + *encephalo-* + *myel-* + *-itis*]. Combined inflammation of the meninges, brain, and spinal cord.
me·nin·go·en·ceph·a·lop·a·thy (me·ning″go·en·sef″uh·lop′uth·ee) *n.* [*meningo-* + *encephalo-* + *-pathy*]. Disease of the brain and meninges.
me·nin·go·my·e·li·tis (me·ning″go·migh″e·lye′tis) *n.* [*meningo-* + *myelitis*]. Inflammation of the spinal cord and its meninges.
me·nin·go·my·e·lo·cele (me·ning″go·migh′e·lo·seel) *n.* [*meningo-* + *myelo-* + *-cele*]. A protrusion of a portion of the spinal cord and membranes through a defect in the vertebral column.
men·in·gop·a·thy (men″ing·gop′uth·ee) *n.* [*meningo-* + *-pathy*]. Any disease of the cerebrospinal meninges.
me·nin·go·ra·chid·i·an (me·ning″go·ra·kid′ee·un) *adj.* [*meningo-* + *rachidian*]. Pertaining to the spinal cord and its membranes.
meningorachidian veins. VERTEBRAL VEINS.
me·nin·go·ra·dic·u·lar (me·ning″go·ra·dick′yoo·lur) *adj.* [*meningo-* + *radicular*]. Pertaining to the meninges and nerve roots (cranial or spinal).
me·nin·gor·rha·gia (me·ning″go·ray′jee·uh) *n.* [*meningo-* + *-rrhagia*]. *Obsol.* Hemorrhage from the meninges.
men·in·go·sis (men″ing·go′sis) *n.* [*mening-* + *-osis*]. The fibrous union of bones.
meningothelial meningioma. A meningioma whose parenchymal cells resemble those of the arachnoid.
me·nin·go·the·li·o·ma (me·ning″go·theel·ee·o′muh) *n.* [*meningothel*ium + *-oma*]. MENINGIOMA. —**meningotheli·om·a·tous** (·om′uh·tus) *adj.*
me·nin·go·the·li·um (me·ning″go·theel′ee·um) *n.* [*meningo-* + epi*thelium*]. The epithelial cells of the arachnoid; the meningocytes. —**meningotheli·al** (·ul) *adj.*
me·nin·go·vas·cu·lar (me·ning″go·vas′kew·lur) *adj.* Involving both the meninges and the cerebral blood vessels.
meningovascular syphilis. A form of neurosyphilis, characterized by syphilitic meningitis in combination with an inflammation and productive fibrosis of the cerebral arteries (Heubner's endarteritis) leading to narrowing and occlusion of the arteries and infarction of the brain or spinal cord.
men·in·gu·ria (men″ing·gew′ree·uh) *n.* [*mening-* + *-uria*]. The passage, or presence, of membranous shreds in the urine.
me·ninx (mee′ninks, men′inks) *n.*, pl. **me·nin·ges** (me·nin′jeez) [Gk. *mēninx*]. A membrane, especially one of the brain or spinal cord; the meninges covering the brain and

spinal cord consist of the dura mater, pia mater, and arachnoid.

meninx pri·mi·ti·va (prim″i·tye′vuh). The layer of mesoderm surrounding the neural tube that forms the neurocranium and meninges.

menisc-, menisco- [Gk. *mēniskos,* crescent]. A combining form meaning (a) *crescentic, sickle-shaped, semilunar;* (b) *meniscus, semilunar cartilage.*

men·is·cec·to·my (men″i·seck′tuh·mee) *n.* [*menisc-* + *-ectomy*]. The surgical excision of a meniscus or semilunar cartilage.

menisci. Plural and genitive singular of *meniscus.*

menisci tac·tus (tack′tus) [NA]. TACTILE DISKS.

men·is·ci·tis (men″i·sigh′tis) *n.* [*menisc-* + *-itis*]. An inflammation of any interarticular cartilage; specifically, of the semilunar cartilages of the knee joint.

menisco-. See *menisc-.*

me·nis·co·cyte (me·nis′ko·site) *n.* [*menisco-* + *-cyte*]. A sickle-shaped erythrocyte.

me·nis·co·cy·to·sis (me·nis″ko·sigh·to′sis) *n.* [*meniscocyte* + *-osis*]. SICKLE CELL ANEMIA.

me·nis·co·fem·o·ral (me·nis″ko·fem′uh·rul) *adj.* Of or pertaining to a meniscus of the knee joint and the femur.

meniscofemoral ligament. Either of the small fibrous bands in the knee joint originating in the posterior end of the lateral meniscus and attached to the medial condyle of the femur near or in conjunction with the posterior cruciate ligament; the anterior meniscofemoral ligament (NA *ligamentum meniscofemorale anterius*) or the posterior meniscofemoral ligament (NA *ligamentum meniscofemorale posterius*), which pass respectively in front of and behind the posterior cruciate ligament.

me·nis·cus (me·nis′kus) *n.*, L. pl. & genit. sing. **menis·ci** (·skye, ·sigh), [Gk. *mēniskos,* crescent]. 1. A crescent-shaped interarticular wedge of fibrocartilage found especially in the sternoclavicular, acromioclavicular, and knee joints. NA *meniscus articularis.* 2. A concavoconvex lens (positive meniscus) or a convexoconcave lens (negative meniscus). 3. The curved surface of a column of liquid.

meniscus ar·ti·cu·la·ris (ahr·tick″yoo·lair′is) [NA]. MENISCUS (1).

meniscus la·te·ra·lis (lat·e·ray′lis) [NA]. LATERAL MENISCUS.

meniscus me·di·a·lis (mee·dee·ay′lis) [NA]. MEDIAL MENISCUS.

meniscus sign. 1. A radiographic sign associated with an ulcerating carcinoma, in which the outline of the stomach is crescentic with overhanging edges. 2. A snapping or clicking associated with a torn meniscus in the knee.

meniscus tac·tus (tack′tus) [NA.]. TACTILE DISK.

Menkes' syndrome [J. H. *Menkes,* U.S. pediatric neurologist, b. 1928]. KINKY HAIR DISEASE.

meno-. See *men-.*

me·noc·tone (me·nock′tone) *n.* 2-(8-Cyclohexyloctyl)-3-hydroxy-1,4-naphthoquinone, $C_{24}H_{32}O_3$, an antimalarial drug.

meno·lip·sis (men″o·lip′sis) *n.* [*meno-* + Gk. *leipsis,* omission]. The retention or absence of the menses.

meno·me·tror·rha·gia (men″o·mee″tro·ray′jee·uh, ·met″ro·) *n.* [*meno-* + *metro-* + *-rrhagia*]. Uterine bleeding of excessive amount at the time of menstruation, plus irregular uterine bleeding at other times.

menopausal flush. HOT FLUSH.

menopausal syndrome. CLIMACTERIC.

meno·pause (men′o·pawz) *n.* [F., from *meno-* + *pause*]. The physiologic cessation of menstruation, usually between the forty-fifth and fifty-fifth years. See also *climacteric.* —**menopaus·ic** (men″o·pawz′ick), **menopaus·al** (·ul) *adj.*

meno·pha·nia (men″o·fay′nee·uh) *n.* [*meno-* + Gk. *phainein,* to appear, + *-ia*]. The first appearance of the menses.

meno·pla·nia (men″o·play′nee·uh) *n.* [*meno-* + *plan-,* wandering, + *-ia*]. A discharge of blood occurring at the menstrual period, but derived from some part of the body other than the uterus; vicarious menstruation, as in endometriosis.

men·or·rha·gia (men″o·ray′jee·uh) *n.* [*meno-* + *-rrhagia*]. An excessive menstrual flow. Syn. *hypermenorrhea.* —**menor·rhag·ic** (·raj′ick) *adj.*

men·or·rhal·gia (men″o·ral′jee·uh) *n.* [*menorrhea* + *-algia*]. Pelvic pain at menstrual periods other than characteristic midline cramp; characteristic of endometriosis.

men·or·rhea, men·or·rhoea (men″o·ree′uh) *n.* [*meno-* + *-rrhea*]. The normal flow of the menses.

me·nos·che·sis (me·nos′ke·sis, men″o·skee′sis) *n.* [*meno-* + Gk. *schesis,* checking, retention]. Retention of the menses.

meno·sta·sia (men″o·stay′zhuh, ·zee·uh) *n.* [*menostasis* + *-ia*]. MENOSTASIS.

me·nos·ta·sis (me·nos′tuh·sis) *n.* [*meno-* + Gk. *stasis,* standstill, stoppage]. Suppression of the menstrual flow.

meno·stax·is (men″o·stack′sis) *n.* [*meno-* + *staxis*]. Prolonged menstruation.

men·o·tro·pins (men″o·tro′pinz) *n.* A purified, standardized extract of postmenopausal urine containing primarily the follicle-stimulating hormone with a trace of luteinizing hormone.

men·o·xe·nia (men″ock·see′nee·uh, men″o·zee′nee·uh) *n.* [*meno-* + Gk. *xenos,* alien, strange, + *-ia*]. Irregularity of menstruation; vicarious menstruation.

mens (menz, mence) *n.*, genit. **men·tis** (men′tis) [L.]. MIND.

men·ses (men′seez) *n.pl.* [L., months]. The recurrent monthly discharge of blood from the genital canal of a woman during reproductive years.

mens sa·na in cor·po·re sa·no (mens sah′nuh in cor′po·re sah′no) [L.]. A sound mind in a sound body.

men·stru·al (men′stroo·ul) *adj.* [L. *menstrualis,* monthly]. Of or pertaining to menstruation.

menstrual age. The age of an embryo or fetus calculated from the first day of the mother's last normal menstruation preceding pregnancy.

menstrual cycle. The periodically recurring series of changes in the uterus, ovaries, and accessory sexual structures associated with menstruation and the intermenstrual periods in primates. See also *endometrial cycle.*

menstrual period. The time of the menses.

men·stru·ant (men′stroo·unt) *adj. & n.* 1. Subject to, or capable of, menstruating. 2. A girl or woman who menstruates.

men·stru·ate (men′stroo·ate) *v.* [L. *menstruare,* from *menstrua,* menses]. To discharge the products of menstruation.

men·stru·a·tion (men″stroo·ay′shun) *n.* [from *menstruate*]. A periodic discharge of a sanguineous fluid from the uterus, occurring during the period of a woman's sexual maturity from puberty to the menopause.

men·stru·um (men′stroo·um) *n.* [L.]. A solvent, commonly one that extracts certain principles from entire plant or animal tissues.

men·su·al (men′shoo·ul, men′sue·ul) *adj.* [L. *mensualis*]. Monthly.

men·su·ra·tion (men″shoo·ray′shun, men″sue·) *n.* [L. *mensuratio,* from *mensura,* measure]. The act or process of measuring.

men·tag·ra (men·tag′ruh) *n.* [*mentum* + *-agra*]. SYCOSIS.

¹men·tal, *adj.* [L. *mentalis,* from *mens,* mind]. 1. Pertaining to the mind, psyche, or inner self, as in mental health. 2. Pertaining to the intellectual or cognitive functions, as distinct from the affective and conative, as in mental test. 3. Imaginary or unreal, as when a pain is said to be merely mental.

²mental, *adj.* [L. *mentum,* chin, + *-al*]. Pertaining to the chin. Syn. *genial.*

mental aberration. A deviation from normal mental function. See also *mental disorders.*

mental adjustment. An adjustment involving an individual's attitudes, traits, or feelings to his social environment. See also *mental health.*

mental age. 1. The degree of mental development of an

individual in terms of the chronological age of the average individual of equivalent mental ability. 2. Specifically, a score, derived from intelligence tests, expressed in terms of the age at which an average individual attains that score. An adult whose score is the equivalent of that of an average child of 12 has a mental age of 12. Abbreviated, MA.

mental artery. NA *arteria mentalis.* See Table of Arteries in the Appendix.

mental chronometry. The study of mental processes in relation to time.

mental deficiency. 1. A defect of intelligence, the degree of which may be indicated by the intelligence quotient for the specific test employed; graded as mild (I.Q. 70 to 85), moderate (I.Q. 50 to 69), and severe (I.Q. below 50). In the United States, the presently preferred term is mental retardation, although some authorities seek to make a distinction between the two terms on the basis of a demonstrable organic lesion in mental deficiency, and the implication that deficiency is a nonremediable state. 2. *In civil law,* the condition as defined by statute, frequently divided into three grades: idiocy, the lowest, imbecility, the intermediate; and moronity, the highest. See also *mental retardation.*

mental disease. MENTAL DISORDER.

mental disorders. Related psychiatric conditions, divided into two major groups: (a) Those in which there is a primary impairment of brain function, generally associated with an organic brain syndrome upon which diagnosis is based; the psychiatric picture is characterized by impairment of intellectual functions, including memory, orientation, and judgment, and by shallowness and lability of affect. Additional disturbances, such as psychosis, neurosis, or behavioral reactions, may be associated with these disorders but are secondary to the diagnosis. (b) Those conditions which are more directly the result of the individual's difficulty in adapting to his environment, and in which any associated impairment of brain function is secondary to the psychiatric disturbance.

mental dynamism. MENTAL MECHANISM.

mental foramen. The external aperture of the mandibular canal; it transmits the mental nerves and vessels to the skin of the face. NA *foramen mentale.*

mental healing. The use of suggestion or faith in the attempt to cure illness, particularly physical illness. Compare *psychotherapy.*

mental health. A relatively enduring state of being in which an individual has effected an integration of his instinctual drives in a way that is reasonably satisfying to himself as reflected in his zest for living and his feeling of self-realization. For most individuals, mental health also implies a large degree of adjustment to the social environment as indicated by the satisfaction derived from their interpersonal relationships as well as their achievements.

mental hygiene. That branch of hygiene dealing with the preservation of mental and emotional health.

mental illness. MENTAL DISORDER.

men·ta·lis (men·tay'lis) *n.* A muscle of the lower lip. NA *musculus mentalis.* See also Table of Muscles in the Appendix.

men·tal·i·ty (men·tal'i·tee) *n.* 1. Mental endowment, capacity, or power; intellect. 2. Outlook, ways of thinking.

mental mechanism. An intrapsychic, largely unconscious process, such as a defense mechanism, memory, perception, or thinking, which is a function of the ego and thus determines behavior.

mental parallax. The phenomenon of two or more individuals observing the same thing somewhat differently, due to their different standpoints.

mental patient. In common usage, any patient who requires psychiatric care and treatment; specifically, those psychiatric cases requiring security accommodations, hospitalization, or institutionalization.

mental point. GNATHION.

mental protuberance. The elevation of the body of the mandible which forms the chin. NA *protuberantia mentalis.*

mental retardation. Subnormal intellectual functioning, often present since birth or apparent in early life; may be primary (hereditary or familial), without demonstrable organic brain lesion or known prenatal cause, or secondary, due to brain tissue anomalies, chromosomal disorder, prenatal, maternal, or postnatally acquired infections, intoxication or trauma, prematurity, disorders of growth, nutrition, or metabolism, degenerative diseases, tumor, or following major psychiatric disorders or associated with psychosocial (environmental) deprivation; classified as borderline, mild, moderate, severe, and profound. See also *mental deficiency, cultural-familial mental retardation, environmental deprivation.* Syn. *mental subnormality.*

mental set. The attitude, interest, or intent of a subject which may influence his perception.

mental spine. The single or double tubercle on each side of the inner surface of the body of the mandible near the midline, for origin of the genioglossus and geniohyoid muscles. Syn. *genial spine.* NA *spina mentalis.*

mental subnormality. MENTAL RETARDATION.

mental tubercle. A raised area on each side of the mental protuberance of the mandible in the midline. Syn. *genial tubercle.* NA *tuberculum mentale mandibulae.* See also *mental spine.*

mental vaginismus. Painful spasm of the vagina due to extreme aversion to the sexual act; PSYCHOLOGIC DYSPAREUNIA.

men·ta·tion (men·tay'shun) *n.* The mechanism of thought; mental activity.

menth-, mentho-. A combining form meaning *menthol.*

Men·tha (men'thuh) *n.* [L., mint]. A genus of plants of the Labiatae; the mints.

Men·tha·ce·ae (men·thay'see·ee) *n.pl.* LABIATAE.

Mentha pip·e·ri·ta (pip''ur·eye'tuh). Peppermint; the dried leaves and flowering tops have been used as an aromatic stimulant and carminative.

Mentha pu·le·gi·um (pew·lee'jee·um). European pennyroyal, the leaves and tops of which have been used as a carminative. See also *hedeoma.*

men·thol (men'thol) *n.* [*Mentha* + *-ol*]. *p*-Menthan-3-ol, $C_{10}H_{19}OH$, an alcohol obtained from peppermint or other mint oils or prepared synthetically. Used externally for its antipruritic, anesthetic, or antiseptic effects.

men·thyl (men'thil) *n.* The monovalent radical $C_{10}H_{19}$— of the alcohol menthol.

men·ti·cide (men'ti·side) *n.* [L. *mens, mentis,* mind, + *-cide*]. BRAINWASHING.

mento- [L. *mentum,* chin]. *In anatomy,* a combining form meaning *chin.*

men·to·an·te·ri·or (men''to·an·teer'ee·ur) *adj.* [*mento-* + *anterior*]. With the chin pointing forward; usually referring to the position of the child's face during parturition.

men·to·hy·oid (men''to·high'oid) *n.* [*mento-* + *hyoid*]. A variant of the digastric muscle extending from the hyoid bone to the chin.

men·ton (men'ton) *n.* [F., chin]. GNATHION.

men·to·pa·ri·etal (men''to·puh·rye'e·tul) *adj.* [*mento-* + *parietal*]. Pertaining to the chin and the parietal bone.

mentoparietal diameter. The diameter joining the chin and the vertex.

men·to·pos·te·ri·or (men''to·pos·teer'ee·ur) *adj.* [*mento-* + *posterior*]. With the chin pointing backward; usually referring to the position of the child's face during parturition.

men·tu·lo·ma·nia (men''tew·lo·may'nee·uh) *n.* [L. *mentula,* penis, + *-mania*]. MASTURBATION.

men·tum (men'tum) *n.,* pl. **men·ta** (·tuh) [L.] [NA]. CHIN.

mep·a·crine (mep'uh·kreen, ·krin) *n.* British name for quinacrine.

Mepadin. A trademark for meperidine, a narcotic analgesic.

me·par·tri·cin (me·pahr'tri·sin) *n.* The methyl ester of partricin, a substance of unknown structure used as an antifungal and antiprotozoal.

mep·a·zine (mep'uh·zeen) *n.* 10-[(1-Methyl-3-piperidyl)-methyl]phenothiazine, $C_{19}H_{22}N_2S$, a tranquilizing and antinauseant drug; used as the hydrochloride salt.

me·pen·zo·late bromide (me·pen'zo·late). *N*-Methyl-3-piperidyl benzilate methyl bromide, $C_{21}H_{26}BrNO_3$, an anticholinergic drug used to relieve gastrointestinal spasm and hypermotility.

me·per·i·dine (me·perr'i·deen, ·din, mep'ur·) *n.* Ethyl 1-methyl-4-phenylisonipecotate, $C_{15}H_{21}NO_2$, a narcotic analgesic; used as the hydrochloride salt. Syn. *isonipecaine, pethidine.*

me·phen·e·sin (me·fen'e·sin) *n.* 3-*o*-(Tolyloxy)-1,2-propanediol, $C_{10}H_{14}O_3$, a skeletal muscle relaxant.

meph·en·ox·a·lone (mef''en·ock'suh·lone) *n.* 5-(*o*-Methoxyphenoxymethyl)-2-oxazolidinone, $C_{11}H_{13}NO_4$, a mild tranquilizer.

me·phen·ter·mine (me·fen'tur·meen) *n.* *N*,α,α-Trimethylphenethylamine, $C_{11}H_{17}N$, a sympathomimetic amine used as the sulfate salt for vasopressor effect in hypotensive conditions and as the base for nasal decongestion.

me·phen·y·to·in (me·fen'ee·to''in) *n.* 5-Ethyl-3-methyl-5-phenylhydantoin, $C_{12}H_{14}N_2O_2$, an anticonvulsant drug effective in generalized seizures. Syn. *methoin.*

me·phit·ic (me·fit'ick) *adj.* [L. *mephiticus,* from *mephitis,* noxious exhalation from the ground]. Foul or noxious; stifling, as mephitic gangrene, necrosis of bone associated with the evolution of offensive odors.

meph·o·bar·bi·tal (mef''o·bahr'bi·tol) *n.* 5-Ethyl-1-methyl-5-phenylbarbituric acid, $C_{13}H_{14}N_2O_3$, a long-acting barbiturate used as an anticonvulsant and sedative; has slight hypnotic action. Syn. *methyl phenobarbital, phemitone.*

Mephyton. A trademark for phytonadione or vitamin K_1, a prothrombogenic vitamin.

me·piv·a·caine (me·piv'uh·kane) *n.* *dl*-1-Methyl-2',6'-pipecoloxylidide, $C_{15}H_{22}N_2O$, an amide-type local anesthetic; used as the hydrochloride salt.

me·pred·ni·sone (me·pred'ni·sone) *n.* 17,21-Dihydroxy-16β-methylpregna-1,4-diene-3,11,20-trione, $C_{22}H_{28}O_5$, an adrenocortical steroid.

me·pro·ba·mate (me·pro'buh·mate, ·pro·bam') *n.* 2-Methyl-2-*n*-propyl-1,3-propanediol dicarbamate, $C_9H_{18}N_2O_4$, a tranquilizer with anticonvulsant, muscle relaxant, and sedative actions.

Meprospan. A trademark for meprobamate, a sedative.

mep·ryl·caine (mep'ril·kane) *n.* 2-Methyl-2-propylaminopropyl benzoate, $C_{14}H_{21}NO_2$, a local anesthetic; used as the hydrochloride salt.

me·pyr·amine (me·pirr'uh·meen) *n.* British name for the antihistaminic drug pyrilamine.

me·pyr·a·pone (me·pirr'uh·pone) *n.* METYRAPONE.

meq, mEq Abbreviation for *milliequivalent.*

meq·ui·dox (meck'wi·docks) *n.* 3-Methyl-2-quinoxalinemethanol 1,4-dioxide, $C_{10}H_{10}N_2O_3$, an antibacterial agent.

-mer [Gk. *-merēs,* from *meros,* part]. A combining form designating *a molecular unit or configuration.*

mer-, mero- [Gk. *meros,* part]. A combining form meaning (a) *part, segment;* (b) *partial.*

me·ral·gia (me·ral'jee·uh) *n.* [Gk. *mēros,* thigh, + *-algia*]. Neuralgic pain in the thigh.

meralgia par·es·thet·i·ca (păr''es·thet'i·kuh). A neuropathy characterized by pain, paresthesias, and sensory disturbances in the area supplied by the lateral femoral cutaneous nerve; usually due to compression of the nerve where it enters the thigh beneath the inguinal ligament, at the level of the anterior superior iliac spine. Syn. *Roth-Bernhardt's disease.*

mer·al·lu·ride (mur·al'yoo·ride, ·rid) *n.* *N*-{[3-(Hydroxymercuri)-2-methoxypropyl] carbamoyl} succinamic acid, and theophylline, in approximately molecular proportions; a mercurial diuretic, the sodium derivative of which is administered parenterally.

mer·a·lo·pia (merr''uh·lo'pee·uh) *n.* Blurring of vision, with halos seen around objects viewed in a bright light; often associated with the administration of oxazolidine derivatives.

mer·am·au·ro·sis (merr·am''aw·ro'sis, merr''uh·maw·ro'sis) *n.* [*mer-* + *amaurosis*]. Partial amaurosis.

M:E ratio. MYELOID:ERYTHROID RATIO.

mer·bro·min (mur·bro'min) *n.* The disodium salt of 2',7'-dibromo-4'-(hydroxymercuri)fluorescein, an organomercurial antibacterial agent applied topically.

mercapt-, mercapto-. A combining form indicating the presence of the thiol, —SH, group.

mer·cap·tal (mur·kap'tal) *n.* A product of the interaction of a mercaptan with an aldehyde, water being eliminated. Syn. *thioacetal.*

mer·cap·tan (mur·kap'tan) *n.* [L. *mer*curium *captan*s, capturing mercury]. 1. An organic compound of the general formula RSH, representing an alcohol ROH, in which oxygen is replaced by sulfur. Syn. *thio alcohol, thiol.* 2. Ethyl mercaptan, C_2H_5SH.

mer·cap·tide (mur·kap'tide) *n.* Any metallic derivative of a mercaptan in which the hydrogen of the SH group of the latter is replaced by metal.

mercapto-. See *mercapt-.*

mer·cap·tol (mur·kap'tol) *n.* A product of the interaction of a ketone and a mercaptan, of the general formula R'R''C(SR)$_2$.

mer·cap·to·mer·in sodium (mur·kap''to·merr'in, mur''kap·tom'ur·in). Disodium *N*-[3-(carboxymethylthiomercuri)-2-methoxypropyl]-α-camphoramate, $C_{16}H_{25}HgNNa_2O_6S$, an organomercurial diuretic drug.

mer·cap·to·pu·rine (mur·kap''to·pew'reen) *n.* 6-Mercaptopurine, $C_5H_4N_4S$, the mercapto analogue of 6-aminopurine or adenine; a cytotoxic agent useful for the treatment of acute leukemia.

mer·cap·tu·ric acid (mur''kap·tew'rick). Any detoxication product in which acetylated cysteine is conjugated with the foreign body undergoing the process of detoxication.

Mer·cier's bar (mehr·syey') [L. A. *Mercier,* French urologist, 1811–1882]. BAR OF THE BLADDER.

Mercloran. A trademark for chlormerodrin, a diuretic.

mer·cu·mat·i·lin (mur''kew·mat'i·lin, mur·kew''muh·til'in) *n.* A mercurial diuretic preparation containing 8-(2'-methoxy-3'-hydroxymercuripropyl)coumarin-3-carboxylic acid (known as mercumallylic acid) and theophylline.

mercuri-. A combining form meaning (a) *mercury;* (b) *mercuric.*

mer·cu·ri·al (mur·kew'ree·ul) *adj.* & *n.* 1. Pertaining to or caused by mercury. 2. Any preparation of mercury or its salts.

mercurial diuretic. An organic mercurial compound which acts primarily by reducing tubular reabsorption of water through binding of mercury with sulfhydryl groups in kidney tubules.

mer·cu·ri·al·ism (mur·kew'ree·ul·iz·um) *n.* Poisoning due to absorption of mercury.

mercurial nephrosis. 1. Nephrotic syndrome occurring in patients treated with mecurial diuretics. 2. Acute tubular necrosis secondary to ingestion of mercuric chloride.

mercurial stomatitis. Stomatitis due to the excessive absorption of mercury.

mercurial tremor. A tremor observed in persons with chronic poisoning by mercury. It may be sudden or gradual in onset and involve the tongue, lips, and hands, next the arms, and then the entire muscular system.

mer·cu·ric (mur·kew'rick) *adj.* Pertaining to, or containing, mercury in the bivalent state.

mercuric chloride. MERCURY BICHLORIDE.

mercuric iodide, red. HgI_2. Scarlet-red amorphous powder; has been used locally as an antiseptic and internally as an antisyphilitic.

mercuric oxide, red. HgO. Orange-red, crystalline powder; has been used locally as an antiseptic.

mercuric oxide, yellow. HgO. Yellow powder, more finely subdivided than red mercuric oxide; used locally as an antibacterial agent, especially for infections of the eye.

Mercurochrome. Trademark for merbromin, an organomercurial antibacterial agent applied topically.

Mercurophen. Trademark for sodium hydroxymercuri-*o*-nitrophenolate, an organomercurial antibacterial agent applied topically.

mer·cu·ro·phyl·line (mur″kew·ro·fil′een, ·in) *n.* The sodium salt of 3-{[3-(hydroxymercuri)-2-methoxypropyl]carbamoyl}-1,2,2-trimethylcyclopentanecarboxylic acid, and theophylline, in approximately molecular proportions; a mercurial diuretic administered orally or intramuscularly.

mer·cu·rous (mur·kew′rus, mur′kew·rus) *adj.* Pertaining to, or containing, mercury in the univalent state.

mercurous chloride. HgCl. White powder, insoluble in water; occasionally used as a cathartic. Syn. *calomel, mild mercurous chloride.*

mer·cu·ry (mur′kew·ree) *n.* [L. *Mercurius,* messenger of the gods]. Hg = 200.59. A shining, silver-white, liquid, volatile metal, having a specific gravity of 13.55. Forms two classes of compounds: (a) mercurous, in which the metal is univalent, and (b) mercuric, in which it is bivalent. Mercuric salts are more soluble and more poisonous than the mercurous. Mercury in the form of its salts was formerly used as a purgative and cholagogue, as an alterative in chronic inflammations, as an antisyphilitic, an antiphlogistic, an intestinal antiseptic, a disinfectant, a parasiticide, a caustic, and an astringent. Absorption of mercury in sufficient quantity causes poisoning, characterized by a coppery taste in the mouth, ptyalism, loosening of the teeth, sponginess of the gums; in more severe cases, ulceration of the cheeks, necrosis of the jaws, marked emaciation; at times neuritis develops, and a peculiar tremor.

mercury bichloride. Mercuric chloride, $HgCl_2$; white crystals or powder, soluble in water. Now used only as a germicide and disinfectant. Syn. *corrosive sublimate.*

mercury vapor lamp. A hollow fused quartz lamp filled with mercury vapor, producing radiations a large proportion of which are at the radiation emission line of 2540 Å, having high germicidal action.

-mere [Gk. *meros*]. A combining form meaning *part, segment.*

mer·er·ga·sia (merr″ur·gay′zhuh, ·zee·uh) *n.* [*mer-* + *ergasia*]. 1. Partial or subnormal ability to function physically or mentally. 2. *In psychobiology,* Meyer's term for a partial disturbance of the personality, as a neurotic or psychoneurotic reaction. Syn. *cacergasia.* —**merer·gas·tic** (·gas′tick) *adj.*

mer·eth·ox·yl·line procaine (mur″eth·ock′si·leen, merr″). A compound of dehydro-2-[*N*-(3′-hydroxymercuri-2′-methoxyethoxy)propylcarbamoyl]phenoxyacetic acid (merethoxylline), procaine, and theophylline; a mercurial diuretic.

me·rid·i·an (me·rid′ee·un) *n.* [L. *meridianus,* of midday]. A great circle surrounding a sphere and intersecting the poles.

meridiani. Plural of *meridianus* (= MERIDIAN).

meridiani bul·bi ocu·li (bul′bye ock′yoo·lye) [NA]. MERIDIANS OF THE EYE.

meridians of the eye. Lines drawn around the globe of the eye and passing through the poles of the vertical axis (vertical meridian), or through the poles of the transverse axis (horizontal meridian). NA *meridiani bulbi oculi.*

me·ri·di·a·nus (me·rid″ee·ay′nus) *n.*, pl. **meridia·ni** (·nigh) [L.]. MERIDIAN.

me·rid·i·o·nal (me·rid′ee·uh·nul) *adj.* Of or pertaining to a meridian.

meridional aniseikonia. Aniseikonia in which one image is larger than the other in one meridian.

meridional cleavage. Vertical cleavage in a plane through the egg axis.

mer·in·tho·pho·bia (merr″in·tho·fo′bee·uh, me·rin″tho·) *n.* [Gk. *mērinthos,* cord, + *-phobia*]. A morbid fear of being tied up.

mer·i·sis (merr′i·sis) *n.*, pl. **meri·ses** (·seez) [Gk., dividing, partition]. HYPERPLASIA.

mer·i·so·prol Hg 197 (merr·eye′so·prole) *n.* 1-(Hydroxymercuri)-2-propanol, $C_3H_8HgO_2$, containing a small quantity of the mercury as radioactive isotope; used as a diagnostic aid for testing renal function.

meri·spore (merr′i·spore) *n.* [Gk. *meris,* part, segment, + *spore*]. A segment or spore of a multicellular spore body.

me·ris·tic (me·ris′tick) *adj.* [Gk. *meristikos,* fit for dividing]. Pertaining to, or divided into, segments.

meristic variations. Variations in the number of parts.

Mer·kel's disk or **corpuscle** (mehr′k^e^l) [F. S. *Merkel,* German anatomist, 1845–1919]. TACTILE DISK.

Merkel's filtrum [K. L. *Merkel,* German anatomist and laryngologist, 1812–1876]. FILTRUM VENTRICULI.

Merkel's tactile disk [F. S. *Merkel*]. TACTILE DISK.

mer·maid fetus. SYMPUS.

mero-. See *mer-.*

mero·acra·nia (merr″o·a·kray′nee·uh) *n.* [*mero-* + *acrania*]. Congenital absence of a part of the cranium.

mero·blas·tic (merr″o·blas′tick) *adj.* [*mero-* + *-blastic*]. Dividing only in part, referring to an egg in which the cleavage divisions are confined to the animal pole, owing to the presence of a large amount of yolk.

meroblastic cleavage. Cleavage restricted to the cytoplasmic part of a yolk-laden ovum. Syn. *partial cleavage.*

mero·crine (merr′o·krin, ·krine) *adj.* [*mero-* + *-crine*]. Pertaining to glands in which the act of secretion leaves the cell itself intact, for example, in salivary and pancreatic glands. Contr. *holocrine, apocrine.*

me·roc·ri·nous (me·rock′ri·nus) *adj.* MEROCRINE.

mero·gen·e·sis (merr″o·jen′e·sis) *n.* [*mero-* + *-genesis*]. Reproduction by segmentation; somite formation.

mero·mi·cro·so·mia (merr″o·mye″kro·so′mee·uh) *n.* [*mero-* + *microsomia*]. Abnormal smallness of some part of the body.

mero·my·o·sin (merr″o·migh′o·sin) *n.* [*mero-* + *myosin*]. A fragment obtained by limited proteolysis of myosin. Two separate meromyosins, designated heavy and light, are obtained.

me·ro·pia (me·ro′pee·uh) *n.* [*mer-* + *-opia*]. Obscuration of vision.

mero·ra·chis·chi·sis (merr″o·ra·kis′ki·sis) *n.* [*mero-* + *rachischisis*]. Partial spina bifida.

me·ros·mia (me·roz′mee·uh, me·ros′) *n.* [*mer-* + *osm-* + *-ia*]. Partial loss of the sense of smell in that certain odors are not perceived.

mero·som·a·tous (merr″o·som′uh·tus, ·so′muh·tus) *adj.* [*mero-* + *somat-* + *-ous*]. Characterizing a monstrosity in which only part of the body is involved. Contr. *pantasomatous.*

mero·some (merr′o·sohm) *n.* [*mero-* + *-some*]. A somite or metamere.

me·rot·o·my (me·rot′um·ee) *n.* [*mero-* + *-tomy*]. 1. The section of a living cell for the study of the ulterior transformation of its segments. 2. The experimental division of unicellular organisms, such as amebas.

mero·zo·ite (merr″o·zo′ite) *n.* [*mero-* + *zo-* + *-ite*]. Any one of the segments resulting from the splitting up of the schizont in the asexual form of reproduction of sporozoa.

Merphenyl. A trademark for certain phenylmercuric salt antiseptic preparations.

Merprane. Trademark for merisoprol Hg 197, a radioactive diagnostic aid for testing renal function.

mer·sal·yl (mur′suh·lil, ·leel, mur·sal′il) *n.* Sodium *o*-{[3-(hydroxymercuri)-2-methoxypropyl] carbamoyl}phenoxyacetate, introduced as a mercurial antisyphilitic but now used as a parenterally administered diuretic; the available preparation contains also theophylline and is called mersalyl and theophylline injection.

Merthiolate. Trademark for thimerosal, a bacteriostatic and fungistatic agent.

Me·ru·li·us (me·roo′lee·us) *n.* [L. *merula*, blackbird]. A genus of fungi of the class Basidiomycetes.

Merulius lac·ri·mans (lack′ri·manz) [L., weeping]. A species of fungus whose mycelium causes dry rot in timber. Chronic bronchitis has been attributed to the inhalation of its spores.

me·ru·tu (me·roo·too′) *n.* MAMPIRRA.

Meruvax. A trademark for live rubella virus vaccine.

mer·y·cism (merr′i·siz·um) *n.* [Gk. *mērykismos*, chewing the cud]. RUMINATION (2).

Merz·bach·er-Pe·li·zae·us disease (mehrts′bakh·ur, peʸ·lee·tseʸ′ŏŏs) [L. *Merzbacher*, German physician, b. 1895; and F. *Pelizaeus*]. PELIZAEUS-MERZBACHER DISEASE.

mes-, meso- [Gk. *mesos*]. A prefix and combining form meaning (a) *mid-, middle, medial;* (b) *medium, moderate, intermediate;* (c) *mesentery;* (d) *mesodermal.* See also *meso-* (2).

mes·ame·boid (mes″uh·mee′boid) *adj.* Minot's term characterizing a primitive ameboid wandering cell of the mesoderm functioning as a hemocytoblast in the embryo and perhaps in the adult.

mes·an·gi·al (mes·an′jee·ul) *adj.* [*mesangium* + *-al*]. Pertaining to or involving the mesangium.

mes·an·gi·um (mes·an′jee·um) *n.* [*mes-* + *-angium*]. The suspensory structure of the renal glomerulus, consisting of a network of sponge fibers and associated cells, which attaches to the hilus of the glomerulus supporting the capillary loops in the fashion of a mesentery.

Mesantoin. Trademark for mephenytoin, an anticonvulsant drug.

mes·aor·ti·tis (mes″ay·or·tye′tis) *n.* [*mes-* + *aortitis*]. Inflammation of the middle coat of the aorta.

mes·a·ra·ic (mes″uh·ray′ick) *adj.* [Gk. *mesaraïkos*]. *Obsol.* MESENTERIC.

mes·ar·te·ri·tis (mes·ahr″te·rye′tis) *n.* [*mes-* + *arteritis*]. Inflammation of the middle coat of an artery.

me·sati·ceph·a·lus (me·sat″i·sef′uh·lus, mes″uh·ti·) *n.* [Gk. *mesatos*, midmost, + *-cephalus*]. *In craniometry,* a person whose skull has a cephalic index of between 75 and 79. —**mesati·ce·phal·ic** (·se·fal′ick) *adj.;* **mesati·ceph·a·ly** (·sef′uh·lee), **mesaticepha·lism** (·liz·um) *n.*

me·sati·pel·lic (me·sat″i·pel′ick, mes″uh·ti·) *adj.* [Gk. *mesatos*, midmost, + *pella*, bowl, cup, + *-ic*]. *In osteometry,* designating a pelvis in which the transverse diameter of the pelvic inlet is nearly equal to the conjugata vera; having a pelvic-inlet index of 90.0 to 94.9.

me·sati·pel·vic (me·sat″i·pel′vick, mes″uh·ti·) *adj.* [Gk. *mesatos*, midmost, + *pelvic*]. MESATIPELLIC.

mes·ax·on (me·zacks′on, me·sacks′on) *n.* [*mes-* + *axon*]. The point where the edges of a Schwann cell come together around an axon to form a paired membrane; seen under the electron microscope.

mes·cal (mes·kal′) *n.* [Sp., from Nahuatl *mexcalli*]. 1. The cactus *Lophophora williamsii,* a potential intoxicant. Syn. *peyote.* See also *mescal buttons.* 2. An intoxicant spirit distilled from Mexican pulque.

mescal buttons. The dried tops from the cactus *Lophophora williamsii;* capable of producing inebriation and hallucinations.

mes·ca·line (mes′kuh·leen) *n.* 3,4,5-Trimethoxyphenethylamine, $C_{11}H_{17}NO_3$, an alkaloid present in mescal buttons; produces unusual psychic effects and visual hallucinations.

mes·ec·to·derm (mez·eck′to·durm, mes·) *n.* That part of the mesenchyme derived from ectoderm, especially from the neural crest in the head region anterior to the somites. It is said to contribute to the formation of meninges; and, in some animals, the pigment cells or melanocytes are derived from it.

mes·en·ce·phal·ic (mez·en″se·fal′ick, mes″en·) *adj.* Of or pertaining to the mesencephalon.

mesencephalic-bulbosacral outflow or **system.** PARASYMPATHETIC NERVOUS SYSTEM.

mesencephalic flexure. A flexure of the embryonic brain concave ventrally occurring in the region of the midbrain. Syn. *cephalic flexure.*

mesencephalic nucleus of the trigeminal nerve. The nucleus of the mesencephalic tract of the trigeminal nerve.

mesencephalic tract of the trigeminal nerve. A slender, sickle-shaped bundle of fibers that arises in cells located in the lateral portion of the central gray matter of the upper fourth ventricle and the cerebral aqueduct (nucleus of the mesencephalic tract) and joins the motor root of the trigeminal nerve. NA *tractus mesencephalicus nervi trigemini.*

mesencephalic tractotomy. MESENCEPHALOTOMY.

mes·en·ceph·a·li·tis (mez″en·sef′uh·lye′tis, mes″) *n.* [*mesencephalon* + *-itis*]. Inflammation of the mesencephalon.

mes·en·ceph·a·lon (mez″en·sef′uh·lon, mes″) *n.*, genit. **mes·encepha·li** (·lye) [*mes-* + *encephalon*] [NA]. The part of the brain developed from the middle cerebral vesicle and consisting of the tectum and cerebral peduncles, and traversed by the cerebral aqueduct. Syn. *midbrain.*

mes·en·ceph·a·lot·o·my (mez″en·sef″uh·lot′um·ee, mes″) *n.* [*mesencephalon* + *-tomy*]. Surgical incision of the spinothalamic tract in the mesencephalon, formerly used to control intractable pain, now in disuse because of resulting dysesthesia.

me·sen·chy·ma (me·seng′ki·muh) *n.* MESENCHYME.

mes·en·chy·mal (me·seng′ki·mul, mes″in·kye′mul, mez″) *adj.* Of or pertaining to mesenchyme.

mesenchymal cell. A large, branched cell found in mesenchyme and believed capable of differentiating into any of the special types of connective tissue. Syn. *fixed undifferentiated mesenchymal cell.*

mesenchymal epithelium. The simple layer of squamous cells lining subdural, subarachnoid, and perilymphatic spaces, and the chambers of the eyeball.

mesenchymal hyalin. A form of hyalin which results from degeneration or necrosis of nonepithelial tissue, usually of muscle, as in Zenker's degeneration, or of blood vessels.

mesenchymal meningioma. MENINGIOMA.

mesenchymal tissue. Undifferentiated embryonic tissue composed of branching cells between which is ground substance of coagulable fluid. See also *mesenchyme.*

mes·en·chyme (mes′in·kime, mez′) *n.* [*mes-* + Gk. *enchyma*, instillation, contents]. The portion of the mesoderm that produces all the connective tissues of the body, the blood vessels, and the blood, the entire lymphatic system proper, and the heart; the nonepithelial portions of the mesoderm.

mes·en·chy·mo·ma (mes″in·kigh·mo′muh, ·ki·mo′muh) *n.* [*mesenchyme* + *-oma*]. 1. A tumor, benign or malignant, whose parenchyma is composed of cells resembling those of the embryonic mesenchyme. 2. A tumor, benign or malignant, whose parenchyma is composed of cells resembling those of the mesenchyme with its derivatives. Syn. *mixed mesenchymal tumor, mixed mesodermal tumor.*

mes·en·ter·ec·to·my (mes″en·tur·eck′tum·ee) *n.* [*mesentery* + *-ectomy*]. Excision of a mesentery or a part of it.

mes·en·ter·ic (mes″un·terr′ick, mez″) *adj.* Of or pertaining to a mesentery.

mesenteric arteries. See Table of Arteries in the Appendix.

mesenteric hernia. A hernia in which a loop of intestine or a portion of omentum or other viscus has passed through an opening in the mesentery.

mesenteric lymphadenitis. Inflammation of the mesenteric lymph nodes.

mes·en·ter·i·co·meso·co·lic (mes·en·terr″i·ko·mes·o·ko′lick, ·kol′ick) *adj.* Pertaining to the mesentery and the mesocolon.

mesenteric plexus. A visceral nerve plexus surrounding the mesenteric arteries. See also *inferior mesenteric plexus, superior mesenteric plexus.*

mesenteric pregnancy. TUBOLIGAMENTARY PREGNANCY.

mesenteric recess. A recess in the primitive gastric mesentery, formed by an invagination of the peritoneum on the right side, that separates the definitive gastric mesentery from the caval mesentery and gives rise to the omental bursa, its vestibule, and the infracardiac bursa.

mes·en·teri·o·lum (mes″en·terr·ee·o′lum, ·terr·eye′o·lum) *n.*, pl. **mesenterio·la** (·luh) [NL., diminutive of *mesenterium*]. A small mesentery.

mesenteriolum pro·ces·sus ver·mi·for·mis (pro·ses′us vur″mi·for′mis) [BNA]. MESOAPPENDIX.

mes·en·ter·io·pexy (mes″un·terr′ee·o·peck″see) *n.* [*mesenterium* + *-pexy*]. MESOPEXY.

mes·en·teri·or·rha·phy (mes″un·terr″ee·or′uh·fee) *n.* [*mesenterium* + *-rrhaphy*]. Surgical repair of a mesentery.

mes·en·ter·i·pli·ca·tion (mes″un·terr″i·pli·kay′shun) *n.* [*mesenterium* + L. *plicatio,* folding]. Mesenteriorrhaphy; reduction of folds of redundant mesentery by overlapping and suture.

mes·en·ter·i·tis (mes″en·ter·eye′tis) *n.* [*mesentery* + *-itis*]. Inflammation of a mesentery.

mes·en·te·ri·um (mes″un·terr′ee·um) *n.*, pl. **mesente·ria** (·ee·uh) [NL., from Gk. *mesenterion*] [NA]. MESENTERY.

mesenterium com·mu·ne (kom·yoo′nee) [BNA]. Mesenterium dorsale commune (= DORSAL MESENTERY).

mesenterium dor·sa·le com·mu·ne (dor·say′lee kom·yoo′nee) [NA]. DORSAL MESENTERY.

mes·en·ter·on (mes·en′tur·on) *n.* [*mes-* + *enteron*]. MIDGUT.

mes·en·tery (mes′un·terr″ee, mez′) *n.* [Gk. *mesenterion*, from *meson,* between, among, + *enteron*]. 1. Any of the peritoneal folds attaching certain organs, especially the intestine, to the abdominal wall. 2. Specifically, that which attaches the small intestine to the posterior abdominal wall. See also Plate 13 and *mesocolon, mesocecum, mesorectum.*

mes·en·to·derm (me·sen′to·durm, me·zen′) *n.* [*mes-* + *entoderm*]. 1. The entodermal division of the mesoderm. 2. The indifferent tissue from which both entoderm and mesoderm are developed. 3. The portion of the mesoderm from which certain digestive tract structures are derived.

mes·en·tor·rha·phy (mes″en·tor′uf·ee, mez″un·) *n.* [*mesentery* + *-rraphy*]. Suture of a mesentery.

me·si·al (mee″zee·ul, ·see·ul, mes′ee·ul) *adj.* 1. MEDIAL. 2. *In dentistry,* toward the sagittal plane along the curve of a dental arch. Contr. *distal.*

mesial angle. The junction of the mesial surface of a crown of a tooth with one of the other surfaces.

mesial drift. The tendency of teeth in proximal contact to move toward the midline as their contact areas become worn.

mesial occlusion. The occlusion occurring when a tooth is more anterior than normal. Contr. *distal occlusion.*

mesial temporal sclerosis. Atrophy and gliosis in the gray and white matter of the medial and inferior portions of the temporal lobe, presumably due to prolapse of the temporal lobe through the incisura of the tentorium during birth, and which may act after a variable period of time as the epileptogenic focus in temporal lobe seizures. Syn. *incisural sclerosis.*

mesio-. *In dentistry,* a combining form meaning *mesial.*

me·sio·an·gu·lar (mee″zee·o·ang′gew·lur) *adj. In dentistry,* characterized by angulation in a mesial direction.

mesioangular impaction. Impaction of a tooth, usually a third molar, with the coronal aspect anterior to the apex. Contr. *distoangular impaction.*

me·sio·buc·cal (mee″zee·o·buck′ul, mee″see·o·) *adj.* Pertaining to the mesial and buccal aspects of the teeth.

me·sio·buc·co·oc·clu·sal (mee″zee·o·buck″o·uh·kloo′zul) *adj.* Pertaining to the mesial, buccal, and occlusal surfaces of a tooth.

me·sio·clu·sion (mee″zee·o·klew′zhun) *n.* [*mesio-* + *occlusion*]. Any malocclusion in which the mandible is anterior to its normal relationship with the maxilla; the mesial groove of the mandibular first permanent molar articulates anteriorly to the mesiobuccal cusp of the maxillary first permanent molar.

me·sio·dens (mee′zee·o·denz″) *n.*, pl. **me·sio·den·tes** (mee″zee·o·den′teez) [*mesio-* + *dens*]. A supernumerary tooth located between the maxillary central incisors.

me·sio·dis·tal (mee″zee·o·dis′tul) *adj.* Pertaining to the mesial and distal surfaces of a tooth.

me·sio·gres·sion (mee″zee·o·gresh′un) *n.* [*mesio-* + *progression*]. The location of teeth anterior to their normal position.

me·sio·in·ci·sal (mee″zee·o·in·sigh′zul) *adj.* Pertaining to the mesial and incisal surfaces of a tooth.

me·sio·la·bi·al (mee″zee·o·lay′bee·ul) *adj.* Pertaining to the mesial and labial surfaces of a tooth.

me·sio·lin·gual (mee″zee·o·ling′gwul) *adj.* Pertaining to the mesial and lingual aspects of a tooth.

me·sio·lin·guo·oc·clu·sal (mee″zee·o·ling″gwo·uh·kloo′zul) *adj.* Pertaining to the mesial, lingual, and occlusal surfaces of a tooth.

me·sio·oc·clu·sal (mee″zee·o·uh·kloo′zul) *adj.* Pertaining to the mesial and occlusal surfaces of a tooth.

mesioocclusal angle. The angle formed by the junction of the mesial and occlusal surfaces of a premolar or molar tooth.

me·sio·oc·clu·sion (mee″zee·o·uh·kloo′zhun) *n.* MESIOCLUSION.

me·sio·ver·sion (mee″zee·o·vur′zhun) *n.* [*mesio-* + *version*]. Greater than normal proximity of a tooth to the median plane of the face along the dental arch.

me·sit·y·lene (me·sit′i·leen) *n.* 1,3,5-Trimethylbenzene, $C_6H_3(CH_3)_3$, a liquid hydrocarbon obtained from coal tar and crude petroleum, and also prepared synthetically.

mes·mer·ism (mez′mur·iz·um) *n.* [F. A. *Mesmer,* German physician, 1734–1815]. Hypnotism induced by animal magnetism, a supposed force passing from operator to man.

meso-. 1. See *mes-.* 2. (italicized) *In chemistry,* a combining form designating (a) an optical isomer that does not rotate polarized light because of internal compensation of its chiral centers; (b) a middle position of a substituent group in certain organic compounds; (c) a porphyrin or other pyrrole derivative in which one or more vinyl groups have been converted to ethyl by hydrogenation; (d) an intermediate hydrated form of an inorganic acid.

meso·ap·pen·di·ci·tis (mes″o·uh·pen″di·sigh′tis) *n.* Inflammation of the mesoappendix.

meso·ap·pen·dix (mes″o·uh·pen′dicks) *n.* [NA]. The mesentery of the vermiform appendix.

meso·bi·lane (mes″o·bye′lane) *n.* One of the products resulting from the reduction of bilirubin in the tissues by an enzyme originating in the reticuloendothelial system. See also *mesobilirubin.*

meso·bil·i·fus·cin (mes″o·bil·i·fus′in) *n.* Either of two isomeric substances, each containing two pyrrole rings but not of definitely known structure, obtained as products of hydrolytic cleavage of mesobilirubinogen when the latter is prepared by reduction of bilirubin. They contribute significantly to the color of normal feces.

meso·bil·i·leu·kan (mes″o·bil·i·lew′kan) *n.* A colorless precursor of mesobilifuscin, apparently identical with promesobilifuscin.

meso·bil·i·rho·din (mes″o·bil·i·ro′din) *n.* A product of dehydrogenation of the urobilin obtained from mesobilirubinogen. Mesobilirhodin is isomeric with mesobiliviolin, these substances differing only in the position of a side methyne bridge.

meso·bil·i·ru·bin (mes″o·bil·i·roo′bin) *n.* A yellow, crystalline substance, $C_{33}H_{40}N_4O_6$, formed by reduction of bilirubin, probably by conversion of two vinyl groups to ethyl groups; it occurs in the small intestine and some claim to have found it in bile.

meso·bil·i·ru·bin·o·gen (mes″o·bil″i·roo·bin′o·jen) *n.* A colorless, crystalline substance, $C_{33}H_{44}N_4O_6$, formed by reduction of bilirubin through conversion of two vinyl groups to ethyl groups and two methyne bridges to methene bridges. By various oxidative processes it may be converted to urobilin, stercobilinogen, or stercobilin.

meso·bil·i·vi·o·lin (mes″o·bil″i·vye·o′lin) *n.* A product of dehydrogenation of the urobilin obtained from mesobilirubinogen. Mesobiliviolin is isomeric with mesobilirhodin, these substances differing only in the position of a side methyne bridge.

meso·blast (mez′o·blast, mes′) *n.* [*meso-* + *-blast*]. 1. The mesoderm during its early development. 2. MESODERM. —**meso·blas·tic** (mez″o·blas′tick) *adj.*

meso·blas·te·ma (mez″o·blas·tee′muh, ·mes″) *n.* [*meso-* + *blastema*]. The mesoderm as a whole.

meso·blas·tem·ic (mez″o·blas·tem′ick, mes″) *adj.* Derived from the mesoblastema.

mesoblastic nephroma. WILMS'S TUMOR.

meso·bran·chi·al (mes″o·brang′kee·ul, mez″) *adj.* [*meso-* + *branchial*]. Pertaining to the medial branchial region.

mesobranchial area. The ventral pharyngeal region between the ventral ends of the visceral arches and grooves.

meso·car·di·um (mes″o·kahr′dee·um, ·mez″) *n.* [*meso-* + *-cardium*]. One of the embryonic mesenteries of the heart.

meso·carp (mez′o·kahrp, mes′) *n.* [*meso-* + *-carp*]. The middle layer of the pericarp.

meso·ce·cum (mes″o·see′kum, mez″) *n.* [*meso-* + *cecum*]. The mesentery that in some cases connects the cecum with the right iliac fossa.

meso·ce·phal·ic (mez″o·se·fal′ick, mes″) *adj.* [*meso-* + *cephalic*]. *In somatometry,* designating a head having a relatively moderate relationship between its greatest length and breadth; having a cephalic index of 76.0 to 80.9.

meso·cne·mic (mez″o·nee′mick, mes″, ·ock·nee′mick) *adj.* [*meso-* + *cnemic*]. *In osteometry,* designating a tibia with a moderate mediolateral flattening of the proximal portion of the diaphysis; having a cnemic index of 65.0 to 69.9.

mesocolic band. MESOCOLIC TAENIA.

mesocolic taenia. The longitudinal muscle band corresponding to the attachment of the mesocolon.

meso·co·lon (mes″o·ko′lun, mez″) *n.* [*meso-* + *colon*] [NA]. The mesentery connecting the colon with the posterior abdominal wall. It may be divided into ascending, descending, and transverse portions. In the adult the transverse portion persists. See also Plate 8. —**meso·co·lic** (·ko′lick, ·kol′ick) *adj.*

mesocolon ascen·dens (a·sen′denz) [NA]. ASCENDING MESOCOLON.

mesocolon de·scen·dens (de·sen′denz) [NA]. DESCENDING MESOCOLON.

mesocolon sig·moi·de·um (sig·moy′dee·um) [NA]. SIGMOID MESOCOLON.

mesocolon trans·ver·sum (trans·vur′sum) [NA]. TRANSVERSE MESOCOLON.

meso·conch (mes′o·konk, mez′) *adj.* [*meso-* + Gk. *konchos,* mussel, shell, eye socket]. *In craniometry,* designating an orbit of medium height; having an orbital index of 76.0 to 84.9.

meso·cra·ni·al (mes″o·kray′nee·ul) *adj.* [*meso-* + *cranial*]. Having a cranial index between 75.0 and 79.9.

meso·derm (mez′o·durm, mes′) *n.* [*meso-* + *-derm*]. The third germ layer, lying between the ectoderm and entoderm. It gives rise to the connective tissues, muscles, urogenital system, vascular system, and the epithelial lining of the coelom. —**meso·der·mal** (mez″o·dur′mul, mes″) *adj.*

mesodermal segment. SOMITE.

mesodermal tumor. A tumor whose parenchyma is composed of elements normally arising from the mesoderm.

meso·di·a·stol·ic (mez″o·dye″uh·stol′ick, mes″o·) *adj.* Of or pertaining to the middle of ventricular diastole.

meso·du·o·de·num (mes″o·dew″o·dee′num, ·dew·od′e·num, mez′) *n.* That part of the mesentery that sometimes connects the duodenum with the posterior wall of the abdominal cavity. Normally in man the true duodenum has no mesentery in its fully developed state.

meso·esoph·a·gus (mes″o·e·sof′uh·gus) *n.* The dorsal mesentery of the lower end of the embryonic esophagus.

meso·gas·ter (mez′o·gas″tur, mes′o·) *n.* [*meso-* + *-gaster*]. The primitive mesentery of the stomach. NA *mesogastrium.*

meso·gas·tri·um (mes″o·gas′tree·um) *n.*, pl. **mesogas·tria** (·tree·uh) [NA]. MESOGASTER.

meso·glea, meso·gloea (mes″o·glee′uh) *n.* [*meso-* + Gk. *gloia,* glue]. The amorphous, gelatinous substance interposed between the entoderm and ectoderm in coelenterates, considered to be more or less homologous to the third germ layer of triploblastic animals. Not to be confused with mesoglia.

me·sog·lia (me·sog′lee·uh) *n.* [*meso-* + *glia*]. *Obsol.* A type of ameboid phagocyte found in the neuroglia, probably of mesodermal origin.

meso·gnath·ic (mes″o·nath′ick, mez″) *adj.* [*meso-* + *gnathic*]. *In craniometry,* designating a condition of the upper jaw in which it has a mild degree of anterior projection with respect to the profile of the facial skeleton, when the skull is oriented on the Frankfort horizontal plane; having a gnathic index of 98.0 to 102.9.

meso·gna·thi·on (mes″o·nayth′ee·on, ·nath′ee·on, mez″) *n.* [NL., from *meso-* + Gk. *gnathos,* jaw]. The hypothetical lateral portion of the premaxilla, considered separate from the medial portion, the endognathion.

me·sog·na·thous (me·zog′nuth·us, me·sog′) *adj.* MESOGNATHIC.

meso·ino·si·tol (mes″o·i·no′si·tol, ·tole) *n.* The most common stereoisomer of inositol. See also *myoinositol.*

meso·lec·i·thal (mes″o·les′i·thul) *adj.* [*meso-* + *lecithal*]. Having a moderate amount of yolk. Syn. *medialecithal.*

meso·mere (mes′o·meer, mez′) *n.* [*meso-* + Gk. *meros,* part]. NEPHROTOME.

meso·me·tri·um (mes″o·mee′tree·um, mez″) *n.*, pl. **mesome·tria** (·tree·uh) [NL., from *meso-* + Gk. *mētra,* womb] [NA]. The portion of the broad ligament directly attached to the uterus.

meso·morph (mez′o·morf, mes′) *n.* In the somatotype, an individual exhibiting relative predominance of mesomorphy.

meso·mor·phy (mez″o·mor·fee, mes′) *n.* [*meso-* + *-morphy*]. Component II of the somatotype, representing relative predominance of somatic structures or the bony and muscular framework of the body, derived from mesoderm. Mesomorphs tend toward massive strength and heavy muscular development. The counterpart on the behavioral level is somatotonia. Contr. *ectomorphy, endomorphy.* —**meso·morph·ic** (mez″o·mor′fick, mes″) *adj.*

mes·on (mez′on, mes′on, mees′on) *n.* [*mes-* + *-on*]. *In nuclear physics,* any of several different elementary particles, having a rest mass typically between that of a proton and an electron.

meso·neph·ric (mes″o·nef′rick) *adj.* Of or pertaining to the mesonephros.

mesonephric cystoma. A cyst, probably of mesonephric origin, at the hilus of the ovary.

mesonephric duct. The duct of the mesonephros or embryonic kidney; becomes the excretory duct of the testis and gives rise to the ureteric bud in both sexes. Syn. *Wolffian duct.* NA *ductus mesonephricus.*

mesonephric fold. MESONEPHRIC RIDGE.

mesonephric rests. Fetal rests of a mesonephric duct.

mesonephric ridge. A ridge or fold of the dorsal coelomic wall in the embryo lateral to the mesentery produced by growth of the mesonephros.

mesonephric tubule. A tubule of the mesonephros.

meso·neph·roid (mes″o·nef′roid) *adj.* Resembling the mesonephros or its adult remnant.

meso·ne·phro·ma (mes″o·nef·ro′muh) *n.* [*mesonephros* + *-oma*]. Any of a variety of rare tumors supposed to be, but not proved to be, derived from mesonephros (Wolffian body), and occurring in the genital tract. Included are extrauterine adenomyomas, cystic or solid tumors of the ovary situated near the hilus, and tumors resembling the adenomyosarcoma of the kidney. Syn. *teratoid adenocystoma.*

mesonephroma ova·rii (o·vair′ee·eye). A malignant tumor of the ovary which microscopically contains structures resembling the primitive mesonephros.

meso·neph·ros (mes″o·nef′ros) *n.*, pl. **mesoneph·roi** (·roy) [*meso-* + *nephros*] [NA]. The middle kidney of higher vertebrates; functional in the embryo, it is replaced by the metanephros. Syn. *Wolffian body.*

meso·pexy (mes′o·peck·see) *n.* [*meso-* + *-pexy*]. The surgical fixation of a mesentery.

meso·phle·bi·tis (mes″o·fle·bye′tis) *n.* [*meso-* + *phlebitis*]. Inflammation of the middle coat of a vein.

meso·phrag·ma (mez″o·frag′muh, mes″) *n.* [*meso-* + Gk. *phragma,* fence, screen]. M DISK.

me·so·pic (me·so′pick, me·sop′ick) *adj.* [*mes-* + Gk. *ōps,* eye, face, + *-ic*]. 1. *In craniometry,* designating a facial skeleton that is moderately wide and flat; having an orbitonasal index of 107.5 to 110.0. 2. *In somatometry,* designating a face that is moderately wide and flat; having an orbitonasal index of 110.0 to 112.9.

Mesopin. A trademark for homatropine methylbromide.

meso·por·phy·rin (mes″o·por′fi·rin) *n.* Any of 15 isomers of the formula $C_{32}H_{36}N_4(COOH)_2$ obtained by addition of hydrogen to the double bond of each vinyl group (thereby forming an ethyl group) in the 15 isomers of protoporphyrin. Mesoporphyrin 9 is the reduced form of the protoporphyrin occurring in hemoglobin.

meso·pul·mo·num (mes″o·pul′mo·num, ·pōōl·mo′num) *n.* [NL., from *meso-* + L. *pulmo, pulmonis,* lung]. The embryonic mesentery of the lung attached to the mesoesophagus.

me·sor·chi·um (me·sor′kee·um) *n.*, pl. **mesor·chia** (·kee·uh) [NL., from *mes-* + Gk. *orchis,* testis] [NA]. The mesentery of the fetal testis by which it is attached to the mesonephros; represented in the adult by a fold between testis and epididymis.

meso·rec·tum (mes″o·reck′tum, mez″o·) *n.* [*meso-* + *rectum*] [BNA]. The narrow fold of the peritoneum connecting the upper part of the rectum with the sacrum.

mes·o·rid·a·zine (mes″o·rid′uh·zeen) *n.* 10-[2-(1-Methyl-2-piperidyl)ethyl]-2-(methylsulfinyl)phenothiazine, $C_{21}H_{26}N_2OS_2$, a tranquilizer.

mes·o·rop·ter (mes″o·rop′tur) *n.* [*mes-* + *horopter*]. The normal position of the eyes when their muscles rest.

mes·or·rha·phy (mes·or′uh·fee) *n.* [*meso-* + *-rrhaphy*]. Suture of a mesentery.

mes·or·rhine (mez′o·rine, mes′) *adj.* [*meso-* + *-rrhine*]. 1. *In craniometry,* designating an apertura piriformis approximately twice as long as it is wide; having a nasal index of 47.0 to 50.9. 2. *In somatometry,* designating a nose that is moderately long and wide; having a height-breadth index of 70.0 to 84.9.

meso·sal·pinx (mes″o·sal′pinks, mez″) *n.*, pl. **meso·sal·pin·ges** (·sal·pin′jeez) [*meso-* + *salpinx*] [NA]. The upper part of the broad ligament that forms the mesentery of the uterine tube. —**meso·sal·pin·ge·al** (·sal·pin′jee·ul, ·sal·pin·jee′ul) *adj.*

meso·sig·moid (mez″o·sig′moid, mes″o·) *n.* [*meso-* + *sigmoid*]. SIGMOID MESOCOLON.

meso·some (mez′o·sohm, mes′) *n.* [*meso-* + *-some*]. In bacteria, invaginations of the cytoplasmic membrane; the site of attachment of the bacterial DNA to the membrane.

meso·tar·tar·ic acid (mes″o·tahr·tăr′ick, ·tahr·tahr′ick, mez″o·). Tartaric acid which is optically inactive by reason of internal compensation.

meso·ten·di·ne·um (mes″o·ten·din′ee·um) *n.* [NA]. MESOTENDON.

meso·ten·don (mes″o·ten′don, mez″o·) *n.* [*meso-* + *tendon*]. The fold of synovial membrane extending to a tendon from its synovial tendon sheath.

mesothelial sarcoma. A malignant mesothelioma.

meso·the·li·o·ma (mes″o·theel″ee·o′muh) *n.* [*mesothelium* + *-oma*]. A primary tumor, either benign or malignant, composed of cells similar to those forming the lining of the peritoneum, pericardium, or pleura. Syn. *celioma, celothelioma.*

mesothelioma of meninges. MENINGIOMA.

meso·the·li·um (mes″o·theel′ee·um, mez″) *n.*, pl. **mesothe·lia** (·ee·uh) [*meso-* + *-thelium*]. 1. The lining of the wall of the primitive body cavity situated between the somatopleure and splanchnopleure. 2. The simple squamous epithelium lining the pleural, pericardial, peritoneal, and scrotal cavities. —**mesotheli·al** (·ul) *adj.*

meso·tho·ri·um (mes″o·tho′ree·um) *n.* Either of the radioactive disintegration products, mesothorium-1 ($MsTh_1$) and mesothorium-2 ($MsTh_2$), formed from thorium and ultimately converted to radiothorium.

me·sot·o·my (me·sot′um·ee) *n.* [*meso-* + *-tomy*]. RESOLUTION (3).

mes·ova·ri·um (mes″o·vair′ee·um) *n.*, pl. **mesova·ria** (·ree·uh) [*mes-* + *ovarium*] [NA]. A peritoneal fold connecting the ovary and the broad ligament. —**mesovari·an** (·un) *adj.*

messenger RNA. A single-stranded ribonucleic acid which arises from, and is complementary to, the double-stranded DNA. It passes from the nucleus to the cytoplasm where its information is translated into protein structure. Abbreviated, mRNA.

mes·ter·o·lone (mes·terr′o·lohn) *n.* 17β-Hydroxy-1α-methyl-5α-androstan-3-one, $C_{20}H_{32}O_2$, an androgenic steroid.

Mestinon Bromide. Trademark for pyridostigmine bromide, a cholinesterase inhibitor used in the treatment of myasthenia gravis.

mes·tra·nol (mes′truh·nol) *n.* 17α-Ethynyl-3-methoxy-1,3,5(10)-estratrien-17β-ol, $C_{21}H_{26}O_2$, an estrogen; used principally, in combination with a progestogen, to inhibit ovulation and control fertility.

mes·u·prine (mes′yoo·preen, mes′oo·) *n.* 2′-Hydroxy-5′-[1-hydroxy-2-[(*p*-methoxyphenethyl)amino]propyl]methanesulfonanilide, $C_{19}H_{26}N_2O_5S$, a vasodilator and uterine relaxant drug; used as the hydrochloride salt.

mes·yl·ate (mes′i·late) *n.* Any salt or ester of methanesulfonic acid, CH_3SO_3H; a methanesulfonate.

met-, meta- [Gk.]. 1. A prefix signifying (a) *behind, beyond, distal to;* (b) *between, among;* (c) *change, transformation;* (d) *after, post-;* (e) *subsequent in development or evolution.* 2. (italicized) *In chemistry,* a prefix indicating the relationship of two atoms in the benzene ring that are separated by one carbon atom in the ring, i.e., the 1,3-position; also any benzene derivative in which two substituents have such a relationship. Symbol, *m*-. 3. *In chemistry,* a prefix designating an acid containing one less molecule of water than the parent acid, commonly designated the ortho-acid; as metaphosphoric acid, HPO_3, from orthophosphoric acid, H_3PO_4.

meta (met′uh) *adj.* [from the prefix *meta-*]. Pertaining to or having two positions in the benzene ring that are separated by one carbon atom in the ring.

meta·bi·o·sis (met″uh·bye·o′sis) *n.* [*meta-* + Gk. *biōsis*, way of life]. A form of commensalism in which only one of the organisms is benefited; the other may remain uninfluenced or be injured. —**metabi·ot·ic** (·ot′ick) *adj.*

me·ta·bi·sul·fite (me″tuh·bye·sul′fite) *n.* A salt containing the anion $S_2O_5^{2-}$, as sodium metabisulfite. Syn. *pyrosulfite.*

met·a·bol·ic (met″uh·bol′ick) *adj.* [Gk. *metabolikos*, mutable, changeable]. Of or pertaining to metabolism.

metabolic acidosis. Acidosis in which the tendency to decreased blood pH results either from renal retention of acid products of metabolism or from injection or ingestion of acids or from excessive losses of bicarbonate from the body, as in diarrhea or pancreatic or biliary fistula. Physiological compensation is by renal retention of bicarbonate and by accelerated pulmonary elimination of carbon dioxide via hyperventilation. See also *respiratory acidosis.*

metabolic alkalosis. Alkalosis in which the tendency to an increased blood pH results either from the addition to body fluids of excess alkali by injection or ingestion or from excessive loss of acid, usually by vomiting or gastric aspiration. Physiological compensation is by pulmonary retention of carbon dioxide via hypoventilation and accelerated renal excretion of sodium bicarbonate. See also *respiratory alkalosis.*

metabolic analog. ANALOGUE (3).

metabolic bed. A bed especially arranged to collect fluid and solid waste of the patient.

metabolic craniopathy. STEWART-MOREL-MORGAGNI SYNDROME.

metabolic equilibrium. NUTRITIVE EQUILIBRIUM.

metabolic ileus. Ileus resulting from interference with the function of the smooth muscle of the intestine, due to metabolic disturbances.

metabolic pigment. A pigment, such as melanin, formed by the metabolic action of cells.

me·tab·o·lim·e·ter (me·tab″o·lim′e·tur, met″uh·bo·) *n.* An apparatus for estimating the rate of basal metabolism.

me·tab·o·lism (me·tab′o·liz·um) *n.* [Gk. *metabolē*, change, + *-ism*]. The sum total of all synthetic (anabolic) and degradative (catabolic) biochemical reactions in the body.

me·tab·o·lite (me·tab′o·lite) *n.* [*metabol*ism + *-ite*]. A product of metabolic change.

me·tab·o·lize (me·tab′o·lize) *v.* To transform by metabolism, to subject to metabolism.

met·a·bol·o·gy (met″uh·bol′uh·jee) *n.* Study of the metabolic processes.

me·tab·o·lous (me·tab′o·lus) *adj.* [Gk. *metabolos*, changeable]. *In zoology*, undergoing metamorphosis, as many insects that pass through a larval, pupal, and adult stage. Compare *hemimetabolous, metamorphosis* (1).

meta·brom·sa·lan (met″uh·brome′suh·lan) *n.* 3,5-Dibromosalicylanilide, $C_{13}H_9Br_2NO_2$, a disinfectant.

meta·bu·teth·a·mine (met″uh·bew·teth′uh·meen) *n.* 2-(Isobutylamino)ethyl *m*-aminobenzoate, $C_{13}H_{20}N_2O_2$, a local anesthetic used in dentistry as the hydrochloride salt.

meta·bu·toxy·caine (met″uh·bew·tock′si·kane) *n.* 2-(Diethylamino)ethyl 3-amino-2-butoxybenzoate, $C_{17}H_{28}N_2O_3$, a local anesthetic used in dentistry as the hydrochloride salt.

meta·car·pal (met″uh·kahr′pul) *adj.* Pertaining to the metacarpus, or to a bone of it.

metacarpal ligament. Any of the ligaments of the intermetacarpal articulations, connecting the adjacent bases of the second, third, fourth, and fifth metacarpal bones on their dorsal, palmar, and apposing surfaces; described respectively as dorsal metacarpal ligaments (NA *ligamenta metacarpea dorsalia*), plamar metacarpal ligaments (NA *ligamenta metacarpea palmaria*), and interosseous metacarpal ligaments (NA *ligamenta metacarpea interossea*).

meta·car·pec·to·my (met″uh·kahr·peck′tum·ee) *n.* [*metacarpal* + *-ectomy*]. Excision of a metacarpal bone.

meta·car·po·pha·lan·ge·al (met″uh·kahr″po·fuh·lan′jee·ul) *adj.* Pertaining to the metacarpus and the phalanges.

metacarpophalangeal articulation. Any of the joints between the heads of the metacarpals and their respective proximal phalanges. NA (pl.) *articulationes metacarpophalangeae.*

metacarpophalangeal ligament. Any of the ligaments connecting the heads of the metacarpals and the bases of the proximal phalanges. See also *collateral ligaments, palmar ligaments.*

meta·car·pus (met″uh·kahr′pus) *n.*, pl. & genit. sing. **metacarpi** (·pye) [NL., from Gk. *metakarpion*] [NA]. The part of the hand between the carpus and the phalanges; it contains five bones.

meta·cen·tric (met″uh·sen′trick). Of a chromosome: having the centromere near the center, resulting in arms of more or less equal length. Contr. *acrocentric, submetacentric, telocentric.*

meta·cer·car·ia (met″uh·sur·kăr′ee·uh) *n.*, pl. **metacercar·i·ae** (·ee·ee) [*meta-* + *cercaria*]. An encysted, maturing stage of a trematode in the tissues of an intermediate host, often representing the infectious part of a parasite's life cycle.

meta·chro·ma·sia (met″uh·kro·may′zee·uh, ·zhuh) *n.* [*meta-* + *-chromasia*]. 1. The property exhibited by certain pure dyestuffs, chiefly basic dyes, of coloring certain tissue elements in a different color, usually of a shorter wavelength absorption maximum, than most other tissue elements. 2. The assumption of different colors or shades by different substances when stained by the same dye. —**metachro·mat·ic** (·mat′ick) *adj.*

meta·chro·ma·sy (met″uh·kro′muh·see) *n.* METACHROMASIA.

metachromatic granules. 1. Granules which take on a color different from that of the dye used to stain them. 2. VOLUTIN GRANULES.

metachromatic leukodystrophy. A heredodegenerative disease due to a deficiency of the enzyme aryl sulfatase A, with increase in sulfated lipids which are normally degraded to cerebrosides; excess cerebroside sulfatides are responsible for metachromasia in cerebral white matter, peripheral nerves, liver and kidney, associated with progressive neurological disease. The disease usually has its onset between 1 and 4 years of age, but variant forms occur in childhood and occasionally in adult life. Variant forms due to other sulfatase deficiencies occur. Autosomal recessive transmission is usual. Abbreviated, MLD. Syn. *sulfatide lipidosis.*

metachromatic stain. A stain which changes apparent color when absorbed by certain cell constituents, as mucin staining red instead of blue with toluidine blue.

meta·chro·ma·tism (met″uh·kro′muh·tiz·um) *n.* METACHROMASIA.

me·tach·ro·nous (me·tack′ruh·nus) *adj.* [Gk. *metachronos*, anachronistic]. Occurring or beginning at different times. Contr. *synchronous.*

meta·chro·sis (met″uh·kro′sis) *n.* [*meta-* + Gk. *chrōsis*, coloring]. *In biology*, the change or play of colors seen in the squid, chameleon, and other animals.

meta·coele (met′uh·seel) *n.* [*meta-* + *-coele*]. The coelom proper, developing in the lateral plate of mesoderm.

meta·cone (met′uh·kone) *n.* [*meta-* + *cone*]. The outer posterior (distobuccal) cusp of an upper molar tooth.

meta·co·nid (met″uh·ko′nid, kon′id) *n.* [*metacone* + *-id*]. The inner anterior (mesiolingual) cusp of a lower molar tooth.

meta·co·nule (met″uh·ko′newl, ·kon′yool) *n.* A small intermediate cusp between the metacone and the protocone on the upper molar teeth of animals.

meta·cre·sol (met″uh·kree′sole, ·sol) *n.* The meta form of cresol, $C_6H_4(CH_3)OH$, a colorless liquid obtained from coal tar. A more powerful germicide than phenol, but less toxic.

meta·cy·e·sis (met″a·sigh·ee′sis) *n.* [*meta-* + Gk. *kyēsis*, pregnancy]. EXTRAUTERINE PREGNANCY.

meta·dra·sis (met″uh·dray′sis) *n.* [*meta-* + Gk. *drasis*, strength, action]. *Obsol.* Overwork of body or mind.

meta·drom·ic (met″uh·drom′ick, ·dro′mick). *adj.* [Gk. *metadromē*, pursuit (from *dromos*, course, running), + *-ic*]. FESTINATING.

meta·fa·cial angle (met″uh·fay′shul). The angle between the base of the skull and the pterygoid process. Syn. *Serres' angle.*

meta·fil·tra·tion (met″uh·fil·tray′shun) *n.* Filtration through superimposed metallic strips with beveled edges, the system depending on the formation of a filter bed in the interstices between the strips.

meta·gen·e·sis (met″uh·jen′e·sis) *n.* [*meta-* + *-genesis*]. ALTERNATION OF GENERATIONS.

Meta·gon·i·mus (met″uh·gon′i·mus) *n.* [*meta-* + Gk. *gonimos*, productive, fertile]. A genus of digenetic trematodes.

Metagonimus yo·ko·ga·wai (yo·ko·gah·wah′eye). A species of trematode found most commonly in the Far East which infects the small intestine of man, dogs, cats, pigs, and mice, producing a mild diarrhea.

meta·gran·u·lo·cyte (met″uh·gran′yoo·lo·site) *n.* [*meta-* + *granulocyte*]. *Rare.* METAMYELOCYTE.

Metahydrin. A trademark for trichlormethiazide, an orally effective diuretic and antihypertensive drug.

meta·karyo·cyte (met″uh·kăr′ee·o·site) *n.* [*meta-* + *karyocyte*]. *Rare.* NORMOBLAST.

meta·ken·trin (met″uh·ken′trin) *n.* [*meta-* + Gk. *kentron*, goad, incentive, + *-in*]. LUTEINIZING HORMONE.

met·al (met′ul) *n.* [Gk. *metallon*, mine]. An elementary substance, or mixture of such substances, usually characterized by hardness, malleability, ductility, fusibility, luster, and conduction of heat and electricity.

metal ague. METAL FUME FEVER.

metal fume fever. A febrile influenza-like occupational disorder following the inhalation of finely divided particles and fumes of metallic oxides. Syn. *brass chills, brass founder's ague, galvo, metal ague, zinc chills, spelter shakes, Teflon shakes, Monday fever.*

Metalid. A trademark for acetaminophen, an analgesic antipyretic.

met·al·ized milk. Milk containing minute traces of iron, copper, and magnesium; has been used in treating anemia.

me·tal·lic (me·tal′ick) *adj.* [Gk. *metallikos*, of mining, of metals]. 1. Of, pertaining to, or resembling metal. 2. *In physical diagnosis,* referring to a sound similar to that produced by metal, high-pitched, short in duration, and with overtones; a form of tympany.

metallic tinkle. A faint, clear, bell-like sound heard after a cough or deep breath in some cases of hydropneumothorax or large pulmonary cavity.

metallo-, metalo-. A combining form meaning *metal, metallic.*

met·al·loid (met′uh·loid) *n. & adj.* 1. An element which has metallic properties in the free state but which behaves chemically as an amphoteric or nonmetallic element. 2. Characteristic of or pertaining to a metalloid.

me·tal·lo·phil·ia (me·tal″o·fil′ee·uh) *n.* [*metallo-* + *-philia*]. The property exhibited by certain tissue elements of binding metal ions, presumably by chelation, which are then identified by inorganic chemical reactions or by binding of dyestuffs which form colored pigments with the bound metal.

met·al·lo·pho·bia (met″uh·lo·fo′bee·uh, me·tal″o·) *n.* A morbid fear of metals or metallic objects.

me·tal·lo·por·phy·rin (me·tal″o·por′fi·rin, met″uh·lo·) *n.* A compound formed by the combination of a porphyrin with a metal such as iron, copper, cobalt, nickel, silver, tin, zinc, manganese, or magnesium. Heme is a metalloporphyrin in which a porphyrin is combined with iron.

me·tal·lo·pro·tein (me·tal″o·pro′tee·in, ·teen) *n.* A protein enzyme containing metal as an inherent portion of its molecule.

metalo-. See *metallo-.*

me·ta·lol (me′tuh·lol) *n.* 4′-[1-Hydroxy-2-(methylamino)propyl]methanesulfonanilide, $C_{11}H_{18}N_2O_3S$, a beta-adrenergic receptor antagonist; used as the hydrochloride salt.

me·talo·phil (me·tal′o·fil) *n.* [*metalo-* + *-phil*]. Any of the reticular cells which stain with metallic salts, as silver carbonate. It may be a fixed or ameboid cell or a monocyte of peripheral blood.

meta·mer (met′uh·mur) *n.* [*meta-* + iso*mer*]. One of two or more compounds having the same number and kind of atoms but with a different distribution of the component radicals.

meta·mere (met′uh·meer) *n.* [*meta-* + *-mere*]. One of the linear series of more or less similar segments of the body of many animals.

meta·mer·ic (met″uh·merr′ick) *adj.* Pertaining to a metamere or metamerism.

metameric syndrome. SEGMENTAL SYNDROME.

me·tam·er·ism (me·tam′ur·iz·um) *n.* 1. *In zoology,* the repetition of more or less similar parts or segments (metameres) in the body of many animals, as exhibited especially by the Annelida, Arthropoda, and Vertebrata. See also *pseudometamerism.* 2. *In chemistry,* the relationship existing between two or more metamers.

Metamine. Trademark for trolnitrate, a vasodilator used as the phosphate salt to reduce the frequency and severity of attacks of angina pectoris.

meta·mor·phic (met″uh·mor′fick) *adj.* Pertaining to metamorphosis.

meta·mor·phop·sia (met″uh·mor·fop′see·uh) *n.* [*metamorpho*sis + *-opsia*]. A visual disturbance in which the image is distorted.

meta·mor·phose (met″uh·mor′foze) *v.* To undergo or cause to undergo metamorphosis.

metamorphosing breath sound. A breath sound which changes in quality or intensity during a respiratory cycle, possibly due to the opening of an occluded bronchus.

meta·mor·pho·sis (met″uh·mor′fuh·sis, ·mor·fo′sis) *n.*, pl. **metamorpho·ses** (·seez) [Gk. *metamorphōsis*, transformation]. 1. A structural change or transformation; usually associated with growth and development of an organism through successive stages, such as egg, larva, pupa, adult. Compare *metabolous.* 2. *In pathology,* a retrogressive change.

Metamucil. Trademark for a laxative composed of the powdered mucilaginous portion of blond psyllium seed and powdered anhydrous dextrose, about 50% of each.

meta·my·e·lo·cyte (met″uh·migh′e·lo·site) *n.* [*meta-* + *myelocyte*]. A cell of the granulocytic series intermediate between the myelocyte and granular leukocyte, having a full complement of specific granules and an indented, bean-shaped (juvenile) nucleus. Syn. *metagranulocyte, juvenile cell.*

Metandren. A trademark for methyltestosterone, a crystalline androgen.

meta·neph·ric (met″uh·nef′rick) *adj.* Of or pertaining to the metanephros.

metanephric blastema. The caudal end of the nephrogenic cord.

metanephric duct. URETER.

meta·neph·rine (met″uh·nef′reen) *n.* [*meta-* + *nephr-* + *-ine*]. An inactive metabolite of epinephrine (3-*O*-methylepinephrine) which is excreted in the urine, where its measurement is used as a test for pheochromocytoma.

meta·neph·ro·gen·ic (met″uh·nef″ro·jen′ick) *adj.* [*metanephros* + *-genic*]. Capable of forming, or giving rise to, the metanephros.

metanephrogenic tissue. The caudal part of the nephrogenic tissue giving rise to the metanephros or definitive kidney.

meta·neph·ros (met″uh·nef′ros) *n.*, pl. **metaneph·roi** (·roy) [*meta-* + *nephros*]. The definitive or permanent kidney of reptiles, birds, and mammals. It develops from the caudal part of the nephrogenic cord in association with the ureteric bud from the mesonephric duct.

meta·phase (met'uh·faze) *n.* [*meta-* + *phase*]. 1. The middle stage of mitosis when the chromosomes lie nearly in a single plane at the equator of the spindle, forming the equatorial plate. It follows the prophase and precedes the anaphase. 2. The middle stage of the first (metaphase I) or second (metaphase II) meiotic division.

Metaphen. Trademark for nitromersol, an organomercurial antibacterial agent used topically.

meta·phos·phor·ic acid (met"uh·fos·for'ick). HPO_3. A clear, viscous liquid or glasslike solid; the commercial product, prepared in stick-form, contains about 17% Na_2O. Used as a reagent.

Metaphyllin. A trademark for aminophylline.

me·taph·y·se·al (me·taf"i·see'ul, met"uh·fiz'ee·ul) *adj.* Pertaining to a metaphysis.

metaphyseal aclasis. MULTIPLE HEREDITARY EXOSTOSES.

metaphyseal chondrodysplasia. METAPHYSEAL DYSOSTOSIS.

metaphyseal dysostosis. A very rare condition in which the roentgenographic appearance of the metaphyses is unique, being largely cartilaginous and irregularly calcified. Many metaphyses appear enlarged and the radiolucent space between the epiphysis and the shaft is markedly widened.

metaphyseal dysplasia. A possibly hereditary condition in which the ends of the long bones become markedly widened, with thin cortices, as a result of failure to become remodeled during endochondral osteogenesis.

meta·phys·i·al (met"uh·fiz'ee·ul) *adj.* METAPHYSEAL.

me·taph·y·sis (me·taf'i·sis) *n.*, pl. **metaphy·ses** (·seez) [*meta-* + Gk. *physis*, growth]. 1. The region of growth between the epiphysis and diaphysis of a bone. Syn. *epiphyseal plate.* 2. The growing end of the diaphysis.

me·taph·y·si·tis (met"uh·fi·sigh'tis, me·taf"i·) *n.* Inflammation of a metaphysis.

meta·pla·sia (met"uh·play'zee·uh, ·zhuh) *n.* [*meta-* + *-plasia*]. Transformation of one form of adult tissue to another, such as replacement of respiratory epithelium by stratified squamous epithelium. —**meta·plas·tic** (·plas'tick) *adj.*

me·tap·la·sis (me·tap'luh·sis) *n.* [*meta-* + Gk. *plasis*, moulding, conformation]. Fulfilled growth and development seen in the stage between anaplasis and cataplasis.

meta·plasm (met'uh·plaz·um) *n.* [*meta-* + *-plasm*]. The lifeless inclusions in protoplasm collectively.

meta·pneu·mon·ic (met"uh·new·mon'ick) *adj.* [*meta-* + *pneumonic*]. Secondary to, or consequent upon, pneumonia.

met·a·poph·y·sis (met"uh·pof'i·sis) *n.* [*met-* + *apophysis*]. Old term for a mamillary process, as seen upon the lumbar vertebrae.

Metaprel. A trademark for metaproterenol, a bronchodilator drug.

meta·pro·tein (met"uh·pro'tee·in, ·teen) *n.* An intermediate product of acid or alkaline hydrolysis of a protein. Soluble in weak acids and alkalis, insoluble in water. See also *protein.*

meta·pro·ter·e·nol (met"uh·pro·terr'e·nol) *n.* 3,5-Dihydroxy-α-[(isopropylamino)methyl]benzyl alcohol, $C_{11}H_{17}NO_3$, a β_2 receptor agonist bronchodilator used as the sulfate salt.

meta·psy·chol·o·gy (met"uh·sigh·kol'uh·jee) *n.* [*meta-* + *psychology*]. Any systematic theory of mental processes which cannot be verified by empirical facts or be disproved by reasoning. See also *parapsychology.*

meta·ram·i·nol (met"uh·ram'i·nol) *n.* *l*-α-(1-Aminoethyl)-*m*-hydroxybenzyl alcohol, $C_9H_{13}NO_2$, a sympathomimetic amine; used as the bitartrate salt.

met·ar·te·ri·ole (met"ahr·teer'ee·ole) *n.* [*met-* + *arteriole*]. PRECAPILLARY.

meta·ru·bri·cyte (met"uh·roo'bri·site) *n.* [*meta-* + *rubricyte*]. NORMOBLAST (1).

Metaspas. Trademark for dihexyverine.

meta·sta·ble (met'uh·stay"bul) *adj.* Of intermediate stability; changing readily either to a more or a less stable state.

metastable state. A state of marginal stability, as the excited state of an atomic system in which its energy of excitation cannot be radiated as electromagnetic energy.

me·tas·ta·sis (me·tas'tuh·sis) *n.*, pl. **metasta·ses** (·seez) [Gk., removal, migration, transference]. The transfer of disease from a primary focus to a distant one by the conveyance of causal agents or cells through the blood vessels or lymph channels. —**meta·stat·ic** (met"uh·stat'ick) *adj.*

me·tas·ta·size (me·tas'tuh·size) *v.* To be transferred to another part of the body by metastasis.

metastasizing leiomyosarcoma. LEIOMYOSARCOMA.

metastasizing struma. An apparently benign goiter which gives rise to metastases.

metastatic abscess. A visceral or brain abscess complicating pyemia or septic embolism.

metastatic anemia. Anemia resulting from bone marrow destruction by metastatic tumor.

metastatic calcification. Pathologic calcification associated with high serum calcium levels and chiefly involving the lungs, stomach, and kidneys.

metastatic choroiditis. Choroiditis due to embolism.

metastatic ophthalmia. A type of suppurative endophthalmitis caused by blood-borne infectious agents which localize in the intraocular structures, producing an exudate which collects in the vitreous chamber.

metastatic parotitis. Parotitis secondary to disease elsewhere; it occurs in infectious disease and usually goes on to suppuration. Syn. *symptomatic parotitis.*

metastatic pneumonia. Pneumonia due to the presence in the lungs of infected emboli.

metastatic tumor. A secondary tumor produced by metastasis.

Meta·stron·gy·lus (met"uh·stron'ji·lus) *n.* [*meta-* + Gk. *strongylos*, round]. A genus of nematode parasites.

Metastrongylus elon·ga·tus (ee"long·gay'tus). A species of nematode common to hogs, occasionally to sheep and cattle, which infects the respiratory tract and produces a pneumonitis and bronchitis often fatal in young animals. A few cases of human infection have been reported.

meta·tar·sal (met"uh·tahr'sul) *adj.* & *n.* 1. Pertaining to the metatarsus. 2. A metatarsal bone.

metatarsal arch. TRANSVERSE ARCH OF THE FOOT.

meta·tar·sal·gia (met"uh·tahr·sal'jee·uh) *n.* [*metatars*us + *-algia*]. Pain and tenderness in the metatarsal region.

metatarsal ligament. Any of the ligaments interconnecting the metatarsal bones, including the dorsal metatarsal ligaments (NA *ligamenta metatarsea dorsalia*), the interosseous metatarsal ligaments (NA *ligamenta metatarsea interossea*), and the plantar metatarsal ligaments (NA *ligamenta metatarsea plantaria*). See also *deep transverse metatarsal ligament, superficial transverse metatarsal ligament.*

meta·tar·sec·to·my (met"uh·tahr·seck'tum·ee) *n.* [*metatars*al + *-ectomy*]. Excision of a metatarsal bone.

meta·tar·so·pha·lan·ge·al (met·uh·tahr"so·fuh·lan'jee·ul) *adj.* Pertaining to the metatarsus and the phalanges.

metatarsophalangeal articulation. Any of the joints between the heads of the metatarsals and their respective proximal phalanges. NA (pl.) *articulationes metatarsophalangeae.*

metatarsophalangeal ligament. Any of the ligaments connecting the heads of the metatarsals and the bases of the proximal phalanges. See also *collateral ligaments, plantar ligaments.*

meta·tar·sus (met"uh·tahr'sus) *n.*, pl. & genit. sing. **metatar·si** (·sigh) [*meta-* + *tarsus*] [NA]. The part of the foot between the tarsus and the phalanges, containing five bones. See also Table of Bones in the Appendix.

metatarsus ab·duc·tus (ab·duck'tus). A congenital deviation of the fore part of the foot away from the midline of the body, the heel remaining in a neutral or slightly valgus position. At birth there is no bone deformity, the deviation of the metatarsals being produced by soft-tissue contracture. In older persons bone deformity may develop due to secondary adaptation.

metatarsus ad·duc·to·va·rus (a·duck"to·vair'us). A congenital deformity of the foot; a deviation of the fore part of the foot toward the midline of the body, associated with an elevation of its inner border, the heel remaining in a neutral or slightly valgus position. It is caused by soft tissue contracture with bony deformity, occurs only in older cases and is due to secondary adaptation.

metatarsus ad·duc·tus (a·duck'tus). A congenital deviation of the fore part of the foot toward the midline of the body, the heel remaining in a neutral or slightly valgus position. At birth there is no bone deformity, the deviation of the metatarsals being produced by soft-tissue contracture. In older persons bone deformity may develop due to secondary adaptation.

metatarsus adductus pri·mus (prye·mus). An abnormality in the developmental process involving the adduction of the first metatarsal. Syn. *metatarsus primus varus.*

metatarsus pri·mus va·rus (prye'mus vair'us). METATARSUS ADDUCTUS PRIMUS.

metatarsus varus. A congenital deformity of the foot; an elevation of the inner border of the fore part of the foot (varus), the heel remaining in a neutral or slightly valgus position.

meta·thal·a·mus (met"uh·thal'uh·mus) *n.* [*meta-* + *thalamus*] [NA]. The lateral and medial geniculate bodies.

me·tath·e·sis (me·tath'e·sis) *n.*, pl. **metathe·ses** (·seez) [Gk., transposition]. A chemical reaction in which there is an exchange of radicals or elements of the type AB + CD = AD + CB with no change in valence. —**meta·thet·ic** (met"uh·thet'ick) *adj.*

meta·troph·ic (met"uh·trof'ick, ·tro'fick) *adj.* [*meta-* + *-trophic*]. 1. Of or pertaining to bacteria that derive sustenance from organic matter. See also *prototrophic.* 2. Modifying nutrition.

metatrophic method. A therapeutic method of modifying the nutrition, with a view of enhancing the action of a drug being administered.

me·tax·a·lone (me·tack'suh·lone) *n.* 5-[(3,5-Dimethylphenoxy)methyl]-2-oxazolidinone, $C_{12}H_{15}NO_3$, a skeletal muscle relaxant.

Meta·zoa (met"uh·zo'uh) *n.pl.* [*meta-* + Gk. *zōa,* living beings, animals]. 1. A subdivision of the animal kingdom which includes all the multicellular forms, and so stands in contrast to the Protozoa. 2. In another classification, a subdivision including all multicellular forms except the Porifera (sponges). —**metazo·an** (·un) *adj. & n.;* **metazo·al** (·ul) *adj.*

Metch·ni·koff's theory (mʸetch'nʸi·kuf) [Élie (Ilya) *Metchnikoff,* Russian biologist in France, 1845–1916]. A theory of development of inflammation and immunity as manifestations of phagocytosis.

me·te·cious, me·toe·cious (me·tee'shus, ·see·us) *adj.* [Gk. *metoikos,* alien resident, sojourner, settler]. HETERECIOUS.

met·em·pir·ic (met"em·pirr'ick) *adj.* [*met-* + *empiric*]. Not derived from experience, but implied or presupposed by it.

met·en·ceph·a·lon (met"en·sef'uh·lon) *n.* [*met-* + *encephalon*] [NA]. The cephalic part of the rhombencephalon, giving rise to the cerebellum and pons.

me·te·or·ic (mee"tee·or'ick) *adj.* [Gk. *meteōros,* off the ground, in mid-air]. 1. Pertaining to atmospheric phenomena. 2. Pertaining to meteors.

me·te·or·ism (mee'tee·ur·iz·um) *n.* [F. *météorisme,* from Gk. *meteōrismos,* being raised, swelling]. Gaseous distention of the abdomen or intestine; tympanites.

me·te·oro·graph (mee"tee·or'o·graf) *n.* [*meteoric* + *-graph*]. An apparatus for securing a continuous and simultaneous record of the pressure, temperature, humidity, and velocity of the wind.

me·te·o·rol·o·gy (mee"tee·ur·ol'uh·jee) *n.* [Gk. *meteōrologia*]. The science that deals with the atmosphere and various atmospheric phenomena, including weather and weather forecasting.

me·te·oro·path·o·log·ic (mee"tee·or"o·path·uh·loj'ick) *adj.* [*meteoric* + *pathologic*]. Pertaining to the influence of weather or climate on incidence, development, and course of disease.

-meter. A combining form designating *an instrument for measuring or recording* the specified kind of phenomena.

me·ter, *n.* [F. *mètre,* from Gk. *metron,* measure]. 1. The basic unit of length in the metric system, originally established as the distance between two scratches on a bar of platinum-iridium alloy kept at the International Bureau of Weights and Measures, near Paris; later defined as 1650763.73 wavelengths, in vacuo, of a specified radiation of the krypton atom of mass 86. Abbreviated, m, m. 2. An instrument for measuring and recording quantities, as of the flow of electricity, liquids, or gases, of intensity of radiation, etc.

meter-angle. The degree of convergence of the eyes when centered on an object one meter distant from each.

met·es·trus, met·oes·trus (met·es'trus) *n.* [*met-* + *estrus*]. The period that follows the estrus when there is marked invasion of the vaginal walls by leukocytes.

met·for·min (met'for·min) *n.* 1,1-Dimethylbiguanide, $C_4H_{11}N_5$, an orally effective hypoglycemic agent.

meth-. A combining form designating *methyl.*

meth·a·cho·line chloride (meth"uh·ko'leen, ·lin). (2-Hydroxypropyl)trimethylammonium chloride acetate, $C_8H_{18}ClNO_2$, a parasympathomimetic drug employed mainly in the management of disorders of the cardiovascular system. The salt is usually administered subcutaneously; for oral administration methacholine bromide is used.

meth·a·cy·cline (meth"uh·sigh'kleen) *n.* 6-Methylene-5-hydroxytetracycline, $C_{22}H_{22}N_2O_8$, a semisynthetic tetracycline antibiotic.

meth·a·done (meth'uh·dohn) *n.* 6-(Dimethylamino)-4,4-diphenyl-3-heptanone, $C_{21}H_{27}NO$, a narcotic analgesic used also for maintenance treatment of heroin addiction; employed as the hydrochloride salt.

meth·a·dyl acetate (meth'uh·dil) *n.* 6-(Dimethylamino)-4,4-diphenyl-3-heptanol acetate(ester), $C_{23}H_{31}NO_2$, a narcotic analgesic.

meth·al·len·es·tril (meth"uh·le·nes'tril) *n.* β-Ethyl-6-methoxy-α,α-dimethyl-2-naphthalenepropionic acid, $C_{18}H_{22}O_3$, an orally effective, nonsteroid estrogen.

meth·al·li·bure (meth·al'i·byoor) *n.* 1-Methyl-6-(1-methylallyl)-2,5-dithiobiurea, $C_7H_{14}N_4S_2$, an anterior pituitary activator used in swine.

meth·al·thi·a·zide (meth"al·thigh'uh·zide) *n.* 3-[(Allylthio)-methyl]-6-chloro-3,4-dihydro-2-methyl-2*H*-1,2,4-benzothiadiazine-7-sulfonamide 1,1-dioxide, a diuretic and antihypertensive drug.

Methalutin. A trademark for normethandrone, an androgen.

meth·am·phet·a·mine (meth"am·fet'uh·meen, ·min) *n.* Deoxyephedrine or *N*, α-dimethylphenethylamine, $C_{10}H_{15}N$, a central stimulant and pressor drug; used as the hydrochloride salt. Syn. *desoxyephedrine, methylamphetamine.*

meth·a·nal (meth'uh·nal) *n.* FORMALDEHYDE.

meth·an·dri·ol (meth·an'dree·ol) *n.* 17-Methylandrost-5-ene-3β,17β-diol, $C_{20}H_{32}O_2$, an anabolic-androgenic steroid.

meth·an·dro·sten·o·lone (meth·an"dro·sten'uh·lone) *n.* Δ^1-17α-Methyltestosterone, $C_{20}H_{28}O_2$, an anabolic-androgenic steroid.

meth·ane (meth'ane) *n.* [*meth-* + *-ane*]. The first member, CH_4, of the homologous series of paraffins having the general formula C_nH_{2n+2}. A colorless, odorless, inflammable gas. Syn. *marsh gas.*

meth·ane·sul·fo·nate (meth"ane·sul'fuh·nate) *n.* MESYLATE.

meth·a·no·ic acid (meth"uh·no'ick). FORMIC ACID (1).

meth·a·nol (meth'uh·nol, ·nole) *n.* METHYL ALCOHOL.

meth·an·the·line bromide (meth·anth'e·leen, ·in). Diethyl(2-hydroxyethyl)methylammonium bromide xanthene-9-carboxylate, $C_{21}H_{26}BrNO_3$, a parasympatholytic drug with the antisecretory and antispasmodic actions of anticholinergic drugs.

meth·a·pyr·i·lene (meth"uh·pirr'i·leen) *n.* 2-{[2-(Dimethylamino)ethyl]-2-thenylamino}pyridine, $C_{14}H_{19}N_3S$, an antihistaminic drug; used as the hydrochloride salt. Syn. *thenylpyramine.*

meth·a·qua·lone (meth"uh·kway'lone, me·thack'wuh·lone) *n.* 2-Methyl-3-*o*-tolyl-4(3*H*)-quinazolinone, $C_{16}H_{14}N_2O$, a nonbarbiturate sedative and hypnotic.

meth·ar·bi·tal (meth·ahr'bi·tawl, ·tal) *n.* 5,5-Diethyl-1-methylbarbituric acid, $C_9H_{14}N_2O_3$, a long-acting barbiturate used mainly for its antiepileptic action.

meth·a·zol·a·mide (meth"uh·zol'uh·mide) *n.* *N*-(4-Methyl-2-sulfamoyl-Δ^2-1,3,4-thiadiazolin-5-ylidene)acetamide, $C_5H_8N_4O_3S_2$, a carbonic anhydrase inhibitor effective orally in lowering intraocular pressure in the treatment of glaucoma.

Methedrine. A trademark for methamphetamine hydrochloride, a central stimulant drug.

meth·dil·a·zine (meth·dil'uh·zine ·dye'luh·zeen) *n.* 10-[(1-Methyl-3-pyrrolidinyl)methyl]phenothiazine, $C_{18}H_{20}N_2S$, an antihistaminic drug used to relieve pruritus.

met·hem·al·bu·min (met"heem·al·bew'min, ·hem·, ·al'bew·min) *n.* [*met-* + *hem-* + *albumin*]. A product of the combination of hematin and serum albumin, comparable to methemoglobin. Syn. *pseudomethemoglobin, Fairley's pigment.*

met·hem·al·bu·mi·ne·mia (met"heem·al·bew"mi·nee'mee·uh, ·al"bew·) *n.* Methemalbumin in the plasma.

met·heme (met'heem) *n.* [*met-* + *heme*]. HEMATIN.

met·he·mo·glo·bin (met"hee'muh·glo"bin) *n.* [*met-* + *hemoglobin*]. The oxidized form of hemoglobin, in which the iron atom is trivalent, and which is not able to combine reversibly with oxygen. Syn. *ferrihemoglobin.*

met·he·mo·glo·bi·ne·mia, met·hae·mo·glo·bi·ne·mia (met·hee"muh·glo·bi·nee'mee·uh) *n.* 1. An excess of methemoglobin in the blood. 2. Any of several hereditary enzyme or hemoglobin abnormalities resulting in elevated methemoglobin levels and characterized clinically by cyanosis. See also *hemoglobin M.*

met·he·mo·glo·bin·uria, met·hae·mo·glo·bin·uria (met·hee"muh·glo·bi·new'ree·uh) *n.* The presence of methemoglobin in the urine.

me·the·na·mine (meth·ee'nuh·meen, ·min, meth'in·uh·meen") *n.* Hexamethylenetetramine, $(CH_2)_6N_4$, a urinary tract antiseptic. Syn. *hexamine.*

meth·ene (meth'een) *n.* 1. The first member, CH_2, of the ethylene (alkene) series of unsaturated hydrocarbons. It has never been isolated. 2. The hydrocarbon radical —CH_2—. Syn. *methylene.*

me·the·no·lone (meth·ee'nuh·lone) *n.* 17β-Hydroxy-1-methyl-5α-androst-1-ene-3-one, $C_{20}H_{30}O_2$, an anabolic steroid; used as the enanthate (heptanoate) ester.

meth·e·nyl (meth'e·nil) *n.* The trivalent radical, CH≡. Syn. *methine, methyne.*

Methergine. Trademark for methylergonovine, an oxytocic agent used as the maleate salt.

meth·et·o·in (meth·et'o·in) *n.* 5-Ethyl-1-methyl-5-phenylhydantoin, $C_{12}H_{14}N_2O_2$, an anticonvulsant drug.

Methiacil. Trademark for methylthiouracil, an antithyroid drug.

meth·i·cil·lin (meth"i·sil'in) *n.* 2,6-Dimethoxyphenylpenicillin, $C_{17}H_{20}N_2O_6S$, a semisynthetic penicillin antibiotic; used as the sodium salt.

meth·im·a·zole (meth·im'uh·zole, me·thigh'muh·zole) *n.* 1-Methyl-2-imidazolethiol, $C_4H_6N_2S$, a thyroid inhibitor drug.

meth·ine, meth·yne (meth'ine, ·een) *n.* METHENYL.

methiodal sodium. SODIUM METHIODAL.

me·thi·o·nine (me·thigh'o·neen, ·nin) *n.* DL-2-Amino-4-(methylthio)butyric acid, $CH_3S(CH_2)_2CHNH_2COOH$, an amino acid essential for growth of animals as it furnishes both labile methyl groups and sulfur necessary for normal metabolism. May be useful for prevention and treatment of certain types of liver damage.

methionine adenosyl transferase. An enzyme that causes methionine to react with ATP to give *S*-adenosyl methionine, an important biological donor of methyl groups.

methionine malabsorption syndrome. A hereditary metabolic disorder in which there appears to be a defect in the transport of methionine across the intestinal and renal tubular epithelium, with high urinary excretion of methionine and α-hydroxybutyric acid resulting from the conversion by *Escherichia coli* of unabsorbed methionine in the colon; manifested clinically by an offensive urinary odor, unpigmented hair, seizures, mental retardation, and episodes of fever, hyperpnea, and edema. Syn. *oasthouse urine disease.*

me·thi·o·nyl (me·thigh'o·nil) *n.* The univalent radical, $CH_3SCH_2CH_2CH(NH_2)CO$—, of the amino acid methionine.

meth·is·a·zone (meth·is'uh·zone, ·iz') *n.* 1-Methylindole-2,3-dione 3-(thiosemicarbazone), $C_{10}H_{10}N_4OS$, an antiviral agent.

Methium Chloride. Trademark for hexamethonium chloride, a ganglionic blocking agent.

me·thix·ene (me·thick'seen) *n.* 1-Methyl-3-(thioxanthen-9-ylmethyl)piperidine, $C_{20}H_{23}NS$, an anticholinergic drug used, as the hydrochloride salt, as an adjunct in the treatment of gastrointestinal hypermotility and spasm associated with functional bowel disorders.

meth·o·car·ba·mol (meth"o·kahr'buh·mol, ·kahr·bam'ol) *n.* 2-Hydroxy-3-*o*-methoxyphenoxypropyl carbamate, $C_{11}H_{15}NO_5$, a skeletal muscle relaxant.

Methocel. Trademark for methyl cellulose.

meth·od, *n.* [Gk. *methodos,* from *met-* + *hodos,* way]. The manner of performance of any act or operation, as a surgical procedure, a maneuver, a treatment, or a test.

method of least squares. LEAST-SQUARES METHOD.

meth·o·hex·i·tal sodium (meth"o·heck'si·tal). Sodium *dl*-5-allyl-1-methyl-5-(1-methyl-2-pentynyl) barbiturate, $C_{14}H_{17}N_2NaO_3$, an ultrashort-acting barbiturate used as a basal and general anesthetic.

meth·o·in (meth'o·in) *n.* MEPHENYTOIN.

metho·ma·nia (meth"o·may'nee·uh) *n.* [Gk. *methē,* strong drink, + *-mania*]. METHYLEPSIA.

me·tho·ni·um (me·tho'nee·um) *n.* A generic name for a homologous series of compounds containing the ion $(CH_3)_3N^+(CH_2)_nN^+(CH_3)_3$. The compounds in which n is 6 (hexamethonium), or 10 (decamethonium) possess therapeutically useful actions.

meth·o·pho·line (meth"o·fo'leen) *n.* 1-(*p*-Chlorophenethyl)-1,2,3,4-tetrahydro-6,7-dimethoxy-2-methylisoquinoline, $C_{20}H_{24}ClNO_2$, an analgesic drug.

meth·o·pyr·a·pone (meth"o·pirr'uh·pone) *n.* METYRAPONE.

Methosarb. A trademark for calusterone.

meth·o·trex·ate (meth"o·treck'sate) *n.* Principally 4-amino-10-methylfolic acid, $C_{20}H_{22}N_8O_5$, with related compounds; an antineoplastic drug that functions as a folic acid antagonist. Used also in the treatment of psoriasis.

meth·o·tri·mep·ra·zine (meth"o·trye·mep'ruh·zeen) *n.* 10-[3-(Dimethylamino)-2-methylpropyl]-2-methoxyphenothiazine, $C_{19}H_{24}N_2OS$, a tranquilizer, nonnarcotic analgesic, and sedative. Syn. *levomepromazine.*

me·thox·a·mine (me·thock'suh·meen) *n.* α-(1-Aminoethyl)-2,5-dimethoxybenzyl alcohol, $C_{11}H_{17}NO_3$, a sympathomimetic amine used for its pressor action to maintain, or restore reduced, blood pressure; employed as the hydrochloride salt.

me·thox·sa·len (me·thock'suh·len) *n.* The δ-lactone of 3-(6-hydroxy-7-methoxybenzofuranyl)acrylic acid, or 8-methoxypsoralen, $C_{12}H_8O_4$. Induces formation of melanin pigment in skin on exposure to sunlight or ultraviolet light; used to treat idiopathic vitiligo.

methoxy-. A combining form designating *the univalent radical* CH_3O—.

me·thoxy·flu·rane (me·thock″see·floo′rane) *n.* 2,2-Dichloro-1,1-difluoroethyl methyl ether, $CHCl_2CF_2OCH_3$, a colorless liquid; used as a general anesthetic.

me·thoxy·phen·a·mine (me·thock″see·fen′uh·meen) *n.* 2-(*o*-Methoxyphenyl)isopropylmethylamine, $C_{11}H_{17}NO$, a sympathomimetic amine with bronchodilatation and inhibition of smooth muscle as predominant actions; used as the hydrochloride salt.

Methral. Trademark for fluperolone, an anti-inflammatory glucocorticoid used as the acetate ester.

meth·sco·pol·a·mine bromide (meth″sko·pol′uh·meen). *N*-Methylscopolammonium bromide, $C_{18}H_{24}BrNO_4$, a quaternary derivative of scopolamine hydrobromide that lacks the central actions of the latter and is used as an anticholinergic drug in the control of peptic ulcers and gastric disorders associated with hyperacidity and hypermotility.

meth·sux·i·mide (meth·suck′si·mide) *n.* *N*,2-Dimethyl-2-phenylsuccinimide, $C_{12}H_{13}NO_2$, an anticonvulsant used to control petit mal and psychomotor seizures.

meth·y·clo·thi·a·zide (meth″ee·klo·thigh′uh·zide) *n.* 6-Chloro-3-(chloromethyl)-3,4-dihydro-2-methyl-2*H*-1,2,4-benzothiadiazine-7-sulfonamide 1,1-dioxide, $C_9H_{11}Cl_2N_3O_4S_2$, an orally effective diuretic and antihypertensive drug.

meth·yl (meth′il) *n.* [from *methylene*]. The univalent hydrocarbon radical CH_3—.

meth·yl·acet·y·lene (meth″il·a·set′i·leen) *n.* ALLYLENE.

meth·yl·al (meth′i·lal) *n.* Dimethoxymethane, $CH_2(OCH_3)_2$, a water-soluble liquid; formerly used as a hypnotic and antispasmodic.

methyl alcohol. CH_3OH. A colorless, toxic liquid, obtained by destructive distillation of wood and by synthesis. Syn. *carbinol, methanol, wood alcohol.*

methyl aldehyde. FORMALDEHYDE.

meth·yl·am·ine (meth″il·am′een, ·a·meen′) *n.* Aminomethane, CH_3NH_2, a colorless gas sometimes produced naturally by certain plant and animal tissues.

meth·yl·ami·no·hep·tane (meth″il·a·mee″no·hep′tane) *n.* 2-Methylaminoheptane, $CH_3(CH_2)_4CH(NHCH_3)CH_3$, a sympathomimetic amine used as the hydrochloride salt to combat hypotension during surgery.

meth·yl·am·phet·a·mine (meth″il·am·fet′uh·meen) *n.* METHAMPHETAMINE.

methyl an·thra·nil·ate (an″thruh·nil′ate). Methyl 2-aminobenzoate, $NH_2C_6H_4COOCH_3$, a fragrant constituent of various essential oils.

meth·yl·ate (meth′i·late) *n.* & *v.* 1. A compound formed from methyl alcohol by substitution of the hydrogen of the hydroxyl by a base. 2. To introduce a methyl group into a compound. —**meth·yl·at·ed** (meth′i·lay·tid) *adj.*

meth·yl·a·tion (meth″i·lay′shun) *n.* The process of introducing a methyl group into a compound.

meth·yl·at·ro·pine bromide (meth″il·at′ro·peen, ·pin). ATROPINE METHYLBROMIDE.

methylatropine nitrate. ATROPINE METHYLNITRATE.

meth·yl·ben·zene (meth″il·ben′zeen) *n.* TOLUENE.

meth·yl·benz·etho·ni·um chloride (meth″il·benz″eth·o′nee·um). Benzyldimethyl {2-[2-(*p*-1,1,3,3-tetramethylbutylcresoxy)ethoxy]ethyl}ammoniumchloride, $C_{28}H_{44}ClNO_2.H_2O$, a quaternary ammonium salt with surface-active and disinfectant properties; used especially for bacteriostasis of urea-splitting organisms causing ammonia dermatitis.

meth·yl·ben·zo·yl·ec·go·nine (meth″il·ben″zo·il·eck′go·neen) *n.* COCAINE.

meth·yl·car·bi·nol (meth″il·kahr′bi·nol) *n.* ETHYL ALCOHOL.

methyl-CCNU. 1-(2-Chloroethyl)-3-(4-methylcyclohexyl)-1-nitrosourea, an antineoplastic agent.

meth·yl·cel·lu·lose (meth″il·sel′yoo·loce) *n.* A methyl ether of cellulose, occurring as a grayish-white fibrous powder, swelling in water to produce a clear to opalescent, viscous, colloidal solution. Used in the treatment of chronic constipation because it imparts bulk and blandness to the stool. Used in pharmacy to produce stable dispersions.

methyl chloride. Chloromethane, CH_3Cl, a gas that may be compressed to a liquid which volatilizes rapidly and produces localized freezing; has been used as a local anesthetic.

meth·yl·chlo·ro·form (meth″il·klor′uh·form) *n.* CH_3CCl_3, a solvent for organic materials.

methyl cyanide. ACETONITRILE.

5-meth·yl·cy·to·sine (meth″il·sigh′to·seen) *n.* A relatively rare pyrimidine base, $C_5H_7N_3O$, found in some nucleic acids, especially transfer RNA; usually obtained from the tubercle bacillus.

meth·yl·do·pa (meth″il·do′puh) *n.* L-3-(3,4-Dihydroxyphenyl)-2-methylalanine, $C_{10}H_{13}NO_4$, an antihypertensive agent. Syn. *alpha methyldopa.*

meth·yl·do·pate (meth″il·do′pate) *n.* Ethyl ester of methyldopa, $C_{12}H_{17}NO_4$, an antihypertensive drug; used as the hydrochloride salt.

meth·yl·ene (meth′i·leen) *n.* [F. *méthylène*, from Gk. *methy*, wine, + *hylē*, wood]. The bivalent hydrocarbon radical, —CH_2—.

methylene bichloride. METHYLENE CHLORIDE.

methylene blue. 3,7-Bis(dimethylamino)phenazathionium chloride, $C_{16}H_{18}ClN_3S.3H_2O$, occurring as dark green crystals or a crystalline powder with a bronzelike luster but forming deep blue solutions. Used as an antidote to cyanide poisoning and, formerly, as a urinary antiseptic; an ingredient of many biologic staining solutions. Syn. *methylthionine chloride.*

methylene blue N or **NN**. A basic dye of the thiazine series, of a greener shade than the true methylene blue.

methylene blue O. TOLUIDINE BLUE O.

methylene blue test. 1. A test for renal function, now seldom used, based on the fact that an injected solution of methylene blue normally appears in the urine in about 30 minutes. A longer interval indicates impaired renal permeability. Syn. *Achard-Castaigne method.* 2. A test for vitamin C. Vitamin C in the unknown is extracted with trichloroacetic acid or sulfosalicylic acid and then determined by its capacity to reduce methylene blue to the leuko-compound. 3. A test for urinary bilirubin. To 5 ml of urine are added 5 drops of 0.2% aqueous methylene blue solution. Green color with transmitted light is positive indication of bilirubin; normal urine is blue; not an absolutely specific test, but valuable as a screening test.

methylene chloride. Dichloromethane, CH_2Cl_2, a volatile liquid; has been used as an inhalation anesthetic for minor operations but is now used as a solvent. Syn. *methylene bichloride.*

methylene violet. A weakly basic thiazine dye, one of the oxidation products of methylene blue, and a constituent of polychrome methylene blue; used in MacNeal's tetrachrome blood stain.

meth·yl·eno·phil (meth″il·en′o·fil, ·een′o·fil) *adj.* & *n.* 1. Readily stainable with methylene blue. 2. A histologic element that is readily stainable with methylene blue. —**methyl·e·noph·i·lous** (·e·nof′i·lus) *adj.*

meth·y·lep·sia (meth″i·lep′see·uh) *n.* [Gk. *methy*, wine, + *lēpsis*, seizure, + *-ia*]. 1. Abnormal desire for intoxicating drink. 2. Hyperexcitability in an alcohol-intoxicated individual.

meth·yl·er·go·no·vine (meth″il·ur″go·no′veen) *n.* *N*-[1-(Hydroxymethyl)propyl]-D-lysergamide, $C_{20}H_{25}N_3O_2$, an oxytocic drug with the actions and uses of ergonovine; employed as the maleate salt.

meth·yl·eth·yl·ace·tic acid (meth″il·eth″il·uh·see′tick). An isomer of valeric acid.

me·thyl·glu·ca·mine (meth″il·gloo′kuh·meen) *n.* MEGLUMINE.

meth·yl·gly·ox·al (meth″il·glye·ock′sal) *n.* CH_3COCHO. The aldehyde of pyruvic acid, capable of transformation into glycogen by the liver.

meth·yl·hex·a·mine (meth″il·heck′suh·meen, ·heck·sam′een) *n.* 1,3-Dimethylamylamine or methylhexaneamine, $C_7H_{17}N$, a volatile sympathomimetic amine used by inhalation as the carbonate salt for its local vasoconstrictor action on the nasal mucosa.

methyl hydrate. METHYL ALCOHOL.

methyl hydride. CH_4. METHANE.

methyl *p*-hy·droxy·ben·zo·ate (păr″uh·high·drock″see·ben′zo·ate). METHYLPARABEN.

meth·yl·ma·lon·ic aciduria (meth″il·ma·lon′ick). An inborn error of metabolism in which there is a block in the conversion of methylmalonic acid to succinic acid, resulting in a chronic metabolic acidosis; inherited as an autosomal recessive.

meth·yl·ma·nia (meth″il·may′nee·uh) *n.* METHYLEPSIA.

meth·yl·mer·cap·tan (meth″il·mur·kap′tan) *n.* Methanethiol, CH_3SH, a gas of disagreeable odor produced in the intestinal tract by decomposition of certain proteins; also occurs in coal tar.

methyl meth·ac·ryl·ate (meth·ack′ri·late). The methyl ester of methacrylic acid, $CH_2{=}C(CH_3)COOCH_3$, a liquid that polymerizes readily to form thermoplastic substances called acrylics.

meth·yl·meth·ane (meth″il·meth′ane) *n.* ETHANE.

meth·yl·mor·phine (meth″il·mor′feen, ·fin) *n.* CODEINE.

methyl orange. Sodium *p*-dimethylaminoazobenzenesulfonate, $C_{14}H_{14}N_3NaO_3S$, occurring as an orange-yellow powder or crystalline scales; used as an indicator in acid-base titrations and occasionally as a histologic counterstain.

meth·yl·par·a·ben (meth″il·păr′uh·ben) *n.* Methyl *p*-hydroxybenzoate, $HOC_6H_4COOCH_3$, an antifungal preservative.

meth·yl·para·fy·nol (meth″il·păr″uh·fye′nol) *n.* 3-Methyl-1-pentyn-3-ol, $C_6H_{10}O$, a liquid; used as a hypnotic.

meth·yl·phen·i·date (meth″il·fen′i·date) *n.* Methyl α-phenyl-2-piperidineacetate, $C_{14}H_{19}NO_2$, a central nervous system stimulant used in the treatment of various types of depression; employed as the hydrochloride salt.

meth·yl·phe·no·bar·bi·tal (meth″il·fee″no·bahr′bi·tawl) *n.* MEPHOBARBITAL.

meth·yl·phe·no·bar·bi·tone (meth″il·fee″no·bahr′bi·tone) *n.* British Pharmacopoeia name for mephobarbital.

meth·yl·phe·nol (meth″il·fee′nol) *n.* CRESOL.

meth·yl·pred·nis·o·lone (meth″il·pred·nis′uh·lone) *n.* 11β,17,21-Trihydroxy-6α-methylpregna-1,4-diene-3,20-dione, $C_{22}H_{30}O_5$. An adrenocortical steroid with the actions and uses of prednisolone; used also in the form of its 21-acetate and 21-(sodium succinate).

methylprednisolone sodium phosphate. 11β,17,20-Trihydroxy-6α-methylpregna-1,4-diene-3,20-dione 21-(disodium phosphate), $C_{22}H_{29}Na_2O_8P$, a progestin.

meth·yl·pu·rine (meth″il·pew′reen, ·rin) *n.* Any compound in which one or more methyl radicals have been introduced into the purine nucleus. Among the more important compounds of this type are caffeine, theobromine, and theophylline.

methyl red. *p*-Dimethylaminoazobenzene-*o*-carboxylic acid, $C_{15}H_{15}N_3O_2$, violet crystals; used as an indicator in titrating weak bases.

methyl red test. A test for the differentiation of Enterobacteriaceae, such as the aerogenes group and the colon group of bacteria, performed by incubating the bacteria in a special medium and testing with methyl red indicator.

meth·yl·ros·an·i·line chloride (meth″il·ro·zan′il·een, ·lin). Hexamethylpararosaniline chloride, $C_{25}H_{30}ClN_3$, usually with more or less pentamethylpararosaniline chloride and tetramethylpararosaniline chloride; a dye mixture used as an antibacterial, antifungal, and anthelmintic agent and also as a biological stain. Crystal violet, gentian violet, and methyl violet are frequently used as synonyms for methylrosaniline chloride but the substances are not absolutely identical, differing in the specific methylpararosanilines present and in their proportions.

methyl salicylate. $C_6H_4(OH)COOCH_3$. A colorless, oily liquid, identical with the essential constituent of wintergreen oil; used externally as a counterirritant and in histology as a clearing agent.

meth·yl·sul·fo·nal (meth″il·sul′fo·nal) *n.* SULFONETHYLMETHANE.

meth·yl·tes·tos·ter·one (meth″il·tes·tos′tur·ohn) *n.* 17β-Hydroxy-17-methylandrost-4-en-3-one, $C_{20}H_{30}O_2$, an orally effective androgenic steroid hormone.

methyl theobromine. CAFFEINE.

meth·yl·thi·o·nine chloride (meth″il·thigh′o·neen, ·nin). METHYLENE BLUE.

meth·yl·thio·ura·cil (meth″il·thigh″o·yoor′uh·sil) *n.* 6-Methyl-2-thiouracil or 4-hydroxy-2-mercapto-6-methylpyrimidine, $C_5H_6N_2OS$, an antithyroid drug.

methyl violet. A form of methylrosaniline chloride.

methyl yellow. DIMETHYLAMINOAZOBENZENE.

meth·yne (meth″ine) *n.* METHENYL.

methy·no·di·ol diacetate (meth″i·no·dye′ole) *n.* 11β-Methyl-19-nor-17α-pregn-4-en-20-yne-3β,17-diol, diacetate, $C_{25}H_{34}O_4$, a progestin.

meth·y·pry·lon (meth″i·prye′lon) *n.* 3,3-Diethyl-5-methyl-2,4-piperidinedione, $C_{10}H_{17}NO_2$, a nonbarbiturate sedative and hypnotic.

meth·y·ser·gide (meth″i·sur′jide) *n.* *N*-[1-(Hydroxymethyl)propyl]-1-methyl-D-lysergamide, a homologue of methylergonovine; used as the bimaleate salt for prophylactic management of migraine headache.

meth·y·sis (meth′i·sis) *n.* [Gk., from *methy,* wine]. INTOXICATION.

me·ti·a·pine (me·tye′uh·peen) *n.* 2-Methyl-11-(4-methyl-1-piperazinyl)dibenzo [*b,f*] [1,4]-thiazepine, $C_{19}H_{21}N_3S$, a drug acting on the central nervous system.

Meticortelone. A trademark for prednisolone, an anti-inflammatory adrenocortical steroid.

Meticorten. A trademark for prednisone, an anti-inflammatory adrenocortical steroid.

met·myo·glo·bin (met″migh′o·glo·bin) *n.* The oxidized form of myoglobin, analogous to methemoglobin.

met·o·clo·pram·ide (met″o·klo·pram′ide) *n.* 4-Amino-5-chloro-*N*-[2-(diethylamino)ethyl]-*o*-anisamide, $C_{14}H_{22}ClN_3O_2$, an antiemetic drug; used as the hydrochloride salt.

met·o·cu·rine (met″o·kew′reen) *n.* (+)-O,O′-Dimethylchondrocurine diiodide, $C_{40}H_{48}I_2N_2O_6$, a skeletal muscle relaxant formerly called dimethyl tubocurarine iodide, possessing the curare action of the parent substance, but less prone to cause respiratory paralysis and of longer duration of action; used to produce muscle relaxation in surgery.

me·toe·cious. HETERECIOUS.

metoestrus. METESTRUS.

met·o·gest (met′o·jest) *n.* 17β-Hydroxy-16,16-dimethylestr-4-en-3-one, $C_{20}H_{30}O_2$, a hormone.

me·to·la·zone (me·to′luh·zone) *n.* 7-Chloro-1,2,3,4-tetrahydro-2-methyl-4-oxo-3-*o*-tolyl-6-quinazolinesulfonamide, $C_{16}H_{16}ClN_3O_3S$, a diuretic drug.

me·top·a·gus (me·top′uh·gus) *n.* [Gk. *metōpon,* forehead, + *-pagus*]. CRANIOPAGUS FRONTALIS.

me·top·ic (me·top′ick, me·to′pick) *adj.* [Gk. *metōpikos,* from *metōpon,* forehead]. 1. Pertaining to the forehead; frontal. 2. Pertaining to a cranium having a frontal suture; characterized by metopism.

metopic suture. The frontal suture, present in infancy, between the two vertical halves of the frontal bone; especially the inferior part or all of it when it persists in the adult skull.

met·o·pim·a·zine (met″o·pim′uh·zeen) *n.* 1-[3-[2-(Methylsulfonyl)phenothiazin-10-yl]propyl]isonipecotamide, $C_{22}H_{27}N_3O_3S_2$, an antiemetic drug.

me·to·pi·on (me·to′pee·on, ·un) *n.* [Gk. *metōpion,* forehead]. *In craniometry,* the point where the line that connects the highest points of the frontal eminences crosses the sagittal plane.

Metopirone. Trademark for metyrapone, a diagnostic aid for determining pituitary function.

met·o·pism (met′o·piz·um) *n.* The condition of having a metopic suture: a frontal suture that persists beyond infancy.

me·to·pi·um (me·to′pee·um) *n.* [L., from Gk. *metōpion*]. Metopon (= FOREHEAD).

Metopium, *n.* A genus of poisonous plants.

¹me·to·pon (me·to′pon, met′o·pon) *n.* [Gk. *metōpon*]. FOREHEAD.

²met·o·pon (met′o·pon) *n.* 6-Methyldihydromorphinone, $C_{18}H_{21}NO_3$, a narcotic analgesic with actions similar to those of morphine; has been used, as the hydrochloride salt, to relieve pain in patients with incurable cancer.

me·to·pro·lol (me·to′pro·lole, ·lol) *n.* 1-(Isopropylamino)-3-[*p*-(2-methoxyethyl)phenoxy]-2-propanol, $C_{15}H_{25}NO_3$, an antiadrenergic.

met·o·qui·zine (met′o·kwi·zeen) *n.* 3,5-Dimethyl-*N*-(4,6,6*a*,7,8,9,10,10*a*-octahydro-4,7-dimethylindolo-[4,3-*fg*]quinolin-9-yl)pyrazole-1-carboxamide, $C_{22}H_{27}N_5O$, an anticholinergic drug.

met·o·ser·pate (met″o·sur′pate) *n.* Methyl 18-epi-reserpate methyl ether, $C_{24}H_{32}N_2O_5$, a veterinary antianxiety drug; used as the hydrochloride salt.

me·tox·e·nous (me·tock′si·nus) *adj.* [*met-* + Gk. *xenos,* foreign, strange]. HETERECIOUS. —**metoxe·ny** (·nee) *n.*

¹metr-, metro- [Gk. *mētra,* womb; *mētēr, mētros,* mother]. A combining form meaning (a) *uterus, uterine;* (b) *mother, maternal.*

²metr-, metro- [Gk. *metron*]. A combining form meaning *measure or distance.*

metraemia. METREMIA.

me·tral·gia (me·tral′jee·uh, ·juh) *n.* [*metr-* + *-algia*]. Pain of uterine origin. Syn. *metrodynia.*

me·tra·pec·tic (mee″truh·peck′tick, met″ruh·) *adj.* [*metr-,* mother, + Gk. *apechein,* to keep away from]. Pertaining to a disease which is transmitted through the mother but which she herself escapes (such as hemophilia).

me·tra·to·nia (mee″truh·to′nee·uh, met″ruh·) *n.* [*metr-* + *atonia*]. Atony of the uterus.

me·tra·tro·phia (mee″truh·tro′fee·uh, met″ruh·) *n.* [*metr-* + Gk. *atrophia*]. Atrophy of the uterus.

me·trauxe (me·trawk′see) *n.* [*metr-* + Gk. *auxē,* increase, growth]. Hypertrophy or enlargement of the uterus.

Metrazol. A trademark for pentylenetetrazol, a central nervous system stimulant.

Metrazol shock therapy. Shock therapy of persons with manic depression or the catatonic form of schizophrenia with an intravenous injection of Metrazol, which causes convulsions and produces temporary brain changes resulting in elevation of the mood to normal levels and promotion of normal mental animation.

me·tre (mee′tur) *n.* METER.

me·trec·ta·sia (mee″treck·tay′zee·uh, ·zhuh, met″reck·) *n.* [*metr-* + *ectasia*]. Enlargement of the nonpregnant uterus.

me·trec·to·pia (mee″treck·to′pee·uh, met″reck·) *n.* [*metr-* + *ectopia*]. Displacement of the uterus.

me·trec·to·py (me·treck′to·pee) *n.* METRECTOPIA.

me·tre·mia, me·trae·mia (me·tree′mee·uh) *n.* [*metr-* + *-emia*]. Hyperemia of the uterus.

me·treu·ryn·ter (mee″troo·rin′tur, met″roo·) *n.* [*metr-* + Gk. *eurynein,* to dilate]. An inflatable bag for dilating the cervical canal of the uterus.

me·treu·ry·sis (me·troo′ri·sis) *n.* [*metr-* + Gk. *eurys,* broad]. Dilatation of the uterine cervix with the metreurynter.

me·tria (mee′tree·uh) *n.* [*metr-* + *-ia*]. 1. Any uterine affection. 2. Any inflammatory condition during the puerperium.

met·ric (met′rick) *adj.* [Gk. *metrikos,* from *metron,* measure]. 1. Of or pertaining to the metric system. 2. Of or for measurement.

metric occupational therapy. A form of occupational therapy in which the amount of work a patient does in a given time is measured to help form a basis for an estimate of the amount of work he can or should do (work tolerance); most useful with chronically ill patients with limited physical capacities. Syn. *measured work therapy.*

metric ophthalmoscopy. Ophthalmoscopy for measuring refraction.

metric system. A decimal system of weights and measures based on the meter as the unit of length, the kilogram as the unit of mass, and the liter as the unit of capacity, the last representing 0.001 cubic meter or 1000 cubic centimeters. See also Tables of Weights and Measures in the Appendix.

met·rio·ce·phal·ic (met″ree·o·se·fal′ick) *adj.* [Gk. *metrios,* moderate, + *cephalic*]. Applied to a skull in which the arch of the vertex is moderate in height, neither acrocephalic (pointed) nor platycephalic (flattened).

metritic synovitis. A synovitis secondary to uterine infection.

me·tri·tis (me·trye′tis) *n.* [*metr-* + *-itis*]. Inflammation of the uterus, involving the endometrium and myometrium. —**me·trit·ic** (me·trit′ick) *adj.*

me·triz·a·mide (me·triz′uh·mide) *n.* 2-[3-Acetamido-2,4,6-triiodo-5-(*N*-Methylacetamido)benzamido]-2-deoxy-D-glucose, $C_{18}H_{22}I_3O_3N_8$, a radiopaque diagnostic medium.

met·ri·zo·ate sodium (met″ri·zo′ate) *n.* Sodium 3-acetamido-2,4,6-triiodo-5-(*N*-methylacetamido)benzoate, $C_{12}H_{10}I_3N_2NaO_4$, a radiopaque diagnostic aid.

metro-. See *metr-.*

me·tro·cele (mee′tro·seel) *n.* [*metro-* + *-cele*]. Hernia of the uterus.

me·tro·clyst (mee′tro·klist) *n.* [*metro-* + Gk. *klystēr,* syringe]. An instrument for giving uterine douches.

me·tro·col·po·cele (mee″tro·kol′po·seel, met″ro·) *n.* [*metro-* + *colpo-* + *-cele*]. Protrusion or prolapse of the uterus into the vagina, with prolapse of the anterior vaginal wall.

me·tro·cys·to·sis (mee″tro·sis·to′sis, met″ro·) *n.* [*metro-* + *cyst* + *-osis*]. 1. The formation of uterine cysts. 2. The condition giving rise to uterine cysts.

me·tro·cyte (mee′tro·site) *n.* [*metro-,* mother, + *-cyte*]. PRONORMOBLAST.

me·tro·dy·na·mom·e·ter (mee″tro·dye″nuh·mom′e·tur) *n.* [*metro* + *dynamometer*]. An instrument for measuring uterine contractions.

me·tro·dyn·ia (mee″tro·din′ee·uh, met″ro·) *n.* [*metr-* + *-odynia*]. METRALGIA.

me·tro·ec·ta·sia (mee″tro·eck·tay′zhuh, ·zee·uh, met″ro·) *n.* METRECTASIA.

me·tro·en·do·me·tri·tis (mee″tro·en″do·me·trye′tis) *n.* [*metro-* + *endometritis*]. Combined inflammation of the uterus and endometrium.

me·trog·ra·phy (me·trog′ruh·fee) *n.* [*metro-* + *-graphy*]. Radiography of the uterus through the injection of contrast media into the uterine cavity; UTEROGRAPHY.

me·trol·o·gy (me·trol′uh·jee) *n.* [Gk. *metrologia,* theory of ratios]. The science that deals with methods of measurement and units of measure.

me·tro·lym·phan·gi·tis (mee″tro·lim″fan·jye′tis, met″ro·) *n.* [*metro-* + *lymphangitis*]. Inflammation of the lymphatic vessels of the uterus; uterine lymphangitis.

me·tro·ma·la·cia (mee″tro·ma·lay′shee·uh, met″ro·) *n.* [*metro-* + *malacia*]. Softening of the tissues of the uterus.

met·ro·ni·da·zole (met″ro·nigh′duh·zole, ·nid′uh·zole) *n.* 1-

(2-Hydroxyethyl)-2-methyl-5-nitroimidazole, $C_6H_9N_3O_3$, a systemic trichomonacide.

met·ro·nome (met'ruh·nome) *n.* An instrument for indicating exact time intervals, usually by means of a pendulum and an audible clicking device.

me·tro·pa·ral·y·sis (mee"tro·puh·ral'i·sis, met"ro·) *n.* [*metro-* + *paralysis*]. Uterine paralysis, usually that which may occur immediately following childbirth.

me·tro·path·ia hem·or·rhag·i·ca (mee"tro·path'ee·uh hem'o·raj'i·kuh). Abnormal uterine bleeding, now generally considered to be of endocrine origin.

me·trop·a·thy (me·trop'uth·ee) *n.* [*metro-* + *-pathy*]. Any uterine disease. —**me·tro·path·ic** (mee"tro·path'ick, met"ro·) *adj.*

me·tro·peri·to·ni·tis (mee"tro·perr"i·tuh·nigh'tis, met"ro·) *n.* [*metro-* + *peritonitis*]. 1. Combined inflammation of uterus and peritoneum. 2. Peritonitis secondary to inflammation of the uterus. 3. Inflammation of the peritoneum about the uterus.

me·tro·pex·ia (mee"tro·peck'see·uh) *n.* HYSTEROPEXY.

me·tro·pexy (mee'tro·peck"see, met'ro·) *n.* [*metro-* + *-pexy*]. HYSTEROPEXY.

me·tro·phle·bi·tis (mee"tro·fle·bye'tis, met"ro·) *n.* [*metro-* + *phlebitis*]. Inflammation of the veins of the uterus.

me·tro·plas·ty (mee'tro·plas"tee, met'ro·) *n.* [*metro-* + *-plasty*]. Plastic surgical repair of the uterus.

me·trop·to·sis (mee"trop·to'sis, mee"tro·to'sis) *n.* [*metro-* + *ptosis*]. PROLAPSE OF THE UTERUS.

me·tror·rha·gia (mee"tro·ray'jee·uh, met"ro·) *n.* [*metro-* + *-rrhagia*]. Uterine hemorrhage independent of the menstrual period. Syn. *intermenstrual flow, polymenorrhea.*

me·tror·rhea, me·tror·rhoea (mee"tro·ree'uh, met"ro·) *n.* [*metro-* + *-rrhea*]. Any pathologic discharge from the uterus.

me·tror·rhex·is (mee"tro·reck'sis) *n.* [*metro-* + *-rrhexis*]. Rupture of the uterus.

me·tro·sal·pin·gi·tis (mee"tro·sal"pin·jye'tis) *n.* [*metro-* + *salping-* + *-itis*]. Inflammation of the uterus and oviducts.

me·tro·sal·pin·gog·ra·phy (mee"tro·sal"ping·gog'ruh·fee) *n.* [*metro-* + *salpingo-* + *-graphy*]. HYSTEROSALPINGOGRAPHY.

me·tro·scope (mee'tro·skope) *n.* [*metro-* + *-scope*]. An instrument for examining the uterus.

me·tro·stax·is (mee"tro·stack'sis) *n.* [*metro-* + *staxis*]. Slight but persistent uterine hemorrhage.

me·tro·ste·no·sis (mee"tro·ste·no'sis) *n.* [*metro-* + *stenosis*]. Abnormal contraction of the cavity of the uterus.

me·tro·tome (mee'tro·tome, met'ro·tome) *n.* [*metro-* + *-tome*]. An instrument for incising the uterine neck.

me·trot·o·my (me·trot'um·ee) *n.* [*metro-* + *-tomy*]. HYSTEROTOMY.

-metry [L. *-metria,* from Gk. *metron,* a measure]. A combining form meaning *science or process of measurement* of a specified object or by a specified means.

me·try·per·ci·ne·sis (me·trye"pur·si·nee'sis) *n.* [*metr-* + *hypercinesis*]. Excessive uterine contraction.

me·try·per·emia (me·trye"pur·ee'mee·uh) *n.* [*metr-* + *hyperemia*]. Hyperemia of the uterus; METREMIA.

me·try·per·es·the·sia (me·trye"pur·es·theez'ee·uh, ·theezh'uh) *n.* [*metr-* + *hyperesthesia*]. Hyperesthesia of the uterus.

me·try·per·tro·phia (me·trye"pur·tro'fee·uh) *n.* [*metr-* + *hypertrophia*]. Hypertrophy of the uterus.

Mett method [E. L. P. *Mett,* German physician, 19th century]. A method for determination of peptic activity in which small glass tubes, filled with coagulated egg albumin, are introduced into the solution to be tested and kept for a definite length of time in the incubator. The protein column is digested at both ends of the tube to an extent depending on the amount of pepsin present.

Metubine Iodide. Trademark for dimethyl tubocurarine iodide, a skeletal muscle relaxant.

me·tu·re·depa (me·tew"re·dep'uh, met"yoo·re·dep'uh) *n.* Ethyl [bis(2,2-dimethyl-1-aziridinyl)phosphinyl]carbamate, $C_{11}H_{22}N_3O_3P$, an antineoplastic agent.

Metycaine. Trademark for piperocaine, an ester local anesthetic used as the hydrochloride salt.

me·tyr·a·pone (me·tirr'uh·pone) *n.* 2-Methyl-1,2-di-3-pyridyl-1-propanone, $C_{14}H_{14}N_2O$, a diagnostic aid for determining pituitary function. Metyrapone blocks 11β-hydroxylation of steroids in the adrenal cortex and causes a compensatory increase in secretion of corticotropin by the normal pituitary as a result of which there is increased urinary excretion of 17-hydroxycorticoids and 17-ketogenic steroids; the quantity excreted is an index of pituitary function. Syn. *mepyrapone, methopyrapone.*

Meu·len·gracht diet [E. *Meulengracht,* Danish physician, b. 1887]. A high calorie, vitamin-rich diet for the treatment of bleeding peptic ulcer.

Meulengracht's method [E. *Meulengracht*]. A method for bile pigment in which the yellow color of serum is compared with a standard potassium dichromate solution. See also *icterus index.*

Meuse fever (mœhz) [after the *Meuse* River valley in northeastern France, site of World War I battles]. TRENCH FEVER.

mev Million electron volts.

mev·a·lon·ic acid (mev"uh·lon'ick). 3,5-Dihydroxy-2-methylvaleric acid, $C_6H_{12}O_4$, a precursor in the biosynthesis of cholesterol and of vitamin A.

Mex·i·can bedbug. ASSASSIN BUG.

Mexican hat cell. TARGET CELL.

Mexican scammony. IPOMEA.

Mexican typhus. MURINE TYPHUS.

mex·ren·o·ate potassium (mecks·ren'o·ate) *n.* 17α-Hydroxy-3-oxopregn-4-ene-7α,21-dicarboxylic acid, 7-methyl ester, monopotassium salt, dihydrate, $C_{24}H_{33}KO_6.2H_2O$, an aldosterone antagonist.

Meyenburg complex. VON MEYENBURG COMPLEX.

Mey·er·hof cycle or **scheme** (migh'ur·hofe) [O. *Meyerhof,* German biochemist, 1884-1951]. A series of enzymatic reactions which have been shown to occur in a variety of animal, plant, and microbial tissues, whereby glucose (or glycogen or starch) is converted to pyruvic acid. Syn. *Embden-Meyerhof scheme.*

Mey·er-Over·ton theory [H. H. *Meyer,* German pharmacologist, 1853-1939; and C. E. *Overton,* German anesthesiologist, b. 1865]. A theory that the degree of anesthetic activity of a compound is correlated with a high oil/water distribution ratio of the anesthetic.

Meyer's loop [A. *Meyer,* U.S. psychiatrist and neurologist, 1866-1950]. The lower portion of the geniculocalcarine radiation which curves around the temporal horn of the lateral ventricle subjacent to the temporal cortex and ends in the calcarine fissure.

Meyer's operation [H. W. *Meyer,* U.S. surgeon, 1854-1932]. A radical excision of the breast.

Meyer's system [A. *Meyer*]. PSYCHOBIOLOGY.

Mey·nert's bundle (migh'nurt) [T. H. *Meynert,* German neurologist and psychiatrist, 1833-1892]. FASCICULUS RETROFLEXUS.

Meynert's commissure [T. H. *Meynert*]. A decussating bundle of fibers, closely applied to the dorsal surface of the optic chiasma. The precise origin of this bundle is obscure. It may arise from the subthalamic nucleus or the hindbrain and it crosses to the globus pallidus of the opposite side. Syn. *dorsal supraoptic decussation.* See also *commissurae supraopticae.*

Mey·net's nodosities (me^h^·ne^h^') [P. C. H. *Meynet,* French physician, 1831-1892]. Nodules attaching to tendon sheaths and joint capsules in rheumatoid diseases.

mez·lo·cil·lin (mez"lo·sil'in) *n.* A penicillin derivative, $C_{21}H_{25}N_5O_8S_2$, with unspecified antibiotic activity.

Mg Symbol for magnesium.

mg, mg. Abbreviation for *milligram.*

mg %, mg. %. MILLIGRAMS PERCENT.

mgh, mgh. MILLIGRAM-HOUR; an older method of expressing radium dosage (exposure) obtained by the application of one milligram of radium element for one hour.

MHC Abbreviation for *major histocompatibility complex.*

mho (mo) *n.* [*ohm* spelled backwards]. The unit of electric conductance; the reciprocal of the ohm.

Mi·a·na or **Mi·a·neh fever** (mee·ah·ne$^{y'}$) [after *Mianeh,* Iran]. RELAPSING FEVER.

mi·an·ser·in (migh·an′sur·in) *n.* 1,2,3,4,10,14b-Hexahydro-2-methyldibenzo[*c,f*]pyrazino[1,2-*a*]azepine, $C_{18}H_{20}N_2$, a substance with antiserotonin and antihistamine activities; used as the hydrochloride salt.

Mi·bel·li's disease (mee·bel′lee) [V. *Mibelli,* Italian dermatologist, 1860–1910]. 1. ANGIOKERATOMA MIBELLI. 2. POROKERATOSIS.

MIBK An abbreviation for *methyl isobutyl ketone,* a solvent.

mi·bo·ler·one (migh·bo′le·rone) *n.* 17β-Hydroxy-7α,17-dimethylestr-4-en-3-one, $C_{20}H_{30}O_2$, an androgen.

mi·ca (migh′kuh) *n.* [L.]. 1. A crumb. 2. A silicate mineral occurring in the form of thin, shining, transparent scales.

mi·ca·ceous (migh·kay′shus) *adj.* 1. Resembling mica. 2. Composed of crumbs; friable.

Micatin. A trademark for miconazole nitrate, an antifungal.

mi·cel·la (mi·sel′uh, migh·) *n.* [L., small crumb, grain]. MICELLE.

mi·celle (mi·sel′, migh·sel′) *n.* [L. *micella,* diminutive of *mica*]. 1. *Obsol.* One of the fundamental submicroscopic structural units of protoplasm. 2. Originally, a highly hydrated and charged colloidal aggregate such as phospholipids dispersed in aqueous media and detergents. 3. More broadly, any unit of structure composed of an aggregate or oriented arrangement of molecules, as in cellulose and rubber. —**mi·cel·lar** (migh·sel′ur, mi·) *adj.*

Mi·cha·e·lis constant (Ger. mi^{k}h·ah·e$^{y'}$lis) [L. *Michaelis,* U.S. chemist, 1875–1949]. The substrate concentration, in moles per liter, at which an enzymic reaction proceeds at one-half the maximal velocity. Symbol, K_m.

Mi·cha·e·lis-Gut·mann bodies or **calcospherules** (goot′ma^{h}n) [L. *Michaelis;* and C. *Gutmann,* German physician, b. 1872]. Basophilic and often concentrically laminated bodies, which may contain iron and calcium, seen in malacoplakia.

Michailow's test. A test for protein in which ferrous sulfate is added to the suspected solution and underlaid with concentrated sulfuric acid; then a drop or two of nitric acid is added. A brown ring and red coloration indicate the presence of protein.

Michel clip. A type of skin clip for closing incisions.

Mi·che·li syndrome (mee·keh′lee) [F. *Micheli,* Italian physician, 1872–1936]. PAROXYSMAL NOCTURNAL HEMOGLOBINURIA.

Michel's flecks or **spots** [J. von *Michel,* German ophthalmologist, 1843–1911]. Atrophic patches in the pigmented posterior portion of the iris epithelium, associated with a minute hyalinized fibrous scar, usually seen in chronic iritis, especially tuberculous.

Micofur. Trademark for nifuroxime, a fungicide.

mi·con·a·zole nitrate (migh·kon′uh·zole) *n.* 1-[2,4-Dichloro-β-[2,4-dichlorobenzyl)oxy]phenethyl] imidazole mononitrate, $C_{18}H_{14}Cl_4N_2O.HNO_3$, an antifungal.

micr-, micro- [Gk. *mikros,* small]. A combining form meaning (a) *small, minute,* as in microinfarct, microwave; (b) *undersized, abnormally small,* as in microcyte, microcephalic; (c) *pertaining to minute objects or quantities,* as in microscope, microanalysis; (d) *microscopic,* as in microanatomy; (e) *one one-millionth,* as in microgram.

micra. A plural of *micron* (= ²MICROMETER).

mi·cra·cous·tic (migh″kruh·koos′tick) *adj.* [*micr-* + *acoustic*]. Pertaining to or adapted to the hearing of very faint sounds.

micracoustic, *n.* An instrument adapted to the audition of very faint sounds.

mi·cren·ceph·a·lon (migh″kren·sef′uh·lon) *n.* [*micr-* + *encephalon*]. 1. An abnormally small brain. 2. *Obsol.* CEREBELLUM.

mi·cren·ceph·a·ly (migh″kren·sef′uh·lee) *n.* [*micr-* + *-encephaly*]. The condition of having an abnormally small brain. —**micrencepha·lous** (·lus) *adj.*

micro-. See *micr-.*

mi·cro·ab·scess (migh″kro·ab′ses) *n.* A very small abscess.

mi·cro·ab·sorp·tion spectroscopy (migh″kro·ub·sorp′shun). Techniques based on absorption spectra whereby the identification and distribution of specific substances can be determined.

mi·cro·aero·phil·ic (migh″kro·ay″ur·o·fil′ick) *adj.* [*micro-* + *aerophil* + *-ic*]. Pertaining to microorganisms which require free oxygen for their growth, but which thrive best when the oxygen is less in amount than that in the atmosphere.

mi·cro·anal·y·sis (migh″kro·uh·nal′i·sis) *n.* Chemical or physical analysis using small quantities of test sample and reagents.

mi·cro·anat·o·my (migh″kro·uh·nat′uh·mee) *n.* MICROSCOPIC ANATOMY. —**microanato·mist** (·mist) *n.*

mi·cro·an·eu·rysm (migh″kro·an′yoo·riz·um) *n.* Aneurysmal dilatation of a capillary, characteristic of diabetic retinopathy, but also seen in the conjunctiva in patients with other diseases.

mi·cro·an·gio·path·ic (migh″kro·an″jee·o·path·ic) *adj.* Characterized by or pertaining to microangiopathy.

microangiopathic hemolytic anemia. THROMBOTIC THROMBOCYTOPENIC PURPURA.

mi·cro·an·gi·op·athy (migh″kro·an″jee·op′uh·thee) *n.* [*micro-* + *angiopathy*]. Any disease of small blood vessels (precapillaries, capillaries, arterioles, or venules). Contr. *macroangiopathy.*

mi·cro·ar·te·rio·gram (migh″kro·ahr·teer′ee·o·gram) *n.* Radiographic visualization of minute arterial branches, usually on material obtained at surgical operations or autopsies. —**microar·te·rio·graph·ic** (·teer″ee·o·graf′ick) *adj.;* **microar·te·ri·og·ra·phy** (·teer″ee·og′ruh·fee) *n.*

mi·cro·au·di·phone (migh″kro·aw′di·fone) *n.* [*micro-* + *audio-* + *-phone*]. An instrument for rendering very slight sounds audible.

Mi·cro·bac·te·ri·um (migh″kro·back·teer′ee·um) *n.* A genus of small, non-spore-forming bacteria commonly found in milk. They are harmless; not readily killed during pasteurization.

mi·crobe (migh′krobe) *n.* [F., from *micro-* + Gk. *bios,* life]. Microorganism; especially, bacterium. —**mi·cro·bi·al** (migh·kro′bee·ul), **mi·cro·bic** (migh·kro′bick) *adj.*

mi·cro·bi·cide (migh·kro′bi·side) *n.* An agent that destroys microbes. Syn. *germicide.* —**mi·cro·bi·ci·dal** (migh·kro″bi·sigh′dul) *adj.*

mi·crob·in·ert (migh″kro·bi·nurt′) *adj.* [*microbe* + *inert*]. Unable to support microbial growth because of absence of necessary nutrients. —**microbinert·ness** (·nis) *n.*

mi·cro·bi·ol·o·gy (migh″kro·bye·ol′uh·jee) *n.* The biology of microorganisms. —**micro·bi·o·log·ic** (·bye″uh·loj′ick) *adj.;* **micro·bi·ol·o·gist** (bye·ol′uh·jist) *n.*

mi·cro·bio·pho·bia (migh″kro·bye″o·fo′bee·uh, migh·kro″bee·o·) *n.* [*microbe* + *-phobia*]. MICROPHOBIA (1).

mi·cro·bi·o·ta (migh″kro·bye·o′tuh) *n.* [*micro-* + *biota*]. The totality of microorganisms normally found in a given area or habitat.

mi·cro·bi·ot·ic (migh″kro·bye·ot′ick) *adj.* [*micro-* + *biotic*]. Pertaining to microscopic forms of life.

mi·cro·bism (migh′kro·biz·um) *n. Obsol.* Infection with microbes.

mi·cro·blast (migh′kro·blast) *n.* [*micro-* + *-blast*]. *Obsol.* 1. An immature blood cell. 2. A small, nucleated, red blood cell. 3. A small, anaplastic leukocyte having the other characteristics of blast cells, but found in the peripheral blood.

mi·cro·ble·pha·ria (migh″kro·ble·fair′ee·uh) *n.* [*micro-* + *blephar-* + *-ia*]. Abnormal smallness of the eyelids.

mi·cro·bleph·a·rism (migh″kro·blef′uh·riz·um) *n.* MICROBLEPHARIA.

mi·cro·bleph·a·ron (migh″kro·blef′uh·ron) *n.* [*micro-* + *blepharon*]. Abnormally small eyelid or eyelids; microblepharia.

mi·cro·body (migh′kro·bod″ee) *n.* [*micro-* + *body*]. PEROXISOME.

mi·cro·bra·chia (migh″kro·bray′kee·uh) *n.* [*micro-* + L. *brachia,* arms]. Abnormally (congenital) small arms.

mi·cro·brachy·ce·pha·lia (migh″kro·brack″ee·se·fay′lee·uh) *n.* Brachycephalia combined with microcephaly.

mi·cro·brachy·ceph·a·ly (migh″kro·brack″ee·sef′uh·lee) *n.* MICROBRACHYCEPHALIA.

mi·cro·bu·ret (migh″kro·bew·ret′) *n.* [*micro-* + *buret*]. An apparatus for delivering or measuring small quantities of liquids or gases.

mi·cro·cal·cu·lus (migh″kro·kal′kew·lus) *n.*, pl. **microcalcu·li** (·lye) [*micro-* + *calculus*]. A concretion of extremely small size; especially, a small focus of renal tubular calcification.

mi·cro·cal·o·rie, mi·cro·cal·o·ry (migh″kro·kal′uh·ree) *n.* A small calorie; for practical purposes, the quantity of heat necessary to raise the temperature of 1 g of water from 15° to 16°C. See also *calorie.*

mi·cro·car·dia (migh″kro·kahr′dee·uh) *n.* [*micro-* + Gk. *kardia,* heart]. Congenital smallness of the heart.

mi·cro·car·di·us (migh″kro·kahr′dee·us) *n.* [*micro-* + *cardi-* + *-us*]. An individual with an abnormally small heart.

mi·cro·cav·i·ta·tion (migh″kro·kav·i·tay′shun) *n.* The presence of minute cavities in a tissue or organ.

mi·cro·cen·trum (migh′kro·sen″trum) *n.* [*micro-* + L. *centrum,* center]. The centrosome or central apparatus typically containing centrioles, microtubules, and Golgi apparatus in a gelated zone of cytoplasm.

mi·cro·ceph·a·lus (migh″kro·sef′uh·lus) *n.*, pl. **microcepha·li** (·lye) [Gk. *mikrokephalos,* small-headed]. An individual with an unusually small head.

mi·cro·ceph·a·ly (migh″kro·sef′uh·lee) *n.* [*micro-* + *cephal-* + *-y*]. A condition characterized by a small head whose circumference is less than two standard deviations below mean for age and sex; may be due to congenital hypoplasia of the cerebrum or be the consequence of severe brain damage in early life; often associated with mental retardation, but may be seen in pituitary dwarfs of normal intelligence. —**micro·ce·phal·ic** (·se·fal′ick), **micro·ceph·a·lous** (·sef′uh·lus) *adj.*

mi·cro·chei·lia (migh″kro·kigh′lee·uh) *n.* [*micro-* + *cheil-* + *-ia*]. Abnormal smallness of the lips.

microchemical analysis. 1. Chemical analysis with the aid of a microscope. 2. Chemical analysis using small quantities of materials, but employing conventional methods.

mi·cro·chem·is·try (migh″kro·kem′is·tree) *n.* 1. The study of chemical reactions, using small quantities of materials, frequently less than 1 mg or 100 μl, and often requiring special small apparatus and microscopical observation. 2. The chemistry of individual cells and minute organisms. —**microchem·i·cal** (·i·kul) *adj.*

mi·cro·chi·ria (migh″kro·kigh′ree·uh) *n.* [*micro-* + *chir-* + *-ia*]. Abnormal smallness of the hand.

mi·cro·cir·cu·la·tion (migh″kro·sur″kew·lay′shun) *n.* The flow of blood or lymph in the vessels of the microcirculatory system.

mi·cro·cir·cu·la·to·ry system (migh″kro·sur′kew·luh·tor·ee). The portion of a blood or lymphatic circulatory system which is made up of minute vessels; especially, the system of arterioles, precapillaries, capillaries, and venules, including that part of the vasculature in which exchange of nutrients, wastes, and other substances occurs between tissues and blood.

Mi·cro·coc·ca·ce·ae (migh″kro·cock·ay′see·ee) *n.pl.* A family of bacteria containing the genera *Micrococcus, Gaffkya, Sarcina,* and *Staphylococcus.*

Mi·cro·coc·cus (migh″kro·kock′us) *n.* [*micro-* + *coccus*]. A genus of bacteria of the family Micrococcaceae.

micrococcus, *n.*, pl. **micrococ·ci** (migh″kro·cock′sigh). A bacterium of the genus *Micrococcus* or any similar small coccus.

Micrococcus al·bus (al′bus) [L., white]. *STAPHYLOCOCCUS EPIDERMIDIS.*

Micrococcus aureus. *STAPHYLOCOCCUS AUREUS.*

Micrococcus catarrhalis. *NEISSERIA CATARRHALIS.*

Micrococcus cit·re·us (sit′ree·us). A common laboratory contaminant. Syn. *Staphylococcus citreus.*

Micrococcus ga·zog·e·nes (ga·zoj′e·neez). *VEILLONELLA ALCALESCENS.*

Micrococcus gonorrheae. *NEISSERIA GONORRHOEAE.*

Micrococcus in·tra·cel·lu·la·ris meningitidis (in″truh·sel·yoo·lair′is). *NEISSERIA MENINGITIDIS.*

Micrococcus lan·ce·o·la·tus (lan″see·o·lay′tus). *STREPTOCOCCUS PNEUMONIAE.*

Micrococcus melitensis. *BRUCELLA MELITENSIS.*

Micrococcus meningitidis. *NEISSERIA MENINGITIDIS.*

Micrococcus par·vu·lus (pahr′vew·lus). *VEILLONELLA PARVULA.*

Micrococcus pneumoniae. *STREPTOCOCCUS PNEUMONIAE.*

Micrococcus py·og·e·nes (pye·oj′e·neez). 1. *STAPHYLOCOCCUS AUREUS.* 2. *STAPHYLOCOCCUS EPIDERMIDIS.*

Micrococcus te·trag·e·nus (te·traj′e·nus). *GAFFKYA TETRAGENA.*

mi·cro·co·lon (migh′kro·ko″lun) *n.* An abnormally small colon.

mi·cro·col·o·ny (migh′kro·kol″uh·nee) *n.* A very small colony of bacteria.

mi·cro·co·nid·i·um (migh″kro·ko·nid′ee·um) *n.*, pl. **microconid·ia** (·ee·uh). *In botany,* a small and single-celled conidium.

mi·cro·co·ria (migh″kro·kor′ee·uh) *n.* [*micro-* + *cor-*, pupil, + *-ia*]. MIOSIS.

mi·cro·cor·nea (migh″kro·kor′nee·uh) *n.* Abnormal smallness of the cornea.

mi·cro·cos·mic salt (migh″kro·koz′mick). SODIUM AMMONIUM PHOSPHATE.

mi·cro·cou·lomb (migh″kro·koo′lom, ·koo·lom′) *n.* The one-millionth part of a coulomb.

mi·cro·cous·tic (migh″kro·koos′tick) *adj. & n.* MICRACOUSTIC.

mi·cro·crys·tal·line (migh″kro·kris′tuh·lin) *adj.* Composed of crystals of microscopic size.

mi·cro·cu·rie (migh′kro·kew″ree) *n.* The amount of a radioactive substance which undergoes 3.7×10^4 disintegrations per second: equivalent to one-millionth of a curie. Symbol, μCi.

mi·cro·cyst (migh′kro·sist) *n.* A cyst of small size. —**mi·cro·cys·tic** (migh″kro·sis′tick) *adj.*

microcystic pseudomucinous cystoma. PSEUDOMUCINOUS CYSTADENOMA.

mi·cro·cyte (migh′kro·site) *n.* [*micro-* + *-cyte*]. 1. An erythrocyte having either a diameter or a mean corpuscular volume (MCV), or both, more than two standard deviations below the mean normal, determined by the same method on the blood of healthy persons of the patient's age and sex group. 2. A cell of the microglia. —**mi·cro·cyt·ic** (migh″kro·sit′ick) *adj.*

mi·cro·cy·the·mia, mi·cro·cy·thae·mia (migh″kro·sigh·theem′ee·uh) *n.* [*microcyte* + *-hemia*]. The presence in blood of abnormally small erythrocytes.

microcytic anemia. Any anemia in which the erythrocytes are smaller than normal.

mi·cro·cy·to·sis (migh″kro·sigh·to′sis) *n.* [*microcyte* + *-osis*]. A condition of the blood characterized by a preponderance of microcytes, as observed microscopically or determined by measurement of cell volume.

mi·cro·cy·to·tox·ic·i·ty (migh″kro·sigh″to·tock·sis′i·tee) *n.* [*micro-* + *cyto* + *toxicity*]. Toxic activity involving cells, observed with the use of minute quantities of the involved materials.

microcytotoxicity test. A test used in transplantation immunology, in which minute quantities of materials are used to detect complement-dependent killing of lymphocytes.

mi·cro·dac·tyl·ia (migh″kro·dack·til′ee·uh) *n.* MICRODACTYLY.

mi·cro·dac·ty·ly (migh″kro·dack′ti·lee) *n.* [*micro-* + *dactyl-* + *-y*]. Abnormal smallness of one or more fingers or toes. —**microdacty·lous** (·lus) *adj.*

mi·cro·dis·sec·tion (migh″kro·di·seck′shun) *n.* Dissection with the aid of a microscope.

mi·cro·don·tia (migh″kro·don′chee·uh) *n.* [*micr-* + *-odontia*]. The condition of having one or more abnormally small teeth. —**mi·cro·dont** (migh′kro·dont) *adj.*

mi·cro·dont·ism (migh′kro·don″tiz·um) *n.* MICRODONTIA.

mi·cro·drep·a·no·cyt·ic (migh″kro·drep″uh·no·sit′ick, ·dre·pan″o·) *adj.* Both microcytic and drepanocytic.

microdrepanocytic disease. SICKLE CELL THALASSEMIA.

mi·cro·drep·a·no·cy·to·sis (migh″kro·drep″uh·no·sigh·to′sis) *n.* [*micro*cyte + *drepanocyte* + *-osis*]. SICKLE CELL THALASSEMIA.

mi·cro·elec·tro·pho·ret·ic (migh″kro·e·lec″tro·fo·ret′ick) *adj.* Pertaining to electrophoresis of minute quantities of solutions.

mi·cro·en·ceph·a·ly (migh″kro·en·sef′ul·ee) *n.* MICRENCEPHALY.

mi·cro·eryth·ro·cyte (migh″kro·e·rith′ro·site, ·err′i·thro·) *n.* MICROCYTE (1).

mi·cro·far·ad (migh″kro·făr′ad) *n.* The one-millionth part of a farad.

mi·cro·fi·bril (migh″kro·figh′bril) *n.* [*micro-* + *fibril*]. An extremely fine fibril. —**microfi·bril·lar** (·bri·lur) *adj.*

microfibrillar collagen hemostat. An absorbable hemostatic agent, prepared from purified bovine corium collagen.

mi·cro·fi·bro·ad·e·no·ma (migh″kro·figh″bro·ad·e·no′muh) *n.* [*micro-* + *fibroadenoma*]. A fibroadenoma detectable only by microscopic examination.

mi·cro·fil·a·ment (migh″kro·fil′uh·munt) *n.* Any of the minute intracellular filaments, about 50 Å in diameter, thought to be composed of actin or a similar protein, and found in virtually every cell type, which are believed to play an important role in cell locomotion, endocytosis, exocytosis, and formation of the contractile ring in cytokinesis.

mi·cro·fi·lar·ia (migh″kro·fi·lăr′ee·uh) *n.*, pl. **microfilar·i·ae** (·ee·ee). The embryonic or prelarval forms of filarial worms; slender motile forms, 150 to 300 μm in length, found in the blood stream and tissues. On ingestion by the proper blood-sucking insects the microfilariae pass through developmental stages in the body of the host and become infective larvae.

mi·cro·flo·ra (migh′kro·flo·ruh) *n.* [*micro-* + *flora*]. 1. The flora of a small area. 2. Microscopic plants.

mi·cro·fol·lic·u·lar (migh″kro·fol·ick′yoo·lur) *adj.* Characterized by very small follicles.

microfollicular adenoma. A thyroid adenoma whose follicles are very small.

mi·cro·frac·ture (migh′kro·frack″chur) *n.* A minute fracture, usually clinically and radiographically obscure.

mi·cro·gam·ete (migh″kro·gam′eet, ·ga·meet′) *n.* [*micro-* + *gamete*]. A male reproductive cell in certain Protozoa, corresponding to the sperm cell in Metazoa.

mi·cro·ga·me·to·cyte (migh″kro·ga·mee′to·site) *n.* [*micro-* + *gametocyte*]. The cell that produces the microgametes in Protozoa.

mi·crog·a·my (migh·krog′uh·mee) *n.* [*micro-* + *-gamy*]. Fusion of male and female reproductive cells in certain Protozoa and Algae.

mi·cro·gas·tria (migh″kro·gas′tree·uh) *n.* [*micro-* + *gastr-* + *-ia*]. Abnormal smallness of the stomach.

mi·cro·gen·e·sis (migh″kro·jen′e·sis) *n.* [*micro-* + *-genesis*]. Abnormally small development of a part.

mi·cro·ge·nia (migh″kro·jee′nee·uh) *n.* [Gk. *mikrogen*eios, small-chinned (from *geneion*, chin), + *-ia*]. Abnormal smallness of the chin.

mi·cro·gen·i·tal·ism (migh″kro·jen′i·tul·iz·um) *n.* Having extremely undersized genital organs. See also *hypogenitalism.*

mi·crog·lia (migh·krog′lee·uh) *n.* [*micro-* + *glia*]. Small neuroglial cells of the central nervous system having long processes and exhibiting ameboid and phagocytic activity under pathologic conditions. Contr. *macroglia.* —**microg·li·al** (·lee·ul) *adj.*

mi·crog·lia·cyte (migh″krog′lee·uh·site) *n.* MICROGLIOCYTE.

mi·crog·lio·blast (migh·krog′lee·o·blast) *n.* [*microgli*a + *-blast*]. The precursor cell of microglia.

mi·crog·lio·blas·to·ma (migh·krog″lee·o·blas·to′muh) *n.* [*microglioblast* + *-oma*]. MICROGLIOMATOSIS.

mi·crog·lio·cyte (migh·krog′lee·o·site) *n.* A microglial cell.

mi·cro·gli·o·ma (migh·krog″lee·o′muh, migh″kro·glye·o′muh) *n.* [*microgli*a + *-oma*]. MICROGLIOMATOSIS.

mi·cro·gli·o·ma·to·sis (migh·krog″lee·o″muh·to′sis, migh″kro·glye″o·) *n.* [*microgli*a + *-oma* + *-osis*]. A brain tumor composed largely, or entirely, of metalophil cells representing varying stages from primitive reticulum cells to mature microglia; it is similar to, or identical with, reticulum-cell sarcoma elsewhere in the body.

mi·cro·glos·sia (migh″kro·glos′ee·uh) *n.* [*micro-* + *gloss-* + *-ia*]. Abnormal smallness of the tongue.

mi·cro·gna·thia (migh″kro·nayth′ee·uh, ·nath′ee·uh, migh″krog·) *n.* [*micro-* + *gnath-* + *-ia*]. Abnormal smallness of the jaws, especially of the lower jaw. —**micro·gnath·ic** (·nath′ick), **mi·crog·na·thous** (migh·krog′nuth·us) *adj.*

mi·cro·gram (migh′kro·gram) *n.* One one-thousandth of a milligram. Abbreviated, mcg. Symbol, μg. Syn. *gamma.*

mi·cro·graph (migh′kro·graf) *n.* 1. A pantographic device for enabling one to draw sketches on a very small scale. 2. An instrument that magnifies the vibrations of a diaphragm and records them on a moving photographic film.

mi·cro·graph·ia (migh″kro·graf′ee·uh) *n.* [*micro-* + *graph-* + *-ia*]. Very small handwriting; particularly the tendency to write smaller than during a state of normal health, seen in certain cerebral disorders, such as parkinsonism.

mi·crog·ra·phy (migh·krog′ruh·fee) *n.* [*micro-* + *-graphy*]. 1. A description of structures studied under the microscope. 2. MICROGRAPHIA.

mi·cro·gy·ria (migh″kro·jye′ree·uh, ·jirr′ee·uh) *n.* [*micro-* + *gyr-* + *-ia*]. Abnormal smallness of the convolutions of the brain.

mi·crohm (migh′krome) *n.* One one-millionth of an ohm.

mi·cro·in·cin·er·a·tion (migh″kro·in·sin″uh·ray′shun) *n.* Reduction of small quantities of organic substances to ash by application of heat.

mi·cro·in·farct (migh″kro·in′fahrkt) *n.* A very small infarct, usually detected only by microscopic examination. —**mi·cro·in·farc·tion** (in·fahrk′shun) *n.*

mi·cro·in·jec·tion (migh′kro·in·jeck″shun) *n.* The injection of materials into tissues by means of a micropipet.

mi·cro·in·va·sion (migh″kro·in·vay′zhun) *n.* Invasion by tumor, especially a squamous cell carcinoma of the uterine cervix, a very short distance into the tissues beneath the point of origin.

mi·cro·ker·a·tome (migh″kro·kerr′uh·tome) *n.* A small keratome used in microsurgery of the cornea.

mi·cro·len·tia (migh″kro·len′tee·uh) *n.* [*micro-* + *lent-* + *-ia*]. MICROPHAKIA.

mi·cro·leu·ko·blast (migh″kro·lew′ko·blast) *n.* A small leukoblast.

mi·cro·li·ter (migh′kro·lee″tur) *n.* A millionth of a liter, or a thousandth of a milliliter.

mi·cro·lith (migh′kro·lith) *n.* [*micro-* + *-lith*]. A microscopic calculus.

mi·cro·li·thi·a·sis (migh″kro·li·thigh′uh·sis) *n.* [*microlith* +

-iasis]. The presence of numerous very minute calculi.

microlithiasis al·ve·o·la·ris pul·mo·num (al″vee·o·lair′is pool·mo′num). A rare form of pulmonary calcification of uncertain cause in which many minute, spherical, concentrically calcified bodies (calcospherites or microliths), and osseous nodules of larger size are found; may simulate pulmonary tuberculosis on radiologic examination.

mi·cro·ma·nia (migh″kro·may′nee·uh) *n.* [*micro-* + *-mania*]. A delusional state in which the patient believes himself diminutive in size and mentally inferior.

mi·cro·ma·nip·u·la·tion (migh″kro·ma·nip″yoo·lay′shun) *n.* Manipulation of minute objects under a microscope; use of a micromanipulator. —**microma·nip·u·la·tive** (·nip′yoo·luh·tiv, ·lay·tiv) *adj.*

micromanipulative technique. 1. A procedure or technique designed to investigate living or preserved biological material on the microscopic level by means of microdissection, microinjection, and other manual maneuvers. 2. Any technique demanding small, careful, and delicate manipulation, usually under a microscope.

mi·cro·ma·nip·u·la·tor (migh″kro·ma·nip′yoo·lay·tur) *n.* A device for moving exceedingly fine instruments, under the magnification of a microscope, for dissection of cells or for other operations involving minute objects.

mi·cro·ma·nom·e·ter (migh″kro·muh·nom′e·tur) *n.* [*micro-* + *manometer*]. A manometer for measuring very small differences of pressure, as in the gasometric determination of the metabolic activity of minute quantities of tissue.

mi·cro·mas·tia (migh″kro·mas′tee·uh) *n.* [*micro-* + *mast-* + *-ia*]. Abnormal smallness of the breasts. Syn. *micromazia.*

mi·cro·ma·zia (migh″kro·may′zee·uh) *n.* [*micro-* + *maz-* + *-ia*]. MICROMASTIA.

mi·cro·me·lia (migh″kro·mee′lee·uh) *n.* [*micro-* + *mel-* + *-ia*]. Abnormal smallness of the limbs.

mi·cro·mel·ic (migh″kro·mel′ick, ·mee′lick) *adj.* [Gk. *mikromelēs*]. Having abnormally small limbs.

mi·crom·e·lus (migh·krom′e·lus) *n.* [*micro-* + *mel-* + *-us*]. An individual with abnormally small limbs.

mi·crom·e·ly (migh·krom′e·lee) *n.* MICROMELIA.

[1]**mi·crom·e·ter** (migh·krom′e·tur) *n.* [*micro-* + *-meter*]. An instrument designed for measuring distances, or apparent diameters; used with a microscope or telescope. —**mi·crome·try** (·tree) *n.*

[2]**mi·cro·me·ter** (migh′kro·mee″tur) *n.* The one-thousandth part of a millimeter, or the one-millionth part of a meter. Symbol, μm.

micrometer disk. A glass disk engraved with a suitable scale, used at the diaphragm of a micrometer ocular. The scale can be focused by the eye lens and seen in the field of view.

mi·cro·meth·od (migh′kro·meth″ud) *n.* A method of laboratory examination in which very small quantities of the substances to be examined are used.

mi·cro·mi·cron (migh″kro·migh′kron) *n. Obsol.* The millionth part of a micron. Symbol, $\mu\mu$.

mi·cro·mil (migh′kro·mil) *n. Obsol.* NANOMETER.

mi·cro·mil·li·me·ter (migh″kro·mil′i·mee·tur) *n. Obsol.* NANOMETER.

mi·cro·mo·to·scope (migh″kro·mo′tuh·skope) *n.* An apparatus for photographing and exhibiting motile microorganisms.

mi·cro·my·e·lia (migh″kro·migh·ee′lee·uh) *n.* [*micro-* + *myel-* + *-ia*]. Abnormal smallness of the spinal cord.

mi·cro·my·e·lo·blast (migh″kro·migh′e·lo·blast) *n.* An extremely small myeloblast.

mi·cro·my·e·lo·lym·pho·cyte (migh″kro·migh″e·lo·lim′fo·site) *n.* [*micro-* + *myelo-* + *lymphocyte*]. A small lymphocyte of myeloid tissue, regarded as a hemocytoblast.

mi·cron (migh′kron) *n.* pl. **microns, mi·cra** (·kruh) [Gk. *mikron,* a little]. [2]MICROMETER. Symbol, μ.

mi·cro·nee·dle (migh′kro·need″ul) *n.* An exceedingly fine glass needle for use in microdissection with a micromanipulator.

mi·cron·e·mous (migh·kron′e·mus) *adj.* [*micro-* + Gk. *nēma,* thread, + *-ous*]. Furnished with short filaments.

mi·cro·nod·u·la·tion (migh″kro·nod″yoo·lay′shun) *n.* The presence of very small nodules in a tissue or organ. —**mi·cro·nod·u·lar** (·nod′yoo·lur) *adj.*

mi·cro·nu·cle·us (migh″kro·new′klee·us) *n.*, pl. **micronu·clei** (·klee·eye). 1. A small or minute nucleus. 2. The reproductive nucleus of protozoa as contrasted with the macronucleus. 3. NUCLEOLUS.

mi·cro·nu·tri·ent (migh″kro·new′tree·unt) *n.* A vitamin or mineral occurring in traces essential for growth, development, and health.

mi·cro·nych·ia (migh″kro·nick′ee·uh) *n.* [*micr-* + *onych-* + *-ia*]. The presence of one or more abnormally small nails which in every other respect seem normal.

mi·cro·or·chism (migh″kro·or′kiz·um) *n.* [*micro-* + *orch-* + *-ism*]. Congenital hypoplasia of the testes; when severe, it may be associated with the eunuchoid state.

mi·cro·or·gan·ism (migh″kro·or′gun·iz·um) *n.* A microscopic organism, either animal or plant, especially a bacterium or protozoan. —**micro·or·gan·ic** (·or·gan′ick) *adj.*

mi·cro·pap·u·lar (migh″kro·pap′yoo·lur) *adj.* Having or pertaining to very small papules.

mi·cro·par·a·site (migh″kro·păr′uh·site) *n.* A parasitic microorganism.

mi·cro·pe·nis (migh″kro·pee′nis) *n.* [*micro-* + *penis*]. MICROPHALLUS.

mi·cro·phage (migh′kro·faij) *n.* [*micro-* + *-phage*]. 1. A neutrophil granulocyte in tissues. 2. A small phagocyte.

mi·cro·pha·kia (migh″kro·fay′kee·uh) *n.* [*micro-* + *phak-* + *-ia*]. A congenital or developmental anomaly in which there is an abnormally small crystalline lens.

mi·cro·phal·lus (migh″kro·fal′us) *n.* [*micro-* + *phallus*]. Abnormal smallness of the penis. Syn. *micropenis.*

mi·cro·pho·bia (migh″kro·fo′bee·uh) *n.* [*micro-* + *-phobia*]. 1. Morbid fear of microbes. 2. Morbid fear of small objects.

mi·cro·phone (migh′kruh·fone) *n.* [*micro-* + *-phone*]. An instrument in which sounds modulate an electric current which can be amplified so that the sounds become audible.

mi·cro·pho·nia (migh″kro·fo′nee·uh) *n.* [*micro-* + *-phonia*]. Weakness of voice.

mi·cro·pho·no·graph (migh″kro·fo′nuh·graf) *n.* [*micro-* + *phono-* + *-graph*]. A combination of microphone and phonograph used for the recording of sounds.

mi·cro·pho·no·scope (migh″kro·fo′nuh·skope) *n.* [*microphone* + steth*oscope*]. A binaural stethoscope with a membrane in the chestpiece to accentuate the sound.

mi·croph·o·ny (migh·krof′uh·nee) *n.* [*micro-* + *-phony*]. MICROPHONIA.

mi·cro·pho·to·graph (migh″kro·fo′tuh·graf) *n.* 1. A photograph of microscopic size. Compare *photomicrograph.* 2. *Erron.* PHOTOMICROGRAPH.

mi·cro·pho·tom·e·ter (migh″kro·fo·tom′e·tur) *n.* [*micro-* + *photometer*]. An instrument that measures the intensity of light reflected or transmitted from a specimen, or that measures the relative densities of spectral lines on a photographic plate or film.

mi·croph·thal·mia (migh″krof·thal′mee·uh) *n.* [*micr-* + *ophthalm-* + *-ia*]. MICROPHTHALMUS (1).

mi·croph·thal·mus (migh″krof·thal′mus) *n.* [Gk. *mikrophthalmos,* small-eyed]. 1. A condition in which the eyeball is abnormally small. Syn. *microphthalmia, nanophthalmus, nanophthalmos, nanophthalmia.* 2. A person manifesting such a condition.

mi·cro·phys·ics (migh″kro·fiz′icks) *n.* A branch of science that deals with elementary particles, atoms, and molecules.

mi·cro·phyte (migh′kro·fite) *n.* [*micro-* + *-phyte*]. Any microscopic plant, especially one that is parasitic.

mi·cro·pia (migh·kro′pee·uh) *n.* [*micr-* + *-opia*]. MICROPSIA.

mi·cro·pi·pet (migh″kro·pye·pet′, ·pi·pet′) *n.* 1. A small pipet with a fine-pointed tip used in microinjection. 2. A pipet for measuring very small volumes.

mi·cro·pleth·ys·mog·ra·phy (migh″kro·pleth″iz·mog′ruf·ee) *n.* [*micro-* + *plethysmography*]. The measurement and recording of minute changes in the size of an organ or limb produced by changes in the volume of blood circulating through it. —**micro·ple·thys·mo·gram** (·ple·thiz′mo·gram), **micro·ple·thys·mo·graph** (·ple·thiz′mo·graph) *n.*

mi·cro·po·dia (migh″kro·po′dee·uh) *n.* [Gk. *mikropous, mikropodos*, small-footed, + *-ia*]. Abnormal smallness of the feet.

mi·crop·o·dy (migh·krop′o·dee) *n.* MICROPODIA.

mi·cro·po·lar·i·scope (migh″kro·po·lăr′i·skope) *n.* A polariscope used in connection with a microscope.

mi·cro·pro·jec·tion (migh′kro·pro·jeck″shun) *n.* The projection of the image of microscopic objects on a screen.

mi·cro·pro·so·pia (migh″kro·pro·so′pee·uh) *n.* [*micro-* + *prosop-* + *-ia*]. Congenital abnormal smallness of the face.

mi·cro·pro·so·pus (migh″kro·pro′suh·pus, ·pro·so′pus) *n.* [*micro-* + *prosop-* + *-us*]. An individual with a small and imperfectly developed face.

mi·cro·pros·o·py (migh″kro·pros′uh·pee, ·pro′suh·pee) *n.* MICROPROSOPIA.

mi·crop·sia (migh·krop′see·uh) *n.* [*micr-* + *-opsia*]. Disturbance of visual perception in which objects appear smaller than their true size. See also *Lilliputian hallucination.*

mi·cro·psy·chia (migh″kro·sigh′kee·uh) *n.* [Gk. *mikropsychia*, pettiness of spirit]. MENTAL DEFICIENCY.

mi·crop·tic (migh·krop′tick) *adj.* [*micr-* + *optic*]. Pertaining to, or affected with, micropsia.

microptic hallucination. LILLIPUTIAN HALLUCINATION.

mi·cro·pus (migh′kro·pus, migh·kro′pus) *n.* [Gk. *mikropous*, small-footed]. MICROPODIA.

mi·cro·pyk·nom·e·ter (migh″kro·pick·nom′e·tur) *n.* [*micro-* + *pyknometer*]. An instrument for determining the specific gravity of minute amounts of liquids or solutions.

mi·cro·pyle (migh′kro·pile) *n.* [*micro-* + Gk. *pylē*, gate]. A minute opening in the investing membrane of many ova, permitting entrance of the sperm.

mi·cro·ra·di·og·ra·phy (migh″kro·ray″dee·og′ruh·fee) *n.* Radiography using a special photographic emulsion so that enlargement (of the order of 100 times) does not reveal silver grains in the emulsion, thereby permitting great magnification of the original image of a very small object.

mi·cro·res·pi·rom·e·ter (migh″kro·res″pi·rom′e·tur) *n.* [*micro-* + *respirometer*]. An apparatus for measuring the respiratory activity of minute amounts of tissue. —**microrespi·ro·met·ric** (·ro·met′rick) *adj.*

mi·cror·rhi·nia, mi·cro·rhi·nia (migh″kro·rye′nee·uh) *n.* [Gk. *mikrorrhin*, small-nosed, + *-ia*]. Congenital smallness of the nose.

mi·cro·ruth·er·ford (migh″kro·ruh′thur·furd) *n.* A unit equivalent to one one-millionth of a rutherford or 1 disintegration per second. Symbol, μrd.

mi·cro·scel·ous (migh″kro·skel′us, migh·kros′ke·lus) *adj.* [Gk. *mikroskelēs*, short-legged, from *skelos*, leg]. Having abnormally small legs.

mi·cro·scope (migh′kruh·skope) *n.* [*micro-* + *-scope*]. An apparatus through which minute objects are rendered visible. It consists of a lens, or group of lenses, by which a magnified image of the object is produced. See also *electron microscope, reflecting microscope, ultramicroscope.*

microscope stage. The platform under the microscope tube which carries the specimen and is usually mounted permanently on the microscope pillar; it may be mounted on a rack and pinion.

mi·cro·scop·ic (migh″kro·skop′ick) *adj.* [*microscope* + *-ic*]. 1. Extremely small; too small to be readily visible to the naked eye. 2. MICROSCOPICAL; pertaining to or done with a microscope.

mi·cro·scop·i·cal (migh″kro·skop′i·kul) *adj.* 1. Pertaining to or done with a microscope. 2. MICROSCOPIC; too small to be readily visible to the naked eye.

microscopical diagnosis. Diagnosis made by means of microscopical examination of tissues or specimens.

microscopic anatomy. The branch of anatomy that deals with the minute structure of tissues; HISTOLOGY. Contr. *gross anatomy.*

microscopic electrophoresis. A method of electrophoresis adapted to the study of particles which may be seen by the microscope or the ultramicroscope. It has been used to great advantage in studying surface and immunologic phenomena in liquids.

mi·cros·co·pist (migh·kros′kuh·pist) *n.* One skilled in microscopy.

mi·cros·co·py (migh·kros′kuh·pee) *n.* The use of the microscope; examination with the microscope.

mi·cros·mat·ic (migh″kroz·mat′ick) *adj.* [*micr-* + *osmatic*]. Having a poorly developed sense of smell. Man is classified as a microsmatic animal.

microsomal electron transport. A membrane-bound microsomal system of enzymes which accomplishes the transport of electrons without the formation of ATP. This system is important in many hydroxylation and desaturation reactions.

mi·cro·some (migh′kro·sohm) *n.* [*micro-* + *-some*]. A small cytoplasmic body composed of fragments of endoplasmic reticulum and associated ribosomes.

mi·cro·so·mia (migh″kro·so′mee·uh) *n.* [*micro-* + *-somia*]. Abnormal smallness of the whole body. Syn. *dwarfism, nanosomia.*

mi·cro·spec·trog·ra·phy (migh″kro·speck·trog′ruf·ee) *n.* Spectrographic methods applied to the study of the composition of minute samples, as, for example, of protoplasm.

mi·cro·spec·tro·pho·tom·e·try (migh″kro·speck″tro·fo·tom′e·tree) *n.* [*micro-* + *spectrophotometry*]. Measurement at different wavelengths of light absorbed, reflected, or emitted by objects in a microscopic field.

mi·cro·spec·tro·scope (migh″kro·speck′truh·skope) *n.* A spectroscope used in connection with the ocular of a microscope, and by means of which the spectra of microscopic objects can be examined.

mi·cro·sphero·cyte (migh″kro·sfeer′o·site) *n.* [*micro-* + *spherocyte*]. A characteristically small, spheroidal erythrocyte observed in hereditary spherocytosis.

mi·cro·sphero·cy·to·sis (migh″kro·sfeer″o·sigh·to′sis) *n.* The presence of microspherocytes in the peripheral blood.

mi·cro·spher·ule (migh″kro·sfeer′yool, ·sferr′yool) *n.* A very small spherule.

mi·cro·sphyg·my (migh′kro·sfig″mee) *n.* [*micro-* + *sphygm-* + *-y*]. MICROSPHYXIA.

mi·cro·sphyx·ia (migh″kro·sfick′see·uh) *n.* [Gk. *mikrosphyxia*, from *sphyxis*, pulse]. Weakness of the pulse.

mi·cro·splanch·nic (migh″kro·splank′nick) *adj.* [*micro-* + *splanchnic*]. HYPOVEGETATIVE.

Mi·cro·spo·rid·ia (migh″kro·spo·rid′ee·uh) *n.pl.* [*micro-* + *sporidia*]. An order of Sporozoa which infect chiefly invertebrates, insects in particular.

Mi·cros·po·ron (migh·kros′pur·on) *n.* *MICROSPORUM.*

mi·cro·spo·ro·sis (migh″kro·spo·ro′sis) *n.* [*Microsporum* + *-osis*]. Dermatophytosis caused by a species of *Microsporum.*

microsporosis nigra. TINEA NIGRA.

Mi·cros·po·rum (migh·kros′puh·rum, migh″kro·spor′um) *n.* [NL., from *micro-* + Gk. *spora*, seed]. A genus of dermatophytes which attack only the hair and the skin.

Microsporum au·dou·i·ni (o·doo′i·nigh) [J. *Audouin*, French physician, 1797–1841]. A species of fungus responsible for epidemic tinea capitis in children; slow growing, producing few spores, with very little growth on polished rice; not found in animals.

Microsporum can·is (kan′is, kay′nis) [L., of the dog]. A species of fungus that causes sporadic tinea capitis in children, generally through contact with infected cats and dogs; grows well on polished rice and other media, with abundant macroconidia and yellow-orange pigmentation of the agar.

Microsporum furfur. MALASSEZIA FURFUR.

Microsporum gyp·se·um (jip'see·um) [L., chalky]. A world-wide soil-inhabiting fungus, fast growing with numerous macroconidia, which produces tinea corporis and tinea capitis in man and animals exposed to soil.

Microsporum la·no·sum (la·no'sum) [L., wooly]. MICROSPORUM CANIS.

Microsporum minutissimus. NOCARDIA MINUTISSIMA.

mi·cro·stetho·phone (migh"kro·steth'uh·fone) *n.* [*microphone* + *stetho*scope]. MICROSTETHOSCOPE.

mi·cro·stetho·scope (migh"kro·steth'uh·skope) *n.* [*micro*phone + *stethoscope*]. A stethoscope which amplifies the sounds heard.

mi·cro·sto·mia (migh"kro·sto'mee·uh) *n.* [*micro-* + *-stomia*]. Abnormal smallness of the mouth.

mi·cro·sur·gery (migh"kro·sur'juh·ree) *n.* Surgery in which a microscope and minute surgical instruments are employed, often on structures as small as an ovum or single living cell.

mi·cro·the·lia (migh"kro·theel'ee·uh) *n.* [*micro-* + *thel-* + *-ia*]. Congenital hypoplasia of the nipple of the breast.

mi·cro·therm (migh'kro·thurm) *n.* [*micro-* + *-therm*]. An organism in which the life processes are carried on at a low temperature.

mi·cro·tia (migh·kro'shee·uh) *n.* [*micr-* + *ot-* + *-ia*]. Abnormal smallness of one or both external ears.

mi·cro·ti·trim·e·try (migh"kro·tye·trim'e·tree) *n.* Titrimetry using small quantities of test sample and standard solution. **—micro·ti·tri·met·ric** (·tye"tri·met'rick) *adj.*

mi·cro·tome (migh'kro·tome) *n.* [*micro-* + *-tome*]. An instrument for making thin sections of tissues for microscopical examination, the tissues usually being embedded in a supporting matrix.

mi·crot·o·my (migh·krot'uh·mee) *n.* [*micro-* + *-tomy*]. The cutting of thin sections of tissue or other substances for microscopic study. **—microto·mist,** *n.*

mi·cro·to·pos·co·py (migh"kro·to·pos'kuh·pee) *n.* [*micro-* + *topo-* + *-scopy*]. Projection of the electrical record of the cerebrum in a three-dimensional visual record.

mi·cro·trau·ma (migh'kro·trow"muh, ·traw"muh) *n.* [*micro-* + *trauma*]. A minor or insignificant injury, in itself not recognized as harmful, which if occurring repeatedly will give rise to an obvious lesion or disorder.

mi·cro·tu·bule (migh"kro·tew'bewl) *n.* Any of the hollow, tubular filaments, composed of repeating subunits of the globular protein tubulin, which play various important structural roles in prokaryotic and eukaryotic cells. Microtubules make up centrioles and cilia, contribute as elements of the cytoskeleton to the formation and maintenance of distinctive, nonsymmetrical cell shapes (as in the axons of neurons), and constitute the distinctive aster and spindle seen in mitosis. See also *neurotubule.*

Mi·cro·tus (migh·kro'tus) *n.* [NL., from *micr-* + Gk. *ous, ōtos,* ear]. A genus of field voles of the Orient that may transmit leptospirosis and rat-bite fever.

mi·cro·unit (migh'kro·yoo"nit) *n.* A unit of minute measurements; the one-millionth part of an ordinary unit.

mi·cro·vas·cu·la·ture (migh"kro·vas'kew·luh·chur) *n.* The sum of minute vessels in a region, part, organ, or organism.

mi·cro·vil·lus (migh"kro·vil'us) *n.*, pl. **microvil·li** (·eye) [*micro-* + *villus*]. Any of the free cell surface evaginations which, depending upon location, may be absorptive or secretory in function.

mi·cro·volt (migh'kro·vohlt) *n.* One one-millionth of a volt.

mi·cro·wave (migh'kro·wave) *n.* An electromagnetic wave having a wavelength between a few tenths of a millimeter and about 30 centimeters, the limits being to some degree arbitrary.

microwave spectroscopy. The study of transitions induced by interactions of matter with microwaves, whereby knowledge of molecular structure and certain properties of matter may be determined.

mi·croxy·cyte (migh·krock'si·site) *n.* [*micr-* + *oxy-* + *-cyte*]. A cell containing fine oxyphil granules and a more or less pigmented nucleus, occurring in the peritoneal fluid of infected subjects.

mi·croxy·phil (migh·krock'si·fil) *n.* [*micr-* + *oxyphil*]. EOSINOPHIL LEUKOCYTE.

mi·cro·zo·on (migh"kro·zo'on) *n.*, pl. **micro·zoa** (·zo'uh) [*micro-* + Gk. *zōon,* living being]. A microscopic animal.

mi·cro·zoo·sper·mia (migh"kro·zo"uh·spur'mee·uh) *n.* [*micro-* + *zoosperm,* spermatozoon, + *-ia*]. Abnormally small living sperms in the semen.

mi·crur·gy (migh'krur·jee) *n.* [*micr-* + Gk. *ourg-,* working, + *-y*]. The art and science of manipulation under the magnification of a microscope, including microdissection, microinjection, and various techniques using the micromanipulator.

Mi·cru·roi·des (migh"kroo·roy'deez) *n.* [*Micrur*us + Gk. *-eidēs,* -like]. A genus of coral snakes. *Micruroides euryxanthus* is the Arizona or Sonora coral snake.

Mi·cru·rus (migh·kroo'rus) *n.* [NL., from *micr-* + Gk. *oura,* tail]. A widespread genus of coral snakes. *Micrurus fulvius* is the common coral snake of southern United States and eastern Mexico.

mic·tion (mick'shun) *n.* [L. *mictio*]. URINATION.

mic·tu·rate (mick'tew·rate) *v.* [L. *micturire,* to urinate, to want to urinate]. To urinate.

mic·tu·ri·tion (mick"tew·rish'un) *n.* [L. *micturire,* to urinate, to want to urinate]. URINATION.

micturition centers. The various neuronal aggregates that govern micturition. Higher centers are located in the cerebral cortex, in the region of the paracentral lobule; the spinal micturition center is located in the second, third, and fourth sacral segments of the spinal cord.

mid-. A combining form meaning *middle.*

mi·da·flur (migh'duh·flure) *n.* 4-Amino-2,2,5,5-tetrakis(trifluoromethyl)-3-imidazoline, $C_7H_3F_{12}N_3$, a sedative.

mid-African sleeping sickness. GAMBIAN TRYPANOSOMIASIS.

mid·ax·il·la (mid"ack·sil'uh) *n.* The center of the axilla. **—mid·ax·il·lary** (mid·ack'si·lerr·ee) *adj.*

midaxillary line. A perpendicular line drawn downward from the apex of the axilla. NA *linea axillaris.*

mid·body, *n.* CELL PLATE.

mid·brain, *n.* MESENCEPHALON. See also Plate 15.

mid·car·pal (mid·kahr'pul) *adj.* MEDIOCARPAL; between the two rows of carpal bones.

midcarpal articulation. MEDIOCARPAL ARTICULATION.

mid·cla·vic·u·lar (mid"kla·vick'yoo·lur) *adj.* Pertaining to or passing through the middle of the clavicle.

midclavicular line. A vertical line parallel to, and midway between, the midsternal line and a vertical line drawn downward through the outer end of the clavicle.

middiaphyseal ring. The ring of bone whose replacement of cartilage at the middiaphysis constitutes the initial stage in the ossification of a long bone.

mid·di·aph·y·sis (mid"dye·af'i·sis) *n.* The midpoint or midportion of a diaphysis. **—mid·di·aph·y·se·al** (mid"dye·af"i·see'ul, mid"dye"uh·fiz'ee·ul) *adj.*

Mid·dle·brook-Du·bos test [G. *Middlebrook,* U.S. pathologist, b. 1915; and R. J. *Dubos*]. A test for antibodies in the human serum against the products of the tubercle bacillus. Washed sheep erythrocytes are sensitized with aqueous extracts of *Mycobacterium tuberculosis.* The treated cells are thereby made agglutinable by the antibodies in the serum of tuberculosis patients.

middle carpal articulation. MEDIOCARPAL ARTICULATION.

middle cerebellar peduncle. One of the bands of white matter joining the pons and the cerebellum. Syn. *pontocerebellar tract, brachium pontis.* NA *pendunculus cerebellaris medius.*

middle clinoid process. Usually a small tubercle situated behind the lateral end of the tuberculum sellae. In some skulls it is not present and in others it is large and joins with the anterior clinoid process. NA *processus clinoideus medius.*

middle coat. The tunica media of a vessel.

middle collateral artery. The posteromedial terminal branch of deep brachial artery, supplying the triceps muscle and anastamosing with the recurrent interosseous artery and other vessels in the rete olecrani. NA *arteria collateralis media.*

middle commissure. *Obsol.* ADHESIO INTERTHALAMICA.

middle cranial fossa. One of the three fossae into which the interior base of each side of the cranium (right and left) is divided; it is deeply concave on a much lower level than the anterior cranial fossa, and lodges the temporal lobe of the cerebrum. NA *fossa cranii media.*

middle ear. The tympanic cavity with associated structures, including the tympanic membrane, the ossicles, the auditory tube, and the mastoid antrum and cells. NA *auris media.*

middle frontal gyrus. A convolution of the frontal lobe lying below and parallel to the superior frontal gyrus and above the inferior frontal gyrus. NA *gyrus frontalis medius.* See also Plate 18.

middle kidney. MESONEPHROS.

middle lobe syndrome. Atelectasis, bronchiectasis, or chronic pneumonitis of the right middle lobe, presumably due to enlarged usually calcified lymph nodes compressing the right middle lobe bronchus. Syn. *Brock's syndrome.*

middle mediastinum. The division of the mediastinum that contains the heart and pericardium, the ascending aorta, the superior vena cava, the bifurcation of the trachea, the pulmonary trunk and pulmonary veins, and the phrenic nerves. NA *mediastinum medium.*

middle medical personnel. Paramedical personnel, such as feldshers, physician's assistants, and sanitarians. See also *syniatrist.*

middle nasal concha. The lower scroll-like projection of the ethmoid bone covered with mucous membrane situated in the lateral wall of the nasal cavity. NA *concha nasalis media.*

middle nasal meatus. The part of the nasal cavity between the middle nasal concha and the inferior nasal concha. NA *meatus nasi medius.*

middle nasal turbinate. MIDDLE NASAL CONCHA.

middle temporal gyrus. A convolution of the temporal lobe which lies between the superior and middle temporal sulci. NA *gyrus temporalis medius.* See also Plate 18.

middle temporal sulcus. A poorly defined furrow lying above the inferior temporal gyrus.

middle thyrohyoid ligament. MEDIAN THYROHYOID LIGAMENT.

mid·epi·gas·tric (mid″ep·i·gas′trick) *adj.* [*mid-* + *epigastric*]. Transversely bisecting the epigastrium.

midepigastric plane. TRANSPYLORIC PLANE.

mid forceps. An obstetric forceps applied when the fetal head is engaged, but has not yet become visible at the introitus and rotated to the occiput anterior position.

mid·fron·tal (mid″frun′tul) *adj.* Pertaining to the middle of the forehead.

midge, *n.* An insect of those Diptera which comprise the families of Ceratopogonidae and Chironomidae; small, delicate forms usually smaller than mosquitoes. The genus *Culicoides* is the most important medically.

midg·et, *n.* An individual who is abnormally small, but otherwise normal.

mid·gut, *n.* The middle portion of the embryonic digestive tube, opening ventrally into the yolk sac.

mid·head, *n.* [*mid-* + *head*]. CENTRICIPUT.

Midicel. A trademark for sulfamethoxypyridazine, an antibacterial sulfonamide.

mid·line, *n.* Any line that bisects a figure symmetrically, as for example the intersection of the median plane with the surface of the body or with structures within the body.

midline cerebellar syndrome. VERMIS SYNDROME.

midline nuclei of the thalamus. Diffusely organized thalamic nuclei, located near the wall of the third ventricle and in the adhesio interthalamica, which are connected mainly to the hypothalamic and intralaminar nuclei.

mid·night croup. SPASMODIC CROUP.

mid·pain, *n.* MITTELSCHMERZ.

mid·pal·mar space (mid″pahl′mur). A deep fascial space beneath the flexor tendons on the ulnar side of the palm. Syn. *medial palmar space.*

mid·rang·er, *n.* MIDRANGE SOMATOTYPE.

midrange somatotype. Any individual whose somatotype includes only the midrange numerical evaluation of the three primary components.

mid·riff, *n.* [OE. *midd* + *hrif,* belly]. 1. The diaphragm. 2. Loosely, the upper part of the abdomen.

mid·sag·it·tal plane (mid″saj′i·tul). MEDIAN PLANE.

mid·ster·nal line (mid″stur′nul). A vertical line through the middle of the sternum.

mid·tar·sal amputation (mid″tahr′sul). MEDIOTARSAL AMPUTATION.

mid·ven·tral (mid″ven′trul) *adj.* Pertaining to the middle portion of the ventral aspect.

mid·ves·i·cal (mid″ves′i·kul) *adj.* [*mid-* + *vesical*]. Pertaining to the middle of a bladder.

mid·wife, *n.* [ME., from OE. *mid,* with, + *wīf,* woman]. A trained or experienced person, especially a woman, who attends women in labor and delivery.

mid·wife·ry (mid′wif·ree, ·wye·free, ·fur·ee) *n.* The practice of a midwife; practical obstetrics.

Mie·scher's granuloma (mee′shur) [G. *Miescher,* Swiss, 1877–1961]. A nodule, seen histologically, composed of histiocytes, granulocytes, and lymphocytes, found in the subcutis in erythema nodosum.

Miescher's tubes [J. F. *Miescher,* Swiss pathologist, 1811–1887]. The elongated tube-like sporocysts of the Sarcosporidia, in the connective tissue between the muscle fibers of the host.

MIF. Abbreviation for *migration inhibitory factor.*

mi·graine (migh′grain) *n.* [F., from Gk. *hēmikrania,* pain on one side of the head]. Recurrent paroxysmal vascular headache; varied in intensity, frequency, and duration; commonly unilateral in onset and often associated with nausea and vomiting; may be preceded by or associated with sensory, motor, or mood disturbances; often familial. Syn. *sick headache.* —**migrain·ous** (·us) *adj.*

migrainous neuralgia. CLUSTER HEADACHE.

migrant sensory neuritis. A chronic form of neuritis involving different noncontiguous sensory nerves at different times.

mi·grate (migh′grate) *v.* [L. *migrare*]. To wander; to shift from one site to another. —**mi·grant** (migh′grunt), **mi·gra·to·ry** (migh′gruh·tor·ee) *adj.;* **mi·gra·tion** (migh·gray′shun) *n.*

migrating testis. A freely movable inguinal testis which may be moved even into the abdominal cavity and predisposes to torsion of the spermatic cord.

migration inhibitory factor. A soluble protein released by sensitized lymphocytes exposed to the proper antigen, which concentrates macrophages at the site of antigen-lymphocyte interaction.

migration of leukocytes. The passage or diapedesis of leukocytes through the vessel wall into the connective tissues; one of the phenomena of inflammation.

migration of ovum. The passage of an ovum following ovulation from the ovary to the oviduct and uterus.

migratory pneumonia. Pneumonic infection which seems to

shift from one part of the lung to another. Syn. *creeping pneumonia.*

Mi·ka·nia (mi·kay'nee·uh) *n.* [J. G. *Mikan,* Czech botanist, d. 1814]. A genus of vines of the Compositae; *Mikania guaco* and other species have been used medicinally.

mikro-. See *micr-.*

mikron. MICRON.

Mi·ku·licz cell (mee'koo·litch) [J. von *Mikulicz*-Radecki, German surgeon, 1850-1905]. A large round or oval phagocytic cell with vacuolated cytoplasm and a small pycnotic nucleus, characteristic of rhinoscleroma.

Mikulicz drain [J. von *Mikulicz*-Radecki]. A tampon made by placing a large layer of gauze so as to line the cavity; strips or wicks of gauze are then packed into the cavity, their ends being left outside so they can be grasped and removed individually.

Mikulicz operation [J. von *Mikulicz*-Radecki]. A multiple-staged enterectomy for obstructive disease of the colon.

Mikulicz's disease or **syndrome** [J. von *Mikulicz*-Radecki]. Salivary and lacrimal gland enlargement from any of a variety of causes, including tuberculosis, sarcoidosis, and malignant lymphoma.

mil·am·me·ter (mil·am'ee·tur) *n.* MILLIAMMETER.

mil·dew, *n.* Any of various minute fungi parasitic on plants, also found on dead vegetable substances such as textiles.

mild mental retardation. Subnormal general intellectual functioning in which the intelligence quotient is approximately 55-69; there may be some impairment of vocational capacities as well as a need for special education.

mild mercurous chloride. MERCUROUS CHLORIDE.

mild silver protein. Silver rendered colloidal by the presence of, or combination with, protein; contains 19 to 23% of silver. Dark brown or almost black, shining scales or granules; freely soluble in water. Used as a local antibacterial in the treatment of infections of mucous membranes.

Miles' operation [W. E. *Miles,* English surgeon, 1869-1947]. A one-stage, radical, abdominoperineal resection of the rectum for carcinoma.

milia. Plural of *milium.*

Mi·lian's ear sign (mee·lyah^{n}') [G. *Milian,* French dermatologist, 1871-1945]. A sign to differentiate facial erysipelas from subcutaneous inflammations; involvement of the ear occurs in the former and not in the latter.

Milian's ninth-day erythema [G. *Milian*]. ERYTHEMA OF NINTH DAY.

mil·i·a·ria (mil''ee·ăr'ee·uh, ·air'ee·uh) *n.* [L. *miliarius,* pertaining to millet]. An acute inflammatory disease of the sweat glands, characterized by lesions of the skin consisting of vesicles and papules, which may be accompanied by a prickling or tingling sensation. It occurs especially in summer and in the tropics, often in the folds of the skin. Syn. *prickly heat, heat rash.*

miliaria crys·tal·li·na (kris''tuh·lye'nuh). SUDAMEN.

miliaria pro·fun·da (pro·fun'duh). The skin reaction seen in the sweat-retention syndrome. The skin is uniformly studded with many discrete normal skin-colored papules located around a sweat pore. There are no subjective symptoms.

miliaria pus·tu·lo·sa (pus''tew·lo'suh). A pustular dermatitis occurring when another dermatitis is complicated by sweat retention.

mil·i·ary (mil'ee·ăr''ee, ·air''ee, mil'yuh·ree) *adj.* [L. *miliarius,* from *milium,* millet]. 1. Of the size of a millet seed, 0.5 to 1.0 mm., as miliary aneurysm, miliary tubercle. 2. Characterized by the formation of numerous lesions the size of a millet seed distributed rather uniformly throughout one or more organs, especially as in miliary tuberculosis.

miliary abscess. A minute embolic abscess.

miliary aneurysm. A minute saclike dilatation of an arteriole.

miliary fever. A febrile illness associated with profuse sweating and characterized by papular, vesicular, and other eruptions attributed to the blockage of the sweat glands.

miliary gumma. A localized lesion of late syphilis differing from the usual gumma in its small size.

miliary tubercles. Tubercles of uniform size, approximating the millet seed, 1.0 to 2.0 mm. in diameter, distributed rather uniformly throughout an organ or series of organs.

Milibis. Trademark for glycobiarsol, an antiamebic drug.

mi·lieu (mee·lyuh', mee·lyoo') *n.,* pl. **mi·lieux** (·lyuh', ·lyoo'), **milieus** [F., from OF. *mi-,* middle, + *lieu,* place]. Environment, surroundings.

milieu ex·té·rieur (ecks·tay·ryur') [F.]. The external environment of an organism, as contrasted with the milieu intérieur.

milieu in·té·rieur (an·tay·ryur') [F., internal environment]. Claude Bernard's concept, now fundamental for modern physiology, postulating that the living organism exists not so much in its gaseous or aqueous external environment (milieu extérieur) as within its aqueous internal environment. Formed by circulating liquid, the blood plasma, interstitial fluid, and lymph, this milieu intérieur bathes all tissue elements, and is the medium in which all elementary exchanges of nutrient and waste materials take place. Its stability is the primary condition for independent existence of the organism, and the mechanisms by which stability is achieved ensure maintenance of all conditions necessary to the life of tissue elements.

milieu therapy. *In psychiatry,* the treatment of a mental disorder or maladjustment by making substantial changes in a patient's immediate life circumstances and environment in a way that will enhance the effectiveness of other forms of therapy. Within a hospital setting, this may involve pleasant physical surroundings, recreational facilities, and the staff. Syn. *situation therapy.*

mil·i·per·tine (mil''i·pur'teen) *n.* 5,6-Dimethoxy-3-[2-[4-(*o*-methoxyphenyl)-1-piperazinyl]ethyl]-2-methylindole, $C_{24}H_{31}N_3O_3$, a tranquilizer.

military medicine. That part of general medicine dealing with the character, epidemiology, prevention, and treatment of diseases and injuries which are brought about by the special conditions incident to military life. Syn. *war medicine.*

military surgery. Surgery in the treatment of gunshot wounds and other usual combat injuries.

mil·i·um (mil'ee·um) *n.,* pl. **mil·ia** (·ee·uh) [L., millet]. A minute epidermal cyst, thought to represent either epidermal inclusion cyst formation or blockage of a pilosebaceous opening.

milk, *n. & v.* 1. The white fluid secreted by the mammary gland for the nourishment of the young. It is composed of carbohydrates, proteins, fats, mineral salts, vitamins, antibodies. 2. Any white fluid resembling milk, as coconut milk. 3. A suspension of certain metallic oxides, as milk of magnesia, iron, bismuth, etc. 4. To express milk from the mammary gland, manually or mechanically. 5. To press a finger along a compressible tube or duct in order to squeeze out the contents.

milk abscess. A mammary abscess occurring during lactation.

milk agent. MILK FACTOR.

milk-alkali syndrome. Hypercalcemia without hypercalcuria or hypophosphaturia, normal or slightly elevated alkaline phosphatase, renal insufficiency with azotemia, mild alkalosis, conjunctivitis, and calcinosis complicating the prolonged excessive intake of milk and soluble alkali. Syn. *Burnett's syndrome, milk-drinker's syndrome.*

milk corpuscle. 1. The detached, fat-drop filled, distal portion of a glandular cell of the mammary gland, constricted off from the rest of the cell body in apocrine secretion. It breaks down, freeing milk globules. 2. A milk globule.

milk crust. CRADLE CAP.

milk cure. GALACTOTHERAPY (1).

milk-drinker's syndrome. MILK-ALKALI SYNDROME.

milk ducts. LACTIFEROUS DUCTS.

milk-duct carcinoma. Ductal carcinoma of the breast.

milk·er's nodes or **nodules.** Papular lesions of paravaccinia on the hands, contracted from affected teats and udders, usually of the cow.

milk factor. A filtrable, noncellular agent in the milk and tissues of certain strains of inbred mice; transmitted from the mother to the offspring by nursing. It seems to be an essential factor in the genesis of mammary cancer in these strains. Syn. *Bittner milk factor.*

milk fever. 1. A fever during the puerperium, once thought to be due to a great accumulation of milk in the breasts, but now generally believed to be due to actual puerperal infection. 2. PARTURIENT PARESIS.

milk intolerance. An intolerance characterized by diarrhea, bloating, abdominal cramps, and vomiting after the ingestion of milk, due to allergy to milk protein or to congenital or acquired lactase deficiency.

milk leg. PHLEGMASIA ALBA DOLENS.

milk line. MAMMARY RIDGE.

Milk·man's syndrome or **disease** [L. A. *Milkman,* U.S. radiologist, 1895–1951]. Decreased tubular reabsorption of phosphate, resulting in osteomalacia which gives a peculiar transverse striped appearance (multiple pseudofractures) to the bones in roentgenograms. Syn. *Looser-Milkman syndrome.*

milk of calcium bile syndrome. LIMY BILE SYNDROME.

milk of magnesia. A suspension of magnesium hydroxide containing 7 to 8.5% of $Mg(OH)_2$; used as an antacid and laxative.

milk plaques. MILK SPOTS.

milk pox. VARIOLA MINOR.

milk ridge. MAMMARY RIDGE.

milk sickness. An acute disease of human beings, characterized by weakness, anorexia, constipation, and vomiting due to ingestion of milk or flesh of animals which have a disease called trembles.

milk spots. Patches of thickening and opacity of the epicardium, found post mortem, usually over the right ventricle; of common occurrence in persons who have passed middle life. Syn. *soldier's patches* or *spots, milk plaques.*

milk sugar. LACTOSE.

milk teeth. DECIDUOUS TEETH.

milk tumor. A swelling of the breast due to the obstruction of milk ducts; not a neoplasm.

milky spots. Small regions of the omentum containing multitudes of fixed and free macrophages.

Mil·lard-Gu·bler syndrome (mee·yar', gue·blehr') [A. L. J. *Millard,* French physician, 1830–1915; and A. *Gubler*]. A form of crossed paralysis due to a pontine lesion, characterized clinically by a peripheral facial paralysis and often also paralysis of the lateral rectus muscle on the side of the lesion and contralateral hemiplegia. Compare *Weber's syndrome.*

Mil·lar's asthma [J. *Millar,* Scottish physician, 1733–1805]. SPASMODIC CROUP.

millepede. MILLIPEDE.

Mil·ler-Ab·bott tube [T. G. *Miller,* U.S. physician, b. 1886; and W. O. *Abbott,* U.S. physician, 1902–1943]. A long, double-lumen, balloon-tipped rubber tube, inserted usually through a nostril and passed through the pylorus; used to locate and treat obstructive conditions of the small intestine.

Miller disk. An ocular micrometer disk containing two squares whose areas have a 1:9 ratio; used in making reticulocyte counts.

Miller ocular disk. MILLER DISK.

mil·let, *n.* [MF., from L. *milium*]. A cereal grass of the genus *Panicum.*

millet seed. The edible seed of millet; frequently used to designate the approximate size of small lesions or tumors, being about 2 mm in diameter.

milli- [L. *mille,* thousand]. A combining form meaning *a thousand* or *a thousandth.*

mil·li·am·me·ter (mil''ee·am'mee·tur) *n.* An ammeter which records electric current in milliamperes. Used in measuring currents passing through the filament circuits of roentgen-ray tubes.

mil·li·am·pere (mil''ee·am'peer) *n.* One one-thousandth of an ampere. Abbreviated, ma.

mil·li·bar (mil'i·bahr) *n.* A unit of atmospheric pressure, the one-thousandth part of a bar. Abbreviated, mb.

mil·li·cu·rie (mil'i·kew·ree) *n.* The amount of a radioactive substance which undergoes 3.7×10^7 disintegrations per second, equivalent to one-thousandth of a curie. Abbreviated, mCi.

millicurie-hour. A dosage unit of radon; the amount of radiation emitted by a millicurie of radon multiplied by time of treatment in hours.

mil·li·equiv·a·lent (mil''ee·e·kwiv'uh·lunt) *n.* One one-thousandth of an equivalent, in specified weight units, of a chemical element, ion, radical, or compound. Abbreviated, meq, mEq.

mil·li·gram (mil'i·gram) *n.* One one-thousandth of a gram. Abbreviated, mg, mg.

milligram-hour. An exposure unit for radium therapy; the amount of radiation emitted by a milligram of radium multiplied by the time of treatment in hours. Abbreviated, mgh, mgh.

milligrams percent. *In biochemistry,* indicating milligrams of a substance per 100 ml of blood. Symbol, mg %, mg. %.

Mil·li·kan rays [R. A. *Millikan,* U.S. physicist, 1868–1953]. COSMIC RAYS.

mil·li·li·ter (mil'i·lee''tur) *n.* The one one-thousandth part of a liter, equivalent to a cubic centimeter. Abbreviated, ml, ml.

mil·li·me·ter (mil'i·mee''tur) *n.* One one-thousandth of a meter. Abbreviated, mm, mm.

mil·li·mi·cro·cu·rie (mil''i·migh'kro·kew·ree) *n.* [*milli-* + *microcurie*]. NANOCURIE.

mil·li·mi·cro·gram (mil''i·migh'kro·gram) *n.* [*milli-* + *microgram*]. NANOGRAM.

mil·li·mi·cron (mil''i·migh'kron) *n.* NANOMETER. Abbreviated, mμ.

mil·li·mi·cro·sec·ond (mil''i·migh'kro·seck·und) *n.* [*milli-* + *micro-* + *second*]. NANOSECOND.

mil·li·mol (mil'i·mol, ·mole) *n.* One one-thousandth of a gram molecule. —**mil·li·mo·lar** (mil''i·mo'lur) *adj.*

Mil·lin·gen's operation [E. Van *Millingen,* English ophthalmologist, 1851–1900]. An operation for trichiasis, in which the wound is covered with mucosa from the patient's lips instead of with skin.

mil·li·nor·mal (mil''i·nor'mul) *adj.* Containing a thousandth part of the quantity designated as normal, as a millinormal solution.

mil·li·os·mol (mil''ee·oz'mol, ·mole) *n.* [*milli-* + *osmol*]. The concentration of an ion in a solution expressed as milligrams per liter divided by atomic weight. In univalent ions, milliosmolar and milliequivalent values are identical; in divalent ions, 1 milliosmol equals 2 milliequivalents. —**milli·os·mo·lar** (·oz·mo'lur) *adj.*

mil·li·pede, mil·le·pede (mil'i·peed) *n.* [L. *millepeda,* wood louse, from *mille,* thousand, + *pes, pedis,* foot]. Wingless, vermiform arthropods with two pairs of legs on each body segment. Some species are incriminated as hosts of *Hymenolepis diminuta.*

mil·li·ruth·er·ford (mil''i·ruh'thur·furd) *n.* [*milli-* + *rutherford*]. A unit of radioactivity representing 10^3 disintegrations per second. Abbreviated, mrd.

mil·li·sec·ond (mil'i·seck''und) *n.* One one-thousandth of a second. Abbreviated, msec.

mil·li·unit (mil'i·yoo''nit) *n.* One one-thousandth of a standard unit.

mil·li·volt (mil'i·vohlt) *n.* One one-thousandth of a volt.

mil·li·volt·me·ter (mil″i·vohlt′mee·tur) *n.* [*milli-* + *voltmeter*]. An instrument for measuring electromotive force in millivolts.

millivolt second. A measurement of an electric current, equal to one one-thousandth of a volt per second.

Millon's reagent. A solution, prepared by dissolving metallic mercury in concentrated nitric acid, that produces a red color with proteins containing tyrosine and also with phenols.

Milontin. Trademark for phensuximide, an anticonvulsant drug primarily useful in the treatment of petit mal epilepsy.

Milovidov method. A staining method for starch using toluidine blue, gentian violet, or methyl green, which give blue, violet, and green colors, respectively.

mil·pho·sis (mil·fo′sis) *n.* [Gk. *milphōsis,* falling out of the eyelashes]. Baldness of the eyebrows.

Mil·roy's disease [W. F. *Milroy,* U.S. physician, 1855–1942]. Familial chronic lymphedema of the lower extremities with onset at birth. Compare *Meige's disease.*

Miltown. A trademark for meprobamate, a tranquilizer drug.

milz·brand (milts′brahnt) *n.* [Ger.]. ANTHRAX.

mim·bane (mim′bane) *n.* 1-Methylyohimbane, $C_{20}H_{26}N_2$, an analgesic; used as the hydrochloride salt.

mi·me·sis (mi·mee′sis, migh·mee′sis) *n.* [Gk. *mimēsis,* imitation]. 1. Mimicry, as of an organic disease. 2. The assumption or imitation of the symptoms of one disease by another disease.

mi·met·ic (mi·met′ick, migh·) *adj.* [Gk. *mimētikos,* able to imitate, imitative]. 1. Characterized by or pertaining to mimesis; false, pseudo-. 2. Pertaining to facial expression.

mimetic labor. FALSE LABOR.

mimetic muscle. Any one of the muscles of facial expression.

mim·ic (mim′ick) *adj.* [Gk. *mimikos,* of or like a mime]. MIMETIC.

mimic spasm. A facial tic.

mim·ma·tion (mim·ay′shun) *n.* [*mīm,* the Arabic letter corresponding to m]. The unduly frequent use of the sound of the letter M in speech.

mi·mo·sis (mi·mo′sis, migh·) *n.* MIMESIS.

min. Abbreviation for (a) *minim;* (b) *minimum;* (c) *minute.*

Minamata disease [after *Minamata* Bay, Japan]. Organic mercurial poisoning from consumption of contaminated fish and shellfish, resulting in constriction of visual fields, ataxia, dysarthria, tremors, mental changes, salivation, sweating, and various signs of extrapyramidal dysfunction.

Mincard. Trademark for the orally effective nonmercurial diuretic aminometradine.

mind (mine′d) *n.* [OE. *gemynd*←Gmc. *gamundi-* (rel. to L. *ment-*)]. 1. The sum total of the neural processes which receive, code, and interpret sensations, recall and correlate stored information, and act on it. 2. The state of consciousness. 3. The understanding, reasoning, and intellectual faculties and processes considered as a whole, often as contrasted with body or with feeling. 4. *In psychiatry,* the psyche, or the conscious, subconscious, and unconscious considered together.

mind cure. MENTAL HEALING.

min·er·al, *n.* & *adj.* [L. *mineralis,* pertaining to mines]. 1. An inorganic chemical compound found in nature, especially one that is solid. 2. Pertaining to, or having characteristics of, a mineral.

mineral acid. An inorganic acid.

mineral balance. The state of dynamic equilibrium in the body, maintained by physiologic processes, between the outgo and intake of any mineral or of any particular mineral constituent such as iron, calcium, or sodium.

mineral glycerin. PETROLEUM.

min·er·al·iza·tion (min″ur·uh·li·zay′shun, ·lye·zay′shun) *n.* Deposition of mineral substances, under either normal or pathologic conditions.

mineral jelly. PETROLATUM.

min·er·alo·cor·ti·coid (min″ur·uh·lo·kor′ti·koid) *n.* An adrenal cortical steroid hormone, such as aldosterone, that primarily regulates mineral metabolism and, indirectly, fluid balance.

mineral oil. A mixture of liquid hydrocarbons obtained from petroleum. When refined to meet U.S.P. standards, it is sometimes known as white mineral oil. The refined oil is sometimes used as a vehicle for medicinal agents to be applied externally, and sometimes for its mechanical action in alleviating constipation. Syn. *liquid petrolatum.*

mineral water. Water naturally or artificially impregnated with sufficient inorganic salts to give it special properties.

mineral wax. CERESIN.

miner's anemia. MINER'S SICKNESS.

miner's asthma. ANTHRACOSILICOSIS.

miner's nystagmus. PENDULAR NYSTAGMUS.

miner's phthisis. ANTHRACOSILICOSIS.

miner's sickness or **anemia.** ANCYLOSTOMIASIS.

miniature fluorography. FLUOROGRAPHY.

min·im (min′im) *n.* [L. *minimus,* least]. A unit of volume in the apothecaries' system; it equals 1/60 fluidram or about 1 drop (of water). Abbreviated, min. Symbol, ♏.

min·i·mal (min′i·mul) *adj.* [*minim*um + *-al*]. The least or smallest; extremely minute.

minimal air. The small amount of air left in the alveoli of an excised or collapsed lung.

minimal brain damage or **injury.** MINIMAL BRAIN DYSFUNCTION SYNDROME.

minimal brain dysfunction syndrome. A complex of learning and behavioral disabilities seen primarily in children of near average to above average intelligence, exhibiting also deviations of function of the central nervous system. The impairment may involve perception, conceptualization, language, memory, and control of attention, impulse, and motor function. Multiple causes, particularly pre- and perinatal disturbances, have been cited. Similar symptoms may complicate the problem of children with more severe brain disease such as epilepsy or blindness.

minimal cerebral damage, dysfunction, injury, or **palsy.** MINIMAL BRAIN DYSFUNCTION SYNDROME.

minimal chronic brain syndrome. MINIMAL BRAIN DYSFUNCTION SYNDROME.

minimal separable acuity. *In ophthalmology,* the minimal angle of separation between two points to produce doubling. At the fovea, the measurements are from 50 to 64 seconds of arc.

minimal stimulus. THRESHOLD STIMULUS.

minimal tuberculosis. Tuberculosis with lesions of slight to moderate density without cavitation and involving one or both lungs, the volume of involved lung tissue not exceeding the volume of lung on one side between the second costochondral junction and the spine of the fourth or the body of the fifth thoracic vertebra.

min·i·mum, *n.,* pl. **mini·ma** (·muh) [L., neuter of *minimus,* smallest, least]. The least quantity or amount; the lowest intensity or level.

minimum cog·no·scib·i·le (kog″no·sib′i·lee) [L.]. *In physiologic optics,* the lowest limit at which recognition of complicated detail of form occurs.

minimum dis·cer·nib·i·le (dis″ur·nib′i·lee) [L.]. MINIMUM DISCERNIBLE.

minimum discernible. *In physiologic optics,* the smallest discernible light difference, i.e., the differential threshold of light sense.

minimum dose. The smallest quantity of a medicine that will produce pharmacologic effects.

minimum le·gib·i·le (le·jib′i·lee) [L.]. *In physiologic optics,* the lowest limit at which recognition of letters or numbers occurs.

minimum lethal dose. 1. That amount of an injurious agent (drug, virus, radiation) which is the average of the smallest dose that kills and the largest dose that fails to kill, when each of a series of animals is given a different dose under controlled conditions. Because of its general lack of accuracy, this measurement has been largely abandoned in favor of *median lethal dose.* Abbreviated, MLD. 2. Formerly, the quantity of a toxin which will kill a guinea pig of 250 g weight in from 4 to 5 days.

minimum sep·a·rab·i·le (sep″uh·rab′i·lee) [L.]. MINIMAL SEPARABLE ACUITY.

minimum separable. MINIMAL SEPARABLE ACUITY.

minimum vi·sib·i·le (vi·zib′i·lee) [L.]. MINIMUM VISIBLE.

minimum visible. *In physiologic optics,* the smallest amount of light (expressed in watts of light energy) just perceptible, i.e., the absolute threshold of light sense.

Minipress. A trademark for prazosin, an antihypertensive agent.

min·i·um (min′ee·um) *n.* [L., red lead]. LEAD ORTHOPLUMBATE.

Min·kow·ski-Chauf·fard hemolytic jaundice (ming·ko[h]f′skee, sho·fahr′) [O. *Minkowski,* Lithuanian pathologist in Germany, 1858–1931; and A. M. E. *Chauffard*]. HEREDITARY SPHEROCYTOSIS.

Min·ne·so·ta multiphasic personality inventory. An empirical scale of an individual's personality based mainly on his own yes-or-no responses to a questionnaire of 550 items; designed to provide scores on all the more important personality traits and adaptations, and including special validating scales which measure the individual's test-taking attitude and degree of frankness. Abbreviated, MMPI.

Minnesota preschool scale. A test for measuring the learning ability of children from 18 months to 6 years of age. Being both verbal and nonverbal, it is particularly valuable in differentiating between the specific kinds of intellectual abilities.

min·o·cy·cline (min″o·sigh′kleen) *n.* A tetracycline derivative, $C_{23}H_{27}N_3O_7$, an antibacterial.

Minocyn. A trademark for minocycline, an antibacterial.

mi·nom·e·ter (mi·nom′e·tur, migh·) *n.* [*mini-,* minute, minimal, + *-meter*]. An instrument for measuring stray radiation from sources of radioactivity.

mi·nor (migh′nur) *adj. & n.* [L.]. 1. Less; lesser; smaller. 2. An individual under legal age; one under the authority of parents or guardians.

minor agglutinin. GROUP AGGLUTININ.

minor alar cartilages. NA *cartilagines alares minores.* See *alar cartilages.*

minor brain damage or **injury.** MINIMAL BRAIN DYSFUNCTION SYNDROME.

minor calices. The 4 to 13 cuplike divisions of the major calices; derived from tubules of the second, third, and fourth orders, each receiving one or more of the renal papillae. NA *calices renales minores.*

minor contusion syndrome. POSTCONCUSSION SYNDROME.

minor cross match. See *cross matching.*

minor duodenal papilla. A minute and variable elevation of the mucosa of the second part of the duodenum where the accessory pancreatic duct empties; when present it is proximal to the major duodenal papilla. NA *papilla duodeni minor.*

minor epilepsy. MINOR MOTOR EPILEPSY.

minor hemisphere. NONDOMINANT HEMISPHERE.

minor lip. LABIUM MINUS.

minor motor epilepsy. Recurrent minor motor seizures as contrasted with recurrent generalized seizures (major motor epilepsy).

minor motor seizure. 1. Any seizure which appears to be less severe than a generalized (grand mal or major motor) attack; in older classifications, petit mal. 2. Specifically, an akinetic, myoclonic, or absence attack, comprising the petit mal triad.

minor operation. An operation which does not threaten life; one in which there is little or no danger.

minor palatine foramen. LESSER PALATINE FORAMEN.

Mi·nor's disease or **syndrome** (mee′nur) [L. S. *Minor,* Russian neurologist, b. 1855]. Hemorrhage into the central spinal cord.

Minor's sweat test [L. S. *Minor*]. A test to demonstrate lesions of the sympathetic nervous system. The adult subject takes 0.5 g of aspirin a half-hour before the test; the skin is painted with iodine solution and after the skin dries, it is dusted with fine starch powder. Sweating is induced by having the patient drink a large amount of usually hot liquid. In dermatomes where sweating is intact, the moisture facilitates the interaction between iodine and starch, producing a blue-black color. Where there is a lack of sweating no color is obtained, but there may be increased sweating in immediately adjacent areas. See also *sweat test.*

Minor's tremor [L. S. *Minor*]. ESSENTIAL TREMOR.

minor surgery. That part of surgery including procedures not involving serious hazard to life and usually not requiring general anesthesia; examples are bandaging, application of splints and casts, suturing of superficial lacerations, excision, incision, and drainage of superficial structures.

Mi·not-Mur·phy diet (migh′nut) [G. R. *Minot,* U.S. physician, 1885–1950; and W. P. *Murphy,* U.S. physician, b. 1892]. A diet high in protein, purines and iron, the chief constituent of which is liver; used in the treatment of pernicious anemia.

min·ox·i·dil (mi·nock′si·dil) *n.* 2,4-Diamino-6-piperidino-pyrimidine-3-oxide, $C_9H_{15}N_5O$, an antihypertensive.

mint, *n.* Any plant belonging to the genus *Mentha.*

Mintezol. A trademark for thiabendazole, an anthelmintic.

minute ventilation or **volume.** The total volume of air breathed in a minute.

mio-, meio- [Gk. *meiōn,* smaller, less]. A combining form meaning (a) *reduced, rudimentary;* (b) *contraction, constriction.*

mio·car·dia (migh″o·kahr′dee·uh) *n.* [*mio-* + *-cardia*]. Diminution of the volume of the heart during systole. Contr. *auxocardia.*

mio·did·y·mus (migh″o·did′i·mus) *n.* [*mio-* + *-didymus*]. A type of dicephalus parasiticus in which a small head is fused occipitally with a large head.

mi·od·y·mus (migh·od′i·mus) *n.* MIODIDYMUS.

Miokon. Trademark for sodium diprotrizoate, a roentgenographic contrast medium.

mio·lec·i·thal, meio·lec·i·thal (migh″o·les′i·thul) *adj.* [*mio-* + *lecithal*]. ALECITHAL.

mi·o·pus (migh·o′pus, migh′o·pus) *n.* [*mio-* + Gk. *ōps,* eye, face]. A type of diprosopus in which one face is rudimentary.

mi·o·sis (migh·o′sis) *n.* [Gk. *meiōsis,* diminution]. 1. Constriction of the pupil of the eye. 2. Specifically, abnormal contraction of the pupil below 2 mm.

mi·ot·ic (migh·ot′ick) *adj. & n.* [Gk. *meiōtikos,* diminishing]. 1. Pertaining to, or characterized by, miosis. 2. Causing contraction of the pupil. 3. Any agent that causes contraction of the pupil of the eye.

mi·ra·cid·i·um (migh″ruh·sid′ee·um) *n.*, pl. **miracid·ia** (·ee·uh) [NL., from Gk. *meirax,* young girl or boy]. The first larval form of the digenetic trematodes which develops from the fertilized ovum and which emerges from the egg as a ciliated, free-swimming, pear-shaped organism. On penetration into the tissue of an appropriate species of snail the miracidium undergoes metamorphosis into a sporocyst.

mir·a·cil D (mirr′uh·sil). LUCANTHONE.

Miradon. Trademark for anisindione, an anticoagulant drug.

Mi·rault's operation (mee·ro′) [G. *Mirault,* French surgeon, 1796–1879]. 1. An operation for the excision of the tongue, in which the lingual arteries were tied as a preliminary step. 2. Plastic repair of unilateral harelip by means of a flap turned down on one side and attached to the opposite side.

mire (meer) *n.* [F., sight, aiming device]. The object on the arc of the ophthalmometer whose reflection from the cornea is employed in determining the amount of corneal astigmatism.

mir·in·ca·my·cin (meer·ing″ka·mye′sin) *n.* An amide of an aminogalactopyranoside and 4-pentyl-2-pyrrolidinecarboxylic acid, $C_{19}H_{35}ClN_2O_5S$, an antimalarial, used as the hydrochloride salt.

mir·ror, *n.* [OF. *mireoir,* from *mirer,* to look at]. 1. A polished surface for reflecting light or forming images of objects placed in front of it. 2. (*Attributive use only*) In a bilaterally symmetrical system, reflecting or imitating the other of a pair, as mirror movements of an infant's hands; in an asymmetrical system, reversed or backward (as: mirror writing).

mirror haploscope. An instrument for observing the effects of varying degrees of convergence of the visual axes.

mirror image. A molecule, crystal, or other object whose parts are arranged in a reverse manner to those of a similar molecule, crystal, or other object with reference to an intervening axis or plane, as in the relationship of an object to its image in a mirror.

mirror movements. Associated movements, or involuntary imitative movements of the opposite side of the body, commonly seen in young children, as when the voluntary wiggling of the fingers of one hand results in similar finger movements in the other. Persistence of these movements in later childhood or in the adult is usually associated with some disturbance of cerebral development or a hemiplegia.

mirror speech. Defective speech characterized by pronouncing words or syllables backward.

mirror vision. The visualization of objects or written words in reverse, as if reflected in a mirror.

mirror writing. Writing in which the letters appear backward, as if seen in a mirror; a not uncommon trait in children first learning to write, but also seen when a person is forced to write with the nondominant hand, following paralysis of the dominant hand.

mi·rya·chit (meer·yah′chit) *n.* [Russian, to be possessed by a *miryak* (or *merek*), a kind of evil spirit]. PALMUS (1).

mis-, miso- [Gk. *misos*]. A combining form meaning *hatred, hating.*

mis·an·thro·py (mi·san′thruh·pee, mi·zan′) *n.* [Gk. *misanthrōpia,* from *mis-,* hatred, + *anthrōpos,* mankind]. An aversion to society; hatred of mankind. —**mis·an·thrope** (mis′un·thrope, miz′) *n.;* **mis·an·throp·ic** (mis″un·throp′ick) *adj.*

mis·car·riage (mis·kăr′ij) *n.* Expulsion of the fetus before it is viable. See also *abortion.* —**miscar·ry** (·ee) *v.*

mis·ce (mis′ee) [L., imperative of *miscere*]. Mix, a direction placed under the ingredients of compound prescriptions. Abbreviated, M. Symbol, M̶.

mis·ce·ge·na·tion (mis″e·je·nay′shun) *n.* [L. *misce*re, to mingle, + *gen*us, kind, + *-ation*]. Intermarriage or interbreeding of different human races.

mis·ci·ble (mis′i·bul) *adj.* [L. *miscibilis*]. Capable of mixing or dissolving in all proportions.

miso-. See *mis-.*

mi·sog·a·my (mi·sog′uh·mee) *n.* [*miso-* + *-gamy*]. Aversion to marriage. —**misoga·mist** (·mist) *n.*

mi·sog·y·ny (mi·soj′i·nee) *n.* [Gk. *misogynia,* from *misos,* hatred, + *gynē,* woman]. Hatred of women. —**misogy·nist** (·nist) *n.*

mi·so·lo·gia (mis″o·lo′jee·uh) *n.* MISOLOGY.

mi·sol·o·gy (mi·sol′uh·jee, migh·sol′) *n.* [Gk. *misologia,* from *misos,* hatred, + *logos,* reason, word]. Unreasoning aversion to intellectual or literary matters, or to argument or speaking.

miso·ne·ism (mis″o·nee′iz·um) *n.* [*miso-* + Gk. *ne*os, new, + *-ism*]. Hatred or horror of novelty or change. —**misone·ist** (·ist) *n.*

miso·pe·dia (mis″o·pee′dee·uh) *n.* [*miso-* + *ped-* + *-ia*]. Morbid hatred of all children, but especially of one's own.

miso·psy·chia (mis″o·sigh′kee·uh) *n.* [*miso-* + Gk. *psychē,* life, + *-ia*]. Morbid disgust with life; hatred of living.

missed abortion. A condition of pregnancy in which a fetus weighing less than 500 g dies in utero with failure of expulsion for an extended period of time.

missed labor. A condition of pregnancy in which the fetus has reached the stage of viability consistent with extrauterine life, but following a transitory episode of uterine contractions, labor ceases, the fetus dies and the uterus fails to empty for an extended period of time.

mis·sense mutation (mis′sence). A mutation in which a codon normally directing the incorporation of one amino acid into a protein is changed into one directing the incorporation of a different amino acid. Compare *nonsense mutation.*

mist. Abbreviation for *mistura* [L.], mixture.

mis·tle·toe, *n.* The woody parasites *Viscum album* (European mistletoe) and *V. flavescens* (American mistletoe). Preparations of the former have been used for treatment of hypertension.

mit-, mito- [Gk. *mitos,* thread, string]. A combining form meaning (a) *filament;* (b) *mitosis.*

Mitch·ell's disease [S. W. *Mitchell,* U.S. neurologist, 1829–1914]. ERYTHROMELALGIA.

mite, *n.* Any representative of a large group of small arachnids, which together with the larger ticks constitute the order Acarina.

mite-borne typhus. TSUTSUGAMUSHI DISEASE.

Mithracin. A trademark for mithramycin, an antibacterial.

mith·ra·my·cin (mith″ruh·migh′sin) *n.* An antibiotic, produced by *Streptomyces argillaceus* and *S. tanashiensis,* that has antineoplastic activity.

mith·ri·da·tism (mith″ri·day′tiz·um, mith·rid′uh·tiz·um) *n.* [*Mithridates,* a king of Pontus]. The practice of taking gradually increasing doses of a poison in order to secure immunity against it.

mi·ti·cide (migh′ti·side) *n.* A substance destructive to mites. —**mi·ti·ci·dal** (migh″ti·sigh′dul) *adj.*

mit·i·gate (mit′i·gate) *v.* [L. *mitigare,* from *mitis,* mild]. To allay, make milder; to moderate.

mi·tis (migh′tis) *adj.* [L.]. Mild.

mito-. See *mit-.*

mi·to·car·cin (migh″to·kahr′sin) *n.* An antineoplastic antibiotic obtained from *Streptomyces.*

mi·to·chon·dria (migh″to·kon′dree·uh, mit″o·) *n.,* sing. **mito·chondri·on** (·un) [*mito-* + Gk. *chondrion,* small granule]. Cytoplasmic organelles in the form of granules, short rods, or filaments which are present in all cells. The fine structure consists of external and internal membrane systems; the inner membrane is folded to form cristae extending into the mitochondrial matrix. Mitochondria supply energy to the cell by stepwise oxidation of substrates. They store the energy in ATP. —**mitochondri·al** (·ul) *adj.*

mitochondrion. Singular of *mitochondria.*

Mitocin-C. A trademark for mitomycin, an antineoplastic.

mi·to·cro·min (migh″to·kro′min) *n.* An antibiotic, produced by *Streptomyces viridochromogenes,* that has antineoplastic activity.

mi·to·gen (migh′to·jin, ·jen) *n.* [*mito-* + *-gen*]. Any substance which induces mitosis.

mi·to·gen·e·sis (migh″to·jen′e·sis, mit″o·) *n.* [*mito-* + *-genesis*]. 1. Initiation of mitosis. 2. Formation as a result of mitosis. —**mito·ge·net·ic** (·je·net′ick) *adj.*

mitogenetic radiation. A kind of radiation said to be produced in cells and tissues, which induces or is induced by the process of mitosis. Syn. *Gurvich radiation.*

mi·to·gen·ic (migh″to·jen′ick) *adj.* [*mito-* + *-genic*]. Promoting mitosis.

mi·to·gil·lin (migh″to·jil′in) *n.* An antibiotic, produced by *Aspergillus restrictus,* that has antineoplastic activity.

mi·to·mal·cin (migh″to·mal′sin) *n.* An antibiotic, produced by *Streptomyces malayensis,* that has antineoplastic activity.

mi·tome (migh′tome) *n.* [*mit-* + *-ome*]. The threads of the reticulum of the cytoplasm of a cell (cytomitome) or of the nucleoplasm (karyomitome).

mi·to·my·cin (migh″to·migh′sin) *n.* A complex of related antibiotic substances (mitomycin A, mitomycin B, mitomycin C) produced by *Streptomyces caespitosus (griseovinaceseus).* Mitomycin C, $C_{15}H_{18}N_4O_5$, is a potent antineoplastic agent.

mi·to·qui·none (migh″to·kwi·nohn′) *n.* UBIQUINONE.

mitoses. Plural of *mitosis.*

mi·to·sis (migh·to′sis, mi·) *n.,* pl. **mito·ses** (·seez) [*mit-* + *-osis*]. 1. Nuclear division; usually divided into a series of stages; prophase, metaphase, anaphase, and telophase. 2. The division of the cytoplasm and nucleus.

mi·to·some (migh′to·sohm, mit′o·) *n.* [*mito-* + *-some*]. A cytoplasmic body derived from the spindle fibers of the preceding mitosis. Syn. *spindle remnant.*

mi·to·sper (migh′to·spur) *n.* An antineoplastic derived from *Aspergillus.*

mi·to·tane (migh′to·tane) *n.* 1,1-Dichloro-2-(*o*-chlorophenyl)-2-(*p*-chlorophenyl)ethane, $C_{14}H_{10}Cl_4$, an antineoplastic agent.

mi·tot·ic (migh·tot′ick, mi·) *adj.* Of or pertaining to mitosis.

mitotic division. MITOSIS.

mitotic figures. Chromosomes observed in one of the stages of mitosis.

mitotic index. The number of dividing cells per thousand cells; used in the estimation of the rate of growth of a tissue.

mi·tral (migh′trul) *adj.* 1. Resembling a bishop's miter. 2. Pertaining to the atrioventricular valve of the left side of the heart. See also *mitral cell.*

mitral buttonhole. Advanced severe mitral stenosis.

mitral cell. One of the large triangular nerve cells in the olfactory bulb.

mitral commissurotomy. An operation for the relief of mitral stenosis, commonly a valvulotomy.

mitral funnel. A funnel-like mitral valve deformation in severe mitral stenosis.

mitral insufficiency or **incompetence.** MITRAL REGURGITATION.

mi·tral·iza·tion (migh″truh·li·zay′shun, ·lye·zay′shun) *n.* Changes in the radiographic outline of the heart seen in mitral stenosis.

mitral murmur. A murmur produced in the mitral valve orifice or heard at the mitral area.

mitral regurgitation. Imperfect closure of the mitral valve during the cardiac systole, permitting blood to reenter the left atrium. Syn. *mitral insufficiency, mitral incompetence.*

mitral stenosis or **obstruction.** Obstruction to the flow of blood through the mitral valve, usually due to narrowing of the valve orifice.

mitral valve. A heart valve containing two cusps, situated between the left atrium and left ventricle. Syn. *left atrioventricular valve, bicuspid valve.* NA *valva atrioventricularis sinistra.* See also Plate 5.

mi·troid (migh′troid) *adj.* Shaped like a miter cap.

Mitronal. Trademark for cinnarizine, an antihistaminic drug.

Mi·tsu·da reaction or **test** [K. *Mitsuda,* Japanese physician, 20th century]. LEPROMIN TEST.

mit·tel·schmerz (mit′ul·shmehrts) *n.* [Ger., middle pain]. Pain or discomfort in the lower abdomen of women occurring midway in the intermenstrual interval, thought to be secondary to the irritation of the pelvic peritoneum by fluid or blood escaping from the point of ovulation in the ovary.

Mit·ten·dorf's dot. A whitish-gray dot on the posterior lens capsule representing the remnant of the fetal hyaloid artery.

mixed anesthesia. Anesthesia produced by two or more anesthetics.

mixed aphasia. Impairment or loss in the use of language characterized by more than one form of aphasia, such as the combination of alexia and motor aphasia; a common clinical situation which occurs when adjacent areas of the brain, each correlated with a specific variety of aphasia, are involved by the same lesion.

mixed arthritis. A combination of features of rheumatoid arthritis and degenerative joint disease seen in the same patient or the same joint.

mixed astigmatism. Astigmatism in which one meridian is myopic and the other hypermetropic.

mixed basosquamous carcinoma. BASOSQUAMOUS CARCINOMA.

mixed carcinoma. Carcinoma of more than one cell type, as in basosquamous carcinoma.

mixed chancre. A lesion due to infection with both *Treponema pallidum* and *Haemophilus ducreyi.*

mixed connective tissue disease. A syndrome with features of several collagen diseases, including synovitis, serositis, myositis, and scleroderma. Characterized by the presence of high concentration of antibodies of ribonucleoprotein.

mixed culture. A culture containing more than one defined species of microorganism.

mixed cyst. CYSTIC TERATOMA.

mixed dentition. Dentition in which there are deciduous and permanent teeth present at the same time. See also *deciduous dentition, permanent dentition.*

mixed gland. A gland containing both serous and mucous components, such as the submandibular. NA *glandula seromucosa.*

mixed hepatic porphyria. PORPHYRIA CUTANEA TARDA HEREDITARIA.

mixed hyperlipemia. FAMILIAL HYPERCHYLOMICRONEMIA WITH HYPERPREBETALIPOPROTEINEMIA.

mixed infection. Concurrent infection with more than one type of organism. Syn. *multiple infection.*

mixed laterality. The tendency, when there is a choice, to prefer to use parts of one side of the body for certain tasks and parts of the opposite side for others, as when a person prefers to use the right eye for sighting, the left hand for writing, and the right foot for kicking.

mixed leukocyte culture test. A matching test to measure the degree of histocompatibility between two individuals by mixing peripheral blood leukocytes of the recipient with the donor's leukocytes treated with mitomycin C; the response of the recipient's leukocytes to those of the donor's being measured as a function of the incorporation of radioactive thymidine into the cells of the recipient; the reactive cells are lymphocytes.

mixed mammary tumor. A neoplasm of the mammary glands of the canine in which cells of the glandular epithelial tissue and the fibrous stroma appear anaplastic.

mixed mastoid. A mastoid process in which solid bone, air sinuses, air cells, and marrow are all found.

mixed mesodermal tumor. MESENCHYMOMA (2).

mixed nerve. A nerve composed of both afferent and efferent fibers.

mixed paralysis. Associated motor and sensory paralysis.

mixed thrombus. STRATIFIED THROMBUS.

mixed tumor. A tumor whose parenchyma is composed of two or more tissue types or cell types.

mixed tumor of the breast. CYSTOSARCOMA PHYLLODES.

mixed vaccine. A vaccine prepared from more than one species of bacteria or viruses.

mix·i·dine (mick′si·deen) *n.* 2-[(3,4-Dimethoxyphenethyl)imino]-1-methylpyrrolidine, $C_{15}H_{22}N_2O_2$, a coronary vasodilator.

mixo·sco·pia (mick″so·sko′pee·uh) *n.* [Gk. *mixis,* intercourse, + *skopos*, watcher, + *-ia*]. A form of sexual perversion in which the orgasm is excited by the sight of coitus. —**mixo·scop·ic** (·skop'ick) *adj.*

mix·ture, *n.* [L. *mixtura*]. 1. *In pharmacy,* a preparation made by incorporating insoluble ingredients in a liquid vehicle, usually with the aid of a suitable suspending agent so that the insoluble substances do not readily settle out. 2. An aqueous solution containing two or more solutes.

Mi·ya·ga·wa·nel·la (mee"yuh·gah"wuh·nel'uh) *n.* [Y. *Miyagawa,* Japanese bacteriologist, 1885–1959]. A genus of the family Chlamydiaceae that includes the causative agents of psittacosis *(Miyagawanella psittaci),* ornithosis *(M. ornithosis),* and lymphogranuloma *(M. lymphogranulomatosis).*

mks. Meter-kilogram-second, a system of units based on the meter as the unit of length, the kilogram as the unit of mass, and the second as the unit of time.

ml, ml. Abbreviation for *milliliter.*

MLD. Abbreviation for (a) *metachromatic leukodystrophy;* (b) *minimum lethal dose.*

M line. A line of relatively high density bisecting the H zone of a striated myofibril, representing a series of projections extending transversely from the centers of the thick myosin filaments.

mm, mm. Abbreviation for *millimeter.*

MMPI. Abbreviation for *Minnesota multiphasic personality inventory.*

Mn Symbol for manganese.

M'Naghten. Listed as if spelled *MacNaghten.*

mnem-, mnemo- [Gk. *mnēmē*]. A combining form meaning *memory.*

mne·mas·the·nia (nee"mas·theen'ee·uh) *n.* [*mnem-* + *asthenia*]. Weakness of memory not due to organic disease.

mne·me (nee'mee) *n.* [Gk. *mnēmē,* memory]. 1. The relatively permanent physiologic basis in an organism or the mind accounting for the recall or recognition of facts, or memory. See also *memory trace.* 2. The enduring modifications produced in an organism by stimulation, which persist even after the stimulus ceases, the change effected being referred to as an engram.

mne·mic (nee'mick) *adj.* [*mneme* + *-ic*]. Pertaining to phenomena resulting from the formation of engrams, i.e., pertaining to memory. Compare *mnemonic.*

mne·mo·der·mia (nee"mo·dur'mee·uh) *n.* [*mnemo-* + *-dermia*]. Pruritis and discomfort of the skin hours and days after the cause of the symptoms has been removed and recovery well established, usually stimulated by scratching or rubbing, sometimes by heat and other stimuli.

mne·mon·ic (ne·mon'ick) *adj. & n.* [Gk. *mnēmonikos,* from *mnēmē,* memory]. 1. Aiding memory. 2. Pertaining to memory. 3. A mnemonic device; any combination of letters, words, pictures, or the like, to help one remember the facts they represent.

mne·mon·ics (ne·mon'icks) *n.* [*mnemonic* + *-s*]. 1. The science of cultivation of the memory by systematic methods. 2. Any technique which makes recall more effective.

mnemonic trace. ENGRAM.

mne·mo·tech·nics (nee"mo·teck'nicks) *n.* [*mnemo-* + *technic* + *-s*]. MNEMONICS.

mne·mo·tech·ny (nee'mo·teck"nee) *n.* MNEMONICS.

-mnesia [Gk. *mnēsis,* memory, + *-ia*]. A combining form designating *a type or condition of memory.*

MNS blood group. A major erythrocyte antigen system defined at first by reactions to immune rabbit sera designated anti-M and anti-N, broadened later to include reactions to sera designated anti-S, anti-s, and certain others.

Mo Symbol for molybdenum.

mobile army surgical hospital. *In military medicine,* a mobile unit designed to provide early surgical treatment for nontransportable cases. It is designed for establishment with, or in the vicinity of, a division clearing station.

mobile hospitalization unit. Any hospital installation whose organization and equipment permit ready movement under field or combat conditions.

mobile septum. The distal, more movable part of the nasal septum. NA *pars mobilis septi nasi.*

mobile spasm. *Obsol.* Posthemiplegic athetosis and dystonia.

mo·bil·i·ty (mo·bil'i·tee) *n.* [L. *mobilitas*]. The condition of being movable.

mo·bi·lize (mo'bi·lize) *v.* [F. *mobiliser*]. 1. To render movable, as an ankylosed part. 2. To free, make accessible, as an organ during surgical operation. 3. To release or liberate in the body, as for example glycogen stored in the liver. —**mo·bi·li·za·tion** (mo"bi·li·zay'shun) *n.*

Mö·bius' disease (mœh'byōōs) [P. J. *Möbius,* German neurologist, 1853–1907]. OPHTHALMOPLEGIC MIGRAINE.

Möbius-Leyden dystrophy. LEYDEN-MÖBIUS DYSTROPHY.

Möbius' sign [P. J. *Möbius*]. Weakness of ocular convergence seen in thyrotoxicosis.

Möbius' syndrome [P. J. *Möbius*]. 1. Congenital, usually bilateral, paralysis of the facial muscles, associated often with abducent paralysis as well as of the oculomotor nerves, but also defects in hearing, musculoskeletal anomalies and mental deficit; presumably due to a lack of nerve cells in the motor nuclei of the brainstem. Syn. *congenital facial diplegia, congenital oculofacial paralysis, infantile nuclear aplasia.* 2. OPHTHALMOPLEGIC MIGRAINE.

moc·ca·sin (mock'uh·sin) *n.* [Algonquian]. Any North American snake of the genus *Agkistrodon;* a cottonmouth or a copperhead.

moccasin venom reaction. An intradermal reaction employing moccasin venom as a test substance. A positive test indicates a purpuric state, usually associated with thrombocytopenia. Also used for prognosis; a positive which becomes negative is favorable.

mock angina. ANGINA PECTORIS VASOMOTORIA.

mod·a·line (mod'uh·leen, mo'duh·) *n.* 2-Methyl-3-piperidinopyrazine, $C_{10}H_{15}N_3$, an antidepressant drug; used as the sulfate salt.

mo·dal·i·ty (mo·dal'i·tee) *n.* A form of sensation, such as touch, pressure, vision, or audition.

mode, *n.* [L. *modus,* a measure]. That value in a series of observations which occurs most frequently. —**mo·dal** (mo'dul) *adj.*

mod·el, *n.* [It. *modello,* from L. *modulus,* measure]. 1. The form or material pattern of anything to be made, or already existing. 2. CAST (2).

mod·er·ate·ly advanced tuberculosis. Tuberculosis with disseminated lesions of slight to moderate density throughout the volume of one lung or the equivalent in both lungs; dense confluent lesions limited to one-third of the volume of one lung; cavitation less than 4 cm in total diameter.

mod·er·ate mental retardation. Subnormal general intellectual functioning, requiring special training and guidance, in which the intelligence quotient is approximately 36-51.

mod·er·a·tor, *n.* A substance, such as water or graphite, used to reduce the velocity of nuclear particles, especially to slow down neutrons to a thermal equilibrium state and thus to promote a chain reaction.

moderator band. A muscle band in the right ventricle of the heart, between the interventricular septum and the base of the right anterior papillary muscle, transporting a fascicle of the atrioventricular bundle. It was once thought to prevent overdistention of the right ventricle. Syn. *septomarginal band.* NA *trabecula septomarginalis.*

Moderil. Trademark for rescinnamine, an antihypertensive and sedative drug.

modified milk. Any milk altered so that its composition approximates human mother's milk.

modified radical mastoidectomy. An operation that exposes and permanently exteriorizes the diseased portions of the mastoid by removal of the superior and posterior osseous meatal wall and the construction of a plastic meatal flap. It differs from the classic operation in that the ossicles and intact pars tensa of the tympanic membrane are left in place and care is taken not to open into the tympanic cavity. Syn. *Bondy operation.*

modified smallpox. VARIOLOID (2).

mo·di·o·lus (mo·dye'o·lus) *n.*, pl. & genit. sing. **modio·li** (·lye) [L., the hub of a wheel]. The central pillar or axis of the cochlea, around which the spiral canal makes two and one-half turns.

mod·u·la·tor (mod'yoo·lay"tur) *n.* 1. A receptive sensory end organ in light-adapted eyes, of relatively infrequent type, occurring in narrow spectral sensitivity curves or absorption bands in three preferential regions of the spectrum: red-sensitive, 5800 to 6000 angstroms; green-sensitive, 5200 to 5400 angstroms; and blue-sensitive, 4500 to 4700 angstroms. Thought to be related to color sensation and discrimination. Contr. *dominator.* 2. ALLOSTERIC EFFECTOR.

mod·u·lus (mod'yoo·lus) *n.* [L., standard of measure]. 1. The measure of a force, of properties of mass, or their effects. 2. A constant which converts a proportionality into an equality.

mo·dus (mo'dus) *n.* [L.]. Mode, method.

modus ope·ran·di (op"uh·ran'dye, ·dee) [L.]. One's method of doing something.

Moebius. See *Möbius.*

Moel·ler-Bar·low disease (mœl'ur) [J. O. L. *Moeller,* German physician, 1819–1887; and T. *Barlow*]. INFANTILE SCURVY.

Moeller's fluid. REGAUD'S FLUID.

Moeller's glossitis [J. O. L. *Moeller*]. A chronic superficial glossitis, occurring mainly in women, characterized by irregular painful red patches on the tongue, sometimes extending to the cheeks and palate.

Mo·ëna anomaly. Factor IX deficiency.

Moenckeberg. See *Mönckeberg.*

mo·e·no·my·cin A (mo·ee"no·migh'sin) *n.* A surface-active glycolipid, approximately $C_{70}H_{121}N_5O_{40}P$; the main component of the antibiotic bambermycins.

Mogadon. Trademark for nitrazepam, an anticonvulsant and hypnotic drug.

mogi·graph·ia (moj"i·graf'ee·uh) *n.* [Gk. *mogis,* with difficulty, + *-graphia*]. *Obsol.* WRITER'S CRAMP.

mogi·la·lia (moj"i·lay'lee·uh) *n.* [Gk. *mogis,* with difficulty, + *-lalia*]. *Obsol.* Difficult or painful speech, as stammering or stuttering.

mogi·pho·nia (moj"i·fo'nee·uh) *n.* [Gk. *mogis,* with difficulty, + *-phonia*]. *Obsol.* Difficulty in speaking, excited by an effort to sing or speak loudly.

Mohr's salt [K. *Mohr,* German chemist, 1806–1879]. Ferrous ammonium sulfate, $Fe(NH_4)_2.6H_2O$, used as a reagent.

moi·e·ty (moy'e·tee) *n.* [MF. *moité,* half]. A part or portion, especially of a molecule, generally complex, having a characteristic chemical or pharmacological property.

moist, *n.* [MF. *moiste,* from L. *mucidus,* moldy]. Damp; slightly wet; characterized by the presence of fluid.

moist chamber. A type of large culture plate made of heavy glass and having a loosely fitting cover; used in bacteriologic work.

moist gangrene. The invasion of necrotic tissue by microorganisms with resultant putrefaction.

moist papule. CONDYLOMA LATUM.

moist wart. CONDYLOMA ACUMINATUM.

mol (mol, mole) *n.* ²MOLE.

mo·lal (mo'lul) *adj.* Pertaining to moles of a solute per 1000 g of solvent. Compare ¹*molar* (2).

molal solution. A solution which contains one gram-molecular weight or mole of reagent dissolved in 1000 g of solvent.

¹mo·lar (mo'lur) *adj.* [L. *moles,* mass, heap, + *-ar*]. 1. Pertaining to masses, in contradistinction to molecular. 2. Pertaining to moles of solute in a definite volume of solution, usually 1 liter. Abbreviated, M. Compare *molal.* —**mo·lar·i·ty** (mo·lăr'i·tee) *n.*

²molar, *n. & adj.* [L. *molaris,* from *mola,* mill]. 1. A molar tooth. 2. Serving to grind or pulverize.

molar glands. A group of mixed buccal glands near the opening of the parotid duct. NA *glandulae molares.*

mo·lar·i·form (mo·lăr'i·form) *adj.* Shaped like a molar tooth.

molar pregnancy. Gestation in which the ovum has been converted into a fleshy tumor mass or mole. See also *hydatidiform mole.*

molar solution. A solution which contains a gram-molecular weight or mole of reagent in 1000 ml of solution.

molar teeth. Multicuspidate, usually multi-rooted, teeth used for crushing, grinding, or triturating food. In the human primary dentition there are two in each quadrant immediately distal to the canine; in the permanent dentition, three, distal to the premolars. NA *dentes molares.*

mo·las·ses (muh·las'iz) *n.* [Pg. *melaço,* from L. *mellaceum,* must]. The syrupy liquid obtained in refining sugar. It contains a considerable quantity of uncrystallizable sugar, and coloring matter.

¹mold, mould, *n.* [ON. *mugla*]. Any of those fungi which form slimy or cottony growths on foodstuffs, leather, etc.

²mold, mould, *n. & v.* [OF. *modle,* from L. *modulus,* measure]. 1. A cavity or form in which a thing is shaped. 2. To make conform to a given shape, as the fetal head in its passage through the birth canal.

¹mole, *n.* [OE. *māl,* spot, stain, blemish]. 1. A mass formed in the uterus by the maldevelopment of all or part of the embryo or of the placenta and membranes. See also *hydatidiform mole.* 2. A fleshy, pigmented nevus.

²mole, *n.* [Ger. *Mol,* from *Molekulargewicht,* molecular weight]. The weight of a chemical in mass units, usually grams, numerically equal to its molecular weight.

mo·lec·to·my (mo·leck'tuh·mee) *n.* [*mole* + *-ectomy*]. Surgical removal of a mole, usually a pigmented nevus of the skin.

mo·lec·u·lar (mo·leck'yoo·lur) *adj.* 1. Pertaining to or consisting of molecules. 2. Individual, piecemeal.

molecular absorption. INTERNAL ABSORPTION.

molecular biology. The study of the relationship between the properties of specific molecules and the structure and function of living things in which these molecules occur.

molecular death. Death of individual cells; ulceration.

molecular distillation. Distillation performed under a very high vacuum and a short path between the distilland and the condenser so that on the average a molecule of distilland will reach the condenser surface without colliding with another molecule; more properly called short-path, high-vacuum distillation.

molecular exclusion chromatography. GEL FILTRATION CHROMATOGRAPHY.

molecular heat. The molecular weight of a compound multiplied by its specific heat.

molecular layer of the cerebellum. The outermost layer of the cerebellar cortex, made up of neuroglia, a few small ganglion cells, and a reticulum of myelinated and unmyelinated nerve fibers. NA *stratum moleculare cerebelli.*

molecular layer of the retina. One of the two layers, inner and outer, of the retina made up of interlacing dendrites. Syn. *plexiform layer.*

molecular movement. BROWNIAN MOVEMENT.

molecular sieve chromatography. GEL FILTRATION CHROMATOGRAPHY.

molecular volume. The volume of one gram molecule of substance; in the gaseous state under the same conditions of temperature and pressure, the molecular volumes of all substances are equal.

molecular weight. The weight of a molecule of any substance, representing the sum of the weights of its constituent atoms. Abbreviated, M.W.

mol·e·cule (mol'e·kyool) *n.* [F., from NL. *molecula,* diminutive of *moles,* mass]. 1. A minute mass of matter. 2. The smallest quantity into which a substance can be divided and retain its characteristic properties; or the smallest quantity that can exist in a free state.

mo·li·la·lia (mol″i·lay′lee·uh) *n.* [Gk. *molis*, with difficulty, + *-lalia*]. *Obsol.* MOGILALIA.

mo·li·men (mo·lye′mun, mo′li·men) *n.*, pl. **mo·lim·i·na** (mo·lim′i·nuh) [L. effort, exertion, from *moliri*, to make an effort]. 1. Effort. 2. *In physiology*, laborious functioning. 3. *In gynecology*, nervous or circulatory symptoms accompanying menstruation.

mo·lin·a·zone (mo·lin′uh·zone) *n.* 3-Morpholino-1,2,3-benzotriazin-4(3*H*)-one, $C_{11}H_{12}N_4O_2$, an analgesic.

mo·lin·done (mo·lin′dohn) *n.* 3-Ethyl-6,7-dihydro-2-methyl-5-(morpholinomethyl)indol-4(5*H*)-one, $C_{16}H_{24}N_2O_2$, a psychotherapeutic agent; used as the hydrochloride salt.

Mo·lisch's test (mo′lish) [H. *Molisch*, Austrian chemist, 1856–1937]. A test for glucose in which an alcoholic solution of naphthol and concentrated sulfuric acid is added to the unknown. The development of a deep violet color and, upon the addition of water, the formation of a violet precipitate indicate the presence of glucose. If a solution of thymol is used instead of naphthol, the color produced is ruby red which changes to carmine on dilution with water.

Mol·la·ret's meningitis (mohʰ·lahʰ·rehʰ′) [P. *Mollaret*, French physician, 20th century]. An unusual form of benign, recurrent aseptic meningitis, which is seen in individuals who are otherwise free of any systemic or neurologic disease, characterized by sudden attacks of fever associated with signs and symptoms of meningeal irritation and generalized myalgia lasting a few days; during the initial phase the cerebrospinal fluid may be under increased pressure and characteristically exhibits a pleocytosis with a mixture of a thousand or more leukocytes and lymphocytes, but there may be only slight or no pleocytosis during the symptom-free intervals. The disease is followed by a spontaneous cure without residual signs. Syn. *benign recurrent meningitis.*

Møller, McIntosh, and Van Slyke's test. UREA CLEARANCE TEST.

Moller test. FABRICUS-MOLLER TEST.

mol·li·ti·es (mo·lish′ee·eez) *n.* [L.]. Softness.

mollities os·si·um (os′ee·um) [L., of the bones]. OSTEOMALACIA.

Moll's glands [Jacob *Moll*, Dutch ophthalmologist, 1832–1914]. CILIARY GLANDS.

Mol·lus·ca (mol·us′kuh) *n.pl.* [L., from *mollis*, soft]. A large phylum of invertebrates with soft, usually unsegmented bodies protected in many forms by a calcareous shell, and including principally the gastropods (snails, slugs, limpets, conchs), the pelecypods or bivalves (clams, mussels, oysters, scallops), and the cephalopods (squid, octopus, cuttlefish, nautilus).

mol·lus·coid (mol·us′koid) *adj.* Resembling molluscum contagiosum.

mol·lus·cum (muh·lus′kum, mol·us′) *n.*, pl. **mollus·ca** (·kuh) [L. *molluscus*, soft]. Any skin disease in which soft, globoid masses occur. —**mollus·cous** (·kus) *adj.*

molluscum bodies. The ovoid or spheroidal keratin bodies formed in the epithelium by the development of the inclusion bodies of molluscum contagiosum. They are much larger than the epithelial cells originally invaded by the virus of molluscum contagiosum.

molluscum con·ta·gi·o·sum (kon·tay″jee·o′sum). A viral, often venereal disease of the skin, characterized by one or more discrete, waxy dome-shaped nodules with frequent umbilication; molluscum bodies are found in the infected epidermal cells.

molluscum ep·i·the·li·a·le (ep″i·theel·ee·ay′lee). MOLLUSCUM CONTAGIOSUM.

molluscum fi·bro·sum (figh·bro′sum). A cutaneous tumor characteristic of neurofibromatosis; it is situated in the dermis and takes the form of a flesh-colored or violaceous papule varying in size from a few millimeters to a centimeter.

molluscum se·ba·ce·um (se·bay′shee·um, ·see·um). KERATOACANTHOMA.

mol·lusk (mol′usk) *n.* Any member of the phylum Mollusca.

Molofac. A trademark for dioctyl sodium sulfosuccinate, a surfactant and stool softener.

Mo·lo·ney test. A test to determine hypersensitivity to diphtheria toxoid performed by the intradermal injection of a small amount of the toxoid. A positive reaction consists in the development of a characteristic erythema and induration more than 1 cm in diameter in 24 hours.

molt, moult, *v.* & *n.* [ME. *mouten*, from L. *mutare*, to change]. 1. To shed skin, feathers, or hair periodically, with the seasons or in stages of growth. 2. An instance of such shedding.

molybd-, molybdo- [Gk. *molybdos*, lead]. A combining form meaning (a) *lead;* (b) in chemistry, *molybdous.*

mo·lyb·date (mo·lib′date) *n.* Any salt of molybdic acid.

mo·lyb·de·no·sis (mo·lib″de·no′sis) *n.* A condition caused by chronic molybdenum poisoning.

mo·lyb·de·num (mo·lib′de·num, mol″lib·dee′num) *n.* [Gk. *molybdaina*, piece of lead]. Mo = 95.94. A hard, silvery-white metallic element, with a density of about 10.2.

mo·lyb·dic (mo·lib′dick) *adj.* Containing or pertaining to hexavalent molybdenum.

molybdic acid. Molybdic hydroxide, H_2MoO_4, a white powder; soluble in alkalis. Used as a reagent.

mo·lyb·do·phos·phate (mo·lib″do·fos′fate) *n.* PHOSPHOMOLYBDATE.

mo·lyb·dous (mo·lib′dus) *adj.* Containing or pertaining to molybdenum in a lower valence state than in molybdic compounds.

mo·lys·mo·pho·bia (mo·liz″mo·fo′bee·uh) *n.* [Gk. *molysmos*, pollution, + *-phobia*]. Abnormal dread of infection or contamination.

mo·ment, *n.* [F., from L. *momentum*, movement, moment]. 1. The tendency or a measure of the tendency to move a body, especially about a point or axis; defined as the product of the force involved and the perpendicular distance from the line of action of the force to the point or axis of rotation. 2. The arithmetic mean of the deviations of the observations in a frequency distribution from any selected value, each raised to the same power. First power for first moment, second power for second moment, etc.

mo·men·tum (mo·men′tum) *n.* [L., movement, from *movere*, to move]. *In physics*, the mass of a body multiplied by its linear velocity.

mon-, mono- [Gk. *monos*, alone]. A combining form meaning (a) *single, one, alone;* (b) in chemistry, the presence of *one atom* or *group* of that to the name of which it is attached.

mo·nad (mo′nad, mon′ad) *n.* [Gk. *monas, monados*, unit]. 1. A univalent element or radical. 2. Any of the small flagellate protozoa. 3. In meiosis, one of the elements of the tetrad produced by the pairing and splitting of homologous chromosomes. Each monad is separated into a different daughter cell as the result of the two meiotic divisions.

Mo·na·kow's bundle, fasciculus, fibers, or **tract** (mah·nah′kuf) [C. von *Monakow*, Russian neurologist, 1853–1930]. RUBROSPINAL TRACT.

Monakow's nucleus [C. von *Monakow*]. ACCESSORY CUNEATE NUCLEUS.

Monakow's striae [C. von *Monakow*]. STRIAE MEDULLARES VENTRICULI QUARTI.

Monakow's syndrome [C. von *Monakow*]. Contralateral hemiplegia, hemianesthesia, and hemianopsia due to occlusion of the anterior choroid artery.

Mo·nal·di drainage or **method** (mo·nahʰl′dee) [V. *Monaldi*, Italian physician, b. 1899]. A method of draining pulmonary cavities in advanced tuberculosis by continuous suction via a rubber catheter passing through the chest wall.

mon·al·kyl·a·mine (mon·al″kil·uh·meen′, ·am′in) *n.* [*mon-* + *alkylamine*]. Primary alkylamine. See *alkylamine.*
mon·am·ide (mon·am′ide) *n.* MONOAMIDE.
mon·am·ine (mon·am′een, ·in) *n.* MONOAMINE.
mon·ar·thric (mon·ahr′thrick) *adj.* [*mon-* + *arthr-* + *-ic*]. Pertaining to one joint.
mon·ar·thri·tis (mon″ahr·thrigh′tis) *n.* [*mon-* + *arthritis*]. Arthritis affecting only a single joint.
mon·ar·tic·u·lar (mon″ahr·tick′yoo·lur) *adj.* [*mon-* + *articular*]. Pertaining to one joint; MONARTHRIC.
mon·as·ter (mon·as′tur) *n.* [*mon-* + *aster*]. 1. The chromosomes in the equatorial plate at the end of the prophase of mitosis; the "mother-star." 2. The single aster formed in an aberrant type of mitosis, in which the chromosomes are doubled but the cell body does not divide.
mon·ath·e·to·sis (mon″ath·e·to′sis) *n.* [*mon-* + *athetosis*]. Athetosis affecting one limb or side.
mon·atom·ic (mon″uh·tom′ick) *adj.* [*mon-* + *atomic*]. 1. Having but one atom of replaceable hydrogen, as a monatomic acid. 2. Having only one atom, as a monatomic molecule. 3. Having the combining power of one atom of hydrogen, as a monatomic radical. 4. Formed by the replacement of one hydrogen atom in a compound by a radical, as a monatomic alcohol.
Möncke·berg's arteriosclerosis or **sclerosis** (mœnk′e·behrk) [J. G. *Mönckeberg,* German pathologist, 1877–1925]. MEDIAL ARTERIOSCLEROSIS.
Monday fever. METAL FUME FEVER.
Monday morning disease of horses. AZOTURIA (2).
Monday morning dyspnea or **fever.** BYSSINOSIS.
Mon·dor's disease or **syndrome** (mohn·dohr′) [H. *Mondor,* French surgeon, 1885–1962]. Thrombophlebitis of an isolated venous segment, chiefly affecting the thoracoepigastric vein, where it may be mistaken for lymphatic permeation by breast cancer.
mo·nel·lin (mo·nel′in) *n.* A polypeptide derived from the fruit of *Dioscoreophyllum cumminsii* Diels, about 3000 times sweeter than sucrose.
mo·nen·sin (mo·nen′sin) *n.* An antibiotic, $C_{36}H_{62}O_{11}$, produced by *Streptomyces cinnamonensis;* it has antiparasitic, antibacterial, and antifungal activity.
mon·es·trous (mon·es′trus) *adj.* [*mon-* + *estrous*]. Having only one estrus period in each sexual season, said of animals.
Mon·ge's disease (mohng′kheh) [Carlos *Monge,* Peruvian physician, b. 1884]. Chronic ALTITUDE SICKNESS.
Mon·go·li·an (mong·go′lee·un) *adj.* 1. Pertaining to Mongolia or to Mongols. 2. MONGOLOID.
Mongolian idiocy. DOWN'S SYNDROME.
Mongolian spot. A focal bluish-grey discoloration of the skin of the lower back, also aberrantly on the face, present at birth and fading gradually.
mon·gol·ism (mong′guh·liz·um) *n.* [*Mongol* + *-ism*]. DOWN'S SYNDROME.
mon·gol·oid (mong′guh·loid) *adj.* [*Mongol* + *-oid*]. 1. Characteristic of the eastern and northern Asian and native American races of man. 2. Having physical characteristics associated with Down's syndrome.
mongoloid forme fruste. PSEUDOMONGOLISM.
mongoloid idiocy. DOWN'S SYNDROME.
mo·nil·e·thrix (mo·nil′e·thricks) *n.* [L. *monile,* necklace, + Gk. *thrix,* hair]. A congenital defect of the hair characterized by dryness and fragility and by nodes which give it a beaded appearance. Syn. *moniliform hair, beaded hair.*
Mo·nil·ia (mo·nil′ee·uh) *n.* [L., necklaces]. *CANDIDA.* —**monil·i·al** (·ee·ul) *adj.*
Mo·nil·i·a·les (mo·nil″ee·ay′leez) *n.pl.* [NL., from *Monilia*]. An order of Fungi Imperfecti that includes a number of important pathogens of man such as *Candida, Blastomyces, Trychophyton,* and *Cryptococcus.*
mon·i·li·a·sis (mon″i·lye′uh·sis) *n.,* pl. **monilia·ses** (·seez) [*Monilia* + *-iasis*]. CANDIDIASIS.
mo·nil·i·form (mo·nil′i·form) *adj.* [L. *monile,* necklace, + *-iform*]. Constricted or jointed at intervals, as antennae; resembling a string of beads.
moniliform hair. MONILETHRIX.
Mo·nil·i·for·mis (mo·nil″i·for′mis) *n.* [NL., moniliform]. A genus of acanthocephalan worms.
Moniliformis moniliformis. An intestinal parasite of wild rodents and rarely dogs and humans.
mo·nil·i·id (mo·nil′ee·id) *n.* [*Monilia* + *-id*]. CANDIDID.
mon·i·tor (mon′i·tur) *n.* & *v.* [L., one who reminds, advises, or warns]. 1. A person or an apparatus whose function is to give continuous or periodic reports based on scanning or measurements, as of a health or security hazard. 2. To determine periodically or continuously the amount of ionizing radiation or radioactive contamination in an occupied area, or in or on personnel, as a safety measure for health protection.
monitor ionization chamber. 1. An ionization chamber employed for checking the constancy of performance of a roentgen-ray tube. 2. An ionization chamber which detects undesirable radiation; used in health protection.
Mo·niz sign (moo·neesh′, mo·neess′) [A. Egas *Moniz,* Portuguese neurologist, 1874–1955]. A sign in which dorsiflexion of the toes follows forceful passive plantar flexion of the foot at the ankle; said to have the same significance as the Babinski sign.
mon·key, *n.* Any primate of the Cercopithecidae or the Cebidae. Compare *ape.* See also *Old World monkey, New World monkey.*
monkey gland. Testis of a monkey, once used as an implant in Voronoff's operation.
monks·hood, *n.* ACONITE.
Mon·ne·ret's pulse (mohn·e·reh′) [J. *Monneret,* French physician, 1810–1868]. The soft, slow, full pulse associated with some cases of jaundice.
mono-. See *mon-.*
mono·ac·id (mon″o·as′id) *adj.* [*mono-* + *acid*]. 1. Having one replaceable hydroxyl group (OH), as a monoacid base. 2. Capable of uniting directly with a molecule of a monobasic acid, with half a molecule of a dibasic acid, etc.
mono·acid·ic (mon″o·a·sid′ick) *adj.* MONOACID.
mono·am·ide (mon″o·am′ide) *n.* An amide formed by the replacement of a hydrogen in one molecule of ammonia by an acid radical.
mono·am·ine (mon″o·am′een, ·in) *n.* An amine containing one amino group.
monoamine oxidase. An enzyme, found within cells of most tissues, that catalyzes oxidative deamination of monoamines such as norepinephrine and serotonin. Abbreviated, MAO.
monoamine oxidase inhibitor. Any drug, such as isocarboxazid and tranylcypromine, that inhibits monoamine oxidase and thereby leads to an accumulation of the amines on which the enzyme normally acts. Abbreviated, MAOI.
mono·am·ni·ot·ic (mon″o·am″nee·ot′ick) *adj.* [*mono-* + *amniotic*]. Having a single amnion.
mono·ar·tic·u·lar (mon″o·ahr·tick′yoo·lur) *adj.* MONARTICULAR.
mono·azo dye (mon″o·az′o, ·ay′zo) [*mono-* + *azo*]. A dye containing one —N=N— group.
mono·bal·lism (mon″o·bal′iz·um) *n.* [*mono-* + *ballism*]. Ballism confined to one limb.
mono·ba·sic (mon″o·bay′sick) *adj.* [*mono-* + *basic*]. Having one hydrogen which can be replaced by a metal or positive radical, as a monobasic acid.
mon·o·ben·zone (mon″o·ben′zone) *n.* *p*-Benzyloxyphenol, $C_{13}H_{12}O_2$, used therapeutically as a melanin pigment-inhibiting agent.
mono·blast (mon′o·blast) *n.* [*mono-* + *-blast*]. The progenitor of the monocytes found in bone marrow. The nucleus has a finely granular to lacy chromatin structure, nucleoli are present, the cytoplasm shows more gray-blue than other blast cells, and may have pseudopods.

mono·blep·sia (mon″o·blep′see·uh) *n.* [*mono-* + Gk. *blepsis*, sight, + *-ia*]. 1. A condition in which either eye has a better visual power than both together. 2. The form of color blindness in which but one color can be perceived.

mono·blep·sis (mon″o·blep′sis) *n.* MONOBLEPSIA.

mono·bra·chi·us (mon″o·bray′kee·us) *n.* & *adj.* [*mono-* + *brachi-* + *-us*]. 1. An individual lacking one arm congenitally. 2. Characterizing a one-armed condition, congenital or acquired.

mono·bro·mat·ed (mon″o·bro′may·tid) *adj.* Containing one atom of bromine in the molecule.

monobromated camphor. $C_{10}H_{15}BrO$. Camphor in which one atom of hydrogen has been replaced by an atom of bromine. Formerly believed to be sedative.

monobasic calcium phosphate. A form of calcium phosphate.

mono·car·box·yl·ic (mon″o·kahr·bock·sil′ick) *adj.* Containing one carboxyl group.

mono·car·di·an (mon″o·kahr′dee·un) *adj.* [*mono-* + *cardi-* + *-an*, adjectival suffix]. Having a heart with a single atrium and ventricle.

mono·car·dio·gram (mon″o·kahr′dee·o·gram) *n.* [*mono-* + *cardiogram*]. VECTORCARDIOGRAM.

mono·cel·lu·lar (mon″o·sel′yoo·lur) *adj.* UNICELLULAR.

mono·ceph·a·lus (mon″o·sef′uh·lus) *n.* [Gk. *monokephalos*, one-headed, from *kephalē*, head]. CEPHALOTHORACOPAGUS.

mono·chlo·ro·phe·nol (mon″o·klor″o·fee′nol) *n.* CHLOROPHENOL.

mono·chord (mon′o·kord) *n.* [*mono-* + *chord*]. A device once used for testing hearing, particularly for the higher tones of speech.

mono·cho·rea (mon″o·ko·ree′uh) *n.* Chorea confined to a single part of the body.

mono·cho·ri·on·ic (mon″o·kor·ee·on′ick) *adj.* [*mono-* + *chorionic*]. Having a common chorion, as monochorionic twins.

monochorionic twins. IDENTICAL TWINS.

mono·chro·ic (mon″o·kro′ick) *adj.* [Gk. *monochroos*, of one color, + *-ic*]. MONOCHROMATIC.

mono·chro·ma·sia (mon″o·kro·may′zee·uh, ·zhuh) *n.* [*mono-* + *-chromasia*]. TOTAL COLORBLINDNESS.

mono·chro·ma·sy (mon″o·kro′muh·see) *n.* Monochromasia (= TOTAL COLORBLINDNESS).

mono·chro·mat (mon″o·kro′mat) *n.* [Gk. *monochrōmatos*, of one color]. A person in whom all the variations of the world of color are reduced to a system of one color. See also *cone-monochromat, rod-monochromat.*

mono·chro·mate (mon″o·kro′mate) *n.* MONOCHROMAT.

mono·chro·mat·ic (mon″o·kro·mat′ick) *adj.* [Gk. *monochrōmatos* + *-ic*]. 1. Pertaining to or possessing one color or substantially one wavelength of light. 2. *In optics,* having no variation in hue and saturation, and varying only in brightness.

monochromatic aberration. SPHERICAL ABERRATION.

monochromatic objective. An objective corrected for use with monochromatic light, as, for example, the quartz objective corrected for the 2750 Å line.

monochromatic radiation. Electromagnetic radiation of a single wavelength or a narrow range of wavelengths, or photons of the same energy level.

mono·chro·ma·tism (mon″o·kro′muh·tiz·um) *n.* [*monochromatic* + *-ism*]. TOTAL COLORBLINDNESS.

mono·chro·mato·phil (mon″o·kro·mat′o·fil) *adj.* [*mono-* + *chromatophil*]. Exhibiting a strong affinity for a single stain.

mono·chro·ma·tor (mon″o·kro′may·tur) *n.* [*monochromatic* + *-or*]. A light-dispersing instrument used to obtain light of substantially one wavelength, or at least of a very narrow band of the spectrum.

mono·chro·mic (mon″o·kro′mick) *adj.* [Gk. *monochrōmos*, of one color, + *-ic*]. MONOCHROMATIC.

mono·clin·ic (mon″o·klin′ick) *adj.* [*mono-* + *clin-* + *-ic*]. Applied to crystals in which the vertical axis is inclined to one, but is at a right angle to the other, or lateral, axis.

mono·clo·nal (mon″o·klo′nul) *adj.* Pertaining to a single group, or clone, of cells, thus involving an identical cell product. Contr. *polyclonal.*

monoclonal gammopathy. M-COMPONENT HYPERGAMMAGLOBULINEMIA.

mono·coc·cus (mon″o·kock′us) *n.*, pl. **monococci** (·sigh) [*mono-* + *coccus*]. A coccus occurring singly, not united in chains, pairs, or groups.

mono·cot·y·le·do·nous (mon″o·kot″i·lee′duh·nus) *adj.* [*mono-* + *cotyledon* + *-ous*]. Pertaining to the plant subclass Monocotyledoneae; having one cotyledon. Contr. *dicotyledonous.*

mono·cra·ni·us (mon″o·kray′nee·us) *n.* [*mono-* + *crani-* + *-us*]. CEPHALOTHORACOPAGUS.

mono·crot·ic (mon″o·krot′ick) *adj.* [*mono-* + *-crotic*]. Having a single beat or impulse; having a single crested wave.

monocrotic pulse. A pulse in which dicrotism is absent; a pulse with one expansion for each cardiac systole.

mon·oc·u·lar (mon·ock′yoo·lur) *adj.* [L. *monoculus*, one-eyed]. 1. Pertaining to or affecting only one eye, as monocular diplopia; performed with one eye only, as monocular vision. 2. Having a single ocular or eyepiece, as a monocular microscope.

monocular diplopia. Diplopia with a single eye; usually due to hysteria, double pupil, beginning cataract, or subluxated lens.

monocular nystagmus. Nystagmus involving one eye only, as may be seen in spasmus nutans or with brainstem lesions involving the medial longitudinal fasciculus. Less pronounced nystagmus is often present in the other eye.

monocular vision. Seeing with one eye, whether as the result of injury to the other eye, or due to central suppression, as in amblyopia ex anopsia.

mon·oc·u·lus (mon·ock′yoo·lus) *n.* [L., one-eyed, from Gk. *monos*, single, + L. *oculus*, eye]. 1. CYCLOPS. 2. *In surgery,* a bandage for covering one eye.

mono·cy·e·sis (mon″o·sigh·ee′sis) *n.* [*mono-* + Gk. *kyēsis*, pregnancy]. Pregnancy with but one fetus.

mono·cys·tic (mon″o·sis′tick) *adj.* [*mono-* + *cystic*]. Composed of, or containing, but one cyst.

mono·cyte (mon′o·site) *n.* [*mono-* + *-cyte*]. A large, mononuclear leukocyte with a more or less deeply indented nucleus, slate-gray cytoplasm, and fine, usually azurophilic granulation; the same as, or related to, the large mononuclear cell, transitional cell, resting wandering cell, clasmatocyte, endothelial leukocyte, or histiocyte of other classifications. It is the precursor of macrophages. —**mono·cyt·ic** (mon″o·sit′ick) *adj.*

monocyte-lymphocyte ratio. The ratio between monocytes and lymphocytes in the blood; has been used as a diagnostic criterion in the study of tuberculosis.

monocytic angina. INFECTIOUS MONONUCLEOSIS.

monocytic leukemia. A form of leukemia in which the predominant cell type belongs to the monocytic series. Two types are differentiated on the basis of the predominant cell present in the peripheral blood; Naegeli (myelomonocytic) type, and the Schilling type.

monocytic series. The cells concerned in the development of the adult monocyte. See also *monoblast, promonocyte.*

mono·cy·to·ma (mon″o·sigh·to′muh) *n.* A tumor whose parenchyma is composed of monocytes, usually anaplastic.

mono·cy·to·pe·nia (mon″o·sigh″to·pee′nee·uh) *n.* [*monocyte* + *-penia*]. Diminution in the number of monocytes per unit volume of peripheral blood.

mono·cy·to·sis (mon″o·sigh·to′sis) *n.* [*monocyte* + *-osis*]. Increase in the number of monocytes per unit volume of peripheral blood.

mono·dac·tyl·ism (mon″o·dack′ti·liz·um) *n.* [*mono-* + *dactyl-* + *-ism*]. The presence of only one toe or finger on the foot or hand.

mono·der·mo·ma (mon″o·dur·mo′muh) *n.* [*mono-* + *-derm* +

-oma]. A teratoma whose parenchyma is composed of derivatives of a single germ layer.

mono·di·plo·pia (mon″o-di-plo′pee-uh) *n.* [*mono-* + *diplopia*]. MONOCULAR DIPLOPIA.

Monodral Bromide. Trademark for the visceral anticholinergic drug penthienate bromide.

mono·en·er·get·ic radiation (mon″o-en″ur-jet′ick). Radiation composed of particles or photons having equal energy.

mono·eth·a·nol·amine (mon″o-eth″uh-nol′uh-meen) *n.* ETHANOLAMINE.

mo·nog·a·my (muh-nog′uh-mee) *n.* [Gk. *monogamia,* from *gamos,* marriage]. Marriage with only one person at a time.

mono·gas·tric (mon″o-gas′trick) *adj.* [*mono-* + *gastric*]. Having one stomach.

mono·ger·mi·nal (mon″o-jur′mi-nul) *adj.* [*mono-* + *germinal*]. Having or developing from a single ovum, as twins with but one chorionic sac.

mo·nog·o·ny (mo-nog′uh-nee) *n.* [*mono-* + *-gony*]. AGAMOGENESIS; asexual reproduction. —**monogo·nous** (-nus) *adj.*

mono·graph (mon′uh-graf) *n.* [*mono-* + *-graph*]. 1. A detailed documented treatise written about a single subject or a limited area of study or inquiry. 2. The standards of purity and strength, tests, assay, and other requirements officially specified by a pharmacopeia or formulary for a drug or drug dosage form.

mono·hy·brid (mon″o-high′brid) *n.* [*mono-* + *hybrid*]. An individual or type heterozygous in respect to a particular pair of genes.

mono·hy·drate (mon″o-high′drate) *n.* [*mono-* + *hydrate*]. A compound containing one molecule of water of hydration. —**monohy·drat·ed** (-dray-tid) *adj.*

mono·hy·dric (mon″-o-high′drick) *adj.* [*mono-* + *hydr-* + *-ic*]. Containing one replaceable hydrogen atom as a monohydric alcohol or a monohydric acid.

mono·hy·drol (mon″o-high′drol) *n.* HYDROL.

mono·ide·ism (mon″o-eye-dee′iz-um) *n.* [*mono-* + *idea* + *-ism*]. A mental condition marked by the domination of a single idea; persistent and complete preoccupation with one idea, seldom complete. May be induced by suggestion or hypnosis, wherein an elementary idea or image is left isolated and is not synthesized or associated with other ideas or impressions.

mono·in·fect·ed (mon″o-in-feck′tid) *adj.* Infected with one and only one strain of a microorganism.

mono·iodo·ace·tic acid (mon″o-eye-o″do-a-see′tic, -eye-o″do-). Iodoacetic acid ICH_2COOH, colorless or white crystals, soluble in water. Salts of the acid markedly inhibit absorption of glucose through interference with the enzyme system involved in phosphorylation of glucose; the sodium salt is used in studies of carbohydrate metabolism.

mono·ke·tone (mon″o-kee′tone) *n.* A ketone containing one CO group.

mono·lay·er (mon′o-lay″ur) *n.* A monomolecular layer.

monolayer viscosimeter. An instrument used for determining the viscosity of monomolecular films.

mono·lep·sis (mon″o-lep′sis) *n.* [*mono-* + Gk. *lēpsis,* taking, receiving]. The transfer of the characteristics of one parent to a child.

mono·lob·u·lar (mon″o-lob′yoo-lur) *adj.* [*mono-* + *lobular*]. Pertaining to a single lobule.

monolobular cirrhosis. Portal cirrhosis in which a single lobule is surrounded by fibrotic portal spaces. Contr. *multilobular cirrhosis.*

mono·loc·u·lar (mon″o-lock′yoo-lur) *adj.* UNILOCULAR.

mono·ma·nia (mon″o-may′nee-uh) *n.* [*mono-* + *mania*]. A form of mental disorder in which the patient's thoughts and actions are dominated by one subject or one idea, as in paranoid states. —**monoma·ni·ac** (-nee-ack) *n.;* **mono·ma·ni·a·cal** (-ma-nigh′uh-kul) *adj.*

mono·mel·ic (mon″o-mel′ick) *adj.* [Gk. *monomelēs,* consisting of a single limb, from *melos,* limb]. Pertaining to one limb.

monomelic hyperostosis. A type of osteosclerosis. See also *melorheostosis.*

mono·mer (mon′uh-mur) *n.* [*mono-* + *-mer*]. The simplest molecular form of a substance. Contr. *dimer, polymer.*

mono·mer·ic (mon″o-merr′ick) *adj.* [Gk. *monomerēs,* from *meros,* part]. 1. Consisting of a single piece or segment. 2. Consisting of or pertaining to a monomer.

mono·mo·lec·u·lar (mon″o-mo-leck′yoo-lur) *adj.* 1. Pertaining to or consisting of one molecule. 2. Composed of many molecules arranged in one molecule thickness.

monomolecular reaction. FIRST-ORDER REACTION.

mono·mo·ria (mon″o-mo′ree-uh) *n.* [*mono-* + Gk. *mōria,* folly]. INVOLUTIONAL MELANCHOLIA.

mono·mor·phic (mon″o-mor′fick) *adj.* [*mono-* + *morph-* + *-ic*]. Having or existing in only one form.

mono·mor·phous (mon″o-mor′fus) *adj.* [*mono-* + *morph-* + *-ous*]. Having a single form or the same appearance; not polymorphous.

mon·om·pha·lus (mon-om′fuh-lus) *n.* [*mon-* + Gk. *omphalos,* navel]. Conjoined twins with a common umbilical cord.

mono·neph·rous (mon″o-nef′rus) *adj.* [*mono-* + *nephr-* + *-ous*]. Pertaining or limited to one kidney.

mono·neu·ral (mon″o-new′rul) *adj.* [*mono-* + *neural*]. 1. Pertaining to a single nerve. 2. Receiving branches from but one nerve; said of muscles.

mono·neu·ri·tis (mon″o-new-rye′tis) *n.* Neuritis affecting a single nerve.

mononeuritis multiplex. Random affection of two or more nerves.

mono·neu·rop·a·thy (mon″o-new-rop′uh-thee) *n.* [*mono-* + *neuropathy*]. Neuropathy affecting a single nerve.

mononeuropathy multiplex. The random affection of two or more individual nerves, as occurs in diabetes mellitus, polyarteritis nodosa, and Wegener's granulomatosis; presumably due to ischemic infarction of nerve.

mono·nu·cle·ar (mon″o-new′klee-ur) *adj.* Having only one nucleus.

mononuclear cell. 1. Any cell with a single nucleus. 2. A lymphocyte, monocyte, plasma cell, or histiocyte.

mono·nu·cle·ate (mon″o-new′klee-ate, -ut) *adj.* MONONUCLEAR.

mono·nu·cle·o·sis (mon″o-new″klee-o′sis) *n.* [*mononuclear* + *-osis*]. 1. A condition of the blood or tissues in which there is an increase in the number of monocytes above the normal. 2. INFECTIOUS MONONUCLEOSIS.

mono·nu·cle·o·tide (mon″o-new′klee-o-tide) *n.* [*mono-* + *nucleotide*]. A product obtained by hydrolytic decomposition of nucleic acid; it is a compound of phosphoric acid, a pentose, and a purine or pyridine base such as guanine, adenine, cytosine, or uracil.

mono·ox·y·gen·ase (mon″o-ock′si-je-nace, -naze) *n.* Any of a group of enzymes which catalyzes the insertion of one oxygen atom into an organic substrate with reduction of the second oxygen atom to water. Contr. *dioxygenase.*

Monopar. Trademark for stilbazium iodide, an anthelmintic.

mono·pa·re·sis (mon″o-pa-ree′sis, -păr′e-sis) *n.* [*mono-* + *paresis*]. Weakness of all the muscles of one limb, whether arm or leg.

mon·o·pha·gia (mon″o-fay′jee-uh) *n.* [*mono-* + *phag-* + *-ia*]. 1. Desire for a single article of food. 2. The eating of a single daily meal.

mo·noph·a·gism (muh-nof′uh-jiz-um) *n.* [*mono-* + *phag-* + *-ism*]. Habitual eating of a single article of food.

mono·pha·sia (mon″o-fay′zhuh, -zee-uh) *n.* [*mono-* + *-phasia*]. A form of aphasia in which speech is limited to a single syllable, word, or phrase.

mono·pha·sic (mon″o-fay′zick) *adj.* [*mono-* + *phasic*]. Having a single phase.

mono·phe·nol (mon″o-fee′nol) *n.* A compound containing one phenolic hydroxyl group, as in phenol (1).

monophenol oxidase. A copper-containing protein enzyme which catalyzes the oxidation of monophenols, including tyrosine. It is probably identical with tyrosinase and perhaps also with polyphenol oxidase.

mono·pho·bia (mon″o·fo′bee·uh) *n.* [*mono-* + *-phobia*]. Abnormal dread of being alone.

mono·phos·phate (mon″o·fos′fate) *n.* A phosphate with but one atom of phosphorus in the molecule.

mon·oph·thal·mia (mon″off·thal′mee·uh) *n.* [Gk. *monophthalmos*, one-eyed, + *-ia*]. Congenital absence of one eye. Syn. *unilateral anophthalmia.*

mono·phy·let·ic (mon″o·figh·let′ick) *adj.* [*mono-* + *phyletic*]. Pertaining to, or derived from, a single original ancestral type. Contr. *polyphyletic.*

monophyletic theory of hemopoiesis. UNITARIAN THEORY.

mono·phy·odont (mon″o·figh′o·dont) *adj.* [Gk. *monophyēs*, singly grown, unpaired, + *-odont*]. Having but a single set of teeth, the permanent ones.

mono·ple·gia (mon″o·plee′jee·uh) *n.* [*mono-* + *-plegia*]. Paralysis of all the muscles of a single limb. It is designated as brachial or crural, when affecting the arm or the leg, respectively, and as central or peripheral, according to the seat of the causal lesion.

mono·po·dia (mon″o·po′dee·uh) *n.* [Gk. *monopous, monopodos*, one-footed, + *-ia*]. The condition of having but one lower limb.

mono·po·lar (mon″o·po′lur) *adj.* [*mono-* + *polar*]. Pertaining to the use of a single active electrode in an electrical recording system, as in electroencephalography, the second electrode being connected to an electrically inactive part, as the ear.

mon·ops (mon′ops) *n.* [Gk. *monōps*, one-eyed]. CYCLOPS.

mon·op·sia (mon·op′see·uh) *n.* [Gk. *monōps*, one-eyed, + *-ia*]. MONOPHTHALMIA.

mono·psy·cho·sis (mon″o·sigh·ko′sis) *n.* [*mono-* + *psychosis*]. MONOMANIA.

mono·pty·chi·al (mon″o·tye′kee·ul) *adj.* [Gk. *monoptychios*, folding once, from *ptyx*, layer, fold]. Arranged in a single layer, as the epithelial cells of some glands.

mono·pus (mon′o·pus) *n.* [Gk. *monopous*, one-footed]. An individual with congenital absence of one foot or leg.

mono·py·ram·i·dal (mon″o·pi·ram′i·dul) *adj.* Having only one (renal) pyramid.

monopyramidal kidney. UNILOBULAR KIDNEY.

mon·or·chid (mon·or′kid) *n.* [Gk. *monorchis*, from *mon-* + *orchis*]. A person who has but one testis, or in whom only one testis has descended into the scrotum.

mon·or·chid·ism (mon·or′kid·iz·um) *n.* [*monorchid* + *-ism*]. Congenital absence of one testis. —**monorchid,** *adj.*

mon·or·chism (mon·or′kiz·um) *n.* MONORCHIDISM.

mon·or·rhi·nous (mon″o·rye′nus) *adj.* [*mono-* + *rhin-* + *-ous*]. Having a single median nasal cavity.

mono·sac·cha·ride (mon″o·sack′uh·ride, ·rid) *n.* [*mono-* + *saccharide*]. A carbohydrate which cannot be hydrolyzed to a simpler carbohydrate, hence called a simple sugar; chemically, a polyhydric alcohol having reducing properties associated with an actual or potential aldehyde or ketone group. It may contain 3 to 10 carbon atoms, and on this basis be classified as a triose, tetrose, pentose, hexose, heptose, octose, nonose, or decose. A diose, glycolaldehyde, is by some classed as a monosaccharide, but does not exhibit the characteristic properties of the class.

mono·scel·ous (mon″o·sel′us, ·skel′us) *adj.* [Gk. *monoskelēs*, on one leg, from *skelos*, leg]. One-legged.

mon·ose (mon′oce) *n.* [*mono*saccharide + *-ose*]. MONOSACCHARIDE.

mono·so·di·um glutamate (mon″o·so′dee·um). Monosodium L-glutamate, $HOOCCHNH_2CH_2CH_2COONa$, used intravenously for symptomatic treatment of hepatic coma in which there is a high blood level of ammonia. It imparts a meat flavor to foods. Abbreviated, MSG. Syn. *sodium glutamate.*

monosodium or·tho·phos·phate (orth″o·fos′fate). SODIUM BIPHOSPHATE.

mono·som·a·tous (mon″o·som′uh·tus) *adj.* [*mono-* + *somat-* + *-ous*]. Pertaining to a monstrosity involving a single body.

mono·some (mon′o·sohm) *n.* [*mono-* + chromo*some*]. 1. An unpaired chromosome. See also *monosomy.* 2. An individual ribosome, which may be obtained from a polyribosome by the action of ribonuclease. —**mono·so·mic** (mon″o·so′mick) *adj.*

mono·so·mus (mon″o·so′mus) *adj.* [*mono-* + Gk. *sōma*, body, + *-us*]. Having a single body, as dicephalus monosomus.

mono·so·my (mon′o·so″mee) *n.* [*monosome* + *-y*]. The state of having one less than the normal diploid number of chromosomes.

mono·spasm (mon′o·spaz·um) *n.* A spasm limited to one limb.

Mono·spo·ri·um (mon″o·spor′ee·um) *n.* [NL., from *mono-* + Gk. *spora*, seed]. A genus of the Fungi Imperfecti. The species *Monosporium apiospermum* and *M. scleriotiale* have been isolated in cases of white-grained mycetoma.

Mono·spot test. A commercial agglutination test to detect heterophile antibodies in patients suspected of having infectious mononucleosis.

mono·stea·rin (mon″o·stee′ur·in, ·steer′in) *n.* [*mono-* + *stearin*]. GLYCERYL MONOSTEARATE.

mon·os·tot·ic (mon″os·tot′ick) *adj.* [*mon-* + *ost-* + *-otic*]. Involving only one bone.

mono·stra·tal (mon″o·stray′tul) *adj.* Arranged in a single layer or stratum.

mono·symp·to·mat·ic (mon″o·simp″tuh·mat′ick) *adj.* Having but a single symptom.

mono·syn·ap·tic (mon″o·si·nap′tick) *adj.* Involving only one synapse.

monosynaptic reflex. Any reflex involving only one synapse and no internuncial neurons, as in the patellar reflex.

mono·ter·pene (mon″o·tur′peen) *n.* A terpene having a composition represented by $C_{10}H_{16}$.

Monotheamin. Trademark for theophylline monoethanolamine.

mono·ther·mia (mon″o·thur′mee·uh) *n.* [*mono-* + *therm-* + *-ia*]. Lack of normal diurnal variation in body temperature.

mon·otic (mon·o′tick, mon·ot′ick) *adj.* [*mon-* + *otic*]. Pertaining to or affecting but one of the ears.

mo·not·o·cous (mo·not′uh·kus) *adj.* [Gk. *monotokos*, from *mono-* + *tokos*, parturition]. Producing one young at a birth.

mono·treme (mon′o·treem) *n.* [*mono-* + Gk. *trēma*, hole]. An egg-laying mammal; a member of the order Monotremata, comprising the platypuses and the echidnas.

mono·trich·ic (mon″o·trick′ick) *adj.* MONOTRICHOUS.

mo·not·ri·chous (mo·not′ri·kus) *adj.* [*mono-* + *trich-* + *-ous*]. Characterizing a unicellular organism in which there is but one flagellum.

mono·trop·ic (mon″o·trop′ick) *adj.* [*mono-* + *-tropic*]. Occurring in one crystalline form only.

mono·typ·ic (mon′o·tip′ick) *adj.* [*mono-* + *typ-* + *-ic*]. Having only one member or subgroup; said especially of genera having a single species.

mono·va·lent (mon″o·vay′lunt, mo·nov′uh·lunt) *adj.* UNIVALENT.

mono·xen·ic (mon″o·zen′ick) *adj.* [*mono-* + *xen-* + *-ic*]. Of laboratory animals, deliberately contaminated with a single species of microorganism but otherwise germ-free (axenic). Contr. *dixenic.*

mo·nox·e·nous (mo·nock′se·nus) *adj.* [*mono-* + *xen-* + *-ous*]. *In parasitology,* confined to a single species of host.

mon·ox·ide (muh·nock′side, mon·ock′) *n.* 1. An oxide containing a single oxygen atom. 2. A popular name for carbon monoxide.

mono·zy·got·ic (mon″o·zye·got′ick, ·go′tick) *adj.* [*mono-* +

zygote + *-ic*]. Developed from a single fertilized egg or zygote, as identical twins.

mono·zy·gous (mon″o·zye′gus) *adj.* [by false analogy to such words as *homozygous*]. MONOZYGOTIC.

Mon·ro's foramen [A. *Monro* (Secundus), Scottish anatomist, 1733–1817]. INTERVENTRICULAR FORAMEN.

mons (monz, monce) *n.*, pl. **mon·tes** (mon′teez) [L., mountain]. *In anatomy*, an eminence.

Mon·sel's salt. Ferric subsulfate, approximately $Fe_4(OH)_2$-$(-SO_4)_5$, a styptic and astringent used in solution.

Mon·son curve. *In prosthodontics*, the curve of occlusion in which each cusp and incisal edge touches or conforms to a segment of the surface of an imaginary sphere 8 inches in diameter; the center of the sphere is in the region of the glabella. See also *compensating curve*.

mons pu·bis (pew′bis) [NA]. The eminence of the lower anterior abdominal wall above the superior rami of the pubic bones.

mon·ster, *n.* [L. *monstrum*, monster, portent, from *monere*, to warn]. A fetus (rarely an adult) which, through congenital faulty development, is incapable of properly performing the vital functions, or which, owing to an excess or deficiency of parts, differs markedly from the normal type of the species; TERATISM.

mon·stri·cide (mon′stri·side) *n.* [*monstri-*, monster, + *-cide*]. The killing of a monster.

mon·strip·a·ra (mon·strip′uh·ruh) *n.* [*monstri-*, monster, + *-para*]. A woman who has given birth to one or more monsters.

mon·stro·cel·lu·lar sarcoma (mon″stro·sel′yoo·lur). A relatively uncommon circumscribed tumor of the brain, derived from the blood vessels, and characterized histologically by dense streams of spindle cells and central areas of bizarre giant cells.

mon·stros·i·ty (mon·stros′i·tee) *n.* [L. *monstrositas*]. 1. The condition of being a monster. 2. MONSTER.

mons ve·ne·ris (ven′e·ris) [L.]. The mound of Venus; MONS PUBIS.

Mon·teg·gia's fracture (mohn·teyj′jah) [G. B. *Monteggia*, Italian surgeon, 1762–1815]. Fracture of the upper shaft of the ulna, with associated dislocation of the radial head.

Mon·te·ne·gro reaction. The intradermal response to the Leishmanin skin test.

Montenegro's test. An intradermal test of aid in the diagnosis of leishmaniasis.

Mont·gom·ery's glands [W. F. *Montgomery*, Irish obstetrician, 1797–1859]. Apocrine sweat glands in the areola of the nipple of the breast.

Montgomery's tubercles [W. F. *Montgomery*]. The elevations due to the apocrine sweat glands in the areola of the nipple which appear more prominent during pregnancy and lactation.

month·ly period. MENSTRUAL PERIOD.

monthly sickness. MENSTRUATION.

mon·tic·u·lus (mon·tick′yoo·lus) *n.* [L., small mountain]. 1. A small elevation. 2. MONTICULUS CEREBELLI.

monticulus ce·re·bel·li (serr″e·bel′eye) [BNA]. The prominent central portion of the superior vermis of the cerebellum including the culmen and declive.

mont·mo·ril·lon·ite (mont″mo·ril′uh·nite) *n.* [after *Montmorillon*, France]. $Al_2Si_4O_{10}(OH)_2.nH_2O$; the principal mineral constituent of bentonite and fuller's earth, occurring as a white or grayish to rose-blue claylike substance with a smooth, greasy texture.

mood, *n.* A sustained emotional or feeling tone, such as excitement, joy, or depression.

moon face. Rounded, full facies characteristic of hyperadrenocorticism.

Moon's molars [H. *Moon*, British surgeon, 19th century]. Maldevelopment of the first molar teeth in congenital syphilis; the cusps are so deformed that they resemble a mulberry.

Moo·ren's ulcer (mo′rᵉn) [A. *Mooren*, German ophthalmologist, 1828–1899]. A rare, progressive condition which develops in the peripheral cornea adjacent to the limbus; characterized by an overhanging anterior margin. Its cause and treatment are presently unknown.

Moore's lightning streaks. An entoptic phenomenon consisting of flashes of light seen on the temporal side of the eye.

Moore's syndrome [M. T. *Moore*, U.S. neurologist, b. 1901]. ABDOMINAL EPILEPSY.

Moo·ser bodies (mo′zur) [H. *Mooser*, Swiss pathologist, b. 1891]. The intracytoplasmic rickettsiae in the serosal cells over the testes observed in the Neill-Mooser reaction.

Mooser reaction or **test** [H. *Mooser*]. NEILL-MOOSER REACTION.

moral idiocy, imbecility, or **insanity.** Inability to understand moral principles and values and to act in accordance with them, apparently without impairment of the reasoning and intellectual faculties. Once used for medicolegal purposes, the concept pertains to aspects of psychopathic and sociopathic personality disturbances.

moral masochism. Masochism in which it is speculated that there is a need for punishment arising from unconscious sexual desires and reactivation of the Oedipus complex, characterized by self-destructive acts or the provocation of punishment from authority figures. Ascetic practices according to this theory are related to moral masochism, the act of mortifying being a distorted expression of blocked sexuality.

moral treatment or **therapy.** A form of treatment of patients hospitalized for mental disorders which was introduced and prevailed in the first half of the nineteenth century, and which emphasized humane care, religious observance, and useful occupational tasks while hospitalized; the forerunner of milieu therapy.

mor·amen·tia (mor″uh·men′shee·uh) *n.* [*mor*al + *amentia*]. MORAL IDIOCY.

mo·ran·tel (mo·ran′tel) *n.* (*E*)-1,4,5,6-Tetrahydro-1-methyl-2-[2-(3-methyl-2-thienyl)vinyl]pyrimidine, $C_{12}H_{16}N_2S$, an anthelmintic agent; used as the tartrate salt.

Moranyl. A trademark for sodium suramin, an antitrypanosomal and antifilarial drug.

Mo·rax-Axen·feld bacillus [V. *Morax*, French ophthalmologist, 1866–1935; and E. *Axenfeld*]. MORAXELLA LACUNATA.

Morax-Axenfeld conjunctivitis [V. *Morax* and E. *Axenfeld*]. Chronic conjunctivitis caused by *Moraxella lacunata*.

Mo·rax·el·la (mor″ack·sel′uh) *n.* [V. *Morax*]. A genus of bacteria, family Brucellaceae.

Moraxella lac·u·na·ta (lack″yoo·nay′tuh) [L., pitted]. A nonmotile, gram-negative, short rod bacterium, occurring singly, in pairs, or in short chains; the type species of its genus. Syn. *Morax-Axenfeld bacillus*.

mor·bi (mor′bye) [L., genitive of *morbus*]. Of a disease, as materies morbi, the agent producing a disease.

mor·bid (mor′bid) *adj.* [L. *morbidus*, from *morbus*, disease]. 1. PATHOLOGIC. 2. Unwholesome; unhealthy.

morbid anatomy. PATHOLOGIC ANATOMY.

morbid hunger syndrome. KLEINE-LEVIN SYNDROME.

morbid impulse. An uncontrollable impulse.

morbid introspection. Unwholesome self-examination; irrational and obsessive dwelling upon one's own thoughts, feelings, impulses, fears, or conduct.

mor·bid·i·ty (mor·bid′i·tee) *n.* [*morbid* + *-ity*]. 1. The quality or state of being diseased. 2. The conditions inducing disease. 3. The ratio of the number of sick individuals to the total population of a community.

morbidity rate. The number of cases of a disease for a certain number of the population in a given time interval.

mor·bif·ic (mor·bif′ick) *adj.* [L. *morb*us, disease, + *-fic*, from L. *-ficus*, producing]. Producing disease; PATHOGENIC.

mor·bil·li (mor·bil'eye, ·ee) *n.* [ML., pl. of *morbillus*, macule]. MEASLES.
mor·bil·li·form (mor·bil'i·form) *adj.* [*morbilli* + *-iform*]. Resembling measles or the fine dusky rose-red, confluent maculopapular eruption seen in measles.
mor·bus (mor'bus) *n.* genit. **mor·bi** (·bye) [L.]. DISEASE.
morbus an·gli·cus (ang'gli·kus) [ML., English]. RICKETS.
morbus ca·du·cus (ka·dew'kus) [L., falling, fallen]. *Obsol.* EPILEPSY.
morbus cae·ru·le·us (se·roo'lee·us) [L., blue]. CYANOTIC CONGENITAL HEART DISEASE.
morbus car·di·a·cus (kahr·dye'uh·kus). Heart disease.
morbus cas·tren·sis (kas·tren'sis) [L., from *castrum*, camp]. EPIDEMIC TYPHUS.
morbus coe·li·a·cus (see·lye'uh·kus). CELIAC SYNDROME.
morbus cor·dis (kor'dis) [L., of the heart]. Heart disease.
morbus cox·ae (kock'see). Hip disease; tuberculous coxitis.
morbus cu·cul·la·ris (kew"kuh·lair'is, kuk"yoo·lair'is) [L., from *cuculus*, cuckoo]. Whooping cough; PERTUSSIS.
morbus di·vi·nus (di·vye'nus). EPILEPSY.
morbus gal·li·cus (gal'i·kus). SYPHILIS.
morbus he·mor·rhag·i·cus neo·na·to·rum (hem"o·raj'i·kus nee"o·nay·to'rum). HEMORRHAGIC DISEASE OF THE NEWBORN.
morbus hun·gar·i·cus (hung·găr'i·kus). EPIDEMIC TYPHUS.
morbus mac·u·lo·sus neo·na·to·rum (mack"yoo·lo'sus nee"o·nay·to'rum). HEMORRHAGIC DISEASE OF THE NEWBORN.
morbus maculosus Werlhofii. IDIOPATHIC THROMBOCYTOPENIC PURPURA.
morbus mag·nus (mag'nus) [L., grand mal]. Recurrent GENERALIZED SEIZURES.
morbus major [L.]. Grand mal epilepsy; recurrent GENERALIZED SEIZURES.
morbus med·i·co·rum (med·i·ko'rum) [L., of physicians]. An abnormal or excessive tendency to seek the advice of physicians, as for imaginary diseases.
morbus mi·ser·i·ae (mi·zerr'ee·ee). Any disease due to poverty and neglect.
morbus Pageti pa·pil·lae (pa·pil'ee). PAGET'S DISEASE (1).
morbus phlyc·te·noi·des (flick"te·noy'deez). PEMPHIGUS.
morbus pu·li·ca·ris (pew"li·kair'is) [L., from *pulex*, flea]. EPIDEMIC TYPHUS.
morbus re·gi·us (ree'jee·us) [L., lit., royal disease]. JAUNDICE.
morbus sa·cer (say'sur, sas'ur) [L., sacred]. EPILEPSY.
morbus sal·ta·to·ri·us (sal"tuh·tor'ee·us). CHOREA.
morbus ve·sic·u·la·ris (ve·sick"yoo·lair'is). PEMPHIGUS.
morbus vir·gin·e·us (vur·jin'ee·us). CHLOROSIS.
morbus vul·pis (vul'pis) [L., of the fox]. ALOPECIA.
mor·cel·la·tion (mor"se·lay'shun) *n.* [F. *morceler*, to divide into pieces, from OF. *morcel*, piece]. A procedure whereby a solid tissue is reduced to fragments.
mor·da·cious (mor·day'shus) *adj.* [L. *mordax*, *mordacis*, from *mordere*, to bite]. Biting, pungent.
mor·dant (mor'dunt) *n.* & *v.* [F., biting]. 1. A substance, such as alum, phenol, aniline, that fixes the dyes used in coloring materials or in staining tissues and bacteria. 2. To treat with a mordent.
Mo·rel ear (moʰ·rel') [F. *Morel*, French psychiatrist, 20th century]. An enlarged, smooth ear with a thin edge.
Morel-Kraepelin disease [B. A. *Morel*, French neuropsychiatrist, 1809–1873; and E. *Kraepelin*]. DEMENTIA PRAECOX.
Morel-Moore syndrome. STEWART-MOREL-MORGAGNI SYNDROME.
Morel's syndrome [F. *Morel*]. STEWART-MOREL-MORGAGNI SYNDROME.
Mor·ga·gni-Adams-Stokes syndrome (mor·gaʰnʸ'ee) [G. B. *Morgagni*, Italian anatomist and pathologist, 1682–1771; R. *Adams*; and W. *Stokes*]. STOKES-ADAMS SYNDROME.
mor·ga·gni·an (mor·gah'nee·un) *adj.* Described by or associated with Giovanni Battista Morgagni, Italian anatomist and pathologist, 1682–1771.
morgagnian cataract. A hypermature cataract in which the lens consists of a sac of milky fluid with a dense nucleus lying at the bottom. May be associated with phacolytic glaucoma.
morgagnian cyst. A vesicle derived from the paramesonephric duct attached to the oviduct or head of the epididymis.
morgagnian globules. Fragments of lens substance seen grossly in cataract, associated microscopically with macrophages.
Morgagni's caruncle [G. B. *Morgagni*]. The middle lobe of the prostate.
Morgagni's concha [G. B. *Morgagni*]. SUPERIOR NASAL CONCHA.
Morgagni's disease [G. B. *Morgagni*]. STOKES-ADAMS SYNDROME.
Morgagni's foramen. FORAMEN OF MORGAGNI.
Morgagni's glands [G. B. *Morgagni*]. URETHRAL GLANDS.
Morgagni's hernia [G. B. *Morgagni*]. Parasternal hernia of the diaphragm.
Morgagni's sinus. SINUS OF MORGAGNI.
Morgagni's syndrome [G. B. *Morgagni*]. STEWART-MOREL-MORGAGNI SYNDROME.
Morgagni-Stewart-Morel syndrome. STEWART-MOREL-MORGAGNI SYNDROME.
Morgagni-Stokes-Adams syndrome. STOKES-ADAMS SYNDROME.
Morgagni's ventricle [G. B. *Morgagni*]. LARYNGEAL VENTRICLE.
Mor·gan's bacillus [H. *Morgan*, British physician, 1863–1931]. *Proteus morganii.* See *Proteus.*
morgue, *n.* [F.]. 1. A place where unknown dead are exposed for identification. 2. A place where dead bodies are stored pending disposition or for autopsy.
mo·ria (mo'ree·uh) *n.* [Gk. *mōria*, folly]. 1. A dementia characterized by talkativeness and silliness. 2. Abnormal desire to joke. See also *witzelsucht.*
mor·i·bund (mor'i·bund) *adj.* [L. *moribundus*]. In a dying condition.
Mor·i·son's pouch [J. R. *Morison*, English surgeon, 1853–1939]. HEPATORENAL POUCH.
Morison-Talma operation [J. R. *Morison* and S. *Talma*]. Omentopexy for the relief of ascites due to cirrhosis of the liver.
Mör·ner's reagent. A solution of formalin, concentrated sulfuric acid, and distilled water, used to test for tyrosine.
Mörner's test. A test for tyrosine, which consists in the development of a green color on boiling with H_2SO_4 containing formaldehyde. See also *Mörner's reagent.*
Mornidine. Trademark for the sedative and antiemetic drug pipamazine.
morn·ing glory syndrome. An unusual congenital anomaly of the optic disk, characterized by a funnel-shaped nerve head containing a dot of whitish tissue in its center, an elevated pigmented ring around the disk, and the retinal blood vessels breaking up into manifold narrow branches at the disk's edge. Visual acuity is seriously diminished.
morning sickness. Nausea and vomiting, usually in the early part of the day; a common symptom of pregnancy from about the end of the first month, usually ceasing by the end of the third month.
mo·ron (mo'ron) *n.* [Gk. *mōros*, dull, stupid]. A mentally defective person with a mental age roughly between 7 and 12 years, or, if a child, an I.Q. between 50 and 69.
mo·ron·i·ty (mo·ron'i·tee) *n.* The condition of being a moron.
Mo·ro reflex, reaction, or **response** [Ernst *Moro*, German pediatrician, 1874–1951]. The startle reflex observed in normal infants from birth through the first few months, consisting in abduction and extension of all extremities with extension and fanning of all digits except for flexion of thumbs and index fingers, followed by flexion and adduction of the extremities as in an embrace; may be elicited by altering the equilibrium or the plane between the child's head and trunk, or by a loud noise. Consistent

failure to respond may indicate diffuse central nervous system damage, while asymmetric responses are seen in palsies of both central and peripheral origin. The presence of the reflex after six months of age usually indicates cerebral cortical disturbance.

mo·ro·sis (mo·ro'sis) *n.* [Gk. *mōrōsis*]. MORONITY.

Moro test. 1. An important test of the integrity of an infant's neurologic responses, consisting in elicitation of the Moro reflex. 2. A skin test performed by inunction of 50% O.T., Koch, in an ointment base. A local erythematous reaction appearing in from 24 to 48 hours indicates present or past infection with tubercle bacilli.

-morph [Gk. *-morphos,* -shaped, from *morphē,* shape]. A combining form designating *a category of individuals or of substances having a* (specified) *form or structure.*

morph-, morpho- [Gk. *morphē,* form, shape]. A combining form meaning *form* or *structure.*

mor·phea (mor'fee·uh) *n.* [ML., from Gk. *morphē,* shape]. Scleroderma in which the changes are limited to local areas of the skin and associated subcutaneous tissue. Syn. *circumscribed scleroderma.*

mor·phia (mor'fee·uh) *n.* MORPHINE.

-morphic [*morph-* + *-ic*]. A combining form meaning *having a* (specified) *form.*

mor·phine (mor'feen, -fin, mor·feen') *n.* [F., from Gk. *Morpheus,* god of dreams, + *-ine*]. $C_{17}H_{19}NO_3.H_2O$. The principal and most active alkaloid of opium; a narcotic analgesic used in the form of the hydrochloride and sulfate salts, especially the latter.

morphine-scopolamine anesthesia. TWILIGHT SLEEP.

mor·phin·ism (mor'fi·niz·um) *n.* 1. Morphine addiction. 2. Morphine poisoning.

mor·phi·no·ma·nia (mor''fi·no·may'nee·uh) *n.* The craving for morphine resulting from its habitual use.

mor·phio·ma·nia (mor''fee·o·may'nee·uh) *n.* MORPHINOMANIA.

morpho-. See *morph-.*

mor·pho·bi·om·e·try (mor''fo·bye·om'e·tree) *n.* [*morpho-* + *bio-* + *-metry*]. The statistics of the shape, size, and structure of living things or parts thereof. —**morpho·bio·met·ric** (·bye''o·met'rick) *adj.*

mor·pho·gen·e·sis (mor''fo·jen'e·sis) *n.* [*morpho-* + *-genesis*]. The morphologic transformations including growth, alterations of germinal layers, and differentiation of cells and tissues during development. Syn. *topogenesis.* —**morpho·ge·net·ic** (·je·net'ick), **morpho·gen·ic** (·jen'ick) *adj.*

morphogenetic hormone. EVOCATOR.

morphogenic hormone. EVOCATOR.

mor·phog·e·ny (mor·foj'e·nee) *n.* MORPHOGENESIS.

mor·pho·line (mor'fuh·leen, ·lin) *n.* Tetrahydro-2*H*-1,4-oxazine, C_4H_9NO, a strongly basic liquid; used as a solvent.

mor·phol·o·gy (mor·fol'uh·jee) *n.* [*morpho-* + *-logy*]. The branch of biology which deals with structure and form. It includes the anatomy, histology, and cytology of the organism at any stage of its life history. —**mor·pho·log·ic** (mor''fuh·loj'ick), **morpholog·i·cal** (·i·kul) *adj.;* **mor·phol·o·gist** (mor·fol'uh·jist) *n.*

mor·phom·e·try (mor·fom'e·tree) *n.* [*morpho-* + *-metry*]. The measurement of the forms of organisms.

-morphosis [Gk. *morphōsis,* process of formation]. A combining form meaning *formation or change of form* of a specified thing or in a specified way.

-morphous [Gk. *-morphos,* from *morphē,* form]. A combining form meaning *having a* (specified) *form.*

-morphy [*morph-* + *-y*]. A combining form designating *the condition or characteristic of having a* (specified) *form.*

Morquio-Brailsford disease [L. *Morquio* and J. F. *Brailsford*]. MORQUIO'S SYNDROME.

Mor·quio's syndrome (mor'kyo) [L. *Morquio,* Uruguayan physician, 1867–1935]. Mucopolysaccharidosis IV, transmitted as an autosomal recessive characterized chemically by the presence of large amounts of keratosulfate in urine, and clinically by severe, distinctive bone changes, including dwarfism due to shortening of the spine and kyphoscoliosis, moderate shortening of the extremities and protruding sternum; the facies is typical with broad mouth, prominent maxilla, short nose, and widely spaced teeth. Clouding of the cornea usually appears later than in Hurler's syndrome, and there may be aortic regurgitation. Mental impairment is variable, but neurologic symptoms frequently result from spinal cord and medullary compression. Syn. *Brailsford-Morquio syndrome, familial osteochondrodystrophy.*

mors, *n.,* genit. **mor·tis** [L.]. DEATH.

mor·sal (mor'sul) *adj.* [L. *morsus,* bite, + *-al*]. Pertaining to the cutting or grinding portion of a tooth; OCCLUSAL.

mors pu·ta·ti·va (pew''tuh·tye'vuh). Apparent death.

mors sub·i·ta (sub'i·tuh, sue'bi·tuh). Sudden death.

mor·sus (mor'sus) *n.* [L., bite, sting]. A bite or sting.

morsus stom·a·chi (stom'uh·kye). Pain in the stomach; HEARTBURN.

morsus ven·tric·u·li (ven·trick'yoo·lye). Pain in the stomach; HEARTBURN.

mor·tal (mor'tul) *adj.* [L. *mortalis,* from *mors,* death]. 1. Liable to death or dissolution. 2. Causing death; fatal.

mor·tal·i·ty (mor·tal'i·tee) *n.* [L. *mortalitas*]. 1. The quality of being mortal. 2. DEATH RATE.

mor·tar (mor'tur) *n.* [L. *mortarium*]. A bowl-shaped vessel of porcelain, iron, glass, or other material; used for pulverizing and mixing substances by means of a pestle.

mort d'amour (mor da·moor') [F., death from love]. Sudden death during sexual intercourse, presumably due to cardiac arrhythmia.

mor·ti·fi·ca·tion (mor''ti·fi·kay'shun) *n.* [L. *mortificatio,* from *mortificare,* to kill, mortify]. 1. GANGRENE. 2. NECROSIS.

Morton's foot. MORTON'S METATARSALGIA.

Mor·ton's metatarsalgia [T. G. *Morton,* U.S. surgeon, 1835–1903]. A specific clinical type of metatarsalgia characterized by severe pain between the heads of the third and fourth metatarsal bones and due to retrogressive changes at the point of union of the digital branches from the medial and lateral plantar nerves.

Morton's neuroma [T.G. *Morton*]. A mass, clinically resembling a neuroma, involving the neurovascular bundle of an intermetatarsal space, especially between the 3rd and 4th metatarsals; it consists of fibrosis and fibronoid degeneration in continuity with the intermetatarsal bursa, and fibrosis of the adjacent fat.

Morton's syndrome [D. J. *Morton,* U.S. orthopedist, 1884–1960]. A condition characterized by tenderness at the head of the second metatarsal bone, callosities beneath the second and third metatarsals, and hypertrophy of the second metatarsal, due to a short first metatarsal bone.

Morton's toe. A painful condition of one or more toes and metatarsalgia characterized by hyperextension deformity at the metatarsophalangeal joint and flexion contracture of the proximal interphalangeal joint.

mor·tu·ary (mor'choo·err''ee) *adj.* & *n.* [L. *mortuarius*]. 1. Pertaining to death or burial. 2. MORGUE. 3. A funeral home.

mor·u·la (mor'yoo·luh, mor'oo·luh) *n.* [diminutive of L. *morum,* blackberry, mulberry]. A type of solid blastula, without a blastocoele but having central cells not reaching the free surface. Frequently used, incorrectly, for the late cleavage stage of the mammalian ovum.

Mor·van's disease or **syndrome** (mor·vahⁿ') [A. M. *Morvan,* French physician, 1819–1917]. A disease in adults, characterized by trophic changes of the distal extremities and particularly the fingers, with painless and very slowly healing lesions, a dissociated type of sensory loss, and muscular atrophy of arms and legs. Now acknowledged to be an example of syringomyelia.

mor·vin (mor'vin) *n.* MALLEIN.

mo·sa·ic (mo·zay'ick) *n.* [ML. *musaicus,* from Gk. *mouseios,* of the Muses]. 1. A pattern made on a surface by the assembly and arrangement of many small pieces. 2. *In genetics,* an individual with adjacent cells of different genetic constitution, as a result of mutation, somatic crossing-over, chromosome elimination, or chimera formation. 3. *In embryology,* an egg in which the cells of the early cleavage stages have already a type of cytoplasm which determines its later fate. Compare *regulative.* 4. In plant pathology, infection with a virus which produces a characteristic spotting, as in tobacco mosaic disease.

mosaic bone. Microscopically, bone appearing as though formed of small pieces fitted together, due to cement lines indicating regional alternating periods of osteogenesis and osteoclasis; characteristic of Paget's disease.

mosaic cleavage. DETERMINATE CLEAVAGE.

mosaic disease. A virus disease of plants.

mosaic fungus. An artifact consisting of a deposition of cholesterol crystals around the borders of epithelial cells, seen in skin scrapings.

mo·sa·i·cism (mo·zay'i·siz·um) *n.* [*mosaic* + *-ism*]. *In genetics,* the presence of cells with differing genetic constitution in the same individual.

Mosch·co·witz's disease or **syndrome** [E. *Moschcowitz,* U.S. physician, 1879–1964]. THROMBOTIC THROMBOCYTOPENIC PURPURA.

Moschcowitz's operation [A. V. *Moschcowitz,* U.S. surgeon, 1865–1933]. 1. A repair of femoral hernia through an inguinal approach. 2. An operation for rectal prolapse, using an abdominal approach and suture of the rectum to the pelvic fascia.

Moschcowitz test or **sign** [E. *Moschcowitz*]. After elevation of the leg and tourniquet application for 5 minutes, tourniquet removal and return of the leg to the horizontal position produces a hyperemic blush to the toes in 2 to 5 seconds. Delayed hyperemia indicates arterial occlusive disease.

Mo·sen·thal test [H. *Mosenthal,* U.S. physician, 1878–1954]. A test for kidney function in which the variability of specific gravity of the urine is measured through a 24-hour period of controlled dietary intake.

mos·qui·to (muh·skee'to) *n.* [Sp., from *mosca,* fly]. Any insect of the subfamily Culicinae of the Diptera. Various species are vectors of important diseases such as filariasis, malaria, dengue, and yellow fever.

mosquito forceps. HALSTED'S FORCEPS (1).

moss, *n.* Any low green bryophytic plant of the class Musci.

Moss·man fever [after *Mossman* District, Australia]. One of the febrile diseases occurring in the rural districts of northern Queensland, Australia, many of which have been identified as mite-transmitted scrub typhus (tsutsugamushi disease).

Moss's groups [W. L. *Moss,* U.S. physician, 1876–1957]. A superseded classification of the ABO group in which type IV = O, III = B, II = A, I = AB.

moss starch. LICHENIN.

mossy fibers. Fibers entering the cerebellum from the inferior cerebellar peduncle to synapse with the granule cell dendrites.

mossy foot. CHROMOBLASTOMYCOSIS.

Mo·tais' operation (mo^{h}·teh') [E. *Motais,* French ophthalmologist, 1845–1913]. An operation for ptosis of the eyelid; part of the tendon of the superior rectus muscle of the eyeball is transplanted to the upper lid.

¹moth·er, *n.* 1. A female parent. 2. The source of anything.

²mother, *n.* A slimy film formed on the surface of fermenting liquid, such as vinegar.

mother cell. 1. The cell from which daughter cells are formed by cell division; PARENT CELL. 2. A chromophobe cell of the adenohypophysis.

mother complex. OEDIPUS COMPLEX.

mother figure. The female parent figure.

mother tincture. *In homeopathy,* a tincture, usually representing 10 percent of the drug, from which the standard dilutions are made.

mother yaw. The primary lesion of yaws. Syn. *maman pian.*

moth fly or **midge.** Any of various small dipteran insects of the family Psychodidae.

moth patches. CHLOASMA.

mo·tile (mo'til) *adj.* Able to move; capable of spontaneous motion, as a motile flagellum. —**mo·til·i·ty** (mo·til'i·tee) *n.*

mo·tion, *n.* [L. *motio,* from *movere,* to move]. 1. The act of changing place; movement. 2. An evacuation of the bowels; the matter evacuated.

motion sickness. A syndrome characterized by nausea, vertigo, and vomiting; occurs in normal persons as the result of random multidirectional accelerations of a ship, airplane, train, or automobile.

mo·ti·va·tion (mo"ti·vay'shun) *n.* [from ML. *motivus,* causing motion]. The comparatively spontaneous drive, force, or incentive which partly determines the direction and strength of the response of a higher organism to a given situation; arising out of the internal state of the organism, this energizing process is differentiated from other determinants of action such as a conditioned response, the situation or stimulus per se, or capability.

mo·to·neu·ron (mo"to·new'ron) *n.* A motor neuron.

mo·to·neu·ro·ni·tis (mo"to·new"ro·nye'tis) *n.* GUILLAIN-BARRÉ DISEASE.

mo·tor, *n.* & *adj.* [L., from *movere,* to move]. 1. That which causes motion. 2. Pertaining to any activity or behavior involving muscular movement, as motor response. 3. Pertaining to the innervation of muscles, especially voluntary muscles; efferent, as motor neuron, motor impulse. Contr. *sensory.*

motor abreaction. Motor or muscular expression of an unconscious impulse.

motor agraphia. *Obsol.* The agraphia characteristic of Broca's aphasia.

motor alexia. *Obsol.* Loss of the ability to read aloud, while understanding of written or printed words is preserved.

motor amusia. *Obsol.* Loss of the power of singing or otherwise reproducing music, while comprehension of musical notes or sounds is preserved.

motor aphasia. BROCA'S APHASIA.

motor apraxia. A division of the apractic syndromes, now largely abandoned, which included those syndromes thought to be due to affection of motor association cortex rather than of an ideation area or pathways connecting it with motor association cortex.

motor area. The area of cerebral cortex from which isolated movements can be evoked by electrical stimuli of minimal intensity. It includes the precentral convolution, containing the Betz cells (Brodmann's area 4) and extends anteriorly into area 6, and posteriorly into sensory areas 1, 2, and 3.

motor ataxia. Inability to coordinate the muscles which becomes apparent only on body movement. Compare *static ataxia.*

motor cell. A motor neuron.

motor cortex. MOTOR AREA.

motor end plate. An area of specialized structure beneath the sarcolemma where a motor nerve fiber makes functional contact with a muscle fiber.

motor nerve. Any nerve composed chiefly or wholly of motor fibers.

motor neuron. See *lower motor neuron, upper motor neuron.*

motor neuron system disease. PROGRESSIVE SPINAL MUSCULAR ATROPHY.

motor nucleus. A nucleus giving origin to a motor nerve.

motor nucleus of the spinal cord. A group of somatic motor cells located in the anterior horn, whose axons project to striated voluntary muscles.

motor nucleus of the trigeminal nerve. An ovoid column of cells in the reticular formation dorsal to the superior olivary nucleus which gives origin to motor fibers of the trigeminal nerve. NA *nucleus motorius nervi trigemini.*

motor paralysis. The loss of voluntary control of skeletal muscle, due to interruption at any point in the motor pathway from the cerebral cortex to, and including, the muscle fiber.

motor paralytic bladder. Atonic bladder caused by interruption of the lower motor neurons that innervate the bladder.

motor point. A point on the skin over a muscle at which electric stimulation will cause contraction of the muscle. Syn. *Ziemssen's point.*

motor root. VENTRAL ROOT.

motor speech area. The cerebral cortical area located in the triangular and opercular portions of the inferior frontal gyrus. In right-handed and most left-handed individuals it is more developed on the left side. Syn. *Brodmann's area 44, Broca's area.*

motor test meal. Ingestion of a meal containing a radiopaque substance, for fluoroscopic or radiographic determination of its speed of passage through the gastrointestinal tract.

motor tract. Any descending tract of the central nervous system, terminating on primary or lower motor neurons.

motor unit. The axon of a single anterior horn cell, or the motor fiber of a cranial nerve, together with all of the striated muscle fibers innervated by its terminal branches. The proportion of muscle fibers innervated by one motor neuron (innervation ratio) varies greatly, muscles carrying out skilled movements having the lowest ratio.

Motrin. A trademark for ibuprofen, an anti-inflammatory.

mottled enamel. CHRONIC DENTAL FLUOROSIS.

mot·tling, *n.* Variability of coloration without distinct pattern.

Mott's law of anticipation [F. W. *Mott,* English neurologist, 1853–1926]. The clinical onset of a hereditary disease tends to be progressively earlier in successive generations.

mouches vo·lantes (moosh' vol·ahnt') [F., flying flies]. Muscae volitantes; FLOATERS.

mou·lage (moo·lahzh') *n.* [F.]. A mold or cast made directly from any portion of the body, used especially to show a surface lesion or defect.

moulage sign. *In radiology,* lack of the normal delicate, feathery appearance of the small intestine after a barium meal; often seen in sprue.

mould. MOLD.

moult. MOLT.

mound·ing (maown'ding) *n.* The rising in a lump of wasting, degenerating muscle fibers when struck by a slight, firm blow. See also *myoedema.*

mound of Venus. MONS PUBIS.

Mou·nier-Kuhn syndrome (moon·yeʸ kuᵉn') [P. *Mounier-Kuhn,* French, 20th century]. TRACHEOBRONCHOMEGALY.

moun·tain fever. 1. ROCKY MOUNTAIN SPOTTED FEVER. 2. COLORADO TICK FEVER.

mountain sickness. ALTITUDE SICKNESS.

moun·tant (maown'tunt) *n.* [*mount,* v., + *-ant,* n. and adj. suffix]. Any medium such as balsam or glycerin in which histological sections or specimens are embedded on slides for microscopic study.

mounting medium. MOUNTANT.

mouse antialopecia factor. INOSITOL.

mouse hepatitis virus. A latent virus commonly found in mouse colonies which may produce mortality in stressed adults and previously unexposed suckling mice. See also *lethal intestinal virus of infant mice.*

mouse poliomyelitis virus. THEILER'S VIRUS.

mouse·pox. A disease of mice caused by a virus very similar to vaccinia which may be latent in many stocks of laboratory mice, but which may result in edema and necrosis leading to a loss of limbs or the tail, and in addition may lead to conjunctivitis, pneumonia, meningitis, and hepatitis. Syn. *infectious ectromelia.*

mouse tapeworm. *HYMENOLEPIS DIMINUTA.*

mouse-tooth forceps. A dressing forceps with interlocking fine teeth at the tips of the blades.

mouse unit. The smallest amount of estrus-producing substance which, when injected into a spayed mouse, will produce a characteristic change in the vaginal epithelium. Syn. *Thayer-Doisy unit.*

mouth, *n.* [OE. *mūth* Gmc. *muntha* (rel. to L. *mandere,* to chew)]. 1. The commencement of the alimentary canal; the cavity in which mastication takes place. In a restricted sense, the aperture between the lips. 2. The entrance to any cavity or canal.

mouth-to-mouth breathing or **insufflation.** A first-aid method of artificial respiration in which the operator places his or her mouth tightly over the patient's and forces air into the lungs in a regular breathing rhythm, allowing passive expiration; the patient's head is kept well back, and the nostrils must be blocked during insufflation.

mouth·wash, *n.* A solution for rinsing the teeth and mouth.

move·able kidney. FLOATING KIDNEY.

move·ment, *n.* [MF.]. 1. The act or process of moving. 2. Bowel movement, defecation.

movement disorder. DYSKINESIA.

movement phosphene. A subjective sensation of light provoked by sudden eye movements in the dark.

moving-boundary electrophoresis. A method of electrophoresis applicable to dissolved substances; used in the study of biologic mixtures in their natural state. It separates, isolates, and defines the homogeneity of various components of the mixture. See also *Tiselius apparatus.*

moxa (mock'suh) *n.* [Jap. *moe kusa,* burning herb]. A combustible material which in Japan has been applied to the skin and ignited for the purpose of producing an eschar or counterirritant effect. It is made with the down of dried leaves of several species of *Artemisia.* Artificial moxa is made from cotton saturated with niter.

mox·i·bus·tion (mock''si·bus'chun) *n.* The application and combustion of moxa.

mox·nid·a·zole (mocks·nid'uh·zole) *n.* 3-[[(1-Methyl-5-nitroimidazol-2-yl)methylene]amino]-5-(morpholinomethyl)-2-oxazolidinone, $C_{13}H_{18}N_6O_5$, an antitrichomonal.

Moy·ni·han's symptom complex [B. A. *Moynihan,* English surgeon, 1865–1936]. Hunger pain three or more hours after eating, thought to be indicative of duodenal ulcer.

Mo·zam·bique ulcer. An endemic skin ulcer of East Africa.

m.p. Abbreviation for *melting point.*

MPI Abbreviation for *multiphasic personality inventory* (= MINNESOTA MULTIPHASIC PERSONALITY INVENTORY).

M protein. Surface protein of group A streptococci which determines their type specificity and is important as a virulence factor.

MPS Abbreviation for *mucopolysaccharidosis.*

M. R. C. P. Member of the Royal College of Physicians.

M. R. C. P. E. Member of the Royal College of Physicians of Edinburgh.

M. R. C. P. I. Member of the Royal College of Physicians of Ireland.

M. R. C. S. Member of the Royal College of Surgeons.

M. R. C. S. E. Member of the Royal College of Surgeons of Edinburgh.

M. R. C. S. I. Member of the Royal College of Surgeons of Ireland.

M. R. C. V. S. Member of the Royal College of Veterinary Surgeons.

mrd Abbreviation for *millirutherford.*

mRNA Abbreviation for *messenger RNA.*

MS Abbreviation for (a) *multiple sclerosis;* (b) *mitral stenosis.*

M.S. Master of Science.

M. Sc. Master of Science.

M.S.D. Master of Science in Dentistry.

msec. Abbreviation for *millisecond.*

MSG Abbreviation for *monosodium glutamate.*

MSH Abbreviation for *melanocyte-stimulating hormone.*

MsTh$_1$ Abbreviation for *mesothorium-1.*

MsTh$_2$ Abbreviation for *mesothorium-2.*

M substance. M PROTEIN.

m. u. Abbreviation for *mouse unit.*

muc-, muci-, muco-. A combining form meaning (a) *mucus;* (b) *mucin;* (c) *mucosa.*

mu·cate (mew'sate) *n.* Any salt of mucic acid.

Mu·cha-Ha·ber·mann's disease (moo'khah, hah'bur·mahn) [V. *Mucha,* Austrian dermatologist, 1877–1919; and R. *Habermann,* German dermatologist, b. 1884]. PITYRIASIS LICHENOIDES ET VARIOLIFORMIS ACUTA.

mu chain, μ chain. The heavy chain of the I_gM immunoglobulin molecule.

Much's granules (moo͞kh) [H. C. R. *Much,* German physician, 1880–1932]. Gram-positive, non-acid-fast granules found in sputum and suspected of being an altered form of tubercle bacillus.

mu·cic acid (mew'sick). Tetrahydroxyadipic acid, $C_6H_{10}O_8$, a dibasic acid resulting from oxidation of D-galactose or from carbohydrates yielding this sugar. Syn. *galactosaccharic acid.*

mucic acid test. A test for galactose in which concentrated nitric acid is added to the unknown, which is heated and let stand overnight. If galactose is present a crystalline precipitate of mucic acid is formed.

mu·ci·car·mine (mew"si·kahr'min) *n.* MAYER'S MUCICARMINE STAIN.

mu·cif·er·ous (mew·sif'e·rus) *adj.* [*muci-* + *-ferous*]. Producing or secreting mucus.

mu·ci·gen (mew'si·jen) *n.* [*muci-* + *-gen*]. A substance from which mucin is produced; it is contained in epithelial cells that form mucus. —**mu·cig·e·nous** (mew·sij'e·nus) *adj.*

mu·ci·lage (mew'si·lij) *n.* [F., from L. *mucilago,* musty juice]. *In pharmacy,* a solution of a gum in water. Mucilages (mucilagines) are employed as applications to irritated surfaces, particularly mucous membranes, as excipients for pills and tablets, and to suspend insoluble substances. The most important are acacia mucilage and tragacanth mucilage. —**mu·ci·lag·i·nous** (mew"si·laj'i·nus) *adj.*

mu·ci·la·go (mew"si·lay'go) *n.,* pl. **muci·lag·i·nes** (laj'i·neez) [L., musty juice]. MUCILAGE.

mu·cin (mew'sin) *n.* A mixture of glycoproteins that forms the basis of mucus. It is soluble in water and precipitated by alcohol or acids.

mucin cell. MUCOUS CELL.

mu·cino·blast (mew'si·no·blast, mew·sin'o·blast) *n.* [*mucin* + *-blast*]. The cell which forms a mucous cell.

mu·cino·gen (mew·sin'o·jen) *n.* [*mucin* + *-gen*]. The antecedent principle from which mucin is derived.

mu·cin·oid (mew'si·noid) *adj.* 1. Resembling mucin. 2. MUCOID (1).

mu·ci·no·sis (mew"si·no'sis) *n.* [*mucin* + *-osis*]. Collections of mucinous material in the skin, with papule and nodule formation in some cases; usually associated with myxedema. See also *follicular mucinosis.*

mu·cin·ous (mew'si·nus) *adj.* Resembling or pertaining to mucin.

mucinous carcinoma. A carcinoma whose parenchymal cells produce mucin.

mucinous cyst. MUCOUS CYST.

mucinous cystadenocarcinoma. An ovarian cancer, the malignant variant of the mucinous cystadenoma.

mucinous cystadenoma. A common benign ovarian tumor composed of columnar mucin-producing cells lining multiocular cysts filled with mucinous material. See also *mucoid cyst.*

mucinous degeneration. MUCOUS DEGENERATION.

mucinous plaque. DENTAL PLAQUE.

mucin reaction. A positive result when any mucin stain is applied.

mucin sugar. LEVULOSE.

mucin therapy. Administration of mucin as therapy for peptic ulcer, to protect the gastric mucosa against the action of pepsin and hydrochloric acid by protective coating and by neutralization of the hydrochloric acid.

mu·cip·a·rous (mew·sip'uh·rus) *adj.* [*muci-* + *-parous*]. Secreting or producing mucus.

muciparous gland. MUCOUS GLAND.

muco-. See *muc-.*

mu·co·al·bu·mi·nous (mew"ko·al·bew'mi·nus) *adj.* [*muco-* + *albuminous*]. MUCOSEROUS.

mu·co·buc·cal (mew"ko·buck'ul) *adj.* [*muco-* + *buccal*]. Pertaining to the oral mucosa and the cheeks.

mucobuccal fold. The reflection of the oral mucosa from the mandible or maxilla to the cheek.

mu·co·cele (mew'ko·seel) *n.* [*muco-* + *-cele*]. A cystic structure filled with mucus; may affect certain viscera which have become obstructed or it may develop without relationship to a recognizable normal structure.

mu·co·co·li·tis (mew"ko·ko·lye'tis) *n.* Mucous colitis; IRRITABLE COLON.

mu·co·col·pos (mew"ko·kol'pos) *n.* [*muco-* + Gk. *kolpos,* vagina]. A collection of mucus in the vagina.

mu·co·cu·ta·ne·ous (mew"ko·kew·tay'nee·us) *adj.* [*muco-* + *cutaneous*]. Pertaining to a mucous membrane and the skin, and to the line where these join.

mucocutaneous junction. The point of transition from skin to mucous membrane at the body orifices.

mucocutaneous leishmaniasis. AMERICAN MUCOCUTANEOUS LEISHMANIASIS.

mucocutaneous lymph node syndrome. An illness of uncertain etiology affecting young children, characterized by high fever, conjunctivitis, strawberry tongue, and nonsuppurative cervical lymphadenitis, followed by characteristic desquamation of the skin of the fingertips. Syn. *Kawasaki disease.*

mu·co·derm (mew'ko·durm) *n.* [*muco-* + *-derm*]. The tunica propria of a mucous membrane.

mu·co·en·ter·i·tis (mew"ko·en"tur·eye'tis) *n.* [*muco-* + *enteritis*]. Inflammation of the mucous membrane of the intestine.

mu·co·epi·der·moid (mew"ko·ep"i·dur'moid) *adj.* [*muco-* + *epiderm-* + *-oid*]. Having both mucous and epidermal characteristics.

mucoepidermoid tumor. A usually benign tumor of salivary glands which contains both mucin-producing elements and squamous epithelium.

mu·co·gin·gi·val (mew"ko·jin'ji·vul, ·jin·jye'vul) *adj.* Pertaining to mucosa and gingiva.

mucogingival junction. The scalloped line between the gingiva and the alveolar mucosa.

mu·co·hem·or·rhag·ic (mew"ko·hem"o·raj'ick) *adj.* [*muco-* + *hemorrhagic*]. Related to, or accompanied by, mucus and blood.

mu·coid (mew'koid) *adj. & n.* [*muc-* + *-oid*]. 1. Resembling mucus. 2. Any of a group of glycoproteins, differing from true mucins in their solubilities and precipitation properties. They are found in cartilage, in the cornea and crystalline lens, in white of egg, and in certain cysts and ascitic fluids.

mucoid adenocarcinoma. MUCINOUS CYSTADENOCARCINOMA.

mucoid carcinoma. MUCINOUS CARCINOMA.

mucoid colony. A glistening smooth colony with gummy or viscoid consistency; often associated with the production of definite capsules or abundant slime-layer material. Abbreviated, M.

mucoid cyst. A mucin-filled cavity produced by mucous degeneration of mesodermal tissues.

mucoid degeneration. MUCOUS DEGENERATION.

mucoid softening. MUCOUS DEGENERATION.

mucoid sputum. MUCOUS SPUTUM.

mucoid tissue. An embryonic subcutaneous connective tissue, as in the umbilical cord (Wharton's jelly). The stellate fibroblast is the dominant cell type. The ground substance is gelatinous in consistency, gives a mucin reaction, and is metachromatic. Collagenous fibers increase with development.

mu·co·i·tin·sul·fu·ric acid (mew·ko''i·tin·sul·few'rick). A component of the mucin of saliva; on hydrolysis, yields sulfuric acid, glucuronic acid, glucosamine, and acetic acid.

mu·co·lyt·ic (mew''ko·lit'ick) *adj.* [*muco-* + *-lytic*]. Dissolving, liquefying, or dispersing mucus.

mu·co·mem·bra·nous (mew''ko·mem'bruh·nus) *adj.* Consisting of or pertaining to mucous membrane.

mu·co·me·tria (mew''ko·mee'tree·uh) *n.* [*muco-* + *metr-* + *-ia*]. An accumulation of mucus in the uterine cavity.

Mucomyst. Trademark for the mucolytic agent acetylcysteine.

mu·co·peri·os·te·um (mew''ko·perr''ee·os'tee·um) *n.* Periosteum with a closely associated mucous membrane.

mu·co·poly·sac·cha·ride (mew''ko·pol''ee·sack'uh·ride, ·rid) *n.* A polysaccharide containing an amino sugar as well as uronic acid units.

mu·co·poly·sac·cha·ri·do·sis (mew''ko·pol''ee·sack''uh·ri·do'sis) *n.* One of several inborn errors in the metabolism of mucopolysaccharides, differentiated on the basis of clinical, genetic, and biochemical findings thus far into six types: MPS I, Hurler's syndrome; MPS II, Hunter's syndrome; MPS III, Sanfillipo's syndrome; MPS IV, Morquio's syndrome; MPS V, Scheie's syndrome; MPS VI, Maroteaux-Lamy's syndrome. May also include MPS VII, a variant of metachromatic leukodystrophy.

mu·co·pro·tein (mew''ko·pro'tee·in, ·teen) *n.* A glycoprotein, particularly one in which the sugar component is chondroitinsulfuric or mucoitinsulfuric acid.

mu·co·pu·ru·lent (mew''ko·pewr'yoo·lunt) *adj.* [*muco-* + *purulent*]. Containing mucus mingled with pus, as mucopurulent sputum.

mu·co·pus (mew'ko·pus'') *n.* A mixture of mucus and pus.

Mu·cor (mew'kore) *n.* [L., moldiness]. A genus of the order Mucorales.

Mu·co·ra·ce·ae (mew''ko·ray'see·ee) *n.pl.* A fungus family in the Mucorales order characterized by thalluses without ramifications or segments.

Mu·co·ra·les (mew''ko·ray'leez) *n.pl.* An order of the nonseptate class of lower fungi, the Phycomycetes, which includes such genera as *Mucor, Rhizopus,* and *Absidia.*

mu·cor·my·co·sis (mew''kor·migh·ko'sis) *n.* [*Mucor* + *mycosis*]. An acute, usually fulminant infection by fungi of the order Mucorales, including such genera as *Absidia, Rhizopus,* and *Mucor,* often associated with underlying disease such as diabetes mellitus, leukemia, or lymphoma. Invasion may be of the brain, lungs, or gastrointestinal tract. Ophthalmoplegia and meningoencephalitis are the most common manifestations. See also *phycomycosis.*

mu·co·sa (mew·ko'suh, ·zuh) *n.*, pl. **muco·sae** (·see, ·zee), **mucosas** [short for *tunica mucosa*]. MUCOUS MEMBRANE. —**muco·sal** (·sul, ·zul) *adj.*

mucosal disease. A viral disease of cattle associated with erosions of the mucosal surfaces.

mucosal graft. A graft of oral mucous membrane or of conjunctiva to repair a defect.

mu·co·sal·pinx (mew''ko·sal'pinks) *n.* [*muco-* + *salpinx*]. Accumulation of mucoid material in a uterine tube.

mucosal prolapse. Protrusion of the mucous membrane of the rectum into the anal canal, or the urethra through the meatus urethrae.

mu·co·san·guin·e·ous (mew''ko·sang·gwin'ee·us) *adj.* [*muco-* + *sanguineous*]. Consisting of mucus and blood.

mucosa of the vagina. The mucous membrane lining the vagina.

mu·co·se·rous (mew''ko·seer'us) *adj.* Mucous and serous; containing mucus and serum.

mucoserous cell. A cell intermediate in characteristics between mucous and serous cells. Syn. *mucoalbuminous cell.*

mu·co·sin (mew·ko'sin, mew'ko·) *n.* A term suggested for mucin from nasal, uterine, and bronchial mucous membranes, because of their special viscous properties, as contrasted with mucins from other regions.

mu·co·sis (mew·ko'sis) *n.* [*muc-* + *-osis*]. CYSTIC FIBROSIS OF THE PANCREAS.

mu·co·si·tis (mew''ko·sigh'tis) *n.* [*mucosa* + *-itis*]. Inflammation of mucous membranes.

mu·cos·i·ty (mew·kos'i·tee) *n.* The quality or condition of being mucous or covered with mucus.

mu·co·stat·ic (mew''ko·stat'ick) *adj.* [*muco-* + *static*]. 1. Arresting the secretion of mucus. 2. Descriptive of the normal, relaxed condition of the mucosal tissues covering the jaws when not in function.

mu·cous (mew'kus) *adj.* Of or pertaining to mucus; secreting mucus, as a mucous gland; depending on the presence of mucus, as mucous rales.

mucous cell. A cell that secretes mucus.

mucous colitis. IRRITABLE COLON.

mucous cyst. A retention cyst of a gland, containing a secretion rich in mucin. Syn. *mucinous cyst.*

mucous cystadenoma. MUCINOUS CYSTADENOMA.

mucous degeneration. Any retrogressive change associated with abnormal production of mucus.

mucous epithelium. 1. The rete mucosum, or germinative layer of a stratified squamous epithelium, especially of the epidermis. 2. The entire embryonic epidermis with the exception of the epitrichium.

mucous gland. A gland that forms mucus. NA *glandula mucosa.*

mucous membrane. The membrane lining those cavities and canals communicating with the air. It is kept moist by the secretions of various types of glands. NA *tunica mucosa.*

mucous neck cells. Mucous cells in the necks of gastric glands.

mucous patch. CONDYLOMA LATUM.

mucous plug. 1. The mass of inspissated mucus which occludes the cervix uteri during pregnancy and is discharged at the beginning of labor. 2. Mucous material obstructing a bronchus.

mucous rale. A sound similar to one heard when blowing through a pipe into soapy water, heard in patients with emphysema, and caused by viscid bubbles bursting in the bronchial tubes.

mucous sheath. TENDON SHEATH.

mucous sputum. Sputum consisting chiefly of mucus, often erroneously designated as mucoid sputum.

mucous tissue. MUCOID TISSUE.

mucous tumor. MYXOMA.

mucous vaginitis. Vaginitis with a profuse mucoid discharge.

mu·co·vis·ci·do·sis (mew''ko·vis''i·do'sis) *n.* [*muco-* + *viscid* + *-osis*]. CYSTIC FIBROSIS OF THE PANCREAS.

mu·cro·nate (mew'kro·nate, ·nut) *adj.* [L. *mucronatus,* pointed]. Tipped with a sharp point.

mu·cu·lent (mew'kew·lunt) *adj.* [L. *muculentus,* sniveling]. Rich in mucus.

Mu·cu·na (mew·kew'nuh) *n.* [Tupi *mucuná*]. A genus of leguminous herbs. The hairs of the pods of *Mucuna pruriens (Stizolobium pruritum),* called cowage or cowitch, were formerly used as a vermifuge and counterirritant.

mu·cus (mew'kus) *n.* [L., nasal mucus (rel. to Gk. *myxa*)]. The viscid liquid secreted by mucous glands, consisting of water, mucin, inorganic salts, epithelial cells, leukocytes, etc., held in suspension. Adj. *mucous.*

Muehr·cke lines. Parallel, paired white bands in the fingernails and toenails of patients with chronic hypoalbuminemia; possibly a sign of mild protein deficiency.

Mueller. See also *Müller.*

Muel·ler's snake. *PSEUDELAPS MUELLERI.*

Mueller's spots. Spots seen sometimes on the iris after an attack of smallpox. Syn. *vitiligo iridis.*

mu·guet (mew″gay′) *n.* [F.]. THRUSH (1).

mu·laire (mew·lair′) *n.* [F.]. A subcutaneous lesion occurring in verruca peruviana which presses against the skin, finally eroding it. This lesion looks very much like that produced by the same disease in mules.

mu·lat·to (mew·lat′o) *n.* [Sp. *mulato*]. 1. A person having one white and one black parent. 2. Any person with mixed Negro and Caucasian ancestry.

mul·ber·ry calculus. A gallstone or urinary calculus with a finely nodular outer surface resembling a mulberry.

mulberry heart disease. Syndrome of young pigs associated with high mortality, sudden onset, and edema. The etiology is unknown.

mulberry mark. NEVUS.

mulberry mass. MORULA.

mulberry molars. MOON'S MOLARS.

mulberry spot. The globular retinal phacoma seen in tuberous sclerosis.

mule spinners' cancer. Squamous cell carcinoma of scrotum or vulva occurring in textile workers, presumably due to exposure to machine oils.

mu·li·e·bria (mew″lee·ee′bree·uh, ·eb′ree·uh) *n.pl.* [L., neuter pl. of *muliebris*, of a woman]. The female genitals.

mu·li·eb·ri·ty (mew″lee·eb′ri·tee) *n.* [L. *muliebritas*]. 1. Womanliness. 2. Puberty in the female. 3. Assumption of female qualities by the male.

mull, *v.* 1. To mix dental amalgam by hand following trituration in order to produce a smoother mass. 2. To reduce a relatively coarse solid to a fine powder by rubbing it, usually in a semifluid dispersion medium, on a flat surface with the flattened area of a piece of glass, stone, or metal.

mul·lein (mul′in) *n.* A plant of the genus *Verbascum*. See *Verbascum*.

mül·le·ri·an (mew·leer′ee·un, ·lerr′) *adj.* 1. Discovered by or associated with Johannes Müller, German anatomist and physiologist, 1801–1858. 2. Pertaining to the müllerian (paramesonephric) duct and its derivatives.

müllerian duct. PARAMESONEPHRIC DUCT.

müllerian duct cyst. A congenital cyst arising from vestiges of the müllerian ducts.

Mül·ler's duct (mueˡ′ur) [J. *Müller*, German anatomist and physiologist, 1801–1858]. PARAMESONEPHRIC DUCT.

Müller's fibers [Heinrich *Müller*, German anatomist, 1820–1864]. Modified neuroglial cells that traverse perpendicularly the layers of the retina, and connect the internal and external limiting membranes.

Müller's fixing fluid [Hermann F. *Müller*, German histologist, 1866–1898]. A mixture of potassium bichromate, sodium sulfate, and distilled water, used for hardening nervous tissue after preliminary fixation.

Müller's hillock [J. *Müller*]. An elevation on the dorsal wall of the embryonic urogenital sinus at the point of entrance of the paramesonephric ducts. Syn. *Müller's tubercle*.

Müller's law of specific nerve energies [J. *Müller*]. A theory that each type of sensory nerve ending gives rise to its own specific sensation, no matter how it is stimulated.

Müller's muscle [Heinrich *Müller*]. MUSCLE OF MÜLLER.

Müller's syndrome [C. *Müller*, Norwegian physician, b. 1886]. A syndrome of hypercholesterolemia, xanthelasma, xanthomas, and angina pectoris.

Müller's test. A test for cystine in which the substance is boiled with potassium hydroxide; when cold, it is diluted with water and a solution of sodium nitroprusside is added. A violet color changing rapidly to yellow is produced if cystine is present.

Müller's tubercle. MÜLLER'S HILLOCK.

mult·an·gu·lar (mul·tang′gyoo·lur) *n.* [L. *multangulus*, many-cornered]. MULTANGULUM.

mult·an·gu·lum (mul·tang′gyoo·lum) *n.* [NL., polygon]. A bone with many angles.

multangulum ma·jus (may′jus). TRAPEZIUM.

multangulum mi·nus (migh′nus). TRAPEZOID.

multi- [L. *multus*]. 1. A combining form meaning *many, much*. 2. *In medicine*, a combining form meaning *affecting many parts*.

mul·ti·cap·su·lar (mul″ti·kap′sue·lur) *adj. In biology*, composed of many capsules.

mul·ti·cel·lu·lar (mul″ti·sel′yoo·lur) *adj.* Having many cells.

mul·ti·cen·tric (mul″ti·sen′trick) *adj.* [*multi-* + *-centric*]. Having many centers.

Mul·ti·ceps (mul′ti·seps) *n.* [NL., many-headed]. A genus of tapeworms.

Multiceps multiceps. A species of tapeworm occurring in the small intestine of dogs and wolves. The larval stage develops in the brain and spinal cord of sheep, goats, cattle, horses, and has also been found in man.

Multiceps se·ri·a·lis (seer·ee·ay′lis). A species of tapeworm which in its adult form infects the intestinal tract of the dog. Human infection is rare.

mul·ti·cip·i·tal (mul″ti·sip′i·tul) *adj.* [*multi-* + *-cipital*, from *-ceps*, -headed]. Many-headed; having multiple origins, as triceps, quadriceps.

multicipital muscle. A muscle with more than two heads or attachments of origin.

mul·ti·clo·nal (mul″ti·klo′nul) *adj.* POLYCLONAL.

mul·ti·cos·tate (mul″ti·kos′tate) *adj.* [*multi-* + *costate*]. Having many ribs.

mul·ti·cus·pid (mul″ti·kus′pid) *adj. & n.* 1. Having several cusps, as the molar teeth. 2. A tooth that has several cusps. —**multicus·pi·date** (·pi·date) *adj.*

mul·ti·cys·tic kidney (mul″ti·sis′tick) [*multi-* + *cystic*]. A congenital anomaly in which one kidney is replaced by a mass of cysts, with atresia or absence of the associated ureter. There is little or no renal parenchyma and there may be an admixture of such mesodermal derivatives as cartilage. Compare *polycystic kidney*.

mul·ti·den·tate (mul″ti·den′tate) *adj.* [*multi-* + *dentate*]. Having many teeth or toothlike processes.

mul·ti·dig·i·tate (mul″ti·dij′i·tate) *adj.* Having many digits or digitate processes.

mul·ti·fac·et·ed (mul″ti·fas′it·id) *adj.* Having many plane surfaces, as certain types of gallstone.

mul·ti·fac·to·ri·al (mul″ti·fack·to′ree·ul) *adj.* Pertaining to an inheritance pattern dependent upon the interaction of multiple genetic and environmental factors.

mul·ti·fa·mil·i·al (mul″ti·fa·mil′ee·ul) *adj.* Affecting several successive generations of a family, as certain diseases.

mul·ti·fe·ta·tion (mul″ti·fe·tay′shun) *n.* SUPERFETATION.

mul·ti·fid (mul′ti·fid) *adj.* [L. *multifidus*]. Divided into many parts.

mul·tif·i·dus (mul·tif′i·dus) *n.*, pl. **multifi·di** (·dye). A deep muscle of the back. See also Table of Muscles in the Appendix.

multifidus spi·nae (spye′nee). MULTIFIDUS.

mul·ti·flag·el·late (mul″ti·flaj′e·late) *adj.* Having many flagella.

mul·ti·fo·cal (mul″ti·fo′kul) *adj.* [*multi-* + *focus* + *-al*]. Having, arising from, or pertaining to many discrete locations or collections.

mul·ti·form (mul′ti·form) *adj.* [L. *multiformis*]. POLYMORPHIC.

multiform layer. LAYER OF FUSIFORM CELLS.

Multifuge. A trademark for the anthelmintic piperazine citrate.

mul·ti·gan·gli·on·ate (mul″ti·gang′glee·uh·nate) *adj.* Having many ganglia.

mul·ti·glan·du·lar (mul″ti·glan′dew·lur) *adj.* Pertaining to several glands, as multiglandular secretions, a mixture of secretions from two or more glands; PLURIGLANDULAR.

mul·ti·grav·i·da (mul″ti·grav′i·duh) *n.* [*multi-* + *gravida*]. A woman who has had one or more previous pregnancies. —**multi·gra·vid·i·ty** (·gra·vid′i·tee) *n.*

mul·ti·he·ma·tin·ic (mul″ti·hee″muh·tin′ick, ·hem″uh·) *n.* A hematinic drug preparation containing several substances concerned with blood formation.

mul·ti·in·fec·tion (mul″tee·in·feck′shun) *n.* MIXED INFECTION.
mul·ti·lo·bar (mul″ti·lo′bahr, ·bur) *adj.* Composed of many lobes.
multilobar kidney. POLYPYRAMIDAL KIDNEY.
mul·ti·lo·bate (mul″ti·lo′bate) *adj.* MULTILOBAR.
multilobate spleen. A splenic anomaly in which that organ is divided into two or more masses, all of them significantly smaller than the normal spleen.
mul·ti·lobed (mul′ti·loabd) *adj.* MULTILOBAR.
multilobed placenta. MULTIPARTITE PLACENTA.
multilobed spleen. MULTILOBATE SPLEEN.
mul·ti·lob·u·lar (mul″ti·lob′yoo·lur) *adj.* Having many lobules.
multilobular cirrhosis. Portal cirrhosis in which several lobules are surrounded by fibrotic portal spaces; the usual form of the disease. Contr. *monolobular cirrhosis.*
mul·ti·loc·u·lar (mul″ti·lock′yoo·lur) *adj.* [*multi-* + *locular*]. Containing or consisting of many loculi or compartments.
multilocular bladder. A sacculated urinary bladder having many pouches.
multilocular crypt. 1. A simple gland with pouched or sacculated walls. 2. The lobule of a racemose gland.
multilocular cyst. A cyst with several more or less separate compartments.
multilocular cyst of ovary. MUCINOUS CYSTADENOMA.
multilocular renal cysts. Rare, unilateral renal cystic lesions the capsules of which may contain smooth muscle and usually collagenized fibrous tissue.
mul·ti·loc·u·lat·ed (mul″ti·lock′yoo·lay·tid) *adj.* MULTILOCULAR.
multiloculated hygroma. HYGROMA.
mul·ti·mam·mae (mul″ti·mam′ee) *n.* [*multi-* + *mammae*]. POLYMASTIA; the presence of more than two breasts in a human being.
mul·ti·nod·u·lar (mul″ti·nod′yoo·lur) *adj.* Having many nodules.
mul·ti·nu·cle·ar (mul″ti·new′klee·ur) *adj.* Having two or more nuclei.
mul·ti·nu·cle·ate (mul″ti·new′klee·ate, ·ut) *adj.* MULTINUCLEAR. **—multinucle·at·ed** (·ay·tid) *adj.*
mul·tip·a·ra (mul·tip′uh·ruh) *n.* [*multi-* + *-para*]. A woman who has already borne one or more children. **—multipa·rous** (·rus) *adj.;* **mul·ti·par·i·ty** (mul″ti·păr′i·tee) *n.*
mul·ti·par·tite (mul″ti·pahr′tite) *adj.* [L. *multipartitus*]. Divided into many parts.
multipartite placenta. A placenta with more than three lobes and vessels which may emerge to form the umbilical cord directly or may first communicate with one or more of the other lobes. Syn. *multilobed placenta, septuplex placenta.*
mul·ti·pen·nate (mul″ti·pen′ate) *adj.* [*multi-* + *pennate*]. Of muscles, exhibiting a structure in which the muscle fibers are inserted into the tendon from several directions.
mul·ti·pha·sic (mul″ti·fay′zick) *adj.* Having numerous phases or facets.
multiphasic personality inventory. MINNESOTA MULTIPHASIC PERSONALITY INVENTORY. Abbreviated, MPI.
mul·ti·ple, *adj.* [F., from L. *multiplex*]. Manifold; affecting many parts at the same time, as multiple sclerosis; repeated two or more times.
multiple alleles. Alleles numbering more than two for a single locus.
multiple benign cystic epithelioma. TRICHOEPITHELIOMA.
multiple bile-duct adenoma. VON MEYENBURG COMPLEX.
multiple birth. The occurrence of two or more offspring at a birth.
multiple cancellous exostoses. MULTIPLE HEREDITARY EXOSTOSES.
multiple cartilaginous exostoses. MULTIPLE HEREDITARY EXOSTOSES.
multiple colloid adenomatous goiter. ADENOMATOUS GOITER.
multiple congenital osteochondromas. MULTIPLE HEREDITARY EXOSTOSES.
multiple enchondromas. ENCHONDROMATOSIS.
multiple endocrine adenomatosis. Hereditary hyperplasia or neoplasia of two or more endocrine glands, usually with increased function. The parathyroid glands, pancreatic islet cells, and pituitary gland are the most frequently affected; transmitted as an autosomal dominant trait.
multiple fission. Cell division in which a series of divisions of the nucleus is followed by a division of the cell body into as many parts as there are daughter nuclei; a form of asexual reproduction in certain classes of unicellular organisms such as the sporozoa. Contr. *binary fission.*
multiple fracture. Simultaneous fracture of two or more parts of a bone, or of more than one bone.
multiple hemorrhagic hemangioma of Kaposi [M. K. *Kaposi*]. MULTIPLE IDIOPATHIC HEMORRHAGIC SARCOMA.
multiple hereditary exostoses. A common heritable disorder of connective tissue, transmitted as a dominant and usually discovered in childhood or adolescence, in which ossified projections capped by proliferating cartilage arise from the cortex of bone within the periosteum, commonly in metaphyseal regions. Syn. *diaphyseal aclasis, hereditary deforming chondrodysplasia.*
multiple idiopathic hemorrhagic sarcoma. A mesodermal tumor characterized by the occurrence of multiple bluish-red or brown nodules and plaques, usually on the extremities. In the early granulomatous lesions, which occasionally involute spontaneously, tumor is not evident; in later stages, the histologic picture resembles angiosarcoma or fibrosarcoma. Syn. *Kaposi's sarcoma, sarcoma cutaneum telangiectaticum multiplex, multiplex angiosarcoma.*
multiple infection. MIXED INFECTION.
multiple intussusception. An enteric intussusception in which there are more than two areas of small intestine involved.
multiple lymphadenoma. LYMPHOMA.
multiple microhamartoma of liver. VON MEYENBURG COMPLEX.
multiple myeloma. A neoplasm that results from a progressive, uncontrolled proliferation of plasma cells in bone marrow. Its clinical manifestations include tumor formation, skeletal and renal disease, abnormal synthesis of immunoglobulins, and bone marrow dysfunction.
multiple neuritis. POLYNEURITIS.
multiple neurofibroma. NEUROFIBROMATOSIS.
multiple neurofibromatosis. NEUROFIBROMATOSIS.
multiple neuroma. NEUROFIBROMATOSIS.
multiple nodular hyperplasia. POSTNECROTIC CIRRHOSIS.
multiple osteocartilaginous exostoses. MULTIPLE HEREDITARY EXOSTOSES.
multiple osteochondritis. DYSPLASIA EPIPHYSIALIS MULTIPLEX.
multiple personality. A personality capable of dissociation into several or many other personalities at the same time, whereby the delusion is entertained that the one person is many separate persons; a symptom in schizophrenic patients.
multiple pregnancy. Gestation with two or more fetuses present within the uterus.
multiple pupil. POLYCORIA.
multiple sclerosis. A common disease of young adults, characterized clinically by episodes of focal disorder of the optic nerves, spinal cord, and brain, which remit to a varying extent and recur over a period of many years; and pathologically by the presence of numerous, scattered, sharply defined demyelinative lesions (plaques) in the white matter of the central nervous system. Syn. *insular sclerosis, disseminated sclerosis, sclérose en plaques.*
multiple serositis. POLYSEROSITIS.
multiple therapy. *In psychoanalysis,* therapy given to one patient by a group of therapists.
multiple vision. POLYOPIA.
mul·ti·plex (mul′ti·plecks) *adj.* [L., from *multi-* + *-plex,* fold]. Multiple.

multiplex angiosarcoma. MULTIPLE IDIOPATHIC HEMORRHAGIC SARCOMA.

multiplication phenomenon of La·vren·tiev (lah·vrent'y'yef) [B. *Lavrentiev,* Russian anatomist, 1892–1944]. The concept that each vagus fiber to the gastrointestinal tract branches terminally to innervate a large number of enteric ganglion cells.

mul·ti·plic·i·ty (mul"ti·plis'i·tee) *n.* 1. The state or quality of being multiple. 2. Increase, reproduction.

multiplicity reactivation. The restoration of phage activity upon the infection of the same bacterium by two inactivated phage particles, neither of which is able to reproduce alone.

mul·ti·po·lar (mul"ti·po'lur) *adj.* Having more than one pole, as multipolar nerve cells, those having more than one process.

mul·ti·pol·yp·oid (mul"ti·pol'i·poid) *adj.* [*multi-* + *polypoid*]. Having more than one polyp.

mul·ti·sep·tate (mul"ti·sep'tate) *adj.* [*multi-* + *septate*]. Divided by more than one septum, as in the case of various fungus conidia.

mul·ti·sys·tem (mul'ti·sis"tum) *adj.* Involving more than one of the major body systems.

mul·ti·va·lent (mul"ti·vay'lunt, mul·tiv'uh·lunt) *adj.* [*multi-* + *valent*]. 1. Capable of combining with more than one atom of a univalent element. 2. POLYVALENT.

multivalent vaccine. A polyvalent vaccine.

mum·mi·fi·ca·tion (mum"i·fi·kay'shun) *n.* [from *mummify*]. 1. The change of a part into a hard, dry mass. 2. DRY GANGRENE.

mum·mi·fied (mum'i·fide) *adj.* [*mummify,* to make into a mummy; to dry]. Dried, as mummified pulp, the condition of the dental pulp when it is affected by dry gangrene.

mumps, *n.* [E. dial., *mump,* lump or bump]. An acute communicable viral disease, usually manifest by painful enlargement of the salivary glands, but frequently invading other tissues, notably testes, pancreas, and meninges. Syn. *epidemic parotitis.*

mumps orchitis. Orchitis due to the mumps virus. It may occur without the usual parotitis associated with mumps.

Mun·chau·sen syndrome (mun'chaow·zun) [Baron K. F. H. von *Münchhausen,* 18th century German traveler and soldier, reputed source of a collection of preposterous adventure stories]. A personality disorder in which the patient describes dramatic but false symptoms or simulates acute illness, happily undergoing numerous examinations, hospitalizations, and diagnostic or therapeutic manipulations, and upon discovery of the real nature of his case, often leaves without notice and moves on to another hospital.

Münch·mey·er's disease (muench'migh·ur) [E. *Münchmeyer,* German physician, 1846–1880]. Myositis ossificans of a progressive nature.

mun·dif·i·cant (mun·dif'ick·unt) *adj. & n.* [L. *mundificare,* to make clean, from *mundus,* clean, neat]. 1. Having the power to cleanse, purge, or heal. 2. A cleansing, purging, or healing agent.

Muracil. Trademark for methylthiouracil, an antithyroid drug.

mu·ral (mew'rul) *adj.* [L *muralis,* from *murus,* wall]. Pertaining to, or located in or on, the wall of a cavity.

mural aneurysm. Aneurysm of the heart wall. See also *cardiac aneurysm.*

mural salpingitis. Chronic INTERSTITIAL SALPINGITIS.

mural thrombus. A thrombus attached to the wall of a blood vessel or mural endocardium. Syn. *lateral thrombus.*

mu·ram·ic acid (mew·ram'ick). A condensation product, $C_9H_{17}NO_7$, of *N*-acetylglucosamine and D(−)-lactic acid; a constituent of certain polysaccharides in the cell walls of some bacteria.

mu·ram·i·dase (mew·ram'i·dace, ·daze) *n.* Term recommended for lysozyme to identify the catalytic action of the enzyme on the hydrolysis of the muramic acid-containing mucopeptide in the cell walls of some bacteria.

Murel. Trademark for valethamate bromide, an anticholinergic drug.

mu·rex·ide (mew·reck'side) *n.* Ammonium purpurate, $C_8H_8N_6O_6$, a purple coloring matter resulting from uric acid by treatment with nitric acid and neutralization with ammonia.

mu·ri·ate (mew'ree·ate) *n.* CHLORIDE. —**muri·at·ed** (·ay·tid) *adj.*

mu·ri·at·ic (mew"ree·at'ick) *adj.* [L. *muriaticus,* from *muria,* brine]. Pertaining to brine.

muriatic acid. HYDROCHLORIC ACID.

mu·rine (mew'rine, ·rin, mew·reen') *adj.* [L. *murinus,* from *mus, muris,* mouse]. Of, resembling, or pertaining to mice, especially to the genus *Mus*; or to mice and rats of the family Muridae in general.

murine arthritis. A fairly common arthritis of rats and mice thought to be due to *Mycoplasma arthritidis.*

murine leprosy. A disease of rats and mice closely resembling human leprosy. The infection has been transmitted by tissue suspensions of acid-fast bacilli, *Mycobacterium lepraemurium.*

murine plague. *Yersinia pestis* infection of the rat, transmitted from rat to rat and from rat to man primarily by the flea.

murine typhus. A relatively mild, acute, febrile illness of worldwide distribution caused by *Rickettsia typhi,* characterized by headache, macular rash, and myalgia; a natural infection of rats, sporadically transmitted to man by the flea. Syn. *endemic typhus, urban typhus, shop typhus, flea-borne typhus, rat typhus.*

mur·mur, *n.* [L., humming, roaring]. A benign or pathologic blowing or roaring sound heard on auscultation, especially having a cardiac or vascular origin.

Mur·phy button [J. B. *Murphy,* U.S. surgeon, 1857–1916]. A double, interlocking metal button used in rapid, end-to-end anastomosis of the intestine.

Murphy drip [J. B. *Murphy*]. RECTOCLYSIS.

Murphy's operation [J. B. *Murphy*]. A surgical approach to the hip joint especially adapted to arthroplasty.

Murphy's sign [J. B. *Murphy*]. 1. A sign for cholecystitis in which pressure is applied over the gallbladder; inspiration produces pain and arrest of respiration as the descending diaphragm causes the inflamed gallbladder to impinge against the examining hand. 2. Punch tenderness at the costovertebral angle in perinephric abscess.

Murphy-Sturm lymphosarcoma. A transplantable malignant lymphoma originally induced in a Wistar rat by dibenzanthracene; it possesses the features of lymphocytic leukemia or lymphosarcoma in accordance with the method of transplantation.

Mur·ray Valley encephalitis [after the *Murray* River *Valley,* Australia]. An acute viral encephalomyelitis, confined to Australia and New Guinea, and occurring predominantly in children. Syn. *Australian X disease.*

mur·ri·na (muh·rye'nuh, muh·ree'nuh) *n.* [Sp. *morriña*]. A form of trypanosomiasis caused by *Trypanosoma hippicum,* seen in horses and mules, with cattle acting as reservoir hosts; characterized by weakness, emaciation, edema, anemia, enlarged spleen, and paralysis.

Mus, *n.* [L., mouse]. A genus of small rodents including the common house mouse (*Mus musculus*) and other small species. Some members of the genus are medically important as intermediate hosts and reservoir hosts of diseases transmissible to man.

Mus·ca (mus'kuh) *n.* [L., fly]. A genus of flies of the family Muscidae.

Musca do·mes·ti·ca (do·mes'ti·kuh). The most important species of *Musca,* the common housefly; it carries and frequently transmits the causal agents of a number of diseases, including typhoid fever, infantile diarrhea, bacillary and amebic dysentery, cholera, trachoma, and tuberculosis.

mus·cae vol·i·tan·tes (mus'ee vol''i·tan'teez, mus'kee) [L., flies flying around]. FLOATERS.

mus·ca·rine (mus'kuh·reen, ·rin, mus·kay'reen) *n.* A poisonous alkaloid obtained from certain mushrooms, as *Amanita muscaria;* a quaternary ammonium compound, the cation of which is trimethyl(tetrahydro-4-hydroxy-5-methylfurfuryl)ammonium, $(C_9H_{20}NO_2)^+$. A parasympathomimetic drug which mimics certain effects of acetylcholine, having the same action as postganglionic cholinergic nerve impulses on endocrine glands, smooth muscle, and heart.

mus·ca·rin·ic (mus''kuh·rin'ick) *adj.* Having, resembling, or subject to the parasympathomimetic actions of muscarine.

mus·ca·rin·ism (mus'kuh·ri·niz·um) *n.* Mushroom poisoning.

Musca ve·tus·tis·si·ma (vet''us·tis'i·muh) [L., most ancient]. The Australian housefly.

Musca vi·ci·na (vi·sigh'nuh) [L., neighboring]. The common housefly of the Orient.

mus·ci·cide (mus'i·side) *n.* [L. *musca*, fly, + *-cide*]. An agent which is poisonous or destructive to flies.

Mus·ci·dae (mus'i·dee) *n.pl.* A family of the Diptera, which includes the common houseflies.

mus·cle, *n.* [L. *musculus,* diminutive of *mus,* mouse]. 1. A tissue composed of contractile fibers or cells. Classified by microscopical appearance as nonstriated (smooth) or striated; by volitional control as voluntary or involuntary; by location in the body as skeletal, cardiac, or visceral. 2. A contractile organ composed of muscle tissue, effecting the movements of the organs and parts of the body; particularly, that composed of a belly of skeletal muscle tissue attached by tendons to bone on either side of a joint effecting movements at the joint by contraction of the belly drawing the more movable attachment, the insertion, toward the more fixed attachment, the origin. For muscles listed by name, see Table of Muscles in the Appendix. See also Plates 3, 4.

muscle adenylic acid. Adenosine 5'-monophosphate. See *adenosine monophosphate.*

muscle-contraction headache. Any headache or sensation of tightness, constriction or pressure, associated with sustained contraction of head and neck muscles in the absence of permanent structural changes, and usually associated with emotional tension; the headache varies widely in intensity, frequency, and duration; frequently suboccipital.

muscle cylinder ratio. The relationship of muscle mass diameter to total extremity cylinder diameter, as determined from roentgenograms of the extremity; it is related to the amount of subcutaneous fat, as opposed to muscle mass.

muscle erotism. The association of the libido with muscular activity.

muscle fiber. Fibers made up of muscle cells. Voluntary muscles consist of transversely striated fibers, involuntary muscles of spindle-shaped fibers or cells.

muscle fiber types. Muscle fibers classified according to their histochemical reactions, and sometimes size. Human muscle falls chiefly into two types: I, rich in oxidative enzymes and poor in phosphorylase, corresponding to red muscle fibers in various other animals; and II, rich in phosphorylase and poor in oxidative enzymes as well as myosin ATPase, and corresponding to white fibers in the other animals.

muscle graft. A portion of muscle sutured in place, for checking hemorrhage where a bleeding vessel cannot be secured.

muscle guarding. MUSCLE SPLINTING.

muscle hemoglobin. MYOGLOBIN.

muscle of Bell [C. *Bell*]. A band of smooth muscle of the urinary bladder, running from the orifice of the ureter toward the median lobe of the prostate gland in the male and toward the neck of the bladder in the female.

muscle of Gantzer [C. F. L. *Gantzer*]. Any of the accessorius muscles of the hand. See Table of Muscles in the Appendix.

muscle of Gegenbaur [C. *Gegenbaur*]. AURICULOFRONTALIS.

muscle of Gruber [W. L. *Gruber*]. PERONEOCALCANEUS EXTERNUS.

muscle of Hall. ISCHIOBULBOSUS.

muscle of Henle [F. G. J. *Henle*]. The anterior auricular muscle. See *auricular* in Table of Muscles in the Appendix.

muscle of Horner [W. E. *Horner*]. The lacrimal part of orbicularis oculi muscle.

muscle of Houston [J. *Houston*]. COMPRESSOR VENAE DORSALIS.

muscle of Jung [C. G. *Jung*]. The pyramidal muscle of the ear. See *pyramidal of ear* in Table of Muscles in the Appendix.

muscle of Klein [E. E. *Klein*]. COMPRESSOR LABII.

muscle of Landström [J. *Landström*]. Smooth muscle fibers in the fascia about the eyeball; the smooth muscle associated with the levator palpebrae superioris muscle is a portion of it.

muscle of Ludwig [W. F. von *Ludwig*]. ARYVOCALIS.

muscle of Mac·al·lis·ter. FIBULOCALCANEUS.

muscle of Müller [Heinrich *Müller*]. 1. ORBITAL (2). 2. The tarsal muscles. 3. The innermost, circular portion of the ciliary muscle.

muscle of Raux. RECTOURETHRALIS.

muscle of Riolan [J. *Riolan*]. The ciliary portion of the palpebral part of the orbicularis oculi muscle.

muscle of Santorini [C. D. *Santorini*]. RISORIUS.

muscle of Sappey [M. P. C. *Sappey*]. MUSCULUS TEMPOROPARIETALIS.

muscle of Treitz [W. *Treitz*]. 1. SUSPENSORY MUSCLE OF THE DUODENUM. 2. RECTOCOCCYGEUS.

muscle of Wood. EXTENSOR CARPI RADIALIS INTERMEDIUS.

muscle phosphorylase deficiency. MCARDLE'S SYNDROME.

muscle plate. MYOTOME (2).

muscle poison. A substance that impairs or destroys the proper functions of muscles.

muscle segment. MYOTOME (2).

muscle sense. PROPRIOCEPTION.

muscle sound. The sound heard through the stethoscope when placed over a muscle while it is contracting; SUSURRUS.

muscle spindle. One of the small fusiform sensory end organs found in almost all the organs of the body. Syn. *neuromuscular spindle.*

muscle splinting. The involuntary limitation of motion of an extremity, or the rigidity of trunk muscles, by muscle spasm.

muscle-splitting incision. An incision in which the muscles are split in the direction of their fibers in order to secure a better line of closure, as the McBurney incision.

muscle stretch reflex. STRETCH REFLEX.

muscle sugar. INOSITOL.

muscle tendon spindle. CORPUSCLE OF GOLGI.

muscle tone. TONUS.

muscle twitch. A single rapid contraction and relaxation of a skeletal muscle following application of a single stimulus.

muscul-, musculo-. A combining form meaning *muscle* or *muscular.*

mus·cu·lar (mus'kew·lur) *adj.* 1. Of or pertaining to muscles. 2. Having well-developed muscles. —**mus·cu·lar·i·ty** (mus''kew·lăr'i·tee) *n.*

muscular anesthesia. Loss of proprioception.

muscular artery. DISTRIBUTING ARTERY.

muscular asthenopia. Asthenopia due to weakness, incoordination (heterophoria), or strain of the external ocular muscles.

muscular atrophy. A loss of muscle bulk due to a lesion

involving either the cell body or axon of the lower motor neuron, or secondary to aging, disuse, deficiency states, or to a variety of degenerative, toxic, inflammatory, vascular, or metabolic disorders of the muscle fibers themselves. Compare *muscular dystrophy*. See also *infantile spinal muscular atrophy, peroneal muscular atrophy, progressive spinal muscular atrophy.*

muscular dystrophy. A hereditary, progressive degeneration of muscle. See *pseudohypertrophic infantile muscular dystrophy.* See also *myotonic dystrophy.*

muscular funnel. The space bounded by the four rectus muscles of the eye (the superior, inferior, lateral, and medial muscles), said to resemble a funnel.

muscular insufficiency. Inability of a muscle to contract sufficiently to produce the normal effect.

muscular irritability. The inherent capacity of a muscle to respond or its capacity to respond to threshold or suprathreshold stimuli by contraction.

mus·cu·la·ris (mus″kew·lair′is) *n.* [short for *tunica muscularis*]. 1. The muscular layer of a tubular or hollow organ. 2. MUSCULARIS MUCOSAE.

muscularis mu·co·sae (mew·ko′see). The single or double thin layer of smooth muscle in the deep portion of some mucous membranes, as in most of the digestive tube.

muscular mesoropter. The angle formed by the visual axes of the eyes when the lateral ocular muscles are at rest.

muscular murmur. The sound heard on auscultation of a contracting muscle.

muscular process. A stout process from the lateral angle of the base of the arytenoid cartilage into which are inserted the cricoarytenoid muscles. NA *processus muscularis cartilaginis arytenoidei.*

muscular rheumatism. FIBROSITIS.

muscular rigidity. Stiffness and generally increased resistance to movements of muscles as seen in a variety of extrapyramidal motor disorders and the catatonic type of schizophrenia.

muscular sense. PROPRIOCEPTION.

muscular subaortic stenosis. IDIOPATHIC HYPERTROPHIC SUBAORTIC STENOSIS.

muscular tension. The state present when muscles are passively stretched or actively contracted.

muscular tone. TONUS.

muscular tremor. Slight, oscillating, rhythmic muscular contractions; FASCICULATIONS.

muscular triangle. INFERIOR CAROTID TRIANGLE.

muscular trophoneurosis. *Obsol.* Trophic changes in the muscles in connection with disease of the nervous system. See also *muscular atrophy.*

mus·cu·la·ture (mus′kew·luh·chur, ·tewr) *n.* The muscular system of the body, or a part of it.

musculi. Plural and genitive singular of *musculus.*

musculi ab·do·mi·nis (ab·dom′i·nis) [NA]. Abdominal muscles.

musculi ar·rec·to·res pi·lo·rum (a·reck·to′reez pi·lo′rum) [NA]. ARRECTORES PILORUM.

musculi bul·bi (bul′bye) [NA]. The muscles of the eyeball, collectively.

musculi ca·pi·tis (kap′i·tis) [NA]. The muscles of the head, collectively.

musculi coc·cy·gei (kock·sij′ee·eye) [NA]. The muscles of the coccyx.

musculi col·li (kol′eye) [NA]. The anterior muscles of the neck, collectively.

musculi dor·si (dor′sigh) [NA]. The muscles of the back, collectively.

musculi ex·tre·mi·ta·tis in·fe·ri·o·ris (eck·strem·i·tay′tis in·feer·ee·o′ris) [BNA]. MUSCULI MEMBRI INFERIORIS.

musculi extremitatis su·pe·ri·o·ris (sue·peer·ee·o′ris) [BNA]. MUSCULI MEMBRI SUPERIORIS.

musculi in·ci·si·vi la·bii in·fe·ri·o·ris (in·si·sigh′vye lay′bee·eye in·feer·ee·o′ris) [BNA]. INCISIVI (sing. INCISIVUS) LABII INFERIORIS.

musculi incisivi labii su·pe·ri·o·ris (sue·peer·ee·o′ris) [BNA]. INCISIVI (sing. INCISIVUS) LABII SUPERIORIS.

musculi in·fra·hy·oi·dei (in″fruh·high·oy′dee·eye) [NA]. INFRAHYOID MUSCLES.

musculi in·ter·cos·ta·les ex·ter·ni (in″tur·kos·tay′leez ecks·tur′nigh) [NA]. The external intercostal muscles. See *intercostal muscles.*

musculi intercostales in·ter·ni (in·tur′nigh) [NA]. The internal intercostal muscles. See *intercostal muscles.*

musculi intercostales in·ti·mi (in′ti·migh) [NA]. The innermost intercostal muscles. See *intercostal muscles.*

musculi in·ter·os·sei dor·sa·les ma·nus (in″tur·os′ee·eye dor·say′leez man′us) [NA]. The dorsal interossei muscles of the hand. See Table of Muscles in the Appendix.

musculi interossei dorsales pe·dis (ped′is) [NA]. The dorsal interossei muscles of the foot. See Table of Muscles in the Appendix.

musculi interossei pal·ma·res (pal·mair′eez) [NA]. The palmar interossei muscles. See Table of Muscles in the Appendix.

musculi interossei plan·ta·res (plan·tair′eez) [NA]. The plantar interossei muscles. See Table of Muscles in the Appendix.

musculi interossei vo·la·res (vo·lair′eez) [BNA]. MUSCULI INTEROSSEI PALMARES.

musculi in·ter·spi·na·les (in″tur·spye·nay′leez) [NA]. INTERSPINALES.

musculi interspinales cer·vi·cis (sur′vi·sis) [NA]. The interspinales muscles of the neck. See Table of Muscles in the Appendix.

musculi interspinales lum·bo·rum (lum·bo′rum) [NA]. The interspinales muscles of the lumbar region. See Table of Muscles in the Appendix.

musculi interspinales tho·ra·cis (tho·ray′sis) [NA]. The interspinales muscles of the thoracic region. See Table of Muscles in the Appendix.

musculi in·ter·trans·ver·sa·rii (in″tur·trans·vur·sair′ee·eye) [NA]. INTERTRANSVERSARII; the intertransverse muscles.

musculi intertransversarii an·te·ri·o·res (an·teer″ee·o′reez) [BNA]. MUSCULI INTERTRANSVERSARII ANTERIORES CERVICIS.

musculi intertransversarii anteriores cer·vi·cis (sur′vi·sis) [NA]. The anterior cervical intertransverse muscles. See Table of Muscles in the Appendix.

musculi intertransversarii la·te·ra·les (lat·e·ray′leez) [BNA]. MUSCULI INTERTRANSVERSARII LATERALES LUMBORUM.

musculi intertransversarii laterales lum·bo·rum (lum·bo′rum) [NA]. The lateral lumbar intertransverse muscles. See Table of Muscles in the Appendix.

musculi intertransversarii me·di·a·les (mee·dee·ay′leez) [BNA]. MUSCULI INTERTRANSVERSARII MEDIALES LUMBORUM.

musculi intertransversarii mediales lum·bo·rum (lum·bo′rum) [NA]. The medial lumbar intertransverse muscles. See Table of Muscles in the Appendix.

musculi intertransversarii pos·te·ri·o·res (pos·teer″ee·o′reez) [BNA]. MUSCULI INTERTRANSVERSARII POSTERIORES CERVICIS.

musculi intertransversarii posteriores cer·vi·cis (sur′vi·sis) [NA]. The posterior cervical intertransverse muscles. See Table of Muscles in the Appendix.

musculi intertransversarii tho·ra·cis (tho·ray′sis) [NA]. The thoracic intertransverse muscles. See Table of Muscles in the Appendix.

musculi la·ryn·gis (la·rin′jis) [NA]. The intrinsic muscles of the larynx, collectively.

musculi le·va·to·res cos·ta·rum (lev·uh·to′reez kos·tair′um) [NA]. LEVATORES COSTARUM.

musculi levatores costarum bre·ves (brev′eez) [NA]. The short levatores costarum muscles. See *levatores costarum.*

musculi levatores costarum lon·gi (long'guy, lon'jye) [NA]. The long levatores costarum muscles. See *levatores costarum.*

musculi lin·guae (ling'gwee) [NA]. The intrinsic and extrinsic muscles of the tongue, collectively.

musculi lum·bri·ca·les (lum·bri·kay'leez) [NA]. LUMBRICALS.

musculi lumbricales ma·nus (man'us) [NA]. The lumbricals of the fingers. See Table of Muscles in the Appendix.

musculi lumbricales pe·dis (ped'is) [NA]. The lumbricals of the toes. See Table of Muscles in the Appendix.

musculi mem·bri in·fe·ri·o·ris (mem'brye in·feer·ee·o'ris) [NA]. The muscles of the inferior member or extremity.

musculi membri su·pe·ri·o·ris (sue·peer·ee·o'ris) [NA]. The muscles of the superior member or extremity.

musculi mul·ti·fi·di (mul·tif'i·dye) [NA]. The multifidus muscles. See Table of Muscles in the Appendix.

musculi ocu·li (ock'yoo·lye) [BNA]. MUSCULI BULBI.

musculi os·si·cu·lo·rum au·di·tus (os·ick"yoo·lo'rum aw·dye'tus) [NA]. The muscles of the ossicles of the ears; the stapedius and tensor tympani.

musculi os·sis hy·oi·dei (os'is high·oy'dee·eye) [BNA]. The muscles of the hyoid; the infrahyoid muscles and the suprahyoid muscles, collectively.

musculi pa·la·ti et fau·ci·um (pa·lay'tye et faw'see·um) [NA]. The muscles associated with the soft palate and fauces.

musculi pa·pil·la·res (pap·i·lair'eez) [NA]. PAPILLARY MUSCLES.

musculi papillares sep·ta·les (sep·tay'leez) [NA]. The septal papillary muscles. See Table of Muscles in the Appendix.

musculi pec·ti·na·ti (peck·ti·nay'tye) [NA]. PECTINATE MUSCLES.

musculi pe·ri·nei (perr·i·nee'eye) [NA]. The muscles of the perineum, collectively.

musculi ro·ta·to·res (ro·tuh·to'reez) [NA]. ROTATORES.

musculi rotatores bre·ves (brev'eez) [BNA]. The rotatores breves muscles. See Table of Muscles in the Appendix.

musculi rotatores cer·vi·cis (sur'vi·sis) [NA]. The rotatores cervicis muscles. See Table of Muscles in the Appendix.

musculi rotatores lon·gi (long'guy, lon'jye) [BNA]. The rotatores longi muscles. See Table of Muscles in the Appendix.

musculi rotatores lum·bo·rum (lum·bo'rum) [NA]. The rotatores lumborum muscles. See Table of Muscles in the Appendix.

musculi rotatores tho·ra·cis (tho·ray'sis) [NA]. The rotatores thoracis muscles. See Table of Muscles in the Appendix.

musculi sub·cos·ta·les (sub"kos·tay'leez) [NA]. SUBCOSTALS.

musculi su·pra·hy·oi·dei (sue"pruh·high·oy'dee·eye) [NA]. SUPRAHYOID MUSCLES.

musculi tho·ra·cis (tho·ray'sis) [NA]. The muscles of the thoracic wall, collectively.

musculo-. See *muscul-.*

mus·cu·lo·apo·neu·rot·ic (mus"kew·lo·ap"o·new·rot'ick) *adj.* [*musculo-* + *aponeurotic*]. Composed of muscle and of fibrous connective tissue in the form of a membrane.

mus·cu·lo·cu·ta·ne·ous (mus"kew·lo·kew·tay'nee·us) *adj.* [*musculo-* + *cutaneous*]. Pertaining to or supplying the muscles and skin.

musculocutaneous nerve of the arm. NA *nervus musculocutaneus.* See Table of Nerves in the Appendix.

mus·cu·lo·fas·cial (mus"kew·lo·fash'ee·ul) *adj.* Consisting of both muscular and fascial elements, as in an amputation flap.

mus·cu·lo·fi·brous (mus"kew·lo·figh'brus) *adj.* Pertaining to a tissue which is partly muscular and partly fibrous connective tissue.

mus·cu·lo·mem·bra·nous (mus"kew·lo·mem'bruh·nus) *adj.* [*musculo-* + *membranous*]. Composed of muscular tissue and membrane.

mus·cu·lo·phren·ic (mus"kew·lo·fren'ick) *adj.* [*musculo-* + *phrenic*]. Pertaining to or supplying the muscles of the diaphragm.

mus·cu·lo·skel·e·tal (mus"kew·lo·skel'e·tul) *adj.* [*musculo-* + *skeletal*]. Pertaining to or composed of the muscles and the skeleton.

mus·cu·lo·spi·ral (mus"kew·lo·spye'rul) *adj.* [*musculo-* + *spiral*]. RADIAL (2).

musculospiral groove or **sulcus.** RADIAL SULCUS.

musculospiral nerve. The radial nerve. See Table of Nerves in the Appendix.

mus·cu·lo·ten·di·nous (mus"kew·lo·ten'di·nus) *adj.* Composed of muscular and tendinous fibers.

musculotendinous cuff. Fibers of the supraspinatus, infraspinatus, teres minor, and subscapularis muscles, which blend with and reinforce the capsule of the shoulder joint. Syn. *rotator cuff.*

mus·cu·lo·tub·al (mus"kew·lo·tew'bul) *adj.* Pertaining to the tensor tympani muscle and the auditory tube.

musculotubal canals. The semicanals in the temporal bone, which transmit the auditory tube and tensor tympani muscle, considered together.

mus·cu·lo·tu·be·ral canals (mus"kew·lo·tew'bur·ul). MUSCULOTUBAL CANALS.

mus·cu·lus (mus'kew·lus) *n.*, pl. & genit. sing. **muscu·li** (·lye) [L.] [NA]. MUSCLE. For muscles listed by name, see Table of Muscles in the Appendix.

musculus abductor di·gi·ti mi·ni·mi (dij'i·tye min'i·migh) [NA]. ABDUCTOR DIGITI MINIMI.

musculus abductor digiti quin·ti (kwin'tye) [BNA]. Musculus abductor digiti minimi (= ABDUCTOR DIGITI MINIMI).

musculus abductor hal·lu·cis (hal'yoo·sis) [NA]. ABDUCTOR HALLUCIS.

musculus abductor pol·li·cis bre·vis (pol'i·sis brev'is) [NA]. ABDUCTOR POLLICIS BREVIS.

musculus abductor pollicis lon·gus (long'gus) [NA]. ABDUCTOR POLLICIS LONGUS.

musculus adductor bre·vis (brev'is) [NA]. ADDUCTOR BREVIS.

musculus adductor hal·lu·cis (hal'yoo·sis) [NA]. ADDUCTOR HALLUCIS.

musculus adductor lon·gus (long'gus) [NA]. ADDUCTOR LONGUS.

musculus adductor mag·nus (mag'nus) [NA]. ADDUCTOR MAGNUS.

musculus adductor mi·ni·mus (min'i·mus) [BNA]. ADDUCTOR MINIMUS.

musculus adductor pol·li·cis (pol'i·sis) [NA]. ADDUCTOR POLLICIS.

musculus an·co·ne·us (ang·ko'nee·us, ang"ko·nee'us) [NA]. ANCONEUS.

musculus an·ti·tra·gi·cus (an"tee·traj'i·kus) [NA]. ANTITRAGICUS.

musculus ar·ti·cu·la·ris (ahr·tick"yoo·lair'is) [NA]. ARTICULAR MUSCLE.

musculus articularis cu·bi·ti (kew'bi·tye) [NA]. The articularis cubiti muscle. See Table of Muscles in the Appendix.

musculus articularis ge·nus (jen'us) [NA]. ARTICULARIS GENUS.

musculus ary·epi·glot·ti·cus (ăr"ee·ep·i·glot'i·kus) [NA]. ARYEPIGLOTTICUS.

musculus ary·te·noi·de·us obli·quus (ăr·i·tee·noy'dee·us ob·lye'kwus) [NA]. The oblique arytenoid muscle. See Table of Muscles in the Appendix.

musculus arytenoideus trans·ver·sus (trans·vur'sus) [NA]. The transverse arytenoid muscle. See Table of Muscles in the Appendix.

musculus au·ri·cu·la·ris anterior (aw·rick"yoo·lair'is) [NA]. The anterior auricular muscle. See Table of Muscles in the Appendix.

musculus auricularis posterior [NA]. The posterior auricular muscle. See Table of Muscles in the Appendix.

musculus auricularis superior [NA]. The superior auricular muscle. See Table of Muscles in the Appendix.

musculus bi·ceps bra·chii (bye'seps bray'kee·eye) [NA]. The biceps brachii. See Table of Muscles in the Appendix.

musculus biceps fe·mo·ris (fem'o·ris) [NA]. The biceps femoris. See Table of Muscles in the Appendix.
musculus bi·pen·na·tus (bye"pen·ay'tus) [NA]. BIPENNATE MUSCLE.
musculus bra·chi·a·lis (bray·kee·ay'lis) [NA]. BRACHIALIS.
musculus bra·chio·ra·di·a·lis (bray"kee·o·ray·dee·ay'lis) [NA]. The brachioradialis muscle. See Table of Muscles in the Appendix.
musculus bron·cho·eso·pha·ge·us (bronk"o·ee·so·faj'ee·us) [NA]. BRONCHOESOPHAGEAL MUSCLE.
musculus buc·ci·na·tor (buck"si·nay'tor) [NA]. BUCCINATOR.
musculus buc·co·pha·ryn·ge·us (buck"o·fa·rin'jee·us) [BNA]. PARS BUCCOPHARYNGEA MUSCULI CONSTRICTORIS PHARYNGIS SUPERIORIS.
musculus bul·bo·ca·ver·no·sus (bul"bo·kav·ur·no'sus) [BNA]. Musculus bulbospongiosus (= BULBOSPONGIOSUS).
musculus bul·bo·spon·gi·o·sus (bul"bo·spon·jee·o'sus) [NA]. BULBOSPONGIOSUS.
musculus ca·ni·nus (ka·nigh'nus) [BNA]. Musculus levator anguli oris (= LEVATOR ANGULI ORIS).
musculus ce·ra·to·cri·coi·de·us (serr"uh·to·kri·koy'dee·us) [NA]. CERATOCRICOID.
musculus ce·ra·to·pha·ryn·ge·us (serr"uh·to·fa·rin'jee·us) [BNA]. PARS CERATOPHARYNGEA MUSCULI CONSTRICTORIS PHARYNGIS MEDII.
musculus chon·dro·glos·sus (kon·dro·glos'us) [NA]. CHONDROGLOSSUS MUSCLE.
musculus chon·dro·pha·ryn·ge·us (kon"dro·fa·rin'jee·us) [BNA]. PARS CHONDROPHARYNGEA MUSCULI CONSTRICTORIS PHARYNGIS MEDII.
musculus ci·li·a·ris (sil·ee·air'is) [NA]. CILIARY MUSCLE.
musculus coc·cy·ge·us (kock·sij'ee·us) [NA]. COCCYGEUS.
musculus con·stric·tor pha·ryn·gis inferior (kon·strick'tor fa·rin'jis) [NA]. The inferior constrictor muscle of the pharynx. See Table of Muscles in the Appendix.
musculus constrictor pharyngis me·di·us (mee'dee·us) [NA]. The middle constrictor muscle of the pharynx. See Table of Muscles in the Appendix.
musculus constrictor pharyngis superior [NA]. The superior constrictor muscle of the pharynx. See Table of Muscles in the Appendix.
musculus co·ra·co·bra·chi·a·lis (kor"uh·ko·bray·kee·ay'lis) [NA]. CORACOBRACHIALIS.
musculus cor·ru·ga·tor su·per·ci·lii (kor·oo·gay'tor sue"pur·sil'ee·eye) [NA]. CORRUGATOR SUPERCILII.
musculus cre·mas·ter (kre·mas'tur) [NA]. CREMASTER.
musculus cri·co·ary·te·noi·de·us la·te·ra·lis (krye"ko·ăr·i·te·noy'dee·us lat·e·ray'lis) [NA]. The lateral cricoarytenoid muscle. See Table of Muscles in the Appendix.
musculus cricoarytenoideus posterior [NA]. The posterior cricoarytenoid muscle. See Table of Muscles in the Appendix.
musculus cri·co·pha·ryn·ge·us (krye"ko·fa·rin'jee·us) [BNA]. PARS CRICOPHARYNGEA MUSCULI CONSTRICTORIS PHARYNGIS INFERIORIS.
musculus cri·co·thy·roi·de·us (krye"ko·thigh·roy'dee·us) [NA]. CRICOTHYROID (2).
musculus cu·ta·ne·us (kew·tay'nee·us) [NA]. CUTANEOUS MUSCLE.
musculus del·toi·de·us (del·toy'dee·us) [NA]. DELTOID MUSCLE.
musculus depressor an·gu·li oris (ang'gew·lye o'ris) [NA]. DEPRESSOR ANGULI ORIS.
musculus depressor la·bii in·fe·ri·o·ris (lay'bee·eye in·feer"ee·o'ris) [NA]. DEPRESSOR LABII INFERIORIS.
musculus depressor sep·ti na·si (sep'tye nay'zye) [NA]. DEPRESSOR SEPTI NASI.
musculus depressor su·per·ci·lii (sue"pur·sil'ee·eye) [NA]. DEPRESSOR SUPERCILII.
musculus di·gas·tri·cus (dye·gas'tri·kus) [NA]. DIGASTRIC MUSCLE.
musculus di·la·ta·tor pu·pil·lae (dil·uh·tay'tor pew·pil'ee) [BNA]. Musculus dilator pupillae (= DILATOR PUPILLAE).
musculus di·la·tor pu·pil·lae (dye·lay'tor pew·pil'ee) [NA]. DILATOR PUPILLAE.
musculus epi·cra·ni·us (ep·i·kray'nee·us) [NA]. EPICRANIUS.
musculus epi·tro·chleo·an·co·nae·us (ep"i·trock"lee·o·ang·ko'nee·us) [BNA]. EPITROCHLEO-OLECRANONIS.
musculus erector spi·nae (spye'nee) [NA]. ERECTOR SPINAE.
musculus ex·ten·sor car·pi ra·di·a·lis bre·vis (ecks·ten'sor kahr'pye ray"dee·ay'lis brev'is) [NA]. EXTENSOR CARPI RADIALIS BREVIS.
musculus extensor carpi radialis lon·gus (long'gus) [NA]. EXTENSOR CARPI RADIALIS LONGUS.
musculus extensor carpi ul·na·ris (ul·nair'is) [NA]. EXTENSOR CARPI ULNARIS.
musculus extensor digiti mi·ni·mi (min'i·migh) [NA]. EXTENSOR DIGITI MINIMI.
musculus extensor digiti quin·ti pro·pri·us (kwin'tye pro'pree·us) [BNA]. Musculus extensor digiti minimi (= EXTENSOR DIGITI MINIMI).
musculus extensor di·gi·to·rum (dij·i·to'rum) [NA]. EXTENSOR DIGITORUM.
musculus extensor digitorum bre·vis (brev'is) [NA]. EXTENSOR DIGITORUM BREVIS.
musculus extensor digitorum com·mu·nis (kom·yoo'nis) [BNA]. Musculus extensor digitorum (= EXTENSOR DIGITORUM).
musculus extensor digitorum lon·gus (long'gus) [NA]. EXTENSOR DIGITORUM LONGUS.
musculus extensor hal·lu·cis bre·vis (hal'yoo·sis brev'is) [NA]. EXTENSOR HALLUCIS BREVIS.
musculus extensor hallucis lon·gus (long'gus) [NA]. EXTENSOR HALLUCIS LONGUS.
musculus extensor in·di·cis (in'di·sis) [NA]. EXTENSOR INDICIS.
musculus extensor indicis pro·pri·us (pro'pree·us) [BNA]. Musculus extensor indicis (= EXTENSOR INDICIS).
musculus extensor pol·li·cis bre·vis (pol'i·sis brev'is) [NA]. EXTENSOR POLLICIS BREVIS.
musculus extensor pollicis lon·gus (long'gus) [NA]. EXTENSOR POLLICIS LONGUS.
musculus fi·bu·la·ris bre·vis (fib"yoo·lair'is brev'is) [NA alt.]. PERONEUS BREVIS. NA alt. *musculus peroneus brevis.*
musculus fibularis lon·gus (long'gus) [NA alt.]. PERONEUS LONGUS. NA alt. *musculus peroneus longus.*
musculus fibularis ter·ti·us (tur'shee·us) [NA alt.]. PERONEUS TERTIUS. NA alt. *musculus peroneus tertius.*
musculus fix·a·tor ba·se·os sta·pe·dis (fick·say'tor bay'see·os stay·pee'dis). STAPEDIUS.
musculus flex·or ac·ces·sor·i·us (fleck'sor ack"se·sor'ee·us) [NA alt.]. MUSCULUS QUADRATUS PLANTAE.
musculus flexor car·pi ra·di·a·lis (kahr'pye ray·dee·ay'lis) [NA]. FLEXOR CARPI RADIALIS.
musculus flexor carpi ul·na·ris (ul·nair'is) [NA]. FLEXOR CARPI ULNARIS.
musculus flexor di·gi·ti mi·ni·mi bre·vis (dij'i·tye min'i·migh brev'is) [NA]. FLEXOR DIGITI MINIMI BREVIS.
musculus flexor digiti quin·ti bre·vis (kwin'tye brev'is) [BNA]. Musculus flexor digiti minimi brevis (= FLEXOR DIGITI MINIMI BREVIS).
musculus flexor di·gi·to·rum bre·vis (dij·i·to'rum brev'is) [NA]. FLEXOR DIGITORUM BREVIS.
musculus flexor digitorum lon·gus (long'gus) [NA]. FLEXOR DIGITORUM LONGUS.
musculus flexor digitorum pro·fun·dus (pro·fun'dus) [NA]. FLEXOR DIGITORUM PROFUNDUS.
musculus flexor digitorum sub·li·mis (sub·lye'mis) [BNA]. Musculus flexor digitorum superficialis (= FLEXOR DIGITORUM SUPERFICIALIS).
musculus flexor digitorum su·per·fi·ci·a·lis (sue"pur·fish"ee·ay'lis) [NA]. FLEXOR DIGITORUM SUPERFICIALIS.
musculus flexor hal·lu·cis bre·vis (hal'yoo·sis brev'is) [NA]. FLEXOR HALLUCIS BREVIS.

musculus flexor hallucis lon·gus (long'gus) [NA]. FLEXOR HALLUCIS LONGUS.

musculus flexor pol·li·cis bre·vis (pol'i·sis brev'is) [NA]. FLEXOR POLLICIS BREVIS.

musculus flexor pollicis lon·gus (long'gus) [NA]. FLEXOR POLLICIS LONGUS.

musculus fron·ta·lis (fron·tay'lis) [BNA]. VENTER FRONTALIS MUSCULI OCCIPITOFRONTALIS.

musculus fu·si·for·mis (few·si·for'mis) [NA]. A spindle-shaped (fusiform) muscle.

musculus gas·tro·cne·mi·us (gas"tro·k'nee'mee·us) [NA]. GASTROCNEMIUS.

musculus ge·mel·lus in·fe·ri·or (je·mel'us in·feer'ee·or) [NA]. The inferior gemellus muscle. See Table of Muscles in the Appendix.

musculus gemellus superior [NA]. The superior gemellus muscle. See Table of Muscles in the Appendix.

musculus ge·nio·glos·sus (jee"nee·o·glos'us) [NA]. GENIOGLOSSUS.

musculus ge·nio·hy·oi·de·us (jee"nee·o·high·oy'dee·us) [NA]. GENIOHYOID.

musculus glos·so·pa·la·ti·nus (glos"o·pal·uh·tye'nus) [BNA]. Musculus palatoglossus (= PALATOGLOSSUS).

musculus glos·so·pha·ryn·ge·us (glos·o·fa·rin'jee·us) [BNA]. PARS GLOSSOPHARYNGEA MUSCULI CONSTRICTORIS PHARYNGIS SUPERIORIS.

musculus glu·te·us max·i·mus (gloo'tee·us mack'si·mus, gloo·tee'us) [NA]. GLUTEUS MAXIMUS.

musculus gluteus me·di·us (mee'dee·us) [NA]. GLUTEUS MEDIUS.

musculus gluteus mi·ni·mus (min'i·mus) [NA]. GLUTEUS MINIMUS.

musculus gra·ci·lis (gras'i·lis) [NA]. GRACILIS MUSCLE.

musculus he·li·cis major (hel'i·sis) [NA]. The helicis major muscle. See *helicis.*

musculus helicis minor [NA]. The helicis minor muscle. See *helicis.*

musculus hyo·glos·sus (high"o·glos'us) [NA]. HYOGLOSSUS.

musculus ili·a·cus (i·lye'uh·kus) [NA]. ILIACUS.

musculus ilio·coc·cy·ge·us (il"ee·o·kock·sij'ee·us) [NA]. ILIOCOCCYGEUS.

musculus ilio·cos·ta·lis (il"ee·o·kos·tay'lis) [NA]. ILIOCOSTALIS.

musculus iliocostalis cer·vi·cis (sur'vi·sis) [NA]. ILIOCOSTALIS CERVICIS.

musculus iliocostalis dor·si (dor'sigh) [BNA]. Musculus iliocostalis thoracis (= ILIOCOSTALIS THORACIS).

musculus iliocostalis lum·bo·rum (lum·bo'rum) [NA]. ILIOCOSTALIS LUMBORUM.

musculus iliocostalis tho·ra·cis (tho·ray'sis) [NA]. ILIOCOSTALIS THORACIS.

musculus ilio·pso·as (il"ee·o·so'us, ·op'so·us) [NA]. ILIOPSOAS.

musculus in·ci·su·rae he·li·cis (in"si·sue'ree hel'i·sis) [NA]. INCISURAE HELICIS.

musculus in·fra·spi·na·tus (in"fruh·spye·nay'tus) [NA]. INFRASPINATUS.

musculus is·chio·ca·ver·no·sus (is"kee·o·kav·ur·no'sus) [NA]. ISCHIOCAVERNOSUS.

musculus la·tis·si·mus dor·si (la·tis'i·mus dor'sigh) [NA]. LATISSIMUS DORSI.

musculus le·va·tor an·gu·li oris (le·vay'tor ang'gew·lye o'ris) [NA]. LEVATOR ANGULI ORIS.

musculus levator ani (ay'nigh) [NA]. LEVATOR ANI.

musculus levator glandulae thy·roi·de·ae (thigh·roy'dee·ee) [NA]. LEVATOR GLANDULAE THYROIDEAE.

musculus levator la·bii su·pe·ri·o·ris (lay'bee·eye sue·peer·ee·o'ris) [NA]. LEVATOR LABII SUPERIORIS.

musculus levator labii superioris alae·que na·si (ay·lee'kwee nay'zye) [NA]. LEVATOR LABII SUPERIORIS ALAEQUE NASI.

musculus levator pal·pe·brae su·pe·ri·o·ris (pal·pee'bree sue·peer"ee·o'ris) [NA]. LEVATOR PALPEBRAE SUPERIORIS.

musculus levator pro·sta·tae (pros'tuh·tee) [NA]. LEVATOR PROSTATAE.

musculus levator sca·pu·lae (skap'yoo·lee) [NA]. LEVATOR SCAPULAE.

musculus levator ve·li pa·la·ti·ni (vee'lye pal·uh·tye'nigh) [NA]. LEVATOR VELI PALATINI.

musculus lon·gis·si·mus (lon·jis'i·mus) [NA]. LONGISSIMUS (2).

musculus longissimus ca·pi·tis (kap'i·tis) [NA]. The longissimus capitis muscle. See Table of Muscles in the Appendix.

musculus longissimus cer·vi·cis (sur'vi·sis) [NA]. The longissimus cervicis muscle. See Table of Muscles in the Appendix.

musculus longissimus dor·si (dor'sigh) [BNA]. MUSCULUS LONGISSIMUS THORACIS.

musculus longissimus tho·ra·cis (tho·ray'sis) [NA]. The longissimus thoracis muscle. See Table of Muscles in the Appendix.

musculus lon·gi·tu·di·na·lis in·fe·ri·or lin·guae (lon"ji·tew·di·nay'lis in·feer'ee·or ling'gwee) [NA]. The inferior longitudinalis muscle of the tongue. See Table of Muscles in the Appendix.

musculus longitudinalis superior linguae [NA]. The superior longitudinalis muscle of the tongue. See Table of Muscles in the Appendix.

musculus lon·gus ca·pi·tis (long'gus kap'i·tis) [NA]. LONGUS CAPITIS.

musculus longus col·li (kol'eye) [NA]. LONGUS COLLI.

musculus mas·se·ter (mas·see'tur) [NA]. MASSETER.

musculus men·ta·lis (men·tay'lis) [NA]. MENTALIS.

musculus mul·ti·fi·dus (mul·tif'i·dus) [BNA]. Singular of *musculi multifidi.*

musculus my·lo·hy·oi·de·us (migh"lo·high·oy'dee·us) [NA]. MYLOHYOID MUSCLE.

musculus my·lo·pha·ryn·ge·us (migh"lo·fa·rin'jee·us) [BNA]. Pars mylopharyngea musculi constrictoris pharyngis superioris (= MYLOPHARYNGEAL).

musculus na·sa·lis (na·say'lis) [NA]. NASALIS.

musculus ob·li·quus au·ri·cu·lae (ob·lye'kwus aw·rick'yoo·lee) [NA]. The oblique auricular muscle. See *auricular* in Table of Muscles in the Appendix.

musculus obliquus ca·pi·tis in·fe·ri·or (kap'i·tis in·feer'ee·or) [NA]. The inferior oblique muscle of the head. See *oblique* in Table of Muscles in the Appendix.

musculus obliquus capitis superior [NA]. The superior oblique muscle of the head. See *oblique* in Table of Muscles in the Appendix.

musculus obliquus ex·ter·nus ab·do·mi·nis (ecks·tur'nus ab·dom'i·nis) [NA]. The external oblique muscle of the abdomen. See *oblique* in Table of Muscles in the Appendix.

musculus obliquus inferior bul·bi (bul'bye) [NA]. The inferior oblique muscle of the eye. See *oblique* in Table of Muscles in the Appendix.

musculus obliquus inferior ocu·li (ock'yoo·lye) [BNA]. MUSCULUS OBLIQUUS INFERIOR BULBI.

musculus obliquus in·ter·nus ab·do·mi·nis (in·tur'nus ab·dom'i·nis) [NA]. The internal oblique muscle of the abdomen. See *oblique* in Table of Muscles in the Appendix.

musculus obliquus superior bul·bi (bul'bye) [NA]. The superior oblique muscle of the eye. See *oblique* in Table of Muscles in the Appendix.

musculus obliquus superior ocu·li (ock'yoo·lye) [BNA]. MUSCULUS OBLIQUUS SUPERIOR BULBI.

musculus ob·tu·ra·tor ex·ter·nus (ob·tew·ray'tur ecks·tur'nus) [BNA]. MUSCULUS OBTURATORIUS EXTERNUS.

musculus obturator in·ter·nus (in·tur'nus) [BNA]. MUSCULUS OBTURATORIUS INTERNUS.

musculus ob·tu·ra·to·ri·us ex·ter·nus (ob·tew·ruh·to'ree·us ecks·tur'nus) [NA]. The obturator externus muscle. See Table of Muscles in the Appendix.

musculus obturatorius in·ter·nus (in·tur'nus) [NA]. The obturator internus muscle. See Table of Muscles in the Appendix.

musculus oc·ci·pi·ta·lis (ock·sip·i·tay'lis) [BNA]. VENTER OCCIPITALIS MUSCULI OCCIPITOFRONTALIS.

musculus oc·ci·pi·to·fron·ta·lis (ock·sip''i·to·fron·tay'lis) [NA]. OCCIPITOFRONTALIS.

musculus omo·hy·oi·de·us (o''mo·high·oy'dee·us) [NA]. OMOHYOID MUSCLE.

musculus op·po·nens di·gi·ti mi·ni·mi (o·po'nenz dij'i·tye min'i·miye) [NA]. OPPONENS DIGITI MINIMI.

musculus opponens digiti quin·ti ma·nus (kwin'tye man'us) [BNA]. Musculus opponens digiti minimi (= OPPONENS DIGITI MINIMI).

musculus opponens digiti quinti pe·dis (ped'is) [BNA]. Opponens digiti quinti of the foot. See Table of Muscles in the Appendix.

musculus opponens pol·li·cis (pol'i·sis) [NA]. OPPONENS POLLICIS.

musculus or·bi·cu·la·ris (or·bick·yoo·lair'is) [NA]. An orbicular muscle.

musculus orbicularis ocu·li (ock'yoo·lye) [NA]. ORBICULARIS OCULI.

musculus orbicularis oris (o'ris) [NA]. ORBICULARIS ORIS.

musculus or·bi·ta·lis (or·bi·tay'lis) [NA]. ORBITAL (2).

musculus pa·la·to·glos·sus (pal''uh·to·glos'us) [NA]. PALATOGLOSSUS.

musculus pa·la·to·pha·ryn·ge·us (pal''uh·to·fa·rin'jee·us) [NA]. PALATOPHARYNGEUS.

musculus pal·ma·ris bre·vis (pal·mair'is brev'is) [NA]. The palmaris brevis muscle. See Table of Muscles in the Appendix.

musculus palmaris lon·gus (long'gus) [NA]. The palmaris longus muscle. See Table of Muscles in the Appendix.

musculus pa·pil·la·ris an·te·ri·or ven·tri·cu·li dex·tri (pap·i·lair'is an·teer'ee·or ven·trick'yoo·lye decks'trye) [NA]. The anterior papillary muscle of the right ventricle. See Table of Muscles in the Appendix.

musculus papillaris anterior ventriculi si·nis·tri (si·nis'trye) [NA]. The anterior papillary muscle of the left ventricle. See Table of Muscles in the Appendix.

musculus papillaris posterior ventriculi dextri [NA]. The posterior papillary muscle of the right ventricle. See Table of Muscles in the Appendix.

musculus papillaris posterior ventriculi sinistri [NA]. The posterior papillary muscle of the left ventricle. See Table of Muscles in the Appendix.

musculus pec·ti·ne·us (peck·tin'ee·us) [NA]. PECTINEUS.

musculus pec·to·ra·lis major (peck·to·ray'lis) [NA]. PECTORALIS MAJOR.

musculus pectoralis minor [NA]. PECTORALIS MINOR.

musculus pe·ro·ne·us bre·vis (perr·o·nee'us brev'is) [NA]. PERONEUS BREVIS. NA alt. *musculus fibularis brevis.*

musculus peroneus lon·gus (long'gus) [NA]. PERONEUS LONGUS. NA alt. *musculus fibularis longus.*

musculus peroneus ter·ti·us (tur'shee·us) [NA]. PERONEUS TERTIUS. NA alt. *musculus fibularis tertius.*

musculus pha·ryn·go·pa·la·ti·nus (fa·ring''go·pal·uh·tye'nus) [BNA]. Musculus palatopharyngeus (= PALATOPHARYNGEUS).

musculus pi·ri·for·mis (pirr''i·for'mis) [NA]. PIRIFORMIS.

musculus plan·ta·ris (plan·tair'is) [NA]. PLANTARIS.

musculus pleu·ro·eso·pha·ge·us (plew''ro·ee·so·faj'ee·us, ·fa·jee'us) [NA]. The pleuroesophageal muscle. See Table of Muscles in the Appendix.

musculus po·pli·te·us (pop·lit'ee·us) [NA]. POPLITEUS (2).

musculus pro·ce·rus (pro·seer'us) [NA]. PROCERUS.

musculus pro·na·tor quad·ra·tus (pro·nay'tor kwah·dray'tus) [NA]. The pronator quadratus. See Table of Muscles in the Appendix.

musculus pronator te·res (teer'eez) [NA]. The pronator teres muscle. See Table of Muscles in the Appendix.

musculus pro·sta·ti·cus (pros·tat'i·kus) [BNA]. SUBSTANTIA MUSCULARIS PROSTATAE.

musculus pso·as major (so'us) [NA]. PSOAS MAJOR.

musculus psoas minor [NA]. PSOAS MINOR.

musculus pte·ry·goi·de·us ex·ter·nus (terr·i·goy'dee·us ecks·tur'nus) [BNA]. MUSCULUS PTERYGOIDEUS LATERALIS.

musculus pterygoideus in·ter·nus (in·tur'nus) [BNA]. MUSCULUS PTERYGOIDEUS MEDIALIS.

musculus pterygoideus la·te·ra·lis (lat·e·ray'lis) [NA]. The lateral pterygoid muscle. See Table of Muscles in the Appendix.

musculus pterygoideus me·di·a·lis (mee·dee·ay'lis) [NA]. The medial pterygoid muscle. See Table of Muscles in the Appendix.

musculus pte·ry·go·pha·ryn·ge·us (terr''i·go·fa·rin'jee·us) [BNA]. PARS PTERYGOPHARYNGEA MUSCULI CONSTRICTORIS PHARYNGIS SUPERIORIS.

musculus pu·bo·coc·cy·ge·us (pew''bo·kock·sij'ee·us) [NA]. PUBOCOCCYGEUS.

musculus pu·bo·pro·sta·ti·cus (pew''bo·pros·tat'i·kus) [NA]. The puboprostatic muscle. See Table of Muscles in the Appendix.

musculus pu·bo·rec·ta·lis (pew''bo·reck·tay'lis) [NA]. PUBORECTALIS.

musculus pu·bo·va·gi·na·lis (pew''bo·vaj·i·nay'lis) [NA]. The pubovaginalis muscle. See Table of Muscles in the Appendix.

musculus pu·bo·ve·si·ca·lis (pew''bo·ves·i·kay'lis) [NA]. The pubovesicalis muscle. See Table of Muscles in the Appendix.

musculus py·ra·mi·da·lis (pi·ram·i·day'lis) [NA]. PYRAMIDALIS (1).

musculus pyramidalis au·ri·cu·lae (aw·rick'yoo·lee) [NA]. The pyramidal muscle of the ear. See Table of Muscles in the Appendix.

musculus qua·dra·tus fe·mo·ris (kwah·dray'tus fem'o·ris) [NA]. QUADRATUS FEMORIS.

musculus quadratus la·bii in·fe·ri·o·ris (lay'bee·eye in·feer·ee·o'ris) [BNA]. Musculus depressor labii inferioris (= DEPRESSOR LABII INFERIORIS).

musculus quadratus labii su·pe·ri·o·ris (sue·peer·ee·o'ris) [BNA]. Musculus levator labii superioris (= LEVATOR LABII SUPERIORIS).

musculus quadratus lum·bo·rum (lum·bo'rum) [NA]. QUADRATUS LUMBORUM.

musculus quadratus plan·tae (plan'tee) [NA]. The quadratus plantae muscle. NA alt. *musculus flexor accessorius.* See Table of Muscles in the Appendix.

musculus qua·dri·ceps fe·mo·ris (kwah'dri·seps fem'o·ris) [NA]. QUADRICEPS FEMORIS.

musculus rec·to·coc·cy·ge·us (reck''to·kock·sij'ee·us) [NA]. RECTOCOCCYGEUS.

musculus rec·to·ure·thra·lis (reck''to·yoo·re·thray'lis) [NA]. RECTOURETHRALIS.

musculus rec·to·ute·ri·nus (reck''to·yoo·te·rye'nus) [NA]. RECTOUTERINE MUSCLE.

musculus rec·to·ve·si·ca·lis (reck''to·ves''i·kay'lis) [NA]. RECTOVESICALIS.

musculus rec·tus ab·do·mi·nis (reck'tus ab·dom'i·nis) [NA]. RECTUS ABDOMINIS.

musculus rectus ca·pi·tis anterior (kap'i·tis) [NA]. The rectus capitis anterior muscle. See Table of Muscles in the Appendix.

musculus rectus capitis la·te·ra·lis (lat·e·ray'lis) [NA]. The rectus capitis lateralis muscle. See Table of Muscles in the Appendix.

musculus rectus capitis posterior major [NA]. The rectus capitis posterior major muscle. See Table of Muscles in the Appendix.

musculus rectus capitis posterior minor [NA]. The rectus capitis posterior minor muscle. See Table of Muscles in the Appendix.

musculus rectus fe·mo·ris (fem'o·ris) [NA]. The rectus femoris muscle. See Table of Muscles in the Appendix.

musculus rectus inferior bul·bi (bul'bye) [NA]. The rectus inferior bulbi muscle. See Table of Muscles in the Appendix.

musculus rectus inferior ocu·li (ock'yoo·lye) [BNA]. MUSCULUS RECTUS INFERIOR BULBI.

musculus rectus la·te·ra·lis bul·bi (lat·e·ray'lis bul'bye) [NA]. The rectus lateralis bulbi muscle. See Table of Muscles in the Appendix.

musculus rectus lateralis ocu·li (ock'yoo·lye) [BNA]. MUSCULUS RECTUS LATERALIS BULBI.

musculus rectus me·di·a·lis bul·bi (mee·dee·ay'lis bul'bye) [NA]. The rectus medialis bulbi muscle. See Table of Muscles in the Appendix.

musculus rectus medialis ocu·li (ock'yoo·lye) [BNA]. MUSCULUS RECTUS MEDIALIS BULBI.

musculus rectus superior bulbi [NA]. The rectus superior bulbi muscle. See Table of Muscles in the Appendix.

musculus rectus superior oculi [BNA]. MUSCULUS RECTUS SUPERIOR BULBI.

musculus rhom·boi·de·us major (rom·boy'dee·us) [NA]. The rhomboideus major muscle. See Table of Muscles in the Appendix.

musculus rhomboideus minor [NA]. The rhomboideus minor muscle. See Table of Muscles in the Appendix.

musculus ri·so·ri·us (ri·so'ree·us) [NA]. RISORIUS.

musculus sa·cro·coc·cy·ge·us an·te·ri·or (say''kro·kock·sij'ee·us an·teer'ee·or) [BNA]. Musculus sacrococcygeus ventralis (= SACROCOCCYGEUS VENTRALIS).

musculus sacrococcygeus dor·sa·lis (dor·say'lis) [NA]. SACROCOCCYGEUS DORSALIS.

musculus sacrococcygeus posterior [BNA]. Musculus sacrococcygeus dorsalis (= SACROCOCCYGEUS DORSALIS).

musculus sacrococcygeus ven·tra·lis (ven·tray'lis) [NA]. SACROCOCCYGEUS VENTRALIS.

musculus sa·cro·spi·na·lis (say''kro·spye·nay'lis) [BNA]. Musculus erector spinae (= ERECTOR SPINAE).

musculus sal·pin·go·pha·ryn·ge·us (sal·ping''go·fa·rin'jee·us) [NA]. SALPINGOPHARYNGEUS.

musculus sar·to·ri·us (sahr·to'ree·us) [NA]. SARTORIUS.

musculus sca·le·nus anterior (skay·lee'nus) [NA]. The anterior scalene muscle. See Table of Muscles in the Appendix.

musculus scalenus me·di·us (mee'dee·us) [NA]. The middle scalene muscle. See Table of Muscles in the Appendix.

musculus scalenus mi·ni·mus (min'i·mus) [NA]. SCALENUS MINIMUS.

musculus scalenus posterior [NA]. The posterior scalene muscle. See Table of Muscles in the Appendix.

musculus se·mi·mem·bra·no·sus (sem''ee·mem·bruh·no'sus) [NA]. SEMIMEMBRANOSUS.

musculus se·mi·spi·na·lis (sem''ee·spye·nay'lis) [NA]. SEMISPINALIS.

musculus semispinalis ca·pi·tis (kap'i·tis) [NA]. The semispinalis capitis muscle. See Table of Muscles in the Appendix.

musculus semispinalis cer·vi·cis (sur'vi·sis) [NA]. The semispinalis cervicis muscle. See Table of Muscles in the Appendix.

musculus semispinalis dor·si (dor'sigh) [BNA]. MUSCULUS SEMISPINALIS THORACIS.

musculus semispinalis tho·ra·cis (tho·ray'sis) [NA]. The semispinalis thoracis muscle. See Table of Muscles in the Appendix.

musculus se·mi·ten·di·no·sus (sem''ee·ten·di·no'sus) [NA]. SEMITENDINOSUS.

musculus ser·ra·tus anterior (serr·ay'tus) [NA]. The serratus anterior muscle. See Table of Muscles in the Appendix.

musculus serratus posterior inferior [NA]. The serratus posterior inferior muscle. See Table of Muscles in the Appendix.

musculus serratus posterior superior [NA]. The serratus posterior superior muscle. See Table of Muscles in the Appendix.

musculus ske·le·ti (skel'e·tye) [NA]. SKELETAL MUSCLE.

musculus so·le·us (so'lee·us) [NA]. SOLEUS.

musculus sphinc·ter (sfink'tur) [NA]. SPHINCTER.

musculus sphincter ampullae (he·pa·to·pan·cre·a·ti·cae) (hep''uh·to·pan·kre·at'i·see) [NA]. SPHINCTER OF THE HEPATOPANCREATIC AMPULLA.

musculus sphincter ani ex·ter·nus (ay'nigh ecks·tur'nus) [NA]. SPHINCTER ANI EXTERNUS.

musculus sphincter ani in·ter·nus (in·tur'nus) [NA]. SPHINCTER ANI INTERNUS.

musculus sphincter duc·tus cho·le·do·chi (duck'tus ko·led'o·kigh) [NA]. SPHINCTER OF THE COMMON BILE DUCT.

musculus sphincter pu·pil·lae (pew·pil'ee) [NA]. SPHINCTER PUPILLAE.

musculus sphincter py·lo·ri (pi·lo'rye) [NA]. PYLORIC SPHINCTER.

musculus sphincter ure·thrae (yoo·ree'three) [NA]. SPHINCTER URETHRAE MEMBRANACEAE.

musculus sphincter urethrae mem·bra·na·ce·ae (mem''bruh·nay'see·ee) [BNA]. Musculus sphincter urethrae (= SPHINCTER URETHRAE MEMBRANACEAE).

musculus spi·na·lis (spye·nay'lis) [NA]. SPINALIS.

musculus spinalis ca·pi·tis (kap'i·tis) [NA]. The spinalis capitis muscle. See Table of Muscles in the Appendix.

musculus spinalis cer·vi·cis (sur'vi·sis) [NA]. The spinalis cervicis muscle. See Table of Muscles in the Appendix.

musculus spinalis dor·si (dor'sigh) [BNA]. MUSCULUS SPINALIS THORACIS.

musculus spinalis tho·ra·cis (tho·ray'sis) [NA]. The spinalis thoracis muscle. See Table of Muscles in the Appendix.

musculus sple·ni·us ca·pi·tis (splee'nee·us kap'i·tis) [NA]. The splenius capitis muscle. See Table of Muscles in the Appendix.

musculus splenius cer·vi·cis (sur'vi·sis) [NA]. The splenius cervicis muscle. See Table of Muscles in the Appendix.

musculus sta·pe·di·us (stay·pee'dee·us) [NA]. STAPEDIUS.

musculus ster·na·lis (stur·nay'lis) [NA]. STERNALIS.

musculus ster·no·clei·do·ma·stoi·de·us (stur''no·klye''do·mas·toy'dee·us) [NA]. STERNOCLEIDOMASTOID.

musculus ster·no·hy·oi·de·us (stur''no·high·oy'dee·us) [NA]. STERNOHYOID.

musculus ster·no·thy·roi·de·us (stur''no·thigh·roy'dee·us) [NA]. STERNOTHYROID (2).

musculus sty·lo·glos·sus (stye''lo·glos'us) [NA]. STYLOGLOSSUS.

musculus sty·lo·hy·oi·de·us (stye''lo·high·oy'dee·us) [NA]. STYLOHYOID MUSCLE.

musculus sty·lo·pha·ryn·ge·us (stye''lo·fa·rin'jee·us) [NA]. STYLOPHARYNGEUS.

musculus sub·cla·vi·us (sub·klay'vee·us) [NA]. SUBCLAVIUS.

musculus sub·sca·pu·la·ris (sub·skap·yoo·lair'is) [NA]. SUBSCAPULARIS.

musculus su·pi·na·tor (sue·pi·nay'tor) [NA]. SUPINATOR.

musculus su·pra·spi·na·tus (sue''pruh·spye·nay'tus) [NA]. SUPRASPINATUS.

musculus sus·pen·so·ri·us du·o·de·ni (sus''pen·so'ree·us dew·o·dee'nigh) [NA]. SUSPENSORY MUSCLE OF THE DUODENUM.

musculus tar·sa·lis inferior (tahr·say'lis) [NA]. The tarsal muscle of the lower eyelid. See Table of Muscles in the Appendix.

musculus tarsalis superior [NA]. The tarsal muscle of the upper eyelid. See Table of Muscles in the Appendix.

musculus tem·po·ra·lis (tem·po·ray'lis) [NA]. TEMPORALIS.

musculus tem·po·ro·pa·ri·e·ta·lis (tem''puh·ro·pa·rye·e·tay'lis) [NA]. The temporoparietalis muscle. See Table of Muscles in the Appendix.

musculus ten·sor fas·ci·ae la·tae (ten'sor fash'ee·ee lay'tee) [NA]. The tensor fasciae latae muscle. See Table of Muscles in the Appendix.

musculus tensor tym·pa·ni (tim'puh·nigh) [NA]. The tensor tympani muscle. See Table of Muscles in the Appendix.

musculus tensor ve·li pa·la·ti·ni (vee'lye pal·uh·tye'nigh) [NA]. TENSOR VELI PALATINI.

musculus te·res major (tee'reez) [NA]. The teres major muscle. See Table of Muscles in the Appendix.

musculus teres minor [NA]. The teres minor muscle. See Table of Muscles in the Appendix.

musculus thy·reo·pha·ryn·ge·us (thigh"ree·o·fa·rin'jee·us) [BNA]. PARS THYROPHARYNGEA MUSCULI CONSTRICTORIS PHARYNGIS INFERIORIS.

musculus thy·ro·ary·te·noi·de·us (thigh"ro·ăr·i·te·noy'dee·us) [NA]. THYROARYTENOID MUSCLE.

musculus thy·ro·epi·glot·ti·cus (thigh"ro·ep·i·glot'i·kus) [NA]. THYROEPIGLOTTIC MUSCLE.

musculus thy·ro·hy·oi·de·us (thigh"ro·high·oy'dee·us) [NA]. THYROHYOID MUSCLE.

musculus ti·bi·a·lis anterior (tib·ee·ay'lis) [NA]. The tibialis anterior muscle. See Table of Muscles in the Appendix.

musculus tibialis posterior [NA]. The tibialis posterior muscle. See Table of Muscles in the Appendix.

musculus tra·che·a·lis (tray·kee·ay'lis) [NA]. The trachealis muscle. See Table of Muscles in the Appendix.

musculus tra·gi·cus (traj'i·kus) [NA]. TRAGICUS.

musculus trans·ver·so·spi·na·lis (trans·vur"so·spye·nay'lis) [NA]. The transversospinalis muscle. See Table of Muscles in the Appendix.

musculus trans·ver·sus ab·do·mi·nis (trans·vur'sus ab·dom'i·nis) [NA]. The transverse abdominal muscle. See Table of Muscles in the Appendix.

musculus transversus au·ri·cu·lae (aw·rick'yoo·lee) [NA]. The transverse auricular muscle. See *auricular* in Table of Muscles in the Appendix.

musculus transversus lin·guae (ling'gwee) [NA]. The transverse lingual muscle. See Table of Muscles in the Appendix.

musculus transversus men·ti (men'tye) [NA]. The transverse mental muscle. See Table of Muscles in the Appendix.

musculus transversus nu·chae (new'kee) [NA]. TRANSVERSE NUCHAL MUSCLE.

musculus transversus pe·ri·nei pro·fun·dus (perr"i·nee'eye pro·fun'dus) [NA]. The deep transverse perineal muscle. See Table of Muscles in the Appendix.

musculus transversus perinei su·per·fi·ci·a·lis (sue"pur·fish·ee·ay'lis) [NA]. The superficial transverse muscle of the perineum. See Table of Muscles in the Appendix.

musculus transversus tho·ra·cis (tho·ray'sis) [NA]. The transverse thoracic muscle. See Table of Muscles in the Appendix.

musculus tra·pe·zi·us (tra·pee'zee·us) [NA]. TRAPEZIUS.

musculus tri·an·gu·la·ris (trye·ang·gew·lair'is) [BNA]. Musculus depressor anguli oris (= DEPRESSOR ANGULI ORIS).

musculus tri·ceps bra·chii (trye'seps bray'kee·eye) [NA]. The triceps brachii muscle. See Table of Muscles in the Appendix.

musculus triceps su·rae (sue'ree) [NA]. The triceps surae muscle. See Table of Muscles in the Appendix.

musculus uni·pen·na·tus (yoo"ni·pen·ay'tus) [NA]. UNIPENNATE MUSCLE.

musculus uvu·lae (yoo'vyoo·lee) [NA]. UVULAE.

musculus vas·tus in·ter·me·di·us (vas'tus in"tur·mee'dee·us) [NA]. The vastus intermedius muscle. See Table of Muscles in the Appendix.

musculus vastus la·te·ra·lis (lat·e·ray'lis) [NA]. The vastus lateralis muscle. See Table of Muscles in the Appendix.

musculus vastus me·di·a·lis (mee·dee·ay'lis) [NA]. The vastus medialis muscle. See Table of Muscles in the Appendix.

musculus ven·tri·cu·la·ris (ven·trick·yoo·lair'is) [BNA]. The ventricular muscle. See Table of Muscles in the Appendix.

musculus ver·ti·ca·lis lin·guae (vur·ti·kay'lis ling'gwee) [NA]. VERTICAL LINGUAL MUSCLE.

musculus vis·ce·rum (vis'e·rum) [BNA]. The muscle of an internal organ.

musculus vo·ca·lis (vo·kay'lis) [NA]. VOCALIS.

musculus zy·go·ma·ti·cus (zye"go·mat'i·kus) [BNA]. MUSCULUS ZYGOMATICUS MAJOR.

musculus zygomaticus major [NA]. The major zygomatic muscle. See Table of Muscles in the Appendix.

musculus zygomaticus minor [NA]. The minor zygomatic muscle. See Table of Muscles in the Appendix.

mush bite. An unfinished bite usually taken in beeswax, showing the correct relationship of the cusps in general, but with little or no reproduction of the outline of the teeth.

mush·room, *n.* [OF. *mousseron*]. Any of numerous fleshy fungi of the Basidiomycetes. See also *Amanita muscaria, Amanita phalloides.*

musical agraphia. Loss of ability to write musical notes.

musical alexia. Loss of ability to read music.

musical deafness. 1. SENSORY AMUSIA. 2. TONE DEAFNESS.

musical therapy. MUSICOTHERAPY.

mu·si·co·gen·ic epilepsy (mew"zi·ko·jen'ick). A form of reflex epilepsy induced by music and sounds within a certain frequency band.

mu·si·co·ma·nia (mew"zi·ko·may'nee·uh) *n.* Monomania for, or insane devotion to, music.

mu·si·co·ther·a·py (mew"zi·ko·therr'uh·pee) *n.* The use of music in the treatment of diseases, particularly of mental disorders.

Mus·ken's tonometer. A tonometer used for measuring the tonicity of the calcaneal tendon.

mus·si·ta·tion (mus"i·tay'shun) *n.* [L. *mussitare,* to mutter to one's self]. Movement of the lips as if speaking but without making speech sounds; frequently observed in silent reading.

mus·tard, *n.* [OF. *moustarde,* from L. *mustum,* must]. 1. A plant of the genus *Brassica.* 2. The dried seed of *Brassica alba* or *B. nigra.* The powdered seed of the latter is used as a rubefacient.

mustard gas. Bis (2-chloroethyl) sulfide, $(ClC_2H_4)_2S$, an oily liquid with deadly vesicant action; has been used as a chemical warfare agent. Syn. *yperite.*

mustard oil. A volatile oil, essentially allyl isothiocyanate, obtained from the dried ripe seed of *Brassica nigra* or *B. juncea.* A powerful rubefacient and blister.

Mustargen Hydrochloride. Trademark for mechlorethamine hydrochloride, a cytotoxic agent used for the treatment of various neoplastic diseases.

mus·tine hydrochloride (mus'teen). MECHLORETHAMINE HYDROCHLORIDE.

mu·ta·cism (mew'tuh·siz·um) *n.* MYTACISM.

mu·ta·gen (mew'tuh·jen) *n.* [*mutation* + *-gen*]. Any substance or agent causing a genetic mutation. —**mu·ta·gen·ic** (mew"tuh·jen'ick) *adj.;* **mu·ta·gen·e·sis** (mew"tuh·jen'e·sis) *n.*

mu·tant (mew'tunt) *adj. & n.* [L. *mutans, mutantis,* changing]. 1. Having undergone or resulting from mutation. 2. An individual with characteristics different from those of the parental type due to a genetic constitution that includes a mutation.

mu·ta·ro·ta·tion (mew"tuh·ro·tay'shun) *n.* [*mutate* + *rotation*]. A change in optical rotation of solutions of certain sugars occurring while standing and continuing until equilibrium between the isomeric forms present in the solution is attained.

mu·tase (mew'tace, ·taze) *n.* 1. An enzyme that simultaneously catalyzes the oxidation of one molecule and reduction of another molecule of the substrate. 2. An enzyme that catalyzes the apparent migration of a phosphate group from one to another hydroxyl group of the same molecule.

mu·ta·tion (mew·tay'shun) *n.* [L. *mutatio,* from *mutare,* to change]. 1. A change of small or moderate extent, which represents a definite stage in the gradual evolution of an organism, such as may be recognized in a series of fossils from successive geologic strata. 2. A change in the characteristics of an organism produced by an alteration of the hereditary material. The alteration in the germ plasm may involve an addition of one or more complete sets of chromosomes, the addition or loss of a whole chromosome, or some change within a chromosome, ranging from a gross rearrangement, loss or addition of a larger or smaller section, down through minute rearrangements to a change at a single locus. The latter are gene mutations, or simply mutation in the restricted use of the term.

mutational equilibrium. A form of genetic equilibrium in which loss of one or more alleles of a gene is just balanced by new mutations.

mute (mewt) *adj.* [L. *mutus*]. Unable to speak.

mute hemisphere. *Obsol.* NONDOMINANT HEMISPHERE.

mu·ti·late (mew'ti·late) *v.* [L. *mutilare*]. To maim or disfigure; to deprive of a member or organ. —**mu·ti·la·tion** (mew"ti·lay'shun) *n.*

mut·ism (mewt'iz·um) *n.* [*mute* + *-ism*]. The condition or state of being speechless.

mut·ton-fat (keratic) precipitates. Large clumps of yellowish epitheloid cells deposited upon the endothelial surface of the cornea that indicate chronic types of uveitis.

mu·tu·al·ism (mew'choo·ul·iz·um) *n.* [*mutual* + *-ism*]. A more or less intimate association between organisms of different species which is beneficial to both parties; SYMBIOSIS (2). Contr. *commensalism, parasitism.*

muz·zle, *n.* [OF. *muzel,* from ML. *musellum*]. The projecting jaws and nose of an animal; a snout.

M. W. Abbreviation for *molecular weight.*

M waves. Microwaves of atrial fibrillation, occurring at a rate of about 40,000 per minute.

my. Abbreviation for *myopia.*

my-, myo- [Gk. *mys, myos,* mouse; muscle]. A combining form meaning *muscle.*

Myagen. Trademark for bolasterone, an anabolic steroid.

my·al·gia (migh·al'juh, ·jee·uh) *n.* [*my-* + *-algia*]. Pain in the muscles. —**myal·gic** (·jick) *adj.*

Myambutol. Trademark for ethambutol, a tuberculostatic drug used as the hydrochloride salt.

Myanesin. A trademark for mephenesin, a skeletal muscle relaxant.

my·as·the·nia (migh"as·theen'ee·uh) *n.* [*my-* + *asthenia*]. 1. Muscular weakness from any cause. 2. Specifically, myasthenia gravis. —**my·as·then·ic** (migh"as·thenn'ick, ·theen'ick) *adj.*

myasthenia grav·is (grav'is). A disorder, characterized by a fluctuant weakness of certain voluntary skeletal muscles, particularly those innervated by the bulbar nuclei, affecting women twice as often as men, and sometimes associated with hyperthyroidism or, in the older age group, with carcinoma, as well as with thymic hyperplasia or with thymic tumor. Recent evidence suggests an autoimmune basis for this disorder resulting in a decreased number of acetylcholine receptors and a simplification of the junctional folds in the postsynaptic membrane of the motor end plate. See also *congenital myasthenia, neonatal myasthenia, myasthenic crisis, cholinergic crisis.*

myasthenic crisis. Profound muscular weakness and respiratory paralysis observed in myasthenia gravis, due to lack of or to insufficient treatment with anticholinesterase drugs. Compare *cholinergic crisis.*

myasthenic reaction. *In electromyography,* the reaction observed in myasthenia gravis, in which there is a rapid reduction in the amplitude of compound muscle action potentials evoked during repetitive stimulation of a peripheral nerve at a rate of 3 per second (decrementing response) and reversal of the response by neostigmine.

myasthenic syndrome. A special form of myasthenia, observed most often in association with oat-cell carcinoma of the lung and affecting the muscles of the trunk, pelvic, and shoulder girdles predominantly. Unlike myasthenia gravis, a single stimulus of nerve may yield a low amplitude muscle action potential, whereas stimulation at the rate of 50 per second yields an increase in amplitude of action potentials (incrementing response). Syn. *Eaton-Lambert syndrome.*

my·a·to·nia con·gen·i·ta (migh"a·to'nee·uh kon·jen'i·tuh). *Obsol.* AMYOTONIA CONGENITA.

myc-, myco- [Gk. *mykēs,* fungus, mushroom]. 1. A combining form meaning (a) *fungus, fungous;* (b) *funguslike* in appearance, *moldlike.* 2. See *muc-.*

mycelial threads. The hyphae of a mycelium.

my·ce·li·oid (migh·see'lee·oid) *adj.* [*mycelium* + *-oid*]. Moldlike, as colonies of bacteria having the appearance of mold colonies.

my·ce·li·um (migh·see'lee·um) *n.,* pl. **myce·lia** (·lee·uh) [NL, from *myc-* + Gk. *hēlos,* nailhead]. The vegetative filaments of fungi, usually forming interwoven masses. —**myceli·al** (·ul) *adj.*

-myces [Gk. *mykēs*]. A combining form meaning *fungus.*

mycet-, myceto- [Gk. *mykēs, mykētos*]. A combining form meaning *fungus.*

-mycete [Gk. *mykēs, mykētos*]. A combining form meaning *fungus.*

my·ce·tes (migh·see'teez) *n.pl.* [Gk. *mykētes*]. FUNGI.

my·ce·tis·mus (migh"se·tiz'mus) *n.* [*mycet-* + L. *-ismus,* -ism]. Fungus poisoning, including mushroom poisoning.

myceto-. See *mycet-.*

my·ce·to·gen·ic (migh·see"to·jen'ick, migh·set"o·) *adj.* [*myceto-* + *-genic*]. Produced or caused by fungi.

my·ce·tog·e·nous (migh"se·toj'e·nus) *adj.* MYCETOGENIC.

my·ce·toid (migh'se·toid) *adj.* [*mycet-* + *-oid*]. Resembling fungus; fungoid.

my·ce·to·ma (migh"se·to'muh) *n.* [*mycet-* + *-oma*]. A chronic infection, usually of the feet, by various fungi or by *Nocardia* or *Streptomyces,* resulting in swelling and sinus tracts. Syn. *maduromycosis.*

Mycifradin. A trademark for the antibiotic neomycin, used as the sulfate salt.

-mycin [*myc-* + *-in*]. A combining form designating *a substance* (usually an antibiotic) *derived from a fungus.*

myco-. 1. See *myc-.* 2. See *muc-.*

my·co·an·gio·neu·ro·sis (migh"ko·an"jee·o·new·ro'sis) *n.* [*myco-,* mucous, + *angioneurosis*]. IRRITABLE COLON.

My·co·bac·te·ri·a·ce·ae (migh"ko·back·teer"ee·ay'see·ee) *n.pl.* A family of the order Actinomycetales; contains one genus, *Mycobacterium.*

my·co·bac·te·ri·o·sis (migh"ko·back·teer·ee·o'sis) *n.* A mycobacterial infection.

My·co·bac·te·ri·um (migh"ko·back·teer'ee·um) *n.* [*myco-* + *bacterium*]. A genus of rod-shaped, aerobic bacteria of the family Mycobacteriaceae. Species of this genus are rarely filamentous and occasionally branch but produce no conidia. They are gram-positive, and stain with difficulty, but are acid-fast. See also *atypical mycobacteria.* —**myco·bacterium,** pl. **mycobacteria,** *com. n.*

Mycobacterium avi·um (ay'vee·um, av'ee·um). The causative organism of tuberculosis in birds which has known pathogenicity for other domestic animals, especially swine and sheep; the organism rarely infects humans or other primates.

Mycobacterium bo·vis (bo'vis). The principal cause of cattle tuberculosis, and, rarely, the cause of human tuberculosis as well; acid-fast rods.

Mycobacterium lep·rae (lep'ree). The causative organism of leprosy; formerly called *Bacillus leprae.*

Mycobacterium lep·rae·mu·ri·um (lep"ree·mew'ree·um). The species of *Mycobacterium* that causes murine leprosy; it is observed within the macrophages in lesions.

Mycobacterium paratuberculosis. The causative agent of a chronic enteritis of cattle, sheep, and deer, nonpathogenic for man. See also *Johne's disease.*

Mycobacterium phlei (flee'eye). A species of *Mycobacterium* found in soil and water.

Mycobacterium tuberculosis. A species of acid-fast bacteria;

the principal cause of tuberculosis in man. Syn. *Bacillus tuberculosis.*

Mycobacterium tuberculosis* var. *mu·ris (mew'ris). VOLE BACILLUS.

Mycobacterium ul·cer·ans (ul'sur·anz). The causative agent of a chronic or subacute ulceration of the skin and subcutaneous tissue on the upper or lower extremity. Syn. *Barnsdale bacillus.*

my·co·ci·din (migh"ko·sigh'din) *n.* [*Myco*bacterium + *-cide* + *-in*]. An antibiotic substance extracted from a mold of the Aspergillaceae family. It is active, in vitro, against *Mycobacterium tuberculosis.*

my·coid (migh'koid) *adj.* [*myc-* + *-oid*]. Resembling, or appearing like, a fungus; fungoid.

α-my·col·ic acid (al'fuh migh·kol'ick). A fatty acid, of high molecular weight, isolated from a human test strain of *Mycobacterium tuberculosis.*

my·col·o·gy (migh·kol'uh·jee) *n.* [*myco-* + *-logy*]. The science of fungi.

my·co·myr·in·gi·tis (migh"ko·mirr"in·jigh'tis, ·migh"rin·) *n.* [*myco-* + *myringitis*]. MYRINGOMYCOSIS.

my·co·phe·no·lic acid (migh"ko·fe·no'lick) *n.* (*E*)-6-(4-Hydroxy-6-methoxy-7-methyl-3-oxo-5-phthalanyl)-4-methyl-4-hexenoic acid, $C_{17}H_{20}O_6$, an antineoplastic.

my·coph·thal·mia (migh"koff·thal'mee·uh) *n.* [*myc-* + *ophthalmia*]. Ophthalmia due to a fungus.

My·co·plas·ma (migh"ko·plaz'muh) *n.* [*myco-* + Gk. *plasma*, form]. A genus of minute microorganisms that lack rigid cell walls, give rise to small colonies on media enriched with body fluids such as serum, and include nonpathogens and pathogens of man and animals.

Mycoplasma ar·thri·ti·dis (ahr·thrit'i·dis). A species of *Mycoplasma* thought to be the causative agent of murine arthritis.

Mycoplasma gal·li·sep·ti·cum (gal"i·sep'ti·kum). The causative agent of air sac disease.

Mycoplasma my·coi·des (migh"koy'deez). The causative agent of bovine pleuropneumonia.

Mycoplasma pneu·mo·ni·ae (new·mo'nee·ee). The causative agent of primary atypical pneumonia of man, often resulting in the appearance of cold agglutinins for human type O red blood cells or of *Streptococcus* MG in the infected individual.

Mycoplasma pul·mo·nis (pōōl·mo'nis). A strain of Mycoplasma isolated from the lungs of rats, with or without demonstrable pulmonary disease.

My·co·plas·ma·ta·ce·ae (migh"ko·plaz"muh·tay'see·ee) *n.pl.* The family of microorganisms that includes the genus *Mycoplasma.*

my·cose (migh'koce, ·koze) *n.* TREHALOSE.

my·co·sis (migh·ko'sis) *n.*, pl. **myco·ses** (·seez) [*myc-* + *-osis*]. Any infection or disease caused by a fungus.

mycosis fun·goi·des (fung·goy'deez). A form of malignant lymphoma, with special cutaneous manifestations, characterized by eczematoid areas, infiltrations, nodules, tumors, and ulcerations. Syn. *granuloma fungoides.*

mycosis fungoides d'em·blée (dahm·blay') [F., at once, suddenly]. The presence of mycosis fungoides without previous erythema or plaques.

Mycostatin. Trademark for the antibiotic substance nystatin, used as an antifungal agent for the treatment of infections caused by *Candida* (*Monilia*) *albicans.*

my·cos·ter·ol (migh·kos'tur·ol, ·ole) *n.* Any sterol occurring in yeast or fungi.

my·co·sub·ti·lin (migh"ko·sub'ti·lin) *n.* [*myco-* + *subtilin*]. An antibiotic derived from a strain of *Bacillus subtilis*, active in vitro against a variety of yeasts and fungi.

my·cot·ic (migh·kot'ick) *adj.* 1. Of or pertaining to mycosis. 2. Fungoid; resembling a fungus in appearance.

mycotic aneurysm. A localized abnormal dilatation of a vessel due to destruction of all or part of its wall by microorganisms.

mycotic keratitis. 1. KERATOMYCOSIS. 2. DENDRITIC KERATITIS.

mycotic otitis ex·ter·na (ecks·tur'nuh). Infection of the external auditory canal due to fungi; an otomycosis.

mycotic splenomegaly. SPLENOGRANULOMATOSIS SIDEROTICA.

mycotic stomatitis. THRUSH (1).

mycotic tonsillitis. Tonsillitis due to fungi.

my·cot·i·za·tion (migh·kot"i·zay'shun) *n.* Superimposition of a mycotic infection on a nonfungous lesion; secondary mycosis.

my·co·tox·i·co·sis (migh"ko·tock"si·ko'sis) *n.* [*myco-* + *toxicosis*]. 1. Poisoning due to a bacterial or fungal toxin. 2. Poisoning from a fungus which is ingested either by itself or in food contaminated by the fungus.

myc·tero·pho·nia (mick"tur·o·fo'nee·uh) *n.* [Gk. *myktēr*, nostril, + *-phonia*]. A nasal quality of the voice.

my·de·sis (migh·dee'sis) *n.* [Gk. *mydēsis*]. 1. PUTREFACTION. 2. A discharge of pus from the eyelids.

Mydriacyl. Trademark for tropicamide, an anticholinergic agent for ophthalmic use.

my·dri·a·sis (mi·drye'uh·sis, migh·) *n.* [Gk.]. Dilatation of the pupil of the eye.

myd·ri·at·ic (mid"ree·at'ick) *adj. & n.* 1. Producing mydriasis; dilating the pupil. 2. An agent that dilates the pupil, such as eucatropine hydrochloride. See also *cycloplegic.*

my·ec·to·my (migh·eck'tuh·mee) *n.* [*my-* + *-ectomy*]. Excision of a portion of muscle.

my·ec·to·py (migh·eck'tuh·pee) *n.* [*my-* + *-ectopy*]. The displacement of a muscle.

myel-, myelo- [Gk. *myelos*, marrow]. A combining form meaning (a) *marrow*; (b) *spinal cord*; (c) *myelin.*

my·el·ap·o·plexy (migh"e·lap'o·pleck·see) *n.* [*myel-* + *apoplexy*]. Hemorrhage into the spinal cord.

my·el·at·ro·phy (migh"e·lat'ruh·fee) *n.* [*myel-* + *atrophy*]. Atrophy of the spinal cord.

my·e·le·mia, my·e·lae·mia (migh"e·lee'mee·uh) *n.* [*myel-* + *-emia*]. GRANULOCYTIC LEUKEMIA.

my·el·en·ceph·a·lon (migh"e·len·sef'uh·lon) *n.* [*myel-* + *encephalon*] [NA]. The caudal part of the embryonic hindbrain, from which the medulla oblongata develops.—**my·elen·ce·phal·ic** (·se·fal'ick) *adj.*

-myelia [*myel-* + *-ia*]. A combining form designating *a condition of the spinal cord.*

my·el·ic (migh·el'ick) *adj.* [*myel-* + *-ic*]. Pertaining to the spinal cord.

my·e·lin (migh'e·lin) *n.* [*myel-* + *-in*]. 1. The white, fatty substance forming a sheath of some nerves. Syn. *white substance of Schwann.* 2. A complex mixture of lipids extracted from nervous tissue; it is doubly refractile and contains phosphatides and cholesterol.

my·e·li·nat·ed (migh'e·li·nay·tid) *adj.* Provided with a myelin sheath; medullated.

my·e·li·na·tion (migh"e·li·nay'shun) *n.* MYELINIZATION.

my·e·lin·ic (migh"e·lin'ick) *adj.* 1. Of or pertaining to myelin. 2. MYELINATED.

myelinic neuroma. A neuroma containing myelinated fibers.

myelin incisure. SCHMIDT-LANTERMANN INCISURE.

my·e·lin·iza·tion (migh"e·li·ni·zay'shun) *n.* The process of elaborating or accumulating myelin during the development, or regeneration of nerves.

my·e·li·noc·la·sis (migh"e·li·nock'luh·sis) *n.* [*myelin* + *-clasis*]. DEMYELINATION; destruction of the myelin.

my·e·lino·gen·e·sis (migh"e·lin·o·jen'e·sis) *n.* [*myelin* + *-genesis*]. MYELINIZATION.

my·e·lin·ol·y·sis (migh"e·lin·ol'i·sis) *n.* [*myelin* + *-lysis*]. Disintegration of myelin.

my·e·li·nop·a·thy (migh"e·li·nop'uth·ee) *n.* [*myelin* + *-pathy*]. Any disease of the myelin.

my·e·li·no·sis (migh"e·li·no'sis) *n.* [*myelin* + *-osis*]. Decomposition of fat with the formation of myelin.

myelin sheath. The short (750 μm) segment of myelin which surrounds the axon and which is enveloped by a Schwann cell plasma membrane.

my·e·li·tis (migh″e·lye′tis) *n.* [*myel-* + *-itis*]. 1. Inflammation of the spinal cord. 2. Inflammation of the bone marrow. See also *osteomyelitis.*—**mye·lit·ic** (·lit′ick) *adj.*

myelo-. See *myel-*.

my·e·lo·blast (migh′e·lo·blast) *n.* [*myelo-* + *-blast*]. The youngest of the precursor cells of the granulocytic series, having a nucleus with a finely granular or homogeneous chromatin structure and nucleoli and intensely basophilic cytoplasm. Syn. *granuloblast.*

my·e·lo·blas·te·mia, my·e·lo·blas·tae·mia (migh″e·lo·blas·tee′mee·uh) *n.* [*myeloblast* + *-emia*]. Presence of myeloblasts in the circulating blood.

my·e·lo·blas·tic (migh″e·lo·blas′tick) *adj.* Originating from, or characterized by, the presence of myeloblasts.

myeloblastic leukemia. Acute granulocytic leukemia, with poorly differentiated cells predominating.

myeloblastic plasma cell. PROPLASMACYTE (1).

my·e·lo·blas·to·ma (migh″e·lo·blas·to′muh) *n.* [*myeloblast* + *-oma*]. A malignant tumor composed of poorly differentiated granulocytes. Syn. *granulocytic sarcoma.*

my·e·lo·blas·to·sis (migh″e·lo·blas·to′sis) *n.* Diffuse proliferation of myeloblasts, with involvement of blood, bone marrow, and other tissues and organs.

my·e·lo·cele (migh′e·lo·seel) *n.* [*myelo-* + *-cele*]. Spina bifida, with protrusion of the spinal cord.

my·e·lo·chlo·ro·ma (migh″e·lo·klo·ro′muh) *n.* GRANULOCYTIC SARCOMA.

my·e·lo·cys·to·cele (migh″e·lo·sis′to·seel) *n.* [*myelo-* + *cysto-* + *-cele*]. A hernial protrusion, in spina bifida, in which there is accumulation of fluid in the central canal of the spinal cord.

my·e·lo·cys·tog·ra·phy (migh″e·lo·sis·tog′ruh·fee) *n.* [*myelo-* + *cysto-* + *-graphy*]. The demonstration of an intramedullary spinal cord cyst by scanning or radiography after percutaneous puncture of the cyst and injection into it of an isotope-labeled substance or contrast material, such as opaque material or air.

my·e·lo·cyte (migh′e·lo·site) *n.* [*myelo-* + *-cyte*]. 1. A granular leukocyte, precursor in the stage of development intermediate between the promyelocyte and metamyelocyte. The staining reactions of the granules differentiate myelocytes into neutrophilic, eosinophilic, and basophilic types. 2. Any cell concerned in development of granular leukocytes. —**my·e·lo·cyt·ic** (migh″e·lo·sit′ick) *adj.*

myelocyte series. GRANULOCYTIC SERIES.

my·e·lo·cy·the·mia, my·e·lo·cy·thae·mia (migh″e·lo·sigh·theem′ee·uh) *n.* [*myelocyte* + *-hemia*]. GRANULOCYTIC LEUKEMIA.

myelocytic leukemia. GRANULOCYTIC LEUKEMIA.

myelocytic sarcoma. A variety of malignant plasmacytoma in which the anaplastic plasma cells resemble myelocytes.

myelocytic series. GRANULOCYTIC SERIES.

my·e·lo·cy·to·ma (migh″e·lo·sigh·to′muh) *n.* [*myelocyte* + *-oma*]. A malignant plasmacytoma.

my·e·lo·cy·to·sis (migh″e·lo·sigh·to′sis) *n.* [*myelocyte* + *-osis*]. Myelocytes in the blood.

my·e·lo·dys·pla·sia (migh″e·lo·dis·play′zhuh, ·zee·uh) *n.* [*myelo-* + *dysplasia*]. Defective development of the spinal cord, especially in its lumbosacral portion.

my·e·lo·en·ceph·a·li·tis (migh″e·lo·en·sef″uh·lye′tis) *n.* [*myelo-* + *encephal-* + *-itis*]. Inflammation of both spinal cord and brain.

my·e·lo·fi·bro·sis (migh″e·lo·figh·bro′sis) *n.* Fibrosis of the bone marrow. It may be a primary disorder of unknown cause, or a complication of bone marrow injury.

my·e·lo·gen·e·sis (migh″e·lo·jen′e·sis) *n.* [*myelo-* + *-genesis*]. MYELINIZATION.

my·e·lo·gen·ic (migh″e·lo·jen′ick) *adj.* [*myelo-* + *-genic*]. Produced in, or by, bone marrow.

my·e·log·e·nous (migh″e·loj′e·nus) *adj.* 1. MYELOGENIC. 2. Pertaining to cells produced in bone marrow.

myelogenous leukemia. GRANULOCYTIC LEUKEMIA.

myelogenous series. GRANULOCYTIC SERIES.

my·e·lo·gone (migh′e·lo·gohn) *n.* [*myelo-* + Gk. *gonē*, offspring, seed]. *Obsol.* A primitive blood cell of the bone marrow from which the myeloblast develops.

my·e·lo·gram (migh′e·lo·gram) *n.* [*myelo-* + *-gram*]. 1. A radiograph of the spinal canal, made after the injection of a contrast medium into the subarachnoid space. 2. A differentiated count of nucleated cells of bone marrow.

my·e·log·ra·phy (migh″e·log′ruh·fee) *n.* [*myelo-* + *-graphy*]. Radiographic demonstration of the spinal subarachnoid space, after the introduction of contrast media such as air, Pantopaque, or absorbable contrast material.

my·e·loid (migh′e·loid) *adj.* [*myel-* + *-oid*]. Pertaining to bone marrow. See also *granulocytic series.*

myeloid cell. One of those cells of myeloid tissue involved in hemopoiesis.

myeloid:erythroid ratio. The ratio of leukocytes of the granulocytic series to nucleated erythrocyte precursors in an aspirated sample of bone marrow. The limits of normal are 0.6:1 to 2.7:1. Syn. *M:E ratio.*

myeloid leukemia. GRANULOCYTIC LEUKEMIA.

myeloid metaplasia. The occurrence of hemopoietic tissue in areas of the body where it is not normally found.

myeloid myeloma. A malignant plasmacytoma in which the anaplastic plasma cells look like myelocytes.

myeloid reaction. Increased numbers of granulocytes in the blood and bone marrow often accompanied by the appearance of immature forms in the blood.

myeloid sarcoma. GIANT-CELL TUMOR (1).

myeloid series. GRANULOCYTIC SERIES.

myeloid tissue. Red bone marrow consisting of reticular cells attached to argyrophile fibers which form wide meshes containing scattered fat cells, erythroblasts, myelocytes, and mature myeloid elements.

myeloid tumor. A malignant plasmacytoma.

my·e·lo·ken·tric acid (migh″e·lo·ken′trick). A keto acid, insoluble in water, in the urine of patients with granulocytic leukemia as a water-soluble conjugate.

my·e·lo·li·po·ma (migh″e·lo·li·po′muh) *n.* [*myelo-* + *lipoma*]. A choristoma, usually of the adrenal gland, composed of adipose tissue and hemopoietic cells.

my·e·lo·lym·phan·gi·o·ma (migh″e·lo·lim·fan·jee·o′muh) *n.* [*myelo-*, soft, marrow-like, + *lymphangioma*]. ELEPHANTIASIS.

my·e·lo·lym·pho·cyte (migh″e·lo·lim′fo·site) *n.* A small lymphocyte formed in the bone marrow.

my·e·lol·y·sis (migh″e·lol′i·sis) *n.* [*myelo-* + *-lysis*]. MYELINOLYSIS.

my·e·lo·ma (migh″e·lo′muh) *n.* [*myel-* + *-oma*]. A malignant plasmacytoma.

myeloma cell. An anaplastic plasma cell composing the parenchyma of a malignant plasmacytoma.

my·e·lo·ma·la·cia (migh″e·lo·ma·lay′shee·uh) *n.* [*myelo-* + *malacia*]. Infarction or softening of the spinal cord.

myeloma protein. Any one of the abnormal globulins found in the blood plasma or urine in malignant plasmacytoma (multiple myeloma).

my·e·lo·ma·to·sis (migh″e·lo·muh·to′sis) *n.* [*myeloma* + *-osis*]. A malignant plasmacytoma.

my·e·lo·ma·tous (migh″e·lo′muh·tus, ·lom′uh·tus) *adj.* Pertaining to or caused by myeloma.

myelomatous neuropathy or **polyneuropathy.** A subacute or chronic sensory or sensorimotor polyneuropathy, occurring as a remote effect of myeloma and characterized pathologically by a noninflammatory degeneration of the peripheral nerves and dorsal root ganglia and roots and by an elevation of cerebrospinal fluid protein.

my·e·lo·men·in·gi·tis (migh″e·lo·men″in·jye′tis) *n.* [*myelo-* +

mening- + *-itis*]. Inflammation of the spinal cord and its meninges.

my·e·lo·me·nin·go·cele (migh″e·lo·me·ning′go·seel) *n.* [*myelo-* + *meningo-* + *-cele*]. Spina bifida with protrusion of a meningeal sac containing elements of the spinal cord or cauda equina.

my·e·lo·mere (migh′e·lo·meer) *n.* [*myelo-* + Gk. *meros*, part, place]. An embryonic segment of the spinal cord.

my·e·lo·mono·cyte (migh″e·lo·mon′o·site) *n.* 1. A monocyte developing in the bone marrow. 2. A blood cell having characteristics of both the monocytic and granulocytic series, seen in the Naegeli type of monocytic leukemia. —**myelo·mono·cyt·ic** (·mon″o·sit′ick) *adj.*

myelomonocytic leukemia. The Naegeli type of monocytic leukemia.

my·e·lon (migh′e·lon) *n.* [Gk.]. SPINAL CORD.

my·e·lo·neu·ri·tis (migh″e·lo·new·rye′tis) *n.* Polyneuritis combined with myelitis. See also *Guillain-Barré disease.*

my·e·lo·pa·ral·y·sis (migh″e·lo·puh·ral′i·sis) *n.* SPINAL PARALYSIS.

my·e·lo·path·ic (migh″e·lo·path′ick) *adj.* [*myelopathy* + *-ic*]. Pertaining to disease of the spinal cord, or of myeloid tissue.

myelopathic anemia. MYELOPHTHISIC ANEMIA.

myelopathic muscular atrophy. PROGRESSIVE SPINAL MUSCULAR ATROPHY.

myelopathic polycythemia. POLYCYTHEMIA VERA.

my·e·lop·a·thy (migh″e·lop′uth·ee) *n.* [*myelo-* + *-pathy*]. Any disease of the spinal cord, or of myeloid tissues.

my·e·lo·per·ox·i·dase (migh″e·lo·pur·ock′si·dace, ·daze) *n.* A green-colored peroxidase in leukocytes.

myeloperoxidase deficiency. A hereditary disorder of leukocytes, characterized by absence or structural alteration of myeloperoxidase associated with decreased anti-*Candida* activity by leukocytes and a resultant enhancement of susceptibility to systemic candidiasis. Inherited as an autosomal recessive trait.

my·e·lop·e·tal (migh″e·lop′e·tul) *adj.* [*myelo-* + *-petal*]. Moving toward the spinal cord.

myelophthisic anemia. An anemia associated with space-occupying disorders of the bone marrow. Syn. *myelopathic anemia, myelosclerotic anemia, osteosclerotic anemia.*

my·e·lo·phthi·sis (migh″e·lo·thigh′sis) *n.* [*myelo-* + *phthisis*]. 1. Loss of bone marrow due to replacement by other tissue, notably fibrous tissue or bone. 2. Spinal cord atrophy in tabes dorsalis.—**myelo·phthis·ic** (·thiz′ick), **myelo·phthis·i·cal** (·i·kul) *adj.*

my·e·lo·plaque (migh′e·lo·plack) *n.* MYELOPLAX.

my·e·lo·plast (migh′e·lo·plast) *n.* [*myelo-* + *-plast*]. A leukocyte of the bone marrow.

my·e·lo·plax (migh′e·lo·placks) *n.* [*myelo-* + Gk. *plax*, flat surface, tablet]. A giant cell of the marrow; an osteoclast.—**my·e·lo·plax·ic** (migh″e·lo·plack′sick) *adj.*

myeloplaxic tumor. GIANT-CELL TUMOR (1).

my·e·lo·ple·gia (migh″e·lo·plee′juh, ·jee·uh) *n.* [*myelo-* + *-plegia*]. SPINAL PARALYSIS.

my·e·lo·poi·e·sis (migh″e·lo·poy·ee′sis) *n.* [*myelo-* + Gk. *poiēsis*, production]. The process of formation and development of the blood cells in the bone marrow.

my·e·lo·pore (migh′e·lo·pore) *n.* [*myelo-* + *pore*]. An opening in the spinal cord.

my·e·lo·pro·lif·er·a·tive disorders or **syndrome** (migh″e·lo·pro·lif′ur·uh·tiv). Proliferation of one or more bone marrow elements without definite evidence of neoplasia, accompanied by extramedullary hemopoiesis and immature cells in the peripheral blood. See also *agnogenic myeloid metaplasia, panmyelosis.*

my·e·lo·ra·dic·u·li·tis (migh″e·lo·ra·dick″yoo·lye′tis) *n.* [*myelo-* + *radicul-* + *-itis*]. Inflammation of the spinal cord and roots of the spinal nerves.

my·e·lo·ra·dic·u·lo·dys·pla·sia (migh″e·lo·ra·dick″yoo·lo·dis·play′zhuh, ·zee·uh) *n.* [*myelo-* + *radiculo-* + *dysplasia*]. Congenital abnormality of the spinal cord and roots of the spinal nerves.

my·e·lo·ra·dic·u·lop·a·thy (migh″e·lo·ra·dick″yoo·lop′uth·ee) *n.* [*myelo-* + *radiculo-* + *-pathy*]. Disease of the spinal cord and roots of the spinal nerves.

my·e·lor·rha·gia (migh″e·lo·ray′jee·uh) *n.* [*myelo-* + *-rrhagia*]. Hemorrhage into the spinal cord.

my·e·lo·sar·co·ma (migh″e·lo·sahr·ko′muh) *n.* [*myelo-* + *sarcoma*]. A malignant plasmacytoma.

my·e·los·chi·sis (migh″e·los′ki·sis) *n.* [*myelo-* + *-schisis*]. Complete or partial failure of the neural plate to form a neural tube, resulting in a cleft spinal cord.

my·e·lo·scin·to·gram (migh″e·lo·sin′tuh·gram) *n.* [*myelo-* + *scintigram*]. A graphic presentation of the distribution of a radioactive tracer introduced into the subarachnoid space.

my·e·lo·scin·tog·ra·phy (migh″e·lo·sin·tog′ruh·fee) *n.* [*myeloscintogram* + *-graphy*]. A technique of introducing a radioactive tracer substance into the spinal subarachnoid space and then of determining the distribution of the radioactive substance by means of a scintiscanner.

my·e·lo·scle·ro·sis (migh″e·lo·skle·ro′sis) *n.* 1. Multiple sclerosis of the spinal cord. 2. MYELOFIBROSIS.

my·e·lo·scle·rot·ic (migh″e·lo·skle·rot′ick) *adj.* [*myelo-* + *sclerotic*]. Of or pertaining to myelophthisis or to myelofibrosis.

myelosclerotic anemia. MYELOPHTHISIC ANEMIA.

my·e·lo·sis (migh″e·lo′sis) *n.* [*myel-* + *-osis*]. 1. MYELOCYTOSIS. 2. A malignant plasmacytoma. 3. GRANULOCYTIC LEUKEMIA.

my·e·lo·spon·gi·um (migh″e·lo·spon′jee·um, ·spun′jee·um) *n.* [NL., from *myelo-* + L. *spongia*, sponge]. A network in the wall of the neural tube of the embryo, composed of protoplasmic fibers of the spongioblasts.

my·e·lo·sup·pres·sive (migh″e·lo·suh·pres′iv) *adj.* Tending to suppress the development of white blood cells and platelets. —**myelosup·pres·sion** (·shun) *n.*

my·e·lo·sy·rin·go·cele (migh″e·lo·si·ring′go·seel) *n.* SYRINGOMYELOCELE.

my·en·ta·sis (migh·en′tuh·sis) *n.* [*my-* + Gk. *entasis*, tension, straining]. The extension or stretching of a muscle.

my·en·ter·ic (migh″en·terr′ick) *adj.* [*my-* + *enteric*]. Pertaining to the muscular coat of the intestine.

myenteric plexus. A visceral nerve plexus situated between the circular and longitudinal muscle layers of the digestive tube. Syn. *Auerbach's plexus.* NA *plexus myentericus.*

myenteric reflex. Contraction of the intestine above and relaxation below a portion of the intestine that is stimulated through the influence of the myenteric nerve plexus. This action occurs during peristalsis. Syn. *intestinal reflex.*

my·en·ter·on (migh·en′tur·on) *n.* [*my-* + *enteron*]. The muscular coat of the intestine.

My·ers and War·dell method. A method for cholesterol in which the serum or plasma is dried on plaster of Paris and extracted with chloroform. The total cholesterol of the extract is determined colorimetrically by the Liebermann-Burchard reaction with acetic anhydride and sulfuric acid.

Myer's method. Urea in blood is converted to ammonium carbonate with urease. The ammonia is collected by aeration and determined by nesslerization.

My·er·son's eye sign or **reflex.** An inability to inhibit blinking in response to repeated tapping over the forehead, nasal bridge, or maxilla; a sign of parkinsonism.

my·es·the·sia (migh″es·theezh′uh, ·theez′ee·uh) *n.* [*my-* + *esthesia*]. The perception or sensibility of impressions coming from the muscles, as of touch, contraction, or direction of movement.

-myia [Gk.]. A combining form meaning *fly.*

my·ia·sis (migh·eye′uh·sis) *n.* [Gk. *myia*, fly, + *-iasis*]. Invasion or infection of a body area or cavity by the larvae of flies.

my·io·de·op·sia (migh·eye″o·dee·op′see·uh, migh″o·) *n.* MYIODESOPSIA.

my·io·des·op·sia (migh·eye″o·dez·op′see·uh, migh″o·des·op′see·uh) *n.* [Gk. *myioeidēs*, flylike, + *opsis*, apparition, + *-ia*]. The condition in which floaters (muscae volitantes) appear.

my·io·sis (migh″eye·o′sis, migh·yo′sis) *n.* [Gk. *myia*, fly, + *-osis*]. MYIASIS.

myl-, mylo- [Gk. *mylē*, millstone]. A combining form meaning *molar*.

my·la·ceph·a·lus (migh″lay·sef′uh·lus) *n.* [Gk. *mylē*, millstone, + *acephalus*]. A placental parasitic twin (omphalosite) which has but vestiges of a head and limbs, hence is only a degree above an amorphic fetus.

Mylaxen. Trademark for hexafluorenium bromide, a drug used with succinylcholine to reduce the dose of the latter and prolong its action as a skeletal muscle relaxant.

Myleran. Trademark for busulfan, an antineoplastic drug.

Mylicon. A trademark for simethicone, an antiflatulent.

mylo-. See *myl-*.

my·lo·hy·oid (migh″lo·high′oid) *adj.* [*mylo-* + *hyoid*]. Pertaining to the region of the lower molar teeth and the hyoid bone.

my·lo·hy·oi·de·an (migh″lo·high·oy′dee·un) *adj.* MYLOHYOID.

mylohyoid groove. A groove running obliquely downward and forward on the medial surface of the ramus of the mandible, below the lingula of the mandible; it lodges the mylohyoid vessels and nerve. NA *sulcus mylohyoideus.*

mylohyoid line or **ridge.** A ridge on the internal surface of the mandible, extending upward and backward from the sublingual fossa to the ramus. NA *linea mylohyoidea.*

mylohyoid muscle. A muscle on the floor of the mouth originating from the mylohyoid line of the mandible and inserted on the hyoid. NA *musculus mylohyoideus.* See also Table of Muscles in the Appendix.

my·lo·pha·ryn·ge·al muscle (migh″lo·fa·rin′jee·ul). The portion of the superior constrictor muscle of the pharynx which arises from the mylohoid line of the mandible. NA *pars mylopharyngea musculi constrictoris pharyngis superioris.*

myo-. See *my-*.

myo·ar·chi·tec·ton·ic (migh″o·ahr″ki·teck·ton′ick) *adj.* [*myo-* + *architectonic*]. Pertaining to the structure and arrangement of muscle fibers.

myo·blast (migh′o·blast) *n.* [*myo-* + *blast*]. A cell which develops into a muscle fiber. —**myo·blas·tic** (migh″o·blas′tick) *adj.*

myoblastic myoma. GRANULAR CELL MYOBLASTOMA.

myo·blas·to·ma (migh″o·blas·to′muh) *n.* [*myoblast* + *-oma*]. GRANULAR CELL MYOBLASTOMA.

myo·car·di·al (migh″o·kahr′dee·ul) *adj.* Of or pertaining to the myocardium.

myocardial insufficiency. HEART FAILURE.

myo·car·di·op·a·thy (migh″o·kahr·dee·op′uth·ee) *n.* Any disease of the myocardium; cardiomyopathy.

myo·car·di·tis (migh″o·kahr·dye′tis) *n.* Inflammation of the myocardium.

myo·car·di·um (migh″o·kahr′dee·um) *n.*, pl. **myocar·dia** (·dee·uh) [*myo-* + *-cardium*] [NA]. The muscular tissue of the heart. See also Plate 5.

myo·car·do·sis (migh″o·kahr·do′sis) *n.* [*myocardium* + *-osis*]. 1. Any noninflammatory disease of the myocardium. 2. MYOCARDIOPATHY; CARDIOMYOPATHY.

Myochrysine. Trademark for gold sodium thiomalate, an antirheumatic drug.

myo·clo·nia (migh″o·klo′nee·uh) *n.* MYOCLONUS.

myoclonia fi·bril·la·ris mul·ti·plex (figh″bri·lair′is mul′ti·plecks). MYOKYMIA.

myo·clon·ic (migh″o·klon′ick) *adj.* Pertaining to or characterized by myoclonus.

myoclonic epilepsy. The association of myoclonus with epilepsy. Included under this title are several seizure states, some relatively benign (idiopathic epilepsy) and others which are associated with intellectual deterioration and a variety of abnormalities of the nervous system.

myoclonic epilepsy with Lafora bodies. PROGRESSIVE FAMILIAL MYOCLONIC EPILEPSY.

myoclonic progressive familial epilepsy. PROGRESSIVE FAMILIAL MYOCLONIC EPILEPSY.

myoclonic status. A state lasting on the order of an hour or more during which myoclonic seizures occur continually. See also *status epilepticus.*

myo·clo·nus (migh″o·klo′nus, migh·ock′luh·nus) *n.* [*myo-* + *clonus*]. Exceedingly abrupt, shocklike contractions of muscles, irregular in rhythm and amplitude and usually asynchronous or asymmetrical in distribution.

myoclonus epilepsy. PROGRESSIVE FAMILIAL MYOCLONIC EPILEPSY.

myo·coele (migh′o·seel) *n.* [*myo-* + *-coele*]. The cavity of a myotome (2).

myo·cyte (migh′o·site) *n.* [*myo-* + *-cyte*]. A muscle cell.

myo·cy·tol·y·sis (migh″o·sigh·tol′i·sis) *n.* [*myo-* + *cytolysis*]. 1. Destruction of muscle cells. 2. Disappearance of cardiac muscle cells without cellular reaction to the loss.

myo·dys·to·nia (migh″o·dis·to′nee·uh) *n.* [*myo-* + *dystonia*]. Any abnormal condition of muscle tone.

myo·dys·tro·phy (migh″o·dis′truh·fee) *n.* [*myo-* + *dystrophy*]. Degeneration of muscles.

myo·ede·ma (migh″o·e·dee′muh) *n.* Edema of a muscle.

myo·elas·tic (migh″o·e·las′tick) *adj.* [*myo-* + *elastic*]. Pertaining to the layer of intimately interrelated smooth muscle cells and elastic fibers in bronchi and bronchioles.

myo·ep·i·the·li·al (migh″o·ep·i·theel′ee·ul) *adj.* Of or pertaining to myoepithelium.

myoepithelial cell. One of the smooth muscle cells of ectodermal origin in sweat, mammary, lacrimal, and salivary glands.

myo·ep·i·the·li·o·ma (my″o·ep·i·theel″ee·o′muh) *n.* [*myoepithelium* + *-oma*]. A slow-growing sweat-gland tumor appearing as a solitary or rarely multiple, firm, well-circumscribed intracutaneous nodule usually less than 2 cm in diameter. The two types of cells found are the secretory and the myoepithelial cells.

myo·ep·i·the·li·um (my″o·ep·i·theel′ee·um) *n.* [*myo-* + *epithelium*]. Collectively, the smooth muscle cells of ectodermal origin.

myo·fa·cial (migh″o·fay′shul) *adj.* Pertaining to the face and related muscles.

myofacial pain-dysfunction syndrome. A unilateral facial pain aggravated by mandibular movement and associated with tenderness of the head and neck muscles and sometimes of the temporomandibular joint on the affected side. The symptoms are presumably related to dysfunction of the temporomandibular joint.

myo·fas·cial (migh″o·fash′ee·ul) *adj.* [*myo-* + *fascial*]. Pertaining to the fasciae of muscles, as myofascial inflammation.

myo·fas·ci·tis (migh″o·fa·sigh′tis) *n.* [*myo-* + *fasci-* + *-itis*]. Musculoskeletal pain of obscure nature; probably due to inflammation of muscle and fascia at its insertion on bone.

myo·fi·ber (migh′o·figh″bur) *n.* MYOFIBRIL.

myo·fi·bril (migh″o·figh′bril, ·fib′ril) *n.* [*myo-* + *fibril*]. A fibril found in the cytoplasm of muscle. —**myo·fi·bril·lar** (migh″o·figh′bril·ur) *adj.*

myo·fi·bro·ma (migh″o·figh·bro′muh) *n.* [*myo-* + *fibroma*]. LEIOMYOMA.

myo·fi·bro·sar·co·ma (migh″o·figh″bro·sahr·ko′muh) *n.* [*myo-* + *fibro-* + *sarcoma*]. Leiomyosarcoma with rich fibromatous component.

myo·fi·bro·si·tis (migh″o·figh″bro·sigh′tis) *n.* [*myo-* + *fibrositis*]. MYOSITIS.

myo·fil·a·ment (migh″o·fil′uh·munt) *n.* One of the filaments constituting the fine structure of a myofibril, seen by means of the electron microscope.

myo·ge·lo·sis (migh″o·je·lo′sis) *n.* [*myo-* + *gelosis*]. A hardened region in a muscle; specifically, hard nodules localized at the origin of a muscle.

myo·gen (migh'o·jen) *n.* [*myo-* + *-gen*]. Collectively, the water-soluble proteins of muscle, largely located in the sarcoplasm and consisting of various enzymes.

myo·gen·ic (migh"o·jen'ick) *adj.* [*myo-* + *-genic*]. 1. Of muscular origin, as myogenic contraction of muscle, in contrast to neurogenic contraction. 2. Giving rise to muscle.

my·og·e·nous (migh·oj'e·nus) *adj.* MYOGENIC (1).

myo·glo·bin (migh'o·glo"bin) *n.* [*myo-* + *globin*]. Myohemoglobin, muscle hemoglobin; the form of hemoglobin occurring in red or mixed muscle fibers. It differs somewhat from blood hemoglobin in showing a displacement of the spectral absorption bands toward the red, a higher oxygen affinity, and a hyperbolic dissociation curve, a smaller Bohr effect, a lower affinity for carbon monoxide, and a lower molecular weight. It serves as a short-time oxygen store, carrying the muscle from one contraction to the next.

myo·glo·bin·uria (migh"o·glo"bi·new'ree·uh) *n.* The presence of free myoglobin in the urine, seen in Haff disease, trauma, ischemia, and other primary lesions of striated muscle which result in muscle necrosis.

my·og·na·thus (migh·og'nuth·us, migh"og·nath'us, migh"o·naith'us) *n.* [*myo-* + *gnath-* + *-us*]. A form of double monster in which a parasitic rudimentary head is joined to the jaw of the autosite by means of muscle and integument only.

myo·gram (migh'o·gram) *n.* [*myo-* + *-gram*]. The recording made by a myograph.

myogranular myopathy. NEMALINE MYOPATHY.

myo·graph (migh'o·graf) *n.* [*myo-* + *-graph*]. An instrument for recording muscular contractions. —**myo·graph·ic** (migh"o·graf'ick) *adj.*

myo·hem·a·tin (migh"o·hem'uh·tin, ·heem') *n.* [*myo-* + *hematin*]. A respiratory enzyme; an iron porphyrin compound allied to hematin; important in animal and plant tissue oxidation. See also *cytochrome.*

myo·he·mo·glo·bin (migh"o·hee'muh·glo"bin) *n.* [*myo-* + *hemoglobin*]. MYOGLOBIN.

myo·he·mo·glo·bin·uria (migh"o·hee"muh·glo·bi·new'ree·uh) *n.* MYOGLOBINURIA.

my·oid (migh'oid) *adj.* Musclelike; resembling muscle.

myoid cells. Polygonal cells, cytologically similar to smooth muscle cells, found in the seminiferous tubules of laboratory rodents; believed to be responsible for the rhythmic contractions observed in the seminiferous tubules of these species.

my·oi·des (migh·oy'deez) *n.* [Gk. *myōdēs,* muscular]. PLATYSMA.

myo·ino·si·tol (migh"o·in·o'si·tole, ·tol) *n.* A name proposed for the common inositol, sometimes called mesoinositol, to distinguish it from the eight other possible stereoisomers.

myo·ki·nase (migh"o·kigh'nace, ·naze, ·kin'ace, migh·ock'i·nace) *n.* [*myo-* + *kinase*]. An enzyme present in muscle tissue which enables myosin to bring about the reaction by which two moles of adenosine diphosphate yield one mole of adenylic acid and one mole of adenosine triphosphate. It also facilitates the action of hexokinase in catalyzing the reaction between glucose or fructose and adenosine triphosphate by which glucose 6-phosphate or fructose 6-phosphate and adenosine diphosphate are formed.

myo·ki·ne·sio·gram (migh"o·ki·nee'zee·o·gram) *n.* The curve obtained in myokinesiography.

myo·ki·ne·si·og·ra·phy (migh"o·ki·nee"zee·og'ruh·fee) *n.* [*myo-* + *kinesio-* + *-graphy*]. 1. A method of recording graphically the movement of muscle either in vivo or in vitro. 2. Specifically, a method for studying muscle action during walking; it reveals disturbances in motor activity and coordination.

myo·ky·mia (migh"o·kigh'mee·uh, ·kim'ee·uh) *n.* [*myo-* + Gk. *kyma*, wave, billow, + *-ia*]. A state of almost continuous fasciculations, which impart a rippling appearance to the overlying skin. It may be transitory or persistent and limited to one muscle or universal, and may be associated with muscle cramps and myotonic-like contractions. Syn. *live flesh, myoclonia fibrillaris multiplex.* See also *facial myokymia.*

myo·lei·ot·ic (migh"o·lye·ot'ick) *adj.* [*myo-* + *leio-* + *-ic*]. Pertaining to or supplying smooth muscle.

myo·li·po·ma (migh"o·li·po'muh) *n.* [*myo-* + *lip-* + *-oma*]. A benign tumor whose parenchyma is composed of adipose and smooth muscle cells.

myo·lo·gia (migh'o·lo'jee·uh) *n.* [NA]. MYOLOGY.

my·ol·o·gy (migh·ol'uh·jee) *n.* [*myo-* + *-logy*]. The science of the nature, structure, functions, and diseases of muscles.

my·o·ma (migh·o'muh) *n.* [*my-* + *-oma*]. 1. A leiomyoma of the uterus. 2. Any tumor derived from muscle. See also *leiomyoma, rhabdomyoma.* —**my·om·a·tous** (migh·om'uh·tus) *adj.*

myo·ma·la·cia (migh"o·ma·lay'shee·uh) *n.* [*myo-* + *malacia*]. Degeneration, with softening, of muscle tissue.

myomalacia cor·dis (kor'dis) [L., of the heart]. Softening of a portion of the heart muscle, usually resulting from myocardial infarction.

myoma strio·cel·lu·la·re (strye"o·sel·yoo·lair'ee). RHABDOMYOMA.

myoma telangiectodes. A myoma with many blood vascular spaces, often cavernous. Syn. *angiomyoma.*

my·o·ma·to·sis (migh·o"muh·to'sis) *n.* [*myoma* + *-osis*]. The presence of multiple leiomyomas, usually uterine.

myoma uteri. LEIOMYOMA UTERI.

my·o·mec·to·my (migh"o·meck'tuh·mee) *n.* [*myoma* + *-ectomy*]. Excision of a uterine or other myoma.

my·ome dar·to·ïque (migh·ome' dahr·to·eek') [F., from *dartos*]. A solitary leiomyoma occurring usually in the external genitalia or rarely in the nipples.

myo·mere (migh'o·meer) *n.* [*myo-* + *-mere*]. MYOTOME (2).

myometrial gland. A collection of cells appearing between the muscle cells of the rabbit's uterus about the middle of pregnancy.

myo·me·tri·tis (migh"o·me·trye'tis) *n.* [*myometrium* + *-itis*]. Inflammation of the uterine muscular tissue.

myo·me·tri·um (migh"o·mee'tree·um) *n.* [NL., from *myo-* + Gk. *mētra,* womb] [NA]. The uterine muscular structure. —**myometri·al** (·ul) *adj.*

myo·neme (migh'o·neem) *n.* [*myo-* + *-neme*]. One of the long contractile fibrillae in protozoa.

myo·neu·ral (migh"o·new'rul) *adj.* [*myo-* + *neural*]. 1. Pertaining to both muscle and nerve. 2. Pertaining to nerve endings in muscle tissue.

myoneural junction. The point of junction of a motor nerve with the muscle which it innervates. Syn. *neuromuscular junction.*

myo·pal·mus (migh"o·pal'mus) *n.* [*myo-* + Gk. *palmos,* quivering, pulsation]. Twitching of the muscles.

myo·pa·ral·y·sis (migh"o·puh·ral'i·sis) *n.* Paralysis of a muscle or muscles.

myo·pa·re·sis (migh"o·pa·ree'sis, ·păr'e·sis) *n.* [*myo-* + *paresis*]. Slight paralysis of muscle.

myo·path·ia (migh"o·path'ee·uh) *n.* MYOPATHY.

myopathia ra·chit·i·ca (ra·kit'i·kuh). Muscle weakness in rickets.

myo·path·ic (migh"o·path'ick) *adj.* [*myo-* + *path-* + *-ic*]. Of or pertaining to disease of the muscles.

myopathic facies. A peculiar facial appearance in patients with myopathies, especially myotonic dystrophy. The brow shows no wrinkling, the face is expressionless or glum, the cheeks are sunken, the lower lip droops. Enophthalmos may be present.

myopathic gait. WADDLING GAIT.

myopathic nystagmus. Nystagmus due to defects or disease of one or more of the extraocular muscles; may be congenital or acquired, as in myasthenia gravis.

myopathic paralysis. Paralysis due to primary muscle disease.

myopathic spasm. Muscular spasm due to a primary disease of the muscles.

my·op·a·thy (migh·op'uth·ee) *n.* [*myo-* + *-pathy*]. Any disease of the muscles.

my·ope (migh'ope) *n.* [Gk. *myōps,* squinting, nearsighted]. A person affected with myopia.

myo·peri·car·di·tis (migh"o·perr"i·kahr·dye'tis) *n.* A combination of pericarditis and myocarditis.

myo·pha·gia (migh"o·fay'jee·uh) *n.* [*myo-* + *-phagia*]. The invasion of degenerated muscle sarcoplasm by histiocytes.

myophosphorylase deficiency glycogenosis. MCARDLE'S SYNDROME.

my·o·pia (migh·o'pee·uh) *n.* [Gk. *myōpia,* from *myōps,* squinting, nearsighted, from *myein,* to close, + *ōps,* eye]. Nearsightedness; an optical defect, usually due to too great length of the anteroposterior diameter of the globe, whereby the focal image is formed in front of the retina. Abbreviated, my. —**my·op·ic** (migh·op'ick, ·o'pick) *adj.*

myopic astigmatism. Astigmatism in which one principal meridian comes to a focus on the retina, while the other is in front of it.

myo·plasm (migh'o·plaz·um) *n.* [*myo-* + *-plasm*]. The cytoplasm of a muscle cell or fiber.

myo·plas·ty (migh'o·plas·tee) *n.* [*myo-* + *-plasty*]. Plastic surgery on a muscle or group of muscles.

my·o·por·tho·sis (migh"o·por·tho'sis) *n.* [*myopia* + Gk. *orthōsis,* straightening, guidance]. The correction of myopia.

myo·psy·chop·a·thy (migh"o·sigh·kop'uth·ee) *n.* [*myo-* + *psychopathy*]. Any myopathy, associated with mental retardation.

myo·psy·cho·sis (migh"o·sigh·ko'sis) *n.* MYOPSYCHOPATHY.

my·or·rha·phy (migh·or'uh·fee) *n.* [*myo-* + *-rrhaphy*]. Suture of a muscle.

my·o·san (migh'o·san) *n.* [*myosin* + *protean*]. A protein derivative of the class of proteans which is formed by the action of dilute acid or water on myosin.

myo·sar·co·ma (migh"o·sahr·ko'muh) *n.* A sarcoma derived from muscle.

myo·schwan·no·ma (migh"o·shwah·no'muh) *n.* [*myo-,* myelin, + *schwannoma*]. NEURILEMMOMA.

myo·scle·ro·sis (migh"o·skle·ro'sis) *n.* [*myo-* + *sclerosis*]. FIBROUS MYOSITIS.

my·o·sin (migh'o·sin, migh'uh·sin) *n.* [Gk. *mys, myos,* mouse; muscle, + *-in*]. One of the principal contractile proteins occurring in muscle, comprising up to one-half of the total muscle protein. It combines reversibly with actin to form actomyosin, and as such is responsible for the birefringent, contractile, and elastic properties of muscle. It is closely associated with the enzyme adenosine triphosphatase (ATPase). Its coagulation with ATP after death is the cause of rigor mortis.

my·o·sino·gen (migh"o·sin'o·jen) *n.* [*myosin* + *-gen*]. MYOGEN.

myosis. MIOSIS.

my·o·si·tis (migh"o·sigh'tis) *n.* [Gk. *mys, myos,* muscle, + *-itis*]. Inflammation of muscle, usually voluntary muscle. —**myo·sit·ic** (·sit'ick) *adj.*

myositis os·sif·i·cans (os·if'i·kanz). Myositis with formation of bone.

myo·spasm (migh'o·spaz·um) *n.* SPASM.

myo·stat·ic (migh"o·stat'ick) *adj.* [*myo-* + *static*]. Pertaining to a muscle of fixed length in relaxation, as in myostatic contracture.

myostatic contracture. Assumption of shortened length after fixation in cast or tendon section with innervation intact.

myo·su·ture (migh'o·sue"chur) *n.* Suture of a muscle; myorrhaphy.

myo·syn·o·vi·tis (migh"o·sin"o·vye'tis) *n.* [*myo-* + *synovitis*]. Inflammation of synovial membranes and surrounding musculature.

myo·tac·tic (migh"o·tack'tick) *adj.* [*myo-* + L. *tactus,* touch, + *-ic*]. Pertaining to the sense of touch of muscle.

my·ot·a·sis (migh·ot'uh·sis) *n.* [*myo-* + Gk. *tasis,* stretching, extension]. Stretching of a muscle.

myo·tat·ic (migh"o·tat'ick) *adj.* Of or pertaining to myotasis.

myotatic contracture. Contracture occurring in a degenerating muscle when tapped or suddenly stretched; may also occur when a fatigued muscle is struck.

myotatic irritability. Contraction of a muscle in response to being stretched.

myotatic reflex. STRETCH REFLEX.

myo·ten·di·nous (migh"o·ten'di·nus) *adj.* Pertaining to both muscle and tendon, especially the junction of the two.

myo·ten·o·si·tis (migh"o·ten"o·sigh'tis) *n.* [*myo-* + *teno-* + *-itis*]. Inflammation of a muscle and its tendon.

myo·te·not·o·my (migh"o·te·not'um·ee) *n.* [*myo-* + *teno-* + *-tomy*]. Surgical division of muscles and tendons.

myo·tome (migh'o·tome) *n.* [*myo-* + *-tome*]. 1. An instrument for performing myotomy. 2. The part of a somite that differentiates into skeletal muscle.

my·ot·o·my (migh·ot'uh·mee) *n.* [*myo-* + *-tomy*]. Division or cutting (dissection) of a muscle, particularly through its belly.

myo·to·nia (migh"o·to'nee·uh) *n.* [*myo-* + *-tonia*]. Continued contraction of muscle, despite attempts at relaxation, characteristic of certain diseases such as myotonia congenita, myotonic dystrophy, and paramyotonia of von Eulenberg.

myotonia ac·qui·si·ta (ack"wi·sigh'tuh, a·kwiz'i·tuh). A form of myotonia which does not become evident until adult years and which may be an expression of a rare, recessive form of congenital myotonia, of hypothyroidism, or of myotonic dystrophy. Syn. *myotonia tarda.*

myotonia atroph·i·ca (a·trof'i·kuh, a·tro'fi·kuh). MYOTONIC DYSTROPHY.

myotonia con·gen·i·ta (kon·jen'i·tuh). A familial disorder of muscle, usually inherited as an autosomal dominant trait, and rarely as a recessive trait, with onset in infancy or childhood, characterized by lack of relaxation of skeletal muscles after initial forceful contraction, often aggravated by cold or emotional stress, and hypertrophy of skeletal muscles. Syn. *Thomsen's disease.*

myotonia congenita in·ter·mit·tens (in"tur·mit'enz). PARAMYOTONIA CONGENITA.

myotonia dys·troph·i·ca (dis·trof'i·kuh, ·tro'fi·kuh). MYOTONIC DYSTROPHY.

myotonia he·red·i·tar·ia (he·red"i·tăr'ee·uh). MYOTONIA CONGENITA.

myotonia par·a·dox·i·ca (păr·uh·dock'si·kuh). A form of myotonia in which the first voluntary movements in a series are less likely to be followed by myotonic spasm than later ones.

myotonia tar·da (tahr'duh). MYOTONIA ACQUISITA.

myo·ton·ic (migh"o·ton'ick) *adj.* Of or characterized by myotonia.

myotonic atrophy. MYOTONIC DYSTROPHY.

myotonic dystrophy. A hereditary disease, transmitted as an autosomal dominant, characterized by lack of normal relaxation of muscles after contraction, slowly progressive muscular weakness and atrophy, especially of the face, neck, and distal muscles of the limbs, cataract formation, early baldness, gonadal atrophy, abnormal glucose tolerance curve, and frequently mental deficiency.

myotonic muscular dystrophy. MYOTONIC DYSTROPHY.

myotonic reaction. *In electromyography,* the high frequency, repetitive discharges which wax and wane in amplitude and frequency, producing a "dive-bomber" sound on the audiomonitor. This electrical picture is also seen following voluntary contraction or electrical stimulation of the muscle via its motor nerve.

my·ot·o·nus (migh·ot'uh·nus) *n.* [*myo-* + Gk. *tonos,* tension, tightening]. Muscle tone; the slight resistance that normal muscle offers to passive movement. This state has no electrical counterpart.

my·ot·ro·phy (migh·ot'ruh·fee) *n.* [*myo-* + *-trophy*]. Nutrition of muscle.

myr·cene (mur'seen) *n.* [*myrc*ia oil + *-ene*]. 7-Methyl-3-methylene-1,6-octadiene, $C_{10}H_{16}$, a terpene hydrocarbon occurring in bay oil and other volatile oils.

myr·cia oil (mur'shuh, ·shee·uh). BAY OIL.

myria- [Gk. *myrias,* ten thousand, myriad]. A combining form meaning (a) *ten thousand;* (b) *very many, numerous.*

myriachit. Miryachit (= PALMUS).

myr·ia·gram (mirr'ee·uh·gram) *n.* [*myria-* + *gram*]. Ten thousand grams.

myr·ia·li·ter (mirr'ee·uh·lee"tur) *n.* [Gk. *myria-* + *liter*]. Ten thousand liters.

myr·ia·me·ter (mirr'ee·uh·mee"tur) *n.* [*myria-* + *meter*]. Ten thousand meters.

myr·ia·pod (mirr'ee·uh·pod) *n.* MYRIOPOD.

myr·i·cyl (mirr'i·sil) *n.* The univalent hydrocarbon radical $CH_3(CH_2)_{29}$—. Syn. *melissyl.*

myring-, myringo- [ML. *myringa,* membrane]. A combining form meaning *tympanic membrane.*

my·rin·ga (mi·ring'guh) *n.* [ML., from Gk. *mēninx, mēningos,* membrane]. TYMPANIC MEMBRANE.

myr·in·gec·to·my (mirr"in·jeck'tuh·mee) *n.* [*myring-* + *-ectomy*]. MYRINGODECTOMY.

myr·in·gi·tis (mirr"in·jye'tis, migh"rin·) *n.* [*myring-* + *-itis*]. Inflammation of the tympanic membrane.

myringitis bul·lo·sa (bul·o'suh, bo͝ol·o'suh). Myringitis with bullous lesions on the tympanic membrane which may contain serum or blood; possibly due to *Mycoplasma pneumoniae.*

my·rin·go·dec·to·my (mi·ring"go·deck'tuh·mee) *n.* [*myringo-* + *-ectomy*]. Excision of a part or of the whole of the tympanic membrane.

my·rin·go·my·co·sis (mi·ring"go·migh·ko'sis) *n.* [*myringo-* + *mycosis*]. An infection of the eardrum due to fungi, usually as the result of spread from the external auditory canal; an otomycosis.

my·rin·go·plas·ty (mi·ring'go·plas"tee) *n.* [*myringo-* + *-plasty*]. A plastic operation to close perforations in the tympanic membrane. —**my·rin·go·plast·ic** (mi·ring"go·plas'tick) *adj.*

my·rin·go·tome (mi·ring'go·tome) *n.* [*myringo-* + *-tome*]. An instrument used in incising tympanic membrane.

myr·in·got·o·my (mirr"in·got'uh·mee) *n.* [*myringo-* + *-tomy*]. Incision of the tympanic membrane for the drainage of fluid or pus in the treatment of otitis media. Syn. *paracentesis of the tympanum, tympanotomy.*

my·rinx (migh'rinks, mirr'inks) *n.* [ML., from Gk. *mēninx,* membrane]. TYMPANIC MEMBRANE.

myr·io·pod (mirr'ee·o·pod) *n.* [Gk. *myriopous, myriopodos,* many-legged]. Any arthropod of certain classes characterized by long, multisegmented bodies and many legs, comprising principally the centipedes and millipedes.

my·ris·ti·ca (mi·ris'ti·kuh, migh·ris') *n.* [Gk. *myristikē,* fragrant]. Nutmeg.

my·ris·tic acid (mi·ris'tick, migh·ris'tick). Tetradecanoic acid, $CH_3(CH_2)_{12}COOH$, a fatty acid occurring in the glycerides of many fats.

my·ris·tin (mi·ris'tin, migh·) *n.* Glyceryl trimyristate, $(C_{14}H_{27}O_2)_3C_3H_5$, a component of spermaceti, nutmeg butter, and other fats.

Myrj. Trademark for several polyoxyl (polyoxyethylene) fatty acid esters individually identified by appending a number to the trademark; the substances are surfactants.

myrrh (mur) *n.* [Gk. *myrra*]. A gum resin obtained from *Commiphora molmol, C. abyssinica,* or other species of *Commiphora.* Contains a volatile oil, a resin myrrhin, and a gum. Has been used as a local protective agent.

Mysoline. Trademark for primidone, an anticonvulsant drug used for control of generalized and psychomotor seizures.

my·so·pho·bia (migh"so·fo'bee·uh) *n.* [Gk. *mysos,* defilement, + *-phobia*]. Abnormal dread of contamination or of dirt.

my·ta·cism (migh'tuh·siz·um) *n.* [Gk. *mytakismos,* fondness for the letter mu]. Excessive or faulty use of the sound of *m,* and its substitution for other sounds.

Mytelase. Trademark for the cholinesterase inhibitor ambenonium chloride.

mytho·ma·nia (mith"o·may'nee·uh) *n.* A pathologic tendency to lie or to exaggerate; a condition seen in certain psychiatric patients.

mytho·pho·bia (mith"o·fo'bee·uh) *n.* A morbid dread of stating what is not absolutely correct.

myt·i·lo·tox·in (mit"i·lo·tock'sin) *n.* [Gk. *mytilos,* mussel, + *toxin*]. A neurotoxic principle found in certain mussels.

myt·i·lo·tox·ism (mit"i·lo·tock'siz·um) *n.* [*mytilotox*in + *-ism*]. Poisoning from eating mussels with paralysis of the central and peripheral nervous system.

my·u·rous (migh·yoor'us) *adj.* [Gk. *myouros,* from *mys,* mouse, + *oura,* tail]. Tapering like the tail of the mouse; said of the pulse when it is progressively growing feeble.

myx-, myxo- [Gk. *myxa*]. A combining form meaning (a) *mucus, mucous;* (b) *mucin, mucinous.*

myx·ad·e·ni·tis (mick·sad"e·nigh'tis) *n.* [*myx-* + *adenitis*]. Inflammation of a mucous gland.

myxadenitis la·bi·a·lis (lay·bee·ay'lis). GLANDULAR CHEILITIS.

myx·ad·e·no·ma (mick·sad"e·no'muh) *n.* MYXOADENOMA.

myx·as·the·nia (micks"as·theen'ee·uh) *n.* [*myx-* + *asthenia*]. Overdryness of the mucosa or impairment of the power to secrete mucus.

myx·ede·ma (mick"se·dee'muh) *n.* [*myx-* + *edema*]. A condition due to inadequacy of thyroid hormone, characterized by hypometabolism, cold sensitivity, dry, coarse skin, hair loss, mental dullness, anemia, and slowed reflexes. See also *Gull's disease, athyreosis.* —**myxedema·tous** (·tus) *adj.*

myxedema cir·cum·scrip·tum thy·ro·tox·i·cum (sur"kum·skrip'tum thigh"ro·tock'si·kum). CIRCUMSCRIBED MYXEDEMA.

myxedematous infantilism. CRETINISM.

myx·id·i·o·cy (mick·sid'ee·uh·see) *n.* [*myx*edematous + *idiocy*]. CRETINISM.

myx·i·o·sis (mick"see·o'sis) *n.* [*myx-* + *-osis*]. A mucous discharge.

myxo-. See *myx-.*

myxo·ad·e·no·ma (mick"so·ad·e·no'muh) *n.* An adenoma of a mucous gland.

myxo·chon·dro·fi·bro·sar·co·ma (mick"so·kon"dro·figh"bro·sahr·ko'muh) *n.* A sarcoma whose parenchyma consists of anaplastic myxoid, chondroid, and fibrous elements.

myxo·chon·dro·ma (mick"so·kon·dro'muh) *n.* A benign tumor whose parenchymal cells are myxoid and chondroid.

myxo·chon·dro·sar·co·ma (mick"so·kon"dro·sahr·ko'muh) *n.* CHONDROMYXOSARCOMA.

myxo·cyte (mick'so·site) *n.* [*myxo-* + *-cyte*]. A large cell, polyhedral or stellate, found in mucous tissue.

myxo·fi·bro·ma (mick"so·figh·bro'muh) *n.* A benign fibroma with a myxomatous component.

myxofibroma of nerve sheath. NEUROFIBROMA.

myxo·fi·bro·sar·co·ma (mick"so·figh"bro·sahr·ko'muh) *n.* A malignant tumor composed of myxosarcomatous and fibrosarcomatous elements.

myxo·gli·o·ma (mick"so·glye·o'muh) *n.* [*myxo-* + *glioma*]. A gelatinous form of glioma.

my·xo·glob·u·lo·sis (mick"so·glob·yoo·lo'sis) *n.* [*myxo-* + *globule* + *-osis*]. A variety of appendiceal mucocele in which opaque globules lie in the mucus.

myx·oid (mick'soid) *adj.* [*myx-* + *-oid*]. Like mucus; MUCOID.

myxo·li·po·ma (mick"so·li·po'muh) *n.* [*myxo-* + *lipoma*]. 1. A benign tumor whose parenchyma contains myxoid and adipose tissue cells. 2. LIPOSARCOMA.

myxo·lipo·sar·co·ma (mick″so·lip″o·sahr·ko′muh) *n.* [*myxo-* + *lipo-* + *sarcoma*]. A sarcoma whose parenchyma is composed of anaplastic myxoid and adipose tissue cells.

myx·o·ma (mick·so′muh) *n.* [*myx-* + *-oma*]. A benign tumor whose parenchyma is composed of mucinous connective tissue.

myxoma cav·er·no·sum (kav″ur·no′sum). A cystic myxoma.

myxoma fi·bro·sum (figh·bro′sum). A myxoma with a fibrous element.

myxoma ge·la·ti·no·sum (je·lat″i·no′sum). MYXOMA.

myxoma li·po·ma·to·des (li·po″muh·to′deez). MYXOLIPOMA.

myxoma med·ul·la·re (med″yoo·lair′ee). MYXOMA.

myxoma simplex. MYXOMA.

myx·o·ma·to·sis (mick″so·muh·to′sis) *n.* [*myxoma* + *-osis*]. 1. A viral disease of rabbits producing fever, myxomatous skin masses, and mucoid swelling of the mucous membranes. 2. The presence of numerous myxomas.

myx·om·a·tous (mick·som′uh·tus) *adj.* Like or pertaining to myxomas.

myxomatous degeneration. MUCOUS DEGENERATION.

Myxo·my·ce·tes (mick″so·migh·see′teez) *n.pl.* [*myxo-* + *mycetes*]. A class of fungi, known as the slime molds, none of which is pathogenic to man; resemble protozoa in some respects.

myxo·neu·ro·ma (mick″so·new·ro′muh) *n.* A neuroma, or more often a neurofibroma, with a myxomatous component, occurring in peripheral nerves.

myxo·pleo·mor·phic epithelium (mick″so·plee″o·mor′fick). PLEOMORPHIC ADENOMA.

myx·or·rhea (mick″so·ree′uh) *n.* [*myxo-* + *-rrhea*]. A copious mucous discharge.

myxo·sar·co·ma (mick″so·sahr·ko′muh) *n.* A sarcoma whose parenchyma is composed of anaplastic myxoid cells. —**myxosar·com·a·tous** (·kom′uh·tus, ·ko′muh·tus) *adj.*

myxo·spore (mick′so·spore) *n.* [*myxo-* + *spore*]. A spore produced in the midst of a gelatinous mass without a distinct ascus or basidium.

Myx·o·spo·rid·ia (mick″so·spo·rid′ee·uh) *n.pl.* An order of sporozoa consisting of intercellular parasites which form nodules in tissue; they affect fishes, amphibians, reptiles, worms, and insects and are transmitted by ingestion of spores.

myxo·vi·rus (mick″so·vye′rus) *n.* [*myxo-* + *virus*]. A member of a group of ether-sensitive, hemagglutinating RNA viruses, including the influenza, mumps, Newcastle, and parainfluenza viruses; so named because of a special affinity for mucins.

My·zo·my·ia (migh″zo·migh′ee·uh) *n.* [Gk. *myzein*, to suck, + *myia*, fly]. A subgenus of the genus *Anopheles*, the mosquito that transmits the malarial parasite.

N

N Symbol for nitrogen.

N, *N* Abbreviation for *normal* (3).

N- *In chemistry,* symbol prefixed to a radical which is attached to the nitrogen atom.

n 1. Symbol for a unit of neutron dosage corresponding to the roentgen. 2. Symbol for refractive index. 3. Symbol for the prefix *nano-*.

n. Abbreviation for *nasal.*

N- *In chemistry,* symbol for *normal.*

NA Abbreviation for *Nomina Anatomica.*

N. A. Abbreviation for *numerical aperture.*

Na [NL. *natrium*]. Symbol for sodium.

Na·bo·thi·an cyst (na·bo'thee·un) [M. *Naboth,* German anatomist, 1675–1721]. Cystic distention of the mucous (Nabothian) glands of the uterine cervix.

Nabothian follicle. NABOTHIAN CYST.

Nabothian glands [M. *Naboth*]. Mucous glands of the cervix of the uterus.

na·cre·ous (nay'kree·us, nack'ree·us) *adj.* Resembling nacre or mother-of-pearl.

Nacton. Trademark for poldine methylsulfate, an anticholinergic drug with actions similar to those of atropine.

N. A. D. No appreciable disease.

NAD Abbreviation for *nicotinamide adenine dinucleotide.*

NAD^{+} Symbol for the oxidized form of nicotinamide adenine dinucleotide.

NADH Symbol for the reduced form of nicotinamide adenine dinucleotide.

NADH dehydrogenase. A flavin-containing mitochondrial enzyme which catalyzes transfer of electrons from NADH to the next member of the electron transport chain.

nad·ide (nad'ide) *n.* A nucleotide composed of one molecule each of adenine and nicotinamide, and two molecules each of D-ribose and phosphoric acid. It is a coenzyme for numerous hydrogenase reactions. Syn. *nicotinamide adenine dinucleotide.*

Nadi reagent [*na*phthol + *di*methyl]. A mixture of β-naphthol with dimethyl-*para*-phenylenediamine, used as a test for indophenol oxidase.

N.A.D.L. National Association of Dental Laboratories.

na·do·lol (nay·do'lole) *n.* 1-(*tert*-Butylamino)-3-[(5,6,7,8-tetrahydro*cis*-6,7-dihydroxy-1-naphthyl)oxy]-2-propanol $C_{17}H_{27}NO_4$, an antiadrenergic (β-receptor).

NADP Abbreviation for *nicotinamide adenine dinucleotide phosphate.*

NADP^{+} Symbol for the oxidized form of nicotinamide adenine dinucleotide phosphate.

NADPH Symbol for the reduced form of nicotinamide adenine dinucleotide phosphate.

Nae·ge·le pelvis (ne^{y}'ge·le^{h}) [F. K. *Naegele,* German obstetrician, 1778–1851]. An obliquely contracted pelvis with ankylosis of one sacroiliac synchondrosis, underdevelopment of the associated sacral ala, and other distorting defects producing an obliquely directed conjugata vera.

Naegele's obliquity [F. K. *Naegele*]. ANTERIOR ASYNCLITISM.

Naegeli test. *Obsol.* SCRATCH-PATCH TEST.

Nae·ge·li type leukemia (ne^{y}'ge·lee) [O. *Naegeli,* Swiss hematologist, 1871–1938]. A variety of monocytic leukemia in which the cells bear certain resemblances to the granulocytic series.

Nae·gle·ria (nay·gleer'ee·uh) *n.* A genus of soil amebas that occasionally cause meningoencephalitis in children who have been swimming in fresh water ponds.

nae·paine (nee'pane) *n.* 2-Pentylaminoethyl *p*-aminobenzoate, $C_{14}H_{22}N_2O_2$, a local anesthetic used as the hydrochloride salt to produce corneal anesthesia.

naevi. NEVI.

naevocarcinoma. A malignant melanoma.

naevoid. NEVOID.

naevomelanoma. A malignant melanoma.

naevose. NEVOSE.

naevoxantho-endothelioma. JUVENILE XANTHOGRANULOMA.

naevus. NEVUS.

naf·cil·lin (naf·sil'in) *n.* 2-Ethoxy-1-naphthylpenicillin, $C_{21}H_{22}N_2O_5S$, a semisynthetic penicillin antibiotic; used as the sodium salt.

na·fen·o·pin (na·fen'o·pin) *n.* 2-Methyl-2-[*p*-(1,2,3,4-tetrahydro-1-naphthyl)phenoxy]propionic acid, $C_{20}H_{22}O_3$, an antihyperlipidemic.

Naff·zig·er's operation [H. C. *Naffziger,* U. S. neurosurgeon, 1884–1961]. Excision of the superior and lateral walls of the orbit for the relief of progressive exophthalmos.

Naffziger's syndrome [H. C. *Naffziger*]. SCALENUS ANTERIOR SYNDROME.

Naffziger's test or **sign** [H. C. *Naffziger*]. 1. Pressure on the jugular veins increases the intraspinal tension which increases the pain in cases of herniated disk. 2. Pressure on the anterior scalene muscles at the root of the neck causes tingling in the hand in the scalenus anterior syndrome.

naf·o·mine (naf'o·meen) *n.* *O*-[(2-Methyl-1-naphthyl)methyl]hydroxylamine, $C_{12}H_{13}NO$, a muscle relaxant used as the malate salt.

naf·ox·i·dine (naf·ock'si·deen) *n.* 1-[2-[*p*-(3,4-Dihydro-6-methoxy-2-phenyl-1-naphthyl)phenoxy]ethyl]pyrrolidine, an antiestrogen; used as the hydrochloride salt.

naf·ro·nyl (naf'ro·nil) *n.* 2-(Diethylamino)ethyl tetrahydro-α-(1-naphthylmethyl)-2-furanpropionate, $C_{24}H_{33}NO_3$, a vasodilator used as the oxalate salt.

naf·ta·lo·fos (naf'tuh·lo·fos) *n.* *N*-Hydroxynaphthalimide diethyl phosphate, $C_{16}H_{16}NO_6P$, a veterinary anthelmintic.

Na·ga·ma·tsu incision. A dorsolumbar approach to the kidney and adrenal gland in which exposure is improved by multiple rib resections creating a movable flap.

na·ga·na (na·gah'nuh) *n.* [Zulu *u-nakane*]. An infectious disease of domestic animals, especially equine animals in East Africa, caused by *Trypanosoma brucei.* It is transmitted by the bite of the tsetse fly.

Naganol. A trademark for suramin sodium, an antitrypanosomal and antifilarial drug.

Na·ga sore (nah'guh) [after *Naga,* on Cebu Is., Philippines]. TROPICAL ULCER.

Na·gel's test. A test for color vision performed by using an instrument in which the patient attempts to match spectral yellow by a mixture of red and green.

Na·geotte-Babinski syndrome (nah·zhoht') [J. *Nageotte,* French pathologist, 1866–1948; and J. F. F. *Babinski*]. BABINSKI-NAGEOTTE SYNDROME.

Nagler's reaction [F. P. O. *Nagler,* Australian bacteriologist, 20th century]. The opalescence produced in human serum when alpha toxin of *Clostridium welchii* is added, due to the splitting of free lecithin into phosphocholine and a diglyceride.

nail, *n.* 1. The horny structure covering the dorsal aspect of the terminal phalanx of each finger and toe. It consists of intimately united, horny epithelial cells probably representing the stratum corneum of the epidermis. NA *unguis.* Comb. form *onych(o)-.* 2. A metallic (usually stainless steel or vitallium) elongated rod with one sharp and one blunt end, used in surgery to anchor bone fragments. Syn. *pin.*

nail bed. Vascular tissue, corresponding to the corium and the germinative layer of the skin, on which a nail rests. NA *matrix unguis.*

nail biting. A nervous habit or neurotic reaction chiefly in children and adolescents, manifested by the habit of biting the fingernails down to the quick.

nail culture. *In bacteriology,* a stab culture showing a growth along the needle track, and on the surface a buttonlike projection, giving the appearance of a nail driven into the gelatin.

nail en ra·quette (ahn ra·ket') [F.]. A dystrophy of the nail in which the nail, usually that of the thumb, appears wider than normal, its transverse curvature diminished so that the nail seems flat, with the appearance of a miniature tennis racket.

nail fold. The fold of skin bounding the sides and proximal portion of a nail.

nail groove. The sulcus between the nail fold and the nail bed.

nail-patella syndrome. A genetic disorder involving tissues of both ectodermal and mesodermal origin, characterized by defects in the nails ranging from complete anonychia to longitudinal ridging, hypoplastic or absent patellae, abnormalities of the elbows, iliac horns and a wide spectrum of other bone, joint, skin, eye, and renal abnormalities. Inherited as an autosomal dominant. Syn. *Fong's lesion.*

nail plate. NAIL (1).

nail root. The part of the body of a nail covered by the proximal nail fold.

nail wall. NAIL FOLD.

Nai·man's test. A test for vitamin B_1, depending upon the production of an orange-red precipitate with vitamin B_1 when bismuth potassium iodide is added.

Nai·ro·bi eye (nye·ro'bee). A conjunctivitis resulting from contact with fluid extracts of the crushed African beetle *Paederus cerebrepunctatus.*

Na·ja (nah'juh, nay'juh) *n.* [Skr. *nāga,* snake]. A genus of the Elapidae comprising the typical cobras; their venom is predominantly neurotoxic.

Naja ha·je (hah'jee, hah'yeh) [Egyptian Ar. *ḥayye,* snake]. The Egyptian cobra, which inhabits most of northern Africa and the drier parts of central Africa.

Naja hannah. *OPHIOPHAGUS HANNAH.*

Naja naja. The hooded cobra of southern Asia; probably accounts for more cases of snakebite than any other snake.

Naj·jar riboflavin method. Riboflavin is extracted with acetic acid-pyridine-butanol mixture after interfering urinary pigments are oxidized with permanganate. The concentration of riboflavin in the extract is measured fluorometrically.

na·ked cell. A cell with no demonstrable cell membrane.

nal·bu·phine (nal'bew·feen) *n.* 17-(Cyclobutylmethyl)-4,5α-epoxymorphinan-3,6α,14-triol, $C_{21}H_{27}NO_4$, an analgesic and narcotic antagonist; used as the hydrochloride salt.

nal·i·dix·ic acid (nal''i·dick'sick). 1-Ethyl-1,4-dihydro-7-methyl-4-oxo-1, 8-naphthyridine-3-carboxylic acid, $C_{12}H_{12}N_2O_3$, an antibacterial agent used clinically for treatment of urinary tract infections caused by gram-negative organisms.

Nalline. Trademark for nalorphine, the hydrochloride salt of which is used as an antidote to narcotic overdosage.

nal·mex·one (nal'meck·sone) *n.* 7,8-Dihydro-14-hydroxy-*N*-(3-methyl-2-butenyl)normorphinone, $C_{21}H_{25}NO_4$, an analgesic and narcotic antagonist; used as the hydrochloride salt.

nal·or·phine (nal'ur·feen, nal·or'feen) *n.* *N*-Allylmorphine, $C_{19}H_{21}NO_3$, a derivative of morphine used, as the hydrochloride salt, principally to counteract severe respiratory depression from overdosage with narcotics and to diagnose addiction to narcotics.

nal·ox·one (nal·ock'sone) *n.* (−)-*N*-Allyl-14-hydroxynordihydromorphinone, $C_{19}H_{21}NO_4$, an antidote for narcotics; used as the hydrochloride salt.

Nalsa. A trademark for proglumide, an anticholinergic.

nal·trex·one (nal·treck'sone) *n.* 17-(Cyclopropylmethyl)-4,5α-epoxy-3,14-dihydroxymorphinan-6-one, $C_{20}H_{23}NO_4$, a narcotic antagonist, also used as the hydrochloride.

nam·bi uvu (nam'bee oo'voo, oo·voo') *n.* [Pg., from Tupi *nambi,* ear, + *u-u,* eats, itches]. A disease of dogs in Brazil; marked by icterus and bleeding from the ear; caused by a blood parasite. Syn. *canine yellow fever, bleeding ear, blood plague.*

nam·ox·y·rate (nam·ock'si·rate) *n.* A compound of 2-(4-biphenylyl)butyric acid with 2-dimethylaminoethanol, $C_{16}H_{16}O_2.C_4H_{11}NO$, an analgesic composition.

nan·dro·lone (nan'druh·lone) *n.* 17β-Hydroxyestr-4-en-3-one, $C_{18}H_{26}O_2$, an androgenic steroid with anabolic activity; used clinically for the latter effect, in the form of the decanoate, phenpropionate, and cyclotate (4-methylbicyclo[2.2.2]oct-2-ene-1-carboxylate) esters.

na·nism (nay'niz·um, nan'iz·um) *n.* [Gk. *nanos,* dwarf, + *-ism*]. Abnormal smallness from arrested development; DWARFISM.

nano- [Gk. *nanos,* dwarf]. A combining form meaning (a) *dwarfed* or *undersized;* (b) *the one-billionth* (10^{-9}) *part* of the unit adjoined. Symbol, n

na·no·ceph·a·lus (nay''no·sef'ul·us, nan''o·) *n.* [*nano-* + *-cephalus*]. A fetus with a dwarfed head.

na·no·cor·mia (nay''no·kor'mee·uh, nan''o·) *n.* [*nano-* + Gk. *kormos,* trunk, + *-ia*]. DWARFISM.

na·no·cor·mus (nay''no·kor'mus, nan''o·) *n.* [*nano-* + Gk. *kormos,* trunk]. NANOSOMUS.

na·no·cu·rie (nay'no·kew''ree) *n.* One billionth (10^{-9}) of a curie; a quantity of a radioactive substance resulting in 37 nuclear disintegrations per second. Abbreviated, nCi Syn. *millimicrocurie.*

na·no·gram (nay'no·gram) *n.* One billionth (10^{-9}) of a gram. Abbreviated, ng Syn. *millimicrogram.*

na·noid (nay'noid, nan'oid) *adj.* [Gk. *nanos,* dwarf, + *-oid*]. Dwarflike.

na·nom·e·lus (nay·nom'e·lus, nan·) *n.* [*nano-* + Gk. *melos,* limb]. An individual characterized by undersized limbs.

na·no·me·ter (nay'no·mee·tur) *n.* [*nano-* + *meter*]. A unit of length equal to one billionth (10^{-9}) of a meter, or to 10 angstroms; the one thousandth part of a micrometer. Abbreviated, nm

nan·oph·thal·mia (nan″off·thal′mee·uh) *n.* [*nano-* + *ophthalm-* + *-ia*]. MICROPHTHALMUS (1).

nan·oph·thal·mos, nan·oph·thal·mus (nan″off·thal′mus) *n.* [*nano-* + Gk. *ophthalmos,* eye]. MICROPHTHALMUS (1).

Na·no·phy·e·tus sal·min·co·la (nay″no·figh·ee′tus sal·mink′o·luh). *TROGLOTREMA SALMINCOLA.*

na·no·sec·ond (nay′no·seck″und) *n.* One billionth (10^{-9}) of a second. Syn. *millimicrosecond.*

na·no·so·ma (nay″no·so′muh, nan″o·) *n.* [*nano-* + Gk. *sōma,* body]. DWARFISM.

na·no·so·mia (nay″no·so′mee·uh, nan″o·) *n.* [*nano-* + *-somia*]. DWARFISM.

na·no·so·mus (nay″no·so′mus, nan″o·) *n.* [*nano-* + Gk. *sōma,* body, + *-us*]. An individual with a dwarfed body.

na·nus (nay′nus, nan′us) *n.* [L., from Gk. *nanos*]. DWARF (1). **—nanous,** *adj.*

na·palm (nay′pahm, ·pahlm) *n.* An aluminum soap, prepared from naphthenic acids and the fatty acids of coconut oil, used for producing gels of gasoline for incendiary munitions.

nape, *n.* The back of the neck; NUCHA.

na·pel·line (na·pel′een, nap′ul·een, ·in) *n.* An alkaloid, $C_{22}H_{33}NO_3$, from aconite; formerly employed as an anodyne and antineuralgic.

na·pex (nay′pecks) *n.* [*nape* + *apex*]. That portion of the scalp just below the occipital protuberance.

na·phaz·o·line (nuh·faz′o·leen, naf·az′o·leen) *n.* 2-(1-Naphthylmethyl)-2-imidazoline, $C_{14}H_{14}N_2$, a sympathomimetic drug; used, as the hydrochloride salt, locally on nasal or ocular mucous membranes for its vasoconstrictor action.

naphth-, naphtho-. A combining form meaning *pertaining to naphthalene or its ring structure.*

naph·tha (naf′thuh) *n.* [Gk.]. 1. Formerly, any strong-smelling, inflammable, volatile liquid. 2. A mixture of low-boiling hydrocarbons distilled from petroleum and bituminous shale. Compare *petroleum, ether, ligroin.*

naphtha jag. A form of intoxication resulting from inhalation of organic solvents, characterized commonly by a feeling of being drunk, with lack of self-control, blurred vision, incoordination, confusion, excitement, and occasionally delirium, usually followed by a sense of depression and hangover.

naph·tha·lene (naf′thuh·leen) *n.* The hydrocarbon, $C_{10}H_8$, a constituent of coal tar; formerly used locally as an antiseptic. Used as a moth repellent and insecticide.

naph·tha·lene·ace·tic acid (naf″thuh·leen·uh·see′tick). Naphthylacetic acid, $C_{10}H_7CH_2COOH$, a plant growth regulator.

naph·thene (naf′theen) *n.* 1. Any cyclic hydrocarbon of the general formula C_nH_{2n}; sometimes called *cycloparaffin.* 2. The naphthalene ring system.

naphtho-. See *naphth-.*

naph·tho·qui·none (naf″tho·kwi·nohn′) *n.* Either of two compounds, $C_{10}H_6O_2$, derived from naphthalene: 1,4-naphthoquinone (α-naphthoquinone), derivatives of which have vitamin-K activity, or 1,2-naphthoquinone (β-naphthoquinone), used as a reagent.

naph·thyl (naf′thil) *n.* $C_{10}H_7$—, the radical of naphthalene.

α-naph·thyl·thio·urea (al″fuh·naf″thil·thigh″o·yoo·ree′uh) *n.* ANTU.

Naphuride Sodium. A trademark for sodium suramin, an antitrypanosomal and antifilarial drug.

na·pi·form (nay′pi·form, nap′i·) *adj.* [L. *napus,* turnip, + *-form*]. Turnip-shaped.

NAPNAP National Association of Pediatric Nurse Associates and Practitioners.

na·prox·en (na·prock′sen) *n.* (+)-6-Methoxy-α-methyl-2-naphthaleneacetic acid, $C_{14}H_{14}O_3$, an analgesic, antipyretic, anti-inflammatory.

na·prox·ol (na·prock′sole) *n.* (−)-6-Methoxy-β-methyl-2-naphthaleneethanol, $C_{14}H_{16}O_2$, an anti-inflammatory, analgesic, antipyretic.

nap·sy·late (nap′si·late) *n.* Any salt or ester of naphthalenesulfonic acid, $C_{10}H_7SO_3H$; a naphthalenesulfonate.

Naqua. A trademark for trichlormethiazide, an orally effective diuretic and antihypertensive drug.

nar·a·nol (năr′uh·nole) *n.* 8,9,10,11,11a,12-Hexahydro-8,10-dimethyl-7a*H*-naphtho[1′,2′:5,6]pyrano[3,2-*c*]pyridin-7a-ol, $C_{18}H_{21}NO_2$, a tranquilizer, used as the hydrochloride salt.

Na·rath's operation (nah′raht) [A. *Narath,* Austrian surgeon, 1864–1924]. Omentopexy for ascites.

Narcan. Trademark for naloxone, a narcotic antidote.

nar·cism (nahr′siz·um) *n.* NARCISSISM.

nar·cis·sism (nahr·sis′iz·um, nahr′si·siz·um) *n.* [Gk. *Narkissos,* a beautiful youth who fell in love with his own reflection]. *In psychoanalysis,* fixation of the libido upon one's self. Some degree of self-love is considered healthy; excessive self-love, however, interferes in one's relations with others. Compare *autoerotism.* **—nar·cis·sis·tic** (nahr″si·sis′tick) *adj.;* **nar·cis·sist** (nahr·sis′ist, nahr′si·sist) *n.*

narcissistic neurosis. *In psychoanalysis,* any neurosis, such as the hypochondriacal or the obsessive-compulsive type, characterized by extreme autoerotism and deficient capacity for transference.

narco- [Gk. *narkoun,* to benumb]. A combining form meaning *narcosis, numbness, or stupor.*

nar·co·anal·y·sis (nahr″ko·uh·nal′uh·sis) *n.* The induction of a quickly reversible sleep by intravenous injections of amobarbital or thiopental sodium during which a trained interrogator elicits memories and feelings not expressed in the patient's wakeful state because of either willful or unconscious resistance; used in the treatment of neuroses and psychophysiologic disorders and occasionally in the investigation of suspected criminals. See also *narcosynthesis.*

nar·co·hyp·no·sis (nahr″ko·hip·no′sis) *n.* HYPNONARCOSIS.

nar·co·lep·sy (nahr′ko·lep″see) *n.* [*narco-* + Gk. *lēpsis,* seizure]. A disorder of sleep mechanism, closely related if not identical with REM sleep, characterized by (1) uncontrollable attacks of drowsiness or sleep in the daytime, (2) cataplectic attacks of loss of muscular power, occurring without warning or during some emotional experience, (3) sleep paralysis, and (4) vivid nocturnal or hypnagogic hallucinations. **—nar·co·lep·tic** (nahr″ko·lep′tick) *adj.*

nar·co·ma (nahr·ko′muh) *n.* Stupor from the use of a narcotic. **—narcoma·tous** (·tus) *adj.*

nar·co·ma·nia (nahr″ko·may′nee·uh) *n.* A pathologic craving for narcotics (medicinal or psychologic). **—narcoma·ni·ac** (·ni·ack) *n.*

nar·co·pep·sia (nahr″ko·pep′see·uh) *n.* [*narco-* + Gk. *pepsis,* digestion, + *-ia*]. Slow or torpid digestion.

nar·co·sis (nahr·ko′sis) *n.* [Gk. *narkōsis,* a benumbing]. A state of profound stupor, unconsciousness, or arrested activity produced by drugs. Adj. & n. *narcotic.*

narcosis therapy. Prolonged sleep as a treatment for certain types of mental disorders, usually induced by drugs such as barbiturates or phenothiazines. Syn. *sleep therapy.*

nar·co·syn·the·sis (nahr″ko·sin′thi·sis) *n.* Psychotherapeutic treatment originally employed in acute combat cases under partial anesthesia as with amobarbital sodium or thiopental sodium, in which abreaction plays an important role in the therapeutic results. See also *narcoanalysis.*

nar·co·ther·a·py (nahr″ko·therr′up·ee) *n.* NARCOANALYSIS.

nar·cot·ic (nahr·kot′ick) *adj. & n.* [Gk. *narkōtikos*]. 1. Pertaining to or producing narcosis. 2. A drug that in therapeutic doses diminishes sensibility, relieves pain, and produces sleep, but in large doses causes stupor, coma, or convulsions. 3. Any drug, with properties similar to morphine, identified as a narcotic drug by federal law. 4. An individual addicted to the use of narcotics.

narcotic blockade. Partial or total inhibition of the euphoria produced by certain drugs through the use of other drugs, such as methadone, which can thus be used in maintenance treatment of addicts without producing the peaks of excitement or elation, withdrawal symptoms, and demands for increasing dosages of the agent to which the patient is addicted.

narcotico-. A combining form meaning *narcotic.*

nar·cot·i·co·ac·rid (nahr·kot″i·ko·ack′rid) *adj.* Both narcotic and irritant. See also *acronarcotic.*

nar·cot·i·co·ir·ri·tant (nahr·kot″i·ko·irr′i·tunt) *adj.* Both narcotic and irritant.

nar·co·tine (nahr′ko·teen, ·tin) *n.* NOSCAPINE.

nar·co·tism (nahr′kuh·tiz·um) *n.* 1. Narcotic poisoning. 2. Narcotic addiction.

nar·co·tize (nahr′kuh·tize) *v.* To put under the influence of a narcotic; to render unconscious through a narcotic.

Nardil. Trademark for the antidepressant drug phenelzine, used as the sulfate salt.

nares [NA]. NOSTRILS; plural of *naris.*

na·ris (nair′is, năr′is) *n.*, pl. **na·res** (·eez) [L.]. NOSTRIL; one of a pair of openings at the anterior part (anterior nares) or at the posterior part (posterior nares; choanae) of the nasal cavities. —**nar·i·al** (năr′ee·ul, nair′ee·ul) *adj.*

narrow-angle glaucoma. Increased intraocular tension due to a block of the angle of the anterior chamber from contact of the iris by the trabecula; begins acutely with extreme eye pain, hyperemia, and sudden visual loss and may resolve spontaneously, medically, or surgically; however, it may become chronic due to repeated acute attacks with the formation of synechial and gradual permanent closure of the angle. May be primary or secondary. Compare *open-angle glaucoma.*

nas-, naso-. A combining form meaning *nose, nasal.*

na·sal (nay′zul) *adj. & n.* [F., from L. *nasus,* nose]. 1. Of or pertaining to the nose. 2. With reference to the eye and its appendages: medial; situated on the side nearer the nose. Contr. *temporal* (1).

nasal area. The ventrolateral thickened ectoderm of the frontonasal process from which the olfactory placode arises.

nasal artery. See Table of Arteries in the Appendix.

nasal bone. NA *os nasale.* See Table of Bones in the Appendix.

nasal canal. 1. NASOLACRIMAL CANAL. 2. An occasional canal found in the posterior portion of the nasal bone; it gives passage to nasal nerves.

nasal capsule. The cartilage around the embryonic nasal cavity.

nasal cavity. One of the pair of cavities between the anterior nares and nasopharynx. NA *cavum nasi.* See also *primary nasal cavity, secondary nasal cavity.*

nasal concha. Any of the three or four medial projections of thin bone from the lateral wall of the nasal cavity, covered by mucous membrane and designated according to position as supreme (NA *concha nasalis suprema*), superior (NA *concha nasalis superior*), middle (NA *concha nasalis media*), and inferior (NA *concha nasalis inferior*). The supreme nasal concha is inconstant and, when present, is situated above the superior nasal concha. See also Plate 12 and *turbinate* in Table of Bones in the Appendix.

nasal crest. 1. The crest on the medial border of the palatal process of the maxilla, articulating with the vomer. NA *crista nasalis maxillae.* 2. The crest on the medial border of the palatine bone, articulating with the vomer. NA *crista nasalis ossis palatini.* 3. The crest on the internal border of the nasal bone and forming part of the septum of the nose.

nasal cycle. Alternating congestion and decongestion of the nasal airways, first one side becoming hyperemic and showing increasing mucosal gland secretion, then the other.

nasal field. 1. NASAL AREA. 2. The medial half of the field of vision, as contrasted with the temporal field.

nasal fossa. 1. OLFACTORY PIT. 2. NASAL CAVITY.

nasal glioma. Heterotopic glial tissue in the nose.

nasal groove. A groove between the median nasal process and maxillary process on either side along the course of a bucconasal membrane.

nasal hemianopsia. Loss of the nasal half of the field of vision. See also *binasal hemianopsia.*

nasal index. *In craniometry,* the ratio of the greatest width of the apertura piriformis wherever it is found, × 100, to the height of the nasal skeleton, which is the distance between nasion and nasospinale. Its values are classified as leptorrhine, x–46.9; mesorrhine, 47.0–50.9; chamaerrhine, 51.0–57.9; hyperchamaerrhine, 58.0–x.

na·sa·lis (nay·zay′lis, na·say′lis) *n.* A muscle of facial expression. NA *musculus nasalis.* See also Table of Muscles in the Appendix.

nasal labyrinth. The irregular cavity formed by the turbinate bones in the nasal passages.

nasal line. A line from the upper margin of the ala nasi curving around the angle of the mouth, ending at the edge of the orbicularis oris; has been noted in diseases of the gastrointestinal tract.

nasal membranous septum. The membranous part of the nasal septum; the anterior inferior portion of the septum. NA *pars membranacea septi nasi.*

nasal nerve. See Table of Nerves in the Appendix.

nasal notch. 1. The concave medial margin of the anterior surface of the maxilla; the lateral margin of the apertura piriformis. NA *incisura nasalis.* 2. An uneven interval between the internal angular process of the frontal bone which articulates with the nasal and maxillary bones.

nasal pit. OLFACTORY PIT.

nasal point. NASION.

nasal polyp. 1. A sessile or pedunculated polypoid mass of edematous connective tissue covered by epithelium and including glands and inflammatory exudate, projecting from the nasal mucosa into the nasal cavity. 2. Any polypoid tumor in the nasal cavity.

nasal process of the frontal bone. The downward projection of the nasal part of the frontal bone which terminates as the nasal spine.

nasal process of the maxilla. The frontal process of the maxilla. See *frontal process.*

nasal reflex. Sneezing induced by stimulation of the nasal mucosa.

nasal septum. The septum between the two nasal cavities. NA *septum nasi.*

nasal sinus. PARANASAL SINUS.

nasal speculum. A small bivalve instrument with handles, which dilates the nostril and allows examination of the nasal passages.

nasal spine. A sharp, medial process projecting downward from the nasal process of the frontal bone into the nasal septum and articulating with the crests of the nasal bones and the perpendicular plate of the ethmoid. NA *spina nasalis ossis frontalis.* See also *anterior nasal spine, posterior nasal spine.*

nasal spine of the palatine bone. POSTERIOR NASAL SPINE.

nasal step. ROENNE'S NASAL STEP.

nasal trephine. An instrument designed for use in the nasal cavity, made of a steel shaft ending in a small, fenestrated tube, having a knife or saw edge.

nasal voice. A peculiar, muffled timbre of the voice, especially marked in cases of perforated palate.

nas·cent (nas′unt, nay′sunt) *adj.* [L. *nascens,* arising, being born, coming forth]. 1. Characterizing an atom or simple compound at the moment of its liberation from chemical combination, when it may have greater activity than in its usual state. 2. Coming into being.

na·sio·al·ve·o·lar (nay″zee·o·al·vee′ul·ur) *adj.* Pertaining to, or connecting, the nasion and the alveolar point.

na·si·on (nay′zee·on, nay′see·on) *n.* [*nas*us + *-ion*]. *In craniometry,* the point where the sagittal plane intersects the frontonasal suture.

na·si·tis (nay·zigh′tis, ·sigh′tis) *n.* [*nas-* + *-itis*]. RHINITIS.

Na·smyth's membrane (nay′smith) [A. *Nasmyth,* Scottish anatomist and dentist, d. 1847]. ENAMEL CUTICLE (1).

naso-. See *nas-.*

na·so·al·ve·o·lar (nay″zo·al·vee′uh·lur) *adj.* [*naso-* + *alveolar*]. Pertaining to the nose and a tooth socket.

na·so·an·tral (nay″zo·an′trul) *adj.* [*naso-* + *antral*]. Pertaining to the nose and the maxillary sinus (antrum).

na·so·bas·i·lar line (nay″zo·bas′i·lur). A line drawn through the basion and the nasion.

na·so·breg·mat·ic arc (nay″zo·breg·mat′ick). A line measured from the root of the nose to the bregma.

na·so·cil·i·ary (nay″zo·sil′ee·err·ee) *adj.* [*naso-* + *ciliary*]. Pertaining to a nerve distributed to the nose, the ethmoid sinuses, and the eyeball.

nasociliary nerve. See Table of Nerves in the Appendix.

nasociliary neuralgia. Pain in the eye, brow, or temple together with pain on the side of the nose and medial canthus with rhinorrhea and sometimes cyclitis or keratitis. Syn. *Charlin's syndrome.*

na·so·fa·cial (nay″zo·fay′shul) *adj.* Pertaining to the nose and the face.

na·so·fron·tal (nay″zo·frun′tul, ·fron′tul) *adj.* Pertaining to the nasal and the frontal bones.

nasofrontal duct. The duct between the frontal sinus and the middle meatus of the nose. Syn. *frontonasal duct.*

nasofrontal fontanel. An abnormal fontanel at the union of the nasal and frontal bones.

nasofrontal process. FRONTONASAL PROCESS.

nasofrontal sulcus. The groove between the frontal process and nasal process in the developing face.

nasofrontal suture. FRONTONASAL SUTURE.

na·so·gas·tric (nay″zo·gas′trick) *adj.* [*naso-* + *gastric*]. Pertaining to the nose and the stomach; used to describe tubes inserted through the nose to end in the stomach.

na·so·gen·i·tal (nay″zo·jen′i·tul) *adj.* [*naso-* + *genital*]. Pertaining to the nose and the genitalia; used to refer to the more or less simultaneous changes which sometimes occur in the nasal mucosa and the endometrium.

na·so·la·bi·al (nay″zo·lay′bee·ul) *adj.* [naso- + *labial*]. Pertaining to the nose and lip.

na·so·la·bi·a·lis (nay″zo·lay·bee·ay′lis) *n.* A portion of the orbicularis oris muscle.

na·so·lac·ri·mal (nay″zo·lack′ri·mul) *adj.* Pertaining to the nose and the lacrimal apparatus.

nasolacrimal canal. The bony canal that lodges the nasolacrimal duct. NA *canalis nasolacrimalis.*

nasolacrimal duct. The membranous duct lodged within the nasolacrimal canal; it gives passage to the tears from the lacrimal sac to the inferior meatus of the nose. NA *ductus lacrimalis.* See also Plates 12, 19.

nasolacrimal groove. The groove or furrow between the embryonic maxillary and lateral nasal processes, the epithelium of which is said to form part of the lacrimal duct.

na·so·lat·er·al process (nay″zo·lat′ur·ul). LATERAL NASAL PROCESS.

na·so·ma·lar (nay″zo·may′lur) *adj.* Pertaining to the nasal and malar (zygomatic) bones.

nasomalar index. Nasomalar width × 100 divided by biorbital breadth.

na·so·max·il·lary (nay″zo·mack′sil·err·ee) *adj.* Pertaining to the nasal and maxillary bones.

nasomaxillary groove. NASOLACRIMAL GROOVE.

nasomaxillary suture. The union between the maxillary and nasal bones. NA *sutura nasomaxillaris.*

na·so·me·di·al process (nay″zo·mee′dee·ul). MEDIAN NASAL PROCESS.

na·so·me·di·an process (nay″zo·mee′dee·un). MEDIAN NASAL PROCESS.

na·so·men·tal (nay″zo·men′tul) *adj.* [*naso-* + *mental,* chin]. Pertaining to the nose and the chin.

nasomental reflex. Contraction of the mentalis muscle with elevation of the lower lip and wrinkling of the skin of the chin in response to a tap on the side of the nose.

na·so-oc·cip·i·tal (nay″zo·ock·sip′i·tul) *adj.* Pertaining to the nose and the occiput.

naso-occipital arc. Measurement from the root of the nose to the lowest point of the occipital protuberance.

na·so-oral (nay″zo·or′ul) *adj.* Pertaining to the nose and the mouth.

na·so-or·bit·al (nay″zo·or′bi·tul) *adj.* Pertaining to the nose and the orbit.

na·so·pal·a·tine (nay″zo·pal′uh·tine, ·tin) *adj.* [*naso-* + *palatine*]. Pertaining to both the nose and the palate.

nasopalatine canal. NASOPALATINE DUCT.

nasopalatine cyst. MEDIAN MAXILLARY CYST.

nasopalatine duct. A duct or canal between the embryonic oral and nasal cavities formed at the site of fusion of the palatine process of the maxillary process of the embryo with the primitive palate. Rarely patent in adults; usually represented by vestigial cords, blind tubes, or cysts.

nasopalatine groove. The groove on the vomer lodging the nasopalatine nerve and vessels.

nasopalatine nerve. See Table of Nerves in the Appendix.

nasopalatine plexus. A plexus uniting the nasopalatine nerves in the incisive foramen.

nasopalatine recess. A depression near the lower margin of the nasal septum above the incisive canal.

na·so·pal·pe·bral (nay″zo·pal′pe·brul) *adj.* [*naso-* + *palpebral*]. Pertaining to the nose and the eyelids.

nasopalpebral reflex. SUPRAORBITAL REFLEX.

na·so·pha·ryn·ge·al (nay″zo·fa·rin′jee·ul) *adj.* Of or pertaining to the nasopharynx.

nasopharyngeal bursitis. PHARYNGEAL BURSITIS.

na·so·phar·yn·gi·tis (nay″zo·făr″in·jye′tis) *n.* [*naso-* + *pharyngitis*]. Inflammation of the nasal passages and pharynx.

na·so·pha·ryn·go·scope (nay″zo·fa·ring′go·skope) *n.* An electrically lighted instrument for inspecting the nasopharynx.

na·so·phar·yn·gos·co·py (nay″zo·făr″ing·gos′kup·ee) *n.* Inspection of the nasopharynx.

na·so·phar·ynx (nay″zo·făr′inks) *n.* [*naso-* + *pharynx*]. The space behind the choanae and above a horizontal plane through the lower margin of the palate. Syn. *epipharynx.* NA *pars nasalis pharyngis.* —**nasopha·ryn·ge·al** (·fa·rin′jee·ul) *adj.*

na·so·scope (nay′zuh·skope) *n.* [*naso-* + *-scope*]. An instrument for examining the nasal cavity.

na·sos·co·py (nay·zos′kup·ee) *n.* [*naso-* + *-scopy*]. Inspection of the nasal cavity.

na·so·spi·na·le (nay″zo·spye·nay′lee, ·nah′lee) *n.* *In craniometry,* a point located in the sagittal plane where it meets a line joining the lowest points on the nasal margins. If this falls within the substance of the anterior nasal spine, a point on the left side wall of the nasal spine is used for taking measurements.

na·so·tra·che·al (nay″zo·tray′kee·ul) *adj.* Pertaining to the nasal cavity and the trachea.

nasotracheal tube. A tube or catheter inserted into the trachea by way of the nasal cavity and pharynx.

na·so·tur·bi·nal (nay″zo·tur′bi·nul) *n.* [*naso-* + *turbinal*]. The ridgelike elevation midway between the anterior extremity of the middle turbinate and the roof of the nose in most lower mammals. In man its rudimentary homologue is the agger nasi.

na·sus (nay′sus, ·zus) *n.,* genit. **na·si** (nay′zye) [NA]. NOSE.

nasus adun·cus (a·dunk′us). Hook nose.

nasus car·ti·la·gi·ne·us (kahr·ti·la·jin′ee·us). The cartilaginous part of the nose.

nasus ex·ter·nus (ecks·tur′nus) [NA]. EXTERNAL NOSE.

nasus in·cur·vus (in·kur'vus). SADDLENOSE.
nasus os·se·us (os'ee·us). The bony part of the nose.
nasus si·mus (sigh'mus). Pug nose.
[1]**na·tal** (nay'tul) *adj.* [L. *natalis,* from *natus,* born]. Of or pertaining to birth.
[2]**natal,** *adj.* Pertaining to the nates or buttocks; GLUTEAL.
na·tal·i·ty (nuh·tal'i·tee, nay·) *n.* [F. *natalité*]. 1. *In medical statistics,* birth rate. 2. Birth.
na·tant (nay'tunt) *adj.* [L. *natans,* from *natare,* to swim]. Swimming or floating on the surface of a liquid.
na·tes (nay'teez) *n.*pl. [L., pl. of *natis,* buttock] [NA]. BUTTOCKS.
National Formulary. A formulary previously published by the American Pharmaceutical Association, now the property of USPC; it is officially recognized by the Federal Food, Drug, and Cosmetic Act. Abbreviated, NF
National Health Service. In Great Britain, a government agency under the Ministry of Health, charged with providing health services for the entire population, such as hospitalization, preventive medicine, family medical, dental, and nursing services, medicines, and appliances; it is financed by the national government. Abbreviated, N.H.S.
National Institutes of Health. A division of the U. S. Department of Health, Education and Welfare that is devoted to research in public health and the diseases of man. Abbreviated, NIH.
na·tive, *adj.* [L. *nativus,* born, native, natural]. 1. Of indigenous origin or growth. 2. Occurring in its natural state; not artificially prepared or altered.
native albumin. Any albumin occurring normally in the tissues.
native immunity. Resistance inherent in the genetic, anatomic, and physiologic attributes of the body, as contrasted with that mediated by operation of specific antibodies or by specific cellular immunity. Contr. *acquired immunity.* See also *active immunity, passive immunity.*
native protein. A protein in its original state; a protein which has not been altered in composition or properties.
natr-, natro-. A combining form meaning *sodium* or *natron.*
na·tre·mia (na·tree'mee·uh) *n.* [*natr-* + *-emia*]. 1. Sodium in the blood. 2. HYPERNATREMIA.
na·tri·um (nay'tree·um) *n.* [NL., from *natr-* + *-ium*]. SODIUM.
na·tri·ure·sis (nay'tri·yoo·ree'sis) *n.* [*natri*um + *uresis*]. The excretion of excessive amounts of sodium in the urine.
na·tri·uret·ic (nay''tree·yoo·ret'ick, nat''ree·) *n. & adj.* [*natr-* + Gk. *ourētikos,* urinary, diuretic]. 1. A medicinal agent which inhibits reabsorption of cations, particularly sodium, from urine. 2. Pertaining to, or characterized by, a natriuretic.
na·tron (nay'tron, ·trun, nat'run) *n.* [Sp. *natrón,* from Ar. *naṭrūn*]. Native sodium carbonate, $Na_2CO_3.10H_2O$.
nat·u·ary (nach'oo·err''ee, nay'choo·) *n.* [L. *natus,* born, birth, + *-ary* as in mortuary]. *Obsol.* A lying-in ward or hospital.
nat·u·ral, *adj.* [L. *naturalis*]. 1. Not abnormal or artificial. 2. Of or pertaining to nature.
natural antibody. An antibody which is not acquired following specific infection or immunization but which arises as a result of cross-reacting antigenic stimuli; for example, an isohemagglutinin.
natural childbirth. A form of childbirth in which psychological, physiological, and emotional aspects are emphasized in order to educate the patient for labor and, when possible, to reduce or eliminate the use of drugs; popular term. The expectant mother is prepared for natural childbirth by gaining an understanding of the anatomy and physiology of the labor process and by a regimen of exercises.
natural healer. An individual supposed to possess personal magnetism capable of overcoming disease.
natural mutation. SPONTANEOUS MUTATION.
natural reflex. UNCONDITIONED REFLEX.
natural resistance. NATIVE IMMUNITY.
natural selection. Darwin's theory of evolution, according to which organisms tend to produce progeny far above the means of subsistence; a struggle for existence ensues which results in the survival of those with favorable variations. Since the favorable variations accumulate as the generations pass, the descendants tend to diverge markedly from their ancestors, and to remain adapted to the conditions under which they live.
Naturetin. Trademark for the diuretic and antihypertensive agent bendroflumethiazide.
na·tur·o·path (nay'chur·o·path) *n.* A person who professes to heal the sick without drugs or surgery, exclusively by the use of natural remedies such as light, heat, cold, water, and fruits. —**na·tur·op·a·thy** (nay''chur·op'uth·ee) *n.*
Nau·heim bath (naow'hime) [after *Nauheim,* Germany, where the bath was popularized]. A process of immersing the body or parts of it in naturally hot carbonated water.
nau·pa·thia (naw·payth'ee·uh, ·path'ee·uh) *n.* [Gk. *naus,* ship, + *-pathia*]. SEASICKNESS.
nau·sea (naw'zhuh, ·zee·uh) *n.* [L., from Gk. *nausia,* from *naus,* ship]. A feeling of discomfort in the region of the stomach, with aversion to food and a tendency to vomit.
nau·se·ant (naw'zee·unt, ·zhee·unt) *adj. & n.* 1. Producing nausea. 2. Any agent that produces nausea.
nau·se·ate (naw'zee·ate, ·zhee·ate) *v.* To induce nausea in (someone).
nau·seous (naw'shus, naw'zee·us) *adj.* [*nause*a + *-ous*]. Producing nausea.
Navane. A trademark for thiothixene, a tranquilizer.
Navaron. Trademark for thiothixene, a tranquilizer.
na·vel (nay'vul) *n.* UMBILICUS.
navel ill. JOINT ILL.
na·vi·cu·la (na·vick'yoo·luh) *n.* [L., small ship]. NAVICULAR FOSSA.
na·vic·u·lar (na·vick'yoo·lur) *adj. & n.* [L. *navicula,* boat]. 1. Boat-shaped. 2. A tarsal bone. NA *os naviculare.* See also Table of Bones in the Appendix.
navicular abdomen. SCAPHOID ABDOMEN.
navicular cells. *In exfoliative cytology,* glycogen-filled, boat-shaped squamous epithelial cells prominent in the cervical exfoliated cells of pregnant women.
navicular disease. NAVICULARTHRITIS.
navicular fossa. 1. VESTIBULAR FOSSA OF THE VAGINA. 2. The dilated distal portion of the urethra in the glans penis. NA *fossa navicularis urethrae.*
navicular fossa of the ear. SCAPHA.
navicular of the hand. SCAPHOID (2).
na·vic·u·lar·thri·tis (na·vick''yoo·lahr·thrigh'tis) *n.* [*navicul*ar + *arthritis*]. Inflammation of the distal sesamoid bone in the horse; causes chronic lameness due to incomplete extension of the joint. Syn. *navicular disease.*
na·vic·u·lo·cu·boid (na·vick''yoo·lo·kew'boid) *adj.* Pertaining to the navicular and cuboid bones, as naviculocuboid ligament.
na·vic·u·lo·cu·ne·i·form (na·vick''yoo·lo·kew·nee'i·form) *adj.* Pertaining to the navicular and cuneiform bones.
Navidrix. Trademark for cyclopenthiazide, an orally effective diuretic and antihypertensive drug.
Nb Symbol for niobium, formerly known as columbium.
NCA Abbreviation for *neurocirculatory asthenia.*
NCI National Cancer Institute, one of the National Institutes of Health.
nCi Abbreviation for *nanocurie.*
Nd Symbol for neodymium.
N.D.A. National Dental Association.
Ne Symbol for neon.
ne-, neo- [Gk. *neos,* young, new]. A combining form meaning (a) *new, newly formed;* (b) *phylogenetically recent;* (c) *young, immature;* (d) *a new chemical compound related to the one to whose name it is prefixed.*

near point. The punctum proximum; the point nearest the eye at which an object can be seen distinctly.

near reflex. ACCOMMODATION REFLEX.

near-sight, *n.* MYOPIA.

near·sight·ed, *adj.* Affected with myopia. —**nearsighted·ness**, *n.*

ne·ar·thro·sis (nee"ahr·thro'sis) *n.*, pl. **nearthro·ses** (·seez) [*ne-* + *arthrosis*]. 1. PSEUDARTHROSIS. 2. An artificial joint constructed surgically in the shaft of a long bone.

near vision chart. Any one of a variety of test cards, using printed letters, numbers, pictures, E's, words, or paragraphs, held at a distance of 14 to 16 inches from the patient and designed to determine the smallest type that can be read comfortably. Compare *Snellen chart.*

Nebcin. A trademark for tobramycin sulfate, an antibacterial.

ne·ben·kern (nay'bin·kairn) *n.* [Ger.]. *Obsol.* PARANUCLEUS.

neb·ra·my·cin (neb"ruh·migh'sin) *n.* A complex of antibiotic substances obtained from *Streptomyces tenebrarius* fermentation broth.

neb·u·la (neb'yoo·luh) *n.*, pl. **nebu·lae** (·lee), **nebulas** [L., mist, fog]. 1. A faint, grayish opacity of the cornea. 2. A spray; a liquid intended for use in an atomizer.

neb·u·lize (neb'yoo·lize) *v.* [from *nebula*]. To convert into a spray or vapor. —**neb·u·li·za·tion** (neb"yoo·lye·zay'shun) *n.*

neb·u·liz·er (neb'yoo·lye"zur) *n.* ATOMIZER.

Ne·ca·tor (ne·kay'tur) *n.* [L., slayer]. A genus of nematode hookworms.

Necator amer·i·ca·nus (uh·merr"i·kay'nus). A species of hookworm widely distributed in tropical America, southern U.S., Africa, southern Asia, Melanesia, and Polynesia; causes necatoriasis.

ne·ca·to·ri·a·sis (ne·kay"tur·eye'uh·sis, nek"uh·to·rye'uh·sis) *n.* [*Necator* + *-iasis*]. Infection of man with the American hookworm, *Necator americanus,* whose infective larvae enter the skin usually at the interdigital regions and may produce a ground itch and vesicular lesions. The adult parasite is found in the small intestine and during the larval migration to the intestine damage to the lungs is commonly incurred.

neck, *n.* 1. The constricted portion of the body connecting the head with the trunk. 2. The narrow portion of any structure serving to join its parts. 3. The area of junction of the crown and root of a tooth.

neck of the bladder. The portion of the urinary bladder immediately surrounding the internal urethral orifice. NA *cervix vesicae.*

neck of the gallbladder. The constricted S-shaped portion of the gallbladder between the fundus and the cystic duct. NA *collum vesicae felleae.*

neck-righting reflex. Any tonic labyrinthine reflex arising in the neck which tends to keep the body oriented in relation to the head.

necr-, necro- [Gk. *nekros,* corpse]. A combining form meaning *pertaining to death.*

nec·ro·bac·il·lo·sis (neck"ro·bas"i·lo'sis) *n.* [*necro-* + *bacillus* + *-osis*]. A disease of animals caused by species of *Sphaerophorus.*

Nec·ro·bac·te·ri·um (neck"ro·back·teer'ee·um) *n.* SPHAEROPHORUS.

Necrobacterium ne·croph·o·rum (ne·krof'ur·um). *SPHAEROPHORUS NECROPHORUS.*

nec·ro·bi·o·sis (neck"ro·bye·o'sis) *n.* [*necro-* + *-biosis*]. Physiologic death of a cell or group of cells, in contrast to necrosis or pathologic death of cells, and to somatic death or death of the entire organism. —**necrobi·ot·ic** (·ot'ick) *adj.*

necrobiosis li·poi·di·ca (li·poy'di·kuh). A cutaneous disease, characterized by multiple yellow to red plaques generally on the extremities, occurring mostly in women, and in about half of the cases in people with diabetes mellitus. There is connective-tissue necrosis with an accumulation of macrophages containing lipids. Syn. *Oppenheim-Urbach disease, necrobiosis lipoidica diabeticorum.*

necrobiosis lipoidica di·a·bet·i·co·rum (dye"uh·bet·i·ko'rum). NECROBIOSIS LIPOIDICA.

necrobiotic atrophy. Atrophy resulting from slow disintegration and loss of cells by necrobiosis.

nec·ro·cy·to·sis (neck"ro·sigh·to'sis) *n.* [*necro-* + *cyt-* + *-osis*]. Death of cells.

nec·ro·cy·to·tox·in (neck"ro·sigh"to·tock'sin) *n.* [*necrocytosis* + *toxin*]. A toxin produced by the death of cells.

nec·ro·gen·ic (neck"ro·jen'ick) *adj.* [*necro-* + *-genic*]. Originating from dead substances.

necrogenic yeast diet. A diet which contains only 7 percent protein and no tocopherol. The yeast used lacks cystine and methionine.

ne·crog·e·nous (ne·kroj'e·nus) *adj.* NECROGENIC.

nec·ro·kid·ney (neck'ro·kid"nee) *n.* [*necro-* + *kidney*]. A kidney removed from a cadaver.

ne·crol·y·sis (ne·krol'i·sis) *n.* [*necro-* + *lysis*]. Dissolution or disintegration of dead tissue. —**nec·ro·lyt·ic** (neck"ro·lit'ick) *adj.*

nec·ro·ma·nia (neck"ro·may'nee·uh) *n.* [*necro-* + *-mania*]. 1. A morbid desire for death. 2. NECROPHILISM.

nec·ro·mi·me·sis (neck"ro·mi·mee'sis, ·migh·mee'sis) *n.* [*necro-* + Gk. *mimēsis,* imitation]. 1. A delusional state in which the patient believes himself to be dead. 2. Simulation of death by a deluded person.

nec·ro·pha·gic (neck"ro·fay'jick, ·faj'ick) *adj.* 1. NECROPHAGOUS. 2. Pertaining to the eating of carrion. —**necropha·gia** (·fay'jee·uh, ·fay'juh) *n.*

ne·croph·a·gous (ne·krof'uh·gus) *adj.* [Gk. *nekrophagos,* from *nekros,* corpse, + *phagein,* to eat]. Eating or subsisting on carrion, or putrid meat.

nec·ro·phile (neck'ro·file) *n.* [*necro-* + *-phile*]. A person affected with necrophilism.

nec·ro·phil·ia (neck"ro·fil'ee·uh) *n.* [*necro-* + *-philia*]. NECROPHILISM. —**necrophil·ic** (·ick) *adj.*

ne·croph·i·lism (ne·krof'il·iz·um) *n.* [*necrophilia* + *-ism*]. 1. Unnatural pleasure in dead bodies and in being in their presence. 2. Sexual perversion in which dead bodies are violated; sexual desire for a corpse.

ne·croph·i·lous (ne·krof'il·us) *adj.* [*necro-* + *phil-* + *-ous*]. Subsisting on dead matter; said of certain bacteria.

ne·croph·i·ly (ne·krof'i·lee) *n.* NECROPHILISM.

nec·ro·pho·bia (neck"ro·fo'bee·uh) *n.* [*necro-* + *-phobia*]. 1. Abnormal dread of dead bodies. 2. Thanatophobia; extreme dread of death.

nec·rop·sy (neck'rop·see) *n.* [*necr-* + *-opsy*]. AUTOPSY.

ne·crose (ne·kroze', ·kroce', neck'roze) *v.* To undergo necrosis or tissue death.

nec·ro·sin (neck'ro·sin) *n.* [*necrosis* + *-in*]. A substance isolated from inflamed areas; said to be capable of injuring body cells.

ne·cro·sis (ne·kro'sis) *n.* [Gk. *nekrōsis,* mortification, death]. The pathologic death of a cell or group of cells in contact with living cells.

nec·ro·sper·mia (neck"ro·spur'mee·uh) *n.* [*necro-* + *sperm* + *-ia*]. NECROZOOSPERMIA.

ne·crot·ic (ne·krot'ick) *adj.* [Gk. *nekrōtikos,* causing necrosis]. Pertaining to, undergoing, or causing necrosis.

necrotic myelitis or **myelopathy**. NECROTIZING MYELITIS.

nec·ro·tize (neck'ro·tize) *v.* [*necrotic* + *-ize*]. 1. To undergo necrosis; to become necrotic. 2. To affect with necrosis, to produce necrosis.

necrotizing arteritis. 1. POLYARTERITIS NODOSA. 2. Any process which involves necrosis of arteries.

necrotizing factor. NECROTOXIN.

necrotizing myelitis or **myelopathy**. A rare disorder of the spinal cord, which may be acute or subacute in onset, characterized by a hemorrhagic necrosis of tissue like that of necrotizing hemorrhagic leukoencephalitis. The subacute variety is also called *Foix-Alajouanine syndrome.*

necrotizing papillitis. PAPILLARY NECROSIS.

necrotizing ulcerative gingivitis. Vincent's infection involving the gingivae. Syn. *trench mouth, Vincent's gingivitis.*

nec·ro·tox·in (neck″ro·tock′sin) *n.* ALPHA HEMOLYSIN.

nec·ro·zoo·sper·mia (neck″ro·zo″o·spur′mee·uh) *n.* [*necro-* + *zoo-* + *sperm* + *-ia*]. A condition in which spermatozoa are present but are immobile and without evidence of life.

nec·tar·e·ous (neck·tăr′ee·us) *adj.* [Gk. *nektareos,* like nectar, fragrant]. Agreeable to the taste.

nec·ta·ry (neck′tur·ee) *n. In biology,* that part of a flower which secretes nectar.

nee·dle, *n.* 1. A sharp-pointed steel instrument, used for puncturing or for sewing tissue; of various shapes, sizes, and edges, the sewing needle has an eye for carrying suture material through the parts. 2. A hollow needle, usually attached to a syringe, for injection or aspiration.

needle bath. A shower bath which throws very fine jets of water at high pressure.

needle biopsy. The securing of biopsy material by means of a hollow needle.

needle carrier. NEEDLE HOLDER.

needle culture. STAB CULTURE.

needle forceps. NEEDLE HOLDER.

needle holder. A handle, usually in the form of a self-locking forceps, for grasping and using a surgical needle.

need·ling, *n.* Discission with a needle, as of a cataract, to afford entrance to the aqueous humor and cause swelling and softening of the lens for either aspiration or absorption.

needling of the kidney. *Informal.* Puncture of the kidney substance for locating a stone.

Neel·sen's method (neʸl′zᵉn) [F. K. A. *Neelsen,* German pathologist, 1854–1894]. A method of staining tubercle bacilli with carbol-fuchsin.

Neelsen stain [F. K. A. *Neelsen*]. CARBOL-FUCHSIN STAIN.

ne·en·ceph·a·lon (nee″en·sef′ul·on) *n.* [*ne-* + *encephalon*]. The neopallium and the phylogenetically new acquisitions of the cerebellum and thalamus collectively. Syn. *neoencephalon.*

nef·o·pam (nef′o·pam) *n.* 3,4,5,6-Tetrahydro-5-methyl-1-phenyl-1*H*-2,5-benzoxazocine, $C_{17}H_{19}NO$, an analgesic, used as the hydrochloride salt.

ne·frens (nee′frenz, nef′renz) *adj.,* pl. **ne·fren·des** (ne·fren′deez) [L., non-biting]. Without teeth, edentate; whether nurslings or aged persons.

Nef·tel's disease [W. B. *Neftel,* U.S. physician, 1830–1906]. ATREMIA.

neg·a·tive, *adj.* [L. negativus, from *negare,* to deny]. 1. Indicating or expressing denial, contradiction, or opposition; in psychiatry, resisting suggestions or advice or reacting with hostility. 2. Indicating failure of response, as to drugs or other therapy. 3. Indicating absence of the entity or condition tested for. 4. Included in a class or range opposite or complementary to that conceived as fundamental or primary, or to that conventionally termed positive, as negative integer, negative pressure, negative pole. Symbol, −. 5. Tending or serving to subtract, retard, or decrease, as negative feedback. 6. Of images (visual, photographic, etc.), having light and dark, or complementary colors, reversed. Contr. *positive.*

negative accommodation. Lessening of the accommodation for distant vision.

negative afterimage. An afterimage that is seen on a bright background and is complementary in color to the initial stimulus. Contr. *positive afterimage.*

negative anxiety. Anxiety which leads to the breakdown of the defense mechanisms of the individual.

negative-contrast radiography or **roentgenography.** Radiographic visualization of a structure or organ by means of a radiolucent contrast agent.

negative electron. The ordinary electron. Syn. *negatron.*

negative empathy. *In psychology,* the empathy which takes place against a certain resistance or unwillingness.

negative eugenics. See *eugenics.*

negative feedback. Feedback which tends to decrease the output; a concept applied in physiology to many bodily processes that tend toward homeostasis, such as the menstrual cycle; analyzed as the result of damped, unself-amplifying fluctuations about a mean value or level. Contr. *positive feedback.*

negative feeling. 1. Aversion, antipathy; coldness. 2. Hostility, antagonism; destructive urge.

negative focus. VIRTUAL FOCUS.

negative ion. ANION.

negative lens. A lens with a negative focal length, the edge of the lens being thicker than the center. The three negative lenses are, according to their figure, planoconcave, double concave or biconcave, and diverging concavoconvex.

negative phase. The temporary lessening of the amount of antibody in the serum immediately following a second inoculation of antigen.

negative pressure. 1. Pressure less than atmospheric pressure. 2. The force of suction.

negative pressure drainage. A closed system for draining an empyema cavity or other closed tissue space.

negative suggestibility. ACTIVE NEGATIVISM.

negative supporting reflex. A proprioceptive reflex causing active inhibition of the muscles involved in positive supporting reflex, elicited by flexion of the finger or the hand, or plantar flexion of the toes; observed in the decerebrate animal.

negative variation. *Obsol.* The diminution of the muscle current during tetanic contraction.

neg·a·tiv·ism (neg′uh·tiv·iz·um) *n.* Indifference, opposition, or resistance to suggestions or commands of another person who is in a position to give these; persistent refusal, without apparent or objective reasons, to do as suggested or asked, seen normally in late infancy and early childhood, but also in adults who feel "pushed around"; in its most pathologic form, it is seen in the catatonic form of schizophrenia as markedly reduced activity, with patients ignoring even inner stimuli.

neg·a·tron (neg′uh·tron) *n.* [blend of *nega*tive + elec*tron*]. A term suggested for electron to distinguish it from its positive counterpart, the positron.

neg·li·gence (neg′li·junce) *n.* [F., from L. *negligentia*]. *In legal medicine,* an act of commission or omission in the care of patients which, without regard to circumstances, violates a statute or is obviously opposed to the dictates of accepted medical practices.

NeGram. Trademark for nalidixic acid, an antibacterial agent used for treatment of urinary tract infections caused by gram-negative organisms.

Ne·gri bodies (neʸ′gree) [A. *Negri,* Italian physician, 1876–1912]. Acidophil inclusion bodies in the cytoplasm of nerve cells, considered diagnostic of rabies; found most often in large cells of the hippocampus and Purkinje cells of the cerebellum, but not limited to these locations.

Negri-Jacod's syndrome. JACOD'S SYNDROME.

Ne·gro (nee′gro) *n.* [Sp., black]. A member of a black-skinned race of people; especially, one of African descent.

Ne·gro's sign. (neʸ′gro) 1. In facial paralysis, when the patient raises his eyes, the eyeball on the paralyzed side deviates outward and elevates more than the normal eye due to overaction of the superior rectus and inferior oblique. 2. COGWHEEL RIGIDITY.

NEI National Eye Institute, one of the National Institutes of Health.

Neill-Mooser bodies. MOOSER BODIES.

Neill-Moo·ser reaction (neel, mo′zur) [M. H. *Neill,* U.S. physician, 1882–1930; and H. *Mooser*]. Reddening and enlargement of the scrotum in male guinea pigs, with adhesions between the testes and the tunica vaginalis, following intraabdominal inoculation of *Rickettsia mooseri.* Occasionally also induced by *R. prowazeki.*

Neil Rob·ert·son stretcher. A canvas litter with bamboo slats used to transport an injured man aboard a vessel.

Neis·se·ria (nigh·seer'ee·uh, nigh·serr'ee·uh) *n.* [A. L. S. *Neisser,* German physician, 1855–1916]. A genus of gram-negative cocci of the family Neisseriaceae.

Neisseria cat·ar·rha·lis (kat''uh·ray'lis, ·ral'is). A species of bacteria found in the respiratory tract; generally not pathogenic.

Neisseria fla·ves·cens (fla·ves'enz). A species of bacteria found in the spinal fluid in rare instances of clinical meningitis, and on the mucous membranes of the respiratory tract.

Neisseria gon·or·rhoe·ae (gon''o·ree'ee). The bacterium that causes gonorrhea; the type species of its genus.

Neisseria in·tra·cel·lu·la·ris (in''truh·sel·yoo·lair'is). NEISSERIA MENINGITIDIS.

Neisseria men·in·git·i·dis (men''in·jit'i·dis). The species of bacteria that causes epidemic cerebrospinal meningitis. Syn. *Diplococcus intracellularis meningitidis, Neisseria intracellularis.*

Neisseria sic·ca (sick'uh). A species of bacteria forming dry, crenated colonies on simple media, found in mucous membranes of the respiratory tract, and generally nonpathogenic.

Neis·ser's coccus (nigh'sur) [A. L. S. *Neisser*]. NEISSERIA GONORRHOEAE.

Neisser's stain [M. *Neisser,* German bacteriologist, 1869–1938]. A stain for demonstration of granules in diphtheria bacilli.

Né·la·ton's fibers or **sphincter** (neʸ·la·tohⁿ') [A. *Nélaton,* French surgeon, 1807–1873]. A variable band of smooth muscle fibers which are said to be present in the rectum about 3 or 4 inches above the anus.

Nélaton's line [A. *Nélaton*]. A line between the tuberosity of the ischium and the anterior superior iliac spine. In dislocated hip, the tip of the greater trochanter is above this line.

Nélaton's tumor [A. *Nélaton*]. A teratoma of the abdominal wall.

n electron. An electron in the n or fourth shell surrounding the nucleus of an atom.

Nel·son's syndrome [D. H. Nelson, U.S. internist, b. 1925]. Skin hyperpigmentation resulting from secretion of melanocyte-stimulating hormone by a pituitary adenoma developing after adrenalectomy for Cushing's disease; adrenocorticotropic hormone is also secreted.

Nel·son's test. *TREPONEMA PALLIDUM* IMMOBILIZATION TEST.

nem, *n.* [Ger. *N*ahrungs *E*inheit *M*ilch, nutritional unit milk]. A unit of nutrition representing the calorific value of 1 gram of breast milk of standard composition; equivalent to approximately ⅔ calorie.

nem-, nema-, nemo- [Gk. *nēma,* thread]. A combining form meaning *filament, filamentous, threadlike.*

-nema, -neme [Gk. *nēma,* thread]. A combining form meaning (a) *filament, thread;* (b) *nematode.*

nem·a·line (nem'uh·line, ·lin) *adj.* [Gk. *nēma,* thread]. Threadlike.

nemaline myopathy. A familial muscular disorder characterized by generalized weakness and skeletal muscular atrophy from the time of birth; there are abnormal rod-shaped structures seen microscopically in affected muscle fibers. The inheritance appears to be autosomal dominant with variable expression of the gene.

nem·a·thel·minth (nem''uh·thel'minth, nee''muh·) *n.* Any roundworm of the phylum Nemathelminthes.

Nem·a·thel·min·thes (nem''uh·thel·min'theez, nee''muh·) *n.pl.* [Gk. *nēma, nēmatos,* thread, + *helmins, helminthos,* worm]. The phylum of the roundworms, which includes the true roundworms or nematodes, the hair snakes, and acanthocephalan worms.

Nem·a·to·da (nem''uh·to'duh, nee''muh·) *n.pl.* [Gk. *nēma, nēmatos,* thread, + *-oda,* modification of *-oidea*]. A class of the phylum Nemathelminthes; the true roundworms. Members of the class are bilaterally symmetrical, unisexual, without a proboscis, and have a body cavity not lined with epithelium.

nem·a·tode (nem'uh·tode, nee'muh·) *n.* Any worm of the class Nematoda.

nem·a·tol·o·gy (nem''uh·tol'uh·jee, nee''muh·) *n.* That portion of the science of parasitology concerned with the study of nematode worms.

Nem·a·to·mor·pha (nem''uh·to·mor'fuh) *n.pl.* [NL., from Gk. *nēma, nēmatos,* thread, + *morphē,* form]. A class of Nemathelminthes (or in some classifications a separate phylum) comprising the hair snakes or horsehair worms. See also *Gordiacea.*

nem·a·to·sper·mia (nem''uh·to·spur'mee·uh, nee''muh·) *n.* [Gk. *nēma, nēmatos,* thread, + *-spermia*]. The characteristic of producing spermatozoa with long, threadlike tails, as those found in human semen.

Nembutal. Trademark for the barbiturate, pentobarbital, commonly used as the sodium salt.

-neme. See *-nema.*

Nemural. Trademark for drocarbil, a veterinary anthelmintic.

Neoantimosan. A trademark for stibophen, an antischistosomal drug.

neo·ars·phen·a·mine (nee''o·ahrs·fen'uh·meen, ·in) *n.* [*neo-* + *arsphenamine*]. Chiefly sodium 3,3′-diamino-4,4′-dihydroxyarsenobenzene-*N*-methylenesulfoxylate, $C_{13}H_{13}As_2N_2NaO_4S$, formerly used for the treatment of spirochetal and some other diseases.

neo·ar·thro·sis (nee''o·ahr·thro'sis) *n.* NEARTHROSIS.

neo·blas·tic (nee''o·blas'tick) *adj.* [*neo-* + *-blast* + *-ic*]. Pertaining to, or of the nature of, new tissue.

neocerebellar syndrome. A syndrome due to a lesion of the posterior lobe(s) of the cerebellum; characterized by hypotonia, intention tremor, and abnormalities in the rate, range, and force of movement of the ipsilateral limb or limbs.

neo·cer·e·bel·lum (nee''o·serr''e·bel'um) *n.* Phylogenetically the most recent part of the cerebellum; consists of the middle portions of the vermis and their large lateral extensions. Practically all of the cerebellar hemispheres fall into this subdivision. It receives cerebral cortex impulses via the corticopontocerebellar tract. —**neocerebel·lar** (·lur) *adj.*

neo·cin·cho·phen (nee''o·sink'o·fen) *n.* [*neo-* + *cinchophen*]. The ethyl ester of 6-methyl-2-phenylquinoline-4-carboxylic acid, $C_{19}H_{17}NO_2$; has been used as an analgesic and antipyretic and to increase urinary excretion of uric acid.

Neo-Cobefrin. Trademark for levonordefrin, a vasoconstrictor.

neo·cor·tex (nee''o·kor'tecks) *n.* That part of the cerebral cortex which is phylogenetically the most recent in development; it includes all of the cortex except the olfactory portions, the hippocampal regions, and the piriform areas. Syn. *isocortex, neopallium.*

neo·cys·tos·to·my (nee''o·sis·tos'tum·ee) *n.* [*neo-* + *cystostomy*]. A surgical procedure whereby a new opening is made into the urinary bladder.

neo·den·ta·tum (nee''o·den·tay'tum) *n.* [*neo-* + *dentatum*]. The phylogenetically new ventrolateral part of the dentate nucleus.

neo·dym·i·um (nee''o·dim'ee·um) *n.* Nd = 144.24. A rare-earth metal occurring in cerium and lanthanum minerals.

Neodyne. Trademark for ethyl dibunate, an antitussive compound.

neo·en·ceph·a·lon (nee''o·en·sef'ul·on) *n.* NEENCEPHALON.

ne·og·a·la (nee·og'uh·luh) *n.* [*neo-* + Gk. *gala*, milk]. COLOSTRUM.

neo·gen·e·sis (nee''o·jen'e·sis) *n.* [*neo-* + *-genesis*]. Growth of tissues or production of a metabolite from a generically different substrate. —**neo·ge·net·ic** (·je·net'ick) *adj.*

neo·ger·mi·trine (nee''o·jur'mi·treen) *n.* A triester alkaloid, hypotensively active, isolated from veratrum viride; on hydrolysis it yields germine, two moles of acetic acid, and one mole of 2-methylbutyric acid.

neo·hes·per·i·din di·hy·dro·chal·cone (nee''o·hes·perr'i·din dye·high''dro·kal'kone). A sweetening agent, $C_{28}H_{36}O_{15}$, prepared from a glycoside occurring naturally in grapefruit; 1000 to 1500 times sweeter than sucrose. Abbreviated, neohesperidin DHC.

Neohetramine. Trademark for thonzylamine, an antihistaminic drug used as the hydrochloride salt.

Neo-Hombreol. A trademark for testosterone propionate, an androgenic hormone ester.

Neo-Hombreol-M. A trademark for methyltestosterone, an androgenic hormone derivative.

neo·ki·net·ic (nee''o·ki·net'ick) *adj.* Pertaining to the motor nervous mechanism that regulates voluntary muscular control; the most recently developed nervous system. Contr. *archeokinetic, paleokinetic.*

ne·ol·o·gism (nee·ol'uh·jiz·um) *n.* [F. *neologisme*, from Gk. *neos*, new, + *logos*, word]. 1. A new word-coinage or unconventional vocabulary innovation. 2. The use of such a coinage or innovation, either rationally to represent a new idea, method, or object, or in disordered neurologic states such as delirium, or in mental disorders such as schizophrenia when the patient wishes to express a highly complex meaning related to his conflicts.

neo·mem·brane (nee''o·mem'brane) *n.* A new or false membrane.

neo·mor·phism (nee''o·mor'fiz·um) *n.* [*neo-* + *morph-* + *-ism*]. *In biology*, the development of a new form.

neo·my·cin (nee''o·migh'sin) *n.* [*neo-* + *-mycin*]. An antibiotic substance isolated from cultures of *Streptomyces fradiae;* a polybasic compound. It is active against a variety of gram-positive and gram-negative bacteria. The sulfate, administered orally, is used as an intestinal antiseptic in surgery of the large bowel and anus; the salt is used for topical application in treatment or prevention of susceptible infections of the skin and the eye.

ne·on (nee'on) *n.* [Gk., new]. Ne = 20.179. A chemically inert, gaseous element occurring, in small amounts, in air.

neo·na·tal (nee''o·nay'tul) *adj.* Pertaining to a newborn infant.

neonatal blennorrhea. INCLUSION CONJUNCTIVITIS.

neonatal edema. SCLEREMA NEONATORUM.

neonatal impetigo. A form of bullous impetigo, occurring in the newborn, usually due to staphylococcal, but occasionally to streptococcal, infection. Syn. *pemphigus neonatorum.*

neonatal isoerythrolysis. ERYTHROBLASTOSIS FETALIS.

neonatal jaundice. JAUNDICE OF THE NEWBORN.

neonatal line. A prominent incremental line formed in the neonatal period in the enamel and dentin of a primary tooth or of a first permanent molar.

neonatal mortality rate. The number of deaths reported among infants under one month of age in a calendar year per 1,000 live births reported in the same year and place.

neonatal myasthenia. Marked muscle weakness, weak cry, ineffective sucking, and difficulties with swallowing in infants born of myasthenic mothers; if properly treated, the myasthenic symptoms disappear within the first weeks of life. See also *congenital myasthenia.*

neonatal subdural hemorrhage. Subdural hematoma due to birth trauma or, rarely, to a blood coagulation disorder.

neonatal tetany. TETANY OF THE NEWBORN.

neo·nate (nee'o·nate) *n.* [NL. *neonatus*, newborn]. A newborn infant; specifically, an infant from birth through its 28th day.

neo·na·ti·cide (nee''o·nay'ti·side) *n.* [*neonate* + *-cide*]. 1. The murder of a newborn. 2. The murderer of a newborn.

neo·na·tol·o·gy (nee''o·nay·tol'uh·jee) *n.* [*neonate* + *-logy*]. The study and science of the newborn up to 2 months of age postnatally. Compare *fetology.* —**neonatolo·gist** (·jist) *n.*

neo·na·to·rum (nee''o·nay·to'rum). Genitive plural of *neonatus;* of the newborn.

neo·na·tus (nee''o·nay'tus) *L. adj. & n.*, pl. & genit. sing. **neona·ti** (·tye), genit. pl. **neo·na·to·rum** (·nay·to'rum) [NL., from *neo-* + L. *natus*, born]. NEWBORN.

neo-ol·ive (nee''o·ol'iv) *n.* The olive with the exception of its small medial portion which is part of the paleo-olive.

neo·pal·li·um (nee''o·pal'ee·um) *n.* [*neo-* + *pallium*]. The cerebral cortex with the exception of the rhinencephalon. —**neopalli·al** (·ul) *adj.*

neo·pen·tane (nee''o·pen'tane) *n.* 2,2-Dimethylpropane or tetramethylmethane, $(CH_3)_4C$, a hydrocarbon, gaseous at room temperature, occurring in petroleum naphtha, and also prepared by synthesis.

ne·oph·il·ism (nee·off'il·iz·um) *n.* [*neo-* + *phil-* + *-ism*]. Morbid or undue desire for novelty.

neo·pho·bia (nee''o·fo'bee·uh) *n.* [*neo-* + *-phobia*]. Dread of new scenes or of novelties.

neo·phre·nia (nee''o·fren'ee·uh, ·free'nee·uh) *n.* [*neo-* + *-phrenia*]. Any psychosis of childhood.

neo·pla·sia (nee''o·play'zhuh, ·zee·uh) *n.* [*neo-* + *-plasia*]. 1. Formation of tumors or neoplasms. 2. Formation of new tissue.

neo·plasm (nee'o·plaz·um) *n.* [*neo-* + Gk. *plasma*, formation]. An aberrant new growth of abnormal cells or tissues; a tumor. —**neo·plas·tic** (nee''o·plas'tick) *adj.*

neo·prene (nee'o·preen) *n.* Generic name for synthetic rubber made by polymerization of 2-chloro-1,3-butadiene. Neoprene vulcanizates are markedly resistant to oils, greases, chemicals, sunlight, ozone, and heat.

Neo·rick·ett·sia hel·minth·i·ca (nee''o·ri·ket'see·uh hel·minth'i·kuh). The causative organism of salmon poisoning in dogs. See also *salmon disease.*

neo·sal·var·san (nee''o·sal'vur·san) *n.* A name given by Ehrlich to the substance later designated neoarsphenamine.

Neo-Silvol. Trademark for a compound of silver iodide with a soluble gelatin base containing silver iodide in colloidal form, a drug employed as an antiseptic on mucous membranes.

Neostibosan. Trademark for the pentavalent antimonial preparation ethylstibamine.

neo·stig·mine (nee''o·stig'meen, ·min) *n.* (*m*-Hydroxyphenyl)trimethylammonium ion, a quaternary ammonium cation with anticholinesterase activity; used as the bromide ($C_{12}H_{19}BrN_2O_2$) or methylsulfate ($C_{13}H_{22}N_2O_6S$) salts for prevention and treatment of postoperative abdominal distention and urinary retention, symptomatic control of myasthenia gravis, as an antidote for excessive curarization with skeletal muscle relaxants, and other conditions.

neo·stri·a·tum (nee''o·strye·ay'tum) *n.* The caudate nucleus and putamen combined; the phylogenetically new part of the corpus striatum.

Neo-Synephrine. Trademark for phenylephrine, a sympathomimetic amine used as the hydrochloride salt to maintain blood pressure and as a local vasoconstrictor.

ne·ot·e·ny (nee·ot'un·ee) *n.* [Gk. *neos*, young, + *teinein*, to stretch, prolong]. *In zoology*, sexual maturity in the larval stage; pedogenesis.

Neothylline. Trademark for dyphylline, a drug with actions characteristic of theophylline.

neo·uni·tar·i·an theory of hematopoiesis (nee''o·yoo''ni·tăr'ee·un). A concept that the lymphocyte of normal blood does not develop into all other cell types but that, under proper environmental conditions as in tissue cultures or in pathologic states, lymphocytes or cells that morphologically resemble lymphocytes can become multipotent.

neo·vas·cu·lar (nee″o·vas′kew·lur) *adj.* Pertaining to newly formed vessels.

neovascular glaucoma. Glaucoma secondary to intraocular neovascularization, as from central retinal vein occlusion or diabetes mellitus.

neo·vas·cu·lar·iza·tion (nee″o·vas″kew·lur·i·zay′shun, ·eye·zay′shun) *n.* 1. New formation of blood vessels in abnormal tissues such as tumors, or in abnormal positions as in diabetic retinopathy. 2. REVASCULARIZATION.

neo·vas·cu·la·ture (nee″o·vas′kew·luh·chur) *n.* [*neo-* + *vasculature*]. A newly formed collection of blood vessels, usually representing an abnormality.

neo-vitamin A. 5-*cis*-Vitamin A, a naturally occurring isomer of vitamin A but less active than the latter.

neph·a·lism (nef′ul·iz·um) *n.* [Gk. *nēphalismos,* soberness, from *nēphalios,* sober]. Total abstinence from alcoholic liquors.

neph·e·lom·e·ter (nef″e·lom′e·tur) *n.* [Gk. *nephelē,* cloud, + *-meter*]. An apparatus for ascertaining the number of bacteria in a suspension, or the turbidity of a fluid.

nephelometric analysis. Quantitative determination of a substance by observation of the degree of turbidity produced by it in a suitable dispersion medium, specifically by measuring the intensity of light scattered by the dispersion relative to a standard.

neph·e·lom·e·try (nef″e·lom′e·tree) *n.* [Gk. *nephelē,* cloud, + *-metry*]. The determination of the degree of turbidity of a fluid. —**nephe·lo·met·ric** (·lo·met′rick) *adj.*

nephr-, nephro- [Gk. *nephros*]. A combining form meaning *kidney, renal.*

ne·phral·gia (ne·fral′juh, ·jee·uh) *n.* [*nephr-* + *-algia*]. Pain in a kidney. —**nephral·gic** (·jick) *adj.*

nephralgic crisis. A ureteral paroxysm of pain observed in tabes dorsalis.

ne·phrec·ta·sia (nef″reck·tay′zhuh, ·zee·uh, nee″freck·) *n.* [*nephr-* + *ectasia*]. Dilatation of a kidney.

ne·phrec·to·mize (ne·freck′tuh·mize) *v.* To remove a kidney.

ne·phrec·to·my (ne·freck′tuh·mee) *n.* [*nephr-* + *-ectomy*]. Excision of a kidney.

neph·ric (nef′rick) *adj.* [Gk. *nephrikos*]. Pertaining to the kidney; RENAL.

nephric tubule. URINIFEROUS TUBULE.

ne·phrid·i·um (ne·frid′ee·um) *n.,* pl. **ne·phrid·ia** (·uh) [*nephr-* + L. *-idium,* from Gk. *-idion,* small, lesser]. One of the segmentally arranged, paired, coiled, excretory tubules of many invertebrates, notably the annelid worms.

ne·phrit·ic (ne·frit′ick) *adj.* [Gk. *nephritikos*]. 1. Pertaining to or affected with nephritis. 2. Pertaining to or affecting the kidney.

ne·phri·tis (ne·frye′tis) *n.,* pl. **ne·phrit·i·des** (ne·frit′i·deez) [Gk. *nephritis*]. Inflammation of the kidney.

neph·ri·to·gen·ic (nef″ri·to·jen′ick, ne·frit″o·) *adj.* [*nephritis* + *-genic*]. Producing nephritis; said especially of certain strains of streptococci.

nephro-. See *nephr-*.

neph·ro·ab·dom·i·nal (nef″ro·ab·dom′i·nul) *adj.* Pertaining to the kidneys and abdomen.

neph·ro·blas·to·ma (nef″ro·blas·to′muh) *n.* [*nephro-* + *blastoma*]. WILMS'S TUMOR.

neph·ro·cal·ci·no·sis (nef″ro·kal″si·no′sis) *n.* Renal calcinosis, marked by radiologically detectable deposits of calcium throughout the renal parenchyma.

neph·ro·cap·sec·to·my (nef″ro·kap·seck′tum·ee) *n.* NEPHROCAPSULECTOMY.

neph·ro·cap·sul·ec·to·my (nef″ro·kap″sue·leck′tum·ee) *n.* [*nephro-* + *capsul-* + *-ectomy*]. Excision of the renal capsule.

neph·ro·cap·su·lot·o·my (nef″ro·kap″sue·lot′um·ee) *n.* [*nephro-* + *capsulo-* + *-tomy*]. Incision of the renal capsule.

neph·ro·car·ci·no·ma (nef″ro·kahr″si·no′muh) *n.* [*nephro-* + *carcinoma*]. Carcinoma of the kidney.

neph·ro·car·di·ac (nef″ro·kahr′dee·ack) *adj.* Pertaining to the kidney and the heart.

neph·ro·coele (nef′ro·seel) *n.* [*nephro-* + *-coele*]. The embryonic cavity in a nephrotome.

neph·ro·co·lic (nef″ro·ko′lick) *adj.* Pertaining to the kidneys and the colon.

nephrocolic ligament. An ill-defined band of connective tissue descending from the right renal capsule to the nearby part of the ascending colon or from the left renal capsule to the nearby part of the descending colon.

neph·ro·co·lo·pexy (nef″ro·kol′o·peck·see, ·ko′luh·) *n.* [*nephro-* + *colo-* + *-pexy*]. The surgical anchoring of a kidney and the nearby part of the colon.

neph·ro·co·lop·to·sis (nef″ro·ko″lop·to′sis) *n.* [*nephro-* + *colo-* + *-ptosis*]. Downward displacement of a kidney and the colon.

neph·ro·cyst·an·as·to·mo·sis (nef″ro·sis″tan·as″tuh·mo′sis) *n.* [*nephro-* + *cyst-* + *anastomosis*]. The surgical formation of an opening between the renal pelvis and the urinary bladder.

neph·ro·cys·ti·tis (nef″ro·sis·tigh′tis) *n.* [*nephro-* + *cyst-* + *-itis*]. Inflammation of both the urinary bladder and kidney.

neph·ro·dys·tro·phy (nef″ro·dis′truh·fee) *n.* [*nephro-* + *dystrophy*]. NEPHROSIS (2).

neph·ro·gen·e·sis (nef″ro·jen′e·sis) *n.* [*nephro-* + *-genesis*]. 1. Formation of a kidney. 2. Formation of a nephron or nephrons.

neph·ro·gen·ic (nef″ro·jen′ick) *adj.* [*nephro-* + *-genic*]. 1. Having the ability to produce kidney tissue. 2. Of renal origin.

nephrogenic cord. The longitudinal, cordlike mass of mesenchyme derived from the mesomere or nephrostomal plate of the mesoderm, from which develop the functional parts of the pronephros, mesonephros, and metanephros.

nephrogenic diabetes insipidus. Diabetes insipidus that is unresponsive to vasopressin, because of inability of the renal tubules to resorb water; it is usually congenital, inherited as a sex-linked trait with variable expression in females, but may occur in chronic renal insufficiency.

nephrogenic dysembryoma. WILMS'S TUMOR.

nephrogenic tissue. The tissue of the nephrogenic cord derived from the nephrotome plate that forms the blastema or primordium from which the embryonic and definitive kidneys develop.

ne·phrog·e·nous (ne·froj′e·nus) *adj.* [*nephro-* + *-genous*]. Of renal origin.

nephrogenous peptonuria. Peptonuria of renal origin.

neph·ro·gram (nef′ro·gram) *n.* [*nephro-* + *-gram*]. Delineation of the kidney parenchyma by radiographic means. —**neph·ro·graph·ic** (nef″ro·graf′ick) *adj.*

nephrographic phase. That early portion of a radiographic contrast study of the kidneys (excretory or arteriographic) in which the renal parenchyma is opacified.

nephroi. Plural of *nephros.*

neph·roid (nef′roid) *adj.* [Gk. *nephroeidēs*]. Kidney-shaped, reniform, resembling a kidney.

neph·ro·lith (nef′ro·lith) *n.* [*nephro-* + *-lith*]. KIDNEY STONE. —**neph·ro·lith·ic** (nef″ro·lith′ick) *adj.*

neph·ro·li·thi·a·sis (nef″ro·li·thigh′uh·sis) *n.* [*nephrolith* + *-iasis*]. The formation of renal calculi, or the disease state characterized by their presence.

neph·ro·li·thot·o·my (nef″ro·li·thot′um·ee) *n.* [*nephrolith* + *-tomy*]. An incision of the kidney for the removal of a calculus.

ne·phrol·o·gy (ne·frol′uh·jee) *n.* [*nephro-* + *-logy*]. The scientific study of the kidney, including its diseases. —**nephrolo·gist,** *n.*

ne·phrol·y·sin (ne·frol′i·sin, nef″ro·lye′sin) *n.* [*nephro-* + *lysin*]. A toxic substance capable of disintegrating kidney cells.

ne·phrol·y·sis (ne·frol′i·sis) *n.* [*nephro-* + *-lysis*]. 1. The disintegration of the kidney by the action of a nephrolysin. 2. The operation of loosening a kidney from surrounding adhesions. —**neph·ro·lyt·ic** (nef″ro·lit′ick) *adj.*

ne·phro·ma (ne·fro′muh) *n.*, pl. **nephromas, nephroma·ta** (·tuh) [*nephr-* + *-oma*]. 1. Any kidney tumor. 2. RENAL CELL CARCINOMA.

neph·ro·meg·a·ly (nef″ro·meg′uh·lee) *n.* [*nephro-* + *-megaly*]. Kidney enlargement.

neph·ro·mere (nef′ro·meer) *n.* [*nephro-* + *-mere*]. NEPHROTOME.

neph·ron (nef′ron) *n.* [*nephr-* + *-on*]. The renal unit, consisting of the glomerular capsule, its glomerulus, and the attached uriniferous tubule.

neph·ro·noph·thi·sis (nef″ro·nof′thi·sis) *n.* [*nephron* + *-phthisis*]. 1. Loss of renal substance. 2. An idiopathic kidney disease, often familial, characterized by loss of renal substance with cyst formation, anemia, and uremia. See also *medullary cystic disease of the kidney.*

ne·phrop·a·thy (ne·frop′uth·ee) *n.* [*nephro-* + *-pathy*]. 1. Any disease of the kidney. 2. NEPHROSIS (2). —**neph·ro·path·ic** (nef″ro·path′ick) *adj.*

neph·ro·pexy (nef′ro·peck″see) *n.* [*nephro-* + *-pexy*]. Surgical fixation of a floating or ptotic kidney.

neph·rop·to·sia (nef″rop·to′shuh, ·zee·uh) *n.* NEPHROPTOSIS.

neph·ro·poi·e·tin (nef″ro·poy′e·tin, ·poy·ee′tin) *n.* [*nephro-* + *-poietic* + *-in*]. A substance supposed to stimulate growth of renal tissue.

neph·rop·to·sis (nef″rop·to′sis) *n.* [*nephro-* + *-ptosis*]. Inferior displacement of the kidney.

neph·ro·py·e·li·tis (nef″ro·pye″e·lye′tis) *n.* [*nephro-* + *pyelitis*]. PYELONEPHRITIS.

neph·ro·py·elo·plas·ty (nef″ro·pye′e·lo·plas″tee) *n.* [*nephro-* + *pyelo-* + *-plasty*]. A plastic operation on the pelvis of the kidney.

ne·phror·rha·phy (ne·fror′uh·fee) *n.* [*nephro-* + *-rrhaphy*]. 1. The stitching of a floating kidney to the posterior wall of the abdomen or to the loin. 2. Suturing a wound in a kidney.

neph·ros (nef′ros) *n.*, pl. **neph·roi** (·roy) [Gk.]. KIDNEY.

neph·ro·scle·ro·sis (nef″ro·skle·ro′sis) *n.* [*nephro-* + *sclerosis*]. Scarring of renal tubules, interstitium, and glomeruli due to arteriosclerotic changes in renal arteries or arterioles; systemic hypertension and sometimes renal failure may be clinically associated.

neph·ro·sid·er·o·sis (nef″ro·sid″ur·o′sis) *n.* [*nephro-* + hemo*siderosis*]. The accumulation of hemosiderin in the kidneys.

ne·phro·sis (ne·fro′sis) *n.* [*nephr-* + *-osis*]. 1. NEPHROTIC SYNDROME. 2. *In pathology,* degenerative or retrogressive renal lesions, distinct from inflammation (nephritis) or vascular involvement (nephrosclerosis), especially as applied to tubular lesions (tubular nephritis). Syn. *nephropathy, nephrodystrophy.*

ne·phro·so·ne·phri·tis (ne·fro″so·ne·frye′tis) *n.* A renal disease having features of nephrosis and nephritis.

neph·ro·so·no·gram (nef″ro·so′nuh·gram) *n.* The graphic or pictorial representation of the kidneys using ultrasonic scanning. —**nephro·so·nog·ra·phy** (·so·nog′ruh·fee) *n.*

ne·phros·to·gram (nef·ros′to·gram) *n.* [*nephrostomy* + *-gram*]. The radiographic depiction of a nephrostomy.

ne·phros·to·ma (ne·fros′tuh·muh, nef″ro·sto′muh) *n.*, pl. **nef·ro·sto·ma·ta** (nef″ro·sto′muh·tuh). NEPHROSTOME.

nephrostomal plate. NEPHROTOME.

neph·ro·stome (nef′ruh·stome) *n.* [*nephro-* + *stoma*]. The opening of a nephron or of a nephridium into the coelom in lower vertebrates and many invertebrates. —**nephro·sto·mal** (·sto′mul) *adj.*

ne·phros·to·my (ne·fros′tum·ee) *n.* [*nephro-* + *-stomy*]. The formation of a fistula leading through the renal parenchyma to the pelvis of a kidney.

ne·phrot·ic (ne·frot′ick) *adj.* Pertaining to or affected by nephrosis.

nephrotic-glycosuric dwarfism. The usually severe growth retardation seen in the Fanconi syndrome.

nephrotic syndrome. Marked proteinuria, hypoproteinemia, anasarca, and hyperlipemia accompanied by normal blood pressure, resulting from any agent damaging the basement membrane of the renal glomerulus.

neph·ro·tome (nef′ruh·tome) *n.* [*nephro-* + *-tome*]. The narrow mass of mesoderm connecting somites and lateral mesoderm, from which the pronephros, mesonephros, metanephros, and their ducts develop.

neph·ro·to·mo·gram (nef″ro·to′muh·gram) *n.* [*nephro-* + *tomogram*]. Radiographic depiction of the kidney by means of tomography and intravenous urography.

neph·ro·to·mog·ra·phy (nef″ro·to·mog′ruh·fee) *n.* [*nephro-* + *tomography*]. A roentgenologic technique combining intravenous urography and sectional radiography.

ne·phrot·o·my (ne·frot′um·ee) *n.* [*nephro-* + *-tomy*]. Incision of the kidney.

neph·ro·tox·ic (nef″ro·tock′sick) *adj.* 1. Pertaining to nephrotoxin. 2. Injurious to the kidney cells; NEPHROLYTIC.

nephrotoxic nephritis. A form of experimental glomerulonephritis in animals produced by the infection of antiglomerular basement membrane antibody.

neph·ro·tox·in (nef″ro·tock′sin) *n.* [*nephro-* + *toxin*]. A cytotoxin that damages the cells of the kidney.

neph·ro·tro·pic (nef″ro·tro′pick, ·trop′ick) *adj.* & *n.* [*nephro-* + *-tropic*]. 1. Affecting the kidney or its function. 2. A medicinal agent that primarily affects the kidney or its function.

neph·ro·tu·ber·cu·lo·sis (nef″ro·tew·bur″kew·lo′sis) *n.* Disease of the kidney due to the tubercle bacillus.

neph·ro·ure·ter·al (nef″ro·yoo·ree′tur·ul) *adj.* Pertaining to the kidney and ureter.

neph·ro·ure·ter·ec·to·my (nef″ro·yoo·ree″tur·eck′tum·ee) *n.* The excision of a kidney and whole ureter at one operation.

nep·i·ol·o·gy (nep″ee·ol′uh·jee, nee″pee·) *n.* [Gk. *nēpios*, infant, + *-logy*]. NEONATOLOGY.

Neptazane. Trademark for methazolamide, a carbonic anhydrase inhibitor used in the treatment of glaucoma.

nep·tu·ni·um (nep·tew′nee·um) *n.* [after the planet *Neptune* (between Uranus and Pluto)]. Np = 237.0482. An element, atomic number 93, obtained by bombarding ordinary uranium with neutrons. Undergoes transformation into plutonium.

ne·quin·ate (ne·kwin′ate) *n.* Methyl 7-(benzyloxy)-6-butyl-1,4-dihydro-4-oxo-3-quinolinecarboxylate, $C_{22}H_{23}NO_4$, a coccidiostat used for poultry.

ne·ral (neer′al) *n.* One of the geometric isomers of citral.

Ne·ri's sign (neh′ree) [B. *Neri,* Italian neurologist, b. 1882]. 1. Combined thigh and leg sign: in cerebral hemiplegia, with the patient standing, flexion of the hips and leaning forward as far as possible results in flexion of the knee on the affected side. With the patient recumbent, alternate raising of the legs results in flexion at the knee of the paretic leg; the normal leg remains straight. 2. Arm sign: in hemiplegia of cerebral origin, with the patient recumbent and his arms pronated on a flat surface, the examiner's hand is placed under one arm and carries out passive flexion at the patient's elbow; the affected arm supinates; the normal arm remains pronated. 3. In sciatic neuritis, forward bending of the trunk with the patient standing results in flexion of the knee on the affected side to avoid stretching the sciatic nerve. 4. In sciatic neuritis, faradic stimulation of the sole of the foot causes extension of the great toe; in a normal condition, it results in flexion.

Nernst lamp (nehrnst) [W. H. *Nernst,* German physicist, 1864–1941]. An electric incandescent lamp with a filament of certain metallic oxides. One form of the lamp, with a filament consisting of a mixture of zirconium oxide with one or more rare-earth oxides, is used as a source of infrared radiation.

Nernst potential [W. H. *Nernst*]. The total difference of potential across a membrane, dependent solely on the difference of activities of the ions on the two sides of the membrane.

ner·o·li oil (nerr'o·lee, neer'o·lee) [It., supposedly after an Italian princess]. ORANGE FLOWER OIL.

nerve, *n.* [L. *nervus,* sinew, tendon; nerve]. A bundle of nerve fibers, usually outside the brain or spinal cord; the nerve fibers are held together by connective tissue called endoneurium inside the nerve bundle and perineurium, the enclosing sheath. A collected bundle of nerve fibers within the brain and spinal cord is usually called a nerve tract. For nerves listed by name, see Table of Nerves in the Appendix. See also Plate 16.

nerve anesthesia. BLOCK ANESTHESIA.

nerve avulsion. Operation of tearing a nerve from its origin by traction.

nerve block. The interruption of the passage of impulses through a nerve, as by chemical, mechanical, or electric means.

nerve bulb. An eminence of protoplasm within the sarcolemma of a muscular fiber, representing the termination of a motor nerve fiber. Syn. *terminal axon.*

nerve cathepsin. An intracellular proteinase enzyme occurring in nervous tissue.

nerve cell. 1. NEURON. 2. The CELL BODY of a neuron.

nerve component. The group of fibers in a nerve having similar functions, as the sensory and motor components of a mixed nerve.

nerve deafness. Deafness due to lesion of the vestibulocochlear nerve.

nerve decompression. Surgical relief of the fibrous or bony constriction of a nerve.

nerve ending. The termination of a nerve at the periphery or in the central nervous system.

nerve epithelium. SENSORY EPITHELIUM.

nerve fiber. The long process of a neuron, usually the axon. Myelinated nerve fibers have a thick layer of myelin surrounding the nerve fiber; unmyelinated nerve fibers contain very little myelin.

nerve gas. Any of a group of chemical compounds, of potential utility as war gases, having a rapid, profound, cumulative, and only slowly reversible effect on the central, peripheral, and parasympathetic nervous system. They act by inhibiting cholinesterase; the effects may be counteracted with atropine. The compounds are mostly derivatives of organic esters of phosphoric acid.

nerve graft. A portion of a nerve sutured in place to restore the continuity of a severed nerve trunk where apposition cannot be secured.

nerve grafting. The transplantation of a portion of a nerve to reestablish the continuity of a severed nerve.

nerve impulse. A transient physicochemical change in the membrane of a nerve fiber which sweeps rapidly along the fiber to its termination, where it causes excitation of other nerves, muscle, or gland cells, depending on the connections and functions of the nerve.

nerve of Arnold [F. *Arnold*]. The auricular branch of the vagus nerve.

nerve of Bell [C. *Bell*]. The long thoracic nerve. See Table of Nerves in the Appendix.

nerve of Co·tun·nius [L., from Domenico *Cotugno,* Italian anatomist, 1736–1822]. The nasopalatine nerve. See Table of Nerves in the Appendix.

nerve of Cruveilhier [J. *Cruveilhier*]. An occasional lingual branch of the facial nerve.

nerve of Cy·on (tsi^h·o^hn') [E. de *Cyon* (I. F. *Tsion*), Russian physiologist, 1843–1912]. In the rabbit, a separate branch of the vagus which carries sensory fibers concerned in cardiac depressor action.

nerve of Eis·ler. The greater coccygeal perforating nerve, only occasionally present, arising from the fourth and fifth sacral nerves.

nerve of Jacobson [L. *Jacobson*]. The tympanic branch of the glossopharyngeal nerve.

nerve of Lancisi [G. *Lancisi*]. MEDIAL LONGITUDINAL STRIA.

nerve of Scarpa [A. *Scarpa*]. The nasopalatine nerve. See Table of Nerves in the Appendix.

nerve of Vi·dius [L., from G. *Guidi*]. The nerve of the pterygoid canal. See Table of Nerves in the Appendix.

nerve of Vieussens [R. *Vieussens*]. ANSA SUBCLAVIA.

nerve of Wrisberg [H. *Wrisberg*]. 1. The intermedius branch of the facial nerve. 2. The medial brachial cutaneous nerve. See Table of Nerves in the Appendix.

nerve retractor. A delicate instrument for isolating nerves during operations.

nerve sheath. PERINEURIUM.

nerve-sheath tumor. NEURILEMMOMA.

nerve supply. The nerves of an organ or structure. See also *extrinsic nerve supply, intrinsic nerve supply.*

nerve tracing. A method used by chiropractors for locating nerves and studying their diseases, dependent on the patient's reports about areas of tenderness or pain when adjoining areas are pressed upon by the operator.

nerve tract. A bundle of nerve fibers having the same general origin and destination within the nervous system; as a rule, all fibers of a nerve tract serve the same or a very similar function.

nervi. Plural and genitive singular of *nervus.*

nervi al·ve·o·la·res su·pe·ri·o·res (al''vee·o·lair'eez sue·peer·ee·o'reez) [NA]. The superior alveolar nerves. See Table of Nerves in the Appendix.

nervi ano·coc·cy·gei (ay''no·kock·sij'ee·eye) [NA]. The anococcygeal nerves. See Table of Nerves in the Appendix.

nervi au·ri·cu·la·res an·te·ri·o·res (aw·rick''yoo·lair'eez an·teer·ee·o'reez) [NA]. The anterior auricular nerves. See Table of Nerves in the Appendix.

nervi car·di·a·ci tho·ra·ci·ci (kahr·dye'uh·sigh tho·ray'si·sigh) [NA]. The cardiac thoracic nerves. See Table of Nerves in the Appendix.

nervi ca·ro·ti·ci ex·ter·ni (ka·rot'i·sigh ecks·tur'nigh) [NA]. EXTERNAL CAROTID NERVES.

nervi ca·ro·ti·co·tym·pa·ni·ci (ka·rot''i·ko·tim·pan'i·sigh) [NA]. The caroticotympanic nerves. See Table of Nerves in the Appendix.

nervi ca·ver·no·si cli·to·ri·dis (kav''ur·no'sigh kli·tor'i·dis) [NA]. The cavernous nerves of the clitoris. See Table of Nerves in the Appendix.

nervi cavernosi clitoridis mi·no·res (mi·no'reez) [BNA]. The lesser cavernous nerves of the clitoris.

nervi cavernosi pe·nis (pee'nis) [NA]. The cavernous nerves of the penis. See Table of Nerves in the Appendix.

nervi cavernosi penis mi·no·res (mi·no'reez) [BNA]. The lesser cavernous nerves of the penis.

nervi ce·re·bra·les (serr·e·bray'leez) [BNA]. Nervi craniales (= CRANIAL NERVES).

nervi cer·vi·ca·les (sur·vi·kay'leez) [NA]. The cervical nerves. See Table of Nerves in the Appendix.

nervi ci·li·a·res bre·ves (sil·ee·air'eez brev'eez) [NA]. The short ciliary nerves. See Table of Nerves in the Appendix.

nervi ciliares lon·gi (long'guy, ·jye) [NA]. The long ciliary nerves. See Table of Nerves in the Appendix.

nervi clu·ni·um in·fe·ri·o·res (klew'nee·um in·feer·ee·o'reez) [NA]. The inferior cluneal nerves. See Table of Nerves in the Appendix.

nervi clunium me·dii (mee'dee·eye) [NA]. The medial cluneal nerves. See Table of Nerves in the Appendix.

nervi clunium su·pe·ri·o·res (sue·peer·ee·o'reez) [NA]. The superior cluneal nerves. See Table of Nerves in the Appendix.

nervi cra·ni·a·les (kray·nee·ay'leez) [NA]. CRANIAL NERVES.

nervi di·gi·ta·les dor·sa·les, hal·lu·cis la·te·ra·lis et di·gi·ti se·cun·di me·di·a·lis (dij·i·tay'leez dor·say'leez, hal'yoo·sis lat'' e·ray'lis et dij'i·tye se·kun'dye mee·dee·ay'lis) [NA]. The dorsal digital nerves of the lateral side of the great toe and of the medial side of the second toe. See Table of Nerves in the Appendix.

nervi digitales dorsales nervi ra·di·a·lis (ray·dee·ay'lis) [NA]. The dorsal digital nerves of the radial nerve. See Table of Nerves in the Appendix.

nervi digitales dorsales nervi ul·na·ris (ul·nair'is) [NA]. The dorsal digital nerves of the ulnar nerve. See Table of Nerves in the Appendix.

nervi digitales dorsales pe·dis (ped'is) [NA]. The dorsal digital nerves of the foot; branches of the superficial peroneal nerve.

nervi digitales pal·ma·res com·mu·nes ner·vi me·di·a·ni (pal·mair'eez kom·yoo'neez nur'vye mee·dee·ay'nigh) [NA]. The common palmar digital nerves of the median nerve. See Table of Nerves in the Appendix.

nervi digitales palmares communes nervi ul·na·ris (ul·nair'is) [NA]. The common palmar digital nerves of the ulnar nerve. See Table of Nerves in the Appendix.

nervi digitales palmares pro·prii ner·vi me·di·a·ni (pro'pree·eye nur'vye mee·dee·ay'nigh) [NA]. The proper palmar digital nerves of the median nerve. See Table of Nerves in the Appendix.

nervi digitales palmares proprii nervi ul·na·ris (ul·nair'is) [NA]. The proper palmar digital nerves of the ulnar nerve. See Table of Nerves in the Appendix.

nervi digitales plan·ta·res com·mu·nes ner·vi plan·ta·ris la·te·ra·lis (plan·tair'eez kom·yoo'neez nur'vye plan·tair'is lat·e·ray'lis) [NA]. The common plantar digital nerves of the lateral plantar nerve. See Table of Nerves in the Appendix.

nervi digitales plantares communes nervi plantaris me·di·a·lis (mee·dee·ay'lis) [NA]. The common plantar digital nerves of the medial plantar nerve. See Table of Nerves in the Appendix.

nervi digitales plantares pro·prii ner·vi plan·ta·ris la·te·ra·lis (pro'pree·eye nur'vye plan·tair'is lat"e·ray'lis) [NA]. The proper plantar digital nerves of the lateral plantar nerve. See Table of Nerves in the Appendix.

nervi digitales plantares proprii nervi plantaris me·di·a·lis (mee·dee·ay'lis) [NA]. The proper plantar digital nerves of the medial plantar nerve. See Table of Nerves in the Appendix.

nervi digitales vo·la·res com·mu·nes ner·vi me·di·a·ni (vo·lair'eez kom·yoo'neez nur'vye mee·dee·ay'nigh) [BNA]. NERVI DIGITALES PALMARES COMMUNES NERVI MEDIANI.

nervi digitales volares communes nervi ul·na·ris (ul·nair'is) [BNA]. NERVI DIGITALES PALMARES COMMUNES NERVI ULNARIS.

nervi digitales volares pro·prii ner·vi me·di·a·ni (pro'pree·eye nur'vye mee·dee·ay'nigh) [BNA]. NERVI DIGITALES PALMARES PROPRII NERVI MEDIANI.

nervi digitales volares proprii nervi ul·na·ris (ul·nair'is) [BNA]. NERVI DIGITALES PALMARES PROPRII NERVI ULNARIS.

nervi eri·gen·tes (err"i·jen'teez) [NA alt.]. PELVIC SPLANCHNIC NERVES. NA alt. *nervi splanchnici pelvini.*

nervi hae·mor·rhoi·da·les in·fe·ri·o·res (hem"o·roy·day'leez in·feer·ee·o'reez) [BNA]. NERVI RECTALES INFERIORES.

nervi haemorrhoidales me·dii (mee'dee·eye) [BNA]. The middle hemorrhoidal nerves. See Table of Nerves in the Appendix.

nervi haemorrhoidales su·pe·ri·o·res (sue·peer·ee·o'reez) [BNA]. The superior hemorrhoidal nerves. See Table of Nerves in the Appendix.

nervi in·ter·cos·ta·les (in·tur·kos·tay'leez) [NA alt.]. INTERCOSTAL NERVES. NA alt. *rami ventrales nervorum thoracicorum.*

nervi in·ter·cos·to·bra·chi·a·les (in"tur·kos"to·bray·kee·ay'leez) [NA]. The intercostobrachial nerves. See Table of Nerves in the Appendix.

nervi la·bi·a·les an·te·ri·o·res (lay·bee·ay'leez an·teer·ee·o'reez) [NA]. The anterior labial nerves. See Table of Nerves in the Appendix.

nervi labiales pos·te·ri·o·res (pos·teer·ee·o'reez) [NA]. The posterior labial nerves. See Table of Nerves in the Appendix.

nervi lum·ba·les (lum·bay'leez) [NA]. The lumbar nerves. See Table of Nerves in the Appendix.

nervi ner·vo·rum (nur·vo'rum). Nerve filaments found in the nerve sheaths.

nervi ol·fac·to·rii (ol·fack·to'ree·eye) [NA]. OLFACTORY NERVES.

nervi pa·la·ti·ni (pal·uh·tye'nigh) [BNA]. The palatine nerves: nervus palatinus major and nervi palatini minores.

nervi palatini mi·no·res (mi·no'reez) [NA]. The lesser palatine nerves. See Table of Nerves in the Appendix.

nervi pe·ri·ne·a·les (perr·i·nee·ay'leez) [NA]. The perineal nerves. See Table of Nerves in the Appendix.

nervi pe·ri·nei (perr·i·nee'eye) [BNA]. NERVI PERINEALES.

nervi phre·ni·ci ac·ces·so·rii (fren'i·sigh ack·se·so'ree·eye) [NA]. The accessory phrenic nerves. See Table of Nerves in the Appendix.

nervi pte·ry·go·pa·la·ti·ni (terr"i·go·pal·uh·tye'nigh) [NA]. PTERYGOPALATINE NERVES.

nervi rec·ta·les in·fe·ri·o·res (reck·tay'leez in·feer·ee·o'reez) [NA]. The inferior rectal nerves. See Table of Nerves in the Appendix.

nervi sa·cra·les (sa·kray'leez) [NA]. SACRAL NERVES.

nervi scro·ta·les an·te·ri·o·res (skro·tay'leez an·teer·ee·o'reez) [NA]. The anterior scrotal nerves. See Table of Nerves in the Appendix.

nervi scrotales pos·te·ri·o·res (pos·teer·ee·o'reez) [NA]. The posterior scrotal nerves. See Table of Nerves in the Appendix.

nervi sphe·no·pa·la·ti·ni (sfee"no·pal·uh·tye'nigh) [BNA]. Nervi pterygopalatini (= PTERYGOPALATINE NERVES).

nervi spi·na·les (spye·nay'leez) [NA]. SPINAL NERVES.

nervi splanch·ni·ci lum·ba·les (splank'ni·sigh lum·bay'leez) [NA]. The lumbar splanchnic nerves. See Table of Nerves in the Appendix.

nervi splanchnici pel·vi·ni (pel·vye'nigh) [NA]. PELVIC SPLANCHNIC NERVES.

nervi splanchnici sa·cra·les (sa·kray'leez) [NA]. The sacral splanchnic nerves. See Table of Nerves in the Appendix.

nervi sub·sca·pu·la·res (sub·skap"yoo·lair'eez) [BNA]. Plural of *nervus subscapularis.*

nervi su·pra·cla·vi·cu·la·res (sue"pruh·kla·vick·yoo·lair'eez) [NA]. The supraclavicular nerves. See Table of Nerves in the Appendix.

nervi supraclaviculares in·ter·me·dii (in·tur·mee'dee·eye) [NA]. The intermediate supraclavicular nerves. See Table of Nerves in the Appendix.

nervi supraclaviculares la·te·ra·les (lat·e·ray'leez) [NA]. The lateral supraclavicular nerves. NA alt. *nervi supraclaviculares posteriores.* See Table of Nerves in the Appendix.

nervi supraclaviculares me·di·a·les (mee·dee·ay'leez) [NA]. The medial supraclavicular nerves. See Table of Nerves in the Appendix.

nervi supraclaviculares me·dii (mee'dee·eye) [BNA]. NERVI SUPRACLAVICULARES INTERMEDII.

nervi supraclaviculares pos·te·ri·o·res (pos·teer·ee·o'reez) [NA alt., BNA]. NERVI SUPRACLAVICULARES LATERALES.

nervi tem·po·ra·les pro·fun·di (tem·po·ray'leez pro·fun'dye) [NA]. The deep temporal nerves. See Table of Nerves in the Appendix.

nervi ter·mi·na·les (tur·mi·nay'leez) [NA]. The terminal nerves. See Table of Nerves in the Appendix.

nervi tho·ra·ca·les (tho·ruh·kay'leez) [BNA]. NERVI THORACICI.

nervi thoracales an·te·ri·o·res (an·teer·ee·o'reez) [BNA]. The anterior thoracic nerves. See Table of Nerves in the Appendix.

nervi thoracales pos·te·ri·o·res (pos·teer·ee·o'reez) [BNA]. The posterior thoracic nerves. See Table of Nerves in the Appendix.

nervi tho·ra·ci·ci (tho·ray'si·sigh, ·kigh) [NA]. The thoracic nerves. See Table of Nerves in the Appendix.

nervi va·gi·na·les (vaj·i·nay'leez) [NA]. The vaginal nerves. See Table of Nerves in the Appendix.

nervi va·so·rum (va·so'rum). Small nerves that innervate the walls of blood vessels.

nervi ve·si·ca·les in·fe·ri·o·res plex·us pu·den·di (ves·i·kay' leez in·feer·ee·o'reez pleck'sus pew·den'dye) [BNA]. The inferior vesical nerves of the pudendal plexus.

nervi vesicales inferiores sys·te·ma·tis sym·pa·thi·ci (sis·tee' ma·tis sim·path'i·sigh) [BNA]. The vesical nerves from the distal part of the sympathetic system.

nervi vesicales su·pe·ri·o·res sys·te·ma·tis sym·pa·thi·ci (sue· peer·ee·o'reez sis·tee'ma·tis sim·path'i·sigh) [BNA]. The superior vesical nerves of the distal part of the sympathetic system.

ner·von (nur'von) *n.* A cerebroside occurring in brain tissue; its characteristic fatty acid is nervonic acid. —**ner·von·ic** (nur·von'ick) *adj.*

nervonic acid. *cis*-15-Tetrocosenic acid, $C_{23}H_{45}COOH$, an unsaturated acid combined in the cerebroside nervon.

ner·vo·sism (nur'vo·siz·um) *n.* [F. *nervosisme*]. 1. Nervousness. 2. An obsolete doctrine that all pathologic phenomena are caused by alterations of nerve force.

ner·vos·i·ty (nur·vos'i·tee) *n.* [L. *nervositas,* strength, thickness]. Nervousness.

ner·vous, *adj.* [L. *nervosus,* sinewy, vigorous]. 1. Of or pertaining to the nerves, as: nervous system, nervous tissue. 2. Affecting or involving a nerve or nerves, as: nervous diseases. 3. Originating in or affected by the nerves; neurogenic. 4. Loosely, psychogenic; pertaining to mental or emotional disorders. 5. In a state of nervousness, afflicted with nervousness. 6. Loosely, NEUROTIC.

nervous bladder. IRRITABLE BLADDER.

nervous breakdown. A nonspecific, nonmedical term for any emotional or mental disorder, particularly when of sudden onset, and when characterized by a predominantly depressive mood. See also *manic-depressive illness, depression, psychotic depressive reaction, involutional melancholia.*

nervous debility. NEURASTHENIA.

nervous diarrhea. Diarrhea as a manifestation of a psychophysiologic disorder.

nervous exhaustion. A state of fatigue and discomfort from emotional causes. See also *neurasthenia.*

nervous headache. PSYCHOGENIC HEADACHE.

nervous irritability. The property of a nerve to respond to stimuli by conducting impulses.

ner·vous·ness, *n.* Excessive excitability of the nervous system, characterized by lack of mental poise, restless, impulsive, or purposeless activity, an uncomfortable awareness of self, and a variety of somatic symptoms such as tremors, fatigue, weight loss, weakness, sleeplessness.

nervous prostration. NEURASTHENIA.

nervous pseudotympany. Pseudotympanites of nervous origin.

nervous shock. An acute nervous collapse, typically accompanied by syncope, produced by severe physical or psychic trauma.

nervous system. 1. The entire nervous apparatus of the body, including the brain, brainstem, spinal cord, cranial and peripheral nerves, and ganglions. NA *systema nervosum.* 2. A functional or anatomic subsystem of this nervous apparatus, as: *autonomic nervous system, central nervous system.*

nervous tissue. The tissue of the nervous system, including the nerve cells, their processes and accessory cells, such as the neuroglia.

ner·vus (nur'vus) *n.*, pl. & genit. sing. **ner·vi** (·vye), genit. pl. **ner·vo·rum** (nur·vo'rum) [NA]. NERVE.

nervus ab·du·cens (ab·dew'senz) [NA]. ABDUCENS NERVE.

nervus ac·ces·so·ri·us (ack·se·so'ree·us) [NA]. ACCESSORY NERVE.

nervus acu·sti·cus (a·koos'ti·kus) [BNA]. Nervus vestibulocochlearis (= VESTIBULOCOCHLEAR NERVE).

nervus al·ve·o·la·ris inferior (al·vee·o·lair'is) [NA]. The inferior alveolar nerve. See Table of Nerves in the Appendix.

nervus am·pul·la·ris anterior (am·pul·air'is) [NA]. The anterior ampullary nerve. See Table of Nerves in the Appendix.

nervus ampullaris inferior [BNA]. NERVUS AMPULLARIS POSTERIOR.

nervus ampullaris la·te·ra·lis (lat·e·ray'lis) [NA]. The lateral ampullary nerve. See Table of Nerves in the Appendix.

nervus ampullaris posterior [NA]. The posterior ampullary nerve. See Table of Nerves in the Appendix.

nervus ampullaris superior [BNA]. NERVUS AMPULLARIS ANTERIOR.

nervus an·te·bra·chii anterior (an·te·bray'kee·eye) [NA alt.]. The anterior interosseous nerve of the forearm. NA alt. *nervus interosseus anterior.* See Table of Nerves in the Appendix.

nervus antebrachii posterior [NA alt.]. The posterior interosseous nerve of the forearm. NA alt. *nervus interosseus posterior.*

nervus ar·ti·cu·la·ris (ahr·tick·yoo·lair'is) [NA]. Any nerve supplying a joint.

nervus au·ri·cu·la·ris mag·nus (aw·rick"yoo·lair'is mag'nus) [NA]. The great auricular nerve. See Table of Nerves in the Appendix.

nervus auricularis posterior [NA]. The posterior auricular nerve. See Table of Nerves in the Appendix.

nervus au·ri·cu·lo·tem·po·ra·lis (aw·rick"yoo·lo·tem·po·ray' lis) [NA]. The auriculotemporal nerve. See Table of Nerves in the Appendix.

nervus ax·il·la·ris (ack·si·lair'is) [NA]. The axillary nerve. See Table of Nerves in the Appendix.

nervus buc·ca·lis (buh·kay'lis) [NA]. BUCCAL NERVE.

nervus buc·ci·na·to·ri·us (buck"si·nuh·to'ree·us) [BNA]. Nervus buccalis (= BUCCAL NERVE).

nervus ca·na·lis pte·ry·goi·dei (ka·nay'lis terr·i·goy'dee·eye) [NA]. The nerve of the pterygoid canal. NA alt. *radix facialis.* See Table of Nerves in the Appendix.

nervus car·di·a·cus cer·vi·ca·lis inferior (kahr·dye'uh·kus sur· vi·kay'lis) [NA]. The inferior cervical cardiac nerve. See Table of Nerves in the Appendix.

nervus cardiacus cervicalis me·di·us (mee'dee·us) [NA]. The middle cervical cardiac nerve. See Table of Nerves in the Appendix.

nervus cardiacus cervicalis superior [NA]. The superior cervical cardiac nerve. See Table of Nerves in the Appendix.

nervus cardiacus inferior [BNA]. NERVUS CARDIACUS CERVICALIS INFERIOR.

nervus cardiacus me·di·us (mee'dee·us) [BNA]. NERVUS CARDIACUS CERVICALIS MEDIUS.

nervus cardiacus superior [BNA]. NERVUS CARDIACUS CERVICALIS SUPERIOR.

nervus ca·ro·ti·co·tym·pa·ni·cus inferior (ka·rot"i·ko·tim·pan' i·kus) [BNA]. The inferior caroticotympanic nerve. See Table of Nerves in the Appendix.

nervus caroticotympanicus superior [BNA]. The superior caroticotympanic nerve. See Table of Nerves in the Appendix.

nervus ca·ro·ti·cus in·ter·nus (ka·rot'i·kus in·tur'nus) [NA]. INTERNAL CAROTID NERVE.

nervus ca·ver·no·sus cli·to·ri·dis major (kav"ur·no'sus kli·tor' i·dis) [BNA]. The greater cavernous nerve of the clitoris.

nervus cavernosus pe·nis major (pee'nis) [BNA]. The greater cavernous nerve of the penis.

nervus coc·cy·ge·us (kock·sij'ee·us) [NA]. COCCYGEAL NERVE.

nervus coch·le·ae (kock'lee·ee) [BNA]. The cochlear nerve. See Table of Nerves in the Appendix.

nervus cu·ta·ne·us (kew·tay'nee·us) [NA]. A cutaneous nerve; any nerve supplying an area of skin.

nervus cutaneus an·te·bra·chii la·te·ra·lis (an''te·bray'kee·eye lat·e·ray'lis) [NA]. The lateral antebrachial cutaneous nerve. See Table of Nerves in the Appendix.

nervus cutaneus antebrachii me·di·a·lis (mee·dee·ay'lis) [NA]. The medial antebrachial cutaneous nerve. See Table of Nerves in the Appendix.

nervus cutaneus antebrachii posterior [NA]. The posterior antebrachial cutaneous nerve. See Table of Nerves in the Appendix.

nervus cutaneus an·ti·bra·chii dor·sa·lis (an''ti·bray'kee·eye dor·say'lis) [BNA]. NERVUS CUTANEUS ANTEBRACHII POSTERIOR.

nervus cutaneus bra·chii la·te·ra·lis (bray'kee·eye lat·e·ray'lis) [BNA]. A lateral brachial cutaneous nerve. See *nervus cutaneus brachii lateralis inferior, nervus cutaneus brachii lateralis superior.*

nervus cutaneus brachii lateralis inferior [NA]. The inferior lateral brachial cutaneous nerve. See Table of Nerves in the Appendix.

nervus cutaneus brachii lateralis superior [NA]. The superior lateral brachial cutaneous nerve. See Table of Nerves in the Appendix.

nervus cutaneus brachii me·di·a·lis (mee·dee·ay'lis) [NA]. The medial brachial cutaneous nerve. See Table of Nerves in the Appendix.

nervus cutaneus brachii posterior [NA]. The posterior brachial cutaneous nerve. See Table of Nerves in the Appendix.

nervus cutaneus col·li (kol'eye) [BNA]. NERVUS TRANSVERSUS COLLI.

nervus cutaneus dor·sa·lis in·ter·me·di·us (dor·say'lis in·tur·mee'dee·us) [NA]. The intermediate dorsal cutaneous nerve of the foot. See Table of Nerves in the Appendix.

nervus cutaneus dorsalis la·te·ra·lis (lat·e·ray'lis) [NA]. The lateral dorsal cutaneous nerve of the foot. See Table of Nerves in the Appendix.

nervus cutaneus dorsalis me·di·a·lis (mee·dee·ay'lis) [NA]. The medial dorsal cutaneous nerve of the foot. See Table of Nerves in the Appendix.

nervus cutaneus fe·mo·ris la·te·ra·lis (fem'o·ris lat·e·ray'lis) [NA]. The lateral femoral cutaneous nerve. See Table of Nerves in the Appendix.

nervus cutaneus femoris posterior [NA]. The posterior femoral cutaneous nerve. See Table of Nerves in the Appendix.

nervus cutaneus su·rae la·te·ra·lis (sue'ree lat·e·ray'lis) [NA]. The lateral sural cutaneous nerve. See Table of Nerves in the Appendix.

nervus cutaneus surae me·di·a·lis (mee·dee·ay'lis) [NA]. The medial sural cutaneous nerve. See Table of Nerves in the Appendix.

nervus dor·sa·lis cli·to·ri·dis (dor·say'lis kli·tor'i·dis) [NA]. The dorsal nerve of the clitoris. See Table of Nerves in the Appendix.

nervus dorsalis pe·nis (pee'nis) [NA]. The dorsal nerve of the penis. See Table of Nerves in the Appendix.

nervus dorsalis sca·pu·lae (skap'yoo·lee) [NA]. The dorsal scapular nerve. See Table of Nerves in the Appendix.

nervus eth·moi·da·lis anterior (eth·moy·day'lis) [NA]. The anterior ethmoid nerve. See Table of Nerves in the Appendix.

nervus ethmoidalis posterior [NA]. The posterior ethmoid nerve. See Table of Nerves in the Appendix.

nervus fa·ci·a·lis (fay·shee·ay'lis) [NA]. FACIAL NERVE.

nervus fe·mo·ra·lis (fem·o·ray'lis) [NA]. FEMORAL NERVE.

nervus fi·bu·la·ris com·mu·nis (fib·yoo·lair'is kom·yoo'nis) [NA alt.]. The common fibular or peroneal nerve. NA alt. *nervus peroneus communis.* See Table of Nerves in the Appendix.

nervus fibularis pro·fun·dus (pro·fun'dus) [NA alt.]. The deep peroneal nerve. NA alt. *nervus peroneus profundus.* See Table of Nerves in the Appendix.

nervus fibularis su·per·fi·ci·a·lis (sue''pur·fish·ee·ay'lis) [NA alt.]. The superficial peroneal nerve. NA alt. *nervus peroneus superficialis.* See Table of Nerves in the Appendix.

nervus fron·ta·lis (fron·tay'lis) [NA]. FRONTAL NERVE.

nervus fur·ca·lis (fur·kay'lis). The fourth lumbar nerve which forks to send fibers to both the lumbar and sacral plexus.

nervus ge·ni·to·fe·mo·ra·lis (jen''i·to·fem·o·ray'lis) [NA]. The genitofemoral nerve. See Table of Nerves in the Appendix.

nervus glos·so·pha·ryn·ge·us (glos''o·fa·rin'jee·us) [NA]. GLOSSOPHARYNGEAL NERVE.

nervus glu·te·us inferior (gloo·tee'us, gloo'tee·us) [NA]. The inferior gluteal nerve. See Table of Nerves in the Appendix.

nervus gluteus superior [NA]. The superior gluteal nerve. See Table of Nerves in the Appendix.

nervus hy·po·gas·tri·cus (dex·ter et si·nis·ter) (high''po·gas'tri·kus decks'tur et si·nis'tur) [NA]. The hypogastric nerve. See Table of Nerves in the Appendix.

nervus hy·po·glos·sus (high''po·glos'us) [NA]. HYPOGLOSSAL NERVE.

nervus ilio·hy·po·gas·tri·cus (il''ee·o·high·po·gas'tri·kus) [NA]. The iliohypogastric nerve. See Table of Nerves in the Appendix.

nervus ilio·in·gui·na·lis (il''ee·o·ing·gwi·nay'lis) [NA]. Ilioinguinal nerve. See Table of Nerves in the Appendix.

nervus in·fra·or·bi·ta·lis (in''fruh·or·bi·tay'lis) [NA]. The infraorbital nerve. See Table of Nerves in the Appendix.

nervus in·fra·tro·chle·a·ris (in''fruh·trock·lee·air'is) [NA]. INFRATROCHLEAR NERVE.

nervus in·ter·me·di·us (in·tur·mee'dee·us) [NA]. The intermediate branch of the seventh cranial or facial nerve. See Table of Nerves in the Appendix.

nervus in·ter·os·se·us anterior (in·tur·os'ee·us) [NA]. The anterior interosseous nerve of the forearm. NA alt. *nervus antebrachii anterior.* See Table of Nerves in the Appendix.

nervus interosseus cru·ris (kroo'ris) [NA]. The crural interosseous nerve. See Table of Nerves in the Appendix.

nervus interosseus dor·sa·lis (dor·say'lis) [BNA]. NERVUS INTEROSSEUS POSTERIOR.

nervus interosseus posterior [NA]. The posterior interosseous nerve of the forearm. NA alt. *nervus antebrachii posterior.* See Table of Nerves in the Appendix.

nervus interosseus vo·la·ris (vo·lair'is) [BNA]. NERVUS INTEROSSEUS ANTERIOR.

nervus is·chi·a·di·cus (is·kee·ad'i·kus) [NA]. SCIATIC NERVE.

nervus ju·gu·la·ris (jug·yoo·lair'is) [NA]. The jugular nerve. See Table of Nerves in the Appendix.

nervus la·cri·ma·lis (lack·ri·may'lis) [NA]. The lacrimal nerve. See Table of Nerves in the Appendix.

nervus la·ryn·ge·us inferior (la·rin'jee·us) [NA]. The inferior laryngeal nerve. See Table of Nerves in the Appendix.

nervus laryngeus re·cur·rens (re·kur'enz) [NA]. The recurrent laryngeal nerve. See Table of Nerves in the Appendix.

nervus laryngeus superior [NA]. The superior laryngeal nerve. See Table of Nerves in the Appendix.

nervus lin·gua·lis (ling·gway'lis) [NA]. The lingual nerve. See Table of Nerves in the Appendix.

nervus lum·bo·in·gui·na·lis (lum''bo·ing·gwi·nay'lis) [BNA]. RAMUS FEMORALIS NERVI GENITOFEMORALIS.

nervus man·di·bu·la·ris (man·dib·yoo·lair'is) [NA]. MANDIBULAR NERVE.

nervus mas·se·te·ri·cus (mas·e·terr'i·kus) [NA]. The masseteric nerve. See Table of Nerves in the Appendix.

nervus mas·ti·ca·to·ri·us (mas''ti·kuh·to'ree·us) [BNA]. MASTICATOR NERVE.

nervus max·il·la·ris (mack·si·lair'is) [NA]. MAXILLARY NERVE.

nervus me·a·tus acu·sti·ci ex·ter·ni (mee·ay'tus a·koos'ti·sigh ecks·tur'nigh) [NA]. The external acoustic meatal nerve. See Table of Nerves in the Appendix.

nervus meatus au·di·to·rii ex·ter·ni (aw·di·to'ree·eye ecks·tur'nigh) [BNA]. NERVUS MEATUS ACUSTICI EXTERNI.

nervus me·di·a·nus (mee·dee·ay'nus) [NA]. The median nerve. See Table of Nerves in the Appendix.

nervus me·nin·ge·us me·di·us (me·nin'jee·us mee'dee·us) [BNA]. RAMUS MENINGEUS MEDIUS NERVI MAXILLARIS.

nervus men·ta·lis (men·tay'lis) [NA]. The mental nerve. See Table of Nerves in the Appendix.

nervus mus·cu·lo·cu·ta·ne·us (mus''kew·lo·kew·tay'nee·us) [NA]. The musculocutaneous nerve of the arm. See Table of Nerves in the Appendix.

nervus my·lo·hy·oi·de·us (migh''lo·high·oy'dee·us) [NA]. The mylohyoid nerve. See Table of Nerves in the Appendix.

nervus na·so·ci·li·a·ris (nay''so·sil·ee·air'is) [NA]. The nasociliary nerve. See Table of Nerves in the Appendix.

nervus na·so·pa·la·ti·nus (nay''so·pal·uh·tye'nus) [NA]. The nasopalatine nerve. See Table of Nerves in the Appendix.

nervus ob·tu·ra·to·ri·us (ob''tew·ruh·to'ree·us) [NA]. The obturator nerve. See Table of Nerves in the Appendix.

nervus oc·ci·pi·ta·lis major (ock·sip·i·tay'lis) [NA]. The greater occipital nerve. See Table of Nerves in the Appendix.

nervus occipitalis minor [NA]. The lesser occipital nerve. See Table of Nerves in the Appendix.

nervus occipitalis ter·ti·us (tur'shee·us) [NA]. The third occipital nerve. See Table of Nerves in the Appendix.

nervus oc·ta·vus (ock·tay'vus) [NA alt.]. The eighth cranial nerve (= VESTIBULOCOCHLEAR NERVE). NA alt. *nervus vestibulocochlearis.*

nervus ocu·lo·mo·to·ri·us (ock''yoo·lo·mo·to'ree·us) [NA]. OCULOMOTOR NERVE.

nervus ol·fac·to·ri·us (ol·fack·to'ree·us). Singular of *nervi olfactorii;* OLFACTORY NERVE.

nervus oph·thal·mi·cus (off·thal'mi·kus) [NA]. OPHTHALMIC NERVE.

nervus op·ti·cus (op'ti·kus) [NA]. OPTIC NERVE.

nervus pa·la·ti·nus anterior (pal·uh·tye'nus) [BNA]. NERVUS PALATINUS MAJOR.

nervus palatinus major [NA]. The greater palatine nerve. See Table of Nerves in the Appendix.

nervus palatinus me·di·us (mee'dee·us) [BNA]. One of the lesser palatine nerves.

nervus palatinus posterior [BNA]. One of the lesser palatine nerves.

nervus pec·to·ra·lis la·te·ra·lis (peck·to·ray'lis lat·e·ray'lis) [NA]. The lateral pectoral nerve. See Table of Nerves in the Appendix.

nervus pectoralis me·di·a·lis (mee·dee·ay'lis) [NA]. The medial pectoral nerve. See Table of Nerves in the Appendix.

nervus pe·ro·ne·us com·mu·nis (perr·o·nee'us kom·yoo'nis) [NA]. The common peroneal nerve. NA alt. *nervus fibularis communis.* See Table of Nerves in the Appendix.

nervus peroneus pro·fun·dus (pro·fun'dus) [NA]. The deep peroneal nerve. NA alt. *nervus fibularis profundus.* See Table of Nerves in the Appendix.

nervus peroneus su·per·fi·ci·a·lis (sue''pur·fish·ee·ay'lis) [NA]. The superficial peroneal nerve. NA alt. *nervus fibularis superficialis.* See Table of Nerves in the Appendix.

nervus pe·tro·sus major (pe·tro'sus) [NA]. The greater petrosal nerve. See Table of Nerves in the Appendix.

nervus petrosus minor [NA]. The lesser petrosal nerve. See Table of Nerves in the Appendix.

nervus petrosus pro·fun·dus (pro·fun'dus) [NA]. The deep petrosal nerve. See Table of Nerves in the Appendix.

nervus petrosus su·per·fi·ci·a·lis major (sue''pur·fish·ee·ay'lis) [BNA]. NERVUS PETROSUS MAJOR.

nervus petrosus superficialis minor [BNA]. NERVUS PETROSUS MINOR.

nervus phre·ni·cus (fren'i·kus) [NA]. PHRENIC NERVE.

nervus plan·ta·ris la·te·ra·lis (plan·tair'is lat·e·ray'lis) [NA]. The lateral plantar nerve. See Table of Nerves in the Appendix.

nervus plantaris me·di·a·lis (mee·dee·ay'lis) [NA]. The medial plantar nerve. See Table of Nerves in the Appendix.

nervus pre·sa·cra·lis (pree·sa·kray'lis) [NA alt.]. Presacral nerve (= SUPERIOR HYPOGASTRIC PLEXUS). NA alt. *plexus hypogastricus superior.*

nervus pte·ry·goi·de·us ex·ter·nus (terr·i·goy'dee·us ecks·tur'nus) [BNA]. NERVUS PTERYGOIDEUS LATERALIS.

nervus pterygoideus in·ter·nus (in·tur'nus) [BNA]. NERVUS PTERYGOIDEUS MEDIALIS.

nervus pterygoideus la·te·ra·lis (lat·e·ray'lis) [NA]. The lateral pterygoid nerve. See Table of Nerves in the Appendix.

nervus pterygoideus me·di·a·lis (mee·dee·ay'lis) [NA]. The medial pterygoid nerve. See Table of Nerves in the Appendix.

nervus pu·den·dus (pew·den'dus) [NA]. PUDENDAL NERVE.

nervus ra·di·a·lis (ray·dee·ay'lis) [NA]. The radial nerve. See Table of Nerves in the Appendix.

nervus re·cur·rens (re·kur'enz) [BNA]. NERVUS LARYNGEUS RECURRENS.

nervus sac·cu·la·ris (sack·yoo·lair'is) [NA]. The saccular nerve. See Table of Nerves in the Appendix.

nervus sa·phe·nus (sa·fee'nus) [NA]. SAPHENOUS NERVE.

nervus sper·ma·ti·cus ex·ter·nus (spur·mat'i·kus eks·tur'nus) [BNA]. RAMUS GENITALIS NERVI GENITOFEMORALIS.

nervus spi·no·sus (spye·no'sus) [BNA]. RAMUS MENINGEUS NERVI MANDIBULARIS.

nervus splanch·ni·cus imus (splank'ni·kus eye'mus) [NA]. LEAST SPLANCHNIC NERVE.

nervus splanchnicus major [NA]. GREATER SPLANCHNIC NERVE.

nervus splanchnicus minor [NA]. LESSER SPLANCHNIC NERVE.

nervus sta·pe·di·us (sta·pee'dee·us) [NA]. The stapedius nerve. See Table of Nerves in the Appendix.

nervus sub·cla·vi·us (sub·klay'vee·us) [NA]. The subclavius nerve. See Table of Nerves in the Appendix.

nervus sub·cos·ta·lis (sub·kos·tay'lis) [NA]. The subcostal nerve. See Table of Nerves in the Appendix.

nervus sub·lin·gua·lis (sub·ling·gway'lis) [NA]. The sublingual nerve. See Table of Nerves in the Appendix.

nervus sub·oc·ci·pi·ta·lis (sub''ock·sip·i·tay'lis) [NA]. The suboccipital nerve. See Table of Nerves in the Appendix.

nervus sub·sca·pu·la·ris (sub·skap''yoo·lair'is) [NA]. The subscapular nerve. See Table of Nerves in the Appendix.

nervus su·pra·or·bi·ta·lis (sue''pruh·or·bi·tay'lis) [NA]. The supraorbital nerve. See Table of Nerves in the Appendix.

nervus su·pra·sca·pu·la·ris (sue''pruh·skap·yoo·lair'is) [NA]. The suprascapular nerve. See Table of Nerves in the Appendix.

nervus su·pra·tro·chle·a·ris (sue''pruh·trock·lee·air'is) [NA]. The supratrochlear nerve. See Table of Nerves in the Appendix.

nervus su·ra·lis (sue·ray'lis) [NA]. The sural nerve. See Table of Nerves in the Appendix.

nervus tem·po·ra·lis pro·fun·dus anterior (tem·po·ray'lis pro·fun'dus) [BNA]. One of the deep temporal nerves.

nervus temporalis profundus posterior [BNA]. One of the deep temporal nerves.

nervus ten·so·ris tym·pa·ni (ten·so'ris tim'puh·nigh) [NA]. The nerve to the tensor tympani. See Table of Nerves in the Appendix.

nervus tensoris ve·li pa·la·ti·ni (vee'lye pal·uh·tye'nigh) [NA]. The nerve to the tensor veli palatini. See Table of Nerves in the Appendix.

nervus ten·to·rii (ten·tor'ee·eye) [BNA]. RAMUS TENTORII NERVI OPHTHALMICI.

nervus tho·ra·ca·lis lon·gus (tho·ruh·kay'lis long'gus) [BNA]. NERVUS THORACICUS LONGUS.

nervus tho·ra·ci·cus lon·gus (tho·ray'si·kus long'gus) [NA].

The long thoracic nerve. See Table of Nerves in the Appendix.

nervus tho·ra·co·dor·sa·lis (thor″a·ko·dor·say′lis) [NA]. The thoracodorsal nerve. See Table of Nerves in the Appendix.

nervus ti·bi·a·lis (tib·ee·ay′lis) [NA]. The tibial nerve. See Table of Nerves in the Appendix.

nervus trans·ver·sus col·li (trans·vur′sus kol′eye) [NA]. The transverse nerve of the neck. See Table of Nerves in the Appendix.

nervus tri·ge·mi·nus (trye·jem′i·nus) [NA]. TRIGEMINAL NERVE.

nervus tro·chle·a·ris (trock·lee·air′is) [NA]. TROCHLEAR NERVE.

nervus tym·pa·ni·cus (tim·pan′i·kus) [NA]. TYMPANIC NERVE.

nervus ul·na·ris (ul·nair′is) [NA]. The ulnar nerve. See Table of Nerves in the Appendix.

nervus utri·cu·la·ris (yoo·trick·yoo·lair′is) [NA]. The utricular nerve. See Table of Nerves in the Appendix.

nervus utri·cu·lo·am·pul·la·ris (yoo·trick″yoo·lo·am″pul·air′is) [NA]. The utriculoampullary nerve. See Table of Nerves in the Appendix.

nervus va·gus (vay′gus) [NA]. VAGUS NERVE.

nervus vas·cu·la·ris (vas·kew·lair′is) [NA]. Any nerve supplying a blood vessel.

nervus ver·te·bra·lis (vur·te·bray′lis) [NA]. The vertebral nerve. See Table of Nerves in the Appendix.

nervus ve·sti·bu·li (ves·tib′yoo·lye) [BNA]. PARS VESTIBULARIS NERVI OCTAVI.

nervus ve·sti·bu·lo·co·chle·a·ris (ves·tib″yoo·lo·kock″lee·air′is) [NA]. VESTIBULOCOCHLEAR NERVE.

nervus zy·go·ma·ti·cus (zye·go·mat′i·kus) [NA]. The zygomatic nerve. See Table of Nerves in the Appendix.

Nesacaine. Trademark for chloroprocaine, a local anesthetic agent used as the hydrochloride salt.

nesidi-, nesidio- [Gk. *nēsidion*, islet]. A combining form meaning *islets of the pancreas.*

ne·sid·i·ec·to·my (ne·sid″ee·eck′tum·ee) *n.* [*nesidi-* + *-ectomy*]. Surgical excision of an islet-cell tumor of the pancreas, or of pancreatic tissue for islet-cell hyperplasia.

ne·sid·io·blast (ne·sid′ee·o·blast) *n.* [*nesidio-* + *-blast*]. The precursor cell of the pancreatic islets parenchyma.

ne·sid·io·blas·to·ma (ne·sid″ee·o·blas·to′muh) *n.* [*nesidioblast* + *-oma*]. ISLET-CELL TUMOR.

ne·sid·io·blas·to·sis (ne·sid″ee·o·blas·to′sis) *n.* [*nesidioblast* + *-osis*]. The differentiation of islet cell precursors from pancreatic ductal epithelium.

ness·ler·ize (nes′lur·ize) *v.* To test with Nessler's reagent. —**ness·ler·iza·tion** (nes″lur·i·zay′shun) *n.*

Ness·ler's reagent [A. *Nessler*, German chemist, 1827–1905]. An aqueous solution of potassium iodide, mercuric chloride, and potassium hydroxide, used in testing for ammonia.

nest, *n.* A group, as of ova or insects.

nes·teia (nes·tye′uh) *n.* [Gk. *nēsteia*, fast]. 1. Fasting. 2. JEJUNUM.

nes·ti·at·ria (nes″tee·at′ree·uh, ·ay′tree·uh) *n.* [*nest*eia + Gk. *iatreia*, treatment, cure]. Treatment by fasting.

nes·ti·os·to·my (nes″tee·os′tum·ee) *n.* [*nestis*, jejunum, + *-stomy*]. JEJUNOSTOMY.

nes·tis (nes′tis) *n.* [Gk. *nēstis*]. 1. Fasting. 2. JEJUNUM.

nes·ti·ther·a·py (nes″ti·therr′up·ee) *n.* NESTIATRIA.

nes·to·ther·a·py (nes″to·therr′up·ee) *n.* NESTIATRIA.

nests of Golgi-Holmgren. HOLMGREN-GOLGI CANALS.

neth·a·lide (neth′uh·lide) *n.* PRONETHALOL.

Neth·er·ton's syndrome [E. W. *Netherton*, U.S. dermatologist, b. 1893]. Erythroderma ichthyosiforme congenitum, abnormality of the hair shaft, and frequent allergic reactions.

ne·tran·eu·rysm (ne·tran′yoo·riz·um) *n.* [Gk. *nētr*on, spindle, + *aneurysm*]. FUSIFORM ANEURYSM.

net·tle rash. URTICARIA.

Neu·berg ester (noy′behrk) [C. *Neuberg*, German biochemist, b. 1877]. FRUCTOSE 6-PHOSPHATE.

Neu·ber's tubes (noy′bur) [G. A. *Neuber*, German surgeon, 1850–1932]. Decalcified bone drainage tubes.

Neu·feld nail. A V-shaped device for internal fixation of intertrochanteric fractures; a nail inserted into the neck of the femur merges with a rounded plate which is fastened to the side of the femur with screws.

Neu·feld quellung test (noy′felt) [F. *Neufeld*, German bacteriologist, 1869–1904]. A test for rapid pneumococcus typing directly from sputum. When pneumococci in dilute suspension are mixed with specific antiserum in the presence of Loeffler's alkaline methylene blue, their capsular swelling appears microscopically as a sharply outlined halo.

Neu·hau·ser's sign [E. B. D. *Neuhauser*, U.S. radiologist, b. 1908]. 1. The bubbly appearance of inspissated meconium seen in roentgenograms of the abdomen of newborns, often a pathognomonic sign of meconium ileus. 2. Absence of adenoid tissue on a lateral roentgenographic view of the nasopharynx, seen in neonates with agammaglobulinemia.

Neu·mann method for total phosphorus. The organic matter is destroyed by digestion with a mixture of sulfuric and nitric acids or some other oxidizing agent. The phosphorus is then precipitated as the phosphomolybdate and determined gravimetrically or volumetrically.

Neu·mann's cells (noy′mahn) [E. *Neumann*, German pathologist, 1834–1918]. The nucleated red cells of the bone marrow.

Neumann's operation [H. *Neumann*, Austrian otolaryngologist, 1873–1939]. *Obsol.* A method of opening the labyrinth of the ear.

Neumann's sheath [E. *Neumann*]. DENTINAL SHEATH.

neur-, neuro- [Gk. *neuron*, sinew, string, nerve]. A combining form meaning *neural, nervous, nerve.*

neu·ral (new′rul) *adj.* [*neur-* + *-al*]. Pertaining to nerves or nervous tissue.

neural arc. A nerve circuit consisting of two or more neurons, the receptor and the effector, with intercalated neurons between them.

neural arch. 1. VERTEBRAL ARCH. 2. *In comparative anatomy,* the dorsal loop of the typical vertebra including the neural canal.

neural axis. CENTRAL NERVOUS SYSTEM.

neural canal. *In embryology,* VERTEBRAL CANAL.

neural crest. A band of ectodermal cells on either side of the neural tube which is the primordium of the cranial, spinal, and autonomic ganglions. Syn. *ganglionic crest.*

neural cyst. A cyst occurring in the brain or the spinal cord.

neural ectoderm. That part of the ectoderm destined to form the neural tube and neural crest. Syn. *neuroblast.*

neural fold. One of the paired, longitudinal folds of the neural plate which unite in the midline to form the neural tube.

neu·ral·gia (new·ral′juh) *n.* [*neur-* + *-algia*]. Severe, sharp, stabbing, paroxysmal pain along the course of a nerve; not associated with demonstrable neurologic signs or structural changes in the nerve. The pain is usually brief; tenderness is often present at the points of exit of the nerve, and the paroxysm can be produced by contact with specific areas (trigger zones). Various forms of neuralgia are named according to their anatomic situation. —**neural·gic** (·jick) *adj.*

neuralgic amyotrophy. A disease of obscure nature, sometimes occurring after an infection or vaccination, beginning with pain in the neck and arm and followed by the rapid development of weakness, and sensory and reflex loss in the territory of supply of the branchial plexus; recovery is the rule. Syn. *brachial neuritis.*

neuralgic torticollis. *Obsol.* Occipital neuralgia.

neu·ral·gi·form (new·ral′ji·form) *adj.* Resembling neuralgia.

neural groove. A longitudinal groove between the neural folds of the embryo before the neural tube is completed.

neural lamina. The lateral portion of the neural arch of a vertebra.

neural leprosy. TUBERCULOID LEPROSY.

neural lobe. INFUNDIBULAR PROCESS.

neural lymphomatosis. A form of the avian leukosis complex affecting primarily the sciatic nerve.

neural plate. The thickened ectodermal plate overlying the head process that differentiates into the neural tube.

neural sheath. MYELIN SHEATH.

neural spine. The spinous process of a vertebra.

neural stalk. The infundibulum of the hypophysis. See *infundibulum.*

neural tube. The embryonic tube formed from the ectodermal neural plate that differentiates into brain and spinal cord.

neur·a·min·ic acid (nur″a·min′ick). An acid, $C_9H_{17}NO_8$, the aldol condensation product of pyruvic acid and *N*-acetyl-D-mannosamine, regarded as the parent acid of a family of widely distributed acyl derivatives known as sialic acids.

neur·amin·i·dase (newr″a·min′i·dace, ·am′in·) *n.* A bacterial enzyme specific for neuraminic acid glycosides, whose action is to split sialic acid from the polymer.

neur·amin-lac·tose (newr″uh·min·lack′toce) *n.* A carbohydrate derivative isolated from the mammary gland of rats; on hydrolysis it yields neuraminic acid and lactose.

neur·apoph·y·sis (newr″uh·pof′i·sis) *n.* Either one of the two apophyses on each embryonic vertebra which blend and form the neural arch, or the dorsal wall of the vertebral canal.

neur·aprax·ia (newr″uh·prack′see·uh, ·ay·prack′) *n.* [*neur-* + *apraxia*]. Paralysis due to impairment of peripheral nerve function without anatomic interruption of the nerve. Recovery is spontaneous, complete, and rapid.

neur·as·the·nia (newr″as·theen′ee·uh) *n.* [*neur-* + *asthenia*]. A group of symptoms formerly considered an important neurosis and ascribed to debility or exhaustion of the nerve centers. —**neuras·then·ic** (·then′ick) *adj.*

neurasthenic asthenopia. Asthenopia due to psychological causes.

neurasthenic neurosis. A neurotic disorder, formerly considered an important neurosis, characterized by chronic complaints of easy fatigability, lack of energy, weakness, various aches and pains, and sometimes exhaustion. Most patients with these complaints are now included in the categories of anxiety neurosis or depression.

neurasthenic stigmas. HYSTERICAL STIGMAS.

neurasthenic vertigo. Dizziness in neurasthenia.

neur·ax·is (newr·ack′sis) *n.* 1. The cerebrospinal axis; NEURAL TUBE. 2. *Obsol.* AXON.

neur·ax·on (newr·acks′on) *n. Obsol.* AXON.

neur·ec·ta·sia (newr″eck·tay′zhuh, ·zee·uh) *n.* NEURECTASIS.

neur·ec·ta·sis (newr·eck′tuh·sis) *n.* [*neur-* + Gk. *ekstasis,* stretching, extension]. Nerve stretching.

neu·rec·to·my (new·reck′tum·ee) *n.* [*neur-* + *-ectomy*]. Excision of a part of a nerve.

neur·ec·to·pia (newr″eck·to′pee·uh) *n.* [*neur-* + *ectopia*]. Displacement or anomalous distribution of a nerve.

neur·ec·to·py (new·reck′tuh·pee) *n.* NEURECTOPIA.

neur·en·ter·ic (newr″en·terr′ick) *adj.* [*neur-* + *-enteric*]. Pertaining to the embryonic neural canal and the intestinal tube.

neurenteric canal. NOTOCHORDAL CANAL.

neurenteric cyst. A cystic epithelium-lined tumor of embryonic origin, resulting from the failure of entodermal tissue to separate from the primitive notochordal plate. The cyst may develop at any point between the lung or gut and the center of the spinal chord, most often in close relation to the lower cervical and upper thoracic portions of the cord.

neur·ep·i·the·li·um (newr·ep″i·theel′ee·um) *n.* NEUROEPITHELIUM.

neu·rer·gic (new·rur′jick) *adj.* [*neur-* + *erg-* + *-ic*]. Pertaining to the activity of a nerve.

neur·ex·ai·re·sis (newr″eck·sigh′re·sis, ·sigh·ree′sis) *n.* NEUREXERESIS.

neur·ex·er·e·sis (newr″eck·serr′e·sis, ·se·ree′sis) *n.* [*neur-* + *exeresis*]. The surgical extraction, or avulsion, of a nerve.

neu·ri·a·sis (new·rye′uh·sis) *n.* [*neur-* + *-iasis*]. *Obsol.* HYPOCHONDRIASIS.

neu·ri·a·try (new·rye′uh·tree) *n.* [*neur-* + *-iatry*]. *Obsol.* The study and treatment of nervous diseases; neurology.

neu·ri·dine (new·ri·deen, ·din) *n.* SPERMINE.

neu·ri·lem·ma, neu·ri·lema (new″ri·lem′uh) *n.* [*neur-* + Gk. *eilēma,* covering, wrapper, veil]. Any of the supporting structures of the nerve fiber, until recently not distinguished from one another. See also *endoneurium, sheath of Schwann, axolemma.* —**neurilem·mal** (·ul) *adj.*

neu·ri·lem·mo·ma, neu·ri·lem·o·ma (new″ri·lem·o′muh) *n.* [*neurilemma* + *-oma*]. A solitary encapsulated benign tumor which originates in the peripheral, cranial, and autonomic nerves, and which is composed of Schwann cells in a collagenous matrix. Syn. *schwannoma, neurinoma.*

neu·ri·lem·mo·sar·co·ma (new″ri·lem″o·sahr·ko′muh) *n.* [*neurilemma* + *sarcoma*]. NEUROFIBROSARCOMA.

neu·rine (new′reen, ·rin) *n.* Trimethylvinylammonium hydroxide, $(CH_3)_3N(OH)CH{=}CH_2$, a product of putrefaction of choline formed in brain, cadavers, and bile.

neu·ri·no·ma (new″ri·no′muh) *n.* 1. NEURILEMMOMA. 2. NEUROFIBROMA.

neu·ri·no·ma·to·sis (new″ri·no″muh·to′sis) *n.* [*neurinoma* + *-osis*]. NEUROFIBROMATOSIS.

neu·rit (new′rit) *n. Obsol.* AXON.

neu·rite (new′rite) *n. Obsol.* AXON.

neuritic muscular atrophy. Atrophy of muscle fibers due to interruption of their nerve supply. Syn. *neuropathic muscular atrophy.*

neu·ri·tis (new·righ′tis) *n.,* pl. **neu·rit·i·des** (new·rit′i·deez) [*neur-* + *-itis*]. An inflammatory disorder of a nerve or nerves, with loss or impairment of motor, sensory, and reflex function in the part supplied. —**neurit·ic** (·rit′ick) *adj.*

neuro-. See *neur-.*

neu·ro·abi·ot·ro·phy (new″ro·ay″bye·ot′ruh·fee, ·ab″ee·ot′) *n.* ABIOTROPHY (1).

neu·ro·anas·to·mo·sis (new″ro·uh·nas″tuh·mo′sis, ·an″us·tuh·) *n.* Surgical anastomosis of nerves.

neu·ro·anat·o·my (new″ro·uh·nat′uh·mee) *n.* The anatomy of the nervous system. —**neuroanato·mist** (·mist) *n.*

neu·ro·ane·mia (new″ro·uh·nee′mee·uh) *n. Obsol.* PERNICIOUS ANEMIA. —**neuroane·mic** (·mick) *adj.*

neuroanemic syndrome. *Obsol.* The various neurological symptoms and deficits associated with pernicious anemia.

neu·ro·ar·thri·tism (new″ro·ahr′thri·tiz·um) *n.* A disease with both neurologic and joint manifestations.

neu·ro·ar·throp·a·thy (new″ro·ahr·throp′uth·ee) *n.* [*neuro-* + *arthropathy*]. A neuropathic joint disease; joint disease related to disease of the nervous system, as Charcot's joint.

neu·ro·as·the·nia (new″ro·as·theen′ee·uh) *n.* NEURASTHENIA.

neu·ro·as·tro·cy·to·ma (new″ro·as″tro·sigh·to′muh) *n.* [*neuro-* + *astrocyte* + *-oma*]. 1. A tumor composed of neurons and glial cells, mainly astrocytes. 2. GANGLIONEUROMA.

neu·ro·ax·on·al (new″ro·ack′suh·nul) *adj.* AXONAL.

neuroaxonal proteid dystrophy. INFANTILE NEUROAXONAL DYSTROPHY.

neu·ro·bi·ol·o·gy (new″ro·bye·ol′uh·jee) *n.* Biology of the nervous system.

neu·ro·bio·tax·is (new″ro·bye″o·tack′sis) *n.* [*neuro-* + *bio-* + *taxis*]. The tendency of nerve cells, during development, to be drawn toward the source of their nutrition and activity.

neu·ro·blast (new′ro·blast) *n.* [*neuro-* + *-blast*]. A formative cell of a neuron, derived from ectoderm of the neural plate.

neu·ro·blas·to·ma (new″ro·blas·to′muh) *n.* A malignant neoplasm composed of primitive neuroectodermal cells, originating in any site in the autonomic nervous system, most commonly in the adrenal medulla of children. Spontaneous remissions may occur. Syn. *sympathicoblastoma.*

neuroblastoma sym·pa·thet·i·cum (sim″puh·thet′i·kum). NEUROBLASTOMA.

neuroblastoma sym·path·i·cum (sim·path′i·kum). NEUROBLASTOMA.

neu·ro·blas·to·ma·to·sis (new″ro·blas″to·muh·to′sis) *n.* 1. Diffuse involvement by neuroblastoma, primary and metastatic. 2. NEUROFIBROMATOSIS.

neu·ro·bru·cel·lo·sis (new″ro·broo″se·lo′sis) *n.* Brucellosis chiefly manifested by the symptoms and signs of meningitis, encephalitis, myelitis, radiculitis, or neuritis; the bizarre complex of neurologic involvement frequently leads to a misdiagnosis of a psychoneurotic disorder.

neu·ro·ca·nal (new″ro·kuh·nal′) *n.* The vertebral canal, containing the spinal cord, cauda equina, and their coverings.

neurocele. NEUROCOELE.

neu·ro·cen·trum (new″ro·sen′trum) *n.* [*neuro-* + *centrum*]. The body of a vertebra. —**neurocen·tral** (·trul) *adj.*

neu·ro·chem·is·try (new″ro·kem′is·tree) *n.* The chemistry of nervous tissue.

neu·ro·cho·rio·ret·i·ni·tis (new″ro·kor″ee·o·ret·i·nigh′tis) *n.* Chorioretinitis combined with optic neuritis.

neu·ro·cho·roid·i·tis (new″ro·kor″oy·dye′tis) *n.* Combined inflammation of the choroid and optic nerve.

neu·ro·cir·cu·la·to·ry (new″ro·sur′kew·luh·tor″ee) *adj.* Pertaining to both the nervous and the circulatory systems.

neurocirculatory asthenia. A form of anxiety neurosis characterized by dyspnea, palpitation, chest pain, fatigue, and faintness. Syn. *soldier's heart.* Abbreviated, NCA.

neurocirculatory syndrome. NEUROCIRCULATORY ASTHENIA.

neu·ro·coele (new′ro·seel) *n.* [*neuro-* + *-coele*]. The system of cavities and ventricles in the central nervous system, comprising the ventricles and central canal of the spinal cord.

neu·ro·cra·ni·um (new″ro·kray′nee·um) *n.* The portion of the cranium which forms the brain case.

neu·ro·cris·top·a·thy (new″ro·kris·top′uh·thee) *n.* [*neuro-* + *crista* + *-pathy*]. A disease arising from defective neural crest elements.

neu·ro·cu·ta·ne·ous (new″ro·kew·tay′nee·us) *adj.* 1. Pertaining to the skin and nerves. 2. Pertaining to the innervation of the skin.

neurocutaneous syndrome. Any heritable disorder or embryologic defect involving both the nervous system and skin, but frequently also other tissues such as bones and the viscera, exemplified by tuberous sclerosis, Hippel-Lindau disease, Sturge-Weber disease, and neurofibromatosis. Syn. *neuroectodermal dysplasia.*

neu·ro·cyte (new′ro·site) *n.* [*neuro-* + *-cyte*]. *Obsol.* NERVE CELL.

neu·ro·cy·tol·y·sin (new″ro·sigh·tol′i·sin) *n.* [*neuro-* + *cytolysin*]. A toxin found in certain snake venoms that produces neurocytolysis.

neu·ro·cy·tol·y·sis (new″ro·sigh·tol′i·sis) *n.* [*neuro-* + *cytolysis*]. Destruction of nerve cells.

neu·ro·de·atro·phia (new·ro″dee·a·tro′fee·uh) *n.* [Gk. *neurōdēs*, neural, + *atrophia*, atrophy]. Atrophy of the retina.

neu·ro·den·drite (new″ro·den′drite) *n.* DENDRITE.

neu·ro·den·dron (new″ro·den′dron) *n.* DENDRITE.

neu·ro·der·ma·ti·tis (new″ro·dur″muh·tigh′tis) *n.* [*neuro-* + *dermatitis*]. A skin disorder characterized by localized, often symmetrical, patches of pruritic dermatitis with lichenification, occurring in patients of nervous temperament.

neurodermatitis cir·cum·scrip·ta (sur″kum·skrip′tuh). LICHEN CHRONICUS SIMPLEX.

neurodermatitis dis·sem·i·na·ta (di·sem″i·nay′tuh). Atopic dermatitis in which psychogenic factors are important.

neu·ro·der·ma·to·sis (new″ro·dur″muh·to′sis) *n.* [*neuro-* + *dermatosis*]. A disease of the skin which is presumed to have a psychogenic component or basis.

neu·ro·der·ma·tro·phia (new″ro·dur″ma·tro′fee·uh) *n.* [*neuro-* + *derm-* + *atrophia*, atrophy]. Atrophy of the skin resulting from neuropathy.

neu·ro·di·as·ta·sis (new″ro·dye·as′tuh·sis) *n.* [*neuro-* + *diastasis*]. Stretching of nerves; neurectasis.

neu·ro·dyn·ia (new″ro·din′ee·uh, ·dye′nee·uh) *n.* [*neur-* + *-odynia*]. NEURALGIA.

neu·ro·ec·to·derm (new″ro·eck′to·durm) *n.* The ectoderm which gives rise to neuroepithelium. —**neuro·ec·to·der·mal** (·eck″to·dur′mul) *adj.*

neuroectodermal dysplasia. NEUROCUTANEOUS SYNDROME.

neu·ro·ef·fec·tor (new″ro·e·feck′tur) *adj.* Pertaining to or involving an efferent nerve and the organ, muscle, or gland innervated.

neu·ro·elec·tro·ther·a·peu·tics (new″ro·e·leck″tro·therr·uh·pew′ticks) *n.* The treatment of nervous affections by means of electricity.

neu·ro·en·do·crine (new″ro·en′duh·krin, ·en′do·krine) *adj.* Pertaining to the nervous and endocrine systems in anatomic or functional relationship; as the hypothalamic nuclei and the hypophysis constitute a neuroendocrine apparatus.

neu·ro·en·ter·ic (new″ro·en·terr′ick) *adj.* NEURENTERIC.

neu·ro·epi·der·mal (new″ro·ep·i·dur′mul) *adj.* Pertaining to the nerves and the epidermis.

neuroepithelial cell. SENSORY CELL.

neuroepithelial layer. Any layer of neuroepithelium, especially the layer of the retina containing the rods and cones. See also *retina.*

neu·ro·ep·i·the·li·o·ma (new″ro·ep″i·theel·ee·o′muh) *n.* [*neuro-* + *epitheli-* + *-oma*]. A tumor resembling primitive medullary epithelium, containing cells of small cuboidal or columnar form with a tendency to form true rosettes, occurring in the retina, where it is also described as a glioma of the retina or retinocytoma, in the central nervous system, and occasionally in peripheral nerves. Syn. *diktyoma, esthesioneuroblastoma, esthesioneuroepithelioma.* See also *retinoblastoma.*

neu·ro·ep·i·the·li·um (new″ro·ep·i·theel′ee·um) *n.*, pl. **neuroepithe·lia** (·lee·uh) [*neuro-* + *epithelium*] [NA]. The highly specialized epithelial structures constituting the terminations of the nerves of special sense, as the rod and cone cells of the retina, the olfactory cells of the nose, the hair cells of the internal ear, and the gustatory cells of the taste buds. —**neuroepitheli·al** (·ul) *adj.*

neu·ro·fi·bril (new″ro·figh′bril) *n.* A fibril of a nerve cell, usually extending from the processes and traversing the cell body, seen by light microscopy after silver or methylene blue staining of fixed tissues. See also *neurofilament, neurotubule.* —**neurofibril·lar** (·ur), **neurofibril·lary** (·err·ee) *adj.*

neu·ro·fi·bro·ma (new″ro·figh·bro′muh) *n.* [*neuro-* + *fibroma*]. A benign, slowly growing, relatively circumscribed but nonencapsulated neoplasm originating in a nerve and composed principally of Schwann cells. The intercellular matrix contains collagen fibrils and a nonorganized mucoid or myxomatous component. The tumor is usually solitary, but may be multiple in patients with neurofibromatosis. Syn. *perineural fibroma, myxofibroma of nerve sheath, neurofibromyxoma.*

neurofibroma gan·glio·cel·lu·la·re (gang″glee·o·sel″yoo·lair′ee). GANGLIONEUROMA.

neurofibroma gan·gli·o·na·re (gang″glee·o·nair′ee). GANGLIONEUROMA.

neu·ro·fi·bro·ma·to·sis (new″ro·figh·bro″muh·to′sis) *n.* A hereditary disease characterized by presence of neurofibromas in the skin or along the course of peripheral nerves. Syn. *von Recklinghausen's disease.*

neu·ro·fi·bro·myx·o·ma (new″ro·figh″bro·mick·so′muh) *n.* [*neuro-* + *fibro-* + *myx-* + *-oma*]. NEUROFIBROMA.

neu·ro·fi·bro·pha·co·ma·to·sis (new″ro·figh″bro·fa·ko″muh·

to'sis, ·fack"o·) *n.* [*neuro-* + *fibro-* + *phacomatosis*]. NEUROFIBROMATOSIS.

neu·ro·fi·bro·sar·co·ma (new"ro·figh"bro·sahr·ko'muh) *n.* [*neuro-* + *fibrosarcoma*]. A malignant tumor composed of interlacing bundles of anaplastic spindle-shaped cells which resemble those of nerve sheaths.

neu·ro·fil·a·ment (new"ro·fil'uh·munt) *n.* [*neuro-* + *filament*]. A structure of indefinite length and about 10 μm in diameter, found throughout the neuron, from the farthest reaches of the dendrites to the tip of the axon. Refined ultrastructural techniques have shown that the neurofilament is a tubular rather than a solid structure.

neu·ro·fil·a·ri·a·sis (new"ro·fil·uh·rye'uh·sis) *n.* [*neuro-* + *filiariasis*]. An infection of the brain or spinal cord with filariae.

neu·ro·gan·gli·itis (new"ro·gang"glee·eye'tis) *n.* [*neuro-* + *gangliitis*]. GANGLIONITIS.

neu·ro·gan·gli·o·ma my·e·lin·i·cum ve·rum (new"ro·gang·glee·o'muh migh·e·lin'i·kum veer'um, vair'um). GANGLIONEUROMA.

neu·ro·gan·gli·on·itis (new"ro·gan"glee·un·eye'tis) *n.* [*neuro-* + *ganglionitis*]. GANGLIONITIS.

neu·ro·gas·tric (new"ro·gas'trick) *adj.* [*neuro-* + *gastric*]. Pertaining to the nerves and the stomach.

neu·ro·gen·e·sis (new"ro·jen'e·sis) *n.* [*neuro-* + *-genesis*]. The formation of nerves.

neu·ro·ge·net·ic (new"ro·je·net'ick) *adj.* NEUROGENIC.

neu·ro·gen·ic (new"ro·jen'ick) *adj.* [*neuro-* + *-genic*]. 1. Of nervous-tissue origin, as neurogenic tumors. 2. Stimulated by nerves, as neurogenic muscular contractions. 3. Caused or affected by a dysfunction, trauma, or disease of nerves or the nervous system, as neurogenic shock, neurogenic bladder. 4. Pertaining to neurogenesis.

neurogenic arthropathy. CHARCOT'S JOINT.

neurogenic bladder. A urinary bladder in a state of dysfunction due to lesions of the central or peripheral nervous system.

neurogenic sarcoma. NEUROFIBROSARCOMA.

neurogenic shock. NEUROPATHIC SHOCK.

neurogenic ulcer. NEUROTROPHIC ULCER.

neu·rog·e·nous (new·roj'e·nus) *adj.* NEUROGENIC.

neurogenous sarcoma. NEUROFIBROSARCOMA.

neu·rog·e·ny (new·roj'e·nee) *n.* NEUROGENESIS.

neu·rog·lia (new·rog'lee·uh) *n.* [*neuro-* + *glia*]. 1. The supporting cells of the central nervous system, consisting of the macroglia (astrocytes and oligodendrocytes), which have an ectodermal origin, and the microglia, the exact origin of which is still not settled. —**neurog·li·al** (·lee·ul) *adj.*

neu·rog·lio·cyte (new·rog'lee·o·site) *n.* A neuroglial cell.

neu·rog·lio·cy·to·ma (new·rog"lee·o·sigh·to'muh) *n.* [*neurogliocyte* + *-oma*]. MEDULLOBLASTOMA.

neu·rog·li·o·ma (new·rog"lee·o'muh) *n.* A tumor composed of neuroglial tissue; a glioma.

neu·rog·li·o·sis (new·rog"lee·o'sis) *n.* A condition of multiple neurogliomas developing diffusely throughout the nervous system.

neu·ro·gram (new'ro·gram) *n.* [*neuro-* + *-gram*]. ENGRAM.

neu·ro·his·tol·o·gy (new"ro·his·tol'uh·jee) *n.* The histology of the nervous system.

neu·ro·hu·mor (new"ro·hew'mur) *n.* [*neuro-* + *humor*]. *Obsol.* NEUROTRANSMITTER. —**neurohumor·al** (·ul) *adj.*

neu·ro·hyp·nol·o·gy (new"ro·hip·nol'uh·jee) *n.* HYPNOLOGY.

neu·ro·hy·poph·y·se·al (new"ro·high·pof"i·see'ul, ·high"po·fiz'ee·ul) *adj.* Pertaining to the neurohypophysis.

neu·ro·hy·po·phys·i·al (new"ro·high·po·fiz'ee·ul) *adj.* Pertaining to the neurohypophysis; NEUROHYPOPHYSEAL.

neu·ro·hy·poph·y·sis (new"ro·high·pof'i·sis) *n.* [NA]. The posterior, neural portion of the hypophysis, which develops as a downward evagination of the neural ectoderm from the floor of the diencephalon and secretes antidiuretic hormone and oxytocin which are produced in the hypothalamus; consists of a main body, the neural lobe or infundibular process, and a stalk, the neural stalk or infundibulum, by which the hypophysis is attached to the hypothalamus. Some classifications also include the pars intermedia. Syn. *posterior pituitary, posterior lobe of the hypophysis.* NA alt. *lobus posterior hypophyseos.* Contr. *adenohypophysis.* See also Plate 26.

neu·roid (new'roid) *adj.* [*neur-* + *-oid*]. Resembling a nerve or nerve substance.

neuroid tube. Nevus cells arranged in thin columns in an intradermal nevus; the columns have the appearance of neural sheaths.

neu·ro·in·duc·tion (new"ro·in·duck'shun) *n.* SUGGESTION (2).

neu·ro·in·su·lar complex (new"ro·in'sue·lur). Small intimate aggregates of islet cells and ganglion cells in the pancreas.

neu·ro·ker·a·tin (new"ro·kerr'uh·tin) *n.* [*neuro-* + *keratin*]. The insoluble protein substance found in the myelin sheath, particularly after fixation in alcohol. It is usually in the form of a network.

neu·ro·lath·y·rism (new"ro·lath'ur·iz·um) *n.* LATHYRISM.

neu·ro·lem·ma (new"ruh·lem'uh) *n.* NEURILEMMA.

neu·ro·lep·tan·al·ge·sia (new"ro·lep"tan·al·jee'zee·uh) *n.* NEUROLEPTOANALGESIA.

neu·ro·lep·tic (new"ro·lep'tic) *adj.* & *n.* [*neuro-* + Gk. *lēptikos*, accepting, assimilative]. 1.Of drug actions: tending to result in overall improvement of patients with mental disorders. 2. A drug that by its characteristic actions and effects is useful in the treatment of mental disorders, especially psychoses. See also *tranquilizer.*

neuroleptic analgesia. NEUROLEPTOANALGESIA.

neu·ro·lep·to·an·al·ge·sia (new"ro·lep"to·an"ul·jee'zee·uh) *n.* A state of altered consciousness produced by a combination of one or more neuroleptic drugs with an analgesic, allowing certain surgical procedures to be carried out on a wakeful subject.

neu·ro·lep·to·an·es·the·sia (new"ro·lep"to·an"es·theezh'uh, ·theez'ee·uh) *n.* NEUROLEPTOANALGESIA.

neu·ro·lo·gia (new·ro·lo'jee·uh) *n.* [BNA]. NEUROANATOMY.

neu·rol·o·gist (new·rol'uh·jist) *n.* A person versed in neurology, usually a physician who specializes in the diagnosis and treatment of disorders of the nervous system and the study of its functioning.

neu·rol·o·gy (new·rol'uh·jee) *n.* [*neuro-* + *-logy*]. The study of the anatomy, physiology, and pathology of the nervous system and treatment of its disorders. —**neu·ro·log·ic** (new"ruh·loj'ick) *adj.*

neu·ro·lo·pho·ma (new"ro·lof·o'muh, ·luh·fo'muh) *n.* [*neuro-* + Gk. *lofos*, crest, + *-oma*]. Any tumor derived from cells of neural crest origin, including neuromas, schwannomas, melanomas, and apudomas.

neu·ro·lu·es (new"ro·lew'eez) *n.* [*neuro-* + *lues*]. NEUROSYPHILIS.

neu·ro·lymph (new'ro·limf) *n.* [*neuro-* + *lymph*]. *Obsol.* CEREBROSPINAL FLUID.

neu·ro·lym·pho·ma·to·sis (new"ro·lim"fo·muh·to'sis) *n.* [*neuro-* + *lymphoma* + *-osis*]. Involvement of nerves by malignant lymphoma.

neurolymphomatosis gal·li·na·rum (gal"i·nair'um) [L. *gallinarum,* of hens, fowl]. NEURAL LYMPHOMATOSIS.

neu·rol·y·sin (new·rol'i·sin, new"ro·lye'sin) *n.* [*neuro-* + *lysin*]. A cytolysin having action upon nerve cells.

neu·rol·y·sis (new·rol'i·sis) *n.* [*neuro-* + *-lysis*]. 1. Stretching of a nerve to relieve anatomical tension. 2. Surgical release of a nerve from harmful fibrous adhesions. 3. Destruction or disintegration of nerve tissue.

neu·ro·ma (new·ro'muh) *n.* [*neur-* + *-oma*]. Any tumor of the nervous system, as originally described by Virchow. These tumors have since been classified into special groups on a histologic basis. See also *neurilemmoma, pseudoneuroma.* —**neu·rom·a·tous** (new·rom'uh·tus, ·ro'muh·tus) *adj.*

neuroma cutis. A cutaneous neurofibroma.

neuroma gan·glio·cel·lu·la·re (gang″glee·o·sel″yoo·lair′ee). GANGLIONEUROMA.

neuroma gangliocellulare ma·lig·num (ma·lig′num). A partly differentiated form of ganglioneuroma.

neu·ro·ma·la·cia (new″ro·ma·lay′shee·uh, ·shuh) *n.* [*neuro-* + *malacia*]. Infarction or softening of nerve tissue.

neuroma telangiectodes. A neuroma with a rich content of blood vessels, often cavernous in type.

neu·ro·ma·toid (new·ro′muh·toid) *adj.* [*neuroma* + *-oid*]. Resembling a neuroma.

neu·ro·ma·to·sis (new″ro·muh·to′sis) *n.* A tendency to form multiple neuromas. See also *neurofibromatosis.*

neuroma ve·rum (vair′um, veer′um) [L., true, real]. GANGLIONEUROMA.

neuroma verum gan·gli·o·sum amy·e·lin·i·cum (gang″glee·o′sum ay″migh·e·lin′i·kum). A form of ganglioneuroma with formation only of axis cylinders.

neu·ro·mech·a·nism (new″ro·meck′uh·niz·um) *n.* The correlated structure and function of the nervous system in relation to a bodily activity.

neu·ro·mere (new′ro·meer) *n.* [*neuro-* + *-mere*]. An embryonic segment of the brain or spinal chord.

neu·rom·ery (new·rom′uh·ree) *n.* [*neuromere* + *-y*]. The segmentation of the central nervous system.

neu·ro·mi·me·sis (new″ro·mi·mee′sis, ·migh·mee′sis) *n.* [*neuro-* + *mimesis*]. A group of phenomena seen in hysterical neurosis resembling neurologic disease. —**neuromi·met·ic** (·met′ick) *adj.*

neu·ro·mo·tor (new″ro·mo′tur) *adj.* 1. Controlling movement. 2. In higher organisms, pertaining to nerves and muscles; neuromuscular.

neu·ro·mus·cu·lar (new″ro·mus′kew·lur) *adj.* Pertaining to both nerves and muscles.

neuromuscular contractility. Contractility mediated by the nervous system, as distinguished from idiomuscular contractility.

neuromuscular junction. MYONEURAL JUNCTION.

neuromuscular spindle. MUSCLE SPINDLE.

neu·ro·my·al (new″ro·migh′ul) *adj.* [*neuro-* + *my-* + *-al*]. NEUROMUSCULAR.

neu·ro·my·as·the·nia (new″ro·migh″as·theen′ee·uh) *n.* [*neuro-* + *myasthenia*]. BENIGN MYALGIC ENCEPHALOMYELITIS.

neu·ro·my·e·li·tis (new″ro·migh·e·ligh′tis) *n.* [*neuro-* + *myel-* + *-itis*]. The conjunction of peripheral nerve and spinal cord inflammation.

neuromyelitis hy·per·al·bu·mi·not·i·ca (high″pur·al·bew″mi·not′i·kuh). GUILLAIN-BARRÉ DISEASE.

neuromyelitis op·ti·ca (op′ti·kuh). A clinical syndrome characterized by simultaneous or successive involvement of the optic nerves and spinal cord; usually a form of mulitple sclerosis, sometimes of another demyelinating disease. Syn. *Devic's disease.*

neu·ro·my·ic (new″ro·migh′ick) *adj.* [*neuro-* + *my-* + *-ic*]. NEUROMUSCULAR.

neu·ro·myo·ar·te·ri·al (new″ro·migh″o·ahr·teer′ee·ul) *adj.* [*neuro-* + *myo-* + *arterial*]. Pertaining to nerves, muscles, and arteries.

neuromyoarterial tumor. GLOMUS TUMOR.

neu·ro·my·on (new″ro·migh′on) *n.* [*neuro-* + *my-* + *-on*]. A functional unit composed of a muscle fiber and its nerve supply. See also *motor unit.* —**neuromy·ic** (·ick) *adj.*

neu·ro·myo·path·ic (new″ro·migh″o·path′ick) *adj.* [*neuro-* + *myo-* + *-pathic*]. Pertaining to disease of both muscles and nerves.

neu·ro·my·o·si·tis (new″ro·migh″o·sigh′tis) *n.* Myositis associated with neuritis.

neu·ron (new′ron) *n.* [Gk., sinew, string, nerve (rel. to L. *nervus* and to E. si*new*)]. The complete nerve cell, including the cell body, axon, and dendrites; specialized as a conductor of impulses. —**neuro·nal** (new′run·ul, new·ro′nul) *adj.*

neuron doctrine. The doctrine (based on the work of van Gehuchten, His, Forel, and Ramón y Cajal) that the basic unit of the central nervous system is a nerve cell with its processes which, having no direct anatomic continuity with other functionally related cells, acts upon another nerve cell solely through a discontinuous interphase, the synapse; opposed to the theory that nerve cells in the central nervous system are united in a syncytium.

neu·rone (new′rone) *n.* NEURON.

neu·ro·ne·vus (new″ro·nee′vus) *n.* 1. A variety of intradermal nevus largely composed of nevus cells possessing neural characteristics. 2. A single neurofibroma.

neu·ron·i·tis (new″ruh·nigh′tis) *n.* [*neuron* + *-itis*]. Inflammation of a neuron or nerve cell; particularly, neuritis involving the cells and roots of spinal nerves.

neu·ro·nog·ra·phy (new″ron·og′ruf·ee, ·ro·nog′) *n.* The study of neuron connections.

neu·ro·nop·a·thy (new″ron·op′uth·ee, ·ro·nop′) *n.* Any disease affecting neurons.

neu·ro·no·pha·gia (new·ro″no·fay′jee·uh) *n.* [*neuron* + *-phagia*]. The removal of injured or diseased nerve cells by phagocytes.

neuron pathway. The successive neurons over which a given impulse is thought to be transmitted.

neuron theory. NEURON DOCTRINE.

neu·ro·oph·thal·mol·o·gy (new″ro·off″thal·mol′uh·jee) *n.* The neurologic aspects of ophthalmology; the study of the physiology and diseases of the visual system as related to the nervous system. —**neuroophthalmolo·gist** (·jist) *n.;* **neu·ro·oph·thal·mo·log·ic** (·off·thal″mo·loj′ick) *adj.*

neu·ro·op·tic (new″ro·op′tick) *adj.* Pertaining to the optic nerve.

neurooptic myelitis. NEUROMYELITIS OPTICA.

neu·ro·pa·ral·y·sis (new″ro·puh·ral′i·sis) *n.* Paralysis or trophic disturbance due to a lesion of the nerve, or the nucleus of the nerve, that supplies the muscle or dermatome involved. —**neuro·par·a·lyt·ic** (·păr″uh·lit′ick) *adj.*

neuroparalytic hyperemia. Hyperemia which is the result of interruption of stimuli through the vasoconstrictor nerves, as in Horner's syndrome.

neuroparalytic keratitis. Keratitis due to corneal anesthesia, as a complication of lesions involving the sensory root of the fifth cranial nerve, or due to other conditions including familial dysautonomia. Syn. *keratitis neuroparalytica.*

neuroparalytic ophthalmia. Disease of the eye from lesion of the trigeminal ganglion or branches of the fifth cranial nerve supplying the eyeball.

neu·ro·path (new′ro·path) *n.* [*neuro-* + *-path*]. An individual with a hereditary predisposition to disorders of the nervous system.

neu·ro·path·ic (new″ro·path′ick) *adj.* [*neuro-* + *-pathic*]. 1. Characterized by a diseased or imperfect nervous system. 2. Depending upon, or pertaining to, nervous disease. 3. Originating in or caused by disease or dysfunction of nerves or the nervous system.

neuropathic arthropathy. CHARCOT'S JOINT.

neuropathic eschar. NEUROTROPHIC ULCER.

neuropathic muscular atrophy. NEURITIC MUSCULAR ATROPHY.

neuropathic shock. A widespread, serious reduction of tissue perfusion due to spinal cord injury, primary autonomic insufficiency, or intoxication with certain drugs, such as anesthetics and ganglion-blocking agents. Syn. *neurogenic shock.*

neu·rop·a·thist (new·rop′uh·thist) *n.* [*neuropathy* + *-ist*]. *Obsol.* NEUROLOGIST.

neu·ro·patho·gen·e·sis (new″ro·path″o·jen′e·sis) *n.* [*neuro-* + *pathogenesis*]. The mechanism or cause of a disease of the nervous system.

neu·ro·pa·thol·o·gy (new″ro·pa·thol′uh·jee) *n.* That part of pathology concerned with diseases of the nervous system. —**neuro·patho·log·ic** (·path·uh·loj′ick) *adj.*

neu·rop·a·thy (new·rop′uth·ee) *n.* [*neuro-* + *-pathy*]. Any noninflammatory disease of peripheral nerves. Compare *neuritis.*

neu·ro·phar·ma·col·o·gy (new″ro·fahr″muh·kol′uh·jee) *n.* The science dealing with the action of drugs on the nervous system.

neu·ro·pho·nia (new″ro·fo′nee·uh) *n.* [*neuro-* + *-phonia*]. A rare form of tic, involving the larynx and muscles of expiration, characterized by the utterance of sharp, spasmodic cries.

neu·ro·phre·nia (new″ro·free′nee·uh) *n.* [*neuro-* + *-phrenia*]. MINIMAL BRAIN DYSFUNCTION SYNDROME.

neu·ro·phys·i·ol·o·gy (new″ro·fiz·ee·ol′uh·jee) *n.* The physiology of the nervous system. —**neurophys·i·o·log·ic** (·ee·o·loj′ick) *adj.*; **neurophysiolo·gist** (·jist) *n.*

neu·ro·pil (new′ro·pil) *n.* [*neuro-* + Gk. *pilos,* felt]. Areas of the central nervous system that contain a feltwork of intermingled and interconnected processes of neurons; in these areas most of the synaptic junctions occur.

neu·ro·pi·tu·i·tary syndrome (new″ro·pi·tew′i·terr·ee). ADIPOSOGENITAL DYSTROPHY.

neu·ro·plasm (new′ro·plaz·um) *n.* The protoplasm filling the interstices of the fibrils of nerve cells.

neu·ro·plas·ty (new′ro·plas″tee) *n.* A plastic operation on the nerves.

neu·ro·ple·gic (new″ro·plee′jick) *adj.* [*neuro-* + *-plegic*]. NEUROLEPTIC.

neu·ro·po·dia (new″ro·po′dee·uh) *n.*, sing. **neuropodi·um** (·um) [*neuro-* + L. *podium,* from Gk. *podion,* small foot]. END FEET.

neu·ro·pore (new′ro·pore) *n.* [*neuro-* + *pore*]. The anterior or posterior terminal aperture of the embryonic neural tube before complete closure occurs (about the 20- to 25-somite stage).

neu·ro·pros·the·sis (new″ro·pros·thee′sis) *n.* [*neuro-* + *prosthesis*]. An artificial device which replaces a neurologic function.

neu·ro·psy·chi·a·try (new″ro·sigh·kigh′uh·tree) *n.* [*neuro-* + *psychiatry*]. The branch of medical science dealing with both nervous and mental diseases. —**neuropsychia·trist** (·trist) *n.*; **neuro·psy·chi·at·ric** (·sigh″kee·at′rick) *adj.*

neu·ro·psy·chol·o·gy (new″ro·sigh·kol′uh·jee) *n. Obsol.* A system of psychology based on neurology.

neu·ro·psy·chop·a·thy (new″ro·sigh·kop′uth·ee) *n.* [*neuro-* + *psychopathy*]. *Obsol.* A mental disease based upon, or manifesting itself in, disorders or symptoms of the nervous system. —**neuro·psy·cho·path·ic** (·sigh″ko·path′ick) *adj.*

neu·ro·psy·cho·sis (new″ro·sigh·ko′sis) *n.* PSYCHOSIS.

neur·op·ti·co·my·e·li·tis (newr·op″ti·ko·migh″e·ligh′tis) *n.* NEUROMYELITIS OPTICA.

neu·ro·ra·di·ol·o·gy (new″ro·ray″dee·ol′uh·jee) *n.* A subspecialty of radiology dealing with the roentgenology of neurologic disease. —**neurora·dio·log·ic** (·dee·o·loj′ick) *adj.*

neu·ro·re·lapse (new″ro·re·laps′) *n.* Subacute syphilitic meningitis, becoming symptomatic during a period of inadequate treatment of early syphilis.

neu·ro·ret·i·ni·tis (new″ro·ret·i·nigh′tis) *n.* Inflammation of both the optic nerve and the retina.

neu·ro·ret·i·nop·a·thy (new″ro·ret″i·nop′uth·ee) *n.* [*neuro-* + *retinopathy*]. Any lesion of the retina not due to inflammation. Compare *neuroretinitis.*

neu·ro·roent·gen·ol·o·gy (new″ro·rent″guh·nol′uh·jee) *n.* NEURORADIOLOGY.

neu·ror·rha·phy (new·ror′uh·fee) *n.* [*neuro-* + *-rrhaphy*]. The operation of suturing a divided nerve.

neu·ror·rhex·is (new″ro·reck′sis) *n.* [*neuro-* + *-rrhexis*]. Avulsion of a nerve, as in the treatment of persistent neuralgia; neurexeresis.

neu·ror·rhyc·tes hy·dro·pho·bi·ae (new″ro·rick′teez high″dro·fo′bee·ee). *Obsol.* NEGRI BODIES.

neu·ro·sal (new·ro′sul) *adj.* Of or pertaining to neurosis.

neu·ro·sar·co·ma (new″ro·sahr·ko′muh) *n.* A sarcoma having features suggesting a nervous system origin.

neu·ro·se·cre·tion (new″ro·se·kree′shun) *n.* [*neuro-* + *secretion*]. 1. The secretory activity of nerve cells. 2. The product of secretory activity of nerve cells. —**neurosecre·to·ry** (·tuh·ree) *adj.*

neu·ro·sen′so·ry (new″ro·sen′suh·ree) *adj.* Of or pertaining to sensory nerves.

neu·ro·sis (new·ro′sis) *n.*, pl. **neuro·ses** (·seez) [*neur-* + *-osis*]. 1. *In psychiatry,* one of the two major categories of emotional maladjustments, classified according to the predominant symptom or defense mechanism. Anxiety is the chief symptom, and though there is no gross disorganization of personality in relation to external reality, there may be some impairment of thinking and judgment. A neurosis usually represents an attempt at resolving unconscious emotional conflicts in a way that diminishes the individual's effectiveness in living. Contr. *psychosis.* See also *anxiety neurosis, hysterical neurosis, depersonalization, depressive neurosis, neurasthenic neurosis, obsessive-compulsive neurosis, phobic neurosis.* 2. *Obsol.* A nervous disorder.

neu·ro·skel·e·tal (new″ro·skel′e·tul) *adj.* Pertaining to nervous and skeletal muscular tissues.

neu·ro·some (new′ro·sohm) *n.* [*neuro-* + *-some*]. 1. The body of a neuron. 2. One of the minute granules of variable size seen by light microscopy in nerve cells.

neu·ro·spasm (new′ro·spaz·um) *n.* Spasm or twitching of a muscle due to or associated with a neurologic disorder.

neu·ro·spon·gi·o·ma (new″ro·spon″jee·o′muh, ·spun″) *n.* [*neurospongium* + *-oma*]. MEDULLOBLASTOMA.

neu·ro·spon·gi·um (new″ro·spun′jee·um, ·spon′jee·um) *n.* [NL., from *neuro-* + L. *spongia,* sponge]. *Obsol.* A meshwork of nerve fibers, as the inner nerve fiber layer of the retina.

Neu·ros·po·ra (new·ros′pur·uh) *n.* A generic name for one of the fungi, more commonly known as the bread mold, which is used as a bioassay organism in enzyme studies.

neu·ro·stea·ric (new″ro·stee′ur·ick, ·stee·ăr′ick) *adj.* [*neuro-* + *stear-* + *-ic*]. Pertaining to nervous tissue and fat.

neu·ro·sthe·nia (new″ro·sthee′nee·uh) *n.* [*neuro-* + Gk. *sthenos,* force, + *-ia*]. *Obsol.* Marked nervous excitement. —**neu·ro·sthen·ic** (·sthen′ick) *adj.*

neu·ro·sur·geon (new″ro·sur′jun) *n.* A physician who specializes in surgery of the central and peripheral nervous system.

neu·ro·sur·gery (new″ro·sur′jur·ee) *n.* Surgery of the nervous system. —**neurosur·gi·cal** (·ji·kul) *adj.*

neu·ro·su·ture (new′ro·sue″chur) *n.* The suture of a nerve.

neu·ro·syph·i·lid (new″ro·sif′i·lid) *n.* [*neurosyphilis* + *-id*]. TERTIARY CIRCINATE ERYTHEMA.

neu·ro·syph·i·lis (new″ro·sif′i·lis) *n.* Syphilitic infection of the nervous system.

neu·ro·ten·di·nal (new″ro·ten′di·nul) *adj.* NEUROTENDINOUS.

neurotendinal spindle. CORPUSCLE OF GOLGI.

neu·ro·ten·di·nous (new″ro·ten′di·nus) *adj.* Pertaining to nerves and tendons.

neurotendinous organ of Golgi. CORPUSCLE OF GOLGI.

neurotendinous xanthomatosis. CEREBROTENDINOUS XANTHOMATOSIS.

neu·ro·ther·a·peu·tics (new″ro·therr″uh·pew′ticks) *n.* NEUROTHERAPY.

neu·ro·ther·a·py (new″ro·therr′up·ee) *n.* The treatment of nervous diseases.

neu·rot·ic (new·rot′ick) *adj.* & *n.* 1. Pertaining to or affected with a neurosis. 2. An individual affected with a neurosis.

neu·rot·i·ca (new·rot′i·kuh) *n.pl. Obsol.* Functional nervous disorders.

neurotic anxiety. Anxiety out of proportion to the apparent cause.

neurotic excoriation. Excoriation from scratching of the skin in response to psychogenic pruritis. See also *acne urticata.*

neurotic personality. An individual who exhibits symptoms or manifestations intermediate between normal character traits and true neurotic features.

neu·rot·i·cism (new·rot'i·siz·um) *n.* A neurotic condition, character, or trait.

neu·roti·gen·ic (new·rot''i·jen'ick, new''ro·ti·) *adj.* NEUROTOGENIC.

neu·roti·za·tion (newr''uh·tye·zay'shun, ·tiz·ay') *n. Obsol.* 1. The regeneration of a divided nerve. 2. Surgical implantation of a nerve into a paralyzed muscle. 3. Providing an anatomic structure with a nerve supply.

neu·rot·me·sis (new''rot·mee'sis) *n.* [*neuro-* + Gk. *tmēsis*, a cutting]. A condition in which the connective-tissue structures and nerve constituents have been interrupted. In the regeneration of new nerve fibers, the new axons and connective tissue grow in misdirected confusion, preventing spontaneous regeneration of the nerve trunk.

neu·roto·gen·ic (new·rot''o·jen'ick) *adj.* Bringing on or favoring the development of a neurosis.

neur·otol·o·gy (new''ro·tol'uh·jee) *n.* [*neur-* + *otology*]. The branch of medical science dealing with the structure and functions of the internal ear, its nervous connections with the brain, and its central pathways within the brain.

neu·ro·tome (new'ro·tome) *n.* [*neuro-* + *-tome*]. 1. An instrument for the division or dissection of a nerve. 2. One of the segments of the embryonic neural tube. Syn. *neuromere.*

neu·rot·o·my (new·rot'um·ee) *n.* [*neuro-* + *-tomy*]. The surgical division or dissection of some or all of the fibers of a nerve.

neu·ro·ton·ic (new''ro·ton'ick) *adj.* Having a tonic effect on the nerves.

neu·ro·tox·ic (new''ro·tock'sick) *adj.* [*neuro-* + *toxic*]. Harmful to nerve tissue. —**neuro·tox·ic·i·ty** (·tock·sis'i·tee) *n.*

neu·ro·tox·in (new''ro·tock'sin) *n.* A toxin capable of damaging nerve tissue.

neu·ro·trans·mit·ter (new''ro·trans·mit'ur) *n.* A chemical agent produced by a nerve cell, usually at the nerve ending, that reacts with a receptor on a neighboring cell or a cell at some distant site, and produces a response in the receptor cell, as, for example, acetylcholine, norepinephrine, vasopressin.

neu·ro·trau·ma (new''ro·traw'muh, ·trow'muh) *n.* [*neuro-* + *trauma*]. Trauma to nervous tissue.

neu·ro·trip·sy (new'ro·trip''see) *n.* [*neuro-* + Gk. *tripsis*, a rubbing]. The crushing of a nerve.

neu·ro·troph·ic (new''ro·trof'ick, ·tro'fick) *adj.* [*neuro-* + *trophic*]. Pertaining to the influence of nerves upon nutrition and maintenance of normal condition in tissues.

neurotrophic arthritis. CHARCOT'S JOINT.

neurotrophic atrophy. Atrophy of muscle and overlying tissue as a result of separation of these tissues from their nerve supply, as seen in the chronic sensory neuropathies.

neurotrophic effect. The effect of one neuron on another neuron, muscle cell, or epithelial cell; removal of this effect leads to atrophic or destructive changes in the dependent cells.

neurotrophic keratitis. NEUROPARALYTIC KERATITIS.

neurotrophic ulcer. Destruction of skin and underlying tissue as a result of separation of these tissues from their nerve supply, as seen in the chronic sensory neuropathies.

neu·ro·tro·pic (new''ro·tro'pick, ·trop'ick) *adj.* [*neuro-* + *-tropic*]. Having an affinity for, or localizing in, nervous tissue.

neurotropic virus. A virus that attacks and has its most serious effects upon nerve tissue.

neu·rot·ro·pism (new·rot'ro·piz·um) *n.* [*neuro-* + *tropism*]. An affinity for nervous tissue, said of certain chemicals, toxins, and viruses.

neu·ro·tu·bule (new''ro·tew'bewl) *n.* [*neuro-* + *tubule*]. An elongated type of microtubule measuring 20 to 26 nm in transverse diameter, observed by electron microscopy in the axon, dendrites, and perikaryon of nerve cells.

neu·ro·var·i·co·sis (new''ro·văr''i·ko'sis) *n.* A varicosity on a nerve fiber, or the formation of one.

neu·ro·vas·cu·lar (new''ro·vas'kew·lur) *adj.* Pertaining to both the nervous and vascular structures.

neu·ro·vis·cer·al (new''ro·vis'ur·ul) *adj.* Pertaining to both nervous tissue and the viscera.

neurovisceral lipidosis. 1. FAMILIAL NEUROVISCERAL LIPIDOSIS. 2. FUCOSIDOSIS.

neu·ru·la (new'ruh·luh) *n.*, pl. **neurulas, neuru·lae** (·lee) [*neur-* + L. *-ula*, small]. *In embryology*, the embryo during the period of neurulation.

neu·ru·la·tion (new''ruh·lay'shun) *n.* [from *neurula*]. *In embryology*, the formation of the neural plate and its subsequent transformation into the neural tube.

Neus·ser's granules (noy'sur) [E. von *Neusser*, Austrian physician, 1852–1912]. Basophilic granules in the vicinity of a leukocyte nucleus.

neutr-, neutro- [L. *neuter, neutr-*, neither one]. A combining form meaning *neutral.*

neu·tral (new'trul) *adj.* [L. *neutralis*, neuter]. 1. Inert, inactive; on neither one side nor the other. 2. Neither alkaline nor acid. —**neutral·i·ty** (new·tral'i·tee) *n.*

neutral acriflavine. ACRIFLAVINE.

neu·tral·iza·tion (new''truh·li·zay'shun, ·lye·zay'shun) *n.* 1. That process or operation which counterbalances or cancels the action of an agent. 2. *In medicine*, the process of checking the functioning of any agent that produces a morbid effect. 3. *In microbiology*, rendering innocuous a toxin or virus by combining it with its corresponding antitoxin or specific antibody. 4. *In chemistry*, a change of medium to that which is neither alkaline nor acid.

neu·tral·ize (new'truh·lize) *v.* To render neutral; render inert; to counterbalance an action or influence.

neutral reaction. The state of a solvent or solution that is neither acid nor alkaline; in aqueous solutions, at 25° C, this is assumed to correspond to pH 7.

neutral red. A water-soluble amino-azine dye used in vital staining and occasionally as an indicator or a general histologic stain.

neutral red bodies. Bodies demonstrated in lymphocytes from peripheral blood supravitally stained with neutral red, closely associated with, if not identical to, the Golgi apparatus.

neutral salt. A salt that in solution has a neutral reaction, as sodium chloride.

neutral stain. A compound produced by the interaction of an acid and a basic dye. It may give a stain differing from that imparted by either component.

neu·tri·no (new·tree'no) *n.* [It., from *neutr-* + *-ino*, small]. A hypothetical atomic particle having the mass of the electron but without an electric charge.

neutro-. See *neutr-.*

neu·tro·clu·sion (new''truh·klew'zhun) *n.* [*neutro-* + *occlusion*]. Occlusion in which the mesiobuccal cusp of the upper first molar interdigitates with the buccal groove of the lower first molar.

neu·tro·cyte (new'tro·site) *n.* A neutrophil granulocyte.

neu·tron (new'tron) *n.* [*neutr-* + *-on*]. An atomic nuclear particle with mass = 1 and charge = 0. A constituent of all atomic nuclei except $^{1}H_1$. (Isotopes differ from one another solely by the number of neutrons in their nuclei.) Free neutrons with various kinetic energies are produced in various nuclear reactions.

neutron capture. A form of nuclear reaction in which a neutron is absorbed by an atomic nucleus.

neutron capture therapy. A technique of internal radiation of an organ or tumor by the administration of a stable compound with an affinity for the organ or tumor and for neutron capture. The area is radiated with neutrons, the stable compound in the target cells becoming radioactive and subsequently undergoing radioactive decay resulting in intense local radiation.

neutron therapy. Irradiation with neutrons for therapeutic purposes.

neu·tro·oc·clu·sion (new″tro·uh·kloo′zhun) *n.* NEUTROCLUSION.

neu·tro·pe·nia (new″tro·pee′nee·uh) *n.* [*neutro-* + *-penia*]. A decrease below normal in the number of neutrophils per unit volume of peripheral blood.

neu·tro·phil (new′truh·fil) *n.* & *adj.* [*neutro-* + *-phil*]. 1. NEUTROPHIL LEUKOCYTE. 2. Any histologic element which, according to Ehrlich's theory, will bind the neutral eosin-azure-methylene blue complex. 3. Stained readily by neutral dyes. —**neu·tro·phil·ic** (new″truh·fil′ick) *adj.*

neutrophil cell. NEUTROPHIL LEUKOCYTE.

neutrophil granules. Granules which take up simultaneously both a basic and an acid dye, assuming a combination tint.

neu·tro·phil·ia (new″tro·fil′ee·uh) *n.* [*neutrophil* + *-ia*]. 1. An affinity for neutral dyes. 2. An increase of neutrophil leukocytes in the blood or tissues.

neutrophilic leukemia. Granulocytic leukemia in which the cells belong almost exclusively to the neutrophilic series.

neutrophilic series. The sequential developmental stages of neutrophilic granulocytes.

neutrophil leukocyte. A highly motile and phagocytic (antimicrobial) leukocyte having numerous fine granules which do not stain definitely either blue (basic dye) or red (acid dye). Its polymorphous nucleus may be ribbonlike, bandlike, or segmented, having two to seven lobules. It has two classes of cytoplasmic granules, one lysosomal, the other smaller and specific.

nevi. Plural of *nevus.*

ne·vi·form (nee′vi·form) *adj.* NEVOID.

ne·vo·car·ci·no·ma, nae·vo·car·ci·no·ma (nee″vo·kahr·si·no′muh) *n.* [*nevus* + *carcinoma*]. A malignant melanoma.

ne·void, nae·void (nee′void) *adj.* 1. Nevuslike. 2. Associated with nevi.

nevoid amentia. STURGE-WEBER DISEASE.

nevoid cyst. A cyst whose walls contain a congeries of blood vessels.

ne·vo·mel·a·no·ma, nae·vo·mel·a·no·ma (nee″vo·mel·uh·no′muh) *n.* [*nevus* + *melanoma*]. A malignant melanoma.

ne·vose, nae·vose (nee′voze, ·voce) *adj.* Spotted; having nevi.

ne·vo·xan·tho·en·do·the·li·o·ma, nae·vo·xan·tho·en·do·the·li·o·ma (nee″vo·zan″tho·en″do·theel·ee·o′muh) *n.* [*nevoid* + *xantho-* + *endothelial* + *-oma*]. JUVENILE XANTHOGRANULOMA.

ne·vus, nae·vus (nee′vus) *n.*, pl. **ne·vi, nae·vi** (·vye) [L., mole]. 1. Any lesion containing melanocytes. 2. *In dermatology,* a cutaneous hamartoma; a birthmark.

nevus ac·ne·i·for·mis uni·lat·e·ra·lis (ack″nee·i·for′mis yoo″ni·lat·ur·ay′lis). NEVUS COMEDONICUS.

nevus an·gio·li·po·ma·to·sus (an″jee·o·li·po″muh·to′sus). FOCAL DERMAL HYPOPLASIA SYNDROME.

nevus arach·noi·de·us (uh·rack·noy′dee·us) [L., from Gk. *arachnoeidēs*]. SPIDER NEVUS.

nevus ara·ne·us (uh·ray′nee·us) [L., pertaining to spiders or spider webs]. SPIDER NEVUS.

nevus cell. MELANOCYTE.

nevus com·e·do·ni·cus (kom″e·do′ni·kus, ·don′i·kus). A unilateral verrucous nevus with hard follicular accretions simulating comedones of acne. Syn. *nevus acneiformis unilateralis, nevus follicularis.*

nevus ep·i·the·li·o·ma·to-cyl·in·dro·ma·to·sus (ep″i·theel·ee·o″muh·to·sil″in·dro″muh·to′sus). CYLINDROMA.

nevus flam·me·us (flam′ee·us) [L., flame-colored]. PORT-WINE NEVUS.

nevus fol·lic·u·la·ris (fol·ick″yoo·lair′is). NEVUS COMEDONICUS.

nevus fus·co·cae·ru·li·us oph·thal·mo·max·il·la·ris of Ota (fus″ko·se·roo′lee·us off·thal′mo·mack″si·lair′is) [L. *fuscus,* dark, + *caerulius,* blue; *ophthalmo-* + L. *maxillaris,* maxillary; M. *Ota,* Japanese, 20th century]. An aberrant Mongolian spot in the region of the eye and upper jaw.

nevus li·po·ma·to·des (li·po″muh·to′deez) [*lipoma* + Gk. *-ōdēs,* of or pertaining to]. An elevated pigmented nevus with connective tissue and fat hypertrophy.

nevus lipomatodes su·per·fi·ci·a·lis (sue″pur·fish″ee·ay′lis). FOCAL DERMAL HYPOPLASIA SYNDROME.

nevus li·po·ma·to·sus (li·po″muh·to′sus). LIPOMA.

nevus pap·il·la·ris (pap″i·lair′is). NEVUS PAPILLOMATOSUS.

nevus pap·il·lo·ma·to·sus (pap″i·lo″muh·to′sus). A papillomatous pigmented nevus.

nevus pel·li·nus (pel·eye′nus) [L., from *pellis,* hide, skin]. A markedly hairy nevus which has the appearance of pelt or fur.

nevus pig·men·to·sus (pig″men·to′sus). PIGMENTED NEVUS.

nevus pi·lo·sus (pi·lo′sus) [L.]. HAIRY NEVUS.

nevus se·ba·ce·us (se·bay′see·us). A single lesion formed by an aggregate of sebaceous glands, usually as a linear streak, most often present since birth on the scalp and face. Syn. *Jadassohn's nevus.*

nevus spi·lus (spye′lus) [L., from Gk. *spilos,* spot, blemish]. A smooth, flat, pigmented nevus devoid of hair.

nevus spon·gi·o·sus al·bus (spon″jee·o′sus al′bus) [L., spongy white]. A rare genodermatosis of the oral and anogenital mucosa, characterized by a white tint and a spongy appearance with numerous small clear follicular openings. Syn. *congenital leukokeratosis mucosae oris, white-sponge nevus of mucosa.*

nevus uni·lat·e·ra·lis (yoo″ni·lat″ur·ay′lis). NEVUS VERRUCOSUS.

nevus uni·us lat·e·ra·lis (yoo′nee·us lat″ur·ay′lis). *Erron.* Nevus unius lateris (= NEVUS VERRUCOSUS).

nevus uni·us lat·e·ris (yoo·nigh′us lat′ur·is, yoo′nee·us) [L., of one side]. NEVUS VERRUCOSUS.

nevus vas·cu·lo·sus (vas″kew·lo′sus). STRAWBERRY MARK.

nevus ver·ru·co·sus (verr″oo·ko′sus, verr′yoo·). A warty brown skin lesion often of linear shape, which is present at birth or appears in early life.

new·born, *adj.* & *n.* 1. Born recently; said of human infants less than a month old, especially of those only a few days old. 2. A newborn infant.

New·burgh's test. LASHMET AND NEWBURGH'S TEST.

New·cas·tle disease. An acute, highly contagious, virus disease of fowls characterized by pneumonia and encephalomyelitis. This virus can cause mild follicular conjunctivitis in humans. Syn. *avian pneumoencephalitis, avian pseudoplague, Philippine fowl disease.*

Newcastle virus. An RNA, hemagglutinating myxovirus responsible for Newcastle disease.

New·com·er method [H. S. *Newcomer,* U.S. physician, b. 1887]. A method for hemoglobin in which hemoglobin is converted to acid hematin with hydrochloric acid and then compared with a yellow ground-glass filter, which approaches the spectroscopic properties of acid hematin, in a balancing type of colorimeter.

new methylene blue. A basic thiazine dye used as a reticulocyte stain for blood and as a nuclear and mucus stain.

new·ton (new′tun) *n.* [I. *Newton,* English natural philosopher and physicist, 1642–1727]. The meter-kilogram-second unit of force, which is the net force that imparts to a mass of one kilogram an acceleration of one meter per second per second.

New·to·ni·an (new·to′nee·un) *adj.* Described or discovered by Sir Isaac Newton, English natural philosopher and physicist, 1642–1727.

Newtonian aberration. CHROMATIC ABERRATION.

Newtonian constant. The gravitation constant *G.* See *G* (1).

Newton method for uric acid determination. Interfering material in the blood filtrate is removed by the acid silver chloride precipitation method. The uric acid remaining is determined colorimetrically by reaction at room temperature in the presence of cyanide with a special arsenotungstate reagent.

Newton's law of cooling. The rate of cooling depends on the difference of temperature between the hot body and its surroundings, so that it steadily diminishes as the temperature difference becomes less.

Newton's method. BENEDICT AND NEWTON'S METHOD.

New World monkey. Any of the monkeys of the Western Hemisphere, classified as the Cebidae, or more broadly, the Ceboidea (including Cebidae and Callitrichidae), considered phylogenetically remote from the Old World monkeys. See also *platyrrhine.*

nex·er·i·dine (neck·serr'i·deen) *n.* 1-[2-(Dimethylamino)-1-methylethyl]-2-phenylcyclohexanol acetate (ester), $C_{19}H_{29}NO_2$, an analgesic.

nex·us (neck'sus) *n.*, pl. **nexuses** [L.]. A tying or binding together, as the grouping of several causes which bring about an infectious disease; interlacing.

Ne·ze·lof's syndrome (nez·lohf') [C. *Nezelof,* French pediatrician, 20th century]. Congenital lymphocytopenia with normal amount of plasma cells and normal immunoglobulins but deficient cellular and humoral responses to some antigens, resulting in frequent virus, fungus, or *Pneumocystis* infections and sometimes early death following the administration of a live vaccine; inherited as an autosomal recessive trait. Syn. *thymic dysplasia.*

NF Abbreviation for *National Formulary.*

ng Abbreviation for *nanogram.*

NHLI National Heart and Lung Institute, one of the Institutes of Health.

N hormone. The factor or factors in adrenocortical secretions having nitrogen-retaining, or protein-anabolic, as well as androgenic activity. Syn. *nitrogen hormone.*

N.H.S. Abbreviation for *National Health Service.*

Ni Symbol for nickel.

NIA National Institute on Aging, one of the National Institutes of Health.

ni·a·cin (nigh'uh·sin) *n.* [*nicotinic acid* + *-in*]. 3-Pyridinecarboxylic acid, $C_6H_5NO_2$, a component of the vitamin B complex; a specific for the treatment of pellagra. Syn. *nicotinic acid.*

ni·a·cin·a·mide (nigh"uh·sin'uh·mide, ·sin·am'ide) *n.* Nicotinic acid amide, $C_6H_6N_2O$; has the vitamin action of niacin but lacks its vasodilator effect. Syn. *nicotinamide.*

ni·a·cin·am·i·do·sis (nigh"uh·sin·am"i·do'sis) *n.* PELLAGRA.

NIAID National Institute of Allergy and Infectious Diseases, one of the National Institutes of Health.

ni·al·a·mide (nigh·al'uh·mide) *n.* 1-[2-(Benzylcarbamyl)-ethyl]-2-isonicotinoylhydrazine, $C_{16}H_{18}N_4O_2$, a monoamine oxidase inhibitor; used clinically as an antidepressant drug.

NIAMD National Institute of Arthritis and Metabolic Disease, former name of the NIAMDD.

NIAMDD National Institute of Arthritis, Metabolic and Digestive Diseases, one of the National Institutes of Health.

ni·brox·ane (nye·brock'sane) *n.* 5-Bromo-2-methyl-5-nitro-*m*-dioxane, $C_5H_8BrNO_4$, a topical antimicrobial.

nic·co·lum (nick'ul·um) *n.* [NL.]. NICKEL.

ni·cer·go·line (nye·sur'go·leen) *n.* 10-Methoxy-1,6-dimethylergoline-8β-methanol, 5-bromonicotinate (ester), a vasodilator.

niche (nitch, neesh) *n.* [F.]. RECESS.

NICHHD National Institute of Child Health and Human Development, one of the National Institutes of Health.

nick·el, *n.* [Swed., from Ger. *Kupfernickel,* niccolite]. Ni = 58.70. A metal of silver-white luster, with a density of 8.9, resembling iron in physical properties.

Nick·er·son-Kveim test. KVEIM TEST.

nick·ing, *n.* 1. Notching. 2. Localized constrictions of retinal veins. 3. Incising of the ventral muscles of the base of a horse's tail, causing the tail to be carried higher.

ni·clo·sa·mide (ni·klo'suh·mide) *n.* 2',5-Dichloro-4'-nitrosalicylanilide, $C_{13}H_8Cl_2N_2O_4$, an anthelmintic.

Ni·co·las-Fa·vre disease (nee·kohn·lah', fahnvr) [J. *Nicolas,* French physician, b. 1868; and M. *Favre*]. LYMPHOGRANULOMA VENEREUM.

Nicolas-Kultschitzsky cells [A. *Nicolas,* French histologist, 19th century; and *N. Kultschitzsky*]. CELLS OF KULTSCHITZSKY.

Ni·co·la's operation [T. *Nicola,* U.S. orthopedist, b. 1894]. An operation for relief of habitual dislocation of the shoulder, by transplant of the long head of the biceps.

Nic·ol prism (nick'ul) [W. *Nicol,* Scottish physicist, 1768–1851]. A prism prepared from two obliquely bisected parts of a rhombohedron of calcite; used for production and analysis of polarized light.

Ni·co·ti·ana (ni·ko"shee·an'uh, ·ay'nuh) *n.* [Jean *Nicot,* French diplomat, 1530–1600]. A genus of plants that includes tobacco.

nic·o·tin·am·ide (nick'uh·tin'uh·mide) *n.* Nicotinic acid amide, $C_6H_6N_2O$; has the vitamin action of nicotinic acid but lacks its vasodilator effect. Syn. *niacinamide.*

nicotinamide adenine dinucleotide. A nucleotide composed of one molecule each of adenine and nicotinamide, and two molecules each of D-ribose and phosphoric acid. It is a coenzyme for numerous hydrogenase reactions. Abbreviated, NAD Syn. *nadide, diphosphophopyridine nucleotide.*

nicotinamide adenine dinucleotide phosphate. A nucleotide composed of one molecule each of adenine and nicotinamide, two molecules of D-ribose, and three molecules of phosphoric acid. It is a coenzyme for oxidation of glucose 6-phosphate to 6-phosphogluconic acid in erythrocytes and is, like nicotinamide adenine dinucleotide, a coenzyme for many other dehydrogenase reactions. Abbreviated, NADP. Syn. *triphosphopyridine nucleotide.*

nic·o·tin·ate (nick'o·tin·ate) *n.* A salt or ester of nicotinic acid.

nic·o·tine (nick'uh·teen) *n.* [F., from *Nicotiana*]. 1-Methyl-2-(3-pyridyl)pyrrolidine, $C_{10}H_{14}N_2$, a colorless, liquid alkaloid in the leaves of the tobacco plant; a toxic substance responsible for many of the effects of tobacco.

nicotine stomatitis. Chronic inflammation and hyperkeratosis around the minor palatal salivary glands; caused by irritation from smoking.

nic·o·tin·ic acid (nick"o·tin'ick). 3-Pyridinecarboxylic acid, $C_6H_5NO_2$, a component of the vitamin B complex; a specific for the treatment of pellagra. Syn. *niacin.*

nicotinic action. Peripheral drug effects similar to those produced by nicotine; small doses result in stimulation of autonomic ganglia and many myoneural junctions, including skeletal muscle; all turn to depression with large doses.

nic·o·tin·yl alcohol (nick"o·tin'il). 3-Pyridinemethanol, C_6H_7NO, a peripheral vasodilator.

nic·ta·tion (nick·tay'shun) *n.* [L. *nictare,* to blink, wink]. The act of blinking.

nic·ti·tate (nick'ti·tate) *n.* [ML. *nictitare,* frequentative of *nictare,* to blink]. To blink, or blink repeatedly. —**nicti·tat·ing** (·tay·ting) *adj. & n.;* **nic·ti·ta·tion** (nick"ti·tay'shun) *n.*

nictitating membrane. The third eyelid of such vertebrates as reptiles and birds, represented vestigially in the human eye by the semilunar fold of the conjunctiva.

ni·da·tion (nigh·day'shun, ni·) *n.* [from L. *nidus,* nest]. The implantation of the fertilized ovum in the endometrium (decidua) of the pregnant uterus.

NIDR National Institute of Dental Research, one of the Institutes of Health.

ni·dus (nigh'dus) *n.*, pl. **ni·di** (·dye) [L., nest]. 1. A locus of production or accumulation, such as a focus of infection or a site at which crystallization or precipitation is initiated. 2. A nestlike structure. —**ni·dal** (·dul) *adj.*

nidus avis ce·re·bel·li (ay'vis serr·e·bel'eye) [L., bird's nest of the cerebellum] [BNA]. A depression between the uvula of the cerebellum and the inferior medullary velum.

NIEHS National Institute of Environmental Health Sciences, one of the National Institutes of Health.

Niel·sen's method. HOLGER NIELSEN METHOD.

Nie·mann-Pick disease (nee'mahn) [A. *Niemann,* German pediatrician, 1880–1921; and L. *Pick*]. A hereditary sphingolipidosis due to the deficiency of an enzyme which catalyzes the hydrolysis of phosphorylcholine from sphingomyelin, resulting in an abnormal accumulation of that substance; manifested in early life by anemia; enlargement of liver, spleen, and lymph nodes; and various neurologic deficits including retinal degeneration and mental retardation.

Niemann-Pick lipid [A. *Niemann* and L. *Pick*]. SPHINGOMYELIN.

Nie·wen·glow·ski's rays (nyeh·væn·glohf·skee') [G. H. *Niewenglowski,* French physicist, 19th century]. Certain luminous rays emitted from phosphorescent substances which have been exposed to sunlight.

ni·fed·i·pine (nye·fed'i·peen) *n.* Dimethyl 1,4-dihydro-2,6-dimethyl-4-(*o*-nitrophenyl)-3,5-pyridinedicarboxylate, $C_{17}H_{18}N_2O_6$, a coronary vasodilator.

ni·fun·gin (nye·fun'jin) *n.* A substance obtained from *Aspergillus giganteus.*

ni·fur·a·trone (nye·fewr'uh·trone) *n.* *N*-(2-Hydroxyethyl)-α-(5-nitro-2-furyl)nitrone, $C_7H_8N_2O_5$, an antibacterial.

ni·fur·da·zil (nye·fewr'duh·zil) *n.* 1-(2-Hydroxyethyl)-3-[(5-nitrofurfurylidene)amino]-2-imidazolidinone, $C_{10}H_{12}N_4O_5$, an antibacterial.

ni·fur·i·mide (nigh·fewr'i·mide) *n.* (±)-4-Methyl-1-[(5-nitrofurfurylidene)amino]-2-imidazolidinone, $C_9H_{10}N_4O_4$, an antibacterial agent.

ni·fur·mer·one (nigh·fewr'mur·ohn, nigh·fewr·merr'ohn) *n.* Chloromethyl 5-nitro-2-furyl ketone, $C_6H_4ClNO_4$, an antifungal agent.

ni·fur·ox·ime (nigh"fewr·ock'seem, ·sim) *n.* *anti*-5-Nitro-2-furaldehyde oxime, $C_5H_4N_2O_4$, a fungicide used in combination with furazolidone for treatment of some types of vaginitis.

ni·fur·pir·i·nol (nye·fewr·pirr'i·nole) *n.* 6-[2-(5-Nitro-2-furyl)vinyl]-2-pyridinemethanol, $C_{12}H_{10}N_2O_4$, an antibacterial.

Ni·ge·ri·an typhus. One of the tick-borne typhus fevers of Africa.

ni·ger·i·cin (nigh·jeer'i·sin, ·jerr') *n.* An antibiotic which acts as an ionophore for K^+ by forming lipid soluble complexes with this cation and thus allowing it to be easily transported across the mitochondrial membrane. Used experimentally as an uncoupler of oxidative phosphorylation.

night blindness. The condition of reduced dark adaptation, resulting temporarily from vitamin A deficiency or permanently from retinitis pigmentosa or other peripheral retinal diseases. Syn. *nyctalopia.* Contr. *day blindness.*

night cry. A shrill cry uttered during sleep; usually of psychic origin, but in a child sometimes symptomatic of a physical disorder.

night guard. A type of bite plate or splint designed to disrupt or prevent a tooth clenching or grinding habit.

night hospital. A hospital or specialized facility within a hospital for psychiatric patients who are able to function in the community during the day, particularly to work, but who require supervision, support, and treatment in a hospital after working hours. Contr. *day hospital.*

night·mare, *n.* [OE. *niht,* night, + *mare,* spirit, goblin, incubus]. A terrifying anxiety dream due to the bursting forth of repressed sexual or aggressive impulses or the fear of death. It is characterized by feelings of helplessness, oppression, or suffocation, and usually awakens the sleeper.

night monkey. DOUROUCOULI.

night pain. Pain, usually in the hip or knee, occurring during muscular relaxation of the limb in sleep; often a symptom of disease of the joints.

night palsy. Numbness of the extremities, sometimes with weakness, occurring during the night, or on waking in the morning, due to positional compression of a part during sleep.

night·shade, *n.* Any of various plants of the family Solanaceae.

night sweat. Drenching perspiration occurring at night or whenever the patient sleeps, in the course of pulmonary tuberculosis or other febrile diseases.

night terrors. NIGHTMARE.

night vision. Vision at light intensities below the threshold at which cones are activated, using the rods and rhodopsin.

night vision tester. A self-recording group testing device for determining the ability to discriminate the break in a Landolt ring at eight different levels of illumination. The testing distance is 20 feet.

NIGMS National Institute of General Medical Sciences, one of the National Institutes of Health.

ni·gral (nigh'grul) *adj.* Pertaining to the substantia nigra.

ni·gran·i·line (nigh·gran'i·leen, ·lin) *n.* Aniline black, a black dye obtained by the oxidation of aniline, used as a histologic stain.

ni·gri·cans (nig'ri·kanz, nigh'gri·) *adj.* [L.]. Black or blackish.

Nigrin. Trademark for streptonigrin, an antibiotic that has antineoplastic activity.

ni·gri·ti·es (nigh·grish'ee·eez) *n.* [L., blackness]. BLACK, HAIRY TONGUE.

ni·gro·re·tic·u·lar (nigh"gro·re·tick'yoo·lur) *adj.* Pertaining to the substantia nigra and to the reticular formation.

ni·gro·ru·bral (nigh"gro·roo'brul) *adj.* [substantia *nigra* + L. *ruber, rubr-,* red]. Pertaining to the substantia nigra and to the red nucleus.

ni·gro·sine (nigh'gro·seen, ·sin) *n.* Any one of several black or dark blue aniline dyes; variously used in bacteriologic and histologic techniques.

ni·gro·stri·a·tal (nigh"gro·strye·ay'tul) *adj.* Pertaining to the substantia nigra and the corpus striatum.

nigrostriatal tract. Nerve fibers which arise in the pars compacta of the substantia nigra and end in the corpus striatum, particularly the putamen.

NIH Abbreviation for *National Institutes of Health.*

ni·hil·ism (nigh'ul·iz·um, ·hil·iz·um) *n.* [L. *nihil,* nothing, + *-ism*]. 1. *In medicine,* pessimism in regard to the efficacy of treatment, particularly the use of drugs; therapeutic nihilism. 2. *In psychiatry,* the content of delusions encountered in depressed or melancholic states. The patient insists that his inner organs no longer exist, and that his relatives have passed away.

NIH swab. A small square of cellophane attached to a glass rod, developed by the National Institutes of Health and used in collecting ova or other material from a mucous surface; the cellophane square is examined directly under a microscope.

nik·eth·a·mide (nick·eth'uh·mide, ·mid) *n.* *N,N*-Diethylnicotinamide, $C_{10}H_{14}N_2O$; stimulates medullary centers. Used, parenterally, as an analeptic, and for its respiratory stimulant effects.

Ni·kol·sky's sign (nyi·kolyʹ·skee) [P. V. *Nikolsky,* Russian dermatologist, b. 1858]. The ready removal of epidermis upon the slightest injury, found between bullae on seemingly unaffected skin in pemphigus and epidermolysis bullosa. It may be disclosed by pulling the ruptured wall of the blister, or rubbing off the epidermis between bullae by slight friction without breaking the surface of the skin.

Nile blue. Diethylaminophenylaminonaphthoxazine chloride, principally used in the staining of lipids and lipid pigments.

Nile blue A. A basic oxazine dye, of value as a fat stain.

Nilevar. Trademark for norethandrolone, an androgenic steroid with anabolic activity used clinically for the latter effect.

Nilodin. Trademark for lucanthone hydrochloride, a drug useful in treating certain types of human schistosomiasis.

ni·met·ti (ni·met'ee) *n.* SIMULIUM GRISEICOLLIS.

NIMH National Institute of Mental Health, one of the National Institutes of Health.

nim·i·dane (nim'i·dane) *n.* *N*-(1,3-Dithietan-2-ylidene)-4-chloro-*o*-toluidine, $C_9H_8ClNS_2$, a veterinary acaricide.

NINDS National Institute of Neurological Diseases and Stroke, one of the National Institutes of Health.

nine mile fever. Q FEVER.

Ninhydrin. Trademark for triketohydrindene hydrate, a reagent that gives a color reaction with proteins and amino acids.

Ninhydrin Schiff reaction. A histochemical test for proteins, depending on deamination of primary amine groups and their replacement by aldehyde which is localized by Schiff's reagent.

ninth (IXth) cranial nerve. GLOSSOPHARYNGEAL NERVE.

ni·o·bi·um (nigh·o'bee·um) *n.* Nb = 92.9064. A steel-gray, lustrous metal, with a density of 8.57. Formerly called *columbium.*

niph·ablep·sia (nif''a·blep'see·uh) *n.* [Gk. *nipha,* snow, + *ablepsia*]. SNOW BLINDNESS.

nipho·typh·lo·sis (nif''o·tif·lo'sis) *n.* [Gk. *nipha,* snow, + *typhlosis*]. SNOW BLINDNESS.

nip·i·ol·o·gy (nip''ee·ol'uh·jee) *n.* [variant of *nepiology*]. NEONATOLOGY.

nip·pers, *n.pl.* 1. An instrument for cutting the cuticle or nail. 2. A small bone-trimming forceps.

nip·ple, *n.* The conical projection in the center of the mamma, containing the outlets of the milk ducts. NA *papilla mammae.* See also Plate 24.

nipple line. MAMILLARY LINE.

nipple protector. A device worn by nursing women to protect the nipple.

nipple shield. NIPPLE PROTECTOR.

ni·rid·a·zole (nigh·rid'uh·zole) *n.* 1-(5-Nitro-2-thiazolyl)-2-imidazolidinone, $C_6H_6N_4O_3S$, an antischistosomal drug.

Nisentil. Trademark for alphaprodine, a narcotic analgesic used as the hydrochloride salt.

ni·sin (nigh'sin) *n.* An antibiotic substance derived from *Streptococcus lactis,* active, in vitro, against a number of bacterial species.

ni·so·bam·ate (nigh''so·bam'ate) *n.* 2-Hydroxymethyl-2,3-dimethylpentyl carbamate isopropylcarbamate, $C_{13}H_{26}N_2O_4$, a tranquilizer, sedative, and hypnotic.

ni·sox·e·tine (ni·sock'se·teen) *n.* (±)-3-(*o*-Methoxyphenoxy)-*N*-methyl-3-phenylpropylamine, $C_{17}H_{21}NO_2$, an antidepressant.

Nissl bodies or **granules** [F. *Nissl,* German neuropathologist, 1860–1919]. Clumps of chromophil substance which represent stocks of rough endoplasmic reticulum in nerve cell cytoplasm. Their staining reactions (basophilia) are due to the ribosomes; CHROMOPHIL GRANULES.

Nissl reaction or **degeneration** [F. *Nissl*]. AXONAL REACTION.

Nissl's acute cell disease. AXONAL REACTION.

Nissl stains [F. *Nissl*]. Stains used to demonstrate the extranuclear ribonucleic acid masses in nerve cells, the tigroid or Nissl substance.

Nissl substance [F. *Nissl*]. The chromophil substance of nerve cells.

Nisulfazole. Trademark for paranitrosulfathiazole, a drug used for the treatment of ulcerative colitis.

ni·sus (nigh'sus) *n.* [L., strain, effort]. 1. Any strong effort or struggle. 2. The periodic desire for procreation manifested in the spring season by certain species of animals. Syn. *nisus formativus.* 3. The contraction of the diaphragm and abdominal muscles for the expulsion of feces, urine, or a fetus.

nisus for·ma·ti·vus (for''muh·tye'vus). NISUS (2).

nit, *n.* The egg or the larva of a louse.

Ni·ta·buch's membrane (nee'tah·bookh) [R. *Nitabuch,* German physician, 19th century]. STRIA OF NITABUCH.

Nitabuch's stria [R. *Nitabuch*]. STRIA OF NITABUCH.

ni·tar·sone (nye·tahr'sone) *n.* *p*-Nitrobenzenearsonic acid, $C_6H_6AsNO_5$, an antiprotozoal effective against *Histomonas.*

ni·ter, ni·tre (nigh'tur) *n.* [Gk. *nitron,* sodium carbonate]. SALTPETER.

ni·thi·amide (nye·thigh'uh·mide) *n.* *N*-(5-Nitro-2-thiazolyl)acetamide, $C_5H_5N_3O_3S$, a veterinary antibiotic.

ni·ton (nigh'ton) *n.* [L. *nitere,* to shine, + *-on*]. RADON.

nitr-, nitro-. A combining form designating (a) *the presence of the monovalent radical* NO_2; (b) *combination with nitrogen.*

ni·trate (nigh'trate) *n.* A salt or ester of nitric acid.

ni·tra·tion (nigh·tray'shun) *n.* The process of combining or reacting with nitric acid.

ni·tra·ze·pam (nigh·tray'ze·pam, ·trah') *n.* 1,3-Dihydro-7-nitro-5-phenyl-2*H*-1,4-benzodiazepin-2-one, $C_{15}H_{11}N_3O_3$, an anticonvulsant and hypnotic drug.

nitre. Niter (= SALTPETER).

ni·tric (nigh'trick) *adj.* [F. *nitrique*]. 1. Containing nitrogen in a higher valence state than in corresponding nitrous compounds. 2. Pertaining to or derived from nitric acid.

nitric acid. A liquid containing about 70% HNO_3, the remainder being water; has a characteristic, highly irritating odor and is very caustic and corrosive. Used externally as an escharotic.

ni·tri·fi·ca·tion (nigh''tri·fi·kay'shun) *n.* [F.]. The conversion of the nitrogen of ammonia and organic compounds into nitrites and nitrates, a process constantly going on in nature under the influence of certain bacteria and other agencies. —**ni·tri·fy** (nigh'tri·figh) *v.*

ni·tri·fi·er (nigh'tri·figh''ur) *n.* A microorganism that participates in the process of nitrification; bacteria of the genus *Nitrosomonas* oxidize ammonium to nitrite; bacteria of the genus *Nitrobacter* oxidize nitrite to nitrate.

ni·trile (nigh'trile, ·tril) *n.* An organic compound containing the monovalent CN group.

ni·trite (nigh'trite) *n.* A salt or ester of nitrous acid.

ni·tri·toid (nigh'tri·toid) *adj.* Like a nitrite or the reaction produced by a nitrite.

ni·tri·tu·ria (nigh''tri·tew'ree·uh) *n.* [*nitrite* + *-uria*]. The presence of nitrates or nitrites, or both, in the urine when voided.

nitro-. See *nitr-.*

ni·tro·cel·lu·lose (nigh''tro·sel'yoo·loce) *n.* Any nitrate ester, or mixture of nitrate esters, of cellulose. See also *pyroxylin.*

ni·tro·dan (nigh'tro·dan) *n.* 3-Methyl-5-[(*p*-nitrophenyl)azo]-rhodanine, $C_{10}H_8N_4O_3S_2$, an anthelmintic drug.

ni·tro·fur·an·to·in (nigh''tro·few·ran'to·in) *n.* 1-[(5-Nitrofurfurylidene)amino]hydantoin, $C_8H_6N_4O_5$, a urinary antibacterial drug.

ni·tro·fur·a·zone (nigh''tro·few'ruh·zone) *n.* 5-Nitro-2-furaldehyde semicarbazone, $C_6H_6N_4O_4$, an antibacterial drug used topically.

ni·tro·gen (nigh'truh·jin) *n.* [F. *nitrogène,* from *nitro-* + *-gène,* generating]. N = 14.0067. A nonmetallic element existing free in the atmosphere, of which it constitutes about 77 percent by weight. A colorless, odorless gas, incapable of sustaining life. Chemically relatively inert, but an important constituent of all animal and vegetable tissues. See also Table of Chemical Constituents of Blood in the Appendix.

nitrogen balance or **equilibrium.** The difference between the nitrogen excreted and the nitrogen taken into the body, excluding respiratory nitrogen.

nitrogen cycle. The fixation of atmospheric nitrogen and the nitrification of inorganic nitrogen compounds by bacteria, the synthesis of these into protein by plants and consumption by animals, with ultimate degradation to inorganic nitrogen compounds and molecular nitrogen.

nitrogen dioxide. NO_2. A toxic gas resulting from the decomposition of nitric acid.

nitrogen fixation. Conversion of free nitrogen in the air into compounds such as ammonia and nitric acid and their salts and derivatives; accomplished naturally through the agency of certain soil organisms and through electrical discharges in the atmosphere, and synthetically by various industrial methods.

nitrogen fixers. Certain bacteria, as of the genus *Azotobacter,* capable of transforming atmospheric nitrogen into nitrogenous compounds in the cell.

nitrogen hormone. N HORMONE.

nitrogen lag. The time elapsing between the ingestion of a protein and the appearance in the urine of an amount of nitrogen equal to that taken in.

nitrogen monoxide. NITROUS OXIDE.

nitrogen mustard. 1. MECHLORETHAMINE HYDROCHLORIDE. 2. Any of a series of nitrogen analogs of bis(2-chloroethyl) sulfide, the chemical warfare agent known as mustard gas. Several nitrogen mustards, including mechlorethamine hydrochloride, melphalan (L-phenylalanine mustard), and uracil mustard, are useful antineoplastic agents.

ni·trog·e·nous (nigh·troj'e·nus) *adj.* [*nitro-* + *-genous*]. Containing nitrogen.

nitrogen pentoxide. The solid substance N_2O_5; reacts with water to form nitric oxide.

nitrogen peroxide. NITROGEN TETROXIDE.

nitrogen retention. AZOTEMIA.

nitrogen tetroxide. N_2O_4. A toxic gas resulting from oxidation of nitrogen dioxide.

ni·tro·glyc·er·in (nigh''tro·glis'ur·in) *n.* Glyceryl trinitrate or glonoin, $C_3H_5(NO_3)_3$, an oily liquid which is explosive but when suitably dispersed may be handled safely. A prompt-acting coronary vasodilator usually administered sublingually.

ni·tro·hy·dro·chlo·ric acid (nigh''tro·high''druh·klor'ick). A mixture of 1 volume of nitric acid and 4 volumes of hydrochloric acid; has been used, well diluted, as a choleretic. Syn. *nitromuriatic acid, aqua regia.*

ni·tro·man·nite (nigh''tro·man'ite) *n.* MANNITOL HEXANITRATE.

ni·tro·man·ni·tol (nigh''tro·man'i·tol) *n.* MANNITOL HEXANITRATE.

ni·tro·mer·sol (nigh''tro·mur'sol) *n.* 4-Nitro-3-hydroxymercuri-*o*-cresol anhydride, $C_7H_5HgNO_3$, an organomercurial antibacterial agent used topically.

ni·trom·e·ter (nigh·trom'e·tur) *n.* [*nitro-* + *-meter*]. An apparatus for collecting and measuring nitrogen evolved during a chemical reaction.

ni·tro·mi·fene (nye·tro'mi·feen) *n.* 1-[2-[*p*-[α-(*p*-Methoxyphenyl)-β-nitrostyryl]phenoxy]ethyl]pyrrolidine, $C_{27}H_{28}N_2O_4$, an antiestrogen, usually used as the citrate salt.

ni·tro·mu·ri·at·ic acid (nigh''tro·mew''ree·at'ick) [*nitro-* + *muriatic*]. NITROHYDROCHLORIC ACID.

ni·tron (nigh'tron) *n.* 4,5-Dihydro-1,4-diphenyl-3,5-phenylamino-1,2,4-triazole, $C_{20}H_{16}N_4$, an analytical reagent for various cations and anions such as boron, nitrate, perchlorate, rhenium, and tungsten.

ni·tro·prus·side (nigh''tro·prus'ide) *n.* Any salt containing the anion $[Fe(CN)_5NO]^{2-}$; a nitroferricyanide.

nitros-, nitroso-. A combining form signifying *combination with nitrosyl,* the univalent radical —NO.

ni·tro·sa·tion (nigh''tro·say'shun) *n. In histochemistry,* treatment with acid solutions of sodium nitrite to destroy primary amino groups, to convert secondary amines to nitrosamines, or to introduce the —NO groups into phenols and form active diazonium compounds. —**ni·tro·sate** (nigh'tro·sate) *v.*

ni·tro·scan·ate (nye·tro·skan'ate) *n.* *p*-(*p*-Nitrophenoxy)phenyl isothiocyanate, $C_{13}H_8N_2O_3S$, a veterinary anthelmintic.

nitroso-. See *nitros-.*

ni·tro·so·urea (nigh·tro''so·yoo·ree'uh) *n.* Any of a class of antineoplastic compounds containing the grouping —NHCON(NO)—, such as carmustine, lomustine, semustine, and streptozocin, which exert their cytotoxicity through the liberation of alkylating moieties.

ni·tro·syl (nigh·tro'sil, nigh'tro·sil) *n.* The univalent radical —NO.

ni·trous (nigh'trus) *adj.* 1. Containing nitrogen in a lower valence state than in corresponding nitric compounds. 2. Pertaining to or derived from nitrous acid.

nitrous acid. HNO_2. An unstable solution prepared by passing N_2O_3 into water.

nitrous ether. Ethyl nitrite, $C_2H_5NO_2$, a very volatile liquid having vasodilative properties similar to those of amyl nitrite.

nitrous oxide. A colorless gas, N_2O, used to produce anesthesia which consists mainly of moderate analgesia and minimum amnesia in dentistry and in surgery. Syn. *hyponitrous oxide, laughing gas, nitrogen monoxide.*

niv·a·zol (niv'uh·zole) *n.* 2'-(*p*-Fluorophenyl)-2'*H*-17α-pregna-2,4-dien-20-yno [3,2-*c*]pyrazol-17-ol, $C_{28}H_{31}FN_2O$, a glucocorticoid.

Nizin. A trademark for zinc sulfanilate, an antibacterial.

NK Nomenklatur Kommission; a committee appointed to revise the BNA. The recommendations of this committee, published in 1935, have not been widely adopted.

N.L.N. National League of Nursing.

nm Abbreviation for *nanometer.*

NNN medium. A medium for culturing *Leishmania donovani,* containing beef extract, agar, neopeptone, sodium chloride, and defibrinated rabbit's blood. Syn. *Senekjie's medium.*

No Symbol for nobelium.

No. *Numero,* number, to the number of.

No·ack's syndrome [M. *Noack*]. See *acrocephalopolysyndactyly.*

no·as·the·nia (no''as·theen'ee·uh) *n.* [Gk. *nous,* mind, + *astheneia,* weakness]. MENTAL DEFICIENCY.

no·bel·i·um (no·bel'ee·um) *n.* [A. B. *Nobel*]. A radioactive element, atomic number 102, produced synthetically. Symbol, No.

No·bel laureate [A. B. *Nobel,* Swedish manufacturer and philanthropist, 1833–1896]. A recipient of one of the annual awards for noteworthy advances in the service of humanity in the physical sciences, physiology or medicine, literature, and in the cause of fraternity among different peoples.

noble gases. The inert gases, helium, neon, argon, krypton, xenon, and radon, so called because they do not generally combine with other elements.

No·ble's posture [C. P. *Noble,* U.S. gynecologist, 1863–1935]. A position for examination of the kidney in which the standing patient's torso is flexed and supported by the extended arms.

No·car·dia (no·kahr'dee·uh) *n.* [E. *Nocard,* French veterinarian, 1850–1903]. A genus of aerobic branching organisms of the family Actinomycetaceae.

Nocardia as·ter·oi·des (as''tur·oy'deez) [Gk. *asteroeidēs,* starlike]. A species of *Nocardia* which is aerobic and acid-fast; causes pulmonary, brain, and subcutaneous lesions, usually without granules.

Nocardia ker·a·to·lyt·i·ca (kerr''uh·to·lit'i·kuh) [NL., keratolytic]. The organism that causes cracked heels in India.

Nocardia ma·du·rae (ma·dew'ree) [L., of Madura]. A species of *Nocardia* which is one of the causes of white-grained mycetoma.

Nocardia mi·nu·tis·si·ma (migh''new·tis'i·muh). A species of *Nocardia* associated with chronic infection of the stratum corneum known as erythrasma.

Nocardia so·ma·li·en·sis (so·mah·lee·en'sis) [NL., Somali]. A species of *Nocardia* which is one of the causes of white-grained mycetoma.

Nocardia ten·u·is (ten'yoo·is) [L., thin]. A species of *Nocardia* which is the causative agent of trichomycosis axillaris.

no·car·di·o·sis (no·kahr″dee·o′sis) *n.* [*Nocardia* + *-osis*]. Infection by certain species of *Nocardia.*

noci- [L. *nocere,* to hurt, injure]. A combining form meaning *pain.*

nociceptive reflex. A reflex initiated by a painful stimulus.

nociceptive reflex of Riddoch and Buzzard [G. *Riddoch* and T. *Buzzard*]. RIDDOCH'S MASS REFLEX.

no·ci·cep·tor (no″si·sep′tur) *n.* [*noci-* + *receptor*]. A high-threshold receptor which responds to stimuli such as burning, crushing, cutting, or pressure sufficiently intense to cause tissue damage. —**nocicep·tive** (·tiv) *adj.*

no·ci·per·cep·tion (no″si·pur·sep′shun) *n.* [*noci-* + *perception*]. Perception of pain.

no·ci·per·cep·tor (no″si·pur·sep′tur) *n.* NOCICEPTOR.

noct-, nocti-, nocto-, noctu- [L. *nox, noctis*]. A combining form meaning *night.*

noc·tal·bu·min·uria (nock″tal·bew″mi·new′ree·uh) *n.* [*noct-* + *albuminuria*]. Excretion of protein in night urine only.

noc·tam·bu·la·tion (nock·tam″bew·lay′shun) *n.* [*noct-* + *ambulation,* walking]. SLEEPWALKING.

noc·ti·pho·bia (nock″ti·fo′bee·uh) *n.* [*nocti-* + *-phobia*]. Morbid fear of night or darkness.

Noc·tu·i·dae (nock·tew′i·dee) *n.pl.* [L. *noctua,* owl]. A family of the Lepidoptera; owlet moths. Caterpillars of this family have irritating hairs which cause caterpillar dermatitis in man.

noc·tu·ria (nock·tew′ree·uh) *n.* [*noct-* + *urinate* + *-ia*]. Frequency of urination at night. Syn. *nycturia.*

noc·tur·nal (nock·tur′nul) *adj.* [L. *nocturnus,* from *nox, noctis,* night]. 1. Occurring or becoming manifest at night. 2. Of animals, active at night.

nocturnal emission. Involuntary seminal discharge occurring during sleep in physiologically normal males beginning with puberty.

nocturnal enuresis. Involuntary urination at night during sleep, by a person in whom bladder control may normally be expected to be present; bed-wetting.

nocturnal pollution. NOCTURNAL EMISSION.

nocturnal proctalgia. PROCTALGIA FUGAX.

noc·u·ous (nock′yoo·us) *adj.* [L. *nocuus,* hurtful, from *nocere,* to hurt]. Injurious, noxious; poisonous.

nod·al points. A pair of axial points of a lens system, one corresponding to each side of the system and its appropriate focal point, locating object and image planes for which the image is the same size as the object and erect. Syn. *Gaussian points.*

nodal rhythm. JUNCTIONAL RHYTHM.

nodal tachycardia. JUNCTIONAL TACHYCARDIA.

nodal tissue. 1. The sinoatrial node, the atrioventricular node and bundle and its branches, which serve for the origin and transmission of impulses in the heart. This system is made up of a dense network of Purkinje fibers. 2. Tissue from a lymph node.

nodding spasm. An obsolete term for spasmus nutans.

node, *n.* [L. *nodus,* knot]. 1. A knob or protuberance. 2. A point of constriction. 3. A small, rounded organ. —**nod·al** (no′dul) *adj.*

node of Keith and Flack [A. *Keith* and M. W. *Flack*]. SINOATRIAL NODE.

node of Ran·vier (rahⁿv·yeʸ′) [L. A. *Ranvier,* French histologist and pathologist, 1835–1922]. The region, in a myelinated nerve, of a local constriction in the myelin sheath at varying intervals on both central and peripheral axons. At each node, the axis cylinder is also constricted. Electron microscopy reveals that the node is formed by the end of one Schwann cell and the beginning of another.

node of Tawara. ATRIOVENTRICULAR NODE.

node of Virchow-Troisier [R. L. K. *Virchow* and E. *Troisier*]. SIGNAL NODE.

nodi. Plural and genitive singular of *nodus.*

nodi lymphatici [NA]. Plural of *nodus lymphaticus.*

nodi lymphatici api·ca·les (ap·i·kay′leez) [NA]. Lymph nodes in the apex of the axilla.

nodi lymphatici axil·la·res (ack·si·lair′reez) [NA]. Lymph nodes in the axilla.

nodi lymphatici bron·cho·pul·mo·na·les (bronk″o·pul″mo·nay′leez) [NA]. Lymph nodes about the root of each lung.

nodi lymphatici buc·ca·les (buh·kay′leez) [NA]. Small lymph nodes in the cheek.

nodi lymphatici ce·li·a·ci (see·lye′uh·sigh) [NA]. Lymph nodes about the celiac trunk.

nodi lymphatici cen·tra·les (sen·tray′leez) [NA]. Lymph nodes in the central part of the axilla.

nodi lymphatici cer·vi·ca·les pro·fun·di (sur·vi·kay′leez pro·fun′dye) [NA]. Deep lymph nodes of the neck.

nodi lymphatici cervicales su·per·fi·ci·a·les (sue″pur·fish·ee·ay′leez) [NA]. Superficial lymph nodes of the neck.

nodi lymphatici co·li·ci dex·tri (ko′li·sigh decks′trye) [NA]. Lymph nodes associated with the right colic artery.

nodi lymphatici colici me·dii (mee′dee·eye) [NA]. Lymph nodes associated with the middle colic artery.

nodi lymphatici colici si·nis·tri (si·nis′trye) [NA]. Lymph nodes associated with the left colic artery.

nodi lymphatici cu·bi·ta·les (kew·bi·tay′leez) [NA]. Small lymph nodes in the cubital fossa.

nodi lymphatici epi·gas·tri·ci (ep·i·gas′tri·sigh) [NA]. Lymph nodes associated with the inferior epigastric artery.

nodi lymphatici gas·tri·ci dex·tri (gas′tri·sigh decks′trye) [NA]. Lymph nodes associated with the right gastric artery.

nodi lymphatici gastrici si·nis·tri (si·nis′trye) [NA]. Lymph nodes associated with the left gastric artery.

nodi lymphatici gas·tro·epi·plo·i·ci dex·tri (gas″tro·ep·i·plo′i·sigh decks′trye) [NA]. Lymph nodes associated with the right gastroepiploic artery.

nodi lymphatici gastroepiploici si·nis·tri (si·nis′trye) [NA]. Lymph nodes associated with the left gastroepiploic artery.

nodi lymphatici he·pa·ti·ci (he·pat′i·sigh) [NA]. Lymph nodes associated with the hepatic artery.

nodi lymphatici ileo·co·li·ci (il·ee·o·ko′li·sigh) [NA]. Lymph nodes associated with the ileocolic branch of the superior mesenteric artery.

nodi lymphatici ili·a·ci com·mu·nes (il·eye′uh·sigh kom·yoo′neez) [NA]. Lymph nodes associated with the common iliac artery.

nodi lymphatici iliaci ex·ter·ni (ecks·tur′nigh) [NA]. Lymph nodes associated with the external iliac artery.

nodi lymphatici iliaci in·ter·ni (in·tur′nigh) [NA]. Lymph nodes associated with the internal iliac artery.

nodi lymphatici in·gui·na·les pro·fun·di (ing·gwi·nay′leez pro·fun′dye) [NA]. Deep lymph nodes of the inguinal region.

nodi lymphatici inguinales su·per·fi·ci·a·les (sue″pur·fish·ee·ay′leez) [NA]. Superficial lymph nodes of the inguinal region.

nodi lymphatici in·ter·cos·ta·les (in·tur·kos·tay′leez) [NA]. Small lymph nodes associated with the intercostal arteries.

nodi lymphatici la·te·ra·les (lat·e·ray′leez) [NA]. Lymph nodes in the lateral part of the axilla.

nodi lymphatici lin·gua·les (ling·gway′leez) [NA]. The deep cervical lymph nodes which receive lymph from the tongue.

nodi lymphatici lum·ba·les (lum·bay′leez) [NA]. Lymph nodes associated with the lower abdominal aorta.

nodi lymphatici man·di·bu·la·res (man·dib·yoo·lair′reez) [NA]. Lymph nodes lying along the lower edge of the posterior part of the mandible.

nodi lymphatici me·di·as·ti·na·les an·te·ri·o·res (mee·dee·as″ti·nay′leez an·teer·ee·o′reez) [NA]. Lymph nodes located in the anterior mediastinum.

nodi lymphatici mediastinales pos·te·ri·o·res (pos·teer·ee·o′

reez) [NA]. Lymph nodes lying in the posterior mediastinum associated with the thoracic aorta.

nodi lymphatici me·sen·te·ri·ci in·fe·ri·o·res (mes·en·terr'i·sigh in·feer·ee·o'reez) [NA]. Lymph nodes associated with the inferior mesenteric artery.

nodi lymphatici mesenterici su·pe·ri·o·res (sue·peer·ee·o'reez) [NA]. Lymph nodes associated with the superior mesenteric artery.

nodi lymphatici oc·ci·pi·ta·les (ock·sip·i·tay'leez) [NA]. Small lymph nodes of the occipital region.

nodi lymphatici pan·cre·a·ti·co·li·e·na·les (pan·kree·at''i·ko·lye''e·nay'leez) [NA]. Lymph nodes associated with the splenic artery.

nodi lymphatici pa·ra·ster·na·les (păr''uh·stur·nay'leez) [NA]. Lymph nodes associated with the internal thoracic artery.

nodi lymphatici pa·ro·ti·dei, su·per·fi·ci·a·les et pro·fun·di (pa·rot·i·dee'eye sue''pur·fish·ee·ay'leez et pro·fun'dye) [NA]. Lymph nodes associated with the parotid gland.

nodi lymphatici pec·to·ra·les (peck·to·ray'leez) [NA]. Axillary lymph nodes associated with the pectoral muscles.

nodi lymphatici phre·ni·ci (fren'i·sigh) [NA]. Small lymph nodes on the upper surface of the diaphragm.

nodi lymphatici po·pli·tei (pop·lit'ee·eye) [NA]. Small lymph nodes located in the popliteal region.

nodi lymphatici pul·mo·na·les (pul·mo·nay'leez) [NA]. Small lymph nodes in each lung lying along the larger bronchi.

nodi lymphatici py·lo·ri·ci (pi·lo'ri·sigh) [NA]. Lymph nodes adjacent to the pylorus.

nodi lymphatici re·tro·au·ri·cu·la·res (ret''ro·aw·rick·yoo·lair'eez) [NA]. Small lymph nodes lying behind the external ear.

nodi lymphatici re·tro·pha·ryn·gei (ret''ro·fa·rin'jee·eye) [NA]. Lymph nodes lying behind the pharynx.

nodi lymphatici sa·cra·les (sa·kray'leez) [NA]. Lymph nodes lying in the hollow of the sacrum.

nodi lymphatici sub·man·di·bu·la·res (sub·man·dib''yoo·lair'eez) [NA]. Lymph nodes associated with the submandibular salivary gland.

nodi lymphatici sub·men·ta·les (sub·men·tay'leez) [NA]. Small lymph nodes located in the submental triangle.

nodi lymphatici sub·sca·pu·la·res (sub·skap·yoo·lair'eez) [NA]. The axillary lymph nodes located along the subscapular artery.

nodi lymphatici tra·che·a·les (tray·kee·ay'leez) [NA]. Lymph nodes associated with the trachea.

nodi lymphatici tra·cheo·bron·chi·a·les in·fe·ri·o·res (tray''kee·o·bronk·ee·ay'leez in·feer·ee·o'reez) [NA]. Lymph nodes situated below the bifurcation of the trachea.

nodi lymphatici tracheobronchiales su·pe·ri·o·res (sue·peer·ee·o'reez) [NA]. Lymph nodes situated above the origin of each main bronchus.

no·dose (no'doce) *adj.* [L. *nodosus*, knotty]. Characterized by nodes or protuberances; jointed or swollen at intervals.

nodose ganglion. INFERIOR GANGLION (2).

no·dos·i·ty (no·dos'i·tee) *n.* 1. The character or state of being nodose. 2. NODE.

nod·u·lar (nod'yoo·lur) *adj.* Of or like a nodule; characterized by nodules.

nodular calcification. DENTICLE (2).

nodular dermal allergid. A dermatosis characterized clinically by nodules and histologically by vasculitis, presumably due to an allergic mechanism.

nodular goiter. ADENOMATOUS GOITER.

nodular headache. MUSCLE-CONTRACTION HEADACHE.

nodular hidradenoma. MYOEPITHELIOMA.

nodular leprosy. LEPROMATOUS LEPROSY.

nodular lymphoma. A variety of malignant lymphoma in which the anaplastic cells grow in such a fashion as to produce nodules superficially resembling the follicles of normal lymph nodes; it is associated with a better prognosis than that of the diffuse form. Syn. *Brill-Symmers disease, follicular lymphoma, giant follicular lymphoblastoma* or *lymphoma, lymphoreticulosis.*

nodular salpingitis. A form of salpingitis marked by formation of solid nodules.

nodular subepidermal fibrosis. DERMATOFIBROMA.

nod·u·la·tion (nod''yoo·lay'shun) *n.* The formation of nodules or the state of being nodular. —**nod·u·lat·ed** (nod'yoo·lay·tid) *adj.*

nod·ule (nod'yool) *n.* [L. *nodulus*, dim. of *nodus*, knot]. 1. A small node. 2. A small aggregation of cells. 3. *In dermatology*, one of the primary skin lesions, a circumscribed solid elevation of varying size but larger than a papule, which is of the order of 1 cm or less.

nodule disease. Oesophagostomiasis in ruminants, characterized by nodules in the mucous membranes of the intestine; the nodules contain the larval form of species of *Oesophagostomum.*

nodule of the cerebellum. NODULUS (2).

nodules of Arantius [G. C. *Arantius*]. NODULES OF THE SEMILUNAR VALVES.

nodules of the semilunar valves. Nodules in the midportion of the pulmonary and aortic semilunar valves, but more pronounced in the latter. NA *noduli valvularum semilunarium.*

noduli. Plural of *nodulus.*

noduli ag·gre·ga·ti pro·ces·sus ver·mi·for·mis (ag·re·gay'tye pro·ses'us vur·mi·for'mis) [BNA]. FOLLICULI LYMPHATICI AGGREGATI APPENDICIS VERMIFORMIS.

noduli Aran·tii (a·ran'shee·eye, ·tee·eye) [G. C. *Arantius*]. NODULES OF THE SEMILUNAR VALVES.

noduli cu·ta·nei (kew·tay'nee·eye) [L., cutaneous nodules]. DERMATOFIBROMA.

noduli lym·pha·ti·ci ag·gre·ga·ti (lim·fat'i·sigh ag·re·gay'tye) [BNA]. FOLLICULI LYMPHATICI AGGREGATI INTESTINI TENUIS.

noduli lymphatici bron·chi·a·les (bronk·ee·ay'leez) [BNA]. Small lymph nodules associated with the bronchi.

noduli lymphatici con·junc·ti·va·les (kon·junk''ti·vay'leez) [BNA]. Lymphatic nodules in the conjunctiva.

noduli lymphatici gas·tri·ci (gas'tri·sigh) [BNA]. FOLLICULI LYMPHATICI GASTRICI.

noduli lymphatici in·te·sti·ni rec·ti (in·tes·tye'nigh reck'tye) [BNA]. FOLLICULI LYMPHATICI RECTI.

noduli lymphatici la·ryn·gei (la·rin'jee·eye) [BNA]. FOLLICULI LYMPHATICI LARYNGEI.

noduli lymphatici li·e·na·les (lye·e·nay'leez) [BNA]. FOLLICULI LYMPHATICI LIENALES.

noduli lymphatici so·li·ta·rii in·te·sti·ni cras·si (sol·i·tair'ee·eye in·tes·tye'nigh kras'eye) [BNA]. FOLLICULI LYMPHATICI SOLITARII INTESTINI CRASSI.

noduli lymphatici solitarii intestini te·nu·is (ten'yoo·is) [BNA]. FOLLICULI LYMPHATICI SOLITERII INTESTINI TENUIS.

noduli lymphatici tu·ba·rii (tew·bair'ee·eye) [BNA]. Lymph follicles associated with the medial end of the auditory tube.

noduli lymphatici va·gi·na·les (vaj·i·nay'leez) [BNA]. Lymph follicles in the mucous membrane of the vagina.

noduli lymphatici ve·si·ca·les (ves·i·kay'leez) [BNA]. Lymph follicles in the mucous membrane of the urinary bladder.

noduli thy·mi·ci ac·ces·so·rii (thigh'mi·sigh ack''se·so'ree·eye) [NA]. Accessory nodules of the thymus.

noduli val·vu·la·rum se·mi·lu·na·ri·um (val·vew·lair'um sem''i·lew·nair'ee·um) [NA]. NODULES OF THE SEMILUNAR VALVES.

no·du·lus (nod'yoo·lus, no'dew·lus) *n.*, pl. **nodu·li** (·lye) [L.]. 1. NODULE. 2. [NA] One of the anterior subdivisions of the vermis of the cerebellum.

nodulus lym·pha·ti·cus (lim·fat'i·kus) [BNA]. Folliculus lymphaticus (= LYMPH NODE).

no·dus (no'dus) *n.*, pl. & genit. sing. **no·di** (·dye) [L., knot]. NODE.

nodus atrio·ven·tri·cu·la·ris (ay″tree·o·ven·trick″yoo·lair′is) [NA]. ATRIOVENTRICULAR NODE.

nodus lym·pha·ti·cus (lim·fat′i·kus), pl. **nodi lymphati·ci** (·sigh) [NA]. LYMPH NODE.

nodus lymphaticus ju·gu·lo·di·gas·tri·cus (jug″yoo·lo·dye·gas′tri·kus) [NA]. A deep cervical lymph node associated with the internal jugular vein beneath the digastric muscle.

nodus lymphaticus ju·gu·lo·omo·hy·oi·de·us (jug″yoo·lo·o″mo·high·oy′dee·us) [NA]. A deep cervical lymph node associated with the internal jugular vein near the omohyoid muscle.

nodus lymphaticus ti·bi·a·lis anterior (tib·ee·ay′lis) [NA]. A lymph node associated with the anterior tibial artery.

nodus si·nu·atri·a·lis (sigh″new·ay″tree·ay′lis) [NA]. SINOATRIAL NODE.

noe·gen·e·sis (no″e·jen′e·sis) *n.* [Gk. *noein*, to think, perceive, + *genesis*]. *In psychology,* the utmost degree of creativeness attainable by the mind, particularly the creation of new knowledge on the basis of a pure feeling.

no·e·ma·ta·chom·e·ter (no·ee′muh·ta·kom′e·tur) *n.* [Gk. *noēma,* perception, + *tachometer*]. An apparatus for estimating the time taken in recording a simple perception.

no·e·mat·ic (no·e·mat′ick) *adj.* [Gk. *noematikos,* rational, from *noēma,* thought, idea]. Pertaining to thought or to any mental process.

no·e·sis (no·ee′sis) *n.* [Gk. *noēsis,* intelligence, understanding]. *In pyschology,* the cognitive process; perception, understanding, and reasoning. —**no·et·ic** (no·et′ick) *adj.*

no·gal·a·my·cin (no·gal″uh·migh′sin) *n.* An antibiotic, produced by *Streptomyces nogalaster,* that has antineoplastic activity.

noisy shoulder. A grating over the scapula on moving the shoulder up and down, believed to be due to a snapping tendon or bursitis.

Noludar. Trademark for methyprylon, a nonbarbiturate sedative and hypnotic.

no·ma (no′muh) *n.* [Gk. *nomē,* spread, spreading ulcer]. Spreading gangrene beginning in the mucous membranes, most frequently in the mouth, but also the nose, external auditory canals, genitalia, or anus, usually following an infectious disease such as measles, and seen most frequently in children under conditions of poor hygiene and nutrition; generally regarded as a malignant form of infection by fusospirochetal organisms. Noma of the mouth is also known as gangrenous stomatitis.

no·mad·ic (no·mad′ick) *adj.* [Gk. *nomadikos,* pastoral, roving]. Spreading; wandering; loose.

noma of the penis. An extremely rare gangrenous ulceration of the penis, seen in young boys.

noma pu·den·di (pew·den′dye). A rare gangrenous ulceration occurring about the genital region of female children.

noma vul·vae (vul′vee). NOMA PUDENDI.

no·men·cla·ture (no′min·klay″chur, no·meng′kluh·chur) *n.* [L. *nomenclatura,* list of names]. A systematic arrangement of the distinctive names employed in any science. See also *BNA, BR, NA, JNA, NK.*

no·mi·fen·sine (no″mi·fen′seen) *n.* 8-Amino-1,2,3,4-tetrahydro-2-methyl-4-phenylisoquinoline, $C_{16}H_{18}N_2$, an antidepressant, usually used as the maleate salt.

No·mi·na An·a·to·mi·ca (nom′i·nuh an″uh·tom′i·kuh, no′mi·nuh). The international anatomical nomenclature in Latin. A revision of the Basle Nomina Anatomica, approved originally in Paris in 1955. Abbreviated, NA.

nom·i·nal (nom′i·nul) *adj.* [L. *nominalis*]. 1. Pertaining to names. 2. In name only; formal, token.

nominal aphasia. ANOMIA.

nomo·gram (nom′o·gram) *n.* NOMOGRAPH.

nomo·graph (nom′o·graf) *n.* [Gk. *nomos,* law, + *-graph*]. A graph on which appear graduated lines for all variables in a formula, arranged in such a manner that the value of one variable can be read on the appropriate line from a knowledge of the values of the other variables.

nomo·top·ic (nom″o·top′ick) *adj.* [Gk. *nomos,* custom, use, + *-topic*]. Occurring at the usual site.

¹non- [L.]. A prefix meaning *not.*

²non- [L. *nonus,* ninth]. A combining form meaning *ninth, nine, nine times.*

no·na (no′nuh) *n.* [It., of obscure origin, perhaps from *nona,* ninth (the disease supposedly coming nine days after onset of influenza)]. An illness which was observed toward the end of the epidemic of influenza of 1889–1890 and which was characterized by profound and prolonged sleep. The illness was often fatal but no neurologic residua were recorded in patients who recovered. A relationship to encephalitis lethargica, suspected by some, has never been established.

non·ab·sorb·able (non″ub·sor′buh·bul) *adj.* Not absorbable.

nonabsorbable ligature. A ligature made of a substance that cannot be absorbed by the tissues, such as nylon, or of slowly or incompletely absorbed substances such as silk or cotton.

non·ac·cess (non″ack′sess) *n. In legal medicine,* the absence of opportunity for, or the lack of, sexual intercourse, especially between husband and wife.

non·ac·tin (non·ack′tin) *n.* An antibiotic ionophore similar to nigericin which allows transport of K^+ into mitochondria and thereby serves to uncouple oxidative phosphorylation.

non·ad·her·ent (non″ad·heer′unt) *adj.* Not connected to an adjacent organ or part.

no·nan (no′nun) *adj.* [L. *nonanus,* of the ninth, from *nonus,* ninth]. Having an exacerbation or recurring every ninth day.

no·na·pep·tide (no″nuh·pep′tide, non″uh·) *n.* A polypeptide composed of nine amino acid groups.

non·aque·ous (non″ay′kwee·us, ·ack′wee·us) *adj.* [*non-* + *aqueous*]. Not consisting of, or pertaining to, water; said of organic solvents.

non·ar·tic·u·lar (non″ahr·tick′yoo·lur) *adj.* [*non-* + *articular*]. Not pertaining to joints.

nonarticular rheumatism. FIBROSITIS.

non·bac·te·ri·al gastroenteritis. An acute illness characterized by nausea, vomiting, and diarrhea, generally assumed to be caused by as yet unknown viruses. Syn. *winter vomiting disease.*

non·chro·maf·fin (non·kro′muh·fin, ·kro·maf′in) *adj.* [*non-* + *chromaffin*]. Not chromaffin; not involving chromaffin cells.

nonchromaffin paraganglioma. CHEMODECTOMA.

nonchromaffin paraganglioma of the middle ear. GLOMUS JUGULARE TUMOR.

noncommunicating hydrocephalus. OBSTRUCTIVE HYDROCEPHALUS.

noncompetitive inhibition. *In biochemistry,* inhibition of enzyme action based solely on the concentration of the inhibitor; substrate concentration is not a factor. Contr. *competitive inhibition, uncompetitive inhibition.*

non com·pos men·tis (non kom′pus men′tis) [L.]. Of unsound mind.

non·con·duc·tor (non″kun·duck′tur) *n.* Any substance not transmitting electricity or heat.

noncongestive glaucoma. OPEN-ANGLE GLAUCOMA.

non·de·form·ing, *adj.* Not deforming.

nondeforming clubfoot. TALIPES CAVUS.

non·dis·junc·tion (non″dis·junk′shun) *n.* [*non-* + *disjunction*]. 1. The failure of homologous material to separate at meiosis. 2. The failure of sister chromosomes to separate in an ordinary mitosis.

non·dom·i·nant (non″dom′i·nunt) *adj.* Not dominant.

nondominant hemisphere. The cerebral hemisphere which does not control the production and/or the comprehension of spoken or written language, or both; usually, even in left-handed individuals, the right hemisphere. Syn. *minor hemisphere, representational hemisphere.*

non·elec·tro·lyte (non″e·leck′tro·lite) *n.* [*non-* + *electrolyte*]. A substance which in solution does not dissociate into ions and is therefore unable to conduct an electric current.

non·en·cap·su·lat·ed (non″en·kap′sue·lay′tid) *adj.* Not encapsulated.

nonencapsulated sclerosing tumor. A small, well-differentiated papillary thyroid carcinoma with marked stromal fibrosis.

nonendemic goitrous cretinism. Cretinism as a result of defective synthesis of thyroid hormone due to defects in the trapping of iodide by the thyroid, iodide organification, coupling, deiodinase activity, or the production of an abnormal serum iodoprotein.

non·equil·i·bra·to·ry (non″e·kwil′i·bruh·tor″ee, ·ee″kwi·lib′) *adj.* 1. Not pertaining to equilibrium. 2. Pertaining to or characterized by disequilibrium.

nonequilibratory ataxia. Disturbance of coordination involving the extremities and sparing equilibrium; usually due to a lesion of one or both cerebellar hemispheres, or of deep sensory pathways.

nonfluent aphasia. Aphasia in which speech is sparse, produced slowly with great effort, poorly articulated, agrammatical, and telegraphic in quality; due to a lesion in Broca's area. Contr. *fluent aphasia.*

non·gran·u·lar (non″gran′yoo·lur) *adj.* Not granular.

nongranular leukocyte. A leukocyte with relatively clear, homogeneous cytoplasm, such as a lymphocyte or monocyte.

no·ni·grav·i·da (no″ni·grav′i·duh, non″i·) *n.* [*non-*, ninth, + *-gravida*]. A woman pregnant for the ninth time.

non·ion·ic (non″eye·on′ick) *adj.* Not ionic.

no·nip·a·ra (no·nip′uh·ruh, non·ip′) *n.* [*non-*, ninth, + *-para*]. A woman who has been in labor nine times.

non·la·mel·lar (non″luh·mel′ur, ·lam′ul·ur) *adj.* Not lamellar.

nonlamellar bone. Bone in which the matrix is not layered.

nonlipid histiocytosis. LETTERER-SIWE DISEASE.

nonlipid reticuloendotheliosis. LETTERER-SIWE DISEASE.

non·lu·et·ic (non″lew·et′ick) *adj.* [*non-* + *luetic*]. Not due to syphilitic infection.

nonluetic Argyll Robertson pupil. ADIE'S PUPIL.

non·med·ul·la·ted (non″med′uh·lay″tid, ·me·dul′) *adj.* [*non-* + *medullated*]. UNMYELINATED.

non·mo·tile (non·mo′til) *adj.* Not motile; not having the power of active motion.

non·my·e·li·nat·ed (non″migh′e·lin·ay″tid) *adj.* UNMYELINATED.

Non·ne-Apelt test (noʰn′eʰ, ah′pᵉlt) [M. *Nonne*, German neurologist, 1861–1959; and F. *Apelt*]. An outmoded test for excess albumin or globulin in spinal fluid in which saturated ammonium sulfate is used as the reagent.

Nonne-Marie syndrome [M. *Nonne* and P. *Marie*]. MARIE'S HEREDITARY CEREBELLAR ATAXIA.

Nonne-Milroy-Meige syndrome [M. *Nonne*, W. *Milroy*, and H. *Meige*]. MILROY'S DISEASE.

Nonne's disease [M. *Nonne*]. MILROY'S DISEASE.

non·nu·cle·at·ed (non″new′klee·ay″tid) *adj.* Without a nucleus, as a mature erythrocyte.

non·opaque (non″o·pake′) *adj.* Radiolucent or relatively permeable to x-rays; not opaque.

non·ose (non′oce) *n.* A monosaccharide which contains nine carbon atoms in the molecule.

non·os·si·fy·ing (non″os′i·figh·ing) *adj.* Not ossifying; non-bone-forming.

nonossifying fibroma. A common benign tumor of bone, exhibiting no osteogenic tendencies, usually found in the shaft of long bones, and histologically characterized by whorls of spindle-shaped connective-tissue cells.

non·os·teo·gen·ic (non″os·tee·o·jen′ick) *adj.* Not producing bone.

nonosteogenic fibroma. NONOSSIFYING FIBROMA.

non·ovu·la·to·ry (non″o′vyoo·luh·tor″ee) *adj.* Not ovulatory; not during ovulation.

non·ox·y·nol (non·ock′si·nol) *n.* A generic name for various nonylphenoxypolyethyleneoxyethanols of the composition $C_9H_{19}{\cdot}C_6H_4(OCH_2CH_2)_nOH$. Specific compounds are identified by appending a number representing the approximate value of *n* in the preceding formula. Nonoxynol 4, nonoxynol 15, and nonoxynol 30 are used as nonionic surfactants; nonoxynol 9 is a spermatocide.

non·par·a·lyt·ic poliomyelitis. Infection by poliomyelitis virus, generally characterized by upper respiratory and/or gastrointestinal symptoms, pain and stiffness in the muscles of the axial skeleton, especially of the neck and back, mild fever, and often increased amounts of protein and number of leukocytes in the cerebrospinal fluid. This may be the clinical maximum of the disease. Definitive diagnosis rests upon isolation of the virus and serological reactions. Contr. *paralytic spinal poliomyelitis, paralytic bulbar poliomyelitis.*

non·par·a·sit·ic sycosis (non″păr″uh·sit′ick). Sycosis due to the presence of coccogenic organisms.

non·par·ous (non″păr′us) *adj.* NULLIPAROUS.

non·patho·gen (non″path′o·jin) *n.* An organism or substance that is not pathogenic. —**non·patho·gen·ic** (non″path″o·jen′ick) *adj.*

non·pa·thog·nom·ic (non″path″ug·nom′ick, ·no′mick) *adj.* NONPATHOGNOMONIC.

non·pa·thog·no·mon·ic (non″path″ug·nuh·mon′ick, ·pa·thog″) *adj.* Not pathognomonic; of symptoms or signs, accessory.

non·pro·pri·e·tary (non″pro·prye′e·terr″ee) *adj.* Not proprietary.

non·pro·tein (non″pro′tee·in, ·teen) *adj.* Not derived from protein, as nonprotein nitrogen; not containing protein, as nonprotein fraction of an extract.

nonprotein nitrogen. The fraction of nitrogen in the blood, tissues, urine, and excreta not precipitated by the usual protein precipitants such as sodium tungstate. Abbreviated, N.P.N.

nonprotein respiratory quotients. The ratio of the volume of carbon dioxide given off to the volume of oxygen consumed after the subtraction from these gas volumes of the amounts utilized in protein metabolism.

non·psy·chot·ic organic brain syndrome (non″sigh·kot′ick). Any organic brain syndrome in which there is no evidence of psychosis. Often referred to in children as minimal brain dysfunction syndrome.

non·pu·ru·lent (non·pewr′yoo·lunt) *adj.* [*non-* + *purulent*]. NONPYOGENIC.

non·pyo·gen·ic (non″pye·o·jen′ick) *adj.* [*non-* + *pyogenic*]. Not inducing the formation of pus.

non·re·frac·tive (non″re·frack′tiv) *adj.* Not possessing properties permitting the refraction of light rays.

non-REM sleep. NREM SLEEP.

non·re·straint (non″re·straint′) *n. In psychiatry*, the treatment of a psychotic, particularly a manic individual, without any forcible means of compulsion.

non·seg·ment·ed (non″seg′men·tid) *adj.* Not segmented.

nonsegmented polymorphonuclear cell. BAND CELL.

nonsense mutation. One of three codons that specify no amino acid, but cause polypeptide chain termination. See also *amber mutation, ochre mutation, opal mutation.*

nonsense syndrome. GANSER SYNDROME.

non·sep·tate (non″sep′tate) *adj.* Not septate; lacking septa.

non·spe·cif·ic (non″spe·sif′ick) *adj.* 1. Not attributable to any one definite cause, as a disease not caused by one particular microorganism, or an immunity not conferred by a specific antibody. 2. Of medicines or therapy, not counteracting any one causative agent.

nonspecific granuloma of the intestine. REGIONAL ENTERITIS.

nonspecific hepatitis. 1. INTERSTITIAL HEPATITIS. 2. Hepatitis not associated with a known cause.

nonspecific immunity. Resistance not assignable to specific antibodies or specific cellular immunity, and including such factors as genetics (innate immunity), age, sex, or hormonal factors.

nonspecific inflammation. Simple inflammation, as opposed to granulomatous inflammation.

nonspecific protein therapy. Treatment which recognizes that stock and autogenous vaccines may owe a part of their value in disease therapy to nonspecific effects; for example, peptone, milk, normal serum, etc., have been employed to replace bacterial products.

nonspecific urethritis. An acute nongonococcal urethritis with a urethral discharge and dysuria; common as a venereal infection; *Chlamidia* and *Mycoplasma* have been implicated in some cases.

non·spo·rog·e·nous (non″spo·roj′e·nus) *adj*. Not sporogenous; not producing spores.

non·strep·to·coc·cal exudative pharyngitis (non·strep″tuh·kock′ul). Exudative pharyngitis which resembles streptococcal pharyngitis but in which group A streptococci are not found. Etiologic agents associated include *Corynebacterium diptheriae*, Epstein-Barr virus, and others.

non·stri·at·ed (non″strye′ay·tid) *adj*. Not striated; smooth.

nonstriated muscle. SMOOTH MUSCLE.

non·sup·pu·ra·tive (non″sup′yoo·ray″tiv) *adj*. [*non-* + *suppurative*]. Uninfected; surgically clean; not forming pus.

nonsuppurative choroiditis. Inflammation of the choroid without necrosis.

nonsuppurative sclerosing osteomyelitis. GARRÉ'S OSTEOMYELITIS.

non·sur·gi·cal (non″sur′ji·kul) *adj*. Not surgical; without surgical operation.

non·sym·bol·ic visual agnosia (non″sim·bol′ick). VISUAL OBJECT AGNOSIA.

non·throm·bo·cy·to·pe·nic (non″throm″bo·sigh·to·pee′nick) *adj*. Not thrombocytopenic.

non·throm·bo·pe·nic (non″throm·bo·pee′nick) *adj*. NONTHROMBOCYTOPENIC.

non·trop·i·cal sprue (non″trop′i·kul). A form of the celiac syndrome seen in adults, which is associated with an intolerance to the gliadin fraction of gluten found in wheat, oats, and rye. Syn. *idiopathic adult steatorrhea*. See also *infantile celiac disease, celiac syndrome*.

non·un·ion (non″yoon′yun) *n*. Failure of union; especially, failure of fractured bone ends to unite firmly.

non·ve·ne·re·al (non″ve·neer′ee·ul) *adj*. Not venereal.

nonvenereal syphilis. 1. Syphilis not acquired during sexual intercourse. 2. BEJEL.

non·vi·a·ble (non″vye′uh·bul) *adj*. Not viable; incapable of surviving.

non·vi·su·al·iza·tion (non″vizh″yoo·ul·i·zay′shun, ·eye·zay′shun) *n*. Failure of an excretory organ to opacify roentgenographically after administration of radiopaque contrast materials which normally opacify that organ.

non·yl (non′il, no′nil) *n*. The univalent hydrocarbon radical $CH_3(CH_2)_8$—.

noo- [Gk. *nous, noos*]. A combining form meaning *mind* or *mentality*.

noo·klo·pia (no″o·klo′pee·uh) *n*. [*noo-* + Gk. *klopeia*, brigandage, thievery]. CASTROPHRENIA.

Noon pollen unit [L. *Noon*, English physician, 1878–1913]. The quantity of pollen extract which contains 0.00001 mg of total nitrogen.

noo·psy·che (no′o·sigh″kee) *n*. [*noo-* + *psyche*]. Mental or reasoning processes.

noo·tro·pic (no″o·tro′pick, ·trop′ick) *adj*. [*noo-* + *-tropic*]. Tending to affect neurons favorably.

N.O.P.H.N. National Organization for Public Health Nursing.

nor- [*nor*mal]. A prefix indicating (a) *removal from a parent compound of a radical* (often methyl) *to form another compound;* (b) *a compound of normal structure isomeric with another compound having the same name but without the prefix,* as norleucine and leucine.

nor·a·cy·meth·a·dol (nor″uh·sigh·meth′uh·dol) *n*. 6-(Methylamino)-4,4-diphenyl-3-heptanol acetate, $C_{22}H_{29}NO_2$, an analgesic; used as the hydrochloride salt.

nor·adren·a·line (nor″uh·dren′uh·lin, ·leen) *n*. Norepinephrine or levarterenol, commonly the *l*- form.

nor·bi·o·tin (nor″bye′uh·tin, nor′bye″) *n*. A homolog of biotin containing one less CH_2 group in the side chain; it is an antagonist of biotin toward some bacteria but is capable of replacing biotin in certain of its functions toward other organisms.

nor·bol·eth·one (nor·bole′eth·ohn) *n*. 13-Ethyl-17-hydroxy-18,19-dinor-17α-pregn-4-en-3-one, $C_{21}H_{32}O_2$, an anabolic steroid.

Nor·dau·ism (nor′daw·iz·um) *n*. [M. S. *Nordau*, German physician and author, 1849–1923]. DEGENERACY (1).

Nor·dau's disease (nor′daw) [M. S. *Nordau*]. DEGENERACY (1).

nor·de·frin (nor′de·frin, nor·def′rin) *n*. *dl*-3,4-Dihydroxynorephedrine, $C_9H_{13}NO_3$, isomeric with epinephrine; a vasoconstrictor used in solutions of local anesthetic agents employed in dentistry.

nor·ephed·rine (nor″e·fed′rin, nor·ef′i·dreen) *n*. Phenylpropanolamine, representing ephedrine in which the methyl radical of the amino group is replaced by hydrogen.

nor·epi·neph·rine (nor·ep″i·nef′reen, ·rin) *n*. α-(Aminomethyl)-3,4-dihydroxybenzyl alcohol, $C_8H_{11}NO_3$, a demethylated epinephrine. The levorotatory isomer (levarterenol) is formed at sympathetic nerve endings as a mediator of functional activity; it is probably the postulated sympathin E. Therapeutically it is useful for maintenance of blood pressure in acute hypotensive states caused by surgical and nonsurgical trauma, central vasomotor depression, and hemorrhage; the bitartrate salt is commonly employed. Syn. *arterenol, noradrenaline*.

nor·eth·an·dro·lone (nor″eth·an′druh·lone) *n*. 17α-Ethyl-17-hydroxy-19-nor-4-androsten-3-one, $C_{20}H_{30}O_2$, an androgenic steroid with anabolic activity used clinically for the latter effect.

nor·eth·in·drone (nor·eth′in·drone) *n*. 17α-Ethinyl-19-nortestosterone, $C_{20}H_{26}O_2$, a potent, orally active progestogen that produces clinical effects similar to those of progesterone; also used, in combination with an estrogen, as an oral contraceptive.

nor·ethy·no·drel (nor″e·thigh′no·drel, ·eth′i·no·) *n*. 17-Hydroxy-19-nor-17α-pregn-5(10)-en-20-yn-3-one, $C_{20}H_{26}O_2$, a progestogen; used principally, in combination with the estrogen mestranol, to inhibit ovulation and control fertility.

Norflex. A trademark for orphenadrine, an antispasmodic and antitremor drug used as the citrate salt.

nor·flu·rane (nor·floo′rane) *n*. 1,1,1,2-Tetrafluoroethane, CH_2FCF_3, a general inhalation anesthetic.

nor·ges·ti·mate (nor·jes′ti·mate) *n*. (+)-13-Ethyl-17-hydroxy-18,19-dinor-17α-pregn-4-en-20-yn-3-one oxime acetate (ester), $C_{23}H_{31}NO_3$, a progestin.

nor·ges·to·met (nor·jes′to·met) *n*. 17-Hydroxy-11β-methyl-19-norpregn-4-ene-3,20-dione acetate, $C_{23}H_{32}O_4$, a progestin.

nor·ges·trel (nor·jes′trel) *n*. (±)-13-Ethyl-17-hydroxy-18,19-dinor-17α-pregn-4-en-20-yn-3-one, $C_{21}H_{28}O_2$, a progestational steroid.

Norisodrine. A trademark for isoproterenol, a sympathomimetic amine used, as the hydrochloride or sulfate salt, principally as a bronchodilator.

nor·leu·cine (nor·lew′seen, ·sin) *n*. 2-Aminohexanoic acid, $C_6H_{13}NO_2$, an amino acid.

nor·leu·cyl (nor·lew′sil) *n*. The univalent radical, $CH_3CH_2CH_2CH_2CH(NH_2)CO$—, of the amino acid norleucine.

Norlutin. Trademark for norethindrone, an orally active progestogen.

norm, *n.* [L. *norma,* rule]. A standard representing the average, typical, or acceptable.

nor·ma (nor'muh) *n.*, pl. **nor·mae** (·mee) [L., rule, model]. *In anatomy,* a view or aspect, essentially of the skull.

norma anterior. NORMA FACIALIS.

norma ba·si·la·ris (bas″i·lair'is). The inferior aspect of the skull.

norma fa·ci·a·lis (fay″shee·ay'lis). The front view or facial aspect of the skull.

norma inferior. The inferior aspect of the skull; the view of the skull from below.

nor·mal, *adj.* [L. *normalis,* from *norma*]. 1. Conforming to some ideal norm or standard; pertaining to the central values of some homogeneous group, as that which is typical of or acceptable to a majority or dominant group; average, common, mean, median, standard, typical, usual, ideal, modal. 2. *In medicine and psychology,* "healthy," i.e., lacking observable or detectable clinical abnormalities, deficiencies, or diseases; also, pertaining to or describing a value or measurement obtained in an ideal group by a particular method, i.e., a value which in itself is not significant of disease; pertaining to the normal variability of an individual's anatomical, physiological, and psychological pattern within the parameters of age, sex, social and physical anthropological factors, population or segment thereof to which the individual belongs, and variability in time, activity, etc. Normal variability frequently is used to cover the values falling within some range, usually the 95-percent range of some factor or factors (mental, physical, emotional, social) measured in a random or selected sample of population or even an individual by standardized methods and recording system during many observations. 3. *In chemistry,* referring to solutions containing the equivalent weight of a substance, in grams, in a liter. Abbreviated, N. 4. *In mathematics,* pertaining to a right angle, i.e., in a perpendicular line or plane.

norma la·te·ra·lis (lat″e·ray'lis). A profile view or lateral aspect of the skull.

normal covalent bond. A bond consisting of a pair of electrons shared by two atoms and thus joining them, one electron being contributed by each atom.

nor·mal·cy (nor'mul·see) *n.* The condition or state of being normal (1,2).

normal distribution. *In statistics,* a frequency distribution, specified by its mathematical form and two constants, the mean and the standard deviation. This distribution is continuous and bell-shaped; 95 percent of the area covered by the distribution curve lies within two standard deviations below and two above the mean. This distribution describes adequately some individual biological measurements and many random sample measurements.

normal dwarf. HYPOPLASTIC DWARF.

normal equivalent deviate. In biological assay, conversion of a percentage response, for example, cases which responded to a certain dose, into the deviation on the normal frequency curve to which the percentage is equivalent, and used to obtain a linear relation between log dose and percentage response. See also *probit.*

normal histology. The microscopic anatomy of healthy tissues.

normal horse serum. Serum obtained from an unimmunized horse. See also *horse serum.*

nor·mal·i·ty (nor·mal'i·tee) *n.* The quality or state of being normal.

normal-pressure hydrocephalus. LOW-PRESSURE HYDROCEPHALUS.

normal probability curve. The curve represented by the equation

$$y = \frac{1}{\sigma\sqrt{2\pi}}\, l - \frac{x^2}{2\sigma^2}$$

in which the ordinate y shows the relative frequency of differences or deviations from the mean represented by the corresponding abscissa x in a large group of observations; σ represents the standard deviation of the distribution; π equals 3.1416 . . . ; e equals 2.7182 . . . .

normal reflex bladder. A reflex bladder with relatively normal capacity and that empties itself automatically at relatively normal intervals.

normal retinal correspondence. The normal condition in which the retinal image formed at the macula of one eye is associated with that formed at the macula of the other eye.

normal saline solution. SODIUM CHLORIDE IRRIGATION; a sterile solution of 0.9 g of sodium chloride in 100 ml of purified water. Isotonic with body fluids; variously used as a physiological salt solution but not to be employed parenterally, for which purpose sodium chloride injection is used. Syn. *normal salt solution.*

normal salt. A salt of an acid and base that have completely neutralized each other. The reaction in solution may be neutral, acid, alkaline, or amphoteric.

normal salt solution. NORMAL SALINE SOLUTION.

normal solution. A solution containing one gram-equivalent weight of reagent in 1,000 ml of solution.

normal tremor. A tremor present in all muscle groups of the body that persists throughout the waking state and sleep. It is so fine that it cannot be recognized by the naked eye and requires special instruments to be detected. It ranges in frequency between 8 and 13 Hz, the usual rate being 10 Hz in adults and somewhat slower in children and in the elderly. Syn. *physiologic tremor.*

Nor·man-Wood disease. CONGENITAL AMAUROTIC FAMILIAL IDIOCY.

norma oc·ci·pi·ta·lis (ock·sip″i·tay'lis). The view of the skull from behind; the posterior aspect of the skull.

norma sa·git·ta·lis (saj·i·tay'lis). The skull seen in a sagittal section.

norma superior. NORMA VERTICALIS.

norma ven·tra·lis (ven·tray'lis). The inferior aspect of the skull; the view of the skull from below.

norma ver·ti·ca·lis (vur·ti·kay'lis). The superior aspect of the skull; the view of the skull from above.

nor·met·a·neph·rine (nor·met″uh·nef'reen) *n.* 3-*o*-Methylnorepinephrine, $C_9H_{13}NO_3$, an inactive metabolite of norepinephrine excreted in the urine, where its measurement is used as a test for pheochromocytoma.

normo-. A combining form meaning *normal.*

nor·mo·blast (nor'mo·blast) *n.* [*normo-* + *-blast*]. 1. The smallest of the nucleated precursors of the erythrocyte, and of slightly larger size than the adult erythrocyte. It has almost a full complement of hemoglobin and shows a small, centrally placed chromatic and pyknotic nucleus. It is usually considered that a single normoblast gives rise to a single erythrocyte. 2. In some terminologies, any nucleated cell of the erythrocytic series.

nor·mo·cal·ce·mia, nor·mo·cal·cae·mia (nor″mo·kal·see'mee·uh) *n.* [*normo-* + *calc-* + *-emia*]. The condition of having a normal blood calcium level. —**normocalce·mic, normocalcae·mic** (·mick) *adj.*

nor·mo·chro·mat·ic (nor″mo·kro·mat'ick) *adj.* [*normo-* + *chromatic*]. Pertaining to the microscopical appearance of cells of the erythrocytic series which show normal staining characteristics, and are considered to have their full complement of hemoglobin and no residual basophilic material in their cytoplasm. —**normochro·ma·sia** (·may'zee·uh) *n.*

nor·mo·chro·mia (nor″mo·kro'mee·uh) *n.* [*normo-* + *-chromia,* coloring, pigmentation]. Normal hemoglobin content of the blood.

nor·mo·chro·mic (nor″mo·kro'mick) *adj.* Pertaining to or characterizing blood in which the erythrocytes have a mean corpuscular hemoglobin (MCH) or color index and a mean corpuscular hemoglobin concentration (MCHC) or saturation index within (plus or minus) two standard deviations of the mean normal as determined by the same method on the blood of healthy persons of the same age and sex group.

normochromic anemia. A type of anemia in which the hemoglobin content of the red blood cell is normal.

nor·mo·cyte (nor'mo·site) *n.* [*normo-* + *-cyte*]. An erythrocyte having both a diameter and a mean corpuscular volume (MCV) within (plus or minus) two standard deviations of the mean normal determined by the same method on the blood of healthy persons of the same age and sex group. —**nor·mo·cyt·ic** (nor''mo·sit'ick) *adj.*

normocytic anemia. Anemia in which the erythrocytes are of normal size.

nor·mo·cy·to·sis (nor''mo·sigh·to'sis) *n.* [*normo-* + *-cyte* + *-osis,* condition]. A normal state of the cells of the blood.

nor·mo·gly·ce·mia (nor''mo·glye·see'mee·uh) *n.* [*normo-* + *glycemia*]. Normal concentration of glucose in the blood.

nor·mo·ka·le·mic (nor''mo·ka·lee'mick) *adj.* [*normo-* + *kalemia* + *-ic*]. Having normal blood potassium levels; not hyperkalemic or hypokalemic.

nor·mo·re·flex·ia (nor''mo·re·fleck'see·uh) *n.* The state of having reflexes of the usual strength.

nor·mo·ten·sion (nor''mo·ten'shun) *n.* Normal blood pressure. Contr. *hypertension.*

nor·mo·ten·sive (nor''mo·ten'siv) *adj.* Pertaining to or having normal blood pressure; not hypertensive or hypotensive.

nor·mo·ther·mia (nor''mo·thur'mee·uh) *n.* [*normo-* + *-thermia*]. A state of normal temperature.

nor·mo·ton·ic (nor''mo·ton'ick) *adj.* Pertaining to or having normal muscular tonus.

nor·mo·to·pia (nor''mo·to'pee·uh) *n.* [*normo-* + *top-* + *-ia*]. Normal location.

nor·mo·vo·le·mia (nor''mo·vo·lee'mee·uh) *n.* [*normo-* + *volume* + *-emia*]. The blood volume found in normal healthy individuals.

Norpramin. A trademark for desipramine, a psychic stimulant drug used as the hydrochloride salt.

Nor·rie's disease [G. *Norrie,* Danish ophthalmologist, 20th century]. A rare form of sex-linked hereditary blindness characterized by peripheral vascular abnormalities, retinal malformations, vitreous opacities, and microphthalmia; sometimes accompanied by mental retardation and loss of hearing. Syn. *congenital oculoacousticocerebral degeneration.*

North African tick-bite fever. One of the tick-borne typhus fevers of Africa.

North American antisnakebite serum. A polyvalent antivenin prepared by the immunization of animals against the venom of North American snakes, principally designed to neutralize the venom of rattlesnakes, copperheads, cottonmouth moccasins, and fer-de-lance.

North American blastomycosis. A primary pulmonary infection, due to *Blastomyces dermatitidis,* that frequently disseminates to the skin and other organs. Syn. *Gilchrist disease.*

North Asian tick-borne rickettsiosis. Infection caused by *Rickettsia siberica* occurring in Siberia, Mongolia, Central Asia, and Armenia, closely related to boutonneuse fever and Rocky Mountain spotted fever.

North Queensland tick typhus. QUEENSLAND TICK TYPHUS FEVER.

nor·trip·ty·line (nor·trip'ti·leen) *n.* 5-(3-Methylaminopropylidene)-10,11-dihydro-5*H*-dibenzo[*a,d*]cycloheptene, $C_{19}H_{21}N$, an antidepressant and tranquilizing drug; used as the hydrochloride salt.

nor·val·ine (nor·val'een, ·vay'leen, ·lin) *n.* α-Amino-*n*-valeric acid, $CH_3CH_2CH_2CHNH_2COOH$, a synthetic amino acid; not found in proteins.

Nor·walk agent. A parvovirus first isolated from stools of children in Norwalk, Ohio, who experienced an outbreak of winter vomiting disease in 1964. The agent appears to cause epidemic outbreaks of acute gastroenteritis in man.

Nor·we·gian itch. A severe variety of scabies; has been seen in many countries, including the United States; scabies crustosa.

nos·ca·pine (nos'kuh·peen) *n.* An alkaloid, $C_{22}H_{23}NO_7$, from opium; used as a nonaddicting antitussive. Syn. *narcotine.*

nose, *n.* The prominent organ in the center of the face; the upper part (regio olfactoria) constitutes the organ of smell, the lower part (regio respiratoria) the beginning of the respiratory tract, in which the inspired air is warmed, moistened, and deprived of impurities. See also Plate 12.

nose·bleed, *n.* A hemorrhage from the nose. Syn. *epistaxis.*

nose clip. 1. A rubberized, spring-steel device worn by swimmers and divers to prevent the passage of water into the nose. 2. A special clamp used to close the nasal air passages in certain tests.

nose drops. A medicated liquid administered by placing drops in the nose.

No·se·ma cu·nic·u·li (no·see'muh kew·nick'yoo·lye). ENCEPHALITOZOON CUNICULI.

no·se·ma·to·sis (no·see''muh·to'sis) *n.* [*Nosema* + *-osis*]. ENCEPHALITOZOONOSIS.

nose·piece, *n.* A mechanical device screwed into the object end of the tube of the microscope, for holding an objective.

nos·er·es·the·sia (nos''ur·es·theezh'uh, ·theez'ee·uh, no·serr'') *n.* [Gk. *noseros,* unhealthy, + *-esthesia*]. Any disorder of perception.

noso- [Gk. *nosos*]. A combining form meaning *disease.*

nos·och·tho·nog·ra·phy (nos·ock''tho·nog'ruh·fee) *n.* [*noso-* + Gk. *chthōn,* earth, land, + *-graphy*]. NOSOGEOGRAPHY.

nos·o·co·mi·al (nos''o·ko'mee·ul) *adj.* [Gk. *nosokomeion,* infirmary, hospital, + *-al*]. 1. Pertaining to a hospital. 2. Of disease, caused or aggravated by hospital life.

noso·gen·e·sis (nos''o·jen'e·sis) *n.* NOSOGENY.

no·sog·e·ny (no·soj'e·nee) *n.* [*noso-* + *-geny*]. The development of diseases; PATHOGENESIS. —**noso·ge·net·ic** (nos''o·je·net'ick) *adj.*

noso·ge·og·ra·phy (nos''o·jee·og'ruh·fee) *n.* [*noso-* + *geography*]. The geographic distribution of illness, including endemic and epidemic diseases. See also *geomedicine.*

no·sol·o·gy (no·sol'uh·jee) *n.* [*noso-* + *-logy*]. The science of the classification of diseases. —**no·so·log·ic** (nos''o·loj'ick, no''so·), **nosolog·i·cal** (·i·kul) *adj.*

noso·ma·nia (nos''o·may'nee·uh) *n.* [*noso-* + *-mania*]. 1. NOSOPHOBIA. 2. A delusion that one is suffering from disease; extreme HYPOCHONDRIASIS.

no·som·e·try (no·som'e·tree) *n.* [*noso-* + *-metry*]. The calculation of morbidity rates.

noso·par·a·site (nos''o·păr'uh·site) *n.* [*noso-* + *parasite*]. A microorganism found in conjunction with a disease process which, while capable of modifying the course of the disease, is not its cause.

noso·phil·ia (nos''o·fil'ee·uh) *n.* [*noso-* + *-philia*]. Love of sickness, a desire to be ill. See also *hypochondriasis.*

noso·pho·bia (nos''o·fo'bee·uh) *n.* [*noso-* + *-phobia*]. An exaggerated fear of disease.

noso·phyte (nos'o·fite) *n.* [*noso-* + *-phyte*]. Any pathogenic vegetable microorganism.

Nos·o·psyl·lus (nos''o·sil'us) *n.* [NL., from *noso-* + Gk. *psylla,* flea]. A genus of fleas.

Nosopsyllus fas·ci·a·tus (fash''ee·ay'tus). A species of rat fleas which may transmit plague.

noso·taxy (nos'o·tack''see) *n.* [*noso-* + *-taxy,* arrangement]. Classification of diseases.

nos·tal·gia (nos·tal'juh, ·jee·uh) *n.* [Gk. *nostos,* return, homecoming, + *-algia*]. 1. A strong desire to return to things or conditions of the past. 2. HOMESICKNESS. —**nostal·gic** (·jick) *adj.*

nos·to·ma·nia (nos''to·may'nee·uh) *n.* [Gk. *nostos,* return, homecoming, + *-mania*]. A pathologic degree of nostalgia, particularly of homesickness.

nos·top·a·thy (nos·top'uh·thee) *n.* [Gk. *nostos,* homecoming, +

-pathy]. Pathogenic homecoming, as observed in veterans discharged from military service or others who have spent a considerable length of time in institutions such as hospitals or prisons. The situational factor of returning home represents a major psychological stress which precipitates illness. The stress may be a fear of assuming adult responsibilities, a reaction against a dependency situation, guilt feelings, or difficulties in controlling instinctual rivalry.

nos·to·pho·bia (nos″to·fo′bee·uh) *n.* [Gk. *nostos*, homecoming, + *-phobia*]. A fear of returning home.

nos·tras (nos′tras, ·trus) *adj.* [L., of our country]. Of a disease: belonging to the country in which it is described, in contradistinction to a similar disease originating elsewhere, as cholera nostras as distinguished from Asiatic cholera.

nos·trate (nos′trate) *adj.* [L. *nostras, nostratis*, of our country]. ENDEMIC; NOSTRAS.

nos·tril (nos′tril) *n.* One of the external orifices of the nose. NA *naris.*

nos·trum (nos′trum) *n.* [neut. sing. of L. *noster*, our]. A quack medicine; a secret medicine.

not-, noto- [Gk. *nōton*]. A combining form meaning *back, dorsal.*

no·tal·gia (no·tal′juh, ·jee·uh) *n.* [*not-* + *-algia*]. *Obsol.* Any pain in the back.

notalgia par·es·thet·i·ca (păr″es·thet′i·kuh) [NL., paresthetic]. A sensory disturbance of the region supplied by the posterior branches of the lumbar nerves; occurs occasionally in vertebral lesions.

no·tan·ce·pha·lia (no″tan·se·fay′lee·uh) *n.* [*not-*, back, + *an-*, lack, without, + *cephal-* + *-ia*]. *Obsol.* Congenital absence of the occipital part of the cranium.

no·tan·en·ce·pha·lia (no″tan·en″se·fay′lee·uh) *n.* [*not-* + *an-encephalia*]. Congenital absence of the cerebellum.

no·ta·tion (no·tay′shun) *n.* [L. *notatio*, a marking, noting]. A system of symbols to indicate in brief form more extensive ideas or data.

notch, *n.* A deep indentation; incisure. —**notched,** *adj.*

notched teeth. Teeth with irregular incisal edges due to imperfect fusion or hypoplasia of the developmental lobes. See also *Hutchinson's teeth.*

notch of Rivinus [A. *Rivinus*]. TYMPANIC NOTCH.

note-blindness, *n.* AMUSIA.

No·te·chis (no·tee′kis) *n.* [Gk. *notos*, south, + *echis*, viper]. A genus of poisonous terrestrial snakes belonging to the family Elapidae.

Notechis scu·ta·tus (skew·tay′tus) [NL., from *scutate*, scaly, from L., armed with a shield]. TIGER SNAKE.

no·ten·ceph·a·lo·cele (no″ten·sef′uh·lo·seel) *n.* [*not-* + *encephalo-* + *-cele*]. *Obsol.* An occipital encephalocele or hydrencephalocele.

no·ten·ceph·a·lus (no″ten·sef′ul·us) *n.* [*not-* + *encephal-* + *-us*]. *Obsol.* An individual with occipital encephalocele, or more usually hydrencephalocele.

Noth·na·gel's acroparesthesia (note′nah·g^el) [C. W. H. *Nothnagel*, German-Austrian physician, 1841-1905]. *Obsol.* ACROPARESTHESIA.

Nothnagel's disease, paralysis, or **syndrome** [C. W. H. *Nothnagel*]. *Obsol.* 1. ACROPARESTHESIA. 2. Unilateral oculomotor paralysis with ipsilateral cerebellar ataxia.

no·ti·fi·a·ble (no″ti·fye′uh·bul) *adj.* Pertaining to a disease which must by law be reported to health authorities.

noto-. See *not-*.

no·to·chord (no′tuh·kord) *n.* [*noto-* + *-chord*, cord]. An elongated cord of cells enclosed in a structureless sheath, which is the primitive axial skeleton of the embryo. It serves as a focal axis about which the vertebral bodies develop and persists as the nuclei pulposi of the intervertebral disks. Syn. *chorda dorsalis.* —**no·to·chord·al** (no″tuh·kor′dul) *adj.*

notochordal canal. A canal formed by a continuation of the primitive pit into the head process of mammals. It perforates the entoderm and opens into the yolk sac, thus forming a temporary connection between yolk sac and amnion.

notochordal plate. A plate of cells representing the root of the head process of the embryo after the latter becomes vesiculated. The plate becomes intercalated in the dorsal wall of the vesicle and later consolidates into the notochord.

notochordal process. HEAD PROCESS.

No·to·ed·res (no″to·ed′reez) *n.* [NL., from *noto-*, back, + Gk. *hedra*, abode]. A genus of mange mites whose species infest cats and rats, producing serious lesions.

no·to·gen·e·sis (no″to·jen′e·sis) *n.* The development of the notochord.

no·tom·e·lus (no·tom′e·lus) *n.* [*noto-* + Gk. *melos*, limb]. An individual in which supernumerary limbs are attached to the back.

Nou·ga·ret type of night blindness (noo·gah·reh′) [J. *Nougaret*, French physician, 1637-1719]. Congenital night blindness without ophthalmoscopic abnormalities, and stationary throughout life, due to an absence of rod function; transmitted as an autosomal dominant trait.

Novatrin. A trademark for homatropine methylbromide.

Novatropine. A trademark for homatropine methylbromide.

no·vo·bi·o·cin (no″vo·bye′o·sin) *n.* An antibiotic, $C_{31}H_{36}N_2O_{11}$, produced by *Streptomyces niveus* (known also as *S. spheroides*). Used as the calcium or sodium salt for treatment of staphylococcic infections.

Novocain. A trademark for procaine hydrochloride.

Novrad. Trademark for levopropoxyphene, an antitussive drug used as the napsylate salt.

nox·ious (nock′shus) *adj.* [L. *noxius*, harmful, from *noxa*, harm, injury]. Harmful, deleterious; poisonous.

Nozinan. Trademark for methotrimeprazine, a tranquilizer, nonnarcotic analgesic, and sedative.

NP In U.S. Army medicine, neuropsychiatric.

Np Symbol for neptunium.

NPD No pathologic diagnosis.

NPH Iletin. Trademark for NPH insulin or isophane insulin suspension.

NPH insulin. *N*eutral *P*rotamine *H*agedorn insulin; a preparation of isophane insulin with intermediate duration of action developed by Hagedorn; consists of crystals containing insulin, protamine, and zinc, suspended in a buffered medium of pH 7.2. Syn. *isophane insulin suspension.*

N.P.N. Abbreviation for *nonprotein nitrogen.*

n-rays, *n.pl.* [initial letter of the French city of *Nancy*]. A nonexistent form of radiant energy once considered to have a variety of properties such as ability to pass through thin metals and to increase the luminosity of phosphorescent bodies. Syn. *Blondot's rays.*

NREM sleep [*no r*apid *e*ye *m*ovements]. The phases of sleep in which neither rapid eye movements nor dreams occur; the first four stages of the normal sleep cycle. Contr. *REM sleep.*

nu·bile (new′bil) *adj.* [L., *nubilis*, from *nubere*, to marry]. Marriageable; of an age for childbearing. —**nu·bil·i·ty** (new·bil′i·tee) *n.*

nu·cel·lus (new·sel′us) *n.* [L. *nucella*, dim. of *nux*, nut, kernel]. *In botany*, the central part or nucleus of an ovule.

nu·cha (new′kuh) *n.* [ML., prob. from misreading of *nucra* (= Ar. *nuqra^h*, nape of the neck) by confusion with Ar. *nu^khā′*, spinal cord] [NA]. The nape of the neck. —**nu·chal** (·kul) *adj.*

nuchal flexure. CERVICAL FLEXURE.

nuchal ligament. An elastic ligament extending from the external occipital protuberance to the spinous process of the seventh cervical vertebra. NA *ligamentum nuchae.*

nuchal plane. PLANUM NUCHALE.

nuchal rigidity. Stiffness of the neck and resistance to passive movements, particularly flexion, usually accompanied by pain and spasm on attempts at motion; recognized widely as the most common sign, after early infancy, of meningeal irritation, notably of meningitis and bleeding into the subarachnoid space.

nuchal tubercle. An elevation projecting beneath the skin, produced by the long spinous process of the seventh cervical vertebra.

Nuck's canal or **diverticulum** (nœck) [A. *Nuck,* Dutch anatomist, 1650-1692]. CANAL OF NUCK.

Nuck's hydrocele [A. *Nuck*]. A hydrocele resulting from incomplete disappearance, in the female, of the vaginal process of the peritoneum.

nucle-, nucleo-. A combining form meaning *nucleus* or *nuclear.*

nu·cle·ar (new'klee·ur) *adj.* Pertaining to, or constituting, a nucleus.

nuclear aplasia. A congenital defect in which certain cranial nerve nuclei are absent or imperfectly developed. See also *Möbius' syndrome.*

nuclear cap. A small mass of chromophilic matter on one side of a cell nucleus.

nuclear cataract. A cataract beginning in the nucleus of the lens.

nuclear chemistry. The branch of chemistry dealing with changes in the nucleus of an atom.

nuclear cisterna. The space between the inner and outer layers of a nuclear membrane.

nuclear disintegration. Any transformation or change involving atomic nuclei.

nuclear disk. EQUATORIAL PLATE.

nuclear division. The production of two nuclei from one, either by karyokinesis in mitosis or by direct separation in amitosis.

nuclear energy. Energy released in reactions involving the nucleus of an atom, especially in quantities sufficient to be of interest in engineering or in astrophysics.

nuclear fast red. 1. A basic dye of the azine class, related to neutral red, used as a nuclear stain. 2. The sodium salt of an aminoanthraquinone sulfonic acid which forms a scarlet lake with calcium and is used as a histochemical reagent for that metal.

nuclear figures. The peculiar arrangement of the chromosomes during mitosis.

nuclear fission. *In chemistry and physics,* the splitting of certain heavy nuclei into two large fragments, accompanied by the emission of neutrons and the release of large amounts of energy.

nuclear fusion. The fusion of the nuclei of two atoms, such as the isotopes of hydrogen, at temperatures of 100 million degrees or more, to produce a single heavier nucleus and either a proton or a neutron along with kinetic energy equivalent to the difference of masses of the reactants and products.

nuclear icterus or **jaundice.** KERNICTERUS.

nuclear juice. NUCLEAR SAP.

nuclear layer. EPENDYMAL LAYER.

nuclear medicine. The branch of medicine that deals with the use of radioisotopes in diagnosis and therapy.

nuclear membrane. The covering structure of a cell nucleus, composed of a fenestrated double-layered membrane and the nuclear cisterna between them. The outer layer may have attached ribosomes and be continous with the endoplasmic reticulum.

nuclear ophthalmoplegia. Inability to move the eye due to a lesion of the nuclei of origin of the motor nerves of the eyeball.

nuclear paralysis. Paralysis from lesions of the nuclei of origin of the nerves.

nuclear physics. The branch of physics dealing with the structure, properties, and interactions of atomic nuclei.

nuclear plate. 1. The metaphase chromosomes arranged along the equatorial plate. 2. The septum which sometimes divides the nucleus in cell division.

nuclear reaction. A reaction involving an atomic nucleus, such as fission, neutron capture, radioactive decay, or fusion.

nuclear reactor. An apparatus in which nuclear fission may be sustained in a self-supporting chain reaction. It includes fissionable material such as uranium or plutonium (referred to as fuel) and generally a moderating material such as carbon or heavy water; also, a reflector to conserve escaping neutrons, and provision for heat removal. Syn. *pile.* See also *reactor.*

nuclear reticulum. The network of linin and chromatin of a nucleus.

nuclear sap. The fluid material with a nucleus, occupying the space not taken by nucleolus, linin, or chromatin. Syn. *nucleochyme.*

nuclear sclerosis. Hardening of the nucleus lentis associated with aging of the ocular lens, which also becomes less pliable, loses its normal clarity, and enlarges. Nuclear sclerosis can give rise to myopia, and in advanced cases can lead to nuclear cataract.

nuclear spindle. A spindle formed from nuclear substance, especially in some types of anastral mitoses.

nuclear stains. Basic or mordant stains devised to stain nuclei selectively.

nuclear threads. Chromatin fibrils of the cell nucleus.

nu·cle·ase (new'klee·ace, ·aze) *n.* An enzyme capable of splitting nucleic acids to nucleotides, nucleosides, or the components of the latter.

nu·cle·at·ed (new'klee·ay·tid) *adj.* [L. *nucleatus,* hardened, kernelly]. Possessing a nucleus.

nu·cle·a·tion (new''klee·ay'shun) *n.* 1. The starting of chemical or physical changes at discrete points in a system, as the formation of nuclei for condensation of vapors or for formation of crystals in a liquid. 2. The formation of cell nuclei.

nuclei. Plural and genitive singular of *nucleus.*

nuclei an·te·ri·o·res tha·la·mi (an·teer·ee·o'reez thal'uh·migh) [NA]. ANTERIOR NUCLEI OF THE THALAMUS.

nuclei ar·cu·a·ti (ahr·kew·ay'tye) [NA]. ARCUATE NUCLEI.

nu·cle·ic acid (new·klee'ick). One of a group of compounds found in nuclei and cytoplasm, which on complete hydrolysis yields pyrimidine and purine bases, a pentose sugar, and phosphoric acid. See also *deoxyribonucleic acid, ribonucleic acid, nucleoside, nucleotide.*

nuclei co·chle·a·res, ven·tra·lis et dor·sa·lis (kock·lee·air'eez ven·tray'lis et dor·say'lis) [NA]. COCHLEAR NUCLEI.

nuclei cor·po·ris ge·ni·cu·la·ti la·te·ra·lis (kor'po·ris je·nick·yoo·lay'tye lat·e·ray'lis) [NA]. The nuclei of the lateral geniculate body.

nuclei corporis ma·mil·la·ris (mam·i·lair'is) [NA]. NUCLEI OF THE MAMILLARY BODY.

nuclei corporis tra·pe·zoi·dei (trap''e·zoy'dee·eye) [NA]. NUCLEI OF THE TRAPEZOID BODY.

nu·cle·ide (new'klee·ide) *n.* A compound of nuclein with some metal, as iron, copper, silver, mercury, etc.

nu·cle·i·form (new'klee·i·form, new·klee') *adj.* Resembling a nucleus.

nuclei ha·be·nu·lae me·di·a·lis et la·te·ra·lis (ha·ben'yoo·lee mee·dee·ay'lis et lat·e·ray'lis) [NA]. HABENULAR NUCLEI.

nuclei in·tra·la·mi·na·res tha·la·mi (in''truh·lam·i·nair'eez thal'uh·migh) [NA]. INTRALAMINAR NUCLEI OF THE THALAMUS.

nuclei la·te·ra·les tha·la·mi (lat·e·ray'leez thal'uh·migh) [NA]. LATERAL NUCLEI OF THE THALAMUS.

nuclei mo·to·rii ner·vi tri·ge·mi·ni (mo·to'ree·eye nur'vye trye·jem'i·nigh) [BNA]. Plural of *nucleus motorius nervi trigemini.*

nu·cle·in (new'klee·in) *n.* Any one of a group of ill-defined complexes of protein and nucleic acid occurring in the nuclei of cells. On hydrolysis, they yield simple proteins and nucleic acid.

nu·cle·in·ase (new'klee·in·ace, ·aze) *n.* NUCLEASE.

nu·clei ner·vi acu·sti·ci (new'klee·eye nur'vye a·koos'ti·sigh) [BNA]. NUCLEI NERVI VESTIBULOCOCHLEARIS.

nuclei nervi co·chle·a·ris (kock·lee·air'ris). COCHLEAR NUCLEI.

nuclei nervi glos·so·pha·ryn·gei (glos"o·fa·rin'jee·eye) [NA]. Nuclei in the brainstem associated with the glossopharyngeal nerve, which are the ambiguus nucleus, the inferior salivatory nucleus, the nucleus of the tractus solitarius, and the nucleus dorsalis nervi glossopharyngei.

nuclei nervi tri·ge·mi·ni (trye·jem'i·nigh) [NA]. Nuclei in the brainstem associated with the trigeminal nerve, which include a motor nucleus, a main sensory nucleus, and a nucleus of the mesencephalic tract and of the spinal tract.

nuclei nervi va·gi (vay'gye) [NA]. The various nuclei associated with the vagus nerve.

nuclei nervi ve·sti·bu·la·ris (ves·tib"yoo·lair'is) [BNA]. NUCLEI VESTIBULARES.

nuclei nervi ve·sti·bu·lo·co·chle·a·ris (ves·tib"yoo·lo·kock"lee·air'is) [NA]. The various sensory nuclei of termination of the fibers of the vestibulocochlear nerve.

nuclei ner·vo·rum ce·re·bra·li·um (nur·vo'rum serr"e·bray'lee·um) [BNA]. NUCLEI NERVORUM CRANIALIUM.

nuclei ner·vo·rum cra·ni·a·li·um (nur·vo'rum kray·nee·ay'lee·um) [NA]. The nuclei of the cranial nerves, collectively.

nu·cle·in·ic acid (new"klee·in'ick). NUCLEIC ACID.

nuclei of the mamillary body. The medial, lateral, and intercalated mamillary nuclei and the premamillary and supramamillary nuclei. NA *nuclei corporis mamillaris.*

nuclei of the trapezoid body. Groups of cells scattered among the fibers of the trapezoid body; there are ventral and dorsal groups. NA *nuclei corporis trapezoidei.*

nuclei ori·gi·nis (o·rye'ji·nis) [NA]. Plural of *nucleus originis* (= NUCLEUS OF ORIGIN).

nuclei pon·tis (pon'tis) [NA]. Various groups of nerve cells situated within the basal part of the pons.

nuclei pulposi. Plural of *nucleus pulposus.*

nuclei sys·te·ma·tis ner·vo·si cen·tra·lis (sis·tee'ma·tis nur·vo'sigh sen·tray'lis) [NA]. The nuclei of the central nervous system.

nuclei teg·men·ti (teg·men'tye) [NA]. TEGMENTAL NUCLEI.

nuclei ter·mi·na·les (tur·mi·nay'leez) [BNA]. NUCLEI TERMINATIONIS.

nuclei ter·mi·na·ti·o·nis (tur"mi·nay"shee·o'nis) [NA]. Plural of *nucleus terminationis* (= NUCLEUS OF TERMINATION).

nuclei tu·be·ra·les (tew·be·ray'leez) [NA]. TUBERAL NUCLEI.

nuclei ves·ti·bu·la·res (ves·tib·yoo·lair'eez) [NA]. VESTIBULAR NUCLEI.

nucleo-. See *nucle-.*

nu·cleo·cap·sid (new"klee·o·kap'sid) *n.* The structure of a virus, composed of the capsid, or the protein coat, and the enclosed viral nucleic acid.

nu·cleo·chy·le·ma (new"klee·o·kigh·lee'muh) *n.* [*nucleo-* + *chyl-*, juice, + Gk. *-ma,* noun suffix]. NUCLEAR SAP.

nu·cleo·chyme (new'klee·o·kime) *n.* [*nucleo-* + Gk. *chymos,* fluid]. NUCLEAR SAP.

nu·cleo·cy·to·plas·mic (new"klee·o·sigh"to·plaz'mick) *adj.* Pertaining to both the nucleus and cytoplasm of a cell.

nucleocytoplasmic ratio. The ratio of the measured cross-sectional area or the estimated volume of the nucleus of a cell to its cytoplasm.

nu·cle·of·u·gal (new"klee·off'yoo·gul, new"klee·o·few'gul) *adj.* [*nucleo-* + *-fugal*]. Moving away from a nucleus.

nu·cleo·his·tone (new"klee·o·his'tone) *n.* [*nucleo-* + *histone*]. A basic protein from cell nuclei.

nu·cleo·hy·a·lo·plasm (new"klee·o·high'uh·lo·plaz·um) *n.* [*nucleo-* + *hyaloplasm*]. NUCLEAR SAP.

nu·cle·oid (new'klee·oid) *adj. & n.* 1. Nucleus-like. 2. A finely granular or fibrillar substance in certain erythrocytes, which resembles a nucleus.

nu·cle·o·lar (new·klee'uh·lur, new"klee·o'lur) *adj.* Pertaining to a nucleolus.

nucleolar organizer. NUCLEOLAR ZONE.

nucleolar zone. A secondary constriction of chromosomes associated with the formation of nucleoli.

nu·cle·ole (new'klee·ole) *n.* NUCLEOLUS.

nucleoli. Plural of *nucleolus.*

nu·cle·o·li·form (new·klee'uh·li·form, new"klee·o') *adj.* Shaped like a nucleolus.

nu·cle·o·loid (new·klee'uh·loid) *adj.* Resembling a nucleolus.

nu·cle·o·lus (new·klee'uh·lus) *n.*, pl. **nucleo·li** (·lye) [L., small kernel]. A small spherical body within the cell nucleus. Syn. *plasmosome.*

nu·cleo·mi·cro·so·ma (new"klee·o·migh"kro·so'muh) *n.* [*nucleo-* + *micro-* + Gk. *sōma,* body]. Any one of the many minute bodies that make up each fiber of the nuclear framework.

nu·cleo·mi·cro·some (new"klee·o·migh'kruh·sohm) *n.* [*nucleo-* + *microsome*]. NUCLEOMICROSOMA.

nu·cle·on (new'klee·on) *n.* An atomic nuclear particle; a proton or a neutron.

nu·cle·on·ics (new"klee·on'icks) *n.* The study of atomic nuclei, including the application of nuclear science in all fields of specialization; nuclear technology.

nu·cle·op·e·tal (new"klee·op'e·tul, new"klee·o·pet'ul) *adj.* [*nucleo-* + L. *pet*ere, to seek, + *-al*]. Seeking the nucleus; said of the movement of the male pronucleus toward the female pronucleus.

Nu·cle·oph·a·ga (new"klee·off'uh·guh) *n.* [NL., from *nucleo-* + Gk. *phagein,* to eat]. A parasite which destroys the nuclei of amebas.

nu·cleo·phil·ic (new"klee·o·fil'ick) *adj.* [*nucleo-* + *-philic*]. Having an affinity for atomic nuclei whereby a bond is formed when an ion or molecule (called the nucleophilic agent) donates a pair of electrons to an electrophilic ion or molecule.

nu·cleo·plasm (new'klee·o·plaz·um) *n.* The protoplasm of the nucleus. Syn. *karyoplasm.*

nu·cleo·plas·mic ratio (new"klee·o·plaz'mick). NUCLEOCYTOPLASMIC RATIO.

nu·cleo·pro·te·id (new"klee·o·pro'tee·id) *n.* NUCLEOPROTEIN.

nu·cleo·pro·tein (new"klee·o·pro'tee·in, ·teen) *n.* A protein constituent of cell nuclei, consisting of nucleic acid and a basic protein, which on hydrolysis yields purine and pyrimidine bases, phosphoric acid, and a pentose sugar, in addition to the protein.

nu·cleo·re·tic·u·lum (new"klee·o·re·tick'yoo·lum) *n.* [*nucleo-* + *reticulum*]. Any network contained within a nucleus.

nu·cleo·sid·ase (new"klee·o·sigh'dace, ·daze, ·o'si·dace) *n.* An enzyme that catalyzes the hydrolysis of a nucleoside into its component pentose and purine or pyrimidine base.

nu·cleo·side (new'klee·o·side) *n.* A glycoside resulting from the removal of phosphate from a nucleotide. It is a combination of a sugar (pentose) with a purine or pyrimidine base.

nucleoside diphosphate. A nucleoside esterified with a pyrophosphate residue on the pentose moiety, usually at the 5′ position; for example, adenosine diphosphate.

nucleoside diphosphate kinase. An enzyme that causes a nucleoside diphosphate to react with adenosine triphosphate, to generate the corresponding nucleoside triphosphate and adenosine diphosphate.

nucleoside monophosphate. Combination of a nucleoside esterified to a single phosphate on the pentose moiety, usually at the 5′ position; for example, adenosine monophosphate.

nucleoside monophosphate kinase. An enzyme that causes a nucleoside monophosphate to react with adenosine triphosphate to generate the corresponding nucleoside diphosphate and adenosine diphosphate.

nucleoside triphosphate. A nucleoside esterified with three consecutive phosphate groups on the pentose moiety, usually at the 5′ position; for example, adenosine triphosphate.

nu·cleo·spin·dle (new'klee·o·spin"dul, new"klee·o·spin'dul) *n.* A mitotic spindle formed from the nuclear substance, as in some forms of anastral mitosis.

nu·cleo·tid·ase (new″klee·o·tye′dace, ·daze, new″klee·ot′i·) *n.* Any of a group of enzymes which split phosphoric acid from nucleotides, leaving nucleosides.

nu·cleo·tide (new′klee·o·tide) *n.* An ester of phosphoric acid and a pentose sugar linked to a pyrimidine or purine base; a phosphorylated nucleoside. The basic structural unit of a nucleic acid.

nu·cleo·tox·in (new″klee·o·tock′sin) *n.* 1. A toxin derived from cell nuclei. 2. Any toxin affecting the nuclei of cells. —**nucleotox·ic** (·ick) *adj.*

nu·cle·us (new′klee·us) *n.*, pl. & genit. sing. **nu·clei** (·klee·eye) [L., kernel, pit, stone, from *nux, nucis,* nut]. 1. The differentiated central protoplasm of a cell; its trophic center. 2. A collection of nerve cells in the central nervous system concerned with a particular function. 3. A stable and characteristic complex of atoms to which other atoms may be attached. 4. The center around which the mass of a crystal aggregates. 5. The core of an atom consisting of protons, neutrons, and alpha particles.

nucleus ac·ces·so·ri·us (ack·se·so′ree·us) [NA]. Any accessory nucleus.

nucleus accessorius ner·vi ocu·lo·mo·to·rii (nur′vye ock·yoo·lo·mo·to′ree·eye) [NA]. AUTONOMIC NUCLEUS OF THE OCULOMOTOR NERVE. NA alt. *nucleus autonomicus nervi oculomotorii.*

nucleus alae ci·ne·re·ae (ay′lee si·neer′ee·ee) [BNA]. Nucleus dorsalis nervi vagi (= DORSAL MOTOR NUCLEUS OF THE VAGUS).

nucleus am·bi·gu·us (am·big′yoo·us) [NA]. A column of cells lying in the lateral half of the reticular formation whose cells give origin to efferent fibers of the glossopharyngeal, vagus, and accessory nerves. Syn. *ambiguus nucleus.*

nucleus amyg·da·lae (a·mig′duh·lee) [BNA]. Corpus amygdaloideum (= AMYGDALOID BODY).

nucleus an·gu·la·ris (ang″gew·lair′is). SUPERIOR VESTIBULAR NUCLEUS.

nucleus anterior tha·la·mi (thal′uh·migh) [BNA]. Singular of *nuclei anteriores thalami.*

nucleus an·te·ro·dor·sa·lis tha·la·mi (an″tur·o·dor·say′lis thal′uh·migh) [NA]. The anterodorsal nucleus of the anterior nuclei of the thalamus.

nucleus an·te·ro·me·di·a·lis tha·la·mi (an″tur·o·mee·dee·ay′lis thal′uh·migh) [NA]. The anteromedial nucleus of the anterior nuclei of the thalamus.

nucleus an·te·ro·ven·tra·lis tha·la·mi (an″tur·o·ven·tray′lis thal′uh·migh) [NA]. The anteroventral nucleus of the anterior nuclei of the thalamus.

nucleus au·to·no·mi·cus ner·vi ocu·lo·mo·to·rii (aw·to·nom′i·kus nur′vye ock·yoo·lo·mo·to′ree·eye) [NA alt.]. AUTONOMIC NUCLEUS OF THE OCULOMOTOR NERVE. NA alt. *nucleus accessorius nervi oculomotorii.*

nucleus ba·sa·lis (ba·say′lis). OLIVARY NUCLEUS.

nucleus cau·da·lis cen·tra·lis (kaw·day′lis sen·tray′lis) [NA]. A part of the nucleus of the oculomotor nerve.

nucleus cau·da·tus (kaw·day′tus) [NA]. CAUDATE NUCLEUS.

nucleus cen·tra·lis tha·la·mi (sen·tray′lis thal′uh·migh) [former NA]. CENTRAL NUCLEUS OF THE THALAMUS.

nucleus cen·tro·me·di·a·nus tha·la·mi (sen″tro·mee·de·ay′nus thal′uh·migh) [NA]. CENTRAL NUCLEUS OF THE THALAMUS. NA alt. *nucleus medialis centralis thalami.*

nucleus co·chle·a·ris dor·sa·lis (kock·lee·air′is dor·say′lis) [NA]. The dorsal cochlear nucleus. See *cochlear nuclei.*

nucleus cochlearis ven·tra·lis (ven·tray′lis) [NA]. The ventral cochlear nucleus. See *cochlear nuclei.*

nucleus col·li·cu·li in·fe·ri·o·ris (kol·ick′yoo·lye in·feer·ee·o′ris) [NA]. NUCLEUS OF THE INFERIOR COLLICULUS.

nucleus con·ter·mi·na·lis (kon·tur·mi·nay′lis). RETROPYRAMIDAL NUCLEUS.

nucleus cor·po·ris ge·ni·cu·la·ti la·te·ra·lis (kor′po·ris je·nick″yoo·lay′tye lat·e·ray′lis) [BNA]. Singular of *nuclei corporis geniculati lateralis.*

nucleus corporis geniculati me·di·a·lis (mee·dee·ay′lis) [NA]. The nucleus of the medial geniculate body.

nucleus corporis ma·mil·la·ris (mam·i·lair′is). Singular of *nuclei corporis mamillaris.*

nucleus cu·ne·a·tus (kew·nee·ay′tus) [NA]. CUNEATE NUCLEUS.

nucleus cuneatus ac·ces·so·ri·us (ack·se·so′ree·us) [NA]. ACCESSORY CUNEATE NUCLEUS.

nucleus den·ta·tus ce·re·bel·li (den·tay′tus serr·e·bel′eye) [NA]. DENTATE NUCLEUS.

nucleus dor·sa·lis (dor·say′lis) [BNA]. Nucleus thoracicus (= THORACIC NUCLEUS).

nucleus dorsalis cor·po·ris tra·pe·zoi·dei (kor′po·ris trap·e·zoy′dee·eye) [NA]. A group of nerve cells in the dorsolateral part of the trapezoid body. See also *superior olive.*

nucleus dorsalis ner·vi glos·so·pha·ryn·gei (nur′vye glos″o·fa·rin′jee·eye) [NA]. The more rostral part of the dorsal motor nucleus of the vagus.

nucleus dorsalis nervi va·gi (vay′guy, ·jye) [NA]. DORSAL MOTOR NUCLEUS OF THE VAGUS.

nucleus dor·so·la·te·ra·lis (dor″so·lat·e·ray′lis) [NA]. The dorsolateral part of the nucleus of the oculomotor nerve.

nucleus dor·so·me·di·a·lis hy·po·tha·la·mi (dor″so·mee·dee·ay′lis high·po·thal′uh·migh) [NA]. DORSOMEDIAL HYPOTHALAMIC NUCLEUS.

nucleus em·bo·li·for·mis ce·re·bel·li (em·bol″i·for′mis serr·e·bel′eye) [NA]. EMBOLIFORM NUCLEUS.

nucleus emi·nen·ti·ae te·re·tis (em″i·nen′shee·ee teer′e·tis, terr′). The lateral extension of the dorsal paramedian nucleus.

nucleus fa·sti·gii (fas·tij′ee·eye, fas·tye′jee·eye) [NA]. FASTIGIAL NUCLEUS.

nucleus fu·ni·cu·li cu·ne·a·ti (few·nick′yoo·lye kew·nee·ay′tye) [BNA]. Nucleus cuneatus (= CUNEATE NUCLEUS).

nucleus funiculi gra·ci·lis (gras′i·lis) [BNA]. Nucleus gracilis (= GRACILIS NUCLEUS).

nucleus glo·bo·sus ce·re·bel·li (glo·bo′sus serr·e·bel′eye) [NA]. GLOBOSE NUCLEUS.

nucleus gra·ci·lis (gras′i·lis) [NA]. GRACILIS NUCLEUS.

nucleus ha·be·nu·lae (ha·ben′yoo·lee) [NA]. HABENULAR NUCLEUS.

nucleus hy·po·tha·la·mi·cus (high″po·thuh·lam′i·kus) [BNA]. Nucleus subthalamicus (= SUBTHALAMIC NUCLEUS).

nucleus inferior pon·tis (pon′tis) [NA]. The inferior nucleus of the pons. See also *pontine nucleus.*

nucleus in·ter·ca·la·tus (in·tur·ka·lay′tus) [NA]. A nucleus of the medulla oblongata in the central gray matter of the ventricular floor located between the hypoglossal nucleus and the dorsal motor nucleus of the vagus. Syn. *intercalated nucleus.*

nucleus in·ter·me·dio·la·te·ra·lis (in·tur·mee″dee·o·lat·e·ray′lis) [NA]. LATERAL SYMPATHETIC NUCLEUS. NA alt. *nucleus lateralis medullae spinalis.*

nucleus in·ter·me·dio·me·di·a·lis (in·tur·mee″dee·o·mee·dee·ay′lis) [NA]. INTERMEDIOMEDIAL NUCLEUS. NA alt. *nucleus medialis medullae spinalis.*

nucleus in·ter·pe·dun·cu·la·ris (in″tur·pe·dunk·yoo·lair′is) [NA]. INTERPEDUNCULAR NUCLEUS.

nucleus in·ter·sti·ti·a·lis (in″tur·stish·ee·ay′lis) [NA]. INTERSTITIAL NUCLEUS.

nucleus la·te·ra·lis dor·sa·lis tha·la·mi (lat·e·ray′lis dor·say′lis thal′uh·migh) [NA]. The dorsal lateral nucleus of the lateral thalamic nuclei.

nucleus lateralis me·dul·lae ob·lon·ga·tae (me·dul′ee ob·long·gay′tee) [NA]. A nucleus in the reticular part of the medulla oblongata.

nucleus lateralis medullae spi·na·lis (spye·nay′lis) [NA alt.]. LATERAL SYMPATHETIC NUCLEUS. NA alt. *nucleus intermediolateralis.*

nucleus lateralis tha·la·mi (thal'uh·migh) [BNA]. Singular of *nuclei laterales thalami.*

nucleus lem·nis·ci la·te·ra·lis (lem·nis'eye lat·e·ray'lis) [NA]. A group of nerve cells in the rostral part of the lateral lemniscus.

nucleus len·ti·for·mis (len·ti·for'mis) [NA]. LENTIFORM NUCLEUS.

nucleus len·tis (len'tis) [NA]. The nucleus of the lens; the harder central portion of the crystalline lens of the eye.

nucleus mag·no·cel·lu·la·ris (mag''no·sel''yoo·lair'is). POSTEROMARGINAL NUCLEUS.

nucleus me·di·a·lis cen·tra·lis tha·la·mi (mee·dee·ay'lis sen·tray'lis thal'uh·migh) [NA]. CENTRAL MEDIAL NUCLEUS OF THE THALAMUS. NA alt. *nucleus centromedianus thalami.*

nucleus medialis dor·sa·lis (dor·say'lis). DORSOMEDIAL NUCLEUS OF THE THALAMUS.

nucleus medialis me·dul·lae spi·na·lis (me·dul'ee spye·nay'lis) [NA alt.]. INTERMEDIOMEDIAL NUCLEUS. NA alt. *nucleus intermediomedialis.*

nucleus medialis pon·tis (pon'tis) [NA]. A nucleus in the medial part of the pons. See also *pontine nucleus.*

nucleus medialis tha·la·mi (thal'uh·migh) [NA]. MEDIAL NUCLEUS OF THE THALAMUS.

nucleus mo·to·ri·us ner·vi tri·ge·mi·ni (mo·to'ree·us nur'vye trye·jem'i·nigh) [NA]. MOTOR NUCLEUS OF THE TRIGEMINAL NERVE.

nucleus ner·vi ab·du·cen·tis (nur'vye ab·dew·sen'tis) [NA]. The nucleus of origin of the fibers of the abducens nerve.

nucleus nervi ac·ces·so·rii (ack·se·so'ree·eye) [NA]. The nucleus of origin of fibers in the accessory nerve. Part are in the nucleus ambiguus and part in the cervical nerve nuclei.

nucleus nervi fa·ci·a·lis (fay·shee·ay'lis) [NA]. FACIAL NUCLEUS.

nucleus nervi hy·po·glos·si (high·po·glos'eye) [NA]. HYPOGLOSSAL NUCLEUS.

nucleus nervi ocu·lo·mo·to·rii (ock''yoo·lo·mo·to'ree·eye) [NA]. OCULOMOTOR NUCLEUS.

nucleus nervi tro·chle·a·ris (trock·lee·air'is) [NA]. TROCHLEAR NERVE NUCLEUS.

nucleus of Bekhterev [V. M. *Bekhterev*]. SUPERIOR VESTIBULAR NUCLEUS.

nucleus of Burdach [K. F. *Burdach*]. CUNEATE NUCLEUS.

nucleus of Darkschewitsch [L. O. *Darkschewitsch*]. NUCLEUS OF THE MEDIAL LONGITUDINAL FASCICULUS.

nucleus of Edinger-Westphal [L. *Edinger* and C. F. O. *Westphal*]. AUTONOMIC NUCLEUS OF THE OCULOMOTOR NERVE.

nucleus of Goll [F. *Goll*, Swiss anatomist, 1829–1904]. GRACILIS NUCLEUS.

nucleus of Monakow [K. *Monakow*]. ACCESSORY CUNEATE NUCLEUS.

nucleus of origin. A collection of nerve cells in the central nervous system giving rise to the fibers of a nerve or a nerve tract. NA *nucleus originis* (pl. *nuclei originis*).

nucleus of Perlia [R. *Perlia*]. A medially placed cell group of the oculomotor nuclei which has been regarded as the mesencephalic center for convergence of the eyes.

nucleus of Rol·ler [C. F. W. *Roller*]. A nucleus that lies ventral to the rostral pole of the hypoglossal nucleus; one of the perihypoglossal nuclei.

nucleus of Schwalbe [G. *Schwalbe*]. MEDIAL VESTIBULAR NUCLEUS.

nucleus of termination. A collection of nerve cells in which the axons of a nerve tract or a nerve root terminate. NA *nucleus terminationis* (pl. *nuclei terminationis*).

nucleus of the ansa lenticularis. ENTOPEDUNCULAR NUCLEUS.

nucleus of the inferior colliculus. An ovoid mass of cells in the body of the inferior colliculus. NA *nucleus colliculi inferioris.*

nucleus of the lateral lemniscus. NUCLEUS LEMNISCI LATERALIS.

nucleus of the lens. The harder central portion of the crystalline lens of the eye. NA *nucleus lentis.*

nucleus of the medial longitudinal fasciculus. An accessory oculomotor nucleus lying dorsal and lateral to the oculomotor complex; its fibers project to the posterior commissure. Syn. *Darkschewitsch's nucleus.*

nucleus of the mesencephalic tract of the trigeminal nerve. A column of large round cells ventrolateral to the aqueduct of the midbrain whose cells give origin to the mesencephalic root of the trigeminal nerve. NA *nucleus tractus mesencephalici nervi trigemini.*

nucleus of the posterior commissure. NUCLEUS OF THE MEDIAL LONGITUDINAL FASCICULUS.

nucleus of the raphe. Any of the collections of nerve cells in the midportion of the reticular formation of the medulla oblongata.

nucleus of the spinal tract of the trigeminal nerve. The column of cells lying medial to the entire length of the spinal tract of the trigeminal nerve in which the fibers of the tract terminate. NA *nucleus tractus spinalis nervi trigemini.*

nucleus of the tegmental field. RETICULAR NUCLEUS OF THE SUBTHALAMUS.

nucleus of the tractus solitarius. A column of cells in the medulla oblongata surrounding the solitary tract and in which part of the fibers of the solitary tract terminate. NA *nucleus tractus solitarii.*

nucleus oli·va·ris (ol·i·vair'is) [NA]. OLIVARY NUCLEUS.

nucleus olivaris ac·ces·so·ri·us dor·sa·lis (ack''se·so'ree·us dor·say'lis) [NA]. DORSAL ACCESSORY OLIVARY NUCLEUS.

nucleus olivaris accessorius me·di·a·lis (mee·dee·ay'lis) [NA]. A mass of cells lying medial to the olivary nucleus.

nucleus olivaris inferior [BNA]. Nucleus olivaris (= OLIVARY NUCLEUS).

nucleus olivaris superior [BNA]. NUCLEUS DORSALIS CORPORIS TRAPEZOIDEI.

nucleus ori·gi·nis (o·rye'ji·nis), pl. **nuclei originis** [NA]. NUCLEUS OF ORIGIN.

nucleus pa·ra·ven·tri·cu·la·ris hy·po·tha·la·mi (păr''uh·ven·trick·yoo·lair'is high·po·thal'uh·migh) [NA]. PARAVENTRICULAR NUCLEUS OF THE HYPOTHALAMUS.

nucleus pig·men·to·sus pon·tis (pig·men·to'sus pon'tis). LOCUS CERULEUS.

nucleus posterior hy·po·tha·la·mi (high·po·thal'uh·migh) [NA]. POSTERIOR HYPOTHALAMIC NUCLEUS.

nucleus posterior tha·la·mi (thal'uh·migh) [NA]. PULVINAR. NA alt. *pulvinar thalami.*

nucleus pre·po·si·tus (pree·poz'i·tus). A group of relatively large cells, extending from the oral limits of the hypoglossal nucleus to the caudal limit of the abducent nucleus. Caudally, it is continuous with the nucleus intercalatus. The connections and functions of this nucleus are not understood.

nucleus pre·tec·ta·lis (pree·teck·tay'lis) [NA]. A nucleus in the tectum of the mesencephalon lateral to the superior colliculus.

nucleus proprius of the anterior horn. Small cells, scattered between the somatic motor cells in the ventral horn, which may serve for intranuclear connections.

nucleus proprius of the posterior horn. A poorly defined cell column in the head and cervix of the dorsal horn, which corresponds to Rexed's laminae III and IV.

nucleus pul·po·sus (pul·po'sus), pl. **nuclei pulpo·si** (·sigh) [NA]. The pulpy body at the center of an intervertebral disk; a remnant of the notochord.

nucleus ra·di·cis de·scen·den·tis ner·vi tri·ge·mi·ni (ra·dye'sis des·en·den'tis nur'vye trye·jem'i·nigh) [BNA]. Nucleus tractus mesencephalici nervi trigemini (= NUCLEUS OF THE MESENCEPHALIC TRACT OF THE TRIGEMINAL NERVE).

nucleus re·ti·cu·la·ris tha·la·mi (re·tick''yoo·lair'is thal'uh·migh) [NA]. RETICULAR NUCLEUS OF THE THALAMUS.

nucleus rhom·boi·da·lis tha·la·mi (rom·boy·day'lis thal'uh·migh) [NA]. RHOMBOID NUCLEUS OF THE THALAMUS.
nucleus ru·ber (roo'bur) [NA]. RED NUCLEUS.
nucleus sa·li·va·to·ri·us inferior (sal''i·vuh·to'ree·us) [NA]. INFERIOR SALIVATORY NUCLEUS.
nucleus salivatorius superior [NA]. SUPERIOR SALIVATORY NUCLEUS.
nucleus sen·so·ri·us in·fe·ri·or ner·vi tri·ge·mi·ni (sen·so'ree·us in·feer'ee·or nur'vye trye·jem'i·nigh) [BNA]. Nucleus tractus spinalis nervi trigemini (= NUCLEUS OF THE SPINAL TRACT OF THE TRIGEMINAL NERVE).
nucleus sensorius prin·ci·pa·lis ner·vi tri·ge·mi·ni (prin·si·pay'lis nur'vye trye·jem'i·nigh) [NA]. MAIN SENSORY NUCLEUS OF THE TRIGEMINAL NERVE.
nucleus sol·i·ta·ri·us (sol·i·tair'ee·us). NUCLEUS OF THE TRACTUS SOLITARIUS.
nucleus spi·na·lis ner·vi ac·ces·so·rii (spye·nay'lis nur'vye ack·se·so'ree·eye) [NA]. SPINAL ACCESSORY NUCLEUS.
nucleus sub·tha·la·mi·cus (sub''thuh·lam'i·kus) [NA]. SUBTHALAMIC NUCLEUS.
nucleus superior pon·tis (pon'tis) [NA]. The superior nucleus of the pons. See also *pontine nucleus.*
nucleus su·pra·op·ti·cus hy·po·tha·la·mi (sue''pruh·op'ti·kus high·po·thal'uh·migh) [NA]. SUPRAOPTIC NUCLEUS OF THE HYPOTHALAMUS.
nucleus sym·pa·thi·cus la·te·ra·lis (sim·path'i·kus lat·e·ray'lis). LATERAL SYMPATHETIC NUCLEUS.
nucleus teg·men·ti (teg·men'tye) [NA]. Singular of *nuclei tegmenti.*
nucleus ter·mi·na·ti·o·nis (tur''mi·nay''shee·o'nis), pl. **nuclei terminationis** [NA]. NUCLEUS OF TERMINATION.
nucleus test. A test for pancreatic function based on the fact that cell nuclei are digested by pancreatic juice and not gastric juice.
nucleus tha·la·mi la·te·ra·lis (thal'uh·migh lat·e·ray'lis). A nucleus in the lateral part of the thalamus.
nucleus tho·ra·ci·cus (tho·ray'si·kus) [NA]. THORACIC NUCLEUS.
nucleus trac·tus me·sen·ce·pha·li·ci ner·vi tri·ge·mi·ni (track'tus mes''en·se·fal'i·sigh nur'vye trye·jem'i·nigh) [NA]. NUCLEUS OF THE MESENCEPHALIC TRACT OF THE TRIGEMINAL NERVE.
nucleus tractus so·li·ta·rii (sol·i·tair'ee·eye) [NA]. NUCLEUS OF THE TRACTUS SOLITARIUS.
nucleus tractus spi·na·lis ner·vi tri·ge·mi·ni (spi·nay'lis nur'vye trye·jem'i·nigh) [NA]. NUCLEUS OF THE SPINAL TRACT OF THE TRIGEMINAL NERVE.
nucleus ven·tra·lis anterior (ven·tray'lis). The anterior ventral nucleus of the thalamus.
nucleus ventralis an·te·ro·la·te·ra·lis tha·la·mi (an·tur·o·lat·e·ray'lis thal'uh·migh) [NA]. The ventral anterolateral nucleus of the lateral thalamic nuclei.
nucleus ventralis cor·po·ris tra·pe·zoi·dei (kor'po·ris trap·e·zoy'dee·eye) [NA]. Cells in the ventral part of the trapezoid body.
nucleus ventralis in·ter·me·di·us tha·la·mi (in·tur·mee'de·us thal'uh·migh) [NA]. The ventral intermediate nucleus of the lateral thalamic nuclei.
nucleus ventralis la·te·ra·lis (lat·e·ray'lis). LATERAL VENTRAL NUCLEUS OF THE THALAMUS.
nucleus ventralis pos·te·ro·la·te·ra·lis tha·la·mi (pos''tur·o·lat'e·ray'lis thal'uh·migh) [NA]. POSTEROLATERAL VENTRAL NUCLEUS OF THE THALAMUS.
nucleus ventralis pos·te·ro·me·di·a·lis tha·la·mi (pos''tur·o·mee·de·ay'lis thal'uh·migh) [NA]. POSTEROMEDIAL VENTRAL NUCLEUS OF THE THALAMUS.
nucleus ventralis tha·la·mi (thal'uh·migh). The ventral part of the lateral nucleus of the thalamus.
nucleus ventralis thalami anterior. The anterior part of the ventral nucleus of the thalamus.
nucleus ventralis thalami in·ter·me·di·us (in''tur·mee'dee·us). The intermediate part of the ventral nucleus of the thalamus.
nucleus ventralis thalami posterior. The posterior part of the ventral nucleus of the thalamus.
nucleus ven·tro·me·di·a·lis hy·po·tha·la·mi (ven''tro·mee·dee·ay'lis high·po·thal'uh·migh) [NA]. VENTROMEDIAL HYPOTHALAMIC NUCLEUS.
nucleus ves·ti·bu·la·ris inferior (ves·tib·yoo·lair'is) [NA]. SPINAL VESTIBULAR NUCLEUS.
nucleus vestibularis la·te·ra·lis (lat·e·ray'lis) [NA]. LATERAL VESTIBULAR NUCLEUS.
nucleus vestibularis me·di·a·lis (mee·dee·ay'lis) [NA]. MEDIAL VESTIBULAR NUCLEUS.
nucleus vestibularis superior [NA]. SUPERIOR VESTIBULAR NUCLEUS.
nu·clide (new'klide) *n.* A species of atom characterized by the constitution of its nucleus, in particular by the number of protons and neutrons in the nucleus.
nud·ism (new'diz·um) *n.* 1. *In psychiatry,* a more or less complete intolerance of clothing; a pathologic tendency to remove the clothing. 2. The practice or cult of those who profess to believe in the benefits of society in which clothes are discarded.
Nu·el's space (nuᵉ·el') [J. *Nuel,* Belgian otologist, 1847–1920]. A space between the outer pillars and the outer hair cells of the spiral organ (of Corti).
NUG Abbreviation for *necrotizing ulcerative gingivitis.*
Nuhn's glands (noon) [A. *Nuhn,* German anatomist, 1814–1889]. *Obsol.* ANTERIOR LINGUAL GLANDS.
nui·sance, *n.* [OF., from L. *nocere,* to harm]. *In legal medicine,* that which is noxious, offensive, or capable of causing distress; applied to persons or things.
nul·lip·a·ra (nuh·lip'ur·uh) *n.* [L. *nullus,* none, + *-para*]. A woman who has never borne a child. —**nullipa·rous** (·rus) *adj.;* **nul·li·par·i·ty** (nul''i·păr'i·tee) *n.*
numb, *adj.* Of a part of the body: anesthetic; having deadened sensation.
num·bered hospital. *In military medicine,* a hospital to which an individual number is assigned. Numbered hospitals may be station hospitals, general hospitals, or other specific types, such as evacuation hospitals.
numb·ness, *n.* Partial or local anesthesia with torpor; deficiency of sensation.
nu·mer·i·cal aperture. A mathematical expression of the resolving power of a microscope objective; specifically, the product of the sine of one-half the angle of aperture of the lens and the refractive index of the medium in front of the lens.
numerical atrophy. Reduction in the number of cells of an organ; NECROBIOTIC ATROPHY.
numerical hypertrophy. HYPERPLASIA.
num·mi·form (num'i·form) *adj.* [L. *nummus,* coin, + *-iform*]. NUMMULAR (1).
num·mu·lar (num'yoo·lur) *adj.* [L. *nummularius,* of money, from *nummulus,* small coin]. 1. Resembling a coin in form, as nummular sputum. 2. Resembling rouleaux or rolls of coin.
nummular dermatitis. Coin-shaped patches of vesicular dermatitis, usually affecting the extensor surfaces of the forearms and legs.
nummular erythema. Discoid lesions of tinea corporis.
nummular sputum. Sputum containing small, round, flattened masses of heavy material resembling coins.
num·mu·la·tion (num''yoo·lay'shun) *n.* The aggregation of blood cells into coinlike rolls or rouleaux.
Numorphan. Trademark for the semisynthetic narcotic analgesic oxymorphone, used as the hydrochloride salt.
nun·na·tion (nuh·nay'shun) *n.* [*nūn,* the Arabic letter n]. The frequent, or abnormal, use of the *n* sound.
Nupercaine. A trademark for dibucaine, a local anesthetic used as the base and as the hydrochloride salt.
¹nurse, *n.* [OF. *nurice,* from L. *nutrix,* nurse, foster-mother].

1. One who cares for a sick person under supervision of a physician. 2. One who cares for an infant or young child; nursemaid.

²nurse, *v.* [ME. *nurishen,* to nourish]. 1. To suckle (an infant). 2. Of an infant: to take milk from the breast. 3. To care for (a sick person).

nurse corps. The nurses in the Armed Services, who have ranks, titles, and status as officers in those services.

nurse·maid's elbow. PULLED ELBOW.

nurse's aide. A worker in a hospital or other medical facility who assists nurses in nonspecialized tasks of patient care, such as bathing, feeding, making beds, taking weights and temperatures.

nurse specialist. SPECIAL NURSE.

nurses' registry. An office listing nurses available for general or special services.

nurses' training school. A technical or vocational school of nursing.

nurse supervisor. A person who has the experience and qualifications for management of a large number of hospital patients and nursing personnel.

nurs·ing, *n.* 1. Care for the ill and infirm. 2. The practice and profession of ¹nurses (1).

nursing bottle. A narrow- or wide-mouthed flask with a rubber nipple attached; used for feeding infants.

nurs·ling, *n.* A nursing infant; an infant that has not been weaned.

nu·ta·tion (new·tay'shun) *n.* [L. *nutare,* to nod]. Nodding or oscillation.

nut·meg liver. Chronic passive hyperemia of the liver; named for the resemblance of the cut surface of such a liver to the cut surface of a nutmeg.

nu·tri·ent (new'tree·unt) *adj. & n.* [L. *nutriens,* from *nutrire,* to nourish]. 1. Affording nutrition. 2. A substance that affords nutrition.

nutrient artery. An artery that supplies blood to a bone.

nutrient artery groove. A linear translucency in a bone caused by a nutrient artery canal which may be mistaken for a fracture on roentgenograms.

nutrient foramen. The opening into the canal which gives passage to the blood vessels of the medullary cavity of a bone. NA *foramen nutricium.*

nu·tri·lite (new'tri·lite) *n.* A substance which, in small amounts, functions in the nutrition of microorganisms.

nu·tri·ment (new'tri·munt) *n.* [L. *nutrimentum,* nourishment]. Anything that nourishes.

nu·tri·tion (new·trish'un) *n.* [L. *nutritio,* from *nutrire,* to nourish]. 1. The sum of the processes concerned in the growth, maintenance, and repair of the living body as a whole, or of its constituent parts. 2. Especially, those processes most directly involved in the intake, metabolism, and utilization of food; nourishment. —**nutrition·al** (·ul) *adj.*

nutritional anemia. Anemia associated with nutritional deficiencies, usually of iron.

nutritional dystrophy. KWASHIORKOR.

nutritional edema. Edema occurring in starvation or in a poorly nourished state. Syn. *famine edema, hunger edema.*

nutritional hypochromic anemia. IRON-DEFICIENCY ANEMIA.

nu·tri·tious (new·trish'us) *adj.* Nourishing; rich in nutritive substances.

nu·tri·tive (new'tri·tiv) *adj.* 1. Of or pertaining to nutrition. 2. Providing nourishment.

nutritive absorption. INTERNAL ABSORPTION.

nutritive canal. HAVERSIAN CANAL.

nutritive equilibrium. A condition of balance between the intake of a nutritive material and the excretion of the products of its metabolism.

nu·tri·to·ry (new'tri·tor·ee) *adj.* Pertaining to the processes of nutrition.

nu·tri·ture (new'tri·chur· ·choor) *n.* Nutritional status.

nu·trix (new'tricks) *n.* [L.]. WET NURSE.

nux vom·i·ca (nucks"vom'i·kuh) [L. *nux,* nut, + *vomica,* from L. *vomere,* to vomit]. The seed of *Strychnos nux-vomica,* an Indian tree of the Loganiaceae. It contains the alkaloid strychnine, for the effects of which nux vomica was formerly used in medicine.

nyct-, nycto- [Gk. *nyx, nyktos*]. A combining form meaning *night.*

nyc·tal·gia (nick·tal'jee·uh) *n.* [*nyct-* + *-algia*]. Pain which occurs chiefly during the night or during sleep.

nyc·ta·lope (nick'tuh·lope) *n.* [Gk. *nyktalōps,* night-blind, from *nyx, nyktos,* night, + *alaos,* blind, + *ōps,* eye]. One who cannot see well in reduced light.

nyc·ta·lo·pia (nick"tuh·lo'pee·uh) *n.* [Gk. *nyktalōps,* night-blind, + *-ia*]. NIGHT BLINDNESS.

nyc·ta·pho·nia (nick"tuh·fo'nee·uh, nikt"a·) *n.* [*nyct-* + *aphonia*]. A conversion type of hysterical neurosis in which there is loss of the voice during the night only. Compare *nyctophonia.*

nyc·ter·ine (nick'tur·ine, ·een, ·in) *adj.* [Gk. *nykterinos,* nightly]. 1. Occurring in the night. 2. Obscure.

nyc·te·ro·hem·er·al (nick"tuh·ro·hem'ur·ul) *adj.* [Gk. *nykteros,* nocturnal, + *hēmera,* day, + *-al*]. NYCTOHEMERAL.

nycto-. See *nyct-.*

nyc·to·hem·er·al (nick"to·hem'ur·ul) *adj.* [Gk. *nyx, nyktos,* night, + *hēmera,* day, + *-al*]. Pertaining to day and night, as in circadian rhythm.

nyc·to·phil·ia (nick"to·fil'ee·uh) *n.* [*nycto-* + *-philia*]. Preference for night or darkness.

nyc·to·pho·bia (nick"to·fo'bee·uh) *n.* [*nycto-* + *-phobia*]. NOCTIPHOBIA.

nyc·to·pho·nia (nick"to·fo'nee·uh) *n.* [*nycto-* + Gk. *phōnē,* voice, + *-ia*]. A conversion type of hysterical neurosis in which there is loss of the voice during the day in one who is capable of speaking during the night. Compare *nyctaphonia.*

nyc·to·typh·lo·sis (nick"to·tif·lo'sis) *n.* [*nycto-* + *typhlosis*]. NIGHT BLINDNESS.

nyc·tu·ria (nick·tew'ree·uh) *n.* [*nyct-* + *urinate* + *-ia*]. NOCTURIA.

Nydrazid. A trademark for isoniazid, a tuberculostatic drug.

Ny·lan·der reagent (nueˈlaʰn·dur) [E. *Nylander,* Swedish chemist, 1835-1907]. A solution of bismuth subnitrate, Rochelle salt (potassium sodium tartrate), and potassium or sodium hydroxide used to test for glucose in urine.

Nylander's test [E. *Nylander*]. A bismuth reduction test used for glucose in the urine.

ny·les·tri·ol (nye·les'tree·ole) *n.* 17α-Ethynylestra-1,3,5(10)-triene-3,16α,17β-triol 3-cyclopentyl ether, $C_{25}H_{32}O_3$, an estrogen.

ny·lic standard (nigh'lick). A standard of weight in accordance with height and age, as adopted by the New York Life Insurance Company.

ny·li·drin (nye'li·drin, nil'i·drin) *n.* 1-(*p*-Hydroxyphenyl)-2-(1-methyl-3-phenylpropylamino)propanol, $C_{19}H_{25}NO_2$, a peripheral vasodilator; used as the hydrochloride salt.

nymph, *n.* [Gk. *nymphē,* maiden]. The immature stage of an insect, during which the wing pads first appear and the reproductive organs have not developed to the functional stage.

nymph-, nympho- [Gk. *nymphē,* maiden, nymph]. A combining form signifying (a) *nymphae, labia minora;* (b) *female sexuality.*

nym·pha (nim'fuh) *n.,* pl. **nym·phae** (·fee) [L., from Gk. *nymphē,* nymph, maiden]. LABIUM MINUS.

nym·phec·to·my (nim·feck'tum·ee) *n.* [*nymph-* + *-ectomy*]. Surgical removal of one or both labia minora of the vulva.

nym·phi·tis (nim·fye'tis) *n.* [*nymph-* + *-itis*]. Inflammation of the labia minora.

nympho-. See *nymph-.*

nym·pho·ca·run·cu·lar (nim"fo·ka·runk'yoo·lur) *adj.* [*nympho-* + *caruncular*]. Pertaining to the nymphae and hymenal caruncles.

nymphocaruncular sulcus. A groove between the labium minus and the hymen.

nym·pho·lep·sy (nim'fo·lep"see) *n.* [*nympho-* + *-lepsy*, from Gk. *nympholēptos*, captured by nymphs]. Ecstasy of an erotic type.

nym·pho·ma·nia (nim"fo·may'nee·uh) *n.* [*nympho-* + *-mania*]. Excessive sexual desire on the part of a woman. Syn. *hysteromania.* —**nymphoma·ni·ac** (·nee·ack) *adj. & n.*

nym·phon·cus (nim·fonk'us) *n.* [*nymph-* + Gk. *onkos*, mass, bulk]. Tumor or swelling of the labium minus.

nym·phot·o·my (nim·fot'um·ee) *n.* [*nympho-* + *-tomy*]. Incision of one or both of the labia minora.

nystagm-, nystagmo-. A combining form meaning *nystagmus.*

nys·tag·mic (nis·tag'mick) *adj.* Pertaining to, or suffering from, nystagmus.

nys·tag·mi·form (nis·tag'mi·form) *adj.* Resembling nystagmus.

nys·tag·mo·graph (nis·tag'mo·graf) *n.* [*nystagmo-* + *-graph*]. An apparatus for recording the movements of the eyeball in nystagmus.

nys·tag·mog·ra·phy (nis"tag·mog'ruf·ee) *n.* [*nystagmo-* + *-graphy*]. The study and recording of the movements of the eyeballs in nystagmus.

nys·tag·moid (nis·tag'moid) *adj.* Resembling nystagmus.

nys·tag·mus (nis·tag'mus) *n.* [Gk. *nystagmos*, drowsiness]. An oscillatory movement of the eyeballs. It may be congenital, acquired, physiologic, or pathologic; due to neurogenic, myopathic, labyrinthine, or ocular causes. See also *dissociated, labyrinthine, lateral, ocular, optokinetic, oscillatory, pendular, positional, retraction,* and *rhythmic nystagmus, palatal myoclonus.*

nystagmus re·trac·to·ri·us (ree·track·tor'ee·us). RETRACTION NYSTAGMUS.

Nys·ten's law (nees·ten') [P. H. *Nysten*, French pediatrician, 1774–1817]. Rigor mortis is first observed in the muscles of mastication, later extends to the facial and cervical muscles, and finally involves the lower extremities.

nys·ta·tin (nis'tuh·tin, nis'tat·in) *n.* [*N*ew *Y*ork *Stat*e + *-in*]. An antibiotic substance, $C_{46}H_{77}NO_{19}$, produced by *Streptomyces noursei;* used as an antifungal agent for the treatment of infections caused by *Candida (Monilia) albicans.*

-nyxis [Gk., a pricking, stabbing]. A combining form meaning *surgical puncture or paracentesis.*

NZB mouse [*N*ew *Z*ealand *B*lack mouse]. An inbred strain of mice which spontaneously develop autoimmune hemolytic anemia. The F_1 hybrid of this mouse and NZW (white) develops a disease which resembles human systemic lupus erythematosus.

INDEX OF ANATOMICAL PLATES

PLATE	SUBJECT
1	The Human Skeleton—Anterior and Posterior Views
2	Joints of the Shoulder, Hip, and Knee
3	Superficial Muscles of the Body—Anterior and Posterior Views
4	Deep Muscles of the Trunk—Lateral and Anterior Views; Topography of the Inguinal and Femoral Regions
5	Blood Circulation—Cardiac and Pulmonary
6	Pre- and Post-natal Blood Circulatory Systems
7	Major Arteries of the Head, Trunk, and Extremities
8	Major Arteries of the Head and Viscera
9	Major Veins of the Head, Trunk, and Extremities
10	Major Veins of the Head and Viscera
11	Superficial Lymphatics of the Body; Deeper Lymphatics of the Neck, Axilla, and Groin
12	Respiratory Tract Showing Air Passages and Sinuses
13	Viscera of the Trunk—Anterior Views
14	Viscera of the Trunk—Posterior Views
15	Autonomic Nervous System Showing Sympathetic and Parasympathetic Distribution
16	Major Pathways of the Spinal Nerves and Distribution of Nerves to the Head and Neck
17	Base of the Brain with the Cranial Nerves
18	Lateral and Mesial Views of the Brain
19	The Orbit and Its Contents
20	The Ear and Its Relationships
21	Deciduous Dentition
22	Mixed and Permanent Dentition
23	Female Genitalia and the Reproductive Cycle
24	Female Urogenital Tract and Mammary Gland
25	Male Urogenital Tract
26	Endocrine Glands: Thyroid, Parathyroid, Pituitary, Adrenal (Suprarenal), Pancreas, and Gonads

PLATE 1

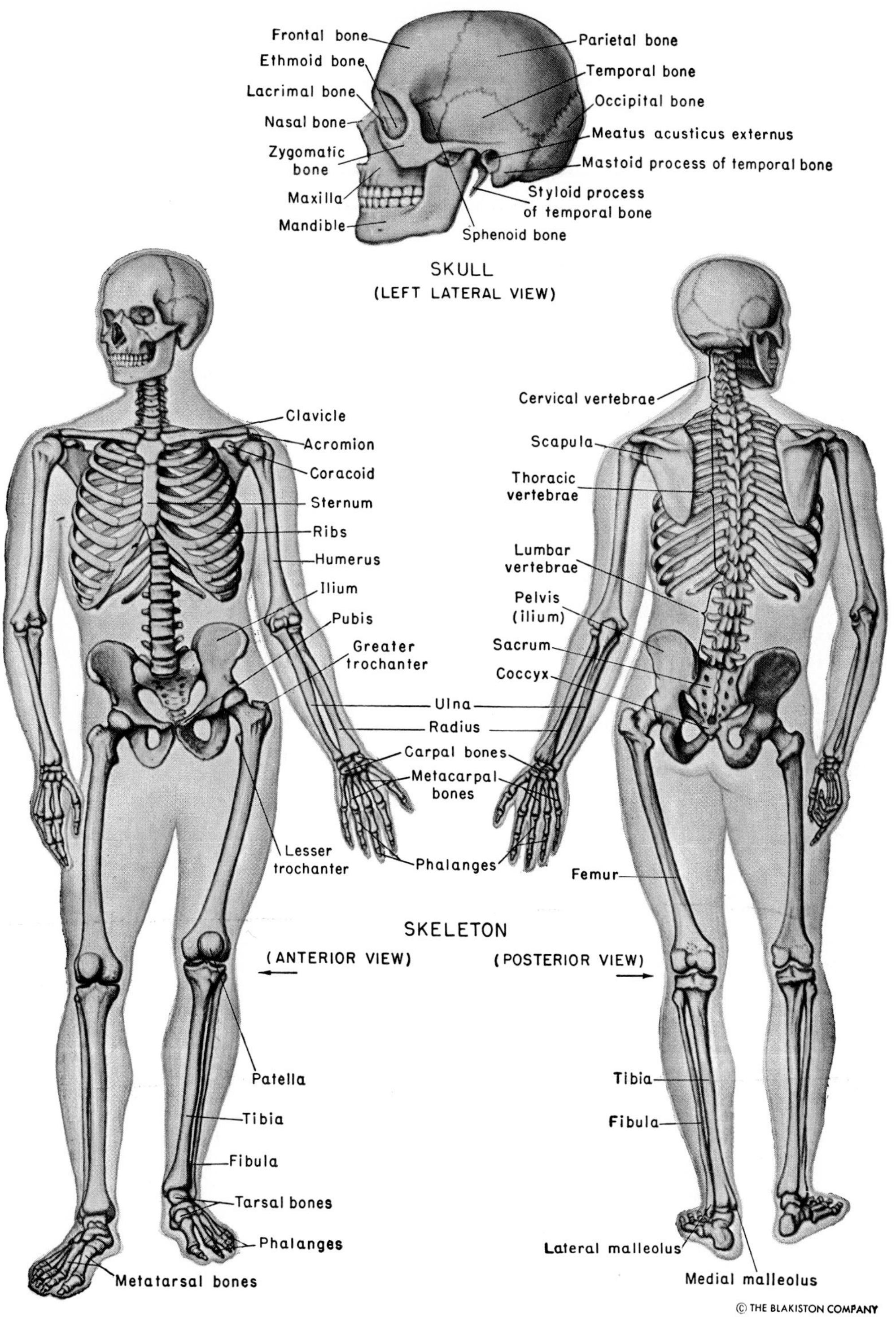

Frontal bone
Ethmoid bone
Lacrimal bone
Nasal bone
Zygomatic bone
Maxilla
Mandible
Parietal bone
Temporal bone
Occipital bone
Meatus acusticus externus
Mastoid process of temporal bone
Styloid process of temporal bone
Sphenoid bone
SKULL
(LEFT LATERAL VIEW)
Clavicle
Acromion
Coracoid
Sternum
Ribs
Humerus
Ilium
Pubis
Greater trochanter
Cervical vertebrae
Scapula
Thoracic vertebrae
Lumbar vertebrae
Pelvis (ilium)
Sacrum
Coccyx
Ulna
Radius
Carpal bones
Metacarpal bones
Phalanges
Lesser trochanter
Femur
SKELETON
(ANTERIOR VIEW)
(POSTERIOR VIEW)
Patella
Tibia
Fibula
Tarsal bones
Phalanges
Metatarsal bones
Tibia
Fibula
Lateral malleolus
Medial malleolus

SKELETON

PLATE 2

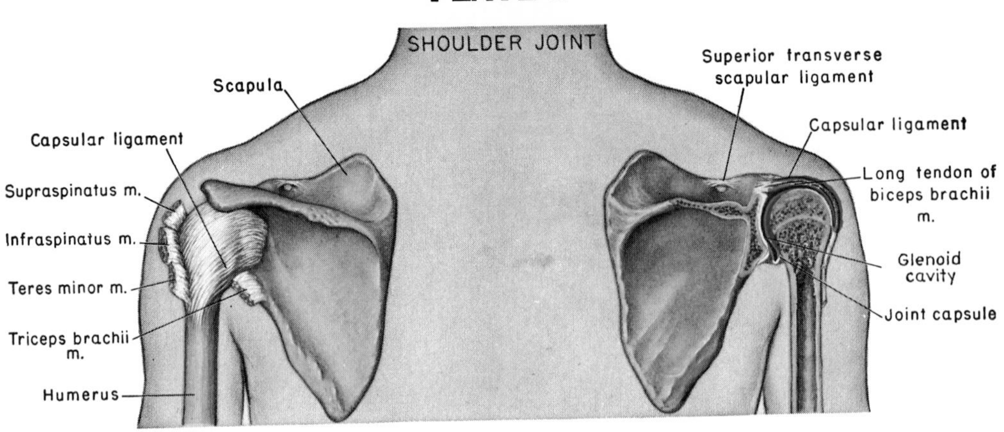
SHOULDER JOINT
Scapula
Capsular ligament
Supraspinatus m.
Infraspinatus m.
Teres minor m.
Triceps brachii m.
Humerus
Superior transverse scapular ligament
Capsular ligament
Long tendon of biceps brachii m.
Glenoid cavity
Joint capsule

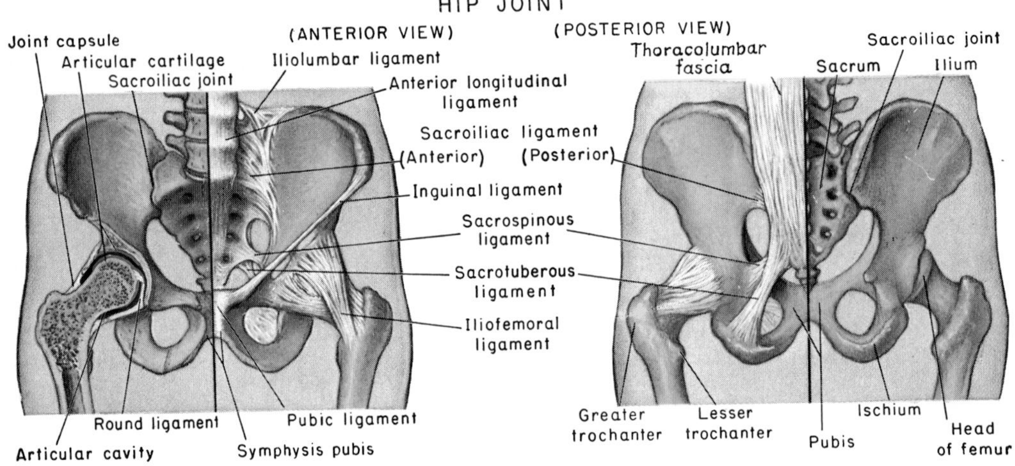
HIP JOINT
(ANTERIOR VIEW)
(POSTERIOR VIEW)
Joint capsule
Articular cartilage
Sacroiliac joint
Iliolumbar ligament
Anterior longitudinal ligament
Sacroiliac ligament
(Anterior)
(Posterior)
Inguinal ligament
Sacrospinous ligament
Sacrotuberous ligament
Iliofemoral ligament
Round ligament
Pubic ligament
Articular cavity
Symphysis pubis
Thoracolumbar fascia
Sacrum
Sacroiliac joint
Ilium
Greater trochanter
Lesser trochanter
Pubis
Ischium
Head of femur

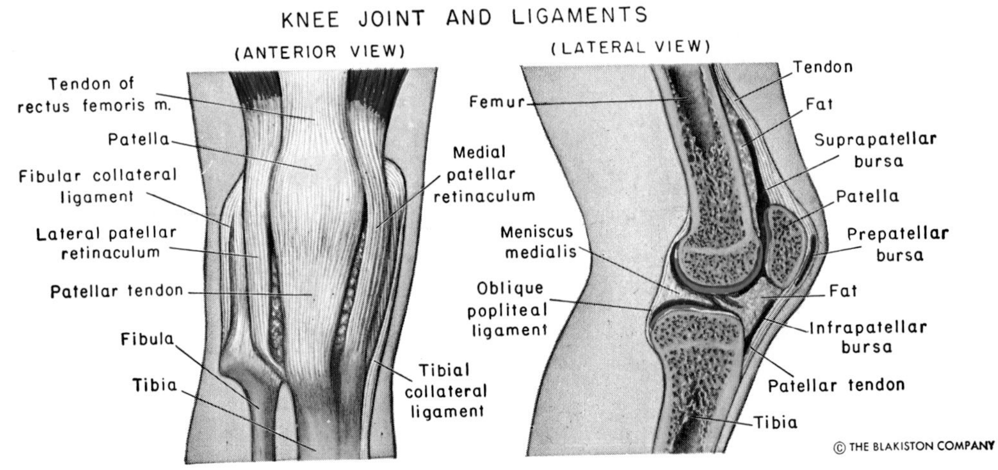
KNEE JOINT AND LIGAMENTS
(ANTERIOR VIEW)
(LATERAL VIEW)
Tendon of rectus femoris m.
Patella
Fibular collateral ligament
Lateral patellar retinaculum
Patellar tendon
Fibula
Tibia
Medial patellar retinaculum
Tibial collateral ligament
Femur
Meniscus medialis
Oblique popliteal ligament
Tendon
Fat
Suprapatellar bursa
Patella
Prepatellar bursa
Fat
Infrapatellar bursa
Patellar tendon
Tibia

JOINTS

PLATE 3

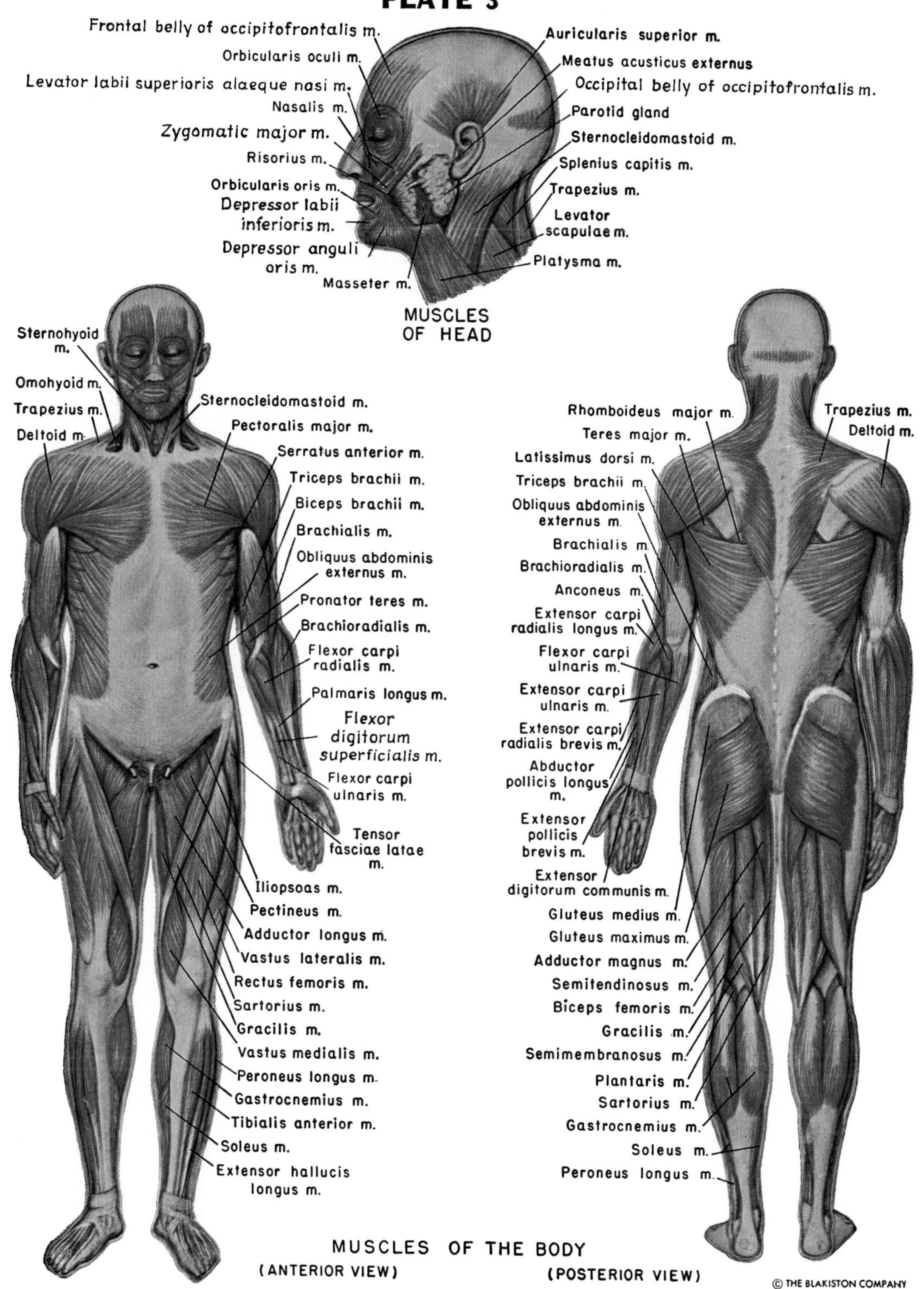

Frontal belly of occipitofrontalis m.
Orbicularis oculi m.
Levator labii superioris alaeque nasi m.
Nasalis m.
Zygomatic major m.
Risorius m.
Orbicularis oris m.
Depressor labii inferioris m.
Depressor anguli oris m.
Masseter m.
Auricularis superior m.
Meatus acusticus externus
Occipital belly of occipitofrontalis m.
Parotid gland
Sternocleidomastoid m.
Splenius capitis m.
Trapezius m.
Levator scapulae m.
Platysma m.
MUSCLES OF HEAD
Sternohyoid m.
Omohyoid m.
Trapezius m.
Deltoid m.
Sternocleidomastoid m.
Pectoralis major m.
Serratus anterior m.
Triceps brachii m.
Biceps brachii m.
Brachialis m.
Obliquus abdominis externus m.
Pronator teres m.
Brachioradialis m.
Flexor carpi radialis m.
Palmaris longus m.
Flexor digitorum superficialis m.
Flexor carpi ulnaris m.
Tensor fasciae latae m.
Iliopsoas m.
Pectineus m.
Adductor longus m.
Vastus lateralis m.
Rectus femoris m.
Sartorius m.
Gracilis m.
Vastus medialis m.
Peroneus longus m.
Gastrocnemius m.
Tibialis anterior m.
Soleus m.
Extensor hallucis longus m.
Rhomboideus major m.
Teres major m.
Latissimus dorsi m.
Triceps brachii m.
Obliquus abdominis externus m.
Brachialis m.
Brachioradialis m.
Anconeus m.
Extensor carpi radialis longus m.
Flexor carpi ulnaris m.
Extensor carpi ulnaris m.
Extensor carpi radialis brevis m.
Abductor pollicis longus m.
Extensor pollicis brevis m.
Extensor digitorum communis m.
Gluteus medius m.
Gluteus maximus m.
Adductor magnus m.
Semitendinosus m.
Biceps femoris m.
Gracilis m.
Semimembranosus m.
Plantaris m.
Sartorius m.
Gastrocnemius m.
Soleus m.
Peroneus longus m.
Trapezius m.
Deltoid m.
MUSCLES OF THE BODY
(ANTERIOR VIEW)
(POSTERIOR VIEW)

MUSCLES

PLATE 4

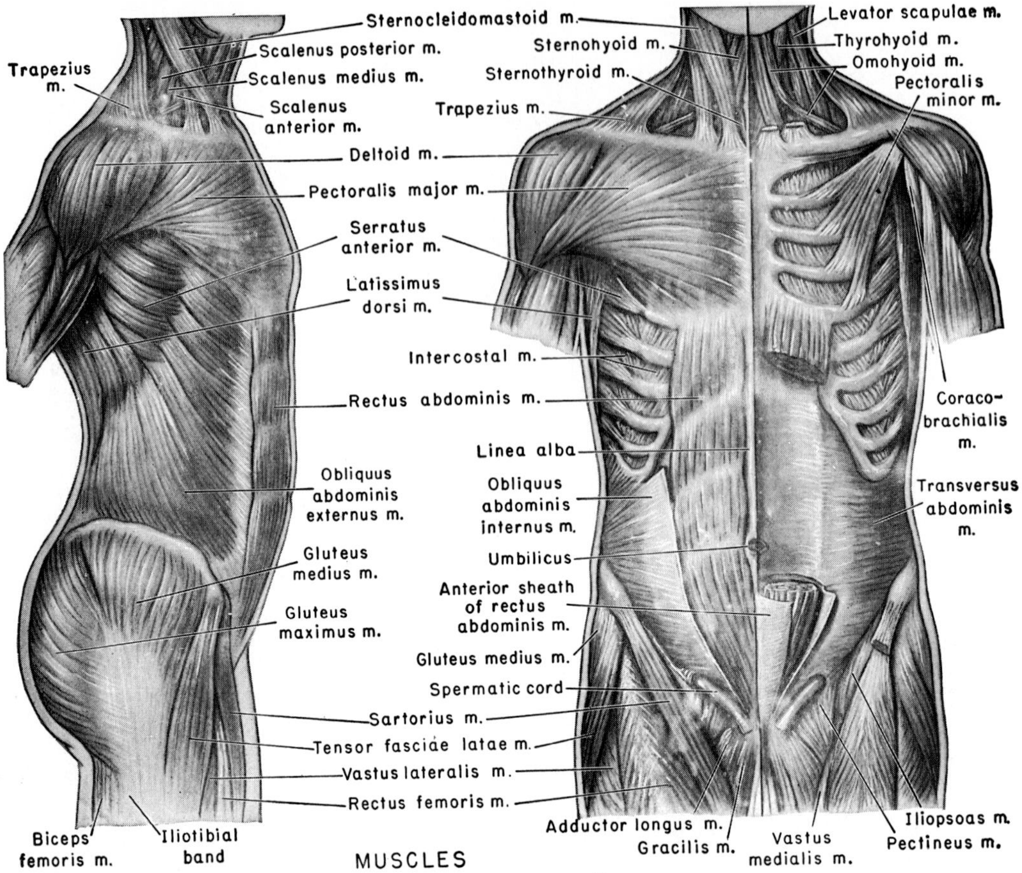

Sternocleidomastoid m.
Scalenus posterior m.
Scalenus medius m.
Trapezius m.
Scalenus anterior m.
Deltoid m.
Pectoralis major m.
Serratus anterior m.
Latissimus dorsi m.
Rectus abdominis m.
Obliquus abdominis externus m.
Gluteus medius m.
Gluteus maximus m.
Sartorius m.
Tensor fasciae latae m.
Vastus lateralis m.
Rectus femoris m.
Biceps femoris m.
Iliotibial band
Levator scapulae m.
Sternohyoid m.
Thyrohyoid m.
Omohyoid m.
Sternothyroid m.
Pectoralis minor m.
Trapezius m.
Intercostal m.
Coraco-brachialis m.
Linea alba
Obliquus abdominis internus m.
Transversus abdominis m.
Umbilicus
Anterior sheath of rectus abdominis m.
Gluteus medius m.
Spermatic cord
Adductor longus m.
Gracilis m.
Vastus medialis m.
Iliopsoas m.
Pectineus m.

MUSCLES OF SHOULDER, TRUNK, AND HIP

(RIGHT LATERAL VIEW) (ANTERIOR VIEW)

Inguinal hernia
Femoral hernia
Deep inguinal ring
Superficial inguinal ring
Femoral v.
Spermatic cord

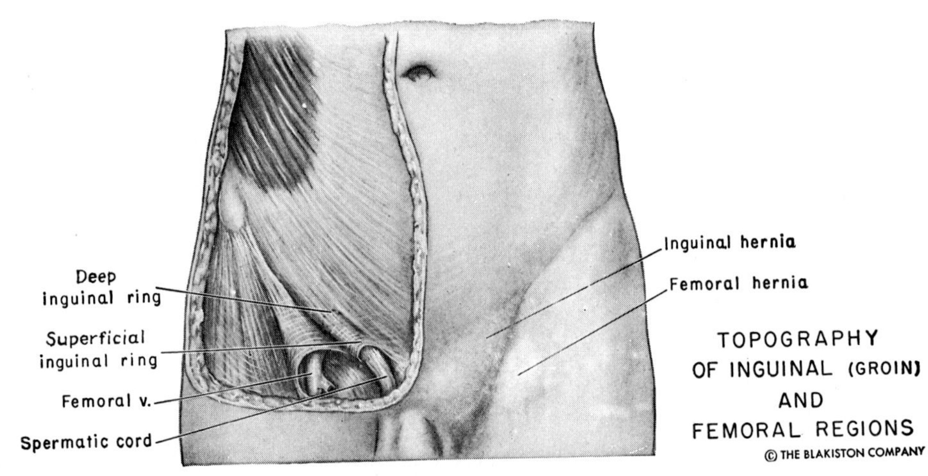

TOPOGRAPHY OF INGUINAL (GROIN) AND FEMORAL REGIONS

MUSCLES

PLATE 5

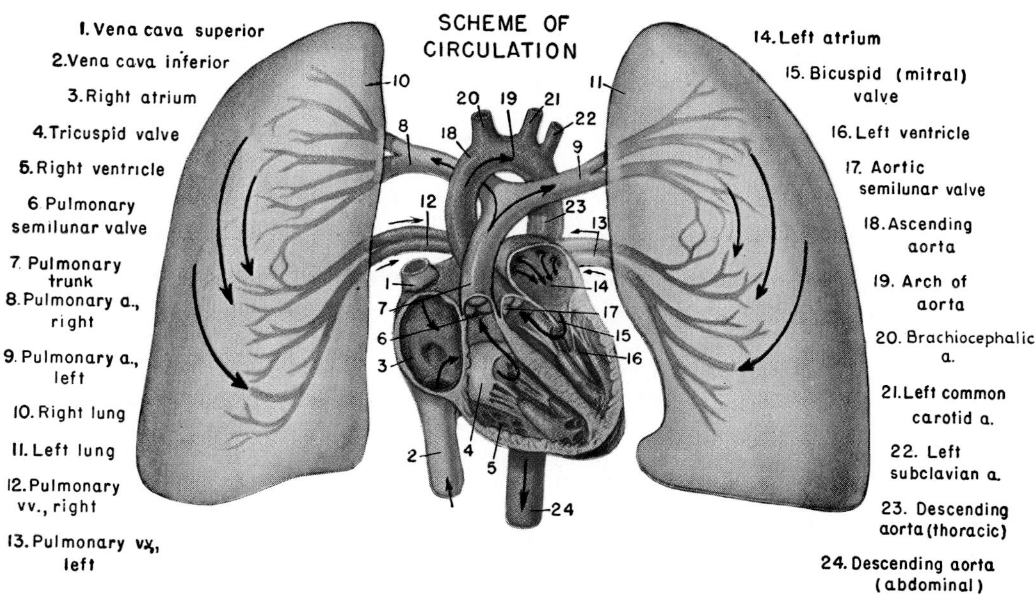

SCHEME OF CIRCULATION
1. Vena cava superior
2. Vena cava inferior
3. Right atrium
4. Tricuspid valve
5. Right ventricle
6. Pulmonary semilunar valve
7. Pulmonary trunk
8. Pulmonary a., right
9. Pulmonary a., left
10. Right lung
11. Left lung
12. Pulmonary vv., right
13. Pulmonary vv., left
14. Left atrium
15. Bicuspid (mitral) valve
16. Left ventricle
17. Aortic semilunar valve
18. Ascending aorta
19. Arch of aorta
20. Brachiocephalic a.
21. Left common carotid a.
22. Left subclavian a.
23. Descending aorta (thoracic)
24. Descending aorta (abdominal)

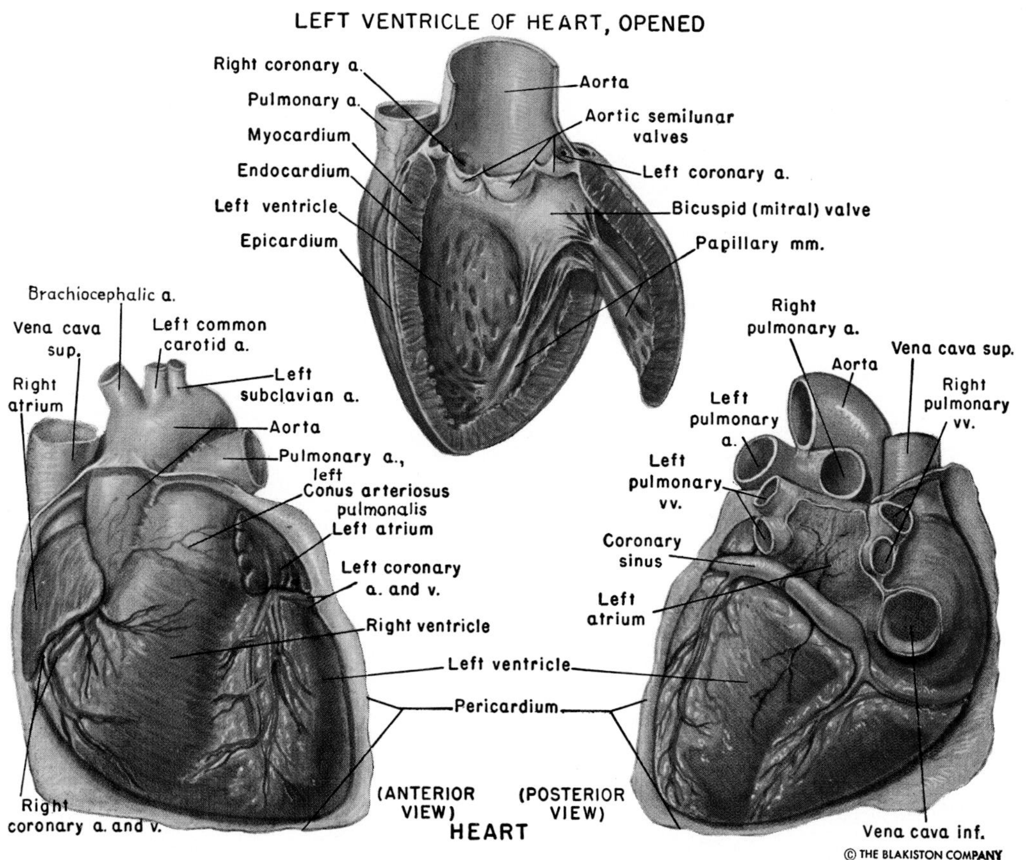

LEFT VENTRICLE OF HEART, OPENED
Right coronary a.
Pulmonary a.
Myocardium
Endocardium
Left ventricle
Epicardium
Aorta
Aortic semilunar valves
Left coronary a.
Bicuspid (mitral) valve
Papillary mm.
Brachiocephalic a.
Vena cava sup.
Left common carotid a.
Right atrium
Left subclavian a.
Aorta
Pulmonary a., left
Conus arteriosus pulmonalis
Left atrium
Left coronary a. and v.
Right ventricle
Left ventricle
Pericardium
Right coronary a. and v.
(ANTERIOR VIEW)
HEART
(POSTERIOR VIEW)
Right pulmonary a.
Aorta
Vena cava sup.
Right pulmonary vv.
Left pulmonary a.
Left pulmonary vv.
Coronary sinus
Left atrium
Vena cava inf.

BLOOD CIRCULATION

PLATE 6

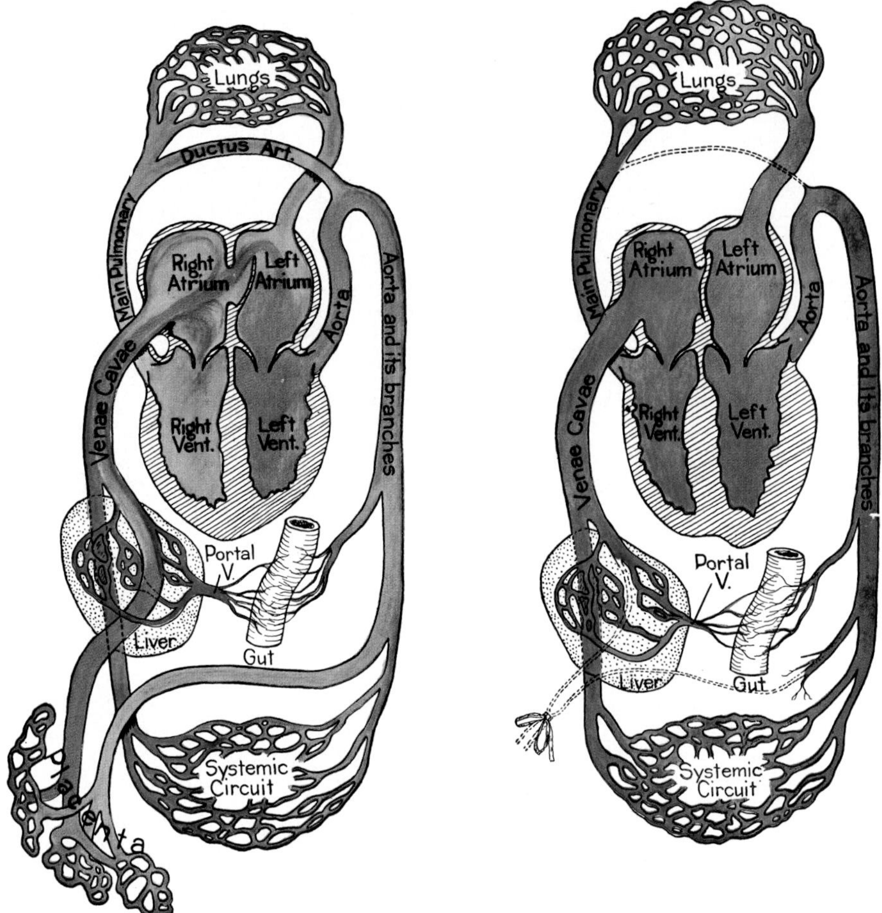

(Left) Prenatal (fetal) circulation. (Right) Postnatal circulation.

(From Patten: "Human Embryology." Copyright, The Blakiston Company.)

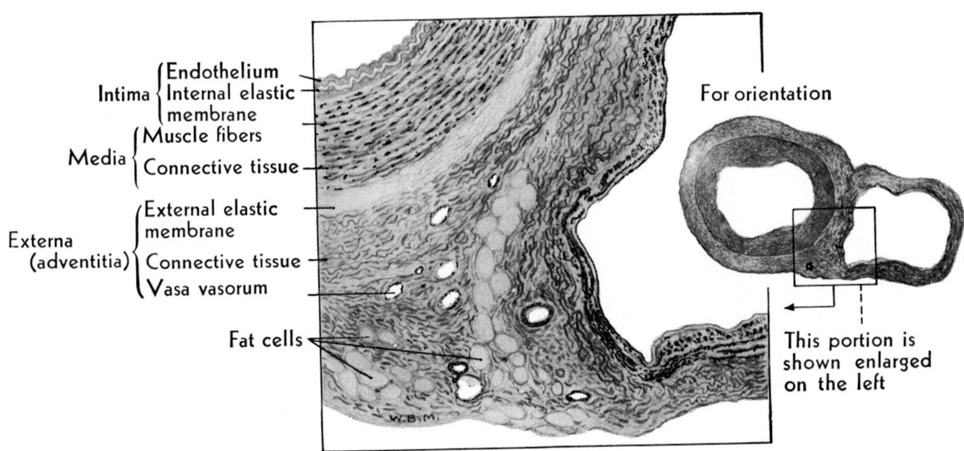

Section through human ulnar artery and vein, showing (left) wall of artery and (right) wall of vein.

(From Bremer-Weatherford: "Textbook of Histology." Copyright, The Blakiston Company.)

PRE- AND POSTNATAL BLOOD CIRCULATORY SYSTEMS

PLATE 7

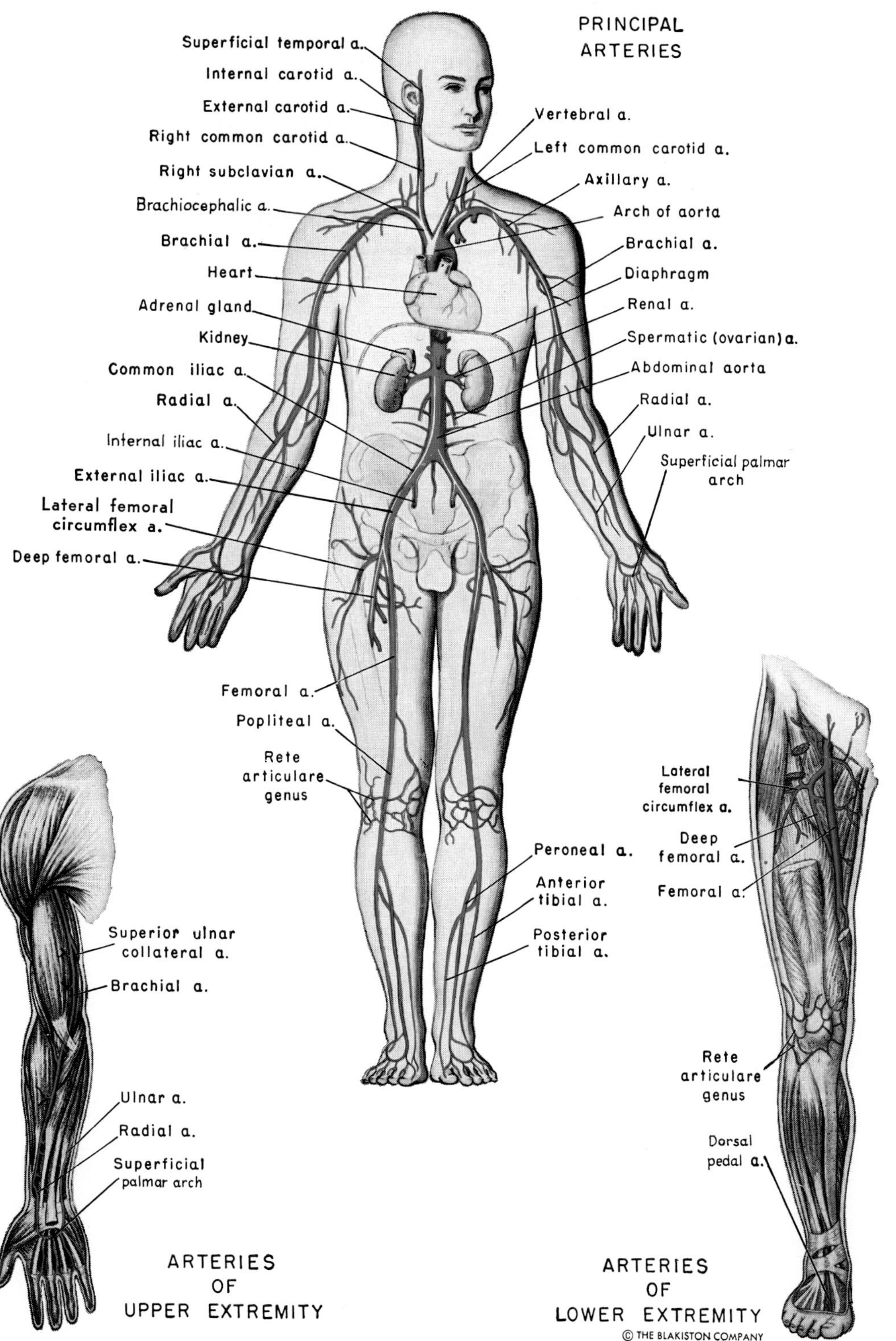
PRINCIPAL ARTERIES
Superficial temporal a.
Internal carotid a.
External carotid a.
Right common carotid a.
Right subclavian a.
Brachiocephalic a.
Brachial a.
Heart
Adrenal gland
Kidney
Common iliac a.
Radial a.
Internal iliac a.
External iliac a.
Lateral femoral circumflex a.
Deep femoral a.
Vertebral a.
Left common carotid a.
Axillary a.
Arch of aorta
Brachial a.
Diaphragm
Renal a.
Spermatic (ovarian) a.
Abdominal aorta
Radial a.
Ulnar a.
Superficial palmar arch
Femoral a.
Popliteal a.
Rete articulare genus
Peroneal a.
Anterior tibial a.
Posterior tibial a.
Superior ulnar collateral a.
Brachial a.
Ulnar a.
Radial a.
Superficial palmar arch
ARTERIES OF UPPER EXTREMITY
Lateral femoral circumflex a.
Deep femoral a.
Femoral a.
Rete articulare genus
Dorsal pedal a.
ARTERIES OF LOWER EXTREMITY

ARTERIES

PLATE 8

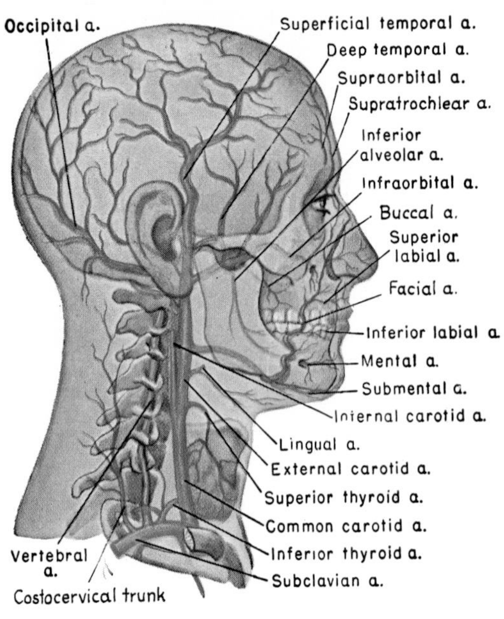

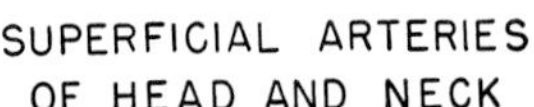
SUPERFICIAL ARTERIES OF HEAD AND NECK

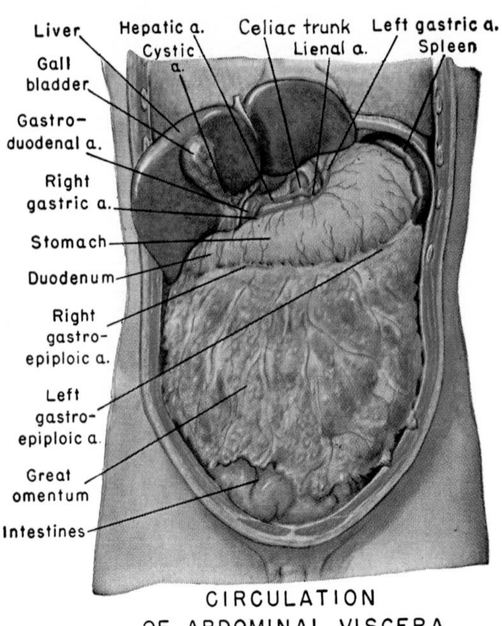

CIRCULATION OF ABDOMINAL VISCERA

CIRCULATION OF DIGESTIVE TRACT

Ileocolic a.
Right colic a.
Middle colic a.
Superior mesenteric a.
Ascending colon
Omentum
Transverse colon
Transverse mesocolon
Left colic a.
Abdominal aorta
Inferior mesenteric a.
Descending colon
Superior rectal a.
Sigmoid a.
Sigmoid colon
Bladder
Rectum

DEEP CIRCULATION OF ABDOMEN

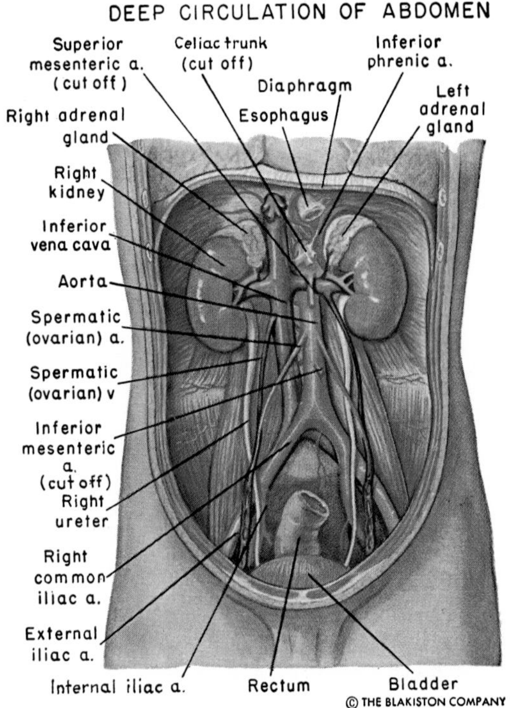

ARTERIES

PLATE 9

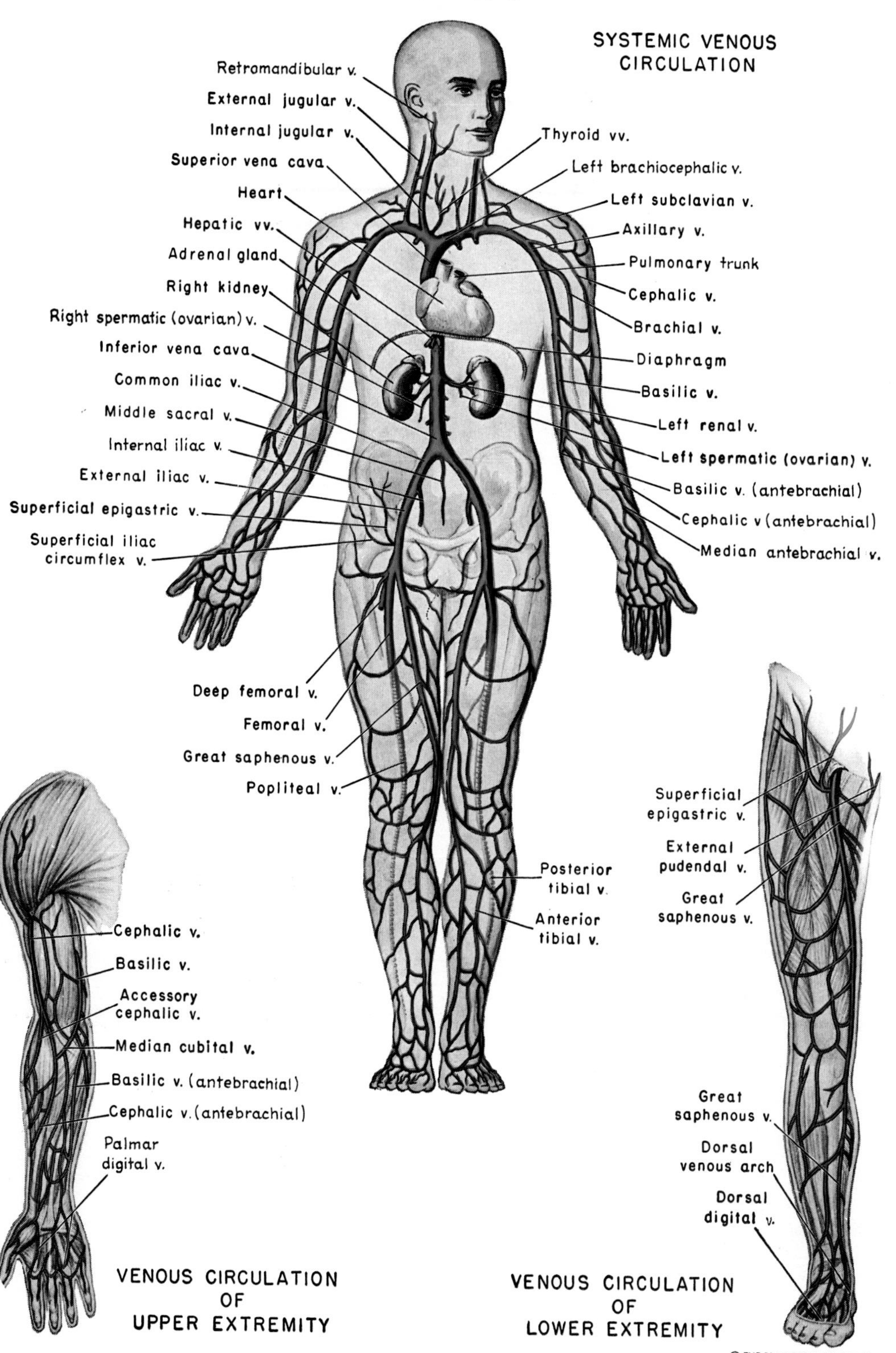

SYSTEMIC VENOUS CIRCULATION
Retromandibular v.
External jugular v.
Internal jugular v.
Superior vena cava
Heart
Hepatic vv.
Adrenal gland
Right kidney
Right spermatic (ovarian) v.
Inferior vena cava
Common iliac v.
Middle sacral v.
Internal iliac v.
External iliac v.
Superficial epigastric v.
Superficial iliac circumflex v.
Thyroid vv.
Left brachiocephalic v.
Left subclavian v.
Axillary v.
Pulmonary trunk
Cephalic v.
Brachial v.
Diaphragm
Basilic v.
Left renal v.
Left spermatic (ovarian) v.
Basilic v. (antebrachial)
Cephalic v (antebrachial)
Median antebrachial v.
Deep femoral v.
Femoral v.
Great saphenous v.
Popliteal v.
Posterior tibial v.
Anterior tibial v.
Cephalic v.
Basilic v.
Accessory cephalic v.
Median cubital v.
Basilic v. (antebrachial)
Cephalic v. (antebrachial)
Palmar digital v.
Superficial epigastric v.
External pudendal v.
Great saphenous v.
Great saphenous v.
Dorsal venous arch
Dorsal digital v.
VENOUS CIRCULATION OF UPPER EXTREMITY
VENOUS CIRCULATION OF LOWER EXTREMITY

VEINS

PLATE 10

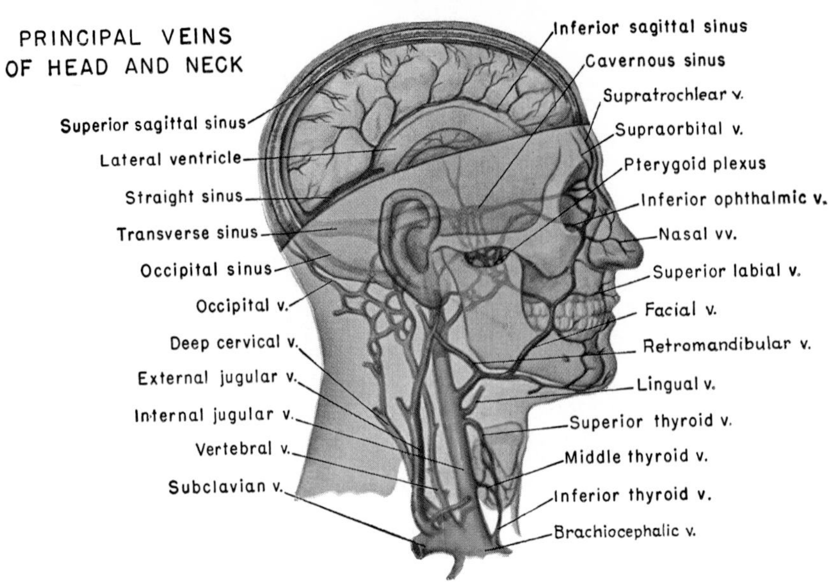
PRINCIPAL VEINS
OF HEAD AND NECK
Superior sagittal sinus
Lateral ventricle
Straight sinus
Transverse sinus
Occipital sinus
Occipital v.
Deep cervical v.
External jugular v.
Internal jugular v.
Vertebral v.
Subclavian v.
Inferior sagittal sinus
Cavernous sinus
Supratrochlear v.
Supraorbital v.
Pterygoid plexus
Inferior ophthalmic v.
Nasal vv.
Superior labial v.
Facial v.
Retromandibular v.
Lingual v.
Superior thyroid v.
Middle thyroid v.
Inferior thyroid v.
Brachiocephalic v.

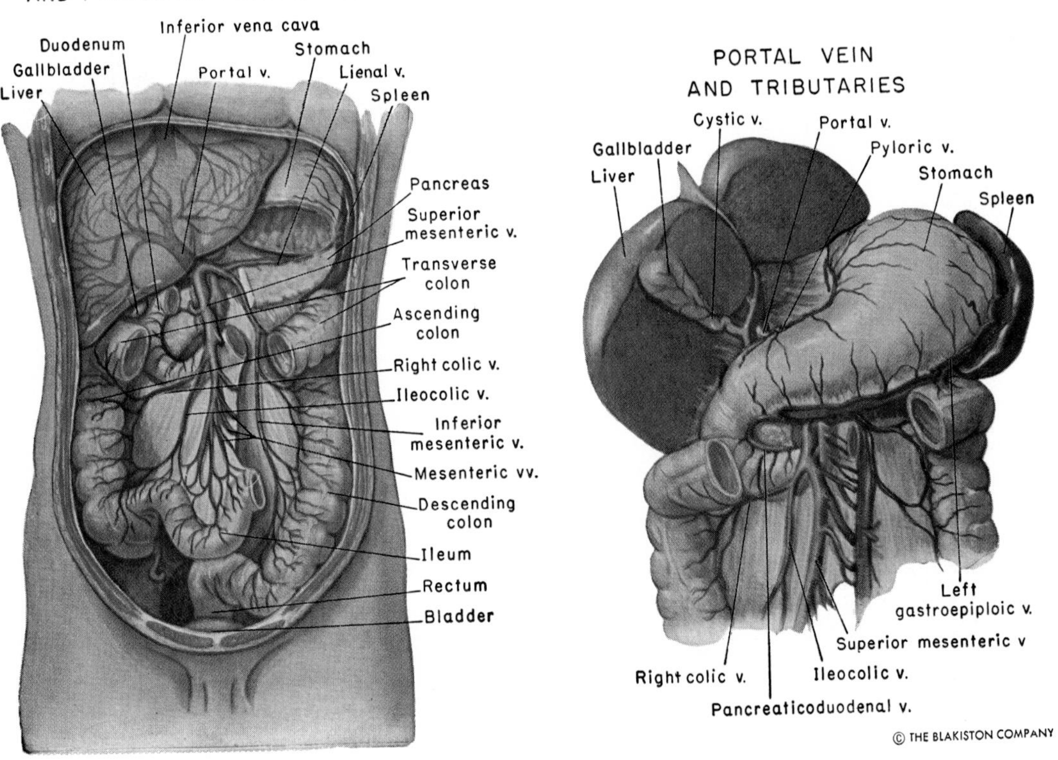
PORTAL VEIN
AND PRINCIPAL TRIBUTARIES
Inferior vena cava
Duodenum
Gallbladder
Liver
Portal v.
Stomach
Lienal v.
Spleen
Pancreas
Superior
mesenteric v.
Transverse
colon
Ascending
colon
Right colic v.
Ileocolic v.
Inferior
mesenteric v.
Mesenteric vv.
Descending
colon
Ileum
Rectum
Bladder
PORTAL VEIN
AND TRIBUTARIES
Cystic v.
Portal v.
Gallbladder
Pyloric v.
Liver
Stomach
Spleen
Left
gastroepiploic v.
Superior mesenteric v
Right colic v.
Ileocolic v.
Pancreaticoduodenal v.

VEINS

PLATE 11

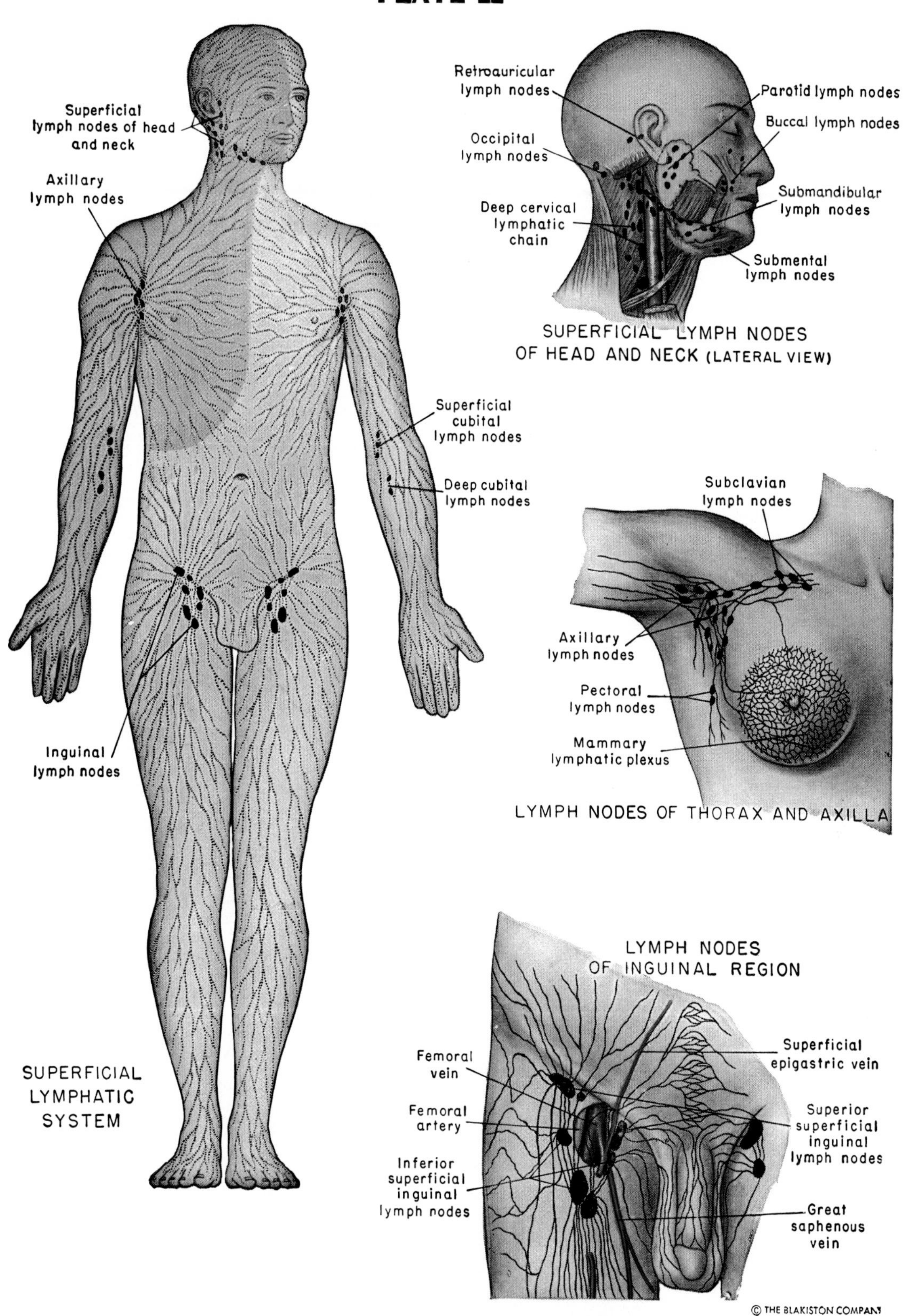

Superficial lymph nodes of head and neck
Axillary lymph nodes
Superficial cubital lymph nodes
Deep cubital lymph nodes
Inguinal lymph nodes
SUPERFICIAL LYMPHATIC SYSTEM
Retroauricular lymph nodes
Parotid lymph nodes
Buccal lymph nodes
Occipital lymph nodes
Submandibular lymph nodes
Deep cervical lymphatic chain
Submental lymph nodes
SUPERFICIAL LYMPH NODES OF HEAD AND NECK (LATERAL VIEW)
Subclavian lymph nodes
Axillary lymph nodes
Pectoral lymph nodes
Mammary lymphatic plexus
LYMPH NODES OF THORAX AND AXILLA
LYMPH NODES OF INGUINAL REGION
Femoral vein
Superficial epigastric vein
Femoral artery
Superior superficial inguinal lymph nodes
Inferior superficial inguinal lymph nodes
Great saphenous vein

LYMPHATIC SYSTEM

PLATE 12

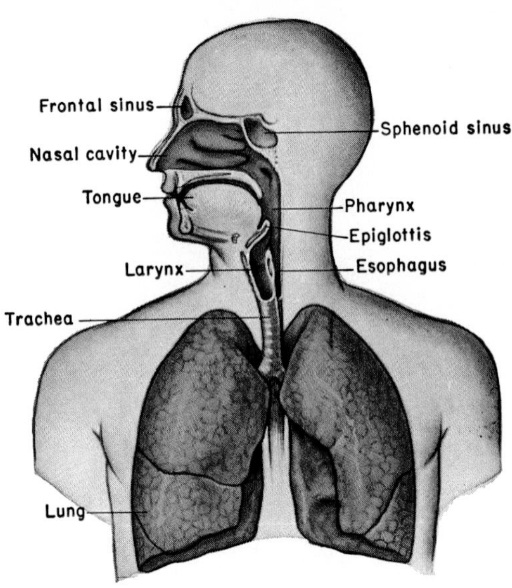

RESPIRATORY TRACT
(SCHEMATIC)

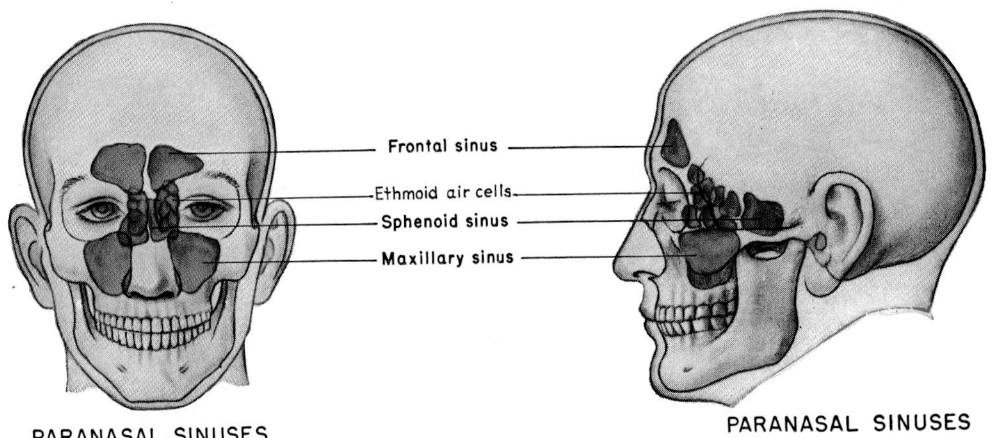

PARANASAL SINUSES
(ANTERIOR VIEW) (SCHEMATIC)

PARANASAL SINUSES
(LATERAL VIEW) (SCHEMATIC)

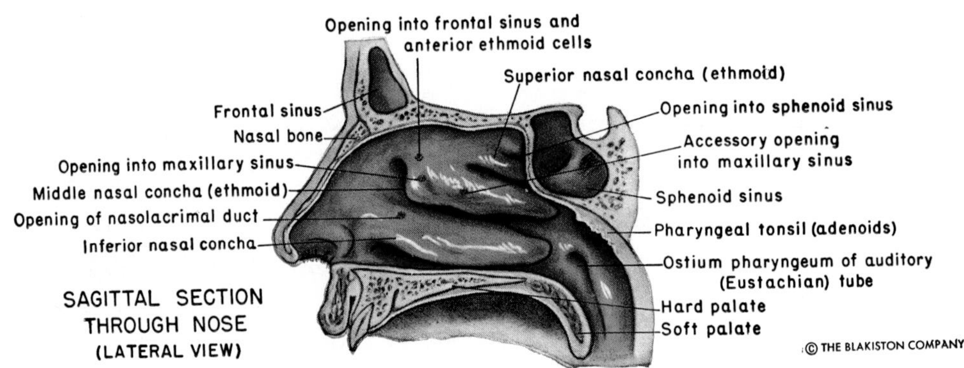

SAGITTAL SECTION
THROUGH NOSE
(LATERAL VIEW)

RESPIRATORY TRACT

PLATE 13

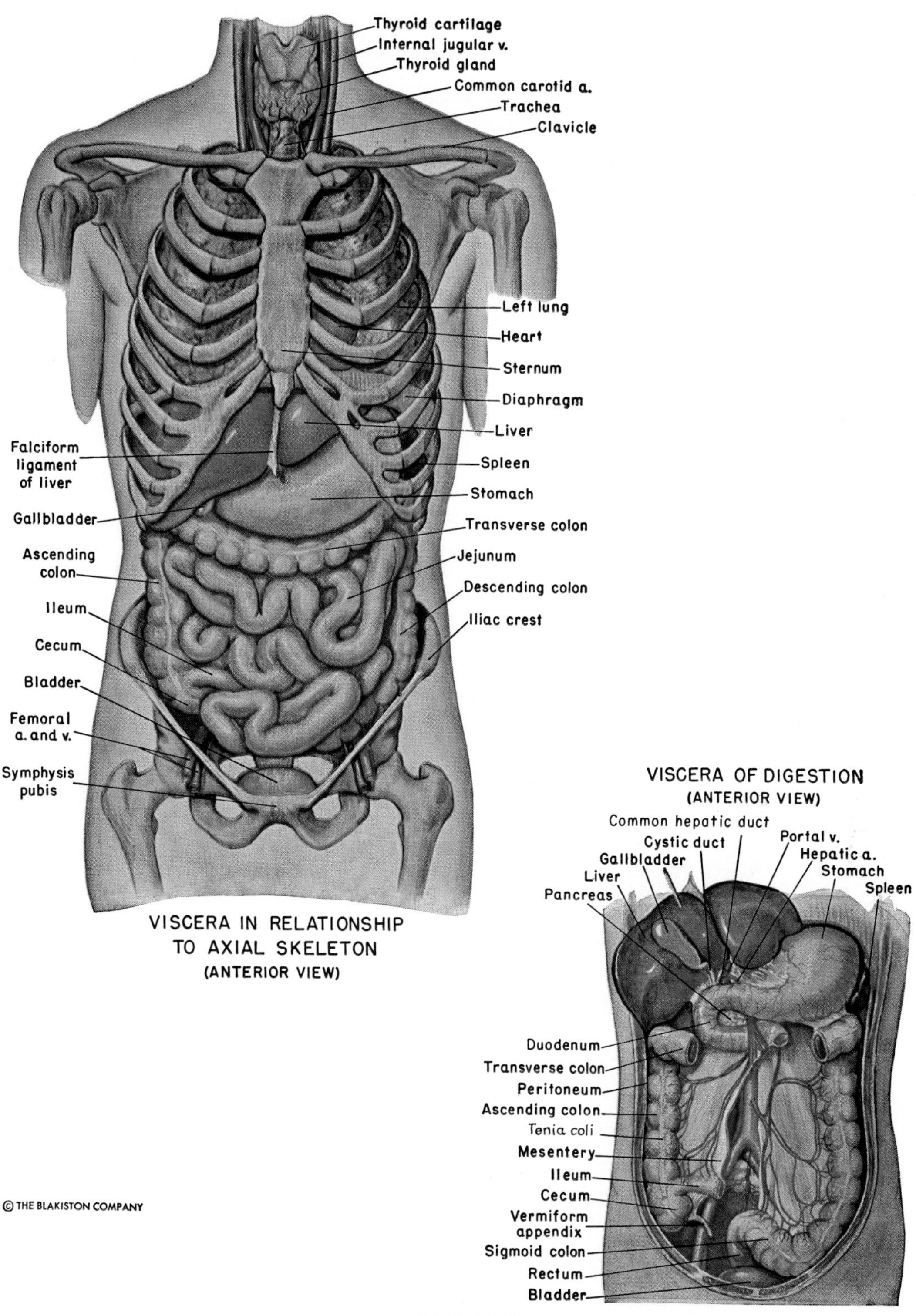

VISCERA IN RELATIONSHIP TO AXIAL SKELETON
(ANTERIOR VIEW)

VISCERA OF DIGESTION
(ANTERIOR VIEW)

VISCERA

PLATE 14

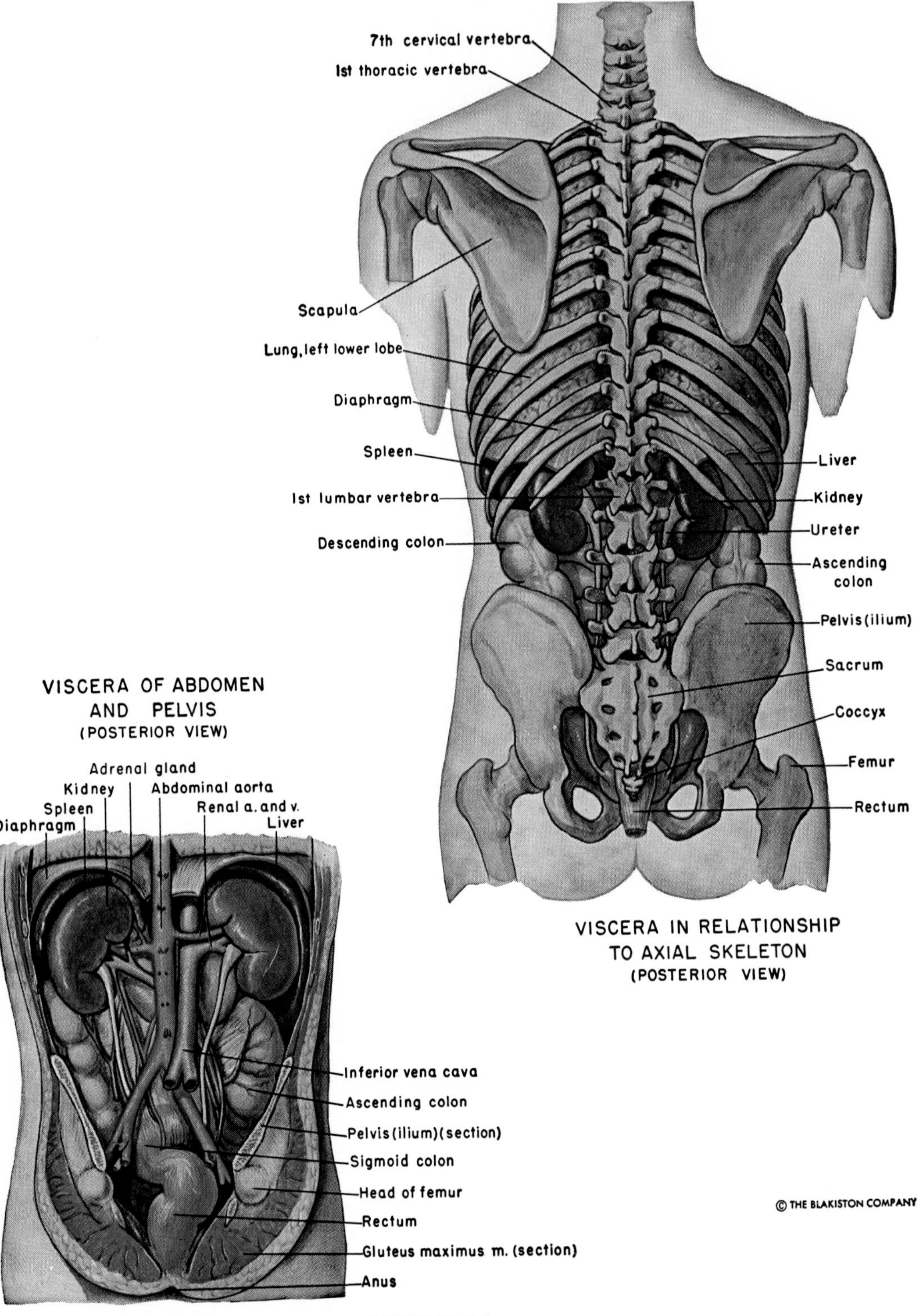

VISCERA IN RELATIONSHIP TO AXIAL SKELETON (POSTERIOR VIEW)

VISCERA OF ABDOMEN AND PELVIS (POSTERIOR VIEW)

VISCERA

PLATE 15

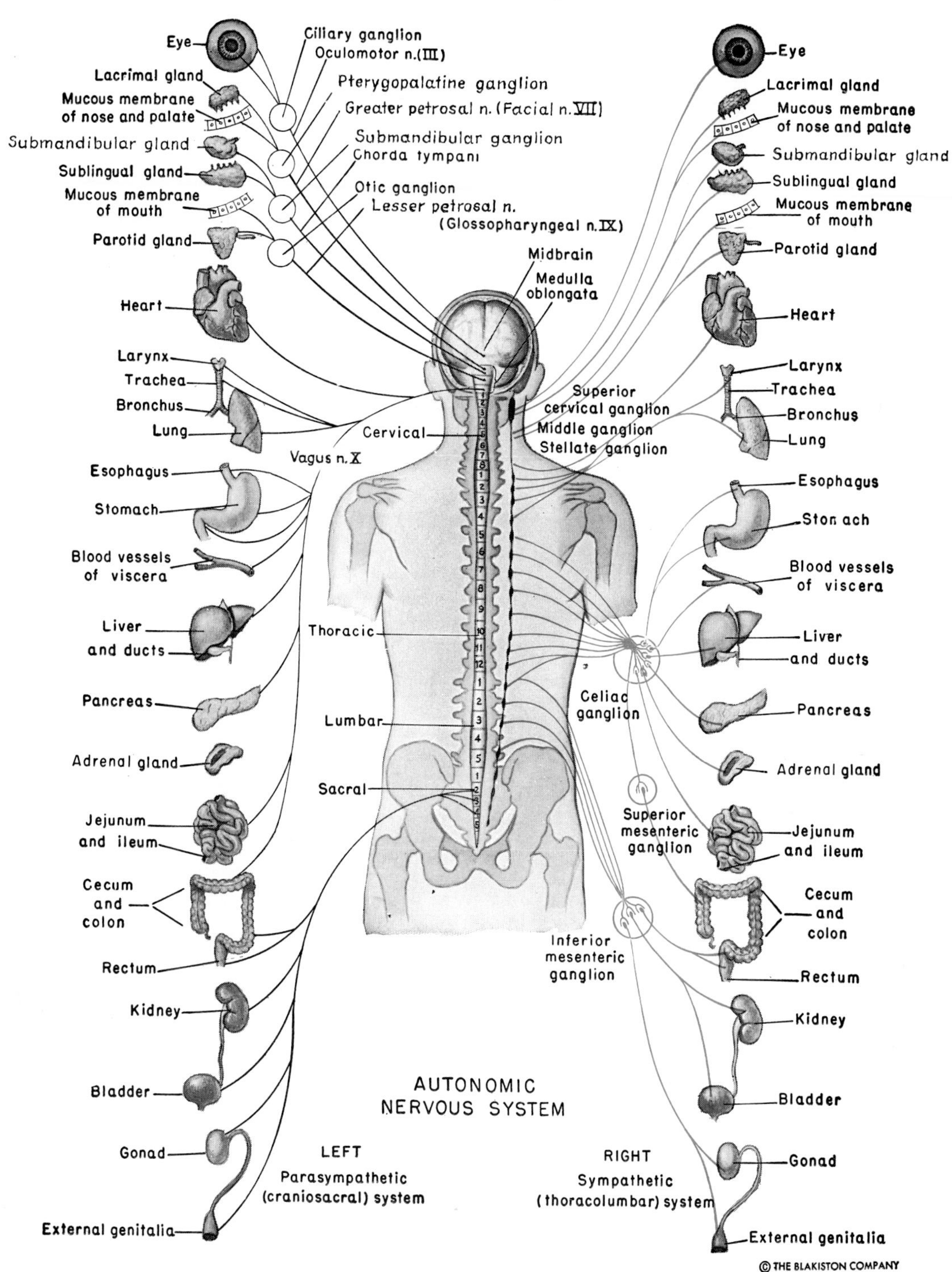

Eye
Lacrimal gland
Mucous membrane of nose and palate
Submandibular gland
Sublingual gland
Mucous membrane of mouth
Parotid gland
Heart
Larynx
Trachea
Bronchus
Lung
Esophagus
Stomach
Blood vessels of viscera
Liver and ducts
Pancreas
Adrenal gland
Jejunum and ileum
Cecum and colon
Rectum
Kidney
Bladder
Gonad
External genitalia
Ciliary ganglion
Oculomotor n.(III)
Pterygopalatine ganglion
Greater petrosal n. (Facial n.VII)
Submandibular ganglion
Chorda tympani
Otic ganglion
Lesser petrosal n.
(Glossopharyngeal n.IX)
Midbrain
Medulla oblongata
Superior cervical ganglion
Middle ganglion
Stellate ganglion
Cervical
Vagus n.X
Thoracic
Lumbar
Sacral
Celiac ganglion
Superior mesenteric ganglion
Inferior mesenteric ganglion
AUTONOMIC NERVOUS SYSTEM
LEFT
Parasympathetic
(craniosacral) system
RIGHT
Sympathetic
(thoracolumbar) system
Eye
Lacrimal gland
Mucous membrane of nose and palate
Submandibular gland
Sublingual gland
Mucous membrane of mouth
Parotid gland
Heart
Larynx
Trachea
Bronchus
Lung
Esophagus
Ston ach
Blood vessels of viscera
Liver
and ducts
Pancreas
Adrenal gland
Jejunum and ileum
Cecum and colon
Rectum
Kidney
Bladder
Gonad
External genitalia

AUTONOMIC NERVOUS SYSTEM

PLATE 16

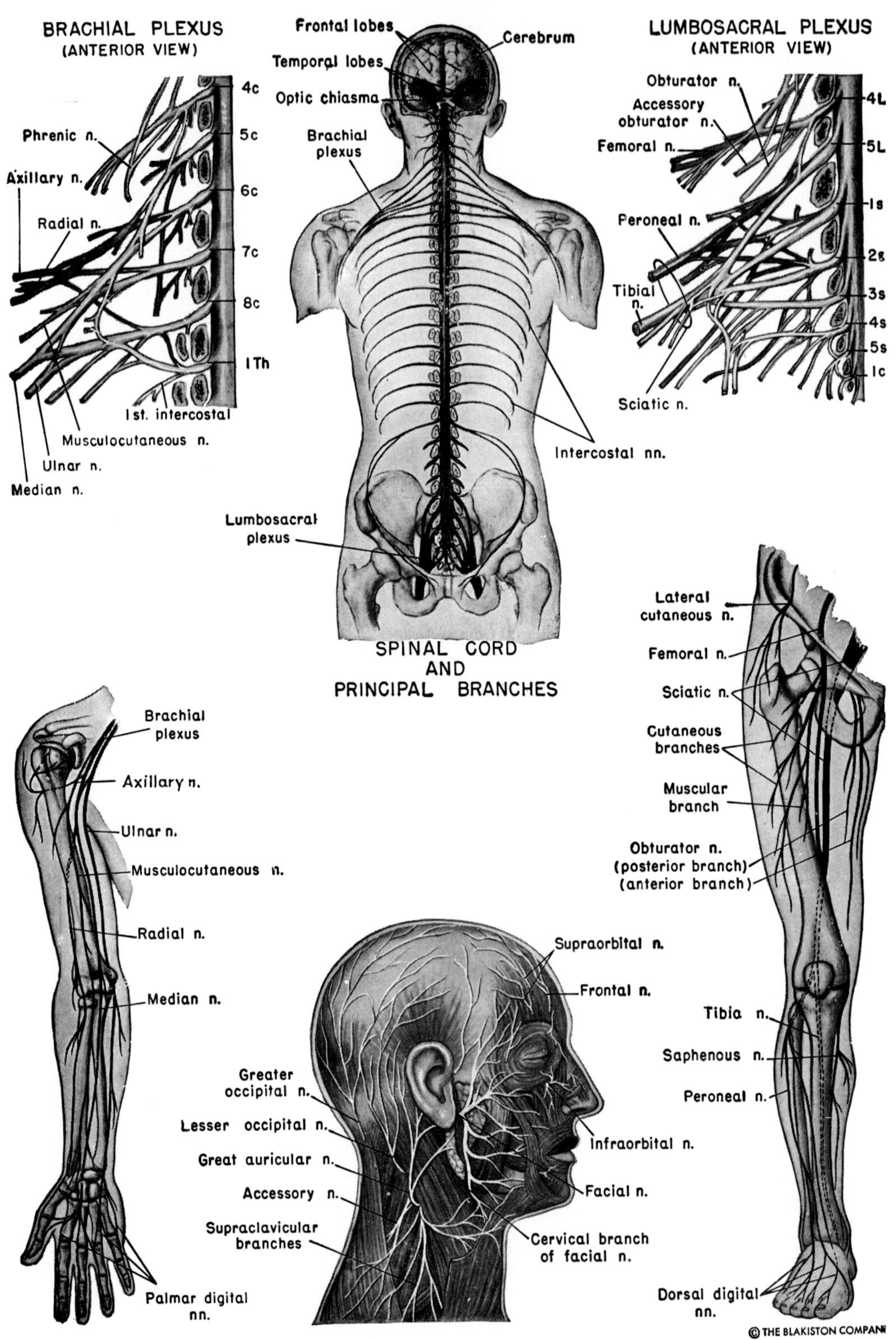

BRACHIAL PLEXUS
(ANTERIOR VIEW)
4c
5c
6c
7c
8c
1Th
Phrenic n.
Axillary n.
Radial n.
1st. intercostal
Musculocutaneous n.
Ulnar n.
Median n.
Frontal lobes
Cerebrum
Temporal lobes
Optic chiasma
Brachial plexus
Intercostal nn.
Lumbosacral plexus
SPINAL CORD
AND
PRINCIPAL BRANCHES
LUMBOSACRAL PLEXUS
(ANTERIOR VIEW)
Obturator n.
Accessory obturator n.
Femoral n.
Peroneal n.
Tibial n.
Sciatic n.
4L
5L
1s
2s
3s
4s
5s
1c
Brachial plexus
Axillary n.
Ulnar n.
Musculocutaneous n.
Radial n.
Median n.
Palmar digital nn.
Supraorbital n.
Frontal n.
Greater occipital n.
Lesser occipital n.
Great auricular n.
Accessory n.
Supraclavicular branches
Infraorbital n.
Facial n.
Cervical branch of facial n.
Lateral cutaneous n.
Femoral n.
Sciatic n.
Cutaneous branches
Muscular branch
Obturator n.
(posterior branch)
(anterior branch)
Tibia n.
Saphenous n.
Peroneal n.
Dorsal digital nn.

NERVOUS SYSTEM

PLATE 17 BASE OF BRAIN

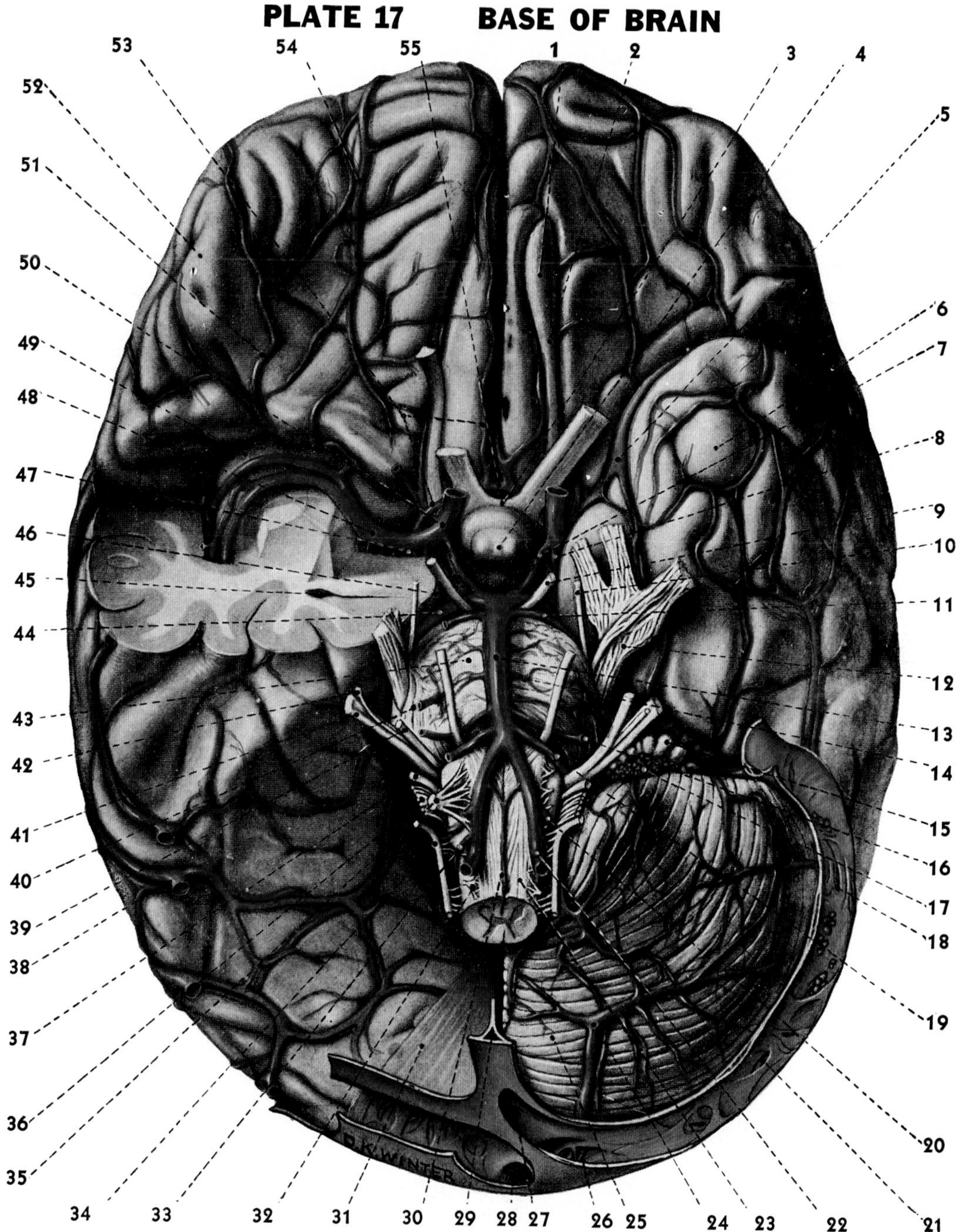

Accessory n. (spinal accessory) (XI), **34.** Vestibulocochlear n. (VIII), **41.** Anterior cerebral a., **53.** Anterior communicating a., **55.** Anterior inferior cerebellar a., **19.** Anterior spinal a., **30.** Basilar a., **13.** Brainstem, **23.** Cerebellar v., **24.** Cerebellar v.—opening of into sinus, **26.** Cerebellum, **25.** Choroid a., **8.** Choroid plexus of 4th ventricle, **17.** Confluens sinuum—opening of straight sinus into, **27.** Facial n. (VII), **39.** Flocculus, **15.** Frontal lobe, **52.** Ganglionic branches, **47.** Glossopharyngeal n. (IX), **37.** Hypoglossal n. (XII), **35.** Inferior frontal v., **54.** Occipital diploic v. to transverse sinus, **38.** Insula (island of Reil), **49.** Intermediary n. (Wrisberg), **42.** Internal auditory a. (a. auditiva interna), **16.** Internal carotid a., **50.** Lateral sinus—junction of with sigmoid sinus, **18.** Lateral sinus—opening of a superficial vein into, **21.** Lateral ventricle—inferior cornu, **45.** Middle cerebral a., **48.** Middle cerebral a.—cortical branch of, **51.** Occipital sinus, **29.** Oculomotor n. (III), **9.** Olfactory bulb, **1.** Olfactory tract, **2.** Optic chiasma, **3.** Hypophysis (pituitary), **4.** Pons, **43.** Pontine branch of basilar a., **14.** Posterior cerebral a., **44.** Posterior cerebral v., **46.** Posterior communicating a., **7.** Posterior inferior cerebellar a., **33.** Posterior spinal a., **20.** Roots of 1st spinal n., **32.** Trigeminal ganglion, **12.** Sigmoid sinus—junction of with transverse sinus, **18.** Sinus—opening of cerebellar v. into, **26.** Straight sinus—opening of into confluens sinuum, **27.** Superior cerebellar a., **11.** Superior sagittal sinus—opening of into confluens sinuum, **28.** Deep middle cerebral v., **5.** Temporal pole, **6.** Tentorium cerebelli, **31.** Trigeminal n. (V)—motor root, **40.** Trochlear n. (IV), **10.** Vagus n. (X), **36.** Vertebral a., **22.**

PLATE 18

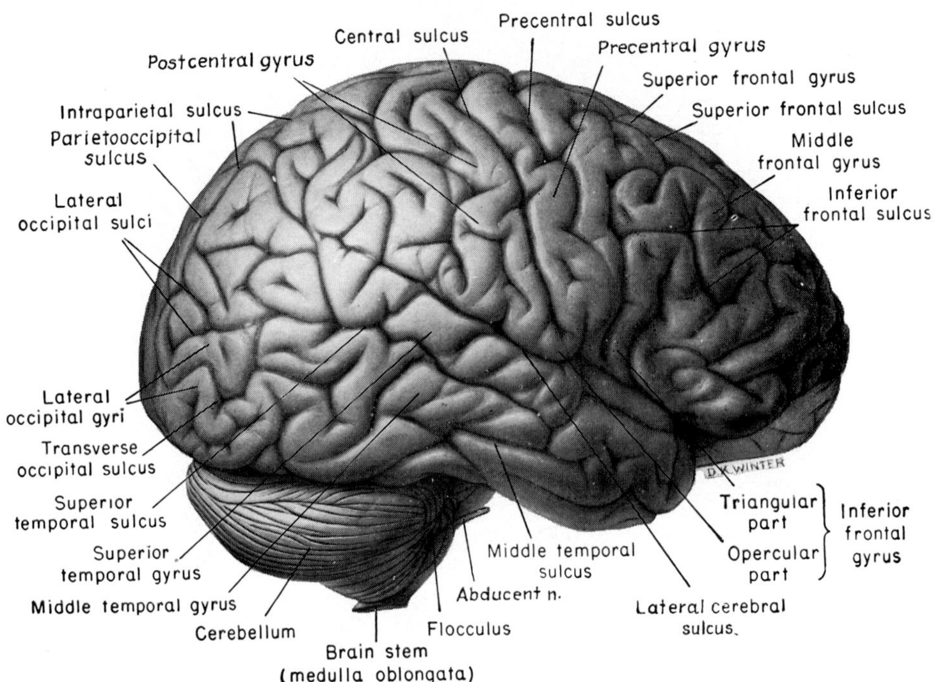

Central sulcus
Precentral sulcus
Precentral gyrus
Postcentral gyrus
Superior frontal gyrus
Superior frontal sulcus
Intraparietal sulcus
Parietooccipital sulcus
Middle frontal gyrus
Inferior frontal sulcus
Lateral occipital sulci
Lateral occipital gyri
Transverse occipital sulcus
D.K. WINTER
Superior temporal sulcus
Triangular part
Opercular part
Inferior frontal gyrus
Superior temporal gyrus
Middle temporal sulcus
Middle temporal gyrus
Abducent n.
Lateral cerebral sulcus
Cerebellum
Flocculus
Brain stem (medulla oblongata)

Lateral View

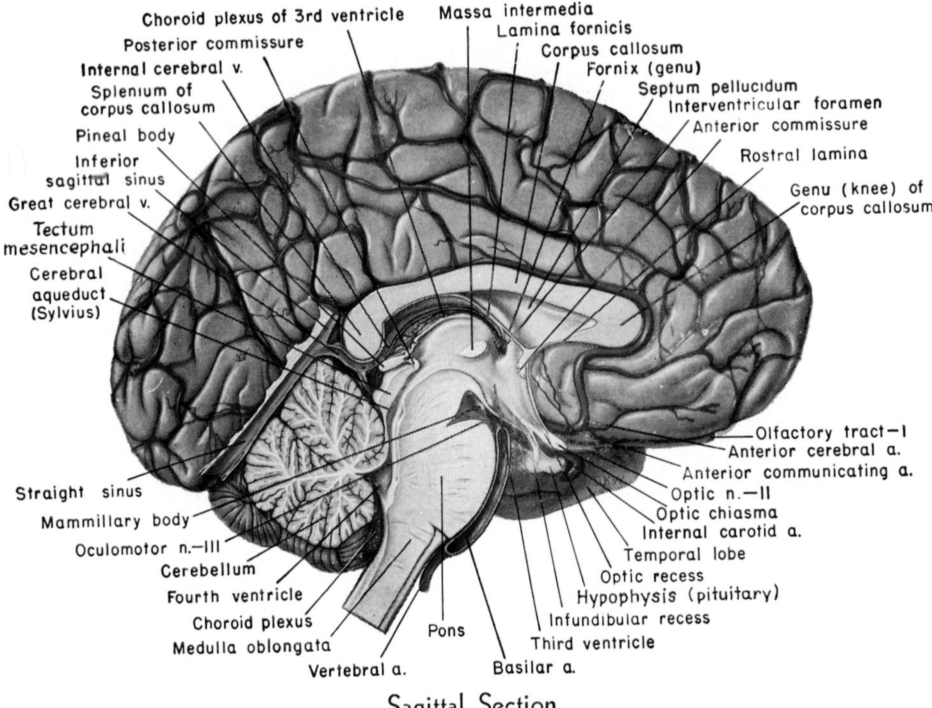

Choroid plexus of 3rd ventricle
Massa intermedia
Lamina fornicis
Posterior commissure
Corpus callosum
Internal cerebral v.
Fornix (genu)
Splenium of corpus callosum
Septum pellucidum
Interventricular foramen
Anterior commissure
Pineal body
Rostral lamina
Inferior sagittal sinus
Great cerebral v.
Genu (knee) of corpus callosum
Tectum mesencephali
Cerebral aqueduct (Sylvius)
Olfactory tract—I
Anterior cerebral a.
Anterior communicating a.
Straight sinus
Optic n.—II
Optic chiasma
Mammillary body
Internal carotid a.
Oculomotor n.—III
Temporal lobe
Cerebellum
Optic recess
Fourth ventricle
Hypophysis (pituitary)
Choroid plexus
Infundibular recess
Pons
Medulla oblongata
Third ventricle
Vertebral a.
Basilar a.

Sagittal Section

BRAIN

PLATE 19

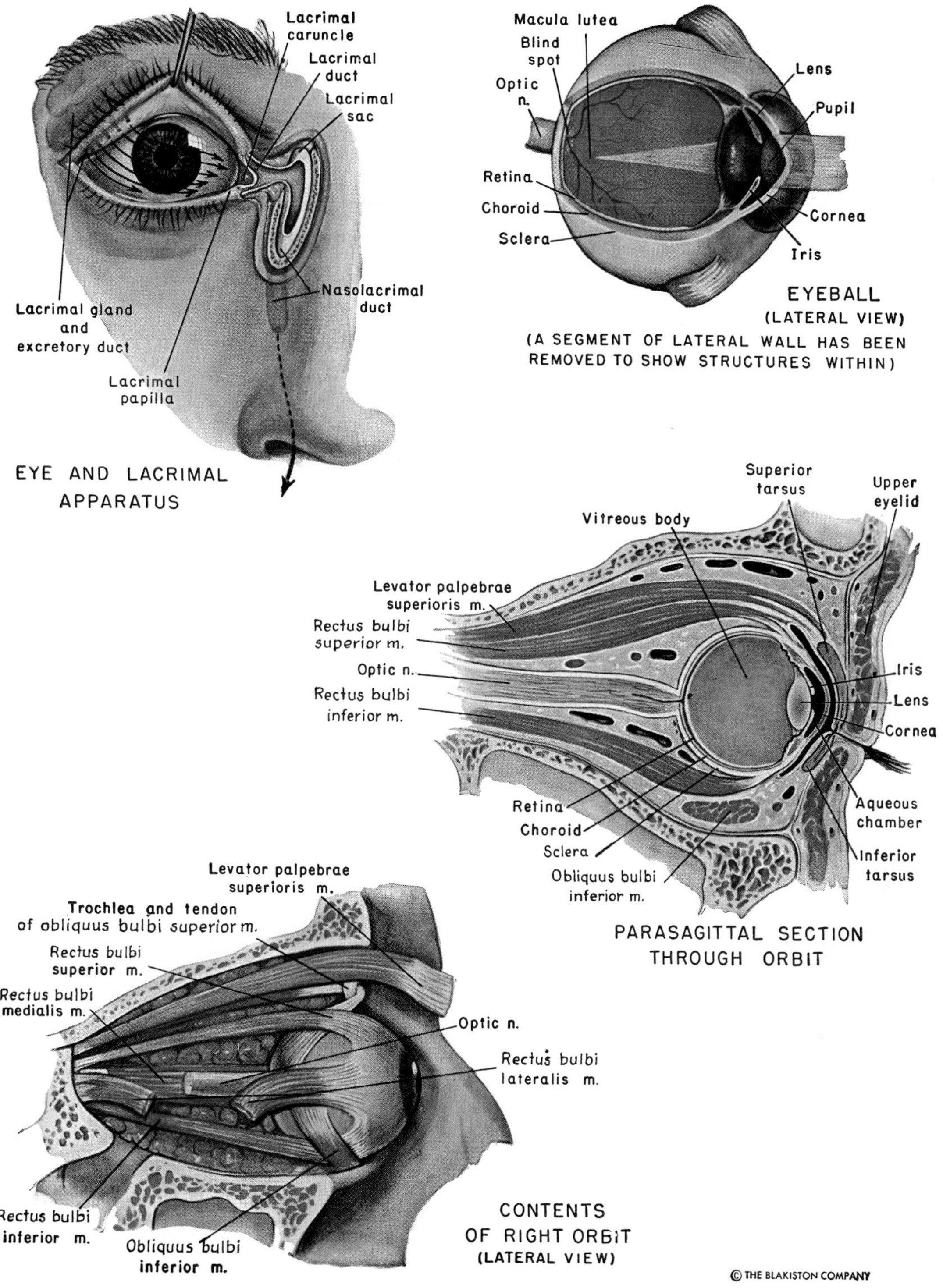
Lacrimal caruncle
Lacrimal duct
Lacrimal sac
Nasolacrimal duct
Lacrimal gland and excretory duct
Lacrimal papilla
EYE AND LACRIMAL APPARATUS
Macula lutea
Blind spot
Optic n.
Retina
Choroid
Sclera
Lens
Pupil
Cornea
Iris
EYEBALL
(LATERAL VIEW)
(A SEGMENT OF LATERAL WALL HAS BEEN REMOVED TO SHOW STRUCTURES WITHIN)
Superior tarsus
Upper eyelid
Vitreous body
Levator palpebrae superioris m.
Rectus bulbi superior m.
Optic n.
Rectus bulbi inferior m.
Iris
Lens
Cornea
Retina
Choroid
Sclera
Obliquus bulbi inferior m.
Aqueous chamber
Inferior tarsus
PARASAGITTAL SECTION THROUGH ORBIT
Levator palpebrae superioris m.
Trochlea and tendon of obliquus bulbi superior m.
Rectus bulbi superior m.
Rectus bulbi medialis m.
Optic n.
Rectus bulbi lateralis m.
Rectus bulbi inferior m.
Obliquus bulbi inferior m.
CONTENTS OF RIGHT ORBIT
(LATERAL VIEW)

EYE

PLATE 20

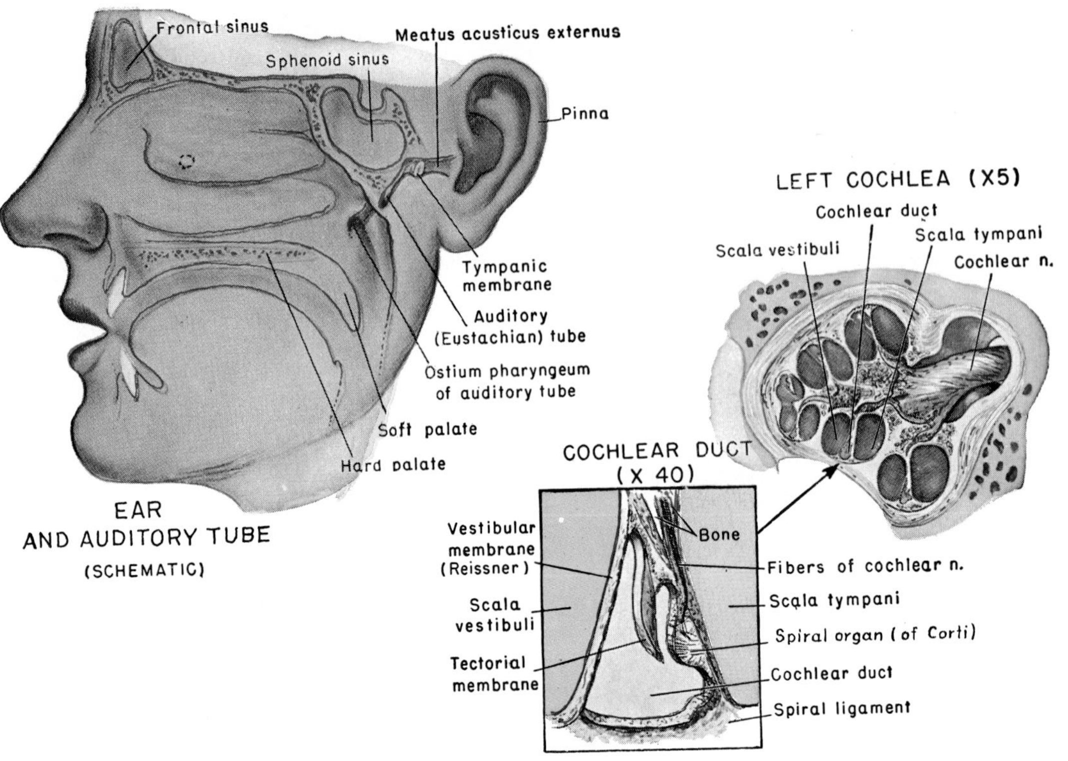
Frontal sinus
Sphenoid sinus
Meatus acusticus externus
Pinna
Tympanic membrane
Auditory (Eustachian) tube
Ostium pharyngeum of auditory tube
Soft palate
Hard palate
EAR AND AUDITORY TUBE (SCHEMATIC)
LEFT COCHLEA (X5)
Cochlear duct
Scala vestibuli
Scala tympani
Cochlear n.
COCHLEAR DUCT (X 40)
Vestibular membrane (Reissner)
Bone
Fibers of cochlear n.
Scala vestibuli
Scala tympani
Spiral organ (of Corti)
Tectorial membrane
Cochlear duct
Spiral ligament

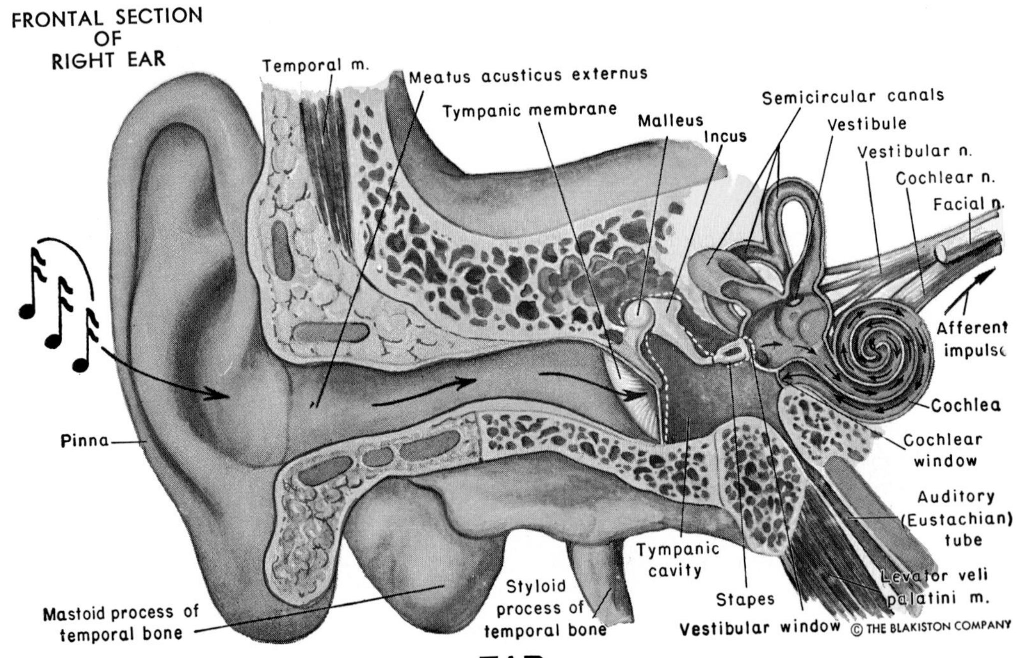
FRONTAL SECTION OF RIGHT EAR
Temporal m.
Meatus acusticus externus
Tympanic membrane
Malleus
Incus
Semicircular canals
Vestibule
Vestibular n.
Cochlear n.
Facial n.
Afferent impulse
Cochlea
Cochlear window
Auditory (Eustachian) tube
Levator veli palatini m.
Pinna
Tympanic cavity
Stapes
Vestibular window
Mastoid process of temporal bone
Styloid process of temporal bone

EAR

PLATE 21

DECIDUOUS DENTITION

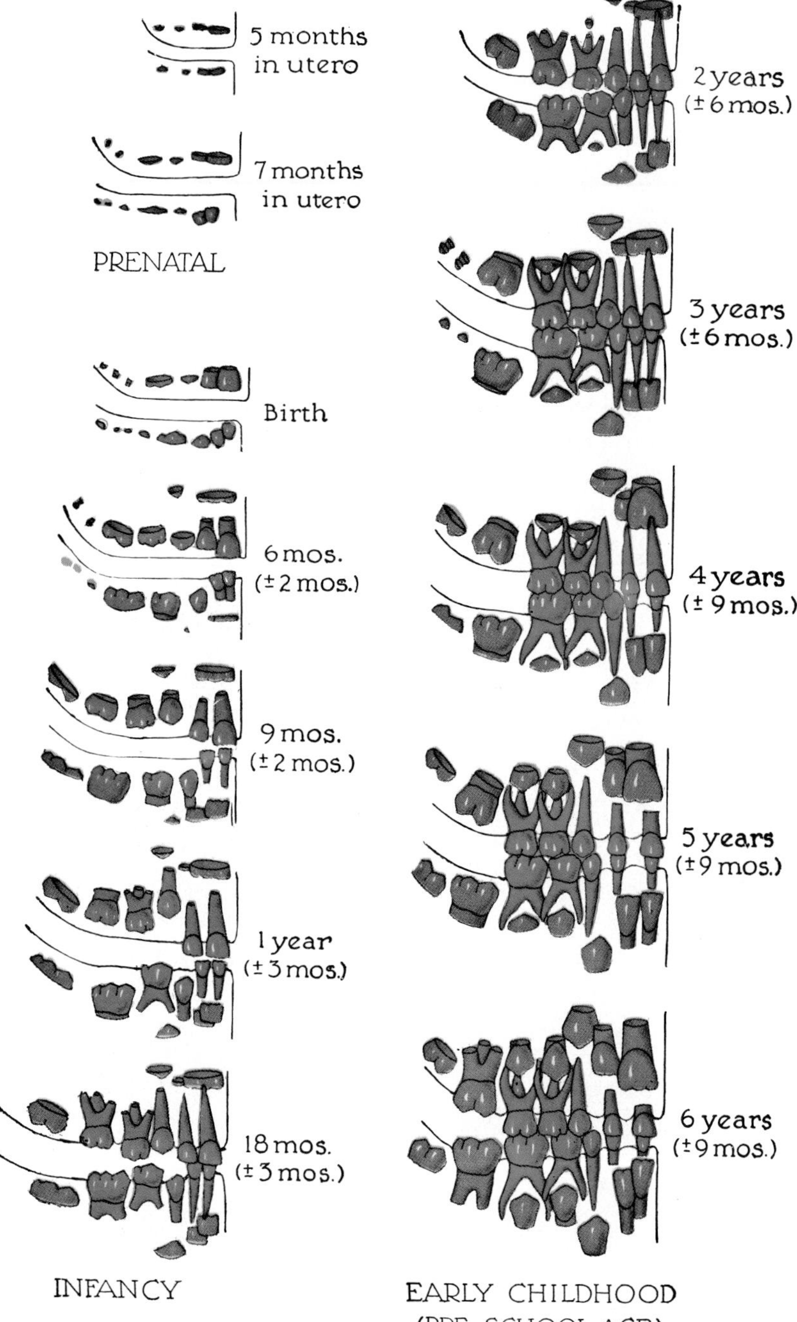

DEVELOPMENT OF HUMAN DENTITION

(Courtesy, Schour and Massler, American Dental Association.)

PLATE 22

MIXED DENTITION

PERMANENT DENTITION

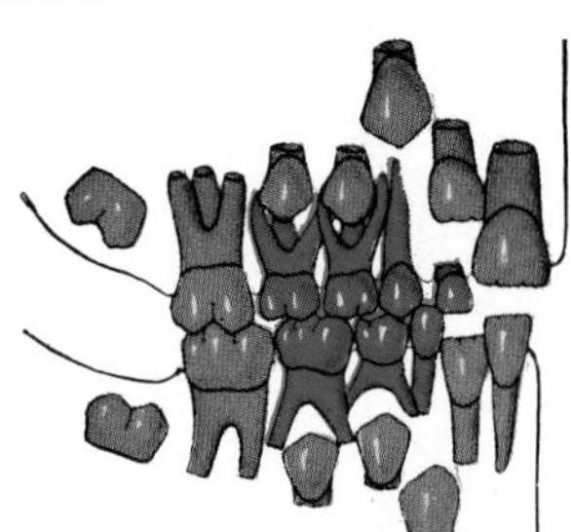

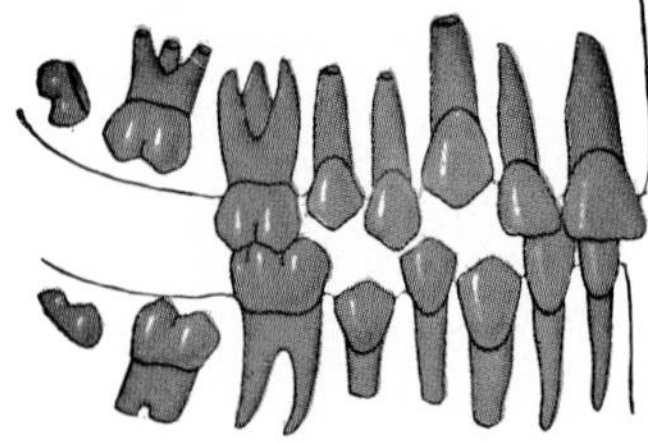

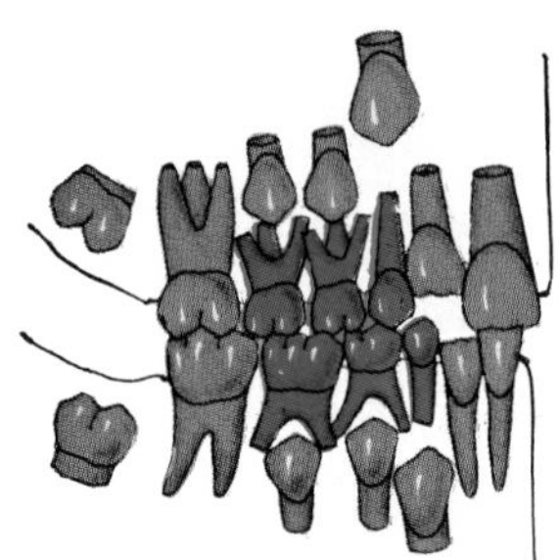

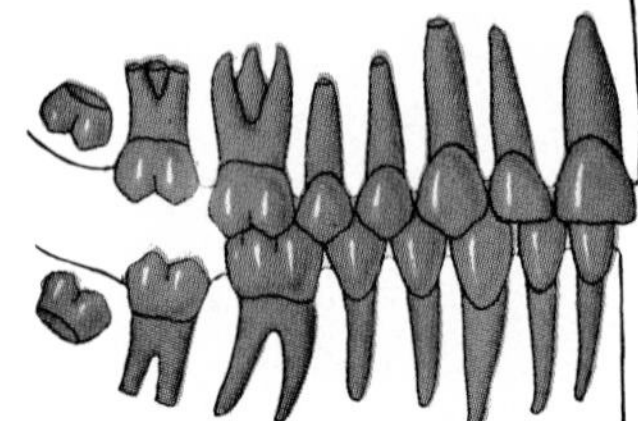

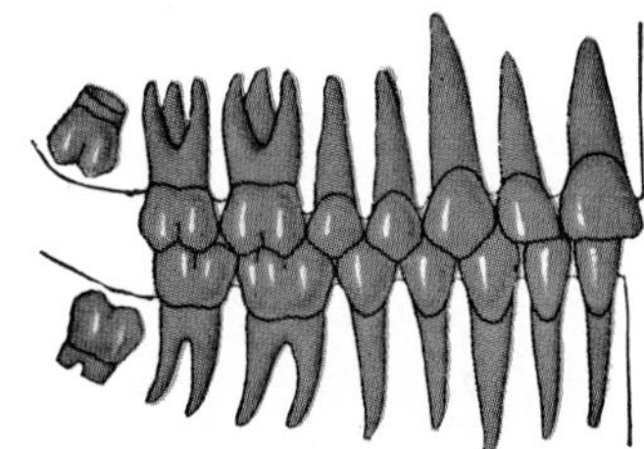

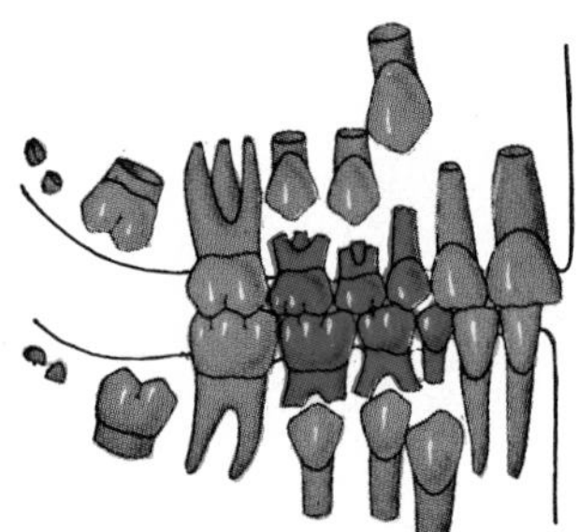

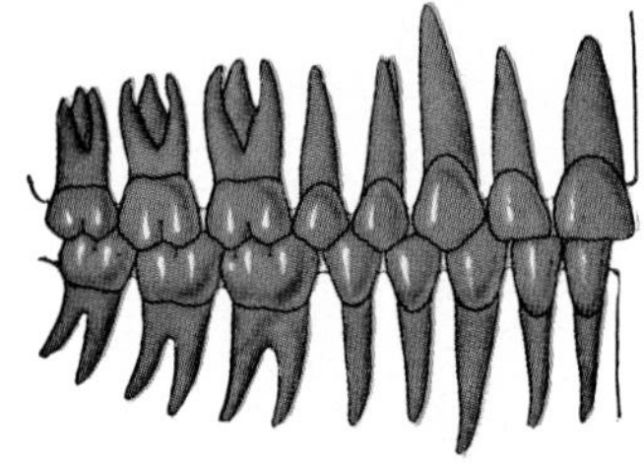

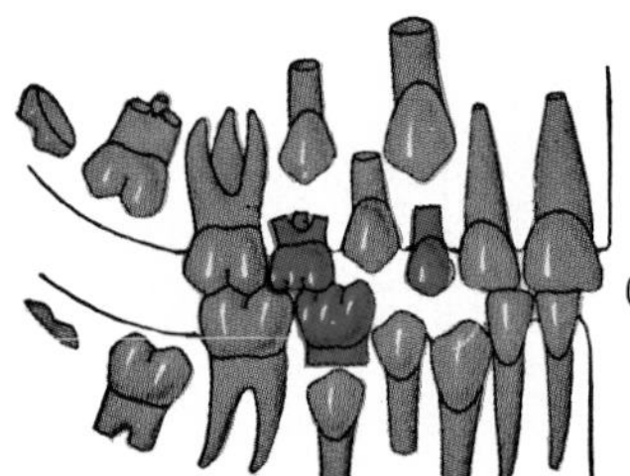

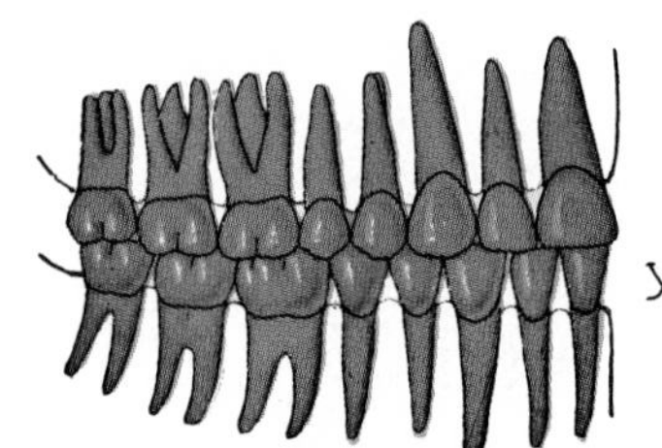

LATE CHILDHOOD
(SCHOOL AGE)

ADOLESCENCE
and ADULTHOOD

DEVELOPMENT OF HUMAN DENTITION

(Courtesy, Schour and Massler, American Dental Association.)

PLATE 23

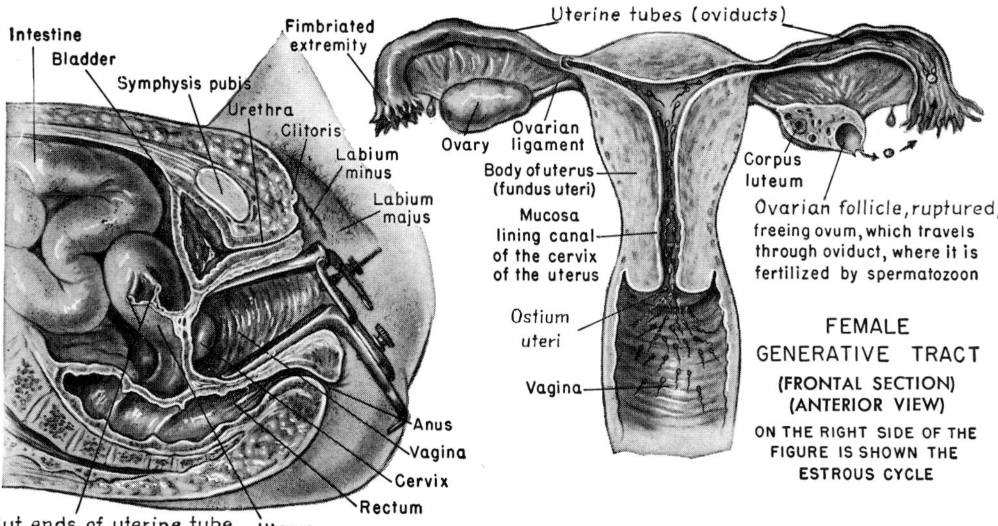

FEMALE GENERATIVE TRACT (FRONTAL SECTION) (ANTERIOR VIEW)

ON THE RIGHT SIDE OF THE FIGURE IS SHOWN THE ESTROUS CYCLE

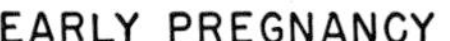

EXTERNAL AND INTERNAL FEMALE GENITALIA

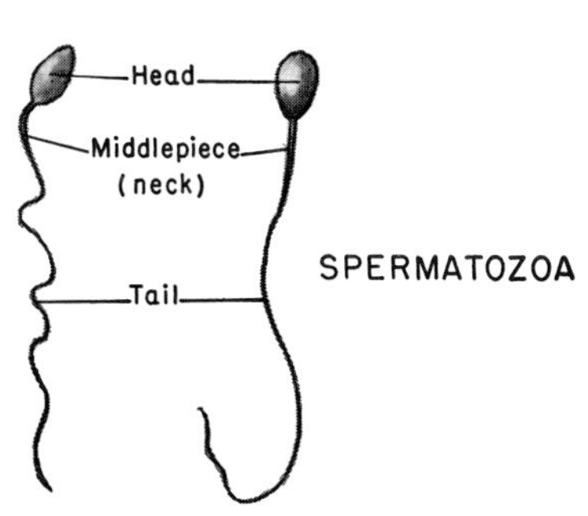

SPERMATOZOA

EARLY PREGNANCY

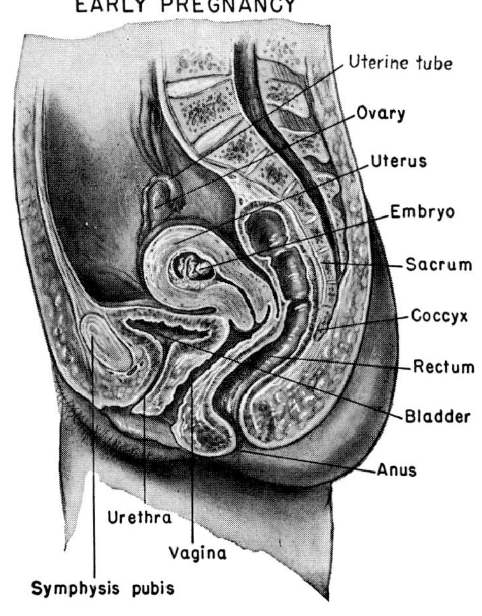

PREGNANT UTERUS AT TERM

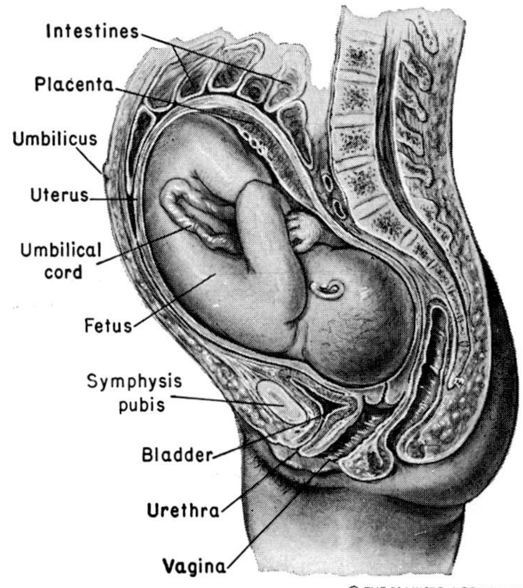

GENITALIA—FEMALE

PLATE 24

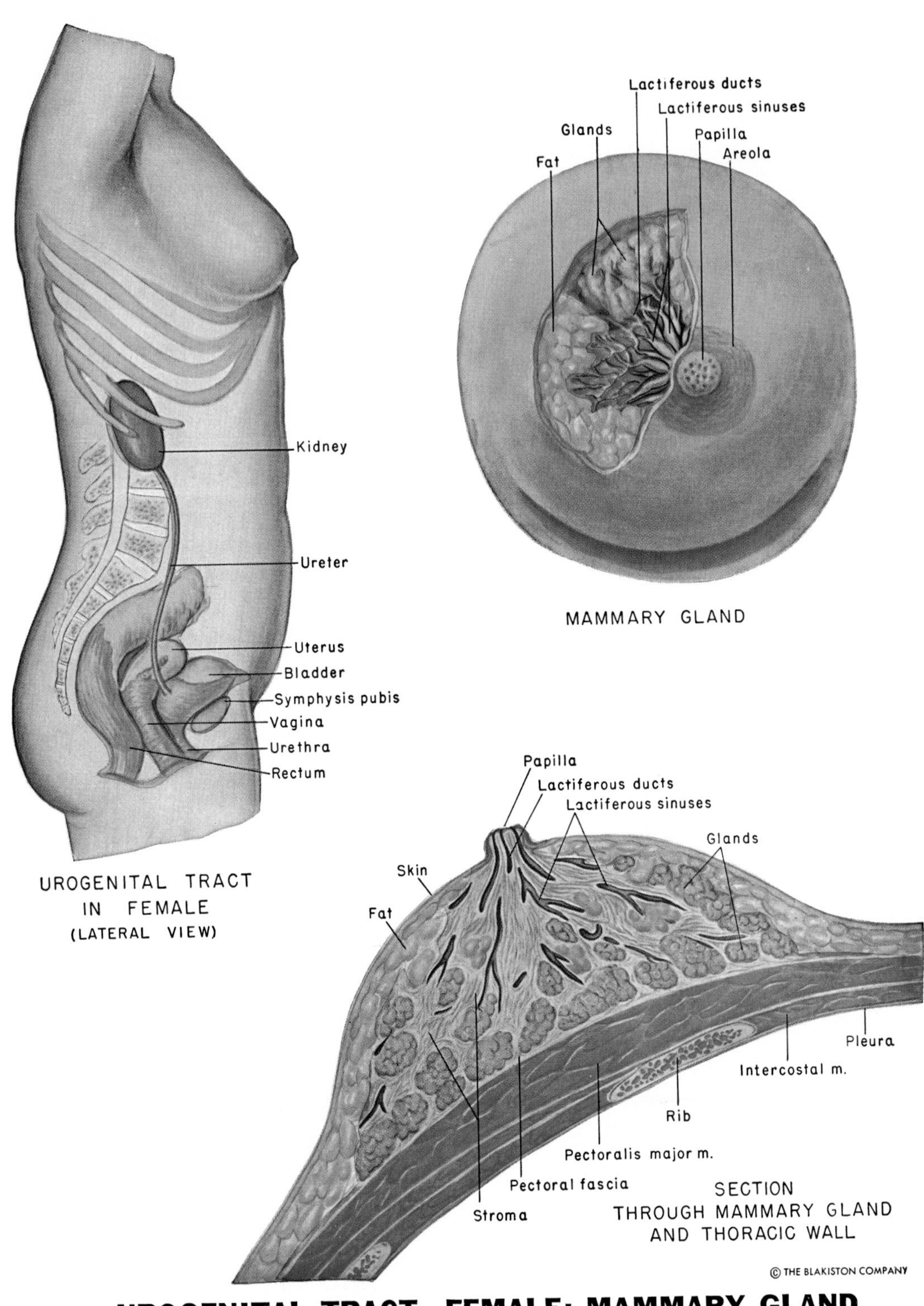

UROGENITAL TRACT—FEMALE; MAMMARY GLAND

PLATE 25

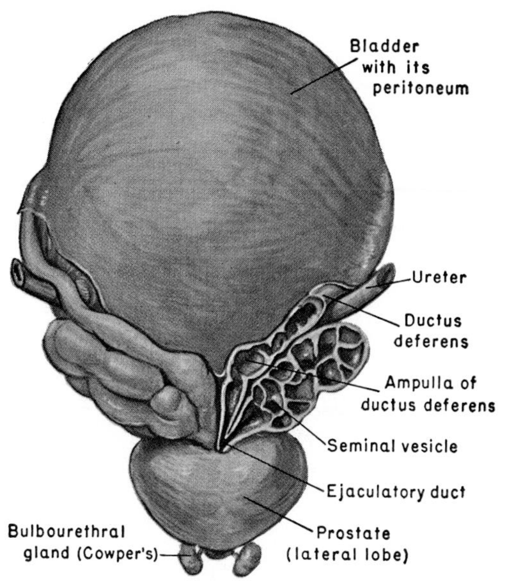

MALE BLADDER, PROSTATE, AND SEMINAL VESICLES
(POSTERIOR VIEW)

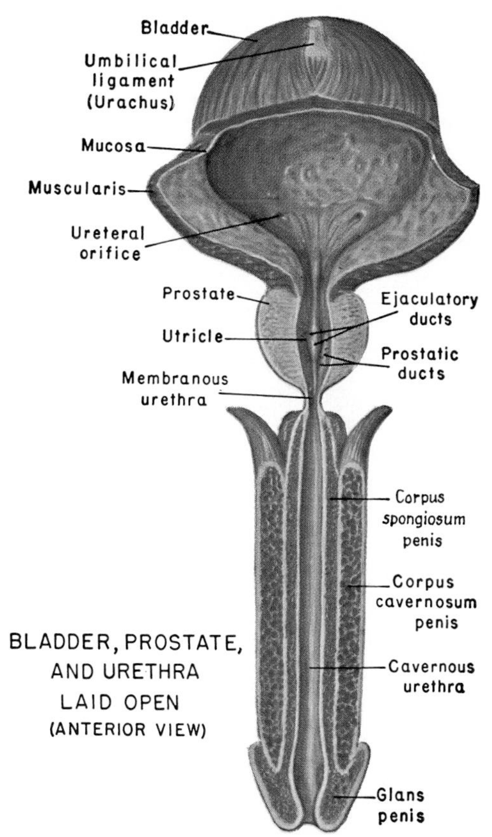

BLADDER, PROSTATE, AND URETHRA LAID OPEN
(ANTERIOR VIEW)

VISCERA OF MALE PELVIS
(LATERAL VIEW)

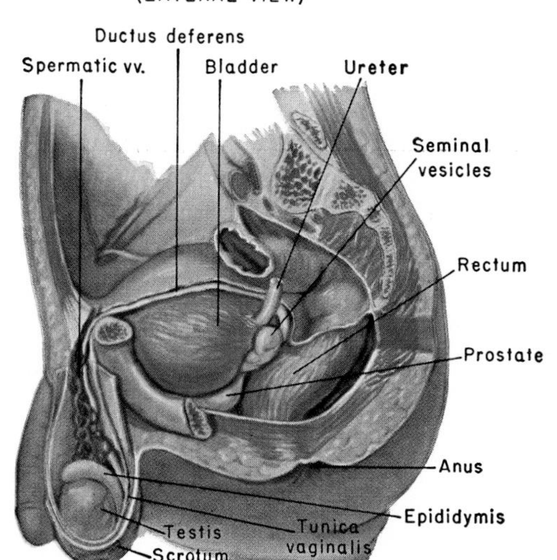

MALE PELVIS
(SAGITTAL SECTION)

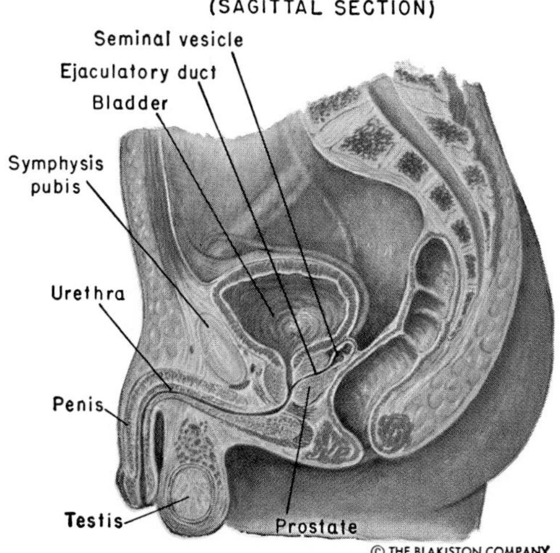

UROGENITAL TRACT—MALE

PLATE 26

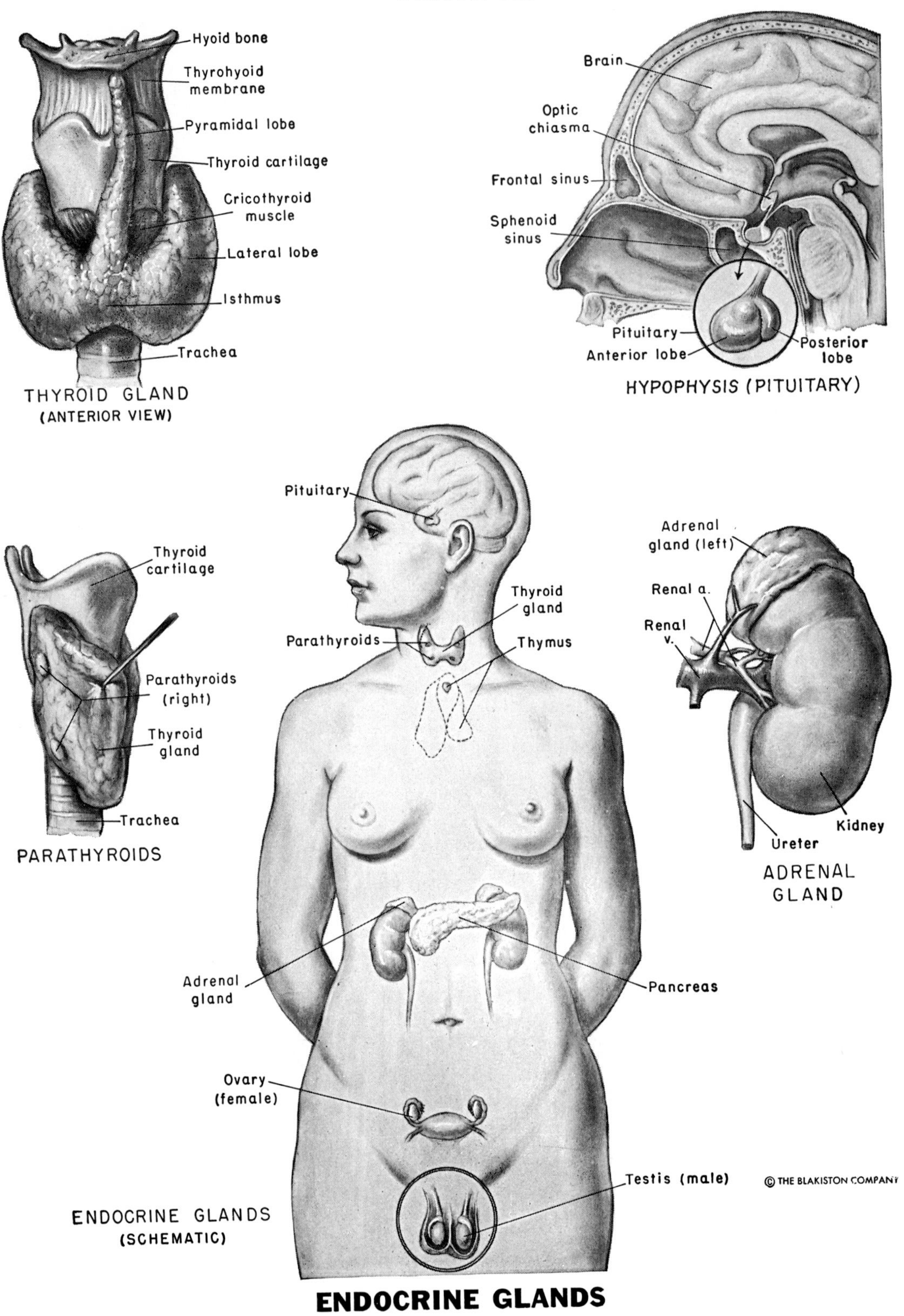

Hyoid bone
Thyrohyoid membrane
Pyramidal lobe
Thyroid cartilage
Cricothyroid muscle
Lateral lobe
Isthmus
Trachea
THYROID GLAND
(ANTERIOR VIEW)
Brain
Optic chiasma
Frontal sinus
Sphenoid sinus
Pituitary
Anterior lobe
Posterior lobe
HYPOPHYSIS (PITUITARY)
Pituitary
Thyroid cartilage
Parathyroids (right)
Thyroid gland
Trachea
PARATHYROIDS
Thyroid gland
Parathyroids
Thymus
Adrenal gland (left)
Renal a.
Renal v.
Kidney
Ureter
ADRENAL GLAND
Adrenal gland
Pancreas
Ovary (female)
Testis (male)
ENDOCRINE GLANDS
(SCHEMATIC)

ENDOCRINE GLANDS

O

O Symbol for oxygen.

O. Abbreviation for (a) *oculus,* eye; (b) *octarius,* pint; (c) *occiput.*

o- *In chemistry,* symbol for ortho-.

O agglutinin. An agglutinin specific for the somatic antigens of a microorganism.

O antigen. The thermostable, somatic antigen of the enteric and related gram-negative bacilli.

oari-, oario- [Gk. *ōarion,* small egg]. See *ovari-; oophor-.*

oa·ri·al·gia (o·ăr″ee·al′jee·uh, o″a·ree·) *n.* [*oari-* + *-algia*]. Ovarian neuralgia; OVARIALGIA.

oario-. See *ovari-; oophor-.*

oast·house urine disease [from the smell suggestive of an *oasthouse,* a building containing kilns in which hops are dried]. METHIONINE MALABSORPTION SYNDROME.

oat-cell carcinoma. A poorly differentiated carcinoma, usually of the lung, in which the anaplastic cells bear a fancied resemblance to oats.

oath of Hip·poc·ra·tes (hi·pock′ruh·teez). HIPPOCRATIC OATH.

ob·ce·ca·tion, ob·cae·ca·tion (ob″se·kay′shun) *n.* [L. *occaecatio,* act of blinding or obscuring, from *caecus,* blind]. Partial blindness.

ob·duc·tion (ob·duck′shun) *n.* [L. *obductio,* a covering]. A postmortem examination; an autopsy; a necropsy.

obe·li·on (o·bee′lee·on, ·un) *n.,* pl. **obe·lia** (·lee·uh) [dim. from Gk. *obelos,* spit]. *In craniometry,* the point where the line which joins the parietal foramens crosses the sagittal suture.

Ober·may·er's test (o′bur·migh″ur) [F. *Obermayer,* Austrian physician, 1861–1925]. A test for indican in which urine is treated with ferric chloride and concentrated hydrochloric acid and then extracted with chloroform. A pale blue to deep blue or violet color indicates indican.

Ober's operations [F. R. *Ober,* U.S. orthopedist, 1881–1960]. Operations for relief of crippling due to paralysis of the quadriceps femoris or gastrocnemius muscles, which utilize the principle of rerouting tendons of other muscles through prepared tunnels.

Ober's sign or **test** [F. R. *Ober*]. A test for contraction of the fascia lata in sciatica or low back pain.

Ober·stei·ner-Red·lich area (o′bur·shtye″nur, reʸt′likh) [H. *Obersteiner,* Austrian neurologist, 1847–1922; and E. *Redlich,* Austrian neurologist, 1866–1930]. ROOT ENTRANCE ZONE.

obese (o·beece′) *adj.* [L. *obesus,* from *ob-,* over-, + *edere, esum,* to eat]. Extremely fat; corpulent.

obe·si·ty (o·bee′si·tee, o·bes′i·tee) *n.* [L. *obesitas,* from *obesus,* obese]. An increase of body weight due to accumulation of fat, 10 to 20 percent beyond the normal range for the particular age, sex, and height. See also *buffalo obesity, hypothalamic obesity.*

obesity diet. REDUCING DIET.

obex (o′becks) *n.* [L., bolt, barrier] [NA]. The thin triangular lamina formed by the meeting of the taeniae choroideae of the fourth ventricle over the caudal limit of the cavity.

ob·fus·ca·tion (ob″fus·kay′shun) *n.* [L. *offuscatio,* a darkening]. 1. Mental confusion. 2. The act of causing mental confusion or the clouding of an issue to confuse the listener.

obi·dox·ime chloride (o″bi·dock′seem) *n.* 1,1′-(Oxydimethylene)bis[4-formylpyridinium]dichloride dioxime, $C_{14}H_{16}Cl_2N_4O_3$, a cholinesterase reactivator.

ob·ject, *n.* [L. *objectus,* lying opposite or against]. 1. Any thing, idea, or person toward which attention is directed; thus, anything which has physical, abstract, or social existence independent of the subject, or knower. 2. Any thing, idea, or person of which a subject (particularly a person) may be aware, toward which an attitude is formed, or toward which a relationship is established.

object choice or **cathexis.** 1. The selection of a real or imaginary person, or object, as a love object. 2. The investment of libido in another person or object.

ob·jec·tive, *adj. & n.* 1. Pertaining to an object or to that which is contemplated or perceived, as distinguished from that which contemplates or perceives. 2. Pertaining to those relations and conditions of the body perceived by another, as objective signs of disease. Contr. *subjective.* 3. The lens or lens system in a compound microscope which is nearest the object and produces the primary inverted magnified image.

objective sign. *In medicine,* a sign which can be detected by someone other than the patient himself. Contr. *subjective sign.*

objective tinnitus. Tinnitus audible to the examiner as well as to the subject, usually caused by organic vascular disease in the head or neck, such as an arteriovenous aneurysm or a venous hum. Syn. *pseudotinnitus.* Contr. *subjective tinnitus.*

objective vertigo. The sensation in which objects seem to revolve around the patient. Contr. *subjective vertigo.*

object libido. The focus of libido upon persons, objects, or things external to the self.

object relationship. *In psychiatry,* the attitudes and responses of one person toward another, chiefly the emotional relationship between them as opposed to the self-interest and self-love exhibited by each individual; in a positive sense, the capacity of an individual to react appropriately to and to accept and love other people.

object space. The space around an optical system each point of which is considered as a possible source of radiation of light.

ob·late (ob'late, ob·late') *adj.* [L. *oblatus,* brought forward]. Having a form or shape that is flattened or depressed at the poles.

oblate spheroid. A spheroid in which the polar axis is less than the equatorial diameter.

ob·li·gate (ob'li·gate, ·gut) *adj.* [L. *obligatus,* bound, obliged]. Able to live only in the way specified, as an obligate anaerobe, an organism that can live only anaerobically. Contr. *facultative.*

obligate aerobe. An organism dependent upon free oxygen at all times.

obligate parasite. A parasite incapable of living without a host.

oblig·a·to·ry (o·blig'uh·tor"ee) *adj.* [LL. *obligatorius*]. 1. Required, necessary. 2. OBLIGATE.

oblique (o·bleek', o·blike') *adj. & n.* [L. *obliquus*]. 1. Not direct; aslant; slanting. 2. *In botany,* unequal-sided. 3. *In anatomy,* an oblique muscle, as the external or internal oblique of the abdomen, or the superior or inferior oblique of the eye. See Table of Muscles in the Appendix. **—oblique·ly** (·lee) *adv.*

oblique astigmatism. Astigmatism correctable by a cylindrical lens whose axes are oblique, that is, neither horizontal nor vertical.

oblique bandage. A bandage which covers a part by oblique turns.

oblique diameter of the pelvic inlet. The line, or the length of the line, joining the iliopectineal eminence to the sacroiliac articulation on the opposite side.

oblique facial cleft. An embryonic fissure between the maxillary and frontonasal processes.

oblique fissure. A fissure separating the superior and inferior lobes of the left lung and the superior and middle lobes of the right lung from the inferior lobe of that lung. NA *fissura obliqua pulmonis.*

oblique hernia. INDIRECT HERNIA.

oblique illumination. Illumination of an object by throwing light upon it, or through it, obliquely. Syn. *lateral illumination.*

oblique light. Light falling obliquely on a surface.

oblique line of the fibula. CRISTA MEDIALIS FIBULAE.

oblique line of the mandible. Continuation of the anterior border of the ramus downward and forward onto the lateral surface of the mandible. NA *linea obliqua mandibulae.*

oblique line of the radius. A ridge of bone extending laterally and downward from the radial tuberosity; it gives origin to the flexor digitorum superficialis and flexor pollicis longus muscles.

oblique line of the thyroid cartilage. A line running downward and forward on the lateral side of each lamina. NA *linea obliqua cartilaginis thyroideae.*

obliquely contracted pelvis. A deformed pelvis with unequal oblique diameters.

oblique popliteal ligament. A broad, fibrous band containing openings for vessels and nerves which passes in the posterior part of the knee joint from the tendon of the semimembranosus muscle and the medial condyle of the tibia obliquely superolaterally to the posterior part of the lateral condyle of the femur. NA *ligamentum popliteum obliquum.*

oblique ridge. 1. A ridge on the occlusal surface of an upper molar tooth, formed by two triangular ridges. 2. TRAPEZOID LINE.

oblique sinus of the pericardium. An arched reflection of pericardium forming a pocket that extends upward on the posterior aspect of the atria. NA *sinus obliquus pericardii.*

oblique vein of Marshall [J. *Marshall,* English surgeon and anatomist, 1818–1891]. OBLIQUE VEIN OF THE LEFT ATRIUM.

oblique vein of the left atrium. The small vein passing downward across the posterior surface of the left atrium and draining into the coronary sinus; it represents the remnant of the left common cardinal vein. NA *vena obliqua atrii sinistri.*

ob·liq·ui·ty (ob·lick'wit·ee) *n.* [L. *obliquitas*]. The state of being oblique.

obliquity of the pelvis. INCLINATION OF THE PELVIS.

ob·li·quus (ob·lye'kwus) *adj.* [L.]. 1. OBLIQUE. 2. Pertaining to an oblique muscle.

obliquus reflex. HYPOGASTRIC REFLEX.

obliterating endarteritis. ENDARTERITIS OBLITERANS.

oblit·er·a·tion (uh·blit"ur·ay'shun, o·blit") *n.* [L. *obliteratio,* from *obliterare,* to blot out]. 1. The complete removal of a part by disease or surgical operation; extirpation. 2. Complete closure of a lumen. 3. The complete loss of memory or consciousness of certain events. **—oblit·er·a·tive** (o·blit' ur·uh·tiv, ·ay·tiv) *adj.*

obliterative appendicitis. Obliteration of the appendiceal lumen by fibrofatty tissue; sometimes ascribed to inflammation. Syn. *appendicitis obliterans.*

oblong fovea. A shallow depression on the external surface of an arytenoid cartilage. NA *fovea oblonga.*

ob·mu·tes·cence (ob"mew·tes'unce) *n.* [L. *obmutescere,* to be or become silent]. The condition of becoming or keeping silent. See also *aphonia, mutism.*

ob·nu·bi·la·tion (ob·new"bi·lay'shun) *n.* [L. *obnubilare,* to cover with clouds]. Mental clouding; may precede loss of consciousness.

ob·ser·va·tion hip. TRANSIENT SYNOVITIS.

ob·ses·sion, *n.* [L. *obsessio,* a besieging]. An idea or emotion that persists in an individual's mind in spite of any conscious attempts to remove it; an imperative idea, as seen in the psychoneurotic disorders. See also *obsessive-compulsive neurosis.* **—obsession·al, ob·ses·sive,** *adj.*

obsessional neurosis. OBSESSIVE-COMPULSIVE NEUROSIS.

obsessive-compulsive neurosis. A neurotic disorder in which anxiety relates to unwanted thoughts and repetitive impulses to perform acts against which the individual usually fights and which he may consider abnormal, inappropriate, or absurd, but which he cannot control and by which he is dominated. The acts often become organized into rituals, and include such forms as touching, counting, hand-washing, and excessive neatness; inability to control the acts or being prevented from performing them often produces extreme distress and anxiety.

obsessive-compulsive personality. An individual who is generally characterized by chronic, excessive concern with adherence to standards of conscience or of conformity resulting in inhibited, rigid, over-dutiful behavior, the inability to relax, and the performance of an inordinate amount of work. This behavioral disturbance may eventually lead to an obsessive-compulsive neurosis.

obsessive-compulsive reaction. OBSESSIVE-COMPULSIVE NEUROSIS.

obsessive personality. OBSESSIVE-COMPULSIVE PERSONALITY.

obsessive ruminative state. A form of neurosis, usually of a depressive character, and similar to the obsessive-compulsive neurosis, characterized by continuous morbid preoccupation with certain ideas, usually trivial or inconsequential, to the exclusion of other interests, but without compulsive acts.

ob·so·les·cent (ob"suh·les'unt) *adj.* [L. *obsolescens,* from *ob-,* away, off, + *solere,* to be accustomed, to be in force]. Becoming obsolete. **—obsoles·cence** (·unce) *n.*

ob·stet·ric (ob·stet'rick) *adj.* [L. *obstetrix,* midwife, from *obstare,* to stand before]. 1. Of or pertaining to pregnancy and childbirth. 2. Of or pertaining to obstetrics. **—obstet·ri·cal** (·ri·kul) *adj.*

obstetric accommodation. Fetal conformation to the cavity of the uterus, particularly during the last third of pregnancy.

obstetrical analgesia. Analgesia induced to relieve the pain of childbirth; perception of pain is diminished or obliterated without necessarily affecting cerebration or motor nerve activity.

obstetrical conjugate. OBSTETRIC CONJUGATE.

obstetrical forceps. OBSTETRIC FORCEPS.

obstetric canal. PARTURIENT CANAL.

obstetric conjugate. The minimum anteroposterior diameter of the pelvic inlet; usually a little shorter than conjugata vera.

obstetric evisceration. Removal of the abdominal or thoracic viscera of a fetus to permit delivery.

obstetric forceps. A large, double-bladed traction forceps; the blades are demountable and are applied separately before interlocking at the handles, in order to fit the fetal head. Employed in difficult labor or to facilitate delivery.

ob·ste·tri·cian (ob″ste·trish′un) *n.* One who practices obstetrics.

obstetric paralysis. BIRTH PALSY.

ob·stet·rics (ob·stet′ricks) *n.* [*obstetric* + *-s*]. The branch of medicine concerning the care of women and their offspring during pregnancy and parturition, with continued care of the women during the puerperium.

ob·sti·pa·tion (ob″sti·pay′shun) *n.* [L. *obstipatio,* close pressure]. Intractable constipation.

obstructed labor. Labor that is mechanically blocked, as from a contracted pelvis or pelvic tumor. Its severity is relative to the size of the fetus and the maternal structures.

ob·struc·tion, *n.* [L. *obstructio*]. 1. The state of being occluded or stenosed, applied especially to hollow viscera, ducts, and vessels. 2. The act of occluding or blocking. 3. An obstacle. —**obstruc·tive,** *adj.;* **ob·struct,** *v.*

obstructive anosmia. See *anosmia.*

obstructive atelectasis. Atelectasis caused by occlusion or obstruction of a bronchus, ascribed to subsequent absorption of the trapped air and collapse of the alveoli. Syn. *absorption atelectasis.*

obstructive dysmenorrhea. MECHANICAL DYSMENORRHEA.

obstructive emphysema. Overdistention of the lung due to partial obstruction of the air passages, which permits air to enter the alveoli but which resists expiration of the air.

obstructive glaucoma. NARROW-ANGLE GLAUCOMA.

obstructive hydrocephalus. Increased volume of cerebrospinal fluid in the ventricular system caused by a blocking of the fluid's passage from the brain ventricles, where it is produced, to the subarachnoid space, where it is absorbed. Obstruction may occur at the interventricular foramens, in the cerebral aqueduct, at the median and lateral apertures of the fourth ventricle, or may be due to arachnoiditis. Syn. *internal hydrocephalus, noncommunicating hydrocephalus.* Compare *occult hydrocephalus.* Contr. *communicating hydrocephalus.*

obstructive jaundice. Jaundice due to interference with the outflow of bile by mechanical obstruction of the biliary passages, as by gallstones, tumor, or fibrosis.

obstructive murmur. DIRECT MURMUR.

ob·stru·ent (ob′stroo·unt) *adj.* & *n.* [L. *obstruens,* blocking up, obstructing]. 1. Obstructive, tending to obstruct. 2. Something which tends or serves to obstruct.

ob·tund (ob·tund′) *v.* [L. *obtundere*]. To blunt or make dull; lessen, as to obtund sensibility. —**ob·tun·da·tion** (ob″tun·day′shun) *n.*

ob·tun·dent (ob·tun′dunt) *adj.* & *n.* 1. Tending to obtund sensibility. 2. A remedy that relieves or overcomes irritation or pain.

ob·tu·ra·tion (ob″tew·ray′shun, ob″tur·ay′shun) *n.* [L. *obturare,* to stop up]. 1. The closing of an opening or passage. 2. A form of intestinal obstruction in which the lumen of the intestine is occupied by its normal contents or by foreign bodies. —**ob·tu·rate** (ob′tew·rate) *v.*

ob·tu·ra·tor (ob′tew·ray″tur, ob′tur·) *adj.* & *n.* [*obturate* + *-or*]. 1. Characterizing that which closes or stops up, as the obturator membrane. 2. Pertaining to various structures associated directly or indirectly with the obturator membrane, as the obturator foramen, obturator muscles. See also Tables of Muscles, Nerves, and Arteries in the Appendix. 3. Any obturator muscle. 4. A solid wire or rod contained within a hollow needle or cannula. Obturators may be bayonet-pointed for piercing tissues, or obliquely faced at the end for fitting, exactly, large aspirating needles. The term includes the metal carriers within urethroscopes and cystoscopes. 5. An appliance that closes a cleft or fissure of the palate.

obturator bursa. The bursa under the tendon of the obturator internus. NA *bursa ischiadica musculi obturatorii.*

obturator canal. A gap in the obturator membrane which closes the obturator foramen in the hipbone; it gives passage to the obturator nerve and vessels. NA *canalis obturatorius.*

obturator crest. A bony ridge running from the pubic tubercle to the acetabular notch. NA *crista obturatoria.*

obturator ex·ter·nus (ecks·tur′nus). The outer obturator muscle. NA *musculus obturatorius externus.* See Table of Muscles in the Appendix.

obturator fascia. The portion of the parietal pelvic fascia overlying the obturator internus muscle. NA *fascia obturatoria.*

obturator foramen. The large oval opening between the ischium and the pubis, anterior, inferior, and medial to the acetabulum, partly closed in by a fibrous membrane; it gives passage to the obturator vessels and nerves. NA *foramen obturatum.*

obturator groove. The furrow at the superior border of the obturator foramen, lodging the obturator vessels and nerves. NA *sulcus obturatorius.*

obturator hernia. A rare hernia through the obturator canal; occurs principally in women. Syn. *pelvic hernia.*

obturator in·ter·nus (in·tur′nus). The inner obturator muscle. NA *musculus obturatorius internus.* See Table of Muscles in the Appendix.

obturator line. A normal radiolucent line seen roentgenologically medial to the acetabulum in an anteroposterior projection of the pelvis.

obturator membrane. 1. The fibrous membrane closing the obturator foramen of the pelvis. NA *membrana obturatoria.* 2. The thin membrane between the crura and foot plate of the stapes. NA *membrana stapedis.*

obturator nerve. NA *nervus obturatorius.* See Table of Nerves in the Appendix.

obturator plexus. SUBSARTORIAL PLEXUS.

obturator sign. A roentgenologic sign sometimes seen in early inflammatory disease of the hip in children, with the obturator line bowed inward into the pelvis.

obturator tubercle. 1. ANTERIOR OBTURATOR TUBERCLE. 2. POSTERIOR OBTURATOR TUBERCLE.

ob·tuse (ob·tewce′) *adj.* [L. *obtusus,* from *obtundere,* to strike against, to dull]. 1. Blunt. 2. Of angles, greater than 90°.

ob·tu·sion (ob·tew′zhun) *n.* [L. *obtusio,* from *obtundere,* to obtund]. The blunting or weakening of normal sensation and perception.

occipit-, occipito-. A combining form meaning *occiput, occipital.*

oc·cip·i·tal (ock·sip′i·tul) *adj.* Of or pertaining to the occiput.

occipital angle. The angle determined by connecting the point in the sagittal curvature of the occipital bone by straight lines with lambda and the point of the external occipital protuberance, respectively. The more convex the occipital bone, the smaller is this angle.

occipital arc. The measurement from the lambda to the opisthion.

occipital arch. *In comparative anatomy,* the ring formed by the basioccipital, exoccipital, and supraoccipital bones.

occipital artery. NA *arteria occipitalis.* See Table of Arteries in the Appendix.

occipital bone. NA *os occipitale.* See Table of Bones in the Appendix.

occipital cross. INTERNAL OCCIPITAL PROTUBERANCE.

occipital emissary vein. A rare venous channel passing through the occipital bone and connecting the confluence of sinuses with the occipital vein. NA *vena emissaria occipitalis.*

occipital eye field. The region (Brodmann's areas 17, 18, and 19) around the calcarine fissure of the occipital lobe where stimulation produces conjugate deviation of the eyes to the opposite side, with stimulation above the fissure resulting in turning of the eyes downward and to the opposite side, while stimulation below the calcarine fissure produces upward movements to the opposite side. Compare *frontal eye field.*

occipital groove. The groove medial to the digastric groove, lodging the occipital artery. NA *sulcus arteriae occipitalis.*

occipital gyri. Two gyri, superior and lateral, on the lateral aspect of the occipital lobe. See also Plate 18.

oc·ci·pi·ta·lis (ock·sip″i·tay′lis) *n.* The posterior belly of the epicranius muscle. NA *venter occipitalis musculi occipitofrontalis.*

occipitalis minor. TRANSVERSE NUCHAL MUSCLE.

oc·cip·i·tal·ize (ock·sip′i·tul·ize) *v.* To incorporate with the occipital bone; to fuse the atlas with the occipital bone.

occipital lobe. One of the lobes of the cerebrum, a triangular area at the occipital extremity, bounded medially by the parieto-occipital fissure and merging laterally with the parietal and the temporal lobes. NA *lobus occipitalis.*

occipital nerve. See Table of Nerves in the Appendix.

occipital pachydermia. A rare disease of the scalp characterized by thickened skin thrown into folds; limited to the occipital region of the scalp.

occipital plane. PLANUM OCCIPITALE.

occipital plexus. A sympathetic network around the occipital artery.

occipital point. The most posterior portion of the occiput in the sagittal plane.

occipital pole. The tip of the occipital lobe of the cerebrum. NA *polus occipitalis.*

occipital sinus. A sinus of the dura mater running in the attached margin of the falx cerebelli from the foramen magnum to the confluence of the sinuses. NA *sinus occipitalis.* See also Table of Veins in the Appendix and Plates 10, 17.

occipital somites. Three or four indistinct somites in the occipital region, part of which form the tongue muscles innervated by the hypoglossal nerve.

occipital suture. LAMBDOID SUTURE.

occipital thalamic peduncles. See *thalamic peduncles.*

occipital torus. TRANSVERSE OCCIPITAL TORUS.

occipital triangle. A triangle bounded in front by the sternocleidomastoid, behind by the trapezius, and below by the omohyoid.

occipito-. See *occipit-.*

oc·cip·i·to·an·te·ri·or (ock·sip″i·to·an·teer′ee·ur) *adj.* [*occipito-* + *anterior*]. Having the occiput directed toward the front, as the occipitoanterior position of the fetus in the uterus.

oc·cip·i·to·ax·i·al (ock·sip″i·to·ack′see·ul) *adj.* [*occipito-* + *axial*]. Pertaining to the occipital bone and the axis.

oc·cip·i·to·cer·vi·cal (ock·sip″i·to·sur′vi·kul) *adj.* Pertaining to the occiput and adjacent cervical regions.

oc·cip·i·to·fron·tal (ock·sip″i·to·frunt′ul) *adj.* [*occipito-* + *frontal*]. Pertaining to the occiput and forehead, the epicranius (occipitofrontalis) muscle, or the occipital and frontal bones.

occipitofrontal circumference. The maximal circumference of the head, measured from the occipital point to around the frontal eminence; useful as an indirect measure of cranial growth. Abbreviated, OFC.

occipitofrontal diameter. The diameter joining the root of the nose and the most prominent point of the occiput.

occipitofrontal fasciculus. A bundle of long association fibers extending from the cortex of the frontal lobe to the cortex of the occipital lobe.

oc·ci·pi·to·fron·ta·lis (ock·sip″i·to·fron·tay′lis) *n.* A part of the epicranius. NA *musculus occipitofrontalis.* See also Table of Muscles in the Appendix.

oc·cip·i·to·lae·vo·an·te·ri·or (ock·sip″i·to·lee″vo·an·teer′ee·ur) *adj.* Left occipitoanterior (position of the fetus). Abbreviated, O.L.A.

oc·cip·i·to·lae·vo·pos·te·ri·or (ock·sip″i·to·lee″vo·pos·teer′ee·ur) *adj.* Left occipitoposterior (position of the fetus). Abbreviated, O.L.P.

oc·cip·i·to·mas·toid (ock·sip″i·to·mas′toid) *adj.* Of or pertaining to the occipital bone and the mastoid process of the temporal bone.

occipitomastoid suture. The union between the mastoid portion of the temporal bone and the occipital bone. NA *sutura occipitomastoidea.*

oc·cip·i·to·men·tal (ock·sip″i·to·men′tul) *adj.* [*occipito-* + *mental,* pertaining to the chin]. Of or pertaining to the occiput and the chin.

occipitomental diameter. The diameter joining the occipital protuberance and the chin.

oc·cip·i·to·pa·ri·e·tal (ock·sip″i·to·pa·rye′e·tul) *adj.* Pertaining to the occipital and parietal bones or lobes.

occipitoparietal suture. LAMBDOID SUTURE.

oc·cip·i·to·pon·tine (ock·sip″i·to·pon′teen, ·tine) *adj.* [*occipito-* + *pontine*]. Pertaining to the occipital lobe of the cerebrum and to the pons.

occipitopontine tract. A tract of nerve fibers which arise in the occipital lobe of the cerebrum, descend from the cortex, pass through the internal capsule, and terminate in the pontine nuclei. NA *tractus occipitopontinus.*

oc·cip·i·to·pos·te·ri·or (ock·sip″i·to·pos·teer′ee·ur) *adj.* Having the occiput directed backward, as the occipitoposterior position of the fetus in the uterus.

oc·cip·i·to·scap·u·la·ris (ock·sip″i·to·skap·yoo·lair′is) *n.* [*occipito-* + L. *scapularis,* scapular]. A variant of the rhomboideus major muscle extending to the occipital bone.

oc·cip·i·to·tem·po·ral (ock·sip″i·to·tem′puh·rul) *adj.* [*occipito-* + *temporal*]. Pertaining to the occipital and temporal regions, lobes, or bones.

occipitotemporal gyrus. Either of two gyri on the medial aspect of the cerebral hemisphere; a lateral and a medial one are present. See also *gyrus occipitotemporalis lateralis, gyrus occipitotemporalis medialis.*

oc·cip·i·to·tha·lam·ic (ock·sip″i·to·tha·lam′ick) *adj.* [*occipito-* + *thalamic*]. Of or pertaining to the occipital lobe and the thalamus.

occipitothalamic fasciculus. A bundle of nerve fibers connecting the thalamus with the occipital lobe.

oc·ci·put (ock′si·put) *n.* [L., from *ob-,* in back, + *caput,* head] [NA]. The back part of the head.

oc·clude (uh·klewd′) *v.* [L. *occludere,* to shut, close in]. To obstruct, stop up; to close; to bring into occlusion.

occluding ligature. A ligature completely obstructing a vessel or channel.

occlus-, occluso- [L.]. A combining form meaning *occlusion, occlusal.*

oc·clu·sal (uh·klew′zul) *adj.* [L. *occlus*us, shut, closed up, + *-al*]. 1. Pertaining to the masticatory surfaces of the teeth or to the plane in which they lie. 2. Of or pertaining to occlusion. —**occlusal·ly** (·ee) *adv.*

occlusal adjustment. OCCLUSAL EQUILIBRATION.

occlusal contact. Areas on opposing teeth which touch in various positions and movements of the jaws.

occlusal disharmony. Any malposition or functional aberration that increases the occlusal force on individual teeth or groups of teeth or alters the direction of occlusal force.

occlusal dystrophy. OCCLUSAL DISHARMONY.

occlusal equilibration. Alteration of occlusal and cuspate forms of teeth by grinding to establish harmonious functional relationships.

occlusal force. The force exerted upon opposing teeth when biting.

occlusal plane. CURVE OF OCCLUSION.

occlusal trauma. Injury to the periodontium associated with abnormal or damaging forces of occlusion.

oc·clu·sio (ock·lew'zee·o) *n.* [L.]. Closure; obliteration.

oc·clu·sion (uh·klew'zhun) *n.* [L. *occlusio*, closure]. 1. A closing or shutting up. 2. The state of being closed or shut. 3. The absorption, by a metal, of gas in large quantities, as of hydrogen by platinum. 4. The relationship of the masticatory surfaces of the maxillary teeth to the masticatory surfaces of the mandibular teeth when the jaws are closed. 5. *In neurophysiology*, the deficit in muscular tension when two afferent nerves that share certain motoneurons in the central nervous system are stimulated simultaneously, as compared to the sum of tensions when the two nerves are stimulated separately.

occlusion nystagmus. LATENT NYSTAGMUS.

occlusion rim. An occluding device made on a temporary or permanent artificial denture base for the development of maxillomandibular relation records and for the arrangement of teeth. Syn. *record rim.*

occlusio pu·pil·lae (pew·pil'ee). Obliteration of the pupil.

oc·clu·sive (uh·klew'siv) *adj.* Closing or shutting up, as an occlusive surgical dressing.

occluso-. See *occlus-.*

oc·clu·som·e·ter (ock''lew·zom'e·tur, ·som'e·tur) *n.* [*occluso-* + *-meter*]. GNATHODYNAMOMETER.

oc·cult (uh·kult', ock'ult) *adj.* [L. *occultus*]. Hidden; concealed; not evident, as an occult disease the nature of which is not readily determined, or occult blood.

occult bifid spine. SPINA BIFIDA OCCULTA.

occult blood. Blood not visible on gross inspection of body products such as feces, and detected only by laboratory tests.

occult blood test. A test for blood not apparent on ordinary inspection of the material concerned.

occult hydrocephalus. A syndrome, usually of middle life, characterized by dementia of variable degree, disturbances of equilibrium and gait, and disorders of praxis and sphincter control, in which there is normal cerebrospinal fluid pressure on lumbar puncture but an enlarged ventricular system on pneumoencephalography. Compare *communicating hydrocephalus, obstructive hydrocephalus.*

occupational acne. Acne artificialis acquired from regular exposure to acnegenic materials in certain industries.

occupational dermatosis. Dermatosis resulting from chemicals or irritations characteristically encountered in an occupation.

occupational disease. Any disease, organic or functional, arising from the particular toxic substances, characteristic hazards, or frequently repeated mechanical operations of a particular industry, trade, or occupation.

occupational injury. Any injury brought about by, or related to, an individual's occupation.

occupational medicine. The branch of medicine which deals with the relationship of people to their occupation, for the purpose of the prevention of disease and injury and the promotion of optimal health, productivity, and social adjustment.

occupational neurosis. Any neurotic disorder manifested by inability to use those parts of the body commonly employed in one's occupation, such as a writer's inability to write due to cramps or painful feeling of fatigue in the hand. The occupation is not the cause of the neurosis, but only an outlet for it.

occupational nystagmus. Ocular nystagmus due to prolonged deficient illumination or retinal fatigue, as seen in miners and telegraphers.

occupational paralysis. Muscular weakness and atrophy due to nerve compression in certain occupations. Compare *occupational neurosis.*

occupational psychiatry. A special field of psychiatry concerned with the diagnosis and treatment of mental illness in business and industry, and dealing with the psychiatric aspects of such problems as hiring, absenteeism, accident proneness, vocational adjustment, and retirement.

occupational therapy. 1.The use of selected occupations for therapeutic purposes. 2. The teaching of trades and arts as a means for the rehabilitation of patients handicapped physically or mentally.

occupational tumor. A tumor resulting from prolonged exposure to some physical or chemical agent in the course of one's occupation.

occupation cramps. OCCUPATION SPASMS.

occupation spasms. Disorders of motility in which a skilled motor act, such as writing or fingering a violin, suddenly requires a conscious and labored effort for its execution. See also *occupational neurosis.*

ocel·lus (o·sel'us) *n.*, pl. **ocel·li** (·eye, ·ee) [L., little eye]. 1. One of the simple eyes or pigmented spots of invertebrate animals. 2. A colored eyelike spot, as on feathers or flowers.

och·e·us (ock'ee·us) *n.* [Gk.]. *Obsol.* SCROTUM.

och·le·sis (ock·lee'sis) *n.* [Gk. *ochlēsis*, disturbance, from *ochlos*, crowd]. A morbid condition produced by or exacerbated by crowding.

och·lo·pho·bia (ock''lo·fo'bee·uh) *n.* [Gk. *ochlos*, crowd, + *-phobia*]. Morbid fear of crowds.

ochre mutation (o'kur). A nonsense mutation in which the codon base sequence is UAA (uracil-adenine-adenine).

ochrom·e·ter (o·krom'e·tur) *n.* [Gk. *ōchros*, paleness, + *-meter*]. An instrument for measuring the capillary blood pressure, which records the force or pressure required to blanch a finger.

ochro·no·sis (o''kruh·no'sis) *n.* [Gk. *ōchros*, yellow, + *-osis*]. A blue or brownish blue pigmentation of cartilage and connective tissue, especially around joints, by a melanotic pigment. The condition is frequently accompanied by alkaptonuria and occurs in those who have had phenol, in large quantities, applied to skin or mucous membrane for a long time. A disturbed metabolism of aromatic compounds is associated with this condition. —**ochro·not·ic** (·not'ick) *adj.*

ochronotic osteoarthritis. A rare degenerative arthropathy associated with the diseased cartilage of ochronosis, accompanied by alkaptonuria.

ochronotic spondylitis. A variety of osteoarthritis and disc degeneration associated with alkaptonuria. The discs are usually heavily calcified.

Ochs·ner-Ma·hor·ner test [A. *Ochsner*, U.S. surgeon, b. 1896; and H. *Mahorner*, U.S. surgeon, b. 1903]. A test for demonstrating the level of incompetent valves in perforating veins between the deep and superficial venous systems of the leg.

oc·i·mene (os'i·meen) *n.* 2,6-Dimethyl-1,5,7-octatriene, $C_{10}H_{16}$, a terpene constituent of many plants.

OCP. Oral contraceptive pill(s).

oc·ry·late (ock'ri·late) *n.* Octyl 2-cyanoacrylate, $C_{21}H_{26}O_3$, a tissue adhesive used in surgery.

oct-, octa-, octo- [Gk. and L. *octō*]. A combining form meaning *eight* or *eighth.*

oc·ta·ben·zone (ock''tuh·ben'zone) *n.* 2-Hydroxy-4-(octyloxy)benzophenone, $C_{21}H_{26}O_3$, an ultraviolet screen.

oc·tad (ock'tad) *n.* [Gk. *oktas, oktados*, a group of eight]. An octavalent element or radical.

oc·ta·meth·yl py·ro·phos·phor·am·ide (ock''tuh·meth'ul pye''ro·fos''for·am'ide). Bis[bisdimethylaminophosphonous]anhydride, $C_8H_{24}N_4O_3P_2$, a systemic insecticide and also a potent anticholinesterase agent, with selective action on peripheral cholinesterase; has been employed in treating myasthenia gravis. Abbreviated, OMPA.

oc·tan (ock'tan) *adj.* [F. *octane*]. Returning or recurring every eighth day, as an octan fever.

oc·tane (ock'tane) *n.* [*oct-* + *-ane*]. C_8H_{18}. The eighth member of the paraffin or marsh gas series.

oc·ta·no·ic acid (ock"tuh·no'ick). CAPRYLIC ACID.

oc·ta·pep·tide (ock"tuh·pep'tide) *n.* A polypeptide composed of eight amino acid groups.

oc·ta·ri·us (ock·tăr'ee·us) *n.* [L.]. An eighth part of a gallon; a pint. Abbreviated, O.

oc·ta·va·lent (ock"tuh·vay'lunt) *adj.* Having a valence of eight.

oc·ta·za·mide (ock·tay'zuh·mide) *n.* 5-Benzoylhexahydro-1*H*-furo[3,4-*c*]pyrrole, $C_{13}H_{15}NO_2$, an analgesic.

oc·tene (ock'teen) *n.* OCTYLENE.

oc·ti·grav·i·da (ock"ti·grav'id·uh) *n.* [*oct-* + L. *gravida*, pregnant]. A woman pregnant for the eighth time.

Octin. Trademark for isometheptene, an antispasmodic and vasoconstrictor drug used as the hydrochloride or mucate salt.

oc·tip·a·ra (ock·tip'ur·uh) *n.* [*oct-* + *-para*]. A woman who has been in labor eight times.

octo-. See *oct-*.

oc·to·drine (ock'to·dreen) *n.* 1,5-Dimethylhexylamine, $C_8H_{19}N$, a vasoconstrictor and local anesthetic.

oc·to·roon (ock"tuh·roon') *n.* [*octo-* + *-roon* as in *quadroon*]. A person with one quadroon and one white parent.

oc·tose (ock'toce) *n.* Any of a group of the monosaccharides with the formula $C_8H_{16}O_8$.

oc·to·xy·nol 9 (ock·to·zye'nole) *n.* Polyethyleneglycol mono-[p-(1,1,3,3-tetramehtylbutyl)phenyl]ether, of average molecular formula $C_{32}H_{58}O_{10}$, a spermatocide.

oc·trip·ty·line (ock·trip'ti·leen) *n.* la,l0*b*-Dihydro-*N*-methyldibenzo[*a,e*]cyclopropa[*c*]cycloheptene-Δ6(1*H*),γ-propylamine, $C_{20}H_{21}N$, an antidepressant used as the phosphate salt.

oc·tyl (ock'til) *n.* The radical C_8H_{17}—.

oc·tyl·ene (ock'til·een) *n.* One of a group of liquid unsaturated hydrocarbons of the formula C_8H_{16}.

octyl nitrite. $C_8H_{17}NO_2$; a liquid used like amyl nitrite, by inhalation, as a vasodilator.

ocul-, oculo- [L. *oculus*]. A combining form meaning *eye* or *ocular*.

oc·u·lar (ock'yoo·lur) *adj.* [L. *ocularis*, from *oculus*, eye]. Of or pertaining to the eye.

ocular, *n.* EYEPIECE.

ocular adnexa. ADNEXA OCULI.

ocular apraxia. PSEUDOOPHTHALMOPLEGIA.

ocular bobbing. Abrupt spontaneous downward jerks of both eyes, followed by a slower return to midposition, at regular or highly irregular intervals; observed in extensive pontine disease, but rarely in otherwise normal newborn infants.

ocular chalcosis. CHALKITIS.

ocular conjunctiva. BULBAR CONJUNCTIVA.

ocular crisis. 1. Any sudden disturbance of eye function. 2. Sudden intense eye pain, tearing, and photophobia. See also *oculogyric crisis.*

ocular dominance. EYE DOMINANCE.

ocular flutter. Quick, multiphasic, usually horizontal oscillations around the point of fixation. This abnormality is associated with cerebellar disease.

ocular fundus. FUNDUS OCULI.

ocular headache. A headache that results from organic disease or impaired function of ocular structures.

ocular herpes. Infection of the eyelids, conjunctivae, or corneas by the virus of herpes simplex.

ocular hypertelorism. A deformity of the frontal region of the cranium, resulting in a conspicuously widened bridge of the nose, and thus increased distance between the eyes and divergent strabismus; may be associated with other cranial or facial deformities and neurologic disturbances. Contr. *ocular hypotelorism.*

ocular hypotelorism. A deformity of the frontal region of the cranium due to deficient development of the lesser wing of the sphenoid bone and premature closure of cranial sutures, resulting in a narrowing of the bridge of the nose, and thus decreased distance between the eyes and convergent strabismus; may be associated with other cranial or facial deformities, particularly microcephaly and neurologic disturbances. Contr. *ocular hypertelorism.*

ocular image. The image that reaches consciousness through the eye; determined by the retinal image, also by the anatomic and physiologic modification imposed upon it before it reaches the brain.

ocular lymphomatosis. A form of the avian leukosis complex affecting primarily the iris of the eye.

ocular micrometer. EYEPIECE MICROMETER.

ocular microscope. SIMPLE MICROSCOPE.

ocular migraine. An attack of migraine accompanied by teichopsia, amblyopia, or other visual disturbances.

ocular motor apraxia. Inability to move the eyes horizontally voluntarily or on command with preservation of reflex eye movements, and lateral rotational jerky thrusts of the head to compensate for the deficiency of eye movements. The congenital form (Cogan's syndrome) is usually seen in boys, who may also have difficulties in reading and in coordination; in the acquired, adult form, compensatory head turning is rarely seen since there is usually an associated apraxia of head turning. The anatomic basis of the condition is not known.

ocular motor dysmetria. An overshooting of the eyes on attempted fixation, followed by several cycles of oscillations of diminishing amplitude until precise fixation is attained. The overshoot may occur on eccentric fixation or on refixation in the primary position of gaze. This sign occurs with disease of the cerebellum and its pathways.

ocular muscles. The extrinsic muscles of the eyeball, including the four recti (superior, inferior, medialis, and lateralis), the two oblique (superior and inferior), and the levator palpebrae superioris.

ocular nystagmus. To-and-fro movements of the eyes when central vision is defective, making fixation difficult or impossible, observed when vision has been deficient since birth or before fixation was achieved (shimmering nystagmus), or when vision becomes impaired due to spending a long time in poorly lit surroundings, as may occur in miners.

ocular paralysis or **palsy.** Paralysis of the extraocular muscles (external ophthalmoplegia) or of the ciliary body and iris (internal ophthalmoplegia).

ocular vertigo. Vertigo due to oculomotor disorders.

oc·u·len·tum (ock"yoo·len'tum) *n.* [*ocul-* + ungu*entum*, ointment]. An ointment for use in the eye.

oculi. Plural and genitive singular of *oculus.*

oculi mar·ma·ry·go·des (mahr"muh·ri·go'deez, mahr·mah") [Gk. *marmarygōdes*, seeing sparks]. METAMORPHOPSIA.

oc·u·list (ock'yoo·list) *n.* [F. *oculiste*]. OPHTHALMOLOGIST.

oculo-. See ocul-.

oc·u·lo·au·ric·u·lo·ver·te·bral (ock"yoo·lo·aw·rick"yoo·lo·vur'te·brul) *adj.* [*oculo-* + *auriculo-* + *vertebral*]. Pertaining to the eyes, the ears, and the vertebral column.

oculoauriculovertebral dysplasia. A syndrome of congenital deformities of the eye, such as epibulbar dermoids; of the ear, such as microtia, auricular appendices, and pretragal blind-ended fistulas; and of the musculoskeletal system, especially the vertebral column. Mild facial and oral hypoplasia and neurologic manifestations may be present. Considered to be due to an abnormal embryonic vascular supply to the first arch. Syn. *Goldenhar's syndrome.*

oc·u·lo·car·di·ac (ock"yoo·lo·kahr'dee·ack) *adj.* [*oculo-* + *cardiac*]. Pertaining to the eyes and the heart.

oculocardiac reflex. Bradycardia or termination of cardiac arrhythmia in response to eyeball pressure; due to the association of the fifth cranial and the vagus nerve. This means of vagal stimulation is employed in the electroencephalographic diagnosis of breath-holding spells, but may be a dangerous maneuver in that retinal detachment may occur.

oc·u·lo·ceph·a·lo·gy·ric (ock″yoo·lo·sef″uh·lo·jye′rick) *adj.* [*oculo-* + *cephalo-* + *gyr-* + *-ic*]. Pertaining to rotatory movements of the eyes and the head.

oculocephalogyric reflex. The associated movements of the eye, head, and body in the process of focusing visual attention upon an object.

oc·u·lo·cer·e·bro·re·nal (ock″yoo·lo·serr″e·bro·ree′nul) *adj.* [*oculo-* + *cerebro-* + *renal*]. Pertaining to the eyes, cerebrum, and kidneys.

oculocerebrorenal syndrome. A familial hereditary affection of males, characterized by growth retardation, mental deficiency, hypotonia, mild or severe metabolic acidosis, generalized hyperaminoaciduria, proteinuria, rickets, and characteristic eye changes, especially bilateral congenital cataracts and glaucoma; believed to be transmitted as an x-linked characteristic. Syn. *Lowe's syndrome.*

oc·u·lo·cu·ta·ne·ous (ock″yoo·lo·kew·tay′nee·us) *adj.* [*oculo-* + *cutaneous*]. Pertaining to both the eyes and skin, as certain congenital or hereditary disorders.

oc·u·lo·den·to·dig·i·tal (ock″yoo·lo·den″to·dij′i·tul) *adj.* Pertaining to the eyes, teeth, and digits, usually the fingers.

oculodentodigital syndrome. An autosomal dominantly inherited disorder characterized by microphthalmia, microcornea, epicanthic folds; enamel hypoplasia, microdontia or anodontia; and camptodactyly of the fifth digit, hypoplasia or absence of the middle phalanx of the second through fifth toes, syndactyly of the forth and fifth fingers, and of the third and fourth toes. The face is unusual with a thin nose and anteversion of the nostrils. Stature and mentality usually are normal. Compare *Hallermann-Streiff-François syndrome.*

oc·u·lo·fa·cial (ock″yoo·lo·fay′shul) *adj.* [*oculo-* + *facial*]. Pertaining to the eyes and face.

oc·u·lo·gas·tric (ock″yoo·lo·gas′trick) *adj.* [*oculo-* + *gastric*]. Pertaining to the eyes and the stomach.

oculogastric reflex. Nausea and mild gastric disturbances as a result of ocular muscular imbalance.

oc·u·lo·glan·du·lar (ock″yoo·lo·glan′dew·lur) *adj.* Pertaining to the eyes and lymph nodes.

oculoglandular syndrome. PARINAUD'S SYNDROME.

oculoglandular tularemia. Infection by *Pasteurella* (*Francisella*) *tularensis* which, in addition to the usual symptoms of tularemia, causes swollen eyelids, conjunctivitis, swollen lymph nodes, and ulcers on the conjunctivae.

oc·u·lo·gy·ra·tion (ock″yoo·lo·jye·ray′shun) *n.* [*oculo-* + *gyration*]. Movement of the eyeballs. **—oculo·gy·ric** (·jye′rick), **oculo·gy·ral** (·jye′rul) *adj.*

oculogyric-auricular reflex. A facial nerve reflex which consists of retraction of the auricle and curling back of the helix of the ear on lateral gaze in the extreme opposite direction, or retraction of both auricles, more on the opposite side, on lateral gaze to one side.

oculogyric crisis or **spasm.** Involuntary tonic spasm of extraocular muscles, lasting minutes to hours, resulting usually in conjugate upward deviation of the eyes, but sometimes in forced conjugate movement in other directions, seen as a sequel of postencephalitic parkinsonism.

oc·u·lo·mo·tor (ock″yoo·lo·mo′tur) *adj.* [*oculo-* + *motor*]. Pertaining to the movement of the eye, or to the oculomotor nerve.

oculomotor nerve. The third cranial nerve, whose motor fibers arise from nuclei in the central gray matter at the level of the superior colliculus and supply the levator palpebrae superioris and all extrinsic eye muscles except the lateral rectus and superior oblique, and whose parasympathetic component goes to the ciliary ganglion, from which short fibers pass to the ciliary and sphincter pupillae muscles. NA *nervus oculomotorius.* See also Table of Nerves in the Appendix.

oculomotor nucleus. A wedge-shaped nucleus lying just rostral to the trochlear nucleus a little below the cerebral aqueduct near the median line. It gives origin to motor fibers of the oculomotor nerve. NA *nucleus nervi oculomotorii.*

oculomotor paralysis. Paralysis of the oculomotor nerve, with pupillary mydriasis and areflexia, ptosis, and external deviation of the eye.

oculomotor sulcus. A longitudinal furrow on the medial surface of the cerebral peduncle from which emerge the roots of the oculomotor nerve. NA *sulcus medialis cruris cerebri.*

oc·u·lo·my·co·sis (ock″yoo·lo·migh·ko′sis) *n.* [*oculo-* + *mycosis*]. Any disease of the eye or its appendages due to a fungus.

oc·u·lo·oto·cu·ta·ne·ous (ock″yoo·lo·o″to·kew·tay′nee·us) *adj.* Pertaining to the eyes, ears, and skin.

oculootocutaneous syndrome of Yuge. UVEOMENINGOENCEPHALITIS.

oc·u·lop·a·thy (ock″yoo·lop′uh·thee) *n.* OPTHALMOPATHY.

oc·u·lo·pha·ryn·ge·al (ock″yoo·lo·fa·rin′jee·ul) *adj.* Involving the eyes and the pharynx.

oculopharyngeal muscular dystrophy. A late-onset muscular dystrophy, usually inherited as an autosomal dominant trait, which is manifested clinically only by a slowly progressive ptosis of the eyelids and dysphagia; the difficulty in swallowing may progress until normal food intake is severely limited.

oculopharyngeal reflex. Rapid movements of deglutition and spontaneous closing of the eyes without apparent contraction of the orbicularis muscle, in response to stimulation of the bulbar conjunctiva.

oc·u·lo·phren·i·co·re·cur·rent (ock″yoo·lo·fren″i·ko·ree·kur′unt) *adj.* [*oculo-* + *phrenico-* + *recurrent*]. Pertaining to the recurrent laryngeal and phrenic nerves associated with Horner's syndrome.

oculophrenicorecurrent paralysis. Paralysis of the recurrent laryngeal and phrenic nerves with associated Horner's syndrome, such as may occur in cancer of the lung with mediastinal extension.

oc·u·lo·pu·pil·lary (ock″yoo·lo·pew′pi·ler″ee) *adj.* [*oculo-* + *pupillary*]. Of or pertaining to the pupil of the eye, or to the pupil in relation to the eye as a whole.

oculopupillary reflex. A variant of the corneal reflex in which a painful stimulus directed towards the eye or its adnexa results in constriction of the pupil or dilatation followed by constriction.

oc·u·lo·sen·so·ry (ock″yoo·lo·sen′suh·ree) *adj.* [*oculo-* + *sensory*]. Pertaining to stimuli to the eye.

oculosensory reflex. OCULOPUPILLARY REFLEX.

oc·u·lo·zy·go·mat·ic (ock″yoo·lo·zye″go·mat′ick) *adj.* Pertaining to the eye and the zygoma.

oc·u·lus (ock′yoo·lus) *n.*, pl. **ocu·li** (·lye) [L.] [NA]. EYE. Abbreviated, O.

oculus cae·si·us (see′zee·us) [L., blue-gray]. GLAUCOMA.

oculus dex·ter (decks′tur) [L.]. The right eye. Abbreviated, O. D.

oculus lac·ri·mans (lack′ri·manz) [L., weeping, shedding tears]. EPIPHORA.

oculus lep·o·ri·nus (lep″o·rye′nus) [L., pertaining to hares]. LAGOPHTHALMOS.

oculus pu·ru·len·tus (pewr″yoo·len′tus) [L.]. HYPOPYON.

oculus simplex. MONOCULUS.

oculus sin·is·ter (sin′is·tur, si·nis′tur) [L.]. The left eye. Abbreviated, O. S.

oculus uni·tas (yoo′ni·tas). OCULUS UTERQUE.

oculus uter·que (yoo·tur′kwee) [L.]. Each eye. Abbreviated, O. U.

ocy·o·din·ic (o″see·o·din′ick, o″sigh·o·) *adj.* [Gk. *ōkys*, swift, + *-ōdis, ōdinos*, pangs of childbirth]. OXYTOCIC.

od (od, ode) *n.* [arbitrary coinage]. The force supposed to produce the phenomena of animal magnetism. **—od·ic** (od′ick) *adj.*

OD, O.D. Abbreviation for *overdose.*

O. D. Abbreviation for *oculus dexter,* right eye.

odax·es·mus (o″dack·sez′mus) *n.* [Gk. *odaxēsmos,* biting, irritation]. Biting the tongue, lip, or cheek during a convulsion.

odont-, odonto- [Gk. *odous, odontos,* tooth]. A combining form meaning (a) *tooth;* (b) *odontoid.*

-odont [Gk. *odous, odontos,* tooth]. A combining form meaning *having teeth of a* (specified) *kind.*

odon·tal·gia (o″don·tal′juh, ·jee·uh) *n.* [Gk.]. TOOTHACHE. **—odontal·gic** (·jick) *adj.*

odon·tec·to·my (o″don·teck′tuh·mee) *n.* [*odont-* + *-ectomy*]. Surgical removal of a tooth.

odon·tex·e·sis (o·don″teck·see′sis) *n.* [*odont-* + Gk. *xesis,* planing, abrasion]. Removal of deposits such as salivary calculi from the teeth.

odon·thy·a·lus (o″don·thigh′uh·lus, o″dont·high′) *n.* [*odont-* + Gk. *hyalos,* glass]. ENAMEL.

-odontia [*odont-* + *-ia*]. A combining form designating a *condition* or a *treatment of the teeth.*

odon·ti·a·sis (o·don·tye′uh·sis) *n.* [Gk., teething]. DENTITION; the cutting of teeth.

odon·tic (o·don′tick) *adj.* [Gk. *odontikos*]. Pertaining to teeth.

odon·tin·oid (o·don′tin·oid) *adj.* [*odont-* + Gk. *-ino-*, of, made of, + *-oid*]. Resembling, or having the nature of, teeth.

odon·ti·tis (o·don·tye′tis) *n.* [*odont-* + *-itis*]. Inflammation associated with a tooth or teeth.

odonto-. See *odont-.*

odon·to·am·e·lo·sar·co·ma (o·don″to·am″e·lo·sahr·ko′muh, ·a·mel″o·) *n.* [*odonto-* + *amelo-* + *sarcoma*]. AMELOBLASTOSARCOMA.

odon·to·at·lan·tal (o·don″to·ut·lan′tul) *adj.* [*odonto-* + *atlantal*]. ATLANTOAXIAL.

odon·to·blast (o·don′to·blast) *n.* [*odonto-* + *-blast*]. One of the cells covering the dental papilla or dental pulp, concerned with the formation of the dentin. **—odon·to·blas·tic** (o·don″to·blas′tick) *adj.*

odontoblastic process. The cytoplasmic process of an odontoblast which lies in a dentinal tubule. Syn. *Tomes's fiber.*

odon·to·blas·to·ma (o·don″to·blas·to′muh) *n.* [*odontoblast* + *-oma*]. AMELOBLASTIC ODONTOMA.

odon·to·cele (o·don′to·seel) *n.* [*odonto-* + *-cele*]. A dentoalveolar cyst.

odon·to·cla·sis (o·don″to·klay′sis, o″don·tock′luh·sis) *n.* [*odonto-* + *-clasis*]. The process of resorption of the dentin of a tooth.

odon·to·clast (o·don′to·klast) *n.* [*odonto-* + *-clast*]. A multinuclear cell, morphologically identical to an osteoclast, which is associated with resorption of tooth roots.

odon·to·gen·e·sis (o·don″to·jen′e·sis) *n.* [*odonto-* + *-genesis*]. 1. Development of a tooth. 2. DENTINOGENESIS.

odontogenesis imperfecta. DENTINOGENESIS IMPERFECTA.

odon·to·gen·ic (o·don″to·jen′ick) *adj.* [*odonto-* + *-genic*]. 1. Pertaining to odontogeny. 2. Originating in tissues associated with teeth.

odontogenic cyst. A cyst originating in tissues associated with teeth; of two main types, dentigerous and radicular.

odontogenic fibroma. A benign tumor formed from the mesenchymal derivatives of the tooth germ, which usually develops at the apex of a tooth.

odontogenic fibrosarcoma. A fibrosarcoma derived from mesenchymal odontogenic tissues.

odontogenic myxoma. A myxoma of the jaws, considered to be of dental origin, and usually seen in young individuals.

odon·tog·e·ny (o″don·toj′e·nee) *n.* [*odonto-* + *-geny*]. The origin and development of teeth.

odon·tog·ra·phy (o″don·tog′ruf·ee) *n.* [*odonto-* + *-graphy*]. The descriptive anatomy of the teeth. **—odon·to·graph·ic** (o·don″to·graf′ick) *adj.*

odon·toid (o·don′toid) *adj.* [Gk. *odontoeidēs*]. 1. Resembling a tooth; toothlike. 2. Pertaining to the dens of the axis, as: odontoid ligament.

odontoid ligament. 1. ALAR ODONTOID LIGAMENT. 2. APICAL DENTAL LIGAMENT.

odontoid process. DENS OF THE AXIS.

odon·tol·o·gist (o″don·tol′uh·jist) *n.* [*odontology* + *-ist*]. DENTIST.

odon·tol·o·gy (o″don·tol′uh·jee) *n.* [*odonto-* + *-logy*]. A branch of science dealing with the formation, development, and abnormalities of the teeth.

odon·to·lox·ia (o·don″to·lock′see·uh) *n.* [*odonto-* + Gk. *loxos,* slanting, + *-ia*]. Irregularity or obliquity of the teeth.

odon·tol·oxy (o″don·tol′uck·see, o·don′to·lock″see) *n.* ODONTOLOXIA.

odon·tol·y·sis (o″don·tol′i·sis) *n.* [*odonto-* + *-lysis*]. The loss of calcified tooth substance by dissolution.

odon·to·ma (o″don·to′muh) *n.,* pl. **odontomas, odontoma·ta** (·tuh) [*odont-* + *-oma*]. A benign tumor representing a developmental excess, composed of mesodermal or ectodermal tooth-forming tissue, alone or in association with the calcified derivatives of these structures.

odon·tome (o·don′tome) *n.* ODONTOMA.

odon·to·pho·bia (o·don″to·fo′bee·uh) *n.* [*odonto-* + *-phobia*]. Morbid fear of teeth (usually animals' teeth).

odon·to·plas·ty (o·don′to·plas″tee) *n.* [*odonto-* + *-plasty*]. The reshaping of a tooth by grinding to produce a more desirable contour in the management of a periodontal problem.

odon·to·pri·sis (o·don″to·prye′sis, o″don·top′ri·sis) *n.* [*odonto-* + Gk. *prisis,* a sawing]. BRUXISM.

odon·to·scope (o·don′tuh·skope) *n.* [*odonto-* + *-scope*]. A dental mirror used for inspecting the teeth.

odon·to·sis (o″don·to′sis, od″un·to′sis) *n.* [*odont-* + *-osis*]. ODONTOGENESIS.

odon·tot·o·my (o″don·tot′uh·mee) *n.* [*odonto-* + *-tomy*]. The cutting into a tooth.

odor, *n.* [L.]. Any stimulus, usually chemical in nature, which adequately results in a sensation of smell; a scent or fragrance. **—odor·ous** (·us) *adj.*

odo·ra·tism (o″duh·ray′tiz·um) *n.* [(*Lathyrus*) *odoratus,* the sweet pea]. LATHYRISM (2).

odor·if·er·ous (o″dur·if′ur·us) *adj.* [L. *odorifer*]. Emitting an odor.

odor·im·e·try (o″dur·im′e·tree) *n.* [*odor* + *-metry*]. The measuring of the effect of odors upon the nasal sensory organs.

odor-of-sweaty-feet syndrome. An inborn error of short-chain fatty acid metabolism, clinically characterized by apparent normality at birth, followed by anorexia, weakness, lethargy, and an unusual odor suggestive of sweaty feet within the first few weeks of life, and severe acidosis and seizures terminally. Butyric and hexanoic acids are found in the exhaled air, blood, and urine. Considered to be an autosomal recessive disorder.

od·yl, od·yle (od′il, o′dil) *n.* [*od* + Gk. *hylē,* material]. OD.

odyn-, odyno- [Gk. *odynē*]. A combining form meaning *pain.*

odyn·a·cou·sis (o·din″uh·koo′sis) *n.* [*odyn-* + *akousis,* hearing]. Hypersensitivity to noise, to the point of being painful.

odyn·a·cu·sis (o·din″uh·kew′sis) *n.* ODYNACOUSIS.

-odynia [*odyn-* + *-ia*]. A combining form designating *a painful condition.*

odyno·pha·gia (o·din″o·fay′juh, ·jee·uh) *n.* [*odyno-* + *-phagia*]. 1. Painful swallowing. 2. DYSPHAGIA.

odyno·pho·bia (o·din″o·fo′bee·uh) *n.* [*odyno-* + *-phobia*]. Abnormal dread of pain.

ody·nu·ria (o″di·new′ree·uh) *n.* [*odyn-* + *-uria*]. Painful urination.

oedema. EDEMA.

oed·i·pal (ed′i·pul, ee′di·pul) *adj.* Pertaining to the Oedipus complex.

oed·i·pism (ed′i·piz·um, ee′di·) *n.* [*Oedipus,* King of Thebes, who put out his own eyes because he unwittingly had killed his father]. Self-inflicted injury to the eyes.

Oed·i·pus complex (ed'i·pus, ee'di·pus) [*Oedipus*, King of Thebes, who unwittingly killed his father and married his mother]. *In psychoanalytic theory*, the attraction and attachment of the child to the parent of the opposite sex, accompanied by feelings of envy and hostility toward the parent of the child's sex, whose displeasure and punishment the child so fears that he represses his feelings. Applied by Freud originally to the male child, the Electra complex referring to the female.

O electron. An electron in the o or fifth shell surrounding the nucleus of an atom.

Oenethyl. Trademark for methylaminoheptane, a sympathomimetic amine used as the hydrochloride salt to combat hypotension during surgery.

oe·no·ma·nia (ee''no·may'nee·uh) *n. Obsol.* OINOMANIA.

Oer·tel's treatment (œr'tᵉl) [M. J. *Oertel*, German physician, 1835–1897]. A regimen for treatment of cardiovascular disease including weight reduction, dietary and fluid regulation, and a system of exercises.

oesophag-, oesophago-. See *esophag-, esophago-*.

oesophagalgia. ESOPHAGALGIA.

oesophageal. ESOPHAGEAL.

oesophagectasia. ESOPHAGECTASIA.

oesophagectasis. Esophagectasis (= ESOPHAGECTASIA).

oesophagectomy. ESOPHAGECTOMY.

oesophagectopy. ESOPHAGECTOPY.

oesophagitis. ESOPHAGITIS.

oesophago-. See *esophag-*.

oesophagobronchial. ESOPHAGOBRONCHIAL.

oesophagocele. ESOPHAGOCELE.

oesophagoduodenostomy. ESOPHAGODUODENOSTOMY.

oesophagoenterostomy. ESOPHAGOENTEROSTOMY.

oesophagogastrectomy. ESOPHAGOGASTRECTOMY.

oesophagogastric. ESOPHAGOGASTRIC.

oesophagogastroplasty. ESOPHAGOGASTROPLASTY.

oesophagogastroscope. ESOPHAGOGASTROSCOPE.

oesophagogastrostomy. ESOPHAGOGASTROSTOMY.

oesophagogram. ESOPHAGOGRAM.

oesophagohiatal. ESOPHAGOHIATAL.

oesophagojejunostomy. ESOPHAGOJEJUNOSTOMY.

oesophagometer. ESOPHAGOMETER.

oesophago-oesophagostomy. ESOPHAGOESOPHAGOSTOMY.

oesophagopathy. ESOPHAGOPATHY.

oesophagoplasty. ESOPHAGOPLASTY.

oesophagoptosis. ESOPHAGOPTOSIS.

oesophagoscope. ESOPHAGOSCOPE.

oesophagospasm. ESOPHAGOSPASM.

oesophagostenosis. ESOPHAGOSTENOSIS.

oesophagostoma. ESOPHAGOSTOMA.

oe·soph·a·go·sto·mi·a·sis, esoph·a·go·sto·mi·a·sis (ee·sof''uh·go·sto·migh'uh·sis, ee·sof''uh·gos''to·) *n.* [*Oesophagostomum* + *-iasis*]. Infection with *Oesophagostomum*.

Oe·soph·a·gos·to·mum (ee·sof''uh·gos'to·mum) *n.* [NL., from *esophago-* + *stoma*]. A genus of nematodes parasitic in the intestines, particularly the cecum, of ruminants, monkeys, and apes; rarely infects man.

oesophagostomy. ESOPHAGOSTOMY.

oesophagotome. ESOPHAGOTOME.

oesophagotomy. ESOPHAGOTOMY.

oesophagus [BNA]. ESOPHAGUS.

oesophogram. ESOPHAGOGRAM.

oestradiol. ESTRADIOL.

oes·tri·a·sis, es·tri·a·sis (es·trye'uh·sis) *n.* [*Oestrus* + *-iasis*]. Myiasis due to the larva of the *Oestrus*.

Oes·tri·dae (es'tri·dee) *n.pl.* [from *Oestrus*]. A family of botflies and warble flies. —**oestrid**, *adj.* & *n.*

oestrin. Estrin (= ESTROGEN).

oestriol. ESTRIOL.

oestrogen. ESTROGEN.

oestrogenic. ESTROGENIC.

oestrogenization. ESTROGENIZATION.

oestrone. ESTRONE.

oestrous. ESTROUS.

oestrual. ESTRUAL.

oestruation. Estruation (= ESTRUS).

oestrum. Estrum (= ESTRUS).

Oes·trus (es'trus) *n.* [NL., from Gk. *oistros*, gadfly]. A genus of botflies.

oestrus. ESTRUS.

Oestrus ovis (o'vis) [L. *ovis*, sheep]. A species of botfly which infects the nose of sheep and sometimes attacks the conjunctiva, the outer nares, and buccal regions of man.

OFC Abbreviation for *occipitofrontal circumference*.

of·fi·cial, *adj.* [L. *officialis*]. Of medicines: recognized by, and conforming to the standards of, the United States Pharmacopeia or the National Formulary.

of·fic·i·nal (o·fis'i·nul, off·i·sign'nul) *adj.* [ML. *officinalis*, pertaining to a storeroom, from *officina*, storeroom]. *Obsol.* On sale without prescription.

off·spring, *n.* A lineal descendent from a known line of forebears.

Og·ston-Luc operation (luᵉk) [A. *Ogston*, Scottish surgeon, 1844–1929; and H. *Luc*, French laryngologist, 1855–1925]. OGSTON'S OPERATION (3).

Ogston's operation [A. *Ogston*]. 1. Removal of a portion of the medial condyle of the femur for knock-knee. 2. Excision of a wedge of the tarsus for flatfoot. 3. Opening the frontal sinus through an anterior approach. Syn. *Ogston-Luc operation*.

Ogu·chi disease [C. *Oguchi*, Japanese ophthalmologist, 1875–1945]. Hereditary night blindness.

Oha·ra's disease [H. *Ohara*, Japanese physician, 20th century]. TULAREMIA.

Ohl·mach·er's fixative solution [A. P. *Ohlmacher*, U.S. pathologist, 1865–1916]. A fixative for animal tissue containing ethanol, chloroform, mercuric chloride, and glacial acetic acid.

ohm, *n.* [G. *Ohm*, German physicist, 1787–1854]. 1. The unit of electric resistance, equal to one thousand million (10^9) units of resistance of the centimeter-gram-second system of electromagnetic units. 2. The international ohm, the resistance of a column of mercury 106.3 cm long and weighing 14.4521 g at 0° C.

ohm-am·me·ter (ome''am'e·tur, ·am'ee·tur) *n.* A combined ohmmeter and ammeter.

ohm·me·ter (ome'mee·tur) *n.* [*ohm* + *meter*]. An apparatus for measuring electric resistance in ohms.

Ohm's law [G. *Ohm*]. The strength of an electric current varies directly as the electromotive force, and inversely as the resistance, that is, $E = I \times R$, in which E = electromotive force (or potential difference between both ends of the conductor, measured in volts); I = current in amperes; R = resistance in ohms.

-oid [Gk. *-oeidēs*, -like, from *eidos*, form]. A suffix meaning *like* or *resembling*.

oid·io·my·cin (o·id''ee·o·migh'sin) *n.* [*Oidium* + *-mycin*]. A vaccine prepared from the fungus *Candida albicans;* also used in a skin test for delayed hypersensitivity.

oidiomycin test. An intradermal test with *Candida albicans* vaccine; said to be of aid in the diagnosis of infections due to *Candida albicans*, but often positive in other fungous infections.

oid·io·my·co·sis (o·id''ee·o·migh·ko'sis) *n.* [*Oidium* + *mycosis*]. CANDIDIASIS.

oid·i·um (o·id'ee·um) *n.*, pl. ***oid·ia*** (·ee·uh) [L., from Gk. *ōon*, egg, + *-idion*, diminutive suffix]. 1. An organism belonging to the former genus *Oidium*, including what are now classified as *Candida, Blastomyces*, etc. 2. The imperfect states of Erysiphaceae, cosmopolitan powdery mildews.

Oidium albicans. *Obsol.* *CANDIDA ALBICANS*.

Oidium dermatitidis. *Obsol.* *BLASTOMYCES DERMATITIDIS*.

oi·kio·ma·nia (oy''kee·o·may'nee·uh) *n.* ECOMANIA.

oi·kol·o·gy (oy·kol'uh·jee) *n.* [Gk. *oikos*, house, + *-logy*]. 1. The science of the home. 2. ECOLOGY.

oi·ko·ma·nia (oy"ko·may'nee·uh) *n.* [Gk. *oikos*, house, + *-mania*]. ECOMANIA.

oi·ko·pho·bia (oy"ko·fo'bee·uh) *n.* [Gk. *oikos*, house, + *-phobia*]. Morbid fear of home, or of a house.

oi·ko·site (oy'ko·site) *n.* [Gk. *oikos*, house, + para*site*]. Parasite fixed to its host; an ectoparasite.

oil, *n.* [L. *oleum*, from Gk. *elaion*]. A liquid, generally viscous, obtained from animal, vegetable, or mineral sources but sometimes synthesized; imiscible with water but miscible with many organic solvents. Most oils are nonvolatile (fixed oils), but some volatilize slowly (volatile oils). The chemical composition of oils varies greatly. **—oily,** *adj.*

oil aspiration pneumonia. LIPID PNEUMONIA (1).

oil gland. SEBACEOUS GLAND.

oil-immersion objective. *In microscopy*, an objective designed for use when oil with a refractive index close to that of glass replaces air between the objective and the object.

oil of vitriol. SULFURIC ACID.

oil red O. An acid monoazo dye which serves as a fat stain.

oil-soluble dyes. A group of naphthol and substituted naphthylamine and aminoanthraquinone dyes which are soluble in fats, less soluble in hydroalcoholic mixtures which do not dissolve fats, and insoluble in water; used as differential stains in histologic techniques for fats in tissue. Syn. *lysochromes.*

oi·no·ma·nia (oy"no·may'nee·uh) *n.* [Gk. *oinos*, wine, + *-mania*]. *Obsol.* A form of mental disorder characterized by an irresistible craving for, and consequent indulgence in, alcoholic drink.

oint·ment, *n.* [L. *unguentum*]. A semisolid preparation used for a protective and emollient effect or as a vehicle for the local or endermic administration of medicaments. Ointment bases are composed of various mixtures of fats, waxes, animal and vegetable oils, and solid and liquid hydrocarbons, or, in the so-called washable or water-soluble bases, there may be from 50 to 75% of water incorporated into an emulsified product.

Oka·mo·to method. A histochemical method for metals based on development of a reddish-violet precipitate by most metals upon their reaction with *p*-dimethylaminobenzylidene rhodanine.

Ok·kels method. A histochemical method for gold using ultraviolet light to obtain black gold granules.

-ol *In organic chemistry*, a suffix designating (a) an *alcohol* or a *phenol*, both characterized by the presence of the OH group; (b) loosely, *oil*.

O.L.A. Abbreviation for *occipitolaevoanterior.*

ola·flur (o'luh·flure) *n.* 2,2'-[[3-[2-Hydroxyethyl)octadecylamino]propyl]imino]diethanol dihydrofluoride, $C_{27}H_{58}N_2O_3$, a dental caries prophylactic.

ol·a·mine (ol'uh·meen) *n.* Contraction for *ethanolamine*, $H_2NCH_2CH_2OH$.

old dislocation. UNREDUCED DISLOCATION.

old sight. PRESBYOPIA.

old tuberculin. A broth culture of tubercle bacilli, sterilized by heat, filtered, and concentrated by evaporation. Abbreviated, O.T., T.O.

Old World hookworm. *ANCYLOSTOMA DUODENALE.*

Old World monkey. Any of the monkeys of the Eastern Hemisphere, classified as the Cercopithecidae and including principally baboons, macaques, guenons, mangabeys, and colobines. Compare *New World monkey.* See also *catarrhine.*

-ole [L. *-olus, -ola, -olum*]. A suffix meaning *small.*

ole-, oleo- [L. *oleum*, oil]. A combining form meaning (a) *oil;* (b) *olein, oleic.*

olea. Plural of *oleum.*

ole·ag·i·nous (o"lee·aj'i·nus) *adj.* [L. *oleagineus*, of the olive tree]. Oily.

ole·an·do·my·cin (o"lee·an"do·migh'sin) *n.* [*oleander* + *-mycin*]. A basic antibiotic, $C_{35}H_{61}NO_{12}$, elaborated by strains of *Streptomyces antibioticus;* used in the treatment of infections due to strains of staphylococci and other gram-positive organisms resistant to penicillin, tetracyclines, and other established antibiotics.

ole·ate (o'lee·ate) *n.* 1. A salt of oleic acid. 2. A pharmaceutical preparation made by a solution of medicinal ingredients in oleic acid.

ole·cra·nar·thri·tis (o"le·kray"nahr·thrye'tis, o·leck"ra·) *n.* [*olecranon* + *arthritis*]. Inflammation of the elbow joint.

ole·cra·nar·throc·a·ce (o"le·kray"nahr·throck'uh·see, o·leck"ran·ahr·) *n.* [*olecranon* + *arthro-* + *-cace*]. Inflammation of the elbow joint.

ole·cra·nar·throp·a·thy (o"le·kray"nahr·throp'uth·ee, o·leck"ran·ahr·) *n.* [*olecranon* + *arthropathy*]. A disease of the elbow joint.

olec·ra·noid (o·leck'run·oid) *adj.* [*olecranon* + *-oid*]. Resembling or pertaining to the olecranon.

olecranoid fossa. OLECRANON FOSSA.

olec·ra·non (o·leck'ruh·non, o"le·kray'non) *n.* [Gk. *ōlekranon*] [NA]. The large process at the upper extremity of the ulna. **—olecra·nal** (·nul) *adj.*

olecranon bursa. A bursa lying between the olecranon process of the ulna and the skin. NA *bursa subcutanea olecrani.*

olecranon fossa. A fossa at the dorsal side of the distal end of the humerus, for the reception of the olecranon. NA *fossa olecrani.*

olecranon process. OLECRANON.

olef·i·ant gas (o·lef'ee·unt, o·leef', o"le·figh'unt) [F.]. ETHYLENE.

ole·fin (o'le·fin, ol'e·fin) *n.* [*olef*iant + *-in*]. Any member of the ethylene series of hydrocarbons; unsaturated compounds of the general formula C_nH_{2n}.

ole·fine (o'le·feen, ·fin) *n.* OLEFIN.

ole·ic acid (o·lee'ick, o'lee·ick) [*ole-* + *-ic*]. An unsaturated acid, $CH_3(CH_2)_7CH{=}CH(CH_2)_7COOH$, present as a glyceride in most fats and fixed oils.

oleic acid series. Unsaturated fatty acids having one double bond and corresponding to the general formula C_nH_{2n-1}-COOH.

ole·in (o'lee·in) *n.* [F. *oléine*]. Glyceryl oleate, $(C_{17}H_{33}COO)_3C_3H_5$, the chief constituent of olive oil and occurring in varying amounts in most other fixed oils. Syn. *triolein.*

oleo-. See *ole-.*

oleo·gran·u·lo·ma (o"lee·o·gran"yoo·lo'muh) *n.* A granuloma resulting from deposits, usually injected, of lipid material.

oleo·mar·ga·rine (o"lee·o·mahr'juh·rin) *n.* [F.]. A butter substitute made by hydrogenation of a mixture of vegetable oils.

ole·om·e·ter (o"lee·om'e·tur) *n.* [*oleo-* + *-meter*]. 1. A hydrometer used to determine the specific gravity of oils, or calibrated in the range of specific gravity of oils. 2. An apparatus for determining the content of oil in a material.

ole·op·tene (o"lee·op'teen) *n.* ELEOPTENE.

oleo·res·in (o"lee·o·rez'in) *n.* A substance consisting chiefly of a mixture of an oil, either fixed or volatile, and a resin, sometimes with other active constituents, extracted from plants by means of a volatile solvent.

oleo·ther·a·py (o"lee·o·therr'uh·pee) *n.* [*oleo-* + *therapy*]. The treatment of disease by the administration of oils. Syn. *eleotherapy.*

oleo·tho·rax (o"lee·o·tho'racks) *n.* [*oleo-* + *thorax*]. A condition in which a lung is compressed in the treatment of tuberculosis by injections of sterile oil.

oleo·vi·ta·min (o"lee·o·vye'tuh·min) *n.* [*oleo-* + *vitamin*]. A solution of a vitamin in oil.

ole·um (o'lee·um) *n.*, pl. **olea** (o'lee·uh) [L.]. 1. OIL. 2. Fuming sulfuric acid; a solution of sulfur trioxide in concentrated sulfuric acid.

oleum suc·ci·ni (suck'si·nigh) [L. *succinum*, amber]. AMBER OIL.

ol·fac·tion (ol·fack'shun, ohl·) *n.* [L. *olfacere*, to smell out, trace by smell, from *olere*, to smell, emit an odor]. 1. The function of smelling. 2. The sense of smell.

ol·fac·to·ha·ben·u·lar tract (ol·fack"to·ha·ben'yoo·lur). Nerve fibers that arise in the basal olfactory nuclei, curve dorsally, and, entering the stria medullaris thalami, project to the habenular nucleus of the same and opposite side.

ol·fac·tom·e·ter (ol"fack·tom'e·tur, ohl") *n.* [*olfac*tion + *-meter*]. An instrument for determining the power of smell.

ol·fac·to·ry (ol·fack'tur·ee, ohl·) *adj.* Of or pertaining to olfaction or the sense of smell.

olfactory anesthesia. ANOSMIA.

olfactory area. ANTERIOR PERFORATED SUBSTANCE.

olfactory aura. A sudden disagreeable sensation of smell preceding or characterizing an epileptic attack. See also *uncinate epilepsy.*

olfactory brain. RHINENCEPHALON.

olfactory bulb. The enlarged distal end of either olfactory tract situated on each side of the longitudinal fissure upon the undersurface of each anterior lobe of the cerebrum. NA *bulbus olfactorius.* See also Plate 17.

olfactory canals. In the embryo, the nasal cavities at an early period of development.

olfactory capsule. NASAL CAPSULE.

olfactory cell. One of the sensory nerve cells in the olfactory epithelium.

olfactory epithelium. The sensory epithelium lining the olfactory region of the nasal cavity.

olfactory esthesioneuroepithelioma. A rare neuroepithelioma occurring in the nasal cavity of adults, which may infiltrate the paranasal sinuses.

olfactory esthesioneuroma. ESTHESIONEUROMA.

olfactory field. The nasal half of the field of vision of the retina.

olfactory foramen. One of numerous foramens in the cribriform plate of the ethmoid, giving passage to the fila olfactoria of the olfactory nerves.

olfactory glands. Serous glands found in the olfactory mucous membrane.

olfactory glomerulus. A structure in the olfactory bulb, formed by the synapse between the primary olfactory fibers and the brushlike terminals of vertically descending dendrites of the mitral cells.

olfactory groove. The groove formed by the cribriform plate of the ethmoid, lodging the olfactory bulb.

olfactory gyrus. GYRUS OLFACTORIUS.

olfactory lobe. An area on the inferior surface of the frontal lobe of the brain and demarcated from the lateral surface of the pallium by the rhinal sulcus. The anterior portion includes the olfactory tract and bulb and the posterior portion includes the anterior perforated substance and other olfactory structures of the anteromedial portion of the temporal lobe, collectively known as the piriform lobe. See also *rhinencephalon.*

olfactory nerve or **nerves.** The first cranial nerve; a plexiform group of sensory nerve fibers, consisting of axons that originate in the olfactory cells of the nasal mucosa, traverse the cribriform plate of the ethmoid bone and end in the glomeruli of the olfactory bulb. NA *nervi olfactorii.*

olfactory neuroepithelioma. OLFACTORY ESTHESIONEUROEPITHELIOMA.

olfactory pit. A pit formed about the olfactory placode in the embryo by the growth of the median and lateral nasal processes; the anlage of part of the nasal cavity. Syn. *nasal pit.*

olfactory placode. The ectodermal anlage of the olfactory region of the nasal cavity.

olfactory pyramid. OLFACTORY TRIGONE.

olfactory region. The area on and above the superior conchae and on the adjoining nasal septum where the mucous membrane has olfactory epithelium and olfactory (Bowman's) glands. NA *regio olfactoria.*

olfactory sac. One of the deepened olfactory pits extending from the embryonic nares to the bucconasal membranes.

olfactory sulcus. A well-defined anteroposterior groove on the medial orbital gyrus for the passage of the olfactory tract. NA *sulcus olfactorius lobi frontalis.*

olfactory tract. A narrow band of white substance originating in the olfactory bulb and extending posteriorly in the olfactory sulcus toward the anterior perforated substance where it divides into lateral and medial olfactory striae. NA *tractus olfactorius.* See also Plates 17, 18.

olfactory trigone. The flattened and splayed caudal end of the olfactory tract. NA *trigonum olfactorium.*

olfactory tubercle. An elevation in the rostral portion of the anterior perforated substance, which is well developed in macrosmatic animals but only rudimentary in the human brain.

olig-, oligo- [Gk. *oligos*, few, little]. A combining form meaning (a) *few, scant;* (b) *deficiency.*

ol·ig·emia, ol·i·gae·mia (ol"ig·ee'mee·uh) *n.* [Gk. *oligaimia*]. A state in which the total quantity of the blood is diminished. See also *hydremia.*

ol·ig·er·ga·sia (ol"i·gur·gay'zhuh, ·zee·uh) *n.* [*olig-* + *ergasia*]. MENTAL DEFICIENCY.

ol·ig·hid·ria (ol"ig·hid'ree·uh, ·high'dree·uh, ol"ig·id'ree·uh) *n.* [*olig-* + *hidr-*, perspiration, + *-ia*]. OLIGOHIDRIA.

ol·ig·hy·dria (ol"ig·high'dree·uh, ·hid'ree·uh, ·id'ree·uh) *n.* [*olig-* + *hydr-* + *-ia*]. OLIGOHYDRIA.

ol·i·gid·ria (ol"i·jid'ree·uh, ol"ig·id'ree·uh) *n.* OLIGOHIDRIA.

oligo-. See *olig-.*

ol·i·go·am·ni·os (ol"i·go·am'nee·os) *n.* [*oligo-* + *amnion*]. OLIGOHYDRAMNIOS.

ol·i·go·blast (ol'i·go·blast) *n.* The precursor cell of the oligodendrocyte.

ol·i·go·blen·nia (ol"i·go·blen'ee·uh) *n.* [*oligo-* + *blenn-* + *-ia*]. A deficient secretion of mucus.

ol·i·go·cho·lia (ol"i·go·ko'lee·uh) *n.* [*oligo-* + *chol-* + *-ia*]. A deficiency of bile.

ol·i·go·chro·ma·sia (ol"i·go·kro·may'zhuh, ·zee·uh) *n.* [*oligo-* + *-chromasia*]. A decreased amount of hemoglobin in the erythrocytes, which present a pale appearance.

ol·i·go·chro·me·mia (ol"i·go·kro·mee'mee·uh) *n.* [*oligo-* + *chrom-* + *-emia*]. Deficiency of hemoglobin in the blood.

ol·i·go·chy·lia (ol"i·go·kigh'lee·uh) *n.* [*oligo-* + *chyl-* + *-ia*]. Deficiency of chyle.

ol·i·go·cy·the·mia (ol"i·go·sigh·theem'ee·uh) *n.* [*oligo-* + *cyt-* + *-hemia*]. A reduction in the total quantity of erythrocytes in the body. —**oligocy·the·mic** (·theem'ick, ·themm'ick) *adj.*

oligocythemic normovolemia. A normal blood volume with a decrease in erythrocytes.

ol·i·go·dac·rya (ol"i·go·dack'ree·uh) *n.* [*oligo-* + *dacry-* + *-ia*]. Deficiency of the tears.

ol·i·go·dac·tyl·ia (ol"i·go·dack·til'ee·uh) *n.* [*oligo-* + *dactyl-* + *-ia*]. Congenital deficiency of fingers or toes.

ol·i·go·den·dro·blas·to·ma (ol"i·go·den"dro·blas·to'muh) *n.* [*oligodendro*glia + *blastoma*]. A glial tumor similar to the oligodendroglioma, but composed of somewhat larger cells showing more cytoplasm, larger nuclei with less dense chromatin, and mitotic figures.

ol·i·go·den·dro·cyte (ol"i·go·den'dro·site) *n.* A cell of the oligodendroglia.

ol·i·go·den·dro·cy·to·ma (ol"i·go·den"dro·sigh·to'muh) *n.* [*oligodendrocyte* + *-oma*]. OLIGODENDROGLIOMA.

ol·i·go·den·drog·lia (ol"i·go·den·drog'lee·uh) *n.* [*oligo-* + *dendro-* + *glia*]. Small supporting cells of the nervous system, located about the nerve cells and between nerve fibers (interfascicular oligodendrocytes) and characterized by spheroidal or polygonal cell bodies and fine cytoplasmic processes with secondary divisions. —**oligodendrog·li·al** (·lee·ul) *adj.*

ol·i·go·den·dro·gli·o·ma (ol″i·go·den″dro·glye·o′muh, ·den·drog″lee·o′muh) *n.* [*oligo-* + *dendro-* + *glioma*]. A slowly growing glioma mainly of the cerebrum, rarely of septum pellucidum, fairly large and well defined, with a tendency to focal calcification. Microscopically, most of the cells are small, with richly chromatic nuclei and scanty, poorly staining cytoplasm without processes. Syn. *oligodendrocytoma, oligodendroma.*

ol·i·go·den·dro·gli·o·ma·to·sis (ol″i·go·den·drog″lee·o″muh·to′sis) *n.* [*oligodendroglioma* + *-osis*]. Diffuse dissemination of oligodendroglioma tumor tissue through the leptomeninges and, sometimes, also into the ependymal lining of the cerebral ventricles.

ol·i·go·den·dro·ma (ol″i·go·den·dro′muh) *n.* OLIGODENDROGLIOMA.

ol·i·go·don·tia (ol″i·go·don′chee·uh) *n.* [*olig-* + *-odontia*]. Congenital deficiency of teeth.

ol·i·go·dy·nam·ic (ol″i·go·dye·nam′ick, ·di·nam′ick) *adj.* [*oligo-* + *dynamic*]. 1. Active in very small quantities. 2. Pertaining to the toxic or other effect of very small quantities of a substance, as a metal, on cells or organisms.

oligodynamic action. Toxicity of heavy metals in very dilute solution for algae and other microorganisms.

ol·i·go·el·e·ment (ol′i·go·el″e·munt) *n.* [*oligo-* + *element*]. An element which, though present in low concentration, possesses a relatively high degree of activity.

ol·i·go·en·ceph·a·ly (ol″i·go·en·sef′ul·ee) *n.* [*oligo-* + *encephal-* + *-y*]. MICROCEPHALY.

ol·i·go·ga·lac·tia (ol″i·go·ga·lack′tee·uh, ·shee·uh) *n.* [*oligo-* + *galact-* + *-ia*]. Deficiency in the secretion of milk.

ol·i·go·gen·ic (ol″i·go·jen′ick) *adj.* [*oligo-* + *-genic*]. Pertaining to hereditary characters determined by one or few genes. —**ol·i·go·gene** (ol′i·go·jeen) *n.*

ol·i·go·gen·ics (ol″i·go·jen′icks) *n.* [*oligo-* + *-genics* as in eugenics]. BIRTH CONTROL.

ol·i·gog·lia (ol″i·gog′lee·uh) *n.* OLIGODENDROGLIA.

ol·i·go·graph·ia (ol″i·go·graf′ee·uh) *n.* [*oligo-* + *-graphia*]. Oligologia as manifested in writing.

ol·i·go·hid·ria (ol″i·go·hid′ree·uh) *n.* [*oligo-* + *hidr-*, perspiration, + *-ia*]. Deficiency of perspiration.

ol·i·go·hy·dram·ni·os (ol″i·go·high·dram′nee·os) *n.* [*oligo-* + *hydr-* + *amnion*]. Deficiency of the amniotic fluid.

ol·i·go·hy·dria (ol″i·go·high′dree·uh, ·hid′ree·uh) *n.* Deficiency of the fluids of the body. Compare *oligohidria.*

ol·i·go·hy·dru·ria (ol″i·go·high·droor′ee·uh) *n.* [*oligo-* + *hydr-* + *-uria*]. Urine with a relative diminution of water; highly concentrated urine.

ol·i·go·la·lia (ol″i·go·lay′lee·uh) *n.* [*oligo-* + *-lalia*]. Oligologia in speech.

ol·i·go·lec·i·thal (ol″i·go·les′i·thul) *adj.* [*oligo-* + *lecithal*]. Having little yolk.

ol·i·go·lo·gia (ol″i·go·lo′jee·uh, ·lo′juh) *n.* [*oligo-* + *log-*, word, + *-ia*]. Fewness of words; a condition in which a person says or writes less than might normally be expected, given his personality, education, and the specific circumstances. Syn. *oligophasia.*

ol·i·go·ma·nia (ol″i·go·may′nee·uh) *n.* [*oligo-* + *-mania*]. Mental disorder on only a few subjects; MONOMANIA.

ol·i·go·mega·ne·phro·nia (ol″i·go·meg″uh·ne·fro′nee·uh) *n.* [*oligo-* + *mega-* + *nephron* + *-ia*]. A rare form of renal hypoplasia associated with chronic renal failure in childhood and characterized by decreased numbers of nephrons with hypertrophy of all nephric elements.

oli·go·méga·né·phro·nie (oʰ·lee·goʰ·meʸ·ga·neʸ·froʰ·nee′) *n.* [F.]. OLIGOMEGANEPHRONIA.

ol·i·go·me·lus (ol″i·go·mee′lus) *n.* [*oligo-* + Gk. *melos*, limb]. Excessive congenital thinness of the limbs, or a deficiency in their number.

ol·i·go·men·or·rhea (ol″i·go·men″o·ree′uh) *n.* [*oligo-* + *menorrhea*]. Abnormally infrequent menstruation. Compare *hypomenorrhea.*

olig·o·mer (o·lig′o·mur) *n.* [*oligo-* + *-mer*]. A short-chain polymer. —**ol·i·go·mer·ic** (ol″i·go·merr′ick, o″li·go·, o·lig″o·) *adj.*

oligomeric protein. A protein composed of two or more polypeptide chains; for example, hemoglobin.

ol·i·go·my·cin (ol″i·go·migh′sin) *n.* Any one of a complex of closely related antibiotics, active against fungi, produced by an actinomycete.

ol·i·go·nu·cleo·tide (ol″i·go·new′klee·o·tide) *n.* [*oligo-* + *nucleotide*]. A depolymerization product of a nucleic acid, characterized by a lower degree of aggregation of nucleotide units.

ol·i·go·pha·sia (ol″i·go·fay′zhuh, ·fay′zee·uh) *n.* [*oligo-* + *-phasia*]. OLIGOLOGIA.

ol·i·go·phos·pha·tu·ria (ol″i·go·fos″fuh·tew′ree·uh) *n.* [*oligo-* + *phosphate* + *-uria*]. A decrease in the amount of phosphates in the urine.

ol·i·go·phre·nia (ol″i·go·free′nee·uh) *n.* [*oligo-* + *-phrenia*]. Mental deficiency. —**oligo·phren·ic** (·fren′ick) *adj.*

ol·i·gop·nea, ol·i·gop·noea (ol″i·gop·nee′uh, ol″i·gop′nee·uh) *n.* [*oligo-* + *-pnea*]. Respiration diminished in depth or frequency.

ol·i·go·psy·chia (ol″i·go·sigh′kee·uh, ol″i·gop·) *n.* [Gk. *oligopsychia*, faint-heartedness]. MENTAL DEFICIENCY.

ol·i·go·pty·a·lism (ol″i·go·tye′uh·liz·um, ol″i·gop·) *n.* [*oligo-* + *ptyal-* + *-ism*]. Deficient secretion of saliva.

ol·i·go·py·rene (ol″i·go·pye′reen) *adj.* [*oligo-* + Gk. *pyrēn*, stone of a fruit]. Of sperm cells, having only a part of the full complement of chromosomes. Contr. *apyrene, eupyrene.*

ol·i·go·ria (ol″i·gor′ee·uh) *n.* [Gk. *oligōria*, contempt, slighting]. An abnormal apathy or indifference to persons or to environment, as in a depressed state.

ol·i·go·sac·cha·ride (ol″i·go·sack′ur·ide) *n.* [*oligo-* + *saccharide*]. Any carbohydrate of a class comprising disaccharides, trisaccharides, tetrasaccharides, and, according to some authorities, pentasaccharides; so named because they yield on hydrolysis a small number of monosaccharides.

ol·i·go·si·al·ia (ol″i·go·sigh·al′ee·uh, ·ay′lee·uh) *n.* [*oligo-* + *sial-* + *-ia*]. Deficiency of saliva.

ol·i·go·sper·mia (ol″i·go·spur′mee·uh) *n.* [*oligo-* + *sperm* + *-ia*]. Scarcity of spermatozoa in the semen; specifically, less then 20 million per ml.

ol·i·go·trich·ia (ol″i·go·trick′ee·uh) *n.* [*oligo-* + *-trichia*]. Scantiness or thinness of hair.

oligotrichia con·gen·i·ta (kon·jen′i·tuh). ALOPECIA CONGENITALIS.

ol·i·go·zoo·sper·mia (ol″i·go·zo″o·spur′mee·uh) *n.* [*oligo-* + *zoo-* + *sperm* + *-ia*]. OLIGOSPERMIA.

ol·i·gu·re·sis (ol″ig·yoo·ree′sis) *n.* [*olig-* + *uresis*]. OLIGURIA.

ol·i·gu·ria (ol″ig·yoo′ree·uh) *n.* [*olig-* + *-uria*]. A diminution in the quantity of urine excreted; specifically, less then 400 ml in a 24-hour period.

ol·i·gyd·ria (ol″ig·id′ree·uh) *n.* [*olig-* + *hydr-* + *-ia*]. OLIGOHYDRIA.

olis·the·ro·chro·ma·tin (o·lis″thur·o·kro′muh·tin) *n.* [Gk. *olisthēros*, slippery, sliding, + *chromatin*]. The material found in the constricted portion of a chromosome.

o·lis·the·ro·zone (o·lis′thur·o·zone) *n.* [Gk. *olisthēros*, slippery, sliding, + *zone*]. An area of constriction of a chromosome, important in identification of chromosomes.

oli·va (o·lye′vuh) *n.* [L.] [NA]. OLIVE (3).

ol·i·vary (ol′i·verr·ee) *adj.* [L. *olivarius*, pertaining to olives]. 1. Olive-shaped. 2. Pertaining to the olivary nucleus.

olivary body. OLIVARY NUCLEUS.

olivary nucleus. A conspicuous convoluted gray band opening medially, dorsal to the pyramids, occupying the entire upper two-thirds of the medulla oblongata, the cells of which give rise to most of the fibers of the olivocerebellar tract. NA *nucleus olivaris.*

ol·ive, *n.* [L. *oliva*, from Gk. *elaia*]. 1. The oil tree, *Olea europaea*, of the Oleaceae. Its fruit yields olive oil, a fixed oil which consists chiefly of olein and palmitin, and is used as a nutritive food; in medicine as a laxative; as an emollient external application to wounds or burns, and as an ingredient of liniments and ointments. 2. OLIVARY NUCLEUS. 3. An oval eminence on the anterior, ventrolateral surface of the medulla oblongata; it marks the location of the olivary nucleus, which lies just beneath the surface. NA *oliva.*

olive baboon. *Chaeropithecus* (or *Papio*) *anubis*, the common baboon of the savannah belt south of the Sahara.

Ol·i·ver-Car·da·rel·li sign or **symptom** (kahr·da·rel′lee) [W. S. *Oliver*, English physician, 1836–1908; and A. *Cardarelli*, Italian physician, 1831–1926]. OLIVER'S SIGN.

Oliver's sign [W. S. *Oliver*]. Laryngeal and tracheal pulsation, synchronous with ventricular systole, elicited by grasping the larynx between thumb and forefinger with the patient erect; a sign of aortic arch aneurysm and certain mediastinal tumors. See also *tracheal tug.*

olive-tipped bougie. A bulbous bougie with an olive- or acorn-shaped tip.

ol·i·vif·u·gal (ol″i·vif′yoo·gul) *adj.* [*oli*vary + *-fugal*]. In a direction away from the olivary nucleus.

ol·i·vip·e·tal (ol″i·vip′e·tul) *adj.* [*oli*vary + *-petal*]. In a direction toward the olivary nucleus.

ol·i·vo·cer·e·bel·lar (ol″i·vo·serr·e·bel′ur) *adj.* Pertaining to the olivary nucleus and the cerebellum.

olivocerebellar tract. A tract of nerve fibers from the olivary nuclei of the same and opposite sides, which reaches the cerebellum by way of the inferior cerebellar peduncle. NA *tractus olivocerebellaris.*

ol·i·vo·pon·to·cer·e·bel·lar (ol″i·vo·pon″to·serr·e·bel′ur) *adj.* Pertaining to the olivary nucleus, pons, and cerebellum.

olivopontocerebellar atrophy, ataxia, or **degeneration**. A heredodegenerative disease occurring in the middle and later decades of life; causes ataxia, hypotonia, and dysarthria. It is characterized pathologically by degeneration of the middle cerebellar white matter, and the pontine, arcuate, and olivary nuclei.

ol·i·vo·spi·nal (ol″i·vo·spye′nul) *adj.* Pertaining to the olivary nucleus and the spinal cord.

olivospinal tract. A bundle of nerve fibers located on the anterior surface of the spinal cord. The evidence is not conclusive that it contains descending fibers from the inferior olivary nucleus, but it may contain ascending spinoolivary fibers. Syn. *Helweg's bundle.*

Ol·lier's disease (oʰl·yeʸ′) [L. *Ollier*, French surgeon, 1830–1900]. ENCHONDROMATOSIS.

-ology. See *-logy.*

olo·pho·nia (ol″o·fo′nee·uh) *n.* [Gk. *oloos*, lost, destroyed, + *phon-* + *-ia*]. Abnormal speech due to a structural defect of the vocal organs.

O.L.P. Abbreviation for *occipitolaevoposterior.*

o·lym·pi·an forehead (o·limp′ee·un). The abnormally high and vaulted forehead seen in children with congenital syphilis and certain types of hydrocephalus.

om-, omo- [Gk. *ōmos*]. A combining form meaning *shoulder.*

-oma [*-o-*, stem vowel, + Gk. *-ma*, resultative nominalizing suffix]. A suffix designating a *tumor* or *neoplasm.*

oma·ceph·a·lus (o″muh·sef′ul·us) *n.* [*om-* + *a-* + *-cephalus*]. A placental parasitic twin in which there is imperfect development of the head and absence of upper extremities.

oma·gra (o·may′gruh, o·mag′ruh) *n.* [*om-* + *-agra*]. Gout in the shoulder.

omar·thral·gia (o″mahr·thral′juh) *n.* [*om-* + *arthralgia*]. Pain in the shoulder joint.

omar·thri·tis (o″mahr·thrigh′tis) *n.* [*om-* + *arthr-* + *-itis*]. Inflammation of the shoulder joint.

oma·sum (o·may′sum) *n.* [L., bullock's tripe]. The third compartment of the stomach of a ruminant. Syn. *manyplies, psalterium.*

om·bro·pho·bia (om″bro·fo′bee·uh) *n.* [Gk. *ombros*, rain, + *-phobia*]. A morbid fear of rain.

-ome [L. *-oma*, from Gk., nominalizing suffix]. A suffix designating a *group* or *mass.*

ome·ga (o·may′guh, o·mee′guh) *n.* [name of the letter Ω, ω, last letter of the Greek alphabet]. The last of a series; as in organic chemistry, an end group of a chain. Symbol, Ω, ω.

omega oxidation. The oxidation of a fatty acid at the end of the chain opposite to that where the carboxyl group occurs, thereby forming a dicarboxylic acid, which may then undergo beta oxidation from both ends of the chain.

oment-, omento-. A combining form meaning *omentum.*

omenta. Plural of *omentum.*

omen·tal (o·men′tul) *adj.* Of or pertaining to an omentum.

omental bursa. The large irregular space lined with peritoneum, lying dorsal to the stomach and lesser omentum, and communicating with the general peritoneal cavity through the epiploic foramen. Syn. *lesser peritoneal cavity, lesser sac.* NA *bursa omentalis.*

omental graft. A portion of greater omentum transplanted to fill a defect, afford blood supply, or check hemorrhage; or placed over a suture line to minimize adhesions and prevent leakage of contents.

omental hernia. A hernia which contains only omentum.

omental recesses. The portions of the omental bursa called, respectively, superior recess, inferior recess, and lienal recess.

omental sac. The sac formed between the ascending and descending portions of the greater omentum.

omen·tec·to·my (o″men·teck′tum·ee) *n.* [*oment-* + *-ectomy*]. Excision of an omentum or any part of it.

omen·ti·tis (o″men·tye′tis) *n.* [*oment-* + *-itis*]. Inflammation of an omentum.

omento-. See *oment-.*

omen·to·cele (o·men′to·seel) *n.* [*omento-* + *-cele*]. A hernia containing omentum only.

omen·to·fix·a·tion (o·men″to·fick·say′shun) *n.* [*omento-* + *fixation*]. OMENTOPEXY.

omen·to·pexy (o·men′to·peck″see) *n.* [*omento-* + *-pexy*]. The surgical operation of suspending the greater omentum, by suturing it to the abdominal wall.

omen·tor·rha·phy (o″men·tor′uh·fee) *n.* [*omento-* + *-rrhaphy*]. Suture of an omentum.

omen·tot·o·my (o″men·tot′um·ee) *n.* [*omento-* + *-tomy*]. Surgical incision of an omentum.

omen·tum (o·men′tum) *n.*, pl. **omen·ta** (·tuh), [L.]. Apron; a fold of the peritoneum connecting abdominal viscera with the stomach. See also *greater omentum, lesser omentum.*

omen·tum·ec·to·my (o·men″tum·eck′tuh·mee) *n.* OMENTECTOMY.

omentum ma·jus (may′jus) [NA]. GREATER OMENTUM.

omentum mi·nus (migh′nus) [NA]. LESSER OMENTUM.

omi·tis (o·migh′tis) *n.* [*om-* + *-itis*]. Inflammation of the shoulder.

om·ma·tid·i·um (om″uh·tid′ee·um) *n.*, pl. **ommatid·ia** (·ee·uh) [L., from Gk. *ommatidion*, dim. of *omma*, eye]. One of the functional prismatic units of a compound eye, as in most arthropods.

om·niv·o·rous (om·niv′ur·us) *adj.* [L. *omnivorus*, from *omnis*, all, + *vorare*, to devour]. Subsisting on a wide variety of food; applied mainly to animals that feed on both animal and vegetable matter.

omo-. See *om-.*

omo·cer·vi·ca·lis (o″mo·sur·vi·kay′lis) *n.* [*omo-* + L. *cervicalis*, of the neck]. LEVATOR CLAVICULAE.

omo·hy·oid (o″mo·high′oid) *adj.* [*omo-* + *hyoid*]. Pertaining conjointly to the scapula and the hyoid bone.

omohyoid muscle. A muscle attached to the scapula and the hyoid bone. NA *musculus omohyoideus.* See also Table of Muscles in the Appendix.

omo·pha·gia (o″mo·fay′jee·uh) *n.* [Gk. *ōmos*, raw, + *-phagia*, eating]. The practice of eating raw foods.

omo·ver·te·bral (o″mo·vur′ti·brul) *adj.* [*omo-* + *vertebral*]. Pertaining to the scapula and vertebrae.

omovertebral bone. SUPRASCAPULA.

OMPA Abbreviation for *octamethyl pyrophosphoramide.*

omphal-, omphalo- [Gk. *omphalos*]. A combining form meaning *navel, umbilicus.*

om·pha·lec·to·my (om″fuh·leck′tum·ee) *n.* [*omphal-* + *-ectomy*]. Excision of the navel.

om·phal·ic (om·fal′ick) *adj.* [*omphal-* + *-ic*]. Pertaining to the umbilicus.

om·pha·li·tis (om″fuh·lye′tis) *n.* [*omphal-* + *-itis*]. Inflammation of the umbilicus.

omphalo-. See *omphal-.*

om·pha·lo·an·gi·op·a·gus (om″fuh·lo·an·jee·op′uh·gus) *n.* [*omphalo-* + *angio-* + *-pagus*]. OMPHALOSITE. —**omphaloangiopagous,** *adj.*

omphaloangiopagous twins. Asymmetric uniovular twins one of which is an omphalosite.

om·pha·lo·cele (om·fal′o·seel, om′fuh·lo·) *n.* [*omphalo-* + *-cele*]. A hernia into the umbilical cord, caused by a congenital midline defect.

om·pha·lo·cho·ri·on (om″fuh·lo·ko′ree·on) *n.* A chorion, or that part of one supplied by the omphalomesenteric blood vessels of the yolk sac. Syn. *chorion omphaloideum, yolk sac placenta.*

om·pha·lo·cra·nio·did·y·mus (om″fuh·lo·kray″nee·o·did′i·mus) *n.* [*omphalo-* + *cranio-* + *-didymus*]. Unequal monochorionic twins in which the parasite is attached to the cranium of the autosite by an umbilical cord.

om·pha·lo·did·y·mus (om″fuh·lo·did′i·mus) *n.* [*omphalo-* + *-didymus*]. OMPHALOPAGUS.

om·pha·lo·gen·e·sis (om″fuh·lo·jen′e·sis) *n.* [*omphalo-* + *-genesis*]. The development of the yolk sac.

om·pha·lo·mes·en·ter·ic (om″fuh·lo·mes″un·terr′ick, ·mez″un·) *adj.* [*omphalo-* + *mesenteric*]. Pertaining conjointly to the umbilicus and mesentery.

omphalomesenteric artery. VITELLINE ARTERY.

omphalomesenteric canal. In the embryo, a canal that connects the cavity of the intestine with the yolk sac.

omphalomesenteric circulation. VITELLINE CIRCULATION.

omphalomesenteric duct. VITELLINE DUCT.

omphalomesenteric veins. Embryonic veins uniting yolk sac and sinus venosus; their proximal fused ends form the portal vein. Syn. *vitelline veins.*

om·pha·lo·mono·did·y·mus (om″fuh·lo·mon″o·did′i·mus) *n.* [*omphalo-* + *mono-* + *-didymus*]. Conjoined twins united at the umbilicus.

om·pha·lop·a·gus (om″fuh·lop′uh·gus) *n.* [*omphalo-* + *-pagus*]. Conjoined twins united at the abdomen.

om·pha·lo·prop·to·sis (om″fuh·lo·prop·to′sis) *n.* [*omphalo-* + *proptosis*]. Abnormal protrusion of the navel.

om·pha·los (om′fuh·los) *n.*, pl. **om·pha·li** (·lye) [Gk.]. UMBILICUS.

om·pha·lo·site (om·fal′o·site, om′fuh·lo·site) *n.* [*omphalo-* + para*site*]. The parasitic member of asymmetric uniovular twins. The parasite has no heart, or only a vestigial one, deriving its blood supply from the placenta of the more or less normal twin (autosite).

om·pha·lo·so·tor (om″fuh·lo·so′tor, ·tur) *n.* [*omphalo-* + Gk. *sōtēr,* preserver]. An instrument for replacing a prolapsed umbilical cord in the uterus.

om·pha·lo·tax·is (om″fuh·lo·tack′sis) *n.* [*omphalo-* + Gk. *taxis,* arrangement]. Reposition of the prolapsed umbilical cord.

om·phalo·tome (om·fal′o·tome) *n.* [*omphalo-* + *-tome*]. An instrument for dividing the umbilical cord.

om·pha·lot·o·my (om·fuh·lot′um·ee) *n.* [*omphalo-* + *-tomy*]. The cutting of the umbilical cord.

om·pha·lo·trip·sy (om′fuh·lo·trip″see) *n.* [*omphalo-* + Gk. *tripsis,* a rubbing]. Separation of the umbilical cord by a crushing instrument.

Omsk hemorrhagic fever. [after *Omsk,* western Siberia, U.S.S.R.]. One of the Russian tick-borne complex of diseases.

-on [Gk. neuter singular suffix]. A suffix designating (a) *an elementary particle or quantum,* as in electron, photon; (b) *a functional unit,* as in nephron; (c) *an inert gas,* as in neon.

onan·ism (o′nuh·niz·um) *n.* [*Onan,* son of Judah]. 1. Incomplete coitus; COITUS INTERRUPTUS. 2. MASTURBATION. —**onan·ist** (·ist) *n.*

oncho-. See *onco-.*

On·cho·cer·ca (onk″o·sur′kuh) *n.* [NL., from *onco-,* hooked, + Gk. *kerkos,* tail]. A genus of filarial worms.

Onchocerca cae·cu·ti·ens (see·kew′shee·enz) [NL., blinding, from *caecus,* blind]. *ONCHOCERCA VOLVULUS.*

Onchocerca vol·vu·lus (vol′vew·lus) [L. *volvulus,* turned, twisted]. A species of filarial worm which infects man, forming fibrous nodular tumors with encapsulation of the adult worms in the subcutaneous connective tissue, and often causing severe ocular disease when microfilariae invade the tissues of the eye.

on·cho·cer·ci·a·sis (onk″o·sur·sigh′uh·sis, ·kigh′uh·sis) *n.* [*Onchocerca* + *-iasis*]. Infection with the filarial worm *Onchocerca volvulus;* produces tumors of the skin, papular dermatitis, and ocular complications in humans. Syn. *river blindness* (in western equatorial Africa).

on·cho·cer·co·ma (onk″o·sur·ko′muh) *n.* [*Onchocerca* + *-oma*]. The fibrous nodular lesion of onchocerciasis which contains the adult worms (*Onchocerca*), usually located at a site at which a bone is close to the surface.

on·cho·cer·co·sis (onk″o·sur·ko′sis) *n.* ONCHOCERCIASIS.

on·cho·der·ma·ti·tis (onk″o·dur″muh·tigh′tis) *n.* [*oncho-* + *dermatitis*]. The cutaneous manifestations of onchocerciasis.

onco-, oncho- [Gk. *onkos,* bulk, heap; curve, hook]. A combining form meaning (a) *tumor;* (b) *bulk, volume;* (c) *hooked, curved.*

on·co·ci·dal (onk″o·sigh′dul) *adj.* [*onco-* + *cide* + *-al*]. Destructive to tumors.

on·co·cyte (onk′o·site) *n.* [*onco-* + *-cyte*]. One of the columnar cells with granular eosinophilic cytoplasm found in salivary and certain endocrine glands, nasal mucosa, and other locations. They represent dedifferentiation of parenchymal cells and may occur singly or in aggregates (oncocytomas).

on·co·cy·to·ma, on·ko·cy·to·ma (onk″o·sigh·to′muh) *n.* [*oncocyte* + *-oma*]. A benign tumor whose parenchyma is composed of large, finely granular eosinophilic cells (oncocytes); it occurs almost exclusively in the salivary glands.

on·co·fe·tal (onk″o·fee′tul) *adj.* [*onco-* + *fetal*]. Pertaining to fetuses and tumors.

oncofetal protein. A protein found in both a tumor and a normal fetus; alpha-fetoprotein is an example.

on·co·gene (onk″o·jeen) *n.* [*once-* + *gene*]. A gene capable of producing a tumor when activated.

on·co·gen·e·sis (onk″o·jen′e·sis) *n.* [*onco-* + *-genesis*]. The process of tumor formation. —**oncogen·ic** (·ick) *adj.*

on·co·graph (onk′o·graf) *n.* An instrument that records the changes of volume of an organ in an oncometer. —**on·cog·ra·phy** (ong·kog′ruh·fee) *n.*

on·col·o·gist (ong·kol′uh·jist) *n.* A specialist in oncology.

on·col·o·gy (ong·kol′uh·jee) *n.* [*onco-* + *-logy*]. The study or science of neoplastic growth.

on·col·y·sis (ong·kol′i·sis) *n.* [*onco-* + *-lysis*]. The destruction or lysis of neoplastic cells, particularly those of carcinoma.

on·co·lyt·ic (ong″ko·lit′ick) *adj.* & *n.* 1. Pertaining to or causing oncolysis. 2. An agent that effects oncolysis.

On·co·me·la·nia (onk″o·me·lay′nee·uh) *n.* A genus of amphibious snails.

Oncomelania for·mo·sa·na (for″mo·sah′nuh, ·say′nuh). A species of amphibious snail; an important intermediate host for *Schistosoma japonicum* in Taiwan. Syn. *Katayama formosana.*

Oncomelania hu·pen·sis (hew·pen′sis). A species of snail found in the Yangtze basin; one of the intermediate hosts of *Schistosoma japonicum.*

Oncomelania hy·dro·bi·op·sis (high″dro·bye·op′sis). A species of snail found in Leyte and other Philippine Islands; an intermediate host of *Schistosoma japonicum.*

Oncomelania no·soph·o·ra (no·sof′uh·ruh). A species of amphibious snail; an intermediate host of *Schistosoma japonicum.* Syn. *Katayama nosophora.*

on·com·e·ter (ong·kom′e·tur) *n.* [*onco-* + *-meter*]. An instrument for measuring variations in the volume of an organ, as of the kidney or spleen, or of an extremity. **—oncome·try** (·tree) *n.;* **on·co·met·ric** (onk″o·met′rick) *adj.*

on·cor·na·vi·rus (ong·kor″nuh·vye′rus) *n.* [*onco-* + *RNA* + *virus*]. An oncogenic RNA virus.

on·co·sis (ong·ko′sis) *n.* [*onco-* + *-osis*]. Any condition marked by the development of tumors.

on·co·sphere (onk′o·sfeer) *n.* [*onco-*, hooked, + *sphere*]. The hexacanth embryo of tapeworms.

on·co·ther·a·py (onk″o·therr′uh·pee) *n.* [*onco-* + *therapy*]. Treatment of tumors, as by surgery, radiation, or chemotherapy.

on·cot·ic (ong·kot′ick, on·) *adj.* 1. Pertaining to oncosis. 2. Pertaining to anything that increases volume or pressure.

oncotic agent. A substance, such as human serum albumin or dextran, that may be used to increase colloidal osmotic pressure and expand plasma volume.

oncotic pressure. 1. The osmotic pressure exerted by colloids in a solution. 2. The pressure exerted by plasma proteins. Syn. *colloidal osmotic pressure.*

Oncovin. Trademark for vincristine, an antineoplastic drug used as the sulfate salt.

On·dine's curse [F., from *Undine,* a water nymph fabled to have caused the human male who loved her to sleep continuously]. PRIMARY ALVEOLAR HYPOVENTILATION SYNDROME.

-one [Gk. *-ōnē,* female descendant]. A suffix in organic chemistry signifying a ketone or certain other compounds that contain oxygen, as a lactone or sulfone.

one-child sterility. Failure of conception in a woman after she has given birth to one child.

oneir-, oneiro- [Gk. *oneiron*]. A combining form meaning *dream.*

onei·ric (o·nigh′rick) *adj.* [*oneir-* + *-ic*]. 1. Of or pertaining to dreams or a dreamlike state. 2. Pertaining to or characterized by oneirism.

onei·rism (o·nigh′riz·um) *n.* [*oneir-* + *-ism*]. An abnormal state of consciousness in which the subject experiences disorders of perception, terrifying hallucinations, vivid dreams, and intense emotions, and imagines involvement in strange and absurd events.

onei·ro·dyn·ia (o·nigh″ro·din′ee·uh) *n.* [*oneir-* + *odyn-*, pain, distress, + *-ia*]. Disquietude of the mind during sleep; somnambulism and nightmare.

oneirodynia ac·ti·va (ack·tye′vuh). SOMNAMBULISM.

onei·rog·mus (o″nigh·rog′mus) *n.* [Gk. *oneirōgmos*]. NOCTURNAL EMISSION.

onei·rol·o·gy (o″nigh·rol′uh·jee) *n.* [*oneiro-* + *-logy*]. The science, or scientific view, of dreams.

onei·ron·o·sus (o″nigh·ron′uh·sus) *n.* [*oneiro-* + Gk. *nosos,* disease]. Disorder manifesting itself in dreams; morbid dreaming.

onei·ros·co·py (o″nigh·ros′kup·ee) *n.* [*oneiro-* + *-scopy,* examination]. Dream interpretation; diagnosis of a mental state by the analysis of dreams.

one-piece bifocals. Bifocals in which greater refractive power is obtained by grinding the two different curvatures on one glass.

one-point discrimination. The act of distinguishing by localization a point of pressure on the surface of the skin.

one-stage method. A method for determination of plasma clotting activity by the addition of thromboplastin and calcium to the decalcified plasma. The clotting time or prothrombin time is an index of the activity of several factors, including prothrombin.

onio·ma·nia (o″nee·o·may′nee·uh) *n.* [Gk. *ōnios,* for sale, + *-mania*]. An irresistible impulse for buying, usually beyond one's needs.

on·ion bulb. *In neuropathology,* a descriptive term for the appearance of a nerve or nerve root seen in cross section, in which a whorl of Schwann cells and fibroblasts encircle naked or finely medullated axons. Onion bulbs are observed in progressive hypertrophic neuropathy (Déjerine-Sottas disease), Refsum's disease, certain instances of peroneal muscular atrophy, and other remitting and relapsing polyneuropathies.

onion-peel dermatomes. The arrangement of the zones or segments of pain and thermal sensibility on the face; the zones have a concentric arrangement centering about the mouth and nose and are said to represent the primitive lamination of the spinal nucleus of the trigeminal nerve.

onir-, oniro-. See *oneir-.*

onk-, onko-. See *onco-.*

on·kino·cele (ong·kin′o·seel) *n.* [*onk-* + *ino-* + *-cele*]. Inflammation of the tendon sheaths, attended by swelling.

onkocytoma. ONCOCYTOMA.

on·lay graft. A bone graft which is laid on the surface of a bone where bone substance has been lost and where conditions are unsuited to inlay grafts. Onlay grafts are fixed in place by vitallium screws.

on·o·mato·ma·nia (on″o·mat″o·may′nee·uh) *n.* [Gk. *onoma, onomatos,* name, word, + *-mania*]. An irresistible impulse to repeat certain words.

on·o·mato·pho·bia (on″o·mat″o·fo′bee·uh) *n.* [Gk. *onoma, onomatos,* name, word, + *-phobia*]. Pathological fear of hearing certain names or words.

on·o·mato·poi·e·sis (on″o·mat″o·poy·ee′sis) *n.* [Gk. *onoma, onomatos,* name, word, + *poiēsis,* production, creation]. 1. The formation of words in imitation of a sound. 2. *In psychiatry,* the extemporaneous formation of words on the basis of sound association; frequently a symptom of schizophrenia.

-ont [Gk. *ōn, ontos,* being, existing]. A combining form meaning *cell* or *organism.*

ont-, onto- [Gk. *ōn, ontos,* being, existing, pres. part. of *einai,* to be]. A combining form meaning (a) *existence, existential;* (b) *an individual being, organism.*

on·to·anal·y·sis (on″to·uh·nal′i·sis) *n.* [*onto-* + *analysis*]. A branch of psychiatry that combines psychoanalysis with existentialism. See also *existential psychiatry.* **—onto·an·a·lyt·ic** (·an·uh·lit′ick) *adj.*

on·to·gen·e·sis (on″to·jen′e·sis) *n.* ONTOGENY.

on·tog·e·ny (on·toj′e·nee) *n.* [*onto-* + *-geny*]. The origin and development of the individual organism from fertilized egg to adult, as distinguished from phylogeny, the evolutionary history of the race or group to which the individual belongs. **—on·to·ge·net·ic** (on″to·je·net′ick) *adj.*

on·y·al·ai (on″ee·al′ay) *n.* A form of acute idiopathic thrombocytopenic purpura occurring in African Negroes and characterized by blood-filled vesicles inside the mouth and on other mucous surfaces. Syn. *tropical thrombocytopenia.*

on·y·al·ia (on″ee·al′ee·uh) *n.* ONYALAI.

onych-, onycho- [Gk. *onyx, onychos*]. A combining form meaning *nail* or *claw.*

on·y·chal·gia ner·vo·sa (on″i·kal′jee·uh nur·vo′suh). Extreme sensitivity of apparently normal nails. Syn. *hyperesthesia unguium.*

on·y·cha·tro·phia (on″i·kuh·tro′fee·uh) *n.* [*onychatrophy* + *-ia*]. 1. Atrophy of nails. 2. Failure of development of the nail.

on·y·chat·ro·phy (on″i·kat′ruh·fee) *n.* [*onych-* + *atrophy*]. ONYCHATROPHIA.

on·ych·aux·is (on″i·kawk′sis) *n.* [*onych-* + *-auxis,* from Gk. *auxein,* to increase]. Hypertrophy of the nail.

on·y·chec·to·my (on″i·keck′tuh·mee) *n.* [*onych-* + *-ectomy*]. Excision of a fingernail or toenail.

on·ych·ex·al·lax·is (on″i·keck″suh·lack′sis) *n.* [*onych-* + Gk. *exallaxis,* alteration]. Degeneration of nails.

onych·ia (o·nick′ee·uh) *n.* [*onych-* + *-ia*]. Inflammation of the nail matrix.

onychia cra·que·lé (krack·lay′) [F.]. Fragility and fracture of the nail.

onychia ma·lig·na (ma·lig′nuh). A form of onychia occurring in debilitated persons; characterized by an ulcer in the matrix of the nail, which becomes discolored and is thrown off.

onychia punc·ta·ta (punk·tay′tuh). A nail characterized by numerous small, punctiform depressions.

onychia sim·plex (sim′plecks). Onychia without much ulceration, with loss of the nail and its replacement by a new one.

onychia su·per·fi·ci·a·lis un·du·la·ta (sue″pur·fish″ee·ay′lis un″due·lay′tuh). A rare type of nail disease seen in secondary syphilis, characterized by superficial waves and ripples across the nail.

on·y·chin (on′i·kin) *n.* [*onych-* + *-in*]. A hard substance found in nails; probably a type of keratin.

onycho-. See *onych-*.

on·y·choc·la·sis (on″i·kock′luh·sis) *n.* [*onycho-* + *-clasis*]. Breaking of a nail.

on·y·cho·cryp·to·sis (on″i·ko·krip·to′sis) *n.* [*onycho-* + Gk. *kryptos,* hidden, + *-osis*]. Ingrowing of a nail. Syn. *unguis incarnatus.*

on·y·cho·dys·tro·phy (on″i·ko·dis′truh·fee) *n.* [*onycho-* + *dystrophy*]. Any distortion of a nail; a symptom seen in several diseases.

on·y·cho·gen·ic (on″i·ko·jen′ick) *adj.* [*onycho-* + *-genic*]. Pertaining to the formation of the nails.

on·y·cho·gry·pho·sis (on″i·ko·grye·fo′sis, ·gri·) *n.* ONYCHOGRYPOSIS.

on·y·cho·gry·po·sis (on″i·ko·grye·po′sis, ·gri·) *n.* [*onycho-* + *gryposis*]. A thickened, ridged, and curved condition of a nail.

on·y·cho·hel·co·sis (on″i·ko·hel·ko′sis) *n.* [*onycho-* + Gk. *helkōsis,* ulceration]. Ulceration of a nail.

on·y·cho·het·ero·to·pia (on″i·ko·het″ur·o·to′pee·uh) *n.* [*onycho-* + *heterotopia*]. An anomaly consisting of the presence of abnormally situated nails, as on the lateral aspect of the terminal phalanges. Most often occurs on the little finger.

on·y·choid (on′i·koid) *adj.* [*onych-* + *-oid*]. Resembling a toenail or fingernail in form or texture.

on·y·chol·y·sis (on″i·kol′i·sis) *n.* [*onycho-* + *-lysis*]. A slow process of loosening of a nail from its bed, beginning at the free edge and progressing gradually toward the root.

on·y·cho·ma (on″i·ko′muh) *n.* [*onych-* + *-oma*]. A tumor of the nail bed.

on·y·cho·ma·de·sis (on″i·ko·muh·dee′sis) *n.* [*onycho-* + Gk. *madēsis,* falling out (of hair)]. Spontaneous separation of a nail from its bed, beginning at the proximal end and progressing rapidly toward the free edge until the nail plate falls off; defluvium unguium.

on·y·cho·ma·la·cia (on″i·ko·ma·lay′shee·uh, ·shuh) *n.* [*onycho-* + *malacia*]. Abnormally soft nails.

on·y·cho·my·co·sis (on″i·ko·migh·ko′sis) *n.* [*onycho-* + *mycosis*]. A disease of the nails due to fungi.

on·y·cho·no·sus (on″i·ko·no′sus) *n.* [*onycho-* + Gk. *nosos,* disease]. ONYCHOSIS.

on·y·cho·os·teo·ar·thro·dys·pla·sia (on″i·ko·os″tee·o·ahr″thro·dis·play′zhuh, ·zee·uh) *n.* [*onycho-* + *osteo-* + *arthro-* + *dysplasia*]. NAIL-PATELLA SYNDROME.

on·y·cho·os·teo·dys·pla·sia (on″i·ko·os″tee·o·dis·play′zhuh, ·zee·uh) *n.* [*onycho-* + *osteo-* + *dysplasia*]. NAIL-PATELLA SYNDROME.

on·y·cho·pac·i·ty (on″i·ko·pas′i·tee) *n.* [*onych-* + *opacity*]. LEUKONYCHIA.

on·y·chop·a·thy (on″i·kop′uth·ee) *n.* [*onycho-* + *-pathy*]. Any disease of the nails. —**ony·cho·path·ic** (·ko·path′ick) *adj.*

on·y·cho·pha·gia (on″i·ko·fay′jee·uh) *n.* [*onycho-* + *phag-* + *-ia*]. NAIL BITING.

on·y·choph·a·gist (on″i·kof′uh·jist) *n.* [*onycho-* + *phag-* + *-ist*]. A person addicted to biting his fingernails.

on·y·chop·to·sis (on″i·kop·to′sis) *n.* [*onycho-* + *-ptosis*]. Downward displacement of the nails.

on·y·cho·phy·ma (on″i·ko·fye′muh) *n.* [*onycho-* + *phyma*]. Enlarged or thickened nails.

on·y·chor·rhex·is (on″i·ko·reck′sis) *n.* [*onycho-* + *-rrhexis*]. Longitudinal striation of the nail plate, with or without the formation of fissures.

on·y·chor·rhi·za (on″i·ko·rye′zuh) *n.* [*onycho-* + Gk. *rhiza,* root]. The root of a nail.

on·y·cho·schiz·ia (on″i·ko·skiz′ee·uh) *n.* [*onycho-* + *schiz-* + *-ia*]. An ungual dystrophy consisting of lamination on the nail in two or more superimposed layers.

on·y·cho·sis (on″i·ko′sis) *n.* [*onych-* + *-osis*]. Any deformity or disease of the nails.

on·y·cho·stro·ma (on″i·ko·stro′muh) *n.* [*onycho-* + *stroma*]. The matrix or bed of a nail.

on·y·chot·il·lo·ma·nia (on″i·kot″i·lo·may′nee·uh) *n.* [*onycho-* + Gk. *tillein,* to pluck at, pull, + *-mania*]. The neurotic picking at a nail until it is permanently altered. See also *nail biting.*

on·y·chot·o·my (on″i·kot′uh·mee) *n.* [*onycho-* + *-tomy*]. Surgical incision into a fingernail or toenail.

on·y·cho·tro·phia (on″i·ko·tro′fee·uh) *n.* ONYCHOTROPHY.

on·y·chot·ro·phy (on″i·kot′ruh·fee) *n.* [*onycho-* + *-trophy*]. Nourishment of the nails.

on·yx (on′icks) *n.* [Gk.]. 1. NAIL; a fingernail or toenail. 2. A collection of pus between the corneal lamellas at the most dependent part.

on·yx·i·tis (on″ick·sigh′tis) *n.* [*onyx* + *-itis*]. ONYCHIA.

oo- [Gk. *ōon*]. A combining form meaning *egg, ovum.*

oo·ceph·a·lus (o″o·sef′uh·lus) *n.* [*oo-* + *-cephalus*]. TRIGONOCEPHALUS.

oo·cyst (o′o·sist) *n.* [*oo-* + *-cyst*]. The encysted zygote in the life history of some sporozoa. Contr. *ookinete.*

oo·cyte (o′o·site) *n.* [*oo-* + *-cyte*]. An egg cell before the completion of the maturation process. Its full history includes its origin from an oogonium, a growth period, and the final meiotic divisions.

oocyte nucleus. The nucleus of the primordial female gamete.

oo·gen·e·sis (o″o·jen′e·sis) *n.* [*oo-* + *genesis*]. The process of the origin, growth, and formation of the ovum in its preparation for fertilization. —**oo·ge·net·ic** (·je·net′ick) *adj.*

oo·go·ni·um (o″o·go′nee·um) *n.*, pl. **oogo·nia** (·nee·uh) [NL., from *oo-* + Gk. *gonē,* seed, generation]. 1. A cell which, by continued division, gives rise to oocytes. 2. An ovum in a primary follicle immediately before the beginning of maturation.

oo·ki·ne·sis (o″o·ki·nee′sis, ·kigh·nee′sis) *n.* [*oo-* + *kinesis*]. The mitotic phenomena in the egg cell during maturation and fertilization.

oo·ki·nete (o″o·kigh′neet, ·ki·neet′) *n.* [*oo-* + Gk. *kinētos,* movable]. The elongated, motile zygote in the life history of some sporozoan parasites; as that of the malaria parasite as it bores through the epithelial lining of the mosquito's intestine, in the wall of which it becomes an oocyst. Contr. *oocyst.* —**oo·ki·net·ic** (·ki·net′ick) *adj.*

oo·lem·ma (o″o·lem′uh) *n.* [*oo-* + *-lemma*]. ZONA PELLUCIDA.

oophor-, oophoro- [Gk. *ōophoros,* egg-bearing, from *ōon,* egg, + *phoros,* bearing]. A combining form meaning *ovary, ovarian.*

oo·pho·rec·to·my (o″uh·fo·reck′tuh·mee, o·off″o·) *n.* [*oophor-* + *-ectomy*]. Excision of an ovary.

oo·pho·ri·tis (o″uh·fo·rye′tis, o·off″uh·rye′tis) *n.* [*oophor-* + *-itis*]. Inflammation of an ovary.

oophoro-. See *oophor-*.

ooph·o·ro·ce·cal, ooph·o·ro·cae·cal (o·off″ur·o·see′kul) *adj.*

[*oophoro-* + *cecal*]. Pertaining to the ovary and the cecum.

ooph·o·ro·cys·tec·to·my (o·off″ur·o·sis·teck′tuh·mee) *n.* [*oophoro-* + *cyst* + *-ectomy*]. Removal of an ovarian cyst.

ooph·o·ro·cys·to·sis (o·off″ur·o·sis·to′sis) *n.* [*oophoro-* + *cyst* + *-osis*]. The formation of ovarian cysts.

ooph·o·ro·cys·tos·to·my (o·off″ur·o·sis·tos′tuh·mee) *n.* [*oophoro-* + *cysto-* + *-stomy*]. OOPHOROSTOMY.

ooph·o·ro·hys·ter·ec·to·my (o·off″ur·o·his·tur·eck′tuh·mee) *n.* [*oophoro-* + *hyster-* + *-ectomy*]. Removal of the uterus and ovaries.

ooph·o·ro·ma (o·off″ur·o′muh) *n.* [*oophor-* + *-oma*]. An ovarian tumor.

oophoroma fol·lic·u·la·re (Brenner) (fol·ick″yoo·lair′ee). BRENNER TUMOR.

ooph·o·ro·ma·la·cia (o·off″ur·o·ma·lay′shee·uh) *n.* [*oophoro-* + *malacia*]. Softening of the ovary.

ooph·o·ro·ma·nia (o·off″ur·o·may′nee·uh) *n.* [*oophoro-* + *-mania*]. Mental disorder related to ovarian dysfunction.

ooph·o·ron (o·off′ur·on) *n.* [*oo-* + Gk. *phoron*, something that bears, carries]. OVARY.

ooph·o·ro·path·i·a (o·off″ur·o·path′ee·uh) *n.* [*oophoro-* + *-pathia*]. Any disease of the ovary.

ooph·o·ro·pex·y (o·off′ur·o·peck″see) *n.* [*oophoro-* + *-pexy*]. Surgical fixation of an ovary.

ooph·o·ro·plas·ty (o·off′ur·o·plas″tee) *n.* [*oophoro-* + *-plasty*]. Plastic surgery on the ovary.

ooph·o·ro·sal·pin·gec·to·my (o·off″ur·o·sal″pin·jeck′tum·ee) *n.* [*oophoro-* + *salping-* + *-ectomy*]. Excision of an ovary and oviduct.

ooph·o·ro·sal·pin·gi·tis (o·off″ur·o·sal″pin·jye′tis) *n.* [*oophoro-* + *salping-* + *-itis*]. Inflammation of an ovary and oviduct.

ooph·o·ros·to·my (o·off″ur·os′tum·ee) *n.* [*oophoro-* + *-stomy*]. The establishment of an opening into an ovarian cyst for drainage. Syn. *oophorocystostomy*.

oo·phor·rha·phy (o″uh·for′uh·fee) *n.* [*oophoro-* + *-rrhaphy*]. Operation of suturing an ovary to the pelvic wall.

oo·plasm (o′o·plaz·um) *n.* [*oo-* + *-plasm*]. The cytoplasm of the egg; it includes the yolk or deuteroplasm as well as the more active cytoplasm.

oo·por·phy·rin (o″o·por′fi·rin) *n.* [*oo-* + *porphyrin*]. A porphyrin occurring in the pigment from the eggshells of certain birds.

Oort's anastomosis. A small branch of the inferior portion of the vestibular nerve that joins the cochlear nerve.

oo·sperm (o′o·spurm) *n.* [*oo-* + *sperm*]. A fertilized egg; a zygote.

Oos·po·ra (o·os′pur·uh) *n.* [*oo-* + Gk. *spora*, seed, procreation]. A genus of fungi which reproduce by mycelial fragmentation.

Oospora madurae. NOCARDIA MADURAE.

Oospora minutissima. NOCARDIA MINUTISSIMA.

oothec-, ootheco- [*oo-* + Gk. *thēkē*, case, box]. A combining form meaning *ovary, ovarian.*

oo·tid (o′uh·tid) *n.* [*oo-* + *-id*]. The ovum after the completion of the maturation divisions, by which one ootid and three polar bodies are found.

oo·type (o′o·tipe) *n.* [*oo-* + Gk. *typos*, form, mold]. A muscular dilatation of the oviduct of certain trematode worms, in which secretory cells furnish shell substance to the ova.

opac·i·fy (o·pas′i·fye) *v.* 1. To make opaque. 2. To become opaque. —**opac·i·fi·ca·tion** (o·pas″i·fi·kay′shun) *n.*

opac·i·ty (o·pas′i·tee) *n.* [F. *opacité*]. 1. The condition of being opaque. 2. An opaque spot, as opacity of the cornea or lens.

opal·es·cent (o″puh·les′unt) *adj.* [*opal* + *-escent*]. Showing a play of colors; reflecting light; iridescent. —**opales·cence** (·unce) *n.*

opal mutation (o′pul). A nonsense mutation in which the codon base sequence is UGA (uracil-guanine-adenine).

Opal·ski cells. Cells with eccentric small nuclei and voluminous cytoplasm filled with fine para-aminosalicylic acid-positive granules and staining light-brown in iron hematoxylin–van Gieson preparations, found scattered in the brainstem ganglia and cerebral cortex of patients with hepatolenticular degeneration, familial (Wilson's disease) or acquired; considered to be degenerating nerve cells.

opaque (o·pake′) *adj.* [L. *opacus*, shaded]. Impervious to light or to other forms of radiation, as: opaque to x-rays. Contr. *transparent, translucent.*

opei·do·scope (o·pye′duh·scope) *n.* [Gk. *ops, opos*, voice, + *eidos*, shape, pattern, + *-scope*]. An instrument for projecting the vibrations of the voice visually onto a screen.

open, *adj.* 1. Exposed to the air, as an open wound. 2. Interrupted, as an open circuit, one through which an electric current cannot pass.

open anesthesia. Inhalation anesthesia with a minimum amount of rebreathing.

open-angle glaucoma. Increased intraocular tension, which is insidious in onset, bilateral, and slowly progressive, with visual loss occurring only when the disease is well advanced, due to diminished aqueous outflow but with the angle open and the aqueous in free contact with the trabecula. Contr. *narrow-angle glaucoma.*

open bite. A condition in which the upper and lower incisors do not occlude.

open chain. A configuration of an organic compound in which the carbon atoms are arranged or linked to form an open chain. Contr. *cyclic* (3).

open chest cardiac massage. Direct manual compression of the heart; usually done in the operating room where the thoracic cavity is opened. Syn. *direct cardiac massage.*

open circulation theory. The theory that in the spleen blood moves from the arteries of the ellipsoids into the tissue of the red pulp, and is transfused back into the vascular system through openings in the walls of the venous sinusoids. Contr. *closed circulation theory.*

open-closed circulation theory. The theory that in the spleen the circulation of blood can be either open or closed, depending on circumstances.

open fracture. COMPOUND FRACTURE.

open hospital. *In psychiatry,* a hospital or part of a hospital in which psychiatric patients are free to come and go, and which has no locked doors or other physical barriers.

open·ing axis. An imaginary line around which the condyles rotate during opening and closing movements of the mandible.

opening snap. A brief heart sound related to the sudden opening of a heart valve, usually the mitral valve. Abbreviated, O. S.

opening the bite. Elevation of the occlusal plane of some or all of the posterior teeth by orthodontic manipulation or prosthetic restorations.

open jump flap. A large flap that begins as a pedicle flap to a movable part and is then transferred to a distant defect directly without tubing.

open pneumothorax. A pneumothorax which communicates with the outside, as through a wound in the thoracic wall.

open reduction. *In surgery,* a reduction performed after making an incision through the soft parts in order to expose the fracture or dislocation.

open-roofed skull. CRANIOSCHISIS.

open tuberculosis. Tuberculosis in which tubercle bacilli are being discharged from the body; tuberculosis capable of transmission to other persons.

op·er·a·ble (op′ur·uh·bul) *adj.* Admitting of an operation with reasonable expectation of favorable results; pertaining to a condition where operation is not contraindicated. —**op·er·a·bil·i·ty** (op″ur·uh·bil′i·tee) *n.*

opera-glass hand. Hand changes including shortening of fingers and/or wrist caused by bone resorption, increased range of motion, and skin redundancy; it may occur after generalized, long-standing, severe rheumatoid arthritis. Syn. *main en lorgnette.*

op·er·ant (op'ur·unt) *adj.* [L. *operans,* working, functioning]. *In psychology,* pertaining to or characterizing behavior or response to a stimulus recognized by its effect on the organism (experimental animal or human subject); the stimulus may or may not be identifiable.

operant conditioning or **learning.** A form of learning in which the subject, human or animal, is taught to make a response or perform a task voluntarily, and this, in turn, determines whether or not the conditioning is reinforced. Syn. *instrumental conditioning, reinforced conditioning.* Compare *conditioning* (1).

op·er·a·tion (op"uh·ray'shun) *n.* [L. *operatio,* from *operari,* to work, from *opera,* work, service]. 1. The mode of action of anything. 2. Anything done or performed, especially with instruments. 3. *In surgery,* a procedure in which the method follows a definite routine. —**operation·al** (·ul), **op·er·a·tive** (op'uh·ruh·tiv) *adj.;* **op·er·ate** (op'uh·rate) *v.*

operational fatigue. FLYING FATIGUE.

operation of election. ELECTIVE OPERATION.

operative ankylosis. ARTHRODESIS.

operative dentistry. The branch of dental science and practice that deals with the prevention and treatment of disease of the hard tissues of the natural teeth.

operative myxedema. POSTOPERATIVE MYXEDEMA.

operative surgery. The branch of surgery dealing with the performance of operations.

op·er·a·tor (op'ur·ay"tur) *n.* [L., worker]. 1. One who performs a surgical operation. 2. One who gives treatments, especially those involving mechanotherapy. 3. The proximal portion of an operon which provides the site for recognition by a repressor protein.

opercular process. A caudal outgrowth of the hyoid arch of an embryo that helps obliterate the cervical sinus.

oper·cu·late (o·pur'kew·lut, ·late) *adj.* Having an operculum.

oper·cu·lat·ed (o·pur'kew·lay·tid) *adj.* OPERCULATE.

oper·cu·lum (o·pur'kew·lum) *n.,* pl. **opercu·la** (·luh), [L., lid]. 1. A lid or cover; a valve. 2. One of the convolutions covering the insula. 3. The soft tissue overlying the crown of a partially erupted tooth, specifically, over a lower third molar. —**opercu·lar** (·lur) *adj.*

operculum fron·ta·le (fron·tay'lee) [NA]. FRONTAL OPERCULUM.

operculum fron·to·pa·ri·e·ta·le (fron"to·puh·rye"e·tay'lee) [NA]. FRONTOPARIETAL OPERCULUM.

operculum ilei (il'ee·eye). ILEOCECAL VALVE.

operculum proper. FRONTOPARIETAL OPERCULUM.

operculum tem·po·ra·le (tem·po·ray'lee) [NA]. TEMPORAL OPERCULUM.

op·er·on (op'ur·on) *n.* A genetic unit consisting of two or more adjacent cistrons which are coordinately regulated via an operator site and whose transcription is initiated at a promotor site.

ophi·a·sis (o·fye'uh·sis) *n.* [Gk., from *ophis,* snake]. Alopecia areata in which the baldness progresses in a serpentine form about the hair margin. Usually seen in children.

ophid·io·pho·bia (o·fid"ee·o·fo'bee·uh) *n.* [Gk. *ophidion,* small snake, + *-phobia*]. Morbid fear of snakes.

ophid·ism (o'fid·iz·um) *n.* [Gk. *ophidion,* small snake, + *-ism*]. Poisoning from snake venom.

Ophi·oph·a·gus (o"fee·off'uh·gus) *n.* [NL., from Gk. *ophiophagus,* snake-eating, from *ophis,* snake]. A monotypic genus of the Elapidae.

Ophiophagus han·nah (han'uh). The king cobra; a large and aggressive snake of southern Asia which has a powerful neurotoxic venom. Formerly called *Naja hannah.*

oph·io·phobe (off'ee·o·fobe, o'fee·o·fobe) *n.* [Gk. *ophis,* snake, + *-phobe*]. A person who has an unusual dread of snakes.

oph·ry·itis (off"ree·eye'tis) *n.* [Gk. *ophrys,* eyebrow, + *-itis*]. Inflammation of the eyebrow.

oph·ry·on (off'ree·on, o'free·on) *n.* [Gk. *ophrys,* eyebrow, + *-on*]. *In craniometry,* the point where the sagittal plane intersects an arc drawn horizontally from the frontotemporalia across the frontal bone.

oph·ry·o·sis (off"ree·o'sis) *n.* [Gk. *ophrys,* eyebrow, + *-osis*]. Spasm of the muscles of the eyebrow.

oph·ryph·thei·ri·a·sis (off"rif·thigh·rye'uh·sis) *n.* [Gk. *ophrys,* eyebrow, + *phtheiriasis*]. Pediculosis of the eyebrows and eyelashes.

oph·rys (off'ris) *n.* [Gk.]. EYEBROW. —**ophryt·ic** (o·frit'ick) *adj.*

Ophthaine. Trademark for proparacaine, a surface anesthetic employed in ophthalmology, as the hydrochloride salt.

ophthalm-, ophthalmo- [Gk. *ophthalmos*]. A combining form meaning *eye.*

oph·thal·ma·cro·sis (off·thal"ma·kro'sis) *n.* [*ophthalm-* + *macr-* + *-osis*]. Enlargement of the eyeball.

oph·thal·ma·gra (off"thal·may'gruh, ·mag'ruh) *n.* [*ophthalm-* + *-agra*]. Sudden pain in the eye.

oph·thal·mal·gia (off"thal·mal'juh, ·jee·uh) *n.* [*ophthalm-* + *-algia*]. Neuralgia of the eye.

oph·thal·mec·chy·mo·sis (off"thal·meck"i·mo'sis) *n.* [*ophthalm-* + *ecchymosis*]. An effusion of blood into the conjunctiva.

oph·thal·mec·to·my (off"thal·meck'tum·ee) *n.* [*ophthalm-* + *-ectomy*]. Excision, or enucleation, of an eye.

oph·thalm·en·ceph·a·lon (off·thal·men·sef'uh·lon) *n.* [*ophthalm-* + *encephalon*]. The visual nervous mechanism; the retina, optic nerves, optic chiasma, optic tract, and visual centers.

oph·thal·mia (off·thal'mee·uh) *n.* [Gk.]. Inflammation of the eye, especially when the conjunctiva is involved.

ophthalmia elec·tri·ca (e·leck'tri·kuh). Conjunctivitis due to intense electric light.

ophthalmia neonatorum. Conjunctivitis in the newborn, which may be from bacterial, viral, or chemical causes.

ophthalmia ni·va·lis (ni·vay'lis). SNOW BLINDNESS.

ophthalmia no·do·sa (no·do'suh). Inflammation of the conjunctiva due to lodging of caterpillar hairs in the conjunctiva, cornea, or iris; characterized by small, semitranslucent, reddish or yellow-gray nodules.

oph·thal·mi·a·ter (off·thal'mee·ay"tur) *n.* [*ophthalm-* + Gk. *iātēr,* surgeon, physician]. OPHTHALMOLOGIST.

oph·thal·mi·at·rics (off·thal'mee·at'ricks) *n.* [*ophthalm-* + *-iatric* + *-s*]. The treatment of eye diseases.

oph·thal·mic (off·thal'mick) *adj.* [Gk. *ophthalmikos*]. Pertaining to the eye.

ophthalmic artery. A main branch of the internal carotid artery supplying the eye and nearby structures. See also Table of Arteries in the Appendix.

ophthalmic migraine. OCULAR MIGRAINE.

ophthalmic nerve. A somatic sensory nerve, a division of the trigeminal nerve, which innervates the skin of the forehead, the upper eyelids, the anterior portion of the scalp, the orbit, the eyeball, the meninges, the nasal mucosa, the frontal, ethmoid, and sphenoid air sinuses. NA *nervus ophthalmicus.*

ophthalmic plexus. A sympathetic nerve plexus surrounding the ophthalmic artery. Syn. *plexus ophthalmicus.*

ophthalmic test or **reaction.** CONJUNCTIVAL TEST.

oph·thal·mi·tis (off"thal·migh'tis) *n.* [*ophthalm-* + *-itis*]. Inflammation of the eye. —**ophthal·mit·ic** (·mit'ick) *adj.*

ophthalmo-. See *ophthalm-.*

oph·thal·mo·blen·nor·rhea (off·thal"mo·blen·or·ee'uh) *n.* [*ophthalmo-* + *blennorrhea*]. Blennorrhea of the conjunctiva.

oph·thal·moc·a·ce (off"thal·mock'uh·see) *n.* [*ophthalmo-* + Gk. *kakē,* badness]. Disease of the eye.

oph·thal·mo·cele (off·thal'mo·seel) *n.* [*ophthalmo-* + *-cele*]. EXOPHTHALMOS.

oph·thal·mo·cen·te·sis (off·thal"mo·sen·tee'sis) *n.* [*ophthalmo-* + *centesis*]. Surgical puncture of the eye. Syn. *paracentesis oculi.*

oph·thal·mo·co·pia, oph·thal·mo·ko·pia (off·thal"mo·ko'pee·

uh) *n.* [*ophthalmo-* + Gk. *kopos,* fatigue, + *-ia*]. ASTHENOPIA.

oph·thal·mo·di·a·stim·e·ter (off·thal″mo·dye″as·tim′e·tur) *n.* [*ophthalmo-* + Gk. *diastasis,* distance, separation, + *-meter*]. An instrument used for determining the proper adjustment of lenses to the axes of the eyes.

oph·thal·mo·do·ne·sis (off·thal″mo·do·nee′sis) *n.* [*ophthalmo-* + Gk. *donēsis,* vibration, shaking]. A tremulous or oscillatory movement of the eye.

oph·thal·mo·dy·na·mom·e·ter (off·thal″mo·dye″nuh·mom′e·tur, ·din″uh·) *n.* [*ophthalmo-* + *dynamometer*]. An instrument which measures the pressure necessary to cause pulsation and collapse the retinal arteries.

oph·thal·mo·dy·na·mom·e·try (off·thal″mo·dye″nuh·mom′e·tree) *n.* Measurement of the systolic and diastolic blood pressure in the retinal circulation by means of an ophthalmodynamometer.

oph·thal·mo·dyn·ia (off·thal″mo·din′ee·uh) *n.* [*ophthalm-* + *-odynia*]. Pain referred to the eye.

ophthalmoeikonometer. OPHTHALMOICONOMETER.

oph·thal·mo·fun·do·scope (off·thal″mo·fun′duh·skope) *n.* [*ophthalmo-* + *fundus* + *-scope*]. OPHTHALMOSCOPE.

oph·thal·mog·ra·phy (off″thal·mog′ruh·fee) *n.* [*ophthalmo-* + *-graphy*]. Descriptive anatomy of the eye.

oph·thal·mo·gy·ric (off·thal″mo·jye′rick) *adj.* [*ophthalmo-* + *gyr-* + *-ic*]. OCULOGYRIC.

oph·thal·mo·ico·nom·e·ter, oph·thal·mo·ei·ko·nom·e·ter (off·thal″mo·eye″kuh·nom′e·tur) *n.* [*ophthalmo-* + *icono-* + *-meter*]. A complex apparatus for the detection and measurement of aniseikonia.

oph·thal·mo·ico·nom·e·try (off·thal″mo·eye″kuh·nom′e·tree) *n.* Measurement of the retinal image with an ophthalmoiconometer.

ophthalmokopia. Ophthalmocopia (= ASTHENOPIA).

oph·thal·mo·leu·ko·scope (off·thal″mo·lew′ko·skope) *n.* [*ophthalmo-* + *leuko-* + *-scope*]. A instrument for testing color sense by means of polarized light.

oph·thal·mo·lith (off·thal′mo·lith) *n.* [*ophthalmo-* + *-lith*]. A calculus of the eye or lacrimal duct.

oph·thal·mol·o·gist (off″thal·mol′uh·jist) *n.* One skilled or specializing in ophthalmology.

oph·thal·mol·o·gy (off″thal·mol′uh·jee) *n.* [*ophthalmo-* + *-logy*]. The science of the anatomy, physiology, diseases, and treatment of the eye. **—oph·thal·mo·log·ic** (off·thal″mo·loj′ick) *adj.*

oph·thal·mo·ma·cro·sis (off·thal″mo·ma·kro′sis) *n.* OPHTHALMACROSIS.

oph·thal·mo·ma·la·cia (off·thal″mo·ma·lay′shee·uh) *n.* [*ophthalmo-* + *malacia*]. Abnormal softness or subnormal tension of the eye.

oph·thal·mom·e·ter (off″thal·mom′e·tur) *n.* [*ophthalmo-* + *-meter*]. 1. An instrument for measuring refractive errors, especially astigmatism. 2. An instrument for measuring the capacity of the chambers of the eye. 3. An instrument for measuring the eye as a whole.

oph·thal·mom·e·try (off″thal·mom′e·tree) *n.* [*ophthalmo-* + *-metry*]. The determination of refractive errors of the eye, mainly by measuring the astigmatism of the cornea.

oph·thal·mo·my·co·sis (off·thal″mo·migh·ko′sis) *n.* [*ophthalmo-* + *mycosis*]. Any disease of the eye or its appendages due to a fungus.

oph·thal·mo·my·ia·sis (off·thal″mo·migh·eye′uh·sis). *n.* [*ophthalmo-* + *myiasis*]. Invasion of the eyes by fly larvae, such as those belonging to the family Oestridae.

oph·thal·mo·my·ot·o·my (off·thal″mo·migh·ot′uh·mee) *n.* [*ophthalmo-* + *myotomy*]. Division of a muscle or muscles of the eye.

oph·thal·mo·neu·ri·tis (off·thal″mo·new·rye′tis) *n.* [*ophthalmo-* + *neuritis*]. OPTIC NEURITIS.

oph·thal·mo·neu·ro·my·e·li·tis (off·thal″mo·new″ro·migh″e·lye′tis) *n.* NEUROMYELITIS OPTICA.

oph·thal·mop·a·thy (off″thal·mop′uth·ee) *n.* [*ophthalmo-* + *-pathy*]. Any disease of the eye.

oph·thal·mo·pha·com·e·ter, oph·thal·mo·pha·kom·e·ter (off·thal″mo·fa·kom′e·tur) *n.* [*ophthalmo-* + *phacometer*]. An instrument for measuring the radius of curvature of the crystalline lens.

oph·thal·mo·phas·ma·tos·co·py (off·thal″mo·faz″muh·tos′kuh·pee) *n.* [*ophthalmo-* + Gk. *phasma, phasmatos,* apparition, + *-scopy*]. Ophthalmoscopic and spectroscopic examination of the interior of an eye.

oph·thal·mo·pho·bia (off·thal″mo·fo′bee·uh) *n.* [*ophthalmo-* + *-phobia*]. Morbid dislike of being stared at.

oph·thal·moph·thi·sis (off″thal·mof′thi·sis, off·thal″mo·tye′sis, off·thal″mof·thigh′sis) *n.* [*ophthalmo-* + *phthisis*]. Shrinking of the eyeball.

oph·thal·mo·phy·ma (off·thal″mo·figh′muh) *n.* [*ophthalmo-* + *phyma*]. Swelling of the eyeball.

oph·thal·mo·plas·ty (off·thal′mo·plas″tee) *n.* [*ophthalmo-* + *-plasty*]. Plastic surgery of the eye or accessory parts. **—oph·thal·mo·plas·tic** (off·thal″mo·plas′tick) *adj.*

oph·thal·mo·ple·gia (off·thal″mo·plee′jee·uh) *n.* [*ophthalmo-* + *-plegia*]. Paralysis of the muscles innervated by the third, fourth, and sixth cranial nerves; may be supranuclear, internuclear, or due to a lesion of individual ocular motor nerves or their nuclei; may be external, internal, or complete. **—ophthalmople·gic** (·jick) *adj.*

ophthalmoplegia externa. EXTERNAL OPHTHALMOPLEGIA.

ophthalmoplegia interna. INTERNAL OPHTHALMOPLEGIA.

ophthalmoplegia plus. Any of the many complex syndromes in which progressive external opthalmoplegia is associated with retinal pigmentation and a variety of myopathic and neurologic abnormalities.

ophthalmoplegic migraine. A form of recurrent, unilateral, vascular headache, accompanied by transient extraocular muscle palsies, usually of the muscles innervated by the third cranial nerve.

oph·thal·mop·to·sis (off·thal″mop·to′sis) *n.* [*ophthalmo-* + *-ptosis*]. EXOPHTHALMOS.

oph·thal·mor·rha·gia (off·thal′mo·ray′jee·uh) *n.* [*ophthalmo-* + *-rrhagia*]. Hemorrhage from the eye.

oph·thal·mor·rhea (off·thal″mo·ree′uh) *n.* [*ophthalmo-* + *-rrhea*]. A watery or sanguineous discharge from the eye.

oph·thal·mor·rhex·is (off·thal″mo·reck′sis) *n.* [*ophthalmo-* + *-rrhexis*]. Rupture of the eyeball.

oph·thal·mos (off·thal′mos) *n.* [Gk.]. EYE.

oph·thal·mo·scope (off·thal′muh·skope) *n.* [*ophthalmo-* + *-scope*]. An instrument for examining the interior of the eye. It consists essentially of a mirror with a hole in it, through which the observer looks, the concavity of the eye being illuminated by light reflected from the mirror into the eye through the pupil and seen by means of the rays reflected from the eye ground back through the hole in the mirror. The ophthalmoscope is fitted with lenses of different powers that may be revolved in front of the observing eye, and these neutralize the ametropia of either the patient's or the observer's eye, thus rendering clear the details of the fundus of the eye. A wide variety of ophthalmoscopes exist, some offering special features, both for direct and indirect ophthalmoscopy.

oph·thal·mos·co·pist (off″thal·mos′kuh·pist) *n.* An individual versed in ophthalmoscopy.

oph·thal·mos·co·py (off″thal·mos′kuh·pee) *n.* The examination of the interior of the eye by means of an ophthalmoscope. **—oph·thal·mo·scop·ic** (off·thal″mo·skop′ick) *adj.*

oph·thal·mo·so·nom·e·try (off·thal″mo·so·nom′e·tree) *n.* A method employing ultrasound for assessing ophthalmic arterial pulsation by applying the transducer over the lid of the closed eye.

oph·thal·mo·spin·ther·ism (off·thal″mo·spin′thur·iz·um) *n.* [*ophthalmo-* + Gk. *spinthēr,* spark, + *-ism*]. A condition of the eye in which there is a visual impression of luminous sparks.

oph·thal·mos·ta·sis (off″thal·mos′tuh·sis) *n.* [*ophthalmo-* + *-stasis*]. Fixation of the eye during an operation upon it.

oph·thal·mo·stat (off·thal′mo·stat) *n.* [*ophthalmo-* + *-stat*]. An instrument used in fixing the eye in any position during an ophthalmic operation.

oph·thal·mo·sta·tom·e·ter (off·thal″mo·sta·tom′e·tur) *n.* [*ophthalmo-* + Gk. *statos*, standing, + *-meter*]. An instrument for determining the position of the eyes.

oph·thal·mo·sta·tom·e·try (off·thal″mo·sta·tom′e·tree) *n.* [*ophthalmo-* + Gk. *statos*, standing, + *-metry*]. The measurement of the position of the eyes.

oph·thal·mo·ste·re·sis (off·thal″mo·ste·ree′sis) *n.* [*ophthalmo-* + Gk. *sterēsis*, loss]. Loss or absence of one or both eyes.

oph·thal·mo·syn·chy·sis (off·thal″mo·sing′ki·sis) *n.* [*ophthalmo-* + Gk. *synchysis*, mixture, disorder]. Effusion into the interior chambers of the eye.

oph·thal·mot·o·my (off″thal·mot′um·ee) *n.* [*ophthalmo-* + *-tomy*]. The dissection or incision of the eye.

oph·thal·mo·to·nom·e·ter (off·thal″mo·to·nom′e·tur) *n.* [*ophthalmo-* + Gk. *tonos*, tension, + *-meter*]. An instrument for measuring intraocular tension.

oph·thal·mo·to·nom·e·try (off·thal″mo·to·nom′e·tree) *n.* [*ophthalmo-* + Gk. *tonos*, tension, + *-metry*]. Measurement of intraocular tension.

oph·thal·mo·trope (off·thal′muh·trope) *n.* [*ophthalmo-* + Gk. *tropos*, turn, direction]. A mechanical eye used for demonstrating the direction and the position that the eye takes under the influence of each of its extraocular muscles, and the position of the false image in the case of paralysis of a given muscle.

oph·thal·mo·tro·pom·e·ter (off·thal″mo·tro·pom′e·tur) *n.* [*ophthalmo-* + Gk. *tropos*, turn, + *-meter*]. An instrument for measuring the movement of the eyeballs.

oph·thal·mo·tro·pom·e·try (off·thal″mo·tro·pom′e·tree) *n.* [*ophthalmo-* + Gk. *tropos*, turn, + *-metry*]. The measurement of the movement of the eyeballs.

oph·thal·mo·xe·ro·sis (off·thal″mo·ze·ro′sis) *n.* [*ophthalmo-* + *xerosis*]. XEROPHTHALMIA.

oph·thal·mus (off·thal′mus) *n.* [NL., from Gk. *ophthalmos*]. The eye.

-opia, -opy [Gk. *-opia*, from *ōps*, eye]. A combining form meaning *a defect of the eye.*

opi·ate (o′pee·ut, ·ate) *n.* [L. *opiatus*, made with opium]. 1. A preparation of opium. 2. Any narcotic or synthetic analgesic. 3. Anything that quiets uneasiness or dulls the feelings.

Opie's paradox [E. L. *Opie*, U.S. pathologist, 1873–1971]. Tissue destruction resulting from the local effects of an anaphylactic reaction may serve as a protection to the host.

opio·ma·nia (o″pee·o·may′nee·uh) *n.* [*opium* + *-mania*]. An uncontrollable desire for opium; opium habit. —**opiomani·ac** (·ack) *n.*

opio·pha·gia (o″pee·o·fay′jee·uh) *n.* [*opium* + *-phagia*]. The eating of opium.

opi·oph·a·gism (o″pee·off′uh·jiz·um) *n.* [*opium* + *phag-* + *-ism*]. OPIOPHAGIA.

opi·oph·a·gy (o″pee·off′uh·jee) *n.* OPIOPHAGIA.

opio·phile (o′pee·o·file) *n.* [*opium* + *-phile*]. An addict of opium; an opium smoker or eater.

opip·ra·mol (o·pip′ruh·mol) *n.* 4-[3-(5*H*-Dibenz[*b,f*]azepin-5-yl)propyl]-1-piperazineethanol, $C_{23}H_{29}N_3O$, a tranquilizer and antidepressant drug; used as the dihydrochloride salt.

opisth-, opistho- [Gk. *opisthe*, after, behind]. A combining form meaning (a) *posterior, dorsal;* (b) *backward.*

opis·then (o·pis′thun) *n.* [Gk., after, behind]. *In biology*, the hind part of the body of an animal.

opis·the·nar (o·pis′thi·nahr) *n.* [*opisth-* + Gk. *thenar*, palm of the hand]. The back of the hand. Contr. *thenar.*

opis·thi·on (o·pis′thee·on) *n.* [Gk., hinder, posterior]. *In craniometry*, the point where the sagittal plane cuts the posterior margin of the foramen magnum.

opistho-. See *opisth-.*

opis·tho·cra·ni·on (o·pis″tho·kray′nee·on) *n.* [*opistho-* + Gk. *cranion*, skull]. *In craniometry*, the point, wherever it may lie in the sagittal plane on the occipital bone, which marks the posterior extremity of the longest diameter of the skull, measured from the glabella.

Op·is·thog·ly·pha (o″pis·thog′li·fluh) *n.pl.* [NL., from *opistho-* + E. *glyph*, vertical groove]. The group of snakes which includes the boomslang and the other venomous species of the Colubridae family, few of which are dangerous to man; distinguished by the presence of grooved rear fangs. Contr. *Aglypha, Proteroglypha, Solenoglypha.*

opis·thog·na·thism (o″pis·thog′nuh·thiz·um, ·tho′nuh·thiz·um, op″is·) *n.* [*opistho-* + *gnath-* + *-ism*]. Recession of the lower jaw.

opis·tho·neph·ros (o·pis″tho·nef′ros) *n.* [*opistho-* + *nephros*]. The mesonephros of certain Anamniota, in which the functional kidney arises from all nephrotomes caudal to the pronephros.

opis·tho·po·reia (o·pis″tho·po·rye′uh) *n.* [*opistho-* + Gk. *poreia*, mode of walking]. Involuntary walking backward in an attempt to go forward; occurs occasionally in postencephalitic parkinsonism.

opis·thor·chi·a·sis (o·pis″thor·kigh′uh·sis, op″is·) *n.* [*Opisthorchis* + *-iasis*]. Infection of the liver with the fluke *Opisthorchis felineus.*

Op·is·thor·chis (op″is·thor′kis, o″pis·) *n.* [*opisth-* + Gk. *orchis*, testis]. A genus of trematodes or flukes.

Opisthorchis fe·lin·e·us (fe·lin′ee·us, fe·lye′nee·us). A species of fluke naturally parasitic to cats, dogs, foxes, and hogs, and accidentally to man. Produces hepatic lesions and extensive hyperplasia of the biliary ducts.

Opisthorchis no·ver·ca (no·vur′kuh). A species of fluke parasitic to dogs and pigs in India, rarely found in man.

Opisthorchis vi·ver·ri·ni (viv″ur·eye′nye). A natural parasite of civet, dog, and cat, and an important human infection in northern Thailand.

op·is·thot·o·nus, op·is·thot·o·nos (op″is·thot′uh·nus) *n.* [Gk. *opisthotonos*, drawn backwards]. A postural abnormality characterized by hypertension of the back and neck muscles, with retraction of the head, and arching forward of the trunk. It is seen in its most dramatic forms in cases of severe meningeal irritation, particularly bacterial meningitis, but also in advanced states of decerebration and spasticity due to various causes. Contr. *orthotonus.*—**opis·thoto·noid** (·noid), **opis·tho·ton·ic** (o·pis″tho·ton′ick) *adj.*

opi·um (o′pee·um) *n.* [L., from Gk. *opion*, poppy juice]. The air-dried juice from unripe capsules of *Papaver somniferum*, or its variety *album.* It contains a number of alkaloids, of which morphine is the most important, since it represents the chief properties of the drug. Crude opium contains 5 to 15% morphine, 2 to 8% narcotine, 0.1 to 2.5% codeine, 0.5 to 2.0% papaverine, 0.15 to 0.5% thebaine, 0.1 to 0.4% narceine, and lesser amounts of cryptopine, laudanine, and other alkaloids. Opium acts as a narcotic, dulls pain and discomfort, and produces deep sleep. The drug is used for the relief of pain of all forms except that due to cerebral inflammation. Used in the form of a standardized powder (10% morphine), extract (20% morphine), and tincture (1% morphine).

opo- [Gk. *opos*]. *In pharmacology*, a combining form meaning *juice.*

opo·ceph·a·lus (op″o·sef′uh·lus) *n.* [Gk. *ōps, ōpos*, eye, + *-cephalus*]. A fetus with cyclopia, arrhinia, agnathia, and synotia; a form of cyclotia.

opo·did·y·mus (op″o·did′i·mus) *n.* [Gk. *ōps, ōpos*, eye, face, + *didymus*]. DIPROSOPUS.

opod·y·mus (o·pod′i·mus) *n.* [Gk. *ōps, ōpos*, eye, face, + *didymus*]. DIPROSOPUS.

O point. The point of the apex cardiogram at the maximum inward motion of the cardiac apex, occurring at the time of opening of the mitral valve.

Op·pen·heim's disease (o^hp'^en·hime) [H. *Oppenheim*, German neurologist, 1858–1919]. 1. *Obsol.* AMYOTONIA CONGENITA. See also *floppy infant syndrome.* 2. DYSTONIA MUSCULORUM DEFORMANS.

Oppenheim's reflex [H. *Oppenheim*]. A great-toe reflex elicited by stroking downward along the medial side of the tibia, a sign of corticospinal-tract lesion.

Oppenheim-Ur·bach disease [M. *Oppenheim*, Austrian dermatologist, b. 1876; and E. *Urbach*, U.S. dermatologist, 1893–1946]. NECROBIOSIS LIPOIDICA.

op·pi·la·tion (op''i·lay'shun) *n.* [L. *oppilatio*, an obstructing]. Obstruction; a closing of the pores. —**op·pi·la·tive** (op'i·lay·tiv) *adj.*

op·po·nens (op·o'nenz) *adj.* [L.]. Opposing; applied to certain muscles that bring one part opposite another.

opponens di·gi·ti mi·ni·mi (dij'i·tye min'i·migh). 1. (of the hand:) An intrinsic muscle of the hand that aids in opposing the little finger to the thumb. NA *musculus opponens digiti minimi.* See also Table of Muscles in the Appendix. 2. (of the foot:) The opponens digiti quinti of the foot. See Table of Muscles in the Appendix.

opponens digiti quin·ti (kwin'tye). 1. (of the hand:) OPPONENS DIGITI MINIMI (1). 2. (of the foot:) See Table of Muscles in the Appendix.

opponens pol·li·cis (pol'i·sis). A muscle that places the thumb opposite the little finger. NA *musculus opponens pollicis.* See also Table of Muscles in the Appendix.

op·por·tun·ist (op''ur·tew'nist) *n. In bacteriology,* an organism incapable of inducing disease in a healthy host, but able to produce infections in a less resistant or injured host; for example, certain types of *Escherichia coli* and the fusospirochetal group of synergistic organisms. —**oppor·tu·nis·tic** (·tew·nis'tick) *adj.*

ops- [Gk. *ōps*, eye]. A combining form meaning *sight, vision.*

-ops [Gk. *ōps*, eye]. *In botany and zoology,* a combining form meaning *-eyed.*

-opsia [Gk., from *opsis*, vision, + *-ia*]. A combining form designating a *condition of vision.*

op·sig·e·nes (op·sij'e·neez) *n.pl.* [Gk. *opsigenēs*, late-born]. Body tissues which come into use long after birth, as the wisdom teeth.

op·sin (op'sin) *n.* [Gk. *opsis*, sight, vision, + *-in*]. One of the colorless proteins in the rods and cones of the retina which, under the influence of light, complex with retinene to form one of the light-sensitive pigments. See also *cone opsin, rod opsin.*

op·sino·gen (op·sin'o·jen) *n.* [*opsonin* + *-gen*]. A substance producing an opsonin. —**opsi·nog·e·nous** (op''si·noj'e·nus) *adj.*

op·si·om·e·ter (op''see·om'e·tur) *n.* [Gk. *opsis*, vision, + *-meter*]. OPTOMETER.

op·si·o·no·sis (op''see·o·no'sis, op''see·on'uh·sis) *n.* [Gk. *opsis*, vision, + *-osis* (influenced by *nosos*, disease)]. A disease of the eye, or of vision.

op·si·uria (op''si·yoo'ree·uh) *n.* [Gk. *opse*, late, + *-uria*]. A condition in which more urine is excreted during fasting than during digestion after a meal.

op·so·clo·nia (op''so·klo'nee·uh) *n.* OPSOCLONUS.

op·so·clo·nus (op''so·klo'nus) *n.* [Gk. *ōps*, eye, + *clonus*]. Rapid, conjugate oscillations of the eyes in a horizontal, rotatory, or vertical direction, made worse by voluntary movement or the need to fixate the eyes, and usually associated with widespread myoclonus of diverse causes.

op·so·gen (op'so·jen) *n.* [*opsonin* + *-gen*]. OPSINOGEN.

op·so·ma·nia (op''so·may'nee·uh) *n.* [Gk. *opson*, rich food, delicacy, + *-mania*]. Intense craving for dainties or some special food. —**opsoma·ni·ac** (·nee·ack) *n.*

opsonic action. The effect produced upon susceptible microorganisms and other cells by opsonins, which renders them vulnerable to phagocytes.

opsonic index. The ratio of the opsonizing power of blood measured by in vitro phagocytosis of a particular organism compared to a normal standard.

op·so·nin (op'suh·nin, op·so'nin) *n.* [Gk. *opsōnion*, provisions, + *-in*]. Any of various substances, including some complement components and specific antibodies, which facilitate phagocytosis of microbial organisms; these substances may be increased by immunization. —**op·son·ic** (op·son'ick) *adj.*

op·so·nize (op'suh·nize) *v.* [*opsonin* + *-ize*]. To render microorganisms susceptible to phagocytosis. —**opso·ni·za·tion** (·zay'shun) *n.*

op·so·no·cy·to·phag·ic (op''suh·no·sigh''to·fay'jick, ·faj'ick) *adj.* [*opsonin* + *cytophagy* + *-ic*]. Pertaining to the phagocytic activity of blood containing serum opsonins and homologous leukocytes.

opsonocytophagic test. A test for brucellosis and tularemia in which the capacity of the leukocytes to phagocytize the causative organisms is determined.

op·so·nom·e·try (op''so·nom'e·tree) *n.* The estimation of the opsonic index.

op·so·no·ther·a·py (op''suh·no·therr'up·ee) *n.* The treatment of disease by increasing the opsonic action of the blood.

-opsy [Gk. *-opsia*, from *opsis*, vision, sight, appearance]. A combining form meaning (a) *examination;* (b) a *condition of vision.*

opt-, opto- [Gk. *optos*, seen, visible]. A combining form meaning *optic* or *vision* or *eye.*

op·tes·the·sia (op''tes·theezh'uh, ·theez'ee·uh) *n.* [*opt-* + *esthesia*]. Visual sensibility.

op·tic (op'tick) *adj.* [Gk. *optikos*]. Pertaining to the eye.

optic agraphia. Inability to copy.

op·ti·cal (op'ti·kul) *adj.* 1. OPTIC. 2. Pertaining to light and the science of optics.

optical activity. The ability of a substance to rotate the plane of vibration of polarized light. It is characteristic of compounds having an asymmetric atom, usually of carbon.

optical antipode. ENANTIOMORPH (1).

optical center. The point where the secondary axes of a refractive system meet and cross the principal axis.

optical cyclophoria. A form of cyclophoria due to uncorrected oblique astigmatism.

optical density. ABSORPTIVITY, as of solutions.

optical flat. A glass or quartz plate or disk, ground flat until any remaining unevenness can be measured only by interferometric methods, the maximum departure from flatness usually being less than $\frac{1}{10}$ of a wavelength of sodium light.

optical glass. An especially fine glass made under the most carefully controlled conditions. There are many kinds, some with low index and high dispersion values and some with high index and low dispersion.

optical index. A constant applied to objectives for purposes of comparison, taking into account the focal length or magnifying power of the lens and also the numerical aperture.

optical isomerism. The isomerism of substances having similar structural formulas and general properties but differing in their rotation of polarized light. See also *stereoisomerism.*

optical manometer. A device for the accurate registration of the details of pressure pulses, in which pressure changes are led through a rigid, fluid-filled system to a tense rubber or metallic membrane on which is mounted a small mirror. The deflections of a beam of light reflected from this mirror are recorded on moving photographic paper.

optical maser. LASER.

optical path difference. The product of the thickness of a specimen times its index of refraction.

optical righting reflex. Righting reflex initiated by the visual perception of an improper orientation of the body in reference to the horizon or to familiar objects.

optical rotation. The angle of rotation of the plane of polarization of polarized light when it passes through an optically active substance.

optic anesthesia. Temporary amaurosis.

optic angle. 1. The angle formed by the optical axes of the two eyes when directed to the same point. 2. VISUAL ANGLE.

optic aphasia. Loss of the ability to name an object clearly seen until it has been perceived through some other sense, such as hearing, touch, smell, or taste; a form of *amnesic aphasia.*

optic atrophy. Atrophy of the optic nerve. On funduscopic examination, the optic disk appears starkly white and sharply demarcated.

optic axis. An imaginary line passing through the midpoint of the cornea (anterior pole) and the midpoint of the retina (posterior pole). NA *axis opticus.*

optic canal. The channel at the apex of the orbit, the anterior termination of the optic groove, just beneath the lesser wing of the sphenoid bone; it gives passage to the optic nerve and ophthalmic artery. NA *canalis opticus.*

optic capsule. The embryonic structure forming the sclera.

optic center. VISUAL CENTER.

optic chiasma. The commissure anterior to the hypophysis where there is a partial decussation of the fibers in the optic nerves. NA *chiasma opticum.* See also Plates 17, 18.

optic chiasm syndrome. CHIASMA SYNDROME.

optic commissure. OPTIC CHIASMA.

optic cup. The double-walled cup formed by invagination of the optic vesicle which differentiates into pigmented and sensory layers of the retina. NA *caliculus ophthalmicus.*

optic disk. The circular area in the retina that is the site of the convergence of fibers from the ganglion cells of the retina to form the optic nerve. NA *discus nervi optici.*

optic evagination. *In embryology,* the development of a hollow diverticulum, the antecedent of the optic cup, along the lateral forebrain.

optic foramen. OPTIC CANAL.

optic groove. CHIASMATIC GROOVE.

op·ti·cian (op·tish'un) *n.* [F. *opticien*]. A maker of optical instruments or lenses.

op·ti·cian·ry (op·tish'un·ree) *n.* The application of the art and science of optics to the compounding, filling, and adapting of ophthalmic prescriptions.

optic lobes. The superior colliculi of lower vertebrates. Syn. *corpora bigemina.*

optic nerve. The second cranial nerve; the sensory nerve that innervates the retina. NA *nervus opticus.* See also Table of Nerves in the Appendix.

optic neuritis. Acute impairment of vision in one eye or both, which may be affected simultaneously or successively, and which may recover spontaneously or leave the patient with a scotoma or scotomas, or even blindness. Usually due to demyelinative disease, sometimes to a toxic or nutritional disorder. See also *axial neuritis, optic neuromyelitis, optic perineuritis, retrobulbar neuritis, transverse optic neuritis.*

optic neuroencephalomyelopathy. NEUROMYELITIS OPTICA.

optic neuromyelitis. NEUROMYELITIS OPTICA.

op·ti·co·chi·as·mat·ic (op"ti·ko·kigh"az·mat'ick) *adj.* Pertaining to the optic nerves and optic chiasma.

opticochiasmatic arachnoiditis. Chronic localized inflammation of the meninges around the optic chiasma and optic nerves, with pressure on these structures by fibrous tissues, resulting in impairment of vision and optic atrophy; occasionally due to syphilis.

op·ti·co·chi·as·mic (op"ti·ko·kigh·az'mick) *adj.* OPTICOCHIASMATIC.

op·ti·co·cil·i·ary (op"ti·ko·sil'ee·err·ee) *adj.* Pertaining to the optic and ciliary nerves.

op·ti·coele (op'ti·seel) *n.* [*optic* + *-coele*]. The cavity of the optic vesicle.

op·ti·co·fa·cial (op"ti·ko·fay'shul) *adj.* Pertaining to the optic and facial nerves.

opticofacial reflex. WINKING REFLEX.

op·ti·co·ki·net·ic (op"ti·ko·ki·net'ick, ·kigh·net'ick) *adj.* OPTOKINETIC.

op·ti·co·pu·pil·lary (op"ti·ko·pew'pil·err·ee) *adj.* Pertaining to the optic nerve and the pupil.

optic papilla. OPTIC DISK.

optic perineuritis. Inflammation of the optic nerve sheaths.

optic radiation. The geniculocalcarine tract, connecting the lateral geniculate body with the calcarine occipital area of the cortex. Syn. *Gratiolet's optic radiation.* NA *radiatio optica.*

optic recess. A recess in front of the infundibular recess which extends downward and forward above the optic chiasma. NA *recessus opticus.* See also Plate 18.

op·tics (op'ticks) *n.* [*optic* + *-s*]. That branch of physics treating of the laws of light, its refraction and reflection, and its relation to vision.

optic stalk. The narrow median part of the optic vesicle and cup which forms a pathway for the developing optic nerve.

optic stratum. The third layer of the superior colliculus, composed mainly of fibers from the ganglion cells of the retina and corticostriate fibers arising from the visual cortex; these fibers enter through the brachium of the superior colliculus and end mainly in the superficial and middle gray layers of the superior colliculus. Syn. *stratum opticum.*

optic tabes. Optic atrophy resulting from syphilis.

optic tectum. OPTIC LOBES.

optic tract. A band of nerve fibers running around the lateral side of a cerebral peduncle from the optic chiasma to the lateral geniculate body and midbrain. NA *tractus opticus.*

optic vesicle. The embryonic evagination of the diencephalon from which are derived the pigment and sensory layers of the retina. NA *vesicula ophthalmica.*

op·ti·mal (op'ti·mul) *adj.* [*optimum* + *-al*]. Most desirable or satisfactory.

op·tim·e·ter (op·tim'e·tur) *n.* OPTOMETER.

op·ti·mum (op'ti·mum) *n.* [L.]. The amount or degree of something, such as temperature, that is most favorable, desirable, or satisfactory for some end or purpose.

opto-. See *opt-.*

op·to·chi·as·mic (op"to·kigh·az'mick) *adj.* OPTICOCHIASMATIC.

optochiasmic arachnoiditis. OPTICOCHIASMATIC ARACHNOIDITIS.

Optochin. Trademark for ethylhydrocupreine, a pneumococcidal agent.

Optochin test. A test for identification of *Streptococcus pneumoniae* in the clinical laboratory.

op·to·gram (op'to·gram) *n.* [*opto-* + *-gram*]. An image made on the retina by the sensitiveness to light of pigment in the eye.

op·to·ki·net·ic (op"to·kigh·net'ick) *adj.* [*opto-* + *kinetic*]. Of or pertaining to eye movements associated with movement of objects in the visual field.

optokinetic nystagmus. Nystagmus which occurs in normal individuals when a succession of moving objects traverses the field of vision, or when the individual moves past a succession of stationary objects. Syn. *train nystagmus.*

op·tom·e·ter (op·tom'e·tur) *n.* [*opto-* + *-meter*]. An instrument for determining the power of vision, especially the degree of refractive error that is to be corrected.

op·tom·e·trist (op·tom'e·trist) *n.* [*optometry* + *-ist*]. One who measures the degrees of visual powers, without the aid of a cycloplegic or mydriatic; a refractionist.

op·tom·e·try (op·tom'e·tree) *n.* [*opto-* + *-metry*]. Measurement of the visual powers.

op·to·my·om·e·ter (op"to·migh·om'e·tur) *n.* [*opto-* + *myo-* +

-meter]. An instrument for measuring the strength of the extrinsic muscles of the eye.

op·to·type (op'to·tipe) *n.* [*opto-* + *type*]. A test type used in determining the acuity of vision.

-or [L.]. A suffix indicating *an agent or doer.*

¹ora (o'ruh) *n.* [L.]. MARGIN.

²ora. Plural of *os* (L., mouth).

orad (or'ad) *adv.* [L. *os, oris*, mouth, + *-ad*, toward]. Toward the mouth, or the oral region.

Oragrafin. Trademark for calcium ipodate (Oragrafin Calcium) and sodium ipodate (Oragrafin Sodium), compounds administered orally for radiographic visualization of the biliary system.

oral (or'ul) *adj.* [L. *os, oris*, mouth, + *-al*]. Pertaining to the mouth.

oral arch. MANDIBULAR ARCH.

oral candidiasis. An infection in the mouth by *Candida albicans*, occurring frequently in young infants.

oral cavity. The cavity of the mouth. NA *cavum oris.* See also *primary oral cavity, secondary oral cavity.*

oral character. A Freudian term applied to persons who, during the developmental period, have undergone an unusual degree of oral stimulation through poor feeding habits and otherwise and who thereby have laid the basis for a particular type of character, usually characterized by a general attitude of carefree indifference and by dependence on a mother or mother substitute to provide for their needs throughout life with little or no effort of their own.

oral contraceptive. Any medication taken by mouth that inhibits fertility in a woman as long as the medication is continued.

oral diaphragm. The diaphragm formed by the mylohyoid and hyoglossus muscles, separating the sublingual from the submandibular region.

ora·le (o·rah'lee, o·ray'lee) *n.* [ML., oral]. *In craniometry*, the point on the anterior portion of the hard palate where the line, drawn tangent to the lingual margins of the alveoli of the medial incisor teeth and projected upon the hard palate, crosses the sagittal plane.

oral erotic stage. *In psychoanalysis*, the first, or receptive, part of the oral phase of psychosexual development, dominated by sucking and lasting for the first 6 to 9 months of life. Compare *oral sadistic stage.*

oral erotism. *In psychiatry*, the primordial pleasurable experience of nursing, reappearing in usually disguised and sublimated form in later life. See also *oral phase, oral personality.*

oral expressive aphasia. BROCA'S APHASIA.

oral medicine. The general area of dental practice concerned with diagnosis, treatment planning, etiology, and medical therapeutics as related to dentistry.

oral membrane. BUCCOPHARYNGEAL MEMBRANE.

oral moniliasis. ORAL CANDIDIASIS.

oral pathology. The branch of dental science concerned with diseases and disorders of the oral cavity, the teeth, and the jaws.

oral personality. An individual who is mouth-centered far beyond the age when the oral phase should have been passed, and who exhibits oral erotism and sadism in disguised and sublimated forms.

oral phase. *In psychoanalysis*, the initial stage in the psychosexual development of a child, extending from birth to about 18 months, in which the mouth is the focus of sensations, interests, and activities and hence the source of gratification and security. It is conceived as progressing from an oral erotic stage to an oral sadistic stage. See also *oral erotism, oral personality.*

oral physiotherapy. The procedures practiced by the individual to maintain mouth hygiene and properly stimulate the soft tissues surrounding the teeth.

oral plate. BUCCOPHARYNGEAL MEMBRANE.

oral sadistic stage. *In psychoanalysis*, the later, or aggressive, part of the oral phase of psychosexual development, lasting from about the eighth to the eighteenth month, in which the pleasure of biting is added to that of sucking. Compare *oral erotic stage.*

oral sinus. STOMODEUM.

oral stage. ORAL PHASE.

oral surgery. That branch of dental science which is concerned with surgical procedures involving the oral cavity, particularly the teeth and jaws.

oral treponemas. Organisms such as *Treponema macrodentium, T. microdentium*, and *T. mucosum*, of no proved pathogenicity, which are found in the mouth.

oral vestibule. VESTIBULE OF THE MOUTH.

orange flower oil. A complex volatile oil distilled from the fresh flowers of *Citrus aurantium* and used for its odor. Syn. *neroli oil.*

orange G. An acid monoazo dye; used as a counterstain with nuclear stains.

orange oil. A volatile oil obtained by expression from the fresh peel of *Citrus sinensis.* Used as a flavor.

ora ser·ra·ta (se·ray'tuh) [NA]. The serrated margin of the sensory portion of the retina, behind the ciliary body.

Or·be·li effect or **phenomenon** (ahr·b^y^e^y^'lee) [L. A. *Orbeli*, Russian physiologist, 1882–1958]. Increased contraction of a fatigued muscle which occurs when its sympathetic nerve supply is stimulated.

Orbenin. A trademark for the sodium salt of cloxacillin, a semisynthetic penicillin antibiotic.

or·bic·u·lar (or·bick'yoo·lur) *adj.* [L. *orbicularis*, circular]. Circular; applied to circular muscles, as the orbicular muscle of the eye (orbicularis oculi) or of the mouth (orbicularis oris).

or·bi·cu·la·re (or·bick"yoo·lair'ee) *n.* [L.]. The orbicular bone, a tubercle at the end of the long process of the incus; it is separate in early fetal life.

or·bi·cu·la·ris (or·bick"yoo·lair'is) *n.* [L.]. An orbicular muscle.

orbicularis ocu·li (ock'yoo·lye). The ring muscle of the eye. NA *musculus orbicularis oculi.* See also Table of Muscles in the Appendix.

orbicularis oculi reflex. SUPRAORBITAL REFLEX.

orbicularis oris (o'ris). The ring muscle of the mouth. NA *musculus orbicularis oris.* See also Table of Muscles in the Appendix.

orbicularis oris reflex. A facial reflex in which percussion over the upper lip or angle of the mouth is followed by a contraction of the levator labii superioris and levator anguli oris on the same side; usually seen in patients with corticobulbar lesions above the facial nucleus.

orbicularis pal·pe·bra·rum (pal"pe·brair'um) [L., of the eyelids]. ORBICULARIS OCULI.

orbicularis sign. REVILLIOD'S SIGN.

or·bi·cu·lus (or·bick'yoo·lus) *n.*, pl. **orbicu·li** (·lye) [L.]. A small disk.

orbiculus ci·li·a·ris (sil·ee·air'is) [NA]. CILIARY RING.

or·bit, *n.* [L. *orbita*, track, course]. The bony cavity containing the eye, which is formed by parts of the frontal, sphenoid, ethmoid, nasal, lacrimal, maxillary, and palatal bones. NA *orbita.* See also Plate 19.

or·bi·ta (or'bi·tuh) *n.*, pl. **orbi·tae** (·tee) [NA]. ORBIT.

or·bi·tal (or'bi·tul) *adj.* & *n.* 1. Of or pertaining to an orbit. 2. Any of certain fibers of smooth muscle bridging the inferior orbital fissure. NA *musculus orbitalis.* 3. Any one of the permissible modes of motion of an electron in an atom or molecule.

orbital canal. ETHMOID CANAL.

orbital cellulitis. An infection of the orbit usually associated with acute sinusitis and characterized by conjunctival edema and proptosis with subsequent motion limitation and diplopia.

orbital decompression. Cranial decompression by an approach in the orbital region.

or·bi·ta·le (or″bi·tah′lee, ·tay′lee) *n.*, pl. **orbi·ta·lia** (·tay′lee·uh, ·tal′ee·uh) [NL., orbital]. *In craniometry,* the lowest point on the inferior margin of the orbit, used in conjunction with the poria to orient the skull on the Frankfort horizontal plane.

orbital fork. FURCA ORBITALIS.

orbital gyri. Four convolutions—the anterior, posterior, lateral, and medial orbital gyri—which compose the inferior surface of the frontal lobe. NA *gyri orbitales.*

orbital height. *In craniometry,* the greatest vertical width of the external opening of the orbit.

orbitalia. Plural of *orbitale.*

orbital index. *In craniometry,* the ratio of the orbital height, taken at right angles to the orbital width between the upper and lower orbital margins, times 100, to the orbital width, taken between the maxillofrontale and lateral margin of the orbit in such a manner that the line of the orbital width bisects the plane of the orbital entrance. Values of the index are classified as follows: chamaeconch, x–75.9; mesoconch, 76.0–84.9; hypsiconch, 85.0–x.

or·bi·ta·lis (or″bi·tay′lis) *n.* An orbital muscle.

orbital lobe. The part of the frontal lobe which rests on the orbital plate of the frontal bone.

orbital operculum. The portion of the orbital gyri of the cerebrum overlying the insula.

orbital plane. 1. *In craniometry,* a plane passing through the two orbital points and perpendicular to the Frankfort horizontal plane. 2. FACIES ORBITALIS MAXILLAE.

orbital plate. One of two thin, triangular plates of the frontal bone which form the vaults of the orbits.

orbital process of the palatine bone. A process directed upward and outward from the upper portion of the palatine bone. NA *processus orbitalis ossis palatini.*

orbital process of the zygomatic bone. The orbital surface of the zygomatic bone, a thick plate projecting backward and medially from the orbital margin.

orbital septum. A sheet of fascia attached to the anterior edge of the orbit where it is continuous with the periosteum. NA *septum orbitale.*

orbital sulci. Several grooves on the inferior surface of the frontal lobe dividing it into four orbital gyri. NA *sulci orbitales.*

or·bi·to·na·sal (or″bi·to·nay′zul) *adj.* Pertaining to the orbit of the skull and the nasal cavity.

orbitonasal index. *In somatometry,* the ratio of the orbitonasal width, taken with a tape measure from the lateral margins of the orbits at the level of the lateral angles of the palpebral fissures, the tape measure passing over the lowest portion of the root of the nose, times 100, to the external orbital width, taken directly with a sliding or spreading caliper from the stated points. Values of the index are classified as follows: platyopic, x–109.9; mesopic, 110.0–112.9; prosopic, 113.0–x.

or·bi·to·nom·e·ter (or″bi·to·nom′e·tur) *n.* [*orbit* + *tonometer*]. A devise used to measure the resistance to pressure of the eye into the orbit in cases of exophthalmic goiter.

or·bi·to·nom·e·try (or″bi·to·nom′e·tree) *n.* The measurement of the resistance of the globe of the eye to retrodisplacement.

or·bi·to·sphe·noid bone (or″bi·to·sfee′noid). The orbital portion of the sphenoid bone, separate in certain lower vertebrates and in embryos, represented by the smaller wing of the sphenoid bone in mammals.

or·bi·to·tem·po·ral (or″bi·to·tem′puh·rul) *adj.* Pertaining to the orbit and the temple.

or·bi·tot·o·my (or″bi·tot′um·ee) *n.* [*orbit* + *-tomy*]. Incision into the orbit.

or·ce·in (or′seen, or·see′in) *n.* A brownish red crystalline powder, containing many components, obtained by oxidation of orcinol; insoluble in water, soluble in alcohol. Used in microscopy as a stain.

orch-. See *orchi-.*

or·che·itis (or″kee·eye′tis) *n.* ORCHITIS.

or·ches·tro·ma·nia (or·kes″tro·may′nee·uh) *n.* [Gk. *orchēstēr,* dancer, + *-mania*]. *Obsol.* SYDENHAM'S CHOREA.

orchi-, orchio-, orchid-, orchido-, orch- [Gk. *orchis, orchios,* testicle]. A combining form meaning *testis.*

or·chi·al·gia (or″kee·al′juh, ·jee·uh) *n.* [*orchi-* + *-algia*]. Testicular pain.

or·chic (or′kick) *adj.* [Gk. *orchikos*]. Pertaining to the testis.

orchid-, orchido-. See *orchi-.*

or·chi·dal·gia (or″ki·dal′juh, ·jee·uh) *n.* ORCHIALGIA.

or·chi·dec·to·my (or″ki·deck′tum·ee) *n.* ORCHIECTOMY.

or·chi·di·tis (or″ki·digh′tis) *n.* ORCHITIS.

orchido-. See *orchi-.*

or·chi·dop·a·thy (or″ki·dop′uth·ee) *n.* [*orchido-* + *-pathy*]. Disease of a testis.

or·chi·do·pexy (or′ki·do·peck″see, or·kid′o·) *n.* ORCHIOPEXY.

or·chi·do·plas·ty (or′ki·do·plas″tee, or·kid′o·) *n.* ORCHIOPLASTY.

or·chi·dor·rha·phy (or″ki·dor′uh·fee) *n.* [*orchido-* + *-rraphy*]. ORCHIOPEXY.

or·chi·dot·o·my (or″ki·dot′um·ee) *n.* [*orchido-* + *-tomy*]. Incision into a testis.

or·chi·ec·to·my (or″kee·eck′tum·ee) *n.* [*orchi-* + *-ectomy*]. Surgical removal of one or both testes; castration.

or·chi·en·ceph·a·lo·ma (or″kee·en·sef″uh·lo′ma) *n.* [*orchi-* + *encephal-* + *-oma*]. An encephaloid carcinoma of the testis.

or·chi·epi·did·y·mi·tis (or″kee·ep″i·did″i·migh′tis) *n.* [*orchi-* + *epididym-* + *-itis*]. Inflammation of both testis and epididymis.

orchio-. See *orchi-.*

or·chio·ca·tab·a·sis (or″kee·o·ka·tab′uh·sis) *n.* [*orchio-* + Gk. *katabasis,* descent]. The normal descent of the testis into the scrotum.

or·chio·cele (or′kee·o·seel) *n.* [*orchio-* + *-cele*]. 1. A complete scrotal hernia. 2. A tumor of the testis. 3. Herniation of a testis. 4. A testis retained in the inguinal canal.

or·chi·op·a·thy (or″kee·op′uth·ee) *n.* [*orchio-* + *-pathy*]. Any disease of the testis.

or·chio·pexy (or′kee·o·peck″see) *n.* [*orchio-* + *-pexy*]. Surgical fixation of a testis, as in a plastic operation for relief of an undescended testis.

or·chio·plas·ty (or′kee·o·plas″tee) *n.* [*orchio-* + *-plasty*]. Plastic surgery of a testis.

or·chi·ot·o·my (or″kee·ot″um·ee) *n.* [*orchio-* + *-tomy*]. ORCHIDOTOMY.

or·chis (or′kis) *n.* [Gk.]. TESTIS.

or·chi·tis (or·kigh′tis) *n.* [*orch-* + *-itis*]. Inflammation of the testis. —**orchit·ic** (·kit′ick) *adj.*

or·chit·o·my (or·kit′um·ee) *n.* [*orchi-* + *-tomy*]. ORCHIDOTOMY.

or·chot·o·my (or·kot′um·ee) *n.* ORCHIDOTOMY.

or·ci·nol (or′si·nol) *n.* 5-Methylresorcinol, $C_7H_8O_2.H_2O$, a constituent of many species of lichens, variously used as a reagent.

or·der, *n.* [L. *ordo*]. 1. Systematic arrangement. 2. *In biology,* the taxonomic group below a class and above a family.

or·der·ly, *n.* A male hospital attendant.

or·di·nate (or′din·ut) *n.* [L. *ordinatus,* ordered]. The vertical line of the two coordinates used in plotting the interrelationship of two sets of data. Contr. *abscissa.*

Orestralyn. A trademark for the estrogen ethynyl estradiol.

Oretic. A trademark for hydrochlorothiazide, an orally effective diuretic and antihypertensive drug.

Oreton. A trademark for certain preparations or derivatives of the androgen testosterone.

Oreton M. A trademark for the androgen methyltestosterone.

-orexia [Gk. *orexis,* appetency, desire, + *-ia*]. A combining form meaning *a condition of the appetite.*

orex·ia (o·reck'see·uh) *n.* OREXIS.

orex·is (o·reck'sis) *n.* [Gk., desire, yearning, appetency]. The aspect of mental functioning or of an act which pertains to feeling, desire, impulse, volition, or purposeful striving as contrasted with its cognitive or intellectual aspect.

orf, *n.* A pox virus disease of sheep and goats that is transmittable to humans, characterized by red vesicular or pustular lesions on the lips, oral mucosa, udder, and feet. Syn. *ecthyma contagiosum.* See also *contagious pustular dermatitis.*

or·gan, *n.* [Gk. *organon,* instrument]. A differentiated part of an organism adapted for a definite function. NA *organum.*

organa. Plural of *organum* and *organon.*

organa ge·ni·ta·lia fe·mi·ni·na (jen''i·tay'lee·uh fem·i·nigh'nuh) [NA]. Female genital organs.

organa genitalia mas·cu·li·na (mas''kew·lye'nuh) [NA]. Male genital organs.

organa genitalia mu·li·e·bria (mew·lee·ee'bree·uh) [BNA]. ORGANA GENITALIA FEMININA.

organa genitalia vi·ri·lia (vi·rye'lee·uh) [BNA]. ORGANA GENITALIA MASCULINA.

organa ocu·li ac·ces·so·ria (ock'yoo·lye ack·se·so'ree·uh) [NA]. ADNEXA OCULI.

organa sen·su·um (sen'sue·um) [NA]. The sensory organs.

organa uro·po·ë·ti·ca (yoo''ro·po·et'i·kuh) [NA]. URINARY SYSTEM.

or·gan·elle (or·guh·nel') *n.* [NL. *organella,* diminutive from *organum,* organ]. A specialized structure or part of a cell presumably having a special function or capacity, as a mitochondrion. —**organel·lar** (·ur) *adj.*

organ erotism. Sexual desire localized in an organ of the body.

or·gan·ic, *adj.* [Gk. *organikos,* instrumental]. 1. Of or pertaining to organs; having organs. 2. Of or pertaining to living organisms. 3. *In chemistry,* of or pertaining to compounds of carbon. 4. Physical, as contrasted with mental, emotional, or psychogenic, particularly as applied to any disorder for which there is a known or hypothesized impairment of structure, biochemistry, or physiology. Contr. *functional.* 5. Pertaining to foods grown and produced without the use of artificial fertilizers or pesticides.

organic absorption. INTERNAL ABSORPTION.

organic acid. Commonly, any acid containing the carboxyl group —COOH.

organic analysis. Analysis of organic chemical substances.

organic brain syndrome or **disorder.** Any nervous disorder either known to have a physical cause or presumed, because it produces physical symptoms, to have one.

organic chemistry. Chemistry of carbon compounds.

organic compound. Any compound containing carbon, exclusive of salts of carbonic acid.

organic contracture. A contracture that persists even when the person is unconscious.

organic disease. A disease associated with recognizable structural changes in the organs or tissues of the body.

organic driv·en·ness (driv'un·nis). The hyperactivity seen in the minimal brain dysfunction syndrome.

organic impotence. Impotence due to some anatomic defect in the sexual organs; may occur in either male or female. Contr. *psychic impotence.*

or·gan·i·cism (or·gan'i·siz·um) *n.* HOLISM.

or·gan·i·cist (or·gan'i·sist) *n.* *In psychiatry,* one who believes that emotional disorders are based upon organic change or disease.

organic murmur. A murmur due to structural changes in the heart, or in other organs such as blood vessels or lungs.

organic psychosis. ORGANIC BRAIN SYNDROME.

organic scoliosis. Scoliosis due to a disease process, as one which affects the spine, such as rickets or infections, or one which affects the muscles which support the spine, such as paralysis; due to deformities of the thoracic cage, as following empyema; or due to disease of the hip or leg.

or·gan·ism (or'guh·niz·um) *n.* [*organ* + *-ism*]. Any living entity having differentiated members with specialized functions that are interdependent, and that is so constituted as to form a unified whole capable of carrying on life processes.

or·ga·ni·za·tion, *n.* 1. The systematic interrelationships of structurally and functionally differentiated parts to form an integrated whole. 2. A part of the repair process occurring in an injury that has destroyed tissue; the ingrowth of capillaries and fibroblasts into thrombi or blood clots.

organization center. ORGANIZER.

or·ga·nize, *v.* 1. To make organic, to form into an organism; to induce to form or develop. 2. To induce to or undergo organization (2).

organized ferment. INTRACELLULAR ENZYME.

or·ga·niz·er, *n.* *In embryology,* the region of the dorsal lip of the blastopore, comprising chordamesoderm, that is self-differentiating and capable of inducing the formation of medullary plate in the adjacent ectoderm; the primary organizer. A second-grade (or higher) organizer, coming into play after the laying down of the main axis of the body induced by the primary organizer is completed, is any part of the embryo which exerts a morphogenetic stimulus on an adjacent part or parts, as in the induction of the lens by the optic vesicle. Syn. *organization center.*

organizing pneumonia. Pneumonia in which the healing process is characterized by organization and cicatrization of the exudate rather than by resolution and resorption. Syn. *unresolved pneumonia.*

organ neurosis. *In psychiatry,* an emotional illness with functional and often anatomic alterations. See also *psychophysiologic disorders.*

organo-. A combining form meaning (a) *organ;* (b) *organic.*

or·ga·no·ax·i·al (or''guh·no·ack'see·ul) *adj.* Rotated around the long axis of the organ, as an organoaxial volvulus.

organ of Corti [A. *Corti*]. SPIRAL ORGAN OF CORTI.

organ of Golgi. CORPUSCLE OF GOLGI.

organ of Jacobson [L. L. *Jacobson*]. VOMERONASAL ORGAN.

or·gano·gel (or·gan'o·jel) *n.* A gel in which the dispersion medium is an organic liquid.

or·ga·no·gen·e·sis (or''guh·no·jen'e·sis) *n.* [*organo-* + *-genesis*]. Development and growth of the various organs of the plant or animal body. —**organo·ge·net·ic** (·je·net'ick) *adj.*

or·ga·nog·e·ny (or''guh·noj'e·nee) *n.* [*organo-* + *-geny*]. ORGANOGENESIS.

or·gan·oid (or'guh·noid) *adj.* Resembling an organ.

organoid tumor. A tumor in which the components are so arranged as to resemble the general structure of an organ, as an adenoma.

or·ga·nol·o·gy (or''guh·nol'uh·jee) *n.* [*organo-* + *-logy*]. The science that treats of the organs of plants and animals.

or·ga·no·meg·a·ly (or''guh·no·meg'uh·lee) *n.* [*organo-* + *-megaly*]. SPLANCHNOMEGALY.

or·gano·mer·cu·ri·al (or·gan''o·mur·kew'ree·ul, or''guh·no·) *n.* An organic compound or substance containing mercury.

or·gano·me·tal·lic (or·gan''o·me·tal'ick, or''guh·no·) *adj.* Pertaining to compounds having a carbon to metal linkage.

or·ga·non (or'guh·non) *n.*, pl. **orga·na** (·nuh) [Gk.] [BNA]. Organum (= ORGAN).

organon au·di·tus (aw·dye'tus) [BNA]. ORGANUM VESTIBULOCOCHLEARE.

organon gus·tus (gus'tus) [BNA]. Organum gustus (= GUSTATORY ORGAN).

organon ol·fac·tus (ol·fack'tus) [BNA]. ORGANUM OLFACTUS.

organon pa·ren·chy·ma·to·sum (pa·reng''ki·muh·to'sum) [BNA]. Any parenchymatous organ.

organon spi·ra·le (spye·ray'lee) [BNA]. Organum spirale (= SPIRAL ORGAN OF CORTI).

organon vi·sus (vye'sus) [BNA]. ORGANUM VISUS.

organon vo·me·ro·na·sa·le (vom''e·ro·na·say'lee) [BNA]. Organum vomeronasale (= VOMERONASAL ORGAN).

or·ga·nos·co·py (or''guh·nos'kuh·pee) *n.* [*organo-* + *-scopy*].

The examination of an organ with a special lens system, such as a cystoscope, esophagoscope, or laryngoscope.

or·gano·sol (or·gan'o·sol) *n.* [*organo-* + *sol*]. A colloidal solution in which the dispersion medium is an organic liquid (alcohol, benzene, ether, etc.).

or·ga·no·ther·a·py (or"guh·no·therr'up·ee) *n.* The treatment of diseases by administration of animal organs or their extracts.

or·ga·no·troph·ic (or"guh·no·trof'ick, ·tro'fick) *adj.* [*organo-* + *trophic*]. Pertaining to the nutrition of living organs.

or·ga·no·trop·ic (or"ga·no·trop'ick, ·tro'pick) *adj.* [*organo-* + *-tropic*]. Pertaining to organotropism. —**orga·not·ro·py** (·not'ruh·pee) *n.*

or·ga·not·ro·pism (or"guh·no·tro'piz·um, or"guh·not'ruh·piz·um) *n.* [*organo-* + *-tropism*]. Ehrlich's theory that certain substances manifest a definite chemical affinity for certain components of cells.

organs of generation. GENERATIVE ORGANS.

organs of Zuckerkandl [E. *Zuckerkandl*]. PARAGANGLIA.

or·ga·num (or'guh·num) *n.*, pl. **orga·na** (·nuh) [L.] [NA]. ORGAN.

organum gus·tus (gus'tus) [NA]. GUSTATORY ORGAN.

organum ol·fac·tus (ol·fack'tus) [NA]. An olfactory organ.

organum spi·ra·le (spye·ray'lee) [NA]. SPIRAL ORGAN (OF CORTI).

organum ve·sti·bu·lo·co·chle·a·re (ves·tib"yoo·lo·kock·lee·air'ee) [NA]. The peripheral organ associated with the sense of equilibrium and hearing; the entire internal ear.

organum vi·sus (vye'sus) [NA]. The peripheral organ associated with the sense of vision; the eyeball and its accessory structures.

organum vo·me·ro·na·sa·le (vom"e·ro·na·say'lee) [NA]. VOMERONASAL ORGAN.

or·gasm (or'gaz·um) *n.* [Gk. *orgasmos*]. The intense, diffuse, and subjectively pleasurable sensation experienced during sexual intercourse or genital manipulation, culminating, for the male, in seminal ejaculation and for the female, in myotonia with uterine contractions, warm suffusion, and pelvic throbbing sensations.

or·gas·mo·lep·sy (or·gaz'mo·lep"see) *n.* [*orgasm* + *-lepsy*]. A sudden loss of muscle tone during sexual orgasm, accompanied by a transitory loss of consciousness.

or·go·tein (or"go·teen) *n.* A water-soluble protein of relatively low molecular weight (about 34,000), obtained from bovine liver, that is chelated with two to four atoms of divalent metals, as magnesium and copper, per molecule of protein; used as an anti-inflammatory agent.

oriental bedbug. *CIMEX HEMIPTERUS.*

oriental sore. CUTANEOUS LEISHMANIASIS.

ori·en·ta·tion (or"ee·en·tay'shun) *n.* 1. *In psychology,* the act of determining one's relation to the environment or a specified aspect of it, such as time, person, or place. 2. The process of helping a person or persons to find their way about in a new situation; orientation program. 3. *In chemistry,* the relative positions of atoms or groups of atoms in certain molecules.

orienting reflex or **response.** 1. A response to a stimulus, such as touch, light, or noise, which results in an animal's or person's altering the position of his head, ears, eyes, or even the entire body, toward that stimulus. 2. A response to a new stimulus which neither is of such a nature as to elicit an unconditioned reflex nor has the background to result in a conditioned reflex.

or·i·fice (or'i·fis) *n.* [L. *orificium,* from *os, oris,* mouth]. An opening, an entrance to a cavity or tube. —**or·i·fi·cial** (or"i·fish'ul) *adj.*

ori·fi·ci·um (or"i·fish'ee·um) *n.*, pl. **orifi·cia** (·ee·uh) [L.]. ORIFICE.

orificium ex·ter·num ute·ri (ecks·tur'num yoo'tur·eye) [BNA]. OSTIUM UTERI.

orificium in·ter·num ute·ri (in·tur'num yoo'tur·eye) [BNA]. The opening between the inner end of the cervix and the uterine cavity.

orificium ure·te·ris (yoo·ree'tur·is) [BNA]. OSTIUM URETERIS.

orificium urethrae in·ter·num (in·tur'num) [BNA]. OSTIUM URETHRAE INTERNUM.

orificium urethrae mu·li·e·bris ex·ter·num (mew"lee·ee'bris ecks·tur'num) [BNA]. OSTIUM URETHRAE FEMINAE EXTERNUM.

orificium urethrae vi·ri·lis ex·ter·num (vi·rye'lis ecks·tur'num) [BNA]. OSTIUM URETHRAE MASCULINAE EXTERNUM.

orificium va·gi·nae (va·jye'nee) [BNA]. OSTIUM VAGINAE.

or·i·gin, *n.* [L. *origo, originis,* from *oriri,* to rise]. 1. The beginning or starting point of anything. 2. *In anatomy,* the end of attachment of a muscle which remains relatively fixed during contraction of the muscle. Contr. *insertion.*

original tuberculin. OLD TUBERCULIN.

Orinase. Trademark for tolbutamide, an orally effective hypoglycemic drug.

Oriodide 131. A trademark for sodium iodide I 131, a diagnostic and therapeutic radioisotope.

Ori·za·ba jalap [*Orizaba,* a mountain in Mexico]. IPOMEA.

Or·mond's syndrome. RETROPERITONEAL FIBROSIS.

Orms·by's method. A method for urea in which a blood filtrate is heated with diacetyl monoxime in acid solution and a yellow color develops. The color is deepened by oxidation with potassium persulfate and compared colorimetrically with a standard urea solution similarly treated.

or·ni·thine (or'ni·theen, ·thin) *n.* [Gk. *ornis, ornithos,* bird, + *-ine*]. α,δ-Diaminovaleric acid, $NH_2(CH_2)_3CHNH_2COOH$; an amino acid occurring in the urine of some birds, but not found in native proteins; an intermediate in the Krebs-Henseleit cycle of urea formation.

ornithine cycle. UREA CYCLE.

ornithine decarboxylase. An enzyme that catalyzes decarboxylation of ornithine to yield the amine putrescine and carbon dioxide.

or·ni·thi·ne·mia (or"ni·thi·nee'mee·uh) *n.* [*ornithine* + *-emia*]. HYPERORNITHINEMIA.

ornithine transaminase. An enzyme that causes ornithine to react with α-ketoglutarate to yield glutamic acid and glutamic acid semialdehyde; important in mammals in the pathway whereby arginine is converted to glutamic acid.

ornithine trans·car·ba·myl·ase (trans"kahr'bam·i·lace, kahr·bam'i·lace, ·laze). The enzyme that catalyzes carbamylation of ornithine to form citrulline, which is the first step in the biochemical synthesis of arginine.

Or·ni·thod·o·rus (or"ni·thod'uh·rus, or"nith·o·dor'us) *n.* [Gk. *ornis, ornithos,* bird, + *doros,* leather bag]. A genus of soft ticks of the family Argasidae including many species parasitic to man, some of which produce painful bites and inflammatory lesions. Several species are vectors of relapsing fever spirochetes, as *Ornithodorus moubata* in Africa, *O. talaje* in tropical America, and *O. rudis* in subtropical regions of the United States.

Ornithonyssus bacoti. *BDELLONYSSUS BACOTI.*

or·ni·tho·sis (or"ni·tho'sis) *n.* [Gk. *ornis, ornithos,* bird, + *-osis*]. Psittacosis contracted from birds other than parrots and parakeets.

or·ni·thyl (or'ni·thil) *n.* The univalent radical $NH_2CH_2CH_2CH_2CHNH_2CO$—, of the amino acid ornithine.

¹oro- [L. *os, oris,* mouth]. A combining form meaning *mouth* or *oral.*

²oro- [Gk. *oros,* whey, serum]. See *orrho-.*

oro·an·tral (or"o·an'trul) *adj.* [*oro-* + *antral*]. Pertaining to the mouth and the maxillary sinus.

oro·di·ag·no·sis (or"o·dye"ug·no'sis) *n.* [*oro-,* serum, + *diagnosis*]. Diagnosis by means of serologic tests.

oro·fa·cial (or"o·fay'shul) *adj.* [*oro-* + *facial*]. Of or pertaining to the mouth and face.

oro·gran·u·lo·cyte (or"o·gran'yoo·lo·site) *n.* [*oro-* + *granulo-*

cyte]. A living polymorphonuclear granulocyte found in saliva.

oro·na·sal (or″o·nay′zul) *adj.* Involving the mouth and the nose.

oronasal membrane. A double layer of epithelium separating the nasal pits from the stomodeum of the embryo. Syn. *bucconasal membrane.*

oron·o·sus (o·ron′uh·sus, or″o·no′sus) *n.* [Gk. *oros*, mountain, + *nosos*, sickness]. ALTITUDE SICKNESS.

oro·phar·ynx (or″o·făr′inks) *n.* The oral pharynx, situated below the level of the lower border of the soft palate and above the larynx, as distinguished from the nasopharynx and laryngeal pharynx. —**oro·pha·ryn·ge·al** (or″o·fa·rin′jee·ul) *adj.*

oro·sin (or′o·sin) *n.* [Gk. *oros*, whey, serum, + *-in*]. The total coagulable protein of serums.

oro·so·mu·coid (or″uh·so·mew′koid) *n.* [Gk. *oros*, whey, serum, + *mucoid*]. An acidic mucoprotein obtained from serum and from nephrotic urine. Syn. *acid seromucoid.*

orot·ic acid (o·rot′ick). 1,2,3,6-Tetrahydro-2,6-dioxo-4-pyrimidinecarboxylic acid or uracil-4-carboxylic acid, $C_5H_4N_2O_4$, a pyrimidine precursor in animal tissues.

Oro·ya fever [La *Oroya*, a town in Peru]. The acute, febrile, anemic stage of bartonellosis in the nonimmune host, characterized by emaciation, prostration, tachycardia, dyspnea, myalgia, and gastrointestinal and neurologic manifestations. Caused by *Bartonella bacilliformis.*

or·phen·a·drine (or·fen′uh·dreen) *n.* 2-(*p*-Chloro-α-methyl-α-phenylbenzyloxy)-*N,N*-dimethylethylamine, $C_{18}H_{23}NO$, an antispasmodic and antitremor drug; used as the citrate and hydrochloride salts.

orrho-, oro- [Gk. *orros* or *oros*, whey, serum]. A combining form meaning *serum.*

or·rho·men·in·gi·tis (or″o·men″in·jye′tis) *n.* [*orrho-* + *mening-* + *-itis*]. Inflammation of a serous membrane.

or·rhos (or′os) *n.* [Gk. *orros*]. SERUM; WHEY.

or·ris·root, *n.* A powder from certain varieties of iris; used in various cosmetics, toothpastes, etc. It is a common sensitizer, both by contact and by inhalation.

Orr-True·ta method (trweʰ′tahʰ) [H. W. *Orr*, U.S. surgeon, 1877–1956; J. *Trueta*, Spanish surgeon in England, 20th century]. Treatment of severe open wounds, especially in compound fractures, by packing with petrolatum gauze after careful debridement and reduction, and applying a plaster cast which is left on for 6 to 8 weeks; formerly used in military surgery.

Ortal. Trademark for hexethal, a barbiturate.

Or·ta·la·ni's click or **sign** (or·tahʰ·lah′nee) [M. *Ortalani*, Italian physician, 20th century]. When a congenitally dislocated hip is forced into the frog or fully abducted position, with pressure applied by the examiner's thumb to the knees to obtain maximal displacement of the femoral head, a snapping sound and thump (jerk of entry) are heard.

orth-, ortho- [Gk. *orthos*, straight]. A combining form meaning (a) *straight;* (b) *direct;* (c) *normal.* See also *ortho-.*

or·ther·ga·sia (or″thur·gay′zhuh, ·zee·uh) *n.* [*orth-* + *ergasia*]. A state of normal functioning.

or·the·sis (orth·ee′sis) *n.* [*orth-* + *-esis* as in *prosthesis*]. An orthopedic brace or device.

or·thet·ics (orth·et′icks) *n.* ORTHOTICS.

or·the·tist (orth′e·tist) *n.* ORTHOTIST.

orthi-, orthio- [Gk. *orthios*]. *In craniometry,* a combining form meaning *steep* or *upright.*

or·thi·auch·e·nus (orth″ee·awk′e·nus) *n.* [*orthi-* + Gk. *auchēn*, neck, + *-us*]. A skull in which the angle formed between the radius fixus and the line joining the basion and the inion is between 38 and 49°.

or·thio·chor·dus (orth″ee·o·kor′dus) *n.* [*orthio-* + *chord-* + *-us*]. A skull in which the angle formed between the radius fixus and the line joining the hormion and the basion is between 33.2 and 52°.

or·thio·cor·y·phus (orth″ee·o·kor′i·fus) *n.* [*orthio-* + Gk. *koryphē*, head, top, + *-us*]. A skull in which the angle formed between the radius fixus and the line joining the bregma and the lambda is between 29 and 41°.

or·thio·don·tus (orth″ee·o·don′tus) *n.* [*orthi-* + *odont-* + *-us*]. A skull in which the angle between the radius fixus and the line joining the alveolar and subnasal points is between 88 and 121°.

or·thio·me·to·pus (orth″ee·o·me·to′pus) *n.* [*orthio-* + Gk. *metōpon*, brow, forehead, + *-us*]. A skull in which the angle between the radius fixus and the line joining the bregma and the nasal point is between 47 and 60°.

or·thi·opis·thi·us (orth″ee·o·pis′thee·us) *n.* [*orthi-* + *opisthion* + *-us*]. A skull in which the angle between the radius fixus and the line joining the lambda and the inion is between 84 and 95°.

or·thi·opis·tho·cra·ni·us (orth″ee·o·pis″tho·kray′nee·us) *n.* [*orthi-* + *opistho-* + *crani-* + *-us*]. A skull in which the angle formed between the radius fixus and the line joining the lambda and the opisthion is 107 to 119°.

or·thio·pro·so·pus (orth″ee·o·pros·o′pus) *n.* [*orthio-* + *prosop-* + *-us*]. A skull in which the angle formed between the radius fixus and the line joining the nasion and the alveolar point is between 89.4 and 100°.

or·thi·op·y·lus (orth″ee·op′i·lus) *n.* [*orthio-* + Gk. *pylē*, gate, opening, + *-us*]. A skull in which the angle formed between the radius fixus and the line joining the middle point of the anterior margin of the foramen magnum and the middle point of the posterior margin of the foramen magnum is between 15.5 and 24°.

or·thi·or·rhi·nus (orth″ee·o·rye′nus) *n.* [*orthio-* + *rhin-* + *-us*]. A skull in which the angle formed between the radius fixus and the line joining the nasion and the subnasal point is between 87.5 and 98°.

or·thi·ura·nis·cus (orth″ee·yoo″ra·nis′kus) *n.* [*orthi-* + *uraniscus*]. A skull in which the angle formed between the radius fixus and a line joining the posterior border of the incisive fossa and the alveolar point is between 40 and 60°.

ortho-. 1. See *orth-.* 2. *In chemistry,* a prefix indicating adjacent relationship of two carbon atoms of the benzene ring, such as the 1,2-position; also any benzene derivative in which two substituents occur at adjacent carbon atoms in the ring. Symbol, *o-*. 3. *In chemistry,* a prefix indicating an acid in fully hydrated or hydroxylated form or, sometimes, in the highest hydrated or hydroxylated form that is stable. Compare *meta-.*

or·tho (orth′o) *adj.* [from prefix *ortho-*]. 1. Of or pertaining to two positions in the benzene ring that are adjacent. 2. Of or pertaining to the state in which the atomic nuclei of a diatomic molecule spin in the same direction.

or·tho·bo·ric acid (orth″o·bor′ick). BORIC ACID.

or·tho·car·di·ac (orth″o·kahr′dee·ack) *adj.* [*ortho-* + *cardiac*]. Pertaining to cardiac effects of assuming an upright posture.

orthocardiac sign. LIVIERATO'S SIGN (2).

or·tho·ceph·a·ly (orth″o·sef′ul·ee) *n.* [*ortho-* + *-cephaly*]. The condition of having a skull with a vertical index of from 70.1 to 75°.

or·tho·chlo·ro·phe·nol (orth″o·klor″o·fee′nol) *n.* [*ortho-* + *chlorophenol*]. A compound, ClC_6H_4OH, of high germicidal activity and high toxicity.

or·tho·cho·rea (orth″o·ko·ree′uh) *n.* [*ortho-* + *chorea*]. Choreic movements in the erect posture.

or·tho·chro·mat·ic (orth″o·kro·mat′ick) *adj.* [*ortho-* + *chromatic*]. 1. *In photography,* correct in the rendering of tones or colors. 2. Of photographic emulsions, not sensitive to red, able to be developed under a red safelight. 3. Having staining characteristics of a normal type.

orthochromatic erythroblast. NORMOBLAST (1).

orthochromatic erythrocyte. An erythrocyte that stains with acid stains only.

orthochromatic normoblast. NORMOBLAST (1).

or·tho·chro·mic (orth″o·kro′mick) *adj.* ORTHOCHROMATIC.

or·tho·cra·sia (orth″o·kray′see·uh, ·zee·uh) *n.* [*ortho-* + *-crasia*]. A condition in which there is no idiosyncrasy; a normal reaction to all drugs, proteins, and the like.

or·tho·cre·sol (orth″o·kree′sol) *n.* One of the isomers of cresol, $CH_3C_6H_4OH$. It has the weakest germicidal activity of the three isomers.

or·tho·dac·ty·lous (orth″o·dack′ti·lus) *adj.* [*ortho-* + *dactyl-* + *-ous*]. Having straight digits.

or·tho·den·tin (orth″o·den′tin) *n.* The mammalian type of dentin; it contains processes, but not cell bodies, of odontoblasts.

or·tho·di·a·gram (orth″o·dye′uh·gram) *n.* [*ortho-* + *diagram*]. A manual tracing of the fluoroscopic image of the heart.

or·tho·di·a·graph (orth″o·dye′uh·graf) *n.* A fluoroscopic apparatus for making orthodiagrams.

or·tho·di·ag·ra·phy (orth″o·dye·ag′ruf·ee) *n.* [*ortho-* + Gk. *diagraphē,* delineation]. A method once used for outlining the heart during fluoroscopy by manually tracing the outline of the heart on thin paper placed on a fluoroscopic screen in order to obtain minimal distortion.

or·tho·dol·i·cho·ceph·a·lous (orth″o·dol″i·ko·sef′uh·lus) *adj.* [*ortho-* + *dolicho-* + *cephal-* + *-ous*]. Having a long and straight head; having a vertical index between 70.1 and 75°.

or·tho·don·tia (orth″o·don′chee·uh) *n.* [*orth-* + *-odontia*]. ORTHODONTICS.

orthodontic band. A metal component of a fixed orthodontic appliance which encircles the tooth and on which a bracket is incorporated, to receive the arch wire which serves as the main force to reposition the tooth.

or·tho·don·tics (orth″o·don′ticks) *n.* [*orthodont*ia + *-ics*]. The branch of dentistry concerned with the treatment and prevention of malocclusion. —**orthodontic,** *adj.*

or·tho·don·tist (orth″o·don′tist) *n.* A specialist in the field of orthodontics.

or·tho·drom·ic (or″tho·drom′ick) *adj.* [Gk. *orthodromein,* to run straight forward, from *ortho-* + *dromos,* race, running]. Conducting nerve impulses in the normal direction. Contr. *antidromic.*—**orthodromi·cal·ly,** *adv.*

or·tho·gen·e·sis (orth″o·jen′e·sis) *n.* [*ortho-* + *genesis*]. The doctrine that phylogenetic evolution takes place according to system in certain well-defined and limited directions, and not by accident in many directions. —**ortho·ge·net·ic** (·je·net′ick) *adj.*

or·tho·gen·ic (orth″o·jen′ick) *adj.* 1. Of or pertaining to orthogenesis. 2. Pertaining to the training and social habilitation of children who behave retardedly because of emotional disturbances. See also *orthopsychiatry.*

or·thog·nath·ic (or″thug·nath′ick, orth″o·nath′ick) *adj.* [*ortho-* + *gnathic*]. *In craniometry,* designating a condition of the upper jaw in which it is in an approximately vertical relationship to the profile of the facial skeleton, when the skull is oriented on the Frankfort horizontal plane; having a gnathic index of 97.9 or less. —**or·thog·na·thism** (or·thog′nuh·thiz·um) *n.*

or·thog·o·nal (or·thog′un·ul) *adj.* [Gk. *orthogōnios,* rectangular]. At right angles, perpendicular to each other.

orthogonal illumination. The system of slit ultramicroscopical arrangement, the line of observation and the line of illumination being at right angles to each other.

or·tho·grade (orth′o·grade) *adj.* [*ortho-* + L. *gradi,* to walk]. Walking or standing in the upright position. Contr. *pronograde.*

or·tho·hy·droxy·ben·zo·ic acid (orth″o·high·drock″see·ben·zo′ick). SALICYLIC ACID.

or·tho·meso·ceph·a·lous (orth″o·mez″o·sef′uh·lus) *adj.* [*ortho-* + *meso-* + *cephal-* + *-ous*]. *In craniometry,* designating a skull with a transversovertical index between 75.1 and 79.9°, and a vertical index between 70.1 and 75°.

or·thom·e·ter (or·thom′e·tur) *n.* [*ortho-* + *-meter*]. An instrument for measuring the relative degree of protrusion of the eyes. Syn. *exophthalmometer.*

or·tho·pe·dic, or·tho·pae·dic (orth″uh·pee′dick) *adj.* [*ortho-* + *ped-,* child, + *-ic*]. Pertaining to orthopedics, as orthopedic surgery.

or·tho·pe·dics, or·tho·pae·dics (orth″uh·pee′dicks) *n.* That branch of surgery concerned with corrective treatment of deformities, diseases, and ailments of the locomotor apparatus, especially those affecting limbs, bones, muscles, joints, and fasciae, whether by apparatus, manipulation, or open operation; originally devoted to the correction and treatment of deformities in children.

orthopedic surgery. The remedy of skeletal deformities by manual and instrumental measures.

or·tho·pe·dist (orth″uh·pee′dist) *n.* One who practices orthopedic surgery; a specialist in orthopedics.

or·tho·per·cus·sion (orth″o·pur·kush′un) *n.* Percussion in which the distal phalanx of the pleximeter finger is flexed at a right angle and held perpendicular to the chest wall; the percussing finger is also held at right angles to the surface.

or·tho·phe·nan·thro·line (orth″o·fe·nan′thro·leen, ·lin) *n.* A compound, $C_{12}H_8N_2.H_2O$, that forms a complex with ferrous ions and is used as an indicator in oxidation-reduction systems in volumetric analysis.

or·tho·pho·ria (orth″o·for′ee·uh) *n.* [*ortho-* + *-phoria*]. 1. A tending of the visual lines to parallelism. 2. Normal balance of eye muscles.

or·tho·phos·phor·ic acid (orth″o·fos·for′ick). PHOSPHORIC ACID.

or·thop·nea (or″thup·nee′uh, or·thop′nee·uh) *n.* [*ortho-* + *-pnea*]. A condition in which there is difficulty in breathing except when sitting or standing upright. —**orthop·ne·ic** (·nee′ick) *adj.*

or·tho·prax·is (orth″o·prack′sis) *n.* [*ortho-* + Gk. *praxis,* action, practice]. ORTHOPRAXY.

or·tho·praxy (orth′o·prack·see) *n.* [*ortho-* + *-praxy*]. Correction of the deformities of the body.

or·tho·psy·chi·a·try (orth″o·sigh·kigh′uh·tree) *n.* Corrective psychiatry; an approach to the study and treatment of behavior which, placing an emphasis on the prevention and early treatment of behavior disorders, involves the collaboration of psychiatry, psychology, pediatrics, social services, and schools to promote healthy emotional growth and development.

Or·thop·tera (or·thop′tur·uh) *n.pl.* [*ortho-* + Gk. *ptera,* wings]. An order of insects including the grasshoppers, crickets, cockroaches, etc.

or·thop·tic (or·thop′tick) *adj.* [*ortho-* + *optic*]. Pertaining to normal binocular vision.

or·thop·tics (or·thop′ticks) *n.* The science of rendering visual reactions and responses right and efficient, usually by some form of exercise or training, as for amblyopia or strabismus.

or·thop·to·scope (or·thop′tuh·skope) *n.* An instrument used in orthoptics.

or·tho·roent·gen·og·ra·phy (orth″o·rent″ge·nog′ruf·ee) *n.* [*ortho-* + *roentgenography*]. ORTHODIAGRAPHY.

or·tho·scope (orth′uh·skope) *n.* 1. An instrument for examination of the eye through a layer of water, whereby the curvature and hence the refraction of the cornea is neutralized, and the cornea acts as a plane medium. 2. An instrument used in drawing the projections of skulls.

or·tho·scop·ic (orth″o·skop′ick) *adj.* 1. Pertaining to an orthoscope or to orthoscopy. 2. Pertaining to lenses cut from near the periphery of a large lens. 3. Having normal vision.

orthoscopic lens. A lens that gives a flat, undistorted field of vision.

or·thos·co·py (orth·os′kuh·pee) *n.* The examination of the eye with an orthoscope.

or·tho·sis (orth·o′sis) *n.* [Gk. *orthōsis,* making straight]. The straightening of a deformity.

or·tho·stat·ic (orth″o·stat′ick) *adj.* [Gk. *orthostatos,* upright, + *-ic*]. Pertaining to, or caused by, standing upright.

orthostatic albuminuria. Proteinuria present only when the patient is in the erect posture.

orthostatic hypotension. A fall of blood pressure which occurs when the erect position is assumed. Syn. *postural hypotension.*

orthostatic hypotension syndrome. PRIMARY ORTHOSTATIC HYPOTENSION.

orthostatic purpura. Purpura which develops in the lower extremities after prolonged standing.

orthostatic syncope. Syncope upon assuming the standing position. See also *orthostatic hypotension.*

or·tho·stat·ism (orth″o·stat′iz·um) *n.* [Gk. *orthostatos,* upright, + *-ism*]. The erect standing posture of the normal body.

or·tho·sym·pa·thet·ic (orth″o·sim″puh·thet′ick) *adj.* SYMPATHETIC (2).

or·tho·tast (orth′o·tast) *n.* [*orthotic* + *-ast,* from Gk. *-(as)tēs,* agentive suffix]. A device for straightening curvatures of long bones. It has also been used as a tourniquet.

or·tho·ter·i·on (orth″o·teer′ee·on) *n.* [*ortho-* + Gk. *tērion,* instrumental noun suffix]. An apparatus for straightening crooked limbs.

or·tho·ther·a·py (orth″o·therr′up·ee) *n.* The treatment of disorders of posture.

or·thot·ic (or·thot′ick) *adj.* Of or pertaining to orthosis or orthotics.

or·thot·ics (or·thot′icks) *n.* The science of orthopedic appliances and their use.

or·tho·tist (orth′uh·tist) *n.* One who practices orthotics.

or·thot·o·nus, or·thot·o·nos (or·thot′un·us) *n.* [*ortho-* + *tonus*]. Tonic spasm in which the body lies rigid and straight. Contr. *opisthotonus.* —**or·tho·ton·ic** (orth″o·ton′ick) *adj.*

or·tho·to·pia (orth″uh·to′pee·uh) *n.* [*ortho-* + Gk. *topos,* place, + *-ia*]. The natural or normal position of a part or organ.

or·tho·top·ic (orth″o·top′ick) *adj.* [*ortho-* + Gk. *topos,* place, + *-ic*]. In the natural or normal position. Contr. *heterotopic.*

orthotopic transplantation. The grafting of a tissue or organ from a donor into its normal anatomic position in the recipient. Contr. *heterotopic transplantation.*

or·thot·ro·pism (or·thot′ruh·piz·um) *n.* [*ortho-* + *tropism*]. Vertical, upward, or downward growth. —**or·tho·trop·ic** (orth″o·trop′ick) *adj.*

or·tho·volt·age (orth′o·vohl″tij) *n.* Roentgen radiation produced by voltages of 200 to 500 kilovolts.

Orthoxine. Trademark for methoxyphenamine, used as the hydrochloride salt as a bronchodilator, antispasmodic, and nasal decongestant.

ory·za·min (o·rye′zuh·min) *n.* [Gk. *oryza,* rice, + vita*min*]. THIAMINE HYDROCHLORIDE.

O.S. Abbreviation for (a) *oculus sinister,* left eye; (b) *opening snap.*

Os Symbol for osmium.

¹os (oce, oss) *n.,* genit. **oris** (o′ris), pl. **ora** (o′ruh) [L.] [NA]. MOUTH.

²os (oss) *n.,* genit. sing. **os·sis** (oss′is), pl. **os·sa** (·uh), genit. pl. **os·si·um** (oss′ee·um) [L.]. BONE.

os ace·ta·bu·li (as″e·tab′yoo·lye). An ossific center in the triradiate cartilage. There is an anterior one between the iliac and pubic portions of the acetabulum and a posterior one between the iliac and ischial portions. Syn. *cotyloid bone.*

os acro·mi·a·le (a·kro″mee·ay′lee). The acromion when not united to the scapula.

os ar·ti·cu·la·re (ahr·tick″yoo·lair′ee) [L.]. The articular bone; ARTICULAR (2).

osa·zone (o′suh·zone) *n.* A compound formed by reaction of a sugar with phenylhydrazine in the presence of acetic acid; used in the identification of sugars.

os ba·si·la·re (bas″i·lair′ee) [BNA]. The basisphenoid and basioccipital bones, collectively.

os ba·si·o·ti·cum (bay″see·ot′i·kum). A separate center of ossification between the basal part of the occipital bone and the sphenoid. Syn. *os prebasioccipitale.*

Osbil. Trademark for iobenzamic acid, a cholecystographic contrast medium.

os breg·ma·ti·cum (breg·mat′i·kum). An occasional sutural bone, caused by the presence of a separate center of ossification in the anterior fontanel.

os bre·ve (brev′ee) [NA]. A short bone.

os cal·cis (kal′sis) [NA alt.]. CALCANEUS (1).

os ca·pi·ta·tum (kap·i·tay′tum) [NA]. CAPITATE BONE.

os car·pi (kahr′pye), *pl.* **ossa carpi** [NA]. CARPAL BONE.

os cen·tra·le (sen·tray′lee) [NA]. An occasional ossicle found on the dorsal aspect of the carpus between any pair of the scaphoid, capitate, and trapezoid bones in many mammals.

osche-, oscheo- [Gk. *oschea*]. A combining form meaning *scrotum.*

os·chea (os′kee·uh) *n.* [Gk.]. SCROTUM. —**osche·al** (·ul) *adj.*

Os·cil·la·ria ma·la·ri·ae (os″i·lair′ee·uh ma·lair′ee·ee). A former species designation that included the malarial plasmodia, *Plasmodium falciparum, P. malariae,* and *P. vivax.*

os·cil·lat·ing bed (os′i·lay″ting). A bed with attached motor which rocks the bed with a set rhythm as a means of artificial respiration in some cases of respiratory paralysis; also used in peripheral vascular disease to prevent decubitus ulcer. Syn. *rocking bed.*

os·cil·la·tion (os″i·lay′shun) *n.* [L. *oscillatio,* from *oscillare,* to swing]. A swinging or vibration; also any tremulous motion. —**os·cil·la·to·ry** (os′i·luh·tor·ee) *adj.*

os·cil·la·tor (os′si·lay′tur) *n.* A mechanical or electronic device that produces electrical vibration; used in physical therapy.

oscillatory nystagmus. OCULAR NYSTAGMUS.

os·cil·lo·graph (os′i·lo·graf, os·il′o·graf) *n.* An apparatus for recording oscillations. —**os·cil·lo·graph·ic** (os″i·lo·graf′ick) *adj.;* **oscil·log·ra·phy** (log′ruh·fee) *n.*

os·cil·lom·e·ter (os″i·lom′e·tur) *n.* An instrument for measuring oscillations, as those seen in taking blood pressures. —**os·cil·lo·met·ric** (os″i·lo·met′rick) *adj.*

oscillometric index. Ratio of the oscillometric reading of the blood pressure at the ankle to that at the wrist.

os·cil·lom·e·try (os″i·lom′e·tree) *n.* Measurement or detection of oscillations of any type, especially circulatory.

os·cil·lop·sia (os″il·op′see·uh) *n.* [*oscill*ation + *-opsia*]. Illusory movement of the environment, in which stationary objects seem to move up or down or from side to side. It may be associated with parietooccipital lesions, with severe nystagmus of any type due to lesions involving the vestibular nuclei, or with labyrinthine lesions.

os·cil·lo·scope (os·il′uh·skope) *n.* A cathode-ray vacuum tube so constructed as to portray visually the deflections or oscillations of electromotive forces as a function of time. Syn. *cathode-ray oscilloscope.* See also *cathode-ray oscillograph.*

Os·cin·i·dae (os·in′i·dee) *n.pl.* A family of the Diptera, which contains many species of small active flies known as eye gnats; contains the medically important genera *Hippelates, Siphunculina,* and *Oscinis.* Syn. *Chloropidae.*

Os·ci·nis (os′in·is) *n.* [NL., of the songbird, from L. *oscen, oscinis,* any bird whose calls were interpreted as omens]. A genus of flies of the family Oscinidae.

Oscinis pal·li·pes (pal′i·peez). *HIPPELATES PALLIPES.*

os·ci·tan·cy (os′i·tun·see) *n.* [L. *oscitare,* to yawn]. The disposition to yawn; drowsiness.

os·ci·ta·tion (os″i·tay′shun) *n.* [L. *oscitatio,* from *oscitare,* to yawn]. YAWNING.

os cli·to·ri·dis (kli·tor′i·dis). A bone in the septum of the clitoris, in some mammals.

os coc·cy·gis (kock′si·jis, kock·sigh′jis) [NA]. COCCYX.

os cor·dis (kor'dis). A bone in the fibrous triangle of the heart, between the atrioventricular and aortic orifices, in some mammals.

os cos·ta·le (kos·tay'lee) [NA]. RIB.

os cox·ae (kock'see) [NA]. HIPBONE.

os cu·boi·de·um (kew·boy'dee·um) [NA]. CUBOID (2).

os·cu·la·tion (os"kew·lay'shun) *n.* [L. *osculatio,* kissing, from *osculum*]. 1. Anastomosis of vessels. 2. Kissing.

os·cu·lum (os'kew·lum) *n.* [L., little mouth]. A small aperture.

os cu·ne·i·for·me in·ter·me·di·um (kew·nee·i·for'mee in·tur·mee'dee·um) [NA]. The intermediate cuneiform bone. See Table of Bones in the Appendix.

os cuneiforme la·te·ra·le (lat·e·ray'lee) [NA]. The lateral cuneiform bone. See Table of Bones in the Appendix.

os cuneiforme me·di·a·le (mee·dee·ay'lee) [NA]. The medial cuneiform bone. See Table of Bones in the Appendix.

os cuneiforme pri·mum (prye'mum) [BNA]. OS CUNEIFORME MEDIALE.

os cuneiforme se·cun·dum (se·kun'dum) [BNA]. OS CUNEIFORME INTERMEDIUM.

os cuneiforme ter·ti·um (tur'shee·um) [BNA]. OS CUNEIFORME LATERALE.

os den·ta·le (den·tay'lee). The bone of the lower beak of birds.

¹-ose [from gluc*ose*]. A suffix meaning (a) *carbohydrate;* (b) *derived by hydrolysis of a protein.*

²-ose [L. *-osus*]. A suffix meaning *having, characterized by.*

os en·to·mi·on (en·to'mee·on). A supernumerary bone situated at the entomion.

os epi·pte·ri·cum (ep"i·terr'i·kum). A supernumerary bone situated near the pterion.

Ose·ret·sky test. A psychologic test designed to measure the motor proficiency of an individual.

os eth·moi·da·le (eth·moy·day'lee) [NA]. ETHMOID BONE.

os fal·ci·for·me (fal·si·for'mee). A sickle-shaped ossicle at the lower end of the radius in moles.

os fron·ta·le (fron·tay'lee) [NA]. FRONTAL BONE.

Os·good-Has·kins test. A test for protein in which acetic acid and saturated sodium chloride solution are added to urine. A precipitate appearing after addition of the acid indicates bile salts, urates, or resin acids. A precipitate appearing after adding the salt solution suggests Bence Jones protein. Upon heating, the Bence Jones protein, if present, will dissolve; if protein or globulin is present, a precipitate will form.

Osgood-Schlat·ter disease [R. B. *Osgood,* U.S. orthopedist, 1873–1956; and C. *Schlatter,* Swiss surgeon, 1864–1934]. A traction avulsion of the tibial tubercle apophysis of chronic nature.

os ha·ma·tum (ha·may'tum) [NA]. HAMATUM.

O'Shaugh·nes·sy's operation [L. *O'Shaughnessy,* British surgeon, 1900–1940]. CARDIOMENTOPEXY.

os hy·oi·de·um (high·oy'dee·um) [NA]. HYOID (1).

os ili·um (il'ee·um) [NA]. ILIUM (2).

os in·ci·si·vum (in"si·sigh'vum) [NA]. INCISIVE BONE.

os in·ter·cu·ne·i·for·me (in"tur·kew·nee·i·for'mee). A rare variant bone occurring between the medial and intermediate cuneiform bones.

os in·ter·fron·ta·le (in"tur·fron·tay'lee). An occasional accessory ossicle in the anterior part of the metopic suture.

os in·ter·me·ta·tar·se·um (in"tur·met"uh·tahr'see·um). An occasional wedge-shaped bone on the dorsal aspect of the foot between the medial cuneiform and first and second metatarsal bones.

os in·ter·pa·ri·e·ta·le (in"tur·pa·rye"e·tay'lee) [NA]. INTERPARIETAL BONE.

2-OS interval. S_2-OS INTERVAL.

-osis [Gk.]. A suffix designating (a) *a process,* as osmosis; (b) *a state,* as narcosis; (c) *a diseased condition of,* as nephrosis; (d) *a disease caused by,* as mycosis; (e) *an increase in,* as leukocytosis.

os is·chii (is'kee·eye) [NA]. ISCHIUM.

os ja·po·ni·cum (ja·pon'i·kum). The divided zygomatic bone, a racial characteristic of the Japanese.

os la·cri·ma·le (lack·ri·may'lee) [NA]. LACRIMAL BONE.

os len·ti·cu·la·re (len·tick"yoo·lair'tee). LENTICULAR PROCESS.

Osler-Libman-Sacks syndrome. LIBMAN-SACKS ENDOCARDITIS.

Osler-Rendu-Weber disease [W. *Osler,* H. *Rendu,* and F. P. *Weber*]. HEREDITARY HEMORRHAGIC TELANGIECTASIA.

Os·ler's disease [W. *Osler,* Canadian physician in U.S. and England, 1849–1919]. POLYCYTHEMIA VERA.

Osler's febrile polyneuritis. GUILLAIN-BARRÉ DISEASE.

Osler's nodes [W. *Osler*]. Painful red indurated areas in the pads of the fingers or toes in bacterial endocarditis.

Osler-Vaquez disease [W. *Osler* and L. *Vaquez*]. POLYCYTHEMIA VERA.

Osler-Vaquez nodes. OSLER'S NODES.

os lon·gum (long'gum) [NA]. LONG BONE.

os lu·na·tum (lew·nay'tum) [NA]. LUNATE.

osm-, osmo- [Gk. *osmē*]. A combining form meaning *smell* or *odor.* See also *osmo-.*

os mag·num (mag'num). CAPITATE (2).

os·mate (oz'mate, os'mate) *n.* A salt of osmic acid.

os·mat·ic (oz·mat"ick) *adj.* [Gk. *osmē,* smell, + *-ic*]. Characterized by a sense of smell.

os·me·sis (oz·mee'sis) *n.* [Gk. *osmēsis,* a smell]. OLFACTION.

os·mes·the·sia (oz"mes·theezh'uh, ·theez'ee·uh) *n.* [*osm-* + *esthesia*]. Olfactory sensibility.

os me·ta·car·pa·le (met"uh·kahr·pay'lee), pl. **ossa metacarpa·lia** (·lee·uh) [NA]. A metacarpal bone. See Table of Bones in the Appendix.

os·mic acid (oz'mick, os'mick). Osmium tetroxide, OsO_4, employed as a histologic stain and reagent, almost universally used as a primary or secondary fixative in electron microscopy; has been used internally, in the form of the potassium salt, in rheumatic affections and in epilepsy.

os·mics (oz'micks) *n.* The study of olfaction.

os·mi·dro·sis (oz"mi·dro'sis) *n.* [*osm-* + Gk. *hidrōsis,* sweating, perspiration]. BROMHIDROSIS.

os·mio·phil·ic (oz"mee·o·fil'ick) *adj.* Having an affinity for osmium tetroxide or osmic acid.

os·mi·um (oz'mee·um, os') *n.* Os = 190.2. A heavy metallic element, with a density of 22.48, belonging to the platinum group. —**os·mic** (oz'mick, os') *adj.*

osmium tetroxide. OSMIC ACID.

¹osmo-. See *osm-.*

²osmo-. A combining form meaning *osmosis.*

os·mo·dys·pho·ria (oz"mo·dis·fo'ree·uh) *n.* [*osmo-,* odor, + *dysphoria*]. Intolerance of certain odors.

os·mol (oz'mol, ·mole) *n.* [*osmo*tic + *mol*e]. The quantity of a solute, existing in solution as molecules and/or ions, commonly stated in grams, that is osmotically equivalent to one mole of an ideally behaving nonelectrolyte. —**os·mo·lal** (oz·mo'lul) *adj.;* **os·mo·lal·i·ty** (oz"mo·lal'i·tee) *n.*

os·mo·lal·i·ty (oz"mo·lal'i·tee) *n.* Osmotic pressure expressed in terms of osmols or milliosmols per kilogram of water. Compare *osmolarity.*

os·mo·lar (oz·mo'lur) *adj.* [*osmo*tic + *molar*]. Of or pertaining to the osmotic property of a solution containing one or more molecular or ionic species, quantitatively expressed in osmol units. —**os·mo·lar·i·ty** (oz"mo·lăr'i·tee) *n.*

os·mo·lar·i·ty (oz"mo·lăr'i·tee) *n.* Osmotic pressure expressed in terms of osmols or milliosmols per kilogram of solution. Compare *osmolality.*

¹os·mol·o·gy (oz·mol'uh·jee) *n.* That part of physical science treating of osmosis.

²osmology, *n.* [*osmo-,* odor, smell, + *-logy*]. OSPHRESIOLOGY.

¹os·mom·e·ter (oz·mom'e·tur) *n.* [*osmo-* + *-meter*]. An instrument for testing the sense of smell; an olfactometer.

²os·mom·e·ter (oz·mom'e·tur) *n.* An apparatus for measuring osmotic pressure.

os·mo·no·sol·o·gy (oz"mo·no·sol'uh·jee) *n.* [*osmo-,* odor, smell, + *nosology*]. The science of olfactory disorders.

os·mo·phil·ic (oz″mo·fil′ick) *adj.* Having an affinity for solutions of high osmotic pressure.

os·mo·pho·bia (oz″mo·fo′bee·uh) *n.* [*osmo-*, odor, + *-phobia*]. An abnormal fear of odors.

os·mo·phor, os·mo·phore (oz′mo·fore) *n.* [*osmo-* + *-phore*]. A group or radical that imparts odor to a compound.

os·mo·re·cep·tors (oz″mo·re·sep′turz) *n.* [*osmo-* + *receptors*]. Structures in the hypothalamus which respond to changes in osmotic pressure of the blood by regulating the secretion of the neurohypophyseal antidiuretic hormone (ADH).

os·mo·sis (oz·mo′sis, os·) *n.* [Gk. *ōsmos*, thrust, pushing, + *-osis*]. The passage of a solvent through a membrane from a dilute solution into a more concentrated one.

os·mot·ic (oz·mot′ick, os·) *adj.* Pertaining to osmosis, particularly to osmotic pressure.

osmotic coefficient. The ratio of observed osmotic pressure to that calculated for a solution of ideal behavior.

osmotic diuretic. A substance producing diuresis because of the osmotic effect of the unabsorbed fraction in the renal tubules with resulting loss of water.

osmotic fragility. The susceptibility of erythrocytes to lysis when placed in hypotonic saline solutions.

osmotic fragility test. ERYTHROCYTE FRAGILITY TEST.

osmotic lysis. Destruction of cells, for example erythrocytes, by hypotonic solutions.

osmotic pressure. The pressure developed when two solutions of different concentrations of the same solute are separated by a membrane permeable to the solvent only.

osmotic shock. The bursting of cells, such as bacteria, suspended in a salt solution when they are subjected to sudden dilution.

os mul·tan·gu·lum ma·jus (mul·tang′gew·lum may′jus) [BNA]. Os trapezium (= TRAPEZIUM).

os multangulum mi·nus (migh′nus) [BNA]. Os trapezoideum (= TRAPEZOID (2)).

os na·sa·le (na·say′lee) [NA]. The nasal bone. See Table of Bones in the Appendix.

os na·vi·cu·la·re (na·vick″yoo·lair′ee) [NA]. NAVICULAR (2).

os naviculare ma·nus (man′us) [BNA]. Os scaphoideum (= SCAPHOID (2)).

os naviculare pe·dis (ped′is) [BNA]. Os naviculare (= NAVICULAR (2)).

os no·vum (no′vum). Bone prepared for grafting by implanting os purum in another site until soft tissues have become associated with it.

os oc·ci·pi·ta·le (ock·sip·i·tay′lee) [NA]. The occipital bone. See Table of Bones in the Appendix.

os odon·toi·de·um (o·don·toy′dee·um). The dens of the axis when it persists as a separate ossicle.

os or·bi·cu·la·re (or·bick″yoo·lair′ee). LENTICULAR PROCESS. See also *orbiculare.*

os or·bi·ta·le (or·bi·tay′lee). The upper of two portions into which the zygomatic bone is sometimes divided by a horizontal suture.

os pa·la·ti·num (pal·uh·tye′num) [NA]. The palatine bone. See Table of Bones in the Appendix.

os pa·ri·e·ta·le (pa·rye″e·tay′lee) [NA]. The parietal bone. See Table of Bones in the Appendix.

os pe·dis (ped′is). COFFIN BONE.

os pe·nis (pee′nis). A bone in the septum of the penis in some mammals, as the dog; seen rarely, as a pathological condition, in man.

os pe·ro·ne·um (perr·o·nee′um). A bone sometimes found in the tendon of the peroneus longus muscle on the lateral aspect of the foot adjacent to the cuboid bone.

os·phre·si·ol·o·gy (os·free″zee·ol′o·jee) *n.* [*osphresis* + *-logy*]. The science of the sense of smell and its organs, and of odors.

os·phre·si·om·e·ter (os·free″zee·om′e·tur) *n.* [*osphresis* + *-meter*]. [1]OSMOMETER; OLFACTOMETER.

os·phre·sis (os·free′sis) *n.* [Gk. *osphrēsis*]. The sense of smell; olfaction.

os·phyo·my·e·li·tis (os″fee·o·migh·e·lye′tis) *n.* [Gk. *osphys*, loins, + *myelitis*]. *Obsol.* Lumbar myelitis.

os pi·si·for·me (pye″si·for′mee) [NA]. PISIFORM (2).

os pla·num (play′num) [NA]. FLAT BONE.

os pneu·ma·ti·cum (new·mat′i·kum) [NA]. PNEUMATIC BONE.

os pre·ba·si·oc·ci·pi·ta·le (pree·bay″see·ock·sip″i·tay′lee). OS BASIOTICUM.

os pu·bis (pew′bis) [NA]. The pubic bone; PUBIS.

os pu·rum (pew′rum). Bone for grafting, processed to remove soft tissue and proteins. It is kept dry and boiled before use.

ossa. Plural of *os* (L., bone).

ossa car·pi (kahr′pye) [NA]. CARPAL BONES.

ossa cra·nii (kray′nee·eye) [NA]. The bones of the braincase, collectively.

os sa·crum (say′krum) [NA]. SACRUM.

ossa di·gi·to·rum ma·nus (dij·i·to′rum man′us) [NA]. The phalanges of the hand. See Table of Bones in the Appendix.

ossa digitorum pe·dis (ped′is) [NA]. The phalanges of the foot. See Table of Bones in the Appendix.

ossa ex·tre·mi·ta·tis in·fe·ri·o·ris (eck·strem·i·tay′tis in·feer·ee·o′ris) [BNA]. OSSA MEMBRI INFERIORIS.

ossa extremitatis su·pe·ri·o·ris (sue·peer·ee·o′ris) [BNA]. OSSA MEMBRI SUPERIORIS.

ossa fa·ci·ei (fay″shee·ee′eye) [NA]. The facial bones. See Table of Bones in the Appendix.

ossa in·ter·ca·la·ria (in″tur·ka·lair′ee·uh). SUTURAL BONES.

ossa mem·bri in·fe·ri·o·ris (mem′brye in·feer·ee·o′ris) [NA]. The bones of the lower limb.

ossa membri su·pe·ri·o·ris (sue·peer·ee·o′ris) [NA]. The bones of the upper limb.

ossa me·ta·car·pa·lia I-V (met″uh·kahr·pay′lee·uh) [NA]. The bones of the metacarpus.

ossa me·ta·tar·sa·lia I-V (met″uh·tahr·say′lee·uh) [NA]. The bones of the metatarsus.

ossa se·sa·moi·dea (ses′uh·moy′dee·uh) [NA]. SESAMOID BONES.

ossa su·pra·ster·na·lia (sue″pruh·stur·nay′lee·uh) [NA]. Small bones occasionally present along the superior border of the manubrium of the sternum.

ossa su·tu·ra·rum (sue·tew·rair′um) [NA]. SUTURAL BONES.

ossa tar·si (tahr′sigh) [NA]. TARSAL BONES.

os sca·phoi·de·um (ska·foy′dee·um) [NA]. SCAPHOID (2).

os·se·in, os·se·ine (os′ee·in) *n.* 1. COLLAGEN. 2. The organic framework of osseous tissue.

os·se·let (os′e·lit) *n.* [F., little bone]. A hard nodule on the inner aspect of a horse's knee. Inflammation of the periosteum at the distal end of the third metacarpal, or at the proximal end of the first phalanx, or both, results in new bone growth.

osseo-. A combining form meaning *osseous* or *bone.*

os·seo·al·bu·min·oid (os″ee·o·al·bew′min·oid) *n.* [*osseo-* + *albuminoid*]. A tough, elastic, and fibrous protein in bone, believed to be a constituent of the lining of the haversian canals.

os·seo·car·ti·lag·i·nous (os″ee·o·kahr·ti·laj′i·nus) *adj.* Pertaining to or composed of both bone and cartilage.

os·seo·fi·brous (os″ee·o·figh′brus) *adj.* Pertaining to or composed of both bone and fibrous tissue.

os·seo·lig·a·men·tous (os″ee·o·lig″uh·men′tus) *adj.* [*osseo-* + *ligamentous*]. Pertaining to the bones and ligaments.

os·seo·mu·coid (os″ee·o·mew′koid) *n.* [*osseo-* + *mucoid*]. A mucin or glycoprotein obtained from bone.

os·se·ous (os′ee·us) *adj.* [L. *osseus*, from *os*, bone]. Bony; composed of or resembling bone.

osseous ampullae. The dilated parts of the three bony semicircular canals of the osseous labyrinth of the internal ear. Each houses a membranous ampulla.

osseous cochlea. OSSEOUS COCHLEAR CANAL.

osseous cochlear canal. The bony canal in which the cochlear duct is housed.

osseous labyrinth. The portion of the petrous part of the temporal bone that surrounds the internal ear. It consists of the vestibule, osseous semicircular canals, and cochlea. NA *labyrinthus osseus.*

osseous semicircular canals. The bony parts of the labyrinth of the ear that house the membranous semicircular canals; three loop-shaped canals in the petrous portion of the temporal bone, the anterior semicircular canal, the posterior semicircular canal, and the lateral or horizontal semicircular canal. They lie at right angles to one another and communicate with the vestibule. NA *canales semicirculares ossei.* See also Plate 20.

osseous sound. The sound heard on percussion over bone.

osseous spiral lamina. The thin spiral shelf of bone projecting from the modiolus and partially subdividing the cochlea; the basilar membrane completes the division. NA *lamina spinalis ossea.*

osseous system. The bony skeleton of the body.

osseous tissue. BONE (1).

ossi- [L. *os, ossis*]. A combining form meaning *bone.*

os·si·cle (os'i·kul) *n.* [from L. *ossiculum,* dim. of *os,* bone]. A small bone; particularly, one of three small bones in the tympanic cavity: the malleus, incus, and stapes.

ossicle of Ber·tin (behr·tæⁿ') [E. *Bertin,* French anatomist, 1712–1781]. CONCHA SPHENOIDALIS.

ossicula. Plural of *ossiculum.*

ossicula au·di·tus (aw·dye'tus, aw'di·tus) [NA]. The bones within the middle ear cavity, collectively; the tympanic ossicles.

os·sic·u·lar (os·ick'yoo·lur) *adj.* Of or pertaining to ossicles.

os·si·cu·lec·to·my (os''i·kew·leck'tuh·mee) *n.* [*ossicul*um + *-ectomy*]. The removal of one or more of the ossicles of the middle ear.

os·si·cu·lot·o·my (os''i·kew·lot'um·ee, os·ick''yoo·) *n.* Surgical incision involving the tissues about the ossicles of the ear.

os·si·cu·lum (os·ick'yoo·lum) *n.*, pl. **ossicu·la** (·luh) [L.]. OSSICLE.

os·sif·er·ous (os·if'ur·us) *adj.* [*ossi-* + *-ferous,* bearing]. Containing or producing bone tissue.

os·sif·ic (os·if'ick) *adj.* [*ossify* + *-ic*]. Producing bone.

os·si·fi·ca·tion (os''i·fi·kay'shun) *n.* [NL. *ossificatio,* from *ossi-* + L. *facere,* to make]. The formation of bone; the conversion of tissue into bone.

os·sif·lu·ence (os·if'lew·unce) *n.* [*ossi-* + *-fluence,* flow]. OSTEOLYSIS.

os·sif·lu·ent (os·if'lew·unt) *adj.* [*ossi-* + *-fluent,* flowing]. Breaking down and softening bony tissue.

ossifluent abscess. An abscess arising from diseased bone.

os·si·form (os'i·form) *adj.* Bonelike.

os·si·fy (os'i·figh) *v.* [*ossi-* + *-fy,* to make]. To turn into bone.

ossifying fibroma. A benign tumor of bone derived from bone-forming connective tissue, seen particularly in the vertebral column, which microscopically appears as vascularized connective tissue interspersed with fibrous bone trabeculae. Syn. *osteogenic fibroma, fibrous osteoma.*

os sphe·noi·da·le (sfee·noy·day'lee) [NA]. SPHENOID (2).

os sty·loi·de·um (stye·loy'dee·um). The styloid process of the third metacarpal when it occurs as a separate ossicle.

os suffraginis. SUFFRAGINIS.

os su·pra·ster·na·le (sue''pruh·stur·nay'lee). Singular of *ossa suprasternalia.*

ost-, oste-, osteo- [Gk. *osteon*]. A combining form meaning *bone.*

os·tal·gia (os·tal'jee·uh) *n.* [*ost-* + *-algia*]. Pain in a bone. Syn. *ostealgia.* —**ostal·gic** (·jick) *adj.*

os·tal·gi·tis (os''tal·jigh'tis) *n.* [*ost-* + *alg-* + *-itis*]. Inflammation of a bone attended by pain.

oste-. See *ost-.*

os·te·al (os'tee·ul) *adj.* [*oste-* + *-al*]. Osseous, bony; pertaining to bone.

os·te·al·gia (os''tee·al'jee·uh) *n.* OSTALGIA.

os·te·al·le·o·sis, os·te·al·loe·o·sis (os''tee·al''ee·o'sis) *n.* [*oste-* + Gk. *alloiōsis,* alteration]. A metamorphosis of the substance of bone, as exemplified in osteosarcoma.

os·te·ana·gen·e·sis (os''tee·an·uh·jen'e·sis) *n.* [*oste-* + *anagenesis*]. Regeneration of bone.

os·te·anaph·y·sis (os''tee·a·naf'i·sis) *n.* [*oste-* + Gk. *anaphysis,* a growing again]. OSTEANAGENESIS.

os·te·ar·throt·o·my (os''tee·ahr·throt'um·ee) *n.* OSTEOARTHROTOMY.

os·tec·to·my (os·teck'tum·ee) *n.* [*ost-* + *-ectomy*]. Excision of a bone or a portion of a bone.

os·tec·to·py (os·teck'tuh·pee) *n.* [*ost-* + *ectopy*]. Displacement of bone. Syn. *osteectopia.*

os·te·ec·to·my (os''tee·eck'tum·ee) *n.* OSTECTOMY.

os·te·ec·to·pia (os''tee·eck·to'pee·uh) *n.* [*oste-* + *ectopia*]. OSTECTOPY.

os·te·in, os·te·ine (os'tee·in) *n.* [Gk. *osteïnos,* of bone]. OSSEIN.

os·te·itis (os''tee·eye'tis) *n.* [*oste-* + *-itis*]. Inflammation of bone. —**oste·it·ic** (·it'ick) *adj.*

osteitis car·no·sa (kahr·no'suh). Inflammation of bone with an excess of granulation tissue.

osteitis con·den·sans il·ii (kun·den'sanz il'ee·eye). A disease of unknown origin characterized by low back pain bilaterally, accompanied by an oval or triangular area of sclerotic opaque bone adjacent to the sacroiliac joints in the ilium.

osteitis cys·ti·ca (sis'ti·kuh). Osseous lesions originally described in sarcoidosis but also seen in normal individuals and in association with other diseases. The phalanges of fingers and toes appear on roentgenograms to have cysts. They represent replacement of bone and marrow by sarcoid nodules. Syn. *Jüngling's disease, osteitis tuberculosa multiplex cystoides.*

osteitis de·for·mans (de·for'manz). PAGET'S DISEASE (2).

osteitis fibrosa. *Informal.* OSTEITIS FIBROSA CYSTICA.

osteitis fi·bro·sa cys·ti·ca (figh·bro'suh sis'ti·kuh). Generalized skeletal demineralization due to an increased rate of bone destruction resulting from hyperparathyroidism, occasionally complicated by large osteoporotic areas resembling cysts. Syn. *von Recklinghausen's disease, Engel-Recklinghausen disease, osteitis fibrosa generalisata.*

osteitis fibrosa cystica dis·sem·i·na·ta (di·sem''i·nay'tuh, ·nah'tuh). FIBROUS DYSPLASIA (1).

osteitis fibrosa disseminata. FIBROUS DYSPLASIA (1).

osteitis fibrosa gen·er·al·i·sa·ta (jen''ur·al·i·zay'tuh, ·sah'tuh). OSTEITIS FIBROSA CYSTICA.

osteitis fra·gil·i·tans (fra·jil'i·tanz). OSTEOGENESIS IMPERFECTA.

osteitis fun·go·sa (fung·go'suh). Inflammatory hyperplasia of the medulla and of the compact substance of bone. It is characterized by fungoid granulation tissue and leads to new ossification or destructive chronic inflammation.

osteitis pubis. Inflammation in the pubic symphysis.

osteitis tu·ber·cu·lo·sa mul·ti·plex cys·toi·des (tew·burk''yoo·lo'suh mul'ti·plecks sis·toy'deez). OSTEITIS CYSTICA.

os·tem·bry·on (os·tem'bree·on) *n.* [*ost-* + *embryon*]. An ossified fetus.

os tem·po·ra·le (tem·po·ray'lee) [NA]. The temporal bone. See Table of Bones in the Appendix.

os·tem·py·e·sis (os''tem·pye·ee'sis, ·pee·ee'sis) *n.* [*ost-* + *empyesis*]. Suppuration of bone.

osteo-. See *ost-.*

os·teo·ana·gen·e·sis (os''tee·o·an·uh·jen'e·sis) *n.* OSTEANAGENESIS.

os·teo·an·eu·rysm (os''tee·o·an'yoo·riz·um) *n.* 1. ANEURYSMAL BONE CYST. 2. The telangiectatic, pulsating form of osteogenic sarcoma.

os·teo·ar·threc·to·my (os''tee·o·ahr·threck'tum·ee) *n.* [*osteo-* + *arthrectomy*]. Surgical excision or partial excision of the bony portion of a joint.

os·teo·ar·thri·tis (os″tee-o-ahr-thrigh′tis) *n.* [*osteo-* + *arthritis*]. DEGENERATIVE JOINT DISEASE.

os·teo·ar·throp·a·thy (os″tee-o-ahr-throp′uth-ee) *n.* [*osteo-* + *arthropathy*]. Any disease of bony articulations.

os·teo·ar·thro·sis (os″tee-o-ahr-thro′sis) *n.* [*osteo-* + *arthrosis*]. DEGENERATIVE JOINT DISEASE.

os·teo·ar·throt·o·my (os″tee-o-ahr-throt′um-ee) *n.* [*osteo-* + *arthrotomy*]. Surgical excision or partial excision of the bony portion of a joint.

os·teo·blast (os′tee-o-blast) *n.* [*osteo-* + *-blast*]. Any one of the cells of mesenchymal origin concerned in the formation of bony tissue. —**os·teo·blas·tic** (os″tee-o-blast′ick) *adj.*

osteoblastic sarcoma. OSTEOGENIC SARCOMA.

os·teo·blas·to·ma (os″tee-o-blas-to′muh) *n.* [*osteoblast* + *-oma*]. 1. A benign tumor of bone, composed of osteoblasts, osteoid and immature bone. It is painless, chiefly affects children and young adults, and is most commonly found in the ilia, the vertebrae, or the medulla of long bones. 2. *Obsol.* OSTEOGENIC SARCOMA.

os·teo·camp·sia (os″tee-o-kamp′see-uh) *n.* [*osteo-* + Gk. *kampsis*, a bending, + *-ia*]. Curvature of a bone without fracture, as in osteomalacia.

os·teo·car·ci·no·ma (os″tee-o-kahr″si-no′muh) *n.* 1. Carcinoma metastatic to bone and associated with osseous hyperplasia. 2. Carcinoma with foci of stromal osseous metaplasia.

os·teo·car·ti·lag·i·nous (os″tee-o-kahr″ti-laj′i-nus) *adj.* Pertaining to or composed of both bone and cartilage.

os·teo·chon·dral (os″tee-o-kon′drul) *adj.* [*osteo-* + *chondral*]. Composed of both bone and cartilage.

os·teo·chon·dri·tis (os″tee-o-kon-drigh′tis) *n.* [*osteo-* + *chondr-* + *-itis*]. 1. Inflammation of both bone and cartilage. 2. OSTEOCHONDROSIS.

osteochondritis de·for·mans cox·ae ju·ve·ni·lis (de-for′manz kock′see joo-ve-nigh′lis). Osteochondrosis of the head of the femur.

osteochondritis deformans juvenilis. Osteochondrosis of the head of the femur.

osteochondritis dis·se·cans (dis′e-kanz). A joint affection characterized by partial or complete detachment of a fragment of articular cartilage and underlying bone. Syn. *osteochondrosis dissecans.*

os·teo·chon·dro·dys·pla·sia (os″tee-o-kon″dro-dis-play′zhuh, -zee-uh) *n.* [*osteo-* + *chondro-* + *dysplasia*]. Abnormal development of bony and cartilaginous structures.

os·teo·chon·dro·dys·tro·phia de·for·mans (os″tee-o-kon″dro-dis-tro′fee-uh de-for′manz). MORQUIO'S SYNDROME.

os·teo·chon·dro·dys·tro·phy (os″tee-o-kon″dro-dis′truh-fee) *n.* [*osteo-* + *chondro-* + *dystrophy*]. MORQUIO'S SYNDROME.

os·teo·chon·dro·ma (os″tee-o-kon-dro′muh) *n.* [*osteo-* + *chondr-* + *-oma*]. 1. A benign hamartomatous tumor originating in bone or cartilage, occasionally from other structure, which histologically contains both bone and cartilage. 2. EXOSTOSIS CARTILAGINEA.

os·teo·chon·dro·ma·to·sis (os″tee-o-kon-dro″muh-to′sis) *n.* MULTIPLE HEREDITARY EXOSTOSES.

os·teo·chon·dro·myx·o·ma (os″tee-o-kon″dro-mick-so′muh) *n.* An osteochondroma with a myxoid component.

os·teo·chon·dro·myxo·sar·co·ma (os″tee-o-kon″dro-mick″so-sahr-ko′muh) *n.* An osteosarcoma with a significant myxosarcomatous element.

os·teo·chon·dro·sar·co·ma (os″tee-o-kon″dro-sahr-ko′muh) *n.* An osteosarcoma with a significant chondrosarcomatous element.

os·teo·chon·dro·sis (os″tee-o-kon-dro′sis) *n.* [*osteo-* + *chondr-* + *-osis*]. A process involving ossification centers chiefly during periods of rapid growth, characterized by avascular necrosis followed by slow regeneration. Compare *osteochondritis.* See also *Calvé's disease* (1), *Kienböck's disease, Köhler's disease, Osgood-Schlatter disease, Scheuermann's disease.*

osteochondrosis de·for·mans ju·ve·ni·lis (de-for′manz joo-ve-nigh′lis). Osteochondrosis of the head of the femur.

osteochondrosis deformans tib·i·ae (tib′ee-ee). Nonrachitic bowing of the legs seen in very young, and less frequently in older, children, which usually improves spontaneously. Syn. *Blount-Barber syndrome.*

osteochondrosis dissecans. OSTEOCHONDRITIS DISSECANS.

os·teo·chon·drous (os″tee-o-kon′drus) *adj.* OSTEOCHONDRAL.

os·te·oc·la·sis (os″tee-ock′luh-sis) *n.* [*osteo-* + *-clasis*]. 1. The fracture of a long bone without resort to open operation, for the purpose of correcting deformity. 2. The destruction of bony tissue; the resorption of bone.

os·teo·clast (os′tee-o-klast) *n.* [*osteo-* + *-clast*]. 1. A powerful surgical apparatus or instrument through which leverage can be brought to bear at the point desired to effect osteoclasis or the forcible fracture of a long bone. 2. One of the large multinuclear cells found in association with the resorption of bone. —**os·teo·clas·tic** (os″tee-o-klast′ick) *adj.*

os·teo·clas·to·ma (os″tee-o-klas-to′muh) *n.* [*osteoclast* + *-oma*]. GIANT-CELL TUMOR.

os·teo·cope (os′tee-o-kope) *n.* [Gk. *osteokopos*, from *osteon*, bone, + *kopos*, pain, fatigue]. OSTEOCOPIC PAIN. —**os·teo·cop·ic** (os″tee-o-kop′ick) *adj.*

osteocopic pain. Severe bone pain, usually referring to syphilitic bone disease.

os·teo·cra·ni·um (os″tee-o-kray′nee-um) *n.* The ossified cranium as distinguished from the chondrocranium.

os·teo·cys·to·ma (os″tee-o-sis-to′muh) *n.* [*osteo-* + *cyst* + *-oma*]. A cystic bone tumor.

os·teo·cyte (os′tee-o-site) *n.* [*osteo-* + *-cyte*]. BONE CELL.

os·teo·den·tin (os″tee-o-den′tin) *n.* [*osteo-* + *dentin*]. A tissue intermediate in structure between bone and dentin.

os·teo·den·tine (os″tee-o-den′teen, -tin) *n.* OSTEODENTIN.

os·teo·der·ma·to·plas·tic (os″tee-o-dur″muh-to-plast′ick) *adj.* [*osteo-* + *dermato-* + *plastic*]. Pertaining to the formation of osseous tissue in dermal structures.

os·teo·der·mia (os″tee-o-dur′mee-uh) *n.* [*osteo-* + *-dermia*]. A condition characterized by bony formations in the skin.

os·teo·di·as·ta·sis (os″tee-o-dye-as′tuh-sis) *n.* [*osteo-* + *diastasis*]. Separation of bone (as an epiphysis) without true fracture, or of two normally contiguous bones.

os·te·o·dyn·ia (os″tee-o-din′ee-uh) *n.* [*oste-* + *-odynia*]. A pain in a bone.

os·teo·dys·tro·phia (os″tee-o-dis-tro′fee-uh) *n.* OSTEODYSTROPHY.

osteodystrophia de·for·mans (de-for′manz). PAGET'S DISEASE (2).

osteodystrophia fi·bro·sa (figh-bro′suh). FIBROUS DYSPLASIA (1).

os·teo·dys·tro·phy (os″tee-o-dis′truh-fee) *n.* [*osteo-* + *dystrophy*]. Any defective bone formation, as in rickets or dwarfism.

os·teo·epiph·y·sis (os″tee-o-e-pif′i-sis) *n.* EPIPHYSIS.

os·teo·fi·bro·chon·dro·ma (os″tee-o-figh″bro-kon-dro′muh) *n.* An osteochondroma with a significant fibrous element.

os·teo·fi·bro·li·po·ma (os″tee-o-figh″bro-li-po′muh) *n.* [*osteo-* + *fibro-* + *lip-* + *-oma*]. A benign tumor with bony, fibrous, and fatty components.

os·teo·fi·bro·ma (os″tee-o-figh-bro′muh) *n.* A benign tumor with fibrous and osseous components. See also *ossifying fibroma.*

os·teo·fi·bro·sar·co·ma (os″tee-o-figh″bro-sahr-ko′muh) *n.* An osteogenic sarcoma with a prominent fibrosarcomatous element.

os·teo·fi·bro·sis (os″tee-o-figh-bro′sis) *n.* Fibrosis of bone; a change involving mainly the red bone marrow.

os·teo·gen (os′tee-o-jen) *n.* The substance from which osteogenic fibers are formed.

os·teo·gen·e·sis (os″tee-o-jen′e-sis) *n.* [*osteo-* + *-genesis*]. The development of bony tissues; ossification; the histogenesis of bone.

osteogenesis im·per·fec·ta (im·pur·feck'tuh). A dominantly heritable disease characterized by hypoplasia of osteoid tissue and collagen, resulting in bone fractures with minimal trauma, hypermotility of joints, blue sclerae, and a hemorrhagic tendency.

osteogenesis imperfecta con·gen·i·ta (kon·jen'i·tuh). A more severe form of osteogenesis imperfecta with onset of multiple fractures in utero and autosomal recessive inheritance in some cases.

osteogenesis imperfecta cys·ti·ca (sis'ti·kuh). A rare form of osteogenesis imperfecta in which cystic changes of bone are found radiographically.

osteogenesis imperfecta tar·da (tahr'duh). Osteogenesis imperfecta in which fractures do not occur until later childhood.

os·teo·ge·net·ic (os''tee·o·je·net'ick) *adj.* OSTEOGENIC.

os·teo·gen·ic (os''tee·o·jen'ick) *adj.* Pertaining to osteogenesis, as osteogenic layer, the deep layer of periosteum from which bone is formed.

osteogenic fibers. The precollagenous fibers that pass between the osteoblasts during bone formation to form the fibrillar component of the bone matrix. Syn. *Korff's fibers.*

osteogenic fibroma. OSSIFYING FIBROMA.

osteogenic layer. The deeper layer of periosteum, connected with the formation of bone.

osteogenic sarcoma. A malignant tumor principally composed of anaplastic cells of mesenchymal derivation. When osteogenesis predominates, it is also called osteoblastic sarcoma, sclerosing osteogenic sarcoma, and osteoblastoma; when osteolysis is the predominating feature, it is called osteolytic sarcoma, telangiectatic sarcoma, malignant bone aneurysm, osteoaneurysm, and malignant bone cyst. Syn. *osteosarcoma.*

osteogenic tumor. Any tumor of bone-forming tissue. See also *osteoma, osteogenic sarcoma.*

os·te·og·e·nous (os''tee·oj'e·nus) *adj.* [Gk. *osteogenēs,* produced in bone]. OSTEOGENIC.

os·te·og·e·ny (os''tee·oj'e·nee) *n.* OSTEOGENESIS.

os·teo·hal·i·ste·re·sis (os''tee·o·hal''i·ste·ree'sis) *n.* [*osteo-* + *halisteresis*]. A loss of the mineral constituents of bone frequently resulting in softening and deformity of the bone.

os·teo·hy·per·troph·ic (os''tee·o·high''pur·trof'ick) *adj.* [*osteo-* + *hypertrophic*]. Pertaining to overgrowth of bone.

os·te·oid (os'tee·oid) *adj. & n.* [*oste-* + *-oid*]. 1. Resembling bone. 2. Of or pertaining to bone. 3. The young hyalin matrix of true bone in which the calcium salts are deposited.

osteoid aneurysm. A pulsating tumor of a bone.

osteoid osteoma. A benign hamartomatous tumor of bone, composed of a nidus of well-vascularized connective tissue and osteoid matrix surrounded by atypical trabeculae of dense new bone, occurring almost exclusively in younger age groups and characteristically accompanied by severe pain.

os·teo·lath·y·rism (os''tee·o·lath'ur·iz·um) *n.* [*osteo-* + *lathyrism*]. Degeneration of collagen in bone, often in the aorta as well, resulting from the experimental administration of beta-aminopropionitrile.

os·teo·lipo·chon·dro·ma (os''tee·o·lip''o·kon·dro'muh) *n.* [*osteo-* + *lipo-* + *chondroma*]. A chondroma with osseous and fatty elements.

os·teo·lith (os'tee·o·lith) *n.* [*osteo-* + *-lith*]. A petrified or fossil bone.

os·teo·lo·gia (os''tee·o·lo'jee·uh) *n.* [NA]. OSTEOLOGY.

os·te·ol·o·gy (os''tee·ol'uh·jee) *n.* [*osteo-* + *-logy*]. The science of anatomy and structure of bones.

os·te·ol·y·sis (os''tee·ol'i·sis) *n.* [*osteo-* + *-lysis*]. 1. Resorption of bone. 2. Degeneration of bone. —**os·teo·lyt·ic** (os''tee·o·lit'ick) *adj.*

osteolytic cancer. A malignant tumor, primary or metastatic, which destroys bone.

osteolytic sarcoma. A variety of osteogenic sarcoma in which bone destruction is prominent.

os·te·o·ma (os''tee·o'muh) *n.* [*oste-* + *-oma*]. 1. A benign bony tumor seen particularly in the membrane bones of the skull and exhibiting a tendency to extend into the orbit or paranasal sinuses. 2. Loosely, a nonneoplastic or neoplastic lesion such as a hyperostosis, a fibrous dysplasia, or an exostosis (osteochondroma). —**osteoma·toid** (·toid) *adj.*

osteoma cutis. Bony metaplasia in the skin and tissue, usually secondary to some other skin lesion.

osteoma du·rum (dew'rum) [L., hard]. A hard, dense osteoma with little marrow. Syn. *osteoma eburneum.*

osteoma ebur·ne·um (e·bur'nee·um) [L., ivory]. OSTEOMA DURUM.

os·teo·ma·la·cia (os''tee·o·muh·lay'shee·uh) *n.* [*osteo-* + *malacia*]. Failure of ossification due to a decrease in the amount of available calcium from any of multiple causes. Syn. *adult rickets.* —**osteomala·ci·al** (·shee·ul), **osteomala·cic** (·sick) *adj.*

osteomalacic pelvis. A distorted pelvis characterized by a lessening of the transverse and oblique diameters, with great increase of the anteroposterior diameter.

osteoma med·ul·la·re (med''uh·lair'ee). An osteoma with conspicuous marrow spaces.

osteoma spon·gi·o·sum (spon·jee·o'sum). An osteoma that is spongy because of coarse bands of cancellous bone.

os·te·o·ma·to·sis (os''tee·o''muh·to'sis) *n.* The presence of multiple osteomas.

os·te·om·e·try (os''tee·om'e·tree) *n.* [*osteo-* + *-metry*]. The study of the proportions and measurements of the skeleton. —**os·teo·met·ric** (os''tee·o·met'rick) *adj.*

os·teo·mu·coid (os''tee·o·mew'koid) *n.* OSSEOMUCOID.

os·teo·my·e·li·tis (os''tee·o·migh''e·lye'tis) *n.* [*osteo-* + *myel-* + *-itis*]. Inflammation of the marrow and hard tissue of bone, usually caused by a bacterial infection. —**osteomye·lit·ic** (·lit'ick) *adj.*

os·teo·myxo·chon·dro·ma (os''tee·o·mick''so·kon·dro'muh) *n.* An osteochondroma with a myxoid component.

os·te·on (os'tee·on) *n.* [*oste-* + *-on*]. A concentric lamellar (haversian) system with its haversian canal.

os·te·one (os'tee·ohn) *n.* OSTEON.

os·teo·ne·cro·sis (os''tee·o·ne·kro'sis) *n.* Necrosis of bone.

os·teo·ne·phrop·a·thy (os''tee·o·nef·rop'uth·ee) *n.* [*osteo-* + *nephro-* + *-pathy*]. Any of a variety of syndromes involving bone changes accompanying renal disease.

os·teo·neu·ral·gia (os''tee·o·new·ral'juh) *n.* [*osteo-* + *neuralgia*]. Bone pain.

os·teo·on·y·cho·dys·tro·phia (os''tee·o·on''i·ko·dis·tro'fee·uh) *n.* [*osteo-* + *onycho-* + *dystrophia*]. NAIL-PATELLA SYNDROME.

osteopaedion. Osteopedion (= LITHOPEDION).

os·teo·path (os'tee·o·path) *n.* One who practices osteopathic medicine.

os·teo·path·ia (os·tee·o·path'ee·uh) *n.* [NL., from *osteo-* + *path-* + *-ia*]. Any bone disease or defect.

osteopathia con·den·sans dis·sem·i·na·ta (kun·den'sanz di·sem'i·nay'tuh, ·nah'tuh). OSTEOPOIKILOSIS.

osteopathia hy·per·os·tot·i·ca mul·ti·plex in·fan·ti·lis (high''pur·os·tot'i·kuh mul'ti·plecks in·fan'ti·lis). PROGRESSIVE DIAPHYSEAL DYSPLASIA.

osteopathia stri·a·ta (strye·ay'tuh). An unusual congenital osseous defect characterized by the roentgenographic finding of striation of the skeleton and particularly cancellous bone. It may be related to osteopoikilosis.

os·te·op·a·thist (os''tee·op'uh·thist) *n.* OSTEOPATH.

osteopathic medicine. The principles and practice of medicine as employed by osteopaths; OSTEOPATHY.

os·te·op·a·thy (os''tee·op'uth·ee) *n.* [NL. *osteopathia*]. 1. A school of healing which teaches that the body is a vital mechanical organism whose structural and functional integrity are coordinate and interdependent, the abnormality of either constituting disease. Its major effort in treatment is in manipulation, but medicine, surgery, and the specialties are also utilized. 2. Any disease of bone. —**os·teo·path·ic** (os″tee·o·path′ick) *adj.*

os·teo·pe·cil·ia (os″tee·o·pe·sil′ee·uh) *n.* [*osteo-* + Gk. *poikilia,* mottling, variegation]. OSTEOPOIKILOSIS.

os·teo·pe·di·on, os·teo·pae·di·on (os″tee·o·pee′dee·un) *n.* [*osteo-* + Gk. *paidion,* little child]. LITHOPEDION.

os·teo·pe·nia (os″tee·o·pee′nee·uh) *n.* [*osteo-* + *-penia*]. Any condition presenting less bone than normal.

os·teo·peri·os·te·al graft (os″tee·o·perr″ee·os′tee·ul). A graft of bone and periosteum.

os·teo·peri·os·ti·tis (os″tee·o·perr″ee·os·tigh′tis) *n.* [*osteo-* + *periostitis*]. Combined inflammation of bone and its periosteum.

os·teo·pe·tro·sis (os″tee·o·pe·tro′sis) *n.* [*osteo-* + *petr-* + *-osis*]. A disorder of bone in which sclerosis obliterates the marrow, leading to bone marrow failure which may cause early death. Clinical features include optic atrophy, deafness, hepatosplenomegaly, and characteristic excess density of bones on x-ray. Syn. *Albers-Schönberg disease.* —**osteope·trot·ic** (·trot′ick) *adj.*

osteopetrosis gal·li·na·rum (gal″i·nair′um) [L., of fowl]. OSTEOPETROTIC LYMPHOMATOSIS.

osteopetrosis gen·er·al·i·sa·ta (jen″ur·al·i·zay′tuh, ·sah′tuh). OSTEOPETROSIS.

osteopetrotic lymphomatosis. A form of the avian leukosis complex affecting bone.

os·teo·phage (os′tee·o·faje) *n.* [*osteo-* + *-phage*]. OSTEOCLAST (2).

os·te·oph·o·ny (os″tee·off′uh·nee) *n.* [*osteo-* + *-phony*]. The transmission of sound through bone.

os·te·oph·thi·sis (os″tee·off′thi·sis) *n.* [*osteo-* + *phthisis*]. Wasting of the bones.

os·teo·phyte (os′tee·o·fite) *n.* [*osteo-* + *-phyte,* growth]. A bony outgrowth.

os·teo·phy·to·sis (os″tee·o·fye·to′sis) *n.* A condition characterized by the presence of osteophytes. —**osteo·phyt·ic** (·fit′ick) *adj.*

os·teo·plaque (os′tee·o·plack) *n.* [*osteo-* + *plaque*]. A layer of bone; a flat osteoma.

os·teo·plast (os′tee·o·plast) *n.* [*osteo-* + *-plast*]. OSTEOBLAST.

os·teo·plas·tic (os″tee·o·plas′tick) *adj.* [*osteo-* + *plastic*]. 1. Pertaining to the formation of bone tissue. 2. Pertaining to reparative operations upon bone.

osteoplastic amputation. An amputation in which there is a portion of bone fitted to the amputated bone end. See also *Gritti-Stokes amputation.*

osteoplastic cancer. A malignant tumor, primary or metastatic, which stimulates bone formation in its immediate neighborhood.

osteoplastic flap. A flap of skin and underlying bone, commonly of scalp and skull, raised for the purpose of exploring the underlying structures.

os·teo·plas·ty (os′tee·o·plas″tee) *n.* [*osteo-* + *-plasty*]. Plastic operations on bone.

os·teo·poi·ki·lo·sis (os″tee·o·poy″ki·lo′sis) *n.* [*osteo-* + Gk. *poikilos,* many-colored, dappled, + *-osis*]. A bone affection of unknown cause, giving rise to no symptoms and discovered by chance on roentgenographic examination when ellipsoidal dense foci are seen in all bones. Syn. *osteopathia condensans disseminata.*

os·teo·po·ro·sis (os″tee·o·po·ro′sis) *n.* [*osteo-* + *porosis*]. Deossification with absolute decrease in bone tissue, resulting in enlargement of marrow and haversian spaces, decreased thickness of cortex and trabeculae, and structural weakness. —**osteopo·rot·ic** (·rot′ick) *adj.*

os·te·op·sath·y·ro·sis (os″tee·op·sath″i·ro′sis, os″·tee·o·sath″i·) *n.* [*osteo-* + Gk. *psathyros,* crumbling, friable, + *-osis*]. OSTEOGENESIS IMPERFECTA.

os·teo·pul·mo·nary arthropathy (os″tee·o·pŏŏl′muh·nerr·ee, ·pul′muh·) [*osteo-* + *pulmonary*]. HYPERTROPHIC PULMONARY OSTEOARTHROPATHY.

os·teo·ra·dio·ne·cro·sis (os″tee·o·ray″dee·o·ne·kro′sis) *n.* [*osteo-* + *radionecrosis*]. Bone necrosis due to irradiation, usually by roentgen or gamma rays.

os·te·or·rha·gia (os″tee·o·ray′jee·uh) *n.* [*osteo-* + *-rrhagia*]. Hemorrhage from a bone.

os·te·or·rha·phy (os″tee·or′uh·fee) *n.* [*osteo-* + *-rrhaphy*]. The suturing or joining of bones.

os·teo·sar·co·ma (os″tee·o·sahr·ko′muh) *n.* OSTEOGENIC SARCOMA. —**osteosarcoma·tous** (·tus) *adj.*

os·teo·scle·ro·sis (os″tee·o·skle·ro′sis) *n.* [*osteo-* + *sclerosis*]. 1. Abnormal increased density of bone, occurring in a variety of pathologic states. 2. OSTEOPETROSIS. —**osteoscle·rot·ic** (·rot′ick) *adj.*

osteosclerosis frag·i·lis gen·er·al·i·sa·ta (fraj′i·lis jen″ur·al·i·zay′tuh, ·sah′tuh) [L.]. OSTEOPETROSIS.

osteosclerotic anemia. MYELOPHTHISIC ANEMIA.

os·te·o·sis (os″tee·o′sis) *n.* [*oste-* + *-osis*]. Metaplastic bone formation.

osteosis cutis. OSTEOMA CUTIS.

os·teo·spon·gi·o·ma (os″tee·o·spon·jee·o′muh, ·spun·jee·o′muh) *n.* [*osteo-* + *spongi-* + *-oma*]. A tumorous mass consisting of cancellous bone.

os·teo·stix·is (os″tee·o·stick′sis) *n.* [*osteo-* + Gk. *stixis,* marking, tattooing]. Surgical puncturing of a bone.

os·teo·su·ture (os′tee·o·sue″chur, os″tee·o·sue′chur) *n.* Suture of bone.

os·teo·syn·o·vi·tis (os″tee·o·sin″o·vye′tis, ·sigh″no·vye′tis) *n.* Synovitis complicated with osteitis of adjacent bones.

os·teo·syn·the·sis (os″tee·o·sin′thi·sis) *n.* Fastening the ends of a fractured bone together by mechanical means, such as a plate.

os·teo·ta·bes (os″tee·o·tay′beez) *n.* [*osteo-* + *tabes*]. Bone degeneration beginning with the destruction of the cells of the bone marrow, which disappears in parts and is replaced by soft gelatinous tissue; later the spongy bone diminishes, and lastly the compact bone.

os·teo·throm·bo·sis (os″tee·o·throm·bo′sis) *n.* Thrombosis of the veins of a bone.

os·teo·tome (os′tee·o·tome) *n.* [*osteo-* + *-tome*]. An instrument for cutting bone; specifically, an instrument somewhat similar to a chisel but without the beveled edge, used for cutting long bones, generally with the aid of a surgical mallet.

os·teo·to·mo·cla·sia (os″tee·o·to″mo·klay′zhuh, ·zee·uh, os″tee·ot″uh·mo·) *n.* OSTEOTOMOCLASIS.

os·teo·to·moc·la·sis (os″tee·ot″o·mock′luh·sis, os″tee·o·to·) *n.* [*osteotome* + *-clasis*]. The correction of a pathologically curved bone by forcible bending following partial division by an osteotome.

os·te·ot·o·my (os″tee·ot′um·ee) *n.* [*osteo-* + *-tomy*]. 1. The division of a bone. 2. Making a section of a bone for the purpose of correcting a deformity.

os·teo·tribe (os′tee·o·tribe) *n.* [*osteo-* + *-tribe*]. A bone rasp.

os·teo·trite (os″tee·o·trite) *n.* [*osteo-* + L. *terere, tritus,* to rub]. OSTEOTRIBE.

os·te·ot·ro·phy (os″tee·ot′ruh·fee) *n.* [*osteo-* + *-trophy*]. Nutrition of bony tissue.

os·teo·tym·pan·ic (os″tee·o·tim·pan′ick) *adj.* [*osteo-* + *tympan-* + *-ic*]. CRANIOTYMPANIC.

osteotympanic conduction. BONE CONDUCTION.

ostia. Plural of *ostium.*

ostia atrio·ven·tri·cu·la·ria dex·trum et si·nis·trum (ay″tree·o·ven·trick″yoo·lair′ee·uh decks′trum et si·nis′trum) [NA]. The right and left atrioventricular openings.

ostia ve·na·rum pul·mo·na·li·um (ve·nair′um pul″mo·nay′lee·um) [NA]. The openings of the pulmonary veins into the left atrium.

os ti·bi·a·le ex·ter·num (tib·ee·ay′lee ecks·tur′num). A small anomalous bone situated in the angle between the navicular bone and the head of the talus.

os·ti·tis (os·tigh′tis) *n.* OSTEITIS.

os·ti·um (os′tee·um) *n.,* genit. **os·tii** (os′tee·eye), pl. **os·tia** (os′

tee·uh) [L., door, mouth, entrance]. A mouth or aperture. —**osti·al** (·ul) *adj.*

ostium ab·do·mi·na·le tu·bae ute·ri·nae (ab·dom″i·nay′lee tew′bee yoo·tur·eye′nee) [NA]. The orifice of the uterine tube communicating with the peritoneal cavity.

ostium aor·tae (ay·or′tee) [NA]. The opening between the left ventricle and the aorta.

ostium ap·pen·di·cis ver·mi·for·mis (a·pen′di·sis vur·mi·for′ mis) [NA]. The opening of the vermiform appendix into the cecum.

ostium ar·te·ri·o·sum cor·dis (ahr·teer·ee·o′sum kor′dis) [BNA]. The opening between the left atrium and the left ventricle.

ostium atrio·ven·tri·cu·la·re (ay″tree·o·ven·trick·yoo·lair′ee). Either the right or left atrioventricular opening.

ostium atrioventriculare dex·trum (decks′trum) [NA]. The right atrioventricular opening.

ostium atrioventriculare si·nis·trum (si·nis′trum) [NA]. The left atrioventricular opening.

ostium car·di·a·cum (kahr·dye′uh·kum) [NA]. CARDIAC ORIFICE.

ostium ileo·ce·ca·le (il″ee·o·see·kay′lee) [NA]. The opening of the ileum into the cecum.

ostium max·il·la·re (mack″si·lair′ee). MAXILLARY HIATUS.

ostium of the uterus. OSTIUM UTERI.

ostium pha·ryn·ge·um tu·bae au·di·ti·vae (fa·rin′jee·um tew′ bee aw·di·tye′vee) [NA]. The opening of the auditory tube into the pharynx.

ostium py·lo·ri·cum (pi·lo′ri·kum) [NA]. The pyloric opening of the stomach into the duodenum.

ostium trun·ci pul·mo·na·lis (trunk′eye pul·mo·nay′lis, trun′ sigh) [NA]. The opening from the right ventricle into the pulmonary trunk.

ostium tym·pa·ni·cum tu·bae au·di·ti·vae (tim·pan′i·kum tew′ bee aw·di·tye′vee) [NA]. The opening of the auditory tube into the middle ear cavity.

ostium ure·te·ris (yoo·ree′tur·is) [NA]. The opening of either ureter into the urinary bladder.

ostium ure·thrae fe·mi·ni·nae ex·ter·num (yoo·ree′three fem·i·nigh′nee ecks·tur′num) [NA]. The external opening of the female urethra.

ostium urethrae in·ter·num [NA]. The opening between the urinary bladder and the urethra.

ostium urethrae mas·cu·li·nae ex·ter·num (mas″kew·lye′nee ecks·tur′num) [NA]. The external opening of the male urethra.

ostium ute·ri (yoo′tur·eye) [NA]. The opening of the cervix of the uterus into the vagina.

ostium ute·ri·num tu·bae (yoo·tur·eye′num tew′bee) [NA]. The opening of either uterine tube into the cavity of the uterus.

ostium va·gi·nae (va·jye′nee) [NA]. The external orifice of the vagina.

ostium ve·nae ca·vae in·fe·ri·o·ris (vee′nee kay′vee in·feer·ee·o′ris) [NA]. The opening of the inferior vena cava into the right atrium.

ostium venae cavae su·pe·ri·o·ris (sue·peer·ee·o′ris) [NA]. The opening of the superior vena cava into the right atrium.

ostium ve·no·sum cor·dis (ve·no′sum kor′dis) [BNA]. OSTIUM ATRIOVENTRICULARE DEXTRUM.

os·to·my (os′tuh·mee) *n.* [by generalization from such terms as col*ostomy*, jejun*ostomy*]. *Informal.* A surgical procedure in which parts of the intestinal or urinary tract are removed from the patient, and an artifical opening or stoma is constructed through the abdominal wall to allow for the passage of urine or feces. See also *colostomy, ileostomy, ureterostomy.*

os·to·sis (os·to′sis) *n.* OSTEOSIS.

os tra·pe·zi·um (tra·pee′zee·um) [NA]. TRAPEZIUM.

os tra·pe·zoi·de·um (trap″e·zoy′dee·um) [NA]. TRAPEZOID (2).

os·treo·tox·ism (os″tree·o·tock′siz·um) *n.* [Gk. *ostreon*, oyster, + *tox-* + *-ism*]. Poisoning from eating diseased or contaminated oysters.

os tri·go·num (trye·go′num). An ossicle due to the separation of the lateral tubercle of the posterior surface of the talus and ossification from a distinct center.

os tri·que·trum (trye·kwee′trum) [NA]. TRIQUETRUM (1).

os ute·ri (yoo′tur·eye). OSTIUM UTERI.

os uteri ex·ter·num (ecks·tur′num). OSTIUM UTERI.

os uteri in·ter·num (in·tur′num). The juncture of the lower end of the isthmus uteri with the endocervical canal.

os Ve·sa·lii (ve·say′lee·eye) [A. *Vesalius*]. 1. An occasional accessory ossicle between the hamate and fifth metacarpal. 2. An occasional accessory ossicle at the base of the fifth metatarsal.

os zy·go·ma·ti·cum (zye″go·mat′i·kum) [NA]. ZYGOMATIC BONE.

OT, O.T. 1. *In anatomy,* old term, in opposition to BNA or NA term. 2. An abbreviation for *original tuberculin* and *old tuberculin.*

ot-, oto- [Gk. *ous, ōtos*]. A combining form meaning *ear.*

otal·gia (o·tal′jee·uh) *n.* [*ot-* + *-algia*]. EARACHE. —**otal·gic** (·jick) *adj.*

otan·tri·tis (o″tan·trye′tis) *n.* [*ot-* + *antr-* + *-itis*]. Inflammation of the mastoid antrum.

Ota ring [T. *Ota*, Jap. gynecologist, 20th century]. An early IUD which has been widely used in Japan and other western Pacific countries.

othel·co·sis (o″thel·ko′sis, oat″hel·ko′sis) *n.* [*ot-* + Gk. *helkōsis*, ulceration]. Ulceration of the ear.

othe·ma·to·ma, othae·ma·to·ma (oat·hee″muh·to′muh, o·theem′uh·) *n.* [*ot-* + *hematoma*]. Hematoma of the external ear, usually the pinna.

ot·hem·or·rha·gia, ot·haem·or·rha·gia (oat″hem·o·ray′juh, ·jee·uh, o·theem′o·) *n.* [*ot-* + *hemo-* + *-rrhagia*]. Hemorrhage from the ear.

ot·hem·or·rhea, ot·haem·or·rhoea (oat″hem·o·ree′uh, oath″ em·o·) *n.* [*ot-* + *hemo-* + *-rrhea*]. A sanguineous discharge from the ear.

-otic [Gk. *-ōtikos*]. A suffix meaning *pertaining to* or *causing the process* or *condition* that is usually designated by a noun ending in *-osis,* as osmotic, narcotic, mycotic, leukocytotic.

otic (o′tick) *adj.* [Gk. *ōtikos,* from *ous, ōtos,* ear.]. Pertaining to the ear.

otic barotrauma. BAROTITIS MEDIA.

otic bulla. TYMPANIC BULLA.

otic capsule. The cartilage capsule that surrounds the developing auditory vesicle and later fuses with the sphenoid and occipital cartilages.

otic cerebral abscess. An abscess of the brain following purulent disease of the ear.

otic duct. ENDOLYMPHATIC DUCT (1).

otic fluid. ENDOLYMPH.

otic ganglion. The nerve ganglion immediately below the foramen ovale of the sphenoid bone, medial to the mandibular nerve; it receives preganglionic fibers from the inferior salivatory nucleus of the ninth cranial nerve by way of the minor petrosal nerve and sends postganglionic parasympathetic fibers to the parotid gland. NA *ganglion oticum.* See also Plate 15.

oti·co·din·ia (o″ti·ko·din′ee·uh) *n.* [*otic* + Gk. *dinē,* whirling, + *-ia*]. *Obsol.* Vertigo from ear disease.

otic pit. AUDITORY PIT.

otic placode. AUDITORY PLACODE.

otic sac. AUDITORY VESICLE.

otic vesicle. AUDITORY VESICLE.

otitic hydrocephalus. A form of benign intracranial hypertension in children, associated with chronic mastoiditis causing a noninfectious thrombotic obstruction of the lateral sinus.

oti·tis (o·tye′tis) *n.*, pl. **otit·i·des** (o·tit′i·deez) [*ot-* + *-itis*]. Inflammation of the ear. —**otit·ic** (o·tit′ick) *adj.*

otitis ex·ter·na (ecks·tur′nuh). Inflammation of the external ear.

otitis in·ter·na (in·tur′nuh). Inflammation of the internal ear.

otitis lab·y·rin·thi·ca (lab·i·rin′thi·kuh). Inflammation of the labyrinth of the inner ear.

otitis mas·toi·dea (mas·toy′dee·uh). Inflammation confined to the mastoid cells.

otitis me·dia (mee′dee·uh). Inflammation of the middle ear.

otitis par·a·sit·i·ca (păr·uh·sit′i·kuh). Inflammation of the ear caused by a parasite.

otitis scle·rot·i·ca (skle·rot′i·kuh). Inflammation of the inner ear with hardening of the tissues. See also *otosclerosis.*

oto-. See *ot-.*

oto·blen·nor·rhea, oto·blen·nor·rhoea (o″to·blen″o·ree′uh) *n.* [*oto-* + *blennorrhea*]. Any discharge of mucus from the ear.

oto·ca·tarrh (o″to·ka·tahr′) *n.* [*oto-* + *catarrh*]. Catarrh of the ear.

oto·ceph·a·lus (o″tuh·sef′ul·us) *n.* [*oto-* + *-cephalus*]. A fetus characterized by a union or close approach of the ears, by absence of the lower jaw, and an ill-developed mouth. See also *synotus, agnathus.* **—otoceph·ly** (·lee) *n.*

oto·clei·sis (o″to·klye′sis) *n.* [*oto-* + Gk. *kleisis,* a closing]. Occlusion of the ear.

oto·co·nia (o″to·ko′nee·uh) *n.,* sing. **otoco·ni·um** (·nee·um) [*oto-* + Gk. *konia,* dust]. Crystals of calcium carbonate, 1 to 5 μm long, contained in the soft substance over the two maculae acusticae. Syn. *statoconia.* See also *otolith.*

oto·cyst (o′to·sist) *n.* [*oto-* + *cyst*]. 1. In invertebrates, an auditory vesicle. 2. In vertebrates, the embryonic auditory vesicle.

oto·dyn·ia (o″to·din′ee·uh) *n.* [*ot-* + *-odynia*]. Pain in the ear.

oto·gen·ic (oto·jen′ick) *adj.* [*oto-* + *-genic*]. Originating or arising within the ear.

otog·e·nous (o·toj′e·nus) *adj.* [*oto-* + *-genous*]. OTOGENIC.

otogenous pyemia. Pyemia originating in the ear.

oto·hemi·neur·as·the·nia (o″to·hem″ee·neur″as·theen′ee·uh) *n.* [*oto-* + *hemi-* + *neur-* + *asthenia*]. A condition in which hearing is limited exclusively to one ear, without the evidence of any material lesion of the auditory apparatus.

oto·lar·yn·gol·o·gist (o″to·lăr″ing·gol′uh·jist) *n.* A person skilled in the practice of otology, rhinology, and laryngology.

oto·lar·yn·gol·o·gy (o″to·lăr″ing·gol′uh·jee) *n.* [*oto-* + *laryngo-* + *-logy*]. A specialty including otology, rhinology, laryngology, and surgery of the head and neck.

oto·lith (o′to·lith) *n.* [*oto-* + *-lith*]. One of the calcareous concretions within the membranous labyrinth of the ear, especially the large ear stones of fishes. See also *otoconia.*

otol·o·gist (o·tol′uh·jist) *n.* A person skilled in otology.

otol·o·gy (o·tol′uh·jee) *n.* [*oto-* + *-logy*]. The science of the ear, its anatomy, functions, and diseases. **—oto·log·ic** (o″tuh·loj′ick), **otolog·i·cal** (·i·kul) *adj.*

oto·my·as·the·nia (o″to·migh″as·theen′ee·uh) *n.* [*oto-* + *myasthenia*]. 1. Weakness of the muscles of the ear. 2. Defective hearing due to a paretic condition of the tensor tympani or stapedius muscle.

oto·my·co·sis (o″to·migh·ko′sis) *n.* [*oto-* + *mycosis*]. Infection of the external auditory meatus and of the ear canal, from which a number of fungi and bacteria can be isolated, but with the weight of evidence favoring the bacteria as the prime agents and the fungi as secondary.

oto·neu·ral·gia (o″to·new·ral′jee·uh) *n.* [*oto-* + *neuralgia*]. Otalgia; EARACHE.

oto·neur·as·the·nia (o″to·newr″as·theen′ee·uh) *n.* [*oto-* + *neur-* + *asthenia*]. A condition of deficient sensitivity of the auditory apparatus.

oto·pal·a·to·dig·i·tal (o″to·pal″uh·to·dij′i·tul) *adj.* Pertaining to the ear, palate, and digits.

otopalatodigital syndrome. Deafness, cleft palate, and generalized bone dysplasia with a pugilistic facies in males.

oto·pha·ryn·ge·al (o″to·fa·rin′jee·ul) *adj.* [*oto-* + *pharyngeal*]. Pertaining to the ear and the pharynx.

oto·plas·ty (o′to·plas″tee) *n.* [*oto-* + *-plasty*]. Plastic surgery of the external ear.

oto·pol·y·pus (o″to·pol′i·pus) *n.* [*oto-* + *polypus*]. A polyp occurring in the ear.

oto·py·or·rhea, oto·py·or·rhoea (o″to·pye″o·ree′uh) *n.* [*oto-* + *pyorrhea*]. A purulent discharge from the ear.

oto·py·o·sis (o″to·pye·o′sis) *n.* [*oto-* + *pyosis*]. Suppuration within the ear.

oto·rhi·no·lar·yn·gol·o·gy (o″to·rye″no·lăr·ing·gol′uh·jee) *n.* [*oto-* + *rhino-* + *laryngo-* + *-logy*]. The study of diseases of the ear, nose, and throat.

oto·rhi·nol·o·gy (o″to·rye·nol′uh·jee) *n.* [*oto-* + *rhino-* + *-logy*]. Literally, the study of diseases of the ears and the nose only. See also *otolaryngology, otorhinolaryngology.*

otor·rha·gia (o″to·ray′jee·uh) *n.* [*oto-* + *-rrhagia*]. A discharge of blood from the external auditory meatus.

otor·rhea, otor·rhoea (o″to·ree′uh) *n.* [*oto-* + *-rrhea*]. A discharge from the external auditory meatus. See also *cerebrospinal otorrhea.*

oto·sal·pinx (o″to·sal′pinks) *n.,* pl. **oto·sal·pin·ges** (·sal·pin′jeez) [*oto-* + *salpinx*]. *Obsol.* AUDITORY TUBE.

oto·scle·ro·sis (o″to·skle·ro′sis) *n.* [*oto-* + *sclerosis*]. A pathologic change in the middle and inner ear resulting in the laying down of new bone around the oval window, the cochlea, or both, and causing progressive impairment of hearing. **—otoscle·rot·ic** (·rot′ick) *adj.*

oto·scope (o′tuh·skope) *n.* [*oto-* + *-scope*]. An apparatus designed for examination of the ear and for rendering the tympanic membrane visible.

otos·co·py (o·tos′kuh·pee) *n.* [*oto-* + *-scopy*]. Visualization of the auditory canal and tympanic membrane by means of the otoscope. **—oto·scop·ic** (o″tuh·skop′ick) *adj.*

otot·o·my (o·tot′uh·mee) *n.* [*oto-* + *-tomy*]. 1. Dissection of the ear. 2. Incision of any of the tissues of the external auditory meatus or the ear proper.

oto·tox·ic (o″to·tock′sick) *adj.* [*oto-* + *toxic*]. Having harmful effects on the ear, especially on its neural parts. **—oto·tox·ic·i·ty** (·tock·sis′i·tee) *n.*

Otrivin. Trademark for xylometazoline, used as the hydrochloride salt as a vasoconstrictor to reduce swelling and congestion of the nasal mucosa.

ot·to (ot′o) *n.* ATTAR.

otto of rose. ROSE OIL.

Ot·to's disease [A. W. *Otto,* German surgeon, 1786–1845]. ARTHROKATADYSIS.

Otto's pelvis [A. W. *Otto*]. ARTHROKATADYSIS.

Ott precipitation test. A test for nucleoprotein in which a solution is mixed with an equal volume of a saturated solution of sodium chloride; Almen's reagent is slowly added. In the presence of nucleoprotein, a precipitate forms.

O. U. Abbreviation for *oculus uterque,* each eye.

oua·ba·in (wah·bah′in, ·bay′in, wah′bah·in) *n.* [*ouabaio,* a kind of African tree]. $C_{29}H_{44}O_{12}.8H_2O$, a steroidal glycoside obtained from seeds of *Strophanthus gratus* and other sources; used clinically for its digitalis-like action.

Ouch·ter·lony technique. Double diffusion in agar wherein solutions of antibodies interact with antigens so as to give readily observable lines of precipitation.

ou·la (oo′luh) *n.* [Gk., gums]. GINGIVA.

ou·loid (oo′loid) *adj.* [Gk. *oulē,* scar, + *-oid*]. Resembling a scar.

ounce, *n.* [L. *uncia,* twelfth part of a pound]. A unit of measure and weight. See also *avoirdupois ounce, troy ounce, fluidounce,* and Tables of Weights and Measures in the Appendix.

ouro-. See *ur-.*

-ous [L. *-osus*]. 1. A general adjective-forming suffix meaning *having, pertaining to.* 2. *In chemistry,* a suffix indicating the lower of two valences assumed by an element. Contr. *-ic.*

outer dental epithelium. The peripheral cells lying at the convexity of the enamel organ.

outer hamstring. The tendon of the biceps femoris muscle.

outer longitudinal arch. NA *pars lateralis arcus pedis longitudinalis.* See *longitudinal arch of the foot.*

outer nuclear layer. The layer of the retina which contains the nucleus of the photoreceptor cells.

outer spiral sulcus. A groove where the basilar membrane is attached to the bony cochlear canal. NA *sulcus spiralis externus.* Contr. *spiral sulcus.*

out·flow, *n. In neurology,* the transmission of efferent impulses, particularly of the autonomic nervous system; these are divided into thoracolumbar and craniosacral outflows.

out·growth, *n.* Growth or development from a preexisting structure or state.

out·let of the pelvis. The lower aperture of the pelvic canal.

outline form. The shape of the area included in a dental cavity preparation.

out·pa·tient, *n.* A patient who comes to the hospital or clinic for diagnosis or treatment but who does not occupy a bed in the institution. Contr. *inpatient.*

out·pouch·ing, *n.* EVAGINATION.

out·put, *n.* Energy or matter leaving a structure or system of structures.

ova. Plural of *ovum.*

oval (o'vul) *adj.* [L. *ovalis,* from *ovum,* egg]. Egg-shaped.

oval area of Flechsig. SEPTOMARGINAL FASCICULUS.

ov·al·bu·min (o''val·bew'min) *n.* [*ovi-* + *albumin*]. The albumin of egg white.

oval area or **bundle of Flechsig** [P. E. *Flechsig*]. SEPTOMARGINAL FASCICULUS.

oval-cell anemia. ELLIPTOCYTOSIS.

ova·le malaria (o·vay'lee). A benign form of malaria occurring in Africa due to *Plasmodium ovale,* characterized by mild recurring tertian paroxysms, and similar to vivax malaria. Red blood cells and trophozoites are both at times oval in shape.

ovalo·cyte (o·val'o·site) *n.* [*oval* + *-cyte*]. ELLIPTOCYTE.

ovalo·cy·to·sis (o·val''o·sigh·to'sis, o''vuh·lo·) *n.* [*ovalocyte* + *-osis*]. ELLIPTOCYTOSIS.

oval window. An oval opening in the medial wall of the middle ear, closed by the foot plate of the stapes. Syn. *vestibular window.* NA *fenestra vestibuli.* See also Plate 20.

ovari-, ovario-. A combining form meaning *ovary* or *ovarian.*

ovaria. Plural of *ovarium.*

ovari·al·gia (o·văr''ee·al'juh, ·jee·uh) *n.* [*ovari-* + *-algia*]. Neuralgic pain in the ovary.

ovar·i·an (o·văr'ee·un, o·vair') *adj.* Pertaining to the ovaries.

ovarian agenesis. Failure of development of the ovaries. See also *Turner's syndrome.*

ovarian appendage. EPOOPHORON.

ovarian artery. The artery in the female that originates in the abdominal aorta and supplies the ovary, also providing ureteric, ligamentous, uterine, and tubal branches; corresponds to the testicular artery in the male. NA *arteria ovarica.*

ovarian bursa. A small pocket containing the ovary; formed by a fold of the broad ligament. Syn. *bursa ovarica.*

ovarian cords. CORTICAL CORDS.

ovarian dwarfism. GONADAL DYSGENESIS.

ovarian dysgenesis, agenesis, or **aplasia.** GONADAL DYSGENESIS.

ovarian dysmenorrhea. That form of dysmenorrhea due to disease of the ovaries.

ovarian follicle. The functional unit of oogenesis and ovulation in the ovary, consisting of an oocyte or ovum with its accessory structures. In the primary follicles (NA *folliculi ovarici primarii*) the growing oocyte is enveloped in increasing layers of follicular cells; the subsequent vesicular follicles (NA *folliculi ovarici vesiculosi*) develop a fluid-filled cavity which (in humans and many animals) displaces the ovum eccentrically. At this stage the follicles produce estrogenic hormones and a few of them progress to the fully mature (graafian follicle) stage, ready for ovulation.

ovarian graft. A portion of ovary implanted anywhere except in its normal bed, usually in the abdominal wall, for the preservation of the hormone production.

ovarian hormones. The two types of hormone produced by the ovary: the follicular or estrogenic hormones, estradiol, estrone, and estriol, which produce estrus in the spayed animal, and the luteal hormone, progesterone, produced by the corpus luteum.

ovarian insufficiency. Deficiency of ovarian function, either primary or secondary, which can result in either amenorrhea, oligomenorrhea, or abnormal dysfunctional uterine bleeding; a clinical term.

ovarian ligament. The terminal portion of the genital ridge uniting the caudal end of the embryonic ovary with the uterus. NA *ligamentum ovarii proprium.*

ovarian plexus. 1. A network of veins in the broad ligament. 2. A nerve plexus distributed to the ovaries. NA *plexus ovaricus.*

ovarian pregnancy. Gestation within the ovary.

ovarian pseudomyxoma. MUCINOUS CYSTADENOMA.

ovarian short-stature syndrome. GONADAL DYSGENESIS.

ovarian varicocele. Varicosity of the veins of an ovary.

ovari·ec·to·my (o·văr''ee·eck'tum·ee) *n.* [*ovari-* + *-ectomy*]. Excision of an ovary; oophorectomy.

ovario-. See *ovari-.*

ovar·io·cele (o·văr'ee·o·seel) *n.* [*ovario-* + *-cele*]. Hernia of an ovary.

ovar·io·cen·te·sis (o·văr''ee·o·sen·tee'sis) *n.* [*ovario-* + *centesis*]. Puncture of an ovary or of an ovarian cyst.

ovar·io·cy·e·sis (o·văr''ee·o·sigh·ee'sis) *n.* [*ovario-* + *cyesis*]. OVARIAN PREGNANCY.

ovar·io·dys·neu·ria (o·văr''ee·o·dis·new'ree·uh) *n.* [*ovario-* + *dys-* + *neur-* + *-ia*]. Ovarian neuralgia.

ovar·io·gen·ic (o·văr''ee·o·jen'ick) *adj.* [*ovario-* + *-genic*]. Arising in the ovary.

ovar·io·hys·ter·ec·to·my (o·văr''ee·o·his·tur·eck'tum·ee) *n.* [*ovario-* + *hyster-* + *-ectomy*]. Surgical removal of one or both ovaries and the uterus.

ovar·io·lyt·ic (o·văr''ee·o·lit'ick) *adj.* [*ovario-* + *-lytic*]. Producing disorganization of ovarian tissue.

ovari·on·cus (o·văr''ee·onk'us) *n.* [*ovari-* + Gk. *onkos,* bulk, mass]. An ovarian tumor.

ovar·i·or·rhex·is (o·văr''ee·o·reck'sis) *n.* [*ovario-* + Gk. *rhēxis,* a breaking]. Rupture of an ovary.

ovar·io·sal·pin·gec·to·my (o·văr''ee·o·sal''pin·jeck'tum·ee) *n.* OOPHOROSALPINGECTOMY.

ovar·io·ste·re·sis (o·văr''ee·o·ste·ree'sis) *n.* [*ovario-* + Gk. *sterēsis,* deprivation]. Extirpation of an ovary.

ovar·i·os·to·my (o·văr''ee·os'tum·ee) *n.* OOPHOROSTOMY.

ovar·i·ot·o·my (o·văr''ee·ot'um·ee) *n.* [*ovario-* + *-tomy*]. Removal of an ovary; oophorectomy.

ovar·io·tu·bal (o·văr''ee·o·tew'bul) *adj.* [*ovario-* + *tubal*]. Pertaining to an ovary and oviduct.

ova·ri·tis (o''vuh·righ'tis) *n.,* pl. **ova·rit·i·des** (·rit'i·deez) [*ovari-* + *-itis*]. OOPHORITIS.

ova·ri·um (o·vair'ee·um) *n.,* genit. **ova·rii** (·ee·eye), pl. **ovar·ia** (·ee·uh) [NA]. OVARY.

ova·ry (o'vur·ee) *n.* [NL. *ovarium,* from *ovum,* egg]. One of a pair of glandular organs which contains and releases ova. It consists of a fibrous framework or stroma, in which are embedded the ovarian follicles, and is surrounded by a serous covering derived from the peritoneum. See also Plates 23, 26.

ova·tes·tic·u·lar (o''vuh·tes·tick'yoo·lur) *adj.* OVOTESTICULAR.

ova·tes·tis (o''vuh·tes'tis) *n.* OVOTESTIS.

over·achiev·er, *n.* 1. A person who performs better than may be expected from certain known characteristics or previous record. 2. Specifically, a pupil or student whose actual scholastic performance is better than predicted from measured aptitude. Contr. *underachiever.* —**overachieve,** *v.;* **overachieve·ment,** *n.*

over·all aniseikonia. A condition in which the image seen by one eye is larger than the image seen by the other in all meridians.

over·bite, *n.* The extent to which the upper anterior teeth overlap the lower when the dentition is in centric occlusion.

over·com·pen·sa·tion, *n. In psychiatry,* a conscious or unconscious mental process in which real or fictitious physical, psychologic, or social deficiencies produce exaggerated correction. Compare *compensation.*

over·cor·rec·tion, *n. In optics,* an aberration of a lens causing the light rays passing the central zones to focus at a point nearer to the lens than rays passing the outer zone.

over·de·pen·den·cy, *n.* A behavioral trait or pattern characterized by seeking support and guidance (advice, decision making) far beyond that sought normally by an individual of a particular age, sex, and social status with average or near-average intelligence. See also *passive-aggressive personality.*

over·de·ter·mi·na·tion, *n. In psychoanalysis,* the state of having more than one cause, applied especially to behavior disorders and dreams. —**over·de·ter·mined,** *adj.*

over·eat·ing disease. INFECTIOUS ENTEROTOXEMIA OF SHEEP.

over·flex·ion, *n.* HYPERFLEXION.

over·flow, *n.* 1. Excessive flow or spread. 2. *In physiology,* the spread of movements after voluntary or involuntary stimulation of one part, as in a mass reflex.

overflow aminoaciduria. A specific enzymatic defect which leads to the presence of excess amounts of one or more amino acids in blood and various body tissues, and excess amounts of amino acids in the urine due to increased glomerular filtration. Compare *renal aminoaciduria.*

over·growth, *n.* Hypertrophy or hyperplasia.

over·jet, *n.* The extent to which the upper incisors project in front of the lower incisors when the dentition is in centric occlusion.

over·lap·ping toe. A congenital variation characterized by dorsal displacement of the fifth toe over the fourth.

over·ly·ing, *adj. & n.* 1. Positioned or resting above or on. 2. A cause of death in infants sleeping with adults; suffocation occurs when one of the adults lies upon the child.

over·max·i·mal (o"vur·mack'si·mul) *adj.* Beyond the normal maximum, as the overmaximal contraction of a muscle.

over·pro·duc·tion theory. WEIGERT'S LAW.

over·pro·tec·tion, *n.* Paying more attention to an infant or child than is necessary for its own safety and well-being; usually implying excessive physical contact with the child, preventing independent behavior or competition by the child with its peers, and forcing the child to act more infantile or dependent than his physical and intellectual development require.

over·reach, *v.* To strike the toe of the hindfoot against the heel or shoe of the forefoot; said of a horse.

over·rid·ing, *adj.* 1. Characterizing a fracture in which broken ends or fragments of the bone slip past each other, with overlapping due to muscular contraction. 2. Characterizing toes which overlap.

over·strain, *v. & n.* 1. To strain to excess. 2. Excessive strain and fatigue resulting from effort beyond capacity.

overt, *adj.* [MF., open]. Evident; manifest, outward.

overt homosexuality. Homosexuality consciously recognized and openly practiced.

over·tone, *n.* A harmonic tone heard above the fundamental tone.

Over·ton theory [C. E. *Overton,* German anesthesiologist, b. 1865]. A theoretical explanation of the action of anesthetics. See also *Meyer-Overton theory.*

over·weight, *adj.* Exceeding normal weight, usually connoting an excess of more than 10 percent.

over·work atrophy. A type of atrophy which follows hypertrophy and is due to excessive use of the part.

ovi-, ovo-. A combining form meaning *egg* or *ovum.*

ovi·cap·sule (o'vi·kap"sewl) *n.* [*ovi-* + *capsule*]. OVARIAN FOLLICLE.

ovi·ci·dal (o"vi·sigh'dul) *adj.* [*ovi-* + *-cide* + *-al*]. Lethal for ova.

ovi·duct (o'vi·dukt) *n.* [*ovi-* + *duct*]. The duct serving to transport the ovum from the ovary to the exterior, or to an organ such as the uterus. In mammals, the oviduct is also called the uterine or fallopian tube. See also Plate 23. —**ovi·du·cal** (o"vi·dew'kul), **ovi·duc·tal** (·duck'tul) *adj.*

ovif·er·ous (o·vif'ur·us) *adj.* [*ovi-* + *-ferous*]. Producing or bearing ova.

ovi·fi·ca·tion (o"vi·fi·kay'shun) *n.* [*ovi-* + *-fication,* from L. *facere,* to make]. The production of ova.

ovi·form (o'vi·form) *adj.* [*ovi-* + *-form*]. Egg-shaped; oval.

ovi·gen·e·sis (o"vi·jen'e·sis) *n.* [*ovi-* + *genesis*]. OOGENESIS.

ovi·ge·net·ic (o"vi·je·net'ick) *adj.* OVIGENOUS.

ovig·e·nous (o·vij'e·nus) *adj.* [*ovi-* + *-genous*]. Producing ova, as the ovigenous layer, the outer layer of the ovary, in which the follicles containing the ova are situated.

ovi·germ (o'vi·jurm) *n.* A cell producing or developing into an ovum.

ovig·er·ous (o·vij'ur·us) *adj.* [*ovi-* + *-gerous*]. Producing or carrying ova.

ovigerous cords. CORTICAL CORDS.

ovigerous disk. CUMULUS OOPHORUS.

ovine (o'vine) *adj.* [L. *ovinus,* from *ovis,* sheep]. 1. Pertaining to or derived from sheep. 2. Sheeplike.

ovine babesiasis. A disease of sheep caused by infection with species of *Babesia;* characterized by fever, anemia, and icterus.

ovine encephalomyelitis. LOUPING ILL.

ovine piroplasmosis. OVINE BABESIASIS.

ovip·a·rous (o·vip'ur·us) *adj.* [L. *oviparus,* egg-laying]. Producing eggs; bringing forth young in the egg stage of development. —**ovipa·ra** (·uh) *n.pl.*

ovi·po·si·tion (o"vi·puh·zish'un) *n.* The act of laying or depositing eggs by the females of oviparous animals. —**ovi·pos·it** (o"vi·poz'it) *v.*

ovi·pos·i·tor (o"vi·poz'i·tur) *n.* [*ovi-* + L. *positor,* from *ponere,* to place]. An organ, common among insects, composed of several modified rings of somites, forming the end of the abdomen, and employed in depositing the eggs.

ovi·sac (o'vi·sack) *n.* [*ovi-* + *sac*]. OVARIAN FOLLICLE.

ovo-. See *ovi-.*

ovo·cen·ter (o'vo·sen"tur) *n.* The centrosome of the ovum during fertilization.

Ovocylin. A trademark for the estrogen estradiol.

ovo·cyte (o'vo·site) *n.* OOCYTE.

ovo·fla·vin (o"vo·flay'vin, ·flav'in) *n.* A flavin separated from eggs, identical with riboflavin.

ovo·gen·e·sis (o"vo·jen'e·sis) *n.* [*ovo-* + *genesis*]. OOGENESIS.

ovo·glob·u·lin (o"vo·glob'yoo·lin) *n.* The globulin of egg white.

ovo·go·ni·um (o"vo·go'nee·um) *n.* OOGONIUM.

ovoid (o'void) *adj.* [*ov-* + *-oid*]. Egg-shaped.

ovo·mu·cin (o"vo·mew'sin) *n.* [*ovo-* + *mucin*]. A glycoprotein component of egg white.

ovo·mu·coid (o"vo·mew'koid) *n.* [*ovo-* + *mucoid*]. A glycoprotein component of egg white.

ovo·plasm (o'vo·plaz·um) *n.* The cytoplasm of the unfertilized ovum.

ovo·tes·tic·u·lar (o"vo·tes·tick'yoo·lur) *adj.* Pertaining to or characterized by an ovotestis or ovotestes.

ovotesticular hermaphroditism. The rare form of hermaphroditism in which an ovotestis is present on one or both sides.

ovo·tes·tis (o"vo·tes"tis) *n.,* pl. **ovotes·tes** (·teez). Ovarian and testicular tissues combined in the same gonad.

ovo·tid (o'vo·tid) *n.* OOCYTE.

ovo·vi·tel·lin (o″vo·vye·tel′in, ·vi·tel′in) *n.* [*ovo-* + *vitellin*]. A protein contained in egg yolk; a white, granular substance, soluble in dilute acids and in alkalies.

ovo·vi·vip·a·rous (o″vo·vye·vip″uh·rus) *adj.* [*ovo-* + *viviparous*]. Reproducing by means of eggs hatched within the body. **—ovovivipa·rism** (·riz·um) *n.*

ovu·lar (o′vyoo·lur) *adj.* Of or pertaining to an ovule or ovum.

ovu·la·tion (o″vyoo·lay′shun, ov″yoo·) *n.* The maturation and discharge of the ovum. **—ovu·late** (o′vyoo·late) *v.*; **ovu·la·to·ry** (o′vyoo·luh·to″ree), **ovu·la·tion·al** (o″vyoo·lay′shun·ul) *adj.*

ovulational age. The age of an embryo or fetus calculated from the time of ovulation.

ovule (o′vyool) *n.* [F., from NL. *ovulum*, diminutive of *ovum*]. 1. A small egg; one in an early stage of development. 2. The egg before its escape from the ovarian follicle. 3. An outgrowth of the ovary in a seed plant that develops, after fertilization, into a seed.

ovu·log·e·nous (o″vyoo·loj′e·nus) *adj.* [*ovule* + *-genous*]. Producing ovules.

ovu·lum (o′vew·lum) *n.*, pl. **ovu·la** (·luh) [BNA]. OVUM.

ovum (o′vum) *n.*, pl. **ova** (o′vuh) [L., egg (rel. to Gk. *ōon, ōion* and to Gmc. *ajjam*→ON. *egg*→E.)]. 1. [NA] A female germ cell; an egg cell; a cell which is capable of developing into a new member of the same species, in animals usually only after maturation and fertilization. The human ovum (see Plate 23) is a large, spheroidal cell containing a large mass of cytoplasm and a large nucleus (germinal vesicle), within which is a nucleolus (germinal spot). 2. The early embryo from the time of fertilization until the bilaminar blastodisk is formed.

ovum tu·ber·cu·lo·sum (tew·bur″kew·lo′sum) [L., tuberous]. BREUS'S MOLE.

Owen's lines [R. *Owen*, English anatomist, 1804–1892]. CONTOUR LINES OF OWEN.

owl-eye cells. Cells appearing in pairs, with large nuclei and prominent nucleoli; the term usually refers to the Aschoff cells of rheumatic carditis.

owl monkey. DOUROUCOULI.

Ow·ren's disease [P. A. *Owren*, Norwegian hematologist, 20th century]. PARAHEMOPHILIA.

ox-. See (a) *oxy-*; (b) *oxal-*.

oxa-. *In chemistry*, a combining form indicating *the presence of oxygen* in place of carbon.

ox·a·cil·lin (ock″suh·sil′in) *n.* 5-Methyl-3-phenyl-4-isoxazolylpenicillin, $C_{19}H_{19}N_3O_5S$, a semisynthetic penicillin antibiotic; used as the sodium salt.

ox·a·fen·da·zole (ock″suh·fen′duh·zole) *n.* Methyl 5-(phenylsulfinyl)-2-benzimidazolecarbamate, $C_{15}H_{13}N_3O_3S$, an anthelmintic.

Oxaine. Trademark for a preparation containing the gastric mucosal anesthetic oxethazaine.

oxal-, oxalo-. A combining form meaning *oxalic* or *oxalate*.

ox·al·ac·e·tate trans·ac·e·tase (ock″sul·as′e·tate tranz·as′e·taze). CITRATE SYNTHASE.

ox·al·ace·tic acid (ock″sul·a·see′tick). OXALOACETIC ACID.

ox·a·late (ock′suh·late) *n.* Any salt or ester of oxalic acid.

ox·a·le·mia, ox·a·lae·mia (ock″suh·lee′mee·uh) *n.* [*oxal-* + *-emia*]. An excess of oxalates in the blood.

ox·al·ic acid (ock·sal′ick) [L. *oxalis*, wood sorrel, from Gk.]. Ethanedioic acid, $HOOCCOOH{\cdot}2H_2O$, found in many plants and vegetables. Used as a reagent.

ox·a·lism (ock′sul·iz·um) *n.* Poisoning by oxalic acid or an oxalate.

oxalo-. See *oxal-*.

ox·alo·ac·e·tate trans·ac·e·tase (ock″sul·o·as′e·tate tranz·as′e·taze). CITRATE SYNTHASE.

ox·alo·ace·tic acid (ock″sul·o·a·see′tick, ock·sal″o·). Ketosuccinic acid, $HOOCCH_2COCOOH$, a participant in the citric acid metabolic cycle. Syn. *oxalacetic acid.*

ox·a·lo·sis (ock·suh·lo′sis) *n.* [*oxal-* + *-osis*]. A rare autosomal recessive metabolic error resulting in impaired glyoxylic acid metabolism with consequent overproduction of oxalic acid and deposition of calcium oxalate in body tissues; in type I, there is hyperoxaluria and hyperglyoxylaturia, while in type II there is hyperoxaluria and hyper-L-glyceric-aciduria. Both types are characterized clinically by renal calculi, nephrocalcinosis, and renal insufficiency. See also *glycolic aciduria, glyceric aciduria.*

ox·alo·suc·cin·ic acid (ock″sul·o·suck·sin′ick, ock·sal″o·) [*oxalo-* + *succinic*]. $HOOCCOHC(COOH)CH_2COOH$; an intermediate substance in the citric acid cycle, formed by dehydrogenation of isocitric acid.

ox·al·uria (ock″suh·lew′ree·uh) *n.* [*oxal-* + *-uria*]. The presence of oxalic acid or oxalates in the urine.

ox·al·uric acid (ock″suh·lew′rick) [*oxal-* + *uric*]. An acid, $NH_2CONHCOCOOH$, occasionally found in traces in normal human urine.

ox·am·i·dine (ock·sam′i·deen, ·din) *n.* AMIDOXIME.

ox·am·ni·quine (ock·sam′ni·kwin) *n.* 1,2,3,4-Tetrahydro-2-[(isopropylamino)methyl]-7-nitro-6-quinolinemethanol, $C_{14}H_{21}N_3O_3$, an antischistosomal.

Oxamycin. Trademark for cycloserine, an antibiotic used for the treatment of tuberculosis.

ox·an·a·mide (ock·san′uh·mide) *n.* 2-Ethyl-3-propylglycidamide, $C_8H_{15}NO_2$, a tranquilizing drug.

ox·an·dro·lone (ock·san′druh·lone) *n.* 17β-Hydroxy-17-methyl-2-oxa-5α-androstane-3-one, $C_{19}H_{30}O_3$, steroidal lactone used to accelerate anabolism or arrest excessive catabolism.

ox·an·tel (ock′san·tel) *n.* (*E*)-*m*-[2-(1,4,5,6-Tetrahydro-1-methyl-2-pyrimidyl)vinyl]phenol, $C_{13}H_{16}N_2O$, an anthelmintic, used as the pamoate salt.

ox·a·pro·zin (ock″suh·pro′zin) *n.* 4,5-Diphenyl-2-oxazolepropionic acid, $C_{18}H_{15}NO_3$, an anti-inflammatory.

ox·a·ze·pam (ock·say′ze·pam, ock·saz′e·pam) *n.* 7-Chloro-1,3-dihydro-3-hydroxy-5-phenyl-2*H*-1,4-benzodiazepin-2-one, $C_{15}H_{11}ClN_2O_2$, a tranquilizing drug.

ox·a·zin (ock′suh·zin) *n.* OXAZINE.

ox·a·zine (ock′suh·zeen) *n.* 1. One of 13 isomeric heterocyclic compounds of the general formula C_4H_5NO, each containing four carbon atoms, one oxygen atom, and one nitrogen atom in the ring; two double bonds are present in each ring. 2. Any derivative, as a dye, of any of the preceding.

ox·a·zol·i·dine (ock″suh·zol′i·deen, ·zo′li·deen) *n.* The heterocyclic compound $\overline{OCH_2NHCH_2CH_2}$, from which medicinal derivatives have been prepared.

ox·eth·a·zaine (ocks·eth′uh·zane) *n.* *N,N*-Bis(*N*-methyl-*N*-phenyl-*tert*-butylacetamide)-β-hydroxyethylamine, $C_{28}H_{39}N_3O_3$, a gastric mucosal anesthetic.

Ox·ford shunt. TRUETA'S SHUNT.

Oxford unit. The minimum quantity of penicillin which, when dissolved in 50 ml of a meat broth, is sufficient to inhibit completely the growth of a test strain of *Micrococcus aureus*; equivalent to the specific activity of 0.6 μg of the master standard penicillin.

ox·i·ben·da·zole (ock″si·ben′duh·zole) *n.* Methyl 5-propoxy-2-benzimidazolecarbamate, $C_{12}H_{15}N_3O_3$, an anthelmintic.

ox·i·dant (ock′sid·unt) *n.* [F.]. An oxidizing agent.

ox·i·dase (ock′si·dace, ·daze) *n.* Any enzyme which promotes an oxidation reaction.

ox·i·da·tion (ock″si·day′shun) *n.* [F.]. 1. An increase in positive valence of an element (or a decrease in negative valence) occurring as a result of the loss of electrons. Each electron so lost is taken on by some other element, thus accomplishing a reduction of that element. 2. Originally, the process of combining with oxygen. **—ox·i·da·tive** (ock′si·day″tiv) *adj.*

oxidation-reduction potential. The electromotive force exerted by a nonreacting electrode in a solution containing the oxidized and reduced forms of a chemical species, relative to a standard hydrogen electrode.

oxidation-reduction reaction. A chemical reaction in which a substance loses electrons and another gains an equal number of electrons.

ox·ide (ock'side) *n.* A binary compound of oxygen and another element or radical.

ox·i·dize (ock'si·dize) *v.* To produce an oxidation or increase in positive valence (or decrease in negative valence) through the loss of electrons. The oxidizing agent is itself reduced in the reaction; that is, it takes on the electrons which have been liberated by the element being oxidized.

oxidized cellulose. Cellulose, in the form of cotton or gauze, which has been oxidized by nitrogen dioxide so as to introduce carboxyl groups into the molecule, thereby imparting to the product a hemostatic effect and also the property of being absorbed when buried in tissues. It is useful for surgical hemostasis. Syn. *absorbable cellulose, cellulosic acid.*

oxidizing enzyme. An enzyme influencing oxidation reactions, as oxidase, dehydrogenase.

ox·i·do·pamine (ock"si·do'puh·meen) *n.* 5-(2-Aminoethyl)-1,2,4-benzenetriol, $C_8H_{11}NO_3$, an opthalmic adrenergic.

ox·i·do·re·duc·tase (ock"si·do·re·duck'tace, ·taze) *n.* An enzyme that catalyzes an oxidation-reduction reaction.

ox·i·lor·phan (ock"si·lor'fan) *n.* (−)-17-(Cyclopropylmethyl)morphinan-3,14-diol, $C_{20}H_{27}NO_2$, a narcotic antagonist.

ox·ime (ock'seem) *n.* Any compound resulting from the action of hydroxylamine upon an aldehyde or ketone; the former yields an oxime having the general formula RCH=NOH, called aldoxime; the latter yields an oxime of the general formula $R_2C{=}NOH$, called ketoxime.

ox·im·e·ter (ock·sim'e·tur) *n.* [*oxygen* + *-meter*]. 1. A photoelectric instrument for measuring the degree of oxygen saturation in a fluid, such as blood. 2. An instrument for measurement of oxygen in a given space, as in an incubator or oxygen tent. —**oxime·try** (·tree) *n.*

ox·i·per·o·mide (ock"si·perr'o·mide) *n.* 1-[1-(2-Phenoxyethyl)-4-piperidyl]-2-benzimidazolinone, $C_{20}H_{23}N_3O_2$, a tranquilizer.

ox·ir·a·mide (ock·sirr'uh·mide) *n.* *N*-[4-(2,6-Dimethylpiperidino)butyl]-2-phenoxy-2-phenylacetamide, $C_{25}H_{34}N_2O_2$, a cardiac depressant.

ox·i·su·ran (ock"si·sue'ran) *n.* (Methylsulfinyl)methyl 2-pyridyl ketone, $C_8H_9NO_2S$, an antineoplastic.

oxo·ges·tone (ock"so·jes'tone) *n.* 20β-Hydroxy-19-norpregn-4-en-3-one, $C_{20}H_{30}O_2$, a progestational steroid; used as the phenpropionate ester.

oxo·isom·er·ase (ock"so·eye·som'ur·ace, ·aze) *n.* PHOSPHOGLUCOSE ISOMERASE.

oxo·phen·ar·sine hydrochloride (ock"so·fen·ahr'seen, ·sin). 2-Amino-4-arsenosophenol hydrochloride, $C_6H_6AsNO_2 \cdot HCl$, an antisyphilitic and antitrypanosomal drug.

ox·pren·o·lol (ocks·pren'o·lol) *n.* 1-[*o*-(Allyloxy)phenoxy]-3-(isopropylamino)-2-propanol, $C_{15}H_{23}NO_3$, a coronary dilator; used as the hydrochloride salt.

Oxsoralen. Trademark for methoxsalen, a compound inducing formation of melanin pigment in the skin.

ox·tri·phyl·line (ocks"trye·fil'een, ocks"tri·fil'een) *n.* Choline theophyllinate, $C_{12}H_{21}N_5O_3$, a drug having the diuretic, myocardial stimulating, vasodilator, and bronchodilator actions of theophylline.

oxy- [Gk. *oxys*]. A combining form meaning (a) *sharp, pointed,* as in oxycephaly; (b) *keen, abnormally acute,* as in oxyopia; (c) *quick, hastening,* as in oxytocic; (d) *acid,* as in oxyphil; (e) *containing oxygen or additional oxygen,* as in oxysteroid; (f) *containing hydroxyl,* as in oxytetracycline.

ox·y·a·coa (ock"see·uh·ko'uh) *n. Obsol.* Oxyakoia (= HYPERACUSIA).

oxy·a·koia (ock"see·uh·koy'uh) *n.* [*oxy-* + Gr. *akoē*, hearing, + *-ia*]. *Obsol.* HYPERACUSIA.

oxy·a·phia (ock"see·ay'fee·uh, ·af'ee·uh) *n.* [*oxy-*, sharp, keen, + Gk. *haphē*, touch, + *-ia*]. 1. Marked or abnormal acuteness of the sense of touch. 2. Extreme sensitivity to touch.

oxy·ben·zone (ock"see·ben'zone) *n.* 2-Hydroxy-4-methoxybenzophenone, $C_{14}H_{12}O_3$, an ultraviolet screen.

oxy·bi·o·tin (ock"see·bye'o·tin) *n.* An analogue of biotin in which oxygen replaces the sulfur atom of biotin.

oxy·blep·sia (ock"see·blep'see·uh) *n.* [Gk.]. Acuteness of vision.

oxy·bu·ty·nin (ock"see·bew'ti·nin) *n.* 4-(Diethylamino)-2-butynyl α-phenylcyclohexaneglycolate, $C_{22}H_{31}NO_3$, an anticholinergic drug; used as the hydrochloride salt.

Oxycel. Trademark for an absorbable oxidized cellulose material used in surgical hemostasis.

oxy·ceph·a·ly (ock"see·sef'ul·ee) *n.* [Gk. *oxykephalos,* having a pointed head]. A condition in which the head is roughly conical in shape; caused by premature closure of the coronal or lambdoid sutures, or both, which induces compensatory development in the region of the bregma. It is also caused by artificial pressure on the frontal and occipital regions of the heads of infants to alter the shape. Syn. *acrocephaly.* See also *scaphocephaly.* —**oxy·ce·phal·ic** (·se·fal'ick) *adj.*

oxy·chlo·ro·sene (ock"si·klor'o·seen) *n.* A complex of hypochlorous acid with long-chain alkyl derivatives of benzenesulfonic acid, a topical antiseptic, usually used as the sodium salt.

oxy·chro·ma·tin (ock"see·kro'muh·tin) *n.* That part of the chromatin having an affinity for acid dyes.

oxy·ci·ne·sis (ock"see·sigh·nee'sis, ·si·nee'sis) *n.* [Gk. *oxykinēsia,* quickness of motion]. Excessive movements, particularly of the limbs, observed in the manic phase of manic-depressive illness.

oxy·co·done (ock"see·ko'dohn) *n.* Dihydrohydroxycodeinone, $C_{18}H_{21}NO_4$, a narcotic analgesic; used principally as the hydrochloride salt.

oxy·cor·ti·co·ste·roid (ock"see·kor"ti·ko·sterr'oid) *n.* An oxysteroid originating in the adrenal cortex.

oxydase. OXIDASE.

oxy·es·the·sia (ock"see·es·theezh'uh, ·theez'ee·uh) *n.* [*oxy-*, sharp, + *esthesia*]. HYPERESTHESIA.

ox·y·gen (ock'si·jin) *n.* [F. *oxygène,* from *oxy-*, acid, + *-gène,* generating]. O = 15.9994. A colorless, tasteless, odorless gas, constituting one-fifth of the atmosphere, eight-ninths of water, and about one-half the crust of the globe; it supports combustion, and is essential to life of animals. It combines with most elements, and is carried by the blood from the lungs to the tissues.

oxygen acid. An acid which contains oxygen.

ox·y·gen·ase (ock'si·ji·naze, ·nace) *n.* An enzyme that makes it possible for atmospheric oxygen to be utilized by the organism or in the system in which it occurs.

ox·y·gen·ate (ock'si·ji·nate) *v.* To combine a substance with oxygen, either by chemical reaction or by mixture. —**oxy·gen·a·tion** (ock"si·ji·nay'shun) *n.*

oxygen bath. An effervescent bath employing oxygen instead of carbon dioxide.

oxygen capacity. The maximum amount of oxygen absorbed by a given amount of blood when it is equilibrated with an excess of oxygen, expressed in volume percent (per 100 ml). See also Table of Chemical Constituents of Blood in the Appendix.

oxygen debt or **deficit.** The volume of oxygen required in addition to the resting oxygen consumption during the period of recovery from intense muscular exertion; it reflects the quantity of excess lactic acid produced during the anaerobic work period, and is required to oxidize this excess as well as to replenish stores of adenosine triphosphate and phosphocreatine that were depleted. Syn. *recovery oxygen.*

oxygen saturation. Oxygen content divided by oxygen capacity expressed in volume percent.

oxygen tent. A transparent airtight chamber, enclosing the patient's head and shoulders, in which the oxygen content can be maintained at a higher than normal atmospheric level.

oxy·geu·sia (ock"si·gyoo'see·uh, ·joo'see·uh) *n.* [*oxy-* + *-geusia*]. Marked acuteness of the sense of taste.

oxy·hem·a·tin (ock"see·hem'uh·tin, ·hee'muh·tin) *n.* $C_{34}H_{32}N_4O_7Fe$. The coloring matter of oxyhemoglobin; on oxidation, it yields hematinic acid; on reduction, hematoporphyrin.

oxy·hem·a·to·por·phy·rin (ock"see·hem"uh·to·por'fi·rin) *n.* A pigment sometimes found in urine; it is related to hematoporphyrin.

oxy·he·mo·glo·bin (ock"si·hee'muh·glo"bin) *n.* Hemoglobin combined with oxygen.

oxy·la·lia (ock"si·lay'lee·uh, ·lal'ee·uh) *n.* [Gk. *oxylalos*, glib, voluble, + *-ia*]. Rapid speech. See also *tachylogia.*

Oxylone. Trademark for fluorometholone, an anti-inflammatory adrenocortical steroid.

oxy·me·taz·o·line (ock"see·me·taz'o·leen, ·met'uh·zo·leen) *n.* 6-*tert*-Butyl-3-(2-imidazolin-2-ylmethyl)-2,4-dimethylphenol, $C_{16}H_{24}N_2O$, a vasoconstrictor used topically to reduce swelling and congestion of the nasal mucosa; employed as the hydrochloride salt.

oxymeter, *n.* OXIMETER. **—oxymetry,** *n.*

oxy·meth·o·lone (ock"see·meth'uh·lone) *n.* 2-Hydroxymethylene-17α-methyldihydrotestosterone, $C_{21}H_{32}O_3$, an anabolic steroid.

oxy·mor·phone (ock"see·mor'fone) *n.* 14-Hydroxydihydromorphinone, $C_{17}H_{19}NO_4$, a semisynthetic narcotic analgesic; used as the hydrochloride salt.

oxy·ner·von (ock"see·nur'von) *n.* A cerebroside occurring in brain tissue; its characteristic acid is oxynervonic acid.

oxy·ner·von·ic acid (ock"see·nur·von'ick). An unsaturated acid, $HOC_{23}H_{44}COOH$, the hydroxy derivative of nervonic acid; a component of oxynervon.

oxy·neu·rine (ock"see·new'reen, ·rin) *n.* BETAINE.

ox·yn·tic (ock·sin'tick) *adj.* [Gk. *oxynein*, to make acid, + *-ic*]. Secreting acid; formerly applied to the parietal cells of the stomach.

oxyntic cell. PARIETAL CELL.

oxy·opia (ock"see·o'pee·uh) *n.* [Gk. *oxyopia,* sharp-sightedness]. Unusual acuity of vision.

oxy·op·ter (ock"see·op'tur) *n.* [Gk. *oxyōpēs*, sharp-sighted, + *-tēr,* agentive noun suffix]. The unit of acuity of vision; it is the reciprocal of the visual angle expressed in degrees.

oxy·o·sis (ock"see·o'sis) *n.* [*oxy-* + *-osis*]. *Obsol.* ACIDOSIS.

oxy·os·mia (ock"see·oz'mee·uh) *n.* [*oxy-*, sharp, acute, + Gk. *osmē*, smell, + *-ia*]. 1. Marked or abnormal sensitivity to smell. 2. Sensitivity to odors to a pathologic extent.

oxy·os·phre·sia (ock"see·os·free'zhuh, ·zee·uh) *n.* [*oxy-*, sharp, acute, + Gk. *osphrēsis*, sense of smell, + *-ia*]. OXYOSMIA.

ox·yp·a·thy (ock·sip'uth·ee) *n.* [*oxy-* + *-pathy*]. A supposed constitutional condition due to faulty elimination of unoxidized acids, which unite with fixed alkalies of the body.

oxy·per·tine (ock"si·pur'teen) *n.* 5,6-Dimethoxy-2-methyl-3-[2-(4-phenyl-1-piperazinyl)ethyl]indole, $C_{23}H_{29}N_3O_2$, a psychotropic agent.

oxy·phen·bu·ta·zone (ock"si·fen·bew'tuh·zone) *n.* 4-Butyl-1-(*p*-hydroxyphenyl)-2-phenyl-3,5-pyrazolidinedione, $C_{19}H_{20}N_2O_3$, a metabolite of phenylbutazone that is used as an antiarthritic and anti-inflammatory drug.

oxy·phen·cy·cli·mine (ock"see·fen·sigh'kli·meen) *n.* (1-Methyl-1,4,5,6-tetrahydro-2-pyrimidyl)methyl α-cyclohexyl-α-phenylglycolate, $C_{20}H_{28}N_2O_3$, an anticholinergic drug employed as an adjunct in the management of peptic ulcer; used as the hydrochloride salt.

oxy·phen·ic acid (ock"see·fen'ick). PYROCATECHOL.

oxy·phen·i·sa·tin (ock"see·fen·eye'suh·tin) *n.* 3,3-Bis(*p*-hydroxyphenyl)-2-indolinone, $C_{20}H_{15}NO_3$, an active cathartic; also used as the diacetate.

oxy·phe·no·ni·um bromide (ock"see·fe·no'nee·um). Diethyl(2-hydroxyethyl)methylammonium bromide α-phenylcyclohexylglycolate, $C_{21}H_{34}BrNO_3$; an anticholinergic agent used in treating peptic ulcer and gastrointestinal hypermotility or spasm.

oxy·phil (ock'si·fil) *adj.* [*oxy-* + *-phil*]. ACIDOPHILIC (1).

oxyphil cell. 1. PARIETAL CELL. 2. An acidophil cell which may be found in the parathyroid, especially in the periphery.

oxy·phile (ock'si·file) *n. & adj.* ACIDOPHIL.

oxyphil granules. Granules that stain with acid dyes.

oxy·phil·ia (ock"si·fil'ee·uh) *n.* [*oxy-* + *-philia*]. 1. ACIDOPHILIA. 2. EOSINOPHILIA.

oxy·phil·ic (ock"si·fil'ick) *adj.* ACIDOPHILIC (1).

oxyphil leukocyte. EOSINOPHIL LEUKOCYTE.

oxy·pho·nia (ock"see·fo'nee·uh) *n.* [*oxy-* + *-phonia*]. Shrillness of voice.

oxy·poly·gel·a·tin (ock"see·pol"ee·jel'uh·tin) *n.* An oxidized, polymerized gelatin used experimentally as a blood plasma substitute.

oxy·pro·line (ock"see·pro'leen) *n.* HYDROXYPROLINE.

oxy·pu·ri·nol (ock"si·pew'ri·nol) *n.* 1*H*-Pyrazolo[3,4-*d*]pyrimidine-4,6-diol, $C_5H_4N_4O_2$, a xanthine oxidase inhibitor.

oxy·quin·o·line (ock"see·kwin'o·leen, ·lin) *n.* HYDROXYQUINOLINE.

oxy·rhine (ock'si·rine) *adj.* [*oxy-* + *-rhine*]. Possessing a sharp-pointed nose or snout.

oxy·ste·roid (ock"see·sterr'oid, ·steer'oid) *n.* A steroid having an oxygen atom, thereby forming an alcohol or a ketone group, at some specified position; for example, an 11-oxysteroid has the oxygen atom present at the number 11 carbon atom of the steroid nucleus.

ox·yt·a·lan fibers (ock·sit'uh·lan) [*oxy-*, acid, + Gk. *tlan,* enduring, resisting]. Acid-resistant connective-tissue fibers morphologically similar to elastin, but resistant to elastase digestion and not stained by the usual specific elastin stains.

oxy·tet·ra·cy·cline (ock"see·tet"ruh·sigh'kleen) *n.* A broad-spectrum antibiotic substance, $C_{22}H_{24}N_2O_9$, produced by the growth of the soil fungus *Streptomyces rimosus,* or by any other means. It represents tetracycline in which a hydrogen atom is replaced by a hydroxyl group, and is active against a number of gram-negative bacteria, rickettsias, and several viruses.

oxy·thi·a·mine (ock"see·thigh'uh·min, ·meen) *n.* A compound differing from thiamine in having an OH group in place of the NH_2 group of thiamine; a powerful antagonist of thiamine.

oxy·to·cia (ock"si·to'shee·uh, ·see·uh) *n.* [Gk. *oxytokia*]. Rapid childbirth.

oxy·to·cic (ock"si·to'sick) *adj. & n.* [Gk. *ōkytokios,* from *ōky-* (=*oxy-*), quick, + *tokos,* childbirth]. 1. Hastening parturition. 2. A drug that hastens parturition.

oxytocic hormone. OXYTOCIN.

ox·y·to·cin (ock"si·to'sin) *n.* [*oxytocic* + *-in*]. An octapeptide, obtained from extracts of the posterior lobe of the pituitary gland and also by synthesis, that is the principal uterine-contracting and lactation-stimulating hormone of the gland. Syn. *alpha-hypophamine.*

oxy·uri·a·sis (ock"see·yoo·rye'uh·sis) *n.* [*Oxyuris* + *-iasis*]. ENTEROBIASIS.

Oxy·uri·dae (ock"see·yoor'i·dee) *n.pl.* [from *Oxyuris,* type genus]. A family of nematode intestinal parasites, including the human pinworm *Enterobius vermicularis.* **—oxy·urid** (ock"see·yoor'id) *adj. & n.*

Oxy·uris (ock"see·yoor'is) *n.* [NL., from *oxy-*, sharp, + Gk. *oura,* tail]. A genus of nematodes, including the horse pinworm, *Oxyuris equi,* and formerly also the human pinworm (*O. vermicularis,* now designated *Enterobius vermicularis*).

-oyl. A suffix indicating a radical formed from an organic acid when OH is removed from the latter, as for example the radical RCO— from RCOOH.

oz. Symbol for avoirdupois ounce.

oze·na, ozae·na (o·zee'nuh) *n.* [Gk. *ozaina,* from *ozein,* to smell]. A disease of the nasal mucosa of uncertain origin, characterized by chronic inflammation with subsequent atrophy, sclerosis, and crusting. Syn. *atrophic rhinitis.*

ozo·chro·tia (o″zo·kro'shee·uh) *n.* [NL., from Gk. *oz*ein, to smell, + *chroa,* skin]. An offensive odor of the skin. —**ozoch·ro·tous** (o·zock″ruh·tus) *adj.*

ozo·ke·rite (o·zo'kur·ite, o″zo·kair'ite) *n.* CERESIN.

ozone (o'zone) *n.* [Gk. *ozōn,* smelling, smelly]. O_3. An allotropic form of oxygen, the molecule of which consists of three atoms; a common constituent of the atmosphere. It is a powerful oxidizing agent and is used as a disinfectant, as for swimming pools.

ozon·ide (o'zo·nide) *n.* A compound of ozone with certain unsaturated organic substances. Such derivatives of fixed oils have been applied locally to infected areas for the bactericidal effect of the nascent oxygen released by the oils.

ozo·sto·mia (o″zo·sto'mee·uh) *n.* [Gk. *ozostom*os, with bad breath (from *ozein,* to smell, + *stoma,* mouth) + *-ia*]. A foul odor of the breath of oral origin; halitosis.

Oz·zard's filariasis. The presence of *Mansonella ozzardi* in humans; the adult worms produce few if any pathologic changes or symptoms.

P

P Symbol for (a) phosphorus; (b) premolar.

P Symbol for radiant flux.

P. Abbreviation for (a) *pharmacopeia;* (b) *position;* (c) *punctum proximum,* near point.

P_2 1. S_{2P}. 2. Symbol for the second heart sound as heard in the second interspace at the left sternal border.

^{32}P. Symbol for phosphorus 32; radiophosphorus. See also Table of Common Radioactive Pharmaceuticals in the Appendix.

p- *In chemistry,* symbol for para-.

PA A posteroanterior projection of x-rays; as those passing from back to front of an anatomic part.

Pa Symbol for protactinium.

PABA Abbreviation for *para-aminobenzoic acid.*

Pablum. Trademark for a soft wheat cereal, used for feeding infants.

pab·u·lum (pab'yoo·lum) *n.* [L.]. Food; any nutrient.

Pacatal. Trademark for mepazine, a tranquilizing and antinauseant drug used as the hydrochloride salt.

Pac·chi·o·ni·an bodies (pack''ee·o'nee·un) [A. *Pacchioni,* Italian anatomist, 1665–1726]. ARACHNOID GRANULATIONS.

pace·mak·er, *n.* 1. Any substance or object that influences the rate at which a process or reaction occurs. 2. Any body part that serves to establish and maintain a rhythmic activity. 3. Specifically, the sinoatrial node, a subsidiary center, or an electrical device functioning to stimulate and pace the heart.

pa·chom·e·ter (pa·kom'e·tur) *n.* [Gk. *pachos,* thickness, + *-meter*]. *In ophthalmology,* an instrument for measuring the thickness of the cornea.

pach·onych·ia (pack''o·nick'ee·uh). PACHYONYCHIA.

pachy- [Gk. *pachys*]. A combining form meaning (a) *thick, thickness;* (b) *coarse;* (c) *dura mater.*

-pachy [*pachy-* + *-y*]. A combining form designating *a condition involving thickening of a part or parts.*

pachy·ac·ria (pack''ee·ack'ree·uh) *n.* [*pachy-* + *acr-* + *-ia*]. ACROPACHYDERMA.

pachy·bleph·a·ron (pack''ee·blef'ur·on) *n.* [*pachy-* + *blepharon*]. Chronic thickening and induration of the eyelids.

pachy·bleph·a·ro·sis (pack''ee·blef''uh·ro'sis) *n.* [*pachy-* + *blephar-* + *-osis*]. PACHYBLEPHARON.

pachy·ce·pha·lia (pack''ee·se·fay'lee·uh) *n.* PACHYCEPHALY. **—pachyce·phal·ic** (·fal'ick) *adj.*

pachy·ceph·a·ly (pack''ee·sef'uh·lee) *n.* [*pachy-* + *-cephaly*]. Unusual thickness of the walls of the skull. **—pachycepha·lous** (·lus) *adj.*

pachy·chei·lia, pachy·chi·lia (pack''i·kigh'lee·uh) *n.* [*pachy-* + *cheil-* + *-ia*]. Increased thickness of one or both lips.

pachy·chro·mat·ic (pack''ee·kro·mat'ick) *adj.* [*pachy-* + *chromatic*]. Having a coarse chromatin network.

pachy·dac·tyl·ia (pack''ee·dack·til'ee·uh) *n.* [Gk. *pachydaktylos,* thick-fingered, + *-ia*]. Abnormal thickness of the fingers.

pachy·dac·ty·ly (pack''ee·dack'ti·lee) *n.* PACHYDACTYLIA.

pachy·der·ma (pack''i·dur'muh) *n.* PACHYDERMIA.

pachyderma ora·lis (o·ray'lis, o·ral'is). Clinical leukoplakia of the oral cavity.

pachy·der·ma·to·cele (pack''i·dur'muh·to·seel) *n.* [*pachy-* + *dermato-* + *-cele*]. A manifestation of von Recklinghausen's neurofibromatosis, taking the form of an overgrowth of subcutaneous tissue, sometimes reaching enormous size. Syn. *plexiform neuroma, elephantiasis neurofibromatosa.*

pachy·der·ma·to·sis (pack''i·dur''muh·to'sis) *n.* [*pachy-* + *dermatosis*]. RHINOPHYMA.

pachy·der·ma·tous (pack''i·dur'muh·tus) *adj.* [*pachy-* + *dermat-* + *-ous*]. Abnormally thick-skinned.

pachy·der·mia (pack''i·dur'mee·uh) *n.* [Gk., thickness of skin, from *pachys,* thick, + *derma,* skin, + *-ia*]. 1. Abnormal thickening of the skin. 2. ELEPHANTIASIS. **—pachyder·mi·al** (·mee·ul), **pachyder·mic** (·mick) *adj.*

pachydermia la·ryn·gis (la·rin'jis). Extensive thickening of the mucous membrane of the larynx, particularly the posterior commissure.

pachydermia lym·phan·gi·ec·tat·i·ca (lim·fan''jee·eck·tat'i·kuh). A diffuse form of lymphangioma.

pachydermic cachexia. Myxedematous cachexia. See *myxedema.*

pachy·der·mo·peri·os·to·sis (pack''ee·dur''mo·perr''ee·os·to'sis) *n.* [*pachy-* + *dermo-* + *periostosis*]. Thickening of the skin over the bones, excess bone growth, and clubbing of fingers and toes which may either result from underlying pulmonary disease or malignancy, or occur in a hereditary form with thickening of the skin of the face and head and increased skin folds.

pachy·glos·sia (pack''ee·glos'ee·uh) *n.* [*pachy-* + *gloss-* + *-ia*]. Abnormal thickness of the tongue.

pachy·gy·ria (pack''i·jye'ree·uh) *n.* [*pachy-* + *gyr-* + *-ia*]. A variety of cerebral malformation characterized by a reduction in the number secondary gyri and an increased depth of the gray matter underlying the smooth part of the cortex. Syn. *lissencephalia, agyria.*

pachy·hem·a·tous, pachy·haem·a·tous (pack''ee·hem'uh·tus) *adj.* [*pachy-* + *hemat-* + *-ous*]. Pertaining to thickening of the blood.

pachy·hy·men·ic (pack''ee·high·men'ick) *adj.* [*pachy-* + *hymen-* + *-ic*]. PACHYDERMATOUS.

pachy·lep·to·men·in·gi·tis (pack''ee·lep''to·men''in·jye'tis) *n.* [*pachy-* + *lepto-* + *meningitis*]. Combined inflammation of the pia-arachnoid and dura mater.

pachy·lo·sis (pack″i·lo′sis) *n.* [Gk. *pachylos*, thickish, + *-osis*]. A thick, dry, harsh, and scaly skin, especially of the legs.

pachy·men·in·gi·tis (pack″ee·men″in·jye′tis) *n.* [*pachy-* + *meningitis*]. Inflammation of the dura mater. —**pachy·menin·git·ic** (·jit′ick) *adj.*

pachymeningitis cer·vi·ca·lis hy·per·troph·i·ca (sur·vi·kay′lis high″pur·trof′i·kuh). HYPERTROPHIC CERVICAL PACHYMENINGITIS.

pachymeningitis ex·ter·na (ecks·tur′nuh). *Obsol.* EPIDURAL ABSCESS.

pachymeningitis in·ter·na hem·or·rha·gi·ca (in·tur′nuh hem·o·ray′ji·kuh). *Obsol.* Chronic SUBDURAL HEMATOMA.

pachy·men·in·gop·a·thy (pack″ee·men″ing·gop′uth·ee) *n.* [*pachy-* + *meningo-* + *-pathy*]. Disease of the dura mater.

pachy·me·ninx (pack″ee·mee′ninks) *n.* [*pachy-* + *meninx*]. DURA MATER.

pachy·ne·ma (pack″i·nee′muh) *n.* [*pachy-* + *-nema*]. PACHYTENE.

pa·chyn·sis (pa·kin′sis) *n.* [Gk.]. A thickening, as of a membrane. —**pachyn·tic** (·tick) *adj.*

pachy·o·nych·ia (pack″ee·o·nick′ee·uh) *n.* [*pachy-* + *onych-* + *-ia*]. Thickening of the nails. Syn. *pachonychia.*

pachyonychia con·gen·i·ta (kon·jen′i·tuh). An ectodermal defect characterized by dystrophic changes of the nails, palmar and plantar hyperkeratosis, anomalies of the hair, follicular keratosis of the knees and elbows, and dyskeratosis of the cornea.

pachy·o·tia (pack″ee·o′shuh, ·shee·uh) *n.* [*pachy-* + *ot-* + *-ia*]. Abnormal thickness of the external ears.

pachy·pel·vi·peri·to·ni·tis (pack″ee·pel″vi·perr″i·to·nigh′tis) *n.* [*pachy-* + *pelvi-* + *peritonitis*]. Pelvic peritonitis with a fibrous deposit over the uterus.

pachy·peri·os·to·sis (pack″ee·perr″ee·os·to′sis) *n.* [*pachy-* + *periostosis*]. Pathologic alteration of the long bones in which the periosteum is greatly thickened.

pachy·peri·to·ni·tis (pack″ee·perr″i·to·nigh′tis) *n.* [*pachy-* + *peritonitis*]. Inflammation, usually chronic, of the peritoneum associated with peritoneal thickening.

pa·chyp·o·dous (pa·kip′uh·dus) *adj.* [Gk. *pachypous, pachypodos,* from *pous, podos,* foot]. Having thick feet.

pachy·rhine (pack′i·rine) *adj.* [Gk. *pachyrin,* from *rhis, rhinos,* nose]. Having a thick or unusually broad and flat nose.

pachy·rhi·nic (pack″i·rye′nick) *adj.* PACHYRHINE.

pachy·sal·pin·go-oo·the·ci·tis (pack″ee·sal·pin″go·o″o·thi·sigh′tis) *n.* [*pachy-* + *salpingo-oothecitis*]. PACHYSALPINGO-OVARITIS.

pachy·sal·pin·go·ova·ri·tis (pack″ee·sal·pin″go·o″vuh·rye′tis) *n.* [*pachy-* + *salpingoovaritis*]. Inflammation of the ovary and oviduct with thickening of the parts.

pachy·tene (pack′i·teen) *n.* [*pachy-* + *-tene*]. The stage in the first meiotic prophase in which tetrads are formed. See also *diplotene, leptotene, zygotene.*

pachy·tes (pack′i·teez) *n.* [Gk. *pachytēs,* thickness]. PACHYBLEPHARON.

pa·chyt·ic (pa·kit′ick) *adj.* [Gk. *pachytēs*, thickness, + *-ic*]. 1. Thick. 2. Tending to thicken, or make viscid.

pachy·vag·i·ni·tis (pack″ee·vaj″i·nigh′tis) *n.* [*pachy-* + *vaginitis*]. Vaginitis accompanied by thickening of the vaginal walls.

pac·i·fi·er (pas′i·figh″ur) *n.* Any article, such as a rubber nipple, placed in the mouths of irritable or teething children to quiet them.

pa·cin·i·an corpuscle (pa·sin′ee·un) [F. *Pacini,* Italian anatomist, 1812–1883]. The largest and most widely distributed of the encapsulated sensory receptors. It differs from other encapsulated organs mainly in the greater development of its perineural capsule, which consists of a large number of concentric lamellae. Syn. *corpuscle of Vater-Pacini.*

pack, *n. & v.* 1. An assemblage of equipment used for a medical procedure, usually of a surgical nature. 2. TAMPON. 3. A dressing or blanket, dry or wet, hot or cold, placed on or wrapped around the body or a part of the body. 4. To fill a cavity; to produce tamponade.

pack·er, *n.* A tapered surgical instrument equipped with a point ending in a shoulder, for inserting gauze or other dressings into a cavity; used generally in conjunction with an aural, vaginal, or other speculum.

packet liver. A type of hepatic cirrhosis, seen in syphilis, characterized by fine fibrous bands enclosing relatively normal collections of lobules.

packing fraction. The difference between the actual mass of an isotope and the nearest whole number divided by this whole number, usually expressed as parts in 10,000; it is related to the loss of energy and therefore loss of mass involved in the formation of atomic nuclei from protons and neutrons.

pack palsy. Brachial plexus palsy as a result of carrying a heavy shoulder pack.

pad, *n.* 1. A small cushion stuffed with cotton, hair, etc., for supporting any part of the body. 2. A compress. 3. Any small circumscribed mass of fatty tissue, as in terminal phalanges of the fingers.

Pad·gett's dermatome [E. C. *Padgett,* U.S. surgeon, 1893–1946]. An instrument for cutting uniform thickness of skin of any desired calibration in large sheets for grafting purposes.

Padgett's operation [E. C. *Padgett*]. Reconstruction of the lip, using transplanted tubular grafts from the scalp and neck.

pad·i·mate A (pad′i·mate). Pentyl *p*-(dimethylamino)benzoate, $C_{14}H_{21}NO_2$, an ultraviolet screen. The pentyl ester is a mixture of 1-pentyl, 2-methylbutyl and 3-methylbutyl esters.

padimate O. 2-Ethylhexyl *p*-(dimethylamino)benzoate, $C_{17}H_{27}NO_2$, an ultraviolet screen.

pad of the corpus callosum. The splenium of the corpus callosum.

paed-, paedo-. See *ped-, pedo-,* child.

paedatrophia. Pedatrophia (= PEDATROPHY).

paedatrophy. PEDATROPHY.

paederasty. PEDERASTY.

paediatrician. PEDIATRICIAN.

paediatrics. PEDIATRICS.

paediatrist. Pediatrist (= PEDIATRICIAN).

paediatry. Pediatry (= PEDIATRICS).

paedicterus. Pedicterus (= PHYSIOLOGIC JAUNDICE OF THE NEWBORN).

paedodontia. Pedodontia (= PEDODONTICS).

paedodontics. PEDODONTICS.

paedodontist. PEDODONTIST.

paedodontology. Pedodontology (= PEDODONTICS).

paedogenesis. Pedogenesis (= NEOTENY).

paedologist. PEDOLOGIST.

paedology. PEDOLOGY.

paedometer. [1]PEDOMETER.

paedonosology. PEDONOSOLOGY.

paedophilia. PEDOPHILIA.

paedophobia. PEDOPHOBIA.

page·ism (pay′jiz·um) *n.* *In psychiatry,* the fantasy of a masochistic male that he is the slave or page of a dominating woman.

Page's syndrome [I. H. *Page,* U.S., 20th century]. ADRENOSYMPATHETIC SYNDROME.

pag·et·oid (paj′e·toid) *adj.* Simulating Paget's disease.

pagetoid malignant melanoma. SUPERFICIAL SPREADING MALIGNANT MELANOMA.

pagetoid reticulosis. WORINGER-KOLOPP DISEASE.

Paget's cancer. PAGET'S DISEASE (1).

Paget's cells. Large epithelial cells with clear cytoplasm, associated with a certain type of breast cancer (Paget's disease (1)) or apocrine gland cancer of the skin (Paget's disease (3)).

Paget-Schroetter's syndrome [J. *Paget* and L. von *Schroetter*].

Acute venous thrombosis with obstruction occurring in the upper extremity of an otherwise healthy person. Syn. *axillary vein thrombosis.*

Paget's disease [J. *Paget,* English surgeon, 1814–1899]. 1. A breast carcinoma involving the nipple or areola and the larger ducts, whose cells are large and have clear cytoplasm (Paget's cells). Syn. *morbus Pageti papillae, Paget's cancer.* 2. A simultaneous osseous hyperplasia and accelerated deossification, resulting in weakness and deformity of various bones. Syn. *osteitis deformans.* 3. A skin cancer associated with apocrine glands, whose parenchyma is composed of Paget's cells.

Pagitane. Trademark for cycrimine, used as the hydrochloride for treatment of parkinsonism.

pa·go·pha·gia (pay″go·fay′jee·uh) *n.* [Gk. *pagos*, frost, + *-phagia*]. Compulsive eating of ice.

pa·go·plex·ia (pay″go·pleck′see·uh) *n.* [Gk. *pagos*, frost, + *plēxis*, stroke, + *-ia*]. Numbness from cold; FROSTBITE.

-pagus [Gk. *pagos,* that which is fixed]. A combining form designating *a pair of conjoined twins joined at a* (specified) *site.*

-pagy [*-pagus* + *-y*]. A combining form designating the state of *conjoined twins joined at a* (specified) *site.*

PAH, PAHA Abbreviation for *para-aminohippuric acid.*

pai·dol·o·gy (pay·dol′uh·jee, pye·dol′) *n.* PEDOLOGY.

pain, *n.* [OF. *peine,* from L. *poena,* penalty, fine, from Gk. *poinē*]. A localized or diffuse abnormal sensation ranging from discomfort to agony; caused by stimulation of functionally specific peripheral nerve endings. It serves as a physiologic protective mechanism. —**pain·ful** (·ful), **pain·less** (·lus) *adj.*

painful feet syndrome. BURNING FEET SYNDROME.

painful heel. Tenderness of the heel, causing severe pain on walking; usually due to bony spurs, rarely due to gonococcal infection.

painful point. Any point on the skin at the exit or along the course of a nerve upon which pressure will cause pain; seen in neuralgia.

pain joy. Masochistic enjoyment of suffering.

pain point. 1. PAINFUL POINT. 2. PAIN SPOT. 3. TRIGGER ZONE.

pain receptor. NOCICEPTOR.

pain reflex. NOCICEPTIVE REFLEX.

pain spots. Small areas of skin overlying the endings of either very small myelinated (delta) or unmyelinated (C) nerve fibers whose stimulation, depending on the intensity and duration, results in the sensation of either pain or itching.

painter's colic. Colic due to lead poisoning.

painter's palsy. LEAD POLYNEUROPATHY.

pain threshold. The lowest limit of perceiving the sensation of pain.

paired allosome. One of a pair of similar allosomes.

pair production. The formation of a positron and a negatron when an x-ray loses its energy in passing close to the nucleus of an atom, occurring only when x-rays have energy of 1 million electron volts or greater.

Pa·jot's hook (pa^h·zho′) [C. *Pajot,* French obstetrician, 1816–1896]. A hook used for decapitation of the fetus in difficult labor.

pal·a·dang (pal′uh·dang) *n.* A pinta-like condition seen in Guam.

palaeo-. See *paleo-.*

palata. Plural of *palatum.*

pal·a·tal (pal′uh·tul) *adj.* Pertaining to the palate.

palatal aponeurosis. APONEUROSIS OF THE SOFT PALATE.

palatal arch. The concavity of the hard palate when seen in transverse section.

palatal bar. A bar of metal extended across a portion of the hard palate for the purpose of joining and strengthening the two sections of a maxillary partial denture.

palatal myoclonus. A rhythmic movement, 30 to 60 per second, of the soft palate, and sometimes the pharynx, facial muscles, diaphragm, vocal cords and even the shoulder muscles. The lesions producing this state are situated in the central tegmental tract, inferior olivary nucleus, or olivocerebellar tract.

palatal nystagmus. PALATAL MYOCLONUS.

palatal process. PALATINE PROCESS (1).

palatal process of the maxilla. PALATINE PROCESS (2).

palatal reflex. 1. Elevation of the soft palate in response to touch. 2. Swallowing produced by irritation of the palate.

pal·ate (pal′ut) *n.* [L. *palatum*]. The roof of the mouth. See also *hard palate, soft palate,* and Plates 12, 20.

palate hook. A surgical instrument for retracting the uvula.

palate myograph. An instrument for taking a tracing of the movements of the soft palate.

pa·lat·ic (pa·lat′ick) *adj.* PALATAL.

pa·lat·i·form (pa·lat′i·form) *adj.* [*palate* + *-iform*]. Resembling the palate.

pal·a·tine (pal′uh·tine) *adj. & n.* 1. PALATAL. 2. The palatine bone. NA *os palatinum.* See Table of Bones in the Appendix.

palatine arches. The palatoglossal and palatopharyngeal arches.

palatine canal. Any of the canals in the palatine bone, giving passage to branches of the descending palatine nerve and artery. The greater palatine canal (NA *canalis palatinus major*) is a continuation of the pterygopalatine canal; the lesser palatine canals (NA *canalis palatini minores*) branch from the greater palatine canal and open separately.

palatine foramen. Any of the lower openings of the palatine canals. See also *greater palatine foramen, lesser palatine foramen.*

palatine fossa. INCISIVE FOSSA (1).

palatine papilla. INCISIVE PAPILLA.

palatine process. 1. A ventromedial outgrowth of the embryonic maxillary process that develops into the definitive palate. 2. A thick process projecting horizontally mediad from the medial aspect of the maxilla, forming part of the floor of the nasal cavity and part of the roof of the mouth. NA *processus palatinus maxillae.*

palatine raphe. The narrow ridge of mucosa in the median line of the palate. NA *raphe palati.*

palatine ridges. The central ridge (raphe) together with the lateral corrugations of the mucosa (rugae) of the hard palate; in man they are especially prominent in the fetus.

palatine spine. POSTERIOR NASAL SPINE.

palatine suture. The median suture joining the bones of the palate. Syn. *median palatine suture.* NA *sutura palatina mediana.*

palatine tonsil. The aggregation of lymph nodules between the palatine arches. NA *tonsilla palantina.*

palatine tubercle. PYRAMIDAL PROCESS OF THE PALATINE BONE.

pal·a·ti·tis (pal″uh·tye′tis) *n.* [*palate* + *-itis*]. Inflammation of the palate.

palato-. A combining form meaning *palate, palatal, palatine.*

pal·a·to·glos·sal (pal″uh·to·glos′ul) *adj.* [*palato-* + *glossal*]. Pertaining to the palate and the tongue.

palatoglossal arch. A fold formed by the projection of the palatoglossal muscle covered by mucous membrane. NA *arcus palatoglossus.*

palatoglossal muscle. PALATOGLOSSUS.

pa·la·to·glos·sus (pal″uh·to·glos′us) *n.* The muscle within the anterior pillar of the fauces; it connects the soft palate with the tongue. NA *musculus palatoglossus.* See also Table of Muscles in the Appendix.

pal·a·to·graph (pal′uh·to·graf) *n.* [*palato-* + *graph*]. An instrument for the recording of palatal movements.

pal·a·to·max·il·lary (pal″uh·to·mack′si·lerr·ee) *adj.* [*palato-* + *maxillary*]. Pertaining to the palate and the maxilla.

palatomaxillary arch. An arch formed by the palatine, maxillary, and premaxillary bones.

palatomaxillary index. An index used to denote the various forms of the dental arch and palate; it is expressed by the following formula: palatomaxillary width multiplied by 100, divided by the palatomaxillary length, when the width is measured between the outer borders of the alveolar arch just above the middle of the second molar tooth, and the length is measured from the alveolar point to the middle of a transverse line touching the posterior borders of the two maxillae.

palatomaxillary suture. A suture between the horizontal part of the palatine bone and the palatine process of the maxilla. NA *sutura palatomaxillaris.*

pal·a·to·myo·graph (pal″uh·to·migh′o·graf) *n.* PALATE MYOGRAPH.

pal·a·to·na·sal (pal″uh·to·nay′zul) *adj.* [*palato-* + *nasal*]. Pertaining to the palate and the nose.

pal·a·top·a·gus par·a·sit·i·cus (pal″uh·top′uh·gus păr″uh·sit′i·kus). EPIPALATUM.

pal·a·to·pha·ryn·ge·al (pal″uh·to·fa·rin′jee·ul, ·făr″in·jee′ul) *adj.* [*palato-* + *pharyngeal*]. Pertaining conjointly to the palate and the pharynx.

palatopharyngeal arch. A fold formed by the projection of the palatopharyngeal muscle covered by mucous membrane. NA *arcus palatopharyngeus.*

pa·la·to·pha·ryn·ge·us (pal″uh·to·fa·rin′jee·us) *n.* The muscle in the palatopharyngeal arch, connecting the soft palate with the lateral wall of the pharynx below. NA *musculus palatopharyngeus.* See also Table of Muscles in the Appendix.

pal·a·to·plas·ty (pal′uh·to·plas″tee) *n.* [*palato-* + *-plasty*]. Plastic surgery of the palate.

pal·a·to·ple·gia (pal″uh·to·plee′jee·uh) *n.* [*palato-* + *-plegia*]. Paralysis of the soft palate.

pal·a·to·pter·y·goid (pal″uh·to·terr′i·goid) *adj.* Pertaining to the palate bone and pterygoid processes of the sphenoid bone; PTERYGOPALATINE.

pal·a·tor·rha·phy (pal″uh·tor′uh·fee) *n.* [*palato-* + *-rrhaphy*]. Suture of a cleft palate.

pal·a·to·sal·pin·ge·us (pal″uh·to·sal·pin′jee·us) *n.* [NL., from *palato-* + *salpinx*]. A portion of the levator veli palatini.

pal·a·tos·chi·sis (pal″uh·tos′ki·sis) *n.* [*palato-* + *-schisis*]. CLEFT PALATE.

pa·la·tum (pa·lay′tum, pa·lah′tum) *n.*, genit. **pala·ti** (·tye), pl. **pala·ta** (·tuh) [L.] [NA]. PALATE.

palatum du·rum (dew′rum) [NA]. HARD PALATE.

palatum fis·sum (fis′um). CLEFT PALATE.

palatum mo·bi·le (mo′bi·lee). SOFT PALATE.

palatum mol·le (mol′ee) [NA]. SOFT PALATE.

palatum os·se·um (os′ee·um) [NA]. HARD PALATE.

pa·le·en·ceph·a·lon (pay″lee·en·sef′uh·lon) *n.* [*paleo-* + *encephalon*]. The brain with the exception of the neencephalon; the phylogenetically old part of the brain.

paleo-, palaeo- [Gk. *palaios,* old, ancient]. A combining form meaning (a) *ancient;* (b) *primitive, phylogenetically early.*

pa·leo·cer·e·bel·lum (pay″lee·o·serr·e·bel′um) *n.* [*paleo-* + *cerebellum*]. Phylogenetically old parts of the cerebellum; the anterior lobe, composed of lingula, central lobule, and culmen, and the posterior part of the posterior lobe, composed of uvula, tonsils, and paraflocculus.

pa·leo·en·ceph·a·lon (pay″lee·o·en·sef′uh·lon) *n.* PALEENCEPHALON.

pa·leo·gen·e·sis (pay″lee·o·jen′e·sis) *n.* [*paleo-* + *-genesis*]. PALINGENESIS.

paleo·ge·net·ics (pay″lee·o·je·net′icks) *n.* [*paleo-* + *genetics*]. The genetics of extinct or ancestral species. See also *chemical paleogenetics.*

pa·leo·ki·net·ic (pay″lee·o·ki·net′ick, ·kigh·net′ick) *adj.* [*paleo-* + *kinetic*]. Pertaining to the motor activities of the older nervous system, represented in mammals by the basal ganglia and brainstem, which are the structures concerned with postural static and automatic movements.

pa·le·on·tol·o·gy (pay″lee·on·tol′uh·jee) *n.* [*paleo-* + *onto-* + *-logy*]. The science and study of fossil remains.

pa·leo·ol·ive (pay″lee·o·ol′iv) *n.* [*paleo-* + *olive*]. The accessory nuclei and the most medial portion of the main nucleus which form, phylogenetically, the oldest part of the olive.

pa·leo·pal·li·um (pay″lee·o·pal′ee·um) *n.* [*paleo-* + *pallium*]. The lateral olfactory lobe, or piriform lobe of lower forms; in the higher mammals, especially in man, it forms the uncus and adjacent anterior part of the parahippocampal gyrus.

pa·leo·pa·thol·o·gy (pay″lee·o·pa·thol′uh·jee) *n.* [*paleo-* + *pathology*]. A branch of pathology dealing with diseases of ancient times demonstrated in human and animal remains.

paleostriatal syndrome. JUVENILE PARALYSIS AGITANS.

pa·leo·stri·a·tum (pay″lee·o·strye·ay′tum) *n.* [*paleo-* + *striatum*]. GLOBUS PALLIDUS; the phylogenetically old part of the corpus striatum. —**paleostria·tal** (·tul) *adj.*

pa·leo·thal·a·mus (pay″lee·o·thal′uh·mus) *n.* [*paleo-* + *thalamus*]. The nuclei of the midline of the thalamus, together with some of the intralaminar nuclei.

pali-, palin- [Gk., back, again]. A prefix indicating *repetition* or *recurrence.*

pali·ci·ne·sia (pal″i·si·nee′zhuh) *n.* PALIKINESIA.

pali·ki·ne·sia (pal″i·ki·nee′zhuh, ·zee·uh, ·kigh·nee′) *n.* [*pali-* + *-kinesia*]. Constant and involuntary repetition of movements.

pali·ki·ne·sis (pal″i·ki·nee′sis, ·kigh·nee′sis) *n.* PALIKINESIA.

pali·la·lia (pal″i·lay′lee·uh) *n.* [*pali-* + *-lalia*]. Pathologic repetition of words or phrases. Compare *palingraphia.* See also *echolalia, perseveration.*

palin-. See *pali-.*

pal·in·dro·mia (pal″in·dro′mee·uh) *n.* [Gk., from *palin,* back, + *dromos,* running, course, + *-ia*]. The recurrence or worsening of a disease; RELAPSE. —**palin·drom·ic** (·drom′ick) *adj.*

palindromic rheumatism. An acute arthritis and periarthritis occurring in multiple, afebrile, irregularly spaced attacks lasting only a few hours or days and disappearing completely; characterized by swelling, redness, and disability of usually only one joint. It attacks adults of either sex. The cause is not known.

pal·in·gen·e·sis (pal″in·jen′e·sis) *n.* [Gk. *palingenesia,* regeneration, reincarnation]. The development of characteristics during ontogeny which are regarded as inherited from ancestral species. Compare *cenogenesis.* See also *recapitulation theory.*

pal·in·graph·ia (pal″ing·graf′ee·uh) *n.* [Gk., rewriting, revision]. Pathologic repetition of syllables, words, or phrases in writing. Compare *palilalia.*

pal·in·ki·ne·sia (pal″ing·ki·nee′zhuh, ·zee·uh, ·kigh·nee′) *n.* [*palin-* + *kinesia*]. PALIKINESIA.

pal·in·ki·ne·sis (pal″ing·ki·nee′sis, ·kigh·nee′) *n.* [*palin-* + *kinesis*]. PALIKINESIA.

pal·in·op·sia (pal″i·nop′see·uh) *n.* [*palin-* + *-opsia*]. The perseveration or recurrence of a visual image after the exciting stimulus object has been removed; a phenomenon of uncertain mechanism which occurs in a defective but not blind homonymous visual field.

pal·in·phra·sia (pal″in·fray′zhuh, ·zee·uh) *n.* [*palin-* + Gk. *phrasis,* expression, phrase, text, + *-ia*]. PALILALIA.

pali·op·sia (pal″ee·op′see·uh) *n.* PALINOPSIA.

pali·phra·sia (pal″i·fray′zhuh, ·zee·uh) *n.* [*pali-* + *phrase* + *-ia*]. PALILALIA.

pal·ir·rhea, pal·ir·rhoea (pal″i·ree′uh) *n.* [Gk. *palirrhoia,* reflux, flowing back, from *pali-* + *rhoia,* flow]. 1. The recurrence of a mucoid discharge. 2. REGURGITATION.

pal·la·di·um (pa·lay′dee·um) *n.* [after the asteroid *Pallas,* from Gk. *Pallas, Pallados,* epithet of Athena]. Pd = 106.4. A silver-white, fairly ductile, hard metal, with a density of 12.02, belonging to the platinum group of metals.

pall·an·es·the·sia (pal″an·es·theezh′uh, ·theez′ee·uh) *n.* [Gk.

*pall*ein, to shake, + *anesthesia*]. Absence of pallesthesia or vibration sense.

pall·es·the·sia, pall·aes·the·sia (pal″es·theezh′uh, ·theez′ee·uh) *n.* [Gk. *pall*ein, to shake, + *esthesia*]. The sense of vibration, involving sensations like those imparted by a vibrating tuning fork.

pallia. A plural of *pallium.*

pal·li·a·tion (pal″ee·ay′shun) *n.* [L. *palliare,* to cloak, from *pallium,* mantle]. Alleviation; the act of soothing or moderating, without really curing. —**pal·li·ate** (pal′ee·ate) *v.*

pal·li·a·tive (pal′ee·uh·tiv, ·ay·tiv) *adj. & n.* [F. *palliatif,* from L. *palliare,* to cloak]. 1. Having a relieving or soothing, but not curative, action. 2. A drug that relieves or soothes the symptoms of a disease without curing it.

pal·li·dal (pal′i·dul) *adj.* Of or pertaining to the globus pallidus.

pallidal atrophy. JUVENILE PARALYSIS AGITANS.

pallido-. A combining form meaning *pallidal, globus pallidus.*

pal·li·dof·u·gal (pal″i·dof′yoo·gul) *adj.* Projecting away from the globus pallidus.

pal·li·do·hy·po·tha·lam·ic (pal″i·do·high″po·thuh·lam′ick) *adj.* [*pallido-* + *hypothalamic*]. *Obsol.* Pertaining to the pallidum and the hypothalamus, with reference to the connections once believed to exist between them.

pallidohypothalamic fibers, tract. *Obsol.* Pallidofugal fibers once believed to connect the pallidum and the hypothalamus, now known to be pallidothalamic.

pal·li·doid·o·sis (pal″i·doy·do′sis) *n.* [(*Treponema*) *pallid*um + *-oid,* -like, + *-osis*]. VENEREAL SPIROCHETOSIS.

pal·li·do·sub·tha·lam·ic fibers or **tract** (pal″i·do·sub″thuh·lam′ick). A topographically-organized group of fibers which arises from the lateral segment of the globus pallidus and projects exclusively to the subthalamic nucleus.

pal·li·do·teg·men·tal fibers (pal″i·do·teg·men′tul). A small group of descending pallidofugal fibers, derived from the medial segment of the globus pallidus. It descends along the ventrolateral border of the red nucleus and terminates upon large cells of the pedunculopontine nucleus.

pal·li·do·tha·lam·ic fibers (pal″i·do·thuh·lam′ick). A system of pallidofugal fibers which arises from the medial segment of the globus pallidus and projects, via the ansa lenticularis and fasciculus lenticularis, to the ventral-anterior and ventral-lateral nuclei of the thalamus, and to a lesser extent to the centromedian nucleus of the thalamus.

pal·li·dot·o·my (pal″i·dot′uh·mee) *n.* [*pallido-* + *-tomy*]. The surgical destruction of the globus pallidus for the treatment of movement disorders such as parkinsonism.

pal·li·dum (pal′i·dum) *n.* [NL., from L. *pallidus,* pale]. The globus pallidus, the medial pale portion of the lenticular nucleus of the brain. —**palli·dal** (·dul) *adj.*

pal·lio·pon·tine fiber (pal″ee·o·pon′tine) [*palli*um + *pontine*]. CORTICOPONTINE FIBER.

pal·li·um (pal′ee·um) *n.,* pl. **pal·lia** (·ee·uh), **palliums** [L., mantle, cloak] [NA]. The cerebral cortex and superficial white matter of a cerebral hemisphere.

pal·lor (pal′ur) *n.* [L.]. Paleness, especially of the skin and mucous membranes.

palm (pahm) *n.* [L. *palma*]. The volar or flexor surface of the hand; the hollow of the hand.

pal·ma (pal′muh) *n.,* pl. **pal·mae** (·mee) [L.]. PALM.

palma ma·nus (man′us) [NA]. The palm of the hand.

palm and sole system. An extension of the Galton identification system to include the imprints of the palmar and plantar surfaces.

pal·mar (pahl′mur, pal′mur, pah′mur) *adj.* Of or pertaining to the palm of the hand.

palmar abscess. An abscess in the palm of the hand, usually beneath the palmar fascia.

palmar aponeurosis. Bundles of dense fibrous connective tissue which radiate from the tendons of the palmaris longus muscle (or deep fascia of the forearm) toward the proximal ends of the fingers. NA *aponeurosis palmaris.*

palmar arches. See *deep palmar arch, superficial palmar arch.*

palmar carpal ligament. A transverse band of deep fascia of the wrist overlying the ulnar artery and nerve; a superficial part of the flexor retinaculum of the wrist. Syn. *volar carpal ligament.*

pal·ma·ris (pal·mair′is) *n.,* pl. **palma·res** (·eez) [NL., palmar]. One of two muscles, palmaris longus and palmaris brevis, inserted into the fascia of the palm. See also Table of Muscles in the Appendix.

palmar ligaments. The fibrocartilaginous plates, one to a joint, on the palmar surfaces of the metacarpophalangeal joints (NA *ligamenta palmaria articulationum metacarpophalangearum*) and the interphalangeal joints of the hand (NA *ligamenta palmaria articulationum interphalangearum manus*).

palmar reflex. Flexion of the fingers when the palm of the hand is irritated.

palmar spaces. The lateral and medial potential fascial spaces in the hand between the thenar and hypothenar areas, separated by a fibrous septum and filled with areolar tissue.

palmar ulnocarpal ligament. A fibrous palmar band in the wrist, passing from the styloid process of the ulna to the capitate and other carpal bones. NA *ligamentum ulnocarpeum palmare.*

pal·mate (pal′mate, pah′mate) *adj.* [L. *palmatus,* from *palma,* palm]. Similar in shape to a hand with fingers spread.

palmate folds. ARBOR VITAE (2).

pal·ma·ture (pal′muh·chur, pahl′) *n.* Union of the fingers; may be congenital or due to burns, wounds, or other trauma.

palm-chin reflex. PALMOMENTAL REFLEX.

pal·mel·lin (pal·mel′in) *n.* A red coloring principle of a freshwater alga, *Palmella cruenta,* resembling hemoglobin.

Palmer method. VAN SLYKE AND PALMER METHOD.

pal·mi·ped (pal′mi·ped) *adj.* [*palm* + *-ped*]. Having webbed feet.

pal·mi·tate (pal′mi·tate) *n.* A salt or ester of palmitic acid.

pal·mit·ic (pal·mit′ick) *adj.* 1. Pertaining to or derived from palm oil. 2. Pertaining to palmitin.

palmitic acid. Hexadecanoic acid, $CH_3(CH_2)_{14}COOH$, a saturated acid occurring in the glycerides of many fats and oils. Syn. *cetic acid.*

pal·mi·tin (pal′mi·tin) *n.* Glyceryl tripalmitate or glyceryl palmitate, $C_{51}H_{98}O_6$, a solid ester of glycerin and palmitic acid occurring in many fats. Syn. *tripalmitin.*

pal·mi·tyl (pal′mi·til) *n.* CETYL.

palmityl alcohol. CETYL ALCOHOL.

pal·mod·ic (pal·mod′ick) *adj.* [Gk. *palmōdēs,* palpitating]. Pertaining to, resembling, or affected with, palmus (1).

pal·mo·men·tal (pal″mo·men′tul, pahl″mo·) *adj.* [*palm* + *mental*]. Pertaining to the palm of the hand and the mentalis muscle.

palmomental reflex (of Marinesco-Radovici) [G. *Marinesco,* Rumanian pathologist; and J. G. *Radovici*]. Contraction of the ipsilateral mentalis and orbicularis oris muscles, with slight elevation and retraction of the angle of the mouth, in response to scratching the thenar area of the hand; occasionally seen in normal individuals, it is present in exaggerated forms in those with corticospinal-tract lesions.

pal·mo·plan·tar (pal″mo·plan′tur, pahl″mo·) *adj.* [*palm* + *plantar*]. Pertaining to both the palms of the hands and the soles of the feet.

palmoplantar sign or **phenomenon.** FILIPOWICZ SIGN.

pal·mus (pal′mus) *n.,* pl. **pal·mi** (·migh) [NL., from Gk. *palmos,* quivering]. Twitching or jerkiness.

pal·pa·ble (pal′puh·bul) *adj.* [L. *palpabilis,* from *palpare,* to touch]. 1. Capable of being touched or palpated. 2. Evident.

pal·pa·tion (pal·pay′shun) *n.* [L. *palpatio,* from *palpare,* to touch gently]. Examination by touch for purposes of diagnosis; application of the hand or fingers to a part, or insertion of a finger into a body orifice, to detect characteristics and conditions of local tissues or of underlying organs or tumors. —**pal·pate** (pal'pate) *v.*; **pal·pa·to·ry** (pal' puh·to''ree) *adj.*

pal·pa·to·per·cus·sion (pal''puh·to·pur·kush'un) *n.* Combined palpation and percussion.

palpatory percussion. Direct percussion with the purpose of obtaining diagnostically relevant information by tactile rather than auditory means.

pal·pe·bra (pal'pe·bruh, pal·pee'bruh) *n.*, pl. & genit. sing. **palpe·brae** (·bree) [L.]. EYELID. —**palpe·bral** (·brul) *adj.*

palpebrae [NA]. Plural and genitive singular of *palpebra.*

palpebra inferior [NA]. The lower eyelid.

palpebral angle. CANTHUS.

palpebral arch. The arterial arcade in each eyelid; the inferior palpebral arch (NA *arcus palpebralis inferior*) or the superior palpebral arch (NA *arcus palpebralis superior*).

palpebral artery. Either of the lateral palpebral arteries (NA *arteriae palpebrales laterales*), which originate in the lacrimal artery, or either of the medial palpebral arteries (NA *arteriae palpebrales mediales*), which originate in the ophthalmic artery; the inferior and superior members of each pair anastamose in the inferior and superior palpebral arches, which supply the eyelids.

palpebral conjunctiva. The conjunctiva of the eyelids. NA *tunica conjunctiva palpebrarum.*

palpebral fascia. The fascia of the eyelids. See also *orbital septum.*

palpebral fissure. The space between the eyelids extending from the outer to the inner canthus. NA *rima palpebrarum.*

palpebral fold. A fold formed by the reflection of the conjunctiva from the eyelids onto the eye. There are two folds, the superior and the inferior.

palpebral follicles. TARSAL GLANDS.

palpebral ligament. A fibrous band running from the extremities of the tarsal plates to the wall of the orbit. There is one medial palpebral ligament (NA *ligamentum palpebrale mediale*) and one lateral palpebral ligament (NA *ligamentum palpebrale laterale*) for each eye.

palpebral-oculogyric reflex. BELL'S PHENOMENON.

palpebra superior [NA]. The upper eyelid.

pal·pe·brate (pal'pe·brate) *adj.* & *v.* [NL. *palpebratus*, from *palpebra*]. 1. Furnished with eyelids. 2. To wink, blink repeatedly.

pal·pe·bra·tion (pal''pe·bray'shun) *n.* [L. *palpebratio*, from *palpebra*, eyelid]. 1. Blinking; nictation. 2. Excessive winking as a form of tic.

pal·pe·bri·tis (pal''pe·brye'tis) *n.* [*palpebra* + *-itis*]. BLEPHARITIS.

pal·pi·tate (pal'pi·tate) *v.* [L. *palpitare*, from *palpare*, to touch, feel]. To flutter, tremble, or beat abnormally fast; applied especially to rapid rate of the heart.

pal·pi·ta·tion (pal''pi·tay'shun) *n.* 1. A fluttering or throbbing, especially of the heart, often associated with a rapid heart rate or irregular heart rhythm. 2. Any heart action that produces a disagreeable awareness in the patient.

pal·sy (pawl'zee) *n.* [OF. *paralisie*, from L. *paralysis*, from Gk.]. Paralysis or weakness; used to designate special types, such as cerebral palsy or Erb's palsy. See also *parkinsonism.* —**pal·sied** (·zeed) *adj.*

Pal·tauf's dwarfism or **nanism** (pahl'taowf) [A. *Paltauf*, Austrian physician, 1860–1893]. Pituitary dwarfism, ascribed by Paltauf to status lymphaticus.

Paltauf-Sternberg disease [R. *Paltauf*, Austrian pathologist, 1858–1924; and C. *Sternberg*]. HODGKIN'S DISEASE.

pa·lu·dal (pal'yoo·dul, pa·lew'dul) *adj.* [L. *palus, paludis*, swamp, + *-al*]. 1. Pertaining to swamps or marshes. 2. MALARIAL.

pal·u·dide (pal'yoo·dide) *n.* [*paludism* + *-ide* (*-id*)]. A cutaneous eruption supposed to be due to malaria.

pal·u·dism (pal'yoo·diz·um) *n.* [L. *palus, paludis*, swamp, + *-ism*]. MALARIA.

Paludrine. A trademark for the antimalarial drug chloroguanide or proguanil, used as the hydrochloride salt.

pa·lus·tral (pa·lus'trul) *adj.* [L. *paluster*, swampy, + *-al*]. PALUDAL.

Pal-Weigert method for nerve tissue [J. *Pal*, Austrian physician, 1863–1936; and C. *Weigert*]. WEIGERT'S METHOD.

pam·a·quine (pam'uh·kween, ·kwin) *n.* 8-{[4-(Diethylamino)-1-methylbutyl]amino}-6-methoxyquinoline, $C_{19}H_{29}N_3O$, an antimalarial drug; used as the pamoate salt.

pam·a·to·lol (pam''uh·to'lole) *n.* Methyl (±)-[*p*-2-hydroxy-3-(isopropylamino)propoxy]phenethylcarbamate, $C_{16}H_{26}N_2O_4$, a *β*-receptor, antiadrenergic, used as the sulfate salt.

Pamine. Trademark for the anticholinergic drug methscopolamine bromide.

pam·o·ate (pam'o·ate) *n.* A contraction for the radical 4,4'-methylenebis(3-hydroxy-2-naphthoate); a salt or ester containing the radical.

pam·pin·i·form (pam·pin'i·form) *adj.* [L. *pampinus*, tendril, + *-iform*]. Having the form of a tendril.

pampiniform plexus. A network of veins in the spermatic cord in the male, and in the broad ligament near the ovary in the female. NA *plexus pampiniformis.*

Pan, *n.* [Gk., god of woods and fields]. A genus of the Pongidae comprising the chimpanzees.

pan- [Gk. *pas, pan*, whole, all]. A combining form meaning *all, every;* in medicine, *general, affecting all or many parts.*

pan·a·cea (pan''uh·see'uh) *n.* [Gk. *panakeia*, from *pan-* + *akos*, remedy]. A cure-all; a quack remedy.

pan·ac·i·nar (pan·as'i·nur) *adj.* [*pan-* + *acinar*]. 1. Involving all acini. 2. Involving all pulmonary alveoli, applied especially to a variety of emphysema.

panacinar emphysema. Emphysema characterized by diffuse destruction of one lung. Syn. *panlobular emphysema.*

Panacur. A trademark for fenbendazole, an anthelmintic.

panaesthesia. Panesthesia (= CENESTHESIA). —**panaesthetic,** *adj.*

pan·ag·glu·ti·nin (pan''uh·gloo'ti·nin) *n.* [*pan-* + *agglutinin*]. Any agglutinating antibody which agglutinates cells of various types; the apparent lack of specificity indicates that it reacts with cell antigens common to cells of different types.

pan·an·es·the·sia (pan''an''es·theezh'uh, ·theez'ee·uh) *n.* [*pan-* + *anesthesia*]. Loss of perception of all sensations, usually a symptom of hysterical neurosis in an otherwise neurologically intact patient.

pan·a·ris (pan'uh·ris, pa·năr'is) *n.* [F., from L. *panaricium, panaritium*, from Gk. *parōnychia*]. PARONYCHIA.

pan·a·ri·ti·um (pan''uh·rish'ee·um) *n.* [L.]. PARONYCHIA.

pan·ar·te·ri·tis (pan''ahr·te·rye'tis) *n.* [*pan-* + *arteritis*]. 1. Inflammation of all the coats of an artery. 2. Inflammation of several arteries at the same time; POLYARTERITIS.

pan·ar·thri·tis (pan''ahr·thrigh'tis) *n.* [*pan-* + *arthritis*]. Inflammation of many joints.

pan·at·ro·phy (pan·at'ruh·fee) *n.* [*pan-* + *atrophy*]. 1. Atrophy affecting every part of a structure. 2. Atrophy affecting every part of the body.

pan·blas·to·trop·ic (pan·blas''to·trop'ick) *adj.* [*pan-* + *blasto-* + *-tropic*]. Pertaining to changes in the ectoderm, mesoderm, and entoderm or in their derivatives.

panblastotropic reaction. A reaction affecting three embryonic layers; it occurs in syphilis.

pan·car·di·tis (pan''kahr·dye'tis) *n.* [*pan-* + *carditis*]. Inflammation of the entire heart, involving endocardium, myocardium, and pericardium.

pan·cav·er·no·si·tis (pan·kav''ur·no·sigh'tis) *n.* [*pan-* + *cavernositis*]. CAVERNITIS.

pan·chrome stain (pan'krome). A stain for blood which is a modification by Pappenheim of the Giemsa stain.

Pan·coast's operation [J. *Pancoast*, U.S. surgeon, 1805–1882].

Section of the mandibular nerve at the foramen ovale for trigeminal neuralgia.

Pancoast's tumor [H. K. *Pancoast*, U.S. radiologist, 1875–1939]. A tumor of the superior pulmonary sulcus. See also *Pancoast syndrome.*

Pancoast syndrome [H. K. *Pancoast*]. The clinical picture of a superior pulmonary sulcus (thoracic inlet) tumor, including ipsilateral Horner's syndrome and brachial motor sensory disturbances due to involvement of the cervical sympathetic chain and brachial plexus; there is usually local bone invasion and destruction. Syn. *Hare's syndrome.*

pan·col·ec·to·my (pan″kol·eck′tuh·mee, ·ko·leck′) *n.* [*pan-* + *colectomy*]. Surgical removal of the entire colon.

pan·col·po·hys·ter·ec·to·my (pan·kol″po·his″tur·eck′tuh·mee) *n.* PANHYSTEROCOLPECTOMY.

pancre-, pancreo-. A combining form meaning *pancreas, pancreatic.*

pan·cre·as (pan′kree·us, pang′kree·us) *n.*, genit. **pan·cre·a·tis** (pan·kree′uh·tis), pl. **pancrea·ta** (·tuh) [Gk. *pankreas*, from *pan-* + *kreas*, meat, flesh]. A compound racemose gland, 6 to 8 inches in length, lying transversely across the posterior wall of the abdomen. Its right extremity, the head, lies in contact with the duodenum; its left extremity, the tail, is in close proximity to the spleen. It secretes a limpid, colorless fluid which contains the enzymes necessary for the digestion of proteins, fats, and carbohydrates. The secretion is conveyed to the duodenum by the pancreatic duct or ducts. It furnishes several important internal secretions, including glucagon and insulin, from the islets of the pancreas. See also Plates 10, 13, 16.

pancreas ac·ces·so·ri·um (ack″se·so′ree·um) [NA]. ACCESSORY PANCREAS.

pancreas of Aselli [G. *Aselli*]. Lymph nodes near the pancreas.

pancreat-, pancreato- [Gk. *pankreas, pankreatos*]. A combining form meaning *pancreas, pancreatic.*

pancreata. Plural of *pancreas.*

pan·cre·a·tec·to·my (pan″kree·uh·teck′tuh·mee) *n.* [*pancreat-* + *-ectomy*]. Excision of the pancreas.

pan·cre·at·ic (pan″kree·at′ick) *adj.* [*pancreat-* + *-ic*]. Pertaining to the pancreas.

pancreatic amylase. An enzyme in pancreatic juice that hydrolyzes starch to maltose. Syn. *amylopsin, pancreatic diastase.*

pancreatic calculus. A calculus situated in the pancreatic duct and composed largely of calcium phosphate.

pancreatic diabetes. 1. DIABETES MELLITUS. 2. Diabetes mellitus due to pancreatic disease.

pancreatic diarrhea. Diarrhea due to deficiency of pancreatic digestive enzymes; characterized by the passage of large, greasy stools having a high fat and nitrogen content.

pancreatic diastase. PANCREATIC AMYLASE.

pancreatic digestion. Digestion by the action of the pancreatic juice.

pancreatic diverticulum. One of two diverticula (dorsal and ventral) from the embryonic duodenum or hepatic diverticulum that form the pancreas and its ducts.

pancreatic dor·nase (dor′naze, ·nace). A preparation of deoxyribonuclease obtained from beef pancreas, used to reduce the tenacity of pulmonary secretions and facilitate expectoration in bronchopulmonary infections.

pancreatic duct. The main duct of the pancreas formed from the dorsal and ventral pancreatic ducts of the embryo. NA *ductus pancreaticus.*

pancreatic fibrosis. CYSTIC FIBROSIS OF THE PANCREAS.

pancreatic fistula. 1. An external opening from the pancreas to the skin of the abdominal wall following the drainage of a pancreatic cyst or other gastric or duodenal operation. 2. An internal opening from the pancreas to the jejunum, duodenum, stomach, or gallbladder, to overcome the formation of an external fistula.

pancreatic glomeruli. ISLETS OF THE PANCREAS.

pancreatic hormones. The hormones formed by the pancreas: insulin, lipocaic, and glucagon.

pancreatic incisure. PANCREATIC NOTCH.

pancreatic infantilism. Growth retardation associated with the chronic undernutrition of infantile celiac disease.

pancreatic insufficiency. Absence of or reduced pancreatic secretion into the duodenum, and resultant poor digestion and absorption of fat, vitamins, nitrogen, and carbohydrates.

pancreatic islet or **island.** ISLET OF THE PANCREAS.

pancreatic juice. The secretion of the pancreas; a thick, transparent, colorless, odorless fluid, of a salty taste, and strongly alkaline, containing proteolytic, lipolytic, and amylolytic enzymes.

pancreatic lipase. An enzyme in pancreatic juice that catalyzes hydrolysis of fats. Syn. *steapsin.*

pancreatic notch. A groove in the pancreas for the superior mesenteric artery and vein, separating the uncinate process from the rest of the head of the pancreas. NA *incisura pancreatis.*

pancreatico-. A combining form meaning *pancreatic.*

pan·cre·at·i·co·du·o·de·nal (pan″kree·at″i·ko·dew″o·dee′nul, ·dew·od′e·nul) *adj.* [*pancreatico-* + *duodenal*]. Pertaining to the pancreas and the duodenum.

pancreaticoduodenal artery. See Table of Arteries in the Appendix.

pancreaticoduodenal plexus. A visceral plexus whose nerve fibers are distributed to the duodenum and the pancreas.

pan·cre·at·i·co·du·o·de·nec·to·my (pan″kree·at″i·ko·dew″o·de·neck′tuh·mee) *n.* [*pancreatico-* + *duoden-* + *-ectomy*]. DUODENOPANCREATECTOMY.

pan·cre·at·i·co·du·o·de·nos·to·my (pan″kree·at″i·ko·dew″o·de·nos′tuh·mee) *n.* PANCREATODUODENOSTOMY.

pan·cre·at·i·co·en·ter·os·to·my (pan″kree·at″i·ko·en″tur·os′tuh·mee) *n.* [*pancreatico-* + *entero-* + *-stomy*]. Anastomosis of the pancreatic duct or a pancreatic fistulous tract with the small intestine.

pan·cre·at·i·co·gas·tros·to·my (pan″kree·at″i·ko·gas·tros′tuh·mee) *n.* [*pancreatico-* + *gastro-* + *-stomy*]. Anastomosis of a pancreatic fistulous tract with the pyloric portion of the stomach.

pan·cre·at·i·co·je·ju·nos·to·my (pan″kree·at″i·ko·jej″oo·nos′tuh·mee) *n.* [*pancreatico-* + *jejuno-* + *-stomy*]. Anastomosis of the pancreatic duct with the jejunum.

pan·cre·at·i·co·li·thot·o·my (pan″kree·at″i·ko·li·thot′uh·mee) *n.* [*pancreatico-* + *lithotomy*]. The surgical removal of a stone in the pancreatic duct.

pan·cre·at·i·co·splen·ic (pan″kree·at″i·ko·splen′ick) *adj.* [*pancreatico-* + *splenic*]. Pertaining to the pancreas and the spleen.

pancreaticosplenic ligament. A fold of peritoneum uniting the tail of the pancreas with the lower part of the medial surface of the spleen.

pancreatic rickets. CELIAC RICKETS.

pancreatic sialorrhea. An abnormal flow of saliva associated with pancreatic disease.

pancreatic succorrhea. A pathologic increase of the pancreatic juice when the secretory activity of the gland is exaggerated.

pan·cre·a·tin (pan′kree·uh·tin) *n.* A substance containing enzymes, principally pancreatic amylase (amylopsin), trypsin, and pancreatic lipase (steapsin), obtained from the fresh pancreas of the hog, *Sus scrofa* var. *domesticus*, or of the ox, *Bos taurus;* it is a cream-colored amorphous powder with a faint odor. Used for its enzymatic action in various forms of digestive failure but of doubtful activity.

pan·cre·a·ti·tis (pan″kree·uh·tye′tis) *n.*, pl. **pancrea·tit·i·des** (·tit′i·deez) [*pancreat-* + *-itis*]. Inflammation of the pancreas, acute or chronic. —**pancrea·tit·ic** (·tit′ick) *adj.*

pancreato-. See *pancreat-.*

pan·cre·a·to·du·o·de·nec·to·my (pan″kree·uh·to·dew″o·de·neck′tuh·mee) *n.* DUODENOPANCREATECTOMY.

pan·cre·a·to·du·o·de·nos·to·my (pan″kree·uh·to·dew″o·de·nos′tuh·mee) *n.* [*pancreato-* + *duodeno-* + *-stomy*]. The anastomosis of a portion of the pancreas, especially a fistulous tract into the duodenum.

pan·cre·a·to·en·ter·os·to·my (pan″kree·uh·to·en″tur·os′tuh·mee) *n.* [*pancreato-* + *entero-* + *-stomy*]. Anastomosis of the pancreatic duct with some part of the small intestine.

pan·cre·a·tog·e·nous (pan″kree·uh·toj′e·nus) *adj.* [*pancreato-* + *-genous*]. Arising in the pancreas.

pan·cre·a·to·li·pase (pan″kree·uh·to·lye′pace) *n.* Lipase found in the pancreatic juice.

pan·cre·ato·lith (pan″kree·at′o·lith) *n.* [*pancreato-* + *-lith*]. A calculus of the pancreas.

pan·cre·a·to·li·thec·to·my (pan″kree·uh·to·li·theck′tuh·mee, pan″kree·at″o·) *n.* [*pancreatolith* + *-ectomy*]. Surgical removal of a pancreatic calculus.

pan·cre·a·to·li·thot·o·my (pan″kree·uh·to·li·thot′uh·mee, pan″kree·at″o·) *n.* [*pancreatolith* + *-tomy*]. Surgical removal of calculus from the pancreas.

pan·cre·a·tol·y·sis (pan″kree·uh·tol′i·sis) *n.* [*pancreato-* + *-lysis*]. Destruction of the pancreas. —**pancre·ato·lyt·ic** (·at″o·lit′ick) *adj.*

pan·cre·a·tot·o·my (pan″kree·uh·tot′uh·mee) *n.* [*pancreato-* + *-tomy*]. Incision of the pancreas.

pan·cre·ec·to·my (pan″kree·eck′tuh·mee) *n.* PANCREATECTOMY.

pan·cre·li·pase (pan″kre·lye′pace) *n.* A concentrate of pancreatic enzymes standardized for lipase content; used as a lipolytic enzyme after diagnosis of exocrine pancreatic insufficiency.

pancreo-. See *pancre-*.

pan·creo·lith (pan′kree·o·lith) *n.* PANCREATOLITH.

pan·creo·li·thot·o·my (pan″kree·o·li·thot′uh·mee) *n.* PANCREATOLITHOTOMY.

pan·cre·ol·y·sis (pan″kree·ol′i·sis) *n.* PANCREATOLYSIS.

pan·creo·path·ia (pan″kree·o·path′ee·uh) *n.* PANCREOPATHY.

pan·cre·op·a·thy (pan″kree·op′uth·ee) *n.* [*pancreo-* + *-pathy*]. Any disease of the pancreas.

pan·creo·zyme (pan′kree·o·zime) *n.* [*pancreo-* + *-zyme*]. A ferment similar to but not identical with secretin.

pan·creo·zy·min (pan″kree·o·zye′min) *n.* A hormone now known to be identical with cholecystokinin.

pan·cu·ro·ni·um bromide (pan″kew·ro′nee·um). $2\beta,16\beta$-Dipiperidino-5α-androstane-$3\alpha,17\beta$-diol diacetate dimethobromide, $C_{35}H_{60}Br_2N_2O_4$, a neuromuscular blocking agent and peripheral muscle relaxant.

pan·cy·to·pe·nia (pan″sigh·to·pee′nee·uh) *n.* [*pan-* + *cyto-* + *-penia*]. Reduction of all three formed elements of the blood: erythrocytes, leukocytes, and blood platelets.

pan·de·mia (pan·dee′mee·uh) *n.* [Gk. *pandēmia,* the whole people]. A widespread epidemic; one affecting the majority of inhabitants of an area.

pan·dem·ic (pan·dem′ick) *adj.* & *n.* [Gk. *pandēmos,* from *pan-,* all, + *dēmos,* country, people]. 1. Epidemic over a wide geographic area, or even worldwide. Contr. *endemic, epidemic, sporadic.* 2. A widespread or worldwide epidemic.

pan·de·my (pan′de·mee) *n.* PANDEMIA.

pan·di·a·stol·ic (pan″dye″uh·stol′ick) *adj.* Pertaining to the entire diastole; HOLODIASTOLIC.

pan·dic·u·la·tion (pan·dick″yoo·lay′shun) *n.* [L. *pandiculari,* to stretch one's self, from *pandere,* to throw open, spread]. The act of stretching the limbs, especially on waking from sleep, accompanied by yawning.

Pan·dy's reagent (pahn′dee) [K. *Pandy,* Hungarian neurologist, b. 1868]. A saturated aqueous solution of phenol used in testing for spinal-fluid protein.

Pandy's test [K. *Pandy*]. A test for protein in which 1 ml of Pandy's reagent is placed in a test tube and one drop of spinal fluid is added. If increased protein is present, a bluish-white ring or cloud is formed.

pan·elec·tro·scope (pan″e·leck′truh·skope) *n.* [*pan-* + *electro-* + *-scope*]. An inspection apparatus for use in such procedures as proctoscopy, esophagoscopy, and urethroscopy. It throws concentrated light through the tube, thus illuminating the spot to be inspected.

pan·en·ceph·a·li·tis (pan″en·sef″uh·lye′tis) *n.* [*pan-* + *encephalitis*]. 1. Generalized inflammation of the brain, involving both gray and white matter. 2. Specifically, SUBACUTE SCLEROSING PANENCEPHALITIS.

pan·en·do·scope (pan·en′duh·skope) *n.* [*pan-* + *endoscope*]. A modification of the cystoscope, utilizing a Foroblique lens system, permitting adequate visualization of both the urinary bladder and the urethra. Compare *urethroscope.*

pan·es·the·sia, pan·aes·the·sia (pan″es·theezh′uh, ·theez′ee·uh) *n.* [Gk. *panaisthēsia,* full vigor of the senses]. CENESTHESIA. —**panes·thet·ic, panaes·thet·ic** (·thet′ick) *adj.*

Pa·neth cells (pah′net) [J. *Paneth,* German physician, 1857–1890]. Coarsely granular secretory cells found in the intestinal glands of the small intestine.

pang, *n.* A momentary, sharp pain; sudden distress.

Pang·born test. A flocculation test for syphilis.

pan·gen·e·sis (pan·jen′e·sis) *n.* [*pan-* + *-genesis*]. Darwin's comprehensive theory of heredity and development, according to which all parts of the body give off gemmules which aggregate in the germ cells. During development, they are sorted out from one another and give rise to parts similar to those of their origin.

pan·glos·sia (pan·glos′ee·uh) *n.* [Gk. *panglōssia,* garrulity, from *glōssa,* tongue]. Excessive or psychotic garrulity. See also *logorrhea.*

pan·hem·a·to·pe·nia, pan·haem·a·to·pe·nia (pan·hem″uh·to·pee′nee·uh, ·hee″muh·to·) *n.* [*pan-* + *hemato-* + *-penia*]. PANCYTOPENIA.

pan·hi·dro·sis (pan″hi·dro′sis) *n.* [*pan-* + *hidrosis*]. Generalized perspiration.

pan·hy·grous (pan·high′grus) *adj.* [Gk. *panygros,* quite damp, from *hygros,* wet, damp]. Damp as to the entire surface.

pan·hy·po·go·nad·ism (pan″high″po·go′nad·iz·um) *n.* [*pan-* + *hypogonadism*]. Underdevelopment of all parts of the genital apparatus.

pan·hy·po·pi·tu·i·ta·rism (pan″high″po·pi·tew′i·ta·riz·um) *n.* Complete absence of all pituitary secretions.

pan·hy·po·pi·tu·i·tary dwarfism (pan″high″po·pi·tew′i·terr″ee). Pituitary dwarfism with deficiencies of all pituitary hormones.

pan·hys·ter·ec·to·my (pan″his″tur·eck′tuh·mee) *n.* [*pan-* + *hysterectomy*]. Total excision of the uterus, including the cervix, body, and associated soft tissue.

pan·hys·tero·col·pec·to·my (pan″his″tur·o·kol·peck′tuh·mee) *n.* [*pan-* + *hystero-* + *colp-* + *-ectomy*]. Complete removal of the uterus and vagina.

pan·hys·tero-oo·pho·rec·to·my (pan″his″tur·o·o·off″uh·reck′tuh·mee) *n.* [*pan-* + *hystero-* + *oophor-* + *-ectomy*]. Excision of the entire uterus and one or both ovaries.

pan·hys·tero·sal·pin·gec·to·my (pan″his″tur·o·sal″pin·jeck′tuh·mee) *n.* [*pan-* + *hystero-* + *salping-* + *-ectomy*]. Excision of the entire uterus and the oviducts.

pan·hys·tero·sal·pin·go-oo·pho·rec·to·my (pan·his″tur·o·sal·ping″go·o·off″uh·reck′tuh·mee) *n.* [*pan-* + *hystero-* + *salpingo-* + *oophor-* + *-ectomy*]. Excision of the uterus, oviducts, and ovaries.

pan·ic, *n.* [Gk. *panikos,* of or caused by the god Pan]. An extreme anxiety attack which may lead to total inaction or more often to precipitate and unreasonable acts; a state of mind frequently spreading rapidly to others in the same situation.

pan·im·mu·ni·ty (pan″i·mew′ni·tee) *n.* [*pan-* + *immunity*]. General immunity to disease or infection.

pa·niv·o·rous (pa·niv′uh·rus) *adj.* [L. *panis,* bread, + *vorare,* to devour, + *-ous*]. Subsisting on bread; bread-eating.

pan·lob·u·lar (pan·lob′yoo·lur) *adj.* [*pan-* + *lobular*]. Involving all lobules; applied especially to a variety of pulmonary emphysema.

panlobular emphysema. PANACINAR EMPHYSEMA.

pan·me·tri·tis (pan″me·trye′tis) *n.* [*pan-* + *metritis*]. Widespread inflammation of the entire uterus, often accompanied by cellulitis of the broad ligaments.

pan·mne·sia (pan·nee′zhuh, ·zee·uh) *n.* [*pan-* + *-mnesia*]. A potential remembrance of all impressions.

Panmycin. A trademark for the antibiotic substance tetracycline and certain of its salts.

pan·my·e·lop·a·thy (pan″migh·e·lop′uth·ee) *n.* [*pan-* + *myelo-* + *-pathy*]. MYELOPROLIFERATIVE DISORDER.

pan·my·e·lo·phthi·sis (pan″migh″e·lo·thigh′sis, ·tee′sis) *n.* [*pan-* + *myelophthisis*]. A general wasting of the bone marrow.

pan·my·e·lo·sis (pan″migh·e·lo′sis) *n.* [*pan-* + *myel-* + *-osis*]. A myeloproliferative disorder affecting all marrow elements.

pan·my·e·lo·tox·i·co·sis (pan·migh″e·lo·tock″si·ko′sis) *n.* [*pan-* + *myelo-* + *toxicosis*]. A toxic condition in which all elements of the bone marrow are affected.

pan·my·o·si·tis (pan″migh·o·sigh′tis) *n.* [*pan-* + *myositis*]. Generalized muscular inflammation.

Pan·ner's disease [H. J. *Panner*, 20th century]. Osteochondrosis of the capitulum humeri.

pan·nic·u·li·tis (pa·nick″yoo·lye′tis) *n.* [*panniculus* + *-itis*]. Inflammation of the panniculus adiposus, especially abdominal.

pan·ni·cu·lus (pa·nick′yoo·lus) *n.*, pl. **pannicu·li** (·lye) [L., thin garment, from *pannus*, garment, piece of cloth]. A membrane or layer.

panniculus adi·po·sus (ad·i·po′sus) [NA]. The layer of subcutaneous fat.

panniculus car·no·sus (kahr·no′sus). The layer of muscles contained in the superficial fascia. It is well developed in some lower animals, but in man is represented mainly by the platysma.

pan·nus (pan′us) *n.*, pl. **pan·ni** (·nigh) [L., cloth]. 1. Vascularization and connective-tissue deposition beneath the epithelium of the cornea. 2. CHLOASMA. 3. Connective tissue overgrowing the articular surface of a diarthrodial joint.

pannus ca·ra·te·us (ka·rah′tee·us) [NL., from *carate*]. PINTA.

pannus car·no·sus (kahr·no′sus). A pannus of the cornea that has acquired a considerable thickness and opacity.

pannus cras·sus (kras′us) [L., thick]. PANNUS CARNOSUS.

pannus de·gen·e·ra·ti·vus (de·jen″e·ruh·tye′vus). Delicate fibrovascular tissue invading the cornea between the epithelium and Bowman's membrane, occurring in blind degenerated eyes following diseases such as cyclitis, glaucoma, or retinal detachment.

pannus he·pat·i·cus (he·pat′i·kus). CHLOASMA HEPATICUM.

pannus sic·cus (sick′us) [L., dry]. The end stage of trachomatous conjunctivitis or pannus, composed of poorly vascularized connective-tissue scarring.

pannus ten·u·is (ten′yoo·is). Slight pannus.

pannus tra·cho·ma·to·sus (tra·ko″muh·to′sus). Pannus occurring with trachoma.

Panolid. Trademark for ethylbenztropine, an anticholinergic compound.

pan·o·pho·bia (pan″o·fo′bee·uh) *n.* PANTOPHOBIA.

pan·oph·thal·mia (pan″off·thal′mee·uh) *n.* [*pan-* + *ophthalmia*]. PANOPHTHALMITIS.

pan·oph·thal·mi·tis (pan″off″thal·migh′tis) *n.* [*pan-* + *ophthalmitis*]. Inflammation of all the tissues of the eyeball.

panophthalmitis pu·ru·len·ta (pewr·yoo·len′tuh). A severe form of panophthalmitis with great protrusion of the eyeball and formation of pus, usually resulting in blindness.

pan·os·te·itis (pan″os·tee·eye′tis) *n.* [*pan-* + *osteitis*]. An inflammation of all parts of a bone.

pan·oti·tis (pan″o·tye′tis) *n.* [*pan-* + *otitis*]. A diffuse inflammation of all parts of the ear, usually beginning in the middle ear.

Panparnit. Trademark for caramiphen, an antispasmodic used as the hydrochloride salt for the treatment of parkinsonism.

pan·phar·ma·con (pan·fahr′muh·kon) *n.* [*pan-* + Gk. *pharmakon*, drug]. PANACEA.

pan·phle·bi·tis (pan″fle·bye′tis) *n.* [*pan-* + *phlebitis*]. 1. Inflammation of all the coats of a vein. 2. Inflammation of several veins simultaneously.

pan·pho·bia (pan·fo′bee·uh) *n.* PANTOPHOBIA.

pan·scle·ro·sis (pan″skle·ro′sis) *n.* [*pan-* + *sclerosis*]. Complete hardening of a part or tissue.

pan·si·nus·itis (pan″sigh·nuh·sigh′tis) *n.* [*pan-* + *sinusitis*]. Inflammation of all the paranasal sinuses. See also *polysinusitis.*

pan·sper·mia (pan·spur′mee·uh) *n.* [*pan-* + *sperm-* + *-ia*]. The hypothesis that life on earth originated from seeds or sperms carried from space by celestial winds.

Pan·stron·gy·lus (pan·stron′ji·lus) *n.* [*pan-* + *Strongylus*, type genus]. A genus of bugs of the family Reduviidae, the assassin or cone-nosed bugs.

Panstrongylus me·gis·tus (me·jis′tus). A species of bug that transmits *Trypanosoma cruzi* in South America.

pan·sys·tol·ic (pan·sis·tol′ick) *adj.* [*pan-* + *systolic*]. Pertaining to the entire phase of systole; HOLOSYSTOLIC.

pant-, panto- [Gk. *pas, pan, pantos*, all, whole]. See *pan-*.

pant, *v.* [OF. *pantaisier*, to be breathless, from L. *phantasia*, fantasy, nightmare]. To breathe hard or to breathe in a labored and spasmodic manner.

pan·ta·mor·phia (pan″tuh·mor′fee·uh) *n.* [*pant-* + *amorphia*]. General deformity. —**pantamor·phic** (·fick) *adj.*

pan·tan·en·ce·pha·lia (pan″tan·en″se·fay′lee·uh) *n.* [*pant-* + *anencephalia*]. Total congenital absence of the brain. —**pantanence·phal·ic** (·fal′ick) *adj.*

pan·tan·en·ceph·a·lus (pan″tan·en·sef′uh·lus) *n.* [*pant-* + *anencephalus*]. An individual showing complete absence of the brain.

pan·tan·ky·lo·bleph·a·ron (pan·tank″i·lo·blef′uh·ron) *n.* [*pant-* + *ankyloblepharon*]. Complete ANKYLOBLEPHARON.

pan·ta·pho·bia (pan″tuh·fo′bee·uh) *n.* [*pant-* + *a-* + *-phobia*]. Total absence of fear.

pan·ta·som·a·tous (pan″tuh·som′uh·tus, ·so′muh·tus) *adj.* Involving the entire body. Syn. *pantosomatous.*

pan·ta·tro·phia (pan″tuh·tro′fee·uh) *n.* PANATROPHY (2).

pan·tat·ro·phy (pan·tat′ruh·fee) *n.* [*pant-* + *atrophy*]. PANATROPHY (2).

pan·te·the·ine (pan″te·thee′een, ·in) *n.* The β-aminoethanethiol ester of pantothenic acid, occurring naturally; a growth factor for *Lactobacillus bulgaricus.*

pan·te·thine (pan′te·theen, ·thin) *n.* The disulfide of pantetheine, occurring naturally. Some lactic acid bacteria show preference for pantethine over pantothenic acid as a growth factor.

pan·the·nol (pan′the·nol) *n.* 2,4-Dihydroxy-*N*-(3-hydroxypropyl)-3,3-dimethylbutyramide, $C_9H_{19}NO_4$, the alcohol derived from pantothenic acid. In the body it is converted to pantothenic acid and is sometimes used for the vitamin activity of the latter compound. Syn. *pantothenyl alcohol.*

pan·ther·a·pist (pan·therr′uh·pist) *n.* [*pan-* + *therapist*]. A person who treats on the basis of any available remedial agent from any system of therapy.

panto- [Gk. *pas, pan, pantos*, all]. See *pan-*.

pan·to·graph (pan′to·graf) *n.* [*panto-* + *-graph*]. 1. An instrument for the mechanical copying of diagrams, maps, or other drawings upon the same scale, or upon an enlarged or a reduced scale. 2. An apparatus for graphically recording the contour of the chest. 3. An apparatus used in dental reconstructive treatment to determine the path of movement of the patient's mandibular condyles. —**pan·to·graph·ic** (pan″to·graf′ick) *adj.*

pan·to·ic acid (pan·to′ick). A pantothenic acid fragment, $HOCH_2C(CH_3)_2CHOHCOOH$, remaining after cleavage of β-alanine; it replaces pantothenic acid as a growth factor for certain organisms.

pan·to·mime (pan'tuh·mime) *n.* [L. *pantomimus,* from Gk. *pantomimos,* actor, mimic]. An expressive sequence of actions or movements unaccompanied by speech, often involving exaggerated or symbolic gestures, and usually for the purpose of conveying information or telling or enacting a story. In medicine, frequently employed as a means of communication by patients suffering from motor aphasia or otherwise incapable of communicating through speech. **pan·to·mim·ic** (pan"tuh·mim'ick) *adj.*

pantomimic spasm. FACIAL HEMISPASM.

Pantopaque. Trademark for iophendylate injection, a radiopaque diagnostic agent.

pan·to·pho·bia (pan"to·fo'bee·uh) *n.* [Gk. *pantophobos,* all-fearing, + *-ia*]. An abnormal fear of everything, including the unknown.

Pantopon. Trademark for a preparation containing all the alkaloids of opium in the form of hydrochlorides, and in the relative proportion in which they occur in the whole gum.

pan·top·to·sis (pan"top·to'sis) *n.* [*panto-* + *ptosis*]. A condition in which several viscera are prolapsed.

pan·to·scop·ic (pan"to·skop'ick) *adj.* [*panto-* + *-scope* + *-ic*]. BIFOCAL.

pan·to·som·a·tous (pan"to·som'uh·tus, ·so'muh·tus) *adj.* [*panto-* + *somat-* + *-ous*]. Involving the entire body. Syn. *pantasomatous.*

pan·to·then·ate (pan"to·thenn'ate) *n.* Any salt or ester of pantothenic acid.

pantothenate kinase. An enzyme that catalyzes the first step in the biosynthesis of coenzyme A from pantothenic acid.

pan·to·then·ic acid (pan"to·thenn'ick) [Gk. *pantothen,* from all sides, everywhere, + *-ic*]. D(+)-*N*-(α,γ-Dihydroxy-β,β-dimethylbutyryl)-β-alanine, $C_9H_{17}NO_5$, widely distributed in animal and plant tissues; a component of coenzyme A and a member of the vitamin-B complex. Essential for nutrition of some animal species, but little is known about its importance in human nutrition. Syn. *chick antidermatitis factor, filtrate factor, pantoyl-β-*alanine.

pan·to·then·yl alcohol (pan"to·thenn'il). PANTHENOL.

pan·to·yl-β-al·a·nine (pan'to·il bay'tuh al'uh·neen) *n.* PANTOTHENIC ACID.

pan·trop·ic (pan·trop'ick) *adj.* [*pan-* + *-tropic*]. POLYTROPIC; having affinity for or affecting many tissues; applied to viruses.

Pa·num's areas (pah'nōōm) [P. L. *Panum,* Danish physiologist, 1820–1885]. The areas of two retinas related physiologically by fusion in spite of different visual directions.

pa·nus (pay'nus) *n.* [L., swelling]. 1. An inflamed, nonsuppurating lymph node. 2. LYMPHOGRANULOMA VENEREUM.

panus fau·ci·um (faw'see·um). An inflamed lymph node in the throat.

panus in·gui·na·lis (ing·gwi·nay'lis). BUBO.

pan·uve·itis (pan"yoo"vee·eye'tis) *n.* [*pan-* + *uveitis*]. An inflammation affecting the entire uveal tract simultaneously.

Panwarfin. Trademark for warfarin, an anticoagulant used as the sodium derivative.

pan·zo·ot·ic (pan"zo·ot'ick) *adj.* [*pan-* + *zo-* + *-otic* (as in biotic)]. Affecting many species of animals.

pap [perhaps from L. *papa,* a word with which infants called for food]. A soft, semisolid food.

pa·pa·in (pa·pay'in) *n.* An enzyme preparation obtained from the juice of the fruit and leaves of *Carica papaya.* Popularly used as a digestant for protein foods; also employed externally for treatment of inflammatory processes. A special preparation of proteolytic enzymes from *Carica papaya* is used internally for reduction of soft tissue inflammation and edema associated with traumatic injury and localized inflammations.

Pa·pa·ni·co·laou classes (pah·pah·nee·koh·laow') [G. N. *Papanicolaou,* U.S. anatomist, 1883–1962]. A system of classifying exfoliated cells, as seen in stained smears, into six groups, as follows: Class O, inadequate for diagnosis; Class I, absence of atypical or abnormal cells (negative); Class II, cytology atypical, but no evidence of malignancy (negative); Class III, cytology suggestive of malignancy, but not conclusive (suspicious); Class IV, cytology strongly suggestive of malignancy (positive); Class V, cytology conclusive for malignancy (positive).

Papanicolaou's stains [G. N. *Papanicolaou*]. A group of stains used for the detailed study of exfoliated cells, particularly those from the vagina.

Papanicolaou's test [G. N. *Papanicolaou*]. A cytological cancer technique mainly for the female genital tract (vagina, cervix, endometrium).

Pa·pa·ver (pa·pay'vur, pa·pav'ur) *n.* [L., poppy]. A genus of herbs of the Papaveraceae; the poppy. See also *opium.*

pa·pav·er·a·mine (pa·pav'ur·uh·meen, pa·pav"ur·am'een) *n.* An alkaloid, $C_{21}H_{25}NO$, from opium.

pa·pav·er·ine (pa·pav'ur·een, ·in, pa·pay'vur·) *n.* An alkaloid, $C_{20}H_{21}NO_4$, obtained from opium, belonging to the benzyl isoquinoline group (it is not a morphine derivative). Relaxes smooth muscle; has weak analgesic activity. Generally used as the hydrochloride salt.

pa·paw (pa·paw', pah'paw) *n.* [Sp. *papayo,* papaya tree]. 1. The seed of the tree *Asimina triloba;* has been used as an emetic. 2. PAPAYA.

pa·pa·ya (pa·pah'yuh, pa·pay'uh) *n.* [Sp., papaya (fruit), from Carib]. Melon tree; papaw; *Carica papaya,* a tree of the Passifloraceae. The unripe fruit yields a milky juice containing papain.

paper chromatography. Chromatography in which paper strips or sheets are employed as the porous solid supporting medium; commonly two immiscible solvents are used, as in *partition chromatography.* Minute quantities of material may be separated by this process.

paper-disk plate. A filter-paper disk soaked with an antibiotic test solution and placed on the surface of seeded agar plates, to determine the zone of inhibition resulting from the diffusion of the antibiotic into the surrounding medium in the course of incubation.

pa·pes·cent (pa·pes'unt) *adj.* Having the consistency of pap.

Papez circuit [J. W. *Papez,* U.S. anatomist, 1883–1958]. The major connections of the limbic system, in which the fornix connects the hippocampus to the mamillary bodies, which in turn are connected to the anterior nuclei of the thalamus by the mamillothalamic tract. The anterior thalamic nuclei project to the cingulate gyri whose connections with the hippocampus complete a complex closed circuit.

papill-, papillo-. A combining form meaning *papilla, papillary.*

pa·pil·la (pa·pil'uh) *n.,* pl. & genit. sing. **papil·lae** (·ee) [L., nipple]. A small, nipplelike eminence.

papilla den·tis (den'tis) [NA]. DENTAL PAPILLA.

papilla du·o·de·ni major (dew·o·dee'nigh) [NA]. MAJOR DUODENAL PAPILLA.

papilla duodeni minor [NA]. MINOR DUODENAL PAPILLA.

papillae. Plural and genitive singular of *papilla.*

papillae co·ni·cae (kon'i·see) [NA]. CONICAL PAPILLAE.

papillae co·rii (ko'ree·eye) [NA]. Small conelike projections of the corium into the epidermis.

papillae fi·li·for·mes (figh·li·for'meez, fil·i·) [NA]. FILIFORM PAPILLAE.

papillae fo·li·a·tae (fo"lee·ay'tee) [NA]. FOLIATE PAPILLAE.

papillae fun·gi·for·mes (fun"ji·for'meez) [NA]. FUNGIFORM PAPILLAE.

papillae la·cri·ma·les (lack"ri·may'leez) [BNA]. Plural of *papilla lacrimalis.*

papillae len·ti·cu·la·res (len·tick"yoo·lair'eez) [BNA]. LENTICULAR PAPILLAE.

papillae lin·gua·les (ling·gway'leez) [NA]. LINGUAL PAPILLAE.

papillae re·na·les (re·nay'leez) [NA]. RENAL PAPILLAE.

papillae val·la·tae (va·lay'tee) [NA]. VALLATE PAPILLAE.

papilla in·ci·si·va (in·si·sigh'vuh) [NA]. INCISIVE PAPILLA.

papilla la·cri·ma·lis (lack·ri·may'lis) [NA]. LACRIMAL PAPILLA.

papilla mam·mae (mam'ee) [NA]. NIPPLE.

papilla ner·vi op·ti·ci (nur'vye op'ti·sigh) [BNA]. Discus nervi optici (= OPTIC DISK).

papilla of Morgagni [G. B. *Morgagni*]. ANAL PAPILLA.

papilla of Santorini [G. D. *Santorini*]. MINOR DUODENAL PAPILLA.

papilla of Vater [A. *Vater*]. MAJOR DUODENAL PAPILLA.

papilla pa·ro·ti·dea (pa·rot·i·dee'uh) [NA]. PAROTID PAPILLA.

papilla pi·li (pye'lye) [NA]. A small, conelike projection of the corium into the bulb of the root of a hair.

pap·il·lary (pap'i·lerr·ee) *adj.* Pertaining to, having, or resembling a papilla or papillae.

papillary adenoma. An adenoma whose parenchymal cells form papillary processes.

papillary carcinoma. A carcinoma with fingerlike outgrowths, a pattern commonly seen in transitional-cell carcinoma of the urinary tract.

papillary cystadenoma lym·pho·ma·to·sum (lim''fo·ma·to'sum). A benign tumor of salivary glands, especially the parotid gland; it is usually cystic, composed of a double layer of eosinophilic cells and has a pronounced lymphoid stroma. Syn. *Warthin's tumor.*

papillary cystadenoma of ovary. SEROUS CYSTADENOMA.

papillary dermis. The portion of the dermis between and just below the rete ridges of the epidermis, consisting of cones made up of narrow, haphazardly arranged collagen bundles; it blends indistinctly with the reticular dermis. Contr. *reticular dermis.*

papillary duct. Any one of the largest collecting tubules of the kidney, opening into the minor calyxes of the renal pelvis. Syn. *duct of Bellini.*

papillary fibroma. A superficial fibroma with papillary projections.

papillary foramens. The orifices of a papillary duct in a minor calyx of the kidney. NA *foramina papillaria renis.*

papillary hidradenoma. A benign sweat-gland tumor occurring most commonly on the labia majores and perineum of women.

papillary layer. The zone of fine-fibered connective tissue within and immediately subjacent to the papillae of the corium. NA *stratum papillare.*

papillary muscles. The muscular eminences in the ventricles of the heart from which the chordae tendineae arise. NA *musculi papillares.* See also Table of Muscles in the Appendix and Plate 5.

papillary necrosis. Renal necrosis occurring in the medulla, particularly in the papillary portion, and affecting one or more papillae in one or both kidneys. It is associated most commonly with urinary tract obstruction, acute pyelonephritis, diabetes mellitus, analgesic abuse, and sickling disorders. Syn. *necrotizing papillitis, medullary necrosis.*

papillary process. A short, rounded process extending inferiorly from the caudate lobe of the liver behind the portal fissure. In the fetus, it is large and is in contact with the pancreas. NA *processus papillaris hepatis.*

papillary serous carcinoma. SEROUS CYSTOADENOCARCINOMA.

papillary serous cyst. SEROUS CYSTADENOMA.

papillary sinusitis. Papillary hypertrophy of the mucosa of any of the paranasal sinuses.

papillary trachoma. A trachoma in which the granulations are red and papillary.

papillary tubercle. An extension of the caudate lobe of the liver into the portal fossa.

papillary varix. A benign cutaneous tumor consisting of a single dilated blood vessel; occurs after middle age. Syn. *angioma senile, Cayenne-pepper spot.*

pap·il·late (pap'i·late, pa·pil'ut) *adj.* [L. *papillatus*]. Having small papillary or nipplelike projections.

pap·il·lec·to·my (pap''i·leck'tuh·mee) *n.* [*papill-* + *-ectomy*]. Surgical removal of a papilla or papillae.

pa·pil·le·de·ma, pa·pil·loe·de·ma (pa·pil''e·dee'muh, pap''i·le·) *n.* [*papill-* + *edema*]. Edema of the optic disk.

pap·il·lif·er·ous (pap''i·lif'ur·us) *adj.* [*papill-* + *-iferous*]. Bearing or containing papillae, as a papilliferous cyst.

papilliferous carcinoma. PAPILLARY CARCINOMA.

pa·pil·li·form (pa·pil'i·form) *adj.* [*papill-* + *-iform*]. Shaped like a papilla.

pap·il·li·tis (pap''i·lye'tis) *n.* [*papill-* + *-itis*]. 1. Inflammation of a papilla. 2. OPTIC NEURITIS. 3. Inflammation of a renal papilla.

papillo-. See *papill-.*

pap·il·lo·cys·to·ma (pap''i·lo·sis·to'muh, pa·pil''o·) *n.* [*papillo-* + *cystoma*]. SEROUS CYSTADENOMA.

papilloedema. PAPILLEDEMA.

pap·il·lo·ma (pap''i·lo'ma) *n.*, pl. **papillomas, papilloma·ta** (·tuh) [*papill-* + *-oma*]. A growth pattern of epithelial tumors in which the proliferating epithelial cells grow outward from a surface, accompanied by vascularized cores of connective tissue, to form a branching structure.

papilloma cho·roi·de·um (ko·roy'dee·um). A neoplasm composed of adult epithelial cells that cover the ventricular choroid plexuses. Since the choroid plexus epithelium is related embryologically to the ependyma, the choroid plexus papillomas are usually grouped with tumors of the ependymal group.

pap·il·lo·mac·u·lar (pap''i·lo·mack'yoo·lur) *adj.* [*papillo-* + *macular*]. Pertaining to the optic disk and macula.

papillomacular bundle. The nerve fibers that pass from the macula of the retina to the outer side of the optic disk where they enter the optic nerve and project, as a distinct bundle, to the lateral geniculate body.

pap·il·lo·ma·to·sis (pap''i·lo''muh·to'sis) *n.* [*papilloma* + *-osis*]. The widespread formation of papillomas; the state of being affected with multiple papillomas.

pap·il·lom·a·tous (pap'i·lom'uh·tus) *adj.* Characterized by or pertaining to a papilloma or papillomas.

Pa·pil·lon-Le·fèvre syndrome. (pa^h·pee·yoh$^{n'}$, luh·fevr') A genodermatosis exhibiting palmar and plantar hyperkeratosis and periodontosis occurring in childhood after the eruption of primary teeth. Asymptomatic ectopic calcification of the choroid plexus and tentorium may occur also. Inherited as an autosomal recessive trait.

pap·il·lo·ret·i·ni·tis (pap'i·lo·ret''i·nigh'tis) *n.* [*papillo-* + *retinitis*]. Inflammation of the optic disk and retina.

pap·il·los·tomy (pap''i·los'tuh·mee) *n.* [(duodenal) *papilla* + *-stomy*]. Surgical section of the common sphincter of the hepaticopancreatic ampulla.

Pa·pio (pay'pee·o) *n.* A genus of the Cercopithecidae comprising the true baboons and including what, in another classification, are divided between the genera *Chaeropithecus* (typical baboons) and *Comopithecus* (hamadryas baboon).

pa·po·va·vi·rus (pa·po''vuh·vye'rus) *n.* [*pa*pilloma + *po*lyoma + *va-* (for *wart*) + *virus*]. A member of a group of ether-resistant deoxyribonucleic acid viruses, including the Shope papilloma, the human papilloma (wart), the polyoma, and the simian virus 40 (SV_{40}).

pap·pa·ta·ci fever (pah''puh·tah'chee) [It., sand fly]. PHLEBOTOMUS FEVER.

Pap·pen·hei·mer bodies [A. M. *Pappenheimer,* U.S. pathologist, b. 1877]. Iron-containing granules sometimes found in the cytoplasm of some normoblasts and erythrocytes, particularly after splenectomy.

pap·pose (pap'ose) *adj.* [*pappus* + *-ose*]. Covered with fine downy hair.

pap·pus (pap'us) *n.* [L., from Gk. *pappos*]. The fine downy hair first appearing on the cheeks and chin.

pa·pri·ka (pa·pree'kuh, pap'ri·kuh) *n.* [Hungarian]. The dried pulverized capsules of *Capsicum annuum.* Contains vitamin C. Syn. *Spanish pepper, Turkish pepper.*

Pap smear [G. N. *Pap*anicolaou]. A vaginal smear prepared for the study of exfoliated cells. See also *Papanicolaou classes.*

Pap test. PAPANICOLAOU'S TEST.

pap·u·la (pap'yoo·luh) *n.*, pl. **papu·lae** (·lee) [L., pimple]. PAPULE.

papular mucinosis. LICHEN MYXEDEMATOSUS.

papular papillomatosis. JUVENILE ACANTHOSIS.

pap·u·la·tion (pap"yoo·lay'shun) *n.* The stage, in certain eruptions, marked by papule formation.

pap·ule (pap'yool) *n.* [L. *papula,* pimple]. A solid circumscribed elevation of the skin varying from less than 0.1 cm to 1 cm in diameter. —**pap·u·lar** (·yoo·lur) *adj.*

pap·u·lif·er·ous (pap"yoo·lif'ur·us) *adj.* [*papule* + *-iferous*]. Covered with papules.

papulo-. A combining form meaning *papule, papular.*

pap·u·lo·er·y·the·ma·tous (pap"yoo·lo·err"i·theem'uh·tus) *adj.* [*papulo-* + *erythematous*]. Having a papular eruption superimposed on a generalized erythema.

pap·u·lo·ne·crot·ic (pap"yoo·lo·ne·krot'ick) *adj.* [*papulo-* + *necrotic*]. Papule formation with a tendency to central necrosis; applied especially to a variety of skin tuberculosis.

papulonecrotic tuberculid. A symmetric eruption of necrotizing papules which appear in crops and heal with scar formation; occurs mostly in children or young adults.

pap·u·lo·pus·tu·lar (pap"yoo·lo·pus'tew·lur) *adj.* [*papulo-* + *pustular*]. Characterized by both papules and pustules.

pap·u·lo·sis (pap"yoo·lo'sis) *n.* [*papul-* + *-osis*]. A condition involving multiple papules.

papulosis atro·phi·cans ma·lig·na (a·trof'i·kanz ma·lig'nuh). DEGOS' DISEASE.

pap·u·lo·squa·mous (pap"yoo·lo·skway'mus) *adj.* [*papulo-* + *squamous*]. Characterized by both papules and scales.

papulosquamous reaction. A skin reaction characterized clinically by discrete lesions, scaling, and, usually, erythema, and microscopically by acanthosis and parakeratosis; seen most commonly in psoriasis, pityriasis rosea, early syphilis, and lichen planus.

pap·u·lo·ve·sic·u·lar (pap"yoo·lo·ve·sick'yoo·lur) *adj.* [*papulo-* + *vesicular*]. Characterized by both papules and vesicles.

pap·y·ra·ce·ous (pap"i·ray'shus, ·see·us) *adj.* [L. *papyraceus,* of papyrus]. Resembling paper, as the papyraceous plate of the ethmoid bone; papery.

papyraceous fetus. FETUS PAPYRACEUS.

Pa·que·lin cautery (pa[h]k·læ[n]) [C. A. *Paquelin,* French surgeon, 1836–1905]. A cauterizing apparatus consisting of a hollow platinum body, in the shape of a knife, which is heated by forcing into it hot hydrocarbon vapor.

par-, para- [Gk. *para*]. A prefix signifying (a) *near;* (b) *beside, adjacent to;* (c) *closely resembling, almost;* (d) *beyond;* (e) *remotely* or *indirectly related to;* (f) *faulty* or *abnormal condition;* (g) *associated in an accessory capacity.*

[1]**para** (păr'uh) *n.* [from the combining form *-para*]. A woman giving birth or having given birth for the time or number of times specified by the following numeral, as: para I (for the first time = primapara), para II (for the second time = secundipara).

[2]**para,** *adj.* [from the prefix *para-*]. 1. Pertaining to the opposite positions in the benzene ring that are separated by two carbon atoms in the ring. 2. Pertaining to the state in which the atomic nuclei of a diatomic molecule spin in opposite directions.

[1]**para-.** See *par-.*

[2]**para-.** A prefix signifying (a) *the relationship of two atoms in the benzene ring that are separated by two carbon atoms in the ring,* i.e., the 1, 4-position; (b) *a benzene derivative in which two substituents have such a relationship.* Symbol, *p-.*

-para [L., from *parere,* to bring forth, bear]. A combining form designating a woman as *having given* (single or multiple) *birth for the* (specified) *time or number of times,* as: primipara (for the first time), secundipara (for the second time).

para-ami·no·ben·zo·ate (păr"uh·a·mee"no·ben'zo·ate) *n.* A salt of para-aminobenzoic acid.

para-ami·no·ben·zo·ic acid (păr"uh·a·mee"no·ben·zo'ick). Aminobenzoic acid, $NH_2C_6H_4COOH$, an off-white, crystalline powder; it has been used as an antirickettsial drug. Abbreviated, PABA. Syn. *vitamin* H', *vitamin* B_x, *vitamin V.*

para-ami·no·hip·pu·rate (păr"uh·a·mee"no·hip'yoo·rate) *n.* A salt of para-aminohippuric acid.

para-ami·no·hip·pu·ric acid (păr"uh·a·mee"no·hi·pew'rick). Aminohippuric acid or *p*-aminobenzoylaminoacetic acid, $C_9H_{10}N_2O_3$, used intravenously as the sodium salt to determine renal function. Abbreviated, PAH, PAHA.

para-aminohippuric acid test. A method for estimating renal plasma flow based on renal clearance of para-aminohippuric acid (PAH), which is normally removed from the plasma and secreted into the urine during a single circulation through the kidney. A known amount of PAH is administered, blood and urine PAH concentrations are determined, and the clearance is calculated.

para-ami·no·sa·lic·y·late (păr"uh·a·mee"no·sa·lis'i·late) *n.* A salt of para-aminosalicylic acid.

para-ami·no·sal·i·cyl·ic acid (păr"uh·a·mee"no·sal"i·sil'ick). 4-Aminosalicylic acid or 4-amino-2-hydroxybenzoic acid, $NH_2C_6H_3OHCOOH$, a tuberculostatic drug. Abbreviated, PAS, PASA.

para-am·y·loid (păr"uh·am'i·loid) *n.* [*para-* + *amyloid*]. An atypical amyloid.

para-am·y·loi·do·sis (păr"uh·am"i·loy·do'sis) *n.* A type of amyloidosis which has some, but not all, of the characteristics of classic amyloidosis. Syn. *atypical amyloidosis.*

para-an·al·ge·sia (păr"uh·an"al·jee'zee·uh) *n.* [*para-* + *analgesia*]. Analgesia of the lower extremities.

para-an·es·the·sia, para-an·aes·the·sia (păr"uh·an"es·theezh'uh, ·theez'ee·uh) *n.* [*para-* + *anesthesia*]. Anesthesia of the lower extremities.

para·aor·tic (păr"uh·ay·or'tick) *adj.* [*para-* + *aortic*]. Adjacent to the aorta.

paraaortic bodies. Small masses of chromaffin tissue scattered along the abdominal aorta; they are macroscopic in size in the fetus and in infancy, but are microscopic in later life. NA *corpora paraaortica.*

para-ap·pen·di·ci·tis (păr"uh·a·pen"di·sigh'tis) *n.* [*para-* + *appendicitis*]. Inflammation of the connective tissue adjacent to that part of the appendix not covered with peritoneum.

para·ba·sal body (păr"uh·bay'sul) [*para-* + *basal*]. In hemoflagellates, the structure, closely associated with the blepharoplast, that serves as the neuromotor apparatus for the flagellum. Syn. *kinetoplast.*

par·ab·du·cent nucleus (păr"ab·dew'sunt) [*para-* + *abducent*]. A group of cells in the reticular formation, near the motor cells of the abducent nucleus, which send fibers to the oculomotor nucleus by way of the medial longitudinal fasciculus.

para·bi·gem·i·nal (păr"uh·bye·jem'i·nul) *adj.* [*para-* + *bigeminal*]. Situated medial and ventral to the superior and inferior colliculi.

parabigeminal nucleus or **body.** A group of cells, ventrolateral to the inferior colliculus and lateral to the lateral lemniscus, which apparently send fibers to the lateral nuclei of the pons.

para·bi·o·sis (păr"uh·bye·o'sis) *n.*, pl. **parabio·ses** (·seez) [*para-* + *-biosis*]. The experimental fusing together of two individuals or embryos so that the effects of one partner upon the other may be studied. —**parabi·ot·ic** (·ot'ick) *adj.*

para·blep·sia (păr"uh·blep'see·uh) *n.* [*parablepsis* + *-ia*]. False or perverted vision.

para·blep·sis (păr"uh·blep'sis) *n.* [Gk., from *parablepein,* to see wrong, from *blepein,* to see]. PARABLEPSIA.

pa·rab·o·loid dark-field condenser (pa·rab'uh·loid). A lens of paraboloid shape, the vertex end being ground back so that its focus can be brought into coincidence with the specimen on the slide. A central stop is provided to block the central rays. It is used chiefly for medium-power work.

para·bu·lia (păr"uh·bew'lee·uh) *n.* [*para-* + Gk. *boulē*, will, + *-ia*]. Abnormality of volitional action; particularly the sudden and seemingly inexplicable substitution of one action or its motive by another, as seen in schizophrenia.

par·ac·an·tho·ma (pa·rack"an·tho'muh, păr"uh·kan·) *n.* [*par-* + *acanthoma*]. A tumor whose parenchyma consists of cells resembling those of the prickle-cell layer of the skin.

par·ac·an·tho·sis (pa·rack"an·tho'sis, păr"uh·kan·) *n.* [*par-* + *acanthosis*]. A process characterized by some disorder of the prickle-cell layer of the epidermis.

para·ca·ri·nal (păr"uh·ka·rye'nul) *adj.* [*para-* + *carina* + *-al*]. Beside a carina, especially the urethral carina.

para·ca·sein (păr"uh·kay'see·in) *n.* A modified form of casein, produced by the action of rennin on milk.

para·ce·cal (păr"uh·see'kul) *adj.* [*para-* + *cecal*]. Adjacent to the cecum.

paracecal fossa. An infrequent peritoneal pouch behind and to one side of the cecum.

paracele. Paracoele (= LATERAL VENTRICLE).

Par·a·cel·sian (păr"uh·sel'see·un, ·shun) *adj.* Pertaining to or originated by Paracelsus (P. A. T. B. von Hohenheim), Swiss alchemist and physician, 1493–1541.

Paracelsian method. The use of chemical agents alone in treating disease.

para·cen·te·sis (păr"uh·sen·tee'sis) *n.*, pl. **paracente·ses** (·seez) [Gk. *parakentēsis*, from *kentein*, to prick, sting]. Puncture; especially the puncture or tapping of a fluid-filled space by means of a hollow needle or trochar, to draw off the contained fluid.

paracentesis ocu·li (ock'yoo·lye). OPHTHALMOCENTESIS.

paracentesis of the bladder. The puncture of the urinary bladder with a vesical trocar for the relief of obstruction or to provide constant drainage.

paracentesis of the chest. The insertion of a needle or trocar into the pleural cavity for the relief of pleural effusion.

paracentesis of the tympanum. MYRINGOTOMY.

para·cen·tral (păr"uh·sen'trul) *adj.* [*para-* + *central*]. Situated near the center.

paracentral lobule. The quadrilateral convolution on the medial surface of the cerebral hemisphere, surrounding the upper end of the central sulcus. NA *lobulus paracentralis.*

paracentral nucleus of the thalamus. One of the intralaminar nuclei of the thalamus, ventrolateral to the dorsomedial nucleus.

paracentral sulcus. A branch of the cingulate sulcus, sometimes reaching the dorsal margin of the cerebral hemisphere.

para·cen·tric inversion (păr"uh·sen'trick). An end-to-end inversion of a chromosome segment that does not involve the centromere.

para·ceph·a·lus (păr"uh·sef'uh·lus) *n.*, pl. **paracepha·li** (·lye) [*para-* + *-cephalus*]. A placental parasitic twin (omphalosite) characterized by a rudimentary, misshapen head and defective trunk and limbs.

para·cer·a·to·sis (păr"uh·serr"uh·to'sis) *n.* PARAKERATOSIS.

para·chlo·ro·phe·nol (păr"uh·klor·o·fee'nol) *n.* 4-Chlorophenol, ClC_6H_4OH, an antibacterial used locally for various purposes.

para·chol·era (păr"uh·kol'ur·uh) *n.* [*para-* + *cholera*]. A disease resembling Asiatic cholera but caused by a different organism from the cholera vibrio.

para·cho·lia (păr"uh·ko'lee·uh) *n.* [*para-* + *chol-* + *-ia*]. 1. Any abnormality in the secretion of bile. 2. The prodrome of disturbed liver-cell activity, in consequence of which bile is present in the blood and lymph.

para·chor·dal (păr"uh·kor'dul) *adj.* & *n.* [*para-* + *chordal*]. 1. Adjoining the cephalochord; situated at the side of the cranial part of the notochord of the embryo. 2. Pertaining to the cartilaginous basis of the cranium in the embryo. 3. One of two bars of cartilage extending alongside the cephalic notochord in the human fetus.

parachordal cartilage. PARACHORDAL (3).

para·chor·da·lia (păr"uh·kor·day'lee·uh) *n.* PARACHORDAL (3).

parachordal plate. PARACHORDAL (3).

para·chro·ma (păr"uh·kro'muh) *n.* [*para-* + Gk. *chrōma*, color]. Change in color, as of the skin.

para·chro·ma·tism (păr"uh·kro'muh·tiz·um) *n.* [*para-* + *chromat-* + *-ism*]. False, or incorrect, perception of color, not true color blindness, which it may approach more or less completely.

para·chro·ma·to·blep·sia (păr"uh·kro"muh·to·blep'see·uh) *n.* [*para-* + *chromato-* + *-blepsia*]. PARACHROMATISM.

para·chro·ma·top·sia (păr"uh·kro"muh·top'see·uh) *n.* [*para-* + *chromat-* + *-opsia*]. COLOR BLINDNESS.

para·chro·ma·to·sis (păr"uh·kro"muh·to'sis) *n.* [*para-* + *chromat-* + *-osis*]. PARACHROMA.

para·chro·mo·phore (păr"uh·kro'mo·fore) *n.* [*para-* + *chromo-* + *-phore*]. Pigment excreted or retained either within cells or in the capsule surrounding the cell. It is not an integral part of the cytoplasm of the cell. The term is applied to bacteria and fungi. —**para·chro·moph·o·rous** (·kro·mof'uh·rus) *adj.*

parachute deformity. A congenital deformity of the mitral valve in which the valve resembles a parachute.

par·ac·mas·tic (par·ack·mas'tick) *adj.* [*par-* + *acmastic*]. PARACMIC.

par·ac·me (păr·ack'mee) *n.* [Gk. *parakmē*, decay, abatement, from *akmē*, culmination]. 1. The degeneration or decadence of a group of organisms after they have reached their acme of development. 2. The period of decline or remission of a disease.

par·ac·mic (păr·ack'mick) *adj.* [*par-* + *acmic*]. Pertaining to the period of abatement of a disease. Contr. *acmic, epacmic.*

paracoccidioidal granuloma. SOUTH AMERICAN BLASTOMYCOSIS.

Para·coc·cid·i·oi·des (păr"uh·kock·sid"ee·oy'deez) *n.* [*para-* + *Coccidioides*]. *BLASTOMYCES.* —**paracoccidioi·dal** (·dul) *adj.*

Paracoccidioides brasiliensis. *BLASTOMYCES BRASILIENSIS.*

para·coc·cid·i·oi·do·my·co·sis (păr"uh·kock·sid"ee·oy"do·migh·ko'sis) *n.* [*Paracoccidioides* + *mycosis*]. SOUTH AMERICAN BLASTOMYCOSIS.

para·coele. (păr'uh·seel) *n.* [*para-* + *-coele*]. *Obsol.* LATERAL VENTRICLE.

para·co·li·tis (păr"uh·ko·lye'tis) *n.* [*para-* + *colitis*]. Inflammation of the tissue adjacent to the colon.

para·co·lon (păr"uh·ko'lun) *n.* [*para-* + *colon*]. A group of bacteria intermediate between the *Escherichia-Aerobacter* genera and the *Salmonella-Shigella* group. Culturally, these organisms may be confused with the non-lactose-fermenting pathogenic bacteria found in the intestinal tract. Some of the paracolon bacilli probably produce disease.

para·col·pi·tis (păr"uh·kol·pye'tis) *n.* [*paracolpium* + *-itis*]. Inflammation of the connective tissue about the vagina.

para·col·pi·um (păr"uh·kol'pee·um) *n.* [NL., from *para-* + Gk. *kolpos*, vagina]. The connective tissue about the vagina.

para·con·dy·lar (păr"uh·kon'di·lur) *adj.* [*para-* + *condylar*]. Situated alongside a condyle or a condylar region.

para·cone (păr'uh·kone) *n.* [*para-* + *cone*]. The mesiobuccal cusp of an upper molar tooth.

para·co·nid (păr"uh·ko'nid) *n.* [*paracone* + *-id*]. The mesiolingual cusp of a lower molar tooth.

Paracort. A trademark for prednisone, an anti-inflammatory adrenocortical steroid.

par·a·cu·sia (păr″uh·kew′zhuh, ·zee·uh) *n.* [*par-* + *-acusia*]. Any perversion of the sense of hearing.

paracusia acris (ay′kris, ack′ris). Excessively acute hearing, rendering the person intolerant of sounds.

paracusia du·pli·ca·ta (dew·pli·kay′tuh). A condition in which all or only certain sounds are heard double.

paracusia lo·ca·lis (lo·kay′lis). Difficulty in estimating the direction of sounds, met with in unilateral deafness, or when the two ears hear unequally.

paracusia ob·tu·sa (ob·tew′suh). Difficulty in hearing.

paracusia Wil·li·sii (wi·lis′ee·eye). A condition of deafness in which the hearing is better in a noisy place, as in a train or factory.

par·a·cu·sis (păr″a·kew′sis) *n.* PARACUSIA.

para·cy·e·sis (păr″uh·sigh·ee′sis) *n.* [*para-* + *cyesis*]. EXTRAUTERINE PREGNANCY.

para·cys·tic (păr″uh·sis′tick) *adj.* [*para-* + *cystic*]. Situated near, or alongside, the urinary bladder.

para·cys·ti·tis (păr″uh·sis·tye′tis) *n.* [*para-* + *cyst-* + *-itis*]. Inflammation of the connective tissue surrounding the urinary bladder.

para·cyt·ic (păr″uh·sit′ick) *adj.* [*para-* + *cyt-* + *-ic*]. Lying among cells.

par·ad·e·ni·tis (păr″ad·e·nigh′tis) *n.* [*par-* + *aden-* + *-itis*]. Inflammation of the tissues about a gland.

para·den·tal (păr″uh·den′tul) *adj.* [*para-* + *dental*]. 1. Near, or beside, a tooth. 2. Associated with dental practice.

para·den·to·sis (păr″uh·den·to′sis) *n.* [*para-* + *dent-* + *-osis*]. PERIODONTOSIS.

para·di·chlo·ro·ben·zene (păr″uh·dye·klo″ro·ben′zeen) *n.* *p*-Dichlorobenzene, $C_6H_4Cl_2$, a crystalline compound used mainly to kill moths and their larvae as well as certain other insects.

para·did·y·mis (păr″uh·did′i·mis) *n.*, pl. **para·di·dy·mi·des** (·di·dim′i·deez) [NL., from *para-* + Gk. *didymos*, testicle] [NA]. The atrophic remains of the paragenital tubules of the mesonephros, which separate from the mesonephric duct and lie near the convolutions of the epididymal duct. Syn. *organ of Giraldes.*

Paradione. Trademark for paramethadione, an anticonvulsant drug.

para·diph·the·ri·al (păr″uh·dif·theer′ee·ul) *adj.* [*para-* + *diphtherial*]. Remotely or indirectly resembling diphtheria, as the membrane covering the pharynx in infectious mononucleosis.

para·diph·the·rit·ic (păr″uh·dif″thi·rit′ick) *adj.* PARADIPHTHERIAL.

para·dis·tem·per (păr″uh·dis·tem′pur) *n.* [*para-* + *distemper*]. HARD PAD.

para·dox·ia sex·u·a·lis (păr″uh·dock′see·uh secks″yoo·ay′lis). Sexual activity occurring outside what is usually regarded as the reproductive period, that is, before puberty or in the senile years.

par·a·dox·ic (păr″uh·dock′sick) *adj.* PARADOXICAL.

par·a·dox·i·cal (păr″uh·dock′si·kul) *adj.* [Gk. *paradoxos*, contrary to expectation, from *para-* + *doxa*, expectation, supposition]. Contrary to the usual or normal kind.

paradoxical embolus. An embolus, usually a venous thrombus, which is transported to the peripheral arterial circulation through a cardiac septal defect or patent ductus arteriosus with a right-to-left shunt, usually a patent foramen ovale. Syn. *crossed embolus.*

paradoxical pulse. PULSUS PARADOXUS.

paradoxical pupillary reaction or **reflex.** Any response of the pupil to a stimulus contrary to the expected one; such responses include dilation of the pupil on exposure to light or constriction when light is withdrawn (as may occur in certain pathologic states or suggest functional exhaustion), convergence and associated dilation of the pupil with near vision or constriction with distant vision, dilation of the pupil by epinephrine following destruction of the superior cervical ganglion, and dilation of the pupil in response to pain in the lower part of the body.

paradoxical respiration. 1. A condition in which the lung fills on expiration and empties on inspiration, seen with open pneumothorax. Syn. *pendelluft respiration.* 2. Elevation of the diaphragm with inspiration and lowering with expiration, seen with diaphragmatic paralysis.

paradoxic flexor reflex. GORDON'S REFLEX (1).

paradoxic patellar reflex. Contraction of the hamstring muscles in response to tapping of the patellar tendon; sometimes observed in tabes dorsalis, poliomyelitis, lesions of the femoral nerve, and other lesions affecting the arc of the patellar reflex.

paradoxic pulse. PULSUS PARADOXUS.

paradoxic triceps reflex. Flexion of the forearm following tapping of the triceps tendon; encountered in lesions involving the arc of the triceps reflex, as may occur with injury to the sixth, seventh, and eighth cervical segments.

para·du·o·de·nal (păr″uh·dew″o·dee′nul, ·dew·od′e·nul) *adj.* [*para-* + *duodenal*]. On either side of the duodenum.

paraduodenal recess or **fossa.** An occasional small pouch of peritoneum situated to the left of the last part of the duodenum. NA *plica paraduodenalis, recessus paraduodenalis.*

para·dys·en·tery (păr″uh·dis′un·terr·ee) *n.* [*para-* + *dysentery*]. 1. A mild form of dysentery. 2. Dysentery due to *Shigella flexneri.*

para·ep·i·lep·sy (păr″uh·ep′i·lep″see) *n.* [*para-* + *epilepsy*]. *Obsol.* An abortive epileptic attack, consisting only of the aura. Consciousness is not lost. Compare *psycholepsy.*

para·eryth·ro·blast (păr″uh·e·rith′ro·blast) *n.* [*para-* + *erythroblast*]. An erythroblast with an indented rather than a spheroid nucleus.

para·esoph·a·ge·al, para-oe·soph·a·ge·al (păr″uh·e·sof″uh·jee′ul) *adj.* [*para-* + *esophageal*]. Situated alongside the esophagus.

paraesophageal cyst. A bronchogenic cyst intimately connected with the esophageal wall, containing cartilage, and usually filled with a mucoid material and desquamated epithelial cells.

paraesthesia. PARESTHESIA.

para·fas·cic·u·lar (păr″uh·fa·sick′yoo·lur) *adj.* In the vicinity of a fasciculus.

parafascicular nucleus of the thalamus. One of the intralaminar nuclei of the thalamus which lies medial to the centromedian nucleus ventral to the caudal portion of the dorsomedial nucleus.

par·af·fin (păr′uh·fin) *n.* [Ger., from L. *parum*, little, insufficient, + *affinis*, having affinity]. 1. Any saturated hydrocarbon having the formula C_nH_{2n+2}. These compounds constitute the paraffin series. Syn. *alkane.* 2. A purified mixture of solid hydrocarbons obtained from petroleum; variously used to impart hardness or stiffness to protective agents, such as ointment bases, suppositories, or bandages.

paraffin bath. 1. An apparatus for the infiltration of pieces of tissues or organs with molten paraffin before embedding them for cutting sections. 2. A container of molten paraffin used for physical therapy.

par·af·fin·oma (păr″uh·fi·no′muh) *n.* [*paraffin* + *-oma*]. A nodular mass of inflammatory, granulation, or scar tissue, due to injection of paraffin into the tissues.

paraffin series. The series of saturated hydrocarbons which have the formula C_nH_{2n+2}.

Paraflex. Trademark for chlorzoxazone, a skeletal muscle relaxant.

para·floc·cu·lus (păr″uh·flock′yoo·lus) *n.* [*para-* + *flocculus*]. A small lobule of the cerebellum, rudimentary in man. It is a subdivision of the paraflocculus ventralis (the tonsilla), and consists of a small group of folia lying adjacent to the posterior surface of the flocculus.

para·fol·lic·u·lar (păr″uh·fol·ick′yoo·lur) *adj.* [*para-* + *follicular*]. In the vicinity of a follicular structure.

parafollicular cells. Argyrophil cells in the thyroid epithelium.

para·form (păr′uh·form) *n.* PARAFORMALDEHYDE.

para·form·al·de·hyde (păr″uh·for·mal′de·hide) *n.* A solid polymer, $(CH_2O)_n$, of formaldehyde, or, more properly, a mixture of polyoxymethylenes, formed when solutions of formaldehyde are allowed to evaporate; has been used as a convenient form for generating small quantities of formaldehyde gas for disinfecting purposes. Syn. *paraform, trioxymethylene.*

Para·fos·sar·u·lus (păr″uh·fos·ăr′yoo·lus) *n.* A genus of snails, species of which are known to transmit the trematode parasite *Clonorchis sinensis.*

para·fuch·sin (păr″uh·fo͝ok′sin, ·fyook′sin) *n.* [*para-* + *fuchsin*]. PARAROSANILINE.

para·func·tion (păr′uh·funk″shun) *n.* [*para-* + *function*]. Abnormal function or use; especially, of the teeth: BRUXISM.

para·gam·ma·cism (păr″uh·gam′uh·siz·um) *n.* [*para-* + *gammacism*]. Inability to pronounce the hard *g* and *k*, other consonants being substituted.

para·gam·ma·cis·mus (păr″uh·gam″uh·siz′mus) *n.* PARAGAMMACISM.

para·gan·glia (păr″uh·gang′glee·uh) *n.*, sing. **paragangli·on** (·on) [*para-* + *ganglion*]. Groups of chromaffin cells scattered along the ventral surface of the aorta, especially in the fetus.

para·gan·gli·o·ma (păr″uh·gang″glee·o′muh) *n.* [*paraganglion* + *-oma*]. A tumor derived from elements that form part of the chemoreceptor system. It originates in the middle ear from the glomus jugulare and consists of a group of cells situated in the adventitia of the jugular bulb or along the ramus tympanicus of the glossopharyngeal nerve.

paraganglion ca·rot·i·cum (ka·rot′i·kum). CAROTID-BODY TUMOR.

paraganglion caroticum sarcoma. CAROTID-BODY TUMOR.

paraganglion ca·rot·i·cus tumor (ka·rot′i·kus). CAROTID-BODY TUMOR.

para·gan·glio·neu·ro·ma (păr″uh·gang″glee·o·new·ro′muh) *n.* [*paraganglion* + *neuroma*]. PARAGANGLIOMA.

para·gan·gli·on·ic (păr″uh·gang″glee·on′ick) *adj.* Pertaining to the paraganglia and their secretions.

para·gan·gli·ons (păr″uh·gang′glee·unz) *n.pl.* PARAGANGLIA.

para·gen·i·tal (păr″uh·jen′i·tul) *adj.* In the vicinity of a genital organ.

para·gen·i·ta·lis (păr″uh·jen″i·tay′lis, ·tal′is) *n.* [*para-* + L. *genitalis*, genital]. 1. The functional part of the mesonephros caudal to the genital part in lower vertebrates. 2. In higher forms, the vestigial paradidymis or paroophoron. See also *caudal mesonephros.*

paragenital mesonephric tubules. Mesonephric tubules that become the efferent ductules of the testis, the appendix of the epididymis, and the paradidymis.

para·geu·sia (păr″uh·gew′see·uh, ·joo′see·uh) *n.* [*para-* + *-geusia*]. Perversion or impairment of the sense of taste. —**parageu·sic** (·sick) *adj.*

para·geu·sis (păr″uh·gew′sis, ·joo′sis) *n.* PARAGEUSIA.

par·ag·glu·ti·na·tion (păr″uh·gloo·ti·nay′shun) *n.* [*par-* + *agglutination*]. Agglutination of colon bacilli and cocci with the serum of patients infected with or recovering from infection with dysentery bacilli. The property of paragglutination disappears when the bacteria are subcultured.

para·gle·noid·al (păr″uh·glee·noy′dul, ·glen·oy′dul) *adj.* In the vicinity of a glenoid cavity.

paraglenoidal sulcus. One of many slight grooves inferior to and in front of the auricular surface of the iliac bone for the attachment of the sacroiliac and interosseous ligaments.

para·glos·sa (păr″uh·glos′uh) *n.* [*para-* + *-glossa*]. Swelling of the tongue; a hypertrophy of the tongue, usually congenital.

para·glos·sia (păr″uh·glos′ee·uh) *n.* [*para-* + *-glossia*]. Inflammation of the muscles and connective tissues under the tongue.

pa·rag·na·thous (pa·rag′nuth·us, păr″ug·nath′us) *adj.* [*para-* + *-gnathous*]. 1. Having upper and lower jaws of equal length, their tips falling together, as in certain birds. 2. Pertaining to or characteristic of a paragnathus.

pa·rag·na·thus (pa·rag′nuth·us, păr″ug·nath′us) *n.* [*para-* + *-gnathus*]. 1. An individual having a supernumerary jaw. 2. A parasitic fetus or part attached to the jaw laterally. See also *epignathus.*

para·gom·pho·sis (par″uh·gom·fo′sis) *n.* [*para-* + *gomphosis*]. Impaction of the fetal head in the pelvic canal.

par·a·gon·i·mi·a·sis (păr″uh·gon″i·migh′uh·sis) *n.*, pl. **paragonimia·ses** (·seez) [*Paragonimus* + *-iasis*]. Infection by species of the genus *Paragonimus*, especially *P. westermani.*

Par·a·gon·i·mus (păr″uh·gon′i·mus) *n.* [NL., from *para-* + Gk. *gonimos*, productive]. A genus of trematode worms.

Paragonimus wes·ter·mani (wes·tur·man′eye). Species of lung flukes which in the adult stage cause tissue destruction, inflammation, and hemorrhage.

para·gram·ma·tism (păr″uh·gram′uh·tiz·um) *n.* AGRAMMATISM.

para·gran·u·lo·ma (păr″uh·gran″yoo·lo′muh) *n.* [*para-* + *granuloma*]. In the Jackson-Parker classification, variety of Hodgkin's disease said to be its least aggressive form.

para·graph·ia (păr″uh·graf′ee·uh) *n.* [*para-* + *graph-* + *-ia*]. 1. Perverted writing; a form of aphasia in which letters or words are misplaced or improperly used. 2. A loss of ability to express ideas in writing or to write from dictation, as the result of a brain lesion. —**paragraph·ic** (·ick) *adj.*

para·he·mo·phil·ia, para·hae·mo·phil·ia (păr″uh·hee″mo·fil′ee·uh, ·hem″o·) *n.* [*para-* + *hemophilia*]. A hemorrhagic disorder characterized by a deficiency of Factor V. Syn. *Owren's disease.*

para·he·pat·ic (păr″uh·he·pat′ick) *adj.* [*para-* + *hepatic*]. About or near the liver.

para·hep·a·ti·tis (păr″uh·hep″uh·tye′tis) *n.* [*para-* + *hepat-* + *-itis*]. Inflammation of structures about or near the liver.

para·hex·yl (păr″uh·heck′sil) *n.* SYNHEXYL.

para·hi·a·tal diaphragmatic hernia (păr″uh·high·ay′tul). A hernia through an opening or defect in the diaphragm other than the esophageal hiatus.

para·hip·po·cam·pal gyrus (păr″uh·hip″o·kam′pul). A gyrus of the medial portion of the temporal lobe, continuous caudally with the cingulate gyrus above the lingual gyrus below and lying between the hippocampal sulcus and the anterior part of the collateral sulcus. NA *gyrus parahippocampalis.*

para·hor·mone (par″uh·hor′mone) *n.* [*para-* + *hormone*]. Any substance which, like carbon dioxide in its effect on the respiratory center, exerts a hormonelike regulatory influence on some organ but which is not synthesized by a specific organ adapted to that purpose, as hormones are.

para·hy·droxy·ben·zo·ic acid (păr″uh·high·drock″see·ben·zo′ick). An isomer, HOC_6H_4COOH, of salicylic acid; its esters are powerful antiseptics used to preserve various medicinal products.

para·hyp·no·sis (păr″uh·hip·no′sis) *n.* [*para-* + *hypnosis*]. Disturbances of sleep, such as somnambulism or night terrors.

para·in·flu·en·za (păr″uh·in″floo·en′zuh) *n.* [*para-* + *influenza*]. A condition similar to or due to influenza.

parainfluenza virus. An RNA virus of the paramyxovirus group; a common cause of respiratory infection, particularly croup.

para·ker·a·to·sis (păr″uh·kerr″uh·to′sis) *n.* [*para-* + *keratosis*]. Incomplete keratinization of epidermal cells characterized by retention of nuclei of cells attaining the level of the stratum corneum; the normal condition of the topmost epithelial cells of mucous membranes. —**parakera·tot·ic** (·tot′ick) *adj.*

parakeratosis gon·or·rhe·i·ca (gon″uh·ree′i·kuh). KERATOSIS BLENNORRHAGICA.

parakeratosis scu·tu·la·ris (skew′tuh·lair′is). Crust formation around scalp hairs which may be a variety of psoriasis.

parakeratosis var·ie·ga·ta (văr″ee·e·gay′tuh). A retiform type of parapsoriasis that is an intermediate between lichen planus and psoriasis; a chronic disease with hyperemia in a patchy network.

para·ki·ne·sia (păr″uh·ki·nee′zhuh, ·zee·uh, ·kigh·nee′) *n.* [*para-* + *-kinesia*]. DYSKINESIA.

para·ki·ne·sis (păr″uh·ki·nee′sis, ·kigh·) *n.* [*para-* + *kinesis*]. DYSKINESIA.

para·lac·tic acid (păr″uh·lack′tick). SARCOLACTIC ACID.

para·la·lia (păr″uh·lay′lee·uh, ·lal′ee·uh) *n.* [*para-* + *-lalia*]. Disturbance of the faculty of speech, characterized by distortion of sounds, or the habitual substitution of one sound for another.

par·al·bu·min (păr″al·bew′min) *n.* [*par-* + *albumin*]. A protein substance found in ovarian cysts.

par·al·de·hyde (păr·al′de·hide) *n.* [*par-* + *aldehyde*]. Paracetaldehyde, $(CH_3CHO)_3$, a colorless liquid with an unpleasant taste. Used as a rapidly acting hypnotic and anticonvulsant but is potentially hazardous as it may be completely oxidized to acetic acid.

para·lep·ro·sis (păr″uh·lep·ro′sis) *n.* [*para-* + Gk. *leprōsis*, leprosy]. An attenuated or modified form of leprosy.

para·lep·ro·sy (păr″uh·lep′ruh·see) *n.* PARALEPROSIS.

para·lep·sy (păr′uh·lep″see) *n.* [*para-* + *-lepsy*]. PSYCHOLEPSY.

para·lex·ia (păr″uh·leck′see·uh) *n.* [*para-* + *-lexia*]. DYSLEXIA. —**paralex·ic** (·sick) *adj.*

par·al·ge·sia (păr″al·jee′zee·uh) *n.* [*par-* + *algesia*]. Painful paresthesia. —**paralge·sic** (·zick) *adj.*

par·al·gia (păr·al′jee·uh) *n.* [*par-* + *-algia*]. PARALGESIA.

para·lipo·pho·bia (păr″uh·lye″po·fo′bee·uh, ·lip″o·) *n.* [Gk. *paralipein*, to neglect (from *lipein*, to leave), + *-phobia*]. Pathologic anxiety or fear of neglecting one's duty or even some trival obligation or matter; seen commonly in obsessive-compulsive neurosis.

par·al·lax (păr′uh·lacks) *n.* [Gk. *parallaxis*, alternation, change of position, from *allassein*, to change, alter]. The apparent displacement of an object, caused by a change in the position of the observer, or by looking at the object alternately first with one eye and then with the other. —**par·al·lac·tic** (păr″uh·lack′tick) *adj.*

parallax test. A test used to locate opacities in the cornea, lens, and vitreous. It is used with the plane mirror at 10 to 12 inches. A body situated anterior to the plane of the nodal point of the eye will move in the direction taken by the eye, while one posterior to the plane of the lens will move against the direction taken by the eye. Bodies lying about the same plane as the nodal point will show little if any movement.

par·al·lel·ism (păr′uh·lel·iz·um) *n.* The state or condition of being parallel; the quality of being similar or of corresponding. See also *isopathy.*

par·al·lel·om·e·ter (păr″uh·lel·om′e·tur) *n.* [*parallel* + *-meter*]. An instrument used for paralleling attachments and abutments for dental prostheses.

parallel technique. In intraoral radiography, the film is placed parallel to the long axes of the teeth and the central rays are directed perpendicularly to it. Syn. *right-angle technique, long-cone technique.*

para·lo·gia (păr″uh·lo′jee·uh) *n.* [Gk., from *para-* + *logos*, reason, reckoning, + *-ia*]. Difficulty in thinking logically; false reasoning.

para·log·i·cal (păr″uh·loj′i·kul) *adj.* [Gk. *paralogos*, beyond reason, incalculable, from *logos*, reason, reckoning]. Illogical.

pa·ral·o·gism (puh·ral′o·jiz·um) *n.* [Gk. *paralogismos*]. *In logic,* the error of considering effects or unrelated phenomena as the cause of a condition. —**pa·ral·o·gis·tic** (puh·ral″o·jis′tick) *adj.*

para·lu·te·in cells (păr″uh·lew′tee·in). The epithelioid cells of the corpus luteum, derived from the theca interna of the ovarian follicle. Syn. *theca lutein cells.* See also *follicular lutein cells.*

paralysant. PARALYZANT.

pa·ral·y·sis (puh·ral′i·sis) *n.*, pl. **paraly·ses** (·seez) [Gk., from *para-*, beside, off, amiss, + *lysis*, loosening, dissolution]. Loss of muscle function or of sensation. Paralyses may be classified according to etiology, as alcoholic or lead; according to part involved, as facial or palatal; according to muscle tone, as flaccid or spastic; according to distribution, as monoplegic or hemiplegic, or according to some other characteristic, as ascending or crossed. Certain types of paralysis are often called palsies; partial paralysis is called paresis.

paralysis ag·i·tans (aj′i·tanz). PARKINSON'S DISEASE.

para·lys·sa (păr″uh·lis′uh) *n.* [*para-* + *lyssa*]. A South American form of rabies, caused by the bite of a rabid vampire bat.

par·a·lyt·ic (păr″uh·lit′ick) *adj. & n.* [Gk. *paralytikos*]. 1. Pertaining to, or affected with, paralysis. 2. A person affected with paralysis.

paralytic abasia. Inability to walk or stand because of organic paralysis of the legs.

paralytic aphonia. Inability to produce sounds because of paralysis of vocal folds.

paralytic bladder. ATONIC BLADDER.

paralytic brachial neuritis. Brachial neuritis with paralysis in the arm and shoulder.

paralytic bulbar poliomyelitis. Poliomyelitis affecting chiefly the medulla oblongata and pons, involving motor cranial nuclei and frequently affecting respiratory and circulatory centers. Contr. *nonparalytic poliomyelitis.*

paralytic bulbospinal poliomyelitis. Both paralytic bulbar and paralytic spinal poliomyelitis.

paralytic dislocation. Dislocation of a joint, most commonly the hip, from paralysis of one group of muscles, usually with overpull by the opposing group.

paralytic ectropion. Ectropion due to paralysis of the facial nerve.

paralytic ileus. ADYNAMIC ILEUS.

paralytic mydriasis. Pupillary dilatation due to paralysis of the oculomotor nerve.

paralytic poliomyelitis. A form of poliomyelitis characterized by muscle weakness or paralysis. Conventionally subdivided, on the basis of the anatomic structures predominantly involved, into spinal, bulbospinal, bulbar, and encephalitic types.

paralytic rabies. A form of rabies confined largely to the spinal cord, or, in dogs, to the spinal cord and brainstem. The chief manifestation in humans is ascending paralysis, with little or no excitation and other signs of brain involvement. In dogs there is also no excitation, but there is usually hydrophobia. The commonest vector of the human infection is the vampire bat. Syn. *dumb rabies.* Compare *furious rabies.* See also *rabies.*

paralytic secretion. The secretion occurring in a gland or organ after denervation, as in the stomach after vagotomy.

paralytic spinal poliomyelitis. A form of paralytic poliomyelitis involving principally the anterior horns of the gray matter of the spinal cord, caused by one or more of the poliomyelitis viruses (type I, Brunhilde; II, Lansing; III, Leon), and producing paralysis of muscle groups, particularly the limbs. Syn. *epidemic paralysis.* Contr. *nonparalytic poliomyelitis.*

paralytic strabismus. A stroke associated with paralysis.

paralytic stroke. Sudden loss of muscular power due to a lesion, usually vascular, of the brain or spinal cord.

paralytic torticollis. SPASMODIC TORTICOLLIS.

paralytic vertigo. Periodic severe vertigo with sudden profound weakness or flaccid paralysis of the neck muscles, levator palpebrae, and occasionally the extraocular and throat muscles, of unknown cause; observed in both epidemic and sporadic form during the summer months in Switzerland, France, and Japan. Syn. *epidemic vertigo, Gerlier's disease, kubisagari.*

par·a·ly·zant, par·a·ly·sant (păr'uh·lye"zunt, puh·ral'i·zunt) *adj. & n.* 1. Causing paralysis. 2. Something which causes paralysis.

par·a·lyze (păr'uh·lize) *v.* 1. To afflict with paralysis. 2. To render powerless or helpless.

par·a·lyz·er (păr'uh·lye"zur) *n.* 1. Anything that will produce paralysis. 2. Any agent that will inhibit a chemical reaction.

paralyzing vertigo. PARALYTIC VERTIGO.

para·mag·net·ic (păr"uh·mag·net'ick) *adj.* [*para-* + *magnetic*]. Pertaining to or characterizing the property of any substance, excluding iron and certain other materials that attract a magnetic field very strongly, which tends to move to the strongest part of a nonuniform magnetic field. —**para·mag·net·ism** (·mag'ne·tiz·um) *n.*

para·mam·ma·ry (păr"uh·mam'uh·ree) *adj.* In the vicinity of a mammary gland.

paramammary route of Gerota [D. *Gerota,* Rumanian surgeon, 1867–1939]. The lymphatic drainage route from mammary glands to the liver or subdiaphragmatic lymph nodes, taken by metastasizing breast carcinoma.

para·ma·nia (păr"uh·may'nee·uh) *n.* [*para-* + *-mania*]. The pleasure or satisfaction derived from complaining; a common neurotic symptom.

para·mas·ti·tis (păr"uh·mas·tye'tis) *n.* [*para-* + *mast-* + *-itis*]. Inflammation of the connective tissue about the mammary gland.

para·mas·toid (păr"uh·mas'toid) *adj.* In the vicinity of the mastoid process.

para·mas·toid·itis (păr"uh·mas"toid·eye'tis) *n.* [*para-* + *mastoiditis*]. Inflammation of the squamous portion of the temporal bone, from extension following mastoiditis.

paramastoid process. In some skulls, a downward projection from the lateral part of the jugular process of the occipital bone which may articulate with the transverse process of the atlas. NA *processus paramastoideus ossis occipitalis.*

Par·a·me·cium, Par·a·moe·cium (păr"uh·mee'shee·um, ·see·um) *n.* [NL., from Gk. *paramēkēs,* oblong]. A genus of ciliate Protozoa, various species of which are used as test and experimental unicellular animals, because of their large size and ease of culture. —**paramecium,** pl. **parame·cia,** *com. n.*

para·me·di·al (păr"uh·mee'dee·ul) *adj.* Situated near a medial structure.

paramedial sulcus. A series of irregular furrows on the lateral surface of the superior frontal gyrus, dividing it into a superior and an inferior part. Compare *paramedian sulcus.*

para·me·di·an (păr"uh·mee'dee·un) *adj.* [*para-* + *median*]. Situated near the median line.

paramedian incision. An incision made to one side of the median line.

paramedian lobule. A rounded lobule on the inferior surface of the cerebellum, medial to the ansiform lobule and lateral to the tonsilla.

paramedian sulcus. A fissure present in the cervical portion of the spinal cord, not far from the posterior median fissure, and separating the fasciculus gracilis from the fasciculus cuneatus. Compare *paramedial sulcus.*

para·med·ic (păr"uh·med'ick) *n.* 1. A person working in a paramedical field. 2. Specifically, a person who assists a physician. See also *syniatrist.*

para·med·i·cal (păr"uh·med'i·kul) *adj.* [*para-* + *medical*]. Pertaining or closely related to the art and practice of medicine; particularly, pertaining to personnel whose work is closely allied to that of practicing physicians.

para·me·nia (păr"uh·mee'nee·uh) *n.* [*para-* + *men-* + *-ia*]. Difficult or disordered menstruation.

para·men·tal (păr"uh·men'tul) *adj.* [*para-* + *mental*]. Adjacent to the chin or mandible.

para·meso·neph·ric (păr"uh·mes"o·nef'rick) *adj.* Situated near a mesonephric duct.

paramesonephric duct. An embryonic genital duct. In the female, the anlage of the oviducts, uterus, and vagina; in the male, it degenerates, leaving the appendix testis. NA *ductus paramesonephricus.*

pa·ram·e·ter (puh·ram'e·tur) *n.* [*para-* + *-meter*]. 1. A constant to which a value is fixed or assigned and by which other values or functions in a given case or system may be defined, such as the definition of an event by the three parameters of space and the parameter of time. 2. *In psychology,* any constant that defines or enters into the equation for some psychological event, such as rate of learning. 3. *In psychiatry,* the difference or variation of a technique of psychoanalysis used for a particular patient or psychiatric disorder, from the theory or model set forth by S. Freud.

para·meth·a·di·one (păr"uh·meth"uh·dye'ohn) *n.* 5-Ethyl-3,5-dimethyl-2,4-oxazolidinedione, $C_7H_{11}NO_3$, an anticonvulsant primarily useful in the treatment of petit mal epilepsy.

para·meth·a·sone (păr"uh·meth'uh·sone) *n.* 6α-Fluoro-16α-methylprednisolone, $C_{22}H_{29}FO_5$, an anti-inflammatory glucocorticoid; used as the 21-acetate ester.

para·me·tri·al (păr"uh·mee'tree·ul) *adj.* [*parametri*um + *-al*]. Pertaining to the tissues about the uterus.

para·me·tric (păr"uh·mee'trick) *adj.* PARAMETRIAL.

para·met·ric (păr"uh·met'rick) *adj.* Pertaining to or in terms of a parameter.

para·me·trism (păr"uh·mee'triz·um) *n.* [*para-* + *metr-* + *-ism*]. Painful spasm of the smooth muscular fibers of the broad ligaments of the uterus.

parametric abscess. An abscess occurring between the folds of the broad ligaments of the uterus or in the neighboring cellular tissue.

para·me·tri·tis (păr"uh·me·trye'tis) *n.* [*parametri*um + *-itis*]. Inflammation of the connective tissue about the uterus. —**para·me·trit·ic** (·trit'ick) *adj.*

parametritis anterior. Parametritis in which the inflammation is limited to the loose, vesicouterine connective tissue, or to that between the symphysis and the bladder. The swelling is anterior, and the pus generally tracks into the bladder, vagina, or inguinal region.

parametritis chron·i·ca atroph·i·cans (kron'i·kuh a·trof'i·kanz). Inflammatory hypertrophy of the connective tissue of the pelvis, progressing to cicatricial atrophy.

parametritis chronica posterior. Chronic, inflammatory processes in the rectouterine ligaments, causing fixation of the uterus at the level of the isthmus, anteflexion by shortening of the folds, and torsion of the uterus when only one fold is shortened.

para·me·tri·um (păr"uh·mee'tree·um) *n.,* pl. **parame·tria** (·tree·uh) [NL., from *para-* + Gk. *mētra,* womb] [NA]. The connective tissue surrounding the uterus.

para·me·trop·a·thy (păr"uh·me·trop'uth·ee) *n.* [*parametri*um + *-pathy*]. Disease of the parametrium.

para·mim·ia (păr"uh·mim'ee·uh) *n.* [*para-* + Gk. *mimia,* mimicry]. A form of aphasia characterized by the faulty use of gestures, inappropriate to the sense expressed.

para·mi·tome (păr"uh·migh'tome) *n.* [*para-* + *mitome*]. HYALOPLASM.

par·am·ne·sia (păr"am·nee'zhuh, ·zee·uh) *n.* [*para-* + *-mnesia*]. Distortion of memory, in which experiences and fantasies are confused; more frequently responsible for erroneous testimony than mere forgetting.

par·am·ne·sis (păr"am·nee'sis) *n.* PARAMNESIA.

Paramoecium. PARAMECIUM.

para·mo·lar (păr"uh·mo'lur) *n.* [*para-* + *molar*]. A usually peg-shaped, occasionally molariform, supernumerary tooth occurring next to the mesiobuccal aspect of a second or third molar.

paramolar tubercle. An accessory lobe or cusp on the mesiobuccal side of a second or third molar tooth, believed to represent a rudimentary paramolar.

para·mor·phine (păr″uh·mor′feen, ·fin) *n.* THEBAINE.

para·mor·phism (păr″uh·mor′fiz·um) *n. In chemistry,* a change of molecular structure without alteration of chemical constitution, as when a mineral changes from one modification to another. —**paramor·phic** (·fick) *adj.*

para·mu·cin (păr″uh·mew′sin) *n.* A colloid isolated from ovarian cysts; it differs from mucin and pseudomucin by reducing Fehling's solution before boiling with acid.

para·mu·sia (păr″uh·mew′zhuh, ·zee·uh) *n.* [Gk. *paramousos*, discordant, + *-ia*]. AMUSIA.

para·mu·ta·tion (păr″uh·mew·tay′shun) *n.* [*para-* + *mutation*]. A mutation in which one allele permanently changes its partner allele.

para·my·e·lo·blast (păr″uh·migh′e·lo·blast) *n.* [*para-* + *myeloblast*]. A myeloblast with an indented rather than spheroid nucleus, present in some leukemias.

par·am·y·loid (pa·ram′i·loid) *n.* [*par-* + *amyloid*]. An atypical amyloid.

par·am·y·loi·do·sis (pa·ram″i·loy·do′sis) *n.* [*paramyloid* + *-osis*]. PARA-AMYLOIDOSIS.

para·my·oc·lo·nus mul·ti·plex (păr″uh·migh·ock′luh·nus, ·migh″o·klo′nus mul′ti·plecks). The name applied by Friedreich, in 1881, to a disorder of unknown cause, predominating in adult life and distinguished by abrupt, irregular, asymmetric clonic contractions of the muscles of the limbs and to a lesser extent of the trunk.

para·myo·to·nia con·gen·i·ta (păr″uh·migh″o·to′nee·uh kon·jen′i·tuh). A heredofamilial condition characterized by recurrent myotonia and muscular weakness on exposure to cold, transmitted as a dominant trait and considered to be a variety of the hyperkalemic form of periodic paralysis. Syn. *von Eulenburg's disease.*

paramyotonia of von Eulenberg. PARAMYOTONIA CONGENITA.

para·myxo·vi·rus (păr″uh·mick″so·vye′rus) *n.* [*para-* + *myxovirus*]. A member of the group of RNA viruses that includes the parainfluenza, mumps, measles, respiratory syncytial, and Newcastle disease viruses.

para·na·sal (păr″uh·nay′zul) *adj.* [*para-* + *nasal*]. Located next to, or near, the nasal cavities.

paranasal cartilage. The embryonic cartilage that gives rise to the inferior nasal conchae and all the ethmoid bone except the perpendicular plate.

paranasal sinuses. Air cavities lined by mucous membrane which communicate with the nasal cavity; the ethmoid, frontal, sphenoid, and maxillary sinuses. NA *sinus paranasales.* See also Plate 12.

para·ne·mic coil (păr″uh·nee′mick) [*para-* + *nem-* + *-ic*]. A chromosome coil in which the subunits are freely separable. Contr. *plectonemic coil.*

para·neo·plas·tic (păr″uh·nee·o·plas′tick) *adj.* [*para-* + *neoplastic*]. Pertaining to changes in tissue structure believed either to presage cancer or to resemble it superficially.

paraneoplastic syndromes. A variety of syndromes in patients with malignant disease which is not due to direct anatomic interference by malignant cells.

para·neph·ric abscess (păr″uh·nef′rick). PERINEPHRIC ABSCESS.

para·ne·phri·tis (păr″uh·ne·frye′tis) *n.* [*para-* + *nephr-* + *-itis*]. 1. Inflammation of the adrenal gland. 2. Inflammation of the connective tissue adjacent to the kidney.

para·neph·ros (păr″uh·nef′ros) *n.*, pl. **paraneph·roi** (·roy) [*para-* + Gk. *nephros,* kidney]. ADRENAL GLAND.

para·neu·ral (păr″uh·new′rul) *adj.* [*para-* + *neural*]. Beside or near a nerve.

paraneural analgesia. Analgesia resulting from injection of an analgesic or anesthetic solution into the immediate vicinity of a nerve trunk.

pa·ran·gi (pa·ran′jee, pa·rang′ghee) *n.* [local name in Ceylon]. YAWS.

para·ni·tro·sul·fa·thi·a·zole (păr″uh·nigh″tro·sul″fuh·thigh′uh·zole) *n.* *p*-Nitro-*N*-(2-thiazolyl)benzenesulfonamide, $C_9H_7N_3O_4S_2$, an antibacterial drug employed by rectal instillation in the treatment of ulcerative colitis and proctitis.

par·a·noia (păr″uh·noy′uh) *n.* [Gk., madness, dementia, from *paranoos,* demented, from *noos,* mind]. A rare form of paranoid psychosis characterized by the slow development of a complex internally logical system of persecutory or grandiose delusions, which is often based on the misinterpretation of an actual event. The delusional thinking is isolated from much of the normal stream of consciousness, the remaining personality being intact despite a chronic course. The patient generally considers himself superior, possessing unique or even divine gifts. Compare *paranoid type of schizophrenia.* —**pa·ra·noi·ac** (păr″uh·noy′ack) *adj.* & *n.*

par·a·noid (păr′uh·noid) *adj.* 1. Resembling paranoia. 2. Characteristic of a paranoid personality.

para·noid·ism (păr′uh·noy·diz·um) *n.* The condition of being paranoid.

paranoid melancholia. INVOLUTIONAL PARANOID STATE.

paranoid personality. An individual characterized by the tendency to be hypersensitive, rigid, extremely self-important, and jealous, to project hostile feelings so that he always is or easily becomes suspicious of others and is quick to blame them or attribute evil motives to them. This behavior may interfere with his ability to maintain any satisfactory interpersonal relations.

paranoid states or **reactions.** Psychotic disorders in which the patients exhibit persistent delusions, usually of persecution or grandeur. Affective responses, behavior, and thinking (including hallucinations) are consistent with the delusions. Compare *paranoid type of schizophrenia, paranoid, paranoid personality.*

paranoid type of schizophrenia. A form of schizophrenia in which delusions of persecution or of grandeur or both, hallucinations, and ideas of reference predominate and sometimes are systematized. The patient is often more intact and less bizarre in other areas, but generally is hostile, grandiose, excessively religious, and sometimes hypochondriacal.

par·a·no·mia (păr″uh·no′mee·uh) *n.* [*para-* + L. *nom*en, name, + *-ia*]. ANOMIA.

par·an·tral (păr·an′trul) *adj.* [*par-* + *antral*]. Situated near an air sinus, as an accessory air cell of a mastoid sinus.

para·nu·cle·in (păr″uh·new′klee·in) *n.* A compound of nucleic acid and protein, derived either by partial degradation of nucleoproteins or by direct combination. Syn. *paranucleoprotein, pseudonuclein.*

para·nu·cleo·pro·tein (păr″uh·new″klee·o·pro′tee·in) *n.* PARANUCLEIN.

para·nu·cle·us (păr″uh·new′klee·us) *n.* [*para-* + *nucleus*]. 1. A small spherical body lying in the cytoplasm of a cell near the nucleus, and perhaps extruded by the latter. 2. A mitochondrial aggregation of a spermatid, which becomes drawn out to form the envelope of the axial filament. Syn. *nebenkern.* —**paranucle·ar** (·ur), **paranucle·ate** (·ate) *adj.*

par·a·ny·line (păr″uh·nigh′leen) *n.* α-Fluoren-9-ylidene-*p*-toluamidine, $C_{21}H_{16}N_2$, an inflammation-counteracting drug; used as the hydrochloride salt.

para·oc·cip·i·tal process (păr″uh·ock·sip′i·tul). PARAMASTOID PROCESS.

para-oesophageal. PARAESOPHAGEAL.

para·oral (păr″uh·o′rul) *adj.* [*para-* + *oral*]. PARENTERAL; said of the administration of nutritive substances and medicines.

par·aor·tic (păr″ay·or′tick) *adj.* PARAAORTIC.

para·os·ti·al (păr″uh·os′tee·ul) *adj.* [*para-* + *ostial*]. Adjacent to an ostium; used to describe atherosclerotic plaques associated with that portion of a coronary artery adjacent to the ostium.

para·pan·cre·at·ic (păr″uh·pan″kree·at′ick) *adj.* [*para-* + *pancreatic*]. Situated beside or near the pancreas.

para·pa·re·sis (păr″uh·pa·ree′sis) *n.* [*para-* + *paresis*]. Partial paralysis or weakness of the lower extremities. —**parapa·ret·ic** (·ret′ick) *adj.*

paraparetic gait. A disorder of gait in which each leg is advanced slowly and stiffly, with restricted motion at the hips and knees and often strong adduction to the thighs (scissors gait).

para·pa·tel·lar (păr″uh·pa·tel′ur) *adj.* [*para-* + *patellar*]. Adjacent to the knee cap.

para·path·ia (păr″uh·path′ee·uh) *n.* [*para-* + *-pathia*]. Psychoneurotic disorder.

par·a·pen·zo·late bromide (păr″uh·pen′zo·late). 4-Hydroxy-1,1-dimethylpiperidinium bromide benzilate, $C_{21}H_{26}BrNO_3$, an anticholinergic drug.

para·per·tus·sis (păr″uh·pur·tus′is) *n.* [*para-* + *pertussis*]. An acute respiratory infection said to resemble mild pertussis, caused by *Bordetella parapertussis.*

para·pha·ryn·ge·al (păr″uh·fa·rin′jee·ul) *adj.* [*para-* + *pharyngeal*]. Adjacent to the pharynx.

par·a·pha·sia (păr″uh·fay′zhuh, ·zee·uh) *n.* [*para-* + *-phasia*]. Aphasic inability to use vocabulary items in relation to objective reality according to their conventional meanings; a pathological tendency to use "the wrong word", often observed in Wernicke's aphasia. —**parapha·sic** (·zick) *adj.*

para·phe·mia (păr″uh·fee′mee·uh) *n.* [*para-* + *-phemia*]. BROCA'S APHASIA.

pa·ra·phia (pa·ray′fee·uh, pa·raf′ee·uh) *n.* [*par-* + Gk. *haphē,* touch, + *-ia*]. Abnormality of the sense of touch.

para·phil·ia (păr″uh·fil′ee·uh) *n.* [*para-* + *-philia*]. SEXUAL DEVIATION. —**paraphil·i·ac** (·ee·ack) *adj. & n.*

para·phi·mo·sis (păr″uh·figh·mo′sis, ·fi·mo′sis) *n.* [*para-* + *phimosis*]. 1. Retraction and constriction, especially of the prepuce behind the glans penis. Syn. *Spanish collar.* Compare *phimosis.* 2. Spastic ectropion from contraction of the palpebral part of the orbicularis oculi muscle. Syn. *paraphimosis palpebrae, paraphimosis oculi, paraphimosis orbicularis.*

paraphimosis or·bic·u·la·ris (or·bick″yoo·lair′is). PARAPHIMOSIS (2).

paraphimosis ocu·li (ock′yoo·lye). PARAPHIMOSIS (2).

paraphimosis pal·pe·brae (pal′pe·bree). PARAPHIMOSIS (2).

para·pho·bia (păr″uh·fo′bee·uh) *n.* [*para-* + *phobia*]. A slight degree of phobia; phobia which can be controlled or overcome by effort.

para·pho·nia (păr″uh·fo′nee·uh) *n.* [*para-* + *phon-* + *-ia*]. Any abnormal condition of the voice.

paraphonia pu·be·rum (pew′bur·um). The change in voice to one more harsh, deep, and irregular noticed in boys at puberty.

paraphonia pu·bes·cen·ti·um (pew″be·sen′tee·um). PARAPHONIA PUBERUM.

pa·raph·o·ra (pa·raf′uh·ruh) *n.* [Gk.]. 1. Slight mental derangement or distraction. 2. Unsteadiness due to intoxication.

para·phra·sia (păr″uh·fray′zhuh, ·zee·uh) *n.* [*para-* + Gk. *phrasis,* speech, + *-ia*]. PARAPHASIA.

para·phre·nia (păr″uh·free′nee·uh) *n.* [*para-* + *-phrenia*]. A term introduced by Kraepelin to describe certain disorders now classed as paranoia or schizophrenia.

para·phre·ni·tis (păr″uh·fre·nigh′tis) *n.* [*para-* + *phren-* + *-itis*]. Inflammation of the tissues adjacent to the diaphragm.

pa·raph·y·se·al (puh·raf″i·see′ul, păr″uh·fiz′ee·ul) *adj.* Pertaining to a paraphysis.

paraphyseal body or **cyst.** PARAPHYSIS (2).

par·a·phys·i·al (păr″uh·fiz′ee·ul) *adj.* PARAPHYSEAL.

pa·raph·y·sis (puh·raf′i·sis) *n.,* pl. **paraphy·ses** (·seez) [Gk., offshoot, from *para-* + *physis,* growth]. 1. *In biology,* one of sterile filaments among reproductive bodies of various kinds in certain cryptogams. 2. A vestigial structure derived from the roof plate of the telencephalon and presumed to give rise to a colloid cyst of the third ventricle. Syn. *paraphyseal body* or *cyst.*

para·pla·sia (păr″uh·play′zhuh, ·zee·uh) *n.* [*para-* + *-plasia*]. PARAPLASM (2).

para·plasm (păr′uh·plaz·um) *n.* [Gk. *paraplasma,* monster]. 1. HYALOPLASM. 2. A malformed substance.

para·plas·tic (păr″uh·plas′tick) *adj.* [Gk. *paraplastos,* counterfeit, forged]. 1. Of the nature of paraplasm. 2. Having morbid formative powers. 3. Misshapen.

para·plas·tin (păr″uh·plas′tin) *n.* A linin-like substance in the nucleus.

para·plec·tic (păr″uh·pleck′tick) *adj.* [Gk. *paraplēktikos,* stricken with paralysis]. PARAPLEGIC.

para·ple·gia (păr″uh·plee′jee·uh) *n.* [Gk. *paraplēgiē,* paralysis, hemiplegia]. Paralysis of the lower limbs.

paraplegia in extension. Paraplegia with extension of the legs.

paraplegia in flexion. Paraplegia with flexion of the legs.

para·ple·gic (păr″uh·plee′jick) *adj. & n.* 1. Affected with or pertaining to paraplegia. 2. An individual affected with paraplegia.

paraplegic headache. A type of pressor headache of brief duration, seen in patients with partial or complete spinal cord transection, following painful stimuli from segments below the lesion or distention of the bladder or rectum; attributed to a pressor reflex undamped by compensatory alterations in peripheral resistance.

para·ple·gi·form (păr″uh·plee′ji·form, ·plej′i·form) *adj.* Resembling paraplegia.

para·pneu·mo·nia (păr″uh·new·mo′nee·uh, ·nyuh) *n.* A disease clinically similar to pneumonia.

par·ap·o·plexy (păr·ap′o·pleck″see) *n.* [*par-* + *apoplexy*]. A masked or slight form of cerebrovascular accident. See also *transient ischemic attack.*

para·prax·ia (păr″uh·prack′see·uh) *n.* [*para-* + *-praxia*]. APRAXIA.

para·prax·is (păr″uh·prack′sis) *n.* [*para-* + *praxis*]. APRAXIA.

para·proc·ti·tis (păr″uh·prock·tye′tis) *n.* [*paraproct*ium + *-itis*]. Inflammation of the connective tissue about the rectum.

para·proc·ti·um (păr″uh·prock′shee·um, ·prock′tee·um) *n.,* pl. **paraproc·tia** (·shee·uh, ·tee·uh) [NL., from *para-* + Gk. *prōktos,* anus]. The connective tissue that surrounds the rectum.

para·pro·fes·sion·al (păr″uh·pro·fesh′uh·nul) *adj. & n.* 1. Pertaining to or performing nonprofessional work that is auxiliary to a given kind of professional work. 2. A paraprofessional worker, as for example a nurse's aide or an orderly.

para·pros·ta·ti·tis (păr″uh·pros″tuh·tye′tis) *n.* [*para-* + *prostat-* + *-itis*]. Inflammation of tissues surrounding the prostate gland.

para·pro·tein (păr″uh·pro′tee·in, ·teen) *n.* 1. Any plasma protein, usually a globulin, which has one or more characteristics unlike those of normal plasma proteins. 2. A modified protein, such as paracasein, which differs slightly from the native protein, as detected by one or more of the standard characterization tests.

para·pro·tein·emia, para·pro·tein·ae·mia (păr″uh·pro″teen·ee′mee·uh) *n.* [*paraprotein* + *-emia*]. The presence in the blood plasma of paraprotein.

para·pso·ri·a·sis (păr″uh·suh·rye′uh·sis) *n.,* pl. **parapsoria·ses** (·seez) [*para-* + *psoriasis*]. Any of a group of rare skin diseases characterized by red, scaly lesions resembling lichen planus or psoriasis. All types are resistant to treatment and usually present no subjective symptoms.

parapsoriasis en plaques (ahn plack) [F.]. Parapsoriasis in which the lesions develop as plaques.

parapsoriasis gut·ta·ta (guh·tay'tuh). Parapsoriasis with scaly, droplike lesions.

parapsoriasis var·i·o·li·for·mis acu·ta (vair"ee·o"li·for'mis a·kew'tuh). PITYRIASIS LICHENOIDES ET VARIOLIFORMIS ACUTA.

para·psy·chol·o·gy (păr"uh·sigh·kol'uh·jee) *n.* [*para-* + *psychology*]. The study of psi phenomena (extrasensory perception and psychokinesis), i.e., the relationships between persons and events which seem to occur without the intervention of the physical senses or physical power.

para·pyk·no·mor·phous (păr"uh·pick"no·mor'fus) *adj.* [*para-* + *pyknomorphous*]. Nissl's term for nerve cells in which the arrangement of the stainable portion of the cell body is intermediate between that of pyknomorphous and apyknomorphous cells.

para·rec·tal (păr"uh·reck'tul) *adj.* [*para-* + *rectal*]. Beside, or near, the rectum.

pararectal fossa. A pouch of the peritoneum on either side of the rectum.

para·rho·ta·cism (păr"uh·ro'tuh·siz·um) *n.* RHOTACISM.

para·ros·an·i·line (păr"uh·ro·zan'i·leen, ·lin) *n.* α-(*p*-Aminophenyl)-α-(4-imino-2,5-cyclohexadien-1-ylidene)-*p*-toluidine, $C_{19}H_{17}N_3$, a dye; used also in the synthesis of other dyes, such as fuchsin. The pamoate salt $[(C_{19}H_{18}N_3)_2 \cdot C_{23}H_{14}O_6] \cdot 2H_2O$, is used as an antischistosomal.

par·ar·rhyth·mia (păr"uh·rith'mee·uh) *n.* [*para-* + *rhythm* + *-ia*]. A dual cardiac rhythm, such as parasystole, in which the independence of the two pacemakers does not result from a disturbance of normal conduction. —**pararrhyth·mic** (·mick) *adj.*

Pa·rá rubber [after Brazilian seaport *Pará* (Belém)]. RUBBER.

para·sa·cral (păr"uh·say'krul) *adj.* [*para-* + *sacral*]. Beside, or near, the sacrum.

parasacral anesthesia. Anesthetization of the sacral nerves near the anterior sacral foramen by injection through the pelvic tissue inferiorly. Syn. *presacral block.*

para·sag·it·tal (păr"uh·saj'i·tul) *adj.* [*para-* + *sagittal*]. Parallel and lateral to the median (midsagittal) plane.

para·sal·pin·gi·tis (păr"uh·sal"pin·jye'tis) *n.* [*para-* + *salping-* + *-itis*]. Inflammation of the tissues around an oviduct.

para·scar·la·ti·na (păr"uh·skahr"luh·tee'nuh) *n.* [*para-* + *scarlatina*]. EXANTHEM SUBITUM.

para·se·cre·tion (păr"uh·se·kree'shun) *n.* [*para-* + *secretion*]. An abnormality of secretion; any substance abnormally secreted.

para·sel·lar (păr"uh·sel'ur) *adj.* [*para-* + *sellar*]. Adjacent to the sella turcica.

para·sep·tal (păr"uh·sep'tul) *adj.* In the vicinity of the nasal septum.

paraseptal cartilages. Embryonic cartilages on either side of the inferior border of the septal cartilage of the nose. The vomeronasal cartilages are the persistent remains.

para·sex·u·al·i·ty (păr"uh·seck"shoo·al'i·tee) *n.* [*para-* + *sexuality*]. Any sexual perversion.

para·si·nus·oi·dal (păr"uh·sigh"nuh·soy'dul) *adj.* In the vicinity of the superior sagittal sinus.

parasit-, parasito-. A combining form meaning *parasite, parasitic.*

par·a·site (păr'uh·site) *n.* [Gk. *parasitos,* one who eats at another's expense, from *para-* + *sitos,* food]. 1. An organism that lives, during all or part of its existence, on or in another organism, its host, at whose expense it obtains nourishment and, in some cases, other benefits necessary for survival. See also *parasitism.* 2. *In teratology,* a fetus or fetal parts attached to or included in another fetus. —**par·a·sit·ic** (păr"uh·sit'ick) *adj.*

parasite index. The percentage of individuals in a community showing malarial parasites in the blood. Syn. *parasite rate.*

par·a·sit·emia (păr"uh·si·tee'mee·uh) *n.* [*parasit-* + *-emia*]. The presence of parasites, especially malarial forms, in circulating blood.

parasite rate. PARASITE INDEX.

parasitic blepharitis. Marginal blepharitis caused by lice and/or mites.

parasitic capture. *In nuclear physics,* any absorption of a neutron which does not result either in fission or formation of another element.

parasitic cyst. A cyst formed by larval stages or cysticerci of animal parasites.

parasitic fetus. A more or less completely formed fetus that is attached to its autosite.

parasitic hemoptysis. A disease caused by the fluke *Paragonimus westermani,* which lodges in the lungs.

par·a·sit·i·ci·dal (păr"uh·sit"i·sigh'dul) *adj.* [*parasiticide* + *-al*]. Destructive to parasites.

par·a·sit·i·cide (păr"uh·sit'i·side) *n.* [*parasit-* + *-cide*]. An agent capable of destroying parasites, especially the parasites living upon or in the skin.

parasitic stomatitis. THRUSH (1).

parasitic sycosis. SYCOSIS PARASITICA.

par·a·sit·ism (păr'uh·sigh·tiz·um, ·si·tiz·um) *n.* [*parasit-* + *-ism*]. The intimate association or union of a parasite with its host, which is beneficial to the parasite and usually detrimental, though not normally fatal, to the host. See also *parasitoid, symbiosis.*

par·a·sit·iza·tion (păr"uh·si·tye·zay'shun, ·sigh·ti·) *n.* Infection with a parasite.

para·sit·ize (păr'uh·si·tize, ·sigh·tize) *v.* To infect or infest as a parasite.

parasito-. See *parasit-.*

par·a·si·to·gen·ic (păr"uh·sigh"to·jen'ick) *adj.* [*parasito-* + *-genic*]. 1. Produced by parasites. 2. Favoring parasitism.

par·a·si·toid (păr'uh·si·toid, ·sigh"toid) *adj. & n.* 1. Resembling a parasite. 2. An organism, such as an insect larva, which lives in or on the tissues of another organism and which, unlike a true parasite, normally causes the death of the host.

par·a·si·toid·ism (păr'uh·si·toy·diz·um, păr"uh·sigh'toy·diz·um) *n.* The association of a parasitoid with its host.

par·a·si·tol·o·gy (păr"uh·sigh·tol'uh·jee, ·si·tol') *n.* [*parasito-* + *-logy*]. The science and study of parasites (1). —**parasi·tolo·gist** (·jist) *n.*

par·a·si·to·pho·bia (păr"uh·sigh"to·fo'bee·uh) *n.* [*parasito-* + *-phobia*]. An abnormal fear of parasites.

par·a·si·to·sis (păr"uh·sigh·to'sis) *n.*, pl. **parasito·ses** (·seez) [*parasit-* + *-osis*]. Infestation or infection with parasites.

par·a·si·to·trope (păr"uh·sigh'tuh·trope) *n. & adj.* [*parasito-* + *-trope*]. PARASITOTROPIC.

par·a·si·to·trop·ic (păr"uh·sigh"to·trop'ick) *adj. & n.* [*parasito-* + *-tropic*]. 1. Having a special affinity for parasites. 2. A substance, such as a drug or a chemical agent, with an affinity for parasites. —**para·si·tot·ro·py** (si·tot'ruh·pee), **parasitot·ro·pism** (ruh·piz·um) *n.*

para·small·pox (păr"uh·smawl'pocks) *n.* A mild form of smallpox.

para·so·ma (păr"uh·so'muh) *n.* PARASOME.

para·some (păr'uh·sohm) *n.* [*para-* + *-some*]. An irregular body found in the cytoplasm near the nucleus. See also *paranucleus.*

para·spa·di·as (păr"uh·spay'dee·us) *n.* [*para-* + *-spadias* (as in hypospadias)]. An acquired condition in which the urethra opens on one side of the penis.

para·spasm (păr'uh·spaz·um) *n.* Spasm involving the lower extremities, as in spastic paraplegia.

para·sprue (păr'uh·sproo") *n.* [*para-* + *sprue*]. A mild form of sprue.

para·ste·a·to·sis (păr"uh·stee"uh·to'sis) *n.* [*para-* + *steat-* + *-osis*]. An altered condition of the sebaceous secretion.

para·ster·nal (păr"uh·stur'nul) *adj.* [*para-* + *sternal*]. Beside or near the sternum, as parasternal line. —**parasternal·ly** (·lee) *adv.*

parasternal line. An imaginary vertical line midway between the lateral margin of the sternum and the mamillary line. Syn. *linea parasternalis.*

parasternal orifice of the diaphragm. FORAMEN OF MORGAGNI.

parasternal region. The region between the sternal margin and the parasternal line.

para·stri·ate (păr″uh·strye′ate) *adj.* Adjacent to the striate area (= VISUAL PROJECTION AREA).

parastriate area. The visual association area of the occipital cortex immediately surrounding the visual projection area. Syn. *Brodmann's area 18.*

para·sym·pa·thet·ic (păr″uh·sim″puh·thet′ick) *adj.* [*para-* + *sympathetic*]. Pertaining to the craniosacral portion of the autonomic nervous system.

parasympathetic nervous system. The craniosacral division of the autonomic nervous system, consisting of preganglionic nerve fibers carried in certain cranial and sacral nerves, outlying ganglions and postganglionic fibers; in general, innervating the same structures and generally having a regulatory function opposite to that of the sympathetic nervous system. Contr. *sympathetic nervous system.*

para·sym·path·i·co·to·nia (păr″uh·sim·path″i·ko·to′nee·uh) *n.* [*parasympathetic* + *-tonia*]. VAGOTONIA.

para·sym·pa·tho·lyt·ic (păr″uh·sim″puh·tho·lit′ick) *adj.* [*parasympathe*tic + *-lytic*]. Blocking the action of parasympathetic nerve fibers.

para·sym·pa·tho·mi·met·ic (păr″uh·sim″puh·tho·mi·met′ick) *adj.* [*parasympathe*tic + *mimetic*]. Of drugs, having an effect similar to that produced when the parasympathetic nerves are stimulated.

para·syn·ap·sis (păr″uh·si·nap′sis) *n.* [*para-* + *synapsis*]. The side-by-side union of homologous chromosomes in preparation for the reduction division of meiosis.

para·syph·i·lis (păr″uh·sif′i·lis) *n.* [*para-* + *syphilis*]. A term for the late manifestations of syphilis, such as tabes dorsalis or general paresis; once considered only indirectly related to syphilis.

para·sys·to·le (păr″uh·sis′tuh·lee) *n.* [*para-* + *systole*]. An arrhythmia characterized by two concurrent independent regular cardiac pacemakers, usually with one normal and one ectopic focus. —**para·sys·tol·ic** (·sis·tol′ick) *adj.*

parasystolic rhythm. PARASYSTOLE.

para·tae·ni·al (păr″uh·tee′nee·ul) *adj.* In the vicinity of the tenia thalami.

parataenial nucleus of the thalamus. One of the midline nuclei of the thalamus, located near the stria medullaris thalami.

para·tax·ia (păr″uh·tack′see·uh) *n.* [*para-* + *tax-* + *-ia*]. 1. Behavior characterized by maladjustment of emotions and desires. 2. A mode of personal experience in which persons, objects, events or other phenomena are seen as separate, in watertight compartments, without relationship to other aspects of one's personality and having only a highly idiosyncratic significance. —**paratax·ic** (·ick) *adj.*

parataxic distortion. *In psychiatry,* one of a number of distortions in perception and judgment, especially as these pertain to interpersonal relations, as a result of the observer's need to see others and his relationship with them in a pattern determined by previous experiences, thus defending himself against anxiety.

para·tax·is (par″uh·tack′sis) *n.* [*para-* + *-taxis*]. PARATAXIA.

para·ten·on (păr″uh·ten′un, ·ten′on) *n.* [*para-* + Gk. *tenōn,* tendon]. The connective tissue that occupies the interstices of fascial compartments containing tendons and their sheaths.

para·te·re·sio·ma·nia (păr″uh·te·ree″see·o·may′nee·uh) *n.* [Gk. *paratērēsis,* observation, surveillance, + *mania*]. A mania for observing, or seeing new sights; uncontrollable inquisitiveness; compulsive peeping.

para·ter·mi·nal (păr″uh·tur′mi·nul) *adj.* Near a terminal.

paraterminal body. The parolfactory area and subcallosal gyrus collectively. Syn. *precommissural area, septal area.*

paraterminal gyrus. GYRUS PARATERMINALIS.

para·the·li·o·ma (păr″uh·theel·ee·o′muh) *n.* [*para-* + *thelioma*]. STROMATOSIS.

Parathion. Trade name for *O,O*-diethyl-*O*-*p*-nitrophenyl thiophosphate, a liquid insecticide having pronounced cholinesterase-inhibiting action.

para·thor·mone (păr″uh·thor′mone) *n.* PARATHYROID HORMONE.

para·thy·mia (păr″uh·thigh′mee·uh) *n.* [*para-* + *-thymia*]. Disturbance of mood in which the emotions are out of harmony with the real situation.

para·thy·reo·pri·val (păr″uh·thigh″ree·o·prye′vul) *adj.* PARATHYROPRIVAL.

par·a·thy·roid (păr″uh·thigh′roid) *adj.* & *n.* [*para-* + *thyroid*]. 1. Adjacent to the thryoid gland. 2. Of or pertaining to the parathyroid glands. 3. PARATHYROID GLAND.

para·thy·roid·ec·to·my (păr″uh·thigh″roy·deck′tuh·mee) *n.* [*parathyroid* + *-ectomy*]. Excision of a parathyroid gland.

parathyroid extract. PARATHYROID INJECTION.

parathyroid gland. One of several (usually four) small endocrine glands lying posterior to the capsule of the thyroid gland, or embedded in the gland, and near the superior and inferior thyroid arteries. See also Plate 26.

parathyroid hormone. A polypeptide hormone in parathyroid glands that regulates blood calcium levels.

parathyroid injection. A sterile aqueous solution of the water-soluble principle or principles of the parathyroid glands, which have the property of relieving the symptoms of parathyroid tetany and of increasing the calcium content of the blood serum in man and other animals. Syn. *parathyroid extract.*

parathyroid osteitis. PARATHYROID OSTEODYSTROPHY.

parathyroid osteodystrophy. Pathologic states in bone associated with hyperparathyroidism, principally including osteitis fibrosa, cysts, and giant-cell tumors; observed most commonly in the hands, clavicles, long bones, and skull. Syn. *parathyroid osteitis.*

parathyroid tetany. Tetany due to parathyroid hormone deficiency.

para·thy·ro·pri·val (păr″uh·thigh″ro·prye′vul) *adj.* [*parathyroid* + L. *privus,* deprived of]. Pertaining to loss of function or removal of the parathyroid glands.

parathyroprival tetany. PARATHYROID TETANY.

para·thy·ro·trop·ic (păr″uh·thigh″ro·trop′ick) *adj.* [*parathyroid* + *-tropic*]. Possessing an affinity for the parathyroid.

parathyrotropic hormone or **principle.** The hypothetical adenohypophyseal hormone regulating the activity of the parathyroid glands.

para·thy·ro·tro·pin (păr″uh·thigh″ro·tro′pin, ·thigh·rot′ro·pin) *n.* PARATHYROTROPIC HORMONE.

para·to·nia (păr″uh·to′nee·uh) *n.* [*para-* + *-tonia*]. Uneven resistance of the limbs to passive movement observed in demented and stuporous patients. Syn. *gegenhalten.*

para·ton·sil·lar (păr″uh·ton′si·lur) *adj.* [*para-* + *tonsillar*]. Near, or around, the tonsil, as paratonsillar abscess.

para·tope (păr′uh·tope) *n.* [*para-* + Gk. *topos,* place site]. COMBINING SITE. Contr. *epitope.*

para·tra·che·al (păr″uh·tray′kee·ul) *adj.* In the vicinity of the trachea.

paratracheal adenitis. Inflammation of the paratracheal lymph nodes.

paratracheal cyst. A bronchogenic cyst attached to the tracheal wall.

para·tra·cho·ma (păr″uh·tra·ko′muh) *n.* [*para-* + *trachoma*]. INCLUSION CONJUNCTIVITIS.

para·tri·cho·sis (păr″uh·tri·ko′sis) *n.* [*para-* + *trichosis*]. A condition in which the hair is either imperfect in growth or develops in abnormal places.

para·tri·gem·i·nal syndrome (păr″uh·trye·jem′i·nul). A rare syndrome due to lesion of the trigeminal ganglion or middle cranial fossa and related sympathetic fibers from the carotid plexus, characterized by trigeminal neuralgia, often followed by sensory loss on the affected side of the face, weakness and atrophy of the muscles of mastication, miosis, and ptosis of the upper eyelid. May be due to an aneurysm of the homolateral internal carotid artery.

para·trip·sis (păr″uh·trip′sis) *n.* [Gk., friction]. *Obsol.* 1. A rubbing or chafing. 2. A retardation of catabolic processes.

para·troph·ic (păr″uh·trof′ick) *adj.* [Gk. *paratrophos*, reared in the same house, from *para-*, alongside, + *trephein*, to nourish]. Obtaining nourishment from living organic matter. See also *metatrophic.*

pa·rat·ro·phy (pa·rat′ruh·fee) *n.* [*para-* + *-trophy*]. Perverted or abnormal nutrition.

para·tub·al (păr″uh·tew′bul) *adj.* In the vicinity of a uterine tube.

paratubal cyst. A mesonephric cyst adjacent to a uterine tube.

para·tu·ber·cu·lin (păr″uh·tew·bur′kew·lin) *n.* [*para-* + *tuberculin*]. JOHNIN.

para·tu·ber·cu·lo·sis (păr″uh·tew·bur″kew·lo′sis) *n.* [*para-* + *tuberculosis*]. JOHNE'S DISEASE.

para·typh·li·tis (păr″uh·tif·lye′tis) *n.* [*para-* + *typhl-* + *-itis*]. Inflammation of the connective tissue near the cecum.

para·ty·phoid fever (păr″uh·tye′foid). A disease of man resembling typhoid fever and caused by *Salmonella* species other than *Salmonella typhi;* the most common etiologic agents are *Salmonella schottmülleri* and *Salmonella typhimurium.*

paratyphoid vaccine. A vaccine made of one or more *Salmonella* cultures, such as *Salmonella paratyphi A* and *S. paratyphi B.*

para·um·bil·i·cal (păr″uh·um·bil′i·kul) *adj.* [*para-* + *umbilical*]. In the region of the umbilicus.

paraumbilical veins. NA *venae paraumbilicales.* See Table of Veins in the Appendix.

para·ure·ter·ic (păr″uh·yoor″e·terr′ick) *adj.* In the vicinity of a ureter.

paraureteric veins. SUPRACARDINAL VEINS.

para·ure·ter·itis (păr″uh·yoo·ree″tur·eye′tis) *n.* [*para-* + *ureter* + *-itis*]. Inflammation of the connective-tissue sheath of a ureter. Syn. *periureteritis.*

para·ure·thral (păr″uh·yoo·ree′thrul) *adj.* [*para-* + *urethral*]. Beside the urethra.

paraurethral duct. A duct of a paraurethral gland. NA *ductus paraurethralis.*

paraurethral glands. Small vestigial glands opening into the posterior wall of the female urethra close to its orifice. The homologue of the distal prostatic glands of the male. Syn. *Skene's glands* or *tubules.*

para·uter·ine (păr″uh·yoo′tur·ine, ·in) *adj.* [*para-* + *uterine*]. Beside or adjacent to the uterus.

para·vac·cin·ia (păr″uh·vack·sin′ee·uh) *n.* [*para-* + *vaccinia*]. A poxlike viral disease (unrelated to vaccinia) affecting the udders of cows and transmissible to humans (and back to other cows) in the process of milking. See also *milker's nodes.*

para·va·gi·nal (păr″uh·vaj′i·nul, ·va·jye′nul) *adj.* [*para-* + *vaginal*]. Beside the vagina.

para·vag·i·ni·tis (păr″uh·vaj″i·nigh′tis) *n.* [*para-* + *vagin-* + *-itis*]. Inflammation of the connective tissue surrounding the vagina.

para·vas·cu·lar (păr″uh·vas′kew·lur) *adj.* [*para-* + *vascular*]. Adjacent to a blood vessel or vessels.

para·ven·tric·u·lar (păr″uh·ven·trick′yoo·lur) *adj.* Situated in the vicinity of the third ventricle.

paraventricular nucleus of the hypothalamus. A thin flat plate of large cells in the anterior hypothalamus whose axons combine with those of the supraoptic nucleus to form the supraopticohypophyseal tract. NA *nucleus paraventricularis hypothalmi.*

paraventricular nucleus of the thalamus. One of the midline nuclei of the thalamus, located in the dorsal ventricular wall.

para·ven·tric·u·lo·hy·poph·y·se·al tract (păr″uh·ven·trick″·yoo·lo·high·pof″i·see′ul). HYPOTHALAMOHYPOPHYSEAL TRACT.

para·ver·te·bral (păr″uh·vur′te·brul) *adj.* [*para-* + *vertebral*]. Occurring or situated near the spinal column, as paravertebral sympathetic nerve block.

paravertebral ganglion. Any of the chain of sympathetic ganglions of the sympathetic trunks; according to location they are grouped into cervical, thoracic (dorsal), lumbar, and sacral.

paravertebral triangle. A triangular area of dullness to percussion on the back on the side opposite to that containing a pleural effusion. Syn. *Grocco's triangle.*

para·ves·i·cal (păr″uh·ves′i·kul) *adj.* [*para-* + *vesical*]. Situated near the urinary bladder.

paravesical fossa. A recess on either side of the urinary bladder.

para·vi·ta·min·osis (păr″uh·vye″tuh·min·o′sis) *n.*, pl. **paravitamino·ses** (·seez) [*para-* + *vitamin* + *-osis*]. 1. A disease associated indirectly with a vitamin deficiency. 2. A disease mimicking vitamin deficiency but not due to avitaminosis.

para·xan·thine (păr″uh·zan′theen, ·thin) *n.* 1,7-Dimethylxanthine, $C_7H_8N_4O_2$, crystalline substance found in normal urine and isomeric with theobromine, which it resembles in its action upon the organism, causing muscular rigidity, dyspnea, and less reflex excitability.

par·ax·i·al (păr·ack′see·ul) *adj.* [*par-* + *axial*]. 1. Lying near the axis of the body. 2. Referring to the space or rays closely surrounding the principal axis of a lens system.

paraxial mesoderm. The medial part of the mesoderm forming a plate-like mass that eventually segments to form the somites.

par·ax·on (păr·acks′on) *n.* [*par-* + *axon*]. A collateral of an axon.

para·zo·on (păr″uh·zo′on) *n.* [*para-* + *-zoon*]. An animal parasite.

par·ben·da·zole (pahr·ben′duh·zole) *n.* Methyl 5-butyl-2-benzimidazolecarbamate, $C_{13}H_{17}N_3O_2$, an anthelmintic.

parchment crackling. The peculiar sound elicited by pressure on the cranial bones of children in diseases where localized thinning (craniotabes) occurs, such as in rickets.

parchment heart. UHL'S ANOMALY.

parchment skin. Atrophy of the skin.

Par·dee T wave [H. E. B. *Pardee*, U.S. cardiologist, b. 1886]. CORONARY T WAVE.

par·ec·ta·sia (păr″eck·tay′zhuh, ·zee·uh) *n.* PARECTASIS.

par·ec·ta·sis (păr·eck′tuh·sis) *n.* [Gk. *parektasis*, stretching out, extension]. Excessive stretching or dilatation.

Paredrine. Trademark for hydroxyamphetamine, the hydrobromide of which is used clinically as a pressor drug, mydriatic, and nasal decongestant.

par·e·gor·ic (păr″e·gor′ick) *n.* [Gk. *parēgorikos*, soothing, gentling]. Camphorated opium tincture, a preparation of opium, camphor, benzoic acid, anise oil, glycerin, and diluted alcohol; used mainly for its antiperistaltic action.

pa·rei·ra (pa·rair′uh) *n.* [Pg. *parreira*, vine]. The root of *Chondodendron tomentosum*, formerly called pareira brava. The plant has been identified as the source of tubocurare, which contains the paralyzant alkaloids *d*-tubocurarine and curine.

par·e·le·i·din (păr″e·lee′i·din) *n.* KERATIN.

pa·ren·chy·ma (pa·renk′i·muh) *n.* [Gk., visceral flesh, from *par-* + *enchyma*, infusion]. The components of an organ or tissue which confer its distinctive function, as contrasted with the stroma, the supporting and nutritive framework.

It is often epithelial although it need not be.—**parenchy·mal** (·mul), *adj.*

parenchymal tissue. The epithelial components of an organ or, in the case of lymphatic organs, the lymphatic tissue, as contrasted with the supporting and nutritive framework of the organ, the stroma.

parenchyma testis [NA]. The parenchyma or glandular portion of a testis.

par·en·chym·a·ti·tis (păr″eng·kim″uh·tye′tis, pa·renk″i·muh·) *n.* [*parenchyma* + *-itis*]. Inflammation of the parenchyma of organs.

par·en·chym·a·tous (păr″un·kim′uh·tus, păr″eng·) *adj.* Consisting of or pertaining to parenchyma.

parenchymatous degeneration. CLOUDY SWELLING.

parenchymatous jaundice. HEPATOCELLULAR JAUNDICE.

parenchymatous keratitis. INTERSTITIAL KERATITIS.

parenchymatous mastitis. Inflammation of the proper glandular substance of the breast.

parenchymatous myositis. Inflammation affecting the muscle fibers.

par·ent (păr′unt) *n.* [L. *parens, parentis,* from *parere,* to give birth]. 1. One who begets young in sexual reproduction. 2. PARENT CELL. 3. *In radiochemistry,* a radioactive nuclide, the disintegration of which gives rise to either a radioactive or stable nuclide, called the daughter. 4. The compound or substance from which another compound or substance is derived. 5. A main trunk or stem from which smaller branches are derived.

parentage test. PATERNITY TEST.

parent cell. The cell from which daughter cells are formed by cell division; MOTHER CELL.

par·en·ter·al (pa·ren′tur·ul) *adj.* [*par-* + *enteral*]. Outside the intestine; not via the alimentary tract, as a subcutaneous, intravenous, intramuscular, or intrasternal injection. —**parenter·al·ly** (·ul·ee) *adv.*

parenteral diarrhea. Diarrhea due to disease outside the intestinal tract.

parent figure. 1. A person who represents within one's emotional life the essential but not necessarily ideal attributes of a father or mother and who is the object of the attitudes and responses, such as respect and love, usually associated with the relationship of a child to his parents. 2. A mature person with whom one identifies and who functions like a parent in providing protection, discipline, love, and comfort. See also *parent image* (1).

parent image. 1. The mental picture a child or adult has formed of his parents at an earlier stage. See also *imago* (2), *father figure, mother figure.* 2. PRIMORDIAL IMAGE.

par·epi·did·y·mis (păr″ep·i·did′i·mis) *n.* [*par-* + *epididymis*]. PARADIDYMIS.

par·epi·gas·tric (păr″ep·i·gas′trick) *adj.* [*par-* + *epigastric*]. Near or adjacent to the epigastric region.

par·ep·i·thym·ia (păr″ep·i·thim′ee·uh, ·thigh′mee·uh) *n.* [*par-* + Gk. *epithymia,* yearning]. An abnormal or perverted desire or craving.

par·ereth·i·sis (păr″e·reth′i·sis) *n.* [*par-* + Gk. *erethizein,* to excite]. Abnormal or perverted excitement.

par·er·ga·sia (păr″ur·gay′zhuh, ·zee·uh) *n.* [*par-* + *ergasia*]. *In psychiatry,* Meyer's term for psychoses manifesting withdrawal, deep regression, delusions, and hallucinations, as schizophrenia and paranoia.

pa·re·sis (pa·ree′sis, păr′e·sis) *n.,* pl. **pare·ses** (·seez) [Gk., slackening, paralysis]. 1. A slight paralysis; incomplete loss of muscular power; weakness of a limb. 2. GENERAL PARALYSIS.

paresis sine pa·re·si (sin′ee pa·ree′sigh). *Obsol.* Late asymptomatic neurosyphilis.

par·es·the·sia, par·aes·the·sia (păr″es·theezh′uh, ·theez′ee·uh) *n.* [*par-* + *-esthesia*]. Abnormal sensations such as tingling, prickling, burning, tightness, pulling and drawing feelings, or a feeling of a band or girdle around the limb or trunk; occurs with disease of the peripheral nerves, roots, or posterior columns of the spinal cord. —**pares·thet·ic, paraes·thet·ic** (·thet′ick) *adj.*

pa·ret·ic (pa·ret′ick) *adj.* Pertaining to, involving, or affected with paresis.

paretic gait. A disorder of gait attributable to weakness of the legs and characterized by shortness of steps, inability to lift the feet, and widening of base of varying degree.

paretic neurosyphilis. GENERAL PARALYSIS.

pa·reu·nia (pa·roo′nee·uh, păr·yoo′nee·uh) *n.* [Gk. *pareunos,* bedfellow (from *eunē,* bed), + *-ia*]. COITUS.

par·fo·cal (pahr·fo′kul) *adj.* [L. *par,* equal, + *focal*]. Pertaining to microscopical oculars and objectives that are so constructed or so mounted that, in changing from higher to lower magnification, the image remains in focus; in changing from lower to higher magnification, only an adjustment with the fine focus control is required to maintain focus.

par·gy·line (pahr′ji·leen) *n.* *N*-Methyl-*N*-(2-propynyl)benzylamine, $C_{11}H_{13}N$, a monoamine oxidase inhibitor employed as an antihypertensive drug; used as the hydrochloride salt.

Par·ham-Mar·tin band [F. W. *Parham,* U.S. surgeon, 1856–1927; and E. D. *Martin*]. A band of aluminum or steel placed around the fractured fragments of long bones for immobilization until union has occurred.

par·hi·dro·sis (păr″hi·dro′sis) *n.* [*par-* + *hidrosis*]. Any abnormal secretion of sweat.

par·i·dro·sis (păr″i·dro′sis) *n.* PARHIDROSIS.

pa·ri·es (păr′ee·eez) *n.,* genit. **pa·ri·e·tis** (pa·rye′e·tis), pl. **parie·tes** (·teez) [L.]. An enveloping or investing structure or wall.

paries anterior. ANTERIOR WALL.

paries anterior va·gi·nae (va·jye′nee) [NA]. The anterior wall of the vagina.

paries anterior ven·tri·cu·li (ven·trick′yoo·lye) [NA]. The anterior or ventral wall of the stomach.

paries ca·ro·ti·cus ca·vi tym·pa·ni (ka·rot′i·kus kay′vye tim′puh·nigh) [NA]. The carotid or anterior wall of the tympanic cavity.

paries ex·ter·nus duc·tus coch·le·a·ris (ecks·tur′nus duck′tus kock·lee·air′is) [NA]. The outer or external wall of the cochlear duct.

paries inferior. Inferior wall.

paries inferior or·bi·tae (or′bi·tee) [NA]. The inferior wall or floor of the orbit.

paries ju·gu·la·ris ca·vi tym·pa·ni (jug·yoo·lair′is kay′vye tim′puh·nigh) [NA]. The jugular wall or floor of the tympanic cavity.

paries la·by·rin·thi·cus ca·vi tym·pa·ni (lab″i·rin′thi·kus kay′vye tim′puh·nigh) [NA]. The labyrinthic or inner wall of the tympanic cavity.

paries la·te·ra·lis (lat·e·ray′lis). Lateral wall.

paries lateralis or·bi·tae (or′bi·tee) [NA]. The lateral wall of the orbit.

paries mas·toi·de·us ca·vi tym·pa·ni (mas·toy′dee·us kay′vye tim′puh·nigh) [NA]. The mastoid or posterior wall of the tympanic cavity.

paries me·di·a·lis (mee·dee·ay′lis). Medial wall.

paries medialis or·bi·tae (or′bi·tee) [NA]. The medial wall of the orbit.

paries mem·bra·na·ce·us ca·vi tym·pa·ni (mem·bruh·nay′see·us kay′vye tim′puh·nigh) [NA]. The membranous or outer wall of the tympanic cavity.

paries membranaceus tra·che·ae (tray′kee·ee) [NA]. The posterior wall of the trachea into which the tracheal cartilages do not extend.

paries posterior. Posterior wall.

paries posterior va·gi·nae (va·jye′nee) [NA]. The posterior wall of the vagina.

paries posterior ven·tri·cu·li (ven·trick′yoo·lye) [NA]. The posterior wall of the stomach.

paries superior. Superior wall.

paries superior or·bi·tae (or'bi·tee) [NA]. The superior wall or roof of the orbit.

paries teg·men·ta·lis ca·vi tym·pa·ni (teg·men·tay'lis kay'vye tim'puh·nigh) [NA]. The tegmental wall of the tympanic cavity.

paries tym·pa·ni·cus duc·tus coch·le·a·ris (tim·pan'i·kus duck'tus kock·lee·air'is) [NA]. The tympanic wall of the cochlear duct which separates the cochlear duct from the scala tympani.

paries ves·ti·bu·la·ris duc·tus coch·le·a·ris (ves·tib"yoo·lair'is duck'tus kock·lee·air'is) [NA]. The anterior wall of the cochlear duct, which separates the cochlear duct from the scala vestibuli. Syn. *vestibular membrane of Reissner.*

pa·ri·e·tal (puh·rye'e·tul) *adj. & n.* [L. *paries, parietis*, wall, + *-al*]. 1. Forming or situated on a wall, as the parietal layer of the peritoneum. 2. Pertaining to, or in relation with, the parietal bone of the skull. 3. The parietal bone. NA *os parietale.* See Table of Bones in the Appendix.

parietal adversive field. The adversive field of the parietal cerebral cortex.

parietal angle. The angle determined by connecting the point in the sagittal curvature that lies highest above the plane passing from right to left through the bregma and lambda, by straight lines with the bregma and lambda, respectively. The greater the angle, the less convex the vault of the skull.

parietal arc. A measurement from the bregma to the lambda.

parietal arch. *In comparative anatomy,* the ring formed by the basisphenoid, alisphenoid, and parietal bones.

parietal block. An intraventricular conduction disturbance, due to myocardial fibrosis of varied causation.

parietal boss. PARIETAL EMINENCE.

parietal cell. One of the cells found in the fundic glands of the stomach. Their function is supposedly the secretion of hydrochloric acid. Syn. *acid cell, delomorphous cell, oxyntic cell.*

parietal diameter. POSTEROTRANSVERSE DIAMETER.

parietal eminence. The rounded part of the parietal bone. This is sometimes bosselated, due to rickets. NA *tuber parietale.*

parietal emissary vein. A venous channel passing through the parietal bone and connecting the superior sagittal sinus with veins of the scalp. NA *vena emissaria parietales.*

parietal foramen. An opening near the posterior superior angle of the parietal bone; inconstant. It gives passage to an emissary vein of the superior longitudinal sinus and occasionally a small branch of the occipital artery. NA *foramen parietale.*

parietal gyri. The postcentral, superior parietal, and inferior parietal convolutions which form the lateral aspect of the parietal lobe of the brain.

parietal lobe. The cerebral lobe above the lateral cerebral sulcus and behind the central sulcus. NA *lobus parietalis.*

parietal lobules. Subdivisions of the parietal lobe of the cerebrum. See also *inferior parietal lobule, superior parietal lobule.*

parietal notch or **incisure.** The angle formed by the squamous and mastoid portions of the temporal bone. NA *incisura parietalis.*

parietal operculum. FRONTOPARIETAL OPERCULUM.

parietal pericardium. The outer wall of the pericardial cavity; it consists of the fibrous pericardium and the parietal serous pericardium.

parietal pleura. The portion of the pleura lining the internal surface of the thoracic cavity. NA *pleura parietalis.*

parietal pregnancy. INTERSTITIAL GESTATION.

parietal protuberance. PARIETAL EMINENCE.

parietal thrombus. A thrombus adherent to the wall of a vessel or a cardiac chamber, not entirely occupying the lumen. Syn. *lateral thrombus.*

parietal tubercle. PARIETAL EMINENCE.

parietes. Plural of *paries.*

parieto-. A combining form meaning *parietal.*

pa·ri·e·to·fron·tal (puh·rye"e·to·frun'tul) *adj.* Pertaining to both the parietal and the frontal bones or lobes; frontoparietal.

pa·ri·e·to·mas·toid (puh·rye"e·to·mas'toid) *adj.* Pertaining to the parietal bone and the mastoid portion of the temporal bone; mastoparietal.

parietomastoid suture. The junction between the mastoid portion of the temporal bone and the parietal bone. NA *sutura parietomastoidea.*

pa·ri·e·to·oc·cip·i·tal (puh·rye"e·to·ock·sip'i·tul) *adj.* Pertaining to the parietal and occipital bones or lobes.

parietooccipital sulcus or **fissure.** The upper limb of the calcarine fissure between the precuneus of the parietal lobe and the cuneus of the occipital lobe. NA *sulcus parietooccipitalis.* See also Plate 18.

parietopontine tract. A tract of nerve fibers which arise in the parietal lobe of the cerebrum, descend from the cortex, pass through the internal capsule, and terminate in the pontine nuclei. NA *tractus parietopontinus.*

pa·ri·e·to·sphe·noid (puh·rye"e·to·sfee'noid) *adj.* Pertaining to the parietal and sphenoid bones.

pa·ri·e·to·splanch·nic (puh·rye"e·to·splank'nick) *adj.* [*parieto-* + *splanchnic*]. PARIETOVISCERAL.

pa·ri·e·to·squa·mo·sal (puh·rye"e·to·skway·mo'sul) *adj.* [*parieto-* + *squamosal*]. Pertaining to the parietal bone and the squamous portion of the temporal bone.

pa·ri·e·to·tem·po·ral (puh·rye"e·to·tem'puh·rul) *adj.* Pertaining to the parietal and temporal bones or to the parietal and temporal lobes of the cerebrum.

pa·ri·e·to·tem·po·ro·pre·oc·ci·pi·tal (puh·rye"e·to·tem"puh·ro·pre"ock·sip'i·tul) *adj.* Parietal, temporal, and preoccipital.

pa·ri·e·to·vis·cer·al (puh·rye"e·to·vis'ur·ul) *adj.* [*parieto-* + *visceral*]. Pertaining to the wall of a body cavity and to the viscera within the cavity.

Parinase. Trademark for the orally effective hypoglycemic compound azepinamide.

Pa·ri·naud's conjunctivitis (pa^{h}·ree·no') [H. *Parinaud,* French ophthalmologist, 1844–1905]. LEPTOTRICHAL CONJUNCTIVITIS.

Parinaud's syndrome [H. *Parinaud*]. 1. Conjunctivitis associated with palpable preauricular lymph nodes. 2. Conjugate paralysis of upward gaze, indicative of a lesion or compression of the corpora quadrigemina of the midbrain, especially the superior colliculi, as from a pineal tumor.

Par·is green. Copper acetoarsenite, $Cu(C_2H_3O_2)_2.3Cu(AsO_2)_2$, a pigment and insecticide. Syn. *imperial, Schweinfurth, Vienna,* or *parrot green.*

par·isth·mi·on (pa·ris'mee·on, pa·rist'mee·on) *n.* [Gk., from *par-*, by, alongside, + *isthmia,* fauces, pharynx, from *isthmos,* neck, isthmus]. TONSIL.

¹par·i·ty (păr'i·tee) *n.* [L. *paritas,* from *par,* like, equal]. Similarity approaching equality; equivalence.

²parity, *n.* [L. *parere,* to bring forth]. The status of a woman with regard to the number of times she has given birth. See also *para* (1), *-para.*

Par·ker's fluid [G. H. *Parker,* American zoologist, 1864–1955]. A hardening and preserving fluid consisting of a formaldehyde solution in 70% alcohol.

Parker's incision [W. *Parker,* U.S. surgeon, 1800–1884]. An incision over the area of dullness in appendiceal abscess.

Parker's method. ASKENSTEDT'S METHOD.

Parkes Weber syndrome [F. *Parkes Weber*]. KLIPPEL-TRÉNAUNAY-WEBER SYNDROME.

par·kin·so·nian (pahr"kin·so'nee·un) *adj.* Pertaining to parkinsonism.

parkinsonian crisis. Sudden severe exacerbation of tremor, rigidity, and dyskinesia in a patient with idiopathic or postencephalitic parkinsonism, accompanied by acute anxiety and its clinical manifestations, and usually the result of psychological stress or sudden withdrawal of antiparkinsonian drugs. In the postencephalitic cases, it may be accompanied by an oculogyric crisis.

parkinsonian mask. The immobile or masklike facies that characterizes parkinsonism.

parkinsonian state or **syndrome.** PARKINSONISM.

par·kin·son·ism (pahr'kin·sun·iz·um) *n.* [J. *Parkinson,* English physician, 1755–1824]. A clinical state characterized by a rhythmic, 3 to 4 per second tremor, poverty of movement (akinesia), rigidity of the muscles, and an impairment or loss of postural reflexes. It may occur in middle or late life from unknown causes, such as idiopathic parkinsonism or paralysis agitans, or as a sequel to encephalitis lethargica or to poisoning with phenothiazine drugs or haloperidol.

Par·kin·son's disease [J. *Parkinson*]. A disease of unknown cause, characterized by an expressionless face, infrequency of blinking, poverty and slowness of voluntary movement, rigidity of muscles, rhythmic 3 to 4 per second tremor most prominent in repose, stooped posture, loss of postural reflexes and festinating gait. Syn. *paralysis agitans, idiopathic parkinsonism.*

Parkinson's syndrome. PARKINSONISM.

Park's aneurysm [H. *Park,* English surgeon, 1744–1831]. A type of arteriovenous aneurysm in which the involved artery communicates with two veins.

Parlodion. Trademark for a shredded form of pure concentrated collodion (cellulose nitrate); used for embedding microscope specimens and preparing semipermeable membranes for dialysis.

Parnate. Trademark for tranylcypromine, an antidepressant drug used as the sulfate salt for the treatment of severe depression.

Par·num's test. A test for protein in which to filtered urine is added one-sixth of its volume of a concentrated solution of magnesium or sodium sulfate. On acidifying with acetic acid and boiling, protein is precipitated.

par·o·don·ti·tis (păr''o·don·tye'tis) *n.* [*parodont*ium + *-itis*]. PERIODONTITIS.

par·o·don·ti·um (păr''o·don'chee·um) *n.* [NL., from *par-* + Gk. *odous, odontos,* tooth]. PERIODONTIUM.

par·o·dyn·ia (păr''o·din'ee·uh) *n.* [L. *par*ere, to bring forth, + *-odynia*]. Difficult parturition.

pa·role (pa·role') *n.* [F., word (of honor)]. *In psychiatry,* the conditional release of a patient from a mental hospital prior to formal discharge so that he may be returned to the hospital, if necessary, without again going through commitment.

pa·rol·ee (pa·ro''lee', pa·ro'lee) *n. In psychiatry,* a patient on parole.

par·ol·fac·to·ry (păr''ol·fack'tur·ee, păr''ohl·) *adj.* Situated near the olfactory area.

parolfactory area. An area of the cerebral cortex just anterior to the gyrus paraterminalis, from which it is separated by the posterior parolfactory sulcus. Syn. *subcallosal area.* NA *area subcallosa*

parolfactory sulcus. Either of the sulci on the medial surface of the frontal lobe which delimit the parolfactory area; specifically, the anterior parolfactory sulcus, which separates the parolfactory area from the superior frontal gyrus, or the posterior parolfactory sulcus, which separates it from the gyrus paraterminalis.

par·ol·i·vary (păr·ol'i·verr·ee) *adj.* [*par-* + *olivary*]. Situated near the olivary body.

par·o·mo·my·cin (păr''o·mo·migh'sin) *n.* A broad-spectrum antibiotic, $C_{23}H_{45}N_5O_{14}$, produced by *Streptomyces rimosus* var. *paromomycinus;* used as the sulfate salt for its antiamebic action.

par·o·ni·ria (păr''o·nigh'ree·uh, ·nirr'ee·uh) *n.* [*par-* + *onir-* + *-ia*]. Morbid dreaming; a nightmare.

paroniria am·bu·lans (am'bew·lanz). SLEEPWALKING.

par·o·nych·ia (păr''o·nick'ee·uh) *n.* [Gk. *parōnychia,* from *para-* + *onyx, onychos,* nail]. A suppurative inflammation about the margin of a nail.

paronychia diph·the·rit·i·ca (dif''the·rit'i·kuh). Paronychia produced by *Corynebacterium diphtheriae.*

par·o·nych·i·um (păr''o·nick'ee·um) *n.* PERIONYCHIUM.

par·on·y·cho·my·co·sis (pa·ron''i·ko·migh·ko'sis) *n.* [*par-* + *onycho-* + *mycosis*]. A fungous infection around the nails.

par·on·y·cho·sis (puh·ron'i·ko'sis) *n.* [*par-* + *onych-* + *-osis*]. 1. A diseased condition of the structures about the nails. 2. Growth of a nail in unusual places.

par·ooph·o·ri·tis (păr''o·off''uh·rye'tis) *n.* [*par-* + *oophor-* + *-itis*]. 1. Inflammation of the epoophoron (parovarium). 2. Inflammation of the tissues about the ovary.

par·ooph·o·ron (păr''o·off'uh·ron) *n.* [*par-* + *oophoron*]. A vestigial, caudal group of mesonephric tubules located in or about the broad ligament of the uterus, homologous with the male paradidymis. They usually disappear in the adult.

par·oph·thal·mia (păr''off·thal'mee·uh) *n.* [*par-* + *ophthalm-* + *-ia*]. Inflammation about the eye.

par·oph·thal·mon·cus (păr''off·thal·mong'kus) *n.* [*par-* + *ophthalm-* + Gk. *onkos,* mass]. A tumor near the eye.

par·op·sia (păr·op'see·uh) *n.* [*par-* + *-opsia*]. Disordered or false vision.

par·op·sis (păr·op'sis) *n.* PAROPSIA.

par·op·tic (păr·op'tick) *adj.* [*par-* + *optic*]. Pertaining to colors produced by the diffraction of light rays.

par·o·ra·sis (păr''o·ray'sis) *n.* [Gk., false vision, from *horasis,* seeing, sight]. Any perversion of vision or of color perception; generally a hallucination.

par·o·rex·ia (păr''o·reck'see·uh) *n.* [*par-* + *-orexia*]. A perverted appetite; PICA.

par·os·mia (păr·oz'mee·uh) *n.* [*par-* + *osm-* + *-ia*]. A perversion of the sense of smell, or the smelling of odors not actually there (olfactory hallucination). See also *cacosmia.*

par·os·phre·sis (păr''os·free'sis) *n.* [*par-* + *osphresis*]. PAROSMIA.

par·os·te·itis (păr·os''tee·eye'tis) *n.* PAROSTITIS.

par·os·te·o·sis (păr·os''tee·o'sis) *n.* PAROSTOSIS.

par·os·ti·tis (păr''os·tye'tis) *n.* [*par-* + *ost-* + *-itis*]. Inflammation of the tissue adjacent to the periosteum.

par·os·to·sis (păr''os·to'sis) *n.* [*par-* + *ost-* + *-osis*]. The abnormal formation of bone outside the periosteum, or in the connective tissue surrounding the periosteum.

par·otic (pa·ro'tick, ·rot'ick) *adj.* [*par-* + *otic*]. Situated near, or about, the ear.

par·otid (pa·rot'id) *adj.* [Gk. *parōtis*]. 1. Situated near the ear, as the parotid gland. 2. Pertaining to, or affecting, the parotid gland.

parotid duct. The duct of the parotid gland. It passes horizontally across the lateral surface of the masseter muscle, pierces the buccinator muscle, and opens into the oral vestibule opposite the second upper molar tooth. NA *ductus parotideus.*

par·ot·i·dec·to·my (pa·rot''i·deck'tuh·mee) *n.* [*parotid* + *-ectomy*]. Excision of a parotid gland.

parotid gland. The salivary gland in front of and below the external ear. It is a compound racemose serous gland. NA *glandula parotis.* See also Plate 3.

pa·rot·id·itis (pa·rot''id·eye'tis) *n.* [*parotid* + *-itis*]. PAROTITIS.

par·ot·i·do·scle·ro·sis (pa·rot''i·do·skle·ro'sis) *n.* [*parotid* + *sclerosis*]. Fibrous induration of the parotid gland.

parotid papilla. The papilla through which the parotid duct empties into the vestibule of the mouth.

parotid plexus. The branches of the facial nerve in close relation to the parotid gland. NA *plexus parotideus.*

parotid region. The area of the face anterior to the ear lying over the parotid gland.

par·o·ti·tis (păr''o·tye'tis) *n.* [*paro*tid + *-itis*]. 1. Inflammation of the parotid gland, as in mumps. —**paro·tit·ic** (·tit'ick) *adj.*

-parous [L. *parere,* to bring forth]. A combining form meaning (a) *producing* or *secreting;* (b) *bearing offspring* of a specified number, as biparous, or in a specified way, as oviparous.

par·ous (păr'us) *adj.* [from the combining form *-parous*]. Having given birth one or more times.

par·ovar·ian (păr″o·văr'ee·un) *adj.* [*par-* + *ovarian*]. 1. Situated near the ovary. 2. Pertaining to the epoophoron (parovarium).

parovarian cyst. A cyst of mesonephric origin arising between the layers of the mesosalpinx, adjacent to the ovary.

par·ovar·i·ot·o·my (păr″o·văr″ee·ot'uh·mee) *n.* [*parovari*an + *-tomy*]. Excision of a parovarian cyst.

par·ova·ri·tis (păr″o·vuh·rye'tis) *n.* [*parovar*ium + *-itis*]. Inflammation of the epoophoron.

par·ovar·i·um (păr″o·văr'ee·um) *n.* [*par-* + *ovarium*]. EPOOPHORON.

par·ox·ysm (păr'uck·siz·um) *n.* [Gk. *paroxysmos*, from *par-* + *oxynein*, to provoke]. 1. The periodic increase or crisis in the progress of a disease; a sudden attack, a sudden reappearance or increase in the intensity of symptoms. 2. A spasm, fit, convulsion, or seizure. 3. A sudden, usually uncontrollable outburst of emotion, as of crying and laughter. 4. *In electroencephalography,* a burst of electrical activity such as spikes, or spikes and waves, denoting cerebral dysrhythmia or epileptic discharges. —**par·ox·ys·mal** (păr″uck·siz'mul) *adj.*

paroxysmal albuminuria. CYCLIC PROTEINURIA.

paroxysmal automatism. EPILEPTIC AUTOMATISM.

paroxysmal choreoathetosis. A syndrome of unknown cause with onset in mid-childhood or early adult life, characterized by attacks of choreoathetoid movements or tonic posturing of limbs, trunk, and face, involving one or both sides of the body, and often triggered by sudden movements; frequently familial, it may be transmitted as a dominant trait with variable penetrance. Syn. *paroxysmal kinesigenic choreoathetosis.*

paroxysmal cold hemoglobinuria. A rare disorder characterized by sudden hemoglobinuria following exposure to cold.

paroxysmal furor. Sudden unprovoked attacks of intense anger and violence occurring in patients with partial complex seizures in psychomotor epilepsy.

paroxysmal hemoglobinuria. A form of hemoglobinuria characterized by repeated acute attacks; it can occur in malaria.

paroxysmal kinesigenic choreoathetosis. PAROXYSMAL CHOREOATHETOSIS.

paroxysmal nocturnal cephalalgia. CLUSTER HEADACHE.

paroxysmal nocturnal hemoglobinuria. A rare disease in which attacks of hemolysis usually occur during sleep; associated with intramuscular thrombosis and its complications.

paroxysmal sleep. NARCOLEPSY.

paroxysmal trepidant abasia. A form of astasia-abasia in which the legs stiffen in spasm when the patient attempts to walk.

parrot-beak nail. A nail curved like a parrot's beak.

parrot fever. PSITTACOSIS.

Par·rot's atrophy of the newborn (paʰ·ro') [J. M. J. *Parrot,* French physician, 1829–1883]. Marasmus of newborn infants.

Parrot's disease or **pseudoparalysis** [J. M. J. *Parrot*]. Syphilitic pseudoparalysis due to osteochondritis with separation of the epiphyses.

Parrot's nodes [J. M. J. *Parrot*]. Nodes on the frontal and parietal bones in congenital syphilis.

parrot tongue. A shriveled, dry tongue that cannot be easily protruded, found with fever.

Par·ry's disease [C. H. *Parry,* English physician, 1775–1822]. HYPERTHYROIDISM.

pars (pahrs) *n.*, genit. **par·tis** (pahr'tis), pl. **par·tes** (pahr'teez) [L.]. A part.

pars ab·do·mi·na·lis eso·pha·gi (ab·dom″i·nay'lis e·sof'uh·jye) [NA]. The distal part of the esophagus lying within the abdominal cavity.

pars abdominalis et pel·vi·na sys·te·ma·tis au·to·no·mi·ci (pel·vye'nuh sis·tee'muh·tis au·to·nom'i·sigh) [NA]. The abdominal and pelvic parts of the autonomic nervous system.

pars abdominalis mus·cu·li pec·to·ra·lis ma·jo·ris (mus'kew·lye peck·to·ray'lis ma·jo'ris) [NA]. The portion of the pectoralis major muscle which arises from the aponeurosis of the external oblique abdominal muscle.

pars abdominalis sys·te·ma·tis sym·pa·thi·ci (sis·tee'muh·tis sim·path'i·sigh) [BNA]. PARS ABDOMINALIS ET PELVINA SYSTEMATIS AUTONOMICI.

pars abdominalis ure·te·ris (yoo·ree'tur·is) [NA]. The abdominal part of the ureter, the portion extending from the renal pelvis to the pelvic cavity.

pars ala·ris mus·cu·li na·sa·lis (ay·lair'is mus'kew·lye na·say'lis) [NA]. Alar part of the nasalis muscle. See also Table of Muscles in the Appendix.

pars al·ve·o·la·ris man·di·bu·lae (al″vee·o·lair'is man·dib'yoo·lee) [NA]. The alveolar process of the mandible. See *alveolar process.*

pars anterior com·mis·su·rae an·te·ri·o·ris ce·re·bri (kom·i·syoor'ee an·teer·ee·o'ris serr'e·brye) [NA]. The anterior part of the anterior cerebral commissure.

pars anterior fa·ci·ei dia·phrag·ma·ti·cae he·pa·tis (fay·shee·ee'eye dye″uh·frag·mat'i·see hep'uh·tis) [NA]. The anterior part of the diaphragmatic surface of the liver.

pars anterior lo·bu·li qua·dran·gu·la·ris (lob'yoo·lye kwah·drang″gew·lair'is) [BNA]. The anterior part of the quadrangular lobule of the cerebellum.

pars anterior rhi·nen·ce·pha·li (rye″nen·sef'uh·lye) [BNA]. The anterior part of the rhinencephalon.

pars anu·la·ris va·gi·nae fi·bro·sae di·gi·to·rum ma·nus (an″yoo·lair'is va·jye'nee figh·bro'see dij·i·to'rum man'us) [NA]. The thick band of transverse fibers of the fibrous sheath of the flexor tendons of each finger, situated at the level of the distal portion of the proximal phalanx.

pars anularis vaginae fibrosae digitorum pe·dis (ped'is) [NA]. The thick band of transverse fibers of the fibrous sheath of the flexor tendons of each toe, situated at the level of the distal portion of the proximal phalanx.

pars ascen·dens du·o·de·ni (a·sen'denz dew·o·dee'nigh) [NA]. The terminal part of the duodenum.

pars ba·sa·lis (ba·say'lis). The portion of each pulmonary artery which sends branches to the pulmonary segments in the base of each lung.

pars basalis ar·te·ri·ae pul·mo·na·lis dex·trae (ahr·teer'ee·ee pul·mo·nay'lis deck'stree) [NA]. The portion of the right pulmonary artery which sends branches to the pulmonary segments in the base of the right lung.

pars basalis arteriae pulmonalis si·nis·trae (si·nis'tree) [NA]. The portion of the left pulmonary artery which sends branches to the pulmonary segments in the base of the left lung.

pars ba·si·la·ris os·sis oc·ci·pi·ta·lis (bas·i·lair'is os'is ock·sip″i·tay'lis) [NA]. Basilar process of the occipital bone.

pars basilaris pon·tis (pon'tis) [BNA]. PARS VENTRALIS PONTIS.

pars buc·ca·lis (buh·kay'lis). ADENOHYPOPHYSIS.

pars buc·co·pha·ryn·gea mus·cu·li con·stric·to·ris pha·ryn·gis su·pe·ri·o·ris (buck″o·fa·rin'jee·uh mus'kew·lye kon·strick·to'ris fa·rin'jis sue·peer″ee·o'ris) [NA]. The portion of the superior constrictor muscle of the pharynx which arises from the pterygomandibular raphe. Syn. *buccopharyngeus.*

pars cal·ca·neo·cu·boi·dea li·ga·men·ti bi·fur·ca·ti (kal·kay″nee·o·kew·boy'dee·uh lig·uh·men'tye bye·fur·kay'tye) [BNA]. Ligamentum calcaneocuboideum (=CALCANEOCUBOID LIGAMENT).

pars cal·ca·neo·na·vi·cu·la·ris li·ga·men·ti bi·fur·ca·ti (kal·kay″nee·o·na·vick″yoo·lay'ris lig″uh·men'tye bye·fur·kay'tye) [BNA]. Ligamentum calcaneonaviculare (=CALCANEOAVICULAR LIGAMENT).

pars car·di·a·ca ven·tri·cu·li (kahr·dye'uh·kuh ven·trick'yoo·

lye) [NA]. The portion of the stomach adjacent to the opening of the esophagus.

pars car·ti·la·gi·nea (kahr″ti·la·jin′ee·uh). A cartilaginous part.

pars cartilaginea sep·ti na·si (sep′tye nay′zye). CARTILAGINOUS SEPTUM OF THE NOSE.

pars cartilaginea tu·bae au·di·ti·vae (tew′bee aw″di·tye′vee) [NA]. The cartilaginous part of the auditory tube.

pars ca·ver·no·sa ure·thrae (kav″ur·no′suh yoo·ree′three) [BNA]. PARS SPONGIOSA URETHRAE MASCULINAE.

pars cen·tra·lis ven·tri·cu·li la·te·ra·lis (sen·tray′lis ven·trick′yoo·lye lat·e·ray′lis) [NA]. The central portion of either lateral ventricle of the cerebrum.

pars ce·pha·li·ca et cer·vi·ca·lis sys·te·ma·tis au·to·no·mi·ci (se·fal′i·kuh et sur·vi·kay′lis sis·tee′muh·tis au·to·nom′i·sigh) [NA]. The cranial and cervical part of the autonomic nervous system.

pars cephalica et cervicalis systematis sym·pa·thi·ci (sim·path′i·sigh) [BNA]. PARS CEPHALICA ET CERVICALIS SYSTEMATIS AUTONOMICI.

pars ce·ra·to·pha·ryn·gea mus·cu·li con·stric·to·ris pha·ryn·gis me·dii (serr″uh·to·fa·rin′jee·uh mus′kew·lye kon·strick·to′ris fa·rin′jis mee′dee·eye) [NA]. The portion of the middle constrictor of the pharynx arising from the cornu of the hyoid bone.

pars cer·vi·ca·lis eso·pha·gi (sur·vi·kay′lis e·sof′uh·jye) [NA]. The upper portion of the esophagus situated in the neck.

pars cervicalis me·dul·lae spi·na·lis (me·dul′ee spye·nay′lis) [NA]. The upper part of the spinal cord containing the cervical segments.

pars chon·dro·pha·ryn·gea mus·cu·li con·stric·to·ris pha·ryn·gis me·dii (kon″dro·fa·rin′jee·uh mus′kew·lye kon·strick·to′ris fa·rin′jis mee′dee·eye) [NA]. The portion of the middle constrictor of the pharynx which arises from the stylohyoid ligament. Syn. *chondropharyngeus muscle.*

pars ci·li·a·ris re·ti·nae (sil·ee·air′is ret′i·nee) [NA]. The part of the retina in front of the ora serrata.

pars cla·vi·cu·la·ris mus·cu·li pec·to·ra·lis ma·jo·ris (kla·vick″yoo·lair′is mus′kew·lye peck″to·ray′lis ma·jo′ris) [NA]. The portion of the pectoralis major muscle which arises from the clavicle.

pars coch·le·a·ris ner·vi oc·ta·vi (kock·lee·air′is nur′vye ock·tay′vye) [NA]. The portion of the eighth cranial nerve subserving the sense of hearing.

pars com·pac·ta (kom·pack′tuh). The dorsal, more compact portion of the substantia nigra.

pars con·vo·lu·ta lo·bu·li cor·ti·ca·lis re·nis (kon″vo·lew′tuh lob′yoo·lye kor·ti·kay′lis ree′nis) [NA]. The convoluted part or labyrinth of the kidney.

pars cos·ta·lis dia·phrag·ma·tis (kos·tay′lis dye″uh·frag′ma·tis) [NA]. The portion of the diaphragm arising from the ribs.

pars cri·co·pha·ryn·gea mus·cu·li con·stric·to·ris pha·ryn·gis in·fe·ri·o·ris (krye″ko·fa·rin′jee·uh mus′kew·lye kon·strick·to′ris fa·rin′jis in·feer·ee·o′ris) [NA]. The portion of the inferior constrictor muscle of the pharynx which arises from the cricoid cartilage.

pars cru·ci·for·mis va·gi·nae fi·bro·sae di·gi·to·rum ma·nus (kroo·si·for′mis va·jye′nee figh·bro′see dij·i·to′rum man′us) [NA]. Interlacing diagonal bands of the fibrous sheath of the flexor tendons of each finger.

pars cruciformis vaginae fibrosae digitorum pe·dis (ped′is) [NA]. Interlacing diagonal bands of the fibrous sheath of the flexor tendons of a toe.

pars cu·pu·la·ris re·ces·sus epi·tym·pa·ni·ci (kew·pew·lair′is re·ses′us ep″i·tim·pan′i·sigh) [NA]. The upper part of the cavity of the middle ear.

pars de·scen·dens du·o·de·ni (de·sen′denz dew·o·dee′nigh) [NA]. The second part of the duodenum.

pars dex·tra fa·ci·ei dia·phrag·ma·ti·cae he·pa·tis (deck′struh fay·shee·ee′eye dye″uh·frag·mat′i·see hep′uh·tis) [NA]. The right part of the diaphragmatic surface of the liver.

pars dis·ta·lis (dis·tay′lis). The distal or anterior portion of the adenohypophysis; the main body of the lobe, separated from the neurohypophysis by the pars intermedia. NA *pars distalis lobi anterioris hypophyseos.*

pars distalis lo·bi an·te·ri·o·ris hy·po·phy·se·os (lo′bye an·teer″ee·o′ris high″po·fiz′ee·os) [NA]. PARS DISTALIS.

pars dor·sa·lis pon·tis (dor·say′lis pon′tis) [NA]. The dorsal or tegmental portion of the pons.

pars fe·ta·lis pla·cen·tae (fee·tay′lis pla·sen′tee) [NA]. The portion of the placenta which is derived from fetal tissue (the chorion).

pars flac·ci·da mem·bra·nae tym·pa·ni (flack′si·duh mem·bray′nee tim′puh·nigh) [NA]. The small triangular upper portion of the tympanic membrane; it is thin and lax.

pars fron·ta·lis cap·su·lae in·ter·nae (fron·tay′lis kap′sue·lee in·tur′nee) [BNA]. CRUS ANTERIUS CAPSULAE INTERNAE.

pars frontalis co·ro·nae ra·di·a·tae (ko·ro′nee ray·dee·ay′tee) [BNA]. The fibers of the corona radiata which are connected with the frontal lobe.

pars frontalis oper·cu·li (o·pur′kew·lye) [BNA]. Operculum frontale (= FRONTAL OPERCULUM).

pars frontalis ra·di·a·ti·o·nis cor·po·ris cal·lo·si (ray·dee·ay″shee·o′nis kor′po·ris ka·lo′sigh) [BNA]. The portion of the radiating fibers of the corpus callosum which go into the frontal lobe.

pars glan·du·la·ris (glan·dew·lair′is). ADENOHYPOPHYSIS.

pars glos·so·pha·ryn·gea mus·cu·li con·stric·to·ris pha·ryn·gis su·pe·ri·o·ris (glos″o·fa·rin′jee·uh mus′kew·lye kon·strick·to′ris fa·rin′jis sue·peer″ee·o′ris) [NA]. The portion of the superior constrictor muscle arising from the side of the tongue.

pars gri·sea hy·po·tha·la·mi (griz′ee·uh high″po·thal′uh·migh) [BNA]. Gray matter of the hypothalamus.

pars ho·ri·zon·ta·lis du·o·de·ni (hor·i·zon·tay′lis dew·o·dee′nigh) [NA]. The transverse or third part of the duodenum. NA alt. *pars inferior duodeni.*

pars horizontalis os·sis pa·la·ti·ni (os′is pal·uh·tye′nigh) [BNA]. LAMINA HORIZONTALIS OSSIS PALATINI.

Parsidol. Trademark for ethopropazine, a parasympatholytic drug used as the hydrochloride salt for the treatment of parkinsonism.

pars ili·a·ca li·ne·ae ter·mi·na·lis (i·lye′uh·kuh lin′ee·ee tur·mi·nay′lis) [BNA]. Linea arcuata (= ARCUATE LINE (1)).

pars inferior du·o·de·ni (dew·o·dee′nigh). 1. [NA alt.] PARS HORIZONTALIS DUODENI. 2. [BNA] The terminal portion of the duodenum; it consists of a horizontal part and a final ascending part.

pars inferior fos·sae rhom·boi·de·ae (fos′ee rom·boy′dee·ee) [BNA]. The inferior part of the floor of the fourth ventricle between the inferior cerebellar peduncles.

pars inferior gy·ri fron·ta·lis me·dii (jye′rye fron·tay′lis mee′dee·eye) [BNA]. The inferior portion of the middle frontal gyrus.

pars inferior par·tis ves·ti·bu·la·ris ner·vi oc·ta·vi (pahr′tis ves·tib″yoo·lair′is nur′vye ock·tay′vye) [NA]. The inferior branch of the vestibular portion of the vestibulocochlear nerve containing fibers from the ampulla of the posterior semicircular canal and from the macula of the saccule.

pars in·fra·cla·vi·cu·la·ris plex·us bra·chi·a·lis (in″fruh·kla·vick·yoo·lair′is pleck′sus bray·kee·ay′lis) [NA]. The portion of the brachial plexus situated distal to the clavicle.

pars in·fun·di·bu·la·ris (in″fun·dib·yoo·lair′is) [former NA]. PARS TUBERALIS.

pars in·ter·ar·ti·cu·la·ris (in″tur·ahr·tick·yoo·lair′is). The isthmic segment of a vertebra (especially a lumbar vertebra) on either side between the superior and inferior articular processes.

pars in·ter·car·ti·la·gi·nea ri·mae glot·ti·dis (in″tur·kahr″ti·la·jin′ee·uh rye′mee glot′i·dis) [NA]. The portion of the rima glottidis between the arytenoid cartilages.

pars in·ter·me·dia (in″tur·mee′dee·uh). 1. The posterior portion of the adenohypophysis, between the pars distalis and the neurohypophysis; sometimes classified as part of the neurohypophysis. NA *pars intermedia lobi anterioris hypophyseos.* 2. The nervus intermedius, the intermediate part of the facial nerve.

pars intermedia fos·sae rhom·boi·de·ae (fos'ee rom·boy'dee·ee) [BNA]. The intermediate part of the floor of the fourth ventricle.

pars intermedia lo·bi an·te·ri·o·ris hy·po·phy·se·os (lo'bye an·teer·ee·o'ris high"po·fiz'ee·os) [NA]. PARS INTERMEDIA (1).

pars in·ter·mem·bra·na·cea ri·mae glot·ti·dis (in"tur·mem·bruh·nay'see·uh rye'mee glot'i·dis) [NA]. The portion of the rima glottidis between the vocal folds.

pars iri·di·ca re·ti·nae (i·rid'i·kuh ret'i·nee) [NA]. UVEAL TRACT.

pars la·bi·a·lis mus·cu·li or·bi·cu·la·ris oris (lay·bee·ay'lis mus'kew·lye or·bick"yoo·lair'is o'ris) [NA]. The central portion of the orbicularis oris muscle.

pars la·cri·ma·lis mus·cu·li or·bi·cu·la·ris ocu·li (lack·ri·may'lis mus·kew·lye or·bick"yoo·lair'is ock'yoo·lye) [NA]. The portion of the orbicularis oculi muscle which is attached to the posterior lacrimal crest of the lacrimal bone.

pars la·ryn·gea pha·ryn·gis (la·rin'jee·uh fa·rin'jis) [NA]. LARYNGOPHARYNX.

pars la·te·ra·lis (lat·e·ray'lis). The lateral part as: 1. The lateral mass of either side of the sacrum. NA *pars lateralis ossis sacri.* 2. The portion of the occipital bone lying on either side of the foramen magnum.

pars la·te·ra·lis ar·cus pe·dis lon·gi·tu·di·na·lis (ahr'kus ped'is lon"ji·tew·di·nay'lis) [NA]. The outer longitudinal arch of the foot. See *longitudinal arch of the foot.*

pars lateralis mus·cu·lo·rum in·ter·trans·ver·sa·ri·o·rum pos·te·ri·o·rum cer·vi·cis (mus·kew·lo'rum in"tur·trans·vur·sair·ee·o'rum pos·teer·ee·o'rum sur'vi·cis) [NA]. The lateral part of the posterior intertransverse muscle of the neck.

pars lateralis os·sis oc·ci·pi·ta·lis (os'is ock·sip"i·tay'lis) [NA]. PARS LATERALIS (2).

pars lateralis ossis sa·cri (say'krye) [NA]. PARS LATERALIS (1).

pars·ley (pahrs'lee) *n.* [OE. *petersilie,* from L. *petrosilium,* from Gk. *petroselinon,* rock parsley]. *Petroselinum crispum,* a plant of the Umbelliferae, containing a volatile oil. From the seed an oily liquid, termed apiol, is obtained. Various parts of the plant have been used as medicinals.

parsley camphor. APIOL.

parsley oleoresin. LIQUID APIOL.

pars lum·ba·lis (lum·bay'lis). 1. The portion of the spinal cord containing the lumbar segments. NA *pars lumbalis medullae spinalis.* 2. The portion of the diaphragm arising from the lumbar vertebrae. NA *pars lumbalis diaphragmatis.*

pars lumbalis di·a·phrag·ma·tis (dye·uh·frag'muh·tis) [NA]. PARS LUMBALIS (2).

pars lumbalis me·dul·lae spi·na·lis (me·dul'ee spye·nay'lis) [NA]. PARS LUMBALIS (1).

pars ma·mil·la·ris hy·po·tha·la·mi (mam·i·lair'is high"po·thal'uh·migh) [BNA]. The mamillary portion of the hypothalamus.

pars mar·gi·na·lis mus·cu·li or·bi·cu·la·ris oris (mahr·ji·nay'lis mus'kew·lye or·bick"yoo·lair'is o'ris) [NA]. The peripheral portion of the orbicularis oris muscle.

pars marginalis sul·ci cin·gu·li (sul'sigh sing'gew·lye) [BNA]. A branch of the cingulate sulcus which curves upward posterior to the central sulcus.

pars mas·toi·dea os·sis tem·po·ra·lis (mas·toy'dee·uh os'is tem·po·ray'lis) [BNA]. The mastoid portion of the temporal bone.

pars me·di·a·lis ar·cus pe·dis lon·gi·tu·di·na·lis (mee·dee·ay'lis ahr'kus ped'is lon·ji·tew·di·nay'lis) [NA]. The inner longitudinal arch of the foot. See *longitudinal arch of the foot.*

pars medialis mus·cu·lo·rum in·ter·trans·ver·sa·ri·o·rum pos·te·ri·o·rum cer·vi·cis (mus'kew·lo'rum in"tur·trans·vur·sair·ee·o'rum pos·teer·ee·o'rum sur'vi·sis) [NA]. The medial part of the posterior intertransverse muscles of the neck.

pars me·di·as·ti·na·lis fa·ci·ei me·di·a·lis pul·mo·nis (mee·dee·as"ti·nay'lis fay·shee·ee'eye mee·dee·ay'lis pul·mo'nis) [NA]. The mediastinal portion of the medial surface of a lung.

pars mem·bra·na·cea sep·ti atri·o·rum (mem·bruh·nay'see·uh sep'tye ay"tree·o'rum) [BNA]. The membranous portion of the interatrial septum.

pars membranacea septi in·ter·ven·tri·cu·la·ris cor·dis (in"tur·ven·trick·yoo·lair'is kor'dis) [NA]. The superior part of the interventricular septum, composed of fibrous connective tissue.

pars membranacea septi na·si (nay·zye) [NA]. The membranous part of the nasal septum; the anterior inferior portion of the septum.

pars membranacea ure·thrae mas·cu·li·nae (yoo·ree'three mas·kew·lye'nee) [NA]. The membranous portion of the male urethra.

pars membranacea urethrae vi·ri·lis (vi·rye'lis) [BNA]. PARS MEMBRANACEA URETHRAE MASCULINAE.

pars mo·bi·lis sep·ti na·si (mo'bi·lis sep'tye nay'zye) [NA]. The distal, more movable part of the nasal septum.

pars mus·cu·la·ris sep·ti in·ter·ven·tri·cu·la·ris cor·dis (mus·kew·lair'is sep'tye in"tur·ven·trick·yoo·lair'is kor'dis) [NA]. The muscular part of the interventricular septum.

pars my·lo·pha·ryn·gea mus·cu·li con·stric·to·ris pha·ryn·gis su·pe·ri·o·ris (migh"lo·fa·rin'jee·uh mus'kew·lye kon·strick·to'ris fa·rin'jis sue·peer"ee·o'ris) [NA]. The mylopharyngeal muscle: the portion of the superior constrictor muscle of the pharynx which arises from the mylohyoid line of the mandible.

pars na·sa·lis os·sis fron·ta·lis (na·say'lis os'is fron·tay'lis) [NA]. The portion of the frontal bone which extends downward in the midline from the squamous portion.

pars nasalis pha·ryn·gis (fa·rin'jis) [NA]. NASOPHARYNX.

pars ner·vo·sa (nur·vo'suh). INFUNDIBULAR PROCESS.

pars neu·ra·lis (new·ray'lis). INFUNDIBULAR PROCESS.

pars obliqua musculi cri·co·thy·roi·dei (krye"ko·thigh·roy'dee·eye) [NA]. The oblique fibers of the cricothyroid muscle.

pars oc·ci·pi·ta·lis cap·su·lae in·ter·nae (ock·sip"i·tay'lis kap'sue·lee in·tur'nee) [BNA]. CRUS POSTERIUS CAPSULAE INTERNAE.

pars occipitalis co·ro·nae ra·di·a·tae (ko·ro'nee ray·dee·ay'tee) [BNA]. The fibers of the corona radiata which are connected with the occipital lobe.

pars occipitalis ra·di·a·ti·o·nis cor·po·ris cal·lo·si (ray·dee·ay"shee·o'nis kor'po·ris ka·lo'sigh) [BNA]. The portion of the radiating fibers of the corpus callosum which go into the occipital lobe.

pars ol·fac·to·ria (ol·fack·to'ree·uh). OLFACTORY REGION.

pars oper·cu·la·ris gy·ri fron·ta·lis in·fe·ri·o·ris (o·pur·kew·lair'is jye'rye fron·tay'lis in·feer·ee·o'ris) [BNA]. Operculum frontale (=FRONTAL OPERCULUM).

pars op·ti·ca hy·po·tha·la·mi (op'ti·kuh high"po·thal'uh·migh) [BNA]. The unpaired anterior portion of the hypothalamus surrounding the anterior part of the third ventricle.

pars optica re·ti·nae (ret'i·nee) [NA]. The portion of the retina which contains the visual receptors.

pars ora·lis pha·ryn·gis (o·ray'lis fa·rin'jis) [NA]. OROPHARYNX.

pars or·bi·ta·lis (or·bi·tay'lis). 1. The portion of the frontal bone which enters into the formation of the roof of the orbits and the floor of the anterior cranial fossa. NA *pars orbitalis ossis frontalis.* 2. The larger upper portion of the lacrimal gland. NA *pars orbitalis glandulae lacrimalis.* 3. The outer portion of the orbicularis oculi muscle. NA *pars orbitalis musculi orbicularis oculi.*

pars orbitalis glan·du·lae la·cri·ma·lis (glan'dew·lee lack·ri·may'lis) [NA]. PARS ORBITALIS (2).

pars orbitalis gy·ri fron·ta·lis in·fe·ri·o·ris (jye'rye fron·tay'lis in·feer″ee·o′ris) [BNA]. The most inferior portion of the inferior frontal gyrus.

pars orbitalis mus·cu·li or·bi·cu·la·ris ocu·li (mus′kew·lye or·bick″yoo·lair′is ock′yoo·lye) [NA]. PARS ORBITALIS (3).

pars orbitalis os·sis fron·ta·lis (os′is fron·tay′lis) [NA]. PARS ORBITALIS (1).

pars os·sea (os′ee·uh). 1. The lateral bony portion of the auditory tube. NA *pars ossea tubae auditivae.* 2. The posterior bony part of the nasal septum. NA *pars ossea septi nasi.*

pars ossea sep·ti na·si (sep′tye nay′zye) [NA]. PARS OSSEA (2).

pars ossea tu·bae au·di·ti·vae (tew′bee aw·di·tye′vee) [NA]. PARS OSSEA (1).

pars pal·pe·bra·lis (pal·pe·bray′lis). 1. The smaller lower portion of the lacrimal gland. NA *pars palpebralis glandulae lacrimalis.* 2. The fibers of the orbicularis oculi muscle which lie within the eyelids. NA *pars palpebralis musculi orbicularis oculi.*

pars palpebralis glan·du·lae la·cri·ma·lis (glan′dew·lee lack·ri·may′lis) [NA]. PARS PALPEBRALIS (1).

pars palpebralis mus·cu·li or·bi·cu·la·ris ocu·li (mus′kew·lye or·bick″yoo·lair′is ock′yoo·lye) [NA]. PARS PALPEBRALIS (2).

pars pa·ra·sym·pa·thi·ca sy·ste·ma·tis ner·vo·si au·to·no·mi·ci (păr″uh·sim·path′i·kuh sis·tee′ma·tis nur·vo′sigh aw·to·nom′i·sigh) [NA]. The parasympathetic portion of the autonomic nervous system.

pars pa·ri·e·ta·lis co·ro·nae ra·di·a·tae (pa·rye″e·tay′lis ko·ro′nee ray·dee·ay′tee) [BNA]. The fibers of the corona radiata which are connected with the parietal lobe.

pars parietalis oper·cu·li (o·pur′kew·lye) [BNA]. Operculum frontoparietale (=FRONTOPARIETAL OPERCULUM).

pars parietalis ra·di·a·ti·o·nis cor·po·ris cal·lo·si (ray·dee·ay″shee·o′nis kor′po·ris ka·lo′sigh) [BNA]. The portion of the radiating fibers of the corpus callosum which go into the parietal lobe.

pars pel·vi·na ure·te·ris (pel·vye′nuh yoo·ree′tur·is) [NA]. The pelvic portion of the ureter.

pars per·pen·di·cu·la·ris os·sis pa·la·ti·ni (pur″pen·dick·yoo·lair′is os′is pal·uh·tye′nigh) [BNA]. Lamina perpendicularis ossis palatini (=PERPENDICULAR PLATE OF THE PALATINE BONE).

pars pe·tro·sa os·sis tem·po·ra·lis (pe·tro′suh os′is tem·po·ray′lis) [NA]. PETROUS PART OF THE TEMPORAL BONE.

pars pla·na (cor·po·ris ci·li·a·ris) (play′nuh kor′po·ris sil·ee·air′is). CILIARY RING.

pars pli·ca·ta (corporis ciliaris) (pli·kay′tuh). CILIARY CROWN.

pars posterior com·mis·su·rae an·te·ri·o·ris ce·re·bri (kom″i·syoor′ee an·teer·ee·o′ris serr′e·brye) [NA]. The posterior part of the anterior cerebral commissure.

pars posterior he·pa·tis (hep′uh·tis) [NA]. The posterior portion of the diaphragmatic surface of the liver.

pars posterior lo·bu·li qua·dran·gu·la·ris (lob′yoo·lye kwah·drang″gew·lair′is) [BNA]. The posterior part of the quadrangular lobule of the cerebellum.

pars posterior rhi·nen·ce·pha·li (rye″nen·sef′uh·lye) [BNA]. The posterior part of the rhinencephalon.

pars postrema. AREA POSTREMA.

pars pro·fun·da (pro·fun′duh). 1. The portion of the masseter muscle arising from the inferior border and deep surface of the zygomatic arch. NA *pars profunda musculi masseteris.* 2. The deepest bundle of fibers of the external anal sphincter muscle. NA *pars profunda musculi sphincteris ani externi.*

pars profunda glan·du·lae pa·ro·ti·dis (glan′dew·lee pa·rot′i·dis) [NA]. The portion of the parotid gland lying deeper than the branches of the facial nerve.

pars profunda musculi mas·se·te·ris (mus′kew·lye mas·e·teer′is) [NA]. PARS PROFUNDA (1).

pars profunda musculi sphinc·te·ris ani ex·ter·ni (sfink·teer′is ay′nigh ecks·tur′nigh) [NA]. PARS PROFUNDA (2).

pars pro·sta·ti·ca ure·thrae mas·cu·li·nae (pros·tat′i·kuh yoo·ree′three mas·kew·lye′nee) [NA]. The prostatic portion of the male urethra.

pars prostatica urethrae vi·ri·lis (vi·rye′lis) [BNA]. PARS PROSTATICA URETHRAE MASCULINAE.

pars pte·ry·go·pha·ryn·gea mus·cu·li con·stric·to·ris pha·ryn·gis su·pe·ri·o·ris (terr″i·go·fa·rin′jee·uh mus′kew·lye kon·strick·to′ris fa·rin′jis sue·peer″ee·o′ris) [NA]. The portion of the superior constrictor muscle of the pharynx which arises from the medial pterygoid process.

pars pu·bi·ca li·ne·ae ter·mi·na·lis (pew′bi·kuh lin′ee·ee tur·mi·nay′lis) [BNA]. The pubic portion of the terminal line, which separates the major pelvis from the minor pelvis, the pecten of the pubic bone.

pars py·lo·ri·ca ven·tri·cu·li (pi·lo′ri·kuh ven·trick′yoo·lye) [NA]. The pyloric portion of the stomach.

pars qua·dra·ta lo·bi he·pa·tis si·nis·tri (kwah·dray′tuh lo′bye hep′uh·tis si·nis′trye) [NA]. The quadrilateral segment of the left lobe of the liver.

pars ra·di·a·ta lo·bu·li cor·ti·ca·lis re·nis (ray·dee·ay′tuh lob′yoo·lye kor·ti·kay′lis ree′nis) [NA]. The radial portion of a cortical lobule of the kidney.

pars rec·ta (reck′tuh). A straight part (of any of various structures).

pars rec·ta mus·cu·li cri·co·thy·roi·dei (reck′tuh mus′kew·lye krye″ko·thigh·roy′dee·eye) [NA]. The straight fibers of the cricothyroid muscle.

pars re·tro·len·ti·for·mis cap·su·lae in·ter·nae (ret″ro·len·ti·for′mis kap′sue·lee in·tur′nee) [NA]. The portion of the posterior limb of the internal capsule which curves around the caudal end of the lentiform nucleus.

pars sa·cra·lis li·ne·ae ter·mi·na·lis (sa·kray′lis lin′ee·ee tur·mi·nay′lis) [BNA]. The sacral portion of the terminal line which separates the major pelvis from the minor pelvis.

pars spon·gi·o·sa ure·thrae mas·cu·li·nae (spon·jee·o′suh yoo·ree′three mas·kew·lye′nee) [NA]. The portion of the male urethra lying within the corpus spongiosum.

pars squa·mo·sa os·sis tem·po·ra·lis (skway·mo′suh os′is tem·po·ray′lis) [NA]. The flat thin portion of the temporal bone forming part of the lateral wall of the skull.

pars ster·na·lis dia·phrag·ma·tis (stur·nay′lis dye·uh·frag′muh·tis) [NA]. The portion of the diaphragm arising from the sternum.

pars ster·no·cos·ta·lis mus·cu·li pec·to·ra·lis ma·jo·ris (stur″no·kos·tay′lis mus′kew·lye peck·to·ray′lis ma·jo′ris) [NA]. The portion of the pectoralis major muscle which arises from the sternum and the rib cartilages.

pars sub·cu·ta·nea mus·cu·li sphinc·te·ris ani ex·ter·ni (sub″kew·tay′nee·uh mus′kew·lye sfink·teer′is ay′nigh eck·stur′nigh) [NA]. The most superficial fibers of the external anal sphincter muscle.

pars sub·fron·ta·lis sul·ci cin·gu·li (sub·fron·tay′lis sul′sigh sing′gew·lye) [BNA]. The continuation of the sulcus cinguli to the under surface of the frontal lobe.

pars sub·len·ti·for·mis cap·su·lae in·ter·nae (sub·len·ti·for′mis kap′sue·lee in·tur′nee) [NA]. The portion of the posterior limb of the internal capsule which lies ventral to the lentiform nucleus.

pars su·per·fi·ci·a·lis (sue″pur·fish·ee·ay′lis). 1. The fibers of the external anal sphincter muscle which are located between the subcutaneous and deep portions. NA *pars superficialis musculi sphincteris ani externi.* 2. The portion of the masseter muscle which arises from the zygomatic arch. NA *pars superficialis musculi masseteris.*

pars superficialis glan·du·lae pa·ro·ti·dis (glan′dew·lee pa·rot′i·dis) [NA]. The portion of the parotid gland which lies superficial to the branches of the facial nerve.

pars superficialis mus·cu·li mas·se·te·ris (mus′kew·lye mas·e·teer′is) [NA]. PARS SUPERFICIALIS (2).

pars superficialis musculi sphinc·te·ris ani ex·ter·ni (sfink·teer′is ay′nigh ecks·tur′nigh) [NA]. PARS SUPERFICIALIS (1).

pars superior du·o·de·ni (dew·o·dee'nigh) [NA]. The first part of the duodenum.

pars superior fa·ci·ei dia·phrag·ma·ti·cae he·pa·tis (fay·shee·ee'eye dye''uh·frag·mat'i·see hep'uh·tis) [NA]. The superior part of the diaphragmatic surface of the liver.

pars superior fos·sae rhom·boi·de·ae (fos'ee rom·boy'dee·ee) [BNA]. The superior part of the fourth ventricle.

pars superior gy·ri fron·ta·lis me·dii (jye'rye fron·tay'lis mee'dee·eye) [BNA]. The upper part of the middle frontal gyrus.

pars superior par·tis ves·ti·bu·la·ris ner·vi oc·ta·vi (pahr'tis ves·tib''yoo·lair'is nur'vye ock·tay'vye) [NA]. The superior branch of the vestibular portion of the vestibulocochlear nerve containing fibers from ampullas of the anterior and lateral semicircular canals and from the macula of the utricle.

pars su·pra·cla·vi·cu·la·ris plex·us bra·chi·a·lis (sue''pruh·kla·vick''yoo·lair'is pleck'sus bray·kee·ay'lis) [NA]. The portion of the brachial plexus lying proximal to the clavicle.

pars su·pra·op·ti·ca (sue''pruh·op'ti·kuh). The anterior region of the hypothalamus.

pars sym·pa·thi·ca sys·te·ma·tis ner·vo·si au·to·no·mi·ci (sim·path'i·kuh sis·tee'ma·tis nur·vo'sigh aw·to·nom'i·sigh) [NA]. The sympathetic (thoracolumbar) portion of the autonomic nervous system.

pars tem·po·ra·lis co·ro·nae ra·di·a·tae (tem·po·ray'lis ko·ro'nee ray·dee·ay'tee) [BNA]. The fibers of the corona radiata connected with the temporal lobe.

pars temporalis oper·cu·li (o·pur'kew·lye) [BNA]. Operculum temporale (= TEMPORAL OPERCULUM).

pars temporalis ra·di·a·ti·o·nis cor·po·ris cal·lo·si (ray''dee·ay·shee·o'nis kor'po·ris ka·lo'sigh) [BNA]. The portion of the radiating fibers of the corpus callosum which go into the temporal lobe.

pars ten·sa mem·bra·nae tym·pa·ni (ten'suh mem·bray'nee tim'puh·nigh) [NA]. All the tympanic membrane except the pars flaccida.

pars tho·ra·ca·lis me·dul·lae spi·na·lis (tho·ra·kay'lis me·dul'ee spye·nay'lis) [BNA]. Pars thoracica medullae spinalis (= PARS THORACICA (2)).

pars thoracalis oe·so·pha·gi (e·sof'uh·jye) [BNA]. Pars thoracica esophagi (= PARS THORACICA (1)).

pars thoracalis sys·te·ma·tis sym·pa·thi·ci (sis·tee'muh·tis sim·path'i·sigh) [BNA]. PARS THORACICA SYSTEMATIS AUTONOMICI.

pars tho·ra·ci·ca (tho·ray'si·kuh, tho·ras'i·kuh). 1. The portion of the esophagus located within the posterior mediastinum. NA *pars thoracica esophagi.* 2. The portion of the spinal cord which contains the thoracic segments. NA *pars thoracica medullae spinalis.*

pars thoracica eso·pha·gi (e·sof'uh·jye) [NA]. PARS THORACICA (1).

pars thoracica me·dul·lae spi·na·lis (me·dul'ee spye·nay'lis) [NA]. PARS THORACICA (2).

pars thoracica sys·te·ma·tis au·to·no·mi·ci (sis·tee'ma·tis aw·to·nom'i·sigh) [NA]. The thoracic portion of the autonomic nervous system.

pars thy·ro·pha·ryn·gea mus·cu·li con·stric·to·ris pha·ryn·gis in·fe·ri·o·ris (thigh''ro·fa·rin'jee·uh mus'kew·lye kon·strick·to'ris fa·rin'jis in·feer·ee·o'ris) [NA]. The portion of the inferior constrictor muscle of the pharynx which arises from the thyroid cartilage.

pars ti·bio·cal·ca·nea li·ga·men·ti me·di·a·lis (tib''ee·o·kal·kay'nee·uh lig·uh·men'tye mee·dee·ay'lis) [NA]. The portion of the medial ligament of the ankle joint which joins the tibia and calcaneus.

pars ti·bio·na·vi·cu·la·ris li·ga·men·ti me·di·a·lis (tib''ee·o·na·vick·yoo·lair'is lig·uh·men'tye mee·dee·ay'lis) [NA]. The portion of the medial ligament of the ankle joint which joins the tibia and navicular bone.

pars ti·bio·ta·la·ris an·te·ri·or li·ga·men·ti me·di·a·lis (tib''ee·o·tay·lair'is an·teer'ee·or lig·uh·men'tye mee·dee·ay'lis) [NA]. The portion of the medial ligament of the ankle joint which joins the anterior portions of the tibia and talus.

pars tibiotalaris posterior ligamenti medialis [NA]. The portion of the medial ligament of the ankle joint which joins the posterior portions of the tibia and talus.

pars trans·ver·sa mus·cu·li na·sa·lis (trans·vur'suh mus'kew·lye na·say'lis) [NA]. Transverse part of the nasalis muscle.

pars tri·an·gu·la·ris gy·ri fron·ta·lis in·fe·ri·o·ris (trye·ang·gew·lair'is jye'rye fron·tay'lis in·feer·ee·o'ris) [BNA]. The triangular portion of the inferior frontal gyrus.

pars tu·be·ra·lis (tew·be·ray'lis) [NA]. The upward extension of the adenohypophysis on the anterior surface of the infundibular stem. Syn. *pars infundibularis.*

pars tym·pa·ni·ca os·sis tem·po·ra·lis (tim·pan'i·kuh os'is tem·po·ray'lis) [NA]. The tympanic portion of the temporal bone.

pars ute·ri·na pla·cen·tae (yoo·te·rye'nuh pla·sen'tee) [NA]. The portion of the placenta derived from the uterine wall.

pars uterina tu·bae ute·ri·nae (tew'bee yoo·te·rye'nee) [NA]. The proximal portion of the uterine tube.

pars ven·tra·lis pon·tis (ven·tray'lis pon'tis) [NA]. The ventral portion of the pons which is characterized by large bundles of transverse fibers.

pars ver·te·bra·lis fa·ci·ei me·di·a·lis pul·mo·nis (vur·te·bray'lis fay·shee·ee'eye mee·dee·ay'lis pul·mo'nis) [NA]. The vertebral part of the medial surface of a lung.

pars ves·ti·bu·la·ris ner·vi oc·ta·vi (ves·tib·yoo·lair'is nur'vye ock·tay'vye) [NA]. The portion of the vestibulocochlear nerve concerned with the sense of equilibrium.

partes. Plural of *pars.*

partes ge·ni·ta·les ex·ter·nae mu·li·e·bres (jen·i·tay'leez ecks·tur'nee mew·lee·ee'breez) [BNA]. PARTES GENITALES FEMININAE EXTERNAE.

partes genitales externae vi·ri·les (vi·rye'leez) [BNA]. PARTES GENITALES MASCULINAE EXTERNAE.

partes genitales fe·mi·ni·nae ex·ter·nae (fem·i·nigh'nee ecks·tur'nee) [NA]. The external genital organs of the female.

partes genitales mas·cu·li·nae ex·ter·nae (mas·kew·lye'nee ecks·tur'nee) [NA]. The external genital organs of the male.

par·the·no·gen·e·sis (pahrth''e·no·jen'e·sis) *n.* [Gk. *parthenos,* virgin, + *-genesis*]. A modification of sexual reproduction, in which the organism develops from an unfertilized egg. It occurs chiefly in certain insects, crustacea, and worms. —**partheno·ge·net·ic** (·je·net'ick) *adj.*

par·the·no·pho·bia (pahrth''e·no·fo'bee·uh) *n.* [Gk. *parthenos,* maiden, virgin, + *-phobia*]. Fear of virgins or girls.

partial abortion. Premature expulsion of one fetus in the presence of multiple gestation.

partial agglutinin. GROUP AGGLUTININ.

partial albuminuria. A form of proteinuria in which it is assumed that only certain nephrons are affected. Syn. *albuminuria parcellaire.*

partial amputation. An amputation in which only a portion of a member, part, or organ has been removed.

partial anesthesia. Anesthesia in which some degree of sensibility is still present.

partial aneurysm. 1. LATERAL ANEURYSM. 2. Aneurysmal dilatation of a portion of the heart.

partial ankylosis. Ankylosis producing limitation of joint motion but not complete fixation.

partial antigen. HAPTEN.

partial birth. In labor, the incomplete expulsion of offspring, as the retention of a portion of a macerated fetus.

partial cleavage. MEROBLASTIC CLEAVAGE.

partial color blindness. A form of color blindness characterized by a decrease or loss of perception of one of the three basic hues. Red-green color blindness is the most common type. Forms of partial color blindness are protanopia, deuteranopia, and tritanopia.

partial complex seizures. TEMPORAL LOBE EPILEPSY.

partial continuous epilepsy. STATUS EPILEPTICUS.

partial denture. A denture that replaces less than the full number of teeth in either arch; it may be either fixed or removable.

partial dislocation. INCOMPLETE DISLOCATION.

partial heart block. ATRIOVENTRICULAR BLOCK.

partial hospitalization. *In psychiatry,* treatment programs for patients within a hospital but not on a full-time basis, such as only during the day or the night time or on weekends.

partial obstruction. Incomplete obstruction.

partial pressure. In a mixture of gases, the pressure exerted by one of the gases is said to be the partial pressure of that gas. In such a mixture, the partial pressures of the gases are exerted independently of each other and the total pressure exerted is the sum of the partial pressures.

partial-thickness burn. A burn of the first or second degree. Contr. *full-thickness burn.* See also *first degree burn, second degree burn.*

partial thromboplastin. Any of several lipid-rich clot accelerators dependent upon factors VIII, IX, and XII for maximum acceleration of clotting.

par·ti·cle (pahr'ti·kul) *n.* [L. *particula,* a little bit]. 1. A small portion or piece of substance. 2. One of the elementary components of atoms and molecules, as the neutron, proton, and electron.

particle accelerator. Any device, such as a betatron or a cyclotron, for accelerating electrically charged atomic particles to high velocities.

par·tic·u·late (pahr·tick'yoo·lut) *adj.* Composed of particles.

par·ti·tion (pahr·tish'un) *n.* [L. *partitio,* from *partire,* to divide, distribute]. The distribution of a substance or ions between two immiscible liquids, or between a liquid and a gas.

partition chromatography. The separation of substances based on countercurrent partition between two immiscible solvents; one immobile solvent is held in the interstices of a column of inert matrix (starch, cellulose, silica); the other, mobile, solvent passes down the column. Each substance moves with the mobile solvent at a unique rate depending on its partition coefficient.

partition coefficient. The ratio of the concentrations of a solute in equilibrium with two immiscible liquids.

par·tri·cin (pahr·trye'sin) *n.* A mixture of two polyenes (heptaenes) of unknown structure having antifungal and antiprotozoal properties.

par·tu·ri·en·cy (pahr·tew'ree·un·see) *n.* The state of being parturient.

par·tu·ri·ent (pahr·tew'ree·unt) *adj.* [L. *parturiens,* from *parturire,* to be in labor, to give birth]. 1. In labor; giving birth. 2. Pertaining to parturition.

parturient canal. BIRTH CANAL.

parturient paresis. A disease of cows, occurring shortly after calving, characterized by motor and sensory nervous paralysis, circulatory collapse, and hypocalcemia. Syn. *milk fever* (2).

par·tu·ri·fa·cient (pahr·tew''ri·fay'shunt) *adj. & n.* [L. *parturire,* to be in labor, + *faciens,* making, producing]. 1. Promoting labor. 2. An agent that induces labor.

par·tu·ri·om·e·ter (pahr·tew''ree·om'e·tur) *n.* [L. *parturire,* to be in labor, + *-meter*]. An instrument to determine the progress of labor by measuring the expulsive force of the uterus.

par·tu·ri·tion (pahr''tew·rish'un) *n.* [L. *parturitio,* from *parturire,* to be in labor, give birth, from *parere,* to bear, produce]. The process of giving birth to young. See also *puerperium.*

par·tus (pahr'tus) *n.,* accus. **par·tum** (pahr'tum) [L., from *parere,* to bring forth]. The bringing forth of offspring; labor.

partus ag·rip·pi·nus (ag''ri·pye'nus) [L., of *Agrippa*]. Labor with breech presentation.

partus cae·sa·re·us (se·zair'ree·us). CESAREAN SECTION.

partus dif·fic·i·lis (di·fis'i·lis). DYSTOCIA.

partus im·ma·tu·rus (im·ma·tewr'us). PREMATURE LABOR.

partus ma·tu·rus (ma·tewr'us). Labor at term.

partus pre·cip·i·ta·tus (pre·sip''i·tay'tus). PRECIPITATE LABOR.

partus se·rot·i·nus (se·rot'i·nus) [L., late]. Labor unduly prolonged.

partus sic·cus (sick'us). DRY LABOR.

pa·ru·lis (pa·roo'lis) *n.,* pl. **paru·li·des** (·li·deez) [Gk. *paroulis,* from *oula,* gums]. A subperiosteal abscess arising from dental structures; a gumboil.

par·um·bil·i·cal (păr''um·bil'i·kul) *adj. & n.* PARAUMBILICAL.

parvi- [L. *parvus*]. A combining form meaning *small, little;* sometimes used instead of the more common *micro-.*

par·vi·cel·lu·lar (pahr''vi·sel'yoo·lur) *adj.* [*parvi-* + *cellular*]. Pertaining to, or composed of, small cells.

par·vi·loc·u·lar (pahr''vi·lock'yoo·lur) *adj.* [*parvi-* + *locular*]. Pertaining to small loculi.

parvilocular pseudomucinous tumor. MUCINOUS CYSTADENOMA.

par·vo·vi·rus (pahr''vo·vye'rus) *n.* [*parvi-* + *virus*]. Any of various small viruses associated with adenoviruses, upon which they may depend for replication in hosts other than their natural ones. Though parvoviruses have been suspected as agents of slow infections and are known to cause specific diseases in laboratory animals, none has yet been identified as pathogenic for humans.

par·vule (pahr'vyool) *n.* [L. *parvulus,* very small]. A small pill or pellet; a granule.

par·vus et tar·dus pulse (pahr'vus et tahr'dus) [L., slight and slow]. PLATEAU PULSE.

Parzine. A trademark for the anthelmintic, piperazine citrate.

PAS Abbreviation for (a) *para-aminosalicylic acid;* (b) *periodic acid Schiff* (reaction).

PASA Abbreviation for *para-aminosalicylic acid.*

Pas·cal's law (pas·kahl') [B. *Pascal,* French scientist and philosopher, 1623–1662]. The pressure exerted anywhere in a mass of fluid is transmitted equally in all directions.

pas·cha·chur·da (pas''kuh·koor'duh) *n.* [term used in central Asia]. CUTANEOUS LEISHMANIASIS.

Pasch·en bodies (pahsh'en) [E. *Paschen,* German bacteriologist, 1860–1936]. Aggregates of smallpox virus, often called elementary bodies, which form the characteristic inclusions seen in smallpox (Guarnieri bodies).

Pa·schu·tin's degeneration (pah·shoo'tyin) [V. V. *Paschutin,* Russian physician, 1845–1901]. The degenerative changes encountered in diabetes mellitus.

pas·sage, *n.* [OF., from *passer,* to pass]. 1. A channel or lumen. 2. The act of passing from one place to another. 3. The introduction of an instrument into a cavity or channel. 4. An evacuation of the bowels.

Pas·sa·vant's cushion or **bar** (pah·sa·vahn') [P. G. *Passavant,* German surgeon, 1815–1893]. The bulging of the posterior pharyngeal wall produced by the contraction of the overlapping superior and middle constrictors of the pharynx.

pas·si·flo·ra (pas''i·flo'ruh) *n.* The rhizome of *Passiflora incarnata* (passionflower); has been used as a sedative and anodyne.

pas·sion, *n.* [OF., from L. *passio,* suffering, from *pati,* to suffer]. 1. An intense emotion of the mind; fervid desire, overpowering emotion. 2. A specific intense excitement, as rage or ardent affection. 3. Pain; suffering. 4. Sexual excitement or love. —**passion·al** (·ul), **passion·ate** (·ut) *adj.*

pas·sive, *adj.* [L. *passivus,* from *pati,* to undergo, allow, suffer]. Not active; not performed or produced by active efforts, but by causes from without.

passive-aggressive personality. An individual whose behavior pattern is characterized by aggressiveness and hostility expressed quietly by such reactions as stubbornness, pouting, procrastination, inefficiency, "doing nothing," or passive obstructionism; a character disorder. Compare *passive-dependent personality.* See also *aggressive personality.*

passive algolagnia. MASOCHISM.

passive anaphylaxis. The elicitation of anaphylaxis by the temporary sensitization of an animal with antibodies and the injection of the corresponding sensitizing antigen.

passive ascites. MECHANICAL ASCITES.

passive congestion. Hyperemia of a part as the result of impairment of return of venous blood.

passive cutaneous anaphylaxis. The vascular reaction at the site of intradermally injected antibody when 3 hours later the specific antigen, usually mixed with Evans blue dye, is injected intravenously.

passive-dependent personality. An individual whose behavioral pattern is characterized by a lack of self-confidence, indecisiveness, and a tendency to cling to and seek support from others; a character disorder. Compare *passive-aggressive personality.*

passive exercise. The moving of parts of the body by another without voluntary help or hindrance by the patient.

passive general anaphylaxis. The introduction of systemic anaphylaxis by the intravenous administration of antibody followed some 48 hours later by the injection of the specific antigen.

passive immunity. 1. Immunity conferred through the parenteral injection of antibodies prepared in the lower animals or other human beings. 2. Immunity acquired by the child in utero by the placental transfer of antibodies from the mother.

passive motion or **movement.** Movement effected by some outside agency.

passive negativism. A form of behavior in which the individual does not do what is expected or usual for him; a normal pattern of many young children, especially between 2 and 5 years of age; it is seen in a mild form in many normally functioning persons.

passive reduction. A form of closed reduction accomplished without manipulative force, but rather by steady traction or the pull of gravity.

passive resistance. *In psychiatry,* PASSIVE NEGATIVISM.

passive spread. *In neurophysiology,* the phenomenon of changes in polarization along one point of an axon, causing changes in polarizations in neighboring regions. Syn. *electronic spread.*

passive transfer test. A method of demonstrating skin-sensitizing antibodies in the blood of an allergic patient, performed by sensitizing a local area of the skin of a nonallergic individual by the intracutaneous injection of the serum of that patient and then challenging the prepared site with corresponding allergen.

passive transport. Transport of a solute across a membrane by simple diffusion, at a rate directly proportional to the difference in concentration of solute on both sides of the membrane. Contr. *active transport.*

passive tremor. RESTING TREMOR.

pas·siv·ism (pas'i·viz·um) *n.* A form of sexual perversion in which one person submits to the will of another in anomalous erotic acts. —**passiv·ist** (·vist) *n.*

pas·ta (pas'tuh) *n.* [L.]. PASTE.

paste, *n.* [OF., from L. *pasta,* paste, dough, from Gk., barley porridge]. An ointmentlike preparation of one or more medicinal substances, such as zinc oxide, coal tar, starch, or sulfur, in a hydrogel or fatty base. Pastes are generally intended for dermatologic use; they are less greasy and better absorbed than ointments.

paste boot. UNNA'S PASTE BOOT.

pas·tern (pas'turn) *n.* [OF. *pasturon,* a hobble]. The part of a horse's leg between the fetlock joint and the coronet of the hoof.

pastern bone. The first phalanx (great pastern bone) or second phalanx (small pastern bone) of a horse's foot.

pastern joint. The articulation between the proximal and second phalanges (great and small pastern bones) of any leg of a horse.

Pas·teur-Cham·ber·land filter (pas·tœr', shah^{n}·be^{h}r·lah^{n}') [L. *Pasteur,* French chemist and bacteriologist, 1822–1895; and C. E. *Chamberland,* French bacteriologist, 1851–1898]. An unglazed porcelain filter, made of kaolin and sand, of graded porosities, L_1 to L_{13}, which permits the recovery of bacteria-free filtrates; used in the study of viruses.

Pasteur effect The inhibition of fermentation when anaerobic conditions are replaced by abundant oxygen supply.

Pas·teu·rel·la (pas"tur·el'uh) *n.* [L. *Pasteur*]. A genus of bipolar staining rods, oxidase-positive and nonmotile, which includes *Pasteurella multocida* and other species causing disease in animals. Formerly this genus included the organisms responsible for plague and other diseases; these are now assigned to the genus *Yersinia.*

Pasteurella avi·sep·ti·ca (av"i·sep'ti·kuh, ay"vi·). A strain of *Pasteurella multocida.*

Pasteurella bol·lin·ge·ri (bol·in'je·rye). A strain of *Pasteurella multocida.*

Pasteurella bo·vi·sep·ti·ca (bo·vi·sep'ti·kuh). A strain of *Pasteurella multocida.*

Pasteurella hae·mo·lyt·i·ca (hee"mo·lit'i·kuh). A hemolytic species of *Pasteurella,* distinct from *Pasteurella multocida,* causing enzootic pneumonia in sheep.

Pasteurella mul·to·ci·da (mul·to'si·duh). A species of small, gram-negative, nonmotile, rod-shaped bacteria, normal inhabitants of the upper respiratory tracts of mammals and birds; the cause of hemorrhagic septicemia in cattle and other animals, a variety of other diseases in mammals, birds, and occasionally man; and occurring as a secondary invader in chicken cholera.

Pasteurella pes·tis (pes'tis). *YERSINIA PESTIS.*

Pasteurella pseu·do·tu·ber·cu·lo·sis (sue"do·tew·bur·kew·lo'sis). A motile species of *Pasteurella* that resembles *Yersinia pseudotuberculosis;* the causative agent of pseudotuberculosis.

Pasteurella sui·sep·ti·ca (soo"i·sep'ti·kuh). The species of *Pasteurella* which is the etiologic agent of swine plague; a strain of *Pasteurella multocida.*

Pasteurella tularensis. *FRANCISELLA TULARENSIS.*

pas·teu·rel·lo·sis (pas"tur·el·o'sis) *n.,* pl. **pasteurello·ses** (·seez) [*Pasteurella* + *-osis*]. Any of several diseases of animals that are associated with organisms in the genus *Pasteurella,* such as shipping fever.

pas·teur·iza·tion (pas"tur·i·zay'shun) *n.* [L. *Pasteur*]. Heat treatment to kill some but not all of the microorganisms in a particular material. In the pasteurization of milk, heating the milk to 62°C for 30 minutes will kill the significant pathogens but leave many harmless bacteria alive. —**pas·teur·ize** (pas'tur·ize) *v.*

pasteurized milk. Milk treated by pasteurization.

pas·teur·iz·er (pas'tur·eye"zur) *n.* An apparatus employed for pasteurization.

Pasteur treatment [L. *Pasteur*]. The original treatment of rabies introduced by Pasteur in which the virus, attenuated by variable periods of drying infected rabbit spinal cords, was administered in doses of progressively increasing virulence during the long incubation period of the disease.

Pastia's lines or **sign** [C. *Pastia,* Rumanian physician, 20th century]. Transverse red streaks in the skin creases, particularly of the antecubital area, seen in scarlet fever.

pas·til (pas'til) *n.* [L. *pastillus,* little roll]. 1. A small mass composed of aromatic substances and employed in fumigation. 2. TROCHE. 3. A paper disk, chemically coated, which changes color on exposure to x-rays; used to determine the dosage.

pas·tille (pas·teel', ·til') *n.* [F.]. PASTIL.

pastoral counseling. The use of psychologic principles and psychotherapeutic techniques by members of the clergy in advising people who come for help with emotional problems.

past pointing. A test in which the patient is asked to point at a fixed object. In cerebellar and labyrinthine disease, there is deviation or past pointing toward the involved side. See also *dysmetria.*

pa·ta·gi·um (puh·tay'jee·um) *n.*, pl. **pata·gia** (·jee·uh) [L., gold edging on a woman's tunic]. PTERYGIUM (3). —**patagi·al** (·ul), **patagi·ate** (·ut) *adj.*

pa·tas monkey (pa·tah'). A slender, long-legged, ground-dwelling African monkey, *Erythrocebus patas,* found in the savannah belt south of the Sahara.

Patau's syndrome [K. *Patau,* U.S. geneticist, 20th century]. TRISOMY 13 SYNDROME.

patch, *n.* [ME. *pacche, peche,* from OF. *pieche, piece,* piece]. An irregular spot or area.

patch graft. *In vascular surgery,* a graft of synthetic material or living vein to close and repair a partial defect in the wall of an artery or large vein.

patch·ou·li, patch·ou·ly (patch'oo·lee, pa·choo'lee) *n.* [Tamil *paccilai,* green leaf]. The herb, *Pogostemon heyneanus,* or other species of *Pogostemon,* the source of patchouli oil; used as a fixative in perfumes.

patch test. A test in which material is applied and left in contact with intact skin surface for 48 hours in order to demonstrate tissue sensitivity.

pate, *n.* The crown or top of the head.

pa·tel·la (pa·tel'uh) *n.*, L. pl. & genit. sing. **patel·lae** (·ee) [L., dish] [NA]. A sesamoid bone in front of the knee, developed in the tendon of the quadriceps femoris muscle; the kneecap. See also Table of Bones in the Appendix and Plates 1, 2. —**patel·lar** (·ur) *adj.*

patella bi·par·ta (bye·pahr'tuh). A developmental variation of the patella, in which a portion (usually the upper lateral part) develops from a distinct center of ossification and remains as a separate ossicle in the adult.

patella cu·bi·ti (kew'bi·tye). An anomalous sesamoid bone lying proximal to the olecranon within the tendon of the triceps brachii muscle.

pa·tel·la·pexy (pa·tel'uh·peck"see) *n.* [*patella* + *-pexy*]. An outmoded operation of fixing the patella to the lower end of the femur to stiffen or stabilize the knee joint in flail joint cases of infantile paralysis, by the production of a partial arthrodesis.

patellar bursa. Any one of a number of variable bursae related to the patella. See also *infrapatellar bursa, prepatellar bursa, suprapatellar bursa.*

patellar clonus. Clonic contraction and relaxation of the quadriceps femoris muscle in response to sharp firm pressure against the upper margin of the patella or on eliciting the patellar reflex; observed with lesions of the corticospinal tract.

patellar ligament. The ligamentous continuation of the tendon of the quadriceps femoris muscle wich attaches the patella to the tuberosity of the tibia. NA *ligamentum patellae.*

patellar plexus. A nerve network situated in front of the patella.

patellar reflex. Contraction of the quadriceps femoris muscle with extension of the leg at the knee in response to a quick tap against the patellar tendon. Syn. *knee jerk, quadriceps reflex.*

patellar retinaculum. Either of the tendinous expansions from the vastus muscles and fascia lata which pass from the lateral and medial margins of the patella to the condyles of the tibia; the lateral patellar retinaculum (NA *retinaculum patellae laterale*) or the medial patellar retinaculum (NA *retinaculum patellae mediale*).

patellar synovial plica. INFRAPATELLAR SYNOVIAL FOLD.

patellar tendon. PATELLAR LIGAMENT.

patellar tendon reflex. PATELLAR REFLEX.

pa·tel·lec·to·my (pat"el·eck'tuh·mee) *n.* [*patella* + *-ectomy*]. The surgical removal or excision of a patella.

pa·tel·lo·ad·duc·tor reflex (pa·tel"o·uh·duck'tur). Adduction of the opposite thigh in response to percussion of one patellar tendon.

pa·tel·lo·fem·o·ral (pa·tel"o·fem'uh·rul) *adj.* Pertaining to the patella and the femur.

patellofemoral joint. The part of the knee joint involving the femur, the patella, and the ligaments connecting them. Contr. *tibiofemoral joint.*

[1]**pa·tent** (pay'tunt, pat'unt) *adj.* [L. *patens,* from *patere,* to be open, accessible]. Open; exposed, noticeable. —**pa·ten·cy** (pay'tun·see, pat'un·see) *n.*

[2]**pat·ent** (pat'unt) *n.* An assignment by a government to an inventor or discoverer of a useful process, composition, formula, machine, or device of the exclusive right, for a specific period of time, to manufacture, use, or sell the product of his invention or discovery or to assign to or license others with that right.

patent ductus arteriosus. A congenital anomaly in which the fetal ductus arteriosus persists after birth.

patent foramen ovale. Persistence of the fetal foramen ovale after birth, usually a functional patency. An anatomic patency is frequent at autopsy without functional patency in life.

patent medicine. A medicine, generally trademarked, whose composition is incompletely disclosed.

patent period. The time in a parasitic disease during which parasites are demonstrable in the body; occasionally used in reference to infection with other microorganisms.

patent urachus. A condition in which the urachus of the embryo does not become obliterated, but persists as a tube from the apex of the urinary bladder to the umbilicus.

pa·ter·nal (puh·tur'nul) *adj.* [L. *paternus*]. Pertaining to a father. —**pater·ni·ty** (·ni·tee) *n.*

paternity test. The determination of the blood groups of an identified mother, an identified child, and a putative father in order to determine hereditary blood characters and to establish the probability of paternity or nonpaternity.

Pat·er·son–Brown Kel·ly syndrome [D. R. *Paterson,* British otolaryngologist, 1863–1939; and A. *Brown Kelly*]. PLUMMER-VINSON SYNDROME.

Paterson-Kelly syndrome [D. R. *Paterson* and A. Brown *Kelly*]. PLUMMER-VINSON SYNDROME.

Paterson's bodies [R. *Paterson,* Scottish physician, 1814–1889]. The microscopic molluscum bodies of molluscum contagiosum.

Paterson's syndrome [D. R. *Paterson*]. PLUMMER-VINSON SYNDROME.

path-, patho- [Gk. *pathos,* experience, misfortune, disease]. A combining form meaning (a) *disease;* (b) *pathologic.*

-path [from *-pathy*]. A combining form designating (a) *specialist in a* (specified) *type of medical treatment;* (b) *individual suffering from a* (specified) *sickness* or *disease.*

path, *n. In neurology,* a nerve fiber pathway.

pa·the·ma (path·ee'muh) *n.* [Gk. *pathēma,* suffering, affection]. Any disease or morbid condition.

path·er·ga·sia (path"ur·gay'zhuh, ·zee·uh) *n.* [*path-* + *ergasia*]. *In psychiatry,* a term applied by Adolf Meyer to personality maladjustments associated with organic or structural changes in the body or with gross functional disturbances.

pa·ther·gia (pa·thur'jee·uh) *n.* PATHERGY.

path·er·gy (path'ur·jee) *n.* [*path-* + *-ergy*]. Either a subnormal response to an allergen or an unusually intense one, in which the individual becomes sensitive not only to the specific substance but to others; hyperergy or hypoergy.

pa·thet·ic (puh·thet'ick) *adj.* [Gk. *pathētikos*]. 1. Pertaining to or causing feelings. 2. *Obsol.* Pertaining to or designating the fourth cranial (trochlear) nerve.

pa·thet·i·cus (pa·thet'i·kus) *n.* [L., from Gk. *pathētikos*]. *Obsol.* TROCHLEAR NERVE.

path·e·tism (path'e·tiz·um) *n.* [Gk. *pathētos,* subject to external influence, + *-ism*]. Hypnotism, mesmerism, animal magnetism.

path·e·tist (path'e·tist) *n.* A mesmerizer, a hypnotist.

-pathia [L., from Gk. *pathos,* experience, misfortune, disease]. A combining form meaning *disease, affection.*

-pathic [*path-* + *-ic*]. A combining form meaning (a) *affected by, depending on, pertaining to,* or *originating in* or *caused by disease of a* (specified) *kind* or *part;* (b) *affected in a* (specified) *way.*

Pathilon Chloride. Trademark for tridihexethyl chloride, an anticholinergic drug used in the treatment of certain gastrointestinal disorders.

patho-. See *path-.*

patho·clis·is (path″o·klis′is) *n.* [*patho-* + Gk. *klisis,* inclination]. 1. A specific sensitivity for certain toxins or viruses. 2. A specific attraction of certain toxins or viruses for a particular organ or organs.

patho·gen (path′uh·jen, path′o·jin) *n.* [*patho-* + *-gen*]. Any agent which is capable of producing disease; usually applied to living agents.

patho·gen·e·sis (path″o·jen′e·sis) *n.* [*patho-* + *-genesis*]. The origin and course of development of disease. —**patho·ge·net·ic** (·je·net′ick) *adj.*

patho·gen·ic (path″uh·jen′ick) *adj.* [*patho-* + *-genic*]. 1. Producing or capable of producing disease. 2. Pertaining to pathogenesis. —**patho·ge·nic·i·ty** (path″o·je·nis′i·tee) *n.*

path·og·nom·ic (path″ug·nom′ick, ·no′mick) *adj.* PATHOGNOMONIC.

pa·thog·no·mon·ic (pa·thog″nuh·mon′ick, path″ug·no·) *adj.* [Gk. *pathognōmonikos,* from *patho-* + *gnōmōn,* discerning; index, pointer]. Characteristic or distinctive of a disease, enabling its recognition and differentiation from other diseases.

path·og·nos·tic (path″ug·nos′tick) *adj.* PATHOGNOMONIC.

patho·ki·ne·si·ol·o·gy (path″o·ki·nee″see·ol′uh·jee) *n.* [*patho-* + *kinesiology*]. The study of the effect of disease states on movement.

patho·le·sia (path″o·lee′zhuh, ·zee·uh) *n.* [*patho-* + Gk. *lēsis,* will, + *-ia*]. Any impairment or weakness of the will.

patho·log·ic (path″uh·loj′ick) *adj.* [Gk. *pathologikos*]. 1. Of or pertaining to pathology. 2. Pertaining to or caused by disease.

patho·log·i·cal (path″uh·loj′i·kul) *adj.* PATHOLOGIC.

pathological chemistry. Chemistry of abnormal tissues and the changes caused by disease.

pathological rigidity of the cervix uteri. Rigidity of the cervix uteri due to organic disease or cicatricial contraction.

pathologic amenorrhea. Amenorrhea due to pathologic conditions, such as hysterectomy, oophorectomy, absence of or damage to endometrium, ovarian failure, debility, or sympathetic vasomotor disturbances.

pathologic amputation. An amputation occurring as a result of some pathologic process.

pathologic anatomy. The study of the changes in structure caused by disease. Syn. *morbid anatomy.*

pathologic anxiety. NEGATIVE ANXIETY.

pathologic atrophy. Atrophy due to disease or other abnormality.

pathologic cramp syndrome. PSEUDOTETANY.

pathologic death. Death of a cell as the result of disease. Contr. *necrobiosis.*

pathologic diagnosis. A diagnosis based on the study of the structural lesions present.

pathologic dislocation. A dislocation resulting from joint disease with destruction of tissue, or from paralysis.

pathologic fracture. A fracture that occurs at the site of a local disease in a bone (as metastatic carcinoma) without significant external violence.

pathologic histology. The microscopic study of diseased tissue.

pathologic intoxication. An unusual reaction to alcoholic intoxication, characterized by an outburst of irrational, combative, and destructive behavior, which terminates when the patient falls into a deep stupor and for which he later has no memory.

pathologic lying or **mendacity.** Persistent habitual lying without external need or actual advantage, involving both falsifications of real events and development of fantasies. The individual may have complete insight, or the condition may be part of a neurosis, organic brain syndrome, personality disorder, or psychosis.

pathologic mitosis. Irregular, atypical, asymmetric, and multipolar mitosis, as often observed in cancer.

pathologic physiology. PATHOPHYSIOLOGY.

pathologic reflex. Any abnormal reflex indicative of a diseased state.

pathologic retraction ring. The abnormally thickened ridge of uterine musculature lying between the upper and lower uterine segments, resulting from obstructed labor and associated with extreme thinning of the lower uterine segment. Syn. *Bandl's ring.* Contr. *physiologic retraction ring.*

pathologic ring. PATHOLOGIC RETRACTION RING.

pa·thol·o·gist (pa·thol′uh·jist) *n.* A person trained and experienced in the study and practice of pathology.

pathologist's wart. TUBERCULOSIS VERRUCOSA.

pa·thol·o·gy (pa·thol′uh·jee) *n.* [Gk. *pathologia,* study of the passions, from *pathos,* experience, feeling, suffering, disease]. 1. The branch of biological science which deals with the nature of disease, through study of its causes, its process, and its effects, together with the associated alterations of structure and function. 2. Laboratory findings of disease, as distinguished from clinical signs and symptoms. 3. *Erron.* DISEASE.

patho·ma·nia (path″o·may′nee·uh) *n.* [*patho-* + *-mania*]. Moral insanity. See also *sociopathic personality disturbance.*

patho·mei·o·sis (path″o·migh·o′sis) *n.* [*patho-* + Gk. *meiōsis,* diminution]. A tendency on the part of a patient to minimize the seriousness of his disease. Contr. *pathopleiosis.*

pa·thom·e·try (pa·thom′e·tree) *n.* [*patho-* + *-metry*]. Estimation of the number of persons suffering from a disease and the conditions that increase or decrease this number. —**patho·met·ric** (path″o·met′rick) *adj.*

patho·mi·me·sis (path″o·mi·mee′sis) *n.* [*patho-* + *mimesis*]. Imitation of the symptoms and signs of a disease; occurs in the conversion type of hysterical neurosis and in malingering.

patho·mim·ic·ry (path″o·mim′i·kree) *n.* [*patho-* + *mimicry*]. PATHOMIMESIS.

patho·phil·ia (path″o·fil′ee·uh) *n.* [*patho-* + *-philia*]. Emotional adaptation by a patient to chronic illness.

patho·pho·bia (path″o·fo′bee·uh) *n.* [*patho-* + *-phobia*]. Exaggerated dread of disease.

patho·phor·ic (path″o·for′ick) *adj.* [*patho-* + *-phoric*]. Carrying or transmitting disease, said of certain insects.

pa·thoph·o·rous (path·off′uh·rus) *adj.* [*patho-* + *-phorous*]. PATHOPHORIC.

patho·phys·i·ol·o·gy (path″o·fiz″ee·ol′uh·jee) *n.* [*patho-* + *physiology*]. The study of disordered functions or of functions modified by disease. —**pathophysi·o·log·ic** (·uh·loj′ick), **pathophysiolog·i·cal** (·i·kul) *adj.*

patho·plei·o·sis (path″o·plye·o′sis) *n.* [*patho-* + *plei-* + *-osis*]. A tendency on the part of a patient to exaggerate the seriousness of his disease. Contr. *pathomeiosis.*

patho·psy·chol·o·gy (path″o·sigh·kol′uh·jee) *n.* [*patho-* + *psychology*]. The branch of science dealing with mental processes, particularly as manifested by abnormal cognitive, perceptual, and intellectual functioning, during the course of mental disorders. See also *psychopathology.*

pa·tho·sis (pa·tho′sis) *n.*, pl. **patho·ses** (·seez) [*path-* + *-osis*]. A diseased condition, abnormality, or pathologic finding.

path·way, *n. In neurophysiology,* a course along nerve fibers which an impulse travels either from the periphery to the center (afferent pathway) or from the center to the effector organ (efferent pathway).

-pathy [L. *-pathia,* from Gk. *-pathia, -patheia,* from *pathos,* experience, sensation; suffering, disease]. A combining form meaning (a) *disease;* (b) *therapy;* (c) *experience, sensation.*

pa·tient (pay'shunt) *n.* [MF., sufferer, suffering, from L. *patiens,* from *pati,* to suffer]. A person under medical care or receiving health care services.

patient vectors. *In psychoanalysis,* immature transference needs expressed between persons when there is some possibility of their satisfaction and resolution.

pat·ri·cide (pat'ri·side) *n.* [L. *patricidium* and *patricida*]. 1. Murder of one's own father. 2. One who murders his own father.

Pat·rick's trigger areas [H. T. *Patrick,* U.S. neurologist, 1860–1938]. Dolorogenic areas of the skin, mucous membrane of the cheeks, sides of the tongue, upper and lower lips, within the area of distribution of the fifth cranial nerve, stimulation of which initiates a paroxysmal attack of trigeminal neuralgia.

pat·ri·lin·e·al (pat"ri·lin'ee·ul) *adj.* [L. *pater, patris,* father, + *lineal*]. Pertaining to descent through the male line.

pat·ten (pat'un) *n.* [OF. *patin,* wooden shoe, clog, from *patte,* paw, hoof]. A metal support serving as a high sole and attached to the shoe on the sound leg, to prevent weight bearing in hip disease and to permit the employment of traction apparatus on the affected leg.

pat·tern, *n.* [OF. *patron,* from L. *patronus,* patron]. 1. A comparatively fully realized model or form proposed or accepted for copying. 2. A functional integration of elements, perceived simultaneously or successively, which together form a design or unit; the parts are separately distinguishable but together form a perceived whole. Syn. *gestalt.* 3. A functional integration of distinguishable elements which operate or respond as a unit, as an action, behavioral, motor, neural, social, or thought pattern. 4. A form, usually of wax, from which a mold is made for casting a dental restoration or appliance.

pat·tern·ing, *n.* 1. Behavior, or the development or imposition thereof, in imitation of a model or in response to a whole set of stimuli. 2. Therapeutic maneuvers and exercises, involving one or more external parts or the whole of the body, imposed on a patient or carried out by him purposefully, and utilizing reflex patterns and various sensory stimuli, designed to facilitate voluntary neuromuscular activity.

pat·ting test. A cerebellar function test in which the patient pats with each hand his other hand, the ipsilateral knee, or the examiner's hand. Normally this is carried out with even amplitude and a smooth rhythm.

Pat·ton-John·ston tube. A four-lumen plastic tube for the treatment of bleeding from esophageal varices. There is one lumen to each of two balloons which inflate separately, one lumen to aspirate the stomach, and one to administer thrombin solution.

pat·u·lin (pat'yoo·lin) *n.* An antibiotic substance originally obtained from cultures of *Penicillium patulum;* CLAVACIN.

pat·u·lous (pat'yoo·lus) *adj.* [L. *patulus,* from *patere,* to stand open]. Expanded; open; loose. —**patulous·ness** (·nus) *n.*

Paul-Bunnell-Davidsohn test. PAUL-BUNNELL TEST.

Paul-Bun·nell test [J. R. *Paul,* U.S. physician, 1893–1971; and W. W. *Bunnell,* U.S. physician, b. 1902]. A test for the presence of heterophil antibodies in the serum produced in infectious mononucleosis and other diseases.

Paul·lin·ia (paw·lin'ee·uh) *n.* [C. F. *Paullini,* German botanist, 1643–1712]. A genus of woody vines. The seeds of *Paullinia cupana* are the source of guarana.

Paul-Mikulicz operation [F. T. *Paul,* English surgeon, 1851–1941; and J. von *Mikulicz*-Radecki]. MIKULICZ' OPERATION.

Paul-Mix·ter tube [F. T. *Paul;* and S. J. *Mixter,* U.S. surgeon, 1855–1926]. PAUL'S TUBE.

pau·lo·car·dia (paw"lo·kahr'dee·uh) *n.* [Gk. *paula,* pause, + *-cardia*]. 1. A subjective sensation of intermission or momentary stoppage of the heartbeat. 2. An abnormally long interval between heartbeats.

Paul's operation [F. T. *Paul*]. MIKULICZ' OPERATION.

Paul's sign (po^{h}l) [C. C. T. *Paul,* French physician, 1833–1896]. A sign for adhesive pericarditis, in which the apex impulse is feeble as compared with the forcible impulse over the rest of the heart.

Paul's test (paowl) [G. *Paul,* Austrian physician, 1859–1935]. A test for smallpox in which the scarified cornea of a rabbit is inoculated with material from a suspected lesion. If the lesion is smallpox, a typical keratitis develops in about 50% of the cases.

Paul's tube [F. T. *Paul*]. A glass drainage tube with flanged edges for temporary use in intestinal operations.

paunch, *n.* [OF. *pance,* from L. *pantex*]. 1. The abdominal cavity and its contents. 2. RUMEN.

pause, *n.* [Of., from L. *pausa,* from Gk. *pausis*]. A temporary stop or rest.

pau·si·me·nia (paw"si·mee'nee·uh) *n.* [Gk. *pausis,* cessation, + *men-* + *-ia*]. MENOPAUSE.

Pau·tri·er's microabscess (po·tree·e^{y}') [L. M. *Pautrier,* French dermatologist, 1876–1959]. A small group of atypical cells occurring in the lower epidermis of patients with mycosis fungoides or reticulum-cell sarcoma of the skin.

pavaex. PAVEX.

pavement epithelium. Simple SQUAMOUS EPITHELIUM.

pave·ment·ing, *n.* A stage in the process of tissue inflammation in which the bloodstream in the capillaries becomes slowed, the leukocytes gravitating out of the central current to become adherent to the vessel walls.

Paveril. Trademark for dioxyline, used as the phosphate salt to relax smooth muscle spasm.

pa·vex, pa·vaex (pay'vecks) *n.* [*pa*ssive *va*scular *ex*ercise]. A positive-negative pressure apparatus for passive exercise in the treatment of thromboangiitis obliterans or other peripheral vascular disease.

paving-stone nevus. COBBLESTONE NEVUS.

Pav·lov·i·an conditioning (pav·lov'ee·un, ·lo'vee·un) [I. P. *Pavlov,* Russian physiologist, 1849–1936]. CONDITIONING (1).

Pav·lov·i·an·ism (pav·lov'ee·un·iz·um) *n.* The experimental methods, involving conditioning or the establishment of conditioned reflexes, and the school of behavioristic psychology based on the work of I. P. Pavlov.

Pav·lov's pouch (pa^{h}v'luf) [I. P. *Pavlov*]. A small portion of stomach, completely separated from the main stomach, but retaining its vagal nerve branches, which communicates with the exterior; used in the long-term investigation of gastric secretion and particularly in the study of conditioned reflexes.

pa·vor (pay'vur, pav'or) *n.* [L., from *pavere,* to fear]. Fright; fear.

pavor di·ur·nus (dye·ur'nus). Daytime attacks of terror or anxiety, especially in children.

pavor noc·tur·nus (nock·tur'nus). Night terror; differing from a nightmare in that it is not recalled on awakening.

Pa·vy's disease [F. W. *Pavy,* English physician, 1829–1911]. Recurrent proteinuria.

Pavy's joint [F. W. *Pavy*]. Arthritis seen in typhoid fever.

Pavy's solution [F. W. *Pavy*]. A modification of Fehling's solution, used to test for such reducing substances as sugars.

Paw·lik's folds (pa^{h}v'lik) [K. J. *Pawlik,* Bohemian surgeon, 1849–1914]. The anterior columns of the vagina which form the lateral boundaries of Pawlik's triangle, and serve as landmarks in locating the openings of the ureters.

Pawlik's triangle [K. J. *Pawlik*]. A triangle on the anterior wall of the vagina which corresponds to the trigonum vesicae.

paw·paw (paw'paw) *n.* PAPAW.

Payr's clamp (pye'ur) [E. *Payr,* German surgeon, 1871–1947].

A crushing forceps used before cutting, in gastrointestinal resection.

Payr's disease [E. *Payr*]. Colonic stasis due to kinking at the hepatic or splenic flexures.

paz·ox·ide (pa·zock'side) *n.* 6,7-Dichloro-3-(3-cyclopenten-1-yl)-2*H*-1,2,4-benzothiadiazine 1,1-dioxide, $C_{12}H_{10}Cl_2N_2O_2S$, an antihypertensive.

Pb [L. *plumbum*]. Symbol for lead.

P. B. E. [*P*erlsucht *B*acillen *E*mulsion]. An original tuberculin prepared from bovine tubercle bacilli, similar to Koch's new tuberculin.

PBI Abbreviation for *protein-bound iodine.*

P blood group. A system of erythrocyte antigens first defined by their reaction with anti-P, an immune rabbit antiserum, and later broadened to include related antigens.

pc Abbreviation for *picocurie.*

P.C. Professional Corporation.

PCB Abbreviation for *polychlorinated biphenyl.*

PCG Abbreviation for *phonocardiogram.*

P_{CO_2} Symbol for the partial pressure of carbon dioxide. See *partial pressure.*

P.D. Doctor of Pharmacy.

Pd Symbol for palladium.

Pé·an's forceps (pe^y·ah$^{n'}$) [J. E. *Péan,* French surgeon, 1830–1898]. One of the earliest hemostats, which provided the basic design for many subsequent modifications.

Péan's position [J. E. *Péan*]. A position used in operations in which the surgeon sits on a stool between the patient's legs, with the patient lying supine on a table.

peanut oil. Refined fixed oil obtained from seed kernels of one or more cultivated varieties of *Arachis hypogaea;* used as a vehicle for injections. Syn. *arachis oil.*

pearl, *n.* 1. A rounded aggregation of squamous epithelial cells, concentrically arranged, seen in certain carcinomas and also in sites of epithelial union of embryonically open hiatuses, e.g., palatine raphe. Syn. *epithelial pearl.* 2. PERLE. 3. A mucous cast of a bronchus or bronchiole in the sputum of asthmatic patients. Syn. *Laennec's perle.*

pearl barley. Husked barley grains, rounded and polished.

pearl disease. A manifestation of tuberculosis in cattle, consisting of small calcified and disseminated lesions commonly found on pleural and peritoneal surfaces.

pearly, *adj.* Resembling a pearl in color or appearance.

pearly eye. OCULAR LYMPHOMATOSIS.

pearly tumor. CHOLESTEATOMA.

pea-soup stools. The peculiar liquid evacuation of some patients with typhoid fever.

peat, *n.* The product of the spontaneous decomposition of plants, especially swamp plants, in many cases mixed with sand, loam, clay, lime, iron pyrites, or ocher.

pec·tase (peck'tace) *n.* An enzyme, found associated with pentose in fruits, which converts the pectose into pectin.

pec·ten (peck'tin) *n.* [L., comb]. 1. *Obsol.* PUBIS. 2. The middle third of the anal canal. 3. A body part which is more or less comblike in structure, as pecten of the pubic bone.

pecten of the pubic bone. A sharp ridge on the anterior surface of the superior ramus extending laterally from the pubic tubercle; it marks the site of attachment of the pectineal fascia, the lacunar ligament, and the lateral extension of the falx inguinalis. NA *pecten ossis pubis.*

pec·te·no·sis (peck''te·no'sis) *n.* [*pecten* + *-osis*]. Induration of the middle third of the anal canal.

pecten os·sis pu·bis (os'is pew'bis) [NA]. PECTEN OF THE PUBIC BONE.

pec·tic acid (peck'tick). A complex acid, partially demethylated, obtained from the pectin of fruits.

pec·tin (peck'tin) *n.* [Gk. *pēktos,* coagulated, + *-in*]. A purified carbohydrate product obtained from the inner portion of the rind of citrus fruits, or from apple pomace; consists chiefly of partially methoxylated polygalacturonic acids. Used as a demulcent and as an emulsifying and thickening agent.

pec·tin·ase (peck'ti·nace) *n.* An enzyme that catalyzes transformation of pectin into sugars and galacturonic acid.

pec·ti·nate (peck'ti·nate) *adj.* [L. *pectinatus,* from *pecten,* comb]. Arranged like the teeth of a comb.

pectinate ligament. Trabecular tissue from the posterior elastic lamina which extends into the substance of the iris. NA *ligamentum pectinatum anguli iridocornealis.*

pectinate line. DENTATE LINE.

pectinate muscles. The small muscular columns traversing the inner surface of the auricles of the heart. NA *musculi pectinati.* See also Table of Muscles in the Appendix.

pec·tin·e·al (peck·tin'ee·ul) *adj.* [L. *pecten, pectinis,* comb, + *-al*]. 1. Comb-shaped. 2. Pertaining to the pecten or pubic bone.

pectineal fascia. The portion of the fascia lata associated with the pectineus muscle. NA *fascia pectinea.*

pectineal ligament. A fibrous lateral extension of the falx inguinalis, attached to the pecten of the pubic bone. NA *ligamentum pectineale.*

pectineal line. 1. The line on the posterior surface of the femur, running downward from the lesser trochanter and giving attachment to the pectineus muscle. NA *linea pectinea.* 2. PECTEN OF THE PUBIC BONE.

pectineal triangle. An area bounded anteriorly by the anterior abdominal wall, laterally by the external iliac vessels, and medially by the pelvic brim.

pec·ti·ne·us (peck·tin'ee·us) *n.* [NL., from *pecten*]. A muscle arising from the pubis and inserted on the femur. NA *musculus pectineus.* See also Table of Muscles in the Appendix.

pec·tin·i·form (peck·tin'i·form) *adj.* [L. *pecten, pectinis,* comb, + *-iform*]. Shaped like a comb.

pectiniform septum. The septum between the corpora cavernosa of the penis or clitoris.

pec·tin·ose (peck'tin·oce) *n.* ARABINOSE.

pectin sugar. ARABINOSE.

pec·ti·za·tion (peck''ti·zay'shun) *n.* [Gk. *pēktikos,* coagulating]. *In colloid chemistry,* the transformation of sols into gels. See also *coagulation, flocculation.*

pec·to·ral (peck'tuh·rul) *adj.* [L. *pectoralis,* from *pectus, pectoris,* breast, chest]. Pertaining to the chest, as the pectoral muscles (pectorales), which connect the arm and the chest.

pectoral fascia. Deep fascia around the pectoralis major muscle on the anterior aspect of the thorax. NA *fascia pectoralis.* See also Plate 24.

pectoral girdle. SHOULDER GIRDLE.

pec·to·ra·lis (peck''to·ray'lis, ·rah'lis) *n.*, pl. **pectora·les** (·leez) [L., pectoral]. One of two muscles, major and minor, on the anterior aspect of the chest.

pectoralis fascia. PECTORAL FASCIA.

pectoralis major. The larger muscle of the anterior thoracic wall. NA *musculus pectoralis major.* See also Table of Muscles in the Appendix.

pectoralis mi·ni·mus (min'i·mus). A variant of the pectoralis minor muscle, extending from the cartilage of the first rib to the coracoid process.

pectoralis minor. The smaller and deeper muscle of the anterior thoracic wall. NA *musculus pectoralis minor.* See also Table of Muscles in the Appendix.

pectoral reflex. Adduction and slight internal rotation of the arm in response to a sharp blow against the humeral insertion of the tendon of the pectoralis major muscle.

pec·to·ril·o·quy (peck''to·ril'uh·kwee) *n.* [L. *pectus, pectoris,* breast, + *loqui,* to speak]. Exaggerated bronchophony, in which there is distinct transmission of articulate speech on auscultation over the lung; indicative of cavitation or consolidation.

pec·tose (peck'toce) *n.* The water-insoluble pectin substance occurring in various unripe fruits. It is converted into the water-soluble pectin by the combined action of weak acid and heat, or, in the fruit, by the enzyme pectase, as the fruit ripens. Syn. *pectinogen, protopectin.*

pec·tous (peck'tus) *adj.* Pertaining to pectin or pectose.

pec·tus (peck'tus) *n.*, genit. **pec·to·ris** (peck'to·ris) [L.] [NA]. The chest or breast.

pectus car·i·na·tum (kăr·i·nay'tum). PIGEON BREAST.

pectus ex·ca·va·tum (ecks·kuh·vay'tum). FUNNEL CHEST.

¹ped-, paed-, pedo-, paedo- [Gk. *pais, paidos*]. A combining form meaning *child.*

²ped-, pedi-, pedo- [L. *pes, pedis*]. A combining form meaning *foot, pedal, hoof.*

-ped, -pede [L. *pes, pedis,* foot]. A combining form meaning *having a* (specified) *number or kind of feet.*

ped·atro·phia, paed·atro·phia (pee"da·tro'fee·uh) *n.* PEDATROPHY.

ped·at·ro·phy, paed·at·ro·phy (pe·dat'ruh·fee) *n.* [*ped-* + *atrophy*]. 1. Any wasting disease of childhood. 2. Mesenteric lymphadenitis associated with tuberculous infection.

-pede. See *-ped.*

ped·er·as·ty, paed·er·as·ty (ped'ur·as"tee, pee'dur·) *n.* [Gk. *paiderastia,* love of boys, from *pais, paidos,* boy, + *erastēs,* lover]. 1. Sexual intercourse between man and boy. 2. Specifically, sodomy between man and boy. —**peder·ast, paeder·ast,** *n.*

pedes. Plural of *pes.*

pe·de·sis (pe·dee'sis) *n.*, pl. **pede·ses** (·seez) [Gk. *pēdēsis,* leaping]. BROWNIAN MOTION.

pedi·al·gia (ped"ee·al'jee·uh, pee"dee·) *n.* [*pedi-* + *-algia*]. Pain in the foot.

pe·di·at·ric, pae·di·at·ric (pee"dee·at'rick) *adj.* Of or pertaining to pediatrics.

pe·di·a·tri·cian, pae·di·a·tri·cian (pee"dee·uh·trish'un) *n.* A physician specializing in pediatrics.

pe·di·at·rics, pae·di·at·rics (pee"dee·at'ricks) *n.* [*ped-* + *-iatrics*]. The branch of medicine that deals with the growth and development of the child through adolescence and with the care, treatment, and prevention of diseases, injuries, and defects of children.

pe·di·at·rist, pae·di·at·rist (pee"dee·at'rist, pe·dye'uh·trist) *n.* PEDIATRICIAN.

pe·di·at·ry, pae·di·at·ry (pee'dee·at"ree, pe·dye'uh·tree) *n.* PEDIATRICS.

ped·i·cel·late (ped'i·se·late, ped"i·sel'ut) *adj.* [NL. *pedicellus,* dim. of *pediculus,* pedicle, + *-ate*]. PEDUNCULATED.

ped·i·cle (ped'i·kul) *n.* [L. *pediculus,* little foot]. A slender process serving as a foot or stem, as the pedicle of a tumor, or a narrow connection, as the pedicle of a vertebra.

pedicle clamp. A clamp for grasping and holding a vascular pedicle during removal of an organ or a tumor.

pedicle flap. A type of flap that obtains its blood supply through a narrow base, or pedicle; used when length is required to fill a remote defect, or on a movable part which can be approximated to the donor site. See also *bipedicled flap, bridge flap, caterpillar flap, compound flap, gauntlet flap, open jump flap, tubed flap, vascular flap.*

pedicle graft. PEDICLE FLAP.

pe·dic·ter·us, pae·dic·ter·us (pe·dick'tur·us) *n.* [*ped-* + *icterus*]. PHYSIOLOGIC JAUNDICE OF THE NEWBORN.

pe·dic·u·lar (pe·dick'yoo·lur) *adj.* [L. *pedicularis,* from *pediculus,* louse]. Of or pertaining to lice.

¹pe·dic·u·la·tion (pe·dick"yoo·lay'shun) *n.* The development or formation of a pedicle.

²pediculation, *n.* [L. *pediculus,* louse]. Infestation with lice; PEDICULOSIS.

pe·dic·u·li·cide (pe·dick'yoo·li·side) *n.* [L. *pediculus,* louse, + *-cide*]. An agent that destroys lice.

Pe·dic·u·loi·des (pi·dick"yoo·loy'deez) *n.* A genus of mites.

Pediculoides ven·tri·co·sus (ven·tri·ko'sus). A small mite which infests straw, stored grain, and cotton. Among laborers handling cereals and cotton it causes outbreaks of a dermatitis (acarodermatitis urticarioides) which may be marked in severe cases by fever and nausea.

pe·dic·u·lo·pho·bia (pe·dick"yoo·lo·fo'bee·uh) *n.* [L. *pediculus,* louse, + *-phobia*]. Abnormal dread of infestation with lice.

pe·dic·u·lo·sis (pe·dick"yoo·lo'sis) *n.* [L. *pediculus,* louse, + *-osis*]. A skin disease due to infestation by lice, characterized by intense pruritis and cutaneous lesions.

pediculosis cap·i·tis (kap'i·tis). Infestation of the scalp with the species *Pediculus humanus* var. *capitis.*

pediculosis cor·po·ris (kor'puh·ris). Infestation of the skin of the body with the species *Pediculus humanus* var. *corporis.*

pediculosis pal·pe·bra·rum (pal"pe·brair'um). Lice infesting the eyebrows and the eyelashes. See also *pediculosis pubis.*

pediculosis pu·bis (pew'bis). An infestation of the pubic hair with *Phthirius pubis,* the crab louse; may spread over the body and involve the axillas, eyebrows, and eyelashes.

pe·dic·u·lous (pe·dick'yoo·lus) *adj.* [L. *pediculus,* louse, + *-ous*]. Infested with lice; lousy.

Pe·dic·u·lus (pe·dick'yoo·lus) *n.* [L., louse]. A genus of lice, species of which produce dermatitis and transmit diseases, such as typhus fever, trench fever, and relapsing fever.

pediculus, *n.* [L., dim. of *pes, pedis,* foot]. PEDICLE.

pediculus ar·cus ver·te·brae (ahr'kus vur'te·bree) [NA]. VERTEBRAL PEDICLE.

Pediculus hu·ma·nus cap·i·tis (hew·may'nus kap'i·tis). HEAD LOUSE.

Pediculus humanus cor·po·ris (kor'puh·ris). BODY LOUSE.

ped·i·cure (ped'i·kewr) *n.* [F. *pédicure,* from *pedi-* + L. *cura,* care]. Care of the feet.

ped·i·gree (ped'i·gree) *n.* A register or chart showing ancestral history; used by geneticists to assist in the analysis of Mendelian inheritance.

ped·i·palp (ped'i·palp) *n.* [*pedi-* + L. *palpus,* feeler]. One of the pincer appendages of *Arachnida* for attaching the animal to its host while sucking.

pe·di·tis (pe·dye'tis) *n.* [*ped-* + *-itis*]. An inflammation of the pedal bone of a horse.

pedo-. See *ped-.*

pe·do·don·tia, pae·do·don·tia (pee"do·don'chee·uh) *n.* PEDODONTICS.

pe·do·don·tics, pae·do·don·tics (pee"do·don'ticks) *n.* [*ped-* + *odont-* + *-ics*]. The branch of dentistry that is concerned with the dental care and treatment of children.

pe·do·don·tist, pae·do·don·tist (pee"do·don'tist) *n.* A dentist who specializes in pedodontics.

pe·do·don·tol·o·gy, pae·do·don·tol·o·gy (pee"do·don·tol'uh·jee) *n.* PEDODONTICS.

pedo·dy·na·mom·e·ter (ped"o·dye"nuh·mom'e·tur) *n.* [*pedo-* + *dynamometer*]. An instrument for measuring the muscular strength of the leg.

pe·do·gen·e·sis, pae·do·gen·e·sis (pee"do·jen'e·sis) *n.* [*pedo-,* child, + *-genesis*]. NEOTENY.

pe·dol·o·gist, pae·dol·o·gist (pee·dol'uh·jist) *n.* [*pedology* + *-ist*]. A specialist in the study of children.

pe·dol·o·gy, pae·dol·o·gy (pee·dol'uh·jee) *n.* [*pedo-,* child, + *-logy*]. The science, or sum of knowledge, regarding childhood, its psychologic as well as physiologic aspects. See also *pediatrics.*

¹pe·dom·e·ter, pae·dom·e·ter (pee·dom'e·tur) *n.* [*pedo-,* child, + *-meter*]. An instrument for weighing and measuring a newborn child. —**pedome·try, paedome·try** (·tree) *n.*

²pe·dom·e·ter (ped·om'e·tur) *n.* [*pedo-,* foot, + *-meter*]. An instrument that registers the number of footsteps in walking. —**pedome·try** (·tree) *n.*

pe·do·no·sol·o·gy, pae·do·no·sol·o·gy (pee"do·no·sol'uh·jee) *n.* [*pedo-,* child, + *nosology*]. The study of diseases peculiar to or predominant in childhood. See also *pediatrics, pedology.*

pe·dop·a·thy (ped·op'uth·ee) *n.* [*pedo-* + *-pathy*]. Any disease of the foot.

pe·do·phil·ia, pae·do·phil·ia (pee"do·fil'ee·uh) *n.* [*pedo-* + *-philia*]. 1. Fondness for children. 2. Love of children by adults for sexual purposes. Compare *pederasty.*

pe·do·pho·bia, pae·do·pho·bia (pee″do·fo′bee·uh) *n.* [*pedo-* + *-phobia*]. Abnormal dislike or fear of children.

pe·do·psy·chi·a·trist (pee″do·sigh·kigh′uh·trist) *n.* [*pedo-* + *psychiatrist*]. A psychiatrist who specializes in treating children.

pe·dun·cle (pe·dunk′ul, ped′unk·ul, pee′dunk·ul) *n.* [NL. *pedunculus,* dim. of L. *pes, pedis,* foot]. 1. A narrow part acting as a support. 2. Any of various bands of nerve fibers connecting various parts of the cerebellum, medulla oblongata, pons, and other parts of the brain. —**pe·dun·cu·lar** (pe·dunk′yoo·lur) *adj.*

peduncle of the pineal body. A delicate white band passing forward from each side of the pineal body along the edge of the third ventricle.

peduncular hallucination or **hallucinosis.** Visual hallucinations, often recognized by the patient as such, composed of a panorama of colorful objects, people, or scenes; frequently combined with altered (nonhallucinatory) mentation; observed in acute lesions of the diencephalon.

peduncular syndrome. Ipsilateral hemiataxia, Weber's syndrome, dysarthria, and conjugate ocular paralysis, in various combinations due to occlusions of a branch of the posterior cerebral artery to the cerebral peduncle which penetrates to the decussation of the superior cerebellar peduncle, oculomotor nucleus, and medial longitudinal fasciculus. If the medial and lateral lemnisci are also affected, there is contralateral reduction in touch and in hearing.

pe·dun·cu·late (pe·dunk′yoo·lut) *adj.* PEDUNCULATED.

pe·dun·cu·lat·ed (pe·dunk′yoo·lay·tid) *adj.* Having a peduncle.

pe·dun·cu·lo·pon·tine (pe·dunk″yoo·lo·pon′tine, ·teen) *adj.* Pertaining to or affecting the cerebral peduncle and the pons.

pe·dun·cu·lot·o·my (pe·dunk″yoo·lot′uh·mee) *n.* [*pedunculus* + *-tomy*]. Surgical interruption of the cerebral peduncles, either unilaterally or bilaterally, for the relief of involuntary movement disorders.

pe·dun·cu·lus (pe·dunk′yoo·lus) *n.,* pl. **pedunculi** (·lye) [NL.]. PEDUNCLE.

pedunculus ce·re·bel·la·ris inferior (serr·e·bel·air′is) [NA]. INFERIOR CEREBELLAR PEDUNCLE.

pedunculus cerebellaris me·di·us (mee′dee·us) [NA]. MIDDLE CEREBELLAR PEDUNCLE.

pedunculus cerebellaris superior [NA]. SUPERIOR CEREBELLAR PEDUNCLE.

pedunculus ce·re·bri (serr′e·brye) [NA]. CEREBRAL PEDUNCLE.

pedunculus cor·po·ris ma·mil·la·ris (kor′po·ris mam·i·lair′is) [NA]. A fiber tract connecting the mamillary body with the tegmentum of the mesencephalon.

pedunculus floc·cu·li (flock′yoo·lye) [NA]. A band connecting the flocculus with the inferior medullary vellum.

pedunculus tha·la·mi inferior (thal′uh·migh) [NA]. Radiating fibers connecting the thalamus and frontal lobe.

peel·ing, *n.* The process of desquamation, as after any inflammation of the skin. It is a result of disturbed keratinization of epidermis.

Peet's operation [M. M. *Peet,* U.S. surgeon, 1885–1949]. Supradiaphragmatic removal of the sympathetic nerves and ganglions for the relief of hypertension.

peg, *n.* 1. A pointed pin of wood, metal, or other material. 2. A wooden leg.

peg·a·nine (peg′uh·neen, ·nin) *n.* *l*-Peganine. An alkaloid, $C_{11}H_{12}N_2O$, from the leaves of *Adhatoda vasica* and *Peganum harmala;* has bronchodilator activity. Syn. *vasicine.*

Peganone. Trademark for ethotoin, an anticonvulsant used in the management of grand mal epilepsy.

peg lateral incisor A form of localized microdontia in which the maxillary lateral incisors are undersized with a tapered, cone-shaped crown.

pe·gly·col 5 oleate (pe·glye′kole). A pharmaceutic emulsifying agent consisting of mixed esters of partially esterified glycerine and polyethylene glycols.

peg·o·ter·ate (peg″o·terr″ate) *n.* A condensation of terephthalic acid and ethylene glycol used as a suspending agent.

pe·gox·ol 7 stearate (pe·gock′sole). A mixture of stearate esters of ethylene glycol and polyethylene glycol used as an emulsifying agent.

peg teeth. HUTCHINSON'S TEETH.

pei·no·ther·a·py (pye″no·therr′uh·pee) *n.* [Gk. *peina,* hunger, + *therapy*]. The cure of disease by deprivation of food.

pel-, pelo- [Gk. *pēlos*]. A combining form meaning *mud.*

pe·la·da (pe·lah′duh) *n.* [Sp., from *pelar,* to remove hair, pluck, from *pelo,* hair]. Alopecia areata of the scalp.

pe·lade (pe·lahd′) *n.* [F., from *peler,* to remove or lose hair; to peel]. PELADA.

pel·age (pel′ij) *n.* [F., from *poil,* hair]. The hairy covering of the body.

pel·a·gism (pel′uh·jiz·um) *n.* [Gk. *pelagos,* sea, + *-ism*]. SEASICKNESS.

pel·ar·gon·ic acid (pel″ahr·gon′ick). The fatty acid, $CH_3(CH_2)_7COOH$, obtained by oxidation of oleic acid; occurs in the glycerides of certain oils.

Pel-Ebstein disease, fever, or **syndrome** [P. K. *Pel,* Dutch physician, 1852–1919; and W. *Ebstein*]. Cyclic fever occasionally associated with malignant lymphoma.

p electron. An electron in the p or sixth shell surrounding the nucleus of an atom.

Pel·ger-Hu·ët anomaly (pel′ghur, huᵉ·et′) [K. *Pelger,* Dutch physician, 1885–1931; and G. *Huët,* Dutch physician, 20th century]. PELGER'S ANOMALY.

Pelger's anomaly [K. *Pelger*]. A hereditary anomaly of granulocytes characterized by small neutrophilic leukocytes in the peripheral blood with no more than one or two nuclear lobes and unusually coarse nuclear chromatin. Syn. *Pelger-Huët anomaly.*

pel·i·com·e·ter (pel″i·kom′e·tur) *n.* [Gk. *pelyx, pelykos,* bowl, + *-meter*]. PELVIMETER.

pel·i·di·si (pel″i·dee′see, ·dee′zee) *n.* [L. *pondus decies lineare divisio sedentis altitudo*]. According to Pirquet, the cube of the sitting height of a person expressed in centimeters is approximately the weight in grams of a normal person. The ratio, as expressed in the following formulas, is called the pelidisi: (10 times the weight)/(sitting height)^3 = 100%, or $\sqrt[3]{10}$ times the weight/(sitting height) = 100%.

pel·i·o·sis (pel″ee·o′sis, pee″lee·) *n.* [Gk. *peliōsis,* extravasation of blood, from *pelios,* black and blue, livid]. PURPURA. —**peli·ot·ic** (·ot′ick) *adj.*

peliosis he·pa·tis (hep′uh·tis). A condition in which small spaces throughout the liver are filled with fluid or clotted blood; seen rarely in patients dead of tuberculosis, or other diseases.

peliosis rheu·mat·i·ca (roo·mat′i·kuh). SCHÖNLEIN'S PURPURA.

Pe·li·zae·us-Merz·bach·er disease (peʸ·lee·tseʸ′o͞os, mehrts′-bakʰh·ur) [F. *Pelizaeus,* German neurologist, 1850–1917; and E. *Merzbacher*]. A slowly progressive X-linked recessive genetic disease characterized pathologically by extensive cerebral and cerebellar demyelination and clinically by various signs, including nystagmus, ataxia, spasticity, and dementia starting in early infancy. Some heterozygous females develop symptoms.

pell- [L. *pellis*]. A combining form meaning *skin.*

pel·lag·ra (pe·lag′ruh, pe·lay′gruh) *n.* [NL., from It. *pelle,* skin, + *agra,* rough]. A syndrome due to a deficiency of niacin or tryptophan, with a characteristic symmetric dermatitis of the exposed parts, stomatitis, glossitis, diarrhea, and, in later stages, dementia. —**pel·lag·rous** (·lag′rus) *adj.*

pellagra-preventive factor. NIACIN. Abbreviated, p-p factor.

pellagra si·ne pellagra (sin′ee). Pellagra without the characteristic skin lesions.

pel·lag·rin (pe·lag′rin) *n.* A person afflicted with pellagra.

Pel·le·gri·ni-Stie·da disease (pel·le·gree′nee, shtee′dah) [A. *Pellegrini,* Italian surgeon, 20th century; and A. *Stieda,* German surgeon, 1869–1945]. Posttraumatic calcification of the medial collateral ligament of the knee.

pel·let (pel′it) *n.* [OF. *pelote,* from L. *pila,* ball]. A small pill.

pel·le·tier·ine (pel″e·teer′een, ·in, pel″e·tye′reen) *n.* [J. *Pelletier,* French chemist, 1782–1842]. An alkaloid or mixture of alkaloids from pomegranate bark; formerly used, mostly as the tannate salt, as a taeniafuge. Syn. *punicine.*

-pellic [Gk. *pella,* bowl, + *-ic*]. A combining form meaning *having a* (specified kind of) *pelvis.*

pel·li·cle (pel′i·kul) *n.* [OF. *pellicule,* from L. *pellicula*]. 1. A thin membrane, or cuticle. 2. A film on the surface of a liquid. 3. A thin brown or gray film of salivary proteins that forms on teeth within minutes after being cleaned. —**pel·lic·u·lar** (pe·lick′yoo·lur), **pellicu·lous** (·lus), **pellicu·late** (·late) *adj.*

pel·lic·u·la (pe·lick′yoo·luh) *n.* [L., dim of *pellis,* skin]. EPIDERMIS.

pel·li·to·ry (pel′i·to″ree) *n.* PYRETHRUM (1).

Pel·li·zi's syndrome (pel·leet′tsee) [G. B. *Pellizi,* Italian, 19th–20th century]. PINEAL SYNDROME.

pel·lo·tine (pel′o·teen, ·tin) *n.* [Sp. *pellote,* variant of *peyote,* + *-ine*]. An alkaloid, $C_{13}H_{19}NO_3$, from the Mexican cactus, *Lophophora williamsii,* that produces central nervous system depression.

pel·lu·cid (pe·lew′sid) *adj.* [L. *pellucidus,* from *per-,* through, + *lucere,* to shine]. Transparent; translucent; not opaque.

pelo-. See *pel-.*

pe·loid (pee′loid) *n.* [*pel-* + *-oid*]. Generic term for mineral or vegetable muds used in physical therapy.

pe·lol·o·gy (pe·lol′o·jee) *n.* [*pelo-* + *-logy*]. The study of mud and similar substances.

pe·lop·sia (pe·lop′see·uh) *n.* [Gk. *pelas,* near, + *-opsia*]. Illusions of abnormal nearness of objects; may occur in psychomotor seizures.

pel·o·sine (pel′o·seen, pe·lo′seen) *n.* [Cissam*pelos* + *-ine*]. BEBEERINE.

pe·lo·ther·a·py (pee″lo·therr′uh·pee) *n.* [*pelo-* + *therapy*]. Treatment with earth or mud.

Pel's crises [P. K. *Pel,* Dutch physician, 1852–1919]. The ocular crises of tabes dorsalis.

Pels-Macht test. The phytopharmacological method of testing the toxicity of human serum for plant protoplasm.

pel·ta·tin (pel·tay′tin) *n.* Either of two related constituents identified as α-peltatin and β-peltatin, obtained from the rhizome and roots of *Podophyllum peltatum.* β-Peltatin, $C_{22}H_{22}O_8$, contains a methoxyl (OCH_3) group in place of a hydroxyl (OH) group in α-peltatin, $C_{21}H_{20}O_8$; both are related to podophyllotoxin. Both are active, when applied topically, against certain wartlike neoplasms.

pelv-, pelvo-. A combining form meaning *pelvis.*

pelves. Plural of *pelvis.*

pelvi-, pelvio-. A combining form meaning *pelvis, pelvic.*

pel·vi·ab·dom·i·nal (pel″vee·ab·dom′i·nul) *adj.* Pertaining to the pelvic and abdominal cavities.

pel·vic (pel′vick) *adj.* Of or pertaining to the pelvis.

pelvic abscess. An abscess involving structures within the pelvis.

pelvic arrest. *In obstetrics,* a condition accompanying labor in which the presenting part of the fetus becomes fixed in its position in the maternal pelvis.

pelvic axis. An imaginary line passing through all the median anteroposterior diameters of the pelvic canal at their centers.

pelvic brim. The margin of the inlet of the pelvis.

pelvic canal. The cavity of the true pelvis from inlet to outlet.

pelvic cavity. 1. The cavity within the bony pelvis including both false and true pelves. NA *cavum pelvis.* 2. *In obstetrics,* the cavity of the true pelvis from inlet to outlet, containing the pelvic viscera.

pelvic diameter. Any one of the diameters of the pelvis, such as the conjugata vera, external conjugate diameter, and obstetric conjugate diameter. See also *diameter obliqua pelvis, diameter transversa pelvis.*

pelvic diaphragm. The muscular partition formed by the levator ani and the coccygeus muscles; the concave floor of the pelvis, separating it from the perineum. NA *diaphragma pelvis.*

pelvic exenteration. Surgical removal of the rectum, internal female organs, and bladder with the performance of a colostomy and urinary diversionary procedure; used in the treatment of pelvic cancer. Anterior pelvic exenteration is similar except that the rectum is spared.

pelvic fascia. A collective name for all the fascia located within the pelvic cavity. It is usually divided into three portions; parietal, diaphragmatic, and visceral or endopelvic. NA *fascia pelvis.*

pelvic ganglions. Groups of ganglion cells located in the pelvic nerve plexus. NA *ganglia pelvina.*

pelvic girdle. The two hipbones united at the pubic symphysis; they support the trunk on the lower extremities. NA *cingulum membri inferioris.*

pelvic hammock. A canvas sling, generally attached to an overhead bed frame, used to suspend the lower part of the trunk and pelvis in pelvic fractures.

pelvic hernia. OBTURATOR HERNIA.

pelvic index. The relation of the anteroposterior diameter to the transverse diameter of the pelvis.

pelvic inflammatory disease. Inflammation of the internal female genital tract; characterized by abdominal pain, fever, and tenderness of the cervix. It may be caused by any of a variety of microorganisms including *Neisseria gonorrhoeae.* Abbreviated, PID.

pelvic inlet. INLET OF THE PELVIS.

pelvic inlet index. The ratio of the sagittal diameter, or conjugata vera of the pelvic inlet, taken between the points where the sagittal plane cuts the sacral promontory and the posterior edge of the superior surface of the symphysis pubis, to the transverse diameter, taken between the points on the arcuate lines that lie farthest lateral from the midline, at right angles to the conjugata vera. When multiplied by 100, values of the index are classified as: platypellic, x-89.9; mesatipellic, 90.0–94.9; dolichopellic, 95.0-x.

pelvic kidney. A kidney abnormally located in the pelvis.

pelvic limb. LOWER EXTREMITY.

pelvic lipomatosis. Fat deposits in the pelvis producing compression and distortion of the bladder, rectum, ureters, and pelvic veins; a rare condition of unknown etiology usually seen in middle-aged men.

pelvic outlet. OUTLET OF THE PELVIS.

pelvic plexus. INFERIOR HYPOGASTRIC PLEXUS.

pelvic region. The region within the true pelvis.

pelvic splanchnic nerves. Sacral parasympathetic fibers which pass through the pelvic plexus to terminal ganglions in the pelvic viscera and are concerned with the emptying mechanisms of the urinary bladder, rectum, and uterus, and with erection of the genital organs. NA *nervi splanchnici pelvini.*

pelvic surgery. Surgical procedures limited to the pelvic area.

pel·vi·ec·ta·sis (pel″vee·eck′tuh·sis) *n.* [*pelvi-* + *ectasis*]. Distention of the renal pelvis by urine, with little or no calyceal distention; HYDROPELVIS.

pel·vi·en·ceph·a·lom·e·try (pel″vee·en·sef″uh·lom′e·tree) *n.* [*pelvi-* + *encephalo-* + *-metry*]. Measurement of the maternal pelvis and fetal skull by means of radiographic examination.

pel·vi·fem·o·ral (pel″vi·fem′ur·ul) *adj.* [*pelvi-* + *femoral*]. Pertaining to the pelvic girdle and the thighs.

pelvifemoral muscular dystrophy. LEYDEN-MÖBIUS DYSTROPHY.

pel·vim·e·ter (pel·vim'e·tur) *n.* [*pelvi-* + *-meter*]. An instrument for measuring the pelvic dimensions.

pel·vim·e·try (pel·vim'e·tree) *n.* [*pelvi-* + *-metry*]. The measurement of the dimensions of the pelvis. Average measurements of the adult female pelvis covered by the soft parts, in centimeters, are as follows:

Between iliac spines	26
Between iliac crests	29
External conjugate diameter	20¼
Internal conjugate diagonal	12¾
True conjugate, estimated	11
Right diagonal	22
Left diagonal	22
Between trochanters	31
Circumference of pelvis	90

pelvio-. See *pelvi-*.

pel·vio·li·thot·o·my (pel''vee·o·li·thot'uh·mee) *n.* [*pelvio-* + *lithotomy*]. Removal of a kidney stone from the renal pelvis. Syn. *pyelolithotomy.*

pel·vio·neo·cys·tos·to·my (pel''vee·o·nee''o·sis·tos'tuh·mee) *n.* [*pelvio-* + *neocystostomy*]. A surgical procedure in which the renal pelvis is anastomosed to the urinary bladder in cases of hydronephrotic ectopic kidneys; rarely used.

pel·vio·ra·di·og·ra·phy (pel''vee·o·ray''dee·og'ruh·fee) *n.* [*pelvio-* + *radiography*]. X-RAY PELVIMETRY.

pel·vi·ot·o·my (pel''vee·ot'uh·mee) *n.* [*pelvio-* + *-tomy*]. 1. Incision of the renal pelvis. 2. PELVISECTION.

pel·vi·rec·tal (pel''vi·reck'tul) *adj.* [*pelvi-* + *rectal*]. Pertaining to the pelvis and the rectum.

pel·vis (pel'vis) *n.*, L. pl. **pel·ves** (·veez) [L., basin]. 1. A basin or basin-shaped cavity, as the pelvis of the kidney. 2. [NA] The bony ring formed by the two hipbones and the sacrum and coccyx. 3. The cavity bounded by the bony pelvis. The cavity consists of the true pelvis and the false pelvis, which are separated by the iliopectineal line. The entrance of the true pelvis, corresponding to this line, is known as the inlet or superior strait; the outlet or inferior strait is bounded by the symphysis pubis, the tip of the coccyx, and the two ischia. See also Plates 1, 14, 25.

pelvis ae·qua·bi·li·ter jus·to ma·jor (ee''kwuh·bil'i·tur jus'to may'jur) [L.]. A generally enlarged pelvis.

pelvis aequabiliter justo minor [L.]. A generally contracted pelvis.

pel·vi·scope (pel'vi·skope) *n.* [*pelvi-* + *-scope*]. An endoscope for examination of the pelvic organs of the female.

pel·vi·sec·tion (pel''vi·seck'shun) *n.* [*pelvi-* + *section*]. A cutting through of one or more of the bones of the pelvis.

pelvis fis·sa (fis'uh). SPLIT PELVIS.

pelvis major [NA]. FALSE PELVIS.

pelvis minor [NA]. TRUE PELVIS.

pelvis na·na (nay'nuh). A generally contracted pelvis tending toward the infantile type, with persistence of cartilage at all the epiphyses; DWARF PELVIS.

pelvis re·na·lis (re·nay'lis) [NA]. RENAL PELVIS.

pelvis spi·no·sa (spye·no'suh). A rachitic pelvis having sharp prominent pelvic crests.

pel·vi·ver·te·bral angle (pel''vi·vur'te·brul). The angle of inclination of the pelvis.

pelvo-. See *pelv-*.

pel·vo·cal·i·ec·ta·sis (pel''vo·kal''ee·eck'tuh·sis) *n.* [*pelvo-* + *calix* + *ectasis*]. Dilatation of the pelvis and calyces of the kidney.

pel·vo·cal·y·ce·al, pel·vo·cal·i·ce·al (pel''vo·kal''i·see'ul) *adj.* [*pelvo-* + *calyceal*]. Pertaining to the pelvis and calyces of the kidney.

pel·vo·cal·y·cec·ta·sis (pel''vo·kal·i·seck'tuh·sis) *n.* PELVOCALIECTASIS.

pem·er·id (pem'e·rid) *n.* 4-[3-(Dimethylamino)propoxy]-1,2,-2,6,6-pentamethylpiperidine, $C_{15}H_{32}N_2O$, an antitussive used as the nitrate salt.

pem·o·line (pem'o·leen) *n.* 2-Imino-5-phenyl-4-oxazolidinone, $C_9H_8N_2O_2$, a central stimulant drug.

pem·phi·goid (pem'fi·goid) *n.* [*pemphigus* + *-oid*]. A skin disease resembling pemphigus. See also *bullous pemphigoid, benign mucosal pemphigoid.*

pem·phi·gus (pem'fi·gus) *n.* [NL., from Gk. *pemphix, pemphigos,* pustule]. An acute or chronic disease of the skin characterized by the appearance of bullae which develop in crops or continuous succession. —**pemphi·goid** (·goid) *adj.*

pemphigus acu·tus (uh·kew'tus). An acute skin disease resembling pemphigus.

pemphigus chron·i·cus (kron'i·kus). PEMPHIGUS VULGARIS.

pemphigus con·ta·gi·o·sus (kon·tay''jee·o'sus). A vesicular dermatitis endemic in tropical areas, chiefly affecting the armpits and groins.

pemphigus er·y·the·ma·to·sus (err''i·theem'uh·to'sis, ·themm''). A form of pemphigus foliaceus, either its beginning or an abortive case. Syn. *Senear-Usher syndrome.*

pemphigus fo·li·a·ce·us (fo''lee·ay'shee·us, ·see·us). A type of pemphigus characterized by crops of flaccid blebs which recur and rupture, producing a marked scaliness and generalized exfoliation.

pemphigus neo·na·to·rum (nee''o·nay·to'rum). NEONATAL IMPETIGO.

pemphigus trop·i·cus (trop'i·kus). A pyoderma in tropical climates.

pemphigus veg·e·tans (vej'e·tanz). A form of pemphigus vulgaris in which the denuded areas are covered by warty epidermis, rather than healing normally. These verrucous outgrowths may include small pustules.

pemphigus vul·ga·ris (vul·gair'is). A form of pemphigus, usually chronic, characterized by flaccid bullae involving the skin and oral mucosa; they rupture and leave enlarging denuded areas of epithelium.

pem·pi·dine (pem'pi·deen) *n.* 1,2,2,6,6-Pentamethylpiperidine, a ganglionic blocking agent used for the treatment of hypertension; employed as the tartrate salt.

pen·al·ge·sia (pen''al·jee'zee·uh) *n.* [Gk. *pen*ia, lack, poverty, + *algesia*]. Reduction in the number of pain and touch spots in the skin.

Penbritin. A trademark for ampicillin, a semisynthetic penicillin antibiotic.

pen·del·luft (pen'dul·lo͝oft'') *n.* [Ger. *Pendel,* pendulum, + *luft,* breath]. The pendulum-like movement of the heart and mediastinal structures with respiration in open pneumothorax, as the air moves in and out of the affected lung.

pendelluft respiration. PARADOXICAL RESPIRATION (1).

Pen·dred's syndrome [V. *Pendred,* English physician, 19th century]. Congenital deafness and familial goiter; nerve deafness is severe and present at birth or in early childhood; the goiter, thought to be due to a defect in the production of thyroid hormone, is present at birth or appears during the first two decades of life, and leads to only mild hypothyroidism with normal growth and intelligence.

pen·du·lar (pen'dew·lur) *adj.* Resembling the swinging of a pendulum.

pendular nystagmus. A form of ocular nystagmus in which the to-and-fro movements of the eyes occur at the same rate in each direction. See also *ocular nystagmus.*

pen·du·lous (pen'dew·lus) *adj.* [L. *pendulus,* from *pendere,* to hang]. 1. Hanging down loosely. 2. Swinging freely; pendular.

pendulous abdomen. A relaxed condition of the abdominal wall in which the anterior abdominal wall hangs down over the pubis.

pendulous nystagmus. OCULAR NYSTAGMUS.

pe·nec·to·my (pee·neck'tuh·mee) *n.* [*penis* + *-ectomy*]. Surgical removal of the penis.

pen·e·trance (pen'e·trunce) *n.* The percentage of organisms having a given genetic constitution which show the corresponding hereditary character. See also *expressivity.*

pen·e·trat·ing, *adj.* Entering beyond the surface, as a penetrating wound that pierces the wall of a cavity or enters an organ.

penetrating fibers. PERFORATING FIBERS.

penetrating keratoplasty. Keratoplasty in which the entire thickness of a portion of the cornea is replaced.

pen·e·tra·tion, *n.* [L. *penetratio,* from *penetrare,* to penetrate]. 1. The act of penetrating or piercing into. 2. The focal depth of a microscope or lens. 3. The entrance of the penis into the vagina.

pen·e·trom·e·ter (pen″e·trom′e·tur) *n.* An instrument for estimating the penetrating power or hardness of an x-ray.

Pen·field's operation [W. G. *Penfield,* Canadian neurosurgeon, b. 1891]. Excision of meningocerebral scar tissue for relief of traumatic epilepsy. Syn. *Foerster-Penfield operation.*

pen·flur·i·dol (pen·floo′ri·dol) *n.* 1-[4,4-Bis(*p*-fluorophenyl)-butyl]-4-(-chloro-α,α,α-trifluoro-*m*-tolyl)-4-piperidinol, $C_{28}H_{27}ClF_5NO$, a tranquilizer.

-penia [Gk. *penia,* poverty, lack]. A combining form meaning *deficiency.*

pe·nic·i·din (pe·nis′i·din, pen″i·sigh′din) *n.* An antibiotic from species of *Penicillium;* active against gram-negative and gram-positive bacteria.

pen·i·cil·la·mine (pen″i·sil′uh·meen, ·sil·am′een) *n.* D-3-Mercaptovaline, $C_5H_{11}NO_2S$, a degradation product of penicillin that chelates heavy metals and is used therapeutically to promote excretion of copper in Wilson's disease. It also reduces urinary cystine concentration and may be used for treatment of cystinuria.

pen·i·cil·lar (pen″i·sil′ur) *adj.* Of or pertaining to a penicillus.

pen·i·cil·lase (pen″i·sil′ace) *n.* PENICILLINASE.

pen·i·cil·late (pen″i·sil′ate) *adj.* [L. *penicillus,* brush, + *-ate*]. Ending in a tuft of hairs.

penicilli. Plural of *penicillus.*

pen·i·cil·lic acid (pen″i·sil′ick). An antibiotic, $C_8H_{10}O_4$, produced by some species of *Penicillium* and *Aspergillus.*

pen·i·cil·li·form (pen″i·sil′i·form) *adj.* PENICILLATE.

penicilli li·e·nis (lye·ee′nis) [NA]. The small tufts of fine twigs formed by the divisions of the arteries of the red pulp of the spleen.

pen·i·cil·lin (pen″i·sil′in) *n.* Generic name for a large group of antibiotic substances derived from several species of *Penicillium;* some are obtained from cultures of the fungus, while others are prepared by biosynthetic manipulation of 6-aminopenicillanic acid produced by the fungus. The penicillins are 6-carboxamido derivatives of 3,3-dimethyl-7-oxo-4-thia-1-azabicyclo[3.2.0]heptane-2-carboxylic acid. The general formula for penicillins is $C_9H_{11}N_2O_4SR$, where R is the radical in the 6-carboxamido group that characterizes specific penicillins; for example, in penicillin G (benzyl penicillin), R is benzyl ($C_6H_5CH_2$—), and in penicillin V (phenoxymethyl penicillin) it is phenoxymethyl ($C_6H_4OCH_2$—). Penicillin G, the first member of the group, continues to be the most widely used; it is employed mainly in the form of its potassium, benzathine, and procaine salts. Penicillin O and its salts, phenoxymethyl penicillin (penicillin V) and its potassium salt, and phenethicillin and its potassium salt are basic variants of penicillin that are used clinically. Methicillin, oxacillin, ampicillin, nafcillin, and cloxacillin are semisynthetic penicillins, certain of which are resistant to penicillinase.

pen·i·cil·lin·ase (pen″i·sil′i·nace) *n.* Any enzyme, found in many bacteria, which antagonizes the antibacterial action of penicillin by hydrolyzing the β-lactam ring.

penicillin N. D-(4-Amino-4-carboxybutyl) penicillin, an antibiotic produced by *Cephalosporium salmosynnematum.* Syn. *synnematin.*

penicillin sensitivity test. A test to determine what bacteria are inhibited by penicillin. The usual method is to place a disk of penicillin in an agar plate. The growth of penicillin-sensitive bacteria will be inhibited in the area around the disk where the penicillin has diffused into the agar. More accurately, serial dilutions of penicillin are incubated with cultures in test tubes.

penicillin-streptomycin blood agar. A bacteria-inhibiting medium for the culture of fungi.

penicillin V. Phenoxymethyl penicillin (see *penicillin*), characterized by stability in acid, including gastric fluid; used in the form of the acid and as the potassium and calcium salts.

pen·i·cil·li·o·sis (pen″i·sil″ee·o′sis) *n.,* pl. **penicillio·ses** (·seez) [*Penicillium* + *-osis*]. Lesions of the ear, skin, and occasionally lungs, presumed to be caused by certain species of *Penicillium.*

Pen·i·cil·li·um (pen″i·sil′ee·um) *n.* [NL., from L. *penicillus,* brush]. A genus of fungi of the Ascomycetes in which the fruiting organs have a brushlike form. The species *Penicillium chrysogenum, P. citrinum, P. claviforme, P. gladioli, P. griseofulvum, P. notatum, P. patulum, P. puberulum, P. spinulosum,* and *P. stoloniferum* are used in the production of antibiotics. Some species are also common allergens.

pen·i·cil·lo·ic acid (pen″i·si·lo′ick). Any one of the dicarboxylic acids formed when the lactam ring in a penicillin is opened by the action of alkalies or penicillinase.

pen·i·cil·lus (pen″i·sil′us) *n.,* pl. **penicil·li** (·eye) [L., brush]. One of the tufts of fine twigs into which the arteries of the spleen subdivide.

pe·nile (pee′nile) *adj.* Of or pertaining to the penis.

penile hypospadias. Hypospadias in which the urethra opens ventrally at some point between the sulcus of the glans and penoscrotal junction.

penile reflex. Contraction of the bulbocavernosus muscle in response to a moderate tap against the dorsum of the penis.

penile strabismus. PEYRONIE'S DISEASE.

penile urethra. The portion of the male urethra contained in the corpus spongiosum penis. Syn. *cavernous urethra.*

pe·nil·lic acid (pe·nil′ick). Any one of the dicarboxylic acids resulting when a penicillin is subjected to a mild acid treatment; the penillic acids are isomeric with the corresponding penicillins.

pe·nis (pee′nis) *n.* [L.] [NA]. The male organ of copulation. Its essential parts consist of the corpus spongiosum penis enclosing the urethra and forming the glans, and the two corpora cavernosa, all covered by fascia and skin. See also Plate 25.

penis cap·ti·vus (kap·tye′vus). Involuntary retention of the penis in the vagina during copulation by spasm of the perineal muscles of the female.

penis clamp. A clamp that is fitted upon the shaft of the penis to retain anesthetic or antiseptic solutions in the urethra, for control of incontinence, or for training an enuretic.

penis envy. *In psychoanalysis,* literally, the envy of the young female child for the penis which she does not possess, or which she thinks she has lost (thus forming a part of the castration complex). More generally, the wish by a female for male attributes and advantages, considered by many to play a significant role in the development of the female character. The wish for a penis may be replaced normally by the wish for a child.

penis plas·ti·cus (plas′ti·kus). PEYRONIE'S DISEASE.

penis reflex. PENILE REFLEX.

penis syringe. URETHRAL SYRINGE.

pen·nate (pen′ate) *adj.* [L. *pennatus,* feathered, winged, from *penna,* feather, wing]. Featherlike; comparable in structure to the arrangement of barbs on the shaft of a feather.

pennate muscle. A muscle whose fibers are inserted obliquely on a tendon.

pen·ni·form (pen′i·form) *adj.* PENNATE.

pen·ny·roy·al (pen″ee·roy′ul) *n.* HEDEOMA.

pen·ny·weight, *n.* A weight of 24 grains. Symbol, dwt.

pen·ny·wort (pen′ee·wurt) *n.* HYDROCOTYLE.

pe·no·scro·tal (pee″no·skro′tul) *adj.* [*penis* + *scrotal*]. Pertaining to the penis and the scrotum, or at the junction or angle between the two.

penoscrotal hypospadias. A form of hypospadias in which the urethra opens at the junction of the penis and the scrotum.

Pen·rose drain [C. B. *Penrose,* U.S. surgeon, 1862–1925]. A thin-walled latex tube used to drain wounds or cavities. See also *cigarette drain.*

pent-, penta- [Gk. *pente*]. A combining form meaning *five.*

pen·ta·bam·ate (pen″tuh·bam′ate) *n.* 3-Methyl-2,4-pentanediol dicarbamate, $C_8H_{16}N_2O_4$, a tranquilizer.

pen·tad (pen′tad) *n.* [Gk. *pentas, pentados,* a group of five]. An element or radical having a valence of five.

pen·ta·dac·tyl (pen″tuh·dack′til) *adj.* [Gk. *pentadaktylos,* from *penta-* + *daktylos,* digit]. Having five fingers or toes upon each hand or foot.

3-pen·ta·dec·yl·cat·e·chol (pen″tuh·des″il·kat′e·chol, ·kol) *n.* Tetrahydrourushiol, $C_{21}H_{36}O_2$, a constituent of the irritant oil of *Rhus toxicodendron* and other species of *Rhus;* used as a standard allergen in patch tests to determine sensitivity to poison ivy.

pen·ta·eryth·ri·tol tet·ra·ni·trate (pen″tuh·e·rith′ri·tol tet″ruh·nigh′trate). PENTAERYTHRITYL TETRANITRATE.

pen·ta·eryth·ri·tyl tetranitrate (pen″tuh·e·rith′ri·til). 2,2-Bis(hydroxymethyl)-1,3-propanediol tetranitrate, $C(CH_2ONO_2)_4$, a coronary vasodilator used in management of angina pectoris.

pen·ta·gas·trin (pen″tuh·gas′trin) *n.* A synthetic pentapeptide with the same sequence of amino acids as in the biologically active component of human gastrin and which stimulates gastric secretion of hydrochloric acid. It is used, parenterally, to measure gastric secretory capacity.

pen·ta·gen·ic (pen″tuh·jen′ick) *adj.* [*penta-* + *-genic*]. Referring to genotypes of polysomic or polyploid organisms which contain five different alleles for any given locus.

pen·tal·o·gy (pen·tal′uh·jee) *n.* [*penta-* + *-logy* (as in tetralogy)]. A combination of five related symptoms or defects that are characteristic of a disease or syndrome.

pentalogy of Fal·lot (fah·lo′) [E. L. A. *Fallot,* French physician, 1850–1911]. A congenital cardiac lesion consisting of the four defects of tetralogy of Fallot plus an atrial septal defect.

pen·ta·me·tho·ni·um (pen″tuh·me·tho′nee·um) *n.* One of a homologous series of polymethylene bis (trimethylammonium) ions, of the general formula $(CH_3)_3N^+$-$(CH_2)_nN^+(CH_3)_3$, in which n is 5. It possesses ganglion-blocking action, effecting reduction in blood pressure. It is used clinically in the form of one of its salts, commonly the bromide or iodide. Also designated *C5.*

pen·ta·meth·yl·ene·tet·ra·zol (pen″tuh·meth″il·een·tet′ruh·zol, ·zole) *n.* PENTYLENETETRAZOL.

pen·ta·meth·yl·ros·an·i·line (pen″tuh·meth″il·ro·zan′i·leen, ·lin) *n.* METHYLROSANILINE CHLORIDE.

pen·tam·i·dine (pen·tam′i·deen, ·din) *n.* A diamidine, 4,4′-(pentamethylenedioxy)dibenzamidine, $C_{19}H_{24}N_4O_2$, used as the dimethylsulfonate and isethionate salts in treatment of African trypanosomiasis and kala azar.

pen·tane (pen′tane) *n.* [*pent-* + *-ane*]. Any one of the three isomeric hydrocarbons of the paraffin series, having the formula C_5H_{12}. All are liquids.

pen·tane·di·o·ic acid (pen″tane·dye·o′ick). GLUTARIC ACID.

pen·ta·pep·tide (pen″tuh·pep′tide) *n.* A polypeptide composed of five amino acid groups.

pen·ta·pip·er·i·um methylsulfate (pen″tuh·pip′ur·ide). 1-Methyl 4-piperidyl-3-methyl-2-phenylvalerate compound with dimethyl sulfate, $C_{18}H_{27}NO_2.C_2H_6O_4S$, an anticholinergic drug.

pen·ta·quine (pen′tuh·kween, ·kwin) *n.* 6-Methoxy-8-(5′-isopropylaminopentylamino)quinoline, $C_{18}H_{27}N_3O$, an antimalarial drug generally given with quinine; used as the phosphate salt.

pen·ta·sac·cha·ride (pen″tuh·sack′uh·ride, ·rid) *n.* A polysaccharide hydrolyzable into five molecules of monosaccharide.

Pen·tas·to·ma (pen·tas′tuh·muh, pen″tuh·sto′muh) *n.* [NL., from Gk. *pente,* five, + *stoma,* mouth]. A genus of the Pentastomida. *Pentastoma najae* has been reported to infect the human upper respiratory tract.

pen·ta·stome (pen′tuh·stome) *n.* Any member of the Pentastomida.

Pen·ta·stom·i·da (pen″tuh·stom′i·duh) *n.pl.* [NL., from *Pentastoma*]. A class of arthropods, known as tongue worms, which infect humans; includes the genera *Linguatula, Armillifer, Pentastoma,* and *Porocephalus.*

Pen·ta·trich·o·mo·nas (pen″tuh·trick″o·mo′nus, ·tri·kom′o·nas) *n.* [*penta-* + *Trichomonas*]. A generic name improperly applied to the five-flagellated variety of *Trichomonas hominis.*

pen·ta·va·lent (pen″tuh·vay′lunt) *n.* [*penta-* + *valent*]. Having a valence of five.

pen·taz·o·cine (pen·taz′o·sin, ·seen) *n.* 1,2,3,4,5,6-Hexahydro-6,11-dimethyl-3-(3-methyl-2-butenyl)-2,6-methano-3-benzazocin-8-ol, $C_{19}H_{27}NO$, a synthetic narcotic analgesic.

pent·dy·o·pent (pent″dye′o·pent) *n.* The red pigment, containing two pyrrole rings, obtained when a propentdyopent is reduced with sodium dithionite.

pen·tene (pen′teen) *n.* [*pent-* + *-ene*]. Any one of the five isomeric hydrocarbons of the olefin series, having the formula C_5H_{10}.

pen·tet·ic acid (pen·tet′ick). Diethyltriaminepentaacetic acid, $C_{14}H_{23}N_3O_{10}$, a diagnostic aid.

pen·tet·ra·zol (pen·tet′ruh·zol, ·zole) *n.* PENTYLENETETRAZOL.

pen·thi·e·nate bromide (pen·thigh′e·nate). Diethyl(2-hydroxyethyl)methylammonium bromide α-cyclopentyl-2-thiopheneglycolate, $C_{18}H_{30}BrNO_3S$, a visceral anticholinergic drug used for antispasmodic effect.

Penthrane. Trademark for methoxyflurane, a general anesthetic.

pen·tiz·i·done sodium (pen·tiz′i·dohn). (*R*)-4-[(1-Methyl-3-oxo-1-butenyl)amino]-3-isoxazolidinone, monosodium salt, $C_8H_{11}N_2NaO_3$, and antibacterial.

pen·to·bar·bi·tal sodium (pen″to·bahr′bi·tol, ·tal). Sodium 5-ethyl-5-(1-methylbutyl)barbiturate, $C_{11}H_{17}N_2NaO_3$, a short- to intermediate-acting barbiturate; used as a hypnotic and sedative drug. Syn. *sodium pentobarbitone* (Brit.).

pen·to·lin·i·um tartrate (pen″to·lin′ee·um). 1,1′-Pentamethylenebis(1-methylpyrrolidinium hydrogen tartrate), $C_{15}H_{32}N_2.2C_4H_5O_6$, a ganglionic blocking agent used in the management of hypertension.

pen·to·san (pen′to·san) *n.* A complex carbohydrate capable of forming a pentose by hydrolysis.

pen·to·sa·zone (pen·to′suh·zone, pen″to·say′zone) *n.* A reaction product of pentose and phenylhydrazine, used to identify and distinguish pentoses from other monosaccharides.

pen·tose (pen′toce, ·toze) *n.* Any one of a class of carbohydrates containing five atoms of carbon.

pentose nucleic acid. RIBONUCLEIC ACID.

pentose phosphate pathway. HEXOSE MONOPHOSPHATE SHUNT.

pen·to·side (pen′to·side, ·sid) *n.* A glycoside in which the sugar component is a pentose; nucleosides are pentosides.

Pentostam. Trademark for a preparation of sodium stibogluconate used for the treatment of leishmaniasis.

pen·tos·uria (pen″to·sue′ree·uh) *n.* [*pentose* + *-uria*]. The presence of pentose in the urine.

Pentothal. PENTOTHAL SODIUM.

pentothal interview. *In psychiatry,* the use of thiopental sodium (Pentothal sodium) as an aid to interview and therapy. See also *narcoanalysis, narcosynthesis.*

Pentothal sodium. Trademark for the ultrashort-acting barbiturate thiopental sodium.

pent·ox·ide (pent·ock'side) *n.* [*pent-* + *oxide*]. An oxide containing five atoms of oxygen.

pent·ox·i·fyl·line (pen''tock·sif'i·leen, pen·tock''si·fil'een) *n.* 1-(5-Oxohexyl)theobromine, $C_{13}H_{18}N_4O_3$, a vasodilator.

pen·tri·ni·trol (pen''trye·nye'trole) *n.* Pentaerythritol trinitrate, $C_5H_9N_3O_{10}$, a coronary vasodilator.

pen·tyl (pen'til) *n.* Any of the eight univalent radicals C_5H_{11}—, derived from the three isomeric pentanes. Syn. *amyl.*

pen·tyl·ene·tet·ra·zol (pen''ti·leen·tet'ruh·zol, ·zole) *n.* 6,7,8,9-Tetrahydro-5*H*-tetrazoloazepine, $C_6H_{10}N_4$, a central nervous system stimulant used as an analeptic.

Pen·zoldt's test (pen'tsoʰlt) [F. *Penzoldt,* German physician, 1849–1927]. 1. A test for urinary glucose using alkaline sodium diazobenzosulfonate. 2. A test for gastric absorption using potassium iodide and testing for iodine in saliva. 3. An *ortho*-nitrobenzaldehyde test for acetone.

peo·til·lo·ma·nia (pee''o·til''o·may'nee·uh) *n.* [Gk. *peos,* penis, + *till*ein, to pull, + *-mania*]. The nervous habit of constantly pulling the penis; not an act of masturbation.

pe·po (pee'po) *n.* Seed of the pumpkin, *Cucurbita pepo;* has been used as a taeniafuge.

pep·per, *n.* [L. *piper,* from Gk. *peperi,* from Skr. *pippalī*]. The dried, unripe fruit of various species of *Piper;* formerly used as a stimulant, carminative, and counterirritant.

pepper-and-salt fundus. A fundus oculi in which yellowish-red, gray, and black spots are present in the choroid; found in congenital rubella syndrome.

pep·per·mint, *n.* The dried leaves and flowering tops of *Mentha piperita.* Preparations or derivatives of peppermint, such as the oil and spirit, are used as flavors and, sometimes, for carminative action.

peppermint oil. The volatile oil from the overground parts of the flowering plant of *Mentha piperita,* containing menthol and its esters; used as a carminative and flavor.

Pep·per syndrome or **type** [W. *Pepper,* Jr., U.S. physician, 1874–1947]. Neuroblastoma with liver metastasis.

Pepper treatment [W. *Pepper,* Sr., U.S. physician, 1843–1898]. The use of large doses of opium to suppress peristalsis in cases of peritonitis.

pep·si·gogue (pep'si·gog) *adj.* [*peps*in + *-agogue*]. Stimulating the discharge of pepsin in the gastric secretion.

pep·sin (pep'sin) *n.* [Gk. *peps*is, digestion, + *-in*]. 1. The proteinase of gastric juice, derived from its zymogen precursor pepsinogen elaborated and secreted by the chief cells of the gastric mucosa. 2. A preparation containing proteinase obtained from the glandular layer of the fresh stomach of the hog and sometimes used medicinally for supposed protein digestant action.

pep·sin·o·gen (pep·sin'o·jen) *n.* [*pepsin* + *-gen*]. The antecedent substance or zymogen of pepsin, present in the cells of the gastric glands, which during digestion is converted into pepsin.

pep·si·no·ther·a·py (pep''si·no·therr'uh·pee) *n.* [*pepsin* + *therapy*]. The employment of pepsin as a digestant.

pep·stat·in (pep·stat'in) *n.* A hexapeptide, $C_{34}H_{63}N_5O_9$, a pepsin inhibitor.

pept-, pepto-. A combining form meaning (a) *pepsin, peptic;* (b) *peptone.*

Peptavlon. A trademark for pentagastrin, a gastric secretion inhibitor.

pep·tic (pep'tick) *adj.* [Gk. *peptikos,* promoting digestion, from *peptein,* to digest]. 1. Pertaining to pepsin. 2. Pertaining to digestion.

peptic cell. CHIEF CELL (1).

peptic digestion. GASTRIC DIGESTION.

peptic glands. The fundic glands of the stomach.

peptic ulcer. A sharply circumscribed loss of tissue, involving chiefly the mucosa, submucosa, and muscular layer in areas of the digestive tract exposed to acid-pepsin gastric juice, particularly the lower esophagus, stomach, and first portion of the duodenum.

pep·ti·dase (pep'ti·dace, ·daze) *n.* An enzyme that splits peptides to amino acids.

pep·tide (pep'tide) *n.* [*pept-* + *-ide*]. A compound of two or more amino acids containing one or more peptide groups, —CONH—. An intermediate between the amino acids and peptones in the synthesis of proteins.

peptide bond. A bond joining two amino acids, in which the amino group of one acid is condensed with the carboxyl group of another with elimination of water and formation of a —CONH— linkage. The amino acids of proteins are joined in this manner.

pep·ti·do·lyt·ic (pep''ti·do·lit'ick) *adj.* [*peptide* + *-lytic*]. Causing the digestion or hydrolysis of peptides into amino acids.

pep·ti·za·tion (pep''ti·zay'shun) *n.* [Gk. *peptein,* to cook, digest, soften]. 1. The liquefaction of a gel to a sol. 2. Dispersion of a solid material as a colloidal suspension. —**pep·tize** (pep'tize) *v.*

pepto-. See *pept-.*

pep·to·gen·ic (pep''to·jen'ick) *adj.* [*pepto-* + *-genic*]. Producing pepsin or peptones.

pep·tog·e·nous (pep·toj'e·nus) *adj.* PEPTOGENIC.

pep·tol·y·sis (pep·tol'i·sis) *n.* PEPTONOLYSIS.

pepton-, peptono-. A combining form meaning *peptone.*

pep·tone (pep'tone) *n.* [Gk. *pepton,* neuter of *peptos,* cooked or digested]. A derived protein produced by partial hydrolysis of natural protein either by an enzyme or by an acid. Peptones, as well as proteoses, which are similar to peptones, are intermediate compounds between proteins and amino acids. Certain peptones are used for the preparation of culture mediums in bacteriologic tests. —**pep·ton·ic** (pep·ton'ick) *adj.*

pep·to·ne·mia, pep·to·nae·mia (pep''to·nee'mee·uh) *n.* [*pepton-* + *-emia*]. The presence of peptone in the blood.

pep·to·nize (pep'to·nize) *v.* 1. To convert into peptones; to predigest. 2. To digest with pepsin.

peptono-. See *pepton-.*

pep·to·nol·y·sis (pep''to·nol'i·sis) *n.* [*peptono-* + *-lysis*]. The hydrolysis or digestion of peptones. Syn. *peptolysis.*

pep·to·nu·ria (pep''to·new'ree·uh) *n.* [*pepton-* + *-uria*]. The presence of peptones in the urine.

per- [L., through, very]. A prefix signifying (a) *throughout, completely, thoroughly, over,* or *very, extremely;* (b) in chemistry, *the highest valence of a series.*

per·aceph·a·lus (pur''a·sef'uh·lus, perr''a·) *n.* [*per-* + *acephalus*]. A placental parasitic twin that lacks head and arms and has a defective or absent thorax, the body being reduced to little more than the pelvis and legs.

per·ace·tic acid (pur''a·see'tick). Peroxyacetic acid, CH_3COOOH, a strong oxidizing agent.

per·ac·id (pur''as'id) *n.* [*per-* + *acid*]. The acid, of a series of acids formed by a particular element, which contains the highest proportion of oxygen.

per·acid·i·ty (pur''a·sid'i·tee) *n.* [*per-* + *acidity*]. Excessive acidity.

per·acute (pur''a·kewt') *adj.* [L. *peracutus*]. Very acute; said of pain or disease.

per anum (pur ay'num) [L.]. By way of or through the anus, as in the administration of drugs or nutrient substances.

per·at·odyn·ia (perr''a·to·din'ee·uh) *n.* [Gk. *peras, peratos,* limit, boundary, + *-odynia*]. Pain at the cardia of the stomach; heartburn.

Perazil. A trademark for chlorcyclizine, an antihistaminic drug used as the hydrochloride salt.

per·bo·rate (pur·bo'rate) *n.* A salt of perboric acid.

per·bo·ric acid (pur·bo'rick). The hypothetical acid, HBO_3, from which perborates are derived.

per·cent, per cent, *n.* [L. *per centum,* per hundred]. An expression, when preceded by a number, of the proportion of a specific article, object, or substance in 100 parts of the entire system.

per·cent·age depth dose (pur·sent'ij). *In radiology,* the amount of radiation delivered at a specific depth in tissue, expressed as a percentage of the dosage to the skin.

per·cen·tile (pur·sen'tile, ·til) *n.* Any of the values of a variable which separate the entire distribution into 100 groups of equal frequency.

per·cept (pur'sept) *n.* The mental image of what is perceived, i.e., the product of perception.

per·cep·tion (pur·sep'shun) *n.* [L. *perceptio*, from *percipere*, to perceive]. Recognition in response to sensory stimuli; the mental act or process by which the memory of certain qualities of an act, experience, or object is associated with other qualities impressing the senses, thereby making possible recognition and interpretation of the new sensory data.

perception or **perceptive deafness**. Deafness caused by a lesion of the cochlea or the cochlear division of the eighth nerve. Syn. *sensorineural deafness.*

per·cep·tive (pur·sep'tiv) *adj.* 1. PERCEPTUAL. 2. Having keen perceptual faculties. —**per·cep·tiv·i·ty** (pur''sep·tiv'i·tee) *n.*

per·cep·to·ri·um (pur''sep·tor'ee·um) *n.* SENSORIUM (1).

per·cep·tu·al (pur·sep'choo·ul) *adj.* Pertaining to perception. —**perceptual·ly** (·lee) *adv.*

perceptual disorder or **dysfunction**. Any disturbance, usually chronic, of the process of perception, most often involving sight or hearing. See also *minimal brain dysfunction syndrome.*

perceptually handicapped. Exhibiting the minimal brain dysfunction syndrome.

per·chlo·rate (pur·klo'rate) *n.* A salt of perchloric acid.

per·chlor·hy·dria (pur''klor·high'dree·uh) *n.* HYPERCHLORHYDRIA.

per·chlo·ric acid (pur·klo'rick). $HClO_4$, a powerful oxidizing acid.

per·chlo·ro·eth·yl·ene (pur·klo''ro·eth'il·een) *n.* TETRACHLOROETHYLENE.

per·clu·sion (pur·kloo'zhun) *n.* [*per-* + L. *claudere*, to be lame]. *Obsol.* Inability to perform any movement.

per·co·la·tion (pur''kuh·lay'shun) *n.* [L. *percolatio*, from *percolare*, to strain through]. The process of extracting the soluble constituents of a substance by allowing a suitable solvent to pass through a column of the powdered substance placed in a long, conical vessel, the percolator. —**per·co·late** (pur'kuh·late) *n. & v.*

per·co·la·tor (pur'ko·lay''tur) *n.* A long, conical vessel with a delivery tube at the lower extremity; used for extracting the soluble constituents of a substance, packed in the percolator, by means of a suitable solvent passing through it.

per·co·morph (pur'ko·morf) *n.* [L. *perca*, perch, + *-morph*]. A fish of the order Acanthopteri (Percomorphi), which includes the genera *Thunnus, Xiphias, Stereolepis, Scomber,* and others. The liver of certain percomorph fishes yields an oil rich in vitamins A and D.

Percorten. A trademark for the salt-regulating adrenocortical steroid deoxycorticosterone, used as the acetate ester.

per·cus·si·ble (pur·kus'i·bul) *adj.* Capable of detection by percussion.

per·cus·sion (pur·kush'un) *n.* [L. *percussio*, from *percutere*, to strike, strike through]. The act of striking or firmly tapping the surface of the body with a finger or a small hammer to elicit sounds, or vibratory sensations, of diagnostic value. —**per·cuss** (pur·kuss') *v.*

percussion area. Any circumscribed surface area of the body which is the site of percussion.

percussion hammer. REFLEX HAMMER.

percussion movements. *In massage,* a series of blows delivered to the surface of a region in rapid succession; called beating, clapping, hacking, slapping and tapping.

percussion note. The sound elicited on percussion.

percussion test. SCHWARTZ TEST.

percussion wave. The initial systolic wave of the bisferiens pulse in idiopathic hypertrophic subaortic stenosis. Contr. *tidal wave.*

per·cus·sor (pur·kus'ur) *n.* [L., one who strikes]. A person who performs percussion; an instrument for use in percussion.

per·cu·ta·ne·ous (pur''kew·tay'nee·us) *adj.* [*per-* + *cutaneous*]. Performed through the skin.

perennial rhinitis. ALLERGIC RHINITIS; year-round in type.

per·fec·tion·ism (pur·feck'shun·iz·um) *n.* The practice of attempting to achieve perfection in all activities of life, no matter how trivial.

per·fo·rans (pur'fo·ranz) *adj.* [L., piercing through]. Penetrating or perforating; a term applied to a muscle, artery, or nerve perforating a part.

¹per·fo·rate (pur'fuh·rut) *adj.* [L. *perforatus*, perforated]. *In biology,* pierced with small holes.

²per·fo·rate (pur'fuh·rate) *v.* [L. *perforare*, from *per-* + *forare*, to bore]. To pierce through. —**perfo·rat·ed** (·ray''tid) *adj.;* **perfo·rat·ing** (·ray''ting) *adj.*

perforated substance. A part of the base of the brain pierced with many small holes for the passage of blood vessels.

perforating arteries. The branches of the deep femoral artery which pass through the adductor magnus muscle. NA *arteriae perforantes.*

perforating fibers. 1. Collagenous fibers of a tendon, ligament, or periosteum buried in the matrix of subperiosteal bone. Syn. *Sharpey's fibers.* 2. Similar fibers in the cementum of a tooth.

per·fo·ra·tion (pur''fuh·ray'shun) *n.* 1. The act or occurrence of piercing or boring into a part, especially into the wall of a hollow organ or viscus. 2. A hole made through a part or wall of a cavity, produced by a variety of means.

per·fo·ra·tor (pur'fuh·ray''tur) *n.* An instrument for perforating, especially one for performing craniotomy on the fetus.

per·fo·ra·to·ri·um (pur''fuh·ruh·to'ree·um) *n.*, pl. **perforato·ria** (·ree·uh) [NL]. The pointed tip differentiated from the acrosome in the spermatozoa of some animals.

per·for·mic acid (pur·for'mick). Peroxyformic acid, HCOOOH, a strong oxidizing agent.

per·fri·ca·tion (pur''fri·kay'shun) *n.* [L. *perfricare*, to rub all over]. INUNCTION; rubbing with an ointment.

per·fus·ate (pur·few'zate) *n.* The fluid that is introduced in perfusion (3).

per·fu·sion (pur·few'zhun) *n.* [L. *perfusio*, from *perfundere*, to pour over]. 1. A pouring of fluid. 2. The passage of a fluid through spaces. 3. The introduction of fluids into tissues by their injection into blood vessels, usually veins. —**per·fuse** (·fuze') *v.*

Pergonal. Trademark for menotropins, a preparation containing primarily follicle-stimulating hormone.

per·hex·i·line (pur·heck'si·leen, perr·) *n.* 2-(2,2-Dicyclohexylethyl) piperidine, $C_{19}H_{35}N$, a coronary vasodilator; used as the maleate salt.

Perhydrol. Trademark for a 30% solution of hydrogen peroxide.

peri- [Gk., about, around]. A prefix signifying *about, beyond, around, near;* especially, *enclosing a part* or *affecting the tissues around a part.*

peri·ac·i·nar (perr''ee·as'i·nur) *adj.* Around an acinus.

periacinar fibroadenoma. A pericanalicular fibroma.

Periactin. Trademark for cyproheptadine, an antagonist of histamine and serotonin used, as the hydrochloride salt, for relief of pruritus.

peri·ad·e·ni·tis (perr''ee·ad''e·nigh'tis) *n.* [*peri-* + *aden-* + *-itis*]. Inflammation of the tissues that surround a gland or lymph node.

periadenitis mu·co·sae ne·crot·i·ca re·cur·rens (mew·ko'see ne·krot'i·kuh re·kur'enz). A disorder characterized by recurring necrotic or ulcerative lesions occurring on the buccal and pharyngeal mucosa. Begins as a small, smooth, hard nodule that sloughs, leaving a deep, crateriform depression. May occur on the tongue or genitalia as well.

peri·ad·ven·ti·tial (perr″ee·ad″ven·tish′ul) *adj.* [*peri-* + *adventitial*]. Around the adventitial coat of a blood vessel.

peri·alien·itis (perr″ee·ay″lee·e·nigh′tis) *n.* [*peri-* + *alien* + *-itis*]. FOREIGN-BODY REACTION.

peri·anal (perr″ee·ay′nul) *adj.* [*peri-* + *anal*]. Situated or occurring around the anus.

perianal abscess. An abscess adjacent to the walls of the anal canal.

peri·an·gi·itis (perr″ee·an″jee·eye′tis) *n.* [*peri-* + *angi-* + *-itis*]. Inflammation of the outer coat of or the tissues surrounding a blood or lymphatic vessel.

peri·an·gio·cho·li·tis (perr″ee·an″jee·o·ko·lye′tis) *n.* PERICHOLANGITIS.

peri·aor·ti·tis (perr″ee·ay″or·tye′tis) *n.* [*peri-* + *aorta* + *-itis*]. Inflammation of the tissues surrounding the aorta.

peri·api·cal (perr″ee·ap′i·kul, ·ay′pi·kul) *adj.* [*peri-* + *apical*]. Around an apex, particularly the apex of a tooth.

periapical abscess. An alveolar abscess originating at the apex of a tooth, usually the result of pulpal disease.

periapical cyst. RADICULAR CYST.

periapical granuloma. A localized mass of chronic granulation tissue formed in response to infection and occurring at the apex of a tooth; often contains islands of epithelial cells (epithelial rests).

peri·ap·pen·di·ci·tis (perr″ee·uh·pen″di·sigh′tis) *n.* [*peri-* + *appendix* + *-itis*]. Inflammation of the tissue around the vermiform process, or of the serosal region of the vermiform appendix.

peri·ap·pen·dic·u·lar (perr″ee·ap″en·dick′yoo·lur) *adj.* [*peri-* + *appendicular*]. Surrounding the vermiform, or any other, appendix.

per·i·apt (perr′ee·apt) *n.* [Gk. *periaption*, from *peri-* + *haptein*, to fasten]. An amulet or charm, sometimes worn to avoid disease.

peri·aq·ue·duc·tal (perr″ee·ack″we·duck′tul) *adj.* Around the cerebral aqueduct.

peri·are·o·lar (perr″ee·a·ree′uh·lur) *adj.* [*peri-* + *areolar*]. Around an areola, usually of the breast.

peri·ar·te·ri·al (perr″ee·ahr·teer′ee·ul) *adj.* [*peri-* + *arterial*]. Surrounding an artery.

peri·ar·te·ri·o·lar (perr″ee·ahr·teer″ee·o′lur) *adj.* [*peri-* + *arteriolar*]. Around an arteriole.

peri·ar·te·ri·tis (perr″ee·ahr″te·rye′tis) *n.* [*peri-* + *arteri-* + *-itis*]. Inflammation of the adventitia of an artery and the periarterial tissues. Contr. *endarteritis.*

periarteritis nodosa. POLYARTERITIS NODOSA.

peri·ar·thri·tis (perr″ee·ahr·thrigh′tis) *n.* [*peri-* + *arthr-* + *-itis*]. Inflammation of the tissues about a joint.

periarthritis cal·ca·rea (kal·kair′ee·uh). Calcification of the musculotendinous cuff of the shoulder joint.

periarthritis of the shoulder. FROZEN SHOULDER.

peri·ar·tic·u·lar (perr″ee·ahr·tick′yoo·lur) *adj.* [*peri-* + *articular*]. About a joint.

peri·atri·al (perr″ee·ay′tree·ul) *adj.* [*peri-* + *atrial*]. Situated around the atria of the heart.

peri·au·ric·u·lar (perr″ee·aw·rick′yoo·lur) *adj.* [*peri-* + *auricular*]. Around the external ear.

peri·ax·i·al (perr″ee·ack′see·ul) *adj.* [*peri-* + *axial*]. Surrounding an axis.

periaxial neuritis. *In ophthalmology,* involvement of the optic nerve outside the papillomacular bundle.

peri·blep·sia (perr″i·blep′see·uh) *n.* PERIBLEPSIS.

peri·blep·sis (perr″i·blep′sis) *n.* [Gk., looking around, from *blepein,* to look]. The wild look of a patient in delirium.

peri·bron·chi·al (perr″i·bronk′ee·ul) *adj.* [*peri-* + *bronchial*]. Surrounding or occurring about a bronchus.

peri·bron·chi·o·lar (perr″i·bronk″ee·o′lur, ·brong·kigh′o·lur) *adj.* [*peri-* + *bronchiolar*]. Surrounding or occurring about a bronchiole.

peri·bron·chi·o·li·tis (perr″i·bronk″ee·o·lye′tis) *n.* [*peri-* + *bronchiole* + *-itis*]. Inflammation of the tissues around the bronchioles.

peri·bron·chi·tis (perr″i·brong·kigh′tis) *n.* [*peri-* + *bronch-* + *-itis*]. Inflammation of the tissues around bronchi; a subacute bronchopneumonia.

peri·bro·sis (perr″i·bro′sis) *n.* [Gk. *peribrōsis,* ulceration, from *brōsis,* eating, corrosion]. Ulceration at the canthus of the eyelid.

peri·bur·sal (perr″i·bur′sul) *adj.* [*peri-* + *bursal*]. Around a bursa.

pericaecal. PERICECAL.

pericaecitis. PERICECITIS.

peri·cal·i·ce·al, peri·cal·y·ce·al (perr″i·kal″i·see′ul) *adj.* [*peri-* + *calyseal*]. Around a kidney calix.

peri·can·a·lic·u·lar (perr″i·kan″uh·lick′yoo·lur) *adj.* [*peri-* + *canalicular*]. Occurring around a canaliculus or canaliculi.

pericanalicular fibroadenoma of the breast. A glandular type of benign breast tumor with large amounts of connective tissue which is often arranged concentrically around the multiplied ductules.

peri·cap·il·lary (perr″i·kap′i·lerr·ee) *adj.* [*peri-* + *capillary*]. Surrounding a capillary.

pericapillary encephalorrhagia. A condition of obscure etiology in which petechial hemorrhages are scattered diffusely in the white matter of the brain. Each lesion is situated around a small blood vessel, usually a capillary, and in this para-adventitial area both the myelin and axis cylinders are destroyed.

pericardi-, pericardio-. A combining form meaning *pericardium, pericardial.*

pericardia. Plural of *pericardium.*

peri·car·di·ac (perr″i·kahr′dee·ack) *adj.* PERICARDIAL.

peri·car·di·a·co·phren·ic (perr″i·kahr·dye″uh·ko·fren′ick) *adj.* [*pericardiac* + *phrenic*]. Pertaining to the pericardium and diaphragm.

pericardiac pleura. The portion of the parietal pleura contiguous to the parietal pericardium.

peri·car·di·al (perr″i·kahr′dee·ul) *adj.* Pertaining to the pericardium; situated around the heart.

pericardial aorta. 1. The part of the aorta within the pericardial cavity. 2. In the embryo, the distal part of the aortic bulb.

pericardial cavity. A space within the pericardium between the serous layer of the pericardium and the epicardium of the heart and roots of the great vessels. NA *cavum pericardii.*

pericardial celomic cyst. PERICARDIAL CYST.

pericardial click. PERICARDIAL KNOCK.

pericardial cyst. A cyst adherent to the parietal pericardium, having a thin fibrous wall and lined by flattened endothelial or mesothelial cells.

pericardial fluid. The fluid in the pericardial cavity. Syn. *liquor pericardii.*

pericardial knock. An early diastolic sound commonly heard in patients with constrictive pericarditis; it occurs in the rapid-filling phase of ventricular diastole.

pericardial murmur. A murmur produced in or by the pericardium.

pericardial sac. The sac formed by the pericardium.

peri·car·di·ec·to·my (perr″i·kahr″dee·eck′tuh·mee) *n.* [*pericardi-* + *-ectomy*]. Excision of a part of the pericardium.

pericardio-. See *pericardi-.*

peri·car·dio·cen·te·sis (perr″i·kahr″dee·o·sen·tee′sis) *n.* [*pericardio-* + *centesis*]. Puncture of the pericardium.

peri·car·di·ol·y·sis (perr″i·kahr″dee·ol′i·sis) *n.* [*pericardio-* + *-lysis*]. CARDIOLYSIS.

peri·car·dio·me·di·as·ti·ni·tis (perr″i·kahr″dee·o·mee″dee·as″ti·nigh′tis) *n.* MEDIASTINOPERICARDITIS.

peri·car·dio·phren·ic (perr″ee·kahr″dee·o·fren′ick) *adj.* [*pericardio-* + *phrenic*]. Pertaining to the pericardium and the diaphragm. Syn. *pericardiacophrenic.*

peri·car·dio·pleu·ral (perr·i·kahr″dee·o·ploor′ul) *adj.* Pertaining to the pericardium and to the pleura.

peri·car·di·or·rha·phy (perr″i·kahr″dee·or′uh·fee) *n.* [*pericar-*

dio- + *-rrhaphy*]. The suturing of a wound in the pericardium.

peri·car·di·os·to·my (perr″i·kahr″dee·os′tuh·mee) *n.* [*pericardio-* + *-stomy*]. The establishing by surgical means of an opening into the pericardium, for repair of wounds of the heart or for drainage of the pericardial sac.

peri·car·di·ot·o·my (perr″i·kahr″dee·ot′uh·mee) *n.* [*pericardio-* + *-tomy*]. Incision of the pericardium.

peri·car·di·tis (perr″i·kahr·dye′tis) *n.*, pl. **pericar·dit·i·des** (·dit′i·deez) [*pericardi-* + *-itis*]. Inflammation of the pericardium, acute or chronic, of varied etiology, with or without effusion or constriction. —**pericar·dit·ic** (·dit′ick) *adj.*

pericarditis obli·te·rans (o·blit′ur·anz). Pericarditis with obliteration of the pericardial cavity by adhesions of the layers.

peri·car·di·um (perr″i·kahr′dee·um) *n.*, genit. **pericar·dii** (·dee·eye), pl. **pericar·dia** (·dee·uh) [NL., from Gk. *perikardios*, around the heart, from *peri-* + *kardia*, heart] [NA]. The closed membranous sac enveloping the heart. Its base is attached to the central tendon of the diaphragm; its apex surrounds, for a short distance, the great vessels arising from the base of the heart. The sac normally contains from 5 to 20 g of clear, serous liquid. The part in contact with the heart (visceral pericardium) is termed the epicardium; the other is the parietal pericardium. See also Plate 5.

pericardium fi·bro·sum (figh·bro′sum) [NA]. FIBROUS PERICARDIUM; the connective tissue on the outer surface of the parietal serous pericardium.

pericardium se·ro·sum (se·ro′sum) [NA]. SEROUS PERICARDIUM.

peri·carp (perr″i·kahrp) *n.* [Gk. *perikarpion*, case of fruit]. *In botany*, the mature ovarian wall.

peri·ca·val (perr″i·kay′vul) *adj.* [*peri-* + *caval*]. Around one of the caval vessels, usually the inferior vena cava.

peri·ce·cal, peri·cae·cal (perr″i·see′kul) *adj.* [*peri-* + *cecal*]. Surrounding the cecum.

peri·ce·ci·tis, peri·cae·ci·tis (perr″i·se·sigh′tis) *n.* [*peri-* + *cec-* + *-itis*]. Inflammation of the serosa of the cecum and the tissues surrounding the cecum.

peri·cel·lu·lar (perr″i·sel′yoo·lur) *adj.* [*peri-* + *cellular*]. Surrounding a cell.

pericellular plexus. *In pathology*, newly formed nerve fibers that arise from the cell body or adjacent axon or cell and grow in circles around the cells in spinal ganglions, forming an interlocking network of fibers.

peri·ce·men·ti·tis (perr″i·see″men·tye′tis, ·sem″en·) *n.* [*pericementum* + *-itis*]. PERIODONTITIS.

peri·ce·men·to·cla·sia (perr″i·se·men″to·klay′zhuh, ·zee·uh) *n.* [*pericementum* + *-clasia*]. PERIODONTITIS.

peri·ce·men·tum (perr″i·se·men′tum) *n.* [*peri-* + *cementum*]. PERIODONTAL LIGAMENT.

peri·cen·tric inversion (perr″i·sen′trick). *In genetics*, an inversion that involves the centromere.

peri·cen·tri·o·lar satellites (perr″i·sen″tree·o′lur). Dense masses of about 700 Å diameter sometimes attached to the wall of a centriole.

peri·cha·reia (perr″i·ka·rye′uh) *n.* [Gk., excessive joyfulness, from *chara*, joy]. Sudden vehement or abnormal rejoicing; seen in certain psychotic brain disorders.

peri·chol·an·gio·lit·ic (perr″i·ko·lan″jee·o·lit′ick) *adj.* [*peri-* + *cholangiole* + *-itic*]. Pertaining to or involving inflammation of tissues around the smaller biliary passages.

pericholangiolitic cirrhosis. Intrahepatic BILIARY CIRRHOSIS.

peri·chol·an·gi·tis (perr″i·kol″an·jye′tis, ·ko″lan·) *n.* [*peri-* + *cholangi-* + *-itis*]. Inflammation of the tissues surrounding the bile ducts or interlobular bile capillaries. —**pericholan·git·ic** (·jit′ick) *adj.*

peri·cho·le·cys·tic (perr″i·kol″e·sis′tick, ·ko″le·) *adj.* [*peri-* + *cholecystic*]. Around the gallbladder.

peri·cho·le·cys·ti·tis (perr″ee·kol″e·sis·tye′tis, ·ko″le·) *n.* [*peri-* + *cholecyst* + *-itis*]. Inflammation of the serosa and tissues around the gallbladder.

peri·chon·dri·tis (perr″i·kon·drye′tis) *n.* [*perichondrium* + *-itis*]. Inflammation of perichondrium. —**perichon·drit·ic** (·drit′ick) *adj.*

peri·chon·dri·um (perr″i·kon′dree·um) *n.*, pl. **perichon·dria** (·dree·uh) [NL., from *peri-* + Gk. *chondros*, cartilage]. The fibrous connective tissue covering cartilage, except articular surfaces. —**perichon·dral** (·drul) *adj.*

peri·chon·dro·ma (perr″i·kon·dro′muh) *n.* [*perichondrium* + *-oma*]. A tumor of the perichondrium.

peri·chord (perr′i·kord) *n.* The sheath of the notochord. —**peri·chor·dal** (perr″i·kor′dul) *adj.*

peri·cho·roid (perr″i·ko′roid) *adj.* [*peri-* + *choroid*]. Surrounding the choroid.

peri·cho·roi·dal (perr″i·ko·roy′dul) *adj.* PERICHOROID.

perichoroidal space. A potential space between the sclera and the choroid. NA *spatium perichoroideale.*

peri·claus·tral (perr″i·klaw′strul) *adj.* [*peri-* + *claustral*]. Situated around the claustrum of the brain.

periclaustral lamina. The layer of white matter between the claustrum and the cortex of the insula.

peri·coc·cyg·e·al (perr″i·kock·sij′ee·ul) *adj.* [*peri-* + *coccygeal*]. Around the coccyx.

peri·co·lic (perr″i·ko′lick, ·kol′ick) *adj.* [*peri-* + *colic*]. Surrounding or about the colon.

peri·co·li·tis (perr″i·ko·lye′tis) *n.* [*peri-* + *col-* + *-itis*]. Inflammation of the peritoneum or tissues around the colon.

peri·co·lon·ic (perr″i·ko·lon′ick) *adj.* [*peri-* + *colonic*]. PERICOLIC.

peri·co·lon·itis (perr″i·ko″lun·eye′tis) *n.* PERICOLITIS.

peri·col·pi·tis (perr″i·kol·pye′tis) *n.* [*peri-* + *colp-* + *-itis*]. PARACOLPITIS.

peri·con·chal (perr″i·kong′kul) *adj.* [*peri-* + *conchal*]. Surrounding the concha of the ear.

peri·con·chi·tis (perr″i·kong·kigh′tis) *n.* [*peri-* + *conchitis*]. Inflammation of the periosteum or lining membrane of the orbit.

peri·cor·ne·al (perr″i·kor′nee·ul) *adj.* [*peri-* + *corneal*]. Surrounding the cornea.

peri·cor·o·nal (perr″i·kor′uh·nul) *adj.* [*peri-* + *coronal*]. 1. Around a tooth crown. 2. Around the corona of the glans penis.

pericoronal cyst. DENTIGEROUS CYST.

peri·cor·o·ni·tis (perr″i·kor″o·nigh′tis) *n.* [*peri-* + *corona* + *-itis*]. Inflammation of the tissue surrounding the coronal portion of the tooth, usually a partially erupted third molar.

peri·cos·tal (perr″i·kos′tul) *adj.* [*peri-* + *costal*]. Around a rib.

peri·cra·ni·um (perr″i·kray′nee·um) *n.* [*peri-* + *cranium*] [NA]. The periosteum on the outer surface of the cranial bones. —**pericrani·al** (·ul) *adj.*

peri·cys·tic (perr″i·sis′tick) *adj.* [*peri-* + *cystic*]. 1. Surrounding a cyst. 2. Surrounding a bladder, either the gallbladder or the urinary bladder.

peri·cys·ti·tis (perr″i·sis·tye′tis) *n.* [*peri-* + *cyst* + *-itis*]. 1. Inflammation surrounding a cyst. 2. Inflammation of the peritoneum or other tissue surrounding the urinary bladder.

peri·cys·ti·um (perr″i·sis′tee·um) *n.*, pl. **pericys·tia** (·tee·uh) [NL., from *peri-* + *cyst*]. 1. The vascular wall of a cyst. 2. The tissues surrounding a bladder.

peri·cyte (perr′i·site) *n.* [*peri-* + *-cyte*]. A cell which is enclosed within the basal membrane of the endothelial cell and which forms a portion of the capillary wall; its functions are presently unknown.

peri·cy·tial (perr″i·sish′ee·ul, ·sish′ul, ·sit′ee·ul) *adj.* [*peri-* + *cyt-* + *-al*]. Surrounding a cell.

peri·cy·to·ma (perr″i·sigh·to′muh) *n.* [*pericyte* + *-oma*]. HEMANGIOPERICYTOMA.

peri·dec·to·my (perr″i·deck′tuh·mee) *n.* [*peri-* + *-ectomy*]. PERITECTOMY.

peri·den·drit·ic (perr″i·den·drit′ick) *adj.* [*peri-* + *dendritic*]. Surrounding a dendrite.

peri·den·tal (perr″i·den′tul) *adj.* [*peri-* + *dental*]. Surrounding a tooth or its root; periodontal.

peridental membrane. PERIODONTAL LIGAMENT.

peri·derm (perr′i·durm) *n.* [*peri-* + *-derm*]. The superficial transient layer of epithelial cells of the embryonic epidermis.

peri·di·ver·tic·u·li·tis (perr″i·dye″vur·tick″yoo·lye′tis) *n.* [*peri-* + *diverticul*um + *-itis*]. Inflammation of the tissues surrounding a diverticulum, particularly of the gastrointestinal tract.

peri·duc·tal (perr″i·duck′tul) *adj.* Around a duct.

periductal sarcoma. CYSTOSARCOMA PHYLLODES.

peri·du·o·de·ni·tis (perr″i·dew″o·de·nigh′tis, ·dew·od″e·nigh′tis) *n.* [*peri-* + *duoden-* + *-itis*]. Inflammation of the tissues surrounding the duodenum.

peri·du·ral (perr″i·dew′rul) *adj.* [*peri-* + *dural*]. EPIDURAL; especially outside the dura mater of the spinal cord.

peridural anesthesia. A form of regional anesthesia resulting from the deposition of a local anesthetic solution, such as procaine, beneath the ligamentum flavum and into the peridural space of the spinal cord.

peri·en·ceph·a·li·tis (perr″ee·en·sef″uh·lye′tis) *n.* [*peri-* + *encephal-* + *-itis*]. *Obsol.* Inflammation of the pia mater and the cortex of the brain; MENINGOENCEPHALITIS.

peri·en·ceph·a·lo·men·in·gi·tis (perr″ee·en·sef″uh·lo·men″in·jye′tis) *n.* [*peri-* + *encephalo-* + *mening-* + *-itis*]. *Obsol.* MENINGOENCEPHALITIS.

peri·en·ter·ic (perr″ee·en·terr′ick) *adj.* [*peri-* + *enteric*]. Situated around the enteron; PERIVISCERAL.

peri·en·ter·i·tis (perr″ee·en″tur·eye′tis) *n.* [*peri-* + *enter-* + *-itis*]. Inflammation of the intestinal peritoneum.

peri·ep·en·dy·mal (perr″ee·e·pen′di·mul) *adj.* [*peri-* + *ependymal*]. Surrounding the ependyma.

periependymal tract. PERIVENTRICULAR TRACT.

peri·epi·did·y·mi·tis (perr″ee·ep″i·did·i·migh′tis) *n.* [*peri-* + *epididym-* + *-itis*]. Inflammation around the epididymis.

peri·epi·glot·tic (perr″ee·ep″i·glot′ick) *adj.* [*peri-* + *epiglottic*]. Around the epiglottis.

peri·esoph·a·ge·al, peri·oesoph·a·ge·al (perr″ee·e·sof″uh·jee′ul) *adj.* [*peri-* + *esophageal*]. Situated or occurring just outside of, or around, the esophagus.

peri·esoph·a·gi·tis, peri·oesoph·a·gi·tis (perr″ee·e·sof″uh·jye′tis) *n.* [*peri-* + *esophagitis*]. Inflammation of the tissues that surround the esophagus.

peri·fis·tu·lar (perr″i·fis′tew·lur) *adj.* [*peri-* + *fistular*]. Around or about a fistula.

peri·fol·lic·u·lar (perr″i·fol·ick′yoo·lur) *adj.* [*peri-* + *follicular*]. Surrounding a follicle.

peri·fol·lic·u·li·tis (perr″i·fol·ick″yoo·lye′tis) *n.* [*peri-* + *folliculus* + *-itis*]. Inflammation around the hair follicles.

perifolliculitis cap·i·tis ab·sce·dens et suf·fod·i·ens (kap′i·tis ab·see′denz et suh·fod′ee·enz, suh·fo′dee·enz). A chronic, recurrent suppurating cicatrizing disease of the scalp.

peri·fu·nic·u·lar (perr″i·few·nick′yoo·lur) *adj.* [*peri-* + *funicular*]. Around the spermatic cord.

peri·gan·gli·itis (perr″i·gang″glee·eye′tis) *n.* [*peri-* + *gangli-* + *-itis*]. Inflammation of the tissues surrounding a ganglion.

peri·gan·gli·on·ic (perr″i·gang″glee·on′ick) *adj.* [*peri-* + *ganglionic*]. Situated, or occurring, around a ganglion.

peri·gas·tric (perr″i·gas′trick) *adj.* [*peri-* + *gastric*]. Surrounding, or in the neighborhood of, the stomach.

peri·gas·tri·tis (perr″i·gas·trye′tis) *n.* [*peri-* + *gastr-* + *-itis*]. Inflammation of the serosa of the stomach.

peri·gem·mal (perr″i·jem′ul) *adj.* [*peri-* + L. *gemma*, bud, + *-al*]. 1. Around a taste bud. 2. Around any bud or developing outcropping of an organ or tissue.

peri·gen·i·tal (perr″i·jen′i·tul) *adj.* [*peri-* + *genital*]. Around the genitalia.

peri·glan·du·lar (perr″i·glan′dew·lur) *adj.* [*peri-* + *glandular*]. Pertaining to the tissue surrounding a gland.

peri·glot·tic (perr″i·glot′ick) *adj.* [*peri-* + *glottic*]. Situated around the base of the tongue and the epiglottis.

peri·glot·tis (perr″i·glot′is) *n.* [*peri-* + *glottis*]. *Obsol.* The mucous membrane of the tongue.

peri·gnath·ic (perr″i·nath′ick, ·nay′thick) *adj.* [*peri-* + *gnathic*]. Situated about the jaws.

peri·he·pat·ic (perr″i·he·pat′ick) *adj.* [*peri-* + *hepatic*]. Surrounding, or occurring around, the liver.

peri·hep·a·ti·tis (perr″i·hep″uh·tye′tis) *n.* [*peri-* + *hepat-* + *-itis*]. Inflammation of the peritoneum and tissues surrounding the liver.

peri·her·ni·al (perr″i·hur′nee·ul) *adj.* [*peri-* + *hernial*]. Around or surrounding a hernia.

peri·hi·lar (perr″i·high′lur) *adj.* [*peri-* + *hilar*]. Around a hilus.

peri·hy·po·glos·sal (perr″ee·high″po·glos′ul) *adj.* Surrounding the hypoglossal nucleus.

perihypoglossal nuclei. A group of nuclei that surround the hypoglossal nucleus, the most important of which are the nucleus intercalatus and the nucleus of Roller.

peri·hy·poph·y·se·al (perr″i·high·pof″i·see′ul, ·high″po·fiz′ee·ul) *adj.* [*peri-* + *hypophyseal*]. Around or near the hypophysis.

peri·hy·po·phys·i·al (perr″i·high″po·fiz′ee·ul) *adj.* PERIHYPOPHYSEAL.

peri·hys·ter·ic (perr″i·his·terr′ick) *adj.* [*peri-* + *hyster-* + *-ic*]. *Obsol.* Around the uterus; PERIUTERINE.

peri·il·i·ac (perr″ee·il′ee·ack) *adj.* [*peri-* + *iliac*]. Surrounding the iliac arteries.

peri·in·farc·tion block (perr″ee·in·fahrk′shun). An intraventricular conduction disturbance associated with myocardial infarction. There is QRS prolongation, the initial force deformity of an infarct, and the terminal forces are opposite in direction to the initial forces.

peri·je·ju·ni·tis (perr″i·jee″joo·nigh′tis, ·jej″oo·nigh′tis) *n.* [*peri-* + *jejun-* + *-itis*]. Inflammation of the peritoneal coat or tissues around the jejunum.

peri·kar·y·on (perr″i·kăr′ee·on) *n.* [*peri-* + *karyon*]. 1. The cytoplasmic mass surrounding the nucleus of a cell; especially, the cell body of a neuron exclusive of the nucleus. 2. The CELL BODY of a neuron.

peri·ke·rat·ic (perr″i·ke·rat′ick) *adj.* [*peri-* + *keratic*]. PERICORNEAL.

peri·ky·ma·ta (perr″i·kigh′muh·tuh) *n.*, sing. **perikyma** [*peri-* + Gk. *kyma*, wave]. Transverse, wavelike grooves on the enamel surface of a tooth, thought to be the external manifestations of the incremental lines of Retzius, which are continuous around the tooth and usually lie parallel to each other and to the cementoenamel junction.

peri·lab·y·rin·thi·tis (perr″i·lab″i·rin·thigh′tis) *n.* [*peri-* + *labyrinth* + *-itis*]. Inflammation in the osseous labyrinth of the internal ear.

peri·la·ryn·ge·al (perr″i·la·rin′jee·ul) *adj.* [*peri-* + *laryngeal*]. Situated, or occurring, around the larynx.

peri·lar·yn·gi·tis (perr″i·lăr″in·jye′tis) *n.* [*peri-* + *laryng-* + *-itis*]. Inflammation of the areolar tissue surrounding the larynx.

peri·len·tic·u·lar (perr″i·len·tick′yoo·lur) *adj.* [*peri-* + *lenticular*]. Around a lens.

perilenticular space. The space surrounding the crystalline lens holding the ciliary zonule.

peri·lymph (perr′i·limf) *n.* [*peri-* + *lymph*]. The fluid separating the membranous from the osseous labyrinth of the internal ear.

pe·ri·lym·pha (perr″i·lim′fuh) *n.* [NA]. PERILYMPH.

peri·lym·phan·ge·al, peri·lym·phan·gi·al (perr″i·lim·fan′jee·ul) *adj.* [*peri-* + *lymphangi-* + *-al*]. Situated, or occurring, around a lymphatic vessel.

peri·lym·phan·gi·tis (perr″i·lim″fan·jye′tis) *n.* [*peri-* + *lymphangi-* + *-itis*]. Inflammation of the tissues surrounding a lymphatic vessel.

peri·lym·phat·ic (perr″i·lim·fat′ick) *adj.* [*peri-* + *lymphatic*].

1. Pertaining to the perilymph. 2. Situated or occurring about a lymphatic vessel.

perilymphatic duct. AQUEDUCT OF THE COCHLEA.

perilymphatic space. Any of the small, irregular cavities filled with perilymph, between the membranous and bony labyrinths of the internal ear. NA *spatium perilymphaticum.*

peri·mac·u·lar (perr″i·mack′yoo·lur) *adj.* [*peri-* + *macular*]. Around the macula of the retina.

peri·mas·ti·tis (perr″i·mas·tye′tis) *n.* [*peri-* + *mast-* + *-itis*]. Inflammation of the fibroadipose tissues around the mammary gland.

peri·men·in·gi·tis (perr″i·men″in·jye′tis) *n.* [*peri-* + *meningitis*]. PACHYMENINGITIS.

pe·rim·e·ter (pe·rim′e·tur) *n.* [Gk. *perimetron,* circumference]. 1. Circumference or border. 2. An instrument for measuring the extent of the field of vision. It consists ordinarily of a flat, narrow, metal plate bent in a semicircle, graduated in degrees, and fixed to an upright at its center by a pivot, on which it is movable. Variously colored disks are moved along the metal plate, and the point noted at which the person, looking directly in front of him, distinguishes the color. Contr. *tangent screen.*

¹peri·met·ric (perr″i·met′rick) *adj.* Pertaining to perimetry.

²peri·me·tric (perr″i·met′rick, ·mee′trick) *adj.* [*peri-* + *metr-,* uterus, + *-ic*]. Situated around the uterus.

perimetric light sense tester. An attachment for a perimeter which may be used for determining the light threshold of the eye at any desired position or positions in the visual field.

pe·rim·e·trist (pe·rim′e·trist) *n.* A person who performs perimetry.

perimetritic abscess. Pus within the peritoneum originating from inflammation of the peritoneal covering of the uterus.

peri·me·tri·tis (perr″i·me·trye′tis) *n.* [*peri-* + *metr-* + *-itis*]. Inflammation of the tissues about the uterus. —**perime·trit·ic** (·trit′ick) *adj.*

peri·me·tri·um (perr″i·mee′tree·um) *n.,* pl. **perime·tria** (·tree·uh) [NL., from *peri-* + Gk. *mētra,* uterus] [NA]. The serous covering of the uterus.

peri·me·tro·sal·pin·gi·tis (perr″i·mee″tro·sal″pin·jye′tis) *n.* [*peri-* + *metro-* + *salping-* + *-itis*]. A collective name for periuterine inflammations.

pe·rim·e·try (pe·rim′e·tree) *n.* [from *perimeter*]. The measuring of the field of vision.

peri·my·e·li·tis (perr″i·migh″e·lye′tis) *n.* [*peri-* + *myel-* + *-itis*]. 1. Inflammation of the pia mater of the spinal cord; MENINGOMYELITIS. 2. Inflammation of the endosteum.

peri·my·o·si·tis (perr″i·migh″o·sigh′tis) *n.* [*peri-* + Gk. *mys, myos,* muscle, + *-itis*]. Inflammation of the connective tissues around muscle.

per·i·my·si·um (perr″i·mis′ee·um, ·miz′ee·um) *n.,* pl. **perimy·sia** (·ee·uh) [NL., from *peri-* + Gk. *mys,* muscle] [NA]. The connective tissue enveloping bundles of muscle fibers. —**perimysi·al** (·ul) *adj.*

perimysium ex·ter·num (ecks·tur′num). EPIMYSIUM.

perimysium in·ter·num (in·tur′num). ENDOMYSIUM.

peri·na·tal (perr″i·nay′tul) *adj.* [*peri-* + *natal*]. Pertaining to the period of viable pregnancy and neonatal life; in medical statistics the period begins when the fetus attains a weight of 500 g and ends after 28 days of neonatal life.

per·i·ne·al (perr″i·nee′ul) *adj.* Pertaining to the perineum.

perineal body. A wedge-shaped mass of intermingled fibrous and muscular tissue situated between the anal canal and the vagina; in the male, the mass lies between the anal canal and the bulb of the corpus spongiosum penis. NA *centrum tendineum perinei.*

perineal crutch. A support or brace attached to an operating table to hold a patient in certain positions.

perineal flexure. A curve of the rectum; its concavity is directed posteriorly. NA *flexura perinealis recti.*

perineal hernia. A hernia passing through the pelvic diaphragm to appear as a rectal hernia, vaginal hernia, or bladder hernia.

perineal hypospadias. A form of hypospadias in which the urethra opens upon the perineum.

perineal lithotomy. A type of lithotomy in which the incision is made through the membranous urethra in the middle of the perineum. The calculus is then removed by means of a lithotrite or suitable forceps.

perineal membrane. The fibrous membrane stretching across the pubic arch and dividing the urogenital triangle into a superficial and a deep portion. NA *fascia diaphragmatis urogenitalis inferior, membrana perinei.*

perineal prostatectomy. The removal of the prostate by a U-shaped or V-shaped incision in the perineum, using a special prostatic retractor or a modification.

perineal raphe. The ridge of skin in the median line of the perineum. NA *raphe perinei.*

perineal region. PERINEUM (2).

perineal section. EXTERNAL URETHROTOMY.

perineal testis. A testis that is situated outside the scrotum in the perineal region.

perineal vaginismus. Vaginismus due to spasm of the perineal muscles.

perineo-. A combining form meaning *perineum, perineal.*

per·i·neo·cele (perr″i·nee′o·seel) *n.* [*perineo-* + *-cele*]. PERINEAL HERNIA.

per·i·ne·om·e·ter (perr″i·nee·om′e·tur) *n.* [*perineo-* + *-meter*]. An instrument used to measure the strength of voluntary muscle contractions about the vagina and urethra.

per·i·neo·plas·ty (perr″i·nee′o·plas″tee) *n.* [*perineo-* + *-plasty*]. Plastic operation upon the perineum.

per·i·neo·rec·tal (perr″i·nee″o·reck′tul) *adj.* [*perineo-* + *rectal*]. Pertaining to the perineum and the rectum.

per·i·ne·or·rha·phy (perr″i·nee·or′uh·fee) *n.* [*perineo-* + *-rrhaphy*]. Suture of the perineum, usually for the repair of a laceration occurring during labor or for the repair of episiotomy.

per·i·neo·scro·tal (perr″i·nee″o·skro′tul) *adj.* [*perineo-* + *scrotal*]. Relating to the perineum and scrotum.

per·i·ne·ot·o·my (perr″i·nee·ot′uh·mee) *n.* [*perineo-* + *-tomy*]. Incision through the perineum; in gynecologic surgery, an incision into and repair of the perineum for the purpose of enlarging the introitus.

per·i·neo·va·gi·nal (perr″i·nee″o·vaj′i·nul, ·va·jye′nul) *adj.* [*perineo-* + *vaginal*]. Pertaining to the perineum and vagina.

per·i·neo·va·gi·no·rec·tal (perr″i·nee″o·vaj″i·no·reck′tul) *adj.* [*perineo-* + *vagino-* + *rectal*]. Relating to the perineum, vagina, and rectum.

peri·neph·ric (perr″i·nef′rick) *adj.* [*peri-* + *nephric*]. Situated or occurring around a kidney.

perinephric abscess. An abscess in the region immediately surrounding the kidney.

peri·ne·phri·tis (perr″i·ne·frye′tis) *n.* [*peri-* + *nephr-* + *-itis*]. Inflammation of the tissues surrounding a kidney. —**perine·phrit·ic** (·frit′ick) *adj.*

peri·neph·ri·um (perr″i·nef′ree·um) *n.,* pl. **perineph·ria** (·ree·uh) [NL., from *peri-* + Gk. *nephros,* kidney]. The connective and adipose tissue surrounding a kidney. —**perinephri·al** (·ul) *adj.*

peri·neph·ros (perr″i·nef′ros) *n.* PERINEPHRIUM.

per·i·ne·um (perr″i·nee′um) *n.,* genit. **peri·nei** (·nee′eye), pl. **peri·nea** (·nee·uh) [NL., from Gk. *perineos*]. 1. [NA] The portion of the body included in the outlet of the pelvis, bounded in front by the pubic arch, behind by the coccyx and sacrotuberous ligaments, and at the sides by the tuberosities of the ischium. In the male it is occupied by the anal canal, membranous urethra, and root of the penis; in the female by the anal canal, urethra, root of the clitoris, and vaginal orifice; in both sexes by the muscles, fasciae, vessels, and nerves of these structures. 2. The region between the anus and the scrotum in the male; between the anus and the posterior commissure of the vulva in the female.

peri·neu·ral (perr″i·new′rul) *adj.* [*peri-* + *neural*]. Situated around nervous tissue or a nerve.

perineural analgesia. Analgesia resulting from injection of an analgesic solution into the immediate vicinity of a nerve trunk to the area.

perineural fibroblastoma. NEURILEMMOMA.

perineural fibroma. NEUROFIBROMA.

perineural satellite. OLIGODENDROGLIA.

perineural spaces. Spaces within the sheaths of nerve roots, through which passes cerebrospinal fluid.

perineurial fibroblastoma. NEURILEMMOMA.

peri·neu·ri·tis (perr″i·new·rye′tis) *n.* [*perineurium* + *-itis*]. Inflammation of the perineurium.

peri·neu·ri·um (perr″i·new′ree·um) *n.*, pl. **perineu·ria** (·ree·uh) [NL., from *peri-* + Gk. *neuron,* nerve]. The connective-tissue sheath investing a fasciculus or primary bundle of nerve fibers. —**perineuri·al** (·ul) *adj.*

peri·neu·ro·nal (perr″i·new′ruh·nul, ·new·ro′nul) *adj.* [*peri-* + *neuronal*]. Around a neuron or neurons.

peri·ne·void (perr″i·nee′void) *adj.* Surrounding a nevus.

perinevoid vitiligo. HALO NEVUS.

peri·nu·cle·ar (perr″i·new′klee·ur) *adj.* [*peri-* + *nuclear*]. Surrounding a nucleus.

perinuclear cisterna. NUCLEAR CISTERNA.

peri·oc·u·lar (perr″ee·ock′yoo·lur) *adj.* [*peri-* + *ocular*]. Surrounding the eye.

periocular hyperpigmentation. MASQUE BILIARE.

periocular space. The space between the globe of the eye and the orbital walls.

pe·ri·od (peer′ee·ud) *n.* [Gk. *periodos,* a going around, cycle, from *peri-* + *hodos,* way]. Duration; measure of time. The space of time during which anything is in progress or an event occurs.

per·io·date (pur·eye′o·date) *n.* A salt of periodic acid.

pe·ri·od·ic (peer″ee·od′ick) *adj.* [Gk. *periodikos*]. Recurring at more or less regular intervals.

per·iod·ic acid (pur″eye·od′ick) [*per-* + *iodic*]. A colorless, crystalline acid, $HIO_4.2H_2O$, used as an oxidizing agent.

periodic acid Schiff reaction. A reaction in which compounds containing two hydroxyl groups or a hydroxyl and an amino group attached to adjacent carbon atoms are cleaved by treatment with periodic acid to form aldehydes, which are then detected by the characteristic color produced with Schiff's aldehyde reagent. The reaction is widely used to test for tissue polysaccharides, mucopolysaccharides with open glycol groups, glycopolids, glycoproteins, and certain hydroxyl-containing fatty acids. Syn. *PAS reaction.*

periodic disease. FAMILIAL MEDITERRANEAN FEVER.

periodic dystonia. PAROXYSMAL CHOREOATHETOSIS.

periodic fever. 1. Fever which recurs according to a certain pattern. 2. FAMILIAL MEDITERRANEAN FEVER. 3. ETIOCHOLANOLONE FEVER.

periodic insanity or **mania.** MANIC-DEPRESSIVE ILLNESS.

pe·ri·od·ic·i·ty (peer″ee·uh·dis′i·tee) *adj.* Recurrence at regular intervals.

periodic law. If the elements are arranged in the sequence of their atomic weights, elements having similar characteristics recur regularly in the series; that is, most of the physical and chemical properties of the elements are periodic functions of their atomic weights. Syn. *Mendeléev's law.*

periodic opthalmia. Iridocyclitis with acute exacerbations at irregular intervals and increasing ocular damage; the principal cause of blindness in horses and mules. Syn. *recurrent iridocyclitis.*

periodic paralysis. A symptom complex, observed in families as an autosomal dominant trait, manifested by recurrent attacks of flaccid muscular weakness which develop abruptly, often on rest after exercise, exposure to cold, or dietary provocation, and which last a few hours to several days. The recognized forms are the hypokalemic, normokalemic, hyperkalemic, and the type associated with hyperthyroidism.

periodic parasite. A parasite that seeks its host periodically to obtain nourishment.

periodic paroxysmal peritonitis. FAMILIAL MEDITERRANEAN FEVER.

periodic peritonitis. FAMILIAL MEDITERRANEAN FEVER.

periodic rhinitis. ALLERGIC RHINITIS.

periodic somnolence syndrome. KLEINE-LEVIN SYNDROME.

periodic table. A table of chemical elements arranged according to the law that chemical and physical properties of elements are periodic functions of their atomic numbers. See also *periodic law.*

period of isovolumetric contraction. ISOVOLUMETRIC INTERVAL.

peri·odon·tal (perr″ee·o·don′tul) *adj.* [*peri-* + *odont-* + *-al*]. 1. Surrounding a tooth, as the periodontal ligament, which covers the cement of a tooth. 2. Pertaining to the periodontium or to periodontics.

periodontal abscess. An accumulation of pus in the gingival wall of a periodontal pocket.

periodontal atrophy. Progressive resorption of alveolar bone with gingival recession and loss of the corresponding part of the periodontal ligament.

periodontal cyst. RADICULAR CYST.

periodontal disease. Any abnormality or pathological state involving the supporting tissues of the teeth; used to designate collectively the inflammatory and degenerative diseases of the periodontium.

periodontal dressing. A protective anodyne material that is placed over an area of periodontal surgery.

periodontal ligament. The connective tissue that surrounds the root of a tooth and attaches it to the alveolar bone; it is continuous with the connective tissue of the gingiva.

periodontal membrane. PERIODONTAL LIGAMENT.

periodontal pack. A dressing placed between and about the teeth in treatment of periodontal disease.

periodontal pocket. A defect between the surface of the tooth and the diseased gingivae associated with an apical migration of the epitheleal attachment.

periodontal probe. An instrument calibrated in millimeters used to measure the depth and determine the outline of a periodontal pocket.

periodontal space. The radiolucent space on a dental radiograph which represents the periodontal ligament.

periodontal traumatism. Injury of the periodontium due to excessive occlusal, operative, accidental, or orthodontic stress.

peri·odon·tic (perr″ee·o·don′tick) *adj.* PERIODONTAL.

peri·odon·tics (perr″ee·o·don′ticks) *n.* The branch of dentistry dealing with the science and treatment and prevention of periodontal disease.

peri·odon·tist (perr″ee·o·don′tist) *n.* A person who specializes in periodontics.

peri·odon·ti·tis (perr″ee·o·don·tye′tis) *n.* [*periodontium* + *-itis*]. Inflammation of the periodontium.

periodontitis complex. An inflammatory periodontal disease associated with systemic etiologic factors.

peri·odon·ti·um (perr″ee·o·don′chee·um) *n.*, pl. **periodon·tia** (·chee·uh) [NL., from *peri-* + Gk. *odous, odontos,* tooth] [NA]. The investing and supporting tissues surrounding a tooth; namely, the periodontal ligament, the gingiva, the cementum, and the alveolar bone.

peri·odon·to·cla·sia (perr″ee·o·don″to·klay′zhuh, ·zee·uh) *n.* [*periodontium* + *-clasia*]. *Obsol.* Any periodontal disease that results in the destruction of the periodontium.

peri·odon·tol·o·gy (perr″ee·o·don·tol′uh·jee) *n.* [*periodontium* + *-logy*]. The science and study of the periodontium and periodontal diseases.

peri·odon·tom·e·ter (perr″ee·o·don·tom′e·tur) *n.* [*periodonti*um + *-meter*]. An instrument used to measure the mobility of teeth.

peri·odon·to·sis (perr″ee·o·don·to′sis) *n.*, pl. **periodonto·ses** (·seez) [*periodont*ium + *-osis*]. A degenerative disturbance of the periodontium, characterized by degeneration of connective-tissue elements of the periodontal ligament and by bone resorption.

pe·ri·odo·scope (peer″ee·od′uh·skope) *n.* [*period* + *-scope*]. A calendar in the form of a movable dial, used in determining the probable date of confinement.

perioesophageal. PERIESOPHAGEAL.

perioesophagitis. PERIESOPHAGITIS.

peri·om·phal·ic (perr″ee·om·fal′ick) *adj.* [*peri-* + *omphalic*]. Around, or near, the umbilicus.

peri·onych·ia (perr″ee·o·nick′ee·uh) *n.* [*peri-* + *onych-* + *-ia*]. Inflammation around the nails.

peri·onych·i·um (perr″ee·o·nick′ee·um) *n.*, pl. **perionych·ia** (·ee·uh) [NL., from *peri-* + Gk. *onyx, onychos,* nail]. The border of epidermis surrounding an entire nail. Syn. *paronychium.*

peri·on·yx (perr″ee·on′icks) *n.* [*peri-* + *onyx*] [NA]. *In embryology,* the remnant of the eponychium which persists for a time across the root of a nail.

peri·ooph·o·ri·tis (perr″ee·o·off″ur·eye′tis) *n.* [*peri-* + *oophor-* + *-itis*]. Inflammation of the peritoneum, the ovary, and the adjacent connective tissues.

peri·ooph·oro·sal·pin·gi·tis (perr″ee·o·off″ur·o·sal″pin·jye′tis) *n.* [*peri-* + *oophoro-* + *salping-* + *-itis*]. Inflammation of the tissues surrounding an ovary and oviduct.

peri·oo·the·ci·tis (perr″ee·o″o·thi·sigh′tis) *n.* [*peri-* + *oothec-* + *-itis*]. PERIOOPHORITIS.

peri·oo·the·co·sal·pin·gi·tis (perr″ee·o″o·theek″o·sal″pin·jye′tis) *n.* [*peri-* + *ootheco-* + *salping-* + *-itis*]. PERIOOPHOROSALPINGITIS.

peri·ople (perr′ee·o″pul) *n.* [*peri-* + Gk. *hoplē,* hoof]. The outer layer of horny tissue of the hoof secreted by the perioplic ring. It extends downward over the wall of the hoof, acting as an impervious protective covering. —**peri·op·lic** (·op′lick) *adj.*

peri·op·tom·e·try (perr″ee·op·tom′e·tree) *n.* [*peri-* + *optometry*]. The measurement of the limits of the visual field.

peri·oral (perr″ee·o′rul) *adj.* [*peri-* + *oral*]. Surrounding the mouth; circumoral.

peri·or·bit (perr″ee·or′bit) *n.* [*peri-* + *orbit*]. The periosteum within the orbit. —**periorbit·al** (·ul) *adj.*

peri·or·bi·ta (perr″ee·or′bi·tuh) *n.* [NA]. PERIORBIT.

peri·or·bi·ti·tis (perr″ee·or″bi·tye′tis) *n.* [*periorbit* + *-itis*]. Inflammation of the periorbit.

periost-, perioste-, periosteo-. A combining form meaning *periosteum, periosteal.*

peri·os·te·al (perr″ee·os′tee·ul) *adj.* Pertaining to or involving the periosteum.

periosteal bone. Membrane bone formed by the periosteum.

periosteal bud. Vascular osteogenic tissue from the cellular layer of the periosteum penetrating cartilage of a growing bone to help form a center of ossification.

periosteal dysplasia. OSTEOGENESIS IMPERFECTA.

periosteal elevator. A surgical instrument designed to separate and preserve the periosteum in osteotomy.

periosteal graft. A graft consisting entirely of periosteum and used for minor bone defects to promote healing or union. See also *bone graft.*

periosteal reflex. Any one of the tendon reflexes, such as the knee jerk, once considered to be a muscular contraction in response to a blow on the periosteum at the point of insertion of the tendon.

periosteal retractor. A toothed instrument for holding periosteum.

peri·os·te·itis (perr″ee·os″tee·eye′tis) *n.* PERIOSTITIS.

periosteo-. See *periost-.*

peri·os·te·o·ma (perr″ee·os″tee·o′muh) *n.*, pl. **periosteomas, periosteoma·ta** (·tuh) [*perioste-* + *-oma*]. PERIOSTOMA.

peri·os·teo·phyte (perr″ee·os′tee·o·fite) *n.* [*periosteo-* + *-phyte*]. A morbid osseous formation upon or proceeding from the periosteum.

peri·os·teo·ra·di·al reflex (perr″ee·os″tee·o·ray′dee·ul). BRACHIORADIALIS REFLEX.

peri·os·te·ot·o·my (perr″ee·os″tee·ot′uh·mee) *n.* [*periosteo-* + *-tomy*]. An incision into periosteum.

peri·os·te·um (perr″ee·os′tee·um) *n.*, pl. **perios·tea** (·tee·uh) [NL., from Gk. *periosteos,* around the bones]. A fibrous membrane investing the surfaces of bones, except at the points of tendinous and ligamentous attachment and on the articular surfaces, where cartilage is substituted.

periosteum al·ve·o·la·re (al·vee·o·lair′ee) [BNA]. PERIODONTIUM.

peri·os·ti·tis (perr″ee·os·tye′tis) *n.* [*periost-* + *-itis*]. Inflammation of periosteum. —**perios·tit·ic** (·tit′ick) *adj.*

peri·os·to·ma (perr″ee·os·to′muh) *n.*, pl. **periostomas, periostoma·ta** (·tuh) [*periost-* + *-oma*]. Any morbid osseous growth occurring on or surrounding a bone.

peri·os·to·sis (perr″ee·os·to′sis) *n.*, pl. **periosto·ses** (·seez) [*periost-* + *-osis*]. Abnormal bone formation on the exterior of a bone.

peri·otic (perr″ee·o′tick, ·ot′ick) *adj.* [*peri-* + *otic*]. 1. Situated about the ear. 2. Of or pertaining to the parts immediately about the internal ear.

periotic capsule. The structure surrounding the internal ear.

periotic duct. AQUEDUCT OF THE COCHLEA.

periotic fluid. PERILYMPH.

periotic spaces. PERILYMPHATIC SPACES.

peri·ova·ri·tis (perr″ee·o″vuh·rye′tis) *n.* [*peri-* + *ovar-* + *-itis*]. PERIOOPHORITIS.

peri·ovu·lar (perr″ee·o′vyoo·lur) *adj.* [*peri-* + *ovular*]. Surrounding the ovum.

peri·pachy·men·in·gi·tis (perr″i·pack″ee·men″in·jye′tis) *n.* [*peri-* + *pachy-* + *mening-* + *-itis*]. *Obsol.* EPIDURAL ABSCESS.

peri·pan·cre·a·ti·tis (perr″i·pang″kree·uh·tye′tis) *n.* [*peri-* + *pancreat-* + *-itis*]. Inflammation of the tissues around the pancreas.

peri·pap·il·lary (perr″i·pap′i·lerr·ee) *n.* [*peri-* + *papillary*]. Occurring or situated around the circumference of a papilla, and especially of the optic disk.

peri·par·tum (perr″i·pahr′tum) *adj.* [*peri-* + L. *partum,* accus. of *partus,* childbirth]. Occurring at or near the time of parturition.

peri·pe·dun·cu·lar nucleus (perr″i·pe·dunk′yoo·lur). The layer of cells covering the dorsal surface of the crus cerebri, lateral to the substantia nigra.

peri·phak·us (perr″i·fack′us, ·fay′kus) *n.* [*peri-* + *-phakus,* from Gk. *phakos,* lens]. The capsule surrounding the crystalline lens.

peri·pha·ryn·ge·al (perr″i·fa·rin′jee·ul) *adj.* [*peri-* + *pharyngeal*]. Surrounding the pharynx.

pe·riph·er·al (pe·rif′e·rul) *adj.* 1. Pertaining to or located at a periphery. 2. Located at or involving a noncentral or outer area or portion. 3. Pertaining to, or located at or near, the surface of the body or of an organ.

peripheral ageusia. Loss or impairment of taste due to a disorder of the nerve endings for taste.

peripheral anesthesia. Loss of sensation due to changes in the peripheral nerves.

peripheral anosmia. See *anosmia.*

peripheral blood. 1. Blood in the systemic circulation; excludes blood in the bone marrow. 2. Occasionally used to designate blood not in the pulmonary circulation and cardiac chambers.

peripheral circulatory failure. SHOCK (1).

peripheral ganglion. TERMINAL GANGLION.

peripheral heart. *Obsol.* The muscular coat of the blood vessels.

peripheral lesion. A lesion in the periphery of the body, especially in the peripheral nerves.

peripheral nerve. Any nerve which is a component of the peripheral nervous system.

peripheral nervous system. The portion of the nervous system consisting of structures which are supported by fibroblasts rather than by astrocytes or oligodendroglia, comprising all nervous structures not enclosed by the piarachnoid membrane of the brain and spinal cord, with the exception of the optic nerve. NA *systema nervosum periphericum.* Contr. *central nervous system.*

peripheral occlusive arteriosclerosis. ARTERIOSCLEROSIS OBLITERANS.

peripheral paralysis. Flaccid paralysis due to disease of peripheral nerves.

peripheral paraplegia. Flaccid paraplegia due to disease of peripheral nerves.

peripheral reference. The condition in which, 10 to 14 weeks following section of a peripheral sensory nerve, tactile and painful stimuli and stimuli of cold, applied within the originally anesthetic area, elicit mixed sensations at the edge of the area of sensory change. This gradually disappears as the true stimulated point becomes perceptible.

peripheral resistance. Impedance to blood flow in the systemic vascular bed. Contr. *pulmonary resistance.*

peripheral vertigo. Vertigo as a symptom of primary disease outside the central nervous system, usually episodic in character, aggravated by postural changes, and accompanied by nystagmus.

peripheral vision. Vision in which the image falls upon parts of the retina outside the macula lutea, less distinct than central vision but important normally in the appreciation of the environment not directly looked at or in lesions involving the macula lutea. Syn. *indirect vision.*

pe·riph·er·aphose (pe·rif′ur·uh·foze, ·af·oze) *n.* An aphose originating in the peripheral organs of vision (the optic nerve or the eyeball).

pe·riph·ero·phose (pe·rif′ur·o·foze) *n.* A phose originating in the peripheral organs of vision (the optic nerve or the eyeball).

pe·riph·ery (pe·rif′ur·ee) *n.* [Gk. *periphereia,* from *peri-* + *pherein,* to carry]. 1. Circumference. 2. The external surface.

peri·phle·bi·tis (perr″i·fle·bye′tis) *n.* [*peri-* + *phleb-* + *-itis*]. Inflammation of the tissues around a vein or of the adventitia of a vein. —**periphle·bit·ic** (·bit′ick) *adj.*

peri·phlo·em (perr′i·flo″em) *n.* [*peri-* + *phloem*]. PHLOEM SHEATH.

pe·riph·ra·sis (pe·rif′ruh·sis) *n.*, pl. **periphra·ses** (·seez) [Gk.]. CIRCUMLOCUTION.

peri·phras·tic (perr″i·fras′tick) *adj.* [Gk. *periphrastikos*]. Characterized by a roundabout or circumlocutory way of speaking which may be pathologic, as in anomia, when a patient uses several words to approximate the word he cannot remember, or psychogenic, by way of being bombastic or because the speaker is uncertain as to whether he has expressed himself adequately.

Peri·pla·ne·ta (perr″i·pla·nee′tuh) *n.* [NL., from Gk. *peri-planēs,* wandering about]. A genus of cockroaches; the species *Periplaneta americana* and *P. orientalis* have served as obligatory hosts for the tapeworm *Hymenolepis diminuta* and may transmit pyogenic bacteria, helminthic ova, and protozoan cysts mechanically.

peri·plas·mic (perr″i·plaz′mick) *adj.* [*peri-* + cyto*plasmic*]. 1. Enclosing cytoplasm (as: periplasmic space). 2. Of or pertaining to the periplasmic space, as: periplasmic proteins.

periplasmic proteins. Proteins (frequently enzymes) localized in the periplasmic space of bacteria.

periplasmic space. The space between the cell membrane and the cell wall of a bacterium.

peri·pleu·ri·tis (perr″i·ploo·rye′tis) *n.* [*peri-* + *pleur-* + *-itis*]. Inflammation of the tissues outside the parietal pleura.

Pe·rip·lo·ca (pe·rip′lo·kuh) *n.* [NL., from Gk. *periplokē,* interlacing, twining]. A genus of Old World wood vines; the species *Periploca graeca,* silk vine, contains the cardioactive glycosides periplocin and periplocymarin.

pe·rip·lo·cin (pe·rip′luh·sin, perr″i·plo′sin) *n.* A cardioactive steroidal glycoside, $C_{36}H_{56}O_{13}$, from *Periploca graeca.*

pe·rip·lo·cy·ma·rin (pe·rip″lo·sigh′muh·rin) *n.* A cardioactive steroidal glycoside, $C_{30}H_{46}O_8$, from *Periploca graeca.*

peri·po·ri·tis (perr″i·po·rye′tis) *n.* [*peri-* + *por-* + *-itis*]. MILIARIA PUSTULOSA.

peri·por·tal (perr″i·por′tul) *adj.* [*peri-* + *portal*]. Surrounding the portal vein and its branches.

peri·proc·tal (perr″i·prock′tul) *adj.* [*peri-* + *proct-* + *-al*]. Surrounding the anus or rectum.

peri·proc·tic (perr″i·prock′tick) *adj.* PERIPROCTAL.

periproctic abscess. An abscess involving the areolar tissue surrounding the lower rectum.

peri·proc·ti·tis (perr″i·prock·tye′tis) *n.* [*peri-* + *proct-* + *-itis*]. Inflammation of the connective tissue about the rectum or anus.

peri·pros·tat·ic (perr″i·pros·tat′ick) *adj.* [*peri-* + *prostatic*]. Situated or occurring around the prostate.

peri·pros·ta·ti·tis (perr″i·pros″tuh·tye′tis) *n.* [*peri-* + *prostat-* + *-itis*]. Inflammation of the tissue situated around the prostate.

peri·py·eli·tis (perr″i·pye″e·lye′tis) *n.* [*peri-* + *pyel-* + *-itis*]. Inflammation about the renal pelvis.

peri·py·e·ma (perr″ee·pye·ee′muh) *n.* [Gk. *peripyēma,* from *peri-* + *pyon,* pus]. Suppuration about an organ or tissue.

peri·py·le·phle·bi·tis (perr″i·pye″le·fle·bye′tis) *n.* [*peri-* + Gk. *pylē,* gate, + *phleb-* + *-itis*]. Inflammation of the tissues surrounding the portal vein.

peri·py·lo·ric (perr″i·pye·lo′rick, ·pi·lo′rick) *adj.* [*peri-* + *pyloric*]. Surrounding the pylorus.

peri·rec·tal (perr″i·reck′tul) *adj.* [*peri-* + *rectal*]. About the rectum.

perirectal abscess. ANORECTAL ABSCESS.

peri·rec·ti·tis (perr″i·reck·tye′tis) *n.* [*peri-* + *rect-* + *-itis*]. PERIPROCTITIS.

peri·re·nal (perr″i·ree′nul) *adj.* [*peri-* + *renal*]. Around a kidney.

perirenal insufflation. *In radiography,* the injection of air or carbon dioxide or other gas into the perirenal tissues to outline the suprarenal glands, kidneys and retroperitoneum tissues.

peri·rhi·nal (perr″i·rye′nul) *adj.* [*peri-* + *rhinal*]. Situated about the nose or nasal cavities.

peri·sal·pin·gi·an cyst (perr″i·sal·pin′jee·un). PAROVARIAN CYST.

peri·sal·pin·gi·tis (perr″i·sal″pin·jye′tis) *n.* [*peri-* + *salping-* + *-itis*]. Inflammation of the peritoneal covering of a uterine tube.

peri·sal·pin·go·ova·ri·tis (perr″i·sal·pin″go·o″vuh·rye′tis) *n.* [*peri-* + *salpingo-* + *ovar-* + *-itis*]. PERIOOPHOROSALPINGITIS.

peri·sal·pinx (perr″i·sal′pinks) *n.* [*peri-* + *salpinx*]. The peritoneum covering the upper border of a uterine tube.

peri·scop·ic lens (perr″i·skop′ick). A lens with concavo-convex or convexo-concave surfaces, the opposite sides being of different curvatures; a meniscus lens.

peri·sig·moid·itis (perr″i·sig″moid·eye′tis) *n.* [*peri-* + *sigmoid* + *-itis*]. Inflammation of the tissues, especially the peritoneum, covering the sigmoid flexure of the colon.

peri·sin·u·ous (perr″i·sin′yoo·us) *adj.* [*peri-* + *sinu-* + *-ous*]. Surrounding a sinus.

peri·si·nus·itis (perr″i·sigh″nuh·sigh′tis) *n.* [*peri-* + *sinus* + *-itis*]. Inflammation of the tissues around a sinus, especially a sinus of the dura mater.

peri·si·nus·oi·dal (perr″i·sigh″nuh·soy′dul) *adj.* [*peri-* + *sinusoid* + *-al*]. Around a sinusoid.

perisinusoidal space. The space in the liver that is bounded on one side by the endothelium of the sinusoids and on the other by the walls of the liver cells. Syn. *space of Disse.*

peri·sper·ma·ti·tis (perr″i·spur″muh·tye′tis) *n.* [*peri-* + *spermat-* + *-itis*]. Inflammation around the spermatic cord, with an effusion of fluid; a funicular hydrocele.

peri·sple·nic (perr″i·splee′nick, ·splen′ick) *adj.* [*peri-* + *splenic*]. Situated near the spleen.

peri·sple·ni·tis (perr″i·sple·nigh′tis) *n.* [*peri-* + *splen-* + *-itis*]. Inflammation of the peritoneum covering the spleen.

perisplenitis car·ti·la·gin·ea (kahr″ti·la·jin′ee·uh). Hyalinization of the capsule of the spleen. Syn. *hyalin capsulitis, zuckerguss.*

peri·spon·dyl·ic (perr″i·spon·dil′ick) *adj.* [*peri-* + *spondyl-* + *-ic*]. Around a vertebra.

peri·spon·dy·li·tis (perr″i·spon″di·lye′tis) *n.* [*peri-* + *spondyl-* + *-itis*]. Inflammation of the tissues around the vertebrae.

peri·stal·sis (perr″i·stal′sis, ·stahl′sis) *n.*, pl. **peristal·ses** (·seez) [NL., from Gk. *peristaltikos,* peristaltic, from *peri-,* around, + *stellein,* to gather, constrict]. A progressive wave of contraction seen in tubes, such as the gastrointestinal tract, provided with longitudinal and transverse muscular fibers. It consists in a narrowing and shortening of a portion of the tube, which then relaxes, while a distal portion becomes shortened and narrowed. By means of this movement the contents of this tube are forced toward the opening. —**peristal·tic** (·tick) *adj.*

peristaltic rush. An exaggerated peristaltic wave that sweeps rapidly along the intestine for a considerable distance.

peri·staph·y·li·tis (perr″i·staf″i·lye′tis) *n.* [*peri-* + *staphyl-* + *-itis*]. Inflammation of the tissues surrounding the uvula.

peri·staph·y·line (perr″i·staf′i·line, ·leen) *adj.* [*peri-* + *staphyline*]. Situated near the uvula.

peri·sta·sis (perr″i·stay′sis, pe·ris′tuh·sis) *n.* [Gk., environment, surroundings, from *peri-* + *stasis,* placement, standing]. 1. An early stage of vascular change in inflammation, chiefly characterized by increased amounts of blood in the affected part, with decreased blood flow. 2. Environment. —**peri·stat·ic** (perr″i·stat′ick) *adj.*

peristatic hyperemia. PERISTASIS.

Peristim. Trademark for casanthranol, a mixture of glycosides from *Cascara sagrada* used as a cathartic.

pe·ris·to·le (pe·ris′tuh·lee) *n.* [Gk. *peristolē*]. Shallow contractions in the gastric wall which serve to mix the contents of the stomach. —**peri·stol·ic** (perr″i·stol′ick) *adj.*

pe·ris·to·ma (pe·ris′to·muh, perr″i·sto′muh) *n.*, pl. **peri·sto·ma·ta** (perr″i·sto′muh·tuh). PERISTOME.

peri·stome (perr′i·stome) *n.* [*peri-* + Gk. *stoma,* mouth]. 1. *In biology,* the parietal region surrounding the mouth, as the oral disk of a polyp. 2. A fringe of hygroscopic teeth, which lines the opening of the capsule in mosses.

peri·stri·ate area (perr″i·strye′ate). The visual association area of the occipital cortex surrounding the parastriate area and extending to the borders of the occipital lobe; the second concentric area around the visual cortex. Syn. *Brodmann's areas* 18 and 19. See also *visuopsychic area.*

peri·syn·o·vi·al (perr″i·si·no′vee·ul) *adj.* [*peri-* + *synovial*]. Situated or occurring around a synovial membrane.

peri·tec·to·my (perr″i·teck′tuh·mee) *n.* [*peri-* + *-ectomy*]. The excision of a ring of conjunctiva around the cornea for the removal of a vascularized pannus. Syn. *peridectomy.* See also *peritomy.*

per·i·ten·din·e·um (perr″i·ten·din′ee·um) *n.*, pl. **peritendin·ea** (·ee·uh) [NL., from *peri-* + *tendo, tendinis,* tendon]. The white, fibrous sheath covering the fiber bundles of tendons.

peri·ten·di·ni·tis (perr″i·ten″di·nigh′tis) *n.* [*peri-* + L. *tendo, tendin*is, tendon + *-itis*]. Inflammation of the sheath and tissues around a tendon.

peritendinitis cal·ca·rea (kal·kair′ree·uh). Calcific deposits in tendons and regional tissues which cause pain and limit motion of the parts.

peri·ten·on (perr″i·ten′un, ·on) *n.* [*peri-* + Gk. *tenōn,* tendon]. 1. The sheath of a tendon. 2. PERITENDINEUM.

peri·ten·o·ni·tis (perr″i·ten·uh·nigh′tis) *n.* PERITENDINITIS.

perithelial cell. ADVENTITIAL CELL.

perithelial endothelioma. HEMANGIOPERICYTOMA.

peri·the·li·o·ma (perr″i·theel″ee·o′muh) *n.* [*perithelium* + *-oma*]. HEMANGIOPERICYTOMA.

peri·the·li·um (perr″i·theel′ee·um) *n.*, pl. **perithe·lia** (·lee·uh) [*peri-* + *-thelium*]. The connective tissue accompanying the capillaries and smaller vessels. —**peritheli·al** (·ul) *adj.*

peri·thy·roid·itis (perr″i·thigh″roy·dye′tis) *n.* [*peri-* + *thyroid* + *-itis*]. Inflammation of the tissue surrounding the thyroid gland.

pe·rit·o·my (pe·rit′uh·mee) *n.* [Gk. *peritomē,* circumcision]. 1. *In ophthalmology,* the incision into the conjunctiva at the corneal scleral margin and the undermining of this half-moon-shaped segment to divide or remove the vessels of a superficial vascularized keratitis; often performed as a preliminary to enucleation and in preparation for a corneal transplant. See also *peritectomy.* 2. CIRCUMCISION.

periton-, peritone-, peritoneo-. A combining form meaning *peritoneum, peritoneal.*

peri·to·nae·um (perr″i·to·nee′um) *n.*, pl. **perito·naea** (·nee′uh) [BNA]. PERITONEUM.

peritonaeum pa·ri·e·ta·le (pa·rye″e·tay′lee) [BNA]. PERITONEUM PARIETALE.

peritonaeum vis·ce·ra·le (vis″e·ray′lee) [BNA]. PERITONEUM VISCERALE.

peritone-. See *periton-.*

peri·to·ne·al, peri·to·nae·al (perr″i·to·nee′ul) *adj.* Pertaining to or affecting the peritoneum.

peritoneal canal. The vaginal process of the peritoneum.

peritoneal cavity. A space between the visceral and parietal layers of the peritoneum. NA *cavum peritonei.*

peri·to·ne·al·iza·tion (perr″i·to·nee″ul·i·zay′shun) *n.* The process of covering with peritoneum.

peri·to·ne·al·ize (perr″i·to·nee′uh·lize) *v.* To cover with peritoneum by operative procedures.

peritoneal recesses. Pockets behind or around organs in the peritoneal cavity, as paraduodenal recesses.

peritoneal sac. A sac formed by the peritoneum.

peritoneal spaces. Spaces within the peritoneum formed by the various reflections from the abdominal wall and abdominal viscera.

peritoneal transfusion. Transfusion into the peritoneal cavity.

peritoneatome. PERITONEOTOME.

peritoneo-. See *periton-.*

peri·to·neo·cen·te·sis (perr″i·to·nee″o·sen·tee′sis) *n.* [*peritoneo-* + *centesis*]. Puncture of the peritoneal cavity, as for the removal of ascitic fluid.

peri·to·ne·op·a·thy (perr″i·to·nee·op′uth·ee) *n.* [*peritoneo-* + *-pathy*]. Any disease or abnormality of the peritoneum.

peri·to·neo·peri·car·di·al (perr″i·to·nee″o·perr″i·kahr′dee·ul) *adj.* Pertaining to the peritoneum and the pericardium.

peri·to·neo·pexy (perr″i·to·nee′o·peck″see) *n.* [*peritoneo-* + *-pexy*]. Fixation of the uterus by the vaginal route in the treatment of retroflexion of this organ.

peri·to·neo·scope (perr″i·to·nee′uh·skope) *n.* [*peritoneo-* + *-scope*]. A long slender endoscope equipped with sheath, obturator, biopsy forceps, a sphygmomanometer bulb and tubing, scissors, and a syringe; introduced into the peritoneal cavity through a small incision in the abdominal wall permitting visualization of the gas-inflated peritoneal cavity for diagnosis of abdominal and pelvic tumors, biliary disease, and other intraabdominal diseases. Syn. *laparoscope.*

peri·to·ne·os·co·py (perr″i·to·nee·os′kuh·pee) *n.* [*peritoneo-* + *-scopy*]. A method of examining the peritoneal cavity by means of a peritoneoscope.

peri·to·neo·sub·arach·noid shunt (perr″i·to·nee″o·sub″uh·rack′noid). A surgical communication between the lumbar subarachnoid space and the peritoneal cavity, for relief of hydrocephalus.

peri·to·neo·the·cal shunt (per″i·to·nee″o·theek′ul). PERITONEOSUBARACHNOID SHUNT.

peri·to·neo·tome, peri·to·nea·tome (perr″i·to·nee′uh·tome) *n.* [*peritoneo-* + *-tome*]. The areas of the peritoneum supplied with sensory fibers from a single spinal nerve.

peri·to·ne·ot·o·my (perr″i·to·nee·ot′uh·mee) *n.* [*peritoneo-* + *-tomy*]. Incision into the peritoneum.

peri·to·ne·um (perr″i·to·nee′um) *n.*, genit. **perito·nei** (·nee′eye), L. pl. **perito·nea** (·nee′uh) [L., from Gk. *peritonaion,* from *peri-,* around, across, + *tonaios,* stretched, from *teinein,* to stretch] [NA]. The serous membrane lining the interior of the abdominal cavity and surrounding the contained viscera. See also Plate 13.

peritoneum pa·ri·e·ta·le (pa·rye″e·tay′lee) [NA]. The parietal peritoneum, the portion lining the abdominal cavity.

peritoneum vis·ce·ra·le (vis″e·ray′lee) [NA]. The visceral peritoneum, the portion covering organs in the abdominal cavity.

peri·to·ni·tis (perr″i·to·nigh′tis) *n.* [*periton-* + *-itis*]. Inflammation of the peritoneum.

peri·to·nize (perr′i·to·nize) *v.* PERITONEALIZE.

peri·ton·sil·lar (perr″i·ton′si·lur) *adj.* [*peri-* + *tonsillar*]. About a tonsil.

peritonsillar abscess. An abscess forming in acute tonsillitis around one or both faucial tonsils; quinsy.

peri·ton·sil·li·tis (perr″i·ton″si·lye′tis) *n.* [*peri-* + *tonsill-* + *-itis*]. Inflammation of the tissues surrounding a tonsil.

peri·tor·cu·lar (perr″i·tork′yoo·lur) *adj.* Around or near the confluence of the sinuses of the cranial dura mater (torcular Herophili).

peri·tra·che·al (perr″i·tray′kee·ul) *adj.* [*peri-* + *tracheal*]. Surrounding the trachea.

peri·tra·che·itis (perr″ee·tray″kee·eye′tis) *n.* [*peri-* + *tracheitis*]. Inflammation of the connective tissue about the trachea.

Peritrate. A trademark for the coronary vasodilator pentaerythrityl tetranitrate.

pe·rit·ri·chal (pe·rit′ri·kul) *adj.* PERITRICHOUS.

peri·trich·i·al (perr″i·trick′ee·ul) *adj.* [*peri-* + *trich-* + *-al*]. Surrounding a hair follicle.

pe·rit·ri·chous (pe·rit′ri·kus) *adj.* [*peri-* + *trich-* + *-ous*]. Having flagella distributed over the entire body surface; said of certain microorganisms.

peri·trun·cal (perr″i·trunk′ul) *adj.* [*peri-* + *truncus* + *-al*]. Perivascular and peribronchial conjointly.

peri·tub·al (perr″i·tew′bul) *adj.* [*peri-* + *tubal*]. 1. Around a uterine tube. 2. Around a tube.

peri·typh·lic (perr″i·tif′lick) *adj.* [*peri-* + *typhl-* + *-ic*]. Surrounding the cecum.

perityphlitic abscess. An abscess involving the tissues surrounding the cecum and vermiform appendix.

peri·typh·li·tis (perr″i·tif·lye′tis) *n.* [*peri-* + *typhl-* + *-itis*]. 1. Inflammation of the peritoneum surrounding the cecum and vermiform appendix. 2. PERICECITIS. —**perityph·lit·ic** (·lit′ick) *adj.*

Perium. A trademark for pentapiperium methylsulfate, an anticholinergic.

peri·um·bil·i·cal (perr″ee·um·bil′i·kul) *adj.* [*peri-* + *umbilical*]. Surrounding or near the umbilicus.

peri·un·gual (perr″ee·ung′gwul) *adj.* [*peri-* + *ungual*]. Around a nail.

peri·ure·ter·ic (perr″i·yoo″re·terr′ick) *adj.* [*peri-* + *ureter* + *-ic*]. Surrounding one or both ureters.

peri·ure·ter·i·tis (perr″i·yoo·ree″tur·eye′tis) *n.* [*peri-* + *ureter* + *-itis*]. Inflammation of the tissues around a ureter. Syn. *paraureteritis.*

peri·ure·thral (perr″i·yoo·ree′thrul) *adj.* [*peri-* + *urethral*]. Surrounding the urethra.

peri·ure·thri·tis (perr″i·yoo″re·thrigh′tis) *n.* [*peri-* + *urethr-* + *-itis*]. Inflammation of the connective tissue about the urethra.

peri·uter·ine (perr″i·yoo′tur·in, ·ine) *adj.* [*peri-* + *uterine*]. About the uterus.

peri·uvu·lar (perr″i·yoo′vew·lur) *adj.* [*peri-* + *uvular*]. Situated near the uvula.

peri·va·gi·nal (perr″i·vaj′i·nul, ·vuh·jye′nul) *adj.* [*peri-* + *vaginal*]. About the vagina.

peri·vag·i·ni·tis (perr″i·vaj″i·nigh′tis) *n.* [*peri-* + *vagin-* + *-itis*]. PARACOLPITIS.

peri·vas·cu·lar (perr″i·vas′kew·lur) *adj.* [*peri-* + *vascular*]. About a vessel.

perivascular foot. The expanded pedicle of a neuroglial cell process attaching it to a blood vessel.

perivascular plexus. A network of nerve fibers that innervates the blood vessels.

perivascular satellites. PERICYTES.

perivascular spaces of Virchow-Robin [R. L. K. *Virchow* and C. P. *Robin*]. Fluid-filled spaces between the adventitia of the blood vessels of the brain substance and the pial limiting membrane, lined with endothelial cells, connecting with the subarachnoid space.

peri·vas·cu·li·tis (perr″i·vas″kew·lye′tis) *n.* Inflammation of the perivascular sheaths and surrounding tissues.

peri·ve·nous (perr″i·vee′nus) *adj.* [*peri-* + *venous*]. Investing a vein; occurring around a vein.

peri·ven·tric·u·lar (perr″i·ven·trick′yoo·lur) *adj.* [*peri-* + *ventricular*]. Around a ventricle, usually of the brain or heart.

periventricular tract. Nerve fibers that arise in the posterior hypothalamic nucleus and tuberal and supraoptic nuclei. Some end in the dorsomedial thalamic nucleus and in some of the midline nuclei. Some descend dorsally to the cerebral aqueduct and end in the tectum of the midbrain. Others presumably descend ventrally to the aqueduct in the subependymal portion of the central gray matter and are relayed to medullary and spinal levels. Syn. *dorsal longitudinal fasciculus (of Schütz).* NA *fasciculus longitudinalis dorsalis.*

peri·ver·te·bral (perr″i·vur′te·brul) *adj.* [*peri-* + *vertebral*]. Around a vertebra or vertebrae.

peri·ves·i·cal (perr″i·ves′i·kul) *adj.* [*peri-* + *vesical*]. Situated about or surrounding the urinary bladder.

peri·ve·sic·u·lar (perr″i·ve·sick′yoo·lur) *adj.* [*peri-* + *vesicular*]. Occurring around a seminal vesicle or vesicles.

peri·ve·sic·u·li·tis (perr″i·ve·sick″yoo·lye′tis) *n.* [*peri-* + *vesicula* + *-itis*]. Inflammation around a seminal vesicle.

peri·vis·cer·al (perr″i·vis′ur·ul) *adj.* [*peri-* + *visceral*]. Surrounding a viscus or viscera.

peri·vis·cer·i·tis (perr″i·vis″ur·eye′tis) *n.* [*peri-* + *viscer-* + *-itis*]. Inflammation around a viscus or viscera.

peri·vi·tel·line (perr″i·vi·tel′ine, ·in) *adj.* [*peri-* + *vitelline*]. Surrounding the vitellus or yolk.

perivitelline space. In mammalian ova, the space formed between the ovum and the zona pellucida at the time of maturation, into which the polar bodies are given off.

peri·vul·var (perr″i·vul′vur) *adj.* [*peri-* + *vulvar*]. Around the vulva.

peri·xe·ni·tis (perr″i·ze·nigh′tis) *n.* [*peri-* + *xen-* + *-itis*]. FOREIGN-BODY REACTION.

per·kin·ism (pur′kin·iz·um) *n.* [E. *Perkins,* U.S. physician, 1741–1799]. The use of metallic tractors or rods, purported to cure disease when drawn over the skin.

per·la·pine (pur′luh·peen) *n.* 6-(4-Methyl-1-piperazinyl)morphanthridine, $C_{19}H_{21}N_3$, a hypnotic.

perle (purl) *n.* [F., pearl]. 1. A soft capsule for administration of a volatile or unpleasant liquid medicine. 2. A thin glass globule that contains a volatile liquid to be inhaled, and that is crushed prior to use.

per·lèche (pur·lesh′) *n.* [F., from a dial. form of (*se*) *pourlécher,* to lick one's lips]. An inflammatory condition occurring at the angles of the mouth with resultant fissuring. In some instances, it appears to be due to overclosure of the mouth in edentulous patients or extreme wearing away of the teeth. Syn. *angular stomatitis.* See also *cheilosis.*

Per·lia's nucleus (pehr'lee·ah) [R. *Perlia,* German ophthalmologist, 19th century]. NUCLEUS OF PERLIA.

Perls's reaction (pehrlss) [M. *Perls,* German pathologist, 1843-1881]. A method of demonstrating hemosiderin in tissues.

perl·sucht (purl'sookt, pehrl'zo͞okht) *n.* [Ger.]. Tuberculosis of cattle.

per·ma·nent callus. A callus which remains as true bone upon completion of the reparative process of which it was a part. See also *definitive callus.*

permanent dentition. 1. The set of PERMANENT TEETH, considered collectively and in place in the dental arch. 2. The eruption of the permanent teeth. Syn. *secondary dentition.* Contr. *primary dentition.* See also *mixed dentition.*

permanent parasite. A parasite that remains in or on the body of the host until maturity and sometimes for its entire life.

permanent teeth. The 32 adult teeth of the second, or permanent, dentition; there are 8 incisors, 4 canines, 8 premolars, and 12 molars. NA *dentes permanentes.* Contr. *deciduous teeth.* See also Plate 22.

per·man·ga·nate (pur·mang'guh·nate) *n.* A salt of permanganic acid.

per·man·gan·ic acid (pur''mang·gan'ick). A monobasic acid, $HMnO_4$, obtained only in solution.

Permapen. A trademark for the antibiotic, benzathine penicillin G.

per·me·abil·i·ty (pur''mee·uh·bil'i·tee) *n. In physiology,* the property of membranes which permits transit of molecules and ions.

per·me·able (pur'mee·uh·bul) *adj.* [L. *permeabilis,* from *permeare,* to pass through]. Affording passage; pervious.

permeable membrane. A membrane that permits the passage of water and certain dissolved substances.

per·me·ase (pur'mee·ace) *n.* A system found in certain bacteria which allows the transport and concentration of galactosides and other solutes within the cell.

per·me·ation (pur''mee·ay'shun) *n.* The process of permeating or passing through; specifically, the extension of a malignant tumor, especially carcinoma, by continuous growth through lymphatics.

permeation analgesia. SURFACE ANALGESIA.

permissible dose. *In radiology,* the amount of radiation an individual may receive during a specific period with no expectation of harmful effects. Compare *tolerance dose.*

Permitil. A trademark for fluphenazine, a tranquilizing drug used as the dihydrochloride salt.

Permutit. Trademark for certain synthetic solid substances used to exchange a component ion, such as sodium, for other ions, such as calcium and magnesium, present in water or an aqueous solution in contact with the solid.

Permutit method. A method for determining the ammonia content of urine in which urine is shaken with a Permutit ion exchanger to remove the ammonia which is set free with alkali, followed by nesslerization and comparison with a standard.

per·ni·cious (pur·nish'us) *adj.* [L. *perniciosus,* from *pernicies,* destruction, ruin, from *nex, necis,* violent death]. Highly destructive; of intense severity; potentially fatal.

pernicious anemia. A megaloblastic, macrocytic anemia resulting from lack of vitamin B_{12} secondary to gastric atrophy and loss of intrinsic factor necessary for vitamin B_{12} absorption, and accompanied by degeneration of the posterior and lateral columns of the spinal cord.

pernicious anemia of pregnancy. A megaloblastic anemia of pregnancy due to folic acid deficiency.

pernicious leukopenia. AGRANULOCYTOSIS (2).

pernicious malaria. FALCIPARUM MALARIA.

pernicious vomiting. Vomiting occasionally occurring in pregnancy and becoming so prolonged and excessive as to threaten life.

per·nio (pur'nee·o) *n.,* pl. **per·ni·o·nes** (pur''nee·o'neez) [L.]. CHILBLAIN.

per·ni·o·sis (pur''nee·o'sis) *n.* [*pernio* + *-osis*]. Any dermatitis resulting from chilblain.

pero- [Gk. *pēros,* maimed]. A combining form meaning *malformed, stunted, defective.*

pe·ro·bra·chi·us (peer''o·bray'kee·us) *n.* [*pero-* + *brachi-* + *-us*]. A developmental defect in which the forearms and hands are malformed or wanting.

pe·ro·ceph·a·lus (peer''o·sef'uh·lus) *n.* [*pero-* + *-cephalus*]. An animal fetus with anomalies of the head.

pe·ro·chi·rus, pe·ro·chei·rus (peer''o·kigh'rus) *n.* [*pero-* + *cheir-* + *-us*]. Congenital absence or stunted growth of the hand.

pe·ro·cor·mus (peer''o·kor'mus) *n.* [NL., from *pero-* + Gk. *kormos,* trunk]. Congenital defect of the trunk.

pe·ro·dac·tyl·ia (peer''o·dack·til'ee·uh) *n.* [*pero-* + *-dactylia*]. Defective development of the fingers or toes.

pe·ro·dac·ty·lus (peer''o·dack'ti·lus) *n.* [*pero-* + *dactyl-* + *-us*]. An individual having congenitally defective and partially absent fingers or toes.

pe·ro·me·lia (peer''o·mee'lee·uh) *n.* [*pero-* + *-melia*]. Teratic malformation of the limbs.

pe·rom·e·lus (pe·rom'e·lus) *n.* [NL., from Gk. *pēromelēs,* maimed, from *pēros,* disabled, + *melos,* limb]. An individual with congenitally deficient, stunted, or misshapen limbs.

pe·rom·e·ly (pe·rom'e·lee) *n.* PEROMELIA.

per·o·ne·al (perr''o·nee'ul) *adj.* [Gk. *peronē,* fibula, + *-al*]. Pertaining to the fibular side of the leg.

peroneal artery. A large branch of the posterior tibial artery which descends close to the fibula through the calf of the ankle, with branches to the heel, ankle, and deep muscles of the calf. NA *arteria peronea, arteria fibularis.* See also Table of Arteries in the Appendix.

peroneal groove. A groove on the lateral aspect of the calcaneus, lodging the tendon of the peroneus longus. NA *sulcus tendinis musculi peronei longi calcanei.*

peroneal muscular atrophy. A chronic familial polyneuropathy usually inherited as an autosomal dominant (or occasionally X-linked dominant, or recessive) trait with onset during late childhood or adolescence. It is characterized by distal muscle atrophy beginning in the feet and legs and later involving the hands. Syn. *Charcot-Marie-Tooth disease.*

peroneal nerve. See Table of Nerves in the Appendix.

peroneal retinaculum. A thickening of deep fascia overlying the tendons of the peroneus longus and peroneus brevis muscles at the ankle. See also *inferior peroneal retinaculum, superior peroneal retinaculum.*

peroneal sign. In tetany, tapping the fibular side of the leg over the peroneal nerve results in eversion and dorsiflexion of the foot.

peroneal trochlea of the calcaneus. A ridge on the lateral aspect of the calcaneus between the grooves for the tendons of the peroneus brevis and peroneus longus muscles. Syn. *trochlear process of the calcaneus.* NA *trochlea peronealis.*

peroneal tubercle. PERONEAL TROCHLEA OF THE CALCANEUS.

peroneo-. A combining form meaning *peroneal* or *peroneus.*

pe·ro·neo·cal·ca·ne·us ex·ter·nus (perr''o·nee''o·kal·kay'nee·us ecks·tur'nus). A variable slip of insertion of the peroneus brevis muscle into the calcaneus.

peroneocalcaneus in·ter·nus (in·tur'nus). An occasional extra slip of the tibialis posterior muscle.

pe·ro·neo·cu·boi·de·us (perr''o·nee''o·kew·boy'dee·us) *n.* An occasional slip of insertion of the peroneus brevis or longus muscle into the cuboid.

pe·ro·neo·ti·bi·a·lis (perr''o·nee''o·tib·ee·ay'lis) *n.* [*peroneo-* + *tibialis*]. An occasional extra slip of the popliteus muscle.

pe·ro·ne·us ac·ces·so·ri·us (perr″o·nee′us ack·se·sor′ee·us). An occasional extra slip of the peroneus longus or brevis muscle.

peroneus accessorius di·gi·ti mi·ni·mi (dij′i·tye min′i·migh). A variant of the peroneus brevis muscle.

peroneus accessorius quar·tus (kwahr′tus). PERONEOCALCANEUS EXTERNUS.

peroneus accessorius ter·ti·us (tur′shee·us). PERONEUS TERTIUS.

peroneus bre·vis (brev′is). The shorter of the peroneal muscles. NA *musculus fibularis brevis, musculus peroneus brevis.* See also Table of Muscles in the Appendix.

peroneus lon·gus (long′gus). The longer peroneal muscle. NA *musculus fibularis longus, musculus peroneus longus.* See also Table of Muscles in the Appendix.

peroneus ter·ti·us (tur′shee·us). The third peroneal muscle. NA *musculus fibularis tertius, musculus peroneus tertius.* See also Table of Muscles in the Appendix.

pe·ro·nia (pe·ro′nee·uh) *n.* [*pero-* + *-ia*]. Mutilation; malformation.

pe·ro·pla·sia (peer″o·play′zhuh, ·zee·uh) *n.* [*pero-* + *-plasia*]. A malformation due to abnormal development.

pe·ro·pus (peer′o·pus) *n.* [*pero-* + Gk. *pous*, foot]. An individual with congenitally malformed feet.

per·oral (pur·o′rul) *adj.* [*per-* + *oral*]. Passed or performed through the mouth.

per os (pur oce, os) [L.]. By way of, or through, the mouth, as in the administration of medicines.

pe·ro·sis (pe·ro′sis) *n.*, pl. **pero·ses** (·seez) [Gk. *pērōsis*, disablement, maiming, from *pēros*, maimed, disabled]. 1. The condition of abnormal or defective formation. 2. Rotation or torsion of the metatarsus of chickens and turkeys associated with either choline, biotin, or manganese deficiency.

pe·ro·so·mus (peer″o·so′mus) *n.* [*pero-* + *-somus*]. An individual presenting malformation of the body.

pe·ro·splanch·nia (peer″o·splank′nee·uh) *n.* [*pero-* + *splanchn-* + *-ia*]. Malformation of the viscera.

per·os·se·ous (pur·os′ee·us) *adj.* [*per-* + *osseous*]. Through bone.

per·ox·i·dase (pur·ock′si·dace, ·daze) *n.* A conjungated, nonporphyrin enzyme, found largely in plant tissues and to a lesser extent in animal tissues, which catalyzes reactions in which hydrogen peroxide is an electron acceptor, i.e., of the following type: $AH_2 + H_2O_2 \rightarrow A + 2H_2O$.

peroxidase reaction. Any reaction indicating the presence of peroxidase in the cytoplasm of cells; usually the enzyme oxidizes the reagent to a deeply colored precipitate manifested as granulations.

peroxidase stain. Any method for detecting peroxidase activity in tissues by means of providing a peroxide and a substance, usually benzidine, which produces a color when oxidized. Chiefly used to differentiate cells of the granulocytic series from other leukocytes.

per·ox·ide (pur·ock′side) *n.* That oxide of any base which contains the most oxygen. —**per·ox·i·da·tion** (pur·ock″si·day′shun) *n.*

per·ox·i·some (pur·ock′si·sohm) *n.* Any of a group of membrane-bound subcellular particles, formed in the cytoplasm of many types of cells, that contain a variety of enzymes, especially relatively high proportions of catalase, D-amino acid oxidase, and other oxidases.

per·pen·dic·u·lar (pur″pun·dick′yoo·lur) *adj.* [L. *perpendicularis*, from *perpendiculum*, plumb line]. At right angles to any given line or plane; at right angles to the horizontal plane.

perpendicular plate of the ethmoid bone. A thin, flat, polygonal lamina of the ethmoid bone which assists in forming the septum of the nose. NA *lamina perpendicularis ossis ethmoidalis.*

perpendicular plate of the palatine bone. The flat, vertical portion of the palatine bone.

per·phen·a·zine (pur·fen′uh·zeen) *n.* 2-Chloro-10-{3-[4-(2-hydroxyethyl)piperazinyl]propyl}phenothiazine, $C_{21}H_{26}ClN_3OS$, a tranquilizer and antiemetic drug.

per pri·mam (pur prye′mum) [L.]. HEALING BY FIRST INTENTION.

per rectum [L.]. By way of the rectum.

Per·rin-Fer·ra·ton's disease (perr·æn′, ferr·ah·tohn′) [M. *Perrin*, French surgeon, 1826–1889; and L. *Ferraton*, French orthopedist, 20th century]. Snapping hip; due to movement of a band of the fascia lata over the greater trochanter.

Perrin's law. Particles constituting the internal phase of a colloidal system, if of sufficiently low concentration, must arrange themselves as a result of the influence of gravity.

Persantine. Trademark for dipyridamole, a vasodilator used for relief of anginal pain.

persecution complex. PARANOIA.

per·sev·er·a·tion (pur·sev″ur·ay′shun) *n.* [L. *perseverare*, to persist]. Involuntary, pathological repetition of words or some activity.

per·sic oil (pur′sick). The oil expressed from kernels of varieties of *Prunus armeniaca* (apricot kernel oil), or from kernels of varieties of *persica* (peach kernel oil); used as an emollient.

persistence time. The time that responses to a stimulus may continue after termination of the stimulus, as persistence of a retinal image.

persistent cloaca. The result of failure of the urorectal septum to develop, leaving a common chamber for rectum and urogenital system. See also *cloacal duct.*

persistent pupillary membrane. An anomaly of the eye, the result of the failure of the pupillary membrane of the fetus to disappear.

persistent war gas. A chemical warfare agent that is normally effective for more than 10 minutes in the open at the point of dispersion.

per·so·na (pur·so′nuh) *n.* [L., a mask]. In the analytic psychology of C. Jung, the personality "mask" or facade that each person presents to the outside world. Compare *anima.*

per·son·al, *adj.* Pertaining to a person, as personal equation, the peculiar difference of individuals in their relation to various orders of stimuli.

personal disorganization. *In psychiatry,* the temporary loss of ability for systematic, harmonious, consequential behavior.

per·son·al·i·ty, *n.* 1. The totality of traits and the habitual modes of behavior of the individual as they impress others; the physical and mental qualities peculiar to the individual, which have social connotations. Regarded by psychoanalysts as the resultant of the interaction of the instincts and the environment. 2. *In psychiatry,* an individual with a certain basic personality pattern which resists efforts at change by either the person himself or others.

personality disorders. *In psychiatry,* a group of disorders characterized by pathological trends in personality structure, with minimal subjective anxiety; in most instances, manifested by a lifelong pattern of abnormal action or behavior (often recognizable by the time of adolescence or earlier) rather than by psychotic, neurotic, or mental disturbances. See also *character disorder, personality pattern disturbance, personality trait disturbance, sociopathic personality disturbances.*

personality formation. *In psychoanalysis,* the arrangement of the basic constituents of personality.

personality pattern disturbance. *In psychiatry,* an abnormal pattern of behavior that can rarely if ever be altered therapeutically in its inherent structure; said of more or less cardinal or arch personality types.

personality test. Any standardized measurement employed in the evaluation of personality.

personality trait disturbance. *In psychiatry,* an inability to maintain emotional equilibrium and independence under more or less severely stressful situations because of the disturbances in emotional development. Psychoneurotic features are relatively insignificant. Sometimes individuals exhibiting these disturbances are called immature, but physical immaturity need not be present.

personal orientation. The act of determining one's relation to other people.

per·son·i·fi·ca·tion (pur·son″i·fi·kay′shun) *n.* The act of giving personal embodiment to an idea, feeling, abstraction, or object, as in art or drama.

per·sorp·tion (pur·sorp′shun) *n.* [*per-* + ab*sorption*]. Direct passage of intact substances through a surface of the body.

per·spi·ra·tion (pur″spi·ray′shun) *n.* 1. The secretion of sweat. 2. SWEAT (2). —**per·spi·ra·to·ry** (pur·spye′ruh·tor·ee) *adj.*

perspiratory gland. SWEAT GLAND.

per·spire (pur·spire′) *v.* [L. *per-,* through, + *spirare,* to breathe]. To sweat.

per·sua·sion (pur·sway′zhun) *n. In psychiatry,* a largely intellectual therapeutic approach, directed toward influencing the patient, his attitudes, behavior, or goals.

per·sul·fate (pur·sul′fate) *n.* A salt of persulfuric acid, $H_2S_2O_8$, an acid obtained by electrolytic oxidation of sulfuric acid. It represents the highest valence of sulfur.

per·sul·fide (pur·sul′fide) *n.* A sulfide that contains more atoms of sulfur than are required by the normal valence of sulfur, as, for example, in Na_2S_2.

Per·thes' disease (pehr′tess) [G. C. *Perthes,* German surgeon, 1869–1927]. OSTEOCHONDRITIS DEFORMANS JUVENILIS.

Perthes' test [G. C. *Perthes*]. A test of adequacy of collateral circulation in the deep veins of the leg; superficial leg veins empty on walking, after a tourniquet is placed below the knee, if there is sufficient collateral circulation in the deep veins.

Per·tik's diverticulum (pehr′tik) [O. *Pertik,* Austro-Hungarian pathologist, 1852–1913]. A diverticulum of the nasopharyngeal space resulting in an abnormally deep lateral pharyngeal fossa.

Pertofrane. A trademark for desipramine, a psychic stimulant drug used as the hydrochloride salt.

per·tur·ba·tion (pur″tur·bay′shun) *n.* [L. *perturbatio,* disturbance]. 1. Restlessness or disquietude; great uneasiness. 2. Abnormal variation in or deviation from the regularity of certain characteristic properties, as in the motions of atoms or planets when a field of force varying with time is applied.

per·tus·sal (pur·tus′ul) *adj.* [*pertuss*is + *-al*]. Resembling or pertaining to pertussis.

per·tus·sis (pur·tus′is) *n.* [*per-* + *tussis*]. A highly infectious inflammatory disease of the air passages, due to *Bordetella pertussis,* characterized at its height by paroxysmal explosive coughing ending in a loud whooping inspiration. Syn. *whooping cough.*

pertussis vaccine. A suspension or fraction of killed pertussis baccilli (*Bordetella pertussis*) prepared in adsorbed or nonadsorbed forms. See also *adsorbed pertussis vaccine.*

per·tus·soid (pur·tus′oid) *adj.* [*pertuss*is + *-oid*]. PERTUSSAL.

Pe·ru·vi·an balsam. A complex mixture of volatile oil and resin obtained by bruising the trunk of the tree *Myroxylon pereirae;* has been used externally as a stimulant and antiseptic application, and internally as an expectorant. Syn. *balsam of Peru, black balsam, Indian balsam.*

Peruvian bark. CINCHONA.

Peruvian wart. VERRUCA PERUVIANA.

per·ve·nous (pur·vee′nus) *adj.* By way of a vein; through veins.

per·ver·sion (pur·vur′zhun) *n.* [L. *perversio,* from *pervertere,* to turn about]. 1. The state of being turned away from the normal or correct. 2. *In psychopathology,* SEXUAL DEVIATION. —**per·vert** (pur·vurt′) *v.;* **per·vert** (pur′vurt) *n.*

perverted appetite. PICA.

per·vi·gil·i·um (pur″vi·jil′ee·um) *n.* [L., vigil, watch]. *Obsol.* 1. INSOMNIA. 2. PSEUDOCOMA.

per·vi·ous (pur′vee·us) *adj.* [L. *pervius*]. PERMEABLE.

pes (peece, pace) *n.*, genit. **pe·dis** (ped′is), pl. **pe·des** (ped′eez) [L.] [NA]. A foot or footlike structure. See also *talipes.*

pes an·se·ri·nus (an·se·rye′nus) [L., lit., goose foot]. 1. The radiate branching of the facial nerve after its exit from the facial canal. 2. The junction of the tendons of the sartorius, gracilis, and semitendinosus muscles at their insertion on the medial aspect of the knee. 3. The distinctive plexiform arrangement of lipoblasts seen in liposarcoma, resembling a goose's foot.

pes ca·vus (kay′vus). A foot deformity characterized by a high plantar arch with retraction of the toes at the metatarsal phalangeal joints and flexion at the interphalangeal joints. Observed frequently in Friedreich's ataxia and peroneal muscular atrophy. See also *talipes cavus.*

pes con·tor·tus (kon·tor′tus). TALIPES.

pes gi·gas (jye′gas). MACROPODIA.

pes pedunculi. CRUS OF THE CEREBRUM.

pes pla·no·val·gus (play″no·val′gus). FLATFOOT.

pes pla·nus (play′nus). FLATFOOT.

pes·sa·ry (pes′uh·ree) *n.* [ML. *pessarium,* from Gk. *pessos*]. 1. An appliance of varied form placed in the vagina for uterine support or contraception. 2. Any suppository or other form of medication placed in the vagina for therapeutic purposes.

pessary cell. An erythrocyte appearing in a stained smear as a pinkish halo with empty or pale centers.

pessary corpuscle. TARGET CELL.

pes·su·lum (pes′yoo·lum) *n.* [NL., from L. *pessulus,* bolt]. PESSARY.

pes·sum (pes′um) *n.* [L.]. PESSARY.

pest, *n.* [F. *peste,* from L. *pestis*]. 1. An annoying, destructive, or infectious organism; often, large numbers of such organisms, as a cockroach or rat pest. 2. A plague; pestilence; in the old medical literature, any major epidemic. 3. BUBONIC PLAGUE.

pes·te lo·ca (pes′teh lo′kah) [Sp., lit., crazy plague]. A form of equine encephalomyelitis, due to the Venezuelan virus.

pest·house, *n.* A hospital for persons sick with pestilential diseases.

pes·ti·cide (pes′ti·side) *n.* [*pest* + *-icide*]. A substance destructive to pests, especially to insects.

pes·ti·lence (pes′ti·lunce) *n.* [L. *pestilentia,* from *pestis,* pest, plague]. 1. Any epidemic contagious disease. 2. Infection with the plague organism *Yersinia pestis.* —**pes·ti·len·tial** (pes″ti·len′shul) *adj.*

pestilential bubo. A bubo associated with the plague.

pes·tis (pes′tis) *n.* [L.]. Pest or plague.

pestis minor. Plague with few systemic manifestations; ambulatory plague.

pes·tle (pes′ul, pes′tul) *n.* [L. *pistillum*]. The device for mixing or powdering substances in a mortar.

-petal [L. *petere,* to seek]. A combining form meaning *moving toward, seeking.*

pet·al, *v.* To place overlapping chevron-shaped pieces of adhesive tape on (the edges of a plaster orthopedic cast) to prevent plaster crumbs from breaking off.

pe·te·chia (pe·tee′kee·uh, pe·teck′ee·uh) *n.*, pl. **pete·chi·ae** (·kee·ee) [NL., from It. *petecchia*]. A minute, rounded spot of hemorrhage on a surface such as skin, mucous membrane, serous membrane, or on a cross-sectional surface of an organ. —**pete·chi·al** (·kee·ul) *adj.*

pe·te·chi·om·e·ter (pe·tee″kee·om′e·tur) *n.* [*petechi*a + *-meter*]. An instrument for the detection of increased capillary fragility by the application of suction to the skin.

Pe·ters' anomaly (peʸ′turss) [A. *Peters*]. Congenital opacity of the cornea caused by dysgenesis of the corneal mesoderm.

Peters' embryo [H. *Peters,* Austrian gynecologist, 1859–

1934]. An early human embryo discovered and described by Peters in 1899.

Pe·ter·sen's bag (pe^y'tur·z^en) [C. F. *Petersen,* German surgeon, 1845–1908]. A rubber bag designed to be placed in the rectum and inflated, to facilitate cystotomy.

Petersen's operation [C. F. *Petersen*]. A method of suprapubic lithotomy.

Peters' method. A procedure for determining urinary creatine under conditions whereby the diluted sample is treated by methods similar to those used for blood filtrates, thus permitting the determination of both blood and urine creatine in essentially the same manner.

peth·i·dine (peth'i·deen, ·din) *n.* Meperidine, an analgesic drug used as the hydrochloride salt.

pet·i·ole (pet'ee·ole) *n.* [L. *petiolus,* small foot, fruitstalk]. A stem or stalk.

pe·ti·o·lus (pe·tye'o·lus) *n.* [L.]. PETIOLE.

petiolus epi·glot·ti·dis (ep''i·glot'i·dis) [NA]. The pointed lower end of the epiglottic cartilage attached to the thyroid cartilage.

pe·tit mal (pet'ee mal', puh·tee') [F., lit., small illness]. ABSENCE ATTACK.

petit mal absence or **seizure.** ABSENCE ATTACK.

petit mal epilepsy. A form of epilepsy characterized by recurrent absence attacks.

petit mal status. ABSENCE STATUS.

petit mal triad. A concept originally proposed by Lennox, but now abandoned, that absence, and myoclonic and akinetic seizures constitute a petit mal triad.

petit mal variant. *In electroencephalography,* a diffuse spike-and-wave pattern that is slower than the 3-per-second spike-and-wave of true petit mal, but which resembles it in many respects; often associated with myoclonic and akinetic seizures, without complete loss of consciousness or postictal manifestations. See also *Lennox syndrome.*

Pe·tit's triangle (p^e·tee') [J. L. *Petit,* French surgeon, 1674–1750]. LUMBAR TRIANGLE.

PETN Abbreviation for *pentaerythrityl tetranitrate.*

petr-, petri-, petro- [Gk. *petros,* stone]. A combining form meaning (a) *stone;* (b) *petroleum;* (c) *pertaining to the petrous portion of the temporal bone.*

pet·ri·fac·tion (pet''ri·fack'shun) *n.* The process of changing to stone, as petrifaction of the fetus.

pe·tri plate or **dish** (pee'tree, Ger. pe^y'tree) [J. *Petri,* German bacteriologist, 1852–1921]. PLATE (3).

pé·tris·sage (pay''tri·sahzh') *n.* [F.]. Kneading massage.

petro-. See *petr-.*

pet·ro·bas·i·lar (pet''ro·bas'i·lur) *adj.* [*petro-* + *basilar*]. Pertaining to the petrous part of the temporal bone and the basilar part of the occipital bone.

pet·ro·chem·i·cal (pet''ro·kem'i·kul) *n.* A chemical obtained from petroleum.

pet·ro·la·tum (pet''ro·lay'tum) *n.* A purified, semisolid mixture of hydrocarbons obtained from petroleum. Occurs as a yellowish to light amber, unctuous mass. Used as a bland, protective dressing and as a base for ointments. Syn. *petroleum jelly, yellow petrolatum.*

petrolatum gauze. Absorbent gauze saturated with white petrolatum to the extent of not less than 4 times the weight of the gauze; used as an emollient dressing, packing, or drain.

pe·tro·le·um (pe·tro'lee·um) *n.* [Gk. *petros,* stone, + L. *oleum,* oil]. A complex mixture of hydrocarbons consisting chiefly of paraffins and cycloparaffins or of cyclic aromatic hydrocarbons, with small amounts of benzene hydrocarbons, sulfur, and oxygenated compounds. Occurs as a dark-yellow to brown or greenish-gray, oily liquid.

petroleum benzin. Benzin, usually a purified grade.

petroleum ether. Benzin, usually a purified grade.

petroleum jelly. PETROLATUM.

petroleum jelly gauze. PETROLATUM GAUZE.

petroleum naphtha. Benzin, usually a purified grade.

pet·ro·mas·toid (pet''ro·mas'toid) *n.* Pertaining to the petrous and mastoid portions of the temporal bone.

pet·ro·oc·cip·i·tal (pet''ro·ock·sip'i·tul) *adj.* Pertaining to the petrous portion of the temporal bone and to the occipital bone.

petrooccipital fissure. The narrow cleft between the petrous part of the temporal bone and the occipital bone. NA *fissura petrooccipitalis.*

petrooccipital suture. The site of union between the occipital bone and the petrous portion of the temporal.

pet·ro·pha·ryn·ge·us (pet''ro·fa·rin'jee·us, ·făr''in·jee'us) *n.* [*petro-* + *pharyngeus*]. A small bundle of muscle fibers arising from the lower surface of the petrous portion of the temporal bone, and blending with the constrictors of the pharynx; a part of the salpingopharyngeus.

pe·tro·sa (pe·tro'suh) *n.,* pl. **petro·sae** (·see) [fem. of L. *petrosus,* rocky; short for *pars petrosa*]. PETROUS PART OF THE TEMPORAL BONE. —**petro·sal** (·sul) *adj.*

petrosal ganglion. INFERIOR GANGLION (1).

petrosal nerve. Any of several small nerves passing through the petrous part of the temporal bone and usually attached to the geniculate ganglion. See also Table of Nerves in the Appendix.

petrosal process. A sharp process of the sphenoid bone located below the notch for the passage of the abducent nerve, which articulates with the apex of the petrous portion of the temporal bone and forms the medial boundary of the foramen lacerum.

pet·ro·si·tis (pet''ro·sigh'tis) *n.* [*petrosa* + *-itis*]. Inflammation of the petrous portion of the temporal bone, usually from extension of a mastoiditis or from middle ear disease.

pet·ro·sphe·noid (pet''ro·sfee'noid) *adj.* Pertaining to the petrous portion of the temporal bone and the sphenoid bone.

petrosphenoid ligament. A thickened portion of the dura mater joining the apex of the petrosal process with the posterior clinoid process. Syn. *Gruber's ligament.*

petrosphenoid space syndrome. JACOD'S SYNDROME.

petrosphenoid suture. The site of union between the great wing of the sphenoid bone and the petrous portion of the temporal bone.

pet·ro·squa·mous (pet''ro·skway'mus) *adj.* Pertaining to the petrous and squamous portions of the temporal bone.

petrosquamous fissure. The narrow cleft formed by incomplete fusion of the petrous and squamous portions of the temporal bone. NA *fissura petrosquamosa.*

petrosquamous sinus. An inconstant sinus of the dura at the junction of the petrous and squamous parts of the temporal bone, opening into the transverse sinus posteriorly.

pet·ro·tym·pan·ic fissure (pet''ro·tim·pan'ick). The narrow slit posterior to the mandibular fossa of the temporal bone, giving passage to the chorda tympani nerve. NA *fissura petrotympanica.*

pet·rous (pet'rus, pee'trus) *adj.* [L. *petrosus,* from Gk. *petra,* stone, rock]. Stony; of the hardness of stone.

petrous part of the temporal bone. The pyramidal dense portion of the temporal bone which projects medially. NA *pars petrosa ossis temporalis.*

petrous pyramid. PETROUS PART OF THE TEMPORAL BONE.

pe·trox·o·lin (pe·trock'so·lin) *n.* A liquid or solid preparation made with a vehicle or base composed of light liquid petrolatum with soft ammonia soap and alcohol and containing medicinal substances. Petroxolins were used as externally applied dermatologic agents.

Pet·te-Dö·ring's disease or **panencephalitis** (pet'e^h, dœh'ring) [H. *Pette,* German, 20th century; and G. *Döring,* German, 20th century]. SUBACUTE SCLEROSING PANENCEPHALITIS.

Pet·ten·ko·fer's test (pet'^en·ko'fur) [M. J. *Pettenkofer,* German chemist, 1818–1901]. A test for bile acids in which urine containing bile acids, mixed with sucrose and sulfuric acid, produces a red color.

Pet·ze·ta·ki's disease (ped·ze^h·tah^h'kee) [M. *Petzetaki,* Greek physician, 20th century]. A viral infection clinically and histopathologically similar to cat-scratch disease, but thought to be due to a different agent.

Petz·val theory (pets'vahl) [J. *Petzval,* Austrian opticist, b. 1891]. A theory which states that the sum of the product of the refractive indexes and focal lengths of two thin lenses must equal zero in order to attain a fairly flat field free from astigmatic conditions.

Peutz-Je·ghers syndrome (pœhts, jay'gurz) [J. L. A. *Peutz,* Dutch physician, 20th century; and H. *Jeghers,* U.S. physician, 20th century]. Familial gastrointestinal polyposis associated with mucocutaneous melanin pigmentation of mouth, hands, and feet. Syn. *hereditary multiple polyposis.*

-pexia. See *-pexy.*

pex·is (peck'sis) *n.* [Gk. *pēxis*]. FIXATION.

-pexy [Gk. *pēxis*]. *In surgery,* a combining form meaning *fixation.*

Pey·er's patches or **glands** (pye'ur) [J. C. *Peyer,* Swiss anatomist, 1653–1712]. AGGREGATE FOLLICLES.

pe·yo·te (pay·o'tee) *n.* [Sp., from Nahuatl *peyotl*]. MESCAL (1).

Pey·ro·nie's disease (peh·roh·nee') [F. de la *Peyronie,* French surgeon, 1678–1747]. A condition of unknown etiology characterized by the development of plaques or masses of dense fibrous tissue in the fascia about the corpus cavernosum of the penis, resulting in deformity of the penis. Syn. *fibrous cavernitis, penile strabismus, penis plasticus.* See also *cavernitis.*

Pey·rot's thorax (peh·ro') [J. J. *Peyrot,* French surgeon, 1843–1918]. The obliquely oval thorax associated with massive pleural effusion.

Pfan·nen·stiel's incision (pfahn'en·shteel) [H. J. *Pfannenstiel,* German gynecologist, 1862–1909]. A low transverse incision through the skin, subcutaneous tissue, and fascia, separating the rectus muscles in the midline vertically, placed below the pubic hair line above the mons pubis, thus making an inconspicuous scar.

Pfaund·ler-Hurler syndrome (pfaownd'lur) [M. von *Pfaundler,* German physician, 1872–1947; and Gertrud *Hurler*]. HURLER'S SYNDROME.

Pfaundler's reaction [M. von *Pfaundler*]. THREAD REACTION.

Pfeif·fer·el·la (figh''fur·el'uh) *n.* [R. F. J. *Pfeiffer,* German bacteriologist, 1858–1945]. *ACTINOBACILLUS.*

Pfeifferella whit·mo·ri (whit·mor'eye). *PSEUDOMONAS PSEUDOMALLEI.*

Pfeif·fer's bacillus (pfigh'fur) [R. F. J. *Pfeiffer*]. *HEMOPHILUS INFLUENZAE.*

Pfeiffer's disease [E. *Pfeiffer,* German physician, 1846–1921]. INFECTIOUS MONONUCLEOSIS.

Pflü·ger's laws (pflueˢgur) [E. F. W. *Pflüger,* German physiologist, 1829–1910]. Laws pertaining to the alteration of excitability and conduction of nerves during and after the application of direct electric current.

Pflüger's tube [E. F. W. *Pflüger*]. One of the cellular cortical sex cords or invaginations of the germinal epithelium of the embryonic ovary.

pg Abbreviation for *picogram.*

PGA Abbreviation for *pteroylglutamic acid* (= FOLIC ACID).

pH A symbol, introduced by Sørensen, used to express hydrogen-ion concentration. It signifies the logarithm, on the base 10, of the reciprocal of the hydrogen-ion concentration. A pH above 7 represents alkalinity in an aqueous medium; below 7, acidity.

Ph¹ Symbol for Philadelphia chromosome.

PHA. Abbreviation for *phytohemagglutinin.*

phac-, phaco- [Gk. *phakos,* lentil, mole, freckle]. A combining form meaning *lens.*

pha·cen·to·cele (fa·sen'to·seel) *n.* [*phac-* + *entocele*]. PHACOCELE.

pha·ci·tis (fa·sigh'tis) *n.* [*phac-* + *-itis*]. Inflammation of the lens of the eye.

phaco-. See *phac-.*

phacoanaphylactic endophthalmitis. The anaphylactic sensitization of the human to his own lens protein by extracapsular cataract extraction; a form of lens-induced uveitis.

phaco·an·a·phy·lax·is (fack''o·an''uh·fi·lack'sis) *n.* [*phaco-* + *anaphylaxis*]. Allergic reaction to crystalline lens protein. —**phacoanaphy·lac·tic** (·lack'tick) *adj.*

phaco·cele (fack'o·seel) *n.* [*phaco-* + *-cele*]. Displacement of the crystalline lens from its proper position; herniation of the lens.

phaco·cyst (fack'o·sist) *n.* [*phaco-* + *-cyst*]. The capsule of the crystalline lens.

phaco·cys·tec·to·my (fack''o·sis·teck'tuh·mee) *n.* [*phacocyst* + *-ectomy*]. Excision of a part of the capsule of the crystalline lens.

pha·co·emul·si·fi·ca·tion (fay''ko·e·mul'si·fi·kay'shun) *n.* [*phaco-* + *emulsification*]. Extracapsular dissolution of a cataract using ultrasonic energy.

phaco·er·y·sis, phaco·er·i·sis (fack''o·err'i·sis) *n.* [*phaco-* + Gk. *erysis,* a pulling, drawing]. An operation for cataract employing suction. Syn. *Barraquer's operation.*

phac·oid (fack'oid, fay'koid) *adj.* [Gk. *phakoeidēs,* from *phakos,* lentil]. Lens-shaped.

pha·col·y·sis (fa·kol'i·sis) *n.* [*phaco-* + *-lysis*]. 1. Dissolution or disintegration of the crystalline lens. 2. An operation for the relief of high myopia, consisting in discission of the crystalline lens followed by extraction. —**phaco·lyt·ic** (fack''o·lit'ick) *adj.*

phacolytic glaucoma. An acute open-angle glaucoma associated with a hypermature cataract in which lens material and macrophages with phagocytosed lens material mechanically block the filtration angle of the eye. See also *phacotoxic uveitis.*

pha·co·ma, pha·ko·ma (fa·ko'muh) *n.,* pl. **phacomas, phacoma·ta** (·tuh), **phakomas, phakoma·ta** (·tuh) [*phac-* + *-oma*]. 1. A lens-shaped retinal hamartoma, occurring in tuberous sclerosis. 2. Any of the hamartomatous masses occurring in familial neurocutaneous diseases such as Hippel-Lindau disease or tuberous sclerosis.

pha·co·ma·to·sis, pha·ko·ma·to·sis (fay''ko·muh·to'sis, fack''o·) *n.,* pl. **phacomato·ses, phakomato·ses** (·seez) [*phacoma* + *-osis*]. A term applied by van der Hoeve (1920) to particular forms of neurocutaneous abnormality, which are often present in minor degree at birth and later evolved as quasineoplastic disorders. The latter include tuberous sclerosis, neurofibromatosis, and cutaneous angiomatosis with central nervous system abnormalities.

phacomatosis of Bourneville [D. M. *Bourneville*]. TUBEROUS SCLEROSIS.

phaco·meta·cho·re·sis (fack''o·met''uh·ko·ree'sis) *n.* [*phaco-* + Gk. *metachōrēsis,* withdrawal]. PHACOCELE.

phaco·met·e·ce·sis (fack''o·met''e·see'sis) *n.* [*phaco-* + *metoikēsis,* migration]. PHACOCELE.

pha·com·e·ter (fa·kom'e·tur) *n.* [*phaco-* + *-meter*]. LENSOMETER.

phaco·pla·ne·sis (fack''o·pla·nee'sis) *n.* [*phaco-* + Gk. *planēsis,* wandering]. Displacement of the crystalline lens of the eye from the posterior to the anterior chamber and back again.

phaco·scle·ro·sis (fack''o·skle·ro'sis) *n.* [*phaco-* + *sclerosis*]. Hardening of the crystalline lens.

phaco·scope (fack'o·skope) *n.* [*phaco-* + *-scope*]. An instrument for observing the accommodative changes of the crystalline lens. —**pha·cos·co·py** (fa·kos'kuh·pee) *n.*

phaco·sco·tas·mus (fack''o·sko·taz'mus) *n.* [NL., from *phaco-* + Gk. *skotasmos,* darkening]. Clouding of the crystalline lens.

phaco·tox·ic (fack''o·tock'sick) *adj.* [*phaco-* + *toxic*]. Being, due to, or pertaining to toxic effects of lenticular material.

phacotoxic uveitis. A form of lens-induced uveitis due to the toxic or allergic effects of lenticular proteins liberated into the eye from a surgical or traumatic break of the lens capsule or from the leaking of a hypermature cataract.

phaenakistoscope. PHENAKISTOSCOPE.

phaeo-. See *pheo-*.
phaeochrome. Pheochrome (= CHROMAFFIN).
phaeochromoblast. PHEOCHROMOBLAST.
phaeochromoblastoma. PHEOCHROMOBLASTOMA.
phaeochromocyte. Pheochromocyte (= CHROMAFFIN CELL).
Phaeo·phy·ce·ae (fee″o·figh′see·ee) *n.pl.* A class of brown algae.
phag-, phago- [Gk. *phagein*, to eat]. A combining form meaning (a) *eating, feeding;* (b) *phagocyte.*
phage (faij, fahzh) *n.* BACTERIOPHAGE.
-phage, -phag [Gk. *phagein*, to eat]. A combining form meaning *eater* or *that which ingests;* used especially to designate *a phagocyte.* See also *bacteriophage.*
phag·e·de·na, phag·e·dae·na (faj″e·dee′nuh) *n.* [Gk. *phagedaina*, cancerous sore]. A rapidly spreading destructive ulceration of soft parts. —**phage·den·ic, phage·daen·ic** (·den′ick) *adj.*
phagedena geo·met·ri·ca (jee·o·met′ri·kuh). Pyoderma gangrenosum with chronic burrowing ulcers.
phagedena trop·i·ca (trop′i·kuh). TROPICAL ULCER.
phagedenic balanitis. A destructive balanitis leading to necrosis of the glans penis.
-phagia [Gk., from *phagein*, to eat]. A combining form designating *a condition involving eating or swallowing.*
phago-. See *phag-*.
phagocaryosis. PHAGOKARYOSIS.
phago·cyt·able (fag″o·sigh′tuh·bul) *adj.* Susceptible to phagocytosis.
phago·cyte (fag′o·site) *n.* [*phago-* + *-cyte*]. A cell having the property of engulfing and digesting foreign or other particles or cells harmful to the body. Fixed phagocytes include the cells of the reticuloendothelial system and fixed macrophages (histiocytes). Free phagocytes include the leukocytes and free macrophages. —**phago·cy·tal** (fag″o·sigh′tul), **phago·cyt·ic** (·sit′ick) *adj.*
phagocytic index. A figure characteristic for a serum, and denoting the average number of bacteria found per leukocyte after a mixture of the serum, a bacterial culture, and washed leukocytes has been incubated.
phago·cyt·ize (fag′o·si·tize) *v.* To consume by enveloping and digesting; to subject to phagocytosis.
phago·cy·to·blast (fag″o·sigh′to·blast) *n.* [*phagocyte* + *-blast*]. A cell giving rise to phagocytes.
phago·cy·tol·y·sis (fag″o·sigh·tol′i·sis) *n.* [*phagocyte* + *-lysis*]. Destruction or dissolution of phagocytes. —**phago·cy·to·lit·ic** (·sigh″to·lit′ick) *adj.*
phago·cy·to·sis (fag″o·sigh·to′sis) *n.*, pl. **phagocyto·ses** (·seez) [*phagocyte* + *-osis*]. Ingestion of foreign or other particles by certain cells. —**phago·cy·tose** (fag″o·sigh′toze) *v.*
phago·dy·na·mom·e·ter (fag″o·dye″nuh·mom′e·tur) *n.* [*phago-* + *dynamometer*]. An apparatus for estimating the force exerted in chewing.
phago·kary·o·sis, phago·cary·o·sis (fag″o·kăr″ee·o′sis) *n.* [*phago-* + *kary-* + *-osis*]. Supposed phagocytic action by the cell nucleus.
pha·gol·y·sis (fa·gol′i·sis) *n.*, pl. **phagoly·ses** (·seez) [*phago-* + *-lysis*]. Destruction or dissolution of phagocytes; phagocytolysis.
phago·ma·nia (fag″o·may′nee·uh) *n.* [*phago-* + *-mania*]. An insatiable craving for food.
phago·some (fag′o·sohm) *n.* [*phago-* + *-some*]. A single-membrane body in the cytoplasm, the result of either phagocytosis.
phago·ther·a·py (fag″o·therr′uh·pee) *n.* [*phago-* + *therapy*]. Treatment by superalimentation; overfeeding.
-phagous [*phag-* + *-ous*]. A combining form meaning *eating* or *subsisting on.*
-phagy [*phag-* + *-y*]. A combining form designating *a* (particular kind of) *eating* or *an eating or swallowing of* (a specific substance).
phak-, phako-. See *phac-*.
phakomatosis. PHACOMATOSIS.
phal·a·cro·sis (fal″uh·kro′sis) *n.* [Gk. *phalakrōsis*, from *phalakros*, bald]. BALDNESS.
phalang-, phalango-. A combining form meaning *phalanx, phalangeal.*
pha·lan·ge·al (fa·lan′jee·ul) *adj.* Pertaining to a phalanx or phalanges.
phalangeal cells. Supporting cells in the spiral organ (of Corti). The inner phalangeal cells are arranged on the inner surface of the pillar cells; the outer phalangeal cells, called Deiters' cells, on the outer surface.
phalangeal process. An outward prolongation of one of the outer rods of the spiral organ (of Corti).
phal·an·gec·to·my (fal″an·jeck′tuh·mee) *n.* [*phalang-* + *-ectomy*]. Surgical excision of a phalanx of a finger or toe.
phalanges. Plural of *phalanx.*
phalanges di·gi·to·rum ma·nus (dij·i·to′rum man′us) [BNA]. OSSA DIGITORUM MANUS.
phalanges digitorum pe·dis (ped′is) [BNA]. OSSA DIGITORUM PEDIS.
phal·an·gi·tis (fal″an·jye′tis) *n.* [*phalang-* + *-itis*]. Inflammation of a phalanx.
phalangitis syphilitica. DACTYLITIS SYPHILITICA.
pha·lan·gi·za·tion (fa·lan″ji·zay′shun) *n.* A plastic operation in which a metacarpal bone is separated from its fellows and surrounded with skin, thus forming a substitute for a finger or thumb.
phalango-. See *phalang-*.
pha·lan·go·pha·lan·ge·al (fa·lang″go·fuh·lan′jee·ul) *adj.* [*phalango-* + *phalangeal*]. Pertaining to the successive phalanges of the digits, as in phalangophalangeal amputation, removal of a finger or toe at an interphalangeal joint.
pha·lanx (fay′lanks, fal′anks) *n.*, genit. **pha·lan·gis** (fa·lan′jis), pl. **phalan·ges** (·jeez) [L., from Gk., lit. row, battle array]. 1. One of the bones of the fingers or toes. See also Table of Bones in the Appendix and Plate 1. 2. One of the delicate processes of the headplate of the outer rod of Corti projecting beyond the inner rod.
phalanx dis·ta·lis di·gi·to·rum ma·nus (dis·tay′lis dij·i·to′rum man′us) [NA]. The distal phalanx of any of the digits of the hand.
phalanx distalis digitorum pe·dis (ped′is) [NA]. The distal phalanx of any of the toes.
phalanx me·dia di·gi·to·rum ma·nus (mee′dee·uh dij·i·to′rum man′us) [NA]. The middle phalanx of any of the fingers.
phalanx media digitorum pe·dis (ped′is) [NA]. The middle phalanx of any of the four lateral toes.
phalanx pri·ma di·gi·to·rum ma·nus (prye′muh dij·i·to′rum man′us) [BNA]. PHALANX PROXIMALIS DIGITORUM MANUS.
phalanx prima digitorum pe·dis (ped′is) [BNA]. PHALANX PROXIMALIS DIGITORUM PEDIS.
phalanx prox·i·ma·lis di·gi·to·rum ma·nus (prock·si·may′lis dij·i·to′rum man′us) [NA]. The proximal phalanx of any of the digits of the hand.
phalanx proximalis digitorum pe·dis (ped′is) [NA]. The proximal phalanx of any of the toes.
phalanx se·cun·da di·gi·to·rum ma·nus (se·kun′duh dij·i·to′rum man′us) [BNA]. PHALANX MEDIA DIGITORUM MANUS.
phalanx secunda digitorum pe·dis (ped′is) [BNA]. PHALANX MEDIA DIGITORUM PEDIS.
phalanx ter·tia di·gi·to·rum ma·nus (tur′shee·uh dij·i·to′rum man′us) [BNA]. PHALANX DISTALIS DIGITORUM MANUS.
phalanx tertia digitorum pe·dis (ped′is) [BNA]. PHALANX DISTALIS DIGITORUM PEDIS.
phalli. A plural of *phallus.*
phal·lic (fal′ick) *adj.* [Gk. *phallikos*, from *phallos*, penis]. Pertaining to the penis or phallus.
phal·li·cism (fal′i·siz·um) *n.* PHALLIC WORSHIP.
phallic phase or **stage**. *In psychoanalysis,* the period in the psychosexual development of a child, usually from about 2 to 6 years, during which sexual interest and pleasure center about the penis in boys, and to a lesser extent about the clitoris in girls.

phallic symbol. *In psychoanalysis,* any form resembling or suggestive of a penis, as a snake, obelisk, tower, or pencil; often employed in dreams and other mental processes to disguise sexual wishes.

phallic urethra. UROGENITAL TUBE.

phallic worship. 1. Adoration and veneration of the penis as symbolic of the creative, death-defying powers of nature; a common practice in certain religious cults, particularly ancient ones. 2. *In psychoanalytic theory,* the penis as the object of libido during the phallic stage of psychosexual development.

phal·lin (fal'in) *n.* A hemolytic nitrogenous glycoside from the poisonous *Amanita* species of mushrooms.

phal·lism (fal'iz·um) *n.* PHALLICISM.

phal·loi·dine (fa·loy'deen, ·din) *n.* A peptide from the poisonous mushroom *Amanita phalloides;* on hydrolysis it yields cystine, alanine, and allohydroxy-L-proline.

phal·lo·plas·ty (fal'o·plas"tee) *n.* [*phall*us + *-plasty*]. Plastic construction or repair of the penis.

phal·lus (fal'us) *n.*, pl. **phal·li** (·lye), **phalluses** [L., from Gk. *phallos,* penis]. 1. The penis, or an analogous organ in certain invertebrates and nonmammalian vertebrates. 2. The indifferent embryonic structure derived from the genital tubercle that, in the male, differentiates into the penis, and, in the female, into the clitoris. —**phal·li·form** (·i·form), **phal·loid** (·oid) *adj.*

-phane [Gk. *phainesthai,* to appear]. A combining form designating *a substance having a* (specified) *form or appearance.*

phaner-, phanero- [Gk. *phaneros,* from *phanein,* to show]. A combining form meaning (a) *visible;* (b) *open, manifest, apparent.*

phan·ero·gam (fan'ur·o·gam) *n.* [*phanero-* + Gk. *gamos,* marriage]. A plant which bears seeds. Compare *cryptogam.* —**phanero·gam·ic** (·gam'ick) *adj.*

phan·ero·ge·net·ic (fan"ur·o·je·net'ick) *adj.* PHANEROGENIC.

phan·ero·gen·ic (fan"ur·o·jen'ick) *adj.* [*phanero-* + *-genic*]. Having a known cause. Contr. *cryptogenic.*

phan·ero·ma·nia (fan"ur·o·may'nee·uh) *n.* [*phanero-* + *-mania*]. A compulsive tendency to handle some external part or growth, such as a pimple, a hair, or a hangnail.

phan·er·o·sis (fan"ur·o'sis) *n.*, pl. **phanero·ses** (·seez) [*phaner-* + *-osis*]. The act of passing from a transparent to a visible state.

Phanodorn. A trademark for the short-acting barbiturate cyclobarbital.

phan·quone (fan'kwone) *n.* 4,7-Phenanthroline-5,6-quinone, $C_{12}H_6N_2O_2$, an antiamebic and antibacterial drug used for the treatment of intestinal and extra-intestinal amebiasis.

phan·tasm (fan'taz·um) *n.* [Gk. *phantasma,* apparition]. 1. An illusive perception of an object that does not exist. 2. An illusion or a hallucination. —**phan·tas·mic** (fan·taz'mick) *adj.*

phan·tas·ma·to·mo·ria (fan·taz"muh·to·mo'ree·uh) *n.* [Gk. *phantasma, phantasmatos,* vision, dream, + *mōria,* folly]. Childishness, or dementia, with absurd fancies or delusions.

phan·tas·mo·pho·bia (fan·taz"mo·fo'bee·uh) *n.* [*phantasm* + *-phobia*]. Fear of ghosts.

phan·tas·mo·sco·pia (fan·taz"mo·sko'pee·uh) *n.* [*phantasm* + Gk. *skop*ein, to watch, + *-ia*]. The seeing of phantasms; hallucinations involving ghosts.

phantasy. FANTASY.

phan·to·geu·sia (fan"to·gew'see·uh, ·joo'see·uh) *n.* [*phantom* + *-geusia*]. PSEUDOGEUSIA.

phan·tom (fan'tum) *n.* [OF. *fantome,* from L. *phantasma,* from Gk.]. 1. An image formed in the mind; a thing or person which takes the place of the real object in a given situation, such as in an experiment. 2. The outward manifestation of a thing or person after the essential or substantive element has been lost. 3. *In radiology,* an object made of substances with densities similar to tissue which simulates tissues in absorbing and scattering radiation and permits determination of the dose of radiation delivered to the surface of and within the simulated tissues through measurements with ionization chambers placed within the phantom material. Also used to establish and check radiographic and other imaging techniques.

phantom cells. GHOST CELLS (1).

phantom hip. TRANSIENT SYNOVITIS.

phantom limb, sensations, or **pain.** A psychological phenomenon frequently occurring in amputees: the patient feels sensations, and often pain, in the missing limb. See also *pseudesthesia.*

phantom odontalgia. Pain felt in the space from which a tooth has been removed.

phantom pregnancy. PSEUDOCYESIS.

phantom tumor. A swelling simulating a tumor; produced usually by the contraction of a muscle or by gaseous distention of the intestine.

phan·tos·mia (fan·toz'mee·uh) *n.* [*phant*om + *osm-* + *-ia*]. PSEUDOSMIA.

phar·a·on·ic circumcision (făr"ay·on'ick). INFIBULATION.

phar·ci·dous (fahr'si·dus) *adj.* [Gk. *pharkis, pharkid*os, wrinkle, + *-ous*]. Wrinkled; rugose; full of wrinkles.

phar·ma·cal (fahr'muh·kul) *adj.* Pertaining to pharmacy.

phar·ma·ceu·tic (fahr"muh·sue'tick) *adj.* [Gk. *pharmakeutikos*]. Pertaining to pharmacy.

phar·ma·ceu·ti·cal (fahr"muh·sue'ti·kul) *adj.* & *n.* 1. PHARMACEUTIC. 2. A medicinal drug.

pharmaceutical chemistry. The chemistry of medicinals, including their composition, synthesis or preparation, and analysis.

phar·ma·ceu·tics (fahr"muh·sue'ticks) *n.* The study of the physical, chemical, and physiological properties of medicinal substances from the standpoint of designing and compounding dosage forms of such substances that will provide an optimum therapeutic response.

phar·ma·ceu·tist (fahr"muh·sue'tist) *n.* PHARMACIST.

phar·ma·cist (fahr'muh·sist) *n.* One engaged in the practice of pharmacy; an apothecary.

pharmaco- [Gk. *pharmakon*]. A combining form meaning *drug.*

phar·ma·co·dy·nam·ics (fahr"muh·ko·dye·nam'icks, ·di·nam'icks) *n.* [*pharmaco-* + *dynamics*]. The science of the action of drugs. —**pharmacodynam·ic** (·ick) *adj.*

phar·ma·co·ge·net·ics (fahr"muh·ko·je·net'icks) *n.* [*pharmaco-* + *genetics*]. The discipline that deals with genetically determined variations in drug responses.

phar·ma·cog·no·sist (fahr"muh·kog'nuh·sist) *n.* One versed in pharmacognosy.

phar·ma·cog·no·sy (fahr"muh·kog'nuh·see) *n.* [*pharmaco-* + *-gnosy*]. The science of crude natural drugs.

phar·ma·col·o·gist (fahr"muh·kol'uh·jist) *n.* One versed in pharmacology.

phar·ma·col·o·gy (fahr"muh·kol'uh·jee) *n.* [*pharmaco-* + *-logy*]. The science of the nature and properties of drugs, particularly their actions. —**pharma·co·log·ic** (·ko·loj'ick), **pharmacologic·al** (·ul) *adj.*

phar·ma·co·ma·nia (fahr"muh·ko·may'nee·uh) *n.* [*pharmaco-* + *-mania*]. 1. An abnormal craving for medicines, or for self-medication. 2. An abnormal desire to administer medications.

phar·ma·co·pe·dics, phar·ma·co·pae·dics (fahr"muh·ko·pee'dicks) *n.* The scientific study of drugs and medicinal substances.

phar·ma·co·pe·ia, phar·ma·co·poe·ia (fahr"muh·ko·pee'uh) *n.* [Gk. *pharmakopoiia,* preparation of drugs, from *pharmakon,* drug, + *poiein,* to make]. A book containing a selected list of medicinal substances and their dosage forms, providing also a description and the standards for purity and strength for each. —**pharmacope·ial, pharmacopoe·ial** (·ul) *adj.*

phar·ma·co·pho·bia (fahr″muh·ko·fo′bee·uh) *n.* [*pharmaco-* + *-phobia*]. Abnormal dislike or fear of medicine.

phar·ma·co·phore (fahr′muh·ko·fore) *n.* [Gk. *pharmakophoros,* drug-producing]. A particular grouping of atoms within a molecule which is considered to confer pharmacological activity to a substance.

phar·ma·co·psy·cho·sis (fahr″muh·ko·sigh·ko′sis) *n.* [*pharmaco-* + *psychosis*]. Any organic brain syndrome associated with ingestion of a drug, alcohol, or poison.

phar·ma·co·ther·a·py (fahr″muh·ko·therr′uh·pee) *n.* [*pharmaco-* + *therapy*]. The treatment of disease by means of drugs.

phar·ma·cy (fahr′muh·see) *n.* [Gk. *pharmakeia,* from *pharmakon,* drug]. 1. The art and science of preparing and dispensing drugs used for the prevention, diagnosis, or treatment of disease. 2. A place where drugs are compounded and dispensed.

Pharm. D. Doctor of Pharmacy.

pharyng-, pharyngo- [Gk. *pharynx, pharyngos*]. A combining form meaning *pharynx, pharyngeal.*

phar·yn·gal·gia (făr″ing·gal′jee·uh) *n.* [*pharyng-* + *-algia*]. Pain in the pharynx.

pha·ryn·ge·al (fa·rin′jee·ul, ·jul, făr″in·jee′ul) *adj.* Pertaining to the pharynx.

pharyngeal aponeurosis. The fibrous submucous layer of the pharynx.

pharyngeal arch. VISCERAL ARCH.

pharyngeal bursa. A small pit caudal to the pharyngeal tonsil, resulting from the ingrowth of epithelium along the course of the degenerating tip of the notochord. NA *bursa pharyngea.*

pharyngeal bursitis. Purulent or mucopurulent inflammation of a pharyngeal bursa.

pharyngeal canal. A passage between the vaginal process of the sphenoid bone and the sphenoid process of the palatine bone for the transmission of pharyngeal branches from the pterygopalatine ganglion and sphenopalatine artery. NA *canalis palatovaginalis.*

pharyngeal diverticulum. PULSION DIVERTICULUM.

pharyngeal groove. VISCERAL GROOVE.

pharyngeal membrane. BUCCOPHARYNGEAL MEMBRANE.

pharyngeal moniliasis. 1. An infection of the throat by *Candida albicans.* 2. A condition of the throat caused by debilitating systemic disease, diabetes, or unhygienic conditions.

pharyngeal plexus. 1. A nerve plexus innervating the pharynx. NA *plexus pharyngeus.* 2. A plexus of veins situated at the side of the pharynx. Syn. *plexus pharyngeus venosus.*

pharyngeal pouch. One of a series of five paired lateral sacculations of the embryonic pharynx corresponding to the ectodermal grooves between the pharyngeal arches.

pharyngeal recess. A lateral mucosal diverticulum of the pharynx situated behind the opening of the auditory tube. Syn. *Rosenmueller's fossa.* NA *recessus pharyngeus.*

pharyngeal reflex. GAG REFLEX.

pharyngeal spine. A small elevation near the middle of the inferior surface of the basilar process of the occipital bone, for the superior attachment of the median raphe of the pharynx.

pharyngeal tonsil. ADENOID (3).

pharyngeal tubercle. The ridge on the undersurface of the basilar process of the occipital bone. NA *tuberculum pharyngeum.*

pharyngeal venous plexus. PHARYNGEAL PLEXUS (2).

phar·yn·gec·to·my (făr″in·jeck′tuh·mee) *n.* [*pharyng-* + *-ectomy*]. Excision of a part of the pharynx.

phar·yn·gem·phrax·is (făr″in·jem·frack′sis) *n.* [*pharyng-* + *emphraxis*]. Obstruction of the pharynx.

pharynges. Plural of *pharynx.*

pha·ryn·ge·us (fa·rin′jee·us) *L. adj.* PHARYNGEAL.

phar·yn·gism (făr′in·jiz·um) *n.* PHARYNGISMUS.

phar·yn·gis·mus (făr″in·jiz′mus) *n.* Spasm of the pharynx.

phar·yn·gi·tis (făr″in·jye′tis) *n.*, pl. **pharyn·git·i·des** (·jit′i·deez) [*pharyng-* + *-itis*]. Inflammation of the pharynx. —**pharyn·git·ic** (·jit′ick) *adj.*

pharyngitis sic·ca (sick′uh). The atrophic form of pharyngitis characterized by a very dry state of the mucous membrane.

pharyngo-. See *pharyng-.*

pha·ryn·go·bran·chi·al (fa·ring″go·brank′ee·ul) *adj.* [*pharyngo-* + *branchial*]. Pertaining to the pharynx and branchial arches.

pharyngobranchial duct. The narrow medial part of a pharyngeal pouch.

pha·ryn·go·cele (fa·ring′go·seel) *n.* [*pharyngo-* + *-cele*]. A hernia or pouch of the pharyngeal mucosa projecting through the pharyngeal wall.

pha·ryn·go·con·junc·ti·val (fa·ring″go·kon″junk·tye′vul) *adj.* Of or pertaining to the pharynx and the conjunctiva.

pharyngoconjunctival fever. An epidemic disease of children, caused by an adenovirus, and characterized by fever, pharyngitis, conjunctivitis, rhinitis, and cervical lymphadenopathy.

pha·ryn·go·dyn·ia (fa·ring″go·din′ee·uh) *n.* [*pharyng-* + *-odynia*]. Pain referred to the pharynx.

pha·ryn·go·epi·glot·tic (fa·ring″go·ep″i·glot′ick) *adj.* Pertaining to the pharynx and the epiglottis.

pharyngoepiglottic fold. One of the paired folds of mucous membrane passing from the pharynx to the epiglottis.

pha·ryn·go·epi·glot·ti·cus (fa·ring″go·ep″i·glot′i·kus) *n.* Muscular fibers derived from the stylopharyngeus and inserted into the side of the epiglottis and the pharyngoepiglottic fold.

pha·ryn·go·esoph·a·ge·al, pha·ryn·go·oesoph·a·ge·al (fa·ring″go·e·sof″uh·jee′ul) *adj.* [*pharyngo-* + *esophageal*]. Pertaining to the pharynx and esophagus.

pharyngoesophageal diverticulum. PULSION DIVERTICULUM.

pha·ryn·go·esoph·a·gus, phar·yn·go·oesoph·a·gus (fa·ring″go·e·sof′uh·gus) *n.* The pharynx and esophagus considered as one organ.

pha·ryn·go·glos·sal (fa·ring″go·glos′ul) *adj.* [*pharyngo-* + *glossal*]. Pertaining conjointly to the pharynx and the tongue.

pha·ryn·go·glos·sus (fa·ring″go·glos′us) *n.* Muscular fibers extending from the superior constrictor of the pharynx to the base of the tongue.

pha·ryn·go·ker·a·to·sis (fa·ring″go·kerr″uh·to′sis) *n.* [*pharyngo-* + *kerat-* + *-osis*]. Thickening of the mucous lining of the pharynx with formation of a tough and adherent exudate.

pha·ryn·go·la·ryn·ge·al (fa·ring″go·la·rin′jee·ul) *adj.* [*pharyngo-* + *laryngeal*]. Pertaining both to the pharynx and to the larynx.

pha·ryn·go·lar·yn·gi·tis (fa·ring″go·lăr″in·jye′tis) *n.* [*pharyngo-* + *laryngitis*]. Simultaneous inflammation of the pharynx and larynx.

pha·ryn·go·lith (fa·ring′go·lith) *n.* [*pharyngo-* + *-lith*]. A calcareous concretion in the walls of the pharynx.

phar·yn·gol·o·gy (far″ing·gol′uh·jee) *n.* [*pharyngo-* + *-logy*]. The science of the pharyngeal mechanism, functions, and diseases.

phar·yn·gol·y·sis (far″ing·gol′i·sis) *n.* [*pharyngo-* + *-lysis*]. *Obsol.* PHARYNGOPLEGIA.

pha·ryn·go·max·il·lary (fa·ring″go·mack′si·lerr·ee) *adj.* [*pharyngo-* + *maxillary*]. Pertaining to the pharynx and the maxilla.

pha·ryn·go·my·co·sis (fa·ring″go·migh·ko′sis) *n.* [*pharyngo-* + *mycosis*]. Disease of the pharynx due to the action of fungi.

pha·ryn·go·na·sal (fa·ring″go·nay′zul) *adj.* [*pharyngo-* + *nasal*]. Pertaining to the pharynx and the nose, as pharyngonasal cavity.

pha·ryn·go·pal·a·tine (fa·ring″go·pal′uh·tine) *adj.* [*pharyngo-* + *palatine*]. PALATOPHARYNGEAL.

pharyngopalatine arch. PALATOPHARYNGEAL ARCH.

pha·ryn·go·pa·la·ti·nus (fa·ring″go·pal″uh·tye′nus) *n.* PALATOPHARYNGEUS.

pha·ryn·go·pa·ral·y·sis (fa·ring″go·puh·ral′i·sis) *n.* [*pharyngo-* + *paralysis*]. PHARYNGOPLEGIA.

phar·yn·gop·a·thy (făr″ing·gop′uth·ee) *n.* [*pharyngo-* + *-pathy*]. Any disease of the pharynx.

pha·ryn·go·pe·ris·to·le (fa·ring″go·pe·ris′tuh·lee) *n.* [*pharyngo-* + *peristole*]. PHARYNGOSTENIA.

pha·ryn·go·plas·ty (fa·ring′go·plas·tee) *n.* [*pharyngo-* + *-plasty*]. Reconstruction of the pharynx by surgery.

pha·ryn·go·ple·gia (fa·ring″go·plee′juh, ·jee·uh) *n.* [*pharyngo-* + *-plegia*]. Paralysis of the muscles of the pharynx.

pha·ryn·go·rhi·ni·tis (fa·ring″go·rye·nigh′tis) *n.* [*pharyngo-* + *rhin-* + *-itis*]. Pharyngitis with rhinitis; inflammation of the pharyngeal and nasal mucosa.

pha·ryn·go·rhi·nos·co·py (fa·ring″go·rye·nos′kuh·pee) *n.* [*pharyngo-* + *rhinoscopy*]. POSTERIOR RHINOSCOPY.

pha·ryn·gor·rha·gia (fa·ring″go·ray′juh, ·jee·uh) *n.* [*pharyngo-* + *-rrhagia*]. Hemorrhage from the pharynx.

pha·ryn·gor·rhea, pha·ryn·gor·rhoea (fa·ring″go·ree′uh) *n.* [*pharyngo-* + *-rrhea*]. A mucous discharge from the pharynx.

pha·ryn·go·scle·ro·ma (fa·ring″go·skle·ro′muh) *n.* Pharyngeal scleroma.

pha·ryn·go·scope (fa·ring′go·skope) *n.* [*pharyngo-* + *-scope*]. An instrument for use in examining the pharynx. —**phar·in·gos·co·py** (făr″ing·gos′kuh·pee) *n.*

pha·ryn·go·spasm (fa·ring′go·spaz·um) *n.* [*pharyngo-* + *spasm*]. Spasmodic contraction of the pharynx. —**pha·ryn·go·spas·mod·ic** (fa·ring″go·spaz·mod′ick) *adj.*

pha·ryn·go·ste·nia (fa·ring″go·stee′nee·uh) *n.* [*pharyngo-* + *sten-* + *-ia*]. Narrowing or stricture of the pharynx. —**phar·yn·gos·te·nous** (făr″ing·gos′te·nus) *adj.*

pha·ryn·go·ther·a·py (fa·ring″go·therr′uh·pee) *n.* [*pharyngo-* + *therapy*]. The treatment of diseases of the pharynx by direct applications or irrigations.

phar·yn·got·o·my (făr″ing·got′uh·mee) *n.* [*pharyngo-* + *tomy*]. Incision into the pharynx.

pha·ryn·go·ton·sil·li·tis (fa·ring″go·ton″si·lye′tis) *n.* [*pharyngo-* + *tonsillitis*]. Inflammation of the pharynx and the tonsils.

pha·ryn·go·tra·che·al canal (fa·ring″go·tray′kee·ul). A narrow opening in the solid dorsal epithelium of the embryonic larynx which enlarges to form the cavity of the larynx.

pha·ryn·go·tym·panic cavity (fa·ring″go·tim·pan′ick). The tubotympanic recess derived from the first and part of the second visceral pouches. The anlage of the middle ear and the auditory tube.

pharyngotympanic tube. AUDITORY TUBE.

pha·ryn·go·xe·ro·sis (fa·ring″go·ze·ro′sis) *n.* [*pharyngo-* + *xerosis*]. Dryness of the pharynx.

phar·ynx (făr′inks) *n.*, genit. **pha·ryn·gis** (fa·rin′jis), pl. **pharyn·ges** (·jeez) [Gk.]. The musculomembranous tube situated back of the nose, mouth, and larynx, and extending from the base of the skull to a point opposite the sixth cervical vertebra, where it becomes continuous with the esophagus. It is lined by mucous membrane, covered in its upper part with pseudostratified ciliated epithelium, in its lower part with stratified squamous epithelium. See also Plate 12.

phase, *n.* [Gk. *phasis*, appearance, from *phainein*, to show]. 1. The condition or stage of a disease or of biologic, chemical, physiologic, and psychologic functions at a given time. 2. A solid, liquid, or gas which is homogeneous throughout and physically separated from another phase by a distinct boundary. 3. A stage or interval in a periodic or developmental cycle.

phase contrast microscopy. PHASE MICROSCOPY.

phase difference microscopy. PHASE MICROSCOPY.

phase microscope. A microscope that permits visualization of the parts of an object by converting phase differences in light transmitted through the object into amplitude differences, thereby providing contrast perceivable by the eye.

phase microscopy. Any procedure that utilizes the phase microscope to provide optional contrast between adjacent parts of an object and thereby improves their visualization.

pha·se·o·lin (fa·see′o·lin) *n.* A simple protein of the globulin type which occurs in kidney beans.

phase variation. BACTERIAL VARIATION.

-phasia, -phasy [Gk. *phasis*, utterance (from *phanai*, to say) + *-ia*]. A combining form meaning *speech disorder.*

pha·sic (fay′zick) *adj.* [*phase* + *-ic*]. Pertaining to a phase; having phases.

phasic blood pressure. The cycle of blood pressure during the cardiac cycle.

phasic sinus arrhythmia. Cyclic speeding of the heart rate during inspiration with a slowing during expiration; occasionally the waxing and waning of the heart rate is independent of respiration.

pha·sin (fay′sin) *n.* A hemagglutinin found in many nonpoisonous plants, such as the Papilionaceae.

phas·mid (faz′mid) *n.* A minute sensory organ the presence or absence of which determines membership in the complementary nematode subclasses Phasmidia and Aphasmidia; thought to be an olfactory receptor.

phas·mo·pho·bia (faz″mo·fo′bee·uh) *n.* [Gk. *phasma*, apparition, + *-phobia*]. PHANTASMOPHOBIA.

-phasy. See *-phasia.*

phel·lan·drene (fe·lan′dreen) *n.* Either of two isomeric substances of the formula $C_{10}H_{16}$: α-phellandrene, *p*-mentha-1,5-diene, or β-phellandrene, *p*-mentha-1(7),2-diene. Both occur in dextrorotatory and levorotatory forms in various volatile oils.

Phemerol Chloride. A trademark for benzethonium chloride, a topical anti-infective agent.

-phemia [Gk. *phēmē*, voice, + *-ia*]. A combining form meaning *speech disorder.*

phem·i·tone (fem′i·tone) *n.* MEPHOBARBITAL.

phen-, pheno- [Gk. *phainein*, to bring to light]. A combining form meaning (a) *light, bright;* (b) *appearing, manifest;* (c) *derivation from benzene.*

phen·a·caine (fen′uh·kane, fee′nuh·) *n.* *N,N′*-Bis(*p*-ethoxyphenyl)acetamidine, $C_{18}H_{22}N_2O_2$, a local anesthetic; used as the hydrochloride salt in ophthalmic practice.

phe·nac·e·mide (fe·nas′e·mide) *n.* Phenylacetylurea, $C_9H_{10}N_2O_2$, an anticonvulsant drug.

phe·nac·e·tin (fe·nas′e·tin) *n.* *p*-Acetophenetidide, $C_2H_5OC_6H_4NHCOCH_3$, an antipyretic and analgesic drug. Syn. *acetophenetidin.*

phe·nac·e·tu·ric acid (fe·nas″e·tew′rick). A glycine conjugate, $C_6H_5CH_2CONHCH_2COOH$, of phenylacetic acid, a form in which the latter is sometimes excreted in animals.

phen·a·dox·one (fen″uh·dock′sone) *n.* 6-Morpholino-4,4-diphenyl-3-heptanone, $C_{23}H_{29}NO$, a narcotic analgesic.

phen·a·gly·co·dol (fen″uh·glye′ko·dol) *n.* 2-*p*-Chlorophenyl-3-methyl-2,3-butanediol, $C_{11}H_{15}ClO_2$, a mild neurosedative with muscle-relaxing property action.

phe·na·kis·to·scope, phae·na·kis·to·scope (fee″nuh·kis′tuh·skope, fen″uh·) *n.* [Gk. *phenakistēs*, deceiver, + *-scope*]. A stroboscope-like device in which figures and slits revolve in the same direction, the moving figures being viewed with a mirror.

phe·nan·threne (fe·nan′threen) *n.* A hydrocarbon, $C_{14}H_{10}$, isomeric with anthracene, and found with it in coal tar. It is considered a carcinogen.

phe·nate (fee′nate) *n.* A salt of phenol (1).

phen·az·o·cine (fen·az′o·seen) *n.* 1,2,3,4,5,6-Hexahydro-8-hydroxy-6,11-dimethyl-3-phenethyl-2,6-methano-3-benzazocine, $C_{22}H_{27}NO$, a synthetic narcotic analgesic; used as the hydrobromide salt.

phen·a·zone (fen′uh·zone) *n.* ANTIPYRINE.

phen·az·o·pyr·i·dine (fen·az″o·pirr′i·deen) *n.* 2,6-Diamino-3-phenylazopyridine, $C_{11}H_{11}N_5$, a urinary analgesic drug; used as the hydrochloride salt.

phen·ben·i·cil·lin (fen·ben″i·sil′in) *n.* α-Phenoxybenzyl penicillin, $C_{22}H_{22}N_2O_5S$, a semisynthetic penicillin that is acid-resistant and absorbed when administered orally.

phen·bu·ta·zone sodium glycerate (fen·bew′tuh·zone). A compound of glycerine with the sodium salt of 4-butyl-3-hydroxy-1,2-diphenyl-3-pyrazolin-5-one, $C_{19}H_{19}N_2NaO_2 \cdot C_3H_8O_3$, an anti-inflammatory.

phen·car·ba·mide (fen·kahr′buh·mide) *n.* *S*-[2-(Diethylamino)ethyl]diphenylthiocarbamate, $C_{19}H_{24}N_2OS$, an anticholinergic drug.

phen·cy·cli·dine (fen·sigh′kli·deen) *n.* 1-(1-Phenylcyclohexyl)piperidine, $C_{17}H_{25}N$, a central nervous system depressant for veterinary use to immobilize primates; administered intramuscularly as the hydrochloride salt.

phen·di·met·ra·zine (fen″dye·met′ruh·zeen) *n.* *d*-3,4-Dimethyl-2-phenylmorpholine, $C_{12}H_{17}NO$, a sympathomimetic drug used as an anorexiant; employed as the bitartrate salt.

phene (feen) *n.* [Gk. *phainein,* to bring to light]. *In chemistry,* benzene; a term sometimes used in naming its derivatives.

phen·el·zine (fen′il·zeen) *n.* β-Phenylethylhydrazine, $C_8H_{12}N_2$, an antidepressant drug; used as the sulfate salt.

Phenergan. Trademark for promethazine, an antihistaminic drug used as the hydrochloride salt.

phen·eth·i·cil·lin (fen·eth″i·sil′in) *n.* α-Phenoxyethylpenicillin, $C_{17}H_{20}N_2O_5S$, a methyl homologue of phenoxymethylpenicillin; relatively resistant to inactivation by the gastric juice. Used, as the potassium salt, like other orally administered penicillin preparations.

phen·eth·yl (fen·eth′il) *n.* PHENYLETHYL.

phenethyl alcohol. PHENYLETHYL ALCOHOL.

phe·net·i·din (fe·net′i·din) *n.* Aminophenetole, $C_8H_{11}NO$, of which three isomers exist. The *para-* isomer frequently appears in the urine following administration of phenacetin.

phe·net·i·din·uria (fe·net″i·di·new′ree·uh) *n.* [*phenetidin* + *-uria*]. The presence of phenetidin in the urine.

phen·for·min (fen·for′min) *n.* 1-Phenethylbiguanide, $C_{10}H_{15}N_5$, an oral hypoglycemic drug; used as the hydrochloride salt.

phen·go·pho·bia (fen″go·fo′bee·uh) *n.* [Gk. *phengos,* daylight, + *-phobia*]. A morbid fear of daylight.

phe·nic acid (fee′nick, fen′ick). PHENOL.

phe·nin·da·mine (fe·nin′duh·meen, ·min) *n.* 2,3,4,9-Tetrahydro-2-methyl-9-phenyl-1*H*-indeno-[2,1-*c*]pyridine, $C_{19}H_{19}N$; an antihistaminic drug used as the tartrate salt.

phen·in·di·one (fen″in·dye′ohn) *n.* 2-Phenyl-1,3-indandione, $C_{15}H_{10}O_2$, an anticoagulant.

phen·ir·a·mine (fen·irr′uh·min) *n.* 2-[α-(2-Dimethylaminoethyl)benzyl]pyridine, $C_{16}H_{20}N_2$, an antihistaminic drug used as the maleate salt. Syn. *prophenpyridamine.*

phen·met·ra·zine (fen·met′ruh·zeen) *n.* 3-Methyl-2-phenylmorpholine, $C_{11}H_{15}NO$, a sympathomimetic drug used as an anorexiant; employed as the hydrochloride salt.

pheno-. See *phen-.*

phe·no·bar·bi·tal (fee″no·bahr′bi·tol) *n.* 5-Ethyl-5-phenylbarbituric acid, $C_{12}H_{12}N_2O_3$, a long-acting sedative and hypnotic barbiturate. Syn. *phenobarbitone.*

phenobarbital sodium. Sodium 5-ethyl-5-phenylbarbiturate, $C_{12}H_{11}N_2NaO_3$, a water-soluble salt of phenobarbital that may be administered also by injection. Syn. *sodium phenobarbital, soluble phenobarbital, phenobarbitone sodium.*

phe·no·bar·bi·tone (fee″no·bahr′bi·tone) *n.* PHENOBARBITAL.

phenobarbitone sodium. PHENOBARBITAL SODIUM.

phe·no·copy (fee′no·kop″ee) *n.* [*pheno-* + *copy*]. An experimentally produced effect on the body which copies the appearance of genetic effects, e.g., tanning produced by ultraviolet light which duplicates hereditary pigmentation.

phe·no·din (fee′no·din) *n.* HEMATIN.

phe·nol (fee′nol) *n.* [*phen-* + *-ol*]. 1. Hydroxybenzene or phenyl hydroxide, C_6H_5OH, colorless to light pink crystals. Used as a disinfectant, topical anesthetic, escharotic, and antipruritic. Syn. *carbolic acid.* 2. Any hydroxy derivative of aromatic hydrocarbons that has the OH group directly attached to the ring.

phe·no·lase (fee′no·lace, ·laze) *n.* Phenol oxidase; an enzyme that catalyzes oxidation of phenolic substances.

phe·no·late (fee′no·late) *n.* A salt of phenol.

phenol coefficient. A number which indicates the germicidal efficiency of a compound relative to phenol. See also *Rideal-Walker method.*

phe·no·lic (fee·no′lick, fee·nol′ick) *adj.* 1. Having the characteristics of phenol or a phenol. 2. Pertaining to, containing, or derived from phenol or a phenol.

phenol oxidase. PHENOLASE.

phe·nol·phthal·ein (fee″nol·thal′een, ·thal′ee·in) *n.* 3,3-Bis(*p*-hydroxyphenyl)phthalide, $C_{20}H_{14}O_4$, a white or faintly yellowish powder; a cathartic drug, also used as an indicator of acidity or alkalinity.

phenolphthalein test. A test for occult blood in which a boiled suspension of feces is added to phenolphthalein reagent (phenolphthalein, potassium hydroxide, powdered zinc, and distilled water). On addition of hydrogen peroxide a pink to red color is a positive test.

phe·nol·phthal·in (fee″nol·thal′in) *n.* 4′,4″-Dihydroxytriphenylmethane-2-carboxylic acid, $C_{20}H_{16}O_4$; used as a reagent for detecting the presence of blood.

phenol red. PHENOLSULFONPHTHALEIN.

phe·nol·sul·fo·nate (fee″nol·sul′fo·nate) *n.* A salt or ester of phenolsulfonic acid.

phe·nol·sul·fon·ic acid (fee″nol·sul·fon′ick). Hydroxybenzenesulfonic acid, $HOC_6H_4SO_3H$, occurring in three isomeric forms: *ortho-, meta-,* and *para-.* Salts of *p*-phenolsulfonic acid have been used as intestinal antiseptics. Syn. *sulfocarbolic acid.*

phe·nol·sul·fon·phthal·ein (fee″nol·sul″fon·thal′een, ·ee·in) *n.* 4,4′-(3*H*-2,1-Benzoxathiol-3-ylidene)diphenol *S,S*-dioxide, $C_{19}H_{14}O_5S$, a bright to dark red crystalline powder. Used as a diagnostic aid, by intramuscular or intravenous injection, to determine kidney function. Syn. *phenol red.*

phenolsulfonphthalein test. A test for kidney function based upon the ability of the kidneys to excrete phenolsulfonphthalein which has been injected intravenously or intramuscularly. From 50 to 70% of the injected P.S.P. is normally excreted in the urine within 2 hours. Abbreviated, P.S.P.

phe·nol·tet·ra·chlo·ro·phthal·ein (fee″nol·tet″ruh·klo·ro·thal′een, ·ee·in) *n.* 3,4,5,6-Tetrachlorophenolphthalein, $C_{20}H_{10}Cl_4O_4$; formerly used, as the sodium salt, in liver function tests.

phenoltetrachlorophthalein test. A test for liver function. After the intravenous injection of phenoltetrachlorophthalein, the feces have a bright color. Delay in the appearance of brightness of the color indicates deficient liver function, as the liver removes phenoltetrachlorophthalein from the blood and excretes it in the bile.

phe·nol·uria (fee″nol·yoo′ree·uh) *n.* The presence of phenols in the urine.

phe·nom·e·nol·o·gy (fe·nom″e·nol′uh·jee) *n.* [*phenomenon* + *-logy*]. That portion of a science in which the phenomena dealt with by the science are described and classified rather than explained or interpreted.

phe·nom·e·non (fe·nom′e·nun, ·non) *n.,* pl. **phenome·na** (·nuh) [Gk. *phainomenon,* from *phainesthai,* to appear, from *phainein,* to show]. An event or manifestation.

-phenone. A combining form meaning *an aromatic ketone that contains a phenyl or substituted phenyl group attached to an acyl group,* as in acetophenone and benzophenone.

phe·no·pho·bia (fee″no·fo′bee·uh) *n.* [*pheno-* + *-phobia*]. Fear of daylight.

phe·no·pro·pa·zine (fee″no·pro′puh·zeen) *n.* Ethopropazine, an anticholinergic drug used as the hydrochloride salt for treatment of parkinsonism.

phe·no·thi·a·zine (fee″no·thigh′uh·zeen, ·zin) *n.* Thiodiphenylamine, $C_{12}H_9NS$, a veterinary anthelmintic drug. Derivatives of phenothiazine are important drugs used in human and veterinary medicine.

phe·no·type (fee′no·tipe) *n.* [*pheno-* + *type*]. 1. The sum total of visible traits which characterize the members of a group. 2. The visible expression of genotype. **—phe·no·typ·ic** (fee″no·tip′ick) *adj.;* **phenotyp·i·cal·ly** (·i·kuh·lee) *adv.*

phe·noxy (fe·nock′see) *n.* The univalent radical C_6H_5O—.

phe·noxy·ace·tic acid (fe·nock″see·a·see′tick). Phenoxyethanoic acid, $C_6H_5OCH_2COOH$, a fungicide.

phe·noxy·ben·za·mine (fe·nock″see·ben′zuh·meen) *n.* *N*-(2-Chloroethyl)-*N*′-(1-methyl-2-phenoxyethyl)benzylamine, $C_{18}H_{22}ClNO$, an adrenergic blocking agent used as the hydrochloride salt as a peripheral vasodilator.

phe·noz·y·gous (fe·noz′i·gus) *adj.* [*pheno-* + *zyg*oma + *-ous*]. Pertaining to an anomaly of development in which the cranium is considerably narrower than the broadest part of the face.

phen·pro·cou·mon (fen″pro·koo′mon) *n.* 3-(α-Ethylbenzyl)-4-hydroxycoumarin, $C_{18}H_{16}O_3$, a synthetic, coumarin-type anticoagulant drug.

phen·pro·pi·o·nate (fen·pro′pee·o·nate) *n.* Any salt or ester of 3-phenylpropionic acid, $C_6H_5CH_2CH_2COOH$; a 3-phenylpropionate.

phen·sux·i·mide (fen·suck′si·mide) *n.* *N*-Methyl-2-phenylsuccinimide, $C_{11}H_{11}NO_2$, an anticonvulsant drug primarily useful in the treatment of petit mal epilepsy.

phen·ter·mine (fen′tur·meen) *n.* α,α-Dimethylphenethylamine, $C_{10}H_{15}N$, an anorexigenic drug used as the base and the hydrochloride salt.

phen·tol·a·mine (fen·tol′uh·meen) *n.* *m*-[*N*-(2-Imidazolin-2-ylmethyl)-*p*-toluidino]phenol, $C_{17}H_{19}N_3O$, an adrenergic blocking drug used in the diagnosis of pheochromocytoma; employed as the hydrochloride and mesylate salts.

Phenurone. Trademark for the anticonvulsant drug phenacemide.

phen·yl (fen′il, fee′nil) *n.* [*phen-* + *-yl*]. The univalent radical C_6H_5—. **—phe·nyl·ic** (fe·nil′ick) *adj.*

phen·yl·acet·a·mide (fen″il·a·set′uh·mide) *n.* ACETANILID.

phen·yl·ace·tic acid (fen″il·a·see′tick). $C_6H_5CH_2COOH$; crystals, soluble in water; a product of apparently faulty metabolism of phenylalanine, also of normal metabolism of phenyl derivatives of fatty acids having an even number of carbon atoms.

phen·yl·ace·tyl·glu·ta·mine (fen″il·a·see″til·gloo′tuh·meen) *n.* $H_2NCO(CH_2)_2(CHNHCOCH_2C_6H_5)COOH$. A conjugated form of phenylacetic acid excreted in man and the chimpanzee.

phen·yl·ace·tyl·urea (fen″il·a·see″til·yoo·ree′uh) *n.* PHENACEMIDE.

phen·yl·al·a·nine (fen″il·al′uh·neen) *n.* α-Amino-β-phenylpropionic acid, $C_6H_5CH_2CH(NH_2)COOH$, an amino acid essential in human nutrition.

phenylalanine hydroxylase. An enzyme that converts phenylalanine to tyrosine, the reaction requiring oxygen and NADPH. Syn. *phenylalanine 4-monooxygenase.* See also *phenylketonuria.*

phen·yl·al·a·nin·emia, phen·yl·al·a·nin·ae·mia (fen″il·al″uh·ni·nee′mee·uh) *n.* [*phenylalanine* + *-emia*]. HYPERPHENYLALANINEMIA.

phenylalanine 4-monooxygenase. PHENYLALANINE HYDROXYLASE.

L-phenylalanine mustard. MELPHALAN.

phenyl alcohol. PHENOL.

phen·yl·am·ine (fen″il·am′een) *n.* ANILINE.

phen·yl·bu·ta·zone (fen″il·bew′tuh·zone) *n.* 4-Butyl-1,2-diphenyl-3,5-pyrazolidinedione, $C_{19}H_{20}N_2O_2$, an analgesic, antipyretic, and anti-inflammatory drug.

phen·yl·car·bi·nol (fen″il·kahr′bi·nol) *n.* BENZYL ALCOHOL.

phen·yl·cin·cho·nin·ic acid (fen″il·sing″ko·nin′ick). CINCHOPHEN.

phen·yl·ene (fen′i·leen, fee′ni·leen) *n.* The bivalent radical —C_6H_4—.

phen·yl·eph·rine (fen″il·ef′reen, ·rin) *n.* *l*-*m*-Hydroxy-α-[(methylamino)methyl]benzyl alcohol, $C_9H_{13}NO_2$, a sympathomimetic amine used as a vasoconstrictor; employed as the hydrochloride salt.

phen·yl·eth·yl (fen″il·eth′il) *n.* The univalent radical $C_6H_5CH_2CH_2$—.

phenylethyl alcohol. 2-Phenylethanol, $C_6H_5CH_2CH_2OH$, a colorless liquid with a roselike odor used as a perfume. Introduced as an antibacterial agent for ophthalmic solutions, but is of limited effectiveness. Syn. *phenethyl alcohol.*

phen·yl·eth·yl·bar·bi·tu·ric acid (fen″il·eth″il·bahr″bi·tew′rick). PHENOBARBITAL.

phen·yl·eth·yl·mal·o·nyl·urea (fen″il·eth″il·mal″o·nil·yoo·ree′uh) *n.* PHENOBARBITAL.

phen·yl·glu·co·sa·zone (fen″il·gloo·ko′suh·zone) *n.* A yellow, crystalline compound, $C_{18}H_{22}N_4O_4$, produced in the phenylhydrazine test for glucose.

phen·yl·hy·dra·zine (fen″il·high′druh·zeen) *n.* Hydrazinobenzene, $C_6H_5NHNH_2$, variously used as a reagent, especially in reactions involving aldehydes and ketones. It is a hemolysin, a property once used therapeutically.

phenylhydrazine test. A test for sugars in which a sugar combines with phenylhydrazine to produce an osazone of definite crystalline form which is typical for that sugar.

phen·yl·hy·dra·zone (fen″il·high′druh·zone) *n.* The product resulting from the interaction of phenylhydrazine with an aldehyde or ketone.

phe·nyl·ic acid (fe·nil′ick). PHENOL.

2-phen·yl·in·dane-1,3-di·one (fen″il·in′dane, dye′ohn) *n.* PHENINDIONE.

phen·yl·ke·to·nu·ria (fen″il·kee″to·new′ree·uh) *n.* [*phenylketone* + *-uria*]. 1. The presence of phenylketone in the urine. 2. A hereditary (autosomal recessive) metabolic disorder in which there is a deficiency of phenylalanine hydroxylase, resulting in increased amounts of phenylalanine in the blood and of excess phenylpyruvic and other acids in the urine; characterized clinically in the typical untreated case by mental retardation, eczema, fair hair, and occasionally seizures; mentally normal untreated cases occur; transmitted as an autosomal recessive trait. Abbreviated, PKU. **—phenylketonu·ric** (·rick) *adj.*

phenyl·mer·cu·ric (fen″il·mur·kew′rick) *adj.* Signifying the monovalent organomercurial cation $C_6H_5Hg^+$, which forms salts (acetate, borate, chloride, nitrate) that have antiseptic, germicidal, and fungicidal action.

phenylmethanol. BENZYL ALCOHOL.

***o*-phen·yl·phe·nol** (or″tho·fen″il·fee′nol) *n.* 2-Hydroxydiphenyl, $C_6H_5C_6H_4OH$, a germicide and fungicide.

phen·yl·pro·pa·nol·amine (fen″il·pro″puh·nol′uh·meen, ·min) *n.* 1-Phenyl-2-aminopropanol, $C_9H_{13}NO$, a sympathomimetic amine used mainly as a bronchodilator; employed as the hydrochloride salt.

phen·yl·pro·pi·o·nate (fen″il·pro′pee·o·nate) *n.* PHENPROPIONATE.

phen·yl·pro·pyl·meth·yl·amine (fen″il·pro″pil·meth′il·uh·meen) *n.* *N*,β-Dimethylphenethylamine, $C_{10}H_{15}N$, a sympathomimetic amine used locally, as the base or hydrochloride salt, to shrink nasal mucosa.

phen·yl·py·ru·vic acid (fen″il·pye·roo′vick, ·pi·roo′vick). A metabolic product, $C_6H_5CH_2COCOOH$, of phenylalanine; the state of mental deficiency known as phenylketonuria is characterized by excretion of the acid.

phenylpyruvic amentia or **oligophrenia.** Mental retardation in phenylketonuria.

phenyl salicylate. $HOC_6H_4COOC_6H_5$, used as an enteric coating for capsules and formerly as an analgesic, antipyretic, antirheumatic, and antibacterial drug. Syn. *salol.*

phen·yl·sul·fate (fen″il·sul′fate) *n.* A salt of phenylsulfuric acid.

phen·yl·sul·fu·ric acid (fen″il·sul·few′rick). A phenol ester, $C_6H_5OSO_3H$, of sulfuric acid.

phen·yl·thio·car·bam·ide (fen″il·thigh″o·kahr·bam′ide, kahr′buh·mide) *n.* PHENYLTHIOUREA. Abbreviated, PTC.

phen·yl·thio·urea (fen″il·thigh″o·yoo·ree′uh) *n.* Phenylthiocarbamide, $C_6H_5NHCSNH_2$, a compound of interest in genetics research because it is bitter to most persons but tasteless to others; non-tasting is recessively inherited.

phen·y·ram·i·dol (fen″i·ram′i·dol) *n.* α-(2-Pyridylaminomethyl)benzyl alcohol, $C_{13}H_{14}N_2$, an analgesic drug; used as the hydrochloride salt.

phe·nyt·o·in (fe·nit′o·in, fen″i·to′in) *n.* 5,5-Diphenyl-2,4-imidazolidinedione, $C_{15}H_{12}N_2O_2$, an anticonvulsant particularly useful in generalized seizures; also used as the sodium derivative. Syn. *diphenylhydantoin.*

pheo-, phaeo- [Gk. *phaios,* grey, dun]. A combining form meaning *brown, brownish.*

pheo·chrome, phaeo·chrome (fee′o·krome) *adj.* [*pheo-* + *-chrome*]. CHROMAFFIN.

pheo·chro·mo·blast, phaeo·chro·mo·blast (fee″o·kro′mo·blast) *n.* A precursor of a pheochromocyte.

pheo·chro·mo·blas·to·ma, phaeo·chro·mo·blas·to·ma (fee″o·kro″mo·blas·to′muh) *n.* [*pheochromoblast* + *-oma*]. A pheochromocytoma made up of less well differentiated cells.

pheo·chro·mo·cyte, phaeo·chro·mo·cyte (fee″o·kro′mo·site) *n.* [*pheochrome* + *-cyte*]. CHROMAFFIN CELL.

pheo·chro·mo·cy·to·ma (fee″o·kro″mo·sigh·to′muh) *n.,* pl. **pheochromocytomas, pheochromocytoma·ta** (·tuh) [*pheochromocyte* + *-oma*]. A tumor of the sympathetic nervous system, found most often in the adrenal medulla but occasionally in other sites such as paraganglia and in the thorax. It is made up largely of pheochromocytes, or chromaffin cells, with a strong affinity for taking up chrome salts. May be accompanied by the adrenal-sympathetic syndrome of spasmodic or persistent hypertension.

pheochromocytoma headache. A transient acute pressor headache associated with paroxysmal hypertension in pheochromocytoma.

pheo·phor·bide (fee″o·for′bide) *n.* [*pheo-* + Gk. *phorbē,* pasture, + *-ide*]. The product resulting when magnesium and the alcohol phytol are removed from chlorophyll by treatment with strong acid.

pheo·phy·tin (fee″o·fye′tin) *n.* The product formed by replacement of magnesium in chlorophyll by hydrogen. The corresponding copper and iron derivatives of chlorophyll, which may be considered magnesium pheophytin, are called copper pheophytin and iron pheophytin. They are sometimes referred to simply as chlorophylls.

-pher [Gk. *pherein,* to carry]. A combining form meaning *carrier.*

phe·re·sis (fe·ree′sis) *n.* [short for *apheresis*]. The removal from a donor's blood of one or more of its components, followed by return of the remainder to the donor. See also *leukapheresis, plateletpheresis.*

pher·o·mone (ferr′o·mone) *n.* [Gk. *pherein,* to carry, convey, + homōn, making alike, uniting]. Any substance, commonly a volatile organic compound, that is secreted by a member of an animal species and that provides communication with other members of the same species to elicit specific or generalized behavior.

Ph.G. Graduate in Pharmacy; German Pharmacopoeia.

Ph.I. International Pharmacopoeia.

phi·al (fye′ul) *n.* [Gk. *phialē*]. VIAL.

Phi·a·loph·o·ra (fye″uh·lof′uh·ruh) *n.* [NL., from Gk. *phialēphoros,* cup-bearer]. A genus of fungi.

Phialophora ver·ru·co·sa (verr″yoo·ko′suh). A species of fungus which is one of the causative agents of chromoblastomycosis.

phil-, philo- [Gk. *philos,* friend, lover of]. A combining form meaning (a) *love of* or *loving;* (b) *affinity for* or *having an affinity for.*

-phil, -phile [Gk. *philos,* friend, lover of]. A suffix designating *a substance having an affinity for,* as acidophil, having an affinity for acid stains.

Phil·a·del·phia chromosome. A number 22 chromosome with a deletion of the long arm found in the hematopoietic cells of many patients with chronic granulocytic leukemia. Symbol, Ph^1.

-philia [Gk. *philia,* friendship, fondness]. A combining form meaning (a) *craving for, abnormal tendency toward;* (b) *affinity for.* Contr. *-phobia.*

phil·i·a·ter (fil′ee·ay″tur, fi·lye′uh·tur) *n.* [Gk. *philiatros,* a friend of the art of medicine]. 1. A student of medicine. 2. A dabbler in medicine.

-philic [*phil-* + *-ic*]. A combining form meaning (a) *having an affinity for;* (b) *loving.*

Phil·ip·pine fowl disease. NEWCASTLE DISEASE.

Phil·lip·son's reflex. Crossed extension reflex, when indicative of an incomplete spinal lesion.

philo-. See *phil-.*

philo·ne·ism (fil″o·nee′iz·um) *n.* [*philo-* + Gk. *neos,* new, + *-ism*]. Abnormal love of novelty. Compare *misoneism.*

philo·pat·ri·do·ma·nia (fil″o·pat″ri·do·may′nee·uh) *n.* [Gk. *philopatris, philopatridos,* loving one's country, + *-mania*]. Abnormal homesickness.

-philous [*phil-* + *-ous*]. A combining form meaning (a) *having an affinity for;* (b) *loving.*

phil·ter, phil·tre (fil′tur) *n.* [Gk. *philtron,* love charm]. A love potion; a preparation supposed to be efficacious in exciting sexual passion.

phil·trum (fil′trum) *n.,* pl. **phil·tra** (·truh) [NL., from Gk. *philtron*] [NA]. The depression on the surface of the upper lip immediately below the septum of the nose.

phi·mo·sis (figh·mo′sis, fi·mo′sis) *n.,* pl. **phimo·ses** (·seez) [*phimōsis,* from *phimos,* muzzle, constriction]. Elongation of the prepuce and constriction of the orifice, so that the foreskin cannot be retracted to uncover the glans penis. —**phi·mot·ic** (·mot′ick) *adj.*

phleb-, phlebo- [Gk. *phleps, phlebos*]. A combining form meaning *vein, venous.*

phleb·an·gi·o·ma (fleb·an″jee·o′muh) *n.* [*phleb-* + *angioma*]. A venous aneurysm.

phleb·ar·te·ri·ec·ta·sia (fleb″ahr·teer″ee·eck·tay′zee·uh, ·zhuh) *n.* [*phleb-* + *ateri-* + *ectasia*]. General arterial and venous dilation.

phleb·ar·te·rio·di·al·y·sis (fleb″ahr·teer″ee·o·dye·al′i·sis) *n.* [*phleb-* + *arterio-* + *dialysis*]. ARTERIOVENOUS FISTULA.

phleb·ec·ta·sia (fleb″eck·tay′zee·uh, ·zhuh) *n.* [*phleb-* + *ectasia*]. Dilatation of a vein; varicosity. —**phlebec·tat·ic** (·tat′ick) *adj.*

phleb·ec·ta·sis (fle·beck′tuh·sis) *n.* [*phleb-* + *ectasis*]. PHLEBECTASIA.

phle·bec·to·my (fle·beck′tuh·mee) *n.* [*phleb-* + *-ectomy*]. Excision of a vein or a portion of a vein.

phleb·ec·to·pia (fleb″eck·to′pee·uh) *n.* [*phleb-* + *ectopia*]. The displacement, or abnormal position, of a vein.

phleb·em·phrax·is (fleb″em·frack′sis) *n.* [*phleb-* + *emphraxis*]. Plugging of a vein, usually by a clot.

phleb·ep·a·ti·tis (fleb″ep·uh·tye′tis) *n.* PHLEBHEPATITIS.

phleb·eu·rys·ma (fleb″yoo·riz′muh) *n.* [NL., from *phleb-* + Gk. *eurynein,* to widen]. VARIX.

phleb·ex·ai·re·sis (fleb″eck·sigh′re·sis) *n.* PHLEBEXERESIS.

phleb·ex·er·e·sis (fleb″eck·serr′e·sis) *n.* [*phleb-* + *exeresis*]. Excision of a vein.

phleb·hep·a·ti·tis (fleb″hep·uh·tye′tis) *n.* [*phleb-* + *hepatitis*]. Inflammation of veins within the liver.

phle·bis·mus (fle·biz′mus) *n.* [*phleb-* + *-ismus*]. Persistent overdistention of a vein, usually caused by obstruction.

phle·bi·tis (fle·bye′tis) *n.,* pl. **phle·bit·i·des** (·bit′i·deez) [*phleb-* + *-itis*]. Inflammation of a vein, with or without infection and thrombus formation. —**phle·bit·ic** (fle·bit′ick) *adj.*

phlebo-. See *phleb-*.

phlebo·car·ci·no·ma (fleb″o·kahr″si·no′muh) *n.* [*phlebo-* + *carcinoma*]. Extension of carcinoma to the walls of a vein.

phle·boc·ly·sis (fle·bock′li·sis, fleb″o·klye′sis) *n.* [*phlebo-* + *clysis*]. The intravenous injection of a large quantity of any solution.

phlebo·gram (fleb′o·gram) *n.* [*phlebo-* + *-gram*]. 1. A radiograph of a vein after the intravascular injection of a radiopaque material. Syn. *venogram.* 2. A tracing or recording of the venous pulse.

phlebo·graph (fleb′o·graf) *n.* [*phlebo-* + *-graph*]. An instrument for recording the venous pulse.

phle·bog·ra·phy (fle·bog′ruh·fee) *n.* [*phlebo-* + *-graphy*]. 1. The radiographic imaging with x-rays of a vein or veins following intravenous injection of a radiopaque substance. 2. Recording of venous pulsations.

phleb·oid (fleb′oid) *adj.* [*phleb-* + *-oid*]. 1. Pertaining to a vein; venous. 2. Resembling a vein.

phlebo·lith (fleb′o·lith) *n.* [*phlebo-* + *-lith*]. A calculus in a vein. —**phlebo·lith·ic** (fleb″o·lith′ick) *adj.*

phlebo·li·thi·a·sis (fleb″o·li·thigh′uh·sis) *n.* [*phlebolith* + *-iasis*]. The formation of phleboliths.

phlebo·ma·nom·e·ter (fleb″o·ma·nom′e·tur) *n.* [*phlebo-* + *manometer*]. An apparatus for the direct measurement of venous pressure.

phlebo·phle·bos·to·my (fleb″o·fle·bos′tuh·mee) *n.* [*phlebo-* + *phlebo-* + *-stomy*]. An operation in which an anastomosis is made between veins.

phlebo·phlo·go·sis (fleb″o·flo·go′sis) *n.* [*phlebo-* + *phlogosis*]. PHLEBITIS.

phlebo·plas·ty (fleb′o·plas″tee) *n.* [*phlebo-* + *-plasty*]. Plastic operation for the repair of veins.

phlebo·ple·ro·sis (fleb″o·ple·ro′sis) *n.* [*phlebo-* + *plerosis*]. Excessive distention of the veins.

phleb·or·rha·gia (fleb″o·ray′jee·uh) *n.* [Gk., from *phleps,* vein, + *rhēgnynai,* to burst forth]. A venous hemorrhage.

phle·bor·rha·phy (fle·bor′uh·fee) *n.* [*phlebo-* + *-rrhaphy*]. Suture of a vein.

phleb·or·rhex·is (fleb″o·reck′sis) *n.* [*phlebo-* + *-rhexis*]. Rupture of a vein.

phlebo·scle·ro·sis (fleb″o·skle·ro′sis) *n.* [*phlebo-* + *sclerosis*]. 1. Sclerosis of a vein. 2. Chronic phlebitis.

phle·bos·ta·sis (fle·bos′tuh·sis) *n.* [*phlebo-* + *stasis*]. 1. Temporary removal of some blood from the general circulation by compression of the veins in the extremities. Syn. *bloodless phlebotomy.* 2. Slowing or cessation of venous blood flow.

phlebo·ste·no·sis (fleb″o·ste·no′sis) *n.* [*phlebo-* + *stenosis*]. Constriction of a vein.

phlebo·strep·sis (fleb″o·strep′sis) *n.* [*phlebo-* + Gk. *strepsis,* a turning round]. Torsion of the cut or torn end of a vein to arrest or control bleeding.

phlebo·throm·bo·sis (fleb″o·throm·bo′sis) *n.* [*phlebo-* + *thrombosis*]. Formation or presence of a thrombus in a vein without associated inflammation. Compare *thrombophlebitis.*

phlebo·tome (fleb′uh·tome) *n.* [L. *phlebotomus,* from Gk. *phlebotomon*]. A cutting instrument used in phlebotomy.

Phle·bot·o·mus (fle·bot′uh·mus) *n.* [NL., from Gk. *phlebotomos,* opening veins]. A genus of small bloodsucking sandflies of the family Psychodidae. The species *Phlebotomus argentipes* transmits the flagellates of kala-azar in India, *P. chinensis* in China; *P. papatasii* is the vector of pappataci fever, phlebotomus sandfly fever of the Balkans. *P. verrucarum* is the vector for *Bartonella bacilliformis,* the causative agent of bartonellosis, or Carrión's disease (Oroya fever and verruca peruviana).

phlebotomus fever. An acute viral infection characterized by fever, headache, ocular pain, conjunctivitis, leukopenia, and malaise, followed by complete recovery. Occurs during the hot dry season in the Mediterranean area, Asia Minor, and India, where the vector fly, *Phlebotomus papatasii,* exists. Syn. *pappataci fever, sandfly fever.*

phle·bot·o·my (fle·bot′uh·mee) *n.* [Gk. *phlebotomia,* from *phleps,* vein, + *tomē,* incision]. The opening of a vein for the purpose of letting blood. —**phleboto·mist** (·mist) *n.*

phlegm (flem) *n.* [Gk. *phlegma*]. 1. A viscid, stringy mucus, secreted by the mucosa of the air passages. 2. One of the four humors of the Hippocratic formulation of general pathology.

phleg·ma·sia (fleg·may′zhuh) *n.* [Gk., turgescence]. INFLAMMATION.

phlegmasia ad·e·no·sa (ad·e·no′suh). ADENITIS.

phlegmasia al·ba do·lens (al′buh do′lenz) [L., white painful]. A painful swelling of the leg usually seen post partum, due to femoral vein thrombophlebitis or lymphatic obstruction. Syn. *milk leg.*

phlegmasia cel·lu·la·ris (sel·yoo·lair′is). CELLULITIS.

phlegmasia ce·ru·lea do·lens (se·roo′lee·uh do′lenz) [L., blue painful]. A severe form of acute thrombophlebitis with extensive thrombosis of deep and superficial veins of the leg, causing pain, edema, and cyanosis, which may result in superficial ischemic necrosis in the distal part of an extremity.

phleg·ma·sia mem·bra·nae mu·co·sae gas·tro·pul·mo·na·lis (fleg·may′zee·uh mem·bray′nee mew·ko′see gas″tro·pul″mo·nay′lis). APHTHAE TROPICAE.

phlegmasia my·o·i·ca (migh·o′i·kuh). MYOSITIS.

phleg·mat·ic (fleg·mat′ick) *adj.* [Gk. *phlegmatikos,* abounding in phlegm]. 1. Of the nature of phlegm or related to phlegm. 2. Characterized by an apathetic, sluggish, dull temperament.

phleg·mon (fleg′mon, ·mun) *n.* [Gk. *phlegmonē,* inflammation, boil]. Pyogenic inflammation with infiltration and spread in the tissues; seen with invasive organisms which produce hyaluronidases and fibrinolysins. Compare *abscess.* —**phleg·mon·ous** (·mun·us) *adj.*

phlegmonous abscess. An acute abscess in connective tissue, especially the subcutaneous.

phlegmonous adenitis. Inflammation of a gland and the adjacent connective tissue.

phlegmonous erysipelas. A form of erysipelas in which there is abscess formation.

phlo·em (flo′em) *n.* [Ger., from Gk. *phloos,* bark]. *In botany,* the portion of a fibrovascular bundle lying beneath the epidermis which consists of sieve tubes, companion cells, and associated fibers or parenchyma; leptome. Contr. *xylem.*

phloem sheath. *In botany,* a layer of thin-walled cells surrounding the phloem tissue. Syn. *bast sheath, periphloem, vascular bundle sheath.*

phlo·gis·tic (flo·jis′tick) *adj.* [Gk. *phlogistos,* inflammable]. Of or pertaining to inflammation or fever.

phlo·gis·ton (flo·jis′tun) *n.* [Gk., neuter of *phlogistos,* inflammable, from *phlox,* flame]. The name, introduced in the 17th century, of the hypothetical component of combustible substances. Such substances were thought to be compounds of phlogiston with another component; on combustion the phlogiston escaped, leaving the other component. The theory was abandoned following the discovery of oxygen and of its role in combustion.

phlogo·gen·ic (flog″o·jen′ick) *adj.* [Gk. *phlox, phlogos,* flame, + *-genic*]. Producing inflammation.

phlo·gog·e·nous (flo·goj′e·nus) *adj.* PHLOGOGENIC.

phlo·go·sis (flo·go′sis) *n.* [Gk. *phlogōsis,* from *phlox,* flame]. 1. INFLAMMATION. 2. ERYSIPELAS.

phlogo·zel·o·tism (flog″o·zel′uh·tiz·um) *n.* [Gk. *phlox, phlogos,* flame, + Gk. *zēlōtēs,* zealot, + *-ism*]. An old craze for ascribing to every disease an inflammatory origin.

phlo·rhi·zin (flo·rye′zin, flor′i·zin) *n.* [Gk. *phloos,* bark, + *rhiza,* root, + *-in*]. A glycoside, $C_{21}H_{24}O_{10}$, obtained from the bark and root of certain fruit trees; used experimentally to produce glycosuria in animals. Syn. *phlorizin, phloridzin, phlorrhizin.*

phlorhizin test. Injected phlorizin blocks renal tubular resorption of glucose and normally produces glycosuria; little or no glycosuria indicates renal insufficiency.

phlo·rid·zin (flo·rid'zin) *n.* PHLORHIZIN.

phlor·o·glu·cine (flor"o·gloo'seen, ·sin) *n.* PHLOROGLUCINOL.

phlor·o·glu·ci·nol (flor"o·gloo'si·nol) *n.* 1,3,5-Benzenetriol, $C_6H_6O_3.2H_2O$, used as a reagent for hydrochloric acid in gastric juice, for lignin, pentosans, pentoses, etc.

phloroglucinol-hydrochloric acid reaction. BIAL'S TEST.

phloroglucinol-hydrochloric acid test. TOLLEN'S TEST.

phlox·ine (flock'seen, ·sin) *n.* [Gk. *phlox*, flame, + *-ine*]. A red acid dye of the xanthine series; used as a counterstain with blue nuclear dyes.

phloxine-methylene blue stain. MALLORY'S PHLOXINE-METHYLENE BLUE STAIN.

phlox·ino·phil·ic (flock"sin·o·fil'ick) *adj.* [*phloxine* + *-philic*]. Having an affinity for phloxine.

phlyc·te·na (flick·tee'nuh) *n.*, pl. **phlycte·nae** (·nee) [Gk. *phlyktaina*, blister]. A vesicle. —**phlyc·te·nar** (flick'te·nur), **phlycte·nous** (·nus) *adj.*

phlyc·ten·u·la (flick·ten'yoo·luh) *n.*, pl. **phlyctenu·lae** (·lee). PHLYCTENULE.

phlyctenular conjunctivitis. PHLYCTENULAR KERATOCONJUNCTIVITIS.

phlyctenular keratitis. PHLYCTENULAR KERATOCONJUNCTIVITIS.

phlyctenular keratoconjunctivitis. Inflammation of the cornea characterized by the formation of pinhead-sized vesicle-like nodules that ulcerate; seen most often in children with evidence of tuberculin sensitivity and general debility; considered to be due to a localized allergic reaction of the conjunctiva, most commonly to tuberculin, but also to other bacterial products. Syn. *eczematous conjunctivitis, scrofulous ophthalmia, strumous ophthalmia.*

phlyctenular ophthalmia. PHLYCTENULAR KERATOCONJUNCTIVITIS.

phlyc·te·nule (flick'te·newl) *n.* A minute phlyctena; a little vesicle or blister. —**phlyc·ten·u·lar** (flick·ten'yoo·lur) *adj.*

phlyc·ten·u·lo·sis (flick·ten"yoo·lo'sis) *n.* [*phlyctenule* + *-osis*]. The presence of phlyctenules.

-phobe. A combining form meaning (a) *resisting, avoiding;* (b) *one having a phobia.*

-phobia [Gk. *phobos*, fear, + *-ia*]. A combining form meaning *fear* or *dread.* Contr. *-philia.*

pho·bia (fo'bee·uh) *n.* [Gk. *phobos*, fear, + *-ia*]. A disproportionate, obsessive, persistent, and unrealistic fear of an external situation or object, symbolically taking the place of an internal unconscious conflict. See also *phobic neurosis.* —**pho·bic** (·bick) *adj.*

phobic avoidance. *In psychiatry,* a psychic process in which intrapsychic or external fear is avoided by displacement onto a particular object or class of objects; avoidance of the object then allows avoidance of anxiety.

phobic neurosis or **reaction.** A neurotic disorder characterized by an intense, persistent fear of some object or situation in which the fear is out of proportion to any real danger, is inconsistent with the patient's general personality, is consciously recognized as unfounded, and frequently interferes with the patient's activities. The tension and apprehension may be manifested by faintness, tremor, sweating, nausea, even panic, and in other ways. In phobias, of which many types are described, the patient's anxiety is fixed to some symbolic object or situation, so that the anxiety may be controlled by avoiding the feared object or situation. The patient may be unconscious of the origin of the anxiety.

pho·bo·dip·sia (fo"bo·dip'see·uh) *n.* [Gk. *phobodipsos*, hydrophobic (from *phobos*, fear, + *dipsa*, thirst) + *-ia*]. HYDROPHOBIA.

pho·bo·pho·bia (fo"bo·fo'bee·uh) *n.* [Gk. *phobos*, fear, + *-phobia*]. An abnormal dread of being afraid or of developing a phobia.

Pho·cas' disease (foʰ·kahs') [B. G. *Phocas*, French physician, 1861–1937]. Mammary dysplasia with chiefly fibrous nodule formation.

pho·co·me·lia (fo"ko·mee'lee·uh) *n.* [Gk. *phōkē*, seal, + *-melia*]. Absence or markedly imperfect development of arms and forearms, thighs and legs, but with hands and feet present. —**phocome·lic** (·lick) *adj.*

phocomelic dwarf. A dwarf with abnormally short diaphyses in the upper and lower extremities.

pho·com·e·lus (fo·kom'e·lus) *n.*, pl. **phocome·li** (·lye). An individual with phocomelia.

pho·com·e·ly (fo·kom'e·lee) *n.* PHOCOMELIA.

phol·co·dine (fol'ko·deen) *n.* 3-(2-Morpholinoethyl)morphine, $C_{23}H_{30}N_2O_4$, an antitussive drug structurally related to codeine.

Pho·ma (fo'muh) *n.* [NL., from Gk. *phōis*, blister]. A genus of fungi whose species may act as common allergens and as laboratory contaminants.

phon-, phono- [Gk. *phōnē*]. A combining form meaning (a) *sound;* (b) *speech, voice.*

pho·nal (fo'nul) *adj.* [*phon-* + *-al*]. Pertaining to the voice or to sound.

phon·as·the·nia (fo"nas·theen'ee·uh) *n.* [*phon-* + *asthenia*]. Weakness of voice, especially that resulting from bodily exhaustion.

pho·na·tion (fo·nay'shun) *n.* The production of vocal sound. Compare *articulation.* —**pho·nate** (fo'nate) *v.;* **pho·na·to·ry** (fo'nuh·tor"ee) *adj.*

phonatory cord. VOCAL FOLD.

phonatory spasm. PHONIC SPASM.

phon·au·to·gram (fo·naw'to·gram) *n.* The tracing produced by a phonautograph.

phon·au·to·graph (fo·naw'to·graf) *n.* [*phon-* + *auto-* + *-graph*]. An apparatus for transforming automatically the vibrations of the air produced by sound, including the voice, into a visible record.

phone (fone) *n.* [Gk. *phōnē*, sound, voice]. A speech sound.

-phone [Gk. *phōnein*, to sound]. A combining form meaning a *sound-transmitting or recording instrument.*

pho·neme (fo'neem) *n.* [Gk. *phōnēma*, sound, utterance]. 1. A speech sound or range of sounds as a structural and functional unit in the sound system of a particular language. 2. An auditory hallucination of hearing speech.

pho·nen·do·scope (fo·nen'duh·skope) *n.* [*phon-* + *endo-* + *-scope*]. A stethoscope which intensifies the ausculatory sounds.

pho·net·ic (fo·net'ick) *adj.* [Gk. *phonētikos*, vocal]. 1. Pertaining to speech sounds. 2. Pertaining to phonetics.

phonetic paralysis. PARALYTIC APHONIA.

pho·net·ics (fo·net'icks) *n.* The analysis and description of speech sounds in terms of the processes by which they are produced (articulatory phonetics), the physical properties of the sounds themselves (acoustic phonetics), and the relation of these properties to the articulatory and auditory processes. Compare *phonics, phonology.*

-phonia, -phony [Gk. *phōnein*, to sound]. A combining form meaning (a) *sound;* (b) *vocal or speech disorder.*

pho·ni·at·rics (fo"nee·at'ricks) *n.* The study and treatment of the voice.

pho·ni·a·try (fo·nigh'uh·tree) *n.* PHONIATRICS.

phon·ic (fon'ick) *adj.* [*phon-* + *-ic*]. 1. Of or pertaining to the voice. 2. Of or pertaining to phonics.

pho·ni·ca (fo'ni·kuh) *n.pl.* Diseases affecting the vocal organs.

phon·ics (fon'icks) *n.* 1. The science of sound. 2. The methodology of teaching reading by the association of letters with phonemes, as opposed to the association of word configurations with spoken words or with concepts. Compare *phonetics.*

phonic spasm. A spasm of the laryngeal muscles occurring on attempting to speak, usually a component of a conversion reaction, but also seen in professional singers and speakers due to faulty voice production.

pho·nism (fo'niz·um) *n.* [*phon-* + *-ism*]. A form of synesthesia in which there is a sensation of sound or hearing, due to the effect of sight, touch, taste, or smell, or even to the thought of some object, person, or general conception. Compare *photism.*

phono-. See *phon-.*

pho·no·car·dio·gram (fo''no·kahr'dee·o·gram) *n.* [*phono-* + *cardiogram*]. A graphic record of heart sounds and murmurs.

pho·no·car·dio·graph (fo''no·kahr'dee·o·graf) *n.* [*phono-* + *cardiograph*]. An instrument for recording heart sounds and murmurs. **—phono·car·dio·graph·ic** (·kahr''dee·o·graf'ick) *adj.*

pho·no·car·di·og·ra·phy (fo''no·kahr''dee·og'ruh·fee) *n.* The graphic recording of heart sounds and murmurs.

pho·no·chor·da (fo''no·kor'duh) *n.*, pl. **phonochor·dae** (·dee) [*phono-* + *chorda*]. VOCAL FOLD.

pho·no·cine·flu·o·ro·car·di·og·ra·phy (fo''no·sin''e·floo''ur·o·kahr''dee·og'ruh·fee) *n.* [*phono-* + *cine-* + *fluorocardiography*]. The use of synchronous cardiac sounds and cinefluorography to study heart form, motion, and function.

pho·no·gram (fo'nuh·gram) *n.* [*phono-* + *-gram*]. A written or graphic record of a sound.

pho·no·graph (fo'nuh·graf) *n.* [*phono-* + *-graph*]. An instrument for recording and reproducing vocal and other sounds.

pho·nol·o·gy (fo·nol'uh·jee) *n.* [*phono-* + *-logy*]. The analysis and description of speech sounds in terms of the linguistic systems in which they function. Compare *phonetics.* See also *phoneme.*

phono·ma·nia (fon''o·may'nee·uh) *n.* [Gk. *phonos*, murder, slaughter, + *mania*]. Homicidal mania.

pho·no·mas·sage (fo''no·muh·sahj') *n.* [*phono-* + *massage*]. Stimulation and exercise of the tympanic membrane and ossicular chain, by alternating pressure and suction in the external auditory meatus.

pho·nom·e·ter (fo·nom'e·tur) *n.* [*phono-* + *-meter*]. An instrument for measuring the pitch and intensity of vocal sounds. **—phonome·try** (·tree) *n.*

pho·no·my·oc·lo·nus (fo''no·migh·ock'luh·nus, ·migh''o·klo'nus) *n.* [*phono-* + *myo-* + *clonus*]. A condition in which a sound is heard on auscultation over a muscle, indicating fibrillary contractions which may be so fine that they are not seen on visual inspection.

pho·no·my·og·ra·phy (fo''no·migh·og'ruh·fee) *n.* [*phono-* + *myo-* + *-graphy*]. Recording of sounds made by the contraction of a muscle.

pho·nop·a·thy (fo·nop'uth·ee) *n.* [*phono-* + *-pathy*]. Any disorder or disease of the voice.

pho·no·pho·bia (fo''no·fo'bee·uh) *n.* [*phono-* + *-phobia*]. 1. A fear of speaking or of one's own voice; may be due to the pain caused by speaking, as in certain organic disorders. 2. Abnormal fear of any sound or noise.

pho·no·pho·tog·ra·phy (fo''no·fuh·tog'ruh·fee) *n.* [*phono-* + *photography*]. Photographic recording of the vibratory characteristics of speech sounds.

pho·nop·sia (fo·nop'see·uh) *n.* [*phon-* + *-opsia*]. The perception of color when certain sounds are heard.

-phony. See *-phonia.*

-phor, -phore [Gk. *phoros,* bearing, bringing]. A combining form meaning *bearer, carrier.*

phor-, phoro- [Gk. *phoros,* bearing, carrying, from *pherein,* to carry, bring, lead]. A combining form meaning (a) *carrying, transmission;* (b) *bearing, supporting;* (c) *directing, turning.*

phor·bin (for'bin) *n.* [Gk. *phorbē,* pasture, + *-in*]. The metal-free ring system characteristic of chlorophylls, composed of four pyrrole rings on one of which is fused a cyclopentane ring. It closely resembles the porphyrin ring system of heme.

-phore. See *-phor.*

-phoresis [Gk. *phorēsis,* transport, being carried]. A combining form meaning *transmission.*

-phoria [*phor-* + *-ia*]. A combining form meaning (a) *tendency;* (b) *turning of the visual axis,* as in exophoria.

-phoric [*phor-* + *-ic*]. A combining form meaning *bearing, carrying.*

Phor·i·dae (for'i·dee) *n.pl.* A family of small flies, some of which cause myiasis. See also *Aphiochaeta.*

Phor·mia (for'mee·uh) *n.* A genus of blowflies.

Phormia re·gi·na (re·jye'nuh). The black blowfly, which normally deposits its eggs or larvae in the decaying flesh of dead animals, but may be a secondary invader of neglected wounds and sores. The maggots may attack living tissue when dead tissue is not available.

phoro-. See *phor-.*

phoro·blast (for'o·blast) *n.* [*phoro-* + *-blast*]. *Obsol.* FIBROBLAST.

phoro·cyte (for'o·site) *n.* [*phoro-* + *-cyte*]. *Obsol.* Any connective-tissue cell.

pho·rol·o·gy (fo·rol'uh·jee) *n.* [*phoro-* + *-logy*]. The science pertaining to disease carriers.

pho·rom·e·ter (fo·rom'e·tur) *n.* [*phoro-* + *-meter*]. An instrument for measuring the relative strength of the ocular muscles.

phoro·op·tom·e·ter (for''o·op·tom'e·tur) *n.* [*phoro-* + *opto-* + *-meter*]. An apparatus for optical testing of muscular defects.

Phoropter. Trademark for a sight-testing device containing 36 lenses; by manipulating the dials, over 61 billion combinations are possible. It adds automatically and rapidly the magnifications of its combinations, thus obviating the tedious shifting of refracting lenses into trial frames by hand.

phoro·scope (for'uh·skope) *n.* [*phoro-* + *-scope*]. An apparatus for testing vision, consisting of a trial frame for lenses, fixed to a bench or table.

phoro·tone (for'uh·tone) *n.* [*phoro-* + *tone*]. An apparatus for exercising the eye muscles.

-phorous [*phor-* + *-ous*]. A combining form meaning *bearing, carrying.*

phos- [Gk. *phōs*]. A combining form meaning *light.*

phose (foze) *n.* [Gk. *phōs,* light]. Any subjective sensation of light or color, as scintillating scotoma of migraine. See also *antrophose, aphose, centrophose, chromophose, cyanophose, erythrophose, peripheraphose, peripherophose.*

phos·gene (fos'jeen, foz') *n.* Carbonyl chloride, $COCl_2$, a colorless gas that has been used in chemical warfare.

phos·gen·ic (fos·jen'ick, foz·) *adj.* [*phos-* + *-genic*]. PHOTOGENIC.

phosph-, phospho-. A combining form meaning *phosphorous* or *phosphoric.*

phos·pha·gen (fos'fuh·jen) *n.* PHOSPHOCREATINE.

phosphataemia. PHOSPHATEMIA.

phos·pha·tase (fos'fuh·tace, ·taze) *n.* An enzyme that catalyzes hydrolysis of esters of phosphoric acid. Numerous phosphatases are known to exist; they play an important role in various metabolic processes, and in bone formation. See also Table of Chemical Constituents of Blood in the Appendix.

phos·phate (fos'fate) *n.* A salt of phosphoric acid.

phosphate cycle. A cycle of continuous phosphorylation and dephosphorylation reactions which provides for conversion of energy derived from certain metabolic processes to useful cellular work.

phosphate diabetes. FAMILIAL HYPOPHOSPHATEMIA.

phos·pha·te·mia, phos·pha·tae·mia (fos''fuh·tee'mee·uh, fos''fay·) *n.* [*phosphate* + *-emia*]. 1. The presence of phosphates in the circulating blood. 2. HYPERPHOSPHATEMIA.

phos·pha·tide (fos'fuh·tide) *n.* PHOSPHOLIPID.

phos·pha·tid·ic acid (fos″fuh·tid′ick). Any ester of glycerin in which two of its alcohol groups are esterified with long-chain fatty acids, and the other alcohol group is esterified with phosphoric acid, with two acidic groups of the phosphoric acid being unsubstituted. Salts of phosphatidic acids have been isolated from plant tissues and beef heart.

phos·pha·ti·dyl·cho·line (fos″fuh·tye′dil·ko′leen) *n.* A phospholipid in which phosphatidic acid is esterified to choline. Syn. *lecithin.*

phos·pha·ti·dyl·eth·a·nol·amine (fos″fuh·tye′dil·eth″uh·nol′uh·meen) *n.* A phospholipid in which phosphatidic is esterified to an ethanolamine base. Syn. *cephalin.*

phos·pha·tu·ria (fos″fuh·tew′ree·uh) *n.* [*phosphate* + *-uria*]. HYPERPHOSPHATURIA.

phos·phene (fos′feen) *n.* [Gk. *phōs,* light, + *phainein,* to show]. A subjective, luminous sensation due to stimulation of the retina by stimuli other than light.

phosphene of accommodation. Accommodation phosphene.

phos·phide (fos′fide) *n.* A compound containing phosphorus in its lowest valence state (−3).

phos·phine (fos′feen, ·fin) *n.* 1. Hydrogen phosphide, PH_3, a poisonous gas with a garlicky odor. 2. A substitution compound of PH_3, bearing the same relation to it that an amine does to ammonia.

phos·phite (fos′fite) *n.* A salt of phosphorous acid.

phospho-. See *phosph-.*

phos·pho·ami·no·lip·id (fos″fo·a·mee″no·lip′id, ·lye″pid, fos″fo·am″i·no·) *n.* A compound lipid that contains phosphorus and an amino group.

phos·pho·ar·gi·nine (fos″fo·ahr′ji·neen, ·nin) *n.* Arginine phosphate. A phosphoric acid derivative of arginine which contains an energy-rich phosphate bond. Phosphoarginine is believed to play a role in invertebrate muscle metabolism similar to that of phosphocreatine in the muscle of vertebrates.

phos·pho·cho·line (fos″fo·ko′leen) *n.* An intermediate in the biosynthesis of phosphatidylcholine in many animal tissues; formed by reaction of choline with ATP in the presence of choline kinase.

phos·pho·cre·a·tine (fos″fo·kree′uh·teen, ·tin) *n.* Creatine phosphate, $C_4H_{10}N_3O_5P$, a phosphoric acid derivative of creatine which contains an energy-rich phosphate bond. Phosphocreatine is present in muscle and other tissues, and during the anaerobic phase of muscular contraction it reacts with ADP to form creatine and ATP and makes energy available for the contractile process.

phos·pho·di·es·ter·ase (fos″fo·dye·es′tur·ace, ·aze) *n.* An enzyme catalyzing hydrolysis of one ester linkage in phosphoric acid esters containing two ester linkages.

phos·pho·enol·py·ru·vic acid (fos″fo·ee″nol·pye·roo′vick). 2-Phosphoenolpyruvic acid; $CH_2{=}COP(O)(OH)_2COOH$; a high-energy phosphate formed by dehydration of 2-phosphoglyceric acid; it reacts with adenosine diphosphate to form adenosine triphosphate and enolpyruvic acid.

phos·pho·fruc·to·ki·nase (fos″fo·fruck″to·kigh′nace, ·naze) *n.* Any enzyme that catalyzes the biochemical conversion of fructose 6-phosphate to fructose 1,6-diphosphate.

phosphofructokinase deficiency disease. TARUI'S DISEASE.

phos·pho·fruc·to·mu·tase (fos″fo·fruck″to·mew′tace, ·taze) *n.* The enzyme that catalyzes the conversion of fructose 1-phosphate to fructose 6-phosphate.

phos·pho·ga·lac·tose uri·dyl transferase (fos″fo·ga·lack′toce yoo′ri·dil). Galactose 1-phosphate uridyl transferase, an enzyme that catalyzes conversion of galactose 1-phosphate to glucose 1-phosphate. Congenital absence of the enzyme results in galactosemia.

phos·pho·glu·co·mu·tase (fos″fo·gloo″ko·mew′tace, ·aze) *n.* The enzyme that catalyzes the reversible conversion of glucose 1-phosphate to glucose 6-phosphate.

phos·pho·glu·co·nate pathway (fos″fo·gloo′ko·nate). HEXOSE MONOPHOSPHATE SHUNT.

phos·pho·glu·con·ic acid (fos″fo·gloo·kon′ick). 6-Phospho-D-gluconic acid, $COOH(CHOH)_4CH_2OPO_3H_2$, a product of the oxidation of glucose 6-phosphate, catalyzed by glucose 6-phosphate dehydrogenase. Triphosphopyridine nucleotide is required as the coenzyme.

phos·pho·glu·cose isomerase (fos″fo·gloo′koce). An enzyme that catalyzes the interconversion of glucose 6-phosphate and fructose 6-phosphate.

phos·pho·glyc·er·al·de·hyde (fos″fo·glis″ur·al′de·hide) *n.* $OHCCHOHCH_2OPO_3H_2$. An intermediate product in carbohydrate metabolism.

2-phos·pho·gly·cer·ic acid (fos″fo·gli·serr′ick). $HOOCCHO\text{-}PO_3H_2CH_2OH$; an intermediate compound in carbohydrate metabolism specifically between 3-phosphoglyceric acid and phosphoenolpyruvic acid.

3-phosphoglyceric acid. $HOOCCHOHCH_2OPO_3H_2$; an intermediate product in carbohydrate metabolism, specifically between 1,3-diphosphoglyceric acid and 2-phosphoglyceric acid.

phos·pho·glyc·ero·mu·tase (fos″fo·glis″ur·o·mew′tace, ·taze) *n.* An enzyme that catalyzes conversion of 3-phosphoglyceric acid to 2-phosphoglyceric acid.

phos·pho-gly·co·gen synthase (fos″fo·glye′ko·jin). The inactive form of glycogen synthase, inactivated by protein kinase. Contr. *dephospho-glycogen synthase.*

phos·pho·hexo·isom·er·ase (fos″fo·heck″so·eye·som′ur·ace) *n.* The enzyme that catalyzes the conversion of glucose 6-phosphate to fructose 6-phosphate.

phos·pho·hexo·ki·nase (fos″fo·heck″so·kigh′nace, ·naze) *n.* The enzyme that catalyzes the formation of fructose 1,6-diphosphate through transfer of phosphate from adenosinetriphosphate to fructose 6-phosphate.

phos·pho·ino·si·tide (fos″fo·i·no′si·tide) *n.* Any of a group of phosphatides, present in the brain, that contain inositol; on hydrolysis they yield glycerin, L-myoinositol, fatty acid, and phosphoric acid.

Phospholine Iodide. Trademark for echothiophate iodide, a cholinesterase inhibitor used in the treatment of glaucoma.

phos·pho·li·pase (fos″fo·lye′pace, ·lip′ace) *n.* [*phospholipid* + *-ase*]. An enzyme that catalyzes a hydrolysis of a phospholipid; especially a lecithinase that acts in this manner on a lecithin.

phos·pho·lip·id (fos″fo·lip′id, ·lye′pid) *n.* A type of lipid compound which is an ester of phosphoric acid and contains, in addition, one or two molecules of fatty acid, an alcohol, and a nitrogenous base. They are widely distributed in nature and include such substances as lecithin, cephalin, and sphingomyelin. See also Table of Chemical Constituents of Blood in the Appendix.

phos·pho·lip·in (fos″fo·lip′in) *n.* PHOSPHOLIPID.

phos·pho·mo·lyb·date (fos″fo·mo·lib′date) *n.* A salt of phosphomolybdic acid.

phos·pho·mo·lyb·dic acid (fos″fo·mo·lib′dick). Approximately $20MoO_3.P_2O_5.51H_2O$, a yellow, crystalline powder; variously used as a reagent.

phos·pho·mono·es·ter·ase (fos″fo·mon″o·es′tur·ace, ·aze, fos″fo·mo″no·) *n.* An enzyme catalyzing hydrolysis of phosphoric acid esters containing one ester linkage.

phos·pho·ne·cro·sis (fos″fo·ne·kro′sis) *n.* [*phospho-* + *necrosis*]. Necrosis of the maxilla and mandible associated with chronic exposure to phosphorus dust. Syn. *phossy jaw.*

phos·pho·ni·um (fos·fo′nee·um) *n.* The hypothetical univalent radical PH_4, analogous to ammonium, NH_4.

phos·pho-phos·pho·ryl·ase kinase (fos″fo·fos′for·i·lace, ·fos·for′i·). The active form of phosphorylase kinase, which has been activated by reaction with adenosine triphosphate and protein kinase. It reacts with inactive phosphorylase b and adenosine triphosphate to convert it to active phosphorylase a, enabling this product to release glucose-1-phosphate from glycogen. Contr. *dephospho-phosphorylase kinase.*

phos·pho·pro·tein (fos″fo·pro′teen, ·tee·in) *n.* A conjugated protein consisting of a compound of protein with a phosphorus-containing substance other than nucleic acid or lecithin.

phos·pho·py·ru·vic acid (fos″fo·pye·roo′vick). An intermediate substance, $CH_2{=}CO(PO_3H_2)COOH$, obtained in the breakdown of glycogen to lactic acid and the resynthesis of glycogen from lactic acid.

phos·phor (fos′for) *n.* A substance that phosphoresces.

phosphor-, phosphoro-. A combining form meaning (a) *phosphorus;* (b) *phosphoric acid;* (c) *phosphorescent.*

phos·pho·res·cence (fos″fuh·res′unce) *n.* 1. The continuous emission of light from a substance without any apparent rise in temperature, produced after exposure to heat, light, or electric discharges. 2. The faint green glow of white phosphorus exposed to air, due to its slow oxidation. 3. *In radiology,* the emission of radiation by a substance as a result of previous absorption of radiation of shorter wavelength. —**phosphores·cent** (·unt) *adj.;* **phospho·resce** (·res′) *v.*

phos·phor·hi·dro·sis (fos″for·hi·dro′sis, ·high·dro′sis) *n.* [*phosphor-* + *hidrosis*]. The secretion of phosphorescent sweat.

phos·pho·ri·bo·mu·tase (fos″fo·rye″bo·mew′tace, ·taze) *n.* An enzyme that catalyzes interconversion of ribose 5-phosphate and ribose 1-phosphate.

phos·pho·ric (fos·fo′rick) *adj.* 1. PHOSPHORESCENT. 2. Of or pertaining to compounds containing phosphorus in the +5 valence state.

phosphoric acid. H_3PO_4. Orthophosphoric acid, a liquid of a syrupy consistency that contains 85% of H_3PO_4.

phos·phor·i·dro·sis (fos″for·i·dro′sis) *n.* PHOSPHORHIDROSIS.

phos·pho·rism (fos′fuh·riz·um) *n.* [*phosphor-* + *-ism*]. Chronic phosphorus poisoning.

phos·phor·ne·cro·sis (fos″for·ne·kro′sis) *n.* PHOSPHONECROSIS.

phosphoro-. See *phosphor-.*

phos·phor·ol·y·sis (fos″for·ol′i·sis) *n.* [*phosphoro-* + *-lysis*]. A chemical reaction by which the elements of phosphoric acid are incorporated into the molecule of a compound.

phos·pho·rous (fos′fuh·rus) *adj.* 1. PHOSPHORESCENT. 2. Containing, resembling, or pertaining to phosphorus.

phos·pho·rous (fos·fo′rus) *adj.* Of or pertaining to compounds containing phosphorous in the +3 valence state.

phosphorous acid. A yellow, crystalline acid, H_3PO_3, used as a reducing agent and as a reagent.

phos·pho·rus (fos′fuh·rus) *n.* [NL., from Gk. *phōsphoros,* light-bearing]. P = 30.9738. A nonmetallic element occurring in two allotropic forms, white or yellow phosphorus and amorphous or red phosphorus; the density of the former is about 1.82, and of the latter about 2.19.

phosphorus 32. A radioactive isotope of phosphorus, which emits beta rays, used in the form of sodium phosphate for locating tumors and in treating polycythemia vera and leukemia; radiophosphorus. Symbol, ^{32}P.

phosphorus-depletion syndrome. Hypophosphatemia, hypophosphaturia, increased gastrointestinal absorption of calcium, hypercalciuria, increased resorption of skeletal calcium and phosphorus, with debility, anorexia, weakness, malaise, and bone pain; produced by prolonged ingestion of nonabsorbable antacids such as magnesium-aluminum hydroxide.

phosphorus necrosis. PHOSPHONECROSIS.

phos·pho·ryl (fos′fuh·ril) *n.* The trivalent radical ≡PO.

phos·pho·ryl·ase (fos′for·i·lace, fos·for′i·lace, ·laze) *n.* An enzyme widely distributed in animals, plants, and microorganisms. It catalyzes the formation of glucose 1-phosphate (Cori ester) from glycogen and inorganic phosphate.

phosphorylating enzymes. Enzymes that catalyze the phosphorylation or dephosphorylation of compounds.

phos·pho·ryl·ation (fos″for·i·lay′shun) *n.* The esterification of compounds with phosphoric acid. —**phos·pho·ryl·ate** (fos′for·i·late) *v.*

phos·pho·trans·acet·y·lase (fos″fo·tranz″uh·set′i·lace, ·laze) *n.* The enzyme that catalyzes the reversible transfer of an acetyl group from acetyl coenzyme A to a phosphate, with formation of acetyl phosphate.

phos·pho·tri·ose isomerase (fos″fo·trye′oce). Triose isomerase, an enzyme in the Meyerhof cycle, catalyzing the interconversion of 3-phosphoglyceraldehyde and dihydroxyacetone phosphate.

phos·pho·tung·state (fos″fo·tung′state) *n.* A salt of phosphotungstic acid.

phos·pho·tung·stic acid (fos″fo·tung′stick). Approximately $P_2O_5.24WO_3.25H_2O$. A white or yellowish-green crystalline acid used as a reagent.

phosphotungstic acid hematoxylin. MALLORY'S PHOSPHOTUNGSTIC ACID HEMATOXYLIN.

phos·sy jaw (fos′ee). PHOSPHONECROSIS.

phos·vi·tin (fos·vye′tin, fos′vye·tin) *n.* A phosphoprotein isolated from the vitellin fraction of egg yolk.

phot-, photo- [Gk. *phōs, phōtos,* light]. A combining form meaning (a) *light;* (b) *photon;* (c) *photographic.*

phot (fote, fot) *n.* [Gk. *phōs, phōtos,* light]. A unit of illumination equivalent to one lumen per square centimeter.

pho·tal·gia (fo·tal′jee·uh) *n.* [*phot-* + *-algia*]. Pain arising from too great intensity of light.

pho·tau·gio·pho·bia (fo·taw″jee·o·fo′bee·uh) *n.* [Gk. *phōtaugeia,* brightness of light (from *phōs,* light, + *augē,* gleam, shine) + *-phobia*]. PHOTOPHOBIA.

pho·tes·the·sia, pho·taes·the·sia (fo″tes·theezh′uh, ·theez′ee·uh) *n.* [*phot-* + *esthesia*]. 1. Sensitiveness to light. 2. PHOTOPHOBIA.

pho·tic (fo′tick) *adj.* [*phot-* + *-ic*]. Pertaining to light.

photic driving. *In electroencephalography,* the production of occipital rhythmic activity by intermittent flashing light stimuli.

photic epilepsy. PHOTOGENIC EPILEPSY.

pho·tism (fo′tiz·um) *n.* [*phot-* + *-ism*]. A form of synesthesia in which there is a visual sensation, as of color or light, produced by hearing, taste, smell, touch, or temperature, or even by the thought of some object, person, or general conception. Compare *phonism.*

photo-. See *phot-.*

pho·to·ac·tin·ic (fo″to·ack·tin′ick) *adj.* [*photo-* + *actinic*]. Emitting both luminous and actinic rays.

pho·to·bac·te·ri·um (fo″to·back·teer′ee·um) *n.,* pl. **photobacte·ria** (·ee·uh) [*photo-* + *bacterium*]. A bacterial organism which is light-producing or phosphorescent.

pho·to·bi·ot·ic (fo″to·bye·ot′ick) *adj.* [*photo-* + *biotic*]. Living in the light exclusively.

pho·to·ca·tal·y·sis (fo″to·kuh·tal′i·sis) *n.* [*photo-* + *catalysis*]. Catalysis of a chemical reaction effected by exposure to light, either in the visible or ultraviolet region.

pho·to·chem·i·cal (fo″to·kem′i·kul) *adj.* [*photo-* + *chemical*]. Pertaining to chemical action produced directly or indirectly by means of radiation.

photochemical radiation. The portion of the visible spectrum that produces chemical reactions.

pho·to·chem·is·try (fo″to·kem′is·tree) *n.* [*photo-* + *chemistry*]. The study of chemical reactions produced directly or indirectly by means of radiation.

pho·to·chro·mat·ic (fo″to·kro·mat′ick) *adj.* [*photo-* + *chromatic*]. 1. Pertaining to colored light. 2. Pertaining to color photography.

pho·to·chro·mo·gen (fo″to·kro′muh·jen) *n.* [*photo-* + *chromogen*]. An atypical pathogenic mycobacterium that produces pigment when grown in light.

pho·to·chro·mo·gen·ic (fo″to·kro″muh·jen′ick) *adj.* [*photo-* + *chromogenic*]. Producing color in response to a light stimulus.

pho·to·co·ag·u·la·tion (fo″to·ko·ag″yoo·lay′shun) *n.* [*photo-* + *coagulation*]. Coagulation of tissue by a controlled and intense beam of light; used in ophthalmology.

pho·to·col·or·im·e·ter (fo″to·kul″ur·im′e·tur) *n.* PHOTOELECTRIC COLORIMETER.

pho·to·con·duc·tive cell (fo″to·kun·duck′tiv). A type of photoelectric cell.

pho·to·con·duc·tiv·i·ty (fo″to·kon″duck·tiv′i·tee) *n.* [*photo-* + *conductivity*]. The increase in electrical conductivity of a substance when illuminated. —**photo·con·duc·tive** (·kun·duck′tiv) *adj.*

pho·to·con·junc·ti·vi·tis (fo″to·kun·junk″ti·vye′tis) *n.* [*photo-* + *conjunctivitis*]. ACTINIC KERATOCONJUNCTIVITIS.

pho·to·der·ma·ti·tis (fo″to·dur·muh·tye′tis) *n.* [*photo-* + *dermatitis*]. Any skin eruption brought on by exposure to light.

pho·to·der·ma·to·sis (fo″to·dur″muh·to′sis) *n.* [*photo-* + *dermatosis*]. PHOTODERMATITIS.

pho·to·dis·in·te·gra·tion (fo″to·di·sin″te·gray′shun) *n.* Nuclear disintegration initiated by an incoming high-energy photon.

pho·tod·ro·my (fo·tod′ruh·mee) *n.* [*photo-* + Gk. *dromos*, running, race, + *-y*]. The movement of particles suspended in a fluid toward light (positive) or away from it (negative).

pho·to·dy·nam·ic (fo″to·dye·nam′ick) *adj.* [*photo-* + *dynamic*]. Pertaining to the energy of light.

pho·to·dyn·ia (fo″to·din′ee·uh) *n.* [*phot-* + *-odynia*]. Pain arising from too great intensity of light. See also *photophobia.*

pho·to·dys·pho·ria (fo″to·dis·fo′ree·uh) *n.* [*photo-* + *dysphoria*]. PHOTOPHOBIA.

photoelectric cell. A cell or vacuum tube whose electrical properties can be modified by the intensity of light; light can vary the resistance (photoconductive cell), cause the emission of electrons (photoemissive cell), or generate an internal electromotive force (photovoltaic cell), depending on the structure of the cell.

photoelectric collision. The impact of a photon with an electron in an atom, whereby the photon gives up all its energy, removes the electron from its place, and imparts a high velocity to the electron.

photoelectric colorimeter. A colorimeter for determining the concentration of the colored component of a solution, consisting of one or more combinations of calibrated filters and photoelectric cells for measurement of the color.

pho·to·elec·tric·i·ty (fo″to·e·leck″tris′i·tee) *n.* [*photo-* + *electricity*]. Electricity produced under the influence of light or other radiations, such as ultraviolet and x-rays. When irradiated by such radiations, certain metals give off photoelectrons. —**photo·elec·tric** (·e·leck′trick) *adj.*

pho·to·elec·tron (fo″to·e·leck′tron) *n.* [*photo-* + *electron*]. An electron set into swift motion by the impact of a photon, and to which the primary photon transmits all its energy.

pho·to·emis·sion (fo″to·e·mish′un) *n.* [*photo-* + *emission*]. Emission of electrons from certain metals by the impact of light or other forms of radiant energy. —**photo·emis·sive** (·e·mis′iv) *adj.*

photoemissive cell. A type of photoelectric cell.

pho·to·flu·o·rog·ra·phy (fo″to·floo″ur·og′ruh·fee) *n.* [*photo-* + *fluorography*]. The process combining x-ray and photography to produce minature films, as of the chest; a photograph of the fluorescing screen is made.

pho·to·flu·o·ros·co·py (fo″to·floo″ur·os′kuh·pee) *n.* [*photo-* + *fluoroscopy*]. PHOTOFLUOROGRAPHY.

pho·to·gen (fo′to·jen) *n.* [*photo-* + *-gen*]. A substance said to exist in certain photogenic microorganisms and to cause phosphorescence.

pho·to·gene (fo′to·jeen) *n.* [*photo-* + *-gene*]. A retinal impression; an afterimage.

pho·to·gen·e·sis (fo″to·jen′e·sis) *n.* [*photo-* + *-genesis*]. The production of light or of phosphorescence.

pho·to·gen·ic (fo″to·jen′ick) *adj.* [*photo-* + *-genic*]. 1. Produced or caused by light. 2. Emitting or producing light. 3. Aesthetically suitable for being photographed.

photogenic epilepsy. A form of reflex epilepsy induced by flicker or intermittent light; the attacks are usually of the myoclonic type, but may be generalized.

pho·to·gram (fo′tuh·gram) *n.* [*photo-* + *-gram*]. 1. A photograph. 2. A photograph of a kymographic record.

pho·to·graph (fo′tuh·graf) *n.* & *v.* 1. A picture obtained by photography. 2. To obtain a picture by photography.

pho·to·graph·ic (fo″tuh·graf′ick) *adj.* Of or pertaining to photography.

photographic density. A measure of the opacity of an exposed film; the greater the exposure, the greater the photographic density.

photographic dosimetry. The determination of radiation dosage by use of photographic film.

pho·tog·ra·phy (fo·tog′ruh·fee) *n.* [*photo-* + *-graphy*]. The process of obtaining pictures by exposure to light of surfaces, usually plated on paper or glass, of substances chromatically altered by the energy of light.

pho·to·ki·net·ic (fo″to·ki·net′ick) *adj.* [*photo-* + *kinetic*]. Causing movement by means of the energy of light.

pho·to·ky·mo·graph (fo″to·kigh′mo·graf) *n.* [*photo-* + *kymograph*]. An instrument for the optical recording of physiologic cycles or actions; a photographic camera having a cylindrical lens, moving photographic paper, and a device for the recording of time intervals simultaneously with the physiologic phenomena.

pho·to·lu·mi·nes·cence (fo″to·lew″mi·nes′unce) *n.* [*photo-* + *luminescence*]. Luminescence induced by visible or invisible light.

pho·tol·y·sis (fo·tol′i·sis) *n.*, pl. **photoly·ses** (·seez) [*photo-* + *-lysis*]. Decomposition by the action of light.

pho·to·lyte (fo′to·lite) *n.* [*photo-* + *-lyte*]. A substance that is decomposed by the action of light.

pho·to·mag·net·ism (fo″to·mag′ne·tiz·um) *n.* [*photo-* + *magnetism*]. Magnetism resulting from absorption by atomic nuclei of electromagnetic radiation such as gamma rays.

pho·to·ma·nia (fo″to·may′nee·uh) *n.* [*photo-* + *mania*]. 1. The increase of maniacal symptoms under the influence of intense light. 2. An abnormal desire for light.

pho·to·mes·on (fo″to·mez′on, ·mees′on) *n.* [*photo-* + *meson*]. A meson ejected from a nucleus by an impinging photon.

pho·tom·e·ter (fo·tom′e·tur) *n.* [*photo-* + *-meter*]. 1. An instrument for measuring the intensity of light. 2. An instrument for testing the sensitiveness of the eye to light, by determining the minimum illumination in which the object is visible. —**pho·to·met·ric** (fo″to·met′rick) *adj;* **photo·met·ri·cal·ly** (·ri·kuh·lee) *adv.*

pho·tom·e·try (fo·tom′e·tree) *n.* [*photo-* + *-metry*]. The measurement of the intensity of light.

pho·to·mi·cro·graph (fo″to·migh′kro·graf) *n.* [*photo-* + *micro-* + *-graph*]. A photograph of a minute or microscopic object, usually made with the aid of a microscope, and magnified to sufficient size for observation with the naked eye. —**photo·mi·crog·ra·phy** (·migh·krog′ruh·fee) *n.*

pho·to·mo·tor (fo″to·mo′tur) *adj.* [*photo-* + *motor*]. Pertaining to a muscular response to light stimuli, as the constriction of the pupil.

pho·to·mul·ti·pli·er tube (fo″to·mul′ti·plye·ur). A vacuum-tube device that converts signals into electrons and amplifies them through a multiple-stage process.

pho·ton (fo′ton) *n.* [*phot-* + *-on*]. A quantum or discrete quantity of energy of visible light or any other electromagnetic radiation.

pho·to·neu·ro·en·do·crine system (fo″to·new″ro·en′do·krin). The neuronal pathway that conveys information concerning light from the retina to the anterior hypothalamus and preoptic region, exerting a physiologic role in the activity of the hypothalamus and hypophysis, especially in nonmammalian vertebrates, as on the reproductive cycle.

pho·to·neu·tron (fo″to·new′tron) *n.* A neutron released from a nucleus in a photonuclear reaction.

pho·ton·o·sus (fo·ton′uh·sus) *n.*, pl. **photono·si** (·sigh) [NL., from *photo-* + Gk. *nosos,* disease]. A diseased condition arising from continued exposure to intense or glaring light, as snow blindness.

pho·to·nu·cle·ar reaction (fo″to·new′klee·ur). A nuclear reaction induced by photons, as of gamma rays or x-rays.

pho·to·par·es·the·sia, pho·to·par·aes·the·sia (fo″to·păr″es·theezh′uh, ·theez′ee·uh) *n.* [*photo-* + *paresthesia*]. Defective, or perverted, retinal sensibility.

pho·to·path·o·log·ic (fo″to·path″uh·loj′ick) *adj.* [*photo-* + *pathologic*]. Pertaining to an abnormality related to light.

pho·top·a·thy (fo·top′uth·ee) *n.* [*photo-* + *-pathy*]. PHOTONOSUS.

pho·to·per·cep·tive (fo″to·pur·sep′tiv) *adj.* [*photo-* + *perceptive*]. Capable of receiving and perceiving rays of light.

pho·to·phil·ic (fo″to·fil′ick) *adj.* [*photo-* + *-philic*]. Seeking or loving light, especially sunlight.

pho·toph·i·lous (fo·tof′i·lus) *adj.* PHOTOPHILIC.

pho·to·pho·bia (fo″to·fo′bee·uh) *n.* [*photo-* + *-phobia*]. 1. Abnormal intolerance of or sensitivity to light. 2. Abnormal fear of light. —**photopho·bic** (·bick) *adj.*

pho·to·phone (fo′to·fone) *n.* [*photo-* + *-phone*]. A device for transmitting sound by a mechanism of modulation of visible or infrared light and subsequent reconversion of the latter to sound.

pho·to·phore (fo′to·fore) *n.* [*photo-* + *-phore*]. An electric light for endoscopes.

pho·toph·thal·mia (fo″toff·thal′mee·uh) *n.* [*phot-* + *ophthalmia*]. ACTINIC KERATOCONJUNCTIVITIS.

pho·to·pia (fo·to′pee·uh) *n.* [*phot-* + *-opia*]. Daylight vision with eyes adapted to normal bright light. —**pho·to·pic** (·to′pick, ·top′ick) *adj.*

photopic dominator curve. A curve plotted from determinations of the sensitivity of elements from the light-adapted eye of animals with cones and also from the dark-adapted eyes of animals having only cones with its maximum at 0.560 μm. Compare *scotopic dominator curve.*

photopic sensitivity curve. PHOTOPIC DOMINATOR CURVE.

photopic vision. Vision with accurate recognition of color, as occurs when the eyes have become properly adapted to good illumination.

pho·to·po·lym·er·iza·tion (fo″to·pol·im″ur·i·zay′shun) *n.* [*photo-* + *polymerization*]. The polymerization of a substance when exposed to light.

pho·to·pro·ton (fo″to·pro′ton) *n.* [*photo-* + *proton*]. A proton released from a nucleus in a photonuclear reaction.

pho·top·sia (fo·top′see·uh) *n.* [*phot-* + *-opsia*]. Subjective sensations of sparks or flashes of light occurring in certain pathologic conditions of the optic nerve, the retina, or the brain. —**photop·tic** (·tick) *adj.*

pho·top·sin (fo·top′sin) *n.* [*phot-* + *opsin*]. CONE OPSIN.

phot·op·tom·e·ter (fo″top·tom′e·tur) *n.* [*phot-* + *optometer*]. An instrument for determining visual acuity.

phot·op·tom·e·try (fo″top·tom′e·tree) *n.* [*phot-* + *opto-* + *-metry*]. The measurement of the perception of light.

pho·to·re·cep·tive (fo″to·re·sep′tiv) *adj.* [*photo-* + *receptive*]. Capable of receiving and perceiving rays of light.

pho·to·re·cep·tors (fo″to·re·sep′turz) *n.* [*photo-* + *receptor*]. The rods and cones of the retina.

pho·to·ret·i·ni·tis (fo″to·ret″i·nigh′tis) *n.* [*photo-* + *retinitis*]. SUN BLINDNESS.

pho·to·scan (fo′to·skan) *n.* [*photo-* + *scan*]. A rectilinear recording, made with photographic technique, of the distribution of radioactivity over a body part.

pho·tos·co·py (fo·tos′kuh·pee) *n.* [*photo-* + *-scopy*]. FLUOROSCOPY.

photosensitive porphyria. ERYTHROPOIETIC PORPHYRIA.

pho·to·sen·si·tiv·i·ty (fo″to·sen″si·tiv′i·tee) *n.* [*photo-* + *sensitivity*]. 1. The capacity of an organ or organism to be stimulated to activity by light, or to react to light. 2. The absorption of a certain portion of the spectrum by a chemical system. —**photo·sen·si·tive** (·sen′si·tiv) *adj.*

pho·to·sen·si·ti·za·tion (fo″to·sen″si·ti·zay′shun) *n.* The development in the skin or mucous membrane of abnormally high reactivity to ultraviolet radiation or natural sunlight; may be produced by the ingestion of such substances as fluorescent dyes, endocrine products, certain drugs, or heavy metals.

pho·to·shock (fo′to·shock″) *n.* [*photo-* + *shock*]. *In psychiatry,* a type of shock treatment in which an intermittently flashing light is used after administration of a sensitizing drug, sometimes precipitating convulsions.

pho·to·syn·the·sis (fo″to·sin′thi·sis) *n.* [*photo-* + *synthesis*]. The process by which simple carbohydrates are synthesized from carbon dioxide and water by the chloroplasts of living plant cells in the presence of light. —**photo·syn·thet·ic** (·sin·thet′ick) *adj.*

photosynthetic autotroph. PHOTOTROPH.

photosynthetic ratio. The ratio of oxygen evolved to the carbon dioxide assimilated during photosynthesis.

photosynthetic reaction. 1. In general, the synthesis of chemical compounds effected by means of radiant energy, especially light. 2. The synthesis of carbohydrate and related substances from carbon dioxide and water in tissues containing chlorophyll.

pho·to·tax·is (fo″to·tack′sis) *n.* [*photo-* + *taxis*]. Response to a stimulus of light. —**photo·tac·tic** (·tack′tick) *adj.*

pho·to·ther·a·py (fo″to·therr′uh·pee) *n.* [*photo-* + *therapy*]. Treatment of disease with light rays.

pho·to·tim·er (fo′to·tye″mur) *n.* An automatic timing device used in radiography and photography which limits the exposure of film by measuring the amount of light or radiation incident in the area of the film.

pho·tot·o·nus (fo·tot′uh·nus) *n.* [NL., from *photo-* + Gk. *tonos,* tension]. State of sensitiveness of any organism to light. —**pho·to·ton·ic** (fo″to·ton′ick) *adj.*

pho·to·to·pia (fo″to·to′pee·uh) *n.* [*photo-* + *-opia*]. A subjective sensation of light.

pho·to·troph (fo′to·trof) *n.* [*photo-* + *-troph*]. An autotrophic bacterium able to utilize light energy for metabolism. —**pho·to·troph·ic** (fo″to·trof′ick) *adj.*

pho·tot·ro·pism (fo·tot′ruh·piz·um) *n.* [*photo-* + *tropism*]. The tendency of most plants and sessile animals to turn or bend toward the greater light. —**photo·trop·ic** (·trop′ick) *adj.*

pho·to·tube (fo′to·tewb) *n.* [*photo-* + *tube*]. A vacuum tube whose electrical properties are altered according to the amount of incident light.

pho·to·vol·ta·ic cell (fo″to·vol·tay′ick, ·vohl·tay′ick). A type of photoelectric cell.

pho·tu·ria (fo·tew′ree·uh) *n.* [*phot-* + *-uria*]. The passage of phosphorescent urine.

phrag·mo·plast (frag′mo·plast) *n.* [Gk. *phragmos*, fence, + *-plast*]. The cytokinetic apparatus in plant cells responsible for the formation of the cell wall.

phren-, phreno- [Gk. *phrēn,* midriff; heart, mind]. A combining form meaning (a) *mind;* (b) *brain;* (c) *diaphragm;* (d) *phrenic nerve.*

phre·nal·gia (fre·nal′jee·uh) *n.* [*phren-,* mind, + *-algia*]. MELANCHOLIA.

phren·as·the·nia (fren″as·theen′ee·uh) *n.* [*phren-* + *asthenia*]. MENTAL DEFICIENCY. —**phrenas·then·ic** (·thenn′ick) *adj. & n.*

phren·atro·phia (fren″a·tro′fee·uh) *n.* [NL., from *phren-* + *atrophy*]. *Obsol.* Atrophy of the brain; idiocy.

phren·em·phrax·is (fren″em·frack′sis) *n.* [*phren-* + *emphraxis*]. Crushing of a phrenic nerve with a hemostat to produce temporary paralysis of the diaphragm.

phre·ne·sia (fre·nee′zhuh, ·zee·uh) *n.* [ML., from L. *phrenesis,* delirium, + *-ia*]. *Obsol.* ENCEPHALITIS. —**phre·ne·si·ac** (fre·nee′zee·ack) *n.*

phre·ne·sis (fre·nee′sis) *n.* [L., from Gk. *phrēn,* mind, + *-esis*]. Frenzy; delirium; insanity. —**phre·net·ic** (fre·net′ick) *adj.*

-phrenia [Gk. *phrēn,* mind, + *-ia*]. A combining form meaning *mental disorder.*

phren·ic (fren′ick) *adj.* [*phren-* + *-ic*]. 1. Pertaining to the diaphragm. 2. Pertaining to the mind.

phrenic artery. See Table of Arteries in the Appendix.

phren·i·cec·to·my (fren″i·seck′tuh·mee) *n.* [*phrenic* + *-ectomy*]. Resection of a section of a phrenic nerve or removal of an entire phrenic nerve.

phrenic emphraxis. PHRENICOEXERESIS.

phrenic ganglion. A ganglion located at the junction of the right phrenic nerve with the phrenic plexus, which sends nerve fibers to the inferior vena cava, right suprarenal gland, and the hepatic plexus. It is a subordinate part of the celiac ganglion. NA (pl.) *ganglia phrenica.*

phren·i·cla·sia (fren″i·klay′zee·uh, ·zhuh) *n.* [*phrenic* + *-clasia*]. PHRENEMPHRAXIS.

phrenic nerve. A nerve, arising from the third, fourth, and fifth cervical (cervical plexus) segments of the cord. It innervates the diaphragm. NA *nervus phrenicus.* See also Table of Nerves in the Appendix.

phrenic neuralgia. Pain referred to the shoulder or arm from diseased viscera, such as pericarditis or a suprarenal tumor.

phrenico-. A combining form meaning *phrenic.*

phren·i·co·col·ic (fren″i·ko·kol′ick, ·ko′lick) *adj.* PHRENOCOLIC.

phrenicocolic ligament. A fold of peritoneum extending from the left colic flexure to the diaphragm and serving to support the spleen. NA *ligamentum phrenicocolicum.*

phren·i·co·cos·tal (fren″i·ko·kos′tul) *adj.* [*phrenico-* + *costal*]. Pertaining to the diaphragm and the ribs.

phrenicocostal sinus. COSTODIAPHRAGMATIC RECESS.

phren·i·co·esoph·a·ge·al, phren·i·co·oesoph·a·ge·al (fren″i·ko·e·sof″uh·jee′ul) *adj.* [*phrenico-* + *esophageal*]. Pertaining to the diaphragm and the esophagus.

phren·i·co·ex·er·e·sis (fren″i·ko·eck·serr′e·sis) *n.* [*phrenico-* + *exeresis*]. Avulsion of a phrenic nerve.

phren·i·co·gas·tric (fren″i·ko·gas′trick) *adj.* PHRENOGASTRIC.

phren·i·co·li·en·al (fren″i·ko·lye′e·nul) *adj.* [*phrenico-* + *lien-* + *-al*]. Pertaining to the diaphragm and the spleen.

phrenicolienal ligament. A fold of peritoneum from the diaphragm, left kidney, and pancreas to the hilus of the spleen. NA *ligamentum phrenicolienale, ligamentum lienorenale.*

phren·i·co·splen·ic (fren″i·ko·splen′ick, splee′nick) *adj.* PHRENOSPLENIC.

phren·i·cot·o·my (fren″i·kot′uh·mee) *n.* [*phrenico-* + *-tomy*]. Surgical division of a phrenic nerve in the neck for the purpose of causing a one-sided paralysis of the diaphragm, with consequent immobilization and compression of a diseased lung.

phren·i·co·trip·sy (fren″i·ko·trip′see) *n.* [*phrenico-* + *-tripsy*]. Crushing of a phrenic nerve.

phrenic plexus. A nerve network that accompanies the inferior phrenic artery to the diaphragm. Syn. *plexus phrenicus.*

phre·ni·tis (fre·nigh′tis) *n.* [Gk., inflammation of the brain]. 1. *Obsol.* Inflammation of the brain. 2. Inflammation of the diaphragm. —**phre·nit·ic** (·nit′ick) *adj.*

phreno-. See *phren-.*

phreno·bla·bia (fren″o·blay′bee·uh) *n.* [Gk. *phrenoblabeia,* from *phrēn,* mind, + *blabē,* harm]. Any mental disorder.

phreno·car·dia (fren″o·kahr′dee·uh) *n.* [*phreno-,* mind, + *-cardia*]. A psychophysiologic disorder characterized by dyspnea and pain in the region of the heart.

phreno·col·ic (fren″o·kol′ick, ·ko′lick) *adj.* [*phreno-* + *colic*]. Pertaining to the diaphragm and the colon.

phreno·esoph·a·ge·al, phreno·oesoph·a·ge·al (fren″o·e·sof″uh·jee′uh) *adj.* [*phreno-* + *esophageal*]. Pertaining to the diaphragm and the esophagus.

phreno·gas·tric (fren″o·gas′trick) *adj.* [*phreno-* + *gastric*]. Pertaining conjointly to the stomach and the diaphragm.

phreno·glot·tic (fren″o·glot′ick) *adj.* [*phreno-* + *glottic*]. Pertaining to the diaphragm and the glottis.

phreno·he·pat·ic (fren″o·he·pat′ick) *adj.* [*phreno-* + *hepatic*]. Pertaining to the diaphragm and the liver.

phreno·lep·sia (fren″o·lep′see·uh) *n.* [Gk. *phrenolēptos,* mad, possessed, + *-ia*]. INSANITY.

phre·nol·o·gy (fre·nol′uh·jee) *n.* [*phreno-* + *-logy*]. A pseudoscience based on the theory that the various faculties of the mind occupy distinct and separate areas in the brain cortex, and that the predominance of certain faculties can be ascertained from modifications of the parts of the skull overlying the areas where these faculties are located.

phreno·pa·ral·y·sis (fren″o·puh·ral′i·sis) *n.* [*phreno-* + *paralysis*]. PHRENOPLEGIA.

phreno·path (fren′o·path) *n.* [*phreno-,* mind, + *-path*]. A psychiatrist. —**phre·nop·a·thy** (fre·nop′uth·ee) *n.*

phreno·ple·gia (fren″o·plee′jee·uh) *n.* [*phreno-* + *-plegia*]. Paralysis of the diaphragm.

phren·o·sin (fren′o·sin) *n.* A complex lipid obtained chiefly from white matter of the central nervous system, and containing sphingosine, cerebronic acid, and a sugar, usually galactose.

phreno·sin·ic acid (fren″o·sin′ick). Cerebronic acid, $C_{24}H_{48}O_3$. A hydroxy fatty acid which is a component of the glycolipid (cerebroside) phrenosin.

phreno·spasm (fren′o·spaz·um) *n.* [*phreno-* + *spasm*]. ACHALASIA (1).

phreno·splen·ic (fren″o·splen′ick) *adj.* [*phreno-* + *splenic*]. Pertaining to the diaphragm and the spleen.

phric·to·path·ic (frick″to·path′ick) *adj.* [Gk. *phrikto-,* from *phrissein,* to shudder, + *path-* + *-ic*]. Pertaining to, or accompanied by, a shuddering sensation.

phron·e·mo·pho·bia (fron″e·mo·fo′bee·uh) *n.* [Gk. *phronēma,* thought, + *-phobia*]. An abnormal fear of thinking or of having an embarrassing thought.

phro·ne·sis (fro·nee′sis) *n.* [Gk. *phronēsis,* practical wisdom]. Soundness of mind or of judgment.

phryg·i·an cap (frij′ee·un). The x-ray appearance of the gallbladder where kinking exists between the fundus and the body; named for its resemblance to the hats of the inhabitants of ancient Phrygia.

phryno·der·ma (frin″o·dur′muh, frye″no·) *n.* [Gk. *phrynos,* toad, + *derma,* skin]. Dryness of the skin with follicular hyperkeratosis; due to vitamin A deficiency.

phry·nol·y·sin (fri·nol′i·sin) *n.* [Gk. *phrynos,* toad, + *lysin*]. The lysin or toxin of the fire toad *Bombinator igneus;* it is hemolytic for the blood of various animals.

phthal-, phthalo-. A combining form meaning *origin from or relationship to phthalic acid.*

phthal·ate (thal′ate) *n.* Any salt or ester of phthalic acid.

phthal·ic acid (thal′ick) [*phthal-,* as in na*phthal*ene, + *-ic*]. *o*-Benzenedicarboxylic acid, $C_6H_4(COOH)_2$, derivatives of which are used in various syntheses, including some of medicinal importance.

phthalic anhydride. The anhydride, $C_6H_4(CO)_2O$, of phthalic acid, used in many organic syntheses.

phthalo-. See *phthal-.*

phthal·o·fyne (thal′o·fine) *n.* 1-Ethyl-1-methyl-2-propynyl phthalate, $C_{14}H_{14}O_4$, a veterinary anthelmintic.

phthal·yl·sul·fa·cet·a·mide (thal″il·sul″fuh·set′uh·mide) *n.* 4′-(Acetylsulfamoyl)phthalanilic acid, $C_{16}H_{14}N_2O_6S$, a poorly absorbed sulfonamide that is used as an intestinal antibacterial drug.

phthal·yl·sul·fa·thi·a·zole (thal″il·sul″fuh·thigh′uh·zole) *n.* 4′-(2-Thiazolylsulfamoyl)phthalanilic acid, $C_{17}H_{13}N_3O_5S_2$, a relatively insoluble sulfonamide sparingly absorbed from the gastrointestinal tract; used as an intestinal antibacterial drug.

phtheiriasis. PHTHIRIASIS.

phthin·oid chest (thin′oid) [Gk. *phthinōdēs,* consumptive, from *phthinein,* to waste away]. PHTHISICAL CHEST.

phthi·o·col (thigh′o·kol) *n.* 2-Hydroxy-3-methyl-1,4-naphthoquinone, $C_{11}H_8O_3$, an antibiotic substance, isomeric with plumbagin, derived from *Mycobacterium tuberculosis;* active, in vitro, against a number of bacteria, and also has some vitamin K activity.

phthi·o·ic acid (thigh·o'ick). A cyclic fatty acid produced by *Mycobacterium tuberculosis.*

phthi·ri·a·sis, phtheiriasis (thigh·rye'uh·sis) *n.,* pl. **phthiria·ses, phtheiria·ses** (·seez) [Gk. *phtheir,* louse, + *-iasis*]. Pediculosis pubis; infestation by the pubic louse *Phthirius pubis.*

phthi·rio·pho·bia (thirr"ee·o·fo'bee·uh, thigh"ree·o·) *n.* [Gk. *phtheir,* louse, + *-phobia*]. An abnormal dread of lice.

Phthir·i·us (thirr'ee·us) *n.* [NL., from Gk. *phtheir,* louse]. A genus of true lice.

Phthirius pu·bis (pew'bis). A species of louse that infests the pubic region of humans; the crab louse.

phthisical chest. A long, narrow, flat chest with winged scapulas, formerly thought to be characteristic of pulmonary tuberculosis.

phthisio- [Gk. *phthisis,* a wasting away]. A combining form meaning *tuberculosis.*

phthis·i·ol·o·gy (tiz"ee·ol'uh·jee, thiz") *n.* [*phthisio-* + *-logy*]. The study or science of tuberculosis.

phthis·io·pho·bia (tiz"ee·o·fo'bee·uh, thiz"ee·o·) *n.* [*phthisio-* + *phobia*]. Abnormal fear of tuberculosis.

phthis·io·ther·a·py (tiz"ee·o·therr'uh·pee, thiz"ee·o·) *n.* [*phthisio-* + *therapy*]. The treatment of tuberculosis.

phthi·sis (tye'sis, thigh'sis) *n.,* pl. **phthi·ses** (·seez) [Gk., from *phthynein,* to waste away, to wane]. 1. Tuberculosis, especially pulmonary tuberculosis. 2. Any disease characterized by emaciation and loss of strength. —**phthis·ic** (tiz'ick), **phthis·i·cal** (·i·kul) *adj.*

-phthisis [Gk. *phthisis,* wasting, waning, decay]. A combining form meaning *loss, diminution.*

phthisis bul·bi (bul'bye). OPHTHALMOPHTHISIS.

phthisis cor·ne·ae (kor'nee·ee). Cicatricial shrinking of the cornea.

phyco- [Gk. *phykos*]. A combining form meaning *algae, seaweed.*

phy·co·bi·lin (figh"ko·bye'lin) *n.* A metal-free pigment, found in algae, in which an open-chain tetrapyrrole group, related to bile pigments, is linked to a globulin-like protein.

phy·co·chrome (figh'ko·krome) *n.* [*phyco-* + *-chrome*]. The complex blue-green pigment that masks the green of the chlorophyll in certain algae.

phy·co·col·loid (figh"ko·kol'oid) *n.* [*phyco-* + *colloid*]. A class name for polysaccharides, derived from brown or red seaweeds, which form colloidal dispersions with water.

phy·co·cy·a·nin (figh"ko·sigh'uh·nin) *n.* [*phyco-* + Gk. *kyanos,* blue, + *-in*]. *In biology,* a blue pigment, characteristic of the Cyanophyceae, blue-green algae. Active in photosynthesis.

phy·co·er·y·thrin (figh"ko·err'i·thrin, ·e·rith'rin) *n.* [*phyco-* + Gk. *erythros,* red, + *-in*]. A red, protein-containing pigment found in the chloroplasts of most red algae.

Phy·co·my·ce·tes (figh"ko·migh·see'teez) *n.pl.* [*phyco-* + *mycetes*]. A class of fungi, with a generally nonseptate mycelium and in which asexual spores are formed endogenously in a saclike structure. This group includes the common black bread mold and water mold.

phy·co·my·co·sis (figh"ko·migh·ko'sis) *n.* [*Phycomycetes* + *-osis*]. Infection of man and of animals caused by members of the class of Phycomycetes, including mucormycosis and the subcutaneous phycomycosis of Africa caused by *Basidiobolus meristosporus.*

phy·go·ga·lac·tic (figh"go·guh·lack'tick) *adj.* & *n.* [Gk. *phygē,* escape, shunning, + *galactic*]. 1. Stopping the secretion of milk. 2. An agent that checks the secretion of milk.

phyl-, phylo- [Gk. *phylon*]. A combining form meaning *descent group, evolutionary taxonomic group.*

phyla. Plural of *phylum.*

phy·lax·is (fi·lack'sis) *n.* [Gk., guarding, from *phylax,* guard]. The activity of the body in defending itself against infection.

phy·let·ic (figh·let'ick) *adj.* [Gk. *phyletikos,* of a tribe, from *phylon,* race, tribe]. Pertaining to a stock or to a race.

phyll-, phyllo- [Gk. *phyllon,* leaf]. A combining form meaning (a) *leaf, leaflike;* (b) *chlorophyll.*

phyl·lo·er·y·thrin (fil"o·err'i·thrin) *n.* A porphyrin pigment resulting from degradation of chlorophyll, found in the bile of ruminants, in bovine gallstones, and in dog feces; claimed to be identical with cholehematin.

phyl·loid (fil'oid) *adj.* [*phyll-* + *-oid*]. Leaflike.

phyl·lo·por·phy·rin (fil"o·por'fi·rin) *n.* A porphyrin obtained by degradation of chlorophyll.

phyl·lo·qui·none (fil"o·kwi·nohn') *n.* PHYTONADIONE.

phylo-. See *phyl-.*

phy·lo·gen·e·sis (figh"lo·jen'e·sis) *n.* [*phylo-* + *-genesis*]. PHYLOGENY.

phy·lo·ge·net·ic (figh"lo·je·net'ick) *adj.* Of or pertaining to phylogeny.

phylogenetic principle. *In Jungian psychology,* the rehearsal in childhood of reminiscences of the prehistory of mankind. See also *recapitulation theory.*

phy·log·e·ny (figh·loj'e·nee) *n.* [*phylo-* + *-geny*]. The origin and development of a group or species of organisms; the evolution of the species. Contr. *ontogeny.*

phy·lum (figh'lum) *n.,* pl. **phy·la** (·luh) [NL., from Gk. *phylon,* tribe, race, class]. A primary division of the animal or vegetable kingdom.

phy·ma (figh'muh) *n.,* pl. **phymas, phyma·ta** (·tuh) [Gk., growth]. 1. A tumor or new growth of varying size, composed of any of the structures of the skin or subcutaneous tissue. 2. A localized plastic exudate larger than a tubercle; a circumscribed swelling of the skin. —**phyma·toid** (·toid) *adj.*

phy·ma·tor·rhy·sin (figh"muh·tor'i·sin) *n.* [Gk. *phyma, phymatos,* growth, + Gk. *rhysis,* flow, yield, + *-in*]. A pigment found in hair and melanotic new growths.

phy·ma·to·sis (figh"muh·to'sis) *n.,* pl. **phymato·ses** (·seez) [*phyma* + *-osis*]. Any disease characterized by the formation of phymas or nodules.

phy·sa·lif·e·rous (fis"uh·lif'e·rus, figh"suh·) *adj.* [Gk. *physallis,* bladder, bubble, + *-ferous*]. PHYSALIPHOROUS.

phy·sal·i·form (fi·sal'i·form) *adj.* [Gk. *physallis,* bubble, + *-iform*]. Bubblelike.

phy·sal·i·phore (fi·sal'i·fore) *n.* [Gk. *physallis,* bubble, + *-phore*]. PHYSALIPHOROUS CELL. —**phy·sa·liph·o·rous** (fis" uh·lif'uh·rus, figh"suh·) *adj.*

physaliphorous cell. The large vacuolated cell found in chordomas, usually surrounded by mucinous material similar to the content of the vacuoles.

Phy·sa·lop·tera (figh"suh·lop'te·ruh) *n.* [Gk. *physallis,* bubble, + *ptera,* wing]. A genus of nematode worms of the family Physalopteridae.

Physaloptera cau·cas·i·ca (kaw·kas'i·kuh). A large nematode of African monkeys, but which has occasionally been recovered from the human intestinal tract in Africa, the Caucasus, India, Panama, and Columbia.

phys·co·nia (fis·ko'nee·uh) *n.* [Gk. *physkōn,* potbelly, + *-ia*]. Any abdominal enlargement.

physi-, physio- [Gk. *physis,* nature]. A combining form meaning (a) *natural;* (b) *physical;* (c) *physiological.*

physi·an·thro·py (fiz"eye·an'thruh·pee, fiz"ee·) *n.* [*physi-* + *anthrop-* + *-y*]. The study of the constitution of man, his diseases, and their remedies.

phys·i·at·rics (fiz"eye·at'ricks, fiz"ee·) *n.* [*physi-* + *-iatrics*]. PHYSICAL MEDICINE.

phys·i·at·rist (fiz"ee·at'rist, fiz·eye'uh·trist) *n.* A physician specializing in physical medicine.

phys·ic (fiz'ick) *n.* & *v.* [L. *physica,* natural science, from Gk. *physikē,* from *physikos,* natural]. 1. The science of medicine and therapeutics. 2. A drug, especially a cathartic. 3. To administer a medicine. 4. To purge.

phys·i·cal (fiz'i·kul) *adj.* & *n.* [ML., *physicalis,* from L. *physicus,* from Gk. *physikos*]. 1. Pertaining to nature; pertaining to the body or material things. 2. Pertaining to physics. 3. *Informal.* A physical examination.

physical allergy. The response of some individuals to various physical factors, as cold, heat, sunlight, or mechanical irritation, manifested by urticaria, edema, and varying systemic reactions.

physical anthropology. The study of prehistoric and contemporary man on a purely biologic basis, including his organic growth, development, and degeneration, inheritance of body traits, the influences of environment, and his physical types and racial differences.

physical chemistry. The branch of science in which the theory and methodology of physics is applied to the study of chemical systems.

physical diagnosis. The part of a physician's clinical study of a patient which utilizes inspection, palpation, percussion, auscultation, and mensuration, including the employment of scopes and other instrumental aids, to assess the patient's physical status or detect his physical abnormalities. It is the counterpart of history-taking and laboratory tests.

physical medicine. A consultative, diagnostic, and therapeutic medical specialty, coordinating and integrating the use of physical and occupational therapy and physical reconditioning in the professional management of the diseased and injured.

physical reconditioning. Progressively graded activities, such as calisthenics or special exercises or treatments, aimed at restoring, maintaining, or improving the physical and psychological fitness of an individual.

physical sign. An objective sign manifested by a patient, or one detected by the physician on inspection, palpation, percussion, auscultation, mensuration, or combinations of these methods.

physical therapist. An individual professionally trained in the utilization of physical agents for therapeutic purposes.

physical therapy. The treatment of disease and injury by physical means, such as light, heat, cold, water, electricity, massage, and exercise.

phy·si·cian (fi·zish'un) *n*. [OF. *fisicien*, from *fisique*, medicine]. A person who is authorized to practice medicine.

physician's assistant. A person who is trained and authorized to provide medical services under the responsibility and supervision of a physician.

phys·i·cist (fiz'i·sist) *n*. A person skilled in physics.

Phys·ick's operation [P. S. *Physick*, U.S. surgeon, 1768–1837]. An operation in which a circular piece of the iris is removed with cutting forceps.

physico-. A combining form meaning *physical*.

phys·i·co·chem·i·cal (fiz''i·ko·kem'i·kul) *adj*. Pertaining to the application of the theory and methodology of physics to the study of chemical systems.

phys·i·co·py·rex·ia (fiz''i·ko·pye·reck'see·uh) *n*. [*physico-* + *pyrexia*]. Artificial fever produced by physical means for its therapeutic effect.

phys·ics (fiz'icks) *n*. [*physic* + *-s*]. The science of the phenomena and laws of nature, especially that treating of the properties of matter and of the forces governing it.

phys·i·no·sis (fiz''i·no'sis) *n*. [*physi-* + Gk. *nosos*, disease (altered in assimilation to suffix *-osis*)]. Any disease due to physical agents.

physio-. See *physi-*.

phys·io·chem·i·cal (fiz''ee·o·kem'i·kul) *adj*. [*physio-* + *chemical*]. BIOCHEMICAL.

phys·i·og·no·my (fiz''ee·og'nuh·mee) *n*. [Gk. *physiognōmonia*]. 1. The countenance; FACIES (1). 2. The science of determining character by a study of the face. 3. PHYSIOGNOSIS.

phys·i·og·no·sis (fiz''ee·og·no'sis) *n*. [*physiognomy* + -gn*osis*]. Diagnosis of disease based on facial characteristics and expression.

phys·i·o·log·ic (fiz''ee·uh·loj'ick) *adj*. [Gk. *physiologikos*, pertaining to natural science]. 1. Pertaining to physiology. 2. Pertaining to natural or normal functional processes in living organisms, as opposed to those that are pathologic. 3. In normal or natural state or quantity, as opposed to pharmacologic.

physiologic age. Age as judged by the functional development.

phys·i·o·log·i·cal (fiz''ee·uh·loj'i·kul) *adj*. PHYSIOLOGIC.

physiological availability. The extent to which the active ingredient of a nutrient or drug dosage can be absorbed and made available in the body in a physiologically active state. Syn. *bioavailability, biological availability*.

physiologic albuminuria. Protein in normal urine, without appreciable coexisting renal lesion or diseased condition.

physiological chemistry. The chemistry of animal and plant systems, especially the former.

physiological dead space. A calculated expression of the anatomical dead space plus whatever degree of overventilation or underperfusion is present. It reflects the relationship between ventilation to pulmonary capillary perfusion. The formula is: physiological dead space = tidal volume $\times$ [(arterial $P\text{CO}_2$ $-$ expired $P\text{CO}_2$ / arterial $P\text{CO}_2$)].

physiological neuronography. The mapping of functional neuron connections by action current recording, after local stimulation of a cortical area.

physiological optics. The branch of optics dealing with the eye.

physiological salt solution. SODIUM CHLORIDE IRRIGATION.

physiological sodium chloride solution. SODIUM CHLORIDE IRRIGATION.

physiologic anatomy. Anatomic study of tissues in respect to their functions.

physiologic anemia. 1. A relative hypochromic microcytic anemia occurring normally in most infants about the third month of life, regardless of the nutritional status of the mother during pregnancy, and representing a normal physiologic adjustment to improved oxygenation of arterial blood. 2. Normocytic normochromic anemia occurring during pregnancy.

physiologic antidote. An antidote that counteracts the physiologic effects of a poison.

physiologic atrophy. Atrophy that affects certain organs at different times of life, as atrophy of the mammary glands and ovaries after menopause, or the thymus after birth.

physiologic availability. PHYSIOLOGICAL AVAILABILITY.

physiologic cup. The normal concavity of the optic disk.

physiologic dead space. PHYSIOLOGICAL DEAD SPACE.

physiologic death. Death of a cell as part of a normal physiologic process, such as maturation of the epidermis.

physiologic diplopia. A normal phenomenon in which there is formation of images on noncorresponding retinal points, giving a perception of depth; normally suppressed during everyday life, it can be demonstrated by fixing the eyes on a distant object and bringing a finger into the field of vision at about one foot, or by placing a prism in front of one eye; it forms the basis of parallax and stereoscopic vision. Syn. *introspective diplopia*.

physiologic dwarf. HYPOPLASTIC DWARF.

physiologic hourglass stomach. CASCADE STOMACH.

physiologic hyperbilirubinemia. Physiologic elevation of the concentration of bilirubin in the serum of neonates. See also *Crigler-Najjar syndrome, Dubin-Johnson syndrome, Gilbert's syndrome, Rotor syndrome*.

physiologic hyperopia. Hyperopia present at birth, corrected as the eyeball reaches its normal anteroposterior diameter at about 8 years of age.

physiologic hypertrophy. Hypertrophy due to natural rather than pathologic causes, as hypertrophy of the pregnant uterus or skeletal muscles following chronic exercise.

physiologic jaundice of the newborn. The yellowness of skin and sclera and hyperbilirubinemia frequently seen in newborn infants in the first 5 days of life and clearing within 7 to 14 days, due to incomplete development of glucuronyl transferase mechanism resulting in a decreased ability to conjugate bilirubin with glucuronic acid. The condition is usually mild and self-limiting, though in premature infants the hyperbilirubinemia may be more severe, last longer, and more frequently result in kernicterus.

physiologic lobule of the liver. The portion of the liver tissue that surrounds and is drained by an interlobular bile duct. Contr. *anatomic lobule of the liver.*

physiologic murmur. INNOCENT MURMUR.

phys·i·o·log·i·co·an·a·tom·ic (fiz″ee·o·loj″i·ko·an″uh·tom′ick) *adj.* Pertaining to physiology and anatomy.

physiologic psychology. A branch of psychology that investigates the structure and functions of the nervous system and bodily organs in their relationship to behavior.

physiologic rest position. The natural position of the mandible when the individual is in an upright position and the condyles are in an unstrained relationship with the mandibular fossae and when the muscles of mastication are in a state of relaxed balance.

physiologic retraction ring. The ridge on the inner uterine surface which constitutes the boundary line between the upper and lower uterine segments. It results from the process of normal labor, which causes thinning of the lower uterine segment and concomitant thickening of the upper uterine segment. Syn. *constriction ring, Braune's ring.* Contr. *pathologic retraction ring.*

physiologic ring. PHYSIOLOGIC RETRACTION RING.

physiologic standardization. BIOLOGICAL STANDARDIZATION.

physiologic tremor. A tremor that is normally present in all muscle groups throughout the waking state and sleep. It ranges in frequency between 8 and 13 Hz and requires special instruments for its detection. Syn. *normal tremor.*

phys·i·ol·o·gist (fiz″ee·ol′uh·jist) *n.* A person skilled in physiology.

phys·i·ol·o·gy (fiz″ee·ol′uh·jee) *n.* [Gk. *physiologia,* the study of nature]. The science that studies the functions of living organisms or their parts, as distinguished from morphology.

phys·io·med·i·cal·ism (fiz″ee·o·med′i·kul·iz·um) *n.* [*physio-* + *medical* + *-ism*]. A system of medicine in which only harmless natural remedies are used.

phys·io·path·o·log·ic (fiz″ee·o·path″uh·loj′ick) *adj.* [*physio-* + *pathologic*]. 1. Pertaining to both physiology and pathology. 2. Involving a pathological modification of normal function. 3. PATHOPHYSIOLOGIC.

phys·io·ther·a·pist (fiz″ee·o·therr′uh·pist) *n.* 1. A person who is competent and qualified to administer physiotherapy. 2. A person who administers physiotherapy.

phys·io·ther·a·py (fiz″ee·o·therr′uh·pee) *n.* [*physio-* + *therapy*]. PHYSICAL MEDICINE.

phy·sique (fi·zeek′) *n.* [F.]. Physical structure or organization; body build.

physo- [Gk. *physa,* breath]. A combining form meaning *presence, accumulation, or formation of gas.*

phy·so·hem·a·to·me·tra, phy·so·haem·a·to·me·tra (figh″so·hem″uh·to·mee′truh, ·hee″muh·to·) *n.* [*physo-* + *hemato-* + *-metra*]. An accumulation of gas, or air, and blood in the uterus, as in decomposition of retained menses, or placental tissue.

phy·so·hy·dro·me·tra (figh″so·high″dro·mee′truh) *n.* [*physo-* + *hydro-* + *-metra*]. An accumulation of gas and fluid in the uterus.

phy·so·me·tra (figh″so·mee′truh) *n.* [*physo-* + *-metra*]. Distention of the uterus with gas.

phy·so·pyo·sal·pinx (figh″so·pye″o·sal′pinks) *n.* [*physo-* + *pyosalpinx*]. Pyosalpinx with formation of gas in the uterine tube.

phy·so·stig·ma (figh″so·stig′muh) *n.* [*physo-* + *stigma*]. The dried ripe seed of *Physostigma venenosum,* the Calabar bean. Of several alkaloids reported present, physostigmine is the most important.

phy·so·stig·mine (figh″so·stig′meen, ·min) *n.* An alkaloid, $C_{15}H_{21}N_3O_2$, obtained from the seeds of *Physostigma venenosum;* a cholinergic drug that functions by inhibiting cholinesterase and has diverse clinical uses. Employed as the base and as the salicylate and sulfate salts. Syn. *eserine.*

phyt-, phyto- [Gk. *phyton*]. A combining form meaning *plant, vegetable.*

phy·tan·ic acid (fye·tan′ick). 3,7,11,15-Tetramethylhexadecanoic acid, a fatty acid found in the tissues of some patients with Refsum's disease.

phytanic acid hydroxylating enzyme deficiency. A metabolic defect associated with Refsum's disease.

phy·tase (figh′tace, ·taze) *n.* An enzyme occurring in plants, especially cereals, which catalyzes hydrolysis of phytic acid to inositol and phosphoric acid.

-phyte [Gk. *phyton,* plant]. A combining form meaning (a) *plant;* (b) *a pathological growth.*

phy·tic acid (figh′tick). Inositolhexaphosphoric acid, or 1,2,-3,4,5,6-cyclohexanehexolphosphoric acid, $C_6H_6[OPO(OH)_2]_6$, a constituent of cereal grains. By combining with ingested calcium, it may prevent absorption of the latter.

Phytin. Trademark for a phytic acid calcium magnesium salt used as a dietary supplement to provide calcium.

phyto-. See *phyt-.*

phy·to·be·zoar (figh″to·bee′zo·ur) *n.* [*phyto-* + *bezoar*]. A bezoar or ball of vegetable fiber sometimes found in the stomach.

phy·to·chem·is·try (figh″to·kem′is·tree) *n.* [*phyto-* + *chemistry*]. The chemistry of plants and their constituents.

phy·to·gen·e·sis (figh″to·jen′e·sis) *n.* [*phyto-* + *-genesis*]. The science of the origin and development of plants. —**phyto·ge·net·ic** (·je·net′ick) *adj.*

phy·tog·e·nous (figh·toj′e·nus) *adj.* [*phyto-* + *-genous*]. Produced by plants.

phy·tog·e·ny (figh·toj′e·nee) *n.* PHYTOGENESIS.

phy·to·hem·ag·glu·ti·nin (figh″to·hee″muh·glew′ti·nin, ·hem″uh·) *n.* [*phyto-* + *hemagglutinin*]. A lectin which agglutinates cells and is mitogenic for lymphocytes. Abbreviated, PHA.

phy·to·hor·mone (figh″to·hor′mone) *n.* [*phyto-* + *hormone*]. Any plant hormone.

phy·toid (figh′toid) *adj.* [Gk. *phytōdēs,* from *phyton,* plant]. Plantlike; referring to certain animals and organs.

phy·tol (figh′tol) *n.* An unsaturated aliphatic alcohol, $C_{20}H_{39}OH$, occurring in chlorophyll as an ester; used in the synthesis of vitamins E and K.

phy·to·na·di·one (figh″to·na·dye′ohn) *n.* 2-Methyl-3-phytyl-1,4-naphthoquinone, $C_{31}H_{46}O_2$, occurring in green plants but usually prepared by synthesis; used therapeutically to promote prothrombin formation. Syn. *phylloquinone, 3-phytylmenadione, vitamin K_1.*

phy·to·par·a·site (figh″to·păr′uh·site) *n.* [*phyto-* + *parasite*]. A vegetable parasite.

phy·to·patho·gen·ic (figh″to·path″uh·jen′ick) *adj.* [*phyto-* + *pathogenic*]. Causing disease in plants.

phy·to·pa·thol·o·gy (figh″to·pa·thol′uh·jee) *n.* [*phyto-* + *pathology*]. The science of diseases of plants.

phy·toph·a·gous (figh·tof′uh·gus) *adj.* [*phyto-* + *-phagous*]. 1. Plant-eating. 2. Vegetarian.

phy·to·phar·ma·col·o·gy (figh″to·fahr″muh·kol′uh·jee) *n.* [*phyto-* + *pharmacology*]. The branch of pharmacology concerned with the effects of drugs on plant growth. —**phytopharma·co·log·i·cal** (·ko·loj′i·kul) *adj.*

phy·to·pho·to·der·ma·ti·tis (figh″to·fo″to·dur·muh·tye′tis) *n.* [*phyto-* + *photo-* + *dermatitis*]. Any skin eruption brought on by certain plants and mediated by exposure to light.

phy·to·pho·to·der·ma·to·sis (figh″to·fo″to·dur″muh·to′sis) *n.* [*phyto-* + *photo-* + *dermatosis*]. PHYTOPHOTODERMATITIS.

phy·to·pneu·mo·co·ni·o·sis (figh″to·new″mo·ko″nee·o′sis) *n.* [*phyto-* + *pneumoconiosis*]. Pulmonary fibrosis due to inhalation of vegetable dust particles.

phy·to·pre·cip·i·tin (figh″to·pre·sip′i·tin) *n.* [*phyto-* + *precipi-*

tin]. A precipitin produced by immunization with protein of vegetable origin.

phy·to·sis (figh·to'sis) *n.*, pl. **phyto·ses** (·seez) [*phyt-* + *-osis*]. 1. Any disease due to the presence of vegetable parasites. 2. The production of disease by vegetable parasites. 3. The presence of vegetable parasites.

phy·to·stea·rin (figh"to·stee'uh·rin) *n.* PHYTOSTEROL.

phy·tos·ter·in (figh·tos'tur·in) *n.* PHYTOSTEROL.

phy·tos·ter·ol (figh·tos'tur·ole, figh"to·steer'ole, ·ol) *n.* Any sterol occurring in a plant oil or fat.

phy·tos·ter·ol·in (figh·tos'tur·o·lin, figh"to·steer') *n.* A glycoside of phytosterol.

phy·to·throm·bo·ki·nase (figh"to·throm"bo·kigh'nace, ·kin'ace, ·aze) *n.* A thrombokinase prepared from yeast or plant sources.

phy·to·tox·ic (figh"to·tock'sick) *adj.* [*phyto-* + *toxic*]. 1. Pertaining to a phytotoxin. 2. Pertaining to or describing a substance poisonous to plants.

phy·to·tox·in (figh"to·tock'sin) *n.* [*phyto-* + *toxin*]. A toxin derived from a plant, such as ricin or crotin.

phy·to·vi·tel·lin (figh"to·vi·tel'in, ·vye·tel'in) *n.* [*phyto-* + *vitellin*]. A vegetable protein resembling vitellin.

3-phy·tyl·men·a·di·one (figh"til·men"uh·dye'ohn) *n.* PHYTONADIONE.

pia (pye'uh, pee'uh) *n.* PIA MATER. —**pi·al** (·ul) *adj.*

pia-arach·noid (pye"uh·uh·rack'noid) *n.* The pia mater and arachnoid considered as one structure. Syn. *leptomeninx*.

pial sheath. The extension of the pia mater which closely invests the surface of the optic nerve.

pia ma·ter (pye'uh may·tur, pee'uh mah'tur) [L., tender mother]. The vascular membrane enveloping the surface of the brain and spinal cord, and consisting of a plexus of blood vessels held in a fine areolar tissue.

pia mater en·ce·pha·li (en·sef'uh·lye) [NA]. The pia mater of the brain.

pia mater spi·na·lis (spye·nay'lis) [NA]. The pia mater of the spinal cord.

pi·an (pee·ahn', pee'an) *n.* [F., from Tupi]. YAWS.

pi·a·rach·noid (pye"uh·rack'noid) *n.* [*pia* + *arachnoid*]. PIA-ARACHNOID.

pi·as·tre·ne·mia, pi·as·tre·nae·mia (pye·as"tre·nee'mee·uh) *n.* THROMBOCYTOSIS.

pi·blok·to (pi·block'to) *n.* [Eskimo]. A hysterical neurosis exhibited by Eskimos, particularly women, in which the individual becomes irrational, often destructive.

pi·ca (pye'kuh, pee'kuh) *n.* [L., magpie]. 1. A desire for strange foods; may occur as a result of emotional disturbance, malnutrition, or during pregnancy. 2. A craving to eat strange articles, as hair, dirt, or sand; the undue persistence or recurrence in later life of the infantile tendency of bringing everything to the mouth.

Pic·co·lo·mi·ni's bands or **striae** (peek·ko·loh'mee·nee) [A. *Piccolomini*, Italian anatomist, 1526-1605]. STRIAE MEDULLARES VENTRICULI QUARTI.

pic·e·ous (pis'ee·us, pye'see·us) *adj.* [L. *piceus*, from *pix*, pitch]. Resembling pitch.

Pick bodies [A. *Pick*]. Argentophilic inclusions in the cytoplasm of neurons seen in [1]Pick's disease.

Pick cell [L. *Pick*, German pathologist, 1868-1935]. FOAM CELL.

[1]Pick's disease [A. *Pick*, Czechoslovakian physician, 1851-1924]. A form of dementia, often familial, characterized pathologically by severe cerebral atrophy usually restricted to the frontal and temporal lobes with less frequent extension to the parietal lobes. Microscopically, there is diffuse loss of neurones, particularly in the outer layers of the cortex, and ballooning of preserved neurones, which frequently contain argentophilic (Pick) bodies within the cytoplasm. Glial proliferation is prominent, and basal ganglions are frequently involved. Syn. *circumscribed cerebral atrophy*. Compare *Alzheimer's disease*.

[2]Pick's disease [F. *Pick*, German physician, 1867-1926]. 1. Recurrent or progressive ascites with little or no edema; postmortem examination shows constrictive pericarditis and atypical cirrhosis of the liver. 2. CONSTRICTIVE PERICARDITIS. 3. POLYSEROSITIS.

[3]Pick's disease [L. *Pick*, German pediatrician, 1868-1935]. NIEMANN-PICK DISEASE.

Pick's syndrome [F. *Pick*]. [2]PICK'S DISEASE (1) and (2).

Pick·wick·i·an syndrome (pick·wick'ee·un). Marked obesity with alveolar hypoventilation, hypoxia, cyanosis, carbon dioxide retention, reduced vital capacity, secondary polycythemia, and somnolence; named for the corpulent, somnolent young man in Dickens' "Pickwick Papers."

Pick·worth method. A benzidine and nitroprussic oxidase method for hemoglobin.

pico- [Sp. *pico*, a little bit]. A combining form signifying the *one trillionth* (10^{-12}) *part* of the unit adjoined.

pi·co·cu·rie (pye'ko·kew"ree) *n.* [*pico-* + *curie*]. One trillionth (10^{-12}) of a curie; the same as a micromicrocurie, a quantity of a radioactive substance resulting in 3.7×10^{-2} nuclear disintegrations per second. Abbreviated, pCi.

pi·co·gram (pye'ko·gram) *n.* [*pico-* + *-gram*]. One trillionth (10^{-12}) of a gram. Abbreviated, pg.

pic·o·lin·ic acid (pick"o·lin'ick) [L. *pix*, *pic*us, pitch, + *-ol* + *-ine* + *-ic*]. 2-Pyridinecarboxylic acid, C_5H_4NCOOH, an isomer of nicotinic acid; used as a metabolite analogue of nicotinic acid.

pi·co·pi·co·gram (pye"ko·pye'ko·gram) *n.* [*pico-* + *picogram*]. One trillionth of a picogram, or 10^{-24} gram. Abbreviated, ppg.

pi·cor·na·vi·rus (pye·kor"nuh·vye'rus) *n.* [*pico-*, very small, + *RNA* + *virus*]. A member of a group of small, ether-resistant RNA viruses including the enteroviruses of poliomyelitis, Coxsackie and echoviruses, the rhinoviruses, and those of nonhuman origin such as foot-and-mouth disease and encephalomyocarditis.

pi·co·sec·ond (pye'ko·seck"und) *n.* [*pico-* + *second*]. One trillionth (10^{-12}) of a second.

pic·ram·ic acid (pick·ram'ick). 4,6-Dinitro-2-aminophenol, $HOC_6H_2(NO_2)_2NH_2$, a reagent for albumin.

Pic·ras·ma (pick·raz'muh) *n.* [NL., from Gk. *pikrasmos*, bitterness]. A genus of the Simarubaceae. The wood of *Picrasma excelsa* is the source of Jamaica quassia, which has been employed in the form of an infusion as an enema for expulsion of seatworms.

pic·rate (pick'rate) *n.* A salt of picric acid.

pic·ric acid (pick'rick) [Gk. *pikros*, bitter, + *-ic*]. TRINITROPHENOL.

pic·ro·car·mine (pick"ro·kahr'min, ·meen) *n.* One of a variety of mixtures of carmine, ammonia, and picric acid, used as a stain for tissues.

pic·ro·lon·ic acid (pick"ro·lon'ick). 3-Methyl-4-nitro-1-(*p*-nitrophenyl)-5-pyrazolone, $C_{10}H_8N_4O_5$; used as a reagent for alkaloids and basic amino acids.

pic·ro·ni·gro·sin (pick"ro·nigh'gro·sin) *n.* A stain for muscle in which, after Bouin or alcohol fixation, sections are stained in a saturated solution of nigrosine in saturated aqueous picric acid. Muscle is stained yellow, connective tissue, black.

pic·ro·podo·phyl·lin (pick"ro·pod"o·fil'in, ·po·dof'i·lin) *n.* A nontoxic substance, $C_{22}H_{22}O_8$, isomeric with podophyllotoxin and formed from it on alkaline hydrolysis; it appears to be physiologically inert.

pic·ro·tox·in (pick"ro·tock'sin) *n.* A glycoside, $C_{30}H_{34}O_{13}$, obtained from the seed of the East Indian woody vine *Anamirta cocculus;* a powerful central nervous system stimulant used to counteract depression from overdosage with barbiturates. Syn. *cocculin*.

PID Abbreviation for *pelvic inflammatory disease*.

pie·bald·ism (pye'bawl·diz·um) *n.* A distinctively patterned hypomelanosis of skin and usually hair (white forelock), inherited as an autosomal dominant trait.

piebald skin. 1. PIEBALDISM. 2. VITILIGO.

pie·dra (pee·ay′druh) *n.* [Sp., stone]. A nodular growth on the hair of the scalp, beard, or mustache. The type known as black piedra is found in tropical regions and is caused by the fungus *Piedraia hortai,* which infests only the hair shafts of the scalp. White piedra, a rarer form, occurs in temperate regions and is caused by the fungus *Trichosporon cutaneum,* which infests the hair of the beard and mustache. Syn. *tinea nodosa, Beigel's disease.*

piedra nostras. Piedra affecting the beard.

pier (peer) *n.* ABUTMENT.

Pierre Ro·bin syndrome (pyehr roʰ·bæⁿ′) [*Pierre Robin,* French, 20th century]. ROBIN SYNDROME.

pi·es·es·the·sia, pi·es·aes·the·sia (pye″es·es·theez′ee·uh, pye″ez·es·) *n.* [Gk. *piesis,* compression, + *esthesia*]. PRESSURE SENSE.

pi·esim·e·ter (pye″e·sim′e·tur) *n.* PIEZOMETER.

pi·esom·e·ter (pye″e·som′e·tur) *n.* PIEZOMETER.

piezo- [Gk. *piezein,* to press, squeeze]. A combining form meaning *pressure, compression.*

pi·ezo·elec·tric·i·ty (pye·ee″zo·e·leck·tris′i·tee) *n.* [*piezo-* + *electricity*]. Electricity or electric charges developed by applying pressure, especially on a crystalline substance such as quartz or Rochelle salt. **—piezo·elec·tric** (·e·leck′trick) *adj.*

pi·ezom·e·ter (pye″e·zom′e·tur) *n.* [*piezo-* + *-meter*]. 1. An apparatus for measuring the degree of compression of gases or fluids. 2. An apparatus for testing the sensitiveness of the skin to pressure. 3. A simple liquid manometer.

Pif·fard's paste [H. G. *Piffard,* U.S. dermatologist, 1842–1910]. *Obsol.* A mixture of sodium tartrate, copper sulfate, and sodium hydroxide used as a paste for testing sugar in urine.

pig·bel (pig′bel) *n.* [Melanesian Pidgin English]. A type of enteritis necroticans occurring among highland peoples of New Guinea in association with pork feasting, and caused by *Clostridium perfringens* type C.

pi·geon breast or **chest.** A chest with a prominent sternum; may be congenital and associated with other malformations; may be due to rickets or obstructed infantile respiration. Syn. *chicken breast, pectus carinatum.*

pigeon-breeder's lung. BIRD-BREEDER'S LUNG.

pigeon-toed, *adj.* Walking with the feet turned in.

pig·ment (pig′munt) *n.* [L. *pigmentum,* from *pingere,* to paint]. 1. A dye; a coloring matter. 2. Any organic coloring matter of the body. 3. Any paintlike medicinal applied externally to the skin. **—pig·men·tary** (pig′mun·terr″ee) *adj.*; **pig·ment·ed** (pig′men·tid) *adj.*

pigmentary cirrhosis. Portal cirrhosis associated with hemosiderosis.

pigmentary degeneration. A retrogressive change, especially in nerve cells, with abnormal deposit of pigmentary substances.

pigmentary degeneration of the globus pallidus. HALLERVORDEN-SPATZ DISEASE.

pig·men·ta·tion (pig″men·tay′shun) *n.* Deposition of or discoloration by pigment.

pigmented basal cell epithelioma. A basal cell tumor in which there is sufficient melanin to produce a brown or black papule.

pigmented cataract. A spurious cataract due to an injury by which the pigment from the posterior surface of the iris has been detached. Syn. *Vossius ring.*

pigmented mole. PIGMENTED NEVUS.

pigmented nevus. A pigmented mole, varying in color from light fawn to blackish, sometimes hairy, frequently papillary and hyperkeratotic, characterized by clear cells, melanocytes, and intermediate forms.

pigmented purpuric lichenoid dermatitis. A form of capillaritis, usually of the lower extremities, though the upper extremities and trunk may be involved, characterized by elevated papules which become purpuric or telangiectatic or pigmented in varying shades. Its course is chronic, leading to lichenification. Syn. *Gougerot-Blum disease.*

pigment layer. The external layer of the embryonic optic cup or retina.

pig·men·to·gen·e·sis (pig·men″to·jen′e·sis) *n.* [*pigment* + *-genesis*]. The process of originating pigment.

pig·men·to·phage (pig·ment′o·faje) *n.* [*pigment* + *-phage*]. A phagocyte which destroys pigment, especially that of hairs.

pig·men·tum ni·grum (pig·men′tum nigh′grum) [L.]. The dark coloring matter which lines the choroid coat of the eye.

pigmy. PYGMY.

pig-tailed macaque. A large, smooth-haired monkey, *Macaca nemestrina,* of Southeast Asia and Indonesia.

pi·itis (pye·eye′tis) *n.* [*pia* + *-itis*]. LEPTOMENINGITIS.

pil-, pilo- [L. *pilus,* a hair]. A combining form meaning *hair.*

pil. Abbreviation for *pilula,* pill.

pi·lar (pye′lur) *adj.* [NL. *pilaris,* from *pilus,* a hair]. Pertaining to the hair or a hair.

pi·la·ry (pye′luh·ree) *adj.* PILAR.

pi·las·tered (pi·last′urd) *adj.* Flanged so as to have a fluted appearance; arranged in pilasters or columns.

pilastered femur. A femur with exaggerated backward concavity and prominent linea aspera.

Pilcz's reflex (pilch) [A. *Pilcz,* Austrian neurologist, b. 1871]. CONSENSUAL LIGHT REFLEX.

¹pile, *n.* [L. *pila,* pillar]. 1. BATTERY (1). 2. NUCLEAR REACTOR.

²pile, *n.* [L. *pilus,* hair]. The hair or hairs collectively of any part of the integument.

³pile, *n.* [L. *pila,* ball]. HEMORRHOID.

pi·le·ous (pye′lee·us, pil′ee·us) *adj.* [*pil-* + *-ous*]. Pertaining to hair; hairy.

piles, *n.pl.* HEMORRHOIDS.

pili. Plural and genitive singular of *pilus.*

pili an·nu·la·ti (an″yoo·lay′tye). RINGED HAIR.

pi·li·a·tion (pye″lee·ay′shun, pil″ee·) *n.* [L. *pilus,* hair]. The formation and production of hair.

pi·li·form (pye′li·form) *adj.* [*pil*us + *-iform*]. Having the appearance of hair; FILIFORM.

pili in·car·na·ti (in·kahr·nay′tye). Ingrown hairs.

pi·li·mic·tion (pye″li·mick′shun) *n.* [*pil*us + *miction*]. The passing of urine containing hairlike filaments.

pili mul·ti·gem·i·ni (mul·ti·jem′i·nigh). Several hairs emerging from a single follicular opening.

pili tac·ti·les (tack′ti·leez). Tactile hairs.

pili tor·ti (tor′tye) [L., twisted]. A congenital deformity of the hair, characterized by short, broken, twisted hairs presenting the appearance of stubble.

pill, *n.* [L. *pilula,* dim. of *pila,* ball]. A small, solid dosage form, of a globular, ovoid, or lenticular shape, containing one or more medicinal substances.

pil·lar cell. Either the inner or outer cell bounding the tunnel in the spiral organ of Corti.

pillar of the fauces. One of the folds of mucous membrane on each side of the fauces. See also *palatoglossal arch, palatopharyngeal arch.*

pil·let (pil′it) *n.* A little pill, or pellet.

pil·le·um (pil′ee·um) *n.* CAUL (1).

pil·le·us (pil′ee·us) *n.* [L., felt cap]. CAUL (1).

pil·lion (pil′yun) *n.* [a kind of cushion or saddle, from Scottish Gaelic *pillean*]. A temporary leg prosthesis.

pillow splint. A pillow support used as an emergency dressing for fractures of the lower leg. The pillow is compressed on either side and posteriorly with board splints held by several straps so as to exert firm pressure upon the leg.

pill-rolling tremor. A parkinsonian tremor which takes the form of flexion-extension of the fingers, combined with adduction-abduction of the thumb.

pilo-. See *pil-.*

pi·lo·car·pine (pye″lo·kahr′peen, ·pin) *n.* An alkaloid, $C_{11}H_{16}N_2O_2$, obtained from various species of *Pilocarpus* (jaborandi); a cholinergic agent that also has ganglionic stimulant activity and is a physiological antagonist of atropine. It contracts the pupil, increases the flow of saliva and perspiration, and stimulates peristalsis; used clinically for these effects as the hydrochloride or nitrate salt.

pi·lo·car·pus (pye″lo·kahr′pus, pil″o·) *n.* [NL., from *pilo-*, felt, + Gk. *karpos*, fruit]. The dried leaflets of *Pilocarpus jaborandi*, or of *P. microphyllus* and other species of *Pilocarpus*. A number of alkaloids have been obtained from various species of pilocarpus, the principal one being pilocarpine. Syn. *jaborandi*.

pi·lo·cys·tic (pye″lo·sis′tick) *adj.* [*pilo-* + *cystic*]. Pertaining to encysted tumors containing hair.

pi·lo·erec·tion (pye″lo·e·reck′shun) *n.* [*pilo-* + *erection*]. Erection of the hair.

pi·lo·ma·tri·co·ma (pye″lo·may″tri·ko′muh, ·mat″ri·) *n.* [*pilo-* + L. *matrix, matricis* + *-oma*]. A benign tumor with differentiation toward hair cells occurring as a solitary lesion usually of the face or upper extremities; varies from 0.5 to 3 cm in diameter; calcification is frequent. Syn. *calcifying epithelioma of Malherbe, hair matrix tumor*.

pi·lo·ma·trix·o·ma (pye″lo·may″trick·so′muh) *n.* PILOMATRICOMA.

pi·lo·mo·tor (pye″lo·mo′tur) *adj.* [*pilo-* + *motor*]. Causing movement of the hair, as the pilomotor muscles.

pilomotor muscle. ARRECTOR PILI.

pilomotor nerve. A nerve causing contraction of one of the arrectores pilorum.

pilomotor reflex. Erection of the hairs of the skin accompanied by gooseflesh in response to chilling or irritation of the skin or to an emotional stimulus.

pi·lo·ni·dal (pye″lo·nigh′dul) *adj.* [*pilo-* + *nidal*]. Pertaining to or containing an accumulation of hairs in a cyst.

pilonidal abscess. An abscess in the sacrococcygeal area within, or resulting from, a pilonidal cyst or sinus.

pilonidal cyst. A hair-containing cavity, in the dermis or subcutaneous tissues, usually connected to the skin surface by a sinus tract; commonly in the sacrococcygeal region. Syn. *sacrococcygeal cyst*.

pilonidal disease. An inclusive term for pilonidal sinus, pilonidal cyst, and combined cyst and sinus.

pilonidal fistula. A form of pilonidal disease characterized by a hair-containing sinus tract emerging on the skin from the subcutaneous tissues, with or without an associated cavity (cyst).

pilonidal sinus. A tract in the sacrococcygeal region; the subcutaneous portion may develop into a pilonidal cyst; when open at the skin surface, it appears as a chronic, recurrently suppurating sinus.

pi·lose (pye′loce) *adj.* [L. *pilosus*]. Hairy; covered with hair.

pi·lo·se·ba·ceous (pye″lo·se·bay′shus) *adj.* [*pilo-* + *sebaceous*]. Pertaining to the hair follicles and sebaceous glands, as the pilosebaceous apparatus, the hair follicle and its attached oil gland.

pi·lo·sis (pye·lo′sis) *n.* [*pil-* + *-osis*]. The abnormal or excessive development of hair.

pi·los·i·ty (pye·los′i·tee) *n.* The state of being pilose or hairy.

pilot fatigue. FLYING FATIGUE.

pi·lous (pye′lus) *adj.* [L. *pilus*, hair, + *-ous*]. PILOSE.

pilous gland. The sebaceous gland of a hair follicle.

pil·u·la (pil′yoo·luh) *n.*, pl. **pilu·lae** (·lee) [L., little ball]. PILL. Abbreviated, pil. —**pilu·lar** (·lur) *adj.*

pilular extract. A soft extract suitable for molding into pills or for incorporation in an ointment.

pil·ule (pil′yool) *n.* [MF., from L. *pilula*]. A small pill.

pi·lus (pye′lus, pil′us) *n.*, pl. & genit. sing. **pi·li** (·lye), genit. pl. **pi·lo·rum** (pi·lo′rum) [L.]. 1. [NA] A hair. 2. *In biology*, a fine, slender, hairlike body.

pilus cu·nic·u·la·tus (kew·nick″yoo·lay′tus). A burrowing hair.

pilus in·car·na·tus (in″kahr·nay′tus). An ingrown hair.

pilus incarnatus re·cur·vus (re·kur′vus). An ingrown hair caused by a curved hair reentering the skin.

pimel-, pimelo- [Gk. *pimelē*, lard]. A combining form meaning *fat, fatty*.

pi·mel·ic acid (pi·mel′ick). Heptanedioic acid, HOOC-$(CH_2)_5COOH$. Biotin may derive part of its molecule from pimelic acid which is interchangeable with biotin for some microorganisms.

pim·e·li·tis (pim″e·lye′tis) *n.* [*pimel-* + *-itis*]. Inflammation of adipose tissue.

pimelo-. See *pimel-*.

pim·e·lo·pte·ryg·i·um (pim″i·lo·te·rij′ee·um) *n.* [*pimelo-* + *pterygium*]. A fatty outgrowth on the conjunctiva.

pim·e·lor·rhea, pim·e·lor·rhoea (pim″e·lo·ree′uh) *n.* [*pimelo-* + *-rrhea*]. 1. An excessive fatty discharge. 2. Diarrhea with excessive fat in the stools.

pim·e·lor·thop·nea, pim·e·lor·thop·noea (pim″e·lor·thop′nee·uh) *n.* [*pimel-* + *orthopnea*]. Orthopnea due to obesity.

pim·e·lu·ria (pim″e·lew′ree·uh) *n.* [*pimel-* + *-uria*]. The excretion of fat in the urine; LIPURIA.

pi·men·ta (pi·men′tuh) *n.* [Pg., pepper, from ML. *pigmentum*, spiced drink]. The nearly ripe fruit of *Pimenta officinalis*, an evergreen tree; the fruit yields a volatile oil. It has been used as a carminative. Syn. *allspice*.

pi·men·to (pi·men′to) *n.* PIMENTA.

pi·min·o·dine (pi·min′o·deen, pye·) *n.* Ethyl 1-(3-anilinopropyl)-4-phenylisonipecotate, $C_{23}H_{30}N_2O_2$, a synthetic narcotic analgesic related to meperidine; used as the esylate (ethanesulfonate) salt.

pim·o·zide (pim′o·zide) *n.* 1-{1-[4,4-Bis(*p*-flurophenyl)butyl]-4-piperidyl}-2-benzimidazolinone, $C_{28}H_{29}F_2N_3O$, a tranquilizer.

pim·pi·nel·la (pim″pi·nel′uh) *n.* The dried rhizome and roots of *Pimpinella saxifraga* or other species; has been variously used in medicine.

pim·ple, *n.* A small pustule or papule.

pin, *n.* 1. NAIL (2). 2. A small metal rod used to aid retention of dental restorations.

pin·a·coid (pin′uh·koid) *adj.* [Gk. *pinakoeidēs*, like a tablet, from *pinax, pinakos*, tablet, board]. Characterizing polyhedral forms having only two parallel faces, as in some condensed systems of large molecules.

pin·a·cy·a·nol (pin″uh·sigh′uh·nol) *n.* A basic quinoline, used as a supravital stain for mitochondria and for the staining of frozen sections.

Pi·nard's maneuver (pee·nahr′) [A. *Pinard*, French obstetrician, 1844–1934]. A technique in breech presentation in which the knee of the fetus is pushed to one side and a foot brought down for traction.

Pinard's sign [A. *Pinard*]. In breech presentation a sharp pain may be elicited by pressure over the uterine fundus after the sixth month of pregnancy.

pince·ment (pance·mahn′) *n.* [F.]. In massage, a pinching or nipping of the tissues.

pin·cers (pin′churz, pin′surz) *n.* [OF. *pinceur*]. FORCEPS.

pinch graft. A small, full-thickness graft lifted from the donor area by a needle and cut free with a razor. Many such small deep grafts are fitted together to cover the defect.

Pin·cus reagent. A solution of antimony trichloride which gives a blue color with most ketosteroids.

pin·do·lol (pin′do·lole) *n.* 1-(Indol-4-yloxy)-3-isopropylamino)-2-propanol, $C_{14}H_{20}N_2O_2$, a vasodilator.

pine, *n.* 1. Any tree of the genus *Pinus*. 2. Loosely, any of various other kinds of coniferous trees.

pi·ne·al (pin′ee·ul, pye′nee·ul) *adj.* [L. *pinea*, pinecone, + *-al*]. Pertaining to the pineal body, or epiphysis cerebri.

pineal appendage. PINEAL BODY.

pi·ne·al·blas·to·ma (pin″ee·ul·blas·to′muh, pye″nee·) *n.* [*pineal* + *blastoma*]. A pinealoma whose cells are less well differentiated.

pineal body. A small cone-shaped structure attached to the roof of the third ventricle between the superior colliculi.

Syn. *epiphysis cerebri.* NA *corpus pineale.* See also Plate 18.

pineal calculus. A small calcified nodule in the pineal body.

pi·ne·al·cy·to·ma (pin″ee·ul·sigh·to′muh, pye″nee·) *n.* [*pineal* + *-cytoma*]. PINEALOMA.

pi·ne·al·ec·to·my (pin″ee·ul·eck′tuh·mee, pye″nee·) *n.* [*pineal* + *-ectomy*]. Surgical removal of the pineal body.

pineal eye. A modification of the pineal body to form a rudimentary dorsal median eye in some lower vertebrates. Syn. *epiphyseal eye.*

pineal germinoma. PINEALOMA.

pineal gland. PINEAL BODY.

pi·ne·al·ism (pin′ee·ul·iz·um, pye′nee·) *n.* [*pineal* + *-ism*]. Disturbances due to abnormality in the secretion of the pineal body.

pi·ne·a·lo·ma (pin″ee·uh·lo′muh, pye″nee·) *n.*, pl. **pinealomas, pinealoma·ta** (·tuh) [*pineal* + *-oma*]. An uncommon, usually small, frequently invasive tumor of the pineal body composed of varying proportions of large, round cells with well defined cell membranes, a pale cytoplasm and conspicuous nuclei and small, darkly stained cells, presumably lymphocytes, distributed along the vascular stroma of the tumor. Syn. *pinealcytoma, pineal germinoma, pineal seminoma, pineal tumor.* See also *pineal syndrome.*

pineal recess. A recess in the roof of the third ventricle extending posteriorly into the stalk of the pineal body. NA *recessus pinealis.*

pineal seminoma. PINEALOMA.

pineal syndrome. A rare syndrome due to a pinealoma or other pathological condition in or about the pineal body, resulting in increased intracranial pressure and associated neurologic disturbances, an inability to look upward (Parinaud's syndrome) and slightly dilated pupils which react in accommodation but not to light.

pineal tumor. PINEALOMA.

pineal ventricle. A cavity found occasionally within the pineal body; the persisting remnant of the fetal cavity.

pine·ap·ple itch. A dermatitis following contact with pineapples, possibly caused by an acarus.

Pi·nel's system (pee·nel′) [P. *Pinel,* French physician, 1745–1826]. The treatment of mental disorders without forcible restraints, such as chains.

pi·nene (pye′neen) *n.* 2,7,7-Trimethyl-Δ^2-bicyclo(1.1.3)-heptene, $C_{10}H_{16}$, a terpene hydrocarbon found in many essential oils.

pin·eo·blas·to·ma (pin″ee·o·blas·to′muh) *n.* PINEALBLASTOMA.

pine tar. A viscid, brownish-black liquid, of terebinthinate odor and sharp taste, obtained by destructive distillation of the wood of *Pinus palustris* or other species of *Pinus;* contains cyclic hydrocarbons and phenols. Has been employed externally as a stimulating and antiseptic application in skin diseases, and sometimes internally as a stimulating expectorant.

pin·guec·u·la (ping·gweck′yoo·luh) *n.*, pl. **pinguecu·lae** (·lee) [NL., from L. *pinguiculus,* dim. of *pinguis,* fat]. A small, slightly elevated yellowish-white patch situated in the conjunctiva, within the interpalpebral fissure, between the cornea and the canthus of the eye; it is the result of the elastotic degeneration of collagen of the connective tissue of the conjectiva.

pin·guid (ping′gwid) *adj.* [L. *pinguis*]. FAT (2); UNCTUOUS.

pin·hole os. An extreme narrowing of the ostium uteri, seen in young and underdeveloped women.

pinhole pupil. PINPOINT PUPIL.

pi·ni·form (pye′ni·form, pin′i·form) *adj.* [L. *pinus,* pine, + *-iform*]. Shaped like a pinecone.

pink disease. ACRODYNIA.

pink·eye, *n.* 1. A contagious, mucopurulent conjunctivitis occurring especially in horses. 2. CATARRHAL CONJUNCTIVITIS.

pink puffer. A person with emphysema, marked dyspnea, debility, and hyperinflation of the lungs. Contr. *blue bloater.*

pink·root, *n.* SPIGELIA.

pin·na (pin′uh) *n.*, L. pl. & genit. sing. **pin·nae** (·ee), [L., feather, wing]. The projecting part of the external ear; AURICLE (1). See also Plate 20. —**pin·nal** (·ul) *adj.*

pi·no·cyte (pin′o·site, pye″no·) *n.* [Gk. *pinein,* to drink, + *-cyte*]. A phagocytic cell exhibiting pinocytosis.

pi·no·cy·to·sis (pin″o·sigh·to′sis, pye″no·) *n.*, pl. **pinocyto·ses** (·seez) [*pinocyte* + *-osis*]. A type of absorption by cells in which the cellular membrane invaginates to form a saccular structure that engulfs extracellular fluid and is then closed at the membrane so that the saccule remains as a vesicle or vacuole (pinosome) within the cell.

pi·no·cy·tot·ic (pin″o·sigh·tot′ick, pye″no·) *adj.* Having the characteristics of pinocytosis.

pi·no·some (pin′uh·sohm, pye′no·) *n.* A vacuole that forms as the result of pinocytosis.

pin·ox·e·pin (pin·ock′se·pin) *n.* *cis*-4-[3-(2-Chlorodibenz-[*b,e*]oxepin-11(6*H*)-ylidene)propyl]-1-piperazineethanol, $C_{23}H_{27}ClN_2O_2$, a tranquilizer; used as the dihydrochloride salt.

pin·point pupil. Contraction of the iris until the pupil is scarcely larger than a pinhead. It is seen in opium poisoning, after the use of miotics, in certain cerebral diseases, and in tabes dorsalis. Syn. *pinhole pupil.*

Pins' sign [E. *Pins,* Austrian physician, 1845–1913]. The disappearance of pleuritic symptoms associated with pericarditis when the patient assumes the knee-chest position.

pint, *n.* [OF. *pinte*]. The eighth part of a gallon; 16 fluidounces. Symbol, 0. (octarius). Abbreviated, pt.

pin·ta (pin′tuh, peen′tah) *n.* [Sp., from *pinto,* spotted, mottled, lit., painted]. A disease of the skin seen most frequently in tropical America, characterized by dyschromic changes and hyperkeratosis in patches of the skin; caused by the spirochete *Treponema carateum,* which is morphologically identical with the spirochetes of syphilis and of yaws. Syn. *carate, mal del pinto, piquite, purupuru, quitiqua.*

pin·tid (pin′tid) *n.* [*pinta* + *-id*]. The characteristic red macular skin eruption of the secondary stage of pinta.

pin·til·lo (pin·til′o) *n.* A patient with pinta.

Pi·nus (pye′nus) *n.* [L., pine]. A genus of coniferous trees of the family Pinaceae. The leaves of *Pinus mugo* yield dwarf pine needle oil; pine tar is derived from the wood of *P. palustris* and other species.

pin·worm, *n.* Any of various oxyurid worms inhabiting the intestinal tracts of mammals, notably *Enterobius vermicularis,* the human pinworm.

pinworm infection. ENTEROBIASIS.

pi·o·ne·mia, pi·o·nae·mia (pye″o·nee′mee·uh) *n.* [Gk. *piōn,* fat, + *-emia*]. The presence of an emulsion of fine oil globules in the blood, sometimes found in diabetes; a form of lipemia.

Pi·oph·i·la (pye·off′i·luh) *n.* [NL., from Gk. *piōn,* fat, + *philos,* lover of]. A genus of small, black, dipterous insects containing the species *Piophila casei,* the cheese fly, which deposits its eggs preferably on cheese but also on ham, bacon, and other fatty foods. The larvae, commonly called cheese skippers, are a cause of intestinal myiasis.

pi·or·thop·nea, pi·or·thop·noea (pye″or·thop′nee·uh, ·or·thup·nee′uh) *n.* [Gk. *piōn,* fat, + *orthopnea*]. PIMELORTHOPNEA.

Pio·trow·ski's anterior tibial reflex or **sign** (pyoʰ·troʰf′skee) [A. *Piotrowski,* German neurologist, b. 1878]. Dorsal flexion of the ankle and foot on percussion of the anterior tibial muscle which, in excess, is indicative of corticospinal tract lesions.

pi·pam·a·zine (pi·pam′uh·zeen) *n.* 10-[3-(4-Carbamoylpiperidino)propyl]-2-chlorophenothiazine, $C_{21}H_{24}ClN_2O$, an antiemetic and sedative drug.

pi·pam·per·one (pi·pam′pur·ohn) *n.* 1′-[3-(*p*-Fluorobenzoyl)-

propyl][1,4′-bipiperidine]-4′-carboxamide, $C_{21}H_{30}FN_3O_2$, a tranquilizer.

pi·paz·e·thate (pi·paz′e·thate) *n.* 2-(2-Piperidinoethoxy) ethyl 10*H*-pyrido[3,2-*b*][1,4]benzothiazine-10-carboxylate, $C_{21}H_{25}N_3O_3S$, an antitussive drug; used as the hydrochloride salt.

pi·pen·zo·late bromide (pi·pen′zo·late) *n.* 1-Ethyl-3-piperidyl benzilate bromide, $C_{22}H_{28}BrNO_3$, an anticholinergic drug used mainly for adjunctive treatment of peptic ulcer.

Pi·per (pye′pur) *n.* [L., pepper]. A genus of tropical plants of the family Piperaceae. Various products, such as betel (from *Piper betel*), cubeb (from *P. cubeba*), kava (from *P. methysticum*), and matico (from *P. agustifolium*), have been used medically. See also *pepper.*

pip·er·a·cet·a·zine (pip″ur·uh·set′uh·zeen) *n.* 10-{3-[4-(2-Hydroxyethyl)piperidino]propyl}phenothiazin-2-yl methyl ketone, $C_{24}H_{30}N_2O_2S$, a tranquilizer.

pip·er·a·mide (pip′ur·uh·mide) *n.* 4′-{4-[3-(Dimethylamino)-propyl]-1-piperazinyl}acetanilide, $C_{17}H_{28}N_4O$, an antiparasitic agent; used as the maleate salt.

pi·per·a·zine (pi·perr′uh·zeen, pip′ur·) *n.* Hexahydropyrazine, $C_4H_{10}O_2$, used in the form of various of its salts (adipate, citrate, tartrate) for treatment of infections caused by certain roundworms. Formerly used for treatment of gout.

pi·per·i·dine (pi·perr′i·deen, ·din, pye·perr′i·) *n.* Hexahydropyridine, $C_5H_{11}N$, a liquid base used as a reagent.

pip·er·i·do·late (pip″ur·i·do′late, pi·perr″i·do′late, pye·perr″) *n.* 1-Ethyl-3-piperidyl diphenylacetate, $C_{21}H_{25}NO_2$, an anticholinergic agent used for treatment of spastic disorders of the upper gastrointestinal tract; employed as the hydrochloride salt.

pip·er·ine (pip′ur·een, ·in) *n.* 1-Piperoylpiperidine, $C_{17}H_{19}NO_3$, an alkaloid in pepper; formerly used as a medicinal.

pip·er·o·caine (pip′ur·o·kane) *n.* 3-(2-Methylpiperidino)propyl benzoate, $C_{16}H_{23}NO_2$, a local anesthetic used as the hydrochloride salt.

pip·er·o·nal (pip′ur·o·nal, pye·perr′o·nal) *n.* Piperonyl aldehyde, $C_8H_6O_3$, used in formulation of perfumes; has been employed as a pediculicide. Syn. *heliotropin.*

pip·er·ox·an (pip″ur·ock′san) *n.* 2-(1-Piperidylmethyl)-1,4-benzodioxan, $C_{14}H_{19}NO_2$, an adrenergic blocking agent that has been used, as the hydrochloride salt, for diagnosis of pheochromocytoma.

pipe·stem artery. An artery with advanced calcification and stiffening.

pipestem cirrhosis. A zooparasitic cirrhosis caused by deposition of the ova of *Schistosoma mansoni* in the portal spaces with reactive fibrosis and granulomatous inflammation.

pi·pet, pi·pette (pi·pet′, pye·pet′) *n.* [OF. *pipette,* dim. of *pipe,* tube]. A graduated open glass or plastic tube used for measuring or transferring definite quantities of liquids.

pip·o·bro·man (pip″o·bro′man) *n.* 1,4-Bis(3-bromopropionyl)piperazine, $C_{10}H_{16}Br_2N_2O_2$, a cytotoxic drug used for treatment of polycythemia vera and chronic granulocytic leukemia.

pip·o·sul·fan (pip″o·sul′fan) *n.* 1,4-Dihydroacryloylpiperazine dimethanesulfonate, $C_{12}H_{22}N_2O_8S_2$, an antineoplastic agent.

pip·o·ti·a·zine (pip″o·tye′uh·zeen) *n.* 10-[3-[4-(2-Hydroxyethyl)piperidino]propyl]-*N,N*-dimethylphenothiazine-2-sulfonamide, palmitate ester, $C_{40}H_{63}N_3O_4S_2$, a tranquilizer.

pip·ra·drol (pip′ruh·drol) *n.* α,α-Diphenyl-2-piperidinemethanol, $C_{18}H_{21}NO$, a central nervous system stimulant; used as the hydrochloride salt.

pip·ro·zol·in (pip″ro·zol′in) *n.* Ethyl 3-ethyl-4-oxo-5-piperidino-$\Delta^{2\alpha}$-thiazolidineacetate, $C_{14}H_{22}N_2O_3S$, a choleretic agent.

pip·syl chloride (pip′sil). *p*-Iodophenylsulfonyl chloride, $IC_6H_4SO_2Cl$, a reagent which reacts nearly quantitatively with free amino groups of amino acids to form pipsylamino acids of the type of $IC_6H_4SO_2NHR$.

Piptal. Trademark for pipenzolate bromide, an anticholinergic drug used mainly for adjunctive treatment of peptic ulcer.

pip·to·nych·ia (pip″to·nick′ee·uh) *n.* [Gk. *pipt*ein, to fall, + *onych-* + *-ia*]. Shedding of the nails.

pi·quite (pi·keet′) *n.* PINTA.

piq·ui·zil (pick′wi·zil) *n.* Isobutyl 4-(6,7-dimethoxy-4-quinazolinyl)-1-piperazinecarboxylate, $C_{19}H_{26}N_4O_4$, a bronchodilator drug; used as the hydrochloride salt.

pi·qûre (pi·kewr′) *n.* [F.]. PUNCTURE.

piqûre diabetes. A form of experimental glycosuria produced by puncturing the floor of the fourth ventricle.

pi·ran·da·mine (pi·ran′duh·meen) *n.* 1,3,4,9-Tetrahydro-*N,N*,1-trimethylindeno[2,1-*c*]pyran-1-ethylamine, $C_{17}H_{23}NO$, an antidepressant, used as the hydrochloride.

pir·ben·i·cil·lin (pirr·ben″i·sil′in) *n.* An isonicotinimidoyl derivative of penicillin, $C_{24}H_{26}N_6O_5S$, an antibacterial used as the sodium salt.

pir·bu·te·rol (pirr·bew′te·role) *n.* α^6-[(*tert*-Butylamino)-methyl]-3-hydroxy-2,6-piperidinedimethanol, $C_{12}H_{20}N_2O_3$, a bronchodilator, usually used as the dihydrochloride salt.

pir·fen·i·done (pirr·fen′i·dohn) *n.* 5-Methyl-1-phenyl-2(1*H*)-pyridone, $C_{12}H_{11}NO$, an analgesic, anti-inflammatory, antipyretic.

pir·i·form, pyr·i·form (pirr′i·form, pye′ri·form) *adj. & n.* [L. *pir*um, pear, + *-iform*]. 1. Pear-shaped. 2. PIRIFORMIS.

piriform area. PIRIFORM LOBE.

pir·i·for·mis (pirr″i·for′mis) *n.* [NL., from L. *pirum,* pear]. A muscle arising from the front of the sacrum and inserted into the greater trochanter of the femur. NA *musculus piriformis.* See also Table of Muscles in the Appendix.

piriform lobe. The lateral olfactory stria, anterior part of the parahippocampal gyrus, and the uncus collectively.

piriform recess or **sinus.** A small space lateral to the laryngeal aditus, bounded laterally by the thyroid cartilage and thyrohyoid membrane and medially by the aryepiglottic fold. NA *recessus piriformis.*

Pi·ro·goff's amputation (p^y^i·rah·go^h^f′) [N. I. *Pirogoff,* Russian surgeon, 1810–1881]. An osteoplastic operation for amputation of the foot, resembling Syme's amputation, in which part of the calcaneus is retained.

pir·o·la·za·mide (pirr″o·lay′zuh·mide) *n.* Hexahydro-α,α-diphenylpyrrolo[1,2-*a*]pyrazine-2(1*H*)-butyramide, $C_{23}H_{29}N_3O$, an antiarrhythmic.

Pir·o·nel·la (pirr″o·nel′uh) *n.* A genus of freshwater snails.

Pironella con·i·ca (kon′i·kuh). The species of snail that serves as the first intermediate host of the fluke *Heterophyes heterophyes* in Egypt.

Pi·ro·plas·ma (pye″ro·plaz′muh) *n.* BABESIA. **—piroplasma,** pl. **piroplasma·ta** (·tuh), *com. n.*

pi·ro·plas·mo·sis (pye″ro·plaz·mo′sis) *n.,* pl. **piroplasmo·ses** (·seez) [*Piroplasm*a + *-osis*]. BABESIOSIS. **—piroplas·mot·ic** (·mot′ick) *adj.*

pir·ox·i·cam (pirr·ock′si·kam) *n.* 4-Hydroxy-2-methyl-*N*-(2-pyridyl)-2*H*-1,2-benzothiazine-3-carboxamide 1,1-dioxide, $C_{15}H_{13}N_3O_4S$, an anti-inflammatory.

pir·pro·fen (pirr·pro′fen) *n.* 3-Chloro-4-(3-pyrrolin-1-yl)hydratropic acid, $C_{13}H_{14}ClNO_2$, an anti-inflammatory.

Pirquet test. VON PIRQUET TEST.

pis·cid·ia (pi·sid′ee·uh) *n.* [NL., from L. *piscis,* fish, + *caedere,* to kill]. The dried bark of *Piscidia piscipula (P. erythrina);* has been used as an anodyne. Syn. *Jamaica dogwood.*

pi·si·an·nu·la·ris (pye″see·an·yoo·lair′is) *n.* A variant of the abductor digiti minimi muscle inserted into the transverse carpal ligament.

pi·si·form (pye′si·form) *adj. & n.* [L. *pis*um, pea, + *-iform*]. 1. Pea-shaped. 2. A small bone on the inner and anterior aspect of the carpus. NA *os pisiforme.* See also Table of Bones in the Appendix.

pisiform articulation. The articulation between the pisiform and the triquetrum. NA *articulatio ossis pisiformis.*

pi·si·me·ta·car·pus (pye″si·met″uh·kahr′pus) *n.* A variant of the abductor digiti minimi muscle inserted into the fifth metacarpal.

pi·si·un·ci·na·tus (pye″see·un″si·nay′tus) *n.* A variant of the abductor digiti minimi muscle inserted into the hamulus of the hamate.

pi·so·ha·mate (pye″so·hay′mate) *adj.* Pertaining to the pisiform and hamate bones.

pisohamate ligament. The ligament connecting the pisiform and hamate bones. NA *ligamentum pisohamatum.*

pi·so·meta·car·pal (pye″so·met″uh·kahr′pul) *adj.* Pertaining to the pisiform and (fifth) metacarpal bones.

pisometacarpal ligament. The ligament connecting the pisiform and the base of the fifth metacarpal. NA *ligamentum pisometacarpeum.*

pi·so·tri·que·tral (pye″so·trye·kwee′trul) *adj.* Pertaining to the pisiform and triquetral bones.

pis·til (pis′til) *n.* [F., from L. *pistillum,* pestle]. The ovule-bearing organ of a seed plant. —**pis·til·late** (·ti·late) *adj.*

pis·tol-shot sound. A loud sound heard on auscultation over the peripheral arteries with each pulsation in aortic regurgitation, severe anemia, hyperthyroidism, arteriovenous fistula, and other conditions; due to rapid arterial distention and collapse. Syn. *Traube's sign.*

pit, *n.* 1. A depression, as the pit of the stomach; the armpit. 2. A sharp, pointed depression in the enamel of a tooth; normally occurring where several developmental grooves join. 3. A microscopic tubular depression in the surface of the mucosa.

pitch, *n.* The quality of sound that depends upon the frequency of the vibrations that produce the sound.

pitch·blende (pitch′blend) *n.* [Ger. *Pechblende,* from *Pech,* pitch, + *Blende,* lustrous ore]. A massive form, having a pitchlike luster, of the mineral uraninite; a native uranium oxide, also containing radium.

pith·i·a·tism (pith′ee·uh·tiz·um, pi·thigh′) *n.* [Gk. *peith*ein, to persuade, + *iat*os, curable, + *-ism*]. 1. A condition caused by suggestion. See also *hysteria.* 2. Treatment of disease by suggestion. —**pith·i·at·ic** (pith″ee·at′ick) *adj.*

pith·i·at·ric (pith″ee·at′rick) *adj.* [Gk. *peith*ein, to persuade, + *iatr-* + *-ic*]. Capable of being relieved by suggestion or persuasion, as certain hysterical conditions.

Pitocin. Trademark for oxytocin injection, an oxytocic posterior pituitary hormone preparation.

pit of the stomach. The part of the abdomen just below the sternum and between the cartilages of the false ribs.

pi·tom·e·ter (pi·tom′e·tur) *n.* [H. *Pitot,* French physicist, 1695–1771]. An instrument that records the rate of flow of liquids.

Pi·tot tube (pee·to′) [H. *Pitot*]. A device for measuring fluid flow by observing the difference in pressure caused by a simple constriction in the tube; used in the construction of certain flowmeters.

Pitres' sections (peet′r) [J. A. *Pitres,* French physician, 1848–1927]. A series of six coronal sections made through the brain for postmortem examinations.

Pitressin. Trademark for antidiuretic hormone injection.

pit·ted, *adj.* Marked by indentations or pits, as from smallpox.

pit·ting, *n.* 1. The formation of pits; in the nails, a consequence and sign of psoriasis. 2. The preservation for a short time of indentations on the skin made by pressing with the finger; seen in pitting edema.

pitting edema. Edema of such degree that the skin can be temporarily indented by pressure with the fingers.

pi·tu·i·cyte (pi·tew′i·site) *n.* [*pituit*ary + *-cyte*]. The characteristic cell of the neurohypophysis.

pi·tu·i·cy·to·ma (pi·tew″i·sigh·to′muh) *n.* [*pituicyt*e + *-oma*]. A benign tumor of the pituicytes of the neurohypophysis.

pi·tu·i·tary (pi·tew′i·terr″ee) *adj.* & *n.* [L. *pituitarius,* from *pituita,* phlegm]. 1. Secreting mucus or phlegm. 2. Pertaining to the hypophysis or pituitary gland. 3. PITUITARY GLAND.

pituitary apoplexy. Hemorrhage into a pituitary adenoma, characterized by the acute onset of ophthalmoplegia, bilateral amaurosis, drowsiness or coma, with either subarachnoid hemorrhage or pleocytosis and elevated protein in the cerebrospinal fluid.

pituitary appendage. PITUITARY GLAND.

pituitary B. LUTEINIZING HORMONE.

pituitary basophilism. CUSHING'S SYNDROME.

pituitary B gonadotropin. LEUTINIZING HORMONE.

pituitary body. PITUITARY GLAND.

pituitary cachexia. SIMMOND'S DISEASE.

pituitary dwarf. An individual afflicted with pituitary dwarfism.

pituitary dwarfism. Stunted growth due to primary growth hormone deficiency, but frequently associated with deficiency of thyrotropic and adrenocorticotropic hormones as detected by appropriate tests and with gonadotropin deficiency which is usually not demonstrable in childhood. The condition may be characterized clinically only by growth failure after the first few years of life, or there may be a childish face, high-pitched voice, small hands and feet, delayed sexual maturation and underdeveloped genitalia, and in older individuals, deficient subcutaneous fat with loose wrinkled skin and precocious senility. The condition may also be secondary to destructive pituitary lesions as from tumor, infection, trauma, or aneurysm.

pituitary eunuchoidism. Eunuchoidism due to a deficiency of pituitary gonadotropin.

pituitary exophthalmos. THYROTROPIC EXOPHTHALMOS.

pituitary fossa. HYPOPHYSEAL FOSSA.

pituitary gland. A small, rounded, bilobate endocrine gland, averaging about 0.5 g in weight, which lies in the sella turcica of the sphenoid bone, is attached by a stalk, the infundibulum, to the floor of the third ventricle of the brain at the hypothalamus, and consists of an anterior lobe, the adenohypophysis, which produces and secretes various important hormones, including several which regulate other endocrine glands, and a less important posterior lobe, the neurohypophysis, which holds and secretes antidiuretic hormone and oxytocin produced in the hypothalamus. Syn. *hypophysis* (NA). NA *glandula pituitaria.* See also *adenohypophysis, neurohypophysis,* and Plates 17, 18, 26.

pituitary hypoadrenocorticism. Hypoplasia and hypofunction of the adrenal cortex resulting from lack of pituitary adrenocorticotropin.

pituitary hypogonadism. Lack of sexual development due to a deficiency of pituitary gonadotropin. See also *pituitary dwarfism, pituitary eunuchoidism.*

pituitary infantilism. PITUITARY DWARFISM.

pituitary insufficiency. HYPOPITUITARISM.

pituitary myxedema. A rare type of myxedema resulting from deficiency of thyrotropic hormone secretion by the adenohypophysis.

pituitary nanism. PITUITARY DWARFISM.

Pituitrin. A trademark for posterior pituitary injection, a preparation of mixed posterior pituitary hormones.

pit viper. Any snake of the family Crotalidae.

pit·y·ri·a·sis (pit″i·rye′uh·sis) *n.* [Gk., from *pityron,* bran, scurf, dandruff]. A fine, branny desquamation of the skin.

pityriasis cap·i·tis (kap′i·tis). SEBORRHEIC DERMATITIS.

pityriasis cir·ci·na·ta (sur″si·nay′tuh). PITYRIASIS ROSEA.

pityriasis li·che·noi·des chron·i·ca (lye″ke·noy′deez kron′i·kuh). A mild form of pityriasis lichenoides et varioliformis acuta.

pityriasis lichenoides et var·i·o·li·for·mis acu·ta (văr″ee·o″li·for′mis a·kew′tuh). A noncommunicable, acute, or subacute skin eruption characterized by vesicles and pustules that form crusts and later scars. Syn. *Mucha-Habermann's disease.*

pityriasis lin·guae (ling'gwee). Transitory benign plaques of the tongue.

pityriasis ni·gra. TINEA NIGRA.

pityriasis pilaris. KERATOSIS PILARIS.

pityriasis ro·sea (ro'zee·uh). An idiopathic self-limited skin disease of the trunk, usually acute; characterized by pale red patches with fawn-colored centers. Syn. *pityriasis circinata, herpes tonsurans maculosus.*

pityriasis ru·bra (roo'bruh). EXFOLIATIVE DERMATITIS.

pityriasis rubra pi·la·ris (pi·lair'is). A chronic, mildly inflammatory skin disease in which firm, acuminate papules form at the mouths of the hair follicles with horny plugs in these follicles. By coalescence scaly patches are formed. Syn. *lichen ruber acuminatus.*

pityriasis sim·plex (sim'plecks). SEBORRHEIC DERMATITIS.

pityriasis ste·a·toi·des (stee''uh·toy'deez). Seborrheic dermatitis when large waxy scales are formed, usually associated with pruritus and alopecia.

pityriasis versicolor. TINEA VERSICOLOR.

pit·y·roid (pit'i·roid) *adj.* [Gk. *pityron*, bran, + *-oid*]. BRANNY.

Pit·y·ro·spo·rum (pit''i·ro·spo'rum, ·ros'puh·rum) *n.* [NL., from Gk. *pityron*, bran, + *spora*, seed]. A genus of fungi which is yeastlike in character, belonging to the Cryptococcaceae.

Pityrosporum fur·fur (fur'fur). The species of fungus that causes tinea versicolor.

Pityrosporum or·bic·u·la·re (or·bick''yoo·lahr'ee). *PITYROSPORUM FURFUR.*

Pityrosporum ovale (o·vay'lee). A species of fungus found in the hair follicles and on the skin in seborrheic dermatitis; of unknown pathogenicity.

pi·val·ate (pi·val'ate, pye·val'ate) *n.* Any salt or ester of pivalic or trimethylacetic acid, $(CH_3)_3CCOOH$; a trimethylacetate.

pi·val·ic acid (pi·val'ick) [*pi*nacolone + *val*eric]. Trimethylacetic acid, $(CH_3)_3CCOOH$, isomeric with normal valeric acid, a weak acid used to form salts with certain medicinal bases.

piv·am·pi·cil·lin (piv·am''pi·sil'in) *n.* The pivalyloxycarbonylmethyl ester of ampicillin, $C_{22}H_{29}N_3O_6S$, an antibacterial, used as the hydrochloride salt; the pamoate salt, $(C_{22}H_{29}N_3O_6S)\cdot C_{23}H_{16}O_6$; and the probenate (*p*-dipropylsulfamoylbenzoic acid) salt, $C_{22}H_{29}N_3O_6S\cdot C_{13}H_{19}NO_4S$.

piv·ot (piv'ut) *n.* [F.]. DOWEL.

pivot crown. A tooth crown of porcelain or other material, attached to the root by means of a pin or post.

pivot joint. A synovial joint in which movement is limited to rotation; the movement is uniaxial, and in the longitudinal axis of the bones. NA *articulatio trochoidea.*

pivot tooth. PIVOT CROWN.

pi·zo·ty·line (pi·zo'ti·leen) *n.* 4-(9,10-Dihydro-4*H*-benzo[4,5]cyclohepta[1,2-*b*]thien-4-ylidene-1-methylpiperidine, $C_{19}H_{21}NS$, an anabolic, antidepressant, serotonin inhibitor, specific in migraine.

pK The negative logarithm of the dissociation constant of an acid or a base; it is equivalent to the hydrogen-ion concentration (expressed in pH units) at which there is an equimolecular concentration of the acidic and basic components of any given buffer system.

PKU Abbreviation for *phenylketonuria* (2).

pla·ce·bo (pla·see'bo) *n.* [L., I shall please]. A preparation, devoid of pharmacologic effect, given for psychological effect, or as a control in evaluating a medicinal believed to have pharmacologic activity.

pla·cen·ta (pluh·sen'tuh) *n.*, L. pl. & genit. sing. **placen·tae** (·tee), E. pl. **placentas** [L., cake] [NA]. The organ on the wall of the uterus to which the embryo is attached by the umbilical cord. Developed from the chorion of the embryo and the decidua basalis of the uterus, it performs the functions of nutrition, respiration, and excretion, as well as secretion of estrogen, progesterone, and other hormones. At term the average human placenta weighs about 1/6 as much as the fetus, and is about 2 cm thick at its center and 15 cm in diameter. See also Plate 23.

placenta ac·cre·ta (a·kree'tuh). A placenta that has partially grown into the myometrium (cleavage zone in basal decidua incompletely developed or absent with chorionic villi in direct contact with the myometrium).

placenta cir·soi·dea (sur·soy'dee·uh). A placenta in which the umbilical vessels have a varicose arrangement.

placenta dif·fu·sa (di·few'suh). PLACENTA MEMBRANACEA.

placenta ex·tra·cho·ri·a·la (ecks''tru·kor''ee·ay'luh). CIRCUMVALLATE PLACENTA.

placenta fe·nes·tra·ta (fen·e·stray'tuh). An irregular, four-sided variety of placenta with an opening near the center.

placenta foe·ta·lis (fee·tay'lis) [BNA]. PARS FETALIS PLACENTAE.

placenta in·cre·ta (in·kree'tuh). A placenta that has grown into the uterine myometrium at all contact areas with no intervening decidua.

pla·cen·tal (pluh·sen'tul) *adj.* Pertaining to or having a placenta.

placental apoplexy. Escape of blood into the placental substance.

placental barrier. The tissues intervening between the maternal and the fetal blood of the placenta, which prevent or hinder certain substances or organisms from passing from mother to fetus.

placental blood spaces. The intervillous lacunae of the placenta.

placental bruit. PLACENTAL MURMUR.

placental circulation. 1. UMBILICAL CIRCULATION. 2. INTERVILLOUS CIRCULATION.

placental membrane. PLACENTAL BARRIER.

placental murmur. A sound attributed to the circulation of the blood in the placenta.

placental parasite. OMPHALOSITE.

placental polyp. A uterine polyp composed of retained placental fragments.

placental respiration. FETAL RESPIRATION.

placental site. The area to which the placenta is attached.

placental stage. The period of labor occupied by the expulsion of the placenta and fetal membranes.

placental thrombosis. Thrombosis of the uterine veins at the site of a placenta.

placental transmission. The conveyance of drug and disease products through the placental circulation from mother to offspring.

placental trophoblast. TROPHODERM (2).

placenta mem·bra·na·cea (mem''bruh·nay'see·uh). A placenta in which the entire ovum is covered by functioning chorionic villi.

placenta nep·pi·for·mis (nep'i·for'mis). CIRCUMVALLATE PLACENTA.

placenta per·cre·ta (pur·kree'tuh). Abnormal penetration of chorionic elements to the serosal layer of the uterus.

placenta pre·via (pree'vee·uh). A placenta superimposed upon and about the os uteri internum, which may produce serious hemorrhage before or during labor.

placenta previa cen·tra·lis (sen·tray'lis). A condition in which the center of the placenta is directly above the os uteri internum.

placenta previa mar·gi·na·lis (mahr·ji·nay'lis). A condition in which the edge of the placenta meets, but does not overlap, the os uteri internum.

placenta previa par·ti·a·lis (pahr·shee·ay'lis). A condition in which the edge of the placenta overlies, but does not completely obstruct, the os uteri internum.

placenta re·flexa (re·fleck'suh). A condition in which a thickening occurs in the peripheral portion of the placenta, giving it a rolled-back appearance.

placenta ren·i·for·mis (ren·i·for'mis). A kidney-shaped placenta.

placenta spu·ria (spew'ree·uh). An adjacent, though separate, portion of placental tissue, apparently serving no role in fetal nourishment.

placenta suc·cen·tu·ri·a·ta (suck"sen·tew"ree·ay'tuh). An anomalous formation in which one or more accessory lobules are developed in the membrane at a greater or lesser distance from the margin of the placenta, but connected with the latter by vascular channels. Syn. *accessory placenta.*

plac·en·ta·tion (plas"en·tay'shun) *n.* Formation and mode of attachment of the placenta.

placenta ute·ri·na (yoo·te·rye'nuh) [BNA]. PARS UTERINA PLACENTAE.

pla·cen·tin (pla·sen'tin) *n.* A desiccated defatted placental extract.

plac·en·ti·tis (plas"en·tye'tis) *n.*, pl. **placen·tit·i·des** (·tit'i·deez) [*placenta* + *-itis*]. Inflammation of the placenta.

plac·en·tog·ra·phy (plas"en·tog'ruh·fee) *n.* [*placenta* + *-graphy*]. Radiography of the placenta after delivery, using a contrast medium.

pla·cen·toid (pluh·sen'toid) *adj.* Resembling a placenta or having a placenta-like structure.

plac·en·tol·y·sin (plas"en·tol'i·sin, pla·sen"to·lye'sin) *n.* [*placenta* + *lysin*]. A cytolysin formed in the blood of an animal which has received injections of placental tissue emulsions from some other animal species.

plac·en·to·sis (plas"en·to'sis) *n.*, pl. **placento·ses** (·seez) [*placenta* + *-osis*]. INTERVILLOUS THROMBOSIS.

pla·cen·to·ther·a·py (pla·sen"to·therr'uh·pee) *n.* [*placenta* + *therapy*]. The remedial use of biological preparations derived from the placenta of animals.

place theory of hearing. The theory that each frequency of sound is detected by a structure having a specific location on the spiral organ of Corti of the inner ear. Compare *resonance theory of hearing.*

Plá·ci·do's disk (plah'si·doo) [A. *Plácido* da Costa, Portuguese ophthalmologist, 1848–1916]. KERATOSCOPE.

Placidyl. Trademark for ethchlorvynol, a sedative-hypnotic with short duration of action.

plac·ing reaction, reflex, or **response.** A postural response, elicited in the early weeks of life, in which the infant is supported by the examiner's hands under the arms and around the chest and lifted so that the dorsal part of the foot lightly touches a protruding edge, such as a table top. Normally, the legs are lifted by simultaneous flexion of the hips and knees, and the feet placed on the table; absent in paralysis of the lower limbs.

placodal stalk. AUDITORY STALK.

plac·ode (plack'ode) *n.* [Gk. *plakōdēs,* laminar, encrusted, from *plax,* plate, slab]. A platelike epithelial thickening, frequently marking, in the embryo, the anlage of an organ or part. —**pla·co·dal** (pla·ko'dul) *adj.*

plad·a·ro·ma (plad"uh·ro'muh) *n.* [Gk. *pladaros,* flaccid, + *-oma*]. A soft wart or tumor of the eyelid.

plad·a·ro·sis (plad"uh·ro'sis) *n.* PLADAROMA.

plagi-, plagio- [Gk. *plagios*]. A combining form meaning *oblique.*

pla·gio·ceph·a·lism (play"jee·o·sef'uh·liz·um) *n.* PLAGIOCEPHALY.

pla·gio·ceph·a·ly (play"jee·o·sef'uh·lee) *n.* [*plagio-* + *-cephaly*]. A type of strongly asymmetric cranial deformation, in which the anterior portion of one side and the posterior portion of the opposite side of the skull are developed more than their counterparts, so that the maximum length of the skull is not in the midline but on a diagonal. Due to a number of causes, such as prenatal, developmental (disordered sequence of suture closure), mechanical (intentional or unintentional). Syn. *wry-head.* —**plagiocepha·lous** (·lus), **plagio·ce·phal·ic** (·se·fal'ick) *adj.*

plague (plaig) *n.* [OF., from L. *plaga,* a blow, wound]. 1. Any contagious, malignant, epidemic disease. 2. An acute disease of rodents due to *Yersinia pestis,* transmitted to humans through the bite of infected fleas, or by inhalation. The human disease is usually divided into three clinical forms: bubonic, septicemic, and pneumonic.

plague spot. The petechial spots seen with plague, probably due to flea bites.

plague vaccine. A vaccine used for active immunization against plague; may be of either killed or attenuated living cultures of *Yersinia pestis.*

plain film. A radiograph made without the use of contrast material. Syn. *scout film.*

plak·al·bu·min (plack·al·bew'min, ·al'bew·min) *n.* A protein derived from egg albumin by the action of a proteinase elaborated by *Bacillus subtilis.*

plan-, plano- [Gk. *planē*]. A combining form meaning *wandering, straying.*

plana. Plural of *planum.*

Planck's constant [M. *Planck,* German physicist, 1858–1947]. The constant *h,* which has the value 6.624×10^{-27} erg second, used in mathematical expressions of the quantum theory.

plane, *n.* [L. *planum,* level ground]. 1. Any flat, smooth surface, especially any assumed or conventional surface, whether tangent to the body or dividing it. 2. A level in any development, process, or existence. —**pla·nar** (play'nur) *adj.*

plane mirror. A mirror with a flat reflecting surface.

plane of Broca [P. P. *Broca*]. ALVEOLOCONDYLEAN PLANE.

plane of incidence. The plane containing a light ray incident to a surface.

plane of inlet of the pelvis. A plane passing through the sacral promontory and the upper border of the symphysis pubis.

plane of outlet of the pelvis. A plane passing through the lower border of the symphysis pubis and the tip of the coccyx.

planes of anesthesia. Subdivisions of the stages of surgical anesthesia, based on Guedel's classification (1937) of the clinical signs of the stages of general anesthesia. The first plane is marked by loss of the eyelid reflex, the second plane by cessation of eyeball movements, the third plane by beginning of intercostal paralysis, and the fourth plane by complete intercostal paralysis and purely diaphragmatic respiration.

plani-, plano- [L. *planus*]. A combining form meaning *flat* or *level.*

-plania [*plan-* + *-ia*]. A combining form indicating *a wandering in or into an anomalous course or pathway.*

pla·ni·ceps (play'ni·seps, plan'i·) *adj.* [*plani-* + L. *-ceps,* from *caput,* head]. Flatheaded.

pla·ni·gram (play'ni·gram, plan'i·) *n.* Radiographic depiction of structure at a particular depth, made by planigraphy; TOMOGRAM.

pla·nig·ra·phy (pla·nig'ruh·fee) *n.* [*plani-* + *-graphy*]. SECTIONAL RADIOGRAPHY.

pla·nim·e·ter (pla·nim'e·tur) *n.* [*plani-* + *-meter*]. An instrument which measures the area of a plane surface by tracing the periphery.

plan·ing (play'ning) *n.* A method of plastic surgery, whereby skin, hardened by freezing, is abraded by means of a burr, sandpaper, or rotating steel-wire brush, to permanently remove scars, pock marks, and superficial skin blemishes.

plank·ton (plank'tun) *n.* [Gk. *planktos,* wandering, from *planasthai,* to wander]. General term for free-floating plants and animals in seawater.

plano-. See (a) *plan-;* (b) *plani-.*

pla·no·cel·lu·lar (play"no·sel'yoo·lur) *adj.* [*plano-* + *cellular*]. Flat-celled.

pla·no·con·cave (play"no·kon'kave, ·kon·kave') *adj.* [*plano-* + *concave*]. Concave on one surface and flat on the opposite side.

pla·no·con·ic (play″no·kon′ick) *adj.* [*plano-* + *conic*]. Having one side flat and the other conical.

pla·no·con·vex (play″no·kon′vecks, ·kun·vecks′) *adj.* [*plano-* + *convex*]. Plane on one side and convex on the other.

plano·cyte (plan′o·site) *n.* [*plano-* + *-cyte*]. WANDERING CELL.

plano·ma·nia (plan″o·may′nee·uh) *n.* [*plano-* + *-mania*]. An abnormal desire for wandering; an impulse to throw off social restraints and live in the wilds.

Pla·nor·bis (pla·nor′bis) *n.* [*plan-*, flat, + L. *orbis*, ring]. A genus of freshwater snails, species of which act as intermediate hosts of the flukes causing schistosomiasis in man.

pla·no·val·gus (play″no·val′gus) *n.* [*plano-* + *valgus*]. The type of flat foot in which the heel, viewed from behind, is lateral to ankle joint; there is no convexity.

plan·ta (plan′tuh) *n.*, pl. & genit. sing. **plan·tae** (·tee) [L.] [NA]. The sole of the foot.

Plan·ta·go (plan·tay′go) *n.* [L.]. Plantain. A genus of weeds, some of which have been used medicinally.

plantago seed. The cleaned, dried, ripe seed of *Plantago psyllium* or of *P. indica*, known as Spanish or French psyllium seed; or of *P. ovata*, known as blonde psyllium or Indian plantago seed. Used as a cathartic.

plan·tar (plan′tur, ·tahr) *adj.* [L. *plantaris*, from *planta*, sole]. Pertaining to the sole of the foot.

plantar aponeurosis. A thick sheet of dense fibrous connective tissue radiating from the medial portion of the undersurface of the tuberosity of the calcaneus toward the heads of the metatarsal bones. NA *aponeurosis plantaris.*

plantar arterial arch. The arch, in the sole of the foot, made by the lateral plantar artery and the deep plantar branch of the dorsalis pedis artery. NA *arcus plantaris.* See also Table of Arteries in the Appendix.

plantar calcaneocuboid ligament. A short, broad, strong ligament attached to the plantar surfaces of the calcaneus and cuboid deep to the long plantar ligament. NA *ligamentum calcaneocuboideum plantare.*

plantar calcaneonavicular ligament. A thick, wide fibroelastic band which connects the sustentaculum tali and the plantar surface of the navicular and which supports the head of the talus. Syn. *spring ligament.* NA *ligamentum calcaneonaviculare plantare.*

plantar cushion. In solipeds, a cuneiform fibrous body lying between the plantar part of the hoof and the perforans tendon.

plantar fascia. PLANTAR APONEUROSIS.

plantar fascitis. An inflammatory process, usually secondary to trauma or chronic strain, involving the plantar fascia, most commonly at its attachment to the calcaneus.

plantar flexion. Bending the foot or toes downward, toward the sole; opposed to dorsiflexion. —**plan·tar·flex** (plan′tur·flecks) *v.*

plan·ta·ris (plan·tair′is) *n.* A small muscle of the calf of the leg. NA *musculus plantaris.* See also Table of Muscles in the Appendix.

plantar ligaments. The ligaments, one to a joint, on the plantar surfaces of the metatarsophalangeal joints (NA *ligamenta plantaria articulationum metatarsophalangearum*) and the interphalangeal joints of the foot (NA *ligamenta plantaria articulationum interphalangearum pedis*). Compare *long plantar ligament.*

plantar process of the navicular bone. The most prominent point on the plantar surface of the navicular bone.

plantar reflex. Flexion of the toes in response to stroking of the outer surface of the sole, from heel to little toe. Compare *Babinski sign* (1), *plantar muscle reflex.*

plantar tubercle. TUBEROSITY OF THE FIRST METATARSAL BONE.

plantar wart. VERRUCA PLANTARIS.

plan·ta·tion (plan·tay′shun) *n.* [L. *plantare*, to plant]. The insertion of a tooth or other material in the human body. See also *implantation, replantation, transplantation.*

plant cancer. CROWN GALL.

plant·er's wart. Plantar wart (= VERRUCA PLANTARIS).

plant insulin. GLUCOKININ.

plant protease concentrate. A mixture of proteolytic enzymes obtained from the stem of the pineapple plant, *Ananus sativus.* On the hypothesis that the enzymes resolve fibrin deposits, the preparation is proposed for oral use in the treatment of inflammation and edema associated with trauma, postoperative tissue reactions, and skin infections. Syn. *bromelains.*

plan·u·la (plan′yoo·luh) *n.*, pl. **planu·lae** (·lee) [NL., dim. of L. *planus*, flat]. *In embryology,* the embryo at the stage of the two primary germ layers of ectoderm and endoderm in coelenterates.

pla·num (play′num) *n.*, pl. **pla·na** (·nuh) [L.]. A plane, or level surface.

planum nu·cha·le (new·kay′lee) [BNA]. The rough, external surface of the squama occipitalis lying below the superior nuchal lines.

planum oc·ci·pi·ta·le (ock·sip·i·tay′lee) [BNA]. The relatively smooth, triangular, external surface of the occipital squama lying above the superior nuchal lines.

planum or·bi·ta·le (or·bi·tay′lee) [BNA]. ORBITAL PLANE.

planum po·pli·te·um (pop·lit′ee·um) [BNA]. Facies poplitea (= POPLITEAL PLANE).

planum ster·na·le (stur·nay′lee) [BNA]. STERNAL PLANE.

planum tem·po·ra·le (tem·po·ray′lee) [BNA]. TEMPORAL PLANE.

plaque (plack) *n.* [F.]. 1. A patch, or an abnormal flat area on any internal or external body surface. 2. A localized area of atherosclerosis. 3. An area of psoriasis. See also *dental plaque.*

plaque jaune (zhone) [F., yellow]. The golden-orange-brown appearance of the meninges and cortex in an area of cerebral contusion in its most chronic stage.

Plaquenil. Trademark for hydroxychloroquine, used as the sulfate salt for the treatment of malaria, lupus erythematosus, and rheumatoid arthritis.

-plasia, -plasy [Gk. *plasis*, molding, + *-ia*]. A combining form meaning *formation, development.*

-plasis [Gk. *plasis*]. A combining form meaning *molding.*

plasm (plaz′um) *n.* [Gk. *plasma*, something formed, molded, from *plassein*, to form, mold]. 1. PLASMA. 2. A part of the substance of a cell.

plasm-, plasmo-. A combining form meaning (a) *plasma;* (b) *protoplasm;* (c) *cytoplasm.*

-plasm, -plasma [Gk. *plasma*]. A combining form meaning (a) *formed material;* (b) *formative material.*

plas·ma (plaz′muh) *n.* [Gk., something formed, from *plassein*, to form, mold]. 1. The fluid portion of blood or lymph, composed of a mixture of many proteins in a crystalloid solution and corresponding closely to the interstitial fluid of the body. 2. *In nuclear technology,* an electrically neutral gaseous mixture of ions, electrons, and neutral particles formed when matter exists at temperatures of 100 million degrees or more.

plasma accelerator globulin. FACTOR V.

plasma bicarbonate. BLOOD BICARBONATE.

plas·ma·blast (plaz′muh·blast) *n.* [*plasma* + *-blast*]. The stem cell of the plasmacytes. Syn. *lymphoblastic plasma cell.*

plasma cell. The antibody-producing leukocyte into which a B lymphocyte differentiates upon stimulation by antigen. See also *humoral immunity.*

plasma cell myeloma. A malignant plasmacytoma.

plas·ma·cules (plaz′muh·kewlz) *n.pl.* [dim. of *plasma*]. HEMOCONIA.

plas·ma·cyte (plaz′muh·site) *n.* [*plasma* + *-cyte*]. PLASMA CELL. —**plasma·cyt·ic** (·sit′ick) *adj.*

plasmacytic leukemia. A type of leukemia characterized by anaplastic plasma cells in the peripheral blood.

plasmacytic myeloma or **sarcoma.** A malignant plasmacytoma.

plasmacytic series. The cells concerned in the development of plasmacytes. See also *plasmablast, proplasmacyte.*

plas·ma·cy·toid (plaz″muh·sigh′toid) *adj.* [*plasmacyte* + *-oid*]. Resembling a plasma cell.

plasmacytoid lymphocyte. PLASMA CELL.

plas·ma·cy·to·ma (plaz″muh·sigh·to′muh) *n.* [*plasmacyte* + *-oma*]. Any benign or malignant tumor of plasma cells.

plas·ma·cy·to·sis (plaz″muh·sigh·to′sis) *n.* [*plasmacyte* + *-osis*]. 1. An increase in the number of plasmacytes in the spleen, lymph nodes, bone marrow, kidney, or liver. 2. An increase in the number of plasmacytes in the peripheral blood.

plas·ma·gel (plaz′muh·jel) *n.* The portion of the cytoplasm of a cell whose physical property is that of a gel. Contr. *plasmasol.*

plas·ma·gene (plaz′muh·jeen) *n.* [*plasma* + *gene*]. CYTOGENE.

plas·mal (plaz′mal) *n.* A long-chain fatty acid aldehyde present in the form of an acetal.

plas·ma·lem·ma (plaz″muh·lem′uh) *n.* [*plasma* + *-lemma*]. PLASMA MEMBRANE.

plasma L.E. test. L.E. CELL TEST.

plas·mal·o·gen (plaz·mal′uh·jen) *n.* One of a group of phosphatides in which the fatty acid at the α' position is replaced by an α, β-unsaturated ether.

plasma membrane. A metabolically active, trilaminar sheet that encloses the cytoplasm and limits the cell, providing selective permeability and containing receptor molecules which form linkages with outside substances. Syn. *plasmalemma, cell membrane.*

plas·ma·pher·e·sis, plas·ma·phaer·e·sis (plaz″muh·fe·ree′sis, ·ferr′e·sis) *n.* [*plasma* + Gk. *aphairesis,* removal]. The withdrawal of blood from a donor to obtain plasma, its components, or the nonerythrocytic formed elements of blood, followed by return of the erythrocytes to the donor.

plasma proteins. The proteins present in blood plasma consisting of fibrinogen, albumins, and globulins.

plasma skimming. The phenomenon of plasma having few erythrocytes flowing into a small side branch of a blood vessel, most of the erythrocytes continuing along the main channel. See also *axial current.*

plas·ma·sol (plaz′muh·sol) *n.* [*plasma* + *sol*]. The more fluid portion of the cytoplasm. Contr. *plasmagel.*

plas·ma·some (plaz′muh·sohm) *n.* [*plasma* + *-some*]. A granule in cytoplasm.

plasma stains. Dyes staining cytoplasmic structures selectively.

plasma substitute. PLASMA VOLUME EXPANDER.

plasmat-, plasmato- [Gk. *plasma, plasmatos,* anything formed]. A combining form meaning (a) *protoplasm;* (b) *cytoplasm;* (c) *plasma.*

plas·ma·ther·a·py (plaz″muh·therr′uh·pee) *n.* [*plasma* + *therapy*]. Treatment by the intravenous injection of blood plasma.

plasma thromboplastic factor A. FACTOR VIII.

plasma thromboplastic factor B. FACTOR IX.

plasma thromboplastin. A procoagulant.

plasma thromboplastin antecedent. FACTOR XI. Abbreviated, PTA.

plasma thromboplastin component. FACTOR IX. Abbreviated, PTC.

plas·mat·ic (plaz·mat′ick) *adj.* Pertaining to plasma.

plasmato-. See *plasmat-.*

plas·ma·tog·a·my (plaz″muh·tog′uh·mee) *n.* [*plasmato-* + *-gamy*]. PLASTOGAMY.

plas·ma·tor·rhex·is (plaz″muh·to·reck′sis) *n.* [*plasmato-* + *-rrhexis*]. PLASMORRHEXIS.

plas·ma·to·sis (plaz″muh·to′sis) *n.* [*plasmat-* + *-osis*]. The liquefaction of cell substance.

plasma volume expander. A solution containing relatively large molecules, such as gelatin, dextran, or serum albumin, which may be administered intravenously, especially as an emergency measure, in hypovolemic shock. Syn. *plasma substitute.*

plas·mic (plaz′mick) *adj.* Of or pertaining to protoplasm or cytoplasm.

plas·min (plaz′min) *n.* [*plasma* + *-in*]. A proteolytic enzyme, present in inactive form as plasminogen, occurring in plasma, and responsible for slow digestion and lysis of fibrin clots. Syn. *fibrinolysin.*

plas·mino·gen (plaz·min′o·jen) *n.* [*plasmin* + *-gen*]. The inactive form of plasmin; when blood is shed over injured tissues, it is converted to plasmin.

plas·mino·geno·pe·nia (plaz·min″o·jen″o·pee′nee·uh) *n.* [*plasminogen* + *-penia*]. A deficiency of plasmin.

plasmo-. See *plasm-.*

plas·mo·ac·an·tho·ma (plaz″mo·ack″an·tho′muh) *n.* [*plasmo-* + *acanthoma*]. ZOON'S BALANITIS.

Plasmochin. A trademark for the antimalarial drug pamaquine, used as the pamoate salt.

plas·mo·crin vacuole (plaz′mo·krin). A crystalloid-filled vacuole in the cytoplasm of a secretory cell.

plas·mo·cyte (plaz′mo·site) *n.* PLASMA CELL. —**plas·mo·cyt·ic** (plaz″mo·sit′ick) *adj.*

plasmocytic leukemia. PLASMACYTIC LEUKEMIA.

plasmocytic myeloma or **sarcoma.** A malignant plasmacytoma.

plas·mo·cy·to·ma (plaz″mo·sigh·to′muh) *n.* PLASMACYTOMA.

plasmod-, plasmodi-. A combining form meaning *plasmodium.*

plasmodesm or **plasmodesma.** Singular of *plasmodesmata.*

plas·mo·des·ma·ta (plaz″mo·dez′muh·tuh) *n.,* sing. **plas·mo·desm** (plaz′mo·dez″um), **plas·mo·des·ma** (plaz″mo·dez′muh) [*plasmo-* + Gk. *desma,* bond]. Tunnels, present in plant cells, which provide avenues of communication through the relatively thick wall.

plasmodi-. See *plasmod-.*

plasmodia. Plural of *plasmodium.*

plas·mo·di·al (plaz·mo′dee·ul) *adj.* Pertaining to or resembling a plasmodium.

plas·mo·di·ate (plaz·mo′dee·ut, ·ate) *adj.* PLASMODIAL.

plas·mo·di·blast (plaz·mo′di·blast) *n.* [*plasmodi-* + *-blast*]. SYNCYTIOTROPHOBLAST.

plas·mod·ic (plaz·mod′ick) *adj.* PLASMODIAL.

plas·mo·di·cide (plaz·mo′di·side) *n.* [*plasmodi-* + *-cide*]. An agent that kills malaria parasites.

Plas·mo·di·i·dae (plaz·mo′dee·i·dee) *n.pl.* A family of the Haemosporidia that contains the genus *Plasmodium.*

plas·mo·di·tro·pho·blast (plaz·mo″di·tro′fo·blast, ·trof′o·) *n.* [*plasmodi-* + *trophoblast*]. SYNCYTIOTROPHOBLAST.

Plas·mo·di·um (plaz·mo′dee·um) *n.* [NL., from *plasm* + Gk. *-ōdēs,* -like]. A genus of protozoa that cause malaria in birds, lower animals, and man. —**plasmodium,** pl. **plasmo·dia,** *com. n.*

Plasmodium fal·cip·a·rum (fal·sip′uh·rum) [L. *falx, falcis,* sickle (from shape of gametocytes), + *-parum,* producing]. The species of *Plasmodium* that is the etiologic agent of falciparum malaria.

Plasmodium ma·la·ri·ae (ma·lair′ee·ee). The species of *Plasmodium* that is the etiologic agent of quartan malaria.

Plasmodium ova·le (o·vay′lee). The species of *Plasmodium* that causes ovale malaria, characterized by an oval distortion of the red blood cells.

Plasmodium vi·vax (vye′vacks). The species of *Plasmodium* that causes vivax or benign tertian malaria.

plas·mog·a·my (plaz·mog′uh·mee) *n.* [*plasmo-* + *-gamy*]. PLASTOGAMY.

plas·mo·gen (plaz′muh·jen) *n.* [*plasmo-* + *-gen*]. 1. GERM PLASM. 2. BIOPLASM.

plas·moid aqueous humor (plaz′moid). The nonphysiological aqueous humor; usually has a higher protein content and can contain a variety of inflammatory cells.

plas·mol·y·sis (plaz·mol′i·sis) *n.,* pl. **plasmoly·ses** (·seez) [*plasmo-* + *-lysis*]. Shrinkage of a cell or its contents, due to withdrawal of water by osmosis when subjected to a hypertonic salt solution. —**plas·mo·lyt·ic** (plaz″mo·lit′ick) *adj.*

plas·mo·lyze (plaz′mo·lize) *v.* To bring about plasmolysis.

plas·mo·ma (plaz·mo′muh) *n.* [*plasm-* + *-oma*]. A malignant plasmacytoma.

plas·mon (plaz′mon) *n.* [Ger.]. The hereditary properties of the egg cytoplasm. Compare *genome.*

plas·mo·nu·cle·ic acid (plaz″mo·new·klee′ick). RIBONUCLEIC ACID.

plas·moph·a·gous (plaz·mof′uh·gus) *adj.* [*plasmo-* + *-phagous*]. Pertaining to certain organisms that decompose organic matter.

plas·mop·ty·sis (plaz·mop′ti·sis) *n.* [*plasmo-* + *ptysis*]. The escape of protoplasm from a cell, due to rupture of the cell wall.

plas·mor·rhex·is (plaz″mo·reck′sis) *n.*, pl. **plasmorrhex·es** (·seez) [*plasmo-* + *-rrhexis*]. The rupture of a cell and the escape or loss of the protoplasm.

plas·mos·chi·sis (plaz·mos′ki·sis) *n.* [*plasmo-* + *-schisis*]. Protoplasmic fragmentation or cleavage.

plas·mo·some (plaz′muh·sohm) *n.* [*plasmo-* + *-some*]. 1. The true nucleolus, distinguished from the karyosomes in the nucleus. 2. Any cytoplasmic granule.

plas·mo·ther·a·py (plaz″mo·therr′uh·pee) *n.* PLASMATHERAPY.

plas·mo·trop·ic (plaz″mo·trop′ick) *adj.* [*plasmo-* + *-tropic*]. Producing excessive hemolysis in the liver, spleen, and bone marrow.

plas·mot·ro·pism (plaz·mot′ruh·piz·um) *n.* [*plasmo-* + *-tropism*]. *Obsol.* Destruction of red cells in the organs producing them.

plas·mo·zyme (plaz′mo·zime) *n.* [*plasmo-* + *-zyme*]. PROTHROMBIN.

-plast [Gk. *plastos,* formed]. A combining form meaning *primitive or formative organized unit of living matter,* such as a granule, organelle, or cell.

plas·te·in (plas′tee·in) *n.* A product of interaction between a protein digest and either pepsin or papain.

plas·ter (plas′tur) *n.* [ML. *plastrum,* from Gk. *emplastron,* from *plassein,* to mold]. 1. A substance intended for external application, made of such materials and of such consistency as to adhere to the skin. 2. Calcined gypsum or calcium sulfate.

plaster bandage. A bandage impregnated with plaster of Paris.

plaster cast. PLASTER OF PARIS CAST.

plaster of Paris. Dried calcium sulfate; used in making bandages and casts to provide mechanical support or to immobilize various parts of the body, and also in various dental procedures.

plaster of Paris cast. A mixture of gypsum and water which becomes hard upon drying; when incorporated into gauze as a binder it may be used to immobilize body parts, such as fractured bones, arthritic joints, or the spine.

plaster of Paris jacket. A casing applied by winding plaster of Paris bandages over padding, so as to encase the body in a hard mold from armpits to groin; used to immobilize the spine.

plas·tic (plas′tick) *adj.* & *n.* [Gk. *plastikos,* fit for molding]. 1. Formative; concerned with building up tissues, restoring lost parts, repairing or rectifying malformations or defects, etc., as plastic surgery, plastic operation, plastic repair. 2. Capable of being molded. 3. Any material of high molecular weight, as acrylics and polystyrene, obtained by various chemical processes, that is solid in its finished state but at some stage of its manufacture or processing can be shaped by flow. 4. Made of or pertaining to plastic.

-plastic [Gk. *plassein,* to form]. A combining form meaning *formative, developmental.*

plastic bronchitis. CROUPOUS BRONCHITIS.

plastic force. *Obsol.* The generative force of the body.

plastic inflammation. PRODUCTIVE INFLAMMATION.

plas·tic·i·ty (plas·tis′i·tee) *n.* The quality or state of being plastic.

plasticity reflex. The reflex property of maintaining a spastic limb in the position of flexion or extension in which it has been placed; a resistance to change, either lengthening or shortening.

plas·ti·ciz·er (plas′ti·sigh″zur) *n.* A substance incorporated in an organic formulation or substance to maintain it in a flexible or plastic condition, preventing or retarding cracking or development of brittleness.

plastic lymph. The inflammatory exudate that covers wounds or inflamed serous surfaces, and becomes organized by the development in it of blood vessels and connective tissues.

plastic motor. A tissue motor fashioned from muscle or tendon covered with skin, in the form of a knob, loop, or tunnel to which is attached a loop or ring; devised in certain kineplastic amputations and used in connection with a prosthesis, notably in amputations of the upper extremity. See also *club motor, loop motor, tunnel motor.*

plastic operation. A reconstructive operation, usually involving transplantation of tissue.

plastic pleurisy. A form of adhesive pleurisy in which there is a layer of semisolid exudate encapsulating the pleura.

plas·tics, *n.pl.* 1. PLASTIC SURGERY. 2. Plastic materials that are used in dentistry or surgery.

plastic splint. A splint made of plastic material that can be molded into the form desired.

plastic surgeon. A surgeon who specializes in plastic surgery.

plastic surgery. Operative repair of defects or deformities, usually involving transference of tissue.

plas·tid (plas′tid) *n.* [Gk. *plastis, plastidos,* fem. of *plastēs,* molder, creator]. 1. A hypothetical elementary organism; a cytode. 2. Any of certain small cytoplasmic bodies in plant cells, regarded as centers of certain metabolic activities of the cells.

plas·tid·ule (plas′ti·dewl) *n.* [dim. of *plastid*]. BIOPHORE.

plas·tin (plas′tin) *n. Obsol.* The substance forming the more solid portion of protoplasm, such as the linin or the cytospongioplasm.

plasto- [Gk. *plastos,* formed]. A combining form meaning (a) *cytoplasm;* (b) *plastid;* (c) *development.*

plas·to·dy·nam·ia (plas″to·dye·nam′ee·uh, ·dye·nay′mee·uh) *n.* [*plasto-* + Gk. *dynam*is, power, + *-ia*]. Growth potential.

plas·tog·a·my (plas·tog′uh·mee) *n.* [*plasto-* + *-gamy*]. Cytoplasmic fusion as contrasted with nuclear fusion.

plas·to·gene (plas′to·jeen) *n.* [*plasto-* + *-gene*]. The basic self-producing unit of the plastids of plants.

plas·to·some (plas′tuh·sohm) *n.* [*plasto-* + *-some*]. *Obsol.* MITOCHONDRION.

-plasty [Gk. *plassein,* to form, mold]. A combining form meaning *plastic surgery.*

-plasy. See *-plasia.*

plat-, platy- [Gk. *platys*]. A combining form meaning *broad, flat.*

plate, *n.* [OF., from Gk. *platys,* broad, flat]. 1. A flattened part, especially a flattened process of bone. 2. A thin piece of metal or some other substance to which artificial teeth are attached. 3. *In microbiology,* a shallow, cylindrical, covered culture dish; also such a dish containing solid cultural medium suitable for the growth of microorganisms; a petri dish. 4. *In orthopedics,* a metallic device used with screws or bolts for internal fixation of bone. 5. ARTIFICIAL DENTURE.

pla·teau (pla·to′) *n.*, pl. **plateaus, plateaux** [F.]. 1. A period, state, or stretch of relative stability, often in contrast to normally prevailing cyclical or fluctuating change. 2. In operating Geiger counter tubes, the voltage range over which the number of impulses recorded is nearly constant.

plateau pulse. A low-amplitude pulse with a slow rate of rise and a prominent anacrotic shoulder, seen in aortic stenosis.

plate culture. A method of obtaining pure cultures by the inoculation of a solid cultural medium in a petri dish with microorganisms. See also *pour plate, streak plate.*

plate·let, *n.* [dim. of *plate*]. BLOOD PLATELET.

platelet cofactor I. FACTOR VIII.

platelet cofactor II. FACTOR IX.

plate·let·phe·re·sis, platelet pheresis (plait″lit·fe·ree′sis) *n.* [*platelet* + Gk. *pherein*, to carry, take away, + *-esis*]. The removal from a donor of a quantity of blood platelets, followed by the return to him of the remaining portions of the donated blood.

platelet thrombosis. A thrombus composed of blood platelets and fibrin, chiefly the former.

plate thrombosis. PLATELET THROMBOSIS.

pla·tin·ic (pla·tin′ick) *adj.* [*platinum* + *-ic*]. Pertaining to a compound containing platinum as a tetravalent element.

plat·i·nous (plat′i·nus) *adj.* [*platinum* + *-ous*]. Pertaining to a compound containing platinum as a divalent element.

plat·i·num (plat′i·num) *n.* [NL., from Sp. *platina*, from *plata*, silver]. Pt = 195.09. A silver-white metal occurring natively or alloyed with other metals; density, approximately 21.4. It is fusible only at very high temperatures, and is insoluble in all acids except nitrohydrochloric. Platinum forms two types of compounds: platinous, in which it is divalent, and platinic, in which it is tetravalent. It is no longer used medicinally.

plat·ode (plat′ode) *n.* A flatworm, as a cestode or trematode.

plat·oid (plat′oid) *adj.* [*plat-* + *-oid*]. Broad or flat, especially as a worm.

plat·onych·ia (plat″o·nick′ee·uh) *n.* [*plat-* + *onych-* + *-ia*]. A dystrophy of the nail; consisting of a modification of its greatest curvature, which, instead of being transverse, as normally, is lengthwise.

platonychia acu·ta abra·ta (uh·kew′tuh uh·bray′tuh). Psoriasiform eruption and lesions of fingernails, consisting of round, whitish, soft, thickened spots in the center of each nail except that of the middle finger.

platy-. See *plat-*.

platy·ba·sia (plat″i·bay′see·uh) *n.* [*platy-* + *base* + *-ia*]. A developmental deformity of the skull and axis in which the base of the skull is flattened, having a basal angle of more than 152°.

platy·ce·lian, platy·coe·lian (plat″i·see′lee·un) *adj.* PLATYCELOUS.

platy·ce·lous, platy·coe·lus (plat″i·see′lus) *adj.* [*platy-* + Gk. *koilos*, hollow]. Concave in front and convex behind.

platy·ce·phal·ic (plat″i·se·fal′ick) *adj.* [*platy-* + *cephalic*]. Having a skull with a relatively flat vertex. —**platy·ceph·a·ly** (·sef′uh·lee) *n.*

platy·cne·mia (plat″ick·nee′mee·uh, plat″i·nee′mee·uh) *n.* [*platy-* + Gk. *knēmē*, leg, + *-ia*]. *In osteometry,* a pronounced mediolateral flattening of the diaphysis of the tibia, determined by a cnemic index of 64.9 or less.

platy·cne·mic (plat″ick·nee′mick, plat″i·nee′mick) *adj.* [*platy-* + *cnemic*]. Designating a tibia with a marked mediolateral flattening.

platy·cne·mism (plat″ick·nee′miz·um, plat″i·) *n.* PLATYCNEMIA.

platy·co·ria (plat″i·ko′ree·uh) *n.* [*platy-* + *cor-* + *-ia*]. MYDRIASIS.

platy·co·ri·a·sis (plat″i·ko·rye′uh·sis) *n.* [*platy-* + *cor-* + *-iasis*]. MYDRIASIS.

Platy·hel·min·thes (plat″i·hel·minth′eez) *n.pl.* [*platy-* + Gk. *helminthes*, pl. of *helmins*, worm]. A phylum of flatworms characterized by bilaterally symmetrical, many-celled, leaf-shaped bodies lacking a body cavity and usually containing both sexual elements. Includes the medically important classes Trematoda and Cestoda.

platy·hi·er·ic (plat″i·high·err′ick) *adj.* [*platy-* + *hier-* + *-ic*]. *In osteometry,* designating a sacrum that is greater in width than in length, with a hieric index of 106 or more.

platy·mer·ic (plat″i·merr′ick, ·meer′ick) *adj.* [*platy-* + *mēros*, thigh, + *-ic*]. *In osteometry,* designating a femur with a moderate anteroposterior compression and an increased mediolateral diameter in the proximal portion of the diaphysis; having a platymeric index of 75.0 to 84.9.

platymeric index. The ratio of the anteroposterior diameter of the proximal diaphysis of the femur × 100 to the transverse diameter taken parallel to the plane of the axis of the femoral neck at the level of the greatest width, from 2 to 5 cm distal from the base of the lesser trochanter. Diameters must be taken at right angles to each other. Values of the index are classified as follows:

hyperplatymeric	x–74.9
platymeric	75.0–84.9
eurymeric	85.0–99.9
stenomeric	100.0–x

Stenomeric femurs are regarded as pathologic.

platy·mor·phia (plat″i·mor′fee·uh) *n.* [*platy-* + *morph-* + *-ia*]. A flatness in the formation of the eye and shortening of the anteroposterior diameter, resulting in hyperopia.

platy·o·nych·ia (plat″ee·o·nick′ee·uh) *n.* PLATONYCHIA.

platy·opia (plat″ee·o′pee·uh) *n.* [*platy-* + *ōps, ōpos*, face, eye, + *-ia*]. Relative flatness of the root of the nose with relation to the biorbital width, designated by craniometric methods by an orbitonasal index of 107.5 or less.

platy·opic (plat″ee·op′ick, ·o′pick) *adj.* [*platy-* + Gk. *ōps, ōpos*, face, + *-ic*]. 1. *In craniometry,* designating a facial skeleton that is flat; having an orbitonasal index of 107.5 or less. 2. *In somatometry,* designating a face that is flat; having an orbitonasal index of 109.9 or less.

platy·pel·lic (plat″i·pel′ick) *adj.* [*platy-* + *-pellic*]. 1. Of a pelvis: having a transverse diameter considerably greater than the anteroposterior diameter. Contr. *android, anthropoid, gynecoid.* Specifically, having a pelvic-inlet index of 89.9 or less.

platy·pel·loid (plat″i·pel′oid) *adj.* PLATYPELLIC.

plat·yr·rhine (plat′i·rine) *adj.* [Gk. *platyrrhis, platyrrhinos*, flat-nosed]. 1. Having a broad nasal septum and nostrils directed to the sides; a characteristic of New World monkeys (Ceboidea) in contrast to Old World monkeys, apes, and human beings. Contr. *catarrhine.* 2. CHAMAERRHINE.

pla·tys·ma (pla·tiz′muh) *n.*, pl. **platysma·ta** (·tuh), **platysmas** [Gk., flat object] [NA]. A subcutaneous muscle in the neck, extending from the face to the clavicle. See also Table of Muscles in the Appendix.

platysma my·oi·des (migh·oy′deez). PLATYSMA.

platysma phenomenon. BABINSKI'S PLATYSMA SIGN.

plat·ys·ten·ce·pha·lia (plat″is·ten·se·fay′lee·uh) *n.* [Gk. *platystos*, broadest, + *encephal-* + *-ia*]. The condition of a skull very wide at the occiput and with prominent jaws.

plat·ys·ten·ceph·a·ly (plat″is·ten·sef′uh·lee) *n.* PLATYSTENCEPHALIA.

Play·fair's treatment [W. S. *Playfair*, English physician, 1836–1903]. The treatment of mental disorders, particularly mild ones, by rest and good food.

play therapy. *In psychiatry and clinical psychology,* a form of treatment, used particularly with children, in which a child's play, as with dolls in the presence of a therapist, is used as a medium for expression and communication.

plea·sure principle. *In psychoanalysis,* the instinctive endeavor to escape from pain, discomfort, or unpleasant situations; the desire to obtain the greatest possible gratification with the smallest possible effort.

pleat·ed sheet. The model of a secondary structure of protein involving side-by-side polypeptide chains in an extended zig-zag pattern, as exemplified by β-keratin.

plec·to·ne·mic (pleck″to·nee′mick) *adj.* [Gk. *plektos*, twisted, + *nema*, thread, + *-ic*]. Resembling or consisting of threads twisted together.

plectonemic coil. A chromosome coil in which the subunits are intertwined and separable only by uncoiling. Contr. *paranemic coil.*

pled·get (plej'it) *n.* A small, flattened compress usually of cotton or gauze.

-plegia [Gk. *plēgē*, blow, stroke (rel. to L. *plaga*→OF. *plague*) + *-ia*]. A combining form meaning *paralysis.*

-plegic [Gk. *plēgē*, blow, stroke, + *-ic*]. A combining form meaning (a) *paralyzed;* (b) *pertaining to paralysis.*

Plegine. Trademark for phendimetrazine, an anorexiant drug used as the bitartrate salt.

plei-, pleio-. See *pleo-.*

plei·ot·ro·pism (plye·ot'ro·piz·um) *n.* [*pleio-* + *-tropism*]. The occurrence of multiple effects produced by a given gene. —**plei·o·trop·ic** (·o·trop'ick) *adj.*

pleo-, pleon-, plei-, pleio- [Gk. *pleiōn*, more]. A combining form meaning (a) *multiple;* (b) *excessive, extra.*

pleo·chro·ic (plee''o·kro'ick) *adj.* [*pleo-* + Gk. *chroia*, color, + *-ic*]. The capacity of a substance to show more than one color.

ple·och·ro·ism (plee·ock'ro·iz·um) *n.* [*pleochroic* + *-ism*]. The property possessed by some bodies, especially crystals, of presenting different colors when viewed in the direction of different axes. —**pleo·chro·it·ic** (plee''o·kro·it'ick), **pleochro·mat·ic** (·mat'ick) *adj.*

pleo·chrome cells (plee'o·krome). CHROMAFFIN CELLS.

pleo·co·ni·al (plee''o·ko'nee·ul) *adj.* [*pleo-* + *coni-* + *-al*]. Of, pertaining to, or characterized by more than the usual number of mitochondria or particles seen in certain muscle cells with the electron microscope.

pleoconial myopathy. A rare disorder of muscle, observed in childhood, characterized by the presence of large quantities of mitochondria throughout the muscle cells, and associated clinically with proximal muscle weakness and wasting, as well as prolonged episodes of flaccid paralysis and craving for salt.

pleo·cy·to·sis (plee''o·sigh·to'sis) *n.*, pl. **pleocyto·ses** (·seez) [*pleo-* + *cyt-* + *-osis*]. Increase of cells in the cerebrospinal fluid.

pleo·mas·tia (plee''o·mas'tee·uh) *n.* [*pleo-* + *-mastia*]. POLYMASTIA.

pleo·ma·zia (plee''o·may'zee·uh) *n.* [*pleo-* + *maz-* + *-ia*]. POLYMASTIA.

pleo·mor·phic (plee''o·mor'fick) *adj.* Pertaining to or characterized by pleomorphism.

pleomorphic adenoma. A mixed tumor of the type usually found in a salivary gland.

pleomorphic carcinoma. A poorly differentiated carcinoma whose parenchymal cells vary widely in size and general appearance.

pleomorphic fibroadenoma. FIBROADENOMA.

pleomorphic granular-cell sarcoma. A malignant GRANULAR CELL MYOBLASTOMA.

pleomorphic lymphosarcoma. HODGKIN'S DISEASE.

pleo·mor·phism (plee''o·mor'fiz·um) *n.* [*pleo-* + *morph-* + *-ism*]. Marked difference in size, shape, or other morphological features, among individuals of a single kind or class, as among bacteria of a particular species or cells of a given type. Mesomorphism in cells may include variation in nuclear characteristics and is seen especially in dysplastic or anaplastic cells, but also in such normal cells as trophoblasts.

pleo·mor·phous (plee''o·mor'fus) *adj.* Pertaining to or characterized by pleomorphism.

pleon-. See *pleo-.*

ple·o·nasm (plee'o·naz·um) *n.* [Gk. *pleonasma*, superfluity]. Any malformation marked by superabundance or excessive size of certain organs or parts. —**ple·o·nas·tic** (plee''o·nas'tick) *adj.*

ple·o·nec·tic (plee''o·neck'tick) *adj.* [Gk. *pleonektikos*, greedy]. 1. Pertaining to or characterized by pleonexia. 2. Pertaining to blood having more than the normal saturation of oxygen.

ple·o·nex·ia (plee''o·neck'see·uh) *n.* [Gk., greediness, from *pleon*, more, + *echein*, to have, hold]. Excessive desire to have or possess; abnormal greed.

ple·o·nexy (plee'o·neck''see) *n.* PLEONEXIA.

ple·on·os·te·o·sis (plee''on·os''tee·o'sis) *n.* [*pleon-* + *osteosis*]. Excessive or premature ossification.

pleonosteosis of Leri [A. *Leri*.]. A rare hereditary condition characterized by thickening and deformity of the digits, limited joint movements, short stature, and mongoloid facies.

ple·o·no·tus (plee''o·no'tus) *n.* [NL., from *pleon-* + Gk. *ous*, *ōtos*, ear]. An earlike appendage located on the neck; cervical auricle.

ple·ro·cer·coid (pleer''o·sur'koid) *n.* [Gk. *plērēs*, full, + *kerkos*, tail, + *-oid*]. The second larval stage in the intermediate host of certain cestodes.

ple·ro·sis (ple·ro'sis) *n.* [Gk. *plērōsis*, a filling]. 1. The restoration of lost tissue. 2. PLETHORA.

plesi-, plesio- [Gk. *plēsios*]. A combining form meaning (a) *near;* (b) *similar.*

ple·sio·gnath·us (plee''see·o·nath'us) *n.* [*plesio-* + *-gnathus*]. An accessory mouth in the parotid region.

ple·sio·mor·phism (plee''see·o·mor'fiz·um) *n.* [*plesio-* + *-morphism*]. Similarity in form.

ple·si·opia (plee''see·o'pee·uh) *n.* [*plesi-* + *-opia*]. Increased convexity of the crystalline lens, producing myopia.

ples·ses·the·sia, ples·saes·the·sia (ples''es·theezh'uh, ·theez'ee·uh) *n.* [Gk. *plessein*, to strike, + *esthesia*]. PALPATORY PERCUSSION.

ples·sim·e·ter (ple·sim'e·tur) *n.* [Gk. *plessein*, to strike, + *-meter*]. PLEXIMETER.

ples·sor (ples'ur) *n.* PLEXOR.

pleth·o·ra (pleth'uh·ruh) *n.* [Gk. *plēthōra*, fullness, from *plēthos*, mass, quantity, bulk]. A state characterized by excess of blood in the body. —**ple·tho·ric** (pleth'uh·rick, ple·tho'rick) *adj.*

plethora apo·cop·ti·ca (ap''o·kop'ti·kuh). A temporary increase in the volume of the blood in other parts of the body, caused by forcing blood from a part to be amputated.

plethoric dysmenorrhea. CONGESTIVE DYSMENORRHEA.

ple·thys·mo·gram (ple·thiz'mo·gram) *n.* A record made by a plethysmograph.

ple·thys·mo·graph (ple·thiz'mo·graf) *n.* [Gk. *plēthysmos*, increase, + *-graph*]. A device for ascertaining rapid changes in volume of an organ or part, through an increase in the quantity of the blood therein. —**ple·thys·mo·graph·ic** (ple·thiz''mo·graf'ick) *adj.*

pleth·ys·mog·ra·phy (pleth''iz·mog'ruh·fee) *n.* [*plēthysmos*, increase, + *-graphy*]. Measurement of volume changes of an extremity or of an organ.

pleur-, pleuro- [Gk. *pleura*, ribs, side]. A combining form meaning (a) *pleura, pleural;* (b) *side, lateral;* (c) *pleurisy.*

pleu·ra (ploor'uh) *n.*, pl. **pleu·rae** (·ree) [Gk., ribs, side] [NA]. The serous membrane enveloping the lung and lining the internal surface of the thoracic cavity. See also *parietal pleura, pulmonary pleura.*

pleu·ra·cen·te·sis (ploor''uh·sen·tee'sis) *n.* PLEUROCENTESIS.

pleura cos·ta·lis (kos·tay'lis) [NA]. COSTAL PLEURA.

pleu·ra·cot·o·my (ploor''uh·kot'uh·mee) *n.* [*pleur-* + *thoracotomy*]. Incision of the thoracic wall and pleura, usually exploratory. Syn. *thoracotomy.*

pleura di·a·phrag·ma·ti·ca (dye''uh·frag·mat'i·kuh) [NA]. DIAPHRAGMATIC PLEURA.

pleu·ral (ploo'rul) *adj.* Of or pertaining to the pleura.

pleural canal. In the embryo, a narrow coelomic passage on either side of the mesentery dorsal to the transverse septum that connects pericardial and general coelom; it later develops into the pleural cavity.

pleural cavity. The potential space, included between the parietal and visceral layers of the pleura. NA *cavum pleurae.*

pleu·ral·gia (ploo·ral'jee·uh) *n.* [*pleur-* + *-algia*]. Pain in the pleura or in the side. —**pleural·gic** (·jick) *adj.*

pleural sac. The sac formed by the pleura.

pleural sarcoma. Malignant mesothelioma of the pleura.

pleural shock. Hypotension, sweating, pallor, and collapse due to pleural irritation, as with a trocar. Syn. *Capp's pleural reflex.*

pleural sinus. 1. COSTOMEDIASTINAL RECESS. 2. COSTODIAPHRAGMATIC RECESS.

pleural space. PLEURAL CAVITY.

pleura me·di·a·sti·na·lis (mee·dee·as·ti·nay'lis) [NA]. MEDIASTINAL PLEURA.

pleur·am·ni·on (ploor·am'nee·on) *n.* [*pleur-* + *amnion*]. An amnion developing by folds, as in sauropsidans and some mammals. Contr. *schizamnion.*

pleura pa·ri·e·ta·lis (pa·rye"e·tay'lis) [NA]. PARIETAL PLEURA.

pleura pe·ri·car·di·a·ca (perr"i·kahr·dye'uh·kuh) [BNA]. PERICARDIAC PLEURA.

pleur·apoph·y·sis (ploor"uh·pof'i·sis) *n.* [*pleur-* + *apophysis*]. One of the lateral processes of a vertebra, corresponding morphologically to a rib. —**pleur·apo·phys·i·al** (·ap·o·fiz'ee·ul), **pleur·apoph·y·se·al** (·a·pof"i·see'ul) *adj.*

pleura pul·mo·na·lis (pul·mo·nay'lis) [NA]. PULMONARY PLEURA.

pleu·ra·tome (ploor'uh·tome) *n.* [*pleura* + *-tome*]. The area of the pleura supplied with sensory fibers from a single spinal nerve.

pleu·rec·to·my (ploo·reck'tuh·mee) *n.* [*pleur-* + *-ectomy*]. Excision of any portion of the pleura.

pleu·ri·sy (ploor'i·see) *n.* [ML. *pleuresis,* from Gk. *pleuritis*]. Inflammation of the pleura. Syn. *pleuritis.*

pleu·rit·ic (ploo·rit'ick) *adj.* [Gk. *pleuritikos,* suffering from pleurisy]. Pertaining to, affected with, or of the nature of pleurisy.

pleu·ri·tis (ploo·rye'tis) *n.,* pl. **pleu·rit·i·des** (ploo·rit'i·deez) [Gk.]. PLEURISY.

pleuro-. See *pleur-.*

pleu·ro·cen·te·sis (ploor"o·sen·tee'sis) *n.* [*pleuro-* + *centesis*]. Puncture of the parietal pleura. See also *thoracentesis.*

pleu·ro·cen·trum (ploor"o·sen'trum) *n.* [*pleuro-* + *centrum*]. The lateral half of a vertebral body, as in a cleft centrum, or when only a lateral half is ossified. Syn. *hemicentrum.* —**pleurocen·tral** (·trul) *adj.*

pleu·ro·cho·le·cys·ti·tis (ploor"o·kol"e·sis·tye'tis, ·ko"le·) *n.* [*pleuro-* + *cholecystitis*]. Inflammation of the gallbladder, with involvement of the diaphragmatic pleura.

pleu·ro·cu·ta·ne·ous (ploor"o·kew·tay'nee·us) *n.* [*pleuro-* + *cutaneous*]. Pertaining to the parietal pleura and the skin, as a pleurocutaneous fistula.

pleur·odont (ploor'o·dont) *n.* [*pleur-* + *-odont*]. Having teeth affixed to the side of the bone which supports them, as in certain lower vertebrates. See also *acrodont, thecodont.*

pleu·ro·dyn·ia (ploor"o·din'ee·uh) *n.* [*pleur-* + *-odynia*]. 1. Severe paroxysmal pain and tenderness of the intercostal muscles. 2. EPIDEMIC PLEURODYNIA.

pleu·ro·gen·ic (ploor"o·jen'ick) *adj.* [*pleuro-* + *-genic*]. Originating in the pleura.

pleu·rog·e·nous (ploo·roj'e·nus) *adj.* [*pleuro-* + *-genous*]. PLEUROGENIC.

pleu·ro·hep·a·ti·tis (ploor"o·hep"uh·tye'tis) *n.* [*pleuro-* + *hepatitis*]. Inflammation of the liver and diaphragmatic part of the pleura.

pleu·ro·lith (ploor'o·lith) *n.* [*pleuro-* + *-lith*]. A calculus in the pleura or the pleural cavity.

pleu·rol·y·sis (ploo·rol'i·sis) *n.* [*pleuro-* + *-lysis*]. Separation of the parietal pleura from the chest wall.

pleu·ro·ma (ploo·ro'muh) *n.* [*pleur-* + *-oma*]. Mesothelioma of the pleura.

pleu·ro·me·lus (ploor"o·mee'lus) *n.* [*pleuro-* + *-melus*]. An individual having a parasitic or accessory limb arising from the thorax laterally.

pleu·ro·peri·car·di·al (ploor"o·perr·i·kahr'dee·ul) *adj.* [*pleuro-* + *pericardial*]. Pertaining to both pleura and pericardium.

pleuropericardial canal or **duct.** The opening in the pleuropericardial membrane temporarily connecting the embryonic pleural and pericardial cavities.

pleuropericardial membrane. The embryonic membrane, derived from the septum transversum, that separates the pericardial coelom from the pleural canal.

pleu·ro·peri·car·di·tis (ploor"o·perr"i·kahr·dye'tis) *n.* [*pleuro-* + *pericarditis*]. Pleurisy associated with pericarditis.

pleu·ro·peri·to·ne·al (ploor"o·perr·i·to·nee'ul) *adj.* [*pleuro-* + *peritoneal*]. Pertaining to the pleura and the peritoneum.

pleuroperitoneal canal or **duct.** The opening in the pleuroperitoneal membrane temporarily connecting the embryonic pleural and peritoneal cavities.

pleuroperitoneal cavity. The coelom or body cavity.

pleuroperitoneal hiatus. A small opening in the diaphragm between pleural and peritoneal cavities in the fetus.

pleuroperitoneal membrane. The embryonic membrane, derived in large measure from the septum transversum, that separates the pleural canal from the peritoneal part of the coelom. It forms a part of the diaphragm.

pleu·ro·pneu·mo·nia (ploor"o·new·mo'nyuh) *n.* [*pleuro-* + *pneumonia*]. 1. Combined pleurisy and pneumonia. 2. An infectious disease of cattle producing pleural and lung inflammation, caused by organisms of the Mycoplasma group.

pleuropneumonia-like organisms. A widely prevalent group of minute, filterable, highly pleomorphic microorganisms belonging to the Mycoplasmataceae; responsible for primary atypical pneumonia in man, for lung disease of cattle and goats, and for mastitis of sheep and goats. Abbreviated, PPLO.

pleu·ro·pros·o·pos·chi·sis (ploor"o·pros"o·pos'ki·sis) *n.* [*pleuro-* + *prosoposchisis*]. PROSOPOSCHISIS.

pleu·ro·pul·mo·nary (ploor"o·pul'muh·nerr"ee, ·pŏŏl') *n.* [*pleuro-* + *pulmonary*]. Pertaining to the pleura and lungs.

pleuropulmonary congestion. 1. WOILLEZ' DISEASE. 2. PULMONARY EDEMA.

pleu·ros·co·py (ploo·ros'kuh·pee) *n.* [*pleuro-* + *-scopy*]. THORACOSCOPY.

pleu·ro·so·ma (ploor"o·so'muh) *n.* [*pleuro-* + *-soma*]. Fissure of both abdomen and thorax with lateral eventration and atrophy or imperfect development of the arm on the side of the eventration.

pleu·ro·so·ma·tos·chi·sis (ploor"o·so"muh·tos'ki·sis) *n.* [*pleuro-* + *somato-* + *-schisis*]. A lateral abdominal fissure.

pleu·ro·so·mus (ploor"o·so'mus) *n.* [*pleuro-* + *-somus*]. An individual exhibiting pleurosoma.

pleu·ro·spasm (ploor'o·spaz·um) *n.* [*pleuro-* + *spasm*]. Cramp, or spasm of the chest wall.

pleu·ro·thot·o·nos, pleu·ro·thot·o·nus (ploo"ro·thot'uh·nus) *n.* [Gk. *pleurothen,* from the side, + *tonos,* tension]. A form of tetanic spasm of the muscles in which the body is bent to one side.

pleu·rot·o·my (ploo·rot'uh·mee) *n.* [*pleuro-* + *-tomy*]. Incision into the pleura.

pleu·ro·ty·phoid (ploor"o·tye'foid) *n.* [*pleuro-* + *typhoid*]. Typhoid fever with pleurisy.

pleu·ro·vis·cer·al (ploor"o·vis'ur·ul) *adj.* [*pleuro-* + *visceral*]. Pertaining to the pleura and to the viscera.

plex·ec·to·my (pleck·seck'tuh·mee) *n.* [*plexus* + *-ectomy*]. Surgical removal of a plexus.

plex·i·form (pleck'si·form) *adj.* [*plexus* + *-iform*]. Resembling a network or plexus.

plexiform angioma. An angioma consisting of tortuous blood vessels.

plexiform layer. MOLECULAR LAYER OF THE RETINA.

plexiform neurofibroma or **neuroma.** 1. A diffuse proliferation of nerve fibers and connective tissue elements producing tortuosity and thickening of the affected segment. 2. PACHYDERMATOCELE.

plex·im·e·ter (pleck·sim'e·tur) *n.* [Gk. *plēxis,* stroke, + *-me-*

ter]. 1. A finger, usually the left third finger, held firmly against the skin to receive the stroke in indirect percussion. 2. A small, thin, oblong plate of hard but flexible material, such as ivory or rubber, used for the same purpose.

plex·om·e·ter (pleck·som'e·tur) *n.* PLEXIMETER.

plex·op·a·thy (pleck·sop'uh·thee) *n.* Any disease of a plexus.

plex·or (pleck'sur) *n.* [Gk. *plēxis*, stroke, + *-or*]. A finger, when used to tap the surface of the body in performing percussion. Syn. *plessor.* See also *reflex hammer.*

plex·us (pleck'sus) *n.*, L. pl. & genit. sing. **plexus,** E. pl. **plexuses** [L., network, from *plectere*, to plait]. A network of interlacing nerves or anastomosing blood vessels or lymphatics. —**plex·al** (·sul) *adj.*

plexus aor·ti·cus ab·do·mi·na·lis (ay·or'ti·kus ab·dom''i·nay'lis) [NA]. A visceral nerve network associated with the abdominal aorta.

plexus aorticus tho·ra·ca·lis (tho·ruh·kay'lis) [BNA]. PLEXUS AORTICUS THORACICUS.

plexus aorticus tho·ra·ci·cus (tho·ray'si·kus) [NA]. A visceral nerve network associated with the thoracic aorta.

plexus ar·te·ri·ae ce·re·bri an·te·ri·o·ris (ahr·teer'ee·ee serr'e·brye an·teer''ee·o'ris) [BNA]. A network of nerve fibers associated with the anterior cerebral artery.

plexus arteriae cerebri me·dii (mee'dee·eye) [BNA]. A network of nerve fibers associated with the middle cerebral artery.

plexus arteriae cho·ri·oi·de·ae (ko·ree·oy'dee·ee) [BNA]. A network of nerve fibers associated with a choroidal artery.

plexus arteriae ova·ri·cae (o·vair'i·see) [BNA]. Plexus ovaricus (= OVARIAN PLEXUS (2)).

plexus au·ri·cu·la·ris posterior (aw·rick''yoo·lair'is) [BNA]. Nerve fibers associated with the posterior auricular artery.

plexus au·to·no·mi·ci (aw·to·nom'i·sigh) [NA]. AUTONOMIC PLEXUSES.

plexus axil·la·ris (ack·si·lair'is) [BNA]. AXILLARY PLEXUS.

plexus ba·si·la·ris (bas·i·lair'is) [NA]. BASILAR PLEXUS.

plexus bra·chi·a·lis (bray·kee·ay'lis) [NA]. BRACHIAL PLEXUS.

plexus car·di·a·cus (kahr·dye'uh·kus) [NA]. CARDIAC PLEXUS.

plexus ca·ro·ti·cus com·mu·nis (ka·rot'i·kus kom·yoo'nis) [NA]. COMMON CAROTID PLEXUS.

plexus caroticus ex·ter·nus (ecks·tur'nus) [NA]. EXTERNAL CAROTID PLEXUS.

plexus caroticus in·ter·nus (in·tur'nus) [NA]. INTERNAL CAROTID PLEXUS.

plexus ca·ver·no·si con·cha·rum (kav''ur·no'sigh kong·kair'um) [NA]. The cavernous plexuses of the conchae. See *cavernous plexus.*

plexus ca·ver·no·sus cli·to·ri·dis (kav''ur·no'sus kli·tor'i·dis) [BNA]. The cavernous plexus of the clitoris; a nerve plexus in the corpus cavernosum.

plexus cavernosus pe·nis (pee'nis) [BNA]. The cavernous plexus of the penis; a nerve plexus in the corpus cavernosum.

plexus ce·li·a·cus (se·lye'uh·kus) [NA]. CELIAC PLEXUS.

plexus cer·vi·ca·lis (sur·vi·kay'lis) [NA]. CERVICAL PLEXUS.

plexus cho·roi·de·us ven·tri·cu·li la·te·ra·lis (ko·roy'dee·us ven·trick'yoo·lye lat·e·ray'lis) [NA]. The choroid plexus of the lateral ventricle.

plexus choroideus ventriculi quar·ti (kwahr'tye) [NA]. The choroid plexus of the fourth ventricle.

plexus choroideus ventriculi ter·tii (tur'shee·eye) [NA]. The choroid plexus of the third ventricle.

plexus coc·cy·ge·us (kock·sij'ee·us) [NA]. COCCYGEAL PLEXUS.

plexus coe·li·a·cus (see·lye'uh·kus) [BNA]. Plexus celiacus (= CELIAC PLEXUS).

plexus co·ro·na·ri·us cor·dis anterior (kor·o·nair'ee·us kor'dis) [BNA]. A network of visceral nerve fibers anterior to the heart. See also *coronary plexus.*

plexus coronarius cordis posterior [BNA]. A network of visceral nerve fibers posterior to the heart. See also *coronary plexus.*

plexus de·fe·ren·ti·a·lis (def·e·ren''shee·ay'lis) [NA]. DEFERENTIAL PLEXUS.

plexus den·ta·lis inferior (den·tay'lis) [NA]. The inferior dental plexus.

plexus dentalis superior [NA]. The superior dental plexus.

plexus en·te·ri·cus (en·terr'i·kus) [NA]. ENTERIC PLEXUS.

plexus eso·pha·ge·us (ee''so·faj'ee·us, e·sof''uh·jee'us) [NA]. ESOPHAGEAL PLEXUS.

plexus fe·mo·ra·lis (fem''o·ray'lis) [NA]. FEMORAL PLEXUS.

plexus gan·gli·o·sus ci·li·a·ris (gang·glee·o'sus sil·ee·air'is) [BNA]. A network of nerve fibers associated with the ciliary ganglion.

plexus gas·tri·ci (gas'tri·sigh) [NA]. GASTRIC PLEXUSES.

plexus gas·tri·cus anterior (gas'tri·kus) [BNA]. RAMI GASTRICI ANTERIORES NERVI VAGI.

plexus gastricus inferior [BNA]. A network of nerve fibers associated with the greater curvature of the stomach.

plexus gastricus posterior [BNA]. RAMI GASTRICI POSTERIORES NERVI VAGI.

plexus gastricus superior [BNA]. A network of nerve fibers associated with the lesser curvature of the stomach.

plexus hae·mor·rhoi·da·lis me·di·us (hem''uh·roy·day'lis mee'dee·us) [BNA]. Plexus rectalis medius (= RECTAL PLEXUS (2b)).

plexus haemorrhoidalis superior [BNA]. Plexus rectalis superior (= RECTAL PLEXUS (2a)).

plexus haemorrhoidalis ve·no·sus (ve·no'sus) [BNA]. Plexus venosus rectalis (= RECTAL PLEXUS (1)).

plexus he·pa·ti·cus (he·pat'i·kus) [NA]. HEPATIC PLEXUS.

plexus hy·po·gas·tri·cus (high·po·gas'tri·kus) [BNA]. The nerve plexus now divided into plexus hypogastricus inferior, plexus hypogastricus superior, and nervus hypogastricus.

plexus hypogastricus inferior [NA]. INFERIOR HYPOGASTRICUS PLEXUS.

plexus hypogastricus superior [NA alt.]. SUPERIOR HYPOGASTRIC PLEXUS. NA alt. *nervus presacralis.*

plexus ili·a·ci (i·lye'uh·sigh) [NA]. ILIAC PLEXUSES.

plexus ili·a·cus (i·lye'uh·kus) [BNA]. Singular of *plexus iliaci.*

plexus iliacus ex·ter·nus (ecks·tur'nus) [BNA]. A network of nerve fibers associated with the external iliac artery.

plexus in·gui·na·lis (ing·gwi·nay'lis) [BNA]. A lymphatic network about the termination of the great saphenous vein.

plexus in·ter·me·sen·te·ri·cus (in''tur·mes·en·terr'i·kus) [NA]. A network of nerve fibers about the abdominal aorta between the superior and inferior mesenteric plexuses.

plexus ju·gu·la·ris (jug·yoo·lair'is) [BNA]. A network of lymphatic vessels around the internal jugular vein.

plexus li·e·na·lis (lye·e·nay'lis) [NA]. SPLENIC PLEXUS.

plexus lin·gua·lis (ling·gway'lis) [BNA]. LINGUAL PLEXUS.

plexus lum·ba·lis (lum·bay'lis) [NA]. LUMBAR PLEXUS.

plexus lum·bo·sa·cra·lis (lum''bo·sa·kray'lis) [NA]. LUMBOSACRAL PLEXUS.

plexus lym·pha·ti·cus (lim·fat'i·kus) [NA]. A general term for any network of lymphatic vessels.

plexus mam·ma·ri·us (ma·mair'ee·us) [BNA]. A network of lymphatic vessels about the internal thoracic artery.

plexus mammarius in·ter·nus (in·tur'nus) [BNA]. A network of nerve fibers associated with the mammary gland.

plexus max·il·la·ris ex·ter·nus (mack·si·lair'is ecks·tur'nus) [BNA]. The external maxillary plexus. See *maxillary plexuses.*

plexus maxillaris in·ter·nus (in·tur'nus) [BNA]. The internal maxillary plexus. See *maxillary plexuses.*

plexus me·nin·ge·us (me·nin'jee·us) [BNA]. MENINGEAL PLEXUS.

plexus mes·en·te·ri·cus inferior (mes·en·terr'i·kus) [NA]. INFERIOR MESENTERIC PLEXUS.

plexus mesentericus superior [NA]. SUPERIOR MESENTERIC PLEXUS.

plexus my·en·te·ri·cus (migh·en·terr'i·kus) [NA]. MYENTERIC PLEXUS.

plexus ner·vo·rum spi·na·li·um (nur·vo'rum spye·nay'lee·um) [NA]. A general term for the intermingling of nerve fibers of more than one spinal nerve.

plexus oc·ci·pi·ta·lis (ock·sip·i·tay'lis) [BNA]. OCCIPITAL PLEXUS.

plexus oe·so·pha·ge·us anterior (e·sof''uh·jee'us, ee''so·faj'ee·us) [BNA]. The anterior part of the esophageal plexus.

plexus oesophageus posterior [BNA]. The posterior part of the esophageal plexus.

plexus of Cruveilhier [J. *Cruveilhier*]. CERVICAL POSTERIOR PLEXUS.

plexus oph·thal·mi·cus (off·thal'mi·kus) [BNA]. OPHTHALMIC PLEXUS.

plexus ova·ri·cus (o·vair'i·kus) [NA]. OVARIAN PLEXUS (2).

plexus pam·pi·ni·for·mis (pam·pin·i·for'mis) [NA]. PAMPINIFORM PLEXUS.

plexus pan·cre·a·ti·cus (pan·kree·at'i·kus) [NA]. A network of visceral nerve fibers associated with the pancreas; it is a subdivision of the celiac plexus.

plexus pa·ro·ti·de·us (pa·rot''i·dee'us) [NA]. PAROTID PLEXUS.

plexus pel·vi·nus (pel·vye'nus) [NA alt.]. INFERIOR HYPOGASTRIC PLEXUS. NA alt. *plexus hypogastricus inferior*.

plexus pe·ri·ar·te·ri·a·lis (perr''ee·ahr·teer·ee·ay'lis) [NA]. A general term for the network of nerve fibers associated with the tunica adventitia of any artery.

plexus pha·ryn·ge·us (fa·rin'jee·us) [NA]. PHARYNGEAL PLEXUS (1).

plexus pharyngeus ascen·dens (a·sen'denz) [BNA]. A network of nerve fibers associated with the ascending pharyngeal artery.

plexus pharyngeus ner·vi va·gi (nur'vye vay'guy) [NA]. A network of nerve fibers in the wall of the pharynx.

plexus pharyngeus ve·no·sus (ve·no'sus) [BNA]. PHARYNGEAL PLEXUS (2).

plexus phre·ni·cus (fren'i·kus) [BNA]. PHRENIC PLEXUS.

plexus po·pli·te·us (pop·lit'ee·us) [BNA]. POPLITEAL PLEXUS.

plexus pro·sta·ti·cus (pros·tat'i·kus) [NA]. PROSTATIC PLEXUS (1).

plexus pte·ry·goi·de·us (terr·i·goy'dee·us) [NA]. PTERYGOID PLEXUS.

plexus pu·den·da·lis ve·no·sus (pew·den·day'lis ve·no'sus) [BNA]. Plexus venosus prostaticus (= PUDENDAL PLEXUS (2)).

plexus pu·den·dus ner·vo·sus (pew·den'dus nur·vo'sus) [BNA]. Nervus pudendus (= PUDENDAL NERVE).

plexus pul·mo·na·lis (pul·mo·nay'lis) [NA]. PULMONARY PLEXUS.

plexus pulmonalis anterior [BNA]. The anterior pulmonary plexus.

plexus pulmonalis posterior [BNA]. The posterior pulmonary plexus.

plexus rec·ta·les inferiores (reck·tay'leez in·feer·ee·o'reez) [NA]. RECTAL PLEXUSES (2c).

plexus rectales me·di·i (mee'dee·eye) [NA]. RECTAL PLEXUSES (2b).

plexus rectalis superior [NA]. RECTAL PLEXUS (2a).

plexus re·na·lis (re·nay'lis) [NA]. RENAL PLEXUS.

plexus sa·cra·lis (sa·kray'lis) [NA]. SACRAL PLEXUS.

plexus sacralis anterior [BNA]. Plexus venosus sacralis (= ANTERIOR SACRAL PLEXUS).

plexus sacralis me·di·us (mee'dee·us) [BNA]. A network of lymphatic vessels on the anterior surface of the sacrum.

plexus sper·ma·ti·cus (spur·mat'i·kus) [BNA]. Plexus testicularis (= SPERMATIC PLEXUS).

plexus sub·cla·vi·us (sub·klay'vee·us) [NA]. SUBCLAVIAN PLEXUS.

plexus sub·mu·co·sus (sub·mew·ko'sus) [NA]. SUBMUCOUS PLEXUS.

plexus sub·se·ro·sus (sub·se·ro'sus) [NA]. A network of nerve fibers situated beneath the tunica serosa of the intestine.

plexus su·pra·re·na·lis (sue·pruh·re·nay'lis) [NA]. SUPRARENAL PLEXUS.

plexus sym·pa·thi·ci (sim·path'i·sigh) [BNA]. Plexus autonomici (= AUTONOMIC PLEXUSES).

plexus tem·po·ra·lis su·per·fi·ci·a·lis (tem·po·ray'lis sue·pur·fish·ee·ay'lis) [BNA]. A network of nerve fibers associated with the superficial temporal artery.

plexus te·sti·cu·la·ris (tes·tick·yoo·lair'is) [NA]. SPERMATIC PLEXUS.

plexus thy·re·oi·de·us im·par (thigh·ree·oy'dee·us im'pahr) [BNA]. Plexus thyroideus impar (= THYROID IMPAR PLEXUS).

plexus thyreoideus inferior [BNA]. The inferior portion of the thyroid plexus.

plexus thyreoideus superior [BNA]. The superior portion of the thyroid plexus.

plexus thy·roi·de·us im·par (thigh·roy'dee·us im'pahr) [NA]. THYROID IMPAR PLEXUS.

plexus tym·pa·ni·cus (tim·pan'i·kus) [NA]. TYMPANIC PLEXUS.

plexus ure·te·ri·cus (yoo·re·terr'i·kus) [NA]. A network of nerve fibers associated with either ureter; a subdivision of the celiac plexus.

plexus ute·ro·va·gi·na·lis (yoo''tur·o·vaj·i·nay'lis) [NA]. UTEROVAGINAL PLEXUS (1).

plexus uterovaginalis ve·no·sus (ve·no'sus) [BNA]. The uterovaginal venous plexus; UTEROVAGINAL PLEXUS (2).

plexus vas·cu·lo·sus (vas·kew·lo'sus) [NA]. A general term for any network of vessels.

plexus ve·no·si ver·te·bra·les an·te·ri·o·res (ve·no'sigh vur·te·bray'leez an·teer·ee·o'reez) [BNA]. The anterior vertebral venous plexuses. See *vertebral plexuses* (2).

plexus venosi vertebrales ex·ter·ni an·te·ri·or et pos·te·ri·or (ecks·tur'nigh an·teer'ee·or et pos·teer'ee·or) [NA]. The anterior and posterior external vertebral plexuses. See *vertebral plexus* (2).

plexus venosi vertebrales in·ter·ni an·te·ri·or et pos·te·ri·or (in·tur'nigh an·teer'ee·or et pos·teer'ee·or) [NA]. The anterior and posterior internal vertebral plexuses. See *vertebral plexus* (2).

plexus venosi vertebrales pos·te·ri·o·res (pos·teer·ee·o'reez) [BNA]. The posterior vertebral venous plexuses. See *vertebral plexuses* (2).

plexus ve·no·sus (ve·no'sus) [NA]. VENOUS PLEXUS.

plexus venosus are·o·la·ris (ăr''e·o·lair'is) [NA]. A venous plexus associated with the areola of the mammary gland.

plexus venosus ca·na·lis hy·po·glos·si (ka·nay'lis high·po·glos'eye) [NA]. A venous network surrounding the hypoglossal nerve in the hypoglossal canal.

plexus venosus ca·ro·ti·cus in·ter·nus (ka·rot'i·kus in·tur'nus) [NA]. A venous plexus associated with the internal carotid artery where it lies in the carotid canal.

plexus venosus fo·ra·mi·nis ova·lis (fo·ram'i·nis o·vay'lis) [NA]. A venous plexus in the foramen ovale connecting the cavernous sinus with the pterygoid plexus.

plexus venosus ma·mil·lae (ma·mil'ee) [BNA]. PLEXUS VENOSUS AREOLARIS.

plexus venosus pro·sta·ti·cus (pros·tat'i·kus) [NA]. PUDENDAL PLEXUS (2).

plexus venosus rec·ta·lis (reck·tay'lis) [NA]. RECTAL PLEXUS (1).

plexus venosus sa·cra·lis (sa·kray'lis) [NA]. ANTERIOR SACRAL PLEXUS.

plexus venosus se·mi·na·lis (sem·i·nay'lis). A venous plexus about the seminal vesicles.

plexus venosus sub·oc·ci·pi·ta·lis (sub·ock·sip·i·tay'lis) [NA]. A venous plexus located in the suboccipital area.

plexus venosus ute·ri·nus (yoo·te·rye'nus) [NA]. UTERINE PLEXUS (1).

plexus venosus va·gi·na·lis (vaj·i·nay'lis) [NA]. VAGINAL PLEXUS (2).

plexus venosus ve·si·ca·lis (ves·i·kay'lis) [NA]. VESICAL PLEXUS (2).

plexus ver·te·bra·lis (vur·te·bray'lis) [NA]. VERTEBRAL PLEXUS (1).

plexus ve·si·ca·lis (ves·i·kay'lis) [NA]. VESICAL PLEXUS (1).

pli·ca (plye'kuh) *n.*, pl. & genit. sing. **pli·cae** (·see) [ML., from L. *plicare*, to fold]. A fold.

plica ary·epi·glot·ti·ca (ăr"ee·ep"i·glot'i·kuh) [NA]. ARYEPIGLOTTIC FOLD.

plica axil·la·ris anterior (ack·si·lair'is) [NA]. The anterior axillary plica. See *axillary plica.*

plica axillaris posterior [NA]. The posterior axillary plica. See *axillary plica.*

plica cae·ca·lis (see·kay'lis) [BNA]. Singular of *plicae caecales.*

plica ce·ca·lis vas·cu·la·ris (see·kay'lis vas·kew·lair'is) [NA]. A fold of peritoneum containing anterior cecal vessels.

plica chor·dae tym·pa·ni (kor'dee tim'puh·nigh) [NA]. A fold of the mucosa of the tympanic cavity overlying the chorda tympani nerve.

plica du·o·de·na·lis inferior (dew·o·de·nay'lis) [NA]. DUODENOMESOCOLIC PLICA.

plica duodenalis superior [NA]. DUODENOJEJUNAL PLICA.

plica du·o·de·no·je·ju·na·lis (dew·o·dee"no·je·joo·nay'lis) [NA alt.]. DUODENOJEJUNAL PLICA. NA alt. *plica duodenalis superior.*

plica du·o·de·no·me·so·co·li·ca (dew·o·dee"no·mes"o·kol'i·kuh) [NA alt.]. DUODENOMESOCOLIC PLICA. NA alt. *plica duodenalis inferior.*

plicae. Plural of *plica.*

plicae adi·po·sae pleu·rae (ad·i·po'see ploo'ree) [BNA]. Folds of pleura containing fat.

plicae ala·res (ay·lair'eez) [NA]. ALAR PLICAE.

plicae am·pul·la·res tu·bae ute·ri·nae (am·pew·lair'eez tew'bee yoo·te·rye'nee) [BNA]. Folds of mucosa in the distal end (ampulla) of the uterine tube.

plicae caecales. PLICAE CECALES.

plicae ce·ca·les (see·kay'leez) [NA]. Folds of peritoneum which when present connect the cecum with the abdominal wall.

plicae ci·li·a·res (sil·ee·air'eez) [NA]. CILIARY PLICAE.

plicae cir·cu·la·res (sur·kew·lair'eez) [NA]. CIRCULAR FOLDS.

plicae gas·tri·cae (gas'tri·see) [NA]. Folds of mucous membrane of the stomach.

plicae gas·tro·pan·cre·a·ti·cae (gas"tro·pan"kree·at'i·see) [NA]. GASTROPANCREATIC PLICAE.

plicae iri·dis (eye'ri·dis) [NA]. Radiating folds on the posterior surface of the iris.

plicae isth·mi·cae tu·bae ute·ri·nae (ist'mi·see tew'bee yoo·te·rye'nee) [BNA]. Folds of peritoneum attached to the uterine tubes where they join the uterus.

plicae pa·la·ti·nae trans·ver·sae (pal·uh·tye'nee trans·vur'see) [NA]. A series of transverse folds of the mucous membrane of the lower anterior part of the hard palate.

plicae pal·ma·tae (pal·may'tee) [NA]. ARBOR VITAE (2).

plica epi·gas·tri·ca (ep·i·gas'tri·kuh) [BNA]. Plica umbilicalis lateralis (= LATERAL UMBILICAL FOLD).

plicae se·mi·lu·na·res co·li (sem"ee·lew·nair'eez ko'lye) [NA]. Crescentic folds of the wall of the colon.

plicae trans·ver·sa·les rec·ti (trans·vur·say'leez reck'tye) [NA]. TRANSVERSE RECTAL FOLDS.

plicae tu·ba·ri·ae (tew·bair'ee·ee) [NA]. TUBAL PLICAE.

plicae tu·ni·cae mu·co·sae ve·si·cae fel·le·ae (tew'ni·see mew·ko'see ve·sigh'see fel'ee·ee) [NA]. Folds of the mucous membrane of the gallbladder.

plicae vil·lo·sae ven·tri·cu·li (vi·lo'see ven·trick'yoo·lye) [NA]. Very small folds of the gastric mucosa which divide the surface into small pits.

plica fim·bri·a·ta (fim·bree·ay'tuh) [NA]. FIMBRIATED FOLD.

plica gas·tro·pan·cre·a·ti·ca (gas"tro·pan·kree·at'i·kuh) [BNA]. Singular of *plicae gastropancreaticae.*

plica glos·so·epi·glot·ti·ca la·te·ra·lis (glos"o·ep·i·glot'i·kuh lat·e·ray'lis) [NA]. LATERAL GLOSSOEPIGLOTTIC FOLD.

plica glossoepiglottica me·di·a·na (mee·dee·ay'nuh) [NA]. MEDIAN GLOSSOEPIGLOTTIC FOLD.

plica ileo·ce·ca·lis (il·ee·o·see·kay'lis) [NA]. ILEOCECAL FOLD.

plica in·cu·dis (ing'kew·dis, ing·kew'dis) [NA]. A variable fold of mucous membrane of the tympanic cavity attached to the incus.

plica in·gui·na·lis (ing·gwi·nay'lis). INGUINAL FOLD.

plica in·ter·ure·te·ri·ca (in"tur·yoo·re·terr'i·kuh) [NA]. BAR OF THE BLADDER.

plica la·cri·ma·lis (lack·ri·may'lis) [NA]. LACRIMAL FOLD.

plica lon·gi·tu·di·na·lis du·o·de·ni (lon"ji·tew·di·nay'lis dew·o·dee'nigh) [NA]. LONGITUDINAL DUODENAL PLICA.

plica mallearis anterior mem·bra·nae tym·pa·ni (mem·bray'nee tim'puh·nigh) [NA]. ANTERIOR MALLEAR FOLD (1).

plica mallearis anterior tu·ni·cae mu·co·sae ca·vi tym·pa·ni (tew'ni·see mew·ko'see kay'vye tim'puh·nigh) [NA]. ANTERIOR MALLEAR FOLD (2).

plica mallearis posterior mem·bra·nae tym·pa·ni (mem·bray'nee tim'puh·nigh) [NA]. POSTERIOR MALLEAR FOLD (1).

plica mallearis posterior tu·ni·cae mu·co·sae ca·vi tym·pa·ni (tew'ni·see mew·ko'see kay'vye tim'puh·nigh) [NA]. POSTERIOR MALLEAR FOLD (2).

plica mal·le·o·la·ris an·te·ri·or mem·bra·nae tym·pa·ni (mal"ee·o·lair'is an·teer'ee·or mem·bray'nee tim'puh·nigh) [BNA]. Plica mallearis anterior membranae tympani (= ANTERIOR MALLEAR FOLD (1)).

plica malleolaris anterior tu·ni·cae mu·co·sae tym·pa·ni·cae (tew'ni·see mew·ko'see tim·pan'i·see) [BNA]. Plica mallearis anterior tunicae mucosae cavi tympani (= ANTERIOR MALLEAR FOLD (2)).

plica malleolaris posterior mem·bra·nae tym·pa·ni (mem·bray'nee tim'puh·nigh) [BNA]. Plica mallearis posterior membranae tympani (= POSTERIOR MALLEAR FOLD (1)).

plica malleolaris posterior tu·ni·cae mu·co·sae tym·pa·ni·cae (tew'ni·see mew·ko'see tim·pan'i·see) [BNA]. Plica mallearis posterior tunicae mucosae cavi tympani (= POSTERIOR MALLEAR FOLD (2)).

plica mu·co·sa (mew·ko'suh) [BNA]. A general term for any fold of mucous membrane.

plica of the ampulla. One of the longitudinal folds of the tunica mucosa of the major duodenal papilla.

plica pal·pe·bro·na·sa·lis (pal·pee·bro·na·say'lis) [NA]. EPICANTHUS (1).

plica pa·ra·du·o·de·na·lis (păr"uh·dew·o·de·nay'lis) [NA]. PARADUODENAL RECESS.

plica po·lon·i·ca (po·lon'i·kuh). A matted condition of the hair caused by filth and neglect.

plica pu·bo·ve·si·ca·lis (pew"bo·ves·i·kay'lis) [BNA]. A fold of peritoneum between the urinary bladder and the pubis.

plica rec·to·ute·ri·na (reck"to·yoo·te·rye'nuh) [NA]. RECTOUTERINE PLICA.

plica sal·pin·go·pa·la·ti·na (sal·ping"go·pal·uh·tye'nuh) [NA]. SALPINGOPALATINE FOLD.

plica sal·pin·go·pha·ryn·gea (sal·ping"go·fa·rin'jee·uh) [NA]. SALPINGOPHARYNGEAL FOLD.

plica se·mi·lu·na·ris (sem"ee·lew·nair'is) [NA]. SEMILUNAR PLICA.

plica semilunaris con·junc·ti·vae (kon·junk·tye'vee) [NA]. SEMILUNAR FOLD.

plica se·ro·sa (se·ro'suh) [BNA]. A general term for any fold of a serous membrane.

plica spi·ra·lis (spye·ray'lis) [NA]. SPIRAL VALVE.

plica sta·pe·dis (sta·pee'dis) [NA]. A fold of the mucous membrane of the tympanic cavity attached to the stapes.

plica sub·lin·gua·lis (sub·ling·gway'lis) [NA]. SUBLINGUAL FOLD.

plica sy·no·vi·a·lis (si·no·vee·ay'lis) [NA]. SYNOVIAL PLICA.

plica synovialis in·fra·pa·tel·la·ris (in″fruh·pat·e·lair′is) [NA]. INFRAPATELLAR SYNOVIAL PLICA.

plica synovialis pa·tel·la·ris (pat·e·lair′is) [BNA]. Plica synovialis infrapatellaris (= INFRAPATELLAR SYNOVIAL PLICA).

plicating suture. A running stitch that is pulled together as a gathering string to shorten the distance between two points.

pli·ca·tion (pli·kay′shun) *n.* [L. *plicare*, to fold]. The state or condition of being folded; the act of folding; any surgical procedure in which folds or tucks are placed in a structure. —**pli·cate** (plye′kate) *v.;* **pli·cate** (plye′kate, ·kut), **pli·cat·ed** (plye′kay·tid) *adj.*

plica tri·an·gu·la·ris (trye·ang·gew·lair′is) [NA]. TRIANGULAR FOLD.

plica um·bi·li·ca·lis la·te·ra·lis (um·bil·i·kay′lis lat·e·ray′lis) [NA]. LATERAL UMBILICAL FOLD.

plica umbilicalis me·dia (mee′dee·uh) [BNA]. Plica umbilicalis mediana (= MEDIAN UMBILICAL FOLD).

plica umbilicalis me·di·a·lis (mee·dee·ay′lis) [NA]. MEDIAL UMBILICAL FOLD.

plica umbilicalis me·di·a·na (mee·dee·ay′nuh) [NA]. MEDIAN UMBILICAL FOLD.

plica ure·te·ri·ca (yoo·re·terr′i·kuh) [BNA]. Plica interureterica (= BAR OF THE BLADDER).

plica ve·nae ca·vae si·nis·trae (vee′nee kay′vee si·nis′tree) [NA]. A small fold of pericardium enclosing the fibrous remains of the embryonic left common cardinal vein.

plica ven·tri·cu·la·ris (ven·trick·yoo·lair′is) [BNA]. Plica vestibularis (= VESTIBULAR FOLD).

plica ve·si·ca·lis trans·ver·sa (ves·i·kay′lis trans·vur′suh) [NA]. TRANSVERSE VESICAL PLICA.

plica ves·ti·bu·la·ris (ves·tib·yoo·lair′is) [NA]. VESTIBULAR FOLD.

plica vo·ca·lis (vo·kay′lis) [NA]. VOCAL FOLD.

pli·cot·o·my (plye·kot′uh·mee) *n.* [*plica* + *-tomy*]. Surgical division of the posterior fold of the tympanic membrane.

-ploid. A suffix indicating a given *multiple of* or *relationship to the haploid number of chromosomes*, as diploid, heteroploid.

plomb, plumb (plum) *n.* [F. *plomb*, lead]. Any plastic or inert material used to close pathologic cavities in the body, as material inserted extrapleurally to collapse the lung in pulmonary tuberculosis or inert and antiseptic preparations used to pack bone cavities.

plom·bage (plom·bahzh′) *n.* [F., the filling of a tooth]. The therapeutic use of plastic or inert materials to close pathologic cavities in the body.

P loop. The vectorcardiographic representation of atrial depolarization.

plo·ra·tion (plo·ray′shun) *n.* [L. *ploratio*, from *plorare*, to cry aloud]. LACRIMATION.

plug, *n.* [MD. *plugge*]. Material that occludes an opening or channel.

plug·ger, *n.* CONDENSER (4).

plug·ging, *n.* Occlusion of an opening by means of a plug. See also *tampon.*

plumb. PLOMB.

plum·ba·gin (plum·bay′jin) *n.* 5-Hydroxy-2-methyl-1,4-naphthoquinone; an antibiotic substance, $C_{11}H_8O_3$, isomeric with phthiocol, found in the root bark of *Plumbago europaea, P. zeylanica,* and *P. rosea,* and also prepared synthetically.

plum·ba·go (plum·bay′go) *n.* [L., a species of lead ore]. Native graphite; black lead. Used in the manufacture of pencils and crucibles, and as a lubricant.

plum·bic (plum′bick) *adj.* [*plumb*um + *-ic*]. Describing or pertaining to a compound of tetravalent lead.

plum·bism (plum′biz·um) *n.* [*plumb*um + *-ism*]. LEAD POISONING.

plum·bite (plum′bite) *n.* A salt derived from lead hydroxide, $Pb(OH)_2$, of the types $MHPbO_2$ or M_2PbO_2.

plum·bum (plum′bum) *n.* [L.]. ²LEAD.

Plum·mer's disease [H. S. *Plummer*, U.S. physician, 1874–1936]. Hyperthyroidism associated with nodular goiter.

Plummer's sign [H. S. *Plummer*]. A sign of thyrotoxic myopathy, in which the patient is unable to sit on a chair.

Plummer's treatment [H. S. *Plummer*]. The use of iodine for the treatment of hyperthyroidism.

Plummer-Vinson syndrome [H. S. *Plummer* and P. P. *Vinson*]. Dysphagia, koilonychia, gastric achlorhydria, glossitis, and hypochromic microcytic anemia, due to an iron deficiency. Syn. *Paterson-Kelly syndrome, sideropenic dysphagia.*

plump·er, *n.* The thickened flange of an artificial denture designed to produce a pleasing contour of the facial outline.

plural birth or **pregnancy.** MULTIPLE BIRTH.

pluri- [L. *plus, pluris,* more]. A combining form meaning *several,* being or having *more than one.*

pluridefìciency syndrome. KWASHIORKOR.

plu·ri·de·fi·cient (ploor″i·de·fish′unt) *adj.* [*pluri-* + *deficient*]. Having many deficiencies, usually of one or more vitamins, hormones, or food factors. —**pluridefi·cien·cy** (·un·see) *n.*

plu·ri·fo·cal (ploor″ri·fo′kul) *adj.* [*pluri-* + *focal*]. MULTIFOCAL.

plu·ri·glan·du·lar (ploor″i·glan′dew·lur) *adj.* [*pluri-* + *glandular*]. Pertaining to more than one gland or to the secretions of more than one gland; MULTIGLANDULAR.

pluriglandular extract. A mixture of extracts from several glands.

plu·ri·grav·i·da (ploor″i·grav′i·duh) *n.* [*pluri-* + *gravida*]. A woman during her third and subsequent pregnancies; multigravida.

plu·ri·loc·u·lar (ploor″i·lock′yoo·lur) *adj.* [*pluri-* + *locular*]. Having more than one compartment or loculus; multilocular.

plu·ri·or·i·fi·cial (ploor″ee·or·i·fish′ul) *adj.* [*pluri-* + *orificial*]. Having many openings or orifices.

plu·rip·a·ra (ploo·rip′uh·ruh) *n.* [*pluri-* + *-para*]. A women who has given birth several times.

plu·ri·par·i·ty (ploor″i·păr′i·tee) *n.* [*pluri-* + *parity*]. The condition of having given birth several times.

plu·rip·o·tent (ploo·rip′uh·tunt) *adj.* [*pluri-* + *potent*]. Characterizing a cell or embryonic tissue capable of producing more than one type of cell or tissue.

plu·to·ma·nia (ploo″to·may′nee·uh) *n.* [Gk. *ploutos*, wealth, + *-mania*]. 1. The delusion of possessing great wealth. 2. Obsessive greed for wealth.

plu·to·nism (ploo′tuh·niz·um) *n.* [*pluto*nium + *-ism*]. A disease caused by exposure to plutonium, manifested in experimental animals by graying of the hair, liver degeneration, and tumor formation.

plu·to·ni·um (ploo·to′nee·um) *n.* [after *Pluto*, the planet beyond Neptune]. Pu = 242. An element, atomic number 94, obtained from neptunium and capable of undergoing fission with release of large amounts of energy.

Pm Symbol for promethium.

P.M.A. Abbreviation for *papillary, marginal, attached*; used to designate the extent of tissue involvement in gingivitis.

P.M.A. index. An epidemiological index used to record the prevalence and severity of gingivitis.

PMI Abbreviation for *point of maximal impulse* (= APEX IMPULSE).

P mi·tra·le wave (migh·tray′lee). A broad, notched P wave in the electrocardiogram, usually indicating left atrial hypertrophy or dilation, as seen in mitral stenosis.

PM & R Abbreviation for physical medicine and rehabilitation.

PMS Abbreviation for *pregnant mare's serum hormone.*

PNA Paris Nomina Anatomica.

-pnea, -pnoea [Gk. *pnoia*, breath]. A combining form meaning *respiration* or *respiratory condition.*

pneo- [Gk. *pnoia,* breath]. A combining form meaning *breathing, respiration.*

pneo·car·di·ac reflex (nee″o·kahr′dee·ack). A change in the cardiac rhythm or the blood pressure, due to the inhalation of an irritating vapor.

pneo·dy·nam·ics (nee″o·dye·nam′icks) *n.* [*pneo-* + *dynamics*]. The dynamics of respiration.

pneo·graph (nee′o·graf) *n.* [*pneo-* + *-graph*]. An instrument for recording the force and character of the current of air during respiration.

pne·om·e·ter (nee·om′e·tur) *n.* [*pneo-* + *-meter*]. SPIROMETER.

pneo·pne·ic reflex (nee″o·nee′ick). A change in the respiratory rhythm, due to the inhalation of an irritating vapor.

pneum-, pneumo- [Gk. *pneuma,* breath]. A combining form meaning (a) *air, gas;* (b) *pulmonary, lung;* (c) *respiratory, respiration;* (d) *pneumonia.*

pneu·mar·thro·sis (new″mahr·thro′sis) *n.* [*pneum-* + *arthrosis*]. Air or gas in a joint.

pneumat-, pneumato- [Gk. *pneuma, pneumatos,* wind, breath]. A combining form meaning (a) *respiration;* (b) in medicine, *the presence of air or gas in a part.*

pneu·mat·ic (new·mat′ick) *adj.* [Gk. *pneumatikos,* of the breath]. 1. Pertaining to or containing air or gas. 2. Functioning by means of air or gas pressure.

pneumatic bone. A bone containing air cells, as the temporal bones, or air sacs, as in flying birds. NA *os pneumaticum.*

pneumatic-hammer disease. Raynaud's phenomenon secondary to the use of a pneumatic hammer or other vibrating tools. Syn. *Loriga's disease, traumatic vasospastic syndrome.*

pneumatic mastoid. A mastoid process completely honeycombed with air spaces.

pneu·mat·ics (new·mat′icks) *n.* The branch of physics treating of the dynamic properties of air and gases.

pneu·ma·ti·za·tion (new″muh·ti·zay′shun) *n.* The progressive development of, or the state of having, air-filled cavities in bones, lined by a mucous membrane, as the accessory nasal sinuses or mastoid air cells. —**pneu·ma·tize** (new′muh·tize) *v.*

pneumato-. See *pneumat-.*

pneu·ma·to·car·dia (new″muh·to·kahr′dee·uh) *n.* [*pneumato-* + *-cardia*]. The presence of air or gas in the chambers of the heart.

pneu·ma·to·cele (new′muh·to·seel, new·mat′o·) *n.* [*pneumato-* + *-cele*]. 1. Herniation of the lung. 2. A sac or tumor containing gas; especially the scrotum filled with gas.

pneu·ma·to·dysp·nea, pneu·ma·to·dysp·noea (new″muh·to·disp′nee·uh) *n.* [*pneumato-* + *dyspnea*]. Dyspnea due to pulmonary emphysema.

pneu·ma·to·gram (new′muh·to·gram, new·mat′o·) *n.* [*pneumato-* + *-gram*]. A tracing showing the frequency, duration, and depth of the respiratory movements.

pneu·ma·to·graph (new′muh·to·graf, new·mat′o·) *n.* [*pneumato-* + *-graph*]. PNEUMOGRAPH.

pneu·ma·tol·o·gy (new″muh·tol′uh·jee) *n.* [*pneumato-* + *-logy*]. The science of pulmonary respiration.

pneu·ma·tom·e·ter (new″muh·tom′e·tur) *n.* [*pneumato-* + *-meter*]. An instrument for measuring the pressure of the inspired and expired air.

pneu·ma·tom·e·try (new″muh·tom′e·tree) *n.* [*pneumato-* + *-metry*]. The measurement of the pressure of the inspired and expired air.

pneu·ma·tor·ra·chis (new″muh·tor′uh·kis) *n.* PNEUMORACHIS.

pneu·ma·to·sis (new″muh·to′sis) *n.,* pl. **pneumato·ses** (·seez) [Gk. *pneumatōsis,* inflation, from *pneuma,* wind, breath]. The presence of air or gas in abnormal situations in the body.

pneumatosis cys·toi·des in·tes·ti·na·lis (sis·toy′deez in·tes·ti·nay′lis). A rare condition characterized by gas-filled cysts in the submucosa or subserosa of the small intestine, usually the terminal ileum.

pneu·ma·tu·ria (new″muh·tew′ree·uh) *n.* [*pneumat-* + *-uria*]. The voiding of urine containing free gas.

pneu·ma·type (new′muh·tipe) *n.* [*pneumat-* + *-type*]. Breath picture. The deposit formed upon a piece of glass by the moist air exhaled through the nostrils when the mouth is closed. It is employed in the diagnosis of nasal obstruction.

pneu·mec·to·my (new·meck′tuh·mee) *n.* [*pneum-* + *-ectomy*]. PNEUMONECTOMY.

pneumo-. See *pneum-.*

pneu·mo·an·gi·og·ra·phy (new″mo·an″jee·og′ruh·fee) *n.* [*pneumo-* + *angiography*]. The outlining of the vessels of the lung by means of a radiopaque material, for roentgenographic visualization.

pneu·mo·ar·throg·ra·phy (new″mo·ahr·throg′ruh·fee) *n.* [*pneumo-* + *arthro-* + *-graphy*]. Radiographic examination of joints into which air or gas has been injected. —**pneumo·ar·thro·gram** (·ahr′thro·gram) *n.*

pneu·mo·ba·cil·lus (new″mo·ba·sil′us) *n.* [*pneumo-* + *bacillus*]. KLEBSIELLA PNEUMONIAE.

pneu·mo·bul·bar (new″mo·bul′bur) *adj.* [*pneumo-* + *bulbar*]. Pertaining to the lungs and to the respiratory center in the medulla oblongata.

pneu·mo·cele (new′mo·seel) *n.* PNEUMATOCELE.

pneu·mo·cen·te·sis (new″mo·sen·tee′sis) *n.* [*pneumo-* + *centesis*]. Puncture of a lung with needle or trocar; usually done to obtain tissue or exudate for diagnostic study, or to establish communication with a cavity.

pneu·mo·ceph·a·lus (new″mo·sef′uh·lus) *n.* [*pneumo-* + *-cephalus*]. The presence of air or gas within the cranial cavity.

pneu·mo·cho·le·cys·ti·tis (new″mo·kol″e·sis·tye′tis, ·ko″le·) *n.* [*pneumo-* + *cholecystitis*]. Cholecystitis associated with gas in the gallbladder.

pneu·mo·coc·cal (new″mo·kock′ul) *adj.* Pertaining to or caused by pneumococci.

pneumococcal fever. A febrile illness seen usually in infants with no clinically apparent focus of infection but from whose blood *Streptococcus pneumoniae* can be isolated.

pneumococcal types. Subdivisions of *Streptococcus pneumoniae,* based on their capsular polysaccharide antigens or specific soluble substance. At present, more than 75 such types have been distinguished.

pneu·mo·coc·ce·mia, pneu·mo·coc·cae·mia (new″mo·kock·see′mee·uh) *n.* [*pneumococcus* + *-emia*]. The presence of pneumococci in the blood.

pneumococci. Plural of *pneumococcus.*

pneu·mo·coc·cic (new″mo·kock′sick) *adj.* PNEUMOCOCCAL.

pneu·mo·coc·ci·dal (new″mo·kock·sigh′dul) *adj.* [*pneumococcus* + *-cide* + *-al*]. Destroying pneumococci.

pneu·mo·coc·co·su·ria (new″mo·kock″o·sue′ree·uh) *n.* The presence of pneumococci in the urine.

pneu·mo·coc·cus (new″mo·kock′us) *n.,* pl. **pneumococ·ci** (·sigh) [*pneumo-* + *coccus*]. A common term for *Streptococcus pneumoniae.*

pneumococcus antibody test. FRANCIS TEST.

pneumococcus type test. A precipitation test performed by layering centrifuged or filtered pneumococcus exudate over immune serum. A turbid ring will form at the junction of the fluids in the tube containing serum homologous with the pneumococcus type causing the infection. See also *Neufeld quellung test.*

pneu·mo·co·lon (new″mo·ko′lun) *n.* [*pneumo-* + *colon*]. 1. The presence of air or gas in the colon. 2. Distention of the colon with air as a diagnostic measure.

pneu·mo·co·ni·o·sis, pneu·mo·ko·ni·o·sis (new″mo·ko″nee·o′sis) *n.* [*pneumo-* + *coniosis*]. Any disease of the lung caused by the inhalation of dust, especially mineral dusts that produce chronic induration and fibrosis.

pneu·mo·cra·ni·um (new″mo·kray′nee·um) *n.* [*pneumo-* + *cranium*]. PNEUMOCEPHALUS.

Pneu·mo·cyst·is (new″mo·sis′tis) *n.* [*pneumo-* + Gk. *kystis,* bag, sac]. A parasite associated with pulmonary infection in hosts with diminished resistance. *Pneumocystis carinii* has received the most attention.

Pneumocystis ca·ri·nii (ka·rye'nee·eye). An extracellular parasite, the taxonomy of which has not been established, consisting of nucleated oval or round organisms 1 to 2 μm in diameter, often with eight cells in a cyst 6 to 9 μm in diameter enclosed in a viscous capsule. It is found in interstitial plasma cell pneumonia of man, and is widely prevalent in animals.

***Pneumocystis carinii* pneumonia.** An infection of the lungs associated with *Pneumocystis carinii,* occurring in debilitated premature infants, sometimes in epidemic form, in children with hypogammaglobulinemia or deficiencies of cell-mediated immunity, and in patients receiving immunosuppressive therapy for cancer or after organ transplantation; treated by pentamidine isethionate. Syn. *interstitial plasma-cell pneumonia.*

pneu·mo·cys·tog·ra·phy (new"mo·sis·tog'ruh·fee) *n.* [*pneumo-* + *cystography*]. Cystography performed after introduction of air or carbon dioxide into the bladder. —**pneumo·cys·to·gram** (·sis'to·gram) *n.*

pneu·mo·cyte (new'mo·site) *n.* PNEUMONOCYTE.

pneu·mo·der·ma (new"mo·dur'muh) *n.* [*pneumo-* + *-derma*]. Air or gas collected under, or in, the skin.

pneu·mo·dy·nam·ics (new"mo·dye·nam'icks) *n.* [*pneumo-* + *dynamics*]. PNEODYNAMICS.

pneu·mo·en·ceph·a·lo·cele (new"mo·en·sef'uh·lo·seel) *n.* [*pneumo-* + *encephalo-* + *-cele*]. PNEUMOCEPHALUS.

pneu·mo·en·ceph·a·lo·gram (new"mo·en·sef'uh·lo·gram) *n.* [*pneumo-* + *encephalogram*]. A radiographic picture of the brain after the replacement of the cerebrospinal fluid with air or gas, which has been injected through a needle into the spinal subarachnoid space.

pneu·mo·en·ceph·a·log·ra·phy (new"mo·en·sef"uh·log'ruh·fee) *n.* [*pneumo-* + *encephalography*]. A method of visualizing the ventricular system and subarachnoid pathways of the brain by radiography after removal of spinal fluid followed by the injection of air or gas into the subarachnoid space.

pneu·mo·en·ter·ic recess (new"mo·en·terr'ick). In certain mammals, an embryonic peritoneal recess between the left lung bud and the esophagus; on the right side it is comparable to the infracardiac bursa.

pneu·mo·en·ter·i·tis (new"mo·en"tur·eye'tis) *n.* [*pneumo-* + *enteritis*]. Inflammation of the lungs and of the intestine.

pneu·mo·gas·tric (new"mo·gas'trick) *adj.* [*pneumo-* + *gastric*]. Pertaining to the lungs and the stomach.

pneumogastric nerve. VAGUS.

pneu·mo·gram (new'mo·gram) *n.* [*pneumo-* + *-gram*]. An x-ray film of an organ inflated with air. Syn. *aerogram.*

pneu·mo·graph (new'mo·graf) *n.* [*pneumo-* + *-graph*]. An apparatus for recording the force and rapidity of the respiratory excursion.

pneu·mog·ra·phy (new·mog'ruh·fee) *n.* [*pneumo-* + *-graphy*]. 1. The recording of the respiratory excursions. 2. PNEUMORADIOGRAPHY.

pneu·mo·he·mo·peri·car·di·um, pneu·mo·hae·mo·peri·car·di·um (new"mo·hee"mo·perr"i·kahr'dee·um) *n.* [*pneumo-* + *hemo-* + *pericardium*]. The presence of air and blood in the pericardial cavity.

pneu·mo·he·mo·tho·rax, pneu·mo·hae·mo·tho·rax (new"mo·hee"mo·tho'racks) *n.* [*pneumo-* + *hemo-* + *thorax*]. The presence of air or gas and blood in the thoracic cavity.

pneu·mo·hy·dro·peri·car·di·um (new"mo·high"dro·perr"i·kahr'dee·um) *n.* [*pneumo-* + *hydro-* + *pericardium*]. An accumulation of air and fluid in the pericardial cavity.

pneu·mo·hy·po·der·ma (new"mo·high"po·dur'muh) *n.* [*pneumo-* + *hypo-* + *-derma*]. SUBCUTANEOUS EMPHYSEMA.

pneumokoniosis. PNEUMOCONIOSIS.

pneu·mo·lip·i·do·sis (new"mo·lip"i·do'sis) *n.* [*pneumo-* + *lipidosis*]. LIPID PNEUMONIA (2).

pneu·mo·lith (new'mo·lith) *n.* [*pneumo-* + *-lith*]. A calculus or concretion occurring in a lung.

pneu·mo·li·thi·a·sis (new"mo·li·thigh'uh·sis) *n.* [*pneumolith* + *-iasis*]. The occurrence of calculi or concretions in a lung.

pneu·mol·y·sis (new·mol'i·sis) *n.* [*pneumo-* + *-lysis*]. PNEUMONOLYSIS.

pneu·mo·me·di·as·ti·num (new"mo·mee"dee·as·tye'num) *n.* [*pneumo-* + *mediastinum*]. 1. The presence of gas or air in the mediastinal tissues. 2. The instillation of air or gas into the mediastinum as a diagnostic measure.

pneu·mom·e·try (new·mom'e·tree) *n.* [*pneumo-* + *-metry*]. Measurement of lung capacity in the living individual, including vital capacity, maximum breathing capacity, tidal volume, and residual volume. See also *spirometry.*

pneu·mo·my·co·sis (new"mo·migh·ko'sis) *n.* [*pneumo-* + *mycosis*]. Any disease of the lungs due to a fungus.

pneumon-, pneumono- [Gk. *pneumōn,* lungs]. A combining form meaning *lung.*

pneu·mo·nec·to·my (new"mo·neck'tuh·mee) *n.* [*pneumon-* + *-ectomy*]. Excision of an entire lung.

pneu·mo·nia (new·mo'nyuh, ·nee·uh) *n.* [Gk., lung disease, from *pneumōn,* lungs]. 1. Inflammation of the lungs associated with exudate in the alveolar lumens. Compare *pneumonitis.* See also *aspiration pneumonia, bronchopneumonia, lobar pneumonia.* 2. Any of various infectious diseases characterized by pneumonia (1); the most common causative agents include pneumococci (*Streptococcus pneumoniae*), pleuropneumonia-like organisms (*Mycoplasma pneumoniae*), and many viruses. See also *pneumocystis carinii pneumonia, primary atypical pneumonia.*

pneumonia al·ba (al'buh). Diffuse interstitial fibrosis of the alveolar walls of the fetal lung due to prenatal syphilis; the lungs are white and often atelectatic at birth.

pneumonia jacket. A padded cotton or wool coat that may contain poultices; once employed in the treatment of pneumonia.

pneu·mon·ic (new·mon'ick) *adj.* [Gk. *pneumonikos,* from *pneumōn,* lungs]. 1. Pertaining to pneumonia. 2. Pertaining to the lungs.

pneumonic plague. An extremely virulent type of plague with lung involvement and a high mortality rate.

pneu·mo·ni·tis (new"mo·nigh'tis) *n.,* pl. **pneumo·nit·i·des** (·nit'i·deez) [*pneumon-* + *-itis*]. 1. Inflammation of the lungs. 2. Inflammation of the lungs in which the exudate is primarily interstitial.

pneumono-. See *pneumon-.*

pneu·mo·no·cele (new'mo·no·seel) *n.* [*pneumono-* + *-cele*]. PNEUMATOCELE.

pneu·mo·no·cen·te·sis (new"mo·no·sen·tee'sis) *n.* PNEUMOCENTESIS.

pneu·mo·no·co·ni·o·sis, pneu·mo·no·ko·ni·o·sis (new"mo·no·ko"nee·o'sis) *n.* PNEUMOCONIOSIS.

pneu·mo·no·cyte (new·mon'o·site, new'muh·no·site) *n.* [*pneumono-* + *-cyte*]. Any of the cells characteristic of a pulmonary alveolus, as a granular pneumonocyte (= GREAT ALVEOLAR CELL), membranous pneumonocyte (= SQUAMOUS ALVEOLAR CELL), or alveolar phagocyte.

pneu·mo·no·li·thi·a·sis (new"mo·no·li·thigh'uh·sis) *n.* PNEUMOLITHIASIS.

pneu·mo·nol·y·sis (new"mo·nol'i·sis) *n.,* pl. **pneumonoly·ses** (·seez) [*pneumono-* + *-lysis*]. The loosening of any portion of lung adherent to the chest wall; a form of collapse therapy used in the treatment of pulmonary tuberculosis.

pneu·mo·no·my·co·sis (new"mo·no·migh·ko'sis) *n.* PNEUMOMYCOSIS.

pneu·mo·nop·a·thy (new"mo·nop'uth·ee) *n.* [*pneumono-* + *-pathy*]. Any abnormality or disease of the lungs.

pneu·mo·no·pexy (new·mo'no·peck"see, ·mon'o·) *n.* [*pneumono-* + *-pexy*]. Fixation of lung tissue to the chest wall.

pneu·mo·nor·rha·phy (new"mo·nor'uh·fee) *n.* [*pneumono-* + *-rrhaphy*]. Suture of a lung.

pneu·mo·no·sis (new"mo·no'sis) *n.,* pl. **pneumono·ses** (·seez) [*pneumon-* + *-osis*]. Any noninfective disease of the lungs; pneumonopathy.

pneu·mo·not·o·my (new″mo·not′uh·mee) *n.* [*pneumono-* + *-tomy*]. Surgical incision of a lung.

pneu·mop·a·thy (new·mop′uth·ee) *n.* [*pneumo-* + *-pathy*]. PNEUMONOPATHY.

pneu·mo·peri·car·di·tis (new″mo·perr″i·kahr·dye′tis) *n.* [*pneumo-* + *pericarditis*]. Pericarditis with the formation of gas in the pericardial cavity.

pneu·mo·peri·car·di·um (new″mo·perr″i·kahr′dee·um) *n.* [*pneumo-* + *pericardium*]. The presence of air in the pericardial cavity.

pneu·mo·peri·to·ne·um (new″mo·perr″i·to·nee′um) *n.* [*pneumo-* + *peritoneum*]. 1. The presence of air or gas in the peritoneal cavity. 2. Injection of a gas into the peritoneal cavity as a diagnostic or therapeutic measure. Syn. *aeroperitoneum.*

pneu·mo·peri·to·ni·tis (new″mo·perr″i·to·nigh′tis) *n.* [*pneumo-* + *peritonitis*]. Peritonitis with the presence of air or gas in the peritoneal cavity.

pneu·mo·pexy (new′mo·peck″see) *n.* PNEUMONOPEXY.

pneu·mo·py·elo·gram (new″mo·pye′e·lo·gram) *n.* [*pneumo-* + *pyelogram*]. A pyelogram in which air or gas is used as the contrast medium instead of an opaque solution.

pneu·mo·pyo·peri·car·di·um (new″mo·pye″o·perr·i·kahr′dee·um) *n.* [*pneumo-* + *pyo-* + *pericardium*]. The presence of air or gas and pus in the pericardial cavity.

pneu·mo·ra·chis (new″mo·ray′kis) *n.* [*pneumo-* + Gk. *rhachis*, spine]. A collection of gas in the spinal canal, accidental or by injection of air for diagnostic purposes.

pneu·mo·ra·di·og·ra·phy (new″mo·ray″dee·og′ruh·fee) *n.* [*pneumo-* + *radiography*]. Radiography of a region, as of a joint or of the abdomen, following the injection of air into a cavity.

pneu·mo·roent·gen·og·ra·phy (new″mo·rent″gun·og′ruh·fee) *n.* [*pneumo-* + *roentgenography*]. PNEUMORADIOGRAPHY.

pneu·mor·rha·chis (new″mo·ray′kis, new·mor′uh·kis) *n.* [*pneumo-* + *-rrhachis*]. PNEUMORACHIS.

pneu·mor·rha·gia (new″mo·ray′jee·uh) *n.* [*pneumo-* + *-rrhagia*]. A pulmonary hemorrhage.

pneu·mor·rha·phy (new·mor′uh·fee) *n.* PNEUMONORRHAPHY.

pneu·mo·scle·ro·sis (new″mo·skle·ro′sis) *n.* [*pneumo-* + *sclerosis*]. Fibrosis of the lungs.

pneu·mo·scro·tum (new″mo·skro′tum) *n.* Air or other gases in the scrotum.

pneu·mo·sid·er·o·sis (new″mo·sid″ur·o′sis) *n.* [*pneumo-* + *sider-* + *-osis*]. The accumulation of iron-containing material in the lungs.

pneu·mo·tacho·graph (new″mo·tack′o·graf) *n.* [*pneumo-* + Gk. *tachos*, speed, quickly, + *-graph*]. An apparatus used to record instantaneous air flow to and from the lungs.

pneumotaxic center. A functional center located in the rostral pons that stimulates the expiratory center in the medulla oblongata, presumably via a negative feedback loop operating between these two areas of the brainstem.

pneu·mo·tax·is (new″mo·tack′sis) *n.* [*pneumo-* + *taxis*]. The control of pulmonary respiration. —**pneumotax·ic** (·ick) *adj.*

pneu·mo·tho·rax (new″mo·tho′racks) *n.* [*pneumo-* + *thorax*]. 1. The presence of air or gas in a pleural cavity from trauma or disease. Syn. *aeropleura.* 2. The introduction of air or gas into the pleural cavity for diagnosis or therapy.

pneu·mot·o·my (new·mot′uh·mee) *n.* PNEUMONOTOMY.

pneu·mo·tox·ic respiration (new″mo·tock′sick). Shallow, rapid, irregular respiration seen with inflammation or disease of the lung.

pneu·mo·tox·in (new″mo·tock′sin) *n.* [*pneumo-* + *toxin*]. An injurious substance liberated upon the autolysis of pneumococci, of rare or minor significance in pathogenicity; includes an oxygen-labile hemolysin and a purpura-producing factor.

pneu·mo·ty·phoid (new″mo·tye′foid) *n.* PNEUMOTYPHUS.

pneu·mo·ty·phus (new″mo·tye′fus) *n.* Typhoid fever with pneumonia. Syn. *typhopneumonia.*

pneu·mo·ven·tri·cle (new″mo·ven′tri·kul) *n.* [*pneumo-* + *ventricle*]. A form of pneumocephalus in which air enters the ventricles of the brain through the accessory sinuses of the skull; sometimes seen as a complication of skull fracture.

pneu·mo·ven·tric·u·log·ra·phy (new″mo·ven·trick″yoo·log′ruh·fee) *n.* [*pneumo-* + *ventriculography*]. A method of depicting the ventricular system of the brain by roentgenography, after cerebrospinal fluid is removed and air injected in appropriate amounts. See also *ventriculography.*

pneu·sis (new′sis) *n.* [Gk., from *pnein*, to breathe]. RESPIRATION.

pnig·ma (nig′muh) *n.* [Gk., from *pnigein*, to choke]. STRANGULATION.

pni·go·pho·bia (nigh″go·fo′bee·uh) *n.* [Gk. *pnigein*, to choke, + *-phobia*]. The fear of choking; sometimes accompanies angina pectoris.

-pnoea. See *-pnea.*

Po Symbol for polonium.

p.o. Abbreviation for *per os*, by mouth.

P_{O_2} Symbol for the partial pressure of oxygen. See *partial pressure.*

pock, *n.* A pustule of an eruptive fever, especially of smallpox.

pocked, *adj.* Pitted; marked with pustules.

pock·et, *n.* 1. *In anatomy*, a blind sac, or sac-shaped cavity. 2. A diverticulum communicating with a cavity.

pocket flap. GAUNTLET FLAP.

pock-marked, *adj.* Pitted with the scars of the smallpox pustule.

pod-, podo- [Gk. *pous, podos*]. A combining form meaning *foot* or *footlike process.*

-pod [Gk. *pous, podos*, foot]. A combining form meaning (a) *having feet of a particular number or kind;* (b) *foot* or *part resembling a foot.*

-poda [NL., from Gk. *pous, podos*, foot]. In zoological taxonomy, a combining form meaning *having feet of a* (specified) *number or kind.*

po·dag·ra (po·dag′ruh) *n.* [Gk., from *pous, podos*, foot, + *agra*, capture, seizure]. GOUT (1).

podagric calculus. A calculus associated with an inflamed joint, usually gouty.

po·dal·gia (po·dal′jee·uh) *n.* [Gk., from *pous, podos*, foot, + *algos*, pain]. Pain in the foot.

po·dal·ic (po·dal′ick) *adj.* [*pod-* + *-al* + *-ic*]. Pertaining to the feet.

podalic version. The operation of changing the position of the fetus in the uterus in which one or both feet are brought down to the outlet.

pod·ar·thri·tis (pod″ahr·thrye′tis) *n.* [*pod-* + *arthritis*]. Inflammation of the joints of the feet.

po·dar·thrum (po·dahr′thrum) *n.*, pl. **podar·thra** (·thruh) [NL., from *pod-* + Gk. *arthron*, joint]. *In biology*, the foot joint or metatarsophalangeal articulation.

pod·ede·ma, pod·oe·de·ma (pod″e·dee′muh) *n.* [*pod-* + *edema*]. Edema of the feet.

pod·el·co·ma, pod·el·ko·ma (pod″el·ko′muh) *n.* [*pod-* + Gk. *helkōma*, ulcer]. MYCETOMA.

pod·en·ceph·a·lus (pod″en·sef′uh·lus) *n.*, pl. **podencepha·li** (·lye) [*pod-* + *-encephalus*]. An individual with partial acrania and protruded brain that hangs by a pedicle.

-podia [*pod-* + *-ia*]. A combining form meaning *a condition of the feet.*

po·di·a·try (po·dye′uh·tree) *n.* [*pod-* + *-iatry*]. Diagnosis and treatment of disorders of the feet. Syn. *chiropody.* —**podia·trist** (·trist) *n.*

podo-. See *pod-.*

podo·brom·hi·dro·sis (pod″o·brome″hi·dro′sis) *n.* [*podo-* + *bromhidrosis*]. Offensive sweating of the feet.

podo·cyte (pod′o·site) *n.* [*podo-* + *-cyte*]. An epithelial cell of the renal glomerulus, so called because of the footlike processes which attach it to the capillary basement membrane of the glomerular tuft. —**podo·cyt·ic** (pod″o·sit′ick) *adj.*

podo·derm (pod′o·durm) *n.* [*podo-* + *-derm*]. The modified, highly vascular corium found under the horny layer of the hoof in ungulates; it furnishes nutrition to the hoof.

podo·der·ma·ti·tis (pod″o·dur·muh·tye′tis) *n.* [*podo-* + *dermatitis*]. Ulcerative dermatitis of the plantar metatarsal or metacarpal surfaces of the hocks of rabbits or of the feet of guinea pigs and other animals.

pod·o·dyn·ia (pod″o·din′ee·uh) *n.* [*pod-* + *-odynia*]. Pain in the foot, especially a neuralgic pain in the heel unattended by swelling or redness.

podoedema. PODEDEMA.

po·dom·e·ter (po·dom′e·tur) *n.* [*podo-* + *-meter*]. PEDOMETER.

podo·phyl·lin (pod″o·fil′in) *n.* Podophyllum resin.

podo·phyl·lo·tox·in (pod″o·fil″o·tock′sin) *n.* A crystalline polycyclic substance, $C_{22}H_{22}O_8$, obtained from the rhizome and roots of *Podophyllum peltatum;* has cathartic properties and, when applied topically, is active against certain wartlike neoplasms.

podo·phyl·lum (pod″o·fil′um) *n.* The dried rhizome and roots of the mayapple, *Podophyllum peltatum,* containing podophyllotoxin, α-peltatin, β-peltatin, and other constituents. Used in the form of an extract called podophyllum resin or podophyllin as a cathartic, and, locally, as a cytotoxic agent for the treatment of certain warts.

-podous [*pod-* + *-ous*]. A combining form meaning *having feet of a* (specified) *number or kind.*

-pody [*pod-* + *-y*]. See *-podia.*

po·go·ni·on (po·go′nee·un) *n.* [Gk. *pōgōnion,* dim. of *pōgōn,* beard]. The most anterior point of the chin on the symphysis of the mandible.

Pohl's test [J. *Pohl,* German pharmacologist, b. 1861]. A test for globulins in which the suspected solution is treated with ammonium sulfate which precipitates the globulins.

-poiesis [Gk. *poiēsis,* from *poiein,* to make, produce]. A combining form meaning *production, making, forming.*

-poietic [Gk. *poiētikos,* productive]. A combining form meaning *producing, formative.*

poikilo- [Gk. *poikilos,* varicolored, diversified]. A combining form meaning *irregular, abnormal, variable.*

poi·kilo·blast (poy′ki·lo·blast, poy·kil′o·) *n.* [*poikilo-* + *-blast*]. A nucleated red blood cell of irregular shape and size.

poi·kilo·cyte (poy′ki·lo·site, poy·kil′o·) *n.* [*poikilo-* + *-cyte*]. An erythrocyte of irregular shape.

poi·kilo·cy·the·mia, poi·kilo·cy·thae·mia (poy″ki·lo·sigh·theem′ee·uh) *n.* [*poikilocyte* + *-hemia*]. The presence of poikilocytes in the blood.

poi·kilo·cy·to·sis (poy″ki·lo·sigh·to′sis) *n.,* pl. **poikilocyto·ses** (·seez) [*poikilocyte* + *-osis*]. Abnormality in shape of circulating erythrocytes.

poi·ki·lo·der·ma (poy″ki·lo·dur′muh) *n.* [*poikilo-* + *-derma*]. A skin syndrome characterized by pigmentation, telangiectasia, and, usually, atrophy.

poikiloderma atro·phi·cans vas·cu·la·re (a·trof′i·kanz vas·kew·lair′ee). A widespread or localized disorder of skin characterized by atrophy, pigmentation, telangiectasia, and purpura; usually observed in association with, or as an end result of, other disorders involving the skin, especially dermatomyositis, but also lupus erythematosus and mycosis fungoides. When observed independently, it is also referred to as Jacobi's type.

poikiloderma con·gen·i·ta·le (kon·jen·i·tay′lee). ROTHMUND-THOMSON SYNDROME.

poikiloderma of Ci·vatte (see·vaʰt′) [A. *Civatte,* French dermatologist, 1877–1956]. RETICULATED PIGMENTED POIKILODERMA.

poikiloderma re·tic·u·la·re of Civatte (re·tick″yoo·lair′ee) [A. *Civatte*]. RETICULATED PIGMENTED POIKILODERMA.

poi·kilo·der·ma·to·my·o·si·tis (poy″ki·lo·dur″muh·to·migh″o·sigh′tis) *n.* Poikiloderma atrophicans vasculare in association with dermatomyositis.

poi·kilo·ther·mal (poy″ki·lo·thur′mul) *adj.* POIKILOTHERMIC.

poi·kilo·ther·mic (poy″ki·lo·thur′mick) *n.* [*poikilo-* + *therm-* + *-ic*]. Having a body temperature that varies with environmental temperature, usually slightly higher than that of the environment, as in all plants and animals except birds and mammals; COLD-BLOODED. Contr. *homeothermic.* —**poikilother·mism** (·miz·um), **poi·kilo·ther·my** (poy′ki·lo·thur″mee, poy·kil′o·) *n.*

poi·kilo·ther·mous (poy″ki·lo·thur′mus) *adj.* POIKILOTHERMIC.

poi·kilo·throm·bo·cyte (poy″ki·lo·throm′bo·site) *n.* [*poikilo-* + *thrombocyte*]. A blood platelet of abnormal shape.

poi·kilo·zoo·sper·mia (poy″ki·lo·zo″o·spur′mee·uh) *n.* [*poikilo-* + *zoo-* + *-spermia*]. Variability in the shapes of spermatozoa.

point angle. The angle formed by the meeting of three surfaces of a tooth.

point·ed ear. An ear with a satyr tubercle.

point·ing, *n.* 1. The coming to a point. 2. The stage of abscess formation when the pus has approached the surface at a localized area.

pointing test. BÁRÁNY'S POINTING TEST.

point of convergence. A conjugate focus upon which the light rays converge.

point of divergence. A conjugate focus from which the light rays proceed.

point of election. *In surgery,* the point at which a certain operation is done by preference.

point of incidence. The point upon which a ray or projectile strikes a reflecting or refracting surface.

point of maximal impulse. APEX IMPULSE. Abbreviated, PMI.

points dou·lou·reux (pwanh″doo·loo·ruh′) [F.]. PAINFUL POINTS.

poise (poiz, pwahz) *n.* [F., from J. L. M. *Poiseuille,* French physiologist, 1799–1869]. The unit of viscosity. The force in dynes necessary to be applied to an area of 1 cm^2 between two parallel planes 1 cm^2 in area and 1 cm apart to produce a difference in streaming velocity between the liquid planes of 1 cm per second.

Poi·seuille's layer or **space** (pwah·zœy′) [J. L. M. *Poiseuille*]. The relatively slow-moving peripheral portion of the bloodstream in minute vessels.

poi·son (poy′zun) *n.* [OF., from L. *potio,* potion]. A substance that in relatively small doses has an action, when it is ingested by, injected into, inhaled or absorbed by, or applied to a living organism, that either destroys life or impairs seriously the functions of one or more organs or tissues.

poison hemlock. CONIUM.

poi·son·ing, *n.* The abnormal condition caused by a toxic substance.

poison ivy. A North American climbing vine, *Toxicodendron radicans* (also called *Rhus toxicodendron* and *R. radicans*); contains an oleoresin (urushiol) which is sensitizing and causes a form of contact dermatitis.

poison nut. NUX VOMICA.

poison oak. *Toxicodendron quercifolium* (also called *Rhus toxicodendron* Linné but not the *R. toxicodendron* of American authors, which is poison ivy); contains an oil which is sensitizing and causes a contact dermatitis similar to that produced by poison ivy. Western poison oak is the *Toxicodendron diversilobum* (also known as *Rhus diversiloba*).

poi·son·ous, *adj.* Having the properties of a poison.

poisonous snakes. The venom-producing snakes, which belong mainly to four families: Elapidae, the cobras and allies; Hydrophidae, the sea snakes; Crotalidae, the pit vipers; and Viperidae, the true vipers. Most have large, hypodermic-like front fangs by which venom is injected.

poison su·mac (sue′mack). A smooth shrub, *Toxicodendron* *vernix* (also called *Rhus vernix* and *R. venenata*); contains an oil which is sensitizing and causes eruptions resembling poison-ivy dermatitis.

Pois·son distribution (pwah·sohⁿ') [S. D. *Poisson*, French mathematician, 1781–1840]. *In statistics*, a discrete mathematical distribution, often called the law of small numbers, that may be regarded as an approximation of the binomial distribution when *p* (probability) is small and *n* (number) large.

po·ker back or **spine.** ANKYLOSING SPONDYLITIS.

Po·land anomaly or **syndrome** [A. *Poland*, British physician, 1820–1872]. Unilateral congenital absence of the sternocostal head of the pectoralis major muscle and ipsilateral syndactyly.

po·lar, *adj.* 1. Pertaining to or having a pole. 2. Of chemical compounds: having molecules composed of atoms that share their common electron pairs unequally and thereby effect a separation of positive and negative centers of electricity to form a dipole.

polar bodies or **cells.** The two minute, abortive cells given off successively by the ovum during the maturation divisions. They mark the animal pole.

polar cataract. A cataract in which the opacity is confined to one pole of the lens. See also *anterior polar cataract, posterior polar cataract.*

polar globules. POLAR BODIES.

po·lar·im·e·ter (po''lur·im'e·tur) *n.* [*polar* + *-meter*]. An instrument for making quantitative studies on the rotation of polarized light by optically active substances.

po·lar·im·e·try (po''lur·im'e·tree) *n.* The use of the polarimeter.

po·lari·scope (po·lăr'i·skope) *n.* [*polar* + *-scope*]. An instrument for studying the properties of or for observing substances in polarized light; a polarimeter.

po·lari·stro·bom·e·ter (po·lăr''i·stro·bom'e·tur) *n.* [*polar* + Gk. *strobos*, whirling, rotation, + *-meter*]. A form of polarimeter or saccharimeter that furnishes a delicate means of fixing the plane of polarization as rotated by the sugar solution under examination.

po·lar·i·ty (po·lăr'i·tee) *n.* 1. The state or quality of having poles or regions of intensity with mutually opposite qualities. 2. The electrically positive or negative condition of a battery, cell, or other electric device with terminals.

polarity mutant. A mutant that causes a reduced rate of polypeptide synthesis beyond its site of action.

po·lar·iza·tion (po''lur·i·zay'shun) *n.* 1. The act of polarizing or the state of being polarized. 2. A condition produced in light or other transverse wave radiation in which the vibrations are restricted and take place in one plane only (plane polarization) or in curves (circular or elliptic polarization). The plane of polarization is altered or rotated when the light is passed through a quartz crystal or solutions of certain substances (rotatory polarization). 3. The deposit of gas bubbles (hydrogen) on the electronegative plate of a galvanic battery, whereby the flow of the current is impeded. 4. Acquisition of electric charges of opposite sign, as across semipermeable cell membranes in living tissues.

polarization of electrodes. Acquisition of charges on electrodes.

po·lar·ize (po'lur·ize) *v.* To endow with polarity; to place in a state of polarization.

polarized light. Light that has undergone polarization.

po·lar·iz·er (po'lur·eye''zur) *n.* An object, such as a Nicol prism, by means of which light is polarized.

po·laro·gram (po·lăr'o·gram) *n.* The current-voltage curve obtained in polarographic analysis.

po·laro·graph (po·lăr'o·graf) *n.* An instrument used in polarography.

po·lar·og·ra·phy (po''lur·og'ruh·fee) *n.* [*polarization* + *-graphy*]. A method of chemical analysis based on the interpretation of the current-voltage curve characteristic of a solution of an electrooxidizable or electroreducible substance when it is electrolyzed with the dropping mercury electrode. —**po·laro·graph·ic** (po·lăr''o·graf'ick, po''lur·o·) *adj.*

Polaroid. Trademark for a film containing an oriented light-polarizing compound. Used as a substitute for Nicol prisms, in polariscopes, and in eyeglasses to prevent glare.

polar sulcus. One of several small grooves at the distal end of the calcarine sulcus.

pol·dine meth·yl·sul·fate (pole'deen meth''il·sul'fate). 2-(Hydroxymethyl)-1,1-dimethylpyrrolidinium methyl sulfate, $C_{22}H_{29}NO_7S$, an anticholinergic drug with actions similar to those of atropine.

pole, *n.* [L. *polus*, from Gk. *polos*]. 1. Either extremity of the axis of a body, as of the fetus or the crystalline lens. 2. One of two points at which opposite physical qualities (of electricity or of magnetism) are concentrated, as either of the electrodes of an electrochemical cell, battery, or dynamo.

pole tubule. *In embryology*, the first two tubules to grow out of the renal pelvis; there is a cranial and a caudal pole tubule.

poli. Plural and genitive singular of *polus* (= POLE).

poli-, polio- [Gk. *polios*]. A combining form meaning (a) *gray;* (b) *gray substance, gray matter.*

po·li·en·ceph·a·li·tis (po''lee·en·sef''uh·lye'tis) *n.* POLIOENCEPHALITIS.

pol·i·gee·nan (pol''i·jee'nun) *n.* A sulfonated polysaccharide produced by hydrolysis of carragheen obtained from red algae, used as an enzyme inhibitor.

po·lig·nate (po·lig'nate) *n.* A sulfonated polymer obtained from coniferous wood used as a pepsin inhibitor.

polio-. See *poli-*.

po·lio (po'lee·o) *n.* POLIOMYELITIS.

po·lio·dys·pla·sia ce·re·bri (po''lee·o·dis·play'zhuh serr'e·brye). PROGRESSIVE CEREBRAL POLIODYSTROPHY.

poliodystrofia. Poliodystrophia (= POLIODYSTROPHY).

po·lio·dys·tro·phia (po''lee·o·dis·tro'fee·uh) *n.* POLIODYSTROPHY.

poliodystrophia cer·ebri pro·gres·si·va in·fan·ti·lis (serr'e·brye pro·gre·sigh'vuh in·fan'ti·lis). PROGRESSIVE CEREBRAL POLIODYSTROPHY.

po·lio·dys·tro·phy (po''lee·o·dis'truh·fee) *n.* [*polio-* + *dystrophy*]. Degeneration of gray matter. See also *progressive cerebral poliodystrophy.*

po·lio·en·ceph·a·li·tis (po''lee·o·en·sef''uh·lye'tis) *n.* [*polio-* + *encephal-* + *-itis*]. Inflammation of the gray matter of the brain.

polioencephalitis acu·ta (a·kew'tuh). POLIOENCEPHALITIS.

polioencephalitis he·mor·rha·gi·ca (hem''o·ray'ji·kuh, ·raj'i·kuh). Inflammation of the gray matter of the brain with hemorrhage.

polioencephalitis hemorrhagica superior. *Obsol.* WERNICKE'S ENCEPHALOPATHY.

po·lio·en·ceph·a·lo·me·nin·go·my·e·li·tis (po''lee·o·en·sef''uh·lo·me·nin''go·migh·e·lye'tis) *n.* [*polio-* + *encephalo-* + *meningo-* + *myel-* + *-itis*]. Inflammation of the gray matter of the brain and spinal cord and of their meninges.

po·lio·en·ceph·a·lo·my·e·li·tis (po'lee·o·en·sef''uh·lo·migh·e·lye'tis) *n.* [*polio-* + *encephalo-* + *myel-* + *-itis*]. Any inflammation of the gray matter of the brain and spinal cord, more specifically paralytic spinal poliomyelitis with encephalitis.

po·lio·en·ceph·a·lop·a·thy (po''lee·o·en·sef''uh·lop'uth·ee) *n.* [*polio-* + *encephalo-* + *-pathy*]. Any disease of the gray matter of the brain.

po·lio·my·el·en·ceph·a·li·tis (po''lee·o·migh''ul·en·sef''uh·lye'tis) *n.* [*polio-* + *myel-* + *encephal-* + *-itis*]. POLIOENCEPHALOMYELITIS.

po·lio·my·e·li·tis (po''lee·o·migh''e·lye'tis) *n.* [*polio-* + *myelitis*]. 1. A common virus disease of man which usually runs a mild or abortive course, characterized by upper respiratory and gastrointestinal symptoms, but which may progress to involve the central nervous system and result in a nonparalytic or paralytic form of the disease, the latter being the classical form of paralytic spinal poliomyelitis. It is endemic with epidemic flare-ups, but is preventable through immunization. 2. Any inflammation of the gray matter of the spinal cord. **—poliomye·lit·ic** (·lit'ick) *adj.*

poliomyelitis vaccine. 1. Officially (USP, USPHS), a sterile suspension of inactivated poliomyelitis virus of types 1, 2, and 3; used for active immunization against poliomyelitis. Syn. *Salk vaccine.* 2. Unofficially and more broadly, any vaccine against poliomyelitis, including preparations of living attenuated poliomyelitis virus, such as Sabin vaccine.

poliomyelitis virus. A small (20 to 25 nm), relatively stable virus which is the causative agent of poliomyelitis. On an immunological basis, three distinct types have been identified, of which the classical prototypes are type 1, Brunhilde; type 2, Lansing; type 3, Leon. Type 1 is the most frequently responsible for the epidemic form of the disease.

po·lio·my·e·lop·a·thy (po''lee·o·migh''e·lop'uth·ee) *n.* [*polio-* + *myelopathy*]. Disease of the gray matter of the spinal cord.

po·li·o·sis (po''lee·o'sis) *n.* [Gk. *poliōsis,* becoming gray, from *polios,* gray]. 1. A condition characterized by the absence of pigment in the hair. Syn. *canities.* 2. Premature graying of the hair.

pol·io·thrix (pol'ee·o·thricks) *n.* [Gk., gray-haired, from *polio-* + *thrix,* hair]. CANITIES.

po·lio·vi·rus (po''lee·o·vye'rus) *n.* POLIOMYELITIS VIRUS.

poliovirus vaccine (live, oral). A preparation of one or all three types of live, attenuated poliomyelitis viruses; administered orally for active immunization against poliomyelitis. Syn. *Sabin oral poliomyelitis vaccine.*

Po·lit·zer bag (po'lit·sur) [A. *Politzer,* Austrian otologist, 1835–1920]. A waterproof bag used to inflate the middle ear. One end is tightly fixed into one nostril while the other is held closed during the act of swallowing water or pronouncing the letter *k.*

po·lit·zer·iza·tion (po''lit·sur·i·zay'shun, pol''it·) *n.* [A. *Politzer*]. The production of sudden increased air pressure in the nasopharynx to inflate the middle ear, by means of compression by a Politzer bag.

Politzer's cone [A. *Politzer*]. CONE OF LIGHT (1).

Politzer's test [A. *Politzer*]. A hearing test in which a tuning fork held in front of the nares will be heard only by the unaffected ear during swallowing.

poll (pole) *n. & v.* [ME. *polle,* from LG.]. 1. *Obsol.* The crown and back of the head. 2. Specifically, the vertex or crest between the ears of a quadruped; in cattle, the part from which the horns grow. 3. To cut off the horns of (cattle).

Pollack method. A histochemical method for the detection of calcium using sodium alizarin sulfonate to give a red precipitate.

pol·la·ki·uria (pol''uh·kee·yoor'ee·uh) *n.* [Gk. *pollakis,* often, + *-uria*]. Abnormally frequent micturition.

Pollak's test. VON JAKSCH-POLLAK'S TEST.

pol·len (pol'un) *n.* [L., fine flour, fine dust]. The fecundating element of flowering plants.

pol·len·osis (pol''e·no'sis) *n.* [*pollen* + *-osis*]. HAY FEVER.

poll evil. A purulent, necrotizing lesion occurring at the occipital attachment of the ligamentum nuchae in horses and usually caused by infection with the bacterium *Brucella abortus.*

pol·lex (pol'ecks) *n.,* genit. **pol·li·cis** (pol'i·sis), pl. **polli·ces** (·seez) [L.] [NA]. THUMB. NA alt. *digitus I.*

pollex val·gus (val'gus). A thumb abnormally bent toward the ulnar side.

pollex va·rus (vair'us). A thumb abnormally bent toward the radial side.

pol·li·ci·za·tion (pol''i·si·zay'shun) *n.* [L. *pollex, pollicis,* thumb]. 1. The freeing of a webbed thumb. 2. A surgically produced substitution of another digit to replace a thumb. **—pol·li·cize** (pol'i·size) *v.*

pol·li·co·men·tal (pol''i·ko·men'tul) *adj.* [L. *pollex, pollicis,* thumb, + *mental*]. Pertaining to the thenar area of the palm and the mentalis muscle.

pollicomental reflex. PALMOMENTAL REFLEX.

Pollister method. MIRSKY-POLLISTER METHOD.

pol·lu·tion, *n.* [L. *pollutio,* from *polluere,* to defile]. 1. The act of defiling or rendering impure, as pollution of drinking water. 2. The discharge of semen without sexual intercourse, as in nocturnal emission.

po·lo·cyte (po'lo·site) *n.* [*pole* + *-cyte*]. One of the polar bodies.

po·lo·ni·um (po·lo'nee·um) *n.* [ML. *Polonia,* Poland]. Po = 210. The first radioactive element isolated by Pierre and Marie Curie from pitchblende (1898); a product of disintegration of radium. Syn. *radium-F.*

pol·ox·a·lene (pol·ock'suh·leen) *n.* A liquid nonionic surfactant of the polyoxypropylene polyoxyethylene type, having a molecular weight of approximately 3,000.

pol·ox·a·mer (pol·ock'suh·mur) *n.* A polymer of ethylene oxide and propylene oxide used for its surface tension reducing action in the treatment of chronic constipation.

pol·toph·a·gy (pol·tof'uh·jee) *n.* [Gk. *poltos,* porridge, + *-phagy*]. Complete chewing of the food to the consistency of porridge before swallowing it.

po·lus (po'lus) *n.,* pl. & genit. sing. **po·li** (·lye) [L.]. POLE.

polus anterior bul·bi ocu·li (bul'bye ock'yoo·lye) [NA]. The central point of the anterior curvature of the eyeball.

polus anterior len·tis (len'tis) [NA]. The central point of the anterior surface of the lens.

polus fron·ta·lis (fron·tay'lis) [NA]. FRONTAL POLE.

polus oc·ci·pi·ta·lis (ock·sip·i·tay'lis) [NA]. OCCIPITAL POLE.

polus posterior bul·bi ocu·li (bul·bye ock'yoo·lye) [NA]. The central point of the posterior curvature of the eyeball.

polus posterior len·tis (len'tis) [NA]. The central point of the posterior surface of the lens.

polus tem·po·ra·lis (tem·po·ray'lis) [NA]. TEMPORAL POLE.

poly- [Gk. *polys,* much, many]. A combining form meaning (a) *multiple, compound, complex;* (b) *various, diverse;* (c) *excessive;* (d) *generalized, disseminated.*

poly·ac·id (pol''ee·as'id) *n.* [*poly-* + *acid*]. 1. An acid, such as phosphoric acid, having more than one replaceable hydrogen atom. 2. A complex acid derived from a number of molecules of one or more inorganic acids by elimination of water.

polyaemia. POLYEMIA.

polyaesthesia. POLYESTHESIA.

poly·am·ine (pol''ee·am'in, pol''ee·uh·meen') *n.* [*poly-* + *amine*]. Any compound having two or more amine groups. **—poly·ami·no** (·am'i·no, ·uh·mee'no) *adj.*

polyamine-formaldehyde resin. POLYAMINE-METHYLENE RESIN.

polyamine-methylene resin. A generic name for a synthetic acid-binding resin obtained by the polymerization of an aromatic amine and formaldehyde or of a polyamine, a phenol, and formaldehyde. Such a resin is useful clinically as a gastric antacid and to prevent acidosis when carbacrylic resin is used for its sodium-depleting effect. See also *carbacrylamine resins, Amberlite.*

poly·an·dry (pol'ee·an''dree) *n.* [Gk. *polyandria,* presence of many men, from *poly-* + *anēr,* man, husband]. A social state in which the marriage of one woman with more than one man at the same time is lawful.

poly·an·gi·i·tis (pol''ee·an''jee·eye'tis) *n.* [*poly-* + *angiitis*]. An inflammatory process involving multiple vascular channels.

poly·ar·te·ri·tis (pol''ee·ahr''te·rye'tis) *n.* [*poly-* + *arteritis*]. 1. Inflammation of a number of arteries at the same time. 2. POLYARTERITIS NODOSA.

polyarteritis no·do·sa (no·do'suh). A systemic disease characterized by widespread inflammation of small and medium-sized arteries in which some of the foci are nodular; complications of the process such as thrombosis lead to retrogressive changes in the tissues and organs supplied by the affected vessels with a correspondingly diverse array of symptoms and signs. Syn. *periarteritis nodosa, disseminated necrotizing periarteritis.*

poly·ar·thric (pol″ee·ahr′thrick) *adj.* [Gk. *polyarthros,* having many joints, from *poly-* + *arthron,* joint]. Pertaining to many joints.

poly·ar·thri·tis (pol″ee·ahr·thrye′tis) *n.* [*poly-* + *arthritis*]. Simultaneous inflammation of several joints.

poly·ar·throp·a·thy (pol″ee·ahr·throp′uth·ee) *n.* [*poly-* + *arthropathy*]. Disease of several joints.

poly·ar·tic·u·lar (pol″ee·ahr·tick′yoo·lur) *adj.* [*poly-* + *articular*]. Pertaining to or affecting several joints.

Pó·lya's operation or **method** (po′yah) [E. *Pólya,* Hungarian surgeon, 1876–1944]. Partial resection of the stomach, followed by posterior end-to-side gastrojejunostomy; a type of Billroth II gastric resection.

poly·atom·ic (pol″ee·uh·tom′ick) *adj.* [*poly-* + *atomic*]. Containing several atoms.

poly·ba·sic (pol″ee·bay′sick) *adj.* [*poly-* + *basic*]. Referring to an acid having several hydrogen atoms replaceable by bases.

poly·blast (pol′ee·blast) *n.* [*poly-* + *blast*]. A free macrophage of inflamed connective tissue derived from blood-borne monocytes.

poly·ble·phar·ia (pol″ee·blef·ăr′ee·uh) *n.* [*poly-* + *blephar-* + *-ia*]. The condition of having a supernumerary eyelid.

poly·bleph·a·ron (pol″ee·blef′uh·ron) *n.* [*poly-* + *blepharon*]. A supernumerary eyelid.

poly·bleph·a·ry (pol″ee·blef′uh·ree) *n.* POLYBLEPHARIA.

poly·bu·ti·late (pol″ee·bew′ti·late) *n.* A poly(oxytetramethyleneoxyadipoyl), $(C_{10}H_{16}O_4)_n$, used as a coating for surgical sutures.

poly·car·bo·phil (pol″ee·kahr′bo·fil) *n.* A granular compound of polyacrylic acid cross-linked with divinyl glycol that is used as a gastrointestinal absorbent.

poly·cel·lu·lar (pol″ee·sel′yoo·lur) *adj.* [*poly-* + *cellular*]. Having many cells.

poly·cen·tric (pol″ee·sen′trick) *adj.* [*poly-* + *-centric*]. Having many centers or nuclear points.

poly·chei·ria (pol″ee·kigh′ree·uh) *n.* [Gk. *polycheir,* many-handed (from *cheir,* hand) + *-ia*]. The state of having a supernumerary hand. —**polychei·rous** (·rus) *adj.*

poly·chlo·ri·nat·ed (pol″ee·klo′rin·ay·tid) *adj.* Having chlorine atoms substituted for more than three hydrogen atoms.

polychlorinated biphenyl. 1. Any biphenyl structure with chlorine atoms attached. 2. Originally, any of a class of pesticides with polychlorinated biphenyl residues. Abbreviated, PCB

poly·cho·lia (pol″ee·ko′lee·uh) *n.* [*poly-* + *chol-* + *-ia*]. Excessive secretion of bile.

poly·chon·dri·tis (pol″ee·kon·drye′tis) *n.* [*poly-* + *chondritis*]. Inflammation of cartilage in various parts of the body. See also *relapsing polychondritis.*

poly·chro·ism (pol″ee·kro′iz·um) *n.* [Gk. *polychroos,* many-colored (from *chroa,* complexion, color) + *-ism*]. A property possessed by certain crystals, under polarized light, of exhibiting different absorption colors which vary as the polarizing instrument is rotated.

poly·chro·ma·sia (pol″ee·kro·may′zhuh) *n.* [*poly-* + *-chromasia*]. POLYCHROMATOPHILIA.

poly·chro·ma·tia (pol″ee·kro·may′shee·uh) *n.* POLYCHROMATOPHILIA.

poly·chro·mat·ic (pol″ee·kro·mat′ick) *adj.* [Gk. *polychrōmatos,* from *poly-* + *chrōma,* color]. 1. Of, pertaining to, or having several colors. 2. POLYCHROMATOPHILIC.

polychromatic erythroblast. An erythroblast containing both hemoglobin and ribosomes both in sufficient concentration to be visualized in stained preparations. The cytoplasm is the polychromatic mixture of red and blue since, in Romanovsky-type stains, hemoglobin is stained red and ribosomes blue.

polychromatic erythrocyte. An erythrocyte formed when a polychromatic erythroblast loses its nucleus.

polychromatic theory. A theory of color vision, postulating seven types of receptors possessing eight response curves: (1) crimson, (2) orange, (3) yellow, (4) green, (5) blue-green, (6) blue, (7) blue-violet.

poly·chro·mato·cyte (pol″ee·kro·mat′o·site, ·kro′muh·to·) *n.* [*poly-* + *chromato-* + *-cyte*]. A cell that will simultaneously assume the color of different dyes.

poly·chro·mato·phil (pol″ee·kro′muh·to·fil, ·kro·mat′o·fil) *n.* [*poly-* + *chromato-* + *-phil*]. A structure stainable with both acidic and basic dyes.

poly·chro·mato·phil·ia (pol″ee·kro″muh·to·fil′ee·uh) *n.* The presence in the blood of polychromatophilic cells.

poly·chro·mato·phil·ic (pol″ee·kro″muh·to·fil′ick) *adj.* [*polychromatophil* + *-ic*]. Susceptible to staining with more than one dye.

polychromatophilic erythrocyte. An erythrocyte that contains variable amounts of basophilic staining material giving an appearance of polychromatophilia on Wright- or Giemsa-stained blood films. See also *polychromatic erythrocyte.*

poly·chrome (pol′ee·krome) *adj.* [Gk. *polychrōmos,* many-colored]. Of or pertaining to many colors.

polychrome methylene blue. Methylene blue partially oxidized into its lower homologues, methylene violet and the azures, with an increase in metachromatic properties; prepared by allowing methylene blue to age or by boiling a methylene blue solution with alkali.

poly·chro·mia (pol″ee·kro′mee·uh) *n.* [*poly-* + *-chromia*]. Increased or abnormal pigmentation.

poly·chro·mo·cy·to·sis (pol″ee·kro″mo·sigh·to′sis) *n.* [*polychromatocyte* + *-osis*]. POLYCHROMATOPHILIA.

poly·chro·mo·phil (pol″ee·kro′mo·fil) *n.* POLYCHROMATOPHIL.

poly·chro·mo·phil·ia (pol″ee·kro″mo·fil′ee·uh) *n.* POLYCHROMATOPHILIA.

poly·chy·lia (pol″ee·kigh′lee·uh) *n.* [*poly-* + *chyl-* + *-ia*]. Excessive formation of chyle. —**polychy·lic** (·lick) *adj.*

Polycillin. A trademark for ampicillin, a semisynthetic penicillin antibiotic.

poly·clin·ic (pol″ee·klin′ick) *n.* [*poly-* + *clinic*]. A hospital in which many types of diseases are treated.

poly·clo·nal (pol′ee·klo′nul) *adj.* [*poly-* + *clone* + *-al*]. Pertaining to or characterizing cells of various different clones, with the implication that the principal proteins or other products manufactured by these cells are different. Contr. *monoclonal.*

polyclonal gammopathy. DIFFUSE HYPERGAMMAGLOBULINEMIA.

poly·co·ria (pol″ee·ko′ree·uh) *n.* [*poly-* + *cor-* + *-ia*]. A hereditary anomaly of the eye characterized by the presence of more than one pupil, each surrounded by a sphincter (true polycoria), the exact mechanism of which is unknown. Similar defects in the periphery of the iris (false polycoria) also occur.

poly·cy·clic (pol″ee·sigh′click, ·sick′lick) *adj.* [*poly-* + *cyclic*]. 1. Describing a molecule that contains two or more groupings of atoms in the form of rings or closed chains. 2. *In dermatology,* pertaining to cutaneous lesions exhibiting many confluent rings or arcs.

poly·cy·e·sis (pol″ee·sigh·ee′sis) *n.* [*poly-* + *cyesis*]. MULTIPLE PREGNANCY.

poly·cys·tic (pol″ee·sis′tick) *adj.* [*poly-* + *cystic*]. Containing many cysts.

polycystic disease or **kidney.** Hereditary bilateral cysts distributed throughout the renal parenchyma, resulting in markedly enlarged kidneys and progressive renal failure.

See also *adult polycystic disease, infantile polycystic disease.*

poly·cy·the·mia, poly·cy·thae·mia (pol″ee·sigh·theem′ee·uh) *n.* [*poly-* + *-cyte* + *-hemia*]. A condition characterized by an increased number of erythrocytes and erythroblasts.

polycythemia hy·per·ton·i·ca (high·pur·ton′i·kuh). GAISBÖCK'S DISEASE.

polycythemia ru·bra ve·ra (roo′bruh veer′uh). POLYCYTHEMIA VERA.

polycythemia ve·ra (veer′uh). An absolute increase in all marrow-derived blood cells, especially erythrocytes and erythroblasts, of unknown cause. Syn. *erythremia, Osler-Vaquez disease, primary polycythemia.*

poly·dac·tyl·ia (pol″ee·dack·til′ee·uh) *n.* POLYDACTYLY.

poly·dac·tyl·ism (pol″ee·dack′til·iz·um) *n.* POLYDACTYLY.

poly·dac·ty·ly (pol″ee·dack′ti·lee) *n.* [*poly-* + *-dactyly*]. The existence of supernumerary fingers or toes.

poly·de·fi·cient (pol″ee·de·fish′unt) *adj.* PLURIDEFICIENT. **—polydefi·cien·cy** (·un·see) *n.*

poly·dip·sia (pol″ee·dip′see·uh) *n.* [Gk. *polydipsios,* very thirsty, from *dipsa,* thirst]. Excessive thirst. Syn. *anadipsia.*

poly·don·tia (pol″ee·don′chee·uh) *n.* POLYODONTIA.

poly·dys·troph·ic (pol″ee·dis·trof′ick) *adj.* [*poly-* + *dystrophic*]. Characterized by or pertaining to many congenital anomalies, especially of connective tissue.

polydystrophic dwarfism. MAROTEAUX-LAMY'S SYNDROME.

polydystrophic oligophrenia. SANFILIPPO'S SYNDROME.

poly·dys·tro·phy (pol″ee·dis′truh·fee) *n.* [*poly-* + *dystrophy*]. The presence of several, usually congenital, structural abnormalities.

poly·elec·tro·lyte (pol″ee·e·leck′tro·lite) *n.* [*poly-* + *electrolyte*]. Any substance of high molecular weight that behaves as an electrolyte, such as proteins.

poly·em·bry·o·ny (pol″ee·em′bree·uh·nee) *n.* [*poly-* + *embryony*]. The instance of a zygote giving rise to more than one embryo.

poly·emia, poly·ae·mia (pol″ee·ee′mee·uh) *n.* [Gk. *polyaimia,* fullness of blood, from *haima,* blood]. An excess of blood over the normal amount in the body.

poly·ene (pol′ee·een) *n.* [*poly-* + *-ene*]. A compound that contains three or more double bonds joining carbon atoms in the compound.

poly·es·the·sia, poly·aes·the·sia (pol″ee·es·theezh′uh, ·theez′ee·uh) *n.* [*poly-* + *-esthesia*]. An abnormality of sensation in which a stimulus such as a single touch or pinprick is felt in two or more places at the same time.

poly·es·trus, poly·oes·trus (pol″ee·es′trus) *n.* [*poly-* + *estrus*]. In animals, the existence of several estrus periods during each sexual season. **—polyestrous,** *adj.*

poly·eth·a·dene (pol″ee·eth′uh·deen) *n.* 1,2:3,4-Diepoxybutane polymer with ethylenimine, $(C_4H_6O_2)_m(C_2H_5N)_n$, an antacid.

poly·eth·yl·ene (pol″ee·eth′il·een) *n.* A long-chain plastic polymer containing hundreds of ethylene units per molecule. In the form of flexible tubing and film, a pure form of the plastic is useful in surgical procedures.

polyethylene glycol. Any one of a series of water-soluble compounds of the general formula $H(OCH_2CH_2)_nOH$, prepared by condensation polymerization of ethylene oxide and water; those with average molecular weights between 200 and 700 are liquids; above 1,000 they are wax-like solids. The liquid compounds are used as solvents and dispersants; the solid glycols are used in the formulation of water-soluble ointment bases.

polyethylene tube. A smooth-walled, flexible, inelastic tube which is comparatively inert in tissues; often used in surgery and in such procedures as transfusions, infusions, and drainage.

Po·lyg·a·la (pol·ig′uh·luh) *n.* [NL., from Gk. *polygalon,* milkwort, from *polygalos,* having much milk]. A genus of herbaceous or shrubby plants, some of which have been used medicinally.

poly·ga·lac·tia (pol″ee·ga·lack′tee·uh, ·shee·uh) *n.* [Gk. *polygalaktos,* having much milk (from *gala,* milk) + *-ia*]. Excessive secretion of milk.

po·lyg·a·mous (pol·ig′uh·mus) *adj.* [Gk. *polygamos,* from *poly-* + *gamos,* marriage]. 1. Having, or allowing, more than one wife or husband at one time, more particularly the former. 2. Having both unisexual and hermaphrodite flowers on one plant. **—polyga·my** (·mee) *n.*

poly·gas·tria (pol″ee·gas′tree·uh) *n.* [*poly-* + *-gastria*]. Excessive secretion of gastric juice.

poly·gas·tric (pol″ee·gas′trick) *adj.* [*poly-* + *gastric*]. 1. Having several bellies, as certain muscles. 2. Having more than one stomach.

poly·gen·ic (pol″ee·jen′ick) *adj.* [*poly-* + *-genic*]. Pertaining to or determined by several different genes.

poly·glac·tin (pol″ee·glack′tin) *n.* A copolymer of glycolic and lactic acids, of approximate molecular weight of 80,000, used as an absorbable suture material.

poly·glan·du·lar (pol″ee·gland′yoo·lur) *adj.* [*poly-* + *glandular*]. Pluriglandular; pertaining to or affecting several glands or their secretions.

poly·glo·bu·lia (pol″ee·glob·yoo′lee·uh) *n.* [*poly-* + *globule* + *-ia*]. POLYCYTHEMIA.

poly·glob·u·lism (pol″ee·glob′yoo·liz·um) *n.* [*poly-* + *globule* + *-ism*]. POLYCYTHEMIA.

pol·y·gly·col·ic acid (pol″ee·glye·kol′ick). Poly(oxycarbonylmethylene), $(OCOCH_2)_n$, a polymer of glycolic acid anhydride units; used as a surgical suture material.

poly·gnath·us (pol″ee·nath′us) *n.* [*poly-* + *-gnathus*]. An individual in which a parasitic twin or part is attached to the jaws of the host.

po·lyg·o·nal (pol·ig′uh·nul) *adj.* [Gk. *polygōnos,* from *poly-* + *gōnia,* angle]. Having many angles.

Po·lyg·o·num (po·lig′o·num) *n.* [NL., from Gk. *polygonon,* knotgrass]. A genus of herbs of the family Polygonaceae. *Polygonum bistorta* is the source of bistort, an astringent.

poly·gram (pol′ee·gram) *n.* The tracing made by a polygraph.

poly·graph (pol′ee·graf) *n.* [*poly-* + *-graph*]. An instrument by means of which tracings can be taken simultaneously of the cardiac movements, the arterial or venous pulse, respiration, and skin resistance. Syn. *polysphygmograph.* See also *Keeler's lie detector, lie detector.* **—poly·graph·ic** (pol″ee·graf′ick) *adj.*

poly·gy·ria (pol″i·jye′ree·uh) *n.* [*poly-* + *gyr-* + *-ia*]. The existence of an excessive number of convolutions in the brain.

poly·he·dral (pol″i·hee′drul) *adj.* [Gk. *polyedros,* having many sides or seats, from *hedra,* seat, facet]. Having many surfaces.

poly·he·mia, poly·hae·mia (pol″ee·hee′mee·uh) *n.* POLYEMIA.

poly·hi·dro·sis (pol″ee·hi·dro′sis) *n.* [*poly-* + *hidrosis*]. HYPERHIDROSIS.

poly·hy·brid (pol″ee·high′brid) *n.* [*poly-* + *hybrid*]. An individual heterozygous for many pairs of genes.

poly·hy·dram·ni·os (pol″ee·high·dram′nee·os) *n.* [*poly-* + *hydr-* + Gk. *amnios,* amnion]. An excessive volume of amniotic fluid.

poly·hy·dric (pol″ee·high′drick) *adj.* [*poly-* + *hydr-* + *-ic*]. 1. In acids, containing more than one replaceable atom of hydrogen. 2. Containing more than one hydroxyl group; polyhydroxy.

poly·hy·droxy (pol″ee·high·drock′see) *adj.* POLYHYDRIC.

poly·hy·dru·ria (pol″ee·high·droor′ee·uh) *n.* [*poly-* + *hydruria*]. A large increase in fluid content of the urine.

poly·idro·sis (pol″ee·i·dro′sis) *n.* Polyhidrosis (= HYPERHIDROSIS).

poly·in·fec·tion (pol″ee·in·feck′shun) *n.* [*poly-* + *infection*]. Infection resulting from the presence of more than one type of organism; mixed infection.

Polykol. A trademark for poloxalkol, a surface-active compound used in the treatment of chronic constipation.

poly·lec·i·thal (pol″ee·les′i·thul) *adj.* [*poly-* + *lecithal*]. Having much yolk.

poly·lep·tic (pol″ee·lep′tick) *adj.* [*poly-* + *-leptic,* from Gk.

lēpsis, attack, seizure]. Characterized by numerous remissions and exacerbations.

poly·lob·u·lar (pol″ee·lob′yoo·lur) *adj.* [*poly-* + *lobular*]. MULTILOBULAR.

poly·ma·con (pol″i·may′kon) *n.* A loosely cross-linked polymer of a small amount of ethyleneglycol dimethacrylate with hydroxyethyl methacrylate used as a hydrophilic contact lens material.

poly·mas·tia (pol″ee·mas′tee·uh) *n.* [*poly-* + *-mastia*]. The presence of more than two breasts.

poly·mas·ti·gate (pol″ee·mas′ti·gate) *adj.* [*poly-* + Gk. *mastix, mastigos*, whip]. Having several flagella.

Poly·mas·ti·gi·da (pol″ee·mas·tij′i·duh) *n.pl.* POLYMASTIGINA.

Poly·mas·ti·gi·na (pol″ee·mas″ti·jye′nuh) *n.pl.* [NL., from *poly-* + Gk. *mastix*, whip]. An order of flagellates all of whose members have three or more flagella.

poly·mas·ti·gous (pol″ee·mas′ti·gus) *adj.* POLYMASTIGATE.

poly·ma·zia (pol″ee·may′zhuh) *n.* [*poly-* + *maz-* + *-ia*]. POLYMASTIA.

poly·me·lia (pol″ee·mee′lee·uh) *n.* [*poly-* + *-melia*]. The presence of more than the normal number of limbs.

poly·me·li·us (pol″ee·mee′lee·us) *n.* POLYMELUS.

poly·me·lus (pol″ee·mee′lus) *n.*, pl. **polyme·li** (·lye) [NL., from Gk. *polymelēs*, many-limbed, from *melos*, limb]. An individual having more than the normal number of limbs.

poly·me·nia (pol″ee·mee′nee·uh) *n.* [*poly-* + *men-* + *-ia*]. MENORRHAGIA.

poly·men·or·rhea, poly·men·or·rhoea (pol″ee·men′o·ree′uh) *n.* [*poly-* + *menorrhea*]. METRORRHAGIA.

poly·mer (pol′i·mur) *n.* [*poly-* + *-mer*]. The product formed by joining together many small molecules (monomers). A polymer may be formed from units of the same monomer (addition polymer) or different monomers (condensation polymer).

poly·mer·ase (pol′i·mur·ace·, ·aze, pol·im′ur·) *n.* Any enzyme that catalyzes polymerization, as of nucleotides.

polymer fume fever. A disease similar to metal fume fever, but associated with inhalation of vaporized polymers.

poly·me·ria (pol″ee·meer′ee·uh) *n.* [*poly-* + *mer-* + *-ia*]. The presence of extra or supernumerary parts of the body.

poly·mer·ic (pol″i·merr′ick) *adj.* [Gk. *polymerēs*, consisting of many parts, from *meros*, part]. 1. Exhibiting polymerism. 2. Of muscles, derived from two or more myotomes.

po·lym·er·ide (pol·im′ur·ide) *n.* POLYMER.

po·lym·er·ism (pol·im′ur·iz·um, pol′i·mur·iz·um) *n.* [*polymeric* + *-ism*]. 1. The existence of more than a normal number of parts. 2. A form of isomerism in which two or more molecules of a simple compound interact to form larger molecules, called polymers, that have repeating structural units of the simple compound.

po·lym·er·iza·tion (pol·im″ur·i·zay′shun, pol″i·mur·) *n.* A reaction in which a complex molecule of relatively high molecular weight is formed by the union of a number of simpler molecules, which may or may not be alike; the reaction may or may not involve elimination of a by-product, such as water or ammonia.

po·lym·er·ize (pol·im′ur·ize, pol′i·mur·ize) *v.* To form a compound from several molecules of the same or different simple molecules. The molecular weight of the polymer may be a simple multiple of the molecular weight of the single simple molecule or the product of the molecular weights of the simple molecules less the molecular weight of the eliminated molecule.

poly·meta·car·pal·ism (pol″ee·met″uh·kahr′pul·iz·um) *n.* [*poly-* + *metacarpal* + *-ism*]. A developmental anomaly in which the metacarpus contains more than the normal five bones.

poly·mi·cro·bic (pol″ee·migh·kro′bick) *adj.* [*poly-* + *microbic*]. Containing many kinds of microorganisms.

poly·mi·cro·gy·ria (pol″ee·migh″kro·jye′ree·uh) *n.* [*poly-* + *microgyria*]. A condition of the cerebral cortex characterized by abnormally numerous but very small convolutions, due to some disturbance during brain development.

poly·morph (pol′ee·morf) *n.* POLYMORPHONUCLEAR LEUKOCYTE.

poly·mor·phic (pol″ee·mor′fick) *adj.* [Gk. *polymorphos* multiform, versatile (from *morphē*, form), + *-ic*]. 1. Having or occurring in several forms, as a substance crystallizing in different forms. 2. *In clinical medicine*, POLYSYMPTOMATIC.

poly·mor·phism (pol″ee·mor′fiz·um) *n.* The state of being polymorphic.

poly·mor·pho·cel·lu·lar (pol″ee·mor″fo·sel′yoo·lur) *adj.* [*polymorphic* + *cellular*]. Having cells of many forms.

poly·mor·pho·cyte (pol″ee·mor′fo·site) *n.* [*polymorphic* + *-cyte*]. A cell having a polymorphic nucleus, especially a granular leukocyte.

poly·mor·pho·nu·cle·ar (pol″ee·mor″fo·new′klee·ur) *adj.* [*polymorphic* + *nuclear*]. Having a nucleus which is lobated, the lobes being connected by more or less thin strands of nuclear substance; for example, the nucleus of a neutrophil leukocyte.

polymorphonuclear leukocyte. The mature neutrophil leukocyte, so-called because of its segmented and irregularly shaped nucleus. See also *granulocyte*.

poly·mor·phous (pol″ee·mor′fus) *adj.* [Gk. *polymorphos*]. POLYMORPHIC.

polymorphous light eruption. An inflammatory dermatosis induced by sunlight presenting pleomorphic or polymorphic clinical patterns.

polymorphous photodermatitis. POLYMORPHOUS LIGHT ERUPTION.

polymorphous sarcoma. A malignant GRANULAR CELL MYOBLASTOMA.

poly·my·al·gia (pol″ee·migh·al′jee·uh, ·juh) *n.* [*poly-* + *myalgia*]. Pain involving many muscles.

polymyalgia rheu·mat·i·ca (roo·mat′i·kuh). Pain and stiffness in the proximal muscle groups occurring in older people, usually related to giant-cell arteritis.

poly·my·oc·lo·nus (pol″ee·migh·ock′luh·nus, ·migh″o·klo′nus) *n.* [*poly-* + *myoclonus*]. Generalized myoclonus.

poly·my·op·a·thy (pol″ee·migh·op′uth·ee) *n.* [*poly-* + *myopathy*]. Any disease affecting several muscles at the same time.

poly·my·o·si·tis (pol″ee·migh″o·sigh′tis) *n.* [*poly-* + *myositis*]. Simultaneous inflammation of many muscles. See also *dermatomyositis*.

poly·myx·in (pol″ee·mick′sin) *n.* A generic term for a group of related polypeptide antibiotic substances derived from cultures of various strains of the spore-forming soil bacterium *Bacillus polymyxa* (*B. aerosporus*); the individual substances are differentiated by affixing A,B,C,D, and E to the name polymyxin. Polymyxin B, the least toxic of the group, is bactericidal against most gram-negative microorganisms; it is used clinically, in the form of the water-soluble sulfate salt, in a variety of infections, especially against *Pseudomonas aeruginosa*.

poly·ne·sic (pol″ee·nee′sick, ·nes′ick) *adj.* [*poly-* + Gk. *nēsos*, island, + *-ic*]. Occurring in several foci.

poly·neu·ral (pol″ee·new′rul) *adj.* [*poly-* + *neural*]. Pertaining to, or supplied by, several nerves.

poly·neu·ral·gia (pol″ee·new·ral′jee·uh, ·juh) *n.* [*poly-* + *neuralgia*]. Neuralgia in which many nerves are involved.

poly·neu·ric (pol″ee·new′rick) *adj.* POLYNEURAL.

polyneuritic spinocerebellar ataxia. REFSUM'S SYNDROME.

poly·neu·ri·tis (pol″ee·new·rye′tis) *n.* [*poly-* + *neuritis*]. Simultaneous inflammatory involvement of multiple nerves, usually symmetrical, as occurs in leprosy and in the Guillain-Barré disease. Syn. *multiple neuritis*. —**polyneu·rit·ic** (·rit′ick) *adj.*

poly·neu·ro·my·o·si·tis (pol″ee·new″ro·migh″o·sigh′tis) *n.* [*poly-* + *neuro-* + *myositis*]. A disease in which there is concurrent polyneuritis and polymyositis.

poly·neu·rop·a·thy (pol″ee·new·rop′uth·ee) *n.* [*poly-* + *neuro-* + *-pathy*]. Simultaneous involvement of many peripheral and/or cranial nerves, usually symmetrical and affecting the distal portions of the limbs more than the proximal ones; a result of metabolic disorders (such as diabetes, uremia, or porphyria), intoxications (arsenic or lead), nutritional defects (beriberi or alcoholism) or a remote effect of carcinoma or myeloma.

poly·neu·ro·ra·dic·u·li·tis (pol″ee·new″ro·ra·dick·yoo·lye′tis) *n.* [*poly-* + *neuro-* + *radiculitis*]. GUILLAIN-BARRÉ DISEASE.

poly·nu·cle·ar (pol″ee·new′klee·ur) *adj.* [*poly-* + *nuclear*]. MULTINUCLEAR.

poly·nu·cle·ate (pol″ee·new′klee·ate) *adj.* MULTINUCLEAR.

poly·nu·cle·o·tid·ase (pol″ee·new″klee·o·tye′dace, ·ot′i·dace) *n.* An enzyme that depolymerizes nucleic acid to form mononucleotides.

poly·nu·cle·o·tide (pol″i·new′klee·o·tide) *n.* A nucleic acid composed of four mononucleotides.

poly·odon·tia (pol″ee·o·don′chee·uh) *n.* [*poly-* + *-odontia*]. The presence of supernumerary teeth.

polyoestrus. POLYESTRUS.

poly·oma virus (pol″ee·o′muh). A small deoxyribonucleic acid virus normally causing inapparent infection in mice, but experimentally capable of producing parotid and a wide variety of other tumors.

poly·onych·ia (pol″ee·o·nick′ee·uh) *n.* [*poly-* + *onych-* + *-ia*]. A condition of supernumerary nails on fingers or toes.

poly·opia (pol″ee·o′pee·uh) *n.* [*poly-* + *-opia*]. A condition in which more than one image of an object is formed upon the retina.

polyopia mo·noph·thal·mi·ca (mon·off·thal′mi·kuh). The phenomenon of multiple vision with a single eye.

poly·op·sia (pol″ee·op′see·uh) *n.* [*poly-* + *-opsia*]. POLYOPIA.

poly·or·chi·dism (pol″ee·or′ki·diz·um) *n.* [*poly-* + *orchid-* + *-ism*]. The presence of more than two testes in one individual.

poly·or·chis (pol″ee·or′kis) *n.* [*poly-* + *orchis*]. An individual who has more than two testes.

poly·or·chism (pol″ee·or′kiz·um) *n.* POLYORCHIDISM.

poly·orex·ia (pol″ee·o·reck′see·uh) *n.* [*poly-* + *-orexia*]. Excessive hunger or appetite; BULIMIA.

poly·or·gano·sil·ox·ane (pol″ee·or″guh·no·sil·ock′sane) *n.* Any synthetic polymer consisting of a chain of alternate links of silicon atoms and oxygen atoms, the two other bonds of the tetravalent silicon atom generally being attached to an organic group. Commonly known as silicones, these substances may be limpid or viscous fluids or semisolid to solid substances. The fluids impart to glass surfaces a water-repellent film.

poly·or·rho·men·in·gi·tis (pol″ee·or″o·men·in·jye′tis) *n.* [*poly-* + *orrhomeningitis*]. POLYSEROSITIS.

poly·or·rhy·men·i·tis (pol″ee·or·high″men·eye′tis, ·or·eye″men·) *n.* [*poly-* + *orr*ho-, serous, + *hymen-*, membrane, + *-itis*]. POLYSEROSITIS.

poly·os·tot·ic (pol″ee·uh·stot′ick) *adj.* [*poly-* + *ost-* + *-otic*]. Involving more than one bone.

polyostotic fibrous dysplasia. FIBROUS DYSPLASIA (1) involving more than one bone.

poly·o·tia (pol″ee·o′shee·uh) *n.* [*poly-* + *ot-* + *-ia*]. A congenital defect in which there is more than one auricle on one or both sides of the head.

poly·ox·yl (pol″ee·ock′sil) *n.* Generic name for various polyoxyethylene diol radicals of esters with fatty acids, of the type of $RCOO(C_2H_4O)_nH$. In polyoxyl 40 stearate, which is a surfactant used in water-soluble ointment and cream bases, n is approximately 40, and RCOO represents stearate.

polyoxyl stearate. Any of several polyoxyethylene stearates that differ in the length of the polymer chain and are identified by number, as polyoxyl 8 stearate, in which the average polymer length is about 8 oxyethylene (C_2H_4O) units, and polyoxyl 40 stearate, in which the average polymer length is about 40 of the same units. They are variously used as surfactants.

pol·yp (pol′ip) *n.* [Gk. *polypous*, octopus; many-footed]. 1. A smooth spherical or oval mass projecting from a membranous surface; may be broad-based or pedunculated. 2. The sessile form of a coelenterate.

poly·pap·il·lo·ma (pol″ee·pap″i·lo′muh) *n.* [*poly-* + *papilloma*]. YAWS.

poly·pa·re·sis (pol″ee·pa·ree′sis, ·păr′e·sis) *n.* [*poly-* + *paresis*]. *Obsol.* GENERAL PARALYSIS.

poly·path·ia (pol″ee·path′ee·uh) *n.* [Gk. *polypatheia*, the suffering of many calamities]. The presence of several diseases at one time, or the frequent recurrence of disease.

pol·yp·ec·to·my (pol″i·peck′tuh·mee) *n.* [*polyp* + *-ectomy*]. Surgical excision of a polyp.

poly·pep·ti·dase (pol″ee·pep′ti·dace, ·daze) *n.* [*polypeptide* + *-ase*]. One of the enzymes that hydrolyze proteins and molecular fragments of proteins.

poly·pep·tide (pol″ee·pep′tide) *n.* [*poly-* + *peptide*]. A compound containing two or more amino acids united through the peptide linkage —CONH—.

poly·pep·tid·emia, poly·pep·ti·dae·mia (pol″ee·pep″ti·dee′mee·uh) *n.* [*polypeptide* + *-emia*]. The presence of polypeptides in the blood.

poly·pep·ti·dor·rha·chia (pol″ee·pep″ti·do·ray′kee·uh, ·rack′ee·uh) *n.* [*polypeptide* + Gk. *rhachis*, spine, + *-ia*]. The presence of polypeptides in the cerebrospinal fluid.

poly·pha·gia (pol″ee·fay′jee·uh) *n.* [Gk., from *poly-* + *phagein*, to eat]. 1. Excessive eating. 2. BULIMIA.

poly·pha·lan·gism (pol″ee·fuh·lan′jiz·um) *n.* [*poly-* + *phalang-* + *-ism*]. An extra phalanx in a finger or toe.

poly·phar·ma·cy (pol″ee·fahr′muh·see) *n.* [Gk. *polypharmakos*, knowing many drugs, using many drugs]. 1. The prescription of many drugs at one time. 2. The excessive use of medication.

poly·phe·nol oxidase (pol″ee·fee′nol). A copper-containing enzyme that catalyzes the oxidation of phenol derivatives to quinones.

poly·pho·bia (pol″ee·fo′bee·uh) *n.* [*poly-* + *-phobia*]. Abnormal fear of many things.

poly·phy·let·ic (pol″ee·fye·let′ick) *adj.* [*poly-* + *phyletic*]. Pertaining to origin from many lines of descent. Contr. *monophyletic.*

polyphyletic theory of hemopoiesis. A hypothesis concerning the mode of origin of blood cells which assumes the development of a specific parental cell for each cell type.

poly·phy·le·tism (pol″ee·fye′le·tiz·um) *n.* The polyphyletic theory of hemopoiesis.

poly·phy·odont (pol″i·fye′o·dont) *adj.* [Gk. *polyphyēs*, manifold, + *-odont*]. Having more than two successive sets of teeth at intervals throughout life.

polypi. Plural of *polypus.*

pol·yp·if·er·ous (pol″i·pif′ur·us) *adj.* [*polyp* + *-iferous*]. Bearing or originating polyps.

poly·plast (pol′i·plast) *adj.* [*poly-* + *-plast*]. 1. Formed of many different structures. 2. Having undergone many modifications during the process of development.

poly·ploid (pol′i·ploid) *adj.* [*poly-* + *-ploid*]. Having more than the somatic number of whole sets of chromosomes characteristic for the species. —**poly·ploi·dy** (pol′i·ploy·dee) *n.*

pol·yp·nea, pol·yp·noea (pol″ip·nee′uh) *n.* [*poly-* + *-pnea*]. Very rapid respiration; panting.

poly·po·dia (pol″i·po′dee·uh) *n.* [Gk., many-footedness, from *poly-* + *pous*, foot]. The condition of having supernumerary feet.

pol·yp·oid (pol″i·poid) *adj.* [*polyp* + *-oid*]. 1. Resembling a polyp. 2. Pertaining to or characterized by polyps.

polypoid adenomatosis. Multiple acquired diffuse polyposis, usually of the large intestine.

polypoid carcinoma. A carcinoma having a polypoid appearance on gross examination, seen commonly on mucous membranes of urinary and gastrointestinal tracts.

polypoid hyperplasia. A hyperplastic state in which the affected tissue resembles a polyp.

polypoid rhinitis. NASAL POLYP.

polypoid urethritis. Nonspecific chronic inflammation of the urethral mucosa, characterized by edematous bullae and blebs that project into the urethral lumen as inflammatory polyps.

po·lyp·o·rous (pol·ip'uh·rus) *adj.* [*poly-* + *porous*]. Having many small openings; cribriform.

Po·lyp·o·rus (po·lip'uh·rus) *n.* [NL., from Gk. *poly-* + *poros,* passage]. A genus of fungi of the family Polyporaceae. *Polyporus officinalis* is the source of agaric; biformin is derived from *Polyporus biformis.*

pol·yp·o·sis (pol''i·po'sis) *n.*, pl. **polypo·ses** (·seez) [*polyp* + *-osis*]. The condition of being affected with polyps.

polyposis co·li (ko'lye). Multiple polyps of the large intestine.

polyposis ven·tric·u·li (ven·trick'yoo·lye). Multiple polyps of the gastric mucosa. See also *état mamelonné.*

pol·yp·ous (pol'i·pus) *adj.* Pertaining to, having, or resembling a polyp or polyps.

poly·pty·chi·al (pol''i·tye'kee·ul) *adj.* [Gk. *polyptychos,* having many folds, from *ptychē,* fold]. Arranged in more than one layer, as the epithelial cells of some glands.

poly·pus (pol'i·pus) *n.*, pl. **poly·pi** (·pye) [L.]. POLYP.

poly·py·ram·i·dal kidney (pol''ee·pi·ram'i·dul). A kidney with more than one renal pyramid. Syn. *multilobar kidney.*

poly·ra·dic·u·li·tis (pol''ee·ra·dick''yoo·lye'tis) *n.* [*poly-* + *radiculitis*]. GUILLAIN-BARRÉ DISEASE.

poly·ra·dic·u·lo·neu·ri·tis (pol''ee·ra·dick''yoo·lo·new·rye'tis) *n.* [*poly-* + *radiculoneuritis*]. GUILLAIN-BARRÉ DISEASE.

poly·ra·dic·u·lo·neu·rop·a·thy (pol''ee·ra·dick''yoo·lo·new·rop'uth·ee) *n.* [*poly-* + *radiculoneuropathy*]. The simultaneous involvement, usually symmetrical, of multiple peripheral nerves and roots.

poly·ri·bo·some (pol''ee·rye'buh·sohm) *n.* [*poly-* + *ribosome*]. An aggregate of ribosomes.

poly·sac·cha·ride (pol''ee·sack'uh·ride, ·rid) *n.* [*poly-* + *saccharide*]. A carbohydrate that is formed by the condensation of two or more, usually many, monosaccharides. Examples are cellulose and starch.

poly·sce·lia (pol''ee·see'lee·uh) *n.* [*poly-* + Gk. *skel*os, leg, + *-ia*]. Excess in the number of legs.

po·lys·ce·lus (pol·iss'e·lus) *n.* [*poly-* + Gk. *skelos,* leg]. An individual having supernumerary legs.

poly·scle·ro·sis (pol''ee·skle·ro'sis) *n.* [*poly-* + *sclerosis*]. MULTIPLE SCLEROSIS.

poly·se·ro·si·tis (pol''ee·seer''o·sigh'tis) *n.* [*poly-* + *serositis*]. Widespread, chronic, fibrosing inflammation of serous membranes, especially in the upper abdomen. Syn. *Pick's disease, multiple serositis, Concato's disease, chronic hyperplastic perihepatitis, polyorrhymenitis.*

poly·si·nus·itis (pol''ee·sigh''nuh''sigh'tis) *n.* [*poly-* + *sinusitis*]. Simultaneous inflammation of several air sinuses. See also *pansinusitis.*

poly·so·ma·tous (pol''ee·so'muh·tus, ·som'uh·tus) *adj.* [Gk. *polysōmatos,* having many bodies, from *sōma,* body]. Of terata, involving more than one body. See also *polysomus.*

poly·some (pol'ee·sohm) *n.* POLYRIBOSOME.

poly·so·mia (pol''ee·so'mee·uh) *n.* [*poly-* + *-somia*]. A polysomatous condition.

poly·so·mic (pol''ee·so'mick) *adj.* [*poly-* + chromo*some* + *-ic*]. 1. Having more than two of any given chromosome. 2. Having more than two sets of chromosomes, as tetraploids, hexaploids. 3. POLYPLOID.

poly·so·mus (pol''ee·so'mus) *n.* [*poly-* + *-somus*]. A general term embracing all grades of duplicity, triplicity, etc. It includes monochorionic twins, conjoined twins, equal or unequal, placental parasitic twins, and all grades of double monsters.

poly·sor·bate (pol''ee·sor'bate) *n.* Any of various polyoxyethylene (20) sorbitan fatty acid esters obtained by copolymerizing the appropriate fatty acid ester of sorbitol and its anhydrides with approximately 20 moles of ethylene oxide for each mole of sorbitol and sorbitol anhydrides. The esters are individually identified by appending a number, as polysorbate 40, which is polyoxyethylene 20 sorbitan monopalmitate, and polysorbate 80, which is polyoxyethylene 20 sorbitan mono-oleate. Polysorbates are used as emulsifying, dispersing, and solubilizing agents.

poly·sper·mia (pol''ee·spur'mee·uh) *n.* [Gk., from *poly-* + *sperma,* seed, semen]. 1. The secretion and discharge of an excessive quantity of seminal fluid. 2. Penetration of the ovum by more than one spermatozoon.

poly·sper·mism (pol''ee·spurm'iz·um) *n.* POLYSPERMIA.

poly·sper·my (pol'ee·spur''mee) *n.* [*poly-* + *sperm* + *-y*]. POLYSPERMIA (2).

poly·sphyg·mo·graph (pol''ee·sfig'mo·graf) *n.* [*poly-* + *sphygmo-* + *-graph*]. POLYGRAPH. —**poly·sphyg·mo·graph·ic** (·sfig''mo·graf'ick) *adj.*

poly·sple·nia (pol''ee·splee'nee·uh) *n.* [*poly-* + *splen-* + *ia*]. A condition in which the spleen is multilobate.

poly·stich·ia (pol''ee·stick'ee·uh) *n.* [*poly-* + Gk. *stich*os, row, + *-ia*]. A condition in which the eyelashes are arranged in more than the normal number of rows.

poly·sto·ma·tous (pol''ee·sto'muh·tus, ·stom'uh·tus) *adj.* [*poly-* + *stomat-* + *-ous*]. Having many mouths or apertures.

poly·sty·rene (pol''ee·stye'reen) *n.* A clear, lightweight plastic prepared by polymerization of styrene and used for the manufacture of various molded articles and sheet materials.

poly·sus·pen·soid (pol''ee·suh·spen'soid) *n.* [*poly-* + *suspensoid*]. A colloid system in which there are several phases in different degrees of dispersion.

poly·symp·to·mat·ic (pol''ee·simp''tuh·mat'ick) *adj.* [*poly-* + *symptomatic*]. *In clinical medicine,* pertaining to a pathological process having manifold symptoms, which may not all occur simultaneously or in the same patient.

poly·syn·ap·tic (pol''ee·si·nap'tick) *adj.* [*poly-* + *synaptic*]. Pertaining to two or more synapses.

poly·syn·dac·tyl·ism (pol''ee·sin·dak'til·iz·um) *n.* [*poly-* + *syndactylism*]. Multiple syndactyly.

poly·ter·pene (pol''ee·tur'peen) *n.* Any of a group of hydrocarbons of the general formula $(C_5H_8)_n$, related to terpene.

poly·the·lia (pol''ee·theel'ee·uh) *n.* [*poly-* + *thel-* + *-ia*]. The presence of supernumerary nipples.

poly·the·lism (pol''ee·theel'iz·um) *n.* POLYTHELIA.

poly·thi·a·zide (pol''ee·thigh'uh·zide) *n.* 6-Chloro-3,4-dihydro-2-methyl-3-{[(2,2,2-trifluoroethyl)thio]methyl}-2*H*-1,2,4-benzothiadiazine-7-sulfonamide 1,1-dioxide, $C_{11}H_{13}ClF_3N_3O_4S_3$, an orally effective diuretic and antihypertensive drug.

po·lyt·o·cous (pol·it'uh·kus) *adj.* [Gk. *polytokos,* prolific, from *poly-* + *tokos,* offspring, birth]. Producing many young at a birth.

poly·trich·ia (pol''ee·trick'ee·uh) *n.* [Gk. *polytrich*os, very hairy (from *thrix, trichos,* hair) + *-ia*]. Excessive development of hair; hypertrichosis.

poly·tri·cho·sis (pol''ee·tri·ko'sis) *n.* POLYTRICHIA.

poly·tro·phia (pol''ee·tro'fee·uh) *n.* [Gk., from *poly-* + *trophē,* nourishment]. Abundant or excessive nutrition.

po·lyt·ro·phy (pol·it'ruh·fee) *n.* POLYTROPHIA.

poly·trop·ic (pol''ee·trop'ick, ·tro'pick) *adj.* [Gk. *polytropos,* versatile (from *tropē,* a turn) + *-ic*]. Having affinity for or affecting more than one type of cell; applied to viruses; pantropic.

poly·typ·ic (pol''ee·tip'ick) *adj.* [*poly-* + *typ-* + *-ic*]. Having more than one member or subgroup. Contr. *monotypic.*

poly·uria (pol''ee·yoo'ree·uh) *n.* [*poly-* + *-uria*]. The passage of an excessive quantity of urine. —**poly·uric** (·yoo'rick) *adj.*

polyuria test. A test for renal insufficiency based on the inability of the diseased kidney to respond with increased urine output to an administered water load. Syn. *Albarrán's test.*

poly·va·lent (pol″ee·vay′lunt) *adj.* [*poly-* + *valent*]. 1. Of antigens, having many combining sites or determinants. 2. Pertaining to vaccines composed of mixtures of different organisms, and to the resulting mixed antiserum. 3. Of a chemical element or group: capable of binding to more than one other element or group.

poly·vi·nyl·pyr·rol·i·done (pol″ee·vye″nil·pirr·ol′i·dohn) *n.* A synthetic polymer of high molecular weight formed by interactions of formaldehyde, ammonia, hydrogen, and acetylene; has been used as a plasma expander and to retard absorption of certain parenterally administered drugs. Abbreviated, PVP.

po·made (po·maid′, po·mahd′) *n.* [F. *pommade*, from It. *pomata*, from *pomo*, apple]. A perfumed ointment, especially one for applying to the scalp.

Pom·pe's disease [J. C. *Pompe*, Dutch, 20th century]. Generalized glycogenosis caused by a deficiency of the lysosomal enzyme, α-1,4-glucosidase, with abnormal storage of glycogen in skeletal muscles, heart, liver, and other organs. The clinical manifestations include marked weakness, cardiomegaly, and cardiac failure with death usually occurring in the first year. Inheritance is autosomal recessive. Syn. *maltase deficiency, cardiomegalia glycogenica diffusa, idiopathic generalized glycogenosis, type II of Cori.* Compare *late infantile acid maltase deficiency.*

pom·pho·ly·he·mia, pom·pho·ly·hae·mia (pom″fo·li·hee″mee·uh) *n.* [Gk. *pompholyx*, bubble, + *-hemia*]. Bubbles in the blood.

pom·pho·lyx (pom′fo·licks) *n.* [Gk., bubble]. CHEIROPOMPHOLYX.

pom·phus (pom′fus) *n.* [Gk. *pomphos*]. WHEAL.

po·mum Ada·mi (po′mum a·day′migh) [L.]. LARYNGEAL PROMINENCE.

pon·ceau B, 2R, 3B (pon·so′) [F., poppy-colored, from OF. *pouncel*, poppy]. Dyes, of various shades of red, used in food, drugs, cosmetics, and histologic stains.

ponceau de xy·li·dine (duh ksee·lee·deen′) [F.]. PONCEAU 2R.

Pon·cet's disease (pohⁿ·seʰ′) [A. *Poncet*, French surgeon, 1849–1913]. An atypical form of generalized tuberculosis chiefly characterized by joint manifestations, with associated disease of different viscera; the usual gross features of tuberculosis infection are lacking, although organisms can be demonstrated by animal inoculation.

Poncet's operation [A. *Poncet*]. 1. Perineal urethrostomy. 2. Lengthening the calcaneal tendon for relief of talipes equinus.

pon·der·a·ble (pon′dur·uh·bul) *adj.* [L. *ponderabilis*, from *pondus*, weight]. Having weight.

pon·der·al (pon′dur·ul) *adj.* [L. *pondus, ponderis*, weight, + *-al*]. Of or pertaining to weight.

ponderal index. The ratio between a person's height and weight, commonly expressed as the height (in inches) divided by the cube root of the weight (in pounds).

Ponderex. Trademark for fenfluramine, an anorexigenic drug used as the hydrochloride salt.

Pon·der-Kin·youn stain. A stain for diphtheria bacilli containing toluidine blue, methylene blue, and azure A dyes.

Pon·fick's shadow [E. *Ponfick*, German pathologist, 1844–1913]. ACHROMACYTE.

Pon·gi·dae (pon′ji·dee) *n.pl.* 1. A family of Primates that includes the genera *Pongo, Pan,* and *Gorilla;* the great apes. 2. In another classification, a family that comprises all the anthropoid apes, including *Hylobates* and *Symphalangus* as well as the great apes. Contr. *Hominidae, Hylobatidae.*

Pon·go (pong′go) *n.* [Kongo *mpungu*, gorilla]. A monotypic genus of the Pongidae that comprises the orangutans.

po·no·graph (po′no·graf) *n.* [Gk. *ponos*, toil, pain, + *-graph*]. An apparatus for determining and registering sensitivity to pain or progressive fatigue of a contracting muscle.

po·no·pal·mo·sis (po″no·pal·mo′sis, pon″o·) *n.* [Gk. *ponos*, exertion, + *palmos*, palpitation, + *-osis*]. *Obsol.* A condition in which slight exertion produces palpitation of the heart; neurocirculatory asthenia.

po·nos (po′nos) *n.* [Gk., trouble, suffering]. KALA AZAR.

pons (ponz) *n.*, genit. **pon·tis** (pon′tis), pl. **pon·tes** (pon′teez) [L., bridge]. 1. A process or bridge of tissue connecting two parts of an organ. 2. [NA] The portion of the brainstem between the midbrain and the medulla oblongata. See also Plates 17, 18. —**pon·tile** (pon′tile), **pon·tine** (·tine, ·teen) *adj.*

pons Va·ro·lii (va·ro′lee·eye) [C. *Varolius*, Italian surgeon, 1543–1575]. PONS (2).

pont-, ponto- [L. *pons, pontis*]. A combining form meaning (a) *bridge;* (b) *pons, pontine.*

pon·tic (pon′tick) *n.* [*pont-* + *-ic*]. The portion of a prosthetic bridge that is between the abutments and serves as the artificial substitute for a lost tooth or teeth. Syn. *dummy.*

pontine cistern. The space in the arachnoid ventral to the pons.

pontine flexure. A flexure of the embryonic brain concave dorsally occurring in the region of the myelencephalon.

pontine myelinosis. CENTRAL PONTINE MYELINOSIS.

pontine nuclei. NUCLEI PONTIS.

pontine septum. RAPHE OF THE PONS.

pon·to·bul·bar (pon″to·bul′bur) *adj.* [*ponto-* + *bulbar*]. Pertaining to the pons and to the medulla oblongata.

pontobulbar nucleus. A small group of medium-sized cells, which caudally are dorsolateral to, and rostrally ventral to, the inferior cerebellar peduncle.

Pontocaine. A trademark for the local anesthetic tetracaine, used as the hydrochloride salt.

pon·to·cer·e·bel·lar (pon″to·serr″e·bel′ur) *adj.* [*ponto-* + *cerebellar*]. Pertaining to the pons and the cerebellum.

pontocerebellar-angle tumor syndrome. CEREBELLOPONTINE-ANGLE TUMOR SYNDROME.

pontocerebellar tract. MIDDLE CEREBELLAR PEDUNCLE.

pon·to·med·ul·lary (pon″to·med′yoo·lerr·ee) *adj.* Pertaining to the pons and the medulla oblongata.

pooled serum. Mixed serum from a number of persons.

Pool-Schle·sing·er's sign (shleʸ′zing·ur) [E. H. *Pool*, U.S. surgeon, 1874–1949; and H. *Schlesinger*]. In tetany, forceful abduction of the arm results in painful spasms of the muscles of the arm and hand; forceful flexion of the thigh on the trunk with the leg extended results in painful spasm of the muscles of the leg and foot.

poplar bud. The air-dried, closed winter leaf bud of *Populus candicans*, known as the balm of Gilead buds, or of *P. tacamahacca* (*P. balsamifera*), known in commerce as balsam poplar buds. Preparations of poplar bud have been used, internally and externally, as medicinals.

po·ples (pop′leez) *n.* genit. **po·pli·tis** (pop′li·tis), pl. **popli·tes** (·teez) [L., the ham] [NA]. The posterior aspect of the knee.

pop·lit·e·al (pop·lit′ee·ul, pop″li·tee′ul) *adj.* [L. *poples, poplitis*, ham, knee, + *-al*]. Pertaining to or situated in the ham, as popliteal artery, popliteal nerve, popliteal space.

popliteal arcuate ligament. ARCUATE POPLITEAL LIGAMENT.

popliteal bursa. RECESSUS SUBPOPLITEUS.

popliteal bursitis. BAKER'S CYST (1).

popliteal fossa. POPLITEAL SPACE.

popliteal ligament. See *arcuate popliteal ligament, oblique popliteal ligament.*

popliteal line. SOLEAL LINE.

popliteal plane. The portion of the posterior surface of the femur which forms the floor of the popliteal fossa. NA *facies poplitea.*

popliteal plexus. A nerve plexus surrounding the popliteal artery.

popliteal space or **region.** A diamond-shaped area behind the knee joint. NA *fossa poplitea.*

po·pli·te·us (pop·lit′ee·us) *n.*, pl. **poplit·ei** (·ee·eye) [NL., from L. *poples*, ham of the knee]. 1. The ham or hinder part of the knee joint. 2. A muscle on the back of the knee joint.

NA *musculus popliteus.* See also Table of Muscles in the Appendix.

popliteus minor. A rare variant of the popliteus muscle arising from the femur medial to the plantaris and inserted into the posterior ligament of the knee joint.

Pop·per method [E. *Popper,* German pathologist, 20th century]. A histochemical method for detecting lipids, using phosphine 3R which gives neutral fats a silver-white fluorescence on a brown background.

pop·py-seed oil. The fixed oil from the seeds of *Papaver somniferum;* used in preparing iodized oil, a radiopaque medium.

population pyramid. A graphic method of representing the age structure of populations. Usually each 5-year age group is represented by a horizontal bar with females shown on one side and males on the other side of the vertical central line. Differences in birth rate and longevity result in pyramid patterns which are distinctively different for different countries, depending on living standards, epidemiology, health care, fertility, and other variables.

por-, poro- [Gk. *poros,* from *peran,* to pass through]. A combining form meaning (a) *passageway, duct;* (b) *pore, opening;* (c) *cavity, tract.*

por·ad·e·ni·tis (por·ad″e·nigh′tis) *n.* [*por-* + *aden-* + *itis*]. LYMPHOGRANULOMA VENEREUM.

por·ad·e·no·lym·phi·tis (por·ad″e·no·lim·fye′tis) *n.* [*por-* + *adeno-* + *lymph* + *-itis*]. LYMPHOGRANULOMA VENEREUM.

P/O ratio. The number of molecules of ATP formed from ADP and inorganic phosphate per atom of oxygen consumed in the process of oxidative phosphorylation. If the complete electron transport chain is involved, the P/O ratio is normally three.

por·cine (por′sine, ·seen) *adj.* [L. *porcinus,* from *porcus,* pig]. Pertaining to or characteristic of swine.

porcine rhinohyperplasia. A syndrome of swine resulting from infection primarily from soil-borne organisms and characterized by irregular proliferations of fibrous and bony tissue over the region of the snout.

-pore [Gk. *poros,* passage]. A combining form meaning *opening.*

pore, *n.* [Gk. *poros,* passage]. 1. A minute opening on a surface. 2. The opening of the duct of a sweat gland. See also *porus.*

por·en·ce·pha·lia (pore″en·se″fay′lee·uh) *n.* PORENCEPHALY.

por·en·ceph·a·li·tis (pore″en·sef·uh·lye′tis) *n.* [*por-* + *encephalitis*]. A term once proposed for encephalitis with a tendency to form cavities in the brain, a pathologic entity now thought not to exist.

por·en·ceph·a·lus (pore″en·sef′uh·lus) *n.* An individual exhibiting porencephaly.

por·en·ceph·a·ly (pore″en·sef′uh·lee) *n.* [*por-* + *-encephaly*]. A term introduced by Heschl, in 1869, to designate a congenital defect extending from the surface of the cerebral hemisphere into the subjacent ventricle, now commonly used to designate any cystic cavity in the brain of an infant or child; may be the result of brain tissue destruction of any causation (encephaloclastic porencephaly) or due to maldevelopment (schizencephaly). —**poren·ce·phal·ic** (·se·fal′ick), **poren·ceph·a·lous** (·sef′uh·lus) *adj.*

pore of Kohn [H. *Kohn*]. ALVEOLAR PORE.

por·firo·my·cin (por″fi·ro·migh′sin) *n.* An antibiotic substance, $C_{16}H_{20}N_4O_5$, produced by *Streptomyces ardus,* that has antitumor activity.

Por·ges-Pol·la·tschek reaction (por′gess, po^hl′ah·check) [O. *Porges,* Austrian physician, b. 1879; and O. *Pollatschek,* Austrian physician]. A test for pregnancy in which an intracutaneous injection of neurohypophysis secretion causes a red area to appear about the injection site if the woman is not pregnant; in a pregnant woman no reaction is observed.

pori. Plural and genitive singular of *porus.*

po·rio·ma·nia (po″ree·o·may′nee·uh) *n.* [Gk. *poreia,* journey, + *-mania*]. A compulsion to wander or travel, usually in a state of impaired consciousness. —**porioma·ni·ac** (·nee·ack) *n.*

po·ri·on (po′ree·on) *n.,* pl. **po·ria** (·ree·uh) [*porus* + *-ion*]. The point of the upper margin of the porus acusticus externus. The two poria and the left orbitale define the Frankfort horizontal plane.

pork tapeworm. TAENIA SOLIUM.

por·nog·ra·phy (por·nog′ruh·fee) *n.* [Gk. *pornē,* prostitute, + *-graphy*]. 1. Obscene writing, drawing, photography, and the like. 2. A treatise on prostitution.

poro-. See *por-.*

po·ro·ceph·a·li·a·sis (po″ro·sef″uh·lye′uh·sis) *n.,* pl. **poroceph·alia·ses** (·seez) [*Porocephalus* + *-iasis*]. An uncommon infection of the lungs, liver, trachea, or nasal cavities of man with any of the varieties of *Porocephalus.*

Po·ro·ceph·a·lus (po″ro·sef′uh·lus) *n.* [*poro-* + *-cephalus*]. A genus of the Pentastomida parasitic in man and reptiles.

po·ro·ker·a·to·sis (po″ro·kerr″uh·to′sis) *n.* [*poro-* + *keratosis*]. A genodermatosis characterized by a collar of elevated hyperkeratosis about an irregular patch of depressed atrophic skin; microscopically, horn plugs or cornoid lamella in the dermis are prominent, but are not necessarily located in the openings of sweat glands as the name "porokeratosis" implies. Syn. *hyperkeratosis excentrica, Mibelli's disease.*

po·ro·ma (po·ro′muh) *n.* [Gk. *pōrōma,* from *pōros,* stone, calculus]. A callosity.

po·ro·plas·tic (po″ro·plas′tick) *adj.* Porous and plastic.

poroplastic felt. A porous, readily molded felt, used in the preparation of splints and jackets.

po·ro·sis (po·ro′sis) *n.,* pl. **poro·ses** (·seez) [*por-* + *-osis*]. Rarefaction; increased roentgen translucency; formation of vacuoles or pores; cavity formation. —**po·rot·ic** (po·rot′ick) *adj.*

po·ros·i·ty (po·ros′i·tee) *n.* The condition or quality of being porous.

po·rous (po′rus) *adj.* [ML. *porosus*]. Having pores.

por·phin (por′fin) *n.* A heterocyclic ring consisting of four pyrrole rings linked by methine (—CH=) bridges; the basic structure of chlorophyll, hemoglobin, the cytochromes, and certain other related substances.

por·pho·bi·lin (por″fo·bye′lin) *n.* A product derived from hemoglobin which may be excreted in urine.

por·pho·bi·lin·o·gen (por″fo·bye·lin′o·jen) *n.* A chromogen intermediate in the biosynthesis of porphyrins and heme; found with its precursor, δ-aminolevulinic acid, in the urine in some forms pf porphyria.

por·phyr·ia (por·firr′ee·uh, ·fye′ree·uh) *n.* [*porphyrin* + *-ia*]. 1. An inborn error of metabolism characterized by the presence of increased quantities of porphyrins or their precursors in the blood and other tissues and in feces and urine, abdominal pain, polyneuropathy, convulsions, and psychosis, as well as dark discoloration of the urine on standing in sunlight. 2. Any disturbance of porphyrin metabolism, congenital or acquired, resulting in porphyrinuria. See also *acute intermittent porphyria, erythropoietic porphyria.*

porphyria cu·ta·nea tar·da he·re·di·ta·ria (kew·tay′nee·uh tahr′duh he·red·i·tair′ee·uh). A hereditary porphyria with constant increased fecal excretion of coproporphyrin and uroporphyrin, characterized clinically by cutaneous lesions and acute attacks of jaundice and abdominal colic. Syn. *porphyria variegata.*

porphyria cutanea tarda symp·to·ma·ti·ca (simp·to·mat′i·kuh). Acquired porphyria appearing in late adulthood, characterized by photosensitivity, cutaneous lesions, and hepatic dysfunction; abdominal pain and neurologic complications do not occur.

porphyria eryth·ro·poi·et·i·ca (e·rith″ro·poy·et′i·kuh). ERYTHROPOIETIC PORPHYRIA.

porphyria he·ma·to·poi·et·i·ca (hee″muh·to·poy·et′i·kuh). ERYTHROPOIETIC PORPHYRIA.

porphyria he·pat·i·ca (he·pat′i·kuh). ACUTE INTERMITTENT PORPHYRIA.

porphyria var·i·e·ga·ta (văr·ee·e·gay′tuh). PORPHYRIA CUTANEA TARDA HEREDITARIA.

por·phy·rin (por′fi·rin) *n.* [Gk. *porphyra*, purple, + *-in*]. A heterocyclic ring derived from porphin by replacing the eight hydrogen atoms attached to the carbon atoms of the pyrrole rings of porphin by various organic groups. In the center of the ring a metal, such as iron (in heme) or magnesium (in chlorophyll), may or may not be present.

por·phy·rin·uria (por″fi·ri·new′ree·uh) *n.* [*porphyrin* + *-uria*]. The excretion of an abnormal amount of a porphyrin, commonly believed to be uroporphyrin I, in the urine.

por·phy·ri·za·tion (por″fi·ri·zay′shun) *n.* Pulverization; reduction to a fine powder, formerly performed on a tablet of porphyry.

por·phy·rop·sin (por″fi·rop′sin) *n.* [Gk. *porphyra*, purple, + *opsin*]. 1. A purple carotenoid protein that occurs in the rods of the retinas of certain freshwater fish. It participates in a retinal cycle identical in arrangement with that of rhodopsin or visual purple. 2. Retinene$_2$ combined with scotopsin.

por·phyr·uria (por″fur·yoo′ree·uh) *n.* PORPHYRINURIA.

por·phy·ry spleen (por′fi·ree). A spleen that is affected by multiple nodular infiltrations.

por·poise heart (por′pus). A heart with preponderance of the right ventricle.

por·ri·go (po·rye′go) *n.* [L. scurf, dandruff]. Any of several diseases of the scalp which have a tendency to spread. —**por·rig·i·nous** (po·rij′i·nus) *adj.*

porrigo de·cal·vans (dee·kal′vanz). ALOPECIA AREATA.

Por·ro's operation (pohʳrro) [E. *Porro*, Italian obstetrician, 1842–1902]. A cesarian section immediately followed by hysterectomy.

port, *n.* [L. *portus*, port]. The area and contour of the beam of radiation directed through the body surface for external radiation therapy.

por·ta (por′tuh) *n.*, pl. & genit. sing. **por·tae** (·tee) [L., gate]. The hilus of an organ through which vessels or ducts enter.

por·ta·ca·val (por″tuh·kay′vul) *adj.* Pertaining to the portal vein and the inferior vena cava.

portacaval anastomosis. A surgical procedure joining the portal vein to the inferior vena cava. Syn. *Eck's fistula.*

portacaval shunt. A surgical connection between the portal vein and inferior vena cava.

porta he·pa·tis (hep′uh·tis) [NA]. The transverse fissure of the liver through which the portal vein and hepatic artery enter the liver and the hepatic ducts leave.

por·tal (por′tul) *adj. & n.* [ML. *portalis*, pertaining to a gate]. 1. Of or pertaining to the porta hepatis. 2. Pertaining to the portal vein or system. 3. The porta or hilus of an organ.

portal canal or **area.** An interlobular artery, vein, bile duct, nerve, and lymph vessel, and the interlobular connective tissue in which they lie, between the corners of the anatomic lobules of the liver.

portal circulation. The passage of blood by a vein from one capillary bed to a second independent set of capillaries; usually, the passage of the blood from the capillaries of the gastrointestinal tract and red pulp of the spleen into the sinusoids of the liver.

portal cirrhosis. Progressive fibrosis centered in the portal areas of the liver; loosely, LAENNEC'S CIRRHOSIS.

portal fissure. TRANSVERSE FISSURE OF THE LIVER.

portal hypertension. Portal venous pressure in excess of 20 mmHg, resulting from intrahepatic or extrahepatic portal venous compression or occlusion, and producing in the late stages large variceal collateral veins, splenomegaly, and ascites.

portal space. PORTAL CANAL.

portal system. The portal circulation, usually the hepatic portal vein and its tributaries. See also *hypophyseoportal circulation.*

portal triad. The three main structures found in each portal canal: a branch of the hepatic artery and of the portal vein, and a tributary to the common bile duct.

por·ta·re·nal shunt (por″tuh·ree′nul). A surgical connection between the left renal vein and the portal system, usually the splenic vein.

porta ves·ti·bu·li (ves·tib′yoo·lye). A narrow orifice between the sinus venosus and the atrium in the embryonic heart.

porte·pol·ish·er (port″pol′i·shur) *n.* An instrument used in dental procedures for holding a polishing point, stick, or brush.

Por·ter-Sil·ber reaction. A reaction used for the quantitative determination of adrenal steroids (cortisone, cortisol, tetrahydrocortisone) in which the dihydroxyacetone side chain of the steroid is reacted with phenylhydrazine in sulfuric acid to produce a yellow color.

Porter's sign [W. H. *Porter*, Irish physician, 1790–1861]. OLIVER'S SIGN.

Portes' operation (port) [L. *Portes*, French obstetrician, 20th century]. Cesarian section followed by temporary exteriorization of the uterus and secondary reintegration.

por·tio (por′shee·o, por′tee·o) *n.*, pl. **por·ti·o·nes** (por″shee·o′neez, por″tee·) [L.]. Portion.

portio major ner·vi tri·ge·mi·ni (nur′vye trye·jem′i·nye) [BNA]. RADIX SENSORIA NERVI TRIGEMINI.

portio minor nervi trigemini [BNA]. RADIX MOTORIA NERVI TRIGEMINI.

portio su·pra·va·gi·na·lis cer·vi·cis (sue″pruh·vaj·i·nay′lis sur′vi·sis) [NA]. The portion of the cervix of the uterus which does not protrude into the vagina.

portio va·gi·na·lis cer·vi·cis (vaj·i·nay′lis sur′vi·sis) [NA]. The portion of the cervix of the uterus which protrudes into the vagina. See also *ectocervix.*

portio vaginalis ute·ri (yoo′te·rye). The vaginal portion of the uterus.

porto-. A combining form meaning *portal.*

por·to·ca·val (por″to·kay′vul) *adj.* PORTACAVAL.

por·to·gram (por″to·gram) *n.* The image produced by portography.

por·tog·ra·phy (por·tog′ruh·fee) *n.* [*porto-* + *-graphy*]. Radiographic depiction of the portal venous system following injection of contrast medium.

por·to·sys·tem·ic (por″to·sis·tem′ick) *adj.* Pertaining to the portal system.

portosystemic encephalopathy. 1. HEPATIC ENCEPHALOPATHY. 2. HEPATIC COMA.

por·to·ve·no·gram (por″to·vee′no·gram) *n.* [*porto-* + *veno-* + *-gram*]. PORTOGRAM.

por·to·ve·nog·ra·phy (por″to·vee·nog′ruh·fee) *n.* PORTOGRAPHY.

port-wine nevus, mark, or **stain.** A congenital hemangioma characterized by one or several red to purplish flat or slightly elevated patches, most often on the face. Syn. *nevus flammeus.*

Portyn. Trademark for benzilonium bromide, an anticholinergic agent.

po·rus (po′rus) *n.*, pl. & genit. sing. **po·ri** (·rye) [L., from Gk. *poros*, passage]. A pore or foramen.

porus acu·sti·cus ex·ter·nus (a·koos′ti·kus eck·stur′nus) [NA]. The opening of the external acoustic meatus.

porus acusticus in·ter·nus (in·tur′nus) [NA]. The opening of the internal acoustic meatus into the cranial cavity.

porus cro·ta·phi·ti·co-buc·ci·na·to·ri·us (kro″tuh·fit″i·ko·buck″si·nuh·to′ree·us). A foramen formed in about 10 percent of skulls by a bar of bone developing between the base of the lateral pterygoid lamina and the undersurface of the greater wing of the sphenoid bone. Syn. *pterygoalar foramen.*

porus gus·ta·to·ri·us (gus·tuh·to′ree·us) [NA]. TASTE PORE.

porus op·ti·cus (op'ti·kus). The opening in the center of the lamina cribrosa transmitting the central artery of the retina.

porus su·do·ri·fe·rus (sue·do·rif'e·rus) [NA]. A sweat pore.

po·sio·ma·nia (po''see·o·may'nee·uh, pos''ee·o·) *n.* [Gk. *posis*, drink, + *-mania*]. DIPSOMANIA.

po·si·tion (puh·zish'un) *n.* [L. *positio*, putting, placement, from *ponere*, to place]. Place; location; attitude; posture. Abbreviated, P. —**position·al** (·ul) *adj.*

positional nystagmus. Nystagmus which occurs only when the patient's head is placed in an abnormal plane. In the central type, the nystagmus appears as soon as the critical or abnormal head position is assumed and while it is maintained, reappearing as soon as the position is resumed; in the paroxysmal type, the nystagmus appears shortly after the abnormal head position is assumed, lasts for up to 10 seconds and does not reappear even if the position is resumed for several minutes.

position effect. The phenomenon whereby the expression of a gene depends upon its position. See also *position pseudoallelism, variegated position effect.*

position of function. An essential primary position of the hand, of importance during prolonged immobilization following injury to the hand or digits. The hand is hyperextended at the wrist at an angle of 45°, the fingers being flexed at 45° at their metacarpophalangeal and interphalangeal joints. The thumb is rotated and adducted so that its flexor surface is opposite the flexor surface of the index finger.

position of the fetus. The relation of the presenting part of the fetus to the cardinal points. For the vertex, the face, and the breech there are four positions each: a right anterior, a right posterior, a left anterior, and a left posterior. For each of the shoulders there is an anterior and a posterior position. In order to shorten and memorize these positions, the initials of the chief words are made use of, as follows: for vertex presentations the word occiput is abbreviated O., and preceded by the letter R. or L. for right or left, and followed by A. or P. according to whether the presenting part is anterior or posterior. Thus the initials L.O.A., left occipitoanterior, indicate that the presenting occiput is upon the anterior left side. In the same way are derived the terms L.O.P., R.O.A., R.O.P. For facial presentations, in the same way, L.F.A., left frontoanterior, L.F.P., R.F.A., R.F.P. For breech or sacral presentations, L.S.A., L.S.P., R.S.A., R.S.P., and for shoulder or dorsal presentations, L.D.A., L.D.P., R.D.A., R.D.P.

position pseudoallelism. The phenomenon whereby the expression of a gene depends on its position with respect to an allele.

pos·i·tive (poz'i·tiv) *adj.* [L. *positivus*, from *ponere*, to lay, place; to assert]. 1. Indicating or expressing affirmation or confirmation; *in psychiatry,* receptive, responsive; warm; constructive. 2. Of a response to a drug or other therapy, satisfactory or as expected. 3. Of results of a test or experiment, confirming the presence or existence of the entity tested for. 4. Included in that one of two classes or ranges which is conceived as fundamental or primary; opposed to negative, as a positive integer. Symbol, +. 5. Of images (visual, photographic, etc.), corresponding to the subject in distribution of light and dark, or in colors with respect to their complements. Contr. *negative.*

positive afterimage. An afterimage persisting after the eyes are closed or turned toward a dark background, and of the same color as the stimulating light. Contr. *negative afterimage.*

positive anxiety. The anxiety for growth.

positive electron. POSITRON.

positive feedback. Feedback that tends to increase the output; a concept applied in physiology to many bodily processes tending away from homeostasis during their duration, such as parturition, urination, and irreversible shock. Contr. *negative feedback.*

positive ion. CATION.

positive lens. Any lens with a positive focal length; it is thicker in the center than around the circumference. There are three types of positive lenses: double convex or biconvex, planoconvex, and converging concavoconvex.

positive pressure breathing. Breathing by introduction of a suitable gas mixture into the lungs at a pressure above the ambient pressure exerted on the external surface of the chest.

positive scotoma. A scotoma perceptible to the patient as a dark spot before his eyes.

positive supporting reflex. EXTENSOR THRUST REFLEX.

pos·i·tron (poz'i·tron) *n.* [*posi*tive + elec*tron*]. An elementary particle having the mass of an electron but carrying a unit positive charge. It is evanescent, dissipating itself as radiation as soon as it encounters an electron, which is annihilated with it.

pos·i·tro·ni·um (poz''i·tro'nee·um) *n.* A combination of a positron and an electron (negatron). The mean life of the combination is about 10^{-7} second, the particle being annihilated by conversion to one or more photons.

po·sol·o·gy (po·sol'uh·jee) *n.* [Gk. *posos*, how much, + *-logy*]. The branch of medical science that deals with the dosage of medicines.

post- [L.]. A prefix meaning *after, behind,* or *subsequent.*

post·abor·tal (pohst''uh·bort'ul) *adj.* [*post-* + *abort-* + *-al*]. Occurring after an abortion.

post·anal (pohst''ay'nul) *adj.* [*post-* + *anal*]. Situated behind the anus.

postanal dimple. COCCYGEAL FOVEOLA.

postanal gut. A transient part of the hindgut caudal to the cloaca.

post·an·es·thet·ic, post·an·aes·thet·ic (pohst''an·es·thet'ick) *adj.* [*post-* + *anesthetic*]. Occurring after anesthesia.

post·ap·o·plec·tic (pohst''ap·o·pleck'tick) *adj.* [*post-* + *apoplectic*]. Occurring after or as a consequence of a cerebral accident.

post·au·di·to·ry (pohst·aw'di·tor·ee) *adj.* Situated posterior to the external auditory meatus.

postauditory fossa. A crescentic notch on the temporal bone separating the temporal ridge from the auditory plate.

postauditory process. A pointed extension of the squamous temporal process which forms the lateral wall of the mastoid antrum and helps form the posterior wall of the external acoustic meatus.

post·ax·i·al (pohst·ack'see·ul) *adj.* [*post-* + *axial*]. Situated behind the axis: in the arm, behind the ulnar aspect; in the leg, behind the fibular aspect.

postaxial muscle. A muscle on the posterior aspect of an extremity.

post·bra·chi·al (pohst·bray'kee·ul) *adj.* [*post-* + *brachial*]. Situated posterior to the arm.

post·bran·chi·al bodies (pohst·brank'ee·ul). ULTIMOBRANCHIAL BODIES.

post·cap·il·lary (pohst·kap'i·lerr''ee) *n.* [*post-* + *capillary*]. VENOUS CAPILLARY.

post·car·di·ac injury syndrome (pohst·kahr'dee·ack). POSTCARDIOTOMY SYNDROME.

post·car·di·nal (pohst·kahr'di·nul) *adj.* Pertaining to the pair of cardinal veins draining the posterior part of the embryo.

post·car·di·ot·o·my (pohst''kahr''dee·ot'uh·mee) *adj.* [*post-* + *cardiotomy*]. Occurring after open-heart surgery.

postcardiotomy syndrome. A syndrome of acute nonspecific pericarditis, which may be recurrent, occurring weeks to months following cardiac surgery, cardiac trauma, or myocardial infarction, responding dramatically to corticosteroid therapy; thought to represent sensitivity to antigens from myocardial necrosis. Syn. *postcardiac injury syndrome.* See also *postcommissurotomy syndrome,* *postmyocardial infarction syndrome, postvalvulotomy syndrome.*

post·ca·va (pohst·kay'vuh) *n.* INFERIOR VENA CAVA. —**postca·val** (·vul) *adj.*

post·cen·tral (pohst·sen'trul) *adj.* [*post-* + *central*]. 1. Situated behind a center. 2. Situated behind the central sulcus of the brain.

postcentral gyrus. The cerebral convolution that lies immediately posterior to the central sulcus and extends from the longitudinal fissure above to the posterior ramus of the lateral sulcus. NA *gyrus postcentralis.*

postcentral sulcus. The first sulcus of the parietal lobe lying behind and roughly parallel to the central sulcus. The upper portion is often called the superior postcentral sulcus and the lower portion, the inferior postcentral sulcus. NA *sulcus postcentralis.*

post·chrom·ing (pohst·kro'ming) *n.* The practice of treating with a potassium dichromate solution after some other primary fixation, to confer on tissue some of the special attributes derived from primary fixations in solutions containing dichromates.

post·ci·bal (pohst·sigh'bul) *adj.* [*post-* + L. *cibus*, food, + *-al*]. Occurring after ingestion of food.

post·cla·vic·u·lar (pohst''kla·vick'yoo·lur) *adj.* [*post-* + *clavicular*]. Situated behind the clavicle.

post·co·i·tal (pohst·ko'it·ul) *adj.* [*post-* + *coital*]. After coitus.

postcoital pill. A high-dose estrogen pill given after coitus to prevent implantation.

post·com·mis·sur·ot·o·my (pohst·kom''i·shur·ot'uh·mee) *adj.* [*post-* + *commissurotomy*]. Following surgical incision of the mitral valve commissure.

postcommissurotomy syndrome. Postcardiotomy syndrome following commissurotomy.

post·con·cep·tu·al (pohst''kun·sep'choo·ul) *adj.* After conception; since conception, calculated from the time of conception.

postconceptual age. FETAL AGE.

post·con·cus·sion syndrome (pohst''kun·kush'un). Symptoms which follow brain concussion: giddiness and occasional vertigo; headache, insomnia, irritability, fatigability, inability to concentrate, tearfulness, and an intolerance of emotional excitement and crowds. Syn. *minor contusion syndrome.*

post·con·dy·lar (pohst''kon'di·lur) *adj.* [*post-* + *condylar*]. Situated behind a condyle.

postcondylar notch. A notch in the lower surface of each side of the occipital bone between the condyle and the foramen magnum.

post·con·i·za·tion (pohst''kon·i·zay'shun, ·ko·ni·) *adj.* [*post-* + *conization*]. Occurring after cervical conization.

post·con·nu·bi·al (pohst''kuh·new'bee·ul) *adj.* [*post-* + L. *conubium*, marriage, + *-al*]. Coming on or occurring after marriage.

post·con·vul·sive (pohst''kun·vul'siv) *adj.* [*post-* + *convulsive*]. Coming on after a convulsion.

post·cor·di·al (pohst·kor'dee·ul) *adj.* [*post-* + L. *cor, cordis*, heart, + *-al*]. Situated behind the heart.

post·cos·tal (pohst''kos'tul) *adj.* [*post-* + *costal*]. Situated behind a rib.

postcostal anastomosis. In the embryo, a longitudinal anastomosis between successive intersegmental arteries, the first through the seventh cervical, which forms the vertebral artery.

post·cri·coid (pohst·krye'koid) *adj.* Behind the cricoid cartilage.

post·dam (pohst'dam) *n.* [*post-* + *dam*]. POSTERIOR PALATAL SEAL.

post·di·crot·ic (pohst''dye·krot'ick) *adj.* [*post-* + *dicrotic*]. Occurring after the dicrotic notch of the arterial pulse tracing, as a postdicrotic wave.

post·di·ges·tive (pohst''di·jes'tiv) *adj.* [*post-* + *digestive*]. Occurring after digestion.

post·diph·ther·ic (pohst''dif·therr'ick) *adj.* POSTDIPHTHERITIC.

post·diph·the·rit·ic (pohst''dif·the·rit'ick) *adj.* [*post-* + *diphtheritic*]. Occurring after or resulting from an attack of diphtheria.

postdiphtheritic paralysis. A form of polyneuropathy that may occur during convalescence from diphtheria. It may affect the ciliary muscles and the palate, and later the muscles of the extremities and trunk.

post·dor·mi·tal (pohst·dor'mi·tul) *adj.* [*post-* + L. *dormire, dormitus*, to sleep, + *-al*]. Pertaining to the period immediately following sleep or the period of awakening.

postdormital paralysis. HYPNOPOMPIC PARALYSIS.

post·em·bry·on·ic (pohst''em·bree·on'ick) *adj.* Occurring after the embryonic stage; FETAL.

post·en·ceph·a·lit·ic (pohst''en·sef''uh·lit'ick) *adj.* [*post-* + *encephalitic*]. Occurring after and presumably as a result of encephalitis.

postencephalitic parkinsonism. The parkinsonian syndrome occurring as a sequel to encephalitis lethargica within a variable period, from days to many years, after the acute process. Clinically distinct, it is characterized by commencing almost exclusively before the age of 40, by a history of varying degrees of lethargy, and very slow but steady evolution of the classical parkinsonian syndrome. Patients frequently exhibit oculogyric and other spasms, tics, breathing arrhythmias, bizarre movements, postures and gaits, and psychopathic behavior. Pathologically, changes in the substantia nigra are demonstrable.

post·ep·i·lep·tic (post''ep·i·lep'tick) *adj.* Occurring after an epileptic attack.

postepileptic automatism. Automatism following an epileptic seizure.

postepileptic paralysis. TODD'S PARALYSIS.

pos·te·ri·ad (pos·teer'ee·ad) *adv.* [*posterior* + *-ad*]. *In anatomy*, from front to back; in an anterior-to-posterior direction. Compare *dorsad.*

pos·te·ri·or (pos·teer'ee·ur) *adj.* [L.]. *In anatomy* (with reference to the human or animal body as poised for its usual manner of locomotion): hind, in back; situated relatively far in the direction opposite to that of normal locomotion. Compare *dorsal.* Contr. *anterior.*

posterior asynclitism. The lateral inclination of the fetal head at the superior pelvic strait which brings the sagittal suture toward the symphysis pubis while the posterior parietal bone occupies most of the superior strait. Syn. *Litzmann's obliquity.*

posterior atlantooccipital membrane. A broad membrane extending from the posterior surface and cranial border of the posterior arch of the atlas to the posterior margin of the foramen magnum. NA *membrana atlantooccipitalis posterior.*

posterior axillary line. A vertical line extending downward from the posterior fold of the axilla on the side of the trunk.

posterior cardinal veins. The paired primary veins of the embryo draining body and mesonephros, located in the dorsolateral part of the urogenital fold; they unite with the anterior cardinal veins to form the common cardinal veins.

posterior central gyrus. POSTCENTRAL GYRUS.

posterior centriole. The centriole forming the annulus of the center piece of the spermatozoon.

posterior cerebellar lobe. The part of the cerebellum which lies posterior to the primary fissure.

posterior cerebellar notch. A narrow notch separating the cerebellar hemispheres posteriorly.

posterior cervical plexus of Cruveilhier [J. *Cruveilhier*]. CERVICAL POSTERIOR PLEXUS.

posterior chamber. The space between the posterior surface of the iris and the ciliary zonule, the lens, and the vitreous body. NA *camera posterior bulbi.*

posterior ciliary artery. See *ciliary artery.*

posterior clinoid process. One of the two short bony extensions from the superior angles of the dorsum sellae which give attachment to the tentorium cerebelli. NA *processus clinoideus posterior.*

posterior column. A division of the longitudinal columns of gray matter in the spinal cord. NA *columna posterior medullae spinalis.*

posterior commissure of the cerebrum. A transverse band of nerve fibers crossing dorsal to the opening of the cerebral aqueduct into the third ventricle. NA *commissura posterior cerebri.* See also Plate 18.

posterior communicating artery. A vessel which passes from the internal carotid artery to the posterior cerebral artery. NA *arteria communicans posterior cerebri.*

posterior condylar canal. CONDYLAR CANAL.

posterior cranial fossa. The lowest in position of the three cranial fossae, lodging the cerebellum, pons, and medulla oblongata. It is formed by the posterior surface of the petrous and inner surface of the mastoid portion of the temporal bone and the inner surface of the occipital bone below the horizontal limb of the confluence of the sinuses. NA *fossa cranii posterior.*

posterior cranial fossa arachnoiditis. CISTERNAL ARACHNOIDITIS.

posterior cricoarytenoid ligament. The ligament which passes posteriorly from the lamina of the cricoid cartilage to the medial part of the arytenoid cartilage. NA *ligamentum cricoarytenoideum posterius.*

posterior elastic lamina. DESCEMET'S MEMBRANE.

posterior embryotoxon. A congenital defect of the eye characterized by an enlarged and anterior location of Schwalbe's line. May be associated with iris processes and hypoplasia of iris stroma; inherited as a recessive trait. Syn. *posterior marginal dysplasia of the cornea.*

posterior embryotoxon of Axenfeld. AXENFELD'S SYNDROME.

posterior ethmoid foramen. A canal between the posterior portions of the frontal and ethmoid bones, transmitting the posterior ethmoid nerve and vessels. NA *foramen ethmoidale posterius.*

posterior focal point. The posterior conjugate focus. See *conjugate foci.*

posterior fontanel. The membranous space at the point of junction of lambdoid and sagittal sutures. May be closed at birth or within a few weeks after birth. NA *fonticulus posterior.*

posterior forceps. FORCEPS MAJOR.

posterior gluteal line. A line beginning near the end of the posterior extremity of the crest of the ilium and curving downward to the posterior part of the greater sciatic notch. NA *linea glutea posterior.*

posterior horn. The posterior column of gray matter as seen in a cross section of the spinal cord. NA *cornu posterius medullae spinalis.*

posterior hypothalamic nucleus. A nucleus found in the posterior region of the hypothalamus. NA *nucleus posterior hypothalami.*

posterior inferior iliac spine. A projection on the posterior border of the ilium, separated from the respective posterior superior spine by a notch. NA *spina iliaca posterior inferior.*

posterior intermediate septum. The septum between the fasciculus gracilis and the fasciculus cuneatus.

posterior intermediate sulcus. A shallow longitudinal furrow on the dorsolateral surface of the cervical and upper thoracic portions of the spinal cord between the fasciculus gracilis and fasciculus cuneatus. NA *sulcus intermedius posterior medullae spinalis.*

posterior interventricular sulcus. A groove situated on the diaphragmatic surface of the heart, between the ventricles. NA *sulcus interventricularis posterior.*

posterior iter. The aperture through which the chorda tympani nerve enters the tympanum. Syn. *iter chordae posterius.* NA *apertura tympanica canaliculi chordae tympani.*

posterior lacrimal crest. A vertical ridge dividing the lateral surface of the lacrimal bone into two parts. Syn. *lacrimal crest.*

posterior lacterocondylar syndrome. COLLET-SICARD SYNDROME.

posterior lateral fontanel. POSTEROLATERAL FONTANEL.

posterior lateral nucleus of the thalamus. The dorsal lateral nucleus of the lateral thalamic nuclei.

posterior ligament of the incus. A short band of fibers connecting the short crus of the incus and the fossa incudis. NA *ligamentum incudis posterius.*

posterior limb of the internal capsule. The portion of the internal capsule that lies between the lentiform nucleus and the thalamus.

posterior lobe of the hypophysis. NEUROHYPOPHYSIS.

posterior longitudinal cardiac sulcus. POSTERIOR INTERVENTRICULAR SULCUS.

posterior longitudinal ligament. A fibrous band connecting the posterior surfaces of the vertebral bodies, passing along the anterior wall of the vertebral canal from the occipital bone to the coccyx, and serving, with the anterior longitudinal ligament and the intervertebral disks, to secure the joints between the vertebral bodies. NA *ligamentum longitudinale posterius.*

posterior mallear fold. 1. A fold on the external surface of the tympanic membrane stretching from the mallear prominence to the posterior portion of the tympanic sulcus of the temporal bone, forming the lower posterior border of the pars flaccida. NA *plica mallearis posterior membrane tympani.* 2. A fold of mucous membrane on the inner aspect of the tympanic membrane over the lateral ligament of the malleus. NA *plica mallearis posterior tunicae mucosae cavi tympani.*

posterior malleolar fold. POSTERIOR MALLEAR FOLD.

posterior marginal dysplasia of the cornea. POSTERIOR EMBRYOTOXON.

posterior median septum. A delicate glial partition, immediately underneath the shallow posterior median sulcus, extending into the spinal cord to a depth of 5 mm and reaching the central gray matter. A structure resulting from fusion of the paired alar plates of the embryonic spinal cord.

posterior median sulcus of the spinal cord. A narrow groove extending the entire length of the spinal cord posteriorly in the midline. NA *sulcus medianus posterior medullae spinalis.*

posterior mediastinum. The division of the mediastinum that contains a part of the aorta, the greater and lesser azygos veins, the vagus and splanchnic nerves, the esophagus, the thoracic duct, and some lymph nodes. NA *mediastinum posterius.*

posterior medullary velum. INFERIOR MEDULLARY VELUM.

posterior nasal spine. A process formed by the united, projecting, medial ends of the posterior borders of the two palate bones, giving attachment to the muscle of the uvula. Syn. *nasal spine of the palatine bone.* NA *spina nasalis posterior ossis palatini.*

posterior neck triangle. An area bounded in front by the sternocleidomastoid muscle, behind by the anterior margin of the trapezius, its base being formed by the middle third of the clavicle, its apex by the occipital bone; divided by the omohyoid into the occipital and subclavian triangles.

posterior neuropore. A neuropore at the caudal end of the neural tube.

posterior nuclei of the thalamus. The pulvinar, medial, and lateral geniculate bodies, and the suprageniculate nucleus.

posterior obturator tubercle. An occasional projection on the medial border of the ischium, immediately anterior to the acetabular notch; the posterior boundary of the obturator groove. NA *tuberculum obturatorium posterius.*

posterior palatal seal. The seal at the posterior border of an upper artificial denture; it is usually established along the junction of the hard and soft palates.

posterior perforated substance. A depressed area at the base of the brain, posterior to the mammillary bodies, containing numerous foramens for the passage of blood vessels. NA *substantia perforata posterior.*

posterior peroneofemoral reflex. EXTERNAL HAMSTRING REFLEX.

posterior pillar of the fauces. PALATOPHARYNGEAL ARCH.

posterior pillar of the fornix. CRUS OF THE FORNIX.

posterior pituitary. NEUROHYPOPHYSIS.

posterior pituitary principle or **substance.** Extracts of the neurohypophysis.

posterior polar cataract. A congenital or acquired cataract at the posterior region of the lens.

posterior process of the talus. A prominent tubercle on the posterior surface of the talus to which the posterior talofibular ligament is attached. NA *processus posterior tali.*

posterior rhinoscopy. Examination of the choanae by means of a rhinoscope or mirror.

posterior rhizotomy. Surgical division of the posterior sensory roots of the spinal nerves within the dura mater for the relief of intractable pain in the distribution of those roots.

posterior root. DORSAL ROOT.

posterior root ganglion. SPINAL GANGLION.

posterior sacral foramen. One of the eight foramina (four on each side) on the posterior surface of the sacrum, external to the articular processes, and giving passage to the posterior branches of the sacral nerves. NA *foramina sacralia dorsalia.*

posterior sclerotomy. Sclerotomy by an incision through the sclera behind the ciliary body, and entering the vitreous chamber.

posterior septum. POSTERIOR MEDIAN SEPTUM.

posterior spinal sclerosis. TABES DORSALIS.

posterior spinocerebellar tract. A nerve tract that arises from the cells of the dorsal nucleus of Clark (thoracic nucleus), ascends the spinal cord in the lateral funiculus, and reaches the cerebellum by way of the inferior cerebellar peduncle; it conveys proprioceptive impulses. NA *tractus spinocerebellaris posterior.*

posterior staphyloma. A backward bulging of the sclera at the posterior pole of the eye.

posterior superior alveolar foramina. FORAMINA ALVEOLARIA MAXILLAE.

posterior superior iliac spine. The projection formed by the posterior extremity of the iliac crest. NA *spina iliaca posterior superior.*

posterior symblepharon. A symblepharon that occurs when the adhesion is near the conjunctival fornix.

posterior synechia. Adhesion between the iris and crystalline lens. See also *annular synechia, synechia.*

posterior thalamic peduncle. See *thalamic peduncles.*

posterior tibiofemoral reflex. INTERNAL HAMSTRING REFLEX.

posterior triangular space. The space lying above the clavicle and between the sternomastoid and the trapezius muscles and the occiput.

posterior tubercle. A tubercle at the posterior part of the extremity of the transverse process of certain cervical vertebrae. NA *tuberculum posterius vertebrarum cervicalium.*

posterior urethritis. Inflammation of the prostatic and membranous portions of the male urethra.

posterior vaginismus. Vaginismus due to spasm of the pubococcygeal portion of the levator ani muscle.

posterior white commissure. The small number of myelinated fibers that cross the midline in the part of the central gray commissure lying posterior to the central canal of the spinal cord. Contr. *anterior white commissure* (= WHITE COMMISSURE (1)).

postero-. A combining form meaning *posterior.*

pos·tero·an·te·ri·or (pos″tur·o·an·teer′ee·ur) *adj.* [*postero-* + *anterior*]. From the back to the front of the body, as in describing the direction of roentgen rays traversing the patient. Abbreviated, PA. Compare *dorsoventral.*

pos·tero·ex·ter·nal (pos″tur·o·ecks·tur′nul) *adj.* [*postero-* + *external*]. Occupying the outer side of a back part, as the posteroexternal column of the spinal cord. —**posteroexter·nad** (·nad) *adv.*

pos·tero·in·ter·nal (pos″tur·o·in·tur′nul) *adj.* [*postero-* + *internal*]. Occupying the inner side of a back part, as the posterointernal column of the spinal cord. —**posterointer·nad** (·nad) *adv.*

pos·tero·lat·er·al (pos″tur·o·lat′ur·ul) *adj.* [*postero-* + *lateral*]. Situated behind and at the side of a part. —**posterolater·ad** (·ad) *adv.*

posterolateral fissure. UVULONODULAR SULCUS.

posterolateral fontanel. The membranous space between the parietal, occipital, and temporal bones; usually closes by 3 months of age.

posterolateral sclerosis. SUBACUTE COMBINED DEGENERATION OF THE SPINAL CORD.

posterolateral spinal sulcus. A narrow deep groove on the posterolateral surface of the spinal cord, corresponding to the line of origin of the dorsal nerve roots. NA *sulcus lateralis posterior medullae spinalis.*

posterolateral sulcus of the medulla oblongata. The extension cephalad of the posterolateral spinal sulcus. NA *sulcus lateralis posterior medullae oblongatae.*

posterolateral ventral nucleus of the thalamus. A column of cells, lying lateral to the posteromedial ventral nucleus, which receives the fibers of the ventral and lateral spinothalamic tracts and medial lemniscus. NA *nucleus ventralis posterolateralis thalami.*

pos·tero·mar·gi·nal nucleus (pos″tur·o·mahr′ji·nul). A thin layer of cells in the zona spongiosa, most prominent in the lumbosacral segments, whose axons go to the lateral white column and bifurcate into ascending and descending fibers, probably forming intersegmental tracts. Syn. *nucleus magnocellularis, marginal nucleus.*

pos·tero·me·di·al (pos″tur·o·mee′dee·ul) *adj.* [*postero-* + *medial*]. Situated posteriorly and toward the midline. —**posteromedi·ad** (·ad) *adv.*

posteromedial ventral nucleus of the thalamus. A sharply defined column of cells ventral to the central nucleus of the thalamus which receives sensory fibers from the nucleus of the spinal tract of the trigeminal nerve and from the main sensory nucleus of the trigeminal nerve. Syn. *arcuate nucleus.* NA *nucleus ventralis posteromedialis thalami.*

pos·tero·me·di·an (pos″tur·o·mee′dee·un) *adj.* [*postero-* + *median*]. Situated posteriorly and in the midline.

pos·tero·su·pe·ri·or (pos″tur·o·sue·peer′ee·ur) *adj.* [*postero-* + *superior*]. Situated behind and above a part.

pos·tero·trans·verse diameter (pos″tur·o·tranz·vurce′, ·trans′vurce). The line joining the parietal eminences of the skull.

post·erup·tive (pohst″e·rup′tiv) *adj.* Following eruption.

post·esoph·a·ge·al, post·oesoph·a·ge·al (pohst″e·sof″uh·jee′ul, ·ee″so·faj′ee·ul) *adj.* [*post-* + *esophageal*]. Situated behind the esophagus.

post·evac·u·a·tion film (pohst″e·vack″yoo·ay′shun). A roentgenogram of the colon obtained just after evacuation of a barium enema to demonstrate the mucosal pattern.

post·ex·an·them·a·tous encephalomyelitis (pohst″eck·santh·em′uh·tus). Acute disseminated encephalomyelitis following an exanthematous disease such as measles, chickenpox, scarlet fever, or rubella.

post·fas·cial abscess (pohst·fash′ee·ul). SUBFASCIAL ABSCESS.

post·fe·brile (pohst·feb′ril, ·fee′bril) *adj.* [*post-* + *febrile*]. Occurring after or resulting from a fever.

post·gan·gli·on·ic (pohst″gang″glee·on′ick) *adj.* [*post-* + *ganglionic*]. Situated beyond a ganglion.

postganglionic neuron. A neuron of the autonomic nervous system having its cell body in a ganglion, the axon extending to an organ or tissue.

postganglionic ramus. GRAY RAMUS COMMUNICANS.

post·gas·trec·to·my (pohst″gas·treck′tuh·mee) *adj.* [*post-* + *gastrectomy*]. Occurring after or resulting from removal of part or all of the stomach.

post·gle·noid (pohst·glee′noid, ·glen′oid) *adj.* [*post-* + *glenoid*]. Situated behind the mandibular (glenoid) fossa of the temporal bone.

postglenoid process. A process of the temporal bone situated immediately in front of the petrotympanic fissure, separating the mandibular fossa from the external acoustic meatus.

postglenoid tubercle. A process of the temporal bone that descends behind the mandibular fossa and prevents backward displacement of the mandible during mastication.

post·grav·id (pohst·grav′id) *adj.* [*post-* + *gravid*]. After pregnancy.

post·hemi·ple·gic (pohst″hem·i·plee′jick) *adj.* [*post-* + *hemiplegic*]. Occurring after or following hemiplegia.

posthemiplegic athetosis. Athetosis following the onset of hemiplegia, most common in children as a result of a cerebrovascular accident involving the capsular and basal ganglionic structures.

posthemiplegic chorea. POSTPARALYTIC CHOREA.

post·hem·or·rhag·ic, post·haem·or·rhag·ic (pohst″hem·o·raj′ick) *adj.* [*post-* + *hemorrhagic*]. Occurring after or resulting from a hemorrhage.

post·he·pat·ic (pohst″he·pat′ick) *adj.* [*post-* + *hepatic*]. Situated or occurring behind the liver.

posthepatic jaundice. OBSTRUCTIVE JAUNDICE.

post·hep·a·tit·ic (pohst·hep″uh·tit′ick) *adj.* [*post-* + *hepatitis* + *-ic*]. Following or resulting from hepatitis.

post·her·pet·ic (pohst″hur·pet′ick) *adj.* [*post-* + *herpetic*]. Occurring after or resulting from herpes zoster or herpes simplex.

postherpetic neuralgia. Neuralgia continuing after healing of the lesions of herpes zoster.

pos·thet·o·my (pos·thet′uh·mee) *n.* [Gk. *posthē*, foreskin, + *-tomy*]. CIRCUMCISION.

pos·thi·tis (pos·thigh′tis) *n.*, pl. **pos·thit·i·des** (·thit′i·deez) [Gk. *posthē*, foreskin, + *-itis*]. Inflammation of the prepuce.

pos·tho·lith (pos′tho·lith) *n.* [Gk. *posthē*, foreskin, + *-lith*]. A preputial calculus.

post·hu·mous (pos′tew·mus) *adj.* [L. *postumus*, last, last born, born after father's death]. 1. Occurring after death. 2. Born after the death of the father, or by cesarean section after the death of the mother. 3. Published after the death of the writer.

post·hyp·not·ic (pohst″hip·not′ick) *adj.* [*post-* + *hypnotic*]. Succeeding the hypnotic state; acting after the hypnotic state has passed off.

posthypnotic amnesia. Loss of memory following hypnosis; may be spontaneous or occur in response to suggestions made during the hypnotic trance.

posthypnotic suggestion. The command to do certain acts given the subject while in the hypnotic stage, and causing him to execute these acts after his return to his normal condition.

post·ic·tal (pohst″ick′tul) *adj.* [*post-* + *ictal*]. Following or resulting from a seizure or a stroke.

postictal automatism. A complex semipurposeful act carried out by the patient after an epileptic attack; usually the consequence of postictal confusion. Contr. *epileptic automatism.*

post·ic·ter·ic (pohst·ick·terr′ick) *adj.* [*post-* + *icteric*]. Of or pertaining to the period or condition following jaundice.

pos·ti·cus (pos·tye′kus) *adj.* [L., hind, back]. POSTERIOR.

post·in·farc·tion syndrome (pohst″in·fahrk′shun). POST-MYOCARDIAL INFARCTION SYNDROME.

post·in·fec·tious (pohst″in·feck′shus) *adj.* [*post-* + *infectious*]. Following an infection.

postinfectious encephalitis or **encephalomyelitis.** ACUTE DISSEMINATED ENCEPHALOMYELITIS.

postinfectious psychosis. Psychosis following an acute infectious disease, such as pneumonia or typhoid fever.

post·in·fec·tive (pohst′in·feck′tiv) *adj.* POSTINFECTIOUS.

postinfective encephalitis or **encephalomyelitis.** ACUTE DISSEMINATED ENCEPHALOMYELITIS.

post·in·flu·en·zal (pohst″in″floo·en′zul) *adj.* [*post-* + *influenzal*]. Occurring after or resulting from influenza.

Post-Lau·der·milk method. A staining method for cellulose in which iodine and lithium chloride are applied to the fibers to obtain a blue, yellow, or green color.

post·ma·lar·i·al (pohst″muh·lăr′ee·ul) *adj.* [*post-* + *malarial*]. Occurring after or as a sequel of malaria.

post·mam·il·lary decussation (pohst″mam′i·lerr″ee). SUPRAMAMILLARY DECUSSATION.

post·mam·mary abscess (pohst·mam′uh·ree). SUBMAMMARY ABSCESS.

post·mas·tec·to·my (pohst″mas·teck′tuh·mee) *adj.* [*post-* + *mastectomy*]. Occurring after or resulting from surgical removal of the breast.

post·ma·ture (pohst″muh·tewr′) *adj.* [*post-* + *mature*]. 1. Of a fetus, having remained in the uterus beyond the normal length of gestation. 2. Overdeveloped. —**postma·tu·ri·ty** (·tewr′i·tee) *n.*

postmaturity syndrome. Failure of birth of an infant after 294 days gestation with resultant change in the appearance of the infant, characterized by absence of vernix caseosa on the skin, meconium staining of the skin, and a freely movable skin over the underlying tissues. Associated with some increase in perinatal mortality and in psychomotor retardation.

post·men·ar·che (pohst″me·nahr′kee) *adj.* [*post-* + *menarche*]. Occurring after the beginning of menstrual cycles.

post·men·o·pau·sal (pohst″men″uh·paw′zul) *adj.* [*post-* + *menopausal*]. Occurring after the menopause.

postmenopausal osteoporosis. A diffuse osteoporosis, often severe, chiefly involving the spine and the pelvis, which may follow artificial or physiological menopause, probably related to gonadal hormonal deficiency and concomitant inadequate bone formation.

post·men·stru·al (pohst·men′stroo·ul) *adj.* [*post-* + *menstrual*]. Following menstruation.

postmenstrual vaginitis. Inflammation of the vagina, usually occurring after the menopause. See also *atrophic vaginitis.*

post·mor·tal (post″mor′tul) *adj.* Occurring after death.

post mor·tem (mor′tum) *adv. phrase* [L.]. After death, as: 2 hours post mortem. Compare *postmortem* (*adj.*). Contr. *ante mortem.*

post·mor·tem (pohst·mor′tum) *adj.* & *n.* [L.]. 1. Following death. 2. An examination of the body after death; AUTOPSY.

postmortem delivery. Extraction of the fetus after the death of the mother.

postmortem rigidity. RIGOR MORTIS.

post·mu·coid (pohst″mew′koid) *adj.* MATT (2).

post-myocardial infarction syndrome. Postcardiotomy syndrome following myocardial infarction. Syn. *Dressler's syndrome, postinfarction syndrome.*

post·na·ris (pohst·nair′is) *n.* [*post-* + *naris*]. The posterior naris; CHOANA (2).

post·na·sal (pohst″nay′zul) *adj.* [*post-* + *nasal*]. Situated behind the nose, or in the nasopharynx.

post·na·tal (pohst·nay′tul) *adj.* [*post-* + *natal*]. Subsequent to birth.

postnatal asphyxia atelectasis. RESPIRATORY DISTRESS SYNDROME OF THE NEWBORN.

postnatal development. Development occurring after birth.

post·ne·crot·ic (pohst″ne·krot′ick) *adj.* [*post-* + *necrotic*].

1. Occurring after the death of a tissue or part. 2. Occurring after death.

postnecrotic cirrhosis. Cirrhosis, usually due to toxic agents or viral hepatitis, characterized by necrosis of liver cells, large regenerating nodules of hepatic tissue, the presence of large bands of connective tissue which course irregularly through the liver, and, in some areas, preservation of the normal hepatic architecture. See also *acute yellow atrophy.*

post·ne·phrec·to·my (post″ne·freck′tuh·mee) *adj.* [*post-* + *nephrectomy*]. Occurring after the removal of a kidney or kidneys.

post·neu·rit·ic (pohst″new·rit′ick) *adj.* [*post-* + *neuritic*]. Occurring after neuritis.

post·nod·u·lar (pohst·nod′yoo·lur) *adj.* [*post-* + *nodular*]. Situated behind the nodulus of the cerebellum.

post·oc·u·lar (pohst·ock′yoo·lur) *adj.* [*post-* + *ocular*]. Behind the eye.

postoesophageal. POSTESOPHAGEAL.

post·ol·i·vary sulcus (pohst·ol′i·verr·ee). A deep groove on the dorsolateral border of the olive; it may be considered as the laterally shifted continuation of the posterolateral sulcus.

post·op·er·a·tive (pohst·op′ur·uh·tiv) *adj.* [*post-* + *operative*]. Occurring after an operation; following closely upon an operation.

postoperative hernia. INCISIONAL HERNIA.

postoperative myxedema. Myxedema resulting from total or partial thyroidectomy. Syn. *operative myxedema.*

post·oral (pohst·o′rul) *adj.* [*post-* + *oral*]. Situated behind the mouth; posterior to the first visceral arch.

postoral arch. Any one of the second to sixth visceral arches.

post·or·bit·al (pohst·or′bi·tul) *adj.* [*post-* + *orbital*]. Behind the orbit.

post·pal·a·tine (pohst″pal′uh·tine) *adj.* [*post-* + *palatine*]. Behind the uvula.

post·pa·lu·dal (pohst″pa·lew′dul, ·pal′yoo·dul) *adj.* [*post-* + *paludal*]. POSTMALARIAL.

post·par·a·lyt·ic (pohst″păr·uh·lit′ick) *adj.* [*post-* + *paralytic*]. Following the onset of paralysis.

postparalytic chorea. Chorea occurring after a cerebrovascular accident or other disorder which results in paralysis.

postparalytic facial spasm. Twitching of facial muscles, mostly combined with their contracture, which occasionally follows facial paralysis (Bell's palsy) after an interval of several months.

post par·tum, *adv. phrase* [L.]. After delivery, as: 24 to 28 hours post partum. Compare *postpartum* (*adj.*). Contr. *ante partum.*

post·par·tum (pohst·pahr′tum) *adj.* [L.]. Following childbirth. Compare *post partum.* Contr. *antepartum, intrapartum.*

postpartum heart disease. POSTPARTUM MYOCARDITIS.

postpartum hemorrhage. Bleeding occurring shortly after childbirth.

postpartum hemorrhagic hypopituitarism. SHEEHAN'S SYNDROME.

postpartum myocarditis or **myocardosis.** Heart failure of obscure etiology occurring in the puerperium, commonly associated with pulmonary embolization.

postpartum panhypopituitary syndrome. SHEEHAN'S SYNDROME.

postpartum pituitary necrosis. SHEEHAN'S SYNDROME.

postpartum psychosis. A psychotic reaction in a woman following childbirth. See also *puerperal psychosis.*

post·per·fu·sion (pohst″pur·few′zhun) *adj.* Following perfusion.

postperfusion psychosis. Psychotic symptoms resulting from diffuse disturbances in cerebral microcirculation occurring 2 to 8 weeks following use of a pump-oxygenator in open-heart surgery or following blood transfusions.

postperfusion syndrome. Fever, splenomegaly, lymphadenopathy, lymphocytosis, and eosinophilia occurring 2 to 8 weeks following use of a pump-oxygenator in open-heart surgery; may represent a reaction to the large amount of blood usually administered during such operations.

post·pha·ryn·ge·al (pohst″fuh·rin′jee·ul) *adj.* RETROPHARYNGEAL.

post·phle·bit·ic (pohst″fle·bit′ick) *adj.* [*post-* + *phlebitic*]. Following or resulting from venous inflammation.

postphlebitic syndrome. The postthrombotic syndrome following thrombophlebitis of deep veins, particularly the ileofemoral vessels.

post·poned labor. Labor delayed beyond 9 months.

post·pran·di·al (pohst·pran′dee·ul) *adj.* [*post-* + *prandial*]. After a meal.

post·pri·ma·ry tuberculosis. CHRONIC TUBERCULOSIS.

post·pros·tat·ic pouch (pohst″pros·tat′ick). The bas-fond in the male.

post·pu·ber·al (pohst·pew′bur·ul) *adj.* [*post-* + *puberal*]. Occurring after puberty.

post·pu·bes·cent (pohst″pew·bes′unt) *adj.* [*post-* + *pubescent*]. Following the onset of puberty.

post·pyc·not·ic (pohst″pick·not′ick) *adj.* [*post-* + *pycnotic*]. Occurring subsequent to pycnosis.

post·py·ram·i·dal (pohst″pi·ram′i·dul) *adj.* [*post-* + *pyramidal*]. Situated behind the pyramidal tract.

post·ra·di·a·tion (pohst″ray·dee·ay′shun) *adj.* [*post-* + *radiation*]. Occurring after exposure to ionizing radiation.

post·re·nal (pohst″ree′nul) *adj.* [*post-* + *renal*]. In the urinary tract, caudal to the kidneys.

postrenal anuria. Anuria because of urinary tract obstruction.

post·rhi·nal (pohst″rye′nul) *adj.* [*post-* + *rhinal*]. POSTNASAL.

post·ro·lan·dic (pohst″ro·lan′dick) *adj.* [*post-* + *rolandic*]. POSTCENTRAL (2).

post·ro·ta·to·ry (pohst·ro′tuh·tor″ee) *adj.* [*post-* + *rotatory*]. After rotation, as postrotatory ocular nystagmus.

post·scar·la·ti·nal (pohst″skahr″luh·tee′nul, ·tye′nul) *adj.* [*post-* + *scarlatinal*]. Occurring after or as a result of scarlet fever.

post·sphyg·mic (pohst″sfig′mick) *adj.* [*post-* + *sphygmic*]. Following the pressure pulse wave.

postsphygmic period. The period of isometric relaxation of the heart muscle at the beginning of ventricular diastole, until the opening of the atrioventricular valves.

post·sple·nec·to·my (pohst″sple·neck′tuh·mee) *adj.* Following or resulting from surgical removal of the spleen.

post·ste·not·ic (pohst″ste·not′ick) *adj.* [*post-* + *stenotic*]. Pertaining to the area beyond an orifice narrowed by disease, or beyond an abnormal constriction of a hollow viscus; usually the area beyond a narrowed heart valve or blood vessel.

post surgeon. The surgeon of an established army post.

post·syn·ap·tic (pohst″si·nap′tick) *adj.* [*post-* + *synaptic*]. Situated behind or occurring after a synapse.

postsynaptic membrane. The chemically excitable membrane bounding the dendritic part of a synapse.

postsynaptic potential. *In neurophysiology,* the transient, graded fluctuation of the dendritic or nerve cell membrane potential that follows, after a brief delay, the arrival of a nerve impulse at an axon terminal.

post·syph·i·lit·ic (pohst″sif·i·lit′ick) *adj.* [*post-* + *syphilitic*]. Following or resulting from syphilis.

post·throm·bot·ic (pohst″throm·bot′ick) *adj.* Occurring after or as a result of thrombosis.

postthrombotic syndrome. Chronic venous insufficiency resulting from deep venous thrombosis of the lower extremity, characterized by edema, pain, stasis dermatitis, stasis cellulitis, varicose veins, pigmentation of the skin, and eventually chronic ulceration of the lower leg.

post-tracheotomy stenosis. Stenosis after tracheotomy.

posttransfusion syndrome. An infectious mononucleosis-like illness brought about by the cytomegalovirus several months after the patient undergoes open heart surgery or blood transfusions; characterized by moderate fever and, frequently, by splenomegaly or hepatomegaly.

post·trans·verse anastomosis (pohst·tranz·vurce′, ·trans′vurce). In the embryo, a longitudinal anastomosis between intersegmental arteries, dorsal to the transverse process, forming the deep cervical artery.

post·trau·mat·ic (pohst″traw·mat′ick) *adj.* [*post-* + *traumatic*]. Pertaining to any process or event following, or resulting from, traumatic injury.

posttraumatic constitution. POSTCONCUSSION SYNDROME.

posttraumatic delirium. TRAUMATIC DELIRIUM.

posttraumatic hernia. INCISIONAL HERNIA.

posttraumatic nervous instability. POSTCONCUSSION SYNDROME.

posttraumatic neurosis. TRAUMATIC NEUROSIS.

posttraumatic osteoporosis. Generalized rarefaction of bone, which follows severe trauma and resultant inactivity of the body and attendant nutritional and metabolic disturbances.

posttraumatic personality disorder. A disorder resulting from direct injury to the head or brain followed by a brief loss of consciousness; manifested by headache, emotional instability, fatigability, insomnia, and memory defects, but usually no demonstrable organic deficits.

posttraumatic psychosis. Psychosis following head trauma.

post·tre·mat·ic (pohst″tre·mat′ick) *adj.* Pertaining to nerves that pass on the hind margin of a trema or gill slit, as the mandibular and lingual nerves do in a masked form in land vertebrates.

post·tus·sive (pohst·tus′iv) *adj.* [*post-* + *tussive*]. Occurring after a cough.

posttussive rale. A rale elicited only after an expiratory cough.

posttussive suction. A sucking sound heard on auscultation over pulmonary cavities during the interval between a cough and the succeeding inspiration.

post·ty·phoid (pohst·tye′foid) *adj.* [*post-* + *typhoid*]. Following or resulting from typhoid fever.

pos·tu·late (pos′tew·late, ·lut) *n.* [L. *postulare*, to demand]. 1. A proposition assumed without proof. 2. A condition that must be fulfilled.

pos·tur·al (pos′tew·rul, pos′chur·ul) *adj.* Pertaining to posture or position; performed by means of a special posture.

postural color test. A test for arterial insufficiency; positive result consists of conspicuous blanching or mottling of the skin of an elevated extremity and delay or failure to flush following dependency.

postural drainage. Removal of bronchial secretions or of the contents of a lung abscess by the use of gravity and position to drain a specific area of the lung.

postural exercise. An activity to correct mild deformities and to improve posture.

postural hypotension. ORTHOSTATIC HYPOTENSION.

postural muscle. ANTIGRAVITY MUSCLE.

postural nystagmus. POSITIONAL NYSTAGMUS.

postural reflex. Any one of many reflexes associated in establishing or maintaining the posture of an individual against the force of gravity.

pos·ture (pos′chur) *n.* [L. *positura*, position]. Position or bearing, especially of the body.

posture sense. The capability of recognizing (without seeing) the position in which a limb has been placed.

post·vac·ci·nal (pohst·vack′si·nul) *adj.* [*post-* + *vaccinal*]. Following, or resulting from, vaccination.

postvaccinal dermatosis. A dermatosis following vaccination, marked by lesions similar to those of urticaria pigmentosa except that desquamation is present and dermographia is absent.

postvaccinal encephalomyelitis. ACUTE DISSEMINATED ENCEPHALOMYELITIS.

postvaccinal hepatitis or **jaundice.** SERUM HEPATITIS.

postvaccinal myelitis. Disseminated perivenous demyelination of the spinal cord that sometimes follows vaccination.

post·val·vu·lot·o·my syndrome (pohst″val″vew·lot′uh·mee). Postcardiotomy syndrome following valvulotomy.

post·ves·i·cal (pohst·ves′i·kul) *adj.* [*post-* + *vesical*]. Behind the urinary bladder.

po·ta·ble (po′tuh·bul) *adj.* [L. *potare*, to drink]. Drinkable; fit to drink.

Po·tain's disease (poh·tæn′) [P. C. E. *Potain*, French physician, 1825–1901]. PULMONARY EDEMA.

Potain's syndrome [P. C. E. *Potain*]. Gastric dilation and dyspepsia with right ventricular dilation and accentuation of the pulmonic component of the second heart sound.

Pot·a·mon (pot′uh·mun) *n.* [NL., from Gk. *potamos*, river]. A genus of freshwater crabs, species of which have been incriminated in the transmission of the fluke, *Paragonimus westermani*.

pot·a·mo·pho·bia (pot″uh·mo·fo′bee·uh) *n.* [Gk. *potamos*, river, + *-phobia*]. Abnormal fear of large rivers or bodies of water.

pot·ash (pot′ash) *n.* [*pot* + *ashes*]. POTASSIUM CARBONATE.

potash alum. POTASSIUM ALUM.

potash lye. POTASSIUM HYDROXIDE.

potash soap. A soft soap. See also *green soap*.

pot·as·se·mia, pot·as·sae·mia (pot″uh·see′mee·uh) *n.* [*potassium* + *-emia*]. HYPERKALEMIA.

po·tas·si·um (puh·tas′ee·um) *n.* [NL., from E. *potash*]. K = 39.102. A light, malleable metallic element formed into ductile lumps, rods, or spheres, which reacts violently with water. A small amount of potassium is physiologically essential. See also Table of Chemical Constituents of Blood in the Appendix.

potassium acetate. CH_3COOK, used medicinally as a source of potassium ion and also as a systemic and urinary alkalizer.

potassium alum. An alum containing potassium, particularly ordinary alum or aluminum potassium sulfate.

potassium bicarbonate. $KHCO_3$, used medicinally as a source of potassium ion, and also as a gastric antacid and to alkalinize urine.

potassium bismuth tartrate. Bismuth and potassium tartrate; formerly used as an antisyphilitic drug.

potassium bitartrate. $KHC_4H_4O_6$, used as a saline cathartic. Syn. *cream of tartar, potassium hydrogen tartrate.*

potassium bromide. KBr, a central nervous system depressant; occasionally used as a sedative.

potassium carb·acry·late (kahrb″a·kril′ate, ·ack′ri·late). The generic name for the potassium form of cross-linked polyacrylic polycarboxylic cation exchange resins. Such a resin, used in combination with carbacrylic resin, is useful clinically for removal of sodium from intestinal fluid with minimum disturbance of potassium ion equilibrium. See also *carbacrylamine resins.*

potassium carbonate. K_2CO_3, used in pharmaceutical and chemical manufacturing.

potassium chlorate. $KClO_3$, formerly used for its supposed disinfectant action, on the assumption that oxygen is released; this reaction does not take place.

potassium chloride. KCl, used for the treatment of potassium deficiency states.

potassium citrate. $K_3C_6H_5O_7$, used for the treatment of potassium deficiency states; also as a systemic alkalizer, diuretic, and expectorant.

potassium glu·cal·drate (gloo·kal′drate). Potassium dihydroxy(gluconato)diaquoaluminate, $C_6H_{16}AlKO_{11}$, an antacid.

potassium guai·a·col·sul·fo·nate (gwye″uh·kol·sul′fo·nate). $HOC_6H_3(OCH_3)SO_3K$, used as an expectorant.

potassium hydrogen tartrate. POTASSIUM BITARTRATE.

potassium hydroxide. KOH, sometimes used as an escharotic. Syn. *caustic potash.*

potassium iodide. KI, used mainly as an expectorant and as a source of iodide ion.

potassium nitrate. KNO_3; has some diuretic properties; SALTPETER.

potassium per·car·bo·nate (pur-kahr′buh-nate, -nut). $K_2C_2O_6.H_2O$, a salt that liberates oxygen in aqueous solution; used as a diagnostic and analytical reagent.

potassium permanganate. $KMnO_4$, used as a disinfectant and cleansing agent; sometimes also as an antidote to certain poisons.

potassium phosphate. DIBASIC POTASSIUM PHOSPHATE.

potassium sodium tartrate. $COOK(CHOH)_2COONa$, used as a saline cathartic. Syn. *Rochelle salt.*

potassium thiocyanate. KSCN, formerly used in the treatment of essential hypertension but produces frequent toxic reactions.

potassium tolerance test. A formerly used test based on the increased rise and duration of the serum potassium in patients with hypoadrenalism as compared to normal after the oral ingestion of a potassium salt.

po·ta·to nose. RHINOPHYMA.

potato tumor. CAROTID-BODY TUMOR.

po·ten·cy (po′tun-see) *n.* [L. *potentia,* power]. 1. Inherent power or strength. 2. Power of the male to perform the sexual act. 3. *In homeopathy,* the degree of dilution of a drug. **—po·tent** (·tunt) *adj.*

po·ten·tial (po·ten′chul) *adj. & n.* [L. *potentialis,* from *potentia,* power]. 1. Possible or probable. 2. Existing in the form of a capacity or disposition as opposed to being realized or overtly manifested; latent. 3. Any inherent possibility, capacity, or power of a thing or a being. 4. In electricity, a state of tension or of difference in energy capable of doing work. If two bodies of different potential are brought into contact, a current is established between them that is capable of producing electric effects.

potential energy. The power possessed by a body at rest, by virtue of its position, as the potential energy of a suspended weight. Syn. *latent energy.*

po·ten·ti·a·tion (po·ten″shee·ay′shun) *n.* 1. The effect of a substance, when added to another, of making the latter more potent. 2. The effect of combination of two drugs resulting in action greater than the total effect of each used separately. **—po·ten·ti·ate** (·ten′shee·ate) *v.*

po·tion (po′shun) *n.* [L. *potio,* from *potare,* to drink]. A drink or draught.

po·to·ma·nia (po″to·may′nee·uh) *n.* [L. *pot*are, to drink, + *-mania*]. *Obsol.* DELIRIUM TREMENS.

Pot·ter-Bucky diaphragm [H. E. *Potter,* U.S. radiologist, b. 1880; and G. *Bucky*]. BUCKY DIAPHRAGM.

pot·ter's asthma, consumption, or **rot.** SILICOSIS.

Pot·ter's disease. A congenital syndrome characterized by various skeletal malformations, renal agenesis, and characteristic facies including low-set malformed ears.

Potter's homogenizer. A glass device consisting of a pestle that rotates inside a close-fitting test tube.

pot·to (pot′o) *n.* A prosimian primate of western and central African rain forests, *Perodicticus potto,* similar to the slow loris of Southeast Asia.

Potts' anastomosis [W. J. *Potts*]. POTTS' OPERATION.

Pott's curvature [P. *Pott,* English surgeon, 1714–1788]. ANGULAR CURVATURE.

Pott's disease [P. *Pott*]. Kyphosis resulting from tuberculous osteitis of the spine.

Pott's fracture [P. *Pott*]. Fibular fracture a few inches above the ankle, sometimes accompanied by fracture of the medial malleolus.

Pott's gangrene [P. *Pott*]. Gangrene resulting from retrogressive vascular changes of old age.

Potts' operation [W. J. *Potts,* U.S. surgeon, b. 1895]. The creation of an aortic-pulmonary artery anastomosis as palliative surgery for tetralogy of Fallot, and other forms of cyanotic heart disease.

Pott's puffy tumor [P. *Pott*]. Posttraumatic osteomyelitis of the skull with edema but without a laceration of the overlying scalp.

Potts-Smith-Gibson operation [W. J. *Potts;* S. *Smith,* U.S. surgeon, b. 1912; and S. *Gibson,* U.S. pediatrician, b. 1883]. POTT'S OPERATION.

pouch, *n.* [OF. *pouche*]. A sac or pocket.

pouch of Douglas [J. *Douglas*]. RECTOUTERINE EXCAVATION.

pouch of Morison [J. R. *Morison*]. HEPATORENAL POUCH.

pou·drage (poo·drahzh′) *n.* [F., powdering]. The therapeutic introduction of an irritating powder on a serous surface to stimulate the formation of adhesions for obliteration of the pleural space, or to stimulate the development of a collateral circulation, as in the pericardial space.

Pou·let's disease (poo·leh′) [A. *Poulet,* French physician, 1848–1888]. Rheumatoid osteoperiostitis.

poul·tice (pohl′tis) *n.* [L. *pultes,* pl. of *puls,* pulse porridge]. A soft, semiliquid mass made of some cohesive substance mixed with water, and used for application to the skin for the purpose of supplying heat and moisture or acting as a local stimulant.

poultry chinch. *Haematosiphon inodora,* a bloodsucking ectoparasite of poultry in southern North America which is closely related to bedbugs (*Cimex*) and often bites man and other mammals.

pound, *n.* [L. *pondo*]. A unit of measure of weight. See Table of Weights and Measures in the Appendix. See also *troy pound, avoirdupois pound.*

Pou·part's ligament (poo·pahr′) [F. *Poupart,* French surgeon, 1616–1708]. INGUINAL LIGAMENT.

pour plate. A bacterial culture in which the culture is incorporated into a medium, poured into a sterile petri dish, and allowed to solidify.

Povan. Trademark for pyrvinium pamoate, a cyanine dye used as an anthelmintic in the treatment of pinworm infections.

po·vi·done (po′vi·dohn) *n.* POLYVINYLPYRROLIDONE.

povidone-iodine, *n.* A water-soluble complex of polyvinylpyrrolidone and iodine used topically for prevention and control of cutaneous infections susceptible to iodine.

Pow·as·san virus [after *Powassan,* Ontario, Canada]. A tick-borne arbovirus, group B, first isolated from a fatal case of encephalitis in Ontario, and also recovered in the United States.

pow·der, *n.* [OF. *poudre,* from L. *pulvis, pulveris,* dust]. 1. A group of pharmaceutical preparations of definite formula, consisting of intimate mixtures of finely divided medicinal substances. 2. *In pharmacy,* a single dose of medicine placed in powder paper, dusting powder, douche powder, or other bulk powder to be administered or used internally or externally.

powder burn. FLASH BURN.

pow·dered, *adj.* Reduced to a powder.

powdered digitalis. Digitalis leaf reduced to powder and standardized to contain 1 U.S.P. Digitalis Unit in each 100 mg.

powdered extract. A powder form of an extract of a vegetable or animal drug; preferred for certain dosage formulations, as capsules.

pow·er, *n.* [F. *pouvoir,* from L. *posse,* to be able]. 1. The ability to produce an effect. 2. *In optics,* the magnification given by a lens or prism.

power reactor. A nuclear reactor designed for use in a nuclear power plant, as distinguished from reactors used primarily for research or for producing radiation or fissionable materials.

Pow·er test [M. H. *Power,* U.S. biochemist, b. 1894]. CUTLER-POWER-WILDER TEST.

pox, *n.* [plural of *pock*]. 1. A vesicular or pustular exanthematic disease, such as smallpox, that may leave pit scars. 2. SYPHILIS.

pox diseases. A group of diseases caused by poxviruses,

characterized clinically usually by vesicles, pustules, and crusting and pathologically by ballooning degeneration and necrosis of the epidermis. Diseases such as chickenpox and herpes simplex show similar skin lesions but are caused by a different group of viruses.

pox·vi·rus (pocks″vye′rus) *n.* [*pox* + *virus*]. A member of a group of large, chemically complex DNA viruses, variably stable to ether, which includes those causing smallpox, vaccinia, ectromelia (mousepox), molluscum contagiosum, and infectious myxomatosis.

Poz·zi's syndrome (poʰd·zee′) [S. J. *Pozzi*, French gynecologist, 1846–1918]. Backache and leukorrhea without enlargement of the uterus, sometimes found in endometritis.

PP An abbreviation for *pellagra-preventive factor* (= NIACIN).

P.p. An abbreviation for *punctum proximum*, near point.

P.P.D. Abbreviation for *purified protein derivative* of tuberculin.

p-p factor [*p*ellagra-*p*reventative factor]. NIACIN.

ppg Abbreviation for *picopicogram*.

PPLO Abbreviation for *pleuropneumonia-like organisms*.

p.p.m., ppm Parts per million.

ppt. Abbreviation for *precipitate*.

P pul·mo·na·le (pul″mo·nay′lee). A tall, peaked P wave, usually indicating right atrial hypertrophy or dilatation.

P-Q interval. P-R INTERVAL.

Pr Symbol for praseodymium.

Pr. Abbreviation for *presbyopia*.

P.r. Abbreviation for *punctum remotum*, far point.

practical nurse. A nurse who is skilled in the care of the sick but who has not been graduated from a regular nursing school or passed an examination to qualify as a graduate nurse.

prac·tice, *v. & n.* [ML. *practicare*, from Gk. *praktikos*, practical, from *prassein*, to practice]. 1. To perform the duties of a physician as regards the diagnosis and treatment of disease. 2. The routine application of the principles of medicine to the diagnosis and treatment of disease. 3. Collectively, the patients of a physician.

prac·ti·tion·er (prack·tish′un·ur) *n.* A qualified person engaged in practicing medicine.

prac·to·lol (prack′to·lole) *n.* 4′-[2-Hydroxy-3-(isopropylamino)propoxy]acetanilide, $C_{14}H_{22}N_2O_3$, an antiadrenergic (β-receptor).

Pra·der-Wil·li syndrome (prah′dur, vil′ee) [A. *Prader*, Swiss pediatrician, 20th century; and H. *Willi*]. A congenital disorder of unknown cause, characterized by hypotonia, small hands and feet, extreme obesity, hypogonadism, and mental retardation.

prae-. See *pre-*.

praecox. PRECOX.

prae·cu·ne·us (pree·kew′nee·us) *n.* [BNA]. PRECUNEUS.

prae·pu·ti·um (pree·pew′shee·um) *n.* [BNA]. Preputium (= PREPUCE).

praevia. PREVIA.

-pragia. See *-praxia*.

prag·mat·ag·no·sia (prag″mat·ag·no′see·uh) *n.* [Gk. *pragma, pragmatos*, thing, + *agnosia*]. Loss of ability to recognize an object formerly known to the patient.

prag·mat·am·ne·sia (prag″mat·am·nee′zhuh, ·zee·uh) *n.* [Gk. *pragma, pragmatos*, thing, + *amnesia*]. Loss of ability to remember the appearance of an object formerly known.

Prague maneuver. Delivery of the aftercoming head by grasping the shoulders from below with two fingers of one hand, while the other hand draws the feet up over the abdomen of the mother.

prai·rie itch. GRAIN ITCH.

pral·i·dox·ime chloride (pral″i·dock′seem). 2-Formyl-1-methylpyridinium chloride oxime, $C_7H_9ClN_2O$, used as a cholinesterase reactivator in the treatment of poisoning by organophosphates, particularly the insecticide parathion.

pra·mox·ine (pra·mock′seen) *n.* 4-[3-(*p*-Butoxyphenoxy)propyl]morpholine, $C_{17}H_{27}NO_3$, a surface anesthetic agent used as the hydrochloride salt.

pran·di·al (pran′dee·ul) *adj.* [L. *prandium*, meal]. Of or pertaining to a meal, especially a dinner.

pran·di·al·i·ty (pran″dee·al′i·tee) *n.* Timing in respect to meals; the fact of being preprandial, prandial, or postprandial.

pra·no·li·um (pray·no′lee·um) *n.* [2-Hydroxy-3-(1-naphthyloxy)propyl]isoproplydimethyl-ammonium chloride, $C_{18}H_{26}ClNO_2$, an antiarrhythmic cardiac depressant.

Prantal Methylsulfate. Trademark for diphemanil methylsulfate, a parasympatholytic agent used to inhibit gastric secretion and motility, relieve pylorospasm, and reduce sweating.

pra·seo·dym·i·um (pray″zee·o·dim′ee·um, pras″ee·o·) *n.* [NL., from Gk. *prasios*, green]. Pr = 140.9077. A lanthanide.

pra·tique (pra·teek′) *n.* [F.]. The bill of health given to incoming vessels by a health officer of a port.

Praus·nitz-Küst·ner reaction (praowss′nits, kuᵉst′nur) [C. *Prausnitz* (Giles), German bacteriologist, b. 1876; and H. *Küstner*, German gynecologist, b. 1897]. A reaction of local hypersensitivity produced by intradermal injection of blood serum from a hypersensitive person followed by injection of the appropriate antigen; a method of passive transfer of hypersensitivity. The reaction forms the basis of the passive transfer test.

Prausnitz-Küstner test [C. W. *Prausnitz* and H. *Küstner*]. PASSIVE TRANSFER TEST.

Pra·vaz's syringe (praʰ·vah′) [C. G. *Pravaz*, French physician, 1791–1853]. A hypodermic syringe fitted with a long slender cannula and trocar.

-praxia [*praxis* + *-ia*]. A combining form designating *a condition involving the performance of movements*.

prax·ino·scope (prack·sin′uh·skope) *n.* [*praxis* + *-scope*]. A modified stroboscope adapted to laryngologic instruction.

prax·i·ol·o·gy (prack″see·ol′uh·jee) *n.* [Gk. *praxis*, action, + *-logy*]. 1. The psychology of acts and of deeds. 2. The science of conduct, as of behavior, in relation to values, such as social, moral, or esthetic ones.

-praxis [Gk.]. A combining form meaning (a) *act, activity;* (b) *practice, use.*

prax·is (prak′sis) *n.* [Gk., doing, action, from *prassein*, to do, act]. 1. The performance of a skilled purposeful movement or series of movements. 2. A skilled purposeful movement.

-praxy. See *-praxis*.

pra·ze·pam (pray′ze·pam) *n.* 7-Chloro-1-(cyclopropylmethyl)-1,3-dihydro-5-phenyl-2*H*-1,4-benzodiazepin-2-one, $C_{19}H_{17}ClN_2O$, a muscle relaxant.

pra·zo·sin (pray′zo·sin) *n.* 1-(4-Amino-6,7-dimethoxy-2-quinazolinyl)-4-(2-furoyl)piperazine, $C_{19}H_{21}N_5O_4$, an antihypertensive drug; used as the hydrochloride salt.

pre- [L. *prae*]. A prefix signifying *before*.

preach·er's hand. Exaggerated extension at the wrist with flexion of the metacarpophalangeal and interphalangeal joints, seen in lesions of the lower cervical cord.

preacher's node. SINGER'S NODE.

pre·ag·o·nal (pree·ag′uh·nul) *adj.* [*pre-* + *agonal*]. Immediately preceding the death agony.

pre·al·bu·min·uric (pree″al·bew′mi·new′rick) *adj.* [*pre-* + *albuminuric*]. Occurring before the appearance of proteinuria.

pre·am·pul·lary (pree·am′pul·err″ee) *adj.* [*pre-* + *ampullary*]. Before an ampulla, as the sphincter muscle of the ductus choledochus proximal to the hepatopancreatic ampulla.

pre·anal (pree·ay′nul) *adj.* [*pre-* + *anal*]. Situated in front of the anus.

pre·an·es·thet·ic, pre·an·aes·thet·ic (pree″an·es·thet′ick) *adj.* [*pre-* + *anesthetic*]. Before anesthesia.

preanesthetic medication. Administration of drugs, such as sedatives and anticholinergic agents, before the patient is anesthetized to facilitate induction of anesthesia.

pre·an·ti·sep·tic (pree″an·ti·sep′tick) *adj.* [*pre-* + *antiseptic*]. Pertaining to that period of time, historically, before antisepsis came into common use.

pre·aor·tic (pree″ay·or′tick) *adj.* [*pre-* + *aortic*]. Situated in front of the aorta.

pre·asep·tic (pree″a·sep′tick) *adj.* [*pre-* + *aseptic*]. Pertaining to the period before the adoption of principles of aseptic surgery.

pre·atax·ic (pree″a·tack′sick) *adj.* [*pre-* + *ataxic*]. Occurring before ataxia.

pre·au·ric·u·lar (pree″aw·rick′yoo·lur) *adj.* [*pre-* + *auricular*]. Situated in front of the auricle.

pre·ax·i·al (pree·ack′see·ul) *adj.* [*pre-* + *axial*]. Situated in front of the axis of the body or of a limb.

preaxial muscle. A muscle on the anterior aspect of an extremity.

pre·beta·lipo·pro·tein (pree″bay″tuh·lip″o·pro′tee·in, ·teen) *n.* [*pre-* + *beta-lipoprotein*]. A lipoprotein which on electrophoretic determination appears before the beta-lipoproteins but behind the alpha-lipoproteins.

pre·beta·lipo·pro·tein·emia (pree·bay″tuh·lip″o·pro″tee·in·ee′mee·uh) *n.* [*prebetalipoprotein* + *-emia*]. The presence of an excessive amount of prebetalipoproteins in the blood.

pre·can·cer·ous (pree·kan′sur·us) *adj.* [*pre-* + *cancerous*]. Pertaining to any pathological condition of a tissue which is likely to develop into cancer.

precancerous dermatosis. A skin disorder that sometimes develops into a malignant skin lesion.

pre·cap·il·lary (pree·kap′i·lerr″ee) *n.* [*pre-* + *capillary*]. A blood vessel intermediate in position and structural characteristics between an arteriole and a true capillary. Syn. *metarteriole, arteriolar capillary.*

precapillary arteriole. PRECAPILLARY.

pre·car·di·ac (pree·kahr′dee·ack) *adj.* [*pre-* + *cardiac*]. Anterior to the heart.

pre·car·di·nal (pree·kahr′di·nul) *adj.* [*pre-* + *cardinal*]. Pertaining to the pair of cardinal veins anterior to the common cardinal vein of the embryo, draining the head and neck.

pre·car·ti·lage (pree·kahr′ti·lij) *n.* [*pre-* + *cartilage*]. Compact, cellular embryonic connective tissue just before it differentiates into cartilage.

pre·ca·va (pree·kay′vuh) *n.* [*pre-* + *cava*]. SUPERIOR VENA CAVA.

pre·cen·tral (pree·sen′trul) *adj.* [*pre-* + *central*]. Situated in front of the central sulcus of the brain.

precentral gyrus. The cerebral convolution that lies between the precentral sulcus and the central sulcus and extends from the superomedial border of the hemisphere to the posterior ramus of the lateral sulcus. NA *gyrus precentralis.*

precentral sulcus. A groove separating the other frontal gyri from the precentral gyrus. NA *sulcus precentralis.* See also Plate 18.

pre·cer·vi·cal (pree·sur′vi·kul) *adj.* [*pre-* + *cervical*]. Pertaining to the anterior or ventral region of the neck.

precervical sinus. CERVICAL SINUS.

pre·chor·dal (pree·kor′dul) *adj.* [*pre-* + *chordal*]. Situated in front of the notochord.

pre·cip·i·tant (pre·sip′i·tunt) *n.* 1. Any reagent causing precipitation. 2. Any action or event which triggers an otherwise latent or dormant event, as a loud sudden noise may act as a precipitant for a startle response or for startle epilepsy.

¹pre·cip·i·tate (pre·sip′i·tate) *v.* & *n.* [L. *praecipitare,* to cast down, from *praeceps,* headlong, precipitous]. 1. To cause a substance to separate in an insoluble form. 2. An insoluble compound deposited in a solution of a substance on the addition of a reagent which produces a chemical reaction or otherwise decreases solubility. Abbreviated, ppt. 3. The product of the reaction between precipitinogen and precipitin.

²pre·cip·i·tate (pre·sip′i·tut, ·tate) *adj.* Headlong; hasty.

precipitated calcium phosphate. TRIBASIC CALCIUM PHOSPHATE.

precipitated sulfur. A form of sulfur that has been refined by a precipitation process.

precipitate labor. An abnormally rapid labor with the rate of cervical dilatation greater than 5 cm per hour in nulliparas or 10 cm per hour in multiparas.

pre·cip·i·ta·tion (pre·sip′i·tay·shun) *n.* The process of making substances insoluble by the addition of a reagent, evaporation, freezing, or electrolysis.

precipitation reaction. *In serology,* the reaction of soluble antigens with antibody resulting in precipitation or flocculation of the complexes under appropriate conditions.

precipitation test. PRECIPITIN TEST.

pre·cip·i·ta·tor (pre·sip′i·tay″tur) *n.* An apparatus that causes precipitation of particles, especially dust particles in the air, which may be counted. Precipitation may be effected by a difference in electrical potential or by a thermal procedure, using a heated wire.

pre·cip·i·tin (pre·sip′i·tin) *n.* An antibody that causes precipitation when combined with a specific soluble antigen.

pre·cip·i·tin·o·gen (pre·sip″i·tin′uh·jen) *n.* [*precipitin* + *-gen*]. *In immunology,* an antigen capable of giving rise to precipitating antibodies when it is injected into an animal.

pre·cip·i·tin·oid (pre·sip′i·ti·noid) *n.* [*precipitin* + *-oid*]. A partial antibody that still combines with its specific antigen, but does not cause precipitation, such as a precipitin modified by heating to 60° C.

precipitin test or **reaction.** An immunologic test in which the reaction between antigen and antibody results in the formation of a visible complex appearing as a precipitate.

pre·clin·i·cal (pree″klin′i·kul) *adj.* [*pre-* + *clinical*]. 1. Occurring prior to the period in a disease in which recognized symptoms or signs make diagnosis possible. 2. Pertaining to medical studies undertaken before the study of patients.

preclinical student nurse. A person who has recently entered nurses' training and has not commenced to give patient care.

pre·coc·cyg·e·al (pree″kock·sij′ee·ul) *adj.* [*pre-* + *coccygeal*]. In front of the coccyx.

pre·co·cious (pre·ko′shus) *adj.* [L. *praecox, praecocis,* from *prae-* + *coquere,* to ripen, cook]. Developing at an age earlier than usual.

precocious puberty. The premature development of somatic changes associated with puberty; arbitrarily, before the age of 8 years in girls and 10 years in boys.

pre·coc·i·ty (pre·kos′i·tee) *n.* 1. Early development or maturity; especially great development of the mental faculties at an early age. 2. PRECOCIOUS PUBERTY.

pre·cog·ni·tion (pree″kog·nish′un) *n.* [*pre-* + *cognition*]. The foreknowledge, apart from rational forecasting or logical inference, of future events. See also *extrasensory perception, psi phenomena.*

pre·co·i·tal (pree″ko′i·tul) *adj.* [*pre-* + *coital*]. Occurring before coitus.

pre·col·lag·e·nous (pree″kol·aj′e·nus) *adj.* [*pre-* + *collagenous*]. Characterizing an incomplete stage in the formation of collagen.

precollagenous fibers. RETICULAR FIBERS.

pre·com·a·tose (pree″kom′uh·toce) *adj.* Characterized by or pertaining to an altered state of consciousness preceding coma.

pre·com·mis·sur·al (pree″kom·ish′ur·ul) *adj.* Situated anterior to a commissure, specifically the anterior commissure of the cerebrum.

precommissural area. PARATERMINAL BODY.

pre·con·scious (pree·kon′shus) *adj.* [*pre-* + *conscious*]. FORECONSCIOUS.

pre·con·vul·sant (pree″kun·vul′sunt) *adj.* [*pre-* + *convulsant*]. PRECONVULSIVE.

pre·con·vul·sive (pree″kun·vul′siv) *adj.* [*pre-* + *convulsive*].

Pertaining to the period just prior to the occurrence of an epileptic seizure.

precordia. Plural of *precordium*.

pre·cor·di·al (pree·kor'dee·ul) *adj.* Of or pertaining to the precordium.

precordial axis. *In electrocardiography,* an electrical axis determined from precordial or chest leads, projected to an approximately horizontal plane through the dipole center.

precordial fright. The precordial sensations of impending physical collapse experienced in the acute panic of an anxiety neurosis.

precordial lead. An exploring unipolar electrocardiographic electrode placed at standard positions across the precordium, usually designated V_1 to V_6; earlier precordial leads were bipolar and were designated CR, CL, CF.

precordial region. The surface of the chest covering the heart.

pre·cor·di·um (pree·kor'dee·um) *n.,* pl. **precor·dia** (·dee·uh) [NL., from *pre-* + L. *cor, cordis,* heart]. The area of the chest overlying the heart.

pre·cos·tal (pree·kos'tul) *adj.* [*pre-* + *costal*]. Situated in front of the ribs.

precostal anastomosis. In the embryo, a longitudinal anastomosis between cervical and thoracic intersegmental arteries, which forms the thyrocervical trunk and the superior intercostal artery.

pre·cox, prae·cox (pree'kocks) *L. adj.* Precocious, developing early.

pre·cri·coid cartilage (pree·krye'koid). INTERARYTENOID CARTILAGE.

pre·cu·ne·us (pree·kew'nee·us) *n.* [*pre-* + *cuneus*] [NA]. A lobule of the parietal lobe, situated in front of the cuneus of the occipital lobe. —**precune·al** (·ul) *adj.*

pre·cur·sor (pree·kur'sur) *n.* [L. *praecursor*]. Something in a stage of a process or development that precedes a later or definitive stage.

pre·den·tin (pree·den'tin) *n.* [*pre-* + *dentin*]. Uncalcified dentinal matrix.

pred·i·cate thinking (pred'i·kut). Thinking organized around adjectives, adverbs, and verbs, rather than around nouns; seen in patients suffering from schizophrenia.

pre·di·crot·ic (pree''dye·krot'ick) *adj.* [*pre-* + *dicrotic*]. Preceding the dicrotic notch of the arterial pulse tracing.

pre·di·gest·ed (pree''di·jes'tid) *adj.* Partly digested before being taken into the stomach.

pre·di·ges·tion (pree''di·jes'chun, ·dye·jes'chun) *n.* The partial digestion of food before it is eaten.

pre·dis·pose (pree''di·spoze') *v.* [*pre-* + L. *disponere,* to arrange]. To incline; to bring about bodily susceptibility to a disease or to render vulnerable to a disorder.

pre·dis·pos·ing (pree''di·spo'zing) *adj.* Rendering susceptible, often referring to vulnerability to disease.

pre·dis·po·si·tion (pree''dis·puh·zish'un) *n.* [*pre-* + *disposition*]. The state of having special susceptibility, as to a disease or condition.

pred·nis·o·lone (pred·nis'uh·lohn) *n.* 11β,17,21-Trihydroxypregna-1,4-diene-3,20-dione, $C_{21}H_{28}O_5$, a glucocorticoid with clinically useful anti-inflammatory action; also used as acetate, butylacetate, sodium phosphate, and succinate esters.

pred·ni·sone (pred'ni·sohn) *n.* 17,21-Dihydroxypregna-1,4-diene-3,11,20-trione, $C_{21}H_{26}O_5$, a glucocorticoid with clinically useful anti-inflammatory action.

pred·ni·val (pred'ni·val) *n.* 11β,17,21-Trihydroxypregna-1,4-diene-3,20-dione 17-valerate, $C_{26}H_{36}O_6$, a topical anti-inflammatory steroid.

pre·dor·mi·tal (pree·dor'mi·tul) *adj.* [*pre-* + L. *dormire, dormitus,* to sleep, + *-al*]. Pertaining to the period immediately preceding sleep or the period of falling asleep.

predormital paralysis. HYPNAGOGIC PARALYSIS.

pre·dor·mi·tion (pree''dor·mish'un) *n.* [*pre-* + L. *dormitio,* sleep, sleeping]. The stage of marked drowsiness and cloudy consciousness immediately preceding deep sleep.

pre·ec·lamp·sia (pree''e·klamp'see·uh) *n.* [*pre-* + *eclampsia*]. A toxemia occurring in the latter half of pregnancy, characterized by an acute elevation of blood pressure and usually by edema and proteinuria, but without the convulsions or coma seen in eclampsia. See also *toxemia of pregnancy.* —**preeclamp·tic** (·tick) *adj.*

preen gland. UROPYGIAL GLAND.

pre·epi·glot·tic (pree·ep''i·glot'ick) *adj.* [*pre-* + *epiglottic*]. Anterior to the epiglottis.

pre·erup·tive (pree''e·rup'tiv) *adj.* [*pre-* + *eruptive*]. Preceding eruption.

preeruptive stage. The period of an exanthematic disease following infection and prior to the appearance of the eruption.

pre-ex·ci·ta·tion syndrome (pree''eck''sigh·tay'shun). WOLFF-PARKINSON-WHITE SYNDROME.

pre·fi·brot·ic (pree''fye·brot'ick) *adj.* Characterizing that stage of an inflammatory process in which the cellular part of the exudate persists while healing is taking place, with associated increase in fibrous tissue.

pre·for·ma·tion (pree''for·may'shun) *n.* [*pre-* + *formation*]. The theory which regards development as merely the unfolding or growth of the organism already fully formed in miniature, and contained in the germ cell (egg or sperm). Contr. *epigenesis.*

pre·fron·tal (pree·frun'tul) *adj.* [*pre-* + *frontal*]. Situated in the anterior part of the frontal lobe of the brain.

prefrontal lobotomy or **leukotomy.** A form of psychosurgery in which the white fibers connecting the prefrontal and frontal lobes with the thalamus are severed.

pre·gan·gli·on·ic (pree''gang·glee·on'ick) *adj.* [*pre-* + *ganglionic*]. Situated in front of or preceding a ganglion.

preganglionic neuron. A neuron of the autonomic nervous system which has its cell body in the brain or spinal cord, its axon terminating in an autonomic ganglion.

preganglionic ramus. WHITE RAMUS COMMUNICANS.

pre·gen·i·tal (pree·jen'i·tul) *adj. In psychoanalysis,* pertaining to the period of psychosexual development, occurring during early childhood, before the genitalia begin to exert their predominant influence in the patterning of sexual behavior and when oral and anal influences are strongest.

pre·gle·noid tubercle (pree·glee'noid, ·glen'oid). A small elevation at the base of the anterior root of the zygomatic process of the temporal bone.

preg·nan·cy (preg'nun·see) *n.* The condition of being pregnant; the state of a woman or any female mammal from conception to parturition. The duration of pregnancy in humans is approximately 280 days from the first day of the last menses or approximately 267 days from conception. To estimate the date of confinement, take the first day of the last menstrual period, count back 3 months, and add 1 year and 7 days. See also Ely's Table of the Duration of Pregnancy in the Appendix and Plate 23.

pregnancy cells. Alpha cells of the adenohypophysis distinguished by their smaller size and finer granules; seen during pregnancy.

pregnancy gingivitis. Changes in the gums seen most frequently during pregnancy; marked by bleeding, hypertrophy of the interdental papillae, inflammation, and, occasionally, a tumorous formation.

pregnancy test. Any procedure, usually biologic or chemical, used to diagnose pregnancy. Biologic tests usually depend upon a significant level of chorionic gonadotropin in the serum or urine.

5-α-preg·nane (preg'nane). ALLOPREGNANE.

preg·nane·di·ol (preg''nain·dye'ol) *n.* A metabolite, $C_{21}H_{36}O_2$, of progesterone, present in urine during the progestational phase of the menstrual cycle and also during pregnancy.

preg·nant (preg'nunt) *adj.* [L. *praegnans,* earlier *praegnas,* from *prae,* before, + *-gnas* as in *(g)nasci,* to be born]. Having potential offspring (fertilized ovum, viable embryo or fetus) within the uterus or analogous organ; said mainly of mammals or other viviparous animals.

pregnant-ewe paralysis. A syndrome affecting pregnant ewes characterized by ketosis and fatty metamorphosis of the liver.

pregnant mare's serum. A source for the manufacture of various sex hormones.

pregnant mare's serum hormone. A placental hormone that has action similar to those of a combination of follicle-stimulating and luteinizing hormones of the adenohypophysis. Abbreviated, PMS.

preg·nen·in·o·lone (preg″nen·in′o·lone, preg″neen·) *n.* ETHISTERONE.

preg·nen·o·lone (preg·nen′uh·lone, preg·neen′) *n.* 3β-Hydroxypregn-5-en-20-one, $C_{21}H_{32}O_2$, a steroid oxidation product of cholesterol and stigmasterol, apparently effective in reducing fatigue and formerly believed of value as an antiarthritic agent.

preg·no·pho·bia (preg″no·fo′bee·uh) *n.* [*pregnant* + *-phobia*]. Morbid fear of becoming pregnant.

Pregnyl. Trademark for a preparation of chorionic gonadotropin.

pre·hal·lux (pree·hal′ucks) *n.* [*pre-* + *hallux*]. A supernumerary digit attached to the great toe on its medial aspect.

pre·hemi·ple·gic (pree″hem·i·plee′jick) *adj.* [*pre-* + *hemiplegic*]. Occurring before hemiplegia.

pre·hen·sile (pre·hen′sil, ·sile) *adj.* [L. *prehendere,* to seize]. Adapted for grasping, as the tail of certain species of monkeys.

pre·hen·sion (pree·hen′shun) *n.* [L. *prehensio*]. The act of grasping or seizing.

pre·he·pat·ic (pree″he·pat′ick) *adj.* [*pre-* + *hepatic*]. 1. In front of the liver. 2. Taking place before the liver is involved, as in certain metabolic activities.

prehepatic jaundice. Jaundice in which there is no apparent liver lesion, as hemolytic jaundice and physiologic hyperbilirubinemia.

pre·ic·ter·ic (pree″ick·terr′ick) *adj.* [*pre-* + *icteric*]. Before the appearance of jaundice.

pre·in·farc·tion (pree″in·fahrk′shun) *adj.* Occurring as an antecedent of infarction.

preinfarction angina. Unstable angina pectoris, occurring more frequently than usual, lasting longer than usual, more severe than usual, or provoked by smaller stimuli than usual. Often an antecedent of myocardial infarction.

pre·in·va·sive (pree″in·vay′siv) *adj.* [*pre-* + *invasive*]. Before invasion of adjacent tissues; said of malignant changes in cells which are confined to their normal location.

Prei·ser's disease (prye′zur) [G. K. F. *Preiser,* German orthopedic surgeon, 1879–1913]. Traumatic osteoporosis of the scaphoid bone of the wrist.

pre·lac·ri·mal (pree·lack′ri·mul) *adj.* Situated in front of the lacrimal sac.

prelacrimal abscess. An abscess caused by caries of a lacrimal or ethmoid bone, producing a swelling at the inner canthus just below the upper margin of the orbit.

pre·lar·val (pree·lahr′vul) *adj.* At or pertaining to a stage prior to the larval one.

pre·leu·ke·mia, pre·leu·kae·mia (pree″lew·kee′mee·uh) *n.* [*pre-* + *leukemia*]. A variety of abnormal maturation patterns of blood cells which sometimes precede a recognizable leukemia.

preliminary film. A plain film preceding a contrast examination.

pre·lo·co·mo·tion (pree″lo·kuh·mo′shun) *n.* [*pre-* + *locomotion*]. The movements of a child who has not yet learned to walk, which indicate the intention of moving from one place to another but show lack of coordination.

Preludin. Trademark for phenmetrazine, an anorexiant drug used as the hydrochloride salt.

pre·lum (pree′lum) *n.* [L., a press]. A squeezing or pressing.

prelum ab·dom·i·na·le (ab·dom″i·nay′lee). The squeezing of the abdominal viscera between the diaphragm and the rigid abdominal wall, as in the processes of defecation, micturition, and parturition.

pre·ma·lig·nant (pree″muh·lig′nunt) *adj.* [*pre-* + *malignant*]. PRECANCEROUS.

pre·mam·il·lary nucleus (pree·mam′i·lerr·ee). A small group of cells on the anterosuperior aspect of the medial mamillary nucleus.

pre·ma·ni·a·cal (pree″ma·nigh′uh·kul) *adj.* [*pre-* + *maniac* + *-al*]. Previous to, or preceding, a psychotic disorder.

Premar. A trademark for ritodrine, a smooth muscle relaxant.

Premarin. Trademark for preparations of conjugated estrogens, chiefly in the form of sodium estrone sulfate.

pre·mar·i·tal (pree″măr′i·tul) *adj.* Occurring before marriage; as of a blood test or sexual relations.

pre·ma·ture (pree″muh·choor′, ·tewr′, prem′uh·tewr) *adj.* [L. *praematurus*]. 1. Occurring before the proper time. 2. Born prematurely. See also *premature infant.*

premature beat or **contraction.** A cardiac contraction arising prematurely from a site other than the normal pacemaker in the atrium, ventricle, or atrioventricular node.

premature delivery. Expulsion of the fetus after the twenty-eighth week and before term.

premature ejaculation. Male orgasm prior to or just upon the penetration by the penis of the vagina; common in males who, because of their immature psychosexual development, unconsciously look on coitus as another form of masturbation and self-gratification, as well as in those who, because of unconscious feelings of guilt or inferiority accompanied by the need for self-punishment, lack the confidence to function well sexually.

premature infant. 1. An infant born before the 37th to 38th week of gestation. 2. Formerly, a neonate weighing less than 2500 g at birth.

premature labor. Labor taking place before the normal period of gestation, but when the fetus is viable.

premature nursery. A nursery for premature infants and other neonates requiring special care or observation.

premature puberty. PRECOCIOUS PUBERTY.

premature senility syndrome. 1. In a child, HUTCHINSON-GILFORD SYNDROME. 2. In an adult, WERNER'S SYNDROME.

premature systole. PREMATURE BEAT.

premature ventricular contraction. An ectopic beat of ventricular origin, dependent on and coupled to the preceding beat, and occurring before the next dominant beat.

pre·ma·tur·i·ty (pree″muh·tewr′i·tee) *n.* [*pre-* + *maturity*]. 1. The state or fact of being premature. 2. An initial point or area of contact of a tooth with an opposing tooth when it limits the opportunity of maximum intercuspation of the teeth in the jaws in any position.

pre·max·il·la (pree″mack·sil′uh) *n.* [*pre-* + *maxilla*]. INCISIVE BONE. —**pre·max·il·lary** (pree·mack′si·lerr·ee) *adj.*

premaxillary palate. PRIMARY PALATE.

pre·med·i·cant (pree″med′i·kunt) *n.* [*pre-* + *medicant*]. PREMEDICATION (2).

pre·med·i·cat·ed (pree″med′i·kay·tid) *adj.* Of a patient or an animal, having received a premedication.

pre·med·i·ca·tion (pree″med·i·kay′shun) *n.* [*pre-* + *medication*]. 1. The administration of drugs before induction of anesthesia, primarily to quiet the patient and to facilitate the administration of the anesthetic. 2. Any drug administered for this purpose. —**pre·med·i·cate** (pree·med′i·kate) *v.*

pre·mel·a·no·some (pree·mel′uh·no·sohm) *n.* [*pre-* + *melanosome*]. Any one of the distinctive particulate stages in the maturation of a melanosome.

pre·men·o·paus·al (pree″men′o·pawz′ul) *adj.* Before the menopause.

premenopausal amenorrhea. A prolongation of the intermenstrual intervals for weeks or months which may occur for a considerable time prior to the menopausal cessation of menstrual flow.

pre·men·stru·al (pree·men'stroo·ul) *adj.* [*pre-* + *menstrual*]. Preceding menstruation.

premenstrual tension. The increased emotional tension and nervous or circulatory symptoms associated with the period in the human menstrual cycle which precedes menstruation.

pre·mo·lar (pree·mo'lur) *adj.* & *n.* [*pre-* + *molar*]. 1. In front of (mesial to) the molars. 2. In each quadrant of the permanent human dentition, one of the two teeth between the canine and the first molar; a bicuspid. NA *dens premolaris* (pl. *dentes premolares*).

pre·mo·ni·tion (prem"uh·nish'un, pree"muh·) *n.* [L. *praemonitio*, forewarning, from *prae-* + *monere*, to warn]. An experience of being intuitively aware of the coming occurrence of some event, usually unpleasant; a foreboding. See also *aura*.

pre·mon·i·to·ry (pre·mon'i·to"ree) *adj.* [L. *praemonere*, to forewarn]. Giving previous warning or notice, as in premonitory symptoms. Syn. *prodromal*.

pre·mon·o·cyte (pree·mon'o·site) *n.* [*pre-* + *monocyte*]. PROMONOCYTE (1).

pre·mor·bid (pree·mor'bid) *adj.* [*pre-* + *morbid*]. Before the appearance of the signs or symptoms of a disease or disorder.

premorbid personality. The behavioral characteristics of a person before the onset of a major mental or physical illness. See also *prepsychotic*.

pre·mor·tal (pree·mor'tul) *adj.* [*pre-* + *mortal*]. ANTEMORTEM.

pre·mo·tor area (pree"mo'tur). The main cortical motor area lying immediately in front of the motor area (Brodmann's area 4) from which it differs histologically by the absence of Betz cells; BRODMANN'S AREA 6.

premotor cortex. PREMOTOR AREA.

premotor syndrome. A syndrome attributed to a lesion of the more anterior part of the motor cortex (Brodmann's area 6) and consisting of spasticity with minimal paresis and a release of grasping reflexes.

pre·mu·ni·tion (pree"mew·nish'un) *n.* [L. *praemunitio*, a fortifying beforehand]. An immunity that depends upon a persistent latent infection, such as an immunity in malaria due to long-continued quiescent infection.

pre·mus·cle mass (pree·mus'ul). *In embryology*, a collection of mesodermal cells, which is the precursor of a muscle or group of muscles.

pre·my·e·lo·blast (pree·migh'e·lo·blast) *n.* A young form of myeloblast.

pre·my·e·lo·cyte (pree·migh'e·lo·site) *n.* PROMYELOCYTE.

pre·nar·co·sis (pree"nahr·ko'sis) *n.* Preliminary, light narcosis produced prior to general anesthesia; PREMEDICATION.

pre·na·tal (pree·nay'tul) *adj.* [*pre-* + *natal*]. 1. Existing or occurring before birth. 2. Loosely: ANTEPARTUM.

prenatal development. The portion of development occurring before birth.

prenatal respiration. FETAL RESPIRATION.

prenatal syphilis. CONGENITAL SYPHILIS.

pre·neo·plas·tic (pree"nee·o·plas'tick) *adj.* [*pre-* + *neoplastic*]. Before the development of a definite tumor. Compare *precancerous*.

pre·nid·a·to·ry (pree·nid'uh·tor·ee, ·nigh'duh·tor·ee) *adj.* Before nidation.

pre·nod·u·lar sulcus (pree·nod'yoo·lur). A groove on the posterolateral surface of the embryonic cerebellum separating the vermis from the flocculus.

pre·nyl·a·mine (pre·nil'uh·meen) *n.* *N*-(3,3-Diphenylpropyl)-α-methylphenethylamine, $C_{24}H_{27}N$, a coronary vasodilator.

pre·oc·cip·i·tal (pree"ock·sip'i·tul) *adj.* [*pre-* + *occipital*]. Situated anterior to the occipital region, as the preoccipital notch, a notch indicating the division between the occipital and temporal lobes of the brain.

pre·ol·i·vary nuclei (pree·ol'i·verr"ee). Two nuclei, the medial (internal) and lateral (external) preolivary nuclei, ventral to the superior olive and intercalated in the secondary auditory pathways.

pre·op·tic area or **region** (pree·op'tick). The most anterior portion of the hypothalamus lying on either side of the third ventricle and above the optic chiasma. See also *hypothalamus*.

preoptic recess. OPTIC RECESS.

pre·op·tic somite (pree·op'tick). Condensation of mesenchyme that forms the eye muscles; believed to represent head somites.

pre·op·ti·cus (pree·op'ti·kus) *n. Obsol.* SUPERIOR COLLICULUS.

pre·par·a·lyt·ic (pree"păr"uh·lit'ick) *adj.* [*pre-* + *paralytic*]. Pertaining to a disease state preceding paralysis.

prep·a·ra·tion (prep"uh·ray'shun) *n.* [L. *praeparare*, to make ready beforehand]. 1. The act of making ready. 2. Anything made ready; especially, in anatomy, any part of the body prepared or preserved for illustrative or other uses. 3. *In pharmacy*, any compound or mixture made according to a formula.

prepared calamine. CALAMINE (2).

prepared chalk. A native form of calcium carbonate freed from most of its impurities by elutriation; a white to grayish-white powder, often prepared in cones; insoluble in water. Used as an antacid and in the treatment of diarrhea.

pre·pa·ret·ic (pree"puh·ret'ick) *adj.* [*pre-* + *paretic*]. Pertaining to a disease state, as of neurosyphilis, preceding the onset of motor weakness or paresis.

preparetic neurosyphilis. ASYMPTOMATIC NEUROSYPHILIS.

pre·par·tal (pree·pahr'tul) *adj.* ANTEPARTUM.

pre·par·tum (pree·pahr'tum) *adj.* ANTEPARTUM.

pre·pa·tel·lar (pree"puh·tel'ur) *adj.* [*pre-* + *patellar*]. Situated in front of the patella.

prepatellar bursa. Any one of three variable bursas situated anterior to the patella. See also *subcutaneous prepatellar bursa, subfascial prepatellar bursa, subtendinous prepatellar bursa*.

pre·pa·tent (pree"pay'tunt) *adj.* [*pre-* + *patent*]. Before becoming observable or demonstrable.

prepatent period. The period in parasitic or other microorganismal disease between the introduction of the organism and its demonstration, as in the blood in malaria.

pre·pel·vic (pree·pel'vick) *adj.* [*pre-* + *pelvic*]. In front of the pelvis.

pre·peri·to·ne·al abscess (pree"perr·i·tuh·nee'ul). SUBPERITONEAL ABSCESS.

pre·pol·lex (pree·pol'ecks) *n.* [*pre-* + *pollex*]. A supernumerary digit attached to the thumb on its radial aspect.

pre·pon·der·ance (pre·pon'dur·unce) *n.* [L. *praeponderare*, to be of greater weight]. 1. The state of being greater in amount or force. 2. *In electrocardiography*, of a cardiac ventricle, superiority over the other in electric force generated; in the normal adult the left ventricular forces are greater than those of the right.

pre·po·tent (pree·po'tunt) *adj.* [*pre-* + *potent*]. 1. Predominant; prior, as of a reflex or response. 2. *In genetics*, having an ability (now explained by reference to Mendelian dominance) as a parent to transmit individual characteristics to offspring to a marked degree. —**prepo·ten·cy** (·tun·see) *n.*

prepotent reflex. The reflex elicited first when two antagonistic stimuli impinge simultaneously upon an organism.

pre·psy·chot·ic (pree"sigh·kot'ick) *adj.* Of or pertaining to the mental state that precedes or is potentially capable of precipitating a psychotic disorder.

pre·pu·ber·al (pree·pew'bur·ul) *adj.* [*pre-* + *puberal*]. Before puberty.

pre·pu·ber·tal (pree"pew'bur·tul) *adj.* PREPUBERAL.

prepubertal panhypopituitarism. PANHYPOPITUITARY DWARFISM.

pre·pu·bes·cent (pree"pew·bes'unt) *adj.* [*pre-* + *pubescent*]. Preceding the onset of puberty.

pre·puce (pree'pewce) *n.* [OF., from L. *praeputium*]. 1. The foreskin of the penis, a fold of skin covering the glans penis. NA *preputium penis.* 2. A similar fold over the glans clitoridis. NA *preputium clitoridis.* —**pre·pu·tial** (pree·pew'shul) *adj.*

pre·pu·cot·o·my (pree"pew·kot'uh·mee) *n.* [*prepuce* + *-tomy*]. An incision into the prepuce; an incomplete circumcision.

preputial glands. Sebaceous glands in the prepuce of the penis. NA *glandulae preputiales.*

preputial space. A potential space between the prepuce and the glans penis represented by two shallow fossae on either side of the frenulum.

pre·pu·ti·um (pree·pew'shee·um) *n.*, pl. **prepu·tia** (·shee·uh) [L. *praeputium*] [NA]. PREPUCE.

preputium cli·to·ri·dis (kli·tor'i·dis) [NA]. PREPUCE (2).

preputium pe·nis (pee'nis) [NA]. PREPUCE (1).

pre·py·lo·ric (pree"pye·lo'rick) *adj.* [*pre-* + *pyloric*]. Placed in front of, or preceding, the pylorus.

pre·py·ram·i·dal (pree"pi·ram'i·dul) *adj.* [*pre-* + *pyramidal*]. Situated anterior to the pyramid.

prepyramidal sulcus of the cerebellum. A groove lying between the middle lobe of the cerebellum and the pyramids.

pre·rec·tal (pree·reck'tul) *adj.* [*pre-* + *rectal*]. Situated in front of the rectum.

pre·re·nal (pree·ree'nul) *adj.* [*pre-* + *renal*]. 1. Situated in front of the kidney. 2. Taking place before the kidney is reached; used especially concerning nitrogen retention in the blood due to decreased blood flow to the kidney, or to increased amounts of nitrogenous metabolites entering the blood.

prerenal anuria. Anuria due to inadequate blood flow to the kidney, as seen in shock.

prerenal uremia. Failure of renal function due to disturbances outside the urinary tract, such as shock, dehydration, hemorrhage, or electrolyte abnormality. Syn. *extra renal uremia.*

pre·re·pro·duc·tive (pree"ree·pruh·duck'tiv) *adj.* [*pre-* + *reproductive*]. Pertaining to the period of life preceding puberty.

pre·ret·i·nal (pree·ret'i·nul) *adj.* [*pre-* + *retinal*]. Anterior to the internal limiting membrane of the retina.

pre·ru·bral (pree·roo'bral) *adj.* [*pre-* + *rubral*]. Located rostral to the red nucleus.

prerubral field. An area of cells, about 2.5 mm thick, which curves over the frontal pole and lateral surface of the red nucleus.

pre·sa·cral (pree·say'krul) *adj.* [*pre-* + *sacral*]. Lying in front of the sacrum.

presacral block. PARASACRAL ANESTHESIA.

presacral nerve. SUPERIOR HYPOGASTRIC PLEXUS.

Pre-Sate. Trademark for chlorphentermine, an anorexigenic drug used as the hydrochloride salt.

presby-, presbyo- [Gk. *presbys*, old man]. A combining form meaning *old age.*

pres·by·acou·sia (prez"bee·a·koo'zhuh) *n.* [*presby-* + *-acousia*]. PRESBYCUSIS.

pres·by·acu·sia (prez"bee·a·kew'zhuh) *n.* [*presby-* + *-acusia*]. PRESBYCUSIS.

pres·by·at·rics (prez"bee·at'ricks) *n.* [*presby-* + *-iatrics*]. GERIATRICS.

pres·by·car·dia (pres"bi·kahr'dee·uh) *n.* [*presby-* + *-cardia*]. Involutional aging changes of the myocardium, with associated pigmentation of the heart. It decreases cardiac reserve but rarely produces heart failure itself. Syn. *senile heart disease.*

pres·by·cou·sis (prez"bi·koo'sis) *n.* PRESBYCUSIS.

pres·by·cu·sis (prez"bi·kew'sis) *n.* [NL., from *presby-* + Gk. *akousis*, hearing]. The lessening of the acuteness of hearing that occurs with advancing age.

pres·by·der·ma (prez"bi·dur'muh) *n.* [*presby-* + *-derma*]. Cutaneous changes associated with the middle and later years of life.

pres·byo·phre·nia (prez"bee·o·free'nee·uh) *n.* [*presbyo-* + *-phrenia*]. Senile dementia, especially that variety in which apparent mental alertness is combined with failure of memory, disorientation, and confabulation. —**presbyo·phren·ic** (·fren'ick) *adj.*

pres·by·opia (prez"bee·o'pee·uh) *n.* [*presby-* + *-opia*]. The condition of vision commonly seen after the middle forties but beginning in late childhood (after age 8), due to diminished power of accommodation from impaired elasticity of the crystalline lens, whereby the near point of distinct vision is removed farther from the eye so that the individual has difficulties in focusing on near objects and in reading fine print. Abbreviated, Pr. —**presby·opic** (·op'ick, ·o'pick) *adj.*; **presby·ope** (prez'bee·ope) *n.*

pres·byo·sphac·e·lus (prez"bee·o·sfas'e·lus) *n.* [*presbyo-* + Gk. *sphakelos*, gangrene]. ARTERIOSCLEROTIC GANGRENE.

pres·by·tia (prez·bish'ee·uh, ·bit'ee·uh) *n.* [*presbytic* + *-ia*]. PRESBYOPIA.

pres·by·ti·at·rics (prez"bi·tee·at'ricks) *n.* [Gk. *presbytēs*, old man, old age, + *-iatrics*]. GERIATRICS.

pres·byt·ic (prez·bit'ick) *adj.* [Gk. *presbytikos*, characteristic of old age]. Suffering from presbyopia.

pres·by·tism (prez'bi·tiz·um) *n.* PRESBYOPIA.

pre·sca·lene (pree·skay'leen) *adj.* In front of the scalene muscles; used to refer to lymph nodes in the fat of this region.

pre·schizo·phren·ic (pree"skiz"o·fren'ick, ·skit"so·) *adj.* [*pre-* + *schizophrenic*]. Pertaining to symptoms and personality characteristics that usually precede schizophrenia.

pre·scle·ro·sis (pree"skle·ro'sis) *n.* [*pre-* + *sclerosis*]. The vascular condition that precedes arteriosclerosis. —**prescle·rot·ic** (·rot'ick) *adj.*

pre·scribe (pre·skribe') *v.* [L. *praescribere*, from *scribere*, to write]. To write an order for a medication and give instructions concerning its use.

pre·scrip·tion (pre·skrip'shun) *n.* [L. *praescriptio*]. Written instructions designating the preparation and use of substances to be administered. See also Table of Latin and Greek Terms Used in Prescription Writing in the Appendix.

pre·se·nile (pree·see'nile) *adj.* [*pre-* + *senile*]. 1. Characterized by or pertaining to a condition occurring in early or middle life that involves characteristics resembling those of old age. 2. Pertaining to presenility.

presenile alopecia. ALOPECIA PREMATURA.

presenile dementia. 1. Any dementia that has its onset in the presenium. 2. ALZHEIMER'S DISEASE.

presenile gangrene. BUERGER'S DISEASE.

presenile psychosis. PRESENILE DEMENTIA.

pre·se·nil·i·ty (pree"se·nil'i·tee) *n.* [*pre-* + *senility*]. 1. Premature old age or the infirmities associated with it. 2. The period of life immediately preceding old age or the senile state.

pre·se·ni·um (pree·see'nee·um, ·sen'ee·um) *n.* [*pre-* + L. *senium*, old age]. The period just before the onset of old age.

pre·sent (pre·zent') *v.* [L. *praesentare*, to place before]. 1. To appear first at the os uteri, applied to a part of the fetus. 2. To give evidence of. 3. To be or become manifest. —**pre·sent·ing** (·ing) *adj.*

pres·en·ta·tion (prez"un·tay'shun, pree"zen·) *n.* [L. *praesentatio*]. 1. *In obstetrics*, the part of the fetus that is palpated through the cervix uteri at the beginning of labor. The relation of the part of the fetus to the birth canal determines the type of presentation. 2. The rather formal oral report of a patient's history made before a group of physicians or a medical teacher by a medical student or a physician.

presentation of the cord. Descent of the umbilical cord between the presenting part and the membranes at the beginning of labor; FUNIC PRESENTATION.

presenting complaints. The symptoms of which the patient is aware and which he discloses to the physician.

pre·ser·va·tive (pre·zur'vuh·tiv) *n.* Any additive used to prevent or retard spoilage or decay, or other chemical or physical change, as in a medicine or food product.

pre·so·mite embryo (pree·so'mite). An embryo from the time of fertilization until the appearance of the first somite, about 21 days.

pre·spas·tic (pree''spas'tick) *adj.* [*pre-* + *spastic*]. Occurring or at a stage prior to the manifestation of spasticity.

pre·sphe·noid (pree·sfee'noid) *n.* [*pre-* + *sphenoid*]. The anterior portion of the body of the sphenoid, ossifying from a separate center. In many reptiles and mammals, it remains a separate bone in the adult.

pre·sphyg·mic (pree·sfig'mick) *adj.* [*pre-* + *sphygmic*]. Pertaining to the period preceding the arterial pulse wave; the isometric contraction phase of systole.

presphygmic interval. ISOVOLUMETRIC INTERVAL.

presphygmic period. The period of isometric contraction of the heart muscle at the beginning of ventricular systole, prior to the opening of the semilunar valves.

pres·sor (pres'ur) *adj.* [L., that which presses, from *premere*, to press]. Producing a rise in blood pressure.

pressor area. The region of the vasomotor center, stimulation of which causes a rise in blood pressure and increased heart rate.

pres·so·re·cep·tor (pres''o·re·sep'tur) *n.* [*pressure* + *receptor*]. BARORECEPTOR.

pressor headache. Any headache produced by a sudden rise in systemic blood pressure, as with pheochromocytoma.

pressor nerve. An afferent nerve, stimulation of which excites the vasomotor center.

pressor reflex. A reflex increase in arterial pressure.

pressor substance. A substance whose pharmacodynamic action results in an elevation of arterial pressure.

pres·so·sen·si·tive (pres''o·sen'si·tiv) *adj.* Stimulated by changes in blood pressure, as nerve endings in the carotid sinus.

pres·sure, *n.* [L. *pressura*, from *premere*, to press]. Physical or mental force, weight, or tension.

pressure anesthesia. Topical use of an anesthetic using pressure to force it into the tissue.

pressure atrophy. The atrophy following prolonged pressure on a part, chiefly the result of local inanition.

pressure bandage. A bandage used to stop hemorrhage, prevent swelling, or support varicose veins by the application of pressure.

pressure compress. A compress that is held in place with a bandage in order to produce pressure on a wound and prevent oozing.

pressure cone. Herniation of either the uncus or the cerebellar tonsils by pressure from above. See also *cerebellar pressure cone, tentorial pressure cone.*

pressure curve. A recording of pressure variations, particularly that of pressure variations in a given heart chamber or blood vessel during the cardiac cycle.

pressure diverticulum. PULSION DIVERTICULUM.

pressure palsy or **paralysis.** Flaccid paralysis due to pressure on a nerve.

pressure phosphene. A subjective sensation of light or of "seeing stars" caused by pressure on the eyeball.

pressure points. Regions of skin and underlying tissue which are maximally sensitive to pressure or weight. Formerly, it was believed that these regions or "points" were morphologically specific receptors that responded to stimulation with only a sensation of pressure.

pressure pulse. The wave form of the pressure wave in a cardiac chamber or blood vessel. Compare *pulse pressure.*

pressure pulse wave. Arterial expansion produced by ejection of blood from the left ventricle into the aorta; marked changes in contour, which may be palpated and recorded, occur as the pulse wave passes to the periphery.

pressure sense. The perception of the amount of weight or of pressure which is exerted upon a part of the body.

pressure sore. DECUBITUS ULCER.

pressure stasis. Localized hyperemia resulting from compression of the venous return from a part of the body.

pressure time per minute. TENSION-TIME INDEX.

pressure ulcer. DECUBITUS ULCER.

pres·tige suggestion (pres·teezh'). *In psychiatry,* the treatment of certain disorders or symptoms by the therapist by assuring the patient directly or indirectly that the problem is being relieved or resolved.

pre·su·bic·u·lum (pree·sue·bick'yoo·lum) *n.* [*pre-* + *subiculum*]. The area of transition between the hippocampus proper and the parahippocampal gyrus.

pre·sump·tive (pre·zum'tiv) *adj.* [L. *praesumptus*, from *praesumere*, to suppose]. 1. Justifying reasonable belief, though not conclusively; based on probable evidence or presumption. 2. Of or pertaining to an embryonic structure, cell, or tissue whose probable later identity in the developed organism is known.

presumptive entoderm. Tissue which is the primordium of the entoderm.

presumptive test. The first step in the bacteriological analysis of water for the coliforms; consists of determining the production of gas in lactose broth. Fermentation tubes containing lactose broth are inoculated with the water to be tested. If more than 10 percent of the fermentation tubes contain gas at the end of 24 hours, the test is positive.

pre·sup·pu·ra·tive (pree''sup'yoo·ruh·tiv) *adj.* [*pre-* + *suppurative*]. Pertaining to an early stage of inflammation, prior to suppuration.

pre·syl·vi·an (pree·sil'vee·un) *adj.* [*pre-* + *sylvian* fissure]. Pertaining to the lateral cerebral sulcus.

presylvian fissure or **sulcus.** The anterior or the ascending ramus of the lateral cerebral sulcus.

pre·symp·to·mat·ic (pree''simp·tuh·mat'ick) *adj.* [*pre-* + *symptomatic*]. Pertaining to a state of mental or physical health before a disorder becomes manifest, as a patient with a diabetic type of glucose-tolerance curve but without clinical signs and symptoms of diabetes mellitus.

pre·syn·ap·tic (pree''si·nap'tick) *adj.* [*pre-* + *synaptic*]. Situated near or occurring before a synapse.

presynaptic membrane. The electrically excitable membrane bounding the axon terminal adjacent to the dendrite.

pre·sys·to·le (pree·sis'tuh·lee) *n.* [*pre-* + *systole*]. The period of the cardiac cycle preceding systole.

pre·sys·tol·ic (pree''sis·tol'ick) *adj.* [*pre-* + *systolic*]. Preceding a cardiac systole, often used in reference to the time immediately preceding the first heart sound.

presystolic extra sound. The heart sound following atrial contraction, immediately preceding the first heart sound, to which it may sometimes contribute. Syn. *fourth heart sound.*

presystolic gallop. ATRIAL GALLOP.

presystolic thrill. A thrill that can sometimes be felt before the systole when the hand is placed over the apex beat (mitral stenosis).

pre·tec·tal (pree·teck'tul) *adj.* [*pre-* + *tectal*]. Situated anterior to the tectum mesencephali.

pretectal area. The area, rostral to the superior colliculus and lateral to the posterior commissure, which receives fibers from the optic tract.

pretectal region. A zone of transition between the thalamus and tectum, rostral to the superior colliculi.

pre·tec·tum (pree·teck'tum) *n.* PRETECTAL AREA.

pre·ter·mi·nal (pree·tur'mi·nul) *adj.* [*pre-* + *terminal*]. Just before the end.

pre·ter·nat·u·ral (pree''tur·nach'ur·ul) *adj.* [L. *praeter*, beyond, + *natural*]. Abnormal.

preternatural anus. An abnormal aperture serving as an anus, whether congenital, made by operation, or due to disease or injury.

preternatural vaginal anus. The rare abnormality of the rectum opening through the vagina or vulva.

pre·thy·roid (pree·thigh'roid) *adj.* PRETHYROIDEAN.

pre·thy·roi·de·al (pree''thigh·roy'dee·ul) *adj.* PRETHYROIDEAN.

pre·thy·roi·de·an (pree''thigh·roy'dee·un) *adj.* In front of the thyroid cartilage or thyroid gland.

pre·tib·i·al (pree·tib'ee·ul) *adj.* [*pre-* + *tibial*]. In front of the tibia.

pretibial fever. An acute infectious disease due to *Leptospira autumnalis* with clinical manifestations of fever, headache, leukopenia, and a cutaneous erythematous eruption on the pretibial aspect of the legs. Syn. *Fort Bragg fever.*

pretibial myxedema. Circumscribed deposition of mucinous material in the pretibial skin, occurring during thyrotoxicosis or treatment for thyrotoxicosis. Syn. *circumscribed myxedema.*

pre·tra·gal (pree·tray'gul) *adj.* Anterior to the tragus.

pre·trans·fer·ence (pree''trans·fur'unce, ·trans'fur·unce) *n.* [*pre-* + *transference*]. *In psychoanalysis,* the arousal of feelings in a patient when he perceives the therapist as a primordial parent or as a part of himself.

pre·tre·mat·ic (pree''tre·mat'ick) *adj.* [*pre-* + *trema* + *-ic*]. Pertaining to nerves that pass on the front margin of a trema or gill slit, as the maxillary nerve does in a masked form in land vertebrates.

pre·ure·thri·tis (pree·yoo''re·thrigh'tis) *n.* [*pre-* + *urethr-* + *-itis*]. Inflammation of the vestibule of the vagina, around the urethral orifice.

prev·a·lence (prev'uh·lunce) *n.* [L. *praevalere,* to prevail]. 1. Frequency of occurrence. 2. PREVALENCE RATE.

prevalence rate. A measure of the prevalence of a disease in a population; usually expressed as the number of cases of a disease present at a given time per 1,000 or 100,000 population.

pre·ven·tive, *adj.* Done, used, or designed for the purpose of prevention rather than correction or cure, as of disease.

preventive dentistry. The branch of dental science dealing with prevention of dental diseases by prophylactic, restorative, and educational methods.

preventive medicine. Any medical activity that seeks to prevent disease, prolong life, and promote physical and mental health and efficiency; especially, the science of the etiology and epidemiology of disease processes, dealing with factors that increase vulnerability, factors that initiate or precipitate a disease, and factors that cause disease progression.

preventive orthodontics. The early management of normal occlusion wherein untoward environmental forces threaten future development; the use of a space maintainer is one example. Syn. *prophylactic orthodontics.*

pre·ven·to·ri·um (pree''ven·to'ree·um) *n.,* pl. **prevento·ria** (·ree·uh), **preventoriums.** 1. A sanatorium devoted to the care of children thought to be predisposed to tuberculosis. 2. Any institution where patients are admitted to prevent the spread of a disease process.

pre·ver·te·bral (pree·vur'te·brul) *adj.* [*pre-* + *vertebral*]. Situated in front of a vertebra or the vertebral column.

prevertebral fascia. The third layer of the deep cervical fascia; a band of connective tissue covering the front of the cervical vertebrae and the prevertebral muscles. It is attached to the esophagus and pharynx by loose connective tissue. NA *lamina prevertebralis fasciae cervicalis.*

prevertebral ganglion. COLLATERAL GANGLION.

prevertebral plexus. The collateral ganglions and nerve fibers of the sympathetic nervous system such as the cardiac, celiac, and hypogastric plexuses.

pre·ver·tig·i·nous (pree''vur·tij'i·nus) *adj.* [*pre-* + *vertiginous*]. Pertaining to a state of vertigo in which the patient has a tendency to fall prone, having the sensation of having been pushed forward.

pre·ves·i·cal (pree·ves'i·kul) *adj.* [*pre-* + *vesical*]. Situated in front of the urinary bladder.

prevesical space. RETROPUBIC SPACE.

pre·via, prae·via (pree'vee·uh) *adj.* [fem. of L. *praevius*]. Coming before, or in front of, as placenta previa.

pre·vil·lous (pree·vil'us) *adj.* [*pre-* + *villous*]. Before the formation of villi; applied to the chorionic vesicle.

previllous embryo. An embryo from the time of fertilization until the development of the chorionic villi.

pre·vi·ral unit (pree·vye'rul). A unit related to early stages of intracellular virus multiplications.

Prey·er's reflex (prye'ur) [W. T. *Preyer,* German physiologist, 1841–1897]. Involuntary movement of the ears in auditory stimulation.

Preyer's test [W. T. *Preyer*]. A spectroscopic test for the presence of carbon monoxide in the blood.

pre·zone (pree'zone) *n.* [*pre-* + *zone*]. PROZONE.

pre·zo·nu·lar (pree·zo'new·lur, ·zon'yoo·lur) *adj.* [*pre-* + *zonular*]. Pertaining to the posterior chamber of the eye.

prezonular space. POSTERIOR CHAMBER.

pre·zyg·apoph·y·sis (pree''zye''guh·pof'i·sis, pree''zig''uh·) *n.* [*pre-* + *zygapophysis*]. An anterior or superior zygapophysis; a superior articular process of a vertebra.

pri·a·pism (prye'uh·piz·um) *n.* [*Priapus,* Greco-Roman god of procreation]. Abnormal, persistent, painful erection of the corpora cavernosa of the penis unrelated to sexual desire, as seen in blood dyscrasia, sickle cell anemia, or lesions of the central nervous system; impotence may result.

Price-Jones curve [C. *Price-Jones,* English hematologist, 1863–1943]. The distribution of erythrocyte diameters as shown by their direct measurement in a stained blood film.

prick·le cell. A cell possessing conspicuous intercellular bridges; especially, a cell of the epidermis lying between the basal layer and the granular layer.

prickle cell carcinoma. Squamous cell carcinoma with parenchymal cells resembling those of the prickle cell layer of the skin.

prickle cell layer. The layer of cells between the granular cell layer and the basal cell layer of the epidermis, notable for intercellular bridges. NA *stratum spinosum epidermidis.*

prickly ash bark or **berries.** XANTHOXYLUM.

prickly heat. MILIARIA.

Priess·nitz bandage (price'nits) [V. *Priessnitz,* German farmer, 1799–1851]. A cold wet compress.

pril·o·caine (pril'o·kane) *n.* 2-(Propylamino)-*o*-propionotoluidide, $C_{13}H_{20}N_2O$, an amide local anesthetic used as the hydrochloride salt. Syn. *propitocaine.*

pri·mal (prye'mul) *adj.* [ML. *primalis,* from L. *primus,* first]. Primordial or fundamental; PRIMARY.

primal depression. *In psychiatry,* the early primordial depressive response in infancy to intense frustration and denial of needs, which establishes an antecedent pattern for depressive reactions in later life.

primal process. PRIMARY PROCESS.

primal repression. PRIMARY REPRESSION.

primal scene. *In psychoanalysis,* the recollection or imagined recollection from childhood of parental or other heterosexual intercourse; frequently the result of a child's fantasy based on fragments of observation plus misinterpretation.

pri·ma·quine (prye'muh·kwin, prim'uh·kween) *n.* 8-(4-Amino-1-methylbutylamino)-6-methoxyquinoline, $C_{15}H_{21}N_3O$, an antimalarial drug used as the diphosphate salt.

pri·ma·ry (prye'merr·ee) *adj.* [L. *primarius,* of the first rank]. 1. First in order of time, development, or derivation (initial, original, primordial, embryonic), in importance (main, principal), or in systematic order (basic, fundamental). 2. Not derivative or mediated; direct. 3. *In chemistry,* first or simplest of a series of related compounds, as that resulting from replacement of one of two or more atoms or groups in a molecule by a substituent, or an alcohol or an amine containing the $—CH_2OH$ or $—NH_2$ group, respectively. See also *alcohol* (1), *amine.* 4. *In pa-*

thology, original as opposed to metastatic (secondary), as a primary tumor or infection.

primary abscess. An abscess originating at the seat of a pyogenic infection.

primary alcohol. An alcohol having the general formula RCH_2OH, where R represents an organic radical.

primary aldosteronism. 1. Primary hyperaldosteronism. See *hyperaldosteronism.* 2. Specifically, hyperaldosteronism due to an adrenal tumor. Syn. *Conn's syndrome.*

primary alveolar hypoventilation syndrome. A disorder in individuals with normal lungs and chest walls, characterized by an elevated alveolar and arterial carbon dioxide tension, cyanosis, polycythemia, and cor pulmonale. It is a result of a functional abnormality of the medullary respiratory neurons, and is associated with subnormal increases in ventilation during exercise and following the inhalation of carbon dioxide-enriched gas mixtures.

primary amenorrhea. Lack of menarche in woman 18 years old or over.

primary ammonium phosphate. AMMONIUM PHOSPHATE, MONOBASIC.

primary amputation. An amputation performed immediately after injury, during the period of reaction from shock and before the onset of suppuration.

primary amyloidosis. A rare disorder of unknown origin characterized by the deposition in various tissues—heart, tongue, gastrointestinal tract, skeletal muscle—of amyloid, a fibrous protein containing sulfated mucopolysaccharides.

primary anal opening. The orifice of the endodermally lined hindgut into the proctodeum of the embryo after rupture of the anal membrane.

primary anemia. PERNICIOUS ANEMIA.

primary anesthesia. The transient anesthesia resulting from a small amount of anesthetic.

primary aneurysm. An aneurysm in which the disease of the arterial wall which predisposes to the dilatation is unknown. Syn. *spontaneous aneurysm.*

primary assimilation. Conversion of food into chyme.

primary atypical pneumonia. 1. An acute respiratory disease caused by infection with *Mycoplasma pneumoniae,* characterized by fever, constitutional symptoms, cough, pulmonary infiltrations, and often prolonged convalescence. 2. Any clinical syndrome simulating primary atypical pneumonia, caused by unknown or known agents, including viruses, bacteria, or rickettsiae.

primary autonomic insufficiency. PRIMARY ORTHOSTATIC HYPOTENSION.

primary bone. The first bone formed in a given location.

primary brain vesicle. One of the first subdivisions of the embryonic brain; the prosencephalon, mesencephalon, or rhombencephalon.

primary bronchus. Either of the two main airways which originate in the bifurcation of the trachea, enter their respective lungs at the hilus, and branch into lobar bronchi. NA *bronchus principalis.* Contr. *secondary bronchus.*

primary care. The care provided at a person's first contact, in any given episode of illness, with the health care system, leading to a decision as to what must be done and including responsibility for the continuum of care, as: appropriate referral, evaluation and management of symptoms, and subsequent maintenance of health.

primary cause. The essential, main, basic, or initial cause without which the effect, such as a specific illness, could not occur. Contr. *ultimate cause.*

primary cell. EMBRYONIC CELL.

primary choana. The embryonic opening between one of the olfactory sacs and the stomodeum. Syn. *primitive choana.*

primary coccidioidomycosis. An asymptomatic or benign self-limited respiratory infection, due to *Coccidioides immitis* with or without erythema nodosum or erythema multiforme and joint manifestations, accompanied by sensitivity to coccidioidin. See also *coccidioidomycosis, disseminated coccidioidomycosis.*

primary coil. The inner coil of an induction apparatus.

primary colors. 1. Any of a group of colors from which all other colors may be obtained, as red, yellow, and blue in painting. 2. *In psychology,* red, yellow-green, and blue.

primary complex. GHON COMPLEX.

primary constriction. The area of chromosomes where the arms (telomeres) of chromosomes meet. The primary constriction precedes the chromosome in its poleward migration during anaphase. Marked angular deviation occurs in this area.

primary cords. MEDULLARY CORDS.

primary degeneration of Nissl [F. *Nissl*]. AXONAL REACTION.

primary degeneration of the corpus callosum. MARCHIAFAVA-BIGNAMI DISEASE.

primary dementia. *Obsol.* SIMPLE TYPE OF SCHIZOPHRENIA.

primary dentition. 1. The first set of teeth, the DECIDUOUS TEETH, considered collectively and in place in the dental arch. 2. The eruption of the deciduous teeth. Syn. *deciduous dentition.* Contr. *permanent dentition.* See also *mixed dentition.*

primary digestion. The phase of digestion that takes place in the gastrointestinal tract, as distinguished from secondary digestion, the assimilation of nutrients by the cells of the body.

primary drive. A drive determined by the species-specific genetic makeup. Contr. *acquired drive.*

primary dysmenorrhea. Dysmenorrhea present from the menarche. Syn. *essential dysmenorrhea, congenital dysmenorrhea.*

primary ectoderm. PRIMITIVE ECTODERM.

primary entoderm. PRIMITIVE ENTODERM.

primary familial xanthomatosis. WOLMAN'S DISEASE.

primary filter. *In radiology,* a thin layer of any one of several materials used to absorb a greater percentage of low-energy rays than of the high-energy rays of a roentgen beam, thus producing a beam with greater average penetrating power. Aluminum filters are used for superficial and medium work, copper or Thoraeus filters for deep therapy, and lead or tin filters for supervoltage work.

primary fissure. A transverse fissure separating the anterior and posterior cerebellar lobes. NA *fissura prima.*

primary focus or **complex.** PRIMARY TUBERCULOSIS.

primary follicle. The immature ovarian follicle in which the ovum is surrounded by a single layer of follicular cells.

primary gain. *In psychiatry,* the unconscious gratification derived by the patient from symptoms or an illness developed largely unconsciously to deal with unresolved conflicts, as when a patient suffers less fear and guilt after compromising an instinctual wish with its social or moral prohibition. The need for such gain is responsible for many of the mental mechanisms and is often responsible for causing mental disorders.

primary genital ducts. The mesonephric and paramesonephric ducts.

primary gonocyte. A primordial germ cell derived from endoderm and found in the germinal epithelium of the gonads.

primary gout. GOUT (1).

primary gut. ARCHENTERON.

primary head veins. The chief veins developing in the head of an early embryo; they are continuous with the anterior cardinal veins and lie medial to the trigeminal, but ventrolateral to the more posterior cranial ganglions.

primary hemorrhage. Hemorrhage as a direct result of trauma.

primary hyperoxaluria. OXALOSIS.

primary hypertension. ESSENTIAL HYPERTENSION.

primary hypothyroidism. Hypothyroidism due to direct loss of functioning thyroid tissue, as by surgical removal, irradiation, inflammation, or atrophy.

primary infection. PRIMARY TUBERCULOSIS.

primary irritant conjunctivitis. Conjunctivitis caused by a topically applied irritant.

primary lateral sclerosis. Degeneration of the descending motor pathways of the spinal cord with spastic weakness of the extremities, hyperreflexia, and Babinski signs, but without muscular atrophy; a variant or early form of amyotrophic lateral sclerosis.

primary lesion. 1. In syphilis, tuberculosis, cowpox, a chancre. 2. *In dermatology,* the earliest clinically recognizable manifestation of a cutaneous disease, such as a macule, papule, vesicle, pustule, or wheal.

primary lymphopenic immunologic deficiency. A primary decrease in the number of circulating lymphocytes and often also of plasma cells, usually with some deficit in the amount of immunoglobulin present, with deficient cellular and humoral immunity, frequently associated clinically with fungus, *Pneumocystis carinii,* or virus infections, leading to early death; inherited both as an X-linked or autosomal recessive trait. Syn. *Gitlin's syndrome.*

primary malabsorption. NONTROPICAL SPRUE.

primary marrow. The fetal marrow, before it becomes hemopoietic.

primary menorrhagia. FUNCTIONAL MENORRHAGIA.

primary myeloid metaplasia. A myeloproliferative disorder.

primary nasal cavity. The part of the nasal cavity derived from the olfactory pit.

primary oocyte. A female germ cell following the oogonial cell and preceding the first meiotic division.

primary oral cavity. The cavity derived from the stomodeum before it contributes to the nasal cavity.

primary orthostatic hypotension. A form of orthostatic hypotension with onset in middle or late adult years, associated with extrapyramidal symptoms (tremor, ataxia, rigidity) and frequently accompanied by impotence, atonicity of the urinary bladder, impaired sweating in the lower part of the body, and other signs of deranged autonomic function. Pathologically, there is a degeneration of preganglionic sympathetic neurons. Syn. *primary autonomic insufficiency, Shy-Drager syndrome.*

primary ovarian follicles. NA *folliculi ovarici primarii.* See *ovarian follicle.*

primary palate. The embryonic palate corresponding approximately to the premaxillary region.

primary perineum. PRIMITIVE PERINEAL BODY.

primary peritonitis. Peritonitis in which the infection is carried directly to the peritoneum by the blood or lymph stream. Syn. *idiopathic peritonitis.*

primary phase. PRIMARY TUBERCULOSIS.

primary polycythemia. POLYCYTHEMIA VERA.

primary process. *In psychoanalysis,* the mental activity characteristic of the id, by which the unconscious strivings and instinctual desires of the individual are satisfied; usually expressed by lack of organization in the mental activity of infancy, and in dreams. Contr. *secondary process.*

primary purpura. IDIOPATHIC THROMBOCYTOPENIC PURPURA.

primary ray. The roentgen ray as it emerges from the roentgen-ray tube.

primary reaction of Nissl [F. *Nissl*]. AXONAL REACTION.

primary refractory anemia. Normocytic normochromic anemia of unknown causation, usually associated with granulocytopenia and thrombocytopenia, unresponsive to treatment other than blood transfusion. Syn. *aregeneratory anemia, cryptogenic anemia, hypoplastic anemia, progressive hypocythemia.*

primary repression. *In psychiatry,* repression that occurs in early life and concerns data which have never really entered into conscious awareness, and that relates to instinctual feelings, drives, and impulses.

primary reticulosis of the brain. MICROGLIOMATOSIS.

primary sequestrum. A sequestrum entirely detached and requiring removal.

primary sex characters. The anatomic structures directly concerned with reproduction, as the gonads and genital apparatus.

primary shock. Shock manifested immediately after an injury.

primary sore. The critical lesion, or chancre, of syphilis. Syn. *hard sore.*

primary spermatocyte. A male germ cell following the spermatogonial cell and preceding the first meiotic division.

primary sprue. CELIAC SYNDROME.

primary structure. The amino acid sequence of a protein or polypeptide chain as determined by peptide bonds between adjacent amino acids. Contr. *secondary, tertiary,* and *quaternary structure.*

primary suture. A suture done at the time of injury or operation.

primary syphilis. The first stage of the disease, characterized clinically by a painless ulcer, or chancre, at the point of infection and equally painless, discrete regional adenopathy.

primary syphilitic adenitis. Enlarged lymph nodes associated with a primary lesion, which follow a slow indolent course of 6 months or more.

primary teeth. DECIDUOUS TEETH; the 20 teeth of the primary dentition, which erupt first and are replaced by succedaneous permanent teeth; there are 8 incisors, 4 canines, and 8 molars. NA *dentes decidui.* See also Plate 21.

primary tuberculosis. The reaction to the first implantation of tubercle bacilli in the body. It consists of a caseous focal reaction in the parenchyma of the organ and in the regional lymph node or nodes. Both foci usually run a benign course and undergo healing, often with calcification. The most frequent site is the lung. Syn. *childhood type tuberculosis.*

primary urethra. The part of the urogenital tube between the embryonic bladder and the urogenital sinus; in the female, it forms the definitive urethra; in the male, the proximal part of the prostatic urethra from urinary bladder to ejaculatory ducts.

primary villi. The earliest villi of the embryonic chorion, consisting of cordlike masses of trophoblast separated by blood lacunas.

primary wandering cell. A primitive wandering cell.

Pri·ma·tes (prye·may'teez) *n.pl.* [plural of L. *primas,* of the highest rank, from *primus,* first]. The order of mammals that includes humans, apes, monkeys, and prosimians. —**pri·mate** (prye'mate) *adj. & n.*

Primbolan. Trademark for methenolone, an anabolic steroid used as the enanthate ester.

pri·mi·done (prye'mi·dohn) *n.* 5-Ethyldihydro-5-phenyl-4,6(1*H*,5*H*)-pyrimidinedione, $C_{12}H_{14}N_2O_2$, an anticonvulsant used primarily for control of generalized and psychomotor seizures.

pri·mi·grav·i·da (prye''mi·grav'i·duh) *n.* [L. *primus,* first, + *gravida*]. A woman who is pregnant for the first time.

pri·mip·a·ra (prye·mip'uh·ruh) *n.* [L. *primus,* first, + *-para*]. A woman who has given birth for the first time. —**primipa·rous** (·rus) *adj.;* **pri·mi·par·i·ty** (prye''mi·păr'i·tee) *n.*

pri·mi·ti·ae (prye·mish'ee·ee) *n.pl.* [L., first things of their kind]. The part of the amniotic fluid discharged before the extrusion of the fetus at birth.

prim·i·tive (prim'i·tiv) *adj.* [L. *primitivus,* from *primus,* first]. 1. Undeveloped; undifferentiated; simple; rudimentary. 2. At a very early stage of development; embryonic. Compare *definitive.* 3. Original; underived.

primitive amenorrhea. PRIMARY AMENORRHEA.

primitive aorta. 1. The part of the aorta extending from its origin to the point where it first branches. 2. Two embryonic vessels which unite to form the aorta.

primitive atrium. The embryonic unpaired chamber of the heart between the sinus venosus and the primitive ventricle.

primitive canal. The vertebral canal of the embryo.
primitive cell. EMBRYONIC CELL.
primitive-cell lipoma. LIPOSARCOMA.
primitive choana. PRIMARY CHOANA.
primitive ectoderm. The undifferentiated external layer of a gastrula or of the bilaminar blastodisk. Syn. *ectoblast.*
primitive entoderm. The internal layer of the gastrula; the group of cells that segregate from the inner cell mass on the ventral surface of the primitive ectoderm and from which are derived the yolk sac and embryonic gut. Syn. *entoblast, hypoblast.*
primitive folds. PRIMITIVE RIDGES.
primitive groove. The longitudinal groove in the primitive streak between the primitive ridges.
primitive gut. ARCHENTERON.
primitive interatrial foramen. FORAMEN PRIMUM.
primitive joint plate. The primary rudiment of a joint which is formed by a separate thickening of mesenchyme between the thickenings that are the forerunners of the bones to be joined.
primitive kidney. PRONEPHROS.
primitive knot. HENSEN'S NODE.
primitive line. PRIMITIVE STREAK.
primitive mouth. BLASTOPORE.
primitive node. HENSEN'S NODE.
primitive olfactory lobe. RHINENCEPHALON.
primitive palate. *In embryology,* the part of the median nasal process that forms the median part of the upper lip and the primary palate.
primitive perineal body. The projecting wedge formed by the urorectal septum, which separates the anus and the orifice of the primitive urogenital sinus after the rupture of the cloacal membrane.
primitive pharynx. The embryonic pharynx with its characteristic visceral arches, grooves, and pouches.
primitive pit. A minute pit at the anterior end of the primitive groove in the embryo just caudal to the primitive node; it may form the opening into the notochordal canal or the site of a neurenteric cyst.
primitive plate. The floor of the primitive groove.
primitive ridges. The ridges bounding the primitive groove.
primitive segment. SOMITE.
primitive stomach. ARCHENTERON.
primitive streak. A dense, opaque band of ectoderm in the bilaminar blastoderm associated with the morphogenetic movements and proliferation of the mesoderm and notochord. It indicates the first trace of the embryo.
primitive thinking. *In psychology and psychiatry,* mental processes characterized by impairment or deficiency of abstraction and generalization, with a tendency toward concrete thinking.
primitive urogenital sinus. The larger part of the cloaca ventral to the urorectal septum. See also *urogenital tube.*
primitive vertebra. PROTOVERTEBRA.
primordia. Plural of *primordium.*
pri·mor·di·al (prye·mor'dee·ul) *adj.* [*primordi*um + *-al*]. Existing in the beginning; first-formed; primitive; original; of the simplest character.
primordial cell. EMBRYONIC CELL.
primordial cyst. A cyst that may form from an epithelial sprout given off of the dental lamina, or in an enamel organ of an early tooth germ before enamel and dentin have been laid down.
primordial dwarf. An individual afflicted with primordial dwarfism.
primordial dwarfism. The condition of being of extremely short stature, usually from birth, but with otherwise normal physical proportions, mental and sexual development, endocrine status, and bone age. There may be a definite genetic history, or it may occur sporadically.
primordial germ cell. One of the large spherical cells found in the germinal epithelium of the gonad, which are frequently considered to be primordia of the ova or spermatozoa.
primordial image or **parent.** *In analytic psychology,* the archetype, primitive, or original parent; the source of all life; the stage prior to the differentiation of mother and father.
primordial ovum. An ovum present in the germinal epithelium of the embryonic ovary, frequently considered to serve as a parent cell for the oogonia.
primordial thinking. PRIMITIVE THINKING.
pri·mor·di·um (prye·mor'dee·um) *n.,* pl. **primor·dia** (·dee·uh) [L., beginning, origin]. The earliest discernible indication of an organ or part, as: acousticofacial primordium; ANLAGE (1).
Prinadol. Trademark for the synthetic narcotic analgesic drug phenazocine, used as the hydrobromide salt.
prin·ceps (prin'seps) *adj.* [L., chief]. First; original; main.
prin·ci·pal (prin'si·pul) *adj.* [L. *principalis,* first, original, chief]. 1. Main, chief. 2. Basic, fundamental.
principal angle. The angle formed by that side of a prism receiving the incident ray with the side from which the refracted ray escapes.
principal axis. 1. *In optics,* a line that extends through the center of a lens at a 90° angle to the surface of its lens. 2. *In ophthalmology,* OPTIC AXIS.
principal cells. CHROMOPHOBE CELLS.
principal plane. A plane normal to the principal axis of a lens, passing through a principal point.
principal point. One of the two points in the optical axis of a lens which are so related that lines drawn from these points to the corresponding points in the object and its image are parallel.
principal vestibular nucleus. MEDIAL VESTIBULAR NUCLEUS.
prin·ci·ple (prin'si·pul) *n.* [L. *principium,* beginning]. 1. A constituent of a compound representing its essential or characteristic properties. 2. A rule or basis of action.
principle of inertia. REPETITION-COMPULSION PRINCIPLE.
Prin·gle's adenoma se·ba·ce·um (se·bay'see·um) [J. J. *Pringle,* British dermatologist, 1855–1922]. The facial cutaneous manifestation of tuberous sclerosis, consisting of hamartomatous malformation principally of fibrovascular tissue, associated in an undetermined way with skin appendages.
printer's palsy. A rare form of neuropathic paralysis allegedly due to chronic antimony poisoning occurring in printers.
P-R interval. The time between the onset of the P wave and the beginning of the QRS complex of the electrocardiogram; represents the duration of impulse conduction from the sinoatrial node to the ventricles.
Priodax. Trademark for iodoalphionic acid, a radiopaque medium for cholecystography.
Pri·on·urus (prye''o·new'rus) *n.* [NL., from Gk. *priōn,* saw, + *oura,* tail]. A genus of scorpions; species of this genus inflict stings that are painful and very poisonous.
Prionurus aus·tra·lis (aw·stray'lis). A well-known species of tropical scorpions found in North Africa. An antivenin has been prepared from members of this species which is effective against the stings of all North African scorpions.
Priscoline. Trademark for tolazoline, an adrenolytic, sympatholytic, and vasodilator drug used as the hydrochloride salt.
pri·sil·i·dene (pri·sil'i·deen) *n.* ALPHAPRODINE.
prism (priz'um) *n.* [Gk. *prisma,* from *priein,* to saw]. 1. A solid whose bases or ends are similar plane figures and whose sides are parallelograms. 2. *In optics,* a transparent solid with triangular ends and two converging sides. It disperses white light into its component colors, bends the rays of light toward the side opposite the angle (the base of the prism), and is used to measure or correct imbalance of the ocular muscles.
pris·ma (priz'muh) *n.,* pl. **prisma·ta** (·tuh) [L., from Gk.]. PRISM.

prism angle. The angle made by the two refracting sides of a prism at its apex.

prismata. Plural of *prisma* (= PRISM).

prismata ada·man·ti·na (ad·uh·man·tye'nuh) [NA]. ENAMEL PRISMS.

pris·mat·ic (priz·mat'ick) *adj.* 1. Of or pertaining to a prism. 2. Prism-shaped. 3. Produced by the action of a prism, as prismatic colors.

prismatic eye. OMMATIDIUM.

prismatic spectacles. Spectacles with prismatic lenses, either alone or combined with spherical or cylindrical lenses; used in insufficiency and paralysis of the ocular muscles.

prism diopter. A unit of prismatic refractive power; the refractive power of a prism that deflects a ray of light 1 cm on a tangent plane situated at a distance of 1 meter.

pris·moid (priz'moid) *adj.* Resembling a prism.

pris·mop·tom·e·ter (priz''mop·tom'e·tur) *n.* [*prism* + *optometer*]. An instrument for estimating refractive defects of the eye by means of two prisms placed base to base.

pris·mo·sphere (priz'muh·sfeer) *n.* [*prism* + *sphere*]. A combination of a prism and a globular lens.

prison psychosis. GANSER SYNDROME.

-prival [L. *-privus* (from *privare,* to deprive) + *-al*]. A combining form meaning (a) *tending to deprive of or remove* a specified thing; (b) *pertaining to deprivation or removal of* a specified thing.

private antigen. An erythrocyte antigen system, defined by specific antisera, found only in a very small number of people, usually members of a given family. Less than 1 percent of the population has such antigens. Syn. *low incidence factors.* Contr. *public antigen.*

private nurse. A nurse who works exclusively for one patient at a time and is employed by him whether in a hospital or a home.

-privic. See *-prival.*

privileged communication. *In legal medicine,* a right existing by statute and belonging to the patient whereby all medical treatment and associated information are confidential, so that the physician cannot be legally compelled to disclose them. Syn. *confidential communication.* See also *confidentiality.*

privileged graft site. A part of the human body which readily accepts foreign tissue with little or no rejection after implantation (such as the cornea of the eye).

Privine. Trademark for naphazoline, a vasoconstrictor used topically as the hydrochloride salt.

p.r.n. Abbreviation for *pro re nata.*

pro- [Gk. and L.]. A prefix signifying (a) *front, forward;* (b) *prior, before;* (c) *precursor;* (d) *promoting, furthering.*

pro·ac·cel·er·in (pro·ack·sel'ur·in) *n.* [*pro-* + *accelerin*]. FACTOR V.

pro·ac·ro·som·al granules (pro·ack''ro·so'mul). Granules in the developing spermatid which by coalescence form the acrosome.

pro·ac·ti·va·tor (pro·ack'ti·vay''tur) *n.* [*pro-* + *activator*]. The inactive precursor of a substance that has the property of activating some other substance or process; applied especially to certain blood-coagulation factors.

pro·ag·glu·ti·noid (pro''uh·gloo'ti·noid) *n.* [*pro-* + *agglutinoid*]. An agglutinoid having a stronger affinity for the agglutinogen than is possessed by the agglutinin.

pro·al (pro'ul) *adj.* [*pro-* + *-al*]. Having a forward direction or movement.

pro·am·ni·on (pro·am'nee·on) *n.* [*pro-* + *amnion*]. The part of the embryonic area at the sides and in front of the head of the developing embryo, which remains without mesoderm for a considerable period.

pro·at·las (pro''at'lus) *n.* [*pro-* + *atlas*]. An accessory vertebral element occasionally present between the atlas and the occipital bone.

probable error. A value that is 0.67449 times the standard error of the mean.

pro·band (pro'band) *n.* [L. *probandus,* from *probare,* to test]. The individual or index case, who is the starting point of a family pedigree or geneological chart. Syn. *propositus.*

pro·bang (pro'bang) *n.* A rod of whalebone or other flexible material, used for making local applications to the esophagus or larynx or for removing foreign bodies.

Pro-Banthine. Trademark for the anticholinergic drug propantheline bromide.

pro·bar·bi·tal (pro·bahr'bi·tal, ·tol) *n.* 5-Ethyl-5-isopropylbarbituric acid, $C_9H_{14}N_2O_3$, a barbiturate with intermediate duration of action; used as a hypnotic and sedative drug, in the form of its calcium and sodium derivatives.

pro·ba·tion·er nurse (pro·bay'shun·ur). PRECLINICAL STUDENT NURSE.

probe, *n.* [L. *proba,* test]. 1. A slender, flexible rod, for exploring or dilating a natural channel, as the lacrimal duct, or for following a sinus or the course of a wound. 2. A stiff rod, usually pointed at one end, used for separating tissues in dissection. 3. An electron stream used to strike a tissue in a scanning electron microscope, generating x-ray spectra which reveal the presence and concentration of various elements. 4. The act of using a probe.

probe gorget. A gorget whose tip is probe-pointed.

pro·ben·e·cid (pro·ben'e·sid) *n.* *p*-(Dipropylsulfamoyl)benzoic acid, $C_{13}H_{19}NO_4S$, a substance that inhibits renal tubular excretion of penicillin, aminosalicylic acid, and phenolsulfonphthalein, and also depresses renal tubular resorption of urate, thereby increasing urinary excretion of uric acid. Useful in prolonging action of penicillin and aminosalicylic acid, and in the treatment of gout.

pro·bit (pro'bit) *n.* [*prob*ability + un*it*]. A statistical unit of probable deviation used in biological assays; equal to the normal equivalent deviate increased by 5, used to make all normal equivalent deviation values positive.

pro·bos·cis (pro·bos'is) *n.,* pl. **proboscises, probos·ci·des** (·i·deez) [Gk. *proboskis,* from *boskein,* to feed, graze]. 1. The cylindrical projection from the face, above or below the orbit, with or without a cavity, which represents the nose in various grades of cyclopia and ethmocephalus. 2. In various invertebrates, especially many insects, an elongate organ, often retractable or extensible and occasionally tactile, which is located at the anterior end of the body; often associated with feeding or, more rarely, defense. —**probos·coid** (·koid) *adj.*

pro·bu·col (pro'bew·kole) *n.* Acetone bis[3,5-di-*tert*-butyl-4-hydroxyphenyl]mercaptole, $C_{31}H_{48}O_2S_2$, an anticholesteremic.

pro·cain·am·ide (pro''kane·am'ide, pro·kay'nuh·mide) *n.* *p*-Amino-*N*-[2-(diethylamino)ethyl]benzamide, $C_{13}H_{21}N_3O$, a cardiac depressant used as the hydrochloride salt for treatment of ventricular and atrial arrhythmias and extrasystoles. Syn. *procaine amide.*

pro·caine (pro'kane) *n.* 2-Diethylaminoethyl *p*-aminobenzoate, $C_{13}H_{20}N_2O_2$, a local anesthetic used as the hydrochloride salt.

procaine penicillin G. The procaine salt of the antibiotic penicillin G; less soluble in water and with a more sustained action than potassium penicillin G.

pro·cal·lus (pro·kal'us) *n.* [*pro-* + *callus*]. The organized blood clot which forms in an early stage of repair of a fractured bone.

pro·car·ba·zine (pro·kahr'buh·zeen) *n.* *N*-Isopropyl-α-(2-methylhydrazino)-*p*-toluamide, $C_{12}H_{19}N_3O$, an antineoplastic agent effective in the management of Hodgkin's disease; used as the hydrochloride salt.

procaryote. PROKARYOTE. —**procaryotic,** *adj.*

pro cell. *Obsol.* Any cell of the second stage of development of a blood cell, without identifying the specific series to which it belongs.

pro·ce·lous (pro·see'lus) *adj.* [*pro-* + Gk. *koilos,* hollow]. Concave in front.

pro·cen·tri·ole (pro·sen′tree·ole) *n.* [*pro-* + *centriole*]. A centriole that arises at an angle from the mother centriole.

pro·ce·phal·ic (pro″se·fal′ick) *adj.* [*pro-* + *cephalic*]. *In biology,* pertaining to the front of the head.

pro·cer·coid (pro·sur′koid) *n.* [*pro-* + Gk. *kerkos*, tail, + *-oid*]. The first larval stage in the first intermediate host of some cestodes.

pro·ce·rus (pro·seer′us) *n.*, pl. **proce·ri** (·eye) [L., slender, long]. A muscle of facial expression. NA *musculus procerus.* See also Table of Muscles in the Appendix.

pro·cess (pro′sess, pros′ess) *n.* [L. *processus*, course, progress]. 1. A course of action or events; a sequence of phenomena, as an inflammatory process. 2. A prominence or outgrowth of tissue, as the spinous process of a vertebra. 3. *In chemistry,* a method of procedure; reaction; test.

pro·ces·so·ma·nia (pro·ses″o·may′nee·uh) *n.* [(legal) *process* + *mania*]. A mania for litigation.

process schizophrenia. Schizophrenia in which an organic brain disorder is considered to be the primary underlying cause; typically gradual in onset and progressive without remission. Contr. *reactive schizophrenia.*

pro·ces·sus (pro·ses′us) *n.*, pl. & genit. sing. **processus** [L.]. PROCESS.

processus ac·ces·so·ri·us ver·te·bra·rum lum·ba·li·um (ack·se·so′ree·us vur·te·brair′um lum·bay′lee·um) [NA]. ACCESSORY PROCESS.

processus ala·ris os·sis eth·moi·da·lis (ay·lair′is os′is eth·moy·day′lis) [BNA]. Ala cristae galli (= ALAR PROCESS).

processus al·ve·o·la·ris max·il·lae (al·vee·o·lair′is mack·sil′ee) [NA]. ALVEOLAR PROCESS of the maxilla.

processus anterior mal·lei (mal′ee·eye) [NA]. ANTERIOR PROCESS OF THE MALLEUS.

processus ar·ti·cu·la·ris inferior (ahr·tick·yoo·lair′is) [NA]. INFERIOR ARTICULAR PROCESS.

processus articularis superior [NA]. SUPERIOR ARTICULAR PROCESS.

processus articularis superior os·sis sa·cri (os′is say′krye) [NA]. Either one of the articular processes of the sacrum which articulate with the inferior articular processes of the fifth lumbar vertebra.

processus cau·da·tus he·pa·tis (kaw·day′tus hep′uh·tis) [NA]. CAUDATE PROCESS (1).

processus ci·li·a·res (sil·ee·air′eez) [NA]. CILIARY PROCESSES.

processus cli·noi·de·us anterior (kli·noy′dee·us) [NA]. ANTERIOR CLINOID PROCESS.

processus clinoideus me·di·us (mee′dee·us) [NA]. MIDDLE CLINOID PROCESS.

processus clinoideus posterior [NA]. POSTERIOR CLINOID PROCESS.

processus co·chle·a·ri·for·mis (kock″lee·ăr·i·for′mis) [NA]. COCHLEARIFORM PROCESS.

processus con·dy·la·ris (kon·di·lair′is) [NA]. CONDYLAR PROCESS.

processus con·dy·loi·de·us man·di·bu·lae (kon·di·loy′dee·us man·dib′yoo·lee) [BNA]. Processus condylaris (= CONDYLAR PROCESS).

processus co·ra·coi·de·us (kor·a·koy′dee·us) [NA]. CORACOID PROCESS.

processus co·ro·noi·de·us man·di·bu·lae (kor·o·noy′dee·us man·dib′yoo·lee) [NA]. CORONOID PROCESS (1).

processus coronoideus ul·nae (ul′nee) [NA]. CORONOID PROCESS (2).

processus cos·ta·ri·us ver·te·brae (kos·tair′ee·us vur′te·bree) [NA]. The anterior portion of the transverse process of a cervical vertebra, lying anterior to the transverse foramen and corresponding to the vertebral end of a rib.

processus eth·moi·da·lis (eth·moy·day′lis) [NA]. ETHMOID PROCESS.

processus fal·ci·for·mis li·ga·men·ti sa·cro·tu·be·ro·si (fal·si·for′mis lig·uh·men′tye say″kro·tew·be·ro′sigh) [NA]. FALCIFORM PROCESS.

processus fron·ta·lis max·il·lae (fron·tay′lis mack·sil′ee) [NA]. FRONTAL PROCESS (1).

processus frontalis os·sis zy·go·ma·ti·ci (os′is zigh·go·mat′i·sigh) [NA]. FRONTOSPHENOID PROCESS.

processus fron·to·sphe·noi·da·lis os·sis zy·go·ma·ti·ci (fron″to·sfee·noy·day′lis os′is zigh·go·mat′i·sigh) [BNA]. Processus frontalis ossis zygomatici (= FRONTAL PROCESS (2)).

processus gra·ci·lis (gras′i·lis). ANTERIOR PROCESS OF THE MALLEUS.

processus in·tra·ju·gu·la·ris os·sis oc·ci·pi·ta·lis (in″truh·jug·yoo·lair′is os′is ock·sip·i·tay′lis) [NA]. INTRAJUGULAR PROCESS (1).

processus intrajugularis ossis tem·po·ra·lis (tem·po·ray′lis) [NA]. INTRAJUGULAR PROCESS (2).

processus ju·gu·la·ris os·sis oc·ci·pi·ta·lis (jug·yoo·lair′is os′is ock·sip·i·tay′lis) [NA]. JUGULAR PROCESS.

processus la·cri·ma·lis (lack·ri·may′lis) [NA]. LACRIMAL PROCESS.

processus la·te·ra·lis mal·lei (lat·e·ray′lis mal′ee·eye) [NA]. LATERAL PROCESS OF THE MALLEUS.

processus lateralis ta·li (tay′lye) [NA]. LATERAL PROCESS OF THE TALUS.

processus lateralis tu·be·ris cal·ca·nei (tew′bur·is kal·kay′nee·eye) [NA]. The elevation on the lateral side of the plantar aspect of the posterior portion of the calcaneus.

processus len·ti·cu·la·ris in·cu·dis (len·tick·yoo·lair′is ing·kew′dis, ink′yoo·dis) [NA]. LENTICULAR PROCESS.

processus ma·mil·la·ris (mam·i·lair′is) [NA]. MAMILLARY PROCESS.

processus mar·gi·na·lis os·sis zy·go·ma·ti·ci (mahr·ji·nay′lis os′is zigh·go·mat′i·sigh) [BNA]. Tuberculum marginale ossis zygomatici (= MARGINAL TUBERCLE OF THE ZYGOMATIC BONE).

processus mas·toi·de·us (mas·toy′dee·us) [NA]. MASTOID PROCESS.

processus max·il·la·ris con·chae na·sa·lis in·fe·ri·o·ris (mack·si·lair′is konk′ee na·say′lis in·feer·ee·o′ris) [NA]. The maxillary process of the inferior nasal concha. See *maxillary process.*

processus me·di·a·lis tu·be·ris cal·ca·nei (mee·dee·ay′lis tew′bur·is kal·kay′nee·eye) [NA]. The elevation on the medial side of the plantar aspect of the posterior portion of the calcaneus.

processus mus·cu·la·ris car·ti·la·gi·nis ary·te·noi·dei (mus·kew·lair′is kahr·ti·laj′i·nis ăr·i·te·noy′dee·eye) [NA]. MUSCULAR PROCESS.

processus or·bi·ta·lis os·sis pa·la·ti·ni (or·bi·tay′lis os′is pal·uh·tye′nigh) [NA]. ORBITAL PROCESS OF THE PALATINE BONE.

processus pa·la·ti·nus max·il·lae (pal·uh·tye′nus mack·sil′ee) [NA]. PALATINE PROCESS (2).

processus pa·pil·la·ris he·pa·tis (pap·i·lair′is hep′uh·tis) [NA]. PAPILLARY PROCESS.

processus pa·ra·ma·stoi·de·us os·sis oc·ci·pi·ta·lis (păr″uh·mas·toy′dee·us os′is ock·sip·i·tay′lis) [NA]. PARAMASTOID PROCESS.

processus posterior sphe·noi·da·lis (sfee·noy·day′lis) [NA]. SPHENOID PROCESS OF THE SEPTAL CARTILAGE.

processus posterior ta·li (tay′lye) [NA]. POSTERIOR PROCESS OF THE TALUS.

processus pte·ry·goi·de·us os·sis sphe·noi·da·lis (terr·i·goy′dee·us os′is sfee·noy·day′lis) [NA]. PTERYGOID PROCESS OF THE SPHENOID BONE.

processus pte·ry·go·spi·no·sus (teer·i·go·spye·no′sus) [NA]. PTERYGOSPINOUS PROCESS.

processus py·ra·mi·da·lis os·sis pa·la·ti·ni (pi·ram·i·day′lis os′is pal·uh·tye′nigh) [NA]. PYRAMIDAL PROCESS OF THE PALATINE BONE.

processus re·tro·man·di·bu·la·ris glan·du·lae pa·ro·ti·dis (ret″ro·man·dib·yoo·lair′is glan′dew·lee pa·rot′i·dis) [BNA]. The portion of the parotid gland lying posterior to the ramus of the mandible.

processus sphe·noi·da·lis os·sis pa·la·ti·ni (sfee·noy·day'lis os'is pal·uh·tye'nigh) [NA]. SPHENOID PROCESS OF THE PALATINE BONE.

processus sphenoidalis sep·ti car·ti·la·gi·nei (sep'tye kahr"ti·la·jin'ee·eye) [BNA]. Processus posterior sphenoidalis (= SPHENOID PROCESS OF THE SEPTAL CARTILAGE).

processus spi·no·sus (spye·no'sus) [NA]. SPINOUS PROCESS OF A VERTEBRA.

processus sty·loi·de·us os·sis me·ta·car·pa·lis III (stye·loy'dee·us os'is met"uh·kahr·pay'lis) [NA]. STYLOID PROCESS OF THE THIRD METACARPAL.

processus styloideus ossis ra·dii (ray'dee·eye) [NA]. STYLOID PROCESS OF THE RADIUS.

processus styloideus ossis tem·po·ra·lis (tem·po·ray'lis) [NA]. STYLOID PROCESS OF THE TEMPORAL BONE.

processus styloidus ul·nae (ul'nee) [NA]. STYLOID PROCESS OF THE ULNA.

processus su·pra·con·dy·la·ris (sue"pruh·kon·di·lair'is) [NA]. SUPRACONDYLAR PROCESS.

processus su·pra·con·dy·loi·de·us (sue"pruh·kon·di·loy'dee·us) [BNA]. Processus supracondylaris (= SUPRACONDYLAR PROCESS).

processus tem·po·ra·lis os·sis zy·go·ma·ti·ci (tem·po·ray'lis os'is zigh·go·mat'i·sigh) [NA]. TEMPORAL PROCESS OF THE ZYGOMATIC BONE.

processus trans·ver·sus (trans·vur'sus) [NA]. TRANSVERSE PROCESS.

processus troch·le·a·ris cal·ca·nei (trock·lee·air'is kal·kay'nee·eye) [BNA]. Trochlea peronealis (= PERONEAL TROCHLEA OF THE CALCANEUS).

processus un·ci·na·tus os·sis eth·moi·da·lis (un·si·nay'tus os'is eth·moy·day'lis) [NA]. UNCINATE PROCESS OF THE ETHMOID BONE.

processus uncinatus pan·cre·a·tis (pan·kree'uh·tis) [NA]. UNCINATE PROCESS OF THE PANCREAS.

processus va·gi·na·lis os·sis sphe·noi·da·lis (vaj·i·nay'lis os'is sfee·noy·day'lis) [NA]. VAGINAL PROCESS OF THE SPHENOID BONE.

processus vaginalis pe·ri·to·nei (perr"i·to·nee'eye) [NA]. VAGINAL PROCESS OF THE PERITONEUM.

processus ver·mi·for·mis (vur·mi·for'mis) [BNA]. Appendix vermiformis (= VERMIFORM APPENDIX).

processus vo·ca·lis (vo·kay'lis) [NA]. VOCAL PROCESS.

processus xi·phoi·de·us (zi·foy'dee·us) [NA]. XIPHOID PROCESS.

processus zy·go·ma·ti·cus max·il·lae (zigh·go·mat'i·kus mack·sil'ee) [NA]. ZYGOMATIC PROCESS OF THE MAXILLA.

processus zygomaticus os·sis fron·ta·lis (os'is fron·tay'lis) [NA]. ZYGOMATIC PROCESS OF THE FRONTAL BONE.

processus zygomaticus ossis tem·po·ra·lis (tem·po·ray'lis) [NA]. ZYGOMATIC PROCESS OF THE TEMPORAL BONE.

pro·chei·lia (pro·kigh'lee·uh) *n.* [Gk. *procheilos*, with prominent lips (from *cheilos*, lip), + *-ia*]. A condition in which a lip is farther forward than is normal. Contr. *retrocheilia*.

pro·chei·lon (pro·kigh'lon) *n.* [Gk., from *pro-* + *cheilos*, lip]. The prominence in the middle of the upper lip.

pro·chlor·per·a·zine (pro"klor·perr'uh·zeen) *n.* 2-Chloro-10-[3-(4-methyl-piperazinyl)propyl]phenothiazine, $C_{20}H_{24}ClN_3S$, an antiemetic and tranquilizing drug; used as the base and as the edisylate (ethanedisulfonate) and maleate salts.

pro·chon·dral (pro·kon'drul) *adj.* [*pro-* + *chondral*]. Prior to the formation of cartilage.

pro·chor·dal (pro·kor'dul) *adj.* [*pro-* + *chordal*]. Situated in front of the notochord.

prochordal plate. A region of thickened endoderm immediately anterior to the notochord and in direct contact with the ectoderm. It forms a part of the buccopharyngeal membrane.

pro·cho·re·sis (pro"kor·ee'sis, pro·kor'e·sis) *n.* [Gk. *prochōrēsis*, a going forth]. The propulsion of food through the gastrointestinal tract.

Pro·chow·nick's method (pro·^{k}ho^{h}v'nick) [L. *Prochownick*, German obstetrician, 1851–1923]. A method for artificial respiration in neonatal asphyxia in which the infant is suspended with the head extended and intermittent pressure is applied to the chest.

pro·ci·den·tia (pro"si·den'chee·uh, pros"i·) *n.* [L., from *procidere*, to fall forward, from *cadere*, to fall]. 1. PROLAPSE. 2. *In gynecology*, PROLAPSE OF THE UTERUS.

pro·clo·nol (pro'klo·nol) *n.* Bis(*p*-chlorophenyl)cyclopropylmethanol, $C_{16}H_{14}Cl_2O$, an acaricide and fungicide.

pro·co·ag·u·lant (pro·ko·ag'yoo·lunt) *n.* [*pro-* + *coagulant*]. Any of several clotting factors (V to XII) present in normal human plasma. These factors, along with thromboplastin and calcium, accelerate the conversion of prothrombin to thrombin.

pro·con·dy·lism (pro·kon'di·liz·um) *n.* [*pro-* + *condyle* + *-ism*]. Forward deviation of the mandibular condyles.

pro·con·ver·tin (pro"kon·vur'tin) *n.* [*pro-* + *convertin*]. FACTOR VII.

pro·cre·ate (pro'kree·ate) *v.* [L. *procreare*, from *creare*, to create]. To beget.

pro·cre·ation (pro"kree·ay'shun) *n.* The begetting of offspring. —**pro·cre·ative** (pro'kree·ay"tiv) *adj.*

proct-, procto- [Gk. *prōktos*, anus]. A combining form meaning (a) *anus*; (b) *rectum*; (c) *anus and rectum*.

proc·tag·ra (prock·tag'ruh) *n.* [*proct-* + *-agra*]. Sudden pain in the anal region.

proc·tal·gia (prock·tal'jee·uh) *n.* [*proct-* + *-algia*]. Pain in the anus or rectum.

proctalgia fu·gax (few'gacks). Acute severe intermittent pain of the anorectal region, more common at night.

proct·atre·sia (prock"ta·tree'zhuh, ·zee·uh) *n.* [*proct-* + *atresia*]. An imperforate condition of the anus or rectum.

proct·ec·ta·sia (prock"teck·tay'zhuh, ·zee·uh) *n.* [*proct-* + *ectasia*]. Dilatation of the anus or rectum.

proc·tec·to·my (prock·teck'tuh·mee) *n.* [*proct-* + *-ectomy*]. Excision of the anus and rectum, usually through the perineal route.

proc·ten·cli·sis (prock·teng'kli·sis) *n.* [*proct-* + Gk. *enklisis*, displacement]. Stricture of the rectum or anus.

proct·eu·ryn·ter (prock"tew·rin'tur) *n.* [*proct-* + Gk. *eurynein*, to dilate]. A baglike device for dilating the anus or rectum.

proc·ti·tis (prock·tye'tis) *n.* [*proct-* + *-itis*]. Inflammation of the anus or rectum.

procto-. See *proct-*.

proc·to·cele (prock'to·seel) *n.* [*procto-* + *-cele*]. The extroversion or prolapse of the mucous coat of the rectum.

proc·to·cly·sis (prock·tock'li·sis) *n.*, pl. **proctocly·ses** (·seez) [*procto-* + *-clysis*]. RECTOCLYSIS.

proc·to·co·li·tis (prock"to·ko·lye'tis) *n.* [*procto-* + *colitis*]. Inflammation of the rectum and colon.

proc·to·co·lon·os·co·py (prock"to·ko"lun·os'kuh·pee) *n.* [*procto-* + *colon* + *-scopy*]. Inspection and examination of the interior of the rectum and lower colon.

proc·to·col·po·plas·ty (prock"to·kol'po·plas"tee) *n.* [*procto-* + *colpo-* + *-plasty*]. Closure of a rectovaginal fistula.

proc·to·cys·to·plas·ty (prock"to·sis'to·plas"tee) *n.* [*procto-* + *cysto-* + *-plasty*]. A plastic operation on the rectum and the urinary bladder for repair of rectovesical fistula.

proc·to·de·um, proc·to·dae·um (prock"to·dee'um) *n.*, pl. **procto·dea, procto·daea** (·dee'uh) [NL., from *proct-* + Gk. *hodaios*, on the way]. A pitlike ectodermal depression formed by the growth of the anal hillocks surrounding the anal part of the cloacal membrane. Upon rupture of the latter, it forms part of the anal canal. Syn. *anal pit*. —**proctode·al, proctodae·al** (·ul) *adj.*

proc·to·dyn·ia (prock"to·din'ee·uh) *n.* [*proct-* + *odyn-* + *-ia*]. Pain about the anus or in the rectum.

proc·tol·o·gist (prock·tol'uh·jist) *n.* A specialist in diseases of the anus and rectum.

proc·tol·o·gy (prock·tol'uh·jee) *n.* [*procto-* + *-logy*]. The science of the anatomy, functions, and diseases of the rectum and anus. —**proc·to·log·ic** (prock"to·loj'ick) *adj.*

proc·to·pa·ral·y·sis (prock"to·puh·ral'i·sis) *n.* [*procto-* + *paralysis*]. Paralysis of the external anal sphincter muscle, usually accompanied by fecal incontinence.

proc·to·pexy (prock'to·peck"see) *n.* [*procto-* + *-pexy*]. The fixation of the rectum by anchoring it into the hollow of the sacrum by means of sutures passing externally across the sacrum. Syn. *rectopexy.*

proc·to·phil·ia (prock"to·fil'ee·uh) *n.* [*procto-* + *-philia*]. A pathological interest in, or liking of, anything connected with the anus.

proc·to·pho·bia (prock"to·fo'bee·uh) *n.* [*procto-* + *-phobia*]. 1. An abnormal fear of anything to do with the anus or rectum. 2. An abnormal dread or apprehension of pain in persons with diseases of the rectum.

proc·to·plas·ty (prock'to·plas"tee) *n.* [*procto-* + *-plasty*]. Plastic surgery of the rectum and anus.

proc·to·ple·gia (prock"to·plee'jee·uh) *n.* [*procto-* + *-plegia*]. PROCTOPARALYSIS.

proc·top·to·sia (prock"top·to'shuh, ·see·uh) *n.* [*procto-* + *ptosis* + *-ia*]. Anal and rectal prolapse.

proc·top·to·sis (prock"top·to'sis) *n.* PROCTOPTOSIA.

proc·tor·rha·phy (prock·tor'uh·fee) *n.* [*procto-* + *-rrhaphy*]. The plaiting of the enlarged and prolapsed rectal walls by suture, to reduce the circumference.

proc·tor·rhea, proc·tor·rhoea (prock"to·ree'uh) *n.* [*procto-* + *-rrhea*]. Discharge of mucus through the anus.

proc·to·scope (prock'tuh·skope) *n.* [*procto-* + *-scope*]. An instrument for inspecting the anal canal and rectum.

proc·tos·co·py (prock·tos'kuh·pee) *n.* Inspection of the anal canal and rectum with a proctoscope.

proc·to·sig·moid·ec·to·my (proc"to·sig"moy·deck'tuh·mee) *n.* [*procto-* + *sigmoid* + *-ectomy*]. The abdominoperineal excision of the anus and rectosigmoid, usually with the formation of an abdominal colostomy.

proc·to·sig·moid·itis (prock"to·sig"moy·dye'tis) *n.* [*procto-* + *sigmoid* + *-itis*]. Inflammation of the rectum and sigmoid colon.

proc·to·sig·moid·os·co·py (proc"to·sig"moy·dos'kuh·pee) *n.* [*procto-* + *sigmoidoscopy*]. Examination of the rectum and sigmoid colon with a sigmoidoscope.

proc·to·spasm (prock'to·spaz·um) *n.* [*procto-* + *spasm*]. Spasm or tenesmus of the rectum; may extend to the anus.

proc·tos·ta·sis (prock·tos'tuh·sis) *n.* [*procto-* + *-stasis*]. Constipation due to nonresponse of the rectum to the defecation stimulus.

proc·to·ste·no·sis (prock"to·ste·no'sis) *n.* [*procto-* + *stenosis*]. Stricture of the anus or rectum.

proc·tos·to·my (prock·tos'tuh·mee) *n.* [*procto-* + *-stomy*]. The establishment of a permanent artificial opening into the rectum.

proc·tot·o·my (prock·tot'uh·mee) *n.* [*procto-* + *-tomy*]. Incision into the rectum or anus, especially for stricture or imperforate anus; described as external if the incision is below the external sphincter, and internal if above it.

pro·cum·bent (pro·kum'bunt) *adj.* [L. *procumbens*, leaning forward]. PRONE; lying face down. —**procum·ben·cy** (·bun·see) *n.*

pro·cur·sive (pro·kur'siv) *adj.* [L. *procurrere*, to rush forward]. Running forward.

procursive epilepsy. A form of epilepsy in which the patient runs at the beginning of the epileptic attack.

pro·cur·va·tion (pro"kur·vay'shun) *n.* [L. *procurvus*, curved forward]. Forward inclination of the body.

pro·cy·cli·dine (pro·sigh'kli·deen) *n.* 1-Cyclohexyl-1-phenyl-3-pyrrolidino-1-propanol, $C_{19}H_{29}NO$, an antiparkinsonian drug; used as the hydrochloride salt.

pro·dig·i·o·sin (pro·dij"ee·o'sin) *n.* An antibiotic substance, $C_{20}H_{25}N_3O$, produced by *Serratia marcescens.*

pro·dil·i·dine (pro·dil'i·deen) *n.* 1,2-Dimethyl-3-phenyl-3-pyrrolidinyl propionate, $C_{15}H_{21}NO_2$, an analgesic; used as the hydrochloride salt.

pro·do·lic acid (pro·do'lic). 1,3,4,9-Tetrahydro 1-propylpyrano[3,4-*b*]indole-1-acetic acid, $C_{16}H_{19}NO_3$, an anti-inflammatory.

pro·dro·ma (pro'dro·muh, prod'ro·muh) *n.*, pl. **prodromas, pro·dro·ma·ta** (pro·dro'muh·tuh) [NL]. PRODROME.

pro·dro·mal (prod'ro·mul, pro·dro'mul) *adj.* [*prodrome* + *-al*]. Pertaining to early manifestations or symptoms of a disease; premonitory.

pro·drome (pro'drome) *n.* [Gk. *prodromos*, precursor, from *pro-* + *dromos*, running]. 1. An early or premonitory manifestation of impending disease, before the specific symptoms begin. 2. AURA.

pro·drom·ic (pro·drom'ick) *adj.* PRODROMAL.

prod·ro·mous (prod'ro·mus) *adj.* PRODROMAL.

prod·uct, *n.* [L. *productum*, from *producere*, to produce]. 1. Effect; result; that which is produced. 2. *In chemistry*, the compound formed by a reaction.

pro·duc·tive, *adj.* 1. Forming or capable of forming new tissue. 2. Raising mucous or secretion, as a productive cough.

productive cough. A cough in which mucus or secretion is removed from the respiratory tract.

productive inflammation. Inflammation in which there is a considerable multiplication of fibroblasts.

pro·en·ceph·a·lus (pro"en·sef'uh·lus) *n.* An individual with proencephaly.

pro·en·ceph·a·ly (pro"en·sef'uh·lee) *n.* [*pro-* + *-encephaly*]. Partial acrania in the frontal region with encephalocele or hydrencephalocele.

pro·en·zyme (pro·en'zime) *n.* An inactive precursor in a living cell from which an enzyme is formed.

pro·eryth·ro·blast (of Fer·ra·ta) (pro"e·rith'ro·blast). PRONORMOBLAST.

pro·eryth·ro·cyte (pro"e·rith'ro·site) *n.* [*pro-* + *erythrocyte*]. RETICULOCYTE (1).

pro·es·tro·gen (pro·es'tro·jin) *n.* [*pro-* + *estrogen*]. A substance, in itself weakly estrogenic, which is converted to a more active estrogen in the body.

pro·es·trus, pro-oes·trus (pro·es'trus) *n.* [*pro-* + *estrus*]. A phase of the estrous cycle in mammals preceding heat; characterized by growth of the endometrium and follicular development in the ovary.

Proetz's treatment (prets) [A. W. *Proetz*, U.S. otolaryngologist, b. 1888]. DISPLACEMENT METHOD.

pro·fen·a·mine (pro·fen'uh·meen) *n.* ETHOPROPAZINE.

pro·fer·ment (pro·fur'ment) *n.* [*pro-* + *ferment*]. PROENZYME.

pro·fes·sion·al (pro·fesh'uh·nul) *adj.* 1. Pertaining to a profession. 2. Of or pertaining to the ethical or technical standards of a profession.

professional neurasthenia. OCCUPATIONAL NEUROSIS.

professional service unit. A mobile unit of the U.S. Army Medical Service composed of professional teams and necessary service elements.

professional spasms. OCCUPATION SPASMS.

Pro·fi·chet's syndrome (proʰ·fee·sheʰ') [G. C. *Profichet*, French physician, b. 1873]. Subcutaneous calcific nodules, especially in the periarticular areas, associated with ulceration of the overlying skin and nervous symptoms.

pro·file, *n.* [It. *profilo* (*proffilo*), from *pro-* + *filare*, to spin out, to draw]. 1. An outline or representation of the distinctive features of something. 2. A graph, curve, or other schema presenting quantitatively or descriptively the chief characteristics of something, as of an organ, process, or person.

pro·fla·vine (pro·flay'vin) *n.* 3,6-Diaminoacridine, $C_{13}H_{11}N_3$, a local antiseptic used as the hydrochloride and sulfate salts.

pro·flu·vi·um (pro·floo'vee·um) *n.*, pl. **proflu·via** (·vee·uh) [L., a flowing forth]. A flux or discharge.

profluvium al·vi (al'vye) [L., of the belly]. DIARRHEA.

profluvium lac·tis (lack'tis). Excessive flow of milk.

profound mental retardation. Subnormal general intellectual functioning to such an extent that the individual cannot profit from training in self-help and requires total nursing care; some motor and speech development may occur. The intelligence quotient is generally below 25.

pro·fun·da (pro·fun'duh) *adj.* [fem. of L. *profundus,* deep]. Deep-seated; a term applied to certain arteries.

pro·fun·dus (pro·fun'dus) *adj.* [L., deep]. Deep-seated; applied to certain muscles and nerves.

pro·gas·ter (pro·gas'tur) *n.* [*pro-* + *-gaster*]. ARCHENTERON.

pro·gen·er·ate (pro·jen'ur·ut) *n.* [*pro-* + *-generate* as in degenerate]. An individual endowed with superior faculties; a genius.

pro·gen·e·sis (pro·jen'e·sis) *n.* [*pro-* + *-genesis*]. The development and fate of the germ cells before fertilization or blastogenesis.

pro·gen·i·tor (pro·jen'i·tur) *n.* [L.]. 1. An ancestor. 2. PRECURSOR.

prog·e·ny (proj'e·nee) *n.* [L. *progenies,* from *progignere,* to beget, produce]. OFFSPRING; descendants.

pro·ge·ria (pro·jeer'ee·uh) *n.* [Gk. *progērōs,* prematurely old (from *pro-* + *gēras,* old age) + *-ia*]. Premature senility. In a child, HUTCHINSON-GILFORD SYNDROME; in an adult, WERNER'S SYNDROME.

pro·ges·ta·gen (pro·jes'tuh·jin) *n.* [*progestational* + *-gen*]. Any progestational hormone; PROGESTOGEN.

pro·ges·ta·tion·al (pro''jes·tay'shun·ul) *adj.* [*pro-* + *gestation* + *-al*]. Pertaining to the second, or luteal, phase of the menstrual cycle, during which the endometrium changes from the proliferative to the secretory state under the influence of progeaterone released from the corpus luteum.

progestational hormone. 1. The natural hormone progesterone, which induces progestational changes of the uterine mucosa. 2. Any derivative or modification of progesterone having similar actions.

pro·ges·ter·one (pro·jes'tur·ohn) *n.* Pregn-4-ene-3,20-dione, $C_{21}H_{30}O_2$, the steroid hormone secreted by the ovary mainly from the corpus luteum. It is essential for nidation of the ovum and maintenance of pregnancy; cessation of its secretion at the end of the menstrual cycle largely determines the time of onset of menstruation. The hormone, now obtained by synthesis, is used for the management of various ovarian disorders.

progesterone receptor. A cytoplasmic protein capable of binding progesterone, found in several tissues including endometrium and breast. Its presence in malignant tissue may be of value in predicting response to hormonal therapy.

pro·ges·tin (pro·jes'tin) *n.* Any progestational hormone; a progestogen. The name has been applied specifically to progesterone.

pro·ges·to·gen (pro·jes'to·jin) *n.* [alteration of *progestagen*]. Any progestational hormone.

pro·glot·tid (pro·glot'id) *n.* [NL. *proglottis,* from Gk. *proglōssis,* tongue tip]. A segment of a tapeworm.

pro·glot·tis (pro·glot'is) *n.,* pl. **proglot·ti·des** (·i·deez). PROGLOTTID.

pro·glu·mide (pro·gloo'mide) *n.* (±)-4-Benzamido-*N,N*-dipropylglutaramic acid, $C_{18}H_{26}N_2O_4$, an anticholinergic.

pro·gnath·ic (pro·nath'ick, ·nay'thick) *adj.* [*pro-* + *gnathic*]. *In craniometry,* designating a condition of the upper jaw in which it projects anteriorly with respect to the profile of the facial skeleton, when the skull is oriented on the Frankfort horizontal plane; having a gnathic index of 103.0 or more.

prog·na·thism (prog'nuh·thiz·um) *n.* [*pro-* + *gnath-* + *-ism*]. The condition of having projecting jaws.

prog·na·thous (prog'nuth·us) *adj.* PROGNATHIC.

prog·nose (prog·noce', ·noze') *v.* PROGNOSTICATE.

prog·no·sis (prog·no'sis) *n.,* pl. **progno·ses** (·seez) [Gk. *prognōsis,* from *pro-,* fore-, + *gnōsis,* knowledge]. A prediction as to the probable course and outcome of a disease, injury, or developmental abnormality in a patient, based on general knowledge of such conditions, as well as on specific information and exercise of clinical judgment in the particular case. —**prog·nos·tic** (·nos'tick) *adj.*

prog·nos·ti·cate (prog·nos'ti·kate) *v.* To give a prognosis.

prog·nos·ti·cian (prog''nos·tish'un) *n.* A physician who is versed in prognosis.

pro·go·nal fold (pro·go'nul). The cephalic part of the genital ridge, in which develops the suspensory ligament of the ovary.

pro·go·no·ma (pro''gon·o'muh, pro''guh·no'muh) *n.* [Gk. *progonos,* ancestor, + *-oma*]. A nodular or tumorlike mass containing structures resembling those of ancestral forms of a species, as exemplified in hairy moles.

pro·gran·u·lo·cyte (pro·gran'yoo·lo·site) *n.* [*pro-* + *granulocyte*]. PROMYELOCYTE.

pro·grav·id (pro·grav'id) *adj.* [*pro-* + *gravid*]. Pertaining to the second, or luteal, phase of the menstrual cycle, when secretion of progesterone changes the endometrium to the secretory state essential for nidation and maintenance of pregnancy. See also *progestational.*

pro·gres·sion (pruh·gresh'un) *n.* [L. *progressio,* from *progredi,* to advance]. The act of advancing or moving forward.

pro·gres·sive (pruh·gres'iv) *adj.* Gradually extending; advancing or increasing in complexity or severity.

progressive arterial occlusive disease (Köhlmeier-Degos). DEGOS' DISEASE.

progressive atrophy of the globus pallidus. JUVENILE PARALYSIS AGITANS.

progressive bulbar paralysis or **palsy.** Progressive symmetrical degeneration of the motor nuclei of the medulla and lower pons, with onset usually in late adult life and occasionally familial, resulting in atrophy, fasciculations, and paralysis of the denervated muscles; related to or associated with progressive spinal muscular atrophy and amyotrophic lateral sclerosis.

progressive bulbar paralysis of childhood. FAZIO-LONDE ATROPHY.

progressive cerebellar asynergy or **dyssynergy.** DYSSYNERGIA CEREBELLARIS PROGRESSIVA.

progressive cerebral poliodystrophy. Cortical degeneration, usually of infants and children, characterized clinically by myoclonic and generalized seizures, ataxia, choreoathetosis, or spasticity, as well as varying degrees of mental deterioration, and pathologically by widespread severe loss of the neurons of the cerebral cortex, accompanied by astrocytic and microglial proliferation, with relative sparing of the white matter; cause or causes are unknown, but slow virus infection may be present. Syn. *Alpers' disease, poliodystrophia cerebri progressiva infantilis.*

progressive coccidioidomycosis. A chronic, often severe and fatal infection with *Coccidioides immitis,* involving viscera, bones, and skin. Syn. *coccidioidal granuloma.*

progressive diaphyseal dysplasia. Cortical thickening of the long bones, beginning in the midshaft and progressing toward the epiphyses; it becomes apparent in infancy or early childhood. Syn. *diaphyseal sclerosis, Engelmann's disease.*

progressive external ophthalmoplegia. Slowly progressive inability to move the eyes, and usually ptosis, with normal pupillary reactions and accommodation. Heart block may be present, and generalized muscular dystrophy may develop; now considered to be a form of muscular dystrophy affecting chiefly the extraocular muscles. See also *ophthalmoplegia plus.*

progressive facial hemiatrophy. Progressive wasting of the muscles of mastication, facial expression, and scalp, with trophic changes in the skin, subcutaneous tissues, and bone, of one half of the face; often beginning in preadolescence but arresting in later life; a form of lipodystrophy of unknown cause. Syn. *Romberg's disease.*

progressive familial myoclonic epilepsy. A heredodegenerative disease beginning in childhood or adolescence, characterized by progressively worsening generalized and myoclonic seizures, cerebellar and extrapyramidal disturbances, and dementia; associated with deposits of relatively insoluble polyglucosans (Lafora bodies) in various sites, and transmitted as an autosomal recessive trait. Syn. *Unverricht's disease.*

progressive hypertrophic interstitial neuropathy. HYPERTROPHIC INTERSTITIAL NEUROPATHY (1).

progressive hypocythemia. PRIMARY REFRACTORY ANEMIA.

progressive infantile spinal muscular atrophy. INFANTILE SPINAL MUSCULAR ATROPHY.

progressive lateral sclerosis. Amyotrophic lateral sclerosis with primary involvement of the corticospinal tracts.

progressive lenticular degeneration. HEPATOLENTICULAR DEGENERATION.

progressive lipodystrophy. A rare disease of unknown cause, occurring mainly in young women, characterized by the symmetrical progressive loss of fat from the face, neck, arms, thorax, and abdomen, associated with an increase of fat in the legs and thighs.

progressive locomotor ataxia. TABES DORSALIS.

progressive multifocal leukoencephalopathy. A rapidly progressive neurological disorder, found in association with diseases of the reticuloendothelial system, carcinomas, and occasionally other debilitating illnesses; clinical findings vary with the loci of demyelination, which are characterized pathologically by bizarre giant cells derived from astrocytes and abnormally large oligodendroglial cells often containing intranuclear inclusions; thought to be due to a papova-like virus, closely resembling the polyoma virus.

progressive muscular dystrophy. Chronic progressive wasting and weakness of skeletal musculature, frequently hereditary and usually associated with elevations of serum creatine kinase and electromyographic abnormalities. There are several variants, named after the age of onset, site of initial muscular involvement, and the severity and distribution of apparent hypertrophy and atrophy. See also *pseudohypertrophic infantile muscular dystrophy, facioscapulohumeral muscular dystrophy, limb-girdle muscular dystrophy, distal muscular dystrophy.*

progressive myopia of children. Continuous increase of myopia, due to increasing growth of the eyeball.

progressive nervous atrophy. Chronic adhesive arachnoiditis of the spine. See *chronic adhesive arachnoiditis.*

progressive neural muscular atrophy. PERONEAL MUSCULAR ATROPHY.

progressive neuropathic muscular atrophy. PERONEAL MUSCULAR ATROPHY.

progressive pallidal atrophy or **degeneration.** JUVENILE PARALYSIS AGITANS.

progressive pallidal degeneration syndrome. HALLERVORDEN-SPATZ DISEASE.

progressive pigmentary dermatosis. A form of capillaritis, characterized by a reddish, purpuric, papular eruption; it is seen principally on the legs and is often progressive in character. Syn. *Schamberg's disease.*

progressive-resistance exercise. An exercise to increase the power of a weakened muscle, or muscles, in which resistance to contraction is progressively increased as muscle power improves. Syn. *graduated-resistance exercise.* See also *load-assisting exercise, load-resisting exercise.*

progressive spastic paraplegia. FAMILIAL SPASTIC PARAPLEGIA.

progressive spinal muscular atrophy. A chronic slowly progressive wasting of individual muscles, or physiologic groups of muscles, and associated weakness and paralysis, usually symmetrical, but more frequently involving the upper extremities than the lower; due to degeneration of the anterior horn cells of the spinal cord, with consecutive degeneration of the anterior nerve roots and muscles, and, occasionally, involvement of bulbar nuclei. It affects adults primarily and may be caused by infections, toxins, avitaminosis, or familial factors. See also *infantile spinal muscular atrophy.*

progressive stroke. A neurological deficit due to occlusive cerebrovascular disease in which the deficit has been present for a day or more and continues to worsen while the patient is under observation.

progressive subcortical encephalopathy. BINSWANGER'S DISEASE.

progressive subcortical gliosis. A rare form of presenile dementia with an insidious progressive course, characterized pathologically by pronounced subcortical gliosis without severe involvement of the cerebral cortex and no significant myelin loss.

progressive supranuclear palsy. A progressive neurologic disorder with onset in late middle life, characterized by a staring facial expression due to impairment of convergence and voluntary, especially vertical, gaze, derangement of optokinetic and vestibular nystagmus, dystonia and other extrapyramidal signs, as well as progressive spasticity and dementia; cause is unknown. Syn. *Steele-Richardson-Olszewski syndrome.*

progressive systemic sclerosis. DIFFUSE SCLERODERMA.

progressive thrombus. A thrombus that continues to grow in the lumen of a vessel.

progressive unilateral facial atrophy. PROGRESSIVE FACIAL HEMIATROPHY.

progressive vaccinia. A complication of smallpox vaccination, observed in patients with impaired immune mechanisms, in which necrotizing and pustular lesions at the original site of vaccination extend and secondary lesions appear elsewhere on the skin and mucous membranes. Syn. *vaccinia gangrenosa, vaccinia necrosum.*

pro·gua·nil (pro·gwah'nil) *n.* Chloroguanide, an antimalarial drug used as the hydrochloride salt.

Progynon. A trademark for certain preparations of estradiol, an estrogenic hormone.

Prohalone. Trademark for haloprogesterone, a progestational drug.

pro·in·su·lin (pro·in'sue·lin) *n.* The precursor of insulin; a single-chain protein, with a molecular weight of approximately 9,000, which is converted to the two-chain insulin molecule by enzyme-catalyzed proteolytic cleavage.

pro·io·sys·to·le (pro''ee·o·sis'tuh·lee) *n.* [Gk. *prōïos*, early, + *systole*]. PREMATURE BEAT.

pro·i·o·tes (pro''ee·o'teez) *n.* PROIOTIA.

pro·i·o·tia (pro''ee·o'shee·uh) *n.* [NL., from Gk. *prōïos*, early]. Sexual precocity.

pro·jec·tile (pro·jeck'til, ·tile) *adj.* Hurled or impelled forward with great force.

projectile vomiting. A form of vomiting in which the stomach contents are suddenly and forcefully shot forth out of the mouth to some distance, usually without nausea.

pro·jec·tion (pro·jeck'shun) *n.* [L. *projectio*, from *projicere*, to throw forward]. 1. The act of throwing forward. 2. A part extending beyond its surroundings. 3. The referring of impressions made on the organs of sense to the position of the object producing them. 4. *In psychology,* the process of unconsciously attributing to other persons or objects one's own qualities or feelings, as a child's assumption that his mother feels as he does. 5. *In psychiatry,* a defense mechanism against feelings of inadequacy or guilt, operating unconsciously, whereby what is emotionally unacceptable to the self is rejected and attributed to others. 6. *In neurology,* the connection of parts of the cerebral cortex (projection area) through projection fibers with subcortical centers which, in turn, are connected with peripheral sense organs.

projection area or **center.** An area of the cortex connected with lower centers by projection fibers. Contr. *association area.*

projection fibers. Fibers joining the cerebral cortex to lower centers, and vice versa.

projection systems. The pathways connecting some structure of the nervous system to some other structure of the nervous system.

pro·jec·tive (pro·jeck'tiv) *adj.* Pertaining to or caused by projection.

projective identification. A form of identification in which the individual does not distinguish between self and object with respect to certain impulses but continues to experience the impulse as well as the fear of that impulse from the person upon whom it is projected. Compare *projection* (4, 5).

projective technique. *In psychology,* any procedure used to discover, estimate, and evaluate a person's characteristic modes of thought and behavior, his personality traits, attitudes, and motivation, by observing his responses to a relatively unstructured situation that does not elicit or require a specific or limited reaction. See also *projective test.*

projective test. *In psychology,* a test given in a relatively unstructured, yet standard situation in which the responses of the subject to the material presented are determined by his prevailing mood and personality characteristics; they may also reveal certain modes of cognition. Test materials include inkblots (Rorschach), pictures of human situations or of clouds, play materials, incomplete sentences to be completed, drawing a human figure, or other drawing tasks.

pro·kary·ote, pro·cary·ote (pro·kăr'ee·ote) *n.* [*pro-* + Gk. *karyon,* kernel, nucleus]. The more primitive type of cellular organism, including bacteria and blue-green algae, which have no membrane-bound nucleus or membrane-bound organelles. Contr. *eukaryote.* —**pro·kary·ot·ic, pro·cary·ot·ic** (·kăr''ee·ot'ick) *adj.*

Proketazine. Trademark for carphenazine, a tranquilizer used as a maleate salt.

pro·ki·nase (pro·kigh'nace, ·kin'ace, ·aze) *n.* A proteolytic enzyme found in extracts of the pancreas and demonstrated to pass into the pancreatic secretion.

pro·la·bi·um (pro·lay'bee·um) *n.* [*pro-* + *labium*]. 1. The exposed part of the lip. 2. The central prominence of the lip.

pro·lac·tin (pro·lack'tin) *n.* A hormone secreted by the adenohypophysis, which stimulates lactation in the mammalian breast and also promotes functional activity of the corpus luteum. Syn. *lactogenic hormone, luteotropic hormone, mammotropin.*

pro·lam·in (pro·lam'in, pro'luh·min) *n.* Any one of a class of simple proteins, such as gliadin or hordein, occurring especially in grains.

pro·lam·ine (pro·lam'een, ·in, pro'luh·meen) *n.* PROLAMIN.

pro·lan (pro'lan) *n.* An old term for follicle-stimulating and luteinizing gonadotropic hormones of the anterior pituitary.

pro·lapse (pro·laps', pro'laps) *n.* & *v.* [L. *prolapsus,* from *pro-,* forward, + *labi,* to fall, slip]. 1. The falling or sinking down of a part or organ; procidentia. 2. To fall or sink down.

prolapsed hemorrhoids. Those in which the enlarged veins protrude through the external anal sphincter.

prolapse of the cord. Premature expulsion of the umbilical cord during parturition, prior to delivery of the fetus.

prolapse of the iris. Protrusion of the iris through a corneal wound.

prolapse of the uterus. Displacement of the uterus downward, sometimes outside the vulva. Syn. *descensus uteri, prolapsus uteri.* See also *frank prolapse.*

prolapse pessary. A ring or cup inserted into the vagina for the purpose of holding up the uterus.

pro·lap·sus (pro·lap'sus) *n.* [L.]. PROLAPSE.

prolapsus ani (ay'nigh). Extrusion of the lower division of the intestinal tract through the external sphincter of the anus.

prolapsus ute·ri (yoo'tur·eye). PROLAPSE OF THE UTERUS.

pro·late (pro'late) *adj.* [L. *prolatus,* brought forward]. Having a form or shape which is elongated along the polar diameter.

prolate spheroid. A spheroid in which the polar axis exceeds the equatorial diameter.

pro·lep·sis (pro·lep'sis) *n.,* pl. **prolep·ses** (·seez) [Gk. *prolēpsis,* anticipation]. In a periodic or recurrent disease, the return of an attack or paroxysm before the expected time or at progressively shorter intervals. —**prolep·tic** (·tick) *adj.*

pro·leu·ko·cyte, pro·leu·co·cyte (pro·lew'ko·site) *n.* [*pro-* + *leukocyte*]. LEUKOBLAST.

pro·lif·er·ate (pro·lif'ur·ate) *v.* To multiply; to generate by increase in number.

pro·lif·er·a·tion (pro·lif''ur·ay'shun) *n.* [ML. *prolifer,* proliferous, from L. *proles,* offspring, + *ferre,* to bear]. Rapid and increased production, as of offspring, or of new parts or cells by repeated cell division. —**pro·lif·er·a·tive** (pro·lif'ur·uh·tiv) *adj.*

proliferative arthritis. RHEUMATOID ARTHRITIS.

proliferative cyst. A cyst in which the lining epithelium proliferates and produces projections from the inner surface of the cyst.

proliferative ileitis. An intestinal infection of unknown etiology that occurs both enzootically and epizootically in hamsters.

proliferative inflammation. PRODUCTIVE INFLAMMATION.

pro·lif·er·ous (pro·lif'ur·us) *adj.* [ML. *prolifer,* from L. *proles,* offspring, + *ferre,* to bear]. 1. Capable of bearing offspring. 2. Reproducing by means of buds.

pro·lif·ic (pro·lif'ick) *adj.* [ML. *prolificus,* from L. *proles,* offspring]. Fruitful; highly productive.

pro·lig·er·ous (pro·lij'ur·us) *adj.* [L. *proles,* offspring, + *gerere,* to carry, bear]. Germinating; producing offspring.

proligerous cyst. Cyst formation in an adenocarcinoma.

pro·lin·ase (pro'lin·ace, ·aze) *n.* The enzyme that hydrolyzes proline peptides to proline and simpler peptides.

pro·line (pro'leen, ·lin) *n.* 2-Pyrrolidinecarboxylic acid, $C_5H_9NO_2$, an amino acid resulting from the hydrolysis of proteins.

pro·lin·emia, pro·lin·ae·mia (pro''lin·ee'mee·uh) *n.* HYPERPROLINEMIA.

pro·lin·tane (pro·lin'tane) *n.* 1-(α-Propylphenethyl)pyrrolidine, $C_{15}H_{23}N$, an antidepressant drug; used as the hydrochloride salt.

pro·lin·uria (pro·lin·yoo'ree·uh) *n.* [*proline* + *-uria*]. The presence of proline in the urine.

pro·li·pase (pro·lye'pace, ·paze) *n.* Inactive form of steapsin found in pancreatic juice.

Prolixin. A trademark for fluphenazine, a tranquilizing drug used as the dihydrochloride salt.

pro·lon·gev·i·ty (pro''lon·jev'i·tee) *n.* The significant extension of the length of life by human action.

pro·lyl (pro'lil) *n.* The univalent radical, $HNCH_2CH_2CH_2CHCO$—, of the amino acid proline.

pro·lym·pho·cyte (pro·lim'fo·site) *n.* [*pro-* + *lymphocyte*]. A cell of the lymphocyte series intermediate in maturity between the lymphoblast and the lymphocyte.

pro·ma·zine (pro'muh·zeen) *n.* 10-[3-(Dimethylamino)propyl]phenothiazine, $C_{17}H_{20}N_2S$, a drug with antiemetic, tranquilizing, and analgesic-potentiating actions; used as the hydrochloride salt.

pro·mega·karyo·cyte (pro·meg''uh·kăr'ee·o·site) *n.* [*pro-* + *megakaryocyte*]. The precursor of a megakaryocyte. It is smaller than the megakaryocyte; the nucleus becomes indented; cytoplasm is lightly basophilic and contains fine granules. Syn. *lymphoid megakaryocyte.*

pro·meg·a·lo·blast (pro·meg'uh·lo·blast) *n.* [*pro-* + *megaloblast*]. The earliest precursor of the abnormal red blood cells in diseases such as pernicious anemia; it is similar to the pronormoblast, but the nuclear chromatin is finer and arranged in a scrollwork pattern.

pro·meg·a·lo·karyo·cyte (pro·meg″uh·lo·kăr′ee·o·site) *n.* PROMEGAKARYOCYTE.

pro·meso·bil·i·fus·cin (pro″mes·o·bil·i·fus′in) *n.* A colorless precursor of mesobilifuscin, apparently identical with mesobilileukan.

pro·meth·a·zine (pro·meth′uh·zeen) *n.* 10-(2-Dimethylaminopropyl)phenothiazine, $C_{17}H_{20}N_2S$, an antihistaminic drug used as the hydrochloride salt.

pro·meth·es·trol, pro·meth·oes·trol (pro·meth′es·trol, pro″me·thes′trol) *n.* 4,4′-(1,2-Diethylethylene)di-*o*-cresol, $C_{20}H_{26}O_2$, a synthetic estrogen used as the dipropionate ester.

pro·me·thi·um (pro·meeth′ee·um) *n.* [*Prometheus,* the Titan pioneer of civilization]. Pm = 147. The name finally adopted for element 61, obtained in radioactive form in certain nuclear reactions.

Prominal. A trademark for the long-acting barbiturate mephobarbital.

prom·i·nence (prom′i·nunce) *n.* [L. *prominentia,* from *pro-* + *minere,* to project]. 1. A projection, especially on a bone. 2. The state of projecting or standing out.

pro·mi·nen·tia (prom″i·nen′shee·uh) *n.,* pl. **prominen·ti·ae** (·shee·ee) [L.]. PROMINENCE.

prominentia ca·na·lis fa·ci·a·lis (ka·nay′lis fay·shee·ay′lis) [NA]. The ridge on the medial wall of the tympanic cavity overlying the facial nerve.

prominentia canalis se·mi·cir·cu·la·ris la·te·ra·lis (sem″i·sur·kew·lair′is lat·e·ray′lis) [NA]. The bulge on the medial wall of the middle ear overlying the lateral semicircular canal.

prominentia la·ryn·gea (la·rin′jee·uh) [NA]. LARYNGEAL PROMINENCE.

prominentia mal·le·a·ris (mal·ee·air′is) [NA]. MALLEAR PROMINENCE.

prominentia mal·le·o·la·ris (mal·ee·o·lair′is) [BNA]. Prominentia mallearis (= MALLEAR PROMINENCE).

prominentia spi·ra·lis (spye·ray′lis) [NA]. A ridge on the outer wall of the cochlear duct.

prominentia sty·loi·dea (stye·loy′dee·uh) [NA]. A variable elevation of the floor of the tympanic cavity overlying the base of the styloid process.

prom·ne·sia (prom·nee′zhuh) *n.* [*pro-* + *-mnesia*]. PARAMNESIA.

pro·mono·cyte (pro·mon′o·site) *n.* [*pro-* + *monocyte*]. 1. An immature monocyte derived from a monoblast. The nucleus is spheroidal or moderately indented, and a nucleolus may be visible. Syn. *young monocyte, premonocyte.* 2. One of the transitional stages between the lymphocyte and monocyte.

pro·mon·to·ri·um (prom″on·to′ree·um) *n.,* pl. **promonto·ria** (·ree·uh) [L.]. PROMONTORY.

promontorium ca·vi tym·pa·ni (kay′vye tim′puh·nigh) [NA]. PROMONTORY OF THE MIDDLE EAR.

promontorium os·sis sa·cri (os′is say′krye) [NA]. PROMONTORY OF THE SACRUM.

prom·on·to·ry (prom′un·to·ree) *n.* [L. *promontorium,* from *prominere,* to project]. A projecting prominence.

promontory of the middle ear. The outward protrusion on the inner wall of the middle ear formed by the basal turn of the cochlea.

promontory of the sacrum. The prominence formed by the angle between the upper extremity of the sacrum and the last lumbar vertebra. NA *promontorium ossis sacri.*

pro·mot·er (pruh·mo′tur) *n.* *In genetics,* the point in an operon at which sequential transcription of two or more cistrons begins.

pro·my·e·lo·cyte (pro·migh′e·lo·site) *n.* [*pro-* + *myelocyte*]. The earliest myelocyte stage derived from the myeloblast; it contains a few granules, some of which may be azurophilic, while others may be characteristic of the type of granulocyte into which the myelocyte develops. In early forms, the nucleus may be covered by the nonspecific granules and still contain small nucleoli.

pro·nate (pro′nate) *v.* [L. *pronare,* to bend forward]. 1. To turn the forearm so that the palm of the hand is down or toward the back. 2. In the foot, to turn the sole outward with the lateral margin of the foot elevated; to evert.

pro·na·tion (pro·nay′shun) *n.* 1. The condition of being prone; the act of placing in the prone position. 2. The turning of the palm of the hand downward.

pronation phenomenon. Immediate return to pronation position of the hand on the affected side of the hemiplegic patient when both hands are passively supinated and suddenly released.

pronation-supination test. A cerebellar function test in which the arms, extended in front, are rapidly pronated and supinated. Normally the movements are of equal amplitude, smooth and even.

pro·na·tor (pro·nay′tur, pro′nay·tur) *n.* That which pronates, as the pronator teres (musculus pronator teres) and pronator quadratus (musculus pronator quadratus), muscles of the forearm attached to the ulna and radius. See also Table of Muscles in the Appendix.

pronator qua·dra·tus (kwah·dray′tus). See Table of Muscles in the Appendix.

pronator ra·dii te·res (ray′dee·eye terr′eez). The pronator teres muscle. See Table of Muscles in the Appendix.

pronator ridge. The bony ridge on the lower anterior surface of the ulna for the attachment of the pronator teres muscle.

pronator te·res (teer′eez, terr′eez). See Table of Muscles in the Appendix.

prone, *adj.* [L. *pronus,* leaning forward]. Lying with the face downward. Contr. *supine.*

pronephric duct. The duct of the pronephros. It becomes the functional mesonephric duct. Syn. *archinephric duct.*

pro·neph·ros (pro·nef′ros) *n.,* pl. **proneph·roi** (·roy) [*pro-* + *nephros*]. The primitive or head kidney, derived from the cranial part of the nephrogenic cord. Vestigial in mammalian embryos, its duct, the pronephric duct, is taken over by the mesonephros and called the mesonephric duct. —**proneph·ric** (·rick) *adj.*

prone pressure method. SCHAFER METHOD.

Pronestyl. Trademark for the antiarrhythmic cardiac depressant procainamide, used as the hydrochloride salt.

pro·neth·al·ol (pro·neth′ul·ol) *n.* α-[(Isopropylamino)methyl]-2-naphthalenemethanol, $C_{15}H_{19}NO$, a beta-adrenergic blocking agent. Syn. *nethalide.*

pro·no·grade (pro′no·grade) *adj.* [L. *pron*us, leaning forward, + *gradi,* to walk]. Walking or standing on all fours, as the quadrupeds. Contr. *orthograde.*

pro·nor·mo·blast (pro·nor′mo·blast) *n.* [*pro-* + *normoblast*]. The earliest erythrocyte precursor; a round or oval cell 12 to 19 microns in diameter, with a large nucleus having fine chromatin and nucleoli, with scanty, basophilic cytoplasm without hemoglobin. Syn. *macroblast, rubriblast, prorubricyte, lymphoid hemoblast (of Pappenheim), proerythroblast (of Ferrata), megaloblast (of Sabin).*

pro·nor·mo·cyte (pro·nor′mo·site) *n.* [*pro-* + *normocyte*]. RETICULOCYTE (1).

pro·nounced, *adj.* Strongly marked, distinct; readily perceivable or recognizable.

Prontosil. Trademark for 2,4-diaminoazobenzene-4′-sulfonamide hydrochloride, the forerunner of the sulfonamide drugs.

pro·nu·cle·us (pro·new′klee·us) *n.* [*pro-* + *nucleus*]. One of the two nuclear bodies of a newly fertilized ovum, the male pronucleus and the female pronucleus, the fusion of which results in the formation of the germinal (cleavage) nucleus.

pro-oestrus. PROESTRUS.

proof gallon. A gallon of proof spirit.

proof spirit. A mixture of ethyl alcohol and water containing 50% by volume of C_2H_5OH.

pro·otic (pro·o'tick, ·ot'ick) *adj.* [*pro-* + *otic*]. In front of the ear.

pro·ovar·i·um (pro"o·văr'ee·um) *n.* [*pro-* + *ovarium*]. EPOOPHORON.

pro·pa·di·ene (pro"pa·dye'een) *n.* ALLENE.

Propadrine. A trademark for the sympathomimetic amine, phenylpropanolamine, used as the hydrochloride salt mainly for bronchodilator action.

pro·pae·deu·tics, pro·pe·deu·tics (pro"pe·dew'ticks) *n.* [*pro-* + Gk. *paideutikos*, of teaching]. Preliminary instruction. —**propaedeu·tic** (·tick) *adj.*

prop·a·gate (prop'uh·gate) *v.* [L. *propagare*, to extend, to generate]. To produce offspring; to multiply; to extend forward. —**prop·a·ga·tion** (prop"uh·gay'shun) *n.*

pro·pal·i·nal (pro·pal'i·nul) *adj.* [*pro-*, forward, + Gk. *palin*, backward, + *-al*]. *In biology*, pertaining to the forward and backward action of the jaws of some animals.

pro·pane (pro'pane) *n.* The gaseous hydrocarbon $CH_3CH_2CH_3$, occurring in natural gas and in solution in crude petroleum.

1,2-pro·pane·di·ol (pro"pane·dye'ol) *n.* PROPYLENE GLYCOL.

pro·pan·i·did (pro·pan'i·did) *n.* Propyl {4-[(diethylcarbamoyl)methoxy]-3-methoxyphenyl}acetate, $C_{18}H_{27}NO_5$, a general anesthetic, administered intravenously.

pro·pa·no·ic acid (pro"pa·no'ick). PROPIONIC ACID.

pro·pa·none (pro'puh·nohn) *n.* ACETONE.

pro·pan·the·line bromide (pro·panth'e·leen). (2-Hydroxyethyl)diisopropylmethylammonium bromide 9-xanthenecarboxylate, $C_{23}H_{30}BrNO_3$, an anticholinergic drug.

pro·par·a·caine (pro·păr'uh·kane) *n.* 2-Diethylaminoethyl 3-amino-4-propoxybenzoate, $C_{16}H_{26}N_2O_3$, a surface anesthetic employed in ophthalmology; used as the hydrochloride salt.

pro·pa·tyl nitrate (pro'puh·til). 2-Ethyl-2-(hydroxymethyl)-1,3-propanediol trinitrate, $C_6H_{11}N_3O_9$, a coronary vasodilator.

propedeutics. PROPAEDEUTICS.

pro·pel·lant 12. Dichlorodifluoromethane, CCl_2F_2, an aerosol propellant.

pro·pene (pro'peen) *n.* PROPYLENE.

propene nitrile. ACRYLONITRILE.

pro·pe·no·ic acid (pro"pe·no'ick). ACRYLIC ACID.

pro·pent·dy·o·pent (pro"pent·dye'o·pent) *n.* Either of the two colorless compounds, each containing two pyrrole rings, obtained when heme, bilirubin, or any other pigment containing four pyrrole rings is oxidized with hydrogen peroxide in alkaline solution. On reduction with sodium dithionite, a propentdyopent is converted to a red pigment known by the generic name pentdyopent.

pro·pe·nyl (pro'pe·nil) *n.* The monovalent radical $CH_3CH=CH—$, derived from propylene.

pro·pen·zo·late (pro·pen'zo·late) *n.* (+)-1-Methyl-3-piperidyl-(±)-α-phenylcyclohexaneglycolate, $C_{20}H_{29}NO_3$, an anticholinergic drug; used as the hydrochloride salt.

pro·pep·sin (pro·pep'sin) *n.* The zymogen of pepsin, found in the cells of the gastric glands. Syn. *pepsinogen.*

pro·pep·tone (pro·pep'tone) *n.* HEMIALBUMOSE.

pro·pep·to·nu·ria (pro"pep·to·new'ree·uh) *n.* [*propeptone* + *-uria*]. The presence of propeptone in the urine.

pro·per·din (pro·pur'din, pro'pur·din) *n.* [*pro-* + L. *per*dere, to destroy, + *-in*]. A macroglobulin of normal plasma capable of killing various bacteria and viruses in the presence of complement and magnesium ions, and involved in the alternate pathway of complement activation.

properdin system. ALTERNATE COMPLEMENT PATHWAY.

proper hepatic artery. The hepatic artery after it gives off the right gastric and gastroduodenal arteries. NA *arteria hepatica propria.* See also Table of Arteries in the Appendix.

pro·peri·to·ne·al (pro"perr·i·to·nee'ul) *adj.* [*pro-* + *peritoneal*]. Situated in front of the peritoneum.

properitoneal hernia. EPIGASTRIC HERNIA.

proper ligament of the ovary. OVARIAN LIGAMENT.

proper ovarian ligament. OVARIAN LIGAMENT.

pro·phase (pro'faze) *n.* [*pro-* + *phase*]. 1. The first stage of mitosis, in which the chromosomes are organized from nuclear materials as elongate spiremes. 2. The first stage of the first (prophase I) or second (prophase II) meiotic divisions; the first meiotic prophase is further divided into leptotene, zygotene, pachytene, diplotene, and diakinesis.

pro·phen·py·rid·a·mine (pro"fen·pi·rid'uh·meen) *n.* PHENIRAMINE.

pro·phy·lac·tic (pro·fi·lack'tick) *adj.* & *n.* [Gk. *prophylaktikos*, from *prophylax*, advance guard, from *phylax*, guard]. 1. Pertaining to prophylaxis; tending to prevent disease. 2. Any agent or device that prevents or helps to prevent the development of disease. 3. CONDOM.

prophylactic forceps operation. The routine delivery by forceps in head presentations as soon as the head has come to rest on the pelvic floor.

prophylactic odontotomy. Opening and filling structural imperfections of the enamel to prevent dental caries.

prophylactic orthodontics. PREVENTIVE ORTHODONTICS.

prophylactic version. Converting a vertex into a breech presentation to avoid prolonged pressure on the head. Formerly employed in moderate dystocia.

pro·phy·lax·is (pro"fi·lack'sis) *n.*, pl. **prophylax·es** (·seez) [NL., from Gk. *prophylaktikos*, prophylactic]. 1. Prevention of disease; measures preventing the development or spread of disease. See also *dental prophylaxis.* 2. *In military medicine*, measures taken to prevent or reduce the harmful effects of chemical agents.

pro·pi·cil·lin (pro"pi·sil'in) *n.* α-Phenoxypropylpenicillin, $C_{18}H_{22}N_2O_5S$, a semisynthetic penicillin that is acid-resistant; administered orally as the potassium salt.

pro·pio·lac·tone (pro"pee·o·lack'tone) *n.* β-Propiolactone, or hydracrylic acid β-lactone, $C_3H_4O_2$, a disinfectant.

pro·pi·o·ma·zine (pro"pee·o'muh·zeen) *n.* 3-Propionyl-10-dimethylaminoisopropylphenothiazine, $C_{20}H_{24}N_2OS$, a sedative especially useful as an adjunct in enhancing the action of analgesics and anesthetics; used as the hydrochloride salt.

propion-, propiono-. *In chemistry*, a combining form meaning *propionic.*

pro·pi·o·nate (pro'pee·o·nate) *n.* A salt of propionic acid.

Pro·pi·oni·bac·te·ri·um (pro"pee·on"i·back·teer'ee·um) *n.* A genus of bacteria of the family Lactobacteriaceae, which ferment hexoses to predominantly propionic and acetic acids.

pro·pi·on·ic acid (pro"pee·on'ick) [*pro-* + Gk. *piōn*, fat, + *-ic*]. Propanoic acid, CH_3CH_2COOH, used as the acid and in the form of its calcium and sodium salts as a topical fungicide.

propiono-. See *propion-.*

pro·pi·ram (pro'pi·ram) *n.* *N*-(1-Methyl-2-piperidinoethyl)-*N*-2-pyridylpropionamide, $C_{16}H_{25}N_3O$, an analgesic; used as the fumarate salt.

pro·pit·o·caine (pro·pit'o·kane) *n.* PRILOCAINE.

pro·plas·ma·cyte (pro·plaz'muh·site) *n.* [*pro-* + *plasmacyte*]. 1. The precursor of the plasmacyte (plasma cell), usually larger than the adult cell, with a nucleus which has a finer chromatin structure and which is not necessarily eccentrically placed. Syn. *lymphoblastic* or *myeloblastic plasma cell.* 2. TÜRK CELL.

pro·pos·i·tus (pro·poz'i·tus) *n.*, pl. **proposi·ti** (·tye) [NL., from L. *propositum*, subject, premise, from *proponere*, to set before]. PROBAND.

pro·poxy·caine (pro·pock'see·kane) *n.* 2-Diethylaminoethyl 4-amino-2-propoxybenzoate, $C_{16}H_{26}N_2O_3$, a local anesthetic used as the hydrochloride salt.

pro·poxy·phene (pro·pock'see·feen) *n.* (+)-α-4-(Dimethylamino)-3-methyl-1,2-diphenyl-2-butanol propionate, $C_{22}H_{29}NO_2$, an analgesic compound, structurally related to methadone, employed for relief of mild to moderate pain; used as the hydrochloride salt.

pro·pran·ol·ol (pro·pran'o·lol) *n.* 1-(Isopropylamino)-3-(1-naphthyloxy)-2-propanol, $C_{16}H_{21}NO_2$, an antiarrhythmic drug used as the hydrochloride salt.

pro·pri·al (pro'pree·ul) *adj.* Pertaining to a lamina propria.

pro·pri·etary (pro·prye'e·terr''ee) *n. & adj.* [L. *proprietarius*, of a proprietor]. 1. Any chemical, drug, or similar preparation used in the treatment of diseases, if such an article is protected against free competition as to name, product, composition, or process of manufacture, by secrecy, patent, copyright, or any other means. 2. Of or pertaining to a proprietary or a proprietor; protected by copyright or patent; made, marketed, or operated by a person or persons having the exclusive right to do so.

proprietary medicine. A medicine, the manufacture of which is limited or controlled by an owner because of a patent, copyright, or secrecy as regards its constitution or method of manufacture.

pro·prio·cep·tion (pro''pree·o·sep'shun) *n.* [L. *proprius*, one's own, + per*ception*]. The normal ongoing awareness, mediated by the action of proprioceptors, of the position, balance, and movement of one's own body or any of its parts. —**propriocep·tive** (·tiv) *adj.*

proprioceptive impulses. Afferent nerve impulses originating in receptors in the muscles, tendons, joints, and vestibular apparatus of the internal ear. Their reflex functions are concerned with movement and maintenance of posture.

proprioceptive reflex. Any reflex elicited by stimulation of a proprioceptor. See also *proprioceptive impulses.*

pro·prio·cep·tor (pro''pree·o·sep'tur) *n.* [L. *proprius*, one's own, + re*ceptor*]. A receptor located in a muscle, tendon, joint, or vestibular apparatus, whose reflex function is locomotor or postural.

pro·pri·us (pro'pree·us) *adj.* [L.]. Individual; special; applied to certain muscles.

prop·tom·e·ter (prop·tom'e·tur) *n.* [*proptosis* + *-meter*]. An instrument for measuring the amount of exophthalmos.

prop·to·sis (prop·to'sis) *n.*, pl. **propto·ses** (·seez) [Gk. *proptōsis*, from *pro-* + *ptōsis*, fall]. 1. A falling downward or forward. 2. PROLAPSE. 3. EXOPHTHALMOS. —**prop·tot·ic** (·tot'ick) *adj.*

pro·pul·sion (pro·pul'shun) *n.* [ML. *propulsio*, from L. *propellere*, to propel]. 1. The act of pushing or driving forward. 2. A leaning and falling forward in walking, as observed in parkinsonism and other disorders of the nervous system. —**propul·sive** (·siv) *adj.*

pro·pyl (pro'pil) *n.* The univalent radical $CH_3CH_2CH_2$—, derived from propane.

pro·pyl·ace·tic acid (pro''pil·a·see'tick). Normal VALERIC ACID.

propyl alcohol. 1-Propanol, or *n*-propyl alcohol, $CH_3CH_2CH_2OH$, used as a solvent.

propyl ami·no·ben·zo·ate (a·mee''no·ben'zo·ate). Propyl *p*-aminobenzoate, $C_{10}H_{13}NO_2$, a topical anesthetic and antipruritic.

pro·pyl·ene (pro'pi·leen) *n.* 1. C_3H_6; the unsaturated hydrocarbon, $CH_3CH{=}CH_2$, a homologue of ethylene and isomer of cyclopropane; a colorless gas. 2. The monovalent radical, $CH_2CH{=}CH$—. 3. The bivalent radical, —$CH(CH_3)CH_2$—.

propylene glycol. 1,2-Propanediol, $CH_3CHOHCH_2OH$, used as a solvent vehicle for many medicinals.

pro·pyl·hex·e·drine (pro''pil·heck'se·dreen) *n.* *N*,α-Dimethylcyclohexaneethylamine, $C_{10}H_{21}N$, a volatile sympathomimetic amine used as a nasal decongestant.

pro·pyl·io·done (pro''pil·eye'o·dohn) *n.* Propyl 3,5-diiodo-4-oxo-1(4*H*)-pyridineacetate, $C_{10}H_{11}I_2NO_3$, a radiopaque contrast medium used in bronchography.

pro·pyl·par·a·ben (pro''pil·păr'a·ben) *n.* Propyl *p*-hydroxybenzoate, $C_{10}H_{12}O_3$, an antifungal preservative agent.

pro·pyl·thio·ura·cil (pro''pil·thigh''o·yoor'uh·sil) *n.* 6-Propyl-2-thiouracil, $C_7H_{10}N_2OS$, a thyroid inhibitor used in the treatment of hyperthyroidism.

pro·pyne (pro'pine) *n.* ALLYLENE.

pro·qua·zone (pro'kwuh·zone) *n.* 1-Isopropyl-7-methyl-4-phenyl-2(1*H*)-quinazolinone, $C_{18}H_{18}N_2O$, an anti-inflammatory.

pro re na·ta (pro ree nay'tuh) [L.]. According to the circumstances of the case, or when necessary. Abbreviated, p.r.n.

pro·ren·nin (pro·ren'in) *n.* RENNINOGEN.

pro·ren·o·ate potassium (pro·ren'o·ate). Potassium 6,7-dihydro-17-hydroxy-3-oxo-3'*H*-cyclopropa[6,7]-17α-pregna-4,6-diene-21-carboxylate, $C_{23}H_{31}KO_4$, an aldosterone antagonist.

pro·ru·bri·cyte (pro·roo'bri·site) *n.* [*pro-* + *rubricyte*]. PRONORMOBLAST.

pros-, proso- [Gk. *pros*, near, toward; *prosō-*, forward, onward]. A prefix meaning (a) *forward, fore-;* (b) *near, close;* (c) *onward, further.*

pro·sce·nio·pho·bia (pro·see''nee·o·fo'bee·uh) *n.* [*proscenium* + *-phobia*]. Stage fright.

pro·scil·lar·i·din (pro''sil·ăr'i·din) *n.* 3β,14β-Dihydroxybufa-4,20,22-trienolide 3-rhamnoside, $C_{30}H_{42}O_8$, a cardioactive steroid glycoside from squill.

pro·se·cre·tin (pro·se·kree'tin) *n.* [*pro-* + *secretin*]. The precursor of secretin; it is secreted by the epithelium of the small intestine.

pro·sect (pro·sekt') *v.* [L. *prosecare*, to cut away]. To dissect a subject or part for purposes of anatomic teaching or demonstration.

pro·sec·tor (pro·seck'tur) *n.* An individual who prepares subjects for anatomic dissection or to illustrate didactic lectures.

prosencephalic dysraphism. Failure in closure of the embryonic prosencephalic vesicle.

prosencephalic vesicle. PROSENCEPHALON.

pros·en·ceph·a·lon (pros''en·sef'uh·lon) *n.* [*pros-* + *encephalon*] [NA]. The forebrain or anterior brain vesicle of the embryo that subdivides into telencephalon and diencephalon. From it are derived the cerebral hemispheres, olfactory lobes, corpus striatum, and various parts of the thalamus, as well as the third and the lateral ventricles. —**prosen·ce·phal·ic** (·se·fal'ick) *adj.*

pro·se·ro·zyme (pro·seer'o·zime) *n.* PROTHROMBIN.

pro·sim·ian (pro·sim'ee·un) *adj. & n.* 1. Of or pertaining to the Prosimii. 2. An animal belonging to the Prosimii. Contr. *anthropoid.*

Pro·sim·ii (pro·sim'ee·eye) *n.pl.* [NL., from *pro-* + L. *simia*, monkey, ape]. The more primitive of the two suborders of Primates, comprising lemurs, lorises, pottos, galagos, tarsiers, and, in some classifications, tree shrews. Contr. *Anthropoidea.*

proso·coele (pros'o·seel) *n.* [*proso-* + *-coele*]. The cavity of the prosencephalon.

proso·dem·ic (pros''o·dem'ick) *adj.* [*proso-* + *dem-* + *-ic*]. Pertaining to disease spread by direct individual contact, as opposed to one spread by general means such as a water or milk supply.

pros·o·dy (pros'uh·dee) *n.* [Gk. *prosōidia*]. *In phonology,* the system of rhythmic and melodic elements in speech, consisting mainly of modulations in pitch, timing, and loudness, which help to organize the segmental elements and supplement their meaning. See also *dysprosody.*

prosop-, prosopo- [Gk. *prosōpon*]. A combining form meaning *face, facial.*

pros·op·ag·no·sia (pros''up·ag·no'see·uh) *n.* [*prosop-* + *agnosia*]. A form of visual agnosia characterized by inability to identify a familiar face either by looking at the person or at a picture, even though the patient knows that it is a face and can point to its separate parts.

pro·sop·a·gus (pro·sop'uh·gus) *n.* PROSOPOPAGUS.

pros·o·pal·gia (pros''o·pal'jee·uh) *n.* [*prosop-* + *-algia*]. *Obsol.* TRIGEMINAL NEURALGIA. —**prosopal·gic** (·jick) *adj.*

pro·sop·ic (pro·sop'ick, ·so'pick) *adj.* [*pros-* + Gk. *ōps, ōpos,* face]. 1. *In craniometry,* designating a facial skeleton that is convex or projects anteriorly in the midline; having an orbitonasal index of 110.0 or more. 2. *In somatometry,* designating a face that is convex or projects anteriorly in the midline; having an orbitonasal index of 113.0 or more.

proso·pla·sia (pros"o·play'zee·uh, ·zhuh) *n.* [Gk. *prosō,* forward, onward, + *-plasia*]. 1. Progressive transformation in the direction of higher orders of differentiation, complexity, or function. 2. Abnormal tissue differentiation. 3. CYTOMORPHOSIS. —**proso·plas·tic** (·plas'tick) *adj.*

prosopo-. See *prosop-.*

pros·o·po·anos·chi·sis (pros"uh·po"a·nos'ki·sis) *n.,* pl. **prosopoanoschi·ses** (·seez) [*prosopo-* + Gk. *anō,* upward, + *-schisis*]. OBLIQUE FACIAL CLEFT.

pros·o·po·di·ple·gia (pros"uh·po·dye·plee'jee·uh) *n.* [*prosopo-* + *diplegia*]. *Obsol.* Bilateral facial paralysis.

pros·o·po·dyn·ia (pros"uh·po·din'ee·uh) *n.* [*prosop-* + *-odynia*]. *Obsol.* Facial pain; TRIGEMINAL NEURALGIA.

pros·o·po·neu·ral·gia (pros"uh·po·new·ral'jee·uh) *n.* [*prosopo-* + *neuralgia*]. *Obsol.* TRIGEMINAL NEURALGIA.

pros·o·pop·a·gus (pros"o·pop'uh·gus) *n.,* pl. **prosopopa·gi** (·guy) [*prosopo-* + *-pagus*]. Unequal conjoined twins in which the parasitic twin, or parts of one, is attached to the face elsewhere than in the region of the jaws.

pros·o·po·ple·gia (pros"uh·po·plee'jee·uh) *n.* [*prosopo-* + *-plegia*]. Peripheral FACIAL PALSY; it may be unilateral (monoplegia facialis) or bilateral (diplegia facialis). —**prosopo·ple·gic** (·plee'jick, ·plej'ick) *adj.*

pros·o·pos·chi·sis (pros"o·pos'ki·sis) *n.,* pl. **prosoposchi·ses** (·seez) [*prosopo-* + *-schisis*]. A congenital facial cleft, from mouth to orbit (oblique facial cleft), or from the mouth to just in front of the auditory meatus (transverse facial cleft).

pros·o·po·spasm (pros'uh·po·spaz·um) *n.* [*prosopo-* + *spasm*]. RISUS SARDONICUS.

pros·o·po·ster·no·did·y·mus (pros"uh·po·stur"no·did'i·mus) *n.* [*prosopo-* + *sterno-* + *-didymus*]. PROSOPOTHORACOPAGUS.

pros·o·po·ster·no·dym·ia (pros"uh·po·stur"no·dim'ee·uh) *n.* [*prosopo-* + *sterno-* + *-dymia*]. The condition exhibited by a prosopothoracopagus.

pros·o·po·thor·a·cop·a·gus (pros"uh·po·thor"uh·kop'uh·gus) *n.,* pl. **prosopothoracopa·gi** (·guy, ·jye) [*prosopo-* + *thoraco-* + *-pagus*]. Conjoined twins united laterally by the thoraces and necks and in some cases by the jaws.

pros·o·po·to·cia (pros"uh·po·to'shee·uh) *n.* [*prosopo-* + Gk. *tok*os, childbirth, + *-ia*]. Face presentation in parturition.

pros·o·pus va·rus (pros'o·pus vair'us, pros·o'pus) [L.]. A congenital hemiatrophy of the face and cranium, resulting in marked facial obliquity.

pros·ta·glan·din (pros"tuh·glan'din) *n.* One of several physiologically potent compounds, of ubiquitous occurrence, that have a unique structure containing 20 carbon atoms and are formed from essential fatty acids, and with activities affecting the nervous system, circulation, female reproductive organs, and metabolism. The highest concentration of prostaglandins has been found in normal human semen.

pros·ta·lene (pros'tuh·leen) *n.* A prostaglandin derivative, $C_{22}H_{36}O_5$.

Prostaphlin. A trademark for the sodium salt of oxacillin, a semisynthetic penicillin antibiotic.

prostat-, prostato-. A combining form meaning *prostate.*

pro·sta·ta (pros'tuh·tuh) *n.* [NA]. PROSTATE.

pros·tate (pros'tate) *n.* [Gk. *prostatēs,* lit., standing before]. The organ surrounding the neck of the urinary bladder and beginning of the urethra in the male (prostatic urethra). It consists of two lateral lobes, an anterior and a posterior lobe, and a middle lobe, and is composed of muscular and glandular tissue; a distinct capsule surrounds it. It is the largest auxiliary gland of the male reproductive system and its secretions comprise approximately 40 percent of the semen. NA *prostata.* See also Plate 25. —**pros·tat·ic** (pros·tat'ick) *adj.*

pros·ta·tec·to·my (pros"tuh·teck'tuh·mee) *n.* [*prostat-* + *-ectomy*]. Excision of part or all of the prostate. See also *transurethral prostatectomy, punch operation.*

prostate gland. PROSTATE.

prostate injury. An injury resulting from unskillful instrumentation, or rarely, from penetrating wounds or pelvic fracture.

prostatic calculus. Calcium phosphate stones of variable size commonly seen in prostatic acini of older men; may be associated with prostatitis.

prostatic concretions. Small masses of waxy material in prostatic acini.

prostatic duct. Any one of the ducts conveying the secretion of the prostate into the urethra. See also Plate 25.

prostatic plexus. 1. A nerve plexus situated at the side of the prostate whose fibers are distributed to the urethra, prostate, and penis. NA *plexus prostaticus.* 2. A venous plexus found in the areolar tissue around the prostate gland. NA *plexus venosus prostaticus.* See also Table of Veins in the Appendix.

prostatic sinus. The groove on each side of the urethral crest into which open the ducts of the prostate gland. NA *sinus prostaticus.*

prostatic tubercle. The middle lobe of the prostate.

prostatic urethra. The portion of the male urethra surrounded by the prostate gland.

prostatic utricle. UTRICLE (2).

pros·ta·tism (pros'tuh·tiz·um) *n.* [*prostat-* + *-ism*]. The condition caused by chronic disorders of the prostate, especially obstruction to urination by prostatic enlargement.

pros·ta·ti·tis (pros"tuh·tye'tis) *n.* [*prostat-* + *-itis*]. Inflammation of the prostate gland. —**prosta·tit·ic** (·tit'ick) *adj.*

prostato-. See *prostat-.*

pros·ta·to·cys·ti·tis (pros"tuh·to·sis·tye'tis) *n.* [*prostato-* + *cyst* + *-itis*]. Inflammation of the prostate, prostatic urethra, and urinary bladder.

pros·tato·gram (pros·tat'o·gram) *n.* [*prostato-* + *-gram*]. A radiograph of the prostate gland, made after injecting a radiopaque substance into the orifices of the tubuloalveolar units through the urethral route.

pros·ta·tog·ra·phy (pros"tuh·tog'ruh·fee) *n.* [*prostato-* + *-graphy*]. Radiography of the prostate gland after injecting a radiopaque substance into the orifices of the tubuloalveolar units through the urethral route.

pros·tato·lith (pros·tat'o·lith) *n.* [*prostato-* + *-lith*]. PROSTATIC CALCULUS.

pros·ta·to·li·thi·a·sis (pros"tuh·to·li·thigh'uh·sis) *n.* [*prostato-* + *lithiasis*]. The presence of calculi in the substance of the prostate.

pros·tato·li·thot·o·my (pros"tuh·to·li·thot'uh·mee, pros·tat"o·) *n.* [*prostato-* + *lithotomy*]. Removal of a stone or calculus from the prostate gland.

pros·ta·tor·rhea, pros·ta·tor·rhoea (pros"tuh·to·ree'uh) *n.* [*prostato-* + *-rrhea*]. A thin urethral discharge coming from the prostate gland.

pros·ta·to·sem·i·no·ve·sic·u·lec·to·my (pros"tuh·to·sem"i·no·ve·sick·yoo·leck'tuh·mee) *n.* Surgical removal of the entire prostate and seminal vesicles.

pros·ta·to·sis (pros"tay·to'sis, pros"tuh·) *n.* Abacterial congestive inflammation of the prostate.

pros·ta·tot·o·my (pros"tuh·tot'uh·mee) *n.* [*prostato-* + *-tomy*]. Incision into the prostate gland.

pros·ta·to·ve·sic·u·li·tis (pros"tuh·to·ve·sick"yoo·lye'tis) *n.* [*prostato-* + *vesicul-* + *-itis*]. Inflammation of the seminal vesicles combined with prostatitis.

pro·ster·num (pro·stur'num) *n.* [*pro-* + *sternum*]. A cartilage bone ventral to the manubrium and attached to the clavicles of some amphibians and primitive mammals. In man, it is occasionally represented by an anomalous pair of suprasternal bones.

pros·the·sis (pros·thee'sis) *n.*, pl. **prosthe·ses** (·seez) [Gk., addition, attachment]. 1. Replacement or substitution. 2. An artificial substitute for a missing part, as denture, hand, leg, or eye. —**pros·thet·ic** (·thet'ick) *adj.*

prosthetic dentistry. PROSTHODONTICS.

prosthetic group. 1. The group formed by a substance that is combined with a simple protein to form a complex protein, as the chromophoric group in chromoproteins. 2. The group formed by an organic radical not derived from an amino acid, that enters into the complex molecule of a conjugated protein. 3. The nonprotein component, or coenzyme, of certain enzyme systems.

pros·thet·ics (pros·thet'icks) *n.* The branch of surgery that deals with prostheses.

prosthetic valve endocarditis. An inflammatory process, of any etiology, affecting a surgically implanted prosthetic cardiac valve.

pros·the·tist (pros'the·tist) *n.* An individual who makes artificial limbs, artificial dentures, or external organs or parts.

pros·thi·on (pros'thee·on) *n.* [Gk. *prosthios*, foremost]. *In craniometry*, the point on the alveolar border of the upper jaw which projects farthest anteriorly in the midsagittal plane, between the central incisor teeth.

pros·tho·don·tia (pros·tho·don'chee·uh) *n.* PROSTHODONTICS.

pros·tho·don·tics (pros"tho·don'ticks) *n.* [*prosthesis* + *odont-* + *-ics*]. The science and practice of the replacement of missing dental and oral structures.

pros·tho·don·tist (pros"tho·don'tist) *n.* A dentist who specializes in prosthodontics.

Prostigmin. Trademark for neostigmine, a quaternary cholinergic drug used as the bromide and methyl sulfate salts.

prostigmin test. A pregnancy test in which the failure of injected prostigmin to bring about menstrual bleeding in a woman who has missed regular menstruation is indicative of pregnancy.

Prostin E_2. A trademark for dinoprostone, an oxytocic.

pros·ti·tu·tion (pros"ti·tew'shun) *n.* [L. *prostitutio*, from *prostituere*, to expose publicly]. The condition or act of using the body for sexual intercourse promiscuously for pay or other considerations.

pros·trate (pros'trate) *adj.* & *v.* [L. *prostratus*, thrown down]. 1. Lying prone or supine; stretched out. 2. Lacking in vitality, powerless, exhausted, stricken down. 3. To render oneself or another prostrate.

pros·trat·ed (pros'tray·tid) *adj.* Exhausted; stricken down.

pros·tra·tion (pros·tray'shun) *n.* The condition of being prostrated; extreme exhaustion; collapse.

prot-, proto- [Gk. *prōtos*, first]. 1. A combining form meaning (a) *first, foremost;* (b) *primitive, early;* (c) *giving rise to, parental to.* 2. *In chemistry,* a combining form meaning *the first or lowest of a series,* as the member of a series of compounds of the same element having the lowest proportion of the element or radical affixed in the name (protochloride, protosulfate).

prot·ac·tin·i·um (pro"tack·tin'ee·um) *n.* [*prot-* + *actinium*]. Pa = 231.0359. A radioactive element occurring in pitchblende and yielding actinium on disintegration. Atomic number, 91.

pro·tag·o·nist (pro·tag'uh·nist) *n.* [Gk. *prōtagōnistēs*, chief actor]. AGONIST (1).

pro·tal (pro'tul) *adj.* [*prot-* + *-al*]. CONGENITAL.

prot·al·bu·mose (pro·tal'bew·moce) *n.* ALBUMOSE.

pro·ta·mine (pro'tuh·meen, ·min) *n.* One of a group of simple proteins occurring in the sperm of fish, as clupeine, iridine, salmine, or sturine.

protamine sulfate. A water-soluble salt of protamine, a protein prepared from the sperm or mature testes of certain species of fish; because it interacts with heparin to inactivate the latter, protamine sulfate is used as an antidote to overdosage with heparin.

protamine zinc insulin. A preparation of insulin modified by addition of zinc chloride and protamine to produce long duration of action.

prot·anom·a·ly (pro"tuh·nom'uh·lee) *n.* [*prot-* + *anomaly*]. PROTANOPIA.

pro·ta·no·pia (pro"tuh·no'pee·uh) *n.* [*prot-* + *an-* + *-opia*]. A form of partial color blindness in which there is defective red vision; green sightedness. See also *dichromatopsia.* —**prota·nop·ic** (·nop'ick, ·no'pick) *adj.*

Protargol. A trademark for strong silver protein, used locally for the germicidal action of the silver component, and also as a biological stain.

prote-, proteo-. A combining form meaning *protein.*

[1]**pro·te·an** (pro'tee·un, pro·tee'un) *adj.* [*Proteus*, Greek god who changed shape]. Taking on many shapes or changing form.

[2]**pro·te·an** (pro'tee·an) *n.* [*protein* + *-an*]. One of a group of derived proteins, insoluble products due to the action of water or enzymes.

pro·te·ase (pro'tee·ace, ·aze) *n.* An enzyme that digests proteins.

protection heart block. ENTRANCE HEART BLOCK.

pro·tec·tive (pruh·teck'tiv) *adj.* & *n.* 1. Affording defense or immunity; PROPHYLACTIC. 2. A covering or shield that protects. 3. A specific dressing, as oiled silk or rubber, used to prevent ingress of water.

protective colloid. A lyophilic colloid which, when added to a lyophobic colloid, confers upon the latter the stability of the former.

protective reflex. Any reflex response to defend the body from harm, as blinking caused by an object rapidly approaching the eye.

protective spectacles. Lenses that shield the eyes from light, dust, heat.

pro·te·ic (pro·tee'ick) *adj.* Pertaining to protein.

pro·teid (pro'tee·id, pro'teed) *n.* PROTEIN.

pro·te·i·form (pro·tee'i·form) *adj.* [*Proteus*, Greek god who changed shape, + *-iform*]. Having various forms.

pro·tein (pro'tee·in, pro'teen) *n.* [F. *protéine*, from Gk. *prōteios*, primary]. One of a group of complex nitrogenous substances of high molecular weight which are found in various forms in animals and plants and are characteristic of living matter. On complete hydrolysis they yield amino acids. See also Table of Chemical Constituents of Blood in the Appendix.

pro·tein·a·ceous (pro"tee·nay'shus, pro"tee·i·nay'shus) *adj.* Of, pertaining to, or characteristic of a protein.

pro·tein·ase (pro'tee·nace, ·naze, pro'tee·i·nace) *n.* One of the subgroups of proteases or proteolytic enzymes which act directly on the native proteins in the first step of their conversion to simpler substances.

protein-bound iodine. Iodine attached to protein; commonly, iodine bound to the protein fraction of the blood; in most instances, it reflects the level of circulating thyroid hormone. Abbreviated, PBI.

pro·tein·emia, pro·tein·ae·mia (pro"tee·nee'mee·uh, ·tee·i·nee') *n.* [*protein* + *-emia*]. 1. Protein in the blood. 2. HYPERPROTEINEMIA.

protein fever. Artificial fever produced by parenteral injection of a foreign protein.

protein fluorochrome tagging. COONS'S FLUORESCENT ANTIBODY TECHNIQUE.

protein hydrolysate. An artificial digest of protein derived by acid, enzymatic, or other hydrolysis of casein, lactalbumin, fibrin, or other suitable proteins that supply the approximate nutritive equivalent of the source protein in the form of its constituent amino acids. See also *amigen.*

pro·tein·ic (pro·teen'ick, pro"tee·in'ick) *adj.* [*protein* + *-ic*]. PROTEINACEOUS.

protein kinase. An allosteric enzyme that is the key to linking cyclic adenosine monophosphate to the phosphorylase system, as cyclic AMP removes the inhibition of enzyme activity that is imposed by the binding of the regulatory subunit to the catalytic subunit.

protein malnutrition. KWASHIORKOR.

protein milk. Milk containing a high percentage of protein, and a low percentage of sugar and fat.

protein nitrogen unit. The quantity of pollen extract which contains 10 ng of protein nitrogen.

pro·teino·chro·mo·gen (pro″tee·in″o·kro′muh·jen, pro″tee·no·) *n.* [*protein* + *chromo-* + *-gen*]. TRYPTOPHAN.

pro·tein·o·sis (pro″teen·o′sis, pro″tee·i·no′sis) *n.* [*protein* + *-osis*]. The accumulation of protein in the tissues.

pro·teino·ther·a·py (pro″tee·no·therr′uh·pee) *n.* PROTEIN THERAPY.

protein quotient. The result of dividing the amount of globulin in the blood plasma by the amount of albumin in it.

protein therapy. 1. The injection of a foreign protein for the therapeutic effect of the resulting reaction. 2. Special alimentation with protein foods.

pro·tein·uria (pro″tee·new′ree·uh, pro″tee·i·new′ree·uh) *n.* [*protein* + *-uria*]. The presence of protein in the urine.

proteinuria of adolescence. CYCLIC PROTEINURIA.

proteo-. See *prote-.*

pro·te·ol·y·sis (pro″tee·ol′i·sis) *n.* [*proteo-* + *-lysis*]. The addition of water to peptide bonds of proteins with resultant fragmentation of the protein molecule. Proteolysis may be enzymatically catalyzed by numerous enzymes, many of which have stereochemically selective points of attack, or it may occur nonenzymatically, especially consequent to the action of mineral acids and heat. —**pro·teo·lyt·ic** (pro″tee·o·lit′ick) *adj.*

proteolytic enzyme. PROTEASE; an enzyme involved in the breaking down of protein, as pepsin, rennin.

pro·teo·me·tab·o·lism (pro″tee·o·me·tab′uh·liz·um) *n.* [*proteo-* + *metabolism*]. The processes of digestion, absorption, and utilization of proteins. —**proteo·meta·bol·ic** (·met″uh·bol′ick) *adj.*

pro·teo·pep·tic (pro″tee·o·pep′tick) *adj.* [*proteo-* + *peptic*]. Pertaining to protein digestion.

pro·te·ose (pro′tee·oce, ·oze) *n.* One of a group of derived proteins intermediate between native proteins and peptones. Soluble in water, not coagulable by heat, but precipitated by saturation with ammonium or zinc sulfate.

pro·teo·su·ria (pro″tee·o·sue′ree·uh) *n.* [*proteose* + *-uria*]. The presence of proteoses in the urine.

Pro·te·rog·ly·pha (pro″tur·o·glif′uh, ·og′li·fuh) *n.pl.* [NL., from Gk. *proteros,* front, + E. *glyph,* vertical groove]. One of the two principal groups of venomous snakes; includes the Elapidae (cobras and allies) and Hydrophiidae (sea snakes); characterized by permanently erect grooved or tubular front fangs. Contr. *Solenoglypha, Aglypha, Opisthoglypha.*

pro·te·uria (pro″tee·yoo′ree·uh) *n.* [*prote-* + *-uria*]. PROTEINURIA.

Pro·teus (pro′tee·us) *n.* [Gk. *Prōteus,* sea god who could change shape]. A genus of bacteria of the family Enterobacteriaceae composed of lactose-negative rods which decompose urea rapidly and actively deaminate phenylalanine to phenylpyruvic acid. Included are *Proteus vulgaris, P. mirabilis, P. rettgeri,* and *P. morganii.* Normal inhabitants of the intestinal tract, they have significant pathogenicity in such conditions as diarrhea in infants, urinary tract infection, and suppurative lesions.

pro·throm·base (pro·throm′bace, ·baze) *n.* PROTHROMBIN.

pro·throm·bin (pro·throm′bin) *n.* [*pro-* + *thrombin*]. A plasma protein precursor of the proteolytic enzyme thrombin, formed in the liver through the action of vitamin K.

pro·throm·bin·emia, pro·throm·bin·ae·mia (pro·throm″bi·nee′mee·uh) *n.* [*prothrombin* + *-emia*]. An excess of prothrombin in the blood plasma.

prothrombin factor. VITAMIN K.

pro·throm·bi·no·gen·ic (pro·throm″bi·no·jen′ick) *adj.* [*prothrombin* + *-genic*]. Having the property of causing or promoting the biosynthesis of prothrombin, an effect characteristic of vitamin K and related compounds.

pro·throm·bi·no·pe·nia (pro·throm″bi·no·pee′nee·uh) *n.* [*prothrombin* + *-penia*]. Decrease in the prothrombin content of the blood.

prothrombin time. A widely used one-stage clotting test devised by A. J. Quick based on the time required for clotting to occur after the addition of tissue thromboplastin and calcium to decalcified plasma.

pro·throm·bo·gen·ic (pro·throm″bo·jen′ick) *adj.* PROTHROMBINOGENIC.

pro·throm·bo·ki·nase (pro·throm″bo·kigh′nace, ·kin′ace) *n.* A hypothetical inactive precursor of thrombokinase.

pro·thy·mia (pro·thigh′mee·uh) *n.* [Gk., readiness, eagerness, from *thymos,* spirit, passion]. Intellectual alertness.

pro·tide (pro′tide) *n.* SIMPLE PROTEIN.

pro·ti·re·lin (pro·tye′re·lin) *n.* 5-Oxo-L-prolyl-L-histidyl-L-prolinamide, $C_{16}H_{22}N_6O_4$, a prothyrotropin.

Pro·tis·ta (pro·tis′tuh) *n.pl.* [Gk. *prōtistos,* very first]. A group of organisms which includes the unicellular plants and animals and, on some classifications, the viruses. —**pro·tist** (pro′tist), *com. n.*

pro·tis·tol·o·gist (pro″tis·tol′uh·jist) *n.* A specialist in the study of the unicellular plants and animals.

pro·tis·tol·o·gy (pro″tis·tol′uh·jee) *n.* [*Protista* + *-logy*]. The study of unicellular plants and animals.

pro·ti·um (pro′tee·um) *n.* [NL., from Gk. *prōtos,* first]. The predominant constituent of ordinary hydrogen; the atom consists of one proton and one electron and therefore has an atomic weight of approximately 1. Symbol, ^{1}H. Syn. *light hydrogen.*

proto-. See *prot-.*

pro·to·al·bu·mose (pro″to·al′bew·moce) *n.* ALBUMOSE.

Pro·to·bi·os bac·te·ri·oph·a·gus (pro″to·bye′os back·teer″ee·off′uh·gus). In some classifications, BACTERIOPHAGE.

pro·to·blast (pro′to·blast) *n.* [*proto-* + *-blast*]. A blastomere produced by mosaic cleavage which is destined to form a particular structure or organ in development. —**proto·blas·tic** (·blas′tick) *adj.*

pro·to·car·di·ac mesoderm (pro″to·kahr′dee·ack). The mesoderm anterior to the buccopharyngeal membrane from which the heart and pericardial coelom develop.

pro·to·chlo·ride (pro″to·klo′ride) *n.* [*proto-* + *chloride*]. The first in a series of chloride compounds, containing the fewest chlorine atoms.

pro·to·col (pro′tuh·kol) *n.* [Gk. *prōtokollon,* first leaf of a papyrus roll]. 1. The original notes or records of an experiment, autopsy, or clinical examination. 2. The records from which a document is prepared. 3. The outline or plan for an experiment or experimental procedure.

pro·to·cone (pro′tuh·kone) *n.* [*proto-* + *cone*]. 1. The primitive single cusp of a reptilian tooth. 2. The mesiolingual cusp on an upper molar.

pro·to·co·nid (pro″to·ko′nid, ·kon′id) *n.* [*protocone* + *-id*]. The mesiobuccal cusp on a molar tooth of the lower jaw.

pro·to·cop·ro·por·phyr·ia he·red·i·ta·ria (pro″to·kop″ro·por·feer′ee·uh he·red″i·tair′ee·uh). PORPHYRIA CUTANEA TARDA HEREDITARIA.

pro·to·derm (pro′tuh·durm) *n.* [*proto-* + *-derm*]. BLASTODERM (2).

pro·to·di·a·stol·ic (pro″to·dye″uh·stol′ick) *adj.* [*proto-* + *diastolic*]. 1. Of or pertaining to the first diastolic action in an embryo. 2. Pertaining to the early part of ventricular diastole, that is, immediately following the second heart sound.

protodiastolic gallop. VENTRICULAR GALLOP.

protodiastolic phase. The interval between the onset of diastole and closure of the aortic semilunar valve; lasts about 20 msec.

pro·to·elas·tose (pro″to·e·las′toce, ·toze) *n.* [*proto-* + *elastose*]. A poorly defined product of the digestion of elastin.

pro·to·fi·bril (pro″to·figh′bril) *n.* [*proto-* + *fibril*]. One of the fine filaments, seen under the electron microscope, of which fibrils are composed.

pro·to·fil·a·ment (pro″to·fil′uh·munt) *n.* PROTOFIBRIL.

pro·tog·a·la (pro·tog′uh·luh) *n.* [Gk., from *proto-* + *gala,* milk]. COLOSTRUM.

pro·to·gas·ter (pro″to·gas′tur) *n.* [*proto-* + *-gaster*]. ARCHENTERON.

pro·to·gen (pro′tuh·jen) *n.* [*protozoa* + *-gen*]. A multiple factor in liver, which has been separated into protogen A and protogen B, essential for growth of certain protozoa. Protogen A appears to be identical with α-lipoic acid, which is a dithiooctanoic acid; protogen B is a thiosulfinyloctanoic acid. See also *lipoic acid, thioctic acid.*

pro·to·glob·u·lose (pro″to·glob′yoo·loce) *n.* [*proto-* + *globulose*]. A poorly defined product of the digestion of globulin.

pro·to·io·dide (pro″to·eye′uh·dide) *n.* [*proto-* + *iodide*]. The first in a series of iodine base compounds, containing the fewest iodine atoms.

pro·tok·yl·ol (pro·tock′i·lol) *n.* α[(α-Methyl-3,4-methylenedioxyphenethylamino)methyl]protocatechuyl alcohol, $C_{18}H_{21}NO_5$, a sympathomimetic amine used principally as a bronchodilator, in the form of the hydrochloride salt.

pro·to·leu·ko·cyte, pro·to·leu·co·cyte (pro″to·lew′ko·site) *n.* [*proto-* + *leukocyte*]. One of the minute lymphoid cells found in the red bone marrow and also in the spleen.

pro·tol·y·sis (pro·tol′i·sis) *n.,* pl. **protoly·ses** (·seez) [*proto-* + *-lysis*]. Any reaction in which a proton (hydrogen ion) is transferred, as: $HCl + H_2O = H_3O^+ + Cl^-$.

pro·to·mer (pro′to·mur) *n.* [*proto-* + *-mer*]. One of the separate polypeptide chains which are subunits of an oligomeric protein.

pro·to·me·rite (pro″to·meer′ite, pro·tom′ur·ite) *n.* [*proto-* + Gk. *meros,* part, + *-ite*]. The anterior portion of a cephaline gregarine.

pro·tom·e·ter (pro·tom′e·tur) *n.* [*proto-* + *-meter*]. PROPTOMETER.

pro·to·me·tro·cyte (pro″to·mee′tro·site) *n.* [*proto-* + *metrocyte*]. Mother cell both of leukocytes and erythrocytes.

Pro·to·mon·a·di·na (pro″to·mon″uh·dye′nuh) *n.pl.* [NL., from *proto-* + Gk. *monas,* unit]. An order of the flagellate Protozoa; it contains many parasitic forms, notably the trypanosomes.

pro·to·my·o·sin·ose (pro″to·migh·o′sin·oce) *n.* [*proto-* + *myosin* + *-ose*]. A poorly defined product of the digestion of myosin.

pro·ton (pro′ton) *n.* [Gk. *prōton,* primary or elemental thing, from *prōtos,* first]. A subatomic particle identical with the nucleus of the hydrogen atom. It has a positive electric charge numerically equal to the negative charge on the electron, but its mass is over 1,800 times that of the electron. The atomic number of an element is equivalent to, and defined by, the number of protons in its nucleus.

pro·ton·at·ed (pro′ton·ay″tid) *adj.* Having a proton or protons added.

pro·to·neu·ron (pro″to·new′ron) *n.* [*proto-* + *neuron*]. A hypothetical unit of the nerve net of the lowest metazoa. Such a unit transmits impulses indiscriminately in all directions, and has none of the polarization of the phylogenetically later synaptic system of neurons of animals in which there is a central nervous system.

proton microscope. A microscope, similar to the electron microscope, utilizing protons rather than electrons and having a magnifying power of 600,000 diameters.

proton-synchrotron, *n.* A synchrotron in which protons are accelerated to have energies in the billion electron volt range. Syn. *bevatron, cosmotron.*

Protopam Chloride. Trademark for the cholinesterase reactivator pralidoxime chloride, used in the treatment of poisoning by organophosphates.

pro·to·path·ic (pro″to·path′ick) *adj.* [*proto-* + Gk. *pathos,* experience, + *-ic*]. A term used by Henry Head to designate a primitive system of cutaneous sensory nerves and end organs, which, he postulated, mediated painful cutaneous stimuli and extremes of heat and cold. According to this theory, an "epicritic" system of nerves has been developed to amplify and control the more primitive protopathic system.

pro·to·pec·tin (pro″to·peck′tin) *n.* [*proto-* + *pectin*]. PECTOSE.

pro·to·pep·sia (pro″to·pep′see·uh) *n.* [*proto-* + Gk. *pepsis,* digestion, + *-ia*]. A primary process of digestion, as that of starches by the saliva.

pro·to·phile (pro′to·file) *n.* [*proto-* + *-phile*]. A substance that has an affinity for, and forms combinations with, protons (hydrogen ions).

Pro·toph·y·ta (pro·tof′i·tuh) *n.pl.* [*proto-* + Gk. *phyta,* pl. of *phyton,* plant]. A group whose boundaries vary with different systems of classification, but which includes the lowest, simplest plants, such as the bacteria and various algae.

pro·to·phyte (pro′to·fite) *n.* [*proto-* + *-phyte*]. Any plant of the lowest and most primitive type. The Schizomycetes, or bacteria, may be classed as protophytes, with other low vegetable forms. They have no visible reproductive organs.

pro·to·pla·sis (pro″to·play′sis) *n.* [*proto-* + Gk. *plasis,* a molding]. The primary formation of tissue.

pro·to·plasm (pro′tuh·plaz·um) *n.* [*proto-* + *-plasm*]. The viscid material constituting the essential substance of living cells, upon which all the vital functions of nutrition, secretion, growth, reproduction, irritability, and motility depend.

pro·to·plas·mat·ic (pro″tuh·plaz·mat′ick) *adj.* PROTOPLASMIC.

pro·to·plas·mic (pro″tuh·plaz′mick) *adj.* Pertaining to, or composed of, protoplasm.

protoplasmic astrocytes. The astrocytes in the gray matter, characterized by numerous, freely branching protoplasmic processes.

protoplasmic astrocytoma. A rare form of astrocytoma which, in pure form, is found almost exclusively in the cerebral hemispheres. Microscopically, the tumor consists of stellate cells with delicate processes devoid of neurofibrils.

protoplasmic process. Any extension of cytoplasm from the body of a cell.

pro·to·plast (pro′tuh·plast) *n.* [Gk. *prōtoplastos,* first-formed]. 1. CELL (1). 2. PROTOPLASM. 3. An osmotically fragile, spherical bacterial cell, consisting of the cytoplasm and the nucleus, but lacking the cell wall.

pro·to·por·phyr·ia (pro″to·por·feer′ee·uh) *n.* [*protoporphyrin* + *-ia*]. The presence of protoporphyrin in red blood cells.

pro·to·por·phy·rin (pro″to·por′fi·rin) *n.* [*proto-* + *porphyrin*]. $C_{32}H_{32}N_4(COOH)_2$. Any of the 15 metal-free porphyrins having as substituents 4 methyl, 2 vinyl, and 2 propionic acid ($-CH_2CH_2COOH$) groups. The particular arrangement of these groups represented by protoporphyrin IX is the one occurring in hemoglobin.

pro·to·por·phy·rin·uria (pro″to·por″fi·ri·new′ree·uh) *n.* [*protoporphyrin* + *-uria*]. The excretion of protoporphyrins in the urine.

pro·to·pro·te·ose (pro″to·pro′tee·oce) *n.* [*proto-* + *proteose*]. A primary proteose; further digestion changes it into deuteroproteose.

pro·to·sid·er·in (pro″to·sid′ur·in) *n.* [*proto-* + *sider-* + *-in*]. A form of iron pigmentation characterized by diffuse nongranular iron staining of cytoplasm and considered as an early stage in hemosiderin formation, seen in spleen cells in acute hemolytic states.

pro·to·spasm (pro′to·spaz·um) *n.* [*proto-* + *spasm*]. A spasm beginning in a limb or part of a limb and extending to others.

pro·to·sul·fate (pro″to·sul′fate) *n.* [*proto-* + *sulfate*]. The salt containing the smallest proportion of sulfate of two or more sulfates of the same base.

pro·to·the·co·sis (pro″to·thee·ko′sis) *n.* An infection produced by achloric algae of the genus *Prototheca.*

pro·to·troph·ic (pro″to·trof′ick ·tro′fick) *adj.* [*proto-* + *-trophic*]. Pertaining to bacteria with the nutritional properties of the wild type, or the strains found in nature. Contr. *auxotrophic.*

pro·tot·ro·py (pro·tot′ruh·pee, pro′to·tro″pee) *n.* [*proto-* + *-tropy*]. The migration of a proton or hydrogen atom within a compound to form an isomer of the compound; a type of change included within the broad scope of tautomerism.

pro·to·ver·a·trine (pro″to·verr′uh·treen) *n.* [*proto-* + *veratrine*]. An ester alkaloid isolated from *Veratrum viride* and *V. album* and subsequently found to consist of protoveratrine A and protoveratrine B. Protoveratrine A is a tetraester and yields, on hydrolysis, protoverine, two moles of acetic acid, and one mole each of 2-methylbutyric acid and methylethylglycolic acid. Protoveratrine B is also a tetraester; on hydrolysis, it yields protoverine, two moles of acetic acid, and one mole each of 2-methylbutyric acid and 2,3-dihydroxy-2-methylbutyric acid. Both protoveratrines possess hypotensive activity.

pro·to·ver·ine (pro″to·verr′een) *n.* A highly hydroxylated alkanolamine steroid base, $C_{27}H_{43}NO_9$, various esters of which constitute certain of the alkaloids of *Veratrum viride* and *V. album.* It is isomeric with germine and cevine, which are also parent bases of other alkaloids in the veratrums.

pro·to·ver·te·bra (pro″to·vur′te·bruh) *n.* [*proto-* + *vertebra*]. 1. Originally, a somite. 2. The condensed caudal half of a sclerotome, from which most of a vertebra is derived. Syn. *primitive vertebra.* —**protoverte·bral** (·brul) *adj.*

pro·tox·in (pro·tock′sin) *n.* [*pro-* + *toxin*]. A substance which is an inactive precursor of a toxin, becoming toxic when acted upon by a proteolytic enzyme or enzymes.

Pro·to·zoa (pro″tuh·zo′uh) *n.pl.* [*proto-* + Gk. *zōa,* creatures, animals]. The phylum of unicellular animals, subdivided into the subphyla Mastigophora, Sarcodina, Sporozoa, and Ciliophora. —**proto·zo·an** (·zo′un) *n. & adj.;* **protozo·al** (·ul) *adj.*

protozoa. Plural of *protozoon.*

pro·to·zo·a·cide (pro″tuh·zo′uh·side) *n.* [*Protozoa* + *-cide*]. An agent that will kill protozoa.

pro·to·zo·ol·o·gist (pro″tuh·zo·ol′uh·jist) *n.* A person versed in protozoology.

pro·to·zo·ol·o·gy (pro″tuh·zo·ol′uh·jee) *n.* [*Protozoa* + *-logy*]. The study of protozoa.

pro·to·zo·on (pro″tuh·zo′on) *n.,* pl. **proto·zoa** (·zo′uh). Any member of the phylum Protozoa.

pro·to·zo·o·phage (pro″tuh·zo′o·faje) *n.* A cell that is phagocytic to protozoa.

pro·tract (pro·trakt′) *v.* [L. *protrahere*]. 1. To extend in time; to prolong. 2. *In anatomy,* to extend or protrude a part of the body, as the tongue or mandible; to draw forward.

protracted labor. Labor prolonged beyond the usual limit (10 to 20 hours in primigravidas, about 8 hours in multiparas).

pro·trac·tion radiation (pro·track′shun). Decrease of the rate of application of a given dose of roentgen rays or radium rays.

pro·trac·tor (pro·track′tur, pro′track·tur) *n.* 1. *In surgery,* an instrument formerly used in debridement. 2. *In anatomy,* EXTENSOR.

pro·trip·ty·line (pro·trip′ti·leen) *n.* *N*-Methyl-5*H*-dibenzo[*a,d*]cycloheptene-5-propylamine, $C_{19}H_{21}N$, an antidepressant drug; used as the hydrochloride salt.

pro·trude (pruh·trood′) *v.* [L. *protrudere,* to thrust forward]. To project; to assume an abnormally prominent position, as a tooth that is thrust forward out of line.

protruded disk. HERNIATED DISK.

pro·tru·sio ac·etab·u·li (pro·troo′zee·o as″e·tab′yoo·lye) [L.]. ARTHROKATADYSIS.

pro·tru·sion (pruh·trew′zhun) *n.* The condition of protruding or being thrust forward, as the protrusion of the incisor teeth. —**protru·sive** (·siv) *adj.*

protrusive occlusion. Occlusion of the teeth with the mandible in a forward position from centric relation.

protrusive position. The position reached when the mandible is thrust forward from centric relation.

pro·tryp·sin (pro·trip′sin) *n.* TRYPSINOGEN.

pro·tu·ber·ance (pro·tew′bur·unce) *n.* [L. *protuberare,* to swell out]. A knoblike projecting part.

pro·tu·be·ran·tia (pro·tew″be·ran′shee·uh) *n.* [L.]. PROTUBERANCE.

protuberantia men·ta·lis (men·tay′lis) [NA]. MENTAL PROTUBERANCE.

protuberantia oc·ci·pi·ta·lis ex·ter·na (ock·sip·i·tay′lis ecks·tur′nuh) [NA]. EXTERNAL OCCIPITAL PROTUBERANCE.

protuberantia occipitalis in·ter·na (in·tur′nuh) [NA]. INTERNAL OCCIPITAL PROTUBERANCE.

pro·ty·ros·in·ase (pro″tye·ros′in·ace, ·ro′sin·ace) *n.* [*pro-* + *tyrosinase*]. An inactive precursor of the enzyme tyrosinase.

proud flesh. EXUBERANT GRANULATION.

Proust-Licht·heim maneuver. The demonstration of mental familiarity with a word by an aphasic patient whereby, though unable to evolve the appropriate term, the patient indicates how many letters or syllables it entails by squeezing the examiner's hand or by tapping the table the appropriate number of times.

pro·ven·tri·cule (pro·ven′tri·kewl) *n.* PROVENTRICULUS.

pro·ven·tric·u·lus (pro″ven·trick′yoo·lus) *n.,* pl. **proventricu·li** (·lye) [*pro-* + *ventriculus*]. The glandular stomach of birds.

Provera. Trademark for medroxyprogesterone acetate, a steroid progestogen.

pro·vi·ta·min (pro·vye′tuh·min) *n.* [*pro-* + *vitamin*]. A precursor of a vitamin. That which assumes vitamin activity upon activation or chemical change within the body, as ergosterol (provitamin D_2), which upon ultraviolet irradiation is converted in part to calciferol (vitamin D_2); or β-carotene, which in the liver is hydrolyzed to vitamin A.

pro·voc·a·tive (pruh·vock′uh·tiv) *adj.* [L. *provocativus,* called forth]. Tending to excite or provoke; arousing signs, symptoms, or reactions.

Pro·wa·zek-Hal·ber·staedt·er bodies (pro^{h}v′a^h·zeck, hal′bur·shtet″ur) [S. J. M. *Prowazek,* German zoologist, 1876–1915; and L. *Halberstaedter*]. Homogeneous irregular inclusion bodies that are near the nuclei of epithelial cells of the conjunctival sac; seen in cases of trachoma. Syn. *trachoma bodies.*

Prow·er factor [*Prower,* a patient in whom factor X deficiency was described]. FACTOR X.

prox·a·zole (prock′suh·zole) *n.* 5-[2-(Diethylamino)ethyl]-3-(α-ethylbenzyl)-1,2,4-oxadiazole,$C_{17}H_{25}N_3O$, a smooth muscle relaxant, anti-inflammatory drug, and analgesic; used as the citrate salt.

prox·i·mal (prock′si·mul) *adj.* [L. *proximus,* nearest]. 1. Nearer or nearest the point of origin along the course of any asymmetrical structure; nearer the beginning; of a limb or appendage, nearer the attached end. Contr. *distal.* 2. In any symmetrical structure, nearer or nearest the center or midline or median plane. 3. *In dentistry,* of the surface of a tooth, next to the adjacent tooth.

proximal contact. The touching of the adjacent surfaces of two teeth in the same arch.

proximal spinal muscular atrophy. WOHLFART-KUGELBERG-WELANDER DISEASE.

prox·i·mate (prock′si·mut) *adj.* [L. *proximare,* to draw near]. Nearest; immediate, as proximate cause.

proximate analysis. Determination of gross constituents, as alkaloids, glycosides, fat, protein, or carbohydrate, in drugs.

proximate cause. The one cause of several causes which is immediately direct and effective.

proximate principle. The active constituent of a drug, as an alkaloid or a glycoside.

proximo-. A combining form meaning *proximal.*

prox·i·mo·atax·ia (prock″si·mo·uh·tack′see·uh) *n.* [*proximo-* + *ataxia*]. Lack of coordination in the muscles of the proximal part of the limbs. Contr. *acroataxia.*

prox·i·mo·buc·cal (prock″si·mo·buck′ul) *adj.* [*proximo-* + *buccal*]. Pertaining to the proximal and buccal surfaces of a tooth.

prox·i·mo·la·bi·al (prock″si·mo·lay′bee·ul) *adj.* [*proximo-* + *labial*]. Pertaining to the proximal and labial surfaces of a tooth.

prox·i·mo·lin·gual (prock″si·mo·ling′gwul) *adj.* [*proximo-* + *lingual*]. Pertaining to the proximal and lingual surfaces of a tooth.

prox. luc. [L.]. Abbreviation for *proxima luce;* the day before.

pro·zone (pro′zone) *n.* [*pro-* + *zone*]. The area of the dilution range in which there is an absence or delay of a reaction at a higher concentration of one of the reactants than at a more dilute level.

pro·zy·go·sis (pro″zye·go′sis, ·zi·) *n.* [*pro-* + Gk. *zygōsis,* yoking, balancing]. The condition of a syncephalus.

P-R segment. The interval on the electrocardiogram between the end of the P wave and the beginning of the QRS complex.

prune-belly syndrome. ABDOMINAL MUSCLE DEFICIENCY SYNDROME.

prune-juice sputum. Dark reddish-brown bloody sputum, resembling prune juice.

Pru·nus (proo′nus) *n.* [L., plum tree]. A genus of trees and shrubs of the Rosaceae family, several species of which yield products of medicinal importance. Among these are *Prunus amygdalus,* the seeds of which yield almond oil; *P. cerasus,* from the fruit of which cherry juice is obtained; and *P. serotina,* the source of wild cherry bark used in making wild cherry syrup.

pru·ri·go (proo·rye′go) *n.* [L., itch]. A chronic inflammatory disease of the skin characterized by small, pale papules and severe itching. It usually begins in childhood and is most prominent on the extensor surfaces of the limbs. There are two forms of the disease: prurigo mitis, comparatively mild, and prurigo agria or ferox, severe. —**pru·rig·i·nous** (proo·rij′i·nus) *adj.*

prurigo aes·ti·va·lis (es″ti·vay′lis). HYDROA VACCINIFORME.

prurigo ag·ria (ag′ree·uh). The severe form of prurigo; PRURIGO FEROX.

prurigo der·mo·graph·i·ca (dur″mo·graf′i·kuh). A type of prurigo seen at friction sites associated with dermographia.

prurigo fer·ox (ferr′ocks). The severe form of prurigo; PRURIGO AGRIA.

prurigo mi·tis (migh′tis, mee′) The comparatively mild form of prurigo.

prurigo nod·u·la·ris (nod″yoo·lair′is). A chronic skin disease which occurs chiefly in women and is characterized by pruritic, nodular, and verrucous lesions. It is regarded as an atypical nodular form of neurodermatitis circumscripta, unrelated to the prurigos. Syn. *lichen obtusus corneus.*

prurigo sim·plex (sim′plecks). URTICARIA PAPULOSA.

pru·ri·tus (proo·rye′tus) *n.* [L., from *prurire,* to itch]. Itching, an uncomfortable sensation due to irritation of a peripheral sensory nerve; a symptom rather than a disease. —**pru·rit·ic** (·rit′ick) *adj.*

pruritus ani (ay′nigh). A common itching condition in and about the anus, especially in men; may be due to several causes.

pruritus hi·e·ma·lis (high″e·may′lis). Itching related to cold, either from the climate or air-conditioning; dryness is also a factor. Syn. *frost-itch, winter itch.*

pruritus se·ni·lis (se·nigh′lis). The pruritus of the aged, probably caused by a lack of oil in the skin; accompanies the atrophy of the skin in old age.

pruritus vul·vae (vul′vee). Intense or mild itching of the vulva and at times adjacent parts. May lead to atrophy, lichenification, and even malignancy. Etiology is varied.

Prus·sak's fibers (proo·sahk′) [A. *Prussak,* Russian otologist, 1839-1907]. Fibers in the tympanic membrane running from the ends of the tympanic notch to the lateral process of the malleus, bounding the lower margin of the pars flaccida of the tympanic membrane.

Prussak's pouch or **space** [A. *Prussak*]. RECESS OF THE TYMPANIC CAVITY (2).

Prus·sian blue. Ferric ferrocyanide, $Fe_4[Fe(CN_6)]_3$.

Prussian blue reaction. Formation of an insoluble dark greenish-blue pigment (Prussian blue) by ferric salts reacting with ferrocyanides; used histochemically for identification of hemosiderin and other iron-bearing pigments.

prus·si·ate (prush′ee·ate, prus′) *n.* Any salt of prussic or hydrocyanic acid; a cyanide; particularly a ferricyanide or ferrocyanide.

prus·sic acid (prus′ick). HYDROCYANIC ACID.

Pryce slide-culture method. A slide microculture technique for demonstrating *Mycobacterium tuberculosis* by drying a film of sputum or other clinical material on glass, treating with acid, washing, incubating with hemolyzed blood for 7 days, and examining directly stained preparations for acid-fast bacilli.

psal·te·ri·um (sawl·teer′ee·um) *n.,* pl. **psal·teria** (·teer′ee·uh) [NL., from L. *psalter,* from the folds which resemble the pages of a book]. 1. OMASUM. 2. COMMISSURE OF THE FORNIX.

psamm-, psammo- [Gk. *psammos*]. A combining form meaning *sand.*

psam·mism (sam′iz·um) *n.* [*psamm-* + *-ism*]. AMMOTHERAPY.

psammo-. See *psamm-.*

psam·mo·ma (sa·mo′muh) *n.,* pl. **psammomas, psammoma·ta** (·tuh) [*psamm-* + *-oma*]. A tumor, usually a meningioma, which contains psammoma bodies. —**psammoma·tous** (·tus) *adj.*

psammoma bodies. Concentric laminae of calcium salts that have been laid down in degenerating tumor cells.

psammomatous meningioma. A meningioma whose parenchyma contains large numbers of psammoma bodies.

psammomatous papilloma. SEROUS CYSTADENOMA.

psam·mo·sar·co·ma (sam″o·sahr·ko′muh) *n.* A psammoma with sarcomatous features, or a sarcoma containing psammoma bodies.

psam·mous (sam′us) *adj.* [*psamm-* + *-ous*]. Sandy or sabulous.

psel·a·phe·sia (sel″uh·fee′zee·uh, ·zhuh) *n.* PSELAPHESIS.

psel·a·phe·sis (sel″uh·fee′sis) *n.* [Gk. *psēlaphēsis,* touching, palpation, from *psēlaphan,* to feel, touch]. The sense of touch.

psel·lism (sel′iz·um) *n.* [Gk. *psellismos,* stammer, from *psellos,* faltering, inarticulate]. *Obsol.* Stuttering or stammering.

psel·lis·mus mer·cu·ri·a·lis (sel·iz′mus mur·kewr″ee·ay′lis). *Obsol.* The unintelligible, hurried, jerking speech accompanying the tremor of mercury poisoning.

pseud-, pseudo- [Gk. *pseudēs*]. A prefix meaning (a) *false, deceptively resembling;* (b) in chemistry, *resembling* or *isomeric with.*

pseud·acous·ma (sue″da·koos′muh, ·kooz′muh) *n.* [*pseud-* + Gk. *akousma,* something heard]. PSEUDACUSIS.

pseud·ac·ro·meg·a·ly (sue·dack″ro·meg′uh·lee) *n.* PSEUDOACROMEGALY.

pseud·acu·sis (sue″da·kew′sis, ·koo′sis) *n.* [*pseud-* + Gk. *akousis,* hearing]. A disturbance of hearing in which sounds are perceived as strange or peculiar, being altered in pitch and quality.

pseudaesthesia. PSEUDESTHESIA.

pseud·agraph·ia (sue″da·graf′ee·uh) *n.* [*pseud-* + *agraphia*]. 1. Incomplete agraphia, in which a person can copy correctly but is unable to write intelligibly or legibly independently. 2. The form of agraphia in which meaningless words are written.

pseud·al·bu·min·uria (sue″dal·bew″mi·new′ree·uh) *n.* [*pseud-* + *albuminuria*]. FALSE PROTEINURIA.

pseud·am·ne·sia (sue″dam·nee′zhuh, ·zee·uh) *n.* [*pseud-* + *amnesia*]. *Obsol.* A fragmentary type of amnesia with scattered loss of memory for unrelated experiences, usually transient and associated with organic brain disease.

pseud·an·gi·na (sue″dan·jye′nuh) *n.* PSEUDOANGINA.

pseud·an·ky·lo·sis (sue·dang″ki·lo′sis) *n.* [*pseud-* + *ankylosis*]. 1. FIBROUS ANKYLOSIS. 2. EXTRACAPSULAR ANKYLOSIS.

pseud·aphe (sue′duh·fee) *n.* [*pseud-* + Gk. *haphē*, touch]. PSEUDESTHESIA.

pseud·aphia (sue·daf′ee·uh) *n.* [*pseudaphe* + *-ia*]. PSEUDESTHESIA.

pseud·ar·thri·tis (sue″dahr·thrye′tis) *n.* [*pseud-* + *arthritis*]. A condition mimicking arthritis.

pseud·ar·thro·sis (sue″dahr·thro′sis) *n.* [*pseud-* + *arthrosis*]. A bony junction that permits abnormal motion, such as a fracture healed by fibrosis or an interspinal articulation that lacks normal rigidity.

Pseud·ech·is (sue·deck′is, sue′de·kis) *n.* [*pseud-* + Gk. *echis*, viper]. A genus of snakes of the Elapidae.

Pseudechis pro·phy·ri·a·cus (por″fi·rye′uh·kus). A poisonous terrestrial snake found in Australia; known as the black snake; possesses a hemolytic venom.

Pseudechis scu·tel·la·tus (skew·te·lay′tus). The giant brown snake or taipan, found in Australia and New Guinea; attains a length of 10 feet.

Pseud·elaps (sue″de·laps) *n.* [*pseud-* + Gk. *elops*, serpent]. A genus of snakes of the Elapidae.

Pseudelaps muel·le·ri (mew′le·rye). A species of venomous snakes found in New Guinea, the Bismarck Islands, and other islands of the southwest Pacific. Syn. *Mueller's snake.*

pseud·el·minth (sue·del′minth) *n.* [*pseud-* + Gk. *helmins*, *helminthos*, worm]. Any wormlike object mistaken for an endoparasitic worm.

pseud·en·ceph·a·ly (sue″den·sef′uh·lee) *n.* [*pseud-* + *-encephaly*]. A type of anencephaly in which the cranial vault is completely, or nearly completely, absent; the upper cervical vertebrae are cleft, and the brain is represented by a mass of membranes, blood vessels, and connective and possibly nervous tissue at the base of the skull.

pseud·es·the·sia, pseud·aes·the·sia (sue″des·theezh′uh, ·theez′ee·uh) *n.* [*pseud-* + *esthesia*]. An imaginary sensation for which there is no corresponding object, as a sensation referred to parts of the body that have been removed by accident or surgical operation. See also *phantom limb.*

pseudo-. See *pseud-.*

pseudo-acanthosis nigricans. Acanthosis nigricans sometimes associated with obesity.

pseu·do·aceph·a·lus (sue″do·a·sef′uh·lus) *n.*, pl. **pseudoacepha·li** (·lye) [*pseudo-* + *acephalus*]. A placental parasitic twin (omphalosite) which is apparently headless, but which has a rudimentary cranium and its contents buried in the superior part of the main mass.

pseu·do·ac·ro·meg·a·ly (sue″do·ack″ro·meg′uh·lee) *n.* [*pseudo-* + *acromegaly*]. 1. Enlargement of the face and extremities not due to disease of the hypophysis. 2. HYPERTROPHIC PULMONARY OSTEOARTHROPATHY.

pseudoaesthesia. PSEUDESTHESIA.

pseu·do·ag·glu·ti·na·tion (sue″do·a·gloo″ti·nay′shun) *n.* [*pseudo-* + *agglutination*]. Rouleau formation and clumping tendency of erythrocytes simulating true agglutination, occurring as a result of the increased concentration of plasma proteins, particularly fibrinogen.

pseu·do·agraph·ia (sue″do·a·graf′ee·uh) *n.* PSEUDAGRAPHIA.

pseu·do·ain·hum (sue″do·eye·nyoom′) *n.* [*pseudo-* + *ainhum*]. A condition in which a circumscribed fissure or inflamed sulcus appears around a digit or limb and the resultant scar tissue or fibrosis forms a constricting band often leading to bloodless amputation of the part. Compare *ainhum.*

pseu·do·al·bu·min·uria (sue″do·al·bew″mi·new′ree·uh) *n.* [*pseudo-* + *albuminuria*]. FALSE PROTEINURIA; the presence in the urine of protein derived from blood, pus, or special secretions and mixed with the urine during its transit through the urinary passages.

pseu·do·al·lele (sue″do·a·leel′, ·lel′) *n.* [*pseudo-* + *allele*]. One of a set of heteroalleles that produce a mutant effect when located on opposite homologous chromosomes (trans position) in the diploid state and a wild-type effect when recombined on one of the homologues (cis position), thereby giving rise to the cis-trans effect. —**pseudoallel·ism** (·iz·um) *n.*

pseu·do·al·ve·o·lar (sue″do·al·vee′uh·lur) *adj.* [*pseudo-* + *alveolar*]. Simulating an alveolus or alveolar structure.

pseu·do·ane·mia, pseu·do·anae·mia (sue″do·uh·nee′mee·uh) *n.* [*pseudo-* + *anemia*]. Pallor and the appearance of anemia without blood changes to support the diagnosis. Syn. *apparent anemia.*

pseu·do·an·eu·rysm (sue″do·an′yoo·riz·um) *n.* [*pseudo-* + *aneurysm*]. FALSE ANEURYSM.

pseu·do·an·gi·na (sue″do·an·jye′nuh) *n.* [*pseudo-* + *angina*]. A psychophysiologic cardiovascular disorder characterized by pain in the chest at the apex of the heart and at times radiating down the left arm, with no evidence of organic disease.

pseu·do·an·gi·o·ma (sue″do·an·jee·o′muh) *n.* [*pseudo-* + *angioma*]. 1. Canalized thrombus of the portal vein. 2. The formation of a temporary angioma, as is sometimes seen in healing stumps.

pseu·do·an·orex·ia (sue″do·an″o·reck′see·uh) *n.* [*pseudo-* + *anorexia*]. Rejection of food because of dysphagia or gastric distress.

pseu·do·apha·kia (sue″do·a·fay′kee·uh) *n.* [*pseudo-* + *aphakia*]. MEMBRANOUS CATARACT.

pseu·do·ap·o·plexy (sue″do·ap′uh·pleck″see) *n.* [*pseudo-* + *apoplexy*]. A condition resembling a cerebrovascular accident, but unaccompanied by cerebral hemorrhage.

pseu·do·ap·pen·di·ci·tis (sue″do·uh·pen″di·sigh′tis) *n.* [*pseudo-* + *appendicitis*]. A condition simulating appendicitis, but with no lesion of the vermiform process.

pseudo Argyll Robertson pupil. ADIE'S PUPIL.

pseu·do·ar·thri·tis (sue″do·ahr·thrye′tis) *n.* PSEUDARTHRITIS.

pseu·do·ar·thro·sis (sue″do·ahr·thro′sis) *n.* PSEUDARTHROSIS.

pseu·do·ath·er·o·ma (sue″do·ath″ur·o′muh) *n.* [*pseudo-* + *atheroma*]. Multiple sebaceous cysts.

pseu·do·ath·e·to·sis (sue″do·ath″e·to′sis) *n.* [*pseudo-* + *athetosis*]. Adventitious movements, particularly of the fingers of the outstretched hand, as a result of the loss of proprioceptive sense; seen in such conditions as tabes dorsalis and subacute combined degeneration.

pseu·do·at·ro·pho·der·ma col·li (sue″do·at″ruh·fo·dur′muh kol′eye). A skin disease characterized by depigmented glossy areas on the neck or, occasionally, elsewhere, surrounded by hyperpigmented skin.

pseu·do·blep·sia (sue″do·blep′see·uh) *n.* [*pseudo-* + Gk. *blepsis*, sight, + *-ia*]. A visual hallucination; a distorted visual image.

pseu·do·blep·sis (sue″do·blep′sis) *n.* PSEUDOBLEPSIA.

pseu·do·bul·bar (sue″do·bul′bur) *adj.* [*pseudo-* + *bulbar*]. Not really bulbar; not concerned with or involving the medulla oblongata.

pseudobulbar palsy or **paralysis.** A weakness or paralysis of the muscle innervated by the motor nuclei of the bulb (the motor nuclei of the fifth, seventh, ninth, tenth, eleventh, and twelfth cranial nerves), due to bilateral interruption of the corticobulbar pathways which project to these nuclei. Clinically, there is impairment of swallowing, articulation and chewing movements, forced laughing or crying, exaggerated facial and jaw jerks, and lack of atrophy and fasciculations of the tongue. Signs of corticospinal tract disease are frequently conjoined. Bilateral lacunar infarction is the commonest cause. Syn. *spastic bulbar palsy* or *paralysis.*

pseu·do·car·ti·lage (sue″do·kahr′ti·lij) *n.* [*pseudo-* + *cartilage*]. An embryonic type of cartilage in which but little matrix is formed, as that of the notochord.

pseu·do·casts (sue′do·kasts) *n.pl.* [*pseudo-* + *casts*]. Urinary structures such as mucous threads, epithelial cells, vegetable fibers, masses of bacteria, or debris which morphologically resemble tubular casts.

pseudocele. PSEUDOCOELE.

pseu·do·chan·cre (sue′do·shank″ur) *n.* [*pseudo-* + *chancre*]. An indurated sore simulating a chancre.

pseu·do·cho·les·tane (sue″do·kol′e·stane, ·ko·les′tane) *n.* COPROSTANE.

pseu·do·cho·les·te·a·to·ma (sue″do·ko·les″tee·uh·to′muh) *n.* [*pseudo-* + *cholesteatoma*]. A cholesteatoma secondary to epithelial ingrowth from the ear canal in chronic otitis media.

pseu·do·cho·lin·es·ter·ase (sue″do·ko″lin·es′tur·ace, ·aze) *n.* [*pseudo-* + *cholinesterase*]. An enzyme that catalyzes the hydrolysis of acetylcholine but that differs from cholinesterase in that it is nonspecific and hydrolyzes esters other than choline esters.

pseu·do·cho·rea (sue″do·ko·ree′uh) *n.* [*pseudo-* + *chorea*]. Spurious chorea, usually a conversion reaction.

pseu·do·chrom·es·the·sia, pseu·do·chrom·aes·the·sia (sue″do·kro″mes·theez′ee·uh, ·theezh′uh) *n.* [*pseudo-* + *chromesthesia*]. A form of synesthesia in which each of the vowels of a word (whether seen, heard, or remembered) seems to have a distinct visual tint. See also *phonism, photism.*

pseu·do·chro·mia (sue″do·kro′mee·uh) *n.* [*pseudo-* + *-chromia*]. A false or incorrect perception of color.

pseu·do·chro·mo·some (sue″do·kro′muh·sohm) *n.* [*pseudo-* + *chromosome*]. One of the filamentous types of mitochondria.

pseu·do·chy·lous (sue″do·kigh′lus) *adj.* [*pseudo-* + *chylous*]. Pertaining to or characterized by a milky fluid, resembling chyle, but containing no fat.

pseu·do·cir·rho·sis (sue″do·si·ro′sis) *n.* [*pseudo-* + *cirrhosis*]. A disease resembling cirrhosis, due to obstruction of the hepatic vein or of inferior vena cava, or to pericarditis.

pseu·do·clau·di·ca·tion syndrome (sue″do·klaw·di·kay′shun). Pain on walking, usually in the thigh and buttocks, which is relieved by rest, caused by herniated disk, osteoarthritis, or spinal cord neoplasm, distinguished from intermittent claudication usually by variation in the walk-pain-rest cycle and by location of the pain.

pseu·do·co·arc·ta·tion (sue″do·ko″ahrk·tay′shun) *n.* [*pseudo-* + *coarctation*]. A condition mimicking coarctation but in which the lumen of the affected structure is not significantly narrowed.

pseudocoarctation of the aorta. A congenital anomaly of the aortic arch in which the kinked aorta resembles aortic coarctation, but the aortic lumen is not significantly narrowed.

pseu·do·coele (sue′do·seel) *n.* [*pseudo-* + *-coele*]. The cavity of the septum pellucidum of the brain.

pseu·do·col·loid (sue″do·kol′oid) *n.* [*pseudo-* + *colloid*]. A mucoid material, found particularly in ovarian cysts.

pseudocolloid ovarian cystoma or **tumor.** MUCINOUS CYSTADENOMA.

pseu·do·col·o·bo·ma (sue″do·kol″o·bo′muh) *n.* [*pseudo-* + *coloboma*]. A scarcely noticeable fissure of the iris, the remains of the embryonic ocular fissure, which has almost, but not perfectly, closed.

pseudocoma. A state in which awareness is normal or nearly so, but capacity for voluntary movement, except possibly that of the eyelids and eyes, is abolished. Syn. *locked-in syndrome, de-efferented state, coma vigile.*

pseu·do·cow·pox (sue″do·kaow′pocks, sue′do·kaow″pocks) *n.* PARAVACCINIA.

pseu·do·cox·al·gia (sue″do·kock·sal′jee·uh) *n.* [*pseudo-* + *coxalgia*]. TRANSIENT SYNOVITIS.

pseu·do·cri·sis (sue″do·krye′sis) *n.* [*pseudo-* + *crisis*]. A false crisis; a sudden fall of temperature resembling the crisis of a disease, subsequently followed by a rise of temperature and a continuation of the fever.

pseu·do·croup (sue′do·kroop) *n.* [*pseudo-* + *croup*]. SPASMODIC CROUP.

pseu·do·cryp·tor·chism (sue″do·krip·tor′kiz·um) *n.* [*pseudo-* + *cryptorchism*]. The condition in which one or both testes are either in the abdomen or in the inguinal canal, but can be brought down by various nonsurgical techniques, including the application of warmth; a common finding in young boys.

pseu·do·cy·e·sis (sue″do·sigh·ee′sis) *n.* [*pseudo-* + *cyesis*]. A condition characterized by amenorrhea, enlargement of the abdomen, and other symptoms simulating gestation, due to an emotional disorder.

pseu·do·cyl·in·droid (sue″do·sil′in·droid) *n.* [*pseudo-* + *cylindroid*]. A band of mucus or any substance in the urine simulating a renal cast.

pseu·do·cyst (sue′do·sist) *n.* [*pseudo-* + *cyst*]. A sac-like space or cavity containing liquid, semiliquid, or gas but without a definite lining membrane.

pseu·do·de·cid·ua (sue″do·de·sid′yoo·uh) *n.* [*pseudo-* + *decidua*]. DECIDUA MENSTRUALIS.

pseu·do·de·men·tia (sue″do·de·men′shuh) *n.* [*pseudo-* + *dementia*]. A condition of apathy resembling dementia, but without the mental degenerative changes.

pseu·do·diph·the·ria (sue″do·dif·theer′ee·uh) *n.* [*pseudo-* + *diphtheria*]. Any membranous formation not due to *Corynebacterium diphtheriae.*

pseu·do·di·ver·tic·u·lum (sue″do·dye″vur·tick′yoo·lum) *n.* [*pseudo-* + *diverticulum*]. A herniation, commonly observed in the large bowel, in which the mucous membrane protrudes through a defect in the muscular layer, producing a pouch the wall of which contains no muscle. Syn. *false diverticulum.*

pseu·do·ede·ma, pseu·do-oe·de·ma (sue″do·e·dee′muh) *n.* [*pseudo-* + *edema*]. A puffy condition simulating edema.

pseu·do·en·do·me·tri·tis (sue″do·en″do·me·trye′tis) *n.* [*pseudo-* + *endometritis*]. A condition resembling endometritis marked by changes in the blood vessels, hyperplasia of the glands, and atrophy.

pseu·do·eo·sin·o·phil (sue″do·ee″o·sin′o·fil) *n.* [*pseudo-* + *eosinophil*]. 1. The polymorphonuclear leukocyte of avian blood which contains elongated red granules. 2. A term sometimes used to describe the neutrophil of rabbit blood because of the bright red staining of the intracytoplasmic granules.

pseu·do·ephed·rine (sue″do·e·fed′rin, ·ef′e·dreen) *n.* [*pseudo-* + *ephedrine*]. One of four stereoisomers of ephedrine equal to ephedrine as a bronchodilator but with less pressor activity than the latter; administered orally, as the hydrochloride salt, in the treatment of nasal congestion.

pseu·do·ep·i·lep·sy (sue″do·ep′i·lep″see) *n.* [*pseudo-* + *epilepsy*]. HYSTEROEPILEPSY.

pseu·do·ep·i·the·li·o·ma·tous hyperplasia (sue″do·ep″i·theel·ee·o′muh·tus). An irregular, penetrating acanthosis accompanied by chronic inflammation in the dermis, found in chronic ulcers of the skin and chronic granulomatous infections. The reaction simulates squamous cell carcinoma.

pseu·do·erec·tile tissue (sue″do·e·reck′til). Tissue with a rich venous plexus, such as the submucosa of the nasal conchae.

pseu·do·es·the·sia, pseu·do·aes·the·sia (sue″do·es·theezh′uh) *n.* PSEUDESTHESIA.

pseu·do·ex·fo·li·a·tion of the lens capsule (sue″do·ecks·fo″lee·ay′shun). A deposition of white, fluffy material on the anterior lens surface, on the zonules, and in the angle; frequently associated with secondary glaucoma.

pseu·do·fluc·tu·a·tion (sue″do·fluck″choo·ay′shun) *n.* [*pseudo-* + *fluctuation*]. A phenomenon simulating fluctuation, sometimes observed on tapping lipomas.

pseu·do·fol·lic·u·lar salpingitis (sue″do·fol·ick′yoo·lur). Adenomyoma originating in the epithelium of the uterine tube.

pseu·do·frac·ture (sue′do·frack″chur) *n.* [*pseudo-* + *fracture*]. A bony defect which in roentgenograms has the appearance of an incomplete fracture with associated periosteal reaction and callus or new bone formation, sometimes observed in osteomalacia.

pseu·do·gan·gli·on (sue″do·gang′glee·un) *n.* [*pseudo-* + *ganglion*]. An enlargement on a nerve trunk which resembles a ganglion in form but which does not contain ganglion cells.

pseu·do·geus·es·the·sia, pseu·do·geus·aes·the·sia (sue″do·gew″ses·theezh′uh) *n.* [*pseudo-* + Gk. *geusis*, taste, + *esthesia*]. COLOR GUSTATION.

pseu·do·geu·sia (sue″do·gew′see·uh) *n.* [*pseudo-* + *-geusia*]. A false perception, or hallucination, of taste independent of any stimulus, often occurring as an aura in psychomotor epilepsy. Syn. *phantogeusia.*

pseu·do·gli·o·ma (sue″do·glye·o′muh) *n.* [*pseudo-* + *glioma*]. A condition in which there are inflammatory changes of the vitreous body, due to iridochoroiditis, and which resembles glioma of the retina.

pseu·do·glob·u·lin (sue″do·glob′yoo·lin) *n.* [*pseudo-* + *globulin*]. A protein, one of the class of globulins; distinguished from the euglobulins by its solubility in distilled water, as well as in dilute salt solutions.

pseu·do·gon·or·rhea, pseu·do·gon·or·rhoea (sue″do·gon·uh·ree′uh) *n.* [*pseudo-* + *gonorrhea*]. NONSPECIFIC URETHRITIS.

pseu·do·gout syndrome (sue″do·gowt′). A condition characterized by acute attacks of arthritis resembling gout and deposition of calcium pyrophosphate crystals in the articular cartilage. Syn. *chondrocalcinosis.*

pseudo-Graefe phenomenon or **sign.** Rapid elevation of the upper eyelid on attempts to move the eye in or down, as a result of aberrant or misregenerated fibers of the oculomotor nerve following trauma or from other causes. Compare *von Graefe's sign.*

pseu·do·gy·ne·co·mas·tia, pseu·do·gy·nae·co·mas·tia (sue″do·jin″e·ko·mas′tee·uh, ·guy″ne·ko·) *n.* [*pseudo-* + *gynecomastia*]. Enlargement of the male breast due to excessive adipose tissue, as opposed to glandular hyperplasia.

Pseu·do·ha·je (sue″do·hah′jee) *n.* [*pseudo-* + *haje* (specific epithet of the Egyptian cobra)]. A genus of arboreal cobras whose species possess a neurotoxic venom; found in the forests of central and western Africa.

pseu·do·hal·lu·ci·na·tion (sue″do·ha·lew″si·nay′shun) *n.* [*pseudo-* + *hallucination*]. A vivid perception without external stimulus (hallucination) recognized by the individual as a hallucinatory, hypnagogic, or hypnopompic experience.

pseu·do·hemi·acar·di·us (sue″do·hem″ee·a·kahr′dee·us) *n.* [*pseudo-* + *hemiacardius*]. A placental parasitic twin (omphalosite) which has no apparent thorax. Syn. *pseudothorax, acephalus athorus.*

pseu·do·he·mo·phil·ia, pseu·do·hae·mo·phil·ia (sue″do·hee″mo·fil′ee·uh, ·hem″o·) *n.* [*pseudo-* + *hemophilia*]. VASCULAR HEMOPHILIA.

pseu·do·her·maph·ro·dite (sue″do·hur·maf′ro·dite) *n.* [*pseudo-* + *hermaphrodite*]. An individual with congenitally malformed external genitalia resembling one sex while the gonads are those of the opposite sex. —**pseudo·her·maph·ro·dit·ic** (·maf″ro·dit′ick) *adj.*

pseu·do·her·maph·ro·dit·ism (sue″do·hur·maf′ro·dye·tiz·um) *n.* The condition of being a pseudohermaphrodite.

pseu·do·her·maph·ro·di·tis·mus fem·i·ni·nus (sue″do·hur·maf″ro·di·tiz′mus fem″i·nye′nus). FEMALE PSEUDOHERMAPHRODITISM.

pseudohermaphroditismus mas·cu·li·nus (mas″kew·lye′nus). MALE PSEUDOHERMAPHRODITISM.

pseu·do·hy·dro·ceph·a·lus (sue″do·high″dro·sef′uh·lee) *n.* False hydrocephalus; a condition in which the head appears disproportionately large as compared to the body; commonly seen in infants who are or were premature and small for their gestational age, the head growing at a faster rate than the body.

pseu·do·hy·dro·ne·phro·sis (sue″do·high″dro·ne·fro′sis) *n.* [*pseudo-* + *hydronephrosis*]. The presence of a cyst near a kidney, which resembles hydronephrosis.

pseu·do·hy·dro·pho·bia (sue″do·high″dro·fo′bee·uh) *n.* [*pseudo-* + *hydrophobia*]. CYNOPHOBIA (2).

pseudohypertrophic infantile muscular dystrophy. A progressive hereditary, sex-linked recessive disorder of muscle, affecting chiefly males, beginning in early childhood; characterized by bulky calf and forearm muscles, which are doughy as a result of infiltration of fat and fibrous tissue, and by progressive weakness and atrophy of the thigh, hip, and back muscles, with resulting waddling gait, inability to rise from the supine position without "climbing-up on oneself" (Gower's sign), and lordosis. There is eventual involvement of the shoulder girdle and the muscles of respiration, as well as of the myocardium and esophagus. Syn. *Duchenne's muscular dystrophy.*

pseudohypertrophic muscular paralysis. PSEUDOHYPERTROPHIC INFANTILE MUSCULAR DYSTROPHY.

pseu·do·hy·per·tro·phy (sue″do·high·pur′truh·fee) *n.* [*pseudo-* + *hypertrophy*]. FALSE HYPERTROPHY; increase in the size of an organ resulting from causes other than increased size of one or more of its normal components. —**pseudo·hy·per·troph·ic** (·high″pur·trof′ick) *adj.*

pseu·do·hy·po·na·tre·mia, pseu·do·hy·po·na·trae·mia (sue″do·high″po·na·tree′mee·uh) *n.* [*pseudo-* + *hyponatremia*]. Low serum sodium concentration due to hyperglycemia or hyperlipemia, which does not mean diminished effective serum osmotic pressure.

pseu·do·hy·po·para·thy·roid·ism (sue″do·high″po·păr″uh·thigh′roy·diz·um) *n.* [*pseudo-* + *hypoparathyroidism*]. A condition exhibiting the signs, symptoms, and chemical findings of hypoparathyroidism, but due to an inability of the body to respond to parathyroid hormone, and not to a deficiency thereof.

pseudo H zone or **band.** The portion of the H zone immediately surrounding the M line, of slightly lower density than the rest of the H zone, representing a region in which bridgelike structures connecting myosin and actin filaments are absent. Syn. *L zone, L band.*

pseu·do·il·e·us (sue″do·il′ee·us) *n.* [*pseudo-* + *ileus*]. ADYNAMIC ILEUS.

pseu·do·iso·chro·mat·ic (sue″do·eye″so·kro·mat′ick) *adj.* [*pseudo-* + *isochromatic*]. Pertaining to the different colors which appear alike to a person who is colorblind. See also *color threshold test, Ishihara's test.*

pseu·do·jaun·dice (sue″do·jawn′dis) *n.* [*pseudo-* + *jaundice*]. Yellow discoloration of the skin from causes other than hepatic disease.

pseu·do·ke·loid (sue″do·kee′loid) *adj.* Keloid-like.

pseu·do·ker·a·tin (sue″do·kerr′uh·tin) *n.* [*pseudo-* + *keratin*]. A keratin that is partly digested by the common proteolytic enzymes, as distinguished from those keratins, classified as eukeratins, which are not digested.

pseu·do·ker·a·to·sis (sue″do·kerr″uh·to′sis) *n.* [*pseudokeratin* + *-osis*]. A condition in which pseudokeratin is present.

pseu·do·lep·ra reaction (sue″do·lep′ruh). A mild lepra reaction in which there are cutaneous hypersensitivity responses, but the patient's general condition is not affected.

pseu·do·leu·ke·mia, pseu·do·leu·kae·mia (sue″do·lew·kee′mee·uh) *n.* [*pseudo-* + *leukemia*]. Any condition simulating leukemia in the absence of that disease.

pseudoleukemia in·fan·tum (in·fan′tum). VON JAKSCH'S ANEMIA.

pseu·do·li·thi·a·sis (sue″do·li·thigh′uh·sis) *n.* [*pseudo-* + *lithiasis*]. A condition in which symptoms mimic those of a calculus in the biliary or urinary passages but where no stone can be demonstrated.

pseu·do·lo·gia fan·tas·ti·ca (sue″do·lo′jee·uh fan·tas′ti·kuh). A syndrome marked by a single, elaborate fantasy, of which the patient gives full details. The fantasy includes real occurrences added to a fantastic basis.

pseu·do·lym·pho·ma (sue″do·lim·fo′muh) *n.* [*pseudo-* + *lymphoma*]. LYMPHOCYTOMA CUTIS.

pseu·do·lys·sa (sue″do·lis′uh) *n.* [*pseudo-* + *lyssa*]. CYNOPHOBIA (2).

pseu·do·mal·a·dy (sue″do·mal′a·dee) *n.* [*pseudo-* + *malady*]. An imaginary or simulated illness.

pseu·do·ma·lar·ia (sue″do·muh·lăr′ee·uh) *n.* [*pseudo-* + *malaria*]. A toxic disease simulating malaria.

pseu·do·mam·ma (sue″do·mam′uh) *n.* [*pseudo-* + *mamma*]. A structure simulating a mammary gland sometimes occurring in dermoid cysts.

pseu·do·ma·nia (sue″do·may′nee·uh) *n.* [*pseudo-* + *-mania*]. 1. A mental disorder in which the patient accuses himself of crimes of which he is innocent. 2. A persistent compulsion for lying. 3. An excited mental state in a conversion type of hysterical neurosis which simulates the true manic phase of manic-depressive illness.

pseu·do·mel·a·no·sis (sue″do·mel·uh·no′sis) *n.* [*pseudo-* + *melanosis*]. The staining of tissues, usually after death, by dark-brown or black pigments commonly derived from hemoglobin.

pseudomelanosis co·li (ko′lye). 1. Brown to black discoloration of all or a part of the colonic mucosa resulting from accumulations of an iron-containing pigment in mucosal macrophages; the presence of iron has been considered the feature distinguishing the pigment in this condition from that found in melanosis coli, but the distinctions are probably less obvious or even nonexistent. 2. Postmortem brown to black discoloration of all or part of the colonic mucosa due to the action of hydrogen sulfide in the bowel on iron in the mucosa.

pseu·do·mem·brane (sue″do·mem′brane) *n.* FALSE MEMBRANE, as in diphtheria. —**pseudomem·bra·nous** (·bruh·nus) *adj.*

pseudomembranous cystitis. An inflammation of the urinary bladder seen mainly in young women, characterized by a thickening irregular appearance of the mucosa of the trigone, suggesting a whitish covering membrane.

pseudomembranous entercolitis. A syndrome believed to be caused by various species of *Staphylococcus* and often appearing postoperatively in patients receiving antibiotics, manifested clinically by severe diarrhea, abdominal pain and distention, and circulatory collapse, often leading to death; and pathologically by the formation of a pseudomembrane over the bowel mucosa with inflammation and necrosis of the mucosa.

pseudomembranous inflammation or **mucositis.** DIPHTHERITIC INFLAMMATION.

pseudomembranous rhinitis. FIBRINOUS RHINITIS.

pseu·do·men·in·gi·tis (sue″do·men·in·jye′tis) *n.* [*pseudo-* + *meningitis*]. MENINGISM.

pseu·do·me·ninx (sue″do·mee′ninks) *n.* [*pseudo-* + *meninx*]. FALSE MEMBRANE.

pseu·do·men·stru·a·tion (sue″do·men″stroo·ay′shun) *n.* [*pseudo-* + *menstruation*]. Bloody vaginal discharge in newborn female infants, ceasing after a few days.

pseu·do·me·tam·er·ism (sue″do·me·tam′ur·iz·um) *n.* [*pseudo-* + *metamerism*]. False metamerism, as seen especially in the linear series of segments of the Cestoda. Each segment, or proglottid, contains a complete set of both male and female reproductive organs.

pseu·do·met·he·mo·glo·bin, pseu·do·met·hae·mo·glo·bin (sue″do·met·hee′muh·glo″bin, ·hem′o·) *n.* [*pseudo-* + *hemoglobin*]. METHEMALBUMIN.

pseu·do·mi·cro·ceph·a·ly (sue″do·migh″kro·sef′uh·lee) *n.* [*pseudo-* + *microcephaly*]. A head that appears to be small in relation to the rest of the body, but whose circumference on measurement falls within two standard deviations below the mean for age and sex. Compare *microcephaly.*

pseu·dom·ne·sia (sue″dom·nee′zhuh, ·zee·uh) *n.* [*pseudo-* + *-mnesia*]. Imaginary memory of events or things that have no basis in fact; CONFABULATION.

Pseu·dom·o·na·da·ce·ae (sue·dom″o·na·day′see·ee, sue″do·mo″na·) *n.pl.* A family of bacteria, usually aerobic, motile, and gram-negative; genera include *Pseudomonas, Acetobacter, Spirillum.*

Pseu·dom·o·nas (sue·dom′o·nas, sue″do·mo′nas) *n.* [*pseudo-* + Gk. *monas*, unit]. A genus of bacteria of the family Pseudomonadaceae; members are small, motile, aerobic, and gram-negative.

Pseudomonas ae·ru·gi·no·sa (e·rue″ji·no′suh). A species of bacteria pathogenic to man; it is the causative agent of various suppurative infections in man. In the multiplication of *Pseudomonas aeruginosa,* pigments are liberated which give pus a blue-green color. Syn. *Pseudomonas pyocyanea, Bacillus pyocyaneus, blue-pus microbe.*

Pseudomonas mal·lei (mal′ee, ·eye). The causative agent of glanders. Formerly called *Actinobacillus mallei, Malleomyces mallei.*

Pseudomonas pseu·do·mal·lei (sue″do·mal′ee·eye). An organism responsible for septicemia, pyemia, and granulomatous nodules in man and in rodents. Syn. *Malleomyces pseudomallei, Bacillus whitmori.*

Pseudomonas pyo·cy·a·nea (pye″o·sigh·ay′nee·uh). *PSEUDOMONAS AERUGINOSA.*

pseu·do·mon·gol·ism (sue″do·mong′guh·liz·um) *n.* [*pseudo-* + *mongolism*]. *Obsol.* A congenital disorder in which the child is a partial phenotype of the Down's syndrome; however, the karyotype may have an extra chromosome fragment presumed to represent a partially deleted 21st chromosome, may show mosaicism, or may be normal. —**pseudomongol·oid** (·loid) *n. & adj.*

pseu·do·mu·cin (sue″do·mew′sin) *n.* [*pseudo-* + *mucin*]. A substance allied to mucin, found in certain cysts. —**pseudomucin·ous** (·us) *adj.*

pseudomucinous adenofibroma. MUCINOUS CYSTADENOMA.

pseudomucinous carcinoma. MUCINOUS CYSTADENOCARCINOMA.

pseudomucinous cyst. MUCINOUS CYSTADENOMA.

pseudomucinous cystadenocarcinoma. MUCINOUS CYSTADENOCARCINOMA.

pseudomucinous cystadenoma. MUCINOUS CYSTADENOMA.

pseudomucinous cystocarcinoma. MUCINOUS CYSTADENOCARCINOMA.

pseudomucinous papillary cystadenocarcinoma. MUCINOUS CYSTADENOCARCINOMA.

pseudomucinous papilloma. MUCINOUS CYSTADENOMA.

pseudomucinous racemose cystoma. MUCINOUS CYSTADENOMA.

pseu·do·myx·o·ma (sue″do·mick·so′muh) *n.* [*pseudo-* + *myxoma*]. An epithelial tumor that contains much mucus but is so interspersed with tissue that grossly it suggests myxoma. —**pseudomyxoma·tous** (·tus) *adj.*

pseudomyxoma pe·ri·to·nei (perr″i·to·nee′eye). A widespread implantation in the peritoneal cavity of nodules secondary to mucinous tumors of the ovary or rupture of a mucocele of the appendix. Syn. *gelatinous ascites, gelatinous peritonitis, Werth's tumor.*

pseudomyxomatous cystadenoma. MUCINOUS CYSTADENOMA.

pseu·do·nar·co·tism (sue″do·nahr′ko·tiz·um) *n.* [*pseudo-* + *narcotism*]. A conversion type of hysterical neurosis simulating narcotism.

pseu·do·neo·plasm (sue″do·nee′o·plaz·um) *n.* [*pseudo-* + *neoplasm*]. 1. PHANTOM TUMOR. 2. A temporary swelling, generally of inflammatory origin. —**pseudo·neo·plas·tic** (·nee″o·plas′tick) *adj.*

pseu·do·neu·ro·ma (sue″do·new·ro′muh) *n.* [*pseudo-* + *neuroma*]. AMPUTATION NEUROMA.

pseu·do·neu·rot·ic (sue″do·new·rot′ick) *adj.* [*pseudo-* + *neu-*

rotic]. Typical of neurosis but stemming from and tending to conceal another disorder, particularly schizophrenia.

pseudoneurotic type of schizophrenia. A form of schizophrenia in which symptoms usually held to be neurotic tend to mask the basic psychotic disorders.

pseu·do·nu·cle·in (sue″do·new′klee·in) *n.* PARANUCLEIN.

pseu·do·nu·cle·o·lus (sue″do·new·klee′o·lus) *n.* [*pseudo-* + *nucleolus*]. KARYOSOME (1).

pseu·do·nys·tag·mus (sue″do·nis·tag′mus) *n.* [*pseudo-* + *nystagmus*]. Any of the symptoms resembling nystagmus but without the regular rhythmic movements of true nystagmus. See also *end-point nystagmus, fatigue nystagmus, labyrinthine nystagmus, ocular nystagmus.*

pseudo-oedema. PSEUDOEDEMA.

pseu·do·oph·thal·mo·ple·gia (sue″do·off·thal″mo·plee′jee·uh) *n.* [*pseudo-* + *ophthalmoplegia*]. A disorder in which eye movements on command or for following an object are unequally affected or even abolished, or in which the patient cannot fix his eyes on an object in the peripheral field, but in which the eyes may follow a slowly moving object or show full excursions with stimulation of the labyrinths. Syn. *ocular apraxia.*

pseu·do·os·teo·ma·la·cia (sue″do·os″tee·o·ma·lay′shee·uh) *n.* [*pseudo-* + *osteomalacia*]. Rachitis in which the pelvic basin is distorted so as to resemble in form that of osteomalacia.

pseu·do·pap·il·le·de·ma, pseu·do·pap·il·loe·de·ma (sue″do·pa·pil″e·dee′muh, ·pap″il·) *n.* [*pseudo-* + *papilledema*]. Apparent swelling of the optic disk, but without elevation of the disk or dilatation of the retinal veins, hyperemia, or enlargement of the blind spot; due to crowding and piling up of the optic nerve fibers and excess glial tissue; seen in extremely hypermetropic eyes, especially in children; may be congenital and familial.

pseu·do·pa·ral·y·sis (sue″do·puh·ral′i·sis) *n.* [*pseudo-* + *paralysis*]. An apparent motor paralysis that is caused by voluntary inhibition of motor impulses because of pain or other organic or psychic causes.

pseu·do·para·ple·gia (sue″do·păr·uh·plee′jee·uh) *n.* [*pseudo-* + *paraplegia*]. HYSTERICAL PARALYSIS.

pseu·do·par·a·site (sue″do·păr′uh·site) *n.* [*pseudo-* + *parasite*]. 1. Any object resembling a parasite. 2. COMMENSAL.

pseu·do·pa·re·sis (sue″do·pa·ree′sis, ·păr′e·sis) *n.* [*pseudo-* + *paresis*]. PSEUDOPARALYSIS.

pseu·do·pa·tient, *n.* 1. An actor or other person who simulates illness for teaching purposes. 2. A person investigating aspects of medical practice by impersonating a patient.

pseu·do·pe·lade (sue″do·pe·lahd′) *n.* [*pseudo-* + *pelade*]. ALOPECIA CICATRISATA.

pseu·do·pep·tone (sue″do·pep′tone) *n.* HEMIALBUMOSE.

pseu·do·phot·es·the·sia (sue″do·fo″tes·theezh′uh, ·theez′ee·uh) *n.* [*pseudo-* + *photesthesia*]. Ability to experience photisms.

pseu·do·pho·to·aes·the·sia (sue″do·fo″to·es·theezh′uh, ·theez′ee·uh) *n.* PSEUDOPHOTESTHESIA.

Pseu·do·phyl·lid·ea (sue″do·fil·lid′ee·uh) *n.pl.* [NL., from *pseudo-* + Gk. *phyllon,* leaf]. An order of the class Cestoda or tapeworms.

pseu·do·ple·gia (sue″do·plee′jee·uh) *n.* [*pseudo-* + *-plegia*]. Simulated paralysis, observed in hysteria or malingering.

pseu·do·pock·et (sue′do·pock″it) *n.* GINGIVAL POCKET.

pseu·do·pod (sue′do·pod) *n.* PSEUDOPODIUM.

pseu·do·po·dio·spore (sue″do·po′dee·o·spore) *n.* [*pseudopodium* + *spore*]. An ameboid swarm spore; AMEBULA.

pseu·do·po·di·um (sue″do·po′dee·um) *n.*, pl. **pseudopo·dia** (·dee·uh) [NL., from *pseudo-* + Gk. *podion,* small foot]. 1. A temporary protrusion of a portion of the cytoplasm of an ameboid cell, as an aid to locomotion or for engulfing particulate matter. 2. An irregular projection of the margin of a wheal.

pseu·do·poly·co·ria (sue″do·pol·ee·kor′ee·uh) *n.* The "false" form of polycoria.

pseu·do·poly·po·sis (sue″do·pol·i·po′sis) *n.* [*pseudo-* + *polyposis*]. An acquired form of polyposis of the colon, secondary to ulcerative colitis or amebic dysentery, in which tufts of mucosa have a pedunculated appearance due to adjacent ulcers or scars.

pseu·do·por·en·ceph·a·ly (sue″do·por″en·sef′uh·lee) *n.* [*pseudo-* + *porencephaly*]. A cavity in the cerebral mantle, usually due to a destructive process, which does not communicate with one of the lateral ventricles.

pseu·do·preg·nan·cy (sue″do·preg′nun·see) *n.* [*pseudo-* + *pregnancy*]. PSEUDOCYESIS.

pseu·do·pseu·do·hy·po·para·thy·roid·ism (sue″do·sue″do·high″po·păr·uh·thigh′roy·diz·um) *n.* [*pseudo-* + *pseudohypoparathyroidism*]. A condition with all the stigmata of pseudohypoparathyroidism, but with normal serum phosphorus and calcium levels.

pseu·dop·sia (sue·dop′see·uh) *n.* [*pseud-* + *-opsia*]. Visual hallucination, or error of visual perception.

pseu·do·psy·cho·path·ic (sue″do·sigh″ko·path′ick) *adj.* Of a condition or symptom, seemingly psychopathic but not so in fact.

pseu·do·pte·ryg·i·um (sue″do·te·rij′ee·um) *n.* [*pseudo-* + *pterygium*]. A false, or cicatricial, pterygium.

pseu·do·pto·sis (sue″do·to′sis, sue″dop·) *n.* [*pseudo-* + *ptosis*]. A condition resembling ptosis, caused by a fold of skin and fat descending below the edge of the eyelid.

pseu·do·pus (sue′do·pus″) *n.* [*pseudo-* + *pus*]. Any fluid resembling a purulent exudate.

pseu·do·ra·bies (sue″do·ray′beez) *n.* [*pseudo-* + *rabies*]. 1. A viral disease chiefly affecting cattle and swine, rarely man, transmitted by wild brown rats. Intense pruritus is followed by various central nervous system signs, including bulbar paralysis. Syn. *Aujeszky's disease.* 2. A disease superficially resembling rabies but hysterical in origin.

pseu·do·re·ac·tion (sue″do·ree·ack′shun) *n.* [*pseudo-* + *reaction*]. 1. A localized reaction following intracutaneous inoculation of a test substance, due to irritating impurities contained in the material. 2. In the Schick test for immunity to diphtheria, a reaction to the toxin and the toxoid which fades within 48 hours, indicating immunity to the toxin and hypersensitivity.

pseu·do·re·tar·da·tion (sue″do·ree″tahr·day′shun) *n.* [*pseudo-* + *retardation*]. A state of slow or defective mentation, in which the patient appears to be mentally retarded when in fact he is not; often due to emotional deprivation or depression or large doses of drugs, such as anticonvulsants or neuroleptics, in which sedation is a major side effect.

pseu·do·ret·i·no·blas·to·ma (sue″do·ret″i·no·blas·to′muh) *n.* Any of a number of conditions that lead to retinal detachment and clinically may be confused with retinoblastoma, such as Coat's disease or retinal dysplasia.

pseu·do·rick·ets (sue′do·rick″its) *n.* [*pseudo-* + *rickets*]. RENAL RICKETS.

pseu·do·rhon·cus (sue″do·ronk′us) *n.* [*pseudo-* + *rhoncus*]. An adventitious sound heard on auscultation of the lungs, mimicking the rhoncus of lung disease.

pseu·do·ro·sette (sue″do·ro·zet′) *n.* [*pseudo-* + *rosette*]. An arrangement of cells in a fashion resembling the primitive ependymal canal, but lacking the open central space of that canal; usually composed of tumor cells arranged around a blood vessel or around necrotic material.

pseu·do·ru·bel·la (sue″do·roo·bel′uh) *n.* [*pseudo-* + *rubella*]. EXANTHEM SUBITUM.

pseu·do·sar·co·ma of the breast (sue″do·sahr·ko′muh). CYSTOSARCOMA PHYLLODES.

pseu·do·scar·la·ti·na (sue″do·skahr·luh·tee′nuh) *n.* [*pseudo-* + *scarlatina*]. A febrile disease with a rash like that of scarlet fever, probably due to an intercurrent viral illness or to drug toxicity.

pseu·do·sci·ence (sue″do·sigh′unce) *n.* [*pseudo-* + *science*].

Any system of theories or methods claiming or appearing to be scientific, but clearly fallacious.

pseu·do·scle·re·ma (sue″do·skle·ree′muh) *n.* [*pseudo-* + *sclerema*]. Induration of the subcutaneous fat of newborn infants.

pseu·do·scle·ro·sis (sue″do·skle·ro′sis) *n.* [*pseudo-* + *sclerosis*]. 1. CREUTZFELDT-JAKOB DISEASE. 2. HEPATOLENTICULAR DEGENERATION.

pseudosclerosis of Westphal and Strümpell [C. F. O. *Westphal* and E. A. G. G. *Strümpell*]. HEPATOLENTICULAR DEGENERATION.

pseu·do·se·rous membrane (sue″do·seer′us). A membrane presenting the moist, glistening surface of a serous membrane, but differing from it in structure, as the endothelium of the blood vessels.

pseu·do·sil·i·cot·i·cum (sue″do·sil″i·kot′i·kum) *n.* TALCUM-POWDER GRANULOMA.

pseu·do·small·pox (sue″do·smawl′pocks) *n.* VARIOLA MINOR.

pseu·dos·mia (sue·doz′mee·uh) *n.* [*pseud-* + *osm-* + *-ia*]. A hallucination of smell; frequently observed in uncinate epilepsy. Syn. *phantosmia.*

pseu·do·sto·ma (sue″do·sto′muh) *n.* [*pseudo-* + *stoma*]. An apparent aperture between endothelial cells whose margins have been stained with silver nitrate.

pseu·do·stra·bis·mus (sue″do·stra·biz′mus) *n.* The false appearance of convergent strabismus even though there is normal alignment of the visual axis, seen in individuals, particularly infants and Orientals, with flat nasal bridges, narrow interpupillary distances, and epicanthic folds, which cause less sclera to be seen nasally than temporally while the eyes look straight ahead; proved by the absence of a shift by either eye during the cover test.

pseu·do·strat·i·fied (sue″do·strat′i·fide) *adj.* [*pseudo-* + *stratified*]. Characterizing an epithelium in which the cells all reach the basement membrane, but are of different lengths, with their nuclei lying at different levels, thus producing the appearance of several layers of cells.

pseu·do·ta·bes (sue″do·tay′beez) *n.* [*pseudo-* + *tabes*]. A neuropathy with symptoms like those of tabes dorsalis (lightning pains, sensory ataxia, atonic bladder), but not due to syphilis. Most often observed with diabetes mellitus. —**pseudo·ta·bet·ic** (·ta·bet′ick) *adj.*

pseu·do·tet·a·nus (sue″do·tet′uh·nus) *n.* [*pseudo-* + *tetanus*]. Tonic spasms of muscles simulating tetanus without the presence of *Clostridium tetani.*

pseu·do·tet·any (sue″do·tet′uh·nee) *n.* A condition resembling tetany, but without measurable hypocalcemia, in which all skeletal muscles may be continuously or intermittently in spasm, and every strong movement leads to cramp. Syn. *pathologic cramp syndrome.*

Pseu·do·thel·phu·sa (sue″do·thel·few′suh) *n.* [*pseudo-* + *Thelphusa* (name of another genus)]. A genus of crayfish, species of which may act as intermediate hosts of the fluke, *Paragonimus westermani.*

pseu·do·tho·rax (sue″do·tho′racks) *n.* [*pseudo-* + *thorax*]. PSEUDOHEMIACARDIUS.

pseu·do·tin·ni·tus (sue″do·tin·eye′tus) *n.* [*pseudo-* + *tinnitus*]. OBJECTIVE TINNITUS.

pseu·do·trich·i·no·sis (sue″do·trick·i·no′sis) *n.* [*pseudo-* + *trichinosis*]. DERMATOMYOSITIS.

pseu·do·tri·loc·u·lar heart (sue″do·trye·lock′yoo·lur). A heart having two atria with a defective interatrial septum and one ventricle, occurring in an individual who would normally have a four-chambered heart.

pseu·do·trun·cus ar·te·ri·o·sus (sue″do·trunk′us ahr·teer″ee·o′sus). A congenital malformation of the heart with high ventricular septal defect, overriding of the aorta, and absent or rudimentary pulmonary artery. Circulation to the lungs is via the bronchial arteries.

pseu·do·tu·ber·cu·lo·sis (sue″do·tew·bur″kew·lo′sis) *n.* [*pseudo-* + *tuberculosis*]. An infection caused by *Yersinia pseudotuberculosis,* occurring in many animals, including rodents and birds, and which in man may produce severe disease with septicemia and sometimes symptoms resembling typhoid fever.

pseu·do·tu·ber·cu·lous enteritis (sue″do·tew·bur′kew·lus). 1. Intestinal inflammation due to *Yersinia pseudotuberculosis.* 2. Intestinal inflammation resembling tuberculosis in some respect, but not due to *Mycobacterium tuberculosis.*

pseu·do·tu·mor (sue″do·tew′mur) *n.* [*pseudo-* + *tumor*]. PSEUDONEOPLASM.

pseudotumor cer·e·bri (serr′e·brye). A syndrome of increased intracranial pressure associated with normal or small cerebral ventricles, of unknown etiology but, in children, sometimes associated with obstruction of the large intracranial sinuses or veins, particularly the lateral sinus. Syn. *benign intracranial hypertension, meningeal hydrops.*

pseu·do·tym·pa·ni·tes (sue″do·tim″puh·nigh′teez) *n.* [*pseudo-* + *tympanites*]. A distension of the abdomen similar to tympanites but not due to accumulation of gas; generally appears and disappears rapidly.

pseu·do·tym·pa·ny (sue″do·tim′puh·nee) *n.* PSEUDOTYMPANITES.

pseu·do·ty·phoid meningitis (sue″do·tye′foid). A nonfatal louse-borne type of meningitis affecting swineherds, characterized by fever, headache, muscular pain, digestive disturbance, and foul diarrhea with occasional rectal hemorrhages.

pseu·do·vac·u·oles (sue″do·vack′yoo·ole′z) *n.pl.* [*pseudo-* + *vacuole*]. Transparent bodies containing pigment, found in blood of malarial patients.

pseu·do·va·gi·nal hypospadias (sue″do·vaj′i·nul, ·va·jye′nul). A form of hypospadias in which the opening of the urethra is upon the perineum, and is funnel-like and wide open; this may be interpreted as a vagina and lead to confusion of sex. See also *pseudohermaphroditism.*

pseu·do·ven·tri·cle (sue″do·ven′tri·kul) *n.* [*pseudo-* + *ventricle*]. The cavity of the septum pellucidum, called the fifth ventricle of the brain, although not a true one.

pseu·do·ver·ti·go (sue″do·vur′ti·go) *n.* [*pseudo-* + *vertigo*]. GIDDINESS.

pseu·do·vom·it·ing (sue″do·vom′i·ting) *n.* [*pseudo-* + *vomiting*]. Passive regurgitation of material from the stomach, without expulsive effort.

pseu·do·xan·tho·ma elas·ti·cum (sue″do·zan·tho′muh e·las′ti·kum). A genodermatosis, usually of recessive inheritance, resulting in deformed and often calcified elastic fibers. There are slightly elevated yellow plaques in the lax skin, accompanied in many cases by degenerative changes in the elastic blood vessels and in the eyes (angioid streaks of the retina). See also *Groenblad-Strandberg syndrome.*

pseu·dy·drops (sue·dye′drops) *n.* [*pseud-* + *hydrops*]. A false dropsy.

psi (sigh) *adj.* [Ψ, 23rd letter of the Greek alphabet]. Psychological or parapsychological.

psi·co·fu·ra·nine (sigh″ko·few′ruh·neen) *n.* 9β-D-Psicofuranosyladenine, $C_{11}H_{15}N_5O_5$, a nucleoside antibiotic produced by *Streptomyces hygroscopicus* var. *decoyicus.* It has antineoplastic and antimicrobial activity.

psi·lo·cin (sigh′lo·sin) *n.* 4-Hydroxy-*N,N*-dimethyltryptamine, $C_{12}H_{16}N_2O$, an active constituent of the hallucinogenic mushroom *Psilocybe mexicana;* a dephosphorylated derivative of psilocybin that is isomeric with bufotenine.

psi·lo·cyb·in (sigh″lo·sib′in, ·sigh′bin) *n.* 4-Phosphoryloxy-*N,N*-dimethyltryptamine, $C_{12}H_{17}N_2O_4P$, an active constituent of the hallucinogenic mushroom *Psilocybe mexicana.*

psi·lo·sis (sigh·lo′sis) *n.,* pl. **psilo·ses** (·seez) [Gk. *psilōsis,* depilation, from *psilos,* bare]. 1. ¹SPRUE. 2. The falling out of the hair. —**psi·lot·ic** (·lot′ick) *adj.*

psi phenomena. *In parapsychology,* personal experiences or events defying physical explanation, such as clairvoyance, precognition, and telepathy.

psit·ta·co·sis (sit″uh·ko′sis) *n.,* pl. **psittaco·ses** (·seez) [Gk.

psittakos, parrot, + *-osis*]. Pneumonia and generalized infection of man and of birds, usually acquired by man from such birds as parrots, parakeets, lovebirds, ducks, pigeons, and turkeys; caused by members of the family Chlamydiaceae. Syn. *parrot fever.*

pso·as (so'us) *n.*, pl. **pso·ai** (·eye), **pso·ae** (·ee) [Gk. *psoa*, muscles of the loins]. One of the two muscles, psoas major and psoas minor.

psoas abscess. An abscess arising from diseased lumbar or lower thoracic vertebrae, the pus gravitating through the sheath of the psoas and pointing finally in the femoral triangle.

psoas mag·nus (mag'nus). PSOAS MAJOR.

psoas major. The greater psoas muscle, which arises from the bodies and transverse processes of the lumbar vertebrae and is inserted into the lesser trochanter of the femur. NA *musculus psoas major.* See also Table of Muscles in the Appendix.

psoas minor. The inconstant smaller psoas muscle, which arises from the bodies and transverse processes of the lumbar vertebrae and is inserted on the pubis. NA *musculus psoas minor.* See also Table of Muscles in the Appendix.

psoas par·vus (pahr'vus). PSOAS MINOR.

psoas sign. Flexion of the hip, or pain on hyperextension of the hip due to an inflammatory process in contact with the psoas muscle on that side.

psod·y·mus (sod'i·mus) *n.* [*psoas* + *-dymus*]. Conjoined twins with two heads and chests and conjoined abdominal and pelvic cavities.

pso·i·tis (so·eye'tis) *n.* [*psoas* + *-itis*]. Inflammation of the psoas major muscle.

pso·mo·pha·gia (so''mo·fay'jee·uh) *n.* [Gk. *psōmos*, bit, morsel, + *-phagia*]. Swallowing chunks of food without thorough chewing. —**psomo·phag·ic** (·faj'ick) *adj.*

pso·moph·a·gy (so·mof'uh·jee) *n.* PSOMOPHAGIA.

pso·ra (so'ruh) *n.* [L., itch, mange, from Gk. *psōra*]. PSORIASIS.

pso·ra·len (sor'uh·len) *n.* Furo[3,2-*g*] coumarin, $C_{11}H_6O_3$, a constituent of *Psoralea corylifolia* Linn. and many other plants, certain derivatives of which, notably methoxsalen (methoxypsoralen) and trioxsalen (trimethylpsoralen), are used as dermal pigmenting agents. The derivatives are often collectively called psoralens.

pso·ra·line (sor'uh·leen, ·lin) *n.* CAFFEINE.

pso·ri·a·si·form (so·rye'uh·si·form, so''rye·as'i·form) *adj.* Like psoriasis.

pso·ri·a·sis (so·rye'uh·sis) *n.* [Gk. *psōriasis*, itch, mange, from *psōra*, from *psēn*, to rub, scratch]. An idiopathic chronic inflammatory skin disease characterized by the development of red patches covered with silvery-white imbricated scales. The disease affects especially the extensor surfaces of the body and the scalp.

psoriasis buc·ca·lis (buh·kay'lis). LEUKOPLAKIA BUCCALIS.

psoriasis cir·ci·na·ta (sur''si·nay'tuh). Psoriasis in which the central part of the lesion disappears and leaves a ring-shaped patch. Syn. *psoriasis orbicularis.*

psoriasis dif·fu·sa (di·few'suh). A form of psoriasis in which there is coalescence of contiguous lesions affecting large areas of the body.

psoriasis dis·coi·dea (dis·koy'dee·uh). A form of psoriasis in which the lesions are the size of small coins. Syn. *psoriasis nummularis.*

psoriasis fol·lic·u·la·ris (fol·ick''yoo·lair'is). A form of psoriasis in which scaly lesions are located at the openings of sweat and sebaceous glands.

psoriasis gut·ta·ta (guh·tay'tuh). PSORIASIS PUNCTATA.

psoriasis gy·ra·ta (jye·ray'tuh). Psoriasis with a serpentine arrangement of the patches.

psoriasis in·vet·e·ra·ta (in·vet''e·ray'tuh). Psoriasis with persistent infiltrated lesions which often fissure and become covered with heavy scales.

psoriasis num·mu·la·ris (num''yoo·lair'is). PSORIASIS DISCOIDEA.

psoriasis or·bic·u·la·ris (or·bick''yoo·lair'is). PSORIASIS CIRCINATA.

psoriasis pal·ma·ris (pal·mair'is, pahl·). Psoriasis affecting the palms of the hands.

psoriasis punc·ta·ta (punk·tay'tuh). A form of psoriasis in which the lesions consist of minute red papules which rapidly become surmounted by pearly scales.

psoriasis ru·pi·oi·des (roo·pee·oy'deez). A variety of psoriasis in which large conical crusts are marked by concentric rings.

psoriasis uni·ver·sa·lis (yoo''ni·vur·say'lis). A form of psoriasis in which the lesions are all over the body.

pso·ri·at·ic (so''ree·at'ick) *adj.* [Gk. *psōriatikos*]. Pertaining to or affected with psoriasis.

psoriatic arthritis or **arthropathy.** Arthritis associated with psoriasis which is either a variant of rheumatoid arthritis or a distinct entity. Inflammatory involvement of the distal interphalangeal joint is frequent.

psor·oph·thal·mia (sor''off·thal'mee·uh) *n.* [Gk. *psōra*, itching, + *ophthalmia*]. MARGINAL BLEPHARITIS.

pso·ro·sperm (sor'o·spurm) *n.* [Gk. *psōros*, rough, scabby, + *sperma*, seed]. 1. Any of the Myxosporidia. 2. CORPS ROND.

pso·ro·sper·mia (sor''o·spur'mee·uh) *n.*, pl. **psorosper·mi·ae** (·mee·ee). The spore phase of a psorosperm.

pso·ro·sper·mi·al (sor''o·spur'mee·ul) *adj.* Pertaining to a psorosperm.

pso·ro·sper·mic (sor''o·spur'mick) *adj.* PSOROSPERMIAL.

pso·ro·sper·mo·sis (sor''o·spur·mo'sis) *n.* [*psorosperm* + *-osis*]. A disease due to psorosperms.

psorospermosis fol·lic·u·la·ris (fol·ick''yoo·lair'is). DARIER'S DISEASE.

P. S. P. Abbreviation for *phenolsulfonphthalein.*

psych-, psycho-. A combining form meaning (a) *psyche, psychic;* (b) *psychology, psychologic.*

psy·cha·go·gia (sigh''kuh·go'jee·uh) *n.* PSYCHAGOGY.

psy·cha·go·gy (sigh'kuh·go''jee) *n.* [Gk. *psychagōgia*, winning over, persuasion, from *psychē*, soul, + *agōgos*, leading]. A reeducational, psychotherapeutic procedure that stresses the proper socialization of the individual. —**psy·cha·gog·ic** (sigh''kuh·goj'ick) *adj.*

psy·chal·gia (sigh·kal'jee·uh) *n.* [*psych-* + *-algia*]. Pains in the head, ascribed by depressed patients to anxiety, or to some psychic rather than physical cause.

psy·cha·lia (sigh·kay'lee·uh) *n.* An abnormal mental state attended by auditory and visual hallucinations.

psych·as·the·nia (sigh''kas·theen'ee·uh) *n.* [*psych-* + *asthenia*]. Any psychoneurotic disorder containing compulsive, obsessive, and phobic tensions. A nervous state characterized by an urge to think, feel, or do something which at the same time is recognized by the patient as being senseless, silly, or irrational. —**psychas·then·ic** (·thenn'ick) *adj.*

psych·atax·ia (sigh''kuh·tack'see·uh) *n.* [*psych-* + *ataxia*]. Impaired power of mental concentration; mental confusion or groping.

psych·au·di·to·ry (sigh·kaw'di·to·ree) *adj.* [*psych-* + *auditory*]. Pertaining to the conscious or intellectual interpretation of sounds.

psy·che (sigh'kee) *n.* [Gk. *psychē*, mind, soul, self]. 1. In Greek philosophy, the personification of the life principle. 2. The mind or self as a functional entity, serving to adjust the total organism to the needs or demands of the environment.

psy·che·del·ic (sigh''ke·del'ick, ·deel'ick) *adj.* [*psyche* + Gk. *dēlos*, manifest]. Pertaining to or producing a psychic state, commonly by use of a hallucinatory drug, in which normally repressed elements are revealed or manifested; mind-revealing or mind-manifesting.

psy·chen·to·nia (sigh''ken·to'nee·uh) *n.* [*psych-* + Gk. *entonia*, tension, from *entonos*, intense]. Mental strain or overwork.

psy·chi·a·ter (sigh·kigh'uh·tur) *n.* PSYCHIATRIST.

psy·chi·at·ric (sigh"kee·at'rick, sick"ee·at'rick) *adj.* Pertaining to psychiatry.

psychiatric abortion. A therapeutic abortion dictated by the aggravation or inception of a mental or an emotional disorder during pregnancy.

psychiatric criminology. *In criminology,* the study of that part of the criminal's personality and experiences which led to the performance of the criminal act.

psychiatric illness. MENTAL DISORDER.

psy·chi·at·rics (sigh"kee·at'ricks) *n.* The theory or practice of psychiatry.

psychiatric social worker. A person with specialized, usually postgraduate, training in social work as well as in certain aspects of psychiatry who utilizes techniques pertinent to both fields, and may to a limited extent conduct psychiatric interviews and therapy.

psy·chi·a·trist (sigh·kigh'uh·trist) *n.* A specialist in psychiatry; specifically, a graduate of a medical school, licensed to practice, with postgraduate training in the diagnosis and treatment of mental and emotional disorders. Compare *psychologist, psychopathologist.*

psy·chi·a·try (sigh·kigh'uh·tree, si·) *n.* [*psych-* + *-iatry*]. The medical science and specialty that deals with the origins, diagnosis, prevention, and treatment of mental and emotional disorders and, by extension, of many problems of personal adjustment. It also includes special fields such as mental retardation and legal psychiatry. See also *descriptive psychiatry, dynamic psychiatry, individual psychology, psychoanalysis, psychobiology.*

psy·chic (sigh'kick) *adj.* [Gk. *psychikos*]. 1. Pertaining to the psyche. 2. Sensitive to nonphysical forces. 3. Mental.

psy·chi·cal (sigh'ki·kul) *adj.* PSYCHIC.

psychic blindness. 1. CORTICAL BLINDNESS. 2. HYSTERICAL AMBLYOPIA.

psychic deafness. 1. CENTRAL DEAFNESS. 2. PSYCHOGENIC DEAFNESS.

psychic energizer. Any drug, as a monoamine oxidase inhibitor or an amphetamine, that produces elevation of mood or mental excitement or stimulation, especially in a depressed person.

psychic energy. PSYCHIC FORCE.

psychic epilepsy. A form of psychomotor or temporal lobe epilepsy in which the seizure consists mainly or solely of psychic aberrations, such as hallucinations, illusions, cognitive aberrations (feelings of increased reality, familiarity, unfamiliarity, depersonalization), or affective experiences (fear, anxiety).

psychic epileptic equivalent. Mental disturbance or excitement which may take the place of epileptic attacks. See also *psychic epilepsy, convulsive equivalent.*

psychic force. Mental power or force generated by thinking; contrasted with physical force. See also *libido.*

psychic impotence. Impotence due to a mental or emotional disturbance. Contr. *organic impotence.*

psychic overtone. An associated impression contributing to a mental image.

psychic profile. PSYCHOGRAM.

psy·chics (sigh'kicks) *n.* PSYCHOLOGY.

psychic trauma. A stressful emotional experience that frequently results in permanent changes in the person.

psychic weeping. The shedding of tears in response to a strong emotion; the physiologic nature of the process is as yet not understood. Contr. *reflex weeping.*

psy·chi·no·sis (sigh"ki·no'sis) *n.* [*psych-* + Gk. *nosos,* disease (assimilated in form to the suffix *-osis*)]. Any disease of the mind.

psy·chlamp·sia (sigh·klamp'see·uh) *n.* [*psych-* + Gk. *lampsis,* shining, illumination, + *-ia*]. *Obsol.* PSYCHOSIS.

psycho-. See *psych-.*

psy·cho·ac·ti·va·tor (sigh"ko·ack'ti·vay·tur) *n.* [*psycho-* + *activator*]. PSYCHIC ENERGIZER.

psy·cho·an·al·ge·sia (sigh"ko·an"ul·jee'zee·uh) *n.* [*psycho-* + *analgesia*]. The relief of pain by psychological means, principally by assurance of and explanations to the patient, suggestion, and therapeutic measures, such as music.

psy·cho·anal·y·sis (sigh"ko·uh·nal'i·sis) *n.* [Ger. *Psychoanalyse*]. 1. The method developed by Sigmund Freud for the exploration and synthesis of patterns in emotional thinking and development; a technique used in the treatment of a wide variety of emotional disorders, particularly the neuroses. Relies essentially upon the free associations of the patient to produce valuable information of which the patient was formerly unaware, by bringing to conscious manipulation ideas and experiences from the unconscious divisions of the psyche. 2. The body of data and theory based on the discoveries of this method; concerned chiefly with the conflict between infantile instinctual striving and parental or social demand, and the manner in which this conflict affects emotional growth, character development, and the formation of mental and emotional disorders.

psy·cho·an·a·lyst (sigh"ko·an'uh·list) *n.* [*psycho-* + *analyst*]. A person who practices psychoanalysis.

psy·cho·an·a·lyt·ic (sigh"ko·an·uh·lit'ick) *adj.* [*psycho-* + *analytic*]. Pertaining to psychoanalysis.

psychoanalytic theory. PSYCHOANALYSIS (2).

psy·cho·au·di·to·ry (sigh"ko·aw'di·tor"ee) *adj.* PSYCHAUDITORY.

psy·cho·bi·ol·o·gist (sigh"ko·bye·ol'uh·jist) *n.* A person who specializes in psychobiology.

psy·cho·bi·ol·o·gy (sigh"ko·bye·ol'uh·jee) *n.* [*psycho-* + *biology*]. The school of psychology and psychiatry originated by Adolf Meyer in the United States in which the individual is considered not only as a physical organism but as the sum of his environment. Mental disorders, like normal behavioral processes, are considered dynamic adaptive reactions of the individual to stress or conflict, and are the understandable results of the development of the individual. See also *distributive analysis and synthesis.* —**psycho·bi·o·log·ic** (·bye"uh·loj'ick), **psychobiolog·i·cal** (·i·kul) *adj.*

psy·cho·car·di·ac reflex (sigh"ko·kahr'dee·ack). Increase in the heart rate induced by recollection of a previous emotional experience.

psy·cho·ci·ne·sia (sigh"ko·si·nee'zhuh, ·zee·uh) *n.* PSYCHOKINESIS.

psy·cho·co·ma (sigh"ko·ko'muh) *n.* [*psycho-* + *coma*]. *Obsol.* STUPOR.

psy·cho·cor·ti·cal (sigh"ko·kor'ti·kul) *adj.* [*psycho-* + *cortical*]. Pertaining to the cerebral cortex as the seat of the mind.

psy·cho·del·ic (sigh"ko·del'ick·, ·deel'ick) *adj.* PSYCHEDELIC.

psy·cho·di·ag·no·sis (sigh"ko·dye"ug·no'sis) *n.* [*psycho-* + *diagnosis*]. Any procedure or means to discover the factors underlying behavior, particularly disordered or abnormal behavior.

psy·cho·di·ag·nos·tics (sigh"ko·dye"ug·nos'ticks) *n.* [*psycho-* + *diagnostics*]. 1. The evaluation of the personality, particularly as furnished by the Rorschach test. 2. PSYCHOGNOSIS (3).

Psy·chod·i·dae (sigh·kod'i·dee) *n.pl.* A family of the Diptera, which includes the moth flies, moth midges, and sand flies. The most important genus medically is *Phlebotomus.*

psy·cho·dom·e·ter (sigh"ko·dom'e·tur) *n.* [*psycho-* + *-dometer* as in speedometer]. 1. An instrument for measuring the rapidity of psychic processes. 2. Any mechanical device for measuring response time.

psy·cho·dom·e·try (sigh"ko·dom'e·tree) *n.* The measurement of the rapidity of the psychic processes, or of response to a stimulus.

psy·cho·dra·ma (sigh'ko·drah"muh) *n.* [*psycho-* + *drama*]. 1. *In psychotherapy,* the reenactment of events from the patient's life, with the patient as either spectator or actor; a technique for obtaining cathartic relief. 2. A form of group psychotherapy in which the patients act out or dramatize their emotional problems.

psy·cho·dy·nam·ic (sigh″ko·dye·nam′ick) *adj.* [*psycho-* + *dynamic*]. 1. Pertaining to any psychological process which is undergoing change or causing change. 2. Pertaining to psychodynamics. 3. Pertaining to psychoanalysis.

psy·cho·dy·nam·ics (sigh″ko·dye·nam′icks) *n.* The study of human behavior from the point of view of motivation and drives, depending largely on the functional significance of emotion, and based on the assumption that an individual's total personality and reactions at any given time are the product of the interaction between his genetic constitution and the environment in which he has lived from conception onward.

psy·cho·ep·i·lep·sy (sigh″ko·ep′i·lep″see) *n.* PSYCHIC EPILEPSY.

psy·cho·gal·van·ic reflex (sigh″ko·gal·van′ick). A variation in the electric conductivity of the skin in response to emotional stimuli; due to changes in blood circulation, secretion of sweat, and skin temperature.

psy·cho·gal·va·nom·e·ter (sigh″ko·gal″vuh·nom′e·tur) *n.* [*psycho-* + *galvanometer*]. A device for recording electrodermal responses to various mental stimuli which provoke emotional reactions. Its practical application is the lie detector, which indicates the emotional reactions of one who is suppressing the truth.

psy·cho·gen·e·sis (sigh″ko·jen′e·sis) *n.* [*psycho-* + *genesis*]. 1. The development of mental characteristics. 2. The process by which activities or ideas originate in the mind, or psyche. 3. The production or causation of a symptom or illness by psychic, rather than organic, factors. The origin of psychic activity contributing to a mental disorder. —**psycho·gen·ic** (·jen′ick), **psycho·ge·net·ic** (·je·net′ick) *adj.*

psychogenic blindness. Blindness of mental or psychic origin; may be a symptom of the hysterical type of conversion neurosis.

psychogenic deafness. Any deafness that has 50 percent or more of a psychic factor. Persons so affected do not know they can hear better than they manifest. It must be distinguished from malingering deafness.

psychogenic dysmenorrhea. Menstrual pain of mental or psychic origin.

psychogenic headache. Headache attributed to tension, anxiety, or a basic personality disorder. See also *muscle-contraction headache.*

psychogenic hyperhidrosis. Increased sweating due to psychogenic factors, most often on the palms, soles, axillas, and forehead.

psychogenic overlay. Exaggeration of complaints and symptoms beyond what one would expect from the organic cause, and therefore presumed to be of functional origin.

psychogenic polydipsia. Polydipsia due to psychological causes; differentiated from organic polydipsia by the patient's ability to concentrate urine.

psychogenic pruritus. Severe itching of skin on a psychogenic basis.

psychogenic torticollis. SPASMODIC TORTICOLLIS.

psychogenic vertigo. Dizziness or giddiness attributed to emotional factors or neurosis.

psy·chog·e·ny (sigh·koj′e·nee) *n.* PSYCHOGENESIS.

psy·cho·geu·sic (sigh″ko·gew′sick, ·joo′sick) *adj.* [*psycho-* + Gk. *geusis*, taste, + *-ic*]. Pertaining to perception of taste.

psy·chog·no·sis (sigh″kog·no′sis) *n.*, pl. **psychogno·ses** (·seez) [*psycho-* + *-gnosis*]. 1. Diagnosis or recognition of mental and psychic conditions. 2. The study of a person by hypnosis. 3. The study of personality and behavior based on the somatotype, facial expressions, and such other signs as posture, gait, and gestures. Compare *characterology.* —**psychog·nos·tic** (·nos′tick) *adj.*

psy·cho·gram (sigh′ko·gram) *n.* [*psycho-* + *-gram*]. A chart, profile, or table of personality traits.

psy·cho·graph·ic (sigh″ko·graf′ick) *adj.* [*psycho-* + *-graphic*]. 1. Pertaining to a chart of the personality traits of an individual. 2. *In psychiatry,* pertaining to the natural history of the mind.

psy·cho·ki·ne·sia (sigh″ko·kigh·nee′zhuh, ·zee·uh) *n.* PSYCHOKINESIS.

psy·cho·ki·ne·sis (sigh″ko·ki·nee′sis, ·kigh·nee′sis) *n.* [*psycho-* + *kinesis*]. 1. Explosive or impulsive maniacal action; a lack of inhibition of primitive instincts leading to violent and hasty actions. 2. *In parapsychology,* the postulated direct action of mind on matter without any intermediate physical energy or instrument, as the supposed determination of how the dice shall fall by mere action of the will.

psy·cho·lag·ny (sigh′ko·lag″nee) *n.* [*psycho-* + Gk. *lagneia,* lust]. Sexual excitement induced by and ending in the imagination.

psy·cho·lep·sy (sigh′ko·lep″see) *n.* [*psycho-* + *-lepsy*]. A sudden intense, usually short decrease in mental tension or mood level, approaching depression. —**psy·cho·lep·tic** (sigh″ko·lep′tick) *adj.*

psycholeptic episode. A strikingly vivid mental experience in the life of the patient from which he cannot free himself and which he believes started his physical illness.

psy·cho·log·ic (sigh″kuh·loj′ick) *adj.* 1. Of or pertaining to psychology. 2. PSYCHIC. 3. Emotional.

psy·cho·log·i·cal (sigh″ko·loj′i·kul) *adj.* PSYCHOLOGIC.

psychological autopsy. The investigation of the psychological and social circumstances which led to suicide or to unnatural death, such as from an accident, and of the manner in which patients contribute to their own deaths.

psychologic dyspareunia. Painful intercourse in the female due to emotional difficulties with no anatomic or pathologic explanation.

psychologic screening. The use of psychologic tests, usually for large groups, as a means of determining general suitability for some specific duty or occupation, such as army service.

psychologic test. A planned and standardized situation in which an individual's behavior can be characterized by his responses to given demands, such as questions or other tasks, with a numerical value or score. See also *aptitude test, intelligence test, personality test.*

psy·chol·o·gist (sigh·kol′uh·jist) *n.* 1. An individual who has made a professional study of, and usually thereafter professionally engages in, psychology. 2. Specifically, an individual with the minimum professional qualifications set forth by an intraprofessionally recognized psychological association, as the American Psychological Association. Compare *psychiatrist.*

psy·chol·o·gy (sigh·kol′uh·jee) *n.* [*psycho-* + *-logy*]. The science that studies the functions of the mind, such as sensation, perception, memory, thought, and, more broadly, the behavior of an organism in relation to its environment. 2. The psychological or mental activity characteristic of a person or a situation, as the psychology of surgeons, or the psychology of dying.

psy·cho·math·e·mat·ics (sigh″ko·math″e·mat′icks) *n.* Mathematics associated with or applied to psychology; specifically, the application of mathematical formulas and procedures to psychology and psychologic tests.

psy·cho·me·tri·cian (sigh″ko·me·trish′un) *n.* 1. A psychologist who specializes in the administration and interpretation of psychologic tests. Compare *psychotechnician.* 2. A specialist in the mathematical and statistical treatment of psychologic data.

psy·cho·met·rics (sigh″ko·met′ricks) *n.* [*psycho-* + *metric* + *-s*]. The measurement of mental and psychological abilities, potentials, and performance; frequently applied specifically to the measurement of intelligence. 2. PSYCHOMATHEMATICS. —**psychomet·ric** (·rick) *adj.*

psy·chom·e·try (sigh·kom′e·tree) *n.* [*psycho-* + *-metry*]. PSYCHOMETRICS.

psy·cho·mo·tor (sigh″ko·mo′tur) *adj.* [*psycho-* + *motor*]. Pertaining to both mental and motor activity, particularly as applied to the development of an infant or a child, to seizures, and to overactivity or underactivity of a confused or delirious patient.

psychomotor development. The progressive acquisition by the infant within a given time period of such motor skills as the ability to turn over at will, sit, crawl, stand, walk, and run, or intellectual skills such as meaningful speech or other ways of communication, of voluntary bladder and bowel control, and of cognitive skills such as the ability to solve problems; in the neurologically and mentally intact child, these developmental milestones are achieved by 3 to 4 years of age, after which there is primarily an increase in cognitive skills due to the child's educational experience.

psychomotor epilepsy. Recurrent multiple psychomotor seizures. Compare *temporal lobe epilepsy.*

psychomotor excitement. Physical and emotional hyperactivity in response to internal or external stimuli, as in hypomania.

psychomotor retardation. 1. Generalized slowness or deficiency in psychomotor development, applied particularly to infants and young children. 2. Generalized lack or diminution of physical and emotional responsiveness to internal or external stimuli, as may be seen in depressive states.

psychomotor seizure. An epileptic attack characterized by an aura which is often a complex hallucination or perceptual illusion, indicating a temporal lobe origin, and by complex semipurposeful activities for which the patient later has no recollection.

psychomotor status. Continuous psychomotor seizures.

psychomotor test. Any standardized test in which the score depends on certain perceptual abilities and some form of motor response and often also the speed of reaction to the stimulus, as aiming at a moving target.

psy·cho·neu·ro·log·ic (sigh″ko·new″ruh·loj′ick) *adj.* [*psycho-* + *neurologic*]. Pertaining to a condition involving both psychic and organic neural components.

psy·cho·neu·ro·log·i·cal (sigh″ko·new″ruh·loj′i·kul) *adj.* PSYCHONEUROLOGIC.

psy·cho·neu·ro·sis (sigh″ko·new·ro′sis) *n.* [*psycho-* + *neurosis*]. NEUROSIS (1).

psy·cho·neu·rot·ic (sigh″ko·new·rot′ick) *adj.* NEUROTIC.

psychoneurotic disorder. NEUROSIS (1).

psychoneurotic paradox. Persistent masochistic behavior not to a person's best self-interest despite his recognition of the harm or damage done; suggestive of self-punishing or self-destructive behavior.

psy·cho·nom·ics (sigh″ko·nom′icks) *n.* [*psycho-* + Gk. *nomikos,* of laws]. 1. PSYCHOLOGY. 2. Psychological development as affected by environmental factors. —**psychonom·ic** (·ick) *adj.*

psy·chon·o·my (sigh·kon′uh·mee) *n.* [*psycho-* + Gk. *nomos,* law, + *-y*]. PSYCHONOMICS.

psy·cho·no·se·ma (sigh″ko·no·see′muh) *n.* [*psycho-* + Gk. *nosēma,* disease]. Any mental disorder.

psy·cho·pa·re·sis (sigh″ko·puh·ree′sis, ·păr′e·sis) *n.* [*psycho-* + *paresis*]. MENTAL DEFICIENCY.

psy·cho·path (sigh′ko·path) *n.* [*psycho-* + *-path*]. A morally irresponsible person; one who continually comes in conflict with accepted behavior and the law. See also *psychopathic personality, sociopathic personality disturbance.*

psy·cho·path·ia (sigh″ko·path′ee·uh) *n.* PSYCHOPATHY.

psychopathia chi·rur·gi·ca·lis (kigh·rur″ji·kay′lis). An uncontrollable urge for being operated upon.

psychopathia sex·u·a·lis (seck″shoo·ay′lis). SEXUAL DEVIATION.

psy·cho·path·ic (sigh″ko·path′ick) *adj.* [*psycho-* + *path-* + *-ic*]. 1. Pertaining to any mental disorder, particularly any disorder not yet diagnosed or not yet severe. 2. Pertaining to a psychopath.

psychopathic personality. An individual characterized by emotional immaturity with marked defects of judgment, prone to impulsive behavior without consideration of others, and without evidence of learning by experience. Though behavior is generally amoral or antisocial, there is little outward evidence of guilt. See also *sociopath, sociopathic personality disturbance.*

psy·chop·a·thist (sigh·kop′uh·thist) *n.* PSYCHIATRIST.

psy·cho·pa·thol·o·gist (sigh″ko·pa·thol′uh·jist) *n.* [*psycho-* + *pathologist*]. An individual who specializes in the pathology of mental disease. Compare *psychiatrist.*

psy·cho·pa·thol·o·gy (sigh″ko·pa·thol′uh·jee) *n.* [*psycho-* + *pathology*]. The systematic study of mental diseases. See also *pathopsychology.*

psy·chop·a·thy (sigh·kop′uth·ee) *n.* [*psycho-* + *-pathy*]. Any disease of the mind.

psy·cho·phar·ma·col·o·gy (sigh″ko·fahr″muh·kol′uh·jee) *n.* [*psycho-* + *pharmacology*]. The science dealing with the action of drugs on mental function.

psy·cho·phon·as·the·nia (sigh″ko·fo″nas·theen′ee·uh) *n.* [*psycho-* + *phonasthenia*]. A speech difficulty of mental origin.

psychophysical law. FECHNER'S LAW.

psy·cho·phys·ics (sigh″ko·fiz′icks) *n.* [*psycho-* + *physics*]. 1. The study of mental processes by physical methods. 2. The study of the relation of stimuli to the sensations they produce, especially the determination of the differences of stimulus required to produce recognizable differences of sensation; experimental psychology. —**psycho-phys·i·cal** (·i·kul) *adj.*

psy·cho·phys·i·o·log·ic (sigh″ko·fiz″ee·o·loj′ick) *adj.* [*psycho-* + *physiologic*]. Pertaining to behavior and its correlation with physiological processes.

psychophysiologic autonomic and visceral disorders. PSYCHOPHYSIOLOGIC DISORDERS.

psychophysiologic disorders. Symptoms arising from chronic and exaggerated forms of the normal physiologic organic components of emotion but with the subjective awareness of the emotion repressed. If long continued, may lead to structural changes in the affected organs, such as peptic ulcer. These disorders differ from conversion types of hysterical neurosis in that they involve overactivity or underactivity of organs and viscera innervated by the autonomic nervous system, fail to alleviate anxiety, and are physiologic rather than symbolic in origin. Syn. *psychosomatic disorders.*

psy·cho·phys·i·ol·o·gy (sigh″ko·fiz·ee·ol′uh·jee) *n.* PHYSIOLOGIC PSYCHOLOGY.

psy·cho·ple·gia (sigh″ko·plee′jee·uh) *n.* [*psycho-* + *-plegia*]. Mental impairment of sudden onset.

psy·cho·ple·gic (sigh″ko·plee′jick) *adj. & n.* 1. Pertaining to psychoplegia. 2. A drug that lessens mental excitability and suppresses mental and sensory receptivity.

psy·cho·rhyth·mia (sigh″ko·rith′mee·uh) *n.* [*psycho-* + *rhythm* + *-ia*]. A mental condition in which there is involuntary repetition of previous volitional behavior.

psy·chor·rha·gia (sigh″ko·ray′jee·uh) *n.* [Gk., from *psychē,* soul, spirit, + *-rrhagia,* from *rhēgnynai,* to break free]. Death agony.

psy·cho·sen·so·ri·al (sigh″ko·sen·so′ree·ul) *adj.* PSYCHOSENSORY.

psy·cho·sen·so·ry (sigh″ko·sen′suh·ree) *adj.* [*psycho-* + *sensory*]. 1. Perceptual. 2. Imaginary or hallucinatory.

psy·cho·sex·u·al (sigh″ko·seck′shoo·ul) *adj.* [*psycho-* + *sexual*]. Pertaining to the mental and emotional aspects of sexuality as contrasted to the strictly physical or endocrine manifestations.

psychosexual development. The changes and stages, such as the oral, anal, and phallic, characterizing the psychological aspects of sexual maturation from birth to adult life.

psychosexual energy. LIBIDO.

psy·cho·sine (sigh′ko·seen) *n.* A compound of sphingosine and galactose believed to be an intermediate in cerebroside synthesis.

psy·cho·sis (sigh·ko'sis) *n.*, pl. **psycho·ses** (·seez) [*psych-* + *-osis*]. *In psychiatry*, an impairment of mental functioning to the extent that it interferes grossly with an individual's ability to meet the ordinary demands of life, characterized generally by severe affective disturbance, profound introspection, and withdrawal from reality with failure to test and evaluate external reality adequately, formation of delusions or hallucinations, and regression presenting the appearance of personality disintegration. In contrast to organic brain syndromes, there is no impairment of orientation, memory, or intellect, though these may be difficult to examine readily, but differentiation from the neuroses may require long and acute observations. Included in this grouping are the affective disorders, paranoid states, and schizophrenias. A psychotic reaction may also accompany a symptomatic clinical picture, as in chronic brain syndromes associated with senile changes or alcohol intoxication. Contr. *neurosis* (1).

psy·cho·so·cial (sigh''ko·so'shul) *adj.* [*psycho-* + *social*]. Pertaining to or involving both psychological and social factors.

psychosocial retardation. Emotional and environmental retardation combined.

psy·cho·so·mat·ic (sigh''ko·so·mat'ick) *adj.* [*psycho-* + *somatic*]. 1. Of or pertaining to the mind and body, as in affections with an emotional background having both mental and bodily components. 2. Pertaining to psychosomatic medicine.

psychosomatic disorders. PSYCHOPHYSIOLOGIC DISORDERS.

psychosomatic medicine. The branch of medicine dealing with psychic and physical components as a unit, and the interrelationship between them.

psychosomatic reaction. SOMATIZATION.

psy·cho·sur·gery (sigh''ko·sur'je·ree) *n.* [*psycho-* + *surgery*]. Treatment of chronic, severe, and medically untreatable mental disorders by surgical interruption or removal of certain areas or pathways in the brain, especially amygdalotomy or prefrontal lobotomy.

psy·cho·tech·ni·cian (sigh''ko·teck·nish'un) *n.* [*psycho-* + *technician*]. A person, not a professionally recognized psychologist, trained in administering psychologic tests. Compare *psychometrician.*

psy·cho·tech·nics (sigh''ko·teck'nicks) *n.* [*psycho-* + *technics*]. The practical application of psychologic principles, as in brainwashing and advertising or other forms of controlling behavior.

psy·cho·ther·a·peu·tics (sigh''ko·therr·uh·pew'ticks) *n.* PSYCHOTHERAPY.

psy·cho·ther·a·pist (sigh''ko·therr'uh·pist) *n.* [*psycho-* + *therapist*]. A person professionally trained and engaged in psychotherapy, usually a psychiatrist, clinical psychologist, or psychiatric social worker.

psy·cho·ther·a·py (sigh''ko·therr'uh·pee) *n.* [*psycho-* + *therapy*]. 1. Treatment of any disease, but particularly emotional maladjustments and mental disorders, by psychological means, i.e., by verbal or nonverbal communication with the patients in distinction to therapy based on physical means. 2. Specifically, treatment of emotional or mental disorders by a psychotherapist. Contr. *somatotherapy.* —**psychothera·peu·tic** (·pew'tick) *adj.*

psy·chot·ic (sigh·kot'ick) *adj. & n.* [*psychosis* + *-ic*]. 1. Pertaining to, marked by, exhibiting, or caused by psychosis. 2. A psychotic individual.

psychotic affective reaction. AFFECTIVE DISORDER.

psychotic depressive reaction. An affective disorder characterized by a depressed mood attributable to or precipitated by some real experience and occurring in an individual with no history of repeated depressions or mood swings. Compare *manic-depressive illness.*

psy·chot·o·gen (sigh·kot'o·jen) *n.* [*psychotic* + *-gen*]. Any natural or synthetic substance that is capable of inducing in man a psychotic-like state. —**psy·chot·o·gen·ic** (sigh·kot''o·jen'ick) *adj.*

psy·choto·mi·met·ic (sigh·kot''o·mi·met'ick) *adj.* 1. Mimicking a psychotic disorder. 2. Pertaining to any drug or compound, such as lysergic acid diethylamide or mescaline, which can induce a psychotic-like state.

psy·cho·trop·ic (sigh''ko·trop'ick) *adj.* [*psycho-* + *-tropic*]. Pertaining to any substance or drug having a special affinity for or effect on the psyche or mind.

psy·cho·vi·su·al sensations (sigh''ko·vizh'yoo·ul). Visions without the stimulation of the retina; visual hallucinations.

psychr-, psychro- [Gk. *psychros*]. A combining form meaning *cold.*

psy·chral·gia (sigh·kral'jee·uh) *n.* [*psychr-* + *-algia*]. A painful subjective sense of cold.

psy·chro·al·gia (sigh''kro·al'jee·uh) *n.* PSYCHRALGIA.

psy·chro·es·the·sia, psy·chro·aes·the·sia (sigh''kro·es·theezh'uh, ·theez'ee·uh) *n.* Subjective sensation of cold.

psy·chro·lu·sia (sigh''kro·lew'see·uh, ·zee·uh) *n.* [Gk. *psychrolousia*, from *psychro-* + *lousis*, bathing]. Cold bathing.

psy·chrom·e·ter (sigh·krom'e·tur) *n.* [*psychro-* + *-meter*]. A hygrometer for determining atmospheric moisture by observing the difference in the indication of two identical thermometers, the bulb of one being kept dry, and the other wet, with a water-soaked wick; both are swung through the air to facilitate evaporation from the wet bulb.

psy·chro·phil·ic (sigh''kro·fil'ick) *adj.* [*psychro-* + *phil-* + *-ic*]. Cold-loving; applied to microorganisms that develop best at temperatures between 15 and 20°C. Syn. *crymophilic.*

psy·chro·pho·bia (sigh''kro·fo'bee·uh) *n.* [Gk. *psychrophobos*, dreading cold (from *psychro-* + *phobos*, fear) + *-ia*]. 1. An abnormal fear of cold. 2. An abnormal sensibility to cold.

psy·chro·phore (sigh'kro·fore) *n.* [Gk. *psychrophoros*, water pipe, from *psychro-* + *phoros*, bearing]. An instrument for applying cold to deeply seated parts, as a double-current catheter for applying cold to the posterior part of the urethra.

psy·chro·ther·a·py (sigh''kro·therr'uh·pee) *n.* [*psychro-* + *therapy*]. The treatment of disease by the application of cold.

psyl·li·um seed (sil'ee·um). PLANTAGO SEED.

Pt Symbol for platinum.

pt. Abbreviation for *pint.*

PTA Abbreviation for *plasma thromboplastin antecedent* (= FACTOR XI).

PTA deficiency. A hemorrhagic disorder due to deficiency of factor XI.

PTAH. Abbreviation for *phosphotungstic acid hematoxylin.*

ptar·mic (tahr'mick) *adj. & n.* [Gk. *ptarmikos*, from *ptarmos*, sneeze, sneezing]. 1. Pertaining to or causing the act of sneezing; sternutatory. 2. A substance that produces sneezing.

ptar·mus (tahr'mus) *n.* [Gk. *ptarmos*]. Sneezing.

PTC Abbreviation for (a) *phenylthiocarbamide;* (b) *plasma thromboplastin component* (= FACTOR IX).

PTC deficiency. A hemorrhagic disorder due to deficiency of factor IX.

ptel·e·or·rhine (tel'ee·o·rine) *adj.* [Gk. *ptelea*, elm, + *-rrhine*]. Pertaining to a facial type in which the nostrils are asymmetric.

pter-, ptero- [Gk. *pteron*]. A combining form meaning (a) *wing;* (b) *feather.*

pter·i·dine (terr'i·din, ·deen) *n.* Any compound, such as folic acid or a pterin, characterized by the presence of a ring system composed of fused pyrimidine and pyrazine rings.

pte·ri·do·phyte (terr'i·do·fite, te·rid'o·) *n.* [Gk. *pteris, pteridos*, fern, + *-phyte*]. A plant of the division Pteridophyta, which includes the ferns and their allies.

pter·in (terr'in) *n.* Any pigment, containing a pteridine ring system, occurring in the wings of butterflies and, by extension, in mammalian tissues.

pter·i·on (terr'ee·on, teer'ee·on) *n.* [Gk., dim. of *pteron*, wing]. *In craniometry*, the region surrounding the sphenoparietal suture where the frontal bone, parietal bone, squama temporalis, and greater wing of the sphenoid bone come together most closely.

ptero-. See *pter-*.

pte·ro·ic acid (te·ro'ick). *p*-[(2-Amino-4-hydroxy-6-pteridyl-methyl)amino]benzoic acid, $C_{14}H_{12}N_6O_3$, representing folic acid without its glutamic acid component.

pter·o·yl·glu·tam·ic acid (terr"o·il·gloo·tam'ick). FOLIC ACID.

pte·ryg·i·um (te·rij'ee·um) *n.*, pl. **pteryg·ia** (·ee·uh) [L., from Gk. *pterygion*, fin, flap, fold, pterygium, from *pteryx*, wing]. 1. A triangular patch of mucous membrane growing on the conjunctiva, usually on the nasal side of the eye. The apex of the patch points toward the pupil, the fan-shaped base toward the canthus. 2. EPONYCHIUM (2). 3. Any fold of skin extending abnormally from one part of the body to another. —**pterygi·al** (·ul) *adj.*

pterygium col·li (kol'eye). WEBBED NECK.

pterygo-. A combining form meaning *pterygoid, pterygoid process.*

pter·y·go·alar foramen (terr"i·go·ay'lur). PORUS CROTAPHITICO-BUCCINATORIUS.

pter·y·goid (terr'i·goid) *adj.* [Gk. *pterygoeidēs*, winglike, from *pteryx*, wing]. 1. Wing-shaped. 2. Pertaining, directly or indirectly, to the pterygoid process of the sphenoid bone.

pterygoid canal. A canal in the sphenoid bone at the base of the medial pterygoid plate; it opens anteriorly into the pterygopalatine fossa. NA *canalis pterygoideus.*

pterygoid fissure. The gap at the inferior portion of the pterygoid fossa between the medial and the lateral laminas. NA *incisura pterygoidea.*

pterygoid fossa. The groove between the medial and lateral laminas of the pterygoid process of the sphenoid bone. NA *fossa pterygoidea.*

pterygoid hamulus. The hooklike process on the lower end of the medial pterygoid plate. NA *hamulus pterygoideus.*

pterygoid plates. Two plates, the lateral pterygoid plate and the medial pterygoid plate, into which the pterygoid process of the sphenoid bone divides.

pterygoid plexus. A plexus of veins which accompanies the maxillary artery between the pterygoid muscles. NA *plexus pterygoideus.* See also Table of Veins in the Appendix and Plate 10.

pterygoid process of the sphenoid bone. A process descending perpendicularly from the point of junction of the body with the greater wing of the sphenoid bone, and consisting of a lateral and a medial plate. NA *processus pterygoideus ossis sphenoidalis.*

pterygoid tubercle. A tubercle on the inner surface of the mandible; it gives attachment to the medial pterygoid muscle. NA *tuberositas pterygoidea.*

pter·y·go·man·dib·u·lar (terr"i·go·man·dib'yoo·lur) *adj.* [*pterygo-* + *mandibular*]. Pertaining to the pterygoid process and the mandible.

pter·y·go·max·il·lary (terr"i·go·mack'si·lerr"ee) *adj.* [*pterygo-* + *maxillary*]. Pertaining to the pterygoid process and the maxilla.

pterygomaxillary fissure. A narrow gap between the lateral pterygoid plate and posterior portion of the maxilla leading into the pterygopalatine fossa. NA *fissura pterygomaxillaris.*

pter·y·go·pal·a·tine (terr"i·go·pal'uh·tine, ·tin) *adj.* [*pterygo-* + *palatine*]. Situated between the pterygoid process of the sphenoid bone and the palatine bone.

pterygopalatine canal. The connection between the pterygopalatine fossa and the mouth; it gives passage to the palatine nerves and vessels. Its inferior opening is the greater palatine foramen. NA *canalis pterygopalatinus.*

pterygopalatine fissure. PTERYGOMAXILLARY FISSURE.

pterygopalatine foramen. SPHENOPALATINE FORAMEN.

pterygopalatine fossa. The gap between the pterygoid process of the sphenoid bone and the maxilla and palatine bone. NA *fossa pterygopalatina.*

pterygopalatine ganglion. A parasympathetic ganglion located in the pterygopalatine fossa. From it, postganglionic fibers arise which project to the lacrimal gland and to the glands in the mucous membrane of the nose and pharynx. NA *ganglion pterygopalatinum.*

pterygopalatine groove. SULCUS PALATINUS MAJOR OSSIS PALATINI.

pterygopalatine nerves. The somatic sensory nerves, branches of the maxillary, which innervate the nose and the palate via the pterygopalatine ganglion and the palatine nerves. NA *nervi pterygopalatini.*

pterygopalatine sulcus. SULCUS PALATINUS MAJOR OSSIS PALATINI.

pter·y·go·pha·ryn·geal (terr"i·go·fa·rin'jee·ul) *adj.* Pertaining to the medial pterygoid plate and the pharynx.

pter·y·go·pha·ryn·ge·us (terr"i·go·fa·rin'jee·us) *n.* PARS PTERYGOPHARYNGEA MUSCULI CONSTRICTORIS PHARYNGIS SUPERIORIS.

pter·y·go·spi·nous (terr"i·go·spye'nus) *adj.* [*pterygo-* + *spinous*]. Pertaining to a pterygoid process and the angular spine of the sphenoid bone.

pterygospinous foramen. A foramen formed by the ossification of the pterygospinous ligament running between the lateral pterygoid lamina and the angular spine of the sphenoid bone.

pterygospinous ligament. A band of fibrous tissue extending from the lateral pterygoid plate to the spine of the sphenoid. NA *ligamentum pterygospinale.*

pterygospinous process. A small spine on the posterior edge of the lateral pterygoid plate which gives attachment to the pterygospinous ligament. NA *processus pterygospinosus.*

pti·lo·sis (ti·lo'sis) *n.*, pl. **ptilo·ses** (·seez) [Gk. *ptilōsis*, from *ptilon*, down, feathers]. Falling out of the eyelashes.

P.T.O. [*P*erlsucht *T*uberculin *o*riginal]. An original tuberculin prepared from bovine tubercle bacilli, in the same manner as Koch's original tuberculin. Syn. *Klemperer's tuberculin.*

pto·maine (to'mane, to'may·een) *n.* [It. *ptomaina* from Gk. *ptōma*, fallen body]. Any of various nitrogenous bases, some of which are poisonous, produced by action of putrefactive bacteria on proteins. Certain ptomaines were formerly believed to cause food poisoning.

pto·mat·i·nu·ria (to·mat"i·new'ree·uh) *n.* The presence of ptomaines in the urine.

pto·sis (to'sis) *n.*, pl. **pto·ses** (·seez) [Gk. *ptōsis*, fall]. Prolapse, abnormal depression, or falling down of an organ or part; applied especially to drooping of the upper eyelid, as from paralysis of the third cranial nerve. —**ptosed** (toazd), **ptot·ic** (tot'ick) *adj.*

-ptosis [Gk. *ptōsis*, fall]. A combining form meaning *a lowered position of an organ.*

ptosis iri·dis (irr'i·dis, eye'ri·dis). PROLAPSE OF THE IRIS.

ptosis sym·pa·thet·i·ca (sim"puh·thet'i·kuh). HORNER'S SYNDROME.

P.T.R. [*P*erlsucht *T*uberculin *R*est]. An original tuberculin prepared from bovine tubercle bacilli.

PTT Partial thromboplastin time.

ptyal-, ptyalo- [Gk. *ptyalon*]. A combining form meaning *saliva, salivary.*

pty·al·a·gogue (tye·al'uh·gog) *n.* [*ptyal-* + *-agogue*]. SIALAGOGUE.

pty·a·lase (tye'uh·lace) *n.* PTYALIN.

pty·a·lec·ta·sis (tye"uh·leck'tuh·sis) *n.* [*ptyal-* + *ectasis*]. Dilatation of the duct of a salivary gland, either spontaneously or surgically.

pty·a·lin (tye'uh·lin) *n.* A diastatic enzyme found in saliva, having the property of hydrolyzing starch to dextrin, maltose, and glucose, and hydrolyzing sucrose to glucose and fructose. Syn. *ptyalase, salivary diastase.*

pty·a·lin·o·gen (tye″uh·lin′o·jen) *n.* The zymogen of ptyalin.
pty·a·lism (tye′uh·liz·um) *n.* [*ptyal-* + *-ism*]. SALIVATION.
pty·a·lith (tye′uh·lith) *n.* Ptyalolith (= SALIVARY CALCULUS).
ptyalo-. See *ptyal-*.
pty·a·lo·cele (tye′uh·lo·seel) *n.* [*ptyalo-* + *-cele*]. A cyst containing saliva; usually due to obstruction of the duct of a salivary gland.
pty·a·lo·gen·ic (tye″uh·lo·jen′ick) *adj.* [*ptyalo-* + *-genic*]. Of salivary origin.
pty·alo·gogue (tye·al′o·gog) *n.* [*ptyalo-* + *-agogue*]. SIALOGOGUE.
pty·a·log·ra·phy (tye″uh·log′ruh·fee) *n.* [*ptyalo-* + *-graphy*]. Radiography of the salivary glands or their ducts; SIALOGRAPHY.
pty·a·lo·lith (tye′uh·lo·lith) *n.* [*ptyalo-* + *-lith*]. SALIVARY CALCULUS.
pty·a·lo·li·thi·a·sis (tye″uh·lo·li·thigh′uh·sis) *n.* [*ptyalolith* + *-iasis*]. The formation, or presence, of a salivary calculus.
pty·a·lor·rhea, pty·a·lor·rhoea (tye″uh·lo·ree′uh) *n.* [*ptyalo-* + *-rrhea*]. Excessive flow of saliva.
pty·a·lose (tye′uh·loce) *n.* [*ptyal-* + *-ose*]. A sugar found in saliva, identical with maltose.
pty·a·lo·sis (tye″uh·lo′sis) *n.* [*ptyal-* + *-osis*]. SALIVATION.
pty·o·crine (tye′o·krin) *adj.* [Gk. *ptyein*, to spit out, disgorge, + *-crine*]. APOCRINE.
pty·oc·ri·nous (tye·ock′ri·nus) *adj.* [*ptyocrine* + *-ous*]. APOCRINE.
pty·sis (tye′sis) *n.*, pl. **pty·ses** (·seez) [Gk.]. The act of spitting.
ptys·ma (tiz′muh) *n.* [Gk., sputum]. SALIVA.
ptys·ma·gogue (tiz′muh·gog) *n.* [*ptysma* + *-agogue*]. A drug that promotes the secretion of saliva.
Pu Symbol for plutonium.
pub·ar·che (pew·bahr′kee) *n.* [*pubes* + Gk. *archē*, beginning]. The onset of pubic hair growth.
pu·ber (pew′bur) *n.* [L.]. One who has arrived at the age of puberty.
pu·ber·al (pew′bur·ul) *adj.* Pubertal. See *puberty*.
pu·ber·tas (pew′bur·tas) *n.* [L.]. PUBERTY.
pubertas ple·na (plee′nuh) [L., full, complete]. The attainment of sexual maturity.
pubertas pre·cox (pree′kocks). PRECOCIOUS PUBERTY.
pu·ber·ty (pew′bur·tee) *n.* [L. *pubertas*, from *puber*, young adult]. The period at which the generative organs become capable of exercising the function of reproduction; signalized in the boy by a change of voice and discharge of semen, in the girl by the appearance of the menses. —**pu·ber·tal** (·tul) *adj.*
pu·ber·u·lon·ic acid (pew·berr″yoo·lon′ick). An antibiotic, $C_8H_4O_7$, from *Penicillium puberulum;* a weak antibiotic agent active largely against gram-positive bacteria.
pu·bes (pew′beez) *n.* [L., the signs of puberty]. 1. [NA] The hairy region covering the pubic bone. 2. The two pubic bones considered together; the portion of the hipbones forming the front of the pelvis.
pu·bes·cence (pew·bes′unce) *n.* [L. *pubescere*, to become pubescent]. 1. Puberty, or the coming on of puberty. 2. Hairiness; the presence of fine, soft hairs. —**pubes·cent** (·unt) *adj.*
pubescent insanity. HEBEPHRENIC TYPE OF SCHIZOPHRENIA.
pubescent uterus. An abnormality of the uterus in which the characters of that organ peculiar to the epoch preceding puberty persist in the adult.
pu·be·trot·o·my (pew″be·trot′uh·mee) *n.* [*pubes* + Gk. *ētron*, lower abdomen, + *-tomy*]. Pelvic section through the pubes.
pu·bic (pew′bick) *adj.* Pertaining to the pubes.
pubic arch. The arch formed by the conjoined rami of the pubis and ischium. NA *arcus pubis.*
pubic crest. A crest extending from the pubic tubercle to the medial extremity of the pubis. NA *crista pubica.*
pubic fascia. PECTINEAL FASCIA.
pubic region. The lowest of the three median abdominal regions, above the symphysis pubis and below the umbilical region. Syn. *hypogastric region, hypogastrium.* NA *regio pubica.*
pubic spine. PUBIC TUBERCLE.
pubic symphysectomy. Removal of the pubic symphysis to afford better exposure in reconstructive or extirpative operations on the anterior pelvic viscera.
pubic symphysis. SYMPHYSIS PUBIS; the fibrocartilaginous union (synchondrosis) of the pubic bones. NA *symphysis pubica.*
pubic tubercle. A prominent bony point on the superior ramus of the pubis for the attachment of the inguinal ligament. NA *tuberculum pubicum ossis pubis.*
pubio-. A combining form meaning *pubis, pubic,* or *pubes.*
pu·bi·ot·o·my (pew″bee·ot′uh·mee) *n.* [*pubio-* + *-tomy*]. Section of the pubic bone lateral to the symphysis. Syn. *hebosteotomy, hebotomy.*
pu·bis (pew′bis) *n.* [L., genitive of *pubes*]. The pubic bone, the portion of the hipbone forming the front of the pelvis. NA *os pubis.* See also Table of Bones in the Appendix and Plates 1, 2.
pub·lic antigen. An erythrocyte antigen system, defined by specific antiserums, found in virtually all people. More than 99 percent of the population have such antigens. Syn. *high incidence factors.* Contr. *private antigen.*
public health. 1. The state of health of a population, as that of a state, nation, or a particular community. 2. The art and science dealing with the protection and improvement of community health through organized community effort, including preventive medicine, health education, communicable disease control, and application of the sanitary and social sciences. See also *social medicine.*
public health nurse. COMMUNITY HEALTH NURSE.
Public Health Service. United States Public Health Service.
pubo-. A combining form meaning *pubis, pubic,* or *pubes.*
pu·bo·ad·duc·tor (pew″bo·a·duck′tur) *adj.* Pertaining to the pubis and the adductor muscles of the hip.
pu·bo·ad·duc·tor reflex (pew″bo·a·duck′tur). With the patient recumbent, his abdominal muscles relaxed and his thighs in slight abduction and internal rotation, tapping the symphysis pubis slightly lateral to the midline is followed by contraction of the adductor muscles on the side stimulated and slight flexion of that hip.
pu·bo·cap·su·lar (pew″bo·kap′sue·lur) *adj.* [*pubo-* + *capsular*]. Pertaining to the os pubis and the capsule of the hip joint.
pubocapsular ligament. PUBOFEMORAL LIGAMENT.
pu·bo·ca·ver·no·sus (pew″bo·kav″ur·no′sus) *n.* A variable part of the ischiocavernosus muscle.
pu·bo·coc·cyg·e·al (pew″bo·kock·sij′ee·ul) *adj.* [*pubo-* + *coccygeal*]. Pertaining to the pubic bone and the coccyx.
pu·bo·coc·cy·ge·us (pew″bo·kock·sij′ee·us) *n.* A part of the levator ani muscle. NA *musculus pubococcygeus.*
pu·bo·fem·o·ral (pew″bo·fem′o·rul) *adj.* [*pubo-* + *femoral*]. Pertaining to the os pubis and the femur.
pubofemoral ligament. A narrow auxiliary band in the hip joint, passing distally from the obturator crest of the pubis and the iliopubic eminence to blend with the articular capsule and iliofemoral ligament near the neck of the femur. NA *ligamentum pubofemorale.*
pu·bo·pe·ri·to·ne·a·lis (pew″bo·perr″i·to·nee·ay′lis) *n.* A variant of the transverse abdominal muscle.
pu·bo·pros·tat·ic (pew″bo·pros·tat′ick) *adj.* [*pubo-* + *prostatic*]. Pertaining to the pubic bone and the prostate gland.
puboprostatic ligament. In the male, a thickening of the pelvic fascia running from the capsule of the prostate gland to the pubic bone; medial and lateral ones on each side are described. NA *ligamentum puboprostaticum.* See also *pubovesical ligament.*
pu·bo·rec·ta·lis (pew″bo·reck·tay′lis) *n.* A part of the levator ani muscle. NA *musculus puborectalis.*
pu·bo·scro·tal testis (pew″bo·skro′tul). A testis situated over the pubic tubercle.

pu·bo·trans·ver·sa·lis (pew″bo·trans·vur·say′lis) *n.* A variant of the transverse abdominal muscle.

pu·bo·tu·ber·ous diameter (pew″bo·tew′bur·us). An external diameter extending perpendicularly from the tuberosity of the ischium to the superior ramus of the pubis.

pu·bo·ves·i·cal (pew″bo·ves′i·kul) *adj.* [*pubo-* + *vesical*]. Pertaining to the pubic bone and the urinary bladder.

pu·bo·ve·si·ca·lis (pew″bo·ves·i·kay′lis) *n.* A portion of the levator ani muscle. NA *musculus pubovesicalis.*

pubovesical ligament. In the female, a thickening of the pelvic fascia running from the urinary bladder to the pubic bone; medial and lateral ones on each side are described. NA *ligamentum pubovesicale.* See also *puboprostatic ligament.*

pudenda. Plural of *pudendum.*

pu·den·dag·ra (pew″den·dag′ruh, ·day′gruh) *n.* [*pudendum* + *-agra*]. Pain in the genital organs, particularly those of the female.

pu·den·dal (pew·den′dul) *adj.* Of, pertaining to, or situated in the region of the pudendum.

pudendal anesthesia. Local anesthesia for obstetrical delivery induced by blocking the pudendal nerve of each side near the spinous process of the ischium.

pudendal artery. See Table of Arteries in the Appendix.

pudendal canal. A passage within the inferior fascia of the obturator internus muscle for the transmission of the pudendal nerve and internal pudendal vessels. NA *canalis pudendalis.*

pudendal gangrene. NOMA PUDENDI.

pudendal nerve. A motor and sensory nerve from the pudendal plexus which supplies the muscles and skin of the perineal region. See also Table of Nerves in the Appendix.

pudendal plexus. 1. A plexus formed by the anterior branches of the second, third, and fourth sacral nerves. 2. PROSTATIC PLEXUS (2).

pudendal plexus neuralgia. Neuralgia of the lower two or three sacral nerves, manifested by pain in the perineum, scrotum, penis, and testes.

pu·den·dum (pew·den′dum) *n.*, pl. **puden·da** (·duh) [NL., from L. *pudendus,* from *pudere,* to be ashamed]. The external genital organs, especially of the female.

pudendum fe·mi·ni·num (fem·i·nigh′num) [NA]. VULVA.

pudendum mu·li·e·bre (mew·lee·ee′bree) [BNA]. Pudendum femininum (= VULVA).

pu·dic (pew′dick) *adj.* [L. *pudicus,* modest]. PUDENDAL.

Puen·te's disease. GLANDULAR CHEILITIS.

pu·er·i·cul·ture (pew′ur·i·kul″chur, pew·err′i·) *n.* [L. *puer,* boy, + *cultura,* cultivation]. The specialty of child training.

pu·er·ile (pew′ur·il) *adj.* [L. *puerilis,* from *puer,* child, boy]. 1. Characteristic of or similar to that of children. 2. Childish. 3. Of or pertaining to childhood.

puerile respiration. Exaggerated prolonged breath sounds, abnormal for the adult but heard in healthy children.

pu·er·il·ism (pew′ur·i·liz·um) *n.* [*puerile* + *-ism*]. Childishness; the reversion particularly in an adult to childlike behavior.

pu·er·i·tia (pew″ur·ish′ee·uh) *n.* [L., boyhood, from *puer,* boy]. SENILE DEMENTIA.

pu·er·pera (pew·ur′pur·uh) *n.*, pl. **puer·per·ae** (·ee) [L., from *puer,* child, + *parere,* to bring forth]. A woman who has recently given birth.

pu·er·per·al (pew·ur′pur·ul) *adj.* [*puerpera* + *-al*]. Pertaining to, caused by, or following childbirth.

puerperal convulsion. See *eclampsia* (1).

puerperal fever. A febrile state caused by infection of the endometrium and septicemia following delivery. Syn. *childbed fever.*

puerperal insanity. PUERPERAL PSYCHOSIS.

pu·er·per·al·ism (pew·ur′pur·ul·iz·um) *n.* [*puerperal* + *-ism*]. The state brought about by pathologic conditions of pregnancy.

puerperal mania. PUERPERAL PSYCHOSIS.

puerperal mastitis. A complication of the early puerperium, in which part or all of the breast becomes indurated from retention of milk and engorgement of the tissues. Syn. *lactation mastitis.*

puerperal metritis. Inflammation of the uterus following childbirth.

puerperal peritonitis. Peritonitis following childbirth; associated with infection of the uterus and adnexa.

puerperal psychosis. Any psychotic reaction in a woman during the postpartum period, usually schizophrenic in nature. Organic or toxic factors may be present.

puerperal sepsis. Sepsis occurring as a complication or sequel of pregnancy; due to infection, usually streptococcal, in the birth canal, especially in the uterus.

puerperal septicemia. A febrile state caused by infection of the bloodstream of the mother through the genital tract following delivery.

puerperal synovitis. Synovitis occurring after childbirth, and due to septic infection.

puerperal thelitis. Postpartum inflammation of the nipple of the breast.

puerperal tubal occlusion. The agglutination of the mucosal folds of the uterine tube occurring about one week after labor, presumably from a mild gonococcal infection and producing one-child sterility.

puerperal venous thrombosis. Thrombosis of the pelvic veins occurring during the puerperium.

pu·er·per·ant (pew·ur′pur·unt) *n.* PUERPERA.

pu·er·pe·ri·um (pew″ur·peer′ee·um) *n.*, pl. **puerpe·ria** (·ree·uh) [L., childbirth, from *puerpera*]. 1. The state of having just given birth. 2. The period from delivery to the time when the uterus has regained its normal size, which is about six weeks.

puff adder. *BITIS LACHESIS.*

puff·ball, *n.* Any of the fungi Lycoperdaceae which discharge their ripe spores like dust when struck. Many are edible when unripe.

Pugh's test. A visual test for fusion in which a stereoscope is used by means of which pictures seen separately by each eye are superimposed.

pu·le·gone (pew′le·gohn) *n.* 1-Methyl-4-isopropylidene-3-cyclohexanone, $C_{10}H_{16}O$, a liquid constituent of many volatile oils from plants of the Labiatae family.

Pu·lex (pew′lecks) *n.* [L., flea]. A genus of fleas.

Pulex ir·ri·tans (irr′i·tanz). The human flea; a species which is the intermediate host and transmitter of *Dipylidium caninum* and *Hymenolepis diminuta,* and may spread plague. It is parasitic on the skin of man and also infests hogs, dogs, and other mammals.

pu·li·ca·ris (pew″li·kair′is) *adj.* [L., of fleas, from *pulex,* flea]. Marked with little spots like flea bites.

pu·li·ca·tio (pew″li·kay′shee·o) *n.* [L. *pulicare,* to produce fleas]. The state of being infested with fleas.

Pu·lic·i·dae (pew·lis′i·dee) *n.pl.* [NL., from L. *pulex, pulicis,* flea]. A family of fleas or Siphonaptera of which the most important to man are the genera *Pulex, Xenopsylla,* and *Ctenocephalides.*

pu·li·cide (pew′li·side) *n.* [L. *pulex, pulicis,* flea, + *-cide*]. An agent capable of killing fleas.

pulled elbow. Subluxation, or partial subluxation, of the head of the radius in small children. Syn. *nursemaid's elbow.*

pul·lo·rum disease (puh·lo′rum). A disease of chickens and other birds caused by *Salmonella pullorum.* Syn. *white diarrhea, bacillary white diarrhea.*

Pul·lu·lar·ia (pul·yoo·lăr′ee·uh) *n.* A genus of thick-walled black fungi with budding spores, common as laboratory contaminants.

pul·lu·late (pul′yoo·late) *v.* [L., *pullulare*]. To germinate, bud.

pul·lu·la·tion (pul″yoo·lay′shun) *n.* The act of sprouting or budding, a mode of reproduction seen in the yeast plant.

pul·mo (pul′mo) *n.*, genit. **pul·mo·nis** (pul·mo′nis), pl. **pulmo·**

nes (·neez) [L. (rel. to Gk. *pleumōn, pneumōn*)] [NA]. LUNG.

pulmo- [L., lung]. A combining form meaning *lung, pulmonic, pulmonary.*

pul·mo·car·di·ac region (pul″mo·kahr′dee·ack). The region of the left thorax in which the left lung overlaps the heart.

pul·mo·gas·tric region (pul′mo·gas′trick). The portion of the left thorax in which the lung overlaps the stomach.

pul·mo·he·pat·ic region (pul″mo·he·pat′ick). The portion of the right thorax in which the lung overlaps the liver.

pulmon-, pulmono-. A combining form meaning *lung, pulmonic, pulmonary.*

pul·mo·nary (pul′muh·nerr″ee, pŏŏl·) *adj.* [L. *pulmonarius,* from *pulmo,* lung]. Pertaining to, or affecting, the lungs or any anatomic component of the lungs. Syn. *pulmonic.*

pulmonary adenomatosis. Progressive overgrowth of alveolar surfaces by columnar cells of uncertain origin, possibly a form of bronchiolar carcinoma, or an infectious disease.

pulmonary alveolar proteinosis. A condition characterized by gradually progressive dyspnea and hypoxia and a productive cough clinically, diffuse perihilar densities on x-ray, and large groups of alveoli filled with eosinophilic proteinaceous material on pathologic examination.

pulmonary alveolus. ALVEOLUS (2).

pulmonary angiothrombosis. Angiothrombosis in the lungs, a common cause of death among drug addicts.

pulmonary apoplexy. Escape of blood into the pulmonary parenchyma.

pulmonary artery. See Table of Arteries in the Appendix.

pulmonary artery wedge pressure. WEDGE PRESSURE.

pulmonary capillary pressure. WEDGE PRESSURE.

pulmonary circulation. The circulation of blood through the lungs by means of the pulmonary arteries and veins, for the purpose of oxygenation and release of carbon dioxide. Syn. *lesser circulation.*

pulmonary decortication. PLEURECTOMY.

pulmonary diffusing capacity. The number of milliliters of a gas transferred across the alveolar-capillary membrane per minute per millimeter difference in partial pressure of the gas in the alveolar air and capillary blood.

pulmonary dysmaturity. WILSON-MIKITY SYNDROME.

pulmonary edema. An effusion of fluid into the air sacs and interstitial tissue of the lungs, producing severe dyspnea; most commonly due to left heart failure. Syn. *Potain's disease.* See also *Woillez' disease.*

pulmonary emphysema. EMPHYSEMA (1).

pulmonary epithelial cell. SQUAMOUS ALVEOLAR CELL. Contr. *alveolar cell* (2) (= GREAT ALVEOLAR CELL).

pulmonary heart. COR PULMONALE.

pulmonary heart disease. COR PULMONALE.

pulmonary ligament. A fold of pleura extending between the lower part of the mediastinal surface of the lung and the pericardium. NA *ligamentum pulmonale.*

pulmonary lobe. One of the five lobes of the lungs, typically two in the left lung and three in the right lung.

pulmonary lobule. A respiratory bronchiole and its branches, the alveolar ducts and alveolar sacs, all with pulmonary alveoli in their walls, constituting a physiologic unit of the lung.

pulmonary murmur. A murmur produced at the pulmonary orifice, or heard in the pulmonary area.

pulmonary overinflation. A pathologic condition of the lung characterized by an increase beyond normal size of the air spaces distal to the terminal nonrespiratory bronchiole, without destructive changes in the alveolar wall.

pulmonary plethora. Hyperemia of the lungs.

pulmonary pleura. The portion of the pleura directly enveloping the lung. NA *pleura pulmonalis.*

pulmonary plexus. A nerve plexus composed chiefly of vagal fibers situated on the anterior and posterior aspects of the bronchi and accompanying them into the substance of the lung. NA *plexus pulmonalis.*

pulmonary reflex. HERING-BREUER REFLEX.

pulmonary resistance. Impedance to blood flow in the pulmonary vascular bed. Contr. *peripheral resistance.*

pulmonary respiration. Respiration in which the interchange of gases between the blood and air occurs in the lungs.

pulmonary ridge. A minor ridge in the embryo on the coelomic surface of the bulging fold formed by the growth of the common cardinal veins, which develops into the pleuropericardial membrane.

pulmonary scleroderma. Interstitial fibrosis of the lungs occurring in diffuse scleroderma.

pulmonary sequestration. A segment or area of lung tissue that derives its blood supply from the systemic circulation.

pulmonary stenosis. Narrowing of the orifice of the pulmonary trunk.

pulmonary transpiration. The exhalation of water vapor from the lungs.

pulmonary trunk. The arterial vessel arising from the right ventricle and giving rise to the right and left pulmonary arteries. NA *truncus pulmonalis.*

pulmonary valve. A valve consisting of three semilunar cusps situated between the right ventricle and the pulmonary trunk. NA *valva trunci pulmonalis.*

pulmonary wedge pressure. WEDGE PRESSURE.

pul·mo·nec·to·my (pul″mo·neck′tuh·mee, pŏŏl·) *n.* [*pulmon-* + *-ectomy*]. PNEUMONECTOMY.

pulmones. Plural of *pulmo.*

pul·mon·ic (pul·mon′ick) *adj.* [*pulmon-* + *-ic*]. PULMONARY.

pulmonic stenosis. PULMONARY STENOSIS.

pul·mo·ni·tis (pul″mo·nigh′tis) *n.* [*pulmon-* + *-itis*]. PNEUMONIA.

pulmono-. See *pulmon-.*

pul·mo·tor (pul′mo″tur, pŏŏl′) *n.* [*pul*mo- + *motor*]. An apparatus for resuscitating persons who have been asphyxiated; it expels the gas from the lungs, introduces oxygen, and provides artificial respiration.

pul·mo·vas·cu·lar region (pul″mo·vas′kew·lur). The part of the thorax in which the lung overlaps the origins of the larger vessels.

pulp, *n.* [L., *pulpa,* flesh, pulp]. 1. The soft, fleshy part of fruit. 2. The soft part in the interior of an organ. —**pulp·al** (·ul), **pulp·ar** (·ur) *adj.*

pul·pa (pul′puh) *n.* [L.]. PULP.

pulpa co·ro·na·le (kor·o·nay′lee) [NA]. The portion of the dental pulp located in the crown portion of the pulp cavity.

pulpa den·tis (den′tis) [NA]. DENTAL PULP.

pulpal horn. The extension of the dental pulp into a cusp of a tooth.

pulpa li·e·nis (lye·ee′nis) [NA]. SPLENIC PULP.

pulpa ra·di·cu·la·ris (ra·dick·yoo·lair′is) [NA]. The portion of the dental pulp contained in the root of a tooth.

pul·pa·tion (pul·pay′shun) *n.* The act or process of reducing to a pulp.

pulp cap. A protective seal composed of various medicaments or agents, applied over an exposed dental pulp prior to the restoration of the tooth.

pulp cavity. The space within the central part of a tooth which contains the dental pulp and comprises the pulp chamber and a root canal for each root. NA *cavum dentis.*

pulp cells. Cells found in the pulp tissue of any organ.

pulp chamber. The coronal portion of the central cavity in a tooth. NA *cavum coronale.*

pulp·ec·to·my (pul·peck′tuh·mee) *n.* [*pulp* + *-ectomy*]. Excision or extirpation of a dental pulp.

pulp·i·tis (pul·pye′tis) *n.*, pl. **pulp·it·i·des** (pul·pit′i·deez) [*pulp* + *-itis*]. An inflammation of the dental pulp.

pulp of the finger. DIGITAL PULP.

pulp of the intervertebral disk. The pulpy body at the center of the intervertebral disk, a remnant of the notochord. NA *nucleus pulposus.*

pulp·ot·o·my (pul·pot′uh·mee) *n.* [*pulp* + *-tomy*]. The surgical removal of the pulp of a tooth.

pulp polyp. HYPERPLASTIC PULPITIS.

pulp·stone, *n.* DENTICLE (2).

pulp traction method. A means of finger extension limited to compound fracture of the phalanges, where the corresponding flexor surfaces of the fingers are wounded. A stainless-steel wire is passed through the pulp in the distal phalanx, and then is attached to a banjo splint, using rubber bands for traction.

pulp vein. One of the veins draining the venous sinuses of the splenic pulp.

pulpy (pulp'ee) *adj.* Resembling pulp; characterized by the formation of a substance resembling pulp.

pulpy kidney disease. INFECTIOUS ENTEROTOXEMIA OF SHEEP.

pul·que (pool'keh) *n.* [Mexican Sp.]. A Mexican fermented beverage prepared from aguamiel.

pul·sate (pul'sate) *v.* [L. *pulsare*]. To beat or throb.

pul·sa·tile (pul'suh·til) *adj.* Pulsating; throbbing.

pulsating empyema. Empyema that has dissected subcutaneously into an intercostal space (empyema necessitatis) and transmits the cardiac pulsation, simulating an aneurysm.

pulsating exophthalmos. Pathologic to-and-fro protrusion of the eyeball, sometimes associated with a bruit, seen in lesions in which the pulse is transmitted to the eye, as in carotid cavernous fistula, aneurysm, or defects of the bony orbit in neurofibromatosis.

pul·sa·tion (pul·say'shun) *n.* [L. *pusatio*]. 1. A beating or throbbing; usually rhythmic. 2. PULSE (2).

pul·sa·tor (pul·say'tur) *n.* An electrical device that produces vibrations to stimulate muscles and nerves.

pulse, *n. & v.* [L. *pulsus,* from *pellere,* to strike]. 1. The regularly recurrent palpable wave of distention in an artery due to blood ejected with each cardiac contraction. 2. A single beat or wave in pulsation from any source. 3. To generate, emit, or modulate energy, as electromagnetic radiation, in the form of pulses.

pulse cycle. The period between the beginning and end of a pulse wave.

pulse deficit. The difference between the auscultatory heart rate and the rate of the peripheral pulse determined by palpation.

pulse-echo diagnosis or **technique.** The use of ultrasonic energy between 1 and 15 megahertz directed into the human body for the purposes of studying alterations of structure. Syn. *ultrasonography.* See also *echoencephalogram, echocardiogram, echorenogram.*

pulse·less, *adj.* Devoid of pulse or pulsation.

pulseless disease. AORTIC ARCH SYNDROME.

pulse pressure. The difference between the systolic and diastolic blood pressure.

pulse rate. The number of pulsations of an artery per minute; same as the heart rate.

pulse wave. PRESSURE PULSE WAVE.

pul·sim·e·ter (pul·sim'e·tur) *n.* [*pulse* + *-meter*]. An instrument for determining the rate or force of the pulse.

pul·sion (pul'shun) *n.* [L., *pulsio,* from *pellere,* to strike, to push]. The act of pushing forward.

pulsion diverticulum. Herniation of the mucous membrane through the muscular coat of an organ, usually the pharynx or esophagus, caused by pressure from within. Contr. *traction diverticulum.*

pul·som·e·ter (pul·som'e·tur) *n.* PULSIMETER.

pul·sus (pul'sus) *n.* [L.]. PULSE.

pulsus al·ter·nans (awl'tur·nanz). A pulse pattern in which the beats occur at regular intervals but with alternating weak and strong beats; commonly seen with left ventricular failure.

pulsus bi·gem·i·nus (bye·jem'i·nus). BIGEMINAL PULSE.

pulsus bis·fer·i·ens (bis·ferr'ee·enz). BISFERIENS PULSE.

pulsus ce·ler (sel'ur) [L., rapid]. A pulse that rises and falls quickly.

pulsus celer et al·tus (al'tus) [L., rapid and high]. A quick, full, bounding pulse, seen especially in aortic regurgitation.

pulsus deb·i·lis (deb'i·lis). A weak pulse.

pulsus du·plex (dew'plecks). DICROTIC PULSE.

pulsus du·rus (dew'rus). A hard, incompressible pulse.

pulsus ir·reg·u·la·ris per·pet·u·us (i·reg''yoo·lair'is pur·pet'yoo·us). The pulse of atrial fibrillation which is completely irregular in rate and amplitude.

pulsus par·a·dox·us (păr''uh·dock'sus). Fall in the systolic blood pressure during inspiration greater than the normal 3 to 10 mmHg; may be seen with conditions such as cardiac tamponade, severe heart failure, emphysema.

pulsus par·vus (pahr'vus). A pulse small in amplitude.

pulsus parvus et tar·dus (tahr'dus). The small, slowly rising pulse characteristic of aortic stenosis.

pulsus tardus. A pulse with a delayed systolic peak.

pul·ta·ceous (pul·tay'shus) *adj.* [from L. *puls, pultis,* pulse porridge, + *-aceous*]. Having the consistency of pulp; mushy; soft.

pulv. Abbreviation for *pulvis.*

pul·ver·ize (pul'vur·ize) *v.* [from L. *pulvis, pulveris,* dust, powder]. To reduce a substance to a powder. —**pul·ver·i·za·tion** (pul''vur·i·zay'shun) *n.*

pul·ver·u·lent (pul·verr'yoo·lunt) *adj.* [L. *pulverulentus,* from *pulvis, pulveris,* dust]. 1. Powdery, dusty, or reducible to a fine powder. 2. Covered with fine powder or dust.

pul·vi·nar (pul·vye'nur) *n.* [L., couch] [NA]. A nuclear mass forming the posterior portion of the thalamus.

pulvinar tha·la·mi (thal'uh·migh) [NA alt.]. POSTERIOR NUCLEUS OF THE THALAMUS. NA alt. *nucleus posterior thalami.*

pul·vis (pul'vis) *n.* [L.]. POWDER.

pulvis an·ti·mo·ni·a·lis (an''ti·mo''nee·ay'lis). ANTIMONY POWDER.

pu·mex (pew'mecks) *n.* [L.]. PUMICE.

pum·ice (pum'is) *n.* [L., *pumex, pumicis*]. A substance of volcanic origin, consisting of complex silicates of aluminum, potassium, and sodium; used as an abrasive.

pump, *n.* [MD. *pompe,* probably from Sp. *bomba*]. An apparatus or machine which, by alternate suction and compression, raises or transfers liquids, or which exhausts or compresses gases.

punch, *n.* [from *puncheon,* from MF. *poinçon,* a sharp tool, from L. *pungere,* to puncture]. A surgical instrument for perforating or cutting out a disk or segment of resistant tissue, as cartilage or bone.

punch-drunk, *adj.* Pertaining to or suffering from the punch-drunk state. —**punch-drunkenness,** *n.*

punch-drunk state. A condition caused by repeated cerebral injury, observed in professional boxers; characterized clinically by dysarthria, ataxia, and impairment of cognition and memory; characterized pathologically by neuronal loss in the substantia nigra and the cerebral and cerebellar cortices and by fibrillary changes in remaining neurons. Syn. *dementia pugilistica, boxer's encephalopathy.*

punch operation. Excision of part or all of the prostate by means of various punches and resectoscope.

puncta. Plural of *punctum.*

puncta do·lo·ro·sa (do·lo·ro'suh). PAINFUL POINTS.

puncta lac·ri·ma·lia (lack·ri·may'lee·uh) [BNA]. Plural of *punctum lacrimale* (= LACRIMAL PUNCTUM).

punc·tate (punk'tate) *adj.* [from L. *punctum,* point]. Dotted; full of minute points.

punctate basophilia. BASOPHILIA (2).

punctate cataract. A form of congenital cataract in which small opacities, appearing light-blue or gray in color, are scattered throughout the lens. There is no loss of vision.

punc·tat·ed (punk'tay·tid) *adj.* PUNCTATE.

punctate pruritus. Patchy areas of itching with no cutaneous lesions; occurs especially over bony prominences.

puncta vas·cu·lo·sa (vas·kew·lo'suh). Minute red spots studding the cut surface of the white central mass of the fresh brain. They are produced by the blood escaping from divided blood vessels.

punc·tic·u·lum (punk·tick'yoo·lum) *n.* [dim. from L. *punctum*, point]. A small point.

punc·ti·form (punk'ti·form) *adj.* [*punctum* + *-iform*]. 1. Having the nature or qualities of a point; seeming to be located at a point, as a punctiform sensation. 2. Of bacterial colonies: very minute.

punc·to·graph (punk'to·graf) *n.* [*punctum* + *-graph*]. *Obsol.* A radiographic instrument for the surgical localization of foreign bodies, as bullets embedded in the tissues.

punc·tum (punk'tum) *n.*, pl. **punc·ta** (·tuh) [L.]. Point.

punctum ce·cum. (see'kum). BLIND SPOT.

punctum lac·ri·ma·le (lack·ri·may'lee) [NA]. LACRIMAL PUNCTUM.

punctum prox·i·mum (prock'si·mum). NEAR POINT. Abbreviated, P., P.p.

punctum re·mo·tum (re·mo'tum). FAR POINT. Abbreviated, P.r.

punc·ture (punk'chur) *n.* [L., *punctura*, from *pungere*, to prick, pierce]. 1. A hole made by the piercing of a pointed instrument. 2. The procedure of making a puncture.

puncture fracture. A fracture in which there is a loss of bone without disruption of continuity, as a hole drilled through a bone by a projectile.

puncture headache. LUMBAR PUNCTURE HEADACHE.

pun·gent (pun'junt) *adj.* [L., *pungere*, to penetrate, sting]. Acrid; penetrating; producing a painful sensation.

pu·ni·cine (pew'ni·seen, ·sin) *n.* PELLETIERINE.

punk·tal lens (punk'tul). A lens that is corrected for astigmatism in all powers throughout the entire field.

pu·nu·dos (poo·noo'doce, pew'new·dos) *n.* A disease resembling leprosy, but apparently not due to the leprosy bacillus, found in Guatemala.

P.U.O. Pyrexia of unknown origin.

pu·pa (pew'puh) *n.*, pl. **pu·pae** (·pee), **pupas** [L., little girl, doll]. The stage, usually quiescent, in the life history of some insects, which follows the larval period and precedes the adult imago. —**pu·pal** (·pul) *adj.*

pu·pil (pew'pil) *n.* [L. *pupilla*, dim. of *pupa*, little girl, doll]. The aperture in the iris of the eye for the passage of light. See also Plate 19.

pu·pil·la (pew·pil'uh) *n.*, pl. & genit. sing. **pupil·lae** (·ee) [L.] [NA]. PUPIL.

pu·pil·lary (pew'pi·lerr·ee) *adj.* Of or pertaining to the pupil of an eye.

pupillary athetosis. HIPPUS.

pupillary axis. An imaginary line through the center of the pupil of the eye and perpendicular to the cornea.

pupillary block glaucoma. Glaucoma which is caused by a pupillary block mechanism, that is, adhesions between the iris and the vitreous.

pupillary cataract. Congenital closure of the pupil.

pupillary membrane. A membrane formed by the mesoderm on the anterior surface of the lens epithelium in the embryo. It combines peripherally with pars iridica retinae to form the iris; centrally it disappears to form the pupil of the eye.

pupillary reflex. 1. Contraction of the pupil in response to stimulation of the retina by light. Syn. *Whytt's reflex*. 2. Contraction of the pupil on accommodation for close vision and dilatation of the pupil on accommodation for distant vision. 3. CONSENSUAL LIGHT REFLEX. 4. Contraction of the pupil on attempted closure of the eye. Syn. *Westphal-Pilcz reflex, Westphal's pupillary reflex*.

pupillary zone. LESSER RING OF THE IRIS.

pupillo-. A combining form meaning *pupil, pupillary*.

pu·pil·lo·con·stric·tor center (pew·pil"o·kun·strick'tur). AUTONOMIC NUCLEUS OF THE OCULOMOTOR NERVE.

pu·pil·lo·di·la·tor center (pew"pi·lo·dye·lay'tur, pew·pil"o·). CILIOSPINAL CENTER.

pu·pil·lom·e·ter (pew"pi·lom'e·tur) *n.* [*pupillo-* + *-meter*]. An instrument for measuring the pupil of the eye. —**pupillome·try** (·tree) *n.*

pu·pil·lo·sta·tom·e·ter (pew·pil"o·sta·tom'e·tur) *n.* [*pupillo-* + Gk. *statos*, fixed, placed, + *-meter*]. An instrument for measuring the exact distance between the centers of the two pupils.

pu·pil·lo·to·nia (pew"pil·o·to'nee·uh) *n.* [*pupillo-* + *-tonia*]. ADIE'S PUPIL. —**pupillo·ton·ic** (·ton'ick) *adj.*

pupillotonic pseudotabes. ADIE'S SYNDROME.

puppet-head phenomenon. DOLL'S-HEAD PHENOMENON.

pure, *adj.* [L. *purus*]. Free from mixture or contact with that which weakens or pollutes; containing no foreign or extraneous material.

pure culture. A culture of a single microorganism.

pure line. 1. All the progeny of a single completely homozygous individual, reproducing by self-fertilization. 2. Organisms with biparental reproduction where the condition of complete homozygosis is realized. 3. Progeny of a single individual reproducing asexually. See also *clone* (1).

pure red-cell anemia. 1. CONGENITAL HYPOPLASTIC ANEMIA. 2. Any anemia involving erythrocytes only.

pure word dumbness. PURE WORD MUTENESS.

pure word muteness. A form of aphasia in which the patient loses all capacity to speak, while retaining the ability to write, understand spoken words, and read silently with comprehension; presumably due to a lesion which separates Broca's convolution from subcortical motor centers. Syn. *aphemia*.

pur·ga·tion (pur·gay'shun) *n.* [L., *purgatio*, a cleansing]. 1. The evacuation of the bowels by means of purgatives. 2. Cleansing.

pur·ga·tive (pur'guh·tiv) *adj.* & *n.* [L., *purgativus*]. 1. Producing purgation. 2. A drug that produces evacuation of the bowel; specifically, a cathartic of moderate potency. Contr. *drastic, laxative*.

purge (purj) *v.* & *n.* [L., *purgare*, to cleanse, purge]. 1. To cause purgation or catharsis. 2. A purgative or cathartic.

purg·ing (pur'jing) *n.* A condition in which there is rapid and continuous evacuation of the bowels.

purging cassia. *Cassia fistula*, the dried fruit of a tree growing in tropical regions. The pulp is a mild laxative.

pu·ri·fied (pewr'i·fide) *adj.* Cleansed; freed from extraneous matter.

purified antidiphtheritic serum. DIPHTHERIA ANTITOXIN.

purified antitetanus serum. TETANUS ANTITOXIN.

purified kieselguhr. DIATOMACEOUS EARTH.

purified protein derivative of tuberculin. A form of dried tuberculin. Abbreviated, P.P.D.

purified siliceous earth. DIATOMACEOUS EARTH.

purified talc. Talc, purified by acid washing. A fine, white, crystalline powder, unctuous to the touch. Used as a filtering medium and as dusting powder.

purified water. The U.S.P. title for water obtained by distillation or by ion-exchange treatment.

pu·ri·form (pew'ri·form) *adj.* [L. *pus, puris*, pus, + *-form*]. In the form of or resembling pus.

pu·rine (pew'reen, ·in) *n.* [L. *purus*, pure, + *uric* + *-ine*]. A heterocyclic compound, $C_5H_4N_4$, in which a pyrimidine ring is fused to an imidazoline ring. Various derivatives of purine, generically called purines and including adenine, guanine, the xanthines, and uric acid, are widely distributed in nature.

purine bases. Generic term for purine and other bases derived from it, as adenine and guanine, which are components of nucleotides, and also caffeine and theobromine, which are alkaloids.

pu·ri·ty (pewr'i·tee) *n. In optics*, the percentage contribution to luminous intensity by the dominant wavelength in a beam of light.

Pur·ki·nje cells (poor'kin·yeʰ) [J. E. *Purkinje*, (Cz. *Purkyně*) Bohemian physiologist, 1787–1869]. Cells of the cerebellar cortex with large, flask-shaped bodies forming a single cell layer between the molecular and granular layers. Their dendrites branch in the molecular layer in a plane at right angles to the long axis of the folia, and their axons run through the granular layer into the white substance to end in the central cerebellar nuclei.

Purkinje fibers [J. E. *Purkinje*]. The modified cardiac muscle fibers that form the terminal part of the conducting system of the heart.

Purkinje images [J. E. *Purkinje*]. Visual sensations on the retina from shadows of blood vessels.

Purkinje network. PURKINJE SYSTEM.

Purkinje-San·son images (sahⁿ·sohⁿ′) [J. E. *Purkinje;* and L. J. *Sanson,* French physician, 1790–1841]. A set of three images which may be seen reflected from the surface of the cornea, the anterior surface of the lens, and the posterior surface of the lens of the eye, respectively.

Purkinje shift [J. E. *Purkinje*]. The change in the sensitivity of the human eye under conditions of light and dark adaptation.

Purkinje system [J. E. *Purkinje*]. The Purkinje fibers as a group.

Purkyně. See *Purkinje.*

Purodigin. A trademark for digitoxin, a cardioactive glycoside.

pu·ro·mu·cous (pew″ro·mew′kus) *adj.* [L., *pus, puris,* pus, + *mucous*]. Consisting of mucus mixed with pus; mucopurulent.

pu·ro·my·cin (pew″ro·migh′sin) *n.* An antibiotic substance, $C_{22}H_{29}N_7O_5$, produced by *Streptomyces alboniger,* that has trypanocidal and amebicidal activity.

pur·pos·ive reflexes (pur′puh·siv). The reflexes that provide the mechanism for the preservation of the individual. See also *protective reflex.*

pur·pu·ra (pur′pew·ruh) *n.* [L., purple]. A condition in which hemorrhages occur in the skin, mucous membranes, serous membranes, and elsewhere. The characteristic skin lesions are petechiae, ecchymoses, and vibices.

purpura an·nu·la·ris te·lan·gi·ec·to·des (an·yoo·lair′is te·lan″jee·eck·to′dees). An eruption of purpuric spots, grouped in ring form and accompanied by telangiectasis. Syn. *Majocchi's disease.*

purpura ful·mi·nans (ful′mi·nanz). Rapidly progressive cutaneous and mucosal bleeding as a result of marked disseminated intravascular clotting with overutilization of platelets, factor V, and other clotting factors, occurring in many overwhelming bacterial and viral infections, especially in children, and best treated with the initiating agent, when possible.

purpura hem·or·rhag·i·ca (hem″o·raj′i·kuh, ·ray′ji·kuh). IDIOPATHIC THROMBOCYTOPENIC PURPURA.

purpura hy·per·glob·u·li·ne·mi·ca (high″pur·glob″yoo·li·nee′mi·kuh). Hemorrhagic diathesis attributed to elevation of the concentration of globulin in the serum.

purpura ne·crot·i·ca (ne·krot′i·kuh). A condition characterized by enormous ecchymotic skin lesions which in later stages become necrotic and gangrenous.

purpura rheu·mat·i·ca (roo·mat′i·kuh). SCHÖNLEIN'S PURPURA.

purpura se·ni·lis (se·nigh′lis). Purpura of unknown cause that occurs in elderly people.

purpura sim·plex (sim′plecks). A mild form of purpura not associated with well-defined defects of blood-clotting mechanisms or mucous-membrane bleeding; often familial and particularly prone to occur in females.

purpura ur·ti·cans (ur′ti·kanz). Purpura associated with urticaria. See also *urticaria hemorrhagica.*

purpura va·ri·o·losa (va·rye″o·lo′suh). A hemorrhagic form of smallpox.

pur·pu·ric (pur·pew′rick) *adj.* Pertaining to or characterized by purpura.

pur·pu·rin (pur′pew·rin) *n.* 1. A dye, $C_{14}H_8O_5$, present with alizarin in madder-root, but also prepared artificially. 2. Uroerythrin, a red pigment sometimes present in urinary deposits.

pur·pu·rin·uria (pur″pew·ri·new′ree·uh) *n.* [*purpurin* + *-uria*]. The presence of purpurin in the urine. Syn. *porphyruria.*

purr, *n.* A low-pitched vibratory murmur, like the purring of a cat.

purse-string suture. A running stitch placed in a circle and pulled together to close an opening.

pu·ru·lence (pewr′yoo·lunce) *n.* [L. *purulentia*]. The quality or state of containing pus.

pu·ru·len·cy (pewr′yoo·lun·see) *n.* PURULENCE.

pu·ru·lent (pewr′yoo·lunt) *adj.* [L. *purulentus,* from *pus, puris,* pus]. Containing, consisting of, or forming pus.

purulent exudate. An exudate containing neutrophils that have undergone necrosis in large numbers; pus.

purulent inflammation. An inflammatory process productive of an exudate rich in neutrophils, which undergoes liquefaction necrosis to produce pus. It is distinguished from suppurative inflammation by the lack of necrosis of fixed tissues, and is exemplified by the exudate often occurring in the common cold.

purulent meningitis. Meningitis due to a pyogenic organism.

purulent ophthalmia. Conjunctivitis with a purulent discharge.

purulent salpingitis. Salpingitis (1) in which there is collection of pus; PYOSALPINX.

purulent sputum. Sputum consisting chiefly of pus.

purulent synovitis. PYARTHROSIS.

pu·ru·loid (pewr′yoo·loid) *adj.* Resembling pus; puriform.

pu·ru·pu·ru (poo·roo″poo·roo′) *n.* PINTA.

pus, *n.* [L. (rel. to Gk. *pyos, pyon*)]. The product of liquefaction necrosis in an exudate rich in neutrophils, giving a viscous, creamy, pale-yellow or yellow-green fluid.

pus blister. A blister containing purulent matter.

pus cell. A degenerate or necrotic granulocyte; the characteristic cell of suppurative and purulent inflammation.

pus organism. PYOGENIC MICROORGANISM.

pus tube. PYOSALPINX.

pus·tu·lant (pus′tyoo·lunt) *adj. & n.* 1. Causing the formation of pustules. 2. An irritant substance giving rise to the formation of pustules.

pustular acrodermatitis. PUSTULOSIS PALMARIS ET PLANTARIS.

pustular bacterid. PUSTULOSIS PALMARIS ET PLANTARIS.

pustular erysipelas. A variety of erysipelas bullosum in which the bullae contain pus.

pustular psoriasis. 1. A variant form of psoriasis occurring in the course of chronic psoriasis, characterized by shiny, dark-red scaly patches bearing superficial pustules. Oral lesions may occur, and chills and fever may be present at onset. 2. ACRODERMATITIS CONTINUA. 3. IMPETIGO HERPETIFORMIS.

pustular tonsillitis. A form of tonsillitis characterized by the formation of pustules.

pus·tu·la·tion (pus″tyoo·lay′shun) *n.* The formation of pustules.

pus·tule (pus′tyool) *n.* [L. *pustula,* blister, pimple (rel. to Gk. *physan,* to blow, puff up; NOT from L. *pus*)]. A small, circumscribed elevation of the skin containing pus. —**pus·tu·lar** (·tyoo·lur) *adj.*

pus·tu·li·form (pus′tyoo·li·form) *adj.* Resembling a pustule.

pus·tu·lo·der·ma (pus″tew·lo·dur′muh) *n.* [*pustule* + *-derma*]. Any skin disease characterized by the formation of pustules.

pus·tu·lo·sis (pus″tew·lo′sis) *n.* [*pustule* + *-osis*]. Any condition characterized by the presence of pustules.

pustulosis pal·ma·ris et plan·ta·ris (pal·mair′is et plan·tair′is). A chronic indolent noninfectious dermatitis chiefly of palms and soles, not related to psoriasis. The pustules are sterile, deep-seated, and appear in continuous crops. Syn. *pustular acrodermatitis, pustular bacterid.*

pu·ta·men (pew·tay′mun) *n.* [L., peel, husk, from *putare,* to prune, cleanse] [NA]. The outer darker part of the lenticular nucleus of the brain. —**pu·tam·i·nal** (pew·tam'i·nul) *adj.*

Put·nam-Da·na syndrome [J. J. *Putnam*, U.S. neurologist, 1846–1918; and C. L. *Dana*]. SUBACUTE COMBINED DEGENERATION OF THE SPINAL CORD.

Putnam's type of spinal sclerosis [J. J. *Putnam*]. SUBACUTE COMBINED DEGENERATION OF THE SPINAL CORD.

pu·tre·fac·tion (pew''tre·fack'shun) *n.* [L. *putrefactio*, from *putrefacere*, to make rotten]. The enzymic decomposition of organic matter, especially proteins, by anaerobic microorganisms, with formation of malodorous substances such as indole and skatole, nitrogenous bases such as cadaverine and putrescine, and many other compounds. See also *ptomaine*.

pu·tre·fac·tive (pew''tre·fack'tiv) *adj.* Pertaining to or causing putrefaction.

pu·tre·fy (pew'tre·figh) *v.* [L. *putrefacere*, from *putrere*, to be rotten]. 1. To render putrid. 2. To become putrid.

pu·tres·cent (pew·tres'unt) *adj.* Undergoing putrefaction. —**putres·cence** (·unce) *n.*

pu·tres·cine (pew·tres'een, ·in) *n.* 1,4-Diaminobutane or tetramethylenediamine, $NH_2(CH_2)_4NH_2$, a product of decarboxylation of ornithine and also found in putrefying flesh; formerly believed to be responsible for food poisoning, and referred to as a ptomaine.

pu·trid (pew'trid) *adj.* [L. *putridus*]. Rotten; characterized by putrefaction.

pu·tro·maine (pew'tro·mane) *n.* A ptomaine developed in putrefactive processes.

Puus·sepp's operation (poos'sep) [L. M. *Puussepp*, Estonian neurologist, 1879–1942]. Incision of the cystic spinal cord in syringomyelia.

Puussepp's reflex [L. M. *Puussepp*]. Slow abduction of the little toe following light stroking of the outer sole of the foot; said to occur in extrapyramidal motor disorders.

PVC. Abbreviation for *premature ventricular contraction.*

PVE Abbreviation for *prosthetic valve endocarditis.*

PVP Abbreviation for *polyvinylpyrrolidone.*

P wave of the electrocardiogram. The electrocardiographic deflection due to depolarization of the atria.

py-, pyo- [Gk. *pyon*, pus]. A combining form meaning *pus* or *suppuration.*

pyaemia. PYEMIA.

py·ar·thro·sis (pye''ahr·thro'sis) *n.* [*py-* + *arthr-* + *-osis*]. Suppuration involving a joint.

pycn-, pycno-. See *pykn-*.

pycnodysostosis. PYKNODYSOSTOSIS.

pycnoepilepsy. PYKNOEPILEPSY (= PYKNOLEPSY).

pycnolepsy. PYKNOLEPSY.

pycnometer. PYKNOMETER.

pycnomorphous. PYKNOMORPHOUS.

pycnophrasia. PYKNOPHRASIA.

pycnosis. PYKNOSIS.

py·ec·chy·sis (pye·eck'i·sis) *n.* [*py-* + Gk. *ekchysis*, outflow]. Effusion of pus.

pyel-, pyelo- [Gk. *pyelos*, trough, pan]. A combining form meaning *renal pelvis, renal pelvic.*

py·el·ec·ta·sia (pye''e·leck·tay'zhuh, ·zee·uh) *n.* PYELECTASIS.

py·el·ec·ta·sis (pye''e·leck'tuh·sis) *n.* [*pyel-* + *ectasis*]. Dilation of a renal pelvis.

py·eli·tis (pye''e·lye'tis) *n.* [*pyel-* + *-itis*]. Inflammation of the pelvis of a kidney. —**py·elit·ic** (pye''e·lit'ick) *adj.*

pyelitis cys·ti·ca (sis'ti·kuh). A nonspecific chronic inflammatory reaction of the renal pelvis, characterized by numerous minute translucent cysts scattered over the surface of the pelvic mucosa.

pyelo-. See *pyel-*.

py·elo·cys·ti·tis (pye''e·lo·sis·tye'tis) *n.* [*pyelo-* + *cyst-* + *-itis*]. Inflammation of the pelvis of the kidney and of the urinary bladder.

py·elo·gen·ic cyst (pye''e·lo·jen'ick). A cyst arising from or associated with the renal pelvis.

py·elo·gram (pye'e·lo·gram) *n.* [*pyelo-* + *-gram*]. A radiograph of the renal pelvis and ureter, employing contrast material.

py·elog·ra·phy (pye''e·log'ruh·fee) *n.* [*pyelo-* + *-graphy*]. Radiography of a renal pelvis and ureter, which have been filled with an opaque solution. See also *urography.*

py·elo·li·thot·o·my (pye''e·lo·li·thot'uh·mee) *n.* [*pyelo-* + *lithotomy*]. Removal of a renal calculus through an incision into the pelvis of a kidney. Syn. *pelviolithotomy.*

py·elo·lym·phat·ic backflow (pye''e·lo·lim·fat'ick). Extravasion of a contrast medium into the renal hilar lymphatics during retrograde pyelography.

py·elo·ne·phri·tis (pye''e·lo·ne·frye'tis) *n.* [*pyelo-* + *nephritis*]. The disease process from the immediate and late effects of bacterial and other infections of the parenchyma and the pelvis of the kidney.

py·elo·plas·ty (pye'e·lo·plas''tee) *n.* [*pyelo-* + *-plasty*]. Plastic repair of the renal pelvis.

py·elo·pli·ca·tion (pye''e·lo·pli·kay'shun) *n.* [*pyelo-* + *plication*]. Reducing an enlarged renal pelvis by plicating or suturing the infolded walls.

py·elos·to·my (pye''e·los'tuh·mee) *n.* [*pyelo-* + *-stomy*]. Incision into the renal pelvis.

py·elot·o·my (pye''e·lot'uh·mee) *n.* [*pyelo-* + *-tomy*]. Incision of the renal pelvis.

py·elo·tu·bu·lar (pye''e·lo·tew'bew·lur) *adj.* [*pyelo-* + *tubular*]. Pertaining to the renal pelvis and tubules.

pyelotubular backflow. Extravasation of opaque media into the tubules of the kidney during retrograde urography.

py·elo·ure·ter·al (py''e·lo·yoo·ree'tur·ul) *adj.* [*pyelo-* + *ureteral*]. Pertaining to the renal pelvis and ureter.

py·elo·ure·ter·ic (pye''e·lo·yoo''re·terr'ick, ·yoo·ree'tur·ick) *adj.* PYELOURETERAL.

py·elo·ure·ter·og·ra·phy (pye''e·lo·yoo·ree''tur·og'ruh·fee) *n.* [*pyelo-* + *uretero-* + *-graphy*]. PYELOGRAPHY.

py·elo·ve·nous (pye''e·lo·vee'nus) *adj.* [*pyelo-* + *venous*]. Pertaining to the renal pelvis and the veins.

pyelovenous backflow or **reflux.** Abnormal passage of fluid from the renal collecting system into renal vein branches, seen during retrograde pyelography.

py·em·e·sis (pye·em'e·sis) *n.* [*py-* + *emesis*]. Vomiting of purulent material.

py·emia, py·ae·mia (pye·ee'mee·uh) *n.* [*py-* + *-emia*]. A disease state due to the presence of pyogenic microorganisms in the blood and the formation, wherever these organisms lodge, of embolic or metastatic abscesses. Compare *bacteremia, septicemia.* —**py·emic, py·ae·mic** (pye·ee'mick) *adj.*

pyemic abscess. An abscess occurring as a complication of pyemia.

py·en·ceph·a·lus (pye''en·sef'uh·lus) *n.* [*py-* + *-encephalus*]. Suppuration within the brain; a brain abscess.

pyg-, pygo- [Gk. *pygē*]. A combining form meaning *buttocks.*

py·gal·gia (pye·gal'juh, ·jee·uh) *n.* [*pyg-* + *-algia*]. Pain in the buttocks.

pyg·ma·li·on·ism (pig·may'lee·un·iz·um) *n.* [*Pygmalion*, Greek legendary sculptor who fell in love with a statue he carved]. The pathological erotic fantasies in which an individual falls in love with a creation of his own.

pyg·my (pig'mee) *n.* [Gk., *pygmaios*, dwarfish, from *pygmē*, a measure of length]. An abnormally small person or dwarf.

pygo-. See *pyg-*.

py·go·amor·phus (pye''go·uh·mor'fus) *n.* [*pygo-* + *amorphus*]. An individual with a teratoma in the sacral region.

py·go·did·y·mus (pye''go·did'i·mus) *n.* [*pygo-* + *-didymus*]. PYGOPAGUS.

py·gom·e·lus (pye·gom'e·lus) *n.*, pl. **pygome·li** (·lye) [*pygo-* + *-melus*]. An individual with an accessory limb or limbs attached to the buttock. Syn. *epipygus.*

py·gop·a·gus (pye·gop'uh·gus) *n.* [*pygo-* + *-pagus*]. Conjoined twins united in a sacral region.

py·go·par·a·si·tus (pye''go·păr''uh·sigh'tus) *n.* [NL., from *pygo-* + Gk. *parasitos*, parasite]. Unequal conjoined twins with the parasite attached to the nates of the autosite.

py·go·ter·a·toi·des (pye″go·terr″uh·toy′deez) *n.* [NL., from *pygo-* + *teratoid*]. An individual with teratoid tumors in the region of the sacrum.

py·ic (pye′ick) *adj.* [*py-* + *-ic*]. PURULENT.

py·in (pye′in) *n.* A proteinaceous substance of complex constitution occurring in pus.

pykn-, pykno-, pycn-, pycno- [Gk. *pyknos*]. A combining form meaning *compact, dense.*

pyk·nic (pick′nick) *adj.* [Gk. *pyknos,* thick, compact]. Pertaining to or characterizing a constitutional body type marked by roundness of contour, amplitude of body cavities, and considerable subcutaneous fat.

pyk·no·dys·os·to·sis, pyc·no·dys·os·to·sis (pick″no·dis″os·to′sis) *n.* [*pykno-* + *dysostosis*]. A heritable disorder of bone, characterized by short stature, a large skull with absence of knitting of the anterior fontanel, receding chin, shortness of fingers and toes, and fragility of bones. Radiographs show an abnormal thickness of bones, which is responsible for the fractures. Transmitted as an autosomal recessive trait. Syn. *Toulouse-Lautrec disease.*

pyk·no·ep·i·lep·sy, pyc·no·ep·i·lep·sy (pick″no·ep′i·lep·see) *n.* PYKNOLEPSY.

pyk·no·lep·sy, pyc·no·lep·sy (pick′no·lep·see) *n.* [*pykno-* + *-lepsy*]. *Obsol.* A form of absence attack in which the episodes of unawareness occur very frequently. —**pyk·no·lep·tic** (pick″no·lep′tick) *adj.*

pyk·nom·e·ter, pyc·nom·e·ter (pick·nom′e·tur) *n.* [*pykno-* + *-meter*]. An instrument for the determination of the specific gravity of fluids.

pyk·no·mor·phous, pyc·no·mor·phous (pick″no·mor′fus) *adj.* [*pykno-* + *-morphous*]. Of or pertaining to nerve cells in which the chromophil substance of the cytoplasm is compactly arranged.

pyk·no·phra·sia, pyc·no·phra·sia (pick″no·fray′zhuh, ·zee·uh) *n.* [*pykno-* + Gk. *phrasis,* expression, phrase, text, + *-ia*]. Thickness of speech.

pyk·no·sis, pyc·no·sis (pick·no′sis) *n.* [*pykn-* + *-osis*]. 1. Thickening; inspissation. 2. A degenerative change in cells whereby the nucleus is condensed and shrinks to a dense, structureless mass of chromatin. —**pyk·not·ic, pyc·not·ic** (·not′ick) *adj.*

pyknotic normoblast. NORMOBLAST (1).

pyl-, pyle-, pylo- [Gk. *pylē,* gate]. A combining form meaning *portal vein.*

py·lem·phrax·is (pye″lem·frack′sis) *n.* [*pyl-* + *emphraxis*]. Obstruction of the portal vein.

py·le·phleb·ec·ta·sia (pye″le·fleb″eck·tay′zhuh, ·zee·uh) *n.* PYLEPHLEBECTASIS.

py·le·phle·bec·ta·sis (pye″le·fle·beck′tuh·sis) *n.* [*pyle-* + *phlebectasis*]. Dilation of the portal vein.

py·le·phle·bi·tis (pye″le·fle·bye′tis) *n.* [*pyle-* + *phlebitis*]. Inflammation of the portal vein, usually secondary to suppuration in tissues drained by its tributaries, or to contiguous tissue suppuration.

py·le·throm·bo·phle·bi·tis (pye″le·throm″bo·fle·bye′tis) *n.* [*pyle-* + *thrombophlebitis*]. Inflammation and thrombosis of the portal vein.

py·le·throm·bo·sis (pye″le·throm·bo′sis) *n.* [*pyle-* + *thrombosis*]. Thrombosis of the portal vein.

pylo-. See *pyl-.*

pylor-, pyloro-. A combining form meaning *pylorus, pyloric.*

py·lo·ral·gia (pye″lo·ral′jee·uh) *n.* [*pylor-* + *-algia*]. Pain in the region of the pylorus.

py·lo·rec·to·my (pye″lo·reck′tuh·mee) *n.* [*pylor-* + *-ectomy*]. Excision of the pylorus; partial gastrectomy.

py·lo·ric (pye·lo′rick) *adj.* Pertaining to or lying in the region of the pylorus.

pyloric antrum. The portion of the stomach lying between the body of the stomach and the pyloric canal. NA *antrum pyloricum.*

pyloric canal or **channel.** That portion of the stomach lying between the pyloric antrum and the base of the duodenal bulb. NA *canalis pyloricus.*

pyloric glands. The glands of the mucous membrane of the pyloric portion of the stomach. NA *glandulae pyloricae.*

pyloric plexus. A nerve plexus found in the region of the pylorus.

pyloric sphincter. The thickened ringlike band of the circular layer of smooth muscle at the lower end of the pyloric canal of the stomach. NA *musculus sphincter pylori.*

pyloric stenosis. Obstruction (usually congenital) of the pyloric orifice of the stomach caused by hypertrophy of the pyloric muscle.

pyloric valve. The fold of mucous membrane at the pyloric end of the stomach together with the underlying pyloric sphincter.

pyloric vestibule. PYLORIC ANTRUM.

py·lo·ri·ste·no·sis (pye·lo″ri·ste·no′sis) *n.* PYLOROSTENOSIS.

pyloro-. See *pylor-.*

py·lo·ro·co·lic (pye·lor″o·ko′lick, ·kol′ick) *adj.* [*pyloro-* + *colic*]. Pertaining to or connecting the pyloric end of the stomach and the transverse colon.

py·lo·ro·di·la·tor (pye·lor″o·dye′lay·tur, ·dye·lay′tur) *n.* [*pyloro-* + *dilator*]. An appliance for dilating the pyloric orifice of the stomach.

py·lo·ro·di·o·sis (pye·lor″o·dye·o′sis) *n.* [*pyloro-* + Gk. *diōsis,* a pushing asunder]. Dilation of the pylorus by the finger or an instrument, as a bougie.

py·lo·ro·du·o·de·nal (pye·lor″o·dew″o·dee′nul, ·dew·od′e·nul) *adj.* [*pyloro-* + *duodenal*]. Pertaining to the pylorus and the duodenum.

py·lo·ro·gas·trec·to·my (pye·lor″o·gas·treck′tuh·mee) *n.* [*pyloro-* + *gastrectomy*]. Resection of the pyloric end of the stomach; pylorectomy.

py·lo·ro·my·ot·o·my (pye·lor″o·migh·ot′uh·mee) *n.* [*pyloro-* + *myotomy*]. The division, anteriorly, of the pyloric muscle, without incision through the mucosa, for congenital pyloric stenosis in infants. Syn. *Ramstedt's operation, Fredet-Ramstedt operation.*

py·lo·ro·plas·ty (pye·lor″o·plas′tee) *n.* [*pyloro-* + *-plasty*]. An operation upon the pylorus, for stenosis due to ulcer, which may involve removal of a portion of the pylorus but which, in principle, divides the pylorus on the gastric and duodenal sides transversely, the wound being closed by sutures which convert it into a transverse incision. It provides a larger opening from the stomach to duodenum. See also *pylorotomy.*

py·lo·rop·to·sia (pye·lor″op·to′zhuh, ·zee·uh) *n.* PYLOROPTOSIS.

py·lo·rop·to·sis (pye·lor″op·to′sis) *n.* [*pyloro-* + *ptosis*]. Downward displacement of the pylorus.

py·lo·ro·sche·sis (pye·lor″o·skee′sis, pye″lo·ros′ki·sis) *n.* [*pyloro-* + Gk. *schesis,* a checking]. Obstruction of the pylorus.

py·lo·ros·co·py (pye″lo·ros′kuh·pee) *n.* [*pyloro-* + *-scopy*]. Inspection of the pylorus.

py·lo·ro·spasm (pye·lor′o·spaz·um) *n.* [*pyloro-* + *spasm*]. Spasm of the pylorus.

py·lo·ro·ste·no·sis (pye·lor″o·ste·no′sis) *n.* [*pyloro-* + *stenosis*]. Narrowing or stricture of the pylorus.

py·lo·ros·to·my (pye″lo·ros′tuh·mee) *n.* [*pyloro-* + *-stomy*]. Incision into the pylorus, as in the formation of a gastric fistula.

py·lo·rot·o·my (pye″lo·rot′uh·mee) *n.* [*pyloro-* + *-tomy*]. An incision into or through the pylorus in the axis of the canal, converting it by sutures from a longitudinal to a transverse wound. Pyloroplasty, Finney's operation, Heineke-Mikulicz operation, gastroduodenostomy are types of pylorotomy.

py·lo·rus (pye·lo′rus, pi·lor′us) *n.,* L. pl. & genit. sing. **pylo·ri** (·rye) [L., from Gk. *pylōros,* porter, gatekeeper, pylorus, from *pylē,* gate]. 1. [NA] The circular opening of the stomach into the duodenum. 2. The fold of mucous membrane and muscular tissue surrounding the aperture between the stomach and the duodenum. 3. PYLORIC CANAL.

pyo-. See *py-*.

pyo·ar·thro·sis (pye″o·ahr·thro′sis) *n.* PYARTHROSIS.

pyo·cele (pye′o·seel) *n.* [*pyo-* + *-cele*]. A pocketing of pus, as in the scrotum.

pyo·ceph·a·lus (pye″o·sef′uh·lus) *n.* [*pyo-* + *-cephalus*]. PYENCEPHALUS.

pyo·che·zia (pye″o·kee′zee·uh) *n.* [*pyo-* + Gk. *chezein*, to defecate, + *-ia*]. Discharge of pus with or in the stool.

pyo·coc·cus (pye″o·kock′us) *n.* [*pyo-* + *coccus*]. Any pus-producing coccus.

pyo·col·po·cele (pye″o·kol′po·seel) *n.* [*pyo-* + *colpocele*]. A suppurating cyst of the vagina.

pyo·col·pos (pye″o·kol′pos) *n.* [*pyo-* + *-colpos*]. An accumulation of pus within the vagina.

pyo·cy·a·nase (pye″o·sigh′uh·nace, ·naze) *n. Obsol.* An early antibiotic preparation, produced by *Pseudomonas aeruginosa,* of variable composition of components, the most active of which was pyocyanin.

pyo·cy·an·ic (pye″o·sigh·an′ick) *adj.* Pertaining to blue pus, or to pyocyanin.

pyo·cy·a·nin (pye″o·sigh′uh·nin) *n.* [*pyo-* + Gk. *kyanos*, dark blue, + *-in*]. An antibiotic substance, $C_{13}H_{10}N_{20}$, forming blue crystals, produced by *Pseudomonas aeruginosa;* active against many bacteria and fungi.

pyo·cy·a·nine (pye″o·sigh′uh·neen, ·nin) *n.* PYOCYANIN.

pyo·cy·a·nol·y·sin (pye″o·sigh″uh·nol′i·sin) *n.* A hemolysin produced by *Pseudomonas aeruginosa.*

pyo·cyst (pye′o·sist) *n.* [*pyo-* + *cyst*]. A cyst containing pus.

pyo·cys·tis (pye″o·sis′tis) *n.* [*pyo-* + Gk. *kystis,* bladder]. Purulent infection in the urinary bladder after diversion of urine inflow.

pyo·der·ma (pye″o·dur′muh) *n.* [*pyo-* + *-derma*]. Any pus-producing skin lesion or lesions, used in referring to groups of furuncles, pustules, or even carbuncles.

pyoderma fa·ci·a·le (fay″shee·ay′lee). An intensely red or cyanotic erythema of the face with superficial and deep abscesses and cystic lesions.

pyoderma gan·gre·no·sum (gang″gre·no′sum). A pyogenic dermatosis usually of the trunk, often with large irregular ulcers; usually associated with ulcerative colitis.

pyo·der·ma·ti·tis (pye″o·dur″muh·tye′tis) *n.* [*pyo-* + *dermatitis*]. Any pustular skin infection.

pyodermatitis vegetans. DERMATITIS VEGETANS.

pyo·der·ma·to·sis (pye″o·dur″muh·to′sis) *n.* [*pyo-* + *dermatosis*]. An inflammation of the skin in which pus formation occurs.

pyo·der·ma·tous (pye″uh·dur′muh·tus) *adj.* Of or pertaining to pyoderma.

pyo·gen (pye′o·jen) *n.* PYOGENIC MICROORGANISM.

py·og·e·nes (pye·oj′e·neez) *adj.* [NL.]. Pus-producing, pyogenic.

pyo·gen·e·sis (pye″o·jen′e·sis) *n.* [*pyo-* + *-genesis*]. The formation of pus. —**pyogen·ic** (·ick), **pyo·ge·net·ic** (·je·net′ick), **py·og·e·nous** (pye·oj′e·nus) *adj.*

pyogenic membrane. The lining of an abscess cavity or a fistula tract.

pyogenic microorganism. A microorganism producing pus; usually staphylococci and streptococci, but many other organisms may produce pus.

pyogenic peptonuria. Peptonuria produced by suppuration in the body.

pyogenic salpingitis. Salpingitis of the uterine tube caused by pus-producing organisms.

pyo·he·mo·tho·rax, py·o·hae·mo·tho·rax (pye″o·hee″mo·tho′racks) *n.* [*pyo-* + *hemo-* + *thorax*]. Pus and blood in the pleural cavity.

py·oid (pye′oid) *adj.* [Gk. *pyoeidēs*]. Resembling pus.

pyo·lab·y·rin·thi·tis (pye″o·lab″i·rin·thigh′tis) *n.* [*pyo-* + *labyrinthitis*]. Suppurative inflammation of the labyrinth of the ear.

pyo·me·tra (pye″o·mee′truh) *n.* [*pyo-* + *-metra*]. A collection of pus in the uterine cavity.

pyo·me·tri·um (pye″o·mee′tree·um) *n.* PYOMETRA.

pyo·my·o·si·tis (pye″ō·migh″o·sigh′tis) *n.* [*pyo-* + *myositis*]. Suppurative myositis.

pyo·ne·phri·tis (pye″o·ne·frye′tis) *n.* [*pyo-* + *nephritis*]. Suppurative inflammation of a kidney.

pyo·neph·ro·li·thi·a·sis (pye″o·nef″ro·li·thigh′uh·sis) *n.* [*pyo-* + *nephrolith* + *-iasis*]. The presence of pus and calculi in a kidney.

pyo·ne·phro·sis (pye″o·ne·fro′sis) *n.* [*pyo-* + *nephrosis*]. Replacement of a substantial portion of the kidney, or all of the kidney, by abscesses. —**pyone·phrot·ic** (·frot′ick) *adj.*

pyo·ovar·i·um (pye″o·o·văr′ee·um) *n.* [*pyo-* + *ovarium*]. An ovarian abscess.

pyo·peri·car·di·tis (pye″o·perr″i·kahr·dye′tis) *n.* [*pyo-* + *pericarditis*]. Purulent pericarditis.

pyo·peri·car·di·um (pye″o·perr″i·kahr′dee·um) *n.* [*pyo-* + *pericardium*]. The presence of pus in the pericardium.

pyo·peri·to·ne·um (pye″o·perr″i·to·nee′um) *n.* [*pyo-* + *peritoneum*]. The presence of pus in the peritoneal cavity.

pyo·peri·to·ni·tis (pye″o·perr″i·to·nigh′tis) *n.* [*pyo-* + *peritonitis*]. Suppurative inflammation of the peritoneum.

pyo·pha·gia (pye″o·fay′jee·uh) *n.* [*pyo-* + *-phagia*]. The swallowing of purulent material.

py·oph·thal·mia (pye″off·thal′mee·uh) *n.* [*py-* + *ophthalmia*]. Purulent ophthalmia.

pyo·phy·lac·tic (pye″o·fi·lack′tick) *n.* [*pyo-* + pro*phylactic*]. A defense or protection against pus or pyogenic organisms.

pyo·phy·so·me·tra (pye″o·figh″so·mee′truh) *n.* [*pyo* + *physo-* + *-metra*]. The presence of pus and gas in the uterus.

pyo·pneu·mo·peri·car·di·tis (pye″o·new″mo·perr″i·kahr·dye′tis) *n.* [*pyo-* + *pneumo-* + *pericarditis*]. Pericarditis complicated by the presence of pus and gas in the pericardium.

pyo·pneu·mo·peri·car·di·um (pye″o·new″mo·perr·i·kahr′dee·um) *n.* [*pyo-* + *pneumo-* + *pericardium*]. Pus and air or gas in the pericardium.

pyo·pneu·mo·peri·to·ne·um (pye″o·new″mo·perr″i·to·nee′um) *n.* [*pyo-* + *pneumo-* + *peritoneum*]. Pus and gas in the peritoneal cavity.

pyo·pneu·mo·peri·to·ni·tis (pye″o·new″mo·perr″i·to·nigh′tis) *n.* [*pyo-* + *pneumo-* + *peritonitis*]. Suppurative inflammation of the peritoneum associated with gas in the abdominal cavity.

pyo·pneu·mo·tho·rax (pye″o·new″mo·tho′racks) *n.* [*pyo-* + *pneumo-* + *thorax*]. The presence of air or gas and pus in the pleural cavity.

pyo·poi·e·sis (pye″o·poy·ee′sis) *n.* [*pyo-* + *-poiesis*]. Pus formation. —**pyopoi·et·ic** (·et′ick) *adj.*

py·op·ty·sis (pye·op′ti·sis) *n.* [*pyo-* + *ptysis*]. The expectoration of pus or purulent material.

py·or·rhea, py·or·rhoea (pye″o·ree′uh) *n.* [Gk. *pyorroia,* discharge of pus]. 1. A purulent discharge. 2. PYORRHEA ALVEOLARIS.

pyorrhea al·ve·o·la·ris (al″vee·o·lair′is). A periodontal disease in which there is a purulent exudate; periodontitis.

pyorrhea pocket. PERIODONTAL POCKET.

pyo·sal·pin·gi·tis (pye″o·sal″pin·jye′tis) *n.* [*pyo-* + *salpingitis*]. Purulent inflammation of the uterus or auditory tube.

pyo·sal·pin·go-oo·pho·ri·tis (pye″o·sal·pin″go·o″uh·fo·rye′tis) *n.* [*pyo-* + *salpingo-* + *oophor-* + *-itis*]. Combined suppurative inflammation of an ovary and oviduct.

pyo·sal·pinx (pye″o·sal′pinks) *n.* [*pyo-* + *salpinx*]. An accumulation of pus in an oviduct.

pyo·sep·ti·ce·mia, pyo·sep·ti·cae·mia (pye″o·sep″ti·see′mee·uh) *n.* [*pyo-* + *septicemia*]. Septicemia coupled with the development of pyemia.

py·o·sis (pye·o′sis) *n.* [Gk. *pyōsis,* from *pyon,* pus]. Suppuration; pus formation.

pyo·sper·mia (pye″o·spur′mee·uh) *n.* [*pyo-* + *-spermia*]. Leukocytes in the seminal fluid.

pyo·stat·ic (pye″o·stat′ick) *adj.* & *n.* [*pyo-* + *-static*]. 1. Arresting or checking the formation of pus. 2. An agent arresting the formation of pus.

pyo·ther·a·py (pye″o·therr′uh·pee) *n.* [*pyo-* + *therapy*]. The use of pus in the treatment of disease.

pyo·tho·rax (pye″o·tho′racks) *n.* [*pyo-* + *thorax*]. EMPYEMA.

pyo·ura·chus (pye″o·yoo′ruh·kus) *n.* [*pyo-* + *urachus*]. The presence of pus in or about the urachus.

pyo·ure·ter (pye″o·yoo·ree′tur, ·yoor′e·tur) *n.* [*pyo-* + *ureter*]. An accumulation of pus in a ureter.

pyo·xan·thin (pye″o·zan′thin) *n.* A yellow pigment sometimes found in pus, and resulting from the oxidation of pyocyanin.

pyo·xan·those (pye″o·zan′thoce) *n.* PYOXANTHIN.

pyr-, pyro- [Gk. *pyr,* (rel. to Gmc. *fūr-* → E. *fire*)]. A combining form meaning (a) *fire;* (b) *heat;* (c) *burning sensation;* (d) *fever;* (e) in chemistry, *derived by the action of heat.*

pyr·a·brom (pirr′uh·brom) *n.* A compound of 8-bromotheophylline with 2-[(2-dimethylamino)ethyl] (*p*-methoxybenzylamino)pyridine, $C_{24}H_{30}BrN_7O_3$, an antihistamine.

py·ra·hex·yl (pye″ra·heck′sil) *n.* SYNHEXYL.

pyr·a·mid (pirr′uh·mid) *n.* [Gk. *pyramis, pyramidos,* pyramid]. 1. Any conical eminence of an organ. 2. A body of the longitudinal nerve fibers of the corticospinal tract on each side of the anterior median fissure of the medulla oblongata. NA *pyramis medullae oblongatae.* 3. A polyhedron whose base is a polygon and whose other faces are triangular with a common vertex. —**py·ram·i·dal** (pi·ram′i·dul) *adj.*

pyramidal area. MOTOR AREA.

pyramidal cataract. A cataract in which the opacity is at the anterior pole and is conoid, the apex extending forward.

pyramidal cell. A nerve cell of the cerebral cortex, somewhat triangular in shape, with one large apical dendrite and several smaller dendrites at the base. The axon is given off from the base of the cell and the upper pointed end of the cell is continued toward the surface of the brain as the apical dendrite.

pyramidal decussation. The oblique crossing in the medulla oblongata of the corticospinal tracts from the opposite sides of the anterior median fissure. NA *decussatio pyramidum.*

pyramidal disease. 1. *In veterinary medicine,* periostitis of the pyramidal process of the os pedis in the horse. 2. Any dysfunction of the corticospinal tracts, resulting in an upper motor neuron lesion.

pyramidal eminence. A bony projection on the posterior wall of the tympanic cavity, having an opening at its tip for the tendon and an elongated cavity for the body of the stapedius muscle. NA *eminentia pyramidalis.*

pyramidal epithelium. Cuboidal or columnar epithelium, the cells of which are modified by pressure of surrounding cells to the form of truncated hexagonal pyramids, as in the acini or tubules of glands.

pyramidal facial fracture. A fracture of the face in which the upper jaw is completely separated from the rest of the skull. The break extends upward through each maxillary sinus to the ethmoid region and the base of the nose, assuming a pyramidal shape with the base upward.

py·ra·mi·da·lis (pi·ram″i·day′lis) *n.* 1. A small inconstant muscle enclosed in the sheath of the rectus abdominis, arising from the pubic crest, and inserted into the linea alba. NA *musculus pyramidalis.* See also Table of Muscles in the Appendix. 2. TRIQUETRUM.

pyramidalis na·si (nay′zye). PROCERUS.

pyramidal lobe. An inconstant portion of the thyroid gland extending upward from the isthmus; it arises from the persisting caudal end of the thyroglossal duct. NA *lobus pyramidalis.* See also Plate 15.

pyramidal process of the palatine bone. A backward and lateral projection from the junction of the vertical and horizontal parts of the palatine bone. NA *processus pyramidalis ossis palatini.*

pyramidal system. The corticospinal and corticobulbar tracts, subserving voluntary motor control.

pyramidal tract. All those fibers which course longitudinally in the pyramid of the medulla oblongata. NA *tractus pyramidales.*

pyramidal tuberosity. PYRAMIDAL PROCESS OF THE PALATINE BONE.

pyramides. Plural of *pyramis* (= PYRAMID).

pyramides re·na·les (re·nay′leez) [NA]. RENAL PYRAMIDS.

pyramid of the cerebellum. PYRAMID OF THE VERMIS.

pyramid of the stapedius muscle. PYRAMIDAL EMINENCE.

pyramid of the tympanum. PYRAMIDAL EMINENCE.

pyramid of the vermis. A subdivision of the cerebellar vermis between the uvula and the tuber. NA *pyramis vermis.*

pyramid of the vestibule. The anterior end of the vestibular crest of the osseous labyrinth. NA *pyramis vestibuli.*

pyr·a·mi·dot·o·my (pirr″a·mi·dot′uh·mee) *n.* [*pyramid* + *-tomy*]. Sectioning of the pyramidal tract in the medulla.

pyr·a·min (pirr′a·min) *n.* 2-Methyl-4-amino-5-hydroxymethylpyrimidine; a hydrolytic cleavage product of thiamine excreted in the urine and also obtained in the presence of the enzyme thiaminase.

py·ra·mis (pirr′uh·mis) *n.*, pl. **py·ra·mi·des** (pi·ram′i·deez) [L., from Gk.]. PYRAMID.

pyramis me·dul·lae ob·lon·ga·tae (me·dul′ee ob·long·gay′tee) [NA]. PYRAMID (2).

pyramis ver·mis (vur′mis) [NA]. PYRAMID OF THE VERMIS.

pyramis ves·ti·bu·li (ves·tib′yoo·lye) [NA]. PYRAMID OF THE VESTIBULE.

py·ran (pye′ran) *n.* The six-membered heterocyclic compound C_5H_6O, of which three isomers are possible. Certain natural compounds are often characterized as derivatives of a pyran, and the pyranose form of certain sugars indicates structural relationship of the latter to a pyran.

py·ra·nis·a·mine (pye″ruh·nis′uh·meen) *n.* *Obsol.* PYRILAMINE.

py·ra·nose (pye′ruh·noce) *n.* The isomeric form of certain sugars and glycosides having a structural analogy to a pyran. See also *furanose.*

py·ran·tel (pye·ran′tel, pye′ran·tel) *n.* 1,4,5,6-Tetrahydro-1-methyl-2-[*trans*-2-(2-thienyl)vinyl]pyrimidine, $C_{11}H_{14}N_2S$, an anthelmintic; used as the tartrate salt.

pyr·a·zin·amide (pirr″uh·zin′uh·mide) *n.* Pyrazinecarboxamide, $C_5H_5N_3O$, a tuberculostatic drug.

pyr·a·zine (pirr′uh·zeen) *n.* 1. The 1,4-isomer of diazine, $C_4H_4N_2$, in which the nitrogen atoms are separated by two carbon atoms; a white, crystalline substance, freely soluble in water. 2. Any derivative of (1).

pyr·azo·fu·rin (pirr·az″o·fyoor′in) *n.* 4-Hydroxy-3-(β-D-ribofuranosyl) pyrazole-5-carboxamide, $C_9H_{13}N_3O_6$, an antineoplastic.

pyr·azole (pirr′uh·zole, ·zol) *n.* $\overline{CH{=}CHNHN{=}CH}$; a heterocyclic compound, isomeric with imidazole, being the ultimate parent compound of certain therapeutically useful analgesic drugs. See also *pyrazolone.*

py·raz·o·lone (pi·raz′uh·lone) *n.* $C_3H_6N_2O$; one of three isomeric derivatives of pyrazole, differentiated as 3-pyrazolone, 4-pyrazolone, and 5-pyrazolone. They differ from pyrazole in containing two additional hydrogen atoms and a keto group.

py·rec·tic (pye·reck′tick) *adj.* [Gk. *pyrektikos,* feverish]. PYRETIC.

py·rene (pye′reen) *n.* A tetracyclic hydrocarbon, $C_{16}H_{10}$, in coal tar, occurring in colorless crystals, insoluble in water.

py·re·nin (pye′re·nin, pye·ree′nin) *n.* [Gk. *pyrēn,* stone of a fruit, + *-in*]. The substance of the plasmosome.

pyret-, pyreto- [Gk. *pyretos,* from *pyr,* fire]. A combining form meaning *fever.*

py·re·thrum (pye·reeth′rum) *n.* [Gk. *pyrethron*]. 1. Pellitory, the root of *Anacyclus pyrethrum;* formerly used as ptyalagogue. 2. Pyrethrum flowers, the flower heads of certain species of *Chrysanthemum;* used as an insecticide.

py·ret·ic (pye·ret'ick) *adj.* [Gk. *pyretikos,* from *pyretos,* fever]. Pertaining to or affected with fever.

pyreto-. See *pyret-.*

py·reto·gen (pye·ret'o·jin) *n.* [*pyreto-* + *-gen*]. PYROGEN.

pyr·e·to·ge·ne·sia (pirr''e·to·je·nee'zee·uh, ·see·uh, pye''re·) *n.* PYRETOGENESIS.

pyr·e·to·gen·e·sis (pirr''e·to·jen'e·sis, pye''re·to·) *n.* [*pyreto-* + *-genesis*]. The origin and causation of fever.

pyr·e·to·ge·net·ic (pirr''e·to·je·net'ick, pye''re·) *adj.* [*pyreto-* + *genetic*]. PYRETOGENIC.

pyr·e·to·gen·ic (pirr''e·to·jen'ick, pye''re·to·) *adj.* [*pyreto-* + *-genic*]. 1. Causing or producing fever. 2. Resulting from fever.

pyr·e·tog·e·nous (pirr''e·toj'e·nus, pye''re·) *adj.* PYRETOGENIC.

pyr·e·tol·o·gist (pirr''e·tol'uh·jist, pye''re·) *n.* A specialist in fevers.

pyr·e·tol·o·gy (pirr''e·tol'uh·jee, pye''re·) *n.* [*pyreto-* + *-logy*]. The science of the nature of fevers.

pyr·e·tol·y·sis (pirr''e·tol'i·sis) *n.* [*pyreto-* + *-lysis*]. 1. Reduction of a fever. 2. A lytic process accelerated by the presence of fever.

pyr·e·to·ther·a·py (pirr''e·to·therr'uh·pee, pye''re·to·) *n.* [*pyreto-* + *therapy*]. 1. Treatment of disease by the induction of fever in the patient. 2. Treatment of fever.

pyr·e·to·ty·pho·sis (pirr''e·to·tye·fo'sis, pye''re·to·) *n.* [*pyreto-* + Gk. *typhos,* delusion, + *-osis*]. The delirium of fever.

py·rex·ia (pye·reck'see·uh) *n.* [noun from Gk. *pyressein,* to be feverish]. Elevation of temperature above the normal; fever. —**pyrex·ial** (·see·ul) *adj.*

py·rex·io·pho·bia (pye·reck''see·o·fo'bee·uh) *n.* [*pyrexia* + *-phobia*]. An abnormal fear of fever.

pyr·go·ceph·a·ly (pur''go·sef'uh·lee) *n.* [Gk. *pyrgos,* tower, + *-cephaly*]. OXYCEPHALY. —**pyrgo·ce·phal·ic** (·se·fal'ick), **pyr·go·ceph·a·lous** (·sef'uh·lus) *adj.*

pyr·he·li·om·e·ter (pyre''hee·lee·om'e·tur) *n.* [*pyr-* + *helio-* + *-meter*]. An instrument for measuring the total intensity of solar radiation.

Pyribenzamine. Trademark for the antihistaminic drug tripelennamine, used as the citrate and hydrochloride salts.

py·rid·a·zine (pye·rid'uh·zeen, pi·) *n.* 1. The 1,2,-isomer of diazine, $C_4H_4N_2$, a liquid in which the two nitrogen atoms are adjacent to each other. 2. Any derivative of (1).

pyr·i·dine (pirr'i·deen, ·din) *n.* A heterocyclic compound, C_5H_5N, first of a series of homologous bases; a colorless liquid with a persistent odor. Used as a solvent and in synthesis; has been used as an antiseptic and germicide.

Pyridium. A trademark for phenazopyridine, a urinary analgesic drug that is used as the hydrochloride salt.

pyr·i·do·stig·mine bromide (pirr''i·do·stig'meen). 3-Hydroxy-1-methylpyridinium bromide dimethylcarbamate, $C_9H_{13}BrN_2O_2$, a cholinesterase inhibitor used in the treatment of myasthenia gravis.

pyr·i·dox·al (pirr''i·dock'sal) *n.* The 4-aldehyde of pyridoxine, an essential component of enzymes concerned with amino acid decarboxylation and with transamination, and therefore with amino acid synthesis.

pyridoxal phosphate. CODECARBOXYLASE.

pyr·i·dox·a·mine (pirr''i·dock'suh·meen) *n.* The amine of pyridoxine in which NH_2 replaces the OH group in position 4; obtained in transamination of pyridoxal.

pyr·i·dox·ic acid (pirr''i·dock'sick). 2-Methyl-3-hydroxy-4-carboxy-5-hydroxymethyl pyridine, a decomposition product occurring in urine following ingestion of pyridoxine by man.

pyr·i·dox·ine (pirr''i·dock'seen, ·sin) *n.* 5-Hydroxy-6-methyl-3,4-pyridinedimethanol, $C_8H_{11}NO_3$; vitamin B_6. Essential in human nutrition, and used for treatment of a variety of conditions, such as vomiting and nausea of pregnancy, or pyridoxine deficiency; employed as the hydrochloride salt.

pyridoxine deficiency. A state of abnormal nervous system activity manifested by seizures, irritability and gastrointestinal distress, and polyneuropathy; of vitamin B_6, as may occur in infants fed a modified milk formula autoclaved in a way that destroys the pyridoxine, or due to the effects of pyridoxine antagonists or compounds that chemically inactivate pyridoxal phosphate, such as the antituberculous agent isonicotinic acid hydrazide and the semicarbazides. Compare *pyridoxine dependency.*

pyridoxine dependency. An inborn error of vitamin B_6 metabolism, manifested chiefly by seizures noted in the neonatal period and even in utero, in which the tryptophan loading test is normal and there is no response to pyridoxine unless very large amounts of the vitamin are given. Compare *pyridoxine deficiency.*

pyr·i·dyl (pirr'i·dil) *n.* The monovalent radical $C_5H_4N—$, from pyridine.

pyriform. PIRIFORM.

pyriform area or **lobe.** PIRIFORM LOBE.

pyriform recess or **sinus.** PIRIFORM RECESS.

py·ril·amine (pye·ril'uh·meen, pi·) *n.* 2-{[2-(Dimethylamino)-ethyl](*p*-methoxybenzyl)amino}pyridine, $C_{17}H_{23}N_3O$, an antihistaminic drug used as the maleate salt. Syn. *mepyramine, pyranisamine.*

pyr·i·meth·a·mine (pirr''i·meth'uh·meen) *n.* 2,4-Diamino-5-(*p*-chlorophenyl)-6-ethylpyrimidine, $C_{12}H_{13}ClN_4$, an antimalarial drug.

py·rim·i·dine (pye·rim'i·deen, pi·) *n.* 1. Any six-membered cyclic compound containing four carbon and two nitrogen atoms in the ring, the nitrogen atoms being separated by one carbon atom. To this group belong barbituric acid and its derivatives, the nucleic acid hydrolysis products thymine, uracil, and cytosine, and many other compounds of physiologic or therapeutic importance. 2. 1,3-Diazine, $C_4H_4N_2$.

pyr·in·o·line (pirr·in'o·leen) *n.* 3-(Di-2-pyridylmethylene)-α,α-di-2-pyridyl-1,4-cyclopentadiene-1-methanol, $C_{27}H_{20}N_4O$, an antiarrhythmic cardiac depressant.

pyr·i·thi·a·mine (pirr''i·thigh'uh·min) *n.* A structural analogue and antimetabolite of thiamine, in which the thiazole ring is replaced by pyridine, that can cause thiamine deficiency in animals.

pyro-. See *pyr-.*

py·ro·cat·e·chase (pye''ro·kat'e·kace) *n.* An enzyme catalyzing oxidative breakdown of pyrocatechol.

py·ro·cat·e·chin (pye''ro·kat'e·chin, ·kin) *n.* PYROCATECHOL.

py·ro·cat·e·chin·uria (pye''ro·kat''e·chi·new'ree·uh) *n.* [*pyrocatechin* + *-uria*]. The presence of pyrocatechol in the urine.

py·ro·cat·e·chol (pye''ro·kat'e·chole, ·kole, ·kol) *n.* *o*-Dihydroxybenzene, $C_6H_4(OH)_2$; has been used topically as an antiseptic. Syn. *pyrocatechin, catechol, oxyphenic acid.*

py·ro·gal·lic acid (pye''ro·gal'ick). PYROGALLOL.

py·ro·gal·lol (pye''ro·gal'ole, ·ol) *n.* 1,2,3-Trihydroxybenzene, $C_6H_3(OH)_3$; has been used topically in the treatment of various skin diseases, especially psoriasis. Syn. *pyrogallic acid.*

py·ro·gen (pye'ro·jen) *n.* [*pyro-* + *-gen*]. Any fever-producing substance; exogenous pyrogens include bacterial endotoxins, especially of gram-negative bacteria; endogenous pyrogen is a thermolabile protein derived from such cells as polymorphonuclear leukocytes which acts on the brain centers to produce fever.

py·ro·gen·ic (pye''ro·jen'ick) *adj.* [*pyro-* + *-genic*]. Producing fever.

py·ro·glob·u·lin (pye''ro·glob'yoo·lin) *n.* [*pyro-* + *globulin*]. A globulin, abnormally present in blood serum, which coagulates on heating.

py·ro·glob·u·lin·emia, py·ro·glob·u·lin·ae·mia (pye''ro·glob''yoo·li·nee'mee·uh) *n.* [*pyroglobulin* + *-emia*]. The abnormal condition in which blood serum contains heat-coagulable globulin (pyroglobulin).

py·ro·glos·sia (pye″ro·glos′ee·uh) *n.* [*pyro-* + *-glossia*]. A burning sensation of the tongue.

py·ro·lag·nia (pye″ro·lag′nee·uh) *n.* [*pyro-* + Gk. *lagneia*, lust]. Sexual gratification attained by the sight of fires; sexual excitement accompanying pyromania.

py·ro·lig·ne·ous (pye″ro·lig′nee·us) *adj.* [*pyro-* + *ligneous*]. Pertaining to the destructive distillation of wood.

py·rol·y·sis (pye·rol′i·sis) *n.* [*pyro-* + *-lysis*]. The decomposition of organic substances by heat. —**py·ro·lyt·ic** (pye″ro·lit′ick) *adj.*

py·ro·ma·nia (pye″ro·may′nee·uh) *n.* [*pyro-* + *mania*]. A monomania for setting or watching fires. —**pyroma·ni·ac** (·nee·ack) *n.*

py·rom·e·ter (pye·rom′i·tur) *n.* [*pyro-* + *-meter*]. An instrument for measuring high temperatures.

py·ro·mu·cic acid (pye″ro·mew′sick). FUROIC ACID.

py·rone (pye′rone) *n.* Any derivative of two of the three possible pyrans in which one or, less frequently, two oxygen atoms are attached to the same number of carbon atoms in the ring; also, certain derivatives of such pyrones, some of which are of medicinal importance.

Pyronil. Trademark for the antihistaminic drug pyrrobutamine, used as the diphosphate salt.

py·ro·nin (pye′ro·nin) *n.* PYRONINE.

py·ro·nine (pye′ro·neen, ·nin) *n.* A histologic stain, tetraethyldiaminoxanthene, used to indicate the presence of ribonucleic acid.

pyronine B. A purplish-red, water and alcohol soluble basic dye, tetraethyldiaminoxanthene chloride, which is used as a stain for nuclei and bacteria, as a basophil cytoplasm stain in the methyl green pyronine technique, and in the alphanaphthol pyronine peroxidase reaction for blood leukocytes.

pyronine G or **Y.** A red, partially water and alcohol soluble basic xanthene dye, tetramethyldiaminoxanthene chloride, which is used as a stain for ribonucleic acid in the methyl green pyronine technique, as counterstain for gram-negative organisms, and in the α-naphthol pyronine leukocyte peroxidase method.

py·ro·nino·phil·ic (pye″ro·nin″o·fil′ick) *adj.* [*pyronine* + *-philic*]. Having an affinity for pyronine.

py·ro·pho·bia (pye″ro·fo′bee·uh) *n.* [*pyro-* + *-phobia*]. An abnormal dread of fire.

py·ro·phos·pha·tase (pye″ro·fos′fuh·tace, ·taze) *n.* An enzyme catalyzing hydrolysis of esters containing two or more molecules of phosphoric acid to form a simpler phosphate ester.

py·ro·phos·phate (pye″ro·fos′fate) *n.* A salt of pyrophosphoric acid.

py·ro·phos·pho·ric acid (pye″ro·fos·fo′rick). $H_4P_2O_7$. A crystalline acid, certain salts of which, notably iron, have been used medicinally.

py·rop·to·thy·mia (pye·rop″to·thigh′mee·uh) *n.* [*pyro-* + Gk. *ptoein*, to frighten, + *-thymia*]. A form of mental disorder in which the person imagines himself enveloped in flame.

py·ro·punc·ture (pye′ro·punk″chur) *n.* [*pyro-* + *puncture*]. Puncturing with hot needles; ignipuncture.

py·ro·ra·ce·mic acid (pye″ro·ra·see′mick). PYRUVIC ACID.

py·ro·scope (pye′ro·scope) *n.* [*pyro-* + *-scope*]. An instrument used for measuring high temperatures.

py·ro·sis (pye·ro′sis) *n.* [Gk. *pyrōsis*, firing]. A substernal or epigastric burning sensation accompanied by eructation of an acrid, irritating fluid; heartburn.

py·ro·sul·fite (pye″ro·sul′fite) *n.* METABISULFITE.

py·rot·ic (pye·rot′ick) *adj.* [Gk. *pyrōtikos*, heating]. 1. Pertaining to pyrosis. 2. Caustic, burning.

py·ro·tox·in (pye″ro·tock′sin) *n.* [*pyro-* + *toxin*]. A toxic agent generated in the course of the febrile process.

py·ro·val·er·one (pye″ro·va·lerr′ohn, ·val′ur·ohn) *n.* 4′-Methyl-2-(1-pyrrolidinyl)valerophenone, $C_{16}H_{23}NO$, a central stimulant drug; used as the hydrochloride salt.

py·rox·a·mine (pye·rock′suh·meen) *n.* 3-[(*p*-Chloro-α-phenylbenzyl)oxy]-1-methylpyrrolidine, $C_{18}H_{20}ClNO$, an antihistaminic drug; used as the maleate salt.

py·rox·y·lin (pye·rock′si·lin) *n.* A product obtained by the action of a mixture of nitric and sulfuric acids on cotton; consists chiefly of cellulose tetranitrate ($C_{12}H_{16}O_6(NO_3)_4$); used as a protective covering in the form of collodion. Syn. *soluble guncotton.*

pyr·rhol cell (pirr′ole). A mononuclear cell found in exudates, which stains supravitally with a dye called pyrrhol blue.

pyr·ro·bu·ta·mine (pirr″o·bew′tuh·meen) *n.* 1-[4-(*p*-Chlorophenyl)-3-phenyl-2-butenyl]pyrrolidine, $C_{20}H_{22}ClN$, an antihistaminic drug used as the diphosphate salt.

pyr·ro·caine (pirr′o·kane) *n.* 1-Pyrrolidineaceto-2′,6′-xylidide, $C_{14}H_{20}N_2O$, a local anesthetic.

pyr·role (pirr′ole) *n.* $\overline{NHCH{=}CHCH{=}CH}$. A colorless liquid occurring in bone oil and to a slight extent in coal tar. Many complex natural compounds, such as hemoglobin and chlorophyll, contain pyrrole components in their structure. See also *porphin, porphyrin.*

pyr·rol·i·done (pirr·ol′i·dohn) *n.* POLYVINYLPYRROLIDONE.

pyr·rol·i·phene (pirr·ol′i·feen) *n.* (+)-α-Benzyl-β-methyl-α-phenyl-1-pyrrolidinepropanol acetate, $C_{23}H_{29}NO_2$, an analgesic; used as the hydrochloride salt.

pyr·rol·ni·trin (pirr″ole·nigh′trin) *n.* 3-Chloro-4-(3-chloro-2-nitrophenyl)pyrrole, $C_{10}H_6Cl_2N_2O_2$, a compound with antifungal activity.

pyr·ro·lo·por·phyr·ia (pirr″uh·lo·por·firr′ee·uh) *n.* ACUTE INTERMITTENT PORPHYRIA.

py·ru·vate (pye·roo′vate, pi·) *n.* A salt or ester of pyruvic acid.

pyruvate-kinase deficiency. Congenital erythrocytic deficiency of the enzyme catalyzing the conversion of phosphoenolpyruvate to pyruvate, associated with hemolytic anemia.

py·ru·vic acid (pye·roo′vick, pi·) [*pyr-* + L. *uva*, grapes, + *-ic*]. 2-Oxopropanoic acid, $CH_3COCOOH$, which is a normal intermediate in carbohydrate and protein metabolism. Excess quantities of pyruvic acid accumulate in blood and tissues in thiamine deficiency. Syn. *ketopropionic acid.*

pyr·vin·i·um pam·o·ate (pirr·vin′ee·um pam′o·ate). 6-Dimethylamino-2-[2-(2,5-dimethyl-1-phenyl-3-pyrrolyl)vinyl]-1-methylquinolinium 4,4′-methylenebis[3-hydroxy-2-naphthoate], $C_{75}H_{70}N_6O_6$, a cyanine dye used as an anthelmintic in the treatment of pinworm infections.

py·uria (pye·yoor′ee·uh) *n.* [*py-* + *-uria*]. The presence of pus in the urine. —**py·uric** (·yoor′ick) adj.

Q

Q_{CO_2} Symbol for the rate of evolution of carbon dioxide, in microliters given off in 1 hour by 1 mg (dry weight) of tissue.

Q_{O_2} Symbol for the oxygen consumption in terms of the number of microliters consumed in 1 hour by 1 mg (dry weight) of tissue; by convention, the consumption of oxygen is given a negative value.

Q disk [Ger. *Querscheibe,* from *quer,* transverse, + *Scheibe,* disk]. A DISK.

q.d.s. Abbreviation for *quater die sumendum,* to be taken four times a day (= q.i.d.).

q electron. An electron in the q or seventh shell surrounding the nucleus of an atom.

Q fever [*q*uery]. An acute infectious disease caused by the filtrable microorganism *Coxiella burnetii,* acquired by inhalation, handling infected material, or drinking contaminated milk; characterized by sudden onset of fever, malaise, headache, and interstitial pneumonitis, but lacking the rash and the agglutinins for *Proteus* bacteria occurring in other rickettsial diseases.

q.h. Abbreviation for *quaque hora;* every hour.

q.2h. Abbreviation for *quaque secunda hora;* every second hour.

q.3h. Abbreviation for *quaque tertia hora;* every third hour.

q.i.d. Abbreviation for *quater in die;* 4 times a day.

q.l. Abbreviation for *quantum libet;* as much as is desired.

q.p. Abbreviation for *quantum placet;* as much as you please.

QRS Q wave, R wave, and S wave.

QRS axis. ELECTRICAL AXIS.

QRS complex of the electrocardiogram. The electrocardiographic deflection representing ventricular depolarization. The initial downward deflection is termed a Q wave; the initial upward deflection, an R wave; and the downward deflection following the R wave, an S wave. Syn. *ventricular depolarization complex.*

QRS interval. The duration of depolarization or excitation of the ventricles, measured from the beginning of Q (or R) wave to the end of S wave of the electrocardiogram; usually 0.10 second or less.

QRS loop. The vectorcardiographic representation of ventricular depolarization.

QRS-T angle. The spatial angle between the mean QRS and T vector axes.

q.s. Abbreviation for *quantum sufficit;* as much as suffices.

Q-S interval. QRS INTERVAL.

QS wave of the electrocardiogram. A totally downward electrocardiographic deflection of ventricular depolarization without an upward R wave.

Q-T interval. The time from the beginning of the QRS complex to the end of the T wave, representing the time from the beginning of ventricular depolarization to the end of repolarization, i.e., ventricular systole.

qt. Abbreviation for *quart.*

Quaalude. Trademark for the nonbarbiturate sedative and hypnotic, methaqualone.

quack, *n.* [short for *quacksalver*]. A pretender to medical skill; a medical charlatan.

quack·ery (kwack'uh·ree) *n.* The practice of medicine by a quack.

quack medicine. A medicine falsely advertised to the laity as being able to cure certain diseases.

quack·sal·ver (kwack'sal·vur) *n.* [D. *kwakzalver*]. A quack or mountebank; a peddler of his own medicines and salves.

qua·dran·gu·lar (kwah·drang'gew·lur) *adj.* [L. *quadrangularis,* from *quadrangulum,* quadrangle]. Having four angles.

quadrangular bandage. A towel or large handkerchief, folded variously and used as a bandage.

quadrangular lobule. The greater portion of the superior surface of each cerebellar hemisphere. NA *lobulus quadrangularis.*

quadrangular membrane. The membrane of the larynx which extends from the aryepiglottic folds above to the level of the vestibular folds below. NA *membrana quadrangularis.*

quadrangular space. The lateral division of the triangular space of the shoulder which contains the axillary nerve and the posterior humeral circumflex artery.

quad·rant (kwah'drunt) *n.* [L. *quadrans,* a fourth part]. 1. The fourth part of a circle, subtending an angle of 90°. 2. One of the four regions into which the abdomen may be divided for purposes of physical diagnosis. 3. A sector of one-fourth of the field of vision of one or both eyes. —**qua·dran·tic** (kwah·dran'tick) *adj.*

quad·ran·ta·no·pia (kwah"dran·tuh·no'pee·uh) *n.* [*quadrant* + *anopia*]. Loss of vision in about one-quarter of the visual field; may be bitemporal or homonymous, upper or lower.

quad·ran·ta·nop·sia (kwah"dran·tuh·nop'see·uh) *n.* [*quadrant* + *anopsia*]. QUADRANTANOPIA.

quadrantic hemianopsia. QUADRANTANOPIA.

quad·rate (kwah'drate) *adj.* [L. *quadratus,* from *quadrare,* to make square]. Square, four-sided.

quadrate cartilages. Several small cartilages extending from the lesser alar cartilages in the external nose.

quadrate foramen. FORAMEN VENAE CAVAE.

quadrate ligament. A thickened band extending from the neck of the radius to the inferior border of the annular ligament below the radial notch. NA *ligamentum quadratum.*

quadrate line. A slight ridge extending downward from the middle of the intertrochanteric crest and giving attachment to the quadratus femoris muscle.

quadrate lobe. An oblong lobe on the inferior surface of the liver. NA *lobus quadratus.* See also Plate 13.

quadrate lobule. PRECUNEUS.

quadrate tubercle. A small elevation on the intertrochanteric line of the femur marking the attachment of the quadratus femoris muscle.

qua·dra·tus (kwah·dray'tus) *L. adj. & n.,* pl. & genit. sing. **quadra·ti** (·tye) 1. Square. 2. A muscle having four sides.

quadratus fe·mo·ris (fem'o·ris). A deep muscle of the posterior part of the thigh attached to the ischial tuber and femur. NA *musculus quadratus femoris.* See also Table of Muscles in the Appendix.

quadratus la·bii in·fe·ri·o·ris (lay'bee·eye in·feer''ee·o'ris). DEPRESSOR LABII INFERIORIS.

quadratus labii su·pe·ri·o·ris (sue·peer''ee·o'ris). LEVATOR LABII SUPERIORIS.

quadratus lum·bo·rum (lum·bo'rum). A muscle of the back attached to the iliac crest and the twelfth rib. NA *musculus quadratus lumborum.* See also Table of Muscles in the Appendix.

quadratus men·ti (men'tye). DEPRESSOR LABII INFERIORIS.

quadratus plan·tae (plan'tee). A muscle of the foot which aids in the flexion of the toes. NA *musculus quadratus plantae.* See also Table of Muscles in the Appendix.

quadri-, quadru- [L.]. A combining form meaning *four.*

quad·ri·ceps (kwah'dri·seps) *adj.* [NL., from *quadri-* + *-ceps,* from L. *caput,* head]. Four-headed.

quadriceps fe·mo·ris (fem'o·ris). The large extensor muscle of the thigh. NA *musculus quadriceps femoris.* See also Table of Muscles in the Appendix.

quadriceps reflex. PATELLAR REFLEX.

quadriceps su·rae (sue'ree). *Obsol.* The muscle mass comprising the gastrocnemius, soleus, and plantaris.

quad·ri·cus·pid (kwah''dri·kus'pid) *adj.* [*quadri-* + L. *cuspis, cuspidis,* point]. Having four cusps.

qua·dri·ge·mi·na (kwah''dri·jem'i·nuh) *n.pl.* CORPORA QUADRIGEMINA.

quad·ri·gem·i·nal (kwah''dri·jem'i·nul) *adj.* [L. *quadrigeminus,* from *quadri-* + *geminus,* twin]. Fourfold; consisting of four parts.

quadrigeminal pulse. A pulse in which a pause occurs after every fourth beat.

quad·ri·lat·e·ral (kwah''dri·lat'ur·ul) *adj.* [L. *quadrilaterus,* from *quadri-* + *latus, lateris,* side]. Having four sides.

quadrilateral space. 1. The anterior and posterior triangles of the neck taken together. 2. The deep fascial space of the wrist beneath the flexor retinaculum and flexor tendons, above the pronator quadratus muscle.

qua·drip·a·ra (kwah·drip'uh·ruh) *n.* [*quadri-* + *-para*]. A woman who has given birth for the fourth time. —**quadripa·rous** (·rus) *adj.*

quad·ri·pa·re·sis (kwah''dri·puh·ree'sis, ·păr'uh·sis) *n.* [*quadri-* + *paresis*]. Weakness of all four limbs.

quad·ri·par·i·ty (kwah''dri·păr'i·tee) *n.* [*quadri-* + *parity,* from *-para*]. The state of having given birth four times.

quad·ri·ple·gia (kwah''dri·plee'jee·uh) *n.* [*quadri-* + *-plegia*]. Paralysis affecting the four extremities of the body; may be spastic or flaccid. —**quadriple·gic,** *adj. & n.*

quad·ri·tu·ber·cu·lar (kwah''dri·tew·bur'kew·lur) *adj.* [*quadri-* + *tubercular*]. Having four tubercles or cusps.

quad·ri·urate (kwah''dri·yoo'rate) *n.* A mixture of a urate with uric acid obtained from urine or blood, formerly believed to be a compound.

quad·ri·va·lent (kwah''dri·vay'lunt) *adj.* [*quadri-* + *valent*]. TETRAVALENT. —**quadriva·lence** (·lunce) *n.*

qua·droon (kwah·droon') *n.* [Sp. *cuarterón,* from *cuarto,* fourth]. The offspring of a white person and a mulatto.

quadru-. See *quadri-.*

quad·ru·ped (kwah'droo·ped) *n.* [*quadrupes, quadrupedis,* from *pes,* foot]. A four-footed animal. —**qua·dru·pe·dal** (kwah·droo'pe·dul, kwah''droo·ped'ul) *adj.*

quadrupedal extensor reflex. An associated movement of extension of the flexed arm in hemiplegia which is sometimes evoked by causing the patient, when standing or kneeling, to lean forward and throw his weight on to the observer's supporting hand placed beneath his chest.

quad·ru·ple rhythm (kwah'druh·pul, kwah·droo'pul). A cardiac cadence in which four sounds recur in each successive cycle.

quad·ru·plet (kwah'druh·plut, kwah·droo'plut) *n.* [L. *quadruplus,* fourfold, + *-et* as in triplet]. Any one of four children born at one birth.

Quain's fatty degeneration [R. *Quain,* English physician, 1816–1898]. Fatty degeneration of the heart.

qua·ker buttons. NUX VOMICA.

qual·i·ta·tive (kwahl'i·tay''tiv) *adj.* Of or pertaining to quality; limited to or concerned with kind as opposed to degree.

qualitative analysis. The detection or identification of the elements or constituents that compose a substance, without regard to their amounts or proportions. Contr. *quantitative analysis.*

qualitative vision. Vision in which there is ability to distinguish objects. Contr. *quantitative vision.*

qual·i·ty, *n.* [L. *qualitas*]. 1. A distinguishing or identifying characteristic. 2. The value of a variable characteristic as, in radiobiology, the approximate characterization of radiation with respect to its penetrating power.

quanta. Plural of *quantum.*

quan·tal summation (kwahn'tul). Excitatory effects produced by the quantity or number of impulses reaching specific structures per unit time. See also *spatial summation, temporal summation.*

quan·tim·e·ter (kwahn·tim'e·tur) *n.* [*quantity* + *-meter*]. An instrument for measuring the quantity of x-rays. See also *dosimeter.*

quan·ti·ta·tive (kwahn'ti·tay''tiv) *adj.* Of or pertaining to quantity; limited to or concerned with degree as opposed to kind.

quantitative analysis. Determination of the amount of an element or constituent in a substance. Contr. *qualitative analysis.*

quantitative vision. Mere perception of light. Contr. *qualitative vision.*

quan·ti·ty, *n.* [L. *quantitas,* from L. *quantus,* how much, how large]. Something measurable or capable of being numerically characterized; amount or degree.

quan·tum (kwahn'tum) *n.,* pl. **quan·ta** (·tuh) [L., how much, as much as]. An elementary, particulate unit of energy. See also *quantum theory.*

quantum constant. PLANCK'S CONSTANT.

quantum lib·et (lib'it) [L.]. As much as is desired. Abbreviated, q.l.

quantum plac·et (plas'it) [L.]. As much as you please. Abbreviated, q.p.

quantum suf·fi·cit (suf'i·sit) [L.]. As much as suffices. Abbreviated, q.s.

quantum theory. A theory, introduced as a hypothesis by Max Planck, that emission and absorption of energy can take place only in discrete units called quanta (singular, quantum), in accordance with the equation $\varepsilon = h\upsilon$, where ε is the magnitude of the quantum of energy, υ is the frequency of the radiation, and h is Planck's constant, which has the value 6.624×10^{-27} erg second.

quantum theory of color vision. The theory of color vision stating that a retinal cone, when stimulated by light, possesses the power of transmitting along its nerve fibers impulses of different kinds, depending upon the quantum number or wavelength of the light; that is, light from the violet end of the spectrum would evoke nerve impulses different from those generated by rays from the red end of the spectrum.

quantum vis [L.]. As much as you wish. Abbreviated, q.v.

quar·an·tine (kwahr'un·teen) *n.* [It. *quarantina,* from L. *quadraginta,* forty]. 1. The limitation of freedom of movement of such susceptible persons or animals as have been exposed to communicable disease, for a period of time (formerly usually 40 days) equal to the longest usual incubation period of the disease to which they have been exposed. 2. The place of detention of such persons. 3. The act of detaining vessels or travelers from suspected ports or places for purposes of inspection or disinfection.

quark, *n.* [from "three quarks for Muster Mark," in James Joyce's *Finnigans Wake*]. *In nuclear physics,* a hypothetical triplet-form of elementary particle, postulated to have a fractional charge of one-third or two-thirds and believed to be capable of forming stable composite particles with nucleons.

quart, *n.* [L. *quartus,* fourth]. In the United States, the fourth part of a gallon; 0.9463 liter. Abbreviated, qt. See also *imperial quart.*

quar·tan (kwor'tun, kwahr'tun) *adj.* [L. *quartanus,* of the fourth]. 1. Recurring at about 72-hour intervals, on the fourth day. 2. Pertaining to quartan malaria.

quartan malaria or **fever.** A form of malaria caused by *Plasmodium malariae,* characterized by paroxysms occurring every 72 hours, that is, on the first, fourth, and seventh days.

quartan malarial nephropathy. MALARIAL NEPHROPATHY.

quar·ter, *n.* [L. *quartarius,* fourth part]. 1. The part of the horse's hoof between the heel and the toe. 2. The fourth part of a slaughtered animal.

quarter crack. A fissuring of the inner or outer aspect of the wall of the hoof in the horse.

quarter evil. BLACKLEG.

quar·tip·a·ra (kwor·tip'uh·ruh, kwahr·) *n.* [L. *quartus,* fourth, + *-para*]. QUADRIPARA. —**quartipa·rous** (·rus) *adj.*

quartz, *n.* [Ger. *Quarz*]. A crystalline silicon dioxide, SiO_2; when pure, in colorless hexagonal crystals. Used in chemical apparatus and for optical and electric instruments.

quartz light. A cold quartz lamp with quartz lens; used for bactericidal therapy.

quartz objective. An objective with quartz lenses for use in fluorescence microscopy and photography with far ultraviolet.

Quarzan Bromide. Trademark for clidinium bromide, an anticholinergic drug.

quas·sia (kwahsh'ee·uh, kwahsh'uh) *n.* [NL., after *Quassi,* a Surinam inhabitant who first used it about 1730]. The wood of *Picrasma excelsa,* known as Jamaica quassia, or of *Quassia amara,* known as Surinam quassia. Has been used as a simple bitter and, in the form of an infusion given as an enema, for expulsion of seatworms.

qua·ter·na·ry (kwah·tur'nuh·ree, kwah'tur·nerr"ee) *adj.* [L. *quaternarius,* consisting of four each]. 1. Consisting of four elements or substances, as quaternary solutions. 2. Fourth in order or stage. 3. Characterizing or pertaining to compounds in which four similar atoms of a radical, as the hydrogen atoms in the ammonium radical, have been replaced by organic radicals.

quaternary ammonium compound. Any compound that may be considered a derivative of an ammonium ion in which the four hydrogen atoms have been replaced by organic radicals; many medicinals are compounds of this kind.

quaternary structure. The arrangement of and linkages between polypeptide chains in any protein molecule containing more than one such chain. Contr. *primary, secondary,* and *tertiary structure.*

quat·tu·or (kwat'oo·or) *n.* [L.]. Four.

quaz·e·pam (kwaz'e·pam) *n.* 7-Chloro-5-(*o*-fluorophenyl)-1,3-dihydro-1-(2,2,2-trifluoroethyl)-2*H*-1,4-benzodiazepin-2-thione, $C_{17}H_{11}ClF_4N_2S$, a sedative-hypnotic.

qua·zo·dine (kway'zo·deen) *n.* 4-Ethyl-6,7-dimethoxyquinazoline, $C_{12}H_{14}N_2O_2$, a cardiac stimulant, pulmonary vasodilator, and bronchodilator.

que·bra·bun·da (kee"bruh·bun'duh, kay"brah·boon'dah) *n.* A tropical disease of horses and swine simulating beriberi of humans.

que·bra·chine (ke·brah'cheen) *n.* [*quebracho* + *-ine*]. YOHIMBINE.

que·bra·cho (ke·brah'cho) *n.* [Sp., from *quebrar,* to break, + *hacha,* axe]. 1. Any one of several hard-wooded trees of South America; the white quebracho is *Aspidosperma quebracho-blanco,* of the family Apocynaceae. 2. ASPIDOSPERMA.

Queck·en·stedt test, sign or **maneuver** (kveck'ᵉn·shtet) [H. H. G. *Queckenstedt,* German neurologist, 1876–1918]. Manual compression of the internal jugular veins with a manometer attached to the lumbar puncture needle to test for the patency of the subarachnoid space. Normally, compression causes a prompt rise in the cerebrospinal fluid pressure with rapid return to resting levels on release of compression; in partial or total subarachnoid block, this does not occur. The maneuver is contraindicated where increased intracranial pressure is present or suspected.

Queens·land coastal fever [after *Queensland,* Australia]. TSUTSUGAMUSHI DISEASE.

Queensland tick typhus fever. Infection caused by *Rickettsia australis,* occurring in Queensland, Australia, transmitted by ixodid ticks with marsupial and wild rodent animal hosts; closely related to boutonneuse fever and to Rocky Mountain spotted fever.

quel·lung (kwel'ung, kvel'ung) *n.* [Ger.]. SWELLING.

quellung phenomenon or **test.** NEUFELD QUELLUNG TEST.

quellung reaction. Swelling of the capsule of a bacterium when in contact with its antigen.

Qué·nu's operation (keʸ·nuᵉ') [E. A. V. A. *Quénu,* French surgeon, 1852–1933]. A method of thoracoplasty involving division of the ribs to promote retraction, for the treatment of empyema.

que·nu·tho·ra·co·plas·ty (kwee"new·tho'ruh·ko·plas"tee) *n.* [E. A. V. A. *Quénu* + *thoracoplasty*]. QUÉNU'S OPERATION.

quer·ce·tin (kwur'se·tin) *n.* 3,3',4',5,7-Pentahydroxyflavone, $C_{15}H_{10}O_7$, the aglycone of quercitrin, rutin, and other glycosides, found especially in varous rinds and barks, but widely distributed in the plant kingdom. Has been used in the expectation of reducing capillary fragility. Syn. *flavin, meletin.*

querci- [L. *quercus,* oak]. A combining form meaning *oak.*

quer·ci·tan·nic acid (kwur"si·tan'ick). The tannic acid from oak bark.

quer·ci·tan·nin (kwur"si·tan'in) *n.* QUERCITANNIC ACID.

quer·cus (kwur'kus) *n.* [L., oak]. The dried inner bark of *Quercus alba,* the white oak.

Quervain's disease. DE QUERVAIN'S DISEASE.

que·ry fever. Q FEVER.

Questran. Trademark for cholestyramine.

Qué·venne's iron (keʸ·ven'). REDUCED IRON.

Quey·rat's erythroplasia (keʰ·rahʰ') [A. *Queyrat,* French dermatologist, b. 1872]. A condition characterized by a circumscribed, erythematous, velvety lesion affecting mucocutaneous junctions or mucosa of the mouth, tongue, vulva, glans penis, or prepuce. Considered precancerous to squamous cell carcinoma.

quick, *adj.* & *n.* [OE. *cwic,* live, alive]. 1. Manifesting life and movement, as a fetus. 2. An exquisitely tender part, as the bed of a nail.

quick·en·ing, *n.* The first feeling on the part of the pregnant woman of fetal movements, occurring between the fourth and fifth months of pregnancy.

quick·lime, *n.* CALCIUM OXIDE.

quick pulse. 1. A pulse that strikes the finger rapidly, but also leaves it rapidly. Syn. *short pulse.* 2. An abnormally rapid heart rate.

quick-section diagnosis. A rapid histologic diagnosis during a surgical operation, of a specimen removed for study, and prepared for microscopy by frozen section.

Quick's hippuric acid synthesis test [A. J. *Quick*, U.S. physician, b. 1894]. HIPPURIC ACID TEST.

quick·sil·ver, *n.* MERCURY.

Quick's test for prothrombin [A. J. *Quick*]. ONE-STAGE METHOD.

Quide. Trademark for piperacetazine, a tranquilizer.

qui·es·cent (kwye·es'unt) *adj.* [L. *quiescens*, from *quiescere*, to rest, to cease activity, from *quies, quietis*, rest]. Inactive, latent, dormant.

quiescent tuberculosis. Inactive cavitary or noncavitary tuberculosis which has negative bacteriologic findings at monthly intervals for 3 consecutive months. By radiography, the noncavitary lesions should be stable, or show some clearing or contraction; in the cavitary disease, the presence of the cavity is permitted, but this should vary only slightly in size.

quiet delirium. Delirium marked by incoherent, scarcely audible mumbling, and generally lacking the usual psychomotor overactivity.

quiet necrosis. ASEPTIC NECROSIS.

Quilene. Trademark for pentapiperium methylsulfate, an anticholinergic drug.

Quil·la·ia (kwi·lay'yuh) *n.* *QUILLAJA.*

Quil·la·ja (kwi·lay'yuh, ·juh) *n.* [NL., from Sp. *quillay*, from Araucanian]. A genus of trees of the family Rosaceae.

quillaja, *n.* The dried inner bark of *Quillaja saponaria;* contains a saponin, quillain (quillaic acid), which is very toxic. Has been used, externally, as a stimulant and detergent.

quill suture. A suture similar to a button suture except that the sutures are tied over a quill, a rubber tube, or a roll of cotton.

quin-, quino- [Sp. *quina*, cinchona]. A combining form meaning (a) *cinchona;* (b) *quinine.*

quin·a·crine (kwin'uh·kreen, ·krin). 6-Chloro-9-{[4-(diethylamino)-1-methylbutyl]amino}-2-methoxyacridine, $C_{23}H_{30}ClN_3O$, formerly an important antimalarial drug but now used in the treatment of giardiasis, tapeworm infections, amebiasis, and a variety of other conditions; employed as the hydrochloride salt. Syn. *mepacrine.*

quin·al·bar·bi·tone (kwin''al·bahr'bi·tone) *n.* British generic name for secobarbital, a barbiturate.

quin·al·dine blue (kwin·al'deen). 1-Ethyl-2-[3-(1-ethyl-2(1*H*)-quinolylidene)propenyl]quinolinium chloride, $C_{25}H_{25}ClN_2$, a stain for use in cytodiagnosis of ruptured fetal membranes.

quin·az·o·sin (kwin·az'o·sin) *n.* 2-(4-Allyl-1-piperazinyl)-4-amino-6,7-dimethoxyquinazoline, $C_{17}H_{23}N_5O_2$, an antihypertensive drug; used as the hydrochloride salt.

quin·bo·lone (kwin'bo·lone) *n.* 17β-(1-Cyclopenten-1-yloxy)-androsta-1,4-dien-3-one, $C_{24}H_{32}O_2$, an anabolic steroid.

Quincke's disease or **edema** (kvink'eʰ) [H. I. *Quincke*, German physician, 1842–1922]. ANGIOEDEMA.

Quincke's pulse [H. I. *Quincke*]. CAPILLARY PULSE.

Quincke's reaction for iron [H. I. *Quincke*]. Hemosiderin forms greenish-black iron sulfides on exposure to ammonium sulfide solution. Reduction to ferrous iron is only partial.

quin·dec·a·mine (kwin·deck'uh·meen) *n.* 4,4'-(Decamethylenediimino)diquinaldine, $C_{30}H_{38}N_4$, an antibacterial agent; used as the diacetate salt.

quin·do·ni·um bromide (kwin·do'nee·um). 2,3,3*a*,5,5,11,12,12*a*-Octahydro-8-hydroxy-1*H*-benzo[*a*]cyclopenta[*f*]quinolizinium bromide, $C_{16}H_{20}BrNO$, an antiarrhythmic cardiac depressant.

quin·es·trol (kwin·es'trol) *n.* 3-Cyclopentyloxy-17α-ethynylestra-1,3,5(10)-trien-17β-ol, $C_{25}H_{32}O_2$, an estrogenic steroid.

quin·eth·a·zone (kwin·eth'uh·zone) *n.* 7-Chloro-2-ethyl-1,2,-3,4-tetrahydro-4-oxo-6-quinazolinesulfonamide, $C_{10}H_{12}ClN_3O_3S$, an orally effective benzothiadiazine diuretic and antihypertensive drug.

quin·ges·ta·nol (kwin·jes'tuh·nol) *n.* 3-(Cyclopentyloxy)-19-nor-17α-pregna-3,5-dien-20-yn-17-ol, $C_{25}H_{34}O_2$, a progestational steroid; used as the acetate ester.

quin·ges·trone (kwin·jes'trone) *n.* 3-(Cyclopentyloxy)pregna-3,5-dien-20-one, $C_{26}H_{38}O_2$, a progestational steroid.

quin·i·dine (kwin'i·deen, ·din) *n.* An alkaloid, $C_{20}H_{24}N_2O_2$, of cinchona, isomeric with quinine; used, as the gluconate and sulfate salts, for the treatment of cardiac arrhythmias.

qui·nine (kwye'nine, kwi·neen') *n.* [Sp. *quina*, cinchona, + *-ine*]. An alkaloid, $C_{20}H_{24}N_2O_2$, of cinchona; used principally as an antimalarial drug, generally as the sulfate salt. Quinine and urea hydrochloride is used as a sclerosing agent.

quinine fever. A drug reaction occurring especially in persons occupationally exposed to quinine; characterized by fever and an exanthema.

qui·nin·ism (kwye'ni·niz·um, kwin'i·) *n.* [*quinine* + *-ism*]. CINCHONISM.

quin·i·no·der·ma (kwin''i·no·dur'muh) *n.* [*quinine* + *-derma*]. A drug dermatitis following the ingestion of quinine or its derivatives.

quin·ism (kwin'iz·um, kwye'niz·um) *n.* CINCHONISM.

quino-. See *quin-.*

quino·chromes (kwin'o·krohmz) *n.pl.* Blue, fluorescent products formed by oxidation of thiamine. See also *thiochrome.*

quin·oid (kwin'oid) *adj.* [*quinone* + *-oid*]. Pertaining to the molecular structure characteristic of quinones and believed to be responsible for the color of certain benzene derivatives.

quin·o·line (kwin'o·leen, ·lin) *n.* 1-Benzazine or benzo[*b*]pyridine, C_9H_7N, used in organic synthesis and, formerly, as an antimalarial; also a structural unit of quinine and other cinchona alkaloids. See also *quinuclidine.*

Quinolor. Trademark for halquinols, a topical anti-infective composition.

qui·none (kwi·nohn', kwin'ohn) *n.* [*quin-* + *-one*]. 1. Either of two known isomers, $C_6H_4O_2$, ortho- or parabenzoquinone, a benzenoid compound of two internal alternating carbon-carbon double bonds and two carbonyl groups. 2. Any derivative of either quinone defined in 1.

quino·tan·nic acid (kwin''o·tan'ick). CINCHOTANNIN.

qui·no·va·tine (kwi·no'vuh·teen) *n.* ARICINE.

Quin·quaud's disease (kaeⁿ·ko') [C. E. *Quinquaud*, French physician, 1841–1894]. FOLLICULITIS DECALVANS.

quin·que·tu·ber·cu·lar (kwin''kwe·tew·bur'kew·lur) *adj.* [L. *quinque*, five, + *tubercular*]. Having five tubercles or cusps.

quin·sy (kwin'zee) *n.* [OF. *quinencie*, from ML. *quinancia*, from Gk. *kynanchē*, dog quinsy, severe sore throat]. PERITONSILLAR ABSCESS.

quin·tan (kwin'tun) *adj. & n.* [L. *quintanus*, of the fifth, from *quintus*, fifth]. 1. Recurring every fifth day. 2. A quintan fever.

quintan fever. 1. An intermittent fever, the paroxysms of which recur every 96 hours; that is, on the fifth, ninth, thirteenth days. 2. TRENCH FEVER.

quin·ter·e·nol (kwin·terr'e·nol) *n.* 8-Hydroxy-α-[(isopropylamino)methyl]-5-quinolinemethanol, $C_{14}H_{18}N_2O_2$, a bronchodilator; used as the sulfate salt.

quin·tip·a·ra (kwin·tip'uh·ruh) *n.* [L. *quintus*, fifth, + *-para*]. A woman who has given birth five times.

quin·tu·plet (kwin'tuh·plit, kwin·tup'lit) *n.* [*quintuple*, fivefold, + *-et* as in triplet]. One of five children who have been born at one birth.

qui·nu·cli·dine (kwi·new'kli·deen) *n.* 1-Azabicyclo[2,2,2]octane or 1,4-ethylenepiperidine, $C_7H_{13}N$, a dicyclic base, representing one of the two principal structural units of quinine and other cinchona alkaloids, the other unit being quinoline.

quip·a·zine (kwip'uh·zeen) *n.* 2-(1-Piperazinyl)quinoline, $C_{13}H_{15}N_3$, an oxytocic drug; used as the maleate salt.

qui·tiq·ua (kwi·tick'wuh) *n.* PINTA.

quit·tor, quit·ter (kwit'ur) *n.* [ME. *quiture*]. *In veterinary medicine,* a disease of the collateral cartilages of the equine foot caused by injury and infection, resulting in the formation of a fistulous tract in the region of the coronet over the quarter.

Quotane. Trademark for dimethisoquin, a surface anesthetic used as the hydrochloride salt.

quo·tid·i·an (kwo·tid'ee·un) *adj.* [L. *quotidianus,* daily]. Recurring every day.

quotidian fever. An intermittent fever, especially malarial, the paroxysms of which recur daily.

quotidian malaria. A form of malaria in which the paroxysms occur every day, as in two concomitant infections with *Plasmodium vivax.*

quo·tient (kwo'shunt) *n.* [L. *quotiens,* how many times]. The result of the process of division.

q.v. Abbreviation for (a) *quantum vis,* as much as you wish; (b) *quod vide,* which see.

Q wave of the electrocardiogram. The initial negative deflection of the (QRS) ventricular depolarization complex, usually preceding an R wave.

R

R Symbol for (a) electrical resistance; (b) any alkyl radical of the general formula C_nH_{2n+1}, where n is the number of carbon atoms in the molecule.
R *In microbiology,* abbreviation for *rough colony.*
R. Abbreviation for (a) *Réaumur*; (b) right.
R [abbreviation of L. *rectus,* right, straight]. According to the Cahn-Ingold-Prelog sequencing rules, a specification of the configuration of a stereoisomeric molecule. Not to be confused with *dextro-*. Contr. *S*
−R. Symbol for Rinne's test negative.
+R. Symbol for Rinne's test positive.
R_f *In chromatography,* a symbol for the ratio of the distance traveled by a substance undergoing diffusion to the distance traveled by the solvent; the ratio is characteristic of the substance.
℞ Symbol for *recipe,* take; used in prescription writing.
r Symbol for roentgen.
Ra Symbol for radium.
rab·bit fever. TULAREMIA.
rab·id (rab'id) *adj.* [L. *rabidus,* mad]. Affected with rabies; pertaining to rabies.
ra·bies (ray'beez) *n.* [L. rage, madness, from *rabere,* to rave]. An acute viral infection mainly of the central nervous system of a variety of animals, occasionally transmitted to man by the bite of a rabid dog, cat, skunk, fox, raccoon, or bat. Symptoms in man generally appear 2 to 12 weeks after infecting contact, and progress from fever, restlessness, and extreme excitability to hydrophobia (1) (with resultant drooling of saliva), generalized seizures, confusional psychosis, and death. A less common paralytic form, due to spinal cord affection, may replace or accompany the state of excitement. Compare *hydrophobia.* See also *furious rabies, paralytic rabies.*
rabies fixed virus. Pasteur's term for a virus that is so high in virulence for rabbits by successive intracerebral transfers that it will kill the animals in a period of 6 or 7 days.
rabies prophylaxis. The inoculation of an exposed person with a rabies vaccine. See also *Pasteur treatment.*
rabies vaccine. 1. A sterile preparation of killed, fixed virus of rabies obtained from brain tissue of rabbits or from duck embryos that have been infected with fixed rabies virus. The vaccine is used as a prophylactic agent against rabies. 2. One of several living modified rabies virus vaccines, such as the Flury strain.
race, *n.* [F., from It. *razza*]. A breed or strain of a species. Adj. *racial.*
Race-Coombs test [R. *Coombs*]. ANTIGLOBULIN TEST.
ra·ce·mic (ra·see'mick, ·sem'ick) *adj.* [L. *racemus,* a bunch of grapes]. Composed of equal parts of dextrorotatory and levorotatory forms of optical isomers and, therefore, optically inactive.
racemic acid. An optically inactive mixture of dextrorotatory and levorotatory forms of tartaric acid.
racemic ephedrine. RACEPHEDRINE.
ra·ce·mi·za·tion (ray''se·mi·zay'shun, ras''e·) *n.* Conversion of the optically active form of a compound to its racemic form, commonly by heating.
rac·e·mose (ras'e·moce) *adj.* [L. *racemosus,* clustered, from *racemus,* a bunch of grapes]. Resembling a bunch of grapes.
racemose aneurysm. CIRSOID ANEURYSM (1).
racemose gland. A compound alveolar or tubuloalveolar gland.
rac·e·phed·rine (ras''e·fed'rin) *n.* Racemic ephedrine, a sympathomimetic amine used, as the hydrochloride salt, like ephedrine. Syn. *dl-ephedrine.*
ra·ce·phen·i·col (ray''se·fen'i·kol) *n.* Racemic thiamphenicol.
rachi-, rachio-, rhachi-, rhachio- [Gk. *rhachis*]. A combining form meaning *vertebral column, spinal.*
ra·chi·an·es·the·sia, ra·chi·an·aes·the·sia (ray''kee·an''es·theezh'uh, ·theez'ee·uh) *n.* [*rachi-* + *anesthesia*]. SPINAL ANESTHESIA.
ra·chi·as·mus (ray''kee·az'mus) *n.* Spasm of the muscles at the back of the neck.
ra·chi·cele (ray'ki·seel) *n.* [*rachi-* + *-cele*]. Hernial protrusion of the contents of the spinal canal in spina bifida. It includes spinal meningocele, myelomeningocele, and myelocystocele (syringomyelocele).
ra·chi·cen·te·sis (ray''ki·sen·tee'sis) *n.* [*rachi-* + *centesis*]. LUMBAR PUNCTURE.
-rachidia, -rrhachidia [NL., from Gk. *rachis,* backbone]. A combining form meaning *condition of the vertebral column.*
ra·chid·i·al (ra·kid'ee·ul) *adj.* RACHIDIAN.
ra·chid·i·an (ra·kid'ee·un) *adj.* [F. *rachidien*]. Pertaining to the rachis or vertebral column.
ra·chil·y·sis (ra·kil'i·sis) *n.,* pl. **rachily·ses** (·seez) [*rachi-* + *-lysis*]. A method of treating lateral curvature of the spine by mechanical counteraction of the abnormal curves.
rachio-. See *rachi-.*
ra·chio·camp·sis (ray''kee·o·kamp'sis) *n.* [*rachio-* + Gk. *kampsis,* a bending]. CURVATURE OF THE SPINE.
ra·chio·cen·te·sis (ray''kee·o·sen·tee'sis) *n.* [*rachio-* + *centesis*]. LUMBAR PUNCTURE.
ra·chi·o·dyn·ia (ray''kee·o·din'ee·uh) *n.* [*rachi-* + *-odynia*]. Pain in the spinal column.
ra·chi·om·e·ter (ray''kee·om'e·tur) *n.* [*rachio-* + *-meter*]. An instrument used to measure the degree of spinal curvature.

ra·chi·op·a·thy (ray″kee·op′uth·ee) *n.* [*rachio-* + *-pathy*]. Any disease of the spine.

ra·chio·ple·gia (ray″kee·o·plee′jee·uh) *n.* [*rachio-* + *-plegia*]. *Obsol.* SPINAL PARALYSIS.

ra·chio·sco·li·o·sis (ray″kee·o·sko″lee·o′sis) *n.* [*rachio-* + *scoliosis*]. Lateral curvature of the spine.

ra·chio·tome (ray′kee·o·tome) *n.* [*rachio-* + *-tome*]. A bone-cutting instrument used in operations upon the vertebrae.

ra·chi·ot·o·my (ray″kee·ot′uh·mee) *n.* [*rachio-* + *-tomy*]. The operation of cutting into the vertebral column.

ra·chip·a·gus (ra·kip′uh·gus) *n.*, pl. **rachipa·gi** (·guy, ·jye) [*rachi-* + *-pagus*]. Conjoined twins united back to back by any portion of the vertebral column.

ra·chi·re·sis·tance (ray″ki·re·zis′tunce) *n.* [*rachi-* + *resistance*]. Resistance of the spinal nerves to the effect of a local anesthetic agent.

ra·chis (ray′kis) *n.*, pl. **rachises, rach·i·des** (rack′i·deez) [Gk.]. VERTEBRAL COLUMN.

ra·chis·chi·sis (ra·kis′ki·sis) *n.*, pl. **rachischi·ses** (·seez) [*rachi-* + *-schisis*]. SPINA BIFIDA.

ra·chit·a·min (ra·kit′uh·min) *n.* [*rachit*is + vit*amin*]. *Obsol.* VITAMIN D.

ra·chi·ter·a·ta (ray″ki·terr′uh·tuh) *n.pl.* [*rachi-* + *terata*]. A collective term for all anomalies involving the spine.

ra·chit·ic (ra·kit′ick) *adj.* [*rachit*is + *-ic*]. Affected with, resembling, or produced by rickets.

rachitic dwarf. An individual whose growth was stunted by severe rickets. See also *Fanconi syndrome.*

rachitic pelvis. A pelvis characterized by a sinking in and forward of the sacrovertebral angle, with a flaring outward of the iliac crests and increased separation of the anterior iliac spines.

rachitic rosary or **beads.** The row of nodules appearing on the ribs at the junctions with their cartilages; often seen in rachitic children.

ra·chi·tis (ra·kye′tis) *n.*, pl. **ra·chit·i·des** (ra·kit′i·deez) [Gk., disease of the spine]. RICKETS.

ra·chi·tism (ray′ki·tiz·um, rack′i·) *n.* [*rachit*is + *-ism*]. RICKETS.

rach·i·to·gen·ic (rack″i·to·jen′ick) *adj.* [*rachit*is + *-genic*]. Producing rickets, as a vitamin-D deficient diet.

ra·cial (ray′shul) *adj.* Of or pertaining to a race or to races.

racial immunity. Relative lack of susceptibility to a disease in certain races of a given species.

racial incidence. The incidence rate according to race.

racial unconscious. COLLECTIVE UNCONSCIOUS.

rack·et amputation. A variety of elliptic or oval amputation with a long cut, like a racket handle, below the elliptic incision.

ra·clage (rah·klahzh′) *n.* [F., from *racler,* to scrape]. The destruction of a soft growth by rubbing, as with a brush or harsh sponge.

ra·cle·ment (rah″kluh·mahn′) *n.* [F.]. RACLAGE.

rac·quet mycelium (rack′it). A hyphal configuration in which the distal end of hyphal cells in many fungi is swollen, as in *Coccidioides immitis.*

RAD Abbreviation for *right axis deviation.*

rad, *n.* [short for radiation]. *In radiology,* the unit of absorbed dose (100 ergs per gram).

ra·dar·ky·mo·gram (ray″dahr·kigh′mo·gram) *n.* A depiction of wave patterns of muscular contraction during a cardiac cycle produced by radarkymography.

ra·dar·ky·mog·ra·phy (ray″dahr·kigh·mog′ruh·fee) *n.* Recording of the horizontal movements of the cardiac silhouette as projected on a television monitor scanning a fluoroscopic screen; the recording is made through a radar device which scans the television image.

ra·dec·to·my (ray·deck′tuh·mee) *n.* [L. *rad*ix, root, + *-ectomy*]. Resection of the root of a tooth, in whole or in part.

ra·di·al (ray′dee·ul) *adj.* [L. *radialis,* from *radius,* spoke, ray]. 1. Radiating; diverging from a common center. 2. Pertaining to, or in relation to, the radius bone of the forearm, as the radial artery.

radial artery. See Table of Arteries in the Appendix.

radial bursa. The synovial sheath of the tendon of the flexor pollicis longus muscle. NA *vagina tendinis musculi flexoris pollicis longi.*

radial carpal collateral ligament. The radial collateral ligament of the wrist. See *radial collateral ligament.*

radial collateral artery. The anterolateral terminal branch of the deep brachial artery, which descends with the radial nerve through the upper arm supplying the brachial, brachioradialis, and triceps muscles, sends a branch to the rete olecrani, and enters the forearm where it anastamoses with the radial recurrent artery. NA *arteria collateralis radialis.*

radial collateral ligament. 1. (of the elbow:) A triangular band on the lateral side of the elbow joint, attached at its narrow end to the lateral condyle of the humerus and passing principally to the lateral side of the annular ligament of the radius. NA *ligamentum collaterale radiale.* 2. (of the wrist:) A short band which passes from the tip of the styloid process of the radius to several points on the scaphoid bone, with a few fibers continuing to the trapezium. NA *ligamentum collaterale carpi radiale.*

radial eminence of the wrist. EMINENTIA CARPI RADIALIS.

radial fossa. The depression on the humerus above the capitulum which accommodates the head of the radius in extreme flexion of the forearm. NA *fossa radialis.*

radial groove. RADIAL SULCUS.

radial immunodiffusion. A technique for measuring concentration of antigen in which a sample is placed in a well and diffuses radially into agar in which the corresponding antibody has been placed.

ra·di·a·lis (ray″dee·ay′lis) *L. adj.* Pertaining to the radius; a term applied to various arteries, nerves, and muscles, as flexor carpi radialis.

radial nerve. NA *nervus radialis.* See Table of Nerves in the Appendix. See also Plate 16.

radial notch. A depression on the lateral surface of the coronoid process of the ulna for articulation with the head of the radius. NA *incisura radialis.*

radial periosteal reflex. BRACHIORADIALIS REFLEX.

radial pulse. The pulse in the radial artery, particularly as felt at the wrist near the base of the thumb.

radial reflex. BRACHIORADIALIS REFLEX.

radial sulcus. A spiral groove on the shaft of the humerus indicating the course of the radial nerve. Syn. *musculospiral groove, radial groove.* NA *sulcus nervi radialis.*

radial tuberosity. The large eminence on the medial side of the upper extremity of the radius, into which the tendon of the biceps brachii muscle is inserted. NA *tuberositas radii.*

ra·di·an (ray′dee·un) *n.* An arc whose length is equal to the radius of the circle of which it is a part.

ra·di·ant (ray′dee·unt) *adj.* [L. *radiare,* to radiate]. Emitting rays or occurring in the form of rays.

radiant energy. Energy propagated in the form of electromagnetic waves.

radiant flux. The rate of transfer of radiant energy. Symbol, *P.*

radiant light therapy. The use in physical therapy of curative rays derived from the sun or artificial sources as ultraviolet and infrared radiation.

radiate carpal ligament. The principal ligament of the mediocarpal articulation, located on the palmar surface of the joint and consisting primarily of groups of fibers passing from the capitate to the scaphoid, lunate, and triquetral bones. NA *ligamentum carpi radiatum.*

radiate ligament. 1. (of the rib:) A fibrous band connecting the anterior part of the head of each rib with the sides of two vertebrae and corresponding intervertebral disk. NA *ligamentum capitis costae radiatum.* 2. (of the carpus or wrist:) RADIATE CARPAL LIGAMENT.

radiate sternocostal ligament. Any of the triangular ligaments in the sternocostal articulations which are composed of fibers radiating from the medial end of a costal cartilage to the sternum. NA (pl.) *ligamenta sternocostalia radiata.*

radiating sensation. SECONDARY SENSATION.

ra·di·a·tio (rad″ee·ay′shee·o, ray″dee·) *n.*, pl. **radiatio·nes** (·neez) [L.]. RADIATION (3).

radiatio acu·sti·ca (a·koos′ti·kuh) [NA]. ACOUSTIC RADIATION.

radiatio cor·po·ris cal·lo·si (kor′po·ris ka·lo′sigh) [NA]. CORPUS CALLOSUM RADIATION.

radiatio corporis stri·a·ti (strye·ay′tye) [BNA]. CORTICOSTRIATE RADIATION.

ra·di·a·tion (ray″dee·ay′shun) *n.* [L. *radiatio,* from *radiare,* to shine, radiate, from *radius,* ray, beam]. 1. The act of radiating or diverging from a central point, as radiation of light; divergence from a center, having the appearance of rays. 2. The emission and propagation of energy through space or through a material medium in a form having certain characteristics of waves, including the energy commonly described as electromagnetic and that of sound; usually, electromagnetic radiation, classified, according to frequency, as Hertzian, infrared, visible, ultraviolet, x-ray, and gamma ray; also, by extension, such corpuscular emissions as alpha and beta particles and cosmic rays. 3. *In neurology,* certain groups of fibers that diverge after leaving their place of origin. —**ra·di·ate** (ray′dee·ate) *v.* & *adj.*

radiation anemia. Aplastic or hypoplastic anemia following excessive exposure to ionizing radiation. Syn. *roentgen-ray anemia.*

radiation burn. A burn resulting from exposure to radiant energy, such as x-ray, radium, or sunlight.

radiation carcinoma. A carcinoma, usually squamous-cell, which is associated with overexposure to radiation.

radiation caries. Demineralization, usually in the cervical areas of the teeth, resembling dental caries and resulting from excessive radiation therapy in the head and neck region.

radiation cataract. IRRADIATION CATARACT.

radiation cystitis. Acute chronic inflammation of the urinary bladder due to radiation therapy; RADIOCYSTITIS.

radiation dermatitis. RADIODERMATITIS.

radiation dosage. The quantity of radiation absorbed; the product of radiation intensity and time also measured as the amount of energy transferred (ergs per gram). See also *median lethal dose.*

radiation dose. The amount of energy absorbed in the form of ionization and excitation per unit of tissue measured in ergs per gram.

radiation myelitis or **myelopathy.** A delayed, progressive myelopathy that follows heavy exposure of the spinal cord to ionizing radiation.

radiation nephritis. Hypertension with or without renal failure due to glomerular, tubular, vascular, and interstitial damage as a result of excessive renal irradiation.

radiation neuropathy. ACTINONEURITIS.

radiation sickness, poisoning, or **syndrome.** 1. Illness due to the effects of therapeutic irradiation, usually manifested by nausea and vomiting. 2. The effect of radiant energy following the explosion of an atomic bomb; the resultant effects may range from a mild white blood cell depression to rapid death with convulsions.

radiation therapy. The treatment of disease with any type of radiation, most commonly with ionizing radiation, such as x-rays, beta rays, and gamma rays.

radiatio oc·ci·pi·to·tha·la·mi·ca (ock·sip″i·to·tha·lam′i·kuh) [BNA]. Radiatio optica (= OPTIC RADIATION).

radiatio op·ti·ca (op′ti·kuh) [NA]. OPTIC RADIATION.

¹rad·i·cal (rad′i·kul) *adj.* [L. *radicalis,* from *radix,* root]. 1. Belonging or relating to a root. 2. Going to the root, or attacking the cause, of a disease. 3. Characterizing or involving extreme measures or treatment to remove the main cause of a disease or condition. Contr. *conservative.*

²radical, *n.* 1. A group of atoms that acts as a unit, but commonly does not exist in the free state, as NH_4^+, ammonium, or C_6H_5, phenyl. 2. *Obsol.* The haptophore group of an antibody.

radical amenorrhea. *Obsol.* PRIMARY AMENORRHEA.

radical cesarean section. Cesarean section followed by hysterectomy; CESAREAN HYSTERECTOMY.

radical mastectomy. Surgical removal of the entire breast and also of adjacent tissue, including the pectoralis minor muscle, part or all of the pectoralis major muscle, and all the lymphatic tissue of chest wall and axilla.

radical mastoidectomy. The complete exenteration of mastoid, epitympanic, perilabyrinthine, and tubal air cells. The tympanic membrane, ossicular chain, middle ear mucous membrane, stapedius muscle, and tensor tympani muscle are also removed.

radical operation. A comparatively extensive operation that seeks to extirpate or remove the causative factor of the disease or condition.

radices. Plural of *radix.*

radices cra·ni·a·les ner·vi ac·ces·so·rii (kray·nee·ay′leez nur′vye ack·se·so′ree·eye) [NA]. The cranial roots of the accessory nerve.

radices spi·na·les ner·vi ac·ces·so·rii (spye·nay′leez nur′vye ack·se·so′ree·eye) [NA]. The spinal roots of the accessory nerve.

radices sym·pa·thi·cae gan·glii ci·li·a·ris (sim·path′i·see gang′glee·eye sil·ee·air′is) [BNA]. RAMUS SYMPATHICUS AD GANGLION CILIARE.

radices vis·ce·ra·les ve·nae ca·vae in·fe·ri·o·ris (vis·e·ray′leez vee′nee kay′vee in·feer·ee·o′ris) [BNA]. Veins from the abdominal viscera to the inferior vena cava.

rad·i·cle (rad′i·kul) *n.* [L. *radicula,* dim. of *radix,* root]. 1. A little root, as the radicle of a nerve, one of the ultimate fibrils of which a nerve is composed; or radicle of a vein, one of the minute vessels uniting to form a vein. 2. ²RADICAL.

rad·i·cot·o·my (rad″i·kot′uh·mee) *n.* [*radix* + *-tomy*]. RHIZOTOMY.

radicul-, radiculo- [L. *radicula,* dim. of *radix,* root]. A combining form meaning *root,* as of a nerve or tooth; specifically, *spinal nerve root or roots.*

ra·dic·u·lar (ra·dick′yoo·lur) *adj.* Pertaining to a root or to a radicle; specifically, pertaining to the roots of the spinal nerves or to those of the teeth.

radicular artery. An artery that supplies the spinal cord, entering with the dorsal and ventral primary roots of the spinal nerves.

radicular cyst. A cyst arising from chronic infection of a granuloma about the root of a tooth.

ra·dic·u·lec·to·my (ra·dick″yoo·leck′tuh·mee) *n.* [*radicul-* + *-ectomy*]. Excision or resection of a spinal nerve root.

ra·dic·u·li·tis (ra·dick″yoo·lye′tis) *n.* [*radicul-* + *-itis*]. Inflammation of a nerve root.

radiculo-. See *radicul-.*

ra·dic·u·lo·my·e·lop·a·thy (ra·dick″yoo·lo·migh″e·lop′uth·ee) *n.* [*radiculo-* + *myelopathy*]. Disease of the spinal cord and roots of the spinal nerves.

ra·dic·u·lo·neu·ri·tis (ra·dick″yoo·lo·new·rye′tis) *n.* [*radiculo-* + *neuritis*]. Inflammation of a peripheral spinal nerve and its root. See also *Guillain-Barré disease.*

ra·dic·u·lo·neu·rop·a·thy (ra·dick″yoo·lo·new·rop′uth·ee) *n.* [*radiculo-* + *neuropathy*]. Disease of the peripheral spinal nerves and their roots. See also *Guillain-Barré disease.*

ra·dic·u·lop·a·thy (ra·dick″yoo·lop′uth·ee) *n.* [*radiculo-* + *-pathy*]. Disease of the roots of spinal nerves.

ra·di·ec·to·my (ray″dee·eck′tuh·mee) *n.* [*radix* + *-ectomy*]. Resection of one of the roots of a tooth.

radii. Plural and genitive singular of *radius.*

radii len·tis (len′tis) [NA]. Faint lines on the anterior and posterior surface of the lens which diverge radially from the poles toward the equator.

radio- [L. *radius,* ray]. A combining form meaning (a) *radiation;* (b) *radium;* (c) *radioactive* or *radioactivity;* (d) *the radius.*

ra·dio·ab·la·tion (ray″dee·o·a·blay′shun) *n.* [*radio-* + *ablation*]. Destruction of tissue by means of radioactive substances.

ra·dio·ac·tin·i·um (ray″dee·o·ack·tin′ee·um) *n.* A radioactive product of actinium. It gives off alpha rays and disintegrates into actinium x.

ra·dio·ac·tive (ray″dee·o·ack′tiv) *adj.* Pertaining to or possessing radioactivity.

radioactive equilibrium. The equilibrium between a radioactive substance and its parent substance, in which at any given moment the rate of disintegration of the former is equal to its rate of formation from the latter.

radioactive isotope. RADIOISOTOPE.

ra·dio·ac·tiv·i·ty (ray″dee·o·ack·tiv′i·tee) *n.* [*radio-* + *activity*]. The spontaneous decay or disintegration of an unstable atomic nucleus, accompanied by emission of alpha particles, beta particles, or gamma rays.

ra·dio·al·ler·go·sor·bent test (ray″dee·o·al″ur·go·sor′bunt) A method of measuring antibodies whereby the antigen is coupled to an insoluble matrix and antibody attaches to the immobilized antigen. The presence of antibody is detected by its reaction with an appropriate (usually heterologous) anti-immunoglobulin. Used to measure specific IgE antibodies. Abbreviated, RAST.

ra·dio·ar·te·rio·gram (ray″dee·o·ahr·teer′ee·o·gram) *n.* [*radio-* + *arteriogram*]. *Obsol.* Radiographic depiction of an artery or series of arteries following injection of a contrast medium.

ra·dio·au·to·gram (ray″dee·o·aw′to·gram) *n.* RADIOAUTOGRAPH.

ra·dio·au·to·graph (ray″dee·o·aw′to·graf) *n.* [*radio-* + *auto-* + *-graph*]. A direct photographic record of the distribution of a radioactive substance in an organism or tissue section.

ra·dio·au·tog·ra·phy (ray″dee·o·aw·tog′ruh·fee) *n.* [*radio-* + *auto-* + *-graphy*]. The technique of locating and measuring the distribution of radioactive elements in a test material, such as tissue, by means of photographic registration of emanations from the radioactive elements.

ra·di·obe (ray′dee·obe) *n.* [*radio-* + *-obe* as in microbe]. A peculiar microscopic formation that is produced in sterilized bouillon by radium radiation, and that has the appearance of bacteria.

radiobiological action. The action of radiation on living things.

ra·dio·bi·ol·o·gy (ray″dee·o·bye·ol′uh·jee) *n.* [*radio-* + *biology*]. The study of the scientific principles, mechanisms, and effects of the interaction of ionizing radiation with living matter. —**radio·bio·log·i·cal** (·bye″uh·loj′i·kul) *adj.*

ra·dio·car·pal (ray″dee·o·kahr′pul) *adj.* Pertaining to the radius and the carpus.

radiocarpal articulation or **joint.** WRIST JOINT.

radiocarpal ligament. Either of two ligaments in the wrist passing from the radius to various carpal bones; the dorsal radiocarpal ligament (NA *ligamentum radiocarpeum dorsale*), connecting the dorsal border of the distal end of the radius and the dorsal surfaces of the proximal carpal bones, attached also to the dorsal intercarpal ligaments, or the palmar radiocarpal ligament (NA *ligamentum radiocarpeum palmare*), which passes from the styloid process and palmar border of the distal end of the radius to the proximal carpal bones and the capitate. See also *wrist* in Table of Synovial Joints and Ligaments in the Appendix.

ra·dio·car·pe·us (ray″dee·o·kahr′pee·us) *n.* FLEXOR CARPI RADIALIS BREVIS.

ra·dio·chem·is·try (ray″dee·o·kem′is·tree) *n.* The branch of chemistry that deals with radioactive phenomena.

ra·dio·co·balt (ray″dee·o·ko′bawlt) *n.* Any radioactive isotope of cobalt, especially that having a mass number of 60 (^{60}C), which has a half-life of 5.2 years and emits a negative beta particle and two gamma rays for each atom of cobalt that decays. In the form of metallic cobalt, its radiation is used in the therapy of malignant tumors.

ra·dio·col·loid (ray″dee·o·kol′oid) *n.* Any colloidal aggregate of radioactive substances.

ra·dio·cur·abil·i·ty (ray″dee·o·kewr·uh·bil′i·tee) *n.* The condition of being susceptible to cure or elimination by irradiation; said of cancer cells.

ra·dio·cys·ti·tis (ray″dee·o·sis·tye′tis) *n.* [*radio-* + *cystitis*]. Inflammation of the bladder following radiation therapy; RADIATION CYSTITIS.

ra·di·ode (ray′dee·ode) *n.* [*radio-* + *-ode* as in electrode]. An electric attachment for the application of radium.

ra·dio·dense (ray″dee·o·dence′) *adj.* Impervious to x-rays at the usual energy levels used in diagnosis.

ra·dio·der·ma·ti·tis (ray″dee·o·dur″muh·tye′tis) *n.* [*radio-* + *dermatitis*]. The retrogressive changes occurring in the skin after excessive exposure to ionizing radiation, especially x-rays and gamma rays.

ra·dio·di·ag·no·sis (ray″dee·o·dye″ug·no′sis) *n.* The diagnosis of disease by means of radiography or radioscopy.

ra·di·o·don·tia (ray″dee·o·don′chee·uh) *n.* [*radio-* + *-odontia*]. RADIODONTICS.

ra·di·o·don·tics (ray″dee·o·don′ticks) *n.* [*radio-* + *odont-* + *-ics*]. The science and practice of radiography of the teeth and associated structures.

ra·di·o·don·tist (ray″dee·o·don′tist) *n.* A specialist in radiodontics.

ra·dio·el·e·ment (ray″dee·o·el′e·munt) *n.* An element that is radioactive.

radio frequency. Any of the electromagnetic frequencies between those of the audible range and the infrared range.

ra·dio·gen·ic (ray″dee·o·jen′ick) *adj.* [*radio-* + *-genic*]. Pertaining to a substance or state resulting from a radioactive transformation, as radiogenic lead resulting from disintegration of radium, or radiogenic heat produced within the earth by disintegration of radioactive substances.

ra·dio·gold (ray″dee·o·gohld′) *n.* Any radioactive isotope of gold, especially that having a mass number of 198 (^{198}Au), which has a half-life of 2.70 days and emits a negative beta particle and a gamma ray for each atom of gold that decays. In the form of a colloidal dispersion of the metal it is used, by injection, in the therapy and palliation of neoplastic disease and in the treatment of neoplastic effusions, and also as a tracer in various studies involving gold.

ra·dio·gram (ray′dee·o·gram) *n.* RADIOGRAPH.

ra·dio·graph (ray′dee·o·graf) *n.* & *v.* [*radio-* + *-graph*]. 1. A photograph made on a sensitive film by projection of x-rays through a part of the body. 2. To make a radiograph.

ra·di·og·ra·pher (ray″dee·og′ruh·fur) *n.* A person skilled in radiography; an x-ray technician.

ra·di·og·ra·phy (ray″dee·og′ruh·fee) *n.* [*radio-* + *-graphy*]. The practice or act of making radiographs. —**ra·dio·gra·phic** (ray″dee·o·graf′ick) *adj.*

ra·dio·hu·mer·al (ray″dee·o·hew′mur·ul) *adj.* [*radio-* + *humeral*]. Pertaining to the radius and the humerus.

radiohumeral bursitis or **epicondylitis.** EPICONDYLITIS (2).

ra·dio·im·mu·no·as·say (ray″dee·o·im″yoo·no·a·say′) *n.* [*radio-* + *immuno-* + *assay*]. The quantitative determination of antigen, antibody, or hapten concentration by the introduction of a radioactively labeled complementary substance which can be expected to bind the molecule in question and the subsequent measurement of resulting radioactive immune complex.

ra·dio·im·mu·no·elec·tro·pho·re·sis (ray″dee·o·im″yoo·no·e·leck″tro·fo·ree′sis) *n.* Immunoelectrophoresis in which either the antigen or the antibody is radioactively labeled.

ra·dio·io·dine (ray″dee·o·eye′uh·dine, ·din) *n.* Any radioactive isotope of iodine, especially that having a mass number of 131 (^{131}I), which has a half-life of 8.08 days and emits two negative beta particles and several gamma rays for each atom of iodine that decays. In the form of sodium iodide, it is used, by intravenous or oral administration, in the treatment of hyperthyroidism and carcinoma of the thyroid, and also for various diagnostic purposes.

ra·dio·iron (ray″dee·o·eye′urn) *n.* Any radioactive isotope of iron, especially that having a mass number of 59 (^{59}Fe), which has a half-life of 45 days and emits two negative beta particles and several gamma rays for each atom of iron that decays. In the form of ferric or ferrous salts, it has been used in the study of iron metabolism.

ra·dio·iso·tope (ray″dee·o·eye′suh·tope) *n.* A radioactive isotope, commonly of an element which is stable. Although certain isotopes of normally stable elements exist naturally in radioactive form, many are prepared only artificially, as by bombarding an element with neutrons, protons, deuterons, or alpha particles in a nuclear reactor or in an accelerating device such as the cyclotron or cosmotron; the bombarded element may form a radioactive isotope of the same element or of another element. By virtue of its radioactivity, a radioisotope is used either for the effect of its radiations, such use often being diagnostic or therapeutic, or as a tracer added to the stable form of a compound to follow the course of the latter in a particular sequence of reactions in living organisms or even in an inanimate system.

radioisotope camera. Any array (one or more) of radiation counters that visualizes a radioisotope deposition and is fixed in relation to the patient.

radioisotope scanner. Any array (one or more) of radiation counters that visualizes a radioisotope deposition and is movable in relation to the patient.

ra·dio·ky·mog·ra·phy (ray″dee·o·kigh·mog′ruh·fee) *n.* [*radio-* + *kymography*]. A method of obtaining a graphic record of movement of the silhouette of an organ or tissue on a single film. Syn. *roentgenokymography.*

ra·di·ol·o·gist (ray″dee·ol′uh·jist) *n.* A physician specializing in radiology.

ra·di·ol·o·gy (ray″dee·ol′uh·jee) *n.* [*radio-* + *-logy*]. The branch of medicine that deals with radioactive substances, x-rays and other ionizing radiations, and with their utilization in the diagnosis and treatment of disease. —**ra·dio·log·ic** (ray″dee·o·loj′ick) *adj.*

ra·dio·lu·cent (ray″dee·o·lew′sunt) *adj.* Partly or wholly transparent to x-rays or other forms of radiation. —**radio·lu·cen·cy** (·sun·see) *n.*

ra·dio·lu·mi·nes·cence (ray″dee·o·lew″mi·nes′unce) *n.* [*radio-* + *luminescence*]. The luminescence brought about by x- or gamma rays striking a suitable crystalline substance.

ra·di·ol·y·sis (ray″dee·ol′i·sis) *n.*, pl. **radioly·ses** (·seez) [*radio-* + *-lysis*]. The dissociation of molecules by radiation as, for example, the dissociation of water into hydrogen and oxygen during operation of certain reactors.

ra·di·om·e·ter (ray″dee·om′e·tur) *n.* [*radio-* + *-meter*]. An instrument for detecting and measuring radiant energy (normally infrared, visible, or ultraviolet). —**ra·dio·met·ric** (ray″dee·o·met′rick) *adj.*

radiometric analysis. Determination of an element that is not itself radioactive by means of an interaction (such as precipitation) with a radioactive element.

ra·dio·mi·crom·e·ter (ray″dee·o·migh·krom′e·tur) *n.* [*radio-* + *micro-* + *-meter*]. A sensitive radiometer used for detection of small intensities of radiant energy.

ra·dio·mi·met·ic (ray″dee·o·mi·met′ick) *adj.* [*radio-* + *mimetic*]. Capable of producing in tissue biologic effects similar to those of ionizing radiation.

radiomimetic agent. Any agent, such as the nitrogen mustards, capable of duplicating many of the radiation-induced effects in tissue.

ra·di·on (ray′dee·on) *n.* A particle ejected by a radioactive substance.

ra·dio·ne·cro·sis (ray″dee·o·ne·kro′sis) *n.* [*radio-* + *necrosis*]. Destruction or ulceration of tissues caused by radiation.

ra·dio·neu·ri·tis (ray″dee·o·new·rye′tis) *n.* A form of neuritis due to exposure to radiation.

ra·dio·neu·rop·a·thy (ray″dee·o·new·rop′uth·ee) *n.* A delayed, progressive, sensorimotor neuropathy that occurs many months or even years after radiation in the vicinity of peripheral nerves or anterior horn cells.

ra·dio·ni·tro·gen (ray″dee·o·nigh′truh·jin) *n.* The radioactive isotope of nitrogen, having a mass number of 13 (^{13}N), which has a half-life of 10.1 minutes and emits a positive beta particle for each atom of nitrogen that decays.

ra·dio·nu·clide (ray″dee·o·new′klide) *n.* A nuclide that is radioactive.

ra·dio·opaque (ray″dee·o·o·pake′) *adj.* RADIOPAQUE. —**radio·opac·i·ty** (·o·pas′i·tee) *n.*

ra·di·opaque (ray″dee·o·pake′) *adj.* [*radio-* + *opaque*]. Not transparent to the x-ray; not permitting total passage of radiant energy. Contr. *radiotransparent.* —**ra·di·opac·i·ty** (ray″dee·o·pas′i·tee) *n.*

ra·dio·pa·thol·o·gy (ray″dee·o·puh·thol′uh·jee) *n.* [*radio-* + *pathology*]. Study of tissue changes brought about by ionizing radiation.

ra·dio·pel·vim·e·try (ray″dee·o·pel·vim′e·tree) *n.* [*radio-* + *pelvimetry*]. A radiographic procedure for making measurements of the maternal pelvis and fetal skull.

ra·dio·phar·ma·ceu·ti·cal (ray″dee·o·fahr″muh·sue′ti·kul) *n.* [*radio-* + *pharmaceutical*]. *In nuclear medicine,* a preparation of a radioactive element or compound containing such an element, commonly used for the diagnosis or treatment of disease.

ra·dio·phos·pho·rus (ray″dee·o·fos′fuh·rus) *n.* The radioactive isotope of phosphorus, having a mass number of 32 (^{32}P), which has a half-life of 14.3 days and emits a negative beta particle for each atom of phosphorus that decays. In the form of sodium phosphate (sodium phosphate P 32) it is used, by intravenous or oral administration, in the treatment of polycythemia vera and as an antineoplastic agent, and in various ways as a diagnostic agent, as in the determination of blood volume, and also as a tracer in various studies involving phosphorus.

ra·dio·prax·is (ray″dee·o·prack′sis) *n.* [*radio-* + *praxis*]. The use of radiant energy either in therapy or for other purposes.

ra·dio·re·sist·ance (ray″dee·o·re·zis′tunce) *n.* The relative resistance of tissues or organisms to the injurious effects of radiation.

ra·di·os·co·py (ray″dee·os′kuh·pee) *n.* [*radio-* + *-scopy*]. The process of securing an image of an object upon a fluorescent screen by means of radiant energy.

ra·dio·sen·si·tiv·i·ty (ray″dee·o·sen″si·tiv′i·tee) *n.* The sensitivity of tissues or organisms to various types of radiations, such as x-rays or rays from radioactive materials. —**radio·sen·si·tive** (·sen′si·tiv) *adj.*

ra·dio·ster·e·os·co·py (ray″dee·o·sterr″ee·os′kuh·pee, ·steer″) *n.* [*radio-* + *stereoscopy*]. The application of the principle of the stereoscope, obtaining a viewpoint for the left eye and one for the right by corresponding displacement of the x-ray tube along the plane of the film, and viewing the two radiographs by one of several methods to obtain a third-dimensional effect.

ra·dio·sur·gery (ray″dee·o·sur′jur·ee) *n.* The use of radium in surgical therapy.

ra·dio·ther·a·peu·tic (ray″dee·o·therr″uh·pew′tick) *adj.* Of or pertaining to the therapeutic use of radiant energy.

ra·dio·ther·a·peu·tics (ray″dee·o·therr″uh·pew′ticks) *n.* RADIATION THERAPY.

ra·dio·ther·a·pist (ray″dee·o·therr′uh·pist) *n.* A physician specializing in, or administering, radiotherapy.

ra·dio·ther·a·py (ray″dee·o·therr′uh·pee) *n.* RADIATION THERAPY.

ra·dio·ther·my (ray′dee·o·thur″mee) *n.* [*radio-* + *-thermy*].

1. Treatment by radiant heat. 2. SHORT-WAVE DIATHERMY.

ra·dio·thy·roid·ec·to·mize (ray″dee-o-thigh″roy-deck′tuh-mize) *v.* [*radio-* + *thyroidectomize*]. To ablate thyroid function by administration of large doses of radioactive iodine.

ra·dio·tox·emia (ray″dee-o-tock-see′mee-uh) *n.* Toxemia induced from overexposure to any radioactive substance.

ra·dio·trans·par·ent (ray″dee-o-trans-păr′unt) *adj.* [*radio-* + *transparent*]. Permitting the passage of radiations; used notably in connection with x-rays. Contr. *radiopaque.*

ra·dio·trop·ic (ray″dee-o-trop′ick, tro′pick) *adj.* [*radio-* + *-tropic*]. Reacting predictably to radiation.

ra·dio·tro·pism (ray″dee-o-tro′piz-um) *n.* [*radio-* + *tropism*]. A tropism related to radiation.

ra·dio·ul·nar (ray″dee-o-ul′nur) *adj.* [*radio-* + *ulnar*]. Pertaining to the radius and the ulna.

radioulnar joint. See Table of Synovial Joints and Ligaments in the Appendix.

ra·di·um (ray′dee-um) *n.* [NL., from L. *radius*, ray, beam]. Ra = 226. A highly radioactive metallic element; atomic number, 88. Discovered in 1898 by Pierre and Marie Curie, who separated it from pitchblende. Radium and its salts emit continuously alpha particles, beta particles, and gamma rays. As the bromide or chloride salt, it has been used as an irradiation source in the treatment of malignant tumors. See also *radon.*

radium emanation. RADON.

radium-F. POLONIUM.

radium needles. Steel or platinum-iridium-walled, needle-shaped containers filled with radium salt and used in radium therapy.

radium therapy. Exposure of a body part to high-voltage radium emanations, usually for their destructive effect on malignant tissues.

ra·di·us (ray′dee-us) *n.*, pl. & genit. sing. **ra·dii** (-dee-eye) [L., spoke, rod] [NA]. *In anatomy*, the outer of the two bones of the forearm. See also Table of Bones in the Appendix and Plate 1.

radius fix·us (fick′sus). A line drawn from the hormion to the inion.

ra·dix (ray′dicks) *n.*, genit. **ra·di·cis** (ray′di-sis, ray-dye′sis), pl. **radi·ces** (-di-seez, -dye′seez) [L.]. ROOT.

radix anterior ner·vo·rum spi·na·li·um (nur-vo′rum spye-nay′lee-um) [BNA]. Radix ventralis nervorum spinalium (= VENTRAL ROOT).

radix aor·tae (ay-or′tee). ROOT OF THE AORTA.

radix ar·cus ver·te·brae (ahr′kus vur′te-bree) [BNA]. Pediculus arcus vertebrae (= VERTEBRAL PEDICLE).

radix bre·vis gan·glii ci·li·a·ris (brev′is gang′glee-eye sil-ee-air′is) [BNA]. RADIX OCULOMOTORIA GANGLII CILIARIS.

radix cli·ni·ca (klin′i-kuh) [NA]. In clinical dentistry, the portion of a tooth which at any given moment is embedded in the surrounding tissues.

radix coch·le·a·ris ner·vi acu·sti·ci (kock-lee-air′is nur′vye a-koos′ti-sigh) [BNA]. RADIX INFERIOR NERVI VESTIBULOCOCHLEARIS.

radix den·tis (den′tis) [NA]. ANATOMIC ROOT OF A TOOTH.

radix de·scen·dens ner·vi tri·ge·mi·ni (de-sen′denz nur′vye trye-jem′i-nigh) [BNA]. Tractus mesencephalicus nervi trigemini (= MESENCEPHALIC TRACT OF THE TRIGEMINAL NERVE).

radix dor·sa·lis ner·vo·rum spi·na·li·um (dor-say′lis nur-vo′rum spye-nay′lee-um) [NA]. DORSAL ROOT.

radix fa·ci·a·lis (fay-shee-ay′lis) [NA alt.]. NERVUS CANALIS PTERYGOIDEI.

radix inferior an·sae cer·vi·ca·lis (an′see sur-vi-kay′lis) [NA]. INFERIOR ROOT OF THE ANSA CERVICALIS.

radix inferior coch·le·a·ris (kock-lee-air′is) [NA alt.]. RADIX INFERIOR NERVI VESTIBULOCOCHLEARIS.

radix inferior ner·vi ves·ti·bu·lo·co·chle·a·ris (nur′vye ves-tib″yoo-lo-kock-lee-air′is) [NA]. The continuation of the cochlear portion of the eighth cranial nerve from the spiral ganglion to the brain. NA alt. *radix inferior cochlearis.*

radix la·te·ra·lis ner·vi me·di·a·ni (lat-e-ray′lis nur′vye mee-dee-ay′nigh) [NA]. The portion of the median nerve arising from the lateral cord of the brachial plexus.

radix lateralis trac·tus op·ti·ci (track′tus op′ti-sigh) [NA]. The fibers from the optic tract to the lateral geniculate body.

radix lin·guae (ling′gwee) [NA]. ROOT OF THE TONGUE.

radix lon·ga gan·glii ci·li·a·ris (long′guh gang′glee-eye sil-ee-air′is) [BNA]. RAMUS COMMUNICANS NERVI NASOCILIARIS CUM GANGLIO CILIARI.

radix me·di·a·lis ner·vi me·di·a·ni (mee-dee-ay′lis nur′vye mee-dee-ay′nigh) [NA]. The portion of the median nerve arising from the medial cord of the brachial plexus.

radix medialis trac·tus op·ti·ci (track′tus op′ti-sigh) [NA]. Fibers from the optic tract to the superior colliculus.

radix me·sen·te·rii (mes-en-terr′ee-eye) [NA]. ROOT OF THE MESENTERY.

radix mo·to·ria ner·vi tri·ge·mi·ni (mo-to′ree-uh nur′vye trye-jem′i-nigh) [NA]. The motor root of the trigeminal nerve; it actually contains proprioceptive sensory fibers in addition to motor fibers.

radix na·si (nay′zye) [NA]. ROOT OF THE NOSE.

radix ner·vi fa·ci·a·lis (nur′vye fay-shee-ay′lis) [BNA]. The root of the facial nerve; the portion of the facial nerve from the facial nucleus to the emergence of the nerve from the pons.

radix ocu·lo·mo·to·ria gan·glii ci·li·a·ris (ock″yoo-lo-mo-to′ree-uh gang′glee-eye sil-ee-air′is) [NA]. The fibers from the inferior branch of the oculomotor nerve to the ciliary ganglion.

radix pe·nis (pee′nis) [NA]. The root of the penis; the proximal attached crura and bulb.

radix pi·li (pye′lye) [NA]. HAIR ROOT.

radix posterior ner·vi spi·na·lis (nur′vye spye-nay′lis) [BNA]. Radix dorsalis nervorum spinalium (= DORSAL ROOT).

radix pul·mo·nis (pul-mo′nis) [NA]. ROOT OF THE LUNG.

radix sen·so·ria ner·vi tri·ge·mi·ni (sen-so′ree-uh nur′vye trye-jem′i-nigh) [NA]. The sensory root of the trigeminal nerve, the thick band of fibers from the trigeminal ganglion to the brain.

radix superior an·sae cer·vi·ca·lis (an′see sur-vi-kay′lis) [NA]. SUPERIOR ROOT OF THE ANSA CERVICALIS.

radix superior ner·vi ves·ti·bu·lo·co·chle·a·ris (nur′vye ves-tib″yoo-lo-kock-lee-air′is) [NA]. The continuation of the vestibular portion of the eighth cranial nerve from the vestibular ganglion to the brain. NA alt. *radix superior vestibularis.*

radix superior ves·ti·bu·la·ris (ves-tib-yoo-lair′is) [NA alt.]. RADIX SUPERIOR NERVI VESTIBULOCOCHLEARIS.

radix sym·pa·thi·ca gan·glii sub·max·il·la·ris (sim-path′i-kuh gang′glee-eye sub-mack-si-lair′is) [BNA]. RAMUS SYMPATHICUS AD GANGLION SUBMANDIBULARE.

radix un·guis (ung′guis) [NA]. ROOT OF THE NAIL.

radix ven·tra·lis ner·vo·rum spi·na·li·um (ven-tray′lis nur-vo′rum spye-nay′lee-um) [NA]. VENTRAL ROOT.

ra·don (ray′don) *n.* [*rad*ium + *-on*]. Rn = 222. A radioactive element, a gas, that is a product of the nuclear disintegration of radium; used as a source of irradiation in the treatment of malignant tumors. Syn. *radium emanation.*

radon seed. A small sealed capillary tube containing radon, suitable for implantation in tissues; the tube may be placed inside a small gold tube.

Ra·do·vi·ci's reflex (rah-doh-vee-see′) [J. *Radovici*, French physician, b. 1868]. PALMOMENTAL REFLEX.

Rae·der's syndrome [J. G. *Raeder*, English neurologist, 20th century]. PARATRIGEMINAL SYNDROME.

Ra-F. Radium-F (= POLONIUM).

raf·fi·nase (raf′i-nace) *n.* An enzyme that hydrolyzes raffinose, fructose being produced in the reaction.

raf·fi·nose (raf′i-noce) *n.* [F., from *raffiner*, to refine]. A trisaccharide, $C_{18}H_{32}O_{16}.5H_2O$, found in sugar beets, cottonseed meal, and molasses. On complete hydrolysis, it yields glucose, fructose, and galactose.

ra·fle (rah'fl) *n.* [F.]. An eruptive pustular disease of cattle in northern France.

ra·fox·a·nide (ra·fock'suh·nide) *n.* 3'-Chloro-4'-(*p*-chlorophenoxy)-3,5-diiodosalicylanilide, $C_{19}H_{11}Cl_2I_2NO_3$, an anthelmintic.

rage, *n.* RABIES.

rage reaction or **response.** An attack of intense and uncontrollable rage which may be encountered: (1) rarely, as part of the behavioral automatism of a psychomotor seizure; (2) as an episodic reaction without recognizable seizures or other neurologic abnormalities; and (3) in the course of some recognizable acute or chronic neurologic disease, particularly one that involves the anteromedial portions of the temporal lobes, the fornices, or the hypothalamus. Compare *sham rage.*

rag·pick·er's disease. ANTHRAX.

rag·weed, *n.* Any of several species of the genus *Ambrosia;* its pollen is the most important allergen in the central and eastern United States, the pollinating period being from the middle of August to the time of frost.

Rail·li·e·ti·na (rye"lee·e·tye'nuh) *n.* [A. *Railliet,* French biologist, 19th century]. A genus of tapeworms, parasites of mammals and birds, and occasionally of man.

Raillietina cel·e·ben·sis (sel·e·ben'sis). A species of tapeworm; infections of man have been reported in Tokyo and in Taiwan.

Raillietina dem·e·rar·i·en·sis (dem"e·răr·ee·en'sis) [after the *Demerara* River, Guyana]. A species of tapeworm; human infections have been reported in Guyana, Cuba, and especially rural Ecuador.

Raillietina qui·ten·sis (kwi·ten'sis). *RAILLIETINA DEMERARIENSIS.*

Raillietina mad·a·gas·car·i·en·sis (mad"uh·gas·kăr"ee·en'sis). A species of tapeworm that infects man.

rail·road nystagmus. OPTOKINETIC NYSTAGMUS.

rail·way fever. SHIPPING FEVER.

railway sickness. MOTION SICKNESS.

railway spine. Traumatic neurosis following concussion injury with spinal symptoms and without demonstrable disease. Frequently, compensation or indemnity neurosis play a major role. Compare *whiplash injury.*

Rai·mist's sign (rye'mist) [J. M. *Raimist,* German neuropsychiatrist, 20th century]. 1. Of the hand: When the patient's hands are held by the examiner so that the forearms are vertical, sudden withdrawal of support of the hands by the examiner is followed by abrupt flexion at the wrist of a paretic hand while the sound hand remains vertical. 2. Of the leg: An associated movement seen in corticospinal tract lesions in which, with the patient in a recumbent position, forceful attempts by the examiner at abduction or adduction of the leg on the normal side are followed by a similar movement of the paretic leg.

Rai·ney's corpuscle [G. *Rainey,* English anatomist, 1801–1884]. Psorosperms forming nodules in the muscles of infected animals.

rake retractor. An instrument shaped like a rake, with sharp or blunt prongs, particularly effective in retracting tissues without slippage.

Ralabol. A trademark for zeranol, an anabolic agent.

rale (rahl) *n.* [F. *râle,* from *râler, racler,* to rattle, scrape, from L. *radere, rasus,* to scrape]. An abnormal sound arising within the lungs or air passages and heard on auscultation over the chest; generally characterized by terms such as coarse, medium, fine, moist, dry.

Ralgro. A trademark for zeranol, an anabolic agent.

Ralph method. A method for the detection of hemoglobin in tissues and erythrocytes by using benzidine and hydrogen peroxide to obtain a blue-black color.

ra·mal (ray'mul) *adj.* Of or pertaining to a ramus.

rami. Plural and genitive singular of *ramus.*

rami ad pon·tem ar·te·ri·ae ba·si·la·ris (ad pon'tem ahr·teer'ee·ee bas·i·lair'is) [NA]. The branches of the basilar artery to the pons.

rami al·ve·o·la·res su·pe·ri·o·res an·te·ri·o·res ner·vi in·fra·or·bi·ta·lis (al·vee·o·lay'reez sue·peer·ee·o·reez an·teer·ee·o'reez nur'vye in·fruh·or·bi·tay'lis) [NA]. The anterior superior alveolar branches of the infraorbital nerve; the anterior superior alveolar nerves. See Table of Nerves in the Appendix.

rami alveolares superiores pos·te·ri·o·res ner·vi in·fra·or·bi·ta·lis (pos·teer·ee·o'reez nur'vye in·fruh·or·bi·tay'lis) [NA]. The posterior superior alveolar branches of the infraorbital nerve; the posterior superior alveolar nerves. See Table of Nerves in the Appendix.

rami alveolares superiores posteriores nervi max·il·la·ris (mack·si·lair'is) [BNA]. RAMI ALVEOLARES SUPERIORES POSTERIORES NERVI INFRAORBITALIS.

rami anas·to·mo·ti·ci ner·vi au·ri·cu·lo·tem·po·ra·lis cum ner·vo fa·ci·a·li (a·nas·to·mot'i·sigh nur'vye aw·rick"yoo·lo·tem"po·ray'lis kum nur'vo fay·shee·ay'lye) [BNA]. RAMI COMMUNICANTES NERVI AURICULOTEMPORALIS CUM NERVO FACIALI.

rami an·te·ri·o·res ar·te·ri·a·rum in·ter·cos·ta·li·um (an·teer·ee·o'reez ahr·teer·ee·ay'rum in·tur·kos·tay'lee·um) [BNA]. The anterior branches of the intercostal arteries.

rami anteriores ner·vo·rum cer·vi·ca·li·um (nur·vo'rum sur·vi·kay'lee·um) [BNA]. RAMI VENTRALES NERVORUM CERVICALIUM.

rami anteriores nervorum lum·ba·li·um (lum·bay'lee·um) [BNA]. RAMI VENTRALES NERVORUM LUMBALIUM.

rami anteriores nervorum tho·ra·ca·li·um (tho·ra·kay'lee·um) [BNA]. Rami ventrales nervorum thoracicorum (= INTERCOSTAL NERVES).

rami ar·te·ri·o·si in·ter·lo·bu·la·res he·pa·tis (ahr·teer·ee·o'sigh in·tur·lob·yoo·lair'eez hep'uh·tis) [BNA]. ARTERIAE INTERLOBULARES HEPATIS.

rami ar·ti·cu·la·res ar·te·ri·ae ge·nus de·scen·den·tis (ahr·tick·yoo·lair'eez ahr·teer'ee·ee jen'us de·sen·den'tis) [NA]. The articular branches of the descending artery of the knee.

rami articulares arteriae ge·nu su·pre·mae (jen'yoo sue·pree'mee) [BNA]. RAMI ARTICULARES ARTERIAE GENUS DESCENDENTIS.

rami au·ri·cu·la·res an·te·ri·o·res ar·te·ri·ae tem·po·ra·lis su·per·fi·ci·a·lis (aw·rick·yoo·lair'eez an·teer·ee·o'reez ahr·teer'ee·ee tem·po·ray'lis sue·pur·fish·ee·ay'lis) [NA]. The anterior auricular branches of the superficial temporal artery.

rami bron·chi·a·les an·te·ri·o·res ner·vi va·gi (brong·kee·ay'leez an·teer·ee·o'reez nur'vye vay'guy, ·jye) [BNA]. RAMI BRONCHIALES NERVI VAGI.

rami bronchiales aor·tae tho·ra·ci·cae (ay·or'tee tho·ray'si·see) [NA]. The bronchial branches of the thoracic aorta.

rami bronchiales ar·te·ri·ae mam·ma·ri·ae in·ter·nae (ahr·teer'ee·ee ma·mair'ee·ee in·tur'nee) [BNA]. RAMI BRONCHIALES ARTERIAE THORACICAE INTERNAE.

rami bronchiales arteriae tho·ra·ci·cae in·ter·nae (tho·ray'si·see in·tur'nee) [NA]. The bronchial branches of the internal thoracic artery.

rami bronchiales bron·cho·rum (brong·ko'rum) [BNA]. The first branches of the main bronchi.

rami bronchiales hyp·ar·te·ri·a·les (hip·ahr·teer·ee·ay'leez) [BNA]. The bronchial branches which take origin below the pulmonary arteries.

rami bronchiales ner·vi va·gi (nur'vye vay'guy, ·jye) [NA]. The bronchial branches of the vagus nerve.

rami bronchiales pos·te·ri·o·res ner·vi va·gi (pos·teer·ee·o'reez nur'vye vay'guy, ·jye) [BNA]. RAMI BRONCHIALES NERVI VAGI.

rami bronchiales seg·men·to·rum (seg·men·to'rum) [NA]. Small bronchial branches arising from the segmental bronchi.

rami buc·ca·les ner·vi fa·ci·a·lis (buh·kay'leez nur'vye fay·shee·ay'lis) [NA]. The buccal branches of the facial nerve.

rami cal·ca·nei ar·te·ri·ae ti·bi·a·lis pos·te·ri·o·ris (kal·kay'nee·eye ahr·teer'ee·ee tib·ee·ay'lis pos·teer·ee·o'ris) [NA]. The calcaneal branches of the posterior tibial artery.

rami calcanei la·te·ra·les ar·te·ri·ae pe·ro·nae·ae (lat·e·ray'leez ahr·teer'ee·ee perr·o·nee'ee) [BNA]. RAMI CALCANEI RAMORUM MALLEOLARIUM LATERALIUM ARTERIAE PERONEAE.

rami calcanei laterales ner·vi su·ra·lis (nur'vye sue·ray'lis) [NA]. The lateral calcaneal branches of the sural nerve.

rami calcanei me·di·a·les ar·te·ri·ae ti·bi·a·lis pos·te·ri·o·ris (mee·dee·ay'leez ahr·teer'ee·ee tib·ee·ay'lis pos·teer·ee·o'ris) [BNA]. The medial calcaneal branches of the posterior tibial artery.

rami calcanei mediales ner·vi ti·bi·a·lis (nur'vye tib·ee·ay'lis) [NA]. The medial calcaneal branches of the tibial nerve.

rami calcanei ra·mo·rum mal·le·o·la·ri·um la·te·ra·li·um ar·te·ri·ae fi·bu·la·ris (ray·mo'rum mal·ee·o·lair'ee·um lat·e·ray'lee·um ahr·teer'ee·ee fib·yoo·lair'is) [NA alt.]. RAMI CALCANEI RAMORUM MALLEOLARIUM LATERALIUM ARTERIAE PERONEAE.

rami calcanei ramorum malleolarium lateralium arteriae pe·ro·ne·ae (perr·o·nee'ee) [NA]. The calcaneal branches of the lateral malleolar branches of the peroneal artery. NA alt. *rami calcanei ramorum malleolarium lateralium arteriae fibularis.*

rami cap·su·la·res ar·te·ri·ae re·nis (kap·sue·lair'eez ahr·teer'ee·ee ree'nis) [NA]. The capsular branches of the renal artery.

rami car·di·a·ci cer·vi·ca·les in·fe·ri·o·res ner·vi va·gi (kahr·dye'uh·sigh sur·vi·kay'leez in·feer·ee·o'reez nur'vye vay'guy, ·jye) [NA]. The inferior cervical cardiac branches of the vagus nerve.

rami cardiaci cervicales su·pe·ri·o·res ner·vi va·gi (sue·peer·ee·o'reez nur'vye vay'guy, ·jye) [NA]. The superior cervical cardiac branches of the vagus nerve.

rami cardiaci in·fe·ri·o·res ner·vi re·cur·ren·tis (in·feer·ee·o'reez nur'vye reck''ur·en'tis) [BNA]. RAMI CARDIACI CERVICALES INFERIORES NERVI VAGI.

rami cardiaci su·pe·ri·o·res ner·vi va·gi (sue·peer·ee·o'reez nur'vye vay'guy, ·jye) [BNA]. RAMI CARDIACI CERVICALES SUPERIORES NERVI VAGI.

rami cardiaci tho·ra·ci·ci ner·vi va·gi (tho·ray'si·sigh nur'vye vay'guy, ·jye) [NA]. The thoracic cardiac branches of the vagus nerve.

rami ca·ro·ti·co·tym·pa·ni·ci ar·te·ri·ae ca·ro·ti·dis in·ter·nae (ka·rot''i·ko·tim·pan'i·sigh ahr·teer'ee·ee ka·rot'i·dis in·tur'nee) [NA]. The caroticotympanic branches of the internal carotid artery.

rami ce·li·a·ci ner·vi va·gi (see·lye'uh·sigh nur'vye vay'guy, ·jye) [NA]. The celiac branches of the vagus nerve.

rami cen·tra·les ar·te·ri·ae ce·re·bri an·te·ri·o·ris (sen·tray'leez ahr·teer'ee·ee serr'e·brye an·teer·ee·o'ris) [NA]. The central branches of the anterior cerebral artery.

rami centrales arteriae cerebri me·di·ae (mee'dee·ee) [NA]. The central branches of the middle cerebral artery.

rami centrales arteriae cerebri pos·te·ri·o·ris (pos·teer·ee·o'ris) [NA]. The central branches of the posterior cerebral artery.

rami cho·roi·dei pos·te·ri·o·res ar·te·ri·ae ce·re·bri pos·te·ri·o·ris (ko·roy'dee·eye pos·teer·ee·o'reez ahr·teer'ee·ee serr'e·brye pos·teer·ee·o'ris) [NA alt.]. RAMUS CHOROIDEUS ARTERIAE CEREBRI POSTERIORIS.

rami coe·li·a·ci ner·vi va·gi (see·lye'uh·sigh nur'vye vay'guy, ·jye) [BNA]. RAMI CELIACI NERVI VAGI.

rami com·mu·ni·can·tes (kom·yoo·ni·kan'teez) [NA]. Plural of *ramus communicans.*

rami communicantes gan·glii sub·man·di·bu·la·ris cum ner·vo lin·gua·li (gang'glee·eye sub·man·dib·yoo·lair'is kum nur'vo ling·gway'lye) [NA]. Nerve fibers connecting the submandibular ganglion with the lingual nerve.

rami communicantes ganglii sub·max·il·la·ris cum ner·vo lin·gua·li (sub·mack·si·lair'is kum nur'vo ling·gway'lye) [BNA]. RAMI COMMUNICANTES GANGLII SUBMANDIBULARE CUM NERVO LINGUALI.

rami communicantes ner·vi au·ri·cu·lo·tem·po·ra·lis cum ner·vo fa·ci·a·li (nur'vye aw·rick·yoo·lo·tem·po·ray'lis kum nur'vo fay·shee·ay'lye) [NA]. Small nerve fibers connecting the auriculotemporal and facial nerves.

rami communicantes nervi lin·gua·lis cum ner·vo hy·po·glos·so (ling·gway'lis kum nur'vo high·po·glos'o) [NA]. Small nerve fibers connecting the lingual and hypoglossal nerves.

rami communicantes ner·vo·rum spi·na·li·um (nur·vo'rum spye·nay'lee·um) [NA]. Communicating branches of the spinal nerves.

rami cor·ti·ca·les ar·te·ri·ae ce·re·bri an·te·ri·o·ris (kor·ti·kay'leez ahr·teer'ee·ee serr'e·brye an·teer·ee·o'ris) [NA]. The cortical branches of the anterior cerebral artery.

rami corticales arteriae cerebri me·di·ae (mee'dee·ee) [NA]. The cortical branches of the middle cerebral artery.

rami corticales arteriae cerebri pos·te·ri·o·ris (pos·teer·ee·o'ris) [NA]. The cortical branches of the posterior cerebral artery.

rami cu·ta·nei an·te·ri·o·res ner·vi fe·mo·ra·lis (kew·tay'nee·eye an·teer·ee·o'reez nur'vye fem·o·ray'lis) [NA]. The anterior cutaneous branches of the femoral nerve.

rami cutanei anteriores [pec·to·ra·les et ab·do·mi·na·les] ra·mo·rum an·te·ri·o·rum ar·te·ri·a·rum in·ter·cos·ta·li·um (peck·to·ray'leez et ab·dom·i·nay'leez ray·mo'rum an·teer·ee·o'rum ahr·teer·ee·air'um in·tur·kos·tay'lee·um) [BNA]. The anterior cutaneous branches of the anterior branches of the intercostal arteries.

rami cutanei ar·te·ri·ae mam·ma·ri·ae in·ter·nae (ahr·teer'ee·ee ma·mair'ee·ee in·tur'nee) [BNA]. The cutaneous branches of the internal thoracic artery.

rami cutanei cru·ris me·di·a·les ner·vi sa·phe·ni (kroo'ris mee·dee·ay'leez nur'vye sa·fee'nigh) [NA]. The medial cutaneous branches of the saphenous nerve.

rami cutanei la·te·ra·les pec·to·ra·les et ab·do·mi·na·les ra·mo·rum an·te·ri·o·rum ar·te·ri·a·rum in·ter·cos·ta·li·um (lat·e·ray'leez peck·to·ray'leez et ab·dom·i·nay'leez ray·mo'rum an·teer·ee·o'rum ahr·teer·ee·air'um in·tur·kos·tay'lee·um) [BNA]. The lateral cutaneous branches (pectoral and abdominal) of the anterior branches of the intercostal arteries.

rami den·ta·les ar·te·ri·ae al·ve·o·la·ris in·fe·ri·o·ris (den·tay'leez ahr·teer'ee·ee al·vee·o·lair'is in·feer·ee·o'ris) [NA]. The dental branches of the inferior alveolar artery.

rami dentales arteriae alveolaris su·pe·ri·o·ris pos·te·ri·o·ris (sue·peer·ee·o'ris pos·teer·ee·o'ris) [NA]. The dental branches of the superior posterior alveolar artery.

rami dentales ar·te·ri·a·rum al·ve·o·la·ri·um su·pe·ri·o·rum an·te·ri·o·rum (ahr·teer·ee·air'um al·vee·o·lair'ee·um sue·peer·ee·o'rum an·teer·ee·o'rum) [NA]. The dental branches of the anterior superior alveolar arteries.

rami dentales in·fe·ri·o·res plex·us den·ta·lis in·fe·ri·o·ris (in·feer·ee·o'reez pleck'sus den·tay'lis in·feer·ee·o'ris) [NA]. The inferior dental branches of the inferior dental plexus.

rami dentales su·pe·ri·o·res plex·us den·ta·lis su·pe·ri·o·ris (sue·peer·ee·o'reez pleck'sus den·tay'lis sue·peer·ee·o'ris) [NA]. The dental branches of the superior dental plexus.

rami dor·sa·les ar·te·ri·ae in·ter·cos·ta·lis su·pre·mae (dor·say'leez ahr·teer'ee·ee in·tur·kos·tay'lis sue·pree'mee) [NA]. The dorsal branches of the highest intercostal artery.

rami dorsales ar·te·ri·a·rum in·ter·cos·ta·li·um pos·te·ri·o·rum [III–XI] (ahr·teer·ee·air'um in·tur·kos·tay'lee·um pos·teer·ee·o'rum). Plural of *ramus dorsalis arteriarum intercostalium posteriorum [III–XI].*

rami dorsales lin·guae ar·te·ri·ae lin·gua·lis (ling'gwee ahr·teer'ee·ee ling·gway'lis) [NA]. The dorsal lingual branches of the lingual artery.

rami dorsales ner·vo·rum cer·vi·ca·li·um (nur·vo'rum sur·vi·kay'lee·um) [NA]. The dorsal branches of the cervical nerves.

rami dorsales nervorum lum·ba·li·um (lum·bay'lee·um) [NA]. The dorsal branches of the lumbar nerves.

rami dorsales nervorum sa·cra·li·um (sa·kray'lee·um) [NA]. The dorsal branches of the sacral nerves.

rami dorsales nervorum tho·ra·ci·co·rum (tho·ray·si·ko'rum) [NA]. The dorsal branches of the thoracic nerves.

rami du·o·de·na·les ar·te·ri·ae pan·cre·a·ti·co·du·o·de·na·lis su·pe·ri·o·ris (dew·o·de·nay'leez ahr·teer'ee·ee pan·kree·at''i·ko·dew·o·de·nay'lis sue·peer·ee·o'ris) [BNA]. The duodenal branches of the superior pancreaticoduodenal artery.

rami duodenales arteriae su·pra·du·o·de·na·les su·pe·ri·o·res (sue''pruh·dew·o·de·nay'leez sue·peer·ee·o'reez) [NA]. The duodenal branches of the superior supraduodenal artery.

rami epi·plo·i·ci ar·te·ri·ae gas·tro·epi·plo·i·cae dex·trae (ep·i·plo'i·sigh ahr·teer'ee·ee gas·tro·ep·i·plo'i·see decks'tree) [NA]. The epiploic branches of the right gastroepiploic artery.

rami epiploici arteriae gastroepiploicae si·nis·trae (si·nis'tree) [NA]. The epiploic branches of the left gastroepiploic artery.

rami eso·pha·gei aor·tae tho·ra·ci·cae (e·sof·uh·jee'eye ay·or'tee tho·ray'si·see) [NA]. The esophageal branches of the thoracic aorta.

rami esophagei ar·te·ri·ae gas·tri·cae si·nis·trae (ahr·teer'ee·ee gas'tri·see si·nis'tree) [NA]. The esophageal branches of the left gastric artery.

rami esophagei arteriae thy·roi·de·ae in·fe·ri·o·ris (thigh·roy'dee·ee in·feer·ee·o'ris) [NA]. The esophageal branches of the inferior thyroid artery.

rami esophagei ner·vi la·ryn·gei re·cur·ren·tis (nur'vye la·rin'jee·eye reck·ur·en'tis) [NA]. The esophageal branches of the recurrent laryngeal nerve.

ram·i·fi·ca·tion (ram''i·fi·kay'shun) *n.* 1. The act or state of branching. 2. A branch.

rami fron·ta·les ar·te·ri·ae ce·re·bri an·te·ri·o·ris (fron·tay'leez ahr·teer'ee·ee serr'e·brye an·teer·ee·o'ris) [NA]. The frontal branches of the anterior cerebral artery.

rami frontales arteriae cerebri me·di·ae (mee'dee·ee) [NA]. The frontal branches of the middle cerebral artery.

ram·i·fy (ram'i·figh) *v.* To form branches; to branch.

rami gas·tri·ci an·te·ri·o·res ner·vi va·gi (gas'tri·sigh an·teer·ee·o'reez nur'vye vay'guy, ·jye) [NA]. The anterior gastric branches of the vagus nerve.

rami gastrici ner·vi va·gi (nur'vye vay'guy, ·jye) [BNA]. The gastric branches of the vagus nerve.

rami gastrici pos·te·ri·o·res ner·vi va·gi (pos·teer·ee·o'reez nur'vye vay'guy, ·jye) [NA]. The posterior gastric branches of the vagus nerve.

rami gin·gi·va·les in·fe·ri·o·res plex·us den·ta·lis in·fe·ri·o·ris (jin·ji·vay'leez in·feer·ee·o·reez pleck'sus den·tay'lis in·feer·ee·o'ris) [NA]. The inferior gingival branches of the inferior dental plexus.

rami gingivales su·pe·ri·o·res plex·us den·ta·lis su·pe·ri·o·ris (sue·peer·ee·o'reez pleck'sus den·tay'lis sue·peer·ee·o'ris) [NA]. The superior gingival branches of the superior dental plexus.

rami glan·du·la·res ar·te·ri·ae fa·ci·a·lis (glan·dew·lair'eez ahr·teer'ee·ee fay·shee·ay'lis) [NA]. The glandular branches of the facial artery.

rami glandulares arteriae max·il·la·ris ex·ter·nae (mack·si·lair'is ecks·tur'nee) [BNA]. RAMI GLANDULARES ARTERIAE FACIALIS.

rami glandulares arteriae thy·re·oi·de·ae su·pe·ri·o·ris (thigh·ree·oy'dee·ee sue·peer·ee·o'ris) [BNA]. The glandular branches of the superior thyroid artery.

rami glandulares arteriae thy·roi·de·ae in·fe·ri·o·ris (thigh·roy'dee·ee in·feer·ee·o'ris) [NA]. The glandular branches of the inferior thyroid artery.

rami glandulares gan·glii sub·man·di·bu·la·ris (gang'glee·eye sub·man·dib·yoo·lair'is) [NA]. The glandular branches of the submandibular ganglion.

rami he·pa·ti·ci ner·vi va·gi (he·pat'i·sigh nur'vye vay'guy, ·jye) [NA]. The hepatic branches of the vagus nerve.

rami in·fe·ri·o·res ner·vi cu·ta·nei col·li (in·feer·ee·o'reez nur'vye kew·tay'nee·eye kol'eye) [BNA]. RAMI INFERIORES NERVI TRANSVERSI COLLI.

rami inferiores nervi trans·ver·si col·li (trans·vur'sigh kol'eye) [NA]. The inferior branches of the transverse nerve of the neck.

rami in·gui·na·les ar·te·ri·ae fe·mo·ra·lis (ing·gwi·nay'leez ahr·teer'ee·ee fem·o·ray'lis) [NA]. The inguinal branches of the femoral artery.

rami in·ter·cos·ta·les an·te·ri·o·res ar·te·ri·ae tho·ra·ci·cae in·ter·nae (in·tur·kos·tay'leez an·teer·ee·o'reez ahr·teer'ee·ee tho·ray'si·see in·tur'nee) [NA]. The anterior intercostal branches of the internal thoracic artery.

rami intercostales ar·te·ri·ae mam·ma·ri·ae in·ter·nae (ahr·teer'ee·ee ma·mair'ee·ee in·tur'nee) [BNA]. RAMI INTERCOSTALES ANTERIORES ARTERIAE THORACICAE INTERNAE.

rami in·ter·gan·gli·o·na·res (in·tur·gang''glee·o·nair'eez) [NA]. A general term for nerve fibers running from one sympathetic ganglion to another.

rami isth·mi fau·ci·um ner·vi lin·gua·lis (ist'migh faw'see·um nur'vye ling·gway'lis) [NA]. The branches of the lingual nerve to the isthmus of the fauces.

rami la·bi·a·les an·te·ri·o·res ar·te·ri·ae fe·mo·ra·lis (lay·bee·ay'leez an·teer·ee·o'reez ahr·teer'ee·ee fem·o·ray'lis) [NA]. The anterior labial branches of the femoral artery.

rami labiales in·fe·ri·o·res ner·vi men·ta·lis (in·feer·ee·o'reez nur'vye men·tay'lis) [NA]. The inferior labial branches of the mental nerve.

rami labiales pos·te·ri·o·res ar·te·ri·ae pu·den·dae in·ter·nae (pos·teer·ee·o'reez ahr·teer'ee·ee pew·den'dee in·tur'nee) [NA]. The posterior labial branches of the internal pudendal artery.

rami labiales su·pe·ri·o·res ner·vi in·fra·or·bi·ta·lis (sue·peer·ee·o'reez nur'vye in·fruh·or·bi·tay'lis) [NA]. The superior labial branches of the infraorbital nerve.

rami la·ryn·go·pha·ryn·gei gan·glii cer·vi·ca·lis su·pe·ri·us (la·ring''go·fa·rin'jee·eye gang'glee·eye sur·vi·kay'lis sue·peer'ee·us) [NA]. The laryngopharyngeal branches of the superior cervical ganglion.

rami laryngopharyngei ner·vi sym·pa·thi·ci (nur'vye sim·path'i·sigh) [BNA]. RAMI LARYNGOPHARYNGEI GANGLII CERVICALIS SUPERIUS.

rami li·e·na·les ar·te·ri·ae li·e·na·lis (lye·e·nay'leez ahr·teer'ee·ee lye·e·nay'lis) [NA]. The splenic branches of the splenic artery.

rami lienales ner·vi va·gi (nur'vye vay'guy, ·jye) [BNA]. The splenic branches of the vagus nerve.

rami lin·gua·les ner·vi glos·so·pha·ryn·gei (ling·gway'leez nur'vye glos·o·fa·rin'jee·eye) [NA]. The lingual branches of the glossopharyngeal nerve.

rami linguales nervi hy·po·glos·si (high·po·glos'eye) [NA]. The lingual branches of the hypoglossal nerve.

rami linguales nervi lin·gua·lis (ling·gway'lis) [NA]. The lingual branches of the lingual nerve.

rami mal·le·o·la·res la·te·ra·les ar·te·ri·ae fi·bu·la·ris (mal·ee·o·lair'eez lat·e·ray'leez ahr·teer'ee·ee fib·yoo·lair'is) [NA alt.]. RAMI MALLEOLARES LATERALES ARTERIAE PERONEAE.

rami malleolares laterales arteriae pe·ro·ne·ae (perr·o·nee'ee) [NA]. The lateral malleolar branches of the peroneal artery. NA alt. *rami malleolares laterales arteriae fibularis.*

rami malleolares me·di·a·les ar·te·ri·ae ti·bi·a·lis pos·te·ri·o·ris (mee·dee·ay'leez ahr·teer'ee·ee tib·ee·ay'lis pos·teer·ee·o'ris) [NA]. The medial malleolar branches of the posterior tibial artery.

rami mammarii ar·te·ri·ae mam·ma·ri·ae in·ter·nae (ahr·teer'ee·ee ma·mair'ee·ee in·tur'nee) [BNA]. RAMI MAMMARII ARTERIAE THORACICAE INTERNAE.

rami mammarii arteriae tho·ra·ci·cae in·ter·nae (tho·ray'si·see in·tur'nee) [NA]. The mammary branches of the internal thoracic artery.

rami mammarii ar·te·ri·a·rum in·ter·cos·ta·li·um pos·te·ri·o·ri·um [III-XI] (ahr·teer″ee·air′um in·tur·kos·tay′lee·um pos·teer·ee·o′ree·um) [NA]. The mammary branches of the posterior intercostal arteries.

rami mammarii ex·ter·ni ar·te·ri·ae tho·ra·ca·lis la·te·ra·lis (ecks·tur′nigh ahr·teer′ee·ee tho·ruh·kay′lis lat·e·ray′lis) [BNA]. RAMI MAMMARII LATERALES ARTERIAE THORACICAE LATERALIS.

rami mammarii la·te·ra·les ar·te·ri·ae tho·ra·ci·cae la·te·ra·lis (lat·e·ray′leez ahr·teer′ee·ee tho·ray′si·see lat·e·ray′lis) [NA]. The lateral mammary branches of the lateral thoracic artery.

rami mammarii laterales ner·vo·rum in·ter·cos·ta·li·um (nur·vo′rum in·tur·kos·tay′lee·um) [BNA]. The lateral mammary branches of the intercostal nerves.

rami mammarii laterales nervorum tho·ra·ci·co·rum (tho·ray·si·ko′rum) [NA]. The lateral mammary branches of the thoracic nerves.

rami mammarii laterales ra·mo·rum cu·ta·ne·o·rum la·te·ra·li·um ra·mo·rum an·te·ri·o·rum ar·te·ri·a·rum in·ter·cos·ta·li·um (ray·mo′rum kew·tay·nee·o′rum lat·e·ray′lee·um ray·mo′rum an·teer·ee·o′rum ahr·teer·ee·air′um in·tur·kos·tay′lee·um) [BNA]. The lateral mammary branches of the lateral cutaneous branches of the anterior branches of the anterior intercostal arteries.

rami mammarii me·di·a·les ar·te·ri·a·rum in·ter·cos·ta·li·um (mee·dee·ay′leez ahr·teer·ee·air′um in·tur·kos·tay′lee·um) [BNA]. The medial mammary branches of the intercostal arteries.

rami mammarii mediales ner·vo·rum in·ter·cos·ta·li·um (nur·vo′rum in·tur·kos·tay′lee·um) [BNA]. The medial mammary branches of the intercostal nerves.

rami mammarii mediales nervorum tho·ra·ci·co·rum (tho·ray·si·ko′rum) [NA]. The medial mammary branches of the thoracic nerves.

rami ma·stoi·dei ar·te·ri·ae au·ri·cu·la·ris pos·te·ri·o·ris (mas·toy′dee·eye ahr·teer′ee·ee aw·rick·yoo·lair′is pos·teer·ee·o′ris) [NA]. The mastoid branches of the posterior auricular artery.

rami mastoidei arteriae sty·lo·ma·stoi·de·ae (stye·lo·mas·toy′dee·ee) [BNA]. The mastoid branches of the stylomastoid artery.

rami me·di·as·ti·na·les aor·tae tho·ra·ca·lis (mee·dee·as·ti·nay′leez ay·or′tee tho·ra·kay′lis) [BNA]. RAMI MEDIASTINALES AORTAE THORACICAE.

rami mediastinales aortae tho·ra·ci·cae (tho·ray′si·see) [NA]. The mediastinal branches of the thoracic aorta.

rami mediastinales aortae thoracicae in·ter·nae (in·tur′nee) [NA]. The mediastinal branches of the internal thoracic artery.

rami men·ta·les ner·vi men·ta·lis (men·tay′leez nur′vye men·tay′lis) [NA]. The mental branches of the mental nerve.

rami mus·cu·la·res ar·te·ri·ae cer·vi·ca·lis ascen·den·tis (mus·kew·lair′eez ahr·teer′ee·ee sur·vi·kay′lis a·sen·den′tis) [BNA]. The muscular branches of the ascending cervical artery.

rami musculares arteriae fe·mo·ra·lis (fem·o·ray′lis) [BNA]. The muscular branches of the femoral artery.

rami musculares arteriae ge·nu su·pre·mae (jee′new sue·pree′mee) [BNA]. The muscular branches of the highest genicular artery.

rami musculares arteriae oc·ci·pi·ta·lis (ock·sip·i·tay′lis) [BNA]. RAMI STERNOCLEIDOMASTOIDEI ARTERIAE OCCIPITALIS.

rami musculares arteriae oph·thal·mi·cae (off·thal′mi·see) [BNA]. The muscular branches of the ophthalmic artery.

rami musculares arteriae ra·di·a·lis (ray·dee·ay′lis) [BNA]. The muscular branches of the radial artery.

rami musculares arteriae ul·na·ris (ul·nair′is) [BNA]. The muscular branches of the ulnar artery.

rami musculares ner·vi ax·il·la·ris (nur′vye ack·si·lair′is) [NA]. The muscular branches of the axillary nerve.

rami musculares nervi fe·mo·ra·lis (fem·o·ray′lis) [NA]. The muscular branches of the femoral nerve.

rami musculares nervi fi·bu·la·ris pro·fun·dus (fib·yoo·lair′is pro·fun′dus) [NA alt.]. RAMI MUSCULARES NERVI PERONEI PROFUNDI.

rami musculares nervi fibularis su·per·fi·ci·a·lis (sue·pur·fish·ee·ay′lis) [NA alt.]. RAMI MUSCULARES NERVI PERONEI SUPERFICIALIS.

rami musculares nervi ilio·hy·po·gas·tri·ci (il″ee·o·high·po·gas′tri·sigh) [BNA]. The muscular branches of the iliohypogastric nerve.

rami musculares nervi ilio·in·gui·na·lis (il″ee·o·ing·gwi·nay′lis) [BNA]. The muscular branches of the ilioinguinal nerve.

rami musculares nervi is·chi·a·di·ci (is·kee·ad′i·sigh) [BNA]. The muscular branches of the sciatic nerve.

rami musculares nervi me·di·a·ni (mee·dee·ay′nigh) [NA]. The muscular branches of the median nerve.

rami musculares nervi mus·cu·lo·cu·ta·nei (mus·kew·lo·kew·tay′nee·eye) [NA]. The muscular branches of the musculocutaneous nerve.

rami musculares nervi ob·tu·ra·to·rii (ob·tew·ruh·to′ree·eye) [NA]. The muscular branches of the obturator nerve.

rami musculares nervi pe·ro·naei com·mu·nis (perr·o·nee′eye kom·yoo′nis) [BNA]. The muscular branches of the common peroneal nerve.

rami musculares nervi peronaei pro·fun·di (pro·fun′dye) [BNA]. RAMI MUSCULARES NERVI PERONEI PROFUNDI.

rami musculares nervi peronaei su·per·fi·ci·a·lis (sue·pur·fish·ee·ay′lis) [BNA]. RAMI MUSCULARES NERVI PERONEI SUPERFICIALIS.

rami musculares nervi pe·ro·nei pro·fun·di (perr·o·nee′eye pro·fun′dye) [NA]. The muscular branches of the deep peroneal nerve. NA alt. *rami musculares nervi fibularis profundus.*

rami musculares nervi peronei su·per·fi·ci·a·lis (sue·pur·fish·ee·ay′lis) [NA]. The muscular branches of the superficial peroneal nerve. NA alt. *rami musculares nervi fibularis superficialis.*

rami musculares nervi ra·di·a·lis (ray·dee·ay′lis) [NA]. The muscular branches of the radial nerve.

rami musculares nervi ti·bi·a·lis (tib·ee·ay′lis) [NA]. The muscular branches of the tibial nerve.

rami musculares nervi ul·na·ris (ul·nair′is) [NA]. The muscular branches of the ulnar nerve.

rami musculares ner·vo·rum in·ter·cos·ta·li·um (nur·vo′rum in·tur·kos·tay′lee·um) [BNA]. The muscular branches of the intercostal nerves.

rami musculares plex·us lum·ba·lis (pleck′sus lum·bay′lis) [BNA]. The muscular branches of the lumbar plexus.

rami musculares ra·mo·rum an·te·ri·o·rum ar·te·ri·a·rum in·ter·cos·ta·li·um (ray·mo′rum an·teer·ee·o′rum ahr·teer·ee·air′um in·tur·kos·tay′lee·um) [BNA]. The muscular branches of the anterior branches of the intercostal arteries.

rami musculares ramorum pos·te·ri·o·rum ar·te·ri·a·rum in·ter·cos·ta·li·um (pos·teer·ee·o′rum ahr·teer·ee·air′um in·tur·kos·tay′lee·um) [BNA]. The muscular branches of the posterior branches of the intercostal arteries.

rami na·sa·les an·te·ri·o·res ner·vi eth·moi·da·lis an·te·ri·o·ris (nay·say′leez an·teer·ee·o′reez nur′vye eth·moy·day′lis an·teer·ee·o′ris) [BNA]. RAMI NASALES NERVI ETHMOIDALIS ANTERIORIS.

rami nasales ex·ter·ni ner·vi in·fra·or·bi·ta·lis (ecks·tur′nigh nur′vye in·fra·or·bi·tay′lis) [NA]. The external nasal branches of the infraorbital nerve.

rami nasales in·ter·ni ner·vi eth·moi·da·lis an·te·ri·o·ris (in·tur′nigh nur′vye eth·moy·day′lis an·teer·ee·o′ris) [NA]. The internal nasal branches of the anterior ethmoid nerve.

rami nasales interni nervi in·fra·or·bi·ta·lis (in·tur′nigh nur′vye in·fra·or·bi·tay′lis) [NA]. The internal nasal branches of the infraorbital nerve.

rami nasales la·te·ra·les ner·vi eth·moi·da·lis an·te·ri·o·ris (lat·e·ray'leez nur'vye eth·moy·day'lis an·teer·ee·o'ris) [NA]. The lateral nasal branches of the anterior ethmoid nerve.

rami nasales me·di·a·les ner·vi eth·moi·da·lis an·te·ri·o·ris (mee·dee·ay'leez nur'vye eth·moy·day'lis an·teer·ee·o'ris) [NA]. The medial nasal branches of the anterior ethmoid nerve.

rami nasales ner·vi eth·moi·da·lis an·te·ri·o·ris (nur'vye eth·moy·day'lis an·teer·ee·o'ris) [NA]. A general term for all the nasal branches of the anterior ethmoid nerve.

rami nasales pos·te·ri·o·res in·fe·ri·o·res la·te·ra·les gan·glii pte·ry·go·pa·la·ti·ni (pos·teer·ee·o'reez in·feer·ee·o'reez lat·e·ray'leez gang'glee·eye terr·i·go·pal·uh·tye'nigh) [NA]. The posterior inferior nasal branches of the pterygopalatine ganglion.

rami nasales posteriores inferiores [laterales] ner·vi pa·la·ti·ni an·te·ri·o·ris (nur'vye pal·uh·tye'nigh an·teer·ee·o'ris) [BNA]. RAMI NASALES POSTERIORES INFERIORES LATERALES GANGLII PTERYGOPALATINI.

rami nasales posteriores su·pe·ri·o·res la·te·ra·les gan·glii pte·ry·go·pa·la·ti·ni (sue·peer·ee·o'reez lat·e·ray'leez gang'glee·eye terr·i·go·pal·uh·tye'nigh) [NA]. The posterior superior lateral nasal branches of the pterygopalatine ganglion.

rami nasales posteriores superiores laterales ganglii sphe·no·pa·la·ti·ni (sfee·no·pal·uh·tye'nigh) [BNA]. RAMI NASALES POSTERIORES SUPERIORES LATERALES GANGLII PTERYGOPALATINI.

rami nasales posteriores superiores me·di·a·les gan·glii pte·ry·go·pa·la·ti·ni (mee·dee·ay'leez gang'glee·eye terr·i·go·pal·uh·tye'nigh) [NA]. The posterior superior medial nasal branches of the pterygopalatine ganglion.

rami nasales posteriores superiores mediales ganglii sphe·no·pa·la·ti·ni (sfee·no·pal·uh·tye'nigh) [BNA]. RAMI NASALES POSTERIORES SUPERIORES MEDIALES GANGLII PTERYGOPALATINI.

rami oc·ci·pi·ta·les ar·te·ri·ae ce·re·bri pos·te·ri·o·ris (ock·sip·i·tay'leez ahr·teer'ee·ee serr'e·brye pos·teer·ee·o'ris) [NA]. The occipital branches of the posterior cerebral artery.

rami occipitales arteriae oc·ci·pi·ta·lis (ock·sip·i·tay'lis) [NA]. The occipital branches of the occipital artery.

rami oe·so·pha·gei aor·tae tho·ra·ca·lis (e·sof·uh·jee'eye ay·or'tee tho·ruh·kay'lis) [BNA]. RAMI ESOPHAGEI AORTAE THORACICAE.

rami oesophagei ar·te·ri·ae gas·tri·cae si·nis·trae (ahr·teer'ee·ee gas'tri·see si·nis'tree) [BNA]. RAMI ESOPHAGEI ARTERIAE GASTRICAE SINISTRAE.

rami oesophagei ner·vi re·cur·ren·tis (nur'vye reck·ur·en'tis) [BNA]. RAMI ESOPHAGEI NERVI LARYNGEI RECURRENTIS.

rami oesophagei nervi va·gi (vay'gye) [BNA]. RAMI ESOPHAGEI NERVI LARYNGEI RECURRENTIS.

rami or·bi·ta·les ar·te·ri·ae ce·re·bri an·te·ri·o·ris (or·bi·tay'leez ahr·teer'ee·ee serr'e·brye an·teer·ee·o'ris) [NA]. The orbital branches of the anterior cerebral artery.

rami orbitales arteriae cerebri me·di·ae (mee'dee·ee) [NA]. The orbital branches of the middle cerebral artery.

rami orbitales gan·glii pte·ry·go·pa·la·ti·ni (gang'glee·eye terr·i·go·pal·uh·tye'nigh) [NA]. The orbital branches of the pterygopalatine ganglion.

rami orbitales ganglii sphe·no·pa·la·ti·ni (sfee·no·pal·uh·tye'nigh) [BNA]. RAMI ORBITALES GANGLII PTERYGOPALATINI.

rami pal·pe·bra·les in·fe·ri·o·res ner·vi in·fra·or·bi·ta·lis (pal·pe·bray'leez in·feer·ee·o'reez nur'vye in·fruh·or·bi·tay'lis) [NA]. The inferior palpebral branches of the infraorbital nerve.

rami palpebrales ner·vi in·fra·troch·le·a·ris (nur'vye in·fruh·trock·lee·air'is) [NA]. The palpebral branches of the infratrochlear nerve.

rami pan·cre·a·ti·ci ar·te·ri·ae li·e·na·lis (pan·kree·at'i·sigh ahr·teer'ee·ee lye·e·nay'lis) [NA]. The pancreatic branches of the splenic artery.

rami pancreatici arteriae pan·cre·a·ti·co·du·o·de·na·lis su·pe·ri·o·ris (pan·kree·at''i·ko·dew·o·de·nay'lis sue·peer·ee·o'ris) [BNA]. The pancreatic branches of the superior pancreaticoduodenal artery.

rami pancreatici arteriae su·pra·du·o·de·na·les su·pe·ri·o·res (sue''pruh·dew·o·de·nay'leez sue·peer·ee·o'reez) [NA]. The pancreatic branches of the supraduodenal artery.

rami pa·ri·e·ta·les aor·tae ab·do·mi·na·lis (pa·rye·e·tay'leez ay·or'tee ab·dom·i·nay'lis) [BNA]. The parietal branches of the abdominal aorta.

rami parietales aortae tho·ra·ca·lis (tho·ra·kay'lis) [BNA]. The parietal branches of the thoracic aorta.

rami parietales ar·te·ri·ae ce·re·bri an·te·ri·o·ris (ahr·teer'ee·ee serr'e·brye an·teer·ee·o'ris) [NA]. The parietal branches of the anterior cerebral artery.

rami parietales arteriae cerebri me·di·ae (mee'dee·ee) [NA]. The parietal branches of the middle cerebral artery.

rami parietales arteriae hy·po·gas·tri·cae (high·po·gas'tri·see) [BNA]. The parietal branches of the hypogastric artery.

rami pa·ro·ti·dei ar·te·ri·ae tem·po·ra·lis su·per·fi·ci·a·lis (pa·rot·i·dee'eye ahr·teer'ee·ee tem·po·ray'lis su·pur·fish·ee·ay'lis) [NA]. The parotid branches of the superficial temporal artery.

rami parotidei ner·vi au·ri·cu·lo·tem·po·ra·lis (nur'vye aw·rick''yoo·lo·tem·po·ray'lis) [NA]. The parotid branches of the auriculotemporal nerve.

rami parotidei ve·nae fa·ci·a·lis (vee'nee fay·shee·ay'lis) [NA]. The parotid tributaries to the facial vein.

rami pec·to·ra·les ar·te·ri·ae tho·ra·co·acro·mi·a·lis (peck·to·ray'leez ahr·teer'ee·ee tho·ra·ko·a·kro·mee·ay'lis) [NA]. The pectoral branches of the thoracoacromial artery.

rami perforantes arteriae mam·ma·ri·ae in·ter·nae (ma·mair'ee·ee in·tur'nee) [BNA]. RAMI PERFORANTES ARTERIAE THORACICAE INTERNAE.

rami perforantes arteriae tho·ra·ci·cae in·ter·nae (tho·ray'si·see in·tur'nee) [NA]. The perforating branches of the internal thoracic artery.

rami per·fo·ran·tes ar·te·ri·a·rum me·ta·car·pa·li·um vo·la·ri·um (pur·fo·ran'teez ahr·teer·ee·air'um met·uh·kahr·pay'lee·um vo·lair'ee·um) [BNA]. RAMI PERFORANTES ARTERIARUM METACARPEARUM PALMARIUM.

rami perforantes arteriarum me·ta·car·pe·a·rum pal·ma·ri·um (met·uh·kahr·pee·air'um pal·mair'ee·um) [NA]. The perforating branches of the palmar metacarpal arteries.

rami perforantes arteriarum me·ta·tar·sa·li·um plan·ta·ri·um (met·uh·tahr·say'lee·um plan·tair'ee·um) [BNA]. RAMI PERFORANTES ARTERIARUM METATARSEARUM PLANTARIUM.

rami perforantes arteriarum me·ta·tar·se·a·rum plan·ta·ri·um (met·uh·tahr·see·air'um plan·tair'ee·um) [NA]. The perforating branches of the plantar metatarsal arteries.

rami pe·ri·car·di·a·ci aor·tae tho·ra·ca·lis (perr·i·kahr·dye'uh·sigh ay·or'tee tho·ra·kay'lis) [BNA]. RAMI PERICARDIACI AORTAE THORACICAE.

rami pericardiaci aortae tho·ra·ci·cae (tho·ray'si·see) [NA]. The pericardial branches of the thoracic aorta.

rami pe·ri·ne·a·les ner·vi cu·ta·nei fe·mo·ris pos·te·ri·o·ris (perr·i·nee·ay'leez nur'vye kew·tay'nee·eye fem'o·ris pos·teer·ee·o'ris) [NA]. The perineal branches of the posterior femoral cutaneous nerve.

rami pha·ryn·gei ar·te·ri·ae pha·ryn·ge·ae ascen·den·tis (fa·rin'jee·eye ahr·teer'ee·ee fa·rin'ji·ee a·sen·den'tis) [NA]. The pharyngeal branches of the ascending pharyngeal artery.

rami pharyngei arteriae thy·roi·de·ae in·fe·ri·o·ris (thigh·roy'dee·ee in·feer·ee·o'ris) [NA]. The pharyngeal branches of the inferior thyroid artery.

rami pharyngei ner·vi glos·so·pha·ryn·gei (nur'vye glos·o·fa·rin'jee·eye) [NA]. The pharyngeal branches of the glossopharyngeal nerve.

rami pharyngei nervi va·gi (vay'guy, vay'jye) [NA]. The pharyngeal branches of the vagus nerve.

rami phre·ni·co·ab·do·mi·na·les ner·vi phre·ni·ci (fren''i·ko·ab·

dom·i·nay'leez nur'vye fren'i·sigh) [NA]. The phrenicoabdominal branches of the phrenic nerve.

rami pos·te·ri·o·res ar·te·ri·a·rum in·ter·cos·ta·li·um (pos·teer·ee·o'reez ahr·teer·ee·ay'rum in·tur·kos·tay'lee·um) [BNA]. RAMI DORSALES ARTERIARUM INTERCOSTALIUM POSTERIORUM [III–XI].

rami posteriores ner·vo·rum cer·vi·ca·li·um (nur·vo'rum sur·vi·kay'lee·um) [BNA]. RAMI DORSALES NERVORUM CERVICALIUM.

rami posteriores nervorum sa·cra·li·um (sa·kray'lee·um) [BNA]. RAMI DORSALES NERVORUM SACRALIUM.

rami posteriores nervorum tho·ra·ca·li·um (tho·ra·kay'lee·um) [BNA]. RAMI DORSALES NERVORUM THORACICORUM.

rami pte·ry·goi·dei ar·te·ri·ae max·il·la·ris (terr·i·goy'dee·eye ahr·teer'ee·ee mack·si·lair'is) [NA]. The pterygoid branches of the maxillary artery.

rami pterygoidei arteriae maxillaris in·ter·nae (in·tur'nee) [BNA]. RAMI PTERYGOIDEI ARTERIAE MAXILLARIS.

rami pul·mo·na·les sy·ste·ma·tis au·to·no·mi·ci (pul·mo·nay'leez sis·tee'ma·tis aw·to·nom'i·sigh) [NA]. The pulmonary branches of the autonomic nervous system.

rami pulmonales systematis sym·pa·thi·ci (sim·path'i·sigh) [BNA]. RAMI PULMONALES SYSTEMATIS AUTONOMICI.

rami re·na·les ner·vi va·gi (ree·nay'leez nur'vye vay'guy, ·jye) [NA]. The renal branches of the vagus nerve.

rami scro·ta·les an·te·ri·o·res ar·te·ri·ae fe·mo·ra·lis (skro·tay'leez an·teer·ee·o'reez ahr·teer'ee·ee fem·o·ray'lis) [NA]. The anterior scrotal branches of the femoral artery.

rami scrotales pos·te·ri·o·res ar·te·ri·ae pu·den·dae in·ter·nae (pos·teer·ee·o'reez ahr·teer'ee·ee pew·den'dee in·tur'nee) [NA]. The posterior scrotal branches of the internal pudendal artery.

rami·sec·tion (ram''i·seck'shun) *n.* [*rami* + *section*]. Surgical division of the rami communicantes of the sympathetic nervous system.

rami·sec·to·my (ram''i·seck'tuh·mee) *n.* RAMISECTION.

rami spi·na·les ar·te·ri·ae cer·vi·ca·lis ascen·den·tis (spye·nay'leez ahr·teer'ee·ee sur·vi·kay'lis a·sen·den'tis) [NA]. The spinal branches of the ascending cervical artery.

rami spinales arteriae ilio·lum·ba·lis (il·ee·o·lum·bay'lis) [NA]. The spinal branches of the iliolumbar artery.

rami spinales arteriae in·ter·cos·ta·lis su·pre·mae (in·tur·kos·tay'lis sue·pree'mee) [NA]. The spinal branches of the highest intercostal artery.

rami spinales arteriae ver·te·bra·lis (vur·te·bray'lis) [NA]. The spinal branches of the vertebral artery.

rami ster·na·les ar·te·ri·ae mam·ma·ri·ae in·ter·nae (stur·nay'leez ahr·teer'ee·ee ma·mair'ee·ee in·tur'nee) [BNA]. RAMI STERNALES ARTERIAE THORACICAE INTERNAE.

rami sternales arteriae tho·ra·ci·cae in·ter·nae (tho·ray'si·see in·tur'nee) [NA]. The sternal branches of the internal thoracic artery.

rami ster·no·clei·do·mas·toi·dei ar·te·ri·ae oc·ci·pi·ta·lis (stur·no·klye·do·mas·toy'dee·eye ahr·teer'ee·ee ock·sip·i·tay'lis) [NA]. The sternocleidomastoid branches of the occipital artery.

rami stri·a·ti ar·te·ri·ae ce·re·bri me·di·ae (strye·ay'tye ahr·teer'ee·ee serr'e·brye mee'dee·ee) [NA]. The striate branches of the middle cerebral artery.

rami sub·max·il·la·res gan·glii sub·max·il·la·ris (sub·mack·si·lair'eez gang'glee·eye sub·mack·si·lair'is) [BNA]. RAMI GLANDULARES GANGLII SUBMANDIBULARIS.

rami sub·sca·pu·la·res ar·te·ri·ae ax·il·la·ris (sub·skap·yoo·lair'eez ahr·teer'ee·ee ack·si·lair'is) [NA]. The subscapular branches of the axillary artery.

rami su·pe·ri·o·res ner·vi cu·ta·nei col·li (sue·peer·ee·o'reez nur'vye kew·tay'nee·eye kol'eye) [BNA]. RAMI SUPERIORES NERVI TRANSVERSI COLLI.

rami superiores nervi trans·ver·si col·li (trans·vur'sigh kol'eye) [NA]. The superior branches of the transverse nerve of the neck.

rami su·pra·re·na·les su·pe·ri·o·res ar·te·ri·ae phre·ni·cae in·fe·ri·o·ris (sue·pruh·re·nay'leez sue·peer·ee·o'reez ahr·teer'ee·ee fren'i·see in·feer·ee·o'ris) [BNA]. ARTERIA SUPRARENALIS SUPERIOR.

rami tem·po·ra·les ar·te·ri·ae ce·re·bri me·di·ae (tem·po·ray'leez ahr·teer'ee·ee serr'e·brye mee'dee·ee) [NA]. The temporal branches of the middle cerebral artery.

rami temporales arteriae cerebri pos·te·ri·o·ris (pos·teer·ee·o'ris) [NA]. The temporal branches of the posterior cerebral artery.

rami temporales ner·vi fa·ci·a·lis (nur'vye fay·shee·ay'lis) [NA]. The temporal branches of the facial nerve.

rami temporales su·per·fi·ci·a·les ner·vi au·ri·cu·lo·tem·po·ra·lis (sue·pur·fish·ee·ay'lis nur'vye aw·rick''yoo·lo·tem·po·ray'lis) [NA]. The superficial temporal branches of the auriculotemporal nerve.

rami thy·mi·ci ar·te·ri·ae tho·ra·ci·cae in·ter·nae (thigh'mi·see ahr·teer'ee·ee tho·ray'si·see in·tur'nee) [NA]. The thymic branches of the internal thoracic artery.

rami ton·sil·la·res ner·vi glos·so·pha·ryn·gei (ton·si·lair'eez nur'vye glos·o·fa·rin'jee·eye) [NA]. The tonsillar branches of the glossopharyngeal nerve.

rami tracheales arteriae thy·roi·de·ae in·fe·ri·o·ris (thigh·roy'dee·ee in·feer·ee·o'ris) [NA]. The tracheal branches of the inferior thyroid artery.

rami tracheales ner·vi la·ryn·gei re·cur·ren·tis (nur'vye la·rin'jee·eye reck·ur·en'tis) [NA]. The tracheal branches of the recurrent laryngeal nerve.

rami tracheales nervi re·cur·ren·tis (reck·ur·en'tis) [BNA]. RAMI TRACHEALES NERVI LARYNGEI RECURRENTIS.

rami ure·te·ri·ci ar·te·ri·ae duc·tus de·fe·ren·tis (yoo·re·terr'i·sigh ahr·teer'ee·ee duck'tus def·e·ren'tis) [NA]. The ureteric branches of the artery of the ductus deferens.

rami ureterici arteriae ova·ri·cae (o·vair'i·see) [NA]. The ureteric branches of the ovarian artery.

rami ureterici arteriae re·na·lis (ree·nay'lis) [NA]. The ureteric branches of the renal artery.

rami ureterici arteriae tes·ti·cu·la·ris (tes·tick·yoo·lair'is) [NA]. The ureteric branches of the testicular artery.

rami ven·tra·les ner·vo·rum cer·vi·ca·li·um (ven·tray'leez nur·vo'rum sur·vi·kay'lee·um) [NA]. The ventral branches of the cervical nerves.

rami ventrales nervorum lum·ba·li·um (lum·bay'lee·um) [NA]. The ventral branches of the lumbar nerves.

rami ventrales nervorum sa·cra·li·um (sa·kray'lee·um) [NA]. The ventral branches of the sacral nerves.

rami ventrales nervorum tho·ra·ci·co·rum (tho·ray·si·ko'rum) [NA]. The ventral branches of the thoracic nerves; INTERCOSTAL NERVES. NA alt. *nervi intercostales.*

rami ves·ti·bu·la·res ar·te·ri·ae au·di·ti·vae in·ter·nae (ves·tib·yoo·lair'eez ahr·teer'ee·ee aw·di·tye'vee in·tur'nee) [BNA]. RAMI VESTIBULARES ARTERIAE LABYRINTHI.

rami vestibulares arteriae la·by·rin·thi (lab·i·rin'thigh) [NA]. The vestibular branches of the labyrinthine artery.

rami vis·ce·ra·les aor·tae ab·do·mi·na·lis (vis·e·ray'leez ay·or'tee ab·dom·i·nay'lis) [BNA]. The visceral branches of the abdominal aorta.

rami viscerales aortae tho·ra·ca·lis (tho·ra·kay'lis) [BNA]. The visceral branches of the thoracic aorta.

rami viscerales ar·te·ri·ae hy·po·gas·tri·cae (ahr·teer'ee·ee high·po·gas'tri·sigh) [BNA]. The visceral branches of the hypogastric artery.

rami zy·go·ma·ti·ci ner·vi fa·ci·a·lis (zye·go·mat'i·sigh nur'vye fay·shee·ay'lis) [NA]. The zygomatic branches of the facial nerve.

ra·mose (ray'moce) *adj.* [L. *ramosus,* from *ramus,* branch]. Having many branches; branching.

ra·mous (ray'mus) *adj.* [L. *ram*us, branch, + *-ous*]. Having many branches; branching.

Ram·say Hunt syndrome [J. *Ramsay Hunt*]. 1. Facial paralysis of lower motor neuron type associated with a painful vesicular eruption in the external auditory canal and other parts of the cranial integument and often with affection of the eighth cranial nerve. This disorder was presumed by Hunt to be due to herpes zoster of the geniculate ganglion. Syn. *geniculate herpes.* 2. DYSSYNERGIA CEREBELLARIS PROGRESSIVA. 3. DYSSYNERGIA CEREBELLARIS MYOCLONICA.

Rams·den ocular [J. *Ramsden,* British optician, 1735–1800]. A positive ocular with two planoconvex lenses, the convex sides facing each other; used in micrometry.

Ram·stedt operation (rahm′shtet) [C. *Ramstedt,* German surgeon, b. 1867]. PYLOROMYOTOMY.

ra·mu·lus (ram′yoo·lus, ray′mew·lus) *n.,* pl. **ramu·li** (·lye) [L., dim. of *ramus,* branch]. A small branch, or ramus.

ra·mus (ray′mus) *n.,* pl. & genit. sing. **ra·mi** (·migh) [L.]. 1. A branch, especially of a vein, artery, or nerve. 2. A process of bone projecting like a branch or twig from a large bone, as the ramus of the lower jaw, or the superior or inferior ramus of the pubis.

ramus ace·ta·bu·la·ris ar·te·ri·ae cir·cum·flex·ae fe·mo·ris me·di·a·lis (as·e·tab·yoo·lair′is ahr·teer′ee·ee sur·kum·fleck′see fem′o·ris mee·dee·ay′lis) [NA]. The acetabular branch of the medial femoral circumflex artery.

ramus acetabularis arteriae ob·tu·ra·to·ri·ae (ob·tew·ruh·to′ree·ee) [NA]. The acetabular branch of the obturator artery.

ramus ace·ta·bu·li ar·te·ri·ae cir·cum·flex·ae fe·mo·ris me·di·a·lis (as·e·tab′yoo·lye ahr·teer′ee·ee sur·kum·fleck′see fem′o·ris mee·dee·ay′lis) [BNA]. RAMUS ACETABULARIS ARTERIAE CIRCUMFLEXAE FEMORIS MEDIALIS.

ramus acro·mi·a·lis ar·te·ri·ae su·pra·sca·pu·la·ris (a·kro·mee·ay′lis ahr·teer′ee·ee sue·pruh·skap·yoo·lair′is) [NA]. The acromial branch of the suprascapular artery.

ramus acromialis arteriae tho·ra·co·acro·mi·a·lis (tho″ruh·ko·a·kro·mee·ay′lis) [NA]. The acromial branch of the thoracoacromial artery.

ramus acromialis arteriae trans·ver·sae sca·pu·lae (trans·vur′see skap′yoo·lee) [BNA]. RAMUS ACROMIALIS ARTERIAE SUPRASCAPULARIS.

ramus al·ve·o·la·ris su·pe·ri·or me·di·us ner·vi in·fra·or·bi·ta·lis (al·vee·o·lair′is sue·peer′ee·or mee′dee·us nur′vye in·fruh·or·bi·tay′lis) [NA]. The middle superior alveolar branch of the infraorbital nerve; the middle superior alveolar nerve. See Table of Nerves in the Appendix.

ramus anas·to·mo·ti·cus (a·nas·to·mot″i·kus) [BNA]. A communicating branch between two arteries.

ramus anastomoticus ar·te·ri·ae me·nin·ge·ae me·di·ae cum ar·te·ria la·cri·ma·li (ahr·teer′ee·ee me·nin′jee·ee mee′dee·ee kum ahr·teer′ee·uh lack·ri·may′lye) [NA]. An anastomatic branch from the middle meningeal artery to the lacrimal artery.

ramus anastomoticus gan·glii oti·ci cum chor·da tym·pa·ni (gang′glee·eye o′ti·sigh kum kor′duh tim′puh·nigh) [BNA]. RAMUS COMMUNICANS GANGLII OTICI CUM CHORDA TYMPANI.

ramus anastomoticus ganglii otici cum ner·vo au·ri·cu·lo·tem·po·ra·li (nur′vo aw·rick″yoo·lo·tem·po·ray′lye) [BNA]. RAMUS COMMUNICANS GANGLII OTICI CUM NERVO AURICULOTEMPORALI.

ramus anastomoticus ganglii otici cum nervo spi·no·so (spye·no′so) [BNA]. RAMUS COMMUNICANS GANGLII OTICI CUM RAMO MENINGEO NERVI MANDIBULARIS.

ramus anastomoticus ner·vi fa·ci·a·lis cum ner·vo glos·so·pha·ryn·geo (nur′vye fay·shee·ay′lis kum nur′vo glos·o·fa·rin′jee·o) [BNA]. RAMUS COMMUNICANS NERVI FACIALIS CUM NERVO GLOSSOPHARYNGEO.

ramus anastomoticus nervi facialis cum plexu tym·pa·ni·co (pleck′sue tim·pan′i·ko) [BNA]. RAMUS COMMUNICANS NERVI FACIALIS CUM PLEXU TYMPANICO.

ramus anastomoticus nervi glos·so·pha·ryn·gei cum ra·mo au·ri·cu·la·ri ner·vi va·gi (glos·o·fa·rin′jee·eye kum ray′mo aw·rick·yoo·lair′eye nur′vye vay′guy, ·jye) [BNA]. RAMUS COMMUNICANS NERVI GLOSSOPHARYNGEI CUM RAMO AURICULARI NERVI VAGI.

ramus anastomoticus nervi la·cri·ma·lis cum ner·vo zy·go·ma·ti·co (lack·ri·may′lis kum nur′vo zye·go·mat′i·ko) [BNA]. RAMUS COMMUNICANS NERVI LACRIMALIS CUM NERVO ZYGOMATICO.

ramus anastomoticus nervi la·ryn·gei su·pe·ri·o·ris cum ner·vo la·ryn·geo in·fe·ri·o·re (la·rin′jee·eye sue·peer·ee·o′ris kum nur′vo la·rin′jee·o in·feer·ee·o′ree) [BNA]. RAMUS COMMUNICANS NERVI LARYNGEI SUPERIORIS CUM NERVO LARYNGEO INFERIORE.

ramus anastomoticus nervi lin·gua·lis cum ner·vo hy·po·glos·so (ling·gway′lis kum nur′vo high·po·glos′o) [BNA]. RAMUS COMMUNICANS NERVI LINGUALIS CUM NERVO HYPOGLOSSO.

ramus anastomoticus nervi me·di·a·ni cum ner·vo ul·na·ri (mee·dee·ay′nigh kum nur′vo ul·nair′eye) [BNA]. RAMUS COMMUNICANS NERVI MEDIANI CUM NERVO ULNARI.

ramus anastomoticus nervi va·gi cum ner·vo glos·so·pha·ryn·geo (vay′guy kum nur′vo glos·o·fa·rin′jee·o) [BNA]. RAMUS COMMUNICANS NERVI VAGI CUM NERVO GLOSSOPHARYNGEO.

ramus anastomoticus pe·ro·nae·us (perr·o·nee′us) [BNA]. RAMUS COMMUNICANS PERONEUS NERVI PERONEI COMMUNIS.

ramus anastomoticus ul·na·ris ra·mi su·per·fi·ci·a·lis ner·vi ra·di·a·lis (ul·nair′is ray′migh sue·pur·fish·ee·ay′lis nur′vye ray·dee·ay′lis) [BNA]. RAMUS COMMUNICANS ULNARIS NERVI RADIALIS.

ramus anterior ar·te·ri·ae ob·tu·ra·to·ri·ae (ahr·teer′ee·ee ob·tew·ruh·to′ree·ee) [NA]. The anterior branch of the obturator artery.

ramus anterior arteriae re·cur·ren·tis ul·na·ris (reck·ur·en′tis ul·nair′is) [NA]. The anterior branch of the ulnar recurrent artery.

ramus anterior arteriae re·na·lis (re·nay′lis) [NA]. The anterior branch of the renal artery.

ramus anterior arteriae thy·roi·de·ae su·pe·ri·o·ris (thigh·roy′dee·ee sue·peer·ee·o′ris) [NA]. The anterior branch of the superior thyroid artery.

ramus anterior ascen·dens ar·te·ri·ae pul·mo·na·lis dex·trae (a·sen′denz ahr·teer′ee·ee pul·mo·nay′lis decks′tree) [NA]. The anterior ascending branch of the right pulmonary artery.

ramus anterior ascendens arteriae pulmonalis si·nis·trae (si·nis′tree) [NA]. The anterior ascending branch of the left pulmonary artery.

ramus anterior ascendens fis·su·rae ce·re·bri la·te·ra·lis (fi·syoo′ree serr′e·brye lat·e·ray′lis) [BNA]. RAMUS ASCENDENS SULCI LATERALIS CEREBRI.

ramus anterior de·scen·dens ar·te·ri·ae pul·mo·na·lis dex·trae (de·sen′denz ahr·teer′ee·ee pul·mo·nay′lis decks′tree) [NA]. The anterior descending branch of the right pulmonary artery.

ramus anterior descendens arteriae pulmonalis si·nis·trae (si·nis′tree) [NA]. The anterior descending branch of the left pulmonary artery.

ramus anterior duc·tus he·pa·ti·ci dex·tri (duck′tus he·pat′i·sigh decks′trye) [NA]. The anterior branch of the right hepatic duct.

ramus anterior ho·ri·zon·ta·lis fis·su·rae ce·re·bri la·te·ra·lis (hor·i·zon·tay′lis fi·syoo′ree serr′e·brye lat·e·ray′lis) [BNA]. RAMUS ANTERIOR SULCI LATERALIS CEREBRI.

ramus anterior ner·vi au·ri·cu·la·ris mag·ni (nur′vye aw·rick·yoo·lair′is mag′nye) [NA]. The anterior branch of the great auricular nerve.

ramus anterior nervi cu·ta·nei an·te·bra·chii me·di·a·lis (kew·tay′nee·eye an·te·bray′kee·eye mee·dee·ay′lis) [NA]. The anterior branch of the medial cutaneous nerve of the forearm.

ramus anterior nervi la·ryn·gei in·fe·ri·o·ris (la·rin′jee·eye in·feer·ee·o′ris) [BNA]. The anterior branch of the inferior laryngeal nerve.

ramus anterior nervi ob·tu·ra·to·rii (ob·tew·ruh·to′ree·eye) [NA]. The anterior branch of the obturator nerve.

ramus anterior nervi spi·na·lis (spye·nay′lis) [BNA]. RAMUS VENTRALIS NERVORUM SPINALIUM.

ramus anterior ra·mi cu·ta·nei la·te·ra·lis ner·vo·rum tho·ra·ca·li·um (ray′migh kew·tay′nee·eye lat·e·ray′lis nur·vo′rum tho·ra·kay′lee·um) [BNA]. The anterior branch of the lateral cutaneous branch of any thoracic nerve.

ramus anterior rami cutanei lateralis rami an·te·ri·o·ris ar·te·ri·ae in·ter·cos·ta·lis (an·teer·ee·o′ris ahr·teer′ee·ee in·tur·kos·tay′lis) [BNA]. The anterior branch of the lateral cutaneous branch of the anterior intercostal artery.

ramus anterior sul·ci la·te·ra·lis ce·re·bri (sul′sigh lat·e·ray′lis serr′e·brye) [NA]. The anterior branch of the lateral cerebral sulcus.

ramus anterior ve·nae pul·mo·na·lis su·pe·ri·o·ris dex·trae (vee′nee pul·mo·nay′lis sue·peer·ee·o′ris decks′tree) [NA]. The anterior tributary of the right superior pulmonary vein.

ramus anterior venae pulmonalis superioris si·nis·trae (si·nis′tree) [NA]. The anterior tributary of the left superior pulmonary vein.

ramus api·ca·lis ar·te·ri·ae pul·mo·na·lis dex·trae (ap·i·kay′lis ahr·teer′ee·ee pul·mo·nay′lis decks′tree) [NA]. The apical branch of the right pulmonary artery.

ramus apicalis arteriae pulmonalis si·nis·trae (si·nis′tree) [NA]. The apical branch of the left pulmonary artery.

ramus apicalis lo·bi in·fe·ri·o·ris ar·te·ri·ae pul·mo·na·lis dex·trae (lo′bye in·feer·ee·o′ris ahr·teer′ee·ee pul·mo·nay′lis decks′tree) [NA]. The branch of the right pulmonary artery to the apical segment of the right inferior lobe. NA alt. *ramus superior lobi inferioris arteriae pulmonalis dextrae.*

ramus apicalis lobi inferioris arteriae pulmonalis si·nis·trae (si·nis′tree) [NA]. The branch of the left pulmonary artery to the apical segment of the left inferior lobe. NA alt. *ramus superior lobi inferioris arteriae pulmonalis sinistrae.*

ramus apicalis ve·nae pul·mo·na·lis in·fe·ri·o·ris dex·trae (vee′nee pul·mo·nay′lis in·feer·ee·o′ris decks′tree) [NA]. The branch of the right inferior pulmonary vein from the apical segment of the inferior lobe of the right lung. NA alt. *ramus superior venae pulmonalis inferioris dextrae.*

ramus apicalis venae pulmonalis inferioris si·nis·trae (si·nis′tree) [NA]. The branch of the left inferior pulmonary vein from the apical segment of the inferior lobe of the left lung. NA alt. *ramus superior venae pulmonalis inferioris sinistrae.*

ramus apicalis venae pulmonalis su·pe·ri·o·ris dex·trae (sue·peer·ee·o′ris decks′tree) [NA]. The branch of the superior right pulmonary vein from the apical segment of the superior lobe of the right lung.

ramus api·co·pos·te·ri·or ve·nae pul·mo·na·lis su·pe·ri·o·ris si·nis·trae (ap·i·ko·pos·teer′ee·or vee′nee pul·mo·nay′lis sue·peer·ee·o′ris si·nis′tree) [NA]. The branch of the left superior pulmonary vein from the apicoposterior segment of the superior lobe of the left lung.

ramus ascen·dens ar·te·ri·ae cir·cum·flex·ae fe·mo·ris la·te·ra·lis (a·sen′denz ahr·teer′ee·ee sur·kum·fleck′see fem′o·ris lat·e·ray′lis) [NA]. The ascending branch of the lateral femoral circumflex artery.

ramus ascendens arteriae circumflexae femoris me·di·a·lis (mee·dee·ay′lis) [NA]. The ascending branch of the medial femoral circumflex artery.

ramus ascendens arteriae circumflexae ilii pro·fun·dae (il′ee·eye pro·fun′dee) [NA]. The ascending branch of the deep circumflex iliac artery.

ramus ascendens arteriae trans·ver·sae col·li (trans·vur′see kol′eye) [BNA]. RAMUS SUPERFICIALIS ARTERIAE TRANSVERSAE COLLI.

ramus ascendens sul·ci la·te·ra·lis ce·re·bri (sul′sigh lat·e·ray′lis serr′e·brye) [NA]. The ascending limb of the lateral cerebral sulcus.

ramus au·ri·cu·la·ris ar·te·ri·ae au·ri·cu·la·ris pos·te·ri·o·ris (aw·rick·yoo·lair′is ahr·teer′ee·ee aw·rick·yoo·lair′is pos·teer·ee·o′ris) [NA]. The auricular branch of the posterior auricular artery.

ramus auricularis arteriae oc·ci·pi·ta·lis (ock·sip·i·tay′lis) [NA]. The auricular branch of the occipital artery.

ramus auricularis ner·vi va·gi (nur′vye vay′guy, vay′jye) [NA]. The auricular branch of the vagus nerve.

ramus ba·sa·lis an·te·ri·or ar·te·ri·ae pul·mo·na·lis dex·trae (ba·say′lis an·teer′ee·or ahr·teer′ee·ee pul·mo·nay′lis decks′tree) [NA]. The branch of the right pulmonary artery to the anterior basal segment of the inferior lobe of the right lung.

ramus basalis anterior arteriae pulmonalis si·nis·trae (si·nis′tree) [NA]. The branch of the left pulmonary artery to the anterior basal segment of the inferior lobe of the left lung.

ramus basalis anterior ve·nae pul·mo·na·lis in·fe·ri·o·ris dex·trae (vee′nee pul·mo·nay′lis in·feer·ee·o′ris decks′tree) [NA]. The branch of the superior right pulmonary vein from the anterior basal segment of inferior lobe of the right lung.

ramus basalis anterior venae pulmonalis inferioris si·nis·trae (si·nis′tree) [NA]. The branch of the left inferior pulmonary vein from the anterior basal segment of the inferior lobe of the left lung.

ramus basalis la·te·ra·lis ar·te·ri·ae pul·mo·na·lis dex·trae (lat·e·ray′lis ahr·teer′ee·ee pul·mo·nay′lis decks′tree) [NA]. The branch of the right pulmonary artery to the basal lateral segment of the inferior lobe of the right lung.

ramus basalis lateralis arteriae pulmonalis si·nis·trae (si·nis′tree) [NA]. The branch of the left pulmonary artery to the basal lateral segment of the inferior lobe of the left lung.

ramus basalis me·di·a·lis ar·te·ri·ae pul·mo·na·lis dex·trae (mee·dee·ay′lis ahr·teer′ee·ee pul·mo·nay′lis decks′tree) [NA]. The branch of the right pulmonary artery to the medial basal segment of the inferior lobe of the right lung. NA alt. *ramus cardiacus arteriae pulmonalis dextrae.*

ramus basalis medialis arteriae pulmonalis si·nis·trae (si·nis′tree) [NA]. The branch of the left pulmonary artery to the medial basal segment of the inferior lobe of the left lung.

ramus basalis posterior arteriae pulmonalis dex·trae (decks′tree) [NA]. The branch of the right pulmonary artery to the posterior basal segment of the inferior lobe of the right lung.

ramus basalis posterior arteriae pulmonalis si·nis·trae (si·nis′tree) [NA]. The branch of the left pulmonary artery to the posterior basal segment of the inferior lobe of the left lung.

ramus bron·chi·a·lis ep·ar·te·ri·a·lis (brong·kee·ay′lis ep·ahr·teer·ee·ay′lis) [BNA]. The eparterial bronchus of the right lung.

ramus car·di·a·cus (kahr·dye′uh·kus). A cardiac branch of the vagus nerve.

ramus cardiacus ar·te·ri·ae pul·mo·na·lis dex·trae (ahr·teer′ee·ee pul·mo·nay′lis decks′tree) [NA alt.]. RAMUS BASALIS MEDIALIS ARTERIAE PULMONALIS DEXTRAE.

ramus ca·ro·ti·co·tym·pa·ni·cus ar·te·ri·ae ca·ro·tis in·ter·nae (ka·rot″i·ko·tim·pan′i·kus ahr·teer′ee·ee ka·rot′is in·tur′nee) [BNA]. RAMI CAROTICOTYMPANICI ARTERIAE CAROTIDIS INTERNAE.

ramus ca·ro·ti·cus (ka·rot′i·kus). A branch of the glossopharyngeal nerve to the carotid sinus.

ramus car·pe·us dor·sa·lis ar·te·ri·ae ra·di·a·lis (kahr′pee·us dor·say′lis ahr·teer′ee·ee ray·dee·ay′lis) [NA]. The dorsal carpal branch of the radial artery.

ramus carpeus dorsalis arteriae ul·na·ris (ul·nair′is) [NA]. The dorsal carpal branch of the ulnar artery.

ramus carpeus pal·ma·ris ar·te·ri·ae ra·di·a·lis (pal·mair′is ahr·teer′ee·ee ray·dee·ay′lis) [NA]. The palmar carpal branch of the radial artery.

ramus carpeus palmaris arteriae ul·na·ris (ul·nair′is) [NA]. The palmar carpal branch of the ulnar artery.

ramus carpeus vo·la·ris ar·te·ri·ae ra·di·a·lis (vo·lair′is ahr·teer′ee·ee ray·dee·ay′lis) [BNA]. RAMUS CARPEUS PALMARIS ARTERIAE RADIALIS.

ramus carpeus volaris arteriae ul·na·ris (ul·nair′is) [BNA]. RAMUS CARPEUS PALMARIS ARTERIAE ULNARIS.

ramus cho·roi·de·us ar·te·ri·ae ce·re·bri pos·te·ri·o·ris (ko·roy'dee·us ahr·teer'ee·ee serr'e·brye pos·teer·ee·o'ris) [NA]. The choroidal branch of the posterior cerebral artery. NA alt. (pl.) *rami choroidei posteriores arteriae cerebri posterioris.*

ramus cir·cum·flex·us ar·te·ri·ae co·ro·na·ri·ae cor·dis si·nis·trae (sur·kum·fleck'sus ahr·teer'ee·ee kor·o·nair'ee·ee kor'dis si·nis'tree) [BNA]. RAMUS CIRCUMFLEXUS ARTERIAE CORONARIAE SINISTRAE.

ramus circumflexus arteriae coronariae sinistrae [NA]. The circumflex branch of the left coronary artery.

ramus circumflexus fi·bu·lae ar·te·ri·ae ti·bi·a·lis pos·te·ri·o·ris (fib'yoo·lee ahr·teer'ee·ee tib·ee·ay'lis pos·teer·ee·o'ris) [NA]. The circumflex fibular branch of the posterior tibial artery.

ramus cla·vi·cu·la·ris ar·te·ri·ae tho·ra·co·acro·mi·a·lis (kla·vick·yoo·lair'is ahr·teer'ee·ee tho·ruh·ko·a·kro·mee·ay'lis) [NA]. The clavicular branch of the thoracoacromial artery.

ramus coch·le·ae ar·te·ri·ae au·di·ti·vae in·ter·nae (kock'lee·ee ahr·teer'ee·ee aw·di·tye'vee in·tur'nee) [BNA]. RAMUS COCHLEARIS ARTERIAE LABYRINTHI.

ramus coch·le·a·ris ar·te·ri·ae la·by·rin·thi (kock·lee·air'is ahr·teer'ee·ee lab·i·rin'thigh) [NA]. The cochlear branch of the labyrinthine artery.

ramus col·la·te·ra·lis ar·te·ri·a·rum in·ter·cos·ta·li·um pos·te·ri·o·rum [III–XI] (ko·lat·e·ray'lis ahr·teer·ee·air'um in·tur·kos·tay'lee·um pos·teer·ee·o'rum) [NA]. The collateral ramus of one of the posterior intercostal arteries.

ramus col·li ner·vi fa·ci·a·lis (kol'eye nur'vye fay·shee·ay'lis) [NA]. The cervical branch of the facial nerve.

ramus com·mu·ni·cans (kom·yoo'ni·kanz), pl. **rami com·mu·ni·can·tes** (kom·yoo·ni·kan'teez) [NA]. A communicating branch; a small nerve or vessel connecting larger ones. See also *gray ramus communicans, white ramus communicans.*

ramus communicans ar·te·ri·ae fi·bu·la·ris (ahr·teer'ee·ee fib·yoo·lair'is) [NA alt.]. RAMUS COMMUNICANS ARTERIAE PERONEAE.

ramus communicans arteriae pe·ro·nae·ae (perr·o·nee'ee) [BNA]. RAMUS COMMUNICANS ARTERIAE PERONEAE.

ramus communicans arteriae pe·ro·ne·ae (perr·o·nee'ee) [NA]. The communicating branch of the peroneal artery with the posterior tibial artery. NA alt. *ramus communicans arteriae fibularis.*

ramus communicans fi·bu·la·ris ner·vi fi·bu·la·ris com·mu·nis (fib·yoo·lair'is nur'vye fib·yoo·lair'is kom·yoo'nis) [NA alt.]. RAMUS COMMUNICANS PERONEUS NERVI PERONEI COMMUNIS.

ramus communicans gan·glii ci·li·a·ris cum ner·vo na·so·ci·li·a·ri (gang'glee·eye sil·ee·air'is kum nur'vo nay''zo·sil·ee·air'eye) [NA]. A communicating nerve branch between the ciliary ganglion and the nasociliary nerve.

ramus communicans ganglii oti·ci cum chor·da tym·pa·ni (o'ti·sigh kum kor'duh tim'puh·nigh) [NA]. A communicating nerve branch between the otic ganglion and the chorda tympani.

ramus communicans ganglii otici cum ner·vo au·ri·cu·lo·tem·po·ra·li (nur'vo aw·rick''yoo·lo·tem·po·ray'lye) [NA]. A communicating nerve branch between the otic ganglion and the auriculotemporal nerve.

ramus communicans ganglii otici cum ra·mo me·nin·geo ner·vi man·di·bu·la·ris (ray'mo me·nin'jee·o nur'vye man·dib·yoo·lair'is) [NA]. A communicating nerve branch between the otic ganglion and the meningeal branch of the mandibular nerve.

ramus communicans ner·vi fa·ci·a·lis cum ner·vo glos·so·pha·ryn·geo (nur'vye fay·shee·ay'lis kum nur'vo glos·o·fa·rin'jee·o) [NA]. A communicating nerve branch between the facial and glossopharyngeal nerves.

ramus communicans nervi facialis cum plexu tym·pa·ni·co (pleck'sue tim·pan'i·ko) [NA]. A communicating nerve branch between the facial nerve and the tympanic plexus.

ramus communicans nervi glos·so·pha·ryn·gei cum ra·mo au·ri·cu·la·ri ner·vi va·gi (glos·o·fa·rin'jee·eye kum ray'mo aw·rick·yoo·lair'eye nur'vye vay'guy, ·jye) [NA]. A communicating nerve branch between the glossopharyngeal nerve and the auricular branch of the vagus nerve.

ramus communicans nervi la·cri·ma·lis cum ner·vo zy·go·ma·ti·co (lack·ri·may'lis kum nur'vo zye·go·mat'i·ko) [NA]. A communicating nerve branch between the lacrimal and zygomatic nerves.

ramus communicans nervi la·ryn·gei re·cur·ren·tis cum ra·mo la·ryn·geo in·ter·no (la·rin'jee·eye reck·ur·en'tis kum ray'mo la·rin'jee·o in·tur'no) [NA]. A communicating nerve branch between the recurrent laryngeal nerve and the internal laryngeal branch of the superior laryngeal nerve.

ramus communicans nervi laryngei su·pe·ri·o·ris cum ner·vo la·ryn·geo in·fe·ri·o·re (sue·peer·ee·o'ris kum nur'vo la·rin'jee·o in·feer·ee·o'ree) [NA]. A communicating nerve branch between the superior laryngeal nerve and the inferior laryngeal nerve.

ramus communicans nervi lin·gua·lis cum chor·da tym·pa·ni (ling·gway'lis kum kor'duh tim'puh·nigh) [NA]. A communicating nerve branch between the lingual nerve and the chorda tympani.

ramus communicans nervi lin·gua·lis cum ner·vo hy·po·glos·so (ling·gway'lis kum nur'vo high·po·glos'o). Singular of *rami communicantes nervi lingualis cum nervo hypoglosso.*

ramus communicans nervi me·di·a·ni cum ner·vo ul·na·ri (mee·dee·ay'nigh kum nur'vo ul·nair'eye) [NA]. A communicating nerve branch between the median and ulnar nerves.

ramus communicans nervi na·so·ci·li·a·ris cum gan·glio ci·li·a·ri (nay·zo·sil·ee·air'is kum gang'lee·o sil·ee·air'eye) [NA]. A communicating nerve branch between the nasociliary nerve and the ciliary ganglion.

ramus communicans nervi spi·na·lis (spye·nay'lis) [BNA]. Singular of *rami communicantes nervorum spinalium.*

ramus communicans nervi va·gi cum ner·vo glos·so·pha·ryn·geo (vay'guy kum ner'vo glos·o·fa·rin'jee·o) [NA]. A communicating nerve branch between the vagus and glossopharyngeal nerves.

ramus communicans pe·ro·ne·us ner·vi pe·ro·nei com·mu·nis (perr·o·nee'us nur'vye perr·o·nee'eye kom·yoo'nis) [NA]. The communicating peroneal branch of the common peroneal nerve. NA alt. *ramus communicans fibularis nervi fibularis communis.*

ramus communicans ul·na·ris ner·vi ra·di·a·lis (ul·nair'is nur'vye ray·dee·ay'lis) [NA]. The communicating ulnar branch of the radial nerve.

ramus cos·ta·lis la·te·ra·lis ar·te·ri·ae mam·ma·ri·ae in·ter·nae (kos·tay'lis lat·e·ray'lis ahr·teer'ee·ee ma·mair'ee·ee in·tur'nee) [BNA]. RAMUS COSTALIS LATERALIS ARTERIAE THORACICAE INTERNAE.

ramus costalis lateralis arteriae tho·ra·ci·cae in·ter·nae (tho·ray'si·see in·tur'nee) [NA]. The lateral costal branch of the internal thoracic artery.

ramus cri·co·thy·re·oi·de·us ar·te·ri·ae thy·re·oi·de·ae su·pe·ri·o·ris (krye''ko·thigh·ree·oy'dee·us ahr·teer'ee·ee thigh·ree·oy'dee·ee sue·peer·ee·o'ris) [BNA]. RAMUS CRICOTHYROIDEUS ARTERIAE THYROIDEAE SUPERIORIS.

ramus cri·co·thy·roi·de·us ar·te·ri·ae thy·roi·de·ae su·pe·ri·o·ris (krye''ko·thigh·roy'dee·us ahr·teer'ee·ee thigh·roy'dee·ee sue·peer'ee·o·ris) [NA]. The cricothyroid branch of the superior thyroid artery.

ramus cu·ta·ne·us an·te·ri·or ner·vi ilio·hy·po·gas·tri·ci (kew·tay'nee·us an·teer'ee·or nur'vye il''ee·o·high·po·gas'tri·sigh) [NA]. The anterior cutaneous branch of the iliohypogastric nerve.

ramus cutaneus anterior [pec·to·ra·lis et ab·do·mi·na·lis] ner·vi in·ter·cos·ta·lis (peck·to·ray'lis et ab·dom·i·nay'lis nur'vye in·tur·kos·tay'lis) [BNA]. RAMUS CUTANEUS ANTERIOR [PECTORALIS ET ABDOMINALIS] NERVI THORACICI.

ramus cutaneus anterior [pectoralis et abdominalis] nervi

tho·ra·ci·ci (tho·ray'si·sigh) [NA]. The anterior cutaneous branch of any thoracic nerve.

ramus cutaneus la·te·ra·lis ar·te·ri·a·rum in·ter·cos·ta·li·um pos·te·ri·o·rum [III–XI] (lat·e·ray'lis ahr·teer·ee·air'um in·tur·kos·tay'lee·um pos·teer·ee·o'rum) [NA]. The lateral cutaneous branch of a posterior intercostal artery.

ramus cutaneus lateralis ner·vi ilio·hy·po·gas·tri·ci (nur'vye il"ee·o·high·po·gas'tri·sigh) [NA]. The lateral cutaneous branch of the iliohypogastric nerve.

ramus cutaneus lateralis [pec·to·ra·lis et ab·do·mi·na·lis] ner·vi tho·ra·ci·ci (peck·to·ray'lis et ab·dom·i·nay'lis nur'vye tho·ray'si·sigh) [NA]. The lateral cutaneous branch of any thoracic nerve.

ramus cutaneus lateralis [pectoralis et abdominalis] ner·vo·rum in·ter·cos·ta·li·um (nur·vo'rum in·tur·kos·tay'lee·um) [BNA]. RAMUS CUTANEUS LATERALIS [PECTORALIS ET ABDOMINALIS] NERVI THORACICI.

ramus cutaneus lateralis ra·mi dor·sa·lis ar·te·ri·a·rum in·ter·cos·ta·li·um pos·te·ri·o·rum [III–XI] (ray'migh dor·say'lis ahr·teer·ee·air'um in·tur·kos·tay'lee·um pos·teer·ee·o'rum) [NA]. The lateral cutaneous branch of the dorsal branch of any posterior intercostal artery.

ramus cutaneus lateralis ra·mo·rum dor·sa·li·um ner·vo·rum tho·ra·ci·co·rum (ray·mo'rum dor·say'lee·um nur·vo'rum tho·ray·si·ko'rum) [NA]. The lateral cutaneous branch of the dorsal branch of any thoracic nerve.

ramus cutaneus lateralis ramorum pos·te·ri·o·rum ar·te·ri·a·rum in·ter·cos·ta·li·um (pos·teer·ee·o'rum ahr·teer·ee·air' um in·tur·kos·tay'lee·um) [BNA]. RAMUS CUTANEUS LATERALIS RAMI DORSALIS ARTERIARUM INTERCOSTALIUM POSTERIORUM [III–XI].

ramus cutaneus lateralis ramorum posteriorum ner·vo·rum tho·ra·ca·li·um (nur·vo'rum tho·ra·kay'lee·um) [BNA]. RAMUS CUTANEUS LATERALIS RAMORUM DORSALIUM NERVORUM THORACICORUM.

ramus cutaneus me·di·a·lis ra·mi dor·sa·lis ar·te·ri·a·rum in·ter·cos·ta·li·um pos·te·ri·o·rum [III–XI] (mee·dee·ay'lis ray' migh dor·say'lis ahr·teer·ee·air'um in·tur·kos·tay'lee·um pos·teer·ee·o'rum) [NA]. The medial cutaneous branch of the dorsal branch of any posterior intercostal artery.

ramus cutaneus medialis ra·mo·rum dor·sa·li·um ner·vo·rum tho·ra·ci·co·rum (ray·mo'rum dor·say'lee·um nur·vo'rum tho·ray·si·ko'rum) [NA]. The medial cutaneous branch of the dorsal branch of any thoracic nerve.

ramus cutaneus medialis ra·mo·rum pos·te·ri·o·rum ar·te·ri·o·rum in·ter·cos·ta·li·um (ray·mo'rum pos·teer·ee·o'rum ahr·teer·ee·o'rum in·tur·kos·tay'lee·um) [BNA]. RAMUS CUTANEUS MEDIALIS RAMI DORSALIS ARTERIARUM INTERCOSTALIUM POSTERIORUM [III–XI].

ramus cutaneus medialis ramorum posteriorum ner·vo·rum tho·ra·ca·li·um (nur·vo'rum tho·ra·kay'lee·um) [BNA]. RAMUS CUTANEUS MEDIALIS RAMORUM DORSALIUM NERVORUM THORACICORUM.

ramus cutaneus ner·vi ob·tu·ra·to·rii (nur'vye ob·tew·ruh·to' ree·eye) [NA]. The cutaneous branch of the obturator nerve.

ramus cutaneus pal·ma·ris ner·vi ul·na·ris (pal·mair'is nur'vye ul·nair'is) [BNA]. RAMUS PALMARIS NERVI ULNARIS.

ramus del·toi·de·us ar·te·ri·ae pro·fun·dae bra·chii (del·toy' dee·us ahr·teer'ee·ee pro·fun'dee bray'kee·eye) [NA]. The deltoid branch of the deep brachial artery.

ramus deltoideus arteriae tho·ra·co·acro·mi·a·lis (tho·ra·ko·a·kro·mee·ay'lis) [NA]. The deltoid branch of the thoracoacromial artery.

ramus de·scen·dens an·te·ri·or ar·te·ri·ae co·ro·na·ri·ae cor·dis si·nis·trae (de·sen'denz an·teer'ee·or ahr·teer'ee·ee kor·o·nair'ee·ee kor'dis si·nis'tree) [BNA]. RAMUS INTERVENTRICULARIS ANTERIOR ARTERIAE CORONARIAE SINISTRAE.

ramus descendens ar·te·ri·ae cir·cum·flex·ae fe·mo·ris la·te·ra·lis (ahr·teer'ee·ee sur·kum·fleck'see fem'o·ris lat·e·ray' lis) [NA]. The descending branch of the lateral femoral circumflex artery.

ramus descendens arteriae oc·ci·pi·ta·lis (ock·sip·i·tay'lis) [NA]. The descending branch of the occipital artery.

ramus descendens arteriae trans·ver·sae col·li (trans·vur'see kol'eye) [BNA]. RAMUS PROFUNDUS ARTERIAE TRANSVERSAE COLLI.

ramus descendens cer·vi·cis (sur'vi·sis). The inferior root of the ansa cervicalis.

ramus descendens hy·po·glos·si (high·po·glos'eye). The superior root of the ansa cervicalis.

ramus descendens ner·vi hy·po·glos·si (nur'vye high·po·glos' eye) [BNA]. RADIX SUPERIOR ANSAE CERVICALIS.

ramus descendens posterior ar·te·ri·ae co·ro·na·ri·ae cor·dis dex·trae (ahr·teer'ee·ee kor·o·nair'ee·ee kor'dis decks'tree) [BNA]. RAMUS INTERVENTRICULARIS POSTERIOR ARTERIAE CORONARIAE DEXTRAE.

ramus dex·ter ar·te·ri·ae he·pa·ti·cae pro·pri·ae (decks'tur ahr·teer'ee·ee he·pat'i·see pro'pree·ee) [NA]. The right branch of the proper hepatic artery; RIGHT HEPATIC ARTERY.

ramus dexter arteriae pul·mo·na·lis (pul·mo·nay'lis) [BNA]. ARTERIA PULMONALIS DEXTRA.

ramus dexter ve·nae por·tae (vee'nee por'tee) [NA]. The right branch of the portal vein.

ramus di·gas·tri·cus ner·vi fa·ci·a·lis (dye·gas'tri·kus nur'vye fay·shee·ay'lis) [NA]. The digastric branch of the facial nerve.

ramus dor·sa·lis ar·te·ri·ae sub·cos·ta·lis (dor·say'lis ahr·teer' ee·ee sub·kos·tay'lis) [NA]. The dorsal branch of the subcostal artery.

ramus dorsalis ar·te·ri·a·rum in·ter·cos·ta·li·um pos·te·ri·o·rum [III–XI] (ahr·teer·ee·air'um in·tur·kos·tay'lee·um pos·teer·ee·o'rum) [NA]. The dorsal branch of any posterior intercostal artery.

ramus dorsalis arteriarum lum·ba·li·um (lum·bay'lee·um) [NA]. The dorsal branch of any lumbar artery.

ramus dorsalis ma·nus ner·vi ul·na·ris (man'us nur'vye ul·nair'is) [BNA]. RAMUS DORSALIS NERVI ULNARIS.

ramus dorsalis ner·vi coc·cy·gei (nur'vye kock·sij'ee·eye) [NA]. The dorsal branch of the coccygeal nerve.

ramus dorsalis ner·vi ul·na·ris (nur'vye ul·nair'is) [NA]. The dorsal branch of the ulnar nerve.

ramus dorsalis ner·vo·rum spi·na·li·um (nur·vo'rum spye·nay' lee·um) [NA]. The dorsal branch of any spinal nerve.

ramus dorsalis ve·na·rum in·ter·cos·ta·li·um (ve·nay'rum in·tur·kos·tay'lee·um) [BNA]. RAMUS DORSALIS VENARUM INTERCOSTALIUM POSTERIORUM [IV–XI].

ramus dorsalis venarum intercostalium pos·te·ri·o·rum [IV–XI] (pos·teer·ee·o'rum) [NA]. The dorsal tributary to any posterior intercostal vein.

ramus ex·ter·nus ner·vi ac·ces·so·rii (ecks·tur'nus nur'vye ack·se·so'ree·eye) [NA]. The external branch of the accessory nerve.

ramus externus nervi la·ryn·gei su·pe·ri·o·ris (la·rin'jee·eye sue·peer·ee·o'ris) [NA]. The external branch of the superior laryngeal nerve.

ramus fe·mo·ra·lis ner·vi ge·ni·to·fe·mo·ra·lis (fem·o·ray'lis nur'vye jen·i·to·fem·o·ray'lis) [NA]. The femoral branch of the genitofemoral nerve.

ramus fi·bu·la·ris ar·te·ri·ae ti·bi·a·lis pos·te·ri·o·ris (fib·yoo·lair'is ahr·teer"ee·ee tib·ee·ay'lis pos·teer·ee·o'ris) [BNA]. RAMUS CIRCUMFLEXUS FIBULAE ARTERIAE TIBIALIS POSTERIORIS.

ramus fron·ta·lis ar·te·ri·ae me·nin·ge·ae me·di·ae (fron·tay' lis ahr·teer'ee·ee me·nin'jee·ee mee'dee·ee) [NA]. The frontal branch of the middle meningeal artery.

ramus frontalis arteriae tem·po·ra·lis su·per·fi·ci·a·lis (tem·po·ray'lis sue·pur·fish·ee·ay'lis) [NA]. The frontal branch of the superficial temporal artery.

ramus frontalis ner·vi fron·ta·lis (nur'vye fron·tay'lis) [BNA]. The frontal branch of the frontal nerve.

ramus ge·ni·ta·lis ner·vi ge·ni·to·fe·mo·ra·lis (jen·i·tay'lis nur' vye jen·i·to·fem·o·ray'lis) [NA]. The genital branch of the genitofemoral nerve.

ramus hy·oi·de·us ar·te·ri·ae lin·gua·lis (high·oy'dee·us ahr·teer'ee·ee ling·gway'lis) [BNA]. RAMUS SUPRAHYOIDEUS ARTERIAE LINGUALIS.

ramus hyoideus arteriae thy·re·oi·de·ae su·pe·ri·o·ris (thigh·ree·oy'dee·ee sue·peer·ee·o'ris) [BNA]. RAMUS INFRAHYOIDEUS ARTERIAE THYROIDEAE SUPERIORIS.

ramus ili·a·cus ar·te·ri·ae ilio·lum·ba·lis (i·lye'uh·kus ahr·teer'ee·ee il"ee·o·lum·bay'lis) [NA]. The iliac branch of the iliolumbar artery.

ramus inferior ar·te·ri·ae glu·tae·ae su·pe·ri·o·ris (ahr·teer'ee·ee gloo'tee·ee sue·peer·ee·o'ris) [BNA]. RAMUS INFERIOR ARTERIAE GLUTEAE SUPERIORIS.

ramus inferior arteriae glu·te·ae su·pe·ri·o·ris (gloo'tee·ee sue·peer·ee·o'ris) [NA]. The inferior branch of the superior gluteal artery.

ramus inferior ner·vi oc·u·lo·mo·to·rii (nur'vye ock"yoo·lo·mo·to'ree·eye) [NA]. The inferior branch of the oculomotor nerve.

ramus inferior os·sis is·chii (os'is is'kee·eye) [BNA]. RAMUS OSSIS ISCHII.

ramus inferior ossis pu·bis (pew'bis) [NA]. The bar of bone extending from the symphyseal portion of the pubis to the ramus of the ischium.

ramus in·fra·hy·oi·de·us ar·te·ri·ae thy·roi·de·ae su·pe·ri·o·ris (in·fruh·high·oy'dee·us ahr·teer'ee·ee thigh·roy'dee·ee sue·peer·ee·o'ris) [NA]. The infrahyoid branch of the superior thyroid artery.

ramus in·fra·pa·tel·la·ris ner·vi sa·phe·ni (in·fruh·pat·e·lair'is nur'vye sa·fee'nigh) [NA]. The infrapatellar branch of the saphenous nerve.

ramus in·ter·nus ner·vi ac·ces·so·rii (in·tur'nus nur'vye ack·se·so'ree·eye) [NA]. The internal ramus of the accessory nerve.

ramus internus nervi la·ryn·gei su·pe·ri·o·ris (la·rin'jee·eye sue·peer·ee·o'ris) [NA]. The internal branch of the superior laryngeal nerve.

ramus in·ter·ven·tri·cu·la·ris an·te·ri·or ar·te·ri·ae co·ro·na·ri·ae si·nis·trae (in·tur·ven·trick·yoo·lair'is an·teer'ee·or ahr·teer'ee·ee kor·o·nair'ee·ee si·nis'tree) [NA]. The anterior interventricular branch of the left coronary artery.

ramus interventricularis posterior arteriae coronariae dex·trae (decks'tree) [NA]. The posterior interventricular branch of the right coronary artery.

ramus la·te·ra·lis ar·te·ri·ae pul·mo·na·lis dex·trae (lat·e·ray'lis ahr·teer'ee·ee pul·mo·nay'lis decks'tree) [NA]. The branch of the right pulmonary artery to the lateral segment of the middle lobe of the right lung.

ramus lateralis duc·tus he·pa·ti·ci si·nis·tri (duck'tus he·pat'i·sigh si·nis'trye) [NA]. The lateral branch of the left hepatic duct.

ramus lateralis ner·vi su·pra·or·bi·ta·lis (nur'vye sue"pruh·or·bi·tay'lis) [NA]. The lateral branch of the supraorbital nerve.

ramus lateralis ra·mi pos·te·ri·o·ris ner·vo·rum cer·vi·ca·li·um (ray'migh pos·teer·ee·o'ris nur·vo'rum sur·vi·kay'lee·um) [BNA]. RAMUS LATERALIS RAMORUM DORSALIUM NERVORUM CERVICALIUM.

ramus lateralis rami posterioris nervorum lum·ba·li·um (lum·bay'lee·um) [BNA]. RAMUS LATERALIS RAMORUM DORSALIUM NERVORUM LUMBALIUM.

ramus lateralis rami posterioris nervorum sa·cra·li·um et ner·vi coc·cy·gei (sa·kray'lee·um et nur'vye kock·sij'ee·eye) [BNA]. RAMUS LATERALIS RAMORUM DORSALIUM NERVORUM SACRALIUM ET NERVI COCCYGEI.

ramus lateralis ra·mo·rum dor·sa·li·um ner·vo·rum cer·vi·ca·li·um (ray·mo'rum dor·say'lee·um nur·vo'rum sur·vi·kay'lee·um) [NA]. The lateral branch of the dorsal branch of any cervical nerve.

ramus lateralis ramorum dorsalium nervorum lum·ba·li·um (lum·bay'lee·um) [NA]. The lateral branch of the dorsal branch of any lumbar nerve.

ramus lateralis ramorum dorsalium nervorum sa·cra·li·um et ner·vi coc·cy·gei (sa·kray'lee·um et nur'vye kock·sij'ee·eye) [NA]. The lateral branch of the dorsal branch of a sacral or coccygeal nerve.

ramus lin·gua·lis ner·vi fa·ci·a·lis (ling·gway'lis nur'vye fay·shee·ay'lis) [NA]. The lingual branch of the facial nerve.

ramus lin·gu·la·ris ar·te·ri·ae pul·mo·na·lis si·nis·trae (ling·gew·lair'is ahr·teer'ee·ee pul·mo·nay'lis si·nis'tree) [NA]. The branch of the left pulmonary artery to the lingula of the superior lobe of the left lung.

ramus lingularis inferior arteriae pulmonalis sinistrae [NA]. The branch of the left pulmonary artery to the inferior segment of the lingula of the superior lobe of the left lung.

ramus lingularis superior arteriae pulmonalis sinistrae [NA]. The branch of the left pulmonary artery to the superior segment of the lingula of the superior lobe of the left lung.

ramus lingularis ve·nae pul·mo·na·lis su·pe·ri·o·ris si·nis·trae (vee'nee pul·mo·nay'lis sue·peer·ee·o'ris si·nis'tree) [NA]. The tributary to the left superior pulmonary vein from the lingula of the superior lobe of the left lung.

ramus lo·bi me·dii ar·te·ri·ae pul·mo·na·lis dex·trae (lo'bye mee'dee·eye ahr·teer'ee·ee pul·mo·nay'lis decks'tree) [NA]. The branch of the right pulmonary artery to the middle lobe of the right lung.

ramus lobi medii ve·nae pul·mo·na·lis su·pe·ri·o·ris dex·trae (vee'nee pul·mo·nay'lis sue·peer·ee·o'ris decks'tree) [NA]. The tributary to the superior right pulmonary vein from the middle lobe of the right lung.

ramus lum·ba·lis ar·te·ri·ae ilio·lum·ba·lis (lum·bay'lis ahr·terr'ee·ee il"ee·o·lum·bay'lis) [NA]. The lumbar branch of the iliolumbar artery.

ramus man·di·bu·lae (man·dib'yoo·lee) [NA]. The heavy flat sheet of bone extending upward from each extremity of the body of the mandible. Syn. *ramus of the mandible.*

ramus mar·gi·na·lis man·di·bu·lae ner·vi fa·ci·a·lis (mahr·ji·nay'lis man·dib'yoo·lee nur'vye fay·shee·ay'lis) [NA]. The branch of the facial nerve passing near the margin of the mandible.

ramus mas·toi·de·us ar·te·ri·ae oc·ci·pi·ta·lis (mas·toy'dee·us ahr·teer'ee·ee ock·sip·i·tay'lis) [NA]. The mastoid branch of the occipital artery.

ramus me·di·a·lis ar·te·ri·ae pul·mo·na·lis dex·trae (mee·dee·ay'lis ahr·teer'ee·ee pul·mo·nay'lis decks'tree) [NA]. The branch of the right pulmonary artery to the medial segment of the middle lobe of the right lung.

ramus medialis duc·tus he·pa·ti·ci si·nis·tri (duck'tus he·pat'i·sigh si·nis'trye) [NA]. The medial branch of the left hepatic duct.

ramus medialis ner·vi su·pra·or·bi·ta·lis (nur'vye sue"pruh·or·bi·tay'lis) [NA]. The medial branch of the supraorbital nerve.

ramus medialis ra·mi pos·te·ri·o·ris ner·vo·rum cer·vi·ca·li·um (ray'migh pos·teer·ee·o'ris nur·vo'rum sur·vi·kay'lee·um) [BNA]. RAMUS MEDIALIS RAMORUM DORSALIUM NERVORUM CERVICALIUM.

ramus medialis rami posterioris nervorum lum·ba·li·um (lum·bay'lee·um) [BNA]. RAMUS MEDIALIS RAMORUM DORSALIUM NERVORUM LUMBALIUM.

ramus medialis rami posterioris nervorum sa·cra·li·um et ner·vi coc·cy·gei (sa·kray'lee·um et nur'vye kock·sij'ee·eye) [BNA]. RAMUS MEDIALIS RAMORUM DORSALIUM NERVORUM SACRALIUM ET NERVI COCCYGEI.

ramus medialis ra·mo·rum dor·sa·li·um ner·vo·rum cer·vi·ca·li·um (ray·mo'rum dor·say'lee·um nur·vo'rum sur·vi·kay'lee·um) [NA]. The medial branch of the dorsal branch of any cervical nerve.

ramus medialis ramorum dorsalium nervorum lum·ba·li·um (lum·bay'lee·um) [NA]. The medial branch of the dorsal branch of any lumbar nerve.

ramus medialis ramorum dorsalium nervorum sa·cra·li·um et

ner·vi coc·cy·gei (sa·kray'lee·um et nur'vye kock·sij'ee·eye) [NA]. The medial branch of the dorsal branch of any sacral or coccygeal nerve.

ramus mem·bra·nae tym·pa·ni ner·vi au·ri·cu·lo·tem·po·ra·lis (mem·bray'nee tim'puh·nigh nur'vye aw·rick"yoo·lo·tem·po·ray'lis) [NA]. The branch of the auriculotemporal nerve to the tympanic membrane.

ramus membranae tympani nervi me·a·tus au·di·to·rii ex·ter·nae (me·ay'tus aw·di·to'ree·eye ecks·tur'nee) [BNA]. RAMUS MEMBRANAE TYMPANI NERVI AURICULOTEMPORALIS.

ramus me·nin·ge·us ac·ces·so·ri·us ar·te·ri·ae max·il·lae (me·nin'jee·us ack·se·so'ree·us ahr·teer'ee·ee mack·sil'ee) [NA]. An occasional accessory meningeal branch of the maxillary artery.

ramus meningeus ar·te·ri·ae oc·ci·pi·ta·lis (ahr·teer'ee·ee ock·sip·i·tay'lis) [NA]. The meningeal branch of the occipital artery.

ramus meningeus arteriae ver·te·bra·lis (vur·te·bray'lis) [NA]. The meningeal branch of the vertebral artery.

ramus meningeus me·di·us ner·vi max·il·la·ris (mee'dee·us nur'vye mack·si·lair'is) [NA]. The middle meningeal branch from the maxillary nerve.

ramus meningeus ner·vi man·di·bu·la·ris (nur'vye man·dib·yoo·lair'is) [NA]. The meningeal branch of the mandibular nerve.

ramus meningeus nervi spi·na·lis (spye·nay'lis) [BNA]. RAMUS MENINGEUS NERVORUM SPINALIUM.

ramus meningeus nervi va·gi (vay'guy, vay'jye) [NA]. The meningeal branch of the vagus nerve.

ramus meningeus ner·vo·rum spi·na·li·um (nur·vo'rum spye·nay'lee·um) [NA]. The meningeal branch of any spinal nerve.

ramus mus·cu·la·ris (mus·kew·lair'is) [NA]. Any muscular branch of a nerve.

ramus mus·cu·li sty·lo·pha·ryn·gei ner·vi glos·so·pha·ryn·gei (mus'kew·lye stye·lo·fa·rin'jee·eye nur'vye glos·o·fa·rin'jee·eye) [NA]. The branch of the glossopharyngeal nerve to the stylopharyngeus muscle.

ramus my·lo·hy·oi·de·us ar·te·ri·ae al·ve·o·la·ris in·fe·ri·o·ris (migh·lo·high·oy'dee·us ahr·teer'ee·ee al·vee·o·lair'is in·feer·ee·o'ris) [NA]. The mylohyoid branch of the inferior alveolar artery.

ramus mylohyoideus arteriae max·il·la·ris in·ter·nae (mack·si·lair'is in·tur'nee) [BNA]. RAMUS MYLOHYOIDEUS ARTERIAE ALVEOLARIS INFERIORIS.

ramus na·sa·lis ex·ter·nus ner·vi eth·moi·da·lis an·te·ri·o·ris (na·say'lis ecks·tur'nus nur'vye eth·moy·day'lis an·teer·ee·o'ris) [NA]. The external nasal branch of the anterior ethmoid nerve.

ramus ob·tu·ra·to·ri·us ar·te·ri·ae epi·gas·tri·cae in·fe·ri·o·ris (ob·tew·ruh·to'ree·us ahr·teer'ee·ee ep·i·gas'tri·see in·feer·ee·o'ris) [NA]. A variable obturator branch of the inferior epigastric artery.

ramus oc·ci·pi·ta·lis ar·te·ri·ae au·ri·cu·la·ris pos·te·ri·o·ris (ock·sip·i·tay'lis ahr·teer'ee·ee aw·rick·yoo·lair'is pos·teer·ee·o'ris) [NA]. The occipital branch of the posterior auricular artery.

ramus occipitalis ner·vi au·ri·cu·la·ris pos·te·ri·o·ris (nur'vye aw·rick·yoo·lair'is pos·teer·ee·o'ris) [NA]. The occipital branch of the posterior auricular nerve.

ramus of the ischium. RAMUS OSSIS ISCHII.

ramus of the mandible. RAMUS MANDIBULAE.

ramus os·sis is·chii (os'is is'kee·eye) [NA]. The bar of bone extending from the ischial tuberosity to the inferior ramus of the pubis; the ramus of the ischium. Syn. *ramus of the ischium.*

ramus ova·ri·cus ar·te·ri·ae ute·ri·nae (o·vair'i·kus ahr·teer'ee·ee yoo·te·rye'nee) [NA]. The ovarian branch of the uterine artery.

ramus ova·rii ar·te·ri·ae ute·ri·nae (o·vair'ee·eye ahr·teer'ee·ee yoo·te·rye'nee) [BNA]. RAMUS OVARICUS ARTERIAE UTERINAE.

ramus pal·ma·ris ner·vi me·di·a·ni (pal·mair'is nur'vye mee·dee·ay'nigh) [NA]. The palmar branch of the median nerve.

ramus palmaris nervi ul·na·ris (ul·nair'is) [NA]. The palmar branch of the ulnar nerve.

ramus palmaris pro·fun·dus ar·te·ri·ae ul·na·ris (pro·fun'dus ahr·teer'ee·ee ul·nair'is) [NA]. The deep palmar branch of the ulnar artery.

ramus palmaris su·per·fi·ci·a·lis ar·te·ri·ae ra·di·a·lis (sue·pur·fish·ee·ay'lis ahr·teer'ee·ee ray·dee·ay'lis) [NA]. The superficial palmar branch of the radial artery.

ramus pal·pe·bra·lis in·fe·ri·or ner·vi in·fra·troch·le·a·ris (pal·pe·bray'lis in·feer'ee·or nur'vye in·fruh·trock·lee·air'is) [BNA]. The inferior ramus palpebralis nervi infratrochlearis; the branch of the infratrochlear nerve to the lower eyelid.

ramus palpebralis ner·vi in·fra·troch·le·a·ris (nur'vye in"fruh·trock·lee·air'is). Singular of *rami palpebrales nervi infratrochlearis.*

ramus palpebralis superior nervi infratrochlearis [BNA]. The superior ramus palpebralis nervi infratrochlearis; the branch of the infratrochlear nerve to the upper eyelid.

ramus pa·ri·e·ta·lis ar·te·ri·ae me·nin·ge·ae me·di·ae (pa·rye·e·tay'lis ahr·teer'ee·ee me·nin'jee·ee mee'dee·ee) [NA]. The parietal branch of the middle meningeal artery.

ramus parietalis arteriae tem·po·ra·lis su·per·fi·ci·a·lis (tem·po·ray'lis sue·pur·fish·ee·ay'lis) [NA]. The parietal branch of the superficial temporal artery.

ramus pa·ri·e·to·oc·ci·pi·ta·lis ar·te·ri·ae ce·re·bri pos·te·ri·o·ris (pa·rye"e·to·ock·sip·i·tay'lis ahr·teer'ee·ee serr'e·brye pos·teer·ee·o'ris) [NA]. The parietooccipital branch of the posterior cerebral artery.

ramus per·fo·rans ar·te·ri·ae fi·bu·la·ris (pur'fo·ranz ahr·teer'ee·ee fib·yoo·lair'is) [NA alt.]. RAMUS PERFORANS ARTERIAE PERONEAE.

ramus perforans arteriae pe·ro·ne·ae (perr·o·nee'ee) [NA]. The perforating branch of the peroneal artery. NA alt. *ramus perforans arteriae fibularis.*

ramus pe·ri·car·di·a·cus ner·vi phre·ni·ci (perr·i·kahr·dye'uh·kus nur'vye fren'i·sigh) [NA]. The pericardial branch of the phrenic nerve.

ramus pe·tro·sus ar·te·ri·ae me·nin·ge·ae me·di·ae (pe·tro'sus ahr·teer'ee·ee me·nin'jee·ee mee'dee·ee) [NA]. The petrosal branch of the middle meningeal artery.

ramus petrosus su·per·fi·ci·a·lis ar·te·ri·ae me·nin·ge·ae me·di·ae (sue·pur·fish·ee·ay'lis ahr·teer'ee·ee me·nin'jee·ee mee'dee·ee) [BNA]. RAMUS PETROSUS ARTERIAE MENINGEAE MEDIAE.

ramus pha·ryn·ge·us gan·glii pte·ry·go·pa·la·ti·ni (fa·rin'jee·eus gang'glee·eye terr"i·go·pal·uh·tye'nigh) [NA]. The pharyngeal branch of the pterygopalatine ganglion.

ramus plan·ta·ris pro·fun·dus ar·te·ri·ae dor·sa·lis pe·dis (plan·tair'is pro·fun'dus ahr·teer'ee·ee dor·say'lis ped'is) [NA]. The deep plantar branch of the dorsalis pedis artery.

ramus posterior ar·te·ri·ae ob·tu·ra·to·ri·ae (ahr·teer'ee·ee ob·tew·ruh·to'ree·ee) [NA]. The posterior branch of the obturator artery.

ramus posterior arteriae pul·mo·na·lis si·nis·trae (pul·mo·nay'lis si·nis'tree) [NA]. The posterior branch of the left pulmonary artery.

ramus posterior arteriae re·cur·ren·tis ul·na·ris (re·kur·en'tis ul·nair'is) [NA]. The posterior branch of the recurrent ulnar artery.

ramus posterior arteriae re·na·lis (re·nay'lis) [NA]. The posterior branch of the renal artery.

ramus posterior arteriae thy·roi·de·ae su·pe·ri·o·ris (thigh·roy'dee·ee sue·peer·ee·o'ris) [NA]. The posterior branch of the superior thyroid artery.

ramus posterior ascen·dens ar·te·ri·ae pul·mo·na·lis dex·trae (a·sen'denz ahr·teer'ee·ee pul·mo·nay'lis decks'tree) [NA]. The posterior ascending branch of the right pulmonary artery.

ramus posterior de·scen·dens ar·te·ri·ae pul·mo·na·lis dex·trae (de·sen'denz ahr·teer'ee·ee pul·mo·nay'lis decks'tree) [NA]. The posterior descending branch of the right pulmonary artery.

ramus posterior duc·tus he·pa·ti·ci dex·tri (duck'tus he·pat'i·sigh decks'trye) [NA]. The posterior branch of the right hepatic duct.

ramus posterior fis·su·rae ce·re·bri la·te·ra·lis (fi·syoo'ree serr'e·brye lat·e·ray'lis) [BNA]. RAMUS POSTERIOR SULCI LATERALIS CEREBRI.

ramus posterior ner·vi au·ri·cu·la·ris mag·ni (nur'vye aw·rick·yoo·lair'is mag'nigh) [NA]. The posterior branch of the great auricular nerve.

ramus posterior nervi coc·cy·gei (kock·sij'ee·eye) [BNA]. RAMUS DORSALIS NERVI COCCYGEI.

ramus posterior nervi la·ryn·gei in·fe·ri·o·ris (la·rin'jee·eye in·feer·ee·o'ris) [BNA]. The posterior branch of the inferior laryngeal nerve.

ramus posterior nervi ob·tu·ra·to·rii (ob·tew·ruh·to'ree·eye) [NA]. The posterior branch of the obturator nerve.

ramus posterior nervi spi·na·lis (spye·nay'lis) [BNA]. RAMUS DORSALIS NERVORUM SPINALIUM.

ramus posterior ra·mi cu·ta·nei la·te·ra·lis ner·vi in·ter·cos·ta·lis (ray'migh kew·tay'nee·eye lat·e·ray'lis nur'vye in·tur·kos·tay'lis) [BNA]. The dorsal branch of the lateral cutaneous branch of any intercostal nerve.

ramus posterior rami cutanei lateralis [pec·to·ra·les et ab·do·mi·na·les] ra·mo·rum an·te·ri·o·rum ar·te·ri·a·rum in·ter·cos·ta·li·um (peck·to·ray'leez et ab·dom·i·nay'leez ray·mo'rum an·teer·ee·o'rum ahr·teer·ee·air'um in·tur·kos·tay'lee·um) [BNA]. The posterior branch of the lateral cutaneous branch of the anterior branch of any intercostal artery.

ramus posterior sul·ci la·te·ra·lis ce·re·bri (sul'sigh lat·e·ray'lis serr'e·brye) [NA]. The posterior branch of the lateral cerebral sulcus.

ramus posterior ve·nae pul·mo·na·lis su·pe·ri·o·ris dex·trae (vee'nee pul·mo·nay'lis sue·peer·ee·o'ris decks'tree) [NA]. The posterior tributary to the right superior pulmonary vein.

ramus pro·fun·dus ar·te·ri·ae cer·vi·ca·lis ascen·den·tis (pro·fun'dus ahr·teer'ee·ee sur·vi·kay'lis a·sen·den'tis) [BNA]. The deep branch of the ascending cervical artery.

ramus profundus arteriae cir·cum·flex·ae fe·mo·ris me·di·a·lis (sur·kum·fleck'see fem'o·ris mee·dee·ay'lis) [NA]. The deep branch of the medial femoral circumflex artery.

ramus profundus arteriae glu·te·ae su·pe·ri·o·ris (gloo'tee·ee sue·peer·ee·o'ris) [NA]. The deep branch of the superior gluteal artery.

ramus profundus arteriae plan·ta·ris me·di·a·lis (plan·tair'is mee·dee·ay'lis) [NA]. The deep branch of the medial plantar artery.

ramus profundus arteriae trans·ver·sae col·li (trans·vur'see kol'eye) [NA]. The deep branch of the transverse artery of the neck; arteria scapularis descendens.

ramus profundus ner·vi plan·ta·ris la·te·ra·lis (nur'vye plan·tair'is lat·e·ray'lis) [NA]. The deep branch of the lateral plantar nerve.

ramus profundus nervi ra·di·a·lis (ray·dee·ay'lis) [NA]. The deep branch of the radial nerve.

ramus profundus nervi ul·na·ris (ul·nair'is) [NA]. The deep branch of the ulnar nerve.

ramus profundus ra·mi vo·la·ris ma·nus ner·vi ul·na·ris (ray'migh vo·lair'is man'us nur'vye ul·nair'is) [BNA]. RAMUS PROFUNDUS NERVI ULNARIS.

ramus pu·bi·cus ar·te·ri·ae epi·gas·tri·cae in·fe·ri·o·ris (pew'bi·kus ahr·teer'ee·ee ep·i·gas'tri·see in·feer·ee·o'ris) [NA]. The pubic branch of the inferior epigastric artery.

ramus pubicus arteriae ob·tu·ra·to·ri·ae (ob·tew·ruh·to'ree·ee) [NA]. The pubic branch of the obturator artery.

ramus re·na·lis ner·vi splanch·ni·ci mi·no·ris (re·nay'lis nur'vye splank'ni·sigh mi·no'ris) [NA]. The renal branch of the lesser splanchnic nerve.

ramus sa·phe·nus ar·te·ri·ae ge·nus de·scen·dens (sa·fee'nus ahr·teer'ee·ee jen'us de·sen'denz) [NA]. The saphenous branch of the descending genicular artery.

ramus saphenus arteriae ge·nu su·pre·mae (jen'yoo sue·pree'mee) [BNA]. RAMUS SAPHENUS ARTERIAE GENUS DESCENDENS.

ramus si·nis·ter ar·te·ri·ae he·pa·ti·cae pro·pri·ae (si·nis'tur ahr·teer'ee·ee he·pat'i·see pro'pree·ee) [NA]. The left branch of the proper hepatic artery; LEFT HEPATIC ARTERY.

ramus sinister arteriae pul·mo·na·lis (pul·mo·nay'lis) [BNA]. ARTERIA PULMONALIS SINISTRA.

ramus sinister ve·nae por·tae (vee'nee por'tee) [NA]. The left branch of the portal vein.

ramus si·nus ca·ro·ti·ci ner·vi glos·so·pha·ryn·gei (sigh'nus ka·rot'i·sigh nur'vye glos·o·fa·rin'jee·eye) [NA]. The branch of the glossopharyngeal nerve to the carotid sinus.

ramus spi·na·lis ar·te·ri·ae ilio·lum·ba·lis (spye·nay'lis ahr·teer'ee·ee il″ee·o·lum·bay'lis) [BNA]. The spinal branch of the iliolumbar artery.

ramus spinalis arteriae sub·cos·ta·lis (sub·kos·tay'lis) [NA]. The spinal branch of the subcostal artery.

ramus spinalis ar·te·ri·a·rum lum·ba·li·um (ahr·teer·ee·air'um lum·bay'lee·um) [NA]. The spinal branch of any lumbar artery.

ramus spinalis ra·mi dor·sa·lis ar·te·ri·a·rum in·ter·cos·ta·li·um pos·te·ri·o·rum [III–XI] (ray'migh dor·say'lis ahr·teer·ee·air'um in·tur·kos·tay'lee·um pos·teer·ee·o'rum) [NA]. The spinal branch of the dorsal branch of a posterior intercostal artery.

ramus spinalis rami pos·te·ri·o·ris ar·te·ri·ae in·ter·cos·ta·lis (pos·teer·ee·o'ris ahr·teer'ee·ee in·tur·kos·tay'lis) [BNA]. RAMUS SPINALIS RAMI DORSALIS ARTERIARUM INTERCOSTALIUM POSTERIORUM [III–XI].

ramus spinalis ve·na·rum in·ter·cos·ta·li·um (vee·nair'um in·tur·kos·tay'lee·um) [BNA]. RAMUS SPINALIS VENARUM INTERCOSTALIUM POSTERIORUM [IV–XI].

ramus spinalis venarum intercostalium pos·te·ri·o·rum [IV–XI] (pos·teer·ee·o'rum) [NA]. The spinal tributary of a posterior intercostal vein.

ramus sta·pe·di·us ar·te·ri·ae sty·lo·mas·toi·de·ae (sta·pee'dee·us ahr·teer'ee·ee stye·lo·mas·toy'dee·ee) [NA]. The stapedial branch of the stylomastoid artery.

ramus ster·no·clei·do·mas·toi·de·us ar·te·ri·ae thy·roi·de·ae su·pe·ri·o·ris (stur″no·klye″do·mas·toy'dee·us ahr·teer'ee·ee thigh·roy'dee·ee sue·peer·ee·o'ris) [NA]. The sternocleidomastoid branch of the superior thyroid artery.

ramus sty·lo·hy·oi·de·us ner·vi fa·ci·a·lis (stye″lo·high·oy'dee·us nur'vye fay·shee·ay'lis) [NA]. The stylohyoid branch of the facial nerve.

ramus sty·lo·pha·ryn·ge·us ner·vi glos·so·pha·ryn·gei (stye·lo·fa·rin'jee·us nur'vye glos·o·fa·rin'jee·eye) [BNA]. RAMUS MUSCULI STYLOPHARYNGEI NERVI GLOSSOPHARYNGEI.

ramus sub·api·ca·lis ar·te·ri·ae pul·mo·na·lis dex·trae (sub·ap·i·kay'lis ahr·teer'ee·ee pul·mo·nay'lis decks'tree) [NA]. The branch of the right pulmonary artery to the subapical segment of the inferior lobe of the right lung. NA alt. *ramus subsuperior arteriae pulmonalis dextrae.*

ramus subapicalis arteriae pulmonalis si·nis·trae (si·nis'tree) [NA]. The branch of the left pulmonary artery to the subapical segment of the inferior lobe of the left lung. NA alt. *ramus subsuperior arteriae pulmonalis sinistrae.*

ramus sub·su·pe·ri·or ar·te·ri·ae pul·mo·na·lis dex·trae (sub·sue·peer'ee·or ahr·teer'ee·ee pul·mo·nay'lis decks'tree) [NA alt.]. RAMUS SUBAPICALIS ARTERIAE PULMONALIS DEXTRAE.

ramus subsuperior arteriae pulmonalis si·nis·trae (si·nis'tree) [NA alt.]. RAMUS SUBAPICALIS ARTERIAE PULMONALIS SINISTRAE.

ramus su·per·fi·ci·a·lis ar·te·ri·ae cir·cum·flex·ae fe·mo·ris me·di·a·lis (sue·pur·fish·ee·ay'lis ahr·teer'ee·ee sur·kum·fleck'see fem'o·ris mee·dee·ay'lis) [BNA]. The superficial ramus of the medial femoral circumflex artery.

ramus superficialis arteriae glu·te·ae su·pe·ri·o·ris (gloo'tee·ee sue·peer·ee·o'ris) [NA]. The superficial branch of the superior gluteal artery.

ramus superficialis arteriae plan·ta·ris me·di·a·lis (plan·tair'is mee·dee·ay'lis) [NA]. The superficial branch of the medial plantar artery.

ramus superficialis arteriae trans·ver·sae col·li (trans·vur'see kol'eye) [NA]. The superficial branch of the transverse artery of the neck.

ramus superficialis ner·vi plan·ta·ris la·te·ra·lis (nur'vye plan·tair'is lat·e·ray'lis) [NA]. The superficial branch of the lateral plantar nerve.

ramus superficialis nervi ra·di·a·lis (ray·dee·ay'lis) [NA]. The superficial branch of the radial nerve.

ramus superficialis nervi ul·na·ris (ul·nair'is) [NA]. The superficial branch of the ulnar nerve.

ramus superficialis ra·mi vo·la·ris ma·nus ner·vi ul·na·ris (ray'migh vo·lair'is man'us nur'vye ul·nair'is) [BNA]. RAMUS SUPERFICIALIS NERVI ULNARIS.

ramus superior ar·te·ri·ae glu·te·ae su·pe·ri·o·ris (ahr·teer'ee·ee gloo'tee·ee sue·peer·ee·o'ris) [NA]. The superior branch of the superior gluteal artery.

ramus superior lo·bi in·fe·ri·o·ris ar·te·ri·ae pul·mo·na·lis dex·trae (lo'bye in·feer·ee·o'ris ahr·teer'ee·ee pul·mo·nay'lis decks'tree) [NA alt.]. RAMUS APICALIS LOBI INFERIORIS ARTERIAE PULMONALIS DEXTRAE.

ramus superior lobi inferioris arteriae pulmonalis si·nis·trae (si·nis'tree) [NA alt.]. RAMUS APICALIS LOBI INFERIORIS ARTERIAE PULMONALIS SINISTRAE.

ramus superior ner·vi ocu·lo·mo·to·rii (nur'vye ock''yoo·lo·mo·to'ree·eye) [NA]. The superior branch of the oculomotor nerve.

ramus superior os·sis is·chii (os'is is'kee·eye) [BNA]. The bar of bone extending upward from the ischial tuberosity toward the acetabulum; now included in the body of the ischium.

ramus superior ossis pu·bis (pew'bis) [NA]. The bar of bone extending from the symphyseal portion of the pubis toward the acetabular portion.

ramus superior ve·nae pul·mo·na·lis in·fe·ri·o·ris dex·trae (vee'nee pul·mo·nay'lis in·feer·ee·o'ris decks'tree) [NA alt.]. RAMUS APICALIS VENAE PULMONALIS INFERIORIS DEXTRAE.

ramus superior venae pulmonalis inferioris si·nis·trae (si·nis'tree) [NA alt.]. RAMUS APICALIS VENAE PULMONALIS INFERIORIS SINISTRAE.

ramus su·pra·hy·oi·de·us ar·te·ri·ae lin·gua·lis (sue·pruh·high·oy'dee·us ahr·teer'ee·ee ling·gway'lis) [NA]. The suprahyoid branch of the lingual artery.

ramus sym·pa·thi·cus ad gan·gli·on ci·li·a·re (sim·path'i·kus ad gang'glee·on sil·ee·air'ee) [NA]. The sympathetic branch to the ciliary ganglion.

ramus sympathicus ad ganglion sub·man·di·bu·la·re (sub·man·dib·yoo·lair'ee) [NA]. The sympathetic branch to the submandibular ganglion.

ramus ten·to·rii ner·vi oph·thal·mi·ci (ten·to'ree·eye nur'vye off·thal'mi·sigh) [NA]. The tentorial branch of the ophthalmic nerve.

ramus thy·reo·hy·oi·de·us ner·vi hy·po·glos·si (thigh·ree·o·high·oy'dee·us nur'vye high·po·glos'eye) [BNA]. RAMUS THYROHYOIDEUS ANSAE CERVICALIS.

ramus thy·ro·hy·oi·de·us an·sae cer·vi·ca·lis (thigh·ro·high·oy'dee·us an·see sur·vi·kay'lis) [NA]. The thyrohyoid branch of the ansa cervicalis.

ramus ton·sil·la·ris ar·te·ri·ae fa·ci·a·lis (ton·si·lair'is ahr·teer'ee·ee fay·shee·ay'lis) [NA]. The tonsillar branch of the facial artery.

ramus tonsillaris arteriae max·il·la·ris ex·ter·nae (mack·si·lair'is ecks·tur'nee) [BNA]. RAMUS TONSILLARIS ARTERIAE FACIALIS.

ramus trans·ver·sus ar·te·ri·ae cir·cum·flex·ae fe·mo·ris la·te·ra·lis (trans·vur'sus ahr·teer'ee·ee sur·kum·fleck'see fem'o·ris lat·e·ray'lis) [NA]. The transverse branch of the lateral femoral circumflex artery.

ramus transversus arteriae circumflexae femoris me·di·a·lis (mee·dee·ay'lis) [NA]. The transverse branch of the medial femoral circumflex artery.

ramus tu·bae plex·us tym·pa·ni·ci (tew'bee pleck'sus tim·pan'i·sigh) [BNA]. RAMUS TUBARIUS PLEXUS TYMPANICI.

ramus tu·ba·ri·us ar·te·ri·ae ute·ri·nae (tew·bair'ee·us ahr·teer'ee·ee yoo·te·rye'nee) [NA]. The branch of the uterine artery to the uterine tube.

ramus tubarius plex·us tym·pa·ni·ci (pleck'sus tim·pan'i·sigh) [NA]. The nerve branch from the tympanic plexus to the auditory tube.

ramus ul·na·ris ner·vi cu·ta·nei an·te·bra·chii me·di·a·lis (ul·nair'is nur'vye kew·tay'nee·eye an·te·bray'kee·eye mee·dee·ay'lis) [NA]. The ulnar branch of the medial cutaneous nerve of the forearm.

ramus ven·tra·lis ner·vo·rum spi·na·li·um (ven·tray'lis nur·vo'rum spye·nay'lee·um) [NA]. The ventral branch of any spinal nerve.

ramus vo·la·ris ma·nus ner·vi ul·na·ris (vo·lair'is man'us nur'vye ul·nair'is) [BNA]. RAMUS PALMARIS NERVI ULNARIS.

ramus volaris ner·vi cu·ta·nei an·ti·bra·chii me·di·a·lis (nur'vye kew·tay'nee·eye an·ti·bray'kee·eye mee·dee·ay'lis) [BNA]. RAMUS ANTERIOR NERVI CUTANEI ANTEBRACHII MEDIALIS.

ramus volaris pro·fun·dus ar·te·ri·ae ul·na·ris (pro·fun'dus ahr·teer'ee·ee ul·nair'is) [BNA]. RAMUS PALMARIS PROFUNDUS ARTERIAE ULNARIS.

ramus volaris su·per·fi·ci·a·lis ar·te·ri·ae ra·di·a·lis (sue·pur·fish·ee·ay'lis ahr·teer'ee·ee ray·dee·ay'lis) [BNA]. RAMUS PALMARIS SUPERFICIALIS ARTERIAE RADIALIS.

ramus zy·go·ma·ti·co·fa·ci·a·lis ner·vi zy·go·ma·ti·ci (zye·go·mat''i·ko·fay·shee·ay'lis nur'vye zye·go·mat'i·sigh) [NA]. The zygomaticofacial branch of the zygomatic nerve.

ramus zy·go·ma·ti·co·tem·po·ra·lis ner·vi zy·go·ma·ti·ci (zye·go·mat''i·ko·tem·po·ray'lis nur'vye zye·go·mat'i·sigh) [NA]. The zygomaticotemporal branch of the zygomatic nerve.

Ra·na (ray'nuh) *n.* [L., frog]. A genus of frogs, species of which are often used as experimental animals and especially in certain pregnancy tests.

ran·cid (ran'sid) *adj.* [L. *rancidus*, rank, stinking]. Having the characteristic odor and taste of fat that has undergone oxidative and/or hydrolytic decomposition. —**ran·cid·i·ty** (ran·sid'i·tee) *n.*

Ran·dall forceps. A surgical instrument for grasping and removing kidney stones.

Ran·dia (ran'dee·uh) *n.* [I. *Rand*, English botanist, 18th century]. A genus of shrubs of the Rubiaceae, several species of which have been variously used as medicinals.

ran·dom mating. A system of breeding in which individuals mate in accordance with the frequency with which they occur in the population; as a first approximation, mating in any human population is of this type.

random process. STOCHASTIC PROCESS.

random sample. A finite number of individuals, cases, or measurements chosen from a larger group in such a manner that each individual, case, or measurement has an equal and independent chance of being selected.

range, *n.* [OF.]. An area or extent over which something varies, or a measure of that extent, as, for example, the difference between the lowest and the highest values in a series of observations.

range of accommodation. The span of clear vision through which the eye can focus (that is, from its far point to its near point).

range paralysis. NEURAL LYMPHOMATOSIS.

ra·ni·my·cin (ray''ni·migh'sin) *n.* An antibiotic substance, $C_{12}H_{18}O_6$, produced by *Streptomyces lincolnensis.*

ra·nine (ray'nine) *adj.* Pertaining to a ranula or to the region in which a ranula occurs.

Ran·ke's theory or **hypothesis** (rahnk'uh) [K. E. *Ranke*, German physician, 1870–1926]. The theory that tuberculosis develops in three stages: primary infection, generalized infection, and chronic isolated organ infection.

Ran·kin's operation [F. W. *Rankin*, U.S. surgeon, 1886–1954]. A two-staged abdominoperineal resection of the rectosigmoid for carcinoma.

rank itch. SCABIES PAPULIFORMIS.

Ran·so·hoff's operation [J. *Ransohoff*, U.S. surgeon, 1853–1921]. Discission of the pulmonary pleura in treatment of chronic empyema.

Ran·son's pyridine silver stain. A modification of a Cajal method for staining nerve fibers, in which the tissue is treated with pyridine before being immersed in the silver nitrate solution.

ran·u·la (ran'yoo·luh) *n.* [L., tadpole, little frog]. A retention cyst of a salivary gland, situated beneath the tongue.

Ra·nun·cu·lus (ra·nunk'yoo·lus) *n.* [L., crowfoot]. A genus of acrid herbs, some species of which have been used as medicinals. **—ra·nun·cu·la·ceous** (ra·nunk"yoo·lay'shus) *adj.*

Ran·vier's node (rahⁿv·yeʸ') [L. A. *Ranvier*]. NODE OF RANVIER.

Ra·oult's law (raʰ·ool') [F. M. *Raoult*, French physicist, 1830–1899]. The vapor pressure of a dilute solution of a nonvolatile nonelectrolyte is proportional to the molecular concentration of solvent in the solution. From this law may be derived equations predicting the freezing-point lowering, boiling-point elevation, and osmotic pressure of the solution.

rape, *n.* [L. *rapere*, to seize]. 1. *In legal medicine*, intimate sexual contact by a male with a female, not his wife, without her valid consent, by compulsion through violence, threats, stealth, or deceit. Laws vary as to whether contact with or penetration of the female genitalia is required to constitute rape; in some laws "without valid consent" means psychologically or physically incapable of resisting the male. Syn. *rape of the first degree.* Compare *statutory rape.* 2. *In veterinary medicine*, the forcible sexual intercourse of the male while the female is not in heat.

rape of the second degree. STATUTORY RAPE.

rape oil. The semidrying oil from the seeds of *Brassica campestris, B. napus*, and other species. Used as a food and for industrial purposes. Syn. *colza oil.*

rape seed. The seed of *Brassica campestris, B. napus*, and other species; the source of rape oil.

ra·pha·nia (ra·fay'nee·uh) *n.* [Gk. *rhaphanos*, radish, + *-ia*]. A disease characterized by spasms of the limbs, attributed to a poison in the seeds of the wild radish which get mixed with grain and thus is ingested over a long period of time.

raph·a·nin (raf'uh·nin) *n.* A liquid antibiotic principle obtained from the seeds of the radish, *Raphanus sativus*, freely soluble in water, and active, in vitro, against several species of bacteria.

ra·phe (ray'fee) *n.* [Gk. *rhaphē*, seam, suture, from *raptein*, to stitch, sew]. A seam or ridge, especially one indicating the line of junction of two symmetric halves.

raphe exterior. 1. LATERAL LONGITUDINAL STRIA. 2. MEDIAL LONGITUDINAL STRIA.

raphe inferior cor·po·ris cal·lo·si (kor'po·ris ka·lo'sigh). The raphe on the inferior surface of the corpus callosum.

raphe me·dul·lae ob·lon·ga·tae (me·dul'ee ob·long·gay'tee) [NA]. In a cross section of the medulla oblongata, the midline seam between the two lateral halves.

raphe of the ampulla. The longitudinal ridge on the roof of the ampulla of a membranous semicircular canal.

raphe of the penis. A continuation of the raphe of the scrotum upon the penis. NA *raphe penis.*

raphe of the pharynx. A fibrous band in the median line of the posterior wall of the pharynx. NA *raphe pharyngis.*

raphe of the pons. The intersection of the fibers at the midline as seen in transection. NA *raphe pontis.*

raphe of the scrotum. A medial ridge dividing the scrotum into two lateral halves; it is continuous posteriorly with the raphe of the perineum, anteriorly with the raphe of the penis. NA *raphe scroti.*

raphe of the tongue. A median furrow on the dorsal surface of the tongue corresponding to the fibrous septum which partially divides it into symmetric halves. NA *sulcus medianus linguae.*

raphe pa·la·ti (pa·lay'tye) [NA]. PALATINE RAPHE.

raphe palati du·ri (dew'rye). PALATINE RAPHE.

raphe pal·pe·bra·lis la·te·ra·lis (pal·pe·bray'lis lat·e·ray'lis) [NA]. A thin band of connecting tissue extending from the lateral palpebral angle to the margin of the orbit.

raphe pe·nis (pee'nis) [NA]. RAPHE OF THE PENIS.

raphe pe·ri·nei (perr·i·nee'eye) [NA]. PERINEAL RAPHE.

raphe pha·ryn·gis (fa·rin'jis) [NA]. RAPHE OF THE PHARYNX.

raphe pon·tis (pon'tis) [NA]. RAPHE OF THE PONS.

raphe post·ob·lon·ga·ta (pohst·ob·long·gay'tuh). The posterior median sulcus of the medulla oblongata.

raphe pte·ry·go·man·di·bu·la·ris (terr"i·go·man·dib·yoo·lair'is) [NA]. A band of connective tissue extending from the hamulus of the medial pterygoid plate to the mandible.

raphe scro·ti (skro'tye) [NA]. RAPHE OF THE SCROTUM.

raphe superior cor·po·ris cal·lo·si (kor'po·ris ka·lo'sigh). The longitudinal raphe in the middle of the superior surface of the corpus callosum.

rap·id ejection phase. The period of early cardiac systole, after opening of the aortic valve, during which the largest volume of blood per unit time is discharged by the ventricles.

rapid eye movement. The rapid, conjugate, usually lateral eye movement which characterizes REM sleep. Abbreviated, REM.

rapid filling wave. The outward deflection of the apex cardiogram immediately following the O point, corresponding to the rapid filling phase of ventricular diastole. Abbreviated, RFW. Contr. *slow filling wave.*

Rap·kine method. A histochemical method for detecting sulfhydryl groups by treating tissue with zinc acetate, nitroprusside, ammonium sulfate, and ammonium hydroxide to obtain a red color.

rap·port (ra·por') *n.* [F., relation, connection]. A comfortable, harmonious, trusting, and mutually responsive relationship between two or more people, of which they are aware, and which in special situations, as between patient and physician or psychiatric therapist, or between testee and tester, contributes to the willingness of the patient or subject to be helped.

rap·tus (rap'tus) *n.* [L., from *rapere*, to seize]. 1. Any sudden attack, intense emotion, or seizure. 2. RAPE.

raptus haem·or·rha·gi·cus (hem"o·ray'ji·kus). A sudden hemorrhage.

raptus impulsive. A sudden attack of extreme agitation, seen most dramatically in catatonic schizophrenia.

raptus ma·ni·a·cus (ma·nigh'uh·kus). A transient maniacal attack.

raptus mel·an·chol·i·cus (mel"un·kol'i·kus). Sudden and vehement melancholy.

raptus ner·vo·rum (nur·vo'rum). *Obsol.* 1. A sudden unprovoked attack of nervous irritability. 2. A cramp or spasm.

rare-earth element or **metal.** LANTHANIDE.

rar·e·fac·tion (rair"e·fack'shun) *n.* [L. *rarefacere*, to make thin]. The act of rarefying or of decreasing the density of a substance.

rarefaction of bone. Any process resulting in loss of mineral content of bone, making it less dense, more liable to fracture, and more radiolucent.

rar·e·fy (rair'i·figh, răr'i·figh) *v.* To make less dense or more porous.

rar·e·fy·ing osteitis (rair'e·fye"ing). OSTEOPOROSIS.

ra·ri·tas (rair'i·tas) *n.* [L.]. Rarity.

ra·sce·ta (ra·see'tuh) *n.pl.* [ML. *raseta*, from Ar. *rāḥa*, palm of the hand]. The transverse lines or creases on the palmar surface of the wrist.

Rasch's sign [H. *Rasch,* German obstetrician, b. 1873]. Detectable fluctuation of amniotic fluid by ballottement as an early indication of pregnancy.

rash, *n.* [probably from OF. *rasche,* scurf]. A lay term used for nearly any skin eruption but more commonly for acute inflammatory dermatoses.

ra·sion (ray'zhun) *n.* [L. *rasio,* from *radere,* to scrape]. The scraping of drugs with a file.

Ras·mus·sen's aneurysm (rahs'moo·sen) [F. W. *Rasmussen,* Danish physician, 1834–1877]. Aneurysm of a terminal pulmonary artery in a tuberculous cavity; rupture results in hemorrhage.

Ra·so·ri·an·ism (ray·zo'ree·un·iz·um) *n.* [G. *Rasori,* Italian physician, 1766–1837]. *Obsol.* The theory of counterstimuli, that is, substances diminish excitability by producing an opposite effect from that of the stimulant.

ra·sor·ite (ray'zur·ite) *n.* [C. M. *Rasor,* U.S. engineer, 20th century]. A native hydrate of borax, $Na_2B_4O_7.4H_2O$; an important source of this chemical.

ras·pa·to·ry (ras'puh·to"ree) *n.* [ML. *raspatorium,* from *raspare,* to rasp]. A rasp or file for trimming rough surfaces or margins of bone or for removing the periosteum.

rasp·ber·ry (raz'berr·ee) *n.* The fruit of *Rubus idaeus,* a plant of the Rosaceae. A syrup is used as a vehicle.

RAST Abbreviation for *radioallergosorbent test.*

rat, *n.* A rodent that lives in close proximity to man, such as in homes, barns, wharves, ships, and garbage dumps. Feral rats are notorious disease carriers, harboring many varieties of intestinal parasites and being responsible especially for the transmission of bubonic plague, as well as a distinct septic disease, rat-bite fever.

rat-bite fever. One of two distinct diseases contracted from the bite of infected rats or other animals. One (Haverhill fever) is caused by *Streptobacillus moniliformis.* The other (sodoku) is due to *Spirillum minus.*

rate, *n.* [OF., from L. *reri, ratum,* to reckon, judge]. The quantity or degree of some property or thing measured or calculated per unit of a reference standard, as the basal metabolic rate, the morbidity rate, or the radioactive decay rate.

rat flea. *XENOPSYLLA CHEOPIS.*

rat growth unit. The amount of vitamin A necessary to maintain a weekly gain of 3g in test rats previously depleted of vitamin A.

Rath·ke's duct (raht'keh) [M. H. *Rathke,* German anatomist, 1783–1810]. A variable persistent remnant of a paramesonephric duct emptying into the prostatic utricle.

Rathke's pouch [M. H. *Rathke*]. CRANIOBUCCAL POUCH.

Rathke's pouch cyst. Cystic distention of the remnants of the craniobuccal (Rathke's) pouch. See also *craniopharyngioma.*

rat·ing, *n.* A systematic, often graded estimate of the qualities or characteristics of a person, process, or thing.

ra·tio (ray'shee·o) *n.* [L., account, reckoning, from *reri,* to reckon, judge]. A proportion.

ra·tion (rash'un, ray'shun) *n.* [F., from L. *ratio,* account]. A daily allowance of food or drink. In the armed services, the term usually means the complete subsistence for one man for one day.

ra·tio·nal (rash'un·ul) *adj.* [L. *rationalis*]. 1. Based upon reason; reasonable. 2. *In therapeutics,* opposed to empirical.

ra·tio·nal·iza·tion (ra"shun·ul·i·zay'shun) *n.* A mode of adjustment to difficult and unpleasant situations; a defense mechanism, operating unconsciously, in which the individual attempts to justify, defend, or make tolerable by plausible means unacceptable attitudes or traits, behavior, feelings, and motives. Not to be confused with conscious misrepresentation or withholding of essential facts.

rat louse. *Polyplax spinulosa,* which carries the organism of murine typhus, *Rickettsia mooseri,* and transmits it to its rat host, but not to man.

rat mite. *BDELLONYSSUS BACOTI.*

rats·bane, *n.* 1. ARSENIC TRIOXIDE. 2. A name given to any rat poison containing arsenic.

rat-tail catheter. A sharp, narrow-ended catheter shaped somewhat like a rat's tail and used in urethral strictures.

rat·tle, *n.* RALE.

rat·tle·snake, *n.* Any snake of the New World pit vipers belonging to the genera *Crotalus* and *Sistrurus.*

rat typhus. MURINE TYPHUS.

Rau·ber's cell (raow'bur) [A. A. *Rauber,* German anatomist, 1845–1917]. One of the trophoblast cells overlying the inner cell mass in many mammals; they disappear, leaving the blastoderm superficial to and continuous with the trophoblast.

Rauwiloid. Trademark for alseroxylon, a fat-soluble alkaloidal fraction from *Rauwolfia serpentina.*

Rau·wol·fia (raw·wol'fee·uh) *n.* [L., after *Rauwolf,* German botanist, 16th century]. A genus of tropical trees and shrubs, mostly poisonous, of the Apocynaceae family. The dried root of *Rauwolfia serpentina,* which contains reserpine and other alkaloids, is used as an antihypertensive and sedative drug.

rau·wol·fine (raw·wol'feen, ·fin) *n.* An alkaloid, $C_{20}H_{26}N_2O_3$, from *Rauwolfia serpentina;* ajmaline.

Ra·va·ton's amputation or **method** (rah·vah·tohn') [H. *Ravaton,* French military surgeon, 18th century]. An external disarticulation of the hip through a racket incision.

Ra·ven Progressive Matrices [J. C. *Raven,* English psychologist, 20th century]. A perceptual test of intelligence.

Ravocaine. Trademark for the local anesthetic propoxycaine, used as the hydrochloride salt.

ray, *n.* [OF. *rai,* from L. *radius*]. 1. A beam of light or other radiant energy. 2. A stream of discrete particles, such as alpha rays or beta rays. 3. A radial streak of different color in an organ, as medullary rays of the kidney.

ray fungus. Formerly, any organism of the genus *Actinomyces* or *Nocardia.*

Ray·gat's test. HYDROSTATIC TEST.

Ray·leigh test (ray'lee). A test for red-green color blindness.

Ray·mond-Ces·tan syndrome (reh·mohn', ses·tahn') [F. *Raymond,* French neurologist, 1844–1910; and R. *Cestan*]. A syndrome characterized by paralysis of lateral gaze, abducens palsy, and contralateral hemiplegia, and ipsilateral hemianesthesia, associated with lesions involving the red nucleus.

Raymond-Foville syndrome. FOVILLE'S PARALYSIS.

Ray·naud's disease (reh·no') [M. *Raynaud,* French physician, 1834–1881]. 1. Episodes of Raynaud's phenomenon, usually bilateral, excited by cold or emotion, with normal arterial pulsations and the absence of other primary causal disease. 2. Primary Raynaud's phenomenon, which occurs more commonly in women.

Raynaud's phenomenon [M. *Raynaud*]. Intermittent pallor, cyanosis, or rubor of the fingers or toes, or both, usually induced by cold or by emotion; secondary to many diseases, but often to chronic arterial occlusive disease.

ray·on, *n.* A purified regenerated cellulose used as a surgical aid.

Ray's mania [I. *Ray,* U.S. physician, 1807–1881]. MORAL INSANITY. See also *sociopathic personality disturbance.*

rays of Sa·gnac (sa·nyahk') [G. *Sagnac,* French physicist]. Secondary beta rays emanating from metals on which roentgen rays fall.

Rb Symbol for rubidium.

RBC, rbc Abbreviation for (a) *red blood cell;* (b) red blood count.

RBE Abbreviation for *relative biological effectiveness* (of radiation).

R body [*r*od-containing]. A spherical structure found within the cytoplasm of human rectal epithelial cells; it is membrane-bound, 0.2–1.5 microns in diameter and contains electron-dense rods. See also *C body.*

R.C.P. Royal College of Physicians.

R.C.S. Royal College of Surgeons.

R.D. Abbreviation for *reaction of degeneration.*

rd Abbreviation for *rutherford.*

R.D.A. The right dorsoanterior position of the fetus.

R.D.P. The right dorsoposterior position of the fetus.

RDS Abbreviation for *respiratory distress syndrome of the newborn.*

Re Symbol for rhenium.

re- [L.]. A prefix signifying *back* or *again.*

re·ac·tant (ree·ack'tunt) *n.* [*react* + *-ant*]. Any substance that reacts chemically with another substance or substances.

re·ac·tion (ree·ack'shun) *n.* 1. A response to stimulus. 2. *In psychiatry,* a behavioral pattern constituting a recognizable clinical disorder. 3. Any chemical change, transformation, or interaction. 4. The state of a system, especially in solution, with reference to the relative proportion of hydrogen and hydroxyl ions, that is, whether neutral, acid, or alkaline. —**re·act** (ree·ackt') *v.*

reaction center. GERMINAL CENTER.

reaction formation. *In psychoanalysis,* a defense mechanism operating unconsciously, characterized by the development of conscious, socially acceptable activity which is the antithesis of repressed or rejected unconscious desires, as excessive prudishness in reaction to strong but repressed erotic wishes.

reaction kinetics. KINETICS (2).

reaction of degeneration. The electric reaction of denervated muscle, developing about 10 days after and varying with the severity of injury; in mild partial degeneration, faradic stimulation of nerve requires more current than normal and galvanic stimulation of nerve and muscle results in normal responses; in severe partial degeneration, faradic stimulation of nerve produces no contraction while galvanic stimulation of nerve and muscle produces normal reactions; in complete or total degeneration, neither faradic nor galvanic stimulation of nerve produces any response, while galvanic stimulation of muscle results in vermicular contractions. Abbreviated, R.D.

reaction period. The time required for the body to respond to some form of stimulation following application of the stimulus; latent or lag period.

reaction time. The interval between the application of a stimulus and the beginning of the response.

re·ac·ti·vate (ree·ack'ti·vate) *v.* 1. To make active again, as by the addition of fresh normal serum containing complement to an immune serum which has lost its complement through age or heat. 2. To restore complementary activity to a serum, deprived of one or several of its C' components, by the addition of these components.

re·ac·ti·va·tion (ree·ack"ti·vay'shun) *n.* Rendering active again, as in the case of the addition of complement or one or several of its components to a serum that has become inactive.

re·ac·tive (ree·ack'tive) *adj.* Pertaining to or marked by reaction. —**re·ac·tiv·i·ty** (ree"ack·tiv'i·tee) *n.*

reactive depression. DEPRESSIVE NEUROSIS.

reactive depressive psychosis. PSYCHOTIC DEPRESSIVE REACTION.

reactive psychosis. PSYCHOTIC DEPRESSIVE REACTION.

reactive schizophrenia. Schizophrenia considered primarily to be due to predisposing or precipitating environmental events, or both; typically manifested by a rapid onset and brief course, with the patient seemingly well before and after the episode. Contr. *process schizophrenia.*

reactive triangle. CODMAN'S TRIANGLE.

re·ac·tor (ree·ack'tur) *n.* 1. A subject that reacts positively to a foreign substance, as in a test for a disease. 2. A subject that reacts to a stimulus in a psychological test. 3. A chemical or organism that reacts. 4. An apparatus in which a chemical or nuclear reaction occurs. See also *nuclear reactor.*

read (reed) *n.* ABOMASUM.

reading epilepsy. A form of sensory epilepsy triggered by reading. See also *reflex epilepsy.*

re·agent (ree·ay'junt) *n.* [L. *reagens,* reacting]. 1. Any substance involved in a chemical reaction. 2. A substance used for the detection or determination of another substance by chemical, microscopical, or other means.

re·agin (ree·ay'jin) *n.* [*reag*ent + *-in*]. An antibody which occurs in human atopy, such as hay fever and asthma, and which readily sensitizes the skin and other tissues by attaching to mast cells and basophils. When combined with the corresponding antigen, it is responsible for the liberation of histamine and other mediators which cause atopic symptoms. See also *gamma-E globulin.* —**re·agin·ic** (ree"uh·jin'ick) *adj.*

reaginic antibody. REAGIN.

real image. An image formed of real foci.

re·al·i·ty principle (ree·al'i·tee). *In psychoanalysis,* the concept that the pleasure principle is normally modified by the demands of the external environment and that the individual adjusts to these inescapable requirements in a way so that he ultimately secures satisfaction of his instinctual wishes.

reality testing. *In psychiatry,* the efforts made by a person to achieve balance between the demands and restrictions of his external environment and his needs for self-recognition, usually in some nonthreatening ways such as fantasy or projection; may be a part of normal adjustment or may become all-absorbing as in the regression of a psychosis.

ream·er (ree'mur) *n.* [OE. *rȳman,* to widen, make room]. 1. A surgical instrument used for gouging out holes or enlarging those already made, especially in bone operations. 2. An endodontic instrument with spiral blades used for cleaning and enlarging root canals.

re·am·i·na·tion (ree·am"i·nay'shun) *n.* [*re-* + *amination*]. The introduction of an amino group into a compound from which an amino group had previously been removed.

re·am·pu·ta·tion (ree·am"pew·tay'shun) *n.* An amputation upon a member on which the operation has already been performed.

re·an·i·mate (ree·an'i·mate) *v.* [*re-* + *animate*]. To revive; resuscitate; to restore to life, as a person apparently dead.

Ré·au·mur thermometer (rey·o·muer') [R. A. F. *Réaumur,* French physiologist, 1683–1757]. A thermometer on which the freezing point of water is 0° and the boiling point 80° with an interval of 80 points or degrees.

re·bound, *n.* [OF. *rebondir,* to spring back]. 1. In reflex activity, a sudden contraction of a muscle following its relaxation; associated with a variety of forms of reflex activity. Seen most typically following the cessation of an inhibitory reflex. 2. The return to health from illness; vigorous recovery.

rebound phenomenon. The normal tendency of a limb whose movement is being resisted to move in the intended direction when resistance is removed and then to jerk back, or rebound, in the opposite direction. The rebound is exaggerated in spastic limbs and is absent in limbs affected by cerebellar disease.

re·breath·ing, *n.* The act of respiring air, or air plus other gases, which has already been exhaled.

rebreathing bag. A flexible rubber bag into and from which breathing takes place for therapeutic or experimental purposes; also, such a bag used in the administration of gas anesthesia.

re·cal·ci·fi·ca·tion (ree·kal"si·fi·kay'shun) *n.* [*re-* + *calcification*]. 1. The restoration of lime salts to bone matrix. 2. The addition of a solution of calcium salts to blood or plasma decalcified by an anticoagulant. —**re·cal·ci·fy** (ree·kal'si·fye) *v.*

recalcification time. RECALCIFIED CLOTTING TIME.

recalcified clotting time. The clotting time of decalcified blood or plasma upon the readdition of calcium ions.

re·cal·ci·trant (re·kal'si·trunt) *adj.* [from L. *recalcitrare,* to be stubbornly disobedient]. Resistant to treatment, whether medical or psychiatric; stubborn.

recalcitrant pustular acrodermatitis. Persistent acrodermatitis.

re·call, *n.* 1. *In psychology,* the complex mental process of bringing the memory trace or engram of a past experience or of material learned into consciousness. 2. *In immunology,* ANAMNESTIC RESPONSE.

Ré·ca·mier's operation (rey·kahm·yey') [J. C. A. *Récamier,* French physician, 1774–1852]. Uterine curettage.

re·ca·pit·u·la·tion (ree''ka·pit''yoo·lay'shun) *n.* [from L. *recapitulare,* to sum up]. The summarizing of the main points of a subject; the repetition of the steps of a process.

recapitulation theory. The theory that the individual organism in its development from the ovum passes through a series of stages that resemble a series of ancestral types through which the species passed in its evolutionary history. This is also called the biogenetic law. Haeckel recognized a difference between those structures which are adaptive to the embryonic, larval, or fetal mode of life and those which may be regarded as inherited from the ancestral types. The former he included under cenogenesis and the latter under palingenesis.

recent memory. Recall of events that occurred in the relatively immediate past. Compare *short-term memory.*

re·cep·tac·u·lum (ree''sep·tack'yoo·lum) *n.,* pl. **receptacu·la** (·luh) [L.]. A receptacle; a small container.

receptaculum chy·li (kye'lye). CISTERNA CHYLI.

re·cep·tive, *adj.* [ML. *receptivus,* from L. *recipere,* to receive]. Having the quality of, or capacity for, receiving. Specifically, pertaining to the mind, open to impressions, ideas, and suggestions from sources other than oneself.

receptive aphasia. SENSORY APHASIA.

receptive centers. *In physiology and psychophysics,* nerve centers which receive influences that may excite sensations or some kind of activity not associated with conscious perception.

receptive field. The area of the retina where spot illumination continues to yield a response in a particular optic nerve fiber.

re·cep·to·ma (ree''sep·to'muh) *n.* [*receptor* + *-oma*]. CHEMODECTOMA.

re·cep·tor (re·sep'tur) *n.* [L., receiver, from *recipere,* to receive]. 1. A specialized structure of sensory nerve terminals characteristically excited by specific stimuli. Contr. *effector.* 2. A molecular structure at the cell surface or within the cell which is capable of combining with molecules such as toxins, hormones, antigens, immunoglobulins and complement components. See also *side-chain theory.* 3. *In pharmacology,* a receptor (2) which combines, with varying degrees of specificity, with a drug or other substance resulting in a given alteration of cell function. See also *alpha-adrenergic receptor, beta-adrenergic receptor.*

α-receptor. Alpha-receptor (= ALPHA-ADRENERGIC RECEPTOR).

β-receptor. Beta-receptor (= BETA-ADRENERGIC RECEPTOR).

receptor of the first order. *Obsol.* According to Ehrlich's side-chain theory, body cells or chemical groups capable of neutralizing toxin.

receptor of the second order. *Obsol.* According to Ehrlich's side-chain theory, body cells or chemical groups which agglutinate or precipitate the antigen.

receptor of the third order. *Obsol.* According to Ehrlich's side-chain theory, body cells or chemical groups which react with the antigen and fix complement.

receptor potential. GENERATOR POTENTIAL.

re·cess, *n.* [L. *recessus,* from *recedere,* to withdraw]. A fossa, ventricle, or ampulla; an anatomic depression.

re·ces·sion (re·sesh'un) *n.* [L. *recessio,* from *recedere,* to withdraw]. The gradual withdrawal of a part from its normal position, as recession of the gums from the necks of teeth.

re·ces·sive (re·ses'iv) *adj.* & *n.* 1. *In genetics,* characterizing the behavior of an allele which is not expressed in the presence of another (dominant) allele. 2. A recessive character or trait.

recessive character or **trait.** The member of a pair of contrasted traits which fails to manifest itself in the heterozygote. Contr. *dominant character.*

recess of the pelvic mesocolon. INTERSIGMOID RECESS.

recess of the tympanic cavity. 1. Anterior and posterior pouches of the mucous membrane covering the lateral wall of the tympanic cavity and found on either side of the manubrium of the malleus. NA *recessus membranae tympani anterior, recessus membranae tympani posterior.* 2. A superior recess situated between the flaccid part of the tympanic membrane and the neck of the malleus. NA *recessus membranae tympani superior.*

recess of Tröltsch [A. F. von *Tröltsch*]. RECESS OF THE TYMPANIC CAVITY (1).

re·ces·sus (ree·ses'us) *n.,* pl. & genit. sing. **recessus** [L.]. RECESS.

recessus anterior fos·sae in·ter·pe·dun·cu·la·ris (fos'ee in·tur·pe·dunk·yoo·lair'is) [BNA]. The anterior part of the interpeduncular fossa.

recessus co·chle·a·ris ve·sti·bu·li (kock·lee·air'is ves·tib'yoo·lye) [NA]. COCHLEAR RECESS.

recessus cos·to·dia·phrag·ma·ti·cus pleu·rae (kos''to·dye·uh·frag·mat'i·kus ploo'ree) [NA]. COSTODIAPHRAGMATIC RECESS.

recessus cos·to·me·di·a·sti·na·lis pleu·rae (kos''to·mee·dee·as·ti·nay'lis ploo'ree) [NA]. COSTOMEDIASTINAL RECESS.

recessus du·o·de·na·lis inferior (dew·o·de·nay'lis) [NA]. An occasional pocket of peritoneum on the left side of the terminal part of the duodenum; the pocket opens cranially.

recessus duodenalis superior [NA]. DUODENOJEJUNAL FOSSA.

recessus du·o·de·no·je·ju·na·lis (dew·o·dee''no·je·joo·nay'lis) [BNA]. Recessus duodenalis superior (= DUODENOJEJUNAL FOSSA).

recessus el·lip·ti·cus ve·sti·bu·li (e·lip'ti·kus ves·tib'yoo·lye) [NA]. ELLIPTICAL RECESS.

recessus epi·tym·pa·ni·cus (ep·i·tim·pan'i·kus) [NA]. EPITYMPANIC RECESS.

recessus he·pa·to·re·na·lis (hep''uh·to·re·nay'lis) [NA]. HEPATORENAL POUCH.

recessus ileo·ce·ca·lis inferior (il''ee·o·see·kay'lis) [NA]. Inferior ileocecal recess. See *ileocecal recesses.*

recessus ileocecalis superior [NA]. Superior ileocecal recess. See *ileocecal recesses.*

recessus inferior omen·ta·lis (o·men·tay'lis) [NA]. INFERIOR RECESS OF THE OMENTAL BURSA.

recessus in·fun·di·bu·li (in·fun·dib'yoo·lye) [NA]. INFUNDIBULAR RECESS.

recessus in·ter·sig·moi·de·us (in''tur·sig·moy'dee·us) [NA]. INTERSIGMOID RECESS.

recessus la·te·ra·lis fos·sae rhom·boi·de·ae (lat·e·ray'lis fos'ee rom·boy'dee·ee) [BNA]. Recessus lateralis ventriculi quarti (= LATERAL RECESS).

recessus lateralis ven·tri·cu·li quar·ti (ven·trick'yoo·lye kwahr'tye) [NA]. LATERAL RECESS.

recessus li·e·na·lis (lye·e·nay'lis) [NA]. LIENAL RECESS.

recessus mem·bra·nae tym·pa·ni anterior (mem·bray'nee tim'puh·nigh) [NA]. RECESS OF THE TYMPANIC CAVITY (1).

recessus membranae tympani posterior [NA]. RECESS OF THE TYMPANIC CAVITY (2).

recessus membranae tympani superior [NA]. RECESS OF THE TYMPANIC CAVITY (2).

recessus op·ti·cus (op'ti·kus) [NA]. OPTIC RECESS.

recessus pa·ra·co·li·ci (păr·uh·ko'li·sigh) [BNA]. SULCI PARACOLICI.

recessus pa·ra·du·o·de·na·lis (păr·uh·dew·o·de·nay'lis) [NA]. PARADUODENAL RECESS.

recessus pha·ryn·ge·us (fa·rin'jee·us) [NA]. PHARYNGEAL RECESS.

recessus phre·ni·co·he·pa·ti·ci (fren·i·ko·he·pat'i·sigh) [BNA]. RECESSUS SUBHEPATICI and RECESSUS SUBPHRENICI.

recessus pi·ne·a·lis (pin·e·ay'lis) [NA]. PINEAL RECESS.

recessus pi·ri·for·mis (pirr·i·for'mis) [NA]. PIRIFORM RECESS.

recessus pleu·ra·les (ploo·ray'leez) [NA]. The recesses of the pleura.

recessus posterior fos·sae in·ter·pe·dun·cu·la·ris (fos'ee in·tur·pe·dunk·yoo·lair'is) [BNA]. The posterior part of the interpeduncular fossa.

recessus re·tro·ce·ca·lis (ret·ro·see·kay'lis) [NA]. RETROCECAL RECESS.

recessus re·tro·du·o·de·na·lis (ret″ro·dew·o·de·nay'lis) [NA]. RETRODUODENAL RECESS.

recessus sac·ci·for·mis ar·ti·cu·la·ti·o·nis cu·bi·ti (sack·si·for'mis ahr·tick″yoo·lay·shee·o'nis kew'bi·tye) [BNA]. The pocket of synovial membrane of the elbow joint which lies between the radius and ulna.

recessus sacciformis articulationis ra·dio·ul·na·ris dis·ta·lis (ray″dee·o·ul·nair'is dis·tay'lis) [NA]. SACCIFORM RECESS OF THE WRIST.

recessus sphae·ri·cus (sfeer'i·kus) [BNA]. Recessus sphericus vestibuli (= SPHERICAL RECESS).

recessus sphe·no·eth·moi·da·lis (sfee″no·eth·moy·day'lis) [NA]. SPHENOETHMOID RECESS.

recessus sphe·ri·cus ves·ti·bu·li (sfeer'i·kus ves·tib'yoo·lye) [NA]. SPHERICAL RECESS.

recessus sub·he·pa·ti·ci (sub·he·pat'i·sigh) [NA]. A pocket of peritoneum beneath the liver.

recessus sub·phre·ni·ci (sub·fren'i·sigh) [NA]. A pocket of peritoneum beneath the diaphragm.

recessus sub·po·pli·te·us (sub·pop·lit'ee·us) [NA]. A pocket of synovial membrane of the knee joint extending beneath the popliteus muscle.

recessus superior omen·ta·lis (o·men·tay'lis) [NA]. SUPERIOR RECESS OF THE OMENTAL BURSA.

recessus su·pra·pi·ne·a·lis (sue″pruh·pin·ee·ay'lis) [NA]. SUPRAPINEAL RECESS.

recessus tri·an·gu·la·ris (trye·ang·gew·lair'is) [BNA]. A triangular area on the anterior wall of the third ventricle.

re·cid·i·va·tion (re·sid″i·vay'shun) *n.* [from *recidivist*]. 1. The relapse of a patient recovering from a disease. 2. *In criminology,* a relapsing into crime.

re·cid·i·vism (re·sid'i·viz·um) *n.* [from *recidivist*]. The repetition of criminal or delinquent acts; repeated bad behavior.

re·cid·i·vist (re·sid'i·vist) *n.* [F. *récidiviste,* from L. *recidivus,* recurring, falling back, from *recidere,* to fall back]. 1. A patient who returns to a hospital for treatment, especially a mentally ill person who so returns. 2. *In criminology,* a confirmed, relapsed, or habitual criminal.

rec·i·div·i·ty (res″i·div'i·tee) *n.* The tendency to relapse in illness or to return to hospital or jail.

rec·i·pe (res'i·pee) *v. & n.* [L., imperative of *recipere,* to receive]. 1. The heading of a physician's prescription, signifying *take.* Symbol, ℞. 2. The prescription itself.

re·cip·i·ent (re·sip'ee·unt) *n.* [L. *recipiens,* receiving]. One who receives blood or other tissue from another, the donor.

re·cip·ro·cal (re·sip'ruh·kul) *adj.* [L. *reciprocus,* returning, going back in the same path, + *-al*]. 1. Complementary. 2. Mutual and equal.

reciprocal articulation. A mode of articulation in which the articular surface is convex on one side and concave on the other. See also *condylar joint.*

reciprocal beating. RECIPROCAL RHYTHM.

reciprocal inhibition and desensitization. *In psychiatry,* a form of behavior therapy in which the patient, while made to relax in comfortable surroundings, is gradually exposed to increasing amounts of anxiety-provoking stimuli. In this way the patient can tolerate these stimuli and may eventually learn to dissociate the anxiety from them.

reciprocal innervation. The state of innervation of certain antagonistic muscles about a joint, as extensors and flexors, by which the one set relaxes as the other contracts.

reciprocal replacement. RETINAL RIVALRY.

reciprocal rhythm. The phenomenon of a retrograde AV junctional impulse reentering an anterograde pathway and reactivating the ventricles; this assumes two functional pathways in the AV junction with unidirectional block in one of them.

reciprocal transfusion. The exchange of approximately equal volumes of blood between two persons; a therapeutic measure used to remove abnormal elements from or add needed elements to the circulation of a patient without altering the blood volume significantly.

reciprocal translocation. Exchange of segments between nonhomologous chromosomes.

rec·i·proc·i·ty (res″i·pros'i·tee) *n. In medicine,* the reciprocal recognition among some states of the U.S. of the validity of examinations and licensures for doctors, nurses, and other professional and paraprofessional personnel.

Recklinghausen's disease. VON RECKLINGHAUSEN'S DISEASE.

rec·li·na·tio (reck″li·nay'shee·o) *n.* [L.]. RECLINATION.

rec·li·na·tion (reck″li·nay'shun) *n.* [L. *reclinare,* to bend back]. An operation for cataract, in which the lens is pushed back into the vitreous chamber. Syn. *couching.*

Re·clus' disease (ruh·klue') [P. *Reclus,* French surgeon, 1847–1914]. Mammary dysplasia of the cystic disease type. See also *cystic disease.*

re·cog·nin (re·kog'nin) *n.* A protein fragment produced from cancer cells.

rec·og·ni·tion time. The time required for recognition of the type of stimulus after its application.

re·coil, *n.* [OF. *reculer,* to recoil, fall back]. 1. The reaction of a body under the impact of force or pressure. 2. The backward or sideways thrust imparted to an object by the ejection of a fragment or component of, or material from, the object.

re·coil atom. The remainder of an atom still in motion after emission of an alpha particle, a beta particle, or a neutron.

recoil electron. An electron removed from its place in an atom and set into motion by impact of a photon; as a result of the collision the photon gives up only part of its energy to the electron and proceeds along a new path. Syn. *Compton electron.*

re·com·bi·nant (re·kom'bi·nunt) *adj.* Pertaining to or resulting from genetic recombination.

re·com·bi·na·tion (ree·kom″bi·nay'shun) *n. In radiobiology,* the coming together of two or more ionized or activated atoms, radicals, or molecules. See also *genetic recombination.*

re·com·po·si·tion (ree·kom″puh·zish'un) *n.* [L. *recomponere,* to put together again]. Reunion of parts or constituents after temporary dissolution.

re·com·pres·sion (ree″kum·presh'un) *n.* Resubjection to increased atmospheric pressure; a procedure used in treating caisson workers or divers who develop decompression sickness returning too rapidly to normal atmospheric pressures.

re·con·stit·u·ent (ree″kun·stich'oo·unt) *n.* A medicine which promotes continuous repair of tissue waste or makes compensation for its loss.

re·con·sti·tu·tion (ree·kon″sti·tew'shun) *n.* Continuous repair of progressive destruction of tissues.

re·con·struc·tion (ree″kun·struck'shun) *n.* 1. In medical history taking and psychoanalysis, the integration into a significant whole of facts which are presented first without consciousness of their relationship. 2. Reproduction, usually with enlargement of the form, of an embryo, organ system, or part by assemblage of properly spaced and oriented outlines of serial sections. 3. *In plastic surgery,* the attempt, often by a series of operations, to restore a disfigured, deformed, or deficient part to more normal appearance or function. —**reconstruc·tive** (·tiv) *adj.*

re·con·struc·tive operation. An operation done to repair a defect, either congenital or acquired.

rec·ord base (reck'urd). BASEPLATE.

record rim. OCCLUSION RIM.

re·cov·ery (re·kuv'ur·ee) *n.* [L. *recuperare*, to recover]. Return to a state of rest, equilibrium, or health from a state of fatigue, stress, or illness.

recovery oxygen. OXYGEN DEBT.

recreation therapy. *In psychiatry*, the use of music, theater, games, and other such group activities which provide the patient relaxation as well as outlets for self-expression and the discharge of aggression and hostility; an adjuvant form of psychotherapy.

rec·re·ment (reck're·munt) *n.* [L. *recrementum*, refuse, from *re-* + *cernere*, to sift]. A substance secreted from a part of the body, as a gland, and again absorbed by the body, as for example saliva or bile. —**rec·re·men·tal** (reck"re·men'tul), **rec·re·men·ti·tial** (reck"re·men·tish'ul), **recremen·ti·tious** (·tish'us) *adj.*

re·cru·des·cence (ree"kroo·des'unce) *n.* [L. *recrudescere*, to become raw again]. An increase or recurrence of the symptoms of a disease after a remission or a short intermission. —**recrudes·cent** (·unt) *adj.*

recrudescent typhus. BRILL'S DISEASE.

re·cruit·ment (re·kroot'munt) *n.* [F. *recrutement*, from *recrue*, recruit, from *recrû*, new growth]. Involvement of increasing numbers of motor units in response to increasing strength of stimulus.

recruitment spasm. In tetanus, the induction, by repetitive voluntary movements, of a gradual increase in tonic contraction and spasms of affected muscles, followed by spread of spasm to neighboring muscle groups.

recruitment test. The measurement of the span between the threshold of a deafened person's hearing and the level of his discomfort. This span is much shorter when there is loss of perception due to a cochlear defect than when there is loss of conduction.

rect-, recto-. A combining form meaning *rectum, rectal.*

recta. A plural of *rectum.*

rec·tal (reck'tul) *adj.* [*rect-* + *-al*]. Pertaining to or affecting the rectum.

rectal aerophagia. Indrawing of air by rectum.

rectal alimentation. The nourishing of a patient by the administration of small quantities of food through the rectum.

rectal ampulla. The dilated part of the rectum situated just above the anal canal.

rectal anesthesia. Anesthesia induced by placing the anesthetic agent, such as avertin, paraldehyde, or barbiturate, in the rectum with a catheter.

rectal columns. ANAL COLUMNS.

rectal crisis. Paroxysmal proctalgia occurring in tabes dorsalis.

rec·tal·gia (reck·tal'jee·uh) *n.* [*rect-* + *-algia*]. PROCTALGIA.

rectal hernia. A condition in which the small bowel, or other abdominal contents, protrudes through the rectovesical excavation or rectouterine pouch, carrying the anterior rectal wall through the anus.

rectal plexus. 1. A venous plexus surrounding the lower part of the rectum. NA *plexus venosus rectalis.* 2. Any of the nerve plexuses supplying the rectum: (a) The superior rectal plexus (NA *plexus rectalis superior*) is part of the inferior mesenteric plexus; (b) the middle rectal plexuses (NA *plexus rectales medii*) are a part of the pelvic nerve plexus; (c) the inferior rectal plexuses (NA *plexus rectales inferiores*) derive from the pudendal nerves.

rectal shelf. BLUMER'S SHELF.

rectal sinus. ANAL CRYPT.

rectal sphincter. NÉLATON'S FIBERS.

rectal triangle. ANAL TRIANGLE.

rectal valves. TRANSVERSE RECTAL FOLDS.

rec·tec·to·my (reck·teck'tuh·mee) *n.* [*rect-* + *-ectomy*]. PROCTECTOMY.

recti. 1. Plural and genitive singular of *rectus.* 2. Genitive singular of *rectum.*

rec·ti·fi·ca·tion (reck"ti·fi·kay'shun) *n.* [L. *rectificare*, to rectify, from *rectus*, straight]. 1. A straightening, as rectification of a crooked limb. 2. The redistillation or fractional distillation of liquids to obtain a product of higher purity or greater concentration of the desired constitutent 3. The conversion of alternating to direct current.

rec·ti·lin·ear (reck"ti·lin'ee·ur) *adj.* [*recti-*, straight, + *linear*]. Describing or characterized by a straight line.

rectilinear lens. APLANATIC LENS.

rec·ti·tis (reck·tye'tis) *n.* [*rect-* + *-itis*]. PROCTITIS.

recto-. See *rect-.*

rec·to·ab·dom·i·nal (reck"to·ab·dom'i·nul) *adj.* Pertaining to the rectum and the abdomen.

rec·to·anal (reck"to·ay'nul) *adj.* Pertaining to the rectum and the anus.

rec·to·cele (reck'to·seel) *n.* [*recto-* + *-cele*]. Protrusion or herniation of the rectum into the vagina. Syn. *vaginal proctocele.*

rec·toc·ly·sis (reck·tock'li·sis) *n.* [*recto-* + *clysis*]. The slow instillation of a liquid into the rectum. Syn. *proctoclysis, Murphy drip.*

rec·to·coc·cyg·e·al (reck"to·cock·sij'ee·ul) *adj.* [*recto-* + *coccygeal*]. Pertaining to the rectum and the coccyx.

rec·to·coc·cy·ge·us (reck"to·kock·sij'ee·us) *n.* A band of mixed smooth and striate muscle fibers extending from the front of the coccyx to the back of the rectum. NA *musculus rectococcygeus.*

rec·to·co·li·tis (reck"to·ko·lye'tis) *n.* [*recto-* + *colitis*]. Inflammation of the mucosa of the rectum and colon.

rec·to·co·lon·ic (reck"to·ko·lon'ick) *adj.* [*recto-* + *colonic*]. Pertaining to the rectum and the colon.

rec·to·cu·ta·ne·ous (reck"to·kew·tay'nee·us) *adj.* [*recto-* + *cutaneous*]. Pertaining to both the rectum and the skin.

rec·to·fis·tu·la (reck"to·fis'tew·luh) *n.* A fistula of the rectum.

rec·to·gen·i·tal (reck"to·jen'i·tul) *adj.* Pertaining to the rectum and the genital organs.

rec·to·la·bi·al (reck"to·lay'bee·ul) *adj.* [*recto-* + *labial*]. Relating to the rectum and the labia pudendi.

rec·to·per·i·ne·al (reck"to·perr·i·nee'ul) *adj.* [*recto-* + *perineal*]. Pertaining to the rectum and the perineum.

rec·to·pexy (reck'to·peck"see) *n.* [*recto-* + *-pexy*]. PROCTOPEXY.

rec·to·pho·bia (reck"to·fo'bee·uh) *n.* [*recto-* + *-phobia*]. PROCTOPHOBIA.

rec·to·plas·ty (reck'to·plas"tee) *n.* [*recto-* + *-plasty*]. PROCTOPLASTY.

rec·to·rec·tos·to·my (reck"to·reck·tos'tuh·mee) *n.* [*recto-* + *recto-* + *-stomy*]. Surgical anastomosis between two parts of the rectum.

rec·to·ro·mano·scope (reck"to·ro·man'uh·skope) *n.* [*recto-* + *romanoscope*]. SIGMOIDOSCOPE.

rec·to·scope (reck'tuh·skope) *n.* [*recto-* + *-scope*]. PROCTOSCOPE. —**rec·tos·co·py** (reck·tos'kuh·pee) *n.*

rec·to·sig·moid (reck"to·sig'moid) *n.* The rectum and sigmoid portion of the colon considered together.

rec·to·sig·moid·ec·to·my (reck"to·sig"moy·deck'tuh·mee) *n.* [*recto-* + *sigmoid* + *-ectomy*]. Surgical excision of the rectum and sigmoid colon.

rec·to·sig·moid·os·co·py (reck"to·sig"moy·dos'kuh·pee) *n.* [*recto-* + *sigmoid* + *-scopy*]. Inspection of the rectum and sigmoid flexure of the colon with the aid of a sigmoidoscope.

rec·to·ste·no·sis (reck"to·ste·no'sis) *n.* [*recto-* + *stenosis*]. Stenosis of the rectum.

rec·tos·to·my (reck·tos'tuh·mee) *n.* [*recto-* + *-stomy*]. PROCTOSTOMY.

rec·tot·o·my (reck·tot'uh·mee) *n.* [*recto-* + *-tomy*]. PROCTOTOMY.

rec·to·ure·thral (reck"to·yoo·ree'thrul) *adj.* [*recto-* + *urethral*]. Pertaining to the rectum and the urethra.

rec·to·ure·thra·lis (reck"to·yoo·ree·thray'lis) *n.* A small band of smooth muscle fibers running from the rectum to the membranous part of the urethra in the male. NA *musculus rectourethralis.*

rec·to·uter·ine (reck"to·yoo'tur·ine) *adj.* [*recto-* + *uterine*]. Pertaining to the rectum and the uterus.

rectouterine excavation or **fossa.** The portion of the peritoneal cavity between the rectum and the posterior surface of the uterus and vagina. Syn. *pouch of Douglas.* NA *excavatio rectouterina.*

rectouterine muscle. A small band of smooth muscle fibers running from the front of the rectum to the uterus, corresponding to the rectovesicalis in the male. NA *musculus rectouterinus.*

rectouterine plica. Either of the two folds of peritoneum extending from the cervix of the uterus on either side of the rectum to the sacrum, and forming the lateral boundaries of the mouth of the rectouterine excavation. NA *plica rectouterina.* See also *uterosacral ligament.*

rectouterine pouch. RECTOUTERINE EXCAVATION.

rec·to·va·gi·nal (reck"to·vaj'i·nul, ·va·jye'nul) *adj.* [*recto-* + *vaginal*]. Pertaining to the rectum and the vagina.

rectovaginal fistula. An opening between the vagina and the rectum.

rectovaginal septum. The tissue forming the partition between the rectum and the vagina. NA *septum rectovaginale.*

rec·to·vag·i·no·ab·dom·i·nal (reck"to·vaj"i·no·ab·dom'i·nul) *adj.* Pertaining to or by way of the rectum, vagina, and abdomen; said of a type of combined pelvic examination.

rec·to·ves·i·cal (reck"to·ves'i·kul) *adj.* [*recto-* + *vesical*]. Pertaining to the rectum and the urinary bladder.

rectovesical excavation. The part of the peritoneal cavity between the urinary bladder and the rectum in the male. NA *excavatio rectovesicalis.*

rectovesical fistula. A congenital or acquired opening between the rectum and the urinary bladder.

rec·to·ves·i·ca·lis (reck"to·ves'i·kay'lis) *n.* Smooth muscle fibers running between the rectum and the base of the urinary bladder. NA *musculus rectovesicalis.*

rectovesical plica. A peritoneal fold extending from the posterior part of the urinary bladder to the rectum and sacrum. Syn. *sacrogenital fold.*

rectovesical pouch or **space.** RECTOVESICAL EXCAVATION.

rec·tum (reck'tum) *n.*, genit. **rec·ti** (·tye), pl. **rec·ta** (·tuh) [L., *intestinum rectum,* the straight or upright intestine] [NA]. The lower part of the large intestine, extending from the sigmoid flexure to the anal canal. It begins opposite the third sacral vertebra and passes downward to terminate at the anal canal. See also Plates 8, 10, 13, 14.

rectum reflex. The mechanism by which feces accumulated in and pressing against the rectum are evacuated, characterized by peristaltic contraction of the rectal musculature and relaxation of the internal and external sphincters of the anus.

rec·tus (reck'tus) *L. adj. & E. n.*, pl. & genit. sing. **rec·ti** (·tye) [lit. ruled, made straight, from *regere,* to rule, direct]. 1. Straight; forward. See also *R.* 2. Vertical or perpendicular. 3. Any of various muscles that are either rectilinear in shape, or oriented along—or perpendicular to—an axis of the body or of a part. See also Table of Muscles in the Appendix.

rectus ab·do·mi·nis (ab·dom'i·nis). The muscle of the anterior abdominal wall which has vertical fibers. NA *musculus rectus abdominis.*

rectus ac·ces·so·ri·us (ack"se·sor'ee·us). A rare variant of the vastus lateralis muscle in which a few fibers arise from the rim of the acetabulum.

rectus incision. An incision made through the rectus abdominis muscle or through its sheath.

re·cum·ben·cy (re·kum'bun·see) *n.* [L. *recumbere,* to recline]. The reclining position.

re·cum·bent (re·kum'bunt) *adj.* Leaning back; reclining.

re·cu·per·ate (re·koo'pur·ate, re·kew') *v.* [L. *recuperare,* to regain]. To regain strength or health.

re·cu·per·a·tion (re·koo"pur·ay'shun, re·kew") *n.* [L. *recuperatio,* from *recuperare,* to regain]. Convalescence; restoration to health.

re·cu·per·a·tive (re·koo'pur·uh·tiv, re·kew") *adj.* Pertaining to, or tending to, recovery or restoration of health or strength.

re·cur·rence (re·kur'unce) *n.* [from *recurrent*]. 1. The return of symptoms or a disease. 2. Reappearance of a neoplasm after apparent complete removal.

re·cur·rent (re·kur'unt) *adj.* [L. *recurrere,* to return, from *re-* + *currere,* to run]. 1. Returning. 2. *In anatomy,* turning back in its course.

recurrent bandage. A bandage in which each turn comes back to the point of starting; used in bandaging the head or an amputation stump.

recurrent dislocation. HABITUAL DISLOCATION.

recurrent fever. RELAPSING FEVER.

recurrent inhibition. *In neurophysiology,* the silencing of the activity of a nerve cell by the discharge of recurrent collateral branches of an efferent neuron terminating on inhibitory interneurons, such as the Renshaw cells.

recurrent insanity. MANIC-DEPRESSIVE ILLNESS.

recurrent iridocyclitis. PERIODIC OPTHALMIA.

recurrent laryngeal nerve. NA *nervus laryngeus recurrens.* See Table of Nerves in the Appendix.

recurrent summer eruption. HYDROA VACCINIFORME.

re·cur·va·tion (ree"kur·vay'shun) *n.* [L. *recurvare,* to curve backward]. The act or process of bending backward.

recurvatum knee. GENU RECURVATUM.

red, *n.* The least refractive of the spectral colors.

red atrophy. Atrophy complicating chronic hyperemia, especially of the liver.

red blindness. PROTANOPIA.

red blood cell. ERYTHROCYTE. Abbreviated, RBC, rbc.

red bone marrow. RED MARROW.

red bug. CHIGGER.

red cell. ERYTHROCYTE.

red corpuscle. ERYTHROCYTE.

red degeneration. Red discoloration of a uterine fibromyoma due to degeneration, necrosis, and edema of the tumor.

red diaper syndrome. Red discoloration of soiled diapers after 24 to 36 hours incubation in a diaper receptacle, due to predominance of *Serratia macrescens* in the bowel flora of newborn infants.

red fever of the Congo. MURINE TYPHUS.

red glass or **lens test.** A test for diplopia and suppression, in which a red glass is placed in front of one eye while the patient looks at a light at a variable distance away, in all cardinal positions of gaze. If diplopia is present, two lights, one red and one white, will be seen.

red gum. STROPHULUS.

red hepatization. A pathologic change in the lungs, usually in pneumococcal lobar pneumonia, in which the lungs have the consistency of the liver and are discolored red.

re·dia (ree'dee·uh) *n.*, pl. **re·di·ae** (·dee·ee) [F. *Redi,* Italian naturalist, 1626–1698]. *In parasitology,* the second larval stage of a trematode, which results from the development of a parthenogenetic egg of the first larval stage.

re·dif·fer·en·ti·a·tion (ree·dif"ur·en"shee·ay'shun) *n.* The return to a position of greater specialization in actual and potential functions.

red induration. 1. Fibrosis of the lung associated with deposit of red oxide of iron; pulmonary hemosiderosis. 2. Marked passive hyperemia of the lung.

red infarct. An infarct in which the necrotic focus is swollen, firm, and either bright or dark red, as the result of hemorrhage.

red·in·te·gra·tion (re·din″te·gray′shun) *n.* [L. *redintegrare,* to make whole again]. 1. Complete restoration of a part that has been injured or destroyed; the reestablishing of a whole. 2. *In psychology,* the principle that the recall of a part of an event or a fraction of the stimulus originally resulting in a certain response will revive the event or response as a whole. See also *reintegration.*

red lead. LEAD ORTHOPLUMBATE.

red lead oxide. LEAD ORTHOPLUMBATE.

red marrow. Marrow of all bones in early life and of restricted locations in adulthood in which active formation of blood cells (hemopoiesis) is taking place; the color is due to the presence of hemoglobin in red blood cells and their precursors. NA *medulla ossium rubra.* Contr. *yellow marrow.*

red mite. Any member of the genus *Trombicula.*

red muscle. A muscle that appears red in the fresh state; in the fibers of red muscles, the longitudinal striation is more prominent and the transverse striation is somewhat irregular. The red color probably is due to myoglobin and cytochrome.

red nucleus. A large oval nucleus, situated in the midbrain ventral to the cerebral aqueduct, which in the fresh brain has a slightly pink color. It receives fibers from the superior cerebellar peduncle and gives fibers to the rubrospinal tract. NA *nucleus ruber.*

red·out (red′owt) *n.* [by analogy from *blackout*]. A condition encountered by flyers as a consequence of centripetal acceleration, causing blood to be driven to the head with resulting severe headache and transient blurring of vision as by a red mist.

re·dox (ree′docks) *n.* [*red*uction + *ox*idation]. An oxidation-reduction reaction, state, or system.

redox potential. The electrical potential developed when a suitable inert electrode is in contact with a solution containing both the oxidized and the reduced forms of one or more substances. The potential is a function of the ratio of the activities (concentrations) of oxidant and reductant, and also provides a measure of the relative oxidizing (or reducing) power of the system.

redox system. A simple oxidation-reduction system in which two substances react reversibly with each other. The oxidized material is a reductant; the reduced material, an oxidant.

red pepper. CAPSICUM.

red precipitate. MERCURIC OXIDE, RED.

red pulp. The red material consisting of anastomosing, cordlike columns of reticular connective tissue separating the venous sinuses of the spleen. Contr. *white pulp.*

red pulp cords. RED PULP.

red reflex. The red glow of light seen to emerge from the pupil when the interior of the eye is illuminated, due to the reflected light having passed through the choroid.

re·dresse·ment (re·dres′munt) *n.* [F.]. 1. A second dressing of a wound. 2. Correction of a deformity.

red softening. Softening of the brain when hemorrhage accompanies the ischemic softening, and the products of disintegration of the blood mingle with the nerve substance, giving it a red hue.

red sweat. A peculiar, red perspiration noted in the axillas and genital region, and due to microorganisms which have developed on the hairs of these warm, moist parts. See also *trichomycosis rubra.*

red test. PHENOLSULFONPHTHALEIN TEST.

red thrombus. A thrombus composed principally of erythrocytes and fibrin intimately mixed, commonly formed by clotting of blood in an occluded vessel.

re·duce (re·dewce′) *v.* [L. *reducere,* to lead back]. 1. To restore a part to its normal relations, as to reduce a hernia or fracture. 2. *In chemistry,* to bring to the metallic form, deprive of oxygen, or add electrons. 3. To lose weight by dietetic regimen.

re·duced, *adj.* 1. Restored to the proper place. 2. *In chemistry,* having undergone reduction, that is, accepted electrons. 3. Diminished in size.

reduced ejection phase. The period of late ventricular systole during which diminishing volumes of blood per unit of time are discharged by the ventricles.

reduced heme. HEME.

reduced iron. A grayish-black powder obtained by the action of hydrogen on ferric oxide or by other means; has been used as a hematinic. Syn. *iron by hydrogen, Quévenne's iron.*

re·duc·ible (re·dew′si·bul) *adj.* Capable of being reduced.

reducible hernia. A hernia whose contents can be replaced through the hernial opening.

reducing diet. A low-caloric diet, used to reduce weight.

reducing sugar. Any of the sugars, including all monosaccharides and certain polysaccharides, which are capable of reducing alkaline solutions.

re·duc·tant (re·duck′tunt) *n.* A reducing agent.

re·duc·tase (re·duck′tace, ·taze) *n.* An enzyme causing reduction.

re·duc·tion (re·duck′shun) *n.* 1. *In chemistry,* an increase in the negative valence of an element (or a decrease in positive valence) occurring as a result of the gain of electrons. Each electron so gained is taken from some other element, thus accomplishing an oxidation of that element. 2. Originally, the process of separation from oxygen, or the combining with hydrogen. 3. The restoration by surgical or manipulative procedures of a dislocated joint or a fractured bone to normal anatomic relationships, or the restoration of an incarcerated hernia to its original location.

reduction division. MEIOSIS.

re·dun·dant (re·dun′dunt) *adj.* [from L. *redundare,* to overflow, be in excess]. Superfluous; characterized by an excess, as of skin. —**redun·dan·cy** (·dun·see) *n.*

re·du·pli·cat·ed (re·dew′pli·kay·tid) *adj.* [L. *reduplicatus,* redoubled]. Doubled, as reduplicated heart sounds.

re·du·pli·ca·tion (re·dew″pli·kay′shun) *n.* [L. *reduplicatio*]. A doubling.

reduplication cyst. Any cyst arising from a duplicated segment of a hollow organ such as intestine or bronchus.

reduplication of the bladder. BILOCULAR BLADDER.

Red·u·vi·idae (red″yoo·vye′i·dee, ree″dew·) *n.pl.* [NL., from L. *reduvia,* hangnail]. A family of the Heteroptera or true bugs, including some 4,000 species, commonly called assassin bugs and kissing bugs. Includes vectors of Chagas' disease, and may cause painful dermatitis at the site of the bite. Syn. *Triatomidae.* —**re·du·vi·id** (re·dew′vee·id) *n. & adj.*

Re·du·vi·us (re·dew′vee·us) *n.* A genus of bugs of the family Reduviidae.

Reduvius per·so·na·tus (pur·so·nay′tus). A reduviid bug that is an avid bloodsucker and has a potent salivary toxin; attacks the face, particularly the lips, often causing pain; found widely distributed in the midwest and eastern United States.

red vision. ERYTHROPSIA.

Reed-Frost theory. *In epidemiology,* a theory, intended to cover acute communicable diseases, based on an expression of the probable number of cases at time $T+1$ in terms of known facts at time T. The theory is one that proceeds stepwise in time and does not give a continuous time curve; it is not expected to describe the course of a particular epidemic, but allows the exploration of a variety of epidemiologic principles.

Reed-Stern·berg cell (shtehrn′behrk) [Dorothy *Reed* Mendenhall, U.S. pathologist, 1874–1964; and C. *Sternberg,*

Austrian pathologist, 1872–1935]. An anaplastic reticuloendothelial cell characteristic of Hodgkin's disease, although found in other conditions as well.

re·ed·u·ca·tion (ree·ej″oo·kay′shun) *n.* The development of the processes of adjustment in an individual who has acquired these processes and then lost them.

reef·ing, *n.* PLICATION.

reef knot. SQUARE KNOT.

Reen·stier·na reaction or **test** (reʸn′steer·naʰ) [J. *Reenstierna,* Swedish dermatologist, 20th century]. ITO-REENSTIERNA TEST.

re·ep·i·the·li·al·iza·tion (ree·ep″i·theel″ee·ul·i·zay′shun) *n.* 1. The regrowth of epithelium over a denuded surface. 2. The placement of epithelium over a denuded surface by surgical means.

re·ep·i·the·lial·ize (ree·ep″i·theel′ee·ul·ize) *v.* To restore an epithelial surface, either surgically or through natural regrowth.

Rees and Eck·er's diluting fluid [E. E. *Ecker*]. A sodium citrate-sucrose solution used as a diluent in blood platelet counting.

re·ev·o·lu·tion (ree·ev″uh·lew′shun) *n.* [*re-* + *evolution*]. According to J. Hughlings Jackson, a symptom following an epileptic attack, which consists of three stages: suspension of power to understand speech (word deafness), perception of words and echolalia without comprehension, return to conscious perception of speech with continued lack of comprehension.

re·ex·cise (ree·eck·size′) *v.* To excise after a previous excision or incomplete excision.

re·ex·ci·ta·tion (ree·eck″si·tay′shun) *n.* Reentrance of the excitation wave into tissue that has recovered from a refractory state.

re·ex·pand (ree″eck·spand′) *v.* To expand again following collapse, as of the lungs.

re·fec·tion (re·feck′shun) *n.* [L. *refectio,* from *reficere,* to restore]. 1. Restoration, refreshment, or recovery, especially after fatigue or hunger. 2. The phenomenon of vitamin B-complex synthesis by the bacterial flora of the intestine in certain animals maintained on a diet devoid of the vitamins.

re·fer, *v.* [L. *referre,* to carry back]. To project to or localize at a distance from the point of origin. **—re·ferred,** *adj.*

reference standard. A substance of defined purity or strength used for comparison in conducting certain assays of the United States Pharmacopeia or National Formulary.

referred pain. Pain whose origin is not in the area in which it is felt; for example, pain felt under the right scapula due to gallbladder disease.

re·fine, *v.* [*re-* + L. *finire,* to finish]. To purify a substance, extract it from raw material, or remove impurities from it.

re·flect, *v.* [L. *reflectere,* to bend, turn]. 1. To bend or turn back, as sound, heat, or a ray of light. 2. *In anatomy,* to bend or fold back upon itself. 3. *In surgery,* to lay or push aside tissue or an organ to gain access to the area to be operated upon.

re·flec·tance (re·fleck′tunce) *n.* The ratio of the light reflected from a surface to that incident upon it. Syn. *reflection coefficient, reflection factor.*

re·flect·ed, *adj.* 1. Cast or thrown back. 2. *In anatomy,* turned back upon itself, as visceral peritoneum from the surface of an organ to become parietal peritoneum.

reflected ligament. An occasional band of fibers of the superior crus of one inguinal ligament which crosses the midline to an attachment on the tubercle of the other pubic bone. Syn. *triangular fascia.* NA *ligamentum reflexum.*

reflected light. Light thrown back from an illuminated object.

re·flect·ing microscope. A microscope using mirror pairs in the objective, thus extending the range of achromatism throughout the optical spectrum.

re·flec·tion (re·fleck′shun) *n.* 1. A bending or turning back; specifically, the turning back of a ray of light from a surface upon which it impinges without penetrating. 2. In membranes, as the peritoneum, the folds which are made in passing from the wall of the cavity over an organ and back again to the wall which bounds such a cavity.

reflection coefficient or **factor.** REFLECTANCE.

re·flec·tor (re·fleck′tur) *n.* A device for reflecting light or sound.

re·flex (ree′flecks) *n.* [L. *reflectere, reflexus,* to turn back, bend back]. A stereotyped involuntary movement or other response of a peripheral organ to an appropriate stimulus, the action occurring immediately, without the aid of the will or without even entering consciousness. **—re·flex·ly,** *adv.*

reflex akinesia. Impairment or loss of reflex action.

reflex arc. The pathway traversed by an impulse during reflex action, extending from a receptor to an effector usually, but not necessarily, via some part of the central nervous system.

reflex arrhythmia. PHASIC SINUS ARRHYTHMIA.

reflex bladder. A urinary bladder whose activity or function is dependent solely upon the primary (simple) reflex arc through the sacral cord, as the result of removal of suprasegmental control secondary to complete transection of the spinal cord, or gross lesions which result in profound disturbance of suprasegmental pathways, comparable to complete transection of the cord. Syn. *automatic bladder, spastic reflex bladder.*

reflex center. Any nerve cell or group of nerve cells in the central nervous system which transforms an afferent impulse into an efferent one.

reflex cough. Cough produced by irritation of a remote organ.

reflex dystrophy. 1. CAUSALGIA. 2. SHOULDER-HAND SYNDROME.

reflex epilepsy. Seizures brought about by sensory stimuli such as music, sudden noise (acousticomotor epilepsy), reading, or an object of touch or sight, often with electroencephalographic changes in the sensory projection area corresponding to the trigger zone.

reflex hammer. A small hammer with a rubber head used to elicit reflexes by tapping on tendons; formerly also used to tap the surface of the body to elicit sounds of diagnostic value. Syn. *percussion hammer.*

reflex hypoxic crisis. BREATH-HOLDING ATTACK.

reflex ileus. ADYNAMIC ILEUS.

reflex inhibition ileus. ADYNAMIC ILEUS.

re·flex·io (re·fleck′see·o) *n.* [L.]. A bending back, turning back, or reflection.

reflexio pal·pe·bra·rum (pal·pe·brair′um). ECTROPION.

re·flexo·gen·ic (re·fleck″so·jen′ick) *adj.* [*reflex* + *-genic*]. Causing or increasing a tendency to reflex action; producing reflexes.

re·flexo·graph (re·fleck′so·graf) *n.* An instrument for graphically recording a reflex, such as the knee jerk or calcaneal tendon reflex.

re·flex·om·e·ter (ree″fleck·som′e·tur) *n.* [*reflex* + *-meter*]. 1. An instrument used to measure the force required to produce a stretch reflex. 2. Any device used to measure the force required to elicit a reflex.

re·flexo·ther·a·py (re·fleck″so·therr′uh·pee) *n.* [*reflex* + *therapy*]. A form of therapeutics based on stimulation by manipulation, anesthetization, or cauterization of areas more or less distant from the affected lesion.

reflex streak. A shining, white streak of light seen reflected along the vessels in the retina on funduscopic examination; wider and more pronounced when the retinal vessels are atherosclerotic.

reflex weeping. Lacrimation in response to stimulation of the trigeminal nerve, especially its conjunctival and corneal endings, strong irritation of the optic nerve, or of the sympathetic or parasympathetic fibers associated with the facial nerve. Contr. *psychic weeping.*

re·flux (ree'flucks) *n.* [L. *refluxum,* from *refluere,* to flow back]. A return flow, as in a reflux condenser, which returns condensate to the original fluid.

reflux esophagitis. Inflammation of the esophagus due to reflux of gastric contents into the esophagus.

reflux menstruation. A backflow through the uterine tubes. Syn. *regurgitant menstruation.*

re·fract (re·frakt') *v.* [L. *refringere, refractus,* to break up]. 1. To change direction by refraction. 2. To estimate the degree of ametropia, heterophoria, and strabismus present in an eye.

re·frac·ta do·si (re·frack'tuh do'sigh) [L.]. In divided doses.

re·fract·ed light. Light rays that have passed from one medium into another and have been bent from their original course.

re·frac·tile (re·frack'til, ·tile) *adj.* REFRACTIVE.

re·frac·tion (re·frack'shun) *n.* [L. *refractio,* from *refringere,* to break up]. 1. The act of refracting or bending back. 2. The deviation of a ray of light from a straight line in passing obliquely from one transparent medium to another of different density. 3. The state of refractive power, especially of the eye; the ametropia, emmetropia, or muscle imbalance present. 4. The act or process of correcting errors of ocular refraction.

re·frac·tion·ist (re·frack'shun·ist) *n.* One who determines the status of ocular refraction.

refraction of the eye. The influence of the ocular media upon a cone or beam of light, whereby a normal or emmetropic eye produces a proper image of the object upon the retina.

refraction point. The point at which a ray of light is refracted.

re·frac·tive (re·frack'tiv) *adj.* 1. Refracting; capable of refracting or bending back. 2. Pertaining to refraction.

refractive error. A defect of the eye which prevents parallel light rays from being brought to a single focus precisely on the retina.

refractive index. The refractive power of any substance as compared with air. It is the quotient of the angle of incidence divided by the angle of refraction of a ray passing through a substance. Symbol, n.

refractive power. A measure of the ability of a substance to refract light, commonly known as refractive index.

re·frac·tiv·i·ty (ree''frack·tiv'i·tee) *n.* The power of refraction; the ability to refract.

re·frac·tom·e·ter (ree''frack·tom'e·tur) *n.* [*refract* + *-meter*]. 1. An instrument for measuring the refraction of the eye. 2. An instrument for measuring the refractive index of a substance.

re·frac·to·ry (re·frack'tuh·ree) *adj.* [L. *refractarius,* from *refragari,* to oppose, thwart]. 1. Resisting treatment. 2. Resisting the action of heat; slow to melt. 3. Unable to respond to appropriate stimulation, as a muscle or nerve immediately after responding to a stimulation.

refractory megaloblastic anemia. Megaloblastic and macrocytic anemia of unknown cause and unresponsive to therapeutic agents such as vitamin B_{12} and folic acid.

refractory period. *In physiology,* the transient period immediately following effective stimulation of an irritable tissue; especially a tissue subject to the all-or-none law. See also *absolute refractory period, relative refractory period.*

refractory rickets. VITAMIN D–REFRACTORY RICKETS.

re·frac·ture (ree·frack'chur) *n.* The breaking again of fractured bones that have united by faulty union.

re·fran·gi·bil·i·ty (re·fran''ji·bil'i·tee) *n.* The capability of undergoing refraction. —**re·fran·gi·ble** (·fran'ji·bul) *adj.*

re·fresh, *v. In surgery,* to give to an old lesion the character of a fresh wound. See also *debridement.*

re·frig·er·ant (re·frij'ur·unt) *adj. & n.* 1. Cooling; lessening fever or thirst. 2. A coolant; a medicine or agent having cooling properties or lowering body temperature.

re·frig·er·a·tion (re·frij''ur·ay'shun) *n.* [L. *refrigeratio,* from *refrigerare,* to cool, from *frigus,* coldness]. The act of lowering the temperature of a body by conducting away its heat to a surrounding cooler substance.

refrigeration anesthesia. A method of rendering a lower limb insensitive by the use of cracked ice applied to the member so as to surround it completely. After 2 to 4 hours of this application, amputation may be performed without medication or anesthesia.

re·frin·gent (re·frin'junt) *adj.* [L. *refringere,* to refract]. REFRACTIVE.

Ref·sum's syndrome or **disease** [S. *Refsum,* Norwegian physician, 20th century]. An autosomal recessive disorder characterized by visual disturbances, ataxia, neuritic changes, and cardiac damage, associated with high blood levels of phytanic acid. Syn. *heredopathia atactica polyneuritiformis.*

re·fu·sion (re·few'zhun) *n.* [*re-* + *-fusion* as in transfusion]. Injection of blood into the circulation after its removal from the same patient.

Re·gaud's fixing fluid (ruh·go') [C. *Regaud,* French surgeon, 1870–1940]. A solution containing 3% aqueous potassium bichromate and formalin.

Regaud's fluid [C. *Regaud*]. A fixative, followed by prolonged chromation, used for the subsequent demonstration of the Golgi apparatus and mitochondria.

Regaud's stain [C. *Regaud*]. An iron hematoxylin method for the demonstration of mitochondria. Tissue must be fixed in Regaud's fixing fluid.

Regaud's theory [C. *Regaud*]. ELECTROSOME THEORY.

re·gen·er·ate (re·jen'er·ate) *v.* [L. *regenerare,* to bring forth again]. 1. To form anew. 2. To reproduce, after loss. —**re·gener·a·ble** (·uh·bul) *adj.*

re·gen·er·a·tion (ree·jen''er·ay'shun) *n.* [L. *regeneratio,* from *regenerare,* to bring forth again]. 1. The new growth or repair of structures or tissues lost by disease or by injury. 2. *In chemistry,* the process of obtaining from the by-products or end products of a process a substance which was employed in the earlier part of the process.

re·gen·er·a·tive (ree·jen'ur·uh·tiv, ·uh·ray·tiv) *adj.* Pertaining to, promoting, or capable of regeneration.

reg·i·men (rej'i·mun) *n.* [L., rule, guidance, from *regere,* to rule]. A systematic course or plan directed toward the improvement of health, the diagnosis of disease, or the investigation of biologic activities. Such a plan is likely to consider diet, drugs, exercise, and therapeutic or experimental procedures.

re·gio (rej'ee·o, ree'jee·o) *n.,* pl. **re·gi·o·nes** (rej''ee·o'neez, ree''jee·) [L.]. REGION.

regio ab·do·mi·na·lis la·te·ra·lis (ab·dom·i·nay'lis lat·e·ray'lis) [BNA]. Regio lateralis abdominis [dextra et sinistra] (= LATERAL REGION OF THE ABDOMEN).

regio acro·mi·a·lis (a·kro·mee·ay'lis) [BNA]. The area over the acromion.

regio ana·lis (ay·nay'lis) [NA]. The area surrounding the anus.

regio an·te·bra·chii anterior (an·te·bray'kee·eye) [NA]. The anterior area of the forearm.

regio antebrachii posterior [NA]. The posterior area of the forearm.

regio an·ti·bra·chii dor·sa·lis (an·ti·bray'kee·eye dor·say'lis) [BNA]. REGIO ANTEBRACHII POSTERIOR.

regio antibrachii ra·di·a·lis (ray·dee·ay'lis) [BNA]. The radial side of the forearm.

regio antibrachii ul·na·ris (ul·nair'is) [BNA]. The ulnar side of the forearm.

regio antibrachii vo·la·ris (vo·lair'is) [BNA]. REGIO ANTEBRACHII ANTERIOR.

regio au·ri·cu·la·ris (aw·rick·yoo·lair'is) [BNA]. The area of the auricle of the external ear.

regio ax·il·la·ris (ack·si·lair'is) [NA]. AXILLARY REGION.

regio bra·chii anterior (bray'kee·eye) [NA]. The anterior area of the arm.

regio brachii la·te·ra·lis (lat·e·ray'lis) [BNA]. The lateral area of the arm.
regio brachii me·di·a·lis (mee·dee·ay'lis) [BNA]. The medial area of the arm.
regio brachii posterior [NA]. The posterior area of the arm.
regio buc·ca·lis (buh·kay'lis) [NA]. The area of the cheek.
regio cal·ca·nea (kal·kay'nee·uh) [NA]. The calcaneal area of the heel.
regio cla·vi·cu·la·ris (kla·vick·yoo·lair'is) [BNA]. The area of the clavicle.
regio col·li anterior (kol'eye) [NA]. The anterior region of the neck.
regio colli la·te·ra·lis (lat·e·ray'lis) [NA]. The lateral region of the neck.
regio colli posterior [NA]. The posterior region of the neck.
regio cos·ta·lis la·te·ra·lis (kos·tay'lis lat·e·ray'lis) [BNA]. The area of the lateral thoracic wall.
regio cox·ae (kock'see) [BNA]. The region of the hip.
regio cru·ris anterior (kroo'ris) [NA]. The anterior region of the leg.
regio cruris la·te·ra·lis (lat·e·ray'lis) [BNA]. The lateral region of the leg.
regio cruris me·di·a·lis (mee·dee·ay'lis) [BNA]. The medial region of the leg.
regio cruris posterior [NA]. The posterior region of the leg, the calf of the leg.
regio cu·bi·ti anterior (kew'bi·tye) [NA]. ANTERIOR CUBITAL REGION.
regio cubiti la·te·ra·lis (lat·e·ray'lis) [BNA]. The lateral cubital region.
regio cubiti me·di·a·lis (mee·dee·ay'lis) [BNA]. The medial cubital region.
regio cubiti posterior [NA]. The posterior cubital region.
regio del·toi·dea (del·toy'dee·uh) [NA]. DELTOID REGION.
regio dor·sa·lis ma·nus (dor·say'lis man'us) [BNA]. DORSUM MANUS.
regio dorsalis pe·dis (ped'is) [BNA]. DORSUM PEDIS.
regio epi·gas·tri·ca (ep·i·gas'tri·kuh) [NA]. EPIGASTRIC REGION.
regio fe·mo·ris anterior (fem'o·ris) [NA]. The anterior region of the thigh.
regio femoris la·te·ra·lis (lat·e·ray'lis) [BNA]. The lateral region of the thigh.
regio femoris me·di·a·lis (mee·dee·ay'lis) [BNA]. The medial region of the thigh.
regio femoris posterior [NA]. The posterior region of the thigh.
regio fron·ta·lis (fron·tay'lis) [NA]. FRONTAL REGION.
regio ge·nus anterior (jen'us) [NA]. The anterior region of the knee.
regio genus posterior [NA]. The posterior region of the knee.
regio glu·tea (gloo'tee·uh, gloo·tee'uh) [NA]. GLUTEAL REGION.
regio hy·oi·dea (high·oy'dee·uh) [BNA]. The hyoid region.
regio hy·po·chon·dri·a·ca (high·po·kon·drye'uh·kuh) [BNA]. Regio hypochondriaca [dextra et sinistra] (= HYPOCHONDRIAC REGIONS).
regio hypochondriaca [dex·tra et si·nis·tra] (decks'truh et si·nis'truh) [NA]. HYPOCHONDRIAC REGIONS.
regio hy·po·gas·tri·ca (high·po·gas'tri·kuh) [BNA]. Hypogastrium (= PUBIC REGION).
regio in·fra·cla·vi·cu·la·ris (in"fruh·kla·vick·yoo'lair'is) [NA]. INFRACLAVICULAR REGION.
regio in·fra·mam·ma·lis (in"fruh·ma·may'lis) [BNA]. INFRAMAMMARY REGION.
regio in·fra·or·bi·ta·lis (in"fruh·or·bi·tay'lis) [NA]. The infraorbital region.
regio in·fra·sca·pu·la·ris (in"fruh·skap·yoo·lair'is) [NA]. INFRASCAPULAR REGION.
regio in·fra·tem·po·ra·lis (in"fruh·tem·po·ray'lis) [NA]. INFRATEMPORAL REGION.
regio in·gui·na·lis (ing·gwi·nay'lis) [BNA]. Regio inguinalis [dextra et sinistra] (= INGUINAL REGION).
regio inguinalis [dex·tra et si·nis·tra] (decks'truh et si·nis'truh) [NA]. INGUINAL REGION.
regio in·ter·sca·pu·la·ris (in"tur·skap·yoo·lair'is) [BNA]. INTERSCAPULAR REGION.
regio la·bi·a·lis inferior (lay·bee·ay'lis) [BNA]. The region of the lower lip.
regio labialis superior [BNA]. The region of the upper lip.
regio la·ryn·gea (la·rin'jee·uh) [BNA]. The region of the larynx.
regio la·te·ra·lis ab·do·mi·nis [dex·tra et si·nis·tra] (lat·e·ray'lis ab·dom'i·nis decks'truh et si·nis'truh) [NA]. LATERAL REGION OF THE ABDOMEN.
regio lum·ba·lis (lum·bay'lis) [NA]. LUMBAR REGION.
regio mal·le·o·la·ris la·te·ra·lis (mal·ee·o·lair'is lat·e·ray'lis) [BNA]. The lateral malleolar region.
regio malleolaris me·di·a·lis (mee·dee·ay'lis) [BNA]. The medial malleolar region.
regio mam·ma·lis (ma·may'lis) [BNA]. Regio mammaria (= MAMMARY REGION).
regio mam·ma·ria (ma·mair'ee·uh) [NA]. MAMMARY REGION.
regio mas·toi·dea (mas·toy'dee·uh) [BNA]. The mastoid region.
regio me·di·a·na dor·si (mee·dee·ay'nuh dor'sigh) [BNA]. Regio vertebralis (= VERTEBRAL REGION).
regio men·ta·lis (men·tay'lis) [NA]. The mental region.
regio me·so·gas·tri·ca (mes·o·gas'tri·kuh) [BNA]. UMBILICAL REGION.
re·gion, *n.* [L. *regio,* direction, region, from *regere,* to direct]. One of the divisions of the body possessing either natural or arbitrary boundaries. —**region·al,** *adj.*
regional anatomy. The study of the anatomy of the body based upon a regional approach.
regional anesthesia. REGIONAL BLOCK ANESTHESIA.
regional block anesthesia. Anesthesia of a region of the body produced by injection of an anesthetic solution into and around the nerve trunks supplying the operative field. The injection may be made at a distance from the site of operation. See also *block anesthesia.*
regional colitis. GRANULOMATOUS COLITIS.
regional differentiation. The appearance of regional differences within an individuation field.
regional enteritis. A chronic, nonspecific, granulomatous process frequently involving the terminal portion of the ileum, but occasionally extending into the colon or arising in the more proximal portions of the small intestine; characterized clinically by recurrent crampy abdominal pain accompanied by diarrhea, fever, anorexia, and weight loss. Syn. *Crohn's disease.*
regional enterocolitis. REGIONAL ENTERITIS.
regional ileitis. Regional enteritis involving the ileum.
regio na·sa·lis (na·say'lis) [NA]. The nasal region.
regiones. Plural of *regio.*
regiones ab·do·mi·nis (ab·dom'i·nis) [NA]. ABDOMINAL REGIONS.
regiones ca·pi·tis (kap'i·tis) [NA]. The regions of the head.
regiones col·li (kol'eye) [NA]. The regions of the neck.
regiones cor·po·ris (kor'po·ris) [NA]. The regions of the body.
regiones corporis hu·ma·ni (hew·may'nigh) [BNA]. REGIONES CORPORIS.
regiones di·gi·ta·les ma·nus (dij·i·tay'leez man'us) [BNA]. The regions of the fingers.
regiones digitales pe·dis (ped'is) [BNA]. The regions of the toes.
regiones dor·sa·les di·gi·to·rum (dor·say'leez dij·i·to'rum) [BNA]. The dorsal regions of the fingers.
regiones dorsales digitorum pe·dis (ped'is) [BNA]. The dorsal regions of the toes.
regiones dor·si (dor'sigh) [NA]. The regions of the back.

regiones ex·tre·mi·ta·tis in·fe·ri·o·ris (eck·strem·i·tay'tis in·feer·ee·o'ris) [BNA]. REGIONES MEMBRI INFERIORIS.

regiones extremitatis su·pe·ri·o·ris (sue·peer·ee·o'ris) [BNA]. REGIONES MEMBRI SUPERIORIS.

regiones fa·ci·ei (fay"shee·ee'eye) [NA]. The regions of the face.

regiones mem·bri in·fe·ri·o·ris (mem'brye in·feer·ee·o'ris) [NA]. The regions of the lower member or extremity.

regiones membri su·pe·ri·o·ris (sue·peer·ee·o'ris) [NA]. The regions of the upper member or extremity.

regiones pec·to·ris (peck'to·ris) [NA]. The regions of the chest.

regiones plan·ta·res di·gi·to·rum pe·dis (plan·tair'eez dij·i·to'rum ped'is) [BNA]. The plantar regions of the toes.

regiones un·gui·cu·la·res ma·nus (ung·gwi·kew·lair'eez man'us) [BNA]. The regions of the nails of the fingers.

regiones unguiculares pe·dis (ped'is) [BNA]. The regions of the nails of the toes.

regiones vo·la·res di·gi·to·rum (vo·lair'eez dij·i·to'rum) [BNA]. The regions of the palmar aspects of the fingers.

region of accommodation. RANGE OF ACCOMMODATION.

regio nu·chae (new'kee) [BNA]. The region of the neck.

regio oc·ci·pi·ta·lis (ock·sip·i·tay'lis) [NA]. The occipital region.

regio ole·cra·ni (o·le·kray'nigh) [BNA]. The olecranon region.

regio ol·fac·to·ria (ol·fack·to'ree·uh) [NA]. OLFACTORY REGION.

regio olfactoria tu·ni·cae mu·co·sae na·si (tew'ni·see mew·ko'see nay'zye) [NA]. The olfactory region of the nose.

regio ora·lis (o·ray'lis) [NA]. The oral region.

regio or·bi·ta·lis (or·bi·tay'lis) [NA]. The orbital region.

regio pal·pe·bra·lis inferior (pal·pe·bray'lis) [BNA]. The region of the lower eyelid.

regio palpebralis superior [BNA]. The region of the upper eyelid.

regio pa·ri·e·ta·lis (pa·rye·e·tay'lis) [NA]. The parietal region.

regio pa·ro·ti·deo·mas·se·te·ri·ca (pa·ro·tid"ee·o·mas·e·terr'i·kuh) [NA]. The region of the parotid gland and masseter muscle.

regio pa·tel·la·ris (pat·e·lair'is) [BNA]. The region of the patella.

regio pec·to·ris anterior (peck'to·ris) [BNA]. The anterior pectoral region.

regio pectoris la·te·ra·lis (lat·e·ray'lis) [BNA]. The lateral pectoral region.

regio pe·ri·ne·a·lis (perr·i·nee·ay'lis) [NA]. PERINEUM (2).

regio plan·ta·ris pe·dis (plan·tair'is ped'is) [BNA]. The plantar region of the foot.

regio pu·bi·ca (pew'bi·kuh) [NA]. PUBIC REGION.

regio pu·den·da·lis (pew·den·day'lis) [BNA]. The pudendal region.

regio re·spi·ra·to·ria (re·spye·ruh·to'ree·uh) [NA]. RESPIRATORY REGION OF THE NOSE.

regio re·tro·mal·le·o·la·ris la·te·ra·lis (ret"ro·mal·ee·o·lair'is lat·e·ray'lis) [BNA]. The region behind the lateral malleolus.

regio retromalleolaris me·di·a·lis (mee·dee·ay'lis) [BNA]. The region behind the medial malleolus.

regio sa·cra·lis (sa·kray'lis) [NA]. The sacral region.

regio sca·pu·la·ris (skap·yoo·lair'is) [NA]. SCAPULAR REGION.

regio ster·na·lis (stur·nay'lis) [BNA]. STERNAL REGION.

regio ster·no·clei·do·mas·toi·dea (stur"no·klye"do·mas·toy'dee·uh) [NA]. The sternocleidomastoid region.

regio sub·hy·oi·dea (sub·high·oy'dee·uh) [BNA]. The subhyoid region.

regio sub·max·il·la·ris (sub·mack·si·lair'is) [BNA]. The submandibular region.

regio sub·men·ta·lis (sub·men·tay'lis) [BNA]. The submental region.

regio su·pra·or·bi·ta·lis (sue"pruh·or·bi·tay'lis) [BNA]. The supraorbital region.

regio su·pra·sca·pu·la·ris (sue"pruh·skap·yoo·lair'is) [BNA]. The suprascapular region.

regio su·pra·ster·na·lis (sue"pruh·stur·nay'lis) [BNA]. SUPRASTERNAL REGION.

regio su·ra·lis (sue·ray'lis) [BNA]. The region of the calf of the leg.

regio tem·po·ra·lis (tem·po·ray'lis) [NA]. The temporal region.

regio thy·re·oi·dea (thigh·ree·oy'dee·uh) [BNA]. The thyroid region.

regio tro·chan·te·ri·ca (tro·kan·terr'i·kuh) [BNA]. The region over the greater trochanter of the femur.

regio um·bi·li·ca·lis (um·bil·i·kay'lis) [NA]. UMBILICAL REGION.

regio uro·ge·ni·ta·lis (yoo·ro·jen·i·tay'lis) [NA]. The urogenital region.

regio ver·te·bra·lis (vur·te·bray'lis) [NA]. VERTEBRAL REGION.

regio vo·la·ris ma·nus (vo·lair'is man'us) [BNA]. PALMA MANUS.

regio zy·go·ma·ti·ca (zye·go·mat'i·kuh) [NA]. The zygomatic region.

reg·is·ter (rej'is·tur) *n.* [ML. *registrum,* from L. *regerere,* to carry back]. 1. The compass of a voice. 2. A subdivision of the compass of a voice, consisting in a series of tones produced in the same way and of a like character.

reg·is·tered nurse. A graduate nurse who has passed the state board examination and is thus qualified to be a nurse, and is legally entitled to add R.N. to his or her name.

reg·is·trar (rej'is·trahr) *n.* 1. An official custodian of records. 2. An officer in charge of hospital registry office. 3. In British hospitals, a resident specialist.

reg·is·tra·tion (rej"is·tray'shun) *n.* 1. The act of recording, as of deaths, births, or marriages. 2. A document certifying an act of registering, as a physician's registration.

reg·is·try (rej'i·stree) *n.* 1. An office listing nurses available for general or special services. 2. A place or central agency where data can be recorded for processing and subsequent retrieval for analysis.

Regitine. Trademark for phentolamine, an adrenergic blocking drug used as the hydrochloride and mesylate salts.

reg·le·men·ta·tion (reg"le·men·tay'shun) *n.* [F. *réglementation,* control]. The legal restriction or regulation of prostitution, as by compulsory medical inspection.

re·gress, *v.* [L. *regredi, regressus,* to go back]. 1. To return to a former state. 2. To subside.

re·gres·sion (re·gresh'un) *n.* [L. *regressio,* from *regredi,* to turn back]. 1. The act or process of regressing. 2. FILIAL REGRESSION. 3. *In psychology,* a mental state and a mode of adjustment to difficult and unpleasant situations, characterized by behavior of a type that had been satisfying and appropriate at an earlier stage of development but which no longer befits the age and social status of the individual. A terminal state in some forms of schizophrenia. 4. *In mathematics,* the tendency for a group equated in one trait to have a mean value closer to the general mean in a related trait. See also *retrogression.*

re·gres·sive (re·gres'iv) *adj.* 1. Going back to a former state, as the return to infantile patterns of behavior in an adult. 2. Subsiding, said of symptoms.

regressive metaplasia. Transformation in the direction of lower orders of differentiation. Syn. *retrogressive atrophy.*

reg·u·lar connective tissue. The densest connective tissue of the body. Collagenous fibers form the main constituent and are arranged in parallel bundles between which are rows of connective-tissue cells. It includes tendons, ligaments, and fibrous membranes, as the dura mater.

regular insulin. AMORPHOUS INSULIN.

reg·u·la·tion (reg"yoo·lay'shun) *n.* The processes by which a given biological phenomenon is maintained within narrow limits compatible with the survival of the organism. Compare *homeostasis.*

reg·u·la·tive (reg'yoo·lay"tiv) *adj. In embryology,* descriptive of development of eggs in which the cells of the early stages can be affected by inducing agents from the surrounding parts; opposed to mosaic development. See also *mosaic* (3).

regulative cleavage. INDETERMINATE CLEAVAGE.

reg·u·la·tor gene (reg'yoo·lay"tur). A gene whose effect is the regulation of another gene. Contr. *structural gene.*

re·gur·gi·tant (re·gur'ji·tunt) *adj.* Flowing backward.

regurgitant menstruation. A backflow through the uterine tubes. Syn. *reflux menstruation.*

regurgitant murmur. A murmur due to regurgitation of blood through an incompetent valvular orifice.

regurgitant wave. The positive-pressure wave in the atrial or venous pulse during ventricular systole, due to atrioventricular valve regurgitation. Syn. *r wave, systolic wave, s wave.* See also *v wave* (2).

re·gur·gi·ta·tion (re·gur"ji·tay'shun) *n.* [ML. *regurgitatio,* from *re-* + L. *gurgitare,* to engulf, flood]. 1. A backflow of blood through a heart valve that is defective. 2. The return of food from the stomach to the mouth without vomiting. —**re·gur·gi·tate** (re·gur'ji·tate) *v.*

regurgitation jaundice. Jaundice due to resorption of conjugated bilirubin into the blood. It may be hepatocellular or obstructive. Syn. *resorptive jaundice.*

re·ha·bil·i·ta·tion (ree"ha·bil"i·tay'shun) *n.* [ML. *rehabilitare,* to rehabilitate, from *habilitare,* to capacitate, make fit, from L. *habilis,* fit, able]. The restoration to a disabled individual of maximum independence commensurate with his limitations by developing his residual capacities. *In medicine,* it implies prescribed training and employment of many different methods and professional workers. —**re·ha·bil·i·tate** (ree"ha·bil'i·tate) *v.*

re·ha·la·tion (ree"ha·lay'shun) *n.* [*re-* + *halare,* to breathe]. Rebreathing; the inhalation of air that has been inspired previously; sometimes used in anesthesia.

Reh·berg's test [P. B. *Rehberg,* Danish physiologist, b. 1895]. A creatinine clearance test of renal function.

Reh·fuss method [M. E. *Rehfuss,* U.S. physician, b. 1887]. REHFUSS TEST MEAL.

Rehfuss test meal [M. E. *Rehfuss*]. A test meal of toast and tea. Specimens of gastric contents are withdrawn at intervals via a stomach tube and tested for acid content.

Rehfuss tube [M. E. *Rehfuss*]. A stomach tube designed for the removal of specimens of gastric contents for analysis after administration of a test meal.

Rehn-De·lorme operation (duh·lorm') [L. *Rehn;* and E. *Delorme,* French surgeon, 1847–1929]. REHN'S OPERATION.

Rehn's operation [L. *Rehn,* German surgeon, 1849–1930]. An operation for rectal prolapse, in which the protruding mucous membrane is resected with infolding of the muscularis by suture. Syn. *Rehn-Delorme operation.*

Rei·chel's duct (rye'kh[e]l) [F. P. *Reichel,* German surgeon, 1858–1934]. CLOACAL DUCT.

Rei·chert's cartilage (rye'khurt) [K. B. *Reichert,* German anatomist, 1811–1883]. The cartilage of the second embryonic visceral (hyoid) arch. It gives rise to the stapes, styloid process, stylohyoid ligament, and lesser horn of the hyoid bone.

Reichert's membrane [K. B. *Reichert*]. BOWMAN'S MEMBRANE.

Reich·mann's disease [M. *Reichmann,* Polish physician, 1851–1918]. Continuous secretion of gastric juice; gastrosuccorrhea. See also *Zollinger-Ellison syndrome.*

Reich·stein's substance Fa (rye'kh'shtine) [T. *Reichstein,* Swiss biochemist, b. 1897]. CORTISONE.

Reichstein's substance M. [T. *Reichstein*]. HYDROCORTISONE.

Rei·fen·stein's syndrome. An inherited form of primary testicular deficiency characterized by hypospadias, gynecomastia, azoospermia, and deficient virilization.

Reilly bodies. The cytoplasmic inclusions of Alder's anomaly.

re·im·plan·ta·tion (ree·im"plan·tay'shun) *n.* Replantation, as of a tooth.

Reincke's crystals (rine'keh) [*Reincke,* German physician, 19th century]. Rod-shaped crystalloids in the interstitial cells of the testis.

rein·deer moss. *CLADONIA RANGIFERINA.*

rei·necke salt (rye'ne·kuh). Ammonium reineckate, $NH_4[Cr(NH_3)_2(SCN)_4].H_2O$. Dark-red crystalline powder; used as a reagent, especially for amines.

re·in·fec·tion (ree"in·feck'shun) *n.* A second infection with the same kind of organism.

reinfection tuberculosis. CHRONIC TUBERCULOSIS.

re·in·force·ment (ree"in·force'munt) *n.* Augmentation or strengthening by addition, repetition, or any action that contributes to a cumulative result. —**reinforce,** *v.*

reinforcement conditioning. OPERANT CONDITIONING.

reinforcement of reflexes. Increased myotatic irritability (or other reflex response) when muscular or mental actions are synchronously carried out, or other stimuli are coincidentally brought to bear upon parts of the body other than that concerned in the reflex arc. See also *Jendrassik's maneuver.*

re·in·fu·sion (ree"in·few'zhun) *n.* [*re-* + *infusion*]. The reinjection of blood, serum, or cerebrospinal fluid.

Rein·hold's method [J. G. *Reinhold,* U.S. biochemist, b. 1900]. LETONOFF AND REINHOLD'S METHOD.

re·in·ner·va·tion (ree·in"ur·vay'shun) *n.* [*re-* + *innervation*]. Restoration of motor or sensory function, either spontaneously or by nerve grafting, to a part that had been deprived of its nerve supply.

re·in·oc·u·la·tion (ree"i·nock"yoo·lay'shun) *n.* Inoculation a second time with the same kind of organism.

Reinsch's test (rye'nsh) [A. *Reinsch,* German physician, 1862–1916]. 1. A test for arsenic in which a piece of bright copper foil is placed into acidified urine which is then heated to the boiling point. If arsenic is present it is deposited on the copper. The copper is then dried, placed in a test tube, and is heated, whereupon the arsenic volatilizes and is condensed upon the upper portion of the tube in the form of arsenic trioxide crystals which may be recognized. 2. A test for mercury similar to the test for arsenic except that the mixture is not heated to boiling and the end product is metallic mercury.

Rein's thermostromuhr. THERMOSTROMUHR OF REIN.

re·in·te·gra·tion (ree"in"te·gray'shun) *n.* [*re-* + *integration*]. *In psychiatry,* the restoration to harmonious mental functioning after disintegration of the personality by a severe mental disorder, as by a psychosis.

re·in·ver·sion (ree"in·vur'zhun) *n.* [*re-* + *inversion*]. The act of reducing an inverted uterus by the application of pressure to the fundus.

Reisinger's method. FARLEY, ST. CLAIR, AND REISINGER'S METHOD.

Reiss·ner's membrane (rice'nur) [E. *Reissner,* German anatomist, 1824–1878]. PARIES VESTIBULARIS DUCTUS COCHLEARIS.

Rei·ter's syndrome or **disease** (rye'tur) [H. *Reiter,* German physician, b. 1881]. The triad of idiopathic nongonococcal urethritis, conjunctivitis, and subacute or chronic polyarthritis; mucocutaneous lesions are common. Syn. *arthritis urethritica, idiopathic blenorrheal arthritis, infectious uroarthritis.*

re·ju·ve·nes·cence (re·joo"ve·nes'unce) *n.* [L. *rejuvenescere,* to be rejuvenated, from *juvenis,* young]. A renewal of youth; a renewal of strength and vigor; specifically a restoration of sexual vigor.

Rela. A trademark for carisoprodol, a centrally acting skeletal muscle relaxant.

re·lapse (re·laps', ree'laps) *n.* [L. *relabi, relapsus,* to fall back]. The return of symptoms and signs of a disease after apparent recovery. Compare *recrudescence.*

relapsing dislocation. HABITUAL DISLOCATION.

relapsing fever. Any of a group of acute arthropod-borne diseases characterized by alternating febrile and afebrile periods; caused by spirochetes, and transmitted by the louse *Pediculus humanus,* and by ticks of the genus *Ornithodorus.* Syn. *famine fever, spirillum fever, recurrent fever.*

relapsing polychondritis. An idiopathic inflammatory disease of cartilage, especially of the ears, trachea, bronchi, larynx, and nose, which tends to recur and to eventuate in deformity; fever, malaise, and polyarthritis are associated; an immunologic basis is suspected.

re·late, *v.* [L. *referre, relatus,* to carry back, refer]. 1. To enter or put into a relationship; to stand in relationship to another. 2. *In psychology and psychiatry,* to be in or establish a meaningful relationship with another individual or individuals, to interact with one's environment, usually on the basis that such interaction will be of significance.

re·la·tion, *n.* [L. *relatio,* a carrying back]. 1. Interdependence; mutual influence or connection between organs or parts. 2. Connection by consanguinity; kinship. 3. *In anatomy,* the position of parts of the body as regards each other. —**relation·al,** *adj.*

relational coil. A coil in which two chromatids are intertwined and separable only by uncoiling.

relational threshold. The ratio between the intensities of two stimuli when their difference is just perceptible.

rel·a·tive, *adj.* [L. *relativus,* from *referre, relatus,* to carry back, refer]. 1. Connected with or considered in reference to something else, as relative accommodation. 2. Comparative or not absolute, as relative sterility, relative scotoma. 3. Not independent; stemming from another condition or state. 4. Of a magnitude, expressed as the ratio of the specified quantity to another magnitude, as relative humidity. 5. Involving a relative magnitude, as relative lymphocytosis.

relative accommodation. Extent of accommodation possible for any particular degree of convergence.

relative alalia. MENTAL ALALIA.

relative biologic effectiveness of radiation. The inverse ratio of tissue doses of two different types of radiation that produces a particular biologic response under identical conditions.

relative humidity. The amount of water vapor in the air as compared with the total amount the air would hold at a given temperature.

relative hyperopia. A high hyperopia in which distinct vision is possible only when excessive convergence is made.

relative lymphocytosis. Increase of lymphocytes in the differential leukocyte count; not necessarily an increase per unit volume of blood.

relative near point. The near point for both eyes at which accommodation is brought into play.

relative permittivity. DIELECTRIC CONSTANT.

relative refractory period. A period of decreased excitability following application of a suitable stimulus to a nerve or muscle. It occurs only in tissues subject to the all-or-none law (such as nerve, striated muscle, heart); during this interval, a suprathreshold stimulus can elicit a second response. Compare *absolute refractory period.*

relative scotoma. A scotoma within which perception of light is only partially impaired.

relative sterility. Inability to produce a viable child.

relative transmittance. In applied spectroscopy, the ratio of the transmittance of the photographic image of a spectrum line to the transmittance of an adjacent clear (unexposed but developed) portion of the photographic emulsion.

re·lax, *v.* [L. *relaxare,* to loosen, from *laxus,* loose]. 1. To loosen or make less tense. 2. To become less tense.

re·lax·ant (ree·lack'sunt) *adj. & n.* 1. Producing relaxation. 2. An agent that lessens or reduces tension, or produces relaxation. 3. *Obsol.* A laxative.

re·lax·a·tion (ree"lack·say'shun) *n.* [L. *relaxatio,* from *relaxare,* to loosen]. A diminution of tension in a part; a diminution in functional activity, as relaxation of the skin or, more specifically, of a muscle.

relaxation heat. Heat evolved by muscle during relaxation.

relaxation response. Deceleration of bodily functions elicited by meditative techniques, which have been developed as a means of coping more adequately with fatigue, anxiety, and stress.

relaxation suture. TENSION SUTURE.

re·lax·in (re·lack'sin) *n.* A water-soluble hormone found in human serum and the serums of certain other animals during pregnancy; probably acting with progesterone and estrogen, it causes relaxation of pelvic ligaments in the guinea pig.

re·lease phenomenon. Any behavior, motor function, or reflex that appears or is exaggerated as a result of the destruction of nerve tissues that normally serve to inhibit the neurons responsible for the particular function or reflex, as the increased tendon reflexes in limbs with interruption of corticospinal tracts.

release syndrome. A symptom complex that follows release of a part from severe crushing injury. See also *crush syndrome.*

releasing factor. A substance produced by one gland which stimulates another to release a specific hormone; especially, any of the hormones secreted by the hypothalamus which act on the adenohypophysis to trigger release of a pituitary hormone, described specifically as corticotropin releasing factor, follicle-stimulating hormone releasing factor, growth hormone releasing factor, luteinizing hormone releasing factor, and thyrotropin releasing factor.

re·lief, *n.* [OF., from *relever,* to relieve]. The partial removal of anything distressing; alleviation of pain or discomfort.

relief chamber. A recess in the impression surface of an artificial denture, designed to relieve undue pressure on the supporting tissues in that area.

re·lieve, *v.* [OF. *relever,* from L. *relevare,* to lighten, from *levis,* light]. To free from pain, discomfort, or distress; to alleviate.

re·lo·my·cin (ree"lo·migh'sin) *n.* An antibacterial antibiotic produced by *Streptomyces hygroscopicus.*

¹REM Abbreviation for *rapid eye movement.* See also *REM sleep.*

²REM, rem Abbreviation for *roentgen equivalent man.*

Re·mak's band (rey'mahk) [R. *Remak,* German physiologist and neurologist, 1815–1865]. *Obsol.* The axis cylinder of a nerve fiber.

Remak's fibers [R. *Remak*]. Peripheral nonmedullated nerve fibers.

Remak's ganglion [R. *Remak*]. A group of nerve cells near the place where the coronary sinus joins the right atrium.

Remak's reflex [E. J. *Remak,* German neurologist, 1849–1911]. Flexion of the toes following irritation of the upper anterior thigh in spinal cord lesions.

re·me·di·al (re·mee'dee·ul) *adj.* [L. *remedialis,* from *remedium,* remedy]. 1. Having the nature of a remedy; relieving; curative. 2. Designed to correct a defect or faulty habit.

rem·e·dy, *n.* [L. *remedium,* from *mederi,* to cure]. Anything used in the treatment of disease.

Re·mij·ia (re·mij'ee·uh) *n.* [*Remijio,* Colombian surgeon, 19th century]. A genus of shrubs and trees of the Rubiaceae closely related to cinchona; some species yield quinine and related alkaloids.

re·min·er·al·iza·tion (ree·min"ur·ul·i·zay'shun) *n.* The restoration of the mineral content of the body or any part, especially of bone.

re·mis·sion (re·mish'un) *n.* [L. *remissio,* from *remittere,* to send back, relieve]. 1. Abatement or subsidence of the symptoms of disease. 2. The period of diminution thereof.

re·mit·tence (re·mit'unce) *n.* Temporary abatement or remission of symptoms. —**remit·tent** (·unt) *adj.*

remittent fever. A paroxysmal fever with exacerbations and remissions, but without return to normal temperature.

re·mote memory. Recall of events that occurred in the relatively distant past. Compare *long-term memory*.

remote parametritis. Parametritis marked by formation of abscesses in places more or less remote from the focus of the disease.

REM sleep [*r*apid *e*ye *m*ovement]. The stage of sleep that follows the deep sleep of stages 3 and 4 and is characterized by bursts of rapid eye movements (REMs), loss of tonic activity of the facial muscles, and desynchronization of the electroencephalogram. Contr. *NREM sleep*. See also *sleep*.

ren, *n*., genit. **re·nis** (ree'nis), pl. **re·nes** (ree'neez) [L.] [NA]. KIDNEY.

ren-, reni-, reno- [L. *ren*]. A combining form meaning *kidney, renal*.

re·nal (ree'nul) *adj*. [L. *renalis*, from *renes*, kidneys]. Pertaining to the kidney.

renal amino acid diabetes. FANCONI SYNDROME.

renal aminoaciduria. Excess amounts of one or more amino acids in the urine due to defective renal tubular reabsorption; the concentration of the relevant amino acids in the blood is normal or low. Compare *overflow aminoaciduria*.

renal anuria. Failure of urine formation due to intrinsic renal disease.

renal artery. See Table of Arteries in the Appendix.

renal autoamputation. The condition in which a kidney is cut off functionally by a diseased or obstructed ureter. Compare *autonephrectomy*.

renal ballottement. Palpation of the kidney by pushing it forward with one hand and pressing from the lumbar area posteriorly against the other hand placed on the anterior abdominal wall.

renal calculus. A concretion in the kidney. Syn. *kidney stone*.

renal calix. One of the divisions or subdivisions of the renal pelvis. The major calices (NA *calices renales majores*) are the two or three (rarely four) primary divisions of the pelvis and the minor calices (NA *calices renales minores*) are the cuplike terminal subdivisions, between 4 and 13 in number, each of which receives one or more of the renal papillae.

renal capsule. FIBROUS CAPSULE OF THE KIDNEY.

renal capsulotomy. Incision of the renal capsule.

renal cell carcinoma. A malignant tumor of the kidney whose parenchyma usually consists of large polygonal cells with abundant, often clear, cytoplasm. Syn. *Grawitz's tumor, clear cell carcinoma, hypernephroma*.

renal columns. The parts of the cortical substance of a kidney lying between the pyramids. NA *columnae renales*.

renal corpuscle. The glomerulus together with its glomerular capsule in the cortex of the kidney. NA *corpuscula renis*.

renal decortication. Decapsulation of the kidney.

renal diabetes. RENAL GLYCOSURIA.

renal dropsy. Anasarca due to nephrotic syndrome.

renal dwarf. An individual suffering from renal dwarfism.

renal dwarfism. Failure to thrive from a certain growth point commonly seen in children with severe chronic renal failure.

renal dyspnea. Dyspnea attributed to the acidosis of renal disease with uremia.

renal failure. A reduction in kidney function, acute or chronic, to a level at which the kidneys are unable to maintain normal biological homeostasis.

renal fascia. The connective-tissue investment of the kidney. There is an anterior and a posterior layer with the kidney and perirenal fat between. The two layers form a pocket; above, below, and laterally they are fused. Syn. *Gerota's fascia*.

renal ganglia. Small, sometimes microscopic ganglia located within the renal plexus. NA *ganglia renalia*.

renal glycosuria. An anomalous condition characterized by a low renal threshold for sugar together with a normal blood sugar level.

renal hilum. HILUS RENALIS.

renal hyperchloremic acidosis. Acidosis associated with an elevated serum chloride as seen in the proximal type of renal tubular acidosis.

renal hypertension. RENOVASCULAR HYPERTENSION.

renal hypoelectrolytemia. BARTTER'S SYNDROME.

renal hypophosphatemia. FAMILIAL HYPOPHOSPHATEMIA.

renal infantilism. RENAL DWARFISM.

renal injury. Damage of the kidney as a result of trauma, crushing, rib fractures, missiles, or muscular action; involves rupture, penetration, and tears of the ureter.

renal insufficiency. A measurable quantitative reduction in renal function, acute or chronic.

renal lobes. The subdivisions of the kidney corresponding to the renal pyramids with their associated cortex; externally visible in the fetus and infant, or throughout life in some mammals. NA *lobi renales*.

renal osteitis. RENAL RICKETS.

renal osteitis fi·bro·sa gen·e·ra·li·sa·ta (figh·bro'suh jen"e·ral·i·say'tuh). RENAL RICKETS.

renal osteodystrophy. RENAL RICKETS.

renal papillae. The summits of the renal pyramids projecting into the renal pelvis. NA *papillae renales*.

renal pelvis. The expansion of the proximal end of the ureter which receives the major and minor calices within the renal sinus. NA *pelvis renalis*.

renal plexus. A nerve plexus derived from the celiac and abdominal aortic plexuses; it accompanies the renal artery, and is distributed to the kidney. NA *plexus renalis*.

renal pressor system. The system whereby renin acts on angiotensinogen to produce angiotensin I, which is converted to angiotensin II, which raises blood pressure by direct arteriolar constrictive effects, and by stimulation of aldosterone release with subsequent sodium retention.

renal pyramids. The conical masses composing the medullary substance of the kidney. NA *pyramides renales*.

renal retinitis. Hypertensive retinopathy due to hypertension caused by renal disease.

renal rickets. A metabolic bone disease due to increased bone resorption resulting from the acidosis and secondary hyperparathyroidism of renal insufficiency. Syn. *renal osteodystrophy, pseudorickets, renal osteitis, renal osteitis fibrosa generalista*.

renal scleroderma. Interstitial nephritis and fibrosis occurring as part of diffuse scleroderma.

renal sclerosis. NEPHROSCLEROSIS.

renal shunt. TRUETA'S SHUNT.

renal sinus. The space surrounded by the mass of the kidney and occupied by the renal pelvis, calices, vessels, and parts of the renal capsule. NA *sinus renalis*.

renal tubular acidosis. A heritable disorder characterized by the inability to acidify the urine. In the proximal renal tubular type, hyperchloremic acidosis results from incomplete reabsorption of bicarbonate in the proximal tubule and excessive base is lost in the urine; the disease is usually confined to males. In the distal type growth, retardation, rickets, nephrocalcinosis, and renal failure are seen predominantly in females, resulting from the inability of the distal tube to establish an acid urine.

renal tubular ectasia. MEDULLARY SPONGE KIDNEY.

renal tubules. The glandular tubules which elaborate the urine in the kidney. NA *tubuli renales*. See also *nephron*.

renal vascular hypertension. RENOVASCULAR HYPERTENSION.

Ren·du-Osler-Weber disease (rahⁿ·dueʼ) [H. J. L. *Rendu*, French physician, 1844–1902; W. *Osler*; and F. P. *Weber*]. HEREDITARY HEMORRHAGIC TELANGIECTASIA.

Rendu's tremor [H. J. L. *Rendu*]. A tremor of psychic origin, provoked or increased by volitional movements.

renes. Plural of *ren*.

Renese. Trademark for polythiazide, an orally effective diuretic and antihypertensive drug.

reni-. See *ren-*.

ren·i·form (ren'i·form) *adj.* [*reni-* + *-form*]. Kidney-shaped.

re·nin (ree'nin) *n.* [*ren-* + *-in*]. A proteolytic enzyme in kidney that acts on renin substrate to liberate angiotensin I.

renin substrate. ANGIOTENSINOGEN.

ren·i·punc·ture (ren"i·punk'chur, ree'ni·punk"chur) *n.* [*reni-* + *puncture*]. Puncture of the capsule of a kidney.

ren mo·bi·lis (mo'bi·lis). FLOATING KIDNEY.

ren·net (ren'it) *n.* 1. RENNIN. 2. A preparation of the lining of the calf stomach used as a source of rennin.

ren·nin (ren'in) *n.* [*rennet* + *-in*]. The milk-coagulating enzyme found in the gastric juice of the fourth stomach of the calf. Syn. *chymosin.*

ren·nin·o·gen (re·nin'o·jen) *n.* [*rennin* + *-gen*]. The zymogen of rennin, found in the wall of the fourth stomach of the calf. Syn. *prorennin.*

ren·no·gen (ren'o·jen) *n.* RENNINOGEN.

reno-. See *ren-.*

Renografin. A trademark for meglumine diatrizoate in injectable dosage forms suitable for excretory urography, retrograde pyelography, and venography.

re·no·gram (ree'no·gram) *n.* [*reno-* + *-gram*]. 1. A continuous recording of the level of radioactivity monitored externally over each kidney after the intravenous injection of an appropriate radiopharmaceutical. 2. NEPHROGRAM.

Ré·non-De·lille syndrome (rey·nohn', duh·leel') [L. *Rénon,* French physician, 1863-1922; and A. *Delille,* French physician, 1876-1950]. Dyspituitarism, characterized by hypotension, tachycardia, oliguria, insomnia, hyperhidrosis, and heat intolerance.

re·no·pri·val (ree"no·prye'vul) *adj.* [*reno-* + L. *privare,* to deprive, + *-al*]. 1. Without kidneys. 2. Pertaining to or caused by absence of kidneys or kidney function.

renoprival hypertension. Systemic arterial hypertension presumed due to the absence of a renal vasodepressor substance in nephrectomized animals or man.

re·no·re·nal (ree"no·ree'nul, ren"o·) *adj.* [*reno-* + *renal*]. Of or pertaining to both kidneys; affecting one kidney and then the other.

renorenal reflex. The mechanism by which disease or injury of one kidney may produce pain in, or impair the function of, the opposite kidney.

re·no·tro·phic (ree"no·tro'fick, ·trof'ick) *adj.* [*reno-* + *-trophic*]. Having the property of promoting enlargement of the kidneys.

re·no·vas·cu·lar (ree"no·vas'kew·lur) *adj.* [*reno-* + *vascular*]. Pertaining to the blood vessels of the kidneys.

renovascular hypertension. Systemic arterial hypertension as a result of intrinsic renal vascular disease; it is usually mediated through the renal pressor system. See also *Goldblatt kidney.*

Ren·shaw cell [B. *Renshaw,* U.S. neurophysiologist, 20th century]. A small interneuron in the ventromedial region of the anterior horn of the spinal cord, innervated by recurrent collaterals from motor neurons and in turn delivering a high-frequency burst of inhibitory impulses to the motor neurons.

Renshaw inhibition [B. *Renshaw*]. RECURRENT INHIBITION.

ren un·gui·for·mis (ung"gwi·for'mis). HORSESHOE KIDNEY.

re·or·ga·ni·za·tion (ree·or"guh·ni·za'shun) *n.* Healing by the development of tissue elements similar to those lost through some morbid process.

reo·vi·rus (ree"o·vye'rus) *n.* [*r*espiratory + *e*nteric + *o*rphan + *virus*]. A member of a group of hemagglutinating, ether-resistant ribonucleic acid viruses, about 72 millimicrons in diameter, producing distinctive intracytoplasmic inclusion bodies in monkey renal cells; parasitic for human and animal species.

REP, rep Abbreviation for *roentgen equivalent physical.*

rep. Abbreviation for *repetatur;* let it be repeated.

re·pair, *v.* [OF. *reparer,* from L. *reparare,* from *parare,* to put in order]. To mend; to restore to a more normal state, artificially as by surgical means, or naturally through the process of healing.

re·par·a·tive (re·păr'uh·tiv) *adj.* Pertaining to or making repairs; repairing.

reparative surgery. PLASTIC SURGERY.

re·pel·lent, re·pel·lant (re·pel'unt) *adj.& n.* 1. Having a tendency or an action to repel or drive away. 2. A substance that repels, as any one of various chemicals used to repel or kill external parasites, such as mosquitoes, chiggers, or ticks.

re·pel·ler (re·pel'ur) *n.* An instrument used in large-animal obstetrics to push back the fetus so head and limbs can be placed for normal delivery.

re·per·co·la·tion (ree·pur"kuh·lay'shun) *n.* Repeated percolation.

re·per·cus·sion (ree"pur·kush'un) *n.* [L. *repercussio,* rebound, reverberation, from *percutere,* to strike, beat]. 1. BALLOTTEMENT. 2. A driving in, or dispersion of, a tumor or eruption.

re·per·cus·sive (ree"pur·kus'iv) *adj.* REPELLENT.

rep·e·ti·tion aphasia (rep"e·tish'un). A form of aphasia characterized by a selective disturbance of repetition of speech, though there is normal comprehension of what was said.

repetition-compulsion principle. A tendency in the unconscious part of the mind to recreate a previously experienced state of affairs in actions or feelings or both, irrespective of any definite advantage to be obtained, but usually in an effort to allay anxiety. The individual may or may not be aware of the tendency.

re·pet·i·tive firing. The ability of a tissue, particularly nerve tissue, to discharge, after suitable excitation, a succession of impulses.

re·place·ment, *n. In psychiatry,* a mental mechanism operating outside of and beyond conscious awareness in which the real object or feeling is replaced by another; as in a phobia, the actual internal but hidden object of fear and dread is replaced by a substitute external one. See also *substitution.*

replacement fibrosis. Fibrosis that replaces destroyed tissues, in part or wholly.

replacement therapy. Therapy in which a natural body constituent or its synthetic equivalent is used to replace a function which has been destroyed surgically or has ceased naturally.

replacement transfusion. EXCHANGE TRANSFUSION.

re·plan·ta·tion (ree"plan·tay'shun) *n.* 1. The act of planting again. 2. The replacement of teeth that have been extracted or otherwise removed from their alveolar sockets, usually after appropriate treatment such as filling the root canals and planing the roots.

re·ple·tion (re·plee'shun) *n.* [L. *repletio,* from *replere,* to fill up]. The condition of being, or the act of making, full. —**re·plete** (re·pleet') *adj.*

rep·li·ca·tion (rep"li·kay'shun) *n.* [L. *replicare,* to fold back, unroll, from *plicare,* to fold]. Multiplication of bacteriophage in bacterium; the phage loses its identity after entering bacterium, and shortly before lysis of the bacterium new phages of adult size and consistency appear. 2. The repetition of an experiment under the same conditions to check for possible error due to personal factors of the observer. 3. A folding back of a part; reduplication. See also *reproduction.* —**rep·li·cate** (rep'li·kate) *v.*

re·po·lar·iza·tion (ree·po"lur·i·zay'shun) *n.* [*re-* + *polarization*]. Restoration of the resting or polarized state in a nerve or muscle fiber during recovery from conduction of an impulse or series of impulses.

re·po·si·tion (ree"puh·zish'un) *n.* [*re-* + *position*]. The return of an abnormally placed part, organ, or fragment to its proper position.

re·pos·i·tor (re·poz'i·tur) *n.* An instrument for replacing parts or organs that have become displaced.

re·pos·i·to·ry (re·poz'i·tor·ee) *adj. & n.* 1. Of a drug: prepared in a form that is slowly absorbed and acts over a prolonged period. 2. A receptacle, place, or substance in which something is stored or deposited.

repository injection. An injection containing the therapeutic agent in slowly absorbable form so as to delay its absorption and prolong the effect.

rep·re·sen·ta·tion·al hemisphere. The cerebral hemisphere that subserves such functions as perception of temporal and spatial relationships. Compare *nondominant hemisphere.* Contr. *categorical hemisphere.*

re·pres·sion (re·presh'un) *n.* [L. *reprimere, repressus,* to hold back, repress, from *premere,* to press]. 1. *In psychiatry,* a defense mechanism whereby ideas, feelings, or desires, in conflict with the individual's conscious self-image or motives, are unconsciously dismissed from consciousness. Compare *suppression.* 2. Sometimes, any defense mechanism.

re·pres·sor (re·pres'ur) *n.* An agent, usually a metabolic end product, which represses the synthesis of the enzymes in the metabolic pathway.

re·pro·duc·tion (ree"pruh·duck'shun) *n.* [*re-* + *production*]. A fundamental property of protoplasm by which organisms give rise to other organisms of the same kind.

re·pro·duc·tive (ree"pruh·duck'tiv) *adj.* Of or pertaining to reproduction.

reproductive system. The generative apparatus, as a whole, consisting in man of the penis, testes, epididymis, deferential ducts, seminal vesicles, and prostate, and in woman of the vagina, uterus, uterine tubes (oviducts), and ovaries together with associated glandular structures.

rep·ro·mi·cin (rep"ro·mye'sin) *n.* A lactone of an unsaturated ketoheptadecanoic acid aldehyde with an aminoxylose substituent, $C_{31}H_{51}NO_8$, an antibiotic of unspecified action.

re·pul·sion (re·pul'shun) *n.* [L. *repulsio,* from *repellere,* to push back]. The act of repelling or driving back or apart.

RER Abbreviation for *rough-surfaced endoplasmic reticulum.*

RES Abbreviation for *reticuloendothelial system.*

res·az·u·rin (res·az'yoo·rin) *n.* So-called diazoresorcinol, a phenoxazine compound, $C_{12}H_7NO_4$; dark-red crystals with a greenish luster. Variously used as a reagent, especially as an oxidation-reduction indicator in the bacteriologic examination of milk.

res·cin·na·mine (re·sin'uh·meen, ·min) *n.* An alkaloid, $C_{35}H_{42}N_2O_9$, in certains species of *Rauwolfia;* an antihypertensive and sedative drug.

re·sect (ree·sekt') *v.* [L. *resecare, resectus* to cut back]. 1. To cut out a portion of a tissue or organ. 2. To cut away the end of one or more of the bones entering into a joint.

re·sec·tion (ree·seck'shun) *n.* [L. *resectio,* from *resecare,* to cut back]. The operation of cutting out, as the removal of a section or segment of an organ.

re·sec·to·scope (ree·seck'tuh·skope) *n.* [*resect* + *-scope*]. A tubular instrument by means of which small structures may be divided or removed within a body cavity without an opening or incision other than that made by the instrument itself; used especially for prostatectomy.

re·ser·pine (re·sur'peen, ·pin) *n.* 3,4,5-Trimethoxybenzoyl methyl reserpate, $C_{33}H_{40}N_2O_9$, an alkaloid in certain species of *Rauwolfia;* an antihypertensive and sedative drug.

re·serve, *n.* [L. *reservare,* to save up]. 1. A remainder. 2. A capacity or potentiality retained as an additional store.

reserve air. EXPIRATORY RESERVE VOLUME.

reserve-cell carcinoma. OAT-CELL CARCINOMA.

reserve cells. 1. Small undifferentiated epithelial cells at the base of the stratified columnar lining of the bronchial tree. 2. CHROMOPHOBE CELLS.

reserve force. Energy latent within an organism or part over and above that required for normal function. See also *cardiac reserve.*

res·er·voir (rez'ur·vwahr) *n.* [F. *réservoir,* from *réserver,* to reserve]. 1. A storage cavity or place. 2. A living organism that supports the growth of an infectious agent although suffering little or no effects from that agent. 3. RESERVOIR HOST.

reservoir host. An animal species on which the parasite depends for its survival in nature and which serves as the source of infection of other species, including man.

res·i·dent, *adj. & n.* [from L. *residere,* to reside, remain, abide]. 1. Dwelling in a given place, often as required by regulation or in connection with professional duties. 2. Stable; fixed. 3. A physician serving a major portion of the time in the hospital for further training after an internship. —**resi·dence, resi·den·cy,** *n.*

resident flora. *In surgery,* the portion of the cutaneous bacterial flora which is relatively stable, and relatively difficult to remove by washing or destroy by means of antiseptics. It consists principally of staphylococci of low pathogenicity.

residua. Plural of *residuum.*

re·sid·u·al (re·zid'yoo·ul) *adj.* [*residue* + *-al*]. Characterizing or pertaining to that which cannot be evacuated or discharged, or which remains.

residual abscess. An abscess forming in or about the residue of a former inflammatory focus.

residual air. RESIDUAL VOLUME.

residual bodies. In the developing spermatid, the anucleate masses that appear in the lumen of tubules after the cytoplasm is shed.

residual cyst. An odontogenic cyst remaining after the loss of the tooth with which it was associated.

residual hearing. In the measurement of hearing loss, the amount of hearing that a person retains irrespective of temporary reductions.

residual lumen. The persisting lumen, or a portion thereof, of the craniobuccal pouch; found in the hypophysis between the pars distalis and pars intermedia.

residual proteinuria or **albuminuria.** Proteinuria which may persist to a slight degree after nephritis.

residual ridge. ALVEOLAR RIDGE.

residual type of schizophrenia. Recognizable residual disturbance of thought, affect, or behavior shown by persons who, after a definite psychotic schizophrenic episode, have improved sufficiently to be able to get along in the general community.

residual urine. The urine remaining in the bladder after urination.

residual valence. The capacity of ions or molecules already apparently saturated as to combining power to form more complex ions or molecules, as in the formation of coordination compounds and associated molecules.

residual volume. Air remaining in the lungs after the most complete expiration possible. It is elevated in diffuse obstructive emphysema and during an attack of asthma. Syn. *residual air* or *capacity.*

res·i·due (rez'i·dew) *n.* [L. *residuum,* from *residere,* to remain]. That which remains after a part has been removed; remainder.

re·sid·u·um (re·zid'yoo·um), pl. **resid·ua** (·yoo·uh) *n.* That which remains; residue.

re·sil·ience (re·zil'yunce) *n.* The quality of being elastic or resilient.

re·sil·ient (re·zil'yunt) *adj.* [L. *resilire,* to spring back]. Rebounding; elastic.

res·in (rez'in) *n.* [L. *resina,* from Gk. *rētinē,* pine resin]. 1. One of a class of vegetable substances exuding from various plants; generally soluble in alcohol and in ether, and insoluble in water. They are composed largely of esters and ethers of organic acids and acid anhydrides. 2. A class of preparations made by extracting resin-containing drugs with alcohol, concentrating the liquid and adding it to water, whereby the resin and other water-insoluble principles precipitate and may be collected and dried. —**resin·ous** (·us) *adj.*

res·in·oid (rez'i·noid) *adj. & n.* 1. Having some of the properties of a resin. 2. A substance which has some of the properties of a resin.

re·sis·tance, *n.* [L. *resistentia,* from *resistere,* to withstand]. 1. Opposition to force or external impression. 2. In electricity, the opposition offered by a conductor to the passage of the current. Abbreviated, R. 3. *In psychiatry,* a defense mechanism characterized by the individual's reluctance to bring repressed material to light and to give up habitual patterns of thinking, feeling, and acting to take on less neurotic and newer modes of adaptation. 4. *In microbiology,* native or acquired immunity. 5. Lack of sensitivity or response to a drug, hormone, or treatment.

re·sis·tant rickets (re·zis'tunt). VITAMIN D–REFRACTORY RICKETS.

re·sis·to·my·cin (re·zis''to·migh'sin) *n.* A weakly acid antibiotic substance, $C_{23}H_{18}O_6$, produced by *Streptomyces resistomycificus.*

Resistopen. A trademark for the sodium salt of oxacillin, a semisynthetic penicillin antibiotic.

res·o·lu·tion (res''uh·lew'shun) *n.* [L. *resolutio,* from *resolvere,* to loosen]. 1. The subsidence of any pathological process, as inflammation, and the return to normal of affected tissues, in some cases occurring by a process of enzymic digestion of an exudate followed by absorption of the products. 2. The ability of the eye or a lens to recognize nearby objects as separate from one another rather than blurred into one apparent object. 3. The separation of an optically inactive mixture of isomers into its optically active components. Syn. *mesotomy.* 4. The analysis of a vector into its component parts. 5. *In psychiatry,* the bringing together or the compromising of opposing views, as in the resolution of emotional conflict.

re·solve, *v.* [L. *resolvere,* to loosen, unbind]. 1. To return to the normal state after some pathologic process. 2. To separate (something) into its component parts.

re·sol·vent (re·zol'vunt) *adj & n.* 1. Capable of dissipating inflammatory processes or effecting absorption of a neoplasm. 2. An agent capable of these actions.

re·solv·ing power. 1. The capability of a photographic film to make clear the finest details of an object. 2. The capability of a lens to make clear the separation of two closely adjacent objects.

res·o·na·tor (rez'uh·nay''tur) *n.* Any physical body capable of being set into vibration in unison with another vibrating body. The thoracic cage, lung, and other human structures possess this capacity in limited degree.

res·o·nance (rez'uh·nunce) *n.* [L. *resonare,* to resound]. 1. The attribute of relatively long duration possessed by certain sounds. 2. Normal resonance; in physical diagnosis, the prolonged, nonmusical, composite sound which results from vibration of the normal chest, usually elicited by percussion. 3. *In chemistry,* the phenomenon of a compound simultaneously having the characteristics of two or more structural forms of the compound, thereby providing additional orbital paths for electrons and conferring greater stability on the compound than if it possessed only one of the structures involved. Benzene represents such a resonance hybrid of forms differing only in the alternation of double bonds in the ring.

resonance theory of hearing. The theory that the inner ear contains tuned resonators that stimulate specific nerve endings when a tone of their resonant frequency enters the ear. Usually associated with the place theory of hearing.

res·o·nant (rez'uh·nunt) *adj.* [L. *resonare,* to resound]. Possessing, or capable of producing, resonance.

re·sorb (re·sorb', ·zorb') *v.* [L. *resorbere,* to suck back, absorb again]. 1. To undergo resorption. 2. To dissolve or lyse.

re·sorb·ent (re·sor'bunt) *adj. & n.* 1. Tending to resorb. 2. A drug that aids in the process of resorption.

re·sor·cin (re·zor'sin) *n.* RESORCINOL.

resorcin-fuchsin. WEIGERT'S STAIN.

re·sor·cin·ol (re·zor'sin·ole) *n.* [*resin* + *orcinol*]. *meta*-Dihydroxybenzene, $C_6H_4(OH)_2$; used in treatment of skin diseases for its antiseptic, keratolytic, exfoliative, and antifungal properties.

resorcinol monoacetate. A viscous liquid, $HOC_6H_4OCOCH_3$, sparingly soluble in water, which slowly liberates resorcinol by hydrolysis; used in treating various diseases of the skin and scalp.

re·sor·cin·ol·phthal·ein (re·zor''sin·ol·thal'een) *n.* FLUORESCEIN SODIUM.

resorcinol test. BOAS' TEST (2).

re·sorp·tion (re·sorp'shun, ·zorp') *n.* [from *resorb*]. The disappearance of all or part of a process, tissue, or exudate by biochemical reactions that may involve dissolution, lysis, absorption, and/or other actions. —**resorp·tive** (·tiv) *adj.*

resorptive jaundice. REGURGITATION JAUNDICE.

re·spi·ra·ble (res'pi·ruh·bul, re·spye'ruh·bul) *adj.* Capable of being inspired and expired; capable of furnishing the gaseous interchange in the lungs necessary for life. —**re·spi·ra·bil·i·ty** (res''pi·ruh·bil'i·tee, re·spye'ruh·bil''i·tee) *n.*

res·pi·ra·tion (res''pi·ray'shun) *n.* [L. *respiratio,* from *respirare,* to breathe]. 1. The physical and chemical processes by which tissues exchange gases with the medium in which they live; generally, aerobic respiration, by which most organisms utilize oxygen in energy-producing reactions and form carbon dioxide and water which is excreted as a waste product; less commonly, anaerobic respiration, by which certain lower organisms can sustain life for some time in the absence of oxygen. 2. The act of breathing with the lungs, consisting of inspiration, or the taking into the lungs of the ambient air, and of expiration, or the expelling of the modified air which contains more carbon dioxide than the air taken in. 3. Transport of respiratory gases (oxygen and carbon dioxide) by the blood.

respiration calorimeter. An apparatus that determines the heat production of an individual by measuring the gaseous exchange of the lungs.

res·pi·ra·tor (res'pi·ray''tur) *n.* A device or apparatus for producing artificial respiration.

res·pi·ra·to·ry (res'pi·ruh·to·ree, re·spye'ruh·to·ree) *adj.* Pertaining to respiration.

respiratory acidosis. Acidosis in which the tendency to decreased blood pH is due to retention of excessive carbon dioxide in the body. Physiologic compensation is largely by renal retention of sodium bicarbonate. Contr. *metabolic acidosis.*

respiratory alkalosis. Alkalosis in which the tendency to increased blood pH is due to accelerated pulmonary elimination of carbon dioxide. Physiologic compensation is largely by accelerated renal excretion of sodium bicarbonate. Contr. *metabolic alkalosis.*

respiratory anosmia. Obstructive anosmia. See *anosmia.*

respiratory arrest. The sudden cessation of spontaneous respiration due to failure of the respiratory center (or centers) of the central nervous system; denotes particularly such failure preceding cardiac arrest.

respiratory arrhythmia. PHASIC SINUS ARRHYTHMIA.

respiratory bronchiole. The last bronchiolar subdivision; one which has pulmonary alveoli in its wall. It is the first portion of the lung capable of gas exchange. NA (pl). *bronchioli respiratorii* (sing. *bronchiolus respiratorius*).

respiratory capacity. 1. VITAL CAPACITY. 2. The ability of the blood to combine with oxygen in the lungs and with the carbon dioxide from the tissues.

respiratory cavity. The thoracic cavity; used as a general term to describe the air passages.

respiratory center. An imperfectly localized aggregate of neurons and synapses in the medullary tegmentum, which receives chemical and neural information from other parts of the brain and from the peripheral nervous system, and controls the rhythmic sequence of breathing.

respiratory chain. The sequence of coenzymes and proteins involved in the process of electron transport in the mitochondria.

respiratory chamber. RESPIRATORY CAVITY.

respiratory coefficient. RESPIRATORY QUOTIENT.

respiratory control index. The ratio of mitochondrial respiration in the presence of high ADP to the respiration in the absence of ADP. A high index is indicative of fresh, intact mitochondria; a low index, of damaged or aged mitochondria. Syn. *acceptor-control index.*

respiratory distress syndrome of the newborn. A disease of unknown cause in the first days of life of premature infants characterized by respiratory distress, cyanosis, easy collapsibility of alveoli, and loss of pulmonary surfactant. A hyaline membrane lines the alveoli and alveolar ducts when the disease persists for more than a few hours. Abbreviated, RDS.

respiratory enzyme. An enzyme, such as cytochrome oxidase, concerned with the mechanism by which molecular oxygen produces oxidation in the living cell.

respiratory epithelium. The pseudostratified, columnar ciliated epithelium lining most of the respiratory tract and distinctive to the respiratory tract.

respiratory insufficiency. Incompetence of the respiratory processes.

respiratory line. The line connecting the bases of the upward strokes in a recorded pulse tracing.

respiratory murmur. The sound produced by the air entering and escaping from the lungs during respiration.

respiratory myoclonus. DIAPHRAGMATIC TIC.

respiratory passage. Any part of the respiratory tract through which breathed air normally passes on its way to and from the lung alveoli. Syn. *airway.*

respiratory period. The interval between two successive inspirations.

respiratory pulse. The modification in the pulse rate produced by respiration.

respiratory quotient. 1. The ratio of the volume of carbon dioxide evolved by respiring cells or tissues to the volume of oxygen consumed in the same time. 2. In respiration, the ratio of the volume of carbon dioxide expired to that of oxygen consumed in a given interval of time. Abbreviated, R.Q.

respiratory region of the nose. The portion of the nasal passages having to do with the act of respiration. NA *regio respiratoria.*

respiratory scleroma. RHINOSCLEROMA.

respiratory standstill. RESPIRATORY ARREST.

respiratory surface. The entire surface of pulmonary tissue coming in contact with the respired air.

respiratory syncytial virus. A large RNA virus named for its ability to cause respiratory disease in humans and its characteristic effect of syncytium formation in tissue cultures; probably the single most important viral respiratory pathogen of infancy throughout the world, causing bronchiolitis and pneumonitis. Abbreviated, RSV, RS virus.

respiratory system. 1. The system of organs or structures involved in respiration. 2. Specifically, the system of organs and structures involved in breathing, including the respiratory tract, the lungs as a whole, the diaphragm, and the muscles and nerves subserving them. NA *apparatus respiratorius.*

respiratory tract. The chain of passages and chambers by means of which breathed air is brought to and from the surfaces where gas exchange with the circulatory system takes place. The tract may be divided clinically into the upper respiratory tract, including the nasal and oral cavities, pharynx, and larynx, and the lower respiratory tract, including the trachea, bronchi, bronchioles, and alveolar structures.

respiratory tree. BRONCHIAL TREE.

respiratory undulation. The variations in the blood pressure related to respiration.

respiratory ventilation meter. A meter that gives a measurement of the minute ventilation. See also *ventilation.*

re·spire, *v.* [L. *respirare,* to breathe, to breathe back, from *spirare,* to breathe, blow]. 1. To move air in and out of the lungs. 2. In animals, to consume oxygen and produce carbon dioxide; in plants, to consume carbon dioxide and produce oxygen.

res·pi·rom·e·ter (res″pi·rom′e·tur) *n.* [*respire* + *-meter*]. A device for measurement of several characteristics of respiration.

res·pi·rom·e·try (res″pi·rom′e·tree) *n.* The quantitative study of respiration.

re·sponse, *n.* [L. *responsum,* a reply, from *respondere,* to reply]. A change in the state of an organism, organ, tissue, or cell succeeding the application of a stimulus.

re·spon·si·bil·i·ty, *n.* 1. The moral, mental, or legal accountability for one's own acts or those of another. 2. The capacity to differentiate right from wrong. 3. *In legal medicine,* the accountability for professional acts.

¹rest, *n.* [OE. *raest*]. 1. Repose; inactivity; cessation of labor or action. 2. A mechanical supportive structure, as: an extension from a dental prosthesis that provides vertical or toothbearing support.

²rest, *n.* [OF. *reste,* from L. *restare,* to stay behind]. 1. Anything remaining or left over. 2. An epithelial remnant persisting after its developmental activity has ceased. Syn. *epithelial debris.* See also *fetal rest.*

re·ste·no·sis (ree″ste·no′sis) *n.* [*re-* + *stenosis*]. Recurrent narrowing, generally referring to the orifice of a heart valve after corrective surgery.

rest force. The cardiac work expended in maintaining the circulation when the body is at rest.

res·ti·form (res′ti·form) *adj.* [L. *restis,* cord, + *-form*]. Corded or cordlike.

restiform body. INFERIOR CEREBELLAR PEDUNCLE.

rest·ing cell. A cell in the interphase or vegetative stage of mitosis.

resting nucleus. KARYOSTASIS.

resting potential. MEMBRANE POTENTIAL.

resting saliva. The saliva produced that is not directly due to a specific stimulus such as mastication.

resting sporangium. *In biology,* a peculiar resting cell formed by the mycelium of a few fungi (such as *Saprolegnia*), in which zoospores are produced.

resting spore. *In biology,* a spore, invested with a firm cell wall, which remains dormant during adverse environmental conditions before it germinates.

resting stage. *In biology,* a period during which reproduction of a microorganism is absent.

resting state. *In biology,* a state of suspended activity, the condition of perennial plants (bulbs, seeds) and spores during their period of dormancy.

resting tremor. A static or parkinsonian tremor, which is maximal in an attitude of repose and which is temporarily diminished by willed movement; with full relaxation, as when the limb is supported against gravity, and with complete rest, as in sleep, the tremor disappears.

resting wandering cell. HISTIOCYTE. See also *fixed macrophage.*

res·ti·tu·tio ad in·te·grum (res″ti·tew′shee·o ad in′te·grum) [L.]. Complete restoration to a healthy condition.

res·ti·tu·tion (res″ti·tew′shun) *n.* [L. *restitutio,* from *restituere,* to restore]. 1. The act of restoring. 2. *In obstetrics,* a rotation of the fetal head immediately after its birth. 3. *In psychiatry,* the psychic mechanism whereby the individual seeks to relieve himself of unconscious guilt by benevolent acts which undo, make good, or repair some harm.

rest·less legs. A condition characterized by creeping, crawling, itching, and sometimes pain of the legs and thighs which impels the patient to seek relief by moving the legs or walking. The state is usually benign but may be a prelude to uremic polyneuropathy. Syn. *restless legs of Ekbom, anxietas tibiarum, Wittmaack-Ekbom syndrome.*

res·to·ra·tion (res″to·ray′shun) *n.* [L. *restauratio,* from *restaurare,* to restore]. 1. The return to a state of health, functioning, or a normal condition. 2. Reconstruction or replacement of a body part. 3. Any structure or appliance that restores or replaces damaged or lost dental parts. —**re·stor·ative** (re·stor′uh·tiv) *adj.*

re·stor·ative (re·stor′uh·tiv) *n.* A tonic.

restorative dentistry. The aspect of clinical dentistry in which the teeth and associated structures are returned to normal form and function by replacement of the missing dental part or parts.

rest position. PHYSIOLOGIC REST POSITION.

re·straint, *n.* [OF. *restrainte,* from L. *restringere,* to draw back tightly]. 1. Hindrance of any action, physical, moral, or mental. 2. The state of being controlled; confinement.

re·stric·tion enzyme. Any specific enzyme that can degrade foreign invading DNA but does not attack host-cell DNA.

restriction of ego. *In psychology,* a defense mechanism for escaping anxiety by avoiding situations consciously perceived as dangerous or uncomfortable, as in the many phobias of childhood and as seen in adults whose sphere of movement is severely limited by their need to avoid anxiety.

re·strin·gent (re·strin′junt) *n.* [L. *restringere,* to draw back tight, restrict]. An astringent or styptic.

re·sul·tant (re·zul′tunt) *n.* [L. *resultare,* to spring back]. 1. That which results; the outcome of any process or action. 2. The product or products of a chemical reaction. 3. A single vector equivalent to a set of vectors.

re·su·pi·nate (ree·sue′pi·nate) *adj.* [L. *resupinare,* to bend backward]. Turned in an abnormal direction.

res·ur·rec·tion·ist (rez″uh·reck′shun·ist) *n.* [L. *resurrectio,* from *resurgere,* to raise oneself again]. One who steals dead bodies from the grave as subjects for dissection.

re·sus·ci·ta·tion (re·sus″i·tay′shun) *n.* [L. *resuscitatio,* from *resuscitare,* to revive]. 1. Restoration to life or consciousness after apparent death. 2. Specifically, restoration of breathing after respiratory arrest or drowning, or of heartbeat after cardiac arrest. —**re·sus·ci·tate** (re·sus′i·tate) *v.*

re·sus·ci·ta·tor (re·sus′i·tay″tur) *n.* A device or apparatus for ventilation of the lungs in resuscitation.

re·su·ture (ree·sue′chur) *n.* Secondary suture; suture of a wound some time after a first suture has been made.

retained placenta. A placenta not expelled by the uterus after labor.

re·tain·er (re·tay′nur) *n.* 1. A dental appliance for holding in position teeth which have been moved orthodontically. 2. Any inlay, crown, clasp, attachment, or other device that provides fixation or stabilization of a fixed or removable dental prosthesis.

re·tar·date (re·tahr′date) *n.* A person with mental retardation.

re·tar·da·tion (ree″tahr·day′shun) *n.* [L. *retardatio,* from *retardare,* to delay, from *tardus,* slow, late]. 1. Slow mental or physical functioning. 2. Specifically, MENTAL RETARDATION.

re·tard·ed depression. A form of depression in which all ordinary activity is inhibited or slowed down, and in which the patient is extremely dejected and self-deprecating, sometimes to the point of painful delusions.

retarded ejaculation. Excessively delayed ejaculation, often due to psychological inhibition of the ejaculatory reflex caused by guilt-induced anxiety or other psychic factors.

re·tard·er, *n.* A negative catalyst, that is, one acting to retard a reaction.

retch, *v.* To make a strong involuntary effort to vomit. —**retch·ing,** *n.*

re·te (ree′tee) *n.,* pl. **re·tia** (·tee·uh) [L., net]. Any network or decussation and interlacing, especially of capillary blood vessels.

rete acro·mi·a·le (a·kro·mee·ay′lee) [NA]. An arterial network about the acromion.

rete ar·te·ri·o·sum (ahr·teer·ee·o′sum) [NA]. Any arterial network.

rete ar·ti·cu·la·re cu·bi·ti (ahr·tick·yoo·lair′ee kew′bi·tye) [NA]. RETE OLECRANI.

rete articulare ge·nu (jen′yoo) [BNA]. RETE ARTICULARE GENUS.

rete articulare ge·nus (jen′us) [NA]. A network formed by the anastomosis of the arteries over the anterior and lateral surfaces of the knee. See also Plate 7.

rete cal·ca·ne·um (kal·kay′nee·um) [NA]. An arterial anastomosis about the calcaneus.

rete ca·na·lis hy·po·glos·si (ka·nay′lis high·po·glos′eye) [BNA]. PLEXUS VENOSUS CANALIS HYPOGLOSSI.

rete car·pi dor·sa·le (kahr′pye dor·say′lee) [NA]. DORSAL CARPAL RETE.

rete cords. The deep, anastomosing region of the medullary cords (1) that forms the rete testis or the rete ovarii.

rete cu·ta·ne·um (kew·tay′nee·um). The network of vessels at the boundary between corium and superficial fascia.

rete dor·sa·le pe·dis (dor·say′lee ped′is). An arterial network on the dorsum of the foot, formed by branches of the tarsal and metatarsal arteries joined by perforating plantar branches.

rete fo·ra·mi·nis ova·lis (fo·ray′mi·nis o·vay′lis) [BNA]. PLEXUS VENOSUS FORAMINIS OVALIS.

rete mal·le·o·la·re la·te·ra·le (mal·ee·o·lair′ee lat·e·ray′lee) [NA]. A vascular network around the lateral malleolus.

rete malleolare me·di·a·le (mee·dee·ay′lee) [NA]. A vascular network around the medial malleolus.

rete mi·ra·bi·le (mi·ray′bi·lee) [NA]. A capillary plexus intercalated in the path of an artery.

rete mu·co·sum (mew·ko′sum). STRATUM GERMINATIVUM.

re·ten·tion (re·ten′shun) *n.* [L. *retentio,* from *retinere,* to hold back]. 1. The act of retaining or holding back, as the holding of urine in the bladder due to some hindrance to urination. 2. The maintenance of orthodontically treated teeth in their reestablished positions until stability of their supporting tissues is established. 3. The fixation and stabilization of a dental prosthesis.

retention band. A thickening of the mesentery which fixes the cranial and the caudal end of the midgut to the dorsal abdominal wall, thus preventing herniation of the foregut and hindgut of the embryo.

retention cyst. A cyst due to obstruction of outflow of secretion from a gland.

retention defect. RETENTIVE MEMORY DEFECT.

retention enema. Liquid injected into the rectum, the expulsion of which is delayed voluntarily in order to liquefy the rectal contents or provide medication.

retention form. The shape given to a prepared dental cavity which provides for stabilization of the restoration in place.

retention hyperlipemia. FAMILIAL FAT-INDUCED HYPERLIPEMIA.

retention jaundice. Jaundice with predominantly unconjugated, or indirect-reacting, serum bilirubin.

retention of urine. A condition in which urine continues to be secreted by the kidneys but is retained in the bladder, as in atonic bladder or other urinary obstruction.

retention toxicosis. Toxicosis with clinical symptoms due to the retention of waste products; uremia or azotemia due to post-renal factors.

retentive memory defect. An impairment or loss of the ability to retain newly presented information, despite an alert state of mind, and intactness of comprehension and registration as demonstrated by the patient's ability to repeat information immediately after it is presented. See also *Korsakoff's syndrome.*

rete ole·cra·ni (o″le·kray′nigh). The network of vessels around the olecranon and at the back of the elbow, formed by the branches of the profunda brachii and other arteries.

rete ova·rii (o·vair'ee·eye). Vestigial tubules or cords of cells near the hilus of the ovary, corresponding with the rete testis, but not connected with the mesonephric duct.

rete pa·tel·lae (pa·tel'ee) [NA]. A plexus of vessels surrounding the patella.

rete peg. The prolongation of the epidermis between the papillae of the corium; the interpapillary epithelium.

rete sub·pa·pil·la·re (sub·pap·i·lair'ee). The network of vessels between the papillary and reticular layers of the corium.

rete tes·tis (tes'tis) [NA]. The network of anastomosing tubules in the mediastinum testis.

rete vas·cu·lo·sum (vas·kew·lo'sum) [BNA]. Any vascular network.

rete ve·no·sum (ve·no'sum) [NA]. Any venous network.

rete venosum dor·sa·le ma·nus (dor·say'lee man'us) [NA]. A venous network in the dorsum of the hand.

rete venosum dorsale pe·dis (ped'is) [NA]. A venous network on the dorsum of the foot.

rete venosum plan·ta·re (plan·tair'ee) [NA]. A venous network in the sole of the foot.

retia. Plural of *rete.*

retia ve·no·sa ver·te·bra·rum (ve·no'suh vur·te·brair'um) [BNA]. The venous networks about the vertebrae.

reticul-, reticulo-. A combining form meaning (a) *reticulum, reticular;* (b) *reticulated.*

reticula. Plural of *reticulum.*

re·tic·u·lar (re·tick'yoo·lur) *adj.* [*reticul*um + *-ar*]. Resembling a net; formed by a network.

reticular activating system. The reticular formation of the superior levels of the brainstem and the adjacent subthalamus, hypothalamus, and medial thalamus, which has been shown in animal experiments to play a basic role in regulating the background activity of the central nervous system. It is connected by collaterals in parallel with long afferent and efferent nervous pathways, and is thus stimulated by and acts upon them. Caudal influences upon spinal cord levels contribute to optimum motor performance; cephalic influences upon the cerebral hemispheres form the basis of the initiation, maintenance, and degree of the state called wakefulness on which higher nervous functions depend. Many hypnotic drugs block transmission of impulses from this area, and lesions of it result in states similar to coma in man. See also *arousal reaction.*

reticular cell. RETICULOCYTE (2).

reticular colliquation. A lesion occurring in vescicular viral diseases in which adjoining cells of the epidermis undergo degenerative changes and coalesce to form reticulated septa separating lobules of fluid.

reticular degeneration. A process in which intracellular edema of the epidermis causes rupture of the cells with formation of multilocular bullae.

reticular dysgenesia. An immunodeficiency disease characterized by marked leukopenia, lymphoid hypoplasia, thymic dysgenesis, bone marrow hypoplasia, and decreased immunoglobulins.

reticular fibers. The delicate, branching connective-tissue fibers forming the reticular framework of lymphatic tissue, myeloid tissue, the red pulp of the spleen, the finest stroma of many glands, and most basement membranes. They differ from collagenous fibers in their response to silver impregnation, in which they are blackened. Syn. *argentaffin fibers, argentophile fibers, lattice fibers, precollagenous fibers.*

reticular formation or **substance.** Any of those portions of the brainstem core that are characterized structurally by a wealth of cells of various sizes and types, arranged in diverse aggregations and enmeshed in a complicated fiber network. Embedded in this matrix are specific nuclei and tracts. NA *formatio reticularis.*

reticular lamina. The hyaline membrane of the inner ear, extending between the heads of the outer rods of Corti and the external row of the outer hair cells.

reticular layer. The deeper layer of the derma, composed of a dense network of collagenous and elastic fibers. NA *stratum reticulare.*

reticular membrane. The membrane covering the space of the outer hair cells of the cochlea. NA *membrana reticularis.*

reticular nuclei. Aggregations of nerve-cell bodies enmeshed in the reticular formation of the central nervous system; they are found in the reticular formation of the spinal cord, medulla oblongata, pontine, tegmentum, mesencephalon, and thalamus.

reticular nucleus of the subthalamus. A nucleus consisting of the nucleus of the tegmental field and cells scattered along the thalamic and lenticular fasciculi.

reticular nucleus of the thalamus. A thin neuronal shell which surrounds the lateral, anterosuperior, and anteroinferior aspects of the dorsal thalamus. NA *nucleus reticularis thalami.*

reticular system. RETICULOENDOTHELIAL SYSTEM.

reticular tissue. Connective tissue in which reticular fibers are the conspicuous element, forming a branching nonelastic network.

re·tic·u·lat·ed (re·tick'yoo·lay"tid) *adj.* [L. *reticulatus,* from *reticulum,* small net]. Having netlike meshes; formed like a web. —**re·tic·u·la·tion** (re·tick"yoo·lay'shun) *n.*

reticulated erythrocyte. RETICULOCYTE (1).

reticulated pigmented poikiloderma. A variety of Riehl's melanosis, located on the neck as a symmetric, pigmented, telangiectatic, and atrophic erythroderma with retiform arrangement. Causes include sunlight and photodynamic substances in cosmetics. Syn. *poikiloderma reticulare of Civatte, Civatte's poikiloderma.*

re·tic·u·late erythema (re·tick'yoo·lut). ERYTHEMA AB IGNE.

re·tic·u·lin (re·tick'yoo·lin) *n.* A protein isolated from the fibers of reticular tissue.

reticulo-. See *reticul-.*

re·tic·u·lo·bul·bar tract (re·tick"yoo·lo·bul'bur). Fibers, derived from the red nucleus, which synapse with cells in the reticular formation, which in turn project onto motor nuclei of the bulb. Not a discrete tract.

re·tic·u·lo·cyte (re·tick'yoo·lo·site) *n.* [*reticulo-* + *-cyte*]. 1. An immature erythrocyte. Retention of ribosomes account for the reticulated appearance when stained supravitally with cresyl blue or when viewed by phase microscopy. It is larger than a normal erythrocyte and usually constitutes less than 1 percent (range: 0.5 to 2.5 percent) of the total. There is an increase during active erythrocytopoiesis. In Wright- or Giemsa-stained blood films, these cells appear as polychromatophilic erythrocytes. 2. RETICULUM CELL. —**re·tic·u·lo·cyt·ic** (re·tick"yoo·lo·sit'ick) *adj.*

reticulocytic sarcoma. RETICULUM-CELL SARCOMA.

re·tic·u·lo·cy·to·pe·nia (re·tick"yoo·lo·sigh"to·pee'nee·uh) *n.* [*reticulocyte* + *-penia*]. Decrease of reticulocytes in the circulating blood.

re·tic·u·lo·cy·to·sis (re·tick"yoo·lo·sigh·to'sis) *n.,* pl. **reticulocy·to·ses** (·seez) [*reticulocyte* + *-osis*]. An excess of reticulocytes in the peripheral blood.

re·tic·u·lo·en·do·the·li·al (re·tick"yoo·lo·en"do·theel'ee·ul) *adj.* [*reticulo-* + *endothelial*]. Of, pertaining to, or involving the reticuloendothelial system or the reticuloendothelium.

reticuloendothelial cell. A cell of the reticuloendothelial system.

reticuloendothelial granulomatosis. A group of rare diseases characterized by generalized reticuloendothelial hyperplasia with or without intracellular lipid deposition. Included in this group are Letterer-Siwe's disease, Hand-Schüller-Christian disease, and eosinophilic granuloma.

reticuloendothelial sarcoma. RETICULUM-CELL SARCOMA.

reticuloendothelial system. The macrophage system, which includes all the phagocytic cells of the body, except the granulocytic leukocytes. These cells, diverse morphologically, all have the capacity for the elective storage of certain colloidal dyes. They include the histiocytes and macrophages of loose connective tissue, the reticular cells of lymphatic and myeloid tissues, the microglia, the blood monocytes, the endothelium-like littoral cells lining lymphatic sinuses and sinusoids of bone marrow, the Kupffer cells of hepatic sinusoids, the cells lining the sinusoids of the adrenal and hypophysis, the pulmonary alveolar macrophages (dust cells), and the microglia cells of the central nervous system. Abbreviated, RES. Syn. *system of macrophages.*

re·tic·u·lo·en·do·the·li·o·ma (re·tick″yoo·lo·en″do·theel·ee·o′muh) *n.* [*reticuloendotheli*um + *-oma*]. RETICULUM-CELL SARCOMA.

re·tic·u·lo·en·do·the·li·o·sis (re·tick″yoo·lo·en″do·theel·ee·o′sis) *n.*, pl. **reticuloendothelio·ses** (·seez) [*reticuloendotheli*um + *-osis*]. HISTIOCYTOSIS X.

re·tic·u·lo·en·do·the·li·um (re·tick″yoo·lo·en″do·theel′ee·um) *n.* [*reticulo-* + *endothelium*]. The basic tissue that forms the reticuloendothelial system.

re·tic·u·lo·ol·i·vary tract (re·tick″yoo·lo·ol′i·verr·ee). Part of the central tegmental tract; nerve fibers that arise in the reticular formation and project to the olive.

re·tic·u·lo·pe·nia (re·tick″yoo·lo·pee′nee·uh) *n.* [*reticulo-* + *-penia*]. RETICULOCYTOPENIA.

re·tic·u·lo·po·dia (re·tick″yoo·lo·po′dee·uh) *n.pl.* Pseudopodia whose brances anastomose.

re·tic·u·lo·re·tic·u·lar fibers (re·tick″yoo·lo·re·tick′yoo·lur). Nerve fibers that arise in the reticular formation and end in it at a different level.

re·tic·u·lo·sar·co·ma (re·tick″yoo·lo·sahr·ko′muh) *n.* RETICULUM-CELL SARCOMA.

re·tic·u·lo·sis (re·tick″yoo·lo′sis) *n.*, pl. **reticulo·ses** (·seez) [*reticul-* + *-osis*]. HISTIOCYTOSIS X.

re·tic·u·lo·spi·nal tract (re·tick″yoo·lo·spye′nul). Nerve fibers descending from two large regions of the brainstem reticular formation and descend into the spinal cord. One region is in the pontine tegmentum and the other in the medulla, giving rise to the pontine and medullary reticulospinal tracts respectively. NA *tractus reticulospinalis.*

re·tic·u·lo·the·li·o·ma (re·tick″yoo·lo·theel″ee·o′muh) *n.* [*reticulotheli*um + *-oma*]. RETICULUM-CELL SARCOMA.

re·tic·u·lo·the·li·um (re·tick″yoo·lo·theel′ee·um) *n.* RETICULOENDOTHELIUM. —**reticulotheli·al** (·ul) *adj.*

re·tic·u·lum (re·tick′yoo·lum) *n.*, pl. **reticu·la** (·luh) [L., dim. of *rete*, net]. 1. A fine network. 2. *In veterinary medicine*, the second division of the ruminant stomach. —**reticu·lose** (·loce) *adj.*

reticulum cell. A cell of reticular tissue. Compare *reticulocyte.*

reticulum-cell lymphosarcoma. RETICULUM-CELL SARCOMA.

reticulum-cell sarcoma. A type of malignant lymphoma in which the predominant cell type is an anaplastic reticulum cell. Multinucleated cells also occur. Syn. *histiocytic sarcoma.* See also *lymphosarcoma.*

re·tif·ism (ree′ti·fiz·um, re·teef′iz·um) *n.* [*Rétif* de la Bretonne, French educator, 1734–1806]. A sexual perversion in which a shoe or foot has the same erotic value as the genital organs.

ret·i·form (ret′i·form, ree′ti·) *adj.* [L. *rete*, net, + *-iform*]. Net-shaped; RETICULAR.

retin-, retino-. A combining form meaning *retina, retinal.*

ret·i·na (ret′i·nuh) *n.*, L. pl. & genit. sing. **reti·nae** (·nee), E. pl. **retinas** [ML., perhaps from *rete*, net]. The light-receptive layer and terminal expansion of the optic nerve in the eye. It extends from the point of exit of the nerve forward to the ora serrata. It consists of the following layers, named from behind forward: the pigment layer; the neuroepithelial layer, comprising the layer of rods and cones (bacillary layer), the outer limiting membrane, and the outer nuclear layer; the outer reticular layer (outer granular or plexiform layer), the inner nuclear layer, the inner reticular layer (inner granular or plexiform layer), the ganglionic layer, the nerve fiber layer. These layers are united and supported by neuroglial elements. See also Plate 19. Adj. *retinal.*

Retin-A. A trademark for tretinoin, a keratolytic.

retinacula. Plural of *retinaculum.*

retinacula cu·tis (kew′tis) [NA]. Fibrous bands connecting the corium with the underlying fascial structure.

retinacula un·guis (ung′gwis) [NA]. The fibers connecting a nail to its underlying structures.

ret·i·nac·u·lum (ret″i·nack′yoo·lum) *n.*, pl. **retinacu·la** (·luh) [L., that which holds back, from *retinere*, to hold back, retain]. A special fascial thickening that holds back an organ or part.

retinaculum cau·da·le (kaw·day′lee) [NA]. The fibrous band extending from the lip of the coccyx to the skin.

retinaculum ex·ten·so·rum ma·nus (ecks·ten·so′rum man′us) [NA]. EXTENSOR RETINACULUM OF THE WRIST.

retinaculum flex·o·rum ma·nus (fleck·so′rum man′us) [NA]. FLEXOR RETINACULUM OF THE WRIST.

retinaculum li·ga·men·ti ar·cu·a·ti (lig·uh·men′tye ahr·kew·ay′tye) [BNA]. A fibrous band from the arcuate popliteal ligament to the fibula.

retinaculum mus·cu·lo·rum ex·ten·so·rum in·fe·ri·us (mus·kew·lo′rum ecks·ten·so′rum in·feer′ee·us) [NA]. INFERIOR EXTENSOR RETINACULUM.

retinaculum musculorum extensorum su·pe·ri·us (sue·peer′ee·us) [NA]. SUPERIOR EXTENSOR RETINACULUM.

retinaculum musculorum fi·bu·la·ri·um in·fe·ri·us (fib·yoo·lair′ee·um in·feer′ee·us) [NA alt.]. INFERIOR PERONEAL RETINACULUM. NA alt. *retinaculum musculorum peroneorum inferius.*

retinaculum musculorum fibularium su·pe·ri·us (sue·peer′ee·us) [NA alt.]. SUPERIOR PERONEAL RETINACULUM. NA alt. *retinaculum musculorum peroneorum superius.*

retinaculum musculorum flex·o·rum pe·dis (fleck·so′rum ped′is) [NA]. FLEXOR RETINACULUM OF THE ANKLE.

retinaculum musculorum pe·ro·ne·o·rum in·fe·ri·us (pe·ro·nee′o·rum in·feer′ee·us) [NA]. INFERIOR PERONEAL RETINACULUM.

retinaculum musculorum peroneorum su·pe·ri·us (sue·peer′ee·us) [NA]. SUPERIOR PERONEAL RETINACULUM.

retinaculum of the hip joint. Any one of three deep longitudinal bands of the articular capsule which reflect upward along the neck of the femur from the femoral attachment toward the articular margin.

retinaculum pa·tel·lae la·te·ra·le (pa·tel′ee lat·e·ray′lee) [NA]. The lateral patellar retinaculum. See *patellar retinaculum.*

retinaculum patellae me·di·a·le (mee·dee·ay′lee) [NA]. The medial patellar retinaculum. See *patellar retinaculum.*

ret·i·nal (ret′i·nul) *adj.* & *n.* 1. Pertaining to or involving the retina. 2. RETINENE.

retinal astigmatism. Astigmatism due to changes in the localization of the fixation point, thought to be caused by changes in light intensity.

retinal cone. CONE (3).

retinal correspondence. The relationship between corresponding points in the retina of both eyes, simultaneous stimulation of which results in the sensation of one image.

retinal detachment. DETACHMENT OF THE RETINA.

retinal dialysis. A disinsertion of the retina from its attachment to the ora serrata.

retinal dysplasia. A developmental anomaly present at birth involving the inner layer of the neuroectoderm forming the optic vesicle; a consistent finding of trisomy 13 syndrome.

retinal glioma. Neuroepithelioma of the retina.

retinal image. The image of external objects as focused on the retina.

retinal incongruity. Lack of correspondence in the situation of the percipient elements of the two retinas. See also *abnormal retinal correspondence.*

retinal periphlebitis. EALES' DISEASE.
retinal pigment. RHODOPSIN.
retinal purple. RHODOPSIN.
retinal reflex. A round or linear light area reflected from the retina when the retinoscope is employed.
retinal rivalry. The continuous physiologic process of alternation in consciousness between stimuli falling on the two eyes. When this process is studied by artificially presenting different stimuli to each eye, the alternation is found to be unpredictable in timing and areas involved and dependent on the strength of stimulus to each eye. Syn. *rivalry of visual fields, strife rivalry, complementary replacement, reciprocal replacement.*
retinal vasculitis. EALES' DISEASE.
ret·i·nene (ret'i·neen) *n.* [*retina* + *-ene*]. A pigment extracted from the retina, turned yellow by light; the chief carotenoid of the retina, appearing in two forms, retinene$_1$ and retinene$_2$, the aldehydes of vitamin A_1 and vitamin A_2. Under the influence of light, retinene$_1$ combines with rod opsin to form rhodopsin, and with cone opsin to form iodopsin, while retinene$_2$ combines with rod opsin to form porphyropsin and with cone opsin to form cyanopsin. Syn. *retinal.*
retinene reductase. The enzyme responsible for the reduction of retinene to retinol (vitamin A); it may be identical with alcohol dehydrogenase.
ret·i·ni·tis (ret"i·nigh'tis) *n.*, pl. **reti·nit·i·des** (·nit'i·deez) [*retin-* + *-itis*]. Inflammation of the retina.
retinitis cir·ci·na·ta (sur·si·nay'tuh). CIRCINATE RETINOPATHY.
retinitis cir·cum·pap·il·la·ris (sur·kum·pap·i·lair'is). A form of syphilitic retinitis in which the retinal changes are localized around the disk.
retinitis dis·ci·for·mis (dis·i·for'mis). *Obsol.* DISCIFORM MACULAR DEGENERATION.
retinitis exu·da·ti·va (eck·sue·da·tye'vuh). The response of histiocytes and fixed tissues to any subretinal hemorrhage, resulting in the production of a pigmented fibrous nodule containing fat-laden histiocytes; it is not a specific disease. Syn. *Coats's disease.*
retinitis ne·phrit·i·ca (ne·frit'i·kuh). Hypertensive retinopathy in persons with hypertension due to renal disease.
retinitis pig·men·to·sa (pig·men·to'suh). A retinal dystrophy of the outer retinal layers characterized by nyctalopia (night blindness), constriction of the visual field, narrowed retinal arterioles, intraretinal pigmentation, and preservation of good visual acuity until late in the course of the disease; occurs in autosomal dominant, autosomal recessive, or x-linked form and in association with a variety of degenerative disorders, including Laurence-Moon-Biedl syndrome, abetalipoproteinemia, and cerebellospinal degenerations.
retinitis pro·li·fer·ans (pro·lif'ur·anz). Neovascularization of retinal vessels with extension into the vitreous; occurs in diabetic retinopathy and retrolental fibroplasia.
retinitis punc·ta·ta al·bes·cens (punk·tay'tuh al·bes'enz). A progressive disorder of the eye characterized by the presence of whitish dots at the level of the retinal pigment epithelium. The degeneration usually follows the pattern of retinitis pigmentosa but without the marked pigmentary change.
retinitis se·ro·sa (se·ro'suh). CENTRAL SEROUS RETINOPATHY.
retinitis sim·plex (sim'plecks). CENTRAL SEROUS RETINOPATHY.
retino-. See *retin-.*
ret·i·no·blas·to·ma (ret"i·no·blas·to'muh) *n.* [*retino-* + *blastoma*]. A hereditary malignant tumor of the sensory portion of the retina transmitted as an autosomal dominant trait.
ret·i·no·cho·roid·i·tis (ret"i·no·ko"roy·dye'tis) *n.* [*retino-* + *choroid* + *-itis*]. Inflammation of the retina and choroid.
retinochoroiditis jux·ta·pa·pil·la·ris (juck"stuh·pap·i·lair'is). JUXTAPAPILLARY CHOROIDITIS.
ret·i·no·cy·to·ma (ret"i·no·sigh·to'muh) *n.* [*retino-* + *-cytoma*]. Neuroepithelioma of the retina.
ret·i·no·di·al·y·sis (ret"i·no·dye·al'i·sis) *n.* [*retino-* + *dialysis*]. DISINSERTION (2).
ret·i·no·ic acid (ret"i·no'ick). Vitamin A acid, $C_{20}H_{28}O_2$, obtained by oxidizing the alcohol group in vitamin A (retinol) to carboxyl. It occurs in two stereoisomeric forms: 9,10-*cis*-retinoic acid and *all-trans*-retinoic acid, the latter used for treatment of scaling dermatoses. See also *tretinoin.*
ret·i·nol (ret'i·nol) *n.* VITAMIN A.
ret·i·no·pap·il·li·tis (ret"i·no·pap"i·lye'tis) *n.* [*retino-* + *papill-* + *-itis*]. Inflammation of the retina and the optic disk.
ret·i·nop·a·thy (ret"i·nop'uth·ee) *n.* [*retino-* + *-pathy*]. Any morbid condition of the retina.
ret·i·no·pexy (ret'i·no·peck"see) *n.* [*retino-* + *-pexy*]. Fixation of a detached retina by operation, or by other methods such as laser, photocoagulation, freezing, or diathermy.
ret·i·nos·chi·sis (ret"i·nos'ki·sis) *n.*, pl. **retinoschi·ses** (·seez) [*retino-* + *-schisis*]. 1. Separation of the retinal layers, with hole formation; usually a degenerative change associated with aging. 2. A congenital anomaly characterized by cleavage of the retina.
ret·i·no·scope (ret'i·nuh·skope) *n.* An instrument employed in retinoscopy.
ret·i·nos·co·py (ret"i·nos'kuh·pee) *n.* [*retino-* + *-scopy*]. A method of determining the refraction of the eye by observation of the movements of the shadow phenomena produced and observed by means of a retinoscope.
ret·i·no·ski·as·co·py (ret"i·no·skye·as'kuh·pee) *n.* [*retino-* + *skiascopy*]. RETINOSCOPY.
re·tort (re·tort') *n.* [ML. *retorta,* from L. *retorquere, retortus,* to twist back]. A distilling vessel consisting of an expanded globular portion and a long neck.
re·to·the·li·o·ma (ree"to·theel·ee·o'muh) *n.* [*retotheli*um + *-oma*]. RETICULUM-CELL SARCOMA.
re·to·the·lio·sar·co·ma (ree"to·theel"ee·o·sahr·ko'muh) *n.* [*retotheli*um + *sarcoma*]. RETICULUM-CELL SARCOMA.
ret·o·the·li·um (ret"o·theel'ee·um) *n.* RETICULOENDOTHELIUM. —**retotheli·al** (·ul) *adj.*
re·tract, *v.* [L. *retrahere, retractus,* from *trahere,* to draw, pull]. To draw back; to contract; to shorten.
retracted nipple. A nipple below the surrounding level of skin.
re·trac·tile testicle. A hypermobile testical which may intermittently migrate into the upper scrotum or inguinal canal.
re·trac·til·i·ty (ree"track·til'i·tee) *n.* The power of retracting or drawing back. —**re·trac·tile** (re·track'til, ·tile) *adj.*
re·trac·tion, *n.* [L. *retractio,* from *retrahere,* to draw back]. The act of retracting or drawing back, as a retraction of the muscles after amputation.
retraction nystagmus. Oscillations of the eyes, which may be horizontal, vertical, or rotatory, accompanied by a drawing of the globes backward into the orbit; may occur spontaneously or on voluntary movements, but usually seen only when there is paresis of upward gaze.
retraction ring. A ridge at the junction of the upper and lower segments of the uterus. Syn. *contraction ring.* See also *pathologic retraction ring, physiologic retraction ring.*
re·trac·tor, *n.* 1. A surgical instrument for holding back the edges of a wound to give access to deeper parts or regions. It consists ordinarily of a handle with a right-angle flange. 2. *In anatomy,* FLEXOR.
re·tra·hens au·rem (ret'ra·henz aw'rem) [L., drawing back the ear]. The posterior auricular muscle.
retro- [L.]. A combining form meaning *back, backward,* or *behind.*
ret·ro·ac·tion (ret"ro·ack'shun) *n.* [L. *retroagere, retroactus,* to reverse, from *agere,* to put in motion]. Reverse action.
ret·ro·an·tero·grade (ret"ro·an'tur·o·grade) *adj.* [*retro-* + *antero-* + *-grade,* from L. *gradi,* to step, go]. Reversing the usual order of a succession.

ret·ro·bul·bar (ret″ro·bul′bur) *adj.* [*retro-* + *bulbar*]. 1. Situated or occurring behind the eyeball. 2. Behind the medulla oblongata.

retrobulbar neuritis or **neuropathy.** Acute impairment of vision in one eye, or in both eyes either simultaneously or successively, due to affection of the optic nerve(s) by demyelinative or nutritional disease or by toxins. The optic disc and retina may appear normal, but if the lesion is near the nerve head there may be swelling of the optic disc (papillitis) and the disc margins may be blurred and surrounded by hemorrhages.

retrocaecal. RETROCECAL.

re·tro·cal·ca·ne·al (ret″ro·kal·kay′nee·ul) *adj.* [*retro-* + *calcaneal*]. Behind the calcaneus.

re·tro·cal·ca·neo·bur·si·tis (ret″ro·kal·kay″nee·o·bur·sigh′tis) *n.* [*retro-* + *calcaneo-* + *bursitis*]. ACHILLOBURSITIS.

ret·ro·car·di·ac (ret″ro·kahr′dee·ack) *adj.* [*retro-* + *cardiac*]. Posterior to the heart.

ret·ro·ca·val (ret″ro·kay′vul) *adj.* [*retro-* + *caval*]. Behind a caval vein, usually the inferior vena cava.

ret·ro·ce·cal, ret·ro·cae·cal (ret″ro·see′kul) *adj.* [*retro-* + *cecal*]. Pertaining to the back of the cecum.

retrocecal recess. An occasional pouch of peritoneum extending upward between the cecum and posterior abdominal wall. NA *recessus retrocecalis.*

ret·ro·cele (ret′ro·seel) *n.* [*retro-* + *-cele*]. Persistence of the postanal part of the embryonic hindgut. Syn. *congenital retrocele.*

ret·ro·ces·sion (ret″ro·sesh′un) *n.* [L. *retrocedere, retrocessus,* to go back, from *cedere,* to go, proceed]. 1. Backward displacement of the entire uterus. 2. Spread of disease from the body surface to deeper areas.

ret·ro·chei·lia (ret″ro·kigh′lee·uh) *n.* [*retro-* + *cheil-* + *-ia*]. A condition in which a lip is farther posterior than is normal. Contr. *procheilia.*

ret·ro·co·lic (ret″ro·ko′lick, ·kol′ick) *adj.* [*retro-* + *colic*]. Behind the colon.

ret·ro·col·lic (ret″ro·kol′ick) *adj.* [*retro-* + L. *collum,* neck, + *-ic*]. Pertaining to the muscles at the back of the neck.

retrocollic spasm. Spasm of the muscles at the back of the neck, causing retraction of the head.

ret·ro·col·lis (ret″ro·kol′is) *n.* Retraction or extension in torticollis.

ret·ro·con·dy·lism (ret″ro·kon′di·liz·um) *n.* [*retro-* + *condyle* + *-ism*]. Posterior deviation of the mandibular condyles.

ret·ro·cop·u·la·tion (ret″ro·kop″yoo·lay′shun) *n.* [*retro-* + *copulation*]. The act of copulating from behind or aversely.

ret·ro·de·vi·a·tion (ret″ro·dee″vee·ay′shun) *n.* [*retro-* + *deviation*]. Any backward displacement; a retroflexion or retroversion.

ret·ro·dis·place·ment (ret″ro·dis·place′munt) *n.* Backward displacement of a part or organ, especially uterine displacement. See also *retroversion of the uterus.*

ret·ro·du·o·de·nal (ret″ro·dew·od′e·nul, ·dew·o·dee′nul) *adj.* [*retro-* + *duodenal*]. Behind the duodenum.

retroduodenal recess or **fossa.** An occasional small pouch of peritoneum situated behind the transverse portion of the duodenum extending upward from below. NA *recessus retroduodenalis.*

ret·ro·esoph·a·ge·al, ret·ro·oe·soph·a·ge·al (ret″ro·e·sof″uh·jee′ul) *adj.* [*retro-* + *esophageal*]. Located behind the esophagus.

ret·ro·flex (ret″ro·flecks) *v.* [L. *retroflectere, retroflexus,* to bend back]. To turn back abruptly.

ret·ro·flexed, *adj.* Bent backward; in a permanent, backward malposition.

ret·ro·flex·ion (ret″ro·fleck′shun) *n.* The state of being bent backward.

retroflexion of the uterus. A condition in which the uterus is bent backward on itself, producing a sharp angle in its longitudinal axis at the junction of the cervix and the fundus.

ret·ro·gas·se·ri·an (ret″ro·ga·seer′ee·un) *adj.* [*retro-* + *gasserian*]. Behind the trigeminal or gasserian ganglion.

ret·ro·gnath·ism (ret″ro·nath′iz·um) *n.* [*retro-* + *gnath-* + *-ism*]. Posterior deviation of the mandible.

ret·ro·grade (ret′ro·grade) *adj.* [L. *retrogradi,* to go backward, from *gradi,* to step, walk]. Going backward; moving contrary to the normal or previous direction or order; characterized by retrogression.

retrograde amnesia. Loss of memory for events that had occurred before the onset of the current injury or illness. Contr. *retrograde memory.*

retrograde beat. RETROGRADE P WAVE.

retrograde conduction. RETROGRADE P WAVE.

retrograde embolism. An embolism in which the embolus has gone against the normal direction of the bloodstream.

retrograde memory. Memory for events in the recent past. Contr. *retrograde amnesia.*

retrograde P wave. Excitation of the atrium by the atrioventricular node or the ventricle; the P wave follows the QRS complex of the electrocardiogram.

retrograde pyelography or **urography.** Visualization of the renal collecting system by instillation of radiographic contrast medium into the ureters through catheters inserted with the aid of a cystoscope.

re·trog·ra·phy, *n.* [*retro-* + *-graphy*]. MIRROR WRITING.

ret·ro·gres·sion, *n.* [L. *retrogradi, retrogressus,* to go backward]. 1. *In biology,* the passing from a higher to a lower type of structure in the development of an animal. 2. *In medicine,* a going backward; degeneration, involution, or atrophy, as of tissue. 3. The subsidence of a disease or its symptoms. 4. *In psychology,* a return to earlier, more infantile behavior. See also *regression.* —**retro·gres·sive** (·gres′iv) *adj.*

retrogressive atrophy. REGRESSIVE METAPLASIA.

ret·ro·in·gui·nal space (ret″ro·ing′gwi·nul). A potential space between the parietal peritoneum and the transversalis fascia, situated in the lower lateral anterior abdominal wall. Syn. *Bogros' space.*

ret·ro·jec·tion (ret″ro·jeck′shun) *n.* [*retro-* + *-jection* as in injection]. The washing out of a cavity from within outward.

ret·ro·jec·tor (ret″ro·jeck′tur) *n.* An instrument for washing out the uterus.

ret·ro·len·tal (ret″ro·len′tul) *adj.* [*retro-* + *lent-* + *-al*]. Behind the lens of the eye.

retrolental fibroplasia. An oxygen-induced retinopathy of premature infants.

ret·ro·len·tic·u·lar (ret″ro·len·tick′yoo·lur) *adj.* [*retro-* + *lenticular*]. RETROLENTAL.

retrolenticular capsule syndrome. Hemiplegia, hemianesthesia and hemianopsia due to infarction of the posterior limb of the internal capsule. It has been attributed on uncertain grounds to occlusion of the anterior choroidal artery.

ret·ro·lin·gual (ret″ro·ling′gwul) *adj.* [*retro-* + *lingual*]. Pertaining to the part of the pharynx behind the tongue.

retrolingual gland. A large salivary gland in certain mammals other than man, the equivalent of the human sublingual gland.

ret·ro·ma·lar (ret″ro·may′lur) *adj.* [*retro-* + *malar*]. Behind the zygoma.

ret·ro·mam·ma·ry (ret″ro·mam′uh·ree) *adj.* [*retro-* + *mammary*]. Behind the breast.

retromammary abscess. SUBMAMMARY ABSCESS.

ret·ro·man·dib·u·lar (ret″ro·man·dib′yoo·lur) *adj.* [*retro-* + *mandibular*]. Behind the mandible.

retromandibular process. The medial, narrow portion of the parotid gland filling the fossa behind the mandible.

re·tro·max·il·lary (ret″ro·mack′si·lerr·ee) *adj.* [*retro-* + *maxillary*]. Behind the maxilla.

retromaxillary region. The potential space behind the maxilla.

ret·ro·mor·pho·sis (ret″ro·mor′fo·sis, ·mor·fo′sis) *n.* [*retro-* +

-morphosis]. 1. CATABOLISM. 2. Retrograde metamorphosis; METAMORPHOSIS (2).

ret·ro·na·sal (ret″ro·nay′zul) *adj.* [*retro-* + *nasal*]. Situated behind the nose or nasal cavities; postnasal.

ret·ro·oc·u·lar (ret″ro·ock′yoo·lur) *adj.* [*retro-* + *ocular*]. Behind the eye.

retrooesophageal. RETROESOPHAGEAL.

ret·ro·or·bi·tal (ret″ro·or′bi·tul) *adj.* [*retro-* + *orbital*]. Behind the orbit.

ret·ro·pa·rot·id (ret″ro·pa·rot′id) *adj.* Behind the parotid gland.

retroparotid space. A potential space situated between the medial surface of the parotid gland and the upper lateral wall of the pharynx.

retroparotid syndrome. VILLARET'S SYNDROME.

ret·ro·per·i·to·ne·al (ret″ro·perr″i·to·nee′ul) *adj.* [*retro-* + *peritoneal*]. Situated behind the peritoneum.

retroperitoneal fibrosis. A benign proliferative disorder of the retroperitoneal connective tissue; it may form a bulky mass and interfere with the function of such structures as the ureters and blood vessels. The ureters are most commonly involved. It has been associated with administration of ergot derivatives in some patients. Syn. *Ormond's syndrome.*

retroperitoneal hernia. A hernia into a recess of the peritoneum, as into a paraduodenal recess.

retroperitoneal space. The space behind the peritoneum, but in front of the vertebral column and lumbar muscles; in it lie the kidneys, the aorta, the inferior vena cava, and the sympathetic trunk. NA *spatium retroperitoneale.*

retroperitoneal veins. Venous plexuses of the posterior abdominal wall which form anastomoses between veins draining into the portal venous return and the phrenic and azygos veins of the systemic venous return.

ret·ro·peri·to·ni·tis (ret″ro·perr·i·tuh·nigh′tis) *n.* [*retroperitoneal* + *-itis*]. Inflammation of the structures in the retroperitoneal space.

ret·ro·pha·ryn·ge·al (ret″ro·fa·rin′jee·ul, ·făr″in·jee′ul) *adj.* [*retro-* + *pharyngeal*]. Situated behind the pharynx.

retropharyngeal space. The space behind the pharynx, containing areolar tissue.

ret·ro·phar·yn·gi·tis (ret″ro·făr″in·jye′tis) *n.* [*retropharyngeal* + *-itis*]. Inflammation of the retropharyngeal tissues.

ret·ro·phar·ynx (ret″ro·făr′inks) *n.* [*retro-* + *pharynx*]. The posterior portion of the pharynx.

ret·ro·pla·cen·tal (ret″ro·pluh·sen′tul) *adj.* [*retro-* + *placental*]. Behind the placenta.

ret·ro·pla·sia (ret″ro·play′zhuh, ·zee·uh) *n.* [*retro-* + *-plasia*]. Retrograde change in a tissue; DEGENERATION.

ret·ro·posed (ret′ro·poazd) *adj.* Displaced backward.

ret·ro·po·si·tion (ret″ro·puh·zish′un) *n.* [*retro-* + *position*]. Backward displacement of the uterus without flexion or version.

ret·ro·pros·tat·ic (ret″ro·pros·tat′ick) *adj.* [*retro-* + *prostatic*]. Behind the prostate.

ret·ro·pu·bic (ret″ro·pew′bick) *adj.* [*retro-* + *pubic*]. Behind the pubis.

retropubic prostatectomy. Removal of the prostate by an approach through the prevesical space.

retropubic space. A space lying immediately above the pubis and between the peritoneum and the posterior surface of the rectus abdominis. Syn. *prevesical space, space of Retzius.* NA *spatium retropubicum.*

ret·ro·pul·sion (ret″ro·pul′shun) *n.* [*retro-* + *pulsion*]. 1. A driving or turning back, as of the fetal head. 2. An involuntary backward walking or running observed in postencephalitic parkinsonism.

ret·ro·py·ram·i·dal (ret″ro·pi·ram′i·dul) *adj.* [*retro-* + *pyramidal*]. Situated behind a pyramid (2).

retropyramidal nucleus. An inconstant mass of gray matter situated between the inferior olivary nucleus and the pyramid. Syn. *nucleus conterminalis.*

ret·ro·spec·tive falsification (ret″ro·speck′tiv). *In psychiatry,* the unconscious alteration of the memory of past events in order to meet present emotional needs.

ret·ro·stal·sis (ret″ro·stal′sis, ·stahl′sis) *n.* REVERSED PERISTALSIS.

ret·ro·tar·sal (ret″ro·tahr′sul) *adj.* [*retro-* + *tarsal*]. Situated behind the tarsus, as the retrotarsal fold of the conjunctiva.

ret·ro·ten·di·nous (ret″ro·ten′di·nus) *adj.* [*retro-* + *tendinous*]. Behind a tendon.

ret·ro·ten·do·achil·lis (ret″ro·ten″do·uh·kil′is) *adj.* [*retro-* + *tendo achillis*]. Behind the calcaneal tendon.

ret·ro·thy·roid (ret″ro·thigh′roid) *adj.* [*retro-* + *thyroid*]. Behind the thyroid gland.

ret·ro·ton·sil·lar (ret″ro·ton′si·lur) *adj.* [*retro-* + *tonsillar*]. Behind a pharyngeal tonsil.

ret·ro·ton·sil·lar abscess (ret″ro·ton′sil·ur). PERITONSILLAR ABSCESS.

ret·ro·tra·che·al (ret″ro·tray′kee·ul) *adj.* [*retro-* + *tracheal*]. Situated or occurring behind the trachea.

ret·ro·ver·sio·flex·ion (ret″ro·vur″see·o·fleck′shun, ·vur″zho·) *n.* Combined retroversion and retroflexion.

ret·ro·ver·sion (ret″ro·vur′zhun) *n.* [L. *retrovertere, retroversus,* to turn backward, from *vertere,* to turn]. A turning back.

retroversion of the uterus. A condition in which the uterus is tilted backward without any change in the angle of its longitudinal axis.

retroversion pessary. Any type of pessary, such as the Smith-Hodge, used to correct a retroverted uterus.

ret·ro·vert·ed (ret″ro·vur′tid) *adj.* Tilted or turned backward, as a retroverted uterus.

ret·ro·ves·i·cal (ret″ro·ves′i·kul·) *adj.* [*retro-* + *vesical*]. Behind the urinary bladder.

retrovesical abscess. An abscess situated behind the urinary bladder in the male or between the urinary bladder and the uterus in the female.

retrovesical hernia. A hernia behind the urinary bladder into the retrovesical space.

re·trude (re·trood′) *v.* [L. *retrudere,* from *trudere,* to push, thrust]. To force inward or backward, as in orthodontically repositioning protruding teeth.

re·tru·sion (re·troo′zhun) *n.* [L. *retrudere, retrusus,* to push back]. 1. The act or process of pressing teeth backward. 2. The condition characterized by the backward or posterior position of the teeth or jaws.

re·tru·sive reflex (re·troo′siv). RUMINATION (1).

Ret·ter·er's stain. A stain for muscle in which sections of tissue are stained with alum carmine, which have previously been fixed in 80% alcohol 10 parts, formic acid 1 part. Muscle will appear bright red; all connective tissue will remain unstained.

returning cycle. COMPENSATORY PAUSE.

Ret·zi·us' lines or **striae** (ret′see·o͞os) [M. G. *Retzius,* Swedish anatomist, 1842–1919]. INCREMENTAL LINES OF RETZIUS.

Retzius' veins [M. G. *Retzius*]. RETROPERITONEAL VEINS.

re·un·ion, *n.* In fractures, the securing of union following its interruption by violence or disease.

re·vac·ci·na·tion (ree″vack·si·nay′shun) *n.* Renewed or repeated vaccination.

re·vas·cu·lar·iza·tion (ree·vas″kew·lur·i·zay′shun) *n.* [*re-* + *vascularization*]. Reestablishment of a blood supply, as after interruption or destruction of the old vessels due to injury or grafting.

rev·e·hent (rev′e·hunt, re·vee′unt) *adj.* [L. *revehens,* from *revehere,* to carry back]. Carrying back.

revehent vein. *In embryology,* the portion of the omphalomesenteric vein between the liver and the sinus venosus. The veins of the two sides join and form the inferior vena cava.

re·vel·lent (re·vel′unt) *adj.* [L. *revellens,* from *revellere,* to pull away]. REVULSIVE.

re·ver·ber·at·ing circuit. Neuronal pathways with branches which turn back on themselves and thus permit reverberation.

re·ver·ber·a·tion (re·vur″bur·ay′shun) *n.* [L. *reverberare,* to beat back, from *verber,* blow, stroke]. Prolonged neuronal activity following a single stimulus, due to transmission of impulses along branches of nerves turning back on themselves, permitting activity to reverberate until unable to cause further propagated transsynaptic response. Such reverberating circuits are common in the brain and spinal cord.

Re·ver·din graft (ruh·vehr·daen′) [J. L. *Reverdin,* Swiss surgeon, 1842–1908]. A pinch graft a few millimeters in diameter sliced off so that the center is of whole skin thickness and the circumferential edge is of epidermis only; similar to a Davis graft.

Reverdin's needle [A. *Reverdin,* Swiss surgeon, 1881–1929]. A suture carrier with a handle, and an eye at the tip which can be opened and closed by means of a lever.

rev·er·ie (rev′ur·ee) *n.* [OF., from *rever,* to dream]. A state of dreamy abstraction; visionary mental or ideational movement, the mind itself, at least so far as volition is concerned, being passive; DAYDREAM.

re·ver·sal, *n.* [L. *reverti, reversus,* to turn back]. 1. A turning around, as the reversal of any pathologic process to a state of healing or health. 2. *In psychiatry,* the change of the content or aim of an instinct or mode of behavior into the opposite, as love into hate, or sadism into masochism.

reversal formation. REACTION FORMATION.

re·verse, *n.* In bandaging, a half-turn employed to change the direction of a bandage.

reverse coarctation. AORTIC ARCH SYNDROME.

reversed bandage. An oblique bandage applied to a limb; for each turn, the roll is given a half twist to make a snug fit over the expanded part of the limb.

reversed dominance of the eyes. In a right-handed person, dominance of the left eye because of disease, operation, or ametropia of the right eye; in a left-handed person, dominance of the right eye. See also *mixed laterality.*

reversed peristalsis. Peristaltic movement opposite to the normal direction.

reversed Prausnitz-Küstner test [C. W. *Prausnitz* and H. *Küstner*]. An urticarial reaction appearing at an injection site when reagin-containing serum is injected into the skin of a person in whom the allergen is already present; the reaction which appears when Prausnitz-Küstner antibody is administered, not before, but after, the administration of the antigen.

reverse mutation. The process whereby a gene reverts or mutates back to its original sequence of bases.

reverse passive anaphylaxis. Hypersensitivity produced when the antigen is injected first, then followed in several hours by the specific antibody, causing shock.

reverse pinocytosis. EMIOCYTOSIS.

reverse transcriptase. An enzyme which catalyzes the synthesis of DNA complementary to an RNA template; found in certain RNA viruses (negative strand viruses) some of which cause neoplastic transformations in infected cells.

re·vers·ible colloid (re·vur′si·bul). A colloid which, on being precipitated or otherwise separated from its dispersion medium, can be restored to its original state merely by adding the dispersion medium.

re·ver·sion (re·vur′zhun) *n.* [L. *reversio,* a turning back, from *reverti,* to turn back]. The reappearance of long-lost ancestral traits; THROWBACK.

Re·vil·liod's sign (ruh·vee·lyo′) [L. *Revilliod,* Swiss physician, 1835–1919]. In hemiplegia, an inability to close the eye on the paralyzed side without closing the opposite eye. Syn. *orbicularis sign.*

re·vi·tal·iza·tion (ree·vye″tul·i·zay′shun) *n.* The act or process of refreshing.

re·vive, *v.* [L. *revivere,* to live again]. To return to life after seeming death; to return to consciousness or strength.

re·viv·i·fi·ca·tion (re·viv″i·fi·kay′shun) *n.* Restoration of life after apparent death.

rev·o·lute (rev′uh·lewt) *adj.* [L. *revolutus,* from *revolvere,* to roll back]. Turned backward or downward.

re·volv·ing nosepiece. A device to be screwed on to the end of the microscope tube to permit the mounting of two to four objectives, any of which may be swung into place, ready for use, by turning the nosepiece into the desired position.

re·vul·sant (re·vul′sunt) *adj. & n.* 1. Tending to revulsion (2). 2. A revulsive agent.

re·vul·sion, *n.* [L. *revulsio,* act of pulling away, from *revellere,* to pull away]. 1. A strong feeling of distaste or dislike. 2. Reduction of local hyperemia or inflammation by means of counterirritation.

re·vul·sive (re·vul′siv) *adj.* 1. Characterized by an altered distribution of blood in one part through congestion or irritation produced elsewhere in the body. 2. Causing revulsion.

Rex·ed's laminae. Ten laminar zones making up the gray matter of the spinal cord in cross section; a descriptive partitioning based on the structural arrangement and cytological characteristics of the nerve cells.

Reye's syndrome [R. D. K. *Reye,* Australian pathologist, d. 1977]. An acute illness of childhood, which usually follows a respiratory or gastrointestinal viral infection, or varicella. It is characterized clinically by fever, vomiting, disturbance of consciousness progressing to coma, and convulsions, and pathologically by fatty infiltration of the parenchymal cells of the liver and kidneys, and brain swelling.

R. F. A. Right frontoanterior position of the fetus.

R. F. P. Right frontoposterior position of the fetus.

RFW *In cardiology,* abbreviation for *rapid filling wave.*

Rh Symbol for rhodium.

Rh [*rh*esus]. Pertaining to or designating an agglutinogen first found in the red blood cells of the rhesus monkey. See also *ABO blood groups, blood groups, Rh factors, Rh genes.*

Rh_o(D) antigen. The major antigen of the Rh blood group.

rhabd-, rhabdo- [Gk. *rhabdos,* rod, stick; stripe; stitch]. A combining form meaning (a) *stick, rod;* (b) *striped, banded, striated.*

Rhab·di·tis (rab·dye′tis) *n.* [NL., from Gk. *rhabdos,* staff, rod]. A genus of phasmid nematodes a few species of which are parasitic in man but of doubtful pathogenicity.

Rhab·di·toi·dea (rab″di·toy′dee·uh) *n.pl.* The name given a superfamily of the Nematoda, of which *Strongyloides stercoralis* is the most important species which infects man.

rhab·do·cyte (rab′do·site) *n.* [*rhabdo-* + *-cyte*]. BAND CELL.

rhab·doid (rab′doid) *adj.* [Gk. *rhabdoeidēs,* striped]. Rodlike.

rhabdoid suture. SAGITTAL SUTURE.

rhab·do·myo·blast·ic mixed tumor (rab″do·migh″o·blas′tick). A malignant mixed mesodermal tumor with a prominent component of anaplastic striated muscle cells.

rhab·do·myo·blas·to·ma (rab″do·migh″o·blas·to′muh) *n.* [*rhabdo-* + *myoblast* + *-oma*]. RHABDOMYOSARCOMA.

rhab·do·my·ol·y·sis (rab″do·migh·ol′i·sis) *n.* [*rhabdo-* + *myo-* + *lysis*]. Destruction or necrosis of skeletal muscle, often accompanied by myoglobinuria.

rhab·do·my·o·ma (rab″do·migh·o′muh) *n.* [*rhabdo-* + *myoma*]. A benign tumor, usually hamartomatous, of striated muscle.

rhabdomyoma ute·ri (yoo′tur·eye). SARCOMA BOTRYOIDES.

rhab·do·myo·sar·co·ma (rab″do·migh″o·sahr·ko′muh) *n.* [*rhabdo-* + *myo-* + *sarcoma*]. A malignant tumor, usually involving the muscles of the extremities or torso, composed of anaplastic striated muscle cells. Syn. *malignant rhabdomyoma, rhabdomyoblastoma.*

rhab·do·pho·bia (rhab″do·fo′bee·uh) *n.* [*rhabdo-* + *-phobia*].

An unwarranted dread of being beaten; unreasoning fear aroused by the sight of a stick.

rhachi-, rhachio-. See *rachi-*.

rha·cous (rack'us, ray'kus) *adj.* [Gk. *rhakē*, tatters, wrinkles, + *-ous*]. Wrinkled; lacerated; fissured.

rhaeboscelia. RHEBOSCELIA. —**rhaebosce·lic,** *adj.*

rhag·a·des (rag'uh·deez) *n.pl.* [Gk., pl. of *rhagas*, crack, fissure]. Linear cracks or fissures occurring in skin that has lost its elasticity through infiltration and thickening; observed in syphilis, intertrigo, keratoderma, and other affections.

rha·ga·dia (ra·gay'dee·uh) *n.pl.* [Gk., pl. of *rhagadion*, dim. of *rhagas*, fissure]. RHAGADES.

rha·gad·i·form (ra·gad'i·form) *adj.* [Gk. *rhagas, rhagados*, fissure, + *-iform*]. Fissured.

-rhagia. See *-rrhagia*.

rhag·i·o·crin, rhag·i·o·crine (raj'ee·o·krin) *adj.* [Gk. *rhagion* (dim. of *rhax*, grape) + *-crine*]. Characterizing or pertaining to colloid-filled vacuoles in the cytoplasm of secretory cells representing a stage in the development of secretory granules.

rha·gio·crine cell (ray'jee·o·krin) [Gk. *rhagia*, small berries, + *krinein*, to pick, separate out]. HISTIOCYTE.

rhag·oid (rag'oid) *adj.* [Gk. *rhagoeidēs*, from *rhax*, grape]. Resembling a grape.

rham·no·glu·co·side (ram''no·gloo'ko·side) *n.* A glycoside, such as rutin, which yields the sugars rhamnose and D-glucose on hydrolysis.

rham·nose (ram'nose) *n.* L-Rhamnose, or 6-deoxy-L-mannose, $C_6H_{12}O_5$, a deoxysugar occurring free in poison sumac and in glycoside combination in many plants. It occurs in α- and β- forms. Syn. *isodulcitol*.

rham·no·side (ram'no·side) *n.* A glycoside, such as quercetin, that yields the sugar rhamnose on hydrolysis.

rham·no·xan·thin (ram''no·zan'thin) *n.* FRANGULIN.

Rham·nus (ram'nus) *n.* [L., from Gk. *rhamnos*, a prickly shrub]. A genus of trees and shrubs that yield cascara (*Rhamnus purshiana*), buckthorn bark (*R. frangula*), and buckthorn berries (*R. cathartica*), all of which are cathartic.

Rh antiserums. Antiserums reacting with one or more of the Rh factors.

rha·pha·nia (ra·fay'nee·uh) *n.* RAPHANIA.

rha·pon·tic (ra·pon'tick) *adj.* [L. *rha ponticum*, Pontic rhubarb, from Gk. *rha*, rhubarb]. Pertaining to rhubarb.

rhat·a·ny (rat'uh·nee) *n.* [Sp. *ratania*, from Quechua]. KRAMERIA.

Rh-blocking serum. A serum that is able to react with blood containing the Rh factor without producing agglutination, though blocking the action of subsequently added anti-Rh serums; i.e., Rh-positive blood treated with Rh-blocking serum can no longer be agglutinated by anti-Rh serum.

Rh-blocking test. A test for the detection of Rh antibody in plasma wherein erythrocytes having the Rh antigen are incubated in the patient's serum so that the antibodies may be adsorbed on these cells, which are then employed in the antiglobulin test. Syn. *indirect developing test, indirect Coombs test*.

Rh blood group. The extensive system of erythrocyte antigens originally defined by reactions with the serum of rabbits immunized with the erythrocytes of rhesus monkeys, and recently by antiserums of human origin.

rhe (ree) *n.* [Gk. *rhein*, to flow]. The unit of fluidity, being the reciprocal of the centipoise or one-hundredth of a poise.

rhe·bo·sce·lia, rhae·bo·sce·lia (ree''bo·see'lee·uh) *n.* [Gk. *rhaiboskelēs* (from *rhaibos*, crooked, + *skelos*, leg) + *-ia*]. The condition of being bowlegged. —**rhebosce·lic, rhaebosce·lic** (·lick) *adj.*

rheg·ma (reg'muh) *n.* [Gk. *rhēgma*, breakage from *rhēgnynai*, to break]. 1. A rupture of the walls of a vessel or of the containing membrane of an organ or region, as the coats of the eye, the walls of the peritoneum. 2. The bursting of an abscess.

rheg·ma·tog·e·nous (reg''muh·toj'e·nus) *adj.* [Gk. *rhēgma, rhēgmatos*, rupture, fracture, + *-genous*]. 1. Producing rupture, bursting, or fracturing. 2. Producing retinal detachment characterized by a hole or tear.

rhem·bas·mus (rem·baz'mus) *n.* [Gk. *rhembasmos*, a roaming about]. Mental distraction; INDECISION.

rhe·ni·um (ree'nee·um) *n.* [NL., from L. *Rhenus*, the Rhine]. Re = 186.2. A metallic element, atomic number 75, of the manganese group; occurs as a minor constituent in many ores.

rheo- [Gk. *rheos*, anything flowing]. A combining form meaning *flow*, as of liquids, or *pertaining to a current*.

rheo·base (ree'o·bace) *n.* [*rheo-* + *base*]. The minimum electric potential necessary for stimulation.

rheo·car·di·og·ra·phy (ree''o·kahr''dee·og'ruh·fee) *n.* [*rheo-* + *cardio-* + *-graphy*]. The recording of differences in electrical conductivity of the body synchronous with the cardiac cycle.

rheo·en·ceph·a·log·ra·phy (ree''o·en·sef''uh·log'ruh·fee) *n.* [*rheo-* + *encephalo-* + *-graphy*]. A method of continuous recording of the changes in an electrical current passed through the head for the purpose of demonstrating cerebral blood flow patterns and their pathologic alterations.

rhe·ol·o·gy (ree·ol'uh·jee) *n.* [*rheo-* + *-logy*]. The science of deformation and flow of matter in such a state that it exhibits a tendency to be deformed by the application of force. —**rhe·o·log·ic** (ree''o·loj'ick) *adj.*

rhe·om·e·ter (ree·om'e·tur) *n.* [*rheo-* + *-meter*]. 1. GALVANOMETER. 2. An apparatus for measuring the velocity of the blood current. 3. An apparatus for measuring the flow of viscous materials.

rheo·nome (ree''o·nome) *n.* [*rheo* + Gk. *nomē*, distribution, from *nemein*, to distribute]. An instrument for the application of electric currents of different intensity to excitable tissues.

rheo·pexy (ree'o·peck''see) *n.* [*rheo-* + *-pexy*]. A special kind of thixotropy consisting of internal-phase particles of a laminar or fibrillar shape, the gelation being greatly hastened by slow but pronounced elliptical stirring or other means of facilitating proper orientation of the particles.

rheo·stat (ree'o·stat) *n.* [*rheo-* + *-stat*]. An apparatus for regulating the amount of electrical current flowing in a circuit by varying the resistance in the circuit.

rhe·os·to·sis (ree''os·to'sis) *n.* [*rheo-* + *ostosis*]. OSTEOPETROSIS.

rheo·ta·chyg·ra·phy (ree''o·ta·kig'ruh·fee) *n.* [*rheo-* + *tachygraphy*]. The registration of the curve of variation in electromotive action of muscles.

rheo·taxis (ree''o·tack'sis) *n.* [*rheo-* + *taxis*]. A taxis in which mechanical stimulation by a current of fluid, as of water, is the directing influence to cause movement of an entire organism against the force of the current.

rheo·trope (ree'o·trope) *n.* [*rheo-* + *-trope*]. An apparatus for reversing the direction of an electric current. Syn. *commutator*.

rhe·ot·ro·pism (ree·ot'ruh·piz·um) *n.* [*rheo-* + *tropism*]. A tropism in which mechanical stimulation by a current of fluid, as of water, is the directing influence and causes movement of a part of an organism against the motion of the force of the current.

rhe·sus monkey (ree'sus) [NL., from Gk. *Rhēsos*, a legendary prince of Thrace]. *Macaca mulatta*, the common macaque of central and Northern India and parts of Southeast Asia.

rheu·mat·ic (roo·mat'ick) *adj. & n.* [Gk. *rheumatikos*, subject to a flux, from *rheuma*, flow, flux; humor]. 1. Pertaining to, of the nature of, or affected with rheumatism. 2. A person suffering from rheumatism.

rheumatic arteritis. Diffuse involvement of small cerebral arteries observed in patients with rheumatic heart disease. The vascular lesions and the microinfarcts that accompany them probably represent multiple cerebral emboli.

rheumatic arthritis. 1. Migratory polyarthritis, particularly of the large joints of the extremities, that is completely reversible; occurs during acute rheumatic fever. 2. RHEUMATOID ARTHRITIS.

rheumatic brain disease. 1. RHEUMATIC ARTERITIS. 2. SYDENHAM'S CHOREA.

rheumatic carditis. Inflammation of the heart associated with rheumatic fever.

rheumatic chorea. SYDENHAM'S CHOREA.

rheumatic encephalopathy or **encephalitis.** RHEUMATIC BRAIN DISEASE.

rheumatic endocarditis. The endocarditis of acute rheumatic fever, usually involving one or more of the heart valves.

rheumatic fever. A febrile disease occurring as a delayed sequel of infections with beta-hemolytic streptococci, group A; characterized by multiple focal inflammatory lesions of connective tissue, notably in the heart, blood vessels, and joints, with such clinical evidence as carditis, arthritis, and skin rash.

rheumatic headache. MUSCLE-CONTRACTION HEADACHE.

rheumatic myocarditis. Myocarditis characterized by the formation of Aschoff nodules in the myocardium, occurring in acute rheumatic fever.

rheumatic nodules. Subcutaneous nonpainful nodules occurring in rheumatic fever over the extensor tendons of the hands, feet, knees, and elbows, and over the spine, scapula, and skull.

rheumatic pericarditis. An inflammation of the pericardium associated with rheumatic fever.

rheumatic pleurisy. Fibrinous pleurisy in acute rheumatic fever.

rheumatic pneumonia. Pneumonia in acute rheumatic fever.

rheumatic pneumonitis. RHEUMATIC PNEUMONIA.

rheumatic purpura. SCHÖNLEIN'S PURPURA.

rheumatic spondylitis. ANKYLOSING SPONDYLITIS.

rheumatic torticollis. A form of stiff neck due to myositis of the sternocleidomastoid or other muscle of the neck.

rheu·ma·tism (roo'muh·tiz·um) *n.* [Gk. *rheumatismos,* flux, rheum, from *rheuma,* flux, flow, stream]. 1. A general term indicating diseases of muscle, tendon, joint, bone, or nerve, that have in common pain and stiffness referable to the musculoskeletal system. 2. RHEUMATIC FEVER.

rheu·ma·toid (roo'muh·toid) *adj.* [*rheumatism* + *-oid*]. Resembling rheumatism.

rheumatoid arthritis. A chronic systemic disease of unknown etiology in which symptoms and inflammatory connective-tissue changes predominate in articular and related structures. Pain, limitation of motion, and joint deformity are common. Syn. *atrophic arthritis, chronic infectious arthritis, proliferative arthritis.* See also *ankylosing spondylitis.*

rheumatoid arthritis of the spine. ANKYLOSING SPONDYLITIS.

rheumatoid factor. An antiglobulin found in the serum of most patients with rheumatoid arthritis.

rheumatoid iritis. Inflammation of the iris of the eye in conjunction with rheumatic fever, rheumatoid arthritis, and other collagen diseases.

rheumatoid myositis. Myositis characterized by focal inflammation, lesions occurring in muscles during the course of rheumatoid arthritis.

rheumatoid nodules. Subcutaneous foci of fibrinoid degeneration or necrosis surrounded by mononuclear cells in a regular palisade arrangement, occurring usually in association with rheumatoid arthritis.

rheumatoid scleritis. An inflammation of the sclera generally associated with rheumatoid arthritis; can be diffuse and progress to scleromalacia perforans, or can be characterized by discrete lesions (rheumatoid nodules).

rheumatoid spondylitis. ANKYLOSING SPONDYLITIS.

rheu·ma·tol·o·gy (roo"muh·tol'uh·jee) *n.* [*rheumatic* + *-logy*]. The study of rheumatic diseases. —**rheuma·to·log·ic** (·tuh·loj'ick) *adj.;* **rheuma·tol·o·gist** (·tol'uh·jist) *n.*

rheu·mo·cri·nol·o·gy (roo"mo·kri·nol'uh·jee) *n.* A study of the endocrine aspects of rheumatic disease, particularly rheumatoid arthritis.

rhex·is (reck·sis) *n.,* pl. **rhex·es** (·seez) [Gk. *rhēxis,* rupture, break, from *rhēgnynai,* to break]. Rupture of a blood vessel or of an organ.

Rh factor. Any of a group of erythrocyte antigens originally described by Landsteiner and Weiner in the blood of rhesus monkeys.

Rh genes. The series of allelic genes which determine the various sorts of Rh agglutinogens and Rh blood types. Eight standard genes have been identified (Wiener): R^0, R^1, R^2, R^Z (Rh-positive), and r, r′, r″, r^y (Rh-negative). See also *blood groups.*

rhin-, rhino- [Gk. *rhis, rhinos*]. A combining form meaning (a) *nose, nasal;* (b) *noselike.*

rhi·nal (rye'nul) *adj.* [*rhin-* + *-al*]. Pertaining to the nose.

rhinal fissure. A shallow groove separating the terminal archipallial part of the hippocampal gyrus from the more lateral neocortex.

rhi·nal·gia (rye·nal'juh, ·jee·uh) *n.* [*rhin-* + *-algia*]. Pain in the nose.

rhi·nan·tral·gia (rye"nan·tral'jee·uh) *n.* [*rhin-* + *antr-* + *-algia*]. Pain in, or referred to, the walls of the cavities of the nose.

-rhine. See *-rrhine.*

rhi·nel·cos (rye·nel'kos) *n.* [*rhin-* + Gk. *helkos,* ulcer]. A nasal ulcer.

rhin·en·ceph·a·lon (rye"nen·sef'uh·lon) *n.* [*rhin-* + *encephalon*] [BNA]. The portions of the central nervous system that receive fibers from the olfactory bulb including the olfactory bulb, tract, tubercle and striae, the anterior olfactory nucleus, parts of the amygdaloid complex and parts of the prepyriform cortex. Syn. *primitive olfactory lobe, olfactory brain.* —**rhin·en·ce·phal·ic** (rye"nen·se·fal'ick) *adj.*

rhi·nen·chy·sis (rye"neng·kigh'sis, rye·neng'ki·sis) *n.* [*rhin-* + Gk. *enchysis,* a pouring in]. Douching of the nasal passages.

rhi·neu·ryn·ter (rye"new·rin'tur) *n.* [*rhin-* + Gk. *eurynein,* to dilate, + *-tēr,* instrumental noun suffix]. A distensible bag or sac which is inflated after insertion into a nostril.

rhin·he·ma·to·ma, rhin·hae·ma·to·ma (rin·hee"muh·to'muh, ·hem"uh·to'muh) *n.* [*rhin-* + *hematoma*]. An effusion of blood around the nasal cartilages.

rhi·ni·a·try (rye·nigh'uh·tree) *n.* [*rhin-* + *-iatry*]. The treatment of diseases and defects of the nose.

rhin·i·on (rin'ee·on) *n.* [Gk., dim. of *rhis,* nose]. *In craniometry,* the point at the distal end of the internasal suture.

rhi·nism (rye'niz·um) *n.* [*rhin-* + *-ism*]. A nasal quality of the voice.

rhi·nis·mus (rye·niz'mus) *n.* RHINISM.

rhi·ni·tis (rye·nigh'tis) *n.,* pl. **rhi·nit·i·des** (·nit'i·deez) [*rhin-* + *-itis*]. Inflammation of the nasal mucous membrane.

rhinitis sic·ca (sick'uh). OZENA.

rhino-. See *rhin-.*

rhi·no·an·tri·tis (rye"no·an·trye'tis) *n.* [*rhino-* + *antr-* + *-itis*]. Inflammation of the nasal mucous membrane and of the maxillary sinus.

rhi·no·by·on (rye"no·bye'on, rye·no'bee·on) *n.* [*rhino-* + Gk. *byein,* to plug]. A nasal plug or tampon.

rhi·no·can·thec·to·my (rye"no·kan·theck'tuh·mee) *n.* [*rhino-* + *canth-* + *-ectomy*]. Excision of the inner canthus of the eye.

rhi·no·ce·pha·lia (rye"no·se·fay'lee·uh) *n.* RHINOCEPHALY.

rhi·no·ceph·a·lus (rye"no·sef'uh·lus) *n.* A fetus exhibiting rhinocephaly.

rhi·no·ceph·a·ly (rye"no·sef'uh·lee) *n.* [*rhino-* + *-cephaly*]. A form of cyclopia in which the nose is a tubular proboscis situated above the fused orbits.

rhi·no·chei·lo·plas·ty (rye"no·kigh'lo·plas"tee) *n.* [*rhino-* + *cheilo-* + *-plasty*]. Plastic surgery of the nose and upper lip.

rhi·no·clei·sis (rye″no·klye′sis) *n.* [*rhino-* + Gk. *kleisis,* a closing]. A nasal obstruction.

rhi·no·cnes·mus (rye″no·k′nez′mus) *n.* [*rhino-* + Gk. *knēsmos,* itching]. Itching of the nose.

rhi·no·dac·ryo·lith (rye″no·dack′ree·o·lith) *n.* [*rhino-* + *dacryo-* + *-lith*]. A calculus in the nasolacrimal duct.

rhi·no·der·ma (rye″no·dur′muh) *n.* [*rhino-* + *-derma*]. KERATOSIS PILARIS.

rhi·no·dym·ia (rye″no·dim′ee·uh) *n.* [*rhino-* + *-dymia*]. A mild form of diprosopia in which, although there is doubling of the skeletal parts of both nose and upper jaw, the face appears only unusually wide with a broad space between the eyes and thick, wide nose.

rhi·nod·y·mus (rye·nod′i·mus) *n.* [*rhino-* + *-dymus*]. An individual exhibiting rhinodymia.

rhi·no·dyn·ia (rye″no·din′ee·uh) *n.* [*rhin-* + *-odynia*]. Any pain in the nose.

Rhi·noes·trus (rye·nes′trus) *n.* [*rhin-* + Gk. *oistros,* gadfly]. A genus of flies of the Oestridae; species of this genus deposit hatched larvae in the nares, on the conjunctiva, and occasionally in the mouths of mammals. The species *Rhinoestrus purpureus,* the Russian gadfly, frequently invades the nasopharyngeal region of horses and cattle and occasionally causes human ophthalmomyiasis.

rhi·nog·e·nous (rye·noj′e·nus) *adj.* [*rhino-* + *-genous*]. Having its origin in the nose.

rhi·no·ky·pho·sis (rye″no·kigh·fo′sis) *n.* [*rhino-* + *kyphosis*]. The condition of having a nose with a prominent bridge.

rhi·no·la·lia (rye″no·lay′lee·uh) *n.* [*rhino-* + *-lalia*]. A nasal tone in the voice.

rhinolalia aper·ta (a·pur′tuh) [L., open]. A nasal tone in the voice due to undue patulousness of the choanae.

rhinolalia clau·sa (klaw′suh) [L., closed]. A nasal tone in the voice due to undue closure of the choanae.

rhi·no·lar·yn·gi·tis (rye″no·lăr″in·jye′tis) *n.* [*rhino-* + *laryng-* + *-itis*]. Simultaneous inflammation of the mucosa of the nose and larynx.

rhi·no·lar·yn·gol·o·gy (rye″no·lăr″in·gol′uh·jee) *n.* [*rhino-* + *laryngo-* + *-logy*]. The science of the anatomy, physiology, and pathology of the nose and larynx.

rhi·no·lite (rye′no·lite) *n.* RHINOLITH.

rhi·no·lith (rye′no·lith) *n.* [*rhino-* + *-lith*]. A nasal calculus.

rhi·no·li·thi·a·sis (rye″no·li·thigh′uh·sis) *n.* [*rhinolith* + *-iasis*]. The formation of nasal calculi.

rhi·nol·o·gist (rye·nol′uh·jist) *n.* A specialist in the treatment of diseases of the nose.

rhi·nol·o·gy (rye·nol′uh·jee) *n.* [*rhino-* + *-logy*]. The science of the anatomy, functions, and diseases of the nose. —**rhi·no·log·ic** (rye·no·loj′ick) *adj.*

rhi·no·ma·nom·e·ter (rye″no·ma·nom′e·tur) *n.* [*rhino-* + *manometer*]. A manometer used for measuring the amount of nasal obstruction.

rhi·nom·e·ter (rye·nom′e·tur) *n.* [*rhino-* + *-meter*]. An instrument for measuring the nose.

rhi·no·mi·o·sis (rye″no·migh·o′sis) *n.* [*rhino-* + Gk. *meiōsis,* diminution]. Operative shortening of the nose.

rhi·nom·mec·to·my (rye″nom·eck′tuh·mee) *n.* [*rhin-* + Gk. *omma,* eye, + *-ectomy*]. RHINOCANTHECTOMY.

rhi·no·my·co·sis (rye″no·migh·ko′sis) *n.* [*rhino-* + *mycosis*]. The presence of fungi in the mucous membrane and secretion of the nose.

rhi·no·ne·cro·sis (rye″no·ne·kro′sis) *n.* [*rhino-* + *necrosis*]. Necrosis of the nasal bones.

rhi·nop·a·thy (rye·nop′uth·ee) *n.* [*rhino-* + *-pathy*]. Any disease of the nose.

rhi·no·pha·ryn·ge·al (rye″no·fa·rin′jee·ul) *adj.* [*rhino-* + *pharyngeal*]. Pertaining to the nose and pharynx, or to the nasopharynx.

rhi·no·phar·yn·gi·tis (rye″no·făr″in·jye′tis) *n.* [*rhino-* + *pharyng-* + *-itis*]. Inflammation of the nose and pharynx, or of the nasopharynx.

rhinopharyngitis mu·ti·lans (mew′ti·lanz). GANGOSA.

rhi·no·pha·ryn·go·lith (rye″no·fa·ring′go·lith) *n.* [*rhino-* + *pharyngo-* + *-lith*]. A nasopharyngeal calculus.

rhi·no·phar·ynx (rye″no·făr′inks) *n.* [*rhino-* + *pharynx*]. NASOPHARYNX.

rhi·no·pho·nia (rye″no·fo′nee·uh) *n.* [*rhino-* + *phon-* + *-ia*]. A nasal tone in the speaking voice.

rhi·no·phy·ma (rye″no·figh′muh) *n.* [*rhino-* + *phyma*]. A form of acne rosacea of the nose characterized by a marked hypertrophy of the blood vessels, sebaceous glands, and connective tissue, producing a lobulated appearance of the end of the nose. May be markedly disfiguring. Syn. *toper's nose, whisky nose.*

rhi·no·plas·ty (rye′no·plas″tee) *n.* [*rhino-* + *-plasty*]. A plastic operation upon the nose. This may be accomplished in a variety of ways, such as the so-called Italian method of rotating bone and skin-lined pedicle flap from the forehead, by flaps from the cheeks, by the transplantation of costal cartilage. See also *rhinorrhaphy.* —**rhi·no·plas·tic** (rye″no·plas′tick) *adj.*

rhi·no·pol·yp (rye″no·pol′ip) *n.* [*rhino-* + *polyp*]. A polyp of the nose.

rhi·no·poly·pus (rye″no·pol′i·pus) *n.* [*rhino-* + *polypus*]. RHINOPOLYP.

rhi·nop·sia (rye·nop′see·uh) *n.* [*rhin-* + *-opsia*]. ESOTROPIA.

rhi·nor·rha·gia (rye″no·ray′jee·uh) *n.* [*rhino-* + *-rrhagia*]. Nosebleed, especially a profuse one.

rhi·nor·rha·phy (rye·nor′uh·fee) *n.* [*rhino-* + *-rrhaphy*]. A plastic reduction in the size of the nose, in which redundant nasal tissue is removed by section, followed by approximation and suture of the wound edges.

rhi·nor·rhea, rhi·nor·rhoea (rye″no·ree′uh) *n.* [*rhino-* + *-rrhea*]. 1. A mucous discharge from the nose. 2. Escape of cerebrospinal fluid through the nose.

rhi·nos·chi·sis (rye·nos′ki·sis) *n.* [*rhino-* + *-schisis*]. A congenital cleft nose.

rhi·no·scle·ro·ma (rye″no·skle·ro′muh) *n.* [*rhino-* + *scleroma*]. A chronic infectious disease caused by *Klebsiella rhinoscleromatis* which begins in the nose and may involve adjacent areas, characterized by hard nodules and plaques of inflamed tissue.

rhi·no·scope (rye′nuh·skope) *n.* [*rhino-* + *-scope*]. An instrument for examining nasal cavities.

rhi·nos·co·py (rye·nos′kuh·pee) *n.* [*rhino-* + *-scopy*]. Examination of the nasal cavities by means of the rhinoscope. See also *anterior rhinoscopy, posterior rhinoscopy.* —**rhi·no·scop·ic** (rye″no·skop′ick) *adj.*

rhi·no·si·nus·itis (rye″no·sigh″nuh·sigh′tis) *n.* [*rhino-* + *sinus* + *-itis*]. Inflammation of the nose and paranasal sinuses.

rhi·no·si·nus·o·path·ia (rye″no·sigh″nus·o·path′ee·uh) *n.* [*rhino-* + *sinus* + *-pathia*]. The diseases of the nose and paranasal sinuses.

rhi·no·spo·rid·i·o·sis (rye″no·spo·rid″ee·o′sis) *n.* [*Rhinosporidium* + *-osis*]. An infection of man and domestic animals, caused by *Rhinosporidium seeberi,* and characterized by the appearance of polyps on mucous membranes, such as the nose, nasopharynx, conjunctiva, or soft palate.

Rhi·no·spo·rid·i·um (rye″no·spo·rid′ee·um) *n.* [NL., from *rhino-* + *spore*]. A genus of organisms pathogenic to man not yet precisely classified but thought to be a fungus.

Rhinosporidium see·be·ri (see′bur·eye). The species of *Rhinosporidium* which is the causative agent of rhinosporidiosis.

rhi·no·ste·no·sis (rye″no·ste·no′sis) *n.* [*rhino-* + *stenosis*]. Permanent constriction of the nose or nasal cavity.

rhi·no·thrix (rye′no·thricks) *n.* [*rhino-* + Gk. *thrix,* hair]. A hair growing in the nostril.

rhi·not·o·my (rye·not′uh·mee) *n.* [*rhino-* + *-tomy*]. Surgical incision of the nose.

rhi·no·vi·rus (rye″no·vye′rus) *n.* [*rhino-* + *virus*]. A member of the picornavirus group which is ether-stable, small, and RNA-containing, and etiologically related to the common cold.

Rhi·pi·ceph·a·lus (rye″pi·sef′uh·lus, rip″i·) *n.* [NL., from Gk.

rhipis, fan, + *kephalos*, head]. A genus of ticks of the superfamily Ixodoidea. Many species act as vectors of such diseases as Rocky Mountain spotted fever, Q fever, and tularemia to man and lower animals.

Rhipicephalus san·guin·e·us (sang·gwin'ee·us). A common species of tick incriminated in the transmission of disease.

rhip·tas·mus (rip·taz'mus) *n.* [Gk. *rhiptazmos*, tossing about]. *Obsol.* BALLISM.

rhitidosis. RHYTIDOSIS.

rhiz-, rhizo- [Gk. *rhiza*]. A combining form meaning *root.*

Rhi·zog·ly·phus (rye·zog'li·fus) *n.* [NL., from *rhizo-* + Gk. *glyphē*, carved work]. A genus of mites, belonging to the family Tyroglyphidae, causing coolie itch.

rhi·zoid (rye'zoid) *adj. & n.* [Gk. *rhizōdēs*, rootlike]. 1. Rootlike; branching irregularly. 2. One of the slender, rootlike filaments which are organs of attachment in many cryptogams. 3. A bacterial plate culture of an irregular branched or rootlike character.

rhi·zome (rye'zome) *n.* [Gk. *rhizōma*, mass of roots]. An underground stem, or rootstock.

rhi·zo·mel·ic (rye''zo·mel'ick) *adj.* [*rhizo-* + Gk. *melos*, limb]. Affecting or pertaining to the roots of the extremities; pertaining to the hip or shoulder joints.

rhizomelic spondylosis. ANKYLOSING SPONDYLITIS.

rhi·zo·mor·phoid (rye''zo·mor'foid) *adj.* [*rhizo-* + *morph-* + *-oid*]. Having the form of a root.

rhi·zo·nych·ia (rye''zo·nick'ee·uh) *n.* [Gk. *rhizonychia*, from *rhiza*, root, + *onyx*, nail]. The root of a nail.

rhi·zo·nych·i·um (rye''zo·nick'ee·um) *n.* [NL.]. RHIZONYCHIA.

rhi·zo·pod (rye''zo·pod) *n.* [*rhizo-* + *-pod*]. A member of the Rhizopoda, a division of Protozoa.

Rhi·zop·o·da (rye·zop'o·duh) *n.pl.* [NL., from Gk. *rhiza*, root, + *poda*, feet]. A class of the Protozoa that includes those amebas, characterized by the possession of pseudopodia, which parasitize man.

rhi·zop·ter·in (ri·zop'tur·in) *n.* The formyl derivative, $C_{15}H_{12}N_6O_4$, of pteroic acid. It appears to be a precursor in the biogenesis of folic acid or of compounds having folic acid activity, possibly by conversion to formylfolic acid through conjugation with glutamic acid. Syn. *formylpteroic acid.*

Rhi·zo·pus (rye'zo·pus) *n.* [NL., from Gk. *rhiza*, root, + *pous*, foot]. A genus of the Phycomycetes whose species may act as common allergens, as the cause of phycomycosis, and as laboratory contaminants.

Rhizopus nig·ri·cans (nig'ri·kans). A species of fungus that causes rots of various fruits and is commonly found as a saprophyte on dung; an important cause of phycomycosis of man.

rhi·zot·o·my (rye·zot'uh·mee) *n.* [*rhizo-* + *-tomy*]. Surgical division of any root, as of a nerve. Syn. *radicotomy.*

Rh-negative, *adj.* Designating the absence of $Rh_o(D)$ antigen from the erythrocytes.

rhod-, rhodo- [Gk. *rhodon*, rose]. A combining form meaning *red.*

rho·da·mine (ro'duh·meen, ·min) *n.* Any of a group of red dyes of the xanthene type, closely related to fluorescein, and used in fluorescence microscopy.

rho·da·nate (ro'duh·nate) *n.* THIOCYANATE.

Rho·de·sian cattle disease. A piroplasmotic disease transmitted by ticks of the genus *Rhipicephalus.*

Rhodesian fever. EAST COAST FEVER.

Rhodesian sleeping sickness. RHODESIAN TRYPANOSOMIASIS.

Rhodesian tick fever. THEILERIASIS.

Rhodesian trypanosomiasis or **sleeping sickness.** The more virulent form of trypanosomiasis, caused by *Trypanosoma brucei rhodesiense*, with which humans may be accidentally infected from wild animals by the tsetse fly vectors in tropical East Africa. The clinical course, which may vary greatly in intensity and duration, is divided into two clinical stages: the first or invasive stage, characterized by fever and lymphadenopathy, and the second, by central nervous system involvement. Compare *Gambian trypanosomiasis.*

Rho·din's fixative [J. A. G. *Rhodin*, Swedish-U.S. electron microscopist, b. 1922]. An osmic acid-dextran solution used as a fixative in electron microscopy.

rho·di·um (ro'dee·um) *n.* [NL., from Gk. *rhodon*, rose]. Rh = 102.905. A rare metal, atomic number 45, of the platinum group.

Rhod·ni·us (rod'nee·us) *n.* A genus of bugs whose species are capable of transmitting *Trypanosoma cruzi.*

rhodo-. See *rhod-.*

rho·do·gen·e·sis (ro''do·jen'e·sis) *n.* [*rhodo-* + *-genesis*]. The reconstitution of visual purple which has been bleached by light.

rho·do·phy·lax·is (ro''do·fi·lack'sis) *n.* [*rhodo-* + *phylaxis*]. The property possessed by the retinal epithelium of producing rhodogenesis. —**rhodophy·lac·tic** (·lack'tick) *adj.*

rho·dop·sin (ro·dop'sin) *n.* [*rhod-* + *ops-* + *-in*]. A deep-red pigment contained in the retinal rods, preserved by darkness but bleached by daylight. Syn. *visual purple.* See also *iodopsin.*

rhoeb·de·sis (reb·dee'sis) *n.* [Gk. *rhoibdēsis*, from *rhoibdein*, to suck down]. Absorption, resorption.

RhoGAM. Trademark for $Rh_o(D)$ immune globulin (human), a sterile, concentrated anti-$Rh_o(D)$ antibody solution.

rhomb-, rhombo- [Gk. *rhombos*, rhomb]. A combining form meaning (a) *rhomboid;* (b) *rhombencephalic.*

rhomb·en·ceph·a·lon (rom''ben·sef'uh·lon) *n.*, pl. **rhomben·cepha·la** (·luh) [*rhomb-* + *encephalon*]. The most caudal of the three primary brain vesicles of the embryo; it divides into myelencephalon and metencephalon. Syn. *hindbrain.* —**rhomben·ce·phal·ic** (·se·fal'ick) *adj.*

rhom·bic (rom'bick) *adj.* [*romb-* + *-ic*]. 1. RHOMBOID. 2. Pertaining to the rhombencephalon.

rhombic groove. One of the seven transverse furrows between the neuromeres of the rhombencephalon.

rhombic lip. The lateral ridge produced by the union of the tela choroidea of the fourth ventricle with the alar plate of the rhombencephalon.

rhombo-. See *rhomb-.*

rhom·bo·coele (rom'bo·seel) *n.* [*rhombo-* + *-coele*]. The cavity of the rhombencephalon.

rhom·boid (rom'boid) *adj. & n.* [Gk. *rhomboeidēs*, from *rhombos*, rhomb]. 1. Having a shape similar to that of a rhomb, a quadrilateral figure with opposite sides equal and parallel and oblique angles. 2. RHOMBOIDEUS.

rhom·boi·de·us (rom·boy'dee·us) *n.* [NL.]. Either of the rhomboid muscles, the rhomboideus major (rhomboid major, greater rhomboid, NA *musculus rhomboideus major*) or the rhomboideus minor (rhomboid minor, lesser rhomboid, NA *musculus rhomboideus minor*), arising from the spines of the lower cervical and upper thoracic vertebrae, and inserted on the vertebral margin of the scapula. See also Table of Muscles in the Appendix.

rhomboideus oc·ci·pi·ta·lis (ock·sip·i·tay'lis). OCCIPITOSCAPULARIS.

rhomboid fossa. The diamond-shaped floor of the fourth ventricle of the brain. NA *fossa rhomboidea.*

rhomboid ligament. COSTOCLAVICULAR LIGAMENT.

rhomboid nucleus. The small, granular cells lying in and superior to the adhesio interthalamica. NA *nucleus rhomboidalis.*

rhomboid sinus. The opening in the extreme posterior end of the embryonic spinal cord which forms the terminal ventricle of the adult.

rhom·bo·mere (rom'bo·meer) *n.* A neuromere of the rhombencephalon.

rhon·chal (ronk'ul) *adj.* RHONCHIAL.

rhonchal fremitus. Vibrations produced by the passage of air through a large bronchial tube containing mucus.

rhonchi. Plural of *rhoncus.*

rhon·chi·al (ronk'ee·ul) *adj.* Pertaining to or caused by rhonchi.

rhon·chus (ronk'us) *n.*, pl. **rhon·chi** (·eye) [Gk. *rhonchos*, wheezing]. A coarse rale produced by the passage of air through a partially obstructed bronchus; vibrations may be also palpated on the chest wall, as fremitus.

rho·pheo·cy·to·sis (ro'fee·o·sigh·to"sis) *n.* [Gk. *rhophein*, to gulp, + *cyt-* + *-osis*]. The direct transfer of ferritin particles from macrophages to erythroblasts in the bone marrow.

rho·ta·cism (ro'tuh·siz·um) *n.* [Gk. *rhōtakizein*, to make overmuch or wrong use of the letter *rho*]. Mispronunciation, or overuse, of the sound of *r*.

Rh-positive, *adj.* Designating the presence of Rh_o(D) antigen in erythrocytes.

rhu·barb, *n.* [L. *rha barbarum*, barbarian rhubarb, from Gk. *rha*, rhubarb]. The dried rhizome and roots of *Rheum officinale* or certain other species of *Rheum;* used as a cathartic.

Rhus (rooce, rus) *n.* [L., sumac, from Gk. *rhous*]. A genus of shrubs or small trees of the Anacardiaceae. Poison ivy, poison oak, and poison sumac were formerly classified under this genus. See also *Toxicodendron.*

rhym·ing mania (rye'ming). CLANG ASSOCIATION.

rhy·poph·a·gy (rye·pof'uh·jee) *n.* [Gk. *rhypos*, filth, + *-phagy*]. SCATOPHAGY.

rhy·po·pho·bia (rye"po·fo'bee·uh) *n.* [Gk. *rhypos*, filth, + *-phobia*]. SCATOPHOBIA.

rhy·se·ma (rye·see'muh) *n.* [Gk. *rhysēma*, wrinkle]. A wrinkle or corrugation.

-rhysis [Gk., flow, course, from *reein*, to flow]. A combining form meaning *flowing out.*

rhythm, *n.* [Gk. *rhythmos*]. 1. Action recurring at regular intervals. 2. A method of contraception, in which continence is practiced during the ovulatory phase of the menstrual cycle.

rhyth·mic (rith'mick) *adj.* [Gk. *rhythmikos*]. Pertaining to or having the quality of rhythm, as rhythmic segmentations.

rhythmic chorea. A tremor with a rate of 2 to 4 per second, irregular intervals between cycles, and on electromyography, the presence of spike potentials whose frequency and voltage exceed those of alternating tremor; due to many different causes, these movements may affect any part of the body and persist in sleep.

rhyth·mic·i·ty (rith·mis'i·tee) *n.* 1. The property of rhythmic periodicity or recurrence. 2. The property of having rhythmic contractions.

rhythmic nystagmus. Ocular nystagmus in which there is a slow phase in one direction and a rapid recovery; may be physiologic, as in optokinetic nystagmus, or labyrinthine, due to lesions of the vestibular apparatus or its connections.

rhyt·i·dec·tom·y (rit"i·deck'tuh·mee) *n.* [Gk. *rhytis, rhytidos*, a wrinkle, + *-ectomy*]. Excision of wrinkles for cosmetic purposes.

rhyt·i·do·plas·ty (rit'i·do·plas"tee) *n.* [Gk. *rhitis, rhytidos*, wrinkle, + *-plasty*]. A plastic operation for the removal of skin wrinkles, particularly those of the face and neck, for cosmetic purposes.

rhyt·i·do·sis, rhit·i·do·sis (rit"i·do'sis) *n.* [Gk. *rhytidōsis*, from *rhytis, rhytidos*, wrinkle]. A wrinkling, particularly of the cornea.

rib, *n.* One of the 24 long, flat, curved bones forming the wall of the thorax. NA *costa.* See also Plate 1. See also Table of Bones in the Appendix.

ri·bam·in·ol (rye·bam'in·ol) *n.* Ribonucleic acid compound with 2-(diethylamino)ethanol; a substance that may have memory-adjuvant activity.

ri·ba·vi·rin (rye"buh·vye'rin) *n.* 1-(β-D-Ribofuranosyl-1*H*-1,2,4-triazole-3-carboxamide, $C_8H_{12}N_4O_5$, an antiviral.

rib·bon stools. LEAD-PENCIL STOOLS.

rib cage. The skeletal framework of the chest, made up of the sternum, the ribs, and the thoracic vertebrae. Syn. *thoracic cage.* See also *thoracic cavity.*

rib-cutting forceps. A type of forceps with one heavy semicircular cutting edge and one heavy hook-shaped blade designed to cut ribs and firm cartilages.

rib notching. Indentation of the ribs, such as that occurring in coarctation of the aorta, secondary to dilatation of the intercostal arteries.

ri·bo·des·ose (ri"bo·des'oce, ·oze) *n.* Deoxyribose; a pentose sugar present in deoxyribonucleic acid.

ri·bo·fla·vin (rye"bo·flay'vin, ·flav'in, rib"o·) *n.* [*ribose* + *flavin*]. 6,7-Dimethyl-9-(D-1'-ribityl)isoalloxazine, $C_{17}H_{20}N_4O_6$, a member of the group of B vitamins; essential in human nutrition. Its deficiency causes characteristic lesions of the tongue, lips, and face, and also certain ocular manifestations. Syn. *vitamin B_2, vitamin G, lactoflavin.*

riboflavin adenine dinucleotide. FLAVIN ADENINE DINUCLEOTIDE.

riboflavin 5'-phosphate. The phosphoric acid ester, $C_{17}H_{21}N_4O_9P$, of riboflavin in which linkage is effected through the CH_2OH group of riboflavin; the prosthetic group of a number of flavoproteins. It functions by being reversibly reduced to a dihydro derivative. Syn. *flavin phosphate, flavin mononucleotide, isoalloxazine mononucleotide, vitamin B_2 phosphate.*

ri·bo·nu·cle·ase (rye"bo·new'klee·ace, ·aze) *n.* An enzyme present in various body tissues which depolymerizes ribonucleic acid.

ri·bo·nu·cle·ic acid (rye"bo·new·klee'ick) [*ribose* + *nucleic*]. Nucleic acid occurring in cell cytoplasm and the nucleolus, first isolated from plants but later found also in animal cells, containing phosphoric acid, D-ribose, adenine, guanine, cytosine, and uracil. Abbreviated, RNA. See also *messenger RNA, ribosomal RNA, transfer RNA.*

ri·bo·nu·cleo·pro·tein (rye"bo·new"klee·o·pro'tee·in, ·teen) *n.* A nucleoprotein that contains a ribonucleic acid moiety.

ri·bo·prine (rye'bo·preen) *n.* *N*-(3-Methyl-2-butenyl)adenosine, $C_{15}H_{21}N_5O_4$, an antineoplastic agent.

ri·bose (rye'boce, ·boze) *n.* [alteration of *arabinose*]. D-ribose, $HOCH_2(CHOH)_3CHO$; a pentose sugar occurring as a structural component of riboflavin, ribonucleic acid, nicotinamide adenine dinucleotide and other nucleotides.

ribose nucleic acid. RIBONUCLEIC ACID.

ri·bo·side (rye'bo·side) *n.* Any glycoside containing ribose as the sugar component.

ribosomal RNA. A type of ribonucleic acid which combines with proteins to form the ribosomes of the cell. More than 80 percent of the total cellular RNA is of this type.

ri·bo·some (rye'bo·sohm) *n.* [*ribo*nucleic + *-some*]. A flattened, spheroidal, cytoplasmic submicroscopic ribonucleoprotein particle, 150 × 250 Å, which in company with other ribosomes linked by messenger RNA into aggregates termed polyribosomes (or polysomes) synthesizes protein. —**ri·bo·so·mal** (rye"bo·so'mul) *adj.*

rib retractor. A strong self-retaining retractor, used to obtain good exposure in intrathoracic operations.

rice, *n.* [OF. *ris*, from It. *riso*, from Gk. *oryza*]. A plant, *Oryza sativa,* of the Gramineae; also its seed. Used as a food and, occasionally, as a demulcent.

rice bodies. Small, free white bodies occurring in the synovial cavity of an arthritic joint (most commonly in tuberculous arthritis), composed of compact masses of fibrin, necrotic villi, or cartilage fragments.

rice-grain medium. A medium of autoclaved rice grains in water, used for the confirmation and identification of the various species of *Microsporum* when microscopy is inconclusive.

rice-water stools. The stools of cholera, in which there is a copious serous exudation containing mucus.

Rich·ter's hernia (rikh'tur) [A. G. *Richter*, German surgeon, 1742–1812]. A form of enterocele in which only a part of the intestinal wall is situated within the hernial sac.

Rich·ter's syndrome [M.N. *Richter,* U.S. physician, 20th century]. Chronic lymphocytic leukemia complicated terminally by fever, cachexia, dysproteinemia and a pleomorphic type of malignant lymphoma.

ri·cin (rye'sin, ris'in) *n.* A highly toxic albumin in the seed of *Ricinus communis.*

ric·in·ism (ris'in·iz·um) *n.* Poisoning from the seeds of *Ricinus communis.* It is marked by hemorrhagic gastroenteritis and icterus.

ric·in·ole·ate (ris''in·o'lee·ate) *n.* A salt or ester of ricinoleic acid.

ric·in·ole·ic acid (ris''i·no·lee'ick). 12-Hydroxy-9-octadecenoic acid, $C_{18}H_{34}O_3$, a hydroxylated fatty acid present as the glyceride in castor oil.

ric·in·ole·in (ris''in·o'lee·in) *n.* Glyceryl ricinoleate, the chief constituent of castor oil.

Ric·i·nus (ris'i·nus) *n.* [L., castor oil plant]. A genus of the Euphorbiaceae. *Ricinus communis* is the source of castor oil.

rick·ets, *n.* [probably from *rachitis*]. A deficiency disease occurring during skeletal growth, due to concurrent lack of vitamin D and insufficient exposure to ultraviolet radiation (sunshine), resulting in altered calcium and phosphorus metabolism, which is reflected in defective bone growth, and, in severe cases, characteristic skeletal deformities. Syn. *Glisson's disease, infantile osteomalacia, juvenile osteomalacia, rachitis.*

Rick·ett·sia (ri·ket'see·uh) *n.* [H. T. *Ricketts,* U.S. pathologist, 1871–1910]. A genus of bacteria of the family Rickettsiaceae, causing the spotted fever group of diseases, characterized by intranuclear and intracytoplasmic multiplication in susceptible animal cells, and transmitted to man by ticks, as in Rocky Mountain spotted fever, or by mites, as in rickettsialpox.

rickettsia, *n.*, pl. **rickett·si·ae** (·see·ee), **rickettsias.** A member of the family Rickettsiaceae. —**rickett·si·al** (·see·ul) *adj.*

Rickettsia aka·mu·shi (ack·uh·moo'shee). RICKETTSIA TSUTSUGAMUSHI.

Rickettsia ak·a·ri (ack'uh·rye). The causative agent of rickettsialpox.

Rickettsia aus·tra·lis (aw·stray'lis). The causative agent of Queensland tick typhus fever.

Rickettsia bur·net·ii (bur·net'ee·eye). COXIELLA BURNETII.

Rick·ett·si·a·ce·ae (ri·ket''see·ay'see·ee) *n.pl.* [NL., from *Rickettsia*]. A family of small, pleomorphic, coccobacillary microorganisms of the order Rickettsiales, principally obligate intracellular parasites, occurring in arthropods and causing a variety of diseases in animals and in man.

Rickettsia co·no·rii (kon·o'ree·eye). The causative agent of boutonneuse fever.

Rickettsia dia·po·ri·ca (dye''uh·por'i·kuh). COXIELLA BURNETII.

rickettsial disease. Any one of the diseases caused by rickettsiae. The most important are typhus fever, caused by *Rickettsia prowazeki;* Rocky Mountain spotted fever, caused by *R. rickettsii;* tsutsugamushi disease, caused by *R. tsutsugamushi;* and Q fever, caused by *Coxiella burnetti.*

rick·ett·si·al·pox (ri·ket'see·ul·pocks'') *n.* [*rickettsial* + *pox*]. A mild, nonfatal, self-limited, acute febrile illness caused by *Rickettsia akari,* which is transmitted from mouse to man by mites. It is characterized by an initial papule at the site of the bite, a week's febrile course, and a papulovesicular rash.

Rickettsia me·loph·a·gi (me·lof'uh·jye). A nonpathogenic species of *Rickettsia* found in the sheep tick *Melophagus ovinus.*

Rickettsia moo·seri (moo'sur·eye). RICKETTSIA TYPHI.

Rickettsia ori·en·ta·lis (or''ee·en·tay'lis). RICKETTSIA TSUTSUGAMUSHI.

Rickettsia pe·dic·u·li (pe·dick'yoo·lye). ROCHALIMAEA QUINTANA.

Rickettsia pro·wa·zek·ii (pro·va·zeck'ee·eye). The causative agent of louse-borne epidemic typhus and Brill's disease.

Rickettsia prowazeki mooseri. RICKETTSIA TYPHI.

Rickettsia prowazeki prowazeki. RICKETTSIA PROWAZEKII.

Rickettsia psittaci. MIYAGAWANELLA PSITTACI.

Rickettsia quintana. ROCHALIMAEA QUINTANA.

Rickettsia rick·ett·sii (ri·ket'see·eye). The causative agent of Rocky Mountain spotted fever.

Rickettsia ru·mi·nan·ti·um (roo·mi·nan'shee·um). The causative agent of heartwater disease.

Rickettsia si·be·ri·ca (sigh·beer'i·kuh). The causative agent of North Asian tick-borne rickettsiosis.

Rickettsia tsu·tsu·ga·mu·shi (tsoo''tsuh·ga·moo'shee). The causative agent of tsutsugamushi disease. Syn. *Rickettsia orientalis.*

Rickettsia ty·phi (tye'fye). The causative agent of murine typhus.

Rickettsia wol·hyn·i·ca (wol·hin'i·kuh). ROCHALIMAEA QUINTANA.

rick·ett·si·o·sis (ri·ket''see·o'sis) *n.*, pl. **rickettsio·ses** (·seez) [*rickettsia* + *-osis*]. A disease of man or animals caused by microorganisms in the family Rickettsiaceae.

Rick·etts' organism [H. T. *Ricketts*]. Any organism of the genus *Rickettsia.*

rick·ety (rick'e·tee) *adj.* Affected with or distorted by rickets; rachitic.

rickety rosary. RACHITIC ROSARY.

Ri·cord's chancre (ree·kohr') [P. *Ricord,* French urologist and dermatologist, 1800–1889]. The initial sore of syphilis.

Ricord's method [P. *Ricord*]. *Obsol.* A technique of circumcision.

Rid·doch's mass reflex [G. *Riddoch,* English neurologist, 1889–1947]. A mass reflex in spinal cord transection, particularly when due to a high cervical lesion. Nociceptive stimuli below the level of the lesion may result in simultaneous flexor spasms of the legs, involuntary emptying of bowel and bladder, and sweating.

Riddoch syndrome [G. *Riddoch*]. Inattention to objects in homonymous half-fields despite the ability to see and recognize objects when attention is directly called to them; observed in persons with lesions of the contralateral parietal lobe.

Rideal-Walker method [S. *Rideal,* English chemist, 1863–1929; and J. T. A. *Walker,* English chemist, 1868–1930]. A procedure for determining the phenol coefficient of disinfectants.

ri·deau phenomenon (ree·do') [F., curtain]. VERNET'S RIDEAU PHENOMENON.

rid·er's bone. An osseous deposit in the adductor muscles of the leg, from long-continued pressure of the leg against the saddle. Syn. *cavalry bone, cavalryman's osteoma.*

rider's bursa. A bursa resulting from pressure on the adductor muscles of the thigh.

rider's legs. Strain of the adductor muscles of the thigh.

rider's sprain. A sprain of the adductor longus muscle of the thigh, resulting from a sudden effort of the horseman to maintain his seat owing to some unexpected movement of his horse.

ridge, *n.* An extended elevation or crest.

ridge·ling (rij'ling) *n.* A domestic animal with cryptorchism.

riding embolus. SADDLE EMBOLUS.

riding of bones. *In surgery,* the displacement of the fractured ends of bones which are forced past each other by muscular contraction, instead of remaining in end-to-end apposition.

riding thrombus. SADDLE THROMBUS.

Rie·del's disease or **struma** (ree'del) [B. M. C. L. *Riedel,* German surgeon, 1846–1916]. A form of chronic thyroiditis with irregular localized areas of stony hard fibrosis; in advanced stages the gland is adherent to surrounding structures.

Riedel's lobe [B. M. C. L. *Riedel*]. A tongue-shaped process extending downward from the costal border of the right lobe of the liver; it occurs infrequently.

Rie·der's cell (ree'dur) [H. *Rieder*, German pathologist, 1858–1932]. An anaplastic leukocyte, considered by some a variety of lymphocyte, by others a type of granulocyte; such cells occur in poorly differentiated acute leukemia.

Rie·gel's test. A test for rennin in which neutralized gastric juice is incubated with fresh milk. Coagulation will occur in 10 to 15 minutes if rennin is present in normal amount.

Rie·ger's anomaly. A rare congenital complex of disorders of the eye, consisting of various manifestations of mesodermal dysgenesis of the cornea and iris, such as posterior embryotoxon, hypoplasia of the anterior stromal layer of the iris, and abnormal tissue in the angle of the anterior chamber, accompanied by secondary glaucoma.

Riehl's melanosis (reel) [G. *Riehl*, Austrian dermatologist, 1855–1943]. An idiopathic inflammatory disease of the skin characterized by hyperpigmentation, chiefly affecting the face.

Ries-Clark operation. A type of radical hysterectomy, similar to Wertheim's operation for carcinoma of the uterus.

Ries·man's myocardosis [D. *Riesman*, U.S. physician, 1867–1940]. Degenerative noninflammatory fibrotic disease of the myocardium.

Riesman's sign [D. *Riesman*]. 1. A bruit heard over the eyeball in hyperthyroidism. 2. Softening of the eyeball in diabetic coma. 3. In gallbladder disease, sharp pain produced in the gallbladder region when the tensed right rectus muscle is struck lightly by the side of the examiner's hand.

Rieux's hernia (ryœh) [L. *Rieux*, French surgeon, 19th century]. A retrocecal hernia.

rif·am·pin (rif'am·pin) *n.* 3-(4-Methylpiperazinyliminomethyl)rifamycin SV, $C_{43}H_{58}N_4O_{12}$, a derivative of rifamycin SV active against isoniazid-resistant strains of tubercle bacilli.

rif·a·my·cin (rif''uh·migh'sin) *n.* Any of a group of related antibiotic substances produced by *Streptomyces mediterranei* and individually identified by suffixing capital letters to the generic name, as rifamycin B, C, D, E, O, S, SV, and X.

Rift Valley fever [*Rift Valley*, Kenya]. A toxic generalized febrile illness of short duration characterized by headache, photophobia conjunctivitis, myalgia, anorexia, leukopenia and thrombocytopenia. Caused by a mosquito-borne arbovirus, epizootic in domestic animals and enzootic in wild game in eastern and southern Africa.

Ri·ga-Fe·de disease (ree'gah, fey'deh) [A. *Riga*, Italian physician, 1832–1919; and F. *Fede*]. FEDE-RIGA DISEASE.

Riga's aphthae [A. *Riga*]. CACHECTIC APHTHAE.

Riga's disease. 1. FEDE-RIGA DISEASE. 2. Riga's aphthae (= CACHECTIC APHTHAE).

Riggs and Stadie method. A method for determining peptic activity in which the enzyme activity is measured photometrically as the decrease in turbidity of a standardized homogenized suspension of coagulated egg white under specified conditions.

Riggs' disease [J. M. *Riggs*, U.S. dentist, 1810–1885]. PERIODONTITIS.

right-angle technique. PARALLEL TECHNIQUE.

right anterior oblique. A position assumed by a patient for x-ray examination, with the anterior aspect of his right side closest to the film so that the x-ray beam passes diagonally through his body.

right atrioventricular valve. TRICUSPID VALVE.

right axis deviation. Mean electrical axis of the QRS complex in the frontal plane of greater than 90°. Abbreviated, RAD.

right axis shift. RIGHT AXIS DEVIATION.

right-eyed, *adj.* Tending to use the right eye when there is a choice rather than the left, as in looking through a monocular telescope.

right-foot·ed, *adj.* Tending to use the right foot when there is a choice rather than the left, as in hopping or kicking.

right-hand·ed, *adj.* Tending to use the right hand when there is a choice rather than the left. —**right-hand·ed·ness,** *n.*

right heart. The part of the heart that furnishes blood to the lungs; the right atrium and right ventricle.

right heart reflex. BAINBRIDGE REFLEX.

right hepatic artery. The right branch of the proper hepatic artery. NA *ramus dexter arteriae hepaticae propriae.*

right·ing reflex. Any of a chain of reflexes that operate to bring, or to maintain, an animal right side up; included are labyrinthine righting reflexes, body righting reflexes acting upon the head, body righting reflexes acting upon the body, neck righting reflexes, and optical righting reflexes.

right lateral. A position assumed by a patient for x-ray examination, with his right side closest to the film and the x-ray beam perpendicular to the film.

right lymphatic duct. The common lymph trunk receiving the right jugular, subclavian, and bronchomediastinal trunks, and emptying into the right subclavian vein at its junction with the right internal jugular vein. NA *ductus lymphaticus dexter, ductus thoracicus dexter.*

right posterior oblique. A position assumed by a patient for x-ray examination, with the posterior aspect of his right side closest to the film so that the x-ray beam passes diagonally through his body.

right-to-left shunt. A cardiac defect characterized by flow of deoxygenated blood from the right side of the heart into the left side of the heart or systemic circulation, without passage through the pulmonary circulation.

right ventricle of the heart. The chamber that pumps blood through the pulmonary trunk and on into the lungs. NA *ventriculus dexter.* See also Plate 5.

rig·id (rij'id) *adj.* [L. *rigidus*]. 1. Stiff, hard, inflexible. 2. Tense, spastic; said of muscles.

ri·gid·i·tas (ri·jid'i·tas) *n.* [L.]. RIGIDITY.

rigiditas ar·tic·u·lo·rum (ahr·tick''yoo·lo'rum). EXTRACAPSULAR ANKYLOSIS.

rigiditas ca·da·ver·i·ca (kad''uh·verr'i·kuh). RIGOR MORTIS.

ri·gid·i·ty (ri·jid'i·tee) *n.* 1. Stiffness; inflexibility; immobility. 2. *In neurology,* a form of hypertonus in which the muscles are continuously or intermittently tense. In contrast to spasticity, the increase in tone has a uniform quality throughout the range of passive movement of the limb. Syn. *lead-pipe rigidity.* Compare *spasticity.* 3. *In psychology,* great resistance and reluctance to change, with fixed patterns of behavior.

rig·or (rig'ur) *n.* [L., stiffness]. 1. CHILL. 2. RIGIDITY (1).

rigor mor·tis (mor'tis) [L., of death]. Temporary stiffening and rigidity of muscle, particularly skeletal and cardiac, which occurs after death.

RIHSA Radioactive iodine-tagged human serum albumin.

Ri·ley-Day syndrome. FAMILIAL DYSAUTONOMIA.

ri·ma (rye'muh) *n.*, pl. & genit. sing. **ri·mae** (·mee) [L.]. A chink or cleft. —**ri·mal** (·mul) *adj.*

rima cor·ne·a·lis (kor·nee·ay'lis) [BNA]. The groove in the sclera into which the edge of the cornea fits.

rima glot·ti·dis (glot'i·dis) [NA]. The space between the true vocal folds.

ri·man·ta·dine (ri·man'tuh·deen) *n.* α-Methyl-1-adamantanemethylamine, $C_{12}H_{21}N$, an antiviral agent.

rima oris (o'ris) [NA]. The line formed by the junction of the lips.

rima pal·pe·bra·rum (pal·pe·brair'um) [NA]. PALPEBRAL FISSURE.

rima pu·den·di (pew·den'dye) [NA]. The fissure between the labia majora.

rima ve·sti·bu·li (ves·tib'yoo·lye) [NA]. The interval between the two vestibular folds of the larynx.

rima vul·vae (vul'vee). RIMA PUDENDI.

Rimifon. A trademark for isoniazid, an antituberculous agent.

rim·i·ter·ol (rim″i·terr′ole) *n. erythro*-α-(3,4-Dihydroxyphenyl)-2-piperidinemethanol, $C_{12}H_{17}NO_3$, a bronchodilator used as the hydrobromide salt.

ri·mose (rye′moce, rye·moce′) *adj.* [L. *rimosus,* from, *rima,* crack]. *In biology,* marked by many crevices or furrows.

rin·der·pest (rin′dur·pest) *n.* [Ger., cattle plague]. A contagious, epidemic disease of cattle and sometimes sheep and goats in Africa and Asia; caused by a filtrable virus and characterized by fever and ulcerative, diphtheritic lesions of the intestinal tract.

Rine·hart and Abul-Haj stain. The Hale dialyzed iron technique for acid mucopolysaccharides is followed by a Van Gieson connective-tissue stain to show mucins in blue, collagen in red, and muscle in yellow.

ring, *n.* 1. A circular opening or the structure surrounding it. 2. A cyclic or closed-chain structure. See also *ring compound.*

ring·bin·den (ring·bin′dun) *n.* [Ger. *Ring,* ring, + *binden,* to tie, encircle]. Abnormal arrangement of myofibrils, best seen in transverse sections as a circular or concentric striated coil entwined about the periphery or penetrating the sarcoplasm at right angles to the usual plane of muscles of aged and prematurely aged individuals, especially in the extraocular muscles where this alteration is occasionally observed in normal younger persons. Syn. *spiral annulet, striated annulet.*

ring biopsy. Surgical excision of the entire circumference of the squamocolumnar junction of the cervix; used in the diagnosis of cancer.

ring bodies. Blue-stained threads arranged in rings and figures of eight, found in the erythrocytes of persons with lead poisoning and other anemias. Syn. *Cabot's rings, Cabot's ring bodies.*

ring·bone, *n.* A chronic, hypertrophic osteitis of the pastern or first, second, or third phalanges of the foot in the horse.

ring cataract. DISC-SHAPED CATARACT.

ring compound. A compound in which the atoms form a ring or closed chain.

ringed hair. A rare form of canities, due to the alternate formation of medulla and no medulla, in which the hairs appear silvery gray and dark in alternating bands. Usually seen in several members of a family. Syn. *pili annulati.*

Ring·er's injection [S. *Ringer,* English physiologist, 1835–1910]. A sterile solution of sodium chloride, potassium chloride, and calcium chloride in sufficient water for injection; used intravenously as a fluid and electrolyte replenisher.

Ringer's lactate solution [S. *Ringer*]. LACTATED RINGER'S INJECTION.

Ringer's solution [S. *Ringer*]. A solution of the same composition as Ringer's injection but prepared with recently boiled purified water and not required to be sterile. Used topically as a physiologic salt solution but not to be administered parenterally, for which purpose Ringer's injection should be employed.

ring finger. The fourth digit of the hand, next to the little finger. NA *digitus anularis, digitus IV.*

ring·hals (ring′hals) *n.* [Afrikaans, ring-necked]. A Southern African cobra of the genus *Haemachates,* family Elapidae.

ring of a heart valve. FIBROUS RING (2). See also *skeleton of the heart.*

ring pessary. A round or ring-shaped pessary.

ring·schwie·le (ring′shvee″luh) *n.* [Ger. *Ring,* ring, + *Schwiele,* wheal, callosity]. The circumferential proliferation of the pigment epithelium of the retina at the ora serrata, resulting in the formation of a large pigmented plaque in eyes with long-standing retinal detachments.

ring scotoma. ANNULAR SCOTOMA.

ring·tail, *n.* A condition in neonatal, poikilothermic rats caused by a low ambient humidity, characterized by edema, inflammation, and annular constrictions and necrosis of the tail.

ring·worm. An infection of the skin, hair, or nails, with various fungi, producing annular lesions with raised borders. Syn. *tinea.* See also *trichophytosis.*

Rin·ne's test (rin′e^h^) [H. A. *Rinne,* German otologist, 1819–1868]. A hearing test in which the duration of bone conduction is compared with that of air conduction. Normally air conduction is longer than bone conduction (Rinne positive; symbol, + R). Alteration in this relationship (Rinne negative; symbol, − R) indicates a lesion of the sound-conducting apparatus.

ri·no·lite (rye′no·lite) *n.* RHINOLITH.

Rio·lan's arc (ryoh·lahn′) [J. *Riolan,* French anatomist and physiologist, 1580–1637]. An arterial arcade which, when present, usually connects the main stem of the superior mesenteric artery with the left colic branch of the inferior mesenteric artery.

Riolan's bones or **ossicles** [J. *Riolan*]. Sutural bones sometimes found in the suture between the occipital bone and the mastoid portion of the temporal bone.

Riolan's muscle [J. *Riolan*]. The ciliary portion of the orbicularis oculi muscle.

Riopan. Trademark for magaldrate, a gastric antacid.

ri·paz·e·pam (ri·paz′e·pam) *n.* 1-Ethyl-4,6-dihydro-3-methyl-8-phenylpyrazolo[4,3-*e*][1,4]diazepin-5(1*H*)-one, $C_{15}H_{16}N_4O$, a minor tranquilizer.

Risa. A trademark for iodinated I 131 serum albumin, a preparation of radioactive iodine used as a diagnostic aid in determining blood or plasma volume, circulation time or cardiac output, and as an adjunct in detecting and localizing brain tumors.

Ris·ley's prism [S. D. *Risley,* U.S. ophthalmologist, 1845–1920]. A pair of prisms of equal strength with the faces apposing, so that by rotation of one, the power is gradually increased from zero to the total of their values.

ri·so·caine (rye′zo·kane) *n.* Propyl *p*-aminobenzoate, $C_{10}H_{13}NO_2$, a local anesthetic.

ri·so·ri·us (ri·so′ree·us) *n.* [NL., from *ridere, risus,* to laugh]. A muscle of the cheek inserted into the angle of the mouth. NA *musculus risorius.* See also Table of Muscles in the Appendix.

ris·to·ce·tin (ris″to·see′tin) *n.* A mixture of two antibiotics, ristocetin A and ristocetin B, produced by the actinomycete *Nocardia lurida.* Used in infections due to streptococci, enterococci, pneumococci, and staphylococci when the infections are resistant to other antibiotics.

ri·sus (rye′sus) *n.* [L., laughter]. A grin or laugh.

risus ca·ni·nus (kay·nigh′nus). RISUS SARDONICUS.

risus sar·don·i·cus (sahr·don′i·kus). The sardonic grin, a peculiar grinning distortion of the face produced by spasm of the muscles about the mouth; characteristically observed in tetanus.

Ritalin. Trademark for methylphenidate, a central nervous system stimulant used as the hydrochloride in the treatment of various types of depression.

Rit·gen's maneuver [F. A. M. F. *Ritgen,* German gynecologist, 1787–1867]. Manual delivery of the head of the fetus by sustained upward pressure through the rectum and perineum with simultaneous downward pressure by the other hand.

rit·o·drine (rit′o·dreen) *n. erythro-p*-Hydroxy-α-[1-[(*p*-hydroxyphenethyl)amino]ethyl]benzyl alcohol, $C_{17}H_{21}NO_3$, a smooth muscle relaxant used as a bronchodilator for the treatment of bronchial asthma.

Rit·ter's disease [G. *Ritter* von Rittershain, Austrian dermatologist, 1820–1883]. DERMATITIS EXFOLIATIVA NEONATORUM.

Ritter-Val·li law (vah^l^′lee) [J. W. *Ritter,* German physiologist, 1776–1810; and E. *Valli,* Italian physiologist, 1755–1816]. *In physiology,* the rule that section of a living nerve is followed first by increased irritability, then by loss of irritability, the reaction moving toward the periphery.

rit·u·al (rich′oo·ul) *n.* [L. *ritualis,* from *ritus,* rite]. 1. A ceremony or system of stereotyped and prescribed activities performed periodically and having special significance relating to religion or other code of belief or behavior. 2. An activity considered by an individual to be a routine, but highly significant part of his life, as reading before bedtime, or, for example, the manner in which parents carry out a child's toilet training, regarding the process as inviolate and imbuing it with special significance. 3. *In psychiatry,* any psychomotor activity other than a tic repeatedly performed, in order to relieve anxiety; usually seen in the obsessive-compulsive neurosis.

ri·val·ry (rye'vul·ree) *n.* A struggle for supremacy. See also *sibling rivalry, retinal rivalry.*

rivalry of colors. Retinal rivalry, where colors are the stimuli.

rivalry of contours. Retinal rivalry, where the contours of two objects are the stimuli.

rivalry of visual fields. RETINAL RIVALRY.

Ri·val·ta's test (ree·vahl'tah) [S. *Rivalta,* Italian veterinarian, 1852–1893]. Exudates are differentiated from transudates by sinking and producing turbidity when a drop of the fluid is allowed to fall into an amount of distilled water to which one drop of 50% acetic acid has been added.

riv·er blindness. In western equatorial Africa: ONCHOCERCIASIS.

riv·et fibers (riv'it). Cytoplasmic processes on the basal surface of the columnar cells of stratified squamous epithelium.

Ri·vi·nus' ducts (ri·vee'nōōs) [A. Q. *Rivinus,* German anatomist and botanist, 1652–1723]. The minor sublingual ducts.

Rivinus' gland [A. Q. *Rivinus*]. SUBLINGUAL GLAND.

Rivinus' notch [A. Q. *Rivinus*]. TYMPANIC NOTCH.

ri·vus (rye'vus) *n.,* pl. **ri·vi** (·vye) [L.]. STREAM.

rivus la·cri·ma·lis (lack·ri·may'lis) [NA]. The stream of tears across the eyeball.

riz·i·form (riz'i·form) *adj.* [F. *riz,* rice, + *-iform*]. Resembling grains of rice.

R.M.A. Right mentoanterior position of the fetus.

R.M.P. Right mentoposterior position of the fetus.

R.N. Abbreviation for *registered nurse.*

Rn Symbol for radon.

RNA Abbreviation for *ribonucleic acid,* nucleic acid occurring in cell cytoplasm and the nucleolus, first isolated from plants but later found also in animal cells, containing phosphoric acid, D-ribose, adenine, guanine, cytosine, and uracil. See also *messenger RNA, ribosomal RNA, transfer RNA.*

RNA polymerase. An enzyme which transcribes an RNA molecule complementary to DNA; required for initiation of DNA replication as well as transcription of RNA.

RNA replicase. An enzyme found in RNA viruses which synthesizes new RNA from an RNA template when the virus infects a host cell.

RNase Abbreviation for *ribonuclease.*

RNA viruses. Viruses, such as picornaviruses, reoviruses, arboviruses, myxoviruses, viruses of mouse tumors, and plant viruses, as well as those implicated in the avian leukosis complex, in which the nucleic acid core consists of ribonucleic acid.

RNP Abbreviation for *ribonucleoprotein.*

R.O.A. Right occipitoanterior position of the fetus.

roar·ing, *n.* A disease of horses, caused by damage to the recurrent laryngeal nerve resulting in paralysis and atrophy of the muscle controlling the arytenoid cartilage of the larynx; the flaccid cartilage impedes normal inspiration and is responsible for the harsh roaring sound heard during vigorous exercise.

Robalate. A trademark for the gastric antacid substance dihydroxyaluminum aminoacetate.

Robaxin. Trademark for methocarbamol, a skeletal muscle relaxant.

ro·ben·i·dine (ro·ben'i·deen) *n.* 1,3-Bis[(*p*-chlorobenzylidene)amino]guanidine, $C_{15}H_{13}Cl_2N_5$, a poultry coccidiostat.

Robenz. A trademark for robenidine, a coccidiostat.

Ro·bert pelvis (ro'behrt) [H. L. F. *Robert,* German gynecologist, 1814–1878]. A transversely contracted pelvis having a rudimentary sacrum, undeveloped sacral alae, and much narrowed oblique and transverse diameters.

Rob·erts' reagent [W. *Roberts,* English physician, 1830–1899]. A solution of 1 part pure nitric acid to 5 parts saturated solution of magnesium sulfate, used to test for urine protein.

Roberts' test [W. *Roberts*]. A test for protein in urine in which urine is overlayed on Roberts' reagent. A white ring at the zone of contact indicates protein.

Rob·in·son-Kep·ler-Pow·er test [F. J. *Robinson,* U.S. physician, 20th century; E. J. *Kepler,* U.S. physician, 20th century; and M. H. *Power,* U.S. physician, 20th century]. A test for adrenal cortical insufficiency or Addison's disease which measures the urea clearance, chloride clearance, and water diuresis.

Robinson's disease [A. R. *Robinson,* U.S. dermatologist, 1845–1924]. HIDROCYSTOMA.

Ro·bin syndrome or **anomalad** (roh·bæn') [*Pierre Robin,* French, 20th century].The association of micrognathia, cleft palate, and glossoptosis, resulting from early mandibular hypoplasia; may occur in otherwise normal infants or as part of a multiple malformation syndrome. There are some familial occurrences but the genetic basis is obscure.

Robinul. Trademark for glycopyrrolate, a drug used in the management of gastrointestinal disorders in which anticholinergic action is indicated.

Robison ester [R. *Robison,* English biochemist, 1883–1941]. GLUCOSE 6-PHOSPHATE.

robo·rant (rob'o·runt, ro'buh·runt) *adj. & n.* [L. *roborare,* to strengthen, from *robur,* hard wood]. 1. Tonic, strengthening. 2. A strengthening agent.

Ro·cha·li·maea (rosh''uh·li·mee'uh, ro''shuh·) *n.* [H. da *Rocha-Lima*]. A genus of the Rickettsiaceae.

Rochalimaea quin·ta·na (kwin·tah'nuh) [L., quintan]. The causative agent of trench fever.

Ro·chelle salt (rosh·el') [after La *Rochelle,* France]. POTASSIUM SODIUM TARTRATE.

rock·er rib. A first rib that is abnormally bent downward at the subclavian sulcus.

rock·et electrophoresis. Electroimmunodiffusion in which the antigen-antibody precipitate is rocket-shaped.

rock·ing bed. OSCILLATING BED.

rocking method. EVE'S METHOD.

Rock·ley's sign. A sign for depression of the zygomatic bone in which there is a difference in the angle on the two sides where two straight edges are placed from the outer edge of the orbit to the prominence of the zygomatic bone.

rock oil. PETROLEUM.

rock salt. Sodium chloride as obtained in solid form by mining.

Rocky Mountain spotted fever. An acute febrile illness caused by *Rickettsia rickettsii,* transmitted to man by ticks. There is the sudden onset of headache, chills, and fever; a characteristic exanthem occurs on the extremities and trunk. Syn. *American spotted fever.*

Rocky Mountain spotted fever vaccine. A vaccine for prophylactic immunization against Rocky Mountain spotted fever. The original method utilizing killed rickettsiae harvested from ground-infected ticks (the Spencer-Parker vaccine) has been supplanted by a formalized vaccine prepared from rickettsiae grown in the yolk sac of the developing chick.

rod, *n.* 1. Any slender, straight structure or object. 2. One of the rod-shaped photosensitive retinal cells concerned with motion and vision at low degrees of illumination (night vision). Contr. *cone* (3). 3. A bacterium shaped like a rod.

rod-body myopathy. NEMALINE MYOPATHY.

rod cell. 1. An elongated microglial cell found in the cerebral cortex in various pathologic conditions, especially paresis. 2. BAND CELL. 3. ROD (2).

ro·den·ti·cide (ro·den'ti·side) *n.* [*rodent* + *-cide*]. A preparation that is poisonous to, or destroys, rodents; used as an agent against rats or mice.

rodent ulcer. BASAL CELL CARCINOMA.

rod epithelium. Striated cells lining certain glands.

Rod·man's incision [W. L. *Rodman,* U.S. surgeon, 1858–1916]. For radical mastectomy, a pear-shaped incision encircling the breast, extending to the axilla.

rod-monochromat, *n.* A person said to have no normal cones in his retina, but only rods, seeing all wavelengths of light as gray; usually photophobic, with low visual acuity and nystagmus. Syn. *achromat.* Contr. *cone-monochromat.*

rod nuclear cell. BAND CELL.

ro·do·caine (ro'do·kane) *n. trans*-6'-Chloro-2,3,4,4a,5,6,7,7a-octahydro-1*H*-1-pyridine-1-propiono-*o*-toluidide, $C_{18}H_{25}ClN_2O$, a local anesthetic.

ro·do·nal·gia (ro''do·nal'jee·uh) *n.* [Gk. *rhodon,* rose, + *-algia*]. ERYTHROMELALGIA.

rod opsin. The protein moiety located in the rods of the retina which, under the influence of light, forms rhodopsin with $retinene_1$ and porphyropsin with $retinene_2$.

rods of Corti [A. *Corti*]. The columnar cells lining the tunnel of Corti. See also *pillar cells, spiral organ* (of Corti).

Roe·de·rer's ecchymoses (rœh'de·rur) [J. G. *Roederer,* German obstetrician, 1727–1763]. Ecchymoses found in the pericardium and pleura of stillborn infants, attributed to intrauterine anoxic capillary damage.

Roederer's obliquity [J. G. *Roederer*]. The position of the fetal head at the brim of the pelvis during normal labor, with occipital presentation favorable for subsequent flexion.

Roe-Kahn method [J. H. *Roe,* U.S. biochemist, 1892–1967]. A method for determining blood calcium in which calcium is precipitated from the protein-free serum filtrate as tricalcium phosphate, which is then determined colorimetrically.

Roen·ne's nasal step (rœn'eʰ) [H. K. T. *Roenne* (*Rønne*), Danish ophthalmologist, b.1878]. A nasal visual field defect typical of glaucoma, caused by asymmetrical nerve fiber damage on either side of the horizontal raphe of the eye, thus appearing like a step.

roent·gen, rönt·gen (rent'gun) *n. & adj.* [W. K. *Röntgen,* German physicist, 1845–1923]. 1. The international unit of x- and gamma radiation. 2. The quantity of x- or gamma radiation which results in associated corpuscular emission of 1 electrostatic unit of electrical charge of either sign per 0.001293 g of air under standard conditions. Abbreviated, r. 3. Of or pertaining to x-rays.

roentgen absorption histospectroscopy. The quantitative estimation of elements in very small histologic specimens by means of roentgen absorption spectra.

roentgen cinematography. Cinematography of x-ray images.

roentgen dermatitis. RADIODERMATITIS.

roentgen equivalent man. The quantity of radiation which, when absorbed by man, produces a biologic effect equivalent to the absorption by man of 1 roentgen of x- or gamma radiation. Abbreviated, REM, rem.

roentgen equivalent physical. The amount of ionizing radiation which is capable of producing 1.615×10^{12} ion pairs per gram of tissue or that will transfer to tissue 93 ergs per gram. This unit is employed primarily to measure beta radiation. Abbreviated, REP, rep.

roentgen kymography. RADIOKYMOGRAPHY.

roent·gen·o·der·ma (rent''gun·o·dur'muh) *n.* [*roentgen* + *-derma*]. RADIODERMATITIS.

roent·gen·o·gram (rent'ge·no·gram) *n.* [*roentgen* + *-gram*]. RADIOGRAPH.

roent·gen·o·graph (rent'ge·no·graf) *v.* To make a roentgenogram.

roent·gen·og·ra·phy (rent''ge·nog'ruh·fee) *n.* [*roentgen* + *-graphy*]. RADIOGRAPHY. —**roentgen·o·graph·ic** (·o·graf'ick) *adj.*

roent·gen·o·ky·mo·gram (rent''ge·no·kigh'mo·gram) *n.* [*roentgen* + *kymogram*]. Radiographic record of the changes in the size or movements of the heart, or the position of the diaphragm.

roent·gen·o·ky·mog·ra·phy (rent''ge·no·kigh·mog'ruh·fee) *n.* [*roentgen* + *kymography*]. RADIOKYMOGRAPHY.

roent·gen·ol·o·gist (rent''ge·nol'uh·jist) *n.* A physician specializing in the practice of roentgenology.

roent·gen·ol·o·gy (rent''ge·nol'uh·jee) *n.* [*roentgen* + *-logy*]. The branch of medical science which deals with the diagnostic and therapeutic application of x-rays. See also *radiology.* —**roentgen·o·log·ic** (·no·loj'ick) *adj.*

roent·gen·o·lu·cent (rent''ge·no·lew'sunt) *adj.* [*roentgen* + *lucent*]. Allowing the passage of x-rays.

roent·gen·os·co·py (rent''ge·nos'kuh·pee) *n.* [*roentgen* + *-scopy*]. Examination with x-rays by means of a fluorescent screen. —**roent·gen·o·scope** (rent'ge·no·skope) *n.*

roent·gen·o·ther·a·py (rent''ge·no·therr'uh·pee) *n.* [*roentgen* + *therapy*]. The treatment of disease by means of x-rays.

roentgen ray. X-RAY.

roentgen-ray anemia. RADIATION ANEMIA.

roentgen tube. An evacuated vessel containing two electrodes, the positive anode and the negative cathode at a considerable potential difference; the cathode contains the source of electrons, as a hot filament, and the anode is of sturdy construction to withstand bombardment by the cathode rays. At the anode the energy of the cathode rays is converted into 98 percent of heat energy and 2 percent of x-rays.

roentgen unit. ROENTGEN.

roe·theln, rö·teln (reh'tuln, ruh'tuln) *n.* [Ger.]. RUBELLA.

ro·flur·ane (ro·floo'rane) *n.* 2-Bromo-1,1,2-trifluoroethyl methyl ether, $C_3H_4BrF_3O$, a general anesthetic, administered by inhalation.

Ro·ger murmur (roʰ·zheʸ') [H. L. *Roger,* French physician, 1809–1891]. A harsh holosystolic murmur, usually accompanied by a thrill, heard best parasternally in the third and fourth left intercostal spaces in patients with ventricular septal defect. Syn. *bruit de Roger.*

Roger's disease [H. L. *Roger*]. VENTRICULAR SEPTAL DEFECT.

Roger's reflex or **syndrome** [G. H. *Roger,* French physiologist, 1860–1946]. Excessive salivation on irritation of the esophagus, as by a tumor.

Rohr's stria [K. *Rohr,* German anatomist, b. 1863]. STRIA OF ROHR.

Ro·ki·tan·sky-Asch·off sinuses (ro·kee·taʰn'skee, aʰsh'oʰf) [C. F. von *Rokitansky,* Austrian pathologist, 1804–1878; and K. A. L. *Aschoff*]. Small outpouchings of the mucosa of the gallbladder extending through the lamina propria and muscular layer.

Rokitansky's disease [C. F. von *Rokitansky*]. POSTNECROTIC CIRRHOSIS.

ro·lan·dic (ro·lan'dick) *adj.* 1. Described by or named for Luigi Rolando, Italian anatomist, 1773–1831. 2. Pertaining to the central sulcus (fissure of Rolando).

rolandic angle The acute angle formed by the central sulcus (fissure of Rolando) with the superior border of the cerebral hemisphere.

rolandic sulcus. CENTRAL SULCUS (1).

Ro·lan·do's area [L. *Rolando,* Italian anatomist, 1773–1831]. The motor area of the cerebral cortex.

Rolando's fibers [L. *Rolando*]. *Obsol.* The external arcuate fibers of the medulla oblongata.

Rolando's fissure [L. *Rolando*]. CENTRAL SULCUS (1).

Rolando's gelatinous substance [L. *Rolando*]. SUBSTANTIA GELATINOSA.

ro·let·a·mide (ro·let'uh·mide) *n.* 3',4',5'-Trimethoxy-3-(3-

pyrrolin-1-yl)acrylophenone, $C_{16}H_{19}NO_4$, a hypnotic drug.

Rolicton. Trademark for the orally effective nonmercurial diuretic amisometradine.

ro·li·cy·prine (ro″li·sigh′preen) *n.* (+)-5-Oxo-*N*-(*trans*-2-phenylcyclopropyl-L-2-pyrrolidinecarboxamide, $C_{14}H_{16}N_2O_2$, an antidepressant drug.

ro·li·tet·ra·cy·cline (ro″li·tet″ruh·sigh′kleen) *n.* *N*-(1-Pyrrolidinylmethyl)tetracycline, $C_{27}H_{33}N_3O_8$, a soluble derivative of tetracycline administered intramuscularly or intravenously when oral administration of tetracycline is impracticable or when a higher blood concentration of antibiotic is required than can be attained orally.

roll·er bandage (ro′lur). A long strip of material ½ to 6 inches in width, rolled on its short axis.

Rol·ler's nucleus (roʰl′ur) [C. F. W. *Roller,* German neurologist, b. 1844]. A nucleus, composed of relatively large cells, which lies ventral to the rostral pole of the hypoglossal nucleus and adjacent to its root fibers.

Rolle·ston's rule (role′stun) [H. D. *Rolleston,* English physician, 1862–1944]. An obsolete method for predicting the effect of age on blood pressure. The optimum systolic blood pressure for an adult was stated to be 100 plus one-half the age; the upper limit of normal was stated as 100 plus the age.

Rol·let's cell [A. *Rollet,* Austrian physiologist, 1834–1903]. PARIETAL CELL.

Rollet's stroma [A. *Rollet*]. STROMA (2).

Rollett's disease [J. P. *Rollett,* French physician, 1824–1894]. MIXED CHANCRE.

Rol·lier's method (roʰl·yeʸ′) [A. *Rollier,* Swiss physician, 1874–1954]. An obsolete method of treating extrapulmonary tuberculosis by use of sunlight.

ro·lo·dine (ro′lo·deen) *n.* 4-(Benzylamino)-2-methyl-7*H*-pyrrolo[2,3-*d*]pyrimidine, $C_{14}H_{14}N_4$, a skeletal muscle relaxant.

Ro·ma·ña's sign [C. *Romaña,* Brazilian physician]. Painless unilateral palpebral edema and conjunctivitis, usually during the first febrile week in acute Chagas' disease.

ro·mano·scope (ro·man′o·skope) *n.* [colon *roman*um, sigmoid colon (referring to the shape of the Roman S as contrasted with the Greek sigma, Σ) + *-scope*]. SIGMOIDOSCOPE.

Ro·ma·nov·sky stains (ruh·mah·noʰf′skee) [D. L. *Romanovsky,* Russian physician and malariologist, 1861–1921]. A generic term applied to stains with nearly balanced mixtures of eosin and oxidation products of methylene blue, used as blood stains.

Rom·berg's disease (roʰm′behrk) [M. H. *Romberg,* German neurologist, 1795–1873]. PROGRESSIVE FACIAL HEMIATROPHY.

Rom·berg's sign [M. H. *Romberg*]. 1. A sign for obturator hernia in which there is pain radiating to the knee. 2. A sign for loss of position sense in which the patient cannot maintain equilibrium when standing with feet together and eyes closed.

Ro·mieu reaction (roʰ·myœh′) A test for tryptophan in proteins. Fixed tissue is treated with a drop of phosphoric acid to give a red or violet color.

Romilar. Trademark for dextromethorphan, a nonaddicting antitussive, used as the hydrobromide salt.

Rompun. A trademark for xylazine hydrochloride, an analgesic.

Rondomycin. Trademark for methacycline, a semisynthetic tetracycline antibiotic.

ron·geur (rohn·zhur′) *n.* [F., from *ronger,* to gnaw]. A bone-cutting forceps.

Roniacol. Trademark for nicotinyl alcohol, a peripheral vasodilator.

ro·ni·da·zole (ro·nigh′duh·zole) *n.* 1-(Methyl-5-nitroimidazol-2-yl)methyl carbamate, $C_6H_8N_4O_4$, an antiprotozoal agent.

ron·nel (ron′ul) *n.* *o*-(2,4,5-Trichlorophenyl) phosphorothioate, $C_8H_8Cl_3O_3PS$, a systemic insecticide.

Rønne's nasal step. ROENNE'S NASAL STEP.

röntgen. ROENTGEN.

roof nuclei of the cerebellum. TECTAL NUCLEI.

roof plate. The dorsal wall of the embryonic neural tube, ependymal in structure.

root, *n.* 1. The descending axis of a plant. 2. The part of an organ embedded in the tissues, as the root of a tooth. 3. The beginning or proximal portion of a structure, especially one of two bundles of nerve fibers, the posterior and anterior emerging from the central nervous system and joining to form a nerve trunk.

root amputation. The removal of a root from a tooth.

root canal. The cavity within the root of a tooth, which contains pulp, nerves, and vessels. NA *canalis radicis dentis.*

root canal filling. The closure and filling of the prepared root canal from the apex to the coronal portion of the tooth with an impervious material to prevent subsequent infection.

root canal treatment. The opening, cleansing, and sterilization of a root canal preparatory to root canal filling.

root cell. ANTERIOR HORN CELL.

root entrance zone. The area of entrance of dorsal roots into the spinal cord, where they are constricted and devoid of myelin. Syn. *Obersteiner-Redlich area.*

root feet. Fine digitations of basal cells of the epidermis into the underlying connective tissue of the corium at the dermoepidermal junction. Syn. *basalzellfüsschen.*

root of the aorta. The site of origin of the aorta at the heart. Syn. *radix aortae.*

root of the lung. The axis formed by the main bronchus, pulmonary vessels, lymphatics, and nerves in the hilus, connecting the lung with the heart and trachea. NA *radix pulmonis.*

root of the mesentery. The parietal attachment of the mesentery extending from the duodenojejunal flexure to the ileocecal junction. NA *radix mesenterii.*

root of the nail. The small proximal region of the nail plate covered entirely by the nail wall. NA *radix unguis.*

root of the nose. The part at the forehead between the eyes, from which emerges the dorsum of the nose. NA *radix nasi.*

root of the tongue. The pharyngeal, fixed part of the tongue, posterior to the sulcus terminalis. NA *radix linguae.*

root plan·ing. The smoothing of roughened tooth-root surfaces by instrumentation.

root resection. Amputation of part of the root of a tooth.

root sheath. The portion of the hair follicle derived from the epidermis; it surrounds the root of the hair and consists of the internal root sheath, three layers of cells immediately surrounding the root, and the external root sheath, a stratified layer adjacent to the dermal portion of the hair follicle.

R.O.P. Right occipitoposterior position of the fetus.

ro·pa·lo·cyte (ro′puh·lo·site, ro·pal′o·) *n.* [Gk. *ropalo*n, club, + *-cyte*]. An erythrocyte with unusual clubbed projections giving it a labyrinthine appearance; seen in transmission electron micrographs of erythrocytes in a variety of hematopoietic diseases.

rope graft. TUBED FLAP.

ro·pi·zine (ro′pi·zeen) *n.* 4-(Diphenylmethyl)-*N*-[(6-methyl-2-pyridinyl)methylene]-1-piperazinamine, $C_{24}H_{26}N_4$, an anticonvulsant.

ropy milk (ro′pee). Milk that becomes viscid so that it may be drawn out into a stringy mass; caused by a growth of bacteria, *Alcaligenes viscosus.*

Ror·schach test or **diagnosis** (rohr′shahᵏh) [H. *Rorschach,* Swiss psychiatrist, 1884–1922]. A psychologic test in which the subject describes what he sees on a series of 10 standard inkblots of varying designs and colors. The subject's responses indicate personality patterns, special interests, originality of thought, emotional conflicts, deviations of effect, and neurotic or psychotic tendencies.

ro·sa·cea (ro·zay'shee·uh, ·see·uh) *n.* [L., of roses]. ACNE ROSACEA.

ro·sa·ce·i·form (ro·zay'shee·i·form) *adj.* [*rosacea* + *-iform*]. Resembling acne rosacea. Having a dusky red, telangiectatic appearance.

ro·sa·lia (ro·say'lee·uh) *n.* [NL., from It. *rosellia,* measles]. 1. SCARLET FEVER. 2. MEASLES. 3. ERYTHEMA.

ro·sa·mi·cin (ro"zuh·mye'sin) *n.* An antibiotic, $C_{31}H_{51}NO_9$, derived from *Micromonospora rosaria.* Also used as the butyrate, propionate and stearate esters, and the sodium phosphate salt.

ros·an·i·line (ro·zan'i·leen, ·lin) *n.* [*rose* + *aniline*]. α^4-(*p*-Aminophenyl)-α^4-(4-imino-2,5-cyclohexadien-1-ylidene)-2,4-xylidine, $C_{20}H_{19}N_3$, a dye; used also in the synthesis of other dyes.

rose, *n.* [L. *rosa*]. Any plant or flower of the genus *Rosa.*

rose ben·gal (beng'gawl). The sodium or potassium salt of 4, 5, 6, 7-tetrachloro-2', 4', 5', 7'-tetraiodofluorescein, used as a bacterial stain and in Lendrum's inclusion-body stain. The rate of disappearance of the dye from the bloodstream following its intravenous administration is a test of liver function.

rose bengal sodium I 131. Sodium 4,5,6,7-tetrachloro-2',4',5',7'-tetraiodofluorescein, in which a portion of the molecules contain radioactive iodine (^{131}I); used in the form of an injection administered intravenously, to test liver function and differentiate various types of jaundice, also for photoscanning of the liver.

rose geranium oil. An odorous volatile oil from *Pelargonium graveolens, P. odoratissimum,* and other species.

ro·se·in (ro'zee·in) *n.* FUCHSIN.

ro·se·ine (ro'zee·een, ·in) *n.* Rosein (= FUCHSIN).

ro·sel·la (ro·sel'uh) *n.* RUBELLA.

rose·mary, *n.* [L. *rosmarinus,* from *ros,* dew, + *marinus,* of the sea]. *Rosmarinus officinalis,* a plant of the Labiatae. The volatile oil of the plant is used as a flavor and perfume.

Ro·sen·bach's disease (ro'z^e^n·bahkh) [O. *Rosenbach,* German physician, 1851–1907]. HEBERDEN'S ARTHRITIS.

Rosenbach's law [O. *Rosenbach*]. In lesions of the anterior horn cells or nerve trunks, paralysis involves the extensor before the flexor muscles.

Rosenbach's sign [O. *Rosenbach*]. 1. Fibrillary tremor of the closed eyelids, sometimes seen in hyperthyroidism. 2. Inability to close the eyes on command; seen with hysteria. 3. Absence of the ipsilateral abdominal skin reflexes in hemiplegia. 4. Absence of abdominal skin reflexes with disease of the abdominal viscera.

Rosenbach's test [O. *Rosenbach*]. A test for bile pigment in which urine is filtered and a drop of concentrated nitric acid is put on the filter paper. If bile pigment is present, a succession of colors will be seen as in Gmelin's test.

Ro·sen·muel·ler's fossa or **recess** (ro'zen·muel"ur) [J. C. *Rosenmueller,* German anatomist, 1771–1826]. PHARYNGEAL RECESS.

Rosenmueller's gland [J. C. *Rosenmueller*]. 1. ACCESSORY LACRIMAL GLAND. 2. ROSENMUELLER'S NODE.

Rosenmueller's node [J. C. *Rosenmueller*]. The highest or most proximal deep inguinal lymph node, located within the femoral ring.

Rosenmueller's organ [J. C. *Rosenmueller*]. EPOOPHORON.

Ro·sen·thal fibers (ro'zen·tahl). Irregular, elongated, or beaded hyaline masses found on microscopic examination in a variety of different central nervous system lesions and in ovarian teratomas.

Rosenthal's canal [I. *Rosenthal,* German physiologist, 1836–1915]. COCHLEAR DUCT.

Rosenthal's vein [F. C. *Rosenthal,* German anatomist, 1780–1829]. BASAL VEIN.

rose oil. The volatile oil distilled from the fresh flowers of *Rosa gallica* and certain other *Rosa* species; used as a perfume. Syn. *attar of rose, otto of rose.*

ro·se·o·la (ro·zee'o·luh) *n.* [NL., from L. *roseus,* rosy]. Any rose-colored eruption. See also *epidemic roseola.*

roseola cho·ler·i·ca (ko·lerr'i·kuh). An eruption sometimes appearing in cholera.

roseola in·fan·tum (in·fan'tum). EXANTHEM SUBITUM.

roseola scarlatiniforme. ERYTHEMA SCARLATINIFORME.

roseola syph·i·lit·i·ca (sif"i·lit'i·kuh). An eruption of rose-colored spots appearing early in secondary syphilis.

roseola ty·pho·sa (tye·fo'suh). The eruption of typhoid or typhus fever.

roseola vac·cin·ia (vack·sin'ee·uh). A general rose-colored eruption occurring about 10 days after vaccination. It is of short duration.

ro·se·o·lous (ro·zee'o·lus) *adj.* Having the character of roseola.

rose rash of infants. EXANTHEM SUBITUM.

Ro·ser-Braun's sign (ro'zur, braown) [W. *Roser,* German surgeon, 1817–1888; and H. *Braun,* German surgeon, 1847–1911]. ROSER'S SIGN.

Roser's sign [W. *Roser*]. Absence of pulsation of the dura mater, indicative of an underlying cerebral tumor.

Rose's operations [W. *Rose,* English surgeon, 1847–1910]. Various operations for harelip.

rose spots. A red, papular eruption which blanches on pressure, occurring mostly on the abdomen and loins during the first 7 days of typhoid fever. Syn. *typhoid roseola, typhoid spots, taches rosées lenticulaires.*

Ro·se's position (ro'zuh) [E. *Rose,* German physician, 1836–1914]. A position taken by the patient on the operating table in which he is dorsally recumbent, the head being over the end of the table in full extension; the object is to prevent body fluids from entering the trachea during operation on the mouth and fauces.

Rose's tamponade [E. *Rose*]. CARDIAC TAMPONADE.

ro·sette (ro·zet') *n.* [F.]. Any structure resembling or suggestive of a rose, such as a cluster of cells in a crowded circle.

ros·in (roz'in) *n.* [variant of *resin*]. The residue left after the volatile oil is distilled from turpentine. It consists chiefly of various modifications of anhydrides of abietic acid with varying quantities of hydrocarbons. Used as a component of plasters. Syn. *colophony.*

ro·sox·a·cin (ro·sock'suh·sin) *n.* 1-Ethyl-1,4-dihydro-4-oxo-7-(4-pyridyl)-3-quinolinecarboxylic acid, $C_{17}H_{14}N_2O_3$, an antibacterial.

Ross·bach's disease (rohss'bahkh) [M. J. *Rossbach,* German physician, 1842–1894]. GASTROXYNSIS.

Ross-Jones test [G. W. *Ross,* Canadian physician, 1841–1931; and E. *Jones,* Canadian psychiatrist, b. 1879]. A test for protein in which spinal fluid is stratified over saturated ammonium sulfate reagent. A turbid ring at the junction of the fluids indicates increased protein.

Ross·man's fluid [I. *Rossman,* U.S. physician, b. 1913]. One part of neutral Formalin and nine parts of saturated picric acid in absolute alcohol; used for fixation of glycogen in tissues.

Ros·so·li·mo's reflex (ruh·sah·lee'muh) [G. I. *Rossolimo,* Russian neurologist, 1860–1928]. A stretch reflex of the plantar muscles of the foot, characterized by flexion of the second to fifth toes in response to tapping of the plantar surfaces of the toes; its intensity varies with the degree of muscle tonus and is most markedly increased in corticospinal tract lesions.

Ross's bodies [E. H. *Ross,* English pathologist, 1875–1928]. Small round structures thought to occur in the blood and tissue fluids in syphilis; described as copper-colored with dark granules and occasional ameboid movements.

Ros·tan's asthma (rohs·tahn') [L. *Rostan,* French physician, 1790–1866]. CARDIAC ASTHMA.

ros·tel·lum (ros·tel'um) *n.* [dim. of L. *rostrum,* beak, snout]. A little beak, especially the hook-bearing portion of the head of certain worms.

rostra. Plural of *rostrum.*

ros·trad (ros'trad) *adv.* [*rostr*um + *-ad*]. Proceeding or projecting toward the beak, snout, or face from another part of the head.

ros·tral (ros'trul) *adj.* 1. Pertaining to or resembling a rostrum. 2. Relatively far advanced in a direction toward the beak, snout, or face (with respect to other parts of the head).

rostral lamina. The thin continuation of the rostrum of the corpus callosum into the lamina terminalis. See also Plate 18.

ros·tral·most (ros'trul·mohst) *adj.* [*rostral* + *most*]. Furthest forward toward the nose, or tip of the frontal lobes.

ros·trum (ros'trum) *n.*, pl. **ros·tra** (·truh) [L.]. A beak; a projection or ridge.

rostrum cor·po·ris cal·lo·si (kor'po·ris ka·lo'sigh) [NA]. The anterior tapering portion of the corpus callosum.

rostrum sphe·noi·da·le (sfee·noy·day'lee) [NA]. The vertical ridge on the inferior aspect of the body of the sphenoid bone, which is received in the upper grooved border of the vomer.

rot, *n.* & *v.* 1. Putrefactive fermentation; decay; decomposition. 2. FOOT ROT. 3. To deteriorate; to undergo decomposition.

ro·tam·e·ter (ro·tam'e·tur, ro'tuh·mee·tur) *n.* [L. *rota,* wheel, + *-meter*]. A device for the measurement of mean flow rate of a liquid or gas.

ro·tate, *adj.* & *v.* [L. *rota*, wheel, + *-ate*]. 1. Wheel-shaped. 2. To undergo or cause rotation.

rotate plane. *In biology,* a wheel-shaped and flat surface.

ro·ta·tion, *n.* [L. *rotatio,* from *rotare,* to turn]. 1. The act of turning about an axis passing through the center of a body, as rotation of the eye, rotation of the head. 2. *In dentistry,* the operation by which a malturned tooth is turned or twisted into its normal position. 3. *In neurophysiology,* the phenomenon whereby every third or fourth impulse is carried over the cochlear nerve when the exciting impulse is above 1,800 hertz (cycles per second). 4. *In obstetrics,* one of the stages of labor, consisting in a rotary movement of the fetal head or other presenting part, whereby it is accommodated to the birth canal. It may be internal, occurring before the birth of the presenting part, or external, occurring afterward.

rotation flap. SLIDING FLAP.

rotation joint. PIVOT JOINT.

rotation stage of labor. ROTATION (4).

rotation test. The study of the reaction of the semicircular canals by rotating the patient with the head fixed in certain planes.

rotation therapy. A technique of radiation therapy in which either the patient is rotated around a central axis with the radiation beam constant, or the radiation source is revolved about the patient.

rotation vertebrae. The first and second cervical vertebrae.

ro·ta·tor cuff (ro'tay·tur). MUSCULOTENDINOUS CUFF.

ro·ta·to·res (ro"tuh·to'reez) *n.pl.* Small deep muscles of the back which extend and rotate the vertebrae, sometimes divided into rotatores breves and longi, depending on their length. NA *musculi rotatores.* See also Table of Muscles in the Appendix.

rotatores spi·nae (spye'nee). ROTATORES.

ro·ta·to·ria (ro"tuh·to'ree·uh) *n.* CURSIVE EPILEPSY.

ro·ta·to·ry (ro'tuh·tor·ee) *adj.* 1. Pertaining to or producing rotation. 2. Occurring in or by rotation. 3. Resembling a body in rotation.

rotatory nystagmus. An oscillatory, partial rolling of the eyeball around the visual axis.

rotatory vertigo. SUBJECTIVE VERTIGO.

Rotch's sign [T. M. *Rotch,* U.S. physician, 1848–1914]. Obliteration of the cardiohepatic angle in pericardial effusion as evidenced by dullness on percussion over the right fifth intercostal space.

rö·teln (reh'tuln, rœh'tuln) *n.* [Ger.]. RUBELLA.

ro·te·none (ro'te·nohn, rot'e·nohn) *n.* An insecticidal principle, $C_{23}H_{22}O_6$, derived from derris root and other plant roots; commonly used as an inhibitor to block the electron transport chain in mitochondria between NADH and ubiquinone.

Roth-Bern·hardt's disease (roht, behrn'hart) [W. K. *Roth* (V. K. *Rot*), Russian neurologist, 1848–1916; and M. *Bernhardt*]. MERALGIA PARESTHETICA.

Roth·era's test (roth'ur·uh) [A. C. H. *Rothera,* Australian biochemist, 1880–1915]. A test for diacetic acid in which to urine saturated with ammonium sulfate, concentrated ammonium hydroxide and sodium nitroprusside are added. The appearance of a purple tinge is a positive test.

Roth-Kva·le test. A test for pheochromocytoma employing the intravenous injection of histamine phosphate, which, in cases of pheochromocytoma, is followed by a very marked elevation in blood pressure and the acute paroxysm typical of the condition.

Roth·mund's syndrome (rote'mŏŏnt) [A. *Rothmund,* German physician, 19th century]. ROTHMUND-THOMSON SYNDROME.

Rothmund-Thomson syndrome [A. *Rothmund;* and M. S. *Thomson,* English dermatologist, b. 1894]. A hereditary oculocutaneous disorder characterized by erythema, atrophy, pigmentation, telangiectasia, and a peculiar marmorization of the skin, particularly in sun-exposed areas, in association with congenital cataracts, short stature, skeletal defects, partial or total alopecia, defective nails and teeth, and hypogonadism; transmitted as a recessive trait.

Roth's disease or **symptom complex** [W. K. *Roth*]. MERALGIA PARESTHETICA.

Roth's spots (rote) [M. *Roth,* Swiss physician, 1839–1914]. Small white spots surrounded by hemorrhage found in the fundus of the eye in subacute bacterial endocarditis and other conditions.

Ro·tor syndrome [A. B. *Rotor*]. Dubin-Johnson syndrome but without hepatic pigmentation.

ro·tox·a·mine (ro·tock'suh·meen) *n.* (−)-2-{*p*-Chloro-α-[2-(dimethylamino)ethoxy]benzyl}pyridine, $C_{16}H_{19}ClN_2O$, an antihistaminic drug.

Rot·ter's test [H. *Rotter,* Hungarian physician, 20th century]. A test for vitamin C deficiency in man, using dichlorophenol-indophenol sodium injected intradermally to color the skin. If decolorization does not occur within 10 minutes, vitamin C deficiency may exist.

Rou·get cell (roo·zheh') [C. M. B. *Rouget,* French physiologist, 1824–1904]. Branched cells on the external walls of capillaries which are contractile in frogs and salamanders, but probably not in mammals.

rough·age (ruf'ij) *n.* Food containing indigestible material, such as bran or cellulose, which stimulates intestinal action and promotes peristalsis.

rough colony. A flat nonglistening bacterial colony with irregular surface and edges. Abbreviated, R.

rough-surfaced endoplasmic reticulum. Intracytoplasmic membranes to which granules of ribonucleoprotein (ribosomes) are adherent, seen by electron microscopy. They represent a complex which synthesizes protein and contains it within membranes. Abbreviated, RER. Contr. *smooth-surfaced endoplasmic reticulum.*

Rough·ton-Scho·lan·der method. A micromethod for determination of gases in capillary blood, using a glass syringe fused to a graduated capillary tube which has a cup-like expansion at its free end. With appropriate procedure and reagents, separate determinations can be made for O_2, CO_2, CO, and N_2. Syn. *syringe-capillary method.*

Rou·gnon-Heb·er·den's disease (roo·nyohn', heb'ur·dun) [N. F. *Rougnon,* French physician, 1727–1799; and W. *Heberden*]. ANGINA PECTORIS.

rou·leau (roo·lo′) *n.* [F.]. A column of red blood cells stacked like a roll of coins.

round cell. Generally, any of the particular cells of an inflammatory exudate which have a round nuclear outline, especially lymphocytes, plasma cells, and macrophages.

round-cell carcinoma. 1. Any poorly differentiated carcinoma with round parenchymal cells. 2. A form of poorly differentiated lung carcinoma.

round-cell infiltration. Generally, an infiltration by such cells as lymphocytes, plasma cells, and macrophages, without specifying cell type.

round ligament. 1. (of the femur:) A flattened band extending from the fovea on the head of the femur to attach on either side of the acetabular notch between which it blends with the transverse ligament. NA *ligamentum capitis femoris.* See also Plate 2. 2. (of the liver:) A fibrous cord running from the umbilicus to the notch in the anterior border of the liver. It represents the remains of the obliterated umbilical vein. NA *ligamentum teres hepatis.* 3. (of the uterus:) A ligament running from the anterior surface of the lateral border of the uterus through the inguinal canal to the labium majus. NA *ligamentum teres uteri.* See also Plate 23.

round needle. Any needle that is circular in cross section without a cutting edge; may be either curved or straight.

round shoulders. Faulty posture in which drooping of the shoulders and increased convexity of the thoracic spine are conspicuous, the postural abnormalities not being limited to the shoulder girdle and chest.

round ulcer. A peptic ulcer of the stomach.

round window. A round opening in the medial wall of the middle ear, closed by the secondary tympanic membrane. Syn. *cochlear window.* NA *fenestra cochleae.* See also Plate 20.

round-window membrane. SECONDARY TYMPANIC MEMBRANE.

round·worm, *n.* A worm of the order Nematoda.

roup (roop) *n.* An infectious disease of fowls, especially pigeons, characterized by infection of the upper digestive tract and cranial sinuses with the protozoan *Trichomonas gallinae.*

Rous sarcoma (rawss) [F. P. *Rous,* U.S. pathologist, 1879–1970]. A fibrosarcoma, transmissible by cell-free filtrates, which originally arose spontaneously in a barred Plymouth Rock hen.

Rous·sy-Dé·je·rine syndrome (roo·see′, deʸzh·reen′) [G. *Roussy,* French pathologist, 1874–1948; and J. J. *Déjerine*]. THALAMIC SYNDROME.

Roussy-Lé·vy disease (leʸ·vee′) [G. *Roussy;* and F. *Lévy,* French neurologist, b. 1881]. A form of hereditary sensory ataxia, pes cavus and areflexia, with atrophy of the muscles of the lower extremities and sometimes of the hands and kyphoscoliosis; beginning in childhood, the disease progresses slowly and often arrests. Compare *Friedreich's ataxia, peroneal muscular atrophy.*

Roux en Y bypass (roo en wye; F. roo ahⁿ·nee·greck′) [César *Roux,* Swiss surgeon, 1857–1926]. ROUX-Y DRAINAGE.

Roux en Y gastroenterostomy [C. *Roux*]. ROUX-Y GASTROJEJUNOSTOMY.

Roux en Y loop [C. *Roux*]. The rearranged segments of jejunum in the Roux-Y drainage.

Roux's gastroenterostomy [C. *Roux*]. ROUX-Y GASTROJEJUNOSTOMY.

Roux's operation [C. *Roux*]. A multistaged operation for excision of the esophagus for carcinoma, in which the esophagus is reattached to the stomach by interposition of a loop of jejunum.

Roux's operation [Jules *Roux,* French surgeon, 1807–1877]. An operation for exstrophy of the bladder, using flaps from the abdominal wall and scrotum.

Roux's serum [P. P. E. *Roux,* French bacteriologist, 1853–1933]. TETANUS ANTITOXIN.

Roux-Y anastomosis [C. *Roux*]. An operation in which the small bowel is divided, the distal end is anastomosed to another organ, such as the stomach or common duct, and the proximal end to the descending limb of the small bowel below the anastomosis. The purpose is to provide drainage for the host organ without reflux of intestinal contents.

Roux-Y drainage or **bypass** [C. *Roux*]. An operation, adapted from the Roux-Y gastrojejunostomy, designed to drain the biliary tract or such organs as the pancreas or esophagus into the jejunum; peristalsis prevents retrograde reflux of intestinal contents into the organ drained.

Roux-Y gastrojejunostomy [C. *Roux*]. An operation in which the jejunum is divided, the distal end is anastomosed to the side of the stomach and the proximal end is anastomosed to the side of the jejunum at a lower level. The result is a Y-shaped double anastomosis which diverts the flow of bile and pancreatic enzymes from the newly made gastric stoma. Syn. *Roux en Y gastroenterostomy.*

rov·ing nystagmus (ro′ving). OCULAR NYSTAGMUS.

Rov·sing's sign (roʰw′sing) [N. T. *Rovsing,* Danish surgeon, 1862–1927]. A sign for acute appendicitis in which pressure over the left iliac fossa causes pain in the right iliac fossa.

Rowapraxin. A trademark for pipoxolan hydrochloride, a muscle relaxant.

Rowe diets [A. H. *Rowe,* U.S. physician, 1889–1971]. A regimen of elimination diets.

row·ing method. A former method of artificial respiration in which the patient's arms are alternately extended above the head and returned to the chest.

roy·al touch. The laying on of hands by a king, formerly believed to be efficacious in scrofula or king's evil.

Rown·tree-Ger·agh·ty test [L. G. *Rowntree,* U.S. physician, b. 1883; and J. T. *Geraghty,* U.S. physician, 1876–1924]. PHENOLSULFONPHTHALEIN TEST.

R.Q. Abbreviation for *respiratory quotient.*

-rrhachidia. See *-rachidia.*

-rrhachis [Gk. *rhachis,* backbone]. A combining form meaning (a) *vertebral column;* (b) *spinal cord.*

-rrhagia, -rrhage [Gk. *-rrhagia,* from *rhēgnynai,* to burst forth]. A combining form meaning *an abnormal or excessive discharge.*

-rrhaphy, -rrhaphia [Gk. *rhaphē,* sewing, suture, from *rhaptein,* to sew]. A combining form meaning *a sewing or suturing,* usually of an immediate or recent injury or laceration.

-rrhea, -rrhoea [Gk. *rhoia,* flow, flux, from *rhein,* to flow]. A combining form meaning *flow, discharge.*

-rrhexis [Gk. *rhēxis,* from *rhēgnynai,* to burst]. A combining form meaning *rupture, splitting.*

-rrhine, -rhine [Gk. *rhis, rhinos,* nose]. A combining form meaning *having a* (specified) *kind of nose.*

-rrhinus [Gk. *rhis, rhinos*]. A combining form meaning *nose, a condition of the nose,* or *an individual exhibiting such a condition.*

-rrhoea. See *-rrhea.*

R-R interval. The period of the electrocardiogram from one R wave to the next.

R.S.A. Right sacroanterior position of the fetus.

R.S.P. Right sacroposterior position of the fetus.

R(S)-T segment. S-T SEGMENT.

RSV, RS virus. Abbreviation for *respiratory syncytial virus.*

R. T. Registered technician; certification awarded to qualified x-ray technicians by the American Registry of Radiologic Technicians.

Ru Symbol for ruthenium.

rub·ber, *n.* 1. The prepared milk juice of several species of *Hevea;* CAOUTCHOUC. Syn. *India rubber, Pará rubber.* 2. *Informal.* CONDOM.

rubber bandage. A broad thin-walled elastic bandage, used to render an extremity bloodless; ESMARCH BANDAGE.

rubber dam. A thin sheet of rubber attached to a frame and used to isolate a tooth to protect it from moisture and contamination during restorative dentistry procedures.

rubbing alcohol. Any of a variety of preparations used as a rubefacient and containing a specially denatured ethyl alcohol, or isopropyl alcohol. It is poisonous.

ru·be·an·ic acid (roo″bee·an′ick). Dithiooxamide, $(CSNH_2)_2$, a histochemical reagent for copper, cobalt, and nickel.

ru·be·do (roo·bee′do) *n.* [L., redness, from *ruber,* red]. Any diffuse redness of the skin.

ru·be·fa·cient (roo″be·fay′shunt) *adj. & n.* [from L. *rubefacere, rubefaciens,* to make red]. 1. Causing redness of the skin. 2. Any substance that causes redness of the skin.

ru·be·fac·tion (roo″be·fack′shun) *n.* [L. *rubefacere,* to redden, from *ruber,* red, + *facere,* to make]. 1. Redness of the skin due to the action of an irritant. 2. The act of causing redness of the skin.

ru·bel·la (roo·bel′uh) *n.* [NL., from L. *rubellus,* reddish, from *ruber,* red]. An acute benign viral contagious disease of children and young adults characterized by fever, a pale pink rash, and posterior cervical lymphadenitis. Associated with fetal abnormalities when maternal infection occurs in early pregnancy. Syn. *epidemic roseola, French measles, German measles, röteln, three-day measles.*

rubella syndrome. Infection of the fetus by the mother with rubella virus during early pregnancy, resulting in a wide variety of severe congenital malformations, including cardiovascular defects, microcephaly, cataracts, deafness, encephalomyelitis, bony changes, and thrombocytopenia.

ru·bel·li·form (roo·bel′i·form) *adj.* [*rubella* + *-iform*]. Resembling rubella.

ru·be·o·la (roo·bee′o·luh) *n.* [NL., dim. of L. *rubeus,* red, reddish]. MEASLES (1).

ru·be·o·sis (roo″bee·o′sis) *n.* [L. *rubeus,* red, + *-osis*]. Redness, in particular red discoloration of the skin.

rubeosis iri·dis (eye′ri·dis). RUBEOSIS OF THE IRIS.

rubeosis iridis di·a·bet·i·ca (dye″a·bet′i·kuh). RUBEOSIS OF THE IRIS, in patients with diabetes.

rubeosis of the iris. Neovascularization present on the anterior surface of the iris, and the filtration angle. Seen in diabetic retinopathy, central retinal vein occlusion, and retinal detachment.

ru·ber (roo′bur) *n.,* fem. **ru·bra,** neut. **ru·brum.** [L.]. Red.

ru·bes·cence (roo·bes′unce) *n.* [L. *rubescere,* to grow red]. The state or quality of redness. —**rubes·cent** (·unt) *adj.*

ru·bid·a·zone (roo·bid′uh·zone) *n.* The antineoplastic agent benzoylhydrazone daunorubicin, a derivative of daunorubicin, active against acute myelogenous leukemia.

ru·bid·i·um (roo·bid′ee·um) *n.* [NL., from *rubidus,* red, reddish]. Rb=85.4678. An alkali metal, atomic number 37, resembling potassium in appearance.

ru·bi·do·my·cin (roo″bi·do·migh′sin) *n.* DAUNORUBICIN.

ru·big·i·nous (roo·bij′i·nus) *adj.* [L. *rubigo, rubiginis,* rust, + *-ous*]. Rust-colored.

ru·bi·jer·vine (roo″bi·jur′veen) *n.* An alkaloidal constituent, $C_{27}H_{43}NO_2$, being an alkanolamine, of *Veratrum viride* and *V. album;* it is practically inert physiologically.

ru·bin (roo′bin) *n.* BASIC FUCHSIN.

Ru·bin·stein-Tay·bi's syndrome [J. H. *Rubinstein,* U.S. pediatrician, b. 1925; and H. *Taybi,* U.S. pediatrician and radiologist, b. 1919]. A complex of multiple congenital defects of unknown cause, characterized by peculiar facies with a relatively small cranium, often a beaked nose, high arched palate, ocular abnormalities including downward slant of the eyes, strikingly broad flat thumbs and great toes, sometimes small stature, and mental and motor retardation.

Ru·bin test [I. C. *Rubin,* U.S. gynecologist, b. 1883]. A test for patency of the uterine tubes by means of insufflation with carbon dioxide.

Rub·ner's laws (roop′nur) [M. *Rubner,* German physiologist, 1854–1932]. 1. The law of constant energy consumption: the rapidity of growth is proportional to the metabolic rate. 2. The law of constant growth quotient: the same fractional part of total body energy (growth quotient) is used for growth.

Rubner's test [M. *Rubner*]. 1. The presence of carbon monoxide in blood is detected by lack of color change on exposure to lead acetate solution. 2. Lactose, maltose, and levulose are detected by their color reactions when urine is boiled with lead acetate solution and alkalinized.

ru·bor (roo′bor) *n.* [L.]. Redness due to inflammation.

rubr-, rubri-, rubro- [L. *ruber*]. A combining form meaning (a) *red;* (b) *pertaining to the red nucleus.*

ru·bres·e·rine (roo·bres′ur·een, ·in) *n.* A red decomposition product of physostigmine; it accounts for part of the color that develops in physostigmine solutions on aging and indicates a decrease in potency.

ru·bri·blast (roo′bri·blast) *n.* [*rubri-* + *-blast*]. PRONORMOBLAST.

ru·bri·cyte (roo′bri·site) *n.* [*rubri-* + *-cyte*]. BASOPHILIC NORMOBLAST.

ru·bri·uria (roo″bri·yoo′ree·uh) *n.* [*rubri-* + *-uria*]. Red discoloration of the urine.

rubro-. See *rubr-.*

ru·bro·bul·bar (roo″bro·bul′bur) *adj.* [*rubro-* + *bulbar*]. Pertaining to the red nucleus and the medulla oblongata.

rubrobulbar tract. A bundle of fibers which arises in the red nucleus, crosses almost immediately in the ventral tegmental decussation and ends in motor nuclei of the fifth and seventh cranial nerves and nucleus ambiguus and the motor centers of the uppermost cord levels. Syn. *crossed rubrospinal tract.*

ru·bro·ol·i·vary (roo″bro·ol′i·verr·ee) *adj.* [*rubro-* + *olivary*]. Pertaining to the red nucleus and the olive.

rubroolivary tract. A bundle of nerve fibers that runs from the red nucleus, via the central tegmental tract, to the homolateral inferior olivary nucleus.

ru·bro·re·tic·u·lar (roo″bro·re·tick′yoo·lur) *adj.* [*rubro-* + *reticular*]. Pertaining to the red nucleus and the reticular formation.

rubroreticular tract. The rubroreticular portion of a pathway which arises from the red nucleus, crosses the midline in the ventral tegmental decussation, swings laterally and caudally through the brainstem and enters the spinal cord ventral to the lateral corticospinal tract. Many of the fibers of this tract end in the reticular region of the brainstem, for relay to the spinal cord and possibly to the motor nuclei of the cranial nerves.

ru·bro·spi·nal (roo″bro·spye′nul) *adj.* [*rubro-* + *spinal*]. Pertaining to the red nucleus and the spinal cord.

rubrospinal tract. A nerve tract descending from the red nucleus into the spinal cord which, in man, has been largely replaced in function by the phylogenetically newer reticulospinal tract. Syn. *Monakow's bundle, fibers,* or *tract.* NA *tractus rubrospinalis.*

ru·bro·sta·sis (roo″bro·stay′sis) *n.* [*rubro-* + *stasis*]. PERISTASIS.

ru·bro·tha·lam·ic tract (roo″bro·thuh·lam′ick). Nerve fibers that arise in the red nucleus and project to the lateral ventral nucleus of the thalamus.

ru·brum scar·la·ti·num (roo′brum skahr″luh·tye′num) [L.]. SCARLET RED.

ru·by spot (roo′bee). PAPILLARY VARIX.

ruc·ta·tion (ruck·tay′shun) *n.* [L. *ructatio,* from *ructare,* to belch]. Eructation; BELCHING.

ruc·tus (ruck′tus) *n.* [L.]. A belching of gas from the stomach.

ructus hys·te·ri·cus (his·terr′i·kus). Hysterical belching, the gas escaping with a loud, sobbing, gurgling noise.

ru·di·ment (roo′di·munt) *n.* [L. *rudimentum,* first try, from *rudis,* rough, untried]. That which is but partially developed.

ru·di·men·ta·ry (roo″di·men′tuh·ree) *adj.* Undeveloped; unfinished; incomplete.

ru·di·men·tum (roo″di·men′tum) *n.*, pl. **rudimen·ta** (·tuh) [L.]. RUDIMENT.

rudimentum pro·ces·sus va·gi·na·lis (pro·ses′us vaj·i·nay′lis) [BNA]. Vestigium processus vaginalis (= VAGINAL LIGAMENT).

Rud's syndrome (roo'th) [E. *Rud*, Danish, 20th century]. SJÖGREN-LARSSON SYNDROME.

rue (roo) *n.* [OF., from L. *ruta*, from Gk. *rhytē*]. A plant, *Ruta graveolens*, of the family Rutaceae, yielding a volatile oil consisting chiefly of methyl nonyl ketone, $CH_3COC_9H_{19}$, and acting as a potent local irritant.

Ruf·fi·ni's cell, corpuscle, or **end organ** (roof·fee′nee) [A. *Ruffini*, Italian anatomist, 1864–1929]. A sensory end organ in the skin and adipose tissue made up of the terminal arborization of nerve fibers within a fibrous framework. It is believed to be a component of the proprioceptive sensory system.

ru·fous (roo′fus) *adj.* [L. *rufus*]. Reddish; ruddy.

ru·ga (roo′guh) *n.*, pl. **ru·gae** (·jee, ·gee) [L.]. A wrinkle, fold, elevation, or ridge, as in the mucosa of the stomach, vagina, and palate.

rugae va·gi·na·les (vaj·i·nay′leez) [NA]. Transverse folds of the mucous membrane of the vagina.

rug·ger jersey sign. The radiographic appearance of dense, transverse bands at the upper and lower margins of vertebral bodies with relatively radiolucent centers, as in renal rickets.

ru·gi·tus (roo′ji·tus) *n.* [L., rumbling, roaring, from *rugire*, to roar]. Rumbling of the intestines; borborygmus.

ru·gose (roo′goce) *adj.* [L. *rugosus*, wrinkled, from *ruga*, wrinkle]. Characterized by many folds.

ru·gos·i·ty (roo·gos′i·tee) *n.* [L. *rugositas*, from *rugosus*, wrinkled]. A condition exhibiting many folds in a tissue or integument.

ru·gous (roo′gus) *adj.* RUGOSE.

Ruhm·korff coil (room′korf) [H. D. *Ruhmkorff*, German physicist, 1823–1887]. An induction coil in which the secondary coil is fixed at the point of maximum intensity.

rule, *n.* [OF. *reule*, from L. *regula*, a model]. An established guide for action or procedure.

rule of impression priority. *In psychiatry,* a rule based on the theory that first impressions ordinarily tend to take emotional priority. This applies to the coloring and influencing of the individual's subsequent attitudes and patterns of reaction to the subject of the impression, or to repetitions of the first experience. See also *theory of antecedent conflicts.*

rule of nines. A rule for the estimate of the percentage of body surface area according to which the head and upper extremities each represent 9 percent, the trunk, anterior and posterior, and the lower extremities, each 18 percent, and the perineum 1 percent; useful in judging the severity and extent of burns.

rum·bling, *n.* BORBORYGMUS.

ru·men (roo′mun) *n.*, pl. **ru·mi·na** (·mi·nuh), **rumens** [L., throat, gullet]. *In veterinary medicine,* the first compartment of the stomach of the ruminant, where food is temporarily stored while undergoing fermentation prior to regurgitation and remastication. Syn. *paunch.*

ru·men·ot·o·my (roo″me·not′uh·mee) *n.* [*rumen* + *-tomy*]. A laparotomy in which the rumen is exposed and incised.

Ru·mex (roo′mecks) *n.* [L., sorrel]. A genus of plants of the Polygonaceae. Yellow dock, the root of *Rumex crispus*, has been used as a mild laxative and astringent.

ru·mi·nant (roo′mi·nunt) *n.* [L. *ruminare*, to chew the cud, from *rumen*, throat]. A cud-chewing animal, characterized by an arrangement of the forestomach whereby food is regurgitated and remasticated. Ruminants include all even-toed ungulates except swine and hippopotamuses.

ru·mi·na·tion (roo″mi·nay′shun) *n.* [L. *ruminatio*]. 1. A characteristic of ruminants in which food is regurgitated and remasticated in preparation for true digestion. 2. The voluntary regurgitation of food which has already reached the stomach, remastication, and swallowing a second time; occurs chiefly in emotionally disturbed younger children, and occasionally in mentally retarded and psychiatric patients. Syn. *merycism.* 3. *In psychiatry,* an obsessional preoccupation with a single idea or system of ideas which dominates the mind despite all efforts to dislodge it. Observed in anxiety states and other psychiatric disorders.

ru·mi·na·tive idea (roo″mi·nay′tiv). An idea pondered repeatedly. See also *fixed idea.*

Rum·mo's disease (roŏm′mo) [G. *Rummo*, Italian physician, 1853–1917]. CARDIOPTOSIS.

rump, *n.* [Scandinavian origin]. The region near the end of the backbone; BUTTOCKS.

Rum·pel-Leede phenomenon, sign, or **test** (roŏm·pel) [T. *Rumpel*, German surgeon, 1862–1923; and C. S. *Leede*, U.S. physician, b. 1882]. The production of an abnormally large number of petechiae on the forearm when a tourniquet is applied at slightly above diastolic pressure for 5 to 10 minutes to the upper arm; positive in disorders where there is an increased bleeding tendency due to increased capillary fragility or decreased number of platelets.

run, *v.* To discharge, as pus or purulent matter from a diseased part.

run-around, *n.* A paronychia extending completely around a nail.

r unit. ROENTGEN.

run·ning fit. CURSIVE EPILEPSY.

running pulse. A very weak, rapid pulse.

runt disease. A syndrome brought about by a graft-versus-host reaction, characterized in animals by runting, failure to thrive, lymph node atrophy, splenomegaly, hepatomegaly and sometimes death. See also *human runt disease.*

runting syndrome. RUNT DISEASE.

Run·yon groups. Four groups into which the atypical mycobacteria have been divided on the basis of growth rate and pigment production: Group I includes the photochromogens, which produce yellow pigment in light, Group II the scotochromogens, which produce orange pigment in light or dark, Group III the nonchromogens, which remain colorless in light or dark, and Group IV the rapid growers, nonchromogens which grow in three days.

Ruotte's operation. VENOPERITONEOSTOMY.

ru·pia (roo′pee·uh) *n.* [NL., from Gk. *rhypos*, filth]. An eruption on the skin characterized by the formation of large, dirty-brown, stratified, conic crusts that resemble oyster shell; commonly seen in syphilis and psoriasis. —**ru·pi·al** (·pee·ul) *adj.*

ru·po·pho·bia (roo″po·fo′bee·uh) *n.* [NL., from Gk. *rhypos*, filth, + *-phobia*]. SCATOPHOBIA.

rup·tio (rup′shee·o) *n.* [L.]. Rupture of a vessel or organ.

rup·ture (rup′chur) *n.* [L. *ruptura*, from *rumpere*, to break]. 1. A forcible tearing of a part, as rupture of the uterus, rupture of the urinary bladder. 2. HERNIA.

rup·tured, *adj.* Burst; broken; forcibly torn; affected with hernia.

ruptured disk. HERNIATED DISK.

ruptured intervertebral disk. HERNIATED DISK.

rural typhus. TSUTSUGAMUSHI DISEASE.

Rus·sell bodies [W. *Russell*, British pathologist, 1852–1940]. Hyaline eosinophilic globules 4 to 5 microns in diameter, occurring in the cytoplasm of plasma cells in chronic inflammatory exudates; once considered etiologic agents of disease, they are now thought to be particles of antibody globulin.

Russell dwarf [A. *Russell*, Scottish pediatrician, 20th century]. A dwarf characterized by low weight and short stature at birth despite normal gestation, anomalies of the head, face, and skeleton resembling those found in Silver's Syndrome but without the asymmetry, lean small muscles, often varying degrees of mental retardation, and sometimes ketotic hypoglycemia.

Russell's method. FRAME, RUSSELL, AND WILHELMI'S METHOD.

Russell's syndrome [A. *Russell*]. 1. DIENCEPHALIC SYNDROME (1). 2. RUSSELL DWARF.

Russell's viper [P. *Russell,* Irish physician, 1727-1805]. *VIPERA RUSSELLII.*

Rus·sel method. A colorimetric method for ammonia based on the reaction of phenol and hypochlorite with ammonia in alkaline solution to give an intense blue product.

Rus·sian autumnal encephalitis. JAPANESE B ENCEPHALITIS.

Russian Far East encephalitis. One of the Russian tick-borne complex.

Russian forest spring encephalitis. One of the Russian tick-borne complex.

Russian intermittent fever. TRENCH FEVER.

Russian spring-summer encephalitis. One of the Russian tick-borne complex.

Russian tick-borne complex or **encephalitides.** An aggregate of viral diseases of men and animals, widely distributed throughout Europe and Asia, transmitted by ticks of the family Ixodidae; characterized by fever, gastrointestinal disturbances, and hemorrhages or by fever and neurologic manifestations. See also *louping ill.*

rust, *n.* 1. A product consisting of the oxide, hydroxide, and carbonate of iron, formed on the surface of iron exposed to moist air. 2. Any of a group of parasitic fungi (Uredinales) causing discoloration on plants. They are common allergens.

Rust's disease (rōōst) [J. N. *Rust,* German surgeon, 1775-1840]. Tuberculous spondylitis of the cervical region.

Rust's phenomenon [J. N. *Rust*]. Use of the hands to support the head during change from recumbent to sitting position; seen in individuals with destructive lesions of the upper cervical vertebrae.

rus·ty sputum (rus'tee). Sputum colored by blood or various decomposition products of blood; seen chiefly in lobar pneumonia.

rut, *n.* [OF. *ruit,* from L. *rugitus,* roaring]. A period of heightened sexual excitement and its accompanying behavior in males, especially that occurring annually in wild ungulates. Compare *heat, estrus.*

Ru·ta·ce·ae (roo·tay'see·ee) *n.pl.* [NL., from L. *ruta,* rue]. A family of herbs, trees, and shrubs that includes the genus *Citrus.*

ru·ta·my·cin (ru"tuh·migh'sin) *n.* An antibiotic produced by *Streptomyces rutgersensis.*

Rut·gers 612. ETHOHEXADIOL.

ru·the·ni·um (roo·theen'ee·um) *n.* [L. *Ruthenia,* Russia]. Ru = 101.07. A metallic element, atomic number 44, of the platinum group.

ruthenium red. Ammoniated ruthenium oxychloride, $Ru(OH)Cl_2.3NH_3.H_2O$, a brownish-red powder used in microscopy as a stain and as a reagent for complexes containing carbohydrate, as pectin and gum.

ruth·er·ford (ruth'ur·furd) *n.* [E. *Rutherford,* British physicist, 1871-1937]. A unit of radioactivity representing 10^6 disintegrations per second. Abbreviated, rd.

Rutherford-Bohr atom model [E. *Rutherford* and N. H. D. *Bohr*]. A concept of atomic structure: the positive charge is located in a centrally located nucleus, negatively charged electrons, in elliptical orbits around the nucleus.

Ruth's method [C. E. *Ruth,* U.S. surgeon, 1861-1930]. A method of reduction of fracture of the femoral neck, a modification of Leadbetter's procedure.

ru·tin (roo'tin) *n.* Quercetin-3-rutinoside, $C_{27}H_{30}O_{16}$, a rhamnoglycoside that occurs in several plants; claimed to decrease capillary fragility in patients with increased fragility. Syn. *eldrin, melin, myrticolorin, phytomelin, violaquercitrin.*

ru·tin·ose (roo'tin·oce, ·oze) *n.* A disaccharide, $C_{12}H_{22}O_{10}$, produced by enzymic or controlled acid hydrolysis of rutin or hesperidin. Rutinose yields one molecule each of glucose and rhamnose on hydrolysis.

r wave. REGURGITANT WAVE.

R wave of the electrocardiogram. The initial positive deflection of the QRS complex of the electrocardiogram.

R' wave. The second positive deflection of the QRS complex of the electrocardiogram, following an R wave (positive) and an S wave (negative).

Ry·a·nia (rye·ay'nee·uh) *n.* A genus of tropical American shrubs and trees, of which the wood of several species is insecticidal.

ry·an·o·dine (rye·an'o·deen, ·din) *n.* An alkaloid, $C_{25}H_{35}NO_9$, isolated from the stem and root of *Ryania speciosa* Vahl.; has insecticidal activity.

Rydygier's operation [L. von *Rydygier,* German surgeon, 1850-1920]. A method of fixation of the spleen in a peritoneal pouch.

rye, *n.* The plant *Secale cereale* and its grain. The grain is used for making bread and whisky.

rye smut. ERGOT.

Ry·tand-Lip·sitch syndrome [D. A. *Rytand,* U.S. internist, b. 1909; L. S. *Lipsitch,* U.S. internist, b. 1912]. Complete atrioventricular block secondary to destruction of the central portion of the cardiac conducting system by extension of a calcific retrogressive process from the mitral valve annulus.

S

S Symbol for sulfur.

S Abbreviation for (a) *signa,* sign; (b) *spherical; (c) spherical lens;* (d) smooth variant in bacteria.

S, s Symbol for Svedberg sedimentation unit.

Ŝ *In electrocardiology,* symbol for spatial vector.

S_1 or **SI.** Symbol for first heart sound.

S_2 or **SII.** Symbol for second heart sound.

S_3 or **SIII.** Symbol for third heart sound.

S_3. VENTRICULAR GALLOP.

S_4 or **SIV.** Symbol for fourth heart sound.

S_4. ATRIAL GALLOP.

S_f Symbol for Svedberg flotation unit.

S [abbreviation of L. *sinister,* left]. According to the Cahn-Ingold-Prelog sequencing rules, a specification of the configuration of a stereoisomeric molecule. Not to be confused with *levo-* (*laevo-*). Contr. *R.*

s. Abbreviation for (a) *sinister,* left; (b) *semis,* half.

-s [plural noun suffix]. A suffix which, when attached to an adjective form ending in -ic, designates *a field of study or practice,* as pediatrics, genetics, obstetrics.

SA, S.A. Abbreviation for *sinoatrial.*

Sa Symbol for samarium.

sab·a·dil·la (sab″uh·dil′uh) *n.* [Sp. *cebadilla,* from *cebada,* barley]. The dried ripe seeds of *Schoenocaulon officinale* (*Asagraea officinalis*) that contain various alkaloids, and preparations of which were formerly used to destroy vermin in the hair.

sa·bad·i·nine (sa·bad′i·neen, ·nin) *n.* CEVINE.

sa·bal (say′bal) *n.* SERENOA.

Sa·ba·ne·ev-Frank operation (suh·bah·nʸe′yᵉf) [I. F. *Sabaneev,* Russian surgeon, 19th century; and R. *Frank*]. FRANK'S OPERATION.

saber tibia or **shin.** Anterior bowing and thickening of the tibia due to periostitis caused by congenital syphilis or yaws.

Sa·be·thes (sa·bee′theez) *n.* A genus of mosquitoes which includes *Sabethes chloropterus,* a species implicated in the transmission of sylvan yellow fever.

Sa·be·thi·ni (sab″e·thigh′nigh, ·theen′ee) *n.pl.* Mosquitoes of a tribe of Diptera known to transmit sylvan yellow fever.

Sa·bin-Feld·man dye test. DYE TEST.

Sabin oral poliomyelitis vaccine [A. B. *Sabin,* U.S. microbiologist, b. 1906]. A poliovirus vaccine (live, oral).

Sa·bou·raud's agar or **broth** (saʰ·boo·ro′) [R. J. A. *Sabouraud,* French dermatologist, 1864–1938]. A liquid medium favorable for the cultivation of fungi, containing 4% glucose or maltose and peptone.

sabre tibia. SABER TIBIA.

sab·u·lous (sab′yoo·lus) *adj.* [L. *sabul*um, coarse sand, + *-ous*]. Gritty; sandy.

sac, *n.* [F., sack, bag]. A pouch; a baglike covering of a natural cavity, or of a hernia, cyst, or tumor.

sacchar-, sacchari-, saccharo- [Gk. *sakchar,* sugar, from Skr. *śarkarā,* sugar, gravel]. A combining form meaning (a) *sugar;* (b) *saccharine.*

sac·cha·rase (sack′uh·race, ·raze) *n.* [*sacchar-* + *-ase*]. An enzyme occurring in plants and microorganisms, particularly yeasts, and capable of hydrolyzing disaccharides to monosaccharides; more specifically, the enzyme which is responsible for hydrolysis of sucrose to dextrose and levulose. Syn. *invertase, invertin, sucrase.*

sac·cha·rate (sack′uh·rate) *n.* A salt of saccharic acid.

sac·cha·rat·ed (sack′uh·ray″tid) *adj.* Containing sugar.

saccharated iron carbonate. A preparation of ferrous carbonate and sugar; has been used as a nonastringent hematinic.

saccharated iron oxide. A water-soluble preparation of ferric oxide and sugar; has been used as a nonastringent hematinic. Syn. *soluble ferric oxide, eisenzucker.*

sac·char·eph·i·dro·sis (sack″ur·ef″i·dro′sis) *n.* [*sacchar-* + *ephidrosis*]. A form of hyperhidrosis, characterized by the excretion of sugar in the sweat.

sacchari-. See *sacchar-.*

sac·char·ic acid (sa·kăr′ick). 1. A product obtained by oxidizing an aldose with nitric acid so that both the aldehyde and primary alcohol groups are converted to carboxyl groups. 2. $HOOC(CHOH)_4COOH$; the saccharic acid obtained by oxidation of D-glucose with nitric acid. Syn. *D-glucosaccharic acid.*

sac·cha·ride (sack′uh·ride) *n.* [*sacchar-* + *-ide*]. A compound of a base with sugar; a sucrate.

sac·char·i·fy (sa·kăr′i·fye) *v.* 1. To make sweet. 2. To convert into sugar. **—sac·char·i·fi·ca·tion** (sa·kar″i·fi·kay′shun) *n.*

sac·cha·rim·e·ter (sack″uh·rim′e·tur) *n.* [*sacchari-* + *-meter*]. An apparatus for determining the amount of sugar in solutions. It may be in the form of a hydrometer, which indicates the concentration of sugar by the specific gravity of the solution; a polarimeter, which indicates the concentration of sugar by the number of degrees of rotation of the plane of polarization; or a fermentation tube, which indicates the concentration of sugar by the amount of gas formed during fermentation.

sac·cha·rim·e·try (sack″uh·rim′e·tree) *n.* [*sacchari-* + *-metry*]. The determination of the sugar content of a solution from its optical activity.

sac·cha·rin (sack′uh·rin) *n.* [*sacchar-* + *-in*]. 1,2-Benzisothiazolin-3-one 1,1-dioxide, $C_7H_5NO_3S$, a noncaloric sweetening agent, generally used in the form of sodium saccharin, which is much more soluble in water than is saccharin. Syn. *benzosulfimide, gluside.*

sac·cha·rine (sack'uh·rin, ·reen, ·rine) *adj.* [*sacchar-* + *-ine*]. 1. Having an excessively sweet taste. 2. Like or pertaining to sugar.

saccharin sodium. SODIUM SACCHARIN.

saccharo-. See *sacchar-*.

sac·cha·ro·ga·lac·tor·rhea, sac·cha·ro·ga·lac·tor·rhoea (sack''uh·ro·guh·lack''to·ree'uh) *n.* [*saccharo-* + *galactorrhea*]. The secretion of milk that contains an excess of sugar.

sac·cha·ro·lyt·ic (sack''uh·ro·lit'ick) *adj.* [*saccharo-* + *-lytic*]. Of or pertaining to metabolic breakdown of sugars.

sac·cha·ro·me·tab·o·lism (sack''uh·ro·me·tab'uh·liz·um) *n.* [*saccharo-* + *metabolism*]. The metabolism of sugars. —**saccharo·met·a·bol·ic** (·met''uh·bol'ick) *adj.*

sac·cha·rom·e·ter (sack''uh·rom'e·tur) *n.* SACCHARIMETER.

Sac·cha·ro·my·ces (sack''uh·ro·migh'seez) *n.* [*saccharo-* + *-myces*]. A genus of yeasts which includes baker's and brewer's yeasts.

Saccharomyces hom·i·nis (hom'i·nis). *CRYPTOCOCCUS NEOFORMANS.*

sac·cha·ro·my·ce·tic (sack''uh·ro·migh·see'tick, ·migh·set'ick) *adj.* Pertaining to or caused by *Saccharomyces.*

sac·cha·ro·my·co·sis (sack''uh·ro·migh·ko'sis) *n.* [*Saccharomyces* + *-osis*]. A pathologic condition due to yeasts or *Saccharomyces.*

sac·char·o·pine (sa·kăr'o·peen) *n.* L-*N*-(5-Amino-5-carboxypentyl)glutamic acid, $C_{11}H_{20}N_2O_6$, an intermediate in the synthesis of lysine in *Saccharomyces,* and also an intermediate in the degradation of lysine by mammalian liver.

sac·cha·ro·pi·nu·ria (sack''uh·ro·pi·new'ree·uh) *n.* [*saccharopine* + *-uria*]. A rare, inborn error of amino acid metabolism, probably of lysine degradation; clinically associated with mental retardation and chemically characterized by an abnormally large amount of saccharopine in the urine.

sac·cha·ror·rhea, sac·cha·ror·rhoea (sack''uh·ro·ree'uh) *n.* [*saccharo-* + *-rrhea*]. GLYCOSURIA.

sac·cha·rose (sack'uh·roce, ·roze) *n.* 1. SUCROSE. 2. A generic term sometimes applied to disaccharides, less frequently to trisaccharides.

sac·cha·ro·su·ria (sack''uh·ro·sue'ree·uh) *n.* [*saccharose* + *-uria*]. The presence of saccharose in the urine.

sac·cha·rum (sack'uh·rum) *n.* [ML., sugar]. SUCROSE.

sacci. Plural of *saccus* (= SAC).

sac·ci·form (sack'si·form) *adj.* [*saccus* + *-iform*]. Resembling a sac.

sacciform recess of the wrist. An elongation of the synovial membrane of the wrist joint extending between the radius and ulna at their distal articulation. NA *recessus sacciformis articulationis radioulnaris distalis.*

sac·cu·lar (sack'yoo·lur) *adj.* [*saccule* + *-ar*]. Sac-shaped.

saccular aneurysm. BERRY ANEURYSM.

saccular gland. ALVEOLAR GLAND.

sac·cu·lat·ed (sack'yoo·lay''tid) *adj.* Divided into small sacs.

sacculated bladder. A condition due to overdistension of the bladder, bladder outlet obstruction, or neurogenic disease of the bladder; pouches in which urine may be held are formed by the forcing out of the mucous coat between the muscular bundles. See also *trabeculated bladder.*

sacculated bronchiectasis. Bronchiectasis characterized by irregularly dilated sacs or pockets.

sac·cu·la·tion (sack''yoo·lay'shun) *n.* 1. The state of being sacculated. 2. The formation of small sacs.

sac·cule (sack'yool) *n.* [L. *sacculus,* small bag]. 1. A small sac. 2. The smaller of two vestibular sacs of the membranous labyrinth of the ear. NA *sacculus.*

saccule of the larynx. A blindly ending diverticulum of mucous membrane extending from the laryngeal ventricle upward between the vestibular fold and the inner surface of the thyroid cartilage. Syn. *appendix of the laryngeal ventricle.* NA *sacculus laryngis.*

sacculi. Plural of *sacculus.*

sacculi al·ve·o·la·res (al·vee·o·lair'eez) [NA]. ALVEOLAR SACS.

sac·cu·lo·coch·le·ar (sack''yoo·lo·kock'lee·ur) *adj.* [*saccule* + *cochlear*]. Pertaining to the saccule of the vestibule and the cochlea.

sacculocochlear canal. DUCTUS REUNIENS.

sac·cu·lus (sack'yoo·lus) *n.,* pl. **saccu·li** (·lye) [L., small sack, dim. of *saccus*]. 1. SACCULE (1). 2. [NA] SACCULE (2).

sacculus la·ryn·gis (la·rin'jis) [NA]. SACCULE OF THE LARYNX.

sac·cus (sack'us) *n.,* pl. **sac·ci** (·sigh) [L., sack, bag, from Gk. *sakkos*]. SAC.

saccus con·junc·ti·vae (kon·junk·tye'vee) [NA]. CONJUNCTIVAL SAC.

saccus en·do·lym·pha·ti·cus (en·do·lim·fat'i·kus) [NA]. ENDOLYMPHATIC SAC.

saccus la·cri·ma·lis (lack·ri·may'lis) [NA]. LACRIMAL SAC.

saccus om·pha·lo·en·te·ri·cus (om·fuh·lo·en·terr'i·kus). YOLK SAC.

saccus va·gi·na·lis (vaj·i·nay'lis). VAGINAL PROCESS OF THE PERITONEUM.

Sachs' disease (sacks) [B. P. *Sachs,* U.S. neurologist, 1858–1944]. TAY-SACHS DISEASE.

Sachs-Ge·or·gi test (zahks, gey·or'gee) [H. *Sachs,* German bacteriologist, 1877–1945; and W. *Georgi,* German bacteriologist, 1889–1920]. A variation of the Wassermann test for the diagnosis of syphilis.

sacr-, sacro-. A combining form meaning *sacrum, sacral.*

sacra. Plural of *sacrum.*

sa·cral (say'krul, sack'rul) *adj.* [*sacr-* + *-al*]. Of or pertaining to the sacrum.

sacral ala. ALA OF THE SACRUM.

sacral block. Anesthesia induced by injection of the anesthetic agent into the sacral canal, usually through the caudal hiatus.

sacral bursa. A bursa found in the aged, over the sacrococcygeal articulation or over the spine of the fourth or fifth sacral vertebra.

sacral canal. The continuation of the vertebral canal in the sacrum. NA *canalis sacralis.*

sacral crest. A series of eminences on the posterior surface of the sacrum. There is a median one representing the spines of the sacral vertebrae, and a lateral one on either side representing the articular facets. See also *crista sacralis intermedia, crista sacralis lateralis, crista sacralis mediana.*

sacral dimple. COCCYGEAL FOVEOLA.

sacral flexure. The curve of the rectum in front of the sacrum; its concavity is directed anteriorly. NA *flexura sacralis recti.*

sa·cral·gia (say·kral'jee·uh) *n.* [*sacr-* + *-algia*]. Pain in the region of the sacrum.

sacral hiatus. The lower or caudal opening of the sacral canal. NA *hiatus sacralis.*

sacral index. HIERIC INDEX.

sa·cral·iza·tion (say''krul·i·zay'shun) *n.* Fusion of the sacrum to the fifth and sometimes the fourth lumbar vertebra, leading to proneness to rupture of the disk between the fourth and fifth lumbar vertebrae. —**sa·cral·ize** (say'krul·ize) *v.*

sacral nerves. The nerves (there are five pairs) attached at the sacral segments of the cord, which innervate by dorsal rami the muscles and skin of the lower back and sacral region. By ventral rami, the sacral plexus supplies muscles and skin of the lower extremity and perineum, and branches to the hypogastric and pelvic plexuses supplying the pelvic viscera and the genitalia. NA *nervi sacrales.* See also Table of Nerves in the Appendix.

sacral perineurial cyst. A cyst found on the posterior sacral or coccygeal nerves or nerve roots in the extradural portion of the cauda, arising as an outpouching between the arachnoid and the perineurium.

sacral plexus. A nerve plexus usually formed from a small part of the ventral ramus of the fourth lumbar nerve, the ventral rami of the fifth lumbar and first sacral nerves, and part of the ventral rami of the second and third sacral nerves. NA *plexus sacralis.*

sacral promontory. PROMONTORY OF THE SACRUM.

sacral tuberosity. A rough area on the posterior surface of the sacrum, bearing three deep, uneven impressions for attachment of the posterior sacroiliac ligaments. NA *tuberositas sacralis.*

sa·crec·to·my (say·kreck'tuh·mee) *n.* [*sacr-* + *-ectomy*]. Excision of part of the sacrum.

sacred bark. CASCARA SAGRADA.

sacro-. See *sacr-*.

sa·cro·an·te·ri·or (say"kro·an·teer'ee·ur) *adj.* [*sacro-* + *anterior*]. Of or pertaining to a fetal position with the sacrum directed forward.

sa·cro·coc·cyg·e·al (say"kro·kock·sij'ee·ul, sack"ro·) *adj.* [*sacro-* + *coccygeal*]. Pertaining to the sacrum and coccyx.

sacrococcygeal cyst. PILONIDAL CYST.

sacrococcygeal fistula. A fistula communicating with a dermoid cyst in the coccygeal region.

sacrococcygeal ligament. Any of the various ligaments connecting the sacrum and coccyx; specifically, the deep dorsal sacrococcygeal ligament (NA *ligamentum sacrococcygeum dorsale profundum*), which is the continuation of the posterior longitudinal ligament, the superficial sacrococcygeal ligament (NA *ligamentum sacrococcygeum dorsale superficiale*), which is the continuation of the supraspinal ligament, the lateral sacrococcygeal ligament (NA *ligamentum sacrococcygeum laterale*), which connects the transverse process of the first coccygeal vertebra with the lateral lower edge of the sacrum, or the ventral sacrococcygeal ligament (NA *ligamentum sacrococcygeum ventrale*), which is the continuation of the anterior longitudinal ligament.

sacrococcygeal notch. The lateral notch at the point of union of the coccyx and sacrum.

sa·cro·coc·cy·ge·us (say"kro·kock·sij'ee·us, sack"ro·) *n.* One of two inconstant thin muscles extending from the lower sacral vertebrae to the coccyx.

sacrococcygeus anterior. SACROCOCCYGEUS VENTRALIS.

sacrococcygeus dor·sa·lis (dor·say'lis). An inconstant thin muscle on the posterior surfaces of the sacrum and coccyx, lying beneath the superficial layer of the sacrotuberous ligament. NA *musculus sacrococcygeus dorsalis.* See also Table of Muscles in the Appendix.

sacrococcygeus posterior. SACROCOCCYGEUS DORSALIS.

sacrococcygeus ven·tra·lis (ven·tray'lis). An inconstant thin muscle on the anterior surfaces of the sacrum and coccyx, inserted into the anterior sacrococcygeal ligament. NA *musculus sacrococcygeus ventralis.* See also Table of Muscles in the Appendix.

sa·cro·cox·al·gia (say"kro·kock·sal'jee·uh, sack"ro·) *n.* [*sacro-* + *cox-* + *-algia*]. SACROILIAC DISEASE.

sa·cro·cox·i·tis (say"kro·kock·sigh'tis, sack"ro·) *n.* [*sacro-* + *cox-* + *-itis*]. SACROILIAC DISEASE.

sa·cro·dyn·ia (say"kro·din'ee·uh, sack"ro·) *n.* [*sacr-* + *-odynia*]. Pain in the sacrum.

sa·cro·gen·i·tal fold (say"kro·jen'i·tul). RECTOVESICAL PLICA.

sa·cro·il·i·ac (sack"ro·il'ee·ack, say"kro·) *adj.* Pertaining to the sacrum and the ilium.

sacroiliac articulation. The joint between the sacrum and the ilium. NA *articulatio sacroiliaca.* See also Table of Synovial Joints and Ligaments in the Appendix.

sacroiliac disease. 1. Inflammatory disease of the sacroiliac articulation. 2. Formerly, chronic tuberculous infection of the joint.

sacroiliac ligament. See *dorsal, interosseous,* and *ventral sacroiliac ligament.*

sa·cro·lum·ba·lis (say"kro·lum·bay'lis, sack"ro·) *n.* ILIOCOSTALIS LUMBORUM.

sa·cro·lum·bar (say"kro·lum'bur, ·bahr, sack"ro·) *adj.* LUMBOSACRAL.

sacrolumbar angle. SACROVERTEBRAL ANGLE.

sa·cro·per·i·ne·al (say"kro·perr"i·nee'ul, sack"ro·) *adj.* Pertaining to the sacrum and the perineum.

sa·cro·pos·te·ri·or (say"kro·pos·teer'ee·ur) *adj.* [*sacro-* + *posterior*]. Characterizing a fetal position with the sacrum directed backward.

sa·cro·pu·bic (say"kro·pew'bick, sack"ro·) *adj.* Pertaining to the sacrum and the pubis.

sacropubic diameter. ANTEROPOSTERIOR DIAMETER (2).

sa·cro·sci·at·ic (say"kro·sigh·at'ick, sack"ro·) *adj.* [*sacro-* + *sciatic*]. Pertaining to the sacrum and the ischium.

sa·cro·spi·na·lis (say"kro·spye·nay'lis, sack"ro·) *n.* ERECTOR SPINAE.

sa·cro·spi·nous (say"kro·spye'nus, sack"ro·) *adj.* Pertaining to the sacrum and the spine of the ischium.

sacrospinous ligament. A thin triangular band running from the spine of the ischium medially to the lateral margin of the sacrum and coccyx. NA *ligamentum sacrospinale.* See also Plate 2.

sa·cro·tu·ber·ous (say"kro·tew'bur·us, sack"ro·) *adj.* Pertaining to the sacrum and the ischial tuberosity.

sacrotuberous ligament. A ligament extending from the sacrum, coccyx, and posterior iliac spines to the tuberosity of the ischium. NA *ligamentum sacrotuberale.* See also Plate 2.

sa·cro·uter·ine (say"kro·yoo'tur·in, ·ine, sack"ro·) *adj.* Pertaining to the sacrum and the uterus; uterosacral.

sa·cro·ver·te·bral (say"kro·vur'te·brul, sack"ro·) *adj.* Of or pertaining to the sacrum and a vertebra or vertebrae.

sacrovertebral angle. The angle the sacrum forms with the last lumbar vertebra.

sa·crum (say'krum, L. sack'rum) *n.*, genit. **sa·cri** (·krye), pl. **sa·cra** (·kruh) [L. *os sacrum,* lit., sacred bone, translation of Gk. *hieron osteon*]. A curved triangular bone composed of five united vertebrae, situated between the last lumbar vertebra above, the coccyx below, and the hipbones on each side, and forming the posterior boundary of the pelvis. NA *os sacrum.* See also Table of Bones in the Appendix and Plates 1, 2, 14.

sac·to·sal·pinx (sack"to·sal'pinks) *n.* [Gk. *saktos,* stuffed, + *salpinx*]. HYDROSALPINX.

sad·dle, *n.* 1. Any of various structures or surfaces shaped like, or suggestive of, a riding saddle. 2. *In dentistry,* the part of the denture that supports the artificial teeth, or receives support, either from the abutment teeth or the residual ridge, or both.

saddle area. The part of the buttocks surrounding the anus, together with the perineum (2) and the upper inner aspects of the thigh.

sad·dle·back, *n.* LORDOSIS.

saddleback temperature curve. A temperature curve characterized by a fever followed by a remission and a second bout of fever.

saddle block. Sensory loss in the saddle area which occurs in spinal or caudal anesthesia.

saddle distribution. Nerve distribution to the saddle area.

saddle embolus. An embolus lodged at the bifurcation of an artery, narrowing or occluding both branches.

saddle joint. A synovial joint in which the opposing surfaces are reciprocally concavoconvex. NA *articulatio sellaris.*

sad·dle·nose, *n.* A nose with a depression in the bridge due to loss of the septum.

saddle thrombus. A U- or Y-shaped thrombus straddling the bifurcation of a vessel. Syn. *riding thrombus.*

saddle ulcer. A peptic ulcer which has become elongated so that it partially encircles the lesser curvature of the stomach.

sa·dism (say'diz·um, sad'iz·um) *n.* [D. A. F. de *Sade,* French author, 1740–1814]. Sexual perversion in which pleasure is derived from inflicting cruelty upon another. Contr. *masochism.* —**sa·dist** (·dist) *n.;* **sa·dis·tic** (sa·dis'tick) *adj.*

sa·do·mas·o·chism (say"do·mas'o·kiz·um, sad"o·) *n.* The coexistence of sadism and masochism, i.e., both aggressiveness and passivity in social and sexual relationships; a strong tendency to hurt others and to invite being hurt.

Saeng·er's operation (zeng'ur) [M. *Saenger,* German gynecologist, 1853-1903]. Classic cesarean section by longitudinal abdominal incision, with exteriorization of the uterus and extraction of the fetus before returning the uterus to the pelvis.

SAF Abbreviation for *serum accelerator factor* (= FACTOR VII).

safe period. The nonovulatory phase of the menstrual cycle, when conception cannot occur. Since the time of ovulation is variable in different women, the safe period is also variable.

safe·ty glasses. Shatter-resistant or nonsplinterable eyeglasses with plastic, heat-treated, or laminated lenses.

saf·fron (saf'run) *n.* [Ar. *za'farān,* saffron]. CROCUS.

saf·ra·nin (saf'ruh·nin) *n.* SAFRANINE.

safranine (saf'ruh·neen, ·nin) *n.* 2,8-Diamino-3,7-dimethyl-10-phenylphenazonium chloride, a water- and alcohol-soluble basic dye used extensively as a nuclear stain and as a counterstain for gram-negative bacteria.

saf·ra·no·phil (saf'ruh·no·fil) *adj.* Staining readily with safranine.

saf·ra·no·phile (saf'ruh·no·fil, ·file) *adj.* SAFRANOPHIL.

saf·rol (saf'rol) *n.* SAFROLE.

saf·role (saf'role) *n.* 4-Allyl-1,2-methylenedioxybenzene, $C_{10}H_{10}O_2$, the preponderant liquid constituent of sassafras oil, present also in other volatile oils; used as a flavor.

sa·fu (sah'foo) *n.* A reticulated vitiligo of the legs, seen in the Pacific area; possibly a form of yaws.

sage, *n.* SALVIA.

sage·brush, *n.* Any of several members of the genus *Artemisia;* its pollen is among the more important causes of seasonal rhinitis in the Mountain and Pacific states.

sage femme (sahzh fam) [F., lit., wise woman]. MIDWIFE.

sag·it·tal (saj'i·tul) *adj.* [L. *sagitta,* arrow, + *-al*]. 1. Comparable to an arrow, as the sagittal suture. 2. Of or pertaining to the sagittal suture. 3. Of a plane or section through the body, median; bisecting the body into a right and a left half. 4. More broadly, either median (midsagittal) or parallel to the median (parasagittal).

sagittal axis of the eye. VISUAL AXIS.

sagittal diameter of the skull. A diameter joining the glabella and the external occipital protuberance. Syn. *inferior longitudinal diameter.*

sagittal fontanel. A fontanel occasionally found in the sagittal suture, about midway between the anterior and posterior fontanels.

sagittal plane. 1. The median plane of a vertebrate body. 2. Any plane parallel to the median plane. 3. *In electrocardiography* and *vectorcardiography,* the projection of the Z or anteroposterior axis.

sagittal sinus. 1. INFERIOR SAGITTAL SINUS. 2. SUPERIOR SAGITTAL SINUS.

sagittal sulcus. A shallow groove in the midline on the cerebral surface of the skull, lodging the superior sagittal sinus.

sagittal suture. The site of union between the superior or sagittal borders of the parietal bones. NA *sutura sagittalis.*

Sagnac rays. RAYS OF SAGNAC.

sa·go (say'go) *n.* [Malay *sagu*]. A starch derived from the pith of certain East Indian and Malaysian palms; used as a food and as a demulcent.

sago spleen. A spleen in which amyloid is present in the follicles showing on section numerous small glassy areas transmitting the red color of the spleen.

sag·u·lum (sag'yoo·lum) *n.* [L., dim. of *sagum,* mantle, cloak]. A cell-poor layer of the superficial gray matter lateral to the inferior colliculus.

Sah·li method (zah'lee) [H. *Sahli,* Swiss physician, 1856-1933]. An acid hematin method for hemoglobin, in which the acid hematin solution is diluted in a special graduated tube by addition of water drop by drop until it matches a glass standard.

Sahli test [H. *Sahli*]. A known mixture of water, salt, flour, and butter is given to a patient, and after an hour his stomach is aspirated. Measurement of volume, acidity, and fat content permit assessment of gastric functional capacity.

Sahyun method. A method for amino acids based on the color developed by the reaction between amino acids and β-naphthoquinone-4-sulfonic acid in alkaline solution. Heating develops the color.

sailor's skin. A condition seen in exposed areas of the skin due to chronic actinic exposure. There is pigmentation and keratosis, frequently leading to squamous cell carcinoma. Syn. *farmer's skin.*

Sai·mi·ri (sigh·mirr'ee) *n.* [Pg. *saimirim,* from Tupi *çai miri,* little monkey]. A genus of the Cebidae comprising the squirrel monkeys.

Saint Agatha's disease. Any disease of the female breast.

Saint Agnan's disease. RINGWORM.

Saint Aman's disease. PELLAGRA.

Saint Anthony's dance. SYDENHAM'S CHOREA.

Saint Anthony's fire. 1. ERYSIPELAS. 2. ERGOTISM.

Saint Avertin's disease. EPILEPSY.

Saint Blaize's disease. PERITONSILLAR ABSCESS.

St. Clair's method. FARLEY, ST. CLAIR, AND REISINGER'S METHOD.

Saint Erasmus' disease. COLIC.

Saint Fiacre's disease. HEMORRHOIDS.

Saint Gervasius' disease. RHEUMATISM.

Saint Giles' disease. LEPROSY.

Saint Gothard's disease. ANCYLOSTOMIASIS.

Saint Guy's dance or **disease.** SYDENHAM'S CHOREA.

Saint Ignatius' itch. PELLAGRA.

St. Louis encephalitis [after *St. Louis,* Missouri, where it occurred as an epidemic]. A mosquito-borne arbovirus infection of the central nervous system, occurring in central and western United States and in Florida.

Saint Main's evil. SCABIES.

Saint Martin's disease. DIPSOMANIA.

Saint Roch's disease. BUBONIC PLAGUE.

Saint Sebastian's disease. PLAGUE.

Saint Valentine's disease. EPILEPSY.

Saint Vitus' dance. SYDENHAM'S CHOREA.

Saint Zachary's disease. MUTISM.

Sakel's method. [M. J. *Sakel,* U.S. psychiatrist, 1900-1957]. INSULIN SHOCK THERAPY.

sal, *n.* [L.]. 1. SALT. 2. Any substance resembling salt.

sa·laam convulsion, seizure, or **spasm** (sa·lahm', sa·lam'). INFANTILE SPASM.

sal am·mo·ni·ac (uh·mo'nee·ack) [L. *sal ammoniacus,* from Gk. *ammōniakos halas,* lit., Ammon's salt, after a temple of Ammon in Egypt near which it was obtained]. AMMONIUM CHLORIDE.

sal·an·tel (sal'an·tel) *n.* 3'-Chloro-4'-(*p*-chlorobenzoyl)-3,5-diiodosalicylanilide, $C_{20}H_{11}Cl_2I_2NO_3$, an antibacterial.

Salbutamol. A trademark for albuterol, a β_2-receptor bronchodilator.

sal·co·lex (sal'ko·lecks) *n.* A 2:1 compound of choline salicylate with magnesium sulfate, used as an analgesic, anti-inflammatory, antipyretic.

sal·ep (sal'ep, suh·lep') *n.* [Ar. *saḥlab,* supposedly from *khuṣa th-tha'lab,* fox's testes]. The dried tubers of various species of the genus *Orchis* and the genus *Eulophia.* Used as a food, like sago and tapioca, or as a demulcent.

sal·eth·a·mide (sal·eth'uh·mide) *n.* *N*-[2-(Diethylamino)ethyl]salicylamide, $C_{13}H_{20}N_2O_2$, an analgesic; used as the maleate salt.

sal·i·cin (sal'i·sin) *n.* Salicyl alcohol glucoside, $C_{13}H_{18}O_7$; has been used as an analgesic.

salicyl-, salicylo-. A combining form meaning *salicylic* or *salicylate.*

sal·i·cyl (sal'i·sil) *n.* [L. *salix, salicis,* willow, + *-yl*]. 1. The radical, $HOC_6H_4CO—$ of salicylic acid. Syn. *salicylyl.*

2. The radical HOC_6H_4— (*ortho*). 3. The radical $HOC_6H_4CH_2$—.

salicyl alcohol. *o*-Hydroxybenzyl alcohol, $HOC_6H_4CH_2OH$, a local anesthetic. Syn. *saligenin.*

sal·i·cyl·am·ide (sal″i-sil-am′ide, sal″i-sil′uh-mide) *n.* *o*-Hydroxybenzamide, $HOC_6H_4CONH_2$, an analgesic, antipyretic, and antirheumatic drug.

sal·i·cyl·an·i·lide (sal″i-sil-an′i-lide) *n.* *N*-Phenylsalicylamide, $C_6H_5NHCOC_6H_4OH$, an antifungal agent useful externally in the treatment of tinea capitis due to *Microsporum audouini.*

sa·li·cy·late (sa-lis′i-late, -lut, sal′i-si-late, sal″i-sil′ate) *n.* A salt or ester of salicylic acid.

salicylate meglumine. *N*-Methylglucamine salicylate, $C_7H_{17}NO_5.C_7H_6O_3$, an antirheumatic analgesic.

sal·i·cyl·azo·sul·fa·pyr·i·dine (sal″i-sil-ay″zo-sul″fuh-pirr′i-deen) *n.* SULFASALAZINE.

sal·i·cyl·ic acid (sal″i-sil′ick) [*salicyl* + *-ic*]. *o*-Hydroxybenzoic acid, HOC_6H_4COOH used topically as a keratoplastic and keratolytic drug, and sometimes for bacteriostatic effect. Its salts, as sodium salicylate, are used mainly as analgesics.

salicylic aldehyde test. BEHRE'S TEST.

sal·i·cyl·ism (sal′i-sil-iz-um) *n.* [*salicyl-* + *-ism*]. A group of symptoms produced by large doses of salicylates; characterized chiefly by tinnitus, dizziness, headache, confusion, nausea, and vomiting.

salicylo-. See *salicyl-.*

sal·i·cyl·uric acid (sal″i-sil-yoo′rick). *o*-$HOC_6H_4CONHCH_2$-COOH. A detoxication product of salicylic acid found in the urine.

sa·lic·y·lyl (sa-lis′i-lil) *n.* SALICYL (1).

sal·i·fy (sal′i-fye) *v.* [F. *salifier*]. To form a salt, as by union with an acid. —**sal·i·fi·a·ble** (sal″i-fye′uh-bul) *adj.*

sal·i·jen·in (sal″i-jen′in, sa-lij′e-nin) *n.* SALICYL ALCOHOL.

sa·lim·e·ter (sa-lim′e-tur) *n.* [*sal* + *-meter*]. A hydrometer used to determine the density of salt solutions.

sa·line (say′leen, say′line) *adj.* & *n.* [L. *salinus*]. 1. Saltlike in character. 2. Containing sodium chloride. 3. Any of various salts of the alkalies or of magnesium; used as hydragogue cathartics. Magnesium sulfate and citrate, sodium sulfate, and Rochelle salt are examples.

saline diuretic. A salt that produces diuresis because of its osmotic effect in the tubules.

Salinidol. A trademark for the fungistatic agent salicylanilide.

Salipyrin. A trademark for antipyrine salicylate, an antipyretic and analgesic.

sa·li·va (suh-lye′vuh) *n.* [L.] [NA]. The secretions of the parotid, submandibular, sublingual, and other glands of the mouth. It is opalescent, tasteless, and has a slightly acid pH (6.8). The functions of saliva are to moisten the food and lubricate the bolus, to dissolve certain substances, to facilitate tasting, to aid in deglutition and articulation, and enzymically to begin the digestion of starches, which it converts into maltose, dextrin, and glucose by the action of ptyalin.

saliva ejector. A suction tube for removing saliva from the mouth during dental operations.

sal·i·vant (sal′i-vunt) *adj.* & *n.* 1. Stimulating the secretion of saliva. 2. A drug that increases the flow of saliva.

sal·i·vary (sal′i-verr-ee) *adj.* 1. Of or pertaining to saliva or the salivary glands. 2. Producing saliva.

salivary amylase. PTYALIN.

salivary calculus. 1. A concretion situated in the duct of a salivary gland. 2. SUPRAGINGIVAL CALCULUS.

salivary corpuscle. A leukocyte in the saliva.

salivary diastase. PTYALIN.

salivary digestion. Digestion by the saliva.

salivary duct. A duct of a salivary gland.

salivary duct cyst. A cyst caused by obstruction of a salivary duct and retention of the secretion of the gland.

salivary fistula. A fistula communicating with a salivary gland or its duct, usually the parotid, with discharge of saliva through an external opening in the skin.

salivary gland. A gland that secretes saliva, as the parotid.

salivary gland virus disease. CYTOMEGALIC INCLUSION DISEASE.

salivary nuclei. SALIVATORY NUCLEI.

salivary reflex. Secretion of saliva following adequate stimulation of the tongue, oral mucosa, pharynx, esophagus, or stomach by physical or chemical means, or any part of the nervous pathways to the salivary glands; it may be a conditioned reflex.

sal·i·va·tion (sal″i-vay′shun) *n.* [L. *salivatio*, from *salivare*, to spit out]. 1. Increased secretion of saliva in response to the usual stimuli. 2. An excessive secretion of saliva; a condition produced by mercury, pilocarpine, and by nervous disturbances. In severe cases of mercurial salivation, ulceration of the gums and loosening of the teeth may occur. 3. Drooling because of inability to swallow saliva, as in parkinsonism. —**sal·i·vate** (sal′i-vate) *v.*

sal·i·va·tor (sal′i-vay″tur) *n.* An agent causing salivation. —**sal·i·va·to·ry** (sal′i-vuh-to″ree, sal″i-vay′tuh-ree) *adj.*

salivatory nuclei. The superior salivatory nucleus and the inferior salivatory nucleus.

sal·i·vo·li·thi·a·sis (sal″i-vo-li-thigh′uh-sis) *n.* [*saliva* + *lithiasis*]. Presence of a salivary calculus.

sa·li·vous (sa-lye′vus) *adj.* [*saliva* + *-ous*]. SALIVARY.

Salk vaccine [J. E. *Salk*, U.S. bacteriologist, b. 1914]. POLIOMYELITIS VACCINE (1).

sal·mine (sal′meen, -min) *n.* A protamine obtained from the spermatozoa of salmon.

sal·mon disease. A disease of dogs and foxes associated with a diet that includes salmon, trout, and other fishes; probably caused by rickettsiae present in a small intestinal fluke that infects the fish.

sal·mone (sal′mone) *n.* A histone obtained from the spermatozoa of salmon.

Sal·mo·nel·la (sal″mo-nel′uh) *n.* [D. E. *Salmon*, U.S. pathologist, 1850–1914]. A genus of serologically related gram-negative, generally motile, rod-shaped bacteria belonging to the family Enterobacteriaceae. All known species are pathogenic for warm-blooded animals, including man, and cause enteric fevers, acute gastroenteritis, and septicemias. A few species are found in reptiles. —**salmonella**, pl. **salmonel·lae** (-ee) *com. n.*

Salmonella abor·ti·vo·equi·na (a-bor″ti-vo-e-kwye′nuh, a-bor-tye″vo-). *SALMONELLA ABORTUS-EQUI.*

Salmonella abor·tus-equi (a-bor′tus eck′wye). A species of *Salmonella* which is a natural pathogen of mares, also infectious for cows, goats, rabbits, and guinea pigs; causes abortion.

Salmonella abor·tus-ovis (a-bor″tus-o′vis). A pathogen causing abortion in sheep, and not known to infect any other animal.

Salmonella aer·trycke (err′tri-kee). *SALMONELLA TYPHIMURIUM.*

Salmonella chol·e·rae-su·is (kol″e-ree-sue′is). A species of *Salmonella* whose natural host is the pig, where it is a secondary invader in the virus disease, hog cholera, and a primary invader in a diphtheritic form of fibrinous inflammation. In man, it is usually involved in localized lesions with or without septicemia, but may also cause enteric fever or gastroenteritis. Syn. *Salmonella suipestifer.*

Salmonella en·te·rit·i·dis (en″te-rit′i-dis). A species of *Salmonella* causing gastroenteritis in man, isolated also from the horse, hog, mouse, rat, and duck. Syn. *Bacterium enteritidis.*

salmonella fever. A disease similar to typhoid, caused by bacteria of the genus *Salmonella.* See also *salmonellosis.*

Salmonella gal·li·na·rum (gal″i-nair′um). A nonmotile species of *Salmonella* causing fowl typhoid, a septicemic disease of domestic fowl, especially adult birds.

Salmonella hirsch·fel·dii (hursh·fel'dee·eye). A species of *Salmonella* causing enteric fever in man. Syn. *Bacterium paratyphosum* C, *Salmonella paratyphi* C.

Salmonella ora·nien·burg (o·rah'nee·un·burg). A species of *Salmonella* isolated from feces of normal carriers and of persons with food poisoning, and from abscesses; often found in dried-egg products.

Salmonella para·ty·phi A (păr"uh·tye'fye). A species of *Salmonella* which is a natural pathogen of man, causing gastroenteritis and enteric fever.

Salmonella paratyphi B. SALMONELLA SCHOTTMÜLLERI.

Salmonella paratyphi C. SALMONELLA HIRSCHFELDII.

Salmonella para·ty·pho·sa (păr"uh·tye·fo'suh). SALMONELLA PARATYPHI A.

Salmonella pul·lo·rum (puh·lo'rum) [L., of chicks]. A species of *Salmonella* causing pullorum disease or bacillary white diarrhea of chicks. Transmission can occur through the egg.

Salmonella schott·mül·leri (shot·mew'lur·eye). A motile species of *Salmonella*; a natural pathogen of man, causing enteric fever; found (rarely) in cattle, sheep, swine, chickens, and lower primates. Syn. *Bacterium paratyphosum B, Salmonella paratyphi B.*

Salmonella sui·pes·ti·fer (sue"ee·pes'ti·fur). SALMONELLA CHOLERAESUIS.

Salmonella ty·phi (tye'fye). SALMONELLA TYPHOSA.

Salmonella ty·phi·mu·ri·um (tye"fi·mew'ree·um). A species of *Salmonella* commonly causing diarrhea in mice, rats, and birds and gastroenteritis in man. The most commonly isolated bacterium in outbreaks of food poisoning in the United States and Great Britain. Syn. *Salmonella aertrycke.*

Salmonella ty·pho·sa (tye·fo'suh). A species of *Salmonella* causing typhoid fever. Syn. *Bacterium typhosum, Eberthella typhosa, Salmonella typhi.*

Sal·mo·nel·le·ae (sal"mo·nel'ee·ee) *n.pl.* A tribe of the family Enterobacteriaceae, including the genera *Salmonella* and *Shigella.*

sal·mo·nel·lo·sis (sal"mo·nel·o'sis) *n.*, pl. **salmonello·ses** (·seez) [*Salmonella* + *-osis*]. Infection with an organism of the genus *Salmonella.* It may be food-poisoning, gastroenteritic, typhoidal, or septicemic.

sal·ol (sal'ol) *n.* PHENYL SALICYLATE.

salping-, salpingo- [Gk. *salpinx, salpingos,* trumpet]. A combining form meaning (a) *auditory tube;* (b) *uterine tube.*

sal·pin·ge·al (sal·pin'jee·ul) *adj.* SALPINGIAN.

sal·pin·gec·to·my (sal"pin·jeck'tuh·mee) *n.* [*salping-* + *-ectomy*]. Excision of a uterine tube.

sal·pin·gem·phrax·is (sal"pin·jem·frack'sis) *n.* [*salping-* + *emphraxis*]. Closure of the auditory or uterine tube.

sal·pin·gi·an (sal·pin'jee·un) *adj.* Of, pertaining to, or involving the auditory tube or the uterine tube.

sal·pin·gi·tis (sal"pin·jye'tis) *n.* [*salping-* + *-itis*]. 1. Inflammation of the uterine tube. 2. Inflammation of the auditory tube. —**salpin·jit·ic** (jit'ick) *adj.*

salpingo-. See *salping-.*

sal·pin·go·cath·e·ter·ism (sal·ping"go·kath'e·tur·iz·um) *n.* [*salpingo-* + *catheter* + *-ism*]. Catheterization of an auditory tube.

sal·pin·go·cele (sal·ping'go·seel) *n.* [*salpingo-* + *-cele*]. Hernia of an oviduct.

sal·pin·go·cy·e·sis (sal·ping"go·sigh·ee'sis) *n.* [*salpingo-* + *cyesis*]. TUBAL PREGNANCY.

sal·pin·go·gram (sal·ping'go·gram) *n.* A radiographic image produced by salpingography.

sal·pin·gog·raphy (sal"ping·gog'ruh·fee) *n.* [*salpingo-* + *-graphy*]. Radiographic demonstration of the uterine tubes after they are filled with a radiopaque liquid.

sal·pin·gol·y·sis (sal"ping·gol'i·sis) *n.* [*salpingo-* + *-lysis*]. The breaking down of adhesions of a uterine tube.

sal·pin·go-oo·pho·rec·to·my (sal·ping"go·o"o·fo·reck'to·mee) *n.* [*salpingo-* + *oophor-* + *-ectomy*]. Excision of a uterine tube and an ovary.

sal·pin·go-oo·pho·ri·tis (sal·ping"go·o"o·fo·rye'tis) *n.* [*salpingo-* + *oophor-* + *-itis*]. Inflammation of the uterine tubes and the ovaries.

sal·pin·go-ooph·o·ro·cele (sal"ping·go·o·off'uh·ro·seel) *n.* [*salpingo-* + *oophoro-* + *-cele*]. Hernial protrusion of an ovary and oviduct.

sal·pin·go-oo·the·cec·to·my (sal·ping"go·o"o·the·seck'tuh·mee) *n.* [*salpingo-* + *oothec-* + *-ectomy*]. SALPINGO-OOPHORECTOMY.

sal·pin·go-oo·the·ci·tis (sal·ping"go·o"o·the·sigh'tis) *n.* [*salpingo-* + *oothec-* + *-itis*]. SALPINGO-OOPHORITIS.

sal·pin·go-oo·the·co·cele (sal·ping"go·o"o·theek'o·seel) *n.* [*salpingo-* + *ootheco-* + *-cele*]. SALPINGO-OOPHOROCELE.

sal·pin·go·ovari·ec·to·my (sal·ping"go·o·văr"ee·eck'tuh·mee) *n.* [*salpingo-* + *ovari-* + *-ectomy*]. SALPINGO-OOPHORECTOMY.

sal·pin·go·ovari·ot·o·my (sal·ping"go·o·văr"ee·ot'uh·mee) *n.* [*salpingo-* + *ovario-* + *-tomy*]. SALPINGO-OOPHORECTOMY.

sal·pin·go·ova·ri·tis (sal·ping"go·o"vuh·rye'tis) *n.* [*salpingo-* + *ovar-* + *-itis*]. SALPINGO-OOPHORITIS.

sal·pin·go·pal·a·tine (sal·ping"go·pal'uh·tine) *adj.* [*salpingo-* + *palatine*]. Pertaining to the auditory tube and the palate.

salpingopalatine fold. A fold of mucous membrane extending from the anterior lip of the torus tubarius to the soft palate. NA *plica salpingopalatina.*

sal·pin·go·peri·to·ni·tis (sal·ping"go·perr"i·to·nigh'tis) *n.* [*salpingo-* + *periton-* + *-itis*]. Inflammation of the peritoneum and uterine tube.

sal·pin·go·pexy (sal·ping'go·peck"see) *n.* [*salpingo-* + *-pexy*]. Operative fixation of one or both uterine tubes.

sal·pin·go·pha·ryn·ge·al (sal·ping"go·fa·rin'jee·ul) *adj.* [*salpingo-* + *pharyngeal*]. Pertaining to the auditory tube and the pharynx.

salpingopharyngeal fold. A vertical fold of mucous membrane extending from the posterior lip of the torus tubarius to the pharynx. NA *plica salpingopharyngea.*

sal·pin·go·pha·ryn·ge·us (sal·ping"go·fa·rin'jee·us) *n.* A muscular bundle passing from the auditory tube downward to the constrictors of the pharynx. NA *musculus salpingopharyngeus.* See also Table of Muscles in the Appendix.

sal·pin·go·plas·ty (sal·ping'go·plas"tee) *n.* [*salpingo-* + *-plasty*]. Surgery of a uterine tube.

sal·pin·gor·rha·phy (sal"ping·gor'uh·fee) *n.* [*salpingo-* + *-rrhaphy*]. Suture of a uterine tube.

sal·pin·go·sal·pin·gos·to·my (sal·ping"go·sal"ping·gos'tuh·mee) *n.* [*salpingo-* + *salpingo-* + *-stomy*]. The operation reuniting an oviduct after removal of an intervening section.

sal·pin·go·scope (sal·ping'go·skope) *n.* [*salpingo-* + *-scope*]. NASOPHARYNGOSCOPE.

sal·pin·go·steno·cho·ria (sal·ping"go·sten"o·ko'ree·uh) *n.* [*salpingo-* + *stenochoria*]. Stenosis or stricture of the auditory tube.

sal·pin·go·sto·mat·o·my (sal·ping"go·sto·mat'uh·mee) *n.* [*salpingo-* + *stomat-* + *-tomy*]. SALPINGOSTOMY.

sal·pin·gos·to·my (sal"ping·gos'tuh·mee) *n.* [*salpingo-* + *-stomy*]. 1. The operation of making an artificial fistula between a uterine tube and the body surface. 2. Any plastic operation for opening the uterine tube.

sal·pin·go·the·cal (sal·ping"go·theek'ul) *adj.* [*salpingo-* + *thecal*]. Pertaining to the oviduct and subarachnoid space.

salpingothecal shunt. Surgical communication between the lumbar subarachnoid space and an oviduct, for drainage of cerebrospinal fluid into the peritoneal cavity.

sal·pin·got·o·my (sal"ping·got'uh·mee) *n.* [*salpingo-* + *-tomy*]. The operation of cutting into a uterine tube.

sal·pin·gys·tero·cy·e·sis (sal"pin·jis"tur·o·sigh·ee'sis) *n.* [*salping-* + *hystero-* + *cyesis*]. INTERSTITIAL PREGNANCY.

sal·pinx (sal'pinks) *n.*, genit. **sal·pin·gis** (sal·pin'jis), pl. **salpin·**

ges (·jeez) [Gk., trumpet]. 1. AUDITORY TUBE. 2. UTERINE TUBE.

sal·sa·late (sal'suh·late) *n.* Salicyl salicylate, $C_{14}H_{10}O_5$, an analgesic anti-inflammatory.

salt, *n.* 1. SODIUM CHLORIDE. 2. *In chemistry,* any of a group of substances that result from the reaction between acids and bases; a compound of a metal or positive radical and a nonmetal or negative radical. 3. A mixture of several salts, especially those occurring in mineral springs.

sal·ta·tion (sal·tay'shun) *n.* [L. *saltatio,* from *saltare,* to dance]. 1. Progression or action by jumps or jerks rather than by smoothly controlled movements. 2. SALTATORY CONDUCTION. 3. A genetic mutation resulting in a very significant difference between parent and offspring.

sal·ta·tor·ic (sal''tuh·tor'ick) *adj.* SALTATORY.

sal·ta·to·ry (sal'tuh·to''ree) *adj.* [L. *saltatorius,* of dancing]. 1. Characterized by jumping or jerky movements. 2. Progressing in a succession of abrupt changes rather than continuously.

saltatory conduction or **transmission.** The passage of the action potential along myelinated nerve axons by skipping from one node of Ranvier to the next, the active node serving electrotonically to depolarize to the firing level the node ahead without significant activation of internodal segments. This process results in conduction of nerve impulses along myelinated axons 50 times faster than in the fastest unmyelinated nerve fibers.

saltatory spasm. A paroxysmal clonic movement of the lower extremities that causes the patient to leap or jump; the cause is not known, although it is sometimes considered to be a tic. See also *jumping Frenchmen of Maine, paroxysmal choreoathetosis.*

salt-depletion syndrome. LOW-SALT SYNDROME.

Sal·ter's lines [S. J. A. *Salter,* English dental surgeon, 1825–1897]. The incremental lines of the dentin.

salt-free diet. 1. A diet low in sodium chloride. 2. A diet without added salt, containing approximately 3 to 5 g NaCl; when salt is not used in cooking, 2 to 3 g; with foods containing a minimum of salt, 0.5 to 1.0 g per day.

salting out. A method of decreasing the solubility, and thereby precipitating, certain substances, such as proteins, by adding to their solutions neutral salts, such as sodium chloride.

salt·pe·ter, salt·pe·tre (sawlt·pee'tur) *n.* [ML. *sal petrae,* rock salt]. Potassium nitrate, KNO_3; has some diuretic properties.

salts, *n.*pl. A saline cathartic, especially magnesium sulfate, sodium sulfate, or Rochelle salt.

salt-sensitive, *adj.* Characterized by a tendency to agglutinate in normal saline solution; said of certain bacteria.

salt sick. Of herbivorous animals: anemic and unthrifty as a result of grazing on grasses of copper-deficient soils.

sa·lu·bri·ous (sa·lew'bree·us) *adj.* [L., *salubris,* from *salus,* health]. Wholesome; in a state of physical well-being. —**salu·bri·ty** (·bri·tee) *n.*

sal·ure·sis (sal''yoo·ree'sis) *n.* [*sal* + *uresis*]. Excretion of salt (specifically, of sodium chloride) in the urine.

sal·uret·ic (sal''yoo·ret'ick) *adj.* Pertaining to or causing saluresis.

Saluron. Trademark for hydroflumethiazide, an orally effective diuretic and antihypertensive drug.

sal·u·tary (sal'yoo·terr·ee) *adj.* [L. *salutaris,* from *salus,* health]. Promoting health.

sal·vage (sal'vij) *v. & n.* [F., from OF. *salver,* to save]. 1. To save through therapeutic or preventive measures, persons, organs, or tissues, that would otherwise be lost. 2. The persons or parts thus saved. 3. The act of salvaging.

Salvarsan. A trademark for arsphenamine, an early antisyphilitic drug.

salve (sav, sahv) *n.* OINTMENT.

sal·via (sal'vee·uh) *n.* [L., the herb sage]. The dried leaves of *Salvia officinalis,* which contain a volatile oil. Formerly used empirically for the treatment of a variety of ailments. Syn. *sage.*

Salz·mann's nodular corneal dystrophy (za^h^lts'ma^h^n) [M. *Salzmann,* Austrian ophthalmologist, 1862–1954]. A nonfamilial disease, probably always a sequel of phlyctenular keratitis, consisting of one to eight dense blue-white nodules on the corneal surface, usually occurring in women.

sa·mar·i·um (sa·măr'ee·um) *n.* [Colonel *Samarski,* Russian mine official, 19th century]. Sm (or Sa) = 150.4. A metallic lanthanide, atomic number 62.

sam·bu·cus (sam·bew'kus) *n.* [L., elder tree]. The dried flowers of *Sambucus canadensis,* or of *Sambucus nigra,* which contain a volatile oil, and also eldrin, which is identical with rutin. Sambucus has been used as a diaphoretic and diuretic. Syn. *elder flowers.*

sam·ple, *n.* [OF. *essample,* from L. *exemplum,* example]. A specimen or part to show the quality of the whole.

sampling variation. *In biostatistics,* variation in the estimates of some biostatistical value, such as mean, between different samples of, or from, the same universe.

Samp·son's cysts [J. A. *Sampson,* U.S. surgeon, 1873–1946]. Cystic endometriosis of the ovary.

Sanamycin. Trademark for cactinomycin, a mixture of antibiotics produced by *Streptomyces chrysomallus.*

Sa·na·rel·li virus (sa^h^·na^h^·rel'lee) [G. *Sanarelli,* Italian bacteriologist, 1864–1940]. The virus of infectious myxomatosis.

san·a·to·ri·um (san''uh·to'ree·um) *n.,* pl. **sanatoriums, sanato·ria** (·ee·uh) [L. *sanatorius,* curative, from *sanare,* to heal, cure]. An establishment for the treatment of patients with chronic diseases or mental disorders; especially, such a private hospital or place.

san·a·to·ry (san'uh·tor''ee) *adj.* [L. *sanatorius*]. Health-giving.

san·da·rac (san'duh·rack) *n.* [Gk. *sandarakē,* realgar]. A white, transparent resin produced by *Callitris quadrivalvis,* a tree of North Africa; sometimes employed as a protective in dentistry.

sandarac varnish. A solution of sandarac in alcohol; used as a separating medium in making dental casts.

sand bath. Immersing the body with warm, dry sand or damp sea sand.

sand bodies. CORPORA ARENACEA.

sand crack. A fissure in the hoof of a horse, from the coronet to the sole; due to disease of the horn-secreting membrane.

San·ders bed [C. E. *Sanders,* U.S. physician, 1885–1949]. OSCILLATING BED.

San·der's disease (za^h^n'dur) [W. *Sander,* German psychiatrist, 1838–1922]. Paranoia appearing in youth.

San·ders-Ho·gan disease or **syndrome** [M. *Sanders,* U.S. bacteriologist, b. 1910]. EPIDEMIC KERATOCONJUNCTIVITIS.

Sanders' sign [J. *Sanders,* English physician, 1777–1843]. An undulating cardiac impulse in the epigastric region, indicating adhesive pericarditis.

sand flea. *TUNGA PENETRANS.*

sand fly. A fly of the genus *Phlebotomus.*

sand-fly fever. PHLEBOTOMUS FEVER.

Sand·hoff's disease. A rare form of G_{M2} gangliosidosis, clinically and pathologically similar to Tay-Sachs disease except for the presence of moderate hepatosplenomegaly and coarse granulations, in bone marrow histiocytes, indicating lipid storage in these organs. It is due to a deficiency of the essential ganglioside-hydrolyzing enzymes hexosaminidase A and hexosaminidase B. See also *amaurotic familial idiocy.*

sand·hog's itch. The patchy mottling of the skin with itching, found in decompression sickness (caisson disease).

Sandoptal. Trademark for butalbital, a sedative and hypnotic with intermediate duration of action.

sand·pa·per gallbladder. Roughness of the lining of the gallbladder, due to deposition of cholesterol crystals.

Sandril. A trademark for reserpine, an antihypertensive and sedative drug.

sand tumor. PSAMMOMA.

sane, *adj.* [L. *sanus,* healthy]. Of sound mind; not insane.

San·fi·lip·po's syndrome [S. J. *Sanfilippo,* U.S. pediatrician, 20th century]. Mucopolysaccharidosis III, transmitted as an autosomal recessive trait, characterized chemically by excessive amounts of heparitin sulfate in urine, and manifested clinically by a facial appearance similar to that seen in the more common Hurler's syndrome, but otherwise less severe skeletal changes and only slight hepatomegaly. Clouding of the cornea and cardiac abnormalities do not appear. Central nervous system deficit with progressive mental deterioration is pronounced.

Sang·er Brown's ataxia [*Sanger Brown,* U.S. neuropsychiatrist, 1852–1928]. A spinal form of hereditary ataxia, with onset between 11 and 45 years of age, characterized by an ataxia that began in the legs and spread to the arms and face, and the muscles of speech and swallowing, occasionally accompanied by choreiform movements, and often by oculomotor paresis and optic atrophy.

sangui-, sanguino- [L. *sanguis, sanguinis,* blood]. A combining form meaning *blood, sanguineous.*

san·guic·o·lous (sang·gwick'o·lus) *adj.* [*sangui-* + L. *colere,* to inhabit, to cultivate]. Living in the blood, as a parasite.

san·guif·er·ous (sang·gwif'ur·us) *adj.* [*sangui-* + *-ferous*]. Carrying, or conveying, blood.

san·gui·fi·ca·tion (sang"gwi·fi·kay'shun) *n.* [*sangui-* + L. *facere,* to make]. The formation of blood; conversion into blood.

san·gui·na·ria (sang"gwi·nair'ee·uh) *n.* [L., from *sanguinarius,* of the blood]. The dried rhizome of *Sanguinaria canadensis,* which contains several alkaloids, including chelerythrine and sanguinarine; has been used as an expectorant. Syn. *bloodroot.*

san·guin·a·rine (sang·gwin'uh·reen, ·rin) *n.* An alkaloid, $C_{20}H_{15}NO_5$, from sanguinaria.

san·gui·nary (sang'gwi·nerr"ee) *adj.* [L. *sanguinarius*]. Pertaining to, consisting of, or derived from blood.

sanguinary calculus. SERUMAL CALCULUS.

san·guine (sang'gwin) *adj.* [L. *sanguineus,* of blood]. 1. Resembling blood; bloody. 2. Hopeful, active, as sanguine temperament.

san·guin·e·ous (sang·gwin'ee·us) *adj.* [L. *sanguineus*]. Pertaining to the blood; containing blood.

sanguineous apoplexy. A cerebral hemorrhage.

sanguineous ascites. A bloody form of ascites affecting sheep and lambs.

sanguineous cyst. A cyst containing blood-stained fluid.

sanguineous exudate. An exudate containing visible blood. Syn. *hemorrhagic exudate.*

sanguino-. See *sangui-.*

san·guin·o·lent (sang·gwin'o·lunt) *adj.* [L. *sanguinolentus*]. Tinged with blood.

san·gui·no·pu·ru·lent (sang"gwi·no·pewr'yoo·lunt) *adj.* [*sanguino-* + *purulent*]. Pertaining to blood and pus.

san·gui·no·se·rous (sang"gwi·no·seer'us, ·serr'us) *adj.* [*sanguino-* + *serous*]. Pertaining to blood and blood serum.

san·guis (sang'gwis) *n.* [L.] [NA]. BLOOD.

san·gui·suc·tion (sang"gwi·suck'shun) *n.* [*sangui-* + *suction*]. Abstraction of blood by suction, as by a leech or other parasite.

san·gui·su·ga (sang"gwi·sue'guh) *n.* [L., from *sanguis,* blood, + *sugere,* to suck]. LEECH.

sa·ni·es (say'nee·eez) *n.* [L., bloody matter]. A thin, fetid, greenish, seropurulent fluid discharged from an ulcer, wound, or fistula. —**sani·ous** (·us) *adj.*

san·i·tar·i·an (san"i·tăr'ee·un) *n.* A person skilled in sanitary science and matters of public health.

san·i·ta·ri·um (san"i·tăr'ee·um) *n.* SANATORIUM.

san·i·tary (san'i·terr·ee) *adj.* [F. *sanitaire,* from L. *sanitas,* health]. Pertaining to health, or to the restoration or maintenance of health, or to the absence of any agent that may be injurious to health.

san·i·ta·tion (san"i·tay'shun) *n.* 1. The act or process of securing a sanitary or healthful condition. 2. The application of sanitary measures.

san·i·tize (san'i·tize) *v.* To make sanitary; to boil instruments, solutions, etc., in order to destroy organisms. Compare *sterilize.*

san·i·ty (san'i·tee) *n.* [L. *sanitas,* health]. Soundness of mind.

San Joa·quin Valley fever (san wah·keen') [after the *San Joaquin* River Valley, California]. COCCIDIOIDOMYCOSIS.

Sansalid. A trademark for uredofos, a veterinary anthelmintic.

Sansert. Trademark for methysergide, a homologue of methylergonovine used as the bimaleate salt for prophylactic management of migraine headache.

San·som's sign [A. E. *Sansom,* English physician, 1838–1907]. 1. Increased dullness parasternally in the second and third interspaces; a sign of pericardial effusion. 2. A rhythmic murmur heard with the stethoscope on the lips; a sign of thoracic aortic aneurysm.

san·ton·i·ca (san·ton'i·kuh) *n.* [L., an herb, probably wormwood]. The dried flower heads of several species of *Artemisia,* which contain santonin. Syn. *wormseed, Levant wormseed.*

san·to·nin (san'to·nin) *n.* A tricyclic constituent, $C_{15}H_{18}O_3$, of the flower heads of certain *Artemisia* species; formerly extensively used as a vermifuge, especially against *Ascaris lumbricoides,* but no longer used because of its potential toxicity.

san·to·nism (san'to·niz·um) *n.* Poisoning produced by santonin.

San·to·ri·ni's cartilages (sa^{h}n·to·ree'nee) [G. D. *Santorini,* Italian anatomist, 1681–1739]. CORNICULATE CARTILAGES.

Santorini's muscle [G. D. *Santorini*]. RISORIUS.

Santorini's tubercle [G. D. *Santorini*]. CORNICULATE TUBERCLE.

San·tos' foreign body remover (san·toosh) [R. dos *Santos,* Portuguese surgeon and radiologist, b. 1880]. An instrument with tiny jaws to remove small particles of metal from tissues, to be used in connection with fluoroscopy.

São Pau·lo fever or **typhus** (saow^{n}paow'loo) [after *São Paulo,* Brazil]. ROCKY MOUNTAIN SPOTTED FEVER.

sap, *n.* Plant juice; the watery solution which circulates through the vascular tissues of a plant.

sa·phe·na (sa·fee'nuh) *n.* [ML., short for *vena saphena*]. SAPHENOUS VEIN.

sa·phe·no·fem·o·ral (sa·fee'no·fem"ur·ul) *adj.* Pertaining to the saphenous and femoral veins.

sa·phe·nous (sa·fee'nus, saf'e·nus) *adj.* [ML. *saphenus* (traditionally associated with Gk. *saphēnēs,* clear, manifest, though actually from Ar. *ṣāfin,* lit., standing)]. 1.See *saphenous vein.* 2. Pertaining to or accompanying a saphenous vein.

saphenous hiatus or **opening.** An opening in the fascia lata of the thigh which gives passage to the great saphenous vein. Syn. *fossa ovalis (femoris).* NA *hiatus saphenus.*

saphenous nerve. The nerve accompanying a great saphenous vein. NA *nervus saphenus.* See also Table of Nerves in the Appendix.

saphenous vein. Either of the two main superficial veins of the lower limb: 1. The great saphenous vein (NA *vena saphena magna*), which begins on the dorsum of the foot, ascends medially along the leg and thigh, and drains into the femoral vein just inside the saphenous hiatus of the fascia lata. 2. The small saphenous vein (NA *vena saphena parva*), which ascends from the outer side of the foot along the middle of the back of the leg and drains into the popliteal vein.

sap·id (sap'id) *adj.* [L. *sapidus,* flavorful, from *sapere,* to taste]. 1. Capable of being tasted. 2. Possessing or giving flavor. 3. Palatable.

sa·po (say'po) *n.* [L.]. SOAP.

sapo-, sapon-, saponi- [L. *sapo, saponis*]. A combining form meaning *soap, soapy.*

sap·o·gen·in (sap″o·jen′in, sa·poj′e·nin) *n.* The nonsugar or aglycone component of a saponin.

sap·o·na·ceous (sap″o·nay′shus) *adj.* [*sapon-* + *-aceous*]. Having the nature of soap.

Sap·o·nar·ia (sap″o·năr′ee·uh) *n.* A genus of plants of the order Caryophylleae. *Saponaria officinalis,* or soapwort, bouncing bet, a species growing wild abundantly in the United States and Europe, was formerly used for the treatment of a variety of ailments.

sa·po·nat·ed (sap′o·nay·tid) *adj.* Combined or treated with soap.

sa·pon·i·fi·ca·tion (sa·pon″i·fi·kay′shun) *n.* [F., from L. *sapo, saponis,* soap]. The conversion of an ester into an alcohol and a salt; in particular, the conversion of a fat into a soap and glycerin by means of an alkali. —**sa·pon·i·fy** (sa·pon′i·fye) *v.*

saponification number or **value.** The number of milligrams of potassium hydroxide required to neutralize the free acids and saponify the esters contained in 1 g of oil, fat, wax, or other substance of similar composition.

sa·pon·i·form (sa·pon′i·form) *adj.* [*sapon-* + *-iform*]. Soaplike in appearance and consistency.

sap·o·nin (sap′o·nin, sa·po′nin) *n.* [*sapon-* + *-in*]. 1. A glycoside usually obtained from *Quillaja* or *Saponaria;* used as a detergent, and a foaming and emulsifying agent. 2. Any of a group of glycosidal principles that foam when shaken with water and lyse red blood cells. Saponins are widely distributed in nature. Because they lower surface tension, they form emulsions with oils and resinous substances. Saponins alter the permeability of cell walls and, therefore, are toxic to all organized tissues.

sapo·tox·in (sap″o·tock′sin) *n.* A name sometimes applied to the more toxic saponins.

Sap·pey's muscle (sah·peh) [M. P. C. *Sappey,* French anatomist, 1810–1896]. The temporoparietalis muscle. See Table of Muscles in the Appendix.

sap·phism (saf′iz·um) *n.* [*Sappho,* Greek poetess of Lesbos]. LESBIANISM.

sapr-, sapro- [Gk. *sapros,* rotten, putrid]. A combining form meaning (a) *dead or decaying organic matter;* (b) *putrefaction, putrefactive.*

sa·pre·mia, sa·prae·mia (sa·pree′mee·uh) *n.* [*sapr-* + *-emia*]. The intoxication supposedly produced by absorption of the products of putrefaction. —**sapre·mic, saprae·mic** (·mick) *adj.*

sap·rine (sap′reen, ·rin) *n.* A product or products of growth when saprophytic or simple parasitic bacteria grow upon diseased or injured tissues.

sapro-. See *sapr-.*

sap·ro·gen (sap′ro·jen) *n.* [*sapro-* + *-gen*]. A putrefactive microorganism.

sap·ro·gen·ic (sap″ro·jen′ick) *adj.* [*sapro-* + *-genic*]. 1. Causing putrefaction. 2. Produced by putrefaction.

sa·prog·e·nous (sa·proj′e·nus) *adj.* SAPROGENIC.

sa·proph·a·gous (sa·prof′uh·gus) *adj.* [*sapro-* + *-phagous*]. Subsisting on decaying matter.

sap·ro·phyte (sap′ro·fite) *n.* [*sapro-* + *-phyte*]. An organism living on dead or decaying organic matter. —**sap·ro·phyt·ic** (sap″ro·fit′ick) *adj.*

sap·ro·zo·ic (sap″ro·zo′ick) *adj.* [*sapro-* + *-zoic*]. Living on decaying organic matter; said mainly of animal organisms, as certain protozoans.

sar·al·a·sin (sahr·al′uh·sin) *n.* A polypeptide of 8 amino acids solvated with acetic acid and water, $C_{42}H_{65}N_{13}O_{10}.x$-$C_2H_4O_2.xH_2O$, an antihypertensive.

sar·a·pus (săr′a·pus) *n.* [Gk. *sarapous,* splay-footed]. A flat-footed person.

sarc-, sarco- [Gk. *sarx, sarkos*]. A combining form meaning (a) *flesh, fleshlike;* (b) *muscle.*

-sarc [Gk. *sarx, sarkos,* flesh]. A combining form meaning *a differentiated substance or tissue of an organism.*

Sar·ci·na (sahr′si·nuh) *n.* [L., bundle]. A genus of bacteria of the family Micrococcaceae. Cell division occurs in three planes forming cubical groups.

sarcina, *n.,* pl. **sarci·nae** (·nee). Any coccus which forms cubical packets of adhering cells by dividing in three perpendicular directions; typified by cocci of the genus *Sarcina.*

sar·ci·tis (sahr·sigh′tis) *n.* [*sarc-* + *-itis*]. Inflammation of fleshy tissue, especially inflammation of muscle; myositis.

sarco-. See *sarc-.*

sar·co·ad·e·no·ma (sahr″ko·ad·e·no′muh) *n.* ADENOSARCOMA.

sar·co·bi·ont (sahr″ko·bye′ont) *n.* [*sarco-* + Gk. *biountes,* living, from *bioun,* to live]. An organism living on flesh.

sar·co·blast (sahr′ko·blast) *n.* [*sarco-* + *-blast*]. MYOBLAST.

sar·co·car·ci·no·ma (sahr″ko·kahr″si·no′muh) *n.* CARCINOSARCOMA.

sar·co·cele (sahr′ko·seel) *n.* [*sarco-* + *-cele*]. A tumor of the testis resembling muscle grossly.

Sar·co·cys·tis (sahr″ko·sis′tis) *n.* [NL., from *sarco-* + Gk. *kystis,* bladder]. A group of presumed protozoa of the order Sarcosporidia, with affinity for the striated and cardiac muscles of vertebrate hosts.

Sarcocystis lin·de·man·ni (lin·de·man′eye). A rare parasite of man, in various muscles.

sar·code (sahr′kode) *n.* [Gk. *sarkōdēs,* fleshy]. The living substance of the cell, the protoplasm.

Sar·co·di·na (sahr″ko·dye′nuh, ·dee′nuh) *n.pl.* [NL., from Gk. *sarkōdēs,* fleshlike]. RHIZOPODA.

sar·co·en·do·the·li·o·ma (sahr″ko·en″do·theel·ee·o′muh) *n.* A sarcoma forming endothelial structures.

sar·co·fe·tal pregnancy (sahr″ko·fee′tul). Gestation with the presence of both a fetus and a mole.

sar·co·gen·ic (sahr″ko·jen′ick) *adj.* [*sarco-* + *-genic*]. Producing muscle.

sarcogenic cell. MYOBLAST.

sar·co·hy·dro·cele (sahr″ko·high′dro·seel) *n.* A sarcocele complicated with hydrocele of the tunica vaginalis.

sar·co·hys·ter·ic pregnancy (sahr″ko·his·terr′ick). Pregnancy productive of a mole.

sar·coid (sahr′koid) *adj.* & *n.* [Gk. *sarkoeidēs,* from *sarx,* flesh]. 1. Resembling flesh. 2. SARCOIDOSIS.

sar·coid·o·sis (sahr·koy·do′sis) *n.,* pl. **sarcoido·ses** (·seez) [*sarcoid* + *-osis*]. A disease of unknown etiology, characterized by granulomatous lesions, somewhat resembling true tubercles, but showing little or no necrosis, affecting lymph nodes, skin, liver, spleen, heart, skeletal muscle, lungs, bones in distal parts of the extremities (osteitis cystica of Jüngling) and other structures, and sometimes by hyperglobulinemia, cutaneous anergy, and hypercalcuria.

sar·co·lac·tic acid (sahr″ko·lack′tick). The L (+) form of lactic acid, $CH_3CHOHCOOH$, occurring in muscle. Syn. *paralactic acid.*

sar·co·lem·ma (sahr″ko·lem′uh) *n.* [*sarco-* + *-lemma*]. The delicate sheath enveloping a muscle fiber. —**sarcolem·mal** (·ul), **sarcolem·mous** (·mus), **sarcolem·mic** (·ick) *adj.*

sar·co·leu·ke·mia, sar·co·leu·kae·mia (sahr″ko·lew·kee′mee·uh) *n.* [*sarco-* + *leukemia*]. LEUKOSARCOMA (1).

L-sar·co·ly·sin (sahr″ko·lye′sin) *n.* MELPHALAN.

sar·co·ma (sahr·ko′muh) *n.,* pl. **sarcomas, sarcoma·ta** (·tuh) [Gk. *sarkōma,* fleshy excrescence, from *sarx,* flesh]. A malignant tumor whose parenchyma is composed of anaplastic cells resembling those of the supportive tissues of the body.

sarcoma bot·ry·oi·des (bot·ree·oy′deez). A malignant mesenchymoma that forms grapelike structures; most common in the vagina of infants.

sarcoma cap·i·tis (kap′i·tis). CYLINDROMA.

sarcoma col·li ute·ri hy·drop·i·cum pap·il·la·re (kol′eye yoo′tur·eye high·drop′i·kum pap·i·lair′ee). SARCOMA BOTRYOIDES.

sarcoma cu·ta·ne·um te·lan·gi·ec·tat·i·cum mul·ti·plex (kew·tay′nee·um te·lan″jee·eck·tat′i·kum mul′ti·plecks). MULTIPLE IDIOPATHIC HEMORRHAGIC SARCOMA.

sarcoma myx·o·ma·to·des (mick·so·muh·to'deez). A sarcoma in which there are foci of mucoid degeneration.

sarcoma of bone. OSTEOGENIC SARCOMA.

sarcoma of peripheral nerve. NEUROFIBROSARCOMA.

sarcoma phylloides. CYSTOSARCOMA PHYLLODES.

sar·co·ma·toid (sahr·ko'muh·toid) *adj.* [*sarcoma* + *-oid*]. Suggesting or bearing some resemblance to sarcoma.

sar·co·ma·to·sis (sahr·ko''muh·to'sis) *n.*, pl. **sarcomato·ses** (·seez) [*sarcoma* + *-osis*]. The formation of multiple sarcomatous growths in various parts of the body.

sar·co·ma·tous (sahr·ko'muh·tus, sahr·kom'uh·tus) *adj.* Of the nature of, or resembling, sarcoma.

sarcomatous goiter. Sarcoma of the thyroid gland.

sar·co·mere (sahr'ko·meer) *n.* [*sarco-* + *-mere*]. One of the segments into which a fibril of striate muscle appears to be divided by Z disks.

sar·co·meso·the·li·o·ma (sahr''ko·mez''o'theel·ee·o'muh) *n.* [*sarco-* + *mesothelioma*]. A malignant mesothelioma.

sar·co·my·ces (sahr''ko·migh'seez) *n.* [*sarco-* + *-myces*]. A fleshy growth of a fungous appearance.

Sar·co·phag·i·dae (sahr''ko·faj'i·dee) *n.pl.* A large cosmopolitan family of the Diptera, commonly known as flesh flies and scavenger flies. They normally deposit their eggs or larvae on the decaying flesh of dead animals, but sometimes also in open wounds and sores of man. The important genera are *Sarcophaga* and *Wohlfahrtia.*

sar·co·plasm (sahr'ko·plaz·um) *n.* [*sarco-* + *-plasm*]. The hyaline or finely granular interfibrillar material of muscle tissue. Compare *myofibril.* —**sar·co·plas·mic** (sahr''ko·plaz' mick) *adj.*

sarcoplasmic cone. One of the conical masses of sarcoplasm at either end of the nucleus of a smooth muscle cell or of a cardiac muscle fiber.

sarcoplasmic reticulum. The specialized endoplasmic reticulum found in muscle cells.

sar·co·plast (sahr'ko·plast) *n.* [*sarco-* + *-plast*]. MYOBLAST.

sar·co·poi·et·ic (sahr''ko·poy·et'ick) *adj.* [*sarco-* + *-poietic*]. Producing muscle.

Sar·cop·tes (sahr·kop'teez) *n.* [*sarc-* + Gk. *koptein,* to cut]. A genus of minute, rounded, short-legged, flattened mites that cause scabies in man and mange in many kinds of animals.

Sarcoptes sca·bi·ei (skay'bee·eye). The mite that causes scabies in man. Syn. *itch mite, sarcoptic mite.*

sar·cop·tic (sahr·kop'tick) *adj.* [*Sarcoptes* + *-ic*]. Pertaining to scabies or mange.

sarcoptic mange. The form of mange most commonly transmitted to man, caused by mites of the genus *Sarcoptes.*

sarcoptic mite. *SARCOPTES SCABIEI.*

Sar·cop·ti·dae (sahr·kop'ti·dee) *n.pl.* A family of the order Acarina, including the genera *Sarcoptes* and *Notoedres.* —**sar·cop·tic** (sahr·kop'tick) *adj.*

sar·cop·toid (sahr·kop'toid) *adj.* Pertaining to the Sarcoptoidea.

Sar·cop·toi·dea (sahr''kop·toy'dee·uh) *n.pl.* A superfamily of the parasitic mites; the mange and itch mites of the genus *Sarcoptes* are included.

sar·co·sine (sahr'ko·seen, ·sin) *n.* *N*-Methylglycine or *N*-methylaminoacetic acid, CH_3NHCH_2COOH, an amino acid obtained on hydrolysis of certain proteins.

sar·co·si·ne·mia (sahr''ko·si·nee'mee·uh) *n.* [*sarcosine* + *-emia*]. An inborn error of metabolism in which there is an increased amount of sarcosine (methylglycine) in plasma and urine due to a deficiency of sarcosine oxidase, and clinically, mental and physical retardation with hypotonia.

sar·co·sis (sahr·ko'sis) *n.* [Gk. *sarkōsis,* growth of flesh, fleshiness]. 1. Multiple tumors of fleshy consistency. 2. Unusual increase in body mass.

Sar·co·spo·rid·ia (sahr''ko·spo·rid'ee·uh) *n.pl.* [*sarco-* + *sporidia*]. An order of sporozoa that questionably includes the genus *Sarcocystis.*

sar·co·spo·rid·i·o·sis (sahr''ko·spo·rid''ee·o'sis) *n.*, pl. **sarcosporidio·ses** (·seez) [*Sarcosporidia* + *-osis*]. A disease of warm-blooded animals presumed to be caused by sporozoa of the order Sarcosporidia; it is rare in man, but common in lower animals, such as sheep. The parasites usually encyst in striated (skeletal or cardiac) muscle and produce few symptoms.

sar·co·style (sahr'ko·stile) *n.* [*sarco-* + Gk. *stylos,* pillar]. MYOFIBRIL.

sar·co·thla·sis (sahr''ko·thlay'sis) *n.* [*sarco-* + Gk. *thlasis,* from *thlan,* to bruise]. A bruise or hematoma.

sar·co·tu·bule (sahr''ko·tew'bewl) *n.* [*sarco-* + *tubule*]. The modified smooth-surfaced endoplasmic reticulum of striated muscle.

sar·cous (sahr'kus) *adj.* [*sarc-* + *-ous*]. Pertaining to flesh or muscle.

sarcous disk. A DISK.

sar·don·ic grin or **laugh** (sahr·don'ick). RISUS SARDONICUS.

sa·rin (za·reen') *n.* [Ger.]. Isopropoxymethylphosphoryl fluoride, $C_4H_{10}FO_2P$, a nerve gas that is an extremely active cholinesterase inhibitor.

sar·men·to·cy·ma·rin (sahr·men''to·sigh'muh·rin) *n.* A cardioactive, steroidal glycoside from the seeds of *Strophanthus sarmentosus;* on hydrolysis it yields sarmentogenin and sarmentose.

sar·men·tog·e·nin (sahr''men·toj'e·nin, sahr·men''to·jen'in) *n.* The steroidal aglycone, $C_{23}H_{34}O_5$, of sarmentocymarin. It is isomeric with digoxigenin and is characterized by having a hydroxyl group at carbon atom number 11.

sar·men·tose (sahr'min·toce, sahr·men'toce) *n.* A sugar, $C_7H_{14}O_4$, the methyl ether of a 2-deoxyhexomethylose; obtained by hydrolysis of sarmentocymarin. It is isomeric with cymarose.

sar·pi·cil·lin (sahr''pi·sil'in) *n.* A phenylimidazole derivative of penicillin, $C_{21}H_{27}N_3O_5S$, used as an antibacterial.

sar·sa (sahr'suh) *n.* SARSAPARILLA.

sar·sa·pa·ril·la (sahr''suh·pa·ril'uh) *n.* [Sp. *zarzaparilla,* briar vine]. The dried root of *Smilax aristolochiaefolia,* or of other species of *Smilax.* The most important principles are at least three saponins: smilasaponin, sarsasaponin, and parillin, which on hydrolysis yield the steroidal sapogenins smilagenin, sarsasapogenin, and parigenin. Sarsaparilla was formerly used in the treatment of chronic rheumatism, skin diseases, and syphilis.

sar·sa·sap·o·gen·in (sahr''suh·sap''o·jen'in, ·sa·poj'e·nin) *n.* The steroidal aglycone, $C_{27}H_{44}O_3$, of sarsasaponin, a glycoside of sarsaparilla; a starting compound for synthesis of deoxycorticosterone, progesterone, and certain other steroid hormones.

sar·sa·sap·o·nin (sahr''suh·sap'o·nin) *n.* A glycoside from sarsaparilla. On hydrolysis it yields the aglycone sarsasapogenin.

sar·to·ri·us (sahr·to'ree·us) *n.*, pl. **sarto·rii** (·ree·eye) [NL., from L. *sartor,* tailor]. The tailor's muscle, so called from being concerned in crossing one leg over the other. NA *musculus sartorius.* See also Table of Muscles in the Appendix.

sas·sa·fras (sas'uh·fras) *n.* [Sp. *sasafrás*]. The dried bark of the root of *Sassafras albidum.* Contains a volatile oil, and has been used as a mild aromatic and carminative.

sassafras oil. The volatile oil from the roots of *Sassafras albidum;* contains about 80% safrol. Used as a flavor and, formerly, as a carminative.

sas·sy bark (sas'ee). CASCA BARK.

sat. Abbreviation for *saturated.*

sat·el·lite (sat'e·lite) *n.* [L. *satelles, satellitis,* attendant]. 1. The part of a telomere of a chromosome distal to the secondary constriction. 2. Any secondary or subsidiary body attached to or controlled by a main body.

satellite cell. 1. Any of the cells which encapsulate nerve cells in ganglia. Syn. *capsular cell, amphicyte.* 2. In muscle, a mononuclear cell, lacking contractile substance, which is enclosed within the basement membrane of the muscle fiber and separated from the muscle fiber by plasma membranes. 3. PERICYTE.

satellite DNA. Short, repetitive sequences of DNA found largely near the centromere region of the chromosomes of higher organisms; thought either to hold no genetic information or to provide structure for the rest of the DNA molecule.

satellite phenomenon. The enhancement of growth of one microorganism in proximity to another, for example, that of the growth of *Hemophilus influenzae* around colonies of staphylococci on a plate.

sat·el·lit·osis (sat″e·li·to′sis) *n.*, pl. **satellito·ses** (·seez) [*satellite* + *-osis*]. *In neuropathology,* a condition in which there is an increase of satellite cells around the nerve cells of the central nervous system in inflammatory and degenerative diseases.

sa·ti·ety (sa·tye′uh·tee, say′shee·uh·tee) *n.* [L. *satietas,* from *satis,* sufficient]. Fullness beyond desire; a condition of gratification beyond desire or need.

satiety center. The region in the ventromedial part of the hypothalamus, near the third ventricle, thought to be concerned with the limitation of food intake.

sat. sol. Abbreviation for *saturated solution.*

Sat·ter·thwaite's method [J. E. *Satterthwaite,* U.S. physician, 1843–1934]. Artificial respiration in which, with the patient on his back, there is alternate pressure upon and relaxation of the abdomen.

sat·u·rat·ed (satch′uh·ray″tid) *adj.* [L. *saturatus*]. 1. Having all the atoms of molecules linked so that only single bonds exist. 2. Having sufficient substance, either solid or gaseous, dissolved in a solution so that no more of that substance can be dissolved. Abbreviated, sat.

saturated compound. An organic compound with no free valence, and in which there are neither double nor triple bonds.

saturated hydrocarbon. A hydrocarbon that contains the maximum number of hydrogen atoms, that is, without double or triple bonds between carbon atoms.

saturated solution. A solution that normally contains the maximum amount of substance able to be dissolved. Abbreviated, sat. sol.

sat·u·ra·tion (satch′uh·ray′shun) *n. In optics,* the quality of visual sensation that distinguishes between colors of the same dominant wavelength but different purities.

saturation index. The amount of hemoglobin per unit volume of red blood cells relative to the normal.

Sat·ur·day night paralysis. DRUNKARD'S ARM PARALYSIS.

sat·ur·nine (sat′ur·nine) *adj.* [L. *Saturnus,* Saturn, identified by alchemists with lead]. 1. Pertaining to or produced by lead. 2. Of gloomy nature.

saturnine breath. The peculiar sweet metallic breath characteristic of lead poisoning.

saturnine encephalopathy. LEAD ENCEPHALOPATHY.

sat·urn·ism (sat′ur·niz·um) *n.* Chronic lead poisoning.

sa·ty·ri·a·sis (sat″i·righ′uh·sis, say″ti·) *n.* [Gk., from *satyros,* satyr]. Excessive sexual desire in males.

sa·ty·ro·ma·nia (sat″i·ro·may′nee·uh, say′ti·ro·) *n.* SATYRIASIS.

sa·tyr tip or **tubercle** (say′tur, sat′ur). A rare pointed projection from the posterior aspect of the helix giving the appearance of pointed ear.

sau·cer·ize (saw′sur·ize) *v.* 1. To convert a cavity or defect into a shallow wound. 2. In chronic osteomyelitis, after removal of diseased bone, to shape the bone cavity so as to eliminate irregularities and overhanging walls, and thus enable soft parts to fill the cavity completely during the healing process. —**sau·cer·iza·tion** (saw″sur·i·zay′shun) *n.*

sau·na (saow′nuh, saw′nuh) *n.* [Finnish]. A type of steam bath originating in Finland. Light whipping of the skin by twigs is an accompaniment.

Saun·ders' disease [E. W. *Saunders,* U.S. physician, 1854–1927]. Acute gastric disturbance in infants caused by carbohydrate excess in the diet.

sau·ria·sis (saw·righ′uh·sis) *n.* [Gk. *sauros,* lizard, + *-iasis*]. ICHTHYOSIS.

sau·ri·o·sis (saw″ree·o′sis) *n.* [Gk. *sauros,* lizard, + *-osis*]. DARIER'S DISEASE.

Sau·rop·si·da (saw·rop′si·duh) *n.pl.* [Gk. *sauros,* lizard, + *opsis,* appearance]. A superclass of vertebrates comprising the birds and reptiles. —**saurop·sid** (·sid), **sauropsi·dan** (·dun) *n. & adj.*

sau·rox·ine (saw·rock′seen, ·sin) *n.* An alkaloid obtained from the plant *Lycopodium saururus.*

sau·ru·rine (saw·roor′een, ·in) *n.* An alkaloid obtained from the plant *Lycopodium saururus.*

sau·sa·rism (saw′suh·riz·um) *n.* [Gk. *sausarismos*]. 1. Paralysis of the tongue. 2. Dryness of the tongue.

Sau·vi·neau's ophthalmoplegia (so·vee·no′) [C. *Sauvineau,* French ophthalmologist, b. 1862]. MEDIAL LONGITUDINAL FASCICULUS SYNDROME.

sav·in (sav′in) *n.* [L. *sabina,* juniper]. The evergreen shrub *Juniperus sabina,* the tops of which contain a volatile oil that was formerly used as an emmenagogue, vermifuge, and antirheumatic.

Savino test. A pyelographic examination to determine renal fixation, made after complete expiration and then after complete inspiration. Perirenal inflammatory diseases fix the kidney, and the radiograph is not blurred.

sa·vory (say′vuh·ree) *adj.* [OF. *savouré,* from L. *sapor,* flavor]. Having a pleasant odor or flavor.

saw, *n.* An instrument having a thin steel blade with sharp teeth on one edge, and used for dividing bones and other hard substances.

Sawah itch. Schistosome dermatitis of the Malay countries.

saw pal·met·to berries (pal·met′o). SERENOA.

Sayre's apparatus [L. A. *Sayre,* U.S. surgeon, 1820–1900]. A device for suspending a patient during the application of a plaster of Paris jacket.

Sb [*stibium*]. Symbol for antimony.

Sc Symbol for scandium.

SCA Abbreviation for *sickle cell anemia.* Compare *SC disease* (= SICKLE CELL–HEMOGLOBIN C DISEASE).

scab, *n.* [ON. *skabb*]. 1. Dried exudate covering an ulcer or wound; crust. 2. A disease of sheep caused by a mite.

scab·bard (skab′urd) *n.* A common term for the prepuce of the horse.

scabbed, *adj.* Crusted.

sca·bi·cide (skay′bi·side) *n.* [*scabies* + *-cide*]. Any agent or drug which kills *Sarcoptes scabiei,* the causative organism of scabies.

sca·bies (skay′beez) *n.* [L., itch, mange, from *scabere,* to scratch]. A contagious disorder of the skin caused by the mite *Sarcoptes scabiei;* characterized by multiform lesions with intense itching which occurs chiefly at night. The female insect, burrowing beneath the skin to lay eggs, causes the irritation. Syn. *seven-year itch.* See also *itch.*

scabies crus·to·sa (krus·to′suh). An extreme form of general scabies of the body resulting in fishscale-like desquamation. Syn. *Boeck's scabies, Norwegian itch.*

scabies pap·u·li·for·mis (pap″yoo·li·for′mis). A form of scabies marked by papular efflorescence. Syn. *rank itch, scabies papulosa.*

scabies pap·u·lo·sa (pap″yoo·lo′suh). SCABIES PAPULIFORMIS.

scabies pus·tu·lo·sa (pus″tew·lo′suh). Scabies complicated by formation of large pustules resembling those of smallpox, occurring on the wrists and buttocks of children.

sca·bi·et·ic (skay″bee·et′ick) *adj.* Pertaining to or affected with scabies.

sca·bio·pho·bia (skay″bee·o·fo′bee·uh) *n.* [*scabies* + *-phobia*]. Abnormal fear of scabies.

sca·bi·ous (skay′bee·us) *adj.* 1. Scabby or scaly. 2. Pertaining to scabies.

sca·bri·ti·es (ska·brish'ee·eez) *n.* [L., from *scaber,* scabby]. Roughness; scabbiness.

scabrities un·gui·um syph·i·lit·i·ca (ung'gwee·um sif"i·lit'i·kuh). Abnormal thickening and roughness of the nails, seen in syphilis.

sca·la (skay'luh) *n.,* pl. **sca·lae** (·lee) [L., ladder]. A subdivision of the cavity of the cochlea; especially, one of the perilymphatic spaces.

scala me·dia (mee'dee·uh). COCHLEAR DUCT.

scala tym·pa·ni (tim'puh·nigh) [NA]. The perilymphatic space below the osseous spiral lamina and the basilar membrane. See also Plate 20.

scala ves·ti·bu·li (ves·tib'yoo·lye) [NA]. The perilymphatic space above the osseous spiral lamina and the vestibular membrane. See also Plate 20.

scald (skawld) *n.* [L. *excaldare,* to wash in hot water]. The burn caused by hot liquids or vapors.

scalded skin syndrome. TOXIC EPIDERMAL NECROLYSIS.

scald head. Any crusting disease of the scalp.

scald·ing (skawl'ding) *n.* Burning pain in urination.

[1]**scale,** *n.* [OF. *escale,* husk]. A visible flake of dead or dying epidermis; squame. —**scaly,** *adj.*

[2]**scale,** *n.* [L. *scala,* ladder, stairs]. 1. A system of measurement based on instruments bearing marks or graduations at regular intervals, as barometric scale, thermometric scale. 2. A system of grading or rating based on tests or other criteria.

sca·lene (skay'leen) *adj.* [Gk. *skalēnos,* uneven]. 1. Having unequal sides, as scalene muscle. 2. Of or pertaining to a scalene muscle.

sca·le·nec·to·my (skay"lee·neck'tuh·mee) *n.* [*scalene* + *-ectomy*]. Excision of the scalene muscles, particularly the anterior scalene muscle.

scalene muscle. See Table of Muscles in the Appendix.

scalene tubercle. A tubercle on the upper surface of the first rib for the insertion of the anterior scalene muscle. Syn. *Lisfranc's tubercle.* NA *tuberculum musculi scaleni anterioris.*

sca·le·not·o·my (skay"lee·not'uh·mee) *n.* [*scalene* + *-tomy*]. Severing of the fibers of a scalene muscle, particularly the anterior scalene muscle.

sca·le·nus (skay·lee'nus) *n.,* pl. **scale·ni** (·nigh) [L., from Gk. *skalēnos,* uneven]. One of three muscles in the neck, an anterior (NA *musculus scalenus anterior*), medial (NA *musculus scalenus medius*), and posterior (NA *musculus scalenus posterior*), arising from the transverse processes of the cervical vertebrae, and inserted on the first two ribs. See also Table of Muscles in the Appendix.

scalenus anterior syndrome. A symptom complex due to compression of the brachial plexus by the scalenus anterior muscle, characterized by pain and numbness, and often by signs of compression of the subclavian artery. Syn. *Naffziger's syndrome, scalenus anticus syndrome.*

scalenus an·ti·cus syndrome (an·tye'kus). SCALENUS ANTERIOR SYNDROME.

scalenus min·i·mus (min'i·mus). An inconstant muscle of the scalene group arising from the anterior tubercle of the sixth or sixth and seventh ribs, inserted into the first rib, and attached to the dome of the pleura. NA *musculus scalenus minimus.*

scalenus pleu·ra·lis (ploo·ray'lis). The part of the scalenus minimus muscle attached to the pleura.

scal·er (skay'lur) *n.* 1. An instrument for removing calcareous deposits from the teeth. 2. An electronic instrument for counting and recording electrical impulses, as those produced by such detectors of radioactivity as the Geiger-Müller tube and the scintillation probe.

scal·ing, *adj.* & *n.* 1. Desquamating; producing scales. 2. A pharmaceutical process consisting of drying concentrated solutions of drugs on glass plates.

scaling circuit. A circuit that permits recording of electrical impulses which are produced at a high frequency, by counting only every 2^n or 10^n impulse; such a circuit is employed in a scaler.

scalp, *n.* The integument covering the cranium.

scal·pel (skal'pul) *n.* [L. *scalpellum,* from *scalpere,* to cut, engrave]. A surgical knife with a short blade, a convex or straight cutting edge, rounded or pointed at the end.

scaly ringworm. TINEA IMBRICATA.

scan, *v.* & *n.* [L. *scandere,* to climb; to scan verses]. 1. To observe (an area or volume) systematically, especially by subjecting it to a series of partial observations by a sensory organ or device. 2. The observation, or the record of the observation, made by such an organ or device.

scan·di·um (skan'dee·um) *n.* [L. *Scandia,* Scandinavia]. Sc=44.9559. A rare metal, atomic number 21, belonging to the aluminum group.

scan·ning electron microscope. An electron microscope which, by scanning an irregularly contoured surface with a concentrated electron beam, provides a high-resolution image possessing a three-dimensional quality; used for examining and photographing cell and tissue surfaces.

scanning micrograph. A micrograph from a scanning electron microscope.

scanning speech. A form of dysarthria, in which speech is slow and words are broken up into syllables, much as verse tends to be pronounced when scanned for meter. Each syllable, after an involuntary pause, may be uttered with less force or more force ("explosive speech") than is natural. Characteristic of lesions of the cerebellum and brainstem. See also *cerebellar speech.*

scan·so·ri·us (skan·so'ree·us) *n.* [L., of or for climbing, from *scandere,* to climb]. A variable small anterior gluteal muscle; a partially separated part of the gluteus minimus muscle.

Scan·zo·ni's maneuver (skah^n·tso'nee) [F. W. *Scanzoni,* German obstetrician, 1821–1891]. Conversion of a posterior vertex presentation to an anterior position by double forceps application.

scaph-, scapho-. A combining form meaning *scaphoid.*

sca·pha (skaf'uh, skay'fuh) *n.* [L., skiff, from Gk. *skaphē*] [NA]. The furrow of the auricle between the helix and anthelix.

scapho-. See *scaph-.*

scapho·ceph·a·ly (skaf"o·sef'uh·lee) *n.* [*scapho-* + *-cephaly*]. A condition of the skull characterized by elongation and narrowing and a projecting, keel-like sagittal suture; due to its premature closure. See also *oxycephaly.* —**scapho·ce·phal·ic** (·se·fal'ick), **scapho·ceph·a·lous** (·sef'uh·lus) *adj.*

scaph·oid (skaf'oid) *adj.* & *n.* [Gk. *skaphoeidēs,* concave, navicular, from *skaphē,* bowl, boat (rel. to L. *scapula*)]. 1. Boat-shaped; CONCAVE. 2. A boat-shaped bone of the carpus. NA *os scaphoideum.* See also Table of Bones in the Appendix.

scaphoid abdomen. A belly characterized by sunken walls, presenting a concavity. Syn. *navicular abdomen.*

scaphoid face. A face that appears concave because of weakly developed nasal and maxillary regions. May occur secondary to midfacial fractures. Syn. *dish-face.*

scaphoid fossa. 1. A depression in the base of the medial pterygoid process of the sphenoid bone. NA *fossa scaphoidea.* 2. SCAPHA.

scaph·oid·itis (skaf"oy·dye'tis) *n.* [*scaphoid* + *-itis*]. Inflammation of the scaphoid bone.

scapul-, scapulo-. A combining form meaning *scapula, scapular.*

scap·u·la (skap'yoo·luh) *n.,* L. pl. & genit. sing. **scapu·lae** (·lee), E. pl. **scapulas** [L. (rel. to Gk. *skaphē,* bowl, boat, whence *scaphoid*)] [NA]. The large, flat, triangular bone forming the back of the shoulder; the shoulder blade. See also Table of Bones in the Appendix and Plates 1, 2, 14.

scapula ala·ta (ay·lay'tuh). WINGED SCAPULA.

scap·u·lal·gia (skap"yoo·lal'jee·uh) *n.* [*scapul-* + *-algia*]. Pain in the region of the scapula.

scap·u·lar (skap'yoo·lur) *adj.* Of or pertaining to the scapula.
scapular artery. See Table of Arteries in the Appendix.
scapular line. A vertical line drawn on the back through the inferior angle of the scapula. NA *linea scapularis.*
scapular notch. The notch in the upper border of the scapula at the base of the coracoid process for the passage of the suprascapular nerve. NA *incisura scapulae.*
scapular reflex. Contraction of the scapular muscles and a retraction and sometimes an elevation of the scapula in response to scratching the skin over the scapula or in the interscapular space.
scapular region. The region of the back corresponding to the position of the scapula, the spine of which divides it into a supraspinous and an infraspinous region. NA *regio scapularis.*
scap·u·lec·to·my (skap"yoo·leck'tuh·mee) *n.* [*scapul-* + *-ectomy*]. Surgical removal of a scapula.
scapulo-. See *scapul-*.
sca·pu·lo·cla·vi·cu·la·ris (skap"yoo·la·kla·vick"yoo·lair'is) *n.* [NL., from *scapulo-* + *clavicular*]. A variable muscle extending from the coracoid process to the lateral third of the clavicle.
scap·u·lo·cos·tal (skap'yoo·lo·kos'tul) *adj.* [*scapulo-* + *costal*]. Of or pertaining to the scapula and the ribs. Syn. *costoscapular.*
scapulocostal syndrome. A syndrome characterized by the insidious onset of pain in the superior or posterior aspect of the shoulder girdle with radiation into the neck, occiput, upper or lower arm, or chest, and often accompanied by tingling and numbness in the fingers. It is due to long-standing alterations in the relationships between the scapula and the posterior thoracic wall. Syn. *fatigue-postural paradox.*
scap·u·lo·hu·mer·al (skap"yoo·lo·hew'mur·ul) *adj.* [*scapulo-* + *humeral*]. Pertaining to the scapula and the humerus, or to the shoulder joint.
scapulohumeral muscular dystrophy (of Erb). A form of limb-girdle muscular dystrophy in which the shoulder girdle is affected earlier and to a greater extent than the pelvic girdle. Compare *Leyden-Möbius dystrophy.*
scapulohumeral periarthritis. FROZEN SHOULDER.
scapulohumeral reflex. Retraction of the scapula, sometimes with adduction and external rotation of the humerus in response to tapping the vertebral border of the scapula. Syn. *scapuloperiosteal reflex.*
scap·u·lo·peri·os·te·al reflex (skap"yoo·lo·perr"ee·os'tee·ul). SCAPULOHUMERAL REFLEX.
scap·u·lo·pexy (skap'yoo·lo·peck"see) *n.* [*scapulo-* + *-pexy*]. Fixation of the scapula to the ribs, as in cases of paralysis of scapular muscles.
sca·pus (skay'pus) *n.*, pl. **sca·pi** (·pye) [L.]. SHAFT.
scapus pi·li (pye'lye) [NA]. HAIR SHAFT.
scar, *n.* [OF. *escare,* from Gk. *eschara,* scab]. A permanent mark resulting from a wound or disease process in tissue, especially the skin.
scar·a·bi·a·sis (skăr"uh·bye'uh·sis) *n.* [L. *scarab*aeus, scarab, dung beetle, + *-iasis*]. A condition occurring usually in children in which the intestine is invaded by the dung beetle. Characterized by anorexia, emaciation, and gastrointestinal disturbances.
scarf·skin, *n.* EPIDERMIS.
scar·i·fi·ca·tion (skăr"i·fi·kay'shun) *n.* [L. *scarificare,* to scratch]. The operation of making numerous small, superficial incisions in skin or other tissue. —**scar·i·fy** (skăr'i·figh) *v.*
scarification test. SCRATCH TEST.
scar·i·fi·ca·tor (skăr'i·fi·kay"tur) *n.* An instrument used in scarification, consisting of a number of small lancets operated by a spring.
scar·la·ti·na (skahr"luh·tee'nuh) *n.* [NL.]. SCARLET FEVER. —**scarla·ti·nal** (·tee'nul), **scarla·ti·nous** (·teen'us) *adj.*
scar·la·ti·nel·la (skahr"luh·ti·nel'uh) *n.* [NL., dim. of *scarlatina*]. EXANTHEM SUBITUM.
scar·la·ti·ni·form (skahr"luh·tee'ni·form, ·tin'i·form) *adj.* [*scarlatina* + *-iform*]. Resembling scarlet fever.
scar·la·ti·noid (skahr"luh·tee'noid, skahr·lat'i·noid) *adj.* [*scarlatina* + *-oid*]. SCARLATINIFORM.
scarlatinoid erythema. ERYTHEMA SCARLATINIFORME.
scarlet fever. An acute contagious febrile disease due to group A hemolytic streptococci, characterized by acute tonsillitis and pharyngitis and a scarlet-red exanthem. Syn. *scarlatina.*
scarlet fever antitoxin. SCARLET FEVER STREPTOCOCCUS ANTITOXIN.
scarlet fever convalescent serum. Human immune serum for scarlet fever. See *human immune serum.*
scarlet fever streptococcus antitoxin. A sterile aqueous solution of antitoxic substances obtained from the blood serum or plasma of a healthy animal which has been immunized against the toxin produced by group A beta hemolytic streptococci. It was formerly used in the treatment of scarlet fever, and occasionally for producing a temporary passive immunity in persons exposed to the infection. It is also used to distinguish the rash of scarlet fever from other rashes.
scarlet fever streptococcus toxin. Toxic filtrates of cultures of *Streptococcus pyogenes* responsible for the characteristic rash of scarlet fever. The toxins are serologically distinct, and are used in the Dick test to establish susceptibility or immunity to scarlet fever.
scarlet fever test. 1. DICK TEST. 2. SCHULTZ-CHARLTON BLANCHING TEST.
scarlet red. The azo dye 1-(4-*o*-tolylazo-*o*-tolylazo)-2-naphthol, $C_{24}H_{20}N_4O$; has been used to stimulate epithelial cell growth in burns, wounds, ulcers.
Scar·pa's fascia [A. *Scarpa,* Italian anatomist and surgeon, 1752–1832]. The deep, membranous layer of the superficial fascia of the lower abdomen.
Scarpa's foramen [A. *Scarpa*]. A median incisive foramen. See also *incisive foramen.*
Scarpa's ganglion [A. *Scarpa*]. VESTIBULAR GANGLION.
Scarpa's triangle [A. *Scarpa*]. FEMORAL TRIANGLE.
scar tissue. Contracted dense connective tissue, the end result of healing.
scat-, scato- [Gk. *skōr, skatos*]. A combining form meaning *excrement, feces, fecal.*
scat·a·cra·tia (skat"uh·kray'shuh, ·shee·uh) *n.* [*scat-* + Gk. *akrateia,* incontinence]. SCORACRATIA.
sca·te·mia (ska·tee'mee·uh) *n.* [*scat-* + *-emia*]. Toxemia of the intestines.
scat·ol (skat'ol, ·ole) *n.* SKATOLE.
scat·o·lo·gia (skat"o·lo'jee·uh) *n.* [*scato-* + *-logia*]. SCATOLOGY.
sca·tol·o·gy (ska·tol'uh·jee) *n.* [*scato-* + *-logy*]. 1. The study of excreta. 2. Preoccupation or obsession with excrement, or with filth and obscenity. —**scat·o·log·ic** (skat"uh·loj'ick), **scatolog·i·cal** (·i·kul) *adj.*
sca·to·ma (ska·to'muh) *n.* [*scat-* + *-oma*]. A mass of fecal matter in the colon resembling, on palpation, an abdominal tumor.
sca·toph·a·gous (ska·tof'uh·gus) *adj.* [Gk. *skatophagos,* from *skōr, skatos,* excrement, + *phagein,* to eat]. Excrement-eating.
sca·toph·a·gy (ska·tof'uh·jee) *n.* [*scato-* + *-phagy*]. The eating of filth or excrement.
scato·pho·bia (skat"o·fo'bee·uh) *n.* [*scato-* + *-phobia*]. An abnormal dread of filth or excrement.
sca·tos·co·py (ska·tos'kuh·pee) *n.* [*scato-* + *-scopy*]. Inspection of the feces.
scat·ter, *n.* 1. The deflection or deviation of x- or gamma rays due to interaction with matter. 2. *In psychology,* the range of levels through which an individual passes on an intelligence test; specifically, the extent to which the individual

tested passes or fails items from widely different levels of ability, as when he does well on verbal and poorly on numerical tests. 3. *In statistics,* the extent to which items in a series are closely grouped about the mean or dispersed over a wide range. —**scat·tered,** *adj.*

scattered ray. A gamma ray or x-ray that has been scattered by a deflecting collision from its original path.

scat·ter·ing, *n.* In nuclear science, the change in direction of a particle or photon as a result of a collision with another particle or system.

scattering collision. Impact of a photon with an electron in an atom, whereby the photon gives up only a part of its energy to set the electron in motion and travels on in a different direction with reduced energy. Syn. *Compton effect.*

scav·en·ger (skav'in-jur) *n.* [ME. *skawager,* toll-collector, from *skawage,* toll, duty, from OF. *escauwage,* inspection]. MACROPHAGE.

scavenger cell. MACROPHAGE.

scav·en·ging (skav'in-jing) *n. In nuclear chemistry,* the formation of an unspecific precipitate to remove from a solution, by adsorption or coprecipitation, a substantial proportion of one or more undesirable radioactive ions.

Sc. D. Doctor of Science.

Sc.D.A. Right scapuloanterior position of the fetus.

SC disease. SICKLE CELL-HEMOGLOBIN C DISEASE. Compare *SS disease.*

Sc.D.P. Right scapuloposterior position of the fetus.

scent, *n.* [OF. *sentir,* to smell]. An effluvium from any body capable of affecting the olfactory sense; odor; fragrance.

Scha·fer method [E. A. Sharpey-*Schafer,* English physician, 1850–1935]. A former method for artificial respiration in which intermittent pressure over the lower thorax of the prone patient promotes a limited degree of exchange of air in the lungs.

Schä·fer's syndrome (she^y'fur) [E. *Schäfer,* German dermatologist, 20th century]. PACHYONYCHIA CONGENITA.

Schäf·fer's reflex (shef'ur) [M. *Schäffer,* German neurologist, 1852–1923]. In spastic paralysis of the lower extremity, extension of the great toe in response to pinching of the calcaneal tendon; similar to Babinski sign (1).

Schales and Schales method [O. *Schales,* U.S. biochemist, b. 1910]. A test for blood chlorides, in which the sample is titrated with standard mercuric nitrate solution at the proper acidity in the presence of diphenylcarbazone as indicator. Chlorides present react with the added mercuric ions to form soluble, but undissociated, mercuric chloride. When an excess of mercuric ion has been added, the indicator turns purple.

Scham·berg's disease [J. F. *Schamberg,* U.S. dermatologist, 1870–1934]. PROGRESSIVE PIGMENTARY DERMATOSIS.

Schanz's syndrome (sha^hnts) [A. *Schanz,* German orthopedist, 1868–1931]. A syndrome of fatigue, pain on pressure over the spinous processes of the vertebrae, pain when lying down, spinal curvature; indicative of spinal weakness.

Schar·lach R stain. A stain utilizing scarlet red solution with subsequent staining with hematoxylin. Used to demonstrate fat in tissue sections. Fat globules stain brilliant red, nuclei dark blue.

Schat·ski ring [R. *Schatski,* U.S. radiologist, b. 1901]. A diaphragmlike localized narrowing in the lower esophagus, sometimes causing dysphagia.

Schau·dinn's fixing fluid (shaow'din) [F. R. *Schaudinn,* German bacteriologist, 1871–1906]. A mixture of 1 part absolute ethanol with 2 parts saturated aqueous mercuric chloride solution; used as a general fixative.

Schau·mann bodies [J. *Schaumann,* Swedish dermatologist, 1879–1953]. Concentrically layered structures with a central core of calcite ($CaCO_3$), surrounded by a protein-calcium complex; they occur as cytoplasmic inclusions in the giant cells of sarcoidosis, berylliosis, and other diseases.

Schau·ta-Wert·heim operation (shaow'tah, vehrt'hime) [F. *Schauta,* Austrian gynecologist, 1849–1919; and E. *Wertheim*]. WERTHEIM-SCHAUTA OPERATION.

Sche·de's method (she^y'de^h) [M. *Schede,* German surgeon, 1844–1902]. A method of treating bone caries by curetting the cavity and allowing it to fill with blood clot.

Schede's operation [M. *Schede*]. EXTRAPLEURAL PNEUMONOLYSIS.

Scheie's syndrome [H. G. *Scheie,* U.S. ophthalmologist, b. 1909]. Mucopolysaccharidosis V, transmitted as an autosomal recessive trait, characterized chemically by the excretion of excessive amounts of chondroitin sulfate B in the urine, and clinically by a facies similar to that seen in the more common Hurler's syndrome though less coarse, hypertrichosis, clouding of the cornea, and aortic valve disease. Stature is usually normal or low-normal, and intellect is little impaired if at all.

Schellong-Strisower phenomenon. A fall of systolic arterial blood pressure on assuming the erect position from recumbency.

sche·ma (skee'muh) *n.,* pl. **schema·ta** (·tuh) [Gk. *schēma,* shape]. 1. A simple design to illustrate a complex mechanism. 2. An outline of a subject. —**sche·mat·ic** (skee·mat'ick) *adj.*

sche·mato·gram (skee·mat'uh·gram, skee'muh·to·) *n.* [*schema* + *-gram*]. *In medicine,* the outline of a person or parts of the body, in which details can be filled in, as after a physical examination or surgery.

sche·mato·graph (skee·mat'uh·graf, skee'muh·to·) *n.* [*schema* + *-graph*]. An instrument for tracing the outline of a person, body part, or other object. Compare *schemograph.*

sche·mo·graph (skee'mo·graf) *n.* [*schema* + *-graph*]. An apparatus for tracing the outline of the field of vision by means of a perimeter.

Schenck's disease [B. R. *Schenck,* U.S. surgeon, 1842–1920]. SPOROTRICHOSIS.

Sche·rer's test (she^y'rur) [J. J. von *Scherer,* German physician, 1814–1869]. A test for inositol, in which ammonium hydroxide and calcium chloride are added to partially evaporated acidified urine and the whole is evaporated. In the presence of inositol, a bright red color is obtained.

sche·ro·ma (ske·ro'muh) *n.* [Gk. *scheros,* dry, + *-oma*]. XEROPHTHALMIA.

Scheu·er·mann's disease [H. W. *Scheuermann,* Danish surgeon, 1877–1960]. Osteochondrosis of the vertebrae, associated with kyphosis in adolescents.

Schick pseudoreaction. PSEUDOREACTION (2).

Schick test [B. *Schick,* U.S. pediatrician, 1877–1967]. A skin test for immunity to diphtheria performed by the intracutaneous injection of an amount of diluted diphtheria toxin equal to one-fiftieth of the minimal lethal dose. A positive reaction is interpreted on the fifth to seventh day. It consists of local erythema with edema, and indicates the lack of immunity.

Schiff's aldehyde reagent [H. *Schiff*]. SCHIFF'S REAGENT.

Schiff-Sherrington phenomenon [M. *Schiff,* German physiologist, 1823–1896; and C. S. *Sherrington*]. Hyperreflexia of the forelimbs after the spinal cord is severed below the cervical enlargement.

Schiff's reagent [H. *Schiff,* German chemist, 1834–1915]. A solution of acid fuchsin in water decolorized by sulfur dioxide; used in testing for aldehydes, the presence of which causes a blue color.

Schil·der-Ad·di·son complex [P. F. *Schilder* and T. *Addison*]. ADRENOLEUKODYSTROPHY.

Schilder's diffuse cerebral sclerosis. SCHILDER'S DISEASE.

Schilder's disease [P. F. *Schilder,* German neuropsychiatrist, 1886–1940]. A nonfamilial disease of children and young adults, characterized clinically by a progressive dementia, homonymous hemianopia, cortical blindness and deafness, and varying degrees of hemiplegia, quadriplegia and pseudobulbar palsy. The typical lesion is a large, sharply outlined, asymmetrical focus of myelin destruction, often involving an entire lobe or cerebral hemisphere, extending across the corpus callosum to affect the opposite hemisphere. In many cases, the optic nerves, brainstem and spinal cord disclose the typical discrete lesions of multiple sclerosis. Syn. *encephalitis periaxalis diffusa.*

Schil·ler-Du·val body [W. *Schiller,* U.S. pathologist, 1887–1960; and M. *Duval,* French anatomist, 19th century]. A convoluted mass of cells resembling a renal glomerulus, characteristic of endodermal sinus tumors of the ovary and similar tumors of the testis; the cells are considered derivatives of yolk sac endoderm.

Schiller's test [W. *Schiller*]. A test using aqueous iodine and potassium iodide solution to delineate areas of squamous epithelium which do not contain glycogen and therefore do not take the stain. It aids in localizing areas of the uterine cervix where biopsy studies should be taken to exclude cancer.

Schil·ling classification, blood count, hemogram, or **method** [V. *Schilling,* Austrian hematologist, 1883–1960]. A system of neutrophilic classification distinguishing myelocytes; metamyelocytes, which have an indented nucleus; band cells, with sharply indented T-, U-, or V-shaped nuclei; and segmented neutrophils.

Schilling test [R. F. *Schilling,* U.S. internist, b. 1919]. A test of the absorption of vitamin B_{12} by the gastrointestinal tract following an oral dose tagged with radioactive cobalt. If absorption is below normal, a repeat oral dose of B_{12} with intrinsic factor tests for its specific lack.

Schilling type leukemia [V. *Schilling*]. Monocytic leukemia in which the cells bear no resemblance to granulocytes.

Schim·mel·busch's disease [C. *Schimmelbusch,* German surgeon, 1860–1895]. A variety of mammary dysplasia; CYSTIC DISEASE OF THE BREAST.

Schimmelbusch's mask [C. *Schimmelbusch*]. A device for administering liquid anesthetic, open drop, for inhalation anesthesia.

schin·dy·le·sis (skin″di·lee′sis) *n.,* pl. **schindyle·ses** (·seez) [Gk. *schindylēsis,* cleavage]. A synarthrosis in which a plate of one bone is fixed in a fissure of another.

Schiötz tonometer (shyœts) [H. *Schiötz,* Norwegian ophthalmologist, 1850–1927]. An indentation tonometer to measure intraocular pressure.

Schir·mer test (shirr′mur) [O. W. A. *Schirmer,* German ophthalmologist, 1864–1917]. A clinical test to evaluate lacrimal secretion. Performed by inserting a strip of filter paper into the lower cul-de-sac (fornix conjunctivae inferior).

-schisis [Gk., cleaving]. A combining form meaning *cleft, split, fissure, splitting.*

schis·ten·ceph·a·ly (skis″ten·sef′uh·lee, shis″) *n.* [*schisto-* + *-encephaly*]. SCHIZENCEPHALY.

schisto- [Gk. *schistos*]. A combining form meaning *split, fissured, cleft.*

schis·to·ce·lia (skis″to·see′lee·uh, shis″) *n.* [*schisto-* + *cel-* + *-ia*]. CELOSOMA.

schis·to·ceph·a·lus (skis″to·sef′uh·lus, shis″) *n.* [*schisto-* + *-cephalus*]. 1. An individual with a fissured skull. 2. A cleft in any part of the head. —**schisto·ce·phal·ic** (·se·fal′ick) *adj.*

schis·to·cor·mus (skis″to·kor′mus, shis″) *n.* [*schisto-* + Gk. *kormos,* trunk]. An individual having a cleft thorax (schistocormus fissisternalis), neck (schistocormus fissicollis), or abdominal wall (schistocormus fissiventralis).

schis·to·cys·tis (skis″to·sis′tis, shis″) *n.* [*schisto-* + Gk. *kystis,* bladder]. EXSTROPHY OF THE BLADDER.

schis·to·cyte (skis′to·site, shis′) *n.* [*schisto-* + *-cyte*]. A fragmented part of an erythrocyte containing hemoglobin.

schis·to·cy·to·sis (skis″to·sigh·to′sis, shis″) *n.* [*schistocyte* + *-osis*]. The presence of large numbers of schistocytes in the blood.

schis·to·glos·sia (skis″to·glos′ee·uh, shis″) *n.* [*schisto-* + *-glossia*]. BIFID TONGUE.

schis·tom·e·lus (skis·tom′e·lus, shis·) *n.* [*schisto-* + *-melus*]. An individual with a cleft extremity.

schis·tom·e·ter (skis·tom′e·tur, shis·) *n.* [*schisto-* + *-meter*]. A device for measuring the distance between the vocal folds.

schis·to·pro·so·pia (skis″to·pro·so′pee·uh, shis″) *n.* [*schisto-* + *prosop-* + *-ia*]. A congenital fissure of the face. —**schisto·pros·o·pous** (·pros′o·pus) *adj.*

schis·to·pros·o·pus (skis″to·pros′o·pus, ·pros·o′pus, shis″) *n.* [*schisto-* + *prosop-* + *-us*]. An individual having a fissure of the face.

schis·to·pros·o·py (skis″to·pros′uh·pee, shis″) *n.* SCHISTOPROSOPIA.

schis·tor·rha·chis, schis·tor·ra·chis (skis·tor′uh·kis, shis·) *n.* [*schisto-* + *-rrhachis*]. SPINA BIFIDA.

schis·to·sis (shis·to′sis) *n.* [*schist,* a kind of laminated rock, + *-osis*]. SILICOSIS.

Schis·to·so·ma (shis″to·so′muh, skis″) *n.* [*schisto-* + Gk. *sōma,* body]. A genus of blood flukes infecting man.

Schistosoma hae·ma·to·bi·um (hee·muh·to′bee·um). A species of flukes the adults of which are found in the vessels of the urinary bladder; common in Africa.

Schistosoma ja·pon·i·cum (ja·pon′i·kum). A species of flukes the adults of which are found in the mesenteric veins; widely distributed in Japan and China.

schis·to·so·mal (shis″to·so′mul) *adj.* Pertaining to or caused by schistosomes.

schistosomal cystitis. A granulomatous urinary cystitis caused by the ova of *Schistosoma haematobium.*

Schistosoma man·so·ni (man·so′nigh). A species of flukes the adults of which are found in the mesenteric veins and portal vein; found in parts of Africa, South America, and the West Indies.

schis·to·some (shis′to·sohm, skis′) *n.* A fluke of the genus *Schistosoma.*

schistosome dermatitis. A dermatitis, sometimes occurring after exposure to freshwater lakes of the United States, Canada, Europe, and Asia, resulting from the penetration of the skin by nonhuman schistosome cercariae, with snails as the intermediate hosts and migratory birds and other animals as the definitive hosts. Syn. *swimmer's itch, swamp itch.*

schis·to·so·mi·a·sis (shis″to·so·mye′uh·sis, skis″) *n.,* pl. **schistosomia·ses** (·seez) [*Schistosoma* + *-iasis*]. Disease produced by digenetic trematodes or blood flukes, *Schistosoma mansoni, S. haemotobium,* and *S. japonicum,* the adult worms inhabiting the circulatory system of man and animals in the tropical and subtropical areas of the world, and constituting one of the most prevalent and important diseases of man. Syn. *bilharziasis.*

Schis·to·so·moph·o·ra (shis″to·so·mof′uh·ruh, skis″) *n.* [NL., from *Schistosoma* + Gk. *phoros,* bearing, carrying]. A genus of freshwater snails.

Schistosomophora hy·dro·bi·op·sis (high″dro·bye·op′sis). A species of freshwater snail, the intermediate host of *Schistosoma japonicum.*

schis·to·so·mus (skis″to·so′mus, shis″) *n.* [*schisto-* + *-somus*]. An individual in which there is a lateral or median eventration extending the whole length of the abdomen, one or both lower extremities being absent or rudimentary.

schis·to·ster·nia (skis″to·stur′nee·uh, shis″) *n.* [*schisto-* + *sternum* + *-ia*]. A congenital fissure of the sternum.

schis·to·tho·rax (skis″to·tho′racks, shis″) *n.* [*schisto-* + *thorax*]. A congenital fissure of the thorax.

schis·to·tra·che·lus (skis″to·tray′ke·lus, shis″) *n.* [NL., from *schisto-* + Gk. *trachelos,* neck]. CERVICAL FISSURE.

schiz-, schizo- [Gk. *schizein,* to split]. A combining form meaning *split* or *cleft.*

schiz·am·ni·on (skiz·am′nee·on) *n.* [*schiz-* + *amnion*]. An amnion developing by cavity formation in the inner cell mass;

as in humans and certain other mammals. Contr. *pleuramnion.*

schiz·ax·on (skiz·acks′on) *n.* [*schiz-* + *axon*]. An axon that divides in its course into equal, or nearly equal, branches.

schiz·en·ceph·a·ly (skiz″en·sef′uh·lee) *n.* [*schiz-* + *-encephaly*]. A form of developmental porencephaly which is characterized by symmetrically placed clefts in the cerebral cortex.

schizo-. See *schiz-*.

schizo·af·fec·tive (skit″so·uh·feck′tiv, skiz″o·) *adj.* Pertaining to psychiatric disorders showing mixtures of schizophrenic and affective or manic-depressive symptoms.

schizoaffective type of schizophrenia. A psychotic disorder in which mental content may be predominantly schizophrenic while mood is markedly excited or depressed.

schizo·ble·phar·ia (skiz″o·ble·făr′ee·uh) *n.* [*schizo-* + *blephar-* + *-ia*]. A fissure of the eyelid.

schizo·cyte (skiz′o·site) *n.* [*schizo-* + *-cyte*]. SCHISTOCYTE.

schizo·cy·to·sis (skiz″o·sigh·to′sis) *n.* SCHISTOCYTOSIS.

schizo·gen·e·sis (skiz″o·jen′e·sis) *n.* [*schizo-* + *-genesis*]. Reproduction by fission.

schi·zog·e·nous (ski·zoj′e·nus) *adj.* [*schizo-* + *-genous*]. Of, pertaining to, or formed by fission. Contr. *lysigenous.*

schizo·gnath·ism (skiz″o·nath′iz·um) *n.* [*schizo-* + *gnath-* + *-ism*]. A condition in which either the upper or lower jaw is cleft. —**schizognath·ous** (·us) *adj.*

schi·zog·o·ny (ski·zog′uh·nee) *n.* [*schizo-* + *-gony*]. 1. SCHIZOGENESIS. 2. Multiple division in which the contents of the oocyst eventually split into swarm spores. —**schizo·gon·ic** (skiz″o·gon′ick) *adj.*

schiz·oid (skit′soid, skiz′oid) *adj.* & *n.* [*schiz-* + *-oid*]. 1. Resembling schizophrenia; often applied to individuals who are extremely shy and introverted. 2. A schizoid individual.

schizoid personality. An individual given to seclusiveness, emotional rigidity, introversion, and unsocial behavior. See also *schizophrenia.*

schizo·ma·nia (skit″so·may′nee·uh, skiz″o·) *n.* [*schizo-* + *mania*]. A schizoaffective type of schizophrenia.

Schizo·my·ce·tes (skiz″o·migh·see′teez) *n.pl.* [*schizo-* + *mycetes*]. A class of fungi; the fission fungi or bacteria.

schiz·ont (skiz′ont) *n.* [*schiz-* + Gk. *ōn, ontos,* being]. A stage in the asexual life cycle of *Plasmodium,* covering the period from beginning of division of nuclear material until the mature merozoites are formed.

schi·zon·ti·cide (ski·zon′ti·side) *n.* [*schizont* + *-cide*]. A substance destructive to schizonts.

schiz·onych·ia (skiz″o·nick′ee·uh) *n.* [*schiz-* + *onych-* + *-ia*]. Disease of the nails characterized by irregular splitting.

schizo·pha·sia (skit″so·fay′zhuh, ·zee·uh, skiz″o·) *n.* [*schizo-* + *-phasia*]. WORD SALAD.

schizo·phre·nia (skit′so·free′nee·uh, ·fren′ee·uh, skiz″o·) *n.* [*schizo-* + *-phrenia*]. A group of psychotic disorders, often beginning after adolescence or in young adulthood, characterized by fundamental alterations in concept formations, with misinterpretation of reality, and associated affective, behavioral, and intellectual disturbances in varying degrees and mixtures. These disorders are marked by a tendency to withdraw from reality, ambivalent, constricted, and inappropriate responses and mood, unpredictable disturbances in stream of thought, regressive tendencies to the point of deterioration, and often hallucinations and delusions. Syn. *dementia praecox.* See also *acute schizophrenic episode, catatonic type of schizophrenia, childhood type of schizophrenia, hebephrenic type of schizophrenia, paranoid type of schizophrenia, residual type of schizophrenia.* —**schizo·phre·nic** (·fren′ick, ·free′nick) *n.* & *adj.*

schizophrenic reaction. SCHIZOPHRENIA.

schizo·so·ma si·re·noi·des (skiz″o·so′muh sigh″re·noy′deez). A lateral abdominal cleft with absence of the leg on that side.

schizo·the·mia (skit″so·theem′ee·uh, skiz′o·) *n.* [*schizo-* + Gk. *thema,* theme, + *-ia*]. Interrupting conversational flow with reminiscenses.

schizo·tho·rax (skiz″o·tho′racks) *n.* SCHISTOTHORAX.

schizo·thy·mic (skit″so·thigh′mick, skiz″o·) *adj.* [*schizo-* + *thym-,* mind, + *-ic*]. Having a schizoid personality or temperament. —**schizothy·mia** (·mee·uh) *n.*

schizo·try·pano·so·mi·a·sis (skiz″o·tri·pan″uh·so·migh′uh·sis) *n.* [*schizo-* + *trypanosomiasis*]. CHAGAS' DISEASE.

schizo·type (skit′so·tipe, skiz′o·) *n.* A schizophrenic phenotype. See also *schizoid personality, schizophrenia.*

Schlaer test. A night vision test using the Hecht-Schlaer adaptometer.

Schlange's sign (shlahng′eh) [H. *Schlange,* German surgeon, 1856–1922]. A sign of intestinal obstruction in which the intestine is dilated above the obstruction and peristalsis is absent below.

Schlatter disease [C. *Schlatter*]. OSGOOD-SCHLATTER DISEASE.

Schlemm's canal [F. S. *Schlemm,* German anatomist, 1795–1858]. An irregular space or plexiform series of spaces at the sclerocorneal junction in the eye. It drains the aqueous humor from the anterior chamber.

Schle·sing·er's sign (shleʸ′zing·ur) [H. *Schlesinger,* Austrian surgeon, 1866–1934]. POOL-SCHLESINGER'S SIGN.

Schlesinger's test [W. *Schlesinger,* Austrian physician, b. 1869]. A test for urobilin, in which Lugol's solution and a saturated alcoholic solution of zinc acetate are added to urine which is then filtered. A greenish fluorescence in the filtrate under strong light indicates urobilin.

Schlof·fer's operation [H. *Schloffer,* German surgeon, 1868–1937]. A method of operating upon pituitary tumors by the nasal route.

Schloffer's tumor [H. *Schloffer*]. An inflammatory swelling of the abdominal wall following surgical repair of inguinal hernia.

Schlös·ser's treatment (shlœs′ur) [C. *Schlösser,* German ophthalmologist, 1857–1925]. Alcohol injection into the peripheral branches of the trigeminal nerve for treatment of trigeminal neuralgia.

Schmidt-Lan·ter·mann incisure or **cleft** (lahn′tur·mahn) [H. D. *Schmidt,* U.S. pathologist, 1823-1888; and A. J. *Lantermann,* Alsatian anatomist, 19th century]. One of the oblique, funnel-shaped clefts in the myelin sheath of peripheral nerves; there may be several such clefts in an internodal segment. Syn. *Lantermann's cleft, myelin incisure.*

Schmidt nuclei test [A. *Schmidt,* German physician, 1865–1918]. A test for pancreatic sufficiency in which beef or thymus, hardened in alcohol, is passed through the intestinal tract. If the nuclei are undigested on microscopic examination, pancreatic insufficiency may be present.

Schmidt's coagulation theory [E. O. *Schmidt,* German anatomist, 1823–1886]. The concept that a soluble protein (fibrinogen) is changed to insoluble fibrin by the action of thrombin.

Schmidt's fibrinoplastin [E. O. *Schmidt*]. SERUM GLOBULIN.

Schmidt's syndrome [A. *Schmidt,* German physician, 1865–1918]. VAGOACCESSORY SYNDROME.

Schmidt's syndrome [M. B. *Schmidt,* German physician, 20th century]. Addison's disease with chronic thyroiditis or diabetes mellitus, or both.

Schmidt's test. [A. *Schmidt*]. A test for urobilin based upon the formation of hydrobilirubin-mercury with the production of a red color.

Schmincke's tumor (shmink′eh) [A. *Schmincke,* German pathologist, 1877–1953]. LYMPHOEPITHELIOMA.

Schmitz's bacillus [K. E. F. *Schmitz,* German physician, b. 1889]. *SHIGELLA AMBIGUA.*

Schmorl's grooves [C. G. *Schmorl,* German pathologist, 1861–1932]. Grooves resulting from emphysematous inflation of those portions of the lungs which lie between the ribs.

Schmorl's nodules [C. G. *Schmorl*]. The herniation of the intervertebral disk into the end plate of a vertebral body; usually identifiable on x-ray examination.

schmutz pyorrhea (shmoots) [Ger. *Schmutz*, dirt, filth]. Periodontitis caused by grossly unhygienic dental conditions.

Schna·bel's atrophy (shnah'bul) [I. *Schnabel*, Austrian ophthalmologist, 1842-1908]. CAVERNOUS OPTIC ATROPHY.

Schnei·der acetocarmine stain [F. C. *Schneider*, German chemist, 1813-1897]. A saturated solution of powdered carmine in 45% acetic acid.

Schnei·de·ri·an membrane (shnye·deer'ee·un) [C. V. *Schneider*, German anatomist, 1614-1680]. The mucosa lining the nasal cavities and paranasal sinuses.

Schneider method. A histochemical method for uranium based on the precipitation of dark brown uranium ferrocyanide.

Schneider's index. A test of general physical and circulatory efficiency, consisting of pulse and blood pressure observations under standard conditions of rest and exercise.

Schoen·bein's test (shœhn'bine) [C. F. *Schoenbein*, German chemist, 1799-1868]. A test for cyanide, in which a strip of filter paper impregnated with guaiac and copper sulfate is suspended over a distillate of the suspected material. No change in color of the paper indicates the absence of cyanide; a blue color indicates that cyanide may be present, and a specific test is then performed.

Schoen·hei·mer and Sper·ry's method or **reaction** [R. *Schoenheimer*, U.S. biochemist, 1898-1941; and W. M. *Sperry*]. A method for cholesterol in the blood, in which the cholesterol is precipitated from an acetone alcohol extract with digitonin. The digitonide undergoes the Liebermann-Burchard reaction and the color is compared with a standard.

Schoenlein. See *Schönlein.*

Scholz-Biel·schow·sky-Hen·ne·berg's disease (shohlts, beel·shohf'skee, hen'e·behrk) [W. *Scholz*, German neuropathologist, b. 1889; M. *Bielschowsky;* and R. *Henneberg*]. METACHROMATIC LEUKODYSTROPHY.

Scholz's disease [W. *Scholz*]. METACHROMATIC LEUKODYSTROPHY.

Schönlein's disease. SCHÖNLEIN'S PURPURA.

Schön·lein's purpura (shœhn'line) [J. L. *Schönlein*, German physician, 1793-1864]. A nonthrombocytopenic purpura marked by tenderness and pain of the joints, often with periarticular effusions, mild fever, and erythematous or urticarial exanthema. Syn. *peliosis rheumatica, rheumatic purpura.* See also *Henoch-Schönlein purpura.*

school nurse. A nurse who provides health supervision, health counseling, and health education in collaboration with other services of a school health program.

school phobia. Avoidance or fear of school, classmates, or teacher; a common reaction of children, particularly in the early years of school life, to separation from the mother or surrogate, reflecting at times displacement of anger toward the mother or siblings onto the teacher or classmates, but more often indicative of covert hostility of the mother toward the child and of acting out of the parent's own dependency conflicts through the child.

Schott·mül·ler's disease (shoht'muel'ur) [H. *Schottmüller*, German physician and bacteriologist, 1867-1936]. PARATYPHOID FEVER.

Schre·ger-Hun·ter bands (shrey'gur) [C. H. T. *Schreger*, German anatomist, 1768-1833; and J. *Hunter*]. HUNTER-SCHREGER BANDS.

Schreger's lines [C. H. T. *Schreger*]. HUNTER-SCHREGER BANDS.

Schrid·de's cancer hairs (shrid'eh) [H. *Schridde*, German pathologist, b. 1875]. Thick, coarse, dark hairs found occasionally in the beard and on the temples of cancerous or cachectic patients.

Schroe·der's method (shrœh'dur) [K. L. E. *Schroeder*, German gynecologist, 1838-1887]. Artificial respiration for asphyxia neonatorum, in which the infant is placed in a bath with its back supported by the operator, who then effects a forceful expiration by bending its body over the belly, thus compressing the thorax.

Schueller. See *Schüller.*

Schüff·ner's dots, granules, or **stippling** (shuef'nur) [W. A. P. *Schüffner*, German pathologist, 1867-1949]. Small, round, pink or red-yellow granules that appear in Romanovsky-stained erythrocytes concomitantly with the developing malarial parasite.

Schül·ler-Chris·tian syndrome or **disease** (shuel'ur) [A. *Schüller*, Austrian neurologist, b. 1874; and H. A. *Christian*]. HAND-SCHÜLLER-CHRISTIAN DISEASE.

Schüller's method [K. H. A. L. M. *Schüller*, German surgeon, 1843-1907]. An obsolete method for artificial respiration in which the thorax is raised rhythmically, the fingers being hooked under the ribs.

Schultz-Charl·ton blanching test (shoolts, charl'tun) [W. *Schultz*, German physician, 1878-1947; and W. *Charlton*]. *Obsol.* An immunologic skin test of aid in the diagnosis of scarlet fever, performed by the intracutaneous injection of human scarlet fever immune serum. A positive reaction which occurs in scarlet fever consists of blanching of the rash in a zone surrounding the point of injection.

Schultz-Dale test or **reaction** [W. *Schultz;* and H. H. *Dale*, British pharmacologist, 1875-1969]. The specific production of contraction of an excised intestinal loop (Schultz) or of the excised (virginal) uterine strip (Dale) of the anaphylactic guinea pig, when the excised tissue is exposed to the anaphylactogen. The intestinal or uterine preparation must also be shown to be susceptible to specific desensitization.

Schult·ze's method (shoolt'seh) [B. S. *Schultze*, German gynecologist, 1827-1919]. An obsolete method of artificial respiration of the newborn. The body is flexed, compressing the chest and abdomen, producing forced expiration, and allowing fluid to drain from the mouth and nose.

Schultze's paresthesia or **syndrome** [F. *Schultze*, German neurologist, 1848-1934]. A form of acroparesthesia characterized by increased electrical and mechanical peripheral nerve irritability but no vasomotor symptoms.

Schultze's placenta [B. S. *Schultze*]. A mechanism in which the retroplacental hematoma forms in the center, causing this portion to present before the periphery.

Schultz's sterol reaction method. SCHULTZ TEST.

Schultz's syndrome [W. *Schultz*]. AGRANULOCYTOSIS (2).

Schultz test. A histochemical adaptation of the Liebermann-Burchard test for cholesterol. Syn. *Schultz's sterol reaction method.*

Schwa·bach's test (shvah'bahkh) [D. *Schwabach*, German otologist, 1846-1920]. A hearing test that compares the duration of bone conduction appreciation of the pathologic ear to the normal.

Schwal·be's line (shvahl'beh) [G. A. *Schwalbe*, German anatomist, 1844-1916]. A thickening of the peripheral margin of Descemet's membrane, formed by a bundle of circular connective fibers.

Schwalbe's nucleus [G. A. *Schwalbe*]. MEDIAL VESTIBULAR NUCLEUS.

Schwalbe's ring. SCHWALBE'S LINE.

Schwalbe's sheath [G. A. *Schwalbe*]. The delicate sheath which covers elastic fibers.

Schwann cell (shvahn) [F. T. *Schwann*, German anatomist, 1810-1882]. A cell that ensheaths one or more peripheral axons. The concentric lamellae of the internodal myelin sheath are derived from the plasma membrane of one Schwann cell.

schwan·no·gli·o·ma (shwah''no·glye·o'muh, shvah'') *n.* [*Schwann* cells + *glioma*]. NEURILEMMOMA.

schwan·no·ma (shwah·no'muh, shvah·) *n.*, pl. **schwannomas, schwannoma·ta** (·tuh) [*Schwann* cells + *-oma*]. NEURILEMMOMA.

schwan·no·sar·co·ma (shwah″no·sahr·ko′muh, shvah″no·) *n.* [*Schwann* cells + *sarcoma*]. NEUROFIBROSARCOMA.

Schwann's sheath [F. T. *Schwann*]. SHEATH OF SCHWANN.

Schwartz-Bartter syndrome [W. B. *Schwartz,* U.S. physician, b. 1922; and F. C. *Bartter,* U.S. physician, b. 1914]. Dilutional hyponatremia resulting from inappropriate secretion of antidiuretic hormone, seen as a complication of oat-cell bronchogenic carcinoma and occasionally in other carcinomas.

Schwartz-Jam·pel syndrome. A syndrome consisting of myotonia, shortness of stature, and hip dysplasia.

Schwartz test [E. *Schwartz,* 19th century]. With the patient standing, the examiner puts one hand along the course of the great saphenous vein in the thigh and percusses the vein in the calf with the other hand. A wave of fluid is palpated in the thigh if the vein is varicose.

Schweig·ger-Sei·del sheath (shvye′gur zye′d^e^l) [F. *Schweigger-Seidel,* German physiologist, 1834–1871]. ELLIPSOID (3).

Schwein·furth green. PARIS GREEN.

Schweizer-Foley Y-plasty. A plastic operation to relieve ureteropelvic stricture.

Schwe·ning·er method (shve^y′ning·ur) [E. *Schweninger,* German physician, 1850–1924]. A method of weight reduction by restricting intake of fluids.

scia-. See *skia-.*

sci·age (see·ahzh′) *n.* [F., sawing]. A sawing movement in massage, practiced with the ulnar border or with the dorsum of the hand.

sci·ap·o·dy (sigh·ap′o·dee, skye·) *n.* [Gk. *Skiapodes,* a mythological people with immense feet]. MACROPODIA.

sci·a·sco·pia (sigh·uh·sko′pee·uh) *n.* [NL., sciascopy]. RETINOSCOPY.

sci·as·co·py (sigh·as′kuh·pee) *n.* [*scia-* + *-scopy*]. RETINOSCOPY.

sci·at·ic (sigh·at′ick) *adj.* [ML. *sciaticus,* from Gk. *ischiadikos,* from *ischion,* hip joint]. 1. Pertaining to the ischium. 2. Pertaining to the sciatic nerve.

sci·at·i·ca (sigh·at′i·kuh) *n.* [ML.]. Pain along the course of the sciatic nerve, dependent upon inflammation or injury to the nerve or its roots, and most commonly due to a herniated disk of the lower lumbar or upper sacral spine. In addition to the pain, there is numbness, tingling, and tenderness along the course of the nerve, and eventually loss of the ankle jerk and superficial sensation in the distribution of the involved root or roots.

sciatic artery. The long, thin branch of the inferior gluteal artery which accompanies and supplies the sciatic nerve; the remnant of the axial artery of the embryonic lower limb. Syn. *companion artery of the sciatic nerve, ischiatic artery.* NA *arteria comitans nervi ischiadici.*

sciatic foramens. The greater sciatic foramen and the lesser sciatic foramen.

sciatic hernia. A hernia through the greater or lesser sciatic notch. Syn. *ischiadic hernia.*

sciatic nerve. A nerve that arises from the sacral plexus, passes out of the pelvis, and extends to the distal third of the thigh where it branches into the tibial and common peroneal nerves. It innervates the skin and muscles of both the foot and the leg. NA *nervus ischiadicus.*

sciatic neuritis. SCIATICA.

sciatic tuberosity. ISCHIAL TUBER.

SCID Abbreviation for *severe combined immunodeficiency.*

sci·ence, *n.* [L. *scientia,* knowledge, from *scire,* to know]. A body or field of systematized knowledge based on observation and experimentation objectively analyzed to determine the basic nature or principles of the subject studied.

sci·en·tif·ic, *adj.* [ML. *scientificus,* producing knowledge, from L. *sciens, scientis,* knowing, aware, + *facere,* to make, produce]. 1. Of or pertaining to science. 2. In accordance with the principles and methods of science.

scientific method. The principles and procedures of science, which seeks to establish knowledge systematically and objectively, and therefore requires the recognition of a phenomenon or problem, the accumulation of pertinent data through observation and experimentation, the formulation of a hypothesis to explain the phenomenon, and the testing and confirmation of the hypothesis based on the accumulated data.

sci·en·tist, *n.* [L. *scien*tia + *-ist*]. An expert in some science; an individual who conducts, or is competent to conduct, scientific research.

sci·e·ro·pia (sigh″e·ro′pee·uh) *n.* [Gk. *skieros,* shady, + *-opia*]. Defective vision in which all objects appear dark.

scil·la (sil′uh) *n.* [L.]. SQUILL.

scil·lism (sil′iz·um) *n.* Poisoning produced by squill or its preparations.

scil·lo·ceph·a·lus (sil″o·sef′uh·lus) *n.* An individual exhibiting scillocephaly.

scil·lo·ceph·aly (sil″o·sef′uh·lee) *n.* [*scilla* + *-cephaly*]. Congenital deformity of the head, in which it is small and conically pointed.

scim·i·tar deformity (sim′i·tur, ·tahr). Congenital anomalous development of the sacrum, resembling a scimitar; pathognomic of or virtually always present with a neurenteric cyst.

scimitar syndrome. Anomalous venous drainage of the lower lobe or all of the right lung into the inferior vena cava at or below the diaphragm, with hypoplasia of the right lung, abnormal right bronchial tree, variable degree of dextroposition of the heart, and other associated vascular, cardiac, and pulmonary anomalies; the diagnosis may frequently be suspected from the plain chest radiograph by a scimitar-shaped shadow in the appropriate position.

scin·ti·gram (sin′ti·gram) *n.* SCINTISCAN.

scin·tig·ra·phy (sin·tig′ruh·fee) *n.* A photographically expressed display of the scintillation scanning of a part of the body. Compare *scintimetry.*

scintillating scotoma. A scotoma with serrated margins extending peripherally and producing a large defect in the visual field.

scin·til·la·tion (sin″ti·lay′shun) *n.* [L. *scintillatio,* from *scintilla,* spark]. 1. An emission of sparks. 2. A subjective visual sensation, as of sparks. 3. Instantaneous emission of light from a substance following the absorption of radiant or particulate energy. —**scin·til·late** (sin′ti·late) *v.;* **scintil·lat·ing** (·lay′ting) *adj.*

scintillation counter. A device that measures radiation by counting flashes of light caused by interaction of rays with certain sensitive crystals.

scintillation probe. A device, in the form of a probe, for detecting radioactive emanations by the flashes of light produced on interaction with a sensitive material in the probe.

scin·tim·e·try (sin·tim′e·tree) *n.* A digitally expressed display of the scintillation scanning of a part of the body. Compare *scintigraphy.*

scin·ti·pho·tog·ra·phy (sint″i·fo·tog′ruh·fee) *n.* [*scinti*llation + *photography*]. Isotopic scanning.

scin·ti·scan (sin′ti·skan) *n.* A recording on film or paper of the distribution of a radioactive tracer in an intact tissue or organ, obtained by an automatic scanning system.

scin·ti·scan·ner (sin′ti·skan″ur) *n.* A directional scintillation counter which automatically scans an object or region of the body to determine the distribution of a radioactive tracer substance and obtain a profile of the radioactive area, simultaneously recording the information in the form of a scintiscan.

scir·rhoid (skirr′oid, sirr′oid) *adj.* Resembling a scirrhous carcinoma.

scir·rhous (skirr′us, sirr′us) *adj.* [Gk. *skiros*]. Hard.

scirrhous carcinoma. A form of poorly differentiated adenocarcinoma in which cords and clusters of anaplastic cells are surrounded by dense collagenous bundles, making the tumor very hard to palpation. Syn. *scirrhus.*

scirrhous cord. Excessive granulation tissue on the stump of the severed spermatic cord of domestic animals following castration.

scirrhous lymphoblastoma. HODGKIN'S DISEASE.

scir·rhus (skirr'us, sirr'us) *n.,* pl. **scir·rhi** (·eye), **schirrhuses** [Gk. *skirrhos, skiros,* hard swelling, induration]. SCIRRHOUS CARCINOMA.

scis·sile (sis'ul, ·ile) *adj.* [L. *scissilis,* from *scindere, scissus,* to split]. Suitable for cutting or dividing, as by scissors.

scis·sion (sizh'un) *n.* [L. *scissio,* from *scindere,* to split]. 1. A splitting or dividing, as of a living cell or a molecule. 2. Fission of the nucleus of an atom.

scis·sor·ing (siz'ur·ing) *n.* The tendency for the legs to cross on standing or lying due to spasm or preponderance of action of the adductors at the hips, seen in spastic diplegia or paraplegia. See also *scissors gait.*

scis·sors, *n.pl.* [MF. *cisoires*]. An instrument consisting of two blades held together on a pivot, and crossing each other so that in closing they cut the object placed between them. The blades may be straight, angular, or curved, blunt, sharp, or probe-pointed.

scissors dissection. *In surgery,* the use of blunt-pointed scissors for dissecting, alternately advancing the closed blades and spreading them, and then cutting the isolated bands of tissue with the scissors.

scissors gait. A spastic gait characteristic of patients with spastic diplegia or paraplegia. The legs are strongly adducted at the thighs, crossing alternately in front of one another with the knees scraping together, resulting in short steps and slow progression.

scis·su·ra (si·sue'ruh) *n.,* pl. **scissu·rae** (·ree) [L.]. A fissure; a splitting.

scis·sure (sizh'ur, sish'ur) *n.* SCISSURA.

scler-, sclero- [Gk. *sklēros,* hard]. A combining form meaning (a) *hard, hardness;* (b) *sclerosis, sclerotic;* (c) *sclera, scleral.*

scle·ra (skleer'uh) *n.,* L. pl. & genit. sing. **scle·rae** (·ree) [NL., from Gk. *sklēros,* hard] [NA]. The sclerotic coat of the eye; the firm, fibrous, outer layer of the eyeball, continuous with the sheath of the optic nerve behind and with the cornea in front. See also Plate 19. **—scle·ral** (·ul) *adj.*

scler·ac·ne (sklerr·ack'nee, skleer·) *n.* [*scler-* + *acne*]. ACNE INDURATA.

scleral buckling. An operative technique for the repair of retinal detachment in which an encircling prosthesis is placed around the eye near the equator to buckle the sclera and choroid inward to make contact with the retina.

scleral ectasia. SCLERECTASIA.

scleral rigidity. A measure of the distensibility of the sclera.

scleral spur. The forward prolongation of the sclera toward the trabecular meshwork.

scleral sulcus. A shallow groove at the junction of the sclera and the cornea. NA *sulcus sclerae.*

scle·ra·ti·tis (sklerr"uh·tye'tis, skleer") *n.* SCLERITIS.

scle·ra·tog·e·nous (skleer"uh·toj'e·nus, sklerr") *adj.* SCLEROGENOUS.

scler·ec·ta·sia (sklerr"eck·tay'zhuh, ·zee·uh, skleer"eck·) *n.* [*scler-* + *ectasia*]. Localized bulging of the sclera.

scle·rec·to·iri·dec·to·my (skle·reck"to·irr"i·deck'tuh·mee) *n.* [*sclerectomy* + *iridectomy*]. Excision of a portion of the sclera and of the iris, for glaucoma.

scle·rec·to·my (skle·reck'tuh·mee) *n.* [*sclera* + *-ectomy*]. Excision of a portion of the sclera.

scler·ede·ma (sklerr"e·dee'muh, skleer") *n.* [*scler-* + *edema*]. An idiopathic skin disease characterized by diffuse nonpitting edema and induration.

scleredema adul·to·rum (ad·ul·to'rum). A disease of unknown cause characterized by benign spreading swelling and induration of the skin and subcutaneous tissues, sparing the hands and feet; often follows an acute infection.

scleredema neonatorum. A milder form of sclerema neonatorum.

scleredema of the newborn. SCLEREDEMA NEONATORUM.

scle·re·ma (skle·ree'muh) *n.* [NL., from Gk. *sklēros,* hard]. Sclerosis, or hardening, especially of the skin.

sclerema ad·i·po·sum (ad·i·po'sum). SCLEREMA NEONATORUM.

sclerema cu·tis (kew'tis). SCLERODERMA.

sclerema edem·a·to·sum (e·dem"uh·to'sum). SCLEREDEMA NEONATORUM.

sclerema ne·o·na·to·rum (nee·o·na·to'rum). A life-threatening disease of the newborn of unknown cause, characterized by a waxy-white hardening of the subcutaneous tissue, especially of the legs and the feet, which does not pit on pressure. Most often seen in premature infants or in those who are undernourished, dehydrated, and debilitated. See also *scleredema neonatorum.*

scle·re·mia (skle·ree'mee·uh) *n.* SCLEREMA.

scle·re·mus (skle·ree'mus) *n.* SCLEREMA.

scle·ren·ce·pha·lia (skleer"en·se·fay'lee·uh) *n.* [*scler-* + *-encephalia*]. Sclerosis of brain tissue.

scle·ren·ceph·a·ly (skleer"en·sef'uh·lee) *n.* [*scler-* + *-encephaly*]. SCLERENCEPHALIA.

scle·ren·chy·ma (skle·reng'ki·muh) *n.,* pl. **sclerenchymas, scle·ren·chym·a·ta** (skleer"eng·kim'uh·tuh) [*scler-* + *-enchyma* as in parenchyma]. The hard, fibrous, woody tissue or covering of plants. **—scle·ren·chym·a·tous** (skleer"eng·kim'uh·tus) *adj.*

scle·ri·a·sis (skle·rye'uh·sis) *n.* [*scler-* + *-iasis*]. SCLERODERMA.

scle·rit·ic (skle·rit'ick) *adj.* SCLEROUS.

scle·ri·tis (skle·rye'tis) *n.* [*scler-* + *-itis*]. Inflammation of the sclerotic coat of the eye. It may exist alone (simple scleritis or episcleritis), or involve the cornea, iris, or choroid.

sclero-. See *scler-.*

scle·ro·atroph·ic (skleer"o·a·trof'ick) *adj.* [*sclero-* + *atrophic*]. Pertaining to fibrosis associated with atrophy.

scle·ro·blas·te·ma (skleer"o·blas·tee'muh) *n.* [*sclero-* + *blastema*]. Embryonic tissue from which bones are formed. **—scleroblas·tem·ic** (·tem'ick) *adj.*

scle·ro·con·junc·ti·val (skleer"o·kon"junk·tye'vul) *adj.* [*sclero-* + *conjunctival*]. Pertaining conjointly to the sclerotic coat of the eye and the conjunctiva.

scle·ro·con·junc·ti·vi·tis (skleer"o·kun·junk"ti·vye'tis) *n.* Simultaneous conjunctivitis and scleritis.

scle·ro·cor·nea (skleer"o·kor'nee·uh) *n.* The sclera and the cornea regarded as one. Syn. *corneosclera.* **—sclerocor·ne·al** (·nee·ul) *adj.*

sclerocorneal junction. The boundary between the white, opaque sclera and the transparent cornea in the eye.

sclerocorneal trephining. The removal of a portion of the sclera by means of a specially devised instrument, for the relief of excessive intraocular tension in chronic open-angle glaucoma.

scle·ro·cys·tic (skeer"o·sis'tick) *adj.* [*sclero-* + *cystic*]. 1. Both hard and cystic. 2. Both fibrous and cystic.

sclerocystic ovaries. The fibrotic ovaries with small cysts found in the Stein-Leventhal syndrome.

scle·ro·dac·tyl·ia (skleer"o·dack·til'ee·uh) *n.* [*sclero-* + *dactyl-* + *-ia*]. Thickening and hardening of the fingers which may occur in scleroderma or as a complication of acrosclerosis.

scle·ro·dac·ty·ly (skleer"o·dack'til·ee) *n.* SCLERODACTYLIA.

scle·ro·der·ma (skleer"o·dur'muh) *n.* [*sclero-* + *-derma*]. An increment in collagenous connective tissue in the skin, either focal or diffuse, the latter form associated with similar changes in the viscera. Syn. *elephantiasis sclerosa, scleriasis, dermatosclerosis, chorionitis.* See also *acrosclerosis, acroscleroderma.*

scle·ro·der·ma·ti·tis (skleer"o·dur"muh·tye'tis) *n.* [*sclero-* + *dermatitis*]. Inflammatory thickening and hardening of the skin.

scle·ro·der·mi·tis (skleer"o·dur·migh'tis) *n.* SCLERODERMATITIS.

scle·rog·e·nous (skle·roj'e·nus) *adj.* [*sclero-* + *-genous*]. Producing a hard substance.

scle·ro·gy·ria (skleer"o·jye'ree·uh, ·jirr'ee·uh) *n.* [*sclero-* + *gyrus* + *-ia*]. Atrophy and scarring of the convolutions of the cerebral cortex. See also *ulegyria.*

scle·roid (skleer'oid) *adj.* [*scler-* + *-oid*]. Hard or bony in texture.

scle·ro·ker·a·ti·tis (skleer"o·kerr"uh·tye'tis) *n.* [*sclero-* + *keratitis*]. Inflammation of the sclera and cornea.

scle·ro·ma (skle·ro'muh) *n.*, pl. **scleromas, scleroma·ta** (·tuh) [Gk. *sklērōma*, from *sklēros*, hard]. Abnormal hardness or induration of a part.

scle·ro·ma·la·cia (skleer"o·ma·lay'shee·uh) *n.* [*sclero-* + *malacia*]. Softening of the sclera.

scleromalacia per·fo·rans (pur'fo·ranz). Softening of the sclera with perforation.

scle·ro·mere (sklee'ro·meer) *n.* [*sclero-* + *-mere*]. PROTOVERTEBRA.

scle·rom·e·ter (skle·rom'e·tur) *n.* [*sclero-* + *-meter*]. An instrument which measures the hardness of substances.

scle·ro·myx·ede·ma (skleer"o·mick"se·dee'muh) *n.* [*sclero-* + *myxedema*]. Diffuse skin thickening with mucoid deposits in the upper dermis.

scle·ro·nych·ia (skleer"o·nick'ee·uh) *n.* [*scler-* + *onych-* + *-ia*]. Induration and thickening of the nails.

scle·ro·nyx·is (skleer"o·nick'sis) *n.* [*sclero-* + Gk. *nyxis*, puncture]. Operative puncture of the sclera.

scle·ro-oo·pho·ri·tis (skleer"o·o"o·fo·rye'tis, ·o·off"o·rye'tis) *n.* [*sclero-* + *oophoritis*]. Sclerosis of the ovary.

scle·ro·plas·ty (skleer'o·plas"tee) *n.* [*sclero-* + *-plasty*]. Plastic surgery on the sclera.

scle·ro·pro·tein (sklee"ro·pro'tee·in) *n.* Any of a class of simple proteins having structural or protective functions, as collagen and keratin, and that are insoluble in aqueous solvents. Syn. *albuminoid.*

scle·ro·sant (skle·ro'sunt, ·zunt) *n.* A chemical irritant producing an inflammatory reaction and subsequent fibrosis.

scle·rose (skle·roze', ·roce', skleer'oze) *v.* To affect with sclerosis; to become affected with sclerosis. —**scle·rosed,** *adj.*; **scle·ros·ing,** *adj.*

sclé·rose en plaque (skleʸ·roze' ahⁿ plaʰck) [F.]. MULTIPLE SCLEROSIS.

sclerosing adenomatosis or **adenosis.** A form of mammary dysplasia in which ductular structures are enclaved in fibrous tissue, simulating invading cancerous ductular structures. Syn. *fibrosing adenosis.*

sclerosing hemangioma. A variety of benign histiocytoma, usually seen in the skin, in which capillary channels and fibrosis are prominent.

sclerosing keratitis. A form of interstitial keratitis associated with scleritis.

sclerosing osteogenic sarcoma. Osteogenic sarcoma with marked dense bone production.

scle·ro·sis (skle·ro'sis) *n.*, pl. **sclero·ses** (·seez) [Gk. *sklērōsis*, from *sklēros*, hard]. Hardening, especially of a part by overgrowth of fibrous tissue; applied particularly to hardening of the nervous system from atrophy or degeneration of the nerve elements and hyperplasia of the interstitial tissue; also to a thickening of the coats of arteries, produced by proliferation of fibrous connective tissue and deposit of lipids and calcium salts.

sclerosis co·rii (ko'ree·eye). SCLERODERMA.

sclerosis der·ma·tis (dur'muh·tis). SCLERODERMA.

sclerosis os·si·um (os'ee·um). CONDENSING OSTEITIS.

scle·ro·ste·no·sis (skleer"o·ste·no'sis) *n.* [*sclero-* + *stenosis*]. Hardening with contracture of a part or closure of an orifice.

sclerostenosis cu·ta·nea (kew·tay'nee·uh). SCLERODERMA.

scle·ros·to·my (skle·ros'tuh·mee) *n.* [*sclero-* + *-stomy*]. Making an artificial opening in the sclera for the relief of glaucoma.

scle·ro·ther·a·py (skleer"o·therr'uh·pee) *n.* [*sclero-* + *therapy*]. Treatment, especially of varicose veins, by injection of chemical agents which cause localized thrombosis and eventual fibrosis and obliteration of the vessels.

scle·ro·thrix (skleer'o·thricks) *n.* [*sclero-* + *-thrix*]. Abnormal brittleness of the hair.

sclerotia. Plural of *sclerotium.*

scle·rot·ic (skle·rot'ick) *adj.* & *n.* [Gk. *sklērotēs*, hardness, + *-ic*]. 1. Hard; indurated. 2. Pertaining to the outer coat of the eye, as the sclerotic coat, or sclera. 3. Pertaining to sclerosis. 4. Related to or derived from ergot. 5. SCLERA.

scle·rot·i·ca (skle·rot'i·kuh) *n.* [ML.]. SCLERA.

sclerotic dentin. Reparative dentin in which the calcium salts are deposited in such a way that the refractive indices are altered and the dentin is transparent.

scle·rot·i·cec·to·my (skle·rot"i·seck'tuh·mee) *n.* [*sclerotica* + *-ectomy*]. SCLEROTOMY.

sclerotic mastoid. A mastoid process composed almost entirely of dense bone.

sclerotic microgyria. ULEGYRIA.

sclerotic nonsuppurating osteomyelitis. GARRÉ'S OSTEOMYELITIS.

scle·rot·i·co·nyx·is (skle·rot"i·ko·nick'sis) *n.* SCLERONYXIS.

scle·rot·i·co·punc·ture (skle·rot"i·ko·punk'chur) *n.* SCLERONYXIS.

sclerotic osteitis. OSTEOPETROSIS.

scle·rot·i·cot·o·my (skle·rot"i·kot'uh·mee) *n.* SCLEROTOMY.

sclerotic zone. A ring of anastomoses of deep, conjunctival vessels around the periphery of the cornea, which perforate the sclera and anastomose with those of the iris and choroid; a condition occurring in iritis.

scle·rot·i·dec·to·my (skle·rot"i·deck'tuh·mee) *n.* SCLERECTOMY.

scle·ro·tis (skle·ro'tis) *n.* [NL., from *sclerotium*]. ERGOT.

scle·ro·ti·tis (skleer"o·tye'tis) *n.* SCLERITIS.

scle·ro·ti·um (skle·ro'shee·um) *n.*, pl. **sclero·tia** (·shee·uh) [NL., from Gk. *sklērotēs*, hardness]. A thick mass of mycelium constituting a resting stage in the development of some fungi, as the ergot.

scle·ro·tome (skleer'o·tome) *n.* [*sclero-* + *-tome*]. 1. A knife used in sclerotomy. 2. The fibrous tissue separating successive myotomes in certain of the lower vertebrates. 3. The part of a mesodermal somite which enters into the formation of the vertebrae. —**scle·ro·to·mic** (skleer"o·to' mick, ·tom'ick) *adj.*

scle·rot·o·my (skle·rot'uh·mee) *n.* [*sclero-* + *-tomy*]. The operation of incising the sclera.

scle·rous (skleer'us) *adj.* [Gk. *sklēros*]. Hard; indurated.

scob·i·nate (skob'i·nate, ·nut) *adj.* [L. *scobina*, rasp, + *-ate*]. Having a rough surface.

sco·lec·i·form (sko·les'i·form) *adj.* Having the form or character of a scolex.

scol·e·coid (skol'e·koid) *adj.* [Gk. *skōlēkoeidēs*, from *skōlēx*, worm]. VERMIFORM.

sco·lex (sko'lecks) *n.*, pl. **scol·i·ces** (skol'i·seez, sko'li·), **sco·le·ces** (sko·lee'seez), **scolexes** [Gk. *skōlēx*, *skōlēkos*, worm, grub]. The head of a tapeworm by means of which it attaches to the intestinal wall.

sco·lio·lor·do·sis (sko"lee·o·lor·do'sis) *n.* Combined scoliosis and lordosis.

sco·li·o·si·om·e·try (sko"lee·o"see·om'e·tree) *n.* [*scoliosis* + *-metry*]. The estimation of the degree of deformity in scoliosis.

sco·li·o·sis, sko·li·o·sis (sko"lee·o'sis) *n.*, pl. **scolio·ses, skolio·ses** (·seez) [Gk. *skoliōsis*, obliquity, crookedness, from *skolios*, bent, crooked]. Lateral curvature of the spine, named according to the location and direction of the convexity, as right thoracic. —**scoli·ot·ic** (·ot'ick) *adj.*

sco·li·o·som·e·ter, sko·li·o·som·e·ter (sko"lee·o·som'e·tur) *n.* [*scoliosis* + *-meter*]. An instrument for measuring the amount of deformity in scoliosis.

sco·li·o·som·e·try (sko"lee·o·som'e·tree) *n.* SCOLIOSIOMETRY.

scoliotic pelvis. A distorted pelvis, its asymmetry depending upon the situation and degree of scoliosis of the vertebral column.

sco·lio·tone (sko'lee·o·tone) *n.* [*scoliosis* + Gk. *tonos*, tension, stretching]. An apparatus for elongating the spine and lessening the rotation in lateral curvature.

S colony. SMOOTH COLONY.

Scol·o·pen·dra (skol"o·pen'druh) *n.* A genus of centipedes.

scom·brine (skom'breen, ·brin) *n.* [Gk. *skombros*, mackerel, + *-ine*]. A protamine obtained from mature spermatozoa of mackerel.

scom·brone (skom'brone) *n.* A histone obtained from spermatozoa of mackerel.

scom·bro·tox·in (skom"bro·tock'sin) *n.* A poison produced by the action of marine bacteria on fish flesh, especially of scombroid fish (including mackerel, tuna, swordfish, etc.); it is a mixture of histamine and other toxic substances.

scoop, *n.* [MD. *schope*]. An instrument resembling a spoon, for the extraction of bodies from cavities, as an ear scoop, a lithotomy scoop.

sco·pa·fun·gin (sko"puh·fun'jin) *n.* A substance obtained from *Streptomyces hygroscopicus* used as an antifungal, antibacterial agent.

sco·pa·rin (sko·păr'in, sko'puh·rin) *n.* A glycosidal principle, $C_{22}H_{22}O_{11}$, from scoparius.

sco·par·i·us (sko·păr'ee·us) *n.* [NL., from L. *scopa*, broom]. The dried tops of *Cytisus scoparius*, a shrub of the family Leguminosae; they contain the alkaloid sparteine, and a glycoside, scoparin. Scoparius has been used as a diuretic and cathartic. Syn. *broom tops.*

-scope [Gk. *skopein*, to examine]. A combining form meaning *an instrument for seeing* or *examining.*

sco·po·la (sko'po·luh) *n.* [G. A. *Scopoli*, Italian naturalist, 1723–1788]. The dried rhizomes of *Scopolia carniolica*, which contain hyoscyamine, scopolamine, and norhyocyamine. It has the actions of belladonna, but is used only as a source of scopolamine and hyoscyamine.

sco·pol·a·mine (sko·pol'uh·meen, ·min, sko"po·lam'in) *n.* An alkaloid, $C_{17}H_{21}NO_4$, from various plants of the Solanaceae. An anticholinergic drug, it resembles atropine in its action on the autonomic nervous system, but whereas the latter stimulates the central nervous system, scopolamine depresses it. Used, generally as the hydrobromide salt, as a sedative, and also as a mydriatic and cycloplegic.

sco·po·phil·ia (sko"po·fil'ee·uh) *n.* [Gk. *skopein*, to look, watch, + *-philia*]. Sexual stimulation derived from looking at the unclad human figure; observed chiefly in normal adolescent and adult males where it takes the aim-inhibited form of "girl watching" or looking at nude or semi-nude females in magazines or as part of some stage performance, or where it may be sublimated as scientific curiosity; when present to a pathologic degree, it is deviant and called voyeurism. **—scopophil·ic** (·ick) *adj.*

sco·po·pho·bia (sko"po·fo'bee·uh) *n.* [Gk. *skopein*, to look, watch, + *-phobia*]. Abnormal fear of being seen.

scop·to·phil·ia (skop"to·fil'ee·uh) *n.* SCOPOPHILIA.

Scop·u·lar·i·op·sis (skop"yoo·lăr"ee·op'sis) *n.* [L. *scopula*, small broom, + Gk. *opsis*, appearance]. A genus of fungi.

Scopulariopsis brev·i·cau·le (brev·i·kaw'lee). One of the species of fungi which are generally considered as contaminants, but have been associated with onychomycosis.

-scopy [Gk. *skopein*, to examine]. A combining form meaning *inspection* or *examination.*

scor·a·cra·tia (skor"uh·kray'shee·uh) *n.* [Gk. *skōr*, feces, + *akrateia*, incontinence]. Fecal incontinence.

scor·bu·tic (skor·bew'tick) *adj.* [*scorbutus* + *-ic*]. Pertaining to or affected with scurvy.

scorbutic stomatitis. Stomatitis associated with scurvy.

scor·bu·tus (skor·bew'tus) *n.* [ML., from MLGer. *schorbūk* (obsc. orig.; supposedly from *schoren*, to break, + *būk*, belly)]. SCURVY.

scor·di·ne·ma (skor"di·nee'muh) *n.* [Gk. *skordinēma*, stretching, yawning]. Yawning, stretching, and lassitude in the prodromal stage of infectious disease.

scor·e·te·mia (skor"e·tee'mee·uh) *n.* [Gk. *skōr*, feces, + *-emia*]. SCATEMIA.

Scor·pio (skor'pee·o) *n.* [L.]. A genus of scorpions of the order Scorpionida.

Scorpio mau·rus (maw'rus). A poisonous species of scorpion found in Egypt and Tunisia.

scor·pi·on (skor'pee·un) *n.* [L. *scorpio, scorpionis*, from Gk. *skorpios*]. An arachnid of the order Scorpionida which injects poison by a sting located on the end of the tail. The venom is a neurotoxin similar in action to cobra venom. See also *Buthus, Centruroides, Euscorpius, Scorpio, Tityus.*

scot-, scoto- [Gk. *skotos*, darkness]. A combining form meaning *of or pertaining to darkness.*

Scotine. Trademark for cotinine, a psychic stimulant used as the fumarate salt.

scoto-. See *scot-.*

sco·to·chro·mo·gen (sko"to·kro'muh·jen, skot"o·) *n.* [*scoto-* + *chromogen*]. 1. Any microorganism which produces pigment when grown without light as well as with light. 2. A member of group II of the "anonymous" or atypical mycobacteria.

sco·to·din·ia (sko"to·din'ee·uh, skot"o·) *n.* [Gk. *skotodinia*, vertigo, from *scoto-* + *dinos*, whirling]. Dizziness and also headache associated with the appearance of black spots before the eyes. See also *vertigo.*

sco·to·gram (sko'to·gram, skot'o·) *n.* [*scoto-* + *-gram*]. An impression made on a photographic plate by a radioactive substance without the intervention of an opaque object.

sco·to·ma (skuh·to'muh, sko·) *n.*, pl. **scotomas, scotoma·ta** (·tuh) [Gk. *skotōma*, dizziness, faintness, from *skotos*, darkness]. An area of absent or depressed vision in the visual field, surrounded by an area of normal or less depressed vision.

sco·to·ma·graph (sco·to'muh·graf) *n.* [*scotoma* + *-graph*]. An instrument for recording the size and shape of a scotoma.

scotomata. A plural of *scotoma.*

sco·tom·e·ter (sko·tom'e·tur) *n.* [*scotoma* + *-meter*]. An instrument for detecting, locating, and measuring scotomas.

sco·to·phil·ia (sko"to·fil'ee·uh, skot"o·) *n.* [*scoto-* + *-philia*]. NYCTOPHILIA.

sco·to·pho·bia (sko"to·fo'bee·uh, skot"o·) *n.* [*scoto-* + *-phobia*]. An abnormal fear of darkness.

sco·to·pho·bin (sko"to·fo'bin, skot"o·) *n.* [*scotophobia* + *-in*]. A substance extracted from the brains of animals conditioned to avoid the dark which, when injected into unconditioned animals, results in increased dark-avoidance by the latter.

sco·to·pia (sko·to'pee·uh) *n.* [*scot-* + *-opia*]. NIGHT VISION. **—sco·to·pic** (·to'pick, ·top'ick) *adj.*

scotopic dominator curve. A curve derived from the measurements of the absolute threshold of the dark-adapted eye for different wavelengths by plotting the reciprocals of these thresholds, which measure sensitivity, against the wavelength; thus the curve represents the relative luminosities of the different wavelengths. Compare *photopic dominator curve.*

scotopic luminosity curve. The curve of sensitivity of the eye to different wavelengths of light taken in the dark.

scotopic sensitivity curve. SCOTOPIC DOMINATOR CURVE.

scotopic vision. Perception of shape and form without recognition of color, as occurs with very dim illumination.

sco·top·sin (sko·top'sin) *n.* [*scot-* + *opsin*]. The protein moiety located in the rods of the retina, functioning in the dark-adapted stage, which combines with retinene$_1$ to form rhodopsin and with retinene$_2$ to form porphyropsin.

sco·tos·co·py (sko·tos'kuh·pee) *n.* [*scoto-* + *-scopy*]. RETINOSCOPY.

sco·to·sis (sko·to'sis) *n.* [Gk. *skotōsis*, darkening, eclipse, from *skotos*, darkness]. SCOTOMA.

scour·ing (skaowr'ing) *n.* Diarrhea in large domestic farm animals, usually caused by bacteria or viruses.

scours (skaowrz) *n.* An infectious diarrhea of large domestic farm animals.

scout film. PLAIN FILM.

scrap·er (skray'pur) *n.* An instrument used to produce an abrasion.

scrap·ie (scrap'ee, skray'pee) *n.* A virus disease of sheep producing a progressive degenerative disorder of central nervous system neurons; named for the tendency of infected sheep to rub or "scrape" against fences to relieve intense pruritus.

scratch-patch test. *Obsol.* A test that consists essentially of the application of patch tests to lightly scarified or abraded skin areas, instead of to normal skin. Often produces reactions when the patch test is negative.

scratch reflex. Reflex scratching movements designed to remove an irritating agent from the surface of the skin.

scratch test. A test performed by severing the stratum corneum of the epidermis with a light scratch and placing an allergen upon the site of the scratch.

screen, *n.* [OF. *escren,* from MD. *scherm*]. A device that cuts off, shelters, or protects.

screening plate. A petri dish using solid media, for distinguishing the effect of some particular agent on bacteria, such as incorporation of antibiotics and notation of zones of inhibition, and susceptibility of *Salmonella typhi* to different bacteriophage types.

screen memory. *In psychoanalysis,* a consciously tolerable but usually unimportant memory recalled in place of an associated important one, which would be painful and disturbing.

screw articulation. A hinge articulation in which the groove of the trochlea is in a plane not at right angles with the axis, and the hinge movement is accompanied by progression at right angles to the hinge plane. Syn. *cochlear articulation, spiral joint.*

screw·fly. The adult form of the screwworm, *Callitroga hominivorax.*

screw micrometer. A fine screw with a scale attached showing the distance passed at each fraction of a revolution.

screw·worm, *n.* The larva of *Callitroga.*

Scrib·ner shunt. A variety of arteriovenous shunt employing a special tube connection outside the body, so as to permit ready hemodialysis. Syn. *Quinton-Scribner shunt.*

scriv·en·er's palsy (skriv'e·nurz). WRITER'S CRAMP.

scro·bic·u·lus (skro·bick'yoo·lus) *n.,* pl. **scrobicu·li** (·lye) [L., little ditch]. A small pit. —**scrobicu·late** (·lut, ·late) *adj.*

scrobiculus cor·dis (kor'dis) [BNA]. Fossa epigastrica (= EPIGASTRIC FOSSA).

scrof·u·la (skrof'yoo·luh) *n.* [L., dim. of *scrofa,* breeding sow]. Tuberculosis of cervical lymph nodes. —**scrofu·lous** (·lus) *adj.*

scrof·u·lo·der·ma (skrof''yoo·lo·dur'muh) *n.* [*scrofula* + *-derma*]. Lesions of the skin produced by the local action of the *Mycobacterium tuberculosis* by direct extension of some focus of infection beneath the skin, usually on the neck from draining lymph nodes, resulting in ulceration, draining sinuses, and scar formation.

scrofulous abscess. A chronic abscess from infected bone or lymph nodes.

scrofulous ophthalmia. PHLYCTENULAR KERATOCONJUNCTIVITIS.

scrota. A plural of *scrotum.*

scro·tal (skro'tul) *adj.* Of or pertaining to the scrotum.

scrotal fistula. A fistula extending from some portion of the testis or epididymis to an external opening in the skin of the scrotum.

scrotal hernia. Any hernia that is found within the scrotum. See also *complete hernia, inguinal hernia, sliding hernia.*

scrotal reaction. Inflammation of the scrotum and tunica vaginalis testis in male guinea pigs, due to infection with spotted fever rickettsiae. Necrosis of the skin frequently occurs.

scrotal reflex. Slow peristaltic contraction of the dartos muscle in response to stimulation of the perineum or thigh by stroking or by cold application.

scrotal tongue. FISSURED TONGUE.

scro·tec·to·my (skro·teck'tuh·mee) *n.* [*scrotum* + *-ectomy*]. Resection of the scrotum or a part of it.

scro·to·plas·ty (skro'to·plas''tee) *n.* [*scrotum* + *-plasty*]. Plastic surgery on the scrotum.

scro·tum (skro'tum) *n.,* pl. **scro·ta** (·tuh), **scrotums** [L.] [NA]. The pouch containing the testes, consisting of skin and subcutaneous tissue, dartos, external spermatic fascia, cremasteric fascia, internal spermatic fascia, and parietal tunica vaginalis propria. See also Plate 25.

scrub nurse. A nurse who is part of an operating team, being scrubbed, gowned, and surgically clean, to assist the operating surgeon.

scrub typhus. A disease characterized by headache, high fever, and a rash, occurring in Japan, Formosa, and islands of the South Pacific; caused by *Rickettsia tsutsugamushi* and transmitted to man by the bite of the larval forms of mites of the genus *Trombicula.* Syn. *tsutsugamushi disease.*

scru·ple (skroo'pul) *n.* [L. *scrupulus,* small stone]. A unit of apothecaries' weight represented by the symbol ℈, and equal to 20 grains.

scru·pu·los·i·ty (skroo''pew·los'i·tee) *n.* [L. *scrupulosus,* careful]. An overprecision, or abnormal conscientiousness as to one's thoughts, words, and deeds. A prominent personality trait in persons predisposed to obsessive-compulsive neurosis and to certain types of schizophrenia.

Scultet's bandage. SCULTETUS' BANDAGE.

Scul·te·tus' bandage or **binder** (skōōl·teʸ'tōōs) [J. *Scultetus* (Schultes, Scultet), German surgeon, 1595–1645]. A short, wide cloth bandage having multiple tails on each end. By overlapping the tails, snug support is obtained, and the bandage can be opened, and closed again, without moving the part.

scurf, *n.* A branlike desquamation of the epidermis, especially from the scalp; DANDRUFF.

scur·vy (skur'vee) *n.* [F. *scorbut* (from ML. *scorbutus,* q.v.) by assimilation to E. adj. *scurvy* (= *scurfy*)]. A nutritional disorder caused by deficiency of vitamin C (ascorbic acid); characterized by extreme weakness, spongy gums, and a tendency to develop hemorrhages under the skin, from the mucous membranes, and under the periosteum, and by mental depression and anemia.

scurvy rickets. INFANTILE SCURVY.

scute (skewt) *n.* [L. *scutum,* shield]. 1. An external plate or scale, as that of reptiles, fish, and certain insects. 2. TEGMEN TYMPANI.

scu·tel·lum (skew·tel'um) *n.,* pl. **scutel·la** (·uh) [dim. of L. *scutum,* shield]. A small plate or squamous structure.

scu·tu·late (skew'chuh·late) *adj.* Shaped like a lozenge.

scu·tu·lum (skew'chuh·lum) *n.,* pl. **scutu·la** (·luh) [L., dim. of *scutum,* shield]. A cup-shaped crust of favus.

scu·tum (skew'tum) *n.,* pl. **scu·ta** (·tuh) [L., shield]. A shield-like plate of bone. —**scu·tate** (·tate) *adj.*

scutum tym·pa·ni·cum (tim·pan'i·kum). The semilunar plate of bone separating the attic of the tympanum from the outer mastoid cells.

scyb·a·lum (sib'uh·lum) *n.,* pl. **scyba·la** (·luh) [NL., from Gk. *skybalon,* dung]. A mass of abnormally hard fecal matter. —**scyba·lous** (·lus) *adj.*

scy·phi·form (sigh'fi·form) *adj.* [Gk. *skyphos,* cup, + *-iform*]. Cup-shaped.

scy·ti·tis (sigh·tye'tis) *n.* [Gk. *skytos,* skin, + *-itis*]. DERMATITIS.

SD Abbreviation for (a) *streptodornase;* (b) *standard deviation.*

SDS Abbreviation for *sodium dodecyl sulfate.*

Se Symbol for selenium.

Sea·bright-Ban·tam syndrome. A phenomenon, first observed in the Seabright-Bantam rooster, in which there is unresponsiveness of the target organ to a hormone; sometimes applied to human physiology, as in the case of pseudohypoparathyroidism.

seal, *n. In prosthodontics,* POSTERIOR PALATAL SEAL.

seal-fin deformity. Ulnar deviation of the fingers, seen in rheumatoid arthritis.

seam, *n.* 1. SUTURE. 2. RAPHE.

seam·less band. A nonadjustable ferrule stamped from a piece of metal; used as a plain or anchor band in an orthodontic appliance.

sea onion. SQUILL.

search·ing nystagmus. OCULAR NYSTAGMUS.

Sea·shore test [C. E. *Seashore,* U.S. psychologist, 1866–1949]. A test to measure native musical aptitude with respect to pitch, loudness, time, timbre, rhythm, and tonal memory.

sea·sick, *adj.* Afflicted with motion sickness in a watercraft; especially, with motion sickness resulting from the pitching and rolling of a ship in a heavy sea. —**seasick·ness,** *n.*

sea snake. Any snake of the family Hydrophidae.

seat·worm, *n.* *ENTEROBIUS VERMICULARIS.*

se·ba·ceo·fol·lic·u·lar (se·bay"shee·o·fol·ick'yoo·lur) *adj.* [*sebaceous* + *follicular*]. Pertaining to a pilosebaceous apparatus.

se·ba·ceous (se·bay'shus) *adj.* [L. *sebaceus,* from *sebum*]. Pertaining to or secreting sebum.

sebaceous crypts. SEBACEOUS GLANDS.

sebaceous cyst. A cyst lined by sebaceous epithelial cells.

sebaceous follicle. A sebaceous gland of the skin.

sebaceous glands. The glands that secrete sebum, an unctuous material composed primarily of fat. NA *glandulae sebaceae.*

sebaceous glands of Zeis. ZEIS'S GLANDS.

se·bac·ic acid (se·bas'ick, se·bay'sick). Decanedioic acid or 1,8-octanedicarboxylic acid, $HOOC(CH_2)_8COOH$, obtained by decomposition of certain fatty acids.

se·bas·to·ma·nia (se·bas"to·may'nee·uh) *n.* [Gk. *sebasto-,* from *sebas,* reverence, + *-mania*]. A psychosis, usually schizophrenia, manifested mainly by religiosity.

se·bif·er·ous (se·bif'ur·us) *adj.* SEBIPAROUS.

se·bip·a·rous (se·bip'ur·us) *adj.* [*sebum* + *-parous*]. Secreting sebum.

se·bo·cys·to·ma·to·sis (see"bo·sis"to·muh·to'sis) *n.* [*sebum* + *cystoma* + *-osis*]. STEATOCYSTOMA MULTIPLEX.

sebo·lith (seb'o·lith) *n.* [*sebum* + *-lith*]. A calculus in a sebaceous gland.

seb·or·rha·gia (seb"o·ray'jee·uh) *n.* [*sebum* + *-rrhagia*]. SEBORRHEA.

seb·or·rhea, seb·or·rhoea (seb"o·ree'uh) *n.* [*sebum* + *-rrhea*]. A functional disease of the sebaceous glands, characterized by an excessive secretion or disturbed quality of sebum, which collects upon the skin in the form of an oily coating or of crusts or scales.

seborrhea cap·i·tis (kap'i·tis). Seborrhea of the scalp.

seborrhea con·ges·ti·va (kon"jes·tye'vuh). CHRONIC DISCOID LUPUS ERYTHEMATOSUS.

seborrhea cor·po·ris (kor'po·ris). Seborrheic dermatitis of the trunk.

seborrhea fur·fu·ra·cea (fur"fuh·ray'see·uh, shee·uh). SEBORRHEIC DERMATITIS.

seborrhea ich·thy·o·sis (ikth"ee·o'sis). A variety of seborrhea characterized by the formation of large, platelike crusts.

seb·or·rhe·al, seb·or·rhoe·al (seb"o·ree'ul) *adj.* SEBORRHEIC.

seborrhea na·si (nay'zye). Seborrhea of the sebaceous glands of the nose.

seborrhea ni·gri·cans (nigh'gri·kanz). Chromhidrosis in which there is a dark, greasy-looking discoloration of the eyelids and adjacent skin.

seborrhea ole·o·sa (o"lee·o'suh). A form of seborrhea characterized by an excessive oiliness of the skin, especially about the forehead and nose.

seborrhea sic·ca (sick'uh). A form of seborrheic dermatitis characterized by dry scaling.

seb·or·rhe·ic, seb·or·rhoe·ic (seb"o·ree'ick) *adj.* Pertaining to or characterized by seborrhea.

seborrheic areas. Areas where sebaceous glands are numerous, as the scalp, sides of the nose, chin, center of the chest, back, axillae, and groins.

seborrheic dermatitis. An acute, inflammatory form of dermatitis, occurring usually on oily skin in areas having large sebaceous glands; characterized by dry, moist, or greasy scales and by crusting yellowish patches, remissions, exacerbations, and itching. Syn. *dermatitis seborrheica, eczema seborrheicum.*

seborrheic keratosis. A benign skin tumor composed of squamous and basaloid cells which are arranged in various patterns to produce a brown papule, studded with yellow collections of keratotic material, giving the lesions a greasy appearance.

seborrhoea. SEBORRHEA.

seborrhoeal. SEBORRHEIC.

seborrhoeic. SEBORRHEIC.

se·bum (see'bum) *n.* [L., tallow, grease]. The secretion of the sebaceous glands, composed of fat, keratohyalin granules, keratin, and cellular debris.

sebum cu·ta·ne·um (kew·tay'nee·um) [BNA]. The fatty secretion of the sebaceous glands of the skin.

sebum pal·pe·bra·le (pal·pe·bray'lee) [BNA]. The secretion of the sebaceous glands of the eyelids.

sebum prae·pu·ti·a·le (pre·pew"shee·ay'lee). SMEGMA PRAEPUTII.

***sec-*.** *In chemistry,* a combining form meaning *secondary.*

se·cern·ment (se·surn'munt) *n.* [L. *secernere,* to separate]. SECRETION, especially of a gland.

Seck·el's syndrome (zeck'ul) [H. P. G. *Seckel,* Swiss pediatrician, b. 1900]. BIRD-HEADED DWARFISM.

sec·la·zone (seck'luh·zone) *n.* 7-Chloro-3, 3a-dihydro-2*H*, 9*H*-isoxazolo[3,2-*b*][1,3]benzoxazine-9-one, $C_{10}H_8ClNO_3$, an anti-inflammatory, uricosuric.

se·clu·sion of pupil. Adhesions of the anterior capsule of the lens and the posterior surface of the iris, with a cyclitic membrane around the lens, as a sequel of iritis.

seco·bar·bi·tal (seck"o·bahr'bi·tol, ·tal, see"ko·) *n.* 5-Allyl-5-(1-methylbutyl)barbituric acid, $C_{12}H_{18}N_2O_3$, a short-acting barbiturate used as a sedative and hypnotic, frequently as the sodium derivative (sodium secobarbital). Syn. *quinalbarbitone.*

sec·o·dont (seck'o·dont, see'ko·) *adj.* [L. *secare,* to cut, + *-odont*]. Possessing molar teeth which have cusps with cutting edges.

Seconal. Trademark for the short-acting barbiturate secobarbital, also used as the sodium derivative.

sec·ond·ary (seck'un·derr"ee) *adj.* [L. *secundarius*]. 1. Second in the order of time or development. 2. Second in relation; subordinate; produced by a cause considered primary.

secondary abscess. EMBOLIC ABSCESS.

secondary amenorrhea. Amenorrhea which occurs after menstruation has been established.

secondary ammonium phosphate. AMMONIUM PHOSPHATE, DIBASIC.

secondary amputation. An amputation performed after suppuration has occurred or for the purpose of improving a temporary circular amputation with flaps left open.

secondary amyloidosis. Amyloidosis that usually follows chronic suppurative inflammatory diseases (tuberculosis, osteomyelitis, bronchiectasis). Amyloid is deposited in fibrous connective tissue, especially in the arterioles, spleen, liver, kidneys, and adrenals.

secondary anal opening. The definitive anal orifice formed by the growth of the external or ectodermal anal part of the cloaca.

secondary anemia. Anemia following or resulting from disease outside the blood-forming organs, such as poisoning, hemorrhage, or visceral cancer.

secondary assimilation. Conversion of absorbed food elements into body tissue.

secondary bone. Bone which replaces primary bone.

secondary bronchus. Any of the bronchi between the primary bronchi and the bronchioles; a lobar bronchus, segmental bronchus, or any of the small bronchi which derive from segmental bronchi and ventilate portions of the lung segments. Contr. *primary bronchus.*

secondary cataract. A capsular cataract appearing after the extraction of the lens. See also *aftercataract.*

secondary cause. A cause or factor or set of conditions which enhances or adds to the primary cause, as pneumonia may be a secondary cause of death in a patient already fatally ill with another disease.

secondary closure. SECONDARY SUTURE.

secondary constriction. Clear areas within a telomere (arm) of a chromosome. Depending upon the presence of a nucleolus, these areas are designated as nucleolar or anucleolar constrictions.

secondary cords. CORTICAL CORDS.

secondary corpuscular irradiation. The interaction of x-rays or gamma rays and atoms of matter to produce high-speed electrons.

secondary cyst. A cyst within a cyst.

secondary degeneration. Ascending or descending degeneration of nerves or tracts. Syn. *Wallerian degeneration.*

secondary dentin. The dentin of repair; that which is deposited on the walls of the pulp chamber by odontoblasts in response to loss of tooth substance from decay or wear.

secondary dentition. PERMANENT DENTITION.

secondary digestion. The assimilation of nutrients by the cells of the body, as distinguished from primary, or gastrointestinal, digestion.

secondary drive. ACQUIRED DRIVE.

secondary dysmenorrhea. Dysmenorrhea associated with organic pelvic disease. Syn. *acquired dysmenorrhea.*

secondary electron. Any photoelectron or recoil electron produced when roentgen rays strike an atom.

secondary emission. Emission of electrons from a metal plate which is being bombarded by a stream of high-energy (primary) electrons.

secondary filter. *In radiology,* a sheet of material of low atomic number relative to that of the primary filter, placed in the path of the filtered beam of radiation to remove the characteristic radiation of the primary filter.

secondary fluorescence. The fluorescence found in nonfluorescent tissues that have been treated with fluorochromes.

secondary gain. *In psychiatry,* the profit reaped from a symptom or illness by a patient, such as increased personal attention, money, or disability benefits. Contr. *primary gain.*

secondary glaucoma. Glaucoma consequent upon other ocular diseases.

secondary gonocyte. A definitive or functional germ cell.

secondary gout. GOUT (2).

secondary hydatid. An echinococcus cyst due to the rupture of another cyst and deposit of germinal cells and scolices in the neighborhood.

secondary hypertension. Hypertension of known organic origin.

secondary hypogonadism. PITUITARY HYPOGONADISM.

secondary hypothyroidism. Hypothyroidism due to inadequate stimulation of the thyroid gland.

secondary infection. Implantation of a new infection upon a preexisting infection.

secondary lesion. A lesion that follows, and is due to, a primary lesion, as the secondary, cutaneous lesions of syphilis or the involvement of mediastinal lymph nodes following pulmonary tuberculosis.

secondary memory. LONG-TERM MEMORY (1).

secondary nasal cavity. The embryonic definitive nasal cavity after formation of the palate.

secondary oocyte. An oocyte preceding the second maturation division.

secondary oral cavity. The definitive oral cavity after the formation of the palate.

secondary palate. The embryonic palate formed by the union of the palatine processes of the maxillary processes; the definitive palate.

secondary peritonitis. The common type of peritonitis, due to extension of infection from neighboring parts, the rupture of a viscus or an abscess, trauma, or as a result of irritation.

secondary polycythemia. Polycythemia resulting from a physiologic response to oxygen unsaturation of arterial blood, as in a fetus, in certain forms of congenital and acquired heart disease, or in chronic pulmonary disease.

secondary process. *In psychoanalysis,* the mental activity characteristic of the ego, and guided by the reality principle. Characterized by organization, intellectualization, and similar conscious processes, it leads to realistic thought and action. Contr. *primary process.*

secondary purpura. SYMPTOMATIC PURPURA.

secondary radiation. In nuclear science, particles or photons produced by the interaction with matter of a radiation that is regarded as primary.

secondary refractory anemia. Anemia alleviated only by transfusion and associated with known infections, chronic kidney disease, or cancer.

secondary repression. *In psychiatry,* repression of information of which a person once was aware, but which has become intolerable to the conscious mind.

secondary response. An immune response evoked in an organism by a previously encountered antigen, characterized by a lower threshold dosage of antigen and prolonged synthesis of greater amounts of antibody.

secondary sensation. 1. The excitation of one sensation by another, or the extension or radiation of unpleasant sensations from an area involved by disease to unaffected parts. 2. SYNESTHESIA (1).

secondary sequestrum. A sequestrum that is partially detached and that, unless very loose, may be pushed into place.

secondary sex characters. Differences between males and females not directly concerned with reproduction, as those of voice, distribution of body hair, patterns of adipose tissue, and of skeletal and muscular development.

secondary spermatocyte. One of the two cells produced by the first meiotic division.

secondary spiral lamina. A short partition projecting from the outer wall of the cochlea in the lower part only. NA *lamina spiralis secundaria.*

secondary structure. The coiled structure of a polypeptide chain determined by non-covalent bonds between its atoms. These bonds include hydrogen bonds, electrostatic attractions between peptide residues, and van der Waals' forces. Contr. *primary, tertiary,* and *quaternary structure.*

secondary suture. A suture done some time after the time of injury or operation. Syn. *delayed suture, secondary closure.*

secondary syphilid. Any syphilid occurring during the early stage of syphilis.

secondary syphilis. Any of the manifestations of syphilis after the primary chancre heals and before the latent stage begins; skin and mucous membrane lesions predominate. During this period, serologic testing is always reactive.

secondary tympanic membrane. The membrane closing the fenestra cochleae. NA *membrana tympani secundaria.*

secondary urethra. The definitive urethra, especially in the male where it includes the primary urethra as well as the urogenital sinus.

secondary villus. A definitive, placental villus having a core of connective tissue and blood vessels. Syn. *true villus.*

second childhood. *Colloq.* Senility or senile dementia.

second (IId) cranial nerve. OPTIC NERVE.

second-degree burn. A burn that is more severe than a first-degree burn and is characterized by blistering as well as reddening of the skin, edema, and destruction of the superficial underlying tissues.

second-degree heart block. ATRIOVENTRICULAR BLOCK.

second heart sound. The heart sound complex related primarily to deceleration of blood in the aorta and pulmonary artery following closure of the aortic and pulmonic valves. Symbol, S_2 or SII.

second-set, *adj.* Characterizing a graft to a recipient which has already rejected a graft of the same genetic constitution.

second stage. *In obstetrics,* EXPULSIVE STAGE.

second-wind angina. Angina pectoris which develops on initial exertion, but disappears if activity continues.

se·cre·ta (se·kree'tuh) *n.pl.* [NL.]. The substances secreted by a gland, follicle, or other organ; the products of secretion.

se·cre·ta·gogue (se·kree'tuh·gog) *n.* [*secrete* + *-agogue*]. A substance promoting or causing secretion, as certain hormones.

Se·cré·tan's disease (suh·kreʸ·tahⁿ') [H. *Secrétan,* Swiss surgeon, 1856–1916]. Posttraumatic hard dorsal edema of the hand or foot.

se·crete (se·kreet') *v.* To separate; specifically, to separate from blood, or form out of materials furnished by the blood, various substances. **—secret·ing** (·ing) *adj.*

se·cre·tin (se·kree'tin) *n.* A basic polypeptide hormone produced in the epithelial cells of the duodenum by the contact of acid. It is absorbed from the cells by the blood and excites the pancreas to activity.

se·cre·tin·ase (se·kree'tin·ace) *n.* An enzyme present in blood serum which inactivates the hormone secretin.

se·cre·tion (se·kree'shun) *n.* [L. *secretio,* from *secernere,* to separate]. 1. The act of secreting or forming, from materials furnished by the blood, various substances either eliminated from the body (excretion) or used in carrying on special functions. 2. The substance secreted.

se·cre·to·gogue (se·kree'to·gog) *n.* SECRETAGOGUE.

se·cre·to·in·hib·i·tor syndrome (se·kree''to·in·hib'i·tur). SJÖGREN'S SYNDROME.

se·cre·tor (se·kree'tur) *n.* A person who secretes demonstrable amounts of the antigen A or B or both in his saliva and gastric juice; a dominant trait.

se·cre·to·ry (se·kree'tuh·ree) *adj.* Pertaining to secretion; performing secretion.

secretory canaliculi or **capillaries.** Fine, intercellular canaliculi formed by grooves in adjoining gland cells, draining the secretion of the cells, and opening into the lumen of the gland.

secretory fibers. Centrifugal nerve fibers exciting secretion.

secretory nerve. An efferent nerve, stimulation of which causes increased activity of the gland to which it is distributed.

secretory otitis media. SEROUS OTITIS MEDIA.

secretory piece. A fourth polypeptide chain found on the exocrine IgA molecule. Of unknown function, though it may serve to enhance the exocrine IgA's resistance to proteolysis.

sec·tar·i·an (seck·tair'ee·un, seck·tăr') *n.* One who, in the practice of medicine, follows a dogma, tenet, or principle based on the authority of its promulgator to the exclusion of demonstration and experience.

sec·tile (seck'tile, ·til) *adj.* [L. *sectilis,* from *secare,* to cut]. Capable of being cut.

sec·tio (seck'shee·o, ·tee·o) *n.,* pl. **sec·ti·o·nes** (seck''shee·o'neez, seck''tee·) [L., a cutting, from *secare,* to cut]. SECTION.

sec·tion, *n.* & *v.* [L. *sectio,* from *secare,* to cut]. 1. A cutting or dividing. 2. A cut or slice. 3. To cut, slice, or divide. **—section·al** (·ul) *adj.*

sectional radiography. The technique of making radiographs of plane sections of objects; its purpose is to show detail in a predetermined plane of the body, while blurring the images of structures in other planes. Syn. *tomography, laminography, planography.*

section cutter. MICROTOME; particularly one to be held in the hand.

sectiones. Plural of *sectio* (= SECTION).

sectiones ce·re·bel·li (serr·e·bel'eye) [NA]. Sections of the cerebellum; usually cross sections.

sectiones cor·po·rum qua·dri·ge·mi·no·rum (kor'po·rum quah''dri·jem·i·no'rum) [BNA]. Sections of the corpora quadrigemina.

sectiones hy·po·tha·la·mi (high·po·thal'uh·migh) [NA]. Sections of the hypothalamus.

sectiones isth·mi (isth'migh) [BNA]. SECTIONES MESENCEPHALI.

sectiones me·dul·lae ob·lon·ga·tae (me·dul'ee ob·long·gay'tee) [NA]. Sections of the medulla oblongata.

sectiones medullae spi·na·lis (spye·nay'lis) [NA]. Sections of the spinal cord.

sectiones me·sen·ce·pha·li (mes·en·sef'uh·lye) [NA]. Sections of the mesencephalon.

sectiones pe·dun·cu·li ce·re·bri (pe·dunk'yoo·lye serr'e·brye) [BNA]. SECTIONES MESENCEPHALI.

sectiones pon·tis (pon'tis) [NA]. Sections of the pons.

sectiones te·len·ce·pha·li (tel·en·sef'uh·lye) [NA]. Sections of the cerebrum.

sectiones tha·la·men·ce·pha·li (thal''uh·men·sef'uh·lye) [NA]. Sections of the thalamic region.

sec·to·ri·al (seck·to'ree·ul) *adj.* [L. *sector,* cutter]. Having cutting edges, as the molar teeth of carnivores.

se·cun·di·grav·i·da (se·kun''di·grav'i·duh) *n.* [L. *secundus,* second, + *gravida*]. A woman pregnant the second time. **—secundigrav·id** (·id) *adj.*

se·cun·di·nae (seck''un·dye'nee) *n.,* sing. **secundi·na** (·nuh) [L.]. SECUNDINES.

se·cun·dines (seck'un·dine'z, ·deenz, se·kun') *n.pl.* [L. *secundinae,* from *secundus,* following]. The placenta and membranes discharged from the uterus after birth.

sec·un·dip·a·ra (seck''un·dip'uh·ruh, see''kun·) *n.* [L. *secundus,* second, + *-para*]. A woman who has borne two children. **—secundipa·rous** (·rus) *adj.;* **se·cun·di·par·i·ty** (se·kun''di·păr'i·tee) *n.*

se·cun·dum ar·tem (se·kun'dum ahr'tem) [L.]. In the approved professional manner.

SED Abbreviation for *skin erythema dose.*

se·da·tion (se·day'shun) *n.* [L. *sedatio,* from *sedare,* to soothe]. 1. A state of lessened functional activity. 2. The production of a state of lessened activity, or the act of allaying anxiety and irritability, or the amelioration of pain by means of a sedative. **—se·date** (se·date') *v.*

sed·a·tive (sed'uh·tiv) *adj.* & *n.* [ML. *sedativus,* from *sedare,* to soothe]. 1. Quieting function or activity. 2. Any drug that can be used to calm anxious and disturbed patients and to produce drowsiness. Compare *hypnotic, narcotic.*

sedative bath. A prolonged, warm, full bath.

sed·en·tary (sed'un·terr''ee) *adj.* [L. *sedentarius,* from *sedere,* to sit]. 1. Occupied in sitting; pertaining to the habit of sitting. 2. Inclined to being physically inactive; pertaining particularly to an occupation or life style in which the individual engages in little physical activity but sits a good part of the time.

sed·i·ment (sed'i·munt) *n.* [L. *sedimentum,* from *sedere,* to sit, settle]. The material settling to the bottom of a liquid. **—sed·i·men·ta·ry** (sed''i·men'tuh·ree) *adj.*

sed·i·men·ta·tion (sed''i·men·tay'shun) *n.* The process of producing the deposition of a sediment, especially the rapid deposition by means of a centrifugal machine.

sedimentation method. A technique of separating any substance by virtue of its differential density from the solution in which it is contained.

sedimentation rate. The rate at which red blood cells settle out of anticoagulated blood.

sedimentation test. 1. AGGLUTINATION TEST. 2. ERYTHROCYTE SEDIMENTATION TEST.

sed·i·men·tom·e·ter (sed″i·men·tom′e·tur) *n.* [*sediment* + *-meter*]. An apparatus for recording the sedimentation rate of blood.

sediment tube. A glass cylinder constricted to a fine point at one end and having both ends open; used in separating precipitates found in urine.

seed, *n.* A fertilized and ripened ovule produced by flowering plants, along with reserve nutritive material and protective covering. It is primarily a sporophyte in a resting stage.

See·lig·muel·ler's neuralgia (zeʸ′lick·muᵉl″ur) [O. L. G. A. *Seeligmueller,* German neurologist, 1837–1912]. Neuralgic pains, particularly on pressure in the cranial region; said by Seeligmueller to characterize systemic syphilis.

Seeligmueller's sign [O. L. G. A. *Seeligmueller*]. In trigeminal neuralgia, mydriasis on the affected side of the face.

seg·ment, *n.* [L. *segmentum,* from *secare,* to cut]. 1. A small piece cut along the radii of anything regarded as circular; a part bounded by a natural or imaginary line. 2. A natural division, resulting from segmentation; one of a series of homologous parts, as a myotome; the part of a limb between two consecutive joints. 3. A subdivision, ring, lobe, somite, or metamere of any cleft or articulated body.

segmenta. Plural of *segmentum.*

segmenta bron·cho·pul·mo·na·lia (bronk″o·pul·mo·nay′lee·uh) [NA]. BRONCHOPULMONARY SEGMENTS.

seg·men·tal, *adj.* 1. Of or pertaining to a segment. 2. Made up of segments. 3. Undergoing or resulting from segmentation.

segmental anesthesia. Loss of sensation of an area supplied by one or a limited group of spinal nerves.

segmental arachnoiditis. A spinal arachnoiditis that extends over a limited vertical extent of the spinal cord and gives rise to symptoms over an area that corresponds to the involved segments.

segmental block. Anesthesia producing a block of both the sensory supply of a visceral organ and the somatic nerves of the region of approach.

segmental bronchus. A bronchus which originates in a lobar bronchus and through its branches ventilates a bronchopulmonary segment. NA (pl.) *bronchi segmentales* (sing. *bronchus segmentalis*).

segmental demyelination. Breakdown of myelin involving one or many internodal segments of peripheral nerves, with preservation of axons and absence of chromatolysis; characteristic of many polyneuropathies. Syn. *Gombault's degeneration.* Compare *secondary degeneration.*

segmental enteritis. REGIONAL ENTERITIS.

segmental fracture. DOUBLE FRACTURE.

segmental nerve. A nerve that supplies the structures from one of the original body somites, as an intercostal nerve.

segmental neuritis. Neuritis affecting a segmental nerve.

segmental reflex. INTRASEGMENTAL REFLEX.

segmental static reflex. A postural reflex involving a whole segment of the body, as both forelimbs or the neck muscles.

segmental syndrome. Signs and symptoms which indicate a lesion of the spinal cord restricted to one or a few adjacent levels.

segmenta re·na·lia (re·nay′lee·uh) [NA]. The segments of the kidney.

seg·men·tary (seg′mun·terr″ee) *adj.* SEGMENTAL.

segmentary neuritis. SEGMENTAL NEURITIS.

segmentary syndrome. SEGMENTAL SYNDROME.

seg·men·ta·tion (seg″men·tay′shun) *n.* 1. The process of cleavage or cell division, especially as applied to the fertilized ovum and blastomeres. 2. The division of an organism into somites or metameres.

segmentation cavity. BLASTOCOELE.

segmentation cell. BLASTOMERE.

segmentation nucleus. The nucleus that appears shortly after the fusion of the male and female pronuclei; the last step in the process of fertilization; it is so called because within it cleavage is first established.

seg·men·tec·to·my (seg″men·teck′tuh·mee) *n.* [*segment* + *-ectomy*]. Surgical removal of a lung segment.

seg·ment·ed cell. Any mature granulocyte (basophil, eosinophil, neutrophil) in which the lobes of the nucleus are connected by a filament. Syn. *lobocyte.*

Seg·men·ti·na (seg″men·tye′nuh) *n.* A genus of freshwater snails; the intermediate host of *Fasciolopsis buski.*

seg·ment·ing body. The sporulating malaria parasite, when the schizont breaks up into the merozoites.

segmenting movements of the small intestine. Spaced and localized constrictions of the intestinal lumen at successive points along the intestine, acting to expose repeatedly new surfaces of the intestinal contents to the action of digestive juices.

seg·men·tum (seg·men′tum) *n.,* pl. **segmen·ta** (·tuh) [L.]. SEGMENT.

segmentum an·te·ri·us in·fe·ri·us re·na·lis (an·teer′ee·us in·feer′ee·us re·nay′lis) [NA]. The anterior inferior segment of the kidney.

segmentum anterius lo·bi he·pa·tis dex·tri (lo′bye hep′uh·tis decks′trye) [NA]. The anterior segment of the right lobe of the liver.

segmentum anterius lobi su·pe·ri·o·ris pul·mo·nis dex·tri (sue·peer·ee·o′ris pul·mo′nis decks′trye) [NA]. The anterior segment of the superior lobe of the right lung.

segmentum anterius lobi superioris pulmonis si·nis·tri (si·nis′trye) [NA]. The anterior segment of the superior lobe of the left lung.

segmentum anterius su·pe·ri·us re·na·lis (sue·peer′ee·us re·nay′lis) [NA]. The anterior superior segment of the kidney.

segmentum api·ca·le lo·bi in·fe·ri·o·ris pul·mo·nis dex·tri (ap·i·kay′lee lo′bye in·feer·ee·o′ris pul·mo′nis decks′trye) [NA]. The apical segment of the inferior lobe of the right lung. NA alt. *segmentum superius lobi inferioris pulmonis dextri.*

segmentum apicale lobi inferioris pulmonis si·nis·tri (si·nis′trye) [NA]. The apical segment of the inferior lobe of the left lung. NA alt. *segmentum superius lobi inferioris pulmonis sinistri.*

segmentum apicale lobi su·pe·ri·o·ris pul·mo·nis dex·tri (sue·peer·ee·o′ris pul·mo′nis decks′trye) [NA]. The apical segment of the superior lobe of the right lung.

segmentum api·co·pos·te·ri·us lo·bi su·pe·ri·o·ris pul·mo·nis si·nis·tri (ap″i·ko·pos·teer′ee·us lo′bye sue·peer·ee·o′ris pul·mo′nis si·nis′trye) [NA]. The apicoposterior segment of the superior lobe of the left lung.

segmentum ba·sa·le an·te·ri·us lo·bi in·fe·ri·o·ris pul·mo·nis dex·tri (ba·say′lee an·teer′ee·us lo′bye in·feer·ee·o′ris pul·mo′nis decks′trye) [NA]. The anterior basal segment of the right lung.

segmentum basale anterius lobi inferioris pulmonis si·nis·tri (si·nis′trye) [NA]. The anterior basal segment of the left lung.

segmentum basale la·te·ra·le lo·bi in·fe·ri·o·ris pul·mo·nis dex·tri (lat·e·ray′lee lo′bye in·feer·ee·o′ris pul·mo′nis decks′trye) [NA]. The lateral basal segment of the inferior lobe of the right lung.

segmentum basale laterale lobi inferioris pulmonis si·nis·tri (si·nis′trye) [NA]. The lateral basal segment of the inferior lobe of the left lung.

segmentum basale me·di·a·le lo·bi in·fe·ri·o·ris pul·mo·nis dex·tri (mee·dee·ay′lee lo′bye in·feer·ee·o′ris pul·mo′nis decks′trye) [NA]. The medial basal segment of the inferior lobe of the right lung. NA alt. *segmentum cardiacum lobi inferioris pulmonis dextri.*

segmentum basale mediale lobi inferioris pulmonis si·nis·tri (si·nis'trye) [NA]. The medial basal segment of the inferior lobe of the left lung. NA alt. *segmentum cardiacum lobi inferioris pulmonis sinistri.*

segmentum basale pos·te·ri·us lo·bi in·fe·ri·o·ris pul·mo·nis dex·tri (pos·teer'ee·us lo'bye in·feer·ee·o'ris pul·mo'nis decks'trye) [NA]. The posterior basal segment of the inferior lobe of the right lung.

segmentum basale posterius lobi inferioris pulmonis si·nis·tri (si·nis'trye) [NA]. The posterior basal segment of the inferior lobe of the left lung.

segmentum car·di·a·cum lo·bi in·fe·ri·o·ris pul·mo·nis dex·tri (kahr·dye'uh·kum lo'bye in·feer·ee·o'ris pul·mo'nis decks'trye) [NA alt.]. SEGMENTUM BASALE MEDIALE LOBI INFERIORIS PULMONIS DEXTRI.

segmentum cardiacum lobi inferioris pulmonis si·nis·tri (si·nis'trye) [NA alt.]. SEGMENTUM BASALE MEDIALE LOBI INFERIORIS PULMONIS SINISTRI.

segmentum in·fe·ri·us re·na·lis (in·feer'ee·us re·nay'lis) [NA]. The inferior segment of the kidney.

segmentum la·te·ra·le lo·bi he·pa·tis si·nis·tri (lat·e·ray'lee lo'bye hep'uh·tis si·nis'trye) [NA]. The lateral segment of the left lobe of the liver.

segmentum laterale lobi me·dii pul·mo·nis dex·tri (mee'dee·eye pul·mo'nis decks'trye) [NA]. The lateral segment of the middle lobe of the right lung.

segmentum lin·gu·la·re in·fe·ri·us lo·bi su·pe·ri·o·ris pul·mo·nis si·nis·tri (ling·gew·lair'ee in·feer'ee·us lo'bye sue·peer·ee·o'ris pul·mo'nis si·nis'trye) [NA]. The inferior lingular segment of the superior lobe of the left lung.

segmentum lingulare su·pe·ri·us lo·bi su·pe·ri·o·ris pul·mo·nis si·nis·tri (sue·peer'ee·us lo'bye sue·peer·ee·o'ris pul·mo'nis si·nis'trye) [NA]. The superior lingular segment of the superior lobe of the left lung.

segmentum me·di·a·le lo·bi he·pa·tis si·nis·tri (mee·dee·ay'lee lo'bye hep'uh·tis si·nis'trye) [NA]. The medial segment of the left lobe of the liver.

segmentum mediale lobi me·dii pul·mo·nis dex·tri (mee'dee·eye pul·mo'nis decks'trye) [NA]. The medial segment of the middle lobe of the right lung.

segmentum pos·te·ri·us lo·bi he·pa·tis dex·tri (pos·teer'ee·us lo'bye hep'uh·tis decks'trye) [NA]. The posterior segment of the right lobe of the liver.

segmentum posterius lobi su·pe·ri·o·ris pul·mo·nis dex·tri (sue·peer·ee·o'ris pul·mo'nis decks'trye) [NA]. The posterior segment of the superior lobe of the right lung.

segmentum posterius re·na·lis (re·nay'lis) [NA]. The posterior segment of the kidney.

segmentum sub·api·ca·le lo·bi in·fe·ri·o·ris pul·mo·nis dex·tri (sub·ap''i·kay'lee lo'bye in·feer·ee·o'ris pul·mo'nis decks'trye) [NA]. The subapical segment of the inferior lobe of the right lung. NA alt. *segmentum subsuperius lobi inferioris pulmonis dextri.*

segmentum subapicale lobi inferioris pulmonis si·nis·tri (si·nis'trye) [NA]. The subapical segment of the inferior lobe of the left lung. NA alt. *segmentum subsuperius lobi inferioris pulmonis sinistri.*

segmentum sub·su·pe·ri·us lo·bi in·fe·ri·o·ris pul·mo·nis dex·tri (sub''sue·peer'ee·us lo'bye in·feer·ee·o'ris pul·mo'nis decks'trye) [NA alt.]. SEGMENTUM SUBAPICALE LOBI INFERIORIS PULMONIS DEXTRI.

segmentum subsuperius lobi inferioris pulmonis si·nis·tri (si·nis'trye) [NA alt.]. SEGMENTUM SUBAPICALE LOBI INFERIORIS PULMONIS SINISTRI.

segmentum su·pe·ri·us lo·bi in·fe·ri·o·ris pul·mo·nis dex·tri (sue·peer'ee·us lo'bye in·feer·ee·o'ris pul·mo'nis decks'trye) [NA alt.]. SEGMENTUM APICALE LOBI INFERIORIS PULMONIS DEXTRI.

segmentum superius lobi inferioris pulmonis si·nis·tri (si·nis'trye) [NA alt.]. SEGMENTUM APICALE LOBI INFERIORIS PULMONIS SINISTRI.

segmentum superius re·na·lis (re·nay'lis) [NA]. The superior segment of the kidney.

Segontin. Trademark for prenylamine, a coronary vasodilator.

seg·re·ga·tion (seg''re·gay'shun) *n.* [L. *segregatio,* from *segregare,* to separate]. 1. The reappearance of contrasted Mendelian characters in the offspring of heterozygotes. 2. The separation of the paired maternal and paternal genes at meiosis in the formation of gametes. —**seg·re·gate** (seg're·gate) *v.*

seg·re·ga·tion·al equilibrium (seg''re·gay'shun·ul). BALANCED POLYMORPHISM.

segregation apparatus. GOLGI APPARATUS.

seg·re·ga·tor (seg're·gay''tur) *n.* An instrument by means of which urine from each kidney may be secured without admixture.

Se·guin's sign or **signal** (se·geen', F. se·gæⁿ') [E. *Seguin,* U.S. psychiatrist, 1812–1880]. Involuntary muscular contraction occurring just before a seizure.

Seid·litz powders (sed'lits) [after *Sedlitz* (Cz. *Sedice*), Czechoslovakia]. Two powders, one commonly in a blue paper, containing potassium sodium tartrate and sodium bicarbonate, the other in a white paper, containing tartaric acid. On mixing solutions of the powders, effervescence occurs; the solution is taken for cathartic effect. Syn. *compound effervescent powders.*

sei·es·the·sia, sei·aes·the·sia (sigh''es·theezh'uh, ·theez'ee·uh) *n.* [Gk. *seiein,* to shake, + *esthesia*]. Perception of jarring of the brain.

seis·mo·ther·a·py (size''mo·therr'uh·pee, sice''mo·) *n.* [Gk. *seismos,* shaking, agitation, + *therapy*]. The treatment of disease using mechanical vibration.

Seitz filter (zights) [E. *Seitz,* German bacteriologist, b. 1885]. A bacterial filter utilizing a matted asbestos filtering pad or disk, the unit being used with either vacuum or pressure.

sei·zure (see'zhur) *n.* [OF. *seisir*]. 1. The sudden onset or recurrence of a disease or an attack. 2. Specifically, an epileptic attack, fit, or convulsion.

seizure equivalent. A form of epilepsy, especially in children, characterized by recurrent paroxysms of autonomic and sometimes behavioral disturbances, usually without specific systemic or intracranial disease, but with frequent abnormalities on the electroencephalogram, and responding to adequate anticonvulsant therapy. Common symptoms include headache, abdominal pain, nausea, vomiting, pallor, flushing, dizziness, faintness, sweating, fever, chills, and temper outbursts; postictal drowsiness and sleep of varying duration may follow. Other forms of epilepsy may be present. Syn. *convulsive equivalent.*

se·junc·tion (se·junk'shun) *n.* [L. *sejunctio,* from *sejungere,* to separate]. *In psychology,* the interruption of the continuity of association processes, tending to break up personality.

se·la·pho·bia (see''luh·fo'bee·uh) *n.* [Gk. *selas,* light, lightning, + *-phobia*]. Abnormal fear of flashing light or lightning.

Seldinger technique [S. I. *Seldinger*]. A technique for the introduction of a fine catheter into a vessel via a percutaneous needle puncture.

se·lec·tion, *n.* [L. *selectio,* from *seligere,* to select]. *In biology,* choosing for survival or elimination. See also *natural selection.*

selective orthopnea. TREPOPNEA.

se·lec·tor, *n.* A device for selecting or separating.

se·le·ne (se·lee'nee) *n.,* pl. **sele·nai** (·nay, ·nigh) [Gk. *selēnē,* moon]. 1. LUNULA (1). 2. Any object resembling the moon in any of its phases.

se·le·nic (se·lee'nick, se·len'ick) *adj.* Of or pertaining to compounds of selenium in which the element has a valence of 6, or sometimes 4.

sel·e·nif·er·ous (sel''e·nif'ur·us) *adj.* [*selenium* + *-ferous*]. Containing selenium.

se·le·ni·ous acid (se·lee'nee·us). H_2SeO_3; the acid formed by tetravalent selenium.

sel·e·nite (sel'e·nite, see'le·nite) *n.* 1. A salt of selenious acid. 2. A translucent form of calcium sulfate.

selenite medium. An enrichment medium, incorporating selenite, which favors the isolation of salmonellae.

se·le·ni·um (se·lee'nee·um) *n.* [NL., from Gk. *selēnē,* moon]. Se = 78.96. An element, atomic number 34, resembling sulfur and existing in several allotropic forms; it is toxic to humans and animals.

selenium sulfide. Selenium disulfide, SeS_2, a bright-orange powder, practically insoluble in water; used for treatment of seborrheic dermatitis and common dandruff of the scalp. Because of its toxicity, absorption should be avoided.

se·len·odont (se·lee'no·dont, se·len'o·) *adj.* [Gk. *selēnē*, moon, + *-odont*]. Possessing molar teeth with crescent-shaped ridges.

sel·e·no·sis (sel''e·no'sis) *n.* [*sele*nium + *-osis*]. Poisoning by selenium.

self-absorption, *n.* Absorption of radiation by the source material itself.

self-abuse, *n.* MASTURBATION.

self-alienation, *n.* The blocking or dissociation of one's own feelings until they seem estranged and depersonalized, and the person considers himself and everything about him unreal.

self-analysis, *n. In psychiatry,* the attempt to gain insight into one's own psychic state and behavior, a practice which, despite Freud's fairly successful one, generally remains rather superficial.

self-curing resin. AUTOPOLYMERIZING RESIN.

self-differentiation, *n.* The differentiation of a tissue, even when isolated, solely as a result of intrinsic factors after determination.

self-digestion, *n.* AUTODIGESTION.

self-fermentation, *n.* AUTOLYSIS.

self-fertilization, *n.* The impregnation of the ovules by pollen of the same flower or of the ova by sperm of the same animal.

self-healing epithelioma. KERATOACANTHOMA.

self-hypnosis, *n.* Hypnosis by autosuggestion.

self-inductance, *n.* The property of a conductor to oppose changes in current by the development of a counter electromotive force.

self-infection, *n.* AUTOINFECTION.

self-inoculation, *n.* AUTOINOCULATION.

self-limited, *adj.* Restricted by its own characteristics rather than by external factors; used to designate a disease which runs a definite course in a specific time.

self-mutilation, *n.* 1. The act of injuring one's own body, as in hyperuricemia or certain mental disorders. 2. Any injury thus sustained.

self-pollution, *n.* MASTURBATION.

self-retaining catheter. A catheter so constructed that, following its introduction, it will be held in position by mechanisms incorporated in its particular structure.

self-retaining retractor. A special instrument having two retractor arms clamped to a bar and adjusted by means of setscrews. Some are equipped with a third arm for retraction of the pubic portion of the urinary bladder during bladder and prostatic operations.

self-suggestibility, *n.* AUTOSUGGESTIBILITY.

self-suggestion, *n.* AUTOSUGGESTION (2).

self-suspension, *n.* Suspension of the body by the head for the purpose of stretching or making extension on the vertebral column.

Se·li·wa·noff's test (se·lee·vah'nuf) [F. F. *Seliwanoff,* Russian chemist, b. 1859]. A test for fructose, in which urine is added to a resorcinol–hydrochloric acid mixture. The production of a red color and the separation of a red precipitate indicate fructose.

sel·la (sel'uh) *n.,* pl. & genit. sing. **sel·lae** (·ee) [L., seat]. SADDLE. —**sel·lar** (·lur) *adj.*

sella tur·ci·ca (tur'si·kuh) [L., Turkish saddle] [NA]. The superior portion of the body of the sphenoid bone that surrounds the hypophyseal fossa. It includes the tuberculum sellae, anterior clinoid processes, and the dorsum sellae with its posterior clinoid processes.

Sel·ter's disease (zel'tur) [P. *Selter,* German pediatrician, 1866–1941]. ACRODYNIA.

Sel·ye's syndrome (zel'yeʰ) [H. *Selye,* Canadian biochemist, b. 1907]. GENERAL ADAPTATION SYNDROME.

se·man·tic (se·man'tick) *adj.* [Gk. *sēmantikos,* signifying, significant]. 1. Pertaining to meaning in language. 2. Pertaining to semantics.

semantic alexia. A form of alexia in which the patient is able to read, but not comprehend, written or printed language.

semantic aphasia. A failure to recognize the full significance of words and phrases apart from their verbal meaning. Although the patient can enumerate many details of what he sees and hears, he fails to integrate them into a general conception.

se·man·tics (se·man'ticks) *n.* [*semantic* + *-s*]. 1. The study of meaning in language or in any system of signs or symbols; especially, analysis of signs in terms of what they signify or denote. 2. More broadly, analysis of the interdependencies of language or symbols with anything outside their own system, such as patterns of behavior and thinking. Compare *general semantics.*

Semb's operation [C. B. *Semb,* Norwegian surgeon, b. 1895]. Thoracoplasty with extrafascial apicolysis for pulmonary tuberculosis.

se·mei·og·ra·phy, se·mi·og·ra·phy (see''migh·og'ruh·fee, see''mee·, sem''ee·) *n.* [Gk. *sēmeion*, sign, symptom, + *-graphy*]. Description of the signs and symptoms of a disease.

se·mei·ol·o·gy, se·mi·ol·o·gy (see''migh·ol'o·jee, see''mee·, sem''ee·) *n.* [Gk. *sēmeion*, sign, symptom, + *-logy*]. SYMPTOMATOLOGY. —**semei·o·log·ic** (·o·loj'ick) *adj.*

se·mei·ot·ics (see''migh·ot'icks, see''mee·, sem''ee·) *n.* [Gk. *sēmeiōtikos,* from *sēmeion,* sign, symptom]. SYMPTOMATOLOGY. See also *semiotics.* —**semeiot·ic** (·ick) *adj.*

se·men (see'mun) *n.,* pl. **semi·na** (sem'i·nuh), **semens** [L.]. 1. SEED. 2. The fluid produced by the male reproductive organs, carrying the male germ cells or spermatozoa.

Semenoff method. A histochemical method for succinic dehydrogenase based on the reduction of methylene blue by the enzyme.

semenuria. SEMINURIA.

semi- [L.]. A prefix meaning (a) *half;* (b) *partial or partially.*

semi·aceph·a·lus (sem''ee·a·sef'uh·lus) *n.* [*semi-* + *acephalus*]. ANENCEPHALUS.

semi·al·lo·ge·ne·ic (sem''ee·al''o·je·nee'ick) *adj.* [*semi-* + *allogeneic*]. Characterizing the genetic makeup of an F_1 hybrid, the offspring of two inbred but genetically different parents. The offspring has the histocompatibility antigens of both parents on each nucleated cell.

semi·ca·nal (sem''ee·kuh·nal') *n.* [*semi-* + *canal*]. A canal open on one side; a sulcus or groove.

se·mi·ca·na·lis (sem''i·ka·nay'lis) *n.,* pl. **semicana·les** (·leez) [NL.]. SEMICANAL.

semicanalis mus·cu·li ten·so·ris tym·pa·ni (mus'kew·lye ten·so'ris tim'puh·nigh) [NA]. SEMICANAL OF THE TENSOR TYMPANI MUSCLE.

semicanalis tu·bae au·di·ti·vae (tew'bee aw·di·tye'vee) [NA]. SEMICANAL OF THE AUDITORY TUBE.

semicanal of the auditory tube. The groove in the temporal bone in which the auditory tube lies. NA *semicanalis tubae auditivae.*

semicanal of the tensor tympani muscle. The groove in the temporal bone in which the tensor tympani muscle lies. NA *semicanalis musculi tensoris tympani.*

semi·car·ba·zide (sem''ee·kahr'buh·zide) *n.* Aminourea,

$NH_2NHCONH_2$, used as the hydrochloride as a reagent for aldehydes and ketones.

semi·car·ba·zone (sem″ee·kahr′buh·zone) *n.* A compound formed by reaction of aldehydes or ketones with semicarbazide.

semi·car·ti·lag·i·nous (sem″ee·kahr″ti·laj′i·nus) *adj.* Gristly; partly cartilaginous.

semi·cir·cu·lar (sem″i·sur′kew·lur) *adj.* Having the shape of half a circle.

semicircular canals. See *membranous semicircular canals, osseous semicircular canals.* See also Plate 20.

semicircular ducts. MEMBRANOUS SEMICIRCULAR CANALS.

semicircular line. The curved lower edge of the internal layer of the aponeurosis of the internal oblique muscle, where it ceases to cover the posterior surface of the rectus muscle. NA *linea arcuata vaginae musculi recti abdominis.*

semi·co·ma (sem″ee·ko′muh) *n.* A state of impaired consciousness in which the patient can be roused and responds with some purposeful movements to strong stimuli, especially to pain.

semi·com·a·tose (sem″ee·kom′uh·toce, ·ko′muh·) *adj.* Being in a state of semicoma.

semi·con·scious (sem″ee·kon′shus) *adj.* Half conscious; partially conscious.

semi·flex·ion (sem″ee·fleck′shun) *n.* Partial flexion; a position about midway between extension and full flexion of a limb or muscle.

semi·le·thal factor (sem″ee·lee′thul). A gene which causes the death of the individual soon after development is completed or before reproductive age.

semi·lu·nar (sem″ee·lew′nur) *adj. & n.* [*semi-* + *lunar*]. 1. Resembling a half moon in shape. 2. LUNATE.

semilunar cartilage or **fibrocartilage.** Either of the menisci of the knee joint. See also *lateral meniscus, medial meniscus.*

semilunar fold. A conjunctival fold in the inner canthus of the eye, the vestigial homologue of the nictitating membrane of Amphibia and Sauropsida. NA *plica semilunaris conjunctivae.*

semilunar ganglion. TRIGEMINAL GANGLION.

semilunar hiatus. 1. A groove in the lateral wall of the middle nasal meatus. The maxillary sinus and anterior ethmoid cells open into it. NA *hiatus semilunaris.* 2. An opening in the deep fascia of the arm for the passage of the basilic vein.

semilunar line. A line, convex laterally, marking the transition of the internal oblique and transverse muscles of the abdomen to aponeuroses. NA *linea semilunaris.*

semilunar lobules. See *inferior semilunar lobule, superior semilunar lobule.*

semilunar notch. TROCHLEAR NOTCH.

semilunar nucleus of the thalamus. POSTEROMEDIAL VENTRAL NUCLEUS OF THE THALAMUS.

semilunar plica. The thin fold of mucous membrane across the supratonsillar fossa, between the palatine arches. NA *plica semilunaris.*

semilunar space. A percussion area on the left anterior portion of the thorax, overlying the stomach. Syn. *Traube's space.*

semilunar valves. The valves situated between the ventricles and the aorta or the pulmonary trunk. See also Plate 5.

semi·lux·a·tion (sem″ee·luck·say′shun) *n.* [*semi-* + *luxation*]. SUBLUXATION.

semi·mem·bra·no·sus (sem″ee·mem″bruh·no′sus) *n.* One of the hamstring muscles, arising from the ischial tuber, and inserted into the tibia. NA *musculus semimembranosus.* See also Table of Muscles in the Appendix.

semimembranosus bursa. A bursa situated between the tendon of the semimembranosus muscle and the medial head of the gastrocnemius muscle and medial meniscus of the knee joint. It frequently communicates with the knee joint cavity.

semimembranosus reflex. INTERNAL HAMSTRING REFLEX.

semi·mem·bra·nous (sem″ee·mem′bruh·nus) *adj.* Partly membranous, applied to a muscle.

sem·i·nal (sem′i·nul) *adj.* [L. *seminalis,* pertaining to seed]. Of or pertaining to semen.

seminal capsule. AMPULLA OF THE DUCTUS DEFERENS.

seminal carcinoma. SEMINOMA.

seminal cyst. A cyst of the epididymis or the spermatic cord containing sperm. Compare *spermatocele.*

seminal duct. The duct of the testis, especially the ductus deferens and the ejaculatory duct.

seminal fluid. SEMEN.

seminal gland. TESTIS.

seminal hillock. COLLICULUS SEMINALIS.

seminal vesicle. The contorted, branched, saccular, glandular diverticulum of each ductus deferens with which its excretory duct unites to form an ejaculatory duct. NA *vesicula seminalis.* See also Plate 25.

seminal vesiculogram. VESICULOGRAM.

seminal vesiculography. VESICULOGRAPHY.

sem·i·na·tion (sem″i·nay′shun) *n.* [L. *seminatio,* sowing, propagation, from *seminare,* to sow]. INSEMINATION.

sem·i·nif·er·ous (sem″i·nif′ur·us, see″mi·) *adj.* [L. *semen, seminis,* seed, semen, + *-ferous*]. Producing or carrying semen.

seminiferous tubule. Any of the tubules of the testes.

sem·i·no·ma (sem″i·no′muh) *n.,* pl. **seminomas, seminoma·ta** (·tuh) [*seminal* + *-oma*]. A malignant testicular tumor made up of characteristic large, uniform cells with clear cytoplasm which resemble spermatogonia. Syn. *seminal carcinoma, spermatocytoma.* See also *dysgerminoma.*

semi·nor·mal (sem″ee·nor′mul) *adj.* Half normal, as seminormal solution, a solution which contains one-half of an equivalent weight of the active reagent, in grams, in one liter of solution. Symbol, 0.5 *N* or *N*/2.

sem·i·nu·ria (see″mi·new′ree·uh, sem″i·) *n.* [L. *semen, seminis,* seed, semen, + *-uria*]. The discharge of semen in the urine.

semiography. SEMEIOGRAPHY.

semiology. SYMPTOMATOLOGY.

semi·open anesthesia (sem″ee·o′pun). Inhalation anesthesia with partial rebreathing.

se·mi·ot·ics (see″mee·ot′icks, see″migh·) *n.* [Gk. *sēmeiōtikos,* from *sēmeion,* sign, symptom]. 1. SYMPTOMATOLOGY. 2. The study or theory of symbol systems.

semi·pen·ni·form (sem″ee·pen′i·form) *adj.* Penniform on one side only; UNIPENNATE.

semipermeable membrane. A membrane that permits water and small solute molecules to diffuse freely, but holds back large molecules, salts, and their ions.

semi·pla·cen·ta (sem″ee·pluh·sen′tuh) *n.* A form of placenta in which the maternal and fetal portions are structurally separate.

semi·ple·gia (sem″i·plee′jee·uh) *n.* [*semi-* + *-plegia*]. *Obsol.* HEMIPLEGIA.

semi·pro·na·tion (sem″ee·pro·nay′shun) *n.* [*semi-* + *pronation*]. The assumption of a semiprone or partly prone position; an attitude of semisupination. —**semi·prone** (·prone′) *adj.*

semi·pto·sis (sem″ee·to′sis) *n.* Partial ptosis.

Se·mir·a·mid·i·an operation (se·mirr″uh·mid′ee·un). *Obsol.* CASTRATION.

se·mis (see′mis) *n.* [L.]. Half. In prescriptions, abbreviated ss, placed after the sign indicating the measure. Sometimes abbreviated, s.

semi·sid·e·ra·tio (sem″ee·sid″e·ray′shee·o) *n.* [*semi-* + L. *sideratio,* blight, stroke]. *Obsol.* HEMIPLEGIA.

semi·som·nus (sem″i·som′nus) *n.* [*semi-* + *somnus*]. *Obsol.* Partial coma. —**semisom·nous** (·nus) *adj.*

semi·so·por (sem″ee·so′por) *n.* [*semi-* + *sopor*]. *Obsol.* Partial coma.

semi·spi·na·lis (sem″ee·spye·nay′lis) *n.* One of the deep longitudinal muscles of the back, attached to the vertebrae. NA *musculus semispinalis.* See also Table of Muscles in the Appendix.

semi·su·pi·na·tion (sem"ee·sue"pi·nay'shun) *n.* A position halfway between supination and pronation.

semi·syn·thet·ic (sem"ee·sin·thet'ick) *adj.* Produced by or pertaining to a process of synthesis that involves chemical alteration of a naturally occurring compound, as the synthesis of certain antibiotics from a natural penicillin or a moiety thereof; partly synthetic.

semi·ten·di·no·sus (sem"ee·ten"di·no'sus) *n.* One of the hamstring muscles, arising from the ischium and inserted into the tibia. NA *musculus semitendinosus.* See also Table of Muscles in the Appendix.

semitendinosus reflex. INTERNAL HAMSTRING REFLEX.

semi·ten·di·nous (sem"ee·ten'di·nus) *adj.* Partly tendinous, as a semitendinous muscle. See also *semitendinosus.*

Semon-Rosenbach law. SEMON'S LAW.

Se·mon's law (see'mun) [F. *Semon,* English laryngologist, 1849–1921]. In progressive organic lesions of the motor laryngeal nerves, the abductor muscles of the vocal cords are the first, and sometimes the only, muscles affected, with only later involvement or sparing of the adductors, while in recovery from complete paralysis the reverse occurs.

Semon's symptom [F. *Semon*]. Impaired mobility of the vocal folds in thyroid carcinoma.

se·mus·tine (se·mus'teen) *n.* 1-(2-Chloroethyl)-3-(4-methylcyclohexyl)-1-nitrosourea, $C_{10}H_{18}ClN_3O_2$, an antineoplastic.

Sen·dai virus (sen'dye). A paramyxovirus–parainfluenza virus which may produce widespread respiratory infections in rodent colonies; used in inactivated form in experimental biology to produce heterokaryons.

Senear-Usher syndrome [F. E. *Senear,* American dermatologist, b. 1889; and B. D. *Usher,* Canadian dermatologist, b. 1899]. PEMPHIGUS ERYTHEMATOSUS.

Se·ne·cio (se·nee'shee·o, ·see·o) *n.* [L.]. Groundsel; a genus of composite-flowered plants, said to contain 960 species, many of which have been used medicinally.

se·nec·ti·tude (se·neck'ti·tude) *n.* [ML. *senectitudo,* from L. *senectus,* from *senex,* old]. Old age.

sen·e·ga (sen'e·guh) *n.* [from *Seneca,* an Iroquois Indian tribe that used the root as a remedy against snakebite]. The dried root of *Polygala senega,* which contains saponin principles such as senegin and polygalic acid. Formerly used as an expectorant.

sen·e·gin (sen'e·jin) *n.* A saponin in senega.

Senekjie's medium [H. *Senekjie,* U.S. parasitologist, 20th century]. NNN MEDIUM.

se·nes·cence (se·nes'unce) *n.* [L. *senescere,* to grow old]. The state of being aged. —**se·nes·cent** (se·nes'unt) *adj.*

senescent arthritis. DEGENERATIVE JOINT DISEASE.

Sengstaken-Blakemore tube [R. W. *Sengstaken,* U.S. surgeon, b. 1923; and A. H. *Blakemore*]. A large three-lumen rubber tube for the treatment of bleeding from esophageal varices. There is one lumen to each of two balloons and a large central lumen for aspiration of the stomach and for feeding.

se·nile (see'nile, sen'ile) *adj.* [L. *senilis,* from *senex,* aged]. 1. Pertaining to, caused by, or characteristic of old age or the infirmities of old age. 2. Afflicted with senile dementia.

senile angioma. PAPILLARY VARIX.

senile arteriosclerosis. MEDIAL ARTERIOSCLEROSIS.

senile arteriosclerotic nephrosclerosis. ARTERIAL NEPHROSCLEROSIS.

senile atrophy. Atrophy of certain organs normally occurring in old age.

senile cataract. The cataract of old persons, the most frequent form.

senile chorea. Chorea with onset late in life and with no familial history of the disease, having a relatively benign course and few, if any, signs of mental deterioration.

senile coxitis. A rheumatoid disease of the hip joint occurring in old people; marked by pain, stiffness, and wasting, with no tendency to suppuration.

senile dementia. A chronic progressive mental disease of late life characterized by failing memory and loss of other intellectual functions. The most common pathologic state underlying this syndrome is Alzheimer's disease. Syn. *senile psychosis.*

senile ectasia. ANGIOECTASIA.

senile ectropion. Ectropion due to changes in the tissues of the lids as a result of old age.

senile emphysema. Changes in the thoracic cage and lungs, seen with aging. See also *aging-lung emphysema.*

senile entropion. Entropion caused by relaxation of a portion of the orbicularis oculi muscle, resulting from senile changes.

senile freckle. LENTIGO MALIGNA.

senile gangrene. ARTERIOSCLEROTIC GANGRENE.

senile guttate keratitis. A form of keratitis characterized by small foci of corneal inflammation, occurring in older people.

senile heart disease. PRESBYCARDIA.

senile involution. The slowly progressive degenerative changes seen with advanced age, often with loss of muscle and subcutaneous tissues and shrinkage of other organs.

senile keratosis. ACTINIC KERATOSIS.

senile miosis. Miosis associated with increase in the connective tissue and hyalinization of the septa of the sphincter pupillae muscle, seen usually in the aged.

senile osteoporosis. Osteoporosis in the aged, due to deficient bone matrix formation probably related to deficiency of gonadal hormones and diminished calcium intake. Blood calcium, phosphorus, and phosphatase levels are all normal or low. See also *postmenopausal osteoporosis.*

senile psychosis or **insanity.** SENILE DEMENTIA.

senile purpura. PURPURA SENILIS.

senile tremor. Essential tremor that becomes evident only in late adult life.

senile vaginitis. POSTMENSTRUAL VAGINITIS.

se·nil·ism (see'nil·iz·um) *n.* Senility, especially when premature, as in progeria.

se·nil·i·ty (se·nil'i·tee) *n.* The state of being senile; physical and mental debility associated with old age.

se·ni·um (see'nee·um) *n.* [L., from *senex,* old, aged]. Old age.

senium prae·cox or **pre·cox** (pree'kocks). *Obsol.* PRESENILE DEMENTIA.

Sen method [K. C. *Sen,* Indian biochemist, 20th century]. A histochemical method for urease, based on decomposition of urea on exposure to urease with formation of carbonic acid which is converted to cobalt carbonate and the latter to a brown or black precipitate of cobalt sulfide.

sen·na (sen'uh) *n.* [Ar. *sanā*]. The dried leaflets of *Cassia acutifolia* or of *C. angustifolia* that contain various anthraquinone derivatives; used as a cathartic.

sen·no·side (sen'o·side) *n.* Either of two anthraquinone glucosides, designated sennoside A and sennoside B, present in senna and which are cathartic.

se·no·pia (se·no'pee·uh) *n.* [*sen*ile + *-opia*]. The change of vision in the aged, in which persons formerly myopic acquire what seems to be normal vision because of presbyopia.

sen·sa·tion (sen·say'shun) *n.* [ML. *sensatio,* from L. *sensus,* sense, perception]. 1. The conscious perception caused by stimulation of an afferent nerve or sensory receptor. See also *sensibility.* 2. A feeling or awareness of an emotional state or psychic activity which may arise within the central nervous system, and not necessarily in immediate response to an external stimulus. 3. A bodily feeling, such as pain experienced in the thalamic syndrome, which is the result of stimuli arising from within, and not from outside of the organism. —**sensation·al** (·ul) *adj.*

sensational-type personality. According to Jung, a person in whom sensations, rather than reflective thinking or feeling, dictate action or attitude.

sensation level. A scale of the strength of a stimulus necessary to produce the minimal or threshold subjective sensation, as in measuring on the decibel scale the sound intensity at which there is an appreciation of hearing. Applicable to light, touch, and other stimuli.

sensation unit. The degree of increase in the intensity of a stimulus just discernible by an individual, chiefly used in audiometry, where the unit measuring an increase in intensity of a tone is not a constant, but the expression of a ratio between two tones whose intensity varies sufficiently to make recognition of difference possible. See also *Fechner's law, Weber's law.*

sense, *n.* [L. *sensus,* from *sentire,* to perceive, feel]. 1. Any one of the faculties by which stimuli from the external world or from within the body are received and transformed into sensations. The faculties receiving impulses from the external world are the senses of sight, hearing, equilibrium, touch, smell, and taste, which are the special senses, and the muscular and dermal senses. Those receiving impulses from the internal organs, the visceral senses, are the hunger sense, thirst sense, sexual sense and others. 2. Judgment; understanding; sound reasoning.

sense capsule. One of the cartilage capsules developing about the sense organs that form a part of the embryonic chondrocranium.

sense organ. An association of tissues, including specialized sensory nerve terminals, giving rise to a specific sensation via impulses transmitted along their afferent nerves to the central nervous system, but responding to any adequate stimulus.

sen·sib·a·mine (sen·sib'uh·meen, ·min, ·sen"si·bam'een) *n.* A name given to an alkaloid of ergot, but later found to be an equimolecular mixture of ergotamine and ergotaminine.

sen·si·bil·i·ty (sen"si·bil'i·tee) *n.* [L. *sensibilitas,* from *sensibilis,* perceivable]. 1. The ability to receive, feel, and appreciate physical and psychological impressions. 2. The ability of a nerve or end organ to receive and transmit impulses.

sen·si·bi·liz·er (sen'si·bi·lye"zur) *n.* 1. An agent that renders an enzyme active. 2. *Obsol.* AMBOCEPTOR.

sen·sib·i·lus pro·pri·us nucleus (sen·sib'i·lis pro'pree·us). A group of cells of varied size, lying ventromedial to the substantia gelatinosa.

sen·si·ble (sen'si·bul) *adj.* [L. *sensibilis,* from *sensus,* sense, perception]. 1. Perceptible by the senses, as by sight or smell. 2. Capable of receiving an impression through the senses; endowed with sensation.

sensible perspiration. Visible drops or beads of sweat.

sen·sim·e·ter (sen·sim'e·tur) *n.* A sensitive galvanometer used to measure skin resistance. See also *galvanic skin response.*

sensitive volume or **region.** *In radiobiology,* a region within a cell containing elements vital to life and normal metabolism. Ionization occurring within it changes these elements and leads to death or metabolic malfunctions.

sen·si·tiv·ity (sen"si·tiv'i·tee) *n.* 1. The capacity to perceive, appreciate, or transmit sensation. 2. Power to react to a stimulus. 3. The capacity of a person to respond emotionally to changes in his environment, particularly his interpersonal or social relationships; thus frequently used synonymously with hypersensitivity. 4. The degree of change or responsiveness of an organism with respect to some specific factor or substance, as antibiotic sensitivity. —**sen·si·tive** (sen'si·tiv) *adj.*

sensitivity training. The enhancement of an individual's sensitivity to his environment and particularly interpersonal relationships by means of various techniques, usually employed in group therapy sessions (t-groups).

sen·si·ti·za·tion (sen"si·ti·zay'shun) *n.* 1. The coating of cells with antibody so that they may be agglutinated, or lysed if complement is added. 2. A greater response to a later stimulus than to the original one. 3. The process of becoming reactive or hypersensitive, especially to pollens, serums, and other antigens.

sen·si·tiz·er (sen'si·tye"zur) *n. In dermatology,* the secondary irritant which makes the susceptible subject sensitive to the same or other irritant. —**sensi·tize** (·tize) *v.;* **sensitiz·ing** (·zing) *adj.*

sensitizing antibody. ANAPHYLACTIC ANTIBODY.

sen·so·mo·tor (sen"so·mo'tur) *adj.* SENSORIMOTOR.

sen·so·pa·ral·y·sis (sen'so·puh·ral'i·sis) *n.* SENSORY PARALYSIS.

sen·sor (sen'sur) *n.* 1. That which senses; a sensory organ or structure. 2. A device that responds to a specific physical stimulus and generates an impulse that may be measured, interpreted, or used to operate a control.

sen·so·ri·mo·tor (sen"suh·ri·mo'tur) *adj.* Concerned with or pertaining to the perception of sensory impulses and the generation of motor impulses, as sensorimotor centers.

sen·so·ri·neu·ral (sen"suh·ri·new'rul) *adj.* Of or pertaining to sensory nerves.

sensorineural deafness. PERCEPTION DEAFNESS.

sen·so·ri·um (sen·so'ree·um) *n.,* pl. **sensoriums, senso·ria** (·ree·uh) [L.]. 1. A center for sensations, especially the part of the brain that receives and combines impressions conveyed to the individual sensory centers. 2. The entire sensory apparatus of an individual, including appreciation and proper interpretation of various sensory stimuli, both external and internal. 3. CONSCIOUSNESS.

sensor site. A region of the chromosome in eukaryotic cells which recognizes specific small-molecular-weight compounds and upon binding allows an adjacent integrator gene to transcribe an activator RNA.

sen·so·ry (sen'suh·ree) *adj.* Pertaining to, or conveying, sensation.

sensory agraphia. Loss of ability to write due to a defect in comprehension of language.

sensory amusia. Amusia characterized chiefly by the loss of the power to comprehend musical sounds; musical deafness. Compare *tone deafness.*

sensory aphasia. Loosely, any loss of comprehension of spoken and written language, including acoustic and visual verbal agnosias as well as the aphasias closely related to these.

sensory apraxia. *Obsol.* IDEATIONAL APRAXIA.

sensory area, center, or **cortex.** Any area of the cerebral cortex associated with the perception of sensations.

sensory cell. 1. A neuron whose terminal processes are connected with sensory nerve endings. 2. An epithelial or Schwann cell adapted and modified for the reception and transmission of sensations to an associated nerve ending such as the specific cells of the taste buds. Syn. *neuroepithelial cell.*

sensory decussation. DECUSSATION OF THE LEMNISCI.

sensory deprivation. The condition of being cut off from external sensory stimuli, as with sudden loss of vision, being placed in a respirator tank, or after a shipwreck; sometimes leading to panic, disorganized thinking, depression, hallucinations, and delusion formation.

sensory discrimination. *In psychology,* the ability to perceive the differences or small variations between similar stimuli, as sounds of the same frequencies but of slightly different intensities, or vice versa.

sensory epilepsy. A form of epilepsy in which various disturbances of sensation occur in paroxysms, and may or may not be followed by focal motor or generalized seizures. See also *reflex epilepsy.*

sensory epithelial cell. One of the modified epithelial cells in a sense organ connected with the nerves of that organ.

sensory epithelium. Modified epithelial or Schwann cells having the functional and staining properties of nerve cells; includes the specific cells of the taste buds, olfactory mucosa, and hair cells of the cochlea and vestibule.

sensory nerve. A nerve that conducts afferent impulses from the periphery to the central nervous system, as those mediating sensations of pain, touch, and temperature.

sensory nerve cell. A nerve cell that receives sensory impulses from a sense organ.

sensory neuron. A neuron that conducts impulses arising in a sense organ or at sensory endings.

sensory neurosis. Abnormality of sensation, such as neurotic pruritus, that is psychoneurotic in origin.

sensory paralysis. Loss of sensation due to disease of sensory nerves, pathways, or centers in the nervous system; anesthesia.

sensory paralytic bladder. Atonic bladder, usually as a result of partial or complete interruption of the sensory limb of the reflex arc, as in tabes dorsalis or diabetes mellitus.

sensory radiation. A diffuse unpleasant lingering pain induced by any stimulus in patients with sensory loss due to a lesion of the thalamus, or of the spinal cord or peripheral nerves. See also *thalamic syndrome.*

sensory root. DORSAL ROOT.

sensory tract. Any tract of fibers conducting sensory impulses to the brain.

sen·su·al (sen'shoo·ul) *adj.* [L. *sensualis,* from *sensus,* sense]. 1. Of, pertaining to, or affecting the senses or sensory organs. 2. Characterized by sensualism.

sen·su·al·ism (sen'shoo·ul·iz·um) *n.* The condition or character of one who is controlled by, or lacks control of, the more primitive bodily appetites or emotions.

sen·sus (sen'sus) *n.* [L.]. Sense; feeling.

sen·tient (sen'chee·unt) *adj.* [L. *sentiens,* from *sentire,* to feel]. Having sensation; capable of feeling.

sen·ti·ment (sen'ti·munt) *n.* [ML. *sentimentum,* from L. *sentire,* to feel]. 1. *In psychology,* a mental attitude characterized by feeling. 2. An emotional disposition toward some object or objects.

sen·ti·nel node (sen'ti·nul). SIGNAL NODE.

sentinel pile. The thickened wall of the anal pocket at the lower end of an anal fissure.

separation anxiety. The apprehension, fear, or psychosomatic complaints observed in children on being separated from significant persons or familiar surroundings; commonly expressed in school phobias, and often the result of an abnormal symbiotic relationship between the parent, usually the mother, and the child; an extension of the stranger anxiety of the infant.

sep·a·ra·tor (sep'uh·ray"tur) *n.* 1. Anything that separates, especially an instrument for separating the teeth. 2. PERIOSTEAL ELEVATOR.

sep·azo·ni·um chloride (sep"uh·zo'nee·um). 1-(2,4-Dichloro-β-[2,4-dichlorobenzyl)oxy]phenethyl]-3-phenethylimidazolium chloride, $C_{26}H_{23}Cl_5N_2O$, a topical anti-infective.

Sephadex. The commercial name of a cross-linked dextran gel used frequently for the gel filtration chromatography separation technique.

sep·sis (sep'sis) *n.*, pl. **sep·ses** (·seez) [Gk. *sēpsis,* decay]. 1. Poisoning by products of putrefaction. 2. The severe toxic, febrile state resulting from infection with pyogenic microorganisms, with or without associated septicemia.

sepsis agran·u·lo·cyt·i·ca (a·gran"yoo·lo·sit'i·kuh). AGRANULOCYTOSIS.

[1]sept-, septi- [L. *septem*]. A combining form meaning *seven.*

[2]sept-, septi-, septo- [L.]. A combining form meaning *septum, septal.*

septa. A plural of *septum.*

septaemia. SEPTICEMIA.

septa in·ter·al·ve·o·la·ria man·di·bu·lae (in·tur·al·vee·o·lair'ee·uh man·dib'yoo·lee) [NA]. The partitions of bone between the dental sockets of the alveolar process of the mandible.

septa interalveolaria max·il·lae (mack·sil'ee) [NA]. The partitions of bone between the dental sockets of the alveolar process of the maxilla.

septa in·ter·ra·di·cu·la·ria man·di·bu·lae (in·tur·ra·dick"yoo·lair'ee·uh man·dib'yoo·lee) [NA]. The plates of bone in the alveolar process of the mandible which subdivide the alveolar socket for a tooth with more than one root.

septa interradicularia max·il·lae (mack·sil'ee) [NA]. The plates of bone of the alveolar process of the maxilla which subdivide the alveolar socket for a tooth with more than one root.

sep·tal (sep'tul) *adj.* Of or pertaining to a septum.

septal area. PARATERMINAL BODY.

septal cartilage of the nose. Cartilage of the nasal septum.

septal cells. Macrophages in the interalveolar septa of the lung. See also *heart-failure cells.*

septal cyst. A cyst of the septum pellucidum.

septal lines. KERLEY LINES.

septal plica. One of several folds occasionally present in the fetus on the posteroinferior portion of the nasal septum.

sep·ta·pep·tide (sep"tuh·pep'tide) *n.* A polypeptide composed of seven amino acid groups.

sep·tate (sep'tate) *adj.* Divided into compartments, as by a membrane.

septate vagina. A vagina more or less completely divided by a longitudinal septum; a congenital abnormality.

sep·ta·tion (sep·tay'shun) *n.* 1. Division by a septum. 2. A septum.

sep·tec·to·my (sep·teck'tuh·mee) *n.* [*sept-* + *-ectomy*]. Surgical excision of part of the nasal septum.

sep·te·mia, sep·tae·mia (sep·tee'mee·uh) *n.* SEPTICEMIA.

sep·tic (sep'tick) *adj.* [Gk. *sēptikos,* putrefactive]. 1. Of or pertaining to sepsis. 2. PUTREFACTIVE.

septic abortion. An abortion complicated by acute infection of the endometrium.

sep·ti·ce·mia, sep·ti·cae·mia (sep"ti·see'mee·uh) *n.* [*septic* + *-emia*]. A clinical syndrome characterized by a severe bacteremic infection, generally involving the significant invasion of the bloodstream by microorganisms from a focus or foci in the tissues, and possibly even with the microorganisms multiplying in the blood. Compare *bacteremia, pyemia.* —**septice·mic, septicae·mic** (·mick) *adj.*

septicemic abscess. An abscess resulting from septicemia.

septic intoxication. A form of poisoning resulting from absorption of products of putrefaction.

sep·ti·co·phle·bi·tis (sep"ti·ko·fle·bye'tis) *n.* [*septicemia* + *phlebitis*]. Inflammation of veins secondary to septicemia.

septic tank. In sewage disposal, a closed chamber through which sewage passes slowly to permit bacterial action.

sep·ti·grav·i·da (sep"ti·grav'i·duh) *n.* [*septi-,* seven, + *gravida*]. A woman who is pregnant for the seventh time.

sep·ti·me·tri·tis (sep"ti·me·trye'tis) *n.* [*septic* + *metritis*]. Infection of the uterus.

sep·tip·a·ra (sep·tip'uh·ruh) *n.* [*septi-,* seven, + *-para*]. A woman who has given birth seven times.

septo-. See *sept-.*

sep·to·mar·gi·nal (sep"to·mahr'ji·nul) *adj.* [*septo-* + *marginal*]. Relating to the margin of a septum.

septomarginal band. MODERATOR BAND.

septomarginal fasciculus. A nerve tract composed of descending fibers of intraspinal and dorsal root origin, located in the posterior funiculus of the lumbar spinal cord, near the middle of the posterior septum. Syn. *oval area of Flechsig.* NA *fasciculus septomarginalis.*

[1]sep·tom·e·ter (sep·tom'e·tur) *n.* [*septo-* + *-meter*]. An instrument for determining the thickness of the nasal septum.

[2]sep·tom·e·ter (sep·tom'e·tur) *n.* [*septic* + *-meter*]. An apparatus for determining organic impurities in the air.

sep·to·plas·ty (sep"to·plas'tee) *n.* [*septo-* + *-plasty*]. Surgical reconstruction of the nasal septum.

sep·tos·to·my (sep·tos'tuh·mee) *n.* [*septo-* + *-stomy*]. The operation of creating a septal defect. Compare *septotomy.*

sep·to·tome (sep'to·tome) *n.* [*septo-* + *-tome*]. An instrument for cutting the nasal septum.

sep·tot·o·my (sep·tot'uh·mee) *n.* [*septo-* + *-tomy*]. The operation of cutting the nasal septum. Compare *septostomy.*

septula. Plural of *septulum.*
septula of the pia mater. Thin septal processes from the pia mater which enter the substance of the white matter of the spinal cord.
septula tes·tis (tes'tis) [NA]. The interlobular septa of the testis.
sep·tu·lum (sep'tew·lum) *n.*, pl. **septu·la** (·luh) [NL.]. A small septum.
sep·tum (sep'tum) *n.*, genit. **sep·ti** (·tye), L. pl. **sep·ta** (·tuh) [L.]. A partition; a dividing wall between two spaces or cavities.
septum atri·o·rum (ay·tree·o'rum) [BNA]. Septum interatriale (= INTERATRIAL SEPTUM).
septum atrio·ven·tri·cu·la·re (ay″tree·o·ven·trick·yoo·lair'ee) [NA]. The portion of the interventricular septum which lies between the left ventricle and the right atrium.
septum bul·bae ure·thrae (bul'bee yoo·ree'three) [BNA]. BULBOURETHRAL SEPTUM.
septum ca·na·lis mus·cu·lo·tu·ba·rii (ka·nay'lis mus″kew·lo·tew·bair'ee·eye) [NA]. SEPTUM OF THE MUSCULOTUBERAL CANAL.
septum car·ti·la·gi·ne·um na·si (kahr·ti·la·jin'ee·um nay'zye) [BNA]. Cartilago septi nasi (= CARTILAGINOUS SEPTUM OF THE NOSE).
septum cer·vi·ca·le in·ter·me·di·um (sur·vi·kay'lee in·tur·mee'dee·um) [NA]. INTERMEDIATE CERVICAL SEPTUM.
septum cor·po·rum ca·ver·no·so·rum (kor'po·rum kav·ur·no·so'rum). SEPTUM PENIS.
septum cor·po·rum ca·ver·no·so·rum cli·to·ri·dis (kor'po·rum kav·ur·no·so'rum kli·tor'i·dis) [NA]. The incomplete septum of the fibrous tissue between the two lateral halves of the clitoris.
septum cru·ra·le (kroo·ray'lee). FEMORAL SEPTUM.
septum fe·mo·ra·le (fem·o·ray'lee) [NA]. FEMORAL SEPTUM.
septum femorale [Clo·que·ti] (klo·ket'eye) [BNA]. Septum femorale (= FEMORAL SEPTUM).
septum glan·dis pe·nis (glan'dis pee'nis) [NA]. A fibrous wall in the midline of the glans of the penis situated below the urethra.
septum in·ter·atri·a·le (in·tur·ay·tree·ay'lee) [NA]. INTERATRIAL SEPTUM.
septum in·ter·mus·cu·la·re an·te·ri·us cru·ris (in″tur·mus·kew·lair'ee an·teer'ee·us kroo'ris) [NA]. The anterior intermuscular septum of the leg.
septum intermusculare anterius fi·bu·la·re (fib·yoo·lair'ee) [BNA]. SEPTUM INTERMUSCULARE ANTERIUS CRURIS.
septum intermusculare bra·chii la·te·ra·le (bray'kee·eye lat·e·ray'lee) [NA]. The lateral intermuscular septum of the arm.
septum intermusculare brachii me·di·a·le (mee·dee·ay'lee) [NA]. The medial intermuscular septum of the arm.
septum intermusculare fe·mo·ris la·te·ra·le (fem'o·ris lat·e·ray'lee) [NA]. The lateral intermuscular septum of the thigh.
septum intermusculare femoris me·di·a·le (mee·dee·ay'lee) [NA]. The medial intermuscular septum of the thigh.
septum intermusculare hu·me·ri la·te·ra·le (hew'me·rye lat·e·ray'lee) [BNA]. SEPTUM INTERMUSCULARE BRACHII LATERALE.
septum intermusculare humeri me·di·a·le (mee·dee·ay'lee) [BNA]. SEPTUM INTERMUSCULARE BRACHII MEDIALE.
septum intermusculare pos·te·ri·us cru·ris (pos·teer'ee·us kroo'ris) [NA]. The posterior intermuscular septum of the leg.
septum intermusculare posterius fi·bu·la·re (fib·yoo·lair'ee) [BNA]. SEPTUM INTERMUSCULARE POSTERIUS CRURIS.
septum in·ter·ven·tri·cu·la·re (in″tur·ven·trick·yoo·lair'ee) [NA]. INTERVENTRICULAR SEPTUM.
septum interventriculare pri·mum (prye'mum). BULBOVENTRICULAR CREST.
septum lin·guae (ling'gwee) [NA]. LINGUAL SEPTUM.
septum lu·ci·dum (lew'si·dum). SEPTUM PELLUCIDUM.
septum mem·bra·na·ce·um na·si (mem·bra·nay'see·um nay'zye) [BNA]. PARS MEMBRANACEA SEPTI NASI.
septum membranaceum ven·tri·cu·lo·rum (ven·trick·yoo·lo'rum) [BNA]. PARS MEMBRANACEA SEPTI INTERVENTRICULARIS CORDIS.
septum mo·bi·le na·si (mo'bi·lee nay'zye) [BNA]. PARS MOBILIS SEPTI NASI.
septum mus·cu·la·re ven·tri·cu·lo·rum (mus·kew·lair'ee ven·trick·yoo·lo'rum) [BNA]. PARS MUSCULARIS SEPTI INTERVENTRICULARIS CORDIS.
septum na·si (nay'zye) [NA]. NASAL SEPTUM.
septum nasi os·se·um (os'ee·um) [NA]. The portion of the nasal septum which is composed of bone.
septum of the musculotuberal canal. A plate of the temporal bone which separates the groove for the auditory tube from the groove for the tensor tympani muscle. NA *septum canalis musculotubarii.*
septum or·bi·ta·le (or·bi·tay'lee) [NA]. ORBITAL SEPTUM.
septum pel·lu·ci·dum (pe·lew'si·dum) [NA]. A thin translucent septum forming the internal boundary of the lateral ventricles of the brain and enclosing between its two laminas the so-called fifth ventricle. See also Plate 18.
septum pe·nis (pee'nis) [NA]. A fibrous septum between the two corpora cavernosa of the shaft of the penis.
septum pri·mum (prye'mum). The first incomplete interatrial septum of the embryo.
septum rec·to·va·gi·na·le (reck″to·vaj·i·nay'lee) [NA]. RECTOVAGINAL SEPTUM.
septum rec·to·ve·si·ca·le (reck″to·ves·i·kay'lee) [NA]. The tissue forming a partition between the rectum and the prostate and seminal vesicles and the urinary bladder.
septum scro·ti (skro'tye) [NA]. The fibrous partition which separates incompletely the scrotal sac into lateral halves.
septum se·cun·dum (se·kun'dum). The second incomplete interatrial septum of the embryo containing the foramen ovale; it develops to the right of the septum primum and fuses with it to form the adult interatrial septum.
septum si·nu·um fron·ta·li·um (sigh'new·um fron·tay'lee·um) [NA]. A thin sheet of bone between the right and left frontal sinuses.
septum sinuum sphe·noi·da·li·um (sfee·noy·day'lee·um) [NA]. A thin sheet of bone between the right and left sphenoidal air sinuses.
septum spu·ri·um (spew'ree·um). A fold on the anterodorsal wall of the embryonic right atrium, formed by the fusion of the ends of the right and left valves of the sinus venosus.
septum trans·ver·sum (trans·vur'sum). TRANSVERSE SEPTUM.
septum ven·tri·cu·lo·rum (ven·trick″yoo·lo'rum) [BNA]. Septum interventriculare (= INTERVENTRICULAR SEPTUM).
sep·tu·plet (sep'tuh·plit, sep·tup'lit) *n.* [L. *septuplum,* group of seven]. One of seven offspring born from a single gestation.
sep·tu·plex placenta (sep'tuh·plecks). MULTIPARTITE PLACENTA.
sep·ul·ture (sep'ul·chur) *n.* [L. *sepultura*]. The disposal of the dead by burial; burial.
se·que·la (se·kwel'uh) *n.*, pl. **seque·lae** (·lee) [L., sequel, from *sequi,* to follow]. 1. An abnormal condition following a disease upon which it is directly or indirectly dependent. 2. A complication of a disease.
se·quence (see'kwence) *n.* [L. *sequentia,* from *sequi,* to follow]. 1. The order of occurrence, as of symptoms. 2. SEQUELA. —**se·quen·tial** (se·kwen'shul) *adj.*
se·ques·ter (se·kwes'tur) *v.* [L. *sequestrare,* from *sequester,* depository]. 1. To separate or to become separated or detached abnormally. 2. To isolate a patient or group of patients. 3. To remove or isolate a constituent of a chemical system, as by binding or chelating. —**sequester·ing,** *adj.*
sequestering agent. Any substance which will inactivate a metallic ion in solution, as by formation of a complex compound, and keep the resulting compound in solution.
sequestra. Plural of *sequestrum.*

se·ques·tra·tion (see″kwes·tray′shun) *n.* [L. *sequestratio,* from *sequestrare,* to give up for safekeeping]. 1. The separation of tissue and formation of a sequestrum. 2. The isolation of persons suffering from disease for purposes of treatment or for the protection of others. 3. The pooling of blood in vascular channels, either physiologically, or therapeutically by means of tourniquets.

se·ques·trec·to·my (see″kwes·treck′tuh·mee) *n.* [*sequestrum* + *-ectomy*]. The operative removal of a sequestrum.

Sequestrene. A trademark for ethylenediaminetetraacetic acid and various of its salts.

se·ques·trot·o·my (see″kwes·trot′uh·mee) *n.* [*sequestrum* + *-tomy*]. An operation to expose a sequestrum.

se·ques·trum (se·kwes′trum) *n.,* pl. **seques·tra** (·truh) [L., deposit]. A detached or dead piece of bone within a cavity, abscess, or wound. —**seques·tral** (·trul) *adj.*

sequestrum forceps. Forceps designed for removing spicules or sequestra of bone.

se·quoi·o·sis (see″kwoy·o′sis) *n.* [*Sequoia,* genus of the California redwood, + *-osis*]. A granulomatous pneumonitis associated with inhalation of redwood sawdust containing fungal particles.

SER Abbreviation for *smooth-surfaced endoplasmic reticulum.*

ser-, seri-, sero-. A combining form meaning *serum, serous.*

sera. Plural of *serum.*

ser·ac·tide acetate (se·rack′tide). A polypeptide of 39 amino acids solvated with acetic acid and water, $C_{207}H_{308}N_{56}O_{58}S \cdot (C_2H_4O_2)_x \cdot xH_2O$, an adrenocorticotropic hormone.

ser·al·bu·min (seer″al·bew′min, serr″) *n.* SERUM ALBUMIN; the albumin fraction of serum.

Serax. Trademark for oxazepam, a tranquilizing drug.

Serc. Trademark for betahistine hydrochloride (dihydrochloride), a drug that has been used to reduce frequency of vertiginous episodes in Ménière's syndrome.

se·rem·pi·on (se·rem′pee·on) *n.* [Sp. *sarampión*]. A form of severe measles occurring especially among children in the West Indies.

Serenium. Trademark for ethoxazene, used as the hydrochloride salt for relief of pain in chronic infections of the urinary tract.

ser·e·noa (serr″e·no′uh, se·ree′no·uh) *n.* [*Sereno* Watson, U.S. botanist, 19th century]. The partially dried ripe fruit of *Serenoa repens,* which contains an oil that is supposed to have a stimulating action on the mucous membranes of the genitourinary tract and for which effect the drug was used in the treatment of chronic and subacute cystitis. Syn. *saw palmetto berries, sabal.*

Serentil. Trademark for mesoridazine, a tranquilizer.

Ser·gent's sign or **line** (sehr·zhahⁿ′) [G. *Sergent,* French physician, 1869–1943]. A white line of the skin of the chest or abdomen appearing shortly after being lightly scratched; seen in hypoadrenal states.

seri-. See *ser-.*

se·ri·al (seer′ee·ul) *adj.* 1. Pertaining to, arranged in, or forming a series. 2. Successive.

serial caudal analgesia. CONTINUOUS CAUDAL ANESTHESIA.

serial caudal anesthesia. CONTINUOUS CAUDAL ANESTHESIA.

serial extractions. Extraction of certain primary or secondary teeth at selected times as partial treatment for malocclusion.

serial sections. A series of histologic preparations made from a single block of tissue, each succeeding section being immediately adjacent to its predecessor. Contr. *step sections.*

ser·i·ceps (serr′i·seps) *n.* [L. *sericum,* silk, + *-ceps* as in forceps]. A device made of loops of ribbon for making traction upon the fetal head.

se·ries (seer′eez) *n.,* pl. **series** [L.]. 1. A succession or a group of compounds, objects, or numbers, arranged systematically according to a rule. 2. *In taxonomy,* the sample of a population which forms the basic working unit in modern systematics. 3. *In hematology,* the succession of cell types in the development of a cell of the circulating blood. See also *monocytic series, thrombocytic series, erythrocytic series, lymphocytic series, granulocytic series.*

ser·i·flux (seer′i·flux, serr′) *n.* [*seri-* + *flux*]. Any serous or watery discharge, or a disease characterized by such a discharge.

ser·ine (seer′een, serr′) *n.* [L. *sericum,* silk, + *-ine*]. β-Hydroxyalanine or 2-amino-3-hydroxypropanoic acid, $HOCH_2CH(NH_2)COOH$, an amino acid component of many proteins.

ser·met·a·cin (sur·met′uh·sin) *n.* *N*-[[1-*p*-Chlorobenzoyl)-5-methoxy-2-methylindol-3-yl]acetyl]-L-serine, $C_{22}H_{21}ClN_2O_6$, an anti-inflammatory.

Sermion. A trademark for nicergoline, a vasodilator.

Sernylan. Trademark for phencyclidine, a veterinary central nervous system depressant used as the hydrochloride salt.

sero-. See *ser-.*

se·ro·al·bu·min·ous (seer″o·al·bew′mi·nus, serr″o·) *adj.* 1. Pertaining to or containing serum and albumin. 2. Containing serum albumin.

Serobacterin. Trademark for emulsions of killed bacteria which have been sensitized by treatment with a specific immune serum and which more rapidly produce immunity.

se·ro·che (se·ro′cheh) *n.* [Sp.]. ALTITUDE SICKNESS.

se·ro·chrome (seer′o·krome) *n.* [*sero-* + *-chrome*]. Gilbert's name for the pigments which serve to give color to normal serum.

se·ro·co·li·tis (seer″o·ko·lye′tis) *n.* [*sero-* + *colitis*]. Inflammation of the serosa of the colon.

se·ro·cul·ture (see′ro·kul″chur) *n.* A bacterial culture on blood serum.

se·ro·cys·tic sarcoma (seer″o·sis′tick). CYSTOSARCOMA PHYLLODES.

se·ro·der·ma·ti·tis (seer″o·dur″muh·tye′tis) *n.* [*sero-* + *dermatitis*]. SERODERMATOSIS.

se·ro·der·ma·to·sis (seer″o·dur″muh·to′sis) *n.* [*sero-* + *dermatosis*]. A skin disease characterized by serous effusion into or onto the skin.

se·ro·der·mi·tis (seer″o·dur·migh′tis) *n.* [*sero-* + *dermitis*]. SERODERMATOSIS.

se·ro·di·ag·no·sis (seer″o·dye″ug·no′sis) *n.* Diagnosis based upon the reactions of blood serum of patients. —**serodiag·nos·tic** (·nos′tick) *adj.*

se·ro·en·ter·i·tis (seer″o·en″tur·eye′tis) *n.* [*sero-* + *enteritis*]. Inflammation of the serosa of the small intestine.

se·ro·fi·brin·ous (seer″o·fye′bri·nus) *adj.* [*sero-* + *fibrinous*]. 1. Composed of serum and fibrin, as a serofibrinous exudate. 2. Characterized by the production of a serofibrinous exudate, as a serofibrinous inflammation.

se·ro·group (seer′o·groop) *n.* An arrangement of serotypes with common antigens.

se·ro·lem·ma (seer″o·lem′uh) *n.* [*sero-* + *-lemma*]. Serosa or false amnion, especially in *Sauropsida.* See also *chorion.*

se·ro·li·pase (seer″o·lye′pace, ·lip′ace) *n.* Lipase as found in blood serum.

serologic test. 1. Any test on serum for the diagnosis of a specified condition. 2. Any test on serum for the diagnosis of syphilis.

se·rol·o·gist (se·rol′uh·jist) *n.* A person versed in serology.

se·rol·o·gy (se·rol′uh·jee) *n.* [*sero-* + *-logy*]. 1. The branch of science that deals with the properties, especially immunologic actions, and reactions of serums. 2. *Informal.* SEROLOGIC TEST. —**se·ro·log·ic** (seer″uh·loj′ick), **serolog·i·cal** (·i·kul) *adj.*

se·rol·y·sin (se·rol′i·sin) *n.* [*sero-* + *-lysin*]. A bactericidal substance contained in normal blood serum.

se·ro·ma (se·ro′muh) *n.* [*ser-* + *-oma*]. An accumulation of blood serum which produces a tumorlike swelling, usually beneath the skin.

se·ro·mem·bra·nous (seer″o·mem′bruh·nus) *adj.* Pertaining to a serous membrane.

se·ro·mu·ci·nous gland (seer″o·mew′si·nus). MIXED GLAND.

se·ro·mu·cous (seer″o·mew′kus) *adj.* [*sero-* + *mucous*]. Having the nature of or containing both serum and mucus, as a glandular cell which has the characteristics of both a serous cell and a mucous cell.

se·ro·mus·cu·lar (seer″o·mus′kew·lur) *adj.* Of or pertaining to the serous and muscular layers of the digestive tract.

Seromycin. Trademark for cycloserine, an antibiotic compound.

se·ro·neg·a·tive (seer″o·neg′uh·tiv) *adj.* 1. Having a negative serologic test for some condition. 2. Specifically, having a negative serologic test for syphilis.

se·ro·peri·to·ne·um (seer″o·perr″i·to·nee′um) *n.* [*sero-* + *peritoneum*]. 1. A membrane which encloses the abdominal viscera. 2. ASCITES.

se·ro·pos·i·tive (seer″o·poz′i·tiv) *adj.* 1. Having a positive serologic test for some condition. 2. Specifically, having a positive serologic test for syphilis.

se·ro·prog·no·sis (seer″o·prog·no′sis) *n.* Prognosis of disease as determined by seroreactions.

se·ro·pu·ru·lent (seer″o·pewr′yoo·lunt) *adj.* [*sero-* + *purulent*]. Composed of serum and pus, as a seropurulent exudate.

se·ro·pus (seer′o·pus″) *n.* [*sero-* + *pus*]. An exudate which has mixed characteristics of serous and purulent nature.

se·ro·re·ac·tion (seer″o·ree·ack′shun) *n.* A reaction performed with serum.

se·ro·re·sis·tance (seer″o·re·zis′tunce) *n.* [*sero-* + *resistance*]. Persistent positive serologic reaction for syphilis despite prolonged intensive treatment. —**seroresis·tant** (·tunt) *adj.*

se·ro·sa (se·ro′suh, ·zuh) *n.*, pl. **serosas, sero·sae** (·see) [short for *tunica serosa*]. 1. A serous membrane composed of mesothelium and subjacent connective tissue, lining the pericardial, pleural, and peritoneal cavities and the cavity of the tunica vaginalis testis and covering their contents. NA *tunica serosa.* 2. The chorion of birds and reptiles. —**sero·sal** (·sul, ·zul) *adj.*

se·ro·sa·mu·cin (se·ro″suh·mew′sin) *n.* [*serosa* + *mucin*]. A protein resembling mucin found in ascitic fluid.

se·ro·san·guin·e·ous (seer″o·sang·gwin′ee·us) *adj.* [*sero-* + *sanguineous*]. Having the nature of, or containing, both serum and blood.

se·ro·se·rous (seer″o·seer′us) *adj.* Of or pertaining jointly to two serous surfaces.

se·ro·si·tis (seer″o·sigh′tis) *n.* [*serosa* + *-itis*]. Inflammation of a serous membrane.

se·ro·syn·o·vi·tis (seer″o·sin″o·vye′tis, ·sigh″no·) *n.* [*sero-* + *synovitis*]. A synovitis with increase of synovial fluid.

se·ro·ther·a·py (seer″o·therr′uh·pee) *n.* [*sero-* + *therapy*]. The treatment of disease by means of human or animal serum containing antibodies.

se·ro·to·nin (seer″o·to′nin, serr″) *n.* [*sero-* + *tonic-* + *-in*]. 5-Hydroxytryptamine, $C_{10}H_{12}N_2O$, present in many tissues, especially blood and nervous tissue; stimulates a variety of smooth muscles and nerves, and is postulated to function as a neurotransmitter.

se·ro·tox·in (seer″o·tock·sin) *n.* [*sero-* + *toxin*]. ANAPHYLATOXIN.

se·ro·type (seer′o·tipe, serr′o·) *n.* A serological type; a type distinguishable on the basis of antigenic composition, used in the subclassification of certain microorganisms, as *Salmonella, Shigella.*

se·rous (seer′us, serr′us) *adj.* 1. Pertaining to, characterized by, or resembling serum. 2. Containing serum. 3. Producing a thin, watery secretion, as a serous gland; may be serozymogenic (pancreas) or not (lacrimal glands).

serous angina. 1. Edema of the glottis. 2. ACUTE PHARYNGITIS.

serous atrophy. Loss of lipid from adipose tissue cells accompanied by collection of serous fluid between the shrunken cells, seen in inanition.

serous cavity. A potential space between two layers of serous membrane, as the pericardial, peritoneal, or pleural cavity or that of the tunica vaginalis testis.

serous circumscribed meningitis. CHRONIC ADHESIVE ARACHNOIDITIS.

serous crescent. DEMILUNE.

serous cystadenocarcinoma. An ovarian tumor, the malignant variant of the serous cystadenoma. Syn. *carcinomatous serous cystoma, papillary serous carcinoma.*

serous cystadenoma. A benign cystic ovarian tumor composed of cylindrical cells resembling those of the uterine tube; the cysts contain clear, watery fluid, and there are often calcific (psammoma) bodies in the wall. Syn. *papillary cystadenoma of ovary, serous cystoma, papillocystoma, psammomatous papilloma.*

serous cystoma. SEROUS CYSTADENOMA.

serous exudate. An exudate composed principally of serum.

serous fat cell. An atrophic fat cell found in serous atrophy of adipose tissue.

serous fluid. 1. Normal lymphatic fluid. 2. Any thin, watery fluid.

serous gland. A gland that secretes a watery, albuminous fluid. NA *glandula serosa.*

serous infiltration. An excess of fluid in tissue spaces, a part of serous inflammation or of edema.

serous inflammation. Inflammation in which the exudate is composed largely of serum.

serous labyrinthitis. Labyrinthitis caused by bacterial infection, toxins, or trauma, marked by increased perilymphatic pressure without suppuration.

serous lingual glands. Serous glands opening into the trenches of the vallate papillae of the tongue. Syn. *Ebner's glands.*

serous membrane. A delicate membrane covered with flat, mesothelial cells lining closed cavities of the body. NA *tunica serosa.*

serous meningitis. PSEUDOTUMOR CEREBRI.

serous otitis media. A common nonpyogenic and often chronic disorder of the middle ear, affecting chiefly children, in which there is an exudate high in protein and in inflammatory cells; may be due to viral infection, allergy, or other factors, and may result in conductive deafness. Syn. *catarrhal otitis media, chronic exudative otitis media, glue ear, secretory otitis media.*

serous pericardium. The thin, smooth lining of the pericardial cavity; its surface is lined with mesothelium. There is a visceral and a parietal portion. NA *pericardium serosum.*

se·ro·zy·mo·gen·ic cell (seer″o·zye″mo·jen′ick). The type of serous cell resembling pancreatic acinous cells and gastric chief cells, found in the parotid gland of most mammals and the submandibular and sublingual glands of man.

Serpasil. Trademark for reserpine, an antihypertensive and sedative alkaloid.

ser·pens (sur′penz) *adj.* [L., serpent]. Serpentine, sinuous; creeping.

ser·pen·tar·ia (sur″pen·tăr′ee·uh) *n.* The dried rhizome and roots of *Aristolochia serpentaria,* Virginia snakeroot, or of *A. reticulata,* Texas snakeroot; has been used as an aromatic bitter and gastric stimulant.

ser·pig·i·nous (sur·pij′i·nus) *adj.* [ML. *serpigo, serpiginis,* a creeping skin lesion, from L. *serpere,* to creep]. Progressing from one surface or part to a contiguous one; applied to skin lesions.

serpiginous angioma. ANGIOMA SERPIGINOSUM.

serpiginous bubo. An ulcerated bubo which changes its seat or in which the ulceration extends in one direction while healing in another.

serpiginous erysipelas. Erysipelas in which the margin between reddened skin and normal skin is wavy, with advancement of involvement along that serpentine line.

serpiginous keratitis. KERATITIS HYPOPYON.

serpiginous ulcer. An ulcer which slowly extends in one area while healing in another. Syn. *creeping ulcer.*

ser·ra (serr'uh) *n.* [L.]. *In biology,* a saw or sawlike structure, as the saw of a sawfish.

ser·rate (serr'ate) *adj.* [L. *serratus,* from *serra,* saw]. SERRATED.

ser·rat·ed (serr'ay·tid) *adj.* Having a toothed margin; having a sawlike edge.

Ser·ra·tia (se·ray'shee·uh) *n.* [S. *Serrati,* Italian entrepreneur, 19th century]. A genus of bacilli commonly found in water, belonging to the family Enterobacteriaceae; about 25 percent of strains are pigmented.

Serratia mar·ces·cens (mahr·ses'enz). A motile, gram-negative organism that occasionally produces a deep red pigment. Found in water, soil, milk, and stools. Long considered a harmless saprophyte, it has recently been incriminated in septicemias, pulmonary disease, hospital epidemics, and even death. Syn. *Bacillus prodigiosus.*

ser·ra·tion (se·ray'shun) *n.* The state or condition of being toothed or having a toothed margin.

ser·ra·tus (se·ray'tus) *L. adj. & n.* [L.]. 1. SERRATED. 2. A muscle arising or inserted by a series of processes like the teeth of a saw. See also Table of Muscles in the Appendix.

serratus mag·nus (mag'nus). The serratus anterior muscle. See Table of Muscles in the Appendix.

Serres' angle (serr) [A. *Serres,* French anatomist, 1786–1868]. METAFACIAL ANGLE.

Sertoli-cell-only syndrome. DEL CASTILLO'S SYNDROME.

Ser·to·li cells (serr'to·lee) [E. *Sertoli,* Italian histologist, 1842–1910]. The sustentacular cells of seminiferous tubules.

Sertoli cell tumor. A well-differentiated form of androblastoma; a common testicular tumor of dogs.

se·rum (seer'um, serr'um) *n.*, pl. **se·ra** (·uh) [L., whey, serum]. 1. The cell and fibrinogen-free amber-colored fluid appearing after blood or plasma clots. 2. IMMUNE SERUM. 3. The clear portion of any biologic fluid. See also Table of Chemical Constituents of Blood in the Appendix.

serum accelerator factor. FACTOR VII. ABBREVIATED, SAF.

serum accelerator globulin. FACTOR V.

serum accident. SERUM SHOCK.

se·rum·al (seer'um·ul, serr') *adj.* Of or pertaining to serum.

serum albumin. The chief protein of blood serum and of serous fluids. See also Table of Chemical Constituents of Blood in the Appendix.

serumal calculus. A dental calculus formerly believed to be a calcareous deposit formed about the teeth by exudation from the gingiva. Syn. *sanguinary calculus.*

serum globulin. The globulin fraction of blood serum; the fraction of serum protein precipitated by half-saturation with ammonium sulfate in contrast to the albumin fraction which is soluble in this salt concentration.

serum gonadotropin. The water-soluble gonad-stimulating substance, by some believed to originate in chorionic tissue, obtained from the serum of pregnant mares.

serum hepatitis. A form of viral hepatitis usually transmitted by the parenteral injection of human blood or blood products contaminated with the hepatitus B virus. Compare *infectious hepatitis.*

serum-hepatitis antigen. HEPATITIS-ASSOCIATED ANTIGEN.

se·rum·nal (se·rum'nul) *adj.* SERUMAL.

serum neuritis. A form of neuritis or neuropathy that follows the administration of heterologous serum. Pain and weakness in the distribution of the brachial plexus are the usual manifestations, but in some cases the neuritis is symmetrical and ascending in type, as in Guillain-Barré disease.

serum protection test. A test in which each animal of a group is given a known immune serum. This is followed by inoculation of these and an equal number of control animals with an organism, the identity of which it is desired to establish. If the animals receiving the immune serum survive, this identifies the organism. The test may also be used to determine the virulence of organisms and the specific activity of products such as toxins and to demonstrate specific antibodies in serum. See also *animal protection tests.*

serum proteins. The proteins present in the serum from clotted blood, differing from plasma proteins only in the absence of fibrinogen. See also Table of Chemical Constituents of Blood in the Appendix.

serum prothrombin conversion accelerator. FACTOR VII. Abbreviated, SPCA.

serum rash. A dermatosis coincident with serum sickness.

serum shock. Anaphylactic shock resulting from the injection of a serum into a sensitive individual. Compare *serum sickness.*

serum sickness. A syndrome originally observed as a sequel of the administration of foreign serum therapeutically, generally resulting in the occurrence in 8 to 12 days of an urticarial rash, edema, enlargement of lymph nodes, arthralgia, fever, and neuritis in some cases. Immunologically, it is related to the formation of circulating antigen-antibody complexes at moderate antigen excess, and possibly to reaginic antibodies. Similar phenomena are noted with purified protein antigens and with chemicals.

serum urticaria. Urticaria following the injection of a foreign serum.

ser·vo·mech·a·nism (sur"vo·meck'uh·niz·um) *n.* [L. *servus,* slave, servant, + *mechanism*]. A means or device for adjusting and controlling the performance of a given system to a desired standard or level through a feedback mechanism.

ser·yl (seer'il, serr'il) *n.* The univalent radical, $HOCH_2CH(NH_2)CO—$, of the amino acid serine.

ses·a·me (ses'uh·mee) *n.* [Gk. *sēsamē*]. An herb, *Sesamum indicum,* the seeds of which yield sesame oil, a fixed oil used as a vehicle for intramuscular injections.

ses·a·moid (ses'uh·moid) *adj.* [Gk. *sēsamoeidēs,* from *sēsamē,* sesame]. Resembling a sesame seed.

sesamoid bones. Small bones developed in tendons subjected to much pressure. NA *ossa sesamoidea.* See also Table of Bones in the Appendix.

sesamoid cartilage. One of a pair of small cartilages lying in the aryepiglottic folds; they are constant in some animals and are occasionally found in man. NA *cartilago sesamoidea.*

ses·a·moid·itis (ses"uh·moy·dye'tis) *n.* [*sesamoid* + *-itis*]. Inflammation of the sesamoid bones which may involve the articular surfaces and cause lameness.

Se·sar·ma (se·sahr'muh) *n.* A genus of freshwater crabs found in Asia. *Sesarma dehaani* and *S. sinensis* are intermediate hosts of the lung fluke, *Paragonimus westermani.*

sesqui- [L., more by a half]. A combining form indicating *one and one-half, the proportion of two* (of one radical or element) *to three* (of another).

ses·qui·chlo·ride (ses"kwi·klo'ride) *n.* [*sesqui-* + *chloride*]. A compound of chlorine and another element containing three atoms of chlorine to two of the other element, as Fe_2Cl_3.

ses·qui·ho·ra (ses"kwi·ho'ruh) *n.* [L., from *sesqui-* + *hora*]. An hour and a half.

ses·qui·ox·ide (ses"kwee·ock'side) *n.* [*sesqui-* + *oxide*]. A compound of three atoms of oxygen to two of another element, as Al_2O_3.

ses·qui·salt (ses'kwi·sawlt) *n.* [*sesqui-* + *salt*]. A salt containing one and one-half times as much of the acid as of the radical or base, as $Fe_2(SO_4)_3$.

ses·qui·sul·fide, ses·qui·sul·phide (ses"kwi·sul'fide) *n.* [*sesqui-* + *sulfide*]. A compound of sulfur and another element containing three atoms of sulfur to two of the other element, as Sb_2S_3.

ses·qui·ter·pene (ses"kwi·tur'peen) *n.* [*sesqui-* + *terpene*]. Any of a group of terpenes of the general formula $C_{15}H_{24}$.

ses·sile (ses'il, ·ile) *adj.* [L. *sessilis,* from *sedere,* to sit]. 1. Attached by a broad base; not pedunculated, as a sessile tumor. 2. Attached, not free moving, as certain invertebrate animals.

set, *v.* 1. To reduce the displacement in a fracture and apply supporting structures suitably arranged for fixation. 2. To harden or solidify, as a cement, amalgam, or plaster. —**set·ting,** *n. & adj.*

se·ta (see'tuh) *n.*, pl. **se·tae** (·tee) [L., bristle]. A stiff, stout, bristlelike appendage; VIBRISSA.

se·ta·ceous (se·tay'shus) *adj.* [L. *seta*, bristle, + *-aceous*]. 1. Having or consisting of bristles or setae. 2. Resembling a bristle.

Se·tar·ia (se·tăr'ee·uh) *n.* 1. A genus of grasses including millet, *Setaria italica.* 2. A genus of filarial nematodes.

se·ton (see'tun) *n.* [ML. *seto, setonis,* from L. *seta,* bristle]. A thread or bundle of threads, passed through an opening in the skin, once used to provide drainage, produce a fistulous tract, or encourage "healing inflammation."

set·ting-sun phenomenon or **sign.** Forced downward deviation of the eyes at rest, exposing the sclera above the partially covered iris, with some paresis of upward gaze; frequently seen with increased intracranial pressure, especially that due to hydrocephalus, in newborns and infants, but seen occasionally for brief periods in normal infants. The mechanism is unknown.

setting-up exercise. Exercise or calisthenics designed for routine use by normal persons to strengthen muscles or promote health.

sev·en-day fever. DENGUE.

sev·enth (VIIth) cranial nerve. FACIAL NERVE.

seventh sense. Visceral sense; the faculty of receiving visceral sensation.

seven-year itch. SCABIES.

severe combined immunodeficiency. Congenital severe deficiency of lymphocytes and absence of plasma cells with marked hypogammaglobulinemia, deficient cellular and humoral responses to all antigens, and early death; inherited as an X-linked or autosomal recessive trait, or may occur sporadically. Abbreviated, SCID. Syn. *alymphocytosis, Glanzmann and Riniker's lymphocytophthisis.*

se·vere mental retardation. Subnormal general intellectual functioning, usually requiring complete protective or custodial care, in which the intelligence quotient is generally about 20 to 39. The person may be able to learn to dress and feed himself and to use the toilet.

Sever's disease [J. W. *Sever,* U.S. orthopedist, b. 1878]. CALCANEUS APOPHYSITIS.

se·vip·a·rous (se·vip'uh·rus) *adj.* [L. *sev*um, tallow, + *-parous*]. SEBIPAROUS; fat-producing.

se·vo·flu·rane (see"vo·floo'rane) *n.* Fluoromethyl 2,2,2-trifluoro-1-(trifluoromethyl)ethyl ether, $C_4H_3F_7O$, an inhalation anesthetic.

se·vum (see'vum) *n.* [L.]. SUET.

sew·age (sue'ij) *n.* [*sewer* + *-age*]. The heterogeneous substances constituting the excreta and waste matter of domestic economy and the contents of sewers.

sew·er (sue'ur) *n.* [OF. *esseouer,* drain, ditch, from L. *ex-* + *aqua,* water, + *-aria*]. A canal for the removal of sewage.

sew·er·age (sue'ur·ij) *n.* 1. The collection and removal of sewage. 2. The system of pipes and sewers for the removal of sewage.

sew·ing spasm (so'ing). An occupation spasm affecting the motions used in sewing.

sex-, sexi- [L. *sex*]. A combining form meaning *six.*

sex, *n.* [L. *sexus, secus* (possibly rel. to *secare,* to divide)]. 1. Either of the two categories, female and male, into which organisms of many species are divided and by the union of whose gametes (ova and spermatozoa) they reproduce. 2. SEXUALITY. 3. *Colloq.* Sexual intercourse; COITUS.

sex chromatin. A condensation of chromatin found in nuclei of cells having more than one X chromosome. It represents the inactive X chromosome and is always equal to the total number of X chromosomes minus one. Syn. *Barr body.*

sex chromosome. A chromosome having a special relation to determining whether a fertilized egg develops into a male or a female; the X chromosome and the Y chromosome. When other conditions are normal, in mammals a fertilized egg with two X's becomes a female; one with the XY combination becomes a male.

sex cords. The cordlike epithelial masses that invaginate from the germinal epithelium of the gonad and form the seminiferous tubules and rete testis, or the primary follicles of the ovary and the rete ovarii.

sex determination. The process which determines the sex of an individual. See also *sex chromosome.*

sex factor. FERTILITY FACTOR.

sex hormone. Any gonadal hormone, whether estrogenic or androgenic, secreted chiefly by the ovaries and the testes but found also in other tissues.

sexi-. See *sex-.*

sexi·dig·i·tal (seck"si·dij'i·tul) *adj.* [*sexi-* + *digital*]. Having six fingers or six toes.

sexi·dig·i·tate (seck"si·dij'i·tate) *adj.* SEXIDIGITAL.

sex infantilism. Continuation of childish sex traits and development beyond puberty.

sex-limited, *adj.* Appearing in, or affecting, one sex only.

sex linkage. The case of linkage in which a gene is located on a sex chromosome. In mammals there are two forms, X-linkage and Y-linkage.

sex-linked, *adj.* Applied to genes located on the X chromosome, and to the characteristics, which may occur in either sex, conditioned by such genes.

sexo·es·thet·ic inversion (seck"so·es·thet'ick). A variety of sexual deviation in which the individual has the feelings and tastes of, and assumes the habits, manners, and costume of the opposite sex. See also *eonism, homosexuality, transvestism.*

sex·ol·o·gy (seck·sol'uh·jee) *n.* [*sex* + *-logy*]. The science or study of sex and sex relations. —**sexo·log·ic** (seck"so·loj'ick) *adj.*

sex organs. The organs pertaining entirely to the sex of the individual; in the male, the external generative organs: penis and testes, and the internal: prostate, deferential ducts, and seminal vesicles; in the female, the external generative organs: vulva, vagina, and clitoris, and the internal: the uterus, uterine tubes, and ovaries.

sex ratio. The relative number of males and females in the population, usually stated as the number of males per 100 females.

sex reflex. GENITAL REFLEX.

sex reversal. Genetic, developmental, or therapeutic conversion of phenotypic sex.

sex surrogate. An extramarital sexual partner used in sexual reconditioning to overcome marital problems or psychogenic sexual dysfunction.

sex·ti·grav·i·da (secks"ti·grav'i·duh) *n.* [L. *sex*tus, sixth, + *gravida*]. A woman who is pregnant for the sixth time.

sex·tip·a·ra (secks·tip'uh·ruh) *n.* [L. *sex*tus, sixth, + *-para*]. A woman who has given birth six times.

sex·tup·let (secks·tup'lit) *n.* [L. *sex*tus, sixth, + *-plet* as in triplet]. One of the six offspring of a single gestation.

sex·u·al (seck'shoo·ul) *adj.* [L. *sexualis*]. Pertaining to or characteristic of sex.

sexual anesthesia. ANAPHRODISIA.

sexual congress. COITUS.

sexual deviant. An individual, and specifically a sociopathic personality, characterized by deviant and aberrant sexual behavior.

sexual deviation. Sexual behavior which is markedly at variance with the generally accepted forms of sexual activities and not part of any more extensive disorder such as schizophrenia or the obsessional neuroses. It includes the various forms and practices of homosexuality, transvestitism, pedophilia, fetishism, and sexual sadism (assault and rape, mutilation).

sexual fold. GENITAL RIDGE.

sexual generation. Reproduction by the union of a male and a female gamete.

sexual gland. GONAD.

sexual hallucination. A false sensory perception of sexual excitement or experience, occurring most frequently in certain types of schizophrenia and often associated with grotesque delusions in which nongenital parts of the body are sexualized.

sexual identity. The chromosomal constitution and, to some extent, the internal genitalia, which make a person biologically a male or a female. This is to be differentiated from gender identity and gender role, which are psychological attributes.

sexual instinct. The biological urge, usually modified by society, toward organ pleasure, which at puberty becomes a function of reproduction.

sexual intercourse. COITUS.

sexual inversion. 1. The condition of having or assuming some of the sex characters of the opposite sex. 2. Assuming the role of the other sex in homosexual acts. 3. HOMOSEXUALITY.

sex·u·al·i·ty (seck″shoo·al′i·tee) *n.* 1. The sum of a person's sexual attributes, behavior, and tendencies. 2. The quality of being sexual, or the degree of a person's sexual attributes, attractiveness, and drives. 3. Excessive preoccupation with sex and sexual functions and behavior. 4. *In psychoanalysis,* the physiological and psychological impulses whose satisfaction affords pleasure, experienced, consciously or unconsciously, even by the infant and young child.

sex·u·al·ize (seck′shoo·ul·ize) *v.* To attribute sex or sexual functions to something not in itself sexual.

sexual metamorphosis. SEXOESTHETIC INVERSION.

sexual passion. EROTISM (1).

sexual reflex. Erection and orgasm in response to direct or psychic stimulation of the genitalia.

sexual selection. Selection by females of certain phenotypic and behavioral features of males, postulated as an evolutionary mechanism to account for the accentuation or generalization of those features in a population.

sexual spore. A spore formed subsequent to the union of two nuclei.

sexual swelling. LABIOSCROTAL SWELLING.

Sé·za·ry cell (se^y·zah^h·ree′) [A. *Sézary,* French dermatologist, 1880–1956]. An atypical mononuclear cell, recently identified as a T lymphocyte, containing mucopolysaccharide-filled cytoplasmic vacuoles, seen in the peripheral blood in Sézary's syndrome. A peripheral arrangement of granules is also characteristic.

Sézary syndrome or **reticulocytosis** [A. *Sézary*]. Exfoliative erythroderma with a cutaneous infiltrate of atypical mononuclear cells; similar cells are also present in the peripheral blood. Bone marrow and lymph nodes are normal. It is thought to be related to mycosis fungoides.

SFW Abbreviation for *slow filling wave.*

S_3 gallop. VENTRICULAR GALLOP.

S_4 gallop. ATRIAL GALLOP.

Sgam·ba·ti's reaction or **test** (zgah^{h}m·bah′tee) [O. *Sgambati,* Italian physician, 20th century]. A test for peritonitis; a persistent red tint, resulting when nitric acid and chloroform are added to urine, is considered a positive result.

SGO Surgeon general's office.

SGOT Serum glutamic oxaloacetic transaminase.

SGPT Serum glutamic pyruvic transaminase.

SH Abbreviation and symbol for *sulfhydryl.*

shad·ow, *n.* 1. SHADOW CELL. 2. *In radiology,* the relatively dark outline seen on a developed x-ray film caused by the interposition of an opaque body and the x-ray beam.

shadow cell. 1. A hemolyzed erythrocyte consisting only of stroma. 2. A cell characteristic of pilomatricoma whose well-outlined cytoplasm stains pink with hematoxylin and eosin, but which shows a central unstained "shadow" in place of the nucleus.

shadow sound. The interference with a sound wave caused by an object being placed between the ear and the source of sound.

shadow test. RETINOSCOPY.

Shaffer method. FOLIN-SHAFFER METHOD.

shaft, *n.* The trunk of any columnar mass, especially the diaphysis of a long bone.

shag·gy chorion. CHORION FRONDOSUM.

shaggy heart. COR VILLOSUM.

sha·green patch, plaque, or **spot** (sha·green′). An area of granular, thickened, grayish-green or brown skin found characteristically in tuberous sclerosis. Syn. *sharkskin spot.*

shak·ing palsy. PARKINSON'S DISEASE.

sham feeding. A type of feeding in which the food is swallowed and then diverted to the exterior of the body via a fistula or other means.

sham rage. A state in which an animal reacts to all stimuli with an expression of intense anger and the signs of autonomic overactivity, produced experimentally by cerebral decortication.

shank, *n.* The leg from the knee to the ankle.

shark skin. DYSSEBACIA.

shark·skin spot. SHAGREEN PATCH.

sharp and slow wave complex. *In electroencephalography,* a complex consisting of a spike followed by a slow wave.

sharp dissection. *In surgery,* the exposure of structures or removal of tissues by cutting. Contr. *blunt dissection.*

Shar·pey's fibers [W. *Sharpey,* English physiologist and anatomist, 1802–1880]. PERFORATING FIBERS (1).

sharp retractor. A toothed retractor, with pointed teeth to prevent slippage during use.

sharp wave. *In electroencephalography,* a transient wave form that is clearly distinguishable from background activity. It has a pointed peak at conventional paper speeds and a duration ranging from 70 to 200 msec.

shaven-beard appearance. MELANOSIS COLI.

Sha·ver's disease [C. G. *Shaver,* 20th century]. BAUXITE FUME PNEUMOCONIOSIS.

shears, *n.pl.* A large pair of scissors.

sheath, *n.* 1. An envelope; a covering. 2. *In anatomy,* the connective tissue covering an organ or structures such as vessels, muscles, nerves, and tendons. 3. CONDOM. —**sheathed,** *adj.*

sheathed artery. The terminal segment of an arteriole in the red pulp of the spleen which is ensheathed by a nodule of phagocytic cells.

sheathed microfilaria. A microfilaria encased in a delicate membrane which usually protrudes beyond the ends of the parasite. The membrane is thought to be the remains of the eggshell. When the membrane or shell breaks, an unsheathed microfilaria results.

sheath·ing canal. The upper end of the vaginal process of peritoneum; it normally closes, leaving the lower end a closed sac, the tunica vaginalis.

sheath of Henle [F. G. J. *Henle*]. ENDONEURIUM.

sheath of Neumann [E. *Neumann*]. DENTINAL SHEATH.

sheath of Schwann [F. T. *Schwann*]. The first cellular layer that intimately encloses an axon or nerve cell in the peripheral nervous system.

sheath of Schweigger-Seidel [F. *Schweigger-Seidel*]. The thickening of the arterial wall in the sheathed arteries of the lienic penicilli.

sheath of the optic nerve. DURAL SHEATH.

sheath of the rectus. The sheath formed by the aponeuroses of the external and internal oblique and transversus abdominis muscles about the rectus abdominis muscle. NA *vagina musculi recti abdominis.* See also Plate 4.

shed, *v.* To throw off, cast off.

shed·ding, *n.* 1. Casting off. 2. The natural process of resorption of the roots and the subsequent loss of deciduous teeth.

Shee·han's syndrome [H. L. *Sheehan,* English pathologist, 20th century]. Hypopituitarism due to postpartum necrosis of the adenohypophysis.

sheep botfly. *OESTRUS OVIS.*

sheep-dung stools. Small, round, fecal masses, similar to the dung of sheep; may occur in such conditions as inanition or spastic colitis.

sheep ked. *MELOPHAGUS OVINUS.*

sheep pox. *In veterinary medicine,* a contagious disease of sheep characterized by vesicopustular lesions of the skin.

sheep tick. *MELOPHAGUS OVINUS.*

sheet bath. A process of cooling the body by sprinkling lukewarm water on a sheet which is spread over the patient's body.

shelf operation. An arthroplastic procedure in the open reduction of a congenitally displaced hip, in which a bony shelf is inserted, by bone grafting, into the upper portion of the acetabulum so as to hold the femoral head and prevent its slipping out of the shallow joint cup.

shell, *n.* 1. A hard outer covering, as for an animal, egg, fruit, or seed. 2. *In ophthalmology,* a temporary prosthesis for an eye. 3. *In physics,* one of several rings of electrons surrounding the nucleus of an atom.

shel·lac (she·lack') *n.* [*shell* + *lac;* translation of F. *laque en écailles*]. A refined form of the resinous substance obtained from several trees growing in India, Thailand, and nearby countries when infested by the sucking insect *Laccifer lacca.*

shell injury. Damage due to shell explosions from artillery fire; due largely to bursting fragments and to secondary missiles set in motion by the burst.

shell·shock, *n.* 1. WAR NEUROSIS. 2. BLAST INJURY.

shell tooth. A form of dentinal dysplasia in which the enamel has a normal appearance, the dentin is very thin, and the pulp chamber is excessively large.

shel·tered workshop. A facility for the treatment of physically, medically, or mentally handicapped ambulatory individuals, where the work, machinery, and tempo are modified so that the handicapped may learn to cope with their jobs successfully.

shel·ter foot. A condition resembling trench foot and immersion foot, but of less severity; seen in persons confined to cold and damp shelters.

Shen·stone's operation [N. S. *Shenstone,* Canadian surgeon, b. 1881]. An operation for the closure of bronchial fistula, in which intercostal muscle is implanted into the fistulous tract.

Shep·herd's fracture [F. J. *Shepherd,* British surgeon, 1851–1929]. A type of fracture of the lateral process of the talus.

Sher·man-Mun·sell unit [H. C. *Sherman,* U.S. chemist, 1875–1955; and Hazel E. *Munsell,* U.S. chemist, b. 1891]. The rat growth unit, which is the daily requirement of vitamin A necessary to maintain a weekly gain of 3 g in test rats previously depleted of vitamin A. Compare *Bourquin-Sherman unit.*

Sherman's plates [H. M. *Sherman,* U.S. orthopedic surgeon, 1854–1921]. Stainless steel bone plates for internal fixation of fractures.

Sherman's screws [H. M. *Sherman*]. Stainless steel tap screws used for attaching Sherman's plates.

Sher·ren's triangle [J. *Sherren,* British surgeon, 1872–1945]. An area of the skin of the anterior abdominal wall bounded by lines joining the umbilicus, pubic tubercle, and anterior superior iliac spine.

Sher·ring·ton's law [C. S. *Sherrington,* English neurophysiologist, 1857–1952]. Each posterior spinal nerve root supplies a specific skin area, though some overlap from the adjacent dermatomes occurs.

Shev·sky's test [Marian C. *Shevsky,* U.S. biochemist, 20th century]. ADDIS AND SHEVSKY'S TEST.

SH group. SULFHYDRYL.

shi·a·tsu (shee'ah·tsoo) *n.* [Jap. *shi,* finger, + *atsu,* pressure]. A therapeutic massage technique, developed in Japan in the 18th century, which involves application of carefully gauged pressure at specific points on the body. The doctrine on which it is based is akin to that of acupuncture.

Shib·ley's sign [G. S. *Shibley,* U.S. internist, b. 1890]. "E" TO "A" SIGN.

shield, *n.* 1. A protective structure or apparatus. 2. *In biology,* a protective plate, scute, lorica, or carapace. 3. A structure having the shape of a shield.

shift, *n.* A change of direction or position.

shift to the left. According to Arneth, a marked increase in the percentage of immature neutrophils (those having a single or bilobed nucleus) in the peripheral blood, occurring in granulocytic leukemia, in acute infective diseases, and also in pernicious anemia.

shift to the right. According to Arneth, a marked increase in the percentage of mature neutrophils (those having nuclei with three or more lobes) in the peripheral blood, frequently occurring in diseases of the liver and in pernicious anemia.

Shi·ga bacillus (shee'guh, Jap. sheeng'ah) [K. *Shiga,* Japanese bacteriologist, 1870–1957]. *SHIGELLA DYSENTERIAE,* subgroup A of *Shigella.*

Shi·gel·la (shi·ghel'uh, shi·jel'uh) *n.* [K. *Shiga*]. A genus of nonmotile, gram-negative bacteria of the Enterobacteriaceae which with few exceptions do not produce gas from fermentable substances and do not ferment lactose; the causative agents of bacillary dysentery. They are antigenically related, and are divided into four major subgroups: (A) *Shigella dysenteriae,* (B) *S. flexneri,* (C) *S. boydii,* and (D) *S. sonnei.*

Shigella al·ka·les·cens (al·kuh·les'enz). Formerly classified with the *Shigella,* now regarded as coliform organisms on the basis of antigenic and biochemical characteristics; cause urinary tract infection but doubtfully involved in dysentery.

Shigella am·big·ua (am·big'yoo·uh). Type 2 of *Shigella dysenteriae.* Syn. *Schmitz bacillus, Shigella schmitzii.*

Shigella dys·en·ter·i·ae (dis''en·terr'ee·ee). Subgroup A of *Shigella,* rarely a cause of dysentery in the United States, but involved in highly virulent epidemics elsewhere. In addition to the endotoxin produced by all *Shigella,* type 1 of *S. dysenteriae* elaborates a potent exotoxin which is neurotoxic for laboratory animals.

Shigella schmitz·ii (shmit'see·eye). *SHIGELLA AMBIGUA.*

shig·el·lo·sis (shig''e·lo'sis) *n.,* pl. **shigello·ses** (·seez) [*Shigella* + *-osis*]. BACILLARY DYSENTERY.

shi·kim·ic acid (shi·kim'ick) *n.* [Jap. *shikimi,* star anise, *Illicium*]. 3,4,5-Trihydroxy-1-cyclohexene-1-carboxylic acid, $C_7H_{10}O_5$, a constituent of plants. It serves as a precursor of phenylalanine, tyrosine, tryptophan, and para-aminobenzoic acid for certain strains of *Escherichia coli* and *Neurospora.*

shi·ma-mu·shi, shi·mu-mushi (shee''muh·moo'shee) *n.* [Jap.]. TSUTSUGAMUSHI DISEASE.

shim·mer·ing nystagmus. A rapid, fine, pendular nystagmus; a form of ocular nystagmus.

shin, *n.* The sharp anterior margin of the tibia and overlying structures.

shin·bone, *n.* TIBIA.

shinbone fever. TRENCH FEVER.

shin·gles, *n.* [ME. *cingules,* from ML. *cingulus,* lit., girdle, translation of Gk. *zōnē* or *zōstēr*]. HERPES ZOSTER.

shin splints. Pain in the anterior tibial compartment of the lower leg brought about by vigorous exercise; caused by ischemia associated with edema secondary to microscopic tears in muscle and connective tissue; considered a mild form of the anterior tibial compartment syndrome.

ship fever. EPIDEMIC TYPHUS.

ship·ping fever. An acute, occasionally subacute, septicemic disease in cattle and sheep, probably caused by a combination of virus and *Pasteurella multocida* or *P. hemolytica.*

ship's surgeon. A physician employed to take responsibility for health matters aboard a ship.

shirt-stud abscess. An abscess near the surface, communicating by means of a sinus with a deeper abscess.

shiv·er, *n.* A tremor or shaking of the body associated with chill or fear; frequently observed also with rapid rises in temperature as in the onset of fever, when the patient has the cutaneous sensation of being cold although actual body temperature is raised, causing reflex contraction of muscles to produce more body heat.

shiv·er·ing reflex. Reflex rhythmic contraction of muscles in response to cold.

shock, *n.* [F. *choc*]. 1. The clinical manifestations of defective venous return to the heart with consequent reduction in cardiac output. Manifestations of this circulatory insufficiency include hypotension, a weak thready pulse, tachycardia, restlessness, pallor, and diminished urinary output. Shock may be classified according to mechanism, as cardiogenic, vasogenic, neurogenic, or hypovolemic. Syn. *peripheral circulatory failure.* See also *countershock, general adaptation syndrome, photoshock, shellshock.* 2. A physical or emotional trauma. 3. *In physiology,* ELECTRIC SHOCK. 4. The first phase of the alarm reaction in the general adaptation syndrome.

Shock and Has·tings method. A procedure for determining the hydrogen-ion concentration of blood by use of a special pipet which not only permits the determination of cell volume as well as plasma pH but also makes possible the transfer of the diluted plasma to the manometric apparatus for carbon dioxide determination.

shock organ. The organ or tissue that exhibits the most marked response to the antigen-antibody interaction in hypersensitivity, as the lungs in allergic asthma, or the skin in allergic contact dermatitis.

shock therapy. The treatment of psychiatric patients by inducing coma, with or without convulsions, by means of carbon dioxide or drugs such as insulin or metrazol, or by passing an electric current through the brain. See also *carbon dioxide therapy, electroshock therapy, insulin shock therapy, metrazol shock therapy, subcoma insulin treatment.*

shoddy fever. A febrile disease with cough and dyspnea; seen in persons who work with shoddy (reclaimed wool).

shoe boil. *In veterinary medicine,* bursitis of the point of the elbow, presumably due to trauma from the horse's shoe hitting the point of the elbow either in motion or when lying down.

Shohl and King method [A. T. *Shohl,* U.S. pediatrician, b. 1889]. A procedure for the colorimetric determination of hydrogen-ion concentration of gastric contents.

shoot·ing pains. Sharp, brief pains that radiate in the distribution of a nerve root.

Shope papilloma [R. E. *Shope,* U.S. pathologist, b. 1902]. A virus-induced, naturally occurring, transmissible papilloma of rabbit skin.

shop typhus. MURINE TYPHUS.

Shorr trichrome stain. A staining method for vaginal epithelium, using an alcoholic solution of Biebrich scarlet, orange G, fast green FCF, and aniline blue stains, phosphomolybdic acid, phosphotungstic acid, and glacial acetic acid. It differentiates between cornified (brilliant orange-red) and noncornified (blue-green) cells.

short bone. A bone having the three dimensions nearly equal.

short circuit. 1. A circuit in which an electric current encounters an abnormally small resistance. 2. *In surgery,* an intestinal anastomosis whereby a segment of bowel, in which is located a tumor or other obstruction, is bypassed, the fecal current being diverted beyond the point of obstruction or pathologic process. It is generally a palliative or temporary procedure.

short crus of the incus. A conical process projecting almost horizontally backward from the body of the incus and attached by ligamentous fibers to the fossa incudis. NA *crus breve incudis.*

shortening reaction. Abnormal reflex contraction of extensor muscles when a flexed limb is extended by some external force, acting to maintain the joints of the limb under a certain degree of tension.

short gyri of the insula. Three to five irregular gyri occupying the anterior portion of the insula, separated from the posterior portion, the long gyrus, by the central sulcus of the insula. NA *gyri breves insulae.*

short-incubation hepatitis. INFECTIOUS HEPATITIS.

short process of the malleus. LATERAL PROCESS OF THE MALLEUS.

short sight. MYOPIA.

short stop. *In radiology and photography,* an acidifier used after a developer in order to arrest the developing process.

short-term memory. Memory store from which information is lost rapidly, usually within 20 to 30 seconds, unless retained through active rehearsal. Syn. *primary memory, immediate memory.* Contr. *long-term memory.*

short-wave diathermy. A process of electrotherapy in which an alternating electric current of extremely high frequency, 10,000 to 100,000 kilohertz per second, at wavelengths of 30 to 3 meters, is run though the body surface for therapeutic heating.

shot·ted suture. A suture in which each end of the suture is passed through a perforated metal shot and then drawn tight and tied.

shoul·der, *n.* The region where the arm joins the trunk, formed by the meeting of the clavicle, scapula, humerus, and the overlying soft parts. See also Table of Synovial Joints and Ligaments in the Appendix and Plates 2, 4.

shoulder blade. SCAPULA.

shoulder girdle. The system of bones supporting an upper limb or arm; it consists of the clavicle, scapula, and, for some authorities, the manubrium of the sternum. NA *cingulum membri superioris.*

shoulder-hand syndrome. A syndrome characterized by pain in the shoulder and arm, limited joint motion, diffuse swelling of the distal part of the upper extremity, atrophy of muscles, cutaneous and subcutaneous structures, and decalcification of underlying bones. The cause is not well understood. It is observed most often following myocardial infarction and self-imposed immobility of the arm. Syn. *hand-shoulder syndrome.*

shoulder-shaking test. A test for extrapyramidal rigidity and cerebellar lesions. When the examiner swings the patient's arms by shaking him at the shoulders, the swinging is lessened by extrapyramidal rigidity and increased by cerebellar affections.

shoulder slip. Upward displacement of the scapula in the horse caused by excessive impact of the front leg with the ground.

show, *n.* A bloody discharge from the birth canal prior to labor or to a menstrual flow.

Shra·dy's saw [G. F. *Shrady,* U.S. surgeon, 1837–1907]. A surgical saw to be used through a cannula which enables the surgeon to cut through bone in a subcutaneous operation.

Shrap·nell's membrane [H. J. *Shrapnell,* English anatomist, 1761–1841]. PARS FLACCIDA MEMBRANAE TYMPANI.

shreds, *n.pl.* Slender strands of mucus visible grossly in urine, denoting inflammation of the urethra, bladder, or prostate.

shriv·el, *v.* To shrink in bulk and wrinkle.

shud·der, *n. & v.* 1. A momentary involuntary tremor, caused by fright or disgust, or occurring as a nervous habit. 2. To shake or tremble.

Shumm test. A test for methemalbumin, which is detected by the appearance of a sharp band in the spectrometer at 558 nm, when plasma mixed with concentrated ammonium sulfide is examined.

Shunk's stain. A staining method for flagella, using a tannic acid-based fixing solution followed by coloring with methylene blue, carbol fuchsin, safranin, or gentian violet.

shunt, *n. & v.* 1. A diversion. 2. *In medicine,* an anomalous natural or surgically created anastamosis or channel, diverting flow from one pathway to another or permitting flow from one part or region to another. Compare *bypass.* 3. In electricity, a branch of a circuit parallel with other parts of it, especially one that provides a low-resistance path for the flow of electricity. 4. To divert, shift.

shunt nephritis. Acute glomerulonephritis associated with infected ventriculoatrial shunts.

SH virus. The virus (hepatitis virus B) associated with serum hepatitis.

Shwartz·man phenomenon or **reaction** [G. *Shwartzman,* U.S. immunologist, b. 1896]. 1. The occurrence of hemorrhage and necrosis at a skin site prepared by the local injection of a bacterial endotoxin when the same or differing material is inoculated intravenously 8 to 24 hours later. Syn. *local Shwartzman phenomenon.* 2. Bilateral cortical renal necrosis and other lesions initiated by intravascular coagulation when both the preparatory and the eliciting materials are administered intravenously. Syn. *generalized Shwartzman phenomenon.*

Shy-Drager syndrome [G. M. *Shy,* U.S. neurologist, 1919–1967; and G. A. *Drager,* U.S. physician, 1917–1967]. PRIMARY ORTHOSTATIC HYPOTENSION.

Si Symbol for silicon.

si·a·go·nag·ra (sigh″uh·go·nag′ruh) *n.* [Gk. *siagōn,* jawbone, + *-agra*]. Gouty pain in the maxilla.

sial-, sialo- [Gk. *sialon*]. A combining form meaning *saliva, salivary.*

si·al·a·den (sigh·al′uh·den) *n.* [*sial-* + Gk. *adēn,* gland]. SALIVARY GLAND.

si·al·ad·e·ni·tis (sigh″ul·ad″e·nigh′tis) *n.* [*sial-* + *aden-* + *-itis*]. Inflammation of a salivary gland.

si·al·ad·e·nog·ra·phy (sigh″ul·ad″e·nog′ruh·fee) *n.* [*sial-* + *adeno-* + *-graphy*]. Radiography of the salivary glands.

si·al·ad·en·on·cus (sigh″ul·ad″e·nonk′us) *n.* [*sial-* + *aden-* + Gk. *onkos,* bulk, heap]. Any salivary gland tumor.

si·al·a·gogue, si·al·a·gog (sigh·al′uh·gog) *n.* [*sial-* + *-agogue*]. A drug which produces a flow of saliva. **—si·al·a·gog·ic** (sigh″ul·uh·goj′ick) *adj. & n.*

si·al·an·gi·og·ra·phy (sigh″uh·lan″jee·og′ruh·fee) *n.* [*sial-* + *angio-* + *-graphy*]. SIALOGRAPHY.

si·al·a·po·ria (sigh″ul·uh·po′ree·uh) *n.* [*sial-* + Gk. *aporia,* difficulty, lack]. Deficiency in the amount of saliva.

si·al·ec·ta·sia (sigh″ul·eck·tay′zhuh, ·zee·uh) *n.* [*sial-* + *ectasia*]. A swelling or enlargement of the salivary glands.

si·al·ic (sigh·al′ick) *adj.* [*sial-* + *-ic*]. Having the nature of saliva.

sialic acid. Any of a family of amino sugars, containing nine or more carbon atoms, that are nitrogen- and oxygen-substituted acyl derivatives of neuraminic acid. As components of lipids, polysaccharides, and mucoproteins, they are widely distributed in bacteria and in animal tissues.

si·al·ine (sigh′uh·line, ·leen) *adj.* SIALIC.

si·a·li·thot·o·my (sigh″uh·li·thot′uh·mee) *n.* SIALOLITHOTOMY.

si·a·li·tis (sigh″uh·lye′tis) *n.* [*sial-* + *-itis*]. 1. SIALADENITIS. 2. Inflammation of a salivary gland or duct.

sialo-. See *sial-.*

si·alo·ad·e·nec·to·my (sigh″uh·lo·ad″e·neck′tuh·mee) *n.* [*sialo-* + *aden-* + *-ectomy*]. Surgical removal of a salivary gland.

si·a·lo·ad·e·ni·tis (sigh″uh·lo·ad″e·nigh′tis) *n.* SIALADENITIS.

si·alo·ad·e·not·o·my (sigh″uh·lo·ad″e·not′uh·mee) *n.* [*sialo-* + *adeno-* + *-tomy*]. Incision of a salivary gland.

si·alo·aer·oph·a·gy (sigh″uh·lo·ay″ur·off′uh·jee) *n.* AEROSIALOPHAGY.

si·alo·an·gi·ec·ta·sis (sigh″uh·lo·an″jee·eck′tuh·sis) *n.* [*sialo-* + *angi-* + *ectasis*]. Dilatation of a salivary gland duct.

si·alo·an·gi·og·ra·phy (sigh″uh·lo·an″jee·og′ruh·fee) *n.* [*sialo-* + *angio-* + *-graphy*]. SIALOGRAPHY.

si·a·lo·an·gi·tis (sigh″uh·lo·an·jye′tis) *n.* [*sialo-* + *angitis*]. Inflammation of a salivary duct.

si·a·lo·dac·ryo·ad·e·ni·tis (sigh″uh·lo·dack″ree·o·ad·e·nigh′tis) *n.* [*sialo-* + *dacryo-* + *adenitis*]. A viral disease of laboratory rats characterized by inflammation and swelling of the lacrimal and salivary glands.

si·alo·do·chi·tis (sigh″uh·lo·do·kigh′tis) *n.* [*sialodoch*ium + *-itis*]. Inflammation of a salivary duct.

si·alo·do·chi·um (sigh″ul·lo·do′kee·um) *n.* [NL., from *sialo-* + Gk. *docheion,* holder]. SALIVARY DUCT.

si·alo·do·cho·li·thi·a·sis (sigh″uh·lo·do″ko·li·thigh′uh·sis) *n.* [*sialodoch*ium + *lithiasis*]. The presence of stones in salivary gland ducts.

si·alo·do·cho·plas·ty (sigh″uh·lo·do′ko·plas″tee) *n.* [*sialodoch*ium + *-plasty*]. Plastic surgery of a salivary duct.

si·alo·gas·trone (sigh″uh·lo·gas′trone) *n.* [*sialo-* + *gastr-* + *-one*]. A gastric inhibitory substance in human saliva, produced mainly in the sublingual glands; it is also present in gastric juice.

si·a·log·e·nous (sigh″uh·loj′e·nus) *adj.* [*sialo-* + *-genous*]. Generating saliva.

sialogogue. SIALAGOGUE.

si·alo·gram (sigh·al′o·gram) *n.* [*sialo-* + *-gram*]. A radiograph of a salivary gland and duct system after the injection of an opaque medium.

si·a·log·ra·phy (sigh″uh·log′ruh·fee) *n.* [*sialo-* + *-graphy*]. Radiographic examination of a salivary gland and its duct following injection of an opaque substance into its duct; PTYALOGRAPHY.

si·a·loid (sigh′uh·loid) *adj.* [*sial-* + *-oid*]. Pertaining to, or like, saliva.

si·alo·lith (sigh·al′o·lith, sigh′uh·lo·lith) *n.* [*sialo-* + *-lith*]. SALIVARY CALCULUS (1).

si·alo·li·thi·a·sis (sigh″uh·lo·li·thigh′uh·sis) *n.* [*sialolith* + *-iasis*]. The occurrence of calcareous concretions in the salivary ducts or glands.

si·alo·li·thot·o·my (sigh″uh·lo·li·thot′uh·mee) *n.* [*sialolith* + *-tomy*]. Surgical incision into a salivary duct or salivary gland for the removal of a calculus.

si·alo·mu·cin (sigh″uh·lo·mew′sin) *n.* An acid mucopolysaccharide whose acidic component is a sialic acid.

si·a·lon (sigh′uh·lon) *n.* [Gk.]. SALIVA.

si·al·or·rhea, si·al·or·rhoea (sigh″uh·lo·ree′uh, sigh·al″o·) *n.* [*sialo-* + *-rrhea*]. SALIVATION (2).

si·a·los·che·sis (sigh″uh·los′ke·sis) *n.* [*sialo-* + Gk. *schesis,* retention]. Suppression of the secretion of saliva.

si·alo·se·mei·ol·o·gy (sigh″uh·lo·see″migh·ol′o·jee) *n.* [*sialo-* + *semeiology*]. Diagnosis based upon examination of the saliva.

si·a·lo·sis (sigh″uh·lo′sis) *n.* [*sial-* + *-osis*]. SALIVATION.

si·alo·ste·no·sis (sigh″uh·lo·ste·no′sis) *n.* [*sialo-* + *stenosis*]. Stricture of a salivary duct.

si·alo·syr·inx (sigh″uh·lo·sirr′inks) *n.* [*sialo-* + *syrinx*]. 1. SALIVARY FISTULA. 2. A syringe for washing out the salivary ducts. 3. A drainage tube for a salivary duct.

Si·a·mese twins (sigh·uh·meez′) [after *Siam* (Thailand), birthplace of Chang and Eng, exhibited in the 19th century]. Viable conjoined twins.

Sia's water test (see′uh) [R. H. P. *Sia,* U.S. physician, 1895–1970]. A test for macroglobulins, in which the patient's serum is mixed with distilled water. The formation of a precipitate constitutes a positive reaction.

sib, *n.* [OE. *sibb*]. 1. *Obsol.* A blood relative. 2. SIBLING. 3. *In cultural anthropology,* a unilateral descent group, as a clan.

Si·be·ri·an cattle plague. ANTHRAX.

sib·i·lant (sib'i·lunt) *adj.* [L. *sibilare,* to hiss]. Hissing or whistling.

sibilant rale. A dry, high-pitched, hissing or whistling sound heard most often in bronchiolar spasm or narrowing.

sib·i·la·tion (sib"i·lay'shun) *n.* [L. *sibilatio,* from *sibilare,* to hiss, whistle]. Pronunciation in which the *s* sound predominates.

sib·i·lis·mus (sib"i·liz'mus) *n.* 1. A hissing sound. 2. SIBILANT RALE.

sibilismus au·ri·um (aw'ree·um). TINNITUS.

sib·i·lus (sib'i·lus) *n.* [L., a hissing]. SIBILANT RALE.

sib·ling, *n.* [OE., kinsman, from *sibb,* kin]. An individual in relation to any other individual having the same parents; a brother or sister.

sibling rivalry. The competition between siblings for the love of one or both parents, or for other recognition or gain which is a rather obvious cover for such competition.

sib·ship, *n.* All the siblings in a family regarded as a single group.

Sib·son's fascia [F. *Sibson,* English anatomist, 1814–1876]. A domelike expansion of fascia strengthening the pleura over the apex of the lung, extending from the first rib to the transverse process of the seventh cervical vertebra. Syn. *suprapleural membrane.* NA *membrana suprapleuralis.*

Si·card's syndrome (see·kahr') [J. A. *Sicard,* French physician and radiologist, 1872–1929]. COLLET-SICARD SYNDROME.

sic·ca (sick'uh) *adj.* [L.]. Feminine of *siccus;* dry.

sic·cant (sick'unt) *adj.* & *n.* [L. *siccare,* to make dry]. 1. Drying; tending to make dry. 2. A substance that speeds up drying.

sicca syndrome. SJÖGREN'S SYNDROME.

sic·ca·tive (sick'uh·tiv) *adj.* & *n.* SICCANT.

sic·cha·sia (si·kay'zhuh, ·zee·uh) *n.* [Gk. *sikchasia,* loathing, from *sikchos,* offensive]. NAUSEA.

sic·cus (sick'us) *adj.* [L.]. Dry.

sick, *adj.* 1. Ill; not well. 2. Nauseated.

Sicka method. A hemoglobinometric method using reduced hemoglobin as pigment and requiring a special comparator.

sick headache. MIGRAINE.

sicklaemia. Sicklemia (= SICKLE CELL ANEMIA).

sick·la·ne·mia (sick"luh·nee'mee·uh) *n.* [*sickle* + *anemia*]. SICKLE CELL ANEMIA.

sickle cell. A crescent-shaped erythrocyte characteristic of sickle cell anemia. Syn. *drepanocyte.*

sickle cell anemia. A chronic hemolytic and thrombotic disorder in which hypoxia causes the erythrocytes to assume a sickled shape; it occurs in persons (usually blacks) homozygous for sickle cell hemoglobin. Syn. *drepanocythemia, sicklanemia, SS disease.*

sickle cell disease. 1. Any disease resulting wholly or in part from the presence of sickle cell hemoglobin, such as sickle cell anemia, sickle cell–hemoglobin C disease, or sickle cell thalassemia. 2. Specifically, SICKLE CELL ANEMIA.

sickle cell hemoglobin. The hemoglobin found in sickle cell anemia, differing in electrophoretic mobility and other physiochemical properties from normal adult hemoglobin. This hemoglobin is especially common in certain populations inhabiting malarious zones of western and central Africa and its occurrence elsewhere is limited mostly to people with ancestry from these zones. Syn. *hemoglobin S.* See also *sickle cell trait.*

sickle cell–hemoglobin C disease. A disorder of hemoglobin formation in which sickle cell hemoglobin, inherited from one parent, and hemoglobin C, from the other, coexist to the exclusion of normal adult hemoglobin. The clinical disease is usually later in onset and often generally milder than homozygous sickle cell disease. Syn. *hemoglobin SC disease.*

sickle cell thalassemia. A congenital disorder of hemoglobin formation in which sickle cell hemoglobin and one of the forms of thalassemia hemoglobin are present in the erythrocytes.

sickle cell trait. The heterozygous genetic constitution in which there is one gene for normal adult hemoglobin and one for sickle cell hemoglobin. Usually no clinical disease is present, and in malarious areas children with the trait are relatively resistant to the more severe forms of *Plasmodium falciparum* infection, possibly because infected cells are selectively sickled and eliminated from the circulation. Compare *sickle cell anemia.*

sickle-hocked, *adj.* Of a horse, having excessive flexion of the hock in the usual stance.

sick·le·mia, sick·lae·mia (sick·lee'mee·uh, sick"ul·ee'mee·uh) *n.* SICKLE CELL ANEMIA.

sick·ness, *n.* Disease; illness.

Sid·bury's syndrome [J. B. *Sidbury,* Jr., U.S. pediatrician, b. 1922]. A disorder of fatty acid metabolism characterized by a deficiency of the acyl dehydrogenase specific for oxidation of 4-carbon and 6-carbon fatty acids, resulting in decreased oxidation of *n*-butyric and *n*-hexanoic acids. The clinical picture resembles that seen in isovaleric acidemia, with familial tendency, malodorous sweat, vomiting, acidosis, lethargy, and coma.

Sid·dall's test [A. C. *Siddall,* U.S. obstetrician, b. 1897]. A pregnancy test by which multiple human serum injections into immature female mice are correlated with enlargement of the mouse uterus and ovaries to yield a positive test.

side, *n.* The lateral aspect of any body or organ.

side·bone, *n.* Ossification of the lateral cartilages of the pedal bone in the horse, resulting in lameness.

side-chain theory. Ehrlich's theory to explain antibody formation and antigen-antibody reaction, in which he postulated the existence of chemical receptors, or side chains, on body cells entering into a chemical union with a corresponding group of the antigen, and which could be stimulated to excess formation resulting in their being cast off in the circulation as antibodies.

sider-, sidero- [Gk. *sidēros*]. A combining form meaning *iron.*

sid·er·a·tion (sid"ur·ay'shun) *n.* [L. *sideratio,* a blight or disease attributed to astral influences, from *sidus, sideris,* constellation]. *Obsol.* 1. A sudden paralysis or stroke. 2. ERYSIPELAS.

sidero-. See *sider-.*

sid·ero·cyte (sid'ur·o·site) *n.* [*sidero-* + *-cyte*]. An erythrocyte which contains granules of hemosiderin which stain blue with the Prussian blue reaction.

sid·ero·cy·to·sis (sid"ur·o·sigh·to'sis) *n.* [*siderocyte* + *-osis*]. The presence in the peripheral blood of significant numbers of siderocytes.

sid·ero·dro·mo·pho·bia (sid"ur·o·dro"mo·fo'bee·uh, sid"ur·od"ro·mo·) *n.* [Modern Gk. *siderodromos,* railway, + *-phobia*]. Abnormal fear of traveling by railway; fear of trains.

sid·ero·fi·bro·sis (sid"ur·o·figh·bro'sis) *n.* [*sidero-* + *fibrosis*]. Fibrosis associated with deposits of iron-bearing pigments.

sid·ero·pe·nia (sid"ur·o·pee'nee·uh) *n.* [*sidero-* + *-penia*]. Deficiency of iron, especially in the blood. —**sidero·pe·nic** (·nick) *adj.*

sideropenic dysphagia. PLUMMER-VINSON SYNDROME.

sid·ero·phage (sid'ur·o·faij) *n.* [*sidero-* + *-phage*]. A macrophage containing granules of iron-containing pigment, especially hemosiderin.

sid·ero·phil (sid'ur·o·fil) *n.* & *adj.* [*sidero-* + *-phil*]. 1. A cell or tissue having affinity for iron. 2. Having an affinity for iron.

sid·ero·phile (sid'ur·o·file, ·fil) *n.* & *adj.* SIDEROPHIL.

sid·ero·phil·ia (sid"ur·o·fil'ee·uh) *n.* The property of being siderophil.

sid·er·oph·i·lin (sid"ur·off'i·lin, sid"ur·o·fil'in) *n.* TRANSFERRIN.

sid·er·oph·i·lous (sid″ur·off′i·lus) *adj.* [*siderophil* + *-ous*]. SIDEROPHIL (2).

sid·ero·phyl·lin (sid″ur·o·fil′in) *n.* TRANSFERRIN.

sid·ero·sil·i·co·sis (sid″ur·o·sil″i·ko′sis) *n.* [*sidero-* + *silicosis*]. A pneumoconiosis due to the prolonged inhalation of dusts containing silica and iron.

sid·er·o·sis (sid″ur·o′sis) *n.* [*sider-* + *-osis*]. 1. The presence or accumulation of stainable iron pigment in the tissues or body fluids or in a particular organ. See also *hemosiderosis.* 2. Pneumoconiosis caused by prolonged inhalation of dust containing iron salt; usually occurring in iron miners and arc welders. Syn. *arc-welder's disease.* **—sider·ot·ic** (·ot′ick) *adj.*

siderosis bul·bi (bul′bye). Degenerative changes in the eyeball resulting from retained ferrous material.

siderotic nodules. Foci of fibrillar material encrusted with iron salts, grossly appearing as brown flecks, usually in spleens with chronic passive hyperemia.

SIDS Abbreviation for *sudden infant death syndrome.*

Sie·gert's sign (zee′gurt) [F. *Siegert,* German pediatrician, 1865–1946]. In Down's syndrome, the terminal phalanges of the little fingers are short and curved inward.

Sie·mens' syndrome (zee′m^e^nss) [H. W. *Siemens,* German dermatologist, b. 1891]. 1. HEREDITARY ANHIDROTIC ECTODERMAL DYSPLASIA. 2. INCONTINENTIA PIGMENTI.

sieve graft (siv). A large skin graft, with openings throughout, corresponding to skin islands left on the donor area.

sig. An abbreviation for (a) *signa,* label it; (b) *signetur,* let it be labeled.

sigh, *n.* A prolonged, deep inspiration followed by a shorter expiration. Syn. *suspirium.*

sight, *n.* 1. The special sense concerned in seeing. 2. That which is seen.

sight-saving class. An educational setup for children with marked defects but not total loss of vision, emphasizing books printed in large type on suitable backgrounds, good lighting, and correct reading posture.

sig·ma (sig′muh) *n.* [name of the letter Σ, σ, eighteenth letter of the Greek alphabet]. 1. A designation used for various categories and quantities, sometimes as one of a series or set along with other Greek letters, and sometimes as a correlate of the Roman letter S. 2. The sum of. Symbol, Σ. 3. STANDARD DEVIATION. Symbol, σ.

sigma angle. The angle between the radius fixus and a line from the hormion to the staphylion.

sigma factor. A subunit of RNA polymerase which can be removed from the enzyme to yield the core polymerase which is completely active; probably regulatory rather than catalytic in function.

sig·ma·tism (sig′muh·tiz·um) *n.* [Gk. *sigma,* Σ, eighteenth letter of the Greek alphabet, + *-ism*]. 1. LISPING. 2. The too frequent use of the *s* sound in speech.

sigmoid-, sigmoido-. A combining form meaning *sigmoid.*

sig·moid (sig′moid) *adj.* & *n.* [Gk. *sigmoeidēs,* shaped like the letter sigma]. 1. Shaped like the letter S. 2. Of or pertaining to the sigmoid colon. 3. SIGMOID COLON.

sigmoid arteries. NA *arteriae sigmoideae.* See Table of Arteries in the Appendix.

sigmoid catheter. A catheter shaped like an S, for passage into the female bladder.

sigmoid colon. The portion of the colon that extends from the descending colon to the rectum. NA *colon sigmoideum.*

sigmoid colostomy. The formation of an artificial anus in the sigmoid colon; SIGMOIDOSTOMY.

sigmoid conduit. A urinary drainage conduit to the skin formed surgically from a defunctionalized segment of the sigmoid colon.

sig·moid·ec·to·my (sig″moy·deck′tuh·mee) *n.* [*sigmoid-* + *-ectomy*]. Excision of a part or all of the sigmoid colon.

sigmoid flexure. SIGMOID COLON.

sigmoid fossa. SULCUS OF THE SIGMOID SINUS.

sigmoid groove. SULCUS OF THE SIGMOID SINUS.

sigmoid gyrus. The S-shaped cerebral fold about and behind the cruciate fissure in carnivora.

sig·moid·itis (sig″moy·dye′tis) *n.* [*sigmoid* + *-itis*]. Inflammation of the sigmoid flexure of the colon.

sigmoid kidney. A congenital anomaly resulting from the fusion of the lower pole of one kidney to the upper pole of the other. Syn. *L-shaped kidney, unilateral fused kidney.*

sigmoid mesocolon. The mesentery of the sigmoid colon. NA *mesocolon sigmoideum.*

sigmoido-. See *sigmoid-.*

sig·moido·pexy (sig·moy′do·peck″see) *n.* [*sigmoido-* + *-pexy*]. An operation for prolapse of the rectum; fixation of the sigmoid colon by obliterating the intersigmoid fossa and shortening the mesosigmoid by suture, through an abdominal incision.

sig·moido·proc·tos·to·my (sig·moy″do·prock·tos′tuh·mee) *n.* [*sigmoido-* + *procto-* + *-stomy*]. Anastomosis of the sigmoid colon with the rectum.

sig·moido·rec·tos·to·my (sig·moy″do·reck·tos′tuh·mee) *n.* [*sigmoido-* + *recto-* + *-stomy*]. Formation by surgical means of an artificial anus at the sigmoid colon, at its junction with the rectum; a low colostomy.

sig·moido·scope (sig·moy′duh·skope) *n.* [*sigmoido-* + *-scope*]. An appliance for the inspection, by artificial light, of the sigmoid colon; it differs from the proctoscope in its greater length and diameter.

sig·moid·os·co·py (sig″moy·dos′kuh·pee) *n.* [*sigmoido-* + *-scopy*]. Visual inspection of the sigmoid colon, with the aid of special instruments.

sig·moido·sig·moid·os·to·my (sig·moy″do·sig″moy·dos′tuh·mee) *n.* [*sigmoido-* + *sigmoido-* + *-stomy*]. Surgical anastomosis between two portions of the sigmoid colon.

sig·moid·os·to·my (sig″moy·dos′tuh·mee) *n.* [*sigmoido-* + *-stomy*]. The formation of an artificial anus in the sigmoid colon; SIGMOID COLOSTOMY.

sig·moid·ot·o·my (sig″moy·dot′uh·mee) *n.* [*sigmoido-* + *-tomy*]. Incision into the sigmoid colon.

sig·moido·ves·i·cal (sig·moy″do·ves′i·kul) *adj.* [*sigmoido-* + *vesical*]. Pertaining to the sigmoid colon and the urinary bladder.

sigmoidovesical fistula. A fistula connecting the sigmoid colon and urinary bladder.

sigmoid septum. A thin membrane that occupies the mandibular notch and separates the masseter from the lateral pterygoid muscles.

sigmoid sinus. The S-shaped part of the transverse sinus which lies on the mastoid portion of the temporal bone and the jugular portion of the occipital bone. NA *sinus sigmoideus.* See also Table of Veins in the Appendix and Plate 17.

sigmoid sulcus. SULCUS OF THE SIGMOID SINUS.

sig·mo·scope (sig′mo·skope) *n.* SIGMOIDOSCOPE.

sign, *n.* [L. *signum*]. An objective evidence or physical manifestation of disease. Compare *symptom.*

signa. 1. Plural of *signum.* 2. Used in prescriptions to mean "write." Abbreviated, S., sig.

sig·nal node. A metastatic tumor in a supraclavicular lymph node, usually on the left side, and most frequently secondary to primary carcinoma in the abdomen or thorax. Syn. *Ewald's node, sentinel node, Virchow's node.*

signal symptom. The first disturbance of sensation preceding a more extensive seizure, as the aura heralding an attack of epilepsy.

sig·na·ture, *n.* [OF., from L. *signare,* to mark]. 1. The part of the prescription that is placed on the label, containing directions to the patient. 2. A distinguishing character.

sig·net-ring cell. A cell with a large cytoplasmic vacuole, containing mucin, fat, or glycogen, which pushes the nucleus to one side, making the cell look like a signet ring.

signet-ring-cell carcinoma. MUCINOUS CARCINOMA.

sig·nif·i·cant difference. A difference between two statistical constants, calculated from two separate samples, which is of such magnitude that it is unlikely to have occurred by chance alone. Usually this probability must be less than 0.05 (5%) before a difference is accepted as significant. The smaller the probability, the more significant is the difference.

signs of pregnancy. The three so-called absolute signs are: (1) hearing fetal heart sounds, (2) perception of fetal movement by the examiner, and (3) recognition of the fetus by radiologic or sonographic examination.

sig·num (sig'num) *n.*, pl. **sig·na** (·nuh) [L.]. A mark, sign, or indication.

sil·an·drone (sil·an'drone) *n.* 17*β*-(Trimethylsiloxy)androst-4-en-3-one, $C_{22}H_{36}O_2Si$, a silicon-containing androgenic steroid.

Si·las·tic stent (si·las'tick). A stent made of a soft, silicone-type material and used with various types of prostheses and plastic supports.

si·lent, *adj.* [L. *silens*, from *silere*, to be silent]. 1. *In medicine*, not exhibiting the usual signs and symptoms of a disorder; characterized by a quiescent state; not manifested clinically. 2. Yielding no response to stimulation. 3. Noiseless.

silent gap. AUSCULTATORY GAP.

sil·i·ca (sil'i·kuh) *n.* [NL., from L. *silex, silicis*, flint]. Silicon dioxide, SiO_2, occurring in nature in the form of quartz, flint, and other minerals.

silica bandage. A bandage impregnated with sodium silicate.

silica gel. A precipitated and dried silicic acid in the form of granules, used as a dehydrating agent and for absorption of various vapors.

sil·i·cate (sil'i·kate, ·kut) *n.* A salt or ester of silicic acid.

sil·i·ca·to·sis (sil''i·kuh·to'sis) *n.* SILICOSIS.

si·li·ceous, si·li·cious (si·lish'us) *adj.* 1. Having the nature of, or containing, silicon. 2. Pertaining to silica.

siliceous granuloma. Any granuloma containing silicon compounds and complexes.

si·lic·ic acid (si·lis'ick). Approximately H_2SiO_3. A white, amorphous powder.

si·li·ci·um (si·lish'ee·um, si·lis'ee·um) *n.* SILICON.

sil·i·co·flu·o·ride (sil''i·ko·floo'uh·ride) *n.* A compound of silicon and fluorine with some other element.

sil·i·co·ma (sil''i·ko'muh) *n.* [*silicone* + *-oma*]. An abnormal swelling or enlargement of an organ resulting from tissue reaction to injected silicone.

sil·i·con (sil'i·kon) *n.* [from *silica*]. Si = 28.086. A nonmetallic element, atomic number 14, of the carbon group. It occurs in several allotropic modifications. Like carbon, it forms many complex compounds that are an essential part of the earth's surface.

silicon carbide. A compound of silicon and carbon next to diamond in hardness; used for cutting hard materials, and as an abrasive.

silicon dioxide. SILICA.

sil·i·cone (sil'i·kone) *n.* Any of a class of synthetic polymers having the composition of a polyorganosiloxane; used as an antiflatulent.

sil·i·co·sid·er·o·sis (sil''i·ko·sid''ur·o'sis) *n.* [*silico-* + *siderosis*]. Pneumoconiosis due to the inhalation of dust containing both silicates and iron.

sil·i·co·sis (sil''i·ko'sis) *n.*, pl. **silico·ses** (·seez) [*silica* + *-osis*]. A chronic pulmonary disease due to inhalation of dust with a high concentration of silica (SiO_2), characterized by widespread fibrosis and clinically by shortness of breath and increased susceptibility to tuberculosis.

Silicote. Trademark for dimethicone, a silicone oil used as a skin protective agent.

sil·i·co·tu·ber·cu·lo·sis (sil''i·ko·tew·bur''kew·lo'sis) *n.* Silicosis with tuberculosis.

sil·i·co·tung·stic acid (sil''i·ko·tung'stick). $SiO_2.12WO_3.26H_2O$, a reagent for alkaloids.

si·lique (si·leek', sil'ick) *n.* [F., from L. *siliqua*, pod]. *In biology*, the slender, two-valved capsule of some plants, as the mustard.

sil·i·quose (sil'i·kwoce) *adj.* Resembling a silique.

sil·o·drate (sil'o·drate) *n.* Magnesium aluminosilicate hydrate, $Al_2Mg_2O_{11}Si_3.xH_2O$, an antacid.

silo-filler's disease. Bronchiolitis obliterans and other lung damage caused by nitrogen dioxide and nitric oxide produced by fermentation of fodder in a silo.

Silubin. Trademark for buformin, an orally effective hypoglycemic agent.

sil·ver, *n.* Ag = 107.868. A white, soft, ductile, and malleable metal; element number 47. Silver compounds are used in medicine for caustic, astringent, and antiseptic effects, which are characteristic of silver ion.

silver amalgam. An amalgam in which silver is the principal ingredient; the kind ordinarily used for dental restoration. See also *dental alloy*.

silver-fork deformity. Displacement of the distal radius and ulna as seen in Colles' fracture.

silver-fork fracture. COLLES' FRACTURE.

silver iodate reagent. Ammoniacal silver iodate added to plasma to precipitate the silver chloride; used in the determination of serum chlorides.

silver nitrate. $AgNO_3$. In aqueous solution, used locally as an astringent and germicide, and also as a prophylactic against ophthalmia neonatorum. In solid form, sometimes used as an escharotic.

silver picrate. $(NO_2)_3C_6H_2OAg.H_2O$; used locally in treatment of urethritis and vaginitis.

silver protein. A compound of protein and silver used for the germicidal effect of the silver component. Two types of preparations, mild silver protein and strong silver protein, have been used; the former contains more silver than the latter but is milder in its effects, presumably because less of the silver is ionized than in strong silver protein.

Silver's syndrome [H. K. *Silver*, U.S. pediatrician, b. 1918]. A congenital, probably sporadic disorder characterized by short stature, asymmetry of part or one side of the body, variations in the pattern of sexual development, including elevated urinary and serum gonadotropins during childhood and precocious sexual development, a triangular-shaped head with broad forehead and narrow jaw, thin mouth with downturned corners, café-au-lait spots, and short, incurved fifth fingers. See also *Russell dwarf*.

silver sul·fa·di·a·zine (sul''fuh·dye'uh·zeen) *n.* The *N*-silver salt of sulfadiazine, $C_{10}H_9AgN_4O_2S$, a topical anti-infective.

Sil·ves·ter's method [H. R. *Silvester*, English physician, 1829–1908]. An obsolete method of artificial respiration in which the arms of a supine person are alternately raised above the head and pressed against the chest.

Silvol. A trademark for mild silver protein.

Sim·a·rou·ba, Sim·a·ru·ba (sim''uh·roo'buh) *n.* [Galabi *simarouba*]. A genus of trees of the family Simarubaceae, several species of which have yielded products used as medicinals.

si·meth·i·cone (si·meth'i·kone) *n.* A mixture of dimethyl polysiloxanes of the composition $(CH_3)_3SiO\text{-}[(CH_3)_2SiO]_n\text{-}OSi(CH_3)_3$, where *n* is between 200 to 300 as an average value, and silica gel; used as an antiflatulent.

Sim·i·ae (sim'ee·ee) *n.pl.* [L., pl. of *simia*, monkey ape]. ANTHROPOIDEA.

sim·i·an (sim'ee·un) *adj.* [L. *simia*, monkey, ape]. Apelike; pertaining to or characteristic of apes or monkeys.

simian crease. A single, continuous, transverse palmar crease; said to be characteristic of Down's syndrome, but also seen as a normal variant.

simian hand. SIMIAN CREASE; a hand with a single, continuous transverse palmar crease.

simian hemorrhagic fever. A severe epizootic disease caused by an RNA virus and characterized by a hemorrhagic diathesis which has resulted in 100 percent mortality in experimental monkey colonies. The virus is not known to infect humans and the disease is thought to be limited to monkeys of the genus *Macaca.*

similar twins. IDENTICAL TWINS.

simile phenomenon. The basis of homeopathy: like is cured by like.

si·mi·lia si·mi·li·bus cu·ran·tur (si·mil'ee·uh si·mil'i·bus kew·ran'tur) [L.]. Likes are cured by likes; a sophism formulated by Hippocrates, then by Paracelsus (simile similis cura, non contrarium). See also *homeopathy.*

si·mil·i·mum (si·mil'i·mum) *n.* [L. *similimus,* superlative of *similis,* like]. The homeopathic remedy that produces a symptom complex most like that of a given disease.

Sim·monds' disease or **cachexia** [M. *Simmonds,* German physician, 1855–1925]. Panhypopituitarism with marked insufficiency of the target glands and profound cachexia. Syn. *hypophyseal cachexia, hypopituitary cachexia.*

Sim·mons' citrate agar [J. S. *Simmons,* U.S. bacteriologist, 1890–1954]. A medium for differentiating among the Enterobacteriaceae on the basis of citrate utilization.

Si·mo·nart's thread (see·moh·nar') [P. J. C. *Simonart,* Belgian obstetrician, 1817–1847]. AMNIOTIC BAND.

Si·mon foci [G. *Simon,* English radiologist, 20th century]. Caseous nodules with a marked tendency to calcification, which develop in children in the apical portions of the lungs due to hematogenous spread of *Mycobacterium tuberculosis* after primary infection is established.

Si·mon·sen phenomenon. A graft-host reaction occurring when adult fowl leukocytes are injected into the chorioallantoic membrane, producing white plaques.

Si·mon's operation (zee'mahn) [G. *Simon,* German surgeon, 1824–1876]. Repair of vesicovaginal fistula and lacerated perineum by colpocleisis.

Simon's position [G. *Simon,* German surgeon, 1824–1876]. The dorsosacral position with the legs and thighs flexed, the hips elevated, and the thighs abducted. Compare *Edebohls' position.*

Simon's septic factor [C. E. *Simon,* U.S. physician, 1866–1927]. The phenomenon of the reduction or disappearance of eosinophils during infections in which neutrophilia occurs; it is now attributed to the action of adrenocortical hormones.

sim·ple, *adj. & n.* [OF., from L. *simplus*]. 1. Consisting of or having only one of some component or structural element that is multiple in certain other things of the same class; single. 2. Without elaborations or complications; minimal or fundamental. 3. A medicinal plant, thought of as possessing a single medicinal substance; also, any drug consisting of but one vegetable medicinal ingredient.

simple adenia. ADENIA.

simple articulation. A synovial joint in which only two bones are involved.

simple bitter. Any medicine that stimulates the gastrointestinal tract without influencing the general system.

simple blepharitis. Mild inflammation of the borders of the eyelids with the formation of moist yellow crusts on the ciliary margins which glue the eyelids together.

simple conjunctivitis. CATARRHAL CONJUNCTIVITIS.

simple cystoma. A dilated ovarian follicle with associated proliferation suggestive of neoplasia.

simple elixir. AROMATIC ELIXIR; a flavored vehicle containing orange and other volatile oils, syrup, alcohol, and water.

simple epithelium. An epithelium with only one layer of cells.

simple flat pelvis. A pelvis in which the only deformity consists in a shortening of the anteroposterior diameter.

simple fracture. A fracture in which the skin is not perforated, from without or within, in such a manner as to expose the fracture site to the environment. Contr. *compound fracture.*

simple gland. 1. A gland which is entirely composed of secretory cells, without a differentiated ductal portion. 2. A gland with but one secretory endpiece and an unbranched duct.

simple glaucoma. OPEN-ANGLE GLAUCOMA.

simple goiter. Diffuse thyroid enlargement, either colloid or hyperplastic in type; usually unassociated with constitutional features.

simple hypertrophy. Hypertrophy occurring without concomitant hyperplasia.

simple inflammation. Inflammation that is not granulomatous. Syn. *nonspecific inflammation.* Contr. *granulomatous inflammation.*

simple lobule. LOBULUS SIMPLEX.

simple lymphangioma. LYMPHANGIOMA.

simple mastectomy. Surgical removal of the breast only.

simple mastoidectomy. Exenteration of the air cells in the mastoid process alone, without disturbing those air cells in the epitympanic space, the external auditory canal, or the perilabyrinthine area, and leaving intact the posterior canal wall.

simple microscope. A microscope of one or more lenses or lens systems acting as a single lens. The rays of light that enter the observer's eye after refraction through these lenses proceed directly from the object itself.

simple necrosis. ASEPTIC NECROSIS.

simple odontoma. A tumor composed of only one histologic element of the tooth germ.

simple protein. One of a group of proteins which, upon hydrolysis, yield exclusively amino acids; included are globulins, glutelins, histones, prolamines, and protamines.

simple scleritis. A form of scleritis that involves only the sclerotic coat of the eye.

simple serous cyst. SEROUS CYSTADENOMA.

simple sugar. MONOSACCHARIDE.

simple syrup. SYRUP (2).

simple translocation. A segment of one chromosome that is transferred to another chromosome.

simple type of schizophrenia. A form of schizophrenia characterized by a slow and insidious general loss of interest in people and external affairs, leading to apathy and typically a progressive course resistant to treatment, with apparent mental deterioration, occasional delusions, and hallucinations.

simple urethritis. *Obsol.* A nonspecific inflammation of the urethra.

Simplotan. A trademark for tinidazole, an antiprotozoal.

Simp·son's forceps [J. Y. *Simpson,* Scottish obstetrician, 1811–1870]. Obstetrical forceps commonly used to aid the second stage of labor.

Simpson's syndrome [L. S. *Simpson*]. A prepuberal endocrine-obesity syndrome characterized by alteration of sexual development and physical habitus, producing a female habitus in boys and accentuated female traits in girls. In boys, also called adipose gynandrism, and in girls, adipose gynism.

Sims's position [J. M. *Sims,* U.S. surgeon and gynecologist, 1813–1883]. The patient lies on the left side and chest with the right knee and thigh drawn up and the left arm along the back.

Sims's speculum [J. M. *Sims*]. DUCKBILL SPECULUM.

sim·tra·zene (sim'truh·zeen) *n.* 1,4-Dimethyl-1,4-diphenyl-2-tetrazene, $C_{14}H_{16}N_4$, an antineoplastic agent.

si·mul (sigh'mul, sim'ul) *adv.* [L.]. At once; at the same time.

sim·u·late, *v.* [L. *simulare*]. To take on the appearance of something else; to feign or imitate.

sim·u·la·tion, *n.* 1. The mimicking of one disease or symptom by another. 2. The feigning or counterfeiting of disease; malingering.

sim·u·la·tor, *n.* 1. MALINGERER. 2. A training device which mimics the conditions and requirements a trainee must meet in reality later, so that he can learn to meet these under controlled circumstances.

Si·mu·li·um (si·mew'lee·um) *n.* A genus of small, robust, humpbacked Diptera with short legs and broad wings, commonly called black flies or buffalo gnats. They are worldwide in distribution. The females are vicious bloodsuckers.

Simulium col·um·bacz·en·se (kol″um·bah·tsen′see). The Columbacz fly, a migratory species of Europe, especially prevalent along the Danube; kills cattle and has been known to kill children.

Simulium dam·no·sum (dam·no′sum). An intermediate host of the nematode worm, *Onchocerca volvulus;* other transmitters of this parasite are *Similium metallicum, S. ochraceum,* and *S. callidum.*

Simulium gris·e·i·col·lis (griz″ee·i·kol′is). A fly known as the nimetti; a pest in the African Sudan.

Simulium pe·cu·a·rum (peck·yoo·air′um). A small black fly which is an important scourge of man and cattle in the Mississippi Valley.

Simulium ve·nus·tum (ve·nus′tum). A small black fly of northern New England, New York, the Midwest, and Canada; most bothersome to man in June and July.

si·mul·tag·no·sia (sigh″mul·tag·no′zhuh, ·no′see·uh) *n.* [*simult-* (as in simultaneous) + *agnosia*]. A form of visual agnosia in which the patient is able to perceive parts of a pattern or picture, but fails to recognize the meaning of the whole.

si·nal (sigh′nul) *adj.* Pertaining to or coming from a sinus.

si·na·pis (si·nay′pis) *n.* [Gk.]. MUSTARD.

sin·a·pism (sin′uh·piz·um) *n.* [Gk. *sinapismos,* from *sinapi,* mustard]. The use or application of a mustard plaster.

sin·ca·lide (sin′kuh·lide) *n.* A polypeptide of 8 amino acids, partially sulfonated, $C_{49}H_{62}N_{10}O_{16}S_3$, a choleretic.

sin·ci·put (sin′si·put) *n.*, pl. **sinciputs, sin·cip·i·ta** (sin·sip′i·tuh) [L., half a head] [NA]. The superior and anterior part of the head. —**sin·cip·i·tal** (sin·sip′i·tul) *adj.*

Sin·ding-Lar·sen disease [C. M. F. *Sinding-Larsen,* Norwegian surgeon, b. 1874]. LARSEN-JOHANSSON DISEASE.

sin·ew (sin′yoo) *n.* TENDON.

Sin·ga·pore ear. OTOMYCOSIS.

sing·er's node or **nodule.** An inflammatory or fibrous nodule on the free margin of the vocal folds.

single blind experiment or **test.** An experiment in which either the subject or the observer does not know which of several forms of treatment the subject is to receive.

single harelip. A congenital cleft in the upper lip on one side only.

single loop wiring. A type of intermaxillary wiring used in repairing fractures of the jaw.

sin·gle·ton (sing′gul·tun) *n.* An offspring born singly; not a twin or one of any multiple pregnancy or litter.

Sin·gle·ton's incision [A. O. *Singleton,* U.S. surgeon, 1882–1947]. An incision for upper abdominal operations.

sing·let oxygen. An electronically excited form of oxygen which emits light as chemiluminescence upon relaxation to the ground state. It is thought to be generated by phagocytizing leukocytes and may be involved in the intraleukocytic killing of bacteria.

single ventricle of the heart. COR TRILOCULARE BIATRIUM.

sin·gul·tus (sing·gul′tus) *n.* [L.]. HICCUP. —**singultous,** *adj.;* **sin·gul·ta·tion** (sing″gul·tay′shun) *n.*

sin·i·grin (sin′i·grin) *n.* Potassium myronate, $KC_{10}H_{16}O_9NS_2 \cdot H_2O$, a glycoside found in black mustard, *Brassica nigra,* which under the influence of myrosin, an albuminous ferment in black mustard, yields allyl isothiocyanate, a powerful rubefacient.

sin·is·ter (sin′is·tur, L. si·nis′tur) *adj.* [L.]. Left. Abbreviated, s. See also *S.*

sinistr-, sinistro-. A combining form meaning *left* or *toward the left side.*

sin·is·trad (sin′is·trad, si·nis′trad) *adv.* [*sinistr-* + *-ad*]. Toward the left.

sin·is·tral (sin′is·trul, si·nis′trul) *adj. & n.* [*sinistr-* + *-al*]. 1. On the left side. 2. Showing preference for the left hand, eye, or foot for certain acts or functions. 3. A left-handed individual.

sin·is·tral·i·ty (sin″is·tral′i·tee) *n.* 1. The condition, often genetically determined, in which, when there is a choice, the left side of the body is more efficient and hence used more than the right. 2. Specifically, LEFT-HANDEDNESS. See also *left-eyed, left-footed.*

sin·is·tra·tion (sin″is·tray′shun) *n.* 1. A turning to the left. 2. Development of dominance of the right side of the cerebral hemisphere in left-handed persons. Contr. *dextralization.*

sin·is·trau·ral (sin″is·traw′rul) *adj.* [*sinistr-* + *aural*]. 1. Left-eared; characterizing an individual who prefers to listen with the left ear, as with a telephone receiver, or who depends more on the left ear in binaural hearing. 2. Pertaining to the left ear.

sinistro-. See *sinistr-.*

si·nis·tro·car·dia (si·nis″tro·kahr′dee·uh) *n.* [*sinistro-* + *-cardia*]. Displacement of the heart to the left.

sin·is·tro·cer·e·bral (sin″is·tro·serr′e·brul) *adj.* [*sinistro-* + *cerebral*]. 1. Located in the left cerebral hemisphere. 2. Functioning preferentially with the left side of the brain. Contr. *dextrocerebral.*

sin·is·troc·u·lar (sin″is·trock′yoo·lur) *adj.* [*sinistr-* + *ocular*]. Left-eyed; characterizing an individual who uses the left eye in preference to the right when there is a choice, as when sighting a gun or looking through a telescope. Contr. *dextrocular.*

sin·is·tro·gy·ra·tion (sin″is·tro·jye·ray′shun, si·nis″tro·) *n.* [*sinistro-* + *gyration*]. Turning or twisting to the left, as the plane of polarization or a movement of the eye. —**sinistro·gy·ric** (·jye′rick) *adj.*

sin·is·tro·man·u·al (sin″is·tro·man′yoo·ul) *adj.* [*sinistro-* + *manual*]. LEFT-HANDED.

sin·is·trop·e·dal (sin″is·trop′e·dul, sin″is·tro·pee′dul) *adj.* [*sinistro-* + *pedal*]. LEFT-FOOTED.

sin·is·trorse (sin′is·trorce) *adj.* [L. *sinistrorsus,* on the left, from *sinistro-* + *versus,* from *vertere,* to turn]. *In biology,* turning from right to left, as certain twining stems.

sin·is·tro·tor·sion (sin″is·tro·tor′shun) *n.* [*sinistro-* + *torsion*]. A twisting or turning toward the left. Contr. *dextrotorsion.*

sin·is·trous (sin′is·trus, sin·is′trus) *adj.* [*sinistr-* + *-ous*]. Awkward; unskilled. Contr. *dextrous.*

sino-, sinu-. A combining form denoting *sinus.*

si·no·atri·al (sigh″no·ay′tree·ul) *adj.* [*sino-* + *atrial*]. Pertaining to the region between the atrium and the sinus venosus.

sinoatrial heart block. Heart block in which the impulses originated in the sinoatrial node are partially or completely prevented from being conducted through the atria.

sinoatrial node. A dense network of Purkinje fibers of the conduction system at the junction of the superior vena cava and the right atrium. NA *nodus sinuatrialis.*

si·no·au·ric·u·lar (sigh″no·aw·rick′yoo·lur) *adj.* [*sino-* + *auricular*]. SINOATRIAL.

si·no·bron·chi·tis (sigh″no·brong·kigh′tis) *n.* [*sino-* + *bronchitis*]. Inflammation of the bronchi and the paranasal sinuses.

si·no·ca·rot·id plexus (sigh″no·ka·rot′id). Nerve fibers supplying the carotid sinus.

si·no·gram (sigh′no·gram) *n.* [*sino-* + *-gram*]. A radiographic depiction of a natural sinus or acquired sinus tract after the introduction of contrast material.

si·nog·ra·phy (sigh·nog′ruh·fee) *n.* [*sino-* + *-graphy*]. The radiographic demonstration of any sinus by the direct injection of contrast medium.

si·no·vag·i·nal bulb (sigh″no·vaj′i·nul). One of the bilateral dorsal evaginations of the urogenital sinus forming the lower fifth of the vagina.

Sintrom. Trademark for acenocoumarol, an anticoagulant.

sinu-. See *sino-.*

sin·u·i·tis (sin″yoo·eye′tis) *n.* SINUSITIS.

sin·u·ot·o·my (sin″yoo·ot′uh·mee) *n.* SINUSOTOMY.

sin·u·ous (sin′yoo·us) *adj.* [L. *sinuosus,* from *sinus,* curve, fold]. Wavy; applied especially to tortuous fistulas and sinuses.

si·nus (sigh′nus) *n.,* L. pl. & genit. sing. **sinus** (sigh′noos, sigh′nus), E. pl. **sinuses** [L.]. 1. A hollow or cavity; a recess or pocket. 2. A large channel containing blood, especially venous blood. 3. A suppurating tract. 4. A cavity within a bone.

si·nus·al (sigh′nus·ul) *adj.* Of or pertaining to a sinus; SINAL.

sinus alae par·vae (ay′lee pahr′vee). SPHENOPARIETAL SINUS.

sinus ana·lis (ay·nay′lis), pl. **sinus ana·les** (·leez) [NA]. ANAL CRYPT.

sinus aor·tae (ay·or′tee) [NA]. AORTIC SINUS.

sinus aortae [Val·sal·vae] (val·sal′vee) [BNA]. Sinus aortae (= AORTIC SINUS).

sinus arrest. Cessation of pacemaker activity of the sinoatrial node.

sinus arrhythmia. Sinus rhythm with variation of at least 0.12 second between the longest and shortest P-P intervals. P waves and P-R intervals are normal and constant. Phasic sinus arrhythmia accelerates with inspiration and slows with expiration; in nonphasic sinus arrhythmia the irregularity is unrelated to respiration.

sinus bradycardia. Sinus rhythm at a rate of less than 60 beats per minute.

sinus ca·ro·ti·cus (ka·rot′i·kus) [NA]. CAROTID SINUS (1).

sinus ca·ver·no·sus (kav·ur·no′sus) [NA]. CAVERNOUS SINUS.

sinus cir·cu·la·ris (sur·kew·lair′is) [BNA]. CIRCULAR SINUS.

sinus co·ro·na·ri·us (kor·o·nair′ee·us) [NA]. CORONARY SINUS.

sinus cos·to·me·di·as·ti·na·lis pleu·rae (kos″to·mee·dee·as·ti·nay′lis ploo′ree) [BNA]. Recessus costomediastinalis pleurae (= COSTOMEDIASTINAL RECESS).

sinus du·rae ma·tris (dew′ree may′tris) [NA]. The sinuses of the dura mater, collectively.

sinus epi·di·dy·mi·dis (ep″i·di·dim′i·dis) [NA]. DIGITAL FOSSA (2).

sinus eth·moi·da·lis (eth·moy·day′lis) [NA]. ETHMOID SINUS.

sinus fron·ta·lis (fron·tay′lis) [NA]. FRONTAL SINUS.

sinus in·ter·ca·ver·no·si (in·tur·kav·ur·no′sigh) [NA]. INTERCAVERNOUS SINUSES.

sinus in·ter·ca·ver·no·sus anterior (in·tur·kav·ur·no′sus) [BNA]. The anterior intercavernous sinus.

sinus intercavernosus posterior [BNA]. The posterior intercavernous sinus.

si·nus·itis (sigh″nuh·sigh′tis) *n.* [*sinus* + *-itis*]. Inflammation of a sinus. May affect any of the paranasal sinuses, as ethmoidal, frontal, maxillary, or sphenoid.

sinus lac·ti·fe·ri (lack·tif′e·rye) [NA]. LACTIFEROUS SINUSES.

sinus li·e·nis (lye·ee′nis) [NA]. Small irregular spaces in the splenic pulp.

sinus max·il·la·ris (mack·si·lair′is) [NA]. MAXILLARY SINUS.

sinus obli·quus pe·ri·car·dii (o·blye′kwus perr·i·kahr′dee·eye) [NA]. OBLIQUE SINUS OF THE PERICARDIUM.

sinus oc·ci·pi·ta·lis (ock·sip·i·tay′lis) [NA]. OCCIPITAL SINUS.

sinus of Morgagni [G. B. *Morgagni*]. 1. The space between the upper border of the levator veli palatini muscle and the base of the skull. 2. ANAL CRYPT.

sinus of the dura mater. Any endothelially lined, venous blood space situated between the periosteal and meningeal layers of the dura mater. One of the channels by which the blood is conveyed from the cerebral veins, and from some of the veins of the meninges and diploë, into the veins of neck. NA *sinus durae matris.*

sinus of the epididymis. DIGITAL FOSSA (2).

sinus of the external jugular vein. The portion of the external jugular vein between two sets of valves in the distal part of the vessel; this area is often dilated.

sinus of the larynx. LARYNGEAL VENTRICLE.

sinus of Valsalva [A. M. *Valsalva*]. AORTIC SINUS.

si·nus·oid (sigh′nuh·soid) *n. & adj.* [*sinus* + *-oid*]. 1. One of the relatively large spaces or tubes constituting part of the venous circulatory system in the suprarenal gland, liver, spleen, and other viscera. 2. SINUSOIDAL (2).

si·nus·oi·dal (sigh″nuh·soy′dul) *adj.* [*sinusoid* + *-al*]. 1. Varying in proportion to the sine of an angle or of a time function. 2. Pertaining to a sinus.

sinusoidal current. A symmetrical alternating current, the rise and fall of which describes a sine curve.

si·nus·oi·dal·iza·tion (sigh″nuh·soy″dul·i·zay′shun, ·eye·zay′shun) *n.* The application of a sinusoidal current.

si·nus·ot·o·my (sigh″nus·ot′uh·mee) *n.* [*sinus* + *-tomy*]. The production of an artificial opening into a paranasal sinus, to promote drainage.

sinus pa·ra·na·sa·les (păr·uh·na·say′leez) [NA]. PARANASAL SINUSES.

sinus pe·tro·sus inferior (pe·tro′sus) [NA]. INFERIOR PETROSAL SINUS.

sinus petrosus superior [NA]. SUPERIOR PETROSAL SINUS.

sinus phre·ni·co·cos·ta·lis pleu·rae (fren″i·ko·kos·tay′lis ploo′ree) [BNA]. Recessus costodiaphragmaticus pleurae (= COSTODIAPHRAGMATIC RECESS).

sinus plate. A median plate of epithelium within the glans penis of the embryo which later takes part in the formation of the external urethral orifice.

sinus pleu·rae (ploo′ree) [BNA]. RECESSUS PLEURALES.

sinus po·cu·la·ris (pock·yoo·lair′is). UTRICLE (2).

sinus posterior ca·vi tym·pa·ni (kay′vye tim′puh·nigh) [NA]. A depression in the posterior wall of the middle ear cavity above the base of the pyramidal eminence.

sinus pro·sta·ti·cus (pros·tat′i·kus) [NA]. PROSTATIC SINUS.

sinus rec·ta·les (reck·tay′leez) [BNA]. Sinus anales (= ANAL CRYPT).

sinus rec·tus (reck′tus) [NA]. STRAIGHT SINUS.

sinus re·na·lis (re·nay′lis) [NA]. RENAL SINUS.

sinus rhythm. The normal heart rhythm in which the sinoatrial node is the dominant pacemaker.

sinus sa·git·ta·lis inferior (saj·i·tay′lis) [NA]. INFERIOR SAGITTAL SINUS.

sinus sagittalis superior [NA]. SUPERIOR SAGITTAL SINUS.

sinus sig·moi·de·us (sig·moy′dee·us) [NA]. SIGMOID SINUS.

sinus sphe·noi·da·lis (sfee·noy·day′lis) [NA]. SPHENOID SINUS.

sinus sphe·no·pa·ri·e·ta·lis (sfee″no·pa·rye·e·tay′lis) [NA]. SPHENOPARIETAL SINUS.

sinus tachycardia. Sinus rhythm at a rate greater than 100 beats per minute.

sinus tar·si (tahr′sigh) [NA]. The space between the talus and calcaneus formed by the calcaneal and talar sulci and containing the interosseous talocalcaneal ligament.

sinus ton·sil·la·ris (ton·si·lair′is) [BNA]. Fossa tonsillaris (= TONSILLAR FOSSA).

sinus trans·ver·sus du·rae ma·tris (trans·vur′sus dew′ree may′tris) [NA]. TRANSVERSE SINUS (1).

sinus transversus pe·ri·car·dii (perr·i·kahr′dee·eye) [NA]. TRANSVERSE SINUS (2).

sinus trun·ci pul·mo·na·lis (trun′sigh pul·mo·nay′lis, trunk′eye) [NA]. The three shallow dilatations of the pulmonary trunk just distal to the three cusps of the pulmonary valve.

sinus tym·pa·ni (tim′puh·nigh) [NA]. TYMPANIC SINUS.

sinus un·guis (ung′gwis) [NA]. The space beneath the free margin of a nail.

sinus uro·ge·ni·ta·lis (yoo″ro·jen·i·tay′lis) [NA]. DEFINITIVE UROGENITAL SINUS.

sinus ve·na·rum ca·va·rum (ve·nair′um ka·vair′um) [NA]. The portion of the adult right atrium behind the crista terminalis.

sinus ve·no·sus (ve·no′sus). 1. The chamber of the lower vertebrate heart to which the veins return blood from the body. 2. [NA] The vessel in the transverse septum of the embryonic mammalian heart into which open the vitelline and allantoic veins, and the common cardinal veins.

sinus venosus scle·rae (skleer′ee) [NA]. VENOUS SINUS OF THE SCLERA.

sinus ver·te·bra·les lon·gi·tu·di·na·les (vur·te·bray′leez lon·ji·

tew·di·nay'leez) [BNA]. The longitudinal venous channels between the spinal cord and its dura mater.

si·phon (sigh'fun) *n.* [Gk. *siphōn*]. A tube bent at an angle, one arm of which is longer than the other; used for the purpose of removing liquids from a cavity or vessel, by means of atmospheric pressure.

si·phon·age (sigh'fuh·nij) *n.* The action of a siphon, such as washing out the stomach or drainage of wounds, by the use of atmospheric pressure.

Si·pho·nap·tera (sigh"fuh·nap'tur·uh) *n.pl.* [NL., from *siphon* + Gk. *apteros,* without wings]. An order of insects, commonly called fleas. They have small, hard, laterally compressed bodies without wings, and the mouth parts are adapted for piercing and sucking. They feed exclusively upon the blood of birds and mammals and so become important disease vectors. The important genera are *Ctenocephalides, Echidnophaga, Pulex, Tunga,* and *Xenopsylla.*

Si·phun·cu·la·ta (sigh·funk"yoo·lay'tuh) *n.pl.* [NL., from L. *siphunculus,* a little pipe]. A suborder of Anoplura; the sucking lice.

Si·phun·cu·li·na (sigh·funk"yoo·lye'nuh) *n.* A genus of flies found in India.

Siphunculina fu·ni·co·la (few"ni·ko'luh, few·nick'o·luh). The common eye fly of India which is responsible for transmitting conjunctivitis.

Sip·ple's syndrome [J. H. *Sipple,* U.S. internist, b. 1930]. Type 2 of multiple endocrine adenomatosis, in which thyroid medullary carcinoma is associated with pheochromocytoma, parathyroid hyperplasia, mucosal neurofibromatosis and autosomal dominant inheritance.

Sip·py diet [B. W. *Sippy,* U.S. physician, 1866–1924]. Dietary treatment of peptic ulcer, consisting first of alternate feedings of Sippy's powders and a milk-cream mixture, with progressive addition of bland foods until a standard diet is reached.

Sippy powder. 1. A mixture of precipitated calcium carbonate 23%, sodium bicarbonate 77%; known as Sippy powder No. 1. Syn. *sodium bicarbonate and calcium carbonate powder.* 2. A mixture of magnesium oxide 50%, sodium bicarbonate 50%, known as Sippy powder No. 2. Syn. *sodium bicarbonate and magnesium oxide powder.* Both powders are used as gastric antacids; Sippy powder No. 2 is also mildly laxative.

si·ren (sigh'rin) *n.* [Gk. *seirēn,* siren]. *In teratology,* SYMPUS.

si·ren·i·form (sigh·ren'i·form) *adj.* Having the form of a siren or sympus.

siren-limb, *n.* SYMPUS.

si·reno·form (sigh·ren'uh·form) *adj.* SIRENIFORM.

sirenoform fetus. SYMPUS.

si·ren·oid (sigh're·noid) *adj.* Like or pertaining to a siren or sympus.

sirenoid monopodia. Congenital absence of a lower limb in gastroschisis.

si·re·no·me·lia (sigh"re·no·mee'lee·uh) *n.* [*siren* + *-melia*]. The condition of having fused lower extremities. See also *sympus.*

si·re·nom·e·lus (sigh"re·nom'e·lus) *n.* [*siren* + *-melus*]. A fetus whose lower extremities are intimately fused. See also *sympus.*

si·re·nom·e·ly (sigh"re·nom'e·lee) *n.* SIRENOMELIA.

si·ri·a·sis (si·rye'uh·sis) *n.,* pl. **siria·ses** (·seez) [Gk. *seiriasis*]. 1. SUNSTROKE. 2. HEATSTROKE.

sir·ih (sirr'ee) *n.* [Malay *sīrih*]. BETEL.

sirih-chewer's carcinoma. BETEL-NUT CARCINOMA.

sir·kari disease (sur·kăr'ee). KALA AZAR.

si·ro·heme (sigh'ro·heem, sirr'o·) *n.* An iron-porphyrin prosthetic group of certain enzymes in which two of the pyrrole rings are reduced.

sirup. SYRUP.

Siseptin. Trademark for sisomicin, an antibiotic.

sis·mo·ther·a·py (sis"mo·therr'uh·pee) *n.* SEISMOTHERAPY.

sis·o·mi·cin (sis"o·mye'sin) *n.* A D-streptamine antibiotic, closely related to gentamicin, derived from *Micromonospora inyoensis.* Also used as the sulfate salt.

sis·ter cell. A cell formed simultaneously with another in the division of a mother cell.

Sis·to's sign (sees'to) [G. *Sisto,* Argentinian pediatrician, d. 1923]. Constant crying as a sign of congenital syphilis in infants, presumably due to cerebral irritation.

Sis·tru·rus (sis·troo'rus) *n.* [NL., from Gk. *seistron,* rattle, + *oura,* tail]. A genus of small rattlesnakes.

site, *n.* [L. *situs,* from *sinere,* to put, set]. The place at which something occurs or the space it occupies.

-site [Gk. *sitos,* grain, food]. A combining form designating (a) *means or manner of nourishment or life support,* as in parasite, coinosite, autosite; (b) *fetal parasite,* as in omphalosite.

sit·fast, *n.* A form of dry gangrene that affects horses, resulting from pressure on a circumscribed area of the skin, with firm adherence of the dead tissue to the living tissue below, through its continuity with fibrous elements of the underlying structures.

sit·i·eir·gia (sit"ee·ire'jee·uh, ·eer'jee·uh) *n.* [Gk. *sitos,* food, + *eirgein,* to shut out, + *-ia*]. ANOREXIA NERVOSA.

sit·i·ol·o·gy (sit"ee·ol'uh·jee, sigh"tee·) *n.* Sitology (= DIETETICS).

sit·io·ma·nia (sit"ee·o·may'nee·uh) *n.* SITOMANIA.

sit·io·pho·bia (sit"ee·o·fo'bee·uh) *n.* SITOPHOBIA.

sito- [Gk. *sitos*]. A combining form meaning (a) *food;* (b) *grain.*

si·tol·o·gy (sigh·tol'uh·jee) *n.* [*sito-* + *-logy*]. DIETETICS.

si·to·ma·nia (sigh"to·may'nee·uh) *n.* [*sito-* + *-mania*]. 1. An abnormal craving for food. 2. Periodic attacks of bulimia.

si·to·pho·bia (sigh"to·fo'bee·uh) *n.* [*sito-* + *-phobia*]. 1. Abnormal aversion to food. 2. Abnormal fear of eating.

si·to·stane (sigh'to·stane, si·tos'tane) *n.* A steroid hydrocarbon, $C_{29}H_{52}$, that may be considered the parent substance of sitosterols.

si·tos·ter·ol (si·tos'tur·ol, sigh"to·steer'ol) *n.* Any one of a group of plant sterols structurally related to sitostane.

sitosterols. A mixture of β-sitosterol (stigmast-5-en-3β-ol) and certain saturated sterols that appears to increase fecal elimination of cholesterol and thereby reduce blood cholesterol levels.

si·to·ther·a·py (sigh"to·therr'uh·pee) *n.* [*sito-* + *therapy*]. DIETOTHERAPY.

sit·ting arch. An arch representing the line of transfer of weight through the pelvis in the sitting position; from the sacrum through the ilia and ischia to the ischial tuberosities.

sitting height. *In anthropometry,* a measurement taken vertically from the table on which the subject is sitting to the vertex, with the anthropometer behind the subject. Enough pressure is applied to compress the hair.

sit·u·a·tion, *n.* [ML. *situatio,* from *situare,* to place, from *situs,* site]. 1. The more or less fixed position and orientation of an object relative to other objects in an area or space. 2. Position relative to circumstances or environment. 3. A set of circumstances. —**situation·al,** *adj.*

situational crisis. *In psychiatry,* any brief, presumably transient period of psychological stress that represents an individual's reaction to or attempts to cope with a specific set of circumstances. External forces predominate, as compared to a developmental crisis.

situational depression. DEPRESSIVE NEUROSIS.

situational psychosis. PSYCHOTIC DEPRESSIVE REACTION.

situation therapy. MILIEU THERAPY.

si·tus (sigh'tus) *n.,* pl. **situs** [L.]. 1. Site, location. 2. Position, orientation.

situs in·ver·sus (in·vur'sus). Reversed location or position.

situs inversus vis·cer·um (vis'ur·um). An anomaly in which the viscera are reversed in position from the normal to the opposite side of the body. Syn. *situs mutatus, situs transversus.*

situs mu·ta·tus (mew·tay'tus). SITUS INVERSUS VISCERUM.

situs per·ver·sus (pur·vur'sus). Malposition of one or more of the viscera.

situs trans·ver·sus (trans·vur'sus). SITUS INVERSUS VISCERUM.

sitz bath. [Ger. *Sitzbad*]. A therapeutic bath in which the patient sits with buttocks and perineal region immersed in warm water.

sixth (VIth) cranial nerve. ABDUCENS NERVE.

sixth disease. EXANTHEM SUBITUM.

sixth sense. 1. *Obsol.* PROPRIOCEPTION. 2. *Colloq.* Very keen intuition or some undefined extrasensory means of perception.

sixth ventricle. CAVUM VERGAE; a misnomer.

six-year molars. The first permanent molar teeth to form and erupt.

Sjö·gren-Lars·son syndrome (shœh'greʸn'', lahr'soʰn) [T. *Sjögren,* Swedish pediatrician, 20th century; and T. *Larsson,* Swedish pediatrician, 20th century]. Mental deficiency, congenital ichthyosis simplex and spastic diplegia, inherited as an autosomal recessive trait. Patients with a probable variant, Rud's syndrome, also exhibit dwarfism, eunuchoidism, seizures, and polyneuropathies.

Sjögren's syndrome [H. S. C. *Sjögren,* Swedish ophthalmologist, b. 1899]. A symptom complex consisting of keratoconjunctivitis sicca, laryngopharyngitis sicca, rhinitis sicca, xerostomia, enlargement of the parotid gland, and polyarthritis. Syn. *xerodermosteosis.*

SK Abbreviation for *streptokinase.*

skat·er's gait. The somewhat abrupt and flinging movements of the arms and legs with flexion and extension of the trunk seen on walking in patients with moderately advanced Huntington's chorea.

skat·ole (skat'ole) *n.* [Gk. *skōr, skat*os, dung, excrement, + *-ole*]. Methylindole, C_9H_9N. A nitrogenous decomposition product of proteins, formed from tryptophan in the intestine. It contributes to the characteristic, disagreeable odor of feces.

skat·ox·yl (skat·ock'sil) *n.* C_9H_9NO. A product of the oxidation of skatole. It occurs as the sulfuric acid ester in the urine in cases of disease of the intestine or in excessive intestinal putrefaction.

skein (skane) *n.* SPIREME.

skein cell. RETICULOCYTE (1).

ske·lal·gia (ske·lal'jee·uh) *n.* [Gk. *skel*os, leg, + *-algia*]. *Obsol.* Pain in the leg.

Skelaxin. Trademark for metaxalone, a skeletal muscle relaxant.

skelet-, skeleto-. A combining form meaning *skeleton, skeletal.*

skel·e·tal (skel'e·tul) *adj.* 1. Pertaining to a skeleton. 2. Resembling a skeleton.

skeletal enchondromatosis. ENCHONDROMATOSIS.

skeletal muscle. A muscle attached to a bone or bones of the skeleton and concerned in body movements; VOLUNTARY MUSCLE.

skeletal traction. Traction exerted directly upon the long bones themselves by means of pins, wire, tongs, and other mechanical devices which are attached to, or passed through, the bones by operative procedures.

skel·e·ti·za·tion (skel''e·ti·zay'shun) *n.* The process of converting into a skeleton; gradual wasting of the soft parts, leaving only the skeleton; emaciation.

skeleto-. See *skelet-.*

skel·e·ton (skel'e·tun) *n.* [Gk., from *skeletos,* dried up]. A supporting structure, especially the bony framework supporting and protecting the soft parts of an organism. See also Plate 1.

skeleton ex·tre·mi·ta·tis in·fe·ri·o·ris li·be·rae (eck·strem·i·tay'tis in·feer·ee·o'ris lib'e·ree) [BNA]. SKELETON MEMBRI INFERIORIS LIBERI.

skeleton extremitatis su·pe·ri·o·ris li·be·rae (sue·peer·ee·o'ris lib'e·ree) [BNA]. SKELETON MEMBRI SUPERIORIS LIBERI.

skeleton mem·bri in·fe·ri·o·ris li·be·ri (mem'brye in·feer·ee·o'ris lib'e·rye) [NA]. The bones of the lower extremity, exclusive of the hipbone.

skeleton membri su·pe·ri·o·ris li·be·ri (sue·peer·ee·o'ris lib'e·rye) [NA]. The bones of the upper extremity, exclusive of the shoulder girdle.

skeleton of the heart. The fibrous rings (annuli fibrosi) surrounding the four valvular orifices of the heart. The four rings are conjoined and attached to the upper membranous part of the interventricular septum (pars membranacea septi interventricularis). All heart muscles arise from the cardiac skeleton and eventually return to be inserted therein.

skene·itis, ske·ni·tis (skee·nigh'tis) *n.* [*Skene* + *-itis*]. Inflammation of the paraurethral (Skene's) glands or ducts.

skene·oscope (skee'nuh·skope) *n.* An endoscope for use in examining the paraurethral (Skene's) glands.

Skene's duct [A. J. C. *Skene,* U.S. gynecologist, 1838–1900]. PARAURETHRAL DUCT.

Skene's glands or **tubules** [A. J. C. *Skene*]. PARAURETHRAL GLANDS.

skenitis. SKENEITIS.

skeo·cy·to·sis (skee''o·sigh·to'sis) *n.* [Gk. *skaios,* left, + *-cyte* + *-osis*]. Shift to the left.

skew deviation. A maintained deviation of one eye above the other, or hypertropia, which may be fixed or variable for different directions of gaze, seen with lesions in the brainstem and cerebellum, particularly when these are unilateral.

skew·foot, *n.* METATARSUS ADDUCTOVARUS.

skia- [Gk. *skia*]. A combining form meaning *shadow.*

skia·gram (skye'uh·gram) *n.* [*skia-* + *-gram*]. An x-ray picture, radiograph.

ski·ag·ra·phy (skye·ag'ruh·fee) *n.* [Gk. *skiagraphia,* shadow-painting, delineation with shadows, from *skia,* shadow]. RADIOGRAPHY.

ski·am·e·try (skye·am'e·tree) *n.* [*skia-* + *-metry*]. RETINOSCOPY.

skia·po·res·co·py (skye''uh·po·res'kuh·pee) *n.* [*skia-* + Gk. *poros,* opening, + *-scopy*]. RETINOSCOPY.

skia·scope (skye'uh·skope) *n.* [*skia-* + *-scope*]. RETINOSCOPE.

skiascope optometer. An optometer designed for the determination of the refraction of the eye by retinoscopy.

ski·as·co·py (skye·as'kuh·pee) *n.* [*skia-* + *-scopy*]. 1. RETINOSCOPY. 2. FLUOROSCOPY.

skim milk. Milk from which the cream has been removed.

skin, *n.* [ON. *skinn*]. The organ that envelops the body, composed of the dermis and epidermis. NA *cutis.*

skin clip. A band of malleable metal with pointed ends, held in a magazine and applied by a special forceps to the apposed edges of a skin wound; a more rapid method of closure than the use of sutures. Syn. *Michel clip, wound clip.*

skin dose. The sum of the air dose and the backscatter from underlying tissues delivered to the skin and measured in roentgens.

skin erythema dose. The least amount of x-ray radiation which will redden the normal skin. Abbreviated, SED.

skin graft. A portion of skin, of any size or thickness, cut from a donor area and transferred to the recipient site where repair is needed.

skin grafting. The application of portions of the skin, either the outer layers or the full thickness, to a granulating wound to promote healing, to fill a defect, or to replace scar tissue for plastic repair.

skin-holding forceps. TOWEL FORCEPS.

skin test. Any test, as for immunity or hypersensitivity, in which the test material is introduced into the skin.

skin traction. Traction exerted by direct attachment to the skin, using adhesive plaster or linen or gauze strips cemented to the skin.

skin writing. DERMOGRAPHIA.

Skiodan. Trademark for sodium methiodal, a radiopaque contrast medium.

skle·ri·a·sis (skle·rye'uh·sis) *n.* [Gk. *sklēros*, hard, + *-iasis*]. SCLERODERMA.

Sklow·sky's symptom (sklohf'skee) [E. L. *Sklowsky*, German physician, 20th century]. A method of differentiating the vesicle of varicella from that of smallpox or herpes. Light pressure of the index finger near and then over the lesion will easily rupture the varicella vesicle; firm pressure is needed for the latter two.

sko·da·ic resonance (sko·day'ick) [J. *Skoda*, Austrian physician, 1805–1881]. Tympanitic resonance to percussion in the area above the region of a lung compressed by pleural effusion.

Sko·da's resonance or **tympany** (sko'dah). SKODAIC RESONANCE.

Skoda's sign. SKODAIC RESONANCE.

skoliosis. SCOLIOSIS.

skoliosometer. SCOLIOSOMETER.

Skop·tsy (skop'tsee) *n.* [Rus., eunuchs]. A religious sect in Czarist Russia whose members practiced castration.

skull, *n.* 1. The entire bony framework of the head, consisting of the cranium and the face. See also Table of Bones in the Appendix and Plate 1. 2. *In embryology,* the neurocranium and visceral cranium.

skull·cap, *n.* CALVARIA.

Skutsch's operation (skōōtch) [F. *Skutsch*, German gynecologist, 1861–1951]. Anastomosis of the uterine tube to the ovary by creation of an artificial ostium.

slake, *v.* 1. To quench or appease. 2. To disintegrate by the action of water.

slaked lime. Lime which has been acted on by water; it consists chiefly of calcium hydroxide.

slant, *n.* A bacterial culture medium in a test tube, poured to produce a slanting surface when solidified.

slant culture. A culture made on the slanting surface of a medium, to get a greater surface for growth.

slap·ping, *n.* 1. *In massage,* percussion movements in which the hands with palms open come down alternately in a sharp series of blows. The movement is carried out chiefly from the wrist. 2. In gait, the striking of the forefoot forcefully due to weakness of the ankle dorsiflexor muscles. See also *steppage gait.*

slav·er (slav'ur, slay'vur) *n.* & *v.* 1. Drivel; saliva, especially that which is discharged involuntarily. 2. To drool, drivel.

sleep, *n.* A transient, reversible, and periodic state of rest in which there is diminution of physiologic activity and of consciousness. The human sleep cycle generally progresses through four stages from the lightest (stage 1) to the deepest (stage 4), followed by an interlude of REM sleep and a repetition of the cycle. See also *REM sleep.*

sleep apnea syndrome. SUDDEN INFANT DEATH SYNDROME.

sleeping sickness. 1. ENCEPHALITIS LETHARGICA. 2. AFRICAN TRYPANOSOMIASIS.

sleep·less·ness, *n.* INSOMNIA.

sleep paralysis. Transient paralysis with spontaneous recovery, clinically resembling cataplexy and often associated with narcolepsy, occurring on falling asleep (hypnagogic paralysis) or more commonly on awakening (hypnopompic paralysis).

sleep spindle. *In electroencephalography,* the bursts of about 14-per-second waves that occur during sleep.

sleep therapy. NARCOSIS THERAPY.

sleep·walk·ing, *n.* A condition in which an individual walks during sleep. Syn. *somnambulism.* —**sleepwalk·er,** *n.*

slide, *n.* A piece of glass on which objects are examined by use of the microscope.

sliding flap. A simple flap that is rotated on a broad base to fill an adjacent defect.

sliding hernia. A variety of indirect, irreducible inguinal hernia in which a section of a viscus, usually cecum or sigmoid colon, forms one wall of the sac; generally a large scrotal hernia.

sling, *n.* A bandage, usually slung from the neck, to support the arm or wrist.

sling and swathe. A dressing for fractures of the humerus at the upper end. It consists of a three-cornered handkerchief sling holding the arm at the side, the forearm flexed at 90°, with an axillary pad, the swathe passing around the body and arm from shoulder to elbow and secured by pins.

sling procedure. A surgical procedure to treat stress incontinence using a strip of fascia or synthetic material to support the neck of the bladder.

slipped disk. HERNIATED DISK.

slipped shoulder. A dislocated humerus.

slipped tendon. 1. HOCK DISEASE. 2. PEROSIS (2).

slipping epiphysis. Displacement of the upper femoral epiphysis; of uncertain etiology. It occurs in children.

slipping rib. Excessive mobility of the lower intercostal joints.

slit, *n.* A narrow opening; a visceral cleft; the separation between any pair of lips.

slit hemorrhage. Orange-colored slits, 1 to 2 cm in length, found in the cerebral hemispheres along the plane between gray and white matter, which represent healed, shrunken, and flattened sites of previous hemorrhages.

slit lamp. An instrument consisting of a light source providing a narrow beam of high intensity and a microscope or binocular magnifier, which makes possible the highly magnified viewing of various parts of the living eye, especially the anterior portions.

Sloan's incision [G. A. *Sloan*, U.S. surgeon, b. 1889]. An incision for upper abdominal surgery.

slotted plate. *In orthopedics,* a steel plate with slots at either end in which screws are placed, allowing for compression of fractured bone fragments while being maintained in contact.

slough (sluf) *n.* & *v.* 1. A mass of necrotic tissue in, or separating from, living tissue, as in a wound or ulcer. 2. To cast off a mass of necrotic tissue. —**slough·ing** (sluf'ing) *n.* & *adj.*

sloughing phagedena. GANGRENE.

slow filling wave. The slower outward deflection of the apex cardiogram, immediately following the rapid filling wave and corresponding to the slower filling phase of ventricular diastole. Abbreviated, SFW. Contr. *rapid filling wave.*

slow infection. Infection of animals or man which have a long initial latency period after transmission lasting from months to years, and a rather regular and usually protracted course after the appearance of clinical signs which ends in serious disability or death. The two general types are those due to conventional viruses such as subacute sclerosing panencephalitis or progressive multifocal leukoencephalopathy, and those due to unconventional agents, such as Kuru and subacute spongiform encephalopathy in man and scrapie in sheep. See also *chronic infectious neuropathic agent.*

slow neutron. THERMAL NEUTRON.

slow reacting substance of anaphylaxis. A substance, known to cause slow contraction of certain smooth muscle tissues, which is synthesized and released in lung and other tissues during anaphylaxis and which may be a major factor in allergic bronchospasm. Abbreviated, SRS-A.

slows, *n.* TREMBLES.

slow virus. Any of the viruses affecting animals or man which have a long latency after being transmitted to the host before clinical manifestations appear and in whom the disease has a rather predictable and usually protracted course. See also *slow infection.*

Slu·der's method or **operation** [G. *Sluder*, U.S. laryngologist, 1865–1928]. *Obsol.* Removal of the tonsil and its capsule by means of a snare.

Sluder's syndrome or **neuralgia** [G. S. *Sluder*]. SPHENOPALATINE NEURALGIA.

sludge, *v.* & *n.* 1. To agglutinate or precipitate from a liquid, forming a semisolid deposit. 2. The deposit formed.

sludged blood. The intravascular aggregation of erythrocytes associated with decreased blood flow in the involved vascular bed.

sluice·way (sloos'way) *n.* SPILLWAY.

slurred speech. A form of dysarthria in which words and syllables are not enunciated clearly or completely, and tend to run into each other; may be due to upper or lower motor neuron weakness of the muscles of articulation, or basal ganglionic or cerebellar disease.

Sm Symbol for samarium.

small alveolar cell. SQUAMOUS ALVEOLAR CELL.

small anterior gluteus. An isolated slip of the gluteus minimus muscle, occasionally present along the anterior margin of the main muscle.

small calorie. CALORIE.

small-cell carcinoma. 1. Any carcinoma with small parenchymal cells. 2. OAT-CELL CARCINOMA.

small fontanel. POSTERIOR FONTANEL.

small intestine. The proximal portion of the intestine, extending from the stomach to the large intestine, and consisting of the duodenum, jejunum, and ileum; it functions primarily in the digestion and absorption of food. NA *intestinum tenue.*

small pastern. CORONARY BONE.

small·pox, *n.* [by contrast with the "great pox" (= syphilis)]. An infectious pox viral disease, characterized by a diphasic severe febrile illness and a generalized vesicular and pustular eruption. It can be prevented by vaccination. Syn. *variola.*

smallpox inoculation. A method formerly used for protecting or attempting to protect against a severe attack of smallpox in adult life, by the direct transfer of the virus from a sick patient to a well person.

smallpox vaccine. A glycerinated suspension of the vesicles of vaccinia, or cowpox, which have been obtained from healthy vaccinated calves or sheep, used in vaccination to confer lifelong immunity against smallpox. Syn. *virus vaccinum, glycerinated vaccine virus, Jennerian vaccine, antismallpox vaccine.* See also *vaccinia.*

smallpox virus. The virus which causes smallpox, one of three major types, all closely related, yet distinguishable by their effects in both man and animals. The viruses are smallpox (variola), alastrim (variola minor), and vaccinia (cowpox). Smallpox and alastrim viruses, by animal passage, become transformed into vaccinia virus. Various strains of vaccinia virus are in use, the dermal strains, used for vaccine, being maintained by passage through calves, sheep, or rabbits. The virus has been grown in tissue cultures and in the egg.

small triangular space. The medial division of the triangular space of the shoulder through which pass the circumflex scapular vessels.

smart, *v.* To be the locus or the cause of a painful burning sensation, as a superficial cut or irritating substance.

smear, *n.* Preparation of secretions or blood or tissue scrapings for microscopical study, made by spreading them on a glass slide or coverslip.

smeg·ma (smeg'muh) *n.* [Gk. *smēgma,* soap, unguent]. SEBUM. —**smeg·mat·ic** (smeg·mat'ick) *adj.*

smegma cli·to·ri·dis (kli·tor'i·dis) [BNA]. The substance secreted by the sebaceous glands of the clitoris.

smegma em·bry·o·num (em·bree·o'num). VERNIX CASEOSA.

smegma prae·pu·tii (pree·pew'shee·eye) [BNA]. The substance secreted by the sebaceous glands of the prepuce.

smell, *n.* 1. The perception of odor, resulting from the adequate stimulation, usually by chemical molecules, of the receptors in the olfactory mucous membrane; a visceral sensation. 2. ODOR.

smell brain. RHINENCEPHALON.

Smel·lie's forceps [W. *Smellie,* English obstetrician, 1697–1763]. Obstetrical forceps for delivery of the aftercoming head in breech presentation.

Smellie's method [W. *Smellie*]. Delivery of the aftercoming head with the infant resting on the physician's forearm in breech presentation.

Smellie's scissors [W. *Smellie*]. Special scissors with external cutting edges used in fetal craniotomy.

smell·ing salts. A preparation containing ammonium carbonate and stronger ammonia water, usually scented with aromatic substances.

smelt·er's chills. METAL FUME FEVER.

Smith-Dietrich method. A method for identifying phospholipids, in which unsaturated phospholipid fatty acids are oxidized, polymerized, and insolubilized by dichromate solutions, from which they at the same time bind chromium in divalent or trivalent form. The bound chromium is then treated with a mordant-free hematoxylin solution which binds to the chromium as a dark blue chelate. The lake bound to phospholipids is differentially resistant to decoloration by alkaline ferricyanide solution.

Smith-Dietrich stain. A staining method for lipids in which the substance is stained in Kultschitzsky's hematoxylin after mordanting in potassium dichromate. Lipid droplets are stained dark blue.

Smith-Hodge pessary [A. J. *Smith,* Irish obstetrician, 19th century; and H. L. *Hodge,* U.S. gynecologist, 1796–1873]. A retroversion pessary.

Smith incision [R. R. *Smith,* U.S. surgeon, 1869–1940]. An incision for radical mastectomy, with wide mobilization of flaps, which facilitates skin closure.

Smith-Lemli-Opitz syndrome [D. W. *Smith,* U.S. pediatrician, 20th century; L. *Lemli,* U.S. physician, 20th century; and J. M. *Opitz,* U.S. geneticist, 20th century]. A rare congenital disorder, presumed to be an autosomal recessive, characterized by small stature, severe mental deficiency, a tendency to vomit frequently in infancy with failure to thrive, facial anomalies including broad upturned nares and broad maxillary alveolar ridges, skeletal anomalies, and cryptorchidism and hypospadias in the male.

Smith-Petersen incision [M. N. *Smith-Petersen,* U.S. orthopedic surgeon, 1886–1953]. An anterior supraarticular subperiosteal approach to the hip joint.

Smith-Petersen nail [M. N. *Smith-Petersen*]. A three-flanged nail used to fix fractures of the neck of the femur. It is inserted from just below the greater trochanter, through the neck, and into the head of the femur.

Smith phenomenon [T. *Smith,* U.S. pathologist, 1859–1934]. *Obsol.* ANAPHYLAXIS.

smith's spasm. A type of occupation spasm affecting the movements used in the work of a smith.

Smith's test [W. G. *Smith,* Irish physician, 1844–1932]. The appearance of a green interface between layered urine and tincture of iodine is a positive test for urinary bilirubin.

Smith·wick's operation [R. H. *Smithwick,* U.S. surgeon, b. 1899]. An operation for hypertension; the greater splanchnic nerve and the sympathetic chain from the ninth thoracic through the first lumbar ganglion are resected through a transdiaphragmatic extrapleural incision. Syn. *lumbodorsal splanchnicectomy.*

smoker's cancer. Squamous cell carcinoma of the lip, usually the lower lip, observed in habitual smokers.

smooth chorion. CHORION LAEVE.

smooth colony. A raised bacterial colony with regular edges and a homogenous-appearing surface.

smooth muscle. Muscle tissue consisting of spindle-shaped, unstriped muscle cells and found in the walls of viscera and blood vessels. See also *involuntary muscle.*

smooth muscle fibers. The straight, or slightly bent, elongated, spindle-shaped, nucleated cells, bearing more or less distinct longitudinal striations, which make up involuntary, or unstriped, muscles. Syn. *involuntary fibers, nonstriated fibers, unstriated fibers, unstriped fibers.*

smooth-surfaced endoplasmic reticulum. Intracytoplasmic membranes devoid of ribosomes, seen by electron microscopy. Abbreviated, SER. Contr. *rough-surfaced endoplasmic reticulum.*

smudge cells. Degenerate leukocytes seen in spreads of blood and bone marrow cells.

smudg·ing (smuj'ing) *n.* A form of defective speech in which the difficult consonants are dropped.

smut, *n.* 1. A fungous disease of plants involving the grains wheat, rye, oats, and corn. 2. A fungus producing such a disease.

Sn [*stannum*]. Symbol for tin.

snail, *n.* An invertebrate of the order Gastropoda, phylum Mollusca. Important as hosts of many of the flukes.

snake·root, *n.* Any of various plants, such as species of *Asarum, Cimicifuga racemosa,* or *Eupatorium rugosum,* most of which have been used as remedies for snakebite.

snake venom. A secretion of the posterior superior labial glands of a poisonous snake, normally yellowish, sometimes colorless, possessing varying degrees of toxicity. Toxic constituents include neurotoxins, cytolysins, hemolysins, and hemocoagulins.

snap, *n.* 1. A short, abrupt sound heard in auscultation of the heart in certain cardiac diseases. 2. The sound made by the action of a tendon on contraction of its muscle.

snap·ping hip. An abnormality caused by the presence of a tendinous band on the surface of the gluteus maximus muscle. Certain movements of the hip cause this band to slip over the greater trochanter.

snapping jaw. A condition characterized by an audible and palpable snap on opening and closing the mouth, usually caused by displacement of the meniscus in the temporomandibular joint.

snapping knee. A condition in which the tibia on sudden extension of the knee rotates outward or glides forward on the femur with an audible snapping sound, occasionally caused by slipping of the biceps femoris tendon or by displacement of one of the menisci.

snare, *n.* An instrument designed to hold a wire loop which can be constricted by means of a mechanism in the handle, and used to remove tonsils, polyps, and small growths having a narrow base or pedicle.

sneeze, *n.* [OE. *fnēosan*]. A sudden, noisy, spasmodic expiration through the nose. It is caused by irritation of nasal nerves or overstimulation of the optic nerve by a very bright light.

sneezing reflex. NASAL REFLEX.

Snel·len chart [H. *Snellen,* Dutch ophthalmologist, 1834–1908]. A chart for the testing of visual acuity, using letters or numbers for literate patients and letter E's in various positions for small children and illiterates, with the symbols varying in size so that at a distance of 20 feet (or 6 meters) the smallest read normally (and therefore recorded as 20/20 or 6/6) subtends an angle of 5 minutes. If the smallest letter or E the patient can read subtends an angle of 5 minutes at 30 feet, vision is recorded as 20/30 and so forth. Compare *near vision chart.* See also *Snellen test.*

Snellen's reflex [H. *Snellen*]. Hyperemia of the ear on the same side in response to stimulation of the distal end of the divided auriculotemporal nerve.

Snellen test [H. *Snellen*]. A test for visual acuity in which the subject stands a certain distance from a standard chart and reads the letters on the chart. It is based upon the fact that objects may be seen by the normal eye when they subtend an angle of one minute.

snore, *v.* To breathe during sleep in such a manner as to cause a vibration of the soft palate, thereby producing a rough, audible sound.

snout reflex. A stretch or myotatic reflex in which sharp tapping of the mid-upper lip results in exaggerated reflex contraction of the lips; a manifestation of bilateral corticobulbar disease.

snow blindness. Impairment of vision and actinic keratoconjunctivitis, both usually transient, due to exposure of the eyes to the reflection of ultraviolet rays from snow.

snuff·box or **snuffbox space.** ANATOMIST'S SNUFFBOX.

snuf·fles, *n.* Serosanguinous nasal discharge containing spirochetes; one of the early clinical manifestations of congenital syphilis.

soap, *n.* A salt of one or more higher fatty acids with an alkali or metal. Soaps may be divided into two classes, soluble and insoluble. Soluble soaps are detergent and usually are prepared from the alkali metals sodium and potassium. Insoluble soaps are salts of the fatty acids and metals of other groups. Soap (soluble) is used chiefly as a detergent. In constipation, a solution of soap forms a useful enema. In skin conditions, soap is useful not only as a detergent but also because it softens the horny layer of the epidermis and is germicidal. In pharmacy, soap is used as an emulsifying agent when the mixture is intended for external use. Soap is also used in making liniments and plasters. See also *green soap, hard soap.*

soap·bark, *n.* QUILLAJA.

soap liniment. CAMPHOR AND SOAP LINIMENT.

soap·wort (soap'wurt) *n.* *SAPONARIA OFFICINALIS.*

sob, *n. & v.* 1. A convulsive inspiration due to contraction of the diaphragm and spasmodic closure of the glottis. 2. To inspire convulsively.

so·cal·o·in (so·kal'o·in) *n.* Aloin obtained from Socotrine aloes.

so·cia (so'shee·uh) *n.* [L., fem. of *socius,* accompanying, companion]. A detached part of an organ.

so·cial (so'shul) *adj.* [L. *socialis,* from *socius,* companion, associate]. 1. Gregarious; growing near, or together. 2. Of or pertaining to society.

social adaptation. The process whereby an individual or group comes to meet without undue strain the usual demands of society at large, so as to survive and function well.

social adjustment. 1. An individual's harmonious relationship, or establishment thereof, with his social environment. 2. The process of modifying the demands and behavior of persons interacting with each other so that a harmonious relationship can be established and maintained.

social anthropology. CULTURAL ANTHROPOLOGY.

social deprivation. The condition of lacking or being deprived of certain cultural and educational experiences and opportunities that are deemed essential for normal social and mental development by the majority of the society of which the individual is a member. This may result in pseudoretardation.

so·cial·iza·tion (so"shul·i·zay'shun) *n.* *In psychology,* the process whereby a child learns to get along with and behave similarly to other people in his group, largely through imitation as well as the pressures of group life; the process of becoming a social being.

socialized drive. A drive which has been converted or channeled as a result of social experience into socially accepted ways. See also *socialization.*

socialized medicine. The control, direction, and financing of the medical care of a population by an organized group, a state, or a nation; assumption of legal, administrative, and financial responsibility for the practice of medicine by professional services and for the total care of the patients, with funds derived usually from assessment, philanthropy, and taxation. Compare *state medicine.*

social maladjustment. The inability of an individual or group to meet the demands of the social environment or of society at large, so that the relationship between them is strained and unsatisfactory.

social medicine. An approach to the maintenance and advancement of health and the prevention, amelioration, and cure of disease, which has its foundation in the study of man, his heredity, and his environment. Compare *socialized medicine.*

social orientation. 1. *In psychology,* the attitude taken by an individual toward the general customs, aspirations, and ethics of a social group. 2. The general direction of the behavior of a social group.

social psychiatry. Psychiatry especially concerned with the study of social influences on the cause and dynamics of emotional and mental illness, the use of the social environment in treatment, and preventive community programs, as well as the application of psychiatry to social issues, industry, law, education, and other such activities and organizations.

social service or **work.** Activity, usually organized and directed by a professionally skilled individual, which seeks to help individuals or groups through their environmental situation.

so·cia pa·rot·i·dis (so'shee·uh, so'see·uh pa·rot'i·dis) [L.]. ACCESSORY PAROTID GLAND.

socia pa·ro·tis (pa·rot'is). ACCESSORY PAROTID GLAND.

socio-. A combining form meaning *social, society.*

so·cio·bi·ol·o·gy (so"see·o·bye·ol'uh·jee, so"shee·o·) *n.* The branch of biology dealing with the biological, especially genetic, determinants of social behavior.

sociological criminology. The study of the criminal in relation to his social environment.

so·ci·ol·o·gy (so"see·ol'uh·jee, so"shee·) *n.* [*socio-* + *-logy*]. The science of mutual relations of people and of social organization. —**so·cio·log·i·cal** (so"see·o·loj'i·kul, so"shuh·) *adj.*

so·cio·med·i·cal (so"see·o·med'i·kul, so"shee·) *adj.* Pertaining to the relationship between social welfare and medicine.

so·cio·path (so'see·o·path, so'shee·) *n.* [*socio-* + *-path*]. An individual with a sociopathic personality disturbance, similar to a psychopathic personality but connoting a pathologic and usually hostile attitude toward society. —**so·cio·path·ic** (so"see·o·path'ick, so"shee·) *adj.*

sociopathic personality disturbance. *In psychiatry,* a personality disorder characterized primarily in terms of the pathologic relationship between the individual and the society and the moral and cultural environment in which he lives, as well as personal discomfort and poor relationships with others. Sociopathic reactions may be symptomatic of severe personality disorders, psychoneurotic or psychotic disorders, or organic brain syndrome, the recognition of which then forms the basic diagnosis. See also *antisocial personality, dyssocial behavior, sexual deviation.*

sock·et, *n.* 1. The concavity into which a movable part is inserted. 2. The space in a jawbone in which a root of a tooth is held.

so·cor·dia (so·kor'dee·uh) *n.* [L., folly]. HALLUCINATION.

So·co·trine aloe (so·ko'trin) [after *Socotra*]. Aloe obtained from *Aloe perryi.*

so·da (so'duh) *n.* [ML., barilla, a plant from which soda is obtained]. SODIUM CARBONATE.

soda ash. Commercial sodium carbonate; essentially anhydrous but containing more or less impurity.

soda lime. A mixture in granular form of calcium hydroxide with sodium hydroxide or potassium hydroxide or both. Used to absorb carbon dioxide in basal metabolism tests, during rebreathing in anesthesia machines, and in oxygen therapy.

soda lye. SODIUM HYDROXIDE.

so·da·mide (so'duh·mide, so·dam'ide) *n.* Sodium amide, $NaNH_2$, prepared by the interaction of sodium and gaseous or liquid ammonia; used in synthesis of various medicinals.

soda niter. SODIUM NITRATE.

soda water. Water charged with carbon dioxide gas.

Sö·der·bergh's pressure reflex. In extrapyramidal motor system disease, firm downward stroking of the ulna may be followed by flexion of the three medial fingers, firm downward stroking of the radius by flexion of the thumb.

sodio-. A combining form meaning *a compound containing sodium.*

so·di·um (so'dee·um) *n.* [NL., from *soda*]. Na = 22.9898. A metallic element, atomic number 11, of the alkali group of metals, which is light, silver-white, and lustrous when freshly cut, but rapidly oxidizes when exposed to air, becoming dull and gray. It violently decomposes water, forming sodium hydroxide and hydrogen. Sodium ion is of great importance biochemically, and sodium salts are extensively employed medicinally. Sodium ion is the least toxic of the metallic ions, and is therefore the base of choice when it is desired to obtain the effects of various acid ions. The majority of sodium salts occur as white or colorless crystals or as a white, crystalline powder, and are freely soluble in water. See also Table of Chemical Constituents of Blood in the Appendix.

sodium acetate. $CH_3COONa.3H_2O$. Used as a systemic and urinary alkalizer and, formerly, as a diuretic and expectorant.

sodium acetrizoate. Sodium 3-acetylamino-2,4,6-triiodobenzoate, $C_9H_5I_3NNaO_3$, a radiopaque contrast medium.

sodium acid phosphate. SODIUM BIPHOSPHATE.

sodium alginate. The sodium salt of alginic acid, a gelatinous substance obtained from various seaweeds. Sodium alginate dissolves in cold water to form a mucilage, and is used in pharmaceutical compounding for preparing suspensions.

sodium amide. SODAMIDE.

sodium ammonium phosphate. $NaNH_4HPO_4.4H_2O$; colorless crystals or white granules, freely soluble in water; used as a reagent for determination of magnesium and zinc. Syn. *microcosmic salt.*

sodium an·azo·lene (an·az'o·leen). 4-[(4-Anilino-5-sulfo-1-naphthyl)azo]-5-hydroxy-2,7-naphthalenedisulfonic acid trisodium salt, $C_{26}H_{16}N_3Na_3O_{10}S_3$, a diagnostic aid for estimating blood volume and cardiac output and a sensitive stain for the detection of proteins on polyacrylamide gels.

sodium an·ti·mo·nyl·glu·co·nate (an"ti·mo"nil·gloo'ko·nate). A trivalent antimony derivative of indefinite composition, prepared by interaction of a trivalent antimony compound, gluconic acid, and sodium hydroxide; a white, amorphous powder. Used in the treatment of schistosomiasis.

sodium antimony tartrate. ANTIMONY SODIUM TARTRATE.

sodium ascorbate. The sodium salt of ascorbic acid, used when parenteral therapy with ascorbic acid is indicated.

sodium au·ro·thio·mal·ate (aw"ro·thigh"o·mal'ate). GOLD SODIUM THIOMALATE.

sodium azide. NaN_3. A compound that has inhibiting action on many gram-negative bacteria and can be used to allow growth of gram-positive organisms in a mixture.

sodium barbital. The sodium salt of barbital.

sodium benzoate. C_6H_5COONa. Used as a diagnostic agent to test for liver function, also as an antimicrobial preservative.

sodium benzoate test. HIPPURIC ACID TEST.

sodium benzosulfimide. SODIUM SACCHARIN.

sodium biborate. SODIUM BORATE.

sodium bicarbonate. $NaHCO_3$. Used as a gastric antacid, to combat systemic acidosis, and to alkalinize urine.

sodium bicarbonate and calcium carbonate powder. SIPPY POWDER (1).

sodium bicarbonate and magnesium oxide powder. SIPPY POWDER (2).

sodium biphosphate. $NaH_2PO_4.H_2O$. Used as a urinary

acidifier. Syn. *sodium dihydrogen phosphate, monosodium orthophosphate, sodium acid phosphate.*

sodium bisulfite. $NaHSO_3$. The commercial article consists mainly of sodium metabisulfite, $Na_2S_2O_4$. Used as a chemical reducing agent.

sodium borate. $Na_2B_4O_7.10H_2O$. A detergent and emulsifier; also a weak antibacterial and astringent. Syn. *borax, sodium tetraborate.*

sodium bromide. NaBr. Formerly extensively used as a hypnotic, sedative, and antiepileptic drug.

sodium butabarbital. BUTABARBITAL SODIUM.

sodium cacodylate. Sodium dimethylarsonate, $Na(CH_3)_2$-$AsO_2.3H_2O$, formerly administered generally parenterally in a variety of ailments in which arsenic was believed beneficial.

sodium carbonate. Na_2CO_3. The anhydrous and monohydrate forms are used in various chemical and pharmaceutical procedures; sometimes for treatment of scaly skin, and as a detergent.

sodium carboxymethylcellulose. $ROCH_2COONa$, where R represents cellulose; a white to light-buff hygroscopic powder that forms viscous solutions with water. A synthetic hydrophilic colloid used to increase viscosity of aqueous systems, as a protective colloid, and in medicine as a colloid laxative and antacid.

sodium chloride. NaCl. Comprises over 90 percent of the inorganic constituents of blood serum; both of its ions are physiologically important. Used medicinally as an electrolyte replenisher.

sodium chloride injection. U.S.P. title for a sterile, isotonic solution of sodium chloride in water for injection, containing 0.9 g of sodium chloride in 100 ml. Used intravenously as a fluid and electrolyte replenisher, also as a solvent for many parenterally administered drugs. Syn. *isotonic sodium chloride injection.*

sodium chloride irrigation. U.S.P. title for a sterile solution of sodium chloride in purified water, containing 0.9 g of sodium chloride in 100 ml. Isotonic with body fluids; variously used as a physiological salt solution but not to be employed parenterally, for which purpose sodium chloride injection is used. Syn. *isotonic sodium chloride solution, normal saline solution, physiological salt solution, physiological sodium chloride solution.*

sodium chromate Cr 51. Sodium chromate in which part of the chromium is the radioactive isotope of mass number 51; used, as an injection, as a diagnostic aid in determining erythrocyte volume, total blood volume, plasma volume, and erythrocyte survival time, and also to detect gastrointestinal bleeding.

sodium citrate. $Na_3C_6H_5O_7.2H_2O$. Used to restore bicarbonate reserve of the blood in acidosis, to overcome excessive acidity of urine, and as a mild diuretic and expectorant. Employed also as an anticoagulant for blood to be fractionated or stored.

sodium cobaltinitrite. Sodium hexanitrocobaltate, Na_3Co-$(NO_2)_6$, used as a reagent for potassium.

sodium colistimethate. COLISTIMETHATE SODIUM.

sodium dehydrocholate. The sodium salt of dehydrocholic acid, used as a choleretic and as a diagnostic agent to determine circulation time.

sodium dextrothyroxine. DEXTROTHYROXINE SODIUM.

sodium diatrizoate. Sodium 3,5-diacetamido-2,4,6-triiodobenzoate, $C_{11}H_8I_3N_2NaO_4$, a roentgenographic contrast medium.

sodium dihydrogen phosphate. SODIUM BIPHOSPHATE.

sodium diphenylhydantoin. See *phenytoin.*

sodium diprotrizoate. Sodium 3,5-dipropionamido-2,4,6-triiodobenzoate, $C_{13}H_{12}I_3N_2NaO_4$, a radiographic contrast medium.

sodium dodecyl sulfate. A detergent commonly employed to dissociate proteins into their protomers. Abbreviated, SDS

sodium eth·a·sul·fate (eth″uh·sul′fate). Sodium 2-ethylhexyl sulfate, $C_8H_{17}NaO_4S$, an anionic surfactant used to facilitate expectoration by reducing the surface tension and viscosity of sputum.

sodium eth·yl·mer·cu·ri·thio·sal·i·cy·late (eth″il·mur·kew″ri·thigh″o·sal′i·si·late). THIMEROSAL.

sodium fluorescein. FLUORESCEIN SODIUM.

sodium fluoride. NaF. Used for fluoridation of water and also applied topically, directly to teeth, to reduce incidence of dental caries.

sodium flu·o·ro·ac·e·tate (floo″ur·o·as′e·tate). FCH_2COONa, a white powder, soluble in water; used as a rodenticide. Syn. *compound 1080.*

sodium fluo·sil·i·cate (floo″o·sil′i·kate). SODIUM SILICOFLUORIDE.

sodium fo·late (fo′late). $C_{19}H_{18}N_7NaO_6$; the form in which folic acid is prepared to obtain water-soluble solutions for injection; has the actions of folic acid.

sodium formaldehyde sulf·ox·y·late (sulf·ock′si·late). $HOCH_2SO_2Na.2H_2O$. It has been used as an antidote for poisoning by mercury bichloride.

sodium fu·si·date (few′si·date). The sodium salt of the steroid antibiotic fusidic acid.

sodium glucosulfone. *p,p′*-Sulfonyldianiline *N,N′*-diglucoside disodium disulfonate, $C_{24}H_{34}N_2Na_2O_{18}S_3$, a leprostatic drug and suppressant for dermatitis herpetiformis.

sodium glutamate. Monosodium L-glutamate, $HOOCCH$-$NH_2CH_2CH_2COONa$, used intravenously for symptomatic treatment of hepatic coma in which there is a high blood level of ammonia. Imparts a meat flavor to foods. Syn. *monosodium glutamate.*

sodium glycerophosphate. $Na_2C_3H_5(OH)_2PO_4.5\frac{1}{2}H_2O$. Formerly used as an ingredient of tonic formulations in the erroneous belief that glycerophosphate was utilized in synthesis of essential phosphorous compounds in nerve tissue.

sodium glycocholate. The sodium salt of glycocholic acid, usually containing also some sodium taurocholate; a constituent of the bile of man and of herbivora; has been used as a choleretic and cholagogue.

sodium gold thiosulfate. GOLD SODIUM THIOSULFATE.

sodium hexametaphosphate. A form of sodium metaphosphate.

sodium hydroxide. NaOH. Occurs as fused masses, small pellets, flakes, or sticks; used as a caustic, and in various chemical and pharmaceutical manipulations. Syn. *caustic soda.*

sodium hy·droxy·di·one suc·ci·nate (high·drock″see·dye′ohn suck′si·nate). Sodium 21-hydroxypregnane-3,20-dione succinate, $C_{25}H_{35}NaO_6$, a steroid that has hypnotic, mild analgesic, and, possibly, some amnesic action.

sodium hypochlorite solution. Contains 5% NaOCl; the solution has the germicidal value of its available chlorine. Used for disinfection of various utensils which are not injured by its bleaching action, such as clinical thermometers, glass, or chinaware. This solution is not suitable for application to wounds; for such use, diluted sodium hypochlorite solution, which contains 0.5% NaOCl and is nearly neutral, is employed.

sodium hypophosphite. $NaH_2PO_2.H_2O$. Formerly used as an ingredient of tonic formulations in the erroneous belief that hypophosphite was utilized in synthesis of essential phosphorus compounds in nerve tissue.

sodium hyposulfite. SODIUM THIOSULFATE.

sodium in·di·go·tin·di·sul·fo·nate (in″di·go·tin·dye·sul′fuh·nate). Disodium 3,3′-dioxo[$\Delta^{2,2'}$-biindoline]-5,5′-disulfonate, $C_{16}H_8N_2Na_2O_8S_2$, a purplish blue powder or blue granules; used parenterally as a diagnostic agent in determining renal function. Syn. *indigo carmine.*

sodium iodide. NaI. Used for the therapeutic effects of iodide ion, especially when intravenous administration is indicated, as in thyroid crisis and paroxysm of asthma.

sodium iodipamide. Sodium 3,3′-(adipoyldiimino)-bis[2,4,6-triiodobenzoate], $C_{20}H_{12}I_6N_2Na_2O_6$, a radiographic contrast medium.

sodium io·do·hip·pur·ate (eye·o″do·hip′yoo·rate). Sodium *o*-iodohippurate, $IC_6H_4CONHCH_2COONa$, a diagnostic agent used for radiography of the urinary tract.

sodium io·do·meth·a·mate (eye·o″do·meth·am′ate, meth′uh·mate). Disodium 1,4-dihydro-3,5-diiodo-1-methyl-4-oxo-2,6-pyridinecarboxylate, $C_8H_3I_2NNa_2O_5$, a radiopaque medium formerly used extensively, especially for intravenous urography and retrograde pyelography. Syn. *iodoxyl.*

sodium io·tha·lam·ate (eye″o·thuh·lam′ate, ·thal′uh·mate). Sodium 5-acetamido-2,4,6-triiodo-*N*-methylisophthalamate, $C_{11}H_8I_3N_2NaO_4$, a radiographic contrast medium.

sodium ip·o·date (eye′o·date). Sodium 3-(dimethylaminomethyleneamino)-2,4,6-triiodohydrocinnamate, $C_{11}H_{12}I_3N_2NaO_2$; administered orally for radiographic visualization of the biliary system. See also *calcium ipodate.*

sodium lactate. $CH_3CHOHCOONa$. For medicinal use prepared by neutralizing a solution of lactic acid with sodium hydroxide; used intravenously, in one-sixth molar solution, as a fluid and electrolyte replenisher. Indicated in the treatment of acidosis.

sodium lauryl sulfate. Chiefly $CH_3(CH_2)_{10}CH_2OSO_3Na$. Used as a wetting agent, emulsifying aid, and detergent; not affected by hard water.

sodium levothyroxine. LEVOTHYROXINE SODIUM.

sodium liothyronine. LIOTHYRONINE SODIUM.

sodium mandelate. $C_6H_5CHOHCOONa$. Formerly used as a urinary antiseptic.

sodium menadiol phosphate. MENADIOL SODIUM DIPHOSPHATE.

sodium mercaptomerin. MERCAPTOMERIN SODIUM.

sodium metabisulfite. $Na_2S_2O_5$; commonly, though incorrectly, called sodium bisulfite. A chemical reducing agent.

sodium metaphosphate. Any of several salts of the composition $(NaPO_3)_n$, where *n* is 2 or more; the most common is sodium hexametaphosphate, where *n* is 6. The salts occur as colorless, hygroscopic sticks, or white flakes or powder, soluble in water to form alkaline solutions. Sodium metaphosphates are used as water softeners.

sodium meth·io·dal (me·thigh′o·dal). Sodium monoiodomethanesulfonate, ICH_2SO_3Na, a radiopaque medium used for intravenous urography or retrograde pyelography.

sodium methohexital. METHOHEXITAL SODIUM.

sodium molybdate. $Na_2MoO_4.2H_2O$. Used as a reagent, especially for alkaloids.

sodium molybdophosphate. SODIUM PHOSPHOMOLYBDATE.

sodium mor·rhu·ate (mor′oo·ate). A mixture of the sodium salts of the saturated and unsaturated fatty acids occurring in cod liver oil; occurs as a pale, yellowish, granular powder; soluble in water. Used as a sclerosing agent for obliteration of varicose veins.

sodium nicotinate. $C_5H_4NCOONa.1\frac{1}{2}H_2O$. It has the actions and is used for the effects of niacin (nicotinic acid), especially when the latter is to be administered by injection.

sodium nitrate. $NaNO_3$. Formerly used in the treatment of dysentery. Syn. *Chile saltpeter, soda niter.*

sodium nitrite. $NaNO_2$. A vasodilator that has been variously used where this action of nitrite ion was indicated. Used as an antidote to cyanide poisoning, by virtue of conversion of hemoglobin by nitrite to methemoglobin, which combines with cyanide to form cyanmethemoglobin. Also used as a reagent.

sodium ni·tro·fer·ri·cy·a·nide (nigh″tro·ferr″i·sigh′uh·nide). Sodium nitrosyl pentacyanoferrate (III), $Na_2Fe(CN)_5NO.2H_2O$, ruby-red transparent crystals. Used as a reagent for the detection of many organic compounds. Formerly used for treatment of hypertensive crises. Syn. *sodium nitroprusside.*

sodium nitroprusside. SODIUM NITROFERRICYANIDE.

sodium oleate. Approximately $C_{17}H_{33}COONa$; formerly used as a choleretic agent.

sodium para-aminobenzoate. The sodium salt of para-aminobenzoic (aminobenzoic) acid.

sodium para-aminosalicylate. The sodium salt of para-aminosalicylic (aminosalicylic) acid.

sodium pentobarbital. PENTOBARBITAL SODIUM.

sodium pentobarbitone. PENTOBARBITAL SODIUM.

sodium Pentothal. PENTOTHAL SODIUM.

sodium perborate. $NaBO_3.4H_2O$. Used as a locally applied anti-infective agent; functions by virtue of decomposition to hydrogen peroxide and release of oxygen.

sodium peroxide. Na_2O_2. The sodium compound analogous to hydrogen peroxide; a powerful oxidizing agent. It has been used for treatment of acne, applied in the form of a paste prepared with liquid petrolatum, or as a soap to remove comedones. Syn. *sodium superoxide.*

sodium phenobarbital. PHENOBARBITAL SODIUM.

sodium phenolsulfonate. $HOC_6H_4SO_3Na.2H_2O$. It has been used internally and externally for supposed antiseptic action. Syn. *sodium sulfocarbolate.*

sodium phosphate. $Na_2HPO_4.7H_2O$. Used as a mild saline cathartic; also beneficial in the treatment of lead poisoning. Syn. *dibasic sodium phosphate, disodium hydrogen phosphate.*

sodium phosphomolybdate. $Na_3PO_4.12MoO_3$. Used as a reagent in various tests. Syn. *sodium molybdophosphate.*

sodium phosphotungstate. $Na_2O.P_2O_5.12WO_3.18H_2O$. Used as a reagent in various tests.

sodium polystyrene sulfonate. A cation exchange resin that exchanges its sodium for potassium and is used in the treatment of hyperkalemia.

sodium-potassium pump. SODIUM PUMP.

sodium propionate. CH_3CH_2COONa. A salt with antibacterial and fungicidal properties; used in the control of athlete's foot, tinea cruris, and other mycoses.

sodium pump. An intramembranous active transport system in most resting cells that selectively expels sodium while allowing the simultaneous concentration of potassium within the cell, using energy derived from hydrolysis of adenosine triphosphate. Syn. *sodium-potassium pump.*

sodium pyrosulfite. The International Pharmacopoeia name for sodium metabisulfite; commonly, though incorrectly, known as sodium bisulfite.

sodium rhodanate. SODIUM THIOCYANATE.

sodium ric·i·nate (ris′i·nate). A mixture of the sodium salts of the fatty acids from castor oil, chiefly ricinoleic acid; has been used to detoxify bacterial toxins in various forms of intestinal intoxication. Syn. *sodium ricinoleate.*

sodium ric·in·ole·ate (ris″in·o′lee·ate). SODIUM RICINATE.

sodium rose bengal I 131. ROSE BENGAL SODIUM I 131.

sodium saccharin. The sodium salt of saccharin.

sodium salicylate. HOC_6H_4COONa. Used as an analgesic, antirheumatic, and antipyretic.

sodium silicate. Any of several compounds representing combinations of Na_2O and SiO_2, as Na_2SiO_3, $Na_6Si_2O_7$, and $Na_2Si_3O_7$, with variable amounts of water. They occur as colorless to white or grayish-white crystal-like pieces or lumps, insoluble or very slightly soluble in cold water, but dissolved by heating with water under pressure. The common sodium silicate solution contains about 40% $Na_2Si_3O_7$. In medicine it has been used as a dressing in fractures, and as a detergent.

sodium silicofluoride. Na_2SiF_6. Used as a source of fluoride in fluoridation of municipal water supplies, and as an insecticide and rodenticide. Syn. *sodium fluosilicate.*

sodium stearate. A soap comprised of varying proportions of sodium stearate ($NaC_{18}H_{35}O_2$) and sodium palmitate

($NaC_{16}H_{31}O_2$). Used as a lubricant in manufacturing tablets, and as a detergent.

sodium stibo·glu·co·nate (stib''o·gloo'ko·nate). A pentavalent antimony derivative, of indefinite composition, prepared by interaction of a pentavalent inorganic antimony compound, gluconic acid, and sodium hydroxide; a colorless powder, soluble in water. Used in the treatment of leishmaniasis.

sodium succinate. $NaOOCCH_2CH_2COONa$. Has been variously used in medicine, formerly in treatment of catarrhal jaundice, gall stones, and infection of gall bladder or bile ducts.

sodium sulfate. $Na_2SO_4.10H_2O$. In large doses, an efficient hydragogue cathartic; in smaller doses, mildly laxative and diuretic. Syn. *Glauber's salt.*

sodium sulfite. $Na_2SO_3.7H_2O$, prepared also in anhydrous form. It has been used for treatment of parasitic skin diseases; variously used as a chemical reducing agent.

sodium sulfobromophthalein. SULFOBROMOPHTHALEIN SODIUM.

sodium sulfocarbolate. SODIUM PHENOLSULFONATE.

sodium sulfocyanate. SODIUM THIOCYANATE.

sodium sulfoxone. SULFOXONE SODIUM.

sodium su·per·ox·ide (sue''pur·ock'side). SODIUM PEROXIDE.

sodium suramin. SURAMIN SODIUM.

sodium tartrate. $Na_2C_4H_4O_6.2H_2O$. Formerly used as a laxative.

sodium taurocholate. The sodium salt of taurocholic acid, usually containing also some sodium glycocholate; a constituent of the bile of carnivora; a yellowish-gray powder, soluble in water: used as a choleretic and cholagogue.

sodium tet·ra·bo·rate (tet''ruh·bo'rate). SODIUM BORATE.

sodium thiamylal. THIAMYLAL SODIUM.

sodium thiocyanate. NaSCN. Formerly employed for the treatment of hypertension but no longer used because of its toxicity. Syn. *sodium rhodanate, sodium sulfocyanate.*

sodium thiopental. THIOPENTAL SODIUM.

sodium thiosulfate. $Na_2S_2O_3.5H_2O$. Used as an antidote, with sodium nitrite, to cyanide poisoning, as a topical application in the treatment of tinea versicolor, and as a prophylactic agent, in foot baths, against ringworm infection. Also used as a reagent. Syn. *sodium hyposulfite.*

sodium tung·state (tung'state). $Na_2WO_4.2H_2O$. Used as a reagent in various tests.

sodium valproate. VALPROATE SODIUM.

sodium warfarin. WARFARIN SODIUM.

so·do·ku (so'do·koo, so·do'koo) *n.* [Japanese *so,* rat, + *doku,* poison]. A disease caused by *Spirillum minus,* usually transmitted by rat bite, and characterized by an indurated ulcer at the site of inoculation, regional lymphadenitis, relapsing fever, and skin rash. Syn. *spirillary rat-bite fever.*

sod·om·ist (sod'um·ist) *n.* A person who practices sodomy.

sod·om·ite (sod'uh·mite) *n.* SODOMIST.

sod·omy (sod'um·ee) *n.* [after *Sodom,* where it is said to have been practiced]. 1. Sexual intercourse by the anus, usually considered as between males. Compare *pederasty.* 2. BESTIALITY (2).

Soem·mer·ing's bone (zœm'ur·ing) [S. T. *Soemmering,* German anatomist, 1755–1830]. MARGINAL PROCESS.

Soemmering's foramen [S. T. *Soemmering*]. FOVEA CENTRALIS.

Soemmering's ganglion [S. T. *Soemmering*]. SUBSTANTIA NIGRA.

Soemmering's nerve [S. T. *Soemmering*]. PUDENDAL NERVE.

Soemmering's ring cataract [S. T. *Soemmering*]. A doughnut-shaped ring behind the pupil consisting of lens remnant and capsule, which can develop following extracapsular lens extraction or following injury to the lens.

Soemmering's spot [S. T. *Soemmering*]. MACULA LUTEA.

Soflens. A trademark for polymacon, a contact lens material.

soft cataract. A cataract, occurring especially in the young, in which the cortex of the lens is of soft consistency and milky in appearance, but the nucleus is relatively unaffected.

soft chancre. CHANCROID.

Softcon. A trademark for vifilcon A, a hydrophilic contact lens material.

soft diet. A diet consisting of easily consumed, easily digested foods.

soft·en·ing, *n.* The process of becoming less cohesive, firm, or resistant.

soft palate. The posterior part of the palate which consists of an aggregation of muscles, the tensor veli palatini, levator veli palatini, azygos uvulae, palatoglossus, and palatopharyngeus, and their covering mucous membrane. NA *palatum molle.*

soft pulse. A pulse that is readily compressed.

soft rays. Roentgen rays coming from a tube operated on a relatively low voltage; they are readily absorbed. Contr. *hard rays.*

soft soap liniment. Green soap tincture. See *green soap.*

soft sore. A lesion of chancroid, caused by *Hemophilus ducreyi.*

soja bean (soy'uh, so'juh). SOYBEAN.

sol, *n.* [from *sol*ution]. A colloidal solution consisting of a suitable dispersion medium, which may be gas, liquid, or solid, and the colloidal substance, the disperse phase, which is distributed throughout the dispersion medium. The disperse phase may be gas, liquid, or solid. See also *hydrosol, alcosol, aerosol.*

sol. Abbreviation for *solution* (1).

So·la·na·ce·ae (so''luh·nay'see·ee, sol''uh·) *n.pl.* A family of herbs, shrubs, and trees comprising approximately 75 genera and 1,800 species and including the potato and tomato plants, and also plants from which are derived such drugs as belladonna, hyoscyamus, scopola, and stramonium. —**solana·ceous** (·shus) *adj.*

So·la·num (so·lay'num) *n.* [L., nightshade]. A genus of the Solanaceae, including the tomato, potato, bittersweet, and black nightshade.

so·lap·sone (so·lap'sone) *n.* A preparation consisting chiefly of the hydrated tetrasodium salt of 4,4'-di(3-phenyl-1,3-disulfopropylamino) diphenylsulfone, $C_{30}H_{28}O_{14}N_2S_5Na_4$, which is related structurally to dapsone. Used in the treatment of leprosy.

so·lar (so'lur) *adj.* [L. *solaris,* from *sol,* sun]. 1. Pertaining to or derived from the sun. 2. Analogous to or resembling the sun.

solar cautery. A glass or lens for concentrating the sun's rays upon tissue to be cauterized.

solar dermatitis. Any skin eruption caused by exposure to the sun, excluding sunburn; it may be plaque-like, eczematous, papular, or erythematous.

solar energy. Energy derived directly from the sun.

so·lar·iza·tion (so''lur·i·zay'shun) *n.* The application of solar or ultraviolet light for therapeutic purposes. —**so·lar·ize** (so'lur·ize) *v.*

solar photophthalmia. SNOW BLINDNESS.

solar plexus. CELIAC PLEXUS.

solar radiation. Radiation from the sun.

solar retinitis. Retinal change from the effect of sunlight.

solar spectrum. The spectrum afforded by the refraction of sunlight.

solar therapy. Treatment of disease by exposing the body to the direct rays of the sun. Syn. *heliotherapy.*

sol·a·tion (sol·ay'shun) *n.* Conversion of a gel into a sol.

soldier fly. *HERMETIA.*

soldier's heart. NEUROCIRCULATORY ASTHENIA.

soldier's patches or **spots.** MILK SPOTS.

sole, *n.* [OF., from L. *solea,* sandal]. The undersurface of the foot between the heel and the toes. NA *planta.*

so·le·al (so'lee·ul) *adj.* Pertaining to the soleus muscle.

soleal line. A rough, oblique line on the upper part of the posterior surface of the shaft of the tibia; it gives attachment to the soleus muscle. Syn. *popliteal line.* NA *linea musculi solei.*

So·le·nog·ly·pha (so″le·nog′li·fuh) *n.* [Gk. *sōlēn,* channel, + E. *glyph,* vertical groove]. One of the two groups of the important venomous snakes; includes the families Crotalidae (pit vipers) and Viperidae (true vipers); characterized by tubular fangs which can be folded back along the upper jaw. Contr. *Proteroglypha, Aglypha, Opisthoglypha.*

sole·plate, *n.* END PLATE.

So·le·ra reaction. A test for thiocyanate in saliva which depends upon the liberation of iodine through the action of thiocyanate upon iodic acid.

so·le·us (so′lee·us) *n.,* L. pl. & genit. sing. **so·lei** (·lee·eye), [NL., from L. *solea,* sole, flatfish]. A flat muscle of the calf. NA *musculus soleus.* See also Table of Muscles in the Appendix.

soleus ac·ces·so·ri·us (ack·se·so′ree·us). A small anomalous muscle running from the head of the fibula to the medial surface of the calcaneus.

Solganol. Trademark for a suspension in oil of aurothioglucose, an antirheumatic gold preparation.

sol·id, *adj.* [L. *solidus*]. 1. Firm; dense; not fluid or gaseous. 2. Not hollow.

solid angle. *In dentistry,* an angle formed by the junction of three surfaces of a tooth or a cavity preparation.

solid carbon dioxide. Carbon dioxide in the solid form, commonly known as dry ice.

solid-cell carcinoma. RENAL CELL CARCINOMA.

so·lid·i·fi·ca·tion (suh·lid″i·fi·kay′shun) *n.* The act of becoming solid.

solid vision. The perception of relief or depth of objects obtained by binocular vision. Syn. *stereoscopic vision.*

sol·i·ped (sol′i·ped) *n.* [L. *sol*us, alone, + *-ped*]. An animal having a solid, undivided hoof, as the horse, donkey, or zebra.

sol·ip·sism (sol′ip·siz·um) *n.* [L. *sol*us, alone, + *ips*e, self, + *-ism*]. The philosophical doctrine that any organism can know only itself and its own conception of its environment, and hence that there is only subjective reality.

sol·i·tary (sol′i·terr″ee) *adj.* [L. *solitarius*]. 1. Single. 2. Existing separately; not collected together.

solitary cells of Meynert [T. H. *Meynert*]. Giant stellate cells arranged in a single row in layer IV of the visual area of the cerebral cortex. Syn. *cells of Meynert, giant stellate cells of Meynert.*

solitary enchondroma. ENCHONDROMA.

solitary exostosis. EXOSTOSIS CARTILAGINEA.

solitary fasciculus or **tract.** A tract in the medulla formed by visceral afferent fibers contributed by the seventh, ninth, and tenth nerves which bends caudally to form a descending bundle and terminates in the dorsal sensory nucleus of the vagus and the nucleus of the solitary tract. NA *tractus solitarius.*

solitary follicles or **nodules.** Minute lymph nodules in the mucous membrane of the small intestine and the colon. NA *folliculi lymphatici solitarii.*

solitary lymphatic follicle or **nodule.** A lymphatic nodule which occurs outside of lymph nodes, in such organs as the small intestine.

sol·lu·nar (sole″loo′nur, sol″) *adj.* Influenced by, or relating to, the sun and the moon.

Sol·o·mon's rule [G. *Solomon,* U.S. pharmacologist, 20th century]. A rule to determine dosage of medicine for children; specifically, dose = age of child in months, multiplied by the adult dose, divided by 150.

Sol·pu·gi·da (sol·pew′ji·duh) *n.pl.* [NL., from L. *solpuga,* a venomous spider]. An order of the Arachnida which are hairy and spiderlike in external appearance but in structure show closer relationship to the scorpions. They lack poison glands, but have powerful fangs capable of inflicting severe wounds that are liable to secondary infections. They live in warm countries in sandy regions, as in the southwestern United States.

sol·u·bil·i·ty (sol″yoo·bil′i·tee) *n.* The extent to which a substance (solute) dissolves in a liquid (solvent) to produce a homogeneous system (solution). The degree of solubility is the concentration of a saturated solution at a given temperature.

solubility product. The product of the concentrations (or activities) of the ions of a substance in a saturated solution of the substance, each concentration term being raised to the power equal to the number of ions represented in a molecule of the substance.

sol·u·bi·lize (sol′yoo·bi·lize) *v.* To make soluble. —**sol·u·bi·li·za·tion** (sol″yoo·bi·li·zay′shun) *n.*

sol·u·ble (sol′yoo·bul) *adj.* [L. *solubilis,* from *solvere,* to loosen]. Capable of mixing with a liquid (dissolving) to form a homogeneous mixture (solution).

soluble barbital. BARBITAL SODIUM.

soluble ferric citrate. FERRIC AMMONIUM CITRATE.

soluble ferric oxide. SACCHARATED IRON OXIDE.

soluble fluorescein. FLUORESCEIN SODIUM.

soluble gluside. SODIUM SACCHARIN.

soluble guncotton. PYROXYLIN.

soluble iron phosphate. Soluble ferric phosphate, a ferric phosphate rendered soluble by sodium citrate; has been used as a hematinic.

soluble iron pyrophosphate. FERRIC PYROPHOSPHATE SOLUBLE.

soluble phenobarbital. PHENOBARBITAL SODIUM.

soluble RNA. TRANSFER RNA.

soluble saccharin. SODIUM SACCHARIN.

soluble starch. Starch transformed into water-soluble dextrins by heating.

so·lum tym·pa·ni (so′lum tim′puh·nigh) *n.* [L.]. The floor of the tympanic cavity.

so·lute (sol′yoot, so′lewt) *n.* [L., *solutus,* from *solvere,* to loosen, dissolve]. The dissolved substance in a solution.

so·lu·tion (suh·lew′shun) *n.* [L. *solutio,* a loosing]. 1. A homogeneous mixture of a solid, liquid, or gaseous substance (the solute) in a liquid (the solvent) from which the dissolved substance can be recovered by crystallization or other physical processes. The formation of a solution is not accompanied by permanent chemical change, and is thus commonly considered a physical phenomenon. Abbreviated, sol. 2. *In physical chemistry,* any homogeneous phase consisting of two or more compounds.

solution pressure. The tendency of molecules or ions to leave the surface of a solute and pass into the solvent. It varies in different solute-solvent combinations.

sol·vate (sol′vate) *n.* [*solv*ent + *-ate*]. A compound formed between solute and solvent in a solution.

sol·va·tion (sol·vay′shun) *n.* The process of forming a solvate.

sol·vent (sol′vunt) *n.* [L. *solvens,* from *solvere,* to loosen, dissolve]. 1. The component of a homogeneous mixture which is in excess. 2. A liquid that dissolves another substance (solute) without any change in chemical composition, such as sugar or salt in water. 3. A liquid that reacts chemically with a solid and brings it into solution, such as acids that dissolve metals.

sol·y·per·tine (sol″i·pur′teen) *n.* 7-{2-[4-(*o*-Methoxyphenyl)-1-piperazinyl]ethyl}-5*H*-1,3-dioxolo[4,5-*f*]indole, $C_{22}H_{25}N_3O_3$, an antiadrenergic compound; used as the tartrate salt.

so·ma (so′muh) *n.,* pl. **soma·ta** (·tuh), **somas** [Gk. *sōma,* body]. 1. The entire body with the exclusion of the germ cells. 2. The body as contrasted with the psyche. —Adj. *somatic.*

Soma. A trademark for carisoprodol, a centrally acting skeletal muscle relaxant.

somaesthesia. SOMESTHESIA.

somaesthetic. SOMESTHETIC.

somaesthetopsychic. SOMESTHETOPSYCHIC.

so·mas·the·nia (so″mas·theen′ee·uh) *n.* [*soma* + *asthenia*]. Bodily deterioration and exhaustion.

somat-, somato- [Gk. *sōma, sōmatos,* body]. A combining form meaning *somatic.*

so·mat·es·the·sia, so·mat·aes·the·sia (so″muh·tes·theezh′uh, ·theez′ee·uh) *n.* [*somat-* + *esthesia*]. SOMESTHESIA. —**soma·tes·thet·ic, somataes·thet·ic** (·thet′ick) *adj.*

so·mat·ic (so·mat′ick) *adj.* [Gk. *sōmatikos*]. 1. Bodily, corporeal. Contr. *psychic* (1). 2. Pertaining to the soma (1). Contr. *germ* (1). 3. Pertaining to the framework of the body and not to the viscera. Contr. *splanchnic.*

somatic agglutinin. Any agglutinin, such as O agglutinin, against somatic antigens.

somatic antigen. 1. Any antigen of gram-negative bacteria, located in the cell wall, consisting of complexes of carbohydrate, lipid, and a protein or polypeptide-like material. The carbohydrate determines the somatic O antigen specificity. 2. Any cellular protein or other component that is antigenic, in contrast to extracellular products or structures, such as capsules or flagella, exterior to the cell wall.

somatic-cell genetics. The study of genetic phenomena by means of somatic cells.

somatic cells. All the cells of the body except the germ cells.

somatic death. Death of the whole organism. Contr. *local death, molecular death.*

somatic layer. SOMATIC MESODERM.

somatic mesoderm. The external layer of the lateral mesoderm associated with ectoderm after formation of the coelom.

somatic mutation. A mutation during the course of development in a somatic cell, resulting in a mosaic condition.

somatic nerve. One of the nerves supplying somatic structures, such as voluntary muscles, skin, tendons, joints, and parietal serous membranes.

somatic nervous system. That part of the nervous system exercising control over skeletal muscle and relating the organism to its environment.

so·mat·i·co·splanch·nic (so·mat″i·ko·splank′nick) *adj.* [*somatic* + *splanchnic*]. SOMATICOVISCERAL.

so·mat·i·co·vis·cer·al (so·mat″i·ko·vis′ur·ul) *adj.* [*somatic* + *visceral*]. Pertaining to the body wall and the viscera.

somatic reduction. A condition in which the rate of somatic cell division exceeds that of chromosomal reduplication, and as a consequence the chromosome number of somatic cells is reduced.

so·ma·tist (so′muh·tist) *n.* A psychiatrist who holds any mental disorder to be of physical origin.

so·ma·ti·za·tion (so″muh·ti·zay′shun) *n.* [from *somatic*]. *In psychiatry,* the neurotic displacement of emotional conflicts onto the body, resulting in various physical symptoms or complaints; this may take the form of a conversion type of hysterical neurosis involving voluntary muscles and the sensory system, or it may express itself as a psychophysiologic disorder involving the autonomic nervous system and the viscera innervated by it. See also *psychophysiologic disorders.* —**so·ma·tize** (so′muh·tize) *v.*

somato-. See *somat-.*

so·ma·to·chrome (so′muh·to·krome, so·mat′o·) *n.* [*somato-* + *-chrome*]. *Obsol.* A nerve cell possessing a well-defined body completely surrounding the nucleus on all sides, the cytoplasm having a distinct contour, and readily taking a stain.

somatochrome cell. SOMATOCHROME.

so·ma·to·did·y·mus (so″muh·to·did′i·mus) *n.* [*somato-* + *didymus*]. SOMATOPAGUS.

so·ma·to·dym·ia (so″muh·to·dim′ee·uh) *n.* [*somato-* + *-dymia*]. The union of the trunks of conjoined twins.

so·ma·tog·e·ny (so″muh·toj′e·nee) *n.* [*somato-* + *-geny*]. The acquirement of bodily characteristics, especially the acquirement of characteristics due to environment. —**soma·to·gen·ic** (·to·jen′ick) *adj.*

so·ma·tol·o·gy (so″muh·tol′uh·jee) *n.* [*somato-* + *-logy*]. The study of the development, structure, and functions of the body. —**soma·to·log·ic** (·to·loj′ick) *adj.*

so·ma·tome (so′muh·tome) *n.* [Gk. *sōma,* body, + *-tome*]. An instrument for cutting transverse sections of an embryo.

so·ma·to·me·din (so″muh·to·mee′din) *n.* A protein formed in the liver which mediates the effects of growth hormone activity; appears to have anabolic and antilipolytic effects similar to those of insulin.

so·ma·to·meg·a·ly (so″muh·to·meg′uh·lee) *n.* [*somato-* + *-megaly*]. GIGANTISM.

so·ma·tom·e·try (so″muh·tom′e·tree) *n.* [*somato-* + *-metry*]. Measurement of the human body with the soft parts intact. —**soma·to·met·ric** (·to·met′rick) *adj.*

so·ma·to·mo·tor (so″muh·to·mo′tur) *adj.* [*somato-* + *motor*]. Pertaining to bodily movements or to the skeletal muscles and their innervation.

so·ma·top·a·gus (so″muh·top′uh·gus) *n.* [*somato-* + *-pagus*]. Conjoined twins with their trunks more or less in common.

so·ma·to·path·ic (so″muh·to·path′ick) *adj.* [*somato-* + *-pathic*]. Pertaining to an organic or bodily disorder.

so·ma·to·plasm (so′muh·to·plaz·um, so·mat′o·) *n.* [*somato-* + *-plasm*]. The protoplasm of the body cells; that form of living matter which composes the mass of the body, as distinguished from germ plasm, which composes the reproductive cells.

so·ma·to·pleure (so′muh·to·ploor, so·mat′o·) *n.* [*somato-* + Gk. *pleura,* side]. The body wall composed of ectoderm and somatic mesoderm. Contr. *splanchnopleure.* —**so·ma·to·pleu·ral** (so″muh·to·ploor′ul) *adj.*

so·ma·to·psy·chic (so″muh·to·sigh′kick) *adj.* [*somato-* + *psychic*]. Pertaining to both the body and mind.

so·ma·to·sen·sory (so″muh·to·sen′suh·ree) *adj.* [*somato-* + *sensory*]. Pertaining to bodily sensation.

somatosensory aura. A sensation of tingling, numbness, or of movement in a part of the body; may represent a focal seizure and be followed by a focal motor or generalized seizure.

so·ma·to·splanch·no·pleu·ric (so″muh·to·splank″no·ploor′ick) *adj.* Pertaining to the somatopleure and the splanchnopleure.

so·ma·to·stat·in (so″muh·to·stat′in, ·tos′tuh·tin) *n.* [*somato-* + *-stat* + *-in*]. A peptide with 14 amino acids connected by a disulfide bridge which inhibits growth hormone secretions in normal humans as well as excess growth hormone secretions found in acromegaly. It has also been found to exhibit suppressive effects on pancreatic insulin and glucagon secretions. Syn. *growth-hormone-release-inhibiting hormone.*

so·ma·to·stat·in·o·ma (so″muh·to·stat″i·no′muh) *n.* A tumor of delta cells of the islets of the pancreas which produces somatostatin; it may metasasize.

so·ma·to·ther·a·py (so″muh·to·therr′uh·pee) *n.* [*somato-* + *therapy*]. *In psychiatry,* the treatment of disease by means such as electric shock, chemotherapy, and other physical means. Contr. *psychotherapy.*

so·ma·to·to·nia (so″muh·to·to′nee·uh) *n.* [*somato-* + *-tonia*]. The behavioral counterpart of component II (mesomorphy) of the somatotype, manifested in desire for expenditure of energy through vigorous bodily assertiveness and the enjoyment of muscular activity. —**somato·ton·ic** (·ton′ick) *adj.*

so·ma·to·top·ag·no·sia (so″muh·to·top″ag·no′zhuh, ·zee·uh) *n.* [*somato-* + *topagnosia*]. AUTOTOPAGNOSIA.

so·ma·to·top·ic (so″muh·to·top′ick) *adj.* [*somato-* + *top-* + *-ic*]. Pertaining to the correspondence between a body part and a particular area of the cerebral cortex, or other region of the brain, to which sensory pathways from the body part are projected, or from which motor pathways to the part take origin.

so·ma·to·trid·y·mus (so″muh·to·trid′i·mus) *n.* [*somato-* + Gk.

tridymos, threefold]. A teratism in which three trunks or bodies are involved.

so·ma·to·tro·phin (so″muh·to·tro′fin, ·tot′ro·fin) *n.* SOMATOTROPIN.

so·ma·to·trop·ic (so″muh·to·trop′ick) *adj.* [*somato-* + *-tropic*]. Promoting growth.

somatotropic hormone. GROWTH HORMONE. Abbreviated, STH.

so·ma·to·tro·pin (so″muh·to·tro′pin, ·tot′ro·pin) *n.* [*somato-* + *tropin*]. 1. GROWTH HORMONE. 2. Purified growth hormone extracted from the human pituitary gland, used to stimulate linear growth in patients with growth hormone deficiency.

somatotropin-release-inhibiting factor. SOMATOSTATIN.

so·ma·to·type (so′muh·to·tipe, so·mat′o·) *n.* [*somato-* + *type*]. 1. The body type. 2. The quantitative description of the morphological structure of an individual by a series of three numerals representing the primary components: I endomorphy; II mesomorphy; III ectomorphy. On the behavioral level, these are termed viscerotonia, somatotonia, and cerebrotonia. See also *aplasia* (2), *dysmorphia, dysplasia, gynandromorphy, t component.*

so·ma·tro·pin (so″muh·tro′pin) *n.* [from *somatotropin*]. An unbranched polypeptide of 191 amino acids, $C_{990}H_{1529}N_{263}O_{299}S_7$, a growth stimulant.

-some [Gk. *sōma*]. A combining form meaning *body.*

som·es·the·sia, som·aes·the·sia (so″mes·theezh′uh, ·theez′ee·uh) *n.* [*soma* + *esthesia*]. Awareness of bodily sensations; consciousness of one's body.

som·es·thet·ic, som·aes·thet·ic (so″mes·thet′ick) *adj.* [*soma* + *esthetic*]. Pertaining to proprioceptive and tactile sensation.

somesthetic area. The receptive center for proprioceptive or tactile sensation in the postcentral gyrus: Brodmann's areas 1, 2, 3.

som·es·the·tog·no·sis (so″mes·theet″og·no′sis, ·es·thet″) *n.* SOMESTHESIA.

som·es·the·to·psy·chic, som·aes·the·to·psy·chic (so″mes·theet″o·sigh′kick, ·es·thet″o·) *adj.* [*somesthetic* + *psychic*]. Pertaining to the somesthetopsychic area.

somesthetopsychic area. The somesthetic association area of the parietal cortex: Brodmann's areas 5 and 7.

-somia [*soma* + *-ia*]. A combining form designating a *condition of the body or soma,* as nanosomia, macrosomia.

so·mite (so′mite) *n.* [Gk. *sōma*, body, + *-ite*]. A segment of the body of an embryo; one of a series of paired segments of the paraxial mesoderm composed of dermatome, myotome, and sclerotome. —**so·mit·ic** (so·mit′ick) *adj.*

somite cavity. The temporary lumen in a somite. Syn. *myocoele.*

somite embryo. An embryo during the period when somites are formed, approximately the twenty-first to the thirty-first days of development.

somn-, somno- [L. *somnus*]. A combining form meaning *sleep.*

som·nam·bu·lance (som·nam′bew·lunce) *n.* SOMNAMBULISM.

som·nam·bu·la·tion (som·nam″bew·lay′shun) *n.* SOMNAMBULISM.

som·nam·bu·la·tor (som·nam′bew·lay″tur) *n.* SOMNAMBULIST.

som·nam·bu·lism (som·nam′bew·liz·um) *n.* [*somn-* + L. *ambulare,* to walk]. 1. SLEEPWALKING. 2. The performance of any fairly complex act while in a sleeplike state or trance. 3. HYPNOTIC SOMNAMBULISM.

som·nam·bu·lis·me pro·vo·qué (som·nam·bew·lees′muh prov·o·kay′). HYPNOTIC SOMNAMBULISM.

som·nam·bu·list (som·nam′bew·list) *n.* One who walks in his sleep.

somni- [L. *somnium,* dream]. A combining form meaning (a) *dream;* (b) *sleep.*

som·ni·al (som′nee·ul) *adj.* [L. *somnialis,* from *somnium,* dream]. Pertaining to sleep or to dreams.

som·ni·a·tion (som″nee·ay′shun) *n.* [L. *somniare,* to dream]. Dreaming. —**som·ni·a·tive** (som′nee·uh·tiv, ·ay″tiv) *adj.*

som·nic·u·lous (som·nick′yoo·lus) *adj.* [L. *somniculosus*]. Drowsy; sleepy.

som·ni·fa·cient (som″ni·fay′shunt) *adj. & n.* 1. Producing sleep; HYPNOTIC (1). 2. A medicine producing sleep; HYPNOTIC (3).

som·nif·er·ous (som·nif′ur·us) *adj.* [L. *somnifer*]. Producing sleep.

som·nif·ic (som·nif′ick) *adj.* [L. *somnificus*]. Causing sleep.

som·nif·u·gous (som·nif′yoo·gus) *adj.* [*somni-* + L. *fugere,* to flee]. Driving away sleep.

som·nil·o·quence (som·nil′o·kwunce) *n.* SOMNILOQUY.

som·nil·o·quism (som·nil′o·kwiz·um) *n.* SOMNILOQUY.

som·nil·o·quist (som·nil′o·kwist) *n.* A person who talks in his sleep.

som·nil·o·quy (som·nil′uh·kwee) *n.* [*somni-* + L. *loqui,* to talk, + *-y*]. Talking in one's sleep.

som·nip·a·thist (som·nip′uh·thist) *n.* 1. A person with a sleep disorder. 2. A person susceptible to hypnotism or who is in a hypnotic state.

som·nip·a·thy (som·nip′uth·ee) *n.* [*somni-* + *-pathy*]. 1. Any disorder of sleep. 2. HYPNOTIC SOMNAMBULISM.

somno-. See *somn-.*

som·no·cin·e·mat·o·graph (som″no·sin″e·mat′o·graf) *n.* [*somno-* + *kinematograph*]. An apparatus for recording movements made during sleep.

som·no·form (som′nuh·form) *n.* An anesthetic formerly used consisting of ethyl chloride 60%, methyl chloride 35%, methyl bromide 5%.

som·no·lence (som′nuh·lunce) *n.* [L. *somnolentia,* from *somnolentus,* sleepy]. Drowsiness; semiconsciousness. —**som·no·lent** (·lunt) *adj.*

som·no·len·tia (som″no·len′chee·uh) *n.* [L.]. 1. The condition of being half awake and unsteady on one's feet, staggering about as if drunk. 2. SOMNOLENCE.

som·no·les·cent (som″no·les′unt) *adj.* 1. Drowsy. 2. Inducing drowsiness.

som·no·lism (som′nuh·liz·um) *n.* 1. HYPNOTISM. 2. A hypnotic trance.

som·nop·a·thist (som·nop′uh·thist) *n.* SOMNIPATHIST.

som·nop·a·thy (som·nop′uth·ee) *n.* SOMNIPATHY.

som·no·vig·il (som″no·vij′il) *n.* PSEUDOCOMA.

som·nus (som′nus) *n.* [L.]. SLEEP.

So·mo·gyi's method or **test** [M. *Somogyi,* U.S. biochemist, 1883–1971]. Either of two methods for detecting serum amylase: (a) Amylase of serum acts upon starch to form a reducing sugar which is determined by a quantitative technique. (b) A rapid clinical method in which the amyloclastic effect of amylase is measured by means of color reaction with iodine.

Somogyi unit [M. *Somogyi*]. A measure of diastase or amylase activity; the amount of diastase in 100 ml of plasma, serum, or urine necessary to produce 1 mg of copper-reducing substance from a starch substrate after 30 minutes of incubation at 40° C.

-somus [Gk. *sōma*, body, + *-us*]. A combining form designating *an individual with a* (specified) *form or condition of the body.*

son-, sono- [L. *sonus*]. A combining form meaning *sound.*

sone, *n.* [L. *sonus,* sound]. The unit of loudness.

son·i·ca·tion (son″i·kay′shun) *n.* Disruption with high-frequency sound.

Sonilyn. Trademark for sulfachlorpyridazine, a sulfonamide used in the treatment of urinary tract infections.

son·i·tus (son′i·tus) *n.* [L., noise]. TINNITUS.

Son·ne dysentery [C. *Sonne,* Danish bacteriologist, 1882–1948]. One of the commonest forms of bacterial intestinal infection, occurring often in epidemic form in children, caused by *Shigella sonnei.*

sono-. See *son-.*

sono·chem·is·try (son″o·kem′is·tree) *n.* The study of chemical reactions brought about by sound waves, especially those in the ultrasonic range. —**sonochem·ical** (·i·kul) *adj.*

sono·en·ceph·a·lo·gram (son″o·en·sef′uh·lo·gram) *n.* [*sono-* + *encephalo-* + *-gram*]. ECHOENCEPHALOGRAM.

sono·gram (son′o·gram) *n.* [*sono-* + *-gram*]. ECHOGRAM.

so·nog·ra·phy (so·nog′ruh·fee) *n.* [*sono-* + *-graphy*]. The making of a record or an anatomic depiction by means of ultrasound.

so·nom·e·ter (so·nom′e·tur) *n.* [*sono-* + *-meter*]. An instrument for determining the pitch of sounds and their relation to the musical scale.

sono·rous (so·no′rus) *adj.* [L. *sonorus*]. 1. RESONANT. 2. Characterized by a loud sound.

sonorous rale. A low-pitched, resonant, snoring sound heard on auscultation of the lungs in asthma and other bronchiolar diseases.

so·nus (so′nus, son′us) *n.* [L.]. SOUND.

soor (soor, sore) *n.* [origin unknown]. THRUSH (1).

so·phis·ti·ca·tion (suh·fis″ti·kay′shun) *n.* [ML. *sophisticare,* to adulterate, from Gk. *sophistikos,* sophistical]. The adulteration or imitation of a substance.

sopho·ma·nia (sof″o·may′nee·uh) *n.* [Gk. *sophos,* wise, + *-mania*]. Megalomania in which the patient believes himself to excel in wisdom.

So·pho·ra (suh·fo′ruh) *n.* [Ar. *ṣufayrā′*]. A genus of the Leguminosae, seeds of several species of which have been variously used medicinally but which are poisonous.

soph·o·rine (sof′o·reen, ·rin, so·fo′) *n.* A paralyzant, poisonous alkaloid, $C_{11}H_{14}N_2O$, which exists in the seeds of some species of *Sophora, Cytisus,* and *Baptisia.*

so·pite syndrome. A subtle variant of motion sickness characterized by yawning, drowsiness, and lack of interest in work and group activities; it may occur with or without associated classic signs of motion sickness.

so·por (so′pur) *n.* [L.]. Sleep, especially the profound sleep symptomatic of an abnormal condition, as in a stupor.

so·po·rate (so′puh·rate, sop′uh·rate) *v.* [L. *soporare,* to put to sleep]. 1. To stupefy. 2. To render drowsy.

so·po·rif·er·ous (so″puh·rif′ur·us) *adj.* [L. *soporifer*]. SOPORIFIC.

so·po·rif·ic (so″puh·rif′ick, sop″uh·) *adj.* & *n.* [F. *soporifique,* from L. *sopor,* sleepiness]. 1. Producing sleep. 2. NARCOTIC (1, 2).

so·po·rose (so′puh·roce) *adj.* [*sopor* + *-ose*]. 1. Sleepy; characterized by abnormal sleep; stuporous. 2. COMATOSE.

sor·be·fa·cient (sor″be·fay′shunt) *n.* & *adj.* [L. *sorbe*re, to suck in, + L. *facere,* to make]. 1. A medicine or agent that induces absorption. 2. Absorption-inducing.

sor·bic acid (sor′bick). 2,4-Hexadienoic acid, $CH_3CH{=}CHCH{=}CHCOOH$, from the berries of *Sorbus aucuparia,* European mountain ash; used as a mold and yeast inhibitor.

sor·bi·tan (sor′bi·tan) *n.* Sorbitol anhydride, $C_6H_{12}O_5$, various fatty acid esters of which, as sorbitan monolaurate and sodium monostearate, are used as surfactants.

sor·bite (sor′bite) *n.* SORBITOL.

sor·bi·tol (sor′bi·tol) *n.* D-Sorbitol or D-glucitol, $C_6H_{14}O_6$, a hexahydric alcohol isomeric with mannitol. Used intravenously as a diuretic; also as a humectant, sweetener, and vehicle for medicinal preparations.

sor·bose (sor′boce, ·boze) *n.* L-Sorbose, $C_6H_{12}O_6$, a ketohexose obtained by oxidative fermentation of D-sorbitol by certain organisms.

Sor·by's cell. A narrow-lumen glass receptacle used for the spectroscopic examination of blood, made of barometer tubing, both ends of which are accurately ground to parallel surfaces, one end being cemented to a small polished glass plate.

sor·des (sor′deez) *n.,* pl. **sordes** [L.]. Filth, dirt; especially the crusts that accumulate on the teeth and lips in continued fevers, consisting of oral debris, epithelium, food, and microorganisms.

sor·did, *adj.* [L. *sordidus,* dirty, from *sordes,* dirt]. *In biology,* of a dull or dirty color.

Sordinol. Trademark for clopenthixol, a tranquilizer.

sore, *adj.* & *n.* 1. Painful; tender. 2. An ulcer or wound.

sore·head, *n.* 1. AVIAN POX. 2. An allergic dermatitis on the forehead or face of sheep due to microfilariae of the species *Elaeophora schneideri.*

sore-mouth, *n.* ORF.

Soret bands. Three distinct absorption bands, designated α, β, and γ, in the visible range characteristic of reduced cytochromes during cellular respiration.

sore throat. Any painful inflammation of the pharynx.

sor·ghum (sor′gum) *n.* [NL., from It. *sorgo*]. A group of annual fodder grasses of the family Gramineae from which a sugar and syrup are obtained.

so·ro·ri·a·tion (so·ror″ee·ay′shun) *n.* [L. *sororiare,* to develop (breasts), from *soror,* sister]. The development that takes place in the female breasts at puberty.

sor·rel (sor′ul) *n.* [OF. *surele,* from *sur,* sour]. A plant of the genus *Rumex,* containing oxalates.

S.O.S. Abbreviation for *si opus sit,* if necessary.

S_2-OS interval. The interval between the second heart sound and the opening snap in mitral stenosis; shorter intervals correlate with more severe mitral stenosis.

so·ta·lol (so′tuh·lol) *n.* 4′-[1-Hydroxy-2-(isopropylamino)-ethyl]methanesulfonanilide, $C_{12}H_{20}N_2O_3S$, a beta adrenergic receptor antagonist; used as the hydrochloride salt.

so·ter·e·nol (so·terr′e·nol) *n.* 2′-Hydroxy-5′-[1-hydroxy-2-(isopropylamino)ethyl]methanesulfonanilide, $C_{12}H_{20}N_2O_4S$, a compound with adrenergic bronchodilator activity; used as the hydrochloride salt.

souf·fle (soo′ful, soofl) *n.* [F.]. A soft blowing sound or murmur heard on auscultation.

sou·ma (soo′muh) *n.* An acute infection in cattle, horses, mules, and sheep, caused by *Trypanosoma vivax,* marked by hemorrhages and serous exudates in the body cavities. It may become chronic, with anemia and subcutaneous edema.

¹sound, *n.* [OF. *sonde,* sounding line]. An instrument for introduction into a channel or cavity, for determining the presence of constriction, foreign bodies, or other abnormal conditions, and for treatment.

²sound, *n.* [OF. *son,* from L. *sonus*]. 1. The aspect of reality perceived by hearing, consisting objectively of vibrations conveyed to and stimulating the inner ear. 2. Any object of sensation peculiar to the sense of hearing.

sound pattern theory. The basilar membrane is supposed to vibrate as a whole, but with nodes, or lines of rest, in different places according to the pitch of the note.

Souques' sign (sook) [A. A. *Souques,* French neurologist, 1860–1944]. 1. Souques' finger sign: active elevation and extension of a paretic arm is followed by involuntary extension and spreading of the fingers. 2. Souques' leg sign: in striatal disease, when a patient seated in a chair is suddenly thrown backwards, the legs fail to extend as they normally do to maintain balance, due to loss of associated movements. 3. Kinesis paradoxica: the sudden and violent overexertion in walking and running observed in patients with parkinsonism who, because of generalized rigidity, are ordinarily inactive or slow to move.

South African genetic porphyria. PORPHYRIA CUTANEA TARDA HEREDITARIA.

South African tick-bite fever. One of the tick-borne typhus fevers of Africa.

South American blastomycosis. A chronic granulomatous disease of the skin and mucous membranes which may involve the lymph nodes and viscera. It is caused by *Blastomyces brasiliensis.*

South American leishmaniasis. AMERICAN MUCOCUTANEOUS LEISHMANIASIS.

Sou·they-Leech tube. SOUTHEY'S TUBE.

Southey's tube [R. S. *Southey,* English physician, 1835–1899].

A small cannula inserted subcutaneously into edematous tissues, usually of the lower extremities, for the purpose of draining fluid.

soy·bean, *n.* [Jap. *shō-yu,* soy]. The seed of *Glycine soja* (*Glycine hispida, Soja hispida*), a legume native to Asia but cultivated in other regions, including the United States, because of the high food value of its seeds. The bean and flour are used in dietetics for their high protein and relatively low carbohydrate content. The enzyme urease is obtained from soybean.

so·zo·io·do·late (so″zo·eye·od′o·late, ·eye′o·do·late) *n.* A salt of sozoiodolic acid.

so·zo·io·dol·ic acid (so″zo·eye″o·dol′ick). 2,6-Diiodophenol-4-sulfonic acid, $C_6H_2I_2(SO_3H)OH$, salts of which have been used as parasiticides and disinfectants.

sp. Abbreviation for (a) *spiritus,* spirit; (b) *species.*

S_{2P} Symbol for the pulmonic valve closure component of the second heart sound.

spa (spah) *n.* [after *Spa,* Belgium, which has mineral springs]. A mineral spring, especially one thought to have medicinal value and visited as a health resort.

space, *n.* [OF. *espace,* from L. *spatium*]. 1. A delimited area or region. 2. The realm outside or beyond the earth's atmosphere.

space maintainer. An orthodontic device used in spaces created by the loss of primary teeth to assure space availability for erupting teeth.

space medicine. A branch of medicine that deals with the physiologic effects, disturbances, and diseases produced in man by high-velocity projection through and beyond the earth's atmosphere, flight through interplanetary space, and return to earth.

space of Burns [A. *Burns,* Scottish anatomist, 1781–1813]. SUPRASTERNAL SPACE.

space of Dis·se [J. *Disse,* German anatomist, 1852–1912]. PERISINUSOIDAL SPACE.

space of Retzius [A. A. *Retzius*]. RETROPUBIC SPACE.

space of Tenon [J. E. *Tenon,* French anatomist and surgeon, 1724–1816]. EPISCLERAL SPACE.

space perception. The awareness of the spatial properties and relations of an object, or of one's own body, in space; especially, the sensory appreciation of position, size, form, distance, and direction of an object, or of the observer himself, in space.

space perception test. A psychological test used to measure the ability to estimate space differences.

space sense. The faculty of orienting environmental objects in space.

spaces of Lit·tré [A. *Littré*]. The spaces between the liver cell cords and the lining cells of the sinusoids; characteristically enlarged and filled with transudate in edema of the liver.

spaces of the iridocorneal angle. A series of small spaces formed by the interlacing of the connective tissue fibers of the framework of the peripheral processes of the iris, situated in the angle of the anterior chamber of the eye, and serving as a medium for the transudation of the aqueous humor from the posterior to the anterior chamber of the eye. Syn. *Fontana's spaces.* NA *spatia anguli iridocornealis.*

spaces of Virchow-Robin. PERIVASCULAR SPACES OF VIRCHOW-ROBIN.

Spacolin. Trademark for alverine, a smooth muscle spasmolytic drug used as the citrate salt.

spa·gyr·ic (spa·jirr′ick) *adj.* Pertaining to the chemical, alchemistic, or Paracelsian school of medicine. —**spag·y·rist** (spaj′i·rist) *n.*

spag·y·rism (spaj′i·riz·um) *n.* The Paracelsian, or spagyric, school or doctrine of medicine.

Spal·ding's sign [A. B. *Spalding,* U.S. gynecologist, b. 1874]. The radiographic finding in a fetus of overlapping of the skull bones at several sutures prior to the onset of labor, associated with the distinct signs of shrinkage of the cerebrum; diagnostic of fetal death.

Spal·lan·za·ni's law (spahl·lahn·tsah′nee) [L. *Spallanzani,* Italian physiologist, 1729–1799]. The regenerative power of cells is inversely related to the age of the individual.

spall·ation (spawl·ay′shun) *n.* [from *spall,* to break up with a hammer]. The process of bombarding various elements with extremely high-energy protons, deuterons, or alpha particles, whereby extensive alterations of the bombarded nucleus result.

Span. Trademark for a group of sorbitan esters used as surfactants and specifically identified by appending a number.

Span·ish collar. PARAPHIMOSIS.

Spanish fly. The beetle *Lytta vesicatoria,* from which the irritant cantharidin is derived, popularly regarded as an aphrodisiac.

Spanish pepper. PAPRIKA.

Spanish pox. SYPHILIS.

Spanish windlass. 1. An improvised tourniquet consisting of a handkerchief knotted around a limb and tightened by means of a stick which is twisted. 2. A temporary emergency method of making traction upon a splinted extremity, pull being provided by twisting the traction cords with a stick.

spar·a·drap (spăr′uh·drap) *n.* [It. *sparadrappo*]. A plaster spread on cotton, linen, silk, leather, or paper; adhesive plaster.

spare, *v.* To preserve from destruction, as in macular sparing.

spargana. Plural of *sparganum.*

spar·ga·no·sis (spahr″guh·no′sis) *n.,* pl. **spargano·ses** (·seez) [*sparganum* + *-osis*]. Infection with sparganum, which is a larval stage of the fish tapeworm *Diphyllobothrium latum.*

spar·ga·num (spahr′guh·num) *n.,* pl. **sparga·na** (·nuh) [NL., from Gk. *sparganon,* swaddling band]. A general name applied to the plerocercoid larva of *Diphyllobothrium,* especially if the adult form is unknown; also used (with initial capital and italicized) as a generic name.

Sparganum man·so·ni (man·so′nigh). A species of larva seen in the Far East, which is frequently found in the eye. Infection probably follows contact with freshly killed frogs.

Sparganum man·son·oi·des (man·sun·oy′deez). A species of larva that infects mice and has also been reported in the muscles and subcutaneous tissues of man.

Sparganum pro·lif·er·um (pro·lif′ur·um). A species of larva that proliferates in the tissues of the host by branching and budding off large numbers of spargana. The adult form is unknown.

spar·go·sis (spahr·go′sis) *n.* [Gk. *spargōsis,* from *spargan,* to swell]. Enlargement or distention, as of the breasts due to accumulation of milk.

Sparine. Trademark for promazine, a drug with antiemetic, tranquilizing, and analgesic-potentiating actions, used as the hydrochloride salt.

spark, *n.* A light flash, usually electric in origin, as that emanating from an electrode through which a current is passing.

spar·so·my·cin (spahr″so·migh′sin) *n.* An antibiotic, produced by *Streptomyces sparsogenes,* that has antineoplastic activity.

spar·te·ine (spahr′tee·een, ·in, spahr′teen) *n.* An alkaloid, $C_{15}H_{26}N_2$, obtained from *Cytisus scoparius;* formerly used, as the sulfate salt, for the treatment of cardiac arrhythmias, as an oxytocic drug for induction of labor at term, and for treatment of uterine inertia following onset of labor.

spasm (spaz′um) *n.* [Gk. *spasmos*]. A sudden involuntary muscular contraction.

spasmo-. A combining form meaning *spasm, spasmodic.*

spas·mod·ic (spaz·mod′ick) *adj.* [Gk. *spasmōdēs*]. 1. Of, pertaining to, or affected by spasm. 2. Occurring intermittently or fitfully. 3. Characterized by periodic outbursts of emotional or physical disturbances.

spasmodic croup. A respiratory disorder of young children with sudden onset at night of severe inspiratory dyspnea with crowing stridor and cough, frequently associated with an upper respiratory infection or external irritant.

spasmodic dysmenorrhea. Dysmenorrhea due to sudden and severe uterine contraction.

spasmodic laryngitis. SPASMODIC CROUP.

spasmodic stricture. A stricture involving the membranous urethra, caused by muscular spasm of the sphincter muscle, and usually associated with urethritis.

spasmodic torticollis. Torticollis occurring without other signs of neurological disease and characterized by an intermittent and arrhythmic or continuous spasm of the muscles of the neck, affecting women more than men, beginning in early or middle adult life, and having no known cause. The sternocleidomastoid and trapezius muscles are the muscles of the neck most prominently involved, causing a turning and tilting of the head, which may be slow and smooth, or jerky. Rarely the spasms spread to involve the muscles of the shoulder girdle, back, and limbs. Thought to be a restricted form of dystonia. Compare *congenital torticollis.*

spasm of accommodation. Excessive or persistent contraction of the ciliary muscle, following the attempt to overcome error of refraction. It simulates myopia.

spasm of the glottis. SPASMODIC CROUP.

spas·mo·lyg·mus (spaz″mo·lig′mus) *n.* [NL., from *spasmo-* + Gk. *lygmos,* hiccup]. 1. HICCUP. 2. Spasmodic sobbing.

spas·mo·lyt·ic (spaz″mo·lit′ick) *n. & adj.* [*spasmo-* + *-lytic*]. ANTISPASMODIC.

spas·mo·phe·mia (spaz″mo·fee′mee·uh) *n.* [*spasmo-* + *-phemia*]. STUTTERING.

spas·mo·phil·ia (spaz″mo·fil′ee·uh) *n.* [*spasmo-* + *-philia*]. A morbid tendency to spasms. —**spasmophil·ic** (·ick) *adj.*

spas·mous (spaz′mus) *adj.* SPASMODIC.

spas·mus (spaz′mus) *n.* [L., from Gk. *spasmos*]. SPASM.

spasmus bron·chi·a·lis (bronk″ee·ay′lis). ASTHMA.

spasmus glot·ti·dis (glot′i·dis). SPASMODIC CROUP.

spasmus mus·cu·la·ris (mus·kew·lair′is). A muscle cramp.

spasmus nic·ti·tans (nick′ti·tanz). WINKING SPASM.

spasmus nu·tans (new′tanz). A specific pendular nystagmus of infants accompanied by head-nodding and occasionally by wry positions of the neck. It affects both sexes, and begins between the fourth and twelfth months of life in most cases, never after the third year. The nystagmus may be horizontal, vertical, or pendular and is more pronounced in or limited to one eye. The cause is unknown and recovery is the rule.

spasmus oc·u·li (ock′yoo·lye). NYSTAGMUS.

spas·tic (spas′tick) *adj. & n.* [Gk. *spastikos,* drawing in]. 1. Pertaining to, or characterized by, recurrent and continuous spasms; produced by spasms. 2. Pertaining to spasticity. 3. Extremely tense, easily agitated, anxious; the opposite of calm and relaxed. 4. A person afflicted with spastic paralysis; particularly, a person suffering from a spastic form of cerebral palsy.

spastic abasia. PAROXYSMAL TREPIDANT ABASIA.

spastic aphonia. PHONIC SPASM.

spastic bladder. SPASTIC REFLEX BLADDER.

spastic bulbar palsy or **paralysis.** PSEUDOBULBAR PALSY.

spastic colon or **colitis.** IRRITABLE COLON.

spastic constipation. Constipation due to spasmodic increased tonus of the colon, as seen in such conditions as neurasthenia and lead poisoning.

spastic diplegia. 1. Spastic paralysis of all four limbs, more marked in the legs; due to cerebral disease. 2. A form of cerebral palsy, due mainly to prenatal or perinatal anoxia, but occasionally to other metabolic disorders of the perinatal period or to malformations or developmental defects; frequently associated with mental retardation and epilepsy. Syn. *cerebral spastic diplegia, Little's disease.*

spastic entropion. Eversion of one or both, and almost always of the lower, eyelids, caused by excessive contraction of the orbicularis muscle due to irritative lesions of the conjunctiva.

spastic flatfoot. A planovalgus deformity of the foot associated with spasm of the peroneal muscles.

spastic gait. 1. HEMIPLEGIC GAIT. 2. SCISSORS GAIT.

spastic hemiplegia. Paralysis of one side of the body characterized by spasticity of the affected extremities.

spastic ileus. A relatively uncommon form of ileus in which temporary obstruction is caused by segmental spasm of the intestine (the colon especially); seen usually in persons having an extremely nervous makeup, or in such conditions as heavy-metal poisoning, porphyria, or uremia. Syn. *dynamic ileus, hyperdynamic ileus.*

spas·tic·i·ty (spas·tis′i·tee) *n.* A state of increased muscular tonus tending to involve the flexors of the arms and extensors of the legs, associated with exaggerated tendon reflexes and a specific two-phased pattern of muscular response to stretch (the "clasp-knife" phenomenon). Compare *rigidity.*

spastic paralysis. A condition in which a group of muscles manifest increased tone, exaggerated tendon reflexes, depressed or absent superficial reflexes, and sometimes clonus, due to an upper motor neuron lesion.

spastic paraplegia. Paralysis of the legs with increased muscular tone and hyperactive tendon reflexes, clonus, and Babinski signs; seen in a variety of diseases that involve the corticospinal pathways in the spinal cord. See also *familial spastic paraplegia.*

spastic pseudosclerosis. CREUTZFELDT-JAKOB DISEASE (1).

spastic quadriplegia. Paralysis of both arms and legs with increased muscular tone and hyperactive deep tendon reflexes.

spastic reflex bladder. A reflex bladder that is contracted and spastic, with a limited capacity, and empties itself automatically at frequent and irregular intervals. See also *neurogenic bladder.*

spastic strabismus. Squint due to contracture of an ocular muscle, as in Duane's retraction syndrome.

spatia. Plural of *spatium.*

spatia an·gu·li iri·dis (ang′gew·lye eye′ri·dis) [BNA]. Spatia anguli iridocornealis (= SPACES OF THE IRIDOCORNEAL ANGLE).

spatia anguli iri·do·cor·ne·a·lis (eye″ri·do·kor·nee·ay′lis) [NA]. SPACES OF THE IRIDOCORNEAL ANGLE.

spatia in·ter·cos·ta·lia (in·tur·kos·tay′lee·uh) [BNA]. Plural of *spatium intercostale;* INTERCOSTAL SPACES.

spatia in·ter·glo·bu·la·ria (in″tur·glob·yoo·lair′ee·uh) [NA]. INTERGLOBULAR SPACES.

spatia in·ter·os·sea me·ta·car·pi (in·tur·os′ee·uh met·uh·kahr′pye) [NA]. Spaces between adjacent metacarpal bones.

spatia interossea me·ta·tar·si (met·uh·tahr′sigh) [NA]. Spaces between adjacent metatarsal bones.

spatia in·ter·va·gi·na·lia (in·tur·vaj·i·nay′lee·uh) [NA]. INTERVAGINAL SPACES.

spa·tial (spay′shul) *adj.* [L. *spati*um, space, + *-al*]. Of, pertaining to, or occupying space.

spatial discrimination. TWO-POINT DISCRIMINATION.

spatial orientation. The act of determining one's relation to space.

spatial summation. The cumulative effect of spatially distributed, virtually simultaneous stimuli converging on an excitable cell or tissue. Compare *temporal summation.*

spatial vectorcardiography. VECTORCARDIOGRAPHY.

spatia zo·nu·la·ria (zon·yoo·lair′ee·uh) [NA]. ZONULAR SPACES.

spa·ti·um (spay′shee·um) *n.,* pl. **spa·tia** (·shee·uh) [L.]. A space.

spatium epi·scle·ra·le (ep·i·skle·ray'lee) [NA]. EPISCLERAL SPACE.

spatium in·ter·co·sta·le (in"tur·kos·tay'lee) [NA]. INTERCOSTAL SPACE.

spatium pe·ri·cho·ri·oi·de·a·le (perr"i·kor·ee·oy"dee·ay'lee) [BNA]. Spatium perichoroideale (= PERICHOROIDAL SPACE).

spatium pe·ri·cho·roi·de·a·le (perr"i·ko·roy"dee·ay'lee) [NA]. PERICHOROIDAL SPACE.

spatium pe·ri·lym·pha·ti·cum (perr"i·lim·fat'i·kum) [NA]. PERILYMPHATIC SPACE.

spatium pe·ri·nei pro·fun·dum (perr·i·nee'eye pro·fun'dum) [NA]. The deep perineal space, a potential space between the superior and inferior fasciae of the urogenital diaphragm.

spatium perinei su·per·fi·ci·a·le (sue"pur·fish·ee·ay'lee) [NA]. The superficial perineal space, a potential space in the perineum superficial to the urogenital diaphragm.

spatium re·tro·pe·ri·to·ne·a·le (ret"ro·perr"i·to·nee·ay'lee) [NA]. RETROPERITONEAL SPACE.

spatium re·tro·pu·bi·cum (ret·ro·pew'bi·kum) [NA]. RETROPUBIC SPACE.

spat·u·la (spatch'oo·luh) *n.* [L., dim. of *spatha,* flat wooden instrument]. A flexible blunt blade; used for mixing or spreading soft materials, or facilitating the mixing of powders in a mortar by scraping. —**spatu·late** (·lut, ·late) *adj.*

spatulate finger. A particular type of broad finger, flattened at the tip.

spav·in (spav'in) *n.* [OF. *espavain*]. Disease of the hock of a horse.

spavin bog. An enlargement due to distention of the capsular ligament of the hock of a horse, prominent on the inner aspect of the joint.

spavin bone. An enlargement due to an exostosis of the tarsal bones of a horse, termed high or low depending on its position.

spay, *v.* [OF. *espeer,* to cut with a sword, from *espee,* sword]. To remove the ovaries of (an animal).

SPCA Abbreviation for *serum prothrombin conversion accelerator* (= FACTOR VII).

S.P.C.A. Society for the Prevention of Cruelty to Animals.

spear·mint, *n.* The dried and flowering tops of *Mentha viridis* or *M. cardiaca* containing a volatile oil (spearmint oil) that imparts a characteristic odor; both spearmint and its oil are used as flavors.

spe·cial·ist, *n.* A physician or surgeon who limits his practice to certain diseases, or to the diseases of a single organ or class, or to a certain type of therapy; in the United States, a diplomate of one of the American specialty boards in medicine, such as the American Board of Surgery.

special nurse. 1. A nurse trained in a particular specialty or field of therapy. Syn. *nurse specialist.* 2. A private duty nurse.

special pathology. Application of the laws of general pathology to individual organs or systems.

special sensation. Any sensation produced by the special senses. See also *sense.*

spe·cial·ty, *n.* A branch of medicine or surgery pursued by a specialist.

spe·cies (spee'sheez) *n.,* pl. **species** [L., appearance, model, kind]. 1. The basic unit of biological taxonomy: For sexually reproducing organisms, a species includes all members of a breeding population together with any other populations that could interbreed freely and productively with it (if geographical, temporal, social, or artificial barriers did not interfere). In the case of asexual organisms, individuals or populations are assigned to species on the basis of similarities—morphological, biochemical, ecological, behavioral, etc.—analogous to those that characterize sexually reproducing species. Compare *genus, subspecies.* 2. A specific kind of atomic nucleus, atom, ion, or molecule. 3. A name sometimes applied to certain mixtures of herbs used in making decoctions and infusions. Abbreviated, sp.

species specificity. The difference in physiologic response to one or more compounds by different species of animals.

spe·cif·ic (spe·sif'ick) *adj. & n.* [ML. *specificus,* from L. *species,* kind]. 1. Of or pertaining to a species, or to that which distinguishes a thing or makes it of the species to which it belongs. 2. Produced by a certain microorganism, as a specific disease. 3. Particularly adapted to its purpose, as a drug with a specific effect on disease. 4. A medicine that has a distinct remedial influence on a particular disease.

specific activity. The activity of a radioactive substance expressed on a unit weight or unit volume basis.

specific agglutination. The reaction between the suspension of an antigen (bacteria or cells) and its specific antiserum, leading to the clumping of the suspended elements. Used in the diagnosis of certain diseases, as the Widal test for typhoid.

specific birth rate. The birth rate calculated for categories such as sex, age of mother, social or economic group of parents, or any other variable or combination of variables.

specific death rate. The death rate calculated for categories such as age, sex, cause, or any other variable or combination of variables.

specific dynamic action. The stimulating effect upon the metabolism produced by the digestion of food, especially proteins, causing the metabolic rate to rise above basal levels.

specific gravity. The measured mass of a substance compared with that of an equal volume of another taken as a standard. For gases, hydrogen or air may be the standard; for liquids and solids, distilled water at a specific temperature. Abbreviated, sp. g., sp. gr. Compare *absolute density.*

specific heat. The amount of heat required to raise the temperature of 1 g of a substance 1°C.

specific immunity. Immunity directed against a specific antigen or disease, such as that conferred by previous exposure.

specific ionization. *In radiobiology,* the number of ion pairs produced per unit length of path of radiation, for example, per centimeter of air, or micrometer of tissue.

spec·i·fic·i·ty (spes"i·fis'i·tee) *n.* The quality of being specific.

specific nerve-sheath tumor. NEURILEMMOMA.

specific parasite. A parasite which lives only on hosts of a single species.

specific phase. *In immunology,* a phase characterized by the presence of flagellar antigens, agglutinated only by the homologous antiserum, for example, "phase one" of *Salmonella.*

specific reading disability. DEVELOPMENTAL DYSLEXIA.

specific rotation. The optical rotation, expressed in angular degrees, of a solution representing 1 g of solute in 1 ml of solution, and referred to a tube 1 dm in length.

specific soluble substance. A soluble, polysaccharide hapten or antigen obtained from the capsule of the pneumococcus; essential for pneumococcal pathogenicity and the basis of the immunological classification of the pneumococci into specific types. Abbreviated, SSS.

specific therapy. Use of a remedy having a selective effect against a specific etiologic factor or having a definite effect upon a particular disease.

specific urethritis. GONOCOCCAL URETHRITIS. Compare *nonspecific urethritis.*

specific volume. The volume occupied by a definite weight of a substance, as the volume in cubic centimeters of 1 g of substance.

spec·i·men (spes'i·mun) *n.* [L., example, model, from *specere,* to look]. A sample of anything that is selected for diagnosis, examination, study, or testing.

spec·ta·cles, *n.pl.* Framed or mounted lenses for aiding vision where there are optical or muscular defects of the eye. See also *lens.*

spec·ti·no·my·cin (speck″ti·no·migh′sin) *n.* A broad-spectrum antibiotic produced by *Streptomyces spectabilis.* Syn. *actinospectocin.*

spectra. A plural of *spectrum.*

spec·tral (speck′trul) *adj.* Of or pertaining to a spectrum.

spectro-. A combining form meaning *spectrum, spectral.*

spec·tro·col·or·im·e·ter (speck″tro·kul″ur·im′e·tur) *n.* [*spectro-* + *color* + *-meter*]. Combination of spectroscope and ophthalmoscope for the detection of color blindness to one spectral color.

spec·tro·gram (speck′tro·gram) *n.* [*spectro-* + *-gram*]. A graphical record of a spectrum.

spec·tro·graph (speck′tro·graf) *n.* A spectroscope which records a spectrum on a photographic plate.

spec·trom·e·ter (speck·trom′e·tur) *n.* [*spectro-* + *-meter*]. 1. Usually, a spectroscope provided with equipment for measuring the deviations of light and other electromagnetic rays, and therewith the wavelengths of spectral lines. 2. MASS SPECTROMETER. —**spectrome·try** (·tree) *n.*

spec·tro·mi·cro·scope (speck″tro·migh′kruh·skope) *n.* MICROSPECTROSCOPE.

spec·tro·pho·tom·e·ter (speck″tro·fo·tom′e·tur) *n.* [*spectro-* + *photo-* + *-meter*]. An apparatus for passing essentially monochromatic radiant energy (visible, ultraviolet, infrared, or other form) through a substance under examination, and measuring the intensity of the transmitted energy. The apparatus includes an energy source, a dispersing device to provide monochromatic radiation, and a sensor that measures the intensity of the incident and transmitted energy. —**spectrophotome·try** (·tree) *n.;* **spectro·pho·to·met·ric** (·fo″to·met′rick) *adj.*

spectrophotometric analysis. Identification and determination of substances through measurement of the absorption of the energy in the ultraviolet, visible, or infrared spectrum.

spec·tro·po·lar·im·e·ter (speck″tro·po″lur·im′e·tur) *n.* Combination of a spectrometer and polariscope; used for measuring optical rotation of solutions at different wavelengths.

spec·tro·scope (speck′truh·skope) *n.* [*spectro-* + *-scope*]. An instrument for dispersing radiations by various methods, such as a prism, diffraction gratings, and crystals, and for observing the resultant spectrum. —**spec·tro·scop·ic** (speck″tro·skop′ick) *adj.*

spec·tros·co·py (speck·tros′kuh·pee) *n.* [*spectro-* + *-scopy*]. 1. Study of spectra. 2. Use of the spectroscope.

spec·trum (speck′trum) *n.*, L. pl. **spec·tra** (·truh) [L., appearance, image, from *specere,* to look at]. 1. The series of components or images resulting when a beam of electromagnetic waves (such as electric waves, infrared, visible light, ultraviolet, or x-rays) is dispersed and the constituent waves are arranged according to their frequencies or wavelengths. 2. Figuratively, any series of entities arranged according to the quantitative variation of a given common property; a range.

spec·u·lum (speck′yoo·lum) *n.*, L. pl. **specu·la** (·luh) [L., mirror (rel. to *specere,* to look, and to *spectrum*)]. An instrument for dilating the opening of a cavity of the body in order that the interior may be more easily visible.

speech, *n.* 1. The production of vocal utterances in a language; the activity of speaking. 2. The utterances produced.

speech apraxia. BROCA'S APHASIA.

speech deafness. 1. AUDITORY APHASIA. 2. AUDITORY VERBAL AGNOSIA.

speech pathologist. A specialist dealing with defects in speech and language.

speech pathology. The science dealing with disorders of speech and language.

speed, *n.* In drug abuse terminology, AMPHETAMINE (2).

Spee's curve (shpey) [F. von *Spee,* German embryologist, 1855–1937]. CURVE OF SPEE.

spe·le·os·to·my (spee″lee·os′tuh·mee) *n.* [Gk. *spēlaion,* cavern, + *-stomy*]. CAVERNOSTOMY.

spel·ter shakes (spel′tur). METAL FUME FEVER.

Spen·cer-Par·ker vaccine [R. R. *Spencer,* U.S. physician, b. 1888; and R. R. *Parker*]. ROCKY MOUNTAIN SPOTTED FEVER VACCINE.

Speng·ler's fragments (shpeng′lur) [C. *Spengler,* Swiss physician, 1861–1937]. Small, spheroidal bodies found in the sputum of tuberculous patients.

Spens's syndrome [T. *Spens,* Scottish physician, 1764–1842]. STOKES-ADAMS SYNDROME.

sperm, *n.*, pl. **sperm, sperms** [Gk. *sperma,* seed]. 1. SPERMATOZOON; SPERMATOZOA. 2. Loosely, SEMEN.

sperm-, sperma-, spermi-, spermio-, spermo- [Gk.]. A combining form meaning *seed, sperm, semen.*

sper·ma·ceti (spur″muh·set′ee, ·see′tee) *n.* [L. *sperma ceti,* whale's sperm]. A waxy substance obtained from the head of the sperm whale *Physeter macrocephalus.* The chief constituents are cetyl palmitate and cetyl alcohol. Used to impart firmness to ointment bases.

sper·ma·cra·sia (spur″muh·kray′zhuh, ·zee·uh) *n.* SPERMATACRASIA.

sperm·al·ist (spur′mul·ist) *n.* A person who held the view that the miniature organism was preformed in the sperm cell rather than in the egg. Syn. *spermist.*

spermat-, spermato-. A combining form meaning (a) *spermatozoa;* (b) *spermatic, seminal.*

sper·ma·ta·cra·sia (spur″muh·tuh·kray′zhuh, ·zee·uh) *n.* [*spermat-* + Gk. *akrasia,* absence of mixture]. Deficiency or decrease of spermatozoa in the semen. Syn. *spermacrasia.*

sper·mat·ic (spur·mat′ick) *adj.* [Gk. *spermatikos*]. 1. Pertaining to the semen or spermatozoa; conveying semen. See also Plate 4. 2. Pertaining to the spermatic cord.

spermatic abscess. An abscess involving the seminiferous tubules.

spermatic artery. See Table of Arteries in the Appendix.

spermatic calculus. A calculus situated in the seminal vesicle, ductus deferens, or epididymis.

spermatic cord. The cord extending from the testis to the deep inguinal ring and consisting of the ductus deferens, the vessels and nerves of the testis and of the epididymis, and the accompanying connective tissue. NA *funiculus spermaticus.* See also Plate 4.

spermatic duct. DUCTUS DEFERENS.

spermatic filament. The axial filament of a spermatozoon.

spermatic hydrocele. Accumulation of spermatic fluid in the tunica vaginalis testis; caused by the rupture of a spermatocele.

sper·ma·ti·ci·dal (spur″muh·ti·sigh′dul) *adj.* SPERMATOCIDAL.

spermatic nerve. See Table of Nerves in the Appendix.

spermatic plexus. A visceral nerve plexus derived from the aortic and renal plexuses and running on each side with the internal spermatic artery to the testis. NA *plexus testicularis.*

sper·ma·tid (spur′muh·tid) *n.* [*spermat-* + *-id*]. A male germ cell immediately before assuming its final typical form.

spermato-. See *spermat-.*

sper·ma·to·cele (spur′muh·to·seel, spur·mat′o·) *n.* [*spermato-* + *-cele*]. Cystic dilatation of a duct in the head of the epididymis or in the rete testis. Rupture into the tunica vaginalis testis produces spermatic hydrocele.

sper·ma·to·ce·lec·to·my (spur″muh·to·se·leck′tuh·mee) *n.* [*spermatocele* + *-ectomy*]. Excision of a spermatocele.

sper·ma·to·ci·dal (spur″muh·to·sigh′dul) *adj.* [*spermato-* + *-cidal*]. Destructive to spermatozoa.

sper·ma·to·cide (spur′muh·to·side) *n.* [*spermato-* + *-cide*]. An agent that destroys spermatozoa.

sper·ma·to·cyst (spur′muh·to·sist, spur·mat′o·) *n.* [*spermato-* + *-cyst*]. SEMINAL VESICLE. —**sper·ma·to·cys·tic** (spur″muh·to·sis′tick) *adj.*

sper·ma·to·cys·tec·to·my (spur″muh·to·sis·teck′tuh·mee) *n.* [*spermatocyst* + *-ectomy*]. VESICULECTOMY.

sper·ma·to·cys·ti·tis (spur″muh·to·sis·tye′tis) *n.* [*spermatocyst* + *-itis*]. Inflammation of the seminal vesicles.

sper·ma·to·cys·tot·o·my (spur″muh·to·sis·tot′uh·mee) *n.* [*spermatocyst* + *-tomy*]. Surgical incision of a seminal vesicle.

sper·ma·to·cyte (spur·mat′o·site, spur′muh·to·) *n.* [*spermato-* + *-cyte*]. A cell of the last or next to the last generation of cells which divide to form spermatozoa.

sper·ma·to·cy·to·ma (spur″muh·to·sigh·to′muh, spur·mat″o·) *n.* [*spermatocyte* + *-oma*]. SEMINOMA.

sper·ma·to·gen·e·sis (spur″muh·to·jen′e·sis) *n.* [*spermato-* + *-genesis*]. The phenomena involved in the production of spermatozoa, sometimes restricted to denote the process of meiosis in the male. Compare *spermiogenesis.*

sper·ma·to·gen·ic (spur″muh·to·jen′ick) *adj.* [*spermato-* + *-genic*]. Producing spermatozoa, as the spermatogenic cells of the testis.

sper·ma·tog·e·nous (spur″muh·toj′e·nus) *adj.* SPERMATOGENIC.

sper·ma·to·go·ni·um (spur″muh·to·go′nee·um) *n.*, pl. **spermatogo·nia** (·nee·uh) [*spermato-* + *gonium*]. One of the primitive male germ cells. The primary spermatocytes arise from the last generation of spermatogonia by an increase in size.

sper·ma·toid (spur′muh·toid) *adj.* [*spermat-* + *-oid*]. Resembling a spermatozoon.

sper·ma·tol·y·sin (spur″muh·tol′i·sin, spur″muh·to·lye′sin) *n.* [*spermato-* + *lysin*]. A substance causing dissolution of spermatozoa.

sper·ma·tol·y·sis (spur″muh·tol′i·sis) *n.* [*spermato-* + *-lysis*]. The process of dissolution of spermatozoa. **—sperma·to·lyt·ic** (·to·lit′ick) *adj.*

sper·ma·top·a·thy (spur″muh·top′uth·ee) *n.* [*spermato-* + *-pathy*]. Disease of the spermatozoa or of their secreting mechanism.

sper·ma·to·phore (spur′muh·to·fore, spur·mat′o·fore) *n.* [*spermato-* + *-phore*]. A special capsule or pocket containing male germ cells; found in certain annelids, crustacea, and vertebrates, but especially remarkable in the cephalopod mollusks.

sper·ma·tor·rhea, sper·ma·tor·rhoea (spur″muh·to·ree′uh) *n.* [*spermato-* + *-rrhea*]. Involuntary discharge of semen without orgasm.

spermatorrhea dor·mi·en·tum (dor″mee·en′tum) [NL., spermatorrhea of the sleeping, from L. *dormire,* to sleep]. NOCTURNAL EMISSION.

sper·ma·to·tox·in (spur″muh·to·tock′sin) *n.* [*spermato-* + *toxin*]. SPERMOLYSIN.

sper·ma·tox·in (spur″muh·tock′sin) *n.* [*sperma-* + *toxin*]. SPERMOLYSIN.

spermatozoa. Plural of *spermatozoon.*

sper·ma·to·zo·i·cide (spur″muh·to·zo′i·side) *n.* [*spermatozoa* + *-cide*]. SPERMATOCIDE.

sper·ma·to·zo·id (spur″muh·to·zo′id) *n.* [*spermatozoon* + *-oid*]. *In botany,* a motile male germ cell found in certain algae, in mosses and ferns, and in certain gymnosperms.

sper·ma·to·zo·oid (spur″muh·to·zo′oid) *n.* SPERMATOZOID.

sper·ma·to·zo·on (spur″muh·to·zo′on, spur·mat″o·) *n.*, pl. **spermato·zoa** (·zo′uh) [*spermato-* + *-zoon*]. The mature male germ cell. See also Plate 23. **—spermatozo·al** (·ul) *adj.*

sper·ma·tu·ria (spur″muh·tew′ree·uh) *n.* [*spermat-* + *-uria*]. The presence of sperm in the urine.

sperm cell. SPERMATOZOON.

sperm center. The centrosome which precedes the sperm nucleus as it advances within the egg. In flagellate spermatozoa it arises from the middle piece.

sper·mec·to·my (spur·meck′tuh·mee) *n.* [*sperm-* + *-ectomy*]. Resection of part of the ductus deferens.

sperm granuloma. A granulomatous inflammatory reaction to extravasion of sperm into the tissues, as may occur after vasectomy.

sperm head. The head of a spermatozoon.

spermi-. See *sperm-.*

-spermia [*sperm* + *-ia*]. A combining form meaning (a) *a form or condition of spermatozoa;* (b) *a condition of the semen.*

sper·mi·cide (spur′mi·side) *n.* [*spermi-* + *-cide*]. SPERMATOCIDE.

sper·mi·dine (spur′mi·deen, ·din) *n.* The triamine $H_2N(CH_2)_3NH(CH_2)_4NH_2$ found in semen and other animal tissues.

sper·min (spur′min) *n.* SPERMINE.

sper·mine (spur′meen) *n.* *N,N′*-Bis(3-aminopropyl-1,4-butanediamine, $C_{10}H_{26}N_4$, a constituent of semen and other animal tissues.

spermio-. See *sperm-.*

sper·mio·gen·e·sis (spur″mee·o·jen′e·sis) *n.* [*spermio-* + *-genesis*]. The morphological transformation of spermatids into spermatozoa. Compare *spermatogenesis.*

sper·mio·gram (spur′mee·o·gram) *n.* [*spermio-* + *-gram*]. Diagrammatic evaluation of spermatogenic morphology as an aid in the evaluation of infertility.

sperm·ism (spur′miz·um) *n.* A form of the theory of preformation, which held that the sperm cell contains the miniature organism.

sperm·ist (spur′mist) *n.* SPERMALIST.

spermo-. See *sperm-.*

sper·mo·lith (spur′mo·lith) *n.* [*spermo-* + *-lith*]. A calculus in a ductus deferens or seminal vesicle.

sper·mol·y·sin (spur·mol′i·sin, spur″mo·lye′sin) *n.* A cytolysin produced by inoculation with spermatozoa. Syn. *spermatoxin.*

sper·mol·y·sis (spur·mol′i·sis) *n.* SPERMATOLYSIS.

sper·mor·rhea, sper·mor·rhoea (spur″mo·ree′uh) *n.* SPERMATORRHEA.

Sper·ry's method [W. M. *Sperry,* U.S. biochemist, b. 1900]. SCHOENHEIMER AND SPERRY'S METHOD.

sp. g., sp. gr. Abbreviations for *specific gravity.*

sph. Abbreviation for *spherical* or *spherical lens.*

sphac·e·la·tion (sfas″e·lay′shun) *n.* [Gk. *sphakelos,* gangrene]. 1. NECROSIS. 2. GANGRENE. **—sphace·late** (·late) *v.*

sphac·e·lism (sfas′e·liz·um) *n.* The condition of being affected by sphacelus.

sphac·e·lo·der·ma (sfas″e·lo·dur′muh) *n.* [*sphacelus* + *-derma*]. Gangrene or ulceration of the skin from any of many different causes.

sphac·e·lus (sfas′e·lus) *n.* [Gk. *sphakelos,* gangrene]. SLOUGH (1). **—sphac·e·loid** (·loid), **sphac·e·lous** (·lus) *adj.*

sphaer-, sphaero-, spher-, sphero-. A combining form meaning *sphere, spherical.*

Sphae·roph·o·rus (sfe·rof′uh·rus) *n.* [NL., from *sphaero-* + Gk. *phoros,* bearing]. A genus of the family Bacteroidaceae, by some not differentiated from the genus *Bacteroides,* consisting of pleomorphic gram-negative nonsporulating rods found in the alimentary and urogenital tracts of man and animals, and responsible for gangrenous and purulent infections of man.

Sphaerophorus ne·croph·o·rus (ne·krof′uh·rus). A species of *Sphaerophorus* found in association with septicemia, puerperal infection, or liver abscess.

spha·gi·as·mus (sfay″jee·az′mus) *n.* [NL., from Gk. *sphagē,* throat]. Spasm of the muscles of the neck in a convulsion.

spha·gi·tis (sfay·jye′tis) *n.* [Gk. *sphagē,* throat, + *-itis*]. 1. Inflammation of a jugular vein. 2. SORE THROAT.

sphen-, spheno- [Gk. *sphēn,* wedge]. A combining form meaning (a) *wedge, wedge-shaped;* (b) *sphenoid* (*bone*).

sphe·ni·on (sfee′nee·on) *n.* [*sphen-* + *-ion*]. *In craniometry,* the point at the anterior extremity of the sphenoparietal suture.

spheno-. See *sphen-.*

sphe·no·bas·i·lar (sfee″no·bas′i·lur) *adj.* [*spheno-* + *basilar*].

Of or pertaining to the sphenoid and occipital bones; SPHENO-OCCIPITAL.

sphenobasilar cartilage. SPHENO-OCCIPITAL CARTILAGE.

sphenobasilar groove. The indefinite depression on the body of the sphenoid bone and the basilar part of the occipital bone, upon which the pons rests.

sphe·no·ceph·a·lus (sfee″no·sef′uh·lus) *n.* [Gk. *sphēnokephalos*, having a wedge-shaped head]. 1. A variety of monster with separated eyes, the ears united under the head, the jaws and mouth distinct, and the sphenoid bone altered in shape. 2. A monster in which the lower jaw is absent or rudimentary, the fauces are occluded, with severe defects in the upper jaw and sphenoid region, and with various degrees of synotia. The upper face is nearly normal. 3. An individual having a wedge-shaped, narrow head, resulting from compensatory enlargement of the anterior fontanel after premature union of the sagittal suture.

sphe·no·ceph·a·ly (sfee″no·sef′uh·lee) *n.* [*spheno-* + *-cephaly*]. The condition of having a wedge-shaped head.

sphe·no·eth·moid (sfee″no·eth′moid) *adj.* Pertaining to both the sphenoid and the ethmoid bones.

sphenoethmoid recess. A small space between the sphenoid bone and the superior nasal concha. NA *recessus sphenoethmoidalis.*

sphenoethmoid suture. The site of union between the sphenoid and ethmoid bones. NA *sutura sphenoethmoidalis.*

sphenofrontal suture. The site of union between the greater wing of a sphenoid bone and the frontal bone.

sphe·noid (sfee′noid) *adj.* & *n.* [Gk. *sphēnoeidēs*, from *sphēn*, wedge]. 1. Wedge-shaped, as the sphenoid bone. 2. The sphenoid bone. NA *os sphenoidale.* See Table of Bones in the Appendix. —**sphe·noi·dal** (sfe·noy′dul) *adj.*

sphenoid air sinus. SPHENOID SINUS.

sphenoid angle. BASAL ANGLE.

sphenoid concha. CONCHA SPHENOIDALIS.

sphenoid crest. A thin ridge of bone in the median line of the anterior surface of the body of the sphenoid bone. NA *crista sphenoidalis.*

sphenoid fissure. SUPERIOR ORBITAL FISSURE.

sphenoid fontanel. ANTEROLATERAL FONTANEL.

sphe·noid·itis (sfee″noid·eye′tis) *n.* [*sphenoid* + *-itis*]. Inflammation of a sphenoid air sinus.

sphe·noid·ot·o·my (sfee″noid·ot′uh·mee) *n.* [*sphenoid* + *-tomy*]. Incision into the sphenoid air sinus.

sphenoid plexus. The upper part of the internal carotid plexus.

sphenoid process of the palatine bone. A thin plate of bone directed upward and inward from the vertical plate of the palatine bone. NA *processus sphenoidalis ossis palatini.*

sphenoid process of the septal cartilage. The posterior extension, variable in size, of the septal cartilage between the vomer and perpendicular plate of the ethmoid. NA *processus posterior sphenoidalis.*

sphenoid sinus. A paranasal sinus in the body of the sphenoid bone; there is a right and a left one. NA *sinus sphenoidalis.* See also Plates 12, 20.

sphenoid spine. A downward projection from the posterior extremity of the greater wing of the sphenoid, giving attachment to the sphenomandibular ligament and a few fibers of the tensor veli palatini muscle. Syn. *angular spine.* NA *spina ossis sphenoidalis.*

sphenoid turbinated process. CONCHA SPHENOIDALIS.

sphe·no·ma·lar (sfee″no·may′lur) *adj.* [*spheno-* + *malar*]. Pertaining to the sphenoid and zygomatic bones.

sphenomalar suture. The site of union between the zygomatic bone and the greater wing of the sphenoid.

sphe·no·man·dib·u·lar (sfee′no·man·dib′yoo·lur) *adj.* Pertaining to the sphenoid and mandibular bones.

sphenomandibular ligament. A fibrous band extending from the sphenoid spine to the lingula of the mandibular foramen. It is derived from the embryonic Meckel's cartilage. NA *ligamentum sphenomandibulare.*

sphe·no·max·il·lary (sfee″no·mack′si·lerr·ee) *adj.* Pertaining to the sphenoid and maxillary bones.

sphenomaxillary fissure. PTERYGOMAXILLARY FISSURE.

sphenomaxillary fossa. PTERYGOPALATINE FOSSA.

sphenomaxillary ligament. SPHENOMANDIBULAR LIGAMENT.

sphenomaxillary process. An inconstant downward prolongation of the greater wing of the sphenoid.

sphe·no-oc·cip·i·tal (sfee″no·ock·sip′i·tul) *adj.* Of or pertaining to the sphenoid and the occipital bones; SPHENOBASILAR.

spheno-occipital cartilage. The cartilage between the sphenoid and basilar part of the occipital bone, permitting growth of basis cranii until the twentieth year.

spheno-occipital groove. SPHENOBASILAR GROOVE.

sphe·nop·a·gus par·a·sit·i·cus (sfe·nop′uh·gus păr″uh·sit′i·kus). EPISPHENOID.

sphe·no·pal·a·tine (sfee″no·pal′uh·tine) *adj.* [*spheno-* + *palatine*]. Pertaining to the sphenoid bone and the palate.

sphenopalatine artery. NA *arteria sphenopalatina.* See Table of Arteries in the Appendix.

sphenopalatine foramen. The space between the sphenoid and orbital processes of the palatine bone; it opens into the nasal cavity and gives passage to branches from the pterygopalatine ganglion and the sphenopalatine branch of the maxillary artery. NA *foramen sphenopalatinum.*

sphenopalatine ganglion. PTERYGOPALATINE GANGLION.

sphenopalatine nerve. PTERYGOPALATINE NERVE.

sphenopalatine neuralgia. A form of facial neuralgia, with pain referred to the root of the nose, upper teeth, eyes, and even to the ears, mastoid regions, and occiput and attributed, on uncertain grounds, to involvement of the sphenopalatine ganglion. Syn. *Sluder's neuralgia.*

sphenopalatine notch. A deep notch separating the orbital and sphenoid processes of the palatine bone. NA *incisura sphenopalatina.*

sphenopalatine suture. A cranial suture between the sphenoid and palatine bones. NA *sutura sphenoorbitalis.*

sphe·no·pa·ri·e·tal (sfee″no·pa·rye′e·tul) *adj.* Pertaining to the sphenoid and parietal bones.

sphenoparietal sinus. A sinus of the dura mater located along the posterior border of the lesser wing of the sphenoid bone. NA *sinus sphenoparietalis.*

sphenoparietal suture. The site of union between the greater wing of the sphenoid bone and the parietal bone. NA *sutura sphenoparietalis.*

sphe·no·pe·tro·sal (sfee″no·pe·tro′sul) *adj.* [*spheno-* + *petrosal*]. Pertaining to the sphenoid and the petrous portion of the temporal bone.

sphenopetrosal fissure. The fissure between the petrous part of the temporal bone and the great wing of the sphenoid. NA *fissura sphenopetrosa.*

sphenopetrosal suture. PETROSPHENOID SUTURE.

sphe·no·sal·pin·go·staph·y·li·nus (sfee″no·sal·ping″go·staf″i·lye′nus) *n.* [*spheno-* + *salpingo-* + *staphylinus*]. TENSOR VELI PALATINI.

sphe·no·sis (sfe·no′sis) *n.* [Gk. *sphēnōsis*, from *sphēn*, wedge]. The wedging of the fetus in the pelvis.

sphe·no·squa·mo·sal (sfee″no·skway·mo′sul) *adj.* [*spheno-* + *squamosa* + *-al*]. Pertaining to the sphenoid and the squamous portion of the temporal bone.

sphenosquamosal suture. The suture between the greater wing of the sphenoid and the squamous portion of the temporal bone. NA *sutura sphenosquamosa.*

sphe·no·tem·po·ral (sfee″no·tem′po·rul) *adj.* Pertaining to the sphenoid and the temporal bone.

sphenotemporal suture. The site of union between the temporal and the sphenoid bones.

sphe·no·tre·sia (sfee″no·tree′zhuh, ·zee·uh) *n.* [*spheno-* + *-tresia*]. A variety of craniotomy in which the basal portion of the fetal skull is perforated.

sphe·no·tribe (sfee′no·tribe) *n.* [*spheno-* + *-tribe*]. An instrument for crushing the basal portion of the fetal skull.

sphe·no·trip·sy (sfee′no·trip″see) *n.* [*spheno-* + *-tripsy*]. Crushing of the fetal skull.

sphe·no·zy·go·mat·ic (sfee″no·zye·go·mat′ick) *adj.* Pertaining to the sphenoid and the zygomatic bone.

sphenozygomatic suture. The site of union between the zygomatic bone and the greater wing of the sphenoid. NA *sutura sphenozygomatica.*

spher-. See *sphaer-.*

sphe·res·the·sia, sphe·raes·the·sia (sfeer″es·theezh′uh, ·theez′ee·uh) *n.* [*sphere* + *esthesia*]. GLOBUS HYSTERICUS.

spher·i·cal aberration. Unequal refraction of monochromatic light in different parts of a spherical lens, producing faulty images that show lack of sharpness or of flatness, or distortion. Syn. *monochromatic aberration.*

spherical lens. A lens in which the curved surface, either concave or convex, is a segment of a sphere. Abbreviated, S, sph.

spherical recess. A depression in the medial wall of the vestibule which lodges the saccule. Small foramina in the recess transmit branches of the eighth cranial nerve to the saccule. NA *recessus sphericus vestibuli.*

spher·ide (sfeer′ide, sferr′) *n.* A cellular inclusion composed of a granular and filamentous substance.

sphero-. See *sphaer-.*

sphero·ceph·a·lus (sfeer″o·sef′uh·lus) *n.* [*sphero-* + *-cephalus*]. A monster with absent or rudimentary lower jaw, occlusion of the fauces, approximation of the ears, lack of the bones of the face, marked deficiencies in the frontal and sphenoid bones, and with a vesicular brain.

sphero·cyl·in·der (sfeer″o·sil′in·dur) *n.* A bifocal lens combining a spherical with a cylindrical surface.

sphero·cyte (sfeer′o·site) *n.* [*sphero-* + *-cyte*]. An erythrocyte which is spherical rather than biconcave. —**sphero·cyt·ic** (sfeer″o·sit′ick) *adj.*

spherocytic anemia. 1. HEREDITARY SPHEROCYTOSIS. 2. Any anemia characterized by large numbers of spherocytes.

sphero·cy·to·sis (sfeer″o·sigh·to′sis) *n.* [*spherocyte* + *-osis*]. 1. A preponderance in the blood of spherocytes. 2. HEREDITARY SPHEROCYTOSIS.

sphe·roid (sfeer′oid, sferr′oid) *n.* & *adj.* [Gk. *sphairoeidēs,* ball-like]. 1. A solid resembling a sphere. 2. SPHEROIDAL.

sphe·roi·dal (sfe·roy′dul) *adj.* Resembling a sphere.

spheroidal-cell carcinoma. CARCINOID.

spheroid articulation. A type of synovial joint, such as that of the hip or shoulder, in which the rounded head of one bone lodges in a concave surface on the other; a ball-and-socket joint. NA *articulatio spheroidea.*

sphe·rom·e·ter (sfe·rom′e·tur) *n.* [*sphero-* + *-meter*]. An instrument for determining the degree of curvature of a sphere or part of a sphere, especially of optical lenses, or of the tools used for grinding them.

sphero·pha·kia (sfeer″o·fay′kee·uh) *n.* [*sphero-* + *phak-* + *-ia*]. A congenital anomaly in which there is a thick spherical ocular lens whose sagittal diameter is increased and equatorial diameter decreased. Contr. *microphakia.*

spher·ule (sfeer′yool, sferr′yool, ·ool) *n.* [L. *sphaerula,* dim. of *sphaera,* sphere]. A minute sphere.

sphinc·ter (sfink′tur) *n.* [Gk. *sphinktēr,* from *sphingein,* to bind tight]. A muscle surrounding and closing an orifice. NA *musculus sphincter.* See also Table of Muscles in the Appendix. —**sphinc·ter·ic** (sfink·terr′ick), **sphinc·ter·al** (sfink′tur·ul) *adj.*

sphincteral achalasia. Failure of relaxation of a gastrointestinal sphincter, practically always at the cardioesophogeal junction.

sphinc·ter·al·gia (sfink″tur·al′jee·uh) *n.* [*sphincter* + *-algia*]. Transient pain in the anal region, due to a spasm of the levator ani muscles. Syn. *proctalgia fugax.*

sphincter am·pul·lae (am·pul′ee). SPHINCTER OF THE HEPATOPANCREATIC AMPULLA.

sphincter ani ex·ter·nus (ay′nigh ecks·tur′nus). The external anal sphincter; bundles of striate muscle fibers surrounding the anus. NA *musculus sphincter ani externus.* See also Table of Muscles in the Appendix.

sphincter ani in·ter·nus (in·tur′nus). The internal anal sphincter; a thickening of the inner circular (smooth) muscle layer of the anal canal. NA *musculus sphincter ani internus.*

sphincter duc·tus cho·le·do·chi (duck′tus ko·led′o·kigh). SPHINCTER OF THE COMMON BILE DUCT.

sphinc·ter·ec·to·my (sfink″tur·eck′tuh·mee) *n.* [*sphincter* + *-ectomy*]. Oblique blepharotomy for the dilatation of the palpebral fissure, or for blepharospasm.

sphinc·ter·is·mus (sfink″tur·iz′mus) *n.* A spasmodic contraction of the anal sphincter, usually attendant upon fissure or ulcer of the anus, but occasionally occurring independently of such lesion.

sphinc·ter·itis (sfink″tur·eye′tis) *n.* [*sphincter* + *-itis*]. Inflammation of a sphincter, especially the anal sphincter.

sphincter of Boyden [E. A. *Boyden*]. SPHINCTER OF THE COMMON BILE DUCT.

sphincter of Od·di (oʰd′dee) [R. *Oddi,* Italian physician, 19th century]. SPHINCTER OF THE HEPATOPANCREATIC AMPULLA.

sphincter of the common bile duct. The circular smooth muscle of the common bile duct just before its junction with the pancreatic duct. NA *musculus sphincter ductus choledochi.*

sphincter of the hepatopancreatic ampulla. The intricate arrangement of smooth muscle about the common bile duct and pancreatic duct in the wall of the duodenum. NA *musculus sphincter ampullae hepatopancreaticae.*

sphincter of the pylorus. PYLORIC SPHINCTER.

sphinc·ter·ol·y·sis (sfink″tur·ol′i·sis) *n.* [*sphincter* + *-lysis*]. The operation of freeing the iris in anterior synechia.

sphinc·tero·plas·ty (sfink′tur·o·plas″tee) *n.* [*sphincter* + *-plasty*]. A plastic or reparative operation on a sphincter muscle.

sphinc·ter·ot·o·my (sfink″tur·ot′uh·mee) *n.* [*sphincter* + *-tomy*]. The operation of incising a sphincter.

sphincter pan·cre·a·ti·cus (pan″kree·at′i·kus). The inconstant band of smooth muscle encircling the pancreatic duct just before it joins the hepatopancreatic duct.

sphincter pupillae. NA *musculus sphincter pupillae.* See Table of Muscles in the Appendix.

sphincter ter·ti·us (tur′shee·us) [L., *third sphincter*]. The muscular component of the middle transverse rectal fold.

sphincter ure·thrae (yoo·ree′three). SPHINCTER URETHRAE MEMBRANACEAE.

sphincter urethrae mem·bra·na·ce·ae (mem″bruh·nay′si·ee). Bundles of voluntary muscle that surround the membranous portion of the urethra in the male; in the female the analogous muscle fibers surround the proximal portion of the urethra. NA *musculus sphincter urethrae.* See also Table of Muscles in the Appendix.

sphincter ve·si·cae (ve·sigh′see, ·kee). Bundles of smooth muscle that are a part of the tunica muscularis of the bladder; the fibers are looped around the neck of the bladder, thus forming an involuntary urethral sphincter; it is not now considered to be a true involuntary sphincter.

sphin·go·lip·id (sfing″go·lip′id) *n.* Any lipid, such as a sphingomyelin, that yields sphingosine or one of its derivatives as a product of hydrolysis.

sphin·go·lip·i·do·sis (sfing″go·lip″i·do′sis) *n.* [*sphingolipid* + *-osis*]. Any one of a group of inherited metabolic disorders characterized by the accumulation of excessive quantities of certain glycolipids and phospholipids in various body tissues. The principal forms include Gaucher's disease, Niemann-Pick disease, metachromatic leukodystrophy, infantile amaurotic familial idiocy (Tay-Sachs disease), familial neurovisceral lipidosis, and angiokeratoma corporis diffusum universale.

sphin·go·my·e·lin (sfing″go·migh′e·lin) *n.* A phospholipid occurring in brain, kidney, liver, and egg yolk. It is composed of choline, sphingosine, phosphoric acid, and a fatty acid.

sphin·go·sine (sfing'go·seen, ·sin) *n.* [Gk. *Sphinx, Sphingos* (from the enigmas it presented to its early investigators) + *-ine*]. 2-Amino-4-octadecene-1,3-diol, $C_{18}H_{37}NO_2$, a moiety of sphingomyelin, cerebrosides, and certain other phosphatides.

sphygm-, sphygmo- [Gk. *sphygmos*]. A combining form meaning *pulse.*

sphyg·mic (sfig'mick) *adj.* [Gk. *sphygmikos,* from *sphygmos,* pulse]. Pertaining to the pulse.

sphyg·mi·cal (sfig'mi·kul) *adj.* SPHYGMIC.

sphygmo-. See *sphygm-.*

sphyg·mo·bo·lom·e·ter (sfig''mo·bo·lom'e·tur) *n.* [*sphygmo-* + Gk. *bolē,* stroke, + *-meter*]. An instrument for measuring and recording the pulse. —**sphygmobolome·try** (·tree) *n.*

sphyg·mo·chrono·graph (sfig''mo·kron'o·graf) *n.* [*sphygmo-* + *chronograph*]. A registering sphygmograph.

sphyg·mo·chro·nog·ra·phy (sfig''mo·kro·nog'ruh·fee) *n.* [*sphygmo-* + *chronography*]. The registration of the time intervals of the pulse wave.

sphyg·mod·ic (sfig·mod'ick, ·mo'dick) *adj.* [Gk. *sphygmōdēs,* from *sphygmos,* pulse]. Like the pulse; throbbing, pulsating.

sphyg·mo·dy·na·mom·e·ter (sfig''mo·dye''nuh·mom'e·tur) *n.* [*sphygmo-* + *dynamo-* + *-meter*]. An instrument for measuring the force of the pulse.

sphyg·mo·gram (sfig'mo·gram) *n.* [*sphygmo-* + *-gram*]. The tracing made by the sphygmograph.

sphyg·mo·graph (sfig'mo·graf) *n.* [*sphygmo-* + *-graph*]. An instrument for recording graphically the pulse wave and the variations in blood pressure. —**sphyg·mo·graph·ic** (sfig''mo·graf'ick) *adj.*

sphyg·mog·ra·phy (sfig·mog'ruh·fee) *n.* [*sphygmo-* + *-graphy*]. 1. A description of the pulse and its pathologic variations. 2. The recording of pulse tracings with the sphygmograph.

sphyg·moid (sfig'moid) *adj.* [*sphygm-* + *-oid*]. Resembling the pulse; having the nature of continuous pulsation.

sphyg·mo·ma·nom·e·ter (sfig''mo·ma·nom'e·tur) *n.* [*sphygmo-* + *manometer*]. An instrument for measuring the arterial blood pressure. —**sphygmomanome·try** (·tree) *n.*

sphyg·mom·e·ter (sfig·mom'e·tur) *n.* [*sphygmo-* + *-meter*]. SPHYGMOGRAPH.

sphyg·mo·os·cil·lom·e·ter (sfig''mo·os''i·lom'e·tur) *n.* [*sphygmo-* + *oscillometer*]. A form of sphygmomanometer in which the systolic and diastolic blood pressures are indicated by an oscillating device.

sphyg·mo·pal·pa·tion (sfig''mo·pal·pay'shun) *n.* [*sphygmo-* + *palpation*]. The palpation of the pulse.

sphyg·mo·phone (sfig'mo·fone) *n.* [*sphygmo-* + *-phone*]. A sphygmograph in which the vibrations of the pulse produce a sound.

sphyg·mo·scope (sfig'mo·skope) *n.* [*sphygmo-* + *-scope*]. A pulse pressure recorder in which the force of arterial pressure is made visible.

sphyg·mos·co·py (sfig·mos'kuh·pee) *n.* 1. The recording of the pulse wave with the sphygmoscope. 2. Examination of the pulse.

sphyg·mo·sys·to·le (sfig''mo·sis'tuh·lee) *n.* [*sphygmo-* + *systole*]. The part of the sphygmogram related to cardiac systole.

sphyg·mo·tech·ny (sfig'mo·teck''nee) *n.* [*sphygmo-* + Gk. *technē,* art]. The art of diagnosis and prognosis by means of the pulse.

sphyg·mo·to·no·graph (sfig''mo·to'nuh·graf) *n.* [*sphygmo-* + *tono-* + *-graph*]. An instrument that records pulsations from an inflatable rubber cuff.

sphyg·mo·to·nom·e·ter (sfig''mo·to·nom'e·tur) *n.* [*sphygmo-* + *tonometer*]. An instrument for measuring the elasticity or tension of the arterial wall.

sphyg·mus (sfig'mus) *n.* [NL., from Gk. *sphygmos*]. PULSE (1); a pulsation. —**sphygmous,** *adj.*

sphynx-neck, *n.* WEBBED NECK.

spi·ca (spye'kuh) *n.,* pl. **spi·cae** (·see), **spicas** [L., head of grain]. 1. A spike or spur. 2. SPICA BANDAGE.

spica bandage. A bandage with successive turns and crosses, as in a modified figure-of-eight bandage; so-called because it resembles the arrangement of grains in the spike (ear) of certain cereal grasses.

spica cast. An orthopedic cast that encases part or all of the trunk and immobilizes one or more of the extremities.

spice, *n.* [L. *species,* kind]. An aromatic vegetable substance used for flavoring; a condiment.

spic·u·la (spick'yoo·luh) *n.,* pl. **spicu·lae** (·lee) [NL.]. SPICULE.

spic·ule (spick'yool) *n.* [L. *spiculum,* sharp point]. 1. A small spike-shaped bone or fragment of bone. 2. A needle-shaped body; a spike. —**spicu·lar** (·lur) *adj.*

spi·der, *n.* [OE. *spīthra,* from *spinnan,* to spin]. 1. An arthropod of the order Araneida of the class Arachnida, characterized by having four pairs of legs, usually eight eyes, and an unsegmented abdomen. See also *Latrodectus, Loxosceles.* 2. (*In attributive use*) Having a form suggestive of a spider or a spider's web.

spider angioma. SPIDER NEVUS.

spider belly. ARACHNOGASTRIA.

spider burst. SPIDER TELANGIECTASIA.

spider cell. ASTROCYTE.

spider fingers. ARACHNODACTYLY.

spider monkey. A slender, prehensile-tailed monkey belonging to the genus *Ateles,* inhabiting tropical forests in South and Central America and coastal southern Mexico.

spider nevus. A type of telangiectasis characterized by a central, elevated, tiny red dot, pinhead in size, from which blood vessels radiate like strands of a spider's web. Syn. *nevus araneus, nevus arachnoideus, stellar nevus.*

spider telangiectasia. Superficial flat telangiectatic areas of the skin of legs associated with venous dilatation.

Spieg·ler-Fendt sarcoid (shpeeg'lur) [E. *Spiegler,* Austrian dermatologist, 1860–1908]. LYMPHOCYTOMA CUTIS.

Spiegler's test [E. *Spiegler*]. A test for protein performed by overlaying clear acidulated urine upon Spiegler's reagent (mercuric chloride, tartaric acid, glycerin, distilled water). Opalescence at the junction of the fluids indicates protein.

Spiegler's tumor [E. *Spiegler*]. CYLINDROMA.

Spiel·mey·er-Vogt disease (shpeel'migh·ur, fohkt) [W. *Spielmeyer,* German neurologist, 1879–1935; and O. *Vogt*]. A hereditary disorder of lipid metabolism, transmitted by both dominant and recessive patterns, characterized by the onset between 4 and 10 years of progressive visual loss and eventual blindness, abnormal pigmentation of the retina, convulsions, extrapyramidal disorders of movement and eventual spasticity, psychotic behavior, and progressive dementia. Syn. *Batten-Mayou disease, juvenile amaurotic familial idiocy.* See also *amaurotic familial idiocy.*

Spi·ge·lia (spye·jee'lee·uh) *n.* [A. van der *Spieghel,* Belgian botanist and anatomist, 1578–1625]. A genus of plants of the family Loganiaceae. The rhizome and rootlets of *Spigelia marilandica,* pinkroot, formerly were used as a vermifuge.

Spi·ge·li·an hernia (spye·jee'lee·un) [A. van der *Spieghel*]. A ventral hernia occurring at the semilunar line.

Spigelian lobe [A. van der *Spieghel*]. CAUDATE LOBE.

Spi·ge·li·us' line [A. van der *Spieghel*]. SEMILUNAR LINE.

spike, *n. In electroencephalography,* a transient wave form that is clearly distinguishable from background activity, having a pointed peak at conventional paper speeds and a duration of 20 to 70 msec.

spike and dome. SPIKE AND SLOW WAVE.

spike and slow wave. *In electroencephalography,* a pattern consisting of a spike followed by a slow wave.

spike and wave. SPIKE AND SLOW WAVE.

spike focus. *In electroencephalography,* a limited region of the scalp, cerebral cortex, or depth of the brain displaying a spike wave form.

spike·nard (spike'nurd, ·nahrd) *n.* [ML. *spica nardi,* lit., spike (ear) of nard]. 1. A name given to the rhizome of various species of *Valeriana* or closely related genera. Used as an aromatic and a perfume among ancient Oriental peoples. 2. American spikenard, *Aralia racemosa,* formerly used as a stimulant and diaphoretic.

spike potential. 1. *In electroencephalography,* SPIKE. 2. ACTION POTENTIAL.

spill, *n.* 1. An overflow, especially that of blood. 2. A form of cellular metastasis in malignant disease.

spill·way, *n.* The physiologic form or contour of a tooth which provides for the escape of food during mastication; an embrasure or a developmental, occlusal, or supplemental groove. Syn. *sluiceway.*

spi·lo·ma (spye·lo'muh) *n.* [*spil*us + *-oma*]. NEVUS.

spi·lo·pla·nia (spye''lo·play'nee·uh) *n.* [Gk. *spilos,* spot, + *plan-* + *-ia*]. A transient skin erythema.

spi·lus (spye'lus) *n.* [NL., from Gk. *spilos,* spot, blemish]. A splotchily colored cutaneous melanocytic nevus.

spin-, spini-, spino-. A combining form meaning *spine, spinal, spinous.*

spi·na (spye'nuh) *n.,* pl. & genit. sing. **spi·nae** (·nee) [L., thorn]. SPINE.

spina an·gu·la·ris (ang·gew·lair'is) [BNA]. Spina ossis sphenoidalis (= SPHENOID SPINE).

spina bi·fi·da (bye'fi·duh, bif'i·duh). A congenital defect in the closure of the vertebral canal with hernial protrusion of the meninges of the cord. The hernial sac contains cerebrospinal fluid and sometimes nervous tissue; most common in the lumbosacral region. It may be diagnosed in mid-pregnancy by aspiration of amniotic fluid which is analyzed for elevation of alpha-fetoprotein.

spina bifida oc·cul·ta (ock·ul'tuh). A defect in the closure of the vertebral canal due to incomplete fusion of the posterior arch without hernial protrusion of the meninges, usually asymptomatic and diagnosed only by radiography.

spinae pa·la·ti·nae (pal·uh·tye'nee) [NA]. Small projections on the lateral margin of the inferior surface of the palatine process of the maxilla.

spina fron·ta·lis (fron·tay'lis) [BNA]. Spina nasalis ossis frontalis (= NASAL SPINE).

spina he·li·cis (hel'i·sis) [NA]. HELICAL SPINE.

spina ili·a·ca anterior inferior (i·lye'uh·kuh) [NA]. ANTERIOR INFERIOR ILIAC SPINE.

spina iliaca anterior superior [NA]. ANTERIOR SUPERIOR ILIAC SPINE.

spina iliaca posterior inferior [NA]. POSTERIOR INFERIOR ILIAC SPINE.

spina iliaca posterior superior [NA]. POSTERIOR SUPERIOR ILIAC SPINE.

spina is·chi·a·di·ca (is·kee·ad'i·kuh) [NA]. SPINE OF THE ISCHIUM.

spi·nal (spye'nul) *adj.* 1. Resembling a spine. 2. Pertaining to, or situated near, the vertebral column.

spinal accessory nerve. ACCESSORY NERVE.

spinal accessory nucleus. A small and discontinuous strand of cells having considerable length in the caudal part of the medulla oblongata and the first five segments of the cervical spinal cord, lying in the motor horn of the cord, lateral to the motor cells of the upper cervical roots. NA *nucleus spinalis nervi accessorii.*

spinal adhesive arachnoiditis. Chronic adhesive arachnoiditis of the spinal cord.

spinal akinesia. Motor impairment due to a lesion of the spinal cord.

spinal anesthesia. 1. Anesthesia due to a lesion of the spinal cord. 2. Anesthesia produced by local anesthetic injected into the spinal subarachnoid space.

spinal animal. An experimental animal surgically prepared by severance of the spinal cord at its junction with the medulla.

spinal apoplexy. A sudden focal neurologic deficit due to infarction of or bleeding into the spinal cord.

spinal ataxia. Motor incoordination due to disease of the posterior columns of the spinal cord.

spinal block. Interference with the flow of cerebrospinal fluid due to blockage of the spinal subarachnoid space.

spinal block syndrome. FROIN'S SYNDROME.

spinal canal. VERTEBRAL CANAL.

spinal cardioaccelerator center. The motor cells in the lateral column of the upper five thoracic segments of the spinal cord from which arise the preganglionic fibers of the accelerator nerves to the heart.

spinal column. VERTEBRAL COLUMN.

spinal cord. The part of the central nervous system contained within the vertebral canal and extending from the medulla oblongata at the level of the foramen magnum to the filum terminale at the level of the first or second lumbar vertebra. NA *medulla spinalis.* See also Plate 16.

spinal cord compression. Deformity of the spinal cord produced by pressure from space-occupying lesions in the subarachnoid, subdural or extradural space, or in the cord itself.

spinal cord concussion. A condition caused by severe shock of the vertebral column, with or without appreciable lesion of the cord; leading to a variety of neurologic symptoms and deficits, varying with the site and severity of the injury.

spinal cord decompression. Laminectomy or other surgical operation to remove pressure upon the spinal cord.

spinal dysraphism. A general term for all manifestations of defective fusion in the dorsal midline whether cutaneous, vertebral, meningeal, or neural.

spinal flexure. CERVICAL FLEXURE.

spinal fluid. CEREBROSPINAL FLUID.

spinal-fluid loss headache. LUMBAR PUNCTURE HEADACHE.

spinal foramen. CENTRAL CANAL OF THE SPINAL CORD.

spinal fusion. The fusion of two or more vertebrae, for immobilization of the spinal column. Used in the treatment of spinal deformities, tuberculosis of the spine, and severe arthritis of the spine.

spinal ganglion. Any one of the sensory ganglions, each associated with the dorsal root of a spinal nerve. NA *ganglion spinale.*

spinal hemiplegia. Paralysis of one side of the body due to a lesion of the cervical spinal cord.

spi·na·lis (spye·nay'lis) *n.* [L.]. A deep muscle of the back attached to the spinous processes of the vertebrae. NA *musculus spinalis.* See also Table of Muscles in the Appendix.

spinal lemniscus. The supposed lateral and ventral spinothalamic tracts combined as they ascend in the brainstem; probably a misconception. NA *lemniscus spinalis.*

spinal man. A patient whose spinal cord has been completely separated from supraspinal influences.

spinal marrow. SPINAL CORD.

spinal meningitis. Inflammation of the meninges of the spinal cord, usually associated with cerebral meningitis. See also *cerebrospinal meningitis.*

spinal meningovascular syphilis. Meningovascular syphilis involving the meninges and blood vessels of the spinal cord predominantly.

spinal micturition center. The spinal neurons, in the second, third and fourth sacral segments, concerned with bladder function.

spinal muscular atrophy. Any of a group of heredodegenerative diseases affecting primarily the anterior horn cells of the spinal cord and brainstem, causing widespread muscular hypotonia and atrophy.

spinal mydriasis. CILIOSPINAL REFLEX.

spinal needle. A hollow needle equipped with an obturator, used for spinal or sacral anesthesia or lumbar puncture.

spinal nerves. Nerves arising from the spinal cord and

exiting through invertebral foramens. There are 31 pairs of spinal nerves: 8 cervical, 12 thoracic, 5 lumbar, 5 sacral, and 1 coccygeal. NA *nervi spinales.*

spinal pachymeningitis. HYPERTROPHIC SPINAL PACHYMENINGITIS.

spinal paralysis. Paralysis caused by a lesion of the spinal cord.

spinal paralytic poliomyelitis. PARALYTIC SPINAL POLIOMYELITIS.

spinal poliomyelitis. PARALYTIC SPINAL POLIOMYELITIS.

spinal puncture. LUMBAR PUNCTURE.

spinal pyramidotomy. Surgical interruption of the corticospinal tract at the level of the second cervical vertebra; formerly used in the treatment of extrapyramidal movement disorders.

spinal reflex. Any reflex mediated through the spinal cord without the necessary participation of more cephalad central nervous system structures.

spinal reflex bladder. REFLEX BLADDER.

spinal sensory-motor seizures. Attacks of unilateral tonic spasm, followed or preceded by contralateral sensory disturbances, presumably due to an irritative lesion in the lateral funiculus of the spinal cord.

spinal shock. A condition of flaccid paralysis and suppression of all reflex activity following immediately upon transection of the spinal cord and involving all segments below the lesion. In most cases, reflex activity returns within 1 to 6 weeks but in a small proportion the state of complete areflexia is permanent.

spinal tap. LUMBAR PUNCTURE.

spinal tract of the trigeminal nerve. A nerve tract located in the medulla, composed of sensory fibers of the trigeminal nerve which terminate in the nucleus of the spinal tract of the trigeminal nerve. NA *tractus spinalis nervi trigemini.*

spinal tractotomy. CHORDOTOMY.

spinal vestibular nucleus. A nucleus dorsolateral to the tractus solitarius the cells of which project to the cerebellum via the juxtarestiform body. NA *nucleus vestibularis inferior.*

spinal vestibular root or **tract.** VESTIBULOSPINAL TRACT.

spina men·ta·lis (men·tay'lis) [NA]. MENTAL SPINE.

spina na·sa·lis an·te·ri·or max·il·lae (na·say'lis an·teer'ee·or mack·sil'ee) [NA]. ANTERIOR NASAL SPINE.

spina nasalis os·sis fron·ta·lis (os'is fron·tay'lis) [NA]. NASAL SPINE.

spina nasalis posterior ossis pa·la·ti·ni (pal·uh·tye'nigh) [NA]. POSTERIOR NASAL SPINE.

spina os·sis sphe·noi·da·lis (os'is sfee·noy·day'lis) [NA]. SPHENOID SPINE.

spina sca·pu·lae (skap'yoo·lee) [NA]. SPINE OF THE SCAPULA.

spina su·pra·me·a·tum (sue·pruh·mee·ay'tum) [NA]. SUPRAMEATAL SPINE.

spina tro·chle·a·ris (trock·lee·air'is) [NA]. TROCHLEAR SPINE.

spina tym·pa·ni·ca major (tim·pan'i·kuh) [NA]. The spine on the anterior margin of the tympanic notch.

spina tympanica minor [NA]. The spine in the posterior margin of the tympanic notch.

spina ven·to·sa (ven·to'suh). Tuberculous infection of the long bones of the hand or foot, involving rarefaction of the compact bone and subperiosteal formation of new bone to produce a spindle-shaped enlargement of the shaft. Syn. *tubercular dactylitis.*

spin·dle, *n.* 1. A tapering rod; a fusiform shape. 2. The part of the achromatic figure in mitosis between the centrosomes or asters, consisting of modified cytoplasm and achromatic fibrils. 3. A group of alphalike synchronized waves which appears in the electroencephalograph during periods of light sleep.

spindle cataract. A cataract characterized by a spindle-shaped opacity extending from the posterior to the anterior portion of the lens capsule.

spindle cell. 1. A fibroblast or smooth muscle cell which is spindle-shaped. 2. A fusiform or spindle-shaped cell, typical of certain tumors.

spindle-cell carcinoma. OAT-CELL CARCINOMA.

spindle-cell sarcoma. A malignant connective-tissue tumor composed of spindle-shaped cells.

spindle fibers. ACHROMATIC FIBRILS.

spindle remnant. MITOSOME.

spine, *n.* [L. *spina*]. 1. A sharp process, especially of bone. See also *tubercle.* 2. VERTEBRAL COLUMN.

spine of the ischium. A pointed eminence on the posterior border of the body of the ischium. It forms the lower border of the greater sciatic notch. NA *spina ischiadica.*

spine of the scapula. The strong, triangular plate of bone attached obliquely to the dorsum of the scapula and dividing it into two unequal parts, the supraspinous and infraspinous fossae. NA *spina scapulae.*

spine of the tibia. INTERCONDYLAR EMINENCE.

spini-. See *spin-.*

spinn·bar·keit (spin'bahr·kite, Ger. shpin') *n.* [Ger., spinnability]. The ability of cervical mucus to form a thin, continuous thread; usually occurs shortly before ovulation.

spino-. See *spin-.*

spi·no·bul·bar (spye"no·bul'bur) *adj.* [*spino-* + *bulbar*]. Pertaining to the spinal cord and the medulla oblongata.

spinobulbar poliomyelitis. PARALYTIC SPINAL and PARALYTIC BULBAR POLIOMYELITIS.

spi·no·cel·lu·lar (spye"no·sel'yoo·lur) *adj.* [*spino-* + *cellular*]. Pertaining to, or like, prickle cells.

spi·no·cer·e·bel·lar (spye"no·serr"e·bel'ur) *adj.* [*spino-* + *cerebellar*]. Pertaining to the spinal cord and the cerebellum.

spinocerebellar degenerations. A group of progressive, heredodegenerative diseases of the central nervous system, characterized clinically chiefly by ataxia and pathologically by affection of the sensory pathways of the spinal cord and of the cerebellum and its major connections. See also *Friedreich's ataxia, cerebellar ataxia, olivopontocerebellar atrophy.*

spinocerebellar nucleus. THORACIC NUCLEUS.

spinocerebellar tract. See *anterior spinocerebellar tract, posterior spinocerebellar tract.*

spi·no·gal·va·ni·za·tion (spye"no·gal"vuh·ni·zay'shun) *n.* An outmoded form of treatment consisting in application of a galvanic current to the spinal column.

spinoolivary tract or **fasciculus.** A tract composed of fibers running from the spinal cord to the olivary nucleus of the medulla oblongata.

spi·no·sal (spye·no'sul) *adj.* Pertaining to or passing through the foramen spinosum of the sphenoid bone.

spinosal nerve. The meningeal branch of the mandibular nerve. NA *ramus meningeus nervi mandibularis.* See also Table of Nerves in the Appendix.

spi·no·spi·nal tracts (spye"no·spye'nul). FASCICULI PROPRII MEDULLAE SPINALIS.

spi·no·sus nerve (spye·no'sus). SPINOSAL NERVE.

spi·no·tec·tal (spye"no·teck'tul) *adj.* [*spino-* + *tectal*]. Pertaining to the spinal cord and the tectum of the mesencephalon.

spinotectal tract. A group of ascending nerve fibers from the lateral funiculus of the spinal cord to the tectum. NA *tractus spinotectalis.*

spi·no·tha·lam·ic (spye"no·tha·lam'ick) *adj.* [*spino-* + *thalamic*]. 1. Pertaining to the spinal cord and the thalamus. 2. Pertaining to a spinothalamic tract.

spinothalamic nucleus. NUCLEUS PROPRIUS OF THE POSTERIOR HORN.

spinothalamic tract. See *anterior spinothalamic tract, lateral spinothalamic tract.*

spi·no·trans·ver·sa·ri·us (spye"no·trans"vur·sair'ee·us) *n.* [*spino-* + L. *transversarius,* transverse]. Any of the rotator muscles of the spine.

spi·nous (spye'nus) *adj.* [L. *spinosus,* thorny, prickly]. 1. Pertaining to a spine or a spinelike process. 2. Having spines or sharp processes.

spinous cell carcinoma. A well-differentiated form of squamous cell carcinoma.

spinous point. A sensitive point over a spinous process.

spinous process. Any slender, sharp-pointed projection.

spinous processes of the ilium. The spines of the ilium, anterior and posterior superior, and anterior and posterior inferior.

spinous process of a vertebra. The prominent backward projection from the middle of the posterior portion of the arch of a vertebra. NA *processus spinosus.*

spin·thar·i·con (spin·thăr'i·kon) *n.* [Gk. *spintharis*, spark, + *icon*]. A direct-viewing radiation imaging system, consisting of a collimator with many pinholes and a spark discharge tube.

spin·ther·ism (spin'thur·iz·um) *n.* [Gk. *spinthēr*, spark, + *-ism*]. Sensation of sparks before the eyes. See also *scintillating scotoma.*

spi·nu·lose (spye'new·loce) *adj.* [L. *spinula*, small spine, + *-ose*]. SPINY.

spi·ny (spye'nee) *adj.* Having or characterized by spines.

spip·er·one (spip'ur·ohn) *n.* 8-[3-(*p*-Fluorobenzoyl)propyl]-1-phenyl-1,3,8-triazaspiro[4.5]decan-4-one, $C_{23}H_{26}FN_3O_2$, a tranquilizer.

spir-, spiro- [Gk. *speira*]. A combining form meaning *coil, spiral.*

spir-, spiro- [L. *spirare*, to breathe]. Combining forms meaning *respiration, breathing.*

spi·rad·e·ni·tis sup·pu·ra·ti·va (spye·rad''e·nigh'tis sup''yoo·ruh·tye'vuh). HIDRADENITIS SUPPURATIVA.

spi·rad·e·no·ma (spye·rad''e·no'muh) *n.* [*spir-* + *adenoma*]. SWEAT GLAND ADENOMA.

spi·ral (spye'rul) *adj.* [ML. *spiralis*, from Gk. *speira*, coil]. 1. Having the two-dimensional form of something wound in a plane around a center. 2. Having the three-dimensional form of something coiled around an axis; HELICAL.

spiral annulet. RINGBINDEN.

spiral bandage. OBLIQUE BANDAGE.

spiral canal of the cochlea. 1. OSSEOUS COCHLEAR CANAL. 2. COCHLEAR DUCT.

spiral canal of the modiolus. An irregular cavity of the bone extending along the line of attachment of the osseous spiral lamina to the modiolus; it lodges the spiral ganglion. NA *canalis spiralis modioli.*

spiral crest. A ridge on the upper border of the spiral lamina of the cochlea.

spiral ganglion of the cochlea. An aggregation of bipolar cells situated in the modiolus of the cochlea and giving rise to fibers of the cochlear division of the vestibulocochlear nerve. NA *ganglion spirale cochleae.*

spiral joint. SCREW ARTICULATION.

spiral lamina. A thin plate in the ear, osseous in the inner part and membranous in the outer, which divides the spiral tube of the cochlea into the scala tympani and scala vestibuli. See also *osseous spiral lamina, basilar membrane.*

spiral ligament. The greatly thickened periosteum of the outer wall of the cochlear duct. NA *ligamentum spirale cochleae.* See also Plate 20.

spiral organ (of Corti) [A. *Corti*]. The sensory portion of the cochlear duct; the end organ of hearing. NA *organum spirale.* See also Plate 20.

spiral plate. SPIRAL LAMINA.

spiral reverse bandage. A bandage in which the oblique turns are reversed and folded back at each turn, to adapt the bandage to the part.

spiral sulcus. A concave groove below the tectorial membrane of the floor of the cochlear duct. Syn. *inner spiral sulcus.* NA *sulcus spiralis internus.* Contr. *outer spiral sulcus.*

spiral valve. The coiled mucomembranous folds in the neck of the gallbladder and cystic duct. Syn. *Heister's valve.* NA *plica spiralis.*

spi·ra·my·cin (spye''ruh·migh'sin) *n.* A complex of related antibiotics, which resemble erythromycin structurally and in antibacterial spectrum, produced by *Streptomyces ambofaciens.*

spi·reme (spye'reem) *n.* [Gk. *speirēma*, coil]. A term applied incorrectly to describe the interphasic condition of chromosomal material. The term implies that chromonemata form a continuous thread.

spirilla. Plural of *spirillum.*

spi·ril·lar (spye·ril'ur) *adj.* [*spirillum* + *-ar*]. Pertaining to spirilla or to the genus *Spirillum.*

spirillar abscess. An abscess containing spirilla.

spi·ril·lary (spye'ri·lerr''ee) *adj.* Caused by spirilla.

spirillary rat-bite fever. SODOKU.

spi·ril·li·ci·dal (spye·ril''i·sigh'dul) *adj.* [*spirillum* + *-cidal*]. Capable of destroying spirilla.

spi·ril·lo·sis (spye''ri·lo'sis, spirr''i·) *n.* [*Spirillum* + *-osis*]. A disease caused by infection with spirilla.

Spi·ril·lum (spye·ril'um) *n.* [dim. of L. *spira*, coil]. A genus of spiral bacilli of the family Pseudomonadaceae. —**spirillum,** pl. **spiril·la,** *com. n.*

spirillum fever. RELAPSING FEVER.

Spirillum mi·nus (migh'nus). A causative agent of rat-bite fever.

spir·it, *n.* [L. *spiritus*, breath]. 1. An alcoholic solution of a volatile principle, formerly prepared by distillation but now generally prepared by dissolving the volatile substance in alcohol. 2. Any distilled liquid. Abbreviated, sp.

spirit of nitrous ether. ETHYL NITRITE SPIRIT.

spirit of wine. ETHYL ALCOHOL.

spiritual healing. FAITH CURE; MENTAL HEALING.

spir·i·tus (spirr'i·tus) *n.* [L.]. SPIRIT. Abbreviated, sp.

spiritus fru·men·ti (froo·men'tye, ·tee) [NL., grain spirit]. Whiskey.

spiro-. See *spir-.*

Spi·ro·chae·ta (spye''ro·kee'tuh) *n.* [NL., from *spiro-*, coil, + Gk. *chaitē*, hair]. A genus of spiral microorganisms of the family Spirochaetaceae, nonpathogenic for man. Formerly included *Treponema, Leptospira,* and others.

Spi·ro·chae·ta·ce·ae (spye''ro·ke·tay'see·ee) *n.pl.* A family of spiral microorganisms which includes the genera *Spirochaeta, Saprospira,* and *Cristispira.* The family is nonpathogenic for man; a few species of *Cristispira* are parasites of crustaceans, all other species are free-living forms.

Spirochaeta cuniculi. *TREPONEMA CUNICULI.*

spirochaetaemia. SPIROCHETEMIA.

Spirochaeta ic·ter·og·e·nes (ick''tur·oj'e·neez). *LEPTOSPIRA ICTEROHAEMORRHAGIAE.*

Spirochaeta ic·tero·hae·mor·rhag·i·ae (ick''tur·o·hem''ur·aj'ee·ee). *LEPTOSPIRA ICTEROHAEMORRHAGIAE.*

spirochaetal. SPIROCHETAL.

Spi·ro·chae·ta·les (spye''ro·ke·tay'leez) *n.pl.* An order of spiral microorganisms which includes the families Spirochaetaceae and Treponemataceae.

Spirochaeta mor·sus mu·ris (mor'sus mew'ris) [L., rat-bite]. *SPIRILLUM MINUS.*

Spirochaeta ober·mei·eri (o''bur·migh'ur·eye). *BORRELIA RECURRENTIS.*

Spirochaeta pal·li·da (pal'i·duh). *TREPONEMA PALLIDUM.*

spirochaete. SPIROCHETE.

spirochaeticide. SPIROCHETICIDE.

spirochaetolysis. SPIROCHETOLYSIS.

spirochaetosis. SPIROCHETOSIS.

spirochaetosis ic·te·ro·hae·mor·rhag·i·ca (ick''tur·o·hee·mo·raj'i·kuh, ·hem·o·). WEIL'S DISEASE.

spirochetal jaundice. WEIL'S DISEASE.

spi·ro·chete, spi·ro·chaete (spye'ro·keet) *n.* [*spiro-* + Gk. *chaitē*, hair]. Any of the spiral microorganisms belonging to the order Spirochaetales. —**spi·ro·che·tal, spi·ro·chae·tal** (spye''ro·kee'tul) *adj.*

spi·ro·chet·emia, spi·ro·chae·tae·mia (spye''ro·ke·tee'mee·uh) *n.* [*spirochete* + *-emia*]. The presence of spirochetes in the blood.

spi·ro·che·ti·cide, spi·ro·chae·ti·cide (spye″ro·keet′i·side) *n.* [*spirochete* + *-cide*]. An agent that kills spirochetes.

spi·ro·che·tol·y·sis, spi·ro·chae·tol·y·sis (spye″ro·kee·tol′i·sis) *n.* [*spirochete* + *-lysis*]. Destruction of spirochetes by lysis.

spi·ro·chet·osis, spi·ro·chaet·osis (spye″ro·ke·to′sis) *n.* [*spirochete* + *-osis*]. Any of the diseases caused by infection with one of the spirochetes. —**spirochet·ot·ic** (·tot′ick) *adj.*

spi·ro·gram (spye′ro·gram) *n.* [*spiro-* + *-gram*]. A recorded tracing of the movements and excursion of the chest during respiration.

spi·ro·graph (spye′ro·graph) *n.* [*spiro-* + *-graph*]. An instrument for registering respiration.

spi·rom·e·ter (spye·rom′e·tur) *n.* [*spiro-* + *meter*]. A device for measuring and recording the amount of air inhaled and exhaled. —**spi·ro·met·ric** (spye″ro·met′rick) *adj.*

spi·rom·e·try (spye·rom′e·tree) *n.* The measurement, by means of a spirometer, of inhaled and exhaled air.

spi·ro·no·lac·tone (spye″ro·no·lack′tone) *n.* 17-Hydroxy-7α-mercapto-3-oxo-17α-pregn-4-ene-21-carboxylic acid γ-lactone 7-acetate, $C_{24}H_{32}O_4S$, a steroid with a lactone ring attached at carbon-17 so that the latter is common to two rings. It is a diuretic drug that blocks the sodium-retaining action of aldosterone.

***Spi·rop·tera* carcinoma** (spye·rop′tur·uh). FIBIGER'S TUMOR.

spi·rox·a·sone (spye·rock′suh·sohn) *n.* 4′,5′-Dihydro-7α-mercaptospiro[androst-4-ene-17,2′(3*H*)-furan]-3-one acetate, $C_{24}H_{34}O_3S$, a diuretic drug.

spis·sat·ed (spis′ay·tid) *adj.* INSPISSATED.

spis·si·tude (spis′i·tewd) *n.* [L. *spissitudo*, thickness, from *spissus*, thick]. The state of being inspissated.

Spitz's nevus or **tumor.** JUVENILE MELANOMA.

splanchn-, splanchno- [Gk. *splanchnon*]. A combining form meaning *viscus, viscera, visceral.*

splanch·na (splank′nuh) *n.pl.* [Gk., pl. of *splanchnon*, viscus, visceral organ]. 1. The intestines. 2. The viscera.

splanch·nec·to·pia (splank″neck·to′pee·uh) *n.* [*splanchn-* + *-ectopia*]. The abnormal position or dislocation of a viscus.

splanch·nem·phrax·is (splank″nem·frack′sis) *n.* [*splanchn-* + *emphraxis*]. Obstruction of a viscus, particularly the intestine.

splanch·nes·the·sia, splanch·naes·the·sia (splank″nes·theez′ee·uh) *n.* [*splanchn-* + *esthesia*]. VISCERAL SENSATION. —**splanchnes·thet·ic, splanchnaes·thet·ic** (·thet′ick) *adj.*

splanch·nic (splank′nick) *adj.* [Gk. *splanchnikos*, from *splanchna*, viscera]. Pertaining to, or supplying, the viscera.

splanch·ni·cec·to·my (splank″ni·seck′tuh·mee) *n.* [*splanchnic* + *-ectomy*]. The surgical excision of the splanchnic nerves.

splanchnic ganglion. A small ganglion located on the greater splanchnic nerve near the twelfth thoracic vertebra. NA *ganglion splanchnicum.*

splanchnic layer. The internal layer of the lateral mesoderm after the formation of the coelom, forming a part of the splanchnopleure.

splanchnic mesoderm. The internal layer of the lateral mesoderm associated with entoderm after formation of the coelom.

splanchnic nerve. Any of the two or sometimes three nerves which arise from the thoracic portion of the sympathetic trunk, pierce the diaphragm, and terminate in the prevertebral ganglia of the mesenteric plexuses. These nerves are made up of preganglionic fibers which merely pass through the paravertebral ganglia en route to the celiac and mesenteric ganglia. See also *greater splanchnic nerve, least splanchnic nerve, lesser splanchnic nerve.*

splanch·ni·cot·o·my (splank″ni·kot′uh·mee) *n.* [*splanchnic* + *-tomy*]. Surgical division of a splanchnic nerve.

splanchno-. See *splanchn-.*

splanch·no·cele (splank′no·seel) *n.* [*splanchno-* + *-cele*]. A hernial protrusion of any abdominal viscus.

splanch·no·coele (splank′no·seel) *n.* [*splanchno-* + *-coele*]. The part of the coelom that persists in the adult, and gives rise to the pericardial, pleural, and abdominal cavities; the ventral coelom, or pleuroperitoneal space. It appears as a narrow fissure in the lateral mesoderm.

splanch·no·di·as·ta·sis (splank″no·dye·as′tuh·sis) *n.* [*splanchno-* + *diastasis*]. Displacement or separation of the viscera.

splanch·nog·ra·phy (splank·nog′ruh·fee) *n.* [*splanchno-* + *-graphy*]. The descriptive anatomy of the viscera.

splanch·no·lith (splank′no·lith) *n.* [*splanchno-* + *-lith*]. A calculus in a viscus.

splanch·no·li·thi·a·sis (splank″no·li·thigh′uh·sis) *n.* [*splanchnolith* + *-iasis*]. The condition of having a calculus of the intestine.

splanch·no·lo·gia (splank·no·lo′jee·uh) *n.* SPLANCHNOLOGY.

splanch·nol·o·gy (splank·nol′uh·jee) *n.* [*splanchno-* + *-logy*]. The branch of medical science pertaining to the viscera.

splanch·no·meg·a·ly (splank″no·meg′uh·lee) *n.* [*splanchno-* + *-megaly*]. Abnormal enlargement of a viscus or the viscera.

splanch·no·mi·cria (splank″no·migh′kree·uh) *n.* [*splanchno-* + *micr-* + *-ia*]. Abnormal smallness of a viscus or the visceral organs.

splanch·nop·a·thy (splank·nop′uth·ee) *n.* [*splanchno-* + *-pathy*]. Any disease of the viscera.

splanch·no·pleure (splank′no·ploor) *n.* [*splanchno-* + Gk. *pleura*, side]. The wall of the embryonic gut, composed of endoderm and the splanchnic layer of lateral mesoderm. —**splanch·no·pleu·ral** (splank″no·ploor′ul) *adj.*

splanch·nop·to·sia (splank″nop·to′zhuh) *n.* [*splanchno-* + *-ptosis* + *-ia*]. VISCEROPTOSIS.

splanch·nop·to·sis (splank″nop·to′sis) *n.* [*splanchno-* + *-ptosis*]. VISCEROPTOSIS.

splanch·no·scle·ro·sis (splank″no·skle·ro′sis) *n.* [*splanchno-* + *sclerosis*]. A visceral induration.

splanch·nos·co·py (splank·nos′kuh·pee) *n.* [*splanchno-* + *-scopy*]. Visual examination of the viscera, as through a peritoneoscope.

splanch·no·skel·e·ton (splank″no·skel′e·tun) *n.* [*splanchno-* + *skeleton*]. VISCERAL SKELETON.

splanch·no·so·mat·ic (splank″no·so·mat′ick) *adj.* [*splanchno-* + *somatic*]. Pertaining to the viscera and the body wall.

splanch·not·o·my (splank·not′uh·mee) *n.* [*splanchno-* + *-tomy*]. Dissection of the viscera.

splanch·no·tribe (splank′no·tribe) *n.* [*splanchno-* + *-tribe*]. An instrument for crushing a segment of the intestine and so occluding its lumen, previous to resecting it.

splay·foot, *n.* Flatfoot with extreme eversion of the forefoot and tarsus.

spleen, *n.* [Gk. *splēn*]. One of the abdominal viscera, located immediately below the diaphragm on the left side. It is the largest lymphatic organ of the body and also functions as a producer of erythrocytes. NA *lien.* See also Plates 8, 10, 13, 14.

spleen rate. The percentage of children aged 2 to 10 years who have enlarged spleens in a community where malaria is endemic.

splen-, spleno-. A combining form meaning *spleen, splenic.*

sple·nal·gia (sple·nal′jee·uh) *n.* [*splen-* + *-algia*]. Pain in the spleen.

Splen·do·re-Hoepp·li phenomenon. Formation of an eosinophilic deposit around *Sporotricum* (Splendore) and ova of *Schistosoma japonicum* (Hoeppli), as well as other fungi, helminths and multifilament silk suture material.

sple·nec·to·my (sple·neck′to·mee) *n.* [*splen-* + *-ectomy*]. Excision of the spleen. —**splenecto·mize** (·mize) *v.*

splen·ec·to·pia (splen″eck·to′pee·uh, splee″neck·) *n.* [*splen-* + *ectopia*]. Displacement of the spleen.

sple·nec·to·py (sple·neck′tuh·pee) *n.* SPLENECTOPIA.

sple·net·ic (sple·net′ick) *adj.* 1. Pertaining to the spleen. 2. Having a diseased spleen. 3. Marked by bad temper or sullen humor.

splenia. Plural of *splenium.*

sple·ni·al (splee'nee·ul) *adj.* Of or pertaining to a splenius muscle.

splen·ic (splen'ick, splee'nick) *adj.* [Gk. *splēnikos,* from *splēn,* spleen]. Of or pertaining to the spleen; lienal.

splenic anemia. Anemia associated with chronic passive splenic hyperemia.

splenic apoplexy. Hemorrhage into the spleen.

splenic artery. The lienal artery. See *lienal* in the Table of Arteries in the Appendix.

splenic corpuscle or **nodule.** MALPIGHIAN CORPUSCLE (1).

splenic fever. ANTHRAX.

splenic flexure. An abrupt turn of the colon beneath the lower end of the spleen, connecting the descending with the transverse colon. NA *flexura coli sinistra.*

splenic-flexure syndrome. Left upper quadrant pain, which may radiate to the left shoulder and inner aspect of the left arm; relieved by passage of feces or gas and presumed due to distention or spasmodic contraction of the colon.

splenic marginal zone. The junctional tissue between the red pulp and white pulp of the spleen, consisting of arterial terminals opening into a reticular meshwork.

splen·i·co·pan·cre·at·ic (splen''i·ko·pan''kree·at'ick) *adj.* [*splenic* + *pancreatic*]. Belonging, or pertaining, to both the spleen and the pancreas.

splenic penicilli. PENICILLI LIENIS.

splenic plexus. A visceral nerve plexus accompanying the splenic artery. NA *plexus lienalis.*

splenic pulp. The proper substance of the spleen. NA *pulpa lienalis.* See also *red pulp, white pulp.*

splenic souffle. A murmur said to be audible over the diseased spleen, as in malaria or leukemia.

splenic puncture. Needle biopsy of the spleen.

splenic tumor. A term sometimes applied to an enlarged spleen, not necessarily neoplastic, and usually only hyperplastic or hyperemic.

splenic vein. VENA LIENALIS.

splenic white pulp. WHITE PULP.

splen·i·form (splen'i·form, splee'ni·form) *adj.* [*splen-* + *-iform*]. Resembling the spleen.

sple·ni·tis (sple·nigh'tis) *n.* [Gk. *splēnitis,* a disease of the spleen]. Inflammation of the spleen.

sple·ni·um (splee'nee·um) *n.,* pl. **sple·nia** (·nee·uh) [NL., from Gk. *splēnion,* bandage]. 1. BANDAGE. 2. The rounded posterior extremity of the corpus callosum. NA *splenium corporis callosi.* See also Plate 18.

splenium cor·po·ris cal·lo·si (kor'po·ris ka·lo'sigh) [NA]. SPLENIUM (2).

sple·ni·us (splee'nee·us) *n.,* pl. **sple·nii** (·nee·eye) [NL., from *splenium*]. One of two muscles of the back of the neck, splenius capitis (NA *musculus splenius capitis*) and splenius cervicis (NA *musculus splenius cervicis*). See also Table of Muscles in the Appendix.

splenius cer·vi·cis ac·ces·so·ri·us (sur'vi·sis ack''se·so'ree·us). A variant of the splenius cervicis muscle.

splen·i·za·tion (splen''i·zay'shun) *n.* The stage of hyperemia and consolidation in pneumonia during which lung tissue grossly resembles the normal spleen or liver.

spleno-. See *splen-.*

sple·no·cele (splee'no·seel) *n.* [*spleno-* + *-cele*]. 1. Hernia of the spleen. 2. A tumor of the spleen.

sple·no·clei·sis (splee''no·klye'sis) *n.* [*spleno-* + *-cleisis*]. 1. Irritation of the surface of the spleen causing the production of new fibrous tissue on the spleen. 2. Explantation of a portion of the spleen underneath the rectus abdominis muscle.

sple·no·cyte (splee'no·site) *n.* [*spleno-* + *-cyte*]. A monocyte, regarded as developing from the pulp of the spleen.

sple·no·dyn·ia (splee''no·din'ee·uh, splen''o·) *n.* [*splen-* + *-odynia*]. Pain in the spleen.

sple·no·gram (splee'no·gram) *n.* [*spleno-* + *-gram*]. 1. A radiographic depiction of the spleen, usually after contrast medium injection. 2. A differential count of the splenic cellular population.

sple·no·gran·u·lo·ma·to·sis sid·er·ot·i·ca (splee''no·gran''yoo·lo''muh·to'sis sid''ur·ot'i·kuh). Slowly progressive splenomegaly, generally considered a form of chronic passive hyperemia. Histologically, the spleen is granulomatous with heavy hemosiderin deposition. Syn. *Gamna's disease, mycotic splenomegaly.*

sple·no·hep·a·to·meg·a·ly (splee''no·hep''uh·to·meg'uh·lee) *n.* [*spleno-* + *hepato-* + *-megaly*]. Englargement of the liver and spleen.

sple·noid (splee'noid) *adj.* [*splen-* + *-oid*]. Resembling the spleen.

sple·nol·y·sis (sple·nol'i·sis) *n.* [*spleno-* + *-lysis*]. Destruction of splenic tissue.

sple·no·ma·la·cia (splee''no·ma·lay'shee·uh) *n.* [*spleno-* + *malacia*]. Softening of the spleen.

sple·no·me·ga·lia (splee''no·me·gay'lee·uh) *n.* SPLENOMEGALY.

sple·no·meg·a·ly (splee''no·meg'uh·lee) *n.* [*spleno-* + *-megaly*]. Enlargement of the spleen.

sple·no·my·e·log·e·nous leukemia (splee''no·migh''e·loj'e·nus). GRANULOCYTIC LEUKEMIA.

sple·nop·a·thy (sple·nop'uth·ee) *n.* [*spleno-* + *-pathy*]. Any disease of the spleen.

sple·no·pexy (splee'no·peck''see) *n.* [*spleno-* + *-pexy*]. Fixation of the spleen to the abdominal wall by means of sutures.

sple·no·pneu·mo·nia (splee''no·new·mo'nyuh) *n.* The stage of pneumonia producing splenization or hepatization of lung tissue.

sple·no·por·tog·ra·phy (splee''no·por·tog'ruh·fee) *n.* [*spleno-* + *portal* + *-graphy*]. Roentgenologic demonstration of the splenic and portal vein system by injection of contrast medium into the spleen. —**spleno·por·to·gram** (·por'to·gram) *n.*

sple·nop·to·sis (splee''nop·to'sis) *n.* [*spleno-* + *-ptosis*]. Downward displacement of the spleen.

sple·no·re·nal (splee''no·ree'nul) *adj.* Pertaining to the spleen and the kidneys, or to the splenic and renal arteries or veins; lienorenal.

splenorenal shunt. An abnormal connection between the splenic vein and the left renal vein; usually it results from a surgical procedure to relieve portal hypertension.

sple·nor·rha·phy (sple·nor'uh·fee) *n.* [*spleno-* + *-rrhaphy*]. Suture of the spleen.

sple·not·o·my (sple·not'uh·mee) *n.* [*spleno-* + *-tomy*]. 1. The operation of incising the spleen. 2. Dissection of the spleen.

sple·no·tox·in (splee''no·tock'sin, splen''o·) *n.* [*spleno-* + *toxin*]. A cytotoxin with specific action on the cells of the spleen.

sple·no·ty·phoid (splee''no·tye'foid) *n.* Typhoid fever with splenic involvement.

splen·u·lus (splen'yoo·lus) *n.,* pl. **splenu·li** (·lye) [NL., dim. of L. *splen,* spleen]. ACCESSORY SPLEEN.

sple·nun·cu·lus (sple·nunk'yoo·lus) *n.,* pl. **splenuncu·li** (·lye). ACCESSORY SPLEEN.

splice, *v.* [MD. *splissen*]. To overlap and join by suture, as to splice a tendon.

splint, *n.* [MD. *splinte*]. 1. A support made of wood, metal, plastic, plaster, or other material for immobilizing the ends of a fractured bone or for restricting the movement of any movable part. 2. *In dentistry,* a device or appliance used to stabilize mobile teeth and redistribute occlusal forces. 3. SPLINT BONE (1). See also *splints.*

splint·age (splin'tij) *n.* The application of splints.

splint bone. 1. A vestigial second or fourth metacarpal or metatarsal of the horse extending, in the forelimb, from the "knee" and, in the hind limb, from the hock, toward the fetlock. 2. FIBULA.

splin·ter hemorrhage. A subungual linear hemorrhage resembling a splinter under the nail; found in patients with bacterial endocarditis and after trauma.

splints. A periostitis of the splint bones in the forelegs of young horses; usually associated with hard training or poor conformation. Compare *shin splints.*

split brain. A mammalian brain in which two independently though not necessarily equally functioning cerebral hemispheres have been created by surgical transection of the corpus callosum and sometimes other commissures; the technique has also been applied to patients with intractable epilepsy or massive lesions of one hemisphere. See also *disconnection syndrome.*

split graft. A free graft of skin using less than full thickness, varying from the very thin epidermal graft to the intermediate split-skin graft and the thick-split graft.

split pelvis. A pelvis in which there is congenital separation of the pubic bones at the symphysis, often associated with exstrophy of the urinary bladder. Syn. *pelvis fissa.*

split personality. The type of human being in whom there is a separation of various components of the normal personality unit, and each component functions as an entity apart from the remaining personality structure; observed in hysteria and schizophrenia. See also *dissociation* (3), *dissociative type of hysterical neurosis.*

split product. A decomposition product, as the aglycone produced by hydrolysis of a glycoside.

split renal function test. HOWARD TEST.

split-skin graft. SPLIT GRAFT.

splitters of Spengler [C. O. *Spengler*]. SPENGLER'S FRAGMENTS.

split-thickness graft. SPLIT GRAFT.

split·ting, *n.* A chemical change in which a compound is changed into two or more simpler bodies, as by hydrolysis. 2. A reduplication of the first or second heart sounds due to asynchronous closure of the mitral and tricuspid valves or aortic and pulmonic valves, respectively. 3. *In psychology,* an ego mechanism that precedes, and in some cases determines the type of, repression.

spo·dio·my·e·li·tis (spo″dee·o·migh″e·lye′tis) *n.* [Gk. *spodios,* gray (from *spodos,* ashes) + *myelitis*]. PARALYTIC SPINAL POLIOMYELITIS.

spodo·gram (spod′o·gram) *n.* [Gk. *spodos*, ashes, + *-gram*]. A photograph or diagram picturing the distribution of mineral ash of a cell or tissue section following microincineration.

spo·dog·ra·phy (spo·dog′ruh·fee) *n.* [Gk. *spodos*, ashes, + *-graphy*]. The microincineration of a cell or tissue section for the study of the distribution of nonvolatile mineral ash.

spondyl-, spondylo- [Gk. *spondylos*]. A combining form meaning *vertebra, vertebral.*

spon·dy·lal·gia (spon″di·lal′jee·uh) *n.* [*spondyl-* + *-algia*]. Pain in a vertebra.

spon·dyl·ar·thri·tis (spon″dil·ahr·thrigh′tis) *n.* [*spondyl-* + *arthritis*]. Arthritis of the vertebrae.

spon·dyl·ar·throc·a·ce (spon″dil·ahr′throck′uh·see) *n.* [*spondyl-* + *arthro-* + *-cace*]. Caries of a vertebra.

spon·dyl·ex·ar·thro·sis (spon″dil·ecks″ăr·thro′sis) *n.* [*spondyl-* + *ex-* + *arthrosis*]. A vertebral dislocation.

spondyli. Plural of *spondylus.*

spon·dy·li·tis (spon″di·lye′tis) *n.* [*spondyl-* + *-itis*]. Inflammation of the vertebrae. —**spondy·lit·ic** (·lit′ick) *adj.*

spondylitis an·ky·lo·poi·et·i·ca (ang″ki·lo·poy·et′i·kuh). ANKYLOSING SPONDYLITIS.

spon·dy·li·ze·ma (spon″di·li·zee′muh) *n.* [*spondyl-* + Gk. *hizēma,* a sinking]. The settling of a vertebra into the place of a subjacent one that has been destroyed.

spondylo-. See *spondyl-.*

spon·dy·lo·ar·thri·tis an·ky·lo·poi·et·i·ca (spon″di·lo·ahr·thrigh′tis ang″ki·lo·poy·et′i·kuh). ANKYLOSING SPONDYLITIS.

spon·dy·loc·a·ce (spon″di·lock′uh·see) *n.* [*spondylo-* + *-cace*]. SPONDYLARTHROCACE.

spon·dy·lo·di·dym·ia (spon″di·lo·di·dim′ee·uh) *n.* [*spondylo-* + *didym-* + *-ia*]. The condition of union of conjoined twins united by their vertebrae.

spon·dy·lod·y·mus (spon″di·lod′i·mus) *n.* [*spondylo-* + *-dymus*]. Conjoined twins united by the vertebrae. See also *rachipagus.*

spon·dy·lo·dyn·ia (spon″di·lo·din′ee·uh) *n.* [*spondyl-* + *-odynia*]. Pain in a vertebra.

spon·dy·lo·lis·the·sis (spon″di·lo·lis·thees′is) *n.* [*spondyl-* + Gk. *olisthēsis,* dislocation]. Forward displacement of a vertebra upon the one below as a result of bilateral defect in the vertebral arch, or erosion of the articular surface of the posterior facets due to degenerative joint disease or elongation of the pedicle. It occurs most commonly between the fifth lumbar vertebra and the sacrum. —**spondylolis·thet·ic** (·thet′ick) *adj.*

spondylolisthetic pelvis. A deformity resulting from a forward displacement of the centrum of the last lumbar vertebra.

spon·dy·lol·y·sis (spon″di·lol′i·sis) *n.* [*spondylo-* + *-lysis*]. A defect or fracture, unilateral or bilateral, through the pars interarticularis of a vertebra which can lead to spondylolisthesis.

spon·dy·lop·a·thy (spon″di·lop′uth·ee) *n.* [*spondylo-* + *-pathy*]. Any disease of the vertebrae.

spon·dy·lo·py·o·sis (spon″di·lo·pye·o′sis) *n.* [*spondylo-* + *pyosis*]. Suppurative inflammation of one or more vertebrae.

spon·dy·lo·sis (spon″di·lo′sis) *n.* [*spondyl-* + *-osis*]. Vertebral ankylosis. —**spondy·lo·lyt·ic** (·lo·lit′ick) *adj.*

spon·dy·lo·syn·de·sis (spon″di·lo·sin·dee′sis) *n.* [*spondylo-* + *syndesis*]. SPINAL FUSION.

spon·dy·lot·o·my (spon″di·lot′uh·mee) *n.* [*spondylo-* + *-tomy*]. Section of a vertebra in correcting a deformity.

spon·dy·lus (spon′di·lus) *n.,* pl. **spondy·li** (·lye) [L., from Gk. *spondylos*]. VERTEBRA. —**spondylous,** *adj.*

sponge (spunj) *n.* [Gk. *spongia*]. 1. A marine animal of the phylum Porifera. 2. The skeleton of the sponge, used as an absorbent. 3. GAUZE SPONGE.

sponge bath. A bath in which the body is sponged or washed one part at a time without being immersed.

sponge-gatherer's disease. A disease of divers due to a secretion of certain species of the sea anemone *Actinia,* found in waters where sponges grow. At the point of contact upon the body, the viscid excretion causes a swelling and intense itching, followed by a papule surrounded by a zone of redness which later becomes black and gangrenous and forms a deep ulcer.

sponge holder. A surgical instrument which clasps a gauze sponge; used to apply antiseptics to skin, cleanse a wound, or sponge away blood from a deep surgical wound.

sponge kidney. MEDULLARY SPONGE KIDNEY.

sponge probang. A probang with a small sponge at one end.

sponge tent. A tent made of compressed sponge, for dilating the os uteri.

spongi-, spongio-. A combining form meaning *sponge, spongy.*

spon·gi·form (spun′ji·form) *adj.* [*spongi-* + *-form*]. Resembling a sponge.

spongiform encephalopathy. SPONGY DEGENERATION (2).

spon·gio·blast (spon′jee·o·blast, spun′jee·o·) *n.* [*spongio-* + *-blast*]. A nonnervous cell derived from the ectoderm of the embryonic neural tube, and later forming the neuroglia, the ependymal cells, the neurilemma sheath cells, the satellite cells of ganglions, and Müller's fibers of the retina.

spon·gio·blas·to·ma (spon″jee·o·blas·to′muh) *n.,* pl. **spongioblastomas, spongioblastoma·ta** (·tuh) [*spongioblast* + *-oma*]. 1. SPONGIOBLASTOMA POLARE. 2. GLIOBLASTOMA MULTIFORME.

spongioblastoma mul·ti·for·me (mul·ti·for′mee). GLIOBLASTOMA MULTIFORME.

spongioblastoma po·la·re (po·lair′ee). A benign glial tumor composed of astrocytes with long polar cytoplasmic fibers.

spongioblastoma prim·i·ti·vum (prim·i·tye′vum). A tumor with the histologic features and natural history of some forms of medulloblastoma.

spongioblastoma uni·po·la·re (yoo″ni·po·lair′ee). SPONGIOBLASTOMA POLARE.

spon·gio·cyte (spon′jee·o·site, spun′) *n.* [*spongio-* + *-cyte*]. A cell, in the fasciculate zone of the adrenal cortex, which appears spongy because of the solution of lipids during preparation of the tissue for microscopical study.

spon·gio·cy·to·ma (spon″jee·o·sigh·to′muh) *n.* [*spongiocyte* + *-oma*]. ASTROCYTOMA.

spon·gio·form (spon′jee·o·form, spun′) *adj.* [*spongio-* + *-form*]. SPONGIFORM; SPONGY.

spon·gi·oid (spon′jee·oid, spun′) *adj.* [*spongi-* + *-oid*]. SPONGIFORM.

spon·gio·plasm (spon′jee·o·plaz·um, spun′) *n.* [*spongio-* + *-plasm*]. The fine protoplasmic threads forming the reticulum of cells after certain fixations.

spon·gi·ose (spon′jee·oce) *adj.* [L. *spongiosus*]. Full of pores, like a sponge.

spon·gi·o·sis (spon″jee·o′sis, spun″) *n.* [*spongi-* + *-osis*]. Accumulation of fluid in the intercellular spaces of the epidermis; an intercellular edema. —**spongi·ot·ic** (·ot′ick) *adj.*

spon·gi·o·si·tis (spon″jee·o·sigh′tis) *n.* [*spongiosum* + *-itis*]. Inflammation of the corpus spongiosum.

-spongium [NL., from L. *spongia*, sponge]. A combining form meaning *a network or reticulum.*

spon·gy (spun′jee) *adj.* Having the texture of sponge; very porous.

spongy body. CORPUS SPONGIOSUM PENIS.

spongy bone. CANCELLOUS BONE.

spongy degeneration. 1. SPONGY DEGENERATION OF INFANCY. 2. Any pathologic state characterized by polymicrocavitation of the central nervous system. Syn. *spongiform encephalopathy.*

spongy degeneration of infancy. A pathologic feature observed in the brains of infants and young children with a variety of conditions disturbing myelination of the brain including some of the aminoacidurias, characterized by the presence of rounded, empty spaces separated by strands of more or less intact neural tissue, resulting in the spongelike appearance. There may be edema, and demyelination may be extensive. Syn. *Canavan's disease, van Bogaert-Bertrand disease.*

spongy degeneration of the central nervous system. SPONGY DEGENERATION OF INFANCY.

spongy layer. The middle zone of the endometrium during the secretory phase of the menstrual cycle, characterized by the dilated portion of the glands and edematous connective tissue.

spongy portion of the urethra. The portion of the urethra contained in the corpus spongiosum penis; PENILE URETHRA. Syn. *cavernous urethra.*

spongy state. SPONGY DEGENERATION (2).

spon·ta·ne·ous (spon·tay′nee·us) *adj.* [L. *spontaneus*, from *sponte*, voluntarily]. 1. Occurring naturally; not induced. 2. Occurring without external cause or influence. 3. Occurring without apparent cause. 4. Unpremeditated; not deliberate.

spontaneous abortion. Unexpected premature expulsion of the product of conception before the 20th completed week of gestation.

spontaneous amputation. 1. CONGENITAL AMPUTATION. 2. Amputation not caused by external trauma or injury, as in ainhum.

spontaneous aneurysm. PRIMARY ANEURYSM.

spontaneous erysipelas. IDIOPATHIC ERYSIPELAS.

spontaneous fracture. A fracture occurring without apparent trauma; occurs in bone diseases.

spontaneous generation. A theory that living organisms can originate from nonliving matter; abiogenesis.

spontaneous labor. Labor requiring no artificial aid.

spontaneous mutation. Mutation in nature which forms the basic materials for evolution. Syn. *natural mutation.*

spontaneous necrosis. ASEPTIC NECROSIS.

spontaneous pneumothorax. Air in a pleural space and consequent lung collapse in the absence of trauma or deliberate introduction of air into the pleural space.

spontaneous subarachnoid hemorrhage. Bleeding confined to the subarachnoid space, due to rupture of a saccular (berry) aneurysm.

spontaneous version. Turning of the fetus without artificial assistance.

spoon, *n.* An instrument, usually made of metal, with a circular or oval bowl attached to a handle. A spoon is considered full when the contained liquid comes up to, but does not show a curve above, the upper edge or rim of the bowl. Teaspoons are popularly used to measure the dose of medicines on the assumption that they hold 5 ml.

spoon·er·ism (spoon′ur·iz·um) *n.* [W. A. *Spooner*, English minister, 1844–1930]. A psychic speech or writing defect characterized by the tendency to transpose sounds or syllables of two or more words.

spoon nail. KOILONYCHIA.

spor-, spori-, sporo- [Gk. *spora*, seed]. A combining form meaning *spore.*

spo·rad·ic (spo·rad′ick) *adj.* [Gk. *sporadikos*, from *speirein*, to sow, scatter]. Scattered; occurring in an isolated manner. Contr. *endemic, epidemic.*

sporadic typhus. BRILL'S DISEASE.

spo·ran·gio·phore (spo·ran′jee·o·fore) *n.* [*sporangium* + *-phore*]. A specialized hyphal branch of a fungus which bears a sporangium.

spo·ran·gio·spore (spo·ran′jee·o·spore) *n.* [*sporangium* + *spore*]. A fungus spore borne within a sporangium.

spo·ran·gi·um (spo·ran′jee·um) *n.*, pl. **sporan·gia** (·jee·uh) [*spor-* + *-angium*]. A specialized structure of a fungus; the enlarged end of a hypha within which spores develop.

spore, *n.* [Gk. *spora*, seed]. 1. *In bacteriology*, a refractile, resting body, highly resistant to heat, toxic chemicals, and dessication, found in the family Bacillaceae. 2. *In mycology and botany*, an asexual or sexual reproductive unit. 3. *In protozoology*, any of various reproductive cells, including the suborder of Eimeriidea; the sporoblasts resulting from nuclear division in the sporocyst.

spori-. See *spor-.*

spo·ri·cide (spo′ri·side) *n.* [*spori-* + *-cide*]. Any agent that destroys spores. —**spo·ri·ci·dal** (spo″ri·sigh′dul) *adj.*

spo·rid·i·um (spo·rid′ee·um) *n.*, pl. **sporid·ia** (·ee·uh) [NL., dim. of *spora*, seed]. A kind of spore occurring in the rusts and the smuts.

sporo-. See *spor-.*

spo·ro·ag·glu·ti·na·tion (spo″ro·uh·gloo″ti·nay′shun) *n.* Agglutination of spores by antiserum.

spo·ro·blast (spo′ro·blast) *n.* [*sporo-* + *-blast*]. Any of two or four daughter cells resulting from nuclear division within the oocyst of a protozoon of the family Eimeriidea.

spo·ro·cyst (spo′ro·sist) *n.* [*sporo-* + *-cyst*]. 1. The oocyst of certain protozoa, e.g., plasmodia and coccidia, in which sporozoites develop. 2. The larval stages of flukes in snails, from which cercariae develop.

spo·ro·cyte (spo′ro·site) *n.* [*sporo-* + *-cyte*]. A single binucleated cell formed in the life cycle of protozoa of the orders Myxosporidia and Actinomyxidia.

spo·ro·gen·e·sis (spo″ro·jen′e·sis) *n.* [*sporo-* + *-genesis*]. Production of spores. —**sporogen·ic** (·ick) *adj.*

spo·rog·e·nous (spo·roj′e·nus) *adj.* [*sporo-* + *-genous*]. Spore-producing.

spo·rog·o·ny (spo·rog′uh·nee) *n.* [*sporo-* + *-gony*]. Reproduction by spores; especially spore formation in Sporozoa following encystment of a zygote.

spo·ront (spo′ront) *n.* [*spor-* + Gk. *ōn, ontos*, being]. In Sporozoa, a cell that forms spores by encystment and subsequent division.

spo·ron·ti·cide (spo·ron'ti·side) *n.* [*sporont* + *-cide*]. A substance destructive to sporonts, such as those used to inhibit the spread of malaria. **—spo·ron·ti·ci·dal** (spo·ron"ti·sigh'dul) *adj.*

spo·ron·to·cide (spo·ron'tuh·side) *n.* SPORONTICIDE.

spo·ro·phyte (spo'ro·fite) *n.* [*sporo-* + *-phyte*]. The asexual, spore-producing phase in plants having alternation of generations.

spo·rot·ri·chin (spo·rot'ri·kin) *n.* An extract of cultures of *Sporotrichum schenckii,* used as a skin test antigen and in the agglutination test for sporotrichosis.

spo·ro·tri·cho·sis (spor"o·tri·ko'sis, ·trye·ko'sis) *n.,* pl. **sporotri·cho·ses** (·seez) [*Sporotrich*um + *-osis*]. A subacute or chronic granulomatous disease caused by the fungus *Sporotrichum.* The lesions are usually cutaneous and spread along lymph channels; occasionally the internal organs and bones may be involved. The disease is reported among farmers, florists, and others working in soil. Syn. *de Beurmann-Gougerot disease, Schenck's disease.*

Spo·rot·ri·chum (spo·rot'ri·kum) *n.* A genus of saprophytic or parasitic fungi.

Sporotrichum beur·man·ni (bewr·man'eye, boyr·). *SPOROTRICHUM SCHENCKII.*

Sporotrichum schenck·ii (shenk'ee·eye). A species of fungi that is the causative agent of sporotrichosis, growing at room temperature and on noncystine-containing media as a leathery, filamentous, brown-to-black colony, but in tissues and exudates of animals, rarely of man, as cigar-shaped, round, or fusiform budding yeast cells.

sporozoa. Plural of *sporozoon.*

Spo·ro·zoa (spo"ruh·zo'uh) *n.pl.* [*sporo-* + Gk. *zōa,* animals]. A class of parasitic Protozoa; the orders Coccidia, Sarcosporidia, and Haemosporidia are parasites of man.

spo·ro·zo·an (spo"ruh·zo'un) *adj.* & *n.* 1. Of or pertaining to the Sporozoa. 2. An organism of the class Sporozoa.

spo·ro·zo·ite (spo"ruh·zo'ite) *n.* The organism resulting from the schizogenesis or sporogony of the Sporozoa.

spo·ro·zo·on (spo"ruh·zo'on) *n.,* pl. **sporo·zoa** [*sporo-* + Gk. *zōon,* animal]. An organism of the class Sporozoa.

sport, *n.* An individual organism that differs from its parents to an unusual degree; a mutant.

spor·u·late (spor'yoo·late) *v.* To eject spores from a sporangium; to form spores.

spor·u·la·tion (spor"yoo·lay'shun) *n.* The formation of spores.

spot film. A small, highly collimated radiograph of an anatomic part, frequently obtained in conjunction with fluoroscopy.

spot grinding. Correction of occlusion by removal of high areas of teeth or prosthetic devices, as disclosed by use of 14192ulating paper.

spotted bones. OSTEOPOIKILOSIS.

spotted fever rickettsiae. A group of rickettsiae which multiply in the nucleus and the cytoplasm of susceptible animal cells, and which are transmitted by ticks and mites. The diseases they cause include Rocky Mountain spotted fever, tick-borne typhus fevers of Africa, and rickettsialpox.

spotted leprosy. LUCIO LEPROSY.

spot test. Any test using small quantities of a reagent and substance tested, as on a plate or sheet of paper, for the determination of the presence of a substance.

spot·ting, *n.* Small amounts of bloody vaginal discharge, usually intermenstrual, and of significance in certain obstetric and gynecologic conditions.

sprain, *n.* A wrenching of a joint, producing a stretching or laceration of the ligaments.

sprain fracture. An injury in which a tendon or ligament, together with a shell of bone, is torn from its attachment; most commonly occurring at the ankle.

spray, *n.* 1. A stream of air and finely divided liquid produced with an atomizer, or other device. 2. A liquid pharmaceutical preparation intended for applying medication to the nose, throat, or other cavities by spraying from an atomizer; may be aqueous or oily in character.

spread·ing, *n.* Growth of bacteria beyond the line of inoculation.

spreading depression. LEÃO'S SPREADING DEPRESSION.

Spreng·el's deformity (shpreng'el) [O. G. K. *Sprengel,* German surgeon, 1852-1915]. Congenital elevation of the scapula; may be due to bony or muscular anomalies.

spring conjunctivitis or **catarrh.** VERNAL CONJUNCTIVITIS.

spring finger. A condition in which there is an obstruction to flexion and extension of one or more fingers; due to injuries or inflammation of the tendinous sheaths.

spring·halt (spring'hawlt) *n.* STRINGHALT.

spring hock. STRINGHALT.

springing mydriasis. ALTERNATING MYDRIASIS.

spring lancet. A lancet in which the blade is thrust out by means of a small spring operating on a trigger; often used to obtain small quantities of blood for laboratory examinations.

spring ligament. PLANTAR CALCANEONAVICULAR LIGAMENT.

spring onion sign. COBRA HEAD SIGN.

spring-water cyst. Any cyst arising from serous membranes, so named because of the clarity of the fluid they contain; applied especially to pericardial cysts.

Spritz bottle. A wash bottle for laboratory use.

¹sprue (sproo) *n.* [D. *spruw*]. Generally a malabsorption syndrome characterized by impaired absorption of foods, minerals, and water by the small bowel; symptoms are due to nutritional deficiencies resulting from impaired absorption or due to altered intestinal activity. See also *celiac syndrome, tropical sprue.*

²sprue, *n.* & *v.* 1. Wax, plastic, or metal that forms the pathway for molten metal in casting procedures; also the hardened metal that fills this pathway. 2. To form a sprue.

spud, *n.* A surgical instrument with a dull flattened blade, used for blunt dissection or removal of foreign bodies.

spur, *n.* 1. A sharp projection. Syn. *calcar.* 2. *In biology,* a pointed, spinelike outgrowth, either of the integument or of a projecting appendage.

spur·gall (spur'gawl) *n.* A calloused and hairless place on the side of a horse, caused by the use of a spur.

spurge (spurj) *n.* [MF., from L. *expurgare,* to purge]. Any of various plants of the genus *Euphorbia.*

spu·ri·ous (spew'ree·us) *adj.* [L. *spurius*]. False; closely resembling a genuine instance functionally or in symptoms but not in pathological or morphological characteristics.

spurious aneurysm. FALSE ANEURYSM.

spurious angina. ANGINA PECTORIS VASOMOTORIA.

spurious ankylosis. EXTRACAPSULAR ANKYLOSIS.

spurious cataract. MITTENDORF'S DOT.

spurious jugular foramen. A foramen in the temporal bone of the embryo; it gives passage to a vein from the lateral sinus to the external jugular vein.

spur of the septum. An outgrowth of the nasal septum.

spurred rye. ERGOT.

spu·tum (spew'tum) *n.,* pl. **spu·ta** (·tuh), **sputums** [L., from *spuere,* to spit out]. Material discharged from the surface of the air passages, throat, or mouth, and removed chiefly by spitting but in lesser degree by swallowing. It may consist of saliva, mucus, or pus, either alone or in any combination. It may also contain microorganisms, fibrin, blood or its decomposition products, or inhaled particulate foreign matter.

sq. cm. (= cm^2) Square centimeter.

squa·lene (squay'leen) *n.* [*Squal*us, a genus of sharks, + *-ene*]. 2,6,10,15,19,23-Hexamethyl-2,6,10,14,18,22-tetracosahexaene, $C_{30}H_{50}$, an unsaturated hydrocarbon occurring in large proportion in shark-liver oil and in smaller proportion in various vegetable oils; an intermediate in the biosynthesis of cholesterol.

squa·ma (skway'muh) *n.,* pl. **squa·mae** (·mee) [L., scale]. 1. A platelike mass, as the squama of the temporal bone. 2. A scale of the skin.

squama fron·ta·lis (fron·tay'lis) [NA]. The vertical portion of the frontal bone.

squama oc·ci·pi·ta·lis (ock·sip·i·tay'lis) [NA]. The posterior part of the occipital bone.

squama tem·po·ra·lis (tem·po·ray'lis) [NA]. The anterior and superior part of the temporal bone which is thin and scalelike.

squame (skwame) *n.* [F.]. SQUAMA.

squamo-. A combining form meaning *squamous.*

squa·mo·ba·sal (skway″mo·bay'sul) *adj.* Pertaining to the basal and squamous cells of a stratified squamous epithelium.

squa·mo·co·lum·nar (skway″mo·kol·um'nur) *adj.* Pertaining to squamous and columnar cells; usually refers to the junction of these two types of epithelium in the uterine cervix.

squa·mo·oc·cip·i·tal (skway″mo·ock·sip'i·tul) *adj.* Pertaining to the squamous portion of the occipital bone, or to the suture between the squamous part of the temporal bone and the occipital bone.

squa·mo·pa·ri·e·tal suture (skway″mo·pa·rye'e·tul). The site of union between the squamous portion of the temporal bone and the parietal bone. NA *sutura squamosa cranii.*

squa·mo·sa (skway·mo'suh) *n.*, pl. **squamo·sae** (·see) [short for *pars squamosa*]. The squamous portion of the temporal bone.

squa·mo·sal (skway·mo'sul) *adj.* 1. SQUAMOUS. 2. Pertaining to the squamosa.

squamosal suture. SQUAMOPARIETAL SUTURE.

squa·mo·sphe·noid (skway″mo·sfee'noid) *adj.* Pertaining to the squamous portion of the temporal bone and to the sphenoid bone.

squamosphenoid suture. SPHENOSQUAMOSAL SUTURE.

squa·mo·tym·pan·ic (skway″mo·tim·pan'ick) *adj.* Pertaining to the squamosal and tympanic parts of the temporal bone.

squa·mous (skway'mus) *adj.* [L. *squamosus,* scaly, from *squama,* scale]. 1. Thin and flat, like a fish's scale. 2. Consisting of or characterized by flat, scalelike cells, as squamous epithelium. 3. Pertaining to or constituting the thin anterior and superior portion of the temporal bone.

squamous alveolar cell. The extremely thin epithelial cell across which respiratory gases pass between air and blood in the wall of a pulmonary alveolus. Syn. *small alveolar cell.* Contr. *great alveolar cell.*

squamous blepharitis. Marginal blepharitis with the formation of branny scales.

squamous cell carcinoma. A carcinoma whose parenchyma is composed of anaplastic squamous cells. Syn. *epidermoid carcinoma.*

squamous cell epithelioma. SQUAMOUS CELL CARCINOMA.

squamous epithelium. Epithelium in which the cells appear as thin plates.

square knot. A double knot in which the free ends of the second knot lie in the same plane as the ends of the first. The knot in most general use in surgery.

squaw root. CAULOPHYLLUM.

squill (skwil) *n.* [L. *squilla,* from Gk. *skilla*]. The cut and dried fleshy inner scale of the bulb of the white variety of *Urginea maritima,* or of *U. indica.* Contains many glycosides, most of them cardioactive. Squill has been used as a diuretic and nauseant and more recently, as a cardiotonic drug, but the uncertainty of the absorption of its active principles has been a deterrent to the use of squill and its preparations and derivatives.

squint, *n.* STRABISMUS.

squint hook. A right-angled or a curved instrument used in the operation for strabismus for exerting traction on tendons.

squir·rel monkey. A very small South and Central American monkey of the genus *Saimiri.*

Sr Symbol for strontium.

^{90}Sr Symbol for strontium 90.

SRIF Abbreviation for *somatotropin-release-inhibiting factor* (= SOMATOSTATIN).

sRNA Abbreviation for *soluble RNA.*

SRS-A Abbreviation for *slow reacting substance of anaphylaxis.*

$\overline{ss}$, ss Abbreviation for *semis,* one-half.

SS disease. Homozygous sickle cell disease: SICKLE CELL ANEMIA. Compare *SC disease.*

SSS Abbreviation for *specific soluble substance.*

$S_1S_2S_3$ pattern. A nonspecific conduction variant seen in an electrocardiogram and characterized by an S wave in standard leads I, II, and III; there are prominent terminal QRS forces directed to the right, superiorly and posteriorly.

stab, *n. & v.* 1. A puncture wound. 2. The path formed by plunging an inoculation needle into nutrient media. 3. BAND CELL. 4. To puncture.

stab cell or **form** (stab, shtahp) [Ger., staff]. BAND CELL.

stab culture. A culture in which the medium is inoculated by means of a needle bearing the microorganisms, which is inserted deeply into the medium.

sta·bile (stay'bil, stay'bile) *adj.* [L. *stabilis*]. 1. Stationary; immobile; maintaining a fixed position. 2. Resistant to chemical change.

stabile current. A current applied with both electrodes in a fixed position.

sta·bi·li·zer (stay'bi·lye″zur) *n.* 1. A retarding agent, or a substance that counteracts the effect of a vigorous accelerator and preserves a chemical equilibrium. 2. A substance added to a solution to render it more stable, as acetanilid to hydrogen peroxide solution.

stab·ker·ni·ge cell (shtahp'kerr″ni·guh) [Ger., from *Stab,* staff, + *Kern,* nucleus]. BAND CELL.

sta·ble, *adj.* [OF. *estable,* from L. *stabilis*]. 1. Steady, regular, not easily moved. 2. Secure; specifically, not subject to sudden alterations in mood. 3. Unlikely to break down or dissolve; in the case of a compound, likely to retain its composition under the application of physical or chemical forces.

stable factor. FACTOR VII.

stable fly. *STOMOXYS.*

stac·ca·to (sta·kah'to) *adj.* [It., detached]. Designating an abrupt, jerky manner of speech with a noticeable interval between words.

stach·y·drine (stack'i·dreen) *n.* *N*-Methylproline methyl betaine, $C_7H_{13}NO_2$, an alkaloid occurring in *Stachys tuberifera* and other plants.

stach·y·ose (stack'ee·oce) *n.* A tetrasaccharide obtained from the tubers of *Stachys tuberifera* and some other plants. On complete hydrolysis, it yields one molecule each of fructose and glucose and two of galactose.

Stader pin. A bicortical pin used with a Stader splint or cast.

Stader's splint [O. *Stader,* U.S. veterinary surgeon]. A metal bar with pins affixed at right angles. The pins are driven into the fragments of a fracture, and the bar maintains the alignment.

Stadie method. RIGGS AND STADIE METHOD.

sta·di·um (stay'dee·um) *n.*, pl. **sta·dia** (·dee·uh) [L., from Gk. *stadion,* a unit of distance, as in a racecourse]. A stage or period in the course of a disease, especially a febrile disease.

stadium ac·mes (ack'meez). The height of a disease.

stadium am·phib·o·les (am·fib'o·leez). The stage of a disease after its height but before it abates.

stadium an·ni·hi·la·ti·o·nis (a·nigh″i·lay·shee·o'nis). The convalescent stage of a disease.

stadium aug·men·ti (awg·men'tye). The period of increase in the intensity of disease.

stadium ca·lo·ris (ka·lo'ris). The period of disease during which there is fever.

stadium con·ta·gii (kon·tay'jee·eye). The prodromal stage of an infectious disease; the period of a disease during which it is contagious.

stadium con·va·les·cen·ti·ae (kon·va·le·sen'shee·ee). The period of recovery from disease.

stadium dec·re·men·ti (deck·re·men'tye). Defervescence of a febrile disease; the period of decrease in the severity of disease.

stadium de·crus·ta·ti·o·nis (dee''krus·tay·shee·o'nis). The stage of an exanthematous disease in which the lesions form crusts.

stadium des·qua·ma·ti·o·nis (des''kwa·may·shee·o'nis). The period of desquamation in an exanthematous disease.

stadium erup·ti·o·nis (e·rup·shee·o'nis). The period of an exanthematous disease in which the exanthem appears.

stadium ex·sic·ca·ti·o·nis (eck''si·kay·shee·o'nis). STADIUM DECRUSTATIONIS.

stadium flo·ri·ti·o·nis (flo·rish·ee·o'nis). The stage of an eruptive disease during which the exanthem is at its height.

stadium frig·o·ris (frig'o·ris). The cold or shivering stage of a febrile disease.

stadium in·cre·men·ti (ing·kre·men'tye). The stage of increase of a fever or disease.

stadium in·cu·ba·ti·o·nis (ing''kew·bay·shee·o'nis). The incubation period of a disease.

stadium ma·ni·a·ca·le (ma·nigh·uh·kay'lee). The stage of greatest excitement and restlessness in a manic illness after which symptoms gradually subside.

stadium ner·vo·sum (nur·vo'sum). The paroxysmal stage of a disease.

stadium pro·dro·mo·rum (pro·dro·mo'rum). The stage immediately prior to the appearance of the signs and symptoms of disease.

stadium su·do·ris (sue·do'ris). The sweating stage of a febrile disease.

stadium sup·pu·ra·ti·o·nis (sup''yoo·ray·shee·o'nis). The period of suppuration in smallpox.

stadium ul·ti·mum (ul'ti·mum). The final stage of a febrile disease.

Staeh·li's pigment line (shte^y'lee) [J. *Staehli,* Swiss ophthalmologist, 20th century]. A pigmented epithelial line across the lower portion of the cornea due to the decomposition of iron; seen in older people. Syn. *Hudson's line, Hudson-Staehli's line.*

staff, *n.* 1. An instrument for passing through the urethra to the urinary bladder, used as a guide in operations on the bladder or for stricture. It is usually grooved. 2. The professional personnel, or a corps of specially trained persons, concerned with the care of patients in a hospital. See also *attending staff, consulting staff, house staff.*

staff cell or **form.** BAND CELL.

stage, *n.* [OF. *estage,* station, standing place (from L. *stare,* to stand), assimilated in meaning to L. *stadium*]. 1. A period or phase of disease characterized by certain symptoms; a condition in the course of a disease. 2. A period or step in a process, activity, or development; or of a surgical operation, or anesthesia. 3. The horizontal plate projecting from the pillar of a microscope for supporting the slide or object.

stage micrometer. A micrometer used for establishing the value of eyepiece micrometer graduations with various microscope lens combinations, and for establishing camera magnifications at specified lens combinations and bellows extension.

stages of general anesthesia. Divisions in the progressive sequence of clinical and physiological responses to general anesthetic agents: Stage 1. Period of repulsive responses to stimuli, loss of self-control, and altered sensibility (effects upon higher cortical centers); from initiation of the anesthesia to loss of consciousness. Stage 2. Period of reflex muscular activity and sometimes delirious excitement (effects upon basal ganglia and cerebellum); from the loss of consciousness to the onset of generalized muscular relaxation. Stage 3. Period of general muscular relaxation, complete anesthesia, abolished reflexes, and deep unconsciousness (effects upon the spinal cord, motor and sensory), which provides ideal conditions for many major surgical procedures; during this time vital functions are controlled by the automatic centers. Stage 4. Period of anesthetic overdosage (medullary paralysis), in which the vital centers are dangerously depressed, first the respiratory and then the cardiac centers. With present-day techniques, multiplicity of potent drugs, and balanced anesthesia, the stages described are not always clearly defined in practice.

stages of labor. Arbitrary divisions of the period of labor; the first begins with the onset of regular uterine contractions, and ends when dilatation of the ostium uteri is complete; the second ends with the expulsion of the child; the third (placental) ends with the expulsion of the placenta.

stag·gers, *n.* Any of various diseases manifested by lack of coordination in movement and a staggering gait, such as gid and sturdy of sheep, encephalomyelitis of horses, botulism, loco poisoning, and some cerebral affections of livestock.

stag·horn calculus. A large, irregularly branched calculus in the renal pelvis.

stag·na·tion (stag·nay'shun) *n.* [L. *stagnare,* to stand, to overflow, from *stagnum,* standing water]. 1. A cessation of motion. 2. *In pathology,* a cessation of motion in any fluid; stasis. —**stag·nate** (stag'nate) *v.*

Stähli. See *Staehli.*

Stahl's ear (shta^hl) [F. K. *Stahl,* German physician, 1811–1879]. A congenital deformity of the ear in which the helix is broad and the fossa of the anthelix and the upper part of the scaphoid fossa are practically invisible.

stain, *n.* [MF. *desteindre,* to discolor, from L. *dis-* + *tingere,* to color]. 1. A discoloration produced by absorption of, or contact with, foreign matter. 2. *In microscopy,* a pigment or dye used to render minute and transparent structures visible, to differentiate tissue elements, or to produce specific microchemical reactions.

staircase phenomenon. The stepwise increases in height of muscle contractions early in a series of responses to artificially applied stimuli of constant intensity. The mechanism of this phenomenon is not fully understood. Syn. TREPPE.

stal·ag·mom·e·ter (stal''ag·mom'e·tur) *n.* [Gk. *stalagma,* drop, + *-meter*]. 1. An instrument for measuring the size of drops, or the number of drops in a given volume of liquid. 2. An instrument for measuring the surface tension of liquids.

stal·ing (stay'ling) *n.* Urination in farm animals.

stalk, *n.* Any lengthened supporting part, as of a plant or an organ.

stalk cell. A cell found in the mesangium.

stalked hydatid. APPENDIX TESTIS.

stalk of the neurohypophysis. INFUNDIBULUM (2).

stal·li·my·cin (stal''i·mye'sin) *n.* N''-(2-Amidinoethyl)-4-formamido-1,1',1''-trimethyl-N,4':N',4''-ter[pyrrole-2-carboxamide], $C_{22}H_{27}N_9O_4$, an antibacterial used as the hydrochloride salt.

sta·men (stay'mun) *n.,* pl. **stamens, sta·mi·na** (stay'mi·nuh) [L., warp (longitudinal) thread in a loom]. The male organ of the flower, consisting of a stalk or filament and an anther containing pollen. —**stam·i·nate** (stam'i·nut) *adj.*

Stamey test [T. A. *Stamey,* U.S. physician, 20th century]. A test of differential urinary excretion designed to detect unilateral renovascular disease.

stam·i·na (stam'i·nuh) *n.* [L., warp of fabric, plural of *stamen,* warp thread]. Natural strength of constitution; vigor; inherent force; endurance.

stam·mer, *n.* & *v.* 1. Any of several irregularities of speech marked by involuntary halting, repetition of words or smaller segments, or transposition or mispronunciation of certain consonants, or by combinations of these defects. 2. To speak with such an irregularity. Compare *stutter.* **—stammer·er,** *n.*

stammering bladder. *Obsol.* A condition in which there is interruption of the urinary stream; may be psychogenic or pathologic in origin.

stamp·er, *n.* A person affected with tabes dorsalis, from the stamping gait incident to this condition.

stan·dard, *n. & adj.* [OF. *estandard,* banner, emblem]. 1. An established form of quality or quantity. 2. A substance of known strength used for determining the strength of an unknown by comparison. 3. Well established.

standard cell. An electrolytic cell having a definite voltage.

standard conditions. In measurements of gases, an atmospheric pressure of 760 mm and a temperature of 0°C. Syn. *standard temperature and pressure.*

standard death certificate. The form of death certificate recommended by the United States Bureau of the Census and in common usage in the United States.

standard deviation. The square root of the arithmetic average of the squares of the differences of each observation in a series from the mean of the series. The most commonly used measure of variation. Symbol, sigma (σ).

standard error. A measure of the variability any statistical constant would be expected to show in taking repeated random samples of a given size from the same universe of observations.

standard extremity lead. STANDARD LIMB LEAD.

standard horizontal plane. HORIZONTAL PLANE.

stan·dard·iza·tion (stan″dur·di·zay′shun) *n.* The procedure whereby a preparation, a process, or a method is evaluated with respect to or brought into conformance with a standard.

standardized death rate. *In biometry,* the number of deaths per 1000 which would have occurred in some standard population with a known age-specific death rate. The rate may be standardized for race, sex, or other variables with known death rates.

standard limb lead. An electrocardiographic connection between electrodes placed on two limbs: lead I, right and left arms; lead II, right arm and left leg; lead III, left arm and left leg. Syn. *bipolar limb lead, standard extremity lead.* Contr. *unipolar limb lead.*

standard million. A population of one million divided into age groups in the same proportion as found in a designated population, as the age distribution of England and Wales in 1901 or the age distribution of the United States as shown in the census of 1940. Used in calculating standardized death rates.

standard solution. A solution that contains an accurately known amount of substance.

standard temperature and pressure. STANDARD CONDITIONS. Abbreviated, STP.

standing arch. The arch representing the line of transfer of weight through the pelvis in the standing position; from the sacrum through the ilia to the acetabulums and heads of the femurs.

stand·still, *n.* A state of quiescence dependent upon suspended action.

Stan·ford achievement test [after *Stanford* University, California]. A group test covering achievement at a variety of school grades. The Primary Examination (grades 2 and 3) includes reading, arithmetic, and spelling; the Advanced Examination (grades 4 to 9), arithmetic computation, arithmetic reasoning, reading, spelling, language usage, literature, history, geography, and health subjects.

Stanford-Binet test. STANFORD REVISIONS OF BINET-SIMON TEST.

Stanford revisions of Binet-Simon test. Revisions of the Binet-Simon test to suit conditions in the United States. The last revision provides for more adequate sampling of intelligence at upper and lower levels by employing two new scales, by procedures for the administration and scoring of the test which have been defined more meticulously, and by standardization based upon larger and more representative samples of the population.

Stanford scientific aptitude test [*Stanford* University]. A test to detect the traits which comprise an aptitude for a science.

stann-, stanno- [L. *stannum*]. A combining form meaning *tin.*

stan·nate (stan′ate) *n.* A salt of stannic acid.

stan·nic (stan′ick) *adj.* [*stann-* + *-ic*]. Pertaining to tin; containing tin in the tetravalent state.

stannic acids. A series of acids that vary in composition from H_2SnO_3 to H_4SnO_4.

stan·nous (stan′us) *adj.* [*stann-* + *-ous*]. Containing tin as a bivalent element.

stannous chloride method for gold. CHRISTELLER METHOD.

stannous sulfur colloid. Colloidal sulfur containing stannous ions, used as a diagnostic aid for bone, liver, and spleen imaging in combination with radioactive techecium.

stan·num (stan′um) *n.* [L.]. TIN.

stan·o·lone (stan′o·lone) *n.* 17β-Hydroxy-5α-androstan-3-one, $C_{19}H_{30}O_2$, a steroid with anabolic and tumor-suppressing effects useful in selected cases of carcinoma of the breast.

stan·o·zo·lol (stan″o·zo′lol) *n.* 17-Methyl-5α-androstano[3,2-c]-pyrazol-17β-ol, $C_{21}H_{32}N_2O$, an anabolic androgen for oral use, with clinical effects similar to those of methyltestosterone.

sta·pe·dec·to·my (stay″pe·deck′tuh·mee) *n.* [NL. *stapes, stapedis,* stapes, + *-ectomy*]. Surgical removal of the stapes and replacement with a prosthesis.

stapedes. A plural of *stapes.*

sta·pe·di·al (stay·pee′dee·ul) *adj.* Pertaining to, or located near, the stapes.

stapedial artery. An artery present in the middle ear of the embryo; the stapes develops around it.

sta·pe·dio·te·not·o·my (sta·pee″dee·o·te·not′uh·mee) *n.* [*stapedius* + *teno-* + *-tomy*]. Cutting of the tendon of the stapedius muscle.

sta·pe·dio·ves·tib·u·lar (sta·pee″dee·o·ves·tib′yoo·lur) *adj.* [*stapedial* + *vestibular*]. Pertaining to the stapes and the vestibule.

sta·pe·di·us (stay·pee′dee·us) *n.,* pl. **stape·dii** (·dee·eye). A muscle in the middle ear, inserted into the stapes. NA *musculus stapedius.* See also Table of Muscles in the Appendix.

sta·pes (stay′peez) *n.,* pl. **stapes, sta·pe·des** (stay·pee′deez) [ML., stirrup] [NA]. The stirrup-shaped bone of the middle ear, articulating with the incus and the fenestra vestibuli. It is composed of the head, the crura or legs, and the footplate. See also Table of Bones in the Appendix and Plate 20.

Staph. An abbreviation for *Staphylococcus.*

Staphcillin. A trademark for the sodium salt of methicillin, a semisynthetic penicillin antibiotic.

staph·i·sa·gria (staf″i·say′gree·uh, ·sag′ree·uh) *n.* [Gk., lit., wild raisin]. The ripe seeds of *Delphinium staphisagria* that contain delphinine and other alkaloids; various preparations of the drug have been used for the destruction of lice in the hair.

staphyl-, staphylo- [Gk. *staphylē,* bunch of grapes; uvula]. A combining form meaning (a) *grapelike* (bunch or single); (b) *pertaining to the uvula, velum palatinum, or the whole soft palate;* (c) *staphylococci, staphylococcal.*

staph·y·le (staf′i·lee) *n.* [Gk.]. UVULA.

staph·y·lec·to·my (staf″i·leck′tuh·mee) *n.* [*staphyl-* + *-ectomy*]. Surgical removal of the uvula.

staph·yl·ede·ma, staph·yl·oe·de·ma (staf″il·e·dee′muh) *n.* [*staphyl-* + *edema*]. Edema of the uvula; any enlargement of the uvula.

staph·y·le·us (staf″i·lee′us) *L. adj.* Pertaining to the uvula.

staph·yl·he·ma·to·ma, staph·yl·hae·ma·to·ma (staf″il·hee″ muh·to′muh, ·hem″uh·to′muh) *n.* [*staphyl-* + *hematoma*]. An extravasation of blood into the uvula.

staph·y·line (staf′i·line, ·leen) *adj.* Pertaining to the uvula or to the entire palate.

sta·phy·li·no·pha·ryn·ge·us (staf″i·lye″no·fa·rin′jee·us) *n.* [*staphylin*us + *pharyngeus*]. PALATOPHARYNGEUS.

staph·y·li·nus (staf″i·lye′nus) *adj.* [NL., from Gk. *staphylē*, uvula]. Pertaining to the soft palate.

staphylinus ex·ter·nus (eck·stur′nus). TENSOR VELI PALATINI.

staphylinus in·ter·nus (in·tur′nus). LEVATOR VELI PALATINI.

staphylinus me·di·us (mee′dee·us). UVULAE.

sta·phyl·i·on (sta·fil′ee·on) *n.* [*staphyl-* + *-ion*]. *In craniometry,* the point where the straight line that is drawn tangent to the two curved posterior borders of the horizontal plates of the palatine bones intersects the interpalatine suture.

staph·y·li·tis (staf″i·lye′tis) *n.* [*staphyl-* + *-itis*]. Inflammation of the uvula.

staphylo-. See *staphyl-*.

staph·y·lo·coc·cal (staf″i·lo·kock′ul) *adj.* Pertaining to or caused by staphylococci.

staphylococcal pneumonia. A potentially serious type of pneumonia caused by *Staphylococcus aureus.*

staph·y·lo·coc·ce·mia, staph·y·lo·coc·cae·mia (staf″i·lo·kock·see′mee·uh) *n.* [*staphylococcus* + *-emia*]. The presence of staphylococci in the blood.

staph·y·lo·coc·cic (staf″i·lo·kock′sick) *adj.* Pertaining to, or caused by, staphylococci.

staph·y·lo·coc·cus (staf″i·lo·kock′us) *n.*, pl. **staphylococ·ci** (·sigh) [Gk. *staphylē*, bunch of grapes, + *coccus*]. A bacterium of the family Micrococcaceae, which is facultatively anaerobic, nonmotile, gram-positive, and tends to grow in irregular clusters.

Staphylococcus, *n.* A genus of cocci officially classified with *Micrococcus* by American bacteriologists.

Staphylococcus al·bus (al′bus). *STAPHYLOCOCCUS EPIDERMIDIS.*

staphylococcus antitoxin. An antitoxin prepared by immunizing horses with staphylococcus toxoid and/or staphylococcus toxin.

Staphylococcus au·re·us (aw′ree·us). A species of staphylococci, developing either yellow or white colonies, that is generally coagulase-positive and elaborates a number of soluble exotoxins and enzymes, and is responsible for a variety of clinical disturbances in man and animals, such as abscesses, endocarditis, pneumonia, osteomyelitis, and septicemia, but also may be found as normal inhabitants of the skin and mucous membranes without disease. Syn. *Staphylococcus pyogenes, Micrococcus aureus.*

Staphylococcus cit·re·us (sit′ree·us). A species of staphylococci developing a lemon-yellow pigment, seldom pathogenic; sometimes classified with *Staphylococcus epidermidis.* Syn. *Micrococcus citreus.*

Staphylococcus epi·der·mi·dis (ep″i·dur′mi·dis). A species of staphylococci, developing white colonies, that is coagulase-negative. It is rarely involved in human disease, such as endocarditis and infection of central nervous system shunts for hydrocephalus. Syn. *Staphylococcus albus, Micrococcus albus.*

Staphylococcus py·og·e·nes (pye·oj′e·neez). *STAPHYLOCOCCUS AUREUS.*

staphylococcus toxin. STAPHYLOTOXIN.

staphylococcus toxoid. Univalent or polyvalent, potently hemolytic and dermonecrotic toxins of *Staphylococcus aureus* altered by a formaldehyde-detoxifying process. Antigenicity is maintained, but toxicity is greatly diminished. Used in the prophylaxis and therapy of various staphylococcic pyodermas and localized pyogenic processes.

staphylococcus vaccine. A vaccine made from *Staphylococcus aureus,* used in the treatment of furunculosis and other infections due to the organism.

staph·y·lo·co·sis (staf″i·lo·ko′sis) *n.* [*staphylococcus* + *-osis*]. Infection by staphylococci.

staph·y·lo·der·ma (staf″i·lo·dur′muh) *n.* [*staphylo-* + *-derma*]. A pyodermatous condition of the skin caused by staphylococci.

staph·y·lo·der·ma·ti·tis (staf″i·lo·dur″muh·tye′tis) *n.* Dermatitis due to staphylococci (*Staphylococcus aureus*).

staph·y·lo·di·al·y·sis (staf″i·lo·dye·al′i·sis) *n.* [*staphylo-* + *dialysis*]. Relaxation of the uvula.

staph·y·lo·ede·ma, staph·y·lo-oe·de·ma (staf″i·lo·e·dee′muh) *n.* [*staphylo-* + *edema*]. STAPHYLEDEMA.

staph·y·lo·ki·nase (staf″i·lo·kigh′nace, ·kin′ace) *n.* [*staphylo-* + *kinase*]. A factor isolated from strains of *Staphylococcus aureus* which can convert plasminogen to plasmin.

staph·y·lol·y·sin (staf″i·lol′i·sin) *n.* [*staphylo-* + *hemolysin*]. A hemolysin produced by staphylococci (*Staphylococcus aureus*).

staph·y·lo·ma (staf″i·lo′muh) *n.* [*staphyl-* + *-oma*]. A bulging of the cornea or sclera of the eye. —**staphy·lo·mat·ic** (·lo·mat′ick), **staphy·lom·a·tous** (·lom′uh·tus) *adj.*

staphyloma cor·ne·ae (kor′nee·ee). A bulging of the cornea due to a thinning of the membrane with or without previous ulceration.

staphyloma uve·a·le (yoo″vee·ay′lee). Thickening of the iris. Syn. *iridoncosis.*

staph·y·lon·cus (staf″i·lonk′us) *n.* [*staphyl-* + Gk. *onkos*, mass]. Swelling of the uvula.

staph·y·lo·pha·ryn·ge·us (staf″i·lo·fa·rin′jee·us) *n.* [*staphylo-* + *pharyngeus*]. PALATOPHARYNGEUS.

staph·y·lo·phar·yn·gor·rha·phy (staf″i·lo·făr″in·gor′uh·fee) *n.* [*staphylo-* + *pharyngo-* + *-rrhaphy*]. A plastic operation on the palate and pharynx, as for repair of a cleft palate.

staph·y·lo·plas·ty (staf′i·lo·plas″tee) *n.* [*staphylo-* + *-plasty*]. A plastic operation on the soft palate or uvula.

staph·y·lop·to·sis (staf″i·lop·to′sis) *n.* [*staphylo-* + *-ptosis*]. Abnormal elongation of the uvula.

staph·y·lor·rha·phy (staf″i·lor′uh·fee) *n.* [*staphylo-* + *-rraphy*]. Repair of a cleft palate by plastic operation and suture.

staph·y·los·chi·sis (staf″i·los′ki·sis) *n.* [*staphylo-* + *-schisis*]. 1. CLEFT UVULA. 2. A cleft soft palate. 3. See *cleft palate.*

staph·y·lot·o·my (staf″i·lot′uh·mee) *n.* [*staphylo-* + *-tomy*]. The operation of incising the uvula. 2. *In ophthalmology,* the operation of incising a staphyloma.

staph·y·lo·tox·in (staf″i·lo·tock′sin) *n.* One of several toxins which may be elaborated by various strains of *Staphylococcus aureus,* such as the alpha hemolysin possessing hemolytic, dermonecrotic, and acutely lethal activities; beta hemolysin with hot-cold activity against sheep erythrocytes; the delta and gamma hemolysins; enterotoxin; and leukocidin.

staph·y·ly·gro·ma (staf″i·li·gro′muh) *n.* [*staphyl-* + *hygroma*]. STAPHYLEDEMA.

star, *n. In biology,* any of various radiate structures, granules, cells, groups of cells, or organisms.

star·blind, *adj.* Half blind; blinking.

star cells. KUPFFER CELLS.

starch, *n.* 1. Any one of a group of carbohydrates or polysaccharides, of the general composition $(C_6H_{10}O_5)_n$, occurring as organized or structural granules of varying size and markings in many plant cells. It hydrolyzes to several forms of dextrin and glucose. Its chemical structure is not completely known, but the granules consist of concentric shells containing at least two fractions: an inner portion called amylose, and an outer portion called amylopectin. 2. CORNSTARCH.

starch bath. A bland bath using starch.

starch-block electrophoresis. Electrophoresis in which a starch block is the supportive medium for the protein solution.

starch-derivative dusting powder. Absorbable dusting powder.

starch sugar. DEXTROSE.

starch syrup. A commercial product obtained by the acid hydrolysis of starch, and containing dextrins, maltose, and dextrose, and variously designated as commercial glucose, glucose syrup, corn syrup.

Star·gardt's disease or **macular degeneration** (shtahr'gart) [K. B. *Stargardt,* German ophthalmologist, 1875–1927]. JUVENILE MACULAR DEGENERATION.

Star·ling's law of the heart. FRANK-STARLING LAW OF THE HEART.

Starr-Edwards valve prosthesis [A. *Starr,* U.S. physician, 20th century; and M. L. *Edwards,* U.S. physician, 20th century]. A prosthetic cardiac valve of the ball-in-cage type.

start·er, *n.* A pure culture of bacteria employed to start a particular fermentation, as sour cream.

star test. A test for determining whether under- or overcorrection exists in the microscope system, and for determining the proper tube length for a microscope.

start·ing pain. Pain caused by a spasmodic contraction of the muscles just before the onset of sleep. It occurs in inflammatory joint diseases.

star·tle, *v.* To arouse unexpectedly and suddenly, causing a more or less involuntary response as of alarm, fear, or surprise.

startle epilepsy. A form of reflex epilepsy in which the precipitant is a sudden, unexpected stimulus, such as a loud noise.

startle response, reaction, reflex, or **pattern.** The complex psychophysiological response of an organism to a sudden unexpected stimulus such as a loud noise or blinding light; usually manifested by involuntary spasmodic movements of the limbs and often of the head and face so as to avoid or escape from the stimulus, but may include feelings of fear and a variety of visceral and autonomic changes; seen as the Moro reaction in infants.

star·va·tion, *n.* 1. Deprivation of food. 2. The state produced by deprivation of food. —**starve,** *v.*

starvation treatment. 1. A former treatment for diabetes; certain days of fasting followed by a limited diet with very little carbohydrate were used to diminish hyperglycemia. Syn. *Allen's treatment.* 2. A similar treatment currently used to treat obesity.

star·wort (stahr'wurt) *n.* ALETRIS.

stasi·basi·pho·bia (stas''i·bas''i·fo'bee·uh, stay''si·bay''si·) *n.* [Gk. *stasis,* standing, + *basis,* stepping, + *-phobia*]. A pathologic fear of one's ability to walk or stand.

stasi·pho·bia (stas''i·fo'bee·uh, stay''si·) *n.* [Gk. *stasis,* standing, + *-phobia*]. A pathologic fear of one's ability to stand upright.

sta·sis (stay'sis) *n.,* pl. **sta·ses** (·seez) [Gk., standing, stoppage]. A cessation of flow in blood or other body fluids.

-stasis [Gk.]. A combining form meaning (a) *stoppage, obstruction;* (b) *arrest, suppression;* (c) *fixation;* (d) *standing, accumulation.*

stasis dermatitis. Chronic inflammation of the skin of the legs, due to vascular stasis.

stasis ulcer. Ulceration, usually of the leg, due to chronic venous insufficiency or venous stasis. Syn. *varicose ulcer.*

stat. Abbreviation for *statim.*

stat, *adv.* [from the abbreviation *stat.*]. *Slang.* Immediately.

-stat [Gk. *-statēs,* from *histanai,* to set up, stand; to check, stop]. A combining form meaning (a) *a substance or device for checking or arresting;* (b) *a device,* such as a servomechanism, *for maintaining a process in a steady state;* (c) *a stand.*

state, *n.* [L. *status,* from *stare,* to stand]. 1. A condition; status. 2. The acme or crisis of a disease.

state medicine. Socialized medicine as exercised by a state or federal government.

stath·mo·ki·net·ic (stath''mo·ki·net'ick, ·kigh·net'ick) *adj.* [Gk. *stathmos,* stage, resting place, + *kinetic*]. Tending to arrest cell division by preventing spindle formation; a property of certain antineoplastic drugs such as vincristine. —**stathmoki·ne·sis** (·nee'sis) *n.*

stat·ic (stat'ick) *adj.* [Gk. *statikos,* causing to stand, from *statos,* standing, placed]. 1. At rest; in equilibrium; nonfluctuating; unchanging. 2. Of or pertaining to static electricity. 3. Pertaining to the laws of statics. 4. CHRONIC.

-static [Gk. *statikos,* causing to stand or stop]. A combining form meaning *arresting, inhibiting.*

static ataxia. Lack of muscular coordination in standing still, or in fixed positions of the limbs, characterized by swaying or oscillating of the body or limbs. Contr. *motor ataxia.*

static breeze. A method of administration of frictional electricity by an electrified air current. Syn. *electric breeze.*

static current. Direct current from a static machine.

static electricity. FRICTIONAL ELECTRICITY.

static occlusion. An occlusion which occurs as the teeth are interdigitated without the imposition of food.

static reflex. Any one of a series of reflexes which are involved in the establishment of muscular tone for maintaining posture against the force of gravity.

static refraction. The refraction of the eye when accommodation is at rest.

stat·ics (stat'icks) *n.* The science that deals with bodies at rest or at equilibrium relative to some given state of reference.

static theory. A theory that every position of the head causes the endolymph of the semicircular canals to exert greatest pressure upon some part of the canals, thus in varying degree exciting the nerve endings of the ampullae.

static tremor. RESTING TREMOR.

stat·im (stat'im, stay'tim) *adv.* [L.]. Immediately; at once. Abbreviated, stat.

sta·tion, *n.* [L. *statio,* from *stare,* to stand]. 1. Standing position or attitude. 2. A place where first aid or treatment is given, as a dressing station, rest station.

sta·tion·ary air. The air remaining in the lungs during normal respiration.

station hospital. In U.S. Army medicine, a fixed military hospital established in or near a post, station, or military installation to give medical and dental care to military personnel.

statistical constant. A value such as the arithmetic mean, the standard error, or any other measure which characterizes a particular series of quantitative observations. Used as an estimate of the corresponding value for the universe from which the observations were chosen.

sta·tis·tics (stuh·tis'ticks) *n.pl.* [NL. *statisticus,* pertaining to matters of state]. 1. A collection of numerical facts relating to any subject. 2. The science dealing with the collection, organization, analysis, and interpretation of numerical facts. —**statis·ti·cal** (ti·kul) *adj.*

stato- [Gk. *statos,* standing]. A combining form meaning *equilibrium* or *steady state.*

stato·acous·tic (stat''o·uh·koos'tick) *adj.* [*stato-* + *acoustic*]. Of or pertaining to equilibrium and hearing.

statoacoustic nerve. VESTIBULOCOCHLEAR NERVE.

stato·co·nia (stat''o·ko'nee·uh) *n.,* sing. **statoco·ni·um** (·nee·um) [*stato-* + Gk. *konia,* dust]. OTOCONIA.

stato·ki·net·ic (stat''o·ki·net'ick) *adj.* [*static* + *kinetic*]. Pertaining to the balance and posture of the body or its parts during movement, as in walking.

statokinetic reflex. ACCELERATORY REFLEX.

stato·lith (stat'o·lith) *n.* [*stato-* + *-lith*]. OTOLITH.

sta·to·lon (stay'to·lone) *n.* A substance, derived from *Penicillium stoloniferum,* that has antiviral activity.

sta·tom·e·ter (sta·tom'e·tur) *n.* [Gk. *statos,* standing, + *-meter*]. An instrument for measuring the degree of exophthalmos.

stat·ure (statch'ur) *n.* [L. *statura*]. The height of any animal when standing. In quadrupeds, it is measured at a point over the shoulders. In humans, it is the measured distance from the sole to the top of the head.

sta·tus (stay'tus, stat'us) *n.* [L., from *stare,* to stand, stay]. A state or condition; often, a severe or intractable condition.

status an·gi·no·sus (an·ji·no'sus). A severe or protracted attack of angina pectoris.

status ar·thrit·i·cus (ahr·thrit'i·kus). *Obsol.* The nervous manifestations preceding an attack of gout.

status asth·mat·i·cus (az·mat'i·kus). Intractable asthma lasting from a few days to a week or longer.

status con·vul·si·vus (kon·vul·sigh'vus, kon·vul'si·vus). STATUS EPILEPTICUS.

status cri·bro·sus (kri·bro'sus). A scarcely macroscopic sievelike condition of the brain or nerve substance, due to a loosening of tissue around thickened vessels; most prominent in the anterior and posterior perforated spaces. Syn. *état criblé.*

status dys·my·e·li·na·tus of O. and C. Vogt (dis·migh"e·li·nay'tus) [Cécile and O. *Vogt*]. A pathologic state of obscure cause in which all myelinated fibers and nerve cells in the lenticular nuclei disappear. The main clinical features are progressive extrapyramidal rigidity, athetosis, and mental decay.

status dys·raph·i·cus (dis·raf'i·kus). A developmental defect in closure of the neural tube, associated with anomalies of midline structures such as the spinal cord, spine, sternum, and palate.

status epi·lep·ti·cus (ep"i·lep'ti·kus). 1. A condition in which generalized convulsions occur at a frequency which does not allow consciousness to be regained in the interval between seizures. Syn. *grand mal status.* 2. Any of various other forms of prolonged seizures with variable degrees of impairment of consciousness, such as absence status, focal status, myoclonic status, or psychomotor status.

status fi·bro·sus (figh·bro'sus). A cerebral abnormality of the neonatal period, affecting the putamen and caudate nucleus bilaterally; characterized by a diffuse loss of nerve cells with gliosis, which causes shrinkage of the tissues and a crowding together of the remaining myelinated fibers and gives the impression of abnormally rich myelination of the area. Syn. *état fibreux.* See also *status marmoratus.*

status lym·phat·i·cus (lim·fat'i·kus). STATUS THYMICOLYMPHATICUS.

status mar·mo·ra·tus (mahr"mo·ray'tus, ·muh·). A cerebral lesion of obscure cause, affecting the thalamus, striatum, and border zones of the cerebral cortex, which are shrunken and have a whitish, marblelike appearance, representing foci of nerve cell loss and gliosis with peculiar condensations of myelinated fibers and even myelination of astroglial fibers (hypermyelination). This lesion does not develop after infancy, after the myelination glia have finished their developmental cycle. The usual clinical features are impairment of psychomotor development, defects in voluntary movement, choreoathetosis, and other extrapyramidal movement disorders. Syn. *état marbré, Vogt disease.*

status mi·grai·nus (migh·gray'nus). Prolonged, intense, intractable migraine, often with repeated vomiting, extending over a day or longer.

status para·thy·reo·pri·vus (păr"uh·thigh"ree·o·prye'vus). A pathologic state caused by complete loss of parathyroid tissue.

status prae·sens (pree'sens, ·zenz). The state of a patient at the time of examination.

status rap·tus (rap'tus). ECSTASY.

status spon·gi·o·sis (spon"jee·o'sis, spun"). SPONGY DEGENERATION (2).

status thy·mi·co·lym·phat·i·cus (thigh"mi·ko·lim·fat'i·kus). An erroneous concept of airway obstruction by an enlarged thymus as a cause of sudden and otherwise unexplained death in infancy.

status thy·mi·cus (thigh'mi·kus). STATUS THYMICOLYMPHATICUS.

status ver·ru·co·sus (verr"oo·ko'sus). A developmental anomaly of the cerebral cortex in which there are numerous small gyri, giving a wartlike appearance to the surface of the brain.

status ver·ti·gi·no·sus (vur·tij"i·no'sus). Persistent vertigo.

stat·u·to·ry rape (statch'oo·tor"ee). The violation of a female under the age of consent as fixed in the state or country in which the attack occurs. Syn. *rape of the second degree.*

sta·tu·vo·lence (sta·tew'vuh·lunce, stat"yoo·vo'lunce) *n.* [*status* + L. *volens,* willing]. 1. AUTOHYPNOTISM. 2. Voluntary somnambulism or clairvoyance. 3. A trance into which one voluntarily enters without aid from another. —**statu·vo·lent** (·lunt) *adj.*

Staub-Trau·gott effect (shtaowp, traow'goht) [H. *Staub,* Swiss physician, b. 1890; and C. *Traugott,* German physician, b. 1885]. The second administration of a dose of glucose 1 hour after the first will not raise the blood sugar level of a normal individual.

stau·ri·on (staw'ree·on) *n.* [Gk., dim. of *stauros,* cross]. *In craniometry,* the point located at the intersection of the median palatine and transverse palatine sutures.

staves·acre (staiv'zay·kur) *n.* STAPHISAGRIA.

stax·is (stack'sis) *n.* [Gk., a dripping, from *stazein,* to drip]. 1. HEMORRHAGE. 2. Dribbling of urine.

STD 1. Skin test dose, a standardized test dose of streptococcal erythrogenic toxin used in the Dick test. 2. Sexually transmitted disease (= VENEREAL DISEASE).

steady state. HOMEOSTASIS.

steady state in muscular exercise. The condition in which the rate of oxygen consumption and the rate of energy release are such that no oxygen debt is incurred.

steal syndrome. Diversion of normal blood flow from a part, due to arterial narrowing or occlusion, which results in rerouting of the usual blood supply by reversal of flow in a large communicating arterial branch. See also *aortoiliac steal syndrome, subclavian steal syndrome.*

steam-fitter's asthma. ASBESTOSIS.

ste·ap·sin (stee·ap'sin) *n.* [*stear-* + *-psin* as in pepsin]. PANCREATIC LIPASE.

stear-, stearo- [Gk. *stear*]. A combining form meaning *fat.*

stea·rate (stee'uh·rate) *n.* An ester or salt of stearic acid, as stearin (glyceryl stearate) or sodium stearate.

stea·ric acid (stee·ăr'ick, stee'ur·ick) [*stear-* + *-ic*]. A mixture of solid acids obtained from fats; consists chiefly of stearic acid, $CH_3(CH_2)_{16}COOH$, and palmitic acid, $CH_3(CH_2)_{14}COOH$. Used in the formulation of many dermatologic creams, in some enteric-coating compositions, and as a lubricant in compressing tablets.

stear·i·form (stee·ăr'i·form) *n.* [*stear-* + *-iform*]. Having the appearance of, or resembling, fat.

stea·rin (stee'uh·rin) *n.* Tristearin, glyceryl tristearate, $C_3H_5O_3(C_{17}H_{35}CO)_3$, the glyceryl ester of stearic acid; occurs in many solid fats.

stearo-. See *stear-.*

stea·ro·der·mia (stee"uh·ro·dur'mee·uh) *n.* [*stearo-* + *-dermia*]. An affection of the sebaceous glands of the skin.

stea·rop·ten (stee·uh·rop'tin) *n.* STEAROPTENE.

stea·rop·tene (stee"uh·rop'teen) *n.* [*stearo-* + Gk. *ptēnos,* flying]. The portion of a volatile oil, usually consisting of oxygenated substances, which is solid at ordinary temperatures. Contr. *eleoptene.*

ste·ar·rhea (stee"uh·ree'uh) *n.* [*stear-* + *-rrhea*]. SEBORRHEA.

stearrhea fla·ves·cens (fla·ves'enz). A seborrhea in which the sebaceous matter turns yellow after being deposited upon the skin.

stearrhea nigricans. CHROMHIDROSIS.

stearrhea sim·plex (sim'plecks). SEBORRHEA OLEOSA.

stea·ryl (stee'uh·ril) *n.* The monovalent radical, $C_{17}H_{35}CO—$, of stearic acid.

stearyl alcohol. Octadecan-1-ol, $CH_3(CH_2)_{16}CH_2OH$, a white unctuous solid. The official substance of this name is a mixture of alcohols. It is an ingredient of ointment bases and creams.

steat-, steato- [Gk. *stear, steatos*]. A combining form meaning *fat.*

ste·a·ti·tis (stee″uh·tye′tis) *n.* [*steat-* + *-itis*]. Inflammation of adipose tissue.

ste·a·to·cryp·to·sis (stee″uh·to·krip·to′sis) *n.* [*steato-* + *crypt-* + *-osis*]. Abnormal function of the sebaceous glands.

ste·a·to·cys·to·ma mul·ti·plex (stee″uh·to·sis·to′muh mul′ti·plecks). A familial skin disorder inherited as a dominant trait, characterized by various-sized epidermal cysts over the trunk, back, arms, or thighs. Both men and women may be affected. Syn. *sebocystomatosis.*

ste·a·tog·e·nous (stee″uh·toj′e·nus) *adj.* [*steato-* + *-genous*]. 1. Producing steatosis or fat. 2. Causing sebaceous gland disease.

ste·a·tol·y·sis (stee″uh·tol′i·sis) *n.* [*steato-* + *-lysis*]. The emulsifying process by which fats are prepared for absorption and assimilation. —**ste·a·to·lyt·ic** (stee″uh·to·lit′ick) *adj.*

ste·atolytic enzyme. An enzyme that catalyzes hydrolysis of a fat.

ste·a·to·ma (stee″uh·to′muh) *n.*, pl. **steatomas, steatoma·ta** (·tuh) [Gk. *steatōma*]. 1. SEBACEOUS CYST. 2. LIPOMA.

ste·a·to·py·gia (stee″uh·to·pij′ee·uh, ·pye′jee·uh) *n.* [*steato-* + *pyg-* + *-ia*]. Excessive accumulation of fat on the buttocks. Syn. *Hottentot bustle.* —**stea·top·y·gous** (·top′i·gus) *adj.*

ste·a·tor·rhea, ste·a·tor·rhoea (stee″uh·to·ree′uh) *n.* [*steato-* + *-rrhea*]. 1. Fatty stools. 2. An increased flow of the secretion of the sebaceous follicles. See also *seborrhea.*

ste·a·to·sis (stee″uh·to′sis) *n.*, pl. **steato·ses** (·seez) [*steat-* + *-osis*]. 1. FATTY DEGENERATION. 2. Disease of sebaceous glands.

Steclin. A trademark for the antibiotic tetracycline hydrochloride.

Steele-Rich·ard·son-Ol·szew·ski syndrome [J. C. *Steele,* neurologist, 20th century; J. C. *Richardson,* U.S. neuropathologist, 20th century; and J. *Olszewski,* neurologist, 20th century]. PROGRESSIVE SUPRANUCLEAR PALSY.

Steen·bock unit [H. *Steenbock,* U.S. biochemist, 1886–1967]. The amount of vitamin D that will produce a line of calcification at the distal ulnar and radial epiphyses of rachitic rats within 10 days.

stee·ple head or **skull.** OXYCEPHALY.

steer·horn stomach. A high, transversely located stomach. Syn. *cow-horn stomach.*

stef·fi·my·cin (stef″i·migh′sin) *n.* An antibiotic substance produced by *Streptomyces steffisburgensis* var. *steffisburgensis* sp. n.

steg·no·sis (steg·no′sis) *n.* [Gk. *stegnōsis,* stoppage]. The closing of a passage; STENOSIS. —**steg·not·ic** (·not′ick) *adj.*

Stego·my·ia (steg″o·migh′ee·uh) *n.* [Gk. *stegos,* roof, + *-myia*]. A subgenus of the genus *Aëdes* of mosquitoes; includes a principal vector of yellow fever, *Aëdes aegypti.*

Stei·nach's method or **operation** (shtye′nahkh) [E. *Steinach,* Austrian physiologist, 1861–1944]. Occlusion of the ductus deferens to promote production of testicular hormones and rejuvenation.

Stein·brinck syndrome (shtine′brink) [W. *Steinbrinck*]. CHÉDIAK-HIGASHI DISEASE.

Steind·ler's operation [A. *Steindler,* U.S. orthopedist, 1878–1959]. 1. Fusion of the shoulder joint. 2. Stripping of the calcaneus. 3. Plastic repair of the elbow paralyzed by poliomyelitis.

Stei·ner's tumor (shtye′nur) [L. *Steiner,* German physician, 20th century]. JUXTA-ARTICULAR NODE (2).

Stei·nert's disease (shtye′nurt) [H. *Steinert,* German physician, 20th century]. MYOTONIC DYSTROPHY.

Stein-Leventhal syndrome [I. F. *Stein,* U.S. gynecologist, b. 1887; and M. L. *Leventhal,* U.S. obstetrician, 1901–1971]. A group of symptoms and findings characterized by amenorrhea or abnormal uterine bleeding or both, enlarged polycystic ovaries, hirsutism frequently, and occasionally retarded breast development and obesity.

Stein·mann pin or **nail** (shtine′mahn) [F. *Steinmann,* Swiss surgeon, 1872–1932]. A surgical nail inserted in distal portions of such bones as the femur or tibia for skeletal tractions.

Stein's test. VON STEIN'S TEST.

Stelazine. Trademark for trifluoperazine, a tranquilizer used as the hydrochloride salt.

stel·la (stel′uh) *n.*, pl. **stel·lae** (·ee) [L.]. STAR.

stella len·tis hy·a·loi·dea (len′tis high″uh·loy′dee·uh). The posterior pole of the lens of the eye.

stella lentis iri·di·ca (eye·rid′i·kuh). The anterior pole of the lens of the eye.

stel·lar nevus (stel′ur). SPIDER NEVUS.

stel·late (stel′ate) *adj.* [L. *stellatus,* starry]. Star-shaped; with parts radiating from a center.

stellate cataract. SUTURAL CATARACT.

stellate cell. Any cell with numerous processes making it appear star-shaped, as a Kupffer cell or an astrocyte.

stellate fracture. A fracture in which numerous fissures radiate from the central point of injury.

stellate ganglion. The ganglion formed by the fusion of the inferior cervical and the first thoracic sympathetic ganglions. NA *ganglion cervicothoracicum, ganglion stellatum.* See also Plate 15.

stellate ligament. RADIATE LIGAMENT (1).

stellate reticulum. The part of the enamel organ of a developing tooth which lies between the inner and outer dental epithelium; the cells are stellate with long processes that anastomose with those of adjacent cells; the spaces between the cells are filled with a mucoid fluid that later supports and protects the enamel-forming cells.

stellate veins. Radially arranged subcapsular veins of the renal cortex which drain into the interlobular veins.

Stellite. Trademark for an acid-resistant alloy, containing cobalt, chromium, tungsten, and molybdenum; used in certain surgical instruments.

Stell·wag's operation (shtel′vah[k]k) [C. *Stellwag* von Carion, Austrian ophthalmologist, 1823–1904]. SPHINCTERECTOMY.

Stellwag's sign [C. *Stellwag* von Carion]. Infrequent blinking; seen in hyperthyroidism.

stem, *n.* 1. The pedicle or stalk of a tumor. 2. A supporting stalk, as of a leaf or plant.

stem bronchus. The continuation of the main bronchus which extends lengthwise in each lung, giving off anterior and posterior branches to the lobes.

stem cell. 1. A totipotential cell in the hematopoietic system, considered by proponents of the unitarian theory of hemopoiesis to be capable of differentiating into each of the blood cell types. 2. A totipotential cell in various systems, as in the intestinal epithelium, capable of differentiating into the various cells of that system. 3. FORMATIVE CELL.

stem cell leukemia. Leukemia in which the type of cell is so poorly differentiated that it is impossible to identify its series.

stem pessary. A device for insertion into the cervical canal, to prevent conception or to stimulate an infantile uterus.

ste·nag·mus (ste·nag′mus) *n.* [NL., from Gk. *stenagmos*]. Sighing.

sten·bo·lone (sten′bo·lone, steen′) *n.* 17β-Hydroxy-2-methyl-5α-androst-1-en-3-one, $C_{20}H_{30}O_2$, an injectable anabolic steroid; used as the acetate ester.

Sten·der dish (shten′dur) [W. B. *Stender,* German manufacturer, 19th century]. A covered cylindrical glass vessel used in histologic technique.

Stenger test. A test for determining actual or simulated unilateral deafness. A tuning fork stem is inserted into a 30-in. length of rubber tubing having an earpiece at the other end. The fork is set in vibration. The earpiece is inserted into the deaf ear and the fork is approximated to the good, or normal, ear. If it is not heard until much closer than was the case in previous tests indicating normal hearing distance, the deafness is simulated. Syn. *Wells-Stenger test.*

ste·ni·on (stee'nee·on, sten'ee·on) *n.*, pl. **ste·nia** (·nee·uh) [Gk. *stenos*, narrow, + *-ion*]. The point on the sphenosquamosal suture which is located most medially.

steno- [Gk. *stenos*]. A combining form meaning *narrow* or *constricted.*

steno·car·dia (sten"o·kahr'dee·uh) *n.* [*steno-* + *-cardia*]. ANGINA PECTORIS.

steno·ce·pha·lia (sten"o·se·fay'lee·uh) *n.* STENOCEPHALY.

steno·ceph·a·ly (sten"o·sef'uh·lee) *n.* [*steno-* + *-cephaly*]. Unusual narrowness of the head. —**steno·ceph·a·lous** (·sef'uh·lus) *adj.*

steno·chas·mus (sten"o·kaz'mus) *n.* [NL., from *steno-* + Gk. *chasma*, opening]. A skull with a small angle, 94 to 74°, of the nasopharynx. The angle is included between two lines drawn, respectively, from the posterior nasal spine and basion to the point on the rostrum of the sphenoid where it is included between the alae of the vomer.

steno·cho·ria (sten"o·ko'ree·uh) *n.* [Gk. *stenochōria*, from *steno-* + *chōros*, space]. A narrowing; partial obstruction, particularly of a lacrimal duct.

steno·co·ri·a·sis (sten"o·ko·rye'uh·sis) *n.* [Gk. *stenokoriasis*, from *steno-* + *korē*, pupil]. Narrowing of the pupil.

steno·crot·a·phy (sten"o·krot'uh·fee) *n.* [*steno-* + Gk. *krotaphos*, temple, + *-y*]. Abnormal narrowness of the skull in the sphenoid of the pterion, probably due to hypoplasia of the sphenoid angles of the parietal bones, and of the great wings of the sphenoid bone.

sten·o·dont (sten'o·dont) *adj.* [*sten-* + *-odont*]. Provided with narrow teeth.

steno·mer·ic (sten"o·merr'ick) *adj.* [*steno-* + Gk. *mēros*, thigh, + *-ic*]. *In osteometry*, designating a femur with no anteroposterior compression of the proximal portion of the diaphysis. There may be considerable mediolateral compression of the same portion as indicated by the platymeric index of 100.0 or more. Stenomeric femurs are abnormal, normal femurs being either platymeric or eurymeric.

steno·myc·te·ria (sten"o·mick·teer'ee·uh) *n.* [*steno-* + Gk. *myktēr*, nostril, + *-ia*]. A nasal stenosis.

Ste·no·ni·an duct (ste·no'nee·un) [N. *Stensen* (*Steno*)]. PAROTID DUCT.

steno·pa·ic (sten"o·pay'ick) *adj.* STENOPEIC.

sten·o·pe·ic, sten·o·pae·ic (sten"o·pee'ick) *adj.* & *n.* [*sten-* + Gk. *opē*, hole, + *-ic*]. 1. Having a narrow slit or minute hole for admitting light. 2. A device of metal or other opaque substance with a very fine slit or minute hole or holes. Held before defective eyes, it facilitates vision. The slitted stenopeic (long used by Eskimos) protects from ultraviolet radiation from sunlight on snow or ice.

stenopeic disk. A lens allowing the passage of light rays only through a straight narrow slit; used for testing astigmatism.

Ste·no's duct (stay'no). Stensen's duct (= PAROTID DUCT).

ste·nose (ste·noce', ste·noze', sten'oze) *v.* [from *stenosis*]. To constrict, narrow. —**ste·nosed** (ste·noazd', ·noast') *adj.*; **ste·nos·ing** (·no'zing, ·no'sing) *adj.*

ste·no·sis (ste·no'sis) *n.*, pl. **steno·ses** (·seez) [Gk. *stenōsis*, from *stenos*, narrow]. Constriction or narrowing, especially of a lumen or orifice; STRICTURE. —**steno·sal** (·sul), **ste·not·ic** (·not'ick) *adj.*

sten·o·sto·mia (sten"o·sto'mee·uh) *n.* STENOSTOMY.

ste·nos·to·my (ste·nos'tuh·mee) *n.* [Gk. *stenostomos*, narrow-mouthed, + *-y*]. Narrowing of any mouth or aperture.

steno·ther·mal (sten"o·thur'mul) *adj.* [*steno-* + *thermal*]. Capable of resisting a small range of temperature.

steno·tho·rax (sten"o·tho'racks) *n.* [Gk. *stenothōrax*, narrow-chested]. An unusually narrow chest.

Sten·sen's duct [N. *Stensen* (*Steno*), Danish anatomist, 1638-1686]. PAROTID DUCT.

Stensen's foramen [N. *Stensen*]. The lateral incisive foramen. See *incisive foramen.*

stent, *n.* [C. R. *Stent*, English dentist, 19th century]. 1. A compound used for immobilizing some forms of skin graft. 2. A mold made of stent, used for immobilizing some forms of skin graft.

sten·to·roph·o·nous (sten"to·rof'o·nus) *adj.* [*Stentōr*, Greek warrior at Troy famous for his loud voice, + *phon-* + *-ous*]. Having a loud voice.

Sten·ver's projection [H. W. *Stenver*, German radiologist, b. 1889]. A PA x-ray of the skull taken with the tip of the nose, the point of the chin, and the outer canthus of the eye in contact with the film and the central ray projected toward the vertex. Designed to demonstrate the petrous pyramid and the mastoid in true frontal projection.

step-down transformer. A transformer to decrease voltage.

ste·pha·ni·on (ste·fay'nee·on, ste·fan'ee·on) *n.* [Gk., dim. of *stephanos*, crown]. *In craniometry*, the point where the coronal suture crosses the inferior temporal line. —**stepha·ni·al** (·ul), **ste·phan·ic** (·fan'ick) *adj.*

Steph·a·no·fi·la·ria (stef"uh·no·fi·lăr'ee·uh) *n.* A genus of filarial nematodes of which some cause dermatitis and granulomatous skin lesions in cattle.

steph·a·no·fil·a·ri·a·sis (stef"uh·no·fil"uh·rye'uh·sis) *n.* [*Stephanofilaria* + *-iasis*]. A nematode dermatitis affecting cattle caused by any of several filarial worms in the genus *Stephanofilaria.*

stephano-zygomatic index. The ratio of the distance between the stephanion points × 100 to that between the zygomatic arches.

steph·a·nu·ri·a·sis (stef"uh·new·rye'uh·sis) *n.* [*Stephanurus* + *-iasis*]. Infection of swine by the kidney worm *Stephanurus dentatus.*

step·page gait (step'ij). The high-stepping gait with exaggerated flexion at the hip and knee, the advancing foot hanging with the toes pointing toward the ground (foot drop). It is seen in various diseases that cause paralysis of the pretibial and peroneal muscles; may be unilateral or bilateral.

step·ping movements or **reflex.** A reflex response of the newborn and young infant, characterized by alternating stepping movements with both legs, as in walking, elicited when the infant is held upright so that both soles touch a flat surface while the infant is moved forward accompanying any step taken; absent in neurologically depressed infants or those with extensive lower motor neuron lesions involving the lower extremities.

step sections. A series of histologic preparations made from a single block of tissue, succeeding sections being a significant distance apart from their predecessor. Contr. *serial sections.*

step-up transformer. A transformer to increase voltage.

Sterane. A trademark for prednisolone, an anti-inflammatory adrenocortical steroid.

sterco- [L. *stercus, stercoris*, dung, manure]. A combining form meaning *feces, fecal.*

ster·co·bi·lin (stur"ko·bye'lin, ·bil'in) *n.* [*sterco-* + *bil-* + *-in*]. Urobilin as a constituent of the brown pigment found in feces; derived from bilirubin by reduction due to bacteria in the intestine.

ster·co·bi·lin·o·gen (stur"ko·bye·lin'o·jen) *n.* A reduction product of stercobilin which occurs in the feces; it is a colorless compound which becomes brown on oxidation, probably identical with urobilinogen.

ster·co·lith (stur'ko·lith) *n.* [*sterco-* + *-lith*]. A calcified fecal concretion.

ster·co·ra·ceous (stur"ko·ray'shus) *adj.* [L. *stercus, stercoris*, dung, + *-aceous*]. FECAL; having the nature of or containing feces.

stercoraceous ulcer. An ulcer of the skin which is contaminated by feces.

stercoraceous vomiting. Ejection of fecal matter in vomit, usually due to intestinal obstruction. Syn. *fecal vomiting.*

ster·co·ral (stur'kuh·rul) *adj.* STERCORACEOUS.

ster·co·rary (stur'kuh·rerr"ee) *adj.* [L. *stercorarius,* of dung]. FECAL.

ster·co·ro·ma (stur"kuh·ro'muh) *n.* [L. *stercus, stercor*is, dung, + *-oma*]. FECALITH; a hard fecal mass usually in the rectum.

ster·co·rous (stur'kuh·rus) *adj.* STERCORACEOUS.

Ster·cu·lia (stur·kew'lee·uh) *n.* [NL., from L. *Sterculius,* god of cultivation and manuring]. A large genus of tropical trees. *Sterculia urens* of India and *S. tragacantha* of Africa yield karaya gum; *S. acuminata* (*Cola nitida*) produces the kola nut.

sterculia gum. KARAYA GUM.

ster·cus (stur'kus) *n.* [L., manure, dung]. FECES.

stere (steer, stair) *n.* [Gk. *stereos,* solid]. A unit of volume equivalent to one cubic meter or one kiloliter.

stere-, stereo- [Gk. *stereos,* solid]. A combining form meaning (a) *involving three dimensions;* (b) *involving depth perception,* especially, *stereoscopic;* (c) *firm, solid.*

ste·reo·ag·no·sis (sterr"ee·o·ag·no'sis, steer"ee·o·) *n.* ASTEREOGNOSIS.

ste·reo·an·es·the·sia, ste·reo·an·aes·the·sia (sterr"ee·o·an"es·theezh'uh, steer"ee·o·) *n.* [*stereo-* + *anesthesia*]. The failure to recognize the shape and form of objects due to interruption of traits transmitting postural and tactile sensation.

ste·reo·ar·throl·y·sis (sterr"ee·o·ahr·throl'i·sis, steer"ee·o·) *n.* [*stereo-* + *arthrolysis*]. Loosening stiff joints by operation or manipulation in cases of ankylosis.

ste·reo·blas·tu·la (sterr"ee·o·blas'tew·luh, steer"ee·o·) *n.* [*stereo-* + *blastula*]. A solid blastula, not having a blastocoele, but having all its cells bounding the external surface.

ste·reo·cam·pim·e·ter (sterr"ee·o·kam·pim'e·tur, steer"ee·o·) *n.* [*stereo-* + *campimeter*]. An instrument for measuring the extent of the visual field of both eyes simultaneously. Syn. *stereoscopic campimeter.*

ste·reo·chem·is·try (sterr"ee·o·kem'is·tree, steer"ee·o·) *n.* [*stereo-* + *chemistry*]. A branch of science that deals with the spatial arrangement of atoms in a molecule. —**stereochem·i·cal** (·i·kul) *adj.*

ste·reo·cil·ia (sterr"ee·o·sil'ee·uh, steer"ee·o·) *n.,* sing. **stereo·cil·i·um** (·ee·um) [*stereo-* + *cilia*]. Irregular, nonmotile tufts of microvilli on the free surface of cells of the male reproductive tract, especially the epididymis, which are secretory in function.

ste·reo·en·ceph·a·lo·tome (sterr"ee·o·en·sef'uh·lo·tome, steer"ee·o·) *n.* [*stereo-* + *encephalotome*]. A device for localizing exactly any point within the brain, for the operation of stereoencephalotomy.

ste·reo·en·ceph·a·lot·o·my (sterr"ee·o·en·sef"uh·lot'uh·mee, steer"ee·o·) *n.* [*stereo-* + *encephalotomy*]. Selective destruction, by cautery or electrolysis, of cerebral tracts or nuclei, using the pineal body or posterior commissure as the point of reference or zero point on the stereotaxic coordinates.

ste·reo·gen·ic (sterr"ee·o·jen'ick, steer"ee·o·) *adj.* [*stereo-* + *-genic*]. Of an atom in a molecule: producing nonidentical compounds if two of the atoms or groups attached to it are interchanged.

ste·re·og·no·sis (sterr"ee·og·no'sis, steer"ee·) *n.* [*stereo-* + *-gnosis*]. The faculty of recognizing the size and shape of objects by palpation. —**stereog·nos·tic** (·nos'tick) *adj.*

stereognostic perception. The recognition of objects by palpation, which includes appreciation of size, shape, weight, and texture.

ste·reo·gram (sterr'ee·o·gram, steer"ee·o·) *n.* [*stereo-* + *-gram*]. 1. A two-dimensional picture which represents an object with the impression of three dimensions, by means of contour lines or shading. 2. A stereoscopic picture.

ste·reo·graph (sterr'ee·o·graf, steer"ee·o·) *n.* [*stereo-* + *-graph*]. An instrument for drawing geometric contours of skulls in various views.

ste·re·og·ra·phy (sterr"ee·og'ruh·fee, steer"ee·) *n.* [*stereo-* + *-graphy*]. The phase of craniometry that consists of making geometric projections of a skull held rigidly in a predetermined plane, thus producing drawings so accurate that lines and angles may be measured on them.

ste·reo·iso·mer (sterr"ee·o·eye'so·mur, steer"ee·o·) *n.* [*stereo-* + *isomer*]. A compound that has the same number and kind of atoms as another compound, and is of similar structure, but with a different arrangement of the atoms in space.

ste·reo·isom·er·ism (sterr"ee·o·eye·som'ur·iz·um, steer"ee·o·) *n.* The state in which two or more compounds are related to each other as stereoisomers.

ste·reo·mono·scope (sterr"ee·o·mon'o·skope, steer"ee·o·) *n.* [*stereo-* + *mono-* + *-scope*]. An instrument which projects two stereoscopic images upon the same spot on a ground-glass screen by means of two lenses, the combined image giving the impression of solidity.

stereo-ophthalmoscope, *n.* An ophthalmoscope with two eyepieces.

ste·reo·par·ent (sterr"ee·o·păr'unt, steer"ee·o·) *n. In chemistry,* the parent molecule that implies specific stereochemical information concerning the configuration of a molecule, as for example, prostane, the stereoparent for the prostaglandins.

ste·reo·phan·to·scope (sterr"ee·o·fan'tuh·skope, steer"ee·o·) *n.* [*stereo-* + Gk. *phantos,* visible, + *-scope*]. A panoramic stereoscope using rotating disks in place of pictures.

ste·reo·phoro·scope (sterr"ee·o·for'uh·skope, steer"ee·o·) *n.* [*stereo-* + *phoroscope*]. A stereoscopic stroboscope, an instrument for producing a series of images apparently in motion; used in tests of visual perception.

ste·reo·plasm (sterr'ee·o·plaz·um, steer"ee·o·) *n.* [*stereo-* + *-plasm*]. The solid part of the protoplasm of cells.

ste·re·op·sis (sterr"ee·op'sis, steer"ee·) *n.* [*stere-* + Gk. *opsis,* vision]. STEREOSCOPIC VISION.

ste·re·op·ter (sterr'ee·op"tur, steer'ee·) *n.* [*stereop*sis + Gk. *-tēr,* instrumental noun suffix]. An instrument to provide a rapid quantitative test for depth perception.

ste·reo·ra·di·og·ra·phy (sterr"ee·o·ray·dee·og'ruh·fee, steer"ee·o·) *n.* [*stereo-* + *radiography*]. The taking of two radiographs with the x-ray tube in two positions, about 6 inches apart, and the viewing of these two films in such a manner that the stereoscopic picture appears three-dimensional.

ste·reo·roent·gen·og·ra·phy (sterr"ee·o·rent·guh·nog'ruh·fee, steer"ee·o·) *n.* [*stereo-* + *roentgenography*]. STEREORADIOGRAPHY.

ste·reo·scope (sterr'ee·o·skope, steer"ee·o·) *n.* [*stereo-* + *-scope*]. An instrument by which two similar pictures of the same object are so mounted that the images are seen as one, thereby giving a three-dimensional impression. —**ste·re·os·co·py** (sterr"ee·os'kuh·pee, steer"ee·) *n.*

ste·reo·scop·ic (sterr"ee·o·skop'ick, steer"ee·o·) *adj.* 1. Of or pertaining to the stereoscope. 2. Pertaining to or characterized by three-dimensional observation of objects.

stereoscopic campimeter. STEREOCAMPIMETER.

stereoscopic parallax. BINOCULAR PARALLAX.

stereoscopic vision. Disparity of retinal images resulting in depth perception.

ste·reo·spe·cif·ic (sterr"ee·o·spe·sif'ick) *adj.* Of a receptor: specific for only one of the possible spatial arrangements of a molecule.

ste·reo·stro·bo·scope (sterr"ee·o·stro'buh·skope, steer"ee·o·) *n.* [*stereo-* + *stroboscope*]. An apparatus for the study of points moving in three dimensions.

ste·reo·tac·tic (sterr"ee·o·tack'tick, steer"ee·o·) *adj.* Pertaining to or involving stereotaxis.

ste·reo·tax·ia (sterr"ee·o·tack'see·uh, steer"ee·o·) *n.* STEREOTAXIS.

ste·reo·tax·ic (sterr"ee·o·tack'sick, steer"ee·o·) *adj.* [*stereo-* + Gk. *tax*is, arrangement, + *-ic*]. Pertaining to or characterized by precise spatial positioning.

stereotaxic apparatus. An apparatus that allows accurate insertion of long electrodes or other probes deep into the brain; may be used in physiologic experimentation or in neurosurgery.

ste·reo·tax·is (sterr″ee·o·tack′sis, steer″ee·o·) *n.* [*stereo-* + *taxis*]. 1. The accurate location of a definite circumscribed area within the brain by moving a probe or electrode along coordinates for measured distances from certain external points or landmarks of the skull. 2. STEREOTROPISM. —**ste·reo·tac·tic** (·tack′tick), **stereotac·ti·cal** (·ti·kul) *adj.*

ste·reo·taxy (sterr′ee·o·tack″see, steer′ee·o·) *n.* STEREOTAXIS.

ste·re·ot·ro·pism (sterr″ee·ot′ro·piz·um, steer″ee·) *n.* [*stereo-* + *-tropism*]. Growth or movement toward a solid body (positive stereotropism) or away from a solid body (negative stereotropism). Syn. *thigmotropism.* —**ste·reo·trop·ic** (sterr″ee·o·trop′ick, steer′ee·o·) *adj.*

ste·reo·ty·py (sterr′ee·o·tye″pee, steer′ee·o·) *n.* [*stereotype* + *-y*]. Persistent repetition of an activity, as the repeatedly similar hallucinations heralding certain psychomotor convulsions, the mannerisms seen in retarded children or the morbidly selfsame movements or ideas encountered in certain psychoses, especially schizophrenia.

ste·reo·vec·tor·car·dio·graph (sterr″ee·o·veck″tur·kahr′dee·o·graf, steer″ee·o·) *n.* [*stereo-* + *vectorcardiograph*]. VECTORCARDIOGRAPH.

ste·ric (steer′ick, sterr′ick) *adj.* [*stere-* + *-ic*]. Pertaining to the arrangement of atoms in space.

steric hindrance. *In chemistry,* the power ascribed to bulky atoms or bulky groups of atoms of interfering with the normal mobility of molecules or parts thereof. According to the theory, if the bulky group is close to the site of the reaction, it may interfere with the attack by a reagent and may retard or prevent the reaction or permit a competing process to occur. The presence of bulky groups in a molecule may also interfere with the free rotation around single bonds. This can increase the number of stable stereoisomeric forms and can decrease the stabilization of the molecule by resonance.

ste·rid (steer″id, sterr′) *n.* A proposed generic name for any substance that is either a sterol or a steroid.

ste·rig·ma (ste·rig′muh) *n.*, pl. **sterigma·ta** (·tuh), **sterigmas** [Gk. *stērigma,* support]. In fungi, specialized cells involved in spore formation, such as those which arise from the vesicle of *Aspergillus.* —**ster·ig·mat·ic** (sterr″ig·mat′ick) *adj.*

Ste·rig·ma·to·cys·tis (ste·rig″muh·to·sis′tis) *n.* A designation, largely obsolete, for some members of the genus *Aspergillus* in which a primary series of sterigmatic cells bear a crown of several sterigmata, which in turn bear chains of spores.

Sterigmatocystis cin·na·mo·mi·nus (sin″uh·mo·migh′nus). *Obsol.* A strain of *Aspergillus terreus.*

ster·ile (sterr′il) *adj.* [L. *sterilis*]. 1. Not fertile; not capable of reproducing. 2. Free from live microorganisms.

sterile cyst. An echinococcus cyst in which the larvae of the worm have died.

sterile hydatid. An Echinococcus cyst in which the germinal layer, brood cysts, and scolices have disappeared; ACEPHALOCYST.

sterile meningitis. Aseptic, usually chemical, meningitis.

sterile regional lymphadenitis. CAT-SCRATCH DISEASE.

sterile water for injection. Water for injection that has been packaged and suitably sterilized. See also *bacteriostatic water for injection, water for injection.*

ste·ril·i·ty (ste·ril′i·tee) *n.* 1. Total inability to reproduce. 2. The condition of freedom from live microorganisms.

sterility clinic. FERTILITY CLINIC.

ster·il·ize (sterr′i·lize) *v.* 1. To render sterile or free from live microorganisms. 2. To render incapable of procreation. —**ster·il·iza·tion** (sterr″il·zay′shun) *n.*

ster·i·li·zer (sterr′i·lye″zur) *n.* An apparatus, such as an autoclave, used to sterilize equipment or other objects by destroying all contaminating microorganisms.

Sterisil. Trademark for hexetidine, a local antibacterial, antifungal, and antitrichomonal agent.

stern-, sterno- [Gk. *sternon,* chest, breast, breastbone]. A combining form meaning (a) *sternum, sternal;* (b) *chest, breast.*

sterna. A plural of *sternum.*

ster·nal (stur′nul) *adj.* Pertaining to, or involving, the sternum.

sternal band. One of the paired mesenchymal anlages of the sternum.

sternal bar. One of the paired cartilaginous bars in the embryo that fuse to form the sternum.

ster·nal·gia (stur·nal′jee·uh, ·juh) *n.* [*stern-* + *-algia*]. 1. Pain in the sternum. 2. ANGINA PECTORIS.

ster·na·lis (stur·nay′lis) *n.* A rare muscle over the sternum. NA *musculus sternalis.* See also Table of Muscles in the Appendix.

sternal line. The median line of the sternum. Syn. *linea sternalis.*

sternal membrane. The fibrous layer ensheathing the sternum in front and behind. NA *membrana sterni.*

sternal plane. The ventral surface of the body of the sternum. Syn. *planum sternale.*

sternal puncture. Insertion of a hollow needle into the sternum to obtain bone marrow specimens.

sternal region. The region overlying the sternum. Syn. *regio sternalis.*

sternal ribs. TRUE RIBS.

sternal transfusion. A transfusion in which the donor's blood is introduced directly into the bone marrow of the recipient by puncture of the sternum.

Stern·berg cell (shtehrn′behrk) [C. *Sternberg,* Austrian pathologist, 1872–1935]. REED-STERNBERG CELL.

Sternberg-Reed cell [C. *Sternberg* and Dorothy M. *Reed*]. REED-STERNBERG CELL.

ster·ne·bra (stur′ne·bruh) *n.*, pl. **sterne·brae** (·bree) [*stern-* + *-ebra* as in vertebra]. An embryologic segment of the body of the sternum; there are usually four, of which the lower two or three arise from paired ossification centers.

Stern·hei·mer-Mal·bin cells. Leukocytes with cytoplasm containing granules agitated by brownian movement, seen in urinary sediments of patients with urological disorders, as in pyelonephritis.

Stern-McCar·thy resectoscope. A bimanual resectoscope used in transurethral surgery. Compare *Iglesias resectoscope.*

sterno-. See *stern-.*

ster·no·chon·dro·scap·u·la·ris (stur″no·kon″dro·skap″yoo·lair′is) *n.* A rare muscle arising from the sternum and the first costal cartilage, and extending to the upper border of the scapula.

ster·no·cla·vic·u·lar (stur″no·kla·vick′yoo·lur) *adj.* [*sterno-* + *clavicular*]. Pertaining to the sternum and the clavicle.

sternoclavicular angle. The angle existing between the clavicle and the sternum.

ster·no·cla·vic·u·la·ris (stur″no·kla·vick″yoo·lair′is) *n.* A rare variant slip of the subclavius muscle.

sternoclavicular joint. The joint between the medial end of the clavicle, the clavicular notch of the sternum, and the first costal cartilage. NA *articulatio sternoclavicularis.* See also Table of Synovial Joints and Ligaments in the Appendix.

sternoclavicular ligament. Either of the flattened bands passing between the medial end of the clavicle and the manubrium sterni on the anterior and posterior surfaces of the sternoclavicular joint, described respectively as the anterior sternoclavicular ligament (NA *ligamentum sternoclaviculare anterius*) and the posterior sternoclavicular ligament (NA *ligamentum sternoclaviculare posterius*).

ster·no·clei·dal (stur″no·klye′dul) *adj.* [*sterno-* + *cleid-* + *-al*]. STERNOCLAVICULAR.

ster·no·clei·do·mas·toid (stur″no·klye″do·mas′toid) *adj.* & *n.*

[*sterno-* + *cleido-* + *mastoid*]. 1. Pertaining to the sternum, the clavicle, and the mastoid process. 2. A muscle of the neck that flexes the head. NA *musculus sternocleidomastoideus.* See also Table of Muscles in the Appendix.

sternocleidomastoid artery. Any of the arterial branches supplying blood to the sternocleidomastoid muscle, arising from the superior thyroid artery (NA *ramus sternocleidomastoideus arteriae thyroideae superioris*), the occipital artery (NA(pl.) *rami sternocleidomastoidei arteriae occipitalis*), and, occasionally, the external carotid artery.

ster·no·cos·tal (stur″no·kos′tul) *adj.* [*sterno-* + *costal*]. Pertaining to the sternum and the ribs.

sternocostal articulation. Any of the articulations between the medial ends of the costal cartilages and the costal notches of the sternum. NA(pl.) *articulationes sternocostales.*

ster·no·cos·ta·lis (stur″no·kos·tay′lis) *n.* A transverse thoracic muscle.

sternocostal ligament. See *intraarticular sternocostal ligament, radiate sternocostal ligament.*

ster·no·dym·ia (stur″no·dim′ee·uh) *n.* [*sterno-* + *-dymia*]. STERNOPAGIA.

ster·nod·y·mus (stur·nod′i·mus) *n.* [*sterno-* + *-dymus*]. STERNOPAGUS.

ster·no·dyn·ia (stur″no·din′ee·uh) *n.* [*stern-* + *-odynia*]. Pain in the sternum.

ster·no·hy·oid (stur″no·high′oid) *adj.* & *n.* 1. Pertaining to the sternum and the hyoid bone. 2. A muscle arising from the manubrium of the sternum and inserted into the hyoid bone. NA *musculus sternohyoideus.* See also Table of Muscles in the Appendix.

ster·no·hy·oi·de·us azy·gos (stur″no·high·oy′dee·us az′i·gos). A rare muscle of the neck extending from the posterior surface of the manubrium of the sternum to the hyoid.

ster·no·mas·toid (stur″no·mas′toid) *n.* STERNOCLEIDOMASTOID (2).

sternomastoid line. A line drawn from a point between the two heads of the sternocleidomastoid muscle to the mastoid process.

sternomastoid sign. Spasm of the sternomastoid muscle with displacement or traction of the mediastinum toward the same side, due to pulmonary disease or local lymph node inflammation.

ster·no-om·pha·lo·dym·ia (stur″no·om″fuh·lo·dim′ee·uh) *n.* [*sterno-* + *omphalo-* + *-dymia*]. A form of conjoined twins in which the union is in both the sternal and the umbilical regions.

ster·no·pa·gia (stur″no·pay′jee·uh) *n.* The condition of being a sternopagus.

ster·nop·a·gus (stur·nop′uh·gus) *n.* [*sterno-* + *-pagus*]. Conjoined twins united at the sternum.

ster·nop·a·gy (stur·nop′uh·jee) *n.* STERNOPAGIA.

ster·no·peri·car·di·al (stur″no·perr″i·kahr′dee·ul) *adj.* [*sterno-* + *pericardial*]. Pertaining to the sternum and the underlying pericardium.

sternopericardial ligament. Any of the fibrous bands connecting the posterior surface of the sternum to the fibrous pericardium. NA (pl.) *ligamenta sternopericardiaca.*

ster·nos·chi·sis (stur·nos′ki·sis) *n.* [*sterno-* + *-schisis*]. A congenital cleft or fissure of the sternum.

ster·no·thy·roid (stur″no·thigh′roid) *adj.* & *n.* 1. Pertaining to the sternum and thyroid cartilage. 2. A muscle arising from the manubrium of the sternum and inserted into the thyroid cartilage. NA *musculus sternothyroideus.* See also Table of Muscles in the Appendix.

ster·not·o·my (stur·not′uh·mee) *n.* [*sterno-* + *-tomy*]. An operation cutting through the sternum.

ster·num (stur′num) *n.*, genit. **ster·ni** (·nye), pl. **sternums, ster·na** (·nuh) [NL., from Gk. *sternon,* chest, breast] [NA]. The flat, narrow bone in the median line in the front of the chest, composed of three portions—the manubrium, the body, and the xiphoid process. See also Table of Bones in the Appendix and Plates 1, 13.

ster·nu·ta·tion (stur″new·tay′shun) *n.* [L. *sternutatio,* from *sternutare,* to sneeze]. The act of sneezing.

ster·nu·ta·tor (stur′new·tay″tur) *n.* [L. *sternutare,* to sneeze, + *-or*]. A substance capable of inducing sneezing, as certain war gases.

ster·nu·ta·to·ry (stur·new′tuh·to″ree) *adj.* & *n.* [ML. *sternutatorius,* from *sternutare,* to sneeze]. 1. Causing or pertaining to sneezing. 2. Anything that causes sneezing.

ste·roid (steer′oid, sterr′oid) *n.* & *adj.* 1. Generally any of the compounds having the cyclopentanoperhydrophenanthrene ring system of sterols but not including the latter. In common usage however, sterols are included. They include the primary sex hormones, androgen and estrogen, and the corticosteroids. 2. Pertaining to or characteristic of a steroid. See also *sterid.* —**steroid·al** (·ul) *adj.*

ste·roid·o·gen·e·sis (ste·roy″do·jen′e·sis) *n.* [*steroid* + *-genesis*]. The production of steroids by living tissue. —**steroid·ogen·ic** (·ick) *adj.*

ste·rol (steer′ol, sterr′ol, ·ole) *n.* [*stere-* + *-ol*]. Any saturated or unsaturated alcohol derived from cyclopentanoperhydrophenanthrene; the alcohols occur both free and combined as esters or glycosides, and often are principal constituents of the nonsaponifiable fraction of fixed oils and fats. See also *mycosterols, phytosterols, zoosterols.*

Sterolone. A trademark for prednisolone, an anti-inflammatory adrenocortical steroid.

ste·rone (steer′ohn, sterr′ohn) *n.* A steroid possessing one or more ketone groups.

ster·tor (sturt′ur) *n.* [NL., from L. *stertere,* to snore]. Sonorous breathing or snoring; the rasping, rattling sound produced when the larynx and the air passages are partially obstructed by mucus. —**stertor·ous** (·us) *adj.*

stertorous respiration. The sound produced by breathing through the nose and mouth at the same time, causing vibration of the soft palate between the two currents of air.

steth-, stetho- [Gk. *stēthos*]. A combining form meaning *breast* or *chest.*

steth·ar·te·ri·tis (steth·ahr″te·rye′tis) *n.* [*steth-* + *arteritis*]. Inflammation of the arteries of the thorax.

stetho·gram (steth′o·gram) *n.* [*stetho-* + *-gram*]. 1. PHONOCARDIOGRAM. 2. Any record of movements of the chest, such as apex cardiogram or kinetocardiogram.

ste·thog·ra·phy (ste·thog′ruh·fee) *n.* [*stetho-* + *-graphy*]. 1. PHONOCARDIOGRAPHY. 2. The recording of chest pulsations and movements. See also *apex cardiogram.*

stetho·phone (steth′uh·fone) *n.* [*stetho-* + *-phone*]. 1. STETHOSCOPE. 2. An electric instrument capable of transmitting stethoscopic sounds to a large group of listeners.

stetho·poly·scope (steth″o·pol′ee·skope) *n.* [*stetho-* + *poly-* + *scope*]. A stethoscope having several tubes for the simultaneous use of several listeners. See also *stethophone* (2).

stetho·scope (steth′uh·skope) *n.* [*stetho-* + *-scope*]. An instrument for mediate auscultation for the detection and study of sounds arising within the body. The sound is conveyed from the body surface to both ears of the examiner simultaneously.

stetho·scop·ic (steth″uh·skop′ick) *adj.* Pertaining to, or detected by means of, a stethoscope.

ste·thos·co·py (ste·thos′kuh·pee) *n.* Examination with the aid of the stethoscope.

Ste·vens-John·son syndrome [A. M. *Stevens,* U.S. pediatrician, 1884–1945; and F. C. *Johnson,* U.S. pediatrician, 1894–1934]. A severe form of erythema multiforme, characterized by constitutional symptoms and marked involvement of the conjunctiva and oral mucosa.

Stew·art-Holmes phenomenon [J. P. *Stewart,* English neurologist, 1869–1949; and G. M. *Holmes*]. REBOUND PHENOMENON.

Stewart-Morel-Morgagni syndrome [J. P. *Stewart,* F. *Morel,* and G. B. *Morgagni*]. Hyperostosis frontalis interna associated with obesity, headache, hypertension, and various endocrine or neurologic and psychologic symptoms.

Stewart-Morel syndrome. STEWART-MOREL-MORGAGNI SYNDROME.

Stewart's incision [F. T. *Stewart,* U.S. surgeon, 1877-1920]. A transverse fusiform skin incision used in radical mastectomy.

Stewart-Treves syndrome. Postmastectomy lymphangiosarcoma.

STH Abbreviation for *somatotropic hormone.*

sthe·nia (sthee'nee·uh) *n.* [Gk. *sthenos,* strength, + *-ia*]. Normal force or vigor. Contr. *asthenia.*

sthen·ic (sthen'ick) *adj.* [Gk. *sthenos,* strength, + *-ic*]. Strong; active.

sthenic fever. A fever with high temperature, hot dry skin, strong pulse, and often delirium.

stib·amine glucoside (stib'uh·meen). A nitrogen glucoside of sodium *p*-aminophenylstibonate, a pentavalent antimony compound used in the treatment of kala azar.

stibi·ac·ne (stib''ee·ack'nee) *n.* [*stibium* + *acne*]. Acne caused by the use of antimony.

stib·i·al·ism (stib'ee·ul·iz·um) *n.* Poisoning by antimony.

stib·ine (stib'een) *n.* Antimonous hydride, SbH_3.

stib·i·um (stib'ee·um) *n.* [L.]. ANTIMONY.

sti·bo·ni·um (sti·bo'nee·um) *n.* The monovalent radical, SbH_4^+, analogous to ammonium.

stib·o·phen (stib'o·fen) *n.* Pentasodium antimony III bis-(pyrocatechol-2,4-disulfonate), $C_{12}H_4Na_5O_{16}S_4Sb$, a trivalent antimony compound used as an antischistosomal drug.

sticho·chrome (stick'o·krome) *n.* [Gk. *stichos,* line, row, + *-chrome*]. A nerve cell in which the chromophilic substance is arranged in striae running in the same direction as, and usually parallel with, the contour of the cell body.

stichochrome cell. STICHOCHROME.

Stick·er's disease (shtick'ur) [G. *Sticker,* German physician, 1860-1960]. ERYTHEMA INFECTIOSUM.

stick·tight flea. *ECHIDNOPHAGA GALLINACEA.*

stic·tac·ne (stick·tack'nee) *n.* [Gk. *stiktos,* pricked, + *acne*]. Acne in which the pustules are tiny and surround a comedo.

Stie·da fracture (shtee'dah) [A. *Stieda,* German surgeon, 1869-1945]. A medial condylar fracture of the femur.

stiff-man syndrome. A particularly malignant and progressive form of painful muscular spasms, of unknown cause but probably of central nervous system origin. Clinically, it resembles tetanus.

stiff neck. NUCHAL RIGIDITY.

stiff skin syndrome. A connective-tissue disorder characterized by localized areas of stony-hard skin, mild hirsutism, and limitation of joint mobility, with abnormal amounts of hyaluronidase-digestible acid mucopolysaccharide in the dermis; thought to be transmitted as an autosomal dominant trait.

sti·fle, *v.* To choke; to kill by impeding respiration.

stifle bone. The patella of the horse.

stifle joint. The true knee joint of the hind leg of the horse, corresponding to the knee joint of man.

stig·ma (stig'muh) *n.,* pl. **stig·ma·ta** (stig·mah'tuh, stig'muh·tuh), **stigmas** [Gk., tattoo-mark, mark, spot]. 1. Any mark, blemish, spot, or scar on the skin. 2. Any one of the marks or features characteristic of a condition, as hysterical stigmas. 3. Specifically, any visible characteristic associated with or diagnostic of a medical disorder, such as café-au-lait spots in neurofibromatosis, the Kayser-Fleischer ring in hepatolenticular degeneration, or the physical appearance commonly seen in Down's syndrome (mongolism). 4. The part of a pistil that receives the pollen. 5. An opening between cells, especially one between the endothelial cells of a capillary, now considered an artifact. —**stig·mal** (·mul), **stig·mat·ic** (stig·mat'ick) *adj.*

stigma of the graafian follicle. The point of rupture through which the ovum escapes.

stig·mas·ter·ol (stig·mas'tur·ol) *n.* A sterol, $C_{29}H_{48}O$, obtained from the soybean.

stigmata ni·gra (nigh'gruh). The black spots due to grains of gunpowder in the skin, produced by firearm discharge close by.

stigmata of Beneke. Erosions and petechial hemorrhages of the gastric mucosa in gastric ulcer. Syn. *stigmata ventriculi.*

stigmata ven·tric·u·li (ven·trick'yoo·lye). STIGMATA OF BENEKE.

stig·ma·tism (stig'muh·tiz·um) *n.* [Gk. *stigma, stigmatos,* mark, point, spot, + *-ism*]. 1. A condition of the refractive media of the eye in which rays of light from a point are accurately brought to a focus on the retina. Contr. *astigmatism.* 2. The condition of having stigmas.

stig·ma·ti·za·tion (stig''muh·ti·zay'shun) *n.* The formation of stigmas.

stig·ma·tose (stig'muh·toce) *adj.* Marked with stigmas.

Stigmonene bromide. Trademark for benzpyrinium bromide, a cholinergic drug.

stil·bam·i·dine (stil·bam'i·deen) *n.* 4,4′-stilbenedicarboxamidine, $C_{16}H_{16}N_4$, an antiprotozoal, used as the 2-hydroxyethanesulfonic acid (isethionate) salt.

stil·baz·i·um iodide (stil·baz'ee·um). 1-Ethyl-2,6-bis[*p*-(1-pyrrolidinyl)styryl]pyridinium iodide, $C_{31}H_{36}IN_3$, an anthelmintic.

stil·bene (stil'been) *n.* The parent hydrocarbon from which diethylstilbestrol and certain other synthetic estrogens may be considered to be derived; *trans*-α,β-Diphenylethylene, $C_6H_5CH{=}CHC_6H_5$.

stil·bes·trol, stil·boes·trol (stil·bes'trole, ·trol) *n.* DIETHYLSTILBESTROL.

Stiles-Craw·ford effect. Light passing through a unit area near the center of the pupil gives rise to a greater sensation of brightness when compared with light passing through a unit area near the margin of the pupil.

sti·let, sti·lette (stye·let', sti·let') *n.* STYLET.

still·birth, *n.* 1. The birth of a dead child. 2. A child born dead.

still·born, *adj.* Born dead. Contr. *liveborn.*

Stil·ler's disease (shtil'ur) [B. *Stiller,* German physician, 1837-1922]. Asthma associated with visceroptosis.

Stiller's sign [B. *Stiller*]. Increased mobility of the tenth rib in neurasthenia and visceroptosis.

stil·li·cid·i·um (stil''i·sid'ee·um) *n.* [L., from *stilla,* drop, + *cadere,* to fall]. The flow of a liquid drop by drop.

stillicidium lac·ri·ma·rum (lack·ri·mair'um). EPIPHORA.

stillicidium uri·nae (yoo·rye'nee). *Obsol.* The dribbling of urine.

stil·lin·gia (sti·lin'jee·uh) *n.* [B. *Stillingfleet,* English botanist, 1702-1771]. The dried root of *Stillingia sylvatica;* preparations of the root have been used for the treatment of various afflictions.

Stil·ling's canal (shtil'ing) [B. *Stilling,* German anatomist, 1810-1879]. 1. CENTRAL CANAL OF THE SPINAL CORD. 2. The hyaloid canal of the vitreous body.

Stilling's raphe [B. *Stilling*]. A narrow band connecting the pyramids of the medulla oblongata.

Stilling's test [J. *Stilling,* German ophthalmologist, 1842-1915]. A color vision test now used as Ishihara's modification.

Still·man's cleft. A slitlike alteration of gingival form; it occurs in the center of the marginal gingiva and extends apically.

Still's disease [G. F. *Still,* English physician, 1868-1941]. Juvenile rheumatoid arthritis in which visceral involvement is prominent. Syn. *Chauffard-Still disease.*

Still's murmur [G. F. *Still*]. An innocent early systolic murmur, vibratory or twanging in character, maximal between the lower left sternal border and the apex; common in children.

Stilphostrol. A trademark for the diphosphate ester of diethylstilbestrol, an estrogen.

Stim·son's method [L. A. *Stimson,* U.S. surgeon, 1844–1917]. A method of passive reduction of dislocation of the humerus or hip.

stim·u·lant (stim'yoo·lunt) *n. & adj.* 1. An agent that stimulates. 2. Producing a temporary increase in activity.

stim·u·late (stim'yoo·late) *v.* [L. *stimulare,* to goad, incite]. To quicken; to stir up; to excite; to increase functional activity. —**stimu·lat·ing** (·lay·ting) *adj.*

stimulating bath. A bath containing tonic, astringent, or aromatic substances that increase the cutaneous and body circulation.

stim·u·la·tion (stim"yoo·lay'shun) *n.* 1. The act of stimulating. 2. The effect of a stimulant. 3. EXCITATION.

stim·u·la·tor (stim'yoo·lay"tur) *n.* A person or thing that stimulates.

stim·u·lin (stim'yoo·lin) *n.* A substance supposed to stimulate the phagocytes to destroy germs.

stim·u·lus (stim'yoo·lus) *n.,* pl. **stimu·li** (·lye) [L., goad]. An excitant or irritant; an alteration in the environment of any living thing (cell, tissue, organism), capable of influencing its activity or of producing a response in or by it. See also *threshold* (1), *adequate stimulus, absolute threshold, suprathreshold stimulus.*

stimulus threshold. ABSOLUTE THRESHOLD.

sting, *n. & v.* 1. The acute burning sensation caused by pricking, striking, or chemically stimulating the skin or a mucous membrane. 2. The wound caused. 3. The organ or part causing the injury, such as the sting of a bee. 4. To prick or pierce with ensuing pain.

S-T interval. The period between the end of the QRS complex and the end of the T wave; the interval representing ventricular repolarization.

stipe, *n.* [L. *stīpes,* log, trunk, post, stake]. A short, stemlike support or stalk.

stip·ple cell. An erythrocyte with numerous fine blue or blue-black dots as seen in Romanovsky-stained preparations; occurs in lead poisoning, thalassemia, and other chronic anemias.

stippled epiphyses. CHONDRODYSTROPHIA CALCIFICANS CONGENITA.

stip·pling, *n.* [D. *stippelen,* to spot]. 1. A change of a surface whereby the presence of tiny nodules produces an appearance like that of a pebbled paper, as slight deposits of fibrin on a serous surface. 2. BASOPHILIA (2). 3. The pitted appearance of the surface of normal gingivae. 4. An effect developed in the surface finishing of artificial dentures to simulate natural tissue. 5. Multiple punctate opacities in radiographs, usually representing calcific deposits. 6. The dotting with basophilic granules in Romanovsky-stained preparations.

stir·rup bone (stur'up, stirr'up). STAPES.

stitch, *n.* 1. A sudden, sharp, lancinating pain, often at a costal margin. 2. SUTURE (2, 3).

stitch abscess. A pustular infection in the skin, about a suture.

stitching instrument. A surgical appliance consisting of a needle holder which utilizes all varieties of surgical needles, the suture material feeding from a continuous spool supply attached to the handle.

S-T junction. J POINT.

sto·chas·tic process (sto·kas'tick) [Gk. *stochastikos,* by guesswork, from *stochos,* guess]. *In statistics,* random process, covering practically all the theory of probability from coin tossing to harmonic analysis; used mostly when a time parameter is introduced.

stock culture. Any identified and characterized microbial culture, such as that maintained and distributed by the American Type Culture Collection.

stock·i·net (stock'i·net") *n.* Cotton material or shirting, woven like a stocking, but of uniform caliber and used according to size to cover extremities or the body preparatory to the application of a fixed dressing, such as a plaster or splints.

stock·ing, *n.* A close-fitting covering for the leg and foot, sometimes designed and fitted for a special hygienic or therapeutic purpose; usually made of knitted or woven goods that sometimes contain an elastic thread.

Stock's pigmentary degeneration or **retinal atrophy** (shtoʰk) [W. *Stock,* German ophthalmologist, b. 1874]. The retinal degeneration seen in juvenile amaurotic familial idiocy.

stock vaccine. A standard mixture of various bacteria.

Stof·fel's operation (shtoʰfʻel) [A. *Stoffel,* German orthopedic surgeon, 1880–1937]. An obsolete operation for the relief of spastic paralysis, in which a portion of the bundles of the nerve trunk supplying the affected area are resected.

stoi·chi·om·e·try (stoy"kee·om'e·tree) *n.* [Gk. *stoicheion,* element, + *-metry*]. The branch of chemistry that deals with the numerical relationship between elements or compounds (atomic weights), the determination of the proportions in which the elements combine (formulas), and the weight relations in reactions (equations). —**stoichi·o·met·ric** (·o·met'rick) *adj.*

Stokes-Adams syndrome [W. *Stokes,* Irish physician, 1804–1878; and R. *Adams*]. Syncope of cardiac origin occurring most frequently in patients with complete atrioventricular block and a pulse rate of 40 or less per minute; during an attack the electrocardiogram will show ventricular standstill, ventricular tachycardia or fibrillation, or slowing of the idioventricular impulses below a critical rate.

Stokes' expectorant [W. *Stokes,* Irish physician]. EXPECTORANT MIXTURE.

Stokes' law [G. G. *Stokes,* English physicist, 1819–1903]. A statement of the relationship between the velocity of fall of a spherical body in a fluid medium and the following variables: density of the sphere and of the medium, radius of the sphere, viscosity of the medium, and gravity.

Stokes' operation [W. *Stokes,* Irish surgeon, 1839–1900]. GRITTI-STOKES AMPUTATION.

Stok·vis' disease [B. J. E. *Stokvis,* Dutch physician, 1834–1902]. ENTEROGENOUS CYANOSIS.

Stoll's method [N. R. *Stoll,* U.S. parasitologist, b. 1892]. A technique for estimating the number of ova in stool specimens in which the solid feces are disintegrated with N/10 sodium hydroxide.

sto·lon (sto'lun) *n.* [L. *stolo, stolonis,* a shoot]. 1. *In biology,* a creeping stem or runner capable of taking root or bearing a bud, where it forms one or more new plants. 2. An analogous budding stock in certain lower animals.

Stoltz's operation [J. *Stoltz,* French gynecologist, 1803–1896]. An operation for cystocele, in which the protrusion is inverted within a purse-string suture.

sto·ma (sto'muh) *n.,* pl. **stoma·ta** (·tuh), **stomas** [Gk., mouth]. 1. A minute opening or pore in a surface. 2. A surgically created opening.

-stoma [Gk. *stoma,* mouth]. A combining form meaning (a) *mouth, opening;* (b) having a (specified) *kind of mouth.*

sto·mac·a·ce (sto·mack'uh·see) *n.* [Gk. *stomakakē,* a disease of the teeth and gums, from *stoma,* mouth, + *kakē,* badness]. ULCERATIVE STOMATITIS.

sto·ma·ceph·a·lus (sto"muh·sef'uh·lus) *n.* [*stoma* + *-cephalus*]. A combination of the ethmocephalic type of cyclopia with agnathia or micrognathia. Microstomia (or astomia) and a variable degree of synotia are associated. Syn. *stomatocephalus.*

stom·ach (stum'uck) *n.* [Gk. *stomachos,* gullet]. The most dilated part of the alimentary canal, in which food is stored immediately after swallowing and is partially digested by the gastric juice. It is situated below the diaphragm in the left hypochondriac, the epigastric, and part of the right hypochondriac regions. It is continuous at the cardiac end with the esophagus, at the pyloric end with the duodenum. Its wall consists of four coats: mucous, submucous, muscular, and serous. NA *ventriculus.*

stomach clamp. A clamp used to grasp an entire segment of the stomach in surgical resection of the organ.

sto·mach·ic (sto·mack'ick) *n.* A substance that may stimulate the secretory activity of the stomach.

stomach tooth. A canine (cuspid) tooth of the lower jaw. Contr. *eye tooth.*

stomach worm disease. Strongyloidiasis of cattle.

sto·mal (sto'mul) *adj.* Pertaining to a stoma.

stomat-, stomato- [Gk. *stoma, stomatos*]. A combining form meaning *mouth.*

sto·ma·tal·gia (sto"muh·tal'jee·uh) *n.* [*stomat-* + *-algia*]. Pain in the mouth.

sto·mat·ic (sto·mat'ick) *adj.* [Gk. *stomatikos*]. Pertaining to the mouth.

sto·ma·ti·tis (sto"muh·tye'tis) *n.*, pl. **stoma·tit·i·des** (·tit'i·deez) [*stomat-* + *-itis*]. Inflammation of the soft tissues of the mouth.

stomatitis med·i·ca·men·to·sa (med"i·kuh·men·to'suh). Inflammation of the mucus membranes of the mouth resulting from a systemic allergic reaction to a drug.

stomatitis ven·e·na·ta (ven·e·nay'tuh). STOMATITIS MEDICAMENTOSA.

sto·ma·toc·a·ce (sto"muh·tock'uh·see) *n.* [*stomato-* + *-cace*]. ULCERATIVE STOMATITIS.

stoma·to·ca·thar·sis (sto"muh·to·ka·thahr'sis) *n.* [*stomato-* + *catharsis*]. The cleaning or disinfection of the mouth.

sto·ma·to·ceph·a·lus (sto"muh·to·sef'uh·lus) *n.* STOMACEPHALUS.

sto·ma·to·dyn·ia (sto"muh·to·din'ee·uh) *n.* [*stomat-* + *-odynia*]. Pain in the mouth.

sto·ma·to·dy·so·dia (sto"muh·to·di·so'dee·uh) *n.* [*stomato-* + Gk. *dysōdia,* foul smell]. Ill-smelling breath.

sto·ma·to·gas·tric (sto"muh·to·gas'trick) *adj.* [*stomato-* + *gastric*]. 1. Pertaining to the mouth and the stomach. 2. Pertaining to the nerves that supply the anterior end of the digestive tract in various invertebrates.

sto·ma·to·glos·si·tis (sto"muh·to·glos·eye'tis) *n.* [*stomato-* + *gloss-* + *-itis*]. Inflammation of the mucous membranes of the mouth and tongue.

sto·ma·to·gnath·ic (sto"muh·to·nath'ick) *adj.* [*stomato-* + *gnathic*]. Pertaining to the mouth, oral cavity, and jaws.

stomatognathic system. The physiological group of organs which perform the functions of mastication, deglutition, and speech.

sto·ma·tol·o·gy (sto"muh·tol'uh·jee) *n.* [*stomato-* + *-logy*]. The branch of medical science concerned with the anatomy, physiology, pathology, therapeutics, and hygiene of the oral cavity, of the tongue, teeth, and adjacent structures and tissues, and of the relationship of that field to the entire body. —**stoma·to·log·ic** (·to·loj'ick) *adj.*

stoma·to·ma·la·cia (sto"muh·to·ma·lay'shee·uh, ·shuh) *n.* [*stomato-* + *malacia*]. Sloughing or degeneration of the structures of the mouth.

sto·ma·to·me·nia (sto"muh·to·mee'nee·uh) *n.* [*stomato-* + *men-* + *-ia*]. STOMENORRHAGIA.

sto·ma·to·mia (sto"muh·to'mee·uh, stom"uh·) *n.* [NL., from Gk. *stoma,* mouth, + *-tomia,* from Gk. *temnein,* to cut]. A general term for the incision of a mouth, as of the uterus.

sto·mat·o·my (sto·mat'uh·mee) *n.* [Gk. *stoma,* mouth, + *-tomy*]. Incision of the ostium uteri.

sto·ma·to·my·co·sis (sto"muh·to·migh·ko'sis) *n.* [*stomato-* + *mycosis*]. THRUSH (1).

sto·ma·to·ne·cro·sis (sto"muh·to·ne·kro'sis) *n.* [*stomato-* + *necrosis*]. Noma of the mouth.

sto·ma·to·no·ma (sto"muh·to·no'muh) *n.* [*stomato-* + *noma*]. Noma of the mouth.

sto·ma·top·a·thy (sto"muh·top'uth·ee) *n.* [*stomato-* + *-pathy*]. Any disease of the mouth.

sto·ma·to·plas·ty (sto'muh·to·plas"tee) *n.* [*stomato-* + *-plasty*]. A plastic operation upon the mouth. —**sto·ma·to·plas·tic** (sto"muh·to·plas'tick) *adj.*

sto·ma·tor·rha·gia (sto"muh·to·ray'jee·uh) *n.* [*stomato-* + *-rrhagia*]. Copious hemorrhage from the mouth.

sto·ma·to·scope (sto'muh·to·skope) *n.* [*stomato-* + *-scope*]. An instrument used for inspecting the cavity of the mouth.

sto·ma·to·sis (sto"muh·to'sis) *n.* [*stomato-* + *-osis*]. Any disease of the mouth.

sto·ma·tot·o·my (sto"muh·tot'uh·mee) *n.* [*stomat-* + *-tomy*]. STOMATOMY.

-stome [Gk. *stoma,* mouth]. A combining form meaning *aperture, opening, mouth.*

sto·men·or·rha·gia (sto·men"o·ray'jee·uh) *n.* [Gk. *stoma,* mouth, + *menorrhagia*]. Vicarious bleeding in the mouth, associated with abnormal menstruation.

-stomia [Gk. *stoma,* mouth, + *-ia*]. A combining form designating *a condition of the mouth.*

stomodeal plate. BUCCOPHARYNGEAL MEMBRANE.

sto·mo·de·um, sto·mo·dae·um (sto"mo·dee'um) *n.* [NL., from Gk. *stoma,* mouth, + *hodaios,* on the way]. The primitive oral cavity of the embryo; an ectodermal fossa formed by the growth of the facial processes about the buccopharyngeal membrane. —**stomode·al, stomodae·al** (·ul) *adj.*

sto·mos·chi·sis (sto·mos'ki·sis) *n.* [*stoma* + *-schisis*]. A fissure of the mouth. See also *harelip, gnathoschisis, cleft palate, staphyloschisis, cleft uvula.*

Sto·mox·ys (sto·mock'sis) *n.* [NL., from Gk. *stoma,* mouth, + *oxys,* sharp]. A genus of bloodsucking flies of the family Muscidae. It is similar to the common housefly.

Stomoxys cal·ci·trans (kal'si·tranz). The common stable fly which aids in the transmission of trypanosomiasis and anthrax, and serves as an intermediate host of the nematode *Habronema,* parasitic in the stomach of the horse.

-stomy [Gk. *stoma,* mouth, + *-y*]. A combining form designating *a surgical operation establishing an opening into a* (specified) *part.*

stone, *n.* 1. CALCULUS. 2. An English unit of weight equal to 14 lb.

Stone clamp [H. B. *Stone,* U.S. surgeon, b. 1882]. A thin-bladed crushing intestinal clamp with detachable handle, used in pairs to facilitate performance of aseptic anastomoses.

stone·cut·ter's disease. Raynaud's phenomenon related to the use of pneumatic or compressed-air tools.

stone oil. PETROLEUM.

Stone operation [H. B. *Stone*]. A plastic operation to restore voluntary anal control. Syn. *Wreden operation, Wreden-Stone operation.*

stone searcher. An instrument equipped with a porcelain tip, formerly used to explore the urinary bladder, bile duct, etc., for concretions.

Stoo·key's reflex [B. P. *Stookey,* U.S. neurosurgeon, 1887–1966]. Flexion of the leg in response to tapping the tendons of the semimembranosus and semitendinosus muscles while the leg is semiflexed at the knee.

stool, *n.* Material evacuated from the bowels; feces.

stop·page (stop'ij) *n.* Cessation of flow or action; closure or stenosis.

stor·age battery. A galvanic cell which can be charged and discharged. On charge, electrical energy is converted into chemical energy; on discharge, the process is reversed.

storage disease. Any metabolic disease, usually due to an inherited enzyme deficiency, characterized by excess deposition of exogenous or endogenous substances within the body. Syn. *thesaurosis.* See also *gangliosidosis, lipid storage diseases, histiocytosis X, mucopolysaccharidosis.*

sto·rax (sto'racks) *n.* [L., from Gk. *styrax*]. A balsam obtained from the wounded trunk of *Liquidambar orientalis,* or of *L. styraciflua;* occurs as a semiliquid, grayish to grayish-brown, sticky, opaque mass, or a semisolid, sometimes solid mass; consists largely of storesin, which is present in two forms—alpha and beta storesin—both free and in the form of a cinnamic ester, and also cinnamic acid and its esters. Has been used as a stimulating expectorant, and externally as a parasiticide.

sto·ri·form (sto'ri·form) *adj.* Having the spiraled, whorled appearance of a nebula.

storm, *n.* Sudden exacerbation of symptoms or crisis in a disease.

Stovarsol. A trademark for acetarsone, a protozoacide.

Stoxil. A trademark for idoxuridine, a topical antiviral agent used for treatment of dendritic keratitis.

¹STP Abbreviation for *standard temperature and pressure.*

²STP [*s*erenity, *t*ranquility and *p*eace, ostensibly brought about by the psychedelic agent]. *Colloq.* DOM.

stra·bi·lis·mus (stray"bi·liz'mus, strab"i·) *n.* STRABISMUS.

stra·bism (stray'biz·um, strab'iz·um) *n.* STRABISMUS.

stra·bis·mom·e·ter (strab"iz·mom'e·tur, stray"biz·) *n.* STRABOMETER.

stra·bis·mom·e·try (strab"iz·mom·e'tree, stray"biz·) *n.* STRABOMETRY.

stra·bis·mus (stra·biz'mus) *n.* [NL., from Gk. *strabismos,* from *strabos,* squinting]. An abnormality of the eyes in which the visual axes do not meet at the desired objective point, in consequence of incoordinate action of the extrinsic ocular muscles. Syn. *squint, heterotropia.* —**strabis·mal** (·mul), **strabis·mic** (·mick) *adj.*

stra·bom·e·ter (stra·bom'e·tur) *n.* [*stra*bismus + *meter*]. An instrument for the measurement of the deviation of the eyes in strabismus. Syn. *strabismometer.*

stra·bom·e·try (stra·bom'e·tree) *n.* The determination of the degree of ocular deviation in strabismus. Syn. *strabismometry.*

strabo·tome (strab'uh·tome) *n.* A knife used for strabotomy.

stra·bot·o·my (stra·bot'uh·mee) *n.* [*stra*bismus + *-tomy*]. An operation for the correction of strabismus.

Strachan's syndrome (strawn) [W. H. W. *Strachan,* British physician, 1857–1921]. A painful neuropathy first observed in Jamaica and now considered to be due to nutritional factors; characterized chiefly by symmetrical loss of sensation and, to a lesser degree, of strength in the distal segments of the limbs, failing vision, occasionally deafness and vertigo, and often accompanied by varying degrees of stomatoglossitis, and genital dermatitis. Syn. *Jamaican neuropathy.*

strad·dling embolus. SADDLE EMBOLUS.

straight arteriole. Any one of the arterioles arising from an arcuate artery of the kidney and passing downward into a renal pyramid. NA (pl.) *arteriolae rectae.*

straight gyrus. GYRUS RECTUS.

straight-leg-raising test. LASÈGUE'S SIGN.

straight-neck paralysis. A common term used to describe the signs of folic acid deficiency of chickens.

straight sinus. A sinus of the dura mater running from the inferior sagittal sinus along the junction of the falx cerebri and tentorium to the transverse sinus. NA *sinus rectus.* See also Table of Veins in the Appendix and Plates 10, 17, 18.

¹strain, *n.* [OE. *strēon,* progeny]. A group of organisms possessing a common characteristic which distinguishes them from other groups within the same species.

²strain, *v.* & *n.* [MF. *estraindre,* from L. *stringere,* to bind tight]. 1. To injure by excessive stretching, overuse, or misuse. 2. To pass through a strainer or other device; to filter. 3. To exert great effort in ejecting something from the body, as when retching or sometimes defecating. 4. Excessive stretching or overuse of a part, as of muscles or joints. 5. The condition produced in a part by overuse or wrong use, as eyestrain. 6. The condition or state of a system exposed to stress; the disturbance of normal and harmonious relationships of one part or person with other parts or persons as a result of such stress; mental tension.

strait, *n.* [OF. *estreit,* from L. *strictus,* close, tight]. A narrow or constricted passage, as the inferior or superior pelvic strait.

strait·jack·et, *n.* A restraining apparatus, not always conforming to the jacket type, used to prevent violent, delirious, or otherwise physically uncontrollable persons from injuring themselves or others.

stra·mo·ni·um (stra·mo'nee·um) *n.* The dried leaves and flowering tops of *Datura stramonium* (including *D. tatula*); contains the alkaloids hyoscyamine and scopolamine. The actions of stramonium are similar to those of belladonna. Stramonium has been used in the treatment of asthma by smoking in cigarettes or by mixing with potassium nitrate and burning and inhaling the vapors, which contain atropine. Syn. *Jamestown weed, Jimson weed.*

stran·ger anxiety. The response, often manifested by apprehension, fear, and crying, of an infant at about 6 to 10 months to a face or person other than the mother or surrogate, marking an important stage in the child's ability to differentiate people, establish object relations, and express anxiety. Syn. *eighth-month anxiety.* See also *separation anxiety.*

stran·gle, *v.* [OF. *estrangler,* from L. *strangulare,* from Gk. *strangalan*]. 1. To choke or throttle by compression of the glottis or trachea. 2. To be choked, to suffocate from tracheal constriction or obstruction.

stran·gles, *n.* An infectious disease of solipeds caused by *Streptococcus equi,* involving the nasal passages and related structures; characterized by a purulent inflammation with involvement of the lymphatic system of the head and, in some instances, accompanied by difficult breathing. Syn. *equine distemper.*

stran·gu·lat·ed hernia (strang'gew·lay"tid). A hernia involving intestine in which circulation of the blood and the fecal current are blocked. If unrelieved, it leads to ileus and necrosis of the intestine.

stran·gu·la·tion (strang"gew·lay'shun) *n.* 1. Asphyxiation due to obstruction of the air passages, as by external pressure on the neck. 2. Constriction of a part producing arrest of the circulation, as strangulation of a hernia. —**stran·gu·lat·ed** (strang'gew·lay"tid) *adj.*

stran·gu·ria (strang·gew'ree·uh) *n.* STRANGURY.

stran·gu·ry (strang'gew·ree) *n.* [Gk. *strangouria,* from *stranx, strangos,* drop, trickle, + *ouron,* urine]. Painful urination, the urine being voided drop by drop.

strap, *n.* & *v.* 1. A long band, as of adhesive plaster. 2. To compress or support a part by means of bands, especially bands of adhesive plaster.

strap procedure. SLING PROCEDURE.

Strass·mann metroplasty. A technique for repair of a bicornuate uterus using a transverse incision.

Strass·mann's phenomenon (shtra^{h}ss'ma^{h}n) [P. F. *Strassmann,* German obstetrician and gynecologist, 1866–1938]. Engorgement of the umbilical vein when pressure is applied to the uterine fundus, indicating that the placenta has not yet separated from the uterus.

strata. Plural of *stratum.*

strat·i·fi·ca·tion (strat"i·fi·kay'shun) *n.* Arrangement in layers or strata.

strat·i·fied (strat'i·fide) *adj.* Arranged in layers or strata.

stratified epithelium. Epithelium in which the cells are arranged in distinct layers.

stratified thrombus. A thrombus in which there are successive layers of fibrin and red blood cells to produce a mixture of colors. Syn. *fibrolaminar thrombus, mixed thrombus.*

stra·tig·ra·phy (stra·tig'ruh·fee) *n.* [*stra*tum + *-graphy*]. SECTIONAL RADIOGRAPHY. —**strat·i·graph·ic** (strat"i·graf'ick) *adj.*

strato·sphere (strat'uh·sfeer) *n.* [*stra*tum + *sphere*]. The atmosphere above the tropopause, where temperature changes are small and winds essentially horizontal.

stra·tum (stray'tum, strah'tum) *n.,* pl. **stra·ta** (·tuh) [L., covering, spread, pavement, from *sternere,* to spread out]. LAYER.

stratum al·bum pro·fun·dum cor·po·rum qua·dri·ge·mi·no·rum (al'bum pro·fun'dum kor'po·rum kwah''dri·jem·i·no'rum) [BNA]. A deep layer of white matter seen in cross section of the superior colliculus.

stratum ba·sa·le (ba·say'lee). BASAL LAYER.

stratum basale epi·der·mi·dis (ep·i·dur'mi·dis) [NA]. STRATUM CYLINDRICUM.

stratum ce·re·bra·le re·ti·nae (serr·e·bray'lee ret'i·nee) [NA]. The layer of the retina which contains the visual and nerve cells.

stratum ci·ne·re·um (si·neer'ee·um). STRATUM GRISEUM COLLICULI SUPERIORIS.

stratum cinereum ce·re·bel·li (serr·e·bel'lye) [BNA]. Stratum moleculare cerebelli (= MOLECULAR LAYER OF THE CEREBELLUM).

stratum cir·cu·la·re mem·bra·nae tym·pa·ni (sur·kew·lair'ree mem·bray'nee tim'puh·nigh) [NA]. The circular fibrous layer of the tympanic membrane.

stratum circulare tu·ni·cae mus·cu·la·ris col·li (tew'ni·see mus·kew·lair'is kol'eye) [NA]. The inner circular layer of the muscular coat of the colon.

stratum circulare tunicae muscularis in·te·sti·ni te·nu·is (in·tes·tye'nigh ten'yoo·is) [NA]. The inner circular layer of the muscular coat of the small intestine.

stratum circulare tunicae muscularis rec·ti (reck'tye) [NA]. The inner circular layer of the muscular coat of the rectum.

stratum circulare tunicae muscularis tu·bae ute·ri·nae (tew'bee yoo·tur·eye'nee) [BNA]. The inner circular layer of the muscular coat of the uterine tube.

stratum circulare tunicae muscularis ure·thrae mu·li·e·bris (yoo·ree'three mew·lee·ee'bris) [BNA]. The inner circular layer of the muscle coat of the female urethra.

stratum circulare tunicae muscularis ven·tri·cu·li (ven·trick'yoo·lye) [NA]. The circular fibers of the muscle coat of the stomach.

stratum com·pac·tum (kom·pack'tum). The surface layer (about one-fourth) of the decidua parietalis.

stratum cor·ne·um (kor'nee·um) [NA]. The layer of keratinized cells of the epidermis. Syn. *horny layer.*

stratum corneum un·guis (ung'gwis) [NA]. The nail proper. Contr. *stratum germinativum unguis.*

stratum cu·ta·ne·um mem·bra·nae tym·pa·ni (kew·tay'nee·um mem·bray'nee tim'puh·nigh) [NA]. The layer covering the lateral aspect of the tympanic membrane.

stratum cy·lin·dri·cum (si·lin'dri·kum). The basal-cell layer of a stratified epithelium, especially of a stratified squamous epithelium, as the epidermis.

stratum dis·junc·tum (dis·junk'tum). The outermost layer of desquamating cells of the stratum corneum of the epidermis.

stratum ex·ter·num tu·ni·cae mus·cu·la·ris duc·tus de·fe·ren·tis (eck·stur'num tew'ni·see mus·kew·lair'is duck'tus def·e·ren'tis) [BNA]. The outer layer of the muscle coat of the ductus deferens.

stratum externum tunicae muscularis ure·te·ris (yoo·ree'tur·is) [BNA]. The outer layer of the muscle coat of the ureter.

stratum externum tunicae muscularis ve·si·cae uri·na·ri·ae (ve·sigh'see yoo·ri·nair'ee·ee) [BNA]. The outer layer of the muscle coat of the urinary bladder.

stratum fi·bro·sum cap·su·lae ar·ti·cu·la·ris (figh·bro'sum kap'sue·lee ahr·tick·yoo·lair'is) [BNA]. MEMBRANA FIBROSA CAPSULAE ARTICULARIS.

stratum gan·gli·o·na·re ner·vi op·ti·ci (gang·glee·o·nair'ee nur'vye op'ti·sigh) [NA]. GANGLIONIC LAYER OF THE OPTIC NERVE.

stratum ganglionare re·ti·nae (ret'i·nee) [NA]. GANGLIONIC LAYER OF THE RETINA.

stratum gan·gli·o·sum ce·re·bel·li (gang·glee·o'sum serr·e·bel'eye) [BNA]. The layer of the cerebellar cortex which contains Purkinje cells.

stratum ger·mi·na·ti·vum (jur''mi·nuh·tye'vum). GERMINATIVE LAYER.

stratum germinativum [Mal·pi·ghii] (mal·peeg'ee·eye) [BNA]. GERMINATIVE LAYER.

stratum ger·mi·na·ti·vum un·guis (jur·mi·nuh·tye'vum ung'gwis) [NA]. The layer of living cells of the nail bed. Contr. *stratum corneum unguis.*

stratum gra·nu·lo·sum (gran·yoo·lo'sum). A layer of minute cells containing many granules. See also *granular layer of the cerebellum, granular layer of the epidermis.*

stratum granulosum ce·re·bel·li (serr·e·bel'eye) [NA]. GRANULAR LAYER OF THE CEREBELLUM.

stratum granulosum epi·der·mi·dis (ep·i·dur'mi·dis) [NA]. GRANULAR LAYER OF THE EPIDERMIS.

stratum granulosum fol·li·cu·li ova·ri·ci ve·si·cu·lo·si (fol·ick'yoo·lye o·vair'i·sigh ve·sick·yoo·lo'sigh) [NA]. The granular cell layer of a vesicular ovarian follicle.

stratum granulosum ova·rii (o·vair'ee·eye) [BNA]. STRATUM GRANULOSUM FOLLICULI OVARICI VESICULOSI.

stratum gri·se·um col·li·cu·li su·pe·ri·o·ris (griz'ee·um kol·ick'yoo·lye sue·peer·ee·o'ris) [NA]. A thin sheet of gray matter seen in cross sections of superior colliculus.

stratum in·ter·me·di·um (in·tur·mee'dee·um). The thin zone of the enamel pulp of an enamel organ which lies next to the ameloblasts and consists of cells that do not become part of the stellate reticulum.

stratum in·ter·num tu·ni·cae mus·cu·la·ris duc·tus de·fe·ren·tis (in·tur'num tew'ni·see mus·kew·lair'is duck'tus def·e·ren'tis) [BNA]. The inner layer of the muscle coat of the ductus deferens.

stratum internum tunicae muscularis ure·te·ris (yoo·ree'tur·is) [BNA]. The inner layer of the muscle coat of the ureter.

stratum internum tunicae muscularis ve·si·cae uri·na·ri·ae (ve·sigh'see yoo·ri·nair'ee·ee) [BNA]. The inner layer of the muscle coat of the urinary bladder.

stratum in·ter·oli·va·re lem·nis·ci (in''tur·ol·i·vair'ee lem·nis'eye) [BNA]. STRATUM LEMNISCI.

stratum lem·nis·ci (lem·nis'eye). The deepest layer of the superior colliculus, composed of cell bodies and nerve fibers, which receives fibers of the spinotectal tract and sends out fibers mainly to the reticular formation, thalamus, and spinal cord.

stratum lon·gi·tu·di·na·le tu·ni·cae mus·cu·la·ris co·li (lon''ji·tew'di·nay'lee tew'ni·see mus·kew·lair'is ko'lye) [NA]. The longitudinal layer of the muscle coat of the colon.

stratum longitudinale tunicae muscularis in·te·sti·ni te·nu·is (in·tes·tye'nigh ten'yoo·is) [NA]. The longitudinal layer of the muscle coat of the small intestine.

stratum longitudinale tunicae muscularis rec·ti (reck'tye) [NA]. The longitudinal layer of the muscle coat of the rectum.

stratum longitudinale tunicae muscularis tu·bae ute·ri·nae (tew'bee yoo·tur·eye'nee) [BNA]. The longitudinal layer of the muscle coat of the uterine tube.

stratum longitudinale tunicae muscularis ure·thrae mu·li·e·bris (yoo·ree'three mew·lee·ee'bris) [BNA]. The longitudinal layer of the muscle coat of the female urethra.

stratum longitudinale tunicae muscularis ven·tri·cu·li (ven·trick'yoo·lye) [NA]. The longitudinal layer of the muscle coat of the stomach.

stratum lu·ci·dum (lew'si·dum) [NA]. A translucent layer of the epidermis consisting of irregular transparent cells with traces of nuclei.

stratum mal·pi·ghii (mal·peeg'ee·eye) [M. *Malpighi*]. PRICKLE-CELL LAYER.

stratum medium tu·ni·cae mus·cu·la·ris duc·tus de·fe·ren·tis (tew'ni·see mus·kew·lair'is duck'tus def·e·ren'tis) [BNA]. The middle layer of the muscle coat of the ductus deferens.

stratum medium tunicae muscularis ure·te·ris (yoo·ree'tur·is) [BNA]. The middle layer of the muscle coat of the ureter.

stratum medium tunicae muscularis ve·si·cae uri·na·ri·ae (ve·

sigh'see yoo·ri·nair'ee·ee) [BNA]. The middle layer of the muscle coat of the urinary bladder.

stratum mo·le·cu·la·re ce·re·bel·li (mo·leck·yoo·lair'ee serr·e·bel'eye) [NA]. MOLECULAR LAYER OF THE CEREBELLUM.

stratum mu·co·sum (mew·ko'sum). PRICKLE CELL LAYER.

stratum mucosum mem·bra·nae tym·pa·ni (mem·bray'nee tim'puh·nigh) [NA]. The mucous membrane covering the inner surface of the tympanic membrane.

stratum neu·ro·epi·the·li·a·le re·ti·nae (new''ro·ep·i·theel·ee·ay'lee ret'i·nee) [NA]. The neuroepithelial layer of the retina, containing the rods and cones.

stratum nu·cle·a·re me·dul·lae ob·lon·ga·tae (new·klee·air'ee me·dul'ee ob·long·gay'tee) [BNA]. *Obsol.* The portion of gray matter in the medulla oblongata where the nuclei of the caudal cranial nerves are located.

stratum op·ti·cum (op'ti·kum). OPTIC STRATUM.

stratum pa·pil·la·re (pap·i·lair'ee ko'ree·eye) [NA]. The zone of fine-fibered connective tissue within and immediately subjacent to the papillae of the corium. Syn. *papillary layer.*

stratum pig·men·ti bul·bi ocu·li (pig·men'tye bul'bye ock'yoo·lye) [NA]. The layer of the eyeball containing pigmented epithelial cells.

stratum pigmenti cor·po·ris ci·li·a·ris (kor'po·ris sil·ee·air'is) [NA]. The pigmented cell layer of the ciliary body.

stratum pigmenti iri·dis (eye'ri·dis) [NA]. The pigmented cell layer of the iris.

stratum pigmenti re·ti·nae (ret'i·nee) [NA]. The layer of the retina containing pigmented epithelial cells.

stratum ra·di·a·tum mem·bra·nae tym·pa·ni (ray·dee·ay'tum mem·bray'nee tim'puh·nigh) [NA]. The radiating connective tissue fibers of the tympanic membrane.

stratum re·ti·cu·la·re (re·tick·yoo·lair'ee) [NA]. RETICULAR LAYER.

stratum spi·no·sum epi·der·mi·dis (spye·no'sum ep·i·dur'mi·dis) [NA]. PRICKLE CELL LAYER.

stratum spon·gi·o·sum (spon·jee·o'sum). SPONGY LAYER.

stratum sub·mu·co·sum (sub·mew·ko'sum). The thin layer of smooth muscle of the myometrium adjacent to the endometrium.

stratum sub·se·ro·sum (sub·se·ro'sum). The thin layer of smooth muscle of the myometrium adjacent to the serous coat.

stratum su·pra·vas·cu·la·re (sue''pruh·vas·kew·lair'ee). The layer of muscle of the myometrium between the stratum vasculare and the stratum subserosum.

stratum sy·no·vi·a·le cap·su·lae ar·ti·cu·la·ris (si·no·vee·ay'lee kap'sue·lee ahr·tick·yoo·lair'is) [BNA]. Membrana synovialis (= SYNOVIAL MEMBRANE).

stratum vas·cu·la·re (vas·kew·lair'ee). The thickest layer of muscle in the myometrium next to the stratum submucosum.

stratum zo·na·le cor·po·rum qua·dri·ge·mi·no·rum (zo·nay'lee kor'po·rum kwah''dri·jem·i·no'rum) [BNA]. STRATUM ZONALE OF THE MIDBRAIN.

stratum zonale of the midbrain. The most superficial layer of the superior colliculus, composed of fibers that arise mainly from the occipital cortex, from the retina via the optic tract, from the spinal cord and the inferior calliculus. Syn. *stratum zonale corporum quadrigeminorum.*

stratum zonale of the thalamus. A thin plate of nerve fibers covering the thalamus and giving it a whitish color. NA *stratum zonale thalami.*

stratum zonale tha·la·mi (thal'uh·migh) [NA]. STRATUM ZONALE OF THE THALAMUS.

Straus reaction or **test** (strohss) [I. *Straus,* French physician, 1845–1896]. Painful swelling of the testes of a rat 2 days after the intraperitoneal injection of *Pseudomonas pseudomallei,* the causative organism of melioidosis.

Strauss's phenomenon (shtraowss) [H. *Strauss,* German physician, 1868–1944]. The administration of fatty foods by mouth results in an increase of fatty constituents in the effusion of chylous ascites.

Strauss's syndrome. MINIMAL BRAIN DYSFUNCTION SYNDROME.

Strauss's test [H. *Strauss*]. A test for lactic acid, in which a solution of ferric chloride is added to an ether extract of gastric juice. A light green or yellow color indicates lactic acid.

straw·ber·ry gallbladder. Deposits of neutral fat and cholesterol in macrophages in the tips of gallbladder folds, producing yellow speckling of the red (when fresh) mucosa, and thereby a resemblance to a strawberry.

strawberry mark. A congenital hemangioma clinically characterized by its raised, bright-red, soft, often lobulated appearance. Syn. *nevus vasculosus.*

strawberry tongue. A strawberry-like appearance of the tongue due to desquamation; seen in about 50 percent of patients with scarlet fever.

streak, *n.* 1. A furrow, line, or stripe. See also *primitive streak.* 2. *In bacteriology,* the process of distributing the inoculum over the surface of a solid culture medium. Cultures thus obtained are called streak cultures.

streak plate. A bacterial culture within a Petri dish formed by streaking across the culture medium with a bacterial suspension.

stream, *n.* A flow, especially in a definite direction.

stream birefringence. The orientation by flow of rod or disk-shaped particles, resulting in double refraction, and characteristic of virus particles.

stream·ing potentials. The electric potentials that result from the streaming of fluids, such as occurs in the flow of blood through the vessels.

stream·line flow. A flow in which particles in the axial stream move more rapidly than those in the periphery, as the blood cells in the capillaries.

street rabies virus. The naturally occurring rabies virus, as contrasted with the fixed virus produced by intracerebral passage in rabbits.

Strep. An abbreviation for *Streptococcus.*

strepho·sym·bo·lia (stref''o·sim·bo'lee·uh) *n.* [Gk. *strephein,* to turn, + *symbol* + *-ia*]. 1. MIRROR VISION. 2. Specifically, the tendency of many children first learning to read to reverse letters in a word or to fail to distinguish between similar letters, as *p* and *q,* or *n* and *u;* abnormal if persisting. 3. Reversal in direction of reading.

strep·i·tus (strep'i·tus) *n.* [L., from *strepere,* to make a loud noise]. A sound; a noise.

strepitus au·ri·um (aw'ree·um). TINNITUS.

strepitus ute·ri (yoo'tur·eye). UTERINE SOUFFLE.

strepitus ute·ri·nus (yoo·tur·eye'nus). UTERINE SOUFFLE.

strepo·gen·in (strep''o·jen'in) *n.* A factor, possibly a peptide derivative of glutamic acid, reported to exist in certain proteins, acting as a growth stimulant to bacteria and mice in the presence of completely hydrolyzed protein. Syn. *streptogenin.*

strept-, strepto- [Gk. *streptos*]. A combining form meaning (a) *twisted, curved;* (b) *streptococcal.*

strep·ta·mine (strep'tuh·meen) *n.* 1,3-diamino-2,4,5-cyclohexanetriol, $C_6H_{14}N_2O_3$, obtained on hydrolytic cleavage of betamicin.

strep·ti·ce·mia, strep·ti·cae·mia (strep''ti·see'mee·uh) *n.* STREPTOSEPTICEMIA.

strep·ti·dine (strep'ti·deen) *n.* 1,3-Diguanidino-2,4,5,6-tetrahydroxycyclohexane, $C_8H_{18}N_6O_4$, obtained when streptomycin undergoes acid hydrolysis; in the streptomycin molecule it is glycosidally linked to streptobiosamine.

strep·to·an·gi·na (strep''to·an·jye'nuh) *n.* [*strepto-* + *angina*]. A streptococcal sore throat; a septic sore throat; a pseudomembranous deposit in the throat due to streptococci.

strep·to·bac·il·lary (strep''to·bas'i·lerr·ee) *adj.* Caused by a streptobacillus.

streptobacillary fever. HAVERHILL FEVER.

strep·to·ba·cil·lus (strep″to·ba·sil′us) *n.*, pl. **streptobacil·li** (·eye) [*strepto-* + *bacillus*]. A bacillus that remains attached end to end, resulting in the formation of chains. It is a constant characteristic of some strains and appears atypically in others.

Streptobacillus, *n.* A genus of bacteria whose medical importance derives principally from *Streptobacillus moniliformis.*

Streptobacillus mo·nil·i·for·mis (mo·nil·i·for′mis). The species of *Streptobacillus* that is the etiologic agent of one type of rat-bite fever; namely, Haverhill fever.

strep·to·bi·o·sa·mine (strep″to·bye·o′suh·meen) *n.* A nitrogen-containing disaccharide, $C_{13}H_{23}NO_9$, obtained when streptomycin undergoes acid hydrolysis; in the streptomycin molecule it is glycosidally linked to streptidine.

strep·to·coc·cal (strep″to·kock′ul) *adj.* Pertaining to or due to streptococci.

streptococcal deoxyribonuclease. STREPTODORNASE.

Strep·to·coc·ce·ae (strep″to·kock′see·ee) *n.pl.* The tribe of gram-positive cocci occurring in pairs or in chains which includes the medically important genera *Diplococcus* and *Streptococcus.*

strep·to·coc·ce·mia, strep·to·coc·cae·mia (strep″to·kock·see′mee·uh) *n.* [*streptococcus* + *-emia*]. The presence of streptococci in the blood.

strep·to·coc·ci (strep″to·kock′sigh) *n.*, sing. **streptococ·cus** (·us). Members of the genus *Streptococcus.* The streptococci have been classified into (1) alpha, beta, and gamma by type of reaction of colonies on blood agar (Brown); (2) groups A through O (Lancefield method) by the specific antigenic complex carbohydrates (C-substance) elaborated; (3) hemolytic streptococci, viridans streptococci, enterococci, and *Streptococcus lactis* by their immunologic, biochemical, and physiologic characters.

strep·to·coc·cic (strep″to·kock′sick) *adj.* STREPTOCOCCAL.

Strep·to·coc·cus (strep″to·kock′us) *n.* [*strepto-* + *coccus*]. A genus of gram-positive, chain-forming bacteria of the tribe Streptococceae, family Lactobacteriaceae.

streptococcus. Singular of *streptococci.*

Streptococcus an·gi·no·sus (an·ji·no′sus). A species of minute, mostly β-hemolytic streptococci growing in pairs or short chains; Lancefield groups F and G. Recovered from abscesses and associated with primary atypical pneumonia. Includes strains designated *Streptococcus MG.*

Streptococcus an·he·mo·lyt·i·cus (an·hee·mo·lit′i·kus). GAMMA STREPTOCOCCI.

Streptococcus dys·ga·lac·ti·ae (dis·ga·lack′tee·ee). An α-hemolytic species of Lancefield group C streptococci causing acute mastitis in cows and possibly polyarthritis in lambs.

Streptococcus epi·dem·i·cus (ep″i·dem′i·kus). HEMOLYTIC STREPTOCOCCI.

Streptococcus eq·ui (eck′wye). A β-hemolytic species of Lancefield group C streptococci; causes equine strangles.

Streptococcus eq·ui·sim·i·lis (eck″wi·sim′i·lis). A β-hemolytic species of Lancefield group C similar to *S. equi;* has been recovered from the upper respiratory tract of healthy and diseased humans and animals.

Streptococcus fae·ci·um (fee′see·um). A species similar to *S. faecalis* in distribution and properties, but distinguishable by several criteria, including inability to grow on tellurite media.

Streptococcus fe·ca·lis (fee·kay′lis). Enterococci, characterized by group D polysaccharide, which are normal inhabitants of the intestinal contents of man and animals, and which are of importance as penicillin-resistant pathogens in endocarditis and in genitourinary and wound infections.

Streptococcus lac·tis (lack′tis). A group all the members of which produce Lancefield group N C-substance and are nonpathogenic for man. They readily coagulate milk and are important in the dairy industry.

Streptococcus MG. See *Streptococcus anginosus.*

Streptococcus mu·tans (mew′tanz). An α-hemolytic streptococcal species similar to *S. salivarius;* dextran-producing strains have been implicated in the etiology of dental caries.

Streptococcus pneu·mo·ni·ae (new·mo′nee·ee). A species of gram-positive, capsulated, nonmotile, facultatively aerobic streptococci which occur singly, in pairs, or in short chains in their natural habitat, the upper respiratory tract of man and other mammals. At least 84 serotypes are now known capable of causing such infectious diseases as pneumonia, meningitis, and otitis media. Formerly called *Diplococcus pneumoniae.* Syn. *pneumococcus.*

Streptococcus py·og·e·nes (pye·oj′e·neez). A species of beta-hemolytic streptococci, Lancefield group A, that causes a variety of suppurative diseases including acute pharyngitis, puerperal sepsis, cellulitis, impetigo, and erysipelas. Nonsuppurative diseases caused by this species include acute glomerulo-nephritis, rheumatic fever, and erythema nodosum.

Streptococcus sal·i·va·ri·us (sal·i·vair′ee·us). An α-hemolytic streptococcal species found in the mouth and upper respiratory tract; involved in subacute bacterial endocarditis.

Streptococcus san·guis (sang′gwis). A species of α-hemolytic streptococci of Lancefield group H; a significant constituent of dental plaque and may cause subacute endocarditis.

strep·to·co·ly·sin (strep″to·ko·lye′sin, ·kol′i·sin) *n.* STREPTOLYSIN.

strep·to·dor·nase (strep″to·dor′nace) *n.* An enzyme, occurring in filtrates of cultures of certain hemolytic streptococci, capable of hydrolyzing deoxyribonucleoproteins and deoxyribonucleic acid; used, along with streptokinase, for enzymic debridement of infected tissues. Abbreviated, SD. Syn. *streptococcal deoxyribonuclease.*

strep·to·gen·in (strep″to·jen′in) *n.* STREPOGENIN.

strep·to·he·mol·y·sin (strep″to·hee·mol′i·sin) *n.* STREPTOLYSIN.

strep·to·ki·nase (strep″to·kigh′nace) *n.* A catalytic enzyme, a component of the fibrinolysin occurring in cultures of certain hemolytic streptococci. The enzyme activates the fibrinolytic system present in the euglobulin fraction of human blood. With streptodornase, it is used for enzymic debridement of infected tissues. Abbreviated, SK.

strep·to·ly·sin (strep″to·lye′sin, strep·tol′i·sin) *n.* A group of hemolysins produced by *Streptococcus pyogenes.* Streptolysin O is oxygen-labile and antigenic. Streptolysin S is an oxygen-stable hemolysin, probably not antigenic, and separable from the streptococcal cells by serum extraction.

Strep·to·my·ces (strep″to·migh′seez) *n.* [*strepto-* + *-myces*]. A genus of aerobic nonacid-fast, nonfragmenting organisms with branching filaments 1 μm or less in diameter, occupying a position intermediate between the bacteria and the fungi, that are primarily saprophytic inhabitants of the soil. Some species (*Streptomyces somaliensis, S. madurae, S. pelletierii, S. paraguayensis*) are causes of localized mycetomas, and several others (*S. aureofaciens, S. erythreus*) are sources of antibiotics.

Streptomyces am·bo·fa·ci·ens (am″bo·fay′see·enz). The organism that produces spiramycin and duazomycin.

Streptomyces au·reo·fa·ci·ens (aw″ree·o·fay′see·enz). The organism that produces the antibiotic chlortetracycline.

Streptomyces eryth·re·us (e·rith′ree·us). The organism from which the antibiotic erythromycin is derived.

Streptomyces fra·di·ae (fray′dee·ee). The organism that produces the antibiotic fradicin.

Streptomyces gris·e·us (griz′ee·us). The organism that produces the antibiotic streptomycin.

Streptomyces hal·sted·ii (hal·sted′ee·ee). The organism that produces the antibiotic carbomycin.

Streptomyces la·ven·du·lae (la·ven′dew·lee). The organism that produces the antibiotic streptothricin.

Streptomyces kan·a·my·ce·ti·cus (kan″uh·migh·see′ti·kus). A species of *Streptomyces* used in the production of the antibiotic kanamycin.

Streptomyces lin·coln·en·sis (link″un·en′sis). The organism that produces the antibiotics lincomycin and raninmycin.

Streptomyces niv·e·us (niv′ee·us). The organism that produces the antibiotic novobiocin.

Streptomyces nour·sei (noor′see·eye). The organism that produces the antibiotic nystatin.

Streptomyces ori·en·ta·lis (o″ree·en·tay′lis). The organism that produces the antibiotic vancomycin.

Streptomyces peu·ce·tius (pew·see′shee·us, ·see′shus). A source of daunorubicin.

Streptomyces prim·pri·na (prim′pri·nuh). The organism that produces the antibiotic hamycin.

Streptomyces ri·mo·sus (rye·mo′sus). A source of the antibiotic oxytetracycline.

Streptomyces sphe·roi·des (sfe·roy′deez). *STREPTOMYCES NIVEUS.*

Streptomyces ven·e·zu·e·lae (ven″e·zoo·ee′lee). A source of the antibiotic chloramphenicol.

Streptomyces ver·ti·cil·lus (vur″ti·sil′us). The organism that produces the antineoplastic bleomycin sulfate.

Strep·to·my·ce·ta·ce·ae (strep″to·migh″se·tay′see·ee) *n.pl.* A family of principally soil-inhabiting organisms that form branching filaments not fragmenting into bacillary and coccoid forms, and which includes the genus *Streptomyces* from which many of the antibiotics have been derived.

strep·to·my·cin (strep″to·migh′sin) *n.* A water-soluble antibiotic, $C_{21}H_{39}N_7O_{12}$, obtained from *Streptomyces griseus.* It consists of a hydroxylated base, streptidine, glycosidally linked to the disaccharide-like molecule streptobiosamine. It is active against a variety of organisms, but its principal therapeutic use is in the treatment of tuberculosis. Resistant strains of organisms have appeared. The antibiotic may produce toxic effects, of which those involving the eighth cranial nerve are the most serious. It is administered, usually as the sulfate salt, by intramuscular injection; sometimes it is given intravenously or intrathecally.

strep·to·nic·o·zid (strep″to·nick′o·zid) *n.* Streptomycylidene isonicotinyl hydrazine sulfate, $(C_{27}H_{44}N_{10}O_{12})_2.(H_2SO_4)_3$, an antitubercular compound combining the effects of streptomycin and isoniazid.

strep·to·ni·grin (strep″to·nigh′grin) *n.* An antibiotic, $C_{25}H_{22}N_4O_8$, produced by *Streptomyces flocculus,* that has antineoplastic activity.

strep·to·sep·ti·ce·mia, strep·to·sep·ti·cae·mia (strep″to·sep″ti·see′mee·uh) *n.* Septicemia due to streptococci.

strep·to·so·mus (strep″to·so′mus) *n.* [*strepto-* + *-somus*]. A nonhuman form of celosoma in which the spine is twisted so that the legs are displaced laterally.

strep·to·thri·cin (strep″to·thrye′sin, ·thris′in) *n.* [*Streptothrix* + *-in*]. An antibiotic substance from *Streptomyces lavendulae;* active against various gram-negative and some gram-positive bacteria.

strep·to·thri·co·sis (strep″to·thri·ko′sis) *n. Obsol.* Any disease caused by microorganisms formerly included in the genus *Streptothrix.*

Strep·to·thrix (strep′to·thricks) *n.* [*strepto-* + *-thrix*]. A former genus including *Actinomyces, Streptomyces, Streptobacillus,* and other such microorganisms.

Streptothrix mu·ris rat·ti (mew′ris rat′eye). *STREPTOBACILLUS MONILIFORMIS.*

strep·to·tri·cho·sis (strep″to·tri·ko′sis) *n.* STREPTOTHRICOSIS.

strep·to·zo·cin (strep″to·zo′sin) *n.* 2-Deoxy-2-(3-methyl-3-nitrosoureido)-α(and β)-D-glucopyranose, $C_8H_{15}N_3O_7$, an antibiotic isolated from *Streptomyces achromogenes* that has antineoplastic activity.

strep·to·zot·o·cin (strep″to·zot′uh·sin) *n.* STREPTOZOCIN.

stress, *n.* [OF. *estrece,* narrowness, oppression, from L. *strictus,* tight]. 1. Force exerted by load, pull, pressure, or other mechanical means; also the exertion of such force. 2. *In medicine,* any stimulus or succession of stimuli of such magnitude as to tend to disrupt the homeostasis of the organism; when mechanisms of adjustment fail or become disproportionate or incoordinate, the stress may be considered an injury, resulting in disease, disability, or death. See also *general adaptation syndrome, injury.* 3. *In dentistry,* the force exerted by the lower teeth against the upper during mastication.

stress fracture. FATIGUE FRACTURE.

stress incontinence. Involuntary loss of urine due to activity causing increased intrabdominal pressure.

stress phenomenon. GENERAL ADAPTATION SYNDROME.

stretch, *v. & n.* 1. To draw out to full length. 2. The act of stretching.

stretch·er, *n.* A litter, particularly one mounted on an easily maneuverable carriage with rubber-shod wheels, used in hospitals for transporting patients.

stretch marks. White or gray, shiny, slightly depressed lines on the anterior abdominal wall skin, or that of the breasts or thighs, following prolonged stretching from such causes as pregnancy, ascites, or obesity. Syn. *striae cutis distensae.*

stretch receptor. A receptor that responds to mechanical deformation wholly brought about by the stretching of the tissue in which the receptor is embedded, such as the stretch receptors stimulated by inflation of the lung which, via ascending vagal nerve fibers, reflexly inhibit the respiratory center. See also *Hering-Breuer reflex.*

stretch reflex. Contraction of a muscle in response to sudden brisk longitudinal stretching of the same muscle. Syn. *myotatic reflex.*

stria (strye′uh) *n.,* pl. **stri·ae** (·ee) [L., *furrow*]. 1. A streak, stripe, or narrow band. 2. FIBRINOID (2).

stria dis·ten·sa (dis·ten′suh). Singular of *striae (cutis) distensae;* STRETCH MARK.

striae. Plural of *stria.*

striae acu·sti·cae (a·koos′ti·see). STRIAE MEDULLARES VENTRICULI QUARTI.

striae al·bi·can·tes gra·vi·da·rum (al·bi·kan′teez grav·i·dair′um). Stretch marks (lineae albicantes) due to pregnancy.

striae atro·phi·cae (a·tro′fi·see). STRETCH MARKS.

striae ce·re·bel·la·ris (serr·e·bel·air′is). STRIAE MEDULLARES VENTRICULI QUARTI.

striae cu·tis dis·ten·sae (kew′tis dis·ten′see). STRETCH MARKS.

striae gra·vi·da·rum (grav·i·dair′um). STRIAE ALBICANTES GRAVIDARUM.

striae me·dul·la·res fos·sae rhom·boi·de·ae (med·yoo·lair′eez fos′ee rhom·boy′dee·ee). STRIAE MEDULLARES VENTRICULI QUARTI.

striae medullares ven·tri·cu·li quar·ti (ven·trick′yoo·lye kwahr′tye) [NA]. Strands of white fibers transversely crossing the intermediate portion of the floor of the fourth ventricle.

striae of Baillarger [J. G. F. *Baillarger*]. STRIPES OF BAILLARGER.

striae of Held [H. *Held,* German anatomist, 1866–1922]. STRIAE MEDULLARES VENTRICULI QUARTI.

striae of Monakov [C. von *Monakov*]. STRIAE MEDULLARES VENTRICULI QUARTI.

striae of Piccolomini [A. *Piccolomini*]. STRIAE MEDULLARES VENTRICULI QUARTI.

striae of Retzius [M. G. *Retzius*]. INCREMENTAL LINES OF RETZIUS.

striae trans·ver·sae cor·po·ris cal·lo·si (trans·vur′see kor′po·ris ka·lo′sigh) [BNA]. Transverse bundles of fibers in the upper surface of the corpus callosum.

stria in·ter·me·dia tri·go·ni ol·fac·to·rii (in·tur·mee′dee·uh trye·go′nigh ol·fack·to′ree·eye) [BNA]. An indistinct band extending from the posterior end of the olfactory trigone and anterior perforated substance.

stria Lan·ci·sii (lan·siz′i·eye) [G. M. *Lancisi*]. MEDIAL LONGITUDINAL STRIA.

stria lon·gi·tu·di·na·lis la·te·ra·lis cor·po·ris cal·lo·si (lon·ji·

tew·di·nay'lis lat·e·ray'lis kor'po·ris ka·lo'sigh). [NA]. LATERAL LONGITUDINAL STRIA.

stria longitudinalis me·di·a·lis cor·po·ris cal·lo·si (mee·dee·ay'lis kor'po·ris ka·lo'sigh) [NA]. MEDIAL LONGITUDINAL STRIA.

stria mal·le·a·ris (mal·ee·air'is) [NA]. A band of connective tissue in the tympanic membrane, extending upward from the umbo.

stria mal·le·o·la·ris (mal·ee·o·lair'is) [BNA]. STRIA MALLEARIS.

stria me·di·a·lis tri·go·ni ol·fac·to·rii (mee·dee·ay'lis trye·go'nigh ol·fack·to'ree·eye) [BNA]. The medial posterior end of the olfactory tract which passes medialward.

stria me·dul·la·ris tha·la·mi (med''yoo·lair'is thal'uh·migh) [NA]. A band of white matter on the dorsal surface of the thalamus.

stria of Gennari [F. *Gennari*]. STRIPE OF GENNARI.

stria of Langhans [T. *Langhans*]. The discontinuous zone of fibrinoid on the chorionic plate present during the first half of pregnancy.

stria of Nitabuch [R. *Nitabuch*]. The first fibrinoid to appear in the placenta, located in the decidua basalis and capsularis below the exposed surface at the boundary of the fetal and maternal tissues.

stria of Rohr [K. *Rohr*]. The fibrinoid found on the maternal surface of the intervillous spaces and on the villi.

stria ol·fac·to·ria (ol·fack·to'ree·uh) [NA]. A band of fibers running from the olfactory region toward the insula.

stria olfactoria la·te·ra·lis (lat·e·ray'lis) [BNA]. STRIA OLFACTORIA.

stria se·mi·cir·cu·la·ris (sem·ee·sur·kew·lair'is). STRIA TERMINALIS.

striata. Plural of *striatum.*

stri·a·tal (strye·ay'tul) *adj.* Pertaining to the corpus striatum.

striatal epilepsy. *Obsol.* Brief epileptic attacks consisting of tonic spasms of one or both limbs on one side, once attributed to a discharging focus in the corpus striatum.

stri·ate (strye'ate) *adj.* STRIATED.

striate area. VISUAL PROJECTION AREA.

stri·at·ed (strye'ay·tid) *adj.* [L. *striare,* to furnish with channels]. Striped, as striated muscle.

striated annulet. RINGBINDEN.

striated border. The layer of modified cytoplasm, showing fine, perpendicular striations, found on the surface of the simple columnar intestinal epithelium.

striated epithelium. Epithelium consisting of striated cells.

striated muscle. Muscle characterized by the banding pattern of cross-striated muscle fibers, seen in skeletal and cardiac muscles. Contr. *smooth muscle.* See also *A band, I band.*

stria ter·mi·na·lis (tur·mi·nay'lis) [NA]. A longitudinal bundle of nerve fibers lying in the terminal sulcus of the thalamus. It arises in the corticomedial group of amygdaloid nuclei and terminates mainly in the preoptic region and medial parts of the anterior hypothalamus, although some fibers cross in the anterior commissure to the amygdaloid nucleus of the opposite side.

stri·a·tion (strye·ay'shun) *n.* 1. The state of being striated. 2. STRIA (1).

stri·a·to·ni·gral degeneration (strye''uh·to·nigh'grul, strye·ay''to·). A degenerative disorder involving principally the corpus striatum and substantia nigra, and sometimes the olivopontocerebellar structures, and characterized clinically by parkinsonism and orthostatic hypotension.

stri·a·to·pal·li·dal (strye''uh·to·pal'i·dul, strye·ay''to·) *adj.* Of or pertaining to the corpus striatum and globus pallidus.

stri·a·to·pal·li·do·ni·gral (strye''uh·to·pal''i·do·nigh'grul, strye·ay''to·) *adj.* Pertaining to the corpus striatum, globus pallidus, and substantia nigra.

striatopallidonigral motor system. The basal ganglionic portion of the extrapyramidal motor system.

stri·a·to·tha·lam·ic radiation (strye''uh·to·thuh·lam'ick, strye·ay''to·). THALAMOSTRIATE RADIATION.

stria·tum (strye·ay'tum) *n.*, pl. **stria·ta** (·tuh). CORPUS STRIATUM.

stria vas·cu·la·ris duc·tus co·chle·a·ris (vas·kew·lair'is duck'tus kock·lee·air'is) [NA]. The vascular upper part of the spiral ligament of the ductus cochlearis.

stria vascularis of Huschke [E. *Huschke*]. STRIA VASCULARIS DUCTUS COCHLEARIS.

stric·ture (strik'chur) *n.* [L. *strictura,* from *stringere, strictus,* to bind together]. A circumscribed narrowing of the lumen of a canal or hollow organ, as the esophagus, pylorus, ureter, or urethra, the result of inflammatory or other changes in its walls, and, occasionally, of external pressure. It may be temporary or permanent, depending upon the cause and the course of the disease producing it.

stri·dor (strye'dur) *n.* [L.]. A high-pitched, harsh, vibrating rale.

stridor den·ti·um (den'shee·um). Grinding of the teeth.

stridor ser·rat·i·cus (serr·at'i·kus). A sound like the sharpening of a saw, sometimes produced by expiration through a tracheotomy tube.

strid·u·lous (strid'yoo·lus) *adj.* [L. *stridulus,* from *stridere,* to creak, grate, hiss]. Characterized by stridor, as stridulous laryngismus.

strife rivalry. RETINAL RIVALRY.

string electrometer. An electrometer consisting of a fine conducting string placed between two conducting plates. An electric field between the plates causes the string to be displaced if a potential is applied to it.

strin·gent (strin'junt) *adj.* [L. *stringere,* to bind]. 1. Rigorous; strict. 2. ASTRINGENT (1). 3. Binding; constricting.

string·halt (string'hawlt) *n.* An involuntary, convulsive movement of the muscles in the hind legs of the horse; the leg is suddenly raised from the ground and lowered again with unnatural force. Syn. *springhalt.*

string operation. A procedure designed for relief of esophageal stricture, consisting of periodic dilatation by bougies over a previously swallowed thread.

string phlebitis. MONDOR'S DISEASE.

strio-. A combining form meaning (a) *stria, striated;* (b) *striatal, corpus striatum.*

strio·cel·lu·lar (strye''o·sel'yoo·lur) *adj.* [*strio-* + *cellular*]. Composed of alternating bands of fibers and cells.

strio·cer·e·bel·lar (strye''o·serr''e·bel'ur) *adj.* Pertaining to the corpus striatum and the cerebellum.

strio·ni·gral tract (strye''o·nigh'grul) [*strio-* + *nigral*]. Nerve fibers that arise in the putamen and caudate nucleus and terminate in the substantia nigra, particularly in the pars compacta.

strip, *v.* 1. To press with a milking movement so as to force out the contents of a canal or duct. 2. To remove lengths of varicose saphenous veins, largely by blind subcutaneous tunneling dissection, using a vein stripper.

strip area. Brodmann's area 4S. See *Brodmann's areas.*

stripe, *n.* A streak; a discolored mark. —**striped,** *adj.*

striped muscle. STRIATED MUSCLE.

stripe of Gen·na·ri (jen·nah'ree) [F. *Gennari,* Italian anatomist, 18th century]. A broad band of white substance seen in vertical sections of the cortex of the visual projection area of the occipital lobe. See also *stripes of Baillarger.*

stripes of Baillarger [J. G. F. *Baillarger*]. Two well-defined, white bands in the cerebral cortex, containing large numbers of myelinated nerve fibers running parallel to the surface of the cortex; in the region of the calcarine fissure, the outer band is known as the stripe of Gennari, the inner band being absent. Syn. *lines of Baillarger, striae of Baillarger.*

strip·per, *n.* VEIN STRIPPER.

strip·ping, *n.* 1. Uncovering; unsheathing. 2. Removal, after ligation and division, of lengths of varicose saphenous veins from a lower extremity by blind, blunt dissection. 3. (pl.) The last and richest milk given at any one milking;

so called because it is slowly removed by the milker, who strips the teats between the fingers.

stripping of the pleura. Removal of the lining membrane of the thorax of an animal used for food, to remove the traces of possible pleurisy and of tuberculosis.

strip region. Brodmann's area 4S. See *Brodmann's areas.*

strob·ic (strob'ick) *adj.* [Gk. *strobos,* a whirling around]. Resembling, or pertaining to, a top.

stro·bi·la (stro·bye'luh) *n.,* pl. **strobi·lae** (·lee) [NL., from Gk. *strobilos,* something rolled up or twisted]. 1. The segmented body of the adult tapeworm. 2. The whole adult tapeworm including the scolex.

strob·i·la·tion (strob"i·lay'shun) *n.* The formation of zooids, disks, or joints by metameric division, gemmation, or fission.

strob·ile (strob'il, ·ile, stro'bil) *n.* [Gk. *strobilos,* pinecone]. 1. A multiple fruit whose seeds are enclosed by prominent scales, as a pinecone. 2. STROBILA.

strob·i·loid (strob'i·loid) *adj.* Like a strobile.

strob·i·lus (strob'i·lus) *n.,* pl. **strobi·li** (·lye). The adult tapeworm.

stro·bo·scope (stro'buh·skope, strob'o·) *n.* [Gk. *strobos,* a whirling, + *-scope*]. A device by which a moving object may appear to be at rest; a rapid motion may appear to be slowed, or motion can be depicted by a series of still pictures. The effect depends upon an accurately controlled, intermittent source of light or periodically interrupted vision. —**strobo·scop·ic** (·skop"ick) *adj.*

stro·bo·ster·eo·scope (stro"bo·sterr'ee·uh·skope) *n.* STEREOSTROBOSCOPE.

Stro·ga·nov's method or **treatment** (straw'guh·nuf) [V. V. *Stroganov,* Russian obstetrician, 1857–1938]. Treatment of eclampsia (1) by the injection of morphine and magnesium sulfate.

stroke, *n. Informal.* CEREBROVASCULAR ACCIDENT.

stroke in evolution. PROGRESSIVE STROKE.

stroke syndrome. The sudden, nonconclusive focal neurologic deficit due to cerebrovascular disease.

stroke volume. The volume of blood ejected by the left ventricle during a single systole.

stro·ma (stro'muh) *n.,* pl. **stroma·ta** (·tuh) [Gk. *strōma,* bed]. 1. [NA] The supporting framework of an organ, including its connective tissue, vessels, and nerves, as contrasted with the epithelial or other tissues performing the special function of the organ, the parenchyma. 2. The internal structure of erythrocytes after extraction of hemoglobin.

stroma glandulae thy·roi·de·ae (thigh·roy'dee·ee) [NA]. The connective-tissue framework of the thyroid gland.

stroma iri·dis (eye'ri·dis) [NA]. The connective tissue of the iris.

stro·mal (stro'mul) *adj.* Of or pertaining to the stroma of an organ.

stromal endometriosis. STROMATOSIS.

stromal myosis. STROMATOSIS.

stroma ova·rii (o·vair'ee·eye) [NA]. The fibrous framework of the ovary.

stroma plexus. A nerve plexus derived from the ciliary nerves found in the substantia propria of the cornea.

stro·ma·tin (stro'muh·tin) *n.* The protein of the stroma of erythrocytes.

stro·ma·to·sis (stro"muh·to'sis) *n.* [*stroma* + *-osis*]. The presence throughout the myometrium of collections of tissue similar to the mesenchymal tissue which forms the bulk of the endometrial stroma. Syn. *stromal myosis, stromal endometriosis, endolymphatic stromal myosis.*

stroma vi·tre·um (vit'ree·um) [NA]. VITREOUS STROMA.

stro·muhr (stro'moor) *n.* [Ger., rheometer, from *Strom,* current, flow, + *Uhr,* clock]. An instrument for measuring the velocity of blood flow.

strong ammonia solution. A 28% solution of ammonia in water; used as a reagent.

stronger ammonia water. STRONG AMMONIA SOLUTION.

strong iodine solution. A solution of 50 g iodine and 100 g potassium iodide in distilled water to 1,000 ml; used for systemic effect of iodine. Syn. *Lugol's solution, compound iodine solution.*

strong iodine tincture. A solution of 70 g iodine and 50 g potassium iodide in 50 ml distilled water and alcohol to 1,000 ml; used as a local anti-infective.

strong silver protein. A preparation of protein and silver containing about 8% silver; used for the germicidal effect of silver. Contains less silver than mild silver protein but produces a higher concentration of silver ion than the latter and hence is more irritating. See also *silver protein.*

Stron·gy·loi·dea (stron"ji·loy'dee·uh) *n.pl.* [from *Strongylus,* a genus, from Gk. *strongylos,* round]. A superfamily of roundworms, of the suborder Strongylinae, order Rhabditida. The genera *Ancylostoma* and *Necator* are included.

Stron·gy·loi·des (stron"ji·loy'deez) *n.* [Gk. *strongyloeidēs,* round in form]. A genus of nematode worms.

Strongyloides in·tes·ti·na·lis (in·tes"ti·nay'lis). *STRONGYLOIDES STERCORALIS.*

Strongyloides ster·co·ra·lis (stur"ko·ray'lis). An intestinal parasite of man with the same distribution as hookworm. Other species are parasites of lower animals. Syn. *Strongyloides intestinalis.*

stron·gy·loi·di·a·sis (stron"ji·loy·dye'uh·sis) *n.* [*Strongyloides* + *-iasis*]. Infection of the intestines with a roundworm of the genus *Strongyloides.*

stron·gy·lo·sis (stron"ji·lo'sis) *n.* [*Strongyloides* + *-osis*]. STRONGYLOIDIASIS.

stron·tia (stron'chee·uh, ·tee·uh) *n.* Strontium oxide.

stron·ti·um (stron'chee·um, ·tee·um) *n.* [NL., after *Strontian,* Scotland, where it was first found]. Sr = 87.62. A silver-white to pale yellow, malleable, ductile metal; atomic number 38; decomposes in water and alcohol. Certain salts of strontium, notably the bromide and salicylate, have been used for the therapeutic effect of the anions; these have no advantage over the corresponding sodium salts.

strontium 90. A radioactive isotope of strontium, a product of uranium fission and dangerous because it concentrates in bone, but in the form of a strontium applicator used for the therapeutic effects of its beta radiation. Symbol, ^{90}Sr.

stro·phan·thi·din (stro·fan'thi·din) *n.* A cardioactive, steroidal aglycone, $C_{23}H_{32}O_6$, obtained by hydrolysis of glycosides found in varieties of *Strophanthus* and related plants. Strophanthin and cymarin are two such glycosides that yield strophanthidin.

stro·phan·thin (stro·fan'thin) *n.* A glycoside or a mixture of glycosides obtained from *Strophanthus kombé;* a cardioactive drug that has been used in the treatment of various heart ailments but, because of variation in potency, is no longer employed.

stro·phan·thus (stro·fanth'us) *n.* [NL., from Gk. *strophos,* twisted band, + *anthos,* flower]. The dried ripe seeds of *Strophanthus kombé,* or of *S. hispidus,* deprived of the awns; formerly used like digitalis, as a cardiotonic drug. See also *strophanthin.*

stropho·ceph·a·lus (strof"o·sef'uh·lus) *n.* An individual exhibiting strophocephaly.

stroph·o·ceph·aly (strof"o·sef'uh·lee) *n.* [Gk. *strophē,* a twist, + *-cephaly*]. A form of otocephaly in which there is marked deformity of the lower face, with partial or complete agnathia and synotia, astomia, and severe disturbance in the maxillary, sphenoid, and temporal regions.

stroph·u·lus (strof'yoo·lus) *n.,* pl. **strophu·li** (·lye). A form of miliaria occurring in infants, and often unilateral.

strophulus pru·ri·gi·no·sus (proo·ri·ji·no'sus). PRURIGO.

struck, *n.* An acute enterotoxemia of sheep occurring in England, caused by *Clostridium perfringens,* type C.

struc·tur·al (struck'chur·ul) *n.* Pertaining to, characterized by, or affecting, a structure.

structural emphysema. EMPHYSEMA (1).

structural formula. A formula which shows the arrangement and relation of every atom in a molecule. One in which the symbols are united by the bonds of affinity according to their valence, as H—O—H.

structural gene. A gene whose product is a functional protein in contrast to a regulator of another gene.

structural isomerism. Isomerism involving compounds with the same molecular formulas but distinctly different structures, as butane, $CH_3CH_2CH_2CH_3$, and isobutane, $(CH_3)_3CH$; propylamine, $CH_3CH_2CH_2NH_2$, and trimethylamine, $(CH_3)_3N$.

structural lesion. A lesion in which there is demonstrable morphologic change.

structural psychology. EXISTENTIAL PSYCHOLOGY (1).

structural scoliosis. A deformity in which a series of vertebrae remain constantly deviated from the normal spinal axis and accompanied by some degree of rotation of the vertebrae with corresponding changes in the thoracic cage. Organic and congenital forms are structural, and the functional type may become so.

struc·ture (struck'chur) *n.* [L. *structura*, from *struere*, to erect]. 1. The manner or method of the building up, arrangement, and formation of the different tissues and organs of the body or of a complete organism. 2. An organ, a part, or a complete organic body.

stru·ma (stroo'muh) *n.*, pl. **stru·mae** (·mee) [L., scrofulous tumor]. GOITER.

struma ab·er·ra·ta (ab''uh·ray'tuh). A goiter of an accessory thyroid gland.

struma androblastoma of the ovary. ADRENOCORTICOID ADENOMA OF THE OVARY.

struma ci·bar·ia (si·băr'ee·uh). Goiter due to the ingestion of goitrogens, such as cabbage and rape seed.

struma con·gen·i·ta (kon·jen'i·tuh). A goiter present at birth.

struma lin·gua·lis (ling·gway'lis). The presence of thyroid glandular tissue in the region of the foramen cecum linguae.

struma lym·pho·ma·to·sa (lim''fo·muh·to'suh). Diffuse thyroid enlargement of unknown origin characterized by retrogressive epithelial changes and lymphoid hyperplasia. Syn. *Hashimoto's struma, lymphadenoid goiter.*

struma ma·lig·na (ma·lig'nuh). Follicular carcinoma of the thyroid.

struma med·i·ca·men·to·sa (med''i·kuh·men·to'suh). Goiter due to medicine, as potassium thiocyanate.

struma ova·rii (o·vair'ee·eye). A rare teratoma of the ovary chiefly or entirely composed of thyroid tissue.

struma ovarii lu·te·ino·cel·lu·la·re (lew·tee''i·no·sel''yoo·lair'ee). LUTEOMA.

struma post·bran·chi·a·lis (post·brank·ee·ay'lis). GETSOWA'S ADENOMA.

Stru·mia's universal stain [M. M. *Strumia*, U.S. pathologist, b. 1896]. A mixture of the Giemsa and May-Grünwald stains in 1% aqueous solution of sodium carbonate.

stru·mi·form (stroo'mi·form) *adj.* [*struma* + *-iform*]. Having the appearance of struma; resembling scrofula or goiter.

stru·mi·pri·val (stroo''mi·priv'ul, ·prye'vul, stroo·mip'riv·ul) *adj.* [*struma* + *-prival*]. THYROPRIVAL.

stru·mi·pri·vic (stroo''mi·prye'vick) *adj.* THYROPRIVAL.

stru·mi·pri·vous (stroo''mi·prye'vus) *adj.* THYROPRIVAL.

stru·mi·tis (stroo·migh'tis) *n.* [*struma* + *-itis*]. Inflammation of a goitrous thyroid gland.

stru·mous (stroo'mus) *adj.* [L. *strumosus*, from *struma*]. 1. GOITROUS. 2. SCROFULOUS.

strumous arthritis. FUNGOUS ARTHRITIS.

strumous ophthalmia. PHLYCTENULAR KERATOCONJUNCTIVITIS.

Strüm·pell-Ma·rie disease (shtru^{e}m'pul, ma·ree') [E. A. G. G. *Strümpell*, German neurologist, 1853–1925; and P. *Marie*]. ANKYLOSING SPONDYLITIS.

Strümpell's sign or **reflex** [E. A. G. G. *Strümpell*]. In a leg showing spastic paralysis, flexion of the thigh results in marked dorsiflexion of the foot. Syn. *tibialis sign.*

Strümpell-West·phal pseudosclerosis [E. A. G. G. *Strümpell* and C. F. O. *Westphal*]. HEPATOLENTICULAR DEGENERATION.

strych·nia (strick'nee·uh) *n.* STRYCHNINE.

strych·nine (strick'nin, ·nine, ·neen) *n.* [F., from Gk. *strychnos*, a kind of nightshade]. An alkaloid, $C_{21}H_{22}N_2O_2$, obtained chiefly from nux vomica; formerly used for central nervous system stimulation in a variety of ailments but of little, if any, therapeutic merit. Various salts were employed.

strych·nin·iza·tion (strick''ni·ni·zay'shun) *n.* 1. The condition produced by large doses of strychnine or nux vomica. 2. Topical application of strychnine to areas of the central nervous system to increase nervous excitability and thus facilitate the study of neuron connections. See also *physiological neuronography.*

Strych·nos (strick'nos) *n.* [Gk., nightshade]. A genus of the Loganiaceae, which includes *Strychnos nux-vomica*, the source of nux vomica.

S.T.S. Serologic test for syphilis.

S-T segment. The interval of the electrocardiogram between the end of the QRS complex and the beginning of the T wave; usually isoelectric. Syn. *R(S)-T segment.*

ST-T wave. The portion of the electrocardiogram that includes the S-T segment and the T-wave.

S.T.U. Skin test unit.

Stu·art factor [*Stuart*, a patient in whom factor X deficiency was first found]. FACTOR X.

Stuart-Prow·er factor [*Stuart* and *Prower*, early patients in whom factor X deficiency was found]. FACTOR X.

stu·dent nurse. A person partaking in some type of nurse training.

study cast. A positive replica of the mouth and teeth used for diagnosis and treatment planning.

stuf·fy nose syndrome. ACUTE RHINITIS OF NEWBORN.

stul·ti·tia (stul·tish'ee·uh) *n.* [L., from *stultus*, foolish]. Foolishness; dullness of intellect.

stump, *n.* The extremity, pedicle, or basis of the part left after surgical amputation, excision, or ablation.

stump neuroma. AMPUTATION NEUROMA.

stump-tailed macaque. A large, shaggy, pink- or red-faced monkey, *Macaca speciosa* (or *M. arctoides*), inhabiting southern China and parts of Southeast Asia.

stun, *v.* [OF. *estoner*]. To render temporarily insensible, as by a blow.

stunt, *v.* To arrest the normal growth and development of an organism. See also *dwarf.*

stu·pe·fa·cient (stew''pe·fay'shunt) *n. & adj.* [L. *stupefacere*, to make senseless]. NARCOTIC.

stu·pe·fac·tion (stew''pe·fack'shun) *n.* 1. STUPOR (1). 2. The process of succumbing to stupor. —**stu·pe·fy** (stew'pe·fye) *v.*

stu·pe·ma·nia (stew''pe·may'nee·uh) *n.* [L. *stupere*, to be struck senseless, + *-mania*]. Mental stupor.

stu·por (stew'pur) *n.* [L.]. 1. A state of depressed consciousness in which mental and physical activity are reduced to a minimum and from which one can be aroused only by vigorous and repeated stimuli, at which time response to spoken commands is either absent or slow and inadequate. 2. *In psychiatry*, a state in which impressions of the external environment are normally received but activity is suspended or marked by negativism, as in catatonic schizophrenia. —**stupor·ous** (·us) *adj.*

stupor me·lan·chol·i·cus (mel''un·kol'i·kus). The stupor associated with a depression.

stuporous insanity. Stupor with immobility.

stupor vig·i·lans (vij'i·lanz). CATALEPSY.

stur·dy (stur'dee) *n.* STAGGERS.

Sturge-Weber disease or **syndrome** [W. A. *Sturge*, English physician, 1850–1919; and F. P. *Weber*]. A form of neurocutaneous dysplasia defined by the presence of a port-wine nevus of the upper part of the face or scalp and leptomeningeal angiomatosis. Rarely, both sides of the face and cortex may be involved and there may be cutaneous angiomatosis of other parts of the body, as well as buphthalmos, seizures, hemianopsia, hemiparesis, and mental retardation. Syn. *encephalofacial angiomatosis.*

Sturm·dorf's operation [A. *Sturmdorf,* U.S. gynecologist, 1861–1934]. Removal of diseased endocervix by conical excision.

stut·ter, *n. & v.* 1. Speech marked by the intermittent inability to enunciate a phonetic segment not more than one syllable in length without repeating it, straining unnaturally, or doing both. 2. To speak in such a manner. Compare *stammer.* **—stutter·er** (·ur) *n.*

stutter spasm. Spasm of the lingual and palatal muscles, psychogenic in origin, resulting in stuttering speech.

Stutt·gart disease. An infectious disease of dogs caused by *Leptospira canicola.*

sty, stye, *n.,* pl. **sties, styes** [OE. *stīgend,* from *stīgan,* to rise]. HORDEOLUM.

styl-, stylo-. A combining form signifying *styloid process of the temporal bone.*

sty·let (stye'lit) *n.* [F., from It. *stiletto,* stiletto, dagger]. 1. A wire inserted into a soft catheter or cannula to insure rigidity. 2. A fine wire inserted into a hollow hypodermic needle or other hollow needle to maintain patency.

sty·lo·glos·sus (stye''lo·glos'us) *n.* A muscle arising from the styloid process of the temporal bone, and inserted into the tongue. NA *musculus styloglossus.* See also Table of Muscles in the Appendix. **—styloglos·sal** (·ul) *adj.*

sty·lo·hy·oid (stye''lo·high'oid) *adj.* Pertaining to the styloid process of the temporal bone and the hyoid bone.

stylohyoid ligament. A fibrous cord attached to the tip of the styloid process of the temporal bone and the lesser horn of the hyoid bone, derived from Reichert's cartilage. NA *ligamentum stylohyoideum.*

stylohyoid muscle. A muscle arising in the stylohyoid process of the temporal bone and inserted into the hyoid bone. NA *musculus stylohyoideus.* See also Table of Muscles in the Appendix.

sty·loid (stye'loid) *adj.* [Gk. *styloeidēs,* like a stylus]. Having one end slender and pointed.

styloid process of the fibula. APEX OF THE HEAD OF THE FIBULA.

styloid process of the radius. A projection from the lateral border of the lower extremity of the radius. NA *processus styloideus ossis radii.*

styloid process of the temporal bone. A sharp spine about an inch in length, descending downward, forward, and inward from the inferior surface of the petrous portion of the temporal bone. NA *processus styloideus ossis temporalis.* See also Plates 1, 20.

styloid process of the third metacarpal. A projection from the lateral side of the base of the third metacarpal. NA *processus styloideus ossis metacarpalis III.*

styloid process of the ulna. A projection from the inner and posterior portion of the lower extremity of the ulna. NA *processus styloideus ulnae.*

sty·lo·man·dib·u·lar (stye''lo·man·dib'yoo·lur) *adj.* Pertaining to the styloid process of the temporal bone and the mandible.

stylomandibular ligament. A thickened band of the cervical fascia passing from the apex of the styloid process of the temporal bone to the angle of the mandible, separating the parotid and submandibular glands. NA *ligamentum stylomandibulare.*

sty·lo·mas·toid (stye''lo·mas'toid) *adj.* Pertaining to the styloid and the mastoid processes of the temporal bone.

stylomastoid foramen. A foramen between the styloid and mastoid processes of the temporal bone; the external aperture of the facial canal. NA *foramen stylomastoideum.*

sty·lo·pha·ryn·ge·us (stye''lo·fa·rin'jee·us) *n.* A muscle arising from the styloid process of the temporal bone, and inserted into the pharynx. NA *musculus stylopharyngeus.* See also Table of Muscles in the Appendix.

sty·lus (stye'lus) *n.* [L. *stilus*]. 1. A pointed device for writing; especially one used with such electrical apparatus as an electrocardiograph or an electroencephalograph. 2. A stylet. 3. A pointed device in the form of a holder for applying medicines, especially caustic ones.

sty·ma·to·sis (stye''muh·to'sis) *n.* [Gk. *styma, stymatos,* priapism, + *-osis*]. A violent erection of the penis attended with hemorrhage.

styp·tic (stip'tick) *adj. & n.* [Gk. *styptikos,* astringent, from *styphein,* to contract]. 1. Having the effect of checking hemorrhage. 2. An agent that checks hemorrhage by causing contraction of the blood vessels, as alum, tannic acid.

sty·ra·mate (stye'ruh·mate) *n.* 2-Hydroxy-2-phenylethyl carbamate, $C_9H_{10}NO_3$, a skeletal muscle relaxant used as an adjunct to reduce spasm in various musculoskeletal disorders.

sty·rene (stye'reen) *n.* Phenylethylene, $C_6H_5CH{=}CH_2$, a liquid hydrocarbon found in storax. Syn. *styrol, cinnamene.*

sty·rol (stye'rol) *n.* STYRENE.

sub- [L., under]. A prefix meaning (a) *under, beneath;* (b) *less than, below;* (c) *just short of, immediately underlying;* (d) *partial, slight, mild;* (e) *subordinate, subsidiary;* (f) in chemistry, *basic;* (g) *containing less of a given radical than another compound of the same elements.*

sub·ab·dom·i·nal (sub''ab·dom'i·nul) *adj.* [*sub-* + *abdominal*]. Beneath the abdomen.

sub·ac·e·tate (sub·as'e·tate) *n.* A basic acetate, as lead subacetate.

sub·acro·mi·al (sub''uh·kro'mee·ul) *adj.* [*sub-* + *acromial*]. Beneath the acromion.

subacromial bursa. A bursa lying beneath the acromion and coracoacromial ligament, separating them from the capsule of the shoulder joint; often continuous with the subdeltoid bursa. NA *bursa subacromialis.*

sub·acute (sub''uh·kewt') *adj.* 1. Somewhat less than acute in severity. 2. Of a disease, intermediate in character between acute and chronic.

subacute appendicitis. Mild acute appendicitis.

subacute bacterial endocarditis. BACTERIAL ENDOCARDITIS.

subacute combined degeneration of the spinal cord. Combined degeneration of posterior and lateral columns of the spinal cord due to deficiency of vitamin B_{12}; the neurological component of pernicious anemia.

subacute combined sclerosis. SUBACUTE COMBINED DEGENERATION OF THE SPINAL CORD.

subacute combined system disease. SUBACUTE COMBINED DEGENERATION OF THE SPINAL CORD.

subacute inclusion body encephalitis. SUBACUTE SCLEROSING PANENCEPHALITIS.

subacute myoclonic spinal neuronitis. A rare disorder characterized clinically by tonic rigidity and intermittent myoclonic jerking and painful spasms of the trunk and limb muscles and pathologically by widespread neuronal loss in the spinal cord, with relative sparing of the anterior horn cells.

subacute necrotizing encephalomyelopathy or **encephalomyelitis.** A heredodegenerative disease of the central nervous system, usually beginning in the early months of life and characterized clinically by poor sucking, anorexia, hypotonia with depressed or absent tendon reflexes, pupillary and ocular disturbances, and arrested development with rapid deterioration; chronic lactic acidosis is usually present. Histopathologic findings resemble those of Wernicke's encephalopathy; may be due to a factor inhibiting the synthesis of thiamine triphosphate, but not exogenous thiamine deficiency. Syn. *Leigh's disease.*

subacute necrotizing myelopathy. A rare disease of unknown cause and pathogenesis, characterized clinically by an ascending reflex and sensory loss and motor impairment progressing from spasticity to flaccidity; characterized pathologically by necrosis of both white and gray matter of the spinal cord. Syn. *Foix-Alajouanine syndrome.*

subacute sclerosing leukoencephalitis. SUBACUTE SCLEROSING PANENCEPHALITIS.

subacute sclerosing panencephalitis. Diffuse inflammation of the brain affecting chiefly children and associated with inclusion bodies in neuronal nuclei or cytoplasm, pursuing an indolent course of months or years, with occasional partial remissions; personality changes, seizures, blindness, and progressive dementia terminate in a febrile, decerebrate state. Now linked etiologically to slow infection with measles virus.

subacute spongiform encephalopathy. A distinctive cerebral disease, in which a profound and rapidly progressive dementia is associated with ataxia and myoclonic jerks. The neuropathologic changes consist of widespread neuronal loss and gliosis accompanied by a striking vacuolation or spongy state in the cerebral and cerebellar cortices. Like kuru, subacute spongiform encephalopathy is due to a transmissible agent, possibly a virus. See also *Creutzfeldt-Jakob disease.*

subacute yellow atrophy. POSTNECROTIC CIRRHOSIS.

sub·ag·glu·ti·nat·ing (sub″uh·gloo′ti·nay·ting) *adj.* Of a concentration of antibody: capable of attaching to a cell or particle surface but insufficient to cause agglutination.

sub·al·i·men·ta·tion (sub·al″i·men·tay′shun) *n.* [*sub-* + *alimentation*]. Inadequate or deficient nourishment.

sub·an·co·ne·us (sub·ang″ko·nee′us, ·ang·ko′nee·us) *n.* [NL., from Gk. *ankōn,* elbow]. A variable muscle arising from the posterior distal surface of the humerus and inserted into the posterior aspect of the capsule of the elbow joint.

sub·aor·tic stenosis (sub·ay·or′tick). Narrowing of the left ventricular outflow tract immediately proximal to the orifice of the aortic valve; it may be localized or diffuse, membranous or muscular. Syn. *subvalvular aortic stenosis.* See also *idiopathic hypertrophic subaortic stenosis.*

sub·ap·i·cal (sub·ap′i·kul, ·ay′pi·kul) *adj.* [*sub-* + *apical*]. Beneath an apex.

sub·ap·o·neu·rot·ic (sub·ap″o·new·rot′ick) *adj.* [*sub-* + *aponeurotic*]. Beneath an aponeurosis.

sub·aque·ous (sub·ay′kwee·us, ·ack′wee·us) *adj.* [*sub-* + L. *aqua*, water, + *-ous*]. Occurring beneath water.

sub·arach·noid (sub″uh·rack′noid) *adj.* Beneath the arachnoid.

subarachnoid anesthesia. The state of conduction nerve block produced by the deposition of a local anesthetic agent in suitable mixture into the cerebrospinal fluid of the vertebral canal. The anesthetic acts upon contact with, and depolarization of, the sensorimotor and vasomotor axons. Syn. *spinal and intrathecal anesthesia.*

subarachnoid block. A condition in which an obstruction in the subarachnoid space prevents the normal flow of cerebrospinal fluid.

subarachnoid fluid. CEREBROSPINAL FLUID.

subarachnoid hemorrhage. 1. Blood in the subarachnoid space from any cause. 2. SPONTANEOUS SUBARACHNOID HEMORRHAGE.

subarachnoid septum. A partition formed by bands of fibroelastic tissue attaching the spinal arachnoid to the pia mater along the dorsal midline.

subarachnoid space. The space between the arachnoid and the pia mater, containing subarachnoid trabeculae and filled with cerebrospinal fluid. NA *cavum subarachnoideale.*

sub·ar·cu·ate (sub·ahr′kew·ate) *adj.* [*sub-* + *arcuate*]. Slightly arched or curved.

subarcuate fossa. An orifice situated in the newborn on the superior margin of the petrous portion of the temporal bone, through which the vessels pass to the temporal bone. This opening disappears after birth and is represented in the adult by a depression beneath the arcuate eminence. NA *fossa subarcuata.*

subarcuate hiatus. A depression on the petrous portion of the temporal bone lodging the flocculus.

sub·are·o·lar (sub″a·ree′o·lur) *adj.* [*sub-* + *areolar*]. Situated, or occurring, beneath the mammary areola.

subareolar abscess. An abscess beneath the pigmented epithelium of the nipple, sometimes draining through the nipple.

sub·as·trag·a·lar (sub″as·trag′a·lur) *adj.* Below the talus.

sub·as·trin·gent (sub″uh·strin′junt) *adj.* [*sub-* + *astringent*]. Only slightly astringent.

sub·atom·ic (sub″uh·tom′ick) *adj.* [*sub-* + *atomic*]. Pertaining to the structure or components of atoms.

sub·au·di·tion (sub″aw·dish′un) *n.* [L. *subauditio,* from *subaudire,* to understand something implied, from *sub-* + *audire,* to hear]. The act or ability of mentally supplying words or ideas not expressed.

sub·au·ral (sub·aw′rul) *adj.* SUBAURICULAR.

sub·au·ric·u·lar (sub″aw·rick′yoo·lur) *adj.* [*sub-* + *auricular*]. Below the auricle or external ear.

sub·au·ric·u·lar fossa (sub″aw·rick′yoo·lur). The depression just below the external ear.

sub·ax·il·lary (sub·ack′si·lerr″ee) *adj.* [*sub-* + *axillary*]. Under the armpit.

sub·brachy·ce·phal·ic (sub·brack″ee·se·fal′ick) *adj.* [*sub-* + *brachycephalic*]. 1. *In craniometry,* once used to characterize the mild degree of brachycephaly embracing cephalic indexes between 80.00 and 83.32. 2. *In cephalometry,* characterizing indexes between 82.01 and 85.33.

sub·cal·car·e·ous (sub″kal·kair′ee·us) *adj.* Somewhat calcareous.

sub·cal·ca·rine (sub·kal′kuh·rine, ·reen) *adj.* Situated beneath the calcarine sulcus.

subcalcarine gyrus. A narrow convolution ventral to the cuneus and lying between the collateral and calcarine sulci.

sub·cal·lo·sal (sub″ka·lo′sul) *adj.* [*sub-* + *callosal*]. Below the corpus callosum.

subcallosal area. PAROLFACTORY AREA.

subcallosal fasciculus. A tract of long association fibers lying under the corpus callosum and connecting the frontal, parietal, and occipital lobes. NA *fasciculus subcallosus.*

subcallosal gyrus. GYRUS PARATERMINALIS.

sub·cap·su·lar (sub·kap′sue·lur) *adj.* [*sub-* + *capsular*]. Beneath a capsule.

subcapsular epithelium. The epithelium-like lining of the internal surface of the capsule of the nerve cells of spinal ganglions; satellite cells.

subcapsular sinus. A lymph sinus between the capsule and the cortex of a lymph node.

sub·car·bon·ate (sub·kahr′buh·nate, ·nut) *n.* A basic carbonate.

sub·car·di·nal veins (sub·kahr′di·nul). Paired longitudinal veins of the embryo partly replacing the postcardinals; the prerenal part of the inferior vena cava develops largely from the right subcardinal.

sub·cer·vi·cal (sub·sur′vi·kul) *adj.* [*sub-* + *cervical*]. Beneath a neck.

sub·cer·vi·cal gland (sub·sur′vi·kul). One of a group of small subsidiary prostatic glands that lie beneath the neck of the urinary bladder. Syn. *Albarrán's gland.*

sub·chlo·ride (sub·klo′ride) *n.* The chloride of a series which contains relatively the least chlorine.

sub·chon·dral (sub·kon′drul) *adj.* [*sub-* + *chondral*]. Situated beneath cartilage.

sub·cho·ri·al (sub·ko′ree·ul) *adj.* [*sub-* + *chorial*]. SUBCHORIONIC.

subchorial closing ring. The remnant of the cytotrophoblast of the chorionic plate found between Langhans' stria and the chorionic connective tissue. Once incorrectly called the decidua subchorialis.

subchorial tuberous hematoma of the decidua. BREUS'S MOLE.

sub·cho·ri·on·ic (sub·ko″ree·on′ick) *adj.* Beneath the chorion.

sub·cho·roi·dal (sub″ko·roy′dul) *adj.* Beneath the choroid membrane of the eye.

sub·chron·ic (sub·kron′ick) *adj.* More nearly chronic than subacute.

sub·class (sub′klass) *n.* 1. The taxonomic category falling just below a class. 2. Subset; a division of a set or group.

sub·cla·vi·an (sub·klay′vee·un) *adj.* [*sub-* + *clav*icle + *-an*]. Lying under the clavicle, as the subclavian artery.

subclavian artery. NA *arteria subclavia.* See Table of Arteries in the Appendix.

subclavian plexus. A nerve plexus found about the subclavian artery. NA *plexus subclavius.*

subclavian steal syndrome. A vascular syndrome due to occlusion of the subclavian artery proximal to the origin of the vertebral artery, with reversal of the normal blood pressure gradient in the vertebral artery and decreased blood flow distal to the occlusion, manifested by pain in the mastoid and posterior head regions, episodes of flaccid paralysis of the arm, and diminished or absent radial pulse on the side involved. See also *steal syndrome.*

subclavian sulcus. A shallow groove on the upper surface of the first rib, lodging the subclavian artery. NA *sulcus arteriae subclaviae.*

subclavian triangle. An area bounded above by the inferior belly of the omohyoid, below by the clavicle, and in front by the posterior border of the sternocleidomastoid.

subclavian trunk. One of two collecting lymph vessels draining the upper extremities. The one on the right empties into the right lymphatic duct, or directly into the right subclavian vein; the one on the left empties into the thoracic duct. NA *truncus subclavius.*

sub·cla·vi·us (sub·klay′vee·us) *n.* A small muscle attached to the clavicle and the first rib. NA *musculus subclavius.* See also Table of Muscles in the Appendix.

subclavius posterior. A variant of the subclavius.

sub·clin·i·cal (sub·klin′i·kul) *adj.* [*sub-* + *clinical*]. Pertaining to a disease in which manifestations are so slight as to be unnoticeable or even not demonstrable.

sub·cli·noid (sub·klye′noid) *adj.* [*sub-* + *clinoid*]. Beneath a clinoid process.

sub·cli·noid aneurysm. INTRACAVERNOUS ANEURYSM.

sub·col·lat·er·al (sub″kuh·lat′ur·ul) *adj.* Ventral to the collateral sulcus of the brain.

sub·co·ma insulin therapy or **treatment** (sub″ko′muh). A form of psychiatric therapy by the injection of insulin in which drowsiness or stupor short of coma is produced. Compare *insulin shock therapy.*

sub·con·junc·ti·val (sub″kon·junk·tye′vul) *adj.* [*sub-* + *conjunctival*]. Situated beneath the conjunctiva.

sub·con·scious (sub·kon′shus) *n.* & *adj.* [*sub-* + *conscious*]. 1. *In psychiatry,* mental material outside the range of clear consciousness, including the preconscious which can be recalled with effort as well as the unconscious, which is nevertheless capable of determining conscious mental or physical reactions. 2. Of, pertaining, or belonging to such mental material.

subconscious memory. CRYPTOMNESIA.

sub·con·scious·ness (sub·kon′shus·nus) *n.* A state or condition in which mental processes take place without the mind being distinctly conscious of its own activity.

sub·con·tin·u·ous (sub″kun·tin′yoo·us) *adj.* Almost continuous.

sub·cor·a·coid (sub·kor′uh·koid) *adj.* Situated below the coracoid process, as subcoracoid dislocation of the humerus.

subcoracoid-pectoralis minor syndrome. WRIGHT'S SYNDROME.

sub·cor·ne·al (sub″kor′nee·ul) *adj.* [*sub-* + *corne*um + *-al*]. Beneath the horny layer of the skin.

sub·cor·ti·cal (sub·kor′ti·kul) *adj.* [*sub-* + *cortical*]. 1. Beneath a cortex. 2. Beneath the cerebral cortex.

subcortical motor aphasia. A form of motor aphasia characterized by a pure loss of spoken speech but with preservation of inner speech and the retained ability to write; pure word mutism.

sub·cos·tal (sub·kos′tul) *adj.* [*sub-* + *costal*]. Lying beneath a rib or the ribs. See also *subcostals.*

subcostal angle. COSTAL ANGLE.

sub·cos·tal·gia (sub″kos·tal′jee·uh) *n.* [*subcost*al + *-algia*]. Pain beneath the ribs, or over a subcostal nerve.

subcostal groove. COSTAL SULCUS.

subcostal line. An imaginary transverse line drawn across the abdomen at the level of the lower border of the tenth costal cartilage.

subcostal nerve. NA *nervus subcostalis.* See Table of Nerves in the Appendix.

subcostal plane. A horizontal plane passing through the lowest points of the costal arch or the lowest points of the tenth costal cartilages. This plane usually lies at the level of the third lumbar vertebra.

subcostals, *n.pl.* Certain variable small muscles associated with the lower ribs. NA *musculi subcostales.* See also Table of Muscles in the Appendix.

sub·crep·i·tant (sub·krep′i·tunt) *adj.* Almost or faintly crepitant.

subcrepitant rale. A fine moist crackling sound similar to a crepitant rale, but coarser and lower pitched. Syn. *crackling rale.*

sub·crep·i·ta·tion (sub·krep″i·tay′shun) *n.* [*sub-* + *crepitation*]. An indistinctly crepitant sound.

sub·cru·re·us (sub·kroo′ree·us) *n.* [*sub-* + *crureus*]. ARTICULARIS GENUS.

sub·cul·ture (sub′kul″chur) *n.* 1. *In microbiology,* the procedure of transferring organisms from one culture to fresh culture medium; also, the resulting culture. 2. *In anthropology and sociology,* the culture that is characteristic of a particular subgroup (community, class, ethnic group, age group, etc.) of a society.

sub·cu·ta·ne·ous (sub″kew·tay′nee·us) *adj.* [*sub-* + *cutaneous*]. Beneath the skin; HYPODERMIC.

subcutaneous acromial bursa. A bursa lying over the acromion, between it and the skin.

subcutaneous emphysema. The accumulation of air or gas in the subcutaneous tissues.

subcutaneous inguinal ring. SUPERFICIAL INGUINAL RING.

subcutaneous necrosis of the newborn. ADIPONECROSIS NEONATORUM.

subcutaneous osteotomy. Osteotomy, usually by Macewen's technique, in which a small incision is made in the skin over the bony area to be divided, the bone itself being unexposed, and the operation completed by the sense of touch.

subcutaneous prepatellar bursa. A bursa situated anterior to the patella between the skin and the fascia lata. NA *bursa subcutanea prepatellaris.*

subcutaneous tissue. The layer of loose connective tissue under the dermis. NA *tela subcutanea.*

sub·cu·tic·u·lar (sub″kew·tick′yoo·lur) *adj.* [*sub-* + *cuticular*]. Beneath the epidermis.

subcuticular suture. A buried, continuous suture in which the needle is passed horizontally into and out of the true skin on each side until the wound is closed. Visible suture scars are thus avoided.

sub·cu·tis (sub·kew′tis) *n.* The superficial fascia below the skin or cutis.

sub·de·lir·ium (sub″de·lirr′ee·um) *n.* A slight or muttering delirium, with lucid intervals.

sub·del·toid (sub·del′toid) *adj.* Beneath the deltoid muscle.

subdeltoid bursa. A bursa lying beneath the deltoid muscle, separating it from the capsule of the shoulder joint. NA *bursa subdeltoidea.* See also *subacromial bursa.*

sub·der·mal (sub·dur′mul) *adj.* [*sub-* + *dermal*]. HYPODERMIC (1, 2).

sub·der·mic (sub·dur′mick) *adj.* [*sub-* + *dermic*]. HYPODERMIC (1, 2).

sub·di·a·phrag·mat·ic (sub″dye″uh·frag·mat′ick) *adj.* [*sub-* + *diaphragmatic*]. Under the diaphragm.

subdiaphragmatic abscess. An abscess situated below the diaphragm and above the dome of the liver.

sub·di·vid·ed (sub″di·vye′did) *adj.* Redivided; making secondary or smaller divisions.

sub·dol·i·cho·ce·phal·ic (sub·dol″i·ko·se·fal′ick) *adj.* [*sub-* + *dolichocephalic*]. 1. *In craniometry,* once used to characterize the lower range of the mesocephalic group, with cephalic indexes between 75.00 and 77.76. 2. *In cephalometry,* characterizing indexes between 77.01 and 79.77.

sub·duct (sub·dukt′) *v.* [L. *subducere, subductus,* to withdraw]. To draw downward.

sub·du·ral (sub·dew′rul) *adj.* [*sub-* + *dura* + *-al*]. Beneath the dura mater.

subdural hematoma. A collection of blood between the dura mater and the arachnoid, involving one or both hemispheres, usually due to head trauma, but also seen in blood dyscrasias and cachexia; classified as neonatal, acute, subacute, or chronic according to time of occurrence and the duration of the symptoms and signs, which vary with the age of the patient and extent of neurologic involvement, but which usually include depression of consciousness, seizures, and focal neurologic deficits such as hemiplegia.

subdural hemorrhage. Hemorrhage between the dura mater and the pia arachnoid. It usually results from injury to the meningeal vessels on the inner side of the dura mater. See also *subdural hematoma.*

subdural space. The space between the dura mater and the arachnoid which usually contains only a capillary layer of fluid.

sub·du·ro·peri·to·ne·al shunt (sub·dew″ro·perr″i·to·nee′ul). Surgical communication between the subdural space and the peritoneal cavity by means of a plastic or rubber tube for the relief of subdural effusion.

sub·du·ro·pleu·ral shunt (sub·dew″ro·ploo′rul). Surgical communication between the subdural space and the pleural cavity by means of a plastic or rubber tube for the relief of subdural effusion.

sub·en·do·car·di·al (sub″en″do·kahr′dee·ul) *adj.* [*sub-* + *endocardial*]. Beneath the endocardium or between the endocardium and myocardium.

subendocardial fibroelastosis. ENDOCARDIAL FIBROELASTOSIS.

subendocardial layer. A layer of loose connective tissue binding the endocardium and myocardium together.

subendocardial sclerosis. ENDOCARDIAL FIBROELASTOSIS.

sub·en·do·the·li·al (sub″en″do·theel′ee·ul) *adj.* [*sub-* + *endothelial*]. Underneath the endothelium.

subendothelial coat. The connective-tissue layer of the tunica intima of the heart and vessels.

subendothelial layer. The middle layer of the tunica intima of veins and of medium and larger arteries, consisting of collagenous and elastic fibers and a few fibroblasts.

sub·en·er·get·ic phonation (sub″en″ur·jet′ick). HYPOPHONIA.

sub·ep·en·dy·mal (sub″ep·en′di·mul) *adj.* Under the ependyma.

subependymal astrocytoma. SUBEPENDYMOMA.

subependymal glomerate astrocytoma. SUBEPENDYMOMA.

sub·ep·en·dy·mo·ma (sub″e·pen″di·mo′muh) *n.* [*sub-* + *ependyma* + *-oma*]. A tumor usually found in the fourth ventricle of the brain, sometimes in relation to other ventricles, and often discovered accidentally at autopsy, due to proliferation of fibrillary subependymal astrocytes.

sub·epi·der·mal (sub″ep″i·dur′mul) *adj.* Beneath the epidermis.

sub·epiph·y·se·al (sub″ep·i·fiz′ee·ul, ·e·pif″i·see′ul) *adj.* [*sub-* + *epiphyseal*]. In the part of a diaphysis next to the epiphysis.

sub·ep·i·the·li·al (sub″ep·i·theel′ee·ul) *adj.* [*sub-* + *epithelial*]. Under the epithelium.

subepithelial plexus. A nerve plexus found beneath the epithelial cells of the cornea; a continuation of the stroma plexus.

su·ber·in (sew′bur·in) *n.* [L. *suber,* cork, + *-in*]. A waxy substance found in the cork cells of plants.

su·ber·o·sis (sue″bur·o′sis) *n.* [L. *suber,* cork, + *-osis*]. A form of pneumoconiosis affecting cork workers, characterized by bronchial asthma or disordered gas exchange in the alveoli.

sub·fal·ci·al (sub·fal′see·ul) *adj.* Beneath the falx cerebri.

subfalcial herniation. A dislocation of the brain beneath the arch of the falx cerebri due to increased pressure.

sub·fam·i·ly, *n.* A taxonomic category falling just below a family.

sub·fas·cial (sub·fash′ee·ul) *adj.* [*sub-* + *fascial*]. Beneath fascia.

subfascial abscess. An abscess beneath a fascia. Syn. *postfascial abscess.*

subfascial prepatellar bursa. A bursa situated anterior to the patella between the fascia lata and the tendon of the quadriceps femoris muscle. NA *bursa subfascialis prepatellaris.*

sub·ga·le·al (sub·gay′lee·ul, ·gal′ee·ul) *adj.* [*sub-* + *galea* + *-al*]. Beneath the galea aponeurotica.

sub·gal·late (sub·gal′ate) *n.* A basic salt of gallic acid.

sub·ger·mi·nal (sub·jur′mi·nul) *adj.* [*sub-* + *germinal*]. Situated beneath a germinal structure or blastoderm.

subgerminal cavity. The enlarged blastocoele of meroblastic ova lying between yolk and blastoderm.

sub·gin·gi·val (sub·jin′ji·vul, ·jin·jye′vul) *adj.* [*sub-* + *gingival*]. Beneath the gingiva.

subgingival calculus. A concretion deposited on the surface of a tooth below the level of the gingival margin.

sub·glan·du·lar (sub·glan′dew·lar) *adj.* Below, or on the inferior aspect of, the glans penis.

subglandular hypospadias. BALANIC HYPOSPADIAS.

sub·gle·noid (sub·glee′noid, ·glen′oid) *adj.* Beneath the glenoid cavity of the scapula, as subglenoid dislocation of the humerus.

sub·glos·si·tis (sub″glos·eye′tis) *n.* [*sub-* + *glossa* + *-itis*]. Inflammation of the tissues under the tongue. See also *ranula.*

sub·gron·da·tion (sub″gron·day′shun) *n.* [F.]. The intrusion of one fragment of a cranial bone beneath another part in a fracture.

sub·grun·da·tion (sub″grun·day′shun) *n.* SUBGRONDATION.

sub·hy·a·loid (sub·high′uh·loid) *adj.* Beneath the hyaloid membrane.

sub·hy·oid (sub·high′oid) *adj.* Beneath the hyoid bone.

subhyoid bursa. A bursa lying between the thyrohyoid membrane and hyoid bone and the conjoint insertion of the omohyoid and sternohyoid muscles. NA *bursa infrahyoidea.*

subhyoid laryngotomy. SUPERIOR LARYNGOTOMY.

su·bic·u·lum (suh·bick′yoo·lum, sue·) *n.,* pl. **subicu·la** (·luh) [NL., from L. *subicere,* to place under]. An underlying structure. —**subicu·lar** (·lur) *adj.*

subiculum pro·mon·to·rii (prom·un·to′ree·eye). [NA] The subiculum of the promontory; a bony ridge in the middle ear posterior to the promontory and the round window, forming the inferior border of the tympanic sinus.

sub·in·ci·sion (sub″in·sizh′un) *n.* [*sub-* + *incision*]. Making a permanent opening into the urethra through the undersurface of the penis, a practice common in some primitive tribes, especially those of central Australia. It does not impair coitus or cause sterility.

sub·in·fec·tion (sub″in·feck′shun) *n.* [*sub-* + *infection*]. Infection with slight or no overt clinical manifestations of disease.

sub·in·gui·nal (sub·ing'gwi·nul) *adj.* Distal to the inguinal region or groin.

subinguinal fossa. The depression of the anterior aspect of the thigh over the femoral triangle.

sub·in·vo·lu·tion (sub''in·vo·lew'shun) *n.* [*sub-* + *involution*]. Imperfect return to normal size after functional enlargement.

subinvolution of the uterus. The imperfect involution of the uterus after delivery.

sub·io·dide (sub·eye'o·dide) *n.* The iodide of a series containing the least iodine.

sub·ja·cent (sub·jay'sunt) *adj.* [L. *subjacens*, from *subjacere*, to lie under]. Lying beneath.

sub·jec·tive, *adj.* 1. Pertaining to or centered on the subject, or that which perceives or observes, as distinguished from the object or that which is observed. 2. Perceived or experienced by an individual himself but not directly observable by others, as sensations in general, or as a patient's symptoms in contrast to objective signs of disease. 3. Originating internally but mimicking to some extent sensations produced by external stimuli, as a ringing in the ears, dizziness, muscae volitantes, or hallucinations. 4. Conceived in terms of an individual's more immediate experiences and responses, with relatively little adjustment for perspective. Contr. *objective.*

subjective angle. *In ophthalmology,* the angle at which the patient's corresponding retinal areas are stimulated as evidenced by his response; may be normal or abnormal.

subjective sensation. A sensation not caused by external stimuli. See also *sensation.*

subjective sign. A sign or symptom recognized only by the patient. Contr. *objective sign.*

subjective sound. PHONISM.

subjective tinnitus. Tinnitus audible only to the subject. Contr. *objective tinnitus.*

subjective vertigo. Giddiness in which the patient has a sensation as if he himself were moving. Syn. *rotatory vertigo.* Contr. *objective vertigo.*

sub·la·tion (sub·lay'shun) *n.* [L. *sublatio*]. Removal; ABLATION.

sub·le·thal (sub·lee'thul) *adj.* [*sub-* + *lethal*]. Less than fatal, as a sublethal dose of poison.

sub·leu·ke·mic, sub·leu·kae·mic (sub''lew·kee'mick) *adj.* Less than leukemic; usually applied to states in which the peripheral blood manifestations of leukemia are temporarily suppressed.

¹sub·li·mate (sub'li·mate) *n.* [L. *sublimare*, to elevate]. A solid or condensed substance obtained by heating a material, which passes directly from the solid to the vapor phase and then back to the solid state.

²sub·li·mate (sub'li·mate) *v.* [L. *sublimare*, to lift up]. *In psychiatry,* to express or externalize instinctual impulses in a socially acceptable or conventional manner. See also *sublimation* (2).

sub·li·ma·tion (sub''li·may'shun) *n.* 1. The transformation of a solid to the gaseous state, followed by condensation to the solid state; used to purify substances such as iodine and mercuric chloride. 2. *In psychiatry,* a defense mechanism, working unconsciously, whereby undesirable instinctual cravings and impulses gain outward expression by converting their energies into socially acceptable activities.

Sublimaze. Trademark for fentanyl, an analgesic used as the citrate salt.

sub·lime (suh·blime') *v.* To successively volatilize and condense a solid. Noun *sublimation.*

sublimed sulfur. The form of sulfur obtained by subliming native sulfur. Syn. *flowers of sulfur.*

sub·lim·i·nal (sub·lim'i·nul) *adj.* [*sub-* + *liminal*]. 1. Below the limit of conscious perception. 2. SUBTHRESHOLD.

subliminal fringe. Neurons that are in close functional association with active neurons the excitability of which is momentarily increased even though they are not directly stimulated.

subliminal stimulus. SUBTHRESHOLD STIMULUS.

sub·li·mis (sub·lye'mis) *adj.* [L.]. Elevated; superficial, a qualification applied to certain muscles, as the flexor digitorum sublimis.

sub·line (sub'line) *n.* A subdivision of a strain.

sub·lin·gual (sub·ling'gwul) *adj.* [*sub-* + *lingual*]. 1. Beneath the tongue. 2. Pertaining to the structures under the tongue.

sublingual caruncle. Any of the small papillae found along the sublingual fold where the ducts of the sublingual and the submandibular glands empty. NA *caruncula sublingualis.*

sublingual cyst. RANULA.

sublingual ducts. The ducts of the sublingual gland opening into the oral cavity. Some unite to form the major sublingual duct (NA *ductus sublingualis major*). Others, the minor sublingual ducts (NA *ductus sublinguales minores*), open separately on the sublingual fold. See also *sublingual gland.*

sublingual fold. The elevation of the mucous membrane of the floor of the mouth, on either side of the tongue, caused by the projection of the sublingual gland. NA *plica sublingualis.*

sublingual fossa. A smooth shallow depression on the internal surface of the body of the mandible above the mylohyoid line which lodges the sublingual gland. NA *fovea sublingualis.*

sublingual gland. A complex of small salivary glands situated in the sublingual fold on each side of the oral floor. The anterior third to half of this complex on each side commonly is drained by a single duct, the major sublingual duct. The remaining glands are drained by the 5 to 15 or more minor sublingual ducts. NA *glandula sublingualis.*

sublingual nucleus. NUCLEUS OF ROLLER.

sublingual plica. SUBLINGUAL FOLD.

sublingual region. The part of the floor of the mouth lying below the tongue.

sub·lin·gui·tis (sub''ling·gwye'tis) *n.* [*sub-* + *lingua* + *-itis*]. Inflammation of sublingual gland.

sub·lob·u·lar (sub''lob'yoo·lur) *adj.* Situated beneath or at the base of a liver lobule or lobules.

sublobular vein. A vein formed by the joining of the central veins of several liver lobules. Syn. *intercalated vein.*

sub·lux (sub·lucks') *v.* To cause subluxation.

sub·lux·a·tion (sub''luck·say'shun) *n.* [*sub-* + *luxation*]. INCOMPLETE DISLOCATION. —**sub·lux·at·ed** (sub·luck'say·tid) *adj.*

sub·mal·le·o·lar (sub''ma·lee'uh·lur) *adj.* [*sub-* + *malleolar*]. Under the malleoli, as submalleolar amputation, removal of the foot at the ankle joint.

sub·mam·ma·ry (sub·mam'uh·ree) *adj.* Situated beneath a mammary gland.

submammary abscess. An abscess lying between the mammary gland and the chest wall. Syn. *postmammary abscess, retromammary abscess.*

sub·man·dib·u·lar (sub''man·dib'yoo·lur) *adj.* [*sub-* + *mandibular*]. Below or beneath the mandible.

submandibular duct. The duct of the submandibular gland which empties into the oral cavity at the side of the frenulum of the tongue. NA *ductus submandibularis.*

submandibular fossa. The oblong depression on the internal surface of the mandible, adjacent to the submandibular gland. NA *fovea submandibularis.*

submandibular ganglion. A parasympathetic ganglion lying between the mylohyoid and hyoglossus muscles and above the duct of the submandibular gland. Its postganglionic fibers go to the submandibular and sublingual glands. NA *ganglion submandibulare.* See also Plate 15.

submandibular gland. A large seromucous or mixed salivary gland situated below the mandible on either side. NA *glandula submandibularis.*

submandibular triangle. An area bounded above by the lower border of the body of the mandible and a line drawn from its angle to the mastoid process, below by the posterior belly of the digastric and the stylohyoid, and in front by the anterior belly of the digastric. Syn. *digastric triangle.* NA *trigonum submandibulare.*

sub·max·il·lar·i·tis (sub"mack·sil"uh·rye'tis) *n.* [*submaxillary* + *-itis*]. Inflammation of a submandibular gland.

sub·max·il·lary (sub·mack'si·lerr"ee) *adj.* [*sub-* + *maxillary*]. SUBMANDIBULAR.

submaxillary duct. SUBMANDIBULAR DUCT.

submaxillary fossa. SUBMANDIBULAR FOSSA.

submaxillary ganglion. SUBMANDIBULAR GANGLION.

submaxillary gland. SUBMANDIBULAR GLAND.

submaxillary region. SUBMANDIBULAR TRIANGLE.

sub·me·di·al (sub·mee'dee·ul) *adj.* [*sub-* + *medial*]. Lying beneath or near the midline.

sub·men·tal (sub·men'tul) *adj.* [*sub-* + *mental*]. Situated under the chin.

submental region. The region just beneath the chin. NA *regio submentalis.*

submental triangle. SUBMENTAL REGION.

sub·mes·a·ti·ce·phal·ic (sub·mes"a·ti·se·fal'ick) *adj. In craniometry,* designating a human skull with a cephalic index between 75 and 76, the lower division of the mesaticephalic skull.

sub·meta·cen·tric (sub"met"uh·sen'trick) *adj.* Of a chromosome: having the centromere near the center but not in the middle, resulting in one long and one short arm. Contr. *acrocentric, metacentric, telocentric.*

sub·me·tal·lic (sub"me·tal'ick) *adj.* Metallic to a certain extent.

sub·mi·cron (sub·migh'kron) *n.* [*sub-* + *micr-* + *-on*]. A colloid particle visible by aid of the ultramicroscope.

sub·mi·cro·scop·ic (sub"migh·kruh·skop'ick) *adj.* [*sub-* + *microscopic*]. Pertaining to a particle that is too small to be resolved by the optical microscope.

sub·mil·i·ary (sub·mil'ee·err·ee) *adj.* Smaller than the usual nodules that are described as miliary, or millet seed, in size.

sub·min·i·mal stimulus (sub·min'i·mul). SUBTHRESHOLD STIMULUS.

sub·mor·phous (sub·mor'fus) *adj.* [*sub-* + *-morphous*]. Having a structure intermediate between amorphous and true crystalline; often applied to the indefinite, partially crystalline structure of calculi.

sub·mu·co·sa (sub"mew·ko'suh) *n.* [short for *tela submucosa*].The layer of fibrous connective tissue that attaches a mucous membrane to its subjacent parts. NA *tela submucosa.* —**submuco·sal** (-sul), **sub·mu·cous** (sub·mew'kus) *adj.*

submucous membrane. SUBMUCOSA.

submucous plexus. A visceral nerve network lying in the submucosa of the digestive tube. Syn. *Meissner's plexus.* NA *plexus submucosus.*

sub·nar·cot·ic (sub"nahr·kot'ick) *adj.* Moderately narcotic.

sub·na·sa·le (sub"na·zay'lee) *n.* SUBNASAL POINT.

sub·na·sal point (sub·nay'zul). The base of the anterior nasal spine.

sub·ni·trate (sub·nigh'trate) *n.* A basic nitrate.

sub·nor·mal (sub·nor'mul) *adj.* Below normal. —**sub·nor·mal·ity** (sub"nor·mal'i·tee) *n.*

sub·no·to·chord·al (sub·no"tuh·kor'dul) *adj.* [*sub-* + *notochordal*]. Below the notochord.

sub·nu·cle·us (sub'new"klee·us) *n.* Any one of the smaller groups of cells into which a large nerve nucleus is divided by the passage through it of nerve bundles.

sub·oc·cip·i·tal (sub"ock·sip'i·tul) *adj.* [*sub-* + *-occipital*]. Situated beneath the occiput.

suboccipital decompression. Cranial decompression by an approach in the occipital region.

suboccipital triangle. An area bounded by the posterior major rectus capitis, the superior oblique, and the inferior oblique muscles.

sub·oc·cip·i·to·breg·mat·ic (sub"ock·sip"i·to·breg·mat'ick) *adj.* [*suboccipital* + *bregmatic*]. Pertaining to the suboccipital area and bregma.

suboccipitobregmatic diameter. The line joining the center of the anterior fontanel to the undersurface of the occipital bone.

sub·oper·cu·lum (sub"o·pur'kew·lum) *n.* ORBITAL OPERCULUM.

sub·or·bit·al (sub·or'bi·tul) *adj.* [*sub-* + *orbital*]. Situated beneath the orbit.

suborbital canal. INFRAORBITAL CANAL.

suborbital fossa. CANINE FOSSA.

sub·or·der (sub'or·dur) *n.* A taxonomic category falling just below an order.

sub·or·di·na·tion, *n.* [ML. *subordinatio,* from L. *sub-* + *ordinare,* to put in order]. 1. The condition of being under subjection or control. 2. The condition of organs that depend upon or are controlled by other organs.

Subose. Trademark for glyhexamide, an orally active hypoglycemic compound.

sub·ox·ide (sub·ock'side) *n.* The oxide of an element which contains the lowest proportion of oxygen.

sub·pap·il·la·ry (sub·pap'i·lerr"ee) *adj.* [*sub-* + *papillary*]. Beneath the stratum papillare.

subpapillary venous plexus. A flat network of small, thin-walled vessels in the deeper part of the papillary layer and in the superficial part of the reticular layer of the dermis.

sub·pap·u·lar (sub·pap'yoo·lur) *adj.* Indistinctly papular.

sub·par·a·lyt·ic (sub"păr"uh·lit'ick) *adj.* Not completely paralytic.

sub·pa·ri·e·tal (sub"puh·rye'e·tul) *adj.* Situated below the parietal lobe.

subparietal sulcus. A groove separating the precuneus of the parietal lobe from the cingulate gyrus. NA *sulcus subparietalis.*

sub·pa·tent (sub·pay'tunt) *adj.* Less than patent; below the threshold of patency.

sub·pec·to·ral (sub·peck'tuh·rul) *adj.* [*sub-* + *pectoral*]. Situated beneath the chest muscles.

subpectoral abscess. An abscess beneath the chest muscles.

sub·peri·car·di·al (sub"perr·i·kahr'dee·ul) *adj.* [*sub-* + *pericardial*]. Situated beneath the pericardium.

sub·peri·os·te·al (sub"perr·ee·os'tee·ul) *adj.* [*sub-* + *periosteal*]. Beneath the periosteum.

subperiosteal amputation. An amputation in which neighboring periosteum is used to cover the divided bone end or ends.

subperiosteal bone. PERIOSTEAL BONE.

subperiosteal fracture. A fracture in which the overlying periosteum is intact.

sub·peri·to·ne·al (sub"perr"i·to·nee'ul) *adj.* [*sub-* + *peritoneal*]. Beneath peritoneum.

subperitoneal abscess. An abscess arising between the parietal peritoneum and the abdominal wall. Syn. *preperitoneal abscess.*

subperitoneal plexus. An arterial plexus, in the extraperitoneal fat of the lumbar region, formed by twigs from the lumbar, inferior phrenic, iliolumbar, hepatic, renal, and colic arteries.

sub·phren·ic (sub·fren'ick) *adj.* [*sub-* + *phrenic*]. SUBDIAPHRAGMATIC.

subphrenic abscess. SUBDIAPHRAGMATIC ABSCESS.

subphrenic space. One of the two spaces, right and left, between the diaphragm and the liver, on either side of the falciform ligament.

sub·phy·lum (sub'fye·lum) *n.* A taxonomic category falling just below a phylum.

sub·pla·cen·ta (sub"pluh·sen'tuh) *n.* [*sub-* + *placenta*]. DECIDUA PARIETALIS.

sub·pla·cen·tal (sub″pluh·sen′tul) *adj.* [*sub-* + *placental*]. 1. Situated beneath the placenta. 2. Pertaining to the decidua parietalis.

sub·plan·ti·grade (sub·plan′ti·grade) *adj.* Incompletely plantigrade; walking with the heel slightly elevated.

sub·platy·hi·er·ic (sub·plat″i·high·err′ick) *adj.* [*sub-* + *platyhieric*]. *In osteometry,* designating a moderately broad sacrum, with a hieric index of 100 to 105.9.

sub·pleu·ral (sub·ploo′rul) *adj.* [*sub-* + *pleural*]. Situated beneath the pleura.

subpleural plexus. An arterial plexus in the mediastinum, derived from small twigs of the pericardiacophrenic and intercostal arteries.

sub·pu·bic (sub·pew′bick) *adj.* Situated beneath the pubic arch or symphysis.

subpubic angle. The angle formed at the pubic arch. NA *angulus subpubicus.*

subpubic ligament. ARCUATE PUBIC LIGAMENT.

sub·sar·to·ri·al (sub″sahr·to′ree·ul) *adj.* [*sub-* + *sartorius* + *-al*]. Situated beneath the sartorius muscle.

subsartorial canal. ADDUCTOR CANAL.

subsartorial plexus. A nerve network situated beneath the sartorius muscle. Syn. *obturator plexus.*

sub·scap·u·lar (sub·skap′yoo·lur) *adj.* 1. Beneath the scapula. 2. Pertaining to the subscapularis muscle.

subscapular aponeurosis. The thin membrane attached to the entire circumference of the subscapular fossa, affording attachment by its inner surface to some of the fibers of the subscapularis muscle.

subscapular bursa. A bursa between the tendon of the subscapularis muscle and the capsule of the shoulder joint; it communicates with the shoulder joint cavity. NA *bursa subtendinea musculi subscapularis.*

subscapular fossa. The ventral (costal) concave surface of the scapula. NA *fossa subscapularis.*

sub·scap·u·la·ris (sub″skap″yoo·lair′is) *n.* A muscle arising from the costal surface of the scapula and inserted on the lesser tubercle of the humerus. NA *musculus subscapularis.* See also Table of Muscles in the Appendix.

subscapular region. INFRASCAPULAR REGION.

sub·scrip·tion, *n.* [L. *subscriptio,* something written underneath]. The part of a prescription containing the directions to the pharmacist, indicating how the ingredients are to be mixed and prepared.

sub·se·rous (sub·seer′us) *adj.* Beneath a serous membrane.

sub·sib·i·lant (sub·sib′i·lunt) *adj.* [*sub-* + *sibilant*]. Having a sound like a muffled whistling.

subsibilant rale. A dull, whistling sound heard over the bronchi; due to viscid secretions.

sub·si·dence (sub·sigh′dunce, sub′si·dunce) *n.* [L. *subsidere,* to settle down]. Gradual cessation and disappearance, as of the manifestations of disease.

sub·sig·moid (sub·sig′moid) *adj.* Under the sigmoid flexure.

subsigmoid fossa. A peritoneal recess at the apex of the attachment of the sigmoid mesocolon. Syn. *intersigmoid fossa.*

sub·spe·cies (sub′spee·sheez) *n.* 1. A taxonomic category falling immediately below a species. 2. Any subdivision of a species, as a variety, type, or race.

sub·spi·nous (sub·spye′nus) *adj.* [*sub-* + *spinous*]. 1. Beneath a spine. 2. Beneath the spinal column.

subspinous dislocation. Luxation of the head of the humerus below the spine of the scapula.

sub·stage, *n.* The parts beneath the stage of a microscope, including the diaphragm, condenser, mirror, and other accessories.

substance Fa (Reichstein's). CORTISONE.

sub·stan·tia (sub·stan′shee·uh) *n.,* pl. & genit. sing. **substan·ti·ae** (·shee·ee) [L.]. Substance; matter.

substantia ada·man·ti·na den·tis (ad·uh·man·tye′nuh den′tis) [BNA]. Enamelum (= ENAMEL).

substantia al·ba (al′buh) [NA]. WHITE SUBSTANCE.

substantia alba me·dul·lae spi·na·lis (me·dul′ee spye·nay′lis) [NA]. The white matter of the spinal cord.

substantia com·pac·ta (kom·pack′tuh) [NA]. COMPACT BONE.

substantia cor·ti·ca·lis (kor·ti·kay′lis) [NA]. A general term for the outer substance of any structure.

substantia corticalis ce·re·bel·li (serr·e·bel′eye) [BNA]. CORTEX CEREBELLI.

substantia corticalis ce·re·bri (serr′e·brye) [BNA]. CORTEX CEREBRI.

substantia corticalis glan·du·lae su·pra·re·na·lis (glan′dew·lee sue·pruh·re·nay′lis) [BNA]. CORTEX GLANDULAE SUPRARENALIS.

substantia corticalis len·tis (len′tis) [BNA]. CORTEX LENTIS.

substantia corticalis lym·pho·glan·du·lae (lim·fo·glan′dew·lee) [BNA]. CORTEX NODI LYMPHATICI.

substantia corticalis os·sis (os′is) [NA]. The hard outer layer of bone.

substantia corticalis re·nis (ree′nis) [BNA]. CORTEX RENIS.

substantia ebur·nea (e·bur′nee·uh) [BNA]. Dentinum (= DENTIN).

substantia fer·ru·gi·nea (ferr·oo·jin′ee·uh). LOCUS CERULEUS.

substantia ge·la·ti·no·sa (je·lat·i·no′suh) [NA]. Translucent, gelatinous gray matter forming the apex of the posterior column of the spinal cord, crescentic or inverted V-shaped in section. A synaptic region for peripheral nerves conveying thermal and pain sensibilities.

substantia gelatinosa cen·tra·lis (sen·tray′lis) [BNA]. SUBSTANTIA GELATINOSA.

substantia gelatinosa Ro·lan·di (ro·lan′dye) [BNA]. SUBSTANTIA GELATINOSA.

substantia glan·du·la·ris pro·sta·tae (glan·dew·lair′is pros′tuh·tee) [NA]. The glandular tissue of the prostate.

substantia gli·o·sa (glye·o′suh). SUBSTANTIA GRISEA CENTRALIS MESENCEPHALI.

substantia gri·sea (gris′ee·uh, griz′) [NA]. GRAY SUBSTANCE.

substantia grisea cen·tra·lis me·dul·lae spi·na·lis (sen·tray′lis me·dul′ee spye·nay′lis) [BNA]. The central gray matter of the spinal cord; the substantia intermedia centralis medullae spinalis and the substantia intermedia lateralis medullae spinalis.

substantia grisea centralis me·sen·ce·pha·li (mes·en·sef′uh·lye) [NA]. The layer of gray matter surrounding the cerebral aqueduct in the midbrain, and continuous with the gray matter surrounding the fourth ventricle and that covering the rhomboid fossa.

substantia grisea me·dul·lae spi·na·lis (me·dul′ee spye·nay′lis) [NA]. The gray matter of the spinal cord.

substantia in·ter·me·dia cen·tra·lis me·dul·lae spi·na·lis (in·tur·mee′dee·uh sen·tray′lis me·dul′ee spye·nay′lis) [NA]. The gray matter surrounding the central canal of the spinal cord.

substantia intermedia la·te·ra·lis me·dul·lae spi·na·lis (lat·e·ray′lis me·dul′ee spye·nay′lis) [NA]. The gray matter of the anterior and posterior horns.

sub·stan·tial emphysema. EMPHYSEMA (1).

substantia len·tis (len′tis) [NA]. The fibrous substance of the lens.

substantia me·dul·la·ris glan·du·lae su·pra·re·na·lis (med·uh·lair′is glan′dew·lee sue·pruh·re·nay′lis) [BNA]. MEDULLA GLANDULAE SUPRARENALIS.

substantia medullaris lym·pho·glan·du·lae (lim·fo·glan′dew·lee) [BNA]. MEDULLA NODI LYMPHATICI.

substantia medullaris re·nis (ree′nis) [BNA]. MEDULLA RENIS.

substantia mus·cu·la·ris pro·sta·tae (mus·kew·lair′is pros′tuh·tee) [NA]. The smooth muscle cells in the stroma of the prostate.

substantia ni·gra (nigh′gruh) [NA]. A broad, thick plate of large, pigmented nerve cells separating the basis pedunculi from the tegmentum and extending from the border of the pons through the mesencephalon into the hypothalamus.

substantia os·sea den·tis (os'ee·uh den'tis) [BNA]. CEMENTUM.

substantia per·fo·ra·ta anterior (pur·fo·ray'tuh) [NA]. ANTERIOR PERFORATED SUBSTANCE.

substantia perforata posterior [NA]. POSTERIOR PERFORATED SUBSTANCE.

substantia pro·pria cor·ne·ae (pro'pree·uh kor'nee·ee) [NA]. SUBSTANTIA PROPRIA OF THE CORNEA.

substantia propria of the cornea. The central, transparent, lamellated layer of dense connective tissue in the cornea. NA *substantia propria corneae.*

substantia propria scle·rae (skleer'ee) [NA]. The connective tissue of the sclera.

substantia re·ti·cu·la·ris (re·tick·yoo·lair'is). Reticular substance. See *reticular formation.*

substantia reticularis al·ba [Ar·nol·di] (al'buh ahr·nol'dye) [BNA]. Reticular white substance.

substantia reticularis alba me·dul·lae ob·lon·ga·tae (me·dul'ee ob·long·gay'tee) [BNA]. The white reticular substance of the medulla oblongata.

substantia reticularis gri·sea me·dul·lae ob·lon·ga·tae (gris'ee·uh me·dul'ee ob·long·gay'tee) [BNA]. The gray reticular substance of the medulla oblongata.

substantia spon·gi·o·sa (spon·jee·o'suh) [NA]. CANCELLOUS BONE.

sub·stan·tive (sub'stun·tiv) *adj.* [L. *substantivus,* having substance, from *substare,* to stand firm]. Pertaining to a dye that requires no mordant.

substantive dye. A dye that combines directly with the substance acted on.

substantive stain. A histologic stain obtained by direct absorption of the pigment from the solution in which the tissue is immersed.

sub·ster·nal (sub"stur'nul) *adj.* [*sub-* + *sternal*]. Beneath the sternum, as substernal pain.

sub·stit·u·ent (sub·stitch'oo·unt) *n.* [L. *substituere,* to substitute]. *In chemistry,* an atom or group of atoms that replaces another atom or group of atoms of different kind in a molecule.

sub·sti·tu·tion, *n.* [L. *substitutio,* from *substituere,* to substitute, from *statuere,* to set up]. 1. The replacement of one thing by another to serve a similar function. 2. *In chemistry,* the replacing of one or more elements or radicals in a compound by other elements or radicals. 3. *In psychiatry,* a defense mechanism whereby alternative or substitutive gratifications are secured to reduce tension resulting from frustration. The substitutes are generally comparable to the pleasures and satisfactions which the individual was frustrated in obtaining.

substitution therapy. The use in treatment of substances the normal secretion of which is deficient or absent.

sub·sti·tu·tive (sub'sti·tew"tiv) *adj.* [L. *substitutivus*]. Effecting a change or substitution.

sub·strate (sub'strate) *n.* [L. *substratus,* spread under, from *substernere,* to spread under]. 1. An underlayer. 2. A substance upon which an enzyme acts.

sub·sul·fate (sub·sul'fate) *n.* A basic sulfate.

sub·sul·to·ry (sub·sul'tuh·ree) *adj.* [from *subsultus*]. Leaping; twitching; convulsive.

sub·sul·tus (sub·sul'tus) *n.* [NL., from L. *subsilire,* to jump up]. A convulsive jerking or twitching.

subsultus clonus. *Obsol.* SUBSULTUS TENDINUM.

subsultus ten·di·num (ten'di·num). *Obsol.* Involuntary twitching of the muscles, especially of the hands and feet, seen with some fevers.

sub·su·pe·ri·or (sub"sue·peer'ee·ur) *adj.* Beneath a superior part; specifically, beneath a superior bronchopulmonary segment.

sub·syn·ap·tic (sub"si·nap'tick) *adj.* [*sub-* + *synaptic*]. POSTSYNAPTIC.

subsynaptic membrane. The region of the postsynaptic membrane juxtaposed against the presynaptic membrane at the synapse.

sub·ta·lar (sub·tay'lur) *adj.* [*sub-* + *talar*]. Beneath the talus.

subtalar articulation. The articulation formed by the posterior articular facets on the inferior surface of the talus and the superior surface of the calcaneus. NA *articulatio subtalaris.* See also Table of Synovial Joints and Ligaments in the Appendix.

sub·tem·po·ral (sub·tem'puh·rul) *adj.* Situated beneath the temporal region of the skull.

subtemporal decompression. Cranial decompression by an approach in the temporal region.

sub·ten·di·nous (sub·ten'di·nus) *adj.* Situated beneath a tendon, as a subtendinous bursa.

subtendinous prepatellar bursa. A bursa between the patella and the tendon of the quadriceps femoris muscle. NA *bursa subtendinea prepatellaris.*

sub·ten·to·ri·al (sub"ten·to'ree·ul) *adj.* [*sub-* + *tentorial*]. Below or beneath the tentorium cerebelli.

sub·ter·mi·nal (sub"tur'mi·nul) *adj.* Located near an end.

sub·ter·tian (sub"tur'shun) *adj.* [*sub-* + *tertian*]. Occurring less frequently than every other day.

subtertian malaria. FALCIPARUM MALARIA.

sub·te·tan·ic (sub"te·tan'ick) *adj.* Not quite tetanic; applied to seizures which are tonic with brief periods of relaxation but not clonic.

sub·tha·lam·ic (sub"thuh·lam'ick) *adj.* Below the thalamus.

subthalamic fasciculus. A bundle of fibers consisting of fibers that emerge from the globus pallidus and pass through the internal capsule into the subthalamic nucleus, and of fibers that project back from the subthalamic nucleus to the globus pallidus.

subthalamic nucleus. A biconvex nucleus between the internal capsule and the cerebral peduncle, having well-developed connections with the globus pallidus. Syn. *corpus Luysii.* NA *nucleus subthalamicus.*

subthalamic region. The region which lies ventral to the thalamus, medial to the internal capsule, and lateral and caudal to the hypothalamus, and which contains the subthalamic nucleus, the zona incerta, and the nuclei of the tegmental fields of Forel. Prominent fiber bundles passing through this region include the ansa lenticularis, the lenticular fasciculus, the thalamic fasciculus, and the subthalamic fasciculus.

subthalamic reticular nucleus. RETICULAR NUCLEUS OF THE THALAMUS.

sub·thal·a·mus (sub·thal'uh·mus) *n.* SUBTHALAMIC REGION.

sub·thresh·old, *adj.* [*sub-* + *threshold*]. Pertaining to a stimulus of insufficient strength to produce a response.

subthreshold stimulus. A stimulus too weak to produce a response that can be perceived or felt or that results in an action potential. Syn. *subliminal stimulus, subminimal stimulus.*

sub·thy·roid·ism (sub"thigh'roid·iz·um) *n.* HYPOTHYROIDISM.

sub·ti·lin (sub'ti·lin) *n.* An antibiotic substance obtained from *Bacillus subtilis,* active against gram-positive bacteria. Compare *subtilisin.*

sub·til·i·sin (sub·til'i·sin) *n.* A proteolytic enzyme obtained from strains of *Bacillus subtilis.* Compare *subtilin.*

sub·to·tal (sub"to'tul) *adj.* [*sub-* + *total*]. Less than complete.

subtotal hysterectomy. SUPRACERVICAL HYSTERECTOMY.

sub·trac·tion technique. A photographic method of eliminating certain unwanted shadows from a roentgenogram made with the use of a contrast medium.

sub·tra·pe·zi·al (sub"tra·pee'zee·ul) *adj.* [*sub-* + *trapezial*]. Located beneath the trapezius muscle.

subtrapezial plexus. A nerve plexus lying beneath the trapezius muscle.

sub·trig·o·nal (sub·trig'uh·nul, ·tri·go'nul) *adj.* [*sub-* + *trigonal*]. Situated beneath the trigone.

subtrigonal gland. One of a group of small subsidiary prostatic glands which lie beneath the mucosa of the trigone. Syn. *Home's gland* or *lobe.*

sub·tro·chan·ter·ic (sub·tro″kan·terr′ick) *adj.* [*sub-* + *trochanteric*]. Below a trochanter.

sub·trop·i·cal (sub·trop′i·kul) *adj.* [*sub-* + *tropical*]. Almost tropical in climate.

sub·uber·es (sub·yoo′bur·eez) *n.pl.* [L., from *sub-* + *uber, uberis,* breast]. Children at the breast; suckling children.

sub·um·bil·i·cal (sub″um·bil′i·kul) *adj.* [*sub-* + *umbilical*]. Situated below the umbilicus.

subumbilical space. A triangular space in the body cavity having its apex at the umbilicus.

sub·un·gual (sub″ung′gwul) *adj.* [*sub-* + *ungual*]. Beneath a nail.

sub·ure·thral (sub″yoo·ree′thrul) *adj.* [*sub-* + *urethral*]. Situated beneath the urethra.

suburethral abscess. An abscess beneath the urethra; in the female it may protrude from the introitus as a bulge in the anterior vaginal wall.

sub·val·vu·lar (sub·val′vew·lur) *adj.* [*sub-* + *valvular*]. Beneath a valve; usually a cardiac semilunar valve.

subvalvular aortic stenosis. SUBAORTIC STENOSIS.

sub·vir·ile (sub·virr′il) *adj.* [*sub-* + *virile*]. Deficient in virility.

sub·vi·ta·min·o·sis (sub·vye″tuh·mi·no′sis) *n.* [*sub-* + *vitamin* + *-osis*]. A state of vitamin deficiency.

sub·vo·lu·tion (sub″vo·lew′shun) *n.* [*sub-* + L. *volvere,* to roll, turn]. A method of operating for pterygium, in which a flap is turned over so that an outer or cutaneous surface comes in contact with a raw, dissected surface. Adhesions are thus prevented.

sub·vo·me·rine (sub·vo′muh·reen) *adj.* [*sub-* + *vomerine*]. Situated beneath the vomer.

subvomerine cartilage. VOMERONASAL CARTILAGE.

sub·wak·ing (sub·way′king) *adj.* Pertaining to the state between sleeping and complete wakefulness.

Sucaryl. Trademark for the noncaloric sweeteners calcium cyclamate (Sucaryl Calcium) and sodium cyclamate (Sucaryl Sodium).

suc·ce·da·ne·ous (suck″se·day′nee·us) *adj.* [L. *succedaneus,* from *succedere,* to come after, to replace]. 1. Pertaining to, or acting as, a substitute. 2. Pertaining to that which follows after.

succedaneous tooth. Any permanent tooth that takes the place of a deciduous tooth.

suc·cen·tu·ri·ate (suck″sen·tew′ree·ut) *adj.* [L. *succenturiare,* to substitute]. ACCESSORY.

succi. Plural of *succus.*

suc·cif·er·ous (suck·sif′ur·us) *adj.* [*succus* + *-ferous*]. Producing sap.

suc·ci·nate (suck′si·nate) *n.* A salt or ester of succinic acid.

suc·cin·ic acid (suck·sin′ick) [L. *succinum,* amber, + *-ic*]. Butanedioic acid, $HOOCCH_2CH_2COOH$, an intermediate in the tricarboxylic acid cycle. Formerly variously used for medicinal purposes. The sodium salt has been used as an analeptic in barbiturate poisoning.

succinic acid dehydrogenase. The enzyme that catalyzes dehydrogenation of succinic acid to fumaric acid in the presence of a hydrogen acceptor.

succinic dehydrogenase. SUCCINIC ACID DEHYDROGENASE.

suc·ci·nyl·cho·line chloride (suck″si·nil·ko′leen). Choline chloride succinate, $C_{14}H_{30}Cl_2N_2O_4$. A powerful inhibitor of neuromuscular transmission, which on intravenous injection produces complete muscular relaxation in about 1 minute, the effect lasting only 2 to 5 minutes because of rapid destruction of the agent in the body by esterases. It is useful clinically in conditions requiring profound but brief muscular relaxation. Syn. *suxamethonium chloride.*

suc·ci·nyl·sul·fa·thi·a·zole (suck″si·nil·sul″fuh·thigh′uh·zole) *n.* 4′-(2-Thiazolylsulfamoyl)succinanilic acid, $C_{13}H_{13}N_3O_5S_2$, a poorly absorbed sulfonamide used as an intestinal antibacterial agent in preoperative preparation of patients for abdominal surgery; also postoperatively to maintain a low bacterial count.

suc·cor·rhea, suc·cor·rhoea (suck″o·ree′uh) *n.* [*succus* + *-rrhea*]. An excessive flow of a secretion, as of saliva or gastric juice.

suc·cu·bus (suck′yoo·bus) *n.,* pl. **succu·bi** (·bye) [ML., from *succubare,* to lie under]. 1. A nightmare. 2. A heavy mental burden. 3. A female demon said to have sexual intercourse with sleeping men. Compare *incubus.*

suc·cu·lent, *adj.* [L. *succulentus,* from *succus,* juice]. Juicy.

suc·cur·sal (suh·kur′sul) *adj.* [L. *succurrere, succursus,* to assist]. Subsidiary.

suc·cus (suck′us) *n.,* pl. **suc·ci** (·sigh) [L.]. 1. A vegetable juice. 2. An animal secretion.

succus en·ter·i·cus (en·terr′i·kus). The intestinal juice, secreted by the glands of the intestinal mucous membrane. It is thin, opalescent, alkaline, and has a specific gravity of 1.011.

succus gas·tri·cus (gas′tri·kus). GASTRIC JUICE.

succus in·te·sti·na·lis (in·tes·ti·nay′lis). SUCCUS ENTERICUS.

succus pan·cre·a·ti·cus (pan·kree·at′i·kus). PANCREATIC JUICE.

succus pro·sta·ti·cus (pros·tat′i·kus). The prostatic fluid, a constituent of the semen.

suc·cuss (suh·kus′) *v.* To make succussion.

suc·cus·sion (suh·kush′un) *n.* [L. *succussio,* from *succutire,* to shake]. A shaking, especially of an individual, to determine the presence of free fluid and gas in a cavity or hollow organ of the body.

succussion sound or **splash.** The splashing sound heard on succussion when there is free fluid and gas in a body cavity or hollow organ.

suck, *v.* 1. To draw up a liquid or gel as by the partial vacuum created by a suction apparatus, or the motions of the mouth, tongue, and lips. 2. Specifically, to nurse at the breast or, in an animal, the udder.

suck·er foot or **apparatus.** The expanded termination of an astrocyte process attached to a capillary wall.

suck·ing, *n.* Nursing; drawing with the mouth.

sucking pad or **cushion.** A fatty pad mass situated between the masseter and the buccinator muscles, well developed in infancy. Syn. *buccal fat pad.* NA *corpus adiposum buccae.*

sucking reflex. Sucking movements of the lips, tongue, and jaw in response to contact of an object with the lips, seen normally in infants, but observed abnormally and often in exaggerated form in patients with bilateral frontal lobe lesions.

sucking wound. A wound in the chest wall through which air is taken in and expelled; seen in traumatopnea.

suck·le, *v.* To nurse at the breast.

suck·ling, *n.* A nursling; especially, a young child or animal that is not yet weaned.

Suc·quet-Hoy·er canal (sueᵉ·kehʰ′) [J. P. *Sucquet,* French anatomist, 1840–1870; and H. F. *Hoyer,* Polish surgeon, 1834–1907]. The afferent arteriole of a glomus. It has a thick wall and a narrow lumen.

su·cral·fate (soo·kral′fate) *n.* A complex of sucrose octakis-(hydrogen sulfate) and aluminum hydroxide, $C_{12}H_xA1_{16}O_yS_8$, a gastrointestinal antiulcerative.

su·crase (sue′krace) *n.* SACCHARASE.

su·crate (sue′krate) *n.* A salt of saccharic acid.

su·crose (sue′kroce, ·kroze) *n.* [F. *sucre,* sugar, + *-ose*]. A sugar, $C_{12}H_{22}O_{11}$, obtained from the plants *Saccharum officinarum, Beta vulgaris,* and other sources; used as a carbohydrate food and as a sweetening agent. Syn. *saccharum, sugar.*

su·cro·su·ria (sue″kro·sue′ree·uh) *n.* [*sucrose* + *-uria*]. A rare condition in which sucrose is not metabolized in the intestine and is excreted in the urine.

suc·tion, *n.* [L. *suctio,* from *sugere,* to suck]. 1. The act of sucking. 2. The act or the force developed by reducing the atmospheric pressure over a surface or a substance.

suction abortion. SUCTION CURETTAGE.

suction apparatus or **device.** A contrivance for evacuating fluid from body cavities, operating by means of negative pressure.

suction cup. CUPPING GLASS.

suction curet. A small hollow tube with a cutting window to which suction may be applied; used for obtaining endometrial biopsy.

suction curettage. Abortion by means of a suction device inserted into the uterus; effective during the first trimester of pregnancy.

suction test. DALLDORF TEST.

Suc·to·ria (suck·to'ree·uh) *n.pl.* 1. Siphonaptera, the fleas. 2. A class of Protozoa, closely related to the Ciliata, without cilia in the mature stage, but possessing processes called tentacles, some of which are suctorial in function. A few species are parasitic on fish and other aquatic animals.

suc·to·ri·al (suck·to'ree·ul) *adj.* Pertaining to, or suitable for, sucking.

sud-, sudo- [L. *sudare,* to sweat]. A combining form meaning *perspiration, sweat.*

su·da·men (sue·day'mun) *n.*, pl. **su·dam·i·na** (·dam'i·nuh) [NL., from L. *sudare,* to sweat]. A skin disease in which sweat accumulates under the superficial horny layers of the epidermis to form small, clear, transparent vesicles.

Su·dan dye or **stain** (soo·dan'). Any one of a number of related fat-soluble dyes used as biological stains. They are related by being oil-soluble and by being aromatic compounds, but fall into at least three chemical groups.

su·dano·phil (soo·dan'o·fil) *adj.* [*Sudan* + *-phil*]. Having an affinity to the Sudan series of fat-soluble dyes; fat-containing.

su·dano·phil·ia (soo·dan''o·fil'ee·uh) *n.* [*sudanophil* + *-ia*]. An affinity for or staining fat-soluble dyes in general, but especially Sudan dyes. —**sudanophil·ic** (·ick) *adj.*

sudanophilic diffuse sclerosis. SUDANOPHILIC LEUKODYSTROPHY.

sudanophilic leukodystrophy. An inherited disease of the nervous system, affecting only males and having its onset between four and sixteen years; characterized by atrophy of the adrenal cortex and widespread degeneration of myelin in the central nervous system associated, in recent lesions, with fat-laden (sudan-positive) macrophages; Originally included under the rubric of Schilder's disease but now considered to be an independent metabolic encephalopathy.

Sudan R. A red neutral dye, $C_{18}H_{16}N_2O_2$, of the monoazo group, used as a stain for lipids.

su·da·tion (sue·day'shun) *n.* [L. *sudatio,* from *sudare,* to sweat]. Sweating.

su·da·to·ria (sue''duh·to'ree·uh) *n.* 1. HYPERHIDROSIS. 2. Plural of *sudatorium.*

su·da·to·ri·um (sue''duh·to'ree·um) *n.*, **sudato·ria** (·ree·uh) [L., a sweating-room]. 1. A hot-air bath. 2. A room for the administration of a hot-air bath.

sudden infant death syndrome. The syndrome of sudden, unexpected death of an apparently healthy infant, occurring almost always during a sleep period and most commonly between the ages of 1 and 4 months. Postmortem examination usually reveals only the results of a fatal apneic episode, and though the etiology remains essentially unknown and perhaps multiple, there is evidence that many such infant deaths are preceded by a period of chronic but subclinical hypoxia. Abbreviated, SIDS. Syn. *crib death, sleep apnea syndrome.*

Su·deck's atrophy, disease, or **dystrophy** (zoo'deck) [P. H. M. *Sudeck,* German surgeon, 1866–1938]. Acute bone atrophy or aseptic necrosis of bone following injury. Syn. *traumatic osteoporosis.*

sudo-. See *sud-.*

su·do·lor·rhea, su·do·lor·rhoea (sue·do''lo·ree'uh) *n.* [*sud-* + L. *ol*eum, oil, + *-rrhea*]. SEBORRHEIC DERMATITIS.

su·do·mo·tor (sue''do·mo'tur) *adj.* [*sudo-* + *motor*]. Pertaining to the efferent nerves that control the activity of sweat glands.

sudomotor nerves. The nerves that excite the sweat glands to activity.

su·dor (sue'dur, ·dor) *n.* [L.] [BNA]. SWEAT. —**sudor·al** (·ul) *adj.*

su·do·re·sis (sue''duh·ree'sis) *n.* [*sudor* + *-esis*]. Excessive sweating.

su·do·rif·er·ous (sue''dur·if'ur·us) *adj.* [L. *sudorifer,* from *sudor*]. Producing sweat.

sudoriferous glands. The sweat glands.

su·do·rif·ic (sue''dur·if'ick) *adj.* & *n.* 1. Inducing sweating. 2. An agent inducing sweating.

su·dor·i·ker·a·to·sis (sue''dur·i·kerr''uh·to'sis) *n.* Keratosis of the sweat glands.

su·do·rip·a·rous (sue''dur·ip'uh·rus) *adj.* [*sudor* + *-parous*]. Secreting sweat.

sudoriparous abscess. An abscess due to inflammation of obstructed sweat glands.

sudoriparous angioma. A soft, pigmented mass, probably hematomatous, characterized clinically by pain and sweating, and histologically by dilated blood vessels, sweat glands, smooth muscle fibers, and fibrous tissues.

sudoriparous gland. SWEAT GLAND.

sudor noc·tur·nus (nock·tur'nus). NIGHT SWEAT.

sudor san·gui·no·sus (sang''gwi·no'sus). HEMATHIDROSIS.

su·dox·i·cam (soo·dock'si·kam) *n.* 4-Hydroxy-2-methyl-*N*-(2-thiazolyl)-2*H*-1,2-benzothiazine-3-carboxamide 1,1-dioxide, $C_{13}H_{11}N_3O_4S_2$, an anti-inflammatory.

su·et (sue'it) *n.* [dim. of OF. *seu,* from L. *sebum,* tallow, suet]. 1. The internal fat of the abdomen of sheep or cattle. 2. Prepared suet.

su·fen·ta·nil (soo·fen'tuh·nil) *n.* *N*-[4-(Methoxymethyl)-1-[(2-thienyl)ethyl]-4-piperidyl]propionanilide, $C_{22}H_{30}N_2O_2S$, an analgesic

suf·fo·cate (suf'uh·kate) *v.* [L. *suffocare,* to choke]. ASPHYXIATE.

suf·fo·ca·tion (suf''uh·kay'shun) *n.* Interference with the entrance of air into the lungs and resultant asphyxiation.

suf·frag·i·nis (suh·fraj'i·nis) *n.* [L. *os suffraginis,* from *suffrago,* hock]. The large pastern or proximal phalangeal bone of the horse.

suf·fu·sion (suh·few'zhun) *n.* [L. *suffusio,* from *suffundere,* to suffuse]. 1. A spreading or flow of any fluid of the body into surrounding tissue; an extensive extravasation of blood. 2. The pouring of water upon a patient as a remedial measure. —**suf·fuse** (·fewz') *v.*

sug·ar, *n.* [OF. *çucre,* from ML. *succarum,* from Ar. *sukkar,* from Per. *shakar,* from Skr. *śarkarā*]. 1. Any carbohydrate having a sweet taste and the general formula $C_nH_{2n}O_n$ or $C_nH_{2n-2}O_{n-1}$. 2. SUCROSE.

sugar-coated spleen. ICED SPLEEN.

sug·ar·ine (shoog'ur·een, ·in) *n.* Methylbenzolsulfinide, a compound said to have 500 times greater sweetening power than sugar.

sugar-loaf head. OXYCEPHALY.

sugar of lead. LEAD ACETATE.

sugar tolerance. The tolerance of a diabetic patient for ingested sugar. It is measured by the maximum amount of sugar intake which does not produce glycosuria.

sug·gest·ibil·i·ty (sug·jes''ti·bil'i·tee) *n.* The condition of being readily influenced by another; an abnormal state when the individual conforms with unusual readiness, as patients who too readily accept ideas of health or illness. Compare *autosuggestibility.*

sug·gest·ible, *adj.* Amenable to suggestion.

sug·ges·tion, *n.* [L. *suggestio,* from *suggerere,* to furnish, put forward]. 1. *In psychiatry,* the influencing of an individual to accept uncritically a belief, attitude, or feeling put forward by the therapist. 2. The artificial production of a certain psychic state in which the individual experiences such sensations as are suggested to him or ceases to experience those which he is instructed not to feel. See also *hypnosis.* 3. The thing suggested.

sug·ges·tion·ist (sug·jes'chun·ist) *n.* A person who treats disease by means of suggestion or who practices hypnotherapy. **—suggestion·ize** (·ize) *v.*

suggestion therapy. Treating disordered states by means of suggestion. See also *hypnotherapy.*

sug·gil·la·tion (sug"ji·lay'shun, suj"i·) *n.* [L. *sugillatio,* from *sugillare,* to beat black and blue]. An ecchymosis or bruise.

sui·cide, *n.* [L. *sui,* of one's self, + *-cide*]. 1. Self-murder; intentionally taking one's own life. 2. One who takes his own life. **—su·i·ci·dal** (sue"i·sigh'dul) *adj.*

su·i·ci·dol·o·gist (sue"i·si·dol'uh·jist) *n.* A person who practices suicidology.

su·i·ci·dol·o·gy (sue"i·si·dol'uh·jee) *n.* [*suicide* + *-logy*]. The science dealing with the study of the causes of suicide and with its prevention.

su·int (sue'int, swint) *n.* [F., from *suer,* to sweat]. A soapy substance rich in potassium salts of higher fatty acids and in cholesterol, derived from sheep's wool. Syn. *wool soap.*

Suker's sign. Inability to maintain fixation on extreme lateral gaze, seen in hyperthyroidism.

Sulamyd. A trademark for sulfacetamide.

sul·a·ze·pam (sul·ay'ze·pam) *n.* 7-Chloro-1,3-dihydro-1-methyl-5-phenyl-2*H*-1,4-benzodiazepine-2-thione, $C_{16}H_{13}ClN_2S$, a tranquilizer.

sul·cal (sul'kul) *adj.* Pertaining to a sulcus.

sul·cate (sul'kate) *adj.* [L. *sulcatus,* from *sulcare,* to furrow]. 1. Pertaining to a sulcus. 2. Furrowed or grooved.

sulcate process. An inconstant process of the palatine bone connecting the orbital process with the sphenoid process.

sulci. Plural and genitive singular of *sulcus.*

sulci ar·te·ri·o·si (ahr·teer·ee·o'sigh) [NA]. Grooves on the inner surface of the cranial bones, in which run the meningeal arteries.

sulci ce·re·bel·li (serr·e·bel'eye) [BNA]. FISSURAE CEREBELLI.

sulci ce·re·bri (serr'e·brye) [NA]. A collective term for the furrows between the gyri of the cerebrum.

sulci cu·tis (kew'tis) [NA]. CUTICULAR SULCI.

sul·ci·form fossa (sul'si·form). A shallow furrow in the inner fore part of the cavity of the vestibule of the ear, behind the elliptical recess and the spherical recess, into which the aqueduct of the vestibule opens.

sulci oc·ci·pi·ta·les la·te·ra·les (ock·sip·i·tay'leez lat·e·ray'leez) [BNA]. LATERAL OCCIPITAL SULCI.

sulci occipitales su·pe·ri·o·res (sue·peer·ee·o'reez) [BNA]. Indefinite grooves in the upper part of the convex surface of the occipital lobe.

sulci or·bi·ta·les (or·bi·tay'leez) [NA]. ORBITAL SULCI.

sulci pa·la·ti·ni max·il·lae (pal·uh·tye'nigh mack·sil'ee) [NA]. Small grooves on the inferior surface of the palatine process of the maxilla for palatine vessels and nerves.

sulci pa·ra·co·li·ci (par·uh·ko'li·sigh) [NA]. Shallow grooves of the posterior wall of the abdominal cavity lying between the lateral side of the ascending and descending colon and lateral abdominal wall.

sulci pa·ra·gle·noi·da·les (par·uh·glee·noy·day'leez) [BNA]. PARAGLENOIDAL SULCI.

sulci tem·po·ra·les trans·ver·si (tem·po·ray'leez trans·vur'sigh) [NA]. TRANSVERSE TEMPORAL SULCI.

sulci ve·no·si (ve·no'sigh) [NA]. Grooves on the inner surface of the bones of the cranial cavity, in which run the meningeal veins.

sul·cus (sul'kus) *n.* pl. & genit. sing. **sul·ci** (·sigh) [L., furrow]. 1. A furrow or linear groove, as in a bone. When applied to linear depressions on the cerebral hemisphere, the term indicates a less deep depression than a fissure. Sulci in the brain separate the convolutions or gyri. See also *fissure* and Plate 18. 2. *In dentistry,* a longitudinal groove in the surface of a tooth the inclines of which meet at an angle; a developmental groove lies at the junction of the inclines. See also *spillway, gingival sulcus.*

sulcus am·pul·la·ris (am·puh·lair'is) [NA]. AMPULLARY SULCUS.

sulcus ant·he·li·cis trans·ver·sus (ant·hel'i·sis trans·vur'sus) [NA]. TRANSVERSE SULCUS OF THE ANTHELIX.

sulcus ar·te·ri·ae oc·ci·pi·ta·lis (ahr·teer'ee·ee ock·sip·i·tay'lis) [NA]. OCCIPITAL GROOVE.

sulcus arteriae sub·cla·vi·ae (sub·klay'vee·ee) [NA]. SUBCLAVIAN SULCUS.

sulcus arteriae tem·po·ra·lis me·di·ae (tem·po·ray'lis mee'dee·ee) [NA]. A groove on the inner surface of the squamous part of the temporal bone for the middle temporal artery.

sulcus arteriae ver·te·bra·lis (vur·te·bray'lis) [NA]. A groove on the posterior arch of the atlas for the vertebral artery.

sulcus au·ri·cu·lae posterior (aw·rick'yoo·lee) [NA]. A shallow depression between the antitragus and the anthelix of the external ear.

sulcus ba·si·la·ris pon·tis (bas·i·lair'is pon'tis) [NA]. BASILAR SULCUS.

sulcus bi·ci·pi·ta·lis la·te·ra·lis (bye·sip·i·tay'lis lat·e·ray'lis) [NA]. A shallow groove on the arm marking the lateral border of the biceps brachii muscle.

sulcus bicipitalis me·di·a·lis (mee·dee·ay'lis) [NA]. A shallow groove on the arm marking the medial border of the biceps brachii muscle.

sulcus bre·vis (brev'is). One of several short furrows seen on the insula of the cerebrum.

sulcus cal·ca·nei (kal·kay'nee·eye) [NA]. CALCANEAL SULCUS.

sulcus cal·ca·ri·nus (kal·kuh·rye'nus) [NA]. CALCARINE SULCUS.

sulcus ca·na·li·cu·li ma·stoi·dei (kan·uh·lick'yoo·lye mas·toy'dee·eye) [BNA]. A small, indefinite groove on the lateral wall of the jugular fossa of the inferior surface of the petrous part of the temporal bone marking the opening of the mastoid canaliculus.

sulcus ca·ro·ti·cus (ka·rot'i·kus) [NA]. CAROTID GROOVE.

sulcus car·pi (kahr'pye) [NA]. The broad groove seen in the articulated carpal bones on the anterior aspect of the wrist between the pisiform and hamulus of the hamate.

sulcus cen·tra·lis (sen·tray'lis) [NA]. CENTRAL SULCUS (1).

sulcus centralis in·su·lae (in'sue·lee) [NA]. CENTRAL SULCUS (2).

sulcus centralis [Ro·lan·di] (ro·lan'dye) [BNA]. Sulcus centralis (= CENTRAL SULCUS (1)).

sulcus chi·as·ma·tis (kigh·az'muh·tis) [NA]. CHIASMATIC GROOVE.

sulcus cin·gu·li (sing'gew·lye) [NA]. CINGULATE SULCUS.

sulcus cir·cu·la·ris in·su·lae (sur·kew·lair'is in'sue·lee) [NA]. CIRCULAR SULCUS.

sulcus circularis [Rei·li] (rye'lye) [BNA]. Sulcus circularis insulae (= CIRCULAR SULCUS).

sulcus col·la·te·ra·lis (ko·lat·e·ray'lis) [NA]. COLLATERAL SULCUS.

sulcus co·ro·na·ri·us (kor·o·nair'ee·us) [NA]. CORONARY SULCUS.

sulcus cor·po·ris cal·lo·si (kor'po·ris ka·lo'sigh) [NA]. CALLOSAL SULCUS.

sulcus cos·tae (kos'tee) [NA]. COSTAL SULCUS.

sulcus cru·ris he·li·cis (kroo'ris hel'i·sis) [NA]. A shallow groove on the medial surface of the pinna.

sulcus eth·moi·da·lis (eth·moy·day'lis) [NA]. A groove on the nasal surface of the nasal bone which lodges the external nasal branch of the anterior ethmoidal nerve.

sulcus fron·ta·lis inferior (fron·tay'lis) [NA]. INFERIOR FRONTAL SULCUS.

sulcus frontalis superior [NA]. SUPERIOR FRONTAL SULCUS.

sulcus glu·tae·us (gloo·tee'us) [BNA]. Sulcus gluteus (= GLUTEAL FOLD).

sulcus glu·te·us (gloo·tee'us, gloo'tee·us) [NA]. GLUTEAL FOLD.

sulcus ha·mu·li pte·ry·goi·dei (ham'yoo·lye terr·i·goy'dee·eye) [NA]. A groove on the lateral aspect of the pterygoid hamulus.

sulcus hip·po·cam·pi (hip·o·kam'pye) [NA]. HIPPOCAMPAL SULCUS.

sulcus ho·ri·zon·ta·lis ce·re·bel·li (hor·i·zon·tay'lis serr·e·bel'eye) [BNA]. Fissura horizontalis cerebelli (HORIZONTAL FISSURE OF THE CEREBELLUM).

sulcus hy·po·tha·la·mi·cus (high·po·thuh·lam'i·kus) [NA]. HYPOTHALAMIC SULCUS.

sulcus hypothalamicus [Mon·roi] (mun·ro'eye) [BNA]. Sulcus hypothalamicus (= HYPOTHALAMIC SULCUS).

sulcus in·fra·or·bi·ta·lis (in"fruh·or·bi·tay'lis) [NA]. INFRAORBITAL SULCUS.

sulcus in·fra·pal·pe·bra·lis (in"fruh·pal·pe·bray'lis) [NA]. An indistinct furrow below the lower eyelid.

sulcus in·ter·me·di·us an·te·ri·or me·dul·lae spi·na·lis (in·tur·mee'dee·us an·teer'ee·or me·dul'ee spye·nay'lis) [BNA]. An occasional shallow groove on the outer lateral aspect of the spinal cord.

sulcus intermedius posterior medullae spinalis [NA]. POSTERIOR INTERMEDIATE SULCUS.

sulcus in·ter·pa·ri·e·ta·lis (in"tur·pa·rye·e·tay'lis) [BNA]. Sulcus intraparietalis (= INTRAPARIETAL SULCUS).

sulcus in·ter·tu·ber·cu·la·ris (in"tur·tew·bur·kew·lair'is) [NA]. INTERTUBERCULAR SULCUS.

sulcus in·ter·ven·tri·cu·la·ris anterior (in"tur·ven·trick·yoo·lair'is) [NA]. ANTERIOR INTERVENTRICULAR SULCUS.

sulcus interventricularis posterior [NA]. POSTERIOR INTERVENTRICULAR SULCUS.

sulcus in·tra·pa·ri·e·ta·lis (in"truh·pa·rye·e·tay'lis) [NA]. INTRAPARIETAL SULCUS.

sulcus la·cri·ma·lis max·il·lae (lack·ri·may'lis mack·sil'ee) [NA]. LACRIMAL SULCUS.

sulcus lacrimalis os·sis la·cri·ma·lis (os'is lack·ri·may'lis) [NA]. The groove on the lateral aspect of the lacrimal bone for the lacrimal sac.

sulcus la·te·ra·lis an·te·ri·or me·dul·lae ob·lon·ga·tae (lat·e·ray'lis an·teer'ee·or me·dul'ee ob·long·gay'tee) [NA]. ANTEROLATERAL SULCUS OF THE MEDULLA OBLONGATA.

sulcus lateralis anterior medullae spi·na·lis (spye·nay'lis) [BNA]. ANTEROLATERAL SPINAL SULCUS.

sulcus lateralis ce·re·bri (serr'e·brye) [NA]. LATERAL CEREBRAL SULCUS.

sulcus lateralis me·sen·ce·pha·li (mes·en·sef'uh·lye) [BNA]. A shallow longitudinal groove on the lateral surface of the mesencephalon.

sulcus lateralis posterior me·dul·lae ob·lon·ga·tae (me·dul'ee ob·long·gay'tee) [NA]. POSTEROLATERAL SULCUS OF THE MEDULLA OBLONGATA.

sulcus lateralis posterior medullae spi·na·lis (spye·nay'lis) [NA]. POSTEROLATERAL SPINAL SULCUS.

sulcus li·mi·tans (lim'i·tanz) [NA]. A longitudinal groove on the middle of the inner surface of the lateral wall of the neural tube, dividing it into a dorsal alar plate and a ventral basal plate.

sulcus limitans ven·tri·cu·li quar·ti (ven·trick'yoo·lye kwahr'tye) [NA]. A longitudinal groove in the floor of the fourth ventricle lying between the medial eminence and the vestibular area.

sulcus limitans ven·tri·cu·lo·rum ce·re·bri (ven·trick·yoo·lo'rum serr'e·brye) [BNA]. *In embryology,* a longitudinal groove on the lateral wall of the neural tube which separates the dorsal, alar plate from the ventral, basal plate.

sulcus lon·gi·tu·di·na·lis an·te·ri·or cor·dis (lon·ji·tew·di·nay'lis an·teer'ee·or kor'dis) [BNA]. Sulcus interventricularis anterior (= ANTERIOR INTERVENTRICULAR SULCUS).

sulcus longitudinalis posterior [BNA]. Sulcus interventricularis posterior (= POSTERIOR INTERVENTRICULAR SULCUS).

sulcus lu·na·tus (lew·nay'tus) [NA]. LUNATE SULCUS.

sulcus mal·le·o·la·ris (mal·ee·o·lair'is) [NA]. MALLEOLAR SULCUS.

sulcus ma·tri·cis un·guis (may'tri·sis ung'gwis) [NA]. A fold in which the base of the nail is embedded.

sulcus me·di·a·lis cru·ris ce·re·bri (mee·dee·ay'lis kroo'ris serr'e·brye) [NA]. OCULOMOTOR SULCUS.

sulcus me·di·a·nus lin·guae (mee·dee·ay'nus ling'gwee) [NA]. MEDIAN LINGUAL SULCUS.

sulcus medianus posterior me·dul·lae ob·lon·ga·tae (me·dul'ee ob·long·gay'tee) [NA]. A narrow groove in the closed portion of the medulla oblongata which is an upward continuation of the posterior median sulcus of the spinal cord.

sulcus medianus posterior medullae spi·na·lis (spye·nay'lis) [NA]. POSTERIOR MEDIAN SULCUS OF THE SPINAL CORD.

sulcus medianus ven·tri·cu·li quar·ti (ven·trick'yoo·lye kwahr'tye) [NA]. MEDIAN SULCUS.

sulcus men·to·la·bi·a·lis (men"to·lay·bee·ay'lis) [NA]. The depression between the lower lip and the chin.

sulcus mus·cu·li flex·o·ris hal·lu·cis lon·gi cal·ca·nei (mus'kew·lye fleck·so'ris hal'yoo·sis long'guy kal·kay'nee·eye) [BNA]. SULCUS TENDINIS MUSCULI FLEXORIS HALLUCIS LONGI CALCANEI.

sulcus musculi flexoris hallucis longi ta·li (tay'lye) [BNA]. SULCUS TENDINIS MUSCULI FLEXORIS HALLUCIS LONGI TALI.

sulcus musculi pe·ro·naei lon·gi cal·ca·nei (perr·o·nee'eye long'guy kal·kay'nee·eye) [BNA]. Sulcus tendinis musculi peronei longi calcanei (= PERONEAL GROOVE).

sulcus musculi peronaei longi os·sis cu·boi·dei (os'is kew·boy'dee·eye) [BNA]. SULCUS TENDINIS MUSCULI PERONEI LONGI OSSIS CUBOIDEI.

sulcus my·lo·hy·oi·de·us (migh"lo·high·oy'dee·us) [NA]. MYLOHYOID GROOVE.

sulcus na·so·la·bi·a·lis (nay"zo·lay·bee·ay'lis) [NA]. A shallow depression between the nose and the upper lip.

sulcus ner·vi ocu·lo·mo·to·rii (nur'vye ock"yoo·lo·mo·to'ree·eye) [BNA]. Sulcus medialis cruris cerebri (= OCULOMOTOR SULCUS).

sulcus nervi pe·tro·si ma·jo·ris (pe·tro'sigh ma·jo'ris) [NA]. A groove on the anterior surface of the petrous part of the temporal bone for the greater petrosal nerve.

sulcus nervi petrosi mi·no·ris (mi·no'ris) [NA]. A groove on the anterior surface of the petrous part of the temporal bone for the lesser petrosal nerve.

sulcus nervi petrosi su·per·fi·ci·a·lis ma·jo·ris (sue"pur·fish·ee·ay'lis ma·jo'ris) [BNA]. SULCUS NERVI PETROSI MAJORIS.

sulcus nervi petrosi superficialis mi·no·ris (mi·no'ris) [BNA]. SULCUS NERVI PETROSI MINORIS.

sulcus nervi ra·di·a·lis (ray·dee·ay'lis) [NA]. RADIAL SULCUS.

sulcus nervi spi·na·lis (spye·nay'lis) [NA]. A groove on the upper surface of the transverse process of each cervical vertebra for the ventral branch of a spinal nerve.

sulcus nervi ul·na·ris (ul·nair'is) [NA]. The groove for the ulnar nerve on the medial epicondyle of the humerus.

sulcus ob·tu·ra·to·ri·us (ob·tew·ruh·to'ree·us) [NA]. OBTURATOR GROOVE.

sulcus oc·ci·pi·ta·lis trans·ver·sus (ock·sip·i·tay'lis trans·vur'sus) [NA]. TRANSVERSE OCCIPITAL SULCUS.

sulcus oc·ci·pi·to·tem·po·ra·lis (ock·sip"i·to·tem·po·ray'lis) [NA]. A sulcus separating the inferior frontal gyrus from the occipitotemporal gyrus.

sulcus of Monro [A. *Monro* (Secundus)]. HYPOTHALAMIC SULCUS.

sulcus of the auditory tube. A groove between the petrous part of the temporal bone and the greater wing of the sphenoid, lodging the cartilaginous part of the auditory tube. NA *sulcus tubae auditivae.*

sulcus of the sigmoid sinus. A deep groove on the inner surface of the skull which lodges the sigmoid sinus. NA *sulcus sinus sigmoidei.*

sulcus ol·fac·to·ri·us ca·vi na·si (ol·fack·to'ree·us kay'vye nay'zye) [NA]. A shallow sulcus in the wall of the nasal cavity adjacent to olfactory mucosa.

sulcus olfactorius lo·bi fron·ta·lis (lo'bye fron·tay'lis) [NA]. OLFACTORY SULCUS.

sulcus or·bi·ta·lis (or·bi·tay'lis). Singular of *sulci orbitales.*

sulcus pa·la·ti·nus ma·jor max·il·lae (pal·uh·tye'nus may'jor mack·sil'ee) [NA]. A groove on the nasal surface of the maxilla, which with a corresponding groove on the perpendicular part of the palatine bone forms the canal for the passage of the greater palatine nerve and accompanying vessels.

sulcus palatinus major os·sis pa·la·ti·ni (os'is pal·uh·tye'nigh) [NA]. A groove on the perpendicular plate of the palatine bone, which together with a corresponding groove on the maxilla forms a canal for the passage of the greater palatine nerve and accompanying vessels.

sulcus pa·la·to·va·gi·na·lis (pal''uh·to·vaj·i·nay'lis) [NA]. A small groove on the upper surface of the vaginal process of the sphenoid bone.

sulcus pa·ri·e·to·oc·ci·pi·ta·lis (pa·rye''e·to·ock·sip·i·tay'lis) [NA]. PARIETOOCCIPITAL SULCUS.

sulcus pa·rol·fac·to·ri·us anterior (păr''ol·fack·to'ree·us) [BNA]. The anterior parolfactory sulcus. See *parolfactory sulcus.*

sulcus parolfactorius posterior [BNA]. The posterior parolfactory sulcus. See *paralfactory sulcus.*

sulcus pe·tro·sus in·fe·ri·or os·sis oc·ci·pi·ta·lis (pe·tro'sus in·feer'ee·or os'is ock·sip·i·tay'lis) [BNA]. SULCUS SINUS PETROSI INFERIORIS OSSIS OCCIPITALIS.

sulcus petrosus inferior ossis tem·po·ra·lis (tem·po·ray'lis) [BNA]. SULCUS SINUS PETROSI INFERIORIS OSSIS TEMPORALIS.

sulcus petrosus superior ossis temporalis [BNA]. SULCUS SINUS PETROSI SUPERIORIS OSSIS TEMPORALIS.

sulcus post·cen·tra·lis (pohst''sen·tray'lis) [NA]. POSTCENTRAL SULCUS.

sulcus prae·cen·tra·lis (pree''sen·tray'lis) [BNA]. Sulcus precentralis (= PRECENTRAL SULCUS).

sulcus pre·cen·tra·lis (pree''sen·tray'lis) [NA]. PRECENTRAL SULCUS.

sulcus pri·ma·ri·us (prye·mair'ee·us). PRIMARY FISSURE.

sulcus pro·mon·to·rii (pro·mon·to'ree·eye) [NA]. A shallow groove on the promontory of the medial wall of the middle ear for the tympanic nerve.

sulcus pte·ry·go·pa·la·ti·nus os·sis pa·la·ti·ni (terr''i·go·pal·uh·tye'nus os'is pal·uh·tye'nigh) [BNA]. SULCUS PALATINUS MAJOR OSSIS PALATINI.

sulcus pul·mo·na·lis (pul·mo·nay'lis) [NA]. The posterior wall of each pleural cavity.

sulcus rhi·na·lis (rye·nay'lis) [NA]. A variable sulcus on the inferior surface of the temporal lobe of the cerebrum.

sulcus sa·git·ta·lis os·sis fron·ta·lis (saj·i·tay'lis os'is fron·tay'lis) [BNA]. SULCUS SINUS SAGITTALIS SUPERIORIS OSSIS FRONTALIS.

sulcus sagittalis ossis oc·ci·pi·ta·lis (ock·sip·i·tay'lis) [BNA]. SULCUS SINUS SAGITTALIS SUPERIORIS OSSIS OCCIPITALIS.

sulcus sagittalis ossis pa·ri·e·ta·lis (pa·rye·e·tay'lis) [BNA]. SULCUS SINUS SAGITTALIS SUPERIORIS OSSIS PARIETALIS.

sulcus scle·rae (skleer'ee) [NA]. SCLERAL SULCUS.

sulcus sig·moi·de·us (sig·moy'dee·us) [BNA]. Sulcus sinus sigmoidei (SULCUS OF THE SIGMOID SINUS).

sulcus si·nus pe·tro·si in·fe·ri·o·ris os·sis oc·ci·pi·ta·lis (sigh'nus pet·ro'sigh in·feer·ee·o'ris os'is ock·sip·i·tay'lis) [NA]. The groove for the inferior petrosal sinus on the occipital bone.

sulcus sinus petrosi inferioris ossis tem·po·ra·lis (tem·po·ray'lis) [NA]. The groove for the inferior petrosal sinus on the temporal bone.

sulcus sinus petrosi su·pe·ri·o·ris os·sis tem·po·ra·lis (sue·peer·ee·o'ris os'is tem·po·ray'lis) [NA]. The groove for the superior petrosal sinus on the temporal bone.

sulcus sinus sa·git·ta·lis su·pe·ri·o·ris os·sis fron·ta·lis (saj·i·tay'lis sue·peer·ee·o'ris os'is fron·tay'lis) [NA]. The groove on the inner surface of the frontal bone which lodges the superior sagittal sinus.

sulcus sinus sagittalis superioris ossis oc·ci·pi·ta·lis (ock·sip·i·tay'lis) [NA]. The groove on the inner surface of the occipital bone which lodges the superior sagittal sinus.

sulcus sinus sagittalis superioris ossis pa·ri·e·ta·lis (pa·rye·e·tay'lis) [NA]. The groove on the inner surface of the skull at the junction of the parietal bones which lodges the superior sagittal sinus.

sulcus sinus sig·moi·dei (sig·moy'dee·eye) [NA]. SULCUS OF THE SIGMOID SINUS.

sulcus sinus sigmoidei os·sis oc·ci·pi·ta·lis (os'is ock·sip·i·tay'lis) [NA]. The portion of the sulcus of the sigmoid sinus on the inner aspect of the occipital bone.

sulcus sinus sigmoidei ossis pa·ri·e·ta·lis (pa·rye·e·tay'lis) [NA]. The portion of the sulcus of the sigmoid sinus on the inner aspect of the parietal bone.

sulcus sinus sigmoidei ossis tem·po·ra·lis (tem·po·ray'lis) [NA]. The portion of the sulcus of the sigmoid sinus on the inner aspect of the temporal bone.

sulcus sinus trans·ver·si (trans·vur'sigh) [NA]. The sulcus of the transverse sinus.

sulcus spi·ra·lis (spye·ray'lis) [BNA]. See *sulcus spiralis externus, sulcus spiralis internus.*

sulcus spiralis ex·ter·nus (ecks·tur'nus) [NA]. OUTER SPIRAL SULCUS.

sulcus spiralis in·ter·nus (in·tur'nus) [NA]. SPIRAL SULCUS.

sulcus sub·cla·vi·ae (sub·klay'vee·ee) [BNA]. Sulcus arteriae subclaviae (= SUBCLAVIAN SULCUS).

sulcus sub·cla·vi·us pul·mo·nis (sub·klay'vee·us pul·mo'nis) [BNA]. A groove on the upper mediastinal surface of a fixed lung made by the subclavian artery.

sulcus sub·pa·ri·e·ta·lis (sub''pa·rye·e·tay'lis) [NA]. SUBPARIETAL SULCUS.

sulcus su·pra·pa·ri·e·ta·lis (sue''pruh·pa·rye·e·tay'lis) [BNA]. Sulcus subparietalis (= SUBPARIETAL SULCUS).

sulcus ta·li (tay'lye) [NA]. TALAR SULCUS.

sulcus tem·po·ra·lis inferior (tem·po·ray'lis) [NA]. The inferior temporal sulcus. See *temporal sulcus.*

sulcus temporalis me·di·us (mee'dee·us) [BNA]. The middle temporal sulcus (= inferior temporal sulcus). See *temporal sulcus.*

sulcus temporalis superior [NA]. The superior temporal sulcus. See *temporal sulcus.*

sulcus ten·di·nis mus·cu·li fi·bu·la·ris lon·gi cal·ca·nei (ten'di·nus mus'kew·lye fib·yoo·lair'is long'guy kal·kay'nee·eye) [NA alt.]. PERONEAL GROOVE. NA alt. *sulcus tendinis musculi peronei longi calcanei.*

sulcus tendinis musculi flex·o·ris hal·lu·cis lon·gi cal·ca·nei (ten'di·nis mus'kew·lye fleck·so'ris hal'yoo·sis long'guy kal·kay'nee·eye) [NA]. The groove on the inferior surface of the sustentaculum of the calcaneus for the tendon of the flexor hallucis longus muscle.

sulcus tendinis musculi flexoris hallucis longi ta·li (tay'lye) [NA]. The groove on posterior surface of the posterior process of the talus for the tendon of the flexor hallucis longus muscle.

sulcus tendinis musculi pe·ro·nei lon·gi cal·ca·nei (perr·o·nee'eye long'guy kal·kay'nee·eye) [NA]. PERONEAL GROOVE.

sulcus tendinis musculi peronei longi os·sis cu·boi·dei (os'is kew·boy'dee·eye) [NA]. The groove on the inferior surface of the cuboid for the tendon of the peroneus longus muscle.

sulcus ter·mi·na·lis atrii dex·tri (tur·mi·nay'lis ay'tree·eye decks'trye) [NA]. TERMINAL CARDIAC SULCUS.

sulcus terminalis lin·guae (ling'gwee) [NA]. TERMINAL LINGUAL SULCUS.

sulcus trans·ver·sus os·sis oc·ci·pi·ta·lis (trans·vur'sus os'is ock·sip·i·tay'lis) [BNA]. SULCUS SINUS TRANSVERSI.

sulcus transversus ossis pa·ri·e·ta·lis (pa·rye·e·tay'lis) [BNA]. SULCUS SINUS SIGMOIDEI OSSIS PARIETALIS.

sulcus tu·bae au·di·ti·vae (tew'bee aw·di·tye'vee) [NA]. SULCUS OF THE AUDITORY TUBE.

sulcus tym·pa·ni·cus (tim·pan'i·kus) [NA]. TYMPANIC SULCUS.

sulcus ve·nae ca·vae (vee'nee kay'vee) [NA]. A groove on the posterior surface of the liver between the caudate and right lobes occupied by the inferior vena cava.

sulcus venae sub·cla·vi·ae (sub-klay'vee-ee) [NA]. A shallow, indistinct groove on the upper orifice of the first rib for the subclavian vein.

sulcus venae um·bi·li·ca·lis (um-bil-i-kay'lis) [NA]. UMBILICAL FOSSA.

sulcus vo·me·ro·va·gi·na·lis (vo"me-ro-vaj-i-nay'lis) [NA]. A medial groove on the superior surface of the vaginal process of the pterygoid process.

sul·fa·ben·za·mide (sul"fuh-ben'zuh-mide) *n.* *N*-Sulfanilylbenzamide, $C_{13}H_{12}N_2O_3S$, an antibacterial.

sul·fa·cet·a·mide (sul"fuh-set'uh-mide) *n.* *N*-Sulfanilylacetamide, $C_8H_{10}N_2O_3S$, used for the treatment of urinary tract infections; the sodium derivative is used for treatment of ophthalmic infections susceptible to sulfonamides.

sul·fa·chlor·py·rid·a·zine (sul"fuh-klor"pye-rid'uh-zeen) *n.* N^1-(6-Chloro-3-pyridazinyl)sulfanilamide, $C_{10}H_9ClN_4O_2S$, a sulfonamide used in the treatment of urinary tract infections.

sul·fa·cy·tine ((sul"fuh-sye'teen) *n.* 1-Ethyl-*N*-sulfanilylcytosine, $C_{12}H_{14}N_4O_3S$, an antibacterial.

sul·fa·di·a·zine (sul"fuh-dye'uh-zeen, -zin, -dye-az'een) *n.* N^1-2-Pyrimidinylsulfanilamide, $C_{10}H_{10}N_4O_2S$, an antibacterial sulfonamide used in the treatment of a variety of infections; frequently given in combination with sulfamerazine and sulfamethazine. Sodium sulfadiazine, which is freely soluble in water, is used when the drug is to be administered intravenously.

sul·fa·di·meth·ox·ine (sul"fuh-dye"meth-ock'seen) *n.* N^1-(2,6-Dimethoxy-4-pyrimidinyl)sulfanilamide, $C_{12}H_{14}N_4O_4S$, a sulfonamide for general use.

sul·fa·di·me·tine (sul"fuh-dye'me-teen) *n.* SULFISOMIDINE.

sul·fa·dox·ine (sul"fuh-dock'seen) *n.* N^1-(5,6-Dimethoxy-4-pyrimidinyl)sulfanilamide, $C_{12}H_{14}N_4O_4S$, an antibacterial sulfonamide.

sul·fa drugs (sul'fuh). A family of drugs of the sulfonamide type which have marked bacteriostatic properties.

sul·fa·eth·i·dole (sul"fuh-eth'i-dole) *n.* N^1-(5-Ethyl-1,3,4-thiadiazol-2-yl)sulfanilamide, $C_{10}H_{12}N_4O_2S_2$, a sulfonamide effective against many gram-positive and gram-negative organisms. Syn. *sulfaethylthiadiazole.*

sul·fa·eth·yl·thia·di·a·zole (sul"fuh-eth"il-thigh-uh-dye'uh-zole) *n.* SULFAETHIDOLE.

sul·fa·gua·ni·dine (sul"fuh-gwah'ni-deen, -gwan'i-deen, -din) *n.* N^1-Amidinosulfanilamide, $C_7H_{10}N_4O_2S$, an intestinal antibacterial sulfonamide proposed for treatment of dysentery and for sterilization of the colon prior to gastrointestinal tract surgery.

sul·fa·lene (sul'fuh-leen) *n.* N^1-(3-Methoxy-2-pyrazinyl)sulfanilamide, $C_{11}H_{12}N_4O_3S$, an antibacterial sulfonamide.

sul·fa·mer·a·zine (sul"fuh-merr'uh-zeen, -zin) *n.* N^1-(4-Methyl-2-pyrimidinyl)sulfanilamide, $C_{11}H_{12}N_4O_2S$; used like sulfadiazine but generally employed in combination with it and with sulfamethazine.

sul·fa·me·ter (sul'fuh-mee"tur) *n.* N^1-(5-Methoxy-2-pyrimidinyl)sulfanilamide, $C_{11}H_{12}N_4O_3S$, an antibacterial sulfonamide. Syn. *sulfamethoxydiazine.*

sul·fa·meth·a·zine (sul"fuh-meth'uh-zeen, -zin) *n.* N^1-(4,6-Dimethyl-2-pyrimidinyl)sulfanilamide, $C_{12}H_{14}N_4O_2S$; used like sulfadiazine but generally employed in combination with it and with sulfamerazine. Syn. *sulphadimidine, sulfamezathine.*

sul·fa·meth·i·zole (sul"fuh-meth'i-zole) *n.* N^1-(5-Methyl-1,3,4-thiadiazol-2-yl)sulfanilamide, $C_9H_{10}N_4O_2S_2$, a sulfonamide used for treatment of infections of the urinary tract.

sul·fa·meth·ox·a·zole (sul"fuh-meth-ock'suh-zole) *n.* 5-Methyl-3-sulfanilamidoisoxazole, $C_{10}H_{11}N_3O_3S$, an antibacterial sulfonamide.

sul·fa·me·thoxy·di·a·zine (sul"fuh-me-thock"see-dye'uh-zeen) *n.* SULFAMETER.

sul·fa·me·thoxy·py·rid·a·zine (sul"fuh-me-thock"see-pi-rid'uh-zeen) *n.* N^1-(6-Methoxy-3-pyridazinyl)sulfanilamide, $C_{11}H_{12}N_4O_3S$, an antibacterial sulfonamide characterized by an exceptionally low rate of excretion.

sul·fa·mez·a·thine (sul"fuh-mez'uh-theen, -thin) *n.* SULFAMETHAZINE.

sul·fa·mono·meth·ox·ine (sul"fuh-mon-o-meth-ock'seen) *n.* N^1-(6-Methoxy-4-pyrimidinyl)sulfanilamide, $C_{11}H_{12}N_4O_3S$, an antibacterial sulfonamide.

sul·fa·mox·ole (sul"fuh-mock'sole) *n.* N^1-(4,5-Dimethyl-2-oxazolyl)sulfanilamide, $C_{11}H_{13}N_3O_3S$, an antibacterial sulfonamide.

Sulfamylon. Trademark for mafenide, an antibacterial sulfonamide.

sul·fa·nil·a·mide (sul"fuh-nil'uh-mide) *n.* *p*-Aminobenzenesulfonamide, $NH_2C_6H_4SO_2NH_2$, the predecessor of a large group of sulfonamides which, by virtue of being more effective and less toxic than sulfanilamide, have supplanted it.

sul·fan·i·late (sul-fan'i-late) *n.* A salt of sulfanilic acid.

sul·fa·nil·ic acid (sul"fuh-nil'ick). *p*-Aminobenzenesulfonic acid, $NH_2C_6H_4SO_3H$; used as a reagent.

sul·fa·pyr·a·zole (sul"fuh-pirr'uh-zole) *n.* SULFAZAMET.

sul·fa·pyr·i·dine (sul"fuh-pirr'i-deen, -din) *n.* N^1-2-Pyridylsulfanilamide, $C_{11}H_{11}N_3O_2S$, a sulfonamide formerly used for the treatment of various infections but found to be too toxic for general use; now employed only as a suppressant for dermatitis herpetiformis.

sulf·ars·phen·a·mine (sulf"ahrs-fen'uh-meen, -min) *n.* Consists chiefly of disodium 3,3'-diamino-4,4'-dihydroxyarsenobenzene-*N*-dimethylenesulfonate; has been used in the treatment of syphilis.

sul·fa·sal·a·zine (sul"fuh-sal'uh-zeen) *n.* 5-[[*p*-(2-Pyridylsulfamoyl)phenyl]azo]salicylic acid, $C_{18}H_{14}N_4O_5S$, an antibacterial.

sul·fa·som·i·zole (sul"fuh-som'i-zole, -so'mi-zole) *n.* N^1-(3-Methyl-5-isothiazolyl)sulfanilamide, $C_{10}H_{11}N_3O_2S_2$, an antibacterial sulfonamide.

sul·fa·tase (sul'fuh-tace, -taze) *n.* Any enzyme that hydrolyzes an ethereal sulfate (ester sulfate).

sulfatase A deficiency. An enzyme deficiency state that may be responsible for metachromatic leukodystrophy.

sul·fate (sul'fate) *n.* A salt or ester of sulfuric acid.

Sulfathalidine. Trademark for phthalysulfathiazole, a poorly absorbed sulfonamide used for suppressing growth of bacteria in the large intestine.

sul·fa·thi·a·zole (sul"fuh-thigh'uh-zole) *n.* N^1-2-Thiazolylsulfanilamide, $C_9H_9N_3O_2S_2$, formerly widely used in the treatment of pneumococcal, staphylococcal, and urinary tract infections; it has been replaced by less toxic sulfonamides.

sul·fa·tide (sul'fuh-tide) *n.* Any cerebroside with a sulfate group esterified to the galactase.

sulfatide lipidosis. METACHROMATIC LEUKODYSTROPHY.

sul·fat·i·do·sis (sul-fat"i-do'sis) *n.* [*sulfatide* + *-osis*]. An excess of sulfatides, such as that occurring in the neural tissues in metachromatic leukodystrophy.

sul·faz·a·met (sul-faz'uh-met) *n.* N^1-(3-Methyl-1-phenylpyrazol-5-yl)sulfanilamide, $C_{16}H_{16}N_4O_2S$, an antibacterial sulfonamide. Syn. *sulfapyrazole.*

sulf·ben·za·mine (sulf-ben'zuh-meen) *n.* MAFENIDE.

sulf·he·mo·glo·bin (sulf-hee'muh-glo"bin) *n.* A greenish substance derived from hemoglobin by the action of hydrogen sulfide. It may appear in the blood following the ingestion of sulfanilamide and other substances. Syn. *sulfmethemoglobin.*

sulf·he·mo·glo·bi·ne·mia (sulf-hee"muh-glo-bi-nee'mee-uh) *n.* [*sulfhemoglobin* + *-emia*]. A condition in which sulfhemoglobin is present in the blood; the symptoms are similar to those present in methemoglobinemia.

sulf·hy·drate (sulf-high'drate) *n.* A compound of a base with the univalent radical sulfhydryl, HS—.

sulf·hy·dryl (sulf-high'dril) *n.* The univalent radical HS—, usually attached to a carbon chain. The presence of active sulfhydryl groups is important for the activity of many enzymes. Syn. *SH group.*

sul·fide (sul'fide) *n.* A compound of sulfur with an element or basic radical.

sul·fine (sul'fine) *n.* SULFONIUM.

sul·fin·pyr·a·zone (sul''fin·pirr'uh·zone, ·pye'ruh·zone) *n.* 1,2-Diphenyl-4-(2'-phenylsulfinethyl)-3,5-pyrazolidinedione, $C_{23}H_{20}N_2O_3S$, a potent uricosuric agent, related to phenylbutazone; used in the management of gout.

sul·fi·som·i·dine (sul''fi·som'i·deen, ·so'mi·deen, ·din) *n.* N^1-(2,6-Dimethyl-4-pyrimidinyl)sulfanilamide, $C_{12}H_{14}N_4O_2S$, a structural isomer of sulfamethazine; useful for the treatment of systemic and urinary tract infections caused by microorganisms susceptible to bacteriostatic effects of sulfonamides. Syn., *sulfadimetine.*

sul·fi·sox·a·zole (sul''fi·sock'suh·zole, sulf''eye·) *n.* N^1-(3,4-Dimethyl-5-isoxazolyl)sulfanilamide, $C_{11}H_{13}N_3O_3S$, a sulfonamide of general therapeutic utility. For parenteral administration the soluble salt sulfisoxazole diethanolamine is used; for pediatric use the tasteless derivative acetyl sulfisoxazole is given. Syn. *sulphafurazole.*

sul·fite (sul'fite) *n.* A salt of sulfurous acid of the type M_2SO_3.

sulf·met·he·mo·glo·bin (sulf''met·hee'muh·glo''bin) *n.* SULFHEMOGLOBIN.

sulfo-. A combining form generally indicating *the presence of divalent sulfur* or *the sulfo- group,* $—SO_3H$.

sul·fo acid (sul'fo). 1. THIOACID. 2. SULFONIC ACID.

sul·fo·bro·mo·phthal·ein sodium (sul''fo·bro''mo·thal'ee·in) *n.* Disodium 3,3'-(tetrabromophthalidylidene)bis (6-hydroxybenzenesulfonate), $C_{20}H_8Br_4Na_2O_{10}S_2$, a diagnostic aid used intravenously to determine the functional capacity of the liver.

sul·fo·car·bo·late (sul''fo·kahr'buh·late) *n.* A salt of phenolsulfonic acid.

sul·fo·car·bol·ic acid (sul''fo·kahr·bol'ick). PHENOLSULFONIC ACID.

sul·fo·cy·a·nate (sul''fo·sigh'uh·nate) *n.* THIOCYANATE.

sul·fo·cy·an·ic acid (sul''fo·sigh·an'ick). THIOCYANIC ACID.

sul·fo·mu·cin (sul''fo·mew'sin) *n.* Any acid mucopolysaccharide characterized by the presence of sulfuric acid ester groups.

Sulfonal. Trademark for sulfonmethane.

sul·fon·amide (sul·fon'uh·mide, sul·fo'nuh·mide, ·mid) *n.* Any of a group of compounds derived from sulfanilamide, $H_2NC_6H_4SO_2NH_2$, and used in the treatment of various bacterial infections. Members of the group vary with respect to activity, degree and rate of absorption, metabolic alteration and excretion, and toxic manifestations produced. Prominent among their adverse effects is renal damage, particularly of the type caused by the crystallization of their N^4-acetyl derivatives in the urinary tract; many other toxic effects have been noted, of which some can be attributed to sensitization.

sul·fo·nate (sul'fuh·nate) *v. & n.* 1. To treat an aromatic hydrocarbon with fuming sulfuric acid. 2. A sulfuric acid derivative. 3. The ester of a sulfonic acid.

sulfonated bitumen. ICHTHAMMOL.

sul·fo·na·tion (sul''fo·nay'shun) *n.* A chemical process resulting in the introduction in a compound of one or more sulfo- groups.

sul·fone (sul'fone) *n.* An oxidation product of thio- compounds containing the group SO_2 attached to a hydrocarbon group, such as RSO_2R.

sul·fone·phthal·ein (sul''fone·thal'ee·in) *n.* Any one of a group of organic compounds made by the interaction of phenols with acid chlorides or anhydrides of orthosulfobenzoic acid and its derivatives, such as thymolsulfonephthalein and phenolsulfonephthalein.

sul·fon·eth·yl·meth·ane (sul''fone·eth''il·meth'ane) *n.* Diethylsulfonemethylethylmethane, $CH_3C_2H_5C(SO_2C_2H_5)_2$, formerly extensively used as a hypnotic. Syn. *methylsulfonal.*

sul·fon·ic acid (sul·fon'ick). An organic acid containing the $—SO_3H$ or $—SO_2OH$ group.

sul·fo·ni·um (sul·fo'nee·um) *n.* The univalent, electropositive radical $R_3S^+—$, in which R is an organic radical. Syn. *sulfine.*

sul·fon·meth·ane (sul''fone·meth'ane) *n.* Diethylsulfonedimethylmethane, $(CH_3)_2C(SO_2C_2H_5)_2$, formerly extensively used as a hypnotic.

sul·fon·ter·ol (sul·fon'tur·ole) *n.* α-[(*tert*-Butylamino)methyl]-4-hydroxy-3-[(methylsulfonyl)methyl]benzyl alcohol, $C_{14}H_{23}NO_4S$, a bronchodilator, used as the hydrochloride salt.

sul·fo·nyl (sul'fo·nil) *n.* The bivalent radical $—SO_2—$.

sul·fo·nyl·urea (sul''fo·nil·yoo·ree'uh) *n.* Any of a number of oral hypoglycemic agents, such as acetohexamide, chlorpropamide, tolazamide and tolbutamide, which act with beta cells in the pancreas to increase the secretion of endogenous insulin.

sul·fo·phe·nate (sul''fo·fee'nate) *n.* 1. Phenolsulfonate, a salt or ester of phenolsulfonic acid, $C_6H_4(OH)SO_3H$. 2. Phenylsulfate, a salt of phenylsulfuric acid, $C_6H_5OSO_3H$.

sul·fo·phen·yl·ate (sul''fo·fen'i·late) *n.* SULFOPHENATE.

sul·fo·sal·i·cyl·ic acid (sul''fo·sal''i·sil'ick). 3-Carboxy-4-hydroxybenzenesulfonic acid, $C_7H_6O_6S$; used as a reagent, mainly for protein in urine, and also for decalcification of bone for histologic study.

sulfosalicylic acid test. A test for urine protein, in which a sulfosalicylic acid solution produces cloudiness in the presence of protein.

sul·fo·salt (sul'fo·sawlt) *n.* A salt of sulfonic acid.

sulf·ox·ide (sulf·ock'side) *n.* 1. The divalent radical $=SO$. 2. An organic compound of the type of R_2SO or $RSOR'$, where R and R' are organic radicals.

sulf·ox·one sodium (sulf·ock'sone) *n.* Disodium [sulfonylbis(*p*-phenyleneimino)]di(methanesulfinate), $C_{14}H_{14}N_2Na_2O_6S_3$, a drug used in the treatment of lepromatous and tuberculoid leprosy, and as a suppressant for dermatitis herpetiformis.

sul·fur, sul·phur (sul'fur) *n.* [L.]. S = 32.06. A solid, nonmetallic element, atomic number 16. Occurs as a yellow, brittle mass or in transparent monoclinic or rhombic crystals and exists in a number of modifications. Sometimes used as a laxative but mainly externally in the treatment of various parasitic and nonparasitic diseases of the skin.

sul·fu·rat·ed (sul'fuh·ray''tid, sul'few·) *n.* Combined with sulfur.

sulfurated lime. Crude CALCIUM SULFIDE.

sulfurated lime solution. A solution of calcium pentasulfide, CaS_5, and calcium thiosulfate, CaS_2O_3, prepared by interaction of lime and sulfur in boiling water. Diluted with water, it is used mainly as a scabicide. Syn. *Vleminckx's solution.*

sulfurated potash. A mixture composed chiefly of potassium polysulfides and potassium thiosulfate; used as a parasiticide and to stimulate and soften the skin in chronic cutaneous diseases. Syn. *liver of sulfur.*

sul·fu·ra·tor (sul'few·ray''tur, sul'fuh·) *n.* An apparatus for applying sulfur dioxide fumes for purposes of disinfection.

sulfur dioxide. A gas, SO_2, with strong reducing action in water. Sometimes employed in preparation of medicinal dosage forms as an antioxidant; has been used as a space disinfectant.

sulfur granules. Yellow flecks composed of masses of densely packed, delicate, branching filaments characteristically exhibiting clublike structures at the periphery; found in tissues infected by *Actinomyces.*

sul·fu·ric acid (sul·few'rick). A solution containing about 96% H_2SO_4, the remainder being water; occurs as a colorless, odorless liquid of oily consistency. Used as a reagent, and in various syntheses, but not employed medicinally. Syn. *oil of vitriol.*

sulfuric ether. ETHER (3).

sul·fu·rous (sul'few·rus) *adj.* 1. Of the nature of sulfur. 2. Combined with sulfur; derived from sulfur dioxide.

sulfurous acid. H_2SO_3. A solution of sulfur dioxide in water; used as a decalcifying agent in histology. Formerly employed as a gastric antiseptic and for treatment of skin diseases.

sulfur trioxide. Sulfuric anhydride, SO_3, existing in three forms, two being solid, and one liquid, at room temperature; an intermediate in the manufacture of sulfuric acid and used in chemical syntheses.

su·lin·dac (suh·lin'dack) *n.* (*Z*)-5-Fluoro-2-methyl-1-[*p*-(methylsulfinyl)benzylidene] indene-3-acetic acid, $C_{20}H_{17}FO_3S$, an anti-inflammatory.

sul·iso·ben·zone (sul·eye"so·ben'zone) *n.* 5-Benzoyl-4-hydroxy-2-methoxybenesulfonic acid, $C_{14}H_{12}O_6S$, an ultraviolet screening agent.

Sul·ko·witch's test [H. W. *Sulkowitch,* U.S. internist, b. 1906]. A test for calcium in the urine, in which equal parts of clear urine and Sulkowitch's reagent (oxalic acid, ammonium oxalate, glacial acetic acid, distilled water) are mixed. A fine white precipitate suggests normal serum calcium, no precipitate suggests reduced calcium, and a milky precipitate suggests increased serum calcium.

Sulla. Trademark for the antibacterial drug sulfameter.

sul·lage (sul'ij) *n.* [MF. *souiller,* to soil]. SEWAGE.

Sul·li·van's test [M. S. *Sullivan,* U.S. biochemist, b. 1875]. A test for cystine, in which, with sodium β-naphthoquinone-4-sulfonate, cysteine develops a red color in the presence of alkali; when treated with sodium cyanide, cystine produces the color.

sul·nid·az·ole (sul·nid'uh·zole) *n.* *O*-Methyl [2-(2-ethyl-5-nitroimidazol-1-yl)ethyl]thiocarbamate, $C_9H_{14}N_4O_3S$, an antiprotozoal effective against *Trichomonas.*

sul·ox·i·fen (sul·ock'si·fen) *n.* *N*-[(2-Diethylamino)ethyl]-*S,S*-diphenylsulfoximine, $C_{18}H_{24}N_2OS$, a bronchodilator, used as the oxalate salt.

sul·pha·dim·i·dine (sul"fuh·dim'i·deen) *n.* SULFAMETHAZINE.

sul·pha·fu·ra·zole (sul"fuh·few'ruh·zole) *n.* SULFISOXAZOLE.

sul·phate (sul'fate) *n.* SULFATE.

sulph·e·mo·glo·bi·ne·mia, sulph·ae·mo·glo·bi·nae·mia (sul·fee"muh·glo"bi·nee'mee·uh, sulf·hee") *n.* SULFHEMOGLOBINEMIA.

Sulphetrone. Trademark for the leprostatic drug solapsone.

sulphur. SULFUR.

Sul-Spansion. Trademark for a suspension of the sulfonamide sulfaethidole.

Sul-Spantab. Trademark for a tablet dosage form of the sulfonamide sulfaethidole.

sul·thi·ame (sul·thigh'ame) *n.* *p*-(Tetrahydro-2*H*-1,2-thiazin-2-yl)benzenesulfonamide *S,S*-dioxide, $C_{10}H_{14}N_2O_4S_2$, an anticonvulsant drug.

Sulz·ber·ger-Garbe disease [M. *Sulzberger,* U.S. dermatologist, b. 1895; and W. *Garbe,* Canadian dermatologist, b. 1908]. A disease, thought to be a neurodermatitis, characterized by discoid, lichenoid, and eczematoid dermatitis.

sum. Abbreviation for (a) *sume,* take; (b) *sumendus,* to be taken; used as a direction in prescriptions.

su·mac, su·mach (sue'mack, shoo'mack) *n.* [OF., from Ar. *summāq*]. A name applied to various species of *Rhus,* especially the nonpoisonous species. See also *poison sumac.*

sum·bul (sum'bul) *n.* [Ar. *sunbul*]. The dried rhizome and roots of *Ferula sumbul,* or other closely related species of *Ferula* possessing a characteristic musklike odor; formerly used as a sedative.

sum·ma·tion (sum·ay'shun) *n.* [ML. *summatio,* from *summa,* sum]. The additory effect of individual events, especially of those of muscular, sensory, or mental stimuli. —**summa·tion·al** (·ul) *adj.*

summation gallop. A gallop sound due to coincidence of the third and fourth heart sounds.

summation of stimuli. 1. SPATIAL SUMMATION. 2. TEMPORAL SUMMATION.

sum·mer diarrhea. An acute diarrhea, usually of children, especially during the summer, associated with an increased prevalence of enteropathogenic bacteria and viruses, as in poorly refrigerated food.

summer diarrhea of children. INFANTILE DIARRHEA.

summer eruption. MILIARIA.

summer prurigo. HYDROA VACCINIFORME.

Sum·mer·son-Bar·ker method [W. H. *Summerson;* and S. B. *Barker,* U.S. physiologist, 20th century]. A method for lactic acid in the blood, in which the glucose and other interfering material of the protein-free blood filtrate are removed by treatment with copper sulfate and calcium hydroxide. An aliquot of the resulting solution is heated with concentrated sulfuric acid to convert lactic acid to aldehyde, which is then determined colorimetrically by reaction with *p*-hydroxydiphenyl in the presence of copper ions.

Sum·ner method [J. B. *Sumner,* U.S. biochemist, 1887–1955]. A method for glucose in the urine, in which urine is heated with dinitrosalicylic acid reagent which is reduced by the sugar, and the resultant color is compared with standards.

Sumner's sign [F. W. *Sumner,* English surgeon, 20th century]. A sign indicative of cystic calculi, appendicitis, or a twisted pedicle of an ovarian cyst. A slight increase in abdominal muscle tonus is detected by very gentle palpation of the iliac fossa.

sump drain. An aspirating tubular drain of rubber, plastic, glass, etc., sometimes with lateral openings and fishtail ends, designed to provide continuous removal of accumulated secretions.

sun bath. The exposure of part or all the body to the sun for actinic effect.

sun blindness. Blindness, either temporary or permanent, caused by retinal injury resulting from gazing at the sun without adequate protection. Syn. *photoretinitis.*

sun·burn, *n.* 1. Erythema, tenderness and vesiculobullous changes of the skin due to exposure to the sun. 2. Inflammation of the skin, due to the action of the sun's rays, which may be of the first or second degree. —**sun·burned, sun·burnt,** *adj.*

sun·cil·lin (sun·sil'in) *n.* An antibacterial sulfamino ampicillin derivative, $C_{16}H_{19}N_3O_7S_2$, used as the disodium salt.

Sun·day morning paralysis. DRUNKARD'S ARM PARALYSIS.

sun lamp. A lamp designed to give off radiations of wavelengths similar to those received from the sun.

sun·shine vitamin. VITAMIN D.

sun·spots, *n.pl.* LENTIGINES.

sun·stroke, *n.* A form of heat stroke occurring on exposure to the sun, characterized by extreme pyrexia, prostration, convulsion, coma. Syn. *insolation, thermic fever.* See also *heatstroke.*

super- [L.]. A prefix meaning (a) *above, upon;* (b) *extreme, in high degree;* (c) *excessive, over-;* (d) *ranking next above, superordinate to.*

su·per·ab·duc·tion (sue"pur·ab·duck'shun) *n.* HYPERABDUCTION.

su·per·ac·id (sue'pur·as"id, sue"pur·as'id) *n.* [*super-* + *acid*]. A highly ionized acid or solution of an acid, as a solution of perchloric acid in glacial acetic acid. Compare *hyperacid.*

su·per·acid·i·ty (sue"pur·a·sid'i·tee) *n.* HYPERACIDITY.

su·per·ac·tiv·i·ty (sue"pur·ack·tiv'i·tee) *n.* HYPERACTIVITY.

su·per·acute (sue"pur·uh·kewt') *adj.* Extremely acute.

su·per·al·bu·mi·no·sis (sue"pur·al·bew"mi·no'sis) *n.* [*super-* + *albumin* + *-osis*]. The overproduction of albumin.

su·per·al·i·men·ta·tion (sue"pur·al"i·men·tay'shun) *n.* [*super-* + *alimentation*]. Overfeeding; the taking in or administration of food or nutritive substances in excess of ordinary metabolic requirements.

su·per·al·ka·lin·i·ty (sue″pur·al″kuh·lin′i·tee) *n.* Excessive alkalinity.

su·per·bus (sue·pur′bus) *n.* MENTALIS.

su·per·cer·e·bel·lar (sue″pur·serr″e·bel′ur) *adj.* [*super-* + *cerebellar*]. Situated in the upper part of the cerebellum.

su·per·cil·ia. 1. Plural of *supercilium.* 2. EYEBROW (2).

su·per·ci·li·ary ridge or **arch.** SUPRAORBITAL RIDGE.

su·per·cil·i·um (sue″pur·sil′ee·um) *n.*, pl. **supercil·ia** (·ee·uh) [L., from *super-* + *cilium,* eyelid] [NA]. EYEBROW (1). —**supercili·ary** (·err″ee) *adj.*

su·per·di·crot·ic (sue″pur·dye·krot′ick) *adj.* HYPERDICROTIC.

su·per·dis·ten·tion (sue″pur·dis·ten′shun) *n.* Excessive distention; HYPERDISTENTION.

su·per·duct (sue″pur·dukt′) *v.* [L. *superducere,* to lead over]. To elevate; to lead upward.

su·per·duc·tion (sue″pur·duck′shun) *n.* [L. *superductio,* from *superducere,* to lead over]. SURSUMDUCTION.

su·per·ego (sue″pur·ee′go) *n.* [*super-* + *ego*]. *In psychoanalysis,* the subdivision of the psyche that acts as the conscience of the unconscious. Its components are derived from both the id and the ego, and are associated with standards of behavior, both personal and social, and self-criticism. It is formed in early life by identification with the individuals, primarily the parents or surrogates, who are esteemed and whose love is sought.

superego lacuna. *In psychiatry,* a gap or defect in superego functioning, resulting from selective inattention to conduct which the parents appear to disregard.

su·per·en·er·get·ic phonation (sue″pur·en″ur·jet′ick). HYPERPHONIA.

su·per·evac·u·a·tion (sue″pur·e·vack″yoo·ay′shun) *n.* Excessive evacuation.

su·per·ex·ci·ta·tion (sue″pur·eck″si·tay′shun) *n.* [*super-* + *excitation*]. Excessive excitement; overstimulation.

su·per·ex·ten·sion (sue″pur·eck·sten′shun) *n.* [*super-* + *extension*]. Excessive extension; HYPEREXTENSION.

su·per·fam·i·ly (sue′pur·fam″i·lee) *n.* A taxonomic category ranking just above a family.

su·per·fe·cun·da·tion (sue″pur·fee″kun·day′shun, ·feck″un·) *n.* [*super-* + *fecundation*]. The fertilization of two or more ova, ovulated more or less simultaneously, by two or more coital acts not necessarily involving the same male.

su·per·fe·cun·di·ty (sue″pur·fe·kun′di·tee) *n.* [*super-* + *fecundity*]. Superabundant fertility.

su·per·fe·ta·tion, su·per·foe·ta·tion (sue″pur·fee·tay′shun) *n.* [*super-* + *fetation*]. The production or development of a second fetus after one is already present in the uterus.

su·per·fi·cial (sue″pur·fish′ul) *adj.* [L. *superficialis,* from *superficies,* surface]. Confined to or pertaining to the surface.

superficial calcaneal bursitis. ACHILLOBURSITIS.

superficial cleavage. Meroblastic cleavage restricted to the peripheral cytoplasm, as in the centrolecithal insect ovum.

superficial fascia. A sheet of subcutaneous tissue. NA *tela subcutanea.*

superficial folliculitis. A type of pustular folliculitis in which the pustule is limited to the distal portion of the hair follicles. Syn. *folliculitis simplex.*

superficial gland. A gland lying entirely within the limits of a mucous membrane.

superficial inguinal ring. An obliquely placed triangular opening in the aponeurosis of the external oblique abdominal muscle forming the external opening of the inguinal canal. Syn. *external inguinal ring.* NA *anulus inguinalis superficialis.*

superficial keratitis. Keratitis affecting primarily the epithelium, Bowman's membrane, and superficial lamellae of the substantia propria of the cornea.

superficial palmar arch. The arterial anastomosis formed by the ulnar artery in the palm with a branch from the radial artery. NA *arcus palmaris superficialis.* See also Table of Arteries in the Appendix and Plate 7.

superficial reflex. Any reflex occurring in response to superficial stimulation, as of the skin.

superficial spreading malignant melanoma. A type of malignant melanoma in which anaplastic melanocytes involve the epidermis primarily, thickening and elevating it; may be confined to the epidermis or invade the dermis; involves skin not exposed to the sun in most cases. Syn. *pagetoid malignant melanoma.*

superficial transverse metacarpal ligament. A group of transverse fibers in the central region of the palm, crossing between the diverging bundles of the plantar aponeurosis. NA *ligamentum metacarpeum transversum superficiale.*

superficial transverse metatarsal ligament. A band of fibers in the plantar aponeurosis running transversely beneath the heads of the metatarsals. NA *ligamentum metatarseum transversum superficiale.*

superficial volar arch. SUPERFICIAL PALMAR ARCH.

su·per·fi·ci·es (sue″pur·fish′ee·eez, ·fish′eez) *n.*, pl. **superficies** [L., from *super-* + *facies,* face]. The outer surface.

superfoetation. SUPERFETATION.

su·per·fu·sion (sue″pur·few′zhun) *n.* [L., *superfusio,* pouring over, from *super-* + *fundere,* to pour]. Metabolic study of an intact organ by allowing medium to flow over it; only extremely small and thin organs are suitable.

su·pe·ri·ad (sue·peer′ee·ad) *adv.* *In anatomy,* upward; in an inferior-to-superior direction. Compare *craniad.*

su·per·im·preg·na·tion (sue″pur·im″preg·nay′shun) *n.* [*super-* + *impregnation*]. 1. SUPERFETATION. 2. SUPERFECUNDATION.

su·per·in·duce (sue″pur·in·dewce′) *v.* [L. *superinducere,* to bring upon]. To add a new factor or a complication of a condition already existing.

su·per·in·fec·tion (sue″pur·in·feck′shun) *n.* A second or subsequent infection by the same microorganism, as seen in tuberculosis, or by a different organism, as seen following antibiotic therapy.

su·per·in·vo·lu·tion (sue″pur·in″vo·lew′shun) *n.* [*super-* + *involution*]. 1. HYPERINVOLUTION. 2. Excessive rolling up.

su·pe·ri·or (sue·peer′ee·ur) *adj.* [L., upper, higher]. *In anatomy* (with reference to the human or animal body as poised for its usual manner of locomotion): upper; farther from the ground or surface of locomotion. Compare *cranial.* Contr. *inferior.*—**superior·ly,** *adv.*

superior alveolar canals. ALVEOLAR CANALS.

superior angle of the scapula. The angle formed by the superior and medial margins of the triangular scapula. NA *angulus superior scapulae.*

superior articular process. One of a pair of processes projecting upward from the side of the vertebral arch and articulating with an inferior articulating process of the vertebra above.

superior bulb of the internal jugular vein. An enlargement of the internal jugular vein at the point of exit from the jugular foramen. NA *bulbus venae jugularis superior.*

superior carotid triangle. A triangle bounded above by the posterior belly of the digastric and the stylohyoid, behind by the sternocleidomastoid, and below by the omohyoid. Syn. *carotid triangle, triangle of election.* NA *trigonum caroticum.*

superior central nucleus. A group of cells in the reticular formation in the upper pontine levels.

superior cerebellar peduncle. A large band of nerve fibers which arise in the dentate and emboliform nuclei of the cerebellum, form the dorsolateral part of the rostral portion of the fourth ventricle, decussate in the region of the inferior colliculi, and end in the red nucleus and ventrolateral thalamus. Syn. *brachium conjunctivum.* NA *pedunculus cerebellaris superior.*

superior cistern. CISTERN OF THE GREAT CEREBRAL VEIN.

superior colliculus. One of the posterior pair of rounded eminences arising from the dorsal portion of the mesencephalon. It contains primary visual centers especially for coordination of eye movement. NA *colliculus superior.*

superior costal facet. The superior facet on the body of a vertebra for articulation with the head of a rib. NA *fovea costalis superior.* See also *costal fossae.*

superior costotransverse ligament. The ligament connecting the superior portion of the neck of a rib to the corresponding transverse process. NA *ligamentum costotransversarium superius.*

superior curved line of the ilium. POSTERIOR GLUTEAL LINE.

superior curved line of the occipital bone. SUPERIOR NUCHAL LINE.

superior dental plexus. A plexus of nerve fibers in the upper jaw formed by branches of the infraorbital (maxillary) nerve. NA *plexus dentalis superior.*

superior duodenal fossa. A small pocket of peritoneum formed on the left of the terminal portion of the duodenum by a triangular fold of peritoneum and having the opening directed downward.

superior duplicity. *In teratology,* duplicity of the superior pole, involving mostly supraumbilical parts; KATADIDYMUS.

superior extensor retinaculum. The broad band which stretches across the front of the leg between the distal parts of the tibia and the fibula, binding the tendons of the tibialis anterior and long extensor muscles of the toes. Syn. *transverse crural ligament, transverse ligament of the leg.* NA *retinaculum musculorum extensorum superius.*

superior fovea. The depression in the floor of the fourth ventricle near the facial colliculus, formed by the widening of the sulcus limitans. NA *fovea superior.*

superior frontal gyrus. A convolution of the frontal lobe situated between the dorsal margin of the hemisphere and the superior frontal sulcus, immediately above the middle frontal gyrus. NA *gyrus frontalis superior.* See also Plate 18.

superior frontal sulcus. A longitudinal groove separating the middle and superior frontal gyri. NA *sulcus frontalis superior.*

superior ganglion. 1. (of the glossopharyngeal nerve:) The upper sensory ganglion of the glossopharyngeal nerve, located in the upper part of the jugular foramen; it is inconstant. NA *ganglion superius nervi glossopharyngei.* 2. (of the vagus nerve:) The upper sensory ganglion of the vagus nerve, located in the jugular foramen. Syn. *jugular ganglion.* NA *ganglion superius nervi vagi.*

superior hemorrhagic polioencephalitis. WERNICKE'S ENCEPHALOPATHY.

superior hypogastric plexus. A large visceral nerve plexus lying just in front of the promontory of the sacrum. Syn. *presacral nerve.* NA *nervus presacralis, plexus hypogastricus superior.*

su·pe·ri·or·i·ty complex (sue·peer″ee·or′i·tee). A general attitude or character trait, often pathologic and usually arising out of an underlying feeling of inferiority, which is characterized by the occurrence of some form of real or assumed ascendancy and by feelings of conceit, vanity, envy, jealousy, or revenge.

superior laryngotomy. Incision of the larynx through the thyrohyoid membrane. Syn. *subhyoid laryngotomy, thyrohyoid laryngotomy.*

superior ligament of the incus. A band connecting the roof of the tympanic recess and the body of the incus. NA *ligamentum incudis superius.*

superior ligamentum of the epididymis. The fold of the tunica vaginalis testis connecting the testis and the head of the epididymis; the upper lip of the digital fossa. NA *ligamentum epididymidis superius.*

superior ligamentum of the malleus. A delicate bundle of fibers connecting the roof of the epitympanic recess and the head of the malleus. NA *ligamentum mallei superius.*

superior longitudinal fasciculus. A bundle of long association fibers in the cerebrum, connecting the frontal lobe with the occipital and temporal lobes. NA *fasciculus longitudinalis superior.*

superior mediastinum. The upper portion of the mediastinum extending from the pericardium to the base of the neck. NA *mediastinum superius.*

superior medullary velum. A thin layer of white substance which forms the anterior portion of the roof of the fourth ventricle. NA *velum medullare superius.*

superior mesenteric ganglion. A collateral sympathetic ganglion lying in the superior mesenteric plexus near the origin of the superior mesenteric artery. NA *ganglion mesentericum superius.* See also Plate 15.

superior mesenteric plexus. A visceral nerve plexus accompanying the superior mesenteric artery, derived from the celiac plexus. NA *plexus mesentericus superior.*

superior nasal concha. The upper scroll-like projection of the ethmoid bone covered with mucous membrane situated in the lateral wall of the nasal cavity. NA *concha nasalis superior.*

superior nasal meatus. The portion of the nasal cavity between the superior nasal concha and the middle nasal concha.

superior nasal turbinate. SUPERIOR NASAL CONCHA.

superior nuchal line. A semicircular line passing outward and forward from the external occipital protuberance. NA *linea nuchae superior.*

superior oblique tendon sheath syndrome. BROWN'S SHEATH SYNDROME.

superior occipital gyri. Convolutions on the upper lateral surface of the occipital lobe of the cerebrum. See also *lateral occipital gyri.*

superior olive. A cellular column, about 4 mm long, extending from the level of the facial nucleus to the motor nucleus of the trigeminal nerve; it is in close contact ventrally with the lateral portion of the trapezoid body.

superior orbital fissure. The elongated opening between the smaller and the greater wing of the sphenoid. NA *fissura orbitalis superior.*

superior parietal lobule. The subdivision of the parietal lobe of the cerebrum that is separated from the inferior parietal lobule by the interparietal sulcus. NA *lobulus parietalis superior.*

superior pelvic aperture or **strait.** The space within the brim of the pelvis; INLET OF THE PELVIS. NA *apertura pelvis superior.*

superior peroneal retinaculum. The retinaculum of the ankle which binds down the tendons of the peroneus longus and the peroneus brevis. NA *retinaculum musculorum peroneorum superius.*

superior petrosal sinus. A sinus of the dura mater running in a groove in the petrous portion of the temporal bone from the cavernous sinus to the transverse sinus. NA *sinus petrosus superior.* See also Table of Veins in the Appendix.

superior pubic ligament. A ligament of the symphysis pubis passing laterally along, and connecting, the upper margins of the pubic bones. NA *ligamentum pubicum superius.*

superior pulmonary sulcus syndrome. PANCOAST SYNDROME.

superior quadrigeminal body. SUPERIOR COLLICULUS.

superior quadrigeminal brachium. BRACHIUM OF THE SUPERIOR COLLICULUS.

superior radix of the ansa cervicalis. SUPERIOR ROOT OF THE ANSA CERVICALIS.

superior recess of the omental bursa. The portion of the omental bursa lying behind the liver. NA *recessus superior omentalis.*

superior rectus. An extrinsic muscle of the eye. See *rectus superior bulbi* in Table of Muscles in the appendix.

superior root of the ansa cervicalis. Fibers from the first and second cervical nerves which travel for a short distance with the hypoglossal nerve and then descend to join fibers from the second and third cervical nerves (the inferior root), forming the ansa cervicalis. Syn. *descendens hypoglossi.* NA *radix superior ansae cervicalis.*

superior sagittal diameter. The line joining the middle of the crest of the frontal bone to the external occipital protuberance.

superior sagittal sinus. A sinus of the dura mater which runs along the upper edge of the falx cerebri, beginning in the front of the crista galli and terminating at the confluence of the sinuses. NA *sinus sagittalis superior.* See also Table of Veins in the Appendix and Plates 10, 17.

superior salivatory nucleus. An ill-defined nucleus in the dorsolateral reticular formation of the pontine tegmentum which sends preganglionic fibers to the submandibular ganglion via the nervus intermedius, facial, and chorda tympani nerves and to the pterygopalatine ganglion via the major superficial petrosal nerve. It is concerned in the regulation of secretion of the submandibular, sublingual, and lacrimal glands. NA *nucleus salivatorius superior.*

superior semilunar lobule. The portion of the posterior lobe of the cerebellum lying just superior to the horizontal cerebellar fissure. NA *lobulus semilunaris superior.*

superior sternal region. The portion of the sternal region lying above the lower margins of the third costal cartilages.

superior strait of the pelvis. INLET OF THE PELVIS.

superior supraoptic decussation (of Meynert). DORSAL SUPRAOPTIC DECUSSATION.

superior temporal gyrus. A convolution of the temporal lobe lying between the lateral cerebral fissure and superior temporal sulcus. NA *gyrus temporalis superior.* See also Plate 18.

superior temporal line. A line arching across the side of the cranium and giving attachment to the temporal fascia. NA *linea temporalis superior ossis parietalis.*

superior thalamic peduncle. See *thalamic peduncles.*

superior thyroid notch. A deep notch in the upper margin of the thyroid cartilage between the two laminae. NA *incisura thyroidea superior.*

superior tracheotomy. Tracheotomy performed above the isthmus of the thyroid gland. The cut may be extended to include the cricoid cartilage. See also *laryngotomy.*

superior transverse ligament of the scapula. The triangular fibrous band which crosses the scapular notch, forming a foramen through which the suprascapular nerve passes. NA *ligamentum transversum scapulae superius.*

superior tympanic canaliculus. CANAL OF THE LESSER PETROSAL NERVE.

superior vena cava. A vein formed by the union of the brachiocephalic veins, and conveying the blood from the head, chest wall, and upper extremities to the right atrium of the heart. NA *vena cava superior.* See also Plates 5, 9.

superior vena cava syndrome. Blockage of the superior vena cava, as by thrombosis, neoplasm, aneurysm, or mediastinitis, resulting in elevation of venous pressure of the upper extremities, head, and neck, with resultant edema, cyanosis, and venous distention.

superior vermis. The anterosuperior part of the cerebellar vermis, consisting of the lingula, the central lobule, and the superior part of the monticulus.

superior vermis syndrome. A disorder of cerebellar function characterized by a wide-based stance and ataxia of gait and normality of coordinated movement of individual limbs.

superior vertebral incisure. A notch on the cranial border of the pedicle of a vertebra. NA *incisura vertebralis superior.*

superior vestibular nucleus. A nucleus dorsal and mostly rostral to the lateral vestibular nucleus in the angle formed by the floor and the lateral wall of the fourth ventricle. NA *nucleus vestibularis superior.*

su·per·lac·ta·tion (sue″pur·lack·tay′shun) *n.* 1. Excess of the secretion of milk. 2. Excessive continuance of lactation.

su·per·le·thal (sue″pur·lee′thul) *adj.* Highly lethal.

su·per·mo·ron (sue″pur·mo′ron) *n.* [*super-* + *moron*]. A person with dull normal or slightly below normal intelligence.

su·per·na·tant (sue″pur·nay′tant) *adj.* & *n.* [L. *supernatans,* from *super-* + *natare,* to swim, float]. 1. Floating on top. 2. The fluid that remains after the removal of suspended matter by centrifugation or other physical or chemical means. —**su·per·nate** (sue′pur·nate) *n.*

su·per·nor·mal (sue″pur·nor′mul) *adj.* 1. Characterizing a faculty or phenomenon that is beyond the level of ordinary experience. 2. Superior to, or greater than, the normal.

su·per·nu·mer·ary (sue″pur·new′mur·err″ee) *adj.* [L. *supernumerarius*]. Existing in more than the usual number.

supernumerary muscle. ACCESSORY MUSCLE.

supernumerary spleen. ACCESSORY SPLEEN.

supernumerary tooth. A tooth which is additional to the normal complement.

su·per·nu·tri·tion (sue″pur·new·trish′un) *n.* [*super-* + *nutrition*]. SUPERALIMENTATION.

supero- [L. *superus,* upper]. A combining form meaning *above, superior.*

su·pe·ro·in·fe·ri·or (sue″pur·o·in·feer′ee·ur) *adj.* [*supero-* + *inferior*]. Pertaining to any dimension extending from above downward.

su·pe·ro·lat·er·al (sue″pur·o·lat′ur·ul) *adj.* [*supero-* + *lateral*]. Above and to the side.

su·pe·ro·me·di·al (sue″pur·o·mee′dee·ul) *adj.* [*supero-* + *medial*]. Above and toward the middle.

su·per·ox·ide (sue″pur·ock′side) *n.* A highly reactive radical which is the product of the univalent reduction of molecular oxygen (O_2^{-}·). Formed in many biological systems, for example, phagocytizing leukocytes.

Superoxol. Trademark for a 30% solution of hydrogen peroxide.

su·per·par·a·site (sue″pur·păr′uh·site) *n. In biology,* a parasite of parasites. —**super·par·a·sit·ic** (·păr″uh·sit′ick) *adj.*

su·per·par·a·sit·ism (sue″pur·păr′uh·sigh·tiz·um) *n.* [*super-* + *parasitism*]. The infestation of parasites by other parasites.

su·per·phos·phate (sue″pur·fos′fate) *n.* ACID PHOSPHATE.

su·per·pig·men·ta·tion (sue″pur·pig″men·tay′shun) *n.* [*super-* + *pigmentation*]. Excessive pigmentation.

su·per·salt (sue′pur·sawlt) *n.* ACID SALT.

su·per·sat·u·rate (sue″pur·satch′uh·rate) *v.* To saturate to excess; to add more of a substance than a liquid can normally and permanently dissolve.

supersaturated solution. A solution that contains a greater quantity of solid than can normally be dissolved at a given temperature. It is an unstable system.

su·per·scrip·tion (sue″pur·skrip′shun) *n.* [L. *superscriptio*]. The sign ℞ (abbreviation of Latin *recipe,* take) at the beginning of a prescription.

su·per·se·cre·tion (sue″pur·se·kree′shun) *n.* Excessive secretion.

su·per·sen·si·tive (sue″pur·sen′si·tiv) *adj.* Abnormally sensitive.

su·per·sen·si·ti·za·tion (sue″pur·sen″si·ti·zay′shun) *n.* [*super-* + *sensitization*]. Excessive susceptibility to the action of a protein following its injection.

su·per·son·ic (sue″pur·son′ick) *adj.* [*super-* + *son-* + *-ic*]. 1. A term, synonymous with ultrasonic but more commonly used than the latter in the physical sciences, describing or pertaining to soundlike waves with a frequency above that of audible sounds, that is, above 20,000 hertz. 2. Of or pertaining to speeds exceeding that of sound in air. —**su·per·sound** (sue′pur·saownd) *n.*

su·per·spi·na·tus (sue″pur·spye·nay′tus) *n.* [NL., from *super-* + *spina*]. *In veterinary medicine,* an extensor muscle of the humerus which has no exact homologue in man.

su·per·ten·sion (sue″pur·ten′shun) *n.* Extreme tension. Compare *hypertension.*

su·per·ve·nos·i·ty (sue″pur·ve·nos′i·tee) *n.* [*super-* + *venosity*].

The condition in which the blood has become venous to a high degree.

su·per·ven·tion (sue″pur·ven′shun) *n.* [L. *superventio,* from *supervenire,* to come upon, to be added to]. That which is added; a new, extraneous, or unexpected condition added to another.

su·per·ver·sion (sue″pur·vur′zhun) *n.* [*super-* + *version*]. SURSUMVERSION.

su·per·vi·sor, *n.* A supervising or head nurse.

su·per·volt·age, *adj.* Pertaining to x-rays produced by a very high-voltage current flow across an x-ray tube or very high-energy radiation produced by other devices, as telecobalt (radioactive cobalt used in telecobalt therapy) and linear accelerators.

supervoltage generator. A generator that produces voltages above 500,000 volts; used in the production of short-wave roentgen rays.

supervoltage radiation. *In radiology,* roentgen radiation produced by voltages above 500,000 volts or equivalent gamma rays.

su·pi·na·tion (sue″pi·nay′shun) *n.* [L. *supinare,* to bend back]. 1. Of the hand: the turning of the palm upward. 2. Of the foot: a turning of the sole inward so that the medial margin is elevated. 3. The condition of being supine; lying on the back. —**su·pi·nate** (sue′pi·nate) *v.*

su·pi·na·tor (sue′pi·nay″tur, sue″pi·nay′tor) *n.* A muscle of the forearm, which rotates the radius outward. NA *musculus supinator.* See also Table of Muscles in the Appendix.

supinator bre·vis (brev′is). SUPINATOR.

supinator crest. A bony ridge on the upper lateral margin of the shaft of the ulna for the origin of the supinator muscle. NA *crista musculi supinatorius.*

supinator longus reflex. BRACHIORADIALIS REFLEX.

supinator reflex. BRACHIORADIALIS REFLEX.

su·pine (suh·pine′, sue′pine) *adj.* [L. *supinus*]. 1. Lying on the back, face upward. Contr. *prone.* 2. Of the hand: palm upward.

supine hypotensive syndrome. Severe hypotension in late pregnancy or during labor caused by compression of the abdominal aorta and vena cava by the gravid uterus when the mother assumes the supine position. The resulting reduction of uterine blood flow may produce fetal distress.

sup·pe·da·ne·ous (sup″e·day′nee·us) *adj.* [L. *suppedaneus,* from *sub-* + *pes, pedis,* foot]. Pertaining to the sole of the foot.

sup·pe·da·ne·um (sup″e·day′nee·um) *n.* [L., footstool]. An application to the sole of the foot.

sup·ple·men·tal (sup″le·men′tul) *adj.* Additional.

supplemental air. EXPIRATORY RESERVE VOLUME.

sup·ple·men·ta·ry (sup″le·men′tur·ee) *adj.* SUPPLEMENTAL.

supplementary articulation. A false articulation in which the ends of the fragments become rounded and covered with a fibrous capsule.

supplementary menstruation. VICARIOUS MENSTRUATION.

supplementary x-ray therapy. The irradiation of affected areas with x-ray in addition to the use of interstitial or intracavitary therapy.

sup·port, *v. & n.* [L. *supportare,* to carry]. 1. To sustain, prop, or hold in position. 2. Any appliance that supports a part or structure, as an arch support. 3. The providing for the needs of another person, particularly for a dependent, such as a child or invalid. 4. *In psychiatry,* the giving of approval, acceptance, sympathy, and encouragement to another person. Adj. *supportive.*

sup·port·er, *n.* An apparatus intended to hold in place a low-hanging or prolapsed organ, as the uterus, the scrotum and its contents, or the abdomen, or to limit the use of certain joints, as the knee or ankle. See also *pessary, jockstrap, binder.*

supporting cell. SUSTENTACULAR CELL.

sup·port·ive, *adj.* Characterizing or pertaining to any device, measure, person, or program which maintains, gives assistance to, sustains, or in any manner helps a patient.

supportive therapy. 1. Any form of treatment designed primarily to bolster and reinforce the patient's own defenses and to suppress disturbing influences or factors in such a way as to allow his own resources to help him back to health. 2. Specifically, a technique of psychotherapy in which the therapist, through encouragement, advice, reassurance, reeducation, and often even environmental manipulation, reinforces the patient's own psychic defenses and helps him suppress disturbing psychologic material; employed particularly in patients whose mental state is too fragile to achieve insight or whose symptoms are not sufficiently severe to justify intensive psychotherapy. Contr. *suppressive psychotherapy.*

sup·pos·i·to·ry (suh·poz′i·tor″ee) *n.* [L. *suppositorius,* that is placed underneath]. A medicated solid body of varying weight and shape, intended for introduction into different orifices of the body, as the rectum, urethra, or vagina. Usually suppositories melt or are softened at body temperature, in some instances release of medication is effected through use of a hydrophilic vehicle. Typical vehicles or bases are theobroma oil (cocoa butter), glycerinated gelatin, sodium stearate, and propylene glycol monostearate.

sup·press, *v.* [L. *supprimere, suppressus,* to press down, hold down]. 1. To hold back, curtail, constrain, arrest; to prevent from functioning. 2. To exclude from overt manifestation or consciousness. —**suppres·sive,** *adj.;* **suppres·sant,** *adj. & n.*

suppressed menstruation. Nonappearance of the menstrual flow in patients who formerly menstruated. Syn. *menostasia.*

sup·pres·sion, *n.* [L. *suppressio,* from *supprimere,* to suppress]. 1. A sudden cessation of secretion, as of the urine, or of a normal process, as the menses. See also *anuria.* 2. *In psychiatry,* the conscious effort to control and cover ideas, feelings, urges, and desires considered to be unacceptable, untenable, or unworthy. Compare *repression.*

suppressive psychotherapy. *In psychiatry,* a form of directive therapy in which the therapist acts as an authority figure who expects to be obeyed and who employs such techniques as firm suggestions, commands, exhortation, and persuasion to help contain or control material leading to emotional conflict or maladaptive behavior. Contr. *supportive therapy* (2).

sup·pres·sor band or **area.** Any area on the cerebral cortex stimulation of which is presumed to suppress the motor response or spontaneous electrical activity of some other part of the cortex. Narrow areas of cortex have been discovered by local stimulation with strychnine near Brodmann's areas 4, 8, 24, 2, and 19, and have been named areas 4S, 8S, 24S, 2S, and 19S.

suppressor cell. A cell, usually of the T lymphocyte lineage, capable of suppressing immune reactions.

suppressor mutation. A mutation at one gene which reverses the effect of a mutation at another gene.

sup·pu·rant (sup′yoo·runt) *adj. & n.* 1. Promoting suppuration. 2. Any agent that promotes suppuration.

sup·pu·ra·tion (sup″yoo·ray′shun) *n.* [L. *suppuratio,* from *suppurare,* to suppurate, from *pus, puris,* pus]. The formation of pus. —**sup·pu·rate** (sup′yoo·rate) *v.*

sup·pu·ra·tive (sup′yoo·ray″tiv) *adj. & n.* 1. Characterized by suppuration. 2. SUPPURANT (2).

suppurative endophthalmitis. Septic inflammation of the uveal tract with pus formation.

suppurative inflammation. An inflammatory process producing a purulent exudate plus death and liquefaction necrosis of the associated fixed tissue. It is distinguished from purulent inflammation by necrosis of fixed tissue.

suppurative labyrinthitis. Labyrinthitis due to bacterial invasion, characterized by all of the diagnostic evidence of infection, including production of pus cells.

suppurative mastitis. Inflammation of the breast with the formation of pus.

suppurative meningitis. Meningitis due to a pyogenic organism, such as *Streptococcus pneumoniae.*

suppurative parotitis. Suppurating inflammation of the parotid gland, usually due to *Staphylococcus aureus* and associated with chronic debilitating disease or blockage of the parotid gland by a calculus; characterized by local pain and swelling, often with fever and chills.

supra- [L.]. A prefix meaning (a) *upon* or *above;* (b) *beyond, transcending, exceeding.*

su·pra·aor·tic (sue″pruh·ay·or′tick) *adj.* [*supra-* + *aortic*]. Above the level of the aortic valve, as supraaortic stenosis.

su·pra·ar·ti·cu·lar (sue″pruh·ahr·tick′yoo·lur) *adj.* [*supra-* + *articular*]. Above an articulation.

su·pra·bony pocket. A periodontal pocket whose base is coronal to the crest of the alveolar process. Contr. *infrabony pocket.*

su·pra·cal·lo·sal (sue″pruh·ka·lo′sul) *adj.* [*supra-* + *callosal*]. Situated above the corpus callosum.

supracallosal gyrus. INDUSIUM GRISEUM.

su·pra·car·di·nal veins (sue″pruh·kahr′di·nul). Paired longitudinal venous channels of the embryo that replace the postcardinal and subcardinal veins and form the azygos-hemiazygos system of veins and, on the right side, most of the postrenal part of the inferior vena cava.

su·pra·cer·vi·cal (sue″pruh·sur′vi·kul) *adj.* [*supra-* + *cervical*]. Situated above the cervix of the uterus.

supracervical hysterectomy. Hysterectomy in which the cervix is not removed.

su·pra·cho·roid (sue″pruh·ko′roid) *adj.* Situated above or upon the choroid coat of the eye.

su·pra·cho·roi·dal (sue″pruh·ko·roy′dul) *adj.* SUPRACHOROID.

suprachoroid layer. LAMINA SUPRACHOROIDEA.

su·pra·cla·vic·u·lar (sue″pruh·kla·vick′yoo·lur) *adj.* [*supra-* + *clavicular*]. Above the clavicle.

supraclavicular fossa. 1. TRIGONUM OMOCLAVICULARE. 2. FOSSA SUPRACLAVICULARIS MINOR.

su·pra·cla·vi·cu·la·ris pro·pri·us (sue″pruh·kla·vick″yoo·lair′is pro′pree·us). A rare muscle extending from the acromial end of the clavicle and lying superficial to the trapezius and sternocleidomastoid muscles.

supraclavicular muscle. CLEIDOOCCIPITAL MUSCLE.

supraclavicular nerves. NA *nervi supraclaviculares.* See Table of Nerves in the Appendix.

supraclavicular point. *In electromyography,* the small area above the clavicle, electrical stimulation of which causes contraction of the arm muscles.

supraclavicular region. The space between the upper margin of the clavicle and lower borders of the omohyoid and sternocleidomastoid muscles.

supraclavicular signal node. SIGNAL NODE.

su·pra·cli·noid (sue″pruh·klye′noid) *adj.* Above the clinoid processes.

supraclinoid aneurysm. An aneurysm occurring just above the sphenoid bone.

su·pra·clu·sion (sue″pruh·klew′zhun) *n.* [*supra-* + *occlusion*]. The position of a tooth that has overerupted in the plane of occlusion.

su·pra·con·dy·lar (sue″pruh·kon′di·lur) *adj.* [*supra-* + *condylar*]. Above a condyle.

supracondylar amputation. An operation in which the femur is sawed through above the condyles. See also *Gritti-Stokes amputation.*

supracondylar eminence. EPICONDYLE.

supracondylar fracture. A fracture of the lower end of the humerus or femur above the condyles.

supracondylar process. A small projection, found in rare instances, about 2 inches above the medial epicondyle of the humerus, with which it connects by a fibrous band, and under which the median nerve and brachial vessels may pass. NA *processus supracondylaris.*

supracondylar ridge. Either of the two ridges, lateral or medial, above the condyle of the humerus, which serve for muscular attachment.

su·pra·cos·ta·lis (sue″pruh·kos·tay′lis) *n.* One of a number of rare variant muscles associated with the serratus muscles; they may be anterior or posterior.

su·pra·cris·tal (sue″pruh·kris′tul) *adj.* [*supra-* + *cristal*]. Above a ridge or crest.

su·pra·di·a·phrag·mat·ic (sue″pruh·dye″uh·frag·mat′ick) *adj.* [*supra-* + *diaphragmatic*]. Above the diaphragm.

su·pra·ge·nic·u·late (sue″pruh·je·nick′yoo·lut) *adj.* [*supra-* + *geniculate*]. Situated above the medial geniculate body.

suprageniculate nucleus. A wedge-shaped nucleus extending dorsomedially from the medial geniculate nucleus, between the pulvinar and the pretectal area.

su·pra·gin·gi·val (sue″pruh·jin′ji·vul, jin·jye′vul) *adj.* [*supra-* + *gingival*]. Located above the gingiva.

supragingival calculus. A concretion deposited on the surface of a tooth above the level of the gingival margin. Syn. *extragingival calculus.*

su·pra·gle·noid (sue″pruh·glee′noid) *adj.* Above the glenoid cavity.

supraglenoid tubercle or **tuberosity.** A slight elevation on the upper margin of the glenoid cavity, which gives attachment to the long head of the biceps brachii muscle. NA *tuberculum supraglenoidale.*

su·pra·glot·tic (sue″pruh·glot′ick) *adj.* [*supra-* + *glottic*]. Above the glottis.

su·pra·gran·u·lar (sue″pruh·gran′yoo·lur) *adj.* [*supra-* + *granular*]. Situated above the external granular layer of the cerebrum.

supragranular layer. The external granular layer and layer of pyramidal cells of the cerebral cortex collectively.

su·pra·hy·oid (sue″pruh·high′oid) *adj.* [*supra-* + *hyoid*]. Above the hyoid bone.

suprahyoid muscles. The muscles attached to the upper margin of the hyoid bone. NA *musculi suprahyoidei.*

suprahyoid region. The region between the mandible and the hyoid bone.

suprahyoid triangle. A triangle limited behind by the anterior belly of the digastric, in front by the middle line of the neck, and below by the body of the hyoid bone.

su·pra·in·gui·nal (sue″pruh·ing′gwi·nul) *adj.* [*supra-* + *inguinal*]. Situated proximal to the inguinal region.

suprainguinal region. The area bounded by the rectus abdominis muscle, the inguinal ligament, and a horizontal line through the iliac crest.

su·pra·le·thal (sue″pruh·lee′thul) *adj.* Above the lethal level.

su·pra·le·va·tor (sue″pruh·le·vay′tur) *adj.* [*supra-* + *levator*]. Situated above a levator ani muscle.

supralevator abscess. An abscess located between the levator ani muscles and the reflection of the peritoneum.

su·pra·lim·i·nal (sue″pruh·lim′i·nul) *adj.* [*supra-* + *liminal*]. Above, or in excess of, a threshold; SUPRATHRESHOLD.

su·pra·mal·le·o·lar (sue″pruh·ma·lee′uh·lur) *adj.* [*supra-* + *malleolar*]. Above a malleolus.

su·pra·ma·mil·lary (sue″pruh·mam′i·lerr·ee) *adj.* [*supra-* + *mamillary*]. Situated above a mamillary body.

supramamillary decussation. The most rostral of the midbrain commissures, lying at the transition between the diencephalon and the tegmentum of the midbrain. It carries a wide range of fibers, including fibers from various levels of the hypothalamus to the tegmentum of the midbrain and connections between the two subthalamic nuclei. Syn. *postmamillary decussation.*

supramamillary nucleus. A layer of large cells on the dorsal aspect of the medial mamillary nucleus, which is not sharply demarcated from the tegmental gray matter.

su·pra·man·dib·u·lar (sue″pruh·man·dib′yoo·lur) *adj.* [*supra-* + *mandibular*]. Situated above the mandible.

su·pra·mar·gin·al (sue″pruh·mahr′jin·ul) *adj.* [*supra-* + *marginal*]. Above an edge or margin.

supramarginal gyrus. A cerebral convolution that forms the anterior portion of the inferior parietal lobule and arches over the upturned end of the lateral cerebral sulcus. NA *gyrus supramarginalis.*

su·pra·mas·toid (sue″pruh·mas′toid) *adj.* Above the mastoid process of the temporal bone.

supramastoid crest. A bony ridge on the squamous part of the temporal bone behind the external acoustic meatus.

su·pra·max·il·lary (sue″pruh·mack′si·lerr·ee) *adj.* [*supra-* + *maxillary*]. Situated above a maxillary alveolar process.

supramaxillary ansa. SUPERIOR DENTAL PLEXUS.

su·pra·me·a·tal (sue″pruh·mee·ay′tul) *adj.* [*supra-* + *meatal*]. Situated above a meatus.

suprameatal spine. A small tubercle projecting from the posterosuperior margin of the external acoustic meatus. NA *spina suprameatum.*

suprameatal triangle. The area between the posterior wall of the external acoustic meatus and the posterior root of the zygomatic process of the temporal bone. Syn. *Macewen's triangle.*

su·pra·nu·cle·ar (sue″pruh·new′klee·ur) *adj.* [*supra-* + *nuclear*]. In the nervous system, central to a nucleus.

supranuclear palsy or **paralysis.** Loss of the motor function in the distribution of a cranial or spinal nerve, due to a lesion in pathways or centers above its nucleus or cells of origin.

su·pra·oc·cip·i·tal (sue″pruh·ock·sip′i·tul) *adj.* [*supra-* + *occipital*]. Situated above the occipital bone.

supraoccipital fontanel. *In comparative embryology,* a cordate membranous space between the occipital cartilage and the more anterior parts of the cranium.

su·pra·oc·clu·sion (use″pruh·o·kloo′zhun) *n.* [*supra-* + *occlusion*]. The condition created by the abnormal elongation of teeth in their sockets.

su·pra·om·pha·lo·dym·ia (sue″pruh·om″fuh·lo·dim′ee·uh) *n.* [*supra-* + *omphalo-* + *-dymia*]. A form of conjoined twins in which the union is in the superior umbilical region. Syn. *gastropagus.*

su·pra·op·tic (sue″pruh·op′tick) *adj.* [*supra-* + *optic*]. Situated above the optic tract.

supraoptic commissures. COMMISSURAE SUPRAOPTICAE.

supraoptic nucleus of the hypothalamus. A well-defined crescent-shaped nucleus that straddles the optic tract lateral to the chiasma. Its efferent fibers combine with those of the paraventricular nucleus to form the supraopticohypophyseal tract. NA *nucleus supraopticus hypothalami.*

su·pra·op·ti·co·hy·poph·y·se·al (sue″pruh·op″ti·ko·high·pof″i·see′ul, ·high″po·fiz′ee·ul) *adj.* [*supraoptic* + *hypophyseal*]. Pertaining to the supraoptic nucleus and the hypophysis.

supraopticohypophyseal system. The supraoptic nucleus with the supraopticohypophyseal tract to the neurohypophysis.

supraopticohypophyseal tract. A part of the hypothalamohypophyseal tract. NA *tractus supraopticohypophysialis.*

su·pra·or·bit·al (sue″pruh·or′bi·tul) *adj.* [*supra-* + *orbital*]. Situated above the orbit.

supraorbital arch. SUPRAORBITAL RIDGE.

supraorbital artery. NA *arteria supraorbitalis.* See Table of Arteries in the Appendix.

supraorbital canal. A canal at the upper margin of the orbit, giving passage to the supraorbital nerve and vessels. It is inconstant.

supraorbital foramen. A notch in the superior orbital margin at the junction of the middle with the inner third, sometimes converted into a foramen by a bony process or a ligamentous band; it gives passage to the supraorbital artery, veins, and nerve. NA *foramen supraorbitalis.*

supraorbital line. A line extending horizontally across the forehead immediately above the zygomatic process of the frontal bone.

supraorbital nerve. NA *nervus supraorbitalis.* See Table of Nerves in the Appendix.

supraorbital notch. The groove in the supraorbital ridge of the frontal bone which is occasionally present in place of a foramen. NA *incisura supraorbitalis.* Compare *supraorbital foramen.*

supraorbital reflex. Contraction of the orbicularis oculi muscle in response to a tap of the outer region of the supraorbital ridge, resulting in closing the eye of the same side or even of both eyes; difficult to elicit normally, the response is exaggerated in lesions above the facial nucleus and absent in lesions of the facial nerve at or below the nucleus. Syn. *McCarthy's reflex, orbicularis oculi reflex.*

supraorbital ridge. The curved and prominent margin of the frontal bone that forms the upper boundary of the orbit. NA *arcus superciliaris.*

supraorbital torus. Extreme development of the supraorbital region.

su·pra·pa·tel·lar (sue″pruh·puh·tel′ur) *adj.* [*supra-* + *patellar*]. Above the patella.

suprapatellar bursa or **pouch.** The bursa situated between the tendon of the quadriceps femoris muscle and the anterior surface of the lower end of the femur; it usually communicates with the knee joint cavity.

suprapatellar reflex. A sudden upward movement of the patella produced by contraction of the quadriceps muscle in response to a sharp blow upon a finger which is placed against the upper border of the patella, with the leg extended.

su·pra·pel·vic (sue″pruh·pel′vick) *adj.* [*supra-* + *pelvic*]. Above the pelvis.

su·pra·pi·ne·al recess (sue″pruh·pin′ee·ul, ·pye′nee·ul). A posterior recess of the third ventricle extending backward as a diverticulum from the ependyma of the roof. NA *recessus suprapinealis.*

su·pra·pleu·ral membrane (sue″pruh·ploo′rul). The extrapleural fascia attached to the inner margin of the first rib and covering the dome of the pleura. Syn. *Sibson's fascia.* NA *membrana suprapleuralis.*

su·pra·pu·bic (sue″pruh·pew′bick) *adj.* [*supra-* + *pubic*]. Above the pubes.

suprapubic lithotomy. A lithotomy in which the incision into the urinary bladder is made through the abdominal wall just above the symphysis, the stone being removed by forceps.

suprapubic prostatectomy. Removal of the prostate by an incision into the urinary bladder through the abdominal (suprapubic) route in a one- or two-stage operation.

suprapubic reflex. Deflection of the linea alba toward the stroked side when the abdomen is stroked above the inguinal ligament.

su·pra·re·nal (sue″pruh·ree′nul) *adj. & n.* [*supra-* + *renal*]. 1. Located above or anterior to the kidneys; ADRENAL (1). 2. A tissue in suprarenal position, especially the adrenal gland.

suprarenal artery. See Table of Arteries in the Appendix.

su·pra·re·nal·ec·to·my (sue″pruh·ree″nul·eck′tuh·mee) *n.* [*suprarenal* + *-ectomy*]. ADRENALECTOMY.

suprarenal gland. ADRENAL GLAND.

Suprarenalin. A trademark for epinephrine.

su·pra·re·na·lis ab·er·ra·ta of the ovary (sue″pruh·re·nay′lis ab″e·ray′tuh). ADRENOCORTICOID ADENOMA OF THE OVARY.

su·pra·re·nal·ism (sue″pruh·ree′nul·iz·um) *n.* [*suprarenal* + *-ism*]. ADRENALISM.

su·pra·re·nal·op·a·thy (sue″pruh·ree″nul·op′uth·ee) *n.* [*suprarenal* + *-pathy*]. A disordered condition resulting from disturbed function of the suprarenal glands.

suprarenal plexus. A sympathetic nerve plexus surrounding the suprarenal gland. NA *plexus suprarenalis.*

Suprarenin. A trademark for epinephrine.

su·pra·scap·u·la (sue″pruh·skap′yoo·luh) *n.* [*supra-* + *scapula*]. An anomalous bone occasionally found between the superior border of the scapula and the spines of the lower cervical or first thoracic vertebrae, present in some cases of congenital elevation of the scapula. Syn. *omovertebral bone.*

su·pra·scap·u·lar (sue″pruh·skap′yoo·lur) *adj.* Above or in the upper part of the scapula, as an artery or nerve.

suprascapular artery. NA *arteria suprascapularis.* See Table of Arteries in the Appendix.

suprascapular nerve. NA *nervus suprascapularis.* See Table of Nerves in the Appendix.

su·pra·scle·ral (sue″pruh·skleer′ul) *adj.* [*supra-* + *scleral*]. Situated at or upon the outer surface of the sclera.

su·pra·sel·lar (sue″pruh·sel′ur) *adj.* [*supra-* + *sellar*]. Situated upon or above the sella turcica of the sphenoid bone.

suprasellar cyst. CRANIOPHARYNGIOMA.

su·pra·son·ic (sue″pruh·son′ick) *adj.* SUPERSONIC.

su·pra·spi·nal (sue″pruh·spye′nul) *adj.* [*supra-* + *spinal*]. Situated above a spine or the spinal column.

supraspinal ligament. A fibrous cord connecting the spinous process of the vertebrae from the sacrum to the seventh cervical vertebra. It continues upward as the nuchal ligament. NA *ligamentum supraspinale.*

supraspinal nucleus. Somatic motor cells of the first cervical nerve, which are located in the ventral gray column of the spinal cord and extend rostrally into the lower medulla.

su·pra·spi·na·tus (sue″pruh·spye·nay′tus) *n.* A muscle originating above the spine of the scapula and inserted on the greater tubercle of the humerus. NA *musculus supraspinatus.* See also Table of Muscles in the Appendix.

su·pra·spi·nous (sue″pruh·spye′nus) *adj.* Above the spinous process of the scapula or of a vertebra.

supraspinous aponeurosis. A thick and dense membranous layer that completes the osseofibrous case in which the supraspinatus muscle is contained, affording attachment by its inner surface to some of the fibers of the muscle.

supraspinous fossa. The triangular depression on the posterior surface of the scapula above the spine. NA *fossa supraspinata.*

supraspinous region. The region corresponding to the supraspinous fossa of the scapula.

su·pra·sple·ni·al (sue″pruh·splee′nee·ul) *adj.* [*supra-* + *splenial*]. Situated above the splenium.

suprasplenial sulcus. SUBPARIETAL SULCUS.

su·pra·ster·nal (sue″pruh·stur′nul) *adj.* [*supra-* + *sternal*]. Above the sternum.

suprasternal bones. Ossified, suprasternal cartilages not attached to the manubrium; anomalous in man, normal in some mammals. NA *ossa suprasternalia.*

suprasternal fossa. The depression in the midline of the base of the neck above the upper border of the sternum and between the insertion of the sternal portions of the two sternocleidomastoid muscles.

suprasternal notch. JUGULAR NOTCH OF THE STERNUM.

suprasternal region. The region just above the jugular notch of the sternum. Syn. *regio suprasternalis.*

suprasternal space. The triangular space above the manubrium, enclosed by the layers of the deep cervical fascia which are attached to the front and back of this bone. Syn. *space of Burns.*

su·pra·ste·rol (sue″pruh·sterr′ol, ·steer′ol) *n.* A type of sterol produced by the irradiation of ergosterol. Suprasterols are toxic.

su·pra·thresh·old (sue″pruh·thresh′hohld) *adj.* Above, or in excess of, a threshold.

suprathreshold stimulus. A stimulus of sufficient intensity to bring about a response during the relative refractory period of a muscle fiber.

su·pra·ton·sil·lar (sue″pruh·ton′si·lur) *adj.* [*supra-* + *tonsillar*]. Above a tonsil.

supratonsillar abscess. An abscess located above a tonsil.

supratonsillar fossa. The upper recess of the tonsillar sinus between the pillars of the fauces and above the palatine tonsil; it is covered by a semilunar fold. NA *fossa supratonsillaris.*

su·pra·tri·gem·i·nal nucleus (sue″pruh·trye·jem′i·nul). A nucleus near the motor nucleus of the trigeminal nerve and functionally similar to the intertrigeminal nucleus.

su·pra·troch·le·ar (sue″pruh·trock′lee·ur) *adj.* Above the trochlea of the superior oblique muscle.

supratrochlear artery. NA *arteria supratrochlearis.* See Table of Arteries in the Appendix.

supratrochlear nerve. NA *nervus supratrochlearis.* See Table of Nerves in the Appendix.

su·pra·um·bil·i·cal (sue″pruh·um·bil′i·kul) *adj.* [*supra-* + *umbilical*]. Above the navel; cranial to a transverse plane at the umbilicus.

su·pra·va·gi·nal (sue″pruh·vaj′i·nul, va·jye′nul) *adj.* [*supra-* + *vaginal*]. Situated above or superior to the vagina.

supravaginal hysterectomy. SUPRACERVICAL HYSTERECTOMY.

su·pra·val·vu·lar (sue″pruh·val′vew·lur) *adj.* [*supra-* + *valvular*]. Above a valve, usually cardiac.

supravalvular aortic stenosis. Narrowing of the ascending aorta immediately distal to the orifice of the aortic valve; localized or diffuse.

su·pra·ven·tric·u·lar (sue″pruh·ven·trick′yoo·lur) *adj.* [*supra-* + *ventricular*]. Occurring or situated above a ventricle.

supraventricular crest. A ridge on the inner wall of the right ventricle delimiting the conus arteriosus, a remnant of the bulboatrial crest. Syn. *infundibuloventricular crest.* NA *crista supraventricularis.*

supraventricular tachycardia. A rapid regular tachycardia with the ectopic pacemaker originating above the ventricles, i.e., in the atria or atrioventricular node.

su·pra·ver·gence (sue″pruh·vur′junce) *n.* [*supra-* + L. *vergere*, to bend, turn]. Divergence of the two eyes in a vertical plane, measured by a prism, of from 2 to 3°; the eye moving upwards is supraverging. Syn. *sursumvergence.* —**supra·verge** (·vurj′) *v.*

su·pra·ves·i·cal fovea (sue″pruh·ves′i·kul). FOSSA SUPRAVESICALIS.

su·pra·vi·tal (sue″pruh·vye′tul) *adj.* [*supra-* + *vital*]. Pertaining to the staining of living cells after removal from a living animal or of still living cells within a recently killed animal. —**supravital·ly** (·lee) *adv.*

su·preme nasal concha. An inconstant concha situated above the superior nasal concha. NA *concha nasalis suprema.*

su·pro·fen (sue·pro′fen) *n.* *p*-2-Thenoylhydratropic acid, $C_{14}H_{12}O_3S$, an anti-inflammatory agent.

su·ra (sue′ruh) *n.* [L.] [NA]. CALF. —**su·ral** (·rul) *adj.*

sur·al·i·men·ta·tion (sur″al″i·men·tay′shun) *n.* [F. *sur*, over, from L. *super*, + *alimentation*]. The method of forced feeding or overalimentation; SUPERALIMENTATION, HYPERALIMENTATION.

sur·a·min sodium (soor′uh·min). Hexasodium *sym*-bis(*m*-aminobenzoyl-*m*-amino-*p*-methylbenzoyl-1-naphthylamino-4,6,8-trisulfonate)carbamide, $C_{51}H_{34}N_6Na_6O_{23}S_6$, an antitrypanosomal and antifilarial drug.

sur·di·tas (sur′di·tas) *n.* [L.]. Deafness.

sur·di·tas ver·ba·lis (sur′di·tas vur·bay′lis) [L., word deafness]. APHASIA.

surd·i·ty (surd′i·tee) *n.* [L. *surditas*]. Deafness.

sur·do·car·di·ac (sur″do·kahr′dee·ack) *adj.* [L. *surd*us, deaf, + *cardiac*]. Characterized by deafness and cardiac abnormalities.

surdocardiac syndrome. CARDIOAUDITORY SYNDROME.

sur·ex·ci·ta·tion (sur″eck·sigh·tay′shun) *n.* [F. *sur*, over, + *excitation*]. Excessive excitement; superexcitation.

Surexin. Trademark for pyrinoline, a cardiac depressant.

Surfacaine. Trademark for cyclomethycaine, a topical anesthetic agent used as the sulfate salt.

sur·face, *n.* [F., modeled on L. *superficies*]. 1. The exterior of a body. 2. The face or faces of a body; a term frequently used in anatomy in the description of various structures.

surface-active, *adj.* Of a substance, such as a detergent: able to change, usually to lower, the interfacial tension between two phases. See also *surfactant.*

surface analgesia. Topical application of local anesthetic on mucous membranes for local analgesia.

surface anatomy. The study of superficial landmarks for the location of internal structures.

surface anesthesia. TOPICAL ANESTHESIA.

surface area. BODY SURFACE AREA.

surface biopsy. Scraping of cells from the surface of tissues, especially from the squamocolumnar junction of the uterine cervix for microscopic examination in cancer diagnosis.

surface-cell biopsy. SURFACE BIOPSY.

surface graft. A graft applied anywhere on the surface of the body where part of the skin is missing.

surface tension. The force operating at surfaces (commonly at the interface of a liquid and a gas) which is due to the unequal molecular attraction on either side of the molecules at the surface. It is the contractile force in the surface of a liquid that causes the surface to shrink and assume the smallest area possible. The surface tension of a liquid is the force in dynes exerted on either side of an imaginary straight line 1 cm long lying on the surface of the liquid.

surface thermometer. A thermometer for registering the surface temperature of any portion of the body.

sur·fac·tant (sur·fack'tunt) *n.* [*surf*ace-*act*ive + *-ant*]. 1. Any surface-active agent which reduces interfacial or surface tension. 2. The surface-active lipoprotein substance, secreted by great alveolar cells and lining the alveolar surface, which serves to maintain the stability of the alveolar mucosa.

surf·er's lumps. Skin nodules developing at points of contact between the bodies of surfboard riders and their boards, usually on the lower extremity.

sur·geon (sur'jun) *n.* [OF. *serurgien*]. A physician who is specially trained and qualified to perform operations and practice surgery.

surgeon general. The chief medical officer of an armed force or public health service unit.

surgeon-in-chief. The surgeon in charge of the entire surgical service in a university hospital; a term often reserved for the chairman of the department of surgery.

surgeon's knot. DOUBLE KNOT.

sur·gery, *n.* [OF. *surgerie, cirurgerie,* from Gk. *cheirourgia,* from *cheirourgein,* to operate, work with the hand, from *cheir,* hand]. 1. The branch of medicine dealing with trauma and diseases requiring operative procedure, including manipulation. See also *chemosurgery.* 2. Any of the treatments and procedures developed and applied in surgery. 3. In British usage, any medical practitioner's place of consultation and treatment. **—sur·gi·cal,** *adj.*

surgical anatomy. Application of anatomy to surgery.

surgical anesthesia. Stage 3 of general anesthesia where muscles are sufficiently relaxed to permit surgical procedures to be carried out readily. See also *stages of general anesthesia.*

surgical aneurysm. An aneurysm which can be treated surgically.

surgical bed. 1. A bed equipped with a double windlass which raises and lowers, independently, the foot and the head of the bed. 2. A hospital bed assigned to a surgical unit.

surgical cleansing. Removal of devitalized tissue and foreign material from traumatic wounds with sterile cutting instruments. See also *debridement.*

surgical decompression. Any operative method to relieve excessive pressure, as in a body cavity, the gastrointestinal tract, or the cranium.

surgical diphtheria. Formation of a diphtheritic membrane on the surface of a wound. Syn. *wound diphtheria.* See also *cutaneous diphtheria.*

surgical erysipelas. Erysipelas occurring in the site of a wound. Syn. *traumatic erysipelas.*

surgical-glove talc granuloma. TALCUM-POWDER GRANULOMA.

surgical hospital. *In military medicine,* a mobile medical unit, attached to an army, that provides special facilities for giving immediate surgical aid to men wounded in combat.

surgical needle. Any sewing needle used in surgical operations.

surgical neck. The constricted part of the humerus just below the tubercles. NA *collum chirurgicum humeri.*

surgical pack. A pack used in an operative wound to secure hemostasis.

surgical pathology. 1. The study of diseases in the realm of surgery. 2. Diagnostic study, gross and microscopic, of tissues removed from the living patient.

surgical scarlet fever. Scarlet fever from infection of a wound or burn by certain hemolytic streptococci.

surgical spoon. CURET.

surgical team. 1. The group of individuals that carries out a surgical operation; it usually consists of a chief surgeon, assistants, surgical nurses, and an anesthesiologist. 2. A team of doctors working as a unit who are proficient in certain surgical procedures.

surgical tetanus. Tetanus following infection of an operative site with *Clostridium tetani.*

surgical third space. THIRD SPACE.

surgical treatment. Treatment requiring manipulation or operative procedure.

surgical triangle. Any triangular area in which surgically important nerves and arteries are found.

Su·ri·nam bark (soor'i·nahm, ·nam) [after *Surinam,* northern South America]. Cabbage tree bark; the bark of *Andira retusa,* which has been used as an anthelmintic.

Surital. Trademark for sodium thiamylal, an ultrashort-acting barbiturate used intravenously as an anesthetic.

Surmontil. Trademark for the antidepressant drug trimipramine.

sur·ra (soor'uh, surr'uh) *n.* [Marathi *sūra,* snort, wheeze]. A type of trypanosomiasis of domestic animals in southern Asia, caused by *Trypanosoma evansi* and transmitted by a number of bloodsucking flies.

sur·ro·gate (sur'uh·gut, ·gate) *n.* [L. *surrogatus,* substitute, alternative, from *surrogare,* to choose as a substitute, from *rogare,* to ask]. 1. Any medicine used as a substitute for a more expensive one, or for one to which there is a special objection in any particular case. 2. *In psychiatry,* an authority figure who takes the place of a parent (father or mother) in the emotional life of the patient.

sursum- [L.]. A combining form meaning *upward.*

sur·sum·duc·tion (sur"sum·duck'shun) *n.* [*sursum* + L. *ducere, ductus,* to lead]. 1. The power of the two eyes of fusing two images when one eye has a prism placed vertically before it. 2. SUPRAVERGENCE. 3. A movement of either eye alone upward.

sur·sum·ver·gence (sur"sum·vur'junce) *n.* [*sursum-* + L. *vergere,* to bend, turn]. SUPRAVERGENCE. **—sursumver·gent** (·junt) *adj.*

sursumvergent strabismus. Strabismus in which the visual axis is directed upward.

sur·sum·ver·sion (sur"sum·vur'zhun) *n.* [*sursum-* + *version*]. The upward movement of both eyes.

survey radiograph. A radiograph of an asymptomatic individual to detect disease; PLAIN FILM.

sus·cep·ti·bil·ity (suh·sep"ti·bil'i·tee) *n.* The inherited or acquired disposition to develop a disease if exposed to the causative agent. Contr. *immunity.*

sus·cep·ti·ble (suh·sep'ti·bul) *adj.* [L. *susceptibilis,* from *suscipere,* to take up, from *capere,* to take, capture]. 1. Sensitive to impression or influence. 2. Characterizing an individual who has neither natural nor acquired immunity to a disease and is liable to infection.

sus·ci·tate (sus'i·tate) *v.* [L. *suscitare,* to arouse, from *ciere,* to shake]. To increase activity; to stimulate.

sus·pend·ed, *adj.* [L. *suspendere,* to hang up, to interrupt, from *pendere,* to hang down]. 1. Hanging; applied to any structure attached to or hanging from another structure, and attached by a pedicle or cord. 2. Interrupted.

suspended animation. A state of interrupted respiration and loss of consciousness; temporary period of apparent death.

sus·pen·sion, *n.* [L. *suspensio,* from *suspendere,* to suspend]. 1. Hanging or fixation in a higher position; a method of treatment, as suspension of the uterus. 2. *In chemistry and pharmacy,* a dispersion of solid particles in a continuous liquid medium.

suspension laryngoscopy. A method of laryngoscopy in which the head is suspended on a combined mouth gag and tongue spatula which are supported by a bar connected with a moving overhead crane. The advantages of the method are that it leaves both hands of the examiner free and gives excellent exposure of the larynx, as in examining laryngeal tumors.

sus·pen·soid (sus·pen'soid) *n.* An apparent solution which is seen, by the microscope, to consist of small particles of solid dispersed material in active Brownian movement.

sus·pen·so·ri·um (sus''pen·so'ree·um) *n.,* pl. **suspenso·ria** (·ree·uh) [NL.]. That upon which anything hangs for support.

suspensorium he·pa·tis (hep'uh·tis). Coronary ligament of the liver. See *coronary ligament.*

suspensorium tes·tis (tes'tis). CREMASTER MUSCLE.

suspensorium ve·si·cae (ve·sigh'see). The superior false ligament of the urinary bladder.

sus·pen·so·ry (su·spen'suh·ree) *adj. & n.* 1. Serving for suspension or support. 2. SUPPORTER. 3. JOCKSTRAP.

suspensory bandage. A bandage for supporting the scrotum.

suspensory ligament. 1. APICAL DENTAL LIGAMENT. 2. (of the duodenum:) A fibrous band extending from the right crus of the diaphragm to the upper margin of the distal part of the duodenum. It usually contains some smooth muscle fibers, the suspensory muscle of the duodenum. Syn. *ligament of Treitz.* 3. (of the lens:) CILIARY ZONULE. 4. (of the ovary:) A small peritoneal fold passing upward from the tubal end of the ovary to the peritoneum over the iliac vessels and psoas muscle. Syn. *infundibulopelvic ligament.* NA *ligamentum suspensorium.* 5. (of the penis:) Fibers from the linea alba and symphysis pubis forming a strong fibrous band which extends to the upper surface of the root to blend with the fascial sheath of the penis. NA *ligamentum suspensorium penis.* 6. (pl.; of the breast:) Fibrous bands that pass through the breast from the overlying skin to the underlying pectoral fascia. Syn. *Cooper's suspensory ligaments.* NA *ligamenta suspensoria mammae.*

suspensory ligament of Lock·wood [C. B. *Lockwood,* English surgeon, 1856–1914]. A thickening of the orbital fascia extending below the eyeball from the cheek ligaments.

suspensory muscle of the duodenum. Muscle tissue sometimes associated with the suspensory ligament of the duodenum; it arises from the right crus of the diaphragm and is inserted on the duodenum at the jejunal junction. NA *musculus suspensorius duodeni.*

sus·pi·ra·tion (sus''pi·ray'shun) *n.* [L. *suspiratio,* from *suspirare,* to sigh]. 1. SIGH. 2. The act of sighing.

sus·pi·ri·um (suh·spye'ree·um) *n.* [L.]. SIGH.

sustentacular cell. One of the supporting cells of an epithelial membrane or tissue as contrasted with other cells with special function, as the nonnervous cells of the olfactory epithelium or the Sertoli cells of the seminiferous tubules. Syn. *Müller's fibers.*

sustentacular fibers. A supporting connective tissue that unites the various layers of the retina.

sus·ten·tac·u·lum (sus''ten·tack'yoo·lum) *n.,* pl. **sustentacu·la** (·luh) [L., from *sustentare,* to hold up, sustain]. A support. —**sustentacu·lar** (·lur) *adj.*

sustentaculum ta·li (tay'lye) [NA]. A process of the calcaneus supporting the talus.

su·sur·ra·tion (sue''sur·ay'shun) *n.* [L. *susurratio,* from *susurrare,* to murmur]. Murmuring, susurrus.

su·sur·rus (suh·sur'us) *n.* [L., murmur, whisper, hum]. A soft murmur.

susurrus au·ri·um (aw'ree·um). [NL, susurrus of the ears]. TINNITUS.

su·ti·lains (soo·ti·lainz') *n.* A preparation of proteolytic enzymes derived from *Bacillus subtilis.*

Sut·ter blood group. An erythrocyte antigen defined by its reaction to anti-Js^a antibody, found in the blood of a Mr. Sutter, who had received transfusions. It occurs in about 20 percent of Negroes and is a Mendelian dominant trait.

su·tu·ra (sue·tew'ruh) *n.,* pl. & genit. sing. **sutu·rae** (·ree), genit. pl. **su·tu·ra·rum** (sue·tew·rair'um) [L.] [NA]. SUTURE.

sutura co·ro·na·lis (kor·o·nay'lis) [NA]. CORONAL SUTURE.

sutura den·ta·ta (den·tay'tuh). SUTURA SERRATA.

suturae cra·nii (kray'nee·eye) [NA]. CRANIAL SUTURES.

sutura eth·moi·deo·max·il·la·ris (eth·moy''dee·o·mack·si·lair'is) [BNA]. SUTURA ETHMOIDOMAXILLARIS.

sutura eth·moi·do·max·il·la·ris (eth·moy''do·mack·si·lair'is) [NA]. The union between the ethmoid and maxilla.

sutura fron·ta·lis (fron·tay'lis) [NA]. FRONTAL SUTURE. NA alt. *sutura metopica.*

sutura fron·to·eth·moi·da·lis (fron''to·eth·moy·day'lis) [NA]. FRONTOETHMOID SUTURE.

sutura fron·to·la·cri·ma·lis (fron''to·lack·ri·may'lis) [NA]. FRONTOLACRIMAL SUTURE.

sutura fron·to·max·il·la·ris (fron''to·mack·si·lair'is) [NA]. FRONTOMAXILLARY SUTURE.

sutura fron·to·na·sa·lis (fron''to·na·say'lis) [NA]. FRONTONASAL SUTURE.

sutura fron·to·zy·go·ma·ti·ca (fron''to·zye·go·mat'i·kuh) [NA]. FRONTOZYGOMATIC SUTURE.

sutura har·mo·nia (hahr·mo'nee·uh). A suture in which there is simple apposition of contiguous rough surfaces.

sutura in·ci·si·va (in·si·sigh'vuh) [NA]. INCISIVE SUTURE.

sutura in·fra·or·bi·ta·lis (in''fruh·or·bi·tay'lis) [NA]. An occasional suture situated between the infraorbital foramen and infraorbital groove.

sutura in·ter·max·il·la·ris (in''tur·mack·si·lair'is) [NA]. INTERMAXILLARY SUTURE.

sutura in·ter·na·sa·lis (in''tur·na·say'lis) [NA]. INTERNASAL SUTURE.

su·tur·al (sue'chur·ul) *adj.* [L. *sutur*ea + *-al*]. Pertaining to, or having the nature of, a suture.

sutura la·cri·mo·con·cha·lis (lack''ri·mo·kong·kay'lis) [NA]. The union between the lacrimal bone and the inferior nasal concha.

sutura la·cri·mo·max·il·la·ris (lack''ri·mo·mack·si·lair'is) [NA]. MAXILLOLACRIMAL SUTURE.

sutura lamb·doi·dea (lam·doy'dee·uh) [NA]. LAMBDOID SUTURE.

sutural bone. Any supernumerary bone occurring in a cranial suture. Syn. *Wormian bone.*

sutural cataract. A congenital cataract in which the opacities involve the embryonic Y-shaped sutures of the eye, usually very thin with a bluish-green line on direct illumination, and causing no visual loss; may be inherited as a dominant trait. Syn. *stellate cataract.*

sutural ligament. A thin layer of fibrous membrane separating bones forming an immovable articulation, as between the bones of the skull.

sutura lim·bo·sa (lim·bo'suh). An interlocking suture, with beveling and overlapping of the articular surfaces, as in the coronal suture.

sutural membrane. Fibrous tissue between the cranial sutures.

sutura me·to·pi·ca (me·top′i·kuh) [NA alt.]. FRONTAL SUTURE. NA alt. *sutura frontalis.*

sutura na·so·fron·ta·lis (nay″zo·fron·tay′lis) [BNA]. Sutura frontonasalis (= FRONTONASAL SUTURE).

sutura na·so·max·il·la·ris (nay″zo·mack·si·lair′is) [NA]. NASOMAXILLARY SUTURE.

sutura no·tha (no′tuh). [NL., from L. *nothus,* false, from Gk. *nothos,* bastard, hybrid, mongrel, false]. A false suture; includes the sutura squamosa and sutura harmonia.

sutura oc·ci·pi·to·ma·stoi·dea (ock·sip″i·to·mas·toy′dee·uh) [NA]. OCCIPITOMASTOID SUTURE.

sutura pa·la·ti·na me·di·a·na (pal·uh·tye′nuh mee·dee·ay′nuh) [NA]. PALATINE SUTURE.

sutura palatina trans·ver·sa (trans·vur′suh) [NA]. The suture between the palatine processes of the maxillae and the horizontal plates of the palatine bones.

sutura pa·la·to·eth·moi·da·lis (pal″uh·to·eth·moy·day′lis) [NA]. The union between the ethmoid and palatine bones.

sutura pa·la·to·max·il·la·ris (pal″uh·to·mack·si·lair′is) [NA]. PALATOMAXILLARY SUTURE.

sutura pa·ri·e·to·mas·toi·dea (pa·rye″e·to·mas·toy′dee·uh) [NA]. PARIETOMASTOID SUTURE.

sutura pla·na (play′nuh) [NA]. A suture in which the edges of the bones are flat.

sutura sa·git·ta·lis (saj·i·tay′lis) [NA]. SAGITTAL SUTURE.

sutura ser·ra·ta (se·ray′tuh) [NA]. A suture in which the edges of the bones are saw-toothed.

sutura sphe·no·eth·moi·da·lis (sfee″no·eth·moy·day′lis) [NA]. SPHENOETHMOID SUTURE.

sutura sphe·no·fron·ta·lis (sfee″no·fron·tay′lis) [NA]. The union between the sphenoid and frontal bones.

sutura sphe·no·max·il·la·ris (sfee″no·mack·si·lair′is) [NA]. The union between the sphenoid and maxilla.

sutura sphe·no·or·bi·ta·lis (sfee″no·or·bi·tay′lis) [BNA]. SPHENOPALATINE SUTURE.

sutura sphe·no·pa·ri·e·ta·lis (sfee″no·pa·rye·e·tay′lis) [NA]. SPHENOPARIETAL SUTURE.

sutura sphe·no·squa·mo·sa (sfee″no·skway·mo′suh) [NA]. SPHENOSQUAMOSAL SUTURE.

sutura sphe·no·zy·go·ma·ti·ca (sfee″no·zye·go·mat′i·kuh) [NA]. SPHENOZYGOMATIC SUTURE.

sutura squa·mo·mas·toi·dea (skway″mo·mas·toy′dee·uh) [NA]. A suture between the squamous and mastoid portions of the temporal bone.

sutura squa·mo·sa (skway·mo′suh) [NA]. A suture formed by the overlapping of contiguous bones by broad, beveled margins.

sutura squamosa cra·nii (kray′nee·eye) [NA]. SQUAMOPARIETAL SUTURE.

sutura tem·po·ro·zy·go·ma·ti·ca (tem″puh·ro·zye·go·mat′i·kuh) [NA]. The union between the temporal and zygomatic bones.

sutura ve·ra (veer′uh). A true suture, one in which the margins of the bones are connected by a series of interlocked processes and indentations.

sutura zy·go·ma·ti·co·fron·ta·lis (zye·go·mat″i·ko·fron·tay′lis) [BNA]. Sutura frontozygomatica (= FRONTOZYGOMATIC SUTURE).

sutura zy·go·ma·ti·co·max·il·la·ris (zye·go·mat″i·ko·mack·si·lair′is) [NA]. The union between the zygomatic bone and the maxilla.

sutura zy·go·ma·ti·co·tem·po·ra·lis (zye·go·mat″i·ko·tem·po·ray′lis) [BNA]. SUTURA TEMPOROZYGOMATICA.

su·ture (sue′chur) *n. & v.* [L. *sutura,* seam, suture, from *suere,* to sew, stitch]. 1. *In osteology,* a line of junction or closure between bones, as a cranial suture. 2. *In surgery,* a fine thread or cordlike absorbable or nonabsorbable material, such as catgut or silk, used to make a repair or close a wound. 3. The method used in suturing, such as interrupted or mattress suture. 4. To close a wound or effect a union of tissues by sewing.

Suvren. Trademark for captodiame, a mild sedative used as the hydrochloride salt.

sux·a·me·tho·ni·um chloride (suck″suh·me·tho′nee·um). SUCCINYLCHOLINE CHLORIDE.

sux·em·er·id (suck·sem′e·rid) *n.* Bis(1,2,2,6,6-pentamethyl-4-piperidyl)succinate, an antitussive employed as the disulfate salt.

sved·berg (sved′burg, Swed. sveʸd′bærʸ) *n.* [T. *Svedberg,* Swedish chemist, 1884–1971]. SVEDBERG SEDIMENTATION UNIT.

Svedberg flotation unit [T. *Svedberg*]. A rate of flotation of a macromolecule, particularly a lipoprotein, in a medium of relatively greater density, of 10^{-13} cm per second under unit centrifugal force. Symbol, S_f.

Svedberg sedimentation unit [T. *Svedberg*]. A rate of sedimentation of a macromolecule, in a specified medium, of 10^{-13} cm per second under unit centrifugal force. Symbol, *s, S.* Syn. *svedberg.*

swab (swahb) *n.* A small stick or clamp with cotton or gauze at the tip, used to clean wounds, clear mucous passageways, take cultures, apply drugs topically, etc.

swage, *n. & v.* [OF. *souage*]. 1. A counter-die used in shaping thin metal. 2. To conform a thin metal plate to the shape of a model, cast, or die with the aid of a counter-die, the swage. 3. To fuse a strand of suture thread onto the end of a suture needle.

swal·low, *v.* 1. To take into the stomach through the esophagus by means of a complex reflex (the swallowing reflex) initiated by voluntary muscles and resulting in esophageal peristalsis. 2. To go through the motions of swallowing something.

swallowing reflex. The chain of reflexes involved in the mechanism of swallowing which may be evoked by stimulation of the palate or pharynx. See also *palatal reflex.*

swamp fever. LEPTOSPIROSIS.

swamp fever of horses. INFECTIOUS EQUINE ANEMIA.

swamp itch. SCHISTOSOME DERMATITIS.

swarm cell or **spore.** ZOOSPORE.

swathe (swahth) *n. & v.* A broad band of cloth used to wrap or bind a part. 2. To wrap or bind in a swathe. See also *sling and swathe.*

s wave. REGURGITANT WAVE.

S wave of the electrocardiogram. The negative deflection of the ventricular depolarization complex, following R (positive) wave.

sway·back, *n.* In humans, increased lumbar lordosis with compensatory increased thoracic kyphosis; in horses, sinking of the back or lordosis.

sweat, *n. & v.* 1. The secretion of the sweat glands, consisting of a transparent, colorless, aqueous fluid, holding in solution neutral fats, volatile fatty acids, traces of albumin and urea, free lactic acid, sodium lactate, sodium chloride, potassium chloride, and traces of alkaline phosphates, sugar, and ascorbic acid. Its excretion, largely by the cooling effect of evaporation, helps regulate the temperature of the body. 2. To produce sweat.

sweat gland. One of the coiled tubular glands of the skin which secrete sweat. NA (pl.) *glandulae sudoriferae.* See also *apocrine glands, eccrine glands.*

sweat gland adenoma. A benign tumor whose parenchyma consists of one or more sweat gland components.

sweat gland carcinoma. A malignant tumor whose parenchymal cells form structures resembling eccrine glands.

sweat·ing sickness. MILIARY FEVER.

sweat-retention syndrome. Inability to sweat because of plugging of sweat pores, followed by the classic clinical and histological signs of prickly heat, which may persist after heat rash has subsided. Syn. *thermogenic anhidrosis.* See also *tropical anhidrotic asthenia.*

sweat test. 1. A test for cystic fibrosis of the pancreas in which sweating is induced by one of several methods, and the sodium and chloride concentrations of the collected sweat are determined. 2. MINOR'S SWEAT TEST.

sweaty-feet syndrome. ODOR-OF-SWEATY-FEET SYNDROME.

Swe·diaur's disease (sveʸd'yaowr) [F. X. *Swediaur,* Austrian physician, 1748–1824]. ACHILLODYNIA.

Swe·dish movements or **gymnastics.** Gymnastics according to a system originating in Sweden and adapted for the treatment of postural deformities; involves a set of movements to be made by a patient against the resistance of an attendant.

Swedish type of porphyria. ACUTE INTERMITTENT PORPHYRIA.

swee·ny (swee'nee, swin'ee) *n.* [Pennsylvania Ger.]. A wasting or atrophy of the scapular muscles of the horse, usually due to an injury of the nerve supply. Syn. *swinney.*

sweet almond oil. ALMOND OIL.

sweet clover disease. A hemorrhagic disease observed in animals after eating spoiled sweet clover; due to a toxic substance (dicoumarin) that lowers the prothrombin content of the blood plasma.

sweet oil. Olive oil. See *olive.*

sweet spirit of niter. ETHYL NITRITE SPIRIT.

swell·ing, *n.* 1. Any morbid enlargement, inflation, or abnormal protuberance. 2. *In embryology,* a small eminence or ridge.

Swift's disease [W. *Swift,* Australian physician, 20th century]. ACRODYNIA.

swim·mer's itch. SCHISTOSOME DERMATITIS.

swim·ming-pool conjunctivitis. INCLUSION CONJUNCTIVITIS.

swine erysipelas. An infectious disease of hogs, caused by *Erysipelothrix insidiosa,* in which skin involvement predominates.

swine fever. HOG CHOLERA.

swine·herd's disease. A form of leptospirosis, ordinarily lasting from three to ten days, which is caused by *Leptospira pomona,* a microorganism typically harbored in swine. The dominant clinical finding is aseptic meningitis.

swine influenza. Disease due to the swine influenza virus, a strain of influenza. A virus having the antigenic marker $H_{sw}1$, N1. The virus causes respiratory-tract inflammation in swine and rarely infects man. The virus is related antigenically to the virus believed to have caused the severe influenza pandemic of 1918–1919.

swine plague. 1. Hemorrhagic septicemia of swine caused by *Pasteurella suiseptica.* The disease is characterized by a pleuropneumonia with focal necrosis and occasionally by septicemia. 2. HOG CHOLERA.

swine pox. A frequent disease of hogs characterized by pox lesions on the body and inner surfaces of the legs. It is a benign infection and usually occurs in young pigs.

swin·ney (swin'ee) *n.* SWEENY.

Swiss type agammaglobulinemia. The autosomal recessive form of severe combined immunodeficiency.

swiv·el stirrup. An apparatus fashioned like a stirrup and used by attaching it to a Steinmann pin for traction in leg fractures.

Sychrocept. A trademark for prostalene, a prostaglandin.

sy·co·ma (sigh·ko'muh) *n.* [Gk. *sykōma,* ulcer resembling a fig, from *sykon,* fig]. A condyloma or wart.

sy·co·si·form (sigh·ko'si·form) *adj.* [*sycosis* + *-iform*]. Resembling sycosis.

sy·co·sis (sigh·ko'sis) *n.* [Gk. *sykōsis,* figlike ulcer, from *sykon,* fig, + *-osis*]. An inflammatory disease affecting the hair follicles, particularly of the beard, and characterized by papules, pustules, and tubercles, perforated by hairs, together with infiltration of the skin and crusting.

sy·co·sis bar·bae (sigh·ko'sis bahr'bee). Inflammation of the hair follicles of the beard.

sycosis cap·il·li·tii (kap''i·lish'ee·eye). KELOID ACNE.

sycosis con·ta·gi·o·sa (kon·tay''jee·o'suh). SYCOSIS PARASITICA.

sycosis fram·boe·si·for·mis (fram·bee''si·for'mis). KELOID ACNE.

sycosis mentagra. TINEA BARBAE.

sycosis pal·pe·brae mar·gi·na·lis (pal'pe·bree mahr''ji·nay' lis). Sycosis affecting the edge of the eyelids.

sycosis par·a·sit·i·ca (păr''uh·sit'i·kuh). Barber's itch; a disease of the hair follicles, usually affecting the region covered by the beard and due to the presence of various trichophyta. See also *tinea barbae.*

sycosis staph·y·log·e·nes (staf''i·loj'e·neez). SYCOSIS VULGARIS.

sycosis vul·ga·ris (vul·gair'is). A pustular, follicular lesion caused by staphylococci.

Syd·en·ham's chorea (sid'ᵉn·um) [T. *Sydenham,* English physician, 1624–1689]. A disorder of childhood characterized by chorea, hypotonia, and hyporeflexia, and frequently by irritability and other psychic disturbances, often insidious in onset, and sometimes more manifest on one side of the body; related to streptococcal infection, with a high incidence of cardiac complications in later life unless prophylaxis against recurrent streptococcal infections is practiced. Syn. *Saint Vitus dance, acute chorea, dancing chorea, chorea minor.*

syl·lab·ic speech or **utterance** (si·lab'ick). SCANNING SPEECH.

syl·la·ble-stumbling. A form of dysphasia wherein each sound and syllable can be distinctly uttered, but the word as a whole is spoken with difficulty; seen in general paresis and other central nervous system disorders.

syl·la·bus (sil'uh·bus) *n.,* pl. **sylla·bi** (·bye), **syllabuses** [L. *sillybus,* label for a book, from Gk. *sillybos* or *sittyba*]. 1. A compendium containing the headings of a discourse. 2. The main propositions of a course of lectures. 3. An abstract.

syl·lep·si·ol·o·gy (si·lep''see·ol'uh·jee) *n.* [*syllepsis* + *-logy*]. The physiologic study of conception and pregnancy.

syl·lep·sis (si·lep'sis) *n.* [Gk. *syllēpsis*]. 1. CONCEPTION (1). 2. PREGNANCY.

syl·van yellow fever (sil'vun). Yellow fever transmitted to man from monkeys by forest mosquitoes.

syl·vat·ic plague (sil·vat'ick). Enzootic and epizootic plague occurring in some 50 rodent species, occurring in many western states of the United States and in many rural and sylvan areas of the world. Man may become infected accidentally by direct contact with these animals or by the bite of vectors, such as the flea.

Syl·vi·an (sil'vee·un) *adj.* 1. Described by or associated with Franciscus Sylvius (François de la Boë), Dutch physician, 1614–1672. 2. Described by or associated with Jacobus Sylvius (Jacques du Bois), French anatomist, 1478–1555.

Sylvian angle. The angle formed by the junction of the posterior ramus of the lateral cerebral sulcus (Sylvian fissure) with a line perpendicular to the superior border of the hemisphere.

Sylvian aqueduct [J. *Sylvius*]. CEREBRAL AQUEDUCT.

Sylvian aqueduct syndrome. Retraction nystagmus, paresis of upward gaze, pupillary abnormalities, and often lid retraction, due to a lesion of the periaqueductal gray matter.

Sylvian artery. The middle cerebral artery. See Table of Arteries in the Appendix.

Sylvian fissure [F. *Sylvius*]. LATERAL CEREBRAL SULCUS.

Sylvian ossicle or **bone** [J. *Sylvius*]. LENTICULAR PROCESS.

Sylvian point. 1. The junction of the anterior rami of the lateral cerebral sulcus (Sylvian fissure) with the posterior ramus of the sulcus. On the lateral surface of the head, it is located about 4.5 cm above the middle point of the zygomatic arch. 2. In cerebral angiography, the point at which the most posterior branch of the middle cerebral artery emerges from the lateral sulcus.

Sylvian triangle. In cerebral angiography, an area on the surface of the insula outlined by five to eight branches of the middle cerebral artery. The apex of the triangle is the Sylvian point; the inferior margin of the triangle is formed by the lower branches of the middle cerebral artery and the superior margin by the looping branches of this artery that are reversing their course.

Sylvian valve [J. *Sylvius*]. CAVAL VALVE.

Sylvian vein. VENA CEREBRI MEDIA SUPERFICIALIS.

sym-. See *syn-*.

sym·bal·lo·phone (sim·bal′o·fone) *n.* [Gk. *symballein*, to throw together, mix, compare, + *-phone*]. A stethoscope equipped with two chest pieces for simultaneous use as a special aid in localizing or in comparing sounds.

sym·bio·gen·ic psychosis (sim″bye·o·jen′ick). SYMBIOTIC PSYCHOSIS.

sym·bi·on (sim′bee·on, ·bye·on) *n.* SYMBIONT.

sym·bi·ont (sim′bee·ont, ·bye·ont) *n.* [Gk. *symbios*, living together]. An organism living in symbiosis.

sym·bi·o·sis (sim″bee·o′sis, ·bye·o′sis) *n.* [Gk. *symbiōsis*, living together, companionship, from *sym-* + *bios*, life, living]. 1. A more or less intimate association between organisms of noncompeting species, such as parasitism, mutalism, or commensalism. Contr. *antibiosis* (1). 2. Specifically, an association or union between organisms of different species which is mutually beneficial or essential to the survival of both parties; MUTUALISM. Contr. *commensalism*, *parasitism*. 3. *In psychiatry*, the more or less mutually advantageous relationship between two or more mentally disturbed individuals who are emotionally dependent on one another. —**symbi·ot·ic** (·ot′ick) *adj.*

symbiotic psychosis. A mental disorder of early childhood characterized by severe developmental and social retardation and profound reactions to separation in a child who appears to be autistic, but whose relationships with his mother or surrogate are abnormally close.

sym·bleph·aron (sim·blef′uh·ron) *n.* [*sym-* + *blepharon*]. Adhesion of the eyelids to the eyeball. See also *anterior symblepharon, posterior symblepharon, total symblepharon.*

sym·bleph·a·ro·sis (sim·blef″uh·ro′sis) *n.* [*sym-* + *blephar-* + *-osis*]. Adhesion of the eyelids to the eyeball or to each other.

sym·bo·lia (sim·bo′lee·uh) *n.* [Gk. *symbolē*, contact, joining, + *-ia*]. The ability to recognize an object by the sense of touch.

sym·bol·ic visual agnosia. Inability to recognize words or fractions of words (agnostic alexia), musical symbols, or numbers and other mathematical symbols, in spite of adequate vision, usually due to a lesion in the angular gyrus or connections thereof with other cortical regions such as Wernicke's and Broca's areas.

sym·bol·ism (sim′bul·iz·um) *n.* [*symbol* + *-ism*]. The delusional or hallucinational interpretation of all events or objects as having a mystic significance, common in certain forms of mental, particularly psychotic, disorders.

sym·bol·iza·tion (sim″bul·i·zay′shun) *n. In psychiatry*, an unconscious mental process by which a feeling, idea, or object is expressed by a substitute device, as in dreams, the meaning of which is not clear to the conscious mind. The symbol contains in disguised form the emotions vested in the initial idea or object.

sym·clo·sene (sim′klo·seen) *n.* Trichloro-*s*-triazine-2,4,-6(1*H*,3*H*,5*H*)trione, $C_3Cl_3N_3O$, a local anti-infective agent.

sy·me·lia (si·mee′lee·uh) *n.* [*sym-* + *-melia*]. A coalescence of the lower extremities. See also *sympodia, sympus.*

sym·e·lus (sim′e·lus) *n.* [*sym-* + *-melus*]. SYMPUS.

Syme's amputation [J. *Syme*, Scottish surgeon, 1799–1870]. Amputation above the ankle joint, the malleoli being sawed through, and a flap made with the skin of the heel.

sym·e·tine (sim′e·teen) *n.* 4,4′-(Ethylenedioxy)bis(*N*-hexyl-*N*-methylbenzylamine), $C_{30}H_{48}N_2O_2$, an anti-amebic drug, used as the dihydrochloride salt.

sym·me·lus (sim′e·lus) *n.* [*sym-* + *-melus*]. SYMPUS.

Symmetrel. Trademark for amantadine, a compound active against influenza virus.

symmetric gangrene. RAYNAUD'S DISEASE.

sym·me·try (sim′e·tree) *n.* [Gk. *symmetria*]. *In anatomy*, a harmonious correspondence of parts; also the relation of homologous parts at opposite sides or ends of the body. —**sym·met·ric** (si·met′rick), **symmet·ri·cal** (·ri·kul) *adj.*

sym·pa·ral·y·sis (sim″puh·ral′i·sis) *n.* [*sym-* + *paralysis*]. CONJUGATE GAZE PARALYSIS.

sym·pa·thec·to·my (sim″puh·theck′tuh·mee) *n.* [*sympathic* + *-ectomy*]. Excision of a portion of the autonomic or sympathetic nervous system.

sym·path·eo·neu·ri·tis (sim·path″ee·o·new·rye′tis) *n.* SYMPATHICONEURITIS.

sym·pa·thet·ic (sim″puh·thet′ick) *adj.* 1. Pertaining to or produced by sympathy. 2. Pertaining to the sympathetic nervous system.

sympathetic abscess. A secondary or metastatic abscess at a distance from the part in which the exciting cause has acted, as a bubo.

sympathetic atrophy. A rarely observed atrophy in one member of paired organs secondary to atrophy of its fellow.

sympathetic cell. A nerve cell of the sympathetic nervous system.

sympathetic dystrophy. 1. CAUSALGIA. 2. SHOULDER-HAND SYNDROME.

sympathetic ganglions. The ganglions of the sympathetic nervous system, including those of the sympathetic trunk and the collateral ganglions.

sympathetic irritation. Inflammation of an organ arising from inflammation of another related organ, as inflammation of an uninjured eye in association with inflammation of the other.

sympathetic meningitis. A form of aseptic meningitis with increased pressure, protein, and cell count in the cerebrospinal fluid in the absence of any infecting organism, due to a septic or necrotic focus in a structure contiguous to the leptomeninges.

sympathetic nerve. A nerve of the sympathetic nervous system.

sympathetic nervous system. 1. The thoracolumbar division of the autonomic nervous system; the ganglionated sympathetic trunk, sympathetic plexuses, and the associated preganglionic and postganglionic nerve fibers. Contr. *parasympathetic nervous system.* 2. *Obsol.* AUTONOMIC NERVOUS SYSTEM.

sympathetic neuroma. GANGLIONEUROMA.

sympathetic neuron. A neuron belonging to the sympathetic nervous system.

sym·pa·thet·i·co·mi·met·ic (sim″puh·thet″i·ko·mi·met′ick, ·migh·met′ick) *adj.* SYMPATHOMIMETIC.

sympathetic ophthalmia. A granulomatous inflammatory condition of the uveal tract which can occur in both eyes following ocular injury or intraocular surgery of one eye.

sympathetic ophthalmitis. Ophthalmitis following injury of the fellow eye. See also *sympathetic ophthalmia.*

sym·pa·thet·i·co·to·nia (sim″puh·thet″i·ko·to′nee·uh) *n.* SYMPATHICOTONIA.

sym·pa·thet·i·co·ton·ic (sim″puh·thet″i·ko·ton′ick) *adj.* Pertaining to the state of sympathicotonia.

sym·pa·thet·i·co·to·nus (sim″puh·thet″i·ko·to′nus) *n.* SYMPATHICOTONIA.

sympathetic plexus. AUTONOMIC PLEXUS.

sympathetic saliva. The saliva produced by stimulation of a sympathetic nerve.

sympathetic symptoms. Symptoms or disease occurring in one part or structure of the body when the actual lesion is in a different part, as in sympathetic meningitis or sympathetic ophthalmia.

sympathetic trunk. The chain of interconnected sympathetic ganglions extending along each side of the vertebral column. NA *truncus sympathicus.*

sym·pa·thet·o·blast (sim″puh·thet′o·blast) *n.* SYMPATHOBLAST.

sym·path·ic (sim·path′ick) *adj.* SYMPATHETIC.

sym·path·i·cec·to·my (sim·path″i·seck′tuh·mee) *n.* SYMPATHECTOMY.

sympathico-. A combining form meaning *sympathetic.*

sym·path·i·co·blast (sim·path′i·ko·blast) *n.* [*sympathico-* + *-blast*]. SYMPATHOBLAST.

sym·path·i·co·blas·to·ma (sim·path″i·ko·blas·to′muh) *n.* [*sympathicoblast* + *-oma*]. NEUROBLASTOMA.

sym·path·i·co·cy·to·ma (sim·path″i·ko·sigh·to′muh) *n.* [*sympathico-* + *-cytoma*]. GANGLIONEUROMA.

sym·path·i·co·go·ni·o·ma (sim·path″i·ko·go″nee·o′muh) *n.* [*sympathogonia* + *-oma*]. NEUROBLASTOMA.

sym·path·i·co·neu·ri·tis (sim·path″i·ko·new·rye′tis) *n.* [*sympathico-* + *neuritis*]. A neuropathy or neuritis involving ganglions and fibers of the sympathetic nervous system.

sym·path·i·cop·a·thy (sim·path″i·kop′uth·ee) *n.* [*sympathico-* + *-pathy*]. A disordered condition resulting from disturbance of the sympathetic nervous system.

sym·path·i·co·to·nia (sim·path″i·ko·to′nee·uh) *n.* [*sympathico-* + *-tonia*]. A condition produced by stimulation of the sympathetic nervous system, manifested by gooseflesh, increased blood pressure, or vascular spasm.

sym·path·i·co·trop·ic (sim·path″i·ko·trop′ick) *adj.* [*sympathico-* + *-tropic*]. Possessing special affinity for the sympathetic nervous system.

sympathicotropic cells. Large, epithelioid, probably chromaffin cells associated with unmyelinated nerves in the hilus of the ovary.

sym·path·i·cus (sim·path′i·kus) *n. Obsol.* SYMPATHETIC NERVOUS SYSTEM.

sym·pa·thin (sim′puh·thin) *n. Obsol.* NOREPINEPHRINE.

sympathin E. *Obsol.* A postulated form of sympathin causing excitation; formed by combination of a chemical mediator released at sympathetic nerve endings with a hypothetical substance in excited effector cells.

sympathin I. *Obsol.* A postulated form of sympathin causing inhibition; formed by combination of a chemical mediator released at sympathetic nerve endings with a hypothetical substance in inhibited effector cells.

sym·pa·thism (sim′puh·thiz·um) *n.* Susceptibility to hypnotic suggestion. See also *suggestibility.* **—sympa·thist** (·thist) *n.*

sym·pa·thi·zer (sim′puh·thigh″zur) *n.* SYMPATHIZING EYE.

sym·pa·thiz·ing eye (sim′puh·thigh″zing). The noninjured eye that becomes involved in sympathetic ophthalmia.

sympatho-. A combining form meaning *sympathetic.*

sym·pa·tho·blast (sim·path′o·blast, sim′puh·tho·) *n.* [*sympatho-* + *-blast*]. An embryonic sympathetic nerve cell which differentiates into the characteristic sympathetic ganglion cell. It is larger than the sympathogonia, with a less dense nucleus, more cytoplasm, and often a short cytoplasmic process.

sym·pa·tho·blas·to·ma (sim″puh·tho·blas·to′muh, sim·path″o·) *n.* [*sympathoblast* + *-oma*]. NEUROBLASTOMA.

sym·pa·tho·chro·maf·fin (sim″puh·tho·kro′muh·fin, sim·path″o·) *n.* [*sympatho-* + *chromaffin*]. Pertaining to sympathetic nerve cells that exhibit a chromaffin reaction.

sympathochromaffin cell. One of the precursors of sympathetic and medullary cells in the adrenal medulla.

sym·pa·tho·gone (sim″puh·tho·gohn, sim·path′o·) *n.* A single cell of the kind referred to collectively as sympathogonia.

sym·pa·tho·go·nia (sim″puh·tho·go′nee·uh, sim·path″o·) *n.pl.* [NL., from *sympatho-* + Gk. *gonē,* seed]. Primitive cells of the sympathetic nervous system derived from neuroblasts of the neural crest. They have dense nuclei, rich in chromatin, and only a thin rim of cytoplasm, and differentiate to form along one line ganglion cells and along another line chromaffin cells.

sym·pa·tho·go·ni·o·ma (sim″puh·tho·go″nee·o′muh, sim·path″o·) *n.* [*sympathogonia* + *-oma*]. NEUROBLASTOMA.

sym·pa·tho·lyt·ic (sim″puh·tho·lit′ick, sim·path″o·) *adj.* [*sympatho-* + *-lytic*]. Having or pertaining to an effect antagonistic to the activity produced by stimulation of the sympathetic nervous system. Contr. *sympathomimetic.*

sympatholytic agent. ADRENERGIC BLOCKING AGENT.

sym·pa·tho·ma (sim″puh·tho′muh) *n.* [*sympatho-* + *-oma*]. NEUROBLASTOMA.

sym·pa·tho·mi·met·ic (sim″puh·tho·mi·met′ick, sim·path″o·) *adj.* [*sympatho-* + *mimetic*]. Having the power to cause physiologic changes similar to those produced by action of the sympathetic nervous system, usually with respect to a drug. Contr. *sympatholytic.*

sym·pa·tho·trop·ic cell (sim″puh·tho·trop′ick, ·tro′pick). HILUS CELL.

sympathotropic-cell tumor. ADRENOCORTICOID ADENOMA OF OVARY.

sym·pa·thy (sim′puth·ee) *n.* [Gk. *sympatheia,* from *sym-* + *pathos,* feeling]. 1. The mutual relation between parts more or less distant, whereby a change in the one has an effect upon the other. 2. Feeling in response to similar feelings of another person; the close sharing of the experiences or feelings of and with another; close identification with another. Compare *empathy.* 3. *Colloq.* The sharing of sad, painful, or unpleasant feelings; commiseration.

sym·pet·al·ous (sim·pet′ul·us) *adj.* [*sym-* + *petal* + *-ous*]. *In botany,* having the petals united.

sym·pex·ion (sim·peck′see·on) *n.* [from *sympexis*]. A concretion found in the seminal vesicles.

sym·pex·is (sim·peck′sis) *n.* [Gk. *sympēxis,* condensation, coagulation]. SYMPEXION.

sym·phal·an·gism (sim·fal′un·jiz·um) *n.* [*syn-* + *phalang-* + *-ism*]. An inherited condition of stiff fingers, or ankylosed finger joints.

sym·phyo·ceph·a·lus (sim″fee·o·sef′uh·lus) *n.* [Gk. *symphyein,* to grow together, + *-cephalus*]. SYNCEPHALUS.

sym·phy·se·al (sim″fi·see′ul, sim·fiz′ee·ul) *adj.* Of or pertaining to a symphysis.

sym·phy·sec·to·my (sim″fi·seck′tuh·mee) *n.* Excision of a symphysis. See also *pubic symphysectomy.*

symphysi-, symphysio-. A combining form meaning *symphysis.*

sym·phys·i·al (sim·fiz′ee·ul) *adj.* Of or pertaining to a symphysis.

sym·phys·ic teratism (sim·fiz′ick). Any congenital anomaly in which certain organs or parts are abnormally fused.

sym·phy·si·ec·to·my (sim″fi·zee·eck′tuh·mee) *n.* [*symphysi-* + *-ectomy*]. *Obsol.* Excision of the symphysis pubis for the purpose of facilitating delivery. Compare *pubic symphysectomy.*

symphysio-. See *symphysi-.*

sym·phys·i·on (sim·fiz′ee·on) *n.* [*symphysi-* + -*ion*]. *In craniometry,* the most anterior point of the alveolar process of the lower jaw.

sym·phy·si·or·rha·phy (sim″fi·zee·or′uh·fee) *n.* [*symphysio-* + *-rrhaphy*]. Suture of a divided symphysis.

sym·phys·io·tome (sim·fiz′ee·o·tome) *n.* An instrument used in performing symphysiotomy.

sym·phy·si·ot·o·my (sim″fi·zee·ot′uh·mee) *n.* [*symphysio-* + *-tomy*]. *Obsol.* The dividing of the symphysis pubis to gain access to or to increase the diameters of the pelvic canal.

sym·phy·sis (sim′fi·sis) *n.,* pl. **symphy·ses** (·seez) [Gk., from *sym-,* together, + *physis,* growth] [NA]. A synchondrosis, especially one in the sagittal plane.

symphysis car·ti·la·gi·no·sa (kahr·ti·laj·i·no′suh). SYNCHONDROSIS.

symphysis li·ga·men·to·sa (lig·uh·men·to′suh). SYNDESMOSIS.

symphysis man·di·bu·lae (man·dib′yoo·lee). The midline osteochondral union of the halves of the mandible.

symphysis os·si·um pu·bis (os′ee·um pew′bis) [BNA]. Symphysis pubica. (= SYMPHYSIS PUBIS).

symphysis pu·bi·ca (pew′bi·kuh) [NA]. SYMPHYSIS PUBIS.

symphysis pu·bis (pew′bis). The fibrocartilaginous union (synchondrosis) of the pubic bones. NA *symphysis pubica.* See also Plates 2, 13.

sym·phy·sis sa·cro·coc·cy·gea (say·kro·kock·sij'ee·uh) [BNA]. JUNCTURA SACROCOCCYGEA.

sym·phy·so·dac·tyl·ia (sim''fi·so·dack·til'ee·uh) *n.* SYNDACTYLY.

sym·phy·sop·sia (sim''fi·zop'see·uh) *n.* [*symphysis* + *-opsia*]. CYCLOPIA.

sym·phy·so·ske·lia (sim''fi·zo·skee'lee·uh) *n.* [*symphysis* + Gk. *skelos*, leg, + *-ia*]. SYMPODIA.

sym·plasm (sim'plaz·um) *n.* [*sym-* + *-plasm*]. A protoplasmic mass resulting from the coalescence of originally separate cells. Compare *syncytium.*

sym·po·dia (sim·po'dee·uh) *n.* [*sym-* + *-podia*]. The condition of united lower extremities. See also *sympus.*

symp·tom (simp'tum) *n.* [Gk. *symptōma,* occurrence, accident; symptom, from *sympiptein,* to occur, from *sym-,* together, + *piptein,* to fall]. A phenomenon of physical or mental disorder or disturbance which leads to complaints on the part of the patient; usually a subjective state, such as headache or pain, in contrast to an objective sign such as papilledema.

symp·tom·at·ic (simp''tuh·mat'ick) *adj.* [Gk. *symptomatikos,* accidental]. 1. Pertaining to, or of the nature of, a symptom. 2. Affecting symptoms, as symptomatic treatment. 3. Characteristic or indicative of a physical or mental disorder, as night sweating may be symptomatic of tuberculosis, or excessive alcoholic intake of emotional disturbance. 4. Pertaining to or having the characteristics of one disorder which reflects a known or diagnosable underlying pathologic cause, as epilepsy may be symptomatic of a brain injury or of a metabolic disorder, in contrast to idiopathic or essential epilepsy where the cause is not known.

symptomatic anthrax. An infection of cattle and sheep characterized by subcutaneous, emphysematous swellings and nodules, due to infection by *Clostridium chauvoei.* Syn. *emphysematous anthrax.*

symptomatic epilepsy. Recurrent seizures due to a diagnosable lesion or agent. Contr. *idiopathic epilepsy.*

symptomatic erythema. Redness of skin as a surface manifestation of an internal cause. A simple form is blushing.

symptomatic parkinsonism. Parkinsonism associated with known factors, such as encephalitis lethargica and intoxications.

symptomatic parotitis. METASTATIC PAROTITIS.

symptomatic purpura. Purpura which may accompany acute infectious diseases or chronic diseases such as malignant tumors, nephritis, and blood dyscrasias, and following administration of certain drugs. Syn. *secondary purpura.*

symp·tom·atol·o·gy (simp''tuh·muh·tol'uh·jee) *n.* 1. The science of symptoms. 2. In common usage, the symptoms of disease taken together as a whole. **—symp·tom·ato·log·ic** (simp''tuh·mat''uh·loj'ick) *adj.*

symptom complex, group, or **grouping.** The ensemble of symptoms of a disease. See also *syndrome.*

symp·to·sis (simp·to'sis) *n.* [Gk. *symptōsis,* a falling together]. Wasting; emaciation; collapse.

sym·pus (sim'pus) *n.* [Gk. *sympous,* with the feet together, from *pous,* foot]. A fetus characterized by greater or less fusion of the legs, rotation of the legs, and marked deficiencies of the pelvic region and genitalia. Syn. *cuspidate fetus, symelus, sirenoform fetus, mermaid fetus.* See also *sirenomelia, sympodia.*

sympus apus (ay'pus). A sympus lacking feet.

sympus di·pus (dye'pus). A sympus with two more or less complete feet.

sympus mono·pus (mon'o·pus). A sympus with but one more or less complete foot.

sym·sep·a·lous (sim·sep'uh·lus) *adj.* [*sym-* + *sepal* + *-ous*]. *In biology,* having the sepals united.

syn-, sym- [Gk.]. A prefix meaning (a) *with, together;* (b) (italicized) in chemistry, the stereoisomeric form of certain compounds, as aldoximes, in which substituent atoms or groups are in cis- relationship. Contr. *anti-.*

Syn-Acthar. A trademark for seractide acetate, an adrenocorticotropic hormone.

syn·ac·to·sis (sin''ack·to'sis) *n.* [Gk. *synaktos,* collected, + *-osis*]. Malformations caused by the abnormal growing together of parts.

syn·a·del·phus (sin''uh·del'fus) *n.* [*syn-* + *-adelphus*]. Equal conjoined twins having eight limbs with but one head and trunk. Not observed in man. Syn. *cephalothoracoiliopagus.*

synaesthesia. SYNESTHESIA.

synaesthesialgia. SYNESTHESIALGIA.

Synalar. Trademark for fluocinolone acetonide, an anti-inflammatory adrenocortical steroid.

syn·al·gia (si·nal'jee·uh, ·juh) *n.* [*syn-* + *-algia*]. REFERRED PAIN. **—syn·al·gic** (si·nal'jick) *adj.*

syn·anas·to·mo·sis (sin''uh·nas''tuh·mo'sis) *n.* [Gk. *synanastomōses,* supposed communications between arteries and veins]. The joining of several blood vessels.

sy·nan·che (si·nang'kee, sigh·) *n.* [Gk. *synanchē,* sore throat]. CYNANCHE.

syn·an·the·ma (sin''an·theem'uh) *n.* [*syn-* + Gk. *anthēma,* blossom, from *anthein,* to bloom]. A group of elementary skin lesions of the same type.

syn·an·throp·ic (sin''an·throp'ick) *adj.* [Gk. *synanthrōp-* (from *synanthrōpeuesthai,* to live with humans, from *syn-,* with, + *anthrōpos,* human being) + *-ic*]. Living in close association with human beings, said of domestic animals, pigeons, rats, mice, cockroaches, etc.

syn·an·throse (sin·an'throce) *n.* FRUCTOSE.

syn·apse (sin'aps, si·naps') *n.* & *v.*, pl. **synap·ses** (·seez) [Gk. *synapsis,* contact, from *syn-* + *haptein,* to join; to touch]. 1. The region of communication between neurons; the point at which an impulse passes from an axon of one neuron to a dendrite or to the cell of another. A synapse is polarized, that is, nerve impulses are transmitted only in one direction, and is characterized by fatigability. 2. The union of the male and female chromosome pairs during meiosis, occurring either side-to-side or end-to-end without either univalent chromosome losing its identity. A bivalent chromosome results and is responsible for transmitting mixed characteristics from the parents to the offspring. 3. To make an interneuronal connection.

syn·ap·sis (sin·ap'sis) *n.*, pl. **synap·ses** (·seez) [Gk.]. SYNAPSE.

syn·ap·tase (si·nap'tace, ·taze) *n.* EMULSIN.

syn·ap·tene (si·nap'teen) *n.* [*synapsis* + *-tene*]. ZYGOTENE.

syn·ap·tic (si·nap'tick) *adj.* [Gk. *synaptikos,* connective, adjustive]. Pertaining to or communicated by a synapse.

synaptic cleft or **gap.** The minute space, usually 200 to 300 angstroms in width but somewhat wider in the myoneural junction, between the presynaptic plasma membrane of an axon terminal and the postsynaptic membranes.

synaptic junction. The specialized presynaptic and postsynaptic membranes together with the synaptic cleft.

synaptic knob. END FEET.

synaptic membrane. The single membrane at the synapse, demonstrated by light microscopy and Cajal's silver methods as separating the cytoplasm of the terminal enlargement of an axon from the cytoplasm of the nerve cell. Syn. *synaptolemma.*

synaptic vesicle. A characteristic circular structure, measuring 300 to 600 angstroms in diameter, found in great numbers adjacent to the presynaptic membrane, and thought to contain a chemical substance or substances important in synaptic transmission.

syn·ap·to·lem·ma (si·nap''to·lem'uh) *n.* [*synaptic* + *-lemma*]. SYNAPTIC MEMBRANE.

syn·ap·to·some (si·nap'tuh·sohm) *n.* [*synaptic-* + *-some*]. The specialized structure observed by means of an electron microscope at synapses, in which synaptic vesicles and mitochondria are enclosed within a thin external membrane.

syn·ar·thro·dia (sin″ahr·thro′dee·uh) *n.* SYNARTHROSIS. —**synarthro·di·al** (·dee·ul) *adj.*

synarthrodial cartilage. The cartilage of any fixed or slightly movable articulation.

syn·ar·thro·phy·sis (sin·ahr″thro·figh′sis) *n.* [*syn-* + *arthro-* + Gk. *physis,* growth]. Progressive ankylosis of the joints.

syn·ar·thro·sis (sin″ahr·thro′sis) *n.,* pl. **synarthro·ses** (·seez) [Gk. *synarthrōsis,* from *syn-* + *arthrōsis,* articulation] [BNA]. A form of articulation in which the bones are immovably bound together without any intervening synovial cavity. The forms are sutura, in which processes are interlocked; schindylesis, in which a thin plate of one bone is inserted into a cleft of another; and gomphosis, in which a conical process is held by a socket. Adj. *synarthrodial.*

syn·can·thus (sin·kan′thus) *n.* [*syn-* + *canthus*]. Adhesions between the orbital tissues and the eyeball.

syncaryon. SYNKARYON.

syn·ceph·a·lus (sin·sef′uh·lus) *n.* [*syn-* + *-cephalus*]. Conjoined twins united by their heads. This group includes the various types of craniopagus (cephalopagus) and cephalothoracopagus.

syncephalus asym·me·tros (a·sim′e·tros). CEPHALOTHORACOPAGUS MONOSYMMETROS.

syn·chei·lia, syn·chi·lia (sin·kigh′lee·uh) *n.* [*syn-* + *cheil-* + *-ia*]. Fusion of the lips.

synchesis. SYNCHYSIS.

synchondroses. Plural of *synchondrosis.*

synchondroses cra·nii (kray′nee·eye) [NA]. Cartilaginous joints between cranial bones.

synchondroses ster·na·les (stur·nay′leez) [NA]. The cartilaginous joints between the parts of the sternum.

syn·chon·dro·sis (sing″kon·dro′sis, sin·) *n.,* pl. **synchondro·ses** (·seez) [Gk. *synchondrōsis,* from *syn-* + *chondros,* cartilage] [NA]. A joint in which the surfaces are connected by a plate of cartilage. —**synchondro·sial** (·zee·ul, ·zhul) *adj.*

synchondrosis ary·cor·ni·cu·la·ta (ăr″i·kor·nick·yoo·lay′tuh) [BNA]. The cartilaginous joint between the corniculate and arytenoid cartilages.

synchondrosis ep·i·phy·se·os (ep·i·fiz′ee·os) [BNA]. Cartilago epiphysialis (= EPIPHYSEAL PLATE (2)).

synchondrosis in·ter·sphe·noi·da·lis (in″tur·sfee·noy·day′lis) [BNA]. In the fetus, the cartilaginous union between parts of the sphenoid.

synchondrosis in·tra·oc·ci·pi·ta·lis anterior (in″truh·ock·sip·i·tay′lis) [NA]. In the fetus, the cartilaginous union between anterior parts of the occipital bone.

synchondrosis intraoccipitalis posterior [NA]. In the fetus, the cartilaginous union between posterior parts of the occipital bone.

synchondrosis ma·nu·brio·ster·na·lis (ma·new″bree·o·stur·nay′lis) [NA]. The cartilaginous union between the manubrium and body of the sternum.

synchondrosis pe·tro·oc·ci·pi·ta·lis (pet″ro·ock·sip·i·tay′lis) [NA]. The cartilaginous union between the petrosal portion of the temporal bone and occipital bone.

synchondrosis sphe·no·oc·ci·pi·ta·lis (sfee″no·ock·sip·i·tay′lis) [NA]. The cartilaginous union between the sphenoid and occipital bones.

synchondrosis sphe·no·pe·tro·sa (sfee·no·pe·tro′suh) [NA]. The cartilaginous union between petrous part of the temporal bone and greater wing of the sphenoid bone.

synchondrosis ster·na·lis (stur·nay′lis) [BNA]. Singular of *synchondroses sternales.*

synchondrosis xi·pho·ster·na·lis (zif″o·stur·nay′lis) [NA]. The cartilaginous union between the xiphoid and body of the sternum.

syn·chon·drot·o·my (sin″kon·drot′uh·mee) *n.* [*synchondrosis* + *-tomy*]. A division of the cartilage uniting bones, especially of that of the symphysis pubis.

syn·cho·pex·ia (sing″ko·peck′se·uh) *n.* TACHYCARDIA.

syn·cho·pexy (sing′ko·peck·see) *n.* TACHYCARDIA.

synchro-. A combining form meaning *synchronous, synchronizing,* or *synchronized.*

syn·chro·cy·clo·tron (sing″kro·sigh′klo·tron) *n.* A cyclotron in which the frequency of the accelerating voltage is decreased with time so as to match exactly the slower revolutions of the accelerated particles resulting from the relativistic increase in mass of the particles.

syn·chro·nia (sing·kro′nee·uh) *n.* [NL.]. SYNCHRONY.

syn·chro·nism (sing′kruh·niz·um) *n.* [Gk. *synchronismos*]. SYNCHRONY.

syn·chro·nous (sing′kruh·nus) *adj.* [Gk. *synchronos,* contemporaneous]. Occurring at the same time; concurrent. Contr. *metachronous.* —**synchro·ny** (·nee) *n.*

syn·chro·tron (sing′kro·tron) *n.* An accelerator in which particles are accelerated around a circular path of essentially constant radius by electrostatic fields.

syn·chy·sis (sing′ki·sis) *n.* [Gk., lit., confusion]. Liquefaction of the vitreous body, due to degenerative changes.

synchysis scin·til·lans (sin′ti·lanz). The presence of bright, shining particles in the vitreous body of the eye.

Syncillin. A trademark for the potassium salt of the antibiotic phenethicillin.

syn·ci·ne·sis (sin″sigh·nee′sis) *n.* SYNKINESIS.

synciput. SINCIPUT.

syn·cli·tism (sing′kli·tiz·um, sin′) *n.* [Gk. *synklinein,* to lean together, + *-ism*]. 1. A condition marked by parallelism or similarity of inclination. 2. Parallelism between the pelvic planes and those of the fetal head. —**syn·clit·ic** (sing·klit′ick, sin·) *adj.*

syn·clon·ic (sin·klon′ick, sing·) *adj.* [*syn-* + *clonic*]. *Obsol.* Pertaining to synclonus.

syn·clo·nus (sing′klo·nus, sin·) *n.* [*syn-* + *clonus*]. *Obsol.* 1. Tremor, or clonic spasm, of several muscles at the same time. 2. A disease thus characterized, as chorea.

synclonus bal·lis·mus (ba·liz′mus). *Obsol.* PARKINSONISM.

synclonus tre·mens (tree′munz). *Obsol.* A general tremor.

syn·co·pe (sing′kuh·pee) *n.* [Gk. *synkopē,* from *synkoptein,* to cut off, cut up]. A faint; an episodic pause in the stream of consciousness due to cerebral hypoxia, of abrupt onset and brief duration and from which recovery is usually complete. —**synco·pal** (·pul), **syn·cop·ic** (sing·kop′ick) *adj.*

syncope an·gi·no·sa (an″ji·no′suh). ANGINA PECTORIS.

Syncurine. Trademark for decamethonium bromide, a skeletal muscle relaxant.

syncytia. Plural of *syncytium.*

syn·cy·tial (sin·sish′ul) *adj.* Pertaining to, or constituting, a syncytium.

syncytial carcinoma. CHORIOCARCINOMA.

syncytial cell. Any cell forming part of a syncytium, as cardiac and skeletal muscle cells, reticular connective-tissue cells, syncytiotrophoblast cells.

syncytial endometritis or **deciduitis.** Excessive proliferation of the syncytiotrophoblastic cells near the site of the placenta with invasion of the endometrium, decidua, and adjacent myometrium by these cells.

syncytial knots. Protuberant masses of syncytiotrophoblast characteristic of the surface of mature placental villi.

syncytial trophoblast. SYNCYTIOTROPHOBLAST.

syn·cy·tio·ly·sin (sin·sish″ee·o·lye′sin, sin·sit″ee·ol′i·sin) *n.* [*syncytium* + *lysin*]. A cytolysin produced by injections of an emulsion made from placental tissue.

syn·cy·ti·o·ma (sin·sish″ee·o′muh, sin·sit″) *n.* [*syncytium* + *-oma*]. CHORIOCARCINOMA.

syn·cy·tio·tox·in (sin·sish″ee·o·tock′sin, sin·sit″) *n.* [*synctium* + *toxin*]. A cytotoxin with specific action on the placenta.

syn·cy·tio·tro·pho·blast (sin·sish″ee·o·tro′fo·blast, sin·sit″) *n.* [*syncytium* + *trophoblast*]. An irregular sheet or net of deeply staining cytoplasm in which nuclei are irregularly scattered; it lies outside the cytotrophoblast from which it is derived by fusion of separate cells. Syn. *plasmoditrophoblast, syncytial trophoblast.*

syn·cy·tium (sin·sish′ee·um, sin·sit′ee·um) *n.,* pl. **syncy·tia**

(·shee·uh, ·tee·uh) [NL., from *syn-*, together, + Gk. *kytos*, vessel, "cell"]. A mass of cytoplasm with numerous nuclei but with no division into separate cells. Compare *symplasm*.

syn·dac·tyl (sin·dack'til) *adj.* [*syn-* + *dactyl*]. Having fingers or toes joined together.

syn·dac·tyl·ia (sin"dack·til'ee·uh) *n.* SYNDACTYLY.

syn·dac·ty·lism (sin·dack'ti·liz·um) *n.* SYNDACTYLY.

syn·dac·ty·lus (sin·dack'ti·lus) *n.* [*syn-* + *dactyl* + *-us*]. A person with webbed fingers or toes.

syn·dac·ty·ly (sin·dack'ti·lee) *n.* [*syndactyl* + *-y*]. Adhesion of fingers or toes; webbed fingers or webbed toes. —**syndacty·lous** (·lus) *adj.*

syn·de·sis (sin'de·sis) *n.* [Gk., from *syndein*, to bind together, from *dein*, to bind]. The state of being bound together.

syndesm-, syndesmo- [Gk. *syndesmos*, bond, fastening; ligament]. A combining form meaning (a) *connective;* (b) *articular, articulation;* (c) *ligament, ligamentous.*

syn·des·mec·to·pia (sin·dez"meck·to'pee·uh) *n.* [*syndesm-* + *-ectopia*]. Displacement of a ligament.

syn·des·mi·tis (sin"dez·migh'tis) *n.* [*syndesm-* + *-itis*]. 1. Inflammation of a ligament. 2. CONJUNCTIVITIS.

syn·des·mo·cho·ri·al (sin·dez"mo·ko'ree·ul) *adj.* [*syndesmo-* + *chorial*]. Pertaining to maternal connective tissue and chorionic ectoderm. See also *placenta.*

syndesmochorial placenta. A placenta in which the chorionic ectoderm is in contact with uterine connective tissue; occurs in ruminants.

syn·des·mo·di·as·ta·sis (sin·dez"mo·dye·as'tuh·sis) *n.* [*syndesmo-* + *diastasis*]. Separation of ligaments.

syn·des·mo·lo·gia (sin·dez"mo·lo'jee·uh) *n.* [NA]. A general heading which includes all joints.

syn·des·mol·ogy (sin"dez·mol'uh·jee) *n.* [*syndesmo-* + *-logy*]. The study of ligaments.

syn·des·mo·pexy (sin·dez'mo·peck"see) *n.* [*syndesmo-* + *-pexy*]. The attachment of a ligament in a new position.

syn·des·mo·phyte (sin·dez'mo·fite) *n.* [*syndesmo-* + *-phyte*]. An osseous outgrowth from a ligament.

syn·des·mor·rha·phy (sin"dez·mor'uh·fee) *n.* [*syndesmo-* + *-rrhaphy*]. Suture or repair of ligaments.

syn·des·mo·sis (sin"dez·mo'sis) *n.*, pl. **syndesmo·ses** (·seez) [*syndesm-* + *-osis*] [NA]. A form of articulation in which the bones are connected by fibrous connective tissue.

syndesmosis ti·bio·fi·bu·la·ris (tib"ee·o·fib·yoo·lair'is) [NA]. TIBIOFIBULAR SYNDESMOSIS. NA alt. *articulatio tibiofibularis.*

syndesmosis tym·pa·no·sta·pe·dia (tim"puh·no·stay·pee'dee·uh) [NA]. TYMPANOSTAPEDIAL SYNDESMOSIS.

syn·des·mot·omy (sin"dez·mot'uh·mee) *n.* [*syndesmo-* + *-tomy*]. The division of a ligament.

syn·det (sin'det) *n.* Any synthetic detergents.

syn·drome (sin'drome, sin'dro·mee) *n.* [Gk. *syndromē*, concurrence, syndrome, from *syn-* + *dromos*, running]. A group of symptoms and signs, which, when considered together, are known or presumed to characterize a disease or lesion. —**syn·dro·mic** (sin·dro'mick, ·drom'ick) *adj.*

syndrome of approximate answers. GANSER SYNDROME.

syndrome of rudimentary ovaries. GONADAL DYSGENESIS.

syn·dro·mol·o·gy (sin"dro·mol'uh·jee) *n.* The study of syndromes; the analysis of constellations of signs or symptoms with a view to determining which of them are significantly linked as probable results of the same underlying cause or causes.

Syndrox. A trademark for methamphetamine, a central stimulant drug used as the hydrochloride salt.

syn·ech·ia (si·neck'ee·uh, si·nee'kee·uh) *n.*, pl. **syn·echiae** (·ee·ee) [Gk. *synecheia*, continuity]. An abnormal union of parts; especially adhesion of the iris to a neighboring part of the eye. See also *annular synechia, posterior synechia.* —**synech·i·al** (·ee·ul) *adj.*

synechia vul·vae (vul'vee). VULVAR FUSION.

syn·ech·o·tome (si·neck'o·tome) *n.* [*synech*ia + *-tome*]. An instrument for the division of adhesions, particularly of the tympanic membrane.

syn·ech·ot·o·my (sin"e·kot'uh·mee) *n.* [*synech*ia + *-tomy*]. The division of a synechia.

syn·en·ceph·a·lo·cele (sin"en·sef'uh·lo·seel) *n.* [*syn-* + *encephalocele*]. An encephalocele with adhesions.

syn·er·e·sis (sin·err'e·sis) *n.*, pl. **synere·ses** (·seez) [Gk. *synairesis*, a drawing together]. 1. Contraction of a clot, as blood, milk. 2. *In colloid chemistry,* the exudation of the liquid constituent of gels irrespective of the vapor pressure imposed upon the system. Lowered vapor pressure aids the process.

syneresis of vitreous. Liquefaction of the vitreous.

syn·er·get·ic (sin"ur·jet'ick) *adj.* [*synergētikos*, cooperative]. Exhibiting synergy; working together; synergic.

syn·er·gia (si·nur'jee·uh, ·juh) *n.* SYNERGY (2).

syn·er·gism (sin'ur·jiz·um) *n.* 1. SYNERGY. 2. The joint action of two types of microorganisms on a carbohydrate medium, leading to the production of gas that is not formed by either organism when grown separately. 3. POTENTIATION (2).

syn·er·gist (sin'ur·jist) *n.* 1. An agent that increases the action or effectiveness of another agent when combined with it. 2. SYNERGISTIC MUSCLE. —**syn·er·gis·tic** (sin"ur·jis'tick) *adj.*

synergistic muscle. A muscle which, though not directly concerned as a prime mover in a particular act, helps some other muscle to perform the movement more efficiently.

syn·er·gy (sin'ur·jee) *n.* [Gk. *synergia*, cooperation, from *syn-* together, + *ergon*, work]. 1. The combined action or effect of two or more organs or agents, often greater than the sum of their individual actions or effects. 2. Coordination of muscular or organ functions by the nervous system in such a way that specific movements and actions can be performed. —**syn·er·gic** (si·nur'jick) *adj.*

syn·es·the·sia, syn·aes·the·sia (sin"es·theezh'uh, ·theez'ee·uh) *n.* [Gk. *synaisthes*is, an accompanying sensation, + *-ia*]. 1. A secondary sensation or subjective impression accompanying an actual perception of a different character, as a sensation of color or sound aroused by a sensation of taste. 2. A sensation experienced in one part of the body following stimulation of another part.

syn·es·thesi·al·gia, syn·aes·the·si·al·gia (sin"es·theez"ee·al'jee·uh, ·juh) *n.* [*synesthesi*a + *-algia*]. A painful sensation secondary to, and of a different quality from, that of a primary irritation.

Syn·ga·mus (sing'guh·mus) *n.* A genus of nematode worms of the family Syngamidae, which inhabits the upper respiratory tract of fowl and mammals.

Syngamus la·ryn·ge·us (la·rin'jee·us). A species which is usually a parasite of ruminants; incidental infection of man has occurred.

Syngamus tra·che·a·lis (tray"kee·ay'lis). The nematode infesting the trachea of avians and causing the condition called gapes of chickens. Syn. *gapeworm.*

syn·ga·my (sing'guh·mee) *n.* [Gk. *syngam*os, married, + *-y*]. Conjugation or union of gametes in fertilization. —**synga·mous** (·mus), **syn·gam·ic** (sing·gam'ick) *adj.*

syn·ge·ne·ic (sin"je·nee'ick) *adj.* SYNGENESIOUS.

syngeneic graft. A transplant between individuals that have been inbred until their genetic similarity allows acceptance of grafts between strain members.

syn·ge·ne·sio·plas·ty (sin"je·nee'zee·o·plas"tee) *n.* [*syngenesi*ous + *-plasty*]. Plastic surgery employing homografts taken from parents, siblings, or offspring. —**synge·ne·sio·plas·tic** (·nee"zee·o·plas'tick) *adj.*

syn·ge·ne·sious (sin"je·nee'zhus, ·zee·us) *adj.* [Gk. *syngenēs*, akin to, + *-ous*]. Of or derived from an individual of the same family or species, as of a tissue transplant.

syn·gig·no·scism (sin·jig'no·siz·um) *n.* [Gk. *syngignōsk*ein, to think with, agree with, + *-ism*] HYPNOTISM.

syn·hex·yl (sin·heck'sil) *n.* 1-Hydroxy-3-*n*-hexyl-6,6,9-trimethyl-7,8,9,10-tetrahydro-6-dibenzopyran, a synthetic analogue of a tetrahydrocannabinol; a pale-yellow, translucent, viscous, and odorless resin. Has been used as a euphoriant in the thalamic syndrome. Syn. *parahexyl, pyrahexyl.*

syn·hi·dro·sis (sin″hi·dro′sis) *n.* [*syn-* + *hidrosis*]. Concurrent sweating; the association of perspiration with another condition.

sy·ni·a·trist (si·nigh′uh·trist) *n.* [*syn-*, with, + Gk. *iatros*, physician, + *-ist*]. A health professional who carries out physician-like tasks and provides significant health care to patients under a physician's supervision and as regulated by law. According to specialty training, the person is designated a family practice syniatrist, a pediatric syniatrist, and the like.

syn·i·dro·sis (sin″i·dro′sis) *n.* [Gk. *synidrōsis*, excessive sweating]. SYNHIDROSIS.

syn·i·ze·sis (sin″i·zee′sis) *n.* [Gk. *synizēsis*, collapse]. SYNIZESIS PUPILLAE.

synizesis pu·pil·lae (pew·pil′ee). Closure of the pupil.

Synkamin. Trademark for 2-methyl-4-amino-1-naphthol hydrochloride, referred to as vitamin K_5, a water-soluble vitamin K compound.

syn·kary·on, syn·cary·on (sing·kăr′ee·on) *n.* [*syn-* + *karyon*]. The diploid zygotic nucleus formed by the fusion of two haploid nuclei, especially in the lower fungi.

Synkayvite. A trademark for menadiol sodium diphosphate, a water-soluble prothrombinogenic compound with the actions and uses of menadione.

syn·ki·ne·sia (sin″kigh·nee′zhuh) *n.* SYNKINESIS.

syn·ki·ne·sis (sin″kigh·nee′sis) *n.* [Gk. *synkinēsis*, movement in the same direction]. Involuntary movement of muscles or limbs coincident with the deliberate or essential movements carried out by another part of the body, such as the swinging of the arms while walking. Syn. *associated automatic movement, accessory movement.* **—synki·net·ic** (·net′ick) *adj.*

synkinetic movement. SYNKINESIS.

syn·ne·ma·tin (si·nee′muh·tin, sin″e·may′tin) *n.* An antibiotic substance, produced by *Cephalosporium salmosynnematum*, found to be D-(4-amino-4-carboxybutyl) penicillin and now generally called *penicillin N.* Syn. *cephalosporin N.*

synnematin B. Synnematin (= PENICILLIN N).

syn·odon·tia (sin″o·don′chee·uh) *n.* [*syn-* + *-odontia*]. Production of one tooth, showing evidence of duplicity, by fusion of two tooth germs.

syn·oph·rys (sin·off′ris) *n.* [Gk., having meeting eyebrows, from *syn-* + *ophrys*, eyebrow]. Meeting of the eyebrows.

syn·oph·thal·mia (sin″off·thal′mee·uh) *n.* [*syn-* + *ophthalm-* + *-ia*]. CYCLOPIA.

syn·oph·thal·mus (sin″off·thal′mus) *n.* [*syn-* + *ophthalmus*]. CYCLOPS.

Synophylate. A trademark for theophylline sodium glycinate.

syn·op·sia (sin·op′see·uh) *n.* [*syn-* + Gk. *ōps*, eye, + *-ia*]. CYCLOPIA.

syn·or·chi·dism (sin·or′ki·diz·um) *n.* [*syn-* + *orchid-* + *-ism*]. Partial or complete fusion of the two testes within the abdomen or scrotum.

syn·or·chism (sin·or′kiz·um) *n.* SYNORCHIDISM.

syn·os·che·os (sin·os′kee·os) *n.* [*syn-* + Gk. *oscheos*, scrotum]. A condition of adherence between the skin of the penis and that of the scrotum.

syn·os·teo·phyte (sin·os′tee·o·fite) *n.* [*syn-* + *osteophyte*]. A congenital bony ankylosis. Syn. *synostosis congenita.*

syn·os·te·o·sis (sin·os″tee·o′sis) *n.* SYNOSTOSIS.

syn·os·tosed (sin′os·tohzd, ·tohst) *adj.* Joined in bony union.

syn·os·to·sis (sin″os·to′sis) *n.*, pl. **synosto·ses** (·seez) [*syn-* + *ostosis*]. A union by osseous material of originally separate bones. **—synos·tot·ic** (·tot′ick) *adj.*

synostosis con·gen·ita (kon·jen′i·tuh). SYNOSTEOPHYTE.

syn·o·tia (si·no′shee·uh) *n.* [*syn-* + *ot-* + *-ia*]. Approximation or union of the ears in the anterior cervical region in the absence, or marked reduction, of the lower jaw.

syn·o·tus (si·no′tus) *n.* An individual with synotia.

syn·o·vec·to·my (sin″o·veck′tuh·mee) *n.* [*synovi-* + *-ectomy*]. Excision of synovial membrane.

synovi-, synovio-. A combining form meaning *synovial.*

syn·o·via (si·no′vee·uh) *n.* [NL., probably from *syn-* + L. *ovum*, egg, from similarity to egg white] [NA]. SYNOVIAL FLUID. **—syno·vi·al** (·vee·ul) *adj.*

synovial bursa. BURSA (1).

synovial capsule. JOINT CAPSULE.

synovial chondromatosis. Synovial hyperplasia with cartilaginous metaplasia and loose body formation.

synovial cyst. A cyst lined by synovial membrane, as in joints or bursae. See also *ganglion* (2).

synovial diverticulum. An abnormal pouch found in a large joint, such as the knee.

synovial fluid. The clear fluid, resembling white of egg, found in various joints, bursas, and sheaths of tendons. NA *synovia.*

synovial hernia. The protrusion of the inner lining of a joint capsule through the outer portion of the capsule.

synovial joint. A freely movable articulation, in which contiguous bone surfaces are covered with collagenous fibrovascular tissue composed of flattened or cuboidal cells. For synovial joints listed by name, see Table of Synovial Joints and Ligaments in the Appendix. NA *junctura synovialis.*

synovial ligament. SYNOVIAL MEMBRANE.

synovial membrane. The sheet of flattened connective tissue cells that lines a synovial bursa, a synovial sheath, or the capsule of a synovial joint. NA *membrana synovialis.*

syn·o·vi·al·o·ma (si·no″vee·uh·lo′muh) *n.* Benign synovioma.

synovial plica. A fold of the synovial membrane of a joint, extending toward or between the articular surfaces; it may contain fat or provide for the course of vessels. NA *plica synovialis.*

synovial sac. The fluid-filled sac formed by the membrane enclosing a synovial joint; its interior constitutes the joint cavity.

synovial sarcoendothelioma. A malignant synovioma.

synovial sarcoma. A malignant synovioma.

synovial sarcomesothelioma. A malignant synovioma.

synovial sheath. A synovial membrane which lines the cavity through which a tendon glides.

synovial villi. The processes extending from a synovial membrane into an articular cavity. NA *villi synoviales.*

synovio-. See *synovi-.*

syn·o·vio·en·do·the·lio·ma (si·no″vee·o·en″do·theel·ee·o′muh) *n.* [*synovio-* + *endothelioma*]. A malignant synovioma.

syn·o·vi·o·ma (si·no″vee·o′muh) *n.* [*synovia* + *-oma*]. Any tumor, benign or malignant, whose parenchyma is composed of cells similar to those covering the synovial membranes.

syn·o·vip·a·rous (sin″o·vip′uh·rus) *adj.* [*synovi-* + *parous*]. Producing or secreting synovia.

synoviparous crypts. Extensions of the synovial membranes sometimes perforating an articular capsule and occasionally becoming shut off from its main sac.

syn·o·vi·tis (sin″o·vye′tis) *n.* [*synovi-* + *-itis*]. Inflammation of a synovial membrane.

synovitis hy·per·plas·ti·ca (high″pur·plas′ti·kuh). FUNGOUS ARTHRITIS.

syn·tac·tic (sin·tack′tick) *adj.* [Gk. *syntaktikos*, putting together, composing]. Pertaining to syntax, or the system whereby linguistic units (especially, words) are combined to form larger units (phrases, sentences).

syn·tac·ti·cal (sin·tack′ti·kul) *adj.* SYNTACTIC.

syntactical or **syntactic aphasia.** A type of Wernicke's aphasia characterized by jargon and impaired comprehension, writing, and reading.

syn·ta·sis (sin'tuh·sis) *n.* [Gk., tension]. A stretching, or tension.

syn·thase (sin'thace, ·thaze) *n.* Any enzyme thus denominated when it is desired to emphasize the synthetic aspect of a reaction catalyzed by the enzyme.

syn·the·sis (sinth'e·sis) *n.*, pl. **synthe·ses** (·seez) [Gk., from *syn-*, together, + *thesis*, setting, placing]. 1. *In chemistry*, the processes and operations necessary to build up a compound. In general, a reaction, or series of reactions, in which a complex compound is obtained from elements or simple compounds. 2. The formation of a complex concept by the combination of separate ideas; the putting together of data to form a whole. 3. *In psychiatry*, the process in which the ego accepts unconscious ideas and feelings and amalgamates them within itself more or less consciously. —**syn·the·size** (sinth'e·size) *v.*

syn·the·tase (sinth'e·tace, ·taze) *n.* LIGASE.

syn·thet·ic (sin·thet'ick) *adj.* [Gk. *synthetikos*, constructive]. Produced by artificial means.

synthetic vitamin K. MENADIONE.

syn·tho·rax (sin·tho'racks) *n.* [*syn-* + *thorax*]. THORACOPAGUS.

Synthroid. A trademark for sodium levothyroxine, used for thyroid hormone replacement therapy.

syn·ton·ic (sin·ton'ick) *adj.* [Gk. *syntonos*, harmonious, from *tonos*, tone]. Characterizing a type of personality in which there is an appropriate harmony of thinking, feeling, and behavior, one in harmony with the environment.

syn·to·nin (sin'to·nin) *n.* 1. A metaprotein obtained by the action of dilute acid on more complex proteins. 2. The specific metaprotein thus obtained from the myosin of muscle.

syn·tro·pho·blast (sin·tro'fo·blast, ·trof'o·) *n.* SYNCYTIOTROPHOBLAST.

syn·tro·phus (sin'tro·fus) *n.* [NL., from Gk. *syntrophos*, brought up with; innate, habitual]. An inherited or congenital disease.

syn·tro·py (sin'truh·pee) *n.* [*syn-* + *-tropy*]. *In psychobiology*, the state of felicitous and mutually satisfactory relationship with other individuals.

Sy·pha·cia (sigh·fay'see·uh) *n.* A genus of nematode worms belonging to the family Oxyuridae.

Syphacia ob·ve·la·ta (ob"ve·lay'tuh). A species of nematode worm commonly found in rats and mice; man is very rarely infected.

syphil-, syphilo-. A combining form meaning *syphilis, syphilitic.*

syph·i·lel·cos (sif"i·lel'kos) *n.* [*syphil-* + Gk. *helkos*, ulcer]. Syphilitic ulcer; CHANCRE (1).

syph·i·lel·cus (sif"i·lel'kus) *n.* [NL.]. SYPHILELCOS.

syph·i·le·mia (sif"i·lee'mee·uh) *n.* [*syphil-* + *-emia*]. The presence of *Treponema pallidum* in the bloodstream.

syph·i·lid (sif'i·lid) *n.* [*syphil-* + *-id*]. Any skin eruption due to syphilis.

syph·i·lide (sif'i·lide) *n.* SYPHILID.

syph·i·li·on·thus (sif"i·lee·onth'us) *n.* [NL., from *syphil-* + Gk. *ionthos*, eruption]. Any copper-colored scaly eruption in syphilis.

syph·i·lis (sif'i·lis) *n.* [after *Syphilus*, a shepherd afflicted with the disease in the poem *Syphilis sive Morbus Gallicus* (1530) by Fracastoro]. A prenatal or acquired systemic infection with *Treponema pallidum*, most often contracted in sexual intercourse. Lesions may occur in any tissue or vascular organ of the body, and the disease may produce various clinical pictures of its own, or give rise to symptoms characteristic of other diseases. See also *primary syphilis, secondary syphilis, tertiary syphilis.*

syphilis d'em·blee [F., at once, immediately]. The invasion of syphilis without a local lesion.

syphilis he·red·i·ta·ria (he·red"i·tair'ee·uh). CONGENITAL SYPHILIS.

syphilis in·son·ti·um (in·son'shee·um). Syphilis acquired in an innocent manner; nonvenereal or congenital syphilis.

syphilis tech·ni·ca (teck'ni·kuh). Syphilis acquired in following one's occupation, as by physicians, midwives, nurses.

syphilis test. Any test for syphilis, such as the Eagle test, Hinton test, Kahn test, Kline test, Kolmer's test, 1., Lange's test, Laughlen test, mastic test, Mazzini test, Meinicke's test, Pangborn test, Wassermann's test, etc.

syph·i·lit·ic (sif"i·lit'ick) *adj.* & *n.* 1. Of, pertaining to, or affected with syphilis. 2. A person affected with syphilis.

syphilitic amyotrophy. A rare disease of questionable syphilitic etiology, characterized by progressive muscular atrophy of the upper limbs and shoulder girdles.

syphilitic cirrhosis. Hepatic fibrosis resulting from syphilitic destruction of liver parenchyma.

syphilitic condyloma. CONDYLOMA LATUM.

syphilitic hyperplastic pachymeningitis. SYPHILITIC SPINAL PACHYMENINGITIS.

syphilitic hypertrophic pachymeningitis or **arachnoiditis.** SYPHILITIC SPINAL PACHYMENINGITIS.

syphilitic keratitis. Interstitial keratitis due to syphilis.

syphilitic meningoencephalitis. GENERAL PARALYSIS.

syphilitic meningomyelitis. A form of spinal syphilis, characterized pathologically by a chronic fibrosing meningitis with subpial loss of myelinated fibers and gliosis, and clinically by signs referable to disease of the lateral and posterior columns of the spinal cord.

syphilitic myelitis. SYPHILITIC MENINGOMYELITIS.

syphilitic node. Localized swelling on bones due to syphilitic periostitis.

syphilitic optic atrophy. Progressive blindness in one eye and then involving the other, due to a syphilitic perioptic meningitis with subpial gliosis and fibrosis replacing degenerated optic nerve fibers.

syphilitic osteochondritis. Syphilitic involvement of the epiphyseal cartilage during infancy, characterized by irregular calcification of the epiphyses and thickening of the distal ends of the long bones. The extremities are usually symmetrically involved.

syphilitic paresis. GENERAL PARALYSIS.

syphilitic retinitis. The retinitis occurring in syphilis; it is chronic, diffuse, and a late manifestation of the systemic disease.

syphilitic spinal muscular atrophy. SYPHILITIC AMYOTROPHY.

syphilitic spinal pachymeningitis. A rare form of neurosyphilis which gives rise to radicular pain and amyotrophy of the hands, and signs of long tract involvement of the legs. Syn. *syphilitic hypertrophic pachymeningitis.*

syphilitic spastic paraplegia. Spastic paraplegia due to spinal syphilis.

syphilitic stomatitis. Inflammation associated with the oral lesions of syphilis.

syphilitic tarsitis. Syphilitic infection of a tarsal bone.

syph·i·li·za·tion (sif"i·li·zay'shun) *n.* 1. Inoculation with *Treponema pallidum*. 2. The occurrence and spread of syphilis in a community.

syphilo-. See *syphil-*.

syph·i·lo·derm (sif'i·lo·durm) *n.* [*syphilo-* + *-derm*]. Any of the skin manifestations of syphilis. —**syph·i·lo·der·ma·tous** (sif"i·lo·dur'muh·tus) *adj.*

syph·i·lo·der·ma (sif"i·lo·dur'muh) *n.* [*syphilo-* + *-derma*]. SYPHILODERM.

syph·i·lo·gen·e·sis (sif"i·lo·jen'e·sis) *n.* [*syphilo-* + *-genesis*]. The origin or development of syphilis.

syph·i·log·ra·pher (sif"i·log'ruh·fer) *n.* One who writes about syphilis.

syph·i·loid (sif'i·loid) *adj.* Resembling syphilis.

syph·i·lol·o·gist (sif"i·lol'uh·jist) *n.* [*syphilology* + *-ist*]. One who has made a study of syphilis; an expert in the diagnosis and treatment of the disease.

syph·i·lol·o·gy (sif"i·lol'uh·jee) *n.* [*syphilo-* + *-logy*]. The sum of knowledge regarding the origin, nature, and treatment of syphilis.

syph·i·lo·ma (sif″i-lo′muh) *n.*, pl. **syphilomas, syphiloma·ta** (·tuh) [*syphil-* + *-oma*]. 1. A syphilitic gumma. 2. A tumor due to syphilis. —**syphi·lom·a·tous** (·lom′uh·tus) *adj.*

syph·i·lo·ma·nia (sif″i·lo·may′nee·uh) *n.* [*syphilo-* + *-mania*]. Extreme syphilophobia.

syph·i·lo·nych·ia (sif″i·lo·nick′ee·uh) *n.* [*syphil-* + *onychia*]. An onychia of syphilitic origin.

syphilonychia ex·ul·ce·rans (eck″sul′se·ranz). Syphilitic onychia with ulceration.

syphilonychia sic·ca (sick′uh). Syphilis of the nail bed.

syph·i·lop·a·thy (sif″i·lop′uth·ee) *n.* [*syphilo-* + *-pathy*]. Any syphilitic disease.

syph·i·lo·phobe (sif′i·lo·fobe) *n.* A person affected with syphilophobia.

syph·i·lo·pho·bia (sif″i·lo·fo′bee·uh) *n.* [*syphilo-* + *-phobia*]. Abnormal fear of syphilis; the delusion of being infected with syphilis.

syph·i·lo·phy·ma (sif″i·lo·fye′muh) *n.* [*syphilo-* + *phyma*]. 1. Syphiloma of the skin. 2. Any growth due to syphilis.

syph·i·lo·ther·a·py (sif″i·lo·therr′uh·pee) *n.* [*syphilo-* + *therapy*]. Treatment for syphilis.

syr. Abbreviation for *syrupus*, syrup.

Syraprim. Trademark for trimethoprim, an antibacterial agent.

Syrette. Trademark for a small hypodermic syringe containing a dose of the drug to be administered.

sy·rig·mo·pho·nia (si·rig″mo·fo′nee·uh) *n.* [*syrigmus* + *-phonia*]. 1. A piping or whistling state of the voice. 2. A sibilant rale.

sy·rig·mus (si·rig′mus) *n., pl.* **syrig·mi** (·mye) [NL., from Gk. *syrigmos*, shrill or sibilant sound]. Any subjective hissing, murmuring, or tinkling sound heard in the ear.

syring-, syringo- [Gk. *syrinx, syringos*, pipe, tube, fistula]. A combining form meaning *long cavity, tube, tubular*, as a sweat gland duct, a fistula, or the spinal cord with its central canal.

syr·ing·ad·e·no·ma (sirr″ing·gad″e·no′muh) *n.* [*syring-* + *adenoma*]. SWEAT GLAND ADENOMA.

syr·ing·ad·e·no·sus (sirr″ing·gad″e·no′sus) *adj.* [NL., from Gk. *syrinx*, pipe, duct, pore, + *adēn*, gland]. Pertaining to the sweat glands.

sy·ringe (suh·rinj′, sirr′inj) *n.* [ML. *syringa*, from Gk. *syrinx, syringos*, tube, pipe]. 1. An apparatus commonly made of glass or plastic, fitted snugly onto a hollow metal needle, used to aspirate or inject fluids for diagnostic or therapeutic purposes. It consists essentially of a barrel, which may be calibrated, and a perfectly matched plunger. 2. A large glass barrel with a fitted rubber bulb at one end and a nozzle at the other, used primarily for irrigation purposes.

syringe-capillary method. ROUGHTON-SCHOLANDER METHOD.

syringe jaundice. SERUM HEPATITIS.

syringo-. See *syring-*.

sy·rin·go·bul·bia (si·ring″go·bul′bee·uh) *n.* [*syringo-* + *bulb* + *-ia*]. An extension of the cavity of syringomyelia into the brainstem, usually into the lateral tegmentum of the medulla and rarely into the pons.

sy·rin·go·car·ci·no·ma (si·ring″go·kahr″si·no′muh) *n.* [*syringo-* + *carcinoma*]. 1. SWEAT GLAND ADENOMA. 2. SWEAT GLAND CARCINOMA.

sy·rin·go·cele, sy·rin·go·coele (si·ring′go·seel) *n.* [*syringo-* + *-coele*]. The cavity or central canal of the spinal cord.

sy·rin·go·coe·lia (si·ring″go·see′lee·uh) *n.* [*syringo-* + Gk. *koilia*, cavity]. SYRINGOCELE.

sy·rin·go·cyst·ad·e·no·ma (si·ring″go·sist″ad·e·no′muh) *n.* [*syringo-* + *cystadenoma*]. SYRINGOMA.

sy·rin·go·cys·to·ma (si·ring″go·sis·to′muh) *n.* [*syringo-* + *cyst-* + *-oma*]. SYRINGOMA.

sy·rin·goid (si·ring′goid) *adj.* [*syring-* + *-oid*]. Like a tube.

syr·in·go·ma (sir″ing·go′muh) *n.* [Gk. *syringōma*, fistula]. A benign tumor of sweat glands, occurring most often in females and developing after puberty. Histologically, the dermis contains numerous small cystic ducts with comma-like tails of epithelium. Syn. *syringocystadenoma, syringocystoma.*

sy·rin·go·me·nin·go·cele (si·ring″go·me·ning′go·seel) *n.* [*syringo-* + *meningocele*]. SYRINGOMYELOCELE.

sy·rin·go·my·e·lia (si·ring″go·migh·ee′lee·uh) *n.* [*syringo-* + *myel-* + *-ia*]. A chronic progressive degenerative disorder of the spinal cord, characterized clinically by brachial amyotrophy and segmental sensory loss of dissociated type, and pathologically by cavitation of the central parts of the cervical spinal cord and extending in some cases into the medulla oblongata or downward into the thoracic and lumbar segments.

sy·rin·go·my·e·lo·cele (si·ring″go·migh′e·lo·seel) *n.* [*syringo-* + *myelocele*]. Spina bifida with protrusion of a meningeal sac containing a portion of the spinal cord whose central canal is greatly distended with cerebrospinal fluid.

syr·inx (sirr′inks) *n.*, pl. **sy·rin·ges** (si·rin′jeez), **syrinxes** [Gk. pipe, duct, fistula]. 1. A fistula or tube. 2. The posterior larynx of birds, found within the thorax at the tracheal bifurcation; the organ of voice in birds. 3. The glial-lined cavity in syringomyelia.

syr·o·sing·o·pine (sirr″o·sing′go·pine) *n.* Carbethoxysyringoyl methylreserpate, $C_{35}H_{42}N_2O_{11}$, a reserpine analogue used as an antihypertensive drug.

syr·up, sir·up (sur′up, sirr′up) *n.* [Ar. *sharāb*, a drink]. 1. A concentrated solution of sugar in aqueous fluids, with the addition of medicating or flavoring ingredients. 2. Simple syrup: the U.S.P. preparation containing sucrose, 850 g and a sufficient quantity of purified water to make 1,000 ml. Used in the preparation of other medicated or flavored syrups and preparations and in pharmaceutical operations where sucrose in solution is required. Abbreviated, syr.

sys-. See *syn-*.

sys·sar·co·sis (sis″ahr·ko′sis) *n.*, pl. **syssarco·ses** (·seez) [Gk. *syssarkōsis*, overgrowth with flesh, from *syn-* + *sarx*, flesh]. The failure of union of bones after fracture by the interposition of muscular tissue. —**syssar·cot·ic** (·kot′ick) *adj.*

sys·so·ma (si·so′muh) *n.* [*sys-* + Gk. *sōma*, body]. DICEPHALISM. —**sysso·mic** (·mick) *adj.*

sys·so·mus (si·so′mus) *n.* [NL., from Gk. *syssōmos*, united in one body, from *syn-*, together, + *sōma*, body]. DICEPHALUS.

sys·tal·tic (sis·tahl′tick, ·tal′tick) *adj.* [Gk. *systaltikos*, contracting, depressing]. Pulsatory; contracting; having a systole.

sys·ta·sis (sis′tuh·sis) *n.* [Gk., from *syn-*, together, + *stasis*, placing, standing]. Consistency, density.

sys·tem, *n.* [Gk. *systēma*, from *syn-*, together, + *hystanai*, to place, to stand]. 1. A methodical arrangement. 2. A combination of parts into a whole, as the digestive system, the nervous system. 3. The body as a functional whole.

sys·te·ma (sis·tee′muh) *L. n.*, genit. **systema·tis** (·tis). SYSTEM.

systema di·ges·to·ri·um (dye·jes·to′ree·um) [NA alt.]. DIGESTIVE SYSTEM. NA alt. *apparatus digestorius.*

systema lym·pha·ti·cum (lim·fat′i·kum) [NA]. LYMPHATIC SYSTEM.

systema ner·vo·rum cen·tra·le (nur·vo′rum sen·tray′lee) [BNA]. Systema nervosum centrale (= CENTRAL NERVOUS SYSTEM).

systema nervorum pe·ri·phe·ri·cum (perr·i·ferr′i·kum) [BNA]. Systema nervosum periphericum (= PERIPHERAL NERVOUS SYSTEM).

systema ner·vo·sum (nur·vo′sum) [NA]. NERVOUS SYSTEM (1).

systema nervosum au·to·no·mi·cum (aw·to·nom′i·kum) [NA]. AUTONOMIC NERVOUS SYSTEM.

systema nervosum cen·tra·le (sen·tray′lee) [NA]. CENTRAL NERVOUS SYSTEM.

systema nervosum pe·ri·phe·ri·cum (perr·i·ferr′i·kum) [NA]. PERIPHERAL NERVOUS SYSTEM.

systema nervosum sym·pa·thi·cum (sim·path′i·kum) [BNA]. Systema nervosum autonomicum (= AUTONOMIC NERVOUS SYSTEM).

systema re·spi·ra·to·ri·um (re·spye·ruh·to'ree·um) [NA alt.]. RESPIRATORY SYSTEM. NA alt. *apparatus respiratorius.*

sys·tem·at·ic (sis''te·mat'ick) *adj.* [Gk. *systēmatikos,* from *systēma,* system]. 1. Pertaining to or constituting a system. 2. Methodical; orderly. 3. Of or pertaining to classification, as in taxonomy. 4. SYSTEMIC (1).

sys·tem·a·tize (sis'te·muh·tize) *v.* 1. To organize into a system. 2. To classify. 3. To render methodical and orderly.

systematized neviform atrophy of the skin. FOCAL DERMAL HYPOPLASIA SYNDROME.

systematized nevus. A widespread nevus with a pattern having an orderly arrangement of some sort.

systematized spinal sclerosis. The systematized degeneration of the lateral and posterior columns of the spinal cord attributed to spinal syphilis.

systema uro·ge·ni·ta·le (yoo''ro·jen·i·tay'lee) [NA alt.]. URO-GENITAL SYSTEM. NA alt. *apparatus urogenitalis.*

sys·tem·ic (sis·tem'ick) *adj.* 1. Of, pertaining to, or involving the body considered as a functional whole. Contr. *local.* 2. Of or pertaining to the systemic circulation.

systemic circulation. The general circulation, as distinct from the pulmonary circulation. Syn. *greater circulation.* See also Plates 7, 9.

systemic emetic. INDIRECT EMETIC.

systemic hyperfibrinolysis. Widespread destruction of fibrinogen and fibrin.

systemic lupus erythematosus. An often fatal disease of unknown cause, characterized clinically by fever, muscle and joint pains, anemia, leukopenia, and frequently by a skin eruption similar to chronic discoid lupus erythematosus. Pathologically it is characterized by alteration in the connective tissue, especially of the arterioles, and the presence of hematoxylin-staining bodies in areas of fibrinoid degeneration of involved tissues. Primarily involved are the kidney, spleen, skin, and endocardium.

systemic multiple lipomas. LIPOBLASTOSIS.

systemic scleroderma. DIFFUSE SCLERODERMA.

systemic symptom. CONSTITUTIONAL SYMPTOM.

systemic vein. One of the veins conveying venous blood from the systemic circuit to the right atrium of the heart.

system of Batson. VERTEBRAL VENOUS SYSTEM.

system of macrophages. RETICULOENDOTHELIAL SYSTEM.

sys·tem·oid (sis'te·moid) *adj.* [*system* + *-oid*]. Characterizing a tumor composed of a number of tissues resembling a system of organs.

sys·to·le (sis'tuh·lee) *n.* [Gk. *systolē,* contraction, from *systellein,* to contract, from *syn-,* together, + *stellein,* gather, fetch]. The contraction phase of the cardiac cycle.

sys·tol·ic (sis·tol'ick) *adj.* Pertaining to the systole; occurring during systole.

systolic blood pressure. The maximum systemic arterial blood pressure during ventricular systole.

systolic click. A single or multiple extra heart sound, occurring in mid- or late systole; usually related to an abnormality of the mitral valve but may occasionally be of extracardiac origin.

systolic shock. The shock occurring in association with a diastolic impact when the heart pounds against the thorax.

systolic thrill. A thrill felt during ventricular systole on palpation of the precordium, as in conditions such as ventricular septal defect and aortic or pulmonic stenosis.

systolic wave. REGURGITANT WAVE.

sys·trem·ma (sis·trem'uh) *n.,* pl. **systremma·ta** (·tuh) [Gk., twist, knot, ball]. A cramp in the muscles of the leg.

syz·y·gy (siz'i·jee) *n.* [Gk. *syzygia,* union, combination, from *syn-,* together, + *zygon,* yoke]. End-to-end union of the sporonts of certain gregarines. —**sy·zyg·i·al** (si·zij'ee·ul) *adj.*

Sza·bo's sign (sob'o) [D. *Szabo,* Hungarian physician, 19th century]. *Obsol.* In sciatica, sensory loss along the lateral surface of the affected foot.

Szent-Györ·gyi test (sen'dʸœr''dʸee) [A. *Szent-Györgyi,* Hungarian biochemist, b. 1893]. A test for ascorbic acid based on the violet coloration upon the addition of ferrous sulfate to an alkaline solution of ascorbic acid.

Szy·ma·now·ski's operation (shi·mah·noʰf'skee) [J. von *Szymanowski,* Russian surgeon, 1829–1868]. 1. A form of blepharoplasty. 2. Operation for the restoration of the auricle; for ectropion; for restoration of the upper lip by lateral flaps brought together in the midline.

T

T 1. Abbreviation for *temperature.* 2. *In molecular biology,* symbol for thymine.

T Symbol for transmittance.

$t^{1/2}$, $t^{1/2}$ *In radiology,* symbol for half-life.

T 1824 EVANS BLUE.

T.A. An abbreviation for *toxin-antitoxin.*

Ta Symbol for tantalum.

Taarn·hoj operation. Surgical decompression of the dorsal root of the trigeminal nerve for the relief of trigeminal neuralgia.

tab·a·co·sis (tab″uh·ko′sis) *n.* [NL. *taba*cum, tobacco, + *-osis*]. A toxic state produced by the excessive use of tobacco, or by the inhalation of tobacco dust.

ta·ba·cum (ta·bay′kum) *n.* [NL.]. TOBACCO.

tab·a·gism (tab′uh·jiz·um) *n.* [F. *tabagisme*]. TABACOSIS.

tab·a·nid (tab′uh·nid) *n.* Any representative of the family Tabanidae.

Ta·ban·i·dae (ta·ban′i·dee) *n.pl.* A family of the Diptera, which includes the horseflies, deerflies, and gadflies. They are medium to large in size, robust and worldwide in distribution. The females of the well-known species are bloodsuckers which attack man and warm-blooded animals generally. Certain species distribute diseases such as anthrax among cattle and sheep; others transmit the trypanosomes of animals, especially the *Trypanosoma evansi,* the cause of surra in horses and cattle. The important genera are *Chrysops, Haematopota, Tabanus,* and *Pangonia.*

ta·bar·di·llo (tah″bahr·dee′yo) *n.* [Sp.]. EPIDEMIC TYPHUS.

ta·ba·tière ana·to·mique (tah·bah·tyair′ an·ah·to·meek′). ANATOMIST'S SNUFFBOX.

ta·bel·la (ta·bel′uh) *n.,* pl. **tabel·lae** (·ee) [L., dim. of *tabula,* board, tablet]. A medicinal troche or tablet.

ta·bes (tay′beez) *n.* [L., from *tabere,* to waste away]. 1. A wasting or consumption of a part of or the whole body. 2. TABES DORSALIS. Adj. *tabetic.*

ta·bes·cense (ta·bes′unce) *n.* [L. *tabescere,* to waste away, from *tabes,* decay, wasting]. Progressive wasting; MARASMUS; EMACIATION. **—tabes·cent** (·unt) *adj.*

tabes cox·a·ria (kock·sair′ree·uh). Wasting from hip disease.

tabes do·lo·ro·sa (do·lo·ro′suh). Tabes dorsalis in which pain is the dominating feature.

tabes dor·sa·lis (dor·say′lis). A form of neurosyphilis which develops 15 to 20 years after the onset of infection. It is characterized clinically by lightning pains, ataxia, urinary incontinence, absent knee and ankle jerks, impaired vibratory and position sense in the feet and legs, and a Romberg posterior sign, and pathologically by a degeneration of the posterior roots and posterior columns of the spinal cord. Syn. *tabetic neurosyphilis, locomotor ataxia.*

tabes er·got·i·ca (ur·got′i·kuh). Ergotism with symptoms resembling those of tabes dorsalis.

tabes mes·en·ter·i·ca (mes″en·terr′i·kuh). Mesenteric lymphadenitis, usually due to infection with *Mycobacterium tuberculosis,* with paroxysmal abdominal symptoms resembling those of tabes dorsalis.

ta·bet·ic (ta·bet′ick) *adj.* [*tab*es + *-ic*]. 1. Affected with tabes; of or pertaining to tabes. 2. Pertaining to, or affected with, tabes dorsalis.

tabetic arthropathy. CHARCOT'S JOINT.

tabetic ataxia. TABES DORSALIS.

tabetic bladder. The atonic bladder seen in tabes dorsalis.

tabetic crisis. Paroxysmal pain occurring in the course of tabes dorsalis.

tabetic cuirass. An anesthetic area encircling the chest, seen in tabes dorsalis.

tabetic gait. The ataxic gait of tabes dorsalis.

tabetic neurosyphilis. TABES DORSALIS.

ta·bet·i·form (ta·bet′i·form) *adj.* [*tab*es + *-iform*]. Resembling tabes.

tab·ic (tab′ick) *adj.* [*tab*es + *-ic*]. TABETIC.

tab·id (tab′id) *adj.* [L. *tabidus,* wasting, decaying, from *tabere,* to waste away]. TABETIC.

ta·ble, *n.* [L. *tabula,* board]. 1. A flat-topped piece of furniture, as an operating table, examining table. 2. A flat plate, especially one of bone, as the inner or outer table (of compact bone) of a flat bone of the cranium. 3. An orderly presentation of numerical data in the form of rows and columns.

ta·ble·spoon, *n.* A large spoon, holding about 15 ml, or 4 fluidrams. Abbreviated, tbsp.

tab·let, *n.* [F. *tablette*]. A solid dosage form of a medicinal substance or substances, with or without suitable diluents, that may be prepared by compression or by molding.

tablet triturate. A small, usually molded but sometimes compressed tablet. Dextrose, or a mixture of sucrose and lactose, is generally employed as the diluent so as to obtain a tablet that is rapidly and completely soluble.

ta·bo·pa·ral·y·sis (tay″bo·puh·ral′i·sis) *n.* [*tab*es + *paralysis*]. TABOPARESIS.

tabo·pa·re·sis (tay″bo·puh·ree′sis, ·păr′e·sis) *n.* [*tab*es + *paresis*]. A form of neurosyphilis in which the symptoms and signs of tabes dorsalis are combined with those of general paresis.

tab·u·lar (tab′yoo·lur) *adj.* [L. *tabularis,* from *tabula,* board]. Having the form of a table.

tabular bone. A flat bone; composed of an outer and an inner table of compact bone with cancellous bone, or diploë, between them.

tabular epithelium. Simple squamous epithelium.

T.A.B. vaccine. Abbreviation for *typhoid-paratyphoid A and B vaccine.*

Tacaryl. Trademark for methdilazine, an antihistaminic drug used to relieve pruritus.

Tace. Trademark for chlorotrianisene, a synthetic estrogen.

tache (tash) *n.*, pl. **taches** (tash) [F.]. A spot, macule, freckle; circumscribed discoloration on the skin or a mucous membrane.

tache bleu·atre (bluh·ahtr', bloo·ahtr'). A spot of a delicate blue tint, sometimes observed in the skin of typhoid fever patients.

tache cé·ré·brale (say·ray·bral'). A red streak, sometimes associated with petechiae, produced by drawing a fingernail over the skin, due to increased vasomotor irritability, occurring in certain neurologic disorders, especially in connection with meningeal irritation. Syn. *Trousseau's sign.*

tache mé·nin·gé·ale (may·nan·zhay·al'). TACHE CÉRÉBRALE.

tache noire (tash nwahr) [F., black spot]. The primary painless lesion of the tick-borne typhus fevers of Africa, manifested by a raised red area with typical black necrotic center which appears at the site of the tick bite.

tach·e·om·e·ter (tack"ee·om'e·tur) *n.* HEMOTACHOMETER.

tache mo·trice (mo·treece'). MOTOR END PLATE.

taches blanches (blahnsh). White spots occurring on the liver, especially on its convex surfaces, in infectious diseases.

taches du café au lait. CAFÉ AU LAIT SPOTS.

tache spi·nale (spee·nal'). A trophic bulla of the skin sometimes seen in diseases of the spinal cord.

taches ro·sées len·ti·cu·laires (ro·zay' lahn·tee·kew·lair'). ROSE SPOTS.

ta·chet·ic (ta·ket'ick) *adj.* [*tache* + *-ic*]. Relating to the formation of reddish blue or purple patches (taches).

ta·chis·to·scope (ta·kis'tuh·skope) *n.* [Gk. *tachistos*, very fast, (from *tachys,* fast) + *-scope*]. 1. An instrument used in physiologic psychology to observe the time rate and time conditions for apperception. 2. Any of several instruments using timed brief flashes of light for testing visual fields or in orthoptic correction procedures. **—ta·chis·to·scop·ic** (ta·kis"tuh·skop'ick) *adj.*

tacho- [Gk. *tachos*]. A combining form meaning *speed.*

tacho·gram (tack'o·gram) *n.* [*tacho-* + *-gram*]. The record made in tachography.

ta·chog·ra·phy (ta·kog'ruh·fee) *n.* [*tacho-* + *-graphy*]. The estimation of the rate of flow of arterial blood by means of a flowmeter.

ta·chom·e·ter (ta·kom'e·tur) *n.* [*tacho-* + *-meter*]. HEMOTACHOMETER. 2. A device for measuring frequency of rotation.

tachy- [Gk. *tachys*]. A combining form meaning *rapid, quick, accelerated.*

tachy·al·i·men·ta·tion (tack"ee·al"i·men·tay'shun) *n.* [*tachy-* + *alimentation*]. Eating more rapidly than normal.

tachy·ar·rhyth·mia (tack"ee·a·rith'mee·uh) *n.* [*tachy-* + *arrhythmia*]. Rapid heart action without control by the sinoatrial node.

tachy·aux·e·sis (tack"ee·awk·see'sis) *n.* [*tachy-* + *auxesis*]. Heterauxesis in which a part grows more rapidly than the whole organism.

tachy·car·dia (tack"i·kahr'dee·uh) *n.* [*tachy-* + *-cardia*]. Excessive rapidity of the heart's action.

tachy·car·di·ac (tack"i·kahr'dee·ack) *adj.* Pertaining to, or suffering from, tachycardia.

tachycardia stru·mo·sa ex·oph·thal·mi·ca (stroo·mo'suh eck"sof·thal'mi·kuh). The tachycardia occurring in hyperthyroidism.

tachy·graph (tack'i·graf) *n.* [*tachy-* + *-graf*]. A blood flowmeter.

ta·chyg·ra·phy (ta·kig'ruh·fee) *n.* [*tachy-* + *-graphy*]. The estimation of the rate of flow of arterial blood by means of a blood flowmeter.

tachy·lo·gia (tack"i·lo'jee·uh) *n.* [*tachy-* + *-logia*]. Extreme rapidity or volubility of speech. See also *cluttering.*

ta·chym·e·ter (ta·kim'e·tur) *n.* [*tachy-* + *-meter*]. An instrument for measuring the speed of a moving object.

tachy·pha·gia (tack"i·fay'jee·uh) *n.* [*tachy-* + *-phagia*]. Rapid eating.

tachy·pha·sia (tack"i·fay'zhuh) *n.* [*tachy-* + *-phasia*]. TACHYLOGIA.

tachy·phe·mia (tach"i·fee'mee·uh) *n.* [*tachy-* + *-phemia*]. TACHYLOGIA.

tachy·phra·sia (tack"i·fray'zhuh) *n.* [*tachy-* + Gk. *phrasis*, expression, phrase, text, + *-ia*]. TACHYLOGIA.

tachy·phy·lax·ia (tack"i·fi·lack'see·uh) *n.* TACHYPHYLAXIS.

tachy·phy·lax·is (tack"i·fi·lack'sis) *n.* [*tachy-* + *phylaxis*]. 1. The rapid desensitization against toxic doses of organ extracts or serum by the previous inoculation of small, subtoxic doses of the same preparation. 2. Decreasing response to stimulation by such substances as hormones or drugs, as doses of the substance are repeatedly given.

tachy·pnea, tachy·pnoea (tack"i·nee'uh, tack"ip·) *n.* [Gk. *tachypnoia,* from *tachys,* quick, + *pnoē,* breathing]. Abnormally rapid rate of breathing. **—tachy·pne·ic, tachy·pnoe·ic** (·nee'ick) *adj.*

tachy·rhyth·mia (tack"i·rith'mee·uh) *n.* [*tachy-* + *rhythm* + *-ia*]. TACHYCARDIA.

ta·chys·ter·ol (ta·kis'tur·ole, ·ol, tack"i·steer'ol) *n.* The precursor of calciferol in the irradiation of ergosterol; an isomer of ergosterol.

tachy·sys·to·le (tack"i·sis'tuh·lee) *n.* [*tachy-* + *systole*]. TACHYCARDIA.

Tacitin. Trademark for benzoctamine, a muscle relaxant and sedative used as the hydrochloride salt.

tac·la·mine (tack'luh·meen) *n.* 2,3,4,4a,8,9,13b,14-Octahydro-1*H*-benzo[6,7]cyclohepta[1,2,3-*de*]pyrido[2,1-*a*]isoquinoline, $C_{21}H_{23}N$, a minor tranquilizer used as the hydrochloride salt.

tac·tile (tack'til) *adj.* [L. *tactilis,* from *tangere,* to touch]. 1. Pertaining to the sense of touch. 2. Capable of being felt.

tactile agnosia. A loss of the capacity to recognize objects by touch, affecting both sides of the body, as a result of a parietal lesion in one (the dominant) cerebral hemisphere. Syn. *bilateral astereognosis.*

tactile alexia. Inability to recognize language symbols by touch, as when a blind person loses the faculty of reading braille.

tactile anesthesia. Loss of sense of touch.

tactile cell. An epithelial cell modified for reception of a tactile stimulus.

tactile corpuscle. Any encapsulated nerve end organ or end bulb having to do with the sense of touch. NA *corpuscula tactus.*

tactile disk. A terminal widening of an axon in contact with a specialized epithelial cell in the epidermis; a receptor for touch. NA *meniscus tactus.*

tactile fremitus. The vibratory sensation conveyed to the hand when applied to the chest of a person speaking.

tactile meniscus. TACTILE DISK.

tactile papilla. A little eminence of the corium containing a tactile corpuscle.

tactile reflexes. Reflex movements resulting from and induced by stimulation of the organs mediating the sense of touch.

tactile sensation. A sensation produced through the sense of touch.

tac·toid (tack'toid) *n.* [Gk. *taktos*, ordered, fixed, (from *tassein,* to arrange) + *-oid*]. A type of colloidal structure showing intense birefringence in which elongated particles are oriented in a group and parallel to a central axis; a cigar-shaped colloidal particle.

tad·pole cells. Anaplastic squamous cells desquamated in cancer of the uterine cervix, appearing with one broad and one narrow end.

tae·di·um vi·tae (tee'dee·um vye'tee) [L.]. Weariness of life, a symptom of depressive illness and sometimes a precursor of suicide.

Tae·nia (tee'nee·uh) *n.* [Gk. *tainia,* band, headband; tapeworm]. A genus of parasitic worms of the class Cestoda; they are ribbonlike segmental flatworms. The adult is an intestinal parasite of vertebrates; the larvae parasitize both vertebrate and invertebrate tissues. The adult consists of a scolex, an undifferentiated germinal neck, and two or more hermaphroditic segments or proglottids that contain fertile ova when mature.

[1]**taenia,** *n.,* pl. **taenias.** 1. A member of the genus *Taenia.* 2. Any tapeworm.

[2]**tae·nia** (tee'nee·uh) *n.,* pl. **tae·ni·ae** (·nee·ee) [NA]. Tenia (= BAND (3)).

taenia cho·ri·oi·dea (ko·ree·oy'dee·uh) [BNA]. TENIA CHOROIDEA.

tae·nia·cide, te·nia·cide (tee'nee·uh·side) *n.* [*taenia* + *-cide*]. Any agent that is destructive of tapeworms.

Taenia echinococcus. *ECHINOCOCCUS GRANULOSUS.*

taeniae co·li (ko'lye) [BNA]. TENIAE COLI.

taenia fim·bri·ae (fim'bree·ee) [BNA]. The line marking the attachment of the choroid plexus of the inferior horn of the lateral ventricle to the fimbria of the hippocampus.

taenia for·ni·cis (for'ni·sis) [BNA]. TENIA FORNICIS.

tae·nia·fuge, te·nia·fuge (tee'nee·uh·fewj) *n.* [*taenia* + *-fuge*]. Any agent that brings about the expulsion of tapeworms.

taenia li·be·ra (lye'be·ruh) [BNA]. TENIA LIBERA.

taenia me·so·co·li·ca (mes·o·kol'i·kuh) [BNA]. TENIA MESOCOLICA.

Taenia nana. *HYMENOLEPIS NANA.*

taenia omen·ta·lis (o·men·tay'lis) [BNA]. TENIA OMENTALIS.

Taenia sag·i·na·ta (saj·i·nay'tuh). A tapeworm that passes its larval stages in cattle, its adult stage in the intestine of man. The human infection is acquired by eating insufficiently cooked infected beef. Syn. *beef tapeworm.*

tae·ni·a·sis (tee·nye'uh·sis) *n.* [*Taenia* + *-iasis*]. The symptoms caused by infection with any of the species of *Taenia.*

Taenia so·li·um (so'lee·um). A tapeworm that passes the larval stages in hogs; the adult is found in the intestine of man. Ingestion of ova may result in larval infection in man; the larva is then called *Cysticercus cellulosae.* Infection is usually acquired by ingestion of viable larvae in pork. Syn. *pork tapeworm.*

taenia te·la·rum (te·lair'um) [BNA]. TENIA TELAE.

taenia tha·la·mi (thal'uh·migh) [BNA]. TENIA THALAMI.

taenia ven·tri·cu·li quar·ti (ven·trick'yoo·lye kwahr'tye) [BNA]. TENIA VENTRICULI QUARTI.

tae·ni·form, te·ni·form (tee'ni·form) *adj.* [*taenia* + *-form*]. Having a ribbonlike form; resembling a tapeworm.

tae·ni·oid, te·ni·oid (tee'nee·oid) *adj.* [Gk. *tainioeidēs*]. TAENIFORM.

taeniola. TENIOLA.

tae·nio·pho·bia, te·nio·pho·bia (tee″nee·o·fo'bee·uh) *n.* [*taenia* + *-phobia*]. An abnormal fear of becoming the host of a tapeworm.

tag, *n. & v.* 1. A flap or appendage. 2. LABEL. **—tagged,** *adj.*

tagged compounds. Chemical compounds into which isotopes have been incorporated, permitting tracing of the isotopes, and therefore the compounds and their products, through an analytic or metabolic sequence. See also *tracer.*

tag·ma (tag'muh) *n.,* pl. **tagma·ta** (·tuh) [Gk., arrangement]. An aggregate of molecules.

tail, *n.* 1. The caudal extremity of an animal. 2. Anything resembling a tail.

tail bud. 1. The anlage of the caudal appendage. 2. END BUD.

tail fold. A fold formed by rapid growth of the caudal end of the embryo over the embryonic disk, resulting in the formation of the hindgut and ventral body wall in this region.

tail gut. POSTANAL GUT.

tail of the epididymus. The inferior extremity of the epididymus.

tail of the pancreas. The splenic end of the pancreas. NA *cauda pancreatis.*

tai·lor's ankle. An abnormal bursa over the lateral malleolus in tailors, due to pressure from sitting on the floor with crossed legs.

tailor's cramp or **spasm.** An occupational cramp affecting the muscles habitually used in sewing.

taint, *n.* [OF. *teint,* color, tint]. 1. Hereditary predisposition to disease; affection by disease without outspoken manifestations. 2. Putrefaction or infestation, as in tainted meat. 3. Local discoloration, as a blemish.

tai·pan (tye'pan) *n. Pseudechis scutellatus,* the giant brown snake, the largest venomous snake of Australia and New Guinea, belonging to the Elapidae.

Taka-diastase. Trademark for a powdered vegetable diastase; obtained by the action of *Aspergillus oryzae* on wheat bran; the substance liquefies starch and is used to correct faulty starch digestion.

Ta·ka·ta-Ara test [M. *Takata,* Japanese pathologist, b. 1892; and K. *Ara,* Japanese pathologist, 20th century]. A test for liver function in which a solution of mercuric chloride is used to determine an imbalance between albumin and globulin in blood plasma or cerebrospinal fluid.

Ta·ka·ya·su's disease or **syndrome** [M. *Takayasu,* Japanese ophthalmologist, b. 1871]. AORTIC ARCH SYNDROME.

take, *n.* 1. *In medicine,* a successful inoculation, as by a vaccine. 2. *In plastic surgery,* the survival of transplanted tissue in its new site, either temporarily or permanently.

tal-, talo-. A combining form meaning *talus, talar, ankle.*

ta·lal·gia (ta·lal'jee·uh) *n.* [*tal-* + *-algia*]. Pain in the ankle.

tal·am·pi·cil·lin (tal·am″pi·sil'in) *n.* An ester of ampicillin with 3-hydroxyphthalide, $C_{24}H_{23}N_3O_6S$, an antibacterial used as the hydrochloride salt.

ta·lar (tay'lur) *adj.* Of or pertaining to the talus.

talar sulcus. A deep groove on the inferior surface of the body of the talus, separating the posterior and middle calcaneal articular surfaces. NA *sulcus tali.*

tal·bu·tal (tal'bew·tal, ·tol) *n.* 5-Allyl-5-*sec*-butylbarbituric acid, $C_{11}H_{16}N_2O_3$, a barbiturate with intermediate duration of action; used as a sedative and hypnotic.

talc, *n.* [Ar. *ṭalq*]. A native hydrous magnesium silicate sometimes containing a little aluminum silicate. Used as a protective and lubricant dusting powder; also, in pharmacy, as a diluent and filter aid.

talc granuloma. TALCUM-POWDER GRANULOMA.

talc·o·sis (tal·ko'sis) *n.,* pl. **talco·ses** (·seez) [*talc* + *-osis*]. Pneumoconiosis caused by talc dust.

tal·cum (tal'kum) *n.* [L.]. TALC.

talcum-powder granuloma. A variety of siliceous granuloma produced by talcum powder. Syn. *surgical-glove talc granuloma, pseudosilicoticum.*

tal·er·a·nol (tal·er'uh·nole) *n.* (6*S*, 10*S*)-6-(6,10-Dihydroxyundecyl)-β-resorcylic acid μ-lactone, $C_{18}H_{26}O_5$, a gonadotropin inhibitor.

tal·i·on principle (tal'ee·un) [OF., retaliation, from L. *talio, talionis*]. *In psychiatry,* the primitive, unrealistic, often unconscious belief that retaliation in kind is the inevitable result of hostility; frequently leads to the expectation of punishment, sometimes even to unconscious self-punishment, for hostile thoughts or words.

tal·i·pes (tal'i·peez) *n.* [NL. from L. *talipedare,* lit., to walk on the ankles, from *talus,* ankle, + *pes,* foot]. Any one of a variety of deformities of the human foot, especially those of congenital origin, such as clubfoot or equinovarus. Also embraces paralytic deformities and the numerous simple varieties of foot distortion, according to whether the forefoot is inverted or everted and whether the calcaneal tendon is shortened or lengthened. Combinations of the various types occur.

talipes ar·cu·a·tus (ahr·kew·ay'tus). TALIPES CAVUS.

talipes cal·ca·neo·ca·vus (kal·kay″nee·o·kay′vus). A calcaneus deformity of the foot in which there is also a cavus; a dorsal rotation of the calcaneus with a relative plantar tilting of the foot.

talipes cal·ca·neo·val·gus (kal·kay″nee·o·val′gus). A calcaneus deformity of the foot with associated valgus deviation.

talipes cal·ca·neo·va·rus (kal·kay′nee·o·vair′us). A calcaneus deformity of the foot with associated varus deviation.

talipes cal·ca·ne·us (kal·kay′nee·us). Talipes in which the patient walks upon the heel alone.

talipes ca·vus (kay′vus). A foot having an abnormally high longitudinal arch, a depression of the metatarsal arch, and dorsal contractures of the toes. It exists in two forms: that in which the outstanding deformity is an exaggeration of the longitudinal arch, and that in which the exaggeration of the longitudinal arch is associated with contraction of the plantar fascia and limitation of dorsiflexion at the ankle. Syn. *hollow foot, contracted foot, nondeforming clubfoot, claw foot.* See also *pes cavus.*

talipes equi·no·ca·vus (e·kwye″no·kay′vus). A deformity of the foot characterized by fixed plantar flexion and a high longitudinal arch.

talipes equi·no·val·gus (e·kwye″no·val′gus, eck″wi·). Faulty development of the foot characterized by elevation and outward rotation of the heel.

talipes equi·no·va·rus (e·kwye″no·vair′us). A deformity of the foot characterized by fixed plantar flexion and a turning inward of the foot; CLUBFOOT.

talipes equi·nus (e·kwye′nus). Talipes in which the heel is elevated and the weight thrown upon the anterior portion of the foot.

talipes per·ca·vus (pur·kay′vus). Excessive plantar curvature.

talipes pla·nus (play′nus). FLATFOOT.

talipes spas·mod·i·ca (spaz·mod′i·kuh). Noncongenital talipes due to muscular spasm.

talipes val·gus (val′gus). Talipes in which the outer border of the foot is everted, with inward rotation of the tarsus and flattening of the plantar arch. Syn. *splayfoot.*

talipes va·rus (vair′us). A variety of talipes in which the foot is inverted, the weight falling on the outer border. If the inversion is extreme, with rotation of the forefoot, the condition is known as clubfoot.

tal·i·pom·a·nus (tal″i·pom′uh·nus, tal″i·po·man′us) *n.* [*talipes* + *manus*]. CLUBHAND.

talk·ing hemisphere. DOMINANT HEMISPHERE.

talking out. The full, spontaneous, and generally nondirected discussion of an emotional problem with another, usually a sympathetic person or counselor.

Tal·ler·man's apparatus [L. A. *Tallerman,* British inventor, 20th century]. An apparatus for the local application of superheated dry air in the treatment of joint diseases, the affected part being enclosed in a cylinder.

Tallerman's treatment. A method of treatment in which Tallerman's apparatus is used.

tal·low (tal′o) *n.* The fat extracted from suet, the solid fat of cattle, sheep, and other ruminants. It consists largely of stearin and palmitin.

Tall·quist's method [T. W. *Tallquist,* Finnish physician, 1871–1927]. Estimation of hemoglobin by comparing the color of a drop of whole blood absorbed on blotting paper with printed color standards.

Tal·ma-Morison operation [S. *Talma,* Dutch surgeon, 1847–1918; and J. R. *Morison*]. MORISON-TALMA OPERATION.

talo-. See *tal-*.

ta·lo·cal·ca·ne·al (tay″lo·kal·kay′nee·ul) *adj.* [*talo-* + *calcaneal*]. Pertaining to the talus and the calcaneus.

talocalcaneal articulation. SUBTALAR ARTICULATION.

talocalcaneal ligament. Any of the ligaments connecting the talus and the calcaneus in the subtalar articulation; the interosseous talocalcaneal ligament (NA *ligamentum talocalcaneum interosseum*) in the sinus tarsi, the lateral talocalcaneal ligament (NA *ligamentum talocalcaneum laterale*), connecting the lateral surfaces of the two bones, the medial talocalcaneal ligament (NA *ligamentum talocalcaneum mediale*), connecting the medial tubercle of the talus and the sustentaculum tali, the anterior talocalcaneal ligament, connecting the neck of the talus and the calcaneus just posterior to the interosseous talocalcaneal ligament, or the posterior talocalcaneal ligament, connecting the lateral tubercle of the talus and the superior and medial surfaces of the calcaneus.

ta·lo·cal·ca·neo·na·vic·u·lar (tay″lo·kal·kay″nee·o·na·vick′yoo·lur) *adj.* [*talo-* + *calcaneo-* + *navicular*]. Pertaining to the talus, calcaneus, and navicular bones.

talocalcaneonavicular articulation. The articulation formed by the head of the talus and the socket defined by the posterior articular surface of the navicular, the plantar calcaneonavicular ligament, and the anterior and middle articular surfaces of the calcaneus. NA *articulatio talocalcaneonavicularis.* See also Table of Synovial Joints and Ligaments in the Appendix.

ta·lo·cru·ral (tay″lo·kroo′rul) *adj.* Pertaining to the talus and the bones of the leg.

talocrural articulation. The ankle joint.

ta·lo·fib·u·lar (tay″lo·fib′yoo·lur) *adj.* Pertaining to the talus and the fibula.

talofibular ligament. Either of the ligaments connecting the talus and the fibula; the anterior talofibular ligament (NA *ligamentum talofibulare anterius*), which connects the anterior margins of the lateral malleolus of the fibula and the lateral articular facet of the talus, or the posterior talofibular ligament (NA *ligamentum talofibulare posterius*), a strong, almost horizontal ligament attached to the posterior medial surface of the lateral malleolus and the lateral tubercle on the posterior projection of the talus.

ta·lo·mal·le·o·lar (tay″lo·ma·lee′uh·lur) *adj.* Pertaining to the talus and a malleolus.

ta·lo·na·vic·u·lar (tay″lo·na·vick′yoo·lur) *adj.* Pertaining to the talus and navicular bones.

talonavicular articulation. That part of the talocalcaneonavicular joint in which the talus articulates with the navicular. See also Table of Synovial Joints and Ligaments in the Appendix.

talonavicular ligament. A ligament of the foot attached to the dorsal surface of the navicular bone and to the dorsal and lateral surfaces of the neck of the talus. NA *ligamentum talonaviculare.*

tal·o·pram (tal′o·pram) *n.* *N*,3,3-Trimethyl-1-phenyl-1-phthalanpropylamine, $C_{20}H_{25}NO$, a catecholamine potantiator, used as the hydrochloride salt.

tal·ose (tal′oce, ·oze) *n.* A monosaccharide, $C_6H_{12}O_6$, isomeric with dextrose.

ta·lus (tay′lus) *n.*, pl. & genit. sing. **ta·li** (·lye) [L.] [NA]. The bone of the ankle which articulates with the bones of the leg. Syn. *astragalus.* See also Table of Bones in the Appendix.

Talwin. Trademark for the synthetic narcotic analgesic pentazocine.

ta·ma (tam′uh, tay′muh) *n.* [L.]. Swelling of the feet and legs.

tam·a·rin (tam′uh·rin) *n.* Any of the small South American primates of the genus *Leontocebus* (or in another classification the genera *Saguinus* and *Leontideus*) which, together with the marmosets, constitute the Callitrichidae.

tam·a·rind (tam′uh·rind) *n.* [Ar. *tamr hindī,* Indian dates]. The fruit of the *Tamarindus indica,* a tree of the Leguminosae. The preserved pulp of the fruit is laxative.

tam·bour (tam′boor, tam·boor′) *n.* [F., from Ar. *ṭanbūr,* from Per. *tabīr*]. A drum; a drumlike instrument used in physiologic experiments for recording. It consists of a metal cylinder over which is stretched an elastic membrane, and to which passes a tube for transmitting changes in air pressure. Recording is done optically by means of a small mirror on the membrane, or mechanically by a stylus attached to the membrane.

Tamm-Hors·fall protein. A high-molecular-weight mucoprotein which is the major protein constitutent of urinary casts.

ta·mox·i·fen (ta·mock'si·fen) *n.* (*Z*)-2-[*p*-(1,2-Diphenyl-1-butenyl)phenoxy]-*N,N*-dimethylethylamine, $C_{26}H_{29}NO$, an anti-estrogen used as the citrate salt.

tam·pan (tam'pan) *n.* An African name for *Ornithodorus moubata*, a parasitic tick infesting birds, small mammals, domestic animals, and occasionally man; an important vector of relapsing fever. Syn. *bibo, mabata.*

tam·pon (tam'pon) *n.* & *v.* [F.]. 1. A plug of cotton, sponge, or other material inserted into the vagina, nose, or other cavity; a pack. 2. To plug with a tampon.

tam·pon·ade (tam"puh·nade') *n.* 1. The act of plugging with a tampon. 2. Compression of a viscus, especially of the heart, by an external agent. See also *cardiac tamponade.*

tam·pon·age (tam'puh·nij) *n.* TAMPONADE.

tam·pon·ing (tam'pon·ing) *n.* The act of inserting a pack or plug within a cavity, as for checking hemorrhage.

tam·pon·ment (tam·pon'munt) *n.* TAMPONING.

tan, *n.* & *v.* [ML. *tannare*, to tan, from *tannum*, oak bark]. 1. The darker color produced by exposure of "white" skin to sun, wind, or, artificially, by use of a sun lamp. 2. To make or become tan.

ta·na·pox (tah'nuh·pocks) *n.* [after the *Tana* River in Kenya, along which the first observed cases were found]. A viral disease, observed in epidemics in Kenya, characterized by a short febrile illness with headache, malaise, and a single pocklike lesion on the upper part of the body, due to a pox virus which is not related to the vaccinia-variola group; probably a zoonosis, transmitted from monkey to man.

tan·da·mine (tan'duh·meen) *n.* 1-[2(Dimethylamino)ethyl]-9-ethyl-1,3,4,9-tetrahydro-1-methylthiopyrano[3,4-*b*]indole, $C_{18}H_{26}N_2S$, an antidepressant, used as the hydrochloride salt.

Tandearil. Trademark for oxyphenbutazone, an antiarthritic and anti-inflammatory drug.

tan·dem gait. A manner of walking in which the heel of the advancing foot is placed directly in front of the toes of the stationary foot; used to test a patient's equilibrium and coordination.

tan·gent screen. *In ophthalmology*, a black or dark gray screen, mapped in circles and diagonals for the examination of the central field of vision, commonly at a distance of 1 meter from the eye of the subject. With one eye occluded and the other fixed on the center of the screen, the patient reports on the appearance and disappearance of test objects of different sizes and colors moved across the field of vision from the periphery to the center at different angles. The areas in which the patient fails to see are plotted. Contr. *perimeter* (2).

Tan·gier disease [*Tangier* Island, Virginia]. Greatly reduced serum alpha-lipoprotein (high-density lipoprotein) and deposition of cholesterol esters in the reticuloendothelial system, manifested clinically by markedly enlarged, strikingly yellow-gray tonsils, lymphadenopathy, splenomegaly, and in adult life by vascular and neurologic involvement.

tan·nase (tan'ace, ·aze) *n.* An enzyme found in cultures of *Penicillium* and *Aspergillus* which converts tannic acid to gallic acid.

tan·nate (tan'ate) *n.* Any salt or ester of tannic acid.

tan·ner's disease. ANTHRAX.

tanner's ulcer. A chronic ulcer occurring on the hands of tanners.

tan·nic acid (tan'ick). A tannin usually obtained from nutgalls, the excrescences formed on the young twigs of *Quercus infectoria* and allied species. Used topically as a styptic and astringent, often in 20% solution in glycerin; has been used for treatment of burns but may be absorbed and cause serious systemic toxicity.

tannic acid test. A test for detecting the presence of carbon monoxide in blood in which blood is mixed with distilled water and a tannic acid solution is added. The development of a cherry red color indicates the presence of carbon monoxide.

tan·nin (tan'in) *n.* 1. TANNIC ACID. 2. Any one of a group of astringent plant principles characterized by their ability to precipitate collagen and to produce dark-colored compounds with ferric salts. The source is frequently identified by a prefix, as gallotannin, quercitannin.

tan·no·phil granules (tan'o·fil). Cell granules that stain specifically by various methods after mordanting with tannin.

Tan·ret-May·er test (tah^n·reh^h') [C. *Tanret*, French physician, 1847–1917; and F. F. *Mayer*, U.S. chemist, 20th century]. A test to determine the presence of quinine in the urine.

Tanret reagent [C. *Tanret*]. A solution of mercuric chloride and potassium iodide in acetic acid and water; used as a reagent for protein in urine, a white precipitate being a positive test.

tan·ta·lum (tan'tuh·lum) *n.* [*Tantalus*, mythical king tortured by thirst, referring to the element's being unaffected by water or acid]. Ta = 180.948. A lanthanide, atomic number 73; very hard, malleable, and ductile. It has been variously used in surgery because of its resistance to corrosion.

tan·trum (tan'trum) *n.* [unkn. orig.]. An expression of uncontrollable anger, sometimes accompanied by acts of violence.

Tao. A trademark for troleandomycin, an antibiotic substance.

tap, *n.* & *v.* 1. A sudden slight blow. 2. Withdrawal of fluid by the use of a trochar or hollow needle. 3. To withdraw fluid by the use of a trochar or hollow needle.

Tapazole. Trademark for the antithyroid drug methimazole.

ta·pei·no·ceph·a·ly (ta·pye"no·sef'uh·lee) *n.* TAPINOCEPHALY.

tapetal reflex. The metallic luster reflected from the back of the eye of certain animals, as the shining green reflex seen in the eyes of cats at night.

ta·pe·to·ret·i·nal (ta·pee"to·ret'i·nul) *adj.* [*tape*tum + *retinal*]. Pertaining to the tapetum and the retina.

tapetoretinal degeneration. Any of the heredodegenerative disorders affecting the retina, pigment epithelium, and choroid; may be "central" and include infantile, juvenile, or adolescent macular degeneration, juvenile disciform macular degeneration, and the infantile and juvenile forms of amaurotic familial idiocy; or may be "peripheral" and include retinitis pigmentosa, retinitis punctata albescens, and peripheral pigmentary degeneration with such diverse disorders as Friedreich's ataxia and the Laurence-Moon-Biedl syndrome.

ta·pe·tum (ta·pee'tum) *n.*, pl. **tape·ta** (·tuh) [NL., from L. *tapete*, carpet, from Gk. *tapēs, tapētos*]. 1. [BNA] The layer forming the roof of the posterior horn of the lateral ventricle of the brain. It is composed of fibers from the corpus callosum. 2. A layer of tissue in the choroid of the eye, between its vascular and capillary layer, usually not present in man; it may be cellular as in carnivores or fibrous as in ruminants and contain crystals which reflect light strongly and which result in the metallic luster seen, as in the cat. In man, it is represented by a layer of fibers. **—tape·tal** (·tul) *adj.*

tapetum al·ve·o·li (al·vee'o·lye). PERIODONTIUM.

tapetum lu·ci·dum (lew'si·dum). TAPETUM (2).

tape·worm, *n.* Any of the species of the class Cestoidea; segmented, ribbonlike flatworms which are parasites of man and other animals. See also *Bertiella, Diphyllobothrium, Dipylidium, Echinococcus, Hymenolepis, Multiceps, Raillietina, Sparganum, Taenia.*

tapeworm anemia. A megaloblastic anemia, possibly identical with pernicious anemia, occurring in persons infected by the fish tapeworm, *Diphyllobothrium latum.*

taph·e·pho·bia, taph·i·pho·bia (taf″e·fo′bee·uh) *n.* [Gk. *taphē*, burial, + *-phobia*]. An abnormal fear of being buried alive.

taph·o·pho·bia (taf″o·fo′bee·uh) *n.* TAPHEPHOBIA.

Ta·pia's syndrome (tah′pyah) [A. G. *Tapia*, Spanish physician, 1875–1950]. Paralysis of the larynx, tongue, and sternocleidomastoid on one side associated with a paralysis of the entire opposite side of the body.

tap·i·no·ceph·a·ly (tap″i·no·sef′uh·lee, ta·pye″no·) *n.* [Gk. *tapeinos*, low-lying, + *-cephaly*]. Flatness of the top of the cranium; flat top. —**tapino·ce·phal·ic** (·se·fal′ick) *adj.*

tap·i·o·ca (tap″ee·o′kuh) *n.* [Pg., from Tupi *tipioca*]. A variety of starch obtained from the cassava or manioc plant, *Jatropha manihot*. Used as a food.

ta·pir mouth or **lip** (tay′pur). The peculiarly loose, thickened, protruding lips of the myopathic facies. The patient is unable to smile or whistle.

ta·pir·oid (tay′pur·oid) *adj.* [*tapir* + *-oid*]. Characterizing pertaining to an elongated cervix of the uterus, so called from its resemblance to a tapir's snout.

tapiroid cervix. A cervix of the uterus with a very elongated anterior lip.

ta·pote·ment (ta·poht′munt, F. ta·poht·mahn′) *n.* [F.]. Percussion movements used in massage.

tap·root, *n.* The main root or downward continuation of a plant axis.

tar, *n.* A thick brown to black liquid consisting of a mixture of hydrocarbons and their derivatives obtained by the destructive distillation of many kinds of carbonaceous matter.

tar·a·ba·gan (tăr′uh·buh·gan″) *n.* TARBAGAN.

Taractan. Trademark for chlorprothixene, a tranquilizing drug with antiemetic activity.

Tar·ak·tog·e·nos (tăr″ack·toj′e·nus) *n.* A genus of trees of India, the seeds of a certain species of which (*Taraktogenos kurzii*) yield chaulmoogra oil.

tar·ant·ism (tăr′un·tiz·um) *n.* [It. *tarantismo*, after *Taranto*, city in southern Italy]. A dancing mania, first described during the 15th to 17th centuries in Southern Europe and ascribed to the bite of a tarantula.

tar·an·tis·mus (tăr″an·tiz′mus) *n.* TARANTISM.

ta·ran·tu·la (tuh·ran′choo·luh) *n.*, pl. **tarantulas, tarantu·lae** (·lee) [after *Taranto*, Italy]. 1. *Lycosa tarentula*, a large spider of southern Europe, whose bite, traditionally supposed to cause tarantism, is now considered innocuous. 2. Any of various very large, hairy New World spiders of the family Theraphosidae, not significantly poisonous to humans. See also *Atrax*.

ta·ran·tu·lism (tuh·ran′choo·liz·um) *n.* TARANTISM.

ta·ras·sis (ta·ras′is) *n.* [Gk. *tarassein*, to disturb]. Hysteria in the male.

ta·rax·a·cum (ta·rack′suh·kum) *n.* [ML., from Ar. *ṭarakhshaqōq*, from Per. *talkh chakōk*, bitter herb]. Dandelion root. The dried rhizomes and roots of *Taraxacum officinale* or *T. laevigatum*, family Compositae; formerly used as a cholagogue and diuretic.

ta·rax·e·in (tah·rack′see·in) *n.* [Gk. *tarax*is, confusion, + prot*ein*]. A protein complex allegedly found in the serum of some actively schizophrenic patients, and presumably related to the acute manifestations.

ta·rax·is (ta·rack′sis) *n.* [Gk., irritation of the eye]. CONJUNCTIVITIS.

tar·ba·gan (tahr′buh·gan) *n.* [Russ., from Turkic]. The marmot *Arctomys bobac*, a disease carrier among fur-bearing animals in northern Asia.

tar cancer. Squamous cell carcinoma associated with prolonged exposure to tar.

Tar·dieu's ecchymoses (tar·dyœh′) [A. A. *Tardieu*, French physician, 1818–1879]. Ecchymotic spots beneath the pleura after death from strangulation or suffocation.

tar·dive (tahr′div) *adj.* Tending to be late; tardy.

tardive dyskinesia. An extrapyramidal disorder manifested by lingual-facial-buccal dyskinesia as well as choreoathetotic movements of the trunk and limbs; occurs as a late and persistent complication of long-term therapy with phenothiazine or haloperidol.

tar·dy median palsy (tahr′dee). CARPAL TUNNEL SYNDROME.

tare, *n.* [OF., from Ar. *ṭarḥa*, that which is thrown away]. 1. A counterweight. 2. A deduction made for the weight of the container. 3. A counterbalance.

tar·get, *n.* [OF. *targette*, from *targe*, light shield]. 1. The anode in a roentgen-ray tube upon which the electrons are directed and from which the roentgen rays arise. 2. MIRE.

target cell. 1. An abnormal erythrocyte with a low mean corpuscular hemoglobin concentration (MCHC) which, when stained, shows a central and peripheral zone of hemoglobin separated by an intermediate unstained area and thus resembles a bull's-eye target. Found after splenectomy and in several types of anemia. Syn. *Mexican hat cell*. 2. A cell bearing a specific surface membrane receptor or antigen which reacts with a given hormone, antibiotic, antibody, sensitized lymphocyte, or other agent and is therefore conceived of as the target of that agent.

target-cell anemia. THALASSEMIA.

target erythrocyte. TARGET CELL (1).

target gland. Any gland directly affected by the hormone of another gland.

target lesion. A vesicular skin lesion with a red rim, characteristic of such diseases as erythema multiforme.

Tar·nier's forceps (tar·nyey′) [E. S. *Tarnier*, French obstetrician, 1828–1897]. Axis-traction forceps, once used in obstetrics.

Tarnier's sign [E. S. *Tarnier*]. Effacement of the angle between the upper and lower segment of the uterus, a sign of inevitable abortion.

ta·ro (tah′ro) *n.* [Tahitian and Maori]. The starchy root of *Colocasia antiquorum* or Indian kale; used as a food in certain Pacific islands.

tar·ry stools (tahr′ee). Stools having the color and consistency of tar, usually due to hemorrhage into the intestinal tract but also produced by iron, bismuth, or other medication.

tars-, tarso-. A combining form meaning *tarsus, tarsal*.

tars·ad·e·ni·tis (tahr·sad″e·nigh′tis) *n.* [*tars-* + *adenitis*]. Inflammation of the tarsal glands and tarsal plate.

tar·sal (tahr′sul) *adj.* 1. Pertaining to the tarsus (1). 2. Pertaining to the tarsus (2), the dense connective tissue forming the support of an eyelid.

tarsal arterial arches. The anastomoses of the palpebral arteries.

tarsal bones. The seven bones of the tarsus. NA *ossa tarsi*.

tarsal conjunctiva. PALPEBRAL CONJUNCTIVA.

tar·sal·gia (tahr·sal′jee·uh) *n.* [*tars-* + *-algia*]. Pain, especially of neuralgic character, in the tarsus of the foot.

tarsal glands. Sebaceous glands in the tarsal plates of the eyelids. Syn. *Meibomian glands*. NA *glandulae tarsales*.

tarsal ligament. PALPEBRAL LIGAMENT.

tarsal muscle. See Table of Muscles in the Appendix.

tarsal plate. Either of the thin, elongated plates, inferior (NA *tarsus inferior palpebrae*) or superior (NA *tarsus superior palpebrae*), which contribute to the form and support of the eyelids.

tarsal tenotomy. Division of the peroneal tendon in the horse for the relief of spavin.

tarsal tunnel syndrome. Pain and sensory loss involving the medial anterior foot and great toe due to compression of the medial plantar nerve by the flexor retinaculum and deep fascia.

tar·sec·to·my (tahr·seck′tuh·mee) *n.* [*tars-* + *-ectomy*]. Excision of a tarsal bone or bones.

tarsi. Plural and genitive singular of *tarsus*.

tar·si·tis (tahr·sigh′tis) *n.* [*tars-* + *-itis*]. 1. Inflammation of the tarsus of the eyelid. 2. BLEPHARITIS. 3. Inflammation of the tarsus of the foot.

tarso-. See *tars-*.

tar·so·chei·lo·plas·ty (tahr″so·kigh′lo·plas″tee) *n.* [*tarso-* + *cheilo-* + *-plasty*]. Plastic surgery of the edge of the eyelid.

tar·so·ma·la·cia (tahr″so·ma·lay′shee·uh, ·see·uh) *n.* [*tarso-* + *malacia*]. Softening of the tarsus of the eyelid.

tar·so·meta·tar·sal (tahr″so·met″uh·tahr′sul) *adj.* [*tarso-* + *metatarsal*]. Pertaining to the tarsus and the metatarsus.

tarsometatarsal articulation. Any of the joints betweeen the bases of the metatarsals and the cuboid or cuniform bones; the cuboideometatarsal, cuneometatarsal, or medial tarsometatarsal articulation. NA (pl.) *articulationes tarsometatarseae.*

tarsometatarsal ligament. Any of the ligaments between the tarsal and metatarsal bones, including the dorsal tarsometatarsal ligaments (NA *ligamenta tarsometatarsea dorsalia*), the plantar tarsometatarsal ligaments (NA *ligamenta tarsometatarsea plantaria*), and the interosseous tarsometatarsal ligaments. See also *interosseous cuneometatarsal ligament.*

Tar·so·nem·i·dae (tahr″so·nem′i·dee) *n.pl.* A family of soft-bodied mites which are parasites of plants, and may cause dermatitis in man.

tar·so·pha·lan·ge·al reflex (tahr″so·fuh·lan′jee·ul). BEKHTEREV-MENDEL REFLEX (1).

tar·so·phy·ma (tahr″so·figh′muh) *n.* [*tarso-* + *phyma*]. Any morbid growth or tumor of the tarsus of the eyelid.

tar·so·pla·sia (tahr″so·play′zhuh, ·zee·uh) *n.* [*tarso-* + *-plasia*]. TARSOPLASTY.

tar·so·plas·ty (tahr′so·plas″tee) *n.* [*tarso-* + *-plasty*]. Plastic surgery of the eyelid; BLEPHAROPLASTY.

tar·sop·to·sia (tahr″sop·to′zhuh, ·zee·uh) *n.* Tarsoptosis (= FLATFOOT).

tar·sop·to·sis (tahr″sop·to′sis) *n.*, pl. **tarsopto·ses** (·seez) [*tarso-* + *ptosis*]. Fallen arches; FLATFOOT.

tar·sor·rha·phy (tahr·sor′uh·fee) *n.* [*tarso-* + *-rrhaphy*]. 1. The operation of sewing the eyelids together for a part or the whole of their extent. 2. Suture of a tarsal plate.

tar·sot·o·my (tahr·sot′uh·mee) *n.* [*tarso-* + *-tomy*]. 1. Operation upon the tarsus of the foot. 2. Operation upon a tarsal plate.

tar·sus (tahr′sus) *n.*, pl. & genit. sing. **tar·si** (·sigh) [Gk. *tarsos,* ankle; edge of the eyelid] [NA]. 1. The instep, or ankle, consisting of the calcaneus, talus, cuboid, navicular, medial, intermediate, and lateral cuneiform bones. See also Table of Bones in the Appendix. 2. The dense connective tissue forming the support of an eyelid; TARSAL PLATE. See also Plate 19.

tarsus inferior pal·pe·brae (pal′pe·bree, pal·pee′bree) [NA]. The tarsal plate of the lower eyelid.

tarsus superior palpebrae [NA]. The tarsal plate of the upper eyelid.

tar·tar (tahr′tur) *n.* [OF. *tartre,* from ML. *tartarum*]. 1. Crude potassium bitartrate, the principal component of argol, yielding cream of tartar when purified. 2. DENTAL CALCULUS.

tartar emetic. ANTIMONY POTASSIUM TARTRATE.

tar·tar·ic acid (tahr·tăr′ick, tahr·tahr′ick). Any of four substances of the composition $HOOC(CHOH)_2COOH$, differentiated as follows: (1) Dextrotartaric acid or *d*-tartaric acid (in accordance with present rules of nomenclature known as L(+)-tartaric acid) is ordinary tartaric acid, dextrorotatory in aqueous solution. (2) Levotartaric acid or *l*-tartaric acid (known also as D(−)-tartaric acid) has the same properties as the preceding, but is levorotatory. (3) Racemic tartaric acid or *dl*-tartaric acid, a mixture of (1) and (2), optically inactive. Syn. *racemic acid.* (4) Mesotartaric acid, optically inactive, in which the dextrorotatory tendency of one of the asymmetric carbon atoms is compensated by the levorotatory tendency of the other; it is not resolvable into optically active components. Ordinary tartaric acid, (1), is variously used in pharmacy as a weak acid.

tart cell [after a patient named *Tart*]. A granulocyte which has ingested the nucleus of another cell, usually a lymphocyte; an important artifact in lupus erythematosus (L.E.) cell preparations.

tartrate (tahr′trate) *n.* Any salt or ester of tartaric acid.

tar·tra·zine (tahr′truh·zeen, ·zin) *n.* The trisodium salt, $C_{16}H_9N_4Na_3O_9S_2$, of 3-carboxy-5-hydroxy-1-*p*-sulfophenyl-4-*p*-sulfophenylazopyrazole, a bright orange-yellow powder used as a dye.

tar·tron·ic acid (tahr·tron′ick). Hydroxymalonic acid, HOOCCHOHCOOH, a product of oxidation, under certain conditions, of dextrose and several other substances.

Tarui's disease. An inborn error of glycogen metabolism, caused by a deficiency of the enzyme phosphofructokinase, with abnormal accumulation of glycogen in muscle.

Tash·kent ulcer [after *Tashkent,* Uzbekistan, U.S.S.R]. CUTANEOUS LEISHMANIASIS.

tasks of emotional development test. *In psychology,* a projective test to assess the emotional and social adjustment of children between 6 and 18 years of age from the stories they tell in response to a series of pictures comprising the test. See also *thematic apperception test.*

taste, *n.* [OF. *taster,* to feel]. A sensation produced by stimulation of special sense organs in the tongue by sweet, sour, bitter, or salty substances.

taste blindness. Inability to recognize the acid, bitter, salty, or sweet flavor of substances, readily detected by others. See also *ageusia.*

taste bud. The end organ of the sense of taste; one of the oval, flask-shaped bodies embedded, most commonly, in the epithelium of the tongue. NA *caliculus gustatorius.*

taste cell. An epithelial cell that receives a gustatory stimulus, as in the taste buds.

taste corpuscle. TASTE BUD.

taste pore. The minute opening through which project the gustatory bristles of a taste bud. Syn. *gustatory pore.* NA *porus gustatorius.*

TAT Abbreviation for (a) *thematic apperception test;* (b) *toxin-antitoxin.*

tat·too·ing, ta·too·ing, *n.* [Tahitian *tatau*]. The production of permanent colors in the skin by the introduction of foreign substances, vegetable or mineral, directly into the corium.

tattooing of the cornea. A method of hiding leukomatous spots.

Tau·ber test [H. *Tauber,* U.S. biochemist, b. 1891]. A test for detecting the presence of pentose in urine using benzidine in glacial acetic acid. The presence of pentose is indicated by the immediate appearance of a pink to red color. If pentoses are absent, the mixture has a yellowish-brown color.

taur-, tauro- [L. *taurus,* bull]. A combining form meaning (a) *bull;* (b) *taurine.*

tau·rine (taw′reen, ·rin) *n.* 2-Aminoethanesulfonic acid, $NH_2CH_2CH_2SO_3H$; occurs in bile combined with cholic acids.

tauro-. See *taur-.*

tau·ro·chol·ano·poi·e·sis (taw″ro·ko·lan″o·poy·ee′sis) *n.* The synthesis of taurocholic acid, which is dependent on a supply of amino acids containing sulfur.

tau·ro·cho·late (taw″ro·ko′late) *n.* A salt of taurocholic acid.

tau·ro·cho·lic acid (taw″ro·ko′lick, ·kol′ick). Cholyltaurine $C_{26}H_{45}NO_7S$, a bile acid resulting from conjugation of cholic acid and taurine.

tau·ro·dont (taw′ro·dont) *adj.* [Gk. *taur,* bull, + *-odont*]. Of or pertaining to teeth having abnormally large pulp chambers that are deepened at the expense of the roots; a characteristic of many of the extinct Neanderthal race and of ungulate animals; sometimes found in modern human teeth.

tau·ryl (taw′ril) *n.* The univalent radical, $H_2NCH_2CH_2SO_2$—, of taurine.

Taus·sig-Bing complex or **malformation** [Helen B. *Taussig,* U.S. pediatrician, b. 1898; and R. R. *Bing,* U.S. surgeon, b.

1909]. A form of congenital incomplete transposition of the great arteries, in which the aorta arises from the right ventricle and is slightly posterior to the pulmonary trunk, which arises anteriorly from both ventricles.

Taussig-Blalock operation [Helen B. *Taussig* and A. *Blalock*]. BLALOCK-TAUSSIG OPERATION.

tau·to·me·ni·al (taw″to·mee′nee·ul) *adj.* [Gk. *tautos*, identical, + *mēn*, month]. Pertaining to the same menstrual period.

tau·tom·er·al (taw·tom′ur·ul) *adj.* [Gk. *tautos*, same, + *meros*, part]. Pertaining to certain nerve fibers involved in the development of the spinal cord and derived from neurons from the same part of the spinal cord.

tau·to·mer·ic (taw″to·merr′ick) *adj.* 1. Pertaining to tautomerism. 2. TAUTOMERAL.

tau·tom·er·ism (taw·tom′ur·iz·um) *n.* [Gk. *tautos*, same, + *mer-* + *-ism*]. The property of existing in a state of equilibrium between two isomeric forms and capable of reacting as either one.

Ta·wa·ra's node [S. *Tawara*, Japanese pathologist, 1873–1952]. ATRIOVENTRICULAR NODE.

Ta wave. The electrocardiographic deflection due to repolarization of the atria; it is usually masked by the QRS complex but may be evident with prolongation of the P-R segment.

tax-, taxi-, taxo- [Gk. *taxis*, from *tassein*, to arrange]. A combining form meaning *arrangement.*

taxa. Plural of *taxon.*

taxi-. See *tax-.*

tax·is (tack′sis) *n.*, pl. **tax·es** (·seez) [Gk., fixing, arrangement]. 1. A manipulation of an organ whereby it is brought into normal position; specifically, the reduction of a hernia by manual methods. 2. The involuntary response of an entire organism involving change of place toward (positive taxis) or away from (negative taxis) a stimulus. See also *tropism.*

-taxis [Gk.]. A combining form meaning (a) *arrangement, order;* (b) *taxis* (2).

taxo-. See *tax-.*

tax·o·di·um (tack·so′dee·um) *n.* [NL., from L. *taxus*, yew]. The common bald or black cypress of the southern United States and Mexico; its resin was formerly used for the treatment of rheumatism and other ailments.

tax·on (tacks′on) *n.*, pl. **taxa** (tack′suh). A taxonomic group.

tax·on·o·my (tacks·on′uh·mee) *n.* [F. *taxonomie*, from Gk. *taxis*, arrangement, + *nomos*, law]. *In biology*, the science of the classification of organisms. **—tax·o·nom·ic** (tack″ suh·nom′ick) *adj.*

-taxy. See *-taxis.*

Tay·lor brace [C. F. *Taylor*, U.S. surgeon, 1827–1899]. A steel back brace for support of the spine.

Tay-Sachs disease (sacks) [W. *Tay*, English physician, 1843–1927; and B. P. *Sachs*, U.S. neurologist, 1858–1944]. A form of G_{M2} gangliosidosis which begins during the first 3 to 6 months of age and is characterized by an abnormal startle reaction, axial hypotonia leading to spasticity, and, in most cases, cherry-red spots in the retinas; death occurs at 3 to 5 years. The disease results from a deficiency of, or defect in, the enzyme hexosaminidase A. Compare *Sandhoff's disease.* See also *amaurotic familial idiocy.*

Tay's choroiditis [W. *Tay*]. CHOROIDITIS GUTTATA.

ta·zo·lol (tay′zo·lole) *n.* (±)-1-(Isopropylamino)-3-(2-thiazolyloxy)-2-propanol, $C_9H_{16}N_2O_2S$, a cardiotonic agent used as the hydrochloride salt.

TB Abbreviation for *tuberculosis.*

Tb Symbol for terbium.

t.b. Abbreviation for *tubercle bacillus.*

T bandage. A bandage with three arms that form a letter T; especially used about the waist and the perineum to hold a dressing.

tbsp Abbreviation for *tablespoon.*

Tc Symbol for technetium.

TCE Abbreviation for *trichloroethylene.*

T cell. T LYMPHOCYTE.

t component. 1. In the somatotype, the textural quality of the body, expressed numerically. 2. Psychologically, the esthetic impression made by the individual's physique.

t.d.s. Abbreviation for *ter die sumendum*, to be taken thrice a day (= t.i.d.).

Te 1. Symbol for tellurium. 2. *Obsol.* Abbreviation for *tetanic contraction.*

tea, *n.* [Amoy Chinese *te*]. 1. The leaves of *Camellia sinensis* (*Thea sinensis*), family Theaceae. Tea contains 1 to 5% caffeine, 5 to 15% tannin, and a fragrant volatile oil. An infusion is used as a stimulating beverage. 2. An infusion or decoction prepared from the leaves of *C. sinensis.* 3. Any vegetable infusion or decoction used as a beverage.

tea·ber·ry, *n.* GAULTHERIA.

teaberry oil. The volatile oil from the leaves of *Gaultheria procumbens*, consisting essentially of methyl salicylate. Syn. *wintergreen oil.*

teach·er's node. SINGER'S NODE.

Teal test. A hearing test to determine actual or simulated air-conduction loss when normal bone conduction is admitted. It is done with two similar tuning forks, one inactive on the mastoid and the other active close to the tested ear. The patient admitting hearing tone actually hears by air, and this is evidence of simulated deafness.

tear (teer) *n.* & *v.* [Gmc. *ta^{k}hr-* (rel. to Gk. *dakryon* and to OL. *dacruma* → Cl.L. *lacrima*)]. 1. A drop of the secretion of the lacrimal glands. 2. A hardened drop or lump of any resinous or gummy drug. 3. To exude tears. 4. More generally, to exude drops or beads of liquid.

tear gas. Substances used to produce physical discomfort without injury by causing inflammation of the mucous membranes of the eyes and nose, followed by lacrimation.

teart disease (teert, turt). Molybdenosis seen especially in cattle.

tease, *v.* To tear or gently separate tissue into its component parts, by the use of needles.

tea·spoon, *n.* A spoon commonly assumed to hold about 5 ml. Abbreviated, tsp.

teat (teet) *n.* [OF. *tete*]. NIPPLE.

te·bu·tate (teb′yoo·tate) *n.* A salt or ester of tertiary butylacetic acid (3,3-dimethylbutyric acid), $(CH_3)_3CCH_2COOH$; a tertiary butylacetate.

tech·ne·ti·um (teck·nee′shee·um) *n.* [NL., from Gk. *technētos*, artificial]. Tc = 98.9062. Element number 43, prepared in 1937 by neutron or deuteron bombardment of molybdenum and later found among the fission products of uranium. Syn. *masurium.*

tech·nic (teck′nick, ·neek, teck·neek′) *n.* TECHNIQUE.

tech·ni·cian (teck·nish′un) *n.* A person trained and expert in the technical details of certain medical fields, as bacteriology, pathology, radiology.

tech·nics (teck′nicks, teck·neeks′) *n.* [*technic* + *-s*]. TECHNOLOGY.

tech·nique (teck·neek′) *n.* [Gk. *technikos*]. The method of procedure in operations or manipulations of any kind.

tech·nol·o·gist (teck·nol′uh·jist) *n.* A specialist in the technology of a particular field.

tech·nol·o·gy (teck·nol′uh·jee) *n.* [Gk. *technologia*, systematic treatment]. Practical application of scientific knowledge.

tec·lo·zan (teck′lo·zan) *n.* *N,N′*-(*p*-Phenylenedimethylene)-bis[2,2-dichloro-*N*-(2-ethoxyethyl)acetamide], $C_{20}H_{28}Cl_4N_2O_4$, an antiamebic drug.

tec·no·cyte, tek·no·cyte (teck′no·site) *n.* [Gk. *teknon*, child, young, + *-cyte*]. A young metamyelocyte.

tecta. Plural of *tectum.*

tec·tal (teck′tul) *adj.* Of or pertaining to a tectum; especially, to the tectum of the mesencephalon.

tectal nuclei. The fastigial nuclei of the cerebellum, one on each side of the midline, in the roof of the fourth ventricle.

tec·ti·form (teck'ti·form) *adj.* [L. *tec*tum, roof, + *-iform*]. Roof-shaped.

tec·to·bul·bar tract (teck"to·bul'bur). A part of the descending tectospinal tract which, at the medullary level, becomes incorporated within the medial longitudinal fasciculus.

tec·to·ceph·a·ly (teck"to·sef'uh·lee) *n.* [L. *tec*tum, roof, + *-cephaly*]. SCAPHOCEPHALY.

tec·to·cer·e·bel·lar (teck"to·serr"e·bel'ur) *adj.* Pertaining to the tectum or roof of the midbrain and the cerebellum.

tec·to·pon·tine tract (teck"to·pon'tine, ·teen). Fibers that arise from the superior colliculus, pass caudally beneath the inferior colliculus, and terminate in the dorsolateral pontine nuclei of the same side.

tec·to·re·tic·u·lar fibers (teck"to·re·tick'yoo·lur). Fibers that arise in the superior colliculus and project diffusely and bilaterally to dorsal regions of the midbrain reticular formation.

tec·to·ri·al (teck·to'ree·ul) *adj.* [L. *tector*ium, covering, + *-al*]. Serving as a roof or covering.

tectorial membrane. 1. A jellylike membrane covering the spiral organ (of Corti). NA *membrana tectoria ductus cochlearis.* 2. A strong sheet of connective tissue running from the basilar part of the occipital bone to the dorsal surface of the bodies of the axis and third cervical vertebra. It is an upward extension of the posterior longitudinal ligament of the vertebral column. NA *membrana tectoria.*

tec·to·ru·bral tract (teck"to·rue'brul) [*tec*tum + *rubr-* + *-al*]. A group of nerve fibers that arises in the superior colliculus and projects in small part to the ipsilateral red nucleus but mainly to the centrolateral red nucleus by way of the dorsal tegmental decussation. Syn. *colliculorubral tract.*

tec·to·spi·nal (teck"to·spye'nul) *adj.* [*tec*tum + *spinal*]. Of or pertaining to the spinal cord and the corpora quadrigemina.

tectospinal tract. A nerve tract that descends from large cells in the tectum of the mesencephalon, decussates, gives off fibers to the motor nuclei of the brainstem, and synapses with motor cells of the spinal cord, chiefly in the cervical region. It includes the tectobulbar tract. NA *tractus tectospinalis.*

tec·to·tha·lam·ic tract (teck"to·thuh·lam'ick). Fibers that arise from the superficial layers of the superior colliculus and project to subdivisions of the ipsilateral pulvinar, dorsal and ventral lateral geniculate nuclei, and perhaps the pretectum.

tec·tum (teck'tum) *n.*, pl. **tec·ta** (·tuh) [L., from *tegere,* to cover]. A roof or covering.

tectum me·sen·ce·pha·li (mes·en·sef'uh·lye) [NA]. The dorsal portion of the mesencephalon, including the superior and inferior colliculi and adjacent areas.

tectum of the mesencephalon. TECTUM MESENCEPHALI.

te·di·ous (tee'dee·us) *adj.* [L. *taediosus*]. Unduly protracted, as tedious labor.

teel oil. SESAME OIL.

teeth. Plural of *tooth.*

teeth·ing (tee'thing) *n.* The eruption of the primary teeth; the process of dentition.

Tee·van's law [W. F. *Teevan,* English surgeon, 1834–1887]. Skull fracture occurs in the line of expansion and not in the line of compression.

Teflon shakes. METAL FUME FEVER.

tef·lur·ane (tef'loo·rane) *n.* 2-Bromo-1,1,1,2-tetrafluoroethane, C_2HBrF_4, a general anesthetic administered by inhalation.

teg·men (teg'mun) *n.*, pl. **teg·mi·na** (·mi·nuh) [L., from *tegere,* to cover]. A cover.

tegmen mas·toi·de·um (mas·toy'dee·um). The roof of the mastoid cells.

tegmenta. Plural of *tegmentum.*

teg·men·tal (teg·men'tul) *adj.* Pertaining to a tegmentum, especially, the tegmentum of the midbrain.

tegmental decussation of Forel [A. H. *Forel*]. VENTRAL TEGMENTAL DECUSSATION.

tegmental fields of Fo·rel (foʰ·rel') [A. H. *Forel*]. A subthalamic area medial and rostral to the red nucleus through which pass important descending extrapyramidal fibers. The area is subdivided into fields H_1 and H_2.

tegmental mesencephalic paralysis. BENEDIKT'S SYNDROME.

tegmental nuclei. Groups of nerve cells located in the tegmentum of the midbrain. NA *nuclei tegmenti.*

teg·men·to·bul·bar tract (teg·men"to·bul'bur) A group of nerve fibers that originates in the deep tegmental or reticular gray matter of the midbrain and projects to the motor nuclei of the brainstem.

teg·men·to·spi·nal tract (teg·men"to·spye'nul). Nerve fibers that connect the large-celled clusters of the midbrain tegmentum with the motor nuclei of the spinal cord.

teg·men·tum (teg·men'tum) *n.*, pl. **tegmen·ta** (·tuh) [L., from *tegere,* to cover]. 1. A covering. 2. [NA] The dorsal portion of the midbrain, exclusive of the corpora quadrigemina and the central gray substance.

tegmentum rhom·ben·ce·pha·li (rom"ben·sef'uh·lye) [NA]. The dorsal part of the pons.

tegmen tym·pa·ni (tim'puh·nigh) [NA]. The roof of the tympanic cavity.

tegmen ven·tri·cu·li quar·ti (ven·trick'yoo·lye kwahr'tye) [NA]. The roof of the fourth ventricle.

tegmina. Plural of *tegmen.*

Tegopen. A trademark for the sodium salt of cloxacillin, a semisynthetic penicillin antibiotic.

Tegretol. Trademark for carbamazepine, an anticonvulsant and antineuralgic drug.

teg·u·ment (teg'yoo·munt) *n.* [L. *tegumentum,* from *tegere,* to cover]. INTEGUMENT.

teg·u·men·ta·ry (teg"yoo·men'tur·ee) *adj.* Pertaining to an integument.

tegumentary epithelium. EPIDERMIS.

Teich·mann's crystals (tye'ᵏh'maʰn)[L. T. S. *Teichmann,* German histologist, 1825–1895]. HEMIN CRYSTALS.

Teichmann's test [L. T. S. *Teichmann*]. A test for detecting the presence of blood in which a crystal of sodium chloride and glacial acetic acid are added to the suspected liquid under a cover glass and the whole is heated without boiling and then cooled. The appearance of rhombic crystals of hemin indicates blood.

tei·cho·ic acids (tye·ko'ick). [Gk. *teix*os, wall, + *-ic*]. Any one of the polymeric esters of glycerol or ribitol with phosphoric acid present in the walls and cell contents of certain bacteria.

tei·chop·sia (tye·kop'see·uh) *n.* [Gk. *teich*os, wall, fortification, + *-opsia*]. Temporary amblyopia, with subjective visual images.

teknocyte. TECNOCYTE.

[1]tel-, tele-, teleo-, telo- [Gk. *tēle*]. A combining form meaning *distant, at a distance, remote.*

[2]tel-, tele-, teleo-, telo- [Gk. *telos*]. A combining form meaning *end, final.*

te·la (tee'luh) *n.*, pl. **te·lae** (·lee) [L., web, from *texere,* to weave]. A web or tissue.

tela adi·po·sa (ad·i·po'suh). ADIPOSE TISSUE.

tela cho·ri·oi·dea ven·tri·cu·li quar·ti (ko·ree·oy'dee·uh ven·trick'yoo·lye kwahr'tye) [BNA]. TELA CHOROIDEA VENTRICULI QUARTI.

tela chorioidea ventriculi ter·tii (tur'shee·eye) [BNA]. TELA CHOROIDEA VENTRICULI TERTII.

tela cho·roi·dea ven·tri·cu·li quar·ti (ko·roy'dee·uh ven·trick'yoo·lye kwahr'tye) [NA]. The membranous roof of the fourth ventricle of the brain, including the choroid plexus.

tela choroidea ventriculi ter·tii (tur"shee·eye) [NA]. The membranous roof of the third ventricle of the brain, including the choroid plexus.

telaesthesia. TELESTHESIA.

tel·al·gia (tel·al'jee·uh) *n.* [*tel-*, distant, + *-algia*]. REFERRED PAIN.

tel·an·gi·ec·ta·sia (tel·an''jee·eck·tay'zhuh, ·zee·uh) *n.* TELANGIECTASIS.

telangiectasia-pigmentation-cataract syndrome. ROTHMUND-THOMSON SYNDROME.

tel·an·gi·ec·ta·sis (tel·an''jee·eck'tuh·sis) *n.* [*tel-*, end, + *angi-* + *ectasis*]. Dilatation of groups of capillaries. They form elevated, dark red, wartlike spots, varying in size from 1 to 7 mm. —**telangi·ec·tat·ic** (·eck·tat'ick) *adj.*

telangiectasis fa·ci·ei (fay''shee·ee'eye). ACNE ROSACEA.

telangiectasis lym·phat·i·ca (lim·fat'i·kuh). LYMPHANGIECTASIS.

telangiectatic angioma. An angioma in which the component vessels are large.

telangiectatic carcinoma. Inflammatory carcinoma with prominent vascularity.

telangiectatic sarcoma. A variety of osteogenic sarcoma with a prominent vascular component.

tel·an·gi·ec·to·des (tel·an''jee·eck·to'deez) *adj.* [*telangiectasis* + Gk. *-ōdēs*, adjectival suffix]. Characterized by telangiectasis.

tel·an·gi·o·ma (tel·an''jee·o'muh) *n.*, pl. **telangiomas, telangioma·ta** (·tuh) [*tel-*, end, + *angi-* + *-oma*]. A mass composed of dilated capillaries.

tel·an·gi·on (tel·an'jee·un) *n.* [*tel-*, end, + Gk. *angeion*, vessel]. A terminal arteriole.

tel·an·gi·o·sis (te·lan''jee·o'sis) *n.* [*tel-*, end, + *angi-* + *-osis*]. Any disease of minute blood vessels.

tel·an·gi·tis (tel''an·jye'tis) *n.* [*tel-*, end, + *angi-* + *-itis*]. Inflammation of capillaries.

tela sub·cu·ta·nea (sub·kew·tay'nee·uh) [NA]. SUBCUTANEOUS TISSUE; SUPERFICIAL FASCIA.

tela sub·mu·co·sa (sub·mew·ko'suh) [NA]. The layer of connective tissue that lies between a mucous membrane and subjacent tissues. Syn. *submucous membrane.*

tela submucosa co·li (ko'lye) [NA]. The tissue underlying the mucous membrane of the colon.

tela submucosa eso·pha·gi (e·sof'uh·jye) [NA]. The layer underlying the mucous membrane of the esophagus.

tela submucosa in·tes·ti·ni rec·ti (in·tes·tye'nigh reck'tye) [BNA]. TELA SUBMUCOSA RECTI.

tela submucosa intestini te·nu·is (ten'yoo·is) [NA]. The layer underlying the mucous membrane of the small intestine.

tela submucosa oe·so·pha·gi (e·sof'uh·jye) [BNA]. TELA SUBMUCOSA ESOPHAGI.

tela submucosa pha·ryn·gis (fa·rin'jis) [NA]. The layer underlying the mucous membrane of the pharynx.

tela submucosa rec·ti (reck'tye) [NA]. The layer underlying the mucous membrane of the rectum.

tela submucosa tra·che·ae et bron·cho·rum (tray'kee·ee et brong·ko'rum) [NA]. The layer underlying the mucous membrane of the trachea and bronchi.

tela submucosa tu·bae ute·ri·nae (tew'bee yoo·te·rye'nee) [BNA]. The layer underlying the mucous membrane of the uterine tube.

tela submucosa ven·tri·cu·li (ven·trick'yoo·lye) [NA]. The layer underlying the mucous membrane of the stomach.

tela submucosa ve·si·cae uri·na·ri·ae (ves'i·see yoo·ri·nair'ee·ee) [NA]. The layer underlying the mucous membrane of the urinary bladder.

tela sub·se·ro·sa (sub·se·ro'suh) [NA]. The layer beneath the outer serous membrane of any organ.

tela subserosa co·li (ko'lye) [NA]. The layer beneath the serous membrane of the colon.

tela subserosa he·pa·tis (hep'uh·tis) [NA]. The layer beneath the serous membrane of the liver.

tela subserosa in·tes·ti·ni te·nu·is (in·tes·tye'nigh ten'yoo·is) [NA]. The layer beneath the serous membrane of the small intestine.

tela subserosa pe·ri·to·naei (perr·i·to·nee'eye) [BNA]. The subserous layer beneath the peritoneum.

tela subserosa pe·ri·to·nei pa·ri·e·ta·lis (perr·i·to·nee'eye pa·rye·e·tay'lis) [NA]. The layer beneath the parietal peritoneum.

tela subserosa peritonei vis·ce·ra·lis (vis·e·ray'lis) [NA]. The layer beneath the visceral peritoneum.

tela subserosa tu·bae ute·ri·nae (tew'bee yoo·te·rye'nee) [NA]. The layer beneath the serous membrane of the uterine tube.

tela subserosa ute·ri (yoo'te·rye) [NA]. The layer beneath the serous membrane of the uterus.

tela subserosa ven·tri·cu·li (ven·trick'yoo·lye) [NA]. The layer beneath the serous membrane of the stomach.

tela subserosa ve·si·cae fel·le·ae (ve·sigh'see fel'ee·ee) [NA]. The layer beneath the serous membrane of the gallbladder.

tela subserosa vesicae uri·na·ri·ae (yoo·ri·nair'ree·ee) [NA]. The layer beneath the serous membrane of the urinary bladder.

tel·au·gic oculars (tel·aw'jick). Oculars with an extremely high exit pupil, so that spectacles can be worn with comfort.

tele-. See *tel-.*

tele·an·gi·ec·ta·sis (tel''ee·an''jee·eck'tuh·sis) *n.* TELANGIECTASIS.

tele·car·dio·gram (tel''e·kahr'dee·o·gram) *n.* TELELECTROCARDIOGRAM.

tele·car·dio·phone (tel''e·kahr'dee·o·fone) *n.* [*tele-* + *cardiophone*]. An apparatus amplifying heart sounds.

tele·cep·tor (tel'e·sep''tur) *n.* [*tele-*, distant, + *receptor*]. A sense organ that is activated by a distant stimulus, for example, the nose, eye, and cochlea. Syn. *teloreceptor.*

tele·ci·ne·sis (tel''e·si·nee'sis) *n.* TELEKINESIS.

tele·co·balt therapy (tel''e·ko'bawlt). External radiation therapy with a radioactive cobalt source at some distance from the skin.

tele·cu·rie therapy (tel''e·kew'ree). Therapy in which the radioactive source is located at some distance from the lesion to be treated.

tele·den·drite (tel''e·den'drite) *n.* TELODENDRON.

tele·di·as·tol·ic (tel''e·dye''us·tol'ick) *adj.* [*tele-* + *diastolic*]. Pertaining to the last phase of a diastole.

tele·flu·or·os·co·py (tel''e·floo''ur·os'kuh·pee) *n.* [*tele-*, end, + *fluoroscopy*]. The procedure by which the usual distortion of a fluoroscopic picture by divergence of the roentgen rays is eliminated by placing the source of the rays 2 meters or more from the body part to be fluoroscoped.

te·leg·o·ny (te·leg'uh·nee) *n.* [*tele-*, distant, + *-gony*]. The erroneous belief that a male once mated with a female will affect the subsequent progeny of the same female mated with a different male.

te·leg·ra·pher's cramp or **spasm.** *Obsol.* The occupational cramp or spasm that affects the arm muscles habitually used by a telegrapher.

telegrapher's nystagmus. OCCUPATIONAL NYSTAGMUS.

tele·graph·ic speech (tel''e·graf'ick). A form of agrammatism in which utterances consist primarily of nouns, verbs of action, and significant modifiers. It is characteristic of Broca's aphasia.

tele·ki·ne·sis (tel''e·ki·nee'sis, ·kigh·nee'sis) *n.* [*tele-*, distant, + *kinesis*]. The power claimed by some people of causing objects to move without touching them.

tel·elec·tro·car·dio·gram (tel''e·leck''tro·kahr'dee·o·gram) *n.* [*tel-* + *electrocardiogram*]. An electrocardiogram taken in a laboratory, the galvonometer being connected by a wire with the patient, who is elsewhere.

tel·elec·tro·ther·a·peu·tics (tel''e·leck''tro·therr·uh·pew'ticks) *n.* [*tel-*, distant, + *electro-* + *therapeutics*]. Treatment of hysterical paralysis by a series of electric discharges near the patient without actual contact.

te·lem·e·try (te·lem'e·tree) *n.* [*tele-*, distant, + *-metry*]. The measurement of a property, such as temperature or pressure, and the transmission of the result to a distant receiving station where it is indicated or recorded.

telencephalic vesicles. CEREBRAL VESICLES.

tel·en·ceph·a·lon (tel″en·sef′uh·lon) *n.* [*tel-*, end, + *encephalon*] [NA]. The anterior subdivision of the primary forebrain that develops into olfactory lobes, cerebral cortex, and corpora striata. —**telen·ce·phal·ic** (·se·fal′ick) *adj.*

tele·neu·rite (tel″e·new′rite) *n.* [*tele-*, end, + Gk. *neuron*, nerve]. One of the terminal filaments of the main stem of an axis cylinder process.

tele·neu·ron (tel″e·new′ron) *n.* [*tele-*, end, + *neuron*]. NERVE ENDING.

teleo-. See *tel-*.

tel·eo·den·dron (tel″ee·o·den′dron) *n.* TELODENDRON.

teleologic hallucination. A hallucination that fits into the delusional scheme of the patient, often directing him to carry out certain acts.

te·le·ol·o·gy (teel″ee·ol′uh·jee, tel″ee·) *n.* [*teleo-*, end, + *-logy*]. The doctrine that explanations of phenomena are to be sought in terms of final causes, purpose, or design in nature. —**tele·o·log·ic** (·o·loj′ick) *adj.*

tele·op·sia (tel″ee·op′see·uh) *n.* [*tele-*, distant, + *-opsia*]. A disorder in visual perception of space characterized by an excess of depth, or the illusion that close objects are far away.

tel·eo·roent·gen·o·gram (tel″ee·o·rent′gen·o·gram) *n.* [*teleo-* + *roentgenogram*]. A radiograph, usually of the heart, made at a distance of 6 or more feet, to minimize distortion.

te·leo·ther·a·peu·tics (teel″ee·o·therr′uh·pew′ticks, tel″ee·o·) *n.* [*teleo-* + *therapeutics*]. SUGGESTION THERAPY.

Telepaque. Trademark for iopanoic acid, a radiopaque diagnostic agent used for oral cholecystography.

te·lep·a·thist (te·lep′uh·thist) *n.* A person versed in telepathy.

te·lep·a·thy (te·lep′uth·ee) *n.* [*tele-*, distant, + *-pathy*]. The direct awareness of what is taking place in another person's mind. See also *extrasensory perception, psi phenomena.* —**tele·path·ic** (tel″e·path′ick) *adj.*

tele·phone theory of hearing. The theory that the auditory nerve transmits nerve impulses to the brain having the same frequency as the sound waves striking the ear.

tele·ra·di·og·ra·phy (tel″e·ray″dee·og′ruh·fee) *n.* [*tele-*, distant, + *radiography*]. Radiography with the tube about 6 feet from the body to avoid distortion and magnification.

tele·ra·di·um (tel′e·ray″dee·um) *n.* [*tele-*, distant, + *radium*]. Radium that is used as the source for telecurie therapy. See also *teleradium therapy.*

teleradium therapy. External radium therapy with the radium source at some distance from the skin.

tele·re·cep·tor (tel″e·re·sep′tur) *n.* TELECEPTOR.

tel·er·gy (tel′ur·jee) *n.* [*tel-*, distant, + *-ergy*]. AUTOMATISM.

tele·roent·gen·og·ra·phy (tel″e·rent″guh·nog′ruh·fee) *n.* [*tele-*, distant, + *roentgenography*]. TELERADIOGRAPHY.

tele·scope nose. Depression below the root of the nose as a result of necrosis of the septum and vomer, seen in leprosy.

tele·scop·ic spectacles (tel″e·skop′ick). Spectacles that magnify the retinal image; useful for persons with cloudy media, partial cataracts, or impaired retinal sensitivity.

tele·ste·reo·roent·gen·og·ra·phy (tel″e·sterr″ee·o·rent″guh·nog′ruh·fee, ·steer″ee·o·) *n.* [*tele-*, distant, + *stereo-* + *roentgenography*]. A stereoscopic x-ray examination made with the x-ray tube a long distance (about 6 feet) from the object.

tel·es·the·sia, tel·aes·the·sia (tel″es·theezh′uh, ·theez′ee·uh) *n.* [*tel-*, distant, + *esthesia*]. 1. Perception of objects or sounds at a distance. 2. A perception of objects or conditions independently of the recognized channels of sense. Compare *telepathy.*

tele·sys·tol·ic (tel″e·sis·tol′ick) *adj.* [*tele-* + *systolic*]. Pertaining to the last phase of systole.

tele·ther·a·py (tel″e·therr′uh·pee) *n.* [*tele-*, distant, + *therapy*]. 1. SUGGESTION THERAPY. 2. Treatment with radiation from a distant source.

tele·vi·sion microscope (tel″e·vizh·un). A television camera fitted to a microscope; large audiences may simultaneously view microscopic preparations.

tel·lu·rite medium (tel′yoo·rite). A medium enriched with blood or serum containing solium tellurite, Na_2TeO_3, used for the isolation and identification of *Corynebacterium diphtheriae* and of certain fungi; it inhibits many species of bacteria.

tel·lu·ri·um (te·lew′ree·um) *n.* [NL., from L. *tellus, telluris*, earth]. Te = 127.60. A nonmetallic element, atomic number 52, of bluish-white color, obtained chiefly as a byproduct in the refining of copper and lead.

telo-. See *tel-*.

telo·cen·tric (tel″o·sen′trick) *adj.* [*telo-* + *-centric*]. Of a chromosome: having the centromere located at the end. Contr. *acrocentric, metacentric, submetacentric.*

telo·coele (tel′o·seel) *n.* [*telo-*, end, + *-coele*]. The cavity of the telencephalon.

telo·den·dron (tel″o·den′dron) *n.*, pl. **teloden·dra** (·druh) [*telo-*, end, + *dendron*]. The branched and variously differentiated terminal of an axon.

tel·o·gen (tel′uh·jen) *n.* [*telo-* + *-genesis*]. The final, quiescent phase of the hair cycle in a follicle, lasting until the fully grown hair is shed and anagen commences. Contr. *anagen, catagen.*

tel·og·no·sis (tel″og·no′sis) *n.* Diagnosis by telephone-transmitted radiographs.

telo·lec·i·thal (tel″o·les′i·thul) *adj.* [*telo-*, end, + *lecithal*]. Pertaining to or characterizing an egg having a large mass of yolk that is concentrated at one pole or in one hemisphere.

telo·lem·ma (tel″o·lem′uh) *n.* [*telo-*, end, + *-lemma*]. The membrane over a motor end plate of a skeletal muscle fiber.

telo·mer (tel′o·mur) *n.* [*telo-*, + end, + *-mer*]. The product of telomerization.

telo·mere (tel′o·meer) *n.* [*telo-*, end, + *-mere*]. An extremity or arm of a chromosome.

telo·mer·iza·tion (te·lom″ur·i·zay′shun, tel″o·mur·) *n.* A type of polymerization and addition reaction in which a compound XY dissociates and unites with another compound R, containing unsaturated groups, to form a large molecule $X(R)_nY$, called a telomer.

telo·phase (tel′o·faze) *n.* [*telo-*, end, + *phase*]. 1. The final stage of mitosis in which the chromosomes reorganize to form an interstage nucleus. 2. The final stage of the first (telophase I) or second (telophase II) meiotic division. 3. The final phase of any process.

telo·phrag·ma (tel″o·frag′muh, tee″lo·) *n.*, pl. **telophragma·ta** (·tuh) [*telo-* + Gk. *phragma*, enclosure]. INTERMEDIATE DISK.

telo·re·cep·tor (tel″o·re·sep′tur) *n.* TELECEPTOR.

Telo·spo·rid·ia (tel″o·spo·rid′ee·uh) *n.pl.* [NL., from *telo-*, end, + Gk. *spora*, seed]. A class of Sporozoa, characterized by spore formation after the sporozoon has completed its growth. The subclasses included are Gregarinida, Coccidia, and Haemosporidia.

telo·syn·ap·sis (tel″o·si·nap′sis) *n.* [*telo-*, end, + *synapsis*]. The end-to-end union of homologous chromosomes at the time of the maturation of the germ cells, in contrast to the side-by-side union as in parasynapsis.

TEM Abbreviation for *triethylenemelamine.*

Temaril. Trademark for trimeprazine, a phenothiazine compound used, as the tartrate salt, to relieve pruritus.

te·maz·e·pam (te·maz′e·pam) *n.* 7-Chloro-1,3-dihydro-3-hydroxy-1-methyl-5-phenyl-2*H*-1,4-benzodiazepin-2-one, $C_{16}H_{13}ClN_2O_2$, a minor tranquilizer.

tem·o·dex (tem′o·decks) *n.* 2-Hydroxyethyl-3-methyl-2-quinoxalinecarboxylate-1,4-dioxide, $C_{12}H_{12}N_2O_5$, a veterinary growth stimulant.

tem·o·fos (tem′o·fos) *n.* 0,0′-(Thiodi-*p*-phenylene)0,0,0′,0′-

tetramethylbis (phosphorothioate), $C_{16}H_{20}O_6O_2S_3$, a veterinary ectoparasiticide.

tem·per, *v. & n.* [L. *temperare,* to mix properly]. 1. To make metals hard and elastic by heating them and then suddenly cooling them. Compare *anneal.* 2. The hardness or brittleness of a metal, as induced by heating and suddenly cooling. 3. Disposition, state of mind, temperament; a show of anger.

tem·per·a·ment (tem'pruh·munt) *n.* [L. *temperamentum,* a mixing in due proportion]. 1. The mixture of physical, intellectual, emotional, and moral qualities which make up a person's personality, his attitudes, and his behavioral responses to varying life situations. See also *personality.* 2. *In constitutional medicine,* the mixture of motivational drives in a personality. The level of personality just above physiologic function and just below acquired attitudes and beliefs. The quantitative patterning of viscerotonia, somatotonia, and cerebrotonia in a personality.

tem·per·ance, *n.* [L. *temperantia*]. Moderation in satisfying desire, especially in the use of alcoholic beverages.

tem·per·ate, *adj.* [L. *temperatus,* from *temperare,* to be moderate]. Moderate; without excess.

tem·per·a·ture, *n.* [L. *temperatura,* mixture, tempering]. The degree of intensity of heat of a body, especially as measured by the scale of a thermometer. Abbreviated, T.

temperature coefficient. A quantitive expression of the effect of an increase in temperature on any chemical or physical process or reaction.

temperature sense. The sense by which differences in temperature are appreciated, consisting of a sense for cold (cryesthesia) and a heat sense (thermesthesia). These are represented on the surface by small areas that respond most consistently to thermal stimuli with a sensation of warmth or cold, the so-called cold and warm points.

temper tantrum. TANTRUM.

tem·plate (tem'plut) *n.* [F. *templet,* temple of a loom]. A preformed macromolecule, usually of DNA but occasionally of RNA, upon which a specific enzyme manufactures a strand complementary to the template in both base composition and sequence.

tem·ple, *n.* [OF., from L. *tempus*]. The portion of the head anterior to the ear and above the zygomatic arch.

tem·po·ra (tem'puh·ruh) *n.pl.* [L., pl. of *tempus,* temple] [NA]. The temporal region on either side of the head.

tem·po·ral (tem'puh·rul) *adj.* 1. Pertaining to, or in the direction of, the temple. 2. Pertaining to the temporal lobe. 3. Pertaining to time.

temporal angle. The outer canthus of the eye.

temporal arteries. See Table of Arteries in the Appendix.

temporal arteritis. GIANT-CELL ARTERITIS (1).

temporal bone. NA *os temporale.* See Table of Bones in the Appendix.

temporal diameter. ANTEROTRANSVERSE DIAMETER.

temporal diplopia. HOMONYMOUS DIPLOPIA.

temporal field. The temporal half of the field of vision.

temporal fossa. The depression that lodges the temporal muscle. NA *fossa temporalis.*

temporal incisure. A small fissure separating the uncus from the apex of the temporal lobe.

tem·po·ra·lis (tem''po·ray'lis) *n.* [L.]. A muscle of mastication, arising from the temporal fossa and inserted into the coronoid process of the mandible. Syn. *temporal muscle.* NA *musculus temporalis.* See also Table of Muscles in the Appendix.

temporalis su·per·fi·ci·alis (sue''pur·fish''ee·ay'lis). A portion of the anterior auricular muscle.

temporal line. The ridge of bone curving upward and backward from the zygomatic process of the frontal bone; it divides into the superior and inferior temporal lines. NA *linea temporalis ossis frontalis.*

temporal lobe. The part of the cerebral hemisphere below the lateral cerebral sulcus, continuous posteriorly with the occipital lobe. NA *lobus temporalis.* See also Plates 16, 18.

temporal lobe epilepsy. Recurrent seizures originating in discharging lesions of the temporal lobe, characterized by hallucinations, illusions, feeling of increased reality or familiarity (déjà vu) or unfamiliarity (jamais vu) and a large variety of affective experiences (fear, anxiety and epigastric sensations). Syn. *partial complex seizures.* Compare *psychomotor epilepsy.*

temporal muscle. TEMPORALIS.

temporal nerve. See *zygomaticotemporal* in the Table of Nerves in the Appendix.

temporal operculum. The portion of the temporal lobe overlying the insula. NA *operculum temporale.*

temporal orientation. The act of determining one's relation to time.

temporal plane. A relatively flat area lying below the linea temporalis inferior and composed of portions of the frontal and parietal bones, great wing of the sphenoid, and squama temporalis. Syn. *planum temporale.*

temporal pole. The tip of the temporal lobe of the cerebrum. NA *polus temporalis.* See also Plate 17.

temporal process of the zygomatic bone. The posterior angle of the zygomatic bone by which it articulates with the zygomatic process of the temporal bone. NA *processus temporalis ossis zygomatici.*

temporal ridge. The ridge extending from the external angular process of the frontal bone, across the frontal and parietal bones, and terminating in the posterior root of the zygomatic process.

temporal space. TEMPORAL FOSSA.

temporal sulcus. Either one of two grooves, superior (NA *sulcus temporalis superior*) and inferior (NA *sulcus temporalis inferior*), that divide the lateral surface of the temporal lobe into superior, middle, and inferior temporal gyri.

temporal summation. The cumulative effect of successive subthreshold stimuli on excitable tissue, resulting in a response. Most phenomena formerly believed to be due to temporal summation can be explained by spatial summation.

tem·po·rary, *adj.* [L. *temporarius,* from *tempus,* time]. Not permanent.

temporary cartilage. A cartilage that is ultimately replaced by bone.

temporary filling. A substance, as cement or gutta percha, used in teeth as a filling which is to be replaced later by a permanent restoration.

temporary magnet. A magnet that derives its magnetism from another magnet or from a galvanic current.

temporary parasite. A parasite that is free-living during part of its life.

temporary prosthesis. An artificial limb used early following amputation and in preparation for the permanent apparatus.

temporary teeth. 1. DECIDUOUS TEETH. 2. A provisional set of artificial teeth.

tem·po·rize (tem'puh·rize) *v.* To provide provisional or temporary treatment for a patient until a definitive diagnosis is established. —**tem·po·ri·za·tion** (tem''puh·ruh·zay'shun) *n.*

temporo-. A combining form meaning *temporal.*

tem·po·ro·fron·tal (tem''puh·ro·frun'tul) *adj.* Pertaining to the temporal and frontal bones or areas.

tem·po·ro·man·dib·u·lar (tem''puh·ro·man·dib'yoo·lur) *adj.* [*temporo-* + *mandibular*]. Pertaining to the temporal bone and the mandible.

temporomandibular joint. NA *articulatio temporomandibularis.* See Table of Synovial Joints and Ligaments in the Appendix.

temporomandibular joint syndrome. MYOFACIAL PAIN-DYSFUNCTION SYNDROME.

temporomandibular syndrome. MYOFACIAL PAIN-DYSFUNCTION SYNDROME.

tem·po·ro·oc·cip·i·tal (tem″puh·ro·ock·sip′i·tul) *adj.* Pertaining to the temporal and occipital bones, regions, or lobes.

tem·po·ro·pa·ri·e·tal (tem″puh·ro·pa·rye′e·tul) *adj.* Pertaining to the temporal and parietal bones, regions, or lobes.

tem·po·ro·pon·tine (tem″puh·ro·pon′tine, ·teen) *adj.* [*temporo-* + *pontine*]. Pertaining to the temporal lobe and the pons.

temporopontine tract. A tract of nerve fibers which arise in the temporal lobe of the cerebrum, descend from the cortex, pass through the anterior limb of the internal capsule, and terminate in the pontine nuclei. NA *tractus temporopontinus.*

tem·u·lence (tem′yoo·lunce) *n.* [L. *temulentia,* from *temetum,* intoxicating drink]. 1. DRUNKENNESS. 2. CHRONIC ALCOHOLISM.

te·mu·len·tia (tem″yoo·len′shee·uh) *n.* [L.]. *Obsol.* TEMULENCE.

ten-, teno- [Gk. *tenon*]. A combining form meaning *tendon.*

te·na·cious (te·nay′shus) *adj.* [L. *tenax, tenacis,* holding fast]. Tough; cohesive, adhesive. **—te·nac·i·ty** (te·nas′i·tee) *n.*

te·nac·u·lum (te·nack′yoo·lum) *n.,* pl. **tenacu·la** (·luh), **tenaculums** [L., holder, from *tenere,* to hold]. A slender, hook-shaped instrument with a long handle for seizing and holding parts or approximating incised edges during surgical operations.

tenaculum forceps. Long-handled forceps with relatively large sharp hooks or teeth, designed to grasp tissues or organs firmly with minimal crushing; adapted especially for gynecologic surgery.

ten·al·gia (ten·al′jee·uh) *n.* [*ten-* + *-algia*]. TENODYNIA.

tenalgia crep·i·tans (krep′i·tanz). TENOSYNOVITIS CREPITANS.

ten·der, *adj.* [OF. *tendre,* from L. *tener*]. Painful to the touch or on palpation. **—tender·ness,** *n.*

tendines. Plural of *tendo.*

ten·di·no·plas·ty (ten′di·no·plas″tee) *n.* [NL. *tendo, tendinis,* tendon, + *-plasty*]. Plastic surgery of tendons. See also *tenoplasty.* **—ten·di·no·plas·tic** (ten″di·no·plas′tick) *adj.*

ten·di·nous (ten′di·nus) *adj.* Pertaining to, or having the nature of, a tendon.

tendinous arch. 1. A fibrous arch formed of thickened fascia, serving as a point of attachment for a muscle or as protection for muscular nerves or vessels. NA *arcus tendineus.* 2. (of the pelvic fascia:) A thickened portion of the parietal pelvic fascia extending from the medial aspect of the body of the pubic bone to the spine of the ischium. NA *arcus tendineus fasciae pelvis.* 3. (of the levator ani:) An arched thickening of the obturator fascia from which the iliococcygeal portion of the levator ani muscle arises. NA *arcus tendineus musculi levatoris ani.* 4. (of the soleus muscle:) A fibrous arch on the deep surface of the upper portion of the soleus muscle overlying the posterior tibial vessels. NA *arcus tendineus musculi solei.*

tendinous cords. The tendons of the papillary muscles of the ventricles of the heart, attached to the atrioventricular valves. NA *chordae tendineae.*

tendinous synovitis. Inflammation of the synovial sheath surrounding a tendon.

ten·do (ten′do) *n.,* genit. **ten·di·nis** (ten′di·nis), pl. **tendi·nes** (·neez) [NL.] [NA]. TENDON.

tendo Achil·lis (a·kil′is) [NA alt.]. CALCANEAL TENDON. NA alt. *tendo calcaneus.*

tendo Achillis reflex. ACHILLES JERK.

tendo cal·ca·ne·us (kal·kay′nee·us) [NA]. CALCANEAL TENDON. NA alt. *tendo Achillis.*

tendo con·junc·ti·vus (kon·junk·tye′vus) [NA alt.] FALX INGUINALIS.

tendo cri·co·eso·pha·ge·us (krye″ko·e·sof·uh·jee′us, ·ee″so·faj′ee·us) [NA]. CRICOESOPHAGEAL TENDON.

ten·dol·y·sis (ten·dol′i·sis) *n.* [*tendon* + *-lysis*]. The freeing of adhesions about a tendon.

ten·do·mu·cin (ten″do·mew′sin) *n.* [*tendon* + *mucin*]. A mucoid found in tendons.

ten·do·mu·coid (ten″do·mew′koid) *n.* [*tendon* + *mucoid*]. TENDOMUCIN.

ten·don (ten′dun) *n.* [ML. *tendo, tendonis,* from Gk. *tenōn,* from *tenein,* to stretch (rel. to L. *tendere,* to stretch, whence by assimilation the *d* in *tendo, tendonis*)]. A band of dense fibrous tissue forming the termination of a muscle and attaching the latter to a bone. NA *tendo.* See also Plate 2.

tendon graft. The graft of tendon to bridge a gap in a tendon. See also *tendon transplantation.*

ten·don·itis (ten″dun·eye′tis) *n.* [*tendon* + *-itis*]. Inflammation of a tendon, usually at the point of its attachment to bone.

tendon of the conus arteriosus. A band of fibrous tissue extending from the fibrous trigone of the heart and fibrous ring about the right atrioventricular opening to the posterior surface of the conus arteriosus.

tendon of Zinn. LIGAMENT OF ZINN.

tendon organ of Golgi. CORPUSCLE OF GOLGI.

tendon palpation test. Decreased resistance to palpation of a tendon as an index of cerebellar or peripheral nervous system disease.

tendon reflex. Contraction of a muscle in response to sudden stretching of the muscle by a brisk tap against its tendon. See also *deep reflex, stretch reflex.*

tendon sheath. In particular, the synovial sheath surrounding a tendon crossing the wrist or ankle joints.

tendon spindle. CORPUSCLE OF GOLGI.

tendon suspension. TENODESIS.

tendon transplantation. The removal of a tendon from its normal attachment and its reinsertion in another place, used to substitute a functioning muscle for a paralyzed one by transplanting its tendon.

ten·do·plas·ty (ten′do·plas″tee) *n.* TENDINOPLASTY.

ten·do·syn·o·vi·tis (ten″do·sin″o·vye′tis, ·sigh″no·) *n.* [*tendon* + *synovitis*]. TENOSYNOVITIS.

ten·do·vag·i·ni·tis (ten″do·vaj″i·nigh′tis) *n.* [*tendon* + *vaginitis*]. Inflammation of a tendon and its sheath; TENOSYNOVITIS.

tendovaginitis crep·i·tans (krep′i·tanz). TENOSYNOVITIS CREPITANS.

tendovaginitis gra·nu·lo·sa (gran″yoo·lo′suh). Tuberculosis of tendon sheaths, the sheaths being filled with granulation tissue.

tendovaginitis ste·no·sans (ste·no′sanz). DE QUERVAIN'S DISEASE.

-tene [L. *taenia,* band, from Gk. *tainia*]. A combining form designating *a chromosome filament in meiosis.*

te·neb·ric (te·neb′rick) *adj.* [L. *tenebrae,* darkness, + *-ic*]. Dark, gloomy.

Te·neb·rio (te·neb′ree·o) *n.* [L., one who shuns the light]. A genus of beetles serving as intermediate hosts of helminth parasites of vertebrates.

Tenebrio mol·i·tor (mol′i·tor). The mealworm. The larva of this species acts as an intermediate host for the tapeworm *Hymenolepis diminuta.*

te·nec·to·my (te·neck′tuh·mee) *n.* [*ten-* + *-ectomy*]. 1. Excision of a lesion, as a ganglion or xanthoma, of a tendon or tendon sheath. 2. TENOPLASTY.

te·nes·mus (tuh·nez′mus) *n.* [L., from Gk. *teinesmos,* a straining]. A straining, especially the painful straining to empty the bowels or bladder without the evacuation of feces or urine. **—tenes·mic** (·mick) *adj.*

¹tenia. ¹TAENIA.

²te·nia. (tee′nee·uh) *n.,* pl. **te·ni·ae** (·nee·ee) [L. *taenia,* band, headband, from Gk. *tainia*] [NA]. BAND (3).

tenia cho·roi·dea (ko·roy′dee·uh) [NA]. The line of attachment of the lateral part of the choroid plexus to the medial side of the cerebral hemisphere in the lateral ventricle.

teniacide. TAENIACIDE.

teniae. Plural of ²*tenia* (BAND (3)).

teniae acu·sti·cae (a·koos′ti·see). STRIAE MEDULLARES VENTRICULI QUARTI.

teniae co·li (ko′lye) [NA]. The three tapelike bands of the longitudinal layer of the tunica muscularis of the colon: the tenia libera, tenia mesocolica, and tenia omentalis. See also Plate 13.

tenia for·ni·cis (for'ni·sis) [NA]. The line of attachment of the choroid plexus of the lateral ventricle to the fornix.

teniafuge. TAENIAFUGE.

tenia li·be·ra (lye'be·ruh) [NA]. The tenia coli midway between the tenia omentalis and the tenia mesocolica.

tenia me·so·co·li·ca (mes·o·ko'li·kuh) [NA]. The tenia coli along the site of attachment of the transverse mesocolon.

tenia of the fourth ventricle. TENIA VENTRICULI QUARTI.

tenia of the third ventricle. TENIA THALAMI.

tenia omen·ta·lis (o·men·tay'lis) [NA]. The tenia coli along the site of attachment of the greater omentum.

tenia pon·tis (pon'tis). *Obsol.* FILUM LATERALIS PONTIS.

tenia te·lae (tee'lee) [NA]. The line of attachment of the ependymal cells of the choroid plexus to various parts of the brain.

tenia tha·la·mi (thal'uh·migh) [NA]. The line of attachment of the choroid plexus to the dorsal margin of the thalamus.

tenia ven·tri·cu·li quar·ti (ven·trick'yoo·lye kwahr'tye) [NA]. The line of attachment of the choroid plexus to the posterior part of the fourth ventricle.

teniform. TAENIFORM.

tenioid. Taenioid (= TAENIFORM).

te·ni·o·la, tae·ni·o·la (te·nigh'o·luh, te·nee'o·luh) *n.* [NL., dim. from Gk. *tainia,* ribbon]. A small ribbon.

teniola ci·ne·rea (si·neer'ee·uh). A thin grayish ridge separating the striae of the fourth ventricle from the cochlear division of the eighth cranial nerve.

teniophobia. TAENIOPHOBIA.

ten·nis elbow or **arm.** EPICONDYLITIS (2).

teno-. See *ten-*.

teno·de·sis (te·nod'e·sis, ten''o·dee'sis) *n.*, pl. **tenode·ses** (·seez) [*teno-* + *-desis*]. Fixation of a tendon, as to a bone.

ten·o·dyn·ia (ten''o·din'ee·uh) *n.* [*ten-* + *-odynia*]. Pain in a tendon.

teno·fi·bril (ten''o·figh'bril) *n.* [Gk. *tein*ein, to extend, reach out, + *fibril*]. A small, delicate fibril connecting one epithelial cell with another; TONOFIBRIL.

te·nol·y·sis (ten·ol'i·sis) *n.* [*teno-* + *-lysis*]. TENDOLYSIS.

te·nom·e·ter (te·nom'e·tur) *n.* [Gk. *tein*ein, to stretch, make taut, + *-meter*]. A device for measuring intraocular tension.

teno·myo·plas·ty (ten'o·migh'o·plas''tee) *n.* TENONTOMYOPLASTY.

teno·my·ot·o·my (ten''o·migh·ot'uh·mee) *n.* [*teno-* + *myo-* + *-tomy*]. *In ophthalmology,* a procedure for the treatment of squint, devised to enfeeble the action of one of the rectus muscles by incising portions of its tendon near the sclerotic insertion.

ten·o·nec·to·my (ten''o·neck'tuh·mee) *n.* [Gk. *tenōn,* tendon, + *-ectomy*]. Excision of a portion of a tendon.

[1]**ten·o·ni·tis** (ten''o·nigh'tis) *n.* TENDONITIS.

[2]**tenonitis,** *n.* [J. R. *Tenon* + *-itis*]. Inflammation of the vagina bulbi (Tenon's capsule).

ten·o·nom·e·ter (ten''o·nom'e·tur) *n.* TENOMETER.

ten·o·nos·to·sis (ten''o·nos·to'sis) *n.* TENOSTOSIS.

Te·non's capsule (tuh·nohⁿ') [J. R. *Tenon,* French anatomist and surgeon, 1724–1816]. VAGINA BULBI.

tenonto- [Gk. *tenōn, tenontos*]. A combining form meaning *tendon.*

te·non·to·myo·plas·ty (te·non''to·migh'o·plas''tee) *n.* [*tenonto-* + *myo-* + *-plasty*]. Reparative surgery involving both tendon and muscle; used particularly for hernia.

te·non·to·my·ot·o·my (te·non''to·migh·ot'uh·mee) *n.* [*tenonto-* + *myo-* + *-tomy*]. Surgical division of tendons and muscles.

te·non·to·the·ci·tis (te·non''to·the·sigh'tis) *n.* [*tenonto-* + *thecitis*]. TENOSYNOVITIS.

tenontothecitis pro·lif·e·ra cal·ca·rea (pro·lif'e·ruh kal·kair'ee·uh). Necrobiosis of a tendon in its sheath with calcareous deposit.

teno·phyte (ten'o·fite) *n.* [*teno-* + *-phyte*]. A bony or cartilaginous growth on a tendon.

tenoplastic transplantation. Surgical repair of a tendon, as in the hand, wherein tendon tissue is transplanted from elsewhere in the body, or from another body.

teno·plas·ty (ten'o·plas''tee) *n.* [*teno-* + *-plasty*]. Reparative or plastic surgery of a tendon. —**teno·plas·tic** (ten''o·plas'tick) *adj.*

te·nor·rha·phy (te·nor'uh·fee) *n.* [*teno-* + *-rrhaphy*]. The uniting of a divided tendon by sutures.

ten·os·to·sis (ten''os·to'sis) *n.*, pl. **tenosto·ses** (·seez) [*ten-* + *oste-* + *-osis*]. Ossification of a tendon.

teno·su·ture (ten'o·sue''chur) *n.* [*teno-* + *suture*]. TENORRHAPHY.

teno·syn·o·vec·to·my (ten''o·sin''o·veck'tuh·mee) *n.* [*teno-* + *synov*ia- + *-ectomy*]. Excision of a tendon sheath.

teno·syn·o·vi·al (ten''o·si·no'vee·ul) *adj.* [*teno-* + *synovial*]. Pertaining to a tendon and a synovial surface.

teno·syn·o·vi·o·ma (ten''o·si·no''vee·o'muh) *n.* A benign synovioma.

teno·syn·o·vi·tis (ten''o·sin''o·vye'tis) *n.* [*teno-* + *synov*ia + *-itis*]. Inflammation of a tendon and its sheath.

tenosynovitis crep·i·tans (krep'i·tanz). Tenosynovitis associated with cracking sounds during muscular activity.

teno·tome (ten'o·tome) *n.* [*teno-* + *-tome*]. A small, narrow-bladed knife mounted on a slender handle; a tenotomy knife.

te·not·o·mize (te·not'uh·mize) *v.* To perform tenotomy.

te·not·o·my (te·not'uh·mee) *n.* [*teno-* + *-tomy*]. The operation of cutting a tendon.

teno·vag·i·ni·tis (ten''o·vaj''i·nigh'tis) *n.* [*teno-* + *vaginitis*]. Inflammation of the sheath of a tendon.

Tensilon Chloride. Trademark for edrophonium chloride, an antagonist of curariform skeletal muscle relaxants.

ten·sion, *n.* [L. *tensio,* from *tendere, tensus,* to stretch]. 1. The act of stretching; the state of being stretched or strained. 2. In electricity, the power of overcoming resistance; electric potential. 3. The partial pressure exerted by a component of a mixture of gases. 4. A state of mental or physical strain.

tension headache. MUSCLE-CONTRACTION HEADACHE.

tension lines. CLEAVAGE LINES.

tension pneumothorax. VALVULAR PNEUMOTHORAX.

tension suture. A suture placed at a distance from the wound edge and through the deeper tissues, to lessen the strain on the more immediate wound sutures. Syn. *relaxation suture.*

tension-time index. The area under the systolic portion of the ventricular pressure curve, i.e., the time integral of the ventricular systolic pressure multiplied by the heart rate per minute. Abbreviated, TTI. Syn. *pressure time per minute.*

ten·si·ty (ten'si·tee) *n.* [ML. *tensitas,* from L. *tensus,* tense]. Tenseness, the condition of being stretched.

ten·sive (ten'siv) *adj.* Giving the sensation of stretching or contraction.

ten·sor (ten'sor, ·sur) *n.* A muscle that serves to make a part tense. See also Table of Muscles in the Appendix.

tensor cap·su·la·ris ar·ti·cu·la·ti·o·nis me·ta·car·po·pha·lan·gei di·gi·ti (kap·sue·lair'is ahr·tick·yoo·lay·shee·o'nis met·uh·kahr''po·fa·lan'jee·eye dij'i·tye kwin'tye). A variant of the opponens digiti minimi muscle.

tensor fas·ci·ae la·tae reflex (fash'ee·ee lay'tee). Tapping over the tensor fasciae latae muscle at its origin near the anterior superior iliac spine, with the patient recumbent, produces slight abduction of the thigh.

tensor la·mi·nae pos·te·ri·o·ris va·gi·nae mus·cu·lae rec·ti ab·do·mi·nis (lam'i·nee pos·teer·ee·o'ris va·jye'nee mus'kew·lee reck'tye ab·dom'i·nis). Rare variant insertion of certain fibers of the transverse abdominal muscle.

tensor li·ga·men·ti an·nu·la·ris (lig·uh·men'tye an·yoo·lair'is).

A variant part of the supinator muscle. There may be anterior or posterior bands.

tensor muscle of the choroid. The outer portion of the ciliary muscle.

tensor pa·la·ti (pa·lay'tye). TENSOR VELI PALATINI.

tensor tym·pa·ni (tim'puh·nye). NA *musculus tensor tympani.* See Table of Muscles in the Appendix.

tensor ve·li pa·la·ti·ni (vee'lye pal·uh·tye'nigh). A muscle of the soft palate arising from the cartilaginous medial end of the auditory tube and a nearby portion of the sphenoid bone and inserted into the palatal aponeurosis. NA *musculus tensor veli palatini.* See also Table of Muscles in the Appendix.

ten·sure (ten'shur) *n.* [L. *tensura,* a stretching]. TENSION (1); a stretching or straining.

ten·ta·tive (ten'tuh·tiv) *adj.* [ML. *tentativus,* from L. *tentare,* to try]. Provisional; not final; offered or proposed for the time being.

tenth (Xth) cranial nerve. VAGUS.

tenth·me·ter (tenth'mee"tur) *n.* One ten-millionth of a millimeter, or one angstrom.

ten·tig·i·nous (ten·tij'i·nus) *adj.* [L. *tentigo, tentiginis,* lust]. Characterized by insane lust.

ten·ti·go (ten·tye'go) *n.* [L.]. Lust; SATYRIASIS.

tentigo ve·ne·rea (ve·neer'ee·uh). NYMPHOMANIA.

tentoria. Plural of *tentorium.*

tentorial notch. INCISURE OF THE TENTORIUM.

tentorial pressure cone or **herniation.** The herniation of the uncus and adjacent structures into the incisure of the tentorium as a result of a sharp pressure gradient from above, as in severe cerebral edema. See also *cerebellar pressure cone.*

ten·to·ri·um (ten·to'ree·um) *n.,* pl. **tento·ria** (·ree·uh) [L., tent]. A partition of dura mater, roofing over the posterior cranial fossa, separating the cerebellum from the cerebral hemispheres. NA *tentorium cerebelli.* See also Plate 17. —**tentori·al** (·ul) *adj.*

tentorium ce·re·bel·li (serr·e·bel'eye) [NA]. TENTORIUM.

tentorium of the hypophysis. DIAPHRAGM OF THE SELLA.

Tenuate. A trademark for diethylpropion hydrochloride, an anorexic.

ten·u·ate (ten'yoo·ate) *v.* [L. *tenuare,* from *tenuis,* thin]. To make thin.

te·nu·i·ty (te·new'i·tee) *n.* [L. *tenuitas*]. Thinness; the condition of being thin.

ten·u·ous (ten'yoo·ous) *adj.* [L. *tenu*is, thin, rare, + *-ous*]. Thin; minute.

teph·ro·my·e·li·tis (tef"ro·migh"e·lye'tis) *n.* [Gk. *tephros,* ash-colored, + *myel-* + *-itis*]. *Obsol.* POLIOMYELITIS.

tep·id, *adj.* [L. *tepidus*]. Moderately warm.

TEPP Abbreviation for *tetraethylpyrophosphate.*

tep·ro·tide (tep'ro·tide) *n.* A nonapeptide angiotensin-covert-ing (inhibiting) enzyme; $C_{53}H_{76}N_{14}O_{12}$.

ter- [L., three times]. A combining form meaning *three* or *threefold.*

ter·ab·del·la (terr"ab·del'uh) *n.* [Gk. *ter*ein, to bore, + *bdella,* leech]. An artificial leech.

tera·mor·phous (terr"uh·mor'fus) *adj.* [*teras* + *-morphous*]. Of the nature of a monstrosity.

te·ras (terr'us) *n.,* pl. **ter·a·ta** (terr'uh·tuh) [Gk.]. MONSTER. —**ter·at·ic** (ter·at'ick) *adj.*

terat-, terato- [Gk. *teras, teratos*]. A combining form meaning *monster.*

terata. Plural of *teras.*

ter·a·tism (terr'uh·tiz·um) *n.* [*terat-* + *-ism*]. A congenital anomaly or monstrosity.

terato-. See *terat-.*

ter·a·to·blas·to·ma (terr"uh·to·blas·to'muh) *n.* [*terato-* + *blastoma*]. TERATOMA.

ter·a·to·car·ci·no·ma (terr"uh·to·kahr"si·no'muh) *n.* [*terato-* + *carcinoma*]. A teratoma with carcinomatous elements.

ter·a·to·gen (terr'uh·to·jen, te·rat'o·jin) *n.* Any agent that brings about teratogenesis, such as a virus, medication, or radiation that can cause maldevelopment of the embryo in the first trimester of pregnancy. —**ter·a·to·gen·ic** (terr"uh·to·jen'ick) *adj.*

ter·a·to·gen·e·sis (terr"uh·to·jen'e·sis) *n.* [*terato-* + *genesis*]. Embryonic maldevelopment leading to teratism or serious congenital defects.

ter·a·tog·e·nous (terr"uh·toj'e·nus) *adj.* [*terato-* + *-genous*]. Arising from totipotential cells, such as those which produce a fetus under normal conditions.

ter·a·tog·e·ny (terr"uh·toj'e·nee) *n.* TERATOGENESIS.

ter·a·toid (terr'uh·toid) *adj.* [*terat-* + *-oid*]. Resembling a monster.

teratoid adenocystoma. MESONEPHROMA.

teratoid carcinoma. A malignant teratoma.

teratoid cyst. A cyst associated with a teratoma.

teratoid tumor. TERATOMA.

ter·a·tol·o·gy (terr"uh·tol'uh·jee) *n.* [*terato-* + *-logy*]. The science of malformations and monstrosities. —**tera·to·log·ic** (·to·loj'ick) *adj.;* **tera·tol·o·gist** (·tol'uh·jist) *n.*

ter·a·to·ma (terr"uh·to'muh) *n.,* pl. **teratomas, teratoma·ta** (·tuh) [*terat-* + *-oma*]. A true neoplasm composed of bizarre and chaotically arranged tissues foreign embryologically as well as histologically to the area in which the tumor is found. —**tera·to·ma·tous** (·muh·tus) *adj.*

teratomatous cyst. TERATOID CYST.

ter·a·to·pho·bia (terr"uh·to·fo'bee·uh) *n.* [*terato-* + *-phobia*]. 1. Abnormal fear of monsters or of deformed people. 2. Abnormal dread, on the part of a pregnant woman, of giving birth to a deformed infant.

ter·a·to·sis (terr"uh·to'sis) *n.,* pl. **terato·ses** (·seez) [*terat-* + *-osis*]. A congenital deformity; TERATISM.

ter·a·to·sper·mia (terr"uh·to·spur'mee·uh) *n.* [*terato-* + *-spermia*]. Abnormal sperm morphology.

ter·a·to·zoo·sper·mia (terr"uh·to·zo·o·spur'mee·uh) *n.* [*terato-* + *zoo-* + *-spermia*]. TERATOSPERMIA.

ter·bi·um (tur'bee·um) *n.* [NL. after *Ytterby,* Sweden]. Tb = 158.9254. A rare metallic element, atomic number 65.

ter·bu·ta·line (tur·bew'tuh·leen) *n.* α-[(*tert*-Butylamino)-methyl]-3,5-dihydroxybenzyl alcohol, $C_{12}H_{19}NO_3$, a bronchodilator used as the sulfate (2:1) salt.

ter·chlor·eth·yl·ene (tur"klor·eth'il·een) *n.* TETRACHLOROETHYLENE.

ter die su·men·dum [L., from *sumere,* to take]. To be taken thrice a day; abbreviated, t.d.s.

te·re (teer'ee) *v.* [L., imperative of *terere,* to rub]. Rub. Used in writing prescriptions.

ter·e·bene (terr'e·been) *n.* A mixture of hydrocarbons, chiefly dipentene and terpinene, prepared by the action of sulfuric acid on turpentine oil followed by steam distillation. It has been used as a stimulant expectorant.

ter·e·bin·thi·nate (terr"e·bin'thi·nate) *adj.* [Gk. *terebinthos,* turpentine, + *-ate*]. Containing or resembling turpentine.

ter·e·bin·thism (terr"e·bin'thiz·um) *n.* [Gk. *terebinthos,* turpentine, + *-ism*]. Poisoning with turpentine oil.

ter·e·bra·che·sis (terr"e·bra·kee'sis) *n.* [L. *teres,* round, + Gk. *brachys,* short, + *-esis*]. The operation of shortening the round ligament of the uterus.

ter·e·brat·ing pain (terr'e·bray"ting). A severe feeling of distress suggesting to the subject the action of a drill or other piercing instrument.

ter·e·bra·tion (terr"e·bray'shun) *n.* [L. *terebrare,* to bore]. TEREBRATING PAIN.

tere·phtha·lic acid (terr·thal'ick). *p*-Benzenedicarboxylic acid, $C_8H_6O_4$, used in the preparation of condensation polymers.

te·res (teer'eez, terr'eez) *adj. & n.,* pl. **ter·e·tes** (teer'e·teez, terr') [L., rounded]. 1. CYLINDRICAL. 2. A muscle having a cylindrical shape. See also Table of Muscles in the Appendix.

teres major. NA *musculus teres major.* See Table of Muscles in the Appendix.

teres minor. NA *musculus teres minor.* See Table of Muscles in the Appendix.

ter·fen·a·dine (tur·fen'uh·deen) *n.* α-(*p-tert*-Butylphenyl)-4-(hydroxydiphenylmethyl)-1-piperidinebutanol, $C_{32}H_{41}O_2$, an antihistaminic.

ter in die. Three times a day; abbreviated, t.i.d.

term, *n.* [OF. *terme,* from L. *terminus,* boundary]. 1. A limit; the time during which anything lasts. 2. The time of expected delivery. 3. A vocabulary item; especially, a word, phrase, or symbol used in specialized or technical language.

Ter·man-Mer·rill revision [L. M. *Terman,* U.S. psychologist, 1877–1956; and M. A. *Merrill,* U.S. psychologist, b. 1888]. STANFORD-BINET TEST.

ter·mi·nal, *adj. & n.* [L. *terminalis,* of a boundary]. 1. Pertaining to the end; placed at or forming the end. 2. The pole of a battery or other electric source, or the end of the conductors or wires connected thereto.

terminal anesthesia. The state of insensitivity produced by the deposition of the local anesthetic agent about the terminal arborizations of the afferent axon. These are designated as anociceptors. This anesthetic works best through very thin mucous membrane surfaces, such as conjunctiva, urethra, urinary bladder, larynx, peritoneum, and pleura.

terminal arborization. 1. The branched end of a sensory nerve fiber. 2. MOTOR END PLATE. 3. The terminal ramifications of the Purkinje system of the heart.

terminal artery. END ARTERY.

terminal axon. NERVE BULB.

terminal bar. An area of occlusion of the lateral surfaces of adjoining epithelial cells, located near the cells' free ends.

terminal boutons. END FEET.

terminal bronchiole. The next to the last bronchiolar subdivision; the last bronchiole without pulmonary alveoli in its wall.

terminal cardiac sulcus. A groove on the external surface of the right atrium, extending from the right side of the superior vena cava to the right side of the inferior vena cava, the embryonic right boundary of the sinus venosus. NA *sulcus terminalis atrii dextri.*

terminal corpuscle. An encapsulated sensory nerve ending.

terminal crest. CRISTA TERMINALIS ATRII DEXTRI.

terminal filament. The end piece or naked axial filament of the tail of a spermatozoon.

terminal ganglion. Any ganglion of the parasympathetic portion of the autonomic nervous system which is located in or near the organ innervated; the preganglionic nerve fibers terminate in these ganglions. NA *ganglion terminale.*

terminal hair. The longer, coarser hair which in humans grows on the scalp, eyebrows, and eyelashes and in the axillae and pubes of adults, and more sparsely and variably (especially in adult males of certain racial groups) on other parts of the body. Contr. *vellus.*

terminal hinge position. The most posterosuperior unstrained position of the mandibular condyle from which opening and lateral movements can be performed.

terminal ileitis. REGIONAL ENTERITIS.

ter·mi·nal·iza·tion (tur''mi·nul·eye·zay'shun) *n.* The process by which the chiasmata of the diplotene stage of meiosis move to the ends of the tetrads in the stage of diakinesis.

terminal line. ILIOPECTINEAL LINE.

terminal lingual sulcus. The shallow, V-shaped groove, with its apex directed backward, on the dorsum of the tongue; it separates the oral and pharyngeal parts of the organ. NA *sulcus terminalis linguae.*

terminal plate. The thin plate of bone of an epiphysis laid down on the metaphyseal surface preceding epiphyseal union.

terminal sinus. The sinus bounding the area vasculosa of the blastoderm of a meroblastic ovum.

terminal sulcus of the thalamus. A groove in the floor of the lateral ventricle of the cerebrum between the thalamus and the caudate nucleus.

terminal ventricle. The dilated portion of the central canal of the spinal cord in the conus medullaris. NA *ventriculus terminalis.*

terminal web. The area of the cytoplasm just beneath the free cell surface traversed by a network of fine filaments.

ter·mi·nat·ing codon. TERMINATION CODON.

ter·mi·na·tio (tur''mi·nay'shee·o) *n.,* genit. **termi·na·ti·o·nis** (·nay''shee·o'nis), pl. **terminatio·nes** (·neez) [L., act of setting bounds]. End, ending.

termination codon. A sequence of three bases on messenger RNA which do not code for an aminoacyl transfer RNA and thus signals termination of growth of the newly synthesized polypeptide chain.

terminationes. Plural of *terminatio.*

terminationes ner·vo·rum li·be·rae (nur·vo'rum lye'be·ree) [NA]. Free nerve endings.

termini. Plural of *terminus.*

termini ad mem·bra spec·tan·tes (ad mem'bruh speck·tan'teez) [NA]. Terms applicable to the extremities.

termini ge·ne·ra·les (jen·e·ray'leez) [NA]. General terms.

termini si·tum et di·rec·ti·o·nem par·ti·um cor·po·ris in·di·can·tes (sigh'tum et di·reck·shee·o'nem pahr'shee·um kor'po·ris in·di·kan'teez) [NA]. Terms indicating the location and direction of parts of the body.

ter·mi·nol·o·gy (tur''mi·nol'uh·jee) *n.* [L. *terminus,* term, + *-logy*]. NOMENCLATURE; a system of technical terms.

ter·mi·nus (tur'mi·nus) *n.,* pl. **termi·ni** (·nigh) [L., boundary]. A term or expression.

terms, *n.pl.* MENSES.

ter·na·ry (tur'nuh·ree) *adj.* [L. *ternarius,* from *terni,* three in a group]. Pertaining to chemical compounds, made up of three elements or radicals.

Ter·ni·dens (tur'ni·denz) *n.* [L. *terni,* three in a group, + *dens,* tooth]. A genus of phasmid nematode worms, a species of which, *Ternidens diminutus,* sometimes infects man and is a common intestinal parasite of simian hosts in Africa, India, and Indonesia.

ter·o·di·line (terr''o·dye'leen) *n.* *N-tert*-Butyl-1-methyl-3,3-diphenylpropylamine, $C_{20}H_{27}N$, a coronary vasodilator.

ter·ox·a·lene (terr·ock'suh·leen) *n.* 1-(3-Chloro-*p*-tolyl)-4-[6-(*p-tert*-pentylphenoxy)hexyl]piperazine, $C_{28}H_{41}ClN_2O$, an antischistosomal drug.

ter·pene (tur'peen) *n.* [*terp*entine (early variant of *turpentine*) + *-ene*]. Any hydrocarbon of the general formula $C_{10}H_{16}$, sometimes represented as a condensation of two isoprene (C_5H_8) units. By extension the term may include compounds representing any multiple of C_5H_8 units. Terpenes occur naturally in volatile oils and other plant sources; they are generally insoluble in water but soluble in alcohol and other organic liquids. Sesquiterpenes are hydrocarbons of the formula $C_{15}H_{24}$ or $(C_5H_8)_3$; diterpenes are hydrocarbons of the formula $C_{20}H_{32}$ or $(C_5H_8)_4$; triterpenes are hydrocarbons of the formula $C_{30}H_{48}$ or $(C_5H_8)_6$; polyterpenes are hydrocarbons of the formula $(C_5H_8)_n$. The term hemiterpene is sometimes applied to the hydrocarbon of the formula C_5H_8 (isoprene).

ter·pe·nism (tur'pe·niz·um) *n.* [*terpene* + *-ism*]. Poisoning by terpene from internal use or inhalation.

ter·pin·e·ol (tur·pin'ee·ol) *n.* A mixture of isomeric alcohols of the formula $C_{10}H_{17}OH$ occurring in many volatile oils; formerly used as an antiseptic.

ter·pin hydrate (tur'pin). *cis-p*-Menthane-1,8-diol hydrate, $C_{10}H_{20}O_2.H_2O$, used as an expectorant.

ter·pi·nol (tur'pi·nol) *n.* An oily liquid, chiefly $C_{10}H_{16}$ and $C_{10}H_{18}O$, obtained by the action of dilute mineral acids on terpin hydrate with heat; formerly used for the treatment of bronchial affections.

Ter-Po·gos·si·an camera (tur·puh·go'see·un) [M. *Ter-Pogossian,* U.S. radiation physicist, b. 1925]. A direct-viewing radiation imaging apparatus consisting of a type of image amplifier tube designed for use with low gamma-ray photon energies.

ter·ra (terr'uh) *n.*, pl. & genit. sing. **ter·rae** (·ee) [L.]. Earth.

terra al·ba (al'buh). KAOLIN.

Terramycin. Trademark for the antibiotic substance oxytetracycline and its hydrochloride salt.

terra si·gil·la·ta (sij·i·lay'tuh). [L.] Sealed earth; KAOLIN. In medieval Europe, earth guaranteed to be genuine through the use of a seal.

ter·ri·to·ri·al matrix (terr″i·to'ree·ul). Matrix in hyalin cartilage differentiated into regions of high basophilia surrounding smaller or larger groups of cells.

Ter·ry's method [B. T. *Terry*, U.S. pathologist, d. 1955]. A method for the rapid preparation of tissue sections by using a slice 0.5 to 1 mm thick and covering the exposed surface with a modified polychrome methylene blue stain.

Terry's stain [B. T. *Terry*]. A thin freehand slice of fresh tissue is stained a few seconds with a drop or two of polychrome methylene blue, and examined by transmitted light.

tert-. A chemical prefix meaning *tertiary.*

ter·tian (tur'shun) *adj.* [L. *tertianus*, of the third]. Recurring every other day, as tertian fever; the initial day is counted as the first, the recurrence taking place on the third.

tertian fever. VIVAX MALARIA.

tertian malaria. VIVAX MALARIA.

ter·ti·ar·ism (tur'shee·ur·iz·um) *n.* TERTIARY SYPHILIS.

ter·ti·ary (tur'shee·err″ee) *adj.* [L. *tertiarius*]. Of the third order or stage.

tertiary alcohol. An alcohol that contains the trivalent group $\equiv$COH.

tertiary amine. An amine of the type R_3N or $R'(R'')NR'''$.

tertiary amyl alcohol. AMYLENE HYDRATE.

tertiary circinate erythema. Pink to red lesions occurring as circular or oval patches with normal or pigmented centers, or in segments of circles which may form gyrate figures by coalescence; occurring several years after syphilitic infection. Syn. *neurosyphilid, circinate syphilitic erythema.*

tertiary sequestrum. A sequestrum that is cracked or partially detached and remaining firmly in place.

tertiary structure. The native folded conformation normally assumed by a specific protein in solution. This conformation is stabilized by hydrogen bonds, hydrophobic bonds, and ionic bonds. Contr. *primary, secondary,* and *quaternary structure.*

tertiary syphilid. Any syphilid occurring during the late (tertiary) stage of syphilis.

tertiary syphilis. Late syphilis, including all the symptoms of disease occurring after the fourth year of infection.

ter·tip·a·ra (tur·tip'uh·ruh) *n.* [L. *terti*us, third, + *-para*]. A woman who has had three viable pregnancies.

ter·va·lence (tur·vay'lunce) *n.* TRIVALENCE.

Teschen disease. A viral neurotropic disease of swine. Syn. *encephalomyelitis of swine.*

tes·i·cam (tess'i·kam) *n.* 4′-Chloro-1,2,3,4-tetrahydro-1,3-dioxo-4-isoquinolinecarboxanilide, $C_{16}H_{11}ClN_2O_3$, an anti-inflammatory agent.

tes·i·mide (tess'i·mide) *n.* 4-Benzylidene-5,6,7,8,-tetrahydro-1,3(2*H*,4*H*)-isoquinolinedione, $C_{16}H_{15}NO_2$, an anti-inflammatory agent.

Teslac. Trademark for testolactone, an antineoplastic steroid.

Tes·la current (tes'luh, Serbo-Croatian tes'lah) [N. *Tesla*, Serbian electrician in U.S., d. 1943]. A high-frequency alternating flow of electricity used in electrotherapy; it is of medium voltage.

Tessalon. Trademark for the antitussive drug benzonatate.

tes·sel·lat·ed epithelium (tes″e·lay'tid). Simple squamous epithelium.

test, *n.* [ME., cupel, from OF., pot, from L. *testum*, earthen vessel]. 1. A trial or examination. 2. A procedure to identify a constituent, to detect changes of a function, or to establish the true nature of a condition. 3. The reagent for producing a special reaction.

tes·ta·ceous (tes·tay'shus) *adj.* [L. *testaceus*, from *testa*, brick, tile; shell]. Pertaining to a shell.

tes·tal·gia (tes·tal'jee·uh) *n.* [*testis* + *-algia*]. Testicular pain.

tes·ta·men·ta·ry capacity (tes″tuh·men'tuh·ree). *In legal medicine*, the mental ability requisite to make a valid will.

test cross. In linkage study, the cross of a double heterozygote with the doubly recessive homozygote parent in order to count the assortment of the two loci.

testes. Plural of *testis.*

tes·ti·cle (tes'ti·kul) *n.* [L. *testiculus*, dim. of *testis*]. A testis; especially, the scrotal testis of larger mammals.

tes·tic·u·lar (tes·tick'yoo·lur) *adj.* Pertaining to the testis.

testicular adenoma. ANDROBLASTOMA (1).

testicular artery. The artery in the male that originates in the abdominal aorta and supplies the testis, also providing branches to the ureter, cremaster, and epididymis; corresponds to the ovarian artery in the female. NA *arteria testicularis.*

testicular compression reflex. Contraction of the abdominal muscles in response to compression or squeezing of the testis. Syn. *Kocher's reflex.*

testicular dysgenesis syndrome. DEL CASTILLO'S SYNDROME.

testicular hormones. The hormones elaborated by the testis; the characteristic substance is testosterone, a steroid that matures and maintains the male genitalia and the secondary sex characters.

tes·tis (tes'tis) *n.*, pl. **tes·tes** (·teez) [L.] [NA]. One of a pair of male reproductive glands, after sexual maturity the source of the spermatozoa; a male gonad. See also Plates 25, 26.

testis cords. MEDULLARY CORDS (1).

testis graft. The grafting by implantation of an entire testis or portion to replace one lost or destroyed.

tes·ti·tis (tes·tye'tis) *n.* [*test*is + *-itis*]. ORCHITIS.

test meal. A specified quantity and type of food given to test the secretory function of the stomach.

tes·toid (tes·toid) *adj.* [*test*is + *-oid*]. Pertaining to any substance, natural or synthetic, which is androgenic, i.e., capable of maintaining or stimulating development of secondary male-sex characters.

tes·to·lac·tone (tes″to·lack'tone) *n.* 17α-Oxa-D-homoandrosta-1,4-diene-3,17-dione, $C_{19}H_{24}O_3$, an antineoplastic steroid.

tes·tos·ter·one (tes·tos'tur·ohn) *n.* [*test*is + *sterone*]. 17-Hydroxyandrost-4-en-3-one, $C_{19}H_{28}O_2$, a male sex hormone; the principal androgen secreted by human testes. May be synthesized from cholesterol and certain other sterols. Used for the treatment of deficiency or absence of testosterone in the male; also for palliation of advanced metastatic carcinoma of the female breast. Employed as the free alcohol and as the following esters: testosterone cypionate, testosterone enanthate, testosterone phenylacetate, and testosterone propionate.

test paper. INDICATOR PAPER.

test solution. A reagent solution. Abbreviated, T.S.

test tube. A cylindrical glass tube with one end open; used for growing cultures of bacteria, or for chemical analysis.

test-tube baby. A child conceived as the result of artificial insemination of the mother.

test type. A chart of letters, most commonly the Snellen chart or its modifications, used to test the acuity of central vision.

tetan-, tetano- [Gk. *tetanos*, rigid]. A combining form meaning (a) *tetanus;* (b) *tetany, tetanic.*

tet·a·nal (tet'uh·nul) *adj.* TETANIC.

te·ta·nia (te·tay'nee·uh) *n.* TETANY.

te·tan·ic (te·tan'ick) *adj.* [Gk. *tetanikos*]. 1. Of, pertaining to, or causing tetanus. 2. Of, pertaining to, or causing tetany.

tetanic cataract. A cataract due to defect in calcium metabolism.

tetanic contraction. 1. *In obstetrics*, a state of continued contraction of the uterine muscle; occurs in prolonged labors, usually in the second stage. Results from a pathologic retraction ring. 2. TETANUS (2).

tetanic convulsions or **seizures.** Paroxysms of tonic contraction or spasm of muscles in the course of tetanus, superimposed on a persistent state of enhanced muscle activity and occurring spontaneously or in response to slight external stimuli. Consciousness is not lost during these paroxysms.

tetanic croup. SPASMODIC CROUP.

tetanic spasm. TETANUS (2).

tetanic spasticity or **rigidity.** In advanced tetanus, the varying degree of continuous involuntary spasm and resistance to passive movement of affected muscles. Syn. *hypertonic contracture.*

te·tan·i·form (te·tan'i·form) *adj.* [*tetan-* + *-iform*]. Resembling either tetanus or tetany.

tet·a·nig·e·nous (tet"uh·nij'e·nus) *adj.* [*tetan-* + *-genous*]. Causing tetanus or tetanic spasms.

tet·a·nil·la (tet"uh·nil'uh) *n.* [NL., dim. from *tetanus*]. *Obsol.* 1. A mild form of tetany. 2. MYOCLONUS.

tet·a·nin (tet'uh·nin) *n.* TETANUS TOXOID.

tet·a·nine (tet'uh·neen, ·nin) *n.* TETANUS TOXOID.

tet·a·ni·za·tion (tet"uh·ni·zay'shun) *n.* Production of tetanus or tetanic spasms. —**tet·a·nize** (tet'uh·nize) *v.*

tetano-. See *tetan-.*

tet·a·no·can·na·bin (tet"uh·no·kan'uh·bin) *n.* A substance found in some samples of cannabis that produces strychnine-like symptoms.

tet·a·node (tet'uh·node) *n.* The quiescent interval in tetanus, between the tonic spasms.

tet·a·noid (tet'uh·noid) *adj.* [*tetan-* + *-oid*]. Resembling the muscular spasms of tetanus or tetany.

tet·a·no·ly·sin (tet"uh·no·lye'sin, tet"uh·nol'i·sin) *n.* [*tetano-* + *lysin*]. The hemolytic toxin of *Clostridium tetani.*

tet·a·no·ly·sis (tet"uh·no·lye'sis, ·nol'i·sis) *n.* [*tetano-* + *-lysis*]. Lysis of erythrocytes in vitro by one of two exotoxins produced by tetanus bacilli.

tet·a·nom·e·ter (tet"uh·nom'e·tur) *n.* [*tetano-* + *-meter*]. An instrument for measuring tetanic spasms.

tet·a·no·mo·tor (tet'uh·no·mo"tur) *n.* [*tetano-* + *motor*]. An instrument for stimulating a nerve mechanically and producing tetanic spasm of the supplied muscle.

tet·a·no·pho·bia (tet"uh·no·fo'bee·uh) *n.* [*tetano-* + *-phobia*]. An abnormal fear of tetanus.

tet·a·no·spas·min (tet"uh·no·spaz'min) *n.* [*tetano-* + *spasm* + *-in*]. The potent exotoxin produced by the vegetative forms of *Clostridium tetani,* responsible for the principal manifestations of tetanus of man and animals.

tet·a·nus (tet'uh·nus) *n.* [L., from Gk. *tetanos,* stretched, rigid, from *teinein,* to stretch, make taut]. 1. An infectious disease characterized by extreme stiffness of the body, painful tonic spasms of the affected muscles including trismus and opisthotonus, exaggeration of reflex activity, and generalized spasms or convulsions without loss of consciousness; due to the exotoxin produced by *Clostridium tetani* which interferes with the function of the reflex arc by suppressing spinal and brainstem inhibitory neurons; results from contamination of a wound not exposed to oxygen. Syn. *lockjaw.* 2. Sustained muscular contraction artificially induced with repeated stimuli of such a frequency that individual contractions fuse.

tetanus antitoxin. Any serum containing specific antibodies that neutralize tetanus toxin; originally produced in horses, now generally produced in humans.

tetanus in·fan·tum (in·fan'tum). TETANUS NEONATORUM.

tetanus ne·o·na·to·rum (nee"o·na·to'rum) [NL.]. Tetanus of the newborn, usually due to infection of the umbilical stump.

tetanus toxoid. Inactivated tetanus toxin which is used to produce active immunity against the disease. See also *adsorbed tetanus toxoid.*

tet·a·ny (tet'uh·nee) *n.* [*tetanus* + *-y*]. A state of increased excitability and spontaneous activity of the central and peripheral nervous system, caused by alkalosis or a decrease of serum calcium, manifested by intermittent numbness and cramps or twitchings of the extremities, carpopedal spasm, laryngospasm, confusion, and such signs of neuromuscular hyperexcitability as the Chvostek, peroneal, Trousseau, and Erb signs. Associated with hypoparathyroidism, vitamin D deficiency, deficiencies in the absorption or utilization of calcium as in rickets or the celiac syndrome, and possibly magnesium deficiency.

tetany of the newborn. A temporary state of neuromuscular hyperirritability seen in the first two months of life, more commonly in infants who are premature, born of diabetic mothers, delivered by cesarian section, recipients of an exchange transfusion, or twins; due to a functional hypoparathyroidism and relatively low renal clearance of phosphorus, resulting in an elevated serum phosphorus and lowered serum calcium; manifested by irritability, muscular twitching, periods of apnea, respiratory distress, and convulsions.

tetart-, tetarto- [Gk. *tetartos*]. A combining form meaning (a) *fourth;* (b) *a quarter, quadrant.*

tet·ar·cone (tet'ahr·kone) *n.* TETARTOCONE.

te·tar·ta·no·pia (te·tahr"tuh·no'pee·uh) *n.* [*tetart-* + *anopia*]. Loss of vision in a homonymous quadrant in each field of vision. See also *quadrantanopia.*

te·tar·ta·nop·sia (te·tahr"tuh·nop'see·uh) *n.* TETARTANOPIA.

tetarto-. See *tetart-.*

te·tar·to·cone (te·tahr'tuh·kone) *n.* [*tetarto-* + *cone*]. The distolingual cone; the fourth or distolingual cusp of an upper molar tooth.

te·tar·to·co·nid (te·tahr"to·ko'nid, ·kon'id) *n.* [*tetartocone* + *-id*]. The distolingual or fourth cusp of a lower molar tooth.

tet·io·thal·ein (tet·eye"o·thal'een) *n.* IODOPHTHALEIN.

tetr-, tetra- [Gk. *tetra-,* from *tessara*]. A combining form meaning *four.*

tet·ra·ba·sic (tet"ruh·bay'sick) *adj.* [*tetra-* + *basic*]. With reference to acids, having four atoms of replaceable hydrogen.

tet·ra·bra·chi·us (tet"ruh·bray'kee·us) *adj.* [NL., from *tetra-* + *brachium*]. Having four arms.

tet·ra·caine (tet'ruh·kane) *n.* 2-(Dimethylamino)ethyl *p*-(butylamino)benzoate, $C_{15}H_{24}N_2O_2$, a potent local anesthetic with many uses; employed as the base and as the hydrochloride salt. Syn. *amethocaine.*

tet·ra·chei·rus (tet"ruh·kigh'rus) *adj.* [Gk. *tetracheir,* from *cheir,* hand]. Having four hands.

tet·ra·chlo·ro·eth·ane (tet"ruh·klo"ro·eth'ane) *n.* 1,1,2,2,-Tetrachloroethane, $CHCl_2CHCl_2$, a nonflammable solvent for fats, oils, and waxes; highly toxic. Syn. *acetylene tetrachloride.*

tet·ra·chlo·ro·eth·yl·ene (tet"ruh·klo"ro·eth'il·ene) *n.* Ethylene tetrachloride, $Cl_2C{=}CCl_2$, a nonflammable liquid; used as an anthelmintic, especially against the hookworm *Necator americanus.* Syn. *perchloroethylene.*

tet·ra·chlo·ro·meth·ane (tet"ruh·klo"ro·meth'ane) *n.* CARBON TETRACHLORIDE.

tet·ra·chrome (tet'ruh·krome) *adj.* [*tetra-* + *-chrome*]. Pertaining to or having four colors.

tet·ra·coc·cus (tet"ruh·kock'us) *n.,* pl. **tetracoc·ci** (·sigh) [*tetra-* + *coccus*]. A coccus that divides in two planes and forms a group of four cells.

tet·ra·cy·cline (tet"ruh·sigh'kleen, ·klin) *n.* [*tetra-* + *cycl-* + *-ine*]. 1. Generic name for a group of biosynthetic antibiotic substances having in common the four-ring structure of chlortetracycline, the first tetracycline to be discovered, and found also in oxytetracycline, the second member of the group to be isolated. 2. The specific antibiotic having the composition $C_{22}H_{24}N_2O_8$; has a wide spectrum of activity.

Tetracyn. A trademark for tetracycline.

tet·rad (tet'rad) *n.* [Gk. *tetras, tetrados*]. 1. A group of four. 2. *In genetics,* a group of four chromatids which arises during meiosis from the pairing and splitting of maternal and paternal homologous chromosomes. 3. *In chemistry,* an element having a valence of four. 4. *Informal.* TETRALOGY OF FALLOT.

tet·ra·dac·tyl (tet"ruh·dack'til) *adj.* [Gk. *tetradaktylos,* four-toed]. Having four digits on each limb.

tetrad of Fallot. TETRALOGY OF FALLOT.

tet·ra·eth·yl·am·mo·ni·um (tet"ruh·eth"il·uh·mo'nee·um) *n.* The univalent cation $(C_2H_5)_4N^+$, used in the form of the bromide or chloride salt, which on intramuscular or intravenous injection produces reversible blockade of impulses of both sympathetic and parasympathetic divisions of the autonomic nervous system. Used diagnostically in treating peripheral vascular diseases, hypertension, and other disorders in which peripheral circulation is disturbed.

tet·ra·eth·yl lead, tet·ra·eth·yl·lead (tet"ruh·eth'il led'). A poisonous liquid, $Pb(C_2H_5)_4$, used in gasoline as an antiknock agent.

tet·ra·eth·yl·py·ro·phos·phate (tet"ruh·eth"il·pye"ro·fos'fate) *n.* $(C_2H_5)_4P_2O_7$; a synthetic substance having the power to inhibit cholinesterase, for which effect it has been used clinically, especially in treatment of myasthenia gravis, and also as an insecticide. Abbreviated, TEPP.

tet·ra·eth·yl·thi·u·ram disulfide (tet"ruh·eth"il·thigh'oo·ram). DISULFIRAM.

tet·ra·fil·con A (tet"ruh·fil'kon) *n.* A copolymer of 2-hydroxyethyl methacrylate, methyl methacrylate, divinylbenzene and 1-vinyl-2-pyrrolidinone, used as a hydrophilic contact lens material.

tet·ra·gen·ic (tet"ruh·jen'ick) *adj.* [*tetra-* + *-genic*]. Pertaining to genotypes of polysomic or polyploid organisms which contain four different alleles for any given locus.

te·trag·e·nous (teh·traj'e·nus) *adj.* [*tetra-* + *-genous*]. *In bacteriology,* pertaining to organisms that divide in two planes and form groups of four cells.

tet·ra·hy·dric (tet"ruh·high'drick) *adj.* [*tetra-* + *hydr-* + *-ic*]. Containing four replaceable atoms of hydrogen.

tet·ra·hy·dro·can·nab·in·ol (tet"ruh·high"dro·ka·nab'i·nol) *n.* Any one of a group of isomeric substances, $C_{21}H_{30}O_2$, obtained from cannabis, that possess to a great degree the activity of that drug. Abbreviated, THC

tet·ra·hy·dro·fo·lic acid (tet"ruh·high"dro·fo'lick). The reduced derivative, $C_{19}H_{23}N_7O_6$, of folic acid that serves as its active metabolite in various biochemical reactions, functioning as a carrier for groups having a single carbon, such as $-CH_3$, $-CH_2OH$, $-CHO$, and $-CH{=}NH$.

tet·ra·hy·dro·zo·line (tet"ruh·high"dro·zo'leen) *n.* 2-(1,2,3,4-Tetrahydro-1-naphthyl)-2-imidazoline, $C_{13}H_{16}N_2$, a sympathomimetic drug used as the hydrochloride salt to produce vasoconstriction of nasal mucosa for relief of nasal congestion.

tet·ra·io·do·phe·nol·phthal·ein (tet"ruh·eye·o"do·fee"nol·tal'een) *n.* IODOPHTHALEIN.

tet·ra·io·do·thy·ro·nine (tet"ruh·eye·o"do·thigh'ro·neen) *n.* THYROXINE.

te·tral·o·gy (te·tral'uh·jee) *n.* [Gk. *tetralogia,* a group of four discourses, from *tetra-* + *-logos,* word, discourse]. The combination of four related symptoms or defects that are characteristic of a disease or syndrome.

tetralogy of Fal·lot (fa^h·lo') [E.-L. A. *Fallot,* French physician, 1850–1911]. A cyanotic congenital cardiac lesion consisting of pulmonary stenosis, ventricular septal defect, right ventricular hypertrophy, and overriding or dextroposition of the aorta. Syn. *tetrad of Fallot.*

tet·ra·mas·tia (tet"ruh·mas'tee·uh) *n.* [*tetra-* + *-mastia*]. The condition of having four breasts.

tet·ra·mas·ti·gote (tet"ruh·mas'ti·gote) *adj.* [*tetra-* + Gk. *mastix, mastigos,* whip]. Having four flagella.

tet·ra·ma·zia (tet"ruh·may'zee·uh) *n.* [*tetra-* + Gk. *maz-* + *-ia*]. TETRAMASTIA.

te·tram·e·lus (te·tram'e·lus) *n.* [*tetra-* + *-melus*]. TETRASCELUS.

tet·ra·mer (tet'ruh·mur) *n.* [*tetra-* + *-mer*]. The compound resulting from combination of four molecules of the same substance and having four times the molecular weight of the single molecule or monomer.

te·tram·er·ism (te·tram'ur·izm) *n.* [Gk. *tetramerēs,* quadripartite (from *meros,* part) + *-ism*]. *In biology,* division into four parts. —**tetramer·ous** (·us) *adj.*

tet·ra·meth·yl·ene·di·am·ine (tet"ruh·meth"il·een·dye'uh·meen, ·min) *n.* PUTRESCINE.

te·tram·i·sole (te·tram'i·sole) *n.* (±)-2,3,5,6-Tetrahydro-6-phenylimidazo[2,1-*b*]thiazole, $C_{11}H_{12}N_2S$, an anthelmintic; used as the hydrochloride salt.

tet·ra·ni·trol (tet"ruh·nigh'trol) *n.* ERYTHRITYL TETRANITRATE.

tet·ra·nop·sia (tet"ra·nop'see·uh) *n.* [*tetr-* + *anopsia*]. QUADRANTANOPIA.

tet·ra·nu·cle·o·tide (tet"ruh·new'klee·o·tide) *n.* 1. *Obsol.* Nucleic acid, which contains four constituent nucleotides. 2. Any molecule composed of four mononucleotides linked by phosphodiester bonds.

tet·ra·oph·thal·mus (tet"ruh·off·thal'mus) *adj.* [NL., from *tetra-* + *ophthalmos*]. Having four eyes. See also *diprosopus.*

tet·ra·otus (tet"ruh·o'tus) *n.* TETROTUS.

tet·ra·pa·ren·tal (tet"ruh·puh·ren'tul) *adj.* [*tetra-* + *parental*]. Having four parents; characterizing animals (usually mice) in which blastocysts of two different strains are fused in vitro and then implanted in foster-parent uteri. The resultant offspring are chimeras containing cells of each strain.

tet·ra·pa·re·sis (tet"ruh·pa·ree'sis, ·păr'e·sis) *n.* [*tetra-* + *paresis*]. Weakness of all four extremities.

tet·ra·pep·tide (tet"ruh·pep'tide) *n.* A polypeptide composed of four amino acid groups.

tet·ra·pho·co·me·lia (tet"ruh·fo"ko·mee'lee·uh) *n.* Phocomelia affecting all four extremities.

tet·ra·ple·gia (tet"ruh·plee'jee·uh) *n.* [*tetra-* + *-plegia*]. QUADRIPLEGIA.

tet·ra·ploid (tet'ruh·ploid) *adj.* [*tetra-* + *-ploid*]. Having four haploid sets of chromosomes.

tet·ra·pus (tet'ruh·pus) *adj.* [Gk. *tetrapous,* from *pous,* foot]. Having four feet.

tet·ra·sac·cha·ride (tet"ruh·sack'uh·ride) *n.* A polysaccharide hydrolyzable into four molecules of monosaccharide.

te·tras·ce·lus (te·tras'e·lus) *adj.* [Gk. *tetraskelēs,* from *skelos,* leg]. Having four legs.

tet·ra·so·mic (tet"ruh·so'mick) *adj.* & *n.* [*tetra-* + *chromosome* + *-ic*]. Having four chromosomes of a given kind, but only two of each of the other chromosomes of a haploid set; hence, having 2n + 2 chromosomes. 2. A tetrasomic organism. —**tet·ra·so·my** (tet'ruh·so"mee) *n.*

tet·ras·ter (tet·ras'tur) *n.* [*tetr-* + *aster*]. The achromatic figure in an abnormal mitosis when four centrosomes are present, as in dispermic eggs.

tet·ra·sti·chi·a·sis (tet"ruh·sti·kigh'uh·sis) *n.* [Gk. *tetrastichos,* in four rows (from *stichos,* row) + *-iasis*]. Arrangement of the eyelashes in four rows.

tet·ra·thi·o·nate (tet"ruh·thigh'o·nate) *n.* The bivalent ion $S_4O_6^{2-}$.

tetrathionate broth base medium. A selective liquid enrichment medium used to isolate *Salmonella typhosa* and other members of the *Salmonella* group in laboratory diagnosis of enteric infections. Syn. *Kaufmann's tetrathionate broth medium.*

tetrathionate reduction. The reduction of a tetrathionate compound; used in bacteriologic isolations.

tet·ra·tom·ic (tet"ruh·tom'ick) *adj.* [*tetr-* + *atomic*]. 1. Containing four atoms. 2. Having four hydroxyl radicals.

tet·ra·vac·cine (tet"ruh·vack'seen) *n.* [*tetra-* + *vaccine*]. A polyvalent vaccine containing four different cultures, as one containing typhoid, paratyphoid A and B, and cholera.

tet·ra·va·lent (tet″ruh·vay′lunt) *adj.* [*tetra-* + *valent*]. *In chemistry,* having a combining power equivalent to that of four hydrogen atoms. Syn. *quadrivalent.*

tet·ra·zole (tet′ruh·zole) *n.* 1. Either of two isomeric heterocyclic compounds in which three nitrogen atoms and one CH and one NH are joined in a ring. 2. Any derivative of the preceding.

tet·ra·zo·li·um salts (tet″ruh·zo′lee·um). A generic term for certain salt-type derivatives of a tetrazole; some are water-soluble, colorless compounds which are reduced to highly pigmented, water-insoluble compounds in the presence of metabolic activity of living cells, or by certain medicinals with reducing groups.

tet·relle (te·trel′, tet′rel) *n.* [F. *téterelle,* from *téter,* to suck]. A device formerly used to enable a weak infant to obtain milk from its mother. It consists of a nipple shield and two tubes; the mother sucks one tube, and the milk flows to the infant's mouth through the other.

tet·ro·do·tox·in (tet″ro·do·tock′sin) *n.* An aminoperhydroquinazoline, $C_{11}H_{17}N_3O_8$, in puffers (family Tetrodontidae) and certain other fishes; a potent neurotoxin, it blocks conduction in nerves and is sometimes used clinically to relax muscular spasms and as a palliative in terminal cancer.

tet·ro·nal (tet′ro·nal) *n.* Diethylsulfonediethylmethane $(C_2H_5)_2C(SO_2C_2H_5)_2$, formerly used as a hypnotic.

tet·roph·thal·mus (tet″rof·thal′mus) *adj.* TETRAOPHTHALMUS.

tet·ro·qui·none (tet″ro·kwi·nohn′) *n.* Tetrahydroxy-*p*-benzoquinone, $C_6H_4O_6$, a systemic keratolytic drug.

tet·rose (tet′roze) *n.* A monosaccharide whose molecule contains four atoms of carbon, as erythrose, $C_4H_8O_4$.

te·tro·tus (te·tro′tus) *n.* [NL., from *tetr-* + Gk. *ous, ōtos,* ear]. Having four ears. See also *diprosopus.*

te·trox·id (te·trock′sid) *n.* TETROXIDE.

te·trox·ide (te·trock′side) *n.* A binary compound containing four atoms of oxygen.

te·tryd·a·mine (te·trid′uh·meen) *n.* 4,5,6,7-Tetrahydro-2-methyl-3-(methylamino)-2*H*-indazole, $C_9H_{15}N_3$, an analgesic and anti-inflammatory agent.

tet·ter (tet′ur) *n.* Any of various skin eruptions, particularly herpes, eczema, and psoriasis.

Tex·as bedbug. ASSASSIN BUG.

Texas fever. An infectious disease of cattle; due to the parasite *Babesia bigemina,* which is transmitted by several species of ticks, now most commonly by *Boophilus microplus,* and which invades the red corpuscles. Characterized by high fever, hemoglobinuria, and enlargement of the spleen.

tex·is (teck′sis) *n.* [Gk., from *tiktein,* to give birth]. CHILDBIRTH.

tex·ti·form (tecks′ti·form) *adj.* [L. *textum,* fabric, + *-iform*]. Reticular, forming a mesh.

tex·to·blas·tic (tecks″to·blas′tick) *adj.* [L. *textum,* fabric, + *-blastic*]. Forming regenerative tissue.

tex·ture (tecks′chur) *n.* [L. *textura,* web, texture, from *texere,* to weave]. 1. Any organized substance or tissue of which the body is composed. 2. The arrangement of the elementary parts of tissue. —**tex·tur·al** (·chur·ul) *adj.*

tex·tus (tecks′tus) *n.* [L., web]. A tissue.

T fracture. A fracture of the end of a long bone, in the form of the letter T; specifically, the intercondylar fracture of the lower end of the humerus or femur, with splitting of the shaft.

t function. T RATIO.

TGA Abbreviation for *thyroglobulin antibodies.*

t-group, *n.* A sensitivity training group. See also *sensitivity training.*

Th Symbol for thorium.

thalam-, thalamo-. A combining form meaning *thalamus, thalamic.*

thal·a·men·ceph·a·lon (thal″uh·men·sef′uh·lon) *n.* [*thalam-* + *encephalon*] [NA]. THALAMUS.

thalami. Plural of *thalamus.*

tha·lam·ic (tha·lam′ick) *adj.* Pertaining to or involving the thalamus.

thalamic animal. An animal with the central nervous system severed just rostral to the thalamus.

thalamic apoplexy. Infarction of or bleeding into the thalamus.

thalamic fasciculus. A complex bundle of nerve fibers containing pallidothalamic as well as dentatothalamic fibers, which ascend through the prerubral region to enter parts of the rostral ventral tier of thalamic nuclei.

thalamic nuclei. The anterior, lateral, medial, and posterior thalamic nuclei. See also *thalamus.*

thalamic pain. HYPERPATHIA.

thalamic peduncles. The four subradiations of the thalamic radiations; specifically, the anterior or frontal peduncle, which connects the frontal lobe with the medial and anterior thalamic nuclei, the superior or centroparietal peduncle, which connects Rolando's area and adjacent frontal and parietal cortex with the ventral tier nuclei, the posterior or occipital peduncle, which connects occipital cortex with caudal portions of the thalamus, and the inferior or temporal peduncle, which includes the auditory radiations.

thalamic radiations. THALAMOCORTICAL FIBERS.

thalamic syndrome. A symptom complex produced by a lesion, usually vascular, of the posterior portion of the lateral nuclear mass of the thalamus. It includes initially contralateral hemianesthesia and sometimes hemiparesis, followed by hypersensitivity to physical stimuli and severe paroxysmal pain over the contralateral half of the body, often aggravated by emotional stress and fatigue, as well as slight hemiataxia, and occasional hemichorea. Syn. *Déjerine-Roussy syndrome, thalamic apoplexy, thalamic hyperesthetic anesthesia.*

thalamo-. See *thalam-.*

thal·a·mo·cor·ti·cal (thal″a·mo·kor′ti·kul) *adj.* [*thalamo-* + *cortical*]. Pertaining to the thalamus and the cortex of the brain.

thalamocortical fibers. Sensory projection fibers passing from the thalamus to the cerebral cortex.

thalamocortical tract. The nerve tract which consists of thalamocortical fibers. See also *thalamic peduncles.*

thal·a·mo·ge·nic·u·late artery (thal″a·mo·je·nick′yoo·lut). Any one of several small branches of the posterior cerebral artery which supply the posterior portion of the thalamus and the lateral geniculate nucleus.

thal·a·mo·len·tic·u·lar (thal″a·mo·len·tick′yoo·lur) *adj.* [*thalamo-* + *lenticular*]. Pertaining to the thalamus and the lentiform nucleus.

thal·a·mo·ma·mil·lary (thal″a·mo·mam′i·lerr·ee) *adj.* [*thalamo-* + *mamillary*]. Pertaining to the thalamus and the mamillary bodies.

thal·a·mo·pa·ri·e·tal (thal″uh·mo·puh·rye′e·tul) *adj.* [*thalamo-* + *parietal*]. Pertaining to the thalamus and the parietal lobe.

thal·a·mo·per·fo·rate arteries (thal″a·mo·pur′fuh·rut). Branches of the posterior cerebral artery to the lateral and more posterior parts of the thalamus.

thal·a·mo·stri·ate radiation (thal″uh·mo·stry′ate). A system of fibers connecting the corpus striatum with the thalamus and the subthalamic region.

thal·a·mo·teg·men·tal (thal″a·mo·teg·men′tul) *adj.* [*thalamo-* + *tegmental*]. Pertaining to the thalamus and the tegmentum.

thal·a·mot·o·my (thal″a·mot′uh·mee) *n.* [*thalamo-* + *-tomy*]. Surgical destruction of parts of the thalamus for the treatment of intractable pain, movement disorders; and rarely mental disorders.

thal·a·mus (thal'uh·mus) *n.*, pl. & genit. sing. **thala·mi** (·migh) [NL., from Gk. *thalamos,* inner chamber]. Either one of two masses of gray matter situated one on either side of the third ventricle, and each forming part of the lateral wall of that cavity. The thalamus sends projection fibers to the primary sensory areas of the cortex and receives fibers from the cortex, the tegmentum, and the optic tract. The internal medullary lamina divides each thalamic mass into groups of nuclei. The anterior thalamic nuclei lie between the diverging anterior sheets of the lamina. Medial to the lamina are the medial and midline thalamic nuclei. Lateral to the lamina are the lateral thalamic nuclei which are further divided into lateral or dorsal groups and ventral groups. The posterior thalamic nuclei include the pulvinar and medial and lateral geniculate bodies.

tha·lass·ane·mia, tha·lass·anae·mia (thuh·las''uh·nee'mee·uh, thal''uh·suh·) *n.* THALASSEMIA.

thal·as·se·mia, thal·as·sae·mia (thal''uh·see'mee·uh) *n.* [Gk. *thalassa* (Mediterranean) sea, + *-emia* (from the occurrence of the disease among Mediterranean peoples)]. A form of hemolytic anemia resulting from a group of hereditary defects in hemoglobin synthesis characterized in common by impaired synthesis of one of its polypeptide chains, resulting in hypochromic, microcytic erythrocytes. Thalassemia major is the homozygous state, with evident clinical disease from early life. Thalassemia minor, the heterozygous state, may or may not be accompanied by clinical illness. There are several variants of the disease, classified according to the globin chains involved.

tha·las·so·pho·bia (thuh·las''o·fo'bee·uh, thal''uh·so·) *n.* [Gk. *thalassa,* sea, + *-phobia*]. An abnormal fear of the sea.

tha·las·so·ther·a·py (tha·las''o·therr''uh·pee) *n.* [Gk. *thalassa,* sea, + *therapy*]. Treatment of disease by sea voyages, sea bathing, sea air.

tha·lid·o·mide (tha·lid'o·mide) *n.* *N*-(2,6-Dioxo-3-piperidyl)-phthalimide, $C_{13}H_{10}N_2O_4$, a sedative and hypnotic; its use has been discontinued because it may produce teratogenic effects when administered during pregnancy.

thalidomide embryopathy. A specific malformation syndrome related to maternal ingestion of thalidomide during the early development of the fetus. It consists of multiple congenital anomalies including one or more of the following: limb-reduction defects ranging from one or more missing digits to absence of all extremities, cardiac defects, deafness, gastrointestinal malformations and hemangiomas.

thal·lei·o·quin (tha·lye'o·kwin) *n.* The green substance produced when quinine (or its salts) is treated with a solution of chlorine or bromine followed by ammonia (the thalleioquin reaction).

thal·le·o·quin (thal''ee·o'kwin) *n.* THALLEIOQUIN.

thal·li·um (thal'ee·um) *n.* [NL., from L. *thallus,* green twig, shoot, from Gk. *thallos* (from the metal's green spectrum line)]. Tl = 204.37 A bluish-white metallic element, atomic number 81, density 11.85. Salts of thallium are highly toxic.

Thal·loph·y·ta (tha·lof'i·tuh) *n.pl.* [NL., from *thallus* + Gk. *phyton,* plant]. The phylum of plants having a thallus and no true roots, stems, and leaves; it includes the algae and the fungi.

thal·lo·phyte (thal'o·fite) *n.* A plant belonging to the phyllum Thallophyta.

thal·lo·spore (thal'o·spore) *n.* An asexual reproductive spore formed by the thallus or mycelium of lower plants. Types of thallospores include arthrospores, blastospores, and chlamydospores.

thal·lo·tox·i·co·sis (thal''o·tock''si·ko'sis) *n.* [*thallium* + *toxicosis*]. Poisoning by thallium or its derivatives.

thal·lus (thal'us) *n.*, pl. **thal·li** (·eye), **thalluses** [L., twig, young shoot, from Gk. *thallos*]. The simple type of plant structure without root, stem, and leaf, characteristic of members of the phylum Thallophyta.

THAM. Trademark for tromethamine, a systemic antacid used for the treatment of metabolic acidosis.

tha·mu·ria (tha·mew'ree·uh) *n.* [Gk. *thama,* often, + *-uria*]. Frequent urination.

thanat-, thanato- [Gk. *thanatos,* death]. A combining form meaning *death.*

than·a·to·gno·mon·ic (than''uh·to·no·mon'ick, than''uh·tog'') *adj.* [*thanato-* + Gk. *gnōmōn,* sign, index, + *-ic*]. Indicative of death.

than·a·tog·ra·phy (than''uh·tog'ruh·fee) *n.* [*thanato-* + *-graphy*]. 1. A dissertation on death. 2. A description of symptoms and feelings experienced in the course of dying.

than·a·toid (than'uh·toid) *adj.* [*thanat-* + *-oid*]. Resembling death.

than·a·tol·o·gy (than''uh·tol'uh·jee) *n.* [*thanato-* + *-logy*]. The study of the phenomena of somatic death.

than·a·to·ma·nia (than''uh·to·may'nee·uh) *n.* [*thanato-* + *-mania*]. Death by autosuggestion, as in individuals who believe they are under the spell of a sorcerer.

than·a·to·pho·bia (than''uh·to·fo'bee·uh) *n.* [*thanato-* + *-phobia*]. An abnormal fear of death.

than·a·to·phor·ic (than''uh·to·for'ick) *adj.* [Gk. *thanatophoros,* from *thanatos,* death, + *pherein,* to carry, bring]. LETHAL.

thanatophoric dwarfism. A form of severe congenital dwarfism, characterized by extreme micromelia, narrow chest, flattened vertebral bodies, and survival for only a short time before death due to respiratory complications.

than·a·top·sy (than'uh·top·see) *n.* [*thanat-* + *-opsy*]. AUTOPSY.

than·a·tos (than'uh·tos) *n.* [Gk., death]. DEATH INSTINCT.

Thap·sia (thap'see·uh) *n.* [L., a poisonous plant, from Gk. *Thapsos,* a town in Sicily]. A genus of plants of the Umbelliferae. The resin of various species has been used as a counterirritant and vesicant.

thas·sa·ne·mia, thas·sa·nae·mia (thas''uh·nee'mee·uh) *n.* THALASSEMIA.

thau·mat·ro·py (thaw·mat'ruh·pee) *n.* [Gk. *thauma,* wonder, + *-tropy*]. METAPLASIA.

Thay·er-Doi·sy unit (thay'ur, doy'zee) [S. A. *Thayer,* U.S. physician, b. 1902; and E. A. *Doisy,* U.S. biochemist, b. 1893]. MOUSE UNIT.

Thay·er-Mar·tin medium. A complex culture medium containing several antibiotics and used to isolate and grow gonococci. Used to screen patients for asymptomatic gonorrhea.

THC Abbreviation for *tetrahydrocannabinol.*

Thea (thee'uh) *n.* [NL., tea]. A genus of plants, now more properly named *Camellia,* from the species of which tea is obtained.

the·ba·ic (the·bay'ick) *adj.* [Gk. *Thēbaikos,* of Thebes, an opium-producing city in ancient Egypt]. Pertaining to, or derived from, opium.

the·ba·ine (theeb'uh·een, thi·bay'een, ·in) *n.* [NL. *thebaia,* Egyptian opium produced at Thebes, + *-ine*]. An alkaloid, $C_{19}H_{21}NO_3$, found in opium; it causes strychnine-like spasms. Syn. *paramorphine.*

the·be·sian valve (thi·beezh'un) [A. C. *Thebesius,* German physician, 1686–1732]. CORONARY VALVE.

thebesian veins [A. C. *Thebesius*]. VENAE CORDIS MINIMAE.

thec-, theci-, theco-. A combining form meaning *theca, sheath.*

the·ca (thee'kuh) *n.*, pl. & genit. sing. **the·cae** (·kee, ·see) [Gk. *thēkē,* chest, case]. A sheath. —**the·cal** (·kul) *adj.*

theca ex·ter·na (ecks·tur'nuh). The outer fibrous layer of the theca folliculi. NA *tunica externa thecae folliculi.*

theca fol·li·cu·li (fol·ick'yoo·lye) [NA]. The capsule of a growing or mature ovarian (graafian) follicle consisting of the theca interna and the theca externa.

theca in·ter·na (in·tur'nuh). The inner vascular, cellular layer of the theca folliculi. NA *tunica interna thecae folliculi.*

thecal abscess. An abscess in the sheath of a tendon.

thecal cyst. Localized distention of a tendon sheath; GANGLION (2).

theca lutein cells. PARALUTEIN CELLS.

theca lutein cyst. A cyst due to distention of the corpus luteum but with well-developed theca in the wall.

theci-. See *thec-*.

the·ci·tis (the·sigh'tis) *n.* [*thec-* + *-itis*]. Inflammation of the sheath of a tendon.

theco-. See *thec-*.

the·co·dont (theek'o·dont) *adj.* [*thec-* + *-odont*]. Characterizing a tooth which is fixed in a separate socket, or a dentition composed of such teeth.

the·co·ma (the·ko'muh) *n.*, L. pl. **thecoma·ta** (·tuh) [*thec-* + *-oma*]. A benign tumor of the ovary composed of cells derived from the ovarian stroma, in some instances resembling the thecal element of the follicle. Syn. *thelioma.*

the·co·steg·no·sis (theek"o·steg·no'sis) *n.* [*theco-* + Gk. *stegnōsis,* narrowing]. The shrinking or contraction of the sheath of a tendon.

the·e·lin (thee'e·lin, theel'in) *n.* ESTRONE.

the·e·lol (thee'e·lole, ·lol) *n.* ESTRIOL.

Thei·le·ria (thigh·leer'ee·uh) *n.* [A. *Theiler,* Swiss bacteriologist, 1867–1936]. A genus of Protozoa, parasites of cattle, transmitted by a tick.

thei·le·ri·a·sis (thigh"le·rye'uh·sis) *n.* [*Theileria* + *-iasis*]. Infection with *Theileria.* A disease of cattle in South Africa. Syn. *East Coast fever, Rhodesian tick fever.*

Thei·ler's virus [M. *Theiler,* U.S. microbiologist, b. 1899]. A neurotropic virus recovered from the intestines of normal laboratory mice. Syn. *mouse poliomyelitis virus.*

the·ine (thee'een, ·in, tee') *n.* [*Thea* + *-ine*]. CAFFEINE.

the·in·ism (thee'in·iz·um) *n.* A toxic condition produced by the excessive drinking of tea.

Theis and Benedict's method [Ruth *Theis,* U.S. biochemist, 20th century; and S. R. *Benedict*]. A method for testing for phenols in blood in which diazotized *p*-nitroaniline reacts with phenols to produce an orange color which is compared with a standard.

the·ism (thee'iz·um) *n.* THEINISM.

Theis method [R. *Theis*]. BENEDICT AND THEIS'S METHOD.

thel-, theli-, thelo- [Gk. *thēlē*]. A combining form meaning *nipple.*

the·lal·gia (the·lal'jee·uh) *n.* [*thel-* + *-algia*]. Pain in a nipple.

the·lar·che (the·lahr'kee) *n.* [*thel-* + Gk. *archē,* beginning]. The onset of female breast development.

the·las·is (the·las'is) *n.* [Gk. *thelazein,* to suck]. The act of sucking.

the·las·mus (the·laz'mus) *n.* THELASIS.

The·la·zia (the·lay'zee·uh) *n.* A genus of threadlike nematodes with a predilection for the eye of their hosts, which include wild and domestic animals and man.

Thelazia ca·li·for·ni·en·sis (kal"i·for"nee·en'sis). A nematode parasite of dogs and cats and other mammals, including man, which is found on the West Coast of the United States.

Thelazia cal·li·pae·da (kal·i·pee'duh). A nematode parasite of dogs, rabbits, and man; found in India and China; the oriental "eyeworm".

thel·a·zi·a·sis (thel"uh·zye'·uh·sis) *n.* [*Thelazia* + *-iasis*]. An affection of the eye produced by infestation by worms of the genus *Thelazia.*

the·le·plas·ty (theel'e·plas·tee) *n.* [*thel-* + *-plasty*]. Plastic surgery of a nipple.

the·ler·e·thism (the·lerr'e·thiz·um) *n.* [*thel-* + *erethism*]. Erection of a nipple, caused by contraction of its smooth muscle.

theli-. See *thel-*.

the·li·o·ma (theel"ee·o'muh) *n.* THECOMA.

the·li·tis (the·lye'tis) *n.* [*thel-* + *-itis*]. MAMILLITIS.

the·li·um (theel'ee·um) *n.* [NL., from Gk. *thēlē*]. 1. NIPPLE. 2. PAPILLA.

-thelium [from *epithelium*]. A combining form designating *a tissue that covers surfaces or lines cavities.*

thelo-. See *thel-*.

the·lon·cus (the·lonk'us) *n.* [NL., from *thel-* + Gk. *onkos,* tumor]. Tumor of a nipple.

the·lo·phleb·o·stem·ma (theel"o·fleb"o·stem'uh) *n.* [*thelo-* + *phlebo-* + Gk. *stemma,* wreath]. Venous circle around a nipple.

the·lor·rha·gia (theel"o·ray'juh, ·jee·uh) *n.* [*thelo-* + *-rrhagia*]. Hemorrhage from a nipple.

the·lo·thism (theel'o·thiz·um) *n.* [*thel-* + Gk. *ōthismos,* a pushing]. THELERETHISM.

thely·gen·ic (thel"i·jen'ick) *adj.* [Gk. *thēlys,* female, + *-genic*]. Producing only female offspring.

thel·y·go·nia (thel"i·go'nee·uh) *n.* [*thēlys,* female, + *gon-* + *-ia*]. Development of female gametes only, as is usual in parthenogenesis.

thel·y·ot·o·ky (thel"ee·ot'uh·kee) *n.* THELYTOKY.

thely·plas·ty (thel'i·plas"tee) *n.* THELEPLASTY.

thel·y·to·cia (thel"i·to'shuh) *n.* THELYTOKY.

the·lyt·o·ky (thel·it'uh·kee) *n.* [Gk. *thēlytokia,* the bearing of females, from *thēlys,* female, + *tokos,* childbearing, offspring]. Parthenogenetic reproduction of females only. —**thelyto·kous** (·kus) *adj.*

the·mat·ic apperception test (the·mat'ick). A projective psychological test using a set of pictures suggesting life situations from which the subject constructs a story, designed to reveal to the trained interpreter some of the dominant drives, emotions, sentiments, complexes, and conflicts of personality. Abbreviated, TAT

thematic paralogia. A mental state in which thought is unduly concentrated on one subject.

Themisone. Trademark for the anticonvulsant drug atrolactamide.

the·nar (theen'ahr) *n. & adj.* [Gk., palm]. 1. The palm of the hand. 2. Of or pertaining to the palm. 3. [NA] The fleshy prominence of the palm corresponding to the base of the thumb. Contr. *opisthenar.*

thenar area. 1. The region of the thenar eminence. 2. The lateral palmar space.

thenar eminence. THENAR (3).

thenar space. 1. The area occupied by the muscles of the thenar eminence and surrounded by deep fascia. 2. A deep fascial space beneath the flexor tendons of the index and occasionally of the middle finger, overlying the adductor muscle of the thumb, and lateral to a fibrous septum separating the thenar space from the midpalmar space.

Thenfadil. Trademark for thenyldiamine.

then·i·um clo·sy·late (then'ee·um klo'si·late). Dimethyl(2-phenoxyethyl)-2-thenylammonium *p*-chlorobenzenesulfonate, $C_{21}H_{24}ClNO_4S_2$, a veterinary anthelmintic.

then·yl·di·a·mine (then"il·dye'uh·meen, ·min) *n.* 2-[(2-Dimethylaminoethyl)-3-thenylamino]pyridine, $C_{14}H_{19}N_3S$, an antihistaminic drug used as the hydrochloride salt.

then·yl·pyr·a·mine (then"il·pirr'uh·meen, ·min) *n.* METHAPYRILENE.

The·o·bro·ma (thee"o·bro'muh) *n.* [Gk. *theos,* god, + *brōma,* food]. A genus of trees of the Sterculiaceae. The seeds of *Theobroma cacao* yield a fixed oil (cocoa butter) and contain the alkaloid theobromine. The seeds are used in the preparation of chocolate and cocoa.

theobroma oil. A yellowish-white solid consisting chiefly of the glycerides of stearic, palmitic, oleic, and lauric acids, obtained from roasted seeds of *Theobroma cacao.* Melts between 30 and 35°C and is used in the preparation of suppositories, in ointments, and as an emollient. Syn. *cocoa butter, cacao butter.*

the·o·bro·mine (thee"o·bro'meen, ·min) *n.* An alkaloid, 3,7-dimethylxanthine, $C_7H_8N_4O_2$, isomeric with theophylline, occurring in cacao beans and kola nuts; used as a diuretic and myocardial stimulant.

Theocin. A trademark for theophylline.

theo·ma·nia (thee″o·may′nee·uh) *n.* [Gk. *theos*, god, + *mania*]. 1. A religious mania. 2. A mental disorder in which the individual believes himself to be a divine being. —**theoma·ni·ac** (·nee·ack) *n.*

theo·pho·bia (thee″o·fo′bee·uh) *n.* [Gk. *theos*, god, + *-phobia*]. An abnormal fear of the deity or of divine punishment.

theo·phyl·line (thee″o·fil′een, thee·off′il·een, ·in) *n.* An alkaloid, 1,3-dimethylxanthine, $C_7H_8N_4O_2$, obtained from tea leaves and also prepared synthetically. It differs chemically from theobromine only in the position of the methyl groups. Used as a diuretic and vasodilator; also to relax bronchial spasms.

theophylline ethylenediamine. AMINOPHYLLINE.

theophylline meth·yl·glu·ca·mine (meth″il·gloo′kuh·meen, ·min). An equimolecular mixture of theophylline and *N*-methylglucosamine; has the action and uses of theophylline. Syn. *theophylline-meglumine.*

theophylline-me·glu·mine (me·gloo′meen, meg′loo·meen). THEOPHYLLINE METHYLGLUCAMINE.

theophylline mono·eth·a·nol·amine (mon″o·eth″uh·nol′uh·meen, ·min). A compound of theophylline and monoethanolamine that contains about 75% theophylline and has the actions and uses of the latter.

theophylline sodium acetate. An approximately equimolecular mixture of theophylline sodium and sodium acetate, representing about 60% theophylline; has the actions and uses of theophylline.

theophylline sodium glycinate. An equilibrium mixture containing theophylline sodium ($C_7H_7N_4NaO_2$) and glycine in approximately molecular proportions buffered with an additional mole of glycine; it has the actions of theophylline but is less irritating than other soluble derivatives.

theories of hemopoiesis. The dualist, neounitarian, polyphyletic, trialist, and unitarian theories of hemopoiesis. See also *extravascular* and *intravascular theory of erythrocyte formation.*

the·o·ry (thee′uh·ree) *n.* [Gk. *theōria*]. The abstract principles of science. Also, a reasonable supposition or assumption, generally better developed and more probable than a mere hypothesis.

theory of antecedent conflicts. *In psychiatry,* a theory that the effect of an emotionally disturbing event in adult life may be greatly multiplied through the conditioning or sensitization effects of events in early life. See also *rule of impression priority.*

theo·ther·a·py (thee″o·therr′uh·pee) *n.* [Gk. *theos*, god, + *therapy*]. The treatment of disease by prayer and religious exercises.

ther·a·peu·sis (therr″uh·pew′sis) *n.* [Gk., treatment]. THERAPEUTICS.

ther·a·peu·tic (therr″uh·pew′tick) *adj.* [Gk. *therapeutikos*]. 1. CURATIVE. 2. Pertaining to therapy or to therapeutics.

therapeutic abortion. 1. Broadly, any abortion induced in a woman for the sake of her physical or mental health or welfare. 2. More narrowly, any such abortion permitted by law.

therapeutic community. *In psychiatry,* the social organization of patients and personnel within a specially structured mental hospital setting which, through various techniques, promotes the patients' functioning within acceptable social bounds and helps the patients to overcome their dependency needs and to assume responsibility for their own rehabilitation and that of other patients.

therapeutic consultation. *In psychiatry,* intervention by a psychiatrist in the care of a medical or surgical patient by consideration of psychiatric problems, planning of proposals, and assistance in the patient's treatment.

therapeutic electrode. ACTIVE ELECTRODE.

therapeutic index. The ratio of the toxic dose of a substance to its therapeutic dose. It is intended to serve as an estimate of the safety of a drug.

therapeutic psychosis. *In psychoanalysis,* a temporary regression during therapy accompanied by primitive means of dealing with drives which provide the basis for the massive resynthesis of personality.

therapeutic ratio. THERAPEUTIC INDEX.

ther·a·peu·tics (therr″uh·pew′ticks) *n.* [*therapeutic* + *-s*]. The branch of medical science dealing with the treatment of disease. See also *therapy.*

therapeutic test. A test in which the response to specific therapy is used to aid in the establishment of a diagnosis.

ther·a·peu·tist (therr″uh·pew′tist) *n.* One skilled in therapeutics.

the·ra·pia ste·ri·li·sans mag·na (the·ray′pee·uh sterr″i·lye′zanz mag′nuh, therr″uh·pye′uh) [L.]. Ehrlich's aim of treatment by destruction of the parasites in the body of a patient without doing serious harm to the patient; it was to be accomplished by the administration, in one large dose, of a sufficient quantity of a drug having a special affinity for the parasite causing the disease.

ther·a·pist (therr′uh·pist) *n.* [*therapy* + *-ist*]. A practitioner of some kind of therapy.

therapist-vector, *n. In psychoanalysis,* the mature affect expressed by a person in response to the immature needs of another person.

ther·a·py (therr′uh·pee) *n.* [Gk. *therapeia,* service, attendance, treatment, from *theraps,* attendant]. The means employed in effecting the cure or management of disease or of diseased patients.

ther·en·ceph·a·lous (therr″en·sef′uh·lus) *adj.* [Gk. *thēr,* wild beast, + *encephal-* + *-ous*]. Pertaining to a skull in which the lines from the inion and nasion to the hormion make an angle of 116 to 129°.

the·ri·ac (theer′ee·ack) *n. Obsol.* Antidote; THERIACA. —**the·ri·a·cal** (the·rye′uh·kul) *adj.*

the·ri·a·ca (the·rye′uh·kuh) *n.* [L., from Gk. *thēriakē,* (antidote to the venom) of beasts]. A formulation of many substances used as an antidote against poisons; especially, theriaca Andromachi (named after Andromachus, the Greek physician to the emperor Nero), which contained nearly 70 ingredients.

Ther·i·di·idae (therr″i·dye′i·dee) *n.pl.* [NL., from Gk. *thēridion,* small animal]. A family of spiders which includes the genus *Latrodectus* or black widow spider.

the·ri·od·ic (theer″ee·od′ick) *adj.* [Gk. *thēriōdēs,* full of wild beasts, malignant]. MALIGNANT.

the·ri·o·ma (theer″ee·o′muh) *n.,* pl. **theriomas, therioma·ta** (·tuh) [Gk. *thēriōma,* malignant ulcer]. A malignant tumor.

therio·mim·ic·ry (theer″ee·o·mim′ick·ree) *n.* [Gk. *thērion,* animal, + *mimicry*]. Imitation of animals.

therm-, thermo- [Gk. *thermē*]. A combining form meaning *heat* or *temperature.*

-therm [Gk. *thermē,* heat]. A combining form designating (a) *an organism having a* (specified) *kind of temperature adaptation;* (b) *a heat-producing device.*

therm, *n.* [Gk. *thermē,* heat]. A unit of heat to which many equivalents have been given, for example, a small calorie, a kilocalorie, 1,000 kilocalories.

thermaesthesia. THERMESTHESIA.

thermaesthesiometer. THERMESTHESIOMETER.

ther·mal (thur′mul) *adj.* [*therm-* + *-al*]. Pertaining to heat.

thermal capacity. HEAT CAPACITY.

thermal death time. The time required to kill microorganisms when kept at a given temperature.

therm·al·ge·sia (thurm″al·jee′zee·uh) *n.* [*therm-* + *algesia*]. Pain caused by heat. Compare *thermohyperalgesia.*

ther·mal·gia (thur·mal′jee·uh) *n.* [*therm-* + *-algia*]. CAUSALGIA.

thermal neutron. A neutron slowed down, following its release by fissioning, to a state of thermal equilibrium with its surrounding medium. Syn. *slow neutron.*

thermal stimulus. A stimulus acting through change in the temperature or heat content of the environment.

thermal unit. The amount of heat required to raise the temperature of a pound of water one degree Fahrenheit or Centigrade.

thermal waters. Hot or warm waters occurring naturally, as in a hot spring.

therm·an·al·ge·sia (thurm·an″al·jee′zee·uh, ·zhuh) *n.* THERMOANALGESIA.

therm·an·es·the·sia, therm·an·aes·the·sia (thurm·an″es·theezh′uh) *n.* THERMOANESTHESIA.

ther·ma·tol·o·gy (thur″muh·tol′uh·jee) *n.* [*therm-* + *-logy*]. The scientific use or understanding of heat or of the waters of thermal springs in the treatment of disease. **—therma·to·log·ic** (·to·loj′ick) *adj.*

therm·es·the·sia, therm·aes·the·sia (thurm″es·theezh′uh) *n.* [*therm-* + *esthesia*]. 1. Temperature sensibility or ability to feel hot and cold or variations in temperature. 2. Sensitiveness to heat.

therm·es·the·si·om·e·ter, therm·aes·the·si·om·e·ter (thurm″es·theez″ee·om′e·tur) *n.* [*therm-* + *esthesio-* + *-meter*]. An instrument for measuring the sensitivity to heat of different regions of the skin.

therm·hy·per·es·the·sia, therm·hy·per·aes·the·sia (thurm″high″pur·es·theezh′uh) *n.* THERMOHYPERESTHESIA.

therm·hyp·es·the·sia, therm·hyp·aes·the·sia (thurm″high″pes·theezh′uh) *n.* THERMOHYPESTHESIA.

-thermia, -thermy [*therm-* + *-ia, -y*]. A combining form meaning (a) *a condition involving heat or temperature;* (b) *treatment by heat.*

ther·mic (thur′mick) *adj.* [*therm-* + *-ic*]. Pertaining to heat.

thermic anesthesia. THERMOANESTHESIA.

thermic balance. BOLOMETER.

thermic fever. SUNSTROKE.

therm·is·tor (thur′mis·tur, thur·mis′tur) *n.* [*therm*al + resis*tor*]. A type of electrical resistance element made of material whose resistance value varies with temperature, allowing its use in temperature-measuring devices.

thermo-. See *therm-*.

thermoaesthesia. THERMESTHESIA.

thermoaesthesiometer. THERMESTHESIOMETER.

ther·mo·al·ge·sia (thur″mo·al·jee′zee·uh) *n.* THERMALGESIA.

ther·mo·an·al·ge·sia (thur″mo·an″al·jee′zee·uh) *n.* [*thermo-* + *analgesia*]. Insensibility to heat or to contact with heated objects.

ther·mo·an·es·the·sia, ther·mo·an·aes·the·sia (thur″mo·an″es·theezh′uh) *n.* [*thermo-* + *anesthesia*]. Loss of temperature sensation, the ability to recognize the difference between hot and cold, or to feel variations in temperature.

ther·mo·bi·ol·o·gy (thur″mo·bye·ol′uh·jee) *n.* [*thermo-* + *biology*]. The study of the effects of thermal energy or heat on living plants, microorganisms, and animals.

ther·mo·cau·tery (thur″mo·kaw′tur·ee) *n.* [*thermo-* + *cautery*]. A cautery that depends for its action upon heat delivered to the metal end of the instrument, either by direct action of flame, aided by the passage of a current of hot air as in the Paquelin cautery, or by the passage of electric current.

ther·mo·chem·is·try (thur″mo·kem′is·tree) *n.* [*thermo-* + *chemistry*]. The branch of chemical science which treats of the mutual relations of heat and chemical changes.

ther·mo·chro·ism (thur″mo·kro′iz·um) *n.* [*thermo-* + Gk. *chro*ia, color, + *-ism*]. The property of some substances of reflecting or transmitting some thermal radiations while absorbing or changing others.

ther·mo·co·ag·u·la·tion (thur″mo·ko·ag″yoo·lay′shun) *n.* [*thermo-* + *coagulation*]. 1. A method of destroying tissue by means of electrocautery or high-frequency current. 2. A method by which one or several layers of the cerebral cortex in a desired area can be destroyed without alteration of the surrounding tissue.

ther·mo·cou·ple (thur′mo·kup″ul) *n.* [*thermo-* + *couple*]. A device for measuring temperature in which plates or wires of two dissimilar metals form a junction that develops a thermoelectric current when heated and the electromotive force of which varies with the temperature at the junction.

ther·mo·di·lu·tion technique (thur″mo·di·lew′shun). A technique to measure volume flow; a cold or warm indicator is injected and sampled by a thermistor.

ther·mo·du·ric (thur″mo·dew′rick) *adj.* [*thermo-* + L. *durus*, hard, enduring, + *-ic*]. Capable of resisting high temperatures.

ther·mo·dy·nam·ics (thur″mo·dye·nam′icks) *n.* [*thermo-* + *dynamics*]. The science that treats of the relations of heat and other forms of energy.

ther·mo·elec·tric pile (thur″mo·e·leck′trick). A number of bars or plates in which two kinds of metal are conjoined (thermocouples). When the junctions are heated, an electric current is generated by which temperature can be measured.

ther·mo·es·the·sia, ther·mo·aes·the·sia (thur″mo·es·theezh′uh) *n.* THERMESTHESIA.

ther·mo·es·the·si·om·e·ter, ther·mo·aes·the·si·om·e·ter (thur″mo·es·theez″ee·om′e·tur) *n.* THERMESTHESIOMETER.

ther·mo·ex·ci·to·ry (thur″mo·eck·sigh′tuh·ree, ·eck′si·to·ree) *adj.* Exciting the production of heat.

ther·mo·gen·ic (thur″mo·jen′ick) *adj.* [*thermo-* + *-genic*]. Pertaining to the production of heat; producing heat.

thermogenic action. The action of various drugs and foods in raising the body temperature. Compare *specific dynamic action.*

thermogenic anhidrosis. SWEAT-RETENTION SYNDROME.

ther·mo·gen·ics (thur″mo·jen′icks) *n.* The science of the production of heat.

ther·mog·e·nous (thur·moj′e·nus) *adj.* [*thermo-* + *-genous*]. THERMOGENIC.

ther·mo·gram (thur′mo·gram) *n.* [*thermo-* + *-gram*]. A visual display of the surface temperatures of the body recorded from the spontaneous infrared emanations, as obtained by thermography.

ther·mog·ra·phy (thur·mog′ruh·fee) *n.* [*thermo-* + *-graphy*]. A diagnostic technique that records infrared radiations spontaneously emanating from the body's surface to provide a thermogram or mathematical recording of its temperature and local thermal differences.

ther·mo·hy·per·al·ge·sia (thur″mo·high″pur·al·jee′zee·uh) *n.* [*thermo-* + *hyperalgesia*]. Hypersensitivity to even moderate degrees of heat, resulting in pain. Compare *thermalgesia.*

ther·mo·hy·per·es·the·sia, ther·mo·hy·per·aes·the·sia (thur″mo·high″pur·es·theezh′uh) *n.* [*thermo-* + *hyperesthesia*]. Increased sensibility to heat or cold, or to variations in temperature.

ther·mo·hyp·es·the·sia, ther·mo·hyp·aes·the·sia (thur″mo·hip″es·theezh′uh, high″pes·) *n.* [*thermo-* + *hypesthesia*]. Reduced perception of heat or cold, or reduced ability to recognize differences in temperatures.

ther·mo·hy·po·es·the·sia, ther·mo·hy·po·aes·the·sia (thur″mo·high″po·es·theezh′uh) *n.* THERMOHYPESTHESIA.

ther·mo·in·hib·i·to·ry (thur″mo·in·hib′i·to·ree) *adj.* Inhibiting the production of heat.

ther·mo·ker·a·to·plas·ty (thur″mo·kerr′uh·to·plas″tee) *n.* [*thermo-* + *keratoplasty*]. Correction of deformed corneal shape by heat.

ther·mo·la·bile (thur″mo·lay′bil, ·bile) *adj.* [*thermo-* + *labile*]. Sensitive to or destroyed or changed by heat.

ther·mol·y·sin (thur·mol′i·sin) *n.* [*thermo-* + *lysin*]. A heat-stable bacterial protease which hydrolyzes peptide bonds involving nonpolar amino acids, particularly valine, leucine, and isoleucine.

ther·mol·y·sis (thur·mol′i·sis) *n.* [*thermo-* + *-lysis*]. 1. Dissipation of animal heat. 2. Chemical decomposition by means of heat. **—ther·mo·lyt·ic** (thur″mo·lit′ick) *adj.*

ther·mo·mas·sage (thur″mo·muh·sahzh′) *n.* [*thermo-* + *massage*]. Massage with application of heat.

ther·mom·e·ter (thur·mom′e·tur) *n.* [*thermo-* + *-meter*]. A device for measuring temperatures or thermal states, generally consisting of a substance capable of expanding and contracting with variation of temperature, and a graduated scale by means of which the expansion or contraction of the substance can be determined.

ther·mo·met·ric (thur″mo·met′rick) *adj.* Pertaining to a thermometer or to thermometry.

thermometric analysis. Analysis by means of observation of the varying temperatures produced by the interaction of substances when mixed.

ther·mom·e·try (thur·mom′e·tree) *n.* [*thermo-* + *-metry*]. Measurement of temperature with the thermometer.

ther·mo·neu·ro·sis (thur″mo·new·ro′sis) *n.* [*thermo-* + *neurosis*]. In a conversion type of hysterical neurosis, fever of vasomotor origin.

ther·moph·a·gy (thur·mof′uh·jee) *n.* [*thermo-* + *-phagy*]. The habit of eating very hot food.

ther·mo·phile (thur′mo·file, ·fil) *n.* [*thermo-* + *-phile*]. A microorganism for which the optimum temperature for growth is between 50 to 55°C; found in soil and water, especially hot springs.

ther·mo·phil·ic (thur″mo·fil′ick) *adj.* [*thermo-* + *-philic*]. Pertaining to a microorganism that grows best at high temperatures.

ther·mo·pho·bia (thur″mo·fo′bee·uh) *n.* [*thermo-* + *-phobia*]. Abnormal dread of heat.

ther·mo·phore (thur′mo·fore) *n.* [*thermo-* + *-phore*]. Any appliance adapted to hold heat; as used in local treatment, a receptacle for hot water.

ther·mo·phy·lic (thur″mo·figh′lick) *adj.* [*thermo-* + Gk. *phylax,* guard]. THERMOSTABLE.

ther·mo·pile (thur′mo·pile) *n.* [*thermo-* + *pile* (accumulation)]. An instrument for measuring temperatures; it consists of a series of thermocouples combined to amplify the effect of each so as to permit measurement of minute temperature effects.

ther·mo·plas·tic (thur″mo·plas′tick) *adj.* [*thermo-* + *plastic*]. Having the property of softening or melting when heated and becoming rigid again when cooled without appreciable chemical change.

ther·mo·ple·gia (thur″mo·plee′jee·uh, ·juh) *n.* [*thermo-* + *-plegia*] SUNSTROKE.

ther·mo·pol·yp·nea (thur″mo·pol″ip·nee′uh) *n.* [*thermo-* + *polypnea*]. Rapid respiration due to fever or exposure to excessive heat.

ther·mo·re·cep·tor (thur″mo·re·sep′tur) *n.* [*thermo-* + *receptor*]. A sensory receptor that responds to alterations in the heat energy of the environment.

ther·mo·reg·u·la·tion (thur″mo·reg″yoo·lay′shun) *n.* Regulation of temperature by regulation of heat production or heat loss, or both.

ther·mo·reg·u·la·tor (thur″mo·reg′yoo·lay″tur) *n.* THERMOSTAT.

ther·mo·scope (thur′muh·skope) *n.* [*thermo-* + *-scope*]. An instrument for detecting changes or differences in temperature by their effect on the volume of some material, as a gas.

ther·mo·sta·ble (thur″mo·stay′bul) *adj.* [*thermo-* + *stable*]. Exhibiting resistance to change in a defined, usually elevated, temperature range. —**thermo·sta·bil·i·ty** (·stuh·bil′i·tee) *n.*

ther·mo·stat (thur′mo·stat) *n.* [*thermo-* + *-stat*]. A device for automatically regulating and maintaining a constant temperature.

ther·mo·ste·re·sis (thur″mo·ste·ree′sis) *n.* [*thermo-* + Gk. *sterēsis,* deprivation]. The removal or deprivation of heat.

ther·mo·stro·muhr of Rein (thur″mo·stro′moor) [*thermo-* + Ger. *Stromuhr,* rheometer]. A flowmeter that indexes flow by measuring the changes in the temperature of the blood resulting from its passage over a small heated coil.

ther·mo·sys·tal·tic (thur″mo·sis·tahl′tick) *adj.* [*thermo-* + Gk. *systaltikos,* depressing]. Contracting under the influence of heat; pertaining to muscular contraction due to heat. —**thermo·sys·tal·tism** (·sis′tul·tiz·um) *n.*

ther·mo·tax·is (thur″mo·tack′sis) *n.* [*thermo-* + *taxis*]. 1. The regulation and correlation of heat production and heat dissipation. 2. Reaction of protoplasm to the stimulus of heat; refers to movement of the organism as a whole. Compare *thermotropism.* —**thermo·tac·tic** (·tack′tick), **ther·mo·tax·ic** (·tack′sick) *adj.*

ther·mo·ther·a·py (thur″mo·therr′uh·pee) *n.* [*thermo-* + *therapy*]. Treatment of disease by heat of any kind.

ther·mo·to·nom·e·ter (thur″mo·to·nom′e·tur) *n.* [*thermo-* + *tono-* + *-meter*]. An apparatus for determining the amount of muscular contraction induced by heat stimuli.

ther·mo·tox·in (thur″mo·tock′sin) *n.* [*thermo-* + *toxin*]. Any poison produced in living tissue under the influence of excessive heat.

ther·mot·ro·pism (thur·mot′ruh·piz·um) *n.* [*thermo-* + *tropism*]. 1. The property possessed by parts of some cells and organisms of moving or growing toward, or away from, heat. 2. Regulation of body temperature. Compare *thermotaxis.*

-thermy. See *-thermia.*

the·ro·morph (theer′o·morf) *n.* [Gk. *thēr,* animal; monster]. 1. A member of an extinct order of reptiles, the Theromorpha, possible ancestors of the mammals. 2. A monster resembling an animal.

the·ro·mor·phia (theer″o·mor′fee·uh) *n.* [Gk. *thēr,* animal, + *morph-* + *-ia*]. A malformation in a human being which resembles or appears to be a reversion to a normal comparable structure in a lower order animal, for example, the presence of a small tail.

the·ro·mor·phism (theer″o·mor′fiz·um) *n.* THEROMORPHIA.

the·sau·ris·mo·sis (the·saw″riz·mo′sis) *n.* [Gk. *thēsaurismos,* storage, collection, + *-osis*]. Thesaurosis (= STORAGE DISEASE).

thesaurismosis he·re·di·ta·ria lipidosis Ruiten-Pompen-Wyers (he·red″i·tair′ee·uh). ANGIOKERATOMA CORPORIS DIFFUSUM UNIVERSALE.

the·sau·ro·sis (thee″saw·ro′sis, thes″aw·) *n.* [Gk. *thēsauros,* store, + *-osis*]. STORAGE DISEASE.

the·ta (thay′tuh) *n.* Name of the letter Θ, θ, eighth letter of the Greek alphabet.

theta antigen, θ antigen. A cell-surface antigen present on thymus cells and thymus-derived cells in mice; serves as a marker for T lymphocytes.

theta rhythm. *In electroencephalography,* a succession of waves with a frequency of 4 to 7 hertz, best recorded from the temporal region.

theta wave. See *theta rhythm.*

the·tin (theet′in) *n.* Any of a group of sulfur compounds structurally resembling the betaines, having the general formula $R_2S^+CH_2COO^-$, where R is commonly an alkyl group.

the·tine (theet′een) *n.* THETIN.

the·ve·tin B (the·veet′in, thev′e·tin) *n.* [A. *Thevet,* French author and traveler, 1502–1590]. A poisonous glycoside, $C_{42}H_{66}O_{18}$, with digitalis-like action, from the seed of *Thevetia neriifolia.*

thi-, thio- [Gk. *theion,* sulfur, brimstone]. A combining form meaning *sulfur.*

thi·a·ben·da·zole (thigh″uh·ben′duh·zole) *n.* 2-(4-Thiazolyl)-benzimidazole, $C_{10}H_7N_3S$, a veterinary anthelmintic that has been beneficial in humans in the treatment of creeping eruption due to larval forms of *Ancylostoma braziliense* and *A. caninum.*

thi·acet·a·zone (thigh″uh·set′uh·zone, ·uh·see′tuh·) *n.* British generic name for amithiozone.

thi·a·min (thigh′uh·min) *n.* THIAMINE.

thi·ami·nase (thigh·am′i·nace, ·naze) *n.* An enzyme, present in raw fish and in certain bacteria, which catalyzes cleavage of thiamine into pyramin (a pyrimidine derivative) and a thiazole derivative.

thi·a·mine (thigh'uh·meen, ·min) *n.* 3-(4-Amino-2-methylpyrimidyl-5-methyl)-4-methyl-5-(β-hydroxyethyl)thiazolium chloride, $C_{12}H_{17}ClN_4OS$, a member of the vitamin B complex that occurs in many natural sources, frequently in the form of the pyrophosphate ester known as cocarboxylase. The commercial product is obtained by synthesis. A deficiency of this vitamin is evidenced chiefly in the nervous system, the circulation, and the alimentary tract. Among the symptoms are irritability, emotional disturbances, multiple neuritis, increased pulse rate, dyspnea, edema, loss of appetite, reduced intestinal motility. Syn. *vitamin* B_1.

thiamine hydrochloride. The salt, $C_{12}H_{17}ClN_4OS.HCl$, produced by neutralization of thiamine with hydrochloric acid; acid in reaction. The form in which thiamine is generally employed.

thiamine mono·ni·trate (mon"o·nigh'trate). 3-(4-Amino-2-methylpyrimidyl-5-methyl)-4-methyl-5-(β-hydroxyethyl)thiazolium nitrate, $C_{12}H_{17}N_5O_4S$, representing thiamine in which the chloride has been replaced by nitrate; neutral in reaction, and in certain formulations more stable than thiamine hydrochloride.

thiamine pyrophosphate. COCARBOXYLASE.

thi·am·i·prine (thigh·am'i·preen) *n.* 2-Amino-6-[(1-methyl-4-nitroimidazol-5-yl)thio]purine, $C_9H_8N_8O_2S$, an antineoplastic agent.

thi·am·phen·i·col (thigh"am·fen'i·kol) *n.* D-(+)-*Threo*-2,2-dichloro-*N*-[β-hydroxy-α-(hydroxymethyl)-*p*-(methylsulfonyl)phenethyl]acetamide, $C_{12}H_{15}Cl_2NO_5S$, an analog of chloramphenicol; an antibacterial agent. Compare *racephenicol.*

thi·am·y·lal sodium (thigh·am'i·lal). Sodium 5-allyl-5-(1-methylbutyl)-2-thiobarbiturate, $C_{12}H_{17}N_2NaO_2S$, an ultrashort-acting barbiturate used intravenously as an anesthetic.

thi·az·e·sim (thigh·az'e·sim) *n.* 5-[2-Dimethylamino)ethyl]-2,3-dihydro-2-phenyl-1,5-benzothiazepin-4(5*H*)-one, $C_{19}H_{22}N_2OS$, an antidepressant drug; used as the hydrochloride salt.

thi·a·zide (thigh'uh·zide) *n.* A diuretic whose main function is to block sodium reabsorption in the first portion of the renal distal tubules, bringing about antihypertensive action.

thi·a·zine (thigh'uh·zeen, ·zin) *n.* Any of a group of heterocyclic compounds containing four carbon atoms, one nitrogen atom, and one sulfur atom in a ring.

thiazine red R. An acid monoazo dye used especially as a counterstain after hematoxylin.

thi·a·zole (thigh'uh·zole) *n.* 1. Either of two isomeric heterocyclic compounds, C_3H_3NS, in which a sulfur atom, a nitrogen atom, and three CH groups are joined in a ring. 2. Any derivative of the preceding.

thick filament. One of two types of interacting protein filaments found in muscle. The thick filaments (diameter approximately 150Å) contain primarily myosin which provides the ATP necessary for muscular contraction. Contr. *thin filament.*

thick-film method. A method for facilitating the search for malarial and other parasites in the blood, by using a large drop of blood, drying and staining with 2% Giemsa stain without prior fixation. Red blood cells are hemolyzed; parasites, white cells, and platelets are retained.

thick-leg disease. OSTEOPETROTIC LYMPHOMATOSIS.

thick-split graft. A split graft in which the grafted skin is relatively thick.

thick·wind, *n.* HEAVES.

Thie·mann-Fleisch·ner disease (tee'mahn, flye'sh'nur). THIEMANN'S DISEASE.

Thiemann's disease. Avascular necrosis of the phalanges of the hand.

Thiersch graft (teersh) [K. *Thiersch,* German surgeon, 1822-1895]. Extensive thin sheets or broad strips of skin, consisting largely of epidermis, sliced with a very sharp knife from healthy surfaces of the body, and transferred to cover large fresh or granulating wounds.

thi·eth·yl·per·a·zine (thigh·eth"il·perr'uh·zeen) *n.* 2-(Ethylthio)-10-[3-(4-methyl-1-piperazinyl)propyl]phenothiazine, $C_{22}H_{29}N_3S_2$, an antiemetic useful in reducing incidence of nausea and vomiting associated with administration of general anesthetics and with vertigo; used as the dimaleate salt.

thigh, *n.* [Gmc. (rel. to L. *tu*ber and *tu*mor)]. The part of the lower extremity from the pelvis to the knee.

thigh amputation. An amputation through the femur below the hip joint.

thigh·bone, *n.* The long bone of the thigh; FEMUR.

thigm-, thigmo- [Gk. *thigma,* touch]. A combining form meaning *touch.*

thig·man·es·the·sia, thig·man·aes·the·sia (thig·man"es·theezh'uh) *n.* [*thigm-* + *anesthesia*]. Loss of tactile sensibility.

thig·mes·the·sia, thig·maes·the·sia (thig"mes·theezh'uh) *n.* [*thigm-* + *esthesia*]. Tactile sensibility.

thigmo-. See *thigm-.*

thig·mo·tax·is (thig"mo·tack'sis) *n.* [*thigmo-* + *taxis*]. STEREOTAXIS.

thig·mot·ro·pism (thig·mot'ruh·piz·um) *n.* [*thigmo-* + *-tropism*]. STEREOTROPISM.

thimble electrode. A device for very rapid localization of motor points, in the form of a long, thin flexible thimble to fit the palpating index finger.

Thimecil. Trademark for methylthiouracil, an antithyroid drug.

thi·mero·sal (thigh·merr'o·sal, ·mur'o·) *n.* Sodium ethylmercurithiosalicylate, $C_6H_4(COONa)SHgC_2H_5$, an organomercurial antiseptic used topically and also as a preservative of certain biological products.

thin filament. One of two types of interacting protein filaments found in muscle. The thin filaments (diameter approximately 70Å) contain the proteins actin, tropomyosin, and troponin which regulate the making and breaking of cross bridges between the two filaments as well as the amount of mechanical force generated by the filaments. Contr. *thick filament.*

thin-film method. The preparation of thin films of blood to facilitate the microscopic observation of all the formed elements and parasites, usually involving subsequent staining, as with the Wright and Giemsa stain.

think·ing, *n. In psychology and psychiatry,* the process of logic and reasoning assumed to exist inside the individual and accessible through a study of the verbalized associations and actions.

thinking-type personality. An individual in whom actions and attitudes are ruled predominantly by deliberation and reflective thought rather than by feeling, intuition, or sensation; the first of the four functional types of personality according to Jung.

thin-layer chromatography. Chromatography in which the porous solid is a thin, uniform layer of material applied over a glass plate, and separation is achieved by adsorption, partition, or a combination of both processes.

thio-. See *thi-.*

thio·ac·e·tal (thigh"o·as'e·tal) *n.* MERCAPTAL.

thio acid (thigh'o). An organic acid in which sulfur replaces oxygen.

thio alcohol. An alcohol in which sulfur replaces oxygen; a mercaptan.

thio·al·de·hyde (thigh"o·al'de·hide) *n.* An aldehyde in which the oxygen of the —CHO radical is replaced by sulfur.

thio·bac·te·ria (thigh"o·back·teer'ee·uh) *n.pl.* [*thio-* + *bacteria*]. Bacteria that grow where decaying organic material releases hydrogen sulfide. Found in stagnant water and at the bottom of the sea. They are not pathogenic to man or animals.

thio·bar·bit·u·rate (thigh″o·bahr·bitch′yoo·rate) *n.* A derivative of thiobarbituric acid, differing from the barbiturates only in the replacement of one oxygen atom by sulfur; they are analogous in their effects.

thio·bar·bi·tu·ric acid (thigh″o·bahr″bi·tew′rick). Malonyl thiourea, $C_6H_4N_2O_2S$, the parent compound of the thiobarbiturates. It represents barbituric acid in which the oxygen atom of the urea component has been replaced by sulfur.

thio·car·bam·ide (thigh″o·kahr·bam′ide, ·kahr′buh·mide) *n.* THIOUREA.

thio·car·ban·i·lide (thigh″o·kahr·ban′i·lide) *n.* Any of a class of compounds of the general formula RC_6H_4-$NHCSNHC_6H_4R'$, where R and R′ are various substituent groups. Several such compounds have antituberculous activity.

thio·chrome (thigh′o·krome) *n.* A fluorescent oxidation product, $C_{12}H_{14}N_4OS$, of thiamine or other derivatives of the vitamin.

Thiocol. A trademark for potassium guaiacolsulfonate.

thi·oc·tic acid (thigh·ock′tick). Any of several cyclized dithio-*n*-octanoic acids, particularly 6,8-thioctic acid which is 1,2-dithiolane-3-valeric acid, all of which function in the oxidative decarboxylation of pyruvic acid by certain bacteria. See also *protogen, lipoic acid.*

thio·cy·a·nate (thigh″o·sigh′uh·nate) *n.* Any compound containing the monovalent radical —SCN. The sodium and potassium salts have been used in the control of hypertension, but are no longer employed because of their toxicity.

thio·cy·an·ic acid (thigh″o·sigh·an′ick). An unstable liquid acid, HCNS, several salts of which are used as chemical reagents. Syn. *sulfocyanic acid.*

thio·es·ter (thigh″o·es′tur) *n.* [*thio-* + *ester*]. A compound formed by reaction of a carboxyl group of one molecule with a sulfhydryl group of another; for example, acetyl coenzyme A.

thio ether. An ether containing sulfur instead of oxygen.

thio·gua·nine (thigh″o·gwah′neen) *n.* 2-Aminopurine-6-thiol, $C_5H_5N_5S$, an antineoplastic agent.

thi·ol (thigh′ol) *n.* 1. The univalent radical —SH, when occurring in organic compounds. 2. Any organic compound containing the —SH radical.

thi·ol·prive (thigh′ol·prive) *n.* [*thiol* + L. *privare,* to deprive]. A substance reacting or interfering with the thiol activity of biologically functional molecules.

Thiomerin. Trademark for the organomercurial diuretic mercaptomerin sodium.

thion-, thiono- [Gk. *theion,* sulfur]. A combining form meaning *sulfur.*

thio·ne·ine (thigh″o·nee′een, ·in) *n.* 1. $C_9H_{15}N_3O_2S$. An amino-acid derivative, the betaine of thiolhistidine, which was first isolated from ergot and later shown to be a normal constituent of blood and especially of blood cells. Syn. *ergothionein.* 2. A water-soluble basic thiazine dye, used for staining nuclei, mast cells, and cartilage.

thi·on·ic (thigh·on′ick) *adj.* [*thion-* + *-ic*]. Pertaining to sulfur.

thi·o·nine (thigh′o·neen, ·nin) *n.* 3,7-Diaminophenothiazonium chloride, $C_{12}H_{10}ClN_3S$, a dark-green powder forming purple solutions; used for staining nuclei, bacteria, cartilage, mucins, and mast cells. Syn. *Lauth's violet.*

thiono-. See *thion-.*

thio·pen·tal sodium (thigh″o·pen′tal, ·tol). Sodium 5-ethyl-5-(1-methylbutyl)-2-thiobarbiturate, $C_{11}H_{17}N_2NaO_2S$, an ultrashort-acting barbiturate used intravenously or by rectal instillation as an anesthetic.

thio·pen·tone sodium (thigh″o·pen′tone). *British Pharmacopoeia.* THIOPENTAL SODIUM.

thi·o·phene (thigh′o·feen) *n.* Thiofuran, C_4H_4S, a heterocyclic constituent of coal tar; used as a solvent and in the manufacture of medicinal agents.

thio·phile (thigh′o·file, ·fil) *n.* & *adj.* [*thio-* + *-phile*]. 1. A microorganism that requires sulfur compounds for metabolism. 2. THIOPHILIC.

thio·phil·ic (thigh″o·fil′ick) *adj.* [*thio-* + *-philic*]. 1. Pertaining to, or characteristic of, a thiophile. 2. Thriving in sulfur.

thio·pro·pa·zate (thigh″o·pro′puh·zate) *n.* 2-Chloro-10-{3-[4-(2-acetoxyethyl)piperazinyl]propyl}phenothiazine, $C_{23}H_{28}ClN_3O_2S$, a tranquilizer employed chiefly in the management of psychoses marked by agitation and aggression; used as the dihydrochloride salt.

Thio·rho·da·ce·ae (thigh″o·ro·day′see·ee) *n.pl.* A family of photosynthetic, anaerobic purple sulfur bacteria.

thio·rid·a·zine (thigh″o·rid′uh·zeen) *n.* 10-[2-(1-Methyl-2-piperidyl)ethyl]-2-(methylthio)phenothiazine, $C_{21}H_{26}N_2S_2$, a tranquilizer used to treat various psychotic conditions; employed as the hydrochloride salt.

thio·sa·lan (thigh′o·suh·lan″) *n.* 3,4′,5-Tribromo-2-mercaptobenzanilide, $C_{13}H_8Br_3NOS$, a germicide.

thio·semi·car·ba·zone (thigh″o·sem″ee·kahr′buh·zone) *n.* A condensation product of an aldehyde or ketone with thiosemicarbazide, $NH_2NHCSNH_2$. Certain thiosemicarbazones, such as amithiozone, have chemotherapeutic activity against tuberculosis.

thio·sin·am·ine (thigh″o·sin·am′een, ·sin′uh·meen) *n.* Allyl thiourea, $CH_2{=}CHCH_2NHCSNH_2$; has been used to promote absorption of cicatrices.

thio·sul·fate (thigh″o·sul′fate) *n.* Any salt or ester of thiosulfuric acid.

Thiosulfil. Trademark for sulfamethizole, a sulfonamide used for treatment of infections of the urinary tract.

thio·sul·fur·ic acid (thigh″o·sul·few′rick). An unstable acid, $H_2S_2O_3$, readily decomposing to sulfurous acid and sulfur.

thio·tepa (thigh″o·tep′uh) *n.* Tris(1-aziridinyl)phosphine sulfide, $C_6H_{12}N_3PS$, an alkylating agent employed for palliation of certain malignant tumors.

thio·thix·ene (thigh″o·thick′seen) *n.* *N,N*-Dimethyl-9-[3-(4-methyl-1-piperazinyl)propylidene]thioxanthene-2-sulfonamide, $C_{23}H_{29}N_3O_2S_2$, a tranquilizer.

thio·ura·cil (thigh″o·yoor′uh·sil) *n.* 2-Mercapto-4-hydroxypyrimidine, $C_4H_4N_2OS$, an antithyroid drug that interferes with synthesis of thyroxine but has adverse effects in many patients; certain of its derivatives are better tolerated.

thio·urea (thigh″o·yoo·ree′uh) *n.* Thiocarbamide, H_2NCSNH_2; has been used as an antithyroid drug in the treatment of hyperthyroidism.

thi·phen·a·mil (thigh·fen′uh·mil) *n.* 2-(Diethylamino)ethyl diphenylthioacetate, $C_{20}H_{25}NOS$, an anticholinergic drug; used as the hydrochloride salt.

thi·ram (thigh′ram) *n.* Bis(dimethylthiocarbamoyl) disulfide, $C_6H_{12}N_2S_4$, an antifungal agent.

third and fourth (III-IV) branchial pouch syndrome. THYMIC APLASIA.

third (IIId) cranial nerve. OCULOMOTOR NERVE.

third-degree burn. A burn that is more severe than a second-degree burn and that destroys the skin and its deeper underlying tissues.

third-degree heart block. A complete atrioventricular block.

third heart sound. The heart sound occurring at the end of rapid ventricular filling, related to the sudden deceleration of blood flow. Symbol, S_3 or SIII. Syn. *ventricular filling sound.* See also *ventricular gallop.*

third space. Any of the regions of the body, such as peritoneal cavity, mesentery, and gastrointestinal tract, viewed as a physiological unit, where excessive amounts of exudates may accumulate and be sequestered, especially in acute peritonitis. Syn. *surgical third space.*

third trochanter. An enlargement of the upper end of the gluteal tuberosity. NA *trochanter tertius.*

third ventricle. The cavity of the diencephalon, a narrow cleft between the two thalami. NA *ventriculus tertius.* See also Plate 18.

third ventriculostomy. INTERNAL VENTRICULOSTOMY.

thirst, *n.* A sensation associated with the need of the body for water. The sensory nerve endings for thirst are principally in the mucous membrane of the pharynx, and less than normal content of water in this region supposedly produces thirst. Prolonged deprivation with dehydration of tissues produces severe unpleasant sensations probably of wide origin.

Thi·ry's fistula (tee'ree) [L. *Thiry,* Austrian physiologist, 1817–1897]. An experimental fistula produced in the dog to obtain secretions from the intestine.

Thixokon. Trademark for a solution of sodium acetrizoate that is used as a radiographic contrast medium.

thix·ot·ro·py (thick·sot'ruh·pee) *n.* [Gk. *thix*is, a touching, + *-tropy*]. The property of some gels, when mechanically agitated, to undergo a reversible isothermal solution and reconversion to a gel when allowed to stand. The tobacco mosaic virus has this property of thixotropy. —**thixo·trop·ic** (thick"so·trop'ick) *adj.*

thlip·sen·ceph·a·lus (thlip"sen·sef'uh·lus) *n.* [Gk. *thlipsis*, a crushing, + *-encephalus*]. A type of anencephalus in which the cranial vault is lacking; there is some degree of cervical spina bifida, and the brain is merely a spongy, vascular mass.

Tho·ma's ampulla (to'mah) [R. *Thoma,* German histologist, 1847–1923]. A dilatation which may occur at the termination of the penicillar arteries of the spleen.

Thomas-Lavollay method. A histochemical method for detecting iron, using hydroxyquinoline and ammonium hydroxide. Iron appears as a greenish-black precipitate.

Thomas method. A histochemical method for determining the presence of arginine and arginine-containing proteins, based on development of an orange-red color when arginine reacts with alphanaphthol and hypobromite or hypochlorite in alkaline medium.

Thom·as' sign [H. O. *Thomas,* English orthopedist, 1834–1891]. A test for flexion fixation of the hip joint in which the examiner flexes the sound hip until the lumbar lordosis is reduced, and then the amount of flexion observed in the affected limb can be estimated.

Thomas skin reaction test. SCRATCH-PATCH TEST.

Thomas's pessary [T. G. *Thomas,* U.S. gynecologist, 1831–1903]. A narrow pessary for use in nulliparous women.

Thomas splint [H. O. *Thomas*]. An appliance designed originally to provide support in the treatment of diseases of the hip or knee, now used chiefly to maintain traction or for emergency transportation in fractures of the femur or humerus. It is made in various sizes and forms, and consists essentially of a padded metal ring which fits around the thigh or upper arm, and long metal rods extending from the ring down each side of the extremity.

Thoma-Zeiss cell [R. *Thoma* and C. *Zeiss*]. THOMA-ZEISS COUNTING CHAMBER.

Thoma-Zeiss counting chamber [R. *Thoma,* German histologist, 1847–1923; and C. *Zeiss,* German optician, 1816–1888]. An early form of hemocytometer. Syn. *Abbe-Zeiss cell, Thoma-Zeiss cell.*

Thom·sen's disease [A. J. T. *Thomsen,* Danish physician, 1815–1896]. MYOTONIA CONGENITA.

Thom·so·ni·an·ism (tom·so'nee·un·iz·um) *n.* [S. *Thomson,* U.S. farmer and healer, 1769–1843]. An empirical system of medicine which insisted on the use of vegetable remedies only.

thon·zyl·a·mine (thon·zil'uh·meen) *n.* 2-[(2-Dimethylaminoethyl)(*p*-methoxybenzyl)amino]pyrimidine, $C_{16}H_{22}N_4O$, an antihistaminic drug used as the hydrochloride salt.

thorac-, thoraci-, thoracico-, thoraco- [Gk. *thōrax, thōrakis,* chest]. A combining form meaning *thorax, thoracic.*

tho·ra·cec·to·my (tho"ruh·seck'tuh·mee) *n.* [*thorac-* + *-ectomy*]. Resection of a rib.

tho·ra·cen·te·sis (tho"ruh·sen·tee'sis) *n.,* pl. **thoracente·ses** (·seez) [*thorac-* + *centesis*]. Aspiration of the chest cavity for the removal of fluid, usually for hydrothorax or empyema.

thoraces. A plural of *thorax.*

thoraci-. See *thorac-.*

tho·rac·ic (tho·ras'ick) *adj.* [*thorac-* + *-ic*]. Pertaining to the thorax.

thoracic aorta. The portion of the descending aorta within the thorax. NA *aorta thoracica.* See also Table of Arteries in the Appendix and Plate 5.

thoracic artery. See Table of Arteries in the Appendix.

thoracic axis. The thoracoacromial artery or vein.

thoracic cage. RIB CAGE.

thoracic cavity. The space within the walls of the thorax, between the base of the neck and the diaphragm, containing the thoracic viscera. NA *cavum thoracis.*

thoracic duct. The common lymph trunk beginning in the cisterna chyli, passing upward, and emptying into the left subclavian vein at its junction with the left internal jugular vein. NA *ductus thoracicus.*

thoracic ganglia. The ganglia of the thoracic sympathetic trunk. NA *ganglia thoracica.*

thoracic index. The ratio of the anteroposterior diameter to the transverse, expressed in percentage.

thoracic inlet. The superior opening of the thoracic cavity, bounded by the first thoracic vertebra, the first ribs, and the manubrium of the sternum. NA *apertura thoracis superior.*

thoracic-inlet tumors. Infiltrating tumors at the thoracic inlet which may produce the symptom complex commonly known as Pancoast syndrome.

thoracic kyphosis. A posterior angular deformity of the spine in the thoracic area.

thoracic limb. An upper extremity.

thoracic nerve. See Table of Nerves in the Appendix.

thoracic nucleus. A prominent round or oval cell column in the medial part of the base of the dorsal gray horn of the spinal cord; contains cells of origin of the uncrossed dorsal spinocerebellar tract. Syn. *dorsal nucleus of Clarke.* NA *nucleus thoracicus.*

thoracico-. See *thorac-.*

tho·rac·i·co·lum·bar (tho·ras'i·ko·lum'bur) *adj.* [*thoracico-* + *lumbar*]. THORACOLUMBAR.

thoracicolumbar autonomic nervous system. SYMPATHETIC NERVOUS SYSTEM (1).

thoracic outlet. 1. The inferior boundary of the thoracic cavity. NA *apertura thoracis inferior.* 2. THORACIC INLET.

thoracic outlet syndrome. SCALENUS ANTERIOR SYNDROME.

thoracic respiration. Respiration caused by contraction of the intercostal and other thoracic muscles. Contr. *abdominal respiration.*

thoracic stomach. Congenital herniation of the stomach above the diaphragm due to imperfect development of the diaphragm.

thoracic surgery. Surgery limited to the thorax, particularly to the rib cage and structures within the thoracic cavity.

thoracic vertebrae. The twelve vertebrae associated with the chest and ribs.

thoraco-. See *thorac-.*

tho·ra·co·ab·dom·i·nal (tho"ruh·ko·ab·dom'i·nul) *adj.* [*thoraco-* + *abdominal*]. Pertaining to the thorax and the abdomen.

tho·ra·co·aceph·a·lus (tho"ruh·ko·a·sef'uh·lus) *n.* [*thoraco-* + *acephalus*]. Thoracopagus parasiticus in which the parasite has no head.

tho·ra·co·acro·mi·al (tho"ruh·ko·a·kro'mee·ul) *adj.* [*thoraco-* + *acromial*]. Pertaining to the acromion and the chest, as the thoracoacromial artery.

thor·a·co·bi·lia (tho"ruh·ko·bye'lee·uh, ·bil'ee·uh) *n.* [*thoraco-* + *bile* + *-ia*]. A syndrome characterized by bile expectoration, fever, and a large, tender liver; it results from a bronchobiliary fistula.

tho·ra·co·ce·li·ot·o·my, tho·ra·co·coe·li·ot·o·my (tho"ruh·ko·see"lee·ot'uh·mee) *n.* [*thoraco-* + *celio-* + *-tomy*]. Surgical opening of the thoracic and abdominal cavities.

tho·ra·co·ce·los·chi·sis, tho·ra·co·coe·los·chi·sis (tho″ruh·ko·se·los′ki·sis) *n.* [*thoraco-* + *celo-* + *schisis*]. THORACOGASTROSCHISIS.

tho·ra·co·cen·te·sis (tho″ruh·ko·sen·tee′sis) *n.* THORACENTESIS.

tho·ra·co·cyl·lo·sis (tho″ruh·ko·sil·o′sis) *n.* [*thoraco-* + Gk. *kyllōsis,* a crippling]. Deformity of the thorax.

tho·ra·co·cyr·to·sis (tho″ruh·ko·sur·to′sis) *n.* [*thoraco-* + *cyrtosis*]. Excessive curvature of the thorax.

tho·ra·co·del·phus (tho″ruh·ko·del′fus) *n.* THORADELPHUS.

tho·ra·co·did·y·mus (tho″ruh·ko·did′i·mus) *n.* [*thoraco-* + *-didymus*]. THORACOPAGUS.

tho·ra·co·dor·sal (tho″ruh·ko·dor′sul) *adj.* [*thoraco-* + *dorsal*]. Pertaining to the thorax and the back, as: thoracodorsal artery.

tho·ra·co·dyn·ia (tho″ruh·ko·din′ee·uh) *n.* [*thorac-* + *-odynia*]. Pain in the chest.

tho·ra·co·gas·tro·did·y·mus (tho″ruh·ko·gas″tro·did′i·mus) *n.* [*thoraco-* + *gastro-* + *-didymus*]. A twin monstrosity united by the thorax and abdomen.

tho·ra·co·gas·tros·chi·sis (thor″uh·ko·gas·tros′ki·sis) *n.* [*thoraco-* + *gastro-* + *-schisis*]. Congenital fissure of the thorax and abdomen. Syn. *thoracoceloschisis.*

tho·ra·co·lap·a·rot·o·my (tho″ruh·ko·lap″uh·rot′uh·mee) *n.* [*thoraco-* + *laparotomy*]. An operation in which both the thorax and the abdomen are opened.

tho·ra·co·lum·bar (tho″ruh·ko·lum′bur) *adj.* [*thoraco-* + *lumbar*]. Pertaining to the thoracic and lumbar portions of the spine, or to thoracic and lumbar ganglions and fibers of the autonomic nervous system.

thoracolumbar autonomic nervous system. SYMPATHETIC NERVOUS SYSTEM (1).

thoracolumbar fascia. Variously described as the sheath of the erector spinae muscle alone, or the sheaths of the erector spinae and the quadratus lumborum muscles. NA *fascia thoracolumbalis.*

thoracolumbar system. SYMPATHETIC NERVOUS SYSTEM (1).

tho·ra·col·y·sis (tho″ruh·kol′i·sis) *n.* [*thoraco-* + *-lysis*]. PNEUMONOLYSIS.

tho·ra·com·e·lus (tho″ruh·kom′e·lus) *n.* [*thoraco-* + *-melus*]. A parasitic limb attached to the thorax of the host.

tho·ra·com·e·try (tho″ruh·kom′e·tree) *n.* [*thoraco-* + *-metry*]. Measurement of the chest.

tho·ra·cop·a·gus (tho″ruh·kop′uh·gus) *n.,* pl. **thoracopa·gi** (·jye, ·guy) [*thoraco-* + *-pagus*]. Conjoined twins united by their thoraxes or epigastric regions. —**thoracopagous,** *adj.*

thoracopagus par·a·sit·i·cus (păr″uh·sit′i·kus). A more or less complete parasitic twin united with the thorax or epigastrium of the host.

thoracopagus tri·bra·chi·us (trye·bray′kee·us). Conjoined thoracopagous twins with two of the upper limbs coalescent.

thoracopagus tri·pus (trye′pus). Conjoined thoracopagous twins with two of the lower limbs coalescent.

tho·ra·co·para·ceph·a·lus (tho″ruh·ko·păr″uh·sef′uh·lus) *n.* [*thoraco-* + *para-* + *-cephalus*]. A thoracopagus parasiticus in which the parasite has a rudimentary head.

thoracoparacephalus pseu·do·acor·mus (sue″do·a·kor′mus). A thoracopagus parasiticus in which the parasite is a little more than a head. See also *heterodymus.*

tho·ra·co·par·a·si·tus (tho″ruh·ko·păr″uh·sigh′tus) *n.* [*thoraco-* + L. *parasitus,* parasite]. Taruffi's term for thoracopagus parasiticus.

tho·ra·co·plas·ty (tho′ruh·ko·plas″tee) *n.* [*thoraco-* + *-plasty*]. The mobilization of the chest wall by the resection of any number of ribs, wholly or in part, in order to produce collapse of the chest wall and obliteration of the pleural cavity or reduction of the thoracic space. The operation is commonly extrapleural and may be partial or complete, the latter involving segments of the first to eleventh ribs. It is also referred to by location, as anterior, lateral, posterior, apical.

tho·ra·co·pneu·mo·plas·ty (tho″ruh·ko·new′mo·plas·tee) *n.* [*thoraco-* + *pneumo-* + *-plasty*]. THORACOPLASTY.

tho·ra·cos·chi·sis (tho″ruh·kos′ki·sis) *n.* [*thoraco-* + *-schisis*]. Congenital fissure of the thorax.

tho·ra·co·scope (tho·ray′kuh·skope, tho·rack″o·) *n.* [*thoraco-* + *-scope*]. An electrically lighted, tubular instrument designed for insertion between ribs into a pneumothorax space. Used for visual examination of the pleural surfaces and for the severance of pleural adhesion bands by electrocautery.

tho·ra·cos·co·py (tho″ruh·kos′kuh·pee) *n.* [*thoraco-* + *-scopy*]. Examination of the pleural cavity in the presence of a pneumothorax by means of a thoracoscope introduced through the thoracic wall. Syn. *pleuroscopy.*

tho·ra·cos·to·my (tho·ruh·kos′tuh·mee) *n.* [*thoraco-* + *-stomy*]. Opening the chest; particularly, the removal of some ribs for drainage, or for access to the pleural cavity.

tho·ra·cot·o·my (tho″ruh·kot′uh·mee) *n.* [*thoraco-* + *-tomy*]. Incision of the thoracic wall.

tho·ra·del·phus (tho″ruh·del′fus) *n.* [*thorac-* + *-adelphus*]. A double monster united above the umbilicus, with one head, four lower and two upper extremities. Syn. *cephalothoracopagus dibrachius.*

Tho·rae·us filter (to·reʸ′o͞os) [R. *Thoraeus,* Swedish physician, 20th century]. A combination filter consisting of tin, copper, and aluminum, used in conventional x-ray therapy.

tho·rax (tho′racks) *n.,* genit. **tho·ra·cis** (tho·ray′sis), pl. **thoraxes, tho·ra·ces** (tho′ruh·seez, tho·ray′seez) [Gk.] [NA]. The chest; the portion of the trunk above the diaphragm and below the neck; the framework of bones and soft tissues bounded by the diaphragm below, the ribs and sternum in front, the ribs and thoracic portion of the vertebral column behind, and above by the structures in the lower part of the neck, and containing the heart enclosed in the pericardium, the lungs invested by the pleura, and mediastinal structures.

Thorazine. Trademark for chlorpromazine, a tranquilizer and antiemetic drug used as the hydrochloride salt.

Tho·rel's bundle. The posterior internodal bundle of the heart.

tho·ri·um (tho′ree·um) *n.* [NL., from *Thor,* Norse god of thunder]. Th = 232.038. A radioactive, grayish-white, lustrous metal, atomic number 90, the parent of a series of radioactive elements.

thorium emanation. THORON.

thorium X. An isotope of radium formed in the disintegration of thorium; has been used in dermatology in treatment of superficial diseases where irradiation is indicated.

Thorn test [G. W. *Thorn,* U.S. physician, b. 1906]. A test of adrenocortical reserve in which the eosinophil count in the fasting patient is compared with the eosinophil count four hours after the intramuscular injection of 25 units of lyophilized adrenocorticotropic hormone (ACTH); a decrease of 50 percent or more is seen in normal individuals, tending to exclude adrenal cortical insufficiency.

Thorn·ton nail. A nail for internal fixation of intertrochanteric fractures; a metallic plate is screwed on to the end of a Smith-Petersen nail and secured to the shaft of the femur with screws.

Thornwald. See *Tornwaldt.*

thorny-headed worms. Intestinal parasites of the phylum Acanthocephela.

tho·ron (tho′ron) *n.* [*Thor,* Norse god of thunder, + *-on*]. Tn = 220. A gaseous, radioactive isotope of radon evolved from thorium X, one of the disintegration products of thorium. Syn. *thorium emanation.*

thor·ough·joint (thur′o·joint) *n.* A synovial joint or diarthrosis.

thor·ough·pin (thur′o·pin) *n.* A bursitis occurring over the tuber calcis of the hock joint of a horse.

Thor·son-Bioerck syndrome (tor′soʰn, byœrk). CARCINOID SYNDROME.

thor·ter ill (thor'tur). LOUPING ILL.
thought reading. TELEPATHY.
thought transference. TELEPATHY.
tho·zal·i·none (tho·zal'i·nohn) *n.* 2-(Dimethylamino)-5-phenyl-2-oxazolin-4-one, $C_{11}H_{12}N_2O_2$, an antidepressant drug.
thread, *n.* 1. The spun and twisted fibers of cotton, linen, or silk. 2. *In surgery,* a fine suture. 3. Any fine filament or natural process resembling a thread.
thread·ed wire. A wire with screw threads. Syn. *Kirschner wire.*
thread reaction. The formation of long chains of bacillary forms of bacteria when grown in immune serum after agglutination.
thread·worm, *n.* ENTEROBIUS VERMICULARIS.
threat·ened abortion. The occurrence of signs and symptoms of impending loss of the embryo or fetus. It may be prevented by treatment or may go on to inevitable abortion.
three-day fever. PHLEBOTOMUS FEVER.
three-day measles. RUBELLA.
three-glass test. GLASS TEST.
threm·ma·tol·o·gy (threm"uh·tol'uh·jee) *n.* [Gk. *thremma, thremmatos,* creature, domestic animal, from *trephein,* to raise, rear, nourish]. The study of heredity and species variation, as in the breeding of plants and animals under domestication.
thre·o·nine (three'o·neen, ·nin) *n.* α-Amino-β-hydroxybutyric acid, $CH_3CHOHCHNH_2COOH$, an amino acid essential to human nutrition.
thre·o·nyl (three'o·nil) *n.* The univalent radical, $CH_3CHOHCHNH_2CO—$, of the amino acid threonine.
thre·ose (three'oce, ·oze) *n.* A monosaccharide, $C_4H_8O_4$, having a spatial configuration similar to that of threonine, the latter having for this reason been named after the former substance.
threp·sol·o·gy (threp·sol'uh·jee) *n.* [Gk. *threpsis,* feeding, nourishment (from *trephein,* to feed, nourish), + *-logy*]. The science of nutrition.
thresh·er's lung. FARMER'S LUNG.
thresh·old, *n.* 1. The lower limit of stimulus capable of producing an impression upon consciousness or of evoking a response in an irritable tissue. 2. The entrance of a canal.
threshold body. Any substance in the blood plasma which, above a certain concentration, is excreted by the kidneys. The critical concentration is called the excretion threshold.
threshold concentration. The molecular concentration of a substance which produces a minimum response when an organ is stimulated by it.
threshold dose. *In therapeutics,* the minimum dose that will produce a detectable response of a specified kind.
threshold stimulus. The least intensity of a stimulus that produces response.
thrill, *n.* A fine vibration felt by the hand or fingertips, and associated in some instances with disease in underlying organs, such as the heart.
-thrix [Gk. *thrix,* hair]. A combining form meaning (a) *hair;* (b) *filament, filamentous.*
thrix an·nu·la·ta (thricks an"yoo·lay'tuh). Hairs with alternating light and dark segments.
throat, *n.* The pharynx and the fauces.
throb, *n.* A pulsation or beating.
Throck·mor·ton reflex [T. B. *Throckmorton,* U.S. neurologist, b. 1885]. A variant of the Babinski sign in which percussion over the dorsal aspect of the metatarsophalangeal joint of the great toe medial to the tendon of the extensor hallucis longus muscle is followed by dorsiflexion of the toes in corticospinal tract lesions.
throes, *n. pl.* The struggle, spasms, or anguish in parturition or preceding death.
thromb-, thrombo- [Gk. *thrombos,* clot, curd]. A combining form meaning (a) *clotting, coagulation;* (b) *blood platelets;* (c) *thrombus, thrombosis.*
throm·base (throm'bace, ·baze) *n.* THROMBIN.
throm·bas·the·nia (throm"bas·theen'ee·uh) *n.* THROMBOASTHENIA.
throm·bec·to·my (throm·beck'tuh·mee) *n.* [*thromb-* + *-ectomy*]. Excision of a thrombus.
thrombi. Plural of *thrombus.*
throm·bic (throm'bick) *adj.* Of or pertaining to a thrombus or thrombi.
throm·bin (throm'bin) *n.* [*thromb-* + *-in*]. An enzyme elaborated in shed blood from an inactive precursor, prothrombin. It induces clotting by converting fibrinogen to fibrin, possibly by proteolysis, and is used therapeutically as a topical hemostatic agent.
throm·bin·o·gen (throm·bin'uh·jen) *n.* [*thrombin* + *-gen*]. PROTHROMBIN.
thrombo-. See *thromb-.*
throm·bo·an·gi·itis (throm"bo·an"jee·eye'tis) *n.* [*thrombo-* + *angiitis*]. Thrombosis associated with inflammation of the vessel wall.
thromboangiitis cu·ta·neo·in·tes·ti·na·lis dis·sem·i·na·ta (kew·tay"nee·o·in·tes·ti·nay'lis di·sem·i·nay'tuh, ·nah'tuh). DEGOS' DISEASE.
thromboangiitis oblit·er·ans (o·blit'ur·anz). BUERGER'S DISEASE.
throm·bo·as·the·nia (throm"bo·as·theen'ee·uh) *n.* [*thrombo-* + *asthenia*]. A rare hereditary disorder in which about 25 percent of the blood platelets are large and poorly granular; it is associated with abnormal posttraumatic bleeding.
throm·bo·blast (throm'bo·blast) *n.* [*thrombo-* + *-blast*]. The precursor of the blood platelet (thrombocyte); MEGAKARYOCYTE.
throm·bo·cav·er·no·si·tis (throm"bo·kav"ur·no·sigh'tis) *n.* [*thrombo-* + *cavernositis*]. Thrombosis combined with inflammation of the corpora cavernosa of the penis.
throm·boc·la·sis (throm·bock'luh·sis) *n.* [*thrombo-* + *-clasis*]. Breaking up or destruction of a thrombus; thrombolysis. —**throm·bo·clas·tic** (throm"bo·klas'tick) *adj.*
throm·bo·cy·ta·pher·e·sis (throm"bo·sigh"tuh·fe·ree'sis, ·ferr'e·sis) *n.* THROMBOCYTOPHERESIS.
throm·bo·cyte (throm'bo·site) *n.* [*thrombo-* + *-cyte*]. BLOOD PLATELET. —**throm·bo·cyt·ic** (throm"bo·sit'ick) *adj.*
throm·bo·cy·the·mia, throm·bo·cy·thae·mia (throm"bo·sigh·theem'ee·uh) *n.* [*thrombocyte* + *-hemia*]. THROMBOCYTOSIS.
thrombocytic series. The series of cells concerned in the origin of blood platelets (thrombocytes), including the megakaryoblasts and megakaryocytes that occur normally in bone marrow.
throm·bo·cy·to·bar·in reaction (throm"bo·sigh"to·băr'in). IMMUNE-ADHERENCE PHENOMENON.
throm·bo·cy·to·crit (throm"bo·sigh'to·krit) *n.* [*thrombocyte* + Gk. *krit-,* from *krinein,* to separate]. A glass tube for counting blood platelets. Blood diluted with sodium oxalate is centrifuged in a special spherical sediment chamber so that the platelets are seen layered above the red cells. This volume can be measured. Normal is 0.35 to 0.67 percent.
throm·bo·cy·tol·y·sin (throm"bo·sigh·tol'i·sin) *n.* [*thrombocyte* + *lysin*]. A substance that disrupts blood platelets.
throm·bo·cy·tol·y·sis (throm"bo·sigh·tol'i·sis) *n.* [*thrombocyte* + *-lysis*]. Destruction of blood platelets. —**thrombo·cy·to·lyt·ic** (·sigh"to·lit'ick) *adj.*
thrombocytolytic purpura. IDIOPATHIC THROMBOCYTOPENIC PURPURA.
throm·bo·cy·to·path·ia (throm"bo·sigh"to·path'ee·uh) *n.* [*thrombocyte* + *-pathia*]. A hemorrhagic state in which the blood platelets are functionally abnormal. —**thrombocyto·path·ic** (·ick) *adj.*
thrombocytopathic purpura. Purpura associated with a normal number of qualitatively defective blood platelets.
throm·bo·cy·to·pe·nia (throm"bo·sigh"to·pee'nee·uh) *n.*

[*thrombocyte* + *-penia*]. A condition in which there is a decrease in the absolute number of platelets below normal. —**thrombocytope·nic** (·nick) *adj.*

thrombocytopenic purpura. Purpura associated with decreased numbers of blood platelets per unit volume of blood.

throm·bo·cy·to·pher·e·sis (throm″bo·sigh″to·ferr′e·sis) *n.* [*thrombocyte* + Gk. *pherein*, to carry off, + *-esis*]. Selective removal of blood platelets from the circulation.

throm·bo·cy·to·sis (throm″bo·sigh·to′sis) *n.*, pl. **thrombocyto·ses** (·seez) [*thrombocyte* + *-osis*]. A condition marked by an absolute increase in the number of blood platelets. Syn. *piastrinemia, thrombocytemia.*

throm·bo·em·bo·lec·to·my (throm″bo·em″bo·leck′tuh·mee) *n.* [*thrombo-* + *embolectomy*]. Surgical removal of an embolus representing a dislodged thrombus or part of a thrombus.

throm·bo·em·bo·lism (throm″bo·em′bo·liz·um) *n.* Embolism due to a dislodged thrombus, or part of a thrombus.

throm·bo·em·bo·li·za·tion (throm″bo·em″bo·li·zay′shun) *n.* The occlusion of a blood vessel by the lodgement of a portion of a thrombus.

throm·bo·em·bo·lus (throm″bo·em′bo·lus) *n.* An embolus composed of a thrombus.

throm·bo·en·dar·ter·ec·to·my (throm″bo·en·dahr″tur·eck′tuh·mee) *n.* ENDARTERECTOMY.

throm·bo·en·do·car·di·tis (throm″bo·en″do·kahr·dye′tis) *n.* [*thrombo-* + *endocarditis*]. Bacterial or nonbacterial thrombotic vegetations on heart valves.

throm·bo·gen (throm′bo·jen) *n.* [*thrombo-* + *-gen*]. PROTHROMBIN.

throm·bo·gen·ic (throm″bo·jen′ick) *adj.* [*thrombo-* + *-genic*]. Producing thrombi.

throm·boid (throm′boid) *adj.* [Gk. *thromboeidēs*, clotted, lumpy]. 1. Pertaining to or characterized by the presence of a thrombus or thrombi. 2. Thrombuslike, clotlike.

throm·bo·ki·nase (throm″bo·kigh′nace, ·kin′ace) *n.* [*thrombo-* + *kinase*]. A proteolytic enzyme in blood plasma that, along with thromboplastin, calcium, and factor V, converts prothrombin to thrombin. May be identical with factor X.

throm·bo·lym·phan·gi·tis (throm″bo·lim″fan·jye′tis) *n.* Lymphangitis with thrombosis.

Thrombolysin. A trademark for a preparation of human fibrinolysin used intravenously with the objective of accelerating intravascular dissolution of clots.

throm·bol·y·sis (throm·bol′i·sis) *n.*, pl. **thromboly·ses** (·seez) [*thrombo-* + *-lysis*]. Destruction or dissolution of a thrombus; thromboclasis. —**throm·bo·lyt·ic** (throm″bo·lit′ick) *adj.*

throm·bop·a·thy (throm·bop′uth·ee) *n.* [*thrombo-* + *-pathy*]. Disease characterized by disturbance of platelet function.

throm·bo·pe·nia (throm″bo·pee′nee·uh) *n.* THROMBOCYTOPENIA. —**thrombope·nic** (·nick) *adj.*

throm·bo·phil·ia (throm″bo·fil′ee·uh) *n.* [*thrombo-* + *-philia*]. A tendency to form thrombi.

throm·bo·phle·bi·tis (throm″bo·fle·bye′tis) *n.* [*thrombo-* + *phlebitis*]. Inflammation of a vein associated with thrombosis.

throm·bo·plas·tic (throm″bo·plas′tick) *adj.* [*thrombo-* + *plastic*]. 1. Causing or hastening the coagulation of the blood. 2. Of or pertaining to a thromboplastin.

throm·bo·plas·tid (throm″bo·plas′tid) *n.* [*thrombo-* + Gk. *plastis, plastidos*, molder, creator]. BLOOD PLATELET.

throm·bo·plas·tin (throm″bo·plas′tin) *n.* [*thromboplastic* + *-in*]. Any of a group of substances that, along with procoagulants and calcium, accelerates the conversion of prothrombin to thrombin. Most such substances are complexes of lipids and proteins.

throm·bo·plas·tin·o·gen (throm″bo·plas·tin′o·jen) *n.* [*thromboplastin* + *-gen*]. FACTOR VIII.

throm·bo·poi·e·sis (throm″bo·poy·e′sis) *n.* [*thrombo-* + *-poiesis*]. The production of blood platelets.

throm·bose (throm′boze) *v.* To form or become a thrombus.

throm·bosed (throm′boze′d) *adj.* 1. Affected with thrombosis. 2. Clotted.

thrombosed hemorrhoid. A hemorrhoid in which the blood within the varicosity has become thrombosed.

throm·bo·sis (throm·bo′sis) *n.*, pl. **thrombo·ses** (·seez) [Gk. *thrombōsis*, from *thrombos*, clot]. The formation of a thrombus. —**throm·bot·ic** (·bot′ick) *adj.*

throm·bo·sta·sis (throm″bo·stay′sis, throm·bos′tuh·sis) *n.* Stasis of blood leading to formation of a thrombus.

throm·bo·sthe·nin (throm·bo·sthee′nin) *n.* [*thrombo-* + Gk. *sthenos*, strength, + *-in*]. A contractile protein present in blood platelets, believed to be essential for clot retraction.

thrombotic endocarditis. MARANTIC ENDOCARDITIS.

thrombotic thrombocytopenic purpura. Thrombi in the vascular channels associated with hyaline deposits in the walls and subendothelial areas of the vessels, and associated thrombocytopenia. Syn. *Moschcowitz's syndrome.*

throm·bo·zym (throm′bo·zim) *n.* A substance, occurring in plasma and in tissue extracts, which is active in bringing about the clotting of blood. It may be identical with, or contain, thrombokinase.

throm·bus (throm′bus) *n.*, pl. **throm·bi** (·bye) [NL., from Gk. *thrombos*, clot, curd, from *trephein*, to curdle, congeal]. A clot of blood formed during life within the heart or blood vessels.

thrombus vul·vae (vul′vee). Hematoma of a labium majus.

throt·tle (throt′ul) *v. & n.* 1. To choke; to suffocate. 2. THROAT.

through drainage. A method of drainage in which a perforated tube is carried through the cavity to be drained, so that the latter can be flushed through and through by the injection of fluid into one end of the tube.

throw·back, *n.* A reversion to an ancestral type. See also *atavism.*

thrush, *n.* 1. A form of candidiasis due to infection by *Candida albicans.* It occurs most often in infants and children and is characterized by small, whitish spots on the tip and sides of the tongue and the buccal mucous membrane. Syn. *mycotic stomatitis, parasitic stomatitis.* 2. A diseased condition of the frog of the horse's foot, with a fetid discharge.

thrush fungus. *CANDIDA ALBICANS*; a fungus of low pathogenicity that inhabits the mucous membranes; produces thrush and other types of candidiasis.

thrust culture. STAB CULTURE.

thryp·sis (thrip′sis) *n.* [Gk., a breaking in pieces]. 1. A comminuted fracture. 2. The hypothetical softening and liquefaction of bone matrix preceding leaching out of bone salt in halisteresis.

Thu·ja (thoo′juh, thoo′yuh) *n.* [Gk. *thyia*, odorous cedar]. A genus of trees of the Pinaceae. The leafy young twigs of *Thuja occidentalis* were formerly used as an antipyretic, expectorant, and anthelmintic.

thuja oil. CEDAR LEAF OIL.

thu·jone (thoo′jone) *n.* A terpene ketone, $C_{10}H_{16}O$, found in several volatile oils; an experimental convulsant.

thu·li·um (thew′lee·um) *n.* [NL., from L. *Thule*, northernmost limit of the habitable world]. Tm = 168.934. A lanthanide, atomic number 69.

thumb, *n.* [Gmc., lit., thick, swollen (rel. to L. *tumor*)]. The digit on the radial side of the hand, differing from the other digits in having but two phalanges, and in that its metacarpal bone is freely movable. NA *pollex, digitus I.*

thumps, *n.* 1. A verminous pneumonia of swine caused by the larvae of *Ascaris lumbricoides* in the lungs. 2. An affection in the horse, similar to hiccup in man, due to spasmodic contraction of the diaphragm.

Thun·berg and Ahl·gren method. A method for the study of tissue oxidations in which finely divided tissue is suspended in a solution containing methylene blue, phosphate solution to regulate the acidity, and the substance whose action it is desired to determine. After subjection to partial vacuum, the tube is placed in a water bath and the time required for the methylene blue to be decolorized is determined. This is a measure of the rate of oxidation in the mixture.

thus (thuss, thooce) *n.* [L.]. 1. True frankincense or olibanum. 2. Turpentine of pine trees.

thy·la·ken·trin (thigh″luh·ken′trin) *n.* [Gk. *thylakos,* sack, + *kentrizein,* to stimulate]. FOLLICLE-STIMULATING HORMONE.

¹thym-, thymo-. A combining form meaning *thymol.*

²thym-, thymo-. A combining form meaning *thymus.*

³thym-, thymo- [Gk. *thymos,* spirit, temper, will]. A combining form meaning (a) *mood;* (b) *affect;* (c) *will.*

thyme (time) *n.* [Gk. *thymon*]. The dried leaves and flowering tops of *Thymus vulgaris* (family Lamiaceae); contains a volatile oil, thyme oil, of which one of the constituents is thymol. It has been used as a diaphoretic, carminative, and expectorant.

thy·mec·to·my (thigh·meck′tuh·mee) *n.* [*thym-,* thymus, + *-ectomy*]. Excision of the thymus. —**thymecto·mize** (·mize) *v.*

thy·mer·ga·sia (thigh″mur·gay′zhuh, ·zee·uh) *n.* [*thym-,* affect, + *ergasia*]. *In psychiatry,* Meyer's term for the affective illnesses. —**thymerga·sic** (·sick) *adj.*

-thymia [*thym-* + *-ia*]. A combining form designating *a condition involving mood or affect.*

¹thy·mic (tigh′mick) *adj.* [*thyme* + *-ic*]. Pertaining to, or derived from, thyme.

²thy·mic (thigh′mick) *adj.* [*thym-,* thymus, + *-ic*]. Pertaining to the thymus.

thymic aplasia. Congenital absence of the thymus and of the parathyroids, and often cardiovascular malformations, with deficient cellular immunity; characterized clinically by frequent virus, fungus, or *Pneumocystis* infections, neonatal tetany, and early death. Syn. *Di George's syndrome, third and fourth (III-IV) branchial pouch syndrome.*

thymic corpuscle. A characteristic, rounded, acidophil body in the medulla of the thymus; composed of hyalinized epithelial cells concentrically arranged about a core which is occasionally calcified.

thymic death. STATUS THYMICOLYMPHATICUS.

thymic dysplasia. NEZELOF'S SYNDROME.

thymic nucleic acid. DEOXYRIBONUCLEIC ACID.

thy·mi·co·lym·phat·ic (thigh″mi·ko·lim·fat′ick) *adj.* [*thymic* + *lymphatic*]. Affecting the thymus and lymphatic structures such as spleen, lymph nodes, and lymphoid aggregates.

thymic sarcoma. 1. A variety of thymoma with prominent spindle cells resembling sarcoma. 2. A sarcoma involving the thymus.

thy·mi·dine (thigh′mi·deen, ·din) *n.* Thymine-2-deoxyriboside, $C_{10}H_{14}N_2O_5$, a nucleoside obtained from deoxyribonucleic acid.

thy·mi·dyl·ic acid (thigh″mi·dil′ick). A mononucleotide component, $C_{10}H_{15}N_2O_8P$, of deoxyribonucleic acid which yields thymine, D-ribose, and phosphoric acid on complete hydrolysis.

thy·mine (thigh′meen, ·min) *n.* 5-Methyluracil or 2,4-dihydroxy-5-methylpyrimidine, $C_5H_6N_2O_2$, one of the pyrimidine components of nucleic acids, first isolated from the thymus.

thy·mi·on (thigh′mee·on) *n.* [Gk., large wart]. WART; CONDYLOMA.

thy·mi·tis (thigh·mye′tis) *n.* [*thym-,* thymus, + *-itis*]. Inflammation of the thymus.

thymo-. See *thym-.*

thy·mo·cyte (thigh′mo·site) *n.* A lymphocyte formed in the thymus.

thy·mo·hy·dro·qui·none (thigh″mo·high″dro·kwi·nohn′, ·kwin′ohn) *n.* A substance occurring in the urine after the ingestion of thymol, coloring the urine green.

thy·mo·ke·sis (thigh″mo·kee′sis) *n.* Abnormal persistence of enlargement of the thymus.

thy·mol (thigh′mol) *n.* 5-Methyl-2-isopropylphenol, $C_{10}H_{14}O$, present in thyme oil and other volatile oils and produced by synthesis; a bactericide and fungicide applied topically.

thy·mo·lep·tic (thigh″mo·lep′tick) *adj. & n.* [*thymo-,* mood, + Gk. *lēptikos,* accepting, assimilative]. 1. Of or pertaining to any action that changes or influences mood or spirit, particularly such action that is favorable in mentally depressed patients. 2. A drug that counteracts mental depression by a mood-elevating or mind-stimulating action; a psychic energizer or stimulant.

thymol flocculation test. A modification of the thymol turbidity test in which the mixture is allowed to stand overnight and the amount of flocculation is measured.

thymol iodide. A mixture of iodine derivatives of thymol, chiefly dithymoldiiodide, $(CH_3C_6H_2C_3H_7OI)_2$; has been used as a topical antiseptic.

thy·mol·phthal·ein (thigh″mol·thal′een, ·ee·in) *n.* A compound, $C_{28}H_{30}O_4$, analogous to phenolphthalein, used as an indicator; colorless below pH 9.3 and blue at pH 10.5.

thymol turbidity test. A test for liver disease based on precipitation of altered serum proteins by a thymol solution.

thy·mo·ma (thigh·mo′muh) *n.,* pl. **thymomas, thymoma·ta** (·tuh) [*thym-,* thymus, + *-oma*]. A primary tumor of the thymus whose parenchyma is composed of mixtures of lymphocytic and epithelial cells, or of either element predominantly; its behavior is usually benign, and some forms are associated with myasthenia gravis or hypoplasia of erythrocyte precursors.

thy·mo·no·ic (thigh″mo·no′ick) *adj.* [*thymo-,* mood, + Gk. *nous,* mind, intellect, + *-ic*]. Pertaining to thoughts and ideas that are strongly influenced by deviations in mood.

thy·mo·nu·cle·ic acid (thigh″mo·new·klee′ick). DEOXYRIBONUCLEIC ACID.

thy·mop·a·thy (thigh·mop′uth·ee) *n.* [*thymo-* + *-pathy*]. Any disease of the thymus.

thy·mo·pha·ryn·ge·al duct (thigh″mo·făr″in·jee′ul, ·fa·rin′jee·ul). The third pharyngobranchial duct which may elongate and persist between the thymus and pharynx.

thy·mo·poi·e·tin (thigh″mo·poy′e·tin) *n.* An extract of thymic tissue similar to thymosin.

thy·mo·priv·ic (thigh″mo·priv′ick) *adj.* [*thymo-,* thymus, + *-privic*]. Related to, or caused by, removal of or premature involution of the thymus.

thy·mop·riv·ous (thigh·mop′riv·us) *adj.* THYMOPRIVIC.

thy·mo·sin (thigh′mo·sin) *n.* An extract of thymic tissue having some properties of a hormone in that it promotes maturation of thymus-derived cells (T lymphocytes).

thy·mus (thy′mus) *n.,* pl. **thymuses, thy·mi** (·migh) [Gk. *thymos*] [NA]. A lymphoepithelial organ developed from the third and fourth branchial pouches and normally situated in the anterior superior mediastinum. It is the site of differentiation of T lymphocytes and is a central lymphoid organ controlling many aspects of immunologic reactivity, particularly delayed hypersensitivity. It is well developed at birth but undergoes gradual involution after puberty. It is lobulated and contains primarily lymphocytes, densely packed in the cortex and more loosely packed in the medulla which also contains concentric arrangements of epithelial cells called thymic corpuscles. See also Plate 26.

thymus nucleic acid. DEOXYRIBONUCLEIC ACID.

thyr-, thyreo-, thyro-. A combining form meaning *thyroid.*

thy·reo·apla·sia con·gen·i·ta (thigh″ree·o·uh·play′zhuh kon·jen′i·tuh). Anomalies found in congenital defects of the thyroid gland and in deficient thyroid secretion.

thy·reo·gen·ic (thigh″ree·o·jen′ick) *adj.* [*thyreo-* + *-genic*]. Of thyroid origin, as thyreogenic obesity.

thy·reo·pri·val (thigh″ree·o·prye′vul) *adj.* THYROPRIVAL.

thyro-. See *thyr-.*

thy·ro·ad·e·ni·tis (thigh″ro·ad″e·nigh′tis) *n.* [*thyro-* + *adenitis*]. Inflammation of the thyroid gland.

thy·ro·ar·y·te·noid (thigh″ro·ăr″i·tee′noid) *adj.* Pertaining to the thyroid and arytenoid cartilages.

thyroarytenoid muscle. A variable muscle that extends between the thyroid and arytenoid cartilages. NA *musculus thyroarytenoideus.* See also Table of Muscles in the Appendix.

thy·ro·cal·ci·to·nin (thigh″ro·kal·si·to′nin) *n.* CALCITONIN.

thy·ro·car·di·ac (thigh″ro·kahr′dee·ack) *adj.* Pertaining to thyroid disease with cardiac symptoms predominating.

thy·ro·cele (thigh′ro·seel) *n.* [*thyro-* + *-cele*]. A tumor affecting the thyroid gland; goiter.

thy·ro·cer·vi·cal (thigh″ro·sur′vi·kul) *adj.* [*thyro-* + *cervical*]. Pertaining to the thyroid gland and the neck.

thyrocervical duct. The fourth branchial duct.

thyrocervical trunk. A main branch of the subclavian artery, dividing into the inferior thyroid, suprascapular, and transverse cervical arteries. NA *truncus thyrocervicalis.*

thy·ro·chon·drot·o·my (thigh″ro·kon·drot′uh·mee) *n.* [*thyro-* + *chondrotomy*]. THYROTOMY.

thy·ro·cri·cot·o·my (thigh″ro·krye·kot′uh·mee, ·kri·) *n.* Tracheotomy performed through the cricothyroid membrane.

thy·ro·epi·glot·tic (thigh″ro·ep″i·glot′ick) *adj.* [*thyro-* + *epiglottic*]. Pertaining to the thyroid cartilage and the epiglottis.

thyroepiglottic ligament. An elastic band between the lower part of the epiglottis and the middle posterior surface of the thyroid cartilage. NA *ligamentum thyroepiglotticum.*

thyroepiglottic muscle. A fairly constant muscle that extends between the thyroid cartilage and the epiglottis. NA *musculus thyroepiglotticus.* See also Table of Muscles in the Appendix.

thy·ro·gen·ic (thigh″ro·jen′ick) *adj.* [*thyro-* + *-genic*]. THYREOGENIC.

thy·rog·e·nous (thigh·roj′e·nus) *adj.* [*thyro-* + *-genous*]. THYREOGENIC.

thy·ro·glob·u·lin (thigh″ro·glob′yoo·lin) *n.* [*thyro-* + *globulin*]. An iodinated protein found in the thyroid follicular lumen and epithelial cells which contains within its structure monoiodotyrosine, diiodotyrosine, triiodothyronine, and tetraiodothyronine. The storage form of the iodinated hormones.

thyroglobulin antibodies. Antibodies, found in the serum of patients with struma lymphomatosa, which react with purified thyroglobulin. Abbreviated, TGA.

thy·ro·glos·sal (thigh″ro·glos′ul) *adj.* [*thyro-* + *glossal*]. Pertaining to the thyroid gland and the tongue.

thyroglossal cyst. Cystic distention of the remnants of the thyroglossal duct, filled with secretion of lining epithelial cells; most often presents over the thyrohyoid membrane in the midline.

thyroglossal duct. A slender temporary duct connecting the thyroid anlage with the surface of the tongue. NA *ductus thyroglossus.* See also *thyroid diverticulum.*

thyroglossal fistula. A developmental abnormality, due to incomplete obliteration of the thyroglossal duct, resulting in a midline cervical fistula.

thy·ro·hy·al (thigh″ro·high′ul) *n.* [*thyro-* + *hy-* + *-al*]. The greater cornu of the hyoid bone.

thy·ro·hy·oid (thigh″ro·high′oid) *adj.* [*thyro-* + *hyoid*]. Pertaining to the thyroid cartilage and the hyoid bone.

thyrohyoid laryngotomy. SUPERIOR LARYNGOTOMY.

thyrohyoid ligament. LATERAL THYROHYOID LIGAMENT. See also *median thyrohyoid ligament.*

thyrohyoid membrane. The membrane joining the thyroid cartilage and hyoid bone. NA *membrana thyrohyoidea.* See also Plate 26.

thyrohyoid muscle. A muscle extending between the thyroid cartilage and the hyoid bone. NA *musculus thyrohyoideus.* See also Table of Muscles in the Appendix.

thyrohyoid region. The region around the thyroid cartilage and the hyoid bone.

[1]thy·roid (thigh′roid) *adj.* & *n.* [earlier *thyreoid,* from Gk. *thyreoeidēs,* shaped like a *thyreos,* a kind of shield]. 1. Shield-shaped, as: thyroid cartilage. 2. Pertaining to the thyroid cartilage, as: thyroid gland. 3. Pertaining to the thyroid gland, its functions and secretions. 4. THYROID GLAND. 5. The cleaned, dried and powdered parenchymal tissue of the thyroid glands of domestic animals, containing about 0.2% iodine in thyroid combination, especially as thyroxine. Used in the treatment of thyroid-deficiency states.

[2]thyroid, *adj.* [Gk. *thyroeidēs,* like a door, from *thyra,* door]. Comparable to a door or doorway, as: thyroid foramen (2).

thyroid cartilage [Gk. *thyreoeidēs chondros,* "shieldlike cartilage" (Galen)]. The largest of the laryngeal cartilages, consisting of two laminas united at an angle in front called the laryngeal prominence. NA *cartilago thyroidea.* See also Plates 13, 26.

thyroid crisis. THYROTOXIC CRISIS.

thyroid diverticulum. An evagination of the ventral floor of the pharynx between the first and second visceral arches which is the primordium of the thyroid gland. The site is marked by the foramen cecum on the tongue.

thyroid dwarfism. 1. CRETINISM. 2. Stunted growth resulting from hypothyroidism.

thy·roid·ec·to·mize (thigh″roy·deck′tuh·mize) *v.* To perform a thyroidectomy.

thy·roid·ec·to·my (thigh″roy·deck′tuh·mee) *n.* [*thyroid* + *-ectomy*]. Partial or complete excision of the thyroid gland.

thyroid foramen. 1. An occasional opening in a lamina of the thyroid cartilage for passage of a superior laryngeal artery. NA *foramen thyroideum.* 2. [Gk. *thyroeides trēma,* "doorway foramen" (Galen)]. OBTURATOR FORAMEN.

thyroid gland. One of the endocrine glands, lying in front of the trachea and consisting of two lateral lobes connected centrally by an isthmus. The organ is composed of follicles lined by epithelium, producing a colloid material. NA *glandula thyroidea.* See also Plates 13, 26.

thyroid heart. GOITER HEART.

thyroid heart disease. Heart disease or cardiac symptoms associated with alteration of thyroid function, either hyperthyroidism or myxedema.

thyroid hormone. Commonly, thyroxine (tetraiodothyronine) or liothyronine (triiodothyronine), or both. See also *calcitonin.*

thyroid impar plexus. A venous plexus found in the substance of the thyroid gland and on its surface beneath the capsule. NA *plexus thyroideus impar.*

thyroid infantilism. Physical and mental underdevelopment resulting from hypothyroidism.

thy·roid·ism (thigh′roid·iz·um) *n.* 1. HYPERTHYROIDISM. 2. A series of phenomena due to continued use of thyroid preparations.

thy·roid·i·tis (thigh″roid·eye′tis) *n.* [*thyroid* + *-itis*]. Inflammation of the thyroid gland.

thy·roid·iza·tion (thigh″roid·i·zay′shun) *n.* Treatment with thyroid gland preparations.

thy·roid·ot·o·my (thigh″roy·dot′uh·mee) *n.* [*thyroid* + *-tomy*]. Incision of the thyroid gland.

thy·roido·tox·in (thigh·roy″do·tock′sin) *n.* [*thyroid* + *toxin*]. A substance specifically toxic for the cells of the thyroid gland.

thyroid plexus. An autonomic nerve plexus in the region of the thyroid gland; the superior part goes to the thyroid gland, and the inferior part surrounds the external carotid and inferior thyroid arteries and is distributed to the larynx and pharynx as well as the thyroid gland.

thyroid retractor. An instrument with a relatively long, narrow blade, used to obtain exposure in thyroid surgery.

thyroid-stimulating hormone. THYROTROPIC HORMONE. Abbreviated, TSH.

thyroid storm. THYROTOXIC CRISIS.

Thyrolar. A trademark for liotrix, a mixture of thyroid hormone salts.

thy·ro·me·dan (thigh·ro'me·dan) *n.* 2-(Diethylamino)ethyl [3,5-diiodo-4-(3-iodo-4-methoxyphenoxy)phenyl]acetate, $C_{21}H_{24}I_3NO_4$, a thyromimetic drug; used as the hydrochloride salt.

thy·ro·meg·a·ly (thigh"ro·meg'uh·lee) *n.* [*thyro-* + *-megaly*]. Enlargement of the thyroid gland.

thy·ro·mi·met·ic (thigh"ro·migh·met'ick, ·mi·) *adj.* [*thyro-* + *mimetic*]. Pertaining to or characterized by thyroid-like action, as of thyroid hormones.

thy·ron·cus (thigh·ronk'us) *n.* [*thyr-* + Gk. *onkos,* tumor]. A thyroid tumor, usually benign goiter.

thy·ro·nyl (thigh'ro·nil) *n.* The univalent radical, *p*-(*p*-HO-$C_6H_4O)C_6H_4CH_2CH(NH_2)CO$—, of thyronine, the amino acid resulting when the iodine atoms in thyroxine are replaced by hydrogen atoms.

thy·ro·para·thy·roid·ec·to·my (thigh"ro·păr"uh·thigh"roy·deck'tuh·mee) *n.* [*thyro-* + *parathyroid* + *-ectomy*]. Excision of the thyroid and parathyroid glands.

thy·ro·pha·ryn·ge·al duct (thigh"ro·făr"in·jee'ul, ·fa·rin'jee·ul). The fourth pharyngobranchial duct.

thy·ro·pha·ryn·ge·us (thy"ro·fa·rin'jee·us) *n.* PARS THYROPHARYNGEA MUSCULI CONSTRICTORIS PHARYNGIS INFERIORIS.

thy·ro·pri·val (thigh"ro·prye'vul) *adj.* [*thyro-* + *-prival*]. Pertaining to the effects of loss of function, or removal, of the thyroid gland.

thyroprival tetany. Tetany following surgical removal of the thyroid gland when the parathyroids have inadvertently been removed also, or have been damaged.

thy·ro·pri·vous (thigh"ro·prye'vus, thigh·rop'ri·vus) *adj.* THYROPRIVAL.

thy·ro·pro·tein (thigh"ro·pro'tee·in, ·teen) *n.* A protein from the thyroid gland.

thy·rop·to·sis (thigh"rop·to'sis) *n.* [*thyro-* + *-ptosis*]. Displacement of a goitrous thyroid so that it is partially or completely concealed in the thorax.

thy·ro·sis (thigh·ro'sis) *n.* [*thyr-* + *-osis*]. Any disorder caused by abnormal functioning of the thyroid gland. See also *hyperthyroidism, hypothyroidism.*

thy·ro·ther·a·py (thigh"ro·therr'uh·pee) *n.* [*thyro-* + *therapy*]. Treatment of disease by thyroid gland preparations.

thy·rot·o·my (thigh·rot'uh·mee) *n.* [*thyro-* + *-tomy*]. Incision or splitting of the thyroid cartilage.

thy·ro·tox·ic (thigh"ro·tock'sick) *adj.* 1. Pertaining to or affected with thyrotoxicosis. 2. Of or pertaining to thyrotoxin.

thyrotoxic crisis. Acute fulminating hyperthyroidism which may lead to extreme tachycardia, muscle weakness, coma, and death. Syn. *thyroid crisis.*

thyrotoxic heart. GOITER HEART.

thy·ro·tox·i·co·sis (thigh"ro·tock"si·ko'sis) *n.* [*thyro-* + *toxicosis*]. HYPERTHYROIDISM.

thyrotoxic storm. THYROTOXIC CRISIS.

thy·ro·tox·in (thigh"ro·tock'sin) *n.* [*thyro-* + *toxin*]. Any substance that is toxic to the thyroid cells.

thy·ro·tro·phic (thigh"ro·tro'fick, ·trof'ick) *adj.* THYROTROPIC.

thy·rot·ro·phin (thigh·rot'ro·fin) *n.* THYROTROPIN.

thy·ro·tro·pic (thigh"ro·trop'ick, ·tro'pick) *adj.* [*thyro-* + *-tropic*]. 1. Stimulating the thyroid gland. 2. Pertaining to thyrotropism (2).

thyrotropic exophthalmos. Exophthalmos associated with either a normal or a low metabolic rate. Asymmetric proptosis is common, often accompanied by chemosis, lid edema, and pareses of extraocular muscles, believed to be due to hypersecretion of a pituitary factor (exophthalmos-producing substance) associated with, but not identical to, thyrotropin. Syn. *pituitary exophthalmos.*

thyrotropic hormone. A hormone of the adenohypophysis which controls the status of the thyroid. Syn. *thyroid-stimulating hormone.*

thy·ro·tro·pin (thigh"ro·tro'pin, thigh·rot'ro·pin) *n.* A thyroid-stimulating hormone produced by the adenohypophysis.

thyrotropin releasing factor or **hormone.** A substance released from the hypothalamus which acts on the pituitary to cause release of thyrotropin. Abbreviated, TRF, TRH

thy·ro·tro·pism (thigh"ro·tro'piz·um, thigh·rot'ro·piz·um) *n.* [*thyro-* + *-tropism*]. 1. An affinity for the thyroid. 2. Constitutional domination by thyroid influence.

thy·rox·in (thigh·rock'sin) *n.* THYROXINE.

thy·rox·ine (thigh·rock'seen, ·sin) *n.* L-3,3′,5,5′-Tetraiodothyronine, $C_{15}H_{11}I_4NO_4$, an active physiologic principle of the thyroid gland; used, in the form of the sodium salt (levothyroxine sodium), as replacement therapy where there is reduced or absent thyroid function. See also *dextrothyroxine sodium.*

thyroxine-binding globulin. A specific glycoprotein found in the circulatory system which serves as a transport molecule for the thyroid hormones.

Ti Symbol for titanium.

TIA Abbreviation for *transient ischemic attack.*

ti·az·u·ril (tye·az'yoo·ril) *n.* 2[4-[(*p*-Chlorophenyl)thio]-3,5-xylyl]-*as*-triazine-3,5(2*H*,4*H*)-dione, $C_{17}H_{14}ClN_3O_2S$, a poultry coccidiostat.

tib·ia (tib'ee·uh) *n.*, L. pl. & genit. sing. **ti·bi·ae** (tib'ee·ee), E. pl. **tibias** [L.] [NA]. The larger of the two bones of the leg, commonly called the shinbone, articulating with the femur, fibula, and talus. See also Table of Bones in the Appendix and Plates 1, 2. —**tib·i·al** (·ee·ul) *adj.*

tibial collateral ligament. A broad, flat ligament on the medial side of the knee joint, connecting the medial condyle of the femur and the medial condyle and surface of the shaft of the tibia, adhering also to the edge of the medial meniscus. NA *ligamentum collaterale tibiale.*

tibial crest. The sharp anterior margin of the shaft of the tibia. NA *margo anterior tibiae.*

tib·i·al·gia (tib"ee·al'jee·uh) *n.* [*tibia* + *-algia*]. Pain in the tibia.

tib·i·a·lis (tib"ee·ay'lis) *n.* [L., of the shinbone]. One of two muscles of the leg, tibialis anterior (NA *musculus tibialis anterior*) and tibialis posterior (NA *musculus tibialis posterior*). See also Table of Muscles in the Appendix.

tibialis phenomenon or **sign.** STRÜMPELL'S SIGN.

tibialis posterior reflex. With the patient prone and the foot in a neutral or slightly everted position and extended beyond the edge of the bed, tapping the tendon of the tibialis posterior muscle just above and behind the medial malleus is followed by inversion of the foot.

tibialis se·cun·dus (se·kun'dus). An occasional small muscle arising from the lower third of the body of the fibula and inserted into the capsule of the ankle joint.

tibial puncture. A puncture method used in children to secure smears of marrow cells. A sternal puncture needle is used in the middle of the shaft of the tibia.

tibio-. A combining form meaning *tibia, tibial.*

tib·io·cal·ca·ne·al (tib"ee·o·kal·kay'nee·ul) *adj.* Pertaining to the tibia and the calcaneus. See also *medial ligament.*

tib·io·fem·o·ral (tib"ee·o·fem'o·rul) *adj.* [*tibio-* + *femoral*]. Pertaining to the tibia and the femur.

tibiofemoral joint. The part of the knee joint involving the femur, the tibia, and the ligaments connecting them. Contr. *patellofemoral joint.*

tib·io·fib·u·lar (tib"ee·o·fib'yoo·lur) *adj.* [*tibio-* + *fibular*]. Pertaining to the tibia and the fibula.

tibiofibular articulation. 1. Either of the articulations between the tibia and the fibula; the proximal or superior tibiofibular articulation (NA *articulatio tibiofibularis*), between the lateral condyle of the tibia and the head of the fibula, or the distal or inferior tibiofibular articulation, the tibiofibular syndesmosis (NA *syndesmosis tibiofibularis*), joining the distal ends of the two bones. 2. Specifically, the proximal tibiofibular articulation, as distinguished from the tibiofibular syndesmosis.

tibiofibular ligament. Either of the two ligaments joining the distal ends of the tibia and the fibula, in the tibiofibular syndesmosis; the anterior tibiofibular ligament (NA *ligamentum tibiofibulare anterius*), connecting the ends of the two bones at their anterior adjacent margins, or the posterior tibiofibular ligament (NA *ligament tibiofibulare posterius*), which passes between them on the posterior face of the syndesmosis. See also *ligamentum capitis fibulae anterius, ligamentum capitis fibulae posterius, interosseous membrane of the leg.*

tibiofibular syndesmosis. The syndesmosis between the distal ends of the tibia and fibula, frequently containing an extension of the talocrural joint cavity; the distal or anterior tibiofibular articulation. NA *syndesmosis tibiofibularis, articulatio tibiofibularis.*

tib·io·na·vic·u·lar (tib″ee·o·na·vick′yoo·lur) *adj.* Pertaining to the tibia and the navicular. See also *medial ligament.*

tib·io·ta·lar (tib″ee·o·tay′lur) *adj.* Pertaining to the tibia and the talus. See also *medial ligament.*

ti·bric acid (tye′brick). 2-Chloro-5-[(*cis*-3,5-dimethylpiperidino)sulfonyl]benzoic acid, $C_{14}H_{18}ClNO_4S$, an antihyperlipidemic.

ti·bro·fan (tye′bro·fan) *n.* 4,4′,5-Tribromo-2-thiophenecarboxanilide, $C_{11}H_6Br_3NOS$, a germicide.

tic, *n.* [F.]. A habitual, irresistible, repetitious, stereotyped movement or complex of movements, of which the patient is aware but feels compelled to make in order to relieve tension. Syn. *habit spasm.*

ti·car·bo·dine (tye·kahr′bo·deen) *n.* α,α,α-Trifluoro-2,6-dimethylthio-1-piperidinecarboxy-*m*-toluidide, $C_{15}H_{19}F_3N_2S$, an anthelmintic.

ti·car·cil·lin (tye″kahr·sil′in) *n.* A penicillin derivative in which the phenoxymethylacetic acid portion is replaced by 3-thienylmalonic acid, $C_{15}H_{16}N_2O_6S_2$, an antibacterial used as the disodium salt.

ti·car·cil·lin cresyl. The *p*-cresylester of ticarcillin, $C_{22}H_{22}N_2O_6S_2$, an antibacterial used as the sodium salt.

tic con·vul·sif (kon·vul·seef′, F. kohⁿ·vuᵉl·seef′) [F.]. GILLES DE LA TOURETTE DISEASE.

tic de sa·laam (duh sa·lahm′) [F.]. Salaam spasm (= INFANTILE SPASM).

tic dou·lou·reux (doo·loo·ruh′) [F., painful spasm]. TRIGEMINAL NEURALGIA.

tick, *n.* An arthropod of the order Acarina infesting vertebrate animals. They are important vectors and reservoirs of rickettsial diseases and also transmit many viral, bacterial, and protozoal diseases. Toxins produced by the female before oviposition produce tick paralysis. The important genera are *Amblyomma, Argas, Boophilus, Dermacentor, Haemaphysalis, Hyalomma, Ixodes, Ornithodorus,* and *Rhipicephalus.*

tick-bite paralysis. A flaccid type of paralysis occurring in animals, and occasionally in man, during the attachment of certain species of ticks. The paralysis will disappear a few hours after removal of the tick. The cause is thought to be a neurotoxin injected by the engorging tick. Syn. *tick paralysis.*

tick-borne typhus fevers of Africa. Infections caused by *Rickettsia conorii,* closely related antigenically to the agent of Rocky Mountain spotted fever, transmitted by the bites of ixodid ticks, occurring in Africa and adjacent territory such as the Mediterranean, Black Sea, and Caspian Sea basins, and India. Includes boutonneuse fever, Marseilles fever, Kenya tick typhus fever, South African tick bite fever.

tick fever. ROCKY MOUNTAIN SPOTTED FEVER.

tick·ling, *n.* A rapid series of light, tactile stimulations of the skin or mucous membrane arousing a tingling sensation.

tick paralysis. TICK-BITE PARALYSIS.

tick typhus. ROCKY MOUNTAIN SPOTTED FEVER.

tic·la·tone (tick′luh·tone) *n.* 6-Chloro-1,2-benzisothiazolin-3-one, C_7H_4ClNOS, an antibacterial, antifungal.

tic of Gilles de la Tourette. GILLES DE LA TOURETTE DISEASE.

tic·po·lon·ga (tick″po·long′guh) *n.* [Sinhalese]. The venomous snake *Vipera russellii.*

tic ro·ta·toire (ro·ta·twahr′). [F.]. SPASMODIC TORTICOLLIS.

ti·cryn·a·fen (tye·krin′uh·fen) *n.* [2,3-Dichloro-4-(2-thenoyl)-phenoxy]acetic acid, $C_{13}H_8Cl_2O_4S$, a diuretic, uricosuric, antihypertensive.

tic·tol·o·gy (tick·tol′uh·jee) *n.* [Gk. *tik*tein, to bring forth, bear, + *-logy*]. OBSTETRICS.

t.i.d. Abbreviation for *ter in die,* three times a day.

tid·al air (tye′dul). TIDAL VOLUME.

tidal drainage. Drainage of a cavity, particularly a paralyzed urinary bladder, with an automatic irrigation apparatus which alternately fills and empties the cavity.

tidal volume. The amount of air moved by a single breath at any level of activity; normally, at rest, approximates 500 ml (resting tidal volume). Syn. *tidal air.*

tidal wave. The second systolic wave in bisferiens pulse. Contr. *percussion wave.*

tide, *n.* [OE. *tīd,* time, season]. A wave of increase in a given factor or constituent of body fluids, as acid tide, alkaline tide.

Tie·de·mann's gland (tee′duh·mahⁿn) [F. *Tiedemann,* German anatomist, 1781–1861]. The greater vestibular gland.

Tiedemann's nerve [F. *Tiedemann*]. A plexus of sympathetic nerve fibers derived from the ciliary nerves, surrounding the central artery of the retina.

Tie·tze's disease or **syndrome** (tee′tsuh) [A. *Tietze,* German surgeon, 1864–1927]. Painful nonsuppurative swelling of the rib cartilages.

Tigan. Trademark for trimethobenzamide, an antiemetic drug used as the hydrochloride salt.

ti·ger lily appearance. The speckled appearance of the myocardium observed in untreated pernicious anemia.

tiger snake. An Australian elapid snake, *Notechis scutatus,* marked with dark bands on yellow-buff and having a very powerful neurotoxic venom.

ti·ges·tol (tye·jes′tol) *n.* 19-Nor-17α-pregn-5(10)-en-20-yn-17-ol, $C_{20}H_{28}O$, a progestational steroid.

ti·gog·e·nin (ti·goj′e·nin) *n.* The steroid aglycone, $C_{27}H_{44}O_3$, of tigonin.

tig·o·nin (tig′o·nin) *n.* A saponin, $C_{56}H_{92}O_{27}$, from *Digitalis purpurea.* On acid hydrolysis it yields the steroid aglycone tigogenin, glucose, galactose, and rhamnose.

ti·groid (tye′groid) *adj.* [Gk. *tigroeidēs,* like a tiger]. 1. Striped or spotted. 2. Being or consisting of the chromophil substance constituting Nissl bodies.

tigroid bodies. The Nissl bodies or chromophil granules of nerve cells.

tigroid retina. The appearance of the retina often seen in darkly pigmented persons, in which darkish streaks or patches of choroidal pigment stand out between the choroidal vessels. It is nonpathological, in contrast to retinitis pigmentosa.

ti·grol·y·sis (tye·grol′i·sis) *n.* [*tigr*oid + *-lysis*]. Disintegration of the chromophil substance in a nerve cell.

ti·ki·ti·ki (tee′kee·tee′kee) *n.* Japanese name for rice polishings, a source of thiamine (vitamin B_1).

ti·let·a·mine (tye·let′uh·meen) *n.* 2-(Ethylamino)-2-(2-thienyl)cyclohexanone, $C_{12}H_{17}NOS$, an anesthetic, anticonvulsant, used as the hydrochloride salt.

til·i·dine (til′i·deen) *n.* (±)-Ethyl *trans*-2-(dimethylamino)-1-phenyl-3-cyclohexene-1-carboxylate, $C_{17}H_{23}NO_2$, an analgesic used as the hydrochloride salt.

Til·laux's disease (tee·yo′) [P. J. *Tillaux,* French surgeon, 1834–1904]. PHOCAS' DISEASE.

til·o·rone (til′o·rone) *n.* 2,7-Bis[2-(diethylamino)ethoxy]fluoren-9-one, $C_{25}H_{34}N_2O_3$, an antiviral used as the dihydrochloride salt.

tilt table. A table top on which a patient lies and which can be rotated to the vertical position, employed for a variety of therapeutic and investigative purposes.

tim·bre (tam'bur, tam'br) *n.* [F.]. The peculiar quality of a tone, other than pitch and intensity, that makes it distinctive. It depends upon the overtones of the vibrating body.

ti·mid·a·zole (tye·mid'uh·zole) *n.* 1-[2-(Ethylsulfonyl)ethyl]-2-methyl-5-nitroimidazole, $C_8H_{13}N_3O_4S$, an antiprotozoal.

ti·mo·lol (tye'mo·lole) *n.* (−)-1-(*tert*-Butylamino)-3-[(4-morpholino-1,2,5-thiadiazol-3-yl)oxy]-2-propanol, $C_{13}H_{24}N_4O_3S$, a β-receptor antiadrenergic used as the maleate salt.

tim·o·thy (tim'uth·ee) *n.* [after *Timothy* Hanson, who brought the seed to Carolina from New York about 1720]. A common name for *Phleum pratense,* the most important meadow grass in America. It flowers during June and July, shedding quantities of pollen, one of the more common causes of the seasonal rhinitis of early summer.

tin, *n.* Sn = 118.69. A silver-white metallic element, atomic number 50; powdered tin was at one time used as a mechanical anthelmintic.

Tinactin. Trademark for tolnaftate, a topically applied antifungal drug.

tin·cal (ting'kul, ·kal) *n.* [Malay *tingkal*]. Crude or native borax.

tin chloride. Stannous chloride, $SnCl_2.2H_2O$; used in chemical procedures as a reducing agent.

tinc·to·ri·al (tink·to'ree·ul) *adj.* [L. *tinctorius,* from *tingere,* to dye]. Pertaining to staining or dyeing.

tinc·tu·ra (tink·tew'ruh) *n.* [L.]. TINCTURE. Abbreviated, tr.

tinc·ture (tink'chur) *n.* [L. *tinctura,* from *tingere,* to dye, to moisten]. Alcoholic or hydroalcoholic solutions of medicinal substances, generally representing 10 or 20% (weight per volume) of drug and usually prepared by maceration or percolation of the drug with suitable menstruum. Abbreviated, tr.

Tindal. Trademark for acetophenazine, a mild tranquilizing agent used as the maleate salt.

tine, *n.* A fine pointed instrument, used in dentistry to explore fine crevices and cavities. Commonly called *explorer.*

tin·ea (tin'ee·uh) *n.* [L., worm, moth larva]. The lesions of dermatophytosis; RINGWORM.

tinea am·i·an·ta·cea (am''ee·an·tay'see·uh). A chronic scalp disease characterized by areas of dry heavy scales binding together the bases of the hairs; it is not a fungus infection.

tinea bar·bae (bahr'bee). Ringworm of the bearded areas of the face and neck, caused by various species of *Trichophyton* and *Microsporum.* Syn. *tinea sycosis.*

tinea cap·i·tis (kap'i·tis). Fungus infection of the scalp and hair. Caused by several species of *Trichophyton* and *Microsporum.* Syn. *tinea tonsurans.*

tinea cir·ci·na·ta (sur''si·nay'tuh). TINEA CORPORIS.

tinea cor·po·ris (kor'po·ris). A fungus infection involving the glabrous skin. Caused by various species of *Trichophyton* and *Microsporum.* Syn. *tinea circinata.* See also *tinea glabrosa.*

tinea cru·ris (kroo'ris). A fungus infection involving the skin of the groin, perineum, and perianal regions. Caused by *Epidermophyton floccosum* and several species of *Trichophyton.* Syn. *gum itch, jockey itch, laundryman's itch.*

tinea de·cal·vans (dee·kal'vanz). ALOPECIA AREATA.

tinea fa·ci·a·le (fay''shee·ay'lee). Fungous infection of the skin of the face, especially of the glabrous skin.

tinea fa·ci·ei (fay''shee·ee'eye, fay'shee·eye). TINEA FACIALE.

tinea fa·vo·sa (fa·vo'suh). FAVUS.

tinea gla·bro·sa (gla·bro'suh). Fungus infection of the nonhairy skin. Included under this heading are tinea corporis, tinea cruris, tinea versicolor, erythrasma, and dermatophytosis of the hands and feet.

tinea im·bri·ca·ta (im''bri·kay'tuh). A superficial fungus disease of the tropics characterized by the presence of concentric rings of pruritic papulosquamous patches scattered over the body. Caused by *Trichophyton concentricum.* Syn. *gogo, scaly ringworm, tropical tinea circinata, Malabar itch.*

tinea kerion. KERION CELSI.

tinea manus. Fungus infection of the hand, usually chronic, due to *Trichophyton purpureum.*

tinea ni·gra (nye'gruh). A contagious cutaneous fungus infection caused by *Cladosporium mansonii* in the East and *Cladosporium werneckii* in the Americas, clinically characterized by its black or dark-brown coloration and its predominant occurrence on the trunk, neck, or palmar regions, though other sites may be involved. Syn. *pityriasis nigra, microsporosis nigra.*

tinea no·do·sa (no·do'suh). PIEDRA.

tinea pedis. A fungus infection of the feet, especially the webs of the toes and the soles. Caused by *Epidermophyton floccosum,* various species of *Trichophyton,* and rarely by *Microsporum.* See also *dermatophytosis.*

tinea sycosis. TINEA BARBAE.

tinea ton·su·rans (ton'sue·ranz). TINEA CAPITIS.

tinea un·gui·um (ung'gwee·um). A chronic fungus infection involving the nails of the hands and feet. Caused by *Epidermophyton floccosum,* various species of *Trichophyton,* and *Candida albicans.*

tinea ver·si·co·lor (vur''si·ko'lor, vur'si·kul''ur). A chronic superficial fungus infection of the skin, usually of the trunk. It is caused by *Malassezia furfur.*

Ti·nel's sign (tee·nel') [J. *Tinel,* French neurosurgeon, 1879–1952]. A tingling sensation in the distal part of an extremity in response to pressure or percussion over the site of a partially divided nerve; it signifies regeneration of a nerve.

tin·gle, *n.* A pricking or stinging sensation; the feeling of a slight, sharp, and sudden thrill, as of pain; acanthesthesia.

ti·nid·a·zole (tye·nid'uh·zole) *n.* 1-[2-(Ethylsulfonyl)ethyl]-2-methyl-5-nitroimidazole, $C_8H_{13}N_3O_4S$, an antiprotozoal.

tin·ni·tus (ti·nigh'tus) *n.* [L., from *tinnire,* to ring, jingle]. A ringing in one or both ears. Buzzing, hissing, humming, whistling, roaring, or clicking sounds are also reported. Syn. *tinnitus aurium.*

tinnitus au·ri·um (aw'ree·um) [NL., ringing of the ears]. TINNITUS.

tinnitus cra·nii (kray'nee·eye). A subjective sound in the head, other than one arising in the ear.

tin oxide. Stannic oxide, SnO_2; formerly used in combination with metallic tin for the treatment of furunculosis.

tint·om·e·ter (tint·om'e·tur) *n.* [*tint* + *-meter*]. An apparatus used in hemoglobinometry. A film of whole blood is arranged between two glass plates, and compared with a series of tinted glasses mounted on a disk.

ti·o·do·ni·um chloride (tye''o·do'nee·um). (*p*-Chlorophenyl)-2-thenyliodonium chloride, $C_{10}H_7Cl_2IS$, an antibacterial.

ti·o·per·i·done (tye''o·perr'i·dohn) *n.* 3-[4-[4-[*o*-(Propylthio)phenyl]-1-piperazinyl]-butyl]-2,4-(1*H*,3*H*)-quinazolinedione, $C_{25}H_{32}N_4O_2S$, a tranquilizer used as the monohydrochloride salt.

ti·pren·o·lol (tye·pren'o·lole) *n.* (±)-1-Isopropylamino)-3-[*o*-(methylthio)phenoxy]-2-propanol, $C_{13}H_{21}NO_2S$, a β-receptor antiadrenergic, used as the hydrochloride salt.

Ti·pu·li·dae (ti·pew'li·dee) *n.pl.* A family of the order Diptera, the crane flies. Their importance as disease vectors is not established.

ti·queur (tee·kur') *n.* [F.]. A person exhibiting tics.

ti·quin·a·mide (tye·kwin'uh·mide) *n.* 5,6,7,8-Tetrahydro-3-methylthio-8-quinolinecarboxamide, $C_{11}H_{14}N_2S$, a gastric anticholinergic, used as the hydrochloride salt.

tire, *v.* To become weary; to become exhausted; used extensively by the medical profession and laymen in reference to muscular and mental fatigue, general bodily and mental exhaustion.

tires. TREMBLES.

ti·sane (tee·zahn′) *n.* [F., from L. *ptisana,* barley groats, from Gk. *ptisanē*]. Any decoction or infusion of leaves or flowers that is used for slight medicinal effect.

Tis·dall method [F. F. *Tisdall,* Canadian pediatrician, b. 1893]. KRAMER-TISDALL METHOD.

Ti·se·li·us apparatus (tee·seʸ′lee·ŏŏs) [A. *Tiselius,* Swedish biochemist, b. 1902]. An apparatus that permits the measurement of electrophoretic mobilities of proteins by use of moving-boundary electrophoresis. The cell is divided into compartments which permit isolation of the components separated by the electric current.

Tis·sot spirometer or **gasometer.** A large bell-type spirometer (capacity 100 liters or more) used for basal metabolism determination. The subject inspires atmospheric air and expires into the spirometer. At the end of the test period, the total volume of expired air is measured and samples are analyzed for CO_2 and O_2. The apparatus can be used to measure maximum breathing capacity.

tis·sue (tish′oo) *n.* [OF. *tissu,* from L. *texere,* to weave]. An aggregation of similar cells and their intercellular substance.

tissue culture. The growing of tissue cells in artificial media.

tissue dose. Radiant energy absorbed by a designated tissue at a point in question, measured in ergs per gram.

tissue equivalent ionization chamber. An ionization chamber in which the materials of the walls and electrodes are so selected as to produce ionization essentially equivalent to that characteristic of the tissue under consideration.

tissue immunity. LOCAL IMMUNITY.

tissue protein. The part of the body protein present in the solid tissues as distinguished from the circulating protein of the blood.

tissue space. A cavity or space in connective tissue.

tissue thromboplastin. Any of several lipid-rich clot accelerators prepared from tissues, particularly from brain or lung. Such preparations are effective in the absence of factors VIII, IX, XI, and XII, but require factors V, VII, and X for maximum acceleration of clotting.

tis·su·lar (tish′yoo·lur) *adj.* Pertaining to the tissues of living organisms.

ti·ta·ni·um (tye·tay′nee·um, ti·tay′nee·um) *n.* [NL., from Gk. *Titanes,* Titans, sons of the earth]. Ti = 47.90. A very hard, dark-gray, lustrous, metallic element, atomic number 22, density 4.51, used in certain alloys to impart toughness.

titanium dioxide. TiO_2; used as a protectant against sunburn.

ti·ter, ti·tre (tye′tur) *n.* [F. *titre,* standard; title]. 1. *In chemistry,* an expression of the strength of a volumetric solution. 2. The amount of one substance that corresponds to, reacts with, or is otherwise equivalent to a stated quantity of another substance.

tit·il·la·tion (tit″i·lay′shun) *n.* [L. *titillatio,* from *titillare,* to tickle]. Tickling; the responses produced by tickling.

ti·tra·tion (tye·tray′shun) *n.* [F. *titrer,* to titrate, from *titre,* titer]. An operation involving the measurement of the concentration or volume of a standard solution required to react chemically or immunologically with a substance being analyzed or standardized. —**ti·trate** (tye′trate) *v.*

titre. TITER.

ti·trim·e·ter (tye·trim′e·tur) *n.* An apparatus or instrument for use in titrimetry.

ti·trim·e·try (tye·trim′e·tree) *n.* [*titr*ation + *-metry*]. Quantitative measurement or analysis by titration. —**ti·tri·met·ric** (tye″tri·met′rick) *adj.*

tit·u·ba·tion (tit′yoo·bay′shun) *n.* [L. *titubatio,* from *titubare,* to stagger]. Unsteadiness of posture, especially in diseases of the cerebellum and its connections; manifested as a rhythmic instability and swaying of the trunk or of the head on the trunk.

Tity·us (tit′ee·us) *n.* [L. *Tityos,* mythical giant]. A genus of Scorpionida.

Tityus ser·ru·la·tus (serr″yoo·lay′tus). A poisonous scorpion of Brazil.

Tityus trin·i·ta·lis (trin″i·tay′lis). A poisonous black scorpion of Trinidad.

tix·a·nox (tick′suh·nocks) *n.* 7-(Methylsulfinyl)-9-oxoxanthene-2-carboxylic acid, $C_{15}H_{10}O_5S$, an antiallergic.

TKD Abbreviation for *tokodynamometer.*

TKG Abbreviation for *tokograph.*

Tl Symbol for thallium.

T loop. The vectorcardiographic representation of ventricular repolarization.

T lymphocyte. A lymphocyte whose differentiation occurs largely in the thymus. It circulates through the blood, lymph, and lymphatic tissue and is primarily responsible for cell-mediated immunity. Syn. *T cell.* See also *cell-mediated immunity.*

Tm Symbol for thulium.

Tn Symbol for thoron.

TNT Abbreviation for *trinitrotoluene.*

T.O. An abbreviation for *original tuberculin* or *old tuberculin.*

toad poisons. The toxic constituents present in the skin glands of various toads, principally bufagin, bufotalin, and bufotoxin.

toad skin. A dry, roughened skin associated with vitamin-A deficiency.

toad test. MALE-TOAD TEST.

to-and-fro murmur. A pericardial murmur heard during both systole and diastole.

to·bac·co (tuh·back′o) *n.,* pl. **tobaccos, tobaccoes** [Sp. *tabaco,* of obscure origin]. A plant, *Nicotiana tabacum,* of the family Solanaceae, the dried leaves of which contain an alkaloid, nicotine. Formerly employed as an enema to overcome intestinal obstruction.

tobacco amblyopia. TOXIC AMBLYOPIA.

tobacco fleck. GAMNA-GANDY BODY.

tobacco mosaic virus. A specific virus causing the mosaic disease of tobacco, frequently used in virus studies.

To·bey-Ay·er test [G. L. *Tobey,* Jr., U.S. otolaryngologist, 1881–1947; and J. B. *Ayer,* U.S. neurologist, b. 1882]. A test for lateral sinus thrombosis, based on changes in the pressure of the spinal fluid during compression of one or both internal jugular veins.

to·bra·my·cin (to″bruh·migh′sin) *n.* A streptamine antibacterial, $C_{18}H_{37}N_5O_9$, produced by *Streptomyces tenebrarius.*

Tobruk plaster. A combination of the long Thomas splint with plaster fixation of the thigh, leg, and foot for the emergency transportation of patients with wounds and fractures of the lower extremity.

to·cam·phyl (to·kam′fil) *n.* Diethanolamine salt of the mono-(+)-camphoric acid ester of *p*-tolylmethylcarbinol, $C_{19}H_{26}O_4.C_4H_{11}NO_2$, a choleretic drug.

Toclase. Trademark for carbetapentane, an antitussive drug used as the citrate salt.

toco-, toko- [Gk. *tokos,* from *tiktein,* to bear, give birth]. A combining form meaning (a) *childbirth, labor;* (b) *offspring.*

toco·al·gog·ra·phy (to″ko·al·gog′ruh·fee, tock″o·) *n.* [*toco-* + *algo-* + *-graphy*]. TOCOGRAPHY.

toco·dy·na·mom·e·ter, toko·dy·na·mom·e·ter (to″ko·dye″nuh·mom′e·tur, tock″o·) *n.* [*toco-* + *dynamometer*]. An instrument for measuring the amplitude, duration, and frequency of uterine muscular contraction, as during labor. Abbreviated, TKD

toco·graph, toko·graph (to′ko·graf, tock″o·) *n.* [*toco-* + *-graph*]. A record taken by a tocodynamometer. Abbreviated, TKG

to·cog·ra·phy, to·kog·ra·phy (to·kog′ruh·fee) *n.* [*toco-* + *-graphy*]. The making and interpreting of graphic recordings of the amplitude, duration, and frequency of uterine muscular contractions during labor. —**toco·graph·ic, toko·graph·ic** (to″ko·graf′ick) *adj.*

to·col·o·gist, to·kol·o·gist (to·kol′uh·jist) *n.* OBSTETRICIAN.

to·col·o·gy, to·kol·o·gy (to·kol'uh·jee) *n.* [*toco-* + *-logy*]. OBSTETRICS.

toco·ma·nia, toko·ma·nia (to''ko·may'nee·uh, tock''o·) *n.* [*toco-* + *-mania*]. PUERPERAL PSYCHOSIS.

to·com·e·try, to·kom·e·try (to·kom'e·tree) *n.* [*toco-* + *-metry*]. A study of the amplitude, duration, and frequency of the uterine muscular contractions, as during labor, with a tocodynamometer. —**tocome·ter, tokome·ter** (·tur) *n.*

to·coph·er·ol (to·kof'ur·ol) *n.* [*toco-* + Gk. *pherein*, to bring, carry, + *-ol*]. Any one of several related substances, occurring naturally in certain oils and also prepared by synthesis, that have vitamin E activity. The most potent of these, alpha tocopherol, is 2,5,7,8-tetramethyl-2-(4',8',12'-trimethyltridecyl)-6-chromanol, $C_{29}H_{50}O_2$; the *d-* form is more active than the *l-* form.

to·coph·er·so·lan (to·kof''ur·so'lan) *n.* (+)-α-Tocopheryl polyethylene glycol 1000 succinate, $C_{33}H_{54}O_5(C_2H_4O)_n$ (n=approximately 22), a water-miscible vitamin E.

toco·pho·bia, toko·pho·bia (to''ko·fo'bee·uh, tock''o·) *n.* [*toco-* + *-phobia*]. Undue dread of childbirth.

to·cus, to·kus (to'kus) *n.* [NL., from Gk. *tokos*]. CHILDBIRTH.

Todd's paralysis [R. B. *Todd*, English physician, 1809–1860]. A temporary localized paralysis that sometimes follows a focal seizure; thought to be due to an exhaustion of the neurons of the epileptic focus.

toe, *n.* [Gmc. *taikhwo* (perhaps rel. to L. *digitus*)]. A digit of the foot.

toe-drop, *n.* DROPPED FOOT.

toe phenomenon. BABINSKI SIGN (1).

to·fen·a·cin (to·fen'uh·sin) *n.* *N*-Methyl-2-[(*o*-methyl-α-phenylbenzyl)oxy] ethylamine, $C_{17}H_{21}NO$, an anticholinergic used as the hydrochloride salt.

Tofranil. Trademark for imipramine, an antidepressant drug used as the hydrochloride salt.

to·ga·vi·rus (to'guh·vye''rus) *n.* [L. *toga*, coat]. A spherical, encapsulated RNA virus that is categorized as either group A or group B. Group A viruses are larger and produce eastern and western equine encephalitis; group B viruses produce various illnesses including encephalitis, hemorrhagic diseases and severe systemic illnesses.

toi·let training. The teaching and encouraging of control of bladder and bowel functions to a child, usually at a critical age of psychosexual development and formation of the child's personality. Since this often marks the first effort by the parents (or surrogates) to control the child, and the child's first good opportunity to resist control, it has been speculated that many adult attitudes about authority, anger, cleanliness, compulsiveness, duty, money, and other restrictive or obligatory life experiences arise from this period.

Toi·son's solution (twahⁿ·zohⁿ') [J. *Toison*, French histologist, 1858–1950]. A diluent for erythrocyte counting containing sodium chloride, sodium sulfate, glycerin, crystal violet, and water.

To·ke·lau ringworm (to''ke·lah'oo) [after *Tokelau* Islands, South Pacific Ocean]. TINEA IMBRICATA.

toko-. See *toco-*.

tokodynamometer. TOCODYNAMOMETER.

tokograph. TOCOGRAPH.

tokography. TOCOGRAPHY.

tokologist. Tocologist (= OBSTETRICIAN).

tokology. Tocology (= OBSTETRICS).

tokomania. Tocomania (= PUERPERAL PSYCHOSIS).

tokometry. TOCOMETRY.

tokophobia. TOCOPHOBIA.

-tokous [Gk. *tokos*, childbirth]. A combining form meaning *producing young* of a specified character, number, or number of kinds.

tokus. Tocus (= CHILDBIRTH).

to·lam·o·lol (to·lam'o·lole) *n.* *p*-[2-[[2-Hydroxy-3-(*o*-tolyloxy)propyl]amino]ethoxy]benzamide, $C_{19}H_{24}N_2O_4$, an antiarrhythmic cardiac depressant and coronary vasodilator.

tol·a·za·mide (to·lay'zuh·mide, ·mid, tol·ay') *n.* 1-(Hexahydro-1*H*-azepin-l-yl)-3-(*p*-tolylsulfonyl)urea, $C_{14}H_{21}N_3O_3S$, an orally effective hypoglycemic drug.

tol·az·o·line (tol·az'o·leen) *n.* 2-Benzyl-2-imidazoline, $C_{10}H_{12}N_2$, a sympathetic blocking and peripheral vasodilator drug; used as the hydrochloride salt.

tol·bu·ta·mide (tol·bew'tuh·mide) *n.* 1-Butyl-3-(*p*-tolylsulfonyl)urea, $C_{12}H_{18}N_2O_3S$, an orally effective hypoglycemic drug.

tol·ci·clate (tohl·sigh'klate) *n.* *o*-(1,2,3,4-Tetrahydro-1,4-methanonaphthalen-6-yl) *m*,*N*-dimethylthiocarbanilate, $C_{20}H_{21}NOS$, a topical antifungal.

Tolectin. A trademark for tolmetin sodium.

tol·er·ance, *n.* [L. *tolerantia*, from *tolerare*, to endure]. 1. The ability of enduring or being less responsive to the influence of a drug or poison, particularly when acquired by continued use of the substance. 2. The allowable deviation from a standard, as the range of variation permitted for the content of a drug in one of its dosage forms. 3. IMMUNOLOGIC TOLERANCE.

tolerance dose. *In radiology*, the radiation dose a tumor bed or adjacent organs will tolerate without gross permanent damage. Compare *permissible dose*.

tol·er·ant, *adj.* 1. Possessing tolerance. 2. Able to survive or grow in a specified environment, as: acid-tolerant.

tol·er·a·tion, *n.* TOLERANCE. —**tol·er·ate,** *v.*

tol·ero·gen·ic (tol''ur·o·jen'ick) *adj.* Able to induce immunologic tolerance.

Toleron. Trademark for ferrous fumarate, used for treatment of iron-deficiency anemias.

Tolinase. Trademark for tolazamide, an orally effective hypoglycemic drug.

to·lin·date (to·lin'date) *n.* *o*-5-indanyl *m*,*N*-dimethylthiocarbanilate, $C_{18}H_{19}NOS$, an antifungal.

to·li·o·di·um chloride (to''lye·o'dee·um). Di-*p*-tolyliodonium chloride, $C_{14}H_{14}ClI$, a veterinary food additive.

Tol·lens' test (tohl'ensss) [B. C. G. *Tollens*, German chemist, 1841–1918]. A test for detecting the presence of galactose, in which phloroglucinol is added to equal volumes of the unknown and hydrochloric acid and the mixture is heated. Galactose, pentose, or glycuronic acid will be indicated by the appearance of a red color. Differentiation is by means of spectroscopic examination.

tol·met·in (tohl'met·in) *n.* 1-Methyl-5-*p*-toluoylpyrrole-2-acetic acid, $C_{15}H_{15}NO_3$, an anti-inflammatory, also used as the sodium salt.

tol·naf·tate (tol·naf'tate) *n.* *O*-2-Naphthyl *m*,*N*-dimethylthiocarbanilate, $C_{19}H_{17}NOS$, a topically applied antifungal drug.

to·lo·ni·um chloride (to·lo'nee·um). 3-Amino-7-dimethylamino-2-methylphenazathionium chloride, the dye toluidine blue O; has been used to reduce the bleeding tendency in certain hemorrhagic conditions associated with excessive amounts of heparinoid substances in the blood.

tol·pyr·ra·mide (tol·pirr'uh·mide) *n.* *N*-*p*-Tolylsulfonyl-1-pyrrolidinecarboxamide, $C_{12}H_{16}N_2O_3S$, an orally effective hypoglycemic agent.

to·lu balsam (to·loo') [after Santiago de *Tolú*, Colombia]. A balsam obtained from *Myroxylon balsamum*, a South American tree of the Leguminosae. It contains cinnamic and benzoic acids, esters of these acids, and resins. Has been used as a mild expectorant.

tol·u·ene (tol'yoo·een) *n.* [*tolu* + *-ene*]. Methylbenzene, $C_6H_5CH_3$, a colorless liquid obtained chiefly from coal tar. Used as a solvent and reagent.

to·lu·ic acid (to·lew'ick). Any of four isomeric, crystalline acids: *o*-toluic, *m*-toluic, *p*-toluic, all represented by the formula $CH_3C_6H_4COOH$, and α-toluic, of the formula $C_6H_5CH_2COOH$, better known as phenylacetic acid.

to·lu·i·dine (to·lew'i·deen, ·din) *n.* Aminotoluene,

$NH_2C_6H_4CH_3$, existing in three isomeric forms. The *o-* and *m-* isomers are liquids; the *p-* is a solid.

toluidine blue O. A basic dye of the thiazine series used in Albert's stain for the diphtheria organism, in the panchrome stain, and for many other purposes. Syn. *methylene blue O.*

tol·u·ol (tol'yoo·ol) *n.* TOLUENE.

tol·u·yl·ene (tol'yoo·i·leen) *n.* STILBENE.

tol·yl (tol'il) *n.* The univalent radical $—C_6H_4CH_3$.

to·ma·tine (to'muh·teen) *n.* A glycosidal alkaloid, isolated from the tomato plant, having antifungal activity.

-tome [Gk. *tomos,* cutting, sharp; a cut, slice]. A combining form designating (a) *a part or a section;* (b) *an instrument for cutting.*

to·men·tum (to·men'tum) *n.* [L., cushion stuffing]. The network of small blood vessels of the pia mater penetrating the cortex of the brain. Syn. *tomentum cerebri.*

tomentum ce·re·bri (serr'e·brye). TOMENTUM.

Tomes's fibers [J. *Tomes,* English dental surgeon, 1815–1895]. ODONTOBLASTIC PROCESSES.

Tomes's granular layer [J. *Tomes*]. GRANULAR LAYER OF TOMES.

Tomes's process [C. S. *Tomes,* English dental surgeon, 1846–1928]. AMELOBLASTIC PROCESS.

Tom·ma·sel·li's syndrome (toʰm·maʰ·zel'lee) [S. *Tommaselli,* Italian physician, 1830–1902]. Hematuria and pyrexia, due to an overdose of quinine.

tomo- [Gk. *tomos,* slice, section]. A combining form meaning (a) *section, sectional;* (b) *surgical operation.*

to·mo·gram (to'muh·gram) *n.* [*tomo-* + *-gram*]. A radiograph obtained by sectional radiography.

to·mog·ra·phy (to·mog'ruh·fee) *n.* [*tomo-* + *-graphy*]. SECTIONAL RADIOGRAPHY. **—to·mo·graph·ic** (to''mo·graf'ick) *adj.*

to·mo·ma·nia (to''mo·may'nee·uh) *n.* [*tomo-* + *mania*]. 1. An abnormal desire to have a surgical procedure performed upon oneself. 2. An abnormal wish to perform surgical procedures.

to·mo·to·cia (to''mo·to'shee·uh, ·see·uh) *n.* [*tomo-* + Gk. *tokos,* birth]. CESAREAN SECTION.

-tomy [Gk. *tomē*]. A combining form meaning *cutting, incision, section.*

ton·al (to'nul) *adj.* Of or pertaining to tone, or to a tone or tones.

tonal discrimination. The auditory perception of pitch differences.

tonal islands. Isolated areas in the range of human hearing in which some persons with practically no hearing have an appreciation of pure tones at maximum intensity.

to·na·pha·sia (to''nuh·fay'zhuh, ·zee·uh, ton''uh·) *n.* [Gk. *tonos,* tone, + *aphasia*]. AMUSIA.

tone, *n.* [L. *tonus,* from Gk. *tonos*]. 1. A sound characterized by a definite pitch or harmonic combination of pitches. 2. The normal state of healthy tension and vigor in the body or in a part; specifically, TONUS. Adj. *tonal, tonic.*

tone deafness. Relative inability to distinguish between musical tones of different pitch; due to abnormalities of the end organ, as opposed to amusia, which is due to lesion of the cerebral cortex. See also *sensory amusia.*

tongue, *n.* [Gmc. *tung-* (rel. to OL. *dingua* → Cl.L. *lingua*)]. The movable muscular organ attached to the floor of the mouth, and concerned in tasting, masticating, swallowing, and speaking. It consists of a number of muscles, and is covered by mucous membrane from which project numerous papillae, and in which are placed the terminal organs of taste. NA *lingua.*

tongue apraxia. Inability to carry out tongue movements, such as protrusion, on command, but preservation of the associated movements in eating or licking; a frequent accompaniment of Broca's aphasia.

tongue depressor. A spatula for pushing down the tongue during the examination of the mouth and throat.

tongue swallowing. The falling back of the mandible and loss of muscle tone of the tongue so that it falls backward, producing respiratory obstruction, seen in states of unconsciousness such as during generalized convulsions and in coma.

tongue thrust. The constant protrusion of the tongue between the gums and teeth; seen normally in early infancy, but pathologically later in many states of mental retardation, notably in Down's syndrome and in cretinism.

tongue-tie, *n.* A congenital abnormality of the frenulum of the tongue, interfering with its mobility.

tongue worm. PENTASTOME.

-tonia. A combining form designating *a condition or degree of tonus.*

ton·ic (ton'ick) *adj. & n.* [Gk. *tonikos,* of stretching]. 1. Pertaining to tone; producing normal tone or tension. 2. Pertaining to or characterized by continuous tension or contraction. Contr. *clonic.* 3. An agent or drug given to improve the normal tone of an organ or of the patient generally.

tonic-clonic, *adj.* Pertaining to muscular spasms, especially as seen in generalized seizures, in which there is a tonic and a clonic phase.

tonic-clonic convulsion or **seizure.** Any convulsive seizure with a phase of tonic contraction and one of clonic contraction; almost always a generalized seizure. See also *generalized seizure.*

tonic contraction. TONIC SPASM.

tonic convulsion. TONIC SEIZURE.

tonic diplegia. SPASTIC DIPLEGIA.

tonic fit. TONIC SEIZURE.

tonic grasp reflex. GRASP REFLEX.

to·nic·i·ty (to·nis'i·tee) *n.* 1. The condition of normal tone or tension of an organ. 2. The condition of a solution with respect to its being hypertonic, isotonic, or hypotonic.

tonic labyrinthine reflexes. The acceleratory and righting reflexes.

tonic neck reflexes. Rotation or deviation of the head causes extension of the limbs on the same side as the chin, and flexion of the opposite extremities. Dorsiflexion of the head produces increased extensor tonus of the upper extremities and relaxation of the lower limbs, and ventroflexion of the head, the reverse. Seen normally in incomplete forms in the very young infant, and thereafter in patients with a lesion at the midbrain level or above.

ton·i·co·clon·ic (ton''i·ko·klon'ick) *adj.* TONIC-CLONIC.

tonic postural epilepsy. Epilepsy characterized by tonic seizures.

tonic pupil. ADIE'S PUPIL.

tonic reflex. 1. Any reflex involved in the establishment and maintenance of the posture or attitude of the individual. 2. Any sustained reflex.

tonic seizure. A major generalized seizure in which the motor manifestations are limited to a tonic spasm of the entire musculature; characterized by a forceful closure of the jaws, often with biting of the tongue, and a piercing cry, as air is forced through closed vocal cords.

tonic spasm. A spasm that persists without relaxation for some time.

tonic treatment. Treatment of disease by tonics.

To·ni-Fan·co·ni syndrome (toʰ'nee, faʰng·ko'nee) [G. de *Toni* and G. *Fanconi*]. FANCONI SYNDROME.

ton·i·tro·pho·bia (ton''i·tro·fo'bee·uh) *n.* [L. *tonitrus,* thunder, + *-phobia*]. Abnormal fear of thunder.

ton·ka bean (tonk'uh). The seed of *Dipteryx odorata,* a tree of South America; it contains coumarin, and is used as a flavoring agent.

tono- [Gk. *tonos,* tension, tone]. A combining form meaning (a) *tone;* (b) *pressure.*

tono·clon·ic (ton''o·klon'ick) *adj.* TONIC-CLONIC.

tono·fi·brils (to''no·figh'brilz) *n.pl.* [*tono-* + *fibrils*]. Delicate fibrils, found particularly in epithelial cells, which converge on desmosomes.

tono·gram (to′nuh·gram, ton′o·) *n.* [*tono-* + *-gram*]. A record made by a tonograph.

tono·graph (to′nuh·graf, ton′o·) *n.* [*tono-* + *-graph*]. A device for determining or recording pressure.

to·nog·ra·phy (to·nog′ruh·fee) *n.* [*tono-* + *-graphy*]. Continuous recording of pressure with an electric tonometer; used especially in measuring intraocular pressure.

to·nom·e·ter (to·nom′e·tur) *n.* [*tono-* + *-meter*]. 1. An instrument to measure tension, as that of the eyeball. 2. An instrument used to equilibrate samples of fluid, as blood, with gases at known concentrations.

to·nom·e·try (to·nom′e·tree) *n.* The measurement of pressure or tension with a tonometer. See also *applanation tonometry, digital tonometry, indentation tonometry.*

tono·plast (to′no·plast, ton′o·) *n.* [*tono-* + *-plast*]. A small intracellular body that builds up strongly osmotic substances within itself and in this way swells to a small vacuole.

ton·os·cil·log·ra·phy (to·nos″si·log′ruh·fee) *n.* [*tono-* + *oscillography*]. A method of automatically recording blood pressure in the extremities.

tono·scope (to′nuh·skope) *n.* [*tono-* + *scope*]. An instrument for examination of the interior of the cranium by means of sound.

ton·sil (ton′sil) *n.* [L. *tonsillae,* tonsils]. 1. Aggregated lymph nodules and associated lymph vessels surrounding crypts or depressions of the pharyngeal mucosa; specifically, the palatine tonsil. See also *lingual tonsil, palatine tonsil, pharyngeal tonsil, tubal tonsil.* 2. The tonsilla of the cerebellum; TONSILLA (1). —**tonsil·lar** (·ur) *adj.*

tonsill-, tonsillo-. A combining form meaning *tonsil.*

ton·sil·la (ton·sil′uh) *n.*, pl. **tonsil·lae** (·ee) [L.]. 1. (of the cerebellum:) A small lobe of the cerebellar hemisphere, on its inferior medial aspect. NA *tonsilla cerebelli.* 2. TONSIL (1).

tonsilla ce·re·bel·li (serr·e·bel′eye) [NA]. The tonsilla of the cerebellum; TONSILLA (1).

tonsilla lin·gua·lis (ling·gway′lis) [NA]. LINGUAL TONSIL.

tonsilla pa·la·ti·na (pal″uh·tye′nuh) [NA]. PALATINE TONSIL.

tonsilla pha·ryn·gea (fa·rin′jee·uh) [NA]. ADENOID (3).

tonsillar arches. The palatoglossal and palatopharyngeal arches.

tonsillar calculus. A calcified mass of detritus in a tonsillar crypt.

tonsillar crypt. A deep epithelium-lined invagination in the palatine or lingual tonsils.

tonsillar fossa. The depression between the palatoglossal and palatopharyngeal arches, in which the palatine tonsil is situated. It is approximately at the site of the second visceral pouch. NA *fossa tonsillaris.*

tonsillar herniation. *Informal.* CEREBELLAR PRESSURE CONE.

tonsillar plexus. A nerve network whose fibers are distributed to the tonsils, fauces, and nearby region of the soft palate.

tonsilla tu·ba·ria (tew·bair′ee·uh) [NA]. TUBAL TONSIL.

ton·sil·lec·tome (ton″si·leck′tome) *n.* An instrument for the performance of tonsillectomy; TONSILLOTOME.

ton·sil·lec·to·my (ton″si·leck′tuh·mee) *n.* [*tonsill-* + *-ectomy*]. Removal of the palatine tonsils.

ton·sil·li·tis (ton″si·lye′tis) *n.* [*tonsill-* + *-itis*]. Inflammation of the tonsils. —**ton·sil·lit·ic** (ton″sil·lit′ick) *adj.*

tonsillo-. See *tonsill-.*

ton·sil·lo·lith (ton·sil′o·lith) *n.* [*tonsillo-* + *-lith*]. A concretion within a tonsil.

ton·sil·lo·phar·yn·gi·tis (ton″si·lo·făr″in·jye′tis) *n.* [*tonsillo-* + *pharyngitis*]. Inflammation of the tonsils and pharynx.

ton·sil·lo·tome (ton·sil′uh·tome) *n.* [*tonsillo-* + *-tome*]. An instrument for removing a tonsil.

ton·sil·lot·o·my (ton″si·lot′uh·mee) *n.* [*tonsillo-* + *-tomy*]. The operation of cutting into or removing part of a tonsil.

ton·sil·lo·ty·phoid (ton″si·lo·tye′foid, ton·sil″o·) *n.* [*tonsillo-* + *typhoid*]. Typhoid fever complicated with a membranous or pseudomembranous deposit on the tonsils.

ton·sil·sec·tor (ton″sil·seck′tur) *n.* [*tonsil* + L. *sector,* cutter]. A tonsillotome consisting of a pair of circular or oval scissor blades moving inside a guarding ring.

ton·sure (ton′shur) *n.* [L. *tonsura,* from *tondere,* to shear, clip, shave]. The shaving or removal of the hair from the crown of the head.

to·nus (to′nus) *n.* [L., tone]. The sustained partial contraction present in relaxed skeletal muscles; the slight resistance that normal, relaxed muscle offers to passive movement. Compare *clonus.*

tooth, *n.*, pl. **teeth.** [Gmc. *tanth-* (rel. to L. *dent-* and to Gk. *odont-*)] One of the calcified organs supported by the alveolar processes and gingivae of both jaws, serving to masticate food, aid speech, and influence facial contour. Each tooth consists of an enamel-covered crown, a single, bifid, or trifid cementum-covered root, a neck (the conjunction of crown and root), and a pulp chamber which contains the dental pulp with its nerves and vessels and is surrounded by a mass of dentin. NA *dens,* pl. *dentes.*

tooth·ache, *n.* Any pain in or about a tooth. Syn. *odontalgia.*

tooth ankylosis. Fixation of the joint formed by a tooth and the alveolus, occurring when the periodontal ligament has been destroyed and the dentin or cementum is directly fused to the alveolar bone.

tooth bud. Primordium of a dental organ; arising from the dental lamina, it is the earliest manifestation of the developing tooth.

toothed, *adj.* Having teeth or indentations.

toothed retractor. An instrument having a broad shallow blade with teeth, to maintain retraction of tissues without slippage.

tooth germ. The dental sac, enamel organ, and dental papilla regarded as a unit; comprising all the formative tissues of a tooth. Syn. *dental germ.*

tooth pulp. DENTAL PULP.

tooth sac. DENTAL SAC.

Tooth's muscular atrophy [H. H. *Tooth,* English physician, 1856–1925]. PERONEAL MUSCULAR ATROPHY.

tooth socket. The alveolus in which the tooth is fixed.

top-, topo- [Gk. *topos,* place]. A combining form meaning (a) *place, part;* (b) *local.*

topaesthesia. TOPESTHESIA.

top·ag·no·sia (top″ag·no′zhuh, ·zee·uh) *n.* 1. Loss of ability to localize a tactile sensation. 2. Difficulty in finding one's way about in familiar surroundings. Syn. *topographical amnesia.*

top·ag·no·sis (top″ag·no′sis) *n.* [*top-* + *agnosis*]. TOPAGNOSIA.

to·pal·gia (to·pal′jee·uh) *n.* [*top-* + *-algia*]. Localized pain, without evident organic basis, common in certain mental disorders, as in the conversion type of hysterical neurosis.

to·pec·to·my (to·peck′tuh·mee) *n.* [*top-* + *-ectomy*]. A form of psychosurgery with excision of a limited portion of the cerebral cortex, usually in the frontal area, as applied in the treatment of certain mental disorders or intractable pain.

top·er's nose (to′purz). RHINOPHYMA.

top·es·the·sia, top·aes·the·sia (top″es·theezh′uh) *n.* [*top-* + *esthesia*]. Ability to localize a tactile sensation.

Töp·fer's reagent (tœp′fur) [A. E. *Töpfer,* German physician, b. 1858]. A 0.5% solution of dimethylaminoazobenzene in 95% alcohol; most commonly used as an indicator to titrate free hydrochloric acid in the gastric contents.

Töpfer's test [A. E. *Töpfer*]. A test for free hydrochloric acid in gastric contents in which a few drops of Töpfer's reagent gives a cherry-red color to a fluid containing free hydrochloric acid.

to·pha·ceous (to·fay′shus) *adj.* [L. *tophaceus*]. Of the nature of tophi; sandy or gritty.

tophaceous gout. Prominent deposits of sodium urate (tophi) in the subcutaneous and periarticular tissues in gout.

to·phus (to'fus) *n.*, pl. **to·phi** (·fye) [L.]. 1. A sodium urate deposit in the skin about a joint, in the ear, or in bone, in gout. 2. A mineral concretion in the body, especially about the joints.

top·ic (top'ick) *adj.* [Gk. *topikos,* from *topos,* place]. LOCAL.

top·i·cal (top'i·kul) *adj.* [Gk. *topik*os (from *topos,* place) + *-al*]. LOCAL.

topical anesthesia. Application of an anesthetic to one of the body surfaces, as with a swab.

To·pi·nard's angle (toh·pee·nahr') [P. *Topinard,* French anthropologist, 1830–1911]. An angle formed at the anterior nasal spine by lines projected from the glabella and the auricular point.

topo-. See *top-.*

topo·al·gia (top''o·al'jee·uh) *n.* TOPALGIA.

topo·an·es·the·sia, topo·an·aes·the·sia (top''o·an''es·theezh' uh) *n.* [*topo-* + *anesthesia*]. TOPAGNOSIA (1).

topo·gen·e·sis (to''po·jen'e·sis, top''o·) *n.* [*topo-* + *-genesis*]. MORPHOGENESIS.

top·og·no·sis (top''og·no'sis) *n.* [*topo-* + *-gnosis*]. TOPESTHESIA.

top·og·nos·tic (top''og·nos'tick) *adj.* [*topo-* + *-gnostic*]. Pertaining to the recognition of changes, positions, or symptoms of parts of the body, as topognostic sensibility.

to·po·graph·ic (top''o·graf'ick, to''po·) *adj.* Of or pertaining to topography.

to·po·graph·i·cal (top''o·graf'i·kul, to''po·) *adj.* TOPOGRAPHIC.

topographical amnesia. TOPAGNOSIA (2).

topographic anatomy. Anatomy of a part in its relation to other parts.

topographic histology. The study of the minute structure of the organs and especially of their formation from the tissues.

to·pog·ra·phy (to·pog'ruh·fee) *n.* [Gk. *topographia,* description of a region, from *topos,* place, region]. A study of the regions of the body or its parts, as cerebral topography.

to·pol·o·gy (to·pol'uh·jee) *n.* [*topo-* + *-logy*]. 1. TOPOGRAPHIC ANATOMY. 2. The relation of the presenting part of a fetus to the pelvic canal.

topo·nar·co·sis (top''o·nahr·ko'sis) *n.* [*topo-* + *narcosis*]. Local insensibility or anesthesia.

topo·neu·ro·sis (top''o·new·ro'sis) *n.* [*topo-* + *neurosis*]. A localized neurosis.

topo·pho·bia (top''o·fo'bee·uh) *n.* [*topo-* + *-phobia*]. An abnormal dread of certain places.

topo·phone (top'o·fone) *n.* [*topo-* + *-phone*]. An instrument to determine the direction of a source of sound.

torch syndrome [acronym for *to*xoplasmosis, *r*ubella, *c*ytomegalic inclusion disease, and *h*erpes simplex]. A group of clinical manifestations that are similar in perinatal infection by the diverse agents *Toxoplasma gondii,* rubella virus, cytomegalovirus, and herpes simplex virus.

tor·cu·lar He·ro·phi·li (tor'kew·lur he·rof'i·lye) [L., the winepress of *Herophilus,* Bithynian surgeon and anatomist at Alexandria, 335–280 B.C.]. CONFLUENS SINUUM.

Torecan. Trademark for thiethylperazine, an antiemetic drug used as the dimaleate salt.

Torek's operation [F. *Torek,* U.S. surgeon, 1861–1938]. 1. An operation for undescended testis. 2. A resection of the thoracic esophagus for cancer.

tori. Plural of *torus.*

to·ric (to'rick) *adj.* Pertaining to or shaped like a torus.

toric lens. A lens wherein the curvatures in two meridians at right angles are different.

Tor·kild·sen procedure [A. *Torkildsen,* Norwegian neurosurgeon, 20th century]. Surgical establishment of a communication between a lateral ventricle and the cisterna magna.

tor·mi·na (tor'mi·nuh) *n.*, sing. **tor·men** (·mun) [L., from *torquere,* to twist]. Griping pains in the bowel.

tormina al·vi (al'vye). COLIC.

tor·mi·nal (tor'mi·nul) *adj.* Affected with tormina.

tor·mi·nous (tor'mi·nus) *adj.* Affected with tormina.

Torn·waldt's abscess (torn'vahlt) [G. L. *Tornwaldt,* German physician, 1843–1910]. An abscess located in the pharyngeal tonsil or surrounding structures and caused by an infection of the pharyngeal bursa.

Tornwaldt's bursitis or **disease** [G. L. *Tornwaldt*]. PHARYNGEAL BURSITIS.

To·ron·to crutch. CANADIAN CRUTCH.

tor·pes·cence (tor·pes'unce) *n.* [L. *torpescere,* to grow stiff]. Growing numbness or torpor.

tor·pid (tor'pid) *adj.* [L. *torpidus*]. Affected with or exhibiting torpor.

tor·pid·i·ty (tor·pid'i·tee) *n.* TORPOR.

tor·por (tor'pur) *n.* [L., from *torpere,* to be sluggish]. Sluggishness; inactivity.

torpor in·tes·ti·no·rum (in·tes''ti·no'rum). CONSTIPATION.

torque, *n.* [L., *torquere,* to twist]. The measure of the effectiveness of a force in producing rotation or torsion of a body about an axis; the moment of force, i.e., the magnitude of the force times the perpendicular distance from the axis to the line of action of the force.

torr, *n.* [E. *Tor*ricelli]. A unit of pressure equivalent to 1 mm-Hg under standard conditions.

torrefied rhubarb. Rhubarb that has had its purgative powers diminished by roasting; its astringency is not affected.

tor·re·fy (tor'e·figh) *v.* [L. *torrere,* to dry]. To dry by roasting. —**torre·fied** (·fide) *adj.*

Tor·ri·cel·li·an vacuum (tor''i·chel'ee·un) [E. *Torricelli,* Italian physicist, 1608–1647]. The vacuum above the mercury in the tube of a barometer.

torsi. A plural of *torso.*

tor·si·oc·clu·sion (tor''see·uh·kloo'zhun) *n.* Occlusion of a tooth that is in torsiversion.

tor·si·om·e·ter (tor''see·om'e·tur) *n.* [*tors*ion + *-meter*]. An instrument for measuring ocular torsion.

tor·sion (tor'shun) *n.* [L. *torsio,* from *torquere,* to twist]. 1. A twisting; also, the rotation of the eye about the visual axis. 2. The tilting of the vertical meridian of the eye.

torsion balance. An instrument that measures small torques by their torsional effect upon elastic fibers or wires.

torsion dystonia. DYSTONIA MUSCULORUM DEFORMANS.

torsion of the testicle. Twisting of the testicle on its mesentery, impairing blood supply and causing pain.

torsion of the umbilical cord. The spontaneous twisting of the umbilical cord. Eight to ten twists are normal; great torsion may occur after the death of the fetus.

torsion spasm. DYSTONIA MUSCULORUM DEFORMANS.

tor·sive (tor'siv) *adj.* Twisted; twisting.

tor·si·ver·sion (tor''si·vur'zhun) *n.* [*tors*ion + *version*]. Rotated position of a tooth in its alveolus.

tor·so (tor'so) *n.*, pl. **torsos, tor·si** (·see), **torsoes** [It.]. The trunk; the body without head or limbs.

tors·oc·clu·sion (tor''suh·kloo'zhun) *n.* TORSIOCCLUSION.

tort, *v.* [L. *torquere, tortus,* to twist]. To tilt the vertical meridian of the eye.

tor·ti·col·lar (tor''ti·kol'ur) *adj.* Affected with torticollis.

tor·ti·col·lis (tor''ti·kol'is, ·kol'ee) *n.* [NL., from L. *tortus,* twisted, + *collum,* neck]. Deformity of the neck due to contraction of cervical muscles or fascia, but most prominently involving the sternocleidomastoid muscle unilaterally, resulting in abnormal position and limitation of movements of the head. Syn. *wryneck.*

torticollis spas·ti·ca (spas'ti·kuh). SPASMODIC TORTICOLLIS.

tor·ti·pel·vis (tor''ti·pel'vis) *n.* [NL., from L. *tort*us, twisted, + *pelvis*]. A manifestation of dystonia, at first phasic but usually becoming persistent, in which the pelvis is involuntarily tilted or twisted.

tor·tu·ous (tor'choo·us) *adj.* [L. *tortuosus*]. Twisted, sinuous. —**tor·tu·os·i·ty** (tor''choo·os'i·tee) *n.*

Tor·u·la (tor'yoo·luh) *n.* [NL., from L. *torulus,* tuft]. *CRYPTOCOCCUS.* —**toru·lar** (·lur) *adj.*

Torula his·to·lyt·i·ca (his″to·lit′i·kuh). CRYPTOCOCCUS NEOFORMANS.

toruli. Plural of *torulus.*

toruli tac·ti·les (tack′ti·leez) [NA]. Small elevations of the skin of the palms and soles, which contain many sensory nerve endings.

tor·u·lo·ma (tor″yoo·lo′muh) *n.* [*Torula* + *-oma*]. A tumorlike nodule resulting from cryptococcal (torular) infection.

Tor·u·lop·sis ne·o·for·mans (tor″yoo·lop′sis nee″o·for′manz). CRYPTOCOCCUS NEOFORMANS.

tor·u·lo·sis (tor″yoo·lo′sis) *n.* [*Torula* + *-osis*]. CRYPTOCOCCOSIS.

tor·u·lus (tor′yoo·lus) *n.*, pl. **toru·li** (·lye) [L., dim. of *torus*]. A minute elevation.

to·rus (to′rus) *n.*, pl. **to·ri** (·rye) [L., mound, bulge]. 1. A surface having a regular curvature with two principal meridians of dissimilar curvature at right angles to each other. 2. An elevation or prominence.

torus ge·ni·ta·lis (jen·i·tay′lis). GENITAL RIDGE.

torus le·va·to·ri·us (lev·uh·to′ree·us) [NA]. An elevation of the lateral part of the upper surface of the soft palate caused by the underlying levator veli palatini muscle.

torus man·dib·u·la·ris (man·dib″yoo·lair′is). An elevation on the lingual surface of the lower jaw, caused by an exostosis.

torus oc·ci·pi·ta·lis (ock·sip·i·tay′lis) [BNA]. TRANSVERSE OCCIPITAL TORUS.

torus pa·la·ti·nus (pal·uh·tye′nus) [NA]. A nodular elevation along the median suture of the hard palate; due to an exostosis.

torus pu·bi·cus (pew′bi·kus). A low vertical elevation overlying the pelvic margin of the fibrocartilaginous disk of the pubic symphysis.

torus tu·ba·ri·us (tew·bair′ee·us) [NA]. The arcuate elevation of the mucous membrane of the pharynx over the medial end of the cartilage of the auditory tube, above and behind the pharyngeal orifice of the tube.

torus ure·te·ri·cus (yoo·re·terr′i·kus). A ridge in the urinary bladder wall connecting the ureteral orifices.

torus ute·ri·nus (yoo·te·rye′nus). A transverse fold on the posterior aspect of the cervix of the uterus formed as an extension of the uterosacral ligaments.

to·si·fen (to′si·fen) *n.* (*S*)-1-(α-Methylphenethyl)-3-(*p*-tolylsulfonyl)urea, $C_{17}H_{20}N_2O_3S$, an anti-anginal.

tos·y·late (tos′i·late) *n.* Any salt or ester of *p*-toluenesulfonic acid, $CH_3C_6H_4SO_3H$; a *p*-toluenesulfonate.

to·tal abduction. The expression in prism diopters of the capacity for turning the eyes outward from the extreme point of inward or positive convergence to the extreme point of outward or negative convergence beyond parallelism. It is measured from relative near point. A test of, and an exercise stimulus for, relaxation of the internal recti and convergence.

total aphasia. GLOBAL APHASIA.

total color blindness. The complete inability to distinguish different hues and saturation. Syn. *monochromatism.* See also *rod monochromat, cone monochromat.*

total hyperopia. The entire amount of hyperopia, both latent and manifest, detected after accommodation has been paralyzed by a mydriatic or during complete relaxation of the ciliary muscle. Symbol, Ht.

total lethal dose. INVARIABLY LETHAL DOSE.

total ophthalmoplegia. COMPLETE OPHTHALMOPLEGIA.

total-push therapy. *In psychiatry,* the simultaneous application in a mental hospital setting of all available forms of psychiatric treatment to speed the rehabilitation of the patient.

total symblepharon. Adhesion of the entire eyelid to the eyeball, or of the eyelids to each other; may be congenital, or due to disease or injury.

total synechia. Adhesion of the entire surface of the iris to the lens. See also *iris bombé.*

total white count. The number of leukocytes in one cubic millimeter of blood.

to·ta·quine (to′tuh·kween, ·kwin) *n.* A mixture of alkaloids from the bark of species of *Cinchona.* It contains not less than 10% of anhydrous quinine and a total of 70 to 80% of the anhydrous alkaloids cinchonidine, cinchonine, quinidine, and quinine. Has been used as an antimalarial.

to·tip·o·tence (to·tip′o·tunce) *n.* [L. *totus,* whole, + *potentia,* power]. The capacity of a precursor stage of a cell or organism to give rise to a full range of types, or a complete organism, at a later stage. **—totipo·tent** (·tunt), **to·ti·po·ten·tial** (to″ti·po·ten′chul) *adj.*

To·ti's operation (toʰ′tee) [A. *Toti,* Italian otolaryngologist, b. 1861]. DACRYOCYSTORHINOSTOMY.

touch, *n.* [OF. *tochier,* to touch]. 1. The tactile sense. 2. PALPATION.

touch corpuscle. TACTILE CORPUSCLE.

tough·ened silver nitrate. A form of silver nitrate.

Tou·louse-Lau·trec disease (too·looz′ lo·treck′) [H. de *Toulouse-Lautrec,* French painter, 1864–1901]. PYKNODYSOSTOSIS.

Tou·raine's aphthosis. Small round or oval ulcers with yellow sloughs in the mouth, vulva, or glans penis, associated with keratitis, conjunctivitis, or scleritis.

tour de mai·tre (toor duh meh′tr) [F., a master's turn]. A method of passing a sound or metal catheter into the male urinary bladder in which it is introduced into the urethra with the convexity upward. The shaft lies obliquely across the left thigh of the patient, and as the point enters the bulb, the handle is swept around toward the abdomen, when the beak passes into the membranous urethra. It is carried into the urinary bladder by depressing the shaft between the patient's thighs.

Tourette's disease or **syndrome.** GILLES DE LA TOURETTE DISEASE.

Tour·nay's sign (toor·neʰ′) [A. *Tournay,* French ophthalmologist, b. 1878] Unilateral dilatation of the pupil of the abducted eye in extreme lateral fixation.

tour·ni·quet (toor′ni·kut, tur′) *n.* [F.]. Any apparatus for controlling hemorrhage from, or circulation in, a limb or part of the body, where pressure can be brought upon the blood vessels by means of straps, cords, rubber tubes, or pads. Tourniquets are made in a multiplicity of forms, from the simplest emergency adaptation to elaborate instruments.

tourniquet paralysis. Pressure paralysis caused by too long application of a tourniquet to a limb while checking hemorrhage. It is most common in the nerves of the arm.

tourniquet test. A test for capillary resistance in which a blood pressure cuff about the upper arm is used to occlude the vein effectively for a measured time, after which the skin of the forearm and hand is examined for petechiae.

Tou·ton cells [K. *Touton,* German dermatologist, b. 1858]. Multinucleated giant cells having foamy, fat-containing cytoplasm which forms a distinct rim outside a wavy row of nuclei; they are associated with disease that destroys adipose tissue.

tow (toe) *n.* The coarse part of flax or hemp; used as an absorbent.

tow·el forceps or **clamp.** A snap, clamp, or forceps with sharp hooked ends which overlap; adapted to holding towels fast to the skin during operations. Syn. *skin-holding forceps.*

tow·er head or **skull.** OXYCEPHALY.

Towne-Cham·ber·lain's projection [E. B. *Towne*]. TOWNE'S PROJECTION.

Towne's projection [E. B. *Towne,* U.S. otolaryngologist, 1883–1957]. An AP x-ray of the skull taken with the occiput positioned on the film and the central ray projected along the slant of the base of the skull (usually 30°

caudally). Designed to demonstrate the foramen magnum, posterior fossa, and the long axis of the calvaria without overlap by the facial bones.

Town·send and Gil·fil·lan plate. A plate used for treating, by open reduction, tibial shatter fractures; the plate is screwed to the tibial shaft, and extends upward to receive a bolt transfixing the condylar fragments.

Townsend operation [D. *Townsend,* U.S. orthopedic surgeon, 1875–1950]. An operation for flatfoot.

tox-, toxi-, toxo-. A combining form meaning *toxic, poisonous, toxin, poison.*

toxaemia. TOXEMIA.

toxaemic. TOXEMIC.

tox·al·bu·min (tock″sal·bew′min) *n.* [*tox-* + *albumin*]. A poisonous protein, obtained from cultures of bacteria and from certain plants.

tox·al·bu·mose (tock·sal′bew·moce, ·moze) *n.* A toxic albumose.

tox·emia, tox·ae·mia (tock·see′mee·uh) *n.* [*tox-* + *-emia*]. A condition in which the blood contains poisonous products, either those produced by the body cells or those resulting from microorganisms.

toxemia of pregnancy. A pathologic condition sometimes occurring in the latter half of pregnancy, manifested by symptoms of eclampsia or preeclampsia.

tox·emic, tox·ae·mic (tock·see′mick) *adj.* Pertaining to, affected with, or caused by toxemia.

toxemic epilepsy. Epilepsy characterized by toxic convulsions.

toxemic vertigo. Vertigo due to some intoxicant in the blood, such as alcohol.

tox·en·zyme (tocks·en′zime) *n.* A toxic enzyme.

toxi-. See *tox-.*

toxic-, toxico-. A combining form meaning *poison, toxic.*

tox·ic (tock′sick) *adj.* [ML. *toxicus,* from L. *toxicum,* poison, from Gk. *toxikon pharmakon,* arrow poison, from *toxikos,* archer's, from *toxon,* bow]. POISONOUS.

toxicaemia. Toxicemia (= TOXEMIA).

toxic amaurosis. TOXIC AMBLYOPIA.

toxic amblyopia. A relative or absolute loss of a portion or all of the visual field caused by a chronic or by an acute toxemia, which may be endogenous, such as uremia, diabetes, or beri beri; or exogenous, such as quinine, lead, tobacco, or methyl alcohol.

toxic anemia. Any hemolytic anemia due to toxins and poisons.

tox·i·cant (tock′si·kunt) *adj. & n.* 1. Poisonous or toxic. 2. A poison or toxin.

toxic atrophy. Atrophy that appears in the course of prolonged wasting and infectious diseases.

toxic blindness. TOXIC AMBLYOPIA.

toxic cirrhosis. POSTNECROTIC CIRRHOSIS.

toxic convulsion or **seizure.** A seizure due to the action of some toxic agent upon the nervous system. The responsible substance may be inorganic (for example, carbon monoxide), organic (for example, alcohol), metallic (for example, lead, arsenic), a foreign protein, or a convulsant substance such as strychnine; or the seizure may be associated with toxemia of pregnancy or uremia.

tox·i·ce·mia, tox·i·cae·mia (tock″si·see′mee·uh) *n.* [*toxic-* + *-emia*]. TOXEMIA.

toxic encephalopathy. 1. Any brain disorder due to toxic factors. 2. A severe, not uncommon, neurologic disorder of infants and children of unknown cause, characterized clinically by rapid onset of fever, depression of consciousness or coma, seizures, and often a fulminant fatal course, and pathologically by acute cerebral edema without other significant histopathological changes. See also *Reye's syndrome.*

toxic epidermal necrolysis. A condition characterized by sudden development of high fever and large, flaccid bullae on the skin generally, and in or about the mucous membranes; in some cases thought to be caused by drugs; in others, due to an exfoliative toxin produced by some strains of *Staphylococcus aureus.* Syn. *scalded skin syndrome, Lyell's syndrome.*

toxic epilepsy. Epilepsy characterized by toxic convulsions.

toxic erythema. Redness of the skin produced by toxic cause.

toxic glycosuria. Glycosuria observed after poisoning by chloral, morphine, or curare, after the inhalation of chloroform or carbon monoxide, or after the ingestion of phlorhizin.

toxic goiter. HYPERTHYROIDISM.

toxic hemoglobinuria. A form of hemoglobinuria due to poisoning.

toxic hepatitis. Inflammation of the liver resulting from the action of toxic compounds. Examples of hepatotoxins include such diverse compounds as the chlorinated hydrocarbons, phosphorus, and certain alkaloids.

toxic hydrocephalus. PSEUDOTUMOR CEREBRI.

tox·i·cide (tock′si·side) *n.* [*toxi-* + *-cide*]. A remedy or principle that destroys toxic agents.

toxic insanity. TOXIC PSYCHOSIS.

tox·ic·i·ty (tock·sis′i·tee) *n.* 1. The quality of being toxic. 2. The kind and amount of poison or toxin produced by a microorganism, or possessed by a chemical substance not of biologic origin.

toxic jaundice. Jaundice associated with toxic hepatitis.

toxic labyrinthitis. Inflammation of the labyrinth due to drugs which cause nausea and vertigo.

toxic myelopathy. Any disease of the spinal cord caused by toxic substances.

toxic neuropathy. Neuropathy due to some poisonous substance; usually a polyneuropathy.

toxic nodular cirrhosis. POSTNECROTIC CIRRHOSIS.

toxico-. See *toxic-.*

tox·i·co·den·drol (tock″si·ko·den′drol) *n.* A toxic nonvolatile oil from poison ivy and poison oak.

Tox·i·co·den·dron (tock″si·ko·den′drun) *n.* [NL., from *toxico-* + Gk. *dendron,* tree]. A genus of plants and shrubs, formerly classified as *Rhus,* including poison ivy, *Toxicodendron radicans;* poison oak, *T. quercifolium;* poison sumac, *T. vernix;* and other species.

tox·i·co·der·ma (tock″si·ko·dur′muh) *n.* [*toxico-* + *-derma*]. Disease of the skin due to poison.

tox·i·co·der·ma·ti·tis (tock″si·ko·dur″muh·tye′tis) *n.* [*toxico-* + *dermatitis*]. Skin inflammation due to poison.

tox·i·co·der·ma·to·sis (tock″si·ko·dur″muh·to′sis) *n.* [*toxico-* + *dermatosis*]. TOXICODERMA.

tox·i·co·gen·ic (tock″si·ko·jen′ick) *adj.* [*toxico-* + *-genic*]. Producing poisons.

tox·i·coid (tock′si·koid) *adj.* [*toxic-* + *-oid*]. Resembling a poison or a toxin.

tox·i·col·o·gist (tock″si·kol′uh·jist) *n.* A person versed in toxicology.

tox·i·col·o·gy (tock″si·kol′uh·jee) *n.* [*toxico-* + *-logy*]. The science of the nature and effects of poisons, their detection, and treatment of their effects. —**toxi·co·log·ic** (·ko·loj′ick), **toxicolog·i·cal** (·i·kul) *adj.*

tox·i·co·ma·nia (tock″si·ko·may′nee·uh) *n.* [*toxico-* + *-mania*]. An abnormal desire to consume poison. —**toxicoma·ni·ac** (·nee·ack) *n.*

tox·i·co·path·ic (tock″si·ko·path′ick) *adj.* [*toxico-* + *-pathic*]. Pertaining to any abnormal condition due to the action of a poison.

tox·i·co·phid·ia (tock″si·ko·fid′ee·uh) *n.pl.* [*toxic-* + Gk. *ophidion,* small serpent]. POISONOUS SNAKES.

tox·i·co·pho·bia (tock″si·ko·fo′bee·uh) *n.* [*toxico-* + *-phobia*]. An abnormal fear of being poisoned.

tox·i·co·sis (tock″si·ko′sis) *n.,* pl. **toxico·ses** (·seez) [*toxic-* + *-osis*]. A state of poisoning.

toxic psychosis. Any acute confusional or delirious state supposedly due to a toxin and associated with medical or surgical diseases, postoperative or posttraumatic states, exogenous intoxications, withdrawal of alcohol or barbiturates, congestive heart failure, or metabolic disorders.

toxic purpura. Purpura caused by various poisons such as arsenic, phosphorus, phenolphthalein, heparin.

toxic spasm. TOXIC CONVULSION.

toxic synovitis. TRANSIENT SYNOVITIS.

toxic tetanus. Generalized muscle spasms produced by an overdose of nux vomica or strychnine.

toxic unit. Any arbitrarily established unit of activity, often expressed in terms of an accepted official reference standard. In the case of diphtheria toxin, the unit is defined as the least amount that will, on the average, kill a 250g guinea pig within 96 hours after subcutaneous injection.

toxic vertigo. TOXEMIC VERTIGO.

toxi·der·ma·to·sis (tock″si·dur″muh·to′sis) *n.* [*toxi-* + *dermatosis*]. TOXICODERMA.

toxi·der·mi·tis (tock″si·dur·migh′tis) *n.* [*toxi-* + *dermitis*]. TOXICODERMATITIS.

tox·if·er·ous (tock·sif′ur·us) *adj.* [*toxi-* + *-ferous*]. Producing or conveying poison.

tox·i·ge·nic·i·ty (tock″see·je·nis′i·tee) *n.* The degree of ability of an organism to produce toxicity or disease.

tox·ig·e·nous (tock·sij′e·nus) *adj.* [*toxi-* + *-genous*]. Producing toxins.

tox·in (tock′sin) *n.* [*tox-* + *-in*]. Any poisonous substance formed by plant or animal cells. Some bacterial toxins, such as diphtheria and tetanus toxins, are readily separable from the cells (exotoxin); others are intimately bound to the cells (endotoxin). Phytotoxins include ricin and abrin. Zootoxins include the venoms of snakes, spiders, scorpions, toads, or sting rays. Many toxins are proteins capable of stimulating the production in man or animals of neutralizing antibodies or antitoxins.

toxin-antitoxin, *n.* A combination of a toxin and an antitoxin for therapeutic use. Abbreviated, T.A., T.A.T. See also *diphtheria toxin-antitoxin.*

toxin-antitoxin reaction. The loss of a toxin's poisonous properties upon mixture with its corresponding antitoxin.

tox·in·fec·tion (tock″sin·feck′shun) *n.* Infection by means of a toxin, the causative microorganism not being recognized.

tox·i·no·sis (tock″si·no′sis) *n.* [*toxin* + *-osis*]. TOXICOSIS.

tox·i·pho·bia (tock″si·fo′bee·uh) *n.* TOXICOPHOBIA.

tox·is·ter·ol (tock·sis′tur·ol) *n.* A product of the excessive irradiation of ergosterol. Although isomeric with calciferol, it has little antirachitic action and is highly toxic.

toxi·ther·a·py (tock″si·therr′uh·pee) *n.* The therapeutic use of antitoxins.

toxi·tu·ber·cu·lide (tock″si·tew·bur′kew·lide) *n.* [*toxi-* + *tuberculide*]. A skin lesion due to the action of tuberculous toxin.

toxo-. See *tox-.*

Tox·o·cara (tock″so·kăr′uh) *n.* [NL., from Gk. *toxon,* bow, arch, + *kara,* head]. A genus of ascarid worms; the larvae of a few species are important causes of human visceral larva migrans.

Toxocara can·is (kan′is, kay′nis). The common ascarid of dogs.

Toxocara cati (kat′eye). The common ascarid of cats.

tox·oid (tock′soid) *n.* [*tox-* + *-oid*]. A toxin detoxified by moderate heat or chemical treatment (formaldehyde) but with antigenic properties intact. The toxoids of diphtheria and tetanus are used frequently for immunization.

toxo·in·fec·tion (tock″so·in·feck′shun) *n.* TOXINFECTION.

toxo·lec·i·thin (tock″so·les′i·thin) *n.* [*toxo-* + *lecithin*]. A mixture of a venom with a lecithin, the latter behaving as a complement for the former.

toxo·no·sis (tock″suh·no′sis) *n.* [*toxo-* + Gk. *nosos,* disease (assimilated to *-osis*)]. An affection resulting from a poison.

toxo·phil (tock′so·fil) *adj.* [*toxo-* + *-phil*]. Having an affinity for toxins or poisons.

toxo·phile (tock′so·file) *adj.* TOXOPHIL.

toxo·phore (tock′so·fore) *n.* [*toxo-* + *-phore*]. The chemical group in a molecule of a toxin which is responsible for its toxic effect. —**tox·oph·o·rous** (tock·sof′uh·rus) *adj.*

Toxo·plas·ma (tock″so·plaz′muh) *n.* [*toxo-* + Gk. *plasma,* anything formed]. A genus of parasitic protozoans.

***Toxoplasma* dye test.** DYE TEST.

Toxoplasma gon·dii (gon′dee·eye). The causative agent of toxoplasmosis.

toxo·plas·mat·ic (tock″so·plaz·mat′ick) *adj.* Pertaining to infection with *Toxoplasma.*

toxo·plas·mic (tock″so·plaz′mick) *adj.* TOXOPLASMATIC.

toxo·plas·min (tock″so·plaz′min) *n.* The *Toxoplasma* antigen, prepared either from infected mouse peritoneal fluid or in embryonated eggs, used in a skin test to demonstrate delayed hypersensitivity to toxoplasmosis.

toxoplasmin test. A cutaneous test for toxoplasmosis by the intradermal injection of toxoplasmin. Observation of a hypersensitivity reaction with a negative reaction in a control injection indicates past or persistent infection.

tox·o·plas·mo·sis (tock″so·plaz·mo′sis) *n.,* pl. **toxoplasmo·ses** (·seez) [*Toxoplasma* + *-osis*]. Infection by the protozoon *Toxoplasma gondii* widely distributed in nature, and causing in man congenital and acquired, often inapparent, illness. The protean clinical manifestations of the congenital form include jaundice, hepatomegaly, and splenomegaly; chorioretinitis, convulsions, hydrocephaly or microcephaly; cerebral calcifications and psychomotor retardation evident at birth or later in life; in acquired form, febrile illness with rash resembling Rocky Mountain spotted fever, lymphadenopathy, hepatosplenomegaly, encephalomyelitis, myocarditis, and granulomatous uveitis may occur.

tox·o·sis (tock·so′sis) *n.* TOXONOSIS.

Toyn·bee's corpuscle [J. *Toynbee,* English otologist, 1815–1866]. CORNEAL CORPUSCLE.

Toynbee's ligament [J. *Toynbee*]. The tensor tympani muscle and its sheath.

TPI *TREPONEMA PALLIDUM* IMMOBILIZATION TEST.

TPI test. Abbreviation for *Treponema pallidum immobilization test.*

TPN Abbreviation for *triphosphopyridine nucleotide* (= NICOTINAMIDE ADENINE DINUCLEOTIDE PHOSPHATE).

TPNH Symbol for the reduced form of triphosphopyridine nucleotide, now more often described as the reduced form of nicotinamide-adenine dinucleotide phosphate and symbolized NADPH.

T.P.R. 1. Total peripheral resistance. 2. Total pulmonary resistance. 3. Temperature, pulse, respiration; also given without periods.

T-P segment. The interval between the end of the T wave and the beginning of the subsequent P wave.

tr. Abbreviation for *tinctura,* tincture.

tra·bec·u·la (tra·beck′yoo·luh) *n.,* pl. **trabecu·lae** (·lee) [NL., dim of L. *trabs,* beam]. 1. Any one of the fibrous bands extending from the capsule into the interior of an organ. 2. One of the variously shaped spicules of bone in cancellous bone.

trabeculae car·ne·ae (kahr′nee·ee) [NA]. The interlacing muscular columns projecting from the inner surface of the ventricles of the heart.

trabeculae cor·dis (kor′dis). TRABECULAE CARNEAE.

trabeculae cor·po·ris spon·gi·o·si (kor′po·ris spon·jee·o′sigh) [NA]. Bands of fibromuscular tissue crossing the corpus spongiosum.

trabeculae cor·po·rum ca·ver·no·so·rum (kor′po·rum kav″ur·no·so′rum) [NA]. Bands of fibromuscular tissue crossing the corpora cavernosa.

trabeculae li·e·nis (lye·ee′nis) [NA]. Fibromuscular bands which pass into the spleen from the capsule.

tra·bec·u·lar (tra·beck′yoo·lur) *adj.* Pertaining to, constituting, or consisting of a trabecula or trabeculae.

trabecular cartilages. The prechordal primordia of the sphenoid, usually single in man.

trabecular syncytial reticulosarcoma. RETICULUM-CELL SARCOMA.

trabecular vein. In the spleen, a tributary of the splenic vein, formed by the confluence of pulp veins.

trabecula sep·to·mar·gi·na·lis (sep″to·mahr·ji·nay′lis) [NA]. MODERATOR BAND.

tra·bec·u·lat·ed bladder. The trabecular-like cystoscopic or radiographic appearance of the bladder when there is hypertrophy of bladder muscle because of obstruction of the urinary flow or neurogenic disease.

trace, *n.* [OF., way, path]. A slight amount, degree, or indication, often barely detectable and often treated as quantitatively indeterminate.

trace-conditioned response. A conditioned response occurring at some interval after the conditioned stimulus; if the interval is less than a minute, it is a short trace response; if over a minute, a long trace response.

trace elements. Substances or elements essential to plant or animal life, but present in extremely small amounts.

trace minerals. Minerals occurring in traces which are essential for growth, development, and health; mineral micronutrients.

trac·er, *n.* An isotope which, because of its unique physical properties, can be detected in extremely minute quantity, and hence is used to trace the chemical behavior of the natural element. As isotopes of the same element differ in physical properties only, but have identical chemical properties (with a few exceptions), an isotope detectable by physical properties may be used to trace the pattern of biochemical reactions. Such use of isotopes is referred to as a tracer study. The isotope itself is a tracer. Stable (by measurement of isotopic ratios) or unstable (by detection of their ionizing radiation) isotopes may be used.

tracer element. TRACER.

trache-, tracheo-. A combining form meaning *trachea, tracheal.*

tra·chea (tray′kee·uh) *n.,* L. pl. & genit. sing. **tra·che·ae** (·kee·ee), E. pl. **tracheas** [ML., from Gk. *(artēria) tracheia,* "rough (artery)"] [NA]. The cartilaginous and membranous tube extending from the lower end of the larynx to its division into the two principal bronchi; the windpipe. See also Plates 12, 13, 26. **—tra·che·al** (·kee·ul) *adj.*

tra·chea·ec·ta·sy (tray″kee·uh·eck′tuh·see) *n.* [*trachea* + Gk. *ektasis,* extension]. Dilatation of the trachea.

tracheal breath sounds. BRONCHIAL BREATH SOUNDS.

tra·che·al·gia (tray″kee·al′jee·uh) *n.* [*trache-* + *-algia*]. Pain in the trachea.

tracheal respiration. The respiratory murmur heard in a normal individual by placing a stethoscope over the suprasternal fossa.

tracheal ring. One of the C-shaped cartilages in the framework of the trachea.

tracheal triangle. INFERIOR CAROTID TRIANGLE.

tracheal tug. The downward tugging movement of the larynx, sometimes observed in aneurysm of the aortic arch. See also *Oliver's sign.*

tra·che·i·tis (tray″kee·eye′tis) *n.* [*trache-* + *-itis*]. Inflammation of the trachea.

trachel-, trachelo- [Gk. *trachēlos,* neck]. A combining form meaning *neck, cervix, cervical.*

trach·e·lec·to·my (track″e·leck′tuh·mee) *n.* [*trachel-* + *-ectomy*]. Excision of the neck of the uterus.

trach·e·le·ma·to·ma (track″e·lee″muh·to′muh) *n.* [*trachel-* + *hematoma*]. A hematoma of the neck, or in the sternocleidomastoid muscle.

trach·e·lis·mus (track″e·liz′mus) *n.* [NL., from Gk. *trachēlismos,* a seizing by the neck]. Spasmodic contraction of the muscles of the neck, with marked retraction of the head, as seen in the tonic phase of a seizure.

trach·e·li·tis (track″e·lye′tis) *n.* [*trachel-* + *-itis*]. Inflammation of the neck of the uterus. See also *cervicitis.*

trachelo-. See *trachel-.*

trach·e·lo·cyl·lo·sis (track″e·lo·si·lo′sis) *n.* [*trachelo-* + Gk. *kyllōsis,* a bending]. *Obsol.* TORTICOLLIS.

trach·e·lo·dyn·ia (track″e·lo·din′ee·uh) *n.* [*trachel-* + *-odynia*]. Pain in the neck.

trach·e·lo·ky·pho·sis (track″e·lo·kigh·fo′sis) *n.* [*trachelo-* + *kyphosis*]. An abnormal anterior curvature of the cervical portion of the spinal column.

trach·e·lo·mas·toid (track″e·lo·mas′toid) *n.* [*trachelo-* + *mastoid*]. The longissimus capitis muscle. See Table of Muscles in the Appendix.

trach·e·lo·par·a·si·tus (track″e·lo·păr″uh·sigh′tus) *n.* [NL., from *trachelo-* + Gk. *parasitos,* parasite]. Any parasitic growth upon the neck or jaws. See also *deromelus, epignathus, pleonotus.*

trach·e·lo·pex·ia (track″e·lo·peck′see·uh) *n.* [*trachelo-* + *-pexia*]. Surgical fixation of the neck of the uterus.

trach·e·lo·plas·ty (track″e·lo·plas′tee) *n.* [*trachelo-* + *-plasty*]. Plastic operation on the neck of the uterus.

trach·e·lor·rha·phy (track″e·lor′uh·fee) *n.* [*trachelo-* + *-rrhaphy*]. Repair of a laceration of the cervix of the uterus.

trach·e·lor·rhec·tes (track″e·lo·reck′teez) *n.* [*trachelo-* + Gk. *rhēktēs,* a breaker]. An instrument for crushing the cervical vertebrae; used in embryotomy.

trach·e·los·chi·sis (track″e·los′ki·sis) *n.* [*trachelo-* + *-schisis*]. CERVICAL FISSURE.

trach·e·lo·syr·in·gor·rha·phy (track″e·lo·sirr″ing·gor′uh·fee) *n.* [*trachelo-* + *syringo-* + *-rrhaphy*]. An operation for vaginal fistula with stitching of the cervix of the uterus.

trach·e·lot·o·my (track″e·lot′uh·mee) *n.* [*trachelo-* + *-tomy*]. Incision into the cervix of the uterus.

tracheo-. See *trache-.*

tra·cheo·blen·nor·rhea, tra·cheo·blen·nor·rhoea (tray″kee·o·blen″o·ree′uh) *n.* [*tracheo-* + *blenno-* + *-rrhea*]. A profuse discharge of mucus from the trachea.

tra·cheo·bron·chi·al (tray″kee·o·bronk′ee·ul) *adj.* [*tracheo-* + *bronchial*]. Pertaining to the trachea and a bronchus or the bronchi.

tracheobronchial groove. LARYNGOTRACHEAL GROOVE.

tra·cheo·bron·chio·meg·a·ly (tray″kee·o·bronk″ee·o·meg′uh·lee) *n.* TRACHEOBRONCHOMEGALY.

tra·cheo·bron·chi·tis (tray″kee·o·brong·kigh′tis) *n.* [*tracheo-* + *bronch-* + *-itis*]. Inflammation of the trachea and bronchi.

tra·cheo·bron·cho·meg·a·ly (tray″kee·o·bronk″o·meg′uh·lee) *n.* [*tracheo-* + *broncho-* + *-megaly*]. Diffuse dilation of the trachea and primary bronchi; may be asymptomatic or associated with major complications. Syn. *Mounier-Kuhn syndrome.*

tra·cheo·bron·chos·co·py (tray″kee·o·brong·kos′kuh·pee) *n.* [*tracheo-* + *broncho-* + *-scopy*]. Inspection of the interior of the trachea and bronchi.

tra·cheo·cele (tray′kee·o·seel) *n.* [*tracheo-* + *-cele*]. An aerocele connected with the trachea.

tra·cheo·esoph·a·ge·al, tra·cheo-oe·soph·a·ge·al (tray″kee·o·e·sof″uh·jee′ul, ·ee″so·faj′ee·ul) *adj.* [*tracheo-* + *esophageal*]. Pertaining to the trachea and the esophagus; usually refers to a congenitial fistulous tract between the two structures.

tra·cheo·fis·sure (tray″kee·o·fish′ur) *n.* [*tracheo-* + *fissure*]. Congenital longitudinal cleft of the trachea.

tra·cheo·gram (tray′kee·o·gram) *n.* [*tracheo-* + *-gram*]. A radiographic depiction of the trachea following the instillation of a contrast medium.

tra·che·og·ra·phy (tray″kee·og′ruh·fee) *n.* [*tracheo-* + *-graphy*]. The process of making a tracheogram.

tra·cheo·la·ryn·ge·al (tray″kee·o·la·rin′jee·ul) *adj.* [*tracheo-* + *laryngeal*]. Pertaining to the trachea and the larynx.

tra·cheo·lar·yn·got·o·my (tray″kee·o·lar″in·got′uh·mee) *n.* [*tracheo-* + *laryngo-* + *-tomy*]. Incision into the larynx and trachea; combined tracheotomy and laryngotomy.

tra·cheo·ma·la·cia (tray"kee·o·ma·lay'shee·uh) *n.* [*tracheo-* + *malacia*]. Softening and destruction of the tracheal wall, especially the cartilaginous rings.

tracheo-oesophageal. TRACHEOESOPHAGEAL.

tra·cheo·path·ia os·teo·plas·ti·ca (tray"kee·o·path'ee·uh os·tee·o·plas'ti·kuh) [L.]. A deposit of cartilage and bone in the mucosa of the trachea.

tra·che·oph·o·ny (tray"kee·off'uh·nee) *n.* [*tracheo-* + *-phony*]. The sound heard over the trachea on auscultation.

tra·cheo·plas·ty (tray'kee·o·plas"tee) *n.* [*tracheo-* + *-plasty*]. Plastic surgery of the trachea.

tra·cheo·py·o·sis (tray"kee·o·pye·o'sis) *n.* [*tracheo-* + *py-* + *-osis*]. Purulent tracheitis.

tra·che·or·rha·gia (tray"kee·o·ray'jee·uh) *n.* [*tracheo-* + *-rrhagia*]. Hemorrhage from the trachea.

tra·che·or·rha·phy (tray"kee·or'uh·fee) *n.* [*tracheo-* + *-rrhaphy*]. Suturing of the trachea.

tra·che·os·chi·sis (tray"kee·os'ki·sis) *n.* [*tracheo-* + *-schisis*]. Congenital fissure of the trachea.

tra·che·os·co·py (tray"kee·os'kuh·pee) *n.* [*tracheo-* + *-scopy*]. Inspection of the interior of the trachea by means of a laryngoscopic mirror and reflected light, or through a bronchoscope. **—trache·o·scop·ic** (·o·skop'ick) *adj.*

tra·cheo·ste·no·sis (tray"kee·o·ste·no'sis) *n.* [*tracheo-* + *stenosis*]. Abnormal constriction or narrowing of the trachea.

tra·che·os·to·ma (tray"kee·os'tuh·muh, ·o·sto'muh) *n.* The opening formed in tracheostomy.

tra·che·os·to·my (tray"kee·os'tuh·mee) *n.* [*tracheo-* + *-stomy*]. The formation of an opening into the trachea, and suturing the edges of the opening to an opening in the skin of the neck, as in laryngectomy.

tra·cheo·tome (tray'kee·o·tome) *n.* [*tracheo-* + *-tome*]. A cutting instrument used in tracheotomy; a tracheotomy knife.

tra·che·ot·o·mist (tray"kee·ot'uh·mist) *n.* A person skilled in tracheotomy.

tra·che·ot·o·mize (tray"kee·ot'uh·mize) *v.* To perform tracheotomy upon a living subject.

tra·che·ot·o·my (tray"kee·ot'uh·mee) *n.* [*tracheo-* + *-tomy*]. The operation of cutting into the trachea.

tracheotomy tube. A metal tube placed in the opening made in a tracheotomy, and through which breathing is carried on.

tra·chi·el·co·sis (tray"kee·el·ko'sis) *n.* [*trache-* + Gk. *helkōsis*, ulceration]. Ulceration of the trachea.

tra·chi·el·cus (tray"kee·el'kus) *n.* [*trache-* + Gk. *helkos*, ulcer]. A tracheal ulcer.

tra·chi·tis (tra·kigh'tis) *n.* [*trache-* + *-itis*]. TRACHEITIS.

tra·cho·ma (tra·ko'muh) *n.* [Gk. *trachōma*, from *trachys*, rough]. An infectious disease of the conjunctiva and cornea, producing photophobia, pain, excessive lacrimation, and sometimes blindness, caused by *Chlamydia trachomatis.* The lesion is characterized initially by inflammation and later by pannus and follicular and papillary hypertrophy of the conjunctiva. Syn. *Egyptian conjunctivitis, Egyptian ophthalmia, conjunctivitis granulosa, granular lids.* **—trachoma·tous** (·tus) *adj.*

trachoma bodies. PROWAZEK-HALBERSTAEDTER BODIES.

trachoma de·for·mans (de·for'manz). A form of kraurosis of the vulva at the stage when it results in diffuse scar tissue.

trachoma of the vocal cords. SINGER'S NODES.

trachomatous conjunctivitis. Conjunctivitis associated with trachoma, characterized by a subepithelial cellular infiltration with a follicular distribution. See also *trachoma.*

trachomatous entropion. Entropion due to trachomatous cicatrization of the conjunctiva.

trachomatous keratitis. PANNUS.

tra·chy·chro·mat·ic (tray"kee·kro·mat'ick, track"i·) *adj.* [Gk. *trachys*, rough, + *chromatic*]. Deeply staining.

tra·chy·onych·ia (tray"kee·o·nick'ee·uh, track"ee·) *n.* [Gk. *trachys*, rough, + *onychia*]. Inflammation of the proximal portion of the nail matrix causing the nail to become covered with an opaque, corrugated, lamellated, grayish superficial layer.

tra·chy·pho·nia (tray"kee·fo'nee·uh, track"i·) *n.* [Gk. *trachys*, rough, + *-phonia*]. Rough or hoarse voice.

trac·ing, *n.* [OF. *trace,* from L. *tractus,* a drawing]. A recording or marking out of a movement, design, or action.

tract, *n.* [L. *tractus,* track, trail, from *trahere,* to draw, pull]. 1. A pathway or course. 2. A bundle or collection of nerve fibers. 3. Any one of the nervous pathways of the spinal cord or brain as an anatomic and functional entity. 4. A group of parts or organs serving some special purpose.

trac·tion, *n.* The act of drawing or pulling.

traction aneurysm. An aneurysm due to traction on an artery, as seen from traction on the aorta by an incompletely atrophied ductus arteriosus.

traction diverticulum. A circumscribed sacculation, usually of the esophagus, with bulging of the full thickness of the wall; due to the pull of adhesions arising from adjacent organs. Contr. *pulsion diverticulum.*

traction headache. Pain arising from traction on sensitive cranial structures, especially on the dura mater at the base of the brain and the arteries within the dura mater and pia-arachnoid, on the skin, subcutaneous tissue, and periosteum of the skull, on the delicate structures of eye, ear, and nasal cavity, on intracranial venous sinuses, and on the sensory cranial nerves.

traction splint. A splint so devised that traction can be exerted on the distal fragment of a fracture to overcome muscle pull and maintain proper alignment of the fractured bone, such as a banjo splint, Thomas splint, or caliper splint.

traction test. Observation of the degree of muscle tone in infancy as judged by resistance to extension of the arms at the elbow, assistance of the shoulders, and maintenance of variable duration of the head in the upright position when the infant is pulled slowly from the symmetrical supine to a sitting position by means of his wrists. Syn. *Knop test.*

tract of Allen. SOLITARY FASCICULUS.

tract of Lissauer. DORSOLATERAL TRACT.

tract of Schütz. PERIVENTRICULAR TRACT.

trac·tor (track'tur) *n.* An instrument or apparatus for making traction.

trac·tot·o·my (track·tot'uh·mee) *n.* [*tract* + *-tomy*]. The surgical resection of a nerve-fiber tract of the central nervous system, usually for relief of pain.

trac·tus (track'tus) *n.*, pl. & genit. sing. **trac·tus** (track'toos, track'tus) [L.]. TRACT.

tractus cen·tra·lis thy·mi (sen·tray'lis thigh'migh) [BNA]. An indefinite core of connective tissue surrounding the blood vessels passing into the thymus.

tractus ce·re·bel·lo·ru·bra·lis (serr·e·bel"o·rew·bray'lis) [NA]. DENTATORUBRAL TRACT.

tractus ce·re·bel·lo·tha·la·mi·cus (serr·e·bel"o·tha·lam'i·kus) [NA]. DENTATOTHALAMIC TRACT.

tractus cor·ti·co·hy·po·tha·la·mi·ci (kor"ti·ko·high·po·thuh·lam'i·sigh) [NA]. CORTICOHYPOTHALAMIC TRACT.

tractus cor·ti·co·pon·ti·ni (kor"ti·ko·pon·tye'nigh). Plural of *tractus corticopontinus.*

tractus cor·ti·co·pon·ti·nus (kor"ti·ko·pon·tye'nus) [NA]. CORTICOPONTINE TRACT.

tractus corticopontinus me·sen·ce·pha·li·cus (mes·en·se·fal'i·kus) [NA]. The corticopontine tract as seen in cross sections of the mesencephalon.

tractus corticopontinus pon·tis (pon'tis) [NA]. The corticopontine tract as seen in cross sections of the pons.

tractus cor·ti·co·spi·na·lis anterior (kor"ti·ko·spye·nay'lis) [NA]. ANTERIOR CORTICOSPINAL TRACT. NA alt. *tractus pyramidalis anterior.*

tractus corticospinalis la·te·ra·lis (lat·e·ray'lis) [NA]. LATERAL CORTICOSPINAL TRACT. NA alt. *tractus pyramidalis lateralis.*

tractus dor·so·la·te·ra·lis (dor·so·lat·e·ray'lis) [NA]. DORSOLATERAL TRACT.

tractus fron·to·pon·ti·nus (fron·to·pon·tye'nus) [NA]. FRONTOPONTINE TRACT.

tractus ge·ni·ta·lis (jen·i·tay'lis). GENITAL CORD.

tractus ilio·ti·bi·a·lis (il''ee·o·tib·ee·ay'lis) [NA]. ILIOTIBIAL TRACT.

tractus iliotibialis [Mais·si·a·ti] (may·see·ay'tye) [BNA]. Tractus iliotibialis (= ILIOTIBIAL TRACT).

tractus me·sen·ce·pha·li·cus ner·vi tri·ge·mi·ni (mes·en·se·fal'i·kus nur'vye trye·jem'i·nigh) [NA]. MESENCEPHALIC TRACT OF THE TRIGEMINAL NERVE.

tractus ner·vo·si as·so·ci·a·ti·o·nis (nur·vo'sigh a·so''see·ay·shee·o'nis) [NA]. A general term to include arcuate fibers of the cerebrum, the uncinate, the superior and inferior longitudinal fasciculi, the cingulum, and the proprius fasciculi of the spinal cord.

tractus nervosi com·mis·su·ra·les (kom·ish·yoo·ray'leez) [NA]. A general term to include the corpus callosum and various commissural pathways of the central nervous system.

tractus nervosi pro·jec·ti·o·nis (pro·jeck·shee·o'nis) [NA]. A general term to include the various projection pathways of the central nervous system that connect one area with another.

tractus oc·ci·pi·to·pon·ti·nus (ock·sip''i·to·pon·tye'nus) [NA]. OCCIPITOPONTINE TRACT.

tractus ol·fac·to·ri·us (ol·fack·to'ree·us) [NA]. OLFACTORY TRACT.

tractus oli·vo·ce·re·bel·la·ris (o·lye''vo·serr·e·be·lair'is, ol''i·vo·) [NA]. OLIVOCEREBELLAR TRACT.

tractus op·ti·cus (op'ti·kus) [NA]. OPTIC TRACT.

tractus pa·ri·e·to·pon·ti·nus (pa·rye''e·to·pon·tye'nus) [NA]. PARIETOPONTINE TRACT.

tractus py·ra·mi·da·les (pi·ram·i·day'leez) [NA]. PYRAMIDAL TRACTS.

tractus py·ra·mi·da·lis anterior (pi·ram·i·day'lis) [NA alt.]. ANTERIOR CORTICOSPINAL TRACT. NA alt. *tractus corticospinalis anterior.*

tractus pyramidalis la·te·ra·lis (lay·e·ray'lis) [NA alt.]. LATERAL CORTICOSPINAL TRACT. NA alt. *tractus corticospinalis lateralis.*

tractus pyramidalis me·dul·lae ob·lon·ga·tae (me·dul'ee ob·long·gay'tee) [NA]. The portion of the pyramidal tract in the medulla oblongata.

tractus pyramidalis me·sen·ce·pha·li·cus (mes·en·se·fal'i·kus) [NA]. The portion of the pyramidal tract in the mesencephalon.

tractus pyramidalis pon·tis (pon'tis) [NA]. The portion of the pyramidal tract in the pons.

tractus re·ti·cu·lo·spi·na·lis (re·tick''yoo·lo·spye·nay'lis) [NA]. RETICULOSPINAL TRACT.

tractus ru·bro·spi·na·lis (roo''bro·spye·nay'lis) [NA]. RUBROSPINAL TRACT.

tractus so·li·ta·ri·us (sol·i·tair'ee·us) [NA]. SOLITARY FASCICULUS.

tractus spi·na·lis ner·vi tri·ge·mi·ni (spye·nay'lis nur'vye trye·jem'i·nigh) [NA]. SPINAL TRACT OF THE TRIGEMINAL NERVE.

tractus spi·no·ce·re·bel·la·ris anterior (spye''no·serr·e·be·lair'is) [NA]. VENTRAL SPINOCEREBELLAR TRACT.

tractus spinocerebellaris posterior [NA]. POSTERIOR SPINOCEREBELLAR TRACT.

tractus spi·no·tec·ta·lis (spye''no·teck·tay'lis) [NA]. SPINOTECTAL TRACT.

tractus spi·no·tha·la·mi·cus anterior (spye''no·thuh·lam'i·kus) [NA]. ANTERIOR SPINOTHALAMIC TRACT.

tractus spinothalamicus la·te·ra·lis (lat·e·ray'lis) [NA]. LATERAL SPINOTHALAMIC TRACT.

tractus spi·ra·lis fo·ra·mi·no·sus (spye·ray'lis fo·ram·i·no'sus) [NA]. A spiral area of the fundus of the internal acoustic meatus overlying the base of the cochlea; it is perforated by many foramina for the passage of the nerve fibers of the eighth cranial nerve.

tractus su·pra·op·ti·co·hy·po·phy·si·a·lis (sue''pruh·op''ti·ko·high·po·fis·ee·ay'lis) [NA]. SUPRAOPTICOHYPOPHYSEAL TRACT.

tractus sys·te·ma·tis ner·vo·si cen·tra·lis (sis·te'muh·tis nur·vo'sigh sen·tray'lis) [NA]. A general term for any nerve tract in the central nervous system.

tractus tec·to·spi·na·lis (teck''to·spye·nay'lis) [NA]. TECTOSPINAL TRACT.

tractus teg·men·ta·lis cen·tra·lis (teg·men·tay'lis sen·tray'lis) [NA]. CENTRAL TEGMENTAL TRACT.

tractus tem·po·ro·pon·ti·nus (tem''po·ro·pon·tye'nus) [NA]. TEMPOROPONTINE TRACT.

tractus ve·sti·bu·lo·spi·na·lis (ves·tib''yoo·lo·spye·nay'lis) [NA]. VESTIBULOSPINAL TRACT.

trade·mark, *n.* A name or mark applied to a substance or product whereby its origin as of a particular producer is indicated; such a name or mark, which may or may not be officially registered, is the property of the producer. A name in this category is frequently called a trademarked name.

trade name. A name, commonly not descriptive or invested with ownership rights, by which a substance or product is known in commerce and industry. If it is intended to indicate the origin of the substance or product as of a particular producer, it is preferably called a trademark or trademarked name.

traf·fic injury. Any injury sustained in traffic, irrespective of whether the injured person is a passenger or a pedestrian.

trag·a·canth (trag'uh·kanth) *n.* [Gk. *tragakantha,* lit., goat's thorn]. A gummy exudation from various Asiatic species of *Astragalus,* of the family Leguminosae. Almost white ribbons or powder; swells with 50 parts of water to make a stiff opalescent mucilage. A soluble portion is said to consist chiefly of uronic acid and arabinose; the insoluble portion that swells in water is largely bassorin, $(C_{11}H_{20}O_{10})_n$. Used as a suspending agent.

tra·gal (tray'gul) *adj.* Of or pertaining to the tragus.

tragi. Plural of *tragus.*

Tra·gia (tray'jee·uh) *n.* A genus of poisonous euphorbiaceous plants; some species have been used in folk medicine as a purgative, diuretic, and caustic.

tra·gi·cus (traj'i·kus, tray'ji·kus) *n.* A vestigial muscle associated with the tragus of the external ear. NA *musculus tragicus.* See also Table of Muscles in the Appendix.

trag·o·mas·chal·ia (trag''o·mas·kal'ee·uh) *n.* [Gk. *tragos,* goat, + *maschalē,* armpit, + *-ia*]. Bromhidrosis of one or both axillae.

trago·pho·nia (trag''o·fo'nee·uh) *n.* [Gk. *tragos,* goat, + *-phonia*]. EGOPHONY.

tra·goph·o·ny (tra·gof'uh·nee) *n.* [Gk. *tragos,* goat, + *-phony*]. EGOPHONY.

tra·gus (tray'gus) *n.,* pl. **tra·gi** (·jye) [NL., from Gk. *tragos,* goat]. 1. [NA] The small prominence of skin-covered cartilage projecting over the meatus of the external ear. 2. One of the coarse hairs at the external auditory meatus.

trail·er, *n.* TRAILING HAND.

trail·ing hand. In synchronous action of both hands, as in playing the piano or drawing with both hands, the hand upon which visual or central attention is not fixed, tends to lag.

train·able, *adj.* 1. Capable of being trained. 2. Specifically, categorizing a mentally retarded individual who can talk and learn to communicate, and who can profit from systematic habit training, learning to feed and dress himself and to take care of his toilet needs, and sometimes able to contribute partially to self-maintenance under complete supervision and in a controlled or sheltered environment. Pertaining largely to individuals with moderate mental retardation (IQ 40 to 54), and often including persons ranked as severely retarded (IQ 25 to 39).

train-dispatcher's nystagmus. OPTOKINETIC NYSTAGMUS.

train nystagmus. OPTOKINETIC NYSTAGMUS.

trait, *n.* [F., from L. *tractus,* trail, track]. Any characteristic, quality, or property of an individual or of a genotype.

Tral. Trademark for hexocyclium methylsulfate, a parasympatholytic agent used for its gastrointestinal antisecretory and antispasmodic effects.

tra·lo·nide (tray'lo·nide) *n.* 9,11β-Dichloro-6α,21-difluoro-16,17-dihydroxypregna-1,4-diene-3,20-dione acetonide, $C_{24}H_{28}Cl_2F_2O_4$, a glucocorticoid.

tram·a·dol (tram'uh·dol) *n.* ($\pm$)-*trans*-2-[(Dimethylamino)methyl]-1-(*m*-methoxyphenyl)cyclohexanol, $C_{16}H_{25}NO_2$, an analgesic; used as the hydrochloride salt.

tra·maz·o·line (tra·maz'o·leen) *n.* 2-[(5,6,7,8-Tetrahydro-1-naphthyl)amino]-2-imidazoline, $C_{13}H_{17}N_3$, an adrenergic, used as the monohydrochloride salt.

trance, *n.* [OF. *transe,* from L. *transire,* to pass over]. 1. The state of hypnosis resembling sleep. 2. The state of being mentally out of touch with the environment. 3. A state of altered consciousness characterized by a prolonged condition of abnormal sleep, in which the vital functions are depressed and from which the patient ordinarily cannot be aroused; breathing is almost imperceptible and sensation abolished; onset and awakening may be sudden.

Trancopal. A trademark for chlormezanone, a tranquilizer.

tran·ex·am·ic acid (tran"eck·sam'ick). *trans*-4-(Aminomethyl)cyclohexanecarboxylic acid, $C_8H_{15}NO_2$, an antifibrinolytic agent; also used in treatment of hereditary angioneurotic edema.

Tranpoise. A trademark for mephenoxalone, a mild tranquilizer.

tran·quil·iz·er, tran·quil·liz·er (tran'kwi·lye"zur, trang') *n.* 1. In popular usage, any agent that brings about a state of peace of mind or relief from anxiety; an ataraxic. 2. Any agent that produces a calming or sedative effect without inducing sleep. 3. Any drug such as chlorpromazine, used primarily for its calming and antipyschotic effects, or meprobamate, used for symptomatic treatment of common psychoneuroses and as an adjunct in somatic disorders complicated by anxiety and tension. —**tranquil·ize, tranquil·lize** (·lize) *v.*

trans- [L., through, across]. A combining form meaning (a) *through* or *across;* (b) (italicized) in chemistry, a prefix indicating that *certain atoms or groups are on opposite sides of a molecule*; usually restricted to cyclic compounds with two stereogenic atoms. Contr. *cis-*.

trans·ab·dom·i·nal (trans"ab·dom'i·nul) *adj.* [*trans-* + *abdominal*]. Through or across the abdomen or abdominal wall.

transabdominal pneumoperitoneum. Injection of gas through the abdominal wall into the peritoneal cavity to outline the organs and boundaries of the abdominal cavity for x-ray examination.

trans·am·i·da·tion (trans·am"i·day'shun) *n.* TRANSDEAMINATION.

trans·am·i·nase (trans·am'i·nace, ·naze) *n.* One of a group of enzymes that catalyze the transfer of the amino group of an amino acid to a keto acid, to form another amino acid. See also *transferase.*

trans·am·i·na·tion (trans·am"i·nay'shun) *n.* 1. The transfer of one or more amino groups from one compound to another. 2. The transposition of an amino group within a single compound.

trans·an·i·ma·tion (trans·an"i·may'shun) *n.* [*trans-* + L. *animare,* to give life to]. MOUTH-TO-MOUTH BREATHING.

trans·aor·tic (trans"ay·or'tick) *adj.* [*trans-* + *aortic*]. Through or across the aorta.

trans·atri·al (trans·ay'tree·ul) *adj.* [*trans-* + *atrial*]. Through or across an atrium.

trans·au·di·ent (trans·aw'dee·unt) *adj.* [*trans-* + L. *audire,* to hear]. Allowing the transmission of sound.

trans·ca·lent (trans·kay'lunt) *adj.* [*trans-* + L. *calere,* to be warm]. Permeable to radiant heat rays.

trans·cav·i·tary (trans·kav'i·terr"ee) *adj.* Through or across a cavity; usually referring to metastasis of tumor cells, most often in the peritoneal cavity.

trans·clo·mi·phene (trans·klo'mi·feen) *n.* A name formerly used for zuclomiphene.

trans·con·dy·lar (trans·kon'di·lur) *adj.* [*trans-* + *condylar*]. Across or through condyles.

trans·cor·ti·cal (trans·kor'ti·kul) *adj.* [*trans-* + *cortical*]. 1. Pertaining to connections between different parts of the cerebral cortex. 2. Through the cortex of an organ.

transcortical motor aphasia. A form of aphasia in which the patient is able to repeat words, but is unable to produce spontaneous speech or to write; thought to be due to a lesion in the third frontal convolution of the dominant hemisphere.

transcortical sensory aphasia. An aphasia characterized by loss of comprehension of the spoken or written word and paraphasic speech, with retention of the ability to read aloud and to write and to repeat words. There is a tendency to echolalia. It is believed by Nielsen to result from the disconnection of the first temporal convolution from the remainder of the cortical language areas.

transcortical syndrome. DISCONNECTION SYNDROME.

trans·cor·tin (trans·kor'tin) *n.* An α_2-globulin in blood that specifically binds hydrocortisone and certain related corticosteroids. Syn. *corticosteroid-binding globulin.*

tran·scrip·tion (tran·skrip'shun) *n.* The deoxyribonucleic acid–directed synthesis of messenger ribonucleic acid.

trans·cul·tur·al psychiatry (trans"kul'chur·ul). CULTURAL PSYCHIATRY.

trans·cu·ta·ne·ous (trans"kew·tay'nee·us) *adj.* [*trans-* + *cutaneous*]. PERCUTANEOUS.

trans·de·am·i·na·tion (trans"dee·am"i·nay'shun) *n.* The transference of amino groups from amino acids to other molecules.

trans·duc·tion (tranz·duck'shun) *n.* [L. *transducere,* to lead across]. 1. The process of transferring energy from one system to another; the transferred energy may be of the same or of a different form, for example, a steam engine converting thermal energy to mechanical energy. 2. The transfer from bacterium to bacterium of genetic material carried by a bacterial virus. —**trans·duc·er** (·dew'sur) *n.*

trans·du·o·de·nal (trans"dew·od'e·nul, ·dew·o·dee'nul) *adj.* [*trans-* + *duodenal*]. Through or across the duodenum.

transduodenal choledocholithotomy. Removal of a biliary calculus in the common bile duct through an opening made into the duodenum.

transduodenal choledochotomy. Incision for the removal of gallstones from the hepaticopancreatic ampulla.

tran·sect (tran·sekt') *v.* [*trans* + L. *secare, sectus,* to cut]. To cut across.

tran·sec·tion (tran·seck'shun) *n.* [*trans-* + *section*]. A section made across the long axis of a part, as transection of the spinal cord.

trans·fer, *n. In prosthodontics,* a nonanatomic cover for a tooth, which may be removed in an impression and used as a receptacle for dies to assure their correct relationship in the poured working cast; usually made of resin, low-fusing metal, or cast gold alloy.

trans·fer·ase (trans'fur·ace, ·aze) *n.* Any of many types of enzymes that catalyze transfer of a chemical group from one molecule to another; among groups that may be transferred are phosphate, methyl, amine, keto.

trans·fer·ence (trans·fur'unce, trans'fur·unce) *n.* [NL. *transferentia,* from L. *transferre,* to carry over]. *In psychiatry,* the unconscious transfer of the patient's feelings and reactions originally associated with important persons in the patient's life, usually father, mother, or siblings, toward others and in the analytic situation, toward the therapist. Transference may be positive, when the feelings and reactions are affectionate, friendly, or loving; it may be negative, when these feelings and reactions are hostile.

transference neurosis. *In psychiatry,* those psychoneurotic disorders, including the anxiety neurosis, obsessive-compulsive neurosis, phobias, and conversion type of hysterical neurosis, grouped together by Freud as most amenable to analytic therapy, because of their basic capacity for developing transference.

transference of sensation. CLAIRVOYANCE.

transfer factor. An uncharacterized low-molecular-weight material extracted from leukocytes of persons with delayed hypersensitivity and apparently capable of transferring such hypersensitivity to unsensitized persons.

trans·fer·rin (trans·ferr'in) *n.* [*trans-* + L. *ferr*um, iron, + *-in*]. A beta-1 globulin of blood serum concerned with binding and transportation of iron. Syn. *siderophilin, siderophyllin.*

transfer RNA. A type of ribonucleic acid that combines with specific amino acids and then with messenger RNA to allow amino acid residues to combine in a certain sequence during protein synthesis. It constitutes 10 to 20 percent of total cellular ribonucleic acid, and its structure is complementary to messenger RNA. Abbreviated, tRNA

trans·fix·ion (trans·fick'shun) *n.* [L. *transfixio,* from *transfigere,* to pierce through]. 1. The act of piercing through and through. 2. A method of amputation in which the knife is passed directly through the soft parts, the cutting being done from within outward. —**trans·fix** (·ficks') *v.*

transfixion suture. 1. A method of closing a wound by the use of a pin or needle which is placed through both wound edges and held by winding suture material over both ends in a figure-of-eight fashion. Syn. *figure-of-eight suture, harelip suture.* 2. A hemostatic suture that does not slip off the bleeding point due to its transfixion of the adjacent tissue.

trans·fo·ra·tion (trans"fo·ray'shun) *n.* [L. *transforatio,* a boring through, from *forare,* to pierce, bore]. The act of perforating the fetal skull. —**trans·fo·rate** (trans'fo·rate) *v.*

trans·fo·ra·tor (trans'fo·ray·tur) *n.* An instrument for perforating the fetal head.

trans·for·ma·tion (trans"for·may'shun) *n.* [L. *transformatio,* from *transformare,* to transform, from *forma,* form]. 1. A marked change in form, structure, or function. 2. *In bacterial genetics,* the acquisition of genetic properties by the uptake and expression of free DNA. 3. *In cell biology and oncology,* the conversion of a normal cell into one which is capable of malignant growth or, by extension, into one exhibiting properties in culture which are those characterizing cultured malignant cells. These may include loss of density-dependent inhibition of growth, ability to form colonies in soft agar; may be spontaneous or induced by viruses of certain chemicals.

trans·form·er (trans·for'mur) *n.* An electrical apparatus for the transformation of lower potentials to higher potentials, or vice versa. It consists of a laminated iron core on which are wound two coils, a primary and a secondary coil, properly insulated from each other. The primary coil is energized by an alternating current at a given voltage, which induces in the secondary coil a voltage related to that in the primary by the ratio of the number of turns of wire in the two coils.

trans·fuse (trans·fewz') *v.* To perform a transfusion of or on.

trans·fu·sion (trans·few'zhun) *n.* [L. *transfusio,* from *transfundere,* to pour from one vessel into another]. The introduction into a blood vessel of blood, saline solution, or other liquid.

tranfusion reaction. Any febrile, allergic, or hemolytic state produced in a patient by a blood transfusion.

trans·fu·sion·ist (trans·few'zhun·ist) *n.* A person skilled in the practice of the transfusion of blood.

transfusion jaundice. SERUM HEPATITIS.

trans·he·pat·ic cholangiography (trans"he·pat'ick). Roentgenologic demonstration of the biliary drainage system by direct injection of contrast medium into the biliary radicles.

tran·sient (tran'shunt, ·zee·unt) *adj.* [L. *transiens,* from *transire,* to go through]. Present for only a short period of time; impermanent; temporary; transitory.

transient dermatozoonosis. Dermatozoonosis in which the parasite attacks, but does not attach itself to, the skin. Syn. *transitozoonosis.*

transient flora. *In surgery,* the loosely attached, easily removed or destroyed portion of the cutaneous bacterial flora, which is acquired largely by contact with germ-laden objects. It is subject to great variations, both quantitative and qualitative.

transient global amnesia. An episode of mental confusion rarely recurrent, observed in middle-aged and elderly persons and lasting several hours; the symptoms have their basis in a defect in memory for events of the present and recent past. During the attack there is no impairment of consciousness, or of motor, sensory, or reflex functions. The pathogenesis is uncertain; it may represent an ischemic attack or a temporal lobe seizure.

transient hypogammaglobulinemia. The temporary deficiency of gamma globulins sometimes seen in infants due to a delay in the onset of gamma-globulin synthesis and occasionally accompanied by increased susceptibility to bacterial infection.

transient ischemic attack. An episode of transient cerebral symptoms, varying from patient to patient but consisting most often of dim vision, hemiparesis, numbness on one side of the body, dizziness and thick speech, that usually lasts 10 minutes or less, but may last as long as 24 hours in some cases. These attacks are usually related to atherosclerotic thrombotic disease; the longer-lasting attacks are probably due to cerebral embolism.

transient neonatal myasthenia. NEONATAL MYASTHENIA.

transient situational disturbances. *In psychiatry,* a form of personality disorder, more or less transient, and generally an acute symptom response to a specific situation, without persistent personality disturbance. The acute symptoms, representing attempts to deal with overwhelming situations, generally recede as stress diminishes; repeated failure to do so indicates more severe disturbance. See also *adjustment reaction, adult situational reaction.*

transient situational personality disorder. TRANSIENT SITUATIONAL DISTURBANCES.

transient synovitis. A common cause of painful hip in children, usually unilateral, affecting boys more than girls, and lasting days to weeks. Cause is unknown, and clinical findings make it difficult to distinguish from osteochondritis deformans juvenilis. Radiographic findings may be normal or show effusion or distention of the capsule of the hip joint. Syn. *transitory synovitis, toxic synovitis.*

trans·il·i·ac (tran·zil'ee·ack) *adj.* [*trans-* + *iliac*]. Passing across from one ilium to the other, as the transiliac diameter.

trans·il·lu·mi·na·ble (trans"i·lew'mi·nuh·bul) *adj.* Capable of being transilluminated.

trans·il·lu·mi·na·tion (trans"i·lew"mi·nay'shun) *n.* 1. Illumination of an object by transmitted light. 2. Illumination of the paranasal sinuses by means of a light placed in the patient's mouth. 3. Illumination of an infant's skull, positive in hydrocephaly, porencephaly, and other brain defects or where there is fluid over the brain.

trans·in·ti·mal (trans·in'ti·mul) *adj.* Through the intima of blood vessels.

tran·sis·tor (tran·zis'tur) *n.* [*trans*fer + re*sistor*]. A solid-state device, considerably smaller than a vacuum tube used similarly, for amplifying electric currents through utilization of a semiconductor such as germanium or silicon.

tran·si·tion·al (tran·zish'un·ul) *adj. & n.* [L. *transitio,* a going across]. 1. Of, pertaining to, or characterized by change.

2. According to Ehrlich, a monocyte having a U-shaped nucleus, which he regarded, incorrectly, as a transitional form in the development of a polymorphonuclear granulocyte; now considered to be an older form of monocyte.

transitional cell. 1. A cell having characteristics of two or more other cell types. 2. An epithelial cell of the urinary collecting system and bladder which assumes different forms under different conditions of distention. 3. MONOCYTE. 4. A large plasma cell, considered transitional between a blast cell and a definitive small plasma cell.

transitional-cell carcinoma. A malignant tumor whose parenchyma is composed of anaplastic transitional epithelial cells.

transitional denture. A removable partial denture to which artificial teeth can be added as natural teeth are lost.

transitional epithelium. The stratified epithelium of the urinary tract. The cells of this form vary in shape between squamous, when the epithelium is stretched, and columnar or cuboidal when not stretched.

transitional leukocyte. MONOCYTE.

transitional vertebra. A vertebra with characteristics that are intermediate between those of a typical vertebra of one group and a typical vertebra of another, as a vertebra intermediate in character between the last thoracic and first lumbar vertebrae.

tran·si·to·ry (tran'si·to·ree) *adj.* TRANSIENT.

transitory arthritis of the hip. TRANSIENT SYNOVITIS.

transitory synovitis. TRANSIENT SYNOVITIS.

tran·si·to·zoo·no·sis (tran''zi·to·zo''uh·no'sis) *n.* TRANSIENT DERMATOZOONOSIS.

trans·la·tion (tranz·lay'shun) *n.* [L. *translatio,* transfer, handing over, from *transferre,* to transfer]. The ribonucleic acid-directed synthesis of protein.

trans·la·to·ry motion or **movement** (tranz·luh·to·ree, ·tor·ee). Movement of all points of an object in the same direction at the same speed, as opposed to movement involving twisting or rotation.

trans·lo·ca·tion (tranz''lo·kay'shun) *n.* The displacement of part or all of one chromosome to another. See also *balanced translocation, reciprocal translocation, simple translocation.*

trans·lu·cent (tranz·lew'sunt) *adj.* [L. *translucere,* to shine through]. Permitting a partial transmission of light; somewhat transparent. Contr. *opaque.*

trans·lu·cid (tranz·lew'sid) *adj.* [*trans-* + L. *lucidus,* shining]. Semitransparent.

trans·lu·mi·nal (trans·lew'mi·nul) *adj.* Across or through a lumen.

transluminal angioplasty. The removal of thrombi or emboli from blood vessels, especially arteries, by catheters inserted through their lumens.

trans·lu·mi·na·tion (trans·lew''mi·nay'shun) *n.* TRANSILLUMINATION.

trans·max·il·lary ethmoidectomy (trans·mack'si·lerr''ee). Ethmoidectomy by incision through the canine fossa and maxillary sinus, preserving the mucous membrane of the lateral nasal wall. Syn. *De Lima's operation.*

trans·meth·yl·a·tion (tranz·meth''i·lay'shun) *n.* A type of metabolic chemical reaction in which a methyl group is transferred from a donor to a receptor compound. Methionine and choline are important sources of methyl groups.

trans·mi·gra·tion (tranz''migh·gray'shun) *n.* [L. *transmigratio,* from *transmigrare,* to transmigrate]. Movement from one place to another which may involve crossing a membrane or other barrier, such as the passage of leukocytes or erythrocytes through the capillary walls (diapedesis).

transmissible gastroenteritis. A highly contagious and frequently fatal viral disease of swine, especially young pigs; characterized by acute diarrhea, vomiting, and severe dehydration.

trans·mis·si·bil·i·ty (tranz·mis''i·bil'i·tee) *n.* The capability of being transmitted or communicated from one person to another. —**trans·mis·si·ble** (·mis'i·bul) *adj.*

trans·mis·sion (tranz·mish'un) *n.* [L. *transmissio,* from *transmittere,* to send across]. The communication or transfer of anything, especially infectious or heritable disease, from one person or place to another.

transmission curve. *In radiology,* a curve showing variation in quantity as a function of thickness of the absorbing material.

trans·mit·tance (tranz·mit'unce) *n.* In applied spectroscopy, the ratio of the radiant power transmitted by a sample to the radiant power incident on the sample, both measurements being made at the same spectral position and with the same slit width. Symbol, *T*

trans·mit·ted light (tranz·mit'id). The light passing through an object.

trans·mit·ter substance (tranz·mit'ur). The chemical released by the arrival of a nerve impulse at an axon terminal which diffuses across the synaptic cleft and results in a dendritic response. See also *neurotransmitter.*

trans·mu·ral (trans·mew'rul) *adj.* [*trans-* + *mural*]. Across a wall, used to describe myocardial infarction involving the full thickness of the myocardium in a given location.

trans·mu·ta·tion (tranz''mew·tay'shun) *n.* [L. *transmutatio,* from *transmutare,* to change]. *In physics,* any process by which an atomic nucleus is converted into another of different atomic number.

trans·oc·u·lar (tranz·ock'yoo·lur) *adj.* [*trans-* + *ocular*]. Extending across the eye.

trans·o·nance (trans'uh·nunce) *n.* [*trans-* + L. *sonare,* to sound]. Transmission of sounds originating in one organ through another organ.

trans·or·bit·al (tranz·or'bit·ul) *adj.* [*trans-* + *orbital*]. Passing through the eye socket.

transorbital lobotomy. A lobotomy performed through the roof of the orbit. See also *psychosurgery.*

trans·par·ent (trans·păr'unt) *adj.* [ML. *transparere,* to show through, from L. *parere,* to appear]. Permitting the passage of light rays without material obstruction, so that objects beyond the transparent body can be seen. Contr. *opaque.*

transparent-chamber method. Insertion of a chamber with a transparent top and bottom into a suitable part of an animal, such as a rat's back or rabbit's ear, to permit microscopic study of enclosed cells or tissues.

transparent media of the eye. The cornea, aqueous humor, lens, and vitreous humor.

trans·peri·to·ne·al (trans·perr''i·to·nee'ul) *adj.* [*trans-* + *peritoneal*]. Passing through or across the peritoneum.

transperitoneal migration. The passage of an ovum from one ovary to the oviduct of the opposite side.

trans·phos·pho·ryl·ase (trans''fos·fo'ri·lace, ·laze) *n.* One of a group of enzymes, widely distributed in living organisms, which catalyze transfer of phosphate from one compound to another.

tran·spir·able (trans·pye'ruh·bul) *adj.* Capable of passing in a gaseous state through the respiratory epithelium or the skin.

tran·spi·ra·tion (tran''spi·ray'shun) *n.* [*trans-* + L. *spirare,* to breathe]. 1. Exhalation of fluid through the skin. 2. PERSPIRATION.

trans·pla·cen·tal (trans''pluh·sen'tul) *adj.* [*trans-* + *placental*]. Across the placenta.

trans·plant (trans'plant) *n.* [L. *transplantare,* to transplant]. Tissue removed from any portion of the body and placed in a different site. —**trans·plant** (trans·plant') *v.*

trans·plan·ta·tion (trans''plan·tay'shun) *n.* The operation of transplanting or of applying to a part of the body tissues taken from another body or from another part of the same body. See also *graft.*

transplantation of the cornea. KERATOPLASTY.

trans·pleu·ral (trans·ploor'ul) *adj.* [*trans-* + *pleural*]. Through the pleura.

trans·port aminoaciduria (trans'port). RENAL AMINOACIDURIA.

trans·pose (trans·poze') *v.* [F. *transposer,* from *poser,* to place]. To displace; to change about, as tissue from one location to another by operation.

trans·po·si·tion (trans"puh·zish'un) *n.* A change of position; a change from the usual order.

transposition of the great arteries or **vessels.** A congenital anomaly in which the aorta arises from the right ventricle and the pulmonary trunk from the left ventricle; this exchange of position may be complete or incomplete. See also *corrected transposition of the great arteries.*

transposition of the heart. A reversal in the position of the heart. See also *dextrocardia, dextroversion, levocardia, levoversion.*

transposition of the pulmonary veins. Drainage of the pulmonary veins into the right rather than left atrium; may be complete or incomplete. Syn. *anomalous pulmonary venous drainage.*

transposition of the viscera. A change in the position of the viscera to the side opposite to that normally occupied; situs inversus viscerum.

trans·py·lor·ic plane (trans"pye·lor'ick). A horizontal plane through the body at the level of the second lumbar vertebra; the pylorus usually lies in this plane.

trans·sa·cral block (trans·say'krul). Anesthesia of the sacral nerves approached through the posterior sacral foramens.

trans·sex·u·al (trans·seck'shoo·ul) *n.* [*trans-* + *sexual*]. An individual whose chromosomes, gonads, and body habitus mark him or her as a member of one sex, but who identifies psychically with the other sex, with an overwhelming desire for sex reassignment through surgical and hormonal intervention. Such an individual may dress and live routinely as a member of the opposite sex.

trans·sex·u·a·lism (trans·seck'shoo·uh·liz·um) *n.* The condition of being a transsexual.

trans·sub·stan·ti·a·tion (trans"sub·stan"shee·ay'shun) *n.* [ML. *transsubstantiatio,* change of one substance into another]. The replacement of tissue of one kind by another.

trans·ten·to·ri·al (trans"ten·to'ree·ul) *adj.* [*trans-* + *tentorial*]. Into the incisure of or across the tentorium.

transtentorial herniation. UNCAL HERNIATION.

trans·tho·rac·ic (trans"tho·ras'ick) *adj.* [*trans-* + *thoracic*]. Across or through the thorax.

transthoracic nephrectomy. Nephrectomy performed through a thoracic approach and an incision through the diaphragm.

trans·tym·pan·ic method (trans"tim·pan'ick). A surgical approach, working backward on the outer wall of the attic, using the external acoustic meatus, to the regions of the middle ear and mastoid process; useful in performing fenestration and radical mastoidectomy.

tran·su·date (tran'sue·date) *n.* A liquid or other substance produced by transudation.

tran·su·da·tion (tran"sue·day'shun) *n.* [*trans* + L. *sudare,* to sweat]. The passing of fluid or a solute through a membrane by means of a hydrostatic or osmotic pressure gradient, especially passage of blood serum through the vessel walls. —**tran·su·da·tory** (tran·sue'duh·tor"ee) *adj.;* **tran·sude** (tran·sue'd') *v.*

trans·uran·ic element (trans"yoo·ran'ick). An element with an atomic number greater than that of uranium (92).

trans·ure·tero·ure·ter·os·to·my (trans"yoo·ree"tur·o·yoo·ree"tur·os'tuh·mee) *n.* [*trans-* + *ureteroureterostomy*]. Suture of one ureter across the midline to the opposite ureter to overcome obstruction.

trans·ure·thral (trans"yoo·ree'thrul) *adj.* [*trans-* + *urethral*]. Via the urethra.

transurethral prostatectomy. Removal of the prostate by means of an operating cystoscope or resectoscope inserted through the urethra.

transurethral resection. Resection of the prostate or a portion of the lower urinary tract by means of a resectoscope passed through the urethra. Abbreviated, TUR

trans·va·gi·nal (trans·vuh·jye'nul, vaj'i·nul) *adj.* [*trans-* + *vaginal*]. Across or through the vagina.

trans·ver·sa·lis (trans"vur·say'lis) *adj.* [NL.]. TRANSVERSE.

transversalis fascia. The thin membrane lying between the transversus abdominis muscle and the peritoneum. NA *fascia transversalis.*

transversalis ster·ni (stur'nigh). The transverse thoracic muscle. See Table of Muscles in the Appendix.

trans·verse (trans·vurce') *adj.* [L. *transversus,* from *vertere, versus,* to turn]. Crosswise; at right angles to the longitudinal axis of the body or of a part.

transverse accessory foramina. Anomalous foramina in the transverse processes of the cervical vertebrae giving passage to an inconstant accessory vertebral artery.

transverse acetabular ligament. The fibrous continuation of the acetabular lip which crosses the acetabular notch, completing the ring formed by the lip and converting the notch into a foramen. NA *ligamentum transversum acetabuli.*

transverse arch of the foot. The transverse hollow on the inner part of the sole of the foot in the line of the tarsometatarsal articulations. NA *arcus pedis transversalis.*

transverse arrest. *In obstetrics,* a faulty condition in the mechanism of labor when a flat type of maternal pelvis causes a fixation of the fetal head in the transverse position.

transverse carpal ligament. FLEXOR RETINACULUM OF THE WRIST.

transverse cerebral fissure. The space between the diencephalon and the cerebral hemispheres. NA *fissura transversa cerebri.*

transverse colon. The portion of the colon between the hepatic flexure and the splenic flexure. NA *colon transversum.*

transverse crural ligament. SUPERIOR EXTENSOR RETINACULUM.

trans·ver·sec·to·my (trans"vur·seck'tuh·mee) *n.* [*transverse* + *-ectomy*]. Excision of a transverse process of a vertebra; specifically, in orthopedics, removal of the transverse process of the fifth lumbar vertebra for pain due to irritation of the lower spinal nerve roots.

transverse diameter of the pelvic inlet. The distance between the two most widely separated points of the pelvic inlet.

transverse diameter of the pelvic outlet. The distance between the two ischial tuberosities.

transverse facial cleft. An embryonic fissure at the angle of the mouth, causing macrostomia.

transverse fissure of the liver. A fissure crossing transversely the lower surface of the right lobe of the liver. It transmits the portal vein, hepatic artery and nerves, and hepatic duct.

transverse foramen. FORAMEN TRANSVERSARIUM.

transverse frontoparietal index. *In craniometry,* the ratio of the minimum frontal diameter, taken between the frontotemporalia, times 100, to the greatest width of the cranium, taken wherever found on the parietal bones or on the squamous parts of the temporal bones, provided the end points of the line of greatest width lie in the same horizontal and frontal planes. Values of the index are classified as:

ultramicroseme	x–54.9
hypermicroseme	55.0–59.9
microseme	60.0–64.9
mesoseme	65.0–69.9
megaseme	70.0–74.9
hypermegaseme	75.0–79.9
ultrahypermegaseme	80.0–x

transverse ligament. 1. (of the atlas:) The thick band which forms the horizontal part of the cruciate ligament of the atlas and which, crossing the ring of the atlas in a curve around the dens, divides the opening of the ring into an anterior portion occupied by the dens and a posterior portion through which the spinal cord passes. NA *ligamentum transverse atlantis.* 2. (of the knee:) The ligament in the knee joint which connects the outer anterior margin of the lateral meniscus and the anterior end of the medial meniscus. NA *ligamentum transversum genus.* 3. (of the acetabulum:) TRANSVERSE ACETABULAR LIGAMENT. 4. (of the perineum:) TRANSVERSE PERINEAL LIGAMENT. 5. (of the wrist:) FLEXOR RETINACULUM OF THE WRIST. 6. (of the leg:) SUPERIOR EXTENSOR RETINACULUM. 7. (of the scapula:) See *inferior transverse ligament of the scapula, superior transverse ligament of the scapula.*

transversely contracted pelvis. A pelvis having a reduced transverse diameter.

transverse mesocolon. The transverse portion of the mesentery connecting the transverse colon with the posterior abdominal wall. NA *mesocolon transversum.* See also Plate 8.

transverse metatarsal ligament. DEEP TRANSVERSE METATARSAL LIGAMENT.

transverse myelitis or **myelopathy.** 1.Paraplegia or quadriplegia due to a sudden total or near-total transection of the spinal cord, occurring most often as a result of trauma, but also as a result of infarction or hemorrhage or rapidly advancing necrotizing, demyelinative or compressive inflammatory or neoplastic lesions. 2. More specifically, the sudden transverse spinal cord lesion of demyelinative disease.

transverse nuchal muscle. An occasional extra slip of the occipitofrontalis muscle. NA *musculus transversus nuchae.*

transverse occipital sulcus. A groove on the lateral superior aspect of the occipital lobe. Frequently it is continuous with the occipital ramus of the intraparietal sulcus. NA *sulcus occipitalis transversus.*

transverse occipital torus. An occasional elevation found on the occipital bone which includes the external occipital protuberance and the adjacent area.

transverse optic neuritis. A form of optic neuritis with loss of the entire visual field.

transverse palatine suture. SUTURA PALATINA TRANSVERSA.

transverse pancreatic artery. INFERIOR PANCREATIC ARTERY.

transverse pelvic ligament. TRANSVERSE PERINEAL LIGAMENT.

transverse perineal ligament. The fibrous anterior margin of the urogenital diaphragm. NA *ligamentum transversum perinei.*

transverse plane. A plane at right angles to the long axis of the body or a part; HORIZONTAL PLANE.

transverse presentation. Presentation in which the child is turned with its long axis across that of the birth canal; the presenting part may be the shoulder, back, or abdomen.

transverse process. A process projecting outward from the side of a vertebra, at the junction of the pedicle and the lamina. NA *processus transversus.*

transverse rectal folds. Large, semilunar folds projecting into the lumen of the rectum. NA *plicae transversales recti.*

transverse section. CROSS SECTION (1).

transverse septum. The embryonic partition between the ventral part of the pericardial cavity and the peritoneal cavity which contributes to the formation of the diaphragm, the capsule and connective tissue of the liver, as well as the lesser omentum.

transverse sinus. 1. A sinus of the dura mater running from the internal occipital protuberance, following for part of its course the attached margin of the tentorium cerebelli, then over the jugular process of the occipital bone to reach the jugular foramen. Syn. *lateral sinus.* NA *sinus transversus durae matris.* See also Table of Veins in the Appendix and Plates 10 and 17. 2. A dorsal communication between the right and left sides of the pericardial cavity between the reflections of the epicardium at the arterial and venous attachments of the heart, passing behind the aorta and pulmonary trunk and in front of the superior vena cava and left atrium. NA *sinus transversus pericardii.*

transverse sulcus of the anthelix. A transverse furrow on the cranial aspect of cartilage of the auricle. NA *sulcus anthelicus transversus.*

transverse tarsal articulation. The calcaneocuboid and talocalcaneonavicular articulations considered as one. NA *articulatio tarsi transversa.*

transverse temporal gyri. Two or three gyri that cross the upper surface of the superior temporal gyrus transversely. Syn. *Heschl's gyri.* NA *gyri temporales transversi.*

transverse temporal sulci. Irregular vertical grooves on the surface of the insula of the temporal lobe. NA *sulci temporales transversi.*

transverse tubule. One of the slender, transversely oriented tubules which are closely associated with the terminal cisternae of the sarcoplasmic reticulum of skeletal muscle cells.

transverse vesical plica. A variable fold of peritoneum extending from the urinary bladder laterally to the pelvic wall; it is seen only when the viscus is empty. NA *plica vesicalis transversa.*

trans·ver·sus (trans·vur'sus) *adj.* [L.]. TRANSVERSE.

transversus nu·chae (new'kee). TRANSVERSE NUCHAL MUSCLE.

trans·ves·tism (trans·ves'tiz·um) *n.* [*transvestite* + *-ism*]. Dressing or masquerading in the clothing of the opposite sex; usually due to an unconscious wish to appear and be accepted as a member of the opposite sex. See also *eonism, sexoesthetic inversion, transsexualism.*

trans·ves·tite (trans·ves'tite) *n.* [*trans-* + L. *vestitus,* dressed, from *vestire,* to dress]. An individual who dresses in the clothes of the opposite sex; usually applied only when this is done rather habitually, as by a homosexual or a transsexual.

trans·ves·ti·tism (trans·ves'ti·tiz·um) *n.* TRANSVESTISM.

tran·yl·cy·pro·mine (tran''il·sigh'pro·meen) *n.* *trans-dl*-2-Phenylcyclopropylamine, $C_9H_{11}N$, a nonhydrazine monoamine oxidase inhibitor used, as the sulfate salt, for the treatment of severe mental depression.

tra·pe·zi·al (tra·pee'zee·ul) *adj.* Pertaining to a trapezium or to a trapezius muscle.

tra·pe·zio·meta·car·pal (tra·pee''zee·o·met''uh·kahr'pul) *adj.* Pertaining to the trapezium and metacarpals.

tra·pe·zi·um (tra·pee'zee·um) *n.*, pl. **trape·zia** (·zee·uh) [NL., from Gk. *trapezion,* dim. of *trapeza,* table]. The first bone of the second row of the carpal bones. NA *os trapezium.* See also Table of Bones in the Appendix.

tra·pe·zi·us (tra·pee'zee·us) *n.* [NL., from *trapezium*]. A muscle arising from the occipital bone, the nuchal ligament, and the spines of the thoracic vertebrae, and inserted into the clavicle, acromion, and spine of the scapula. NA *musculus trapezius.* See also Table of Muscles in the Appendix.

trap·e·zoid (trap'e·zoid) *n.* [Gk. *trapezoeidēs,* trapezium-shaped]. 1. A geometric, four-sided figure having two parallel and two diverging sides. 2. The second bone of the second row of the carpus. NA *os trapezoideum.* See also Table of Bones in the Appendix.

trapezoid body. Transverse decussating fibers in the ventral tegmental part of the pons, which connect the ventral cochlear nucleus of one side with the lateral lemniscus of the other side. NA *corpus trapezoideum.*

trapezoid ligament. A broad quadrilateral ligament extending from the upper surface of the coracoid process to the oblique ridge on the undersurface of the clavicle, the trapezoid line; a part of the coracoclavicular ligament. NA *ligamentum trapezoideum.*

trapezoid line or **ridge.** A line on the inferior surface of the acromial end of the clavicle to which the trapezoid portion of the coracoclavicular ligament is attached. NA *linea trapezoidea.*

Trapp's formula [J. *Trapp,* Russian pharmacist, 1815-1908].

Obsol. The last two digits of the urine specific gravity value are multiplied by 2 (Trapp's coefficient) or 2.33 (Haeser's coefficient) to approximate the weight in grains of solids in 1 liter of urine. See also *Haeser's formula.*

Trasentine. Trademark for adiphenine, an antispasmodic drug used as the hydrochloride salt.

Trasylol. Trademark for the proteinase inhibitor aprotinin.

t ratio. The ratio of a statistical constant to its standard error. Syn. *t function.*

Trau·be-He·ring curves or **waves** (traow'buh, heʸr'ing) [L. *Traube,* German physician, 1818–1876; and K. E. K. *Hering*]. TRAUBE WAVES.

Traube's membrane [L. *Traube*]. A film formed at the interface of a solution of potassium ferrocyanide with a solution of a copper salt.

Traube's rule [L. *Traube*]. The extent to which members of homologous series are adsorbed from aqueous solution increases as the number of CH_2 groups in the molecule increases or as the molecular weight increases.

Traube's semilunar space [L. *Traube*]. An area of the lower left lateral and anterior chest wall which is tympanitic to percussion because of gas in the underlying stomach.

Traube's sign [L. *Traube*]. PISTOL-SHOT SOUND.

Traube's space [L. *Traube*]. SEMILUNAR SPACE.

Traube waves [L. *Traube*]. Prominent high deflection of the sphygmograph seen in complete respiratory arrest.

trau·ma (traw'muh, traow'muh) *n.*, pl. **trauma·ta** (·tuh), **traumas** [Gk.]. 1. An injury caused by a mechanical or physical agent. 2. A severe psychic injury.

traumat-, traumato-. A combining form meaning *trauma, traumatic.*

trau·mat·ic (traw·mat'ick) *adj.* [Gk. *traumatikos,* from *trauma,* wound]. Pertaining to or caused by a wound or injury.

traumatic acid. $HOOCCH{=}CH(CH_2)_8COOH$, 2-Dodecenedioic acid, a dibasic acid found in certain plants after they have been cut or bruised; stimulates resumption of division of mature cells.

traumatic amenorrhea. ASHERMAN'S SYNDROME.

traumatic amputation. An amputation resulting from direct trauma.

traumatic anesthesia. Loss of sensation due to injury of a nerve.

traumatic aneurysm. An aneurysm produced by injury, as crushing, or following a stab or gunshot wound, as distinguished from one resulting from disease.

traumatic asphyxia or **apnea.** Cyanosis of the head and neck from sudden compression of the thorax or upper abdomen or both.

traumatic convulsion. A seizure associated with or due to an acute brain injury, such as a concussion or contusion. See also *traumatic epilepsy.*

traumatic cyanosis. COMPRESSION CYANOSIS.

traumatic delirium. Acute delirium resulting from head or brain injury.

traumatic dementia. 1. Chronic brain disorder with loss of intellectual functioning due to severe cerebral injury. 2. PUNCH-DRUNK STATE.

traumatic dislocation. A dislocation as a result of violence.

traumatic epilepsy. Recurrent seizures due to or associated with brain injury, such as a laceration and subsequent meningocerebral scarring; may be focal, psychomotor, or generalized.

traumatic erysipelas. Erysipelas occurring as a complication of skin trauma.

traumatic glycosuria. ARTIFICIAL GLYCOSURIA.

traumatic intrauterine synechiae. ASHERMAN'S SYNDROME.

traumatic keratitis. Keratitis resulting from wounds or injury of the cornea.

traumatic labyrinthitis. Inflammation of the labyrinth due to trauma, as a fractured skull or such functional labyrinthine surgery as a fenestration operation.

traumatic marginal alopecia. Partial alopecia involving the marginal area of the scalp above and anterior to the ears, usually caused by continued traction on the hair from braiding or hair-straightening procedures.

traumatic meningitis. Meningitis resulting from the invasion of organisms after injuries to the head or spine.

traumatic myoglobinuria. Myoglobinuria following severe physical damage to striated muscle as the result of crushing injuries, high-voltage currents, or even extreme punishment.

traumatic neuroma. AMPUTATION NEUROMA.

traumatic neurosis. Any neurotic reaction in which an injury is the precipitating cause; encompasses combat, compensation, and occupational neuroses. The traumatic event usually has specific symbolic significance for the patient, which may be further enforced by secondary gain.

traumatic occlusion. An abnormal occlusion stress leading to injury of the periodontium.

traumatic osteoporosis. SUDECK'S ATROPHY.

traumatic pneumocephalus. The presence of air in the ventricles of the brain following an injury, chiefly to the frontal part of the skull.

traumatic pneumonosis. *In aerospace medicine,* acute noninflammatory pathologic changes produced in the lungs by large momentary deceleration. The principal changes are hemorrhage, emphysema, and laceration.

traumatic suggestion. A suggestion mechanism whereby a person in a highly suggestible state of mind after an accident may have hysterical pain, paralysis, or other disorders triggered by a very slight injury. Compare *autosuggestion.*

traumatic vasospastic syndrome. PNEUMATIC-HAMMER DISEASE.

trau·ma·tism (traw'muh·tiz·um, traow') *n.* [Gk. *traumatismos,* wounding]. The general or local condition produced by a wound or injury. —**trauma·tize** (·tize) *v.*

traumato-. See *traumat-.*

trau·ma·tol·o·gy (traw''muh·tol'uh·jee, traow'') *n.* [*traumato-* + *-logy*]. The science or description of wounds and injuries, especially as they occur as disability in industry.

trau·ma·top·a·thy (traw''muh·top'uth·ee, traow'') *n.* [*traumato-* + *-pathy*]. Pathologic condition due to wounds or other violence.

trau·ma·top·nea, trau·ma·top·noea (traw''muh·top·nee'uh, traow'') *n.* [*traumato-* + *-pnea*]. The passage of respiratory air through a wound in the chest wall.

trau·ma·to·sis (traw'muh·to'sis, traow'') *n.* [*traumat-* + *-osis*]. TRAUMATISM.

Traut·mann's triangle (traowt'mahn) [M. F. *Trautmann,* German aural surgeon, 1832–1902]. In mastoidectomy, the triangular area bounded anteriorly by the osseous wall of the inner ear, posteriorly by the bony wall covering the sigmoid sinus, and superiorly by the osseous roof of the mastoid air cells.

tra·vail (trav'ail, truh·vail') *n.* [F.]. Labor of parturition.

trav·el·er's diarrhea. Transitory diarrhea and abdominal cramping often encountered by travelers to foreign countries. Enterotoxin-producing strains of *Escherichia coli* are thought to be etiologically important in many cases.

tray, *n.* A flat, shallow vessel of glass, hard rubber, or metal, for holding instruments during a surgical operation.

tra·zo·done (tray'zo·dohn) *n.* 2-[3-[4-(*m*-Chlorophenyl)-1-piperazinyl]propyl]-*S*-triazolo[4,3-*a*]-pyridin-3(2*H*)-one, an antidepressant, used as the monohydrochloride salt.

Trea·cher Col·lins syndrome [E. *Treacher Collins,* English ophthalmologist, 1862–1932]. MANDIBULOFACIAL DYSOSTOSIS.

tread, *n. In veterinary medicine,* injury to the coronet of a horse's hoof, due to striking with the shoe of the opposite side.

treat, *v.* [L. *tractare,* to manage, treat]. To combat disease by the application of remedies; to care for medically or surgically.

treat·ment, *n.* 1. Application of therapeutic measures; therapy. 2. Application of a chemical agent or a physical process to a substance or object to render it fit for use or disposal.

tre·ben·zo·mine (tre·ben'zo·meen) *n.* (±)-*N*,*N*,2-Trimethyl-3-chromanamine, $C_{12}H_{17}NO$, an antidepressant, used as the hydrochloride salt.

Trecator. Trademark for ethionamide, a tuberculostatic drug.

tree, *n.* 1. A perennial woody plant with one main stem and numerous branches. 2. *In medicine,* a structure resembling a tree; a system or organ with many branches.

tree shrew. A small, predominantly aboreal mammal of the family Tupaiidae (comprising 4 or 5 genera), found in Southeast Asia, India, Indonesia, and the Philippines, classified by some authorities as a primate, and by some as an insectivore or as a link between insectivores and primates.

tre·foil tendon (tree'foil, tref'oil). CENTRAL TENDON.

tre·ha·la (tre·hah'luh) *n.* [Turkish *tigala*]. A variety of manna derived from cocoons of *Larinus maculatus,* an insect that feeds upon an Asiatic thistle, *Echinops persicus;* Turkish manna.

tre·ha·lose (tree'huh·loce, tre·hal'oce) *n.* 1-α-D-Glucopyranosyl-α-D-glucopyranoside, $C_{12}H_{22}O_{11}$, a disaccharide in trehala manna and also widely distributed in fungi; on hydrolysis yields two molecules of D-glucose.

Treitz's fossa (trite's) [W. *Treitz,* Austrian physician, 1819–1872]. INFERIOR DUODENAL FOSSA.

Treitz's hernia [W. *Treitz*]. A retroperitoneal hernia through the duodenojejunal fossa.

Treitz's muscle [W. *Treitz*]. MUSCLE OF TREITZ.

tre·lox·i·nate (tre·lock'si·nate) *n.* Methyl 2,10-dichloro-12*H*-dibenzo[*d,g*][1,3]dioxocin-6-carboxylate, $C_{16}H_{12}Cl_2O_4$, an anticholesteremic.

tre·ma (tree'muh) *n.* [Gk. *trēma,* hole]. 1. FORAMEN. 2. *Obsol.* VULVA. 3. In a fish or tadpole, a hole from the pharynx to the outside for the passage of water; a gill slit. —**tre·mat·ic** (tre·mat'ick) *adj.*

Trem·a·to·da (trem''uh·to'duh) *n.pl.* [NL., from Gk. *trēmatōdēs,* having holes, from *trēma,* hole]. The flukes; a class of flat worms of which the digenetic species are endoparasites of man. The life cycle is complex, involving sexual and asexual reproduction; two intermediate hosts are required. Some of the genera seen most often are *Clonorchis, Fasciola, Fasciolopsis, Opisthorchis, Paragonimus, Schistosoma,* and *Troglotrema.* —**trem·a·tode** (trem'uh·tode) *adj. & n.*

trem·a·to·di·a·sis (trem''uh·to·dye'uh·sis) *n.*, pl. **trematodia·ses** (·seez) [*trematode* + *-iasis*]. Infection with a trematode.

trem·bles, *n.pl.* 1. A disease of cattle and sheep, manifest by weakness and falling, presumed due to ingestion of white snakeroot, *Eupatorium urticaefolium,* or the rayless goldenrod, *Aplopappus heterophyllus.* 2. MILK SICKNESS. 3. A congenital disease of neonatal pigs of unknown etiology, characterized by severe trembling, difficulty in nursing, and occasionally death.

trem·bling abasia. Incapacity to walk because of marked trembling of the legs.

trembling ill. LOUPING ILL.

trem·el·loid (trem'e·loid) *adj.* 1. GELATINOUS. 2. Resembling the spore-producing organ of the fungus *Tremella.*

trem·el·lose (trem'e·loce) *adj.* GELATINOUS.

trem·e·tol (trem'e·tol) *n.* A toxic unsaturated alcohol from white snakeroot; produces trembles in cattle and sheep that eat the plant.

tremo·gram (trem'o·gram, tree'mo·) *n.* [*tremor* + *-gram*]. The tracing of tremor made by means of a special device such as a tremograph.

tremo·graph (trem'o·graf, tree'mo·) *n.* [*tremor* + *-graph*]. A device for recording tremor.

tremo·la·bile (trem''o·lay'bil, tree''mo·) *adj.* [*tremor* + *labile*]. Easily inactivated or destroyed by agitation.

trem·o·lo (trem'uh·lo) *n.* [It.]. An irregular, exaggerated vibrato; a voice tremor, symptomatic of psychogenic disturbance, old age, or diseases affecting the organs of respiration and phonation or their nervous control.

tremo·pho·bia (trem''o·fo'bee·uh, tree''mo·) *n.* [*tremor* + *-phobia*]. An abnormal fear of trembling.

trem·or (trem'ur) *n.* [L.]. A more or less regular, rhythmic oscillation of a part of the body around a fixed point involving alternate contraction of agonist and antagonist muscles.

tremor ar·tu·um (ahr'tew·um). *Obsol.* PARKINSONISM.

tremor ca·pi·tis (kap'i·tis). Tremor affecting the muscles of the neck and head.

tremor cor·dis (kor'dis). *Obsol.* Palpitation of the heart.

tremor me·tal·li·cus (me·tal'i·kus). A tremor associated with chronic poisoning from a heavy metal, e.g., mercurial tremor.

tremor po·ta·to·rum (po·ta·to'rum). *Obsol.* DELIRIUM TREMENS.

tremor sa·tur·ni·nus (sat·ur·nigh'nus). The tremor associated with lead poisoning.

tremor ten·di·num (ten'di·num). *Obsol.* SUBSULTUS TENDINUM.

tremo·sta·ble (trem''o·stay'bul, tree''mo·) *adj.* [*tremor* + *stable*]. Not easily inactivated or destroyed by agitation.

trem·u·la·tion (trem''yoo·lay'shun) *n.* [L. *tremulare,* to tremble]. A tremulous condition.

trem·u·lous (trem'yoo·lus) *adj.* [L. *tremulus*]. Trembling, quivering, as tremulous iris; affected by tremor.

trench back. Dorsolumbar pain and rigidity experienced by troops engaged in trench warfare.

trench fever. A louse-borne infection caused by *Rochalimaea quintana,* epidemic during World Wars I and II but rare now; characterized by headache, chills, rash, pain in the legs and back, and frequently by a relapsing fever.

trench foot. A condition of the feet, somewhat like immersion foot, due to exposure to cold and dampness.

trench mouth. NECROTIZING ULCERATIVE GINGIVITIS.

Tren·de·len·burg's position (tren'de·len·boork) [F. *Trendelenburg,* German surgeon, 1844–1924]. The posture of a patient lying supine on a table which is tilted head downward 45° or less.

Trendelenburg's test [F. *Trendelenburg*]. 1. A test of competence of the saphenous vein valves; the legs are raised to empty the veins and quickly lowered; the veins become immediately distended if the valves are incompetent. 2. A test for abnormality of the pelvis seen in congenital hip dislocation, poliomyelitis, etc.; when the patient stands on the involved foot, the opposite (normal) gluteal fold falls rather than rises.

tre·pan (tre·pan') *n.* [Gk. *trypanon,* auger, borer]. TREPHINE.

trep·a·na·tion (trep''uh·nay'shun) *n.* The operation of trephining.

trep·a·nize (trep'uh·nize) *v.* TREPHINE (2).

tre·pan·ning (tre·pan'ing) *n.* Boring; using the trephine.

tre·phine (tre·fine', tre·feen') *n. & v.* [L. *tres fines,* three ends]. 1. A circular instrument with a sawlike edge for cutting out a disk of bone, usually from the skull. 2. To cut with a trephine.

treph·one (tref'ohn) *n.* [Gk. *trephein,* to nourish, make grow, + *-one* as in hormone]. A postulated growth-promoting hormone produced by leukocytes, said to stimulate fibroblastic activity.

trep·i·dant (trep'i·dant) *adj.* [L. *trepidare,* to be agitated]. Trembling.

tre·pi·da·tio (trep''i·day'shee·o) *n.* [L., from *trepidus,* agitated]. 1. A state of agitation. 2. TREPIDATION.

trepidatio cor·dis (kor'dis). Palpitation of the heart.

trep·i·da·tion (trep''i·day'shun) *n.* [L. *trepidatio*]. 1. Trembling. 2. A state of fear, alarm, or anxiety.

Trep·o·ne·ma (trep"o·nee'muh) *n.* [NL., from Gk. *trep*ein, to turn, + *-nema*]. A genus of spirochetes of the family Treponemataceae.

treponema, *n.*, pl. **treponema·ta** (·tuh), **treponemas.** A spirochete of the genus *Treponema.*

Treponema amer·i·ca·num (uh·merr"i·kay'num). TREPONEMA CARATEUM.

Treponema buc·ca·le (buh·kay'lee). BORRELIA BUCCALIS.

Treponema ca·ra·te·um (ka·rah'tee·um). The organism that causes pinta. Syn. *Treponema americanum, T.* herrijoni, T. pictor, T. pintae.

Treponema cu·nic·u·li (kew·nick'yoo·lye). The organism that causes pallidoidosis, a venereal disease of rabbits.

Treponema her·re·jo·ni (herr·e·jo'nye). TREPONEMA CARATEUM.

trep·o·ne·mal (trep"o·nee'mul) *adj.* Pertaining to *Treponema.*

Treponema pal·li·dum (pal'i·dum). The organism that causes syphilis.

***Treponema pallidum* immobilization test.** A specific serologic test for syphilis involving antibodies differing from the Wassermann antibody, in which suspensions of *Treponema pallidum* are immobilized in the presence of the syphilitic serum and complement. Abbreviated, TPI test.

Treponema per·ten·ue (pur·ten'yoo·ee). The organism that causes yaws.

Treponema pic·tor (pick'tor). TREPONEMA CARATEUM.

Treponema pin·tae (pin'tee). TREPONEMA CARATEUM.

Treponema refringens. BORRELIA REFRINGENS.

Trep·o·ne·ma·ta·ce·ae (trep"o·nee"muh·tay'see·ee) *n.pl.* The family of spiral microorganisms which includes the genera *Borrelia, Leptospira,* and *Treponema.*

trep·o·ne·ma·to·sis (trep"o·nee"muh·to'sis) *n.*, pl. **treponema·to·ses** (·seez) [*Treponema* + *-osis*]. Infection caused by a spirochete of the genus *Treponema.*

Treponema vincentii. BORRELIA VINCENTII.

trep·o·ne·mi·a·sis (trep"o·ne·migh'uh·sis) *n.*, pl. **treponemia·ses** (·seez) [*Treponema* + *-iasis*]. Infection caused by a spirochete of the genus *Treponema.*

trep·o·ne·mi·ci·dal (trep"o·nee"mi·sigh'dul) *adj.* [*Treponema* + *-cide* + *-al*]. 1. Destructive to any organism of the genus *Treponema.* 2. ANTISYPHILITIC.

trep·o·ne·min (trep"o·nee'min) *n.* An antigen prepared from formalin-killed *Treponema pallidum;* formerly used in a skin test for syphilis.

tre·pop·nea, tre·pop·noea (tre·pop'nee·uh) *n.* [Gk. *trep*ein, to turn, + *-pnea*]. A respiratory distress present in one posture and absent in another. Syn. *selective orthopnea.*

trep·pe (trep'eh) *n.* [Ger., stairs]. STAIRCASE PHENOMENON.

-tresia [Gk. *trēsis*]. A combining form meaning *perforation.*

Tre·sil·ian's sign (tre·sil'yun) [F. J. *Tresilian,* English physician, 1862–1926]. *Obsol.* A sign of mumps, in which the opening of the parotid duct on the inner surface of the cheek, opposite the second upper molar, appears as a bright-red papilla.

Trest. Trademark for methixene, an anticholinergic drug used as the hydrochloride salt.

tres·to·lone acetate (tres'to·lone) *n.* 17β-Hydroxy-7α-methylester-4-en-3-one acetate, $C_{21}H_{30}O_3$, an androgen and antineoplastic.

tre·tin·o·in (tre·tin'o·in) *n.* The *all-trans* stereoisomer of retinoic acid, $C_{20}H_{28}O_2$, a keratolytic.

Treves's bloodless fold (treevz) [F. *Treves,* English surgeon, 1853–1923]. ILEOCECAL FOLD.

TRF Abbreviation for *thyrotropin releasing factor.*

TRH Abbreviation for *thyrotropin releasing hormone* (= THYROTROPIN RELEASING FACTOR).

tri- [Gk. and L.]. A combining form meaning *three.*

tri·ac·e·tin (trye·as'e·tin) *n.* GLYCERYL TRIACETATE.

tri·ac·e·tyl·ole·an·do·my·cin (trye·as"e·til·o"lee·an"do·migh'oin) *n.* TROLEANDOMYCIN.

tri·ac·yl·glyc·er·ol (trye·as"il·glis'ur·ole) *n.* An ester of glycerin in which all three hydroxyl groups of the latter are esterified with an acid; animal and vegetable fixed oils are composed chiefly of triacylglycerols of fatty acids. Syn. *triglyceride.*

tri·ad (trye'ad) *n.* [Gk. *trias, triados*]. 1. A set of three related elements, objects, or symptoms. 2. *In chemistry,* a trivalent element, atom, or radical.

triad of Whipple [A. O. *Whipple*]. WHIPPLE'S TRIAD.

tri·age (tree·ahzh') *n.* [F. from *trier,* to sort]. 1. *In military medicine,* the process of sorting sick and wounded on the basis of urgency and type of condition presented, so that they can be properly routed to medical installations appropriately situated and equipped; with large numbers of wounded, it may become a process of concentrating limited resources on those who have a reasonable chance of survival. 2. More broadly, any of various comparable processes of screening patients in civilian institutions such as hospitals or community health clinics.

tria·kai·deka·pho·bia (trye"uh·kye"deck·uh·fo'bee·uh) *n.* [Gk. *tria kai deka,* thirteen, + *-phobia*]. TRISKAIDEKAPHOBIA.

tri·al (trye'ul) *n.* [Norman French, from *trier,* to sort, pick out]. The act of trying or testing.

trial base. BASEPLATE.

tri·al·ist theory (trye'ul·ist). A polyphyletic theory of hemopoiesis involving three stem cells, each having different potencies; usually, lymphoblast, myeloblast, monoblast.

tri·al·kyl·a·mine (trye·al"kil·uh·meen', ·am'in) *n.* Tertiary alkylamine.

trial visit. PAROLE.

tri·am·cin·o·lone (trye"am·sin'o·lone) *n.* 9α-Fluoro-16α-hydroxyprednisolone, $C_{21}H_{27}FO_6$, a potent glucocorticoid with anti-inflammatory, hormonal, and metabolic effects similar to those of prednisolone. Administered orally as the free alcohol or its diacetate ester; topically or by intraarticular, intrasynovial, or intrabursal injection as the acetonide derivative.

tri·am·py·zine (try·am'pi·zeen) *n.* 2-(Dimethylamino)-3,5,6-trimethylpyrazine, $C_9H_{15}N_3$, an anticholinergic drug; used as the sulfate salt.

tri·am·ter·ene (trye·am'tur·een) *n.* 2,4,7-Triamino-6-phenylpteridine, $C_{12}H_{11}N_7$, a diuretic drug.

tri·an·gle (trye'ang·gul) *n.* [L. *triangulus,* having three corners]. 1. A geometrical figure having three sides and three angles. 2. A three-sided area or region having natural or arbitrary boundaries. —**tri·an·gu·lar** (trye·ang'gew·lur) *adj.*

triangle of auscultation. An area limited above by the trapezius, below by the latissimus dorsi, and laterally by the vertebral border of the scapula.

triangle of Calot [J. F. *Calot*]. A triangle formed by the cystic duct, the hepatic duct, and the liver. The cystic artery can usually be found in it, often running posterior to the hepatic duct.

triangle of election. SUPERIOR CAROTID TRIANGLE.

triangle of Gom·bault-Phi·lippe (gohⁿbo', fee·leep') [F. A. A. *Gombault* and C. *Philippe*]. A small triangle, in the dorsomedian border of the spinal cord at the sacral level, occupied by the descending dorsal root fibers. Syn. *triangle of Philippe-Gombault.*

triangle of necessity. INFERIOR CAROTID TRIANGLE.

triangle of Phillipe-Gombault. TRIANGLE OF GOMBAULT-PHILLIPE.

triangle of the vagus nerve. TRIGONUM NERVI VAGI.

triangular area. *In embryology,* the portion of the median nasal process between the nasofrontal sulcus and the future tip of the nose; forms the dorsum, or bridge, of the nose.

triangular bandage. A bandage made from a square of muslin cut or folded diagonally to make a triangle, used as a sling, and for inclusive dressing of a part, as a whole hand.

triangular fascia. REFLECTED LIGAMENT.

triangular fold. A triangular membrane extending from the upper posterior portion of the palatoglossal arch backward and downward, until lost in the tissues at the base of the tongue. NA *plica triangularis.*

triangular fossa. The fossa of the anthelix. NA *fossa triangularis auriculae.*

triangular fovea. A deep depression on the external surface of an arytenoid cartilage. NA *fovea triangularis cartilaginis arytenoideae.*

triangular foveola. A triangular depression between the anterior columns of the fornix.

tri·an·gu·la·ris (trye·ang″gew·lair′is) *n.* 1. TRIQUETRUM (1). See also Table of Bones in the Appendix. 2. A muscle of facial expression. See also Table of Muscles in the Appendix.

triangular ligament. 1. UROGENITAL DIAPHRAGM. 2. (of the liver:) Either of the extensions of the coronary ligament which connect the right and left lobes of the liver with the diaphragm, designated respectively the right triangular ligament (NA *ligamentum triangulare dextrum*) and the left triangular ligament (NA *ligamentum triangulare sinistrum*).

triangular nucleus. MEDIAL VESTIBULAR NUCLEUS.

triangular space. A space of triangular form in the posterior wall of the axilla, bounded by the latissimus dorsi, teres minor, and subscapular muscles and the surgical neck of the humerus; it is divided by the long head of the triceps into the quadrangular and small triangular spaces.

Tri·at·o·ma (trye·at′o·muh) *n.* A genus of bloodsucking Hemiptera, commonly called conenose bugs. The most important species is *Triatoma megista,* the chief carrier of *Trypanosoma cruzi.* Other species are *Triatoma sordida, T. dimidiata,* and *T. infestans.*

Tri·a·tom·i·dae (trye″uh·tom′i·dee) *n.pl.* [from *Triatoma*]. REDUVIIDAE. **—tri·at·o·mid** (trye·at′o·mid) *adj. & n.*

tri·atri·al (trye·ay′tree·ul) *adj.* [*tri-* + *atrial*]. The anomalous condition of having three atria.

tri·ax·i·al reference system (trye·ack′see·ul). Superimposition of the lead axes of electrocardiographic leads I, II, and III so that their midpoints coincide. A reference frame for frontal plane vectors.

tri·a·zo·lam (trye·ay′zo·lam) *n.* 8-Chloro-6-(*o*-chlorophenyl)-1-methyl-4*H*-*S*-triazolo [4,3-*a*]benzodiazepine, $C_{17}H_{12}Cl_2N_4$, a sedative-hypnotic.

trib·ade (trib′ud, tri·bahd′) *n.* [F., from Gk. *tribas, tribados,* from *tribein,* to rub]. A woman who plays the role of the male in lesbian practices. **—trib·a·dism** (trib′uh·diz·um) *n.*

tri·ba·sic (trye·bay′sick) *adj.* [*tri-* + *basic*]. Having three hydrogen atoms replaceable by bases.

tribasic calcium phosphate. $Ca_3(PO_4)_2$. A white powder almost insoluble in water; used as an antacid in gastric hyperacidity. Syn. *precipitated calcium phosphate.*

tribasic magnesium phosphate. $Mg_3(PO_4)_2$. A gastric antacid; almost insoluble in water.

tri·bas·i·lar (trye·bas′i·lur) *adj.* [*tri-* + *basilar*]. Having three bases.

tribasilar synostosis. Shortening of the base of the skull and consequent curvature of the basal parts of the brain caused by fusion in infancy of the three bones at the base of the skull.

tribe, *n.* [L. *tribus,* tribe]. A taxonomic category intermediate in the hierarchy between a genus and a family.

-tribe [Gk. *tribein,* to rub]. A combining form designating *an instrument for crushing or compressing.*

tri·ben·o·side (trye·ben′o·side) *n.* Ethyl 3,5,6-tri-*O*-benzyl-D-glucofuranoside, $C_{29}H_{34}O_6$, a sclerosing agent.

tribo·lu·mi·nes·cence (trye″bo·lew″mi·nes′unce, trib″o·) *n.* [Gk. *tribein,* to rub, + *luminescence*]. Luminosity induced by friction, as by grinding and pulverizing of solids.

tri·bra·chi·us (trye·bray′kee·us) *adj.* [NL., from *brachium,* arm]. Having three arms.

tri·bro·mo·eth·a·nol (trye·bro″mo·eth′uh·nol) *n.* 2,2,2-Tribromoethanol, Br_3CCH_2OH; used as a basal anesthetic when dissolved in amylene hydrate.

tri·bro·mo·meth·ane (trye·bro″mo·meth′ane) *n.* BROMOFORM.

tri·brom·sa·lan (trye·brohm′suh·lan) *n.* 3,4′,5-Tribromosalicylanilide, $C_{13}H_8Br_3NO_2$, a disinfectant.

tri·bu·ty·rin (trye·bew′ti·rin) *n.* BUTYRIN.

tri·car·box·yl·ic acid (trye·kahr″bock·sil′ick). An organic compound with three —COOH groups.

tricarboxylic acid cycle. CITRIC ACID CYCLE.

tri·cel·lu·lar (trye·sel′yoo·lur) *adj.* [*tri-* + *cellular*]. Having three cells.

tri·ceph·a·lus (trye·sef′uh·lus) *n.,* pl. **tricepha·li** (·lye) [NL., from Gk. *trikephalos,* three-headed, from *kephalē,* head]. An individual with three heads.

tri·ceps (trye′seps) *adj. & n.* [L., from *tri-* + *caput, capitis,* head]. 1. Three-headed. 2. A muscle having three heads, as the triceps brachii muscle. See also Table of Muscles in the Appendix.

triceps ex·ten·sor cu·bi·ti (ecks·ten′sor kew′bi·tye). The triceps brachii muscle. See Table of Muscles in the Appendix.

triceps reflex or **jerk.** Extension of the forearm in response to a brisk tap against the triceps tendon, with the forearm at right angles to the arm.

triceps surae jerk or **reflex.** ACHILLES JERK.

Tri·cer·com·o·nas (trye″sur·kom′o·nas) *n.* *ENTEROMONAS.*

tri·cet·a·mide (try·set′uh·mide) *n.* *N*-[(Diethylcarbamoyl)-methyl]-3,4,5-trimethoxybenzamide, $C_{16}H_{24}N_2O_5$, a sedative drug.

trich-, tricho- [Gk. *thrix, trichos*]. A combining form meaning (a) *hair;* (b) *filament.*

trich·an·gi·ec·ta·sia (trick·an″jee·eck·tay′zhuh, ·zee·uh) *n.* [*trich-* + *angiectasia*]. Dilatation of the capillaries.

trich·an·gi·ec·ta·sis (trick·an″jee·eck′tuh·sis) *n.* [*trich-* + *angiectasis*]. TRICHANGIECTASIA.

trich·atro·phia (trick″a·tro′fee·uh) *n.* [*trich-* + *atrophy* + *-ia*]. A brittle state of the hair from atrophy of the hair bulbs.

trich·es·the·sia, trich·aes·the·sia (trick″es·theezh′uh, ·theez′ee·uh) *n.* [*trich-* + *esthesia*]. 1. A particular form of tactile sensibility in regions covered with hairs. 2. TRICHOESTHESIA.

-trichia [*trich-* + *-ia*]. A combining form designating (a) *a condition of the hair;* (b) *hairiness.*

tri·chi·a·sis (tri·kigh′uh·sis) *n.* [Gk., from *thrix, trichos,* hair]. 1. An abnormal position of the eyelashes which produces irritation by friction upon the globe. The acquired type usually follows an inflammatory condition that produces distortion. 2. The presence of minute hairlike filaments in the urine.

trichiasis of the anus. An incurvation of the hairs about the anus, consequently irritating the mucous membrane.

Tri·chi·na (tri·kigh′nuh) *n.* *TRICHINELLA.*

Trich·i·nel·la (trick″i·nel′uh) *n.* [NL., from Gk. *trichinos,* of hair]. A genus of nematode worms that are parasites of man, hogs, rats, dogs, cats, and many other mammals.

Trichinella spi·ra·lis (spye·ray′lis). The species of nematode responsible for trichinosis in man.

trich·i·ni·a·sis (trick″i·nigh′uh·sis) *n.* [*Trichina* + *-iasis*]. TRICHINOSIS.

trich·i·no·pho·bia (trick″i·no·fo′bee·uh) *n.* [*Trichina* + *-phobia*]. An abnormal fear of trichinosis.

trich·i·no·sis (trick″i·no′sis) *n.,* pl. **trichino·ses** (·seez) [*Trichina* + *-osis*]. A disease produced by the ingestion of uncooked or insufficiently cooked pork containing *Trichinella spiralis.* It is characterized by eosinophilia, nausea, fever, diarrhea, stiffness and painful swelling of muscles, and edema of the face. The intestinal symptoms are due to the development of the adult stage of the organisms; the muscular and systemic symptoms are due to the larval migration of the organisms through the tissues.

trich·i·nous (trick′i·nus, tri·kigh′nus) *adj.* [*Trichina* + *-ous*]. Pertaining to, or containing, *Trichinella.*

trichinous myositis. Myositis due to *Trichinella spiralis* in the muscle.

tri·chi·tis (tri·kigh'tis) *n.* [*trich-* + *-itis*]. Inflammation of the hair bulbs.

tri·chlor·me·thi·a·zide (trye"klor·me·thigh'uh·zide) *n.* 6-Chloro-3-(dichloromethyl)-3,4-dihydro-2*H*-1,2,4-benzothiadiazine-7-sulfonamide 1,1-dioxide, $C_8H_8Cl_3N_3O_4S_2$, an orally effective diuretic and antihypertensive drug.

tri·chlo·ro·ac·et·al·de·hyde (trye·klo"ro·as"e·tal'de·hide) *n.* CHLORAL (1).

tri·chlo·ro·ace·tic acid (trye·klor"o·uh·see'tick). Cl_3CCOOH. A crystalline, deliquescent acid, very corrosive; used topically as a caustic and astringent, and also as a protein precipitant.

tri·chlo·ro·bu·tyl alcohol (trye·klo"ro·bew'til). CHLOROBUTANOL.

tri·chlo·ro·eth·yl·ene (trye·klo"ro·eth'il·een) *n.* $CHCl{=}CCl_2$. A liquid anesthetic and analgesic often self-administered by inhalation to relieve facial neuralgias.

tri·chlo·ro·meth·ane (trye·klo"ro·meth'ane) *n.* CHLOROFORM.

tricho-. See *trich-*.

trichoaesthesia. TRICHOESTHESIA.

tricho·an·es·the·sia, tricho·an·aes·the·sia (trick"o·an"es·theezh'uh, ·theez'ee·uh) *n.* [*tricho-* + *anesthesia*]. Lack of sensation when the hair is stimulated or moved.

tricho·be·zoar (trick"o·bee'zo·ur) *n.* [*tricho-* + *bezoar*]. A hair ball or concretion in the stomach or intestine.

Tricho·bil·har·zia oc·el·la·ta (trick"o·bil·hahr'zee·uh os·el·ay'tuh). A parasite of wild and domesticated ducks in Europe and North America whose cercaria (*Cercaria elvae*) may cause schistosome dermatitis.

tricho·car·dia (trick"o·kahr'dee·uh) *n.* [*tricho-* + *-cardia*]. COR VILLOSUM.

tricho·ceph·a·li·a·sis (trick"o·sef"uh·lye'uh·sis) *n.* [*Trichocephalus* + *-iasis*]. TRICHURIASIS.

Tricho·ceph·a·lus (trick"o·sef'uh·lus) *n.* [*tricho-* + *-cephalus*]. *TRICHURIS.*

Trichocephalus dis·par (dis'pahr). *TRICHURIS TRICHIURA.*

Trichocephalus trich·i·u·rus (trick"ee·yoo'rus). *TRICHURIS TRICHIURA.*

tricho·cla·sia (trick"o·klay'zee·uh, ·zhuh) *n.* [*tricho-* + *-clasia*]. TRICHORRHEXIS NODOSA.

tri·choc·la·sis (tri·kock'luh·sis) *n.* [*tricho-* + *-clasis*]. TRICHORRHEXIS NODOSA.

tricho·clas·ma·nia (trick"o·klaz·may'nee·uh) *n.* [*tricho-* + Gk. *klasis*, breaking, pruning, + *-mania*]. An abnormal desire to pull out the hair, usually of the scalp.

tricho·cryp·to·sis (trick"o·krip·to'sis) *n.* [*tricho-* + *crypt-* + *-osis*]. Any disease of the hair follicles.

tricho·cyst (trick'o·sist) *n.* [*tricho-* + *-cyst*]. *In biology*, a small vesicle containing a thread, which can be shot out rapidly; found in the ectoplasm of the Infusoria and in some of the Flagellata.

Trich·o·dec·tes (trick"o·deck'teez) *n.* [*tricho-* + Gk. *dektēs*, beggar]. A genus of the suborder Mallophaga or biting lice. They do not infest man.

Trichodectes can·is (kan'is, kay'nis). The dog louse; one of the intermediate hosts of the dog tapeworm, *Dipylidium caninum.*

Tricho·der·ma (trick"o·dur'muh) *n.* [*tricho-* + *-derma*]. A genus of fungi which is a common laboratory contaminant.

tricho·ep·i·the·li·o·ma (trick"o·ep"i·theel"ee·o'muh) *n.* [*tricho-* + *epithelioma*]. A benign tumor characterized by many pin-headed to pea-sized, round, yellow, or skin-colored papules chiefly on the central face. It may be associated with syringoma or cylindroma.

trichoepithelioma pa·pu·lo·sum mul·ti·plex (pap"yoo·lo'sum mul'ti·plecks). TRICHOEPITHELIOMA.

tricho·es·the·sia, tricho·aes·the·sia (trick"o·ee·theezh'uh, ·theez'ee·uh) *n.* [*tricho-* + *esthesia*]. 1. The sensation received when a hair is touched. 2. A type of paresthesia wherein there is a sensation as of uticaria on the skin, on the oral mucosa, or on the conjunctiva.

tricho·es·the·si·om·e·ter (trick"o·es·theez"ee·om'e·tur) *n.* [*tricho-* + *esthesiometer*]. An electric appliance for determining the amount of sensation when a hair is touched.

tricho·fol·lic·u·lo·ma (trick"o·fol·ick"yoo·lo'muh) *n.* [*tricho-* + *folliculus* + *-oma*]. A rare, benign, hamartomatous mass of tissue which may form a multiloculated cyst in the subcutaneous tissue of man and animals; characterized by a cyst wall that is composed of stratified squamous epithelium and numerous abortive hair follicles.

tricho·gen (trick'o·jen) *n.* [*tricho-* + *-gen*]. A substance that stimulates growth of hair.

tricho·glos·sia (trick"o·glos'ee·uh) *n.* [*tricho-* + *-glossia*]. Hairy tongue, a lengthening of the filiform papillae, producing an appearance as if the tongue were covered with hair.

tricho·hy·a·lin (trick"o·high'uh·lin) *n.* [*tricho-* + *hyalin*]. The hyalin of the hair which is like keratohyalin.

trich·oid (trick'oid) *adj.* [Gk. *trichoiedēs*, from *thrix, trichos*, hair]. Resembling hair.

tricho·kryp·to·ma·nia (trick"o·krip"to·may'nee·uh) *n.* [*tricho-* + *krypto-* + *-mania*]. TRICHORRHEXOMANIA.

tricho·lith (trick'o·lith) *n.* [*tricho-* + *-lith*]. A calcified hair ball within the stomach or intestines.

tricho·lo·gia (trick"o·lo'jee·uh) *n.* [*tricho-* + Gk. *legein*, to pick, gather]. 1. CARPHOLOGY. 2. The plucking out of one's hair.

tri·chol·o·gy (tri·kol'uh·jee) *n.* [*tricho-* + *-logy*]. 1. TRICHOLOGIA. 2. The study of hair.

tri·cho·ma (tri·ko'muh) *n.* [Gk. *trichōma*, growth of hair]. 1. TRICHOMATOSIS. 2. TRICHIASIS.

tricho·ma·de·sis (trick"o·ma·dee'sis) *n.* [*tricho-* + Gk. *madēsis*, shedding]. The falling out of hair which may lead to alopecia.

tricho·ma·nia (trick"o·may'nee·uh) *n.* TRICHOTILLOMANIA.

tri·cho·ma·tose (tri·ko'muh·toze) *adj.* Matted together.

tricho·ma·to·sis (trick"o·muh·to'sis, tri·ko") *n.* [Gk. *trichōma*, growth of hair, + *-osis*]. An affection of the hair characterized by a matted condition, a result of neglect, filth, and the invasion of parasites.

trich·ome (trick'ome, trye'kome) *n.* [Gk. *trichōma*, growth of hair]. A hair or other appendage of the epidermis.

trichome dermatitis. Dermatitis due to irritation by spicules, hairs, and scales of the epidermis of plants.

trich·o·mo·na·ci·dal (trick"o·mo"nuh·sigh'dul) *adj.* [*trichomonad* + *-cide* + *-al*]. Lethal for trichomonads.

trich·o·mo·na·cide (trick"o·mo'nuh·side) *n.* [*Trichomonas* + *-cide*]. Any drug that destroys *Trichomonas* parasites.

trich·o·mo·nad (trick"o·mo'nad, ·mon'ad) *n. & adj.* A flagellate belonging to the genus *Trichomonas.* 2. Belonging or pertaining to the genus *Trichomonas.*

trich·o·mo·nad·i·ci·dal (trick"o·mo·nad"i·sigh'dul) *adj.* TRICHOMONACIDAL.

Trich·o·mo·nas (trick"o·mo'nas) *n.* [*tricho-* + Gk. *monas*, unit]. A genus of flagellate protozoa, belonging to the subphylum Mastigophora. Three to five flagella, a thick rodlike axostyle extending throughout the pear-shaped body, and an undulating membrane characterize members of the genus.

Trichomonas gal·li·nae (ga·lye'nee) The species of *Trichomonas* that causes roup in fowls.

Trichomonas hom·i·nis (hom'i·nis). The species found in the human intestine; it is not pathogenic.

Trichomonas vag·i·na·lis (vaj·i·nay'lis). The species of flagellate protozoa that has been implicated in vaginitis.

***Trichomonas* vaginitis**. Vaginitis associated with, and caused by, *Trichomonas vaginalis.*

trich·o·mo·ni·a·sis (trick"o·mo·nigh'uh·sis) *n.*, pl. **trichomonia·ses** (·seez) [*Trichomonas* + *-iasis*]. Infection with *Trichomonas.*

trich·o·mo·ni·cide (trick"o·mo'ni·side) *adj.* TRICHOMONACIDE.

Tricho·my·ce·tes (trick"o·migh·see'teez) *n.pl.* [*tricho-* + *mycetes*]. *Obsol.* A group of delicate, filamentous organisms, including *Actinomyces, Nocardia,* and *Leptothrix.*

tricho·my·co·sis (trick″o·migh·ko′sis) *n.* [*tricho-* + *mycosis*]. A disease of the hair produced by fungi.

trichomycosis ax·il·la·ris (ack″si·lair′is). Nodules formed on the axillary hairs by the saprophytic growth of species of *Nocardia* and bacteria. Syn. *trichonocardiosis axillaris, chromotrichomycosis.*

trichomycosis bar·bae (bahr′bee). SYCOSIS PARASITICA.

trichomycosis cap·il·li·tii (kap″i·lish′ee·eye). TRICHOMYCOSIS CIRCINATA.

trichomycosis cir·ci·na·ta (sur″si·nay′tuh). Ringworm of the scalp.

trichomycosis fa·vo·sa (fay·vo′suh). FAVUS.

trichomycosis fla·va ni·gra (flay′vuh nye′gruh). A yellow-red variety of trichomycosis nodosa.

trichomycosis no·do·sa (no·do′suh). The growth of masses of fungous and bacterial material along the axillary and scrotal hair to form nodules; lepothrix.

trichomycosis pal·mel·li·na (pal″me·lye′nuh). Fungal infection of the hairy parts of the trunk; a variety of trichomycosis nodosa.

trichomycosis pus·tu·lo·sa (pus″tew·lo′suh). A pustular, parasitic disease affecting hairy regions.

trichomycosis ru·bra (roo′bruh). A red variety of trichomycosis nodosa. Red cocci are found in the gelatinous nodules.

tri·chon (trye′kon) *n.* A substance produced by autolysis of fungi of the genus *Trichophyton.*

tricho·no·car·di·o·sis (trick″o·no·kahr″dee·o′sis) *n.* [*tricho-* + *nocardiosis*]. Nodular appearance of the hair due to a species of *Nocardia;* axillary hair is most often affected.

trichonocardiosis axillaris. TRICHOMYCOSIS AXILLARIS.

tricho·no·do·sis (trick″o·no·do′sis) *n.* [*tricho-* + L. *nod*us, knot, + *-osis*]. Fraying of the hair, with formation of true and false knots, associated with thinning and breaking of the hair shaft. Syn. *knotting hair.*

tricho·no·sis (trick″o·no′sis) *n.* [*tricho-* + Gk. *nosos,* disease (assimilated to the suffix *-osis*)]. Any disease of the hair.

trichonosis ca·na (kay′nuh). CANITIES.

trichonosis discolor. CANITIES.

tricho·patho·pho·bia (trick″o·path″o·fo′bee·uh) *n.* [*tricho-* + *patho-* + *-phobia*]. Undue anxiety and fear regarding the hair, its growth, color, or diseases.

tri·chop·a·thy (tri·kop′uth·ee) *n.* [*tricho-* + *-pathy*]. Any disease of the hair. —**tricho·path·ic** (trick″o·path′ick) *adj.*

tricho·pha·gia (trick″o·fay′jee·uh) *n.* [*tricho-* + *-phagia*]. TRICHOPHAGY.

trich·oph·a·gy (trick·off′uh·jee) *n.* [*tricho-* + *-phagy*]. The eating of hair.

tricho·pho·bia (trick″o·fo′bee·uh) *n.* [*tricho-* + *-phobia*]. 1. An abnormal fear of hair. 2. TRICHOPATHOPHOBIA.

trichophyta. Plural of *trichophyton.*

tricho·phyte (trick′o·fite) *n.* [*tricho-* + *-phyte*]. A fungus of the genus *Trichophyton.*

tricho·phy·tid (trick″o·figh′tid, tri·kof′i·tid) *n.* [*Trichophyt*on + *-id*]. A dermatophytid caused by dead *Trichophyton* fungi or their breakdown products.

trich·o·phy·tin (trick″o·figh′tin, tri·kof′i·tin) *n.* A group antigen generally derived from filtrates of *Trichophyton mentagrophytes,* used in a skin test to determine past or present infection with the dermatophytes. Immediate and delayed hypersensitivity reactions occur; the test is of limited value diagnostically but is useful in confirming or disproving the diagnosis of a dermatophytid reaction.

tricho·phy·to·be·zoar (trick″o·figh″to·bee′zo·ur) *n.* [*tricho-* + *phyto-* + *bezoar*]. A ball or concretion in the stomach or intestine, made of hair and fibers of vegetable matter and food detritus.

Trich·o·phy·ton (trick″o·figh′ton, tri·kof′i·ton) *n.* [*tricho-* + Gk. *phyton,* plant]. A principal genus of keratophilic fungi, attacking the hair, skin, and nails, causing dermatophytosis of man and animals. The genus has distinctive macroconidia, and the many species are distinguished by cultural and nutritional characteristics. When involving the hair, some species are called ectothrix, in which a prominent sheath of spore forms outside the hair shaft in addition to the invasion of the interior of the hair (e.g. *Trichophyton mentagrophytes, T. rubrum, T. verrucosum*); others are called endothrix, in which invasion of the hair shaft is not accompanied by the formation of the outside sheath of spores (e.g., *T. schoenleinii, T. tonsurans*).

trichophyton, *n.,* pl. **trichophy·ta** (·tuh), **trichophytons.** Any fungus of the genus *Trichophyton;* trichophyte.

Trichophyton gal·li·nae (ga·lye′nee). The causative agent of comb disease in fowl.

trich·o·phy·to·sis (trick″o·figh·to′sis) *n.* [*Trichophyt*on + *-osis*]. A contagious disease of skin and hair, occurring mostly in children, and due to skin invasion by the *Trichophyton* fungus. It is characterized by circular scaly patches and partial loss of hair.

trichophytosis barbae. TINEA BARBAE.

trichophytosis cruris. Tinea cruris caused by *Trichophyton.*

tricho·po·lio·dys·tro·phy (trick″o·po″lee·o·dis′truh·fee) *n.* [*tricho-* + *poliodystrophy*]. KINKY HAIR DISEASE.

tricho·po·li·o·sis (trich″o·po″lee·o′sis) *n.* [*tricho-* + *poliosis*]. CANITIES.

tricho·pti·lo·sis (trick″o·ti·lo′sis, tri·kop″ti·lo′sis) *n.* [*tricho-* + *ptilosis*]. TRICHORRHEXIS NODOSA.

tricho·rhi·no·pha·lan·ge·al syndrome (trick″o·rye″no·fa·lan′jee·ul). A congenital disorder of connective tissue, characterized by sparse fine hair, pear-shaped nose, and multiple cone-shaped epiphyses of the digits of the hands and feet. Other anomalies and increased susceptibility to respiratory infection may be present. Probably transmitted as an autosomal recessive trait.

trich·or·rhea (trick″o·ree′uh) *n.* [*tricho-* + *-rrhea*]. Rapid loss of the hair.

trich·or·rhex·is (trick″o·reck′sis) *n.* [*tricho-* + *-rrhexis*]. Brittleness of the hair.

trichorrhexis no·do·sa (no·do′suh). An atrophic condition of the hair, affecting more often the male beard, and characterized by irregular thickenings resembling nodes on the hair shaft that are really partial fractures of the hair. The hairs often break, leaving a brush-like end; a certain amount of alopecia is thus produced.

trich·or·rhexo·ma·nia (trick″o·reck″so·may′nee·uh) *n.* [*tricho-* + *-rrhex*is + *-mania*]. A compulsion to break off hairs of the scalp or beard with the fingernails.

tricho·sid·er·in (trick″o·sid′ur·in) *n.* [*tricho-* + *sider-* + *-in*]. An iron-containing pigment found in human red hair.

tri·cho·sis (tri·ko′sis) *n.* [*trich-* + *-osis*]. Any morbid affection of the hair.

Trich·o·spo·ron (trick″o·spor′on, trick·os′po·ron) *n.* [NL., from *tricho-* + *spore*]. A genus of fungi which grow on hair shafts. A causative agent of piedra. *Trichosporon beigelii* (*T. giganteum*) is the principal cause of white piedra.

trich·o·spo·ro·sis (trich″o·spo·ro′sis) *n.* [*Trichospor*on + *-osis*]. A fungous infection of the hair shaft. See also *piedra.*

tricho·sta·sis spi·nu·lo·sa (trick″o·stay′sis spye″new·lo′suh, spin″yoo·). A disease of hair follicles characterized by dark comedo-like plugs in the follicles over the trunk, composed of bundles of many tiny hairs.

trich·o·stron·gy·li·a·sis (trick″o·stron″ji·lye′uh·sis) *n.* [*Tricho-strongyl*us + *-iasis*]. Infection with *Trichostrongylus.*

Trich·o·stron·gy·lus (trick″o·stron′ji·lus) *n.* [NL., from *tricho-* + Gk. *strongylos,* round]. A genus of nematode worms which usually are parasites of ruminants. Man is infected by consuming raw plants grown in contaminated soil. The species identified from human cases are *Trichostrongylus colubriformis, T. orientalis, T. probolurus, T. vitrinus.*

trich·o·the·cin (trick″o·thees′in) *n.* An antifungal substance produced in cultures of *Trichothecium roseum,* a bright pink mold found on fruit, wood, and soil.

tricho·til·lo·ma·nia (trick″o·til″o·may′nee·uh) *n.* [*tricho-* + Gk. *tille*in, to pluck, + *-mania*]. An uncontrollable impulse to pull out one's hair.

tri·chot·o·my (trye·kot'uh·mee) *n.* [Gk. *trichotom*ein, to trisect, from *tricha,* in three parts, + *temnein,* to cut]. Division into three parts.

tri·chro·ism (trye'kro·iz·um) *n.* [Gk. *trichro*os, three-colored, + *-ism*]. The property of exhibiting three different colors when viewed in three different aspects. —**tri·chro·ic** (trye·kro'ick) *adj.*

tri·chro·mat (trye'kro·mat) *n.* [*tri-* + *chromat*ic]. A person with normal color vision.

tri·chro·mat·ic (trye"kro·mat'ick) *adj.* [Gk. *trichrōmatos,* three-colored]. Having three standard colors.

tri·chro·ma·top·sia (trye"kro·muh·top'see·uh) *n.* [*tri-* + *chromat-* + *-opsia*]. Normal color vision; ability to see the three primary colors.

tri·chrome (trye'krome) *adj.* [*tri-* + *-chrome*]. Three-colored.

tri·chro·mic (trye·kro'mick) *adj.* [*tri-* + *chrom-* + *-ic*]. 1. Able to distinguish the three colors red, blue, and green. 2. Having three colors, as in a histologic stain.

trich·ter·brust (trikh'tur·broost) *n.* [Ger.]. FUNNEL CHEST.

trich·u·ri·a·sis (trick"yoo·rye'uh·sis) *n.*, pl. **trichuria·ses** (·seez) [*Trichur*is + *-iasis*]. Infection by *Trichuris trichiura.*

Trich·u·ris (trick·yoo'ris) *n.* [NL., from *trich-* + Gk. *oura,* tail]. A genus of nematodes of the superfamily Trichuroidea, parasitic in the digestive tracts of mammals.

Trichuris trich·i·u·ra (trick"ee·yoo'ruh). The species infecting man. Transmission is from man to man by ingestion of mature ova. Syn. *Trichocephalus dispar, Trichocephalus trichiurus, whipworm.*

tri·cip·i·tal (trye·sip'i·tul) *adj.* [L. *triceps, tricipit*is, + *-al*]. 1. Having three heads. 2. Pertaining to a triceps muscle.

tricipital muscle. A triceps muscle.

tri·clo·bi·son·i·um chloride (trye"klo·bi·son'ee·um). *N,N'*-Bis[1-methyl-3-(2,2,6-trimethylcyclohexyl)propyl]-*N,N'*-dimethyl-1,6-hexanediamine bis(methochloride), $C_{36}H_{74}Cl_2N_2$, a synthetic drug for topical treatment of superficial infections of the skin and vagina.

tri·clo·car·ban (trye·klo·kahr'ban) *n.* 3,4,4'-Trichlorocarbanilide, $C_{13}H_9Cl_3N_2O$, a disinfectant.

tri·clo·fen·ol piperazine (trye"klo·fen'ol). A compound, $2C_6H_3Cl_3O.C_4H_{10}N_2$, of 2,4,5-trichlorophenol and piperazine, used as an anthelmintic.

tri·clo·nide (trye·klo'nide) *n.* 9,11β,21-Trichloro-6α-fluoro-16α,17-dihydroxypregna-1,4-diene-3,20-dione acetonide, $C_{24}H_{28}Cl_3FO_4$, an anti-inflammatory.

tri·clo·san (trye·klo'san) *n.* 2,4,4'-Trichloro-2'-hydroxydiphenyl ether, $C_{12}H_7Cl_3O_2$, a disinfectant.

Tricoloid. A trademark for tricyclamol, an anticholinergic drug used as the methochloride salt.

tri·cre·sol (trye·kree'sole, ·sol) *n.* CRESOL, a mixture of three isomeric compounds of the composition $HOC_6H_4CH_3$.

tricrotic pulse. A pulse in which the three waves are palpated during each cardiac cycle.

tri·cro·tism (trye'kro·tiz·um) *n.* [*tri-* + Gk. *krot*os, beat, + *-ism*]. The condition of having three waves corresponding to one pulse beat. —**tri·crot·ic** (trye·krot'ick) *adj.*

tri·cus·pid (trye·kus'pid) *adj.* [L. *tricuspis, tricuspidis,* three-pointed, from *cuspis,* point]. 1. Having three cusps. 2. Pertaining to or affecting the tricuspid valve.

tricuspid atresia. A complex cogenital cardiac anomaly with failure of development of the tricuspid valve, underdevelopment of the right ventricle, an atrial septal defect, and a large but normal mitral valve and left ventricle; there is usually also a ventricular septal defect and pulmonary artery hypoplasia.

tricuspid insufficiency. TRICUSPID REGURGITATION.

tricuspid murmur. A murmur produced at the tricuspid orifice.

tricuspid regurgitation. Reflux of blood into the right atrium during ventricular systole, due to incomplete or inadequate closure of the tricuspid valve.

tricuspid stenosis. Narrowing of the tricuspid valve, with resultant elevation of right atrial and venous pressure.

tricuspid valve. The three-cusped valve situated between the right atrium and right ventricle. Syn. *right atrioventricular valve, valva atrioventricularis dextra.* See also Plate 5.

tri·cy·cla·mol (trye·sigh'kluh·mol) *n.* 1-Cyclohexyl-1-phenyl-3-pyrrolidino-1-propanol, $C_{19}H_{29}NO$, an anticholinergic drug employed in gastrointestinal disorders; used as the methochloride salt.

tri·dac·tyl (trye·dack'til) *adj.* [*tri-* + *dactyl*]. Having three digits.

tri·dent (trye'dunt) *adj.* [L. *tridens, tridentis,* from *tri-* + *dens,* tooth]. TRIDENTATE.

tri·den·tate (trye·den'tate) *adj.* [*tri-* + *dentate*]. Three-pronged.

trident hand. A hand whose fingers cannot be completely approximated when extended.

tri·der·mic (trye·dur'mick) *adj.* [*tri-* + *derm-* + *-ic*]. Derived from or pertaining to all three germ layers of the embryo.

tri·der·mo·ma (trye"dur·mo'muh) *n.* [*tri-* + *derm-* + *-oma*]. TERATOMA.

tri·di·hex·eth·yl chloride (trye"dye·hecks·eth'il). (3-Cyclohexyl-3-hydroxy-3-phenylpropyl)triethylammonium chloride, $C_{21}H_{36}ClNO$, an anticholinergic drug used in the treatment of certain gastrointestinal disorders.

Tridione. Trademark for trimethadione, an anticonvulsant drug used for the treatment of petit mal and akinetic epilepsy.

trid·y·mite (trid'i·mite) *n.* A very hard native silica occurring in volcanic rocks.

trid·y·mus (trid'i·mus) *n.* [NL., from Gk. *tridymos*]. A triplet.

tri·en·ceph·a·lus (trye"en·sef'uh·lus) *n.* [NL., from *tri-* + Gk. *enkephalos,* brain]. TRIOCEPHALUS.

tri·eth·a·nol·am·ine (trye·eth"uh·nol'uh·meen, ·min) *n.* Trihydroxytriethylamine, $N(CH_2CH_2OH)_3$, a strongly basic, hygroscopic liquid; used as a solvent, emulsifying agent, and intermediate in many syntheses. Syn. *trolamine.*

tri·eth·yl·a·mine (trye·eth"il·uh·meen', ·am'een, ·am'in) *n.* A liquid base, $(C_2H_5)_3N$, formed in certain putrefactive processes; used in the synthesis of quaternary ammonium compounds.

tri·eth·yl·ene·mel·a·mine (trye·eth"il·een·mel'uh·meen, ·min) *n.* 2,4,6-Tris(1-aziridinyl)-*s*-triazine, $C_9H_{12}N_6$, an antineoplastic drug that forms ethyleneammonium ion in the body, as does nitrogen mustard, and is effective for palliative treatment of certain cancers. Abbreviated, TEM

tri·fa·cial nerve (trye·fay'shul). The fifth cranial or trigeminal nerve, so called because it divides into three main branches that supply the face.

trifacial neuralgia. TRIGEMINAL NEURALGIA.

tri·fid (trye'fid) *adj.* [L. *trifidus,* from *tri-* + *findere,* to split]. Three-cleft, tripartite.

tri·flo·cin (trye·flo'sin) *n.* 4-(α,α,α-Trifluoro-*m*-toluidino)nicotinic acid, $C_{13}H_9F_3N_2O_2$, a diuretic.

tri·flu·ba·zam (trye·floo'buh·zam) *n.* 1-Methyl-5-phenyl-7-(trifluoromethyl-1*H*-1,5-benzodiazepine-2,4(3*H*,5*H*)-dione, $C_{17}H_{13}F_3N_2O_2$, a minor tranquilizer.

tri·flu·mi·date (trye·floo'mi·date) *n.* Ethyl *m*-benzoyl-*N*-[(trifluoromethyl)sulfonyl]carbanilate, $C_{17}H_{14}F_3NO_5S$, an anti-inflammatory drug.

tri·flu·o·per·a·zine (trye·floo"o·perr'uh·zeen) *n.* 10-[3-(4-Methyl-1-piperazinyl)propyl]-2-trifluoromethylphenothiazine, $C_{21}H_{24}F_3N_3S$, a tranquilizer used as the hydrochloride salt principally to control acute and chronic psychoses marked by psychomotor activity.

tri·flu·per·i·dol (trye"floo·perr'i·dol) *n.* 4'-Fluoro-4-[4-hydroxy-4-(α,α,α-trifluoro-*m*-tolyl)piperidino]butyrophenone, $C_{22}H_{23}F_4NO_2$, a tranquilizer.

tri·flu·pro·ma·zine (trye"floo·pro'muh·zeen) *n.* 10-(3-Dimethylaminopropyl)-2-(trifluoromethyl)phenothiazine, $C_{18}H_{19}F_3N_2S$, a tranquilizer used, as the hydrochloride salt, to treat various psychiatric disorders and psychoses; also employed as an antiemetic.

tri·flu·ri·dine (trye·floo'ri·deen) *n.* 2'-Deoxy-5-(trifluoromethyl)uridine, $C_{10}H_{11}F_3N_2O_5$, an ophthalmic antiviral.

tri·fo·cal glasses or **spectacles** (trye·fo'kul). Glasses or spectacles having three refractive powers to correct for distant, intermediate, and near vision.

tri·fo·li·o·sis (trye·fo"lee·o'sis, tri·) *n.*, pl. **trifolio·ses** (·seez) [L. *trifoli*um, clover, + *-osis*]. *In veterinary medicine,* a superficial necrosis of the white markings, caused by exposure to the sun after the animals have been sensitized to light by eating certain substances, chiefly the legumes.

Tri·fo·li·um (trye·fo'lee·um, tri·) *n.* [L., from *tri-* + *folium,* leaf]. A genus of herbs including the clovers.

tri·fur·ca·tion (trye"fur·kay'shun) *n.* [*tri-* + L. *furca,* fork]. Division into three prongs. —**tri·fur·cate** (trye'fur·kate) *adj. & v.*

tri·gas·tric (trye·gas'trick) *adj.* [*tri-* + Gk. *gastēr,* belly, + *-ic*]. Having three fleshy bellies, as certain muscles.

tri·gas·tri·cus (tri·gas'tri·kus) *n.* A variant form of the digastric muscle.

tri·gem·i·nal (trye·jem'i·nul) *adj.* [L. *trigeminus,* three-fold, from *tri-* + *geminus,* twin]. Triple; dividing into three parts.

trigeminal cave. CAVUM TRIGEMINALE.

trigeminal ganglion. The large ganglion of the sensory portion of the trigeminal nerve; the ophthalmic, maxillary, and mandibular divisions of the fifth nerve are attached to it. NA *ganglion trigeminale.*

trigeminal ghost or **phantom.** Unpleasant dysesthesias on the side of the face following trigeminal rhizotomy.

trigeminal impression of the temporal bone. IMPRESSIO TRIGEMINI OSSIS TEMPORALIS.

trigeminal lemniscus. The secondary fibers from the main sensory nucleus of the trigeminal nerve and spinal nucleus of the trigeminal nerve, terminating in the posteromedial ventral nucleus of the thalamus. NA *lemniscus trigeminalis.*

trigeminal nerve. The fifth cranial nerve with central attachment at the lateral aspect of the pons. At the trigeminal (semilunar or Gasserian) ganglion it divides into three divisions: mandibular, maxillary, and ophthalmic. Syn. *nervus trigeminus,* See also *mandibular nerve, maxillary nerve, ophthalmic nerve.*

trigeminal neuralgia. Sudden, severe, lancinating pains in the distribution of one or more divisions of the trigeminal nerve, generally of unknown cause, but triggered by irritation of a fairly constant zone, such as the angle of the mouth or the side of the nose.

trigeminal nuclei. Main sensory nucleus of the trigeminal nerve, mesencephalic nucleus of the trigeminal nerve, motor nucleus of the trigeminal nerve, and nucleus of the spinal tract of the trigeminal nerve.

trigeminal pulse. A pulse in which a pause occurs after every third beat.

trigeminal rhythm. TRIGEMINY.

tri·gem·i·no·tha·lam·ic tract (trye·jem"i·no·thuh·lam'ick). TRIGEMINAL LEMNISCUS.

tri·gem·i·nus (trye·jem'i·nus) *n.* [L., threefold]. TRIGEMINAL NERVE.

tri·gem·i·ny (trye·jem'i·nee) *n.* [L. *trigemin*us, triple, + *-y*]. 1. Any grouping in threes. 2. Grouping of arterial pulse beats in groups of three.

tri·gen·ic (trye·jen'ick) *adj.* [*tri-* + *-genic*]. Pertaining to genotypes of polysomic or polyploid organisms which contain three different alleles for any given locus.

trig·ger action. A sudden stimulus that initiates a physiologic or pathologic process that may have nothing in common with the action that started it.

trigger finger. A condition in which flexion or extension of a finger is at first obstructed, but finally accomplished with a jerk or sweep. It is due to chronic tenosynovitis.

trigger zone. Any area of hyperexcitability, stimulation of which will precipitate a specific response such as the lancinating pain of trigeminal neuralgia. See also *pain point.*

tri·glyc·er·ide (trye·glis'ur·ide) *n.* An ester of glycerin in which all three hydroxyl groups of the latter are esterified with an acid; animal and vegetable fixed oils are composed chiefly of triglycerides of fatty acids; TRIACYLGLYCEROL.

trigona. Plural of *trigonum.*

trigona fi·bro·sa cor·dis (figh·bro'suh, kor'dis) [NA]. FIBROUS TRIGONES OF THE HEART.

tri·gone (trye'gohn) *n.* [Gk. *trigōnon,* from *trigōnos,* three-cornered]. 1. Any of various triangular anatomic areas or structures. 2. The smooth triangular area on the inner surface of the urinary bladder between the openings of the two ureters and the internal urethral opening. NA *trigonum vesicae.* —**trig·o·nal** (trig'uh·nul) *adj.*

Trig·o·nel·la (trig"o·nel'uh) *n.* A genus of the Leguminosae, certain species of which have been used medicinally.

trigone of Lieu·taud (lyœh·to') [J. *Lieutaud,* French physician, 1703–1780]. TRIGONE (2).

trigone of the hypoglossal nerve. The triangular area of the floor of the fourth ventricle overlying the nucleus of the hypoglossal nerve. NA *trigonum nervi hypoglossi.*

trigone of the urinary bladder. TRIGONE (2).

trigone of the vagus nerve. TRIGONUM NERVI VAGI.

tri·go·nid (trye'go·nid, trye·gon'id, trig'o·) *n.* The first three cusps (viewed as one) of a lower molar tooth.

tri·go·ni·tis (trye"go·nigh'tis) *n.* [*trigone* + *-itis*]. Inflammation of the trigone of the urinary bladder.

trig·o·no·ceph·a·lus (trig"uh·no·sef'uh·lus, tri·go"no·) *n.* [Gk. *trigōnos*, triangular, + *-cephalus*]. An individual exhibiting trigonocephaly.

trig·o·no·ceph·a·ly (trig"uh·no·sef'uh·lee, tri·go"no·) *n.* [*trigōnos* + *-cephaly*]. Triangular or egg-shaped head, due to early synostosis of the metopic suture.

tri·go·num (trye·go'num) *n.*, pl. **trigo·na** (·nuh) [L.]. TRIGONE.

trigonum acu·sti·ci (a·koos'ti·sigh). VESTIBULAR AREA.

trigonum ca·ro·ti·cum (ka·rot'i·kum) [NA]. SUPERIOR CAROTID TRIANGLE.

trigonum col·la·te·ra·le (ko·lat·e·ray'lee) [NA]. COLLATERAL TRIGONE.

trigonum del·toi·deo·pec·to·ra·le [BNA]. INFRACLAVICULAR FOSSA.

trigonum fe·mo·ra·le (fem·o·ray'lee) [NA]. FEMORAL TRIANGLE.

trigonum fi·bro·sum cor·dis [dextrum et si·nis·trum] (figh·bro'sum kor'dis decks'trum et si·nis'trum). FIBROUS TRIGONES OF THE HEART.

trigonum ha·be·nu·lae (ha·ben'yoo·lee) [NA]. HABENULAR TRIGONE.

trigonum in·gui·na·le (ing·gwi·nay'lee) [NA]. INGUINAL TRIANGLE.

trigonum in·ter·pe·dun·cu·la·re (in"tur·pe·dunk·yoo·lair'ee). INTERPEDUNCULAR FOSSA.

trigonum lem·nis·ci (lem·nis'eye, ·kigh) [BNA]. A slightly elevated area of the tegmentum overlying the lateral lemniscus.

trigonum lum·ba·le (lum·bay'lee) [NA]. LUMBAR TRIANGLE.

trigonum lumbale [Pe·ti·ti] (pet'i·tye) [BNA]. LUMBAR TRIANGLE.

trigonum ner·vi hy·po·glos·si (nur'vye high·po·glos'eye) [NA]. TRIGONE OF THE HYPOGLOSSAL NERVE.

trigonum nervi va·gi (vay'guy) [NA]. The trigone of the vagus nerve; the area in the floor of the fourth ventricle overlying the dorsal motor nucleus of the vagus nerve. Syn. *ala cinerea, trigonum vagi, vagal triangle.*

trigonum ol·fac·to·ri·um (ol·fack·to'ree·um) [NA]. OLFACTORY TRIGONE.

trigonum omo·cla·vi·cu·la·re (o"mo·kla·vick"yoo·lair'ee) [NA]. The depression in the base of the neck located above the clavicle and lateral to the sternocleidomastoid muscle.

trigonum sub·man·di·bu·la·re (sub"man·dib·yoo·lair'ee) [NA]. SUBMANDIBULAR TRIANGLE.

trigonum uro·gen·i·ta·le (yoor"o·jen"i·tay'lee). UROGENITAL DIAPHRAGM.

trigonum vagi. TRIGONUM NERVI VAGI.

trigonum ve·si·cae (ve·sigh'see, ·kee) [NA]. TRIGONE (2).

tri·hex·y·phen·i·dyl (trye"heck·si·fen'i·dil) *n.* α-Cyclohexyl-α-phenyl-1-piperidinepropanol, $C_{20}H_{31}NO$, an anticholinergic drug used as the hydrochloride salt; also used for the treatment of parkinsonism.

tri·hy·brid (trye·high'brid) *n.* [*tri-* + *hybrid*]. The offspring of parents differing in three pairs of Mendelian characteristics.

tri·hy·dric (trye·high'drick) *adj.* Containing three atoms of hydrogen replaceable by metals.

tri·hy·drol (trye·high'drol) *n.* An associated form of water having the composition $(H_2O)_3$.

tri·hy·droxy·ben·zo·ic acid (trye"high·drock"see·ben·zo'ick). GALLIC ACID.

tri·hy·droxy·pro·pane (trye"high·drock"see·pro'pane) *n.* GLYCERIN.

tri·in·i·od·y·mus (trye·in"ee·od'i·mus) *n.* [*tri-* + *inion* + *-dymus*]. A monster having three heads united posteriorly and attached to a single body.

tri·io·do·eth·i·on·ic acid (trye·eye"o·do·eth"eye·on'ick). IOPHENOXIC ACID.

tri·io·do·meth·ane (trye·eye"o·do·meth'ane) *n.* IODOFORM.

tri·io·do·thy·ro·nine (trye·eye"o·do·thigh'ro·neen, ·nin) *n.* Either of two isomeric hormones present in thyroid, specifically identified as L-3,3'5-triiodothyronine and L-3,3',5'-triiodothyronine. The former, now called liothyronine, is more active than thyroxine and also more rapid in action, and is used for the treatment of hypothyroid states in the form of its sodium salt.

tri·ke·to·cho·lan·ic acid (trye·kee"to·ko·lan'ick). DEHYDROCHOLIC ACID.

tri·ke·to·hy·drin·dene hydrate (trye·kee"to·high·drin'deen). 1,2,3-Indantrione monohydrate, $C_9H_4O_3.H_2O$, a reagent for proteins and amino acids.

tri·ke·to·pu·rine (trye·kee"to·pew'reen) *n.* URIC ACID.

Trilafon. Trademark for the tranquilizer and antiemetic drug perphenazine.

tri·lam·i·nar (trye·lam'i·nur) *adj.* [*tri-* + *laminar*]. Three-layered.

trilaminar blastodisk or **blastoderm.** The early embryo at the time of formation of the mesoderm and the head process.

Trilene. A trademark for trichloroethylene, a liquid anesthetic and analgesic.

tri·li·no·le·in (trye"li·no'lee·in) *n.* Glyceryl linoleate, $(C_{18}H_{31}O_2)_3C_3H_5$, occurring in many vegetable oils.

tri·lo·bate (trye·lo'bate) *adj.* [*tri-* + *lobate*]. Three-lobed.

tri·loc·u·lar (trye·lock'yoo·lur) *adj.* [*tri-* + *locular*]. *In biology,* having three chambers or cells.

trilocular heart. A three-chambered heart; in humans, a congenital anomaly in which there is either a single atrium or single ventricle. Syn. *cor triloculare.*

tri·lo·stane (trye'lo·stane) *n.* 4α,5-Epoxy-17β-hydroxy-3-oxo-5α-androstane-2α-carbonitrile, $C_{20}H_{27}NO_3$, an adrenocortical suppressant.

tri·mal·le·o·lar fracture (trye"ma·lee'o·lur). A fracture in which the medial and lateral malleoli and the posterior lip of the tibia are fractured, usually associated with a posterior dislocation of the talus. Syn. *Cotton's fracture.*

tri·man·u·al (trye·man'yoo·ul) *adj.* [*tri-* + *manual*]. Accomplished by the aid of three hands.

tri·mas·ti·gate (trye·mas'ti·gut) *adj.* [*tri-* + Gk. *mastix, mastigos,* whip]. Having three flagella; triflagellate.

tri·ma·zo·sin (trye·may'zo·sin) *n.* 2-Hydroxy-2-methylpropyl-4-(4-amino-6,7,8-trimethoxy-2-quinazolinyl)-1-piperazinecarboxylate, $C_{20}H_{29}N_5O_6$, an antihypertensive, used as the hydrochloride salt.

tri·men·su·al (trye·men'syoo·ul, shoo·ul) *adj.* [*tri-* + *mensual*]. Occurring at periods of 3 months.

tri·mep·ra·zine (trye·mep'ruh·zeen) *n.* 10-(3-Dimethylamino-2-methylpropyl)phenothiazine, $C_{18}H_{22}N_2S$, a phenothiazine compound that is used, as the tartrate salt, to relieve pruritus.

Trim·er·e·su·rus (trim"ur·e·sue'rus) *n.* [NL. from Gk. *trimerēs,* having three parts, + *oura,* tail]. A genus of Asiatic pit vipers. *Trimeresurus flavoviridis* or habu, *T. gramineus,* and *T. macrosquamosus* are representative species.

tri·mes·ter (trye·mes'tur) *n.* [L. *trimestris,* of three months]. A stage or period of 3 months.

tri·meth·a·di·one (trye"meth·uh·dye'ohn) *n.* 3,5,5-Trimethyl-2,4-oxazolidinedione, $C_6H_9NO_3$, an anticonvulsant drug used for the treatment of petit mal and akinetic epilepsy.

tri·meth·a·phan cam·syl·ate (try·meth'uh·fan kam'zil·ate). (+)-1,3-Dibenzyldecahydro-2-oxoimidazo[4,5-*c*]thieno[1,2-*a*]thiolium 2-oxo-10-bornanesulfonate, $C_{32}H_{40}N_2O_5S_2$, a ganglionic blocking agent used as an antihypertensive drug.

tri·meth·i·din·i·um metho·sul·fate (trye·meth"i·din'ee·um meth"o·sul'fate). 1,3,8,8-Tetramethyl-3-[3-(trimethylammonio)propyl]-3-azoniabicyclo[3.2.1]octane bis(methyl sulfate), $C_{19}H_{42}N_2O_8S_2$, a ganglionic blocking agent used in the treatment of hypertension.

tri·metho·benz·a·mide (trye·meth"o·benz'uh·mide) *n.* *N*-{*p*-[2-(Dimethylamino)ethoxy]benzyl}-3,4,5-trimethoxybenzamide, $C_{21}H_{28}N_2O_5$, an antiemetic drug used as the hydrochloride salt.

tri·meth·o·prim (trye·meth'o·prim) *n.* 2,4-Diamino-5-(3,4,5-trimethoxybenzyl)pyrimidine, $C_{14}H_{18}N_4O_3$, an antibacterial agent.

tri·meth·yl·ace·tic acid (trye·meth"il·uh·see'tick). VALERIC ACID (4).

tri·meth·yl·a·mine (trye·meth"il·uh·meen', ·am'een, ·am'in) *n.* $(CH_3)_3N$. A degradation product, often by putrefaction, of various plant and animal substances; used in the synthesis of quaternary ammonium compounds.

tri·meth·yl·ene (trye·meth'il·een) *n.* CYCLOPROPANE.

tri·meth·yl·gly·cine (trye·meth"il·glye'seen, ·sin) *n.* BETAINE.

tri·meth·yl·xan·thine (trye·meth"il·zan'theen, ·thin) *n.* CAFFEINE.

tri·met·o·zine (trye·met'o·zeen) *n.* 4-(3,4,5-Trimethoxybenzoyl)morpholine, $C_{14}H_{19}NO_5$, a sedative drug.

tri·mip·ra·mine (trye·mip'ruh·meen) *n.* 5-[3-(Dimethylamino)-2-methylpropyl]-10,11-dihydro-5*H*-dibenz[*b,f*]azepine, an antidepressant drug.

tri·mo·pam (trye'mo·pam) *n.* (+)2,3,4,5-Tetrahydro-7,8-dimethoxy-3-methyl-1-phenyl-1*H*-3-benzazepine, $C_{19}H_{23}NO_2$, a tranquilizer, used as the maleate salt.

tri·mor·phism (trye·mor'fiz·um) *n.* [*tri-* + *-morphism*]. 1. *In biology,* occurrence of hermaphrodite flowers of three kinds (short-styled, mid-styled, and long-styled) produced on the same species of plant. 2. Occurrence in three distinct forms, as certain insects. —**trimor·phic** (·fick) *adj.*

tri·mox·a·mine (trye·mock'suh·meen) *n.* α-Allyl-3,4,5-trimethoxy-*N*-methylphenethylamine, $C_{15}H_{23}NO_3$, an antihypertensive drug; used as the hydrochloride salt.

tri·ni·tro·glyc·er·in (trye·nigh"tro·glis'ur·in) *n.* Glyceryl trinitrate; NITROGLYCERIN.

tri·ni·tro·phe·nol (trye·nigh"tro·fee'nol) *n.* 2,4,6-Trinitrophenol, $C_6H_2(NO_2)_3OH$, a yellow, crystalline solid; has been used topically as an antiseptic, astringent, and epithelization stimulant. Syn. *picric acid.*

tri·ni·tro·tol·u·ene (trye·nigh"tro·tol'yoo·een) *n.* $(NO_2)_3C_6H_2CH_3$; any of six isomers of this formula, but especially 1-methyl-2,4,6-trinitrobenzene, occurring as pale-yellow crystals; used in explosives. Abbreviated, TNT.

tri·no·mi·al (trye·no'mee·ul) *n.* [*tri-* + *-nomial* as in binomial]. 1. A botanical or zoological name consisting of three terms, the first designating the genus, the second the species, and the third the subspecies or variety. 2. A mathematical expression consisting of three terms.

tri·nu·cle·ate (trye·new'klee·ut) *adj.* Having three nuclei.

tri·nu·cle·o·tide (trye·new'klee·o·tide) *n.* A molecule composed of three mononucleotides linked by phosphodiester bonds.

trio·ceph·a·lus (trye"o·sef'uh·lus) *n.*, pl. **triocepha·li** (·lye) [*tri-* + *-cephalus*]. A monster characterized by an absence of the ocular, nasal, and oral apparatus, the head being merely a small spheroidal mass with no brain.

tri·o·le·in (trye·o'lee·in) *n.* OLEIN.

trio·lism (trye'o·liz·um, tree'o·) *n.* [*triole*, triplet (of musical notes), + *-ism*]. Sexual interests or practices involving three persons of both sexes, as when one of the heterosexual partners is also involved in a homosexual relationship, or may indulge in voyeurism by watching his or her partner in the sexual act with a third party.

trio·list (trye'o·list, tree') *n.* One partner of a sexual trio. See also *triolism.*

tri·oph·thal·mos (trye"off·thal'mus) *adj.* [*tri-* + *ophthalmos*]. Characterizing that variety of diprosopus in which three eyes are present.

tri·o·pod·y·mus (trye"o·pod'i·mus) *n.* [*tri-* + Gk. *ōps, ōpos*, face, + *-dymus*]. An individual with three faces and a single head.

tri·or·chid (trye·or'kid) *adj.* & *n.* [*tri-* + Gk. *orchis*, testis]. 1. Having three testes. 2. An individual having three testes. —**trior·chidy** (·ki·dee) *n.*

tri·or·chis (trye·or'kis) *n.* TRIORCHID (2).

tri·or·tho·cres·yl phosphate (trye·or"tho·kres'il). A mixture of esters of the composition $(CH_3C_6H_4)_3PO_4$; a colorless or pale-yellow liquid used in industry as a plasticizer and solvent and for other purposes. It is neurotoxic.

triorthocresyl phosphate neuropathy. A polyneuropathy resulting from the ingestion of grain, cooking oil, or ginger extract contaminated with triorthocresyl phosphate. The neural effects are mainly those of a motor polyneuropathy, but the spinal cord, particularly the corticospinal tracts, is also affected. The effects on the latter are usually permanent. Syn. *Jamaica ginger paralysis, jake palsy.*

tri·ose (trye'oce, ·oze) *n.* A monosaccharide containing three carbon atoms in the molecule.

tri·ose·phos·pho·ric acid (trye"oce·fos·fo'rick). Triose phosphate. A phosphorylated three-carbon sugar. Several of these compounds are intermediaries in the breakdown of glycogen to pyruvic acid in carbohydrate metabolism.

Triostam. Trademark for sodium antimonylgluconate, a trivalent antimony compound used in the treatment of schistosomiasis.

tri·o·tus (trye·o'tus) *adj.* [NL., from *tri-* + Gk. *ous, ōtos*, ear]. Having three ears.

tri·ox·sa·len (trye·ock'suh·len) *n.* 6-Hydroxy-β,2,7-trimethyl-5-benzofuranacrylic acid δ-lactone, or 4,5,8-trimethylpsoralen, $C_{14}H_{12}O_3$, a drug that enhances dermal repigmentation.

tri·oxy·meth·yl·ene (trye·ock'see·meth'il·een) *n.* PARAFORMALDEHYDE.

tri·oxy·pu·rine (trye·ock"see·pew'reen, ·rin) *n.* URIC ACID.

tri·pal·mi·tin (trye·pal'mi·tin) *n.* PALMITIN.

trip·a·ra (trip'uh·ruh) *n.* [*tri-* + *-para*]. A woman who has had three viable pregnancies.

tri·par·tite placenta (trye·pahr'tite). A three-lobed placenta connected by vessels, membranes, and a thinned portion of placenta.

tri·pel·en·na·mine (trye"pel·en'uh·meen, ·min) *n.* 2-{Benzyl[2-(dimethylamino)ethyl]amino}pyridine, $C_{16}H_{21}N_3$, an antihistaminic drug used as the citrate and hydrochloride salts.

tri·pep·tid (trye·pep'tid) *n.* TRIPEPTIDE.

tri·pep·tide (trye·pep'tide) *n.* A protein hydrolysis product representing condensation of three molecules of amino acids, or a natural or synthetic peptide containing three amino acids.

Triperidol. Trademark for trifluperidol, a tranquilizer.

tri·pha·lan·gia (trye"fa·lan'jee·uh) *n.* TRIPHALANGISM.

tri·pha·lan·gism (trye"fa·lan'jiz·um) *n.* [*tri-* + *phalang-* + *-ism*]. The presence of three phalanges in the thumb or great toe. See also *hyperphalangism.*

tri·pha·lan·gy (trye"fa·lan'jee) *n.* TRIPHALANGISM.

tri·phar·ma·con (trye·fahr'muh·kon) *n.* [*tri-* + Gk. *pharmakon*, drug]. A medicine made up of three ingredients.

tri·phar·ma·cum (trye·fahr'muh·kum) *n.* TRIPHARMACON.

tri·pha·sic (trye·fay'zick) *adj.* [*tri-* + *phase* + *-ic*]. Having three phases or variations.

tri·phos·pho·pyr·i·dine nucleotide (trye·fos"fo·pirr'i·deen). NICOTINAMIDE ADENINE DINUCLEOTIDE PHOSPHATE. Abbreviated, TPN

tri·ple·gia (trye·plee'jee·uh) *n.* [*tri-* + *-plegia*]. Hemiplegia with the additional paralysis of one limb on the opposite side.

triple kidney. A developmental condition in which one of the kidneys is subdivided into three parts.

triple phosphate crystals. Coffin-lid shaped or feathery crystals of ammonium magnesium phosphate occurring in alkaline urine.

triple point. The single temperature and pressure at which the solid, liquid, and vapor forms of a substance may coexist.

triple quartan fever. A form of intermittent malarial fever in which there are three concurrent cycles of quartan fever, not synchronous with each other, resulting in paroxysms every day.

triple response. The three stages of normal vasomotor reaction resulting when a pointed instrument is drawn heavily across the skin. They are: reddening of the area stimulated, wide spreading of flush to adjacent skin, and development of wheals. The response is said to be due to a histamine-like substance liberated from injured tissue by a noxious stimulus.

triple rhythm. A cardiac cadence in which three sounds recur in successive cycles; it may be normal or abnormal. See also *gallop rhythm.*

triple stain. 1. MALLORY'S TRIPLE STAIN. 2. MASSON'S TRICHROME STAIN.

trip·let *n.* [*triple* + *-et* as in doublet]. 1. One of three children born at one birth. 2. *In optics*, a system consisting of three lenses.

triple vaccine for typhoid. TYPHOID-PARATYPHOID A AND B VACCINE.

triple-X syndrome. A human chromosomal abnormality in which somatic cells contain 47 chromosomes, with X-trisomy; subjects are phenotypic females, often mentally retarded.

trip·lo·blas·tic (trip"lo·blas'tick) *adj.* [*triple* + *-blastic*]. Possessing three germ layers, ectoderm, entoderm, and mesoderm.

trip·lo·co·ria, trip·lo·ko·ria (trip"lo·ko'ree·uh) *n.* [*triple* + *cor-* + *-ia*]. The existence of three pupillary openings in one eye. See also *multiple pupil.*

trip·loid (trip'loid) *adj.* [*tri-* + *-ploid*]. Having triple the haploid or gametic number of chromosomes. —**trip·loi·dy** (·loy·dee) *n.*

tri·plo·pia (trip·lo'pee·uh) *n.* [*triple* + *-opia*]. A disturbance of vision in which three images of a single object are seen.

tri·prol·i·dine (trye·prol'i·deen) *n.* *trans*-2-[3-(1-Pyrrolidinyl)-1-(*p*-tolyl)propenyl]pyridine, $C_{19}H_{22}N$, an antihistaminic agent used as the hydrochloride salt.

tri·pro·so·pus (trye"pro·so'pus, trye·pro'so·pus) *n.* [NL., from *tri-* + Gk. *prosōpon*, face]. An individual in which there is a fusion of three faces in one.

trip·sis (trip'sis) *n.* [Gk., a rubbing]. 1. TRITURATION. 2. MASSAGE.

-tripsy [Gk. *tripsis*, from *tribein*, to rub, grind, crush]. A combining form meaning *a crushing.*

Trip·te·ryg·i·um (trip"te·rij'ee·um) *n.* A genus of twining vines the root bark of certain species of which, notably *Tripterygium wilfordi* Hook, or thunder-god vine, has long been used in China as an insecticide.

tri·que·trum (trye·kwee'trum, trye·kwet'rum) *n.*, pl. **trique·tra** (·truh) [L. *triquetrus*, three-cornered]. 1. The third carpal bone from the radial side in the proximal row. NA *os triquetrum*. See also Table of Bones in the Appendix. 2. Any of the Wormian bones.

tri·ra·di·ate cartilage (trye·ray'dee·ut). The Y-shaped cartilage in the acetabulum between the ilium, pubis, and ischium; it disappears when the three bones fuse to form the adult hipbone.

tri·sac·cha·ride (trye·sack'uh·ride, ·rid) *n.* A carbohydrate which, on hydrolysis, yields three molecules of monosaccharides.

tri·sect (trye'sekt) *v.* [*tri-* + L. *secare, sectus*, to cut]. To cut into three parts.

tris·kai·deka·pho·bia (tris·kigh''deck·uh·fo'bee·uh) *n.* [Gk. *triskaideka*, thirteen, + *-phobia*]. Superstitious fear of thirteen.

tris·mus (triz'mus) *n.* [NL., from Gk. *trismos*, rasping, grating]. Tonic spasms of the muscles of the jaw; a frequent and sensitive sign of tetanus.

tri·so·mic (trye·so'mick) *adj. & n.* [*tri-* + *-some* (as in chromosome) + *-ic*]. 1. Having three chromosomes of a given kind, but otherwise only two of each of the other chromosomes of a haploid set. 2. A trisomic individual, having three chromosomes of a given kind in an otherwise diploid set.

tri·so·mus (trye·so'mus) *n.* [*tri-* + *-somus*]. More or less conjoined triplets from a single ovum, as a tricephalus.

trisomus omphaloangiopagus. Monochorionic triplets of which two are more or less normal autosites and the third is an omphalosite.

tri·so·my (trye'so·mee) *n.* [*trisom*ic + *-y*]. The occurrence of three of a given chromosome rather than the normal diploid number of two; often followed by a specification of the aberrant chromosome or chromosome group, as trisomy 13 (Patau's) syndrome, trisomy 18 (Edwards') syndrome, and trisomy 21 syndrome.

trisomy 13 syndrome. A congenital disorder due to trisomy of the number 13 chromosome (D trisomy) and rarely of an unbalanced translocation (D/D), characterized by the infant's failure to thrive, severe mental retardation, seizures, arhinencephalia, sloping forehead, deformities of the eyes, low-set ears, cleft lip and palate, rocker-bottom shaped feet, congenital heart defects, and multiple other anomalies. Syn. *Patau's syndrome.*

trisomy 18 syndrome. A congenital disorder due to trisomy for all, or a large part of, the 18 chromosome, characterized by severe mental deficiency, hypertonicity with clenched hands, anomalies of the hands, sternum, and pelvis, abnormal facies with low-set malformed ears and prominent occiput, ventricular septal defect with or without patent ductus arteriosus, and renal anomalies; the majority of infants are female, and most infants fail to thrive. Syn. *Edwards' syndrome.*

trisomy 21 syndrome. DOWN'S SYNDROME.

Trisoralen. Trademark for trioxsalen, a drug that enhances dermal repigmentation.

tri·stea·rin (trye·stee'uh·rin) *n.* STEARIN.

tris·ti·chi·a·sis (tris''ti·kigh'uh·sis) *n.* [*tri-* + Gk. *stichos*, row, + *-iasis*]. The arrangement of the cilia (eyelashes) in three rows.

tris·ti·ma·nia, tris·te·ma·nia (tris''ti·may'nee·uh) *n.* [L. *tristis*, sad, + *-mania*]. MELANCHOLIA. See also *manic-depressive illness.*

tris·tis (tris'tis) *adj.* [L.]. 1. Sad; gloomy. 2. Dull in color.

trit·an·o·pia (trit''an·o'pee·uh, trye''tan·) *n.* [Gk. *tritos*, third, + *anopia*]. A defect in a third constituent essential for color vision, as in violet blindness. See also *dichromatopsia.*

tri·ter·pene (trye·tur'peen) *n.* Any of a group of hydrocarbons of the general formula $C_{30}H_{48}$ or $(C_5H_8)_6$, related to terpene.

trit·i·a·tion (trit''ee·ay'shun) *n.* The process of introducing into a chemical compound one or more atoms of the hydrogen isotope tritium in place of a like number of atoms of ordinary hydrogen (protium) commonly existing in the compound.

tri·ti·ceo·glos·sus (tri·tish''ee·o·glos'us) *adj.* [NL., from *triticeous* + Gk. *glōssa*, tongue]. Pertaining to the triticeous cartilage and tongue.

triticeoglossus muscle. See Table of Muscles in the Appendix.

tri·ti·ceous (tri·tish'us) *adj.* [L. *triticeus*, of wheat, from *triticum*, wheat]. Having the shape of a grain of wheat.

triticeous cartilage or **nodule.** A small, oblong cartilaginous nodule often found in the lateral thyrohyoid membrane. NA *cartilago triticea.*

tri·ti·co·nu·cle·ic acid (trit''ti·ko·new·klee'ick). A nucleic acid from wheat and having ribose as the sugar component.

Trit·i·cum (trit'i·kum) *n.* [L., wheat]. A genus of the family Gramineae. *Triticum sativum* is wheat.

triticum, *n.* The dried rhizome and roots of *Agropyron repens*, family Gramineae; formerly used as a diuretic.

trit·i·um (trit'ee·um, trish'ee·um) *n.* The radioactive isotope of hydrogen of mass 3; used as a tracer. Symbol, ^3H

trit·o·cone (trit'o·kone) *n.* [Gk. *tritos*, third, + *cone*]. The distobuccal cusp on a premolar tooth of the upper jaw; not found in man.

trit·o·co·nid (trit''o·ko'nid) *n.* The distolingual cusp on a premolar tooth of the lower jaw; not found in man.

tri·ton (trye'ton) *n.* The nucleus of the tritium atom. It contains two neutrons and one proton, and thus bears unit positive charge.

trit·o·pine (trit'o·peen, ·pin, trye·to'pin) *n.* An alkaloid, $C_{20}H_{25}NO_4$, of opium. Syn. *laudanine.*

tri·tu·ber·cu·lar (trye''tew·bur'kew·lur) *adj.* [*tri-* + *tubercular*]. Having three tubercles or cusps; TRICUSPID.

tritubercular theory. The theory that mammalian molar teeth are derived phylogenetically from primitive three-cusped teeth.

trit·u·ra·ble (trit'yoo·ruh·bul) *adj.* Capable of being powdered or triturated.

trit·u·rate (trit'yoo·rate) *v. & n.* [L. *triturare*, to thresh]. 1. To reduce to a fine powder. 2. To mix powdered substances in a mortar with the aid of a pestle. 3. A finely divided powder. 4. TRITURATION (2).

trit·u·ra·tion (trit''yoo·ray'shun) *n.* [L. *trituratio*, act or process of threshing]. 1. The process of reducing a solid substance to a powder by rubbing. 2. The product obtained by triturating a potent medicinal substance with powdered lactose or other diluent. 3. The process of amalgamation.

tri·va·lence (trye·vay'lunce, triv'uh·) *n.* [*tri-* + *valence*]. The quality of having a valence of three. —**triva·lent** (·lunt) *adj.*

tri·valve (trye'valv) *adj.* [*tri-* + *valve*]. Having three valves or blades, as a speculum.

tri·val·vu·lar (trye·val'vyoo·lur) *adj.* [*tri-* + *valvular*]. Having three valves.

tRNA Abbreviation for *transfer RNA.*

Trobicin. Trademark for the antibiotic spectinomycin.

tro·car (tro'kahr) *n.* [F. *trocart*, from *trois*, three, + *carre*, side of a sword blade]. A sharp-pointed surgical instrument, fitted with a hollow cannula, used to puncture a body cavity for withdrawal of fluid. When the instrument is withdrawn the cannula is left in place to act as a drainage outlet.

troch. Abbreviation for *trochiscus*, a troche.

troch-, trocho- [Gk. *trochos*, wheel]. A combining form meaning (a) *round, resembling a wheel;* (b) *rotation;* (c) *trochoid.*

tro·chan·ter (tro·kan'tur) *n.* [Gk., *trochantēr*, from *trechein*, to run]. One of two processes on the upper extremity of the femur below the neck, the greater trochanter and the lesser trochanter. See also Plates 1, 2. —**tro·chan·ter·ic** (tro''kan·terr'ick). *adj.*

trochanteric bursa. 1. (of the gluteus maximus muscle:) A large, often multilocular bursa between the fascial tendon of the gluteus maximus and the posterior lateral surface of the greater trochanter. Syn. *gluteotrochanteric bursa.* NA *bursa trochanterica musculi glutei maximi.* 2. (of the gluteus medius muscle:) Either of two bursae between the tendon of the gluteus medius and adjacent parts, one separating that tendon from the lateral surface of the greater trochanter and the other (inconstant) between the tendons of the gluteus medius and piriform muscles. NA (pl.) *bursae trochantericae musculi glutei medii.* 3. (of the gluteus minimus muscle:) A bursa between the tendon of the gluteus minimus and the greater trochanter. NA *bursa trochanterica musculi glutei minimi.*

trochanteric fossa. A hollow at the base of the inner surface of the greater trochanter of the femur. NA *fossa trochanterica.*

trochanter major [NA]. GREATER TROCHANTER.

trochanter minor [NA]. LESSER TROCHANTER.

trochanter ter·ti·us (tur'shee·us) [NA]. THIRD TROCHANTER.

tro·chan·tin (tro·kan'tin) *n.* 1. LESSER TROCHANTER. 2. The proximal segment of the trochanter of an insect's leg.

tro·chan·tin·i·an (tro"kan·tin'ee·un) *adj.* Pertaining to the trochantin.

tro·char (tro'kahr) *n.* TROCAR.

tro·che (tro'kee) *n.* [earlier *trochisk,* from L. *trochiscus,* from Gk. *trochiskos,* dim of *trochos,* wheel]. LOZENGE.

tro·chis·ca·tion (tro"kis·kay'shun) *n.* The process of making troches from fine powder obtained by elutriation.

tro·chis·cus (tro·kis'kus) *n.,* pl. **trochis·ci** (·kigh, ·eye). [L.]. A troche; LOZENGE. Abbreviated, troch.

troch·lea (trock'lee·uh) *n.,* pl. & genit. sing. **troch·le·ae** (·lee·ee) [L., block and tackle, from Gk. *trochileia*]. A part or process having the nature of a pulley.

trochlea fi·bu·la·ris (fib·yoo·lair'is) [NA alt.]. PERONEAL TROCHLEA OF THE CALCANEUS. NA alt. *trochlea peronealis.*

trochlea hu·me·ri (hew'mur·eye) [NA]. TROCHLEA OF THE HUMERUS.

trochlea mus·cu·la·ris (mus·kew·lair'is) [NA]. Any anatomic attachment which serves to change the direction of pull of a muscle.

trochlea mus·cu·li ob·li·qui ocu·li su·pe·ri·o·ris (mus'kew·lye ob·lye'kwye ock'yoo·lye sue·peer·ee·o'ris) [BNA]. Trochlea musculi obliqui superioris (= TROCHLEA OF THE OBLIQUUS OCULI SUPERIOR).

trochlea musculi obliqui superioris [NA]. TROCHLEA OF THE OBLIQUUS OCULI SUPERIOR.

trochlea of the astragalus. TROCHLEA TALI.

trochlea of the femur. INTERCONDYLAR FOSSA.

trochlea of the humerus. The medial portion of the distal articulation of the humerus; the surface which articulates with the trochlear or semilunar notch of the ulna. NA *trochlea humeri.*

trochlea of the obliquus oculi superior. The ligamentous ring or pulley, attached to the upper medial margin of the orbit, which transmits the tendon of the superior oblique muscle of the eye. NA *trochlea musculi obliqui superioris.* See also Plate 19.

trochlea pe·ro·ne·a·lis (pe·ro·nee·ay'lis) [NA]. PERONEAL TROCHLEA OF THE CALCANEUS. NA alt. *trochlea fibularis.*

trochlea pha·lan·gis (fa·lan'jis) [BNA]. The head of any phalanx.

troch·le·ar (trock'lee·ur) *adj.* 1. Of or pertaining to a trochlea. 2. Of or pertaining to the trochlear nerve.

trochlear decussation. The crossing of the fibers that emerge from the trochlear nerve nuclei in the superior medullary velum. NA *decussatio nervorum trochlearium.*

trochlear fossa or **fovea.** A hollow in the frontal bone, below the internal angular process, furnishing attachment to the trochlea, or pulley, of the superior oblique muscle. NA *fovea trochlearis.*

troch·le·a·ris (trock"lee·air'is) *n.* The superior oblique muscle of the eyeball.

trochlear nerve. The fourth cranial nerve, whose fibers emerge from the brainstem on the dorsal surface just caudal to the inferior colliculus and go to supply the superior oblique muscle of the eye. NA *nervus trochlearis.* See also Table of Nerves in the Appendix.

trochlear nerve nucleus. A nucleus in the midbrain ventral to the central canal and dorsal to the medial longitudinal fasciculus giving rise to motor fibers of the trochlear nerve. NA *nucleus nervi trochlearis.*

trochlear notch. The concavity on the proximal end of the ulna for articulation with the trochlea of the humerus. NA *incisura trochlearis.*

trochlear process of the calcaneus. PERONEAL TROCHLEA OF THE CALCANEUS.

trochlear spine. An inconstant small projection on the upper medial wall of the orbit, for attachment of the fibrocartilaginous pulley for the superior oblique muscle. NA *spina trochlearis.*

trochlea ta·li (tay'lye) [NA]. The surface of the talus articulating with the tibia.

trocho-. See *troch-.*

tro·cho·car·dia (trock"o·kahr'dee·uh, tro"ko·) *n.* [*trocho-* + *-cardia*]. Displacement of the heart by rotation on its long axis.

tro·cho·ceph·a·lus (trock"o·sef'uh·lus) *n.* [*trocho-* + *-cephalus*]. A rounded appearance of the head, due to early partial synostosis of the frontal and parietal bones.

tro·cho·gin·gly·mus (trock"o·jing'gli·mus, ·ging'gli·mus) *n.* [*trocho-* + *ginglymus*]. A combination of a hinge joint and a pivot joint, as in the humeroradial articulation.

tro·choid (tro'koid) *adj.* [Gk. *trochoeidēs,* wheel-like]. Serving as a pulley or pivot; involving a pivotal action.

trochoid articulation. A type of rotary joint in which a pivot-like process rotates within a ring, or a ring rotates around a pivot, the ring being formed partly of bone, partly of ligament.

trochoid joint. PIVOT JOINT.

tro·cho·phore (trock'o·fore) *n.* [*trocho-* + *-phore*]. The typical, primitive larval form of annelids.

troch·o·ri·zo·car·dia (trock"o·rye"zo·kahr'dee·uh) *n.* [*troch-* + *horizontal* + *-cardia*]. A form of displacement of the heart characterized by trochocardia and change to horizontal position.

Trocinate. Trademark for thiphenamil, an anticholinergic drug.

Trog·lo·tre·ma (trog"lo·tree'muh) *n.* A genus of flukes that are common parasites of fish-eating mammals and birds.

Troglotrema sal·min·co·la (sal·mink'o·luh). A species of fluke that has been found in cases of human infection, and transmits a severe and often fatal infection to dogs by serving as a vector for *Neorickettsia helmintheca,* and causing acute salmon poisoning. Syn. *Nanophyetus salmincola.*

Trog·lo·tre·mat·i·dae (trog"lo·tre·mat'i·dee) *n.pl.* A family of flukes which includes the genera *Paragonimus* and *Troglotrema.*

Troi·sier's sign (trwa^{h}z·ye$^{y'}$) [C. E. *Troisier,* French physician, 1844–1919]. Enlargement of the supraclavicular lymph nodes; a sign of advanced abdominal or thoracic neoplasm.

Troisier's syndrome [C. E. *Troisier*]. Diabetic cachexia with bronzed skin. See also *hemochromatosis.*

trol·a·mine (trol'uh·meen) *n.* TRIETHANOLAMINE.

tro·le·an·do·my·cin (tro"lee·an"do·migh'sin) *n.* Triacetyloleandomycin, $C_{41}H_{67}NO_{15}$, the triacetyl ester of the antibiotic substance oleandomycin.

Trolene. A trademark for ronnel, a systemic insecticide.

trol·ni·trate (trol·nigh'trate) *n.* Triethanolamine trinitrate, $N(CH_2CH_2ONO_2)_3$, a vasodilator used as the phosphate salt to reduce the frequency and severity of attacks of angina pectoris.

Tröltsch's corpuscles (trœlch) [A. F. von *Tröltsch,* German otologist, 1829–1890]. Small spaces seen among the radial fibers of the tympanic membrane.

Tröltsch's recesses or **spaces** [A. F. von *Tröltsch*]. Two small pockets of the mucous membrane which envelop the chorda tympani in the middle ear.

Tromal. Trademark for butacetin, an analgesic and antidepressant drug.

Trom·bic·u·la (trom·bick'yoo·luh) *n.* A genus of mites; the larvae are blood suckers and cause a severe dermatitis.

Trombicula aka·mu·shi (ack''uh·moosh'ee). A vector of *Rickettsia tsutsugamushi,* the cause of tsutsugamushi disease.

Trombicula alfreddugesi. *EUTROMBICULA ALFREDDUGESI.*

Trombicula ir·ri·tans (irr'i·tanz). *EUTROMBICULA ALFREDDUGESI.*

trom·bic·u·lo·sis (trom·bick''yoo·lo'sis) *n.* [*Trombicula* + *-osis*]. Infestation with *Trombicula.*

trom·bid·i·o·sis (trom·bid''ee·o'sis) *n.* [*Trombidium* + *-osis*]. TROMBICULOSIS.

Trom·bid·i·um (trom·bid'ee·um) *n.* A genus of mites that formerly included chiggers (*Trombicula* and related genera) but which now includes no medically significant species.

tro·meth·a·mine (tro·meth'uh·meen) *n.* Tris(hydroxymethyl)aminomethane, $C_4H_{11}NO_3$, a systemic antacid.

Tromexan. Trademark for the anticoagulant drug ethyl biscoumacetate.

Trom·mer's test [K. E. *Trommer,* German chemist, 1806–1879]. A test for reducing sugars involving copper sulfate in a solution of potassium hydroxide. Fehling's test is similar but can detect smaller concentrations of sugar.

Tröm·ner's sign (trœm'nur) [E. L. O. *Trömner,* German neurologist, b. 1868]. A variant of Rossolimo's reflex.

tromo·ma·nia (trom''o·may'nee·uh) *n.* [Gk. *tromos,* a trembling, + *mania*]. *Obsol.* DELIRIUM TREMENS.

-tron [Gk., instrumental noun suffix]. A suffix designating *an electronic or atomic apparatus.*

tro·na (tro'nuh) *n.* [Swed., from Ar. *ṭrōn,* from *naṭrūn,* natron]. A native compound of sodium carbonate and sodium bicarbonate. $Na_2CO_3.NaHCO_3.2H_2O$.

Tronothane. Trademark for the surface anesthetic drug pramoxine, used as the hydrochloride salt.

trop-, tropo- [Gk. *tropos,* from *trepein,* to turn]. A combining form meaning (a) *turn, turning, change;* (b) *tendency, affinity.*

tro·pa·co·caine (tro''puh·ko·kain', ·ko'kain) *n.* Benzoylpseudotropine, $C_{15}H_{19}NO_2$, an alkaloid in Java coca leaves; the hydrochloride salt has been used as a local anesthetic.

tro·pae·o·lin, tro·pe·o·lin (tro·pee'o·lin, tro·pay'o·lin) *n.* An indefinite name for several dyes used as pH indicators; so called because their colors resemble the flowers of *Tropaeolum,* the garden nasturtium.

tro·pane (tro'pane) *n.* 2,3-Dihydro-8-methylnortropidine, $C_8H_{15}N$, a two-ring heterocyclic liquid hydrocarbon from which tropine is derived. Many ester alkaloids, including atropine and cocaine, are referred to as belonging to the tropane group.

-trope [Gk. *tropos,* turn, direction, way]. A combining form meaning (a) *tendency, tending, having an affinity for;* (b) *reflecting, turning, reversing;* (c) *changing, alternating.*

tro·pe·ine (tro'pee·een, ·in) *n.* An ester of tropine and an organic acid, as atropine and homatropine.

tro·pe·sis (tro·pee'sis) *n.* [Gk. *tropē,* a turning, + *-esis*]. INCLINATION (1).

troph-, tropho- [Gk. *trophē,* from *trephein,* to nourish]. A combining form meaning *nutrition, nutritive, nourishment.*

-troph [Gk. *trophos,* feeder, from *trephein,* to feed]. A combining form meaning *an organism nourishing itself in a* (specified) *way or having* (specified) *nutritional requirements.*

troph·ede·ma, troph·oe·de·ma (tro''fe·dee'muh, trof''e·) *n.* [*troph-* + *edema*]. *Obsol.* Localized chronic edema of the feet or legs due to damaged nourishment or nerve supply.

troph·e·sy (trof'e·see) *n. Obsol.* TROPHONEUROSIS. **—tro·phe·si·al** (tro·fee'zee·ul), **trophe·sic** (·sick) *adj.*

troph·ic (trof'ick) *adj.* [Gk. *trophikos,* nursing, tending, alimentary]. Pertaining to the functions concerned in nutrition, digestion, assimilation, and growth.

-trophic [Gk. *trophē,* nutrition]. A combining form designating (a) *a specified type of nutrition;* (b) *a specified nutritional requirement.* Compare *-tropic.*

trophic center. Any part of the central nervous system whose proper functioning is thought to be necessary for the nutrition, growth, or maintenance of a peripheral part of the body, as the parietal lobe for the development of the muscles of an extremity.

tro·phic·i·ty (tro·fis'i·tee) *n.* A trophic influence or state.

trophic keratitis. Keratitis due to chronic or repeated infections of the cornea by herpesvirus.

trophic ulcer. NEUROTROPHIC ULCER.

troph·ism (trof'iz·um) *n.* [*troph-* + *-ism*]. 1. NUTRITION. 2. TROPHICITY.

tropho-. See *troph-.*

tro·pho·blast (trof'o·blast, tro'fo·) *n.* [*tropho-* + *-blast*]. The outer, ectodermal epithelium of the mammalian blastocyst or chorion and chorionic villi. See also *cytotrophoblast, syncytiotrophoblast.* **—tro·pho·blas·tic** (trof''o·blas'tick, tro''fo·) *adj.*

trophoblastic knob. In rodents, the mass of trophoblast cells opposite to, and resembling, the embryonic knob from which the placenta develops.

trophoblastic operculum. The operculum, formed from the trophoblast, closing the wound in the endometrium made by the implanting ovum.

tro·pho·blas·to·ma (trof''o·blas·to'muh, tro''fo·) *n.* [*trophoblast* + *-oma*]. CHORIOCARCINOMA.

tro·pho·chrome cell (trof'o·krome, tro'fo·). MUCOSEROUS CELL.

tro·pho·chro·mid·ia (trof''o·kro·mid'ee·uh, tro''fo·) *n.* [*tropho-* + *chromidia*]. The nutritional chromatin of the cell.

tro·pho·cyte (trof'o·site, tro'fo·) *n.* [*tropho-* + *-cyte*]. A Sertoli or sustentacular cell of the testis.

tro·pho·derm (trof'o·durm, tro'fo·) *n.* [*tropho-* + *-derm*]. 1. The trophoblast or chorionic ectoderm. 2. The growing, active part of the trophoblast in the placental region. Syn. *placental trophoblast, ectoplacenta.* **—tro·pho·der·mal** (trof''o·dur'mul, tro''fo·) *adj.*

tro·pho·der·ma·to·neu·ro·sis (trof''o·dur''muh·to·new·ro'sis, tro''fo·) *n.* [*tropho-* + *dermato-* + *neur-* + *-osis*]. *Obsol.* ACRODYNIA.

tro·pho·dy·nam·ics (trof''o·dye·nam'icks, tro''fo·) *n.* [*tropho-* + *dynamics*]. The branch of medical science dealing with the forces governing nutrition.

trophoedema. TROPHEDEMA.

tro·phol·o·gy (tro·fol'uh·jee) *n.* [*tropho-* + *-logy*]. The science of nutrition.

tro·pho·neu·ro·sis (trof''o·new·ro'sis, tro''fo·) *n.*, pl. **tropho·neuro·ses** (·seez) [*tropho-* + *neur-* + *-osis*]. Any disease of a part due to disturbance of the nerves or nerve centers with which it is connected. **—trophoneu·rot·ic** (·rot'ick) *adj.*

trophoneurosis of Romberg [M. H. *Romberg*]. PROGRESSIVE FACIAL HEMIATROPHY.

tro·pho·no·sis (trof''o·no'sis, tro''fo·) *n.* TROPHOPATHY.

tro·pho·nu·cle·us (trof''o·new'klee·us, tro''fo·) *n.* [*tropho-* + *nucleus*]. The nucleus which is concerned with the nutrition of a unicellular organism and not with its reproduction.

tro·phop·a·thy (tro·fop'uth·ee) *n.* [*tropho-* + *-pathy*]. A disorder of nutrition; for example, a vitamin deficiency.

tro·pho·plasm (trof'o·plaz·um, tro'fo·) *n.* [*tropho-* + *plasm*]. The alveolar nutritive protoplasm in contrast to the filar, active kinoplasm of a cell.

tro·pho·spon·gia (trof''o·spon'jee·uh, tro''fo·) *n.* [*tropho-* + L. *spongia,* sponge]. The vascular endometrium forming the outer or maternal layer of the placenta.

tro·pho·spon·gi·um (trof″o·spon′jee·um, tro″fo·) *n.* [*tropho-* + *-spongium*]. Holmgren-Golgi canals whose number and distribution vary with the amount and distribution of Golgi material.

tro·pho·tax·is (trof″o·tack′sis, tro″fo·) *n.* [*tropho-* + *taxis*]. TROPHOTROPISM.

tro·pho·ther·a·py (trof″o·therr′uh·pee, tro″fo·) *n.* [*tropho-* + *therapy*]. Dietary therapy.

tro·pho·trop·ic (trof″o·trop′ick, tro″fo·) *adj.* Exhibiting trophotropism.

tro·phot·ro·pism (tro·fot′ruh·piz·um) *n.* [*tropho-* + *-tropism*]. The attraction or repulsion exhibited by certain organic cells to various nutritive substances. Syn. *trophotaxis.*

tro·pho·zo·ite (trof″o·zo′ite, tro″fo·) *n.* [*tropho-* + *zo-* + *-ite*]. The active, motile, feeding stage of a protozoon. In ameba, the motile feeding stage forms in contrast to the nonmotile cysts; in the plasmodia of malaria, the motile stage between the signet rings and the schizonts during development in the red blood cells of the vertebrate host.

-trophy [Gk. *trophē*]. A combining form meaning *nutrition, nourishment, growth.*

tro·pia (tro′pee·uh) *n.* [Gk. *tropē*, turn, + *-ia*]. 1. A deviation of an eye from the normal position when both eyes are uncovered and open. 2. STRABISMUS. See also *esotropia, exotropia.*

-tropia [*trop-* + *-ia*]. A combining form designating *a* (specified) *deviation in the line of vision.*

-tropic [*trop-* + *-ic*]. A combining form meaning *turning toward, having an affinity for.* Compare *-trophic.*

trop·ic acid (trop′ick). α-Phenyl-β-hydroxypropionic acid, $C_9H_{10}O_3$, a product of acid hydrolysis of atropine.

trop·i·cal (trop′i·kul) *adj.* [Gk. *tropikos*]. Pertaining to the zone of the earth lying between the Tropic of Cancer and the Tropic of Capricorn.

tropical abscess. AMEBIC ABSCESS.

tropical adenitis. LYMPHOGRANULOMA VENEREUM.

tropical anhidrotic asthenia. Heat exhaustion due to inability to sweat.

tropical eosinophilia. A condition of unknown cause, described in India and the South Pacific area, which is similar to Loeffler's syndrome; characterized clinically by cough, asthmatic attacks, a pulmonary infiltrate on x-ray, splenomegaly, and eosinophilia.

tropical hen flea. *ECHIDNOPHAGA GALLINACEA.*

tropical impetigo. BULLOUS IMPETIGO.

tropical macrocytic anemia. Macrocytic anemia resembling pernicious anemia, but without nervous system changes or achlorhydria, and occurring in the indigenous peoples of tropical and subtropical regions.

tropical medicine. The branch of medical science concerned chiefly with problems of health and disease found commonly or exclusively in the tropical or subtropical regions.

tropical sore. CUTANEOUS LEISHMANIASIS.

tropical sprue. A disease found primarily in areas of the Far East, India, and the Caribbean, characterized by fatigue, asthenia, and bulky stools leading to anemia, megaloblastosis, and pronounced weight loss. The etiology is uncertain.

tropical thrombocytopenia. ONYALAI.

tropical tinea circinata. TINEA IMBRICATA.

tropical typhus. TSUTSUGAMUSHI DISEASE.

tropical ulcer. A chronic, often progressive, sloughing ulcer, usually on the lower extremities and occasionally extending deeply with destruction of underlying muscles, tendons, and bones. Etiology is uncertain but spirochetes, fusiform bacilli and other bacteria are generally present in the lesions.

tro·pic·a·mide (tro·pick′uh·mide) *n.* *N.*-Ethyl-*N*-(γ-picolyl) tropamide, $C_{17}H_{20}N_2O_2$, an anticholinergic agent used topically to produce mydriasis and cycloplegia.

tro·pin (tro′pin) *n.* [*trop-* + *-in*]. Any one of the substances in the blood serum which make bacteria susceptible to phagocytosis. See also *bacteriotropin, opsonin.*

tro·pine (tro′peen, ·pin) *n.* 3α-Tropanol, $C_8H_{15}NO$, a two-ring heterocyclic hydrolysis product of atropine and certain other alkaloids.

tro·pism (tro′piz·um) *n.* [*trop-* + *-ism*]. The involuntary bending, turning, or orientation of an organism or a part toward (positive tropism), or away from (negative tropism), a stimulus. Various types, depending upon the directing influence, include chemotropism, galvanotropism, geotropism, phototropism, rheotropism, stereotropism, thermotropism.

-tropism [*trop-* + *-ism*]. A combining form meaning (a) *a tendency to turn;* (b) *an affinity for.*

tropo-. See *trop-.*

tro·po·chrome (tro′puh·krome, trop′o·) *adj.* [*tropo-* + *-chrome*]. Pertaining to serous cells of the salivary glands which do not stain with mucin stains after fixation in a Formalin-bichromate mixture. Compare *homeochrome.*

tro·po·col·la·gen (tro″po·kol′uh·jin, trop″o·) *n.* The fundamental unit of collagen fibrils, obtained by prolonged extraction of insoluble collagen with dilute acid.

trop·o·lone (trop′uh·lone) *n.* 1. Hydroxycycloheptatrienone, $C_7H_5O(OH)$, a 7-membered cyclic compound, certain derivatives of which occur naturally, notably in plants. 2. Any derivative of $C_7H_5O(OH)$.

tro·pom·e·ter (tro·pom′e·tur) *n.* [*tropo-* + *-meter*]. 1. An instrument for measuring the various rotations of the eyeball. 2. An instrument for estimating the amount of torsion in long bones.

tro·po·my·o·sin (tro″po·migh′o·sin) *n.* [*tropo-* + *myosin*]. A regulatory protein which is found as a portion of the thin filament of mammalian skeletal muscle and which binds specifically to the actin molecules.

tro·po·nin (tro′po·nin) *n.* A regulatory protein found as a portion of the thin filament of mammalian skeletal muscle. Each troponin molecule is attached both to a tropomyosin molecule and to an actin molecule.

tro·po·pause (trop′o·pawz, tro′po·) *n.* [*tropo-* + *pause*]. The top of the troposphere, just below the stratosphere.

tro·po·sphere (tro′po·sfeer, trop′o·) *n.* [*tropo-* + *sphere*]. The atmosphere that lies between the stratosphere and the earth's surface, a zone of marked changes in temperature, with ascending and descending air currents and cloud formations.

-tropy [Gk. *-tropia,* from *tropos,* turn]. A combining form meaning (a) *tendency, tropism;* (b) *turning, reflecting.*

Trous·seau's disease (troo·so′) [A. *Trousseau,* French physician, 1801–1867]. HEMOCHROMATOSIS.

Trousseau's mark or **spot** [A. *Trousseau*]. TACHE CÉRÉBRALE.

Trousseau's sign or **phenomenon** [A. *Trousseau*]. 1. A sign of tetany in which carpal spasm can be elicited by compressing the upper arm. 2. TACHE CÉRÉBRALE.

trox·i·done (trock′si·dohn) *n.* TRIMETHADIONE.

troy ounce. The twelfth part of the troy pound, or 480 grains (31.10 g). Symbol, ℥.

troy pound. Twelve troy ounces, or 5,760 grains; equivalent to 5,760/7,000 of an avoirdupois pound.

troy weight. A system of weights in which a pound is twelve ounces or 5,760 grains.

true, *adj.* 1. Real; not false. 2. Typical, as true vipers.

true albuminuria. Proteinuria associated with renal disease.

true amnion. The inner amniotic folds of avian, reptilian, and certain mammalian embryos; the amnion proper.

true aneurysm. An aneurysm in which the sac is formed of one, two, or all of the arterial coats.

true ankylosis. BONY ANKYLOSIS.

true apophysis. An apophysis that has never been an epiphysis.

true bulbar palsy. PROGRESSIVE BULBAR PALSY.

true conjugate. CONJUGATA VERA.

true cramp bark. *VIBURNUM OPULUS.*

true hernia. A hernia having a sac, usually of peritoneum, covering the hernial contents.

true image. In diplopia, the image received by the undeviated eye, projected on the macula.

true knot. A knot of the umbilical cord formed by the fetus slipping through a loop in the cord.

true lateral ligament of the bladder. A thickening of the pelvic fascia extending laterally on either side from the lower part of the urinary bladder or prostate gland.

truem·mer·feld zone (trōōm′ur·felt, Ger. trueᵉm′) [Ger. *Trümmerfeld*, a field strewn with debris, from *Trümmer*, fragments]. In scurvy, a zone of increased fragmentation in the diaphysis just below the epiphysis, and proximal to the dense white line of Fraenkel.

true mole. A mole that is the remains of a fetus or fetal membranes.

true nucleolus. PLASMOSOME (1).

true pelvis. The part of the pelvic cavity situated below the iliopectineal line. NA *pelvis minor*.

true ribs. The seven upper ribs on each side that are attached to the sternum. NA *costae verae*.

true skin. DERMIS.

True·ta's shunt (Sp. trwehʰ′tahʰ). A part of the renal circulation in which blood passes through the juxtamedullary glomeruli into the capillary beds of the medulla, bypassing the cortex. It results in greatly decreased production of urine and may be of special significance under certain abnormal circulatory conditions, as hemorrhage and shock. Syn. *Oxford shunt, renal shunt*.

true vertebra. One of the cervical, thoracic, or lumbar vertebrae.

true villus. SECONDARY VILLUS.

true vocal cord. VOCAL FOLD.

trun·cal (trunk′ul) *adj*. [L. *truncus*, trunk, + *-al*]. Pertaining to the trunk.

truncal ataxia. Incoordination of the axial musculature, so that there is swaying; seen in cerebellar disturbances.

trun·cat·ed (trunk′ay·tid) *adj*. [L. *truncatus*, from *truncare*, to cut off]. 1. With the top cut off; shortened in height. 2. Deprived of limbs or accessory parts.

trunci. Plural and genitive singular of *truncus*.

trunci in·tes·ti·na·les (in·tes·ti·nay′leez) [NA]. INTESTINAL TRUNKS.

trunci lum·ba·les (lum·bay′leez) [BNA]. Trunci lumbales [dexter et sinister] (= LUMBAR TRUNKS).

trunci lumbales [dex·ter et si·nis·ter] (decks′tur et si·nis′ter) [NA]. LUMBAR TRUNKS.

trunci plex·us bra·chi·a·lis (pleck′sus bray·kee·ay′lis) [NA]. The trunks of the brachial plexus considered collectively.

trun·co·co·nal (trunk″o·ko′nul) *adj*. [*trunc*us + *con*us + *-al*]. Pertaining to both the truncus arteriosus and the conus of the developing heart.

truncoconal ridge. One of a pair of ridges bounding the interventricular orifice in the developing heart. They share in closure of that orifice and in formation of the aorticopulmonary septum.

truncoconal septum. AORTICOPULMONARY SEPTUM.

trun·cus (trunk′us) *n*., pl. & genit. sing. **trun·ci** (·sigh) [L.] [NA]. TRUNK.

truncus ar·te·ri·o·sus (ahr·teer·ee·o′sus). The embryonic arterial trunk arising from the heart which develops into the definitive aorta and pulmonary trunk. It may persist as an anomalous cardiac defect in which it receives blood from both ventricles and supplies the coronary, pulmonary, and systemic circulations.

truncus bra·chio·ce·pha·li·cus (bray″kee·o·se·fal′i·kus) [NA]. BRACHIOCEPHALIC TRUNK.

truncus bron·cho·me·di·a·sti·na·lis (bronk″o·mee·dee·as·ti·nay′lis) [NA]. BRONCHOMEDIASTINAL TRUNK.

truncus bronchomediastinalis dex·ter (decks′tur) [BNA]. The bronchomediastinal trunk on the right.

truncus ce·li·a·cus (see·lye′uh·kus) [NA]. CELIAC TRUNK.

truncus cor·po·ris cal·lo·si (kor′po·ris ka·lo′sigh) [NA]. The central portion of the corpus callosum.

truncus cos·to·cer·vi·ca·lis (kos″to·sur·vi·kay′lis) [NA]. COSTOCERVICAL TRUNK.

truncus fas·ci·cu·li atrio·ven·tri·cu·la·ris (fa·sick′yoo·lye ay″tree·o·ven·trick·yoo·lair′is) [NA]. The proximal undivided portion of the atrioventricular bundle.

truncus inferior plex·us bra·chi·a·lis (pleck′sus bray·kee·ay′lis) [NA]. The inferior trunk of the brachial plexus formed from the ventral rami of the eighth cervical and first thoracic nerves.

truncus in·tes·ti·na·lis (in·tes·ti·nay′lis) [BNA]. Singular of *trunci intestinales*. (= INTESTINAL TRUNKS).

truncus ju·gu·la·ris (jug·yoo·lair′is) [NA]. JUGULAR TRUNK.

truncus lin·guo·fa·ci·a·lis (ling″gwo·fay·shee·ay′lis) [NA]. The vessel present when the lingual and facial arteries arise from a common branch of the external carotid artery.

truncus lum·bo·sa·cra·lis (lum″bo·sa·kray′lis) [NA]. LUMBOSACRAL TRUNK.

truncus me·di·us plex·us bra·chi·a·lis (mee′dee·us pleck′sus bray·kee·ay′lis) [NA]. The middle trunk of the brachial plexus formed from the ventral ramus of the seventh cervical nerve.

truncus pul·mo·na·lis (pul·mo·nay′lis) [NA]. PULMONARY TRUNK.

truncus sub·cla·vi·us (sub·klay′vee·us) [NA]. SUBCLAVIAN TRUNK.

truncus superior plex·us bra·chi·a·lis (pleck′sus bray′kee·ay′lis) [NA]. The superior trunk of the brachial plexus formed from the ventral rami of the fifth and sixth cervical nerves.

truncus sym·pa·thi·cus (sim·path′i·kus) [NA]. SYMPATHETIC TRUNK.

truncus thy·reo·cer·vi·ca·lis (thigh″ree·o·sur·vi·kay′lis) [BNA]. Truncus thyrocervicalis (= THYROCERVICAL TRUNK).

truncus thy·ro·cer·vi·ca·lis (thigh″ro·sur·vi·kay′lis) [NA]. THYROCERVICAL TRUNK.

truncus trans·ver·sus (trans·vur′sus). COMMON CARDINAL VEIN.

truncus va·ga·lis anterior (va·gay′lis) [NA]. A fairly distinct bundle of nerve fibers situated on the anterior aspect of the lower end of the esophagus and formed from the esophageal plexus.

truncus vagalis posterior [NA]. A fairly distinct bundle of nerve fibers situated on the posterior aspect of the lower end of the esophagus and formed from the esophageal plexus.

trunk, *n*. [L. *truncus*]. 1. The torso; the body without head or limbs. NA *truncus*. See also Plate 4. 2. The main stem of a blood vessel, lymphatic, or nerve.

trunk-thigh sign of Babinski [J. F. F. *Babinski*]. The patient, lying flat on his back and with legs abducted, tries to rise to the sitting position while keeping his arms crossed in front of his chest. Normally, the legs stay motionless and the heels are pressed down. In the patient with hemiplegia, there is flexion of the thigh in association with flexion of the trunk, resulting in an involuntary elevation of the paretic limb; the normal limb is either not raised or only slightly. In paraplegia, both legs are raised. In hysterical hemiplegia, the normal leg may be elevated, while in hysterical paraplegia neither leg is raised. The sign may also be elicited by having the patient attempt to sit up from the recumbent position with his legs hanging over the edge of the bed, at which time the thigh is flexed and the lower leg extended on the paretic side.

truss, *n*. [OF. *trousse*]. Any mechanical apparatus for preventing the recurrence of a hernial protrusion which has been reduced. The term includes simple devices such as a yarn truss for the control of infantile hernia, as well as complicated pieces of apparatus with pressure pads designed to hold large inguinal or abdominal hernias.

truth serum. An intravenous solution of a barbiturate used in narcoanalysis; sodium amytal or thiopental are the most common ones.

Trypaflavin. A trademark for acriflavine.

tryp·an blue (trip'an, trye'pan). An acid diazo dye of the benzopurpurin series used in vital staining, and also as a trypanocide.

try·pa·no·cide (tri·pan'o·side, trip'uh·no·side) *n.* [*trypanosome* + *-cide*]. An agent that destroys trypanosomes. **—trypano·ci·dal** (tri·pan''o·sigh'dul) *adj.*

Try·pa·no·so·ma (tri·pan''o·so''muh, trip''uh·no·) *n.* [Gk. *trypanon*, auger, borer, + *sōma*, body]. A genus of protozoa belonging to the subphylum Mastigophora, which are slender, elongate organisms with a central nucleus, posterior blepharoplast, and an undulatory membrane, from which flagellum projects forward; transmitted by insect vectors, and responsible for such infections as trypanosomiasis and Chagas' disease in man and dourine, nagana, and surra in animals.

Trypanosoma bru·cei (broo'see·eye, broo'sigh). The species of *Trypanosoma* that causes nagana, Gambian trypanosomiasis (subspecies *T. brucei gambiense*), and Rhodesian trypanosomiasis (subsp. *T. brucei rhodesiense*).

Trypanosoma cru·zi (kroo'zye). The causative agent of Chagas' disease.

Trypanosoma equi·per·dum (eck''wee·pur'dum). The causative agent of dourine.

Trypanosoma evan·si (ev''un·zye). The parasite that causes surra.

Trypanosoma gam·bi·en·se (gam·bee·en'see). *Trypanosoma brucei gambiense.* See *Trypanosoma brucei.*

Trypanosoma hip·pi·cum (hip'i·kum). The species of *Trypanosoma* that causes murrina.

try·pa·no·so·mal (tri·pan''o·so'mul, trip''uh·no·) *adj.* Caused by a trypanosome.

Trypanosoma lew·i·si (lew'i·sigh). The nonpathogenic parasite transmitted by the rat flea.

Trypanosoma rho·de·si·en·se (ro·dee''zee·en'see). *Trypanosoma brucei rhodesiense.* See *Trypanosoma brucei.*

Try·pa·no·so·mat·i·dae (tri·pan''o·so·mat'i·dee, trip''uh·no·) *n.pl.* A family of parasitic protozoons which includes the genera *Crithidia, Herpetomonas, Leishmania, Leptomonas,* and *Trypanosoma.*

Trypanosoma vi·vax (vye'vacks). The species of *Trypanosoma* that causes soma.

try·pa·no·some (tri·pan'o·sohm, trip'uh·no·) *n.* One of any species of *Trypanosoma,* a flagellated protozoan living in the blood and tissues of its host. **—trypano·som·ic** (·so'mick) *adj.*

try·pa·no·so·mi·a·sis (tri·pan''o·so·migh'uh·sis, trip''uh·no·) *n.*, pl. **trypanosomia·ses** (·seez) [*trypanosome* + *-iasis*]. Any of many diseases of man and animals caused by infection with species of *Trypanosoma* and transmitted by tsetse flies or other insects. See also *Chagas' disease, dourine, Gambian trypanosomiasis, nagana, Rhodesian trypanosomiasis, surra.*

try·pano·so·mide (tri·pan'o·so·mide, ·mid) *n.* A skin lesion in any disease caused by a trypanosome.

try·pa·no·tox·yl (trip''uh·no·tock'sil) *n.* A substance (thought to be a reduced glutathione) in the liver or blood, which transforms atoxyl into a trypanocidal agent.

tryp·ar·sa·mide (tri·pahr'suh·mide, ·id) *n.* Monosodium *N*-(carbamoylmethyl)arsanilate, $C_8H_{10}AsN_2NaO_4$; an effective therapeutic agent for the treatment of trypanosomiasis.

tryp·sin (trip'sin) *n.* The proteolytic enzyme resulting from the action of the enterokinase of intestinal juice upon the trypsinogen secreted in the pancreatic juice. It catalyzes the hydrolysis of peptide linkages in proteins and partially hydrolyzed proteins, more readily on the latter. Syn. *tryptase.* **—tryp·tic** (·tick) *adj.*

tryp·sin·o·gen (trip·sin'uh·jen) *n.* The zymogen of trypsin, occurring in the pancreatic juice and converted to trypsin by enterokinase in the small intestine. Syn. *protrypsin.*

tryp·ta·mine (trip'tuh·meen, ·min) *n.* 3-(2-Aminoethyl)indole, $C_{10}H_{12}N_2$, the decarboxylation product of tryptophan; an intermediate substance in certain metabolic processes in plants and animals.

tryp·tase (trip'tace) *n.* TRYPSIN.

tryp·to·lyt·ic (trip''to·lit'ick) *adj.* Of or pertaining to the hydrolysis of proteins caused by trypsin.

tryp·to·phan (trip'to·fan) *n.* *l*-α-Aminoindole-3-propionic acid, $C_{11}H_{12}N_2O_2$, an amino acid component of casein and other proteins that is essential in human nutrition but is not synthesized by the human body.

tryp·to·pha·nase (trip'to·fa·nace, trip·tof'uh·) *n.* A bacterial enzyme that catalyzes degradation of tryptophan to indole, pyruvic acid, and ammonia.

tryp·to·phane (trip'to·fane) *n.* TRYPTOPHAN.

tryp·to·phan·emia, tryp·to·pha·nae·mia (trip''to·fa·nee'mee·uh) *n.* [*tryptophan* + *-emia*]. TRYPTOPHANURIA (2).

tryptophan test. An obsolete test for tuberculous meningitis in which on sodium nitrate solution is overlaid a mixture of spinal fluid, hydrochloric acid, and Formalin. A violet ring at the junction of the fluids is said to be a positive reaction.

tryp·to·phan·uria (trip''to·fan·yoo'ree·uh) *n.* [*tryptophan* + *-uria*]. 1. The presence of tryptophan in the urine. 2. A rare inborn error of metabolism characterized by an increase in urinary tryptophan and delayed clearing of tryptophan from the plasma following an oral load. Clinical manifestations include mental retardation, dwarfism, photosensitivity, ataxia, telangiectasis, and hyperpigmentation. The nature of the basic defect is unknown.

tryp·to·phyl (trip''to·fil) *n.* The univalent radical, $C_8H_6NCH_2CH(NH_2)CO$—, of the amino acid tryptophan.

T.S. Abbreviation for *test solution.*

Tscher·ning's theory of accommodation [M. H. E. *Tscherning,* Danish ophthalmologist, b. 1854]. By the contraction of the anterior part of both the radiating and circular fibers of the ciliary muscle, the ciliary processes are drawn backward and the suspensory ligament is pulled backward and outward; pressure of the anterior portion of the muscle causes increased convexity of the lens.

tset·se fly (tset'see, tsee'tsee) *n.* [Tswana]. Any dipterous insect of the genus *Glossina,* almost wholly restricted to Africa. *Glossina* flies carry the flagellate trypanosomes, the causative agents of nagana in cattle and of trypanosomiasis in man.

TSH Abbreviation for *thyroid-stimulating hormone.*

tsp Abbreviation for *teaspoon.*

T splint. A splint used to hold back the shoulders, and adapted by bandaging to hold the fragments in apposition in fractures of the clavicle.

TSTA Tumor-specific transplantation antigens: antigens on the surfaces of tumor cells capable of intiating a rejection phenomenon.

Tsu·chi·ya's reagent. A reagent containing phosphotungstic acid, alcohol, and concentrated hydrochloric acid, used to test for urine protein.

Tsu·ga (tsoo'guh) *n.* [Jap., larch]. The generic name of the hemlock tree that belongs to the pine family (Pinaceae). Not to be confused with the poison hemlock (*Conium*) which is an herb (Umbelliferae).

tsu·tsu·ga·mu·shi disease or **fever** (tsoo''tsuh·ga·moo'shee) [Jap., from *tsutuga,* small and dangerous, + *mushi,* mite]. A disease characterized by headache, high fever, and a rash, occurring in Japan, Formosa, and islands of the South Pacific; caused by *Rickettsia tsutsugamushi* and transmitted to man by the bite of the larval forms of mites of the genus *Trombicula.*

***t* test.** A test of significance of differences between statistical constants calculated from small samples.

TTI Abbreviation for *tension-time index.*

T tube. A rubber or glass tube in the form of the letter T.

T-tube cholangiography. Roentgenologic demonstration of the biliary drainage system by injecting contrast material via a surgically placed tube in the hepatic and common duct.

Tuamine. Trademark for the sympathomimetic amine tuaminoheptane.

tu·ami·no·hep·tane (too″uh·mee·no·hep′tane, too·am″i·no·) *n*. 1-Methylhexylamine, also known as a 2-aminoheptane, $C_7H_{17}N$, a sympathomimetic amine used for local vasoconstrictive action by inhalation of the vapor of the base and by application of a solution of the sulfate.

tu·ba (tew′buh) *n*., pl. & genit. sing. **tu·bae** (·bee) [L., trumpet]. TUBE.

tuba au·di·ti·va (aw·di·tye′vuh) [NA]. AUDITORY TUBE.

tuba auditiva [Eu·sta·chii] (yoo·stay′kee·eye) [BNA]. Tuba auditiva (= AUDITORY TUBE).

tu·bage (tew′bij) *n*. [F.]. The introduction of a tube or catheter.

tubage of the glottis. *Obsol*. INTUBATION.

tub·al (tew′bul)· *adj*. Pertaining to a tube, especially the uterine or the auditory.

tubal abortion. Escape of the products of conception through the abdominal opening of the oviduct into the peritoneal cavity in cases of tubal pregnancy.

tubal block. 1. Obstruction of the lumen of a tube. 2. EAR BLOCK.

tubal cartilage. A rolled triangular cartilage running from the osseous part of the auditory tube to the pharynx.

tubal dysmenorrhea. Dysmenorrhea associated with salpingitis.

tubal elevation. TORUS TUBARIUS.

tubal insufflation. RUBIN TEST.

tubal mole. The remains of a fetus or fetal membranes and placenta in incomplete tubal abortion which have become infiltrated with blood.

tubal occlusion. Loss of patency of the oviduct.

tubal plicae. Folds of the tunica mucosa in the uterine tubes. NA *plicae tubariae*.

tubal pregnancy. Gestation within an oviduct.

tubal process. An occasional spur of bone projecting backward from the middle portion of the posterior border of the medial pterygoid lamina.

tubal septum. COCHLEARIFORM PROCESS.

tubal tonsil. Minor and variable aggregations of lymphatic tissue about the pharyngeal orifice of each pharyngotympanic (auditory) tube. Syn. *Gerlach's tubal tonsil*. NA *tonsilla tubaria*.

tuba ute·ri·na (yoo·te·rye′nuh) [NA]. UTERINE TUBE.

tuba uterina [Fal·lop·pii] (fa·lop′ee·eye) [BNA]. Tuba uterina (= UTERINE TUBE).

tub bath. Any bath in which the body is immersed in a tub.

tube, *n*. [L. *tubus*]. A hollow, cylindrical structure, especially a uterine tube or an auditory tube.

tu·bec·to·my (tew·beck′tuh·mee) *n*. [*tube* + *-ectomy*]. SALPINGECTOMY; excision of a tube, specifically a uterine tube.

tube curare. TUBOCURARE.

tubed flap. A long pedicle flap, usually tubed or rolled on itself with the free edges sutured together.

tube length. In a microscope, the distance between the upper focal point of the objective and the lower focal point of the eyepiece. The tube length of a monocular microscope is measured from the top of the eyepiece tube to the bottom of the nosepiece. In the binocular microscope, a correction is introduced to compensate for the distance added by the system of prisms.

tu·ber (tew′bur) *n*., pl. **tubers, tu·be·ra** (·be·ruh) [L., hump, protuberance]. 1. A thickened portion of an underground stem. 2. Any rounded swelling. See also *tuberosity, eminence*. **—tu·ber·al** (·ul) *adj*.

tuberal nuclei. Circular cell groups, in the lateral part of the tuber cinereum, which often produce small eminences on the basal surface of the hypothalamus. NA *nuclei tuberales*.

tuber cal·ca·nei (kal·kay′nee·eye) [NA]. CALCANEAL TUBEROSITY.

tuber cal·cis (kal′sis), pl. **tubera cal·ci·um** (kal′see·um) [L.]. CALCANEAL TUBEROSITY.

tuber ci·ne·re·um (si·nee′ree·um) [NA]. An area of gray matter extending from the optic chiasma to the mamillary bodies and forming part of the floor of the third ventricle. The stalk of the neurohypophysis is attached to it.

tu·ber·cle (tew′bur·kul) *n*. [L. *tuberculum*, dim. of *tuber*]. 1. A small nodule. 2. A rounded prominence on a bone. 3. The specific lesion produced by the tubercle bacillus, consisting of a collection of lymphocytes and epithelioid cells, at times with giant cells.

tubercle bacillus. *MYCOBACTERIUM TUBERCULOSIS*. Abbreviated, t.b.

tubercul-, tuberculo-. A combining form meaning *tuberculous, tuberculosis, tubercle bacillus*.

tubercula. Plural of *tuberculum*.

tubercula co·ro·nae den·tis (ko·ro′nee den′tis) [BNA]. Singular of *tuberculum coronae dentis* (= CUSP (1)).

tu·ber·cu·lar (tew·bur′kew·lur) *adj*. [*tubercul-* + *-ar*]. 1. Characterized by the presence of small nodules or tubercles. 2. Of or pertaining to a tubercle. 3. *Erron*. TUBERCULOUS.

tubercular dactylitis. SPINA VENTOSA.

tubercular process. DIAPOPHYSIS.

tu·ber·cu·lat·ed (tew·bur′kew·lay″tid) *adj*. Having tubercles; TUBERCULAR.

tu·ber·cu·la·tion (tew·bur″kew·lay′shun) *n*. 1. The formation, development, or arrangement of tubercles. 2. The process of affecting a part with tubercles.

tu·ber·cu·lid (tew·bur′kew·lid) *n*. [*tubercul-* + *-id*]. Any of a group of varied skin manifestations, always free of tubercle bacilli, presumed to be reactions of hypersensitivity to a focus of tuberculous infection elsewhere in the body. Included are papular and papulonecrotic skin lesions, lichen scrofulosus, and erythema induratum.

tu·ber·cu·lide (tew·bur′kew·lide) *n*. TUBERCULID.

tu·ber·cu·lin (tew·bur′kew·lin) *n*. [*tubercul-* + *-in*]. A preparation containing tuberculoproteins derived from *Mycobacterium tuberculosis* which elicit reactions of delayed hypersensitivity, namely erythema, induration, and even necrosis in human or animal hosts with past or present sensitization to tubercle bacilli. Similar preparations may be derived from mycobacteria other than *M. tuberculosis*.

tuberculin reaction. The prototype of delayed hypersensitivity upon the introduction of tuberculin in an individual with prior or present sensitization with *Mycobacterium tuberculosis*. Locally, induration and erythema, with or without necrosis, reaches its height in 48 to 72 hours. Focal reactions at the site of tuberculous lesions, and constitutional reactions, including fever and malaise, may also occur.

tuberculin test. A test for past or present infection with tubercle bacilli, based on a delayed hypersensitivity reaction of edema, erythema, or necrosis at the site, reaching its height in 48 to 72 hours. It is elicited by such products as old tuberculin or purified protein derivative, usually introduced into the skin. See also *Calmette test, Mantoux test, Moro test, Vollmer patch test, Von Pirquet test*.

tuberculin-type allergy. DELAYED HYPERSENSITIVITY.

tuberculin-type sensitivity. TUBERCULIN REACTION.

tuberculo-. See *tubercul-*.

tu·ber·cu·lo·der·ma (tew·bur″kew·lo·dur′muh) *n*. [*tuberculo-* + *-derma*]. TUBERCULID.

tu·ber·cu·lo·fi·broid (tew·bur″kew·lo·figh′broid) *adj*. [*tuberculo-* + *fibr-* + *-oid*]. Pertaining to a tubercle (3) that has undergone dense fibrosis.

tu·ber·cu·loid (tew·bur′kew·loid) *adj*. Resembling tuberculosis or a tubercle.

tuberculoid leprosy. A principal form of leprosy, characterized by a paucity or absence of *Mycobacterium leprae* in the tissues, a positive lepromin reaction, and principally by asymmetric maculoanesthetic skin lesions, with involvement of peripheral nerve trunks leading to sensorimotor deficit in the distribution of the involved nerve in addition to the patch of cutaneous anesthesla. Contr. *lepromatous leprosy.*

tu·ber·cu·lo·ma (tew·bur″kew·lo′muh) *n.*, pl. **tuberculomas, tuberculoma·ta** (·tuh) [*tubercul-* + *-oma*]. A conglomerate caseous tubercle, usually solitary, whose size and sharp circumscription resemble that of a neoplasm.

tuberculoma en plaque. A rare type of chronic tuberculous meningoencephalitis, characterized by a flat plaque of a granulomatous reaction in the meninges.

tu·ber·cu·lo·ma·nia (tew·bur″kew·lo·may′nee·uh) *n.* [*tuberculo-* + *-mania*]. An unalterable and unfounded conviction that one is suffering from tuberculosis.

tu·ber·cu·lo·pho·bia (tew·bur″kew·lo·fo′bee·uh) *n.* [*tuberculo-* + *-phobia*]. An abnormal fear of tuberculosis.

tu·ber·cu·lo·pro·tein (tew·bur″kew·lo·pro′teen, ·tee·in) *n.* [*tuberculo-* + *protein*]. A variety of protein not exerting appreciable toxic effect upon the normal body but highly toxic for the tuberculous, hypersensitive individual, leading to necrosis, fever, and severe constitutional symptoms. Smaller, standardized doses elicit the tuberculin reaction of delayed hypersensitivity.

tu·ber·cu·lose (tew·bur′kew·loce) *adj.* TUBERCULATED.

tu·ber·cu·lo·sil·i·co·sis (tew·bur″kew·lo·sil″i·ko′sis) *n.* SILICOTUBERCULOSIS.

tu·ber·cu·lo·sis (tew·bur″kew·lo′sis) *n.* [L. *tubercul*um, tubercle, + *-osis*]. A chronic infectious disease with protean manifestations, primarily involving the lungs but capable of attacking most organs of the body, caused by *Mycobacterium tuberculosis.* Usually the primary infection becomes arrested, but widespread tuberculous disease occasionally occurs. Severe clinical manifestations may include fever, weight loss, cough, chest pain, sputum, and hemoptysis. The pathological response may include tubercle formation, exudation, necrosis, and fibrosis, depending on local biochemical factors, the hypersensitive state, the number and virulence of the organisms, and the resistance of the host. Abbreviated, TB. Syn. *phthisis, consumption.* See also *quiescent tuberculosis.*

tuberculosis cutis. Tuberculosis of the skin. See also *lupus vegetans, tuberculosis lichenoides, tuberculid.*

tuberculosis cutis in·du·ra·ti·va (in·dew″ruh·tye′vuh). ERYTHEMA INDURATUM.

tuberculosis cutis ori·fi·ci·a·lis (o″ri·fish″ee·ay′lis). Ulcerative tuberculosis of the skin at the body orifices.

tuberculosis li·chen·oi·des (lye″ke·noy′deez). A skin eruption consisting of groups of papules, usually on the trunk, seen especially in subjects suffering from tuberculosis of the lymph nodes and bone. Syn. *lichen scrofulosus.*

tuberculosis lu·po·sa (loo·po′suh). LUPUS VULGARIS.

tuberculosis ver·ru·co·sa (verr″oo·ko′suh). A type of warty skin eruption, usually on the hands and arms, due to inoculation with the tubercle bacillus from handling meat of infected cattle or infected human material. Syn. *anatomic tubercle, dissection tubercle, verruca necrogenica.*

tu·ber·cu·lo·stat·ic (tew·bur″kew·lo·stat′ick) *adj.* [*tuberculo-* + *-static*]. Inhibiting the growth of tubercle bacilli.

tu·ber·cu·lo·stear·ic acid (tew·bur″kew·lo·stee′uh·rick). 10-Methylstearic acid, obtained from tubercle bacilli.

tu·ber·cu·lous (tew·bur′kew·lus) *adj.* Affected with, or caused by, tuberculosis. Compare *tubercular.*

tuberculous cirrhosis. Cirrhosis secondary to tuberculosis of the liver.

tuberculous keratitis. Keratitis associated with tuberculous infection.

tuberculous laryngitis. Laryngitis usually secondary to active tuberculosis of the lung. It usually attacks the vocal folds and arytenoid region and later extends as a markedly destructive lesion.

tuberculous rheumatism. Arthritis associated with tuberculous infection.

tuberculous salpingitis. Salpingitis marked by the development in the lining membrane and walls of a uterine tube of tubercles caused by *Mycobacterium tuberculosis.*

tuberculous spondylitis. Tuberculosis of the vertebral bodies leading to bone destruction, vertebral collapse, and kyphosis, healing by fusion of adjacent vertebrae. There may be accompanying psoas abscess and, rarely, compression of the spinal cord.

tuberculous synovitis. Synovitis due to tuberculosis.

tuberculous tarsitis. Tuberculous infection of a tarsal bone.

tuberculous tenosynovitis. A slow and progressively destructive tuberculosis of the sheaths of the tendons. The tendons of the wrist are the ones most commonly involved.

tu·ber·cu·lum (tew·bur′kew·lum) *n.*, pl. **tubercu·la** (·luh) [L.]. TUBERCLE.

tuberculum acu·sti·cum (a·koos′ti·kum). AREA VESTIBULARIS.

tuberculum ad·duc·to·ri·um (a·duck·to′ree·um) [NA]. ADDUCTOR TUBERCLE.

tuberculum an·te·ri·us at·lan·tis (an·teer′ee·us at·lan′tis) [NA]. The conical prominence on the anterior arch of the atlas.

tuberculum anterius tha·la·mi (thal′uh·migh) [NA]. The frontal extremity of the thalamus.

tuberculum anterius ver·te·bra·rum cer·vi·ca·li·um (vur·te·brair′um sur·vi·kay′lee·um) [NA]. ANTERIOR TUBERCLE (of the cervical vertebrae).

tuberculum ar·ti·cu·la·re os·sis tem·po·ra·lis (ahr·tick·yoo·lair′ee os′is tem·po·ray′lis) [NA]. ARTICULAR TUBERCLE.

tuberculum au·ri·cu·lae (aw·rick′yoo·lee) [NA]. AURICULAR TUBERCLE (1).

tuberculum auriculae [Dar·wi·ni] (dahr′win·eye) [BNA]. Tuberculum auriculae (= AURICULAR TUBERCLE (1)).

tuberculum ca·ro·ti·cum ver·te·brae cer·vi·ca·lis VI (ka·rot′i·kum vur′te·bree sur·vi·kay′lis) [NA]. CAROTID TUBERCLE.

tuberculum cau·da·tum (kaw·day′tum). CAUDATE LOBE.

tuberculum ci·ne·re·um (si·neer′ee·um). 1. [BNA] A longitudinal elevation between the cuneate fasciculus and tubercle on the one hand and the roots of the ninth, tenth, and eleventh cranial nerves on the other. It is formed by the expansion of the substantia gelatinosa extending into the medulla oblongata and descending fibers derived from the sensory root of the trigeminal nerve. 2. TUBER CINEREUM.

tuberculum co·noi·de·um (ko·noy′dee·um) [NA]. CONOID TUBERCLE.

tuberculum cor·ni·cu·la·tum (kor·nick·yoo·lay′tum) [NA]. CORNICULATE TUBERCLE.

tuberculum corniculatum [San·to·ri·ni] (san·to·ree′nee) [BNA]. Tuberculum corniculatum (= CORNICULATE TUBERCLE).

tuberculum co·ro·nae den·tis (ko·ro′nee den′tis) [NA]. CUSP (1).

tuberculum cos·tae (kos′tee) [NA]. COSTAL TUBERCLE.

tuberculum cu·ne·i·for·me (kew·nee·i·for′mee) [NA]. CUNEIFORM TUBERCLE.

tuberculum cuneiforme [Wris·ber·gi] (vris·bur′gye) [BNA]. Tuberculum cuneiforme (= CUNEIFORM TUBERCLE).

tuberculum epi·glot·ti·cum (ep·i·glot′i·kum) [NA]. EPIGLOTTIC TUBERCLE; CUSHION OF THE EPIGLOTTIS.

tuberculum ge·ni·ta·le (jen·i·tay′lee). GENITAL TUBERCLE.

tuberculum im·par (im′pahr). The unpaired mass of tissue between the anterior lingual swellings and the copula in the developing tongue.

tuberculum in·fra·gle·noi·da·le (in·fruh·glee·noy·day′lee) [NA]. INFRAGLENOID TUBERCLE.

tuberculum in·ter·con·dy·la·re la·te·ra·le (in·tur·kon·di·lair′ee lat·e·ray′lee) [NA]. LATERAL INTERCONDYLAR TUBERCLE.

tuberculum intercondylare me·di·a·le (mee·dee·ay′lee) [NA]. MEDIAL INTERCONDYLAR TUBERCLE.

tuberculum in·ter·con·dy·loi·de·um la·te·ra·le (in·tur·kon·di·loy′dee·um lat·e·ray′lee) [BNA]. Tuberculum intercondylare laterale (= LATERAL INTERCONDYLAR TUBERCLE).

tuberculum intercondyloideum me·di·a·le (mee·dee·ay'lee) [BNA]. Tuberculum intercondylare mediale (= MEDIAL INTERCONDYLAR TUBERCLE).

tuberculum in·ter·ve·no·sum (in·tur·vee·no'sum) [NA]. INTERVENOUS TUBERCLE.

tuberculum intervenosum [Lo·we·ri] (low'e·rye) [BNA]. Tuberculum intervenosum (= INTERVENOUS TUBERCLE).

tuberculum ju·gu·la·re os·sis oc·ci·pi·ta·lis (jug·yoo·lair'ee os'is ock·sip·i·tay'lis) [NA]. JUGULAR TUBERCLE.

tuberculum la·bii su·pe·ri·o·ris (lay'bee·eye sue·peer·ee·o'ris) [NA]. LABIAL TUBERCLE.

tuberculum la·te·ra·le pro·ces·sus pos·te·ri·o·ris ta·li (lat·e·ray'lee pro·ses'us pos·teer·ee·o'ris tay'lye) [NA]. An elevation in the lateral side of the margin of the posterior process of the talus.

tuberculum lin·gua·le la·te·ra·le (ling·gway'lee lat·e·ray'lee). The lateral lingual swelling in the embryo.

tuberculum linguale me·di·a·le (mee·dee·ay'lee). TUBERCULUM IMPAR.

tuberculum ma·jus hu·me·ri (may'jus hew'mur·eye) [NA]. GREATER TUBERCLE OF THE HUMERUS.

tuberculum mar·gi·na·le os·sis zy·go·ma·ti·ci (mahr·ji·nay'lee os'is zye·go·mat'i·sigh) [NA]. MARGINAL TUBERCLE OF THE ZYGOMATIC BONE.

tuberculum me·di·a·le pro·ces·sus pos·te·ri·o·ris ta·li (mee·dee·ay'lee pro·ses'us pos·teer·ee·o'ris tay'lye) [NA]. An elevation on the medial side of the margin of the posterior process of the talus.

tuberculum men·ta·le man·di·bu·lae (men·tay'lee man·dib'yoo·lee) [NA]. MENTAL TUBERCLE.

tuberculum mi·nus hu·me·ri (migh'nus hew'mur·eye) [NA]. LESSER TUBERCLE OF THE HUMERUS.

tuberculum mus·cu·li sca·le·ni an·te·ri·o·ris (mus'kew·lye ska·lee'nye an·teer·ee·o'ris) [NA]. SCALENE TUBERCLE.

tuberculum nu·clei cu·ne·a·ti (new'klee·eye kew·nee·ay'tye) [NA]. CUNEATE TUBERCLE.

tuberculum nuclei gra·ci·lis (gras'i·lis) [NA]. CLAVA.

tuberculum ob·tu·ra·to·ri·um an·te·ri·us (ob·tew·ruh·to'ree·um an·teer'ee·us) [NA]. ANTERIOR OBTURATOR TUBERCLE.

tuberculum obturatorium pos·te·ri·us (pos·teer'ee·us) [NA]. POSTERIOR OBTURATOR TUBERCLE.

tuberculum of Santorini [G. D. *Santorini*]. CUNEIFORM TUBERCLE.

tuberculum of the second rib. A rough eminence on the lateral surface of the second rib for attachment of part of the first and all of the second digitation of the serratus anterior muscle.

tuberculum os·sis mul·tan·gu·li ma·jo·ris (os'is mul·tang'gew·lye ma·jo'ris) [BNA]. TUBERCULUM OSSIS TRAPEZII.

tuberculum ossis na·vi·cu·la·ris (na·vick·yoo·lair'is) [BNA]. Tuberositas ossis navicularis (= TUBEROSITY OF THE NAVICULAR BONE).

tuberculum ossis sca·phoi·dei (ska·foy'dee·eye) [NA]. A small elevation on the distal part of the palmar surface of the scaphoid bone.

tuberculum ossis tra·pe·zii (tra·pee'zee·eye) [NA]. A ridge on the lateral part of the palmar surface of the trapezium bone.

tuberculum pha·ryn·ge·um (fa·rin'jee·um) [NA]. PHARYNGEAL TUBERCLE.

tuberculum pos·te·ri·us at·lan·tis (pos·teer'ee·us at·lan'tis) [NA]. The rudimentary spinous process of the atlas.

tuberculum posterius ver·te·bra·rum cer·vi·ca·li·um (vur·te·brair'um sur·vi·kay'lee·um) [NA]. POSTERIOR TUBERCLE.

tuberculum pu·bi·cum os·sis pu·bis (pew'bi·kum os'is pew'bis) [NA]. PUBIC TUBERCLE.

tuberculum sca·le·ni [Lis·fran·ci] (ska·lee'nigh lis·fran'sigh) [BNA]. Tuberculum musculi scaleni anterioris (= SCALENE TUBERCLE).

tuberculum sel·lae tur·ci·cae (sel'ee tur'si·see) [NA]. The anterior boundary of the sella turcica.

tuberculum su·pra·gle·noi·da·le (sue''pruh·glee·noy·day'lee) [NA]. SUPRAGLENOID TUBERCLE.

tuberculum su·pra·tra·gi·cum (sue·pruh·tray'ji·kum) [NA]. A small elevation occasionally present on the upper part of the tragus.

tuberculum thy·re·oi·de·um in·fe·ri·us (thigh·ree·oy'dee·um in·feer'ee·us) [BNA]. TUBERCULUM THYROIDEUM INFERIUS.

tuberculum thyreoideum su·pe·ri·us (sue·peer'ee·us) [BNA]. TUBERCULUM THYROIDEUM SUPERIUS.

tuberculum thy·roi·de·um in·fe·ri·us (thigh·roy'dee·um in·feer'ee·us) [NA]. An occasional, indistinct elevation on the lower posterior part of the lateral aspect of either lamina of the thyroid cartilage.

tuberculum thyroideum su·pe·ri·us (sue·peer'ee·us) [NA]. An occasional, indistinct elevation on the upper posterior part of the lateral aspect of either lamina of the thyroid cartilage.

tuber fron·ta·le (fron·tay'lee) [NA]. FRONTAL EMINENCE.

tu·ber·in (tew'bur·in) *n.* A simple protein of the globulin type which occurs in potatoes.

tuber is·chi·a·di·cum (is·kee·ad'i·kum) [NA]. ISCHIAL TUBEROSITY.

tuber max·il·lae (mack·sil'ee) [NA]. MAXILLARY TUBEROSITY.

tuber max·il·la·re (mack·si·lair'ee) [BNA]. Tuber maxillae (= MAXILLARY TUBEROSITY).

tu·bero·hy·poph·y·se·al tract (tew''bur·o·high·pof·i·see'ul). A part of the hypothalamohypophyseal tract.

tuber omen·ta·le he·pa·tis (o·men·tay'lee hep'uh·tis) [NA]. A prominence on the left lobe of the liver, corresponding to the lesser curvature of the stomach.

tuber omentale pan·cre·a·tis (pan·kree'uh·tis) [NA]. A prominence of the middle part of the pancreas, corresponding to the lesser omentum.

tu·be·ro·si·tas (tew·bur·os'i·tas) *n.*, pl. **tube·ro·si·ta·tes** (·os·i·tay'teez) [L.]. TUBEROSITY.

tuberositas co·ra·coi·dea cla·vi·cu·lae (kor·uh·koy'dee·uh kla·vick'yoo·lee) [BNA]. Tuberculum conoideum (= CONOID TUBERCLE) and linea trapezoidea (= TRAPEZOID LINE).

tuberositas cos·tae II (kos'tee) [BNA]. Tuberositas musculi serrati anterioris (= TUBEROSITY OF THE SECOND RIB).

tuberositas cos·ta·lis cla·vi·cu·lae (kos·tay'lis kla·vick'yoo·lee) [BNA]. Impressio ligamenti costoclavicularis (= COSTAL TUBEROSITY).

tuberositas del·toi·dea (del·toy'dee·uh) [NA]. DELTOID TUBEROSITY.

tuberositas glu·taea (gloo'tee·uh, gloo·tee'uh) [BNA]. Tuberositas glutea (= GLUTEAL TUBEROSITY).

tuberositas glu·tea (gloo'tee·uh, gloo·tee'uh) [NA]. GLUTEAL TUBEROSITY.

tuberositas ili·a·ca (i·lye'uh·kuh) [NA]. ILIAC TUBEROSITY.

tuberositas in·fra·gle·noi·da·lis (in·fruh·glee·noy·day'lis) [BNA]. Tuberculum infraglenoidale (= INFRAGLENOID TUBERCLE).

tuberositas mas·se·te·ri·ca (mas·e·terr'i·kuh) [NA]. An indefinite series of low ridges on the lower part of the lateral aspect of either ramus of the mandible.

tuberositas mus·cu·li ser·ra·ti an·te·ri·o·ris (mus'kew·lye se·ray'tye an·teer·ee·o'ris) [NA]. TUBEROSITY OF THE SECOND RIB.

tuberositas os·sis cu·boi·dei (os'is kew·boy'dee·eye) [NA]. TUBEROSITY OF THE CUBOID BONE.

tuberositas ossis me·ta·tar·sa·lis I (met·uh·tahr·say'lis) [NA]. TUBEROSITY OF THE FIRST METATARSAL.

tuberositas ossis metatarsalis V [NA]. TUBEROSITY OF THE FIFTH METATARSAL.

tuberositas ossis na·vi·cu·la·ris (na·vick·yoo·lair'is) [NA]. TUBEROSITY OF THE NAVICULAR BONE.

tuberositas pha·lan·gis dis·ta·lis (fa·lan'jis dis·tay'lis) [NA]. UNGUAL TUBEROSITY.

tuberositas pte·ry·goi·dea (terr·i·goy'dee·uh) [NA]. PTERYGOID TUBERCLE.

tuberositas ra·dii (ray'dee·eye) [NA]. RADIAL TUBEROSITY.

tuberositas sa·cra·lis (sa·kray'lis) [NA]. SACRAL TUBEROSITY.

tuberositas su·pra·gle·noi·da·lis (sue·pruh·glee·noy·day'lis) [BNA]. Tuberculum supraglenoidale (= SUPRAGLENOID TUBERCLE).

tuberositas ti·bi·ae (tib'ee·ee) [NA]. TUBEROSITY OF THE TIBIA.

tuberositas ul·nae (ul'nee) [NA]. TUBEROSITY OF THE ULNA.

tuberositas un·gui·cu·la·ris (ung·gwick·yoo·lair'is) [BNA]. Tuberositas phalangis distalis (= UNGUAL TUBEROSITY).

tu·ber·os·i·ty (tew"bur·os'i·tee) *n.* A protuberance on a bone.

tuberosity of the cuboid bone. An eminence on the lateral side of the cuboid bone; it bears an oval facet on which glides the sesamoid bone or cartilage often found in the tendon of the peroneus longus muscle. NA *tuberositas ossis cuboidei.*

tuberosity of the fifth metatarsal. A rough projection from the lateral surface of the base of the bone, giving attachment to the peroneus brevis muscle on its dorsal surface, and to the flexor digiti minimi brevis muscle on its plantar surface. NA *tuberositas ossis metatarsalis V.*

tuberosity of the first metatarsal bone. An oval prominence on the lateral side of the base of the bone, into which part of the tendon of the peroneus longus muscle is inserted. Syn. *plantar tubercle.* NA *tuberositas ossis metatarsalis I.*

tuberosity of the ischium. ISCHIAL TUBER or TUBEROSITY.

tuberosity of the navicular bone. A rounded eminence on the medial surface of the navicular bone into which part of the tendon of the tibialis posterior muscle is inserted. NA *tuberositas ossis navicularis.*

tuberosity of the palatine bone. PYRAMIDAL PROCESS OF THE PALATINE BONE.

tuberosity of the second rib. A rough eminence on the lateral surface of the second rib for attachment of part of the first and all of the second digitation of the serratus anterior muscle. NA *tuberositas musculi serrati anterioris.*

tuberosity of the tibia. An oblong elevation on the anterior surface of the upper extremity of the tibia, to which the patellar ligament is attached. NA *tuberositas tibiae.*

tuberosity of the ulna. A rough eminence below the coronoid process on the anterior surface of the ulna, which gives insertion to part of the brachialis muscle. NA *tuberositas ulnae.*

tu·ber·ous (tew'bur·us) *adj.* [*tuber* + *-ous*]. 1. Resembling a tuber. 2. Having, or characterized by the presence of, tubers or tuberosities.

tuberous cystic tumor of the breast. CYSTOSARCOMA PHYLLODES.

tuberous mole. BREUS'S MOLE.

tuberous sclerosis. A familial neurocutaneous syndrome characterized in its complete form by epilepsy, adenoma sebaceum, and mental deficiency and pathologically by nodular sclerosis of the cerebral cortex. Retinal phacoma, other skin lesions such as areas of depigmentation, hyperpigmentation and shagreen patches, intracranial calcification, and hamartomas of different viscera are frequently present.

tuberous subchorial hematoma. BREUS'S MOLE.

tuberous tumor. Any tumor, such as an angioma, which grossly resembles a tuber.

tuber pa·ri·e·ta·le (pa·rye·e·tay'lee) [NA]. PARIETAL EMINENCE.

tuber ver·mis (vur'mis) [NA]. A portion of the inferior vermis just caudal to the horizontal fissure of the cerebellum.

tubi. Plural and genitive singular of *tubus.*

tubo-. A combining form meaning *tube.*

tu·bo·ab·dom·i·nal (tew"bo·ab·dom'i·nul) *adj.* [*tubo-* + *abdominal*]. Pertaining to a uterine tube and to the abdomen.

tuboabdominal pregnancy. Gestation that develops in the ampulla of the uterine tube and extends into the peritoneal cavity.

tu·bo·ad·nexo·pexy (tew"bo·ad·neck'so·peck"see) *n.* [*tubo-* + *adnexa* + *-pexy*]. Surgical fixation of the uterine adnexa.

tu·bo·cu·ra·re (tew"bo·kew·rah'ree) *n.* Curare so named because of its tube shape, the result of being packed in hollow bamboo canes.

***d*-tu·bo·cu·ra·rine** (tew"bo·kew·rah'reen, ·rin) *n.* TUBOCURARINE CHLORIDE.

tubocurarine chloride. The chloride of a quaternary base obtained from the bark and stems of plants of the genus *Chondodendron*, $C_{38}H_{44}Cl_2N_2O_6$; a skeletal muscle relaxant used as an adjunct in surgical anesthesia to soften convulsions in electroshock therapy, to reduce muscle spasm in fractures, and for diagnosis of myasthenia gravis. Syn. *d-tubocurarine.*

tu·bo·lig·a·men·ta·ry pregnancy (tew"bo·lig"uh·men'tuh·ree). Gestation arising in a uterine tube with extension into the broad ligament.

tu·bo·lig·a·men·tous (tew"bo·lig"uh·men'tus) *adj.* [*tubo-* + *ligamentous*]. Pertaining to the uterine tube and the broad ligament.

tu·bo·ovar·i·an (tew"bo·o·văr'ee·un) *adj.* [*tubo-* + *ovarian*]. Pertaining to the uterine tube and the ovary.

tuboovarian cyst. A cyst involving an ovary and its uterine tube.

tuboovarian pregnancy. Gestation arising in a uterine tube and extending into the ovary.

tu·bo·ovar·i·ot·o·my (tew"bo·o·văr"ee·ot'uh·mee) *n.* [*tubo-* + *ovario-* + *-tomy*]. Excision of a uterine tube and ovary.

tu·bo·peri·to·ne·al (tew"bo·perr"i·to·nee'ul) *adj.* [*tubo-* + *peritoneal*]. Pertaining to the uterine tubes and the peritoneum.

tu·bo·plas·ty (tew'bo·plas"tee) *n.* [*tubo-* + *-plasty*]. Plastic repair of a uterine tube.

tu·bo·tym·pan·ic (tew"bo·tim·pan'ick) *adj.* Pertaining to the auditory tube and the tympanic cavity.

tubotympanic recess. The dorsal wing of the first pharyngeal pouch and possibly part of the second, which forms the tympanic cavity of the middle ear and the auditory tube.

tu·bo·uter·ine (tew"bo·yoo'tur·in, ·ine) *adj.* [*tubo-* + *uterine*]. Pertaining to the uterine tube and the uterus.

tubouterine pregnancy. INTERSTITIAL PREGNANCY.

tu·bo·va·gi·nal (tew"bo·vuh·jye'nul, ·vaj'i·nul) *adj.* [*tubo-* + *vaginal*]. Pertaining to a uterine tube and the vagina.

tu·bu·lar (tew'bew·lur) *adj.* 1. Shaped like a tube. 2. Pertaining to or affecting tubules, as tubular nephritis. 3. Produced in a tube, as tubular breathing.

tubular acidosis. RENAL TUBULAR ACIDOSIS.

tubular adenoma. An adenoma in which the parenchymal cells form tubules.

tubular gland. A secreting gland, tubelike or cylindrical in shape.

tubular hamartoma of the ovary. ADRENOCORTICOID ADENOMA OF THE OVARY.

tubular vision. A hysterical phenomenon in which the constricted visual field defies the laws of physical projection and maintains a uniform small size, despite a change in distance of the patient from the tangent screen or the size of the test object. Syn. *gun-barrel vision, tunnel vision.*

tu·bule (tew'bewl) *n.* [L. *tubulus*, dim. of *tubus*]. 1. A small tube. 2. *In anatomy,* any minute, tube-shaped structure.

tubuli. Plural and genitive singular of *tubulus.*

tubuli lac·ti·fe·ri (lack·tif'e·rye). The excretory ducts of the mammary glands.

tu·bu·lin (tew'bew·lin) *n.* [*tubule* + *-in*]. A globular protein containing two protomers; 10 to 14 tubulin molecules are arranged in a helix to form the microtubules of cells.

tubuli re·na·les (re·nay'leez) [NA]. RENAL TUBULES.

tubuli renales con·tor·ti (kon·tor'tye) [NA]. The convoluted renal tubules; CONVOLUTED TUBULES (2).

tubuli renales rec·ti (reck'tye) [NA]. The straight renal tubules; COLLECTING TUBULES.

tubuli se·mi·ni·fe·ri con·tor·ti (sem·i·nif'e·rye kon·tor'tye) [NA]. The convoluted seminiferous tubules.

tubuli seminiferi rec·ti (reck'tye) [NA]. The straight seminiferous tubules.

tu·bu·li·za·tion (tew"bew·li·zay'shun) *n.* Protection of the ends of nerves, after neurorrhaphy, by an absorbable cylinder.

tu·bu·lo·ac·i·nous (tew"bew·lo·as'i·nus) *adj.* [*tubulo-* + *acinous*]. TUBULOALVEOLAR.

tu·bu·lo·al·ve·o·lar (tew"bew·lo·al·vee'o·lur) *adj.* [*tubulo-* + *alveolar*]. Consisting of a system of branching tubules that terminate in alveoli, as in the salivary glands.

tubuloalveolar gland. A gland whose secretory endpieces are tubular and alveolar. To this group belong most of the larger exocrine glands.

tu·bu·lo·cyst (tew'bew·lo·sist") *n.* [*tubulo-* + *-cyst*]. A cystic dilatation in an occluded canal or duct.

tu·bu·lo·in·ter·sti·tial (tew"bew·lo·in·tur·stish'ul) *adj.* Pertaining to renal tubules and interstitial tissues.

tubulointerstitial nephritis. Renal interstitial disease characterized by the presence of interstitial inflammatory cells and tubular destruction.

tu·bu·lo·rac·e·mose (tew"bu·lo·ras'e·moce) *adj.* Characterizing a gland that is both tubular and racemose.

tu·bu·lus (tew'bew·lus) *n.*, pl. & genit. sing. **tubu·li** (·lye) [L.]. TUBULE.

tu·bus (tew'bus) *n.*, pl. & genit. sing. **tu·bi** (·bye) [L.]. TUBE, CANAL.

tubus di·ges·to·ri·us (dye·jes·to'ree·us) [BNA]. Canalis alimentarius (= ALIMENTARY CANAL).

tubus me·dul·la·ris (med·yoo·lair'is). CENTRAL CANAL OF THE SPINAL CORD.

tubus ver·te·bra·lis (vur·te·bray'lis). VERTEBRAL CANAL.

Tuf·fier's inferior ligament (tueᵉf·yeʸ') [T. *Tuffier,* French surgeon, 1857–1929]. A mesenterioparietal fold, a portion of the mesentery extending into the right iliac fossa.

tu·la·re·mia (tew"luh·ree'mee·uh) *n.* [after *Tulare* county, Calif.]. An infectious disease caused by *Francisella tularensis* (*Pasteurella tularensis*) widely prevalent in wild animals, birds, and ancillary hosts, primarily transmitted to man by contact with infected tissues or fluids (for example, skinning rabbits), or by insect bites, but also by ingestion and inhalation. Depending on the host response and point of entry, a variety of forms are recognized, such as ulceroglandular, oculoglandular, typhoidal, pneumonic, or gastrointestinal. Syn. *deer-fly fever, rabbit fever.*

tum·bu fly (tŏŏm'boo) *n.* An African species of the Diptera, *Cordylobia anthropophaga,* whose larvae develop in the skin of man and various mammals, such as rats, dogs, cats, monkeys.

tu·me·fa·cient (tew"me·fay'shunt) *adj.* [L. *tumefacere,* to cause to swell, from *tumere,* to be swollen]. Tending to cause swelling.

tu·me·fac·tion (tew"me·fack'shun) *n.* [L. *tumefacere,* to cause to swell]. 1. A swelling. 2. The act or process of swelling.

tu·me·fy (tew'me·fye) *v.* [MF. *tumefier,* from L. *tumefacere,* to cause to swell]. To swell or cause to swell.

tu·men·tia (tew·men'shee·uh) *n.* [L., from *tumere,* to swell]. 1. Swelling. 2. Particularly, vasomotor disturbance characterized by irregular edematous swellings in the legs and arms.

tu·mer·ic (tew'mur·ick) *n.* CURCUMA.

tu·mes·cence (tew·mes'unce) *n.* [L. *tumescere,* to be swelling, begin to swell]. 1. The condition of growing tumid. 2. A swelling. 3. The vascular congestion of the sex organs, as the swelling of the penis, associated with heightened emotional and physical excitement, characteristic of the readiness to engage in copulation. —**tumes·cent** (·unt) *adj.*

tu·meur ro·yale (tueᵉ·mœr' rwa·yahˡ') [F., lit., royal tumor]. PACHYDERMATOCELE.

tu·mid (tew'mid) *adj.* [L. *tumidus*]. Swollen.

tu·mid·i·ty (tew·mid'i·tee) *n.* [L. *tumidus,* swollen]. The state of being swollen.

tu·mor, tu·mour (tew'mur) *n.* [L., from *tumere,* to swell]. 1. Any abnormal mass resulting from the excessive multiplication of cells. 2. A swelling. —**tumor·al** (·ul) *adj.*

tu·mor·af·fin (tew"mur·af'in) *adj.* [*tumor-* + L. *affinis,* allied by marriage]. Being or pertaining to something, as a drug or radiant energy, that has some special affinity for tumor cells.

tumoral calcinosis. LIPOCALCIGRANULOMATOSIS.

tumor blush. TUMOR STAIN.

tu·mori·gen·ic (tew"mur·i·jen'ick) *adj.* [*tumor* + *-genic*]. Tumor-forming.

tu·mor·let (tew'mur·lit) *n.* 1. A tumorlike proliferation of cells in scarred lung tissue; thought to be of bronchial epithelial origin. 2. A small tumor.

tu·mor·ous (tew'mur·ous) *adj.* Of the nature of a neoplasm or tumor.

tumor stain. An angiographic appearance of contrast media in very small vessels and vascular spaces of a highly vascular tumor, usually resulting in diffuse, prolonged opacification. Syn. *tumor blush.*

tumour. TUMOR.

tu·mul·tus cor·dis (tew·mul'tus kor'dis). [L., tumult of the heart]. Irregular heart action.

tumultus ser·mo·nis (sur·mo'nis). *Obsol.* STUTTERING.

Tun·ga (tung'guh) *n.* [Tupi]. A genus of fleas that burrow beneath the skin to lay their eggs; serious local inflammation results.

Tunga pen·e·trans (pen'e·tranz). A flea prevalent in the tropical regions of Africa and America; often attacks between the toes or on the foot; a chigoe or a jigger.

tun·gi·a·sis (tung·guy'uh·sis, tun·jye') *n.* [*Tunga* + *-iasis*]. The cutaneous pustular inflammation caused by the gravid female sandflea, *Tunga penetrans.*

tung·sten (tung'stun) *n.* [Swed., from *tung,* heavy, + *sten,* stone]. W = 183.85. A heavy metallic element, atomic number 74, density 19.3. Used in steel to increase hardness and tensile strength, in the manufacture of filaments for electric lamps, in contact points, and other products where hardness and toughness are demanded. Syn. *wolfram.*

tu·nic (tew'nick) *n.* [L. *tunica*]. A coat, layer, membrane, or sheath.

tu·ni·ca (tew'ni·kuh) *n.*, pl. & genit. sing. **tuni·cae** (·see) [L.]. A coat, layer, membrane, or sheath.

tunica ad·ven·ti·tia (ad·ven·tish'ee·uh) [NA]. The outer connective tissue coat of an organ where it is not covered by a serous membrane.

tunica adventitia duc·tus de·fe·ren·tis (duck'tus def·e·ren'tis) [NA]. The outer connective-tissue coat of the ductus deferens.

tunica adventitia eso·pha·gi (e·sof'uh·jye) [NA]. The outer connective-tissue coat of the esophagus.

tunica adventitia oe·so·pha·gi (e·sof'uh·jye) [BNA]. TUNICA ADVENTITIA ESOPHAGI.

tunica adventitia tu·bae ute·ri·nae (tew'bee yoo·te·rye'nee) [BNA]. TELA SUBSEROSA TUBAE UTERINAE.

tunica adventitia ure·te·ris (yoo·ree'tur·is) [NA]. The outer connective-tissue coat of the ureter.

tunica adventitia ve·si·cae se·mi·na·lis (ve·sigh'see sem·i·nay'lis) [BNA]. TUNICA ADVENTITIA VESICULAE SEMINALIS.

tunica adventitia ve·si·cu·lae se·mi·na·lis (ve·sick'yoo·lee sem·i·nay'lis) [NA]. The outer connective-tissue coat of the seminal vesicle.

tunica al·bu·gi·nea (al·bew·jin'ee·uh) [NA]. A general term for a dense connective-tissue covering layer.

tunica albuginea cor·po·ris spon·gi·o·si (kor'po·ris spon·jee·o'sigh) [NA]. The dense fibroelastic sheath of the corpus spongiosum.

tunica albuginea cor·po·rum ca·ver·no·so·rum (kor'po·rum kav·ur·no·so'rum) [NA]. The dense fibroelastic sheath of the corpora cavernosa.

tunica albuginea li·e·nis (lye·ee'nis) [BNA]. TUNICA FIBROSA LIENIS.

tunica albuginea ocu·li (ock'yoo·lye). SCLERA.

tunica albuginea ova·rii (o·vair'ee·eye). The compact connective tissue immediately under the germinal epithelium of the cortex of the ovary.

tunica albuginea pe·nis (pee'nis). The outer layer of the corpora cavernosa of the penis.

tunica albuginea tes·tis (tes'tis) [NA]. The dense fibrous capsule of the testis, deep to the tunica vaginalis propria.

tunica con·junc·ti·va (kon·junk·tye'vuh) [NA]. CONJUNCTIVA.

tunica conjunctiva bul·bi (bul'bye) [NA]. BULBAR CONJUNCTIVA.

tunica conjunctiva pal·pe·bra·rum (pal·pe·brair'um) [NA]. PALPEBRAL CONJUNCTIVA.

tunica dar·tos (dahr'tos) [NA]. DARTOS.

tunica decidua. DECIDUA.

tunicae. Plural and genitive singular of *tunica*.

tunicae fu·ni·cu·li sper·ma·ti·ci (few·nick'yoo·lye spur·mat'i·sigh) [BNA]. The coverings of the spermatic cord.

tunicae funiculi spermatici et testis (tes'tis) [NA]. The coverings of the spermatic cord and testis.

tunica elas·ti·ca (e·las'ti·kuh). TUNICA INTIMA.

tunica ex·ter·na (ecks·tur'nuh) [NA]. The outermost coat of a blood or lymph vessel.

tunica externa the·cae fol·li·cu·li (thees'ee fol·ick'yoo·lye) [NA]. THECA EXTERNA.

tunica externa va·so·rum (va·so'rum) [BNA]. TUNICA EXTERNA.

tunica fi·bro·sa (figh·bro'suh) [NA]. Any connective-tissue coat of an organ.

tunica fibrosa bul·bi (bul'bye) [NA]. The sclera and cornea, the outer covering of the eyeball.

tunica fibrosa he·pa·tis (hep'uh·tis) [NA]. The fibroelastic layer beneath the peritoneum covering the liver.

tunica fibrosa li·e·nis (lye·ee'nis) [NA]. The fibroelastic coat of the spleen.

tunica fibrosa ocu·li (ock'yoo·lye) [BNA]. TUNICA FIBROSA BULBI.

tunica fibrosa re·nis (ree'nis) [BNA]. The fibroelastic coat of the kidney, the proper renal capsule.

tunica in·ter·na (in·tur'nuh). TUNICA INTIMA.

tunica interna bul·bi (bul'bye) [NA]. RETINA.

tunica interna the·cae fol·li·cu·li (thees'ee fol·ick'yoo·lye) [NA]. THECA INTERNA.

tunica in·ti·ma (in'ti·muh) [NA]. The inner coat of a blood or lymph vessel.

tunica me·dia (mee'dee·uh) [NA]. The middle coat of a blood or lymph vessel, composed of varying amounts of smooth muscle and elastic tissue.

tunica mu·co·sa (mew·ko'suh) [NA]. MUCOUS MEMBRANE.

tunica mucosa ca·vi tym·pa·ni (kay'vye tim'puh·nigh) [NA]. The mucous membrane lining of the tympanic cavity.

tunica mucosa co·li (ko'lye) [NA]. The mucous membrane lining the colon.

tunica mucosa duc·tus de·fe·ren·tis (duck'tus def·e·ren'tis) [NA]. The mucous membrane of the ductus deferens.

tunica mucosa eso·pha·gi (e·sof'uh·jye) [NA]. The mucous membrane lining the esophagus.

tunica mucosa in·tes·ti·ni cras·si (in·tes·tye'nigh kras'eye) [BNA]. The mucous membrane lining the large intestine.

tunica mucosa intestini rec·ti (reck'tye) [BNA]. TUNICA MUCOSA RECTI.

tunica mucosa intestini te·nu·is (ten'yoo·is) [NA]. The mucous membrane of the small intestine.

tunica mucosa la·ryn·gis (la·rin'jis) [NA]. The mucous membrane of the larynx.

tunica mucosa lin·guae (ling'gwee) [NA]. The mucous membrane covering of the tongue.

tunica mucosa na·si (nay'zye) [NA]. The mucous membrane of the nasal cavity.

tunica mucosa oe·so·pha·gi (e·sof'uh·jye) [BNA]. TUNICA MUCOSA ESOPHAGI.

tunica mucosa oris (o'ris) [NA]. The mucous membrane of the oral cavity.

tunica mucosa pha·ryn·gis (fa·rin'jis) [NA]. The mucous membrane of the pharynx.

tunica mucosa rec·ti (reck'tye) [NA]. The mucous membrane of the rectum.

tunica mucosa tra·che·ae et bron·cho·rum (tray'kee·ee et brong·ko'rum) [NA]. The mucous membrane of the trachea and bronchi.

tunica mucosa tu·bae au·di·ti·vae (tew'bee aw·di·tye'vee) [NA]. The mucous membrane of the auditory tube.

tunica mucosa tubae ute·ri·nae (yoo·te·rye'nee) [NA]. The mucous membrane of the uterine tube.

tunica mucosa tym·pa·ni·ca (tim·pan'i·kuh) [BNA]. TUNICA MUCOSA CAVI TYMPANI.

tunica mucosa ure·te·ris (yoo·ree'tur·is) [NA]. The mucous membrane of the ureter.

tunica mucosa ure·thrae fe·mi·ni·nae (yoo·ree'three fem·i·nigh'nee) [NA]. The mucous membrane of the female urethra.

tunica mucosa urethrae mu·li·e·bris (mew·lee·ee'bris) [BNA]. TUNICA MUCOSA URETHRAE FEMININAE.

tunica mucosa ute·ri (yoo'te·rye) [NA]. ENDOMETRIUM.

tunica mucosa va·gi·nae (va·jye'nee) [NA]. The mucous membrane of the vagina.

tunica mucosa ven·tri·cu·li (ven·trick'yoo·lye) [NA]. The mucous membrane of the stomach.

tunica mucosa ve·si·cae fel·le·ae (ve·sigh'see fel'ee·ee) [NA]. The mucous membrane of the gallbladder.

tunica mucosa vesicae uri·na·ri·ae (yoo·ri·nair'ree·ee) [NA]. The mucous membrane of the urinary bladder.

tunica mucosa ve·si·cu·lae se·mi·na·lis (ve·sick'yoo·lee sem·i·nay'lis) [NA]. The mucous membrane of the seminal vesicle.

tunica mus·cu·la·ris (mus·kew·lair'ris) [NA]. The muscular coat of certain hollow organs, for example, the bronchi.

tunica muscularis bron·cho·rum (brong·ko'rum) [NA]. The muscular coat of the bronchi.

tunica muscularis cer·vi·cis ute·ri (sur'vi·sis yoo'te·rye) [BNA]. The muscular coat of the cervix of the uterus.

tunica muscularis co·li (ko'lye) [NA]. The muscular coat of the colon.

tunica muscularis duc·tus de·fe·ren·tis (duck'tus def·e·ren'tis) [NA]. The muscular coat of the ductus deferens.

tunica muscularis eso·pha·gi (e·sof'uh·jye) [NA]. The muscular coat of the esophagus.

tunica muscularis in·tes·ti·ni cras·si (in·tes·tye'nigh kras'eye) [BNA]. The muscular coat of the large intestine.

tunica muscularis intestini rec·ti (reck'tye) [BNA]. TUNICA MUSCULARIS RECTI.

tunica muscularis intestini te·nu·is (ten'yoo·is) [NA]. The muscular coat of the small intestine.

tunica muscularis oe·so·pha·gi (e·sof'uh·jye) [BNA]. TUNICA MUSCULARIS ESOPHAGI.

tunica muscularis pha·ryn·gis (fa·rin'jis) [NA]. The muscular coat of the pharynx.

tunica muscularis rec·ti (reck'tye) [NA]. The muscular coat of the rectum.

tunica muscularis tra·che·ae et bron·cho·rum (tray'kee·ee et brong·ko'rum) [BNA]. The smooth muscle of the trachea and bronchi.

tunica muscularis tu·bae ute·ri·nae (tew'bee yoo·te·rye'nee) [NA]. The muscular coat of the uterine tube.

tunica muscularis ure·te·ris (yoo·ree'tur·is) [NA]. The muscular coat of the ureter.

tunica muscularis ure·thrae fe·mi·ni·nae (yoo·ree'three fem·i·nigh'nee) [NA]. The muscular coat of the female urethra.

tunica muscularis urethrae mu·li·e·bris (mew·lee·ee'bris) [BNA]. TUNICA MUSCULARIS URETHRAE FEMININAE.

tunica muscularis ute·ri (yoo'te·rye) [NA]. MYOMETRIUM.

tunica muscularis va·gi·nae (va·jye'nee) [NA]. The muscular coat of the vagina.

tunica muscularis ven·tri·cu·li (ven·trick'yoo·lye) [NA]. The muscular coat of the stomach.

tunica muscularis ve·si·cae fel·le·ae (ve·sigh'see fel'ee·ee) [NA]. The muscular coat of the gallbladder.

tunica muscularis vesicae uri·na·ri·ae (yoo·ri·nair'ee·ee) [NA]. The muscular coat of the urinary bladder.

tunica muscularis ve·si·cu·lae se·mi·na·lis (ve·sick'yoo·lee sem·i·nay'lis) [NA]. The muscular coat of the seminal vesicle.

tunica pro·pria co·rii (pro'pree·uh ko'ree·eye) [BNA]. Stratum reticulare (= RETICULAR LAYER).

tunica propria mu·co·sa (mew·ko'suh). LAMINA PROPRIA MUCOSAE.

tunica propria tu·bu·li se·mi·ni·fe·ri (tew'bew·lye sem·i·nif'e·rye) [BNA]. The connective tissue of the mucous membrane of the seminiferous tubules.

tunica reaction. Enlargement of the scrotum of male guinea pigs, with reddening of the scrotal skin and adhesions between testes and tunica vaginalis, due to infection with epidemic or murine typhus.

tunica se·ro·sa (se·ro'suh) [NA]. SEROUS MEMBRANE; the mesothelium and underlying connective tissue forming the visceral and parietal pericardium, pleura, peritoneum, and tunica vaginalis propria testis.

tunica serosa co·li (ko'lye) [NA]. The serous membrane of the colon.

tunica serosa he·pa·tis (hep'uh·tis) [NA]. The serous membrane of the liver.

tunica serosa in·tes·ti·ni cras·si (in·tes·tye'nigh kras'eye) [BNA]. TUNICA SEROSA COLI.

tunica serosa intestini te·nu·is (ten'yoo·is) [NA]. The serous membrane of the small intestine.

tunica serosa li·e·nis (lye·ee'nis) [NA]. The serous membrane covering the spleen.

tunica serosa pe·ri·to·naei (perr·i·to·nee'eye) [BNA]. The serous membrane lining the abdominal cavity (NA *tunica serosa peritonei parietalis*) and covering the organs within the abdominal cavity (NA *tunica serosa peritonei visceralis*).

tunica serosa pe·ri·to·nei pa·ri·e·ta·lis (perr·i·to·nee'eye pa·rye·e·tay'lis) [NA]. The serous membrane lining the abdominal cavity.

tunica serosa peritonei vis·ce·ra·lis (vis·e·ray'lis) [NA]. The serous membrane covering the organs within the abdominal cavity.

tunica serosa tu·bae ute·ri·nae (tew'bee yoo·te·rye'nee) [NA]. The serous membrane of the uterine tube.

tunica serosa ute·ri (yoo'te·rye). [NA]. PERIMETRIUM.

tunica serosa ven·tri·cu·li (ven·trick'yoo·lye) [NA]. The serous membrane of the stomach.

tunica serosa ve·si·cae fel·le·ae (ve·sigh'see fel'ee·ee) [NA]. The serous membrane of the gallbladder.

tunica serosa vesicae uri·na·ri·ae (yoo·ri·nair'ee·ee) [NA]. The serous membrane of the urinary bladder.

tunica sub·mu·co·sa (sub·mew·ko'suh). TELA SUBMUCOSA.

tunica submucosa ure·thrae mu·li·e·bris (yoo·ree'three mew·lee·ee'bris) [BNA]. The connective tissue outside the mucous membrane of the female urethra.

tunica tes·tis (tes'tis) [BNA]. TUNICAE FUNICULI SPERMATICI ET TESTIS.

tunica uvea (yoo'vee·uh). TUNICA VASCULOSA BULBI.

tunica va·gi·na·lis com·mu·nis (vaj·i·nay'lis kom·yoo'nis) [BNA]. The external and internal spermatic fasciae considered as one.

tunica vaginalis pro·pria tes·tis (pro'pree·uh tes'tis) [BNA]. TUNICA VAGINALIS TESTIS.

tunica vaginalis tes·tis (tes'tis) [NA]. The serous membrane covering the testis and epididymis and lining the serous cavity of the scrotum.

tunica vas·cu·lo·sa bul·bi (vas·kew·lo'suh bul'bye) [NA]. The choroid, ciliary body, and iris of the eye.

tunica vasculosa len·tis (len'tis). A mesodermal lens capsule in the embryo, vascularized by the hyaloid and annular arteries; the anterior part is the pupillary membrane.

tunica vasculosa ocu·li (ock'yoo·lye) [BNA]. TUNICA VASCULOSA BULBI.

tunica vasculosa tes·tis (tes'tis). A layer of loose connective tissue containing many blood vessels, on the inner surface of the tunica albuginea testis.

tun·ing fork. A two-tined metallic fork capable of vibrating at a rate which will produce a pure tone of a specific frequency.

tuning-fork test. The testing of hearing acuity or loss by use of a tuning fork. See also *bone conduction test, Rinne's test, Schwabach's test, Teal test, Weber's test.*

tun·nel anemia. ANCYLOSTOMIASIS.

tunnel disease. 1. DECOMPRESSION SICKNESS. 2. ANCYLOSTOMIASIS.

tunnel flap. GAUNTLET FLAP.

tunnel graft. A skin graft with the epithelial side inward, introduced into tissues under a contracted scar, etc. The tunnel is split later, and the epithelial surface becomes superficial or is left in place to replace a part, such as the urethra.

tunnel motor. A plastic motor formed by tunneling through a muscle.

tunnel murmur. CONTINUOUS MURMUR.

tunnel of Cor·ti (kor'tee) [A. *Corti*, Italian anatomist, 1822–1888]. The triangular canal formed by the pillar cells of the spiral organ (of Corti) and the lamina basilaris. It extends over the entire length of the lamina basilaris. Syn. *canal of Corti, tunnel space.*

tunnel space. TUNNEL OF CORTI.

tunnel vision. TUBULAR VISION.

Tuo·hy needle (too'hee, too'ee). A needle with a directional bevel for accurately inserting and positioning a small catheter into the subarachnoid or peridural space.

Tu·paia (too·pye'uh) *n.* [NL., from Malay *tūpai*, squirrel]. An Indonesian and Malaysian genus of tree shrews.

TUR Abbreviation for *transurethral resection.*

tu·ran·ose (tew'ran·oce) *n.* A reducing disaccharide, $C_{12}H_{22}O_{11}$, yielding on hydrolysis glucose and fructose.

tur·ban tumor (tur'bun). CYLINDROMA.

tur·bid (tur'bid) *adj.* [L. *turbidus*, confused]. Cloudy. —**tur·bid·i·ty** (tur·bid'i·tee) *n.*

tur·bi·dim·e·ter (tur"bi·dim'e·tur) *n.* [*turbid* + *-meter*]. An instrument for measuring the degree of turbidity of a liquid. —**turbi·di·met·ric** (·di·met'rick) *adj.*; **turbi·dim·e·try** (·dim'e·tree) *n.*

tur·bid·i·ty (tur·bid'i·tee) *n.* [ML. *turbiditas*, from L. *turbidus*, turbid, confused]. The characteristic of being turbid.

tur·bi·nal (tur'bi·nul) *adj.* TURBINATE.

tur·bi·nate (tur'bin·ut, ·ate) *adj.* & *n.* [NL. *turbinatus*, from *turbo, turbinis*, top, spindle]. 1. Shaped like a top. 2. NASAL CONCHA. 3. Pertaining to a concha.

turbinate crest. CONCHAL CREST.

tur·bi·nat·ed (tur'bi·nay"tid) *adj.* Top-shaped; scroll-shaped.

tur·bi·nec·to·my (tur"bi·neck'tuh·mee) *n.* [*turbin*al + *-ectomy*]. Excision of a nasal concha.

tur·bi·no·tome (tur'bi·no·tome) *n.* An instrument used in turbinotomy.

tur·bi·not·o·my (tur"bi·not'uh·mee) *n.* [*turbin*al + *-tomy*]. Cutting of a turbinated bone.

tur·bu·lent flow. The occurrence of eddies and vortices within fluid that has exceeded critical velocity, as in arterial blood flow. Compare *streamline flow.*

Türck's bundle (tuerk) [L. *Türck*, Austrian neurologist and laryngologist, 1810–1868]. TEMPOROPONTINE TRACT.

Türck's column [L. *Türck*]. The direct corticospinal tract.

Türck's trachoma [L. *Türck*]. *Obsol.* DRY LARYNGITIS.

tur·ges·cense (tur·jes'unce) *n.* [L. *turgescere*, to begin to swell, to be swelling, from *turgere*, to be swollen]. Swelling.

tur·ges·cent (tur·jes'unt) *adj.* [L. *turgescens*, from *turgescere*, to be swelling]. Becoming or being swollen, tumid.

tur·gid (tur'jid) *adj.* [L. *turgidus,* from *turgere,* to be swollen]. 1. Swollen. 2. CONGESTED.
tur·gor (tur'gur) *n.* [L., from L. *turgere,* to be swollen]. Active hyperemia; turgescence.
turgor vi·ta·lis (vye·tay'lis). The normal fullness of the capillaries.
Türk cell (tuerk) [W. *Türk,* Austrian physician, 1871-1916]. An abnormal cell of the peripheral blood closely resembling a plasma cell in nuclear placement and cytoplasmic staining, but having a chromatin pattern roughly intermediate between a lymphocyte and plasma cell.
Turk·el and Beth·ell needle. An instrument that consists of an outer guiding, or splitting, needle and an inner trephine needle and a stylet for bone-marrow biopsy or for the infusion of solutions into the marrow.
Turk·ish bath. A bath in which the bather is placed in steam rooms or cabinets of successively higher temperature, then is rubbed and massaged and finally stimulated by a cold shower.
Turkish manna. TREHALA.
Turkish pepper. PAPRIKA.
Turkish saber syndrome. SCIMITAR SYNDROME.
Türk's irritation cell or **leukocyte** [W. *Türk*]. TÜRK CELL.
Tur·ling·ton's balsam. COMPOUND BENZOIN TINCTURE.
Turloc. Trademark for meturedepa, an antineoplastic agent.
tur·mer·ic (tur'mur·ick) *n.* [OF. *terre merite,* lit., meritorious earth]. CURCUMA.
turn, *v.* [L. *tornare,* to turn in a lathe]. 1. To cause to revolve about an axis. 2. To change the position of the fetus so as to facilitate delivery.
Tur·ner's sign [G. G. *Turner,* English surgeon, 1877-1951]. Local discoloration of the abdominal wall in the flanks as a sign of acute pancreatitis.
Tur·ner's syndrome [H. H. *Turner,* U.S. physician, b. 1892]. GONADAL DYSGENESIS.
Turner's tooth. Hypoplasia, usually of a single tooth, most commonly involving the permanent maxillary incisor or a premolar.
turn·ing *n.* VERSION (1).
turn·over number. An expression of enzyme activity designating the number of molecules of substrate modified per molecule of enzyme per minute.
TURP Transurethral resection of the prostate.
tur·pen·tine (tur'pun·tine) *n.* [L. *terebinthina,* from Gk. *terebinthos,* terebinth]. 1. A concrete or liquid oleoresin obtained from coniferous trees. 2. The concrete oleoresin from *Pinus palustris* and other species of *Pinus.* Yellow-orange, opaque masses of characteristic odor and taste; contains a volatile oil. Has been used for local irritant effect. Syn. *gum thus, gum turpentine.*
turpentine oil. The volatile oil distilled from turpentine; consists essentially of terpenes, principally varieties of pinene. The rectified oil has been used as a stimulant expectorant in chronic bronchitis, a carminative in flatulent colic, and externally as a rubefacient. Syn. *turpentine spirits.*
tur·ri·ceph·a·ly (tur''i·sef'uh·lee) *n.* [L. *turris,* tower, + *-cephaly*]. OXYCEPHALY.
tur·tle-neck nail. Marked distortion of the nail with exaggerated convexity.
tusk, *n.* A large, projecting tooth; in man, usually an upper canine tooth; in animals, a tooth that projects outside the mouth, as in the elephant, walrus, or boar.
tus·se·do (tuh·see'do) *n.* [L.]. TUSSIS.
tus·sic·u·la·tion (tuh·sick''yoo·lay'shun) *n.* A hacking cough.
Tus·si·la·go (tus''i·lay'go) *n.* [L., coltsfoot]. A genus of plants of the Compositae. The leaves of *Tussilago farfara,* coltsfoot, and also other parts of the plant have been used as a demulcent in the treatment of cough.
tus·sis (tus'is) *n.* [L., from *tussire,* to cough]. COUGH.
tussis con·vul·si·va (kon''vul·sigh'vuh). PERTUSSIS.
tus·sive (tus'iv) *adj.* [from *tussis*]. Pertaining to, or caused by, a cough.
tussive fremitus. A thrill felt by the hand when applied to the chest of a person coughing.
tussive syndrome or **syncope.** COUGH SYNCOPE.
Tut·hill's method. BUTLER AND TUTHILL'S METHOD.
Tut·tle operation [J. P. *Tuttle,* U.S. surgeon, 1857-1913]. A one-stage operation for rectal cancer.
Tuttle's proctoscope [J. P. *Tuttle*]. A rectal speculum with an electric light and a device for inflation of the rectum.
T wave of the electrocardiogram. The electrocardiographic deflection due to repolarization of the ventricles; it may be positive, negative, or both in succession. Syn. *ventricular repolarization complex.*
Tween. Trademark for any of several polysorbate fatty acid esters individually identified by appending a number to the trademark; the substances are surfactants.
Tween 80. Trademark for polysorbate 80, a surfactant.
tweez·ers, *n.pl.* [F. *étui,* instrument case]. Delicate surgical forceps that are capable of seizing without crushing easily damaged structures, as nerves; they are also used for removing eyelashes or hairs.
twelfth (XIIth) cranial nerve. HYPOGLOSSAL NERVE.
twelve-year molars. The second permanent molars.
twig, *n.* A small branch, especially a nerve filament, or an arteriole.
twi·light sleep. *In obstetrics,* an injection of scopolamine and morphine to produce amnesia and analgesia.
twilight state. DREAMY STATE.
twin, *n.* One of two born at the same birth.
twin brain. SPLIT BRAIN.
twinge, *n.* A sudden short, sharp pain.
Twi·ning's line [E. W. *Twining,* British radiologist, 20th century]. *In radiology,* a line extending from the tuberculum sellae to the internal occipital protuberance, the midpoint of which normally falls within the rostral aspect of the fourth ventricle.
twin·ning, *n.* 1. Production of like structures by division. 2. The occurrence of twin pregnancies.
twin pregnancy. Gestation with two fetuses.
Twiston. Trademark for rotoxamine, an antihistaminic drug.
twitch, *n.* 1. A brief phasic contraction of a muscle fiber or the short, sudden, visible contractile response of a small muscular unit to a single maximal stimulus. 2. A spasmodic jerk of a muscle or group of muscles.
two-glass test. GLASS TEST.
two-joint muscle. A muscle that crosses two joints and effects the movements at each joint.
two-layered ectoderm. The epidermis of young embryos, consisting of a germinal layer and the epitrichium.
two-point discrimination or **sensibility.** The ability to discriminate between two punctate stimuli applied simultaneously to the skin. The minimal separation at which discrimination is possible is proportional to the distance between the points, and varies in different skin areas.
two-stage amputation. An amputation of an extremity performed in two stages because of infection or dangerous ischemia. In the first stage, a circular amputation is performed with the flaps left open. In the second stage, after infection has been controlled or circulation has improved, the stump is repaired and closed.
two-stage method. A method of determination of plasma prothrombic activity by the addition of thromboplastin and calcium to decalcified and defibrinated plasma (first stage) and the estimation of the thrombin which evolves by the addition of fibrinogen (second stage).
two-step test. Repeated ascents over two 9-inch steps as a simple exercise test of cardiovascular function. Syn. *Master's two-step test.*
two-way catheter. A double-current uterine catheter. Syn. *Bozeman's catheter.*
ty·bam·ate (tye·bam'ate) *n.* 2-(Hydroxymethyl)-2-methyl-

pentyl butylcarbamate carbamate, $C_{13}H_{26}N_2O_4$, a tranquilizer.

ty·lec·to·my (tye·leck'tuh·mee) *n.* [Gk. *tylos*, knot, + *-ectomy*]. Excision of a lump of tissue.

tyl·i·on (til'ee·on, tye'lee·on) *n.*, pl. **tyl·ia** (·ee·uh) [Gk. *tylē*, a swelling, + *-ion*]. *In craniometry,* a point in the midline on the anterior border of the optic or chiasmatic groove.

ty·lo·ma (tye·lo'muh) *n.* [Gk. *tylōma,* from *tylos,* callus]. CALLOSITY.

ty·lo·sis (tye·lo'sis) *n.*, pl. **tylo·ses** (·seez) [Gk. *tylōsis,* a making callous, from *tylos,* callus]. 1. A localized patch of hyperkeratotic skin due to chronic pressure and friction. 2. A form of blepharitis with thickening and hardening of the edge of the lid. **—ty·lot·ic** (·lot'ick) *adj.*

tylosis pal·ma·ris et plan·ta·ris (pal·mair'is et plan·tair'is). KERATOSIS PALMARIS ET PLANTARIS.

ty·lox·a·pol (tye·lock'suh·pol) *n.* Oxyethylated *tert*-octylphenol formaldehyde polymer, a detergent.

tympan-, tympano-. A combining form meaning (a) *tympanum, tympanic;* (b) *tympanites, tympanitic.*

tym·pa·nal (tim'puh·nul) *adj.* TYMPANIC.

tym·pa·nec·to·my (tim''puh·neck'tuh·mee) *n.* [*tympan-* + *-ectomy*]. Excision of the tympanic membrane.

tym·pan·ia (tim·pan'ee·uh) *n.* TYMPANITES.

tym·pan·ic (tim·pan'ick) *adj.* [*tympan-* + *-ic*]. 1. Of, pertaining to, or associated with the tympanum. 2. RESONANT.

tympanic antrum. MASTOID ANTRUM.

tympanic bulla. The bullous accessory tympanic bone housing an expansion of the cavity of the middle ear; found in certain mammals but not in humans.

tympanic canaliculus. A small canal that opens on the lower surface of the petrous portion of the temporal bone between the carotid canal and the jugular fossa. It gives passage to the tympanic branch of the glossopharyngeal nerve. NA *canaliculus tympanicus.*

tympanic cavity. The cavity of the middle ear; an irregular, air-containing, mucous membrane–lined space in the temporal bone. The chain of auditory ossicles extends from its lateral wall, the tympanic membrane, to its medial wall, the bony labyrinth. It communicates anteriorly with the nasopharynx through the auditory tube and posterosuperiorly with the mastoid cells through the mastoid antrum. NA *cavum tympani.* See also Plate 20.

tympanic cell. MASTOID CELL.

tympanic covering layer. The connective-tissue layer covering the lower surface of the basilar membrane of the cochlea.

tympanic ganglion. A small swelling of the tympanic nerve. NA *ganglion tympanicum.*

tympanic incisure. TYMPANIC NOTCH.

tympanic lip. The upper margin of the internal spiral sulcus in the cochlea.

tympanic membrane. The membrane separating the external from the middle ear. It consists of three layers: an outer or skin layer, a fibrous layer, and an inner mucous layer. Syn. *eardrum.* NA *membrana tympani.* See also Plate 20.

tympanic nerve. A visceral sensory and parasympathetic nerve attached to the glossopharyngeal. It innervates the mucosa of the middle ear, mastoid air cells, and auditory tube, and sends filaments to the otic ganglion and parotid gland. NA *nervus tympanicus.* See also Table of Nerves in the Appendix.

tympanic neuralgia. Neuralgia in the distribution of the tympanic branch of the glossopharyngeal nerve, manifested by pain in the ear and neck.

tympanic notch. The gap in the tympanic sulcus occupied by the flaccid, highest portion of the tympanic membrane. NA *incisura tympanica.*

tympanic plate. The bony sides and floor of the external auditory meatus.

tympanic plexus. A nerve network formed by the tympanic branch of the glossopharyngeal and tympanopetrosal branches of the facial and sympathetic nerves derived from the internal carotid plexus. NA *plexus tympanicus.*

tympanic ring. At the time of birth, an incomplete osseous ring that develops into the tympanic part of the temporal bone. NA *anulus tympanicus.*

tympanic sinus. A deep recess in the labyrinthine wall of the tympanic cavity whose inferior border is formed by the subiculum promontorii. NA *sinus tympani.*

tympanic sulcus. The groove in the osseous portion of the external auditory meatus in which the circumference of the tympanic membrane is attached; it is deficient superiorly at the tympanic notch. NA *sulcus tympanicus.*

tympanic trephine. An instrument made of a small steel shaft ending in a small, polished tube, 2 mm in diameter, with a cutting edge.

tym·pa·nism (tim'puh·niz·um) *n.* [*tympan-* + *-ism*]. Distention with gas; TYMPANITES.

tym·pa·ni·tes (tim''puh·nigh'teez) *n.* [Gk. *tympanitēs,* from *tympanon,* drum]. A distention of the abdomen from accumulation of gas in the intestine or peritoneal cavity.

tym·pa·nit·ic (tim''puh·nit'ick) *adj.* [*tympanites* + *-ic*]. 1. Caused by, or of the nature of, tympanites. 2. Tympanic or resonant to percussion.

tympanitic abscess. An abscess containing gas. Syn. *abscessus flatuosus, gas abscess.*

tympanitic resonance. 1. The prolonged musical sound heard on percussion over an air-containing cavity with flexible walls. Its sounds vary widely in pitch. 2. A percussion note which exhibits in varying proportion the characteristics of both resonance and tympany. Syn. *bandbox resonance, Skoda's resonance.*

tym·pa·ni·tis (tim''puh·nigh'tis) *n.* [*tympan-* + *-itis*]. Inflammation of the tympanum; OTITIS MEDIA.

tympano-. See *tympan-.*

tym·pa·no·mas·toid (tim''puh·no·mas'toid) *adj.* [*tympano-* + *mastoid*]. Pertaining to the tympanum and the mastoid process or the mastoid cells.

tym·pa·no·mas·toid·itis (tim''puh·no·mas''toy·dye'tis) *n.* [*tympano-* + *mastoid* + *-itis*]. Inflammation of the tympanum and mastoid cells.

tym·pa·no·plas·ty (tim'puh·no·plas''tee) *n.* [*tympano-* + *-plasty*]. 1. Surgical repair of the eardrum. 2. Surgical repair of the eardrum and reconstruction of the bony pathway of the middle ear.

tym·pa·no·scle·ro·sis (tim''puh·no·skle·ro'sis) *n.* [*tympano-* + *sclerosis*]. Fibrosis and sclerosis of the mucous membrane of the middle ear secondary to infection.

tym·pa·no·sis (tim''puh·no'sis) *n.* [*tympan-* + *-osis*]. TYMPANITES.

tym·pa·no·squa·mous (tim''puh·no·skway'mus) *adj.* Pertaining to the tympanic and squamous parts of the temporal bone.

tympanosquamous suture. FISSURA TYMPANOSQUAMOSA.

tym·pa·no·sta·pe·di·al (tim''puh·no·stay·pee'dee·ul) *adj.* [*tympano-* + *stapedial*]. Pertaining to the tympanum and stapes.

tympanostapedial syndesmosis. The joint between the foot plate of the stapes and fenestra vestibuli. NA *syndesmosis tympanostapedia.*

tym·pa·not·o·my (tim''puh·not'uh·mee) *n.* [*tympano-* + *-tomy*]. MYRINGOTOMY.

tym·pa·nous (tim'puh·nus) *adj.* [*tympan-* + *-ous*]. Distended with gas; pertaining to tympanism.

tym·pa·num (tim'puh·num) *n., genit.* **tympa·ni** (·nye), pl. **tym·pa·na** (·nuh) [ML., from Gk. *tympanon,* drum]. MIDDLE EAR.

tym·pa·ny (tim'puh·nee) *n.* 1. TYMPANITES. 2. A tympanitic percussion note. 3. BLOAT (2).

Tyn·dall effect (tin'dul) [J. *Tyndall,* English physicist, 1820–1893]. The scattering of a beam of light by small particles suspended in a liquid or gas, thereby rendering the path of the beam luminous. The diffused light often appears blue.

Tyn·dal·li·za·tion (tin″dul·i·zay′shun) *n.* [J. *Tyndall*]. Fractional sterilization by the use of steam at atmospheric pressure. A sufficient period is permitted to elapse between treatments to allow spores of microorganisms to germinate.

Tyndall phenomenon [J. *Tyndall*]. TYNDALL EFFECT.

typ-, typo- [Gk. *typos*]. A combining form meaning *image, model.*

type, *n. & v.* [Gk. *typos,* impression]. 1. A category or subcategory based on specified characteristics. 2. An example of such a category taken as a standard. 3. *In pathology,* the grouping of the distinguishing features of a fever, disease, etc., whereby it is referred to its proper class. 4. *In bacteriology,* members of a species having some further characteristic in common. 5. To identify or classify, as a blood group or a bacterial culture.

type A encephalitis. *Obsol.* ENCEPHALITIS LETHARGICA.

type B encephalitis. *Obsol.* JAPANESE B ENCEPHALITIS.

type C encephalitis. *Obsol.* ST. LOUIS ENCEPHALITIS.

type I of Cori [C. F. *Cori* and Gerty T. *Cori*]. VON GIERKE'S DISEASE.

type II of Cori [C. F. *Cori* and Gerty T. *Cori*]. POMPE'S DISEASE.

type III of Cori [C. F. *Cori* and Gerty T. *Cori*]. LIMIT DEXTRINOSIS.

type IV of Cori [C. F. *Cori* and Gerty T. *Cori*]. AMYLOPECTINOSIS.

type V of Cori [C. F. *Cori* and Gerty T. *Cori*]. MCARDLE'S DISEASE.

type VI of Cori [C. F. *Cori* and Gerty T. *Cori*]. HERS' DISEASE.

typh-, typho-. A combining form meaning (a) *typhus;* (b) *typhoid.*

typhl-, typhlo- [Gk. *typhlos*]. A combining form meaning (a) *blind, blindness;* (b) *cecum.*

typh·la·to·nia (tif″luh·to′nee·uh) *n.* TYPHLATONY.

typh·lat·o·ny (tif·lat′uh·nee) *n.* [*typhl-,* cecum, + *atony*]. An atonic condition of the wall of the cecum.

typh·lec·ta·sia (tif″leck·tay′zhuh, ·zee·uh) *n.* [*typhl-,* cecum, + *ectasia*]. Dilatation of the cecum.

typh·lec·to·my (tif·leck′tuh·mee) *n.* [*typhl-,* cecum, + *-ectomy*]. Excision of the cecum.

typh·len·ter·i·tis (tif·len″tur·eye′tis) *n.* [*typhl-* + *enteritis*]. CECITIS.

typh·li·tis (tif·lye′tis) *n.* [*typhl-,* cecum, + *-itis*]. CECITIS.

typhlo-. See *typhl-.*

typh·lo·cele (tif′lo·seel) *n.* [*typhlo-,* cecum, + *-cele*]. CECOCELE.

typh·lo·dic·li·di·tis (tif″lo·dick″li·dye′tis, ·dye″kli·) *n.* [*typhlo-* + Gk. *diklis,* double-folding, + *-itis*]. Inflammation of the ileocecal valve.

typh·lo·em·py·e·ma (tif″lo·em″pye·ee′muh) *n.* [*typhlo-,* cecum, + *empyema*]. Abscess attending cecitis or appendicitis.

typh·lo·en·ter·i·tis (tif″lo·en″tur·eye′tis) *n.* [*typhlo-* + *enteritis*]. CECITIS.

typh·loid (tif′loid) *adj.* [*typhl-,* blind, + *-oid*]. Having defective vision.

typh·lo·lex·ia (tif″lo·leck′see·uh) *n.* [*typhlo-,* blind, + *-lexia*]. *Obsol.* ALEXIA.

typh·lo·li·thi·a·sis (tif″lo·li·thigh′uh·sis) *n.* [*typhlo-,* cecum, + *lithiasis*]. The formation of calculi in the cecum.

typh·lo·meg·a·ly (tif″lo·meg′uh·lee) *n.* [*typhlo-,* cecum, + *-megaly*]. Enlargement or hypertrophy of the cecum.

typh·lo·pto·sis (tif″lo·to′sis, tif″lop·to′sis) *n.* [*typhlo-* + *-ptosis*]. Downward displacement or prolapse of the cecum.

typh·lo·sis (tif·lo′sis) *n.* [*typhl-,* blind, + *-osis*]. BLINDNESS.

typh·lo·sole (tif′lo·sole) *n.* [*typhlo-,* cecum, + Gk. *sōlēn,* channel]. A longitudinal internal ridge or fold of the dorsal intestinal wall of certain worms, such as the common earthworm, and of certain cyclostomes.

typh·lo·spasm (tif′lo·spaz·um) *n.* [*typhlo-,* cecum, + *spasm*]. Spasm of the cecum.

typh·lo·ste·no·sis (tif″lo·ste·no′sis) *n.* [*typhlo-* + *stenosis*]. Stenosis of the cecum.

typh·los·to·my (tif·los′tuh·mee) *n.* [*typhlo-,* cecum, + *-stomy*]. A cecal colostomy.

typho-. See *typh-.*

ty·pho·ba·cil·lo·sis of Landouzy (tye″fo·bas·il·o′sis). Fulminating septicemia caused by *Mycobacterium tuberculosis,* without the formation of miliary tubercles.

ty·pho·bac·ter·in (tye″fo·back′tur·in) *n.* [*typho-* + *bacterin*]. A vaccine prepared from the typhoid bacillus.

ty·phoid (tye′foid) *adj. & n.* [*typh*us + *-oid*]. 1. Resembling typhus fever, as: typhoid fever. 2. TYPHOID FEVER. 3. Of or pertaining to typhoid fever; typhoidal.

ty·phoid·al (tye·foy′dul) *adj.* Of or pertaining to typhoid fever.

typhoid bacillus. *SALMONELLA TYPHOSA.*

typhoid fever. An acute systemic infection caused by *Salmonella typhosa;* characterized clinically by fever, headache, cough, toxemia, abnormal pulse, rose spots on the skin, leukopenia, and bacteremia and pathologically by hyperplasia and ulceration of intestinal lymph follicles, mesenteric lymphadenopathy, and splenomegaly.

typhoid nodules. Characteristic lesions found in the liver after fatal typhoid.

typhoid-paratyphoid A and B vaccine. A vaccine containing organisms of typhoid, and paratyphoid A and B strains, for simultaneous immunization against all three diseases. Abbreviated, T.A.B. vaccine.

typhoid roseola. ROSE SPOTS.

typhoid spots. ROSE SPOTS.

typhoid state. A condition of stupor and hebetude, with dry, brown tongue, sordes on the teeth, rapid, feeble pulse, incontinence of feces and urine, and rapid wasting; seen in typhoid fever and other continued fevers.

typhoid vaccine. A sterile suspension of killed typhoid bacilli (*Salmonella typhosa*) of a strain selected for high antigenic efficiency. The vaccine contains not less than 1 billion typhoid organisms in each milliliter. An active immunizing agent against typhoid fever.

ty·pho·ma·lar·i·al (tye″fo·muh·lăr′ee·ul) *adj.* Of malarial origin, with symptoms that resemble typhoid.

typhomalarial fever. Malaria with symptoms resembling those of typhoid fever.

ty·pho·pneu·mo·nia (tye″fo·new·mo′nyuh) *n.* [*typho-* + *pneumonia*]. PNEUMOTYPHUS.

ty·phus (tye′fus) *n.* [Gk. *typhos,* fever]. TYPHUS FEVER.

typhus ex·an·thé·ma·tique (eg·zahn·tay·ma·teek′). EPIDEMIC TYPHUS.

typhus fever. An acute infectious disease caused by a rickettsia and characterized by severe headache, sustained high fever, generalized macular or maculopapular rash, and termination by lysis in about 2 weeks. See also *epidemic typhus, Brill-Zinsser disease, murine typhus.*

typhus nodule. A focal collection of lymphocytes, plasmacytes, and large mononuclear cells around or near small blood vessels; a common feature of rickettsial diseases. Syn. *Fraenkel's nodule.*

typhus vaccine. 1. COX VACCINE. 2. CASTAÑEDA VACCINE.

typ·i·cal (tip′i·kul) *adj.* [Gk. *typikos,* from *typos,* replica, impression]. 1. Constituting a characteristic type or form for comparison. 2. Illustrative. 3. Complete.

typo-. See *typ-.*

ty·po·scope (tye′puh·skope) *n.* A small device to exclude extraneous light, for the use of cataract patients and amblyopes in reading.

ty·pus de·gen·e·ra·ti·vus am·ste·lo·da·men·sis (tye′pus de·jen″e·ruh·tye′vus am″ste·lo·da·men′sis). CORNELIA DE LANGE'S SYNDROME (1).

tyr-, tyro- [Gk. *tyros*]. A combining form meaning *cheese* or *cheeselike substance.*

tyr·an·nism (tirr′uh·niz·um) *n.* [Gk. *tyrannos,* tyrant, + *-ism*].

Cruelty of abnormal inception, of which sadism is an erotic variety.

ty·ra·mine (tye'ruh·meen) *n.* 4-Hydroxyphenethylamine, $HOC_6H_4CH_2NH_2$, a decarboxylation product of tyrosine; occurs in putrefied animal tissue, ripe cheese, and ergot. Has been used as a sympathomimetic agent. Syn. *tyrosamine.*

ty·rem·e·sis (tye·rem'e·sis) *n.* [*tyr-* + *emesis*]. The vomiting of caseous or curdy matter, often seen in infants.

tyro-. See *tyr-.*

ty·ro·ci·dine, ty·ro·ci·din (tye"ro·sigh'din) *n.* An antibiotic substance that is a major component of tyrothricin.

Ty·rode solution [M. V. *Tyrode,* U.S. pharmacologist, 1878–1930]. A solution containing sodium chloride, calcium chloride, potassium chloride, sodium bicarbonate, glucose, magnesium chloride, and sodium diphosphate; used in certain pharmacological experiments.

ty·rog·e·nous (tye·roj'e·nus) *adj.* [*tyro-* + *-genous*]. Produced by or in cheese.

Ty·rog·ly·phus (tye·rog'li·fus, tye"ro·glif'us) *n.* [NL., from *tyro-* + Gk. *glyphein,* to carve]. A genus of sarcoptoid mites that usually infest dried vegetable products, cheese, and dead or living plants. Occasionally, they produce a temporary pruritus which is named by the occupation of the host. *Tyroglyphus farinor* causes grocer's itch; *T. siro* causes vanillism among handlers of vanilla pods; and *T. longior* causes copra itch and grocer's itch.

ty·roid (tye'roid) *adj.* [*tyr-* + *-oid*]. Cheeselike.

ty·ro·pa·no·ate (tye"ro·pa·no'ate) *n.* 3-Butyramido-α-ethyl-2,4,6-triiodohydrocinnamate, $C_{15}H_{18}I_3NO_3$, a cholecystographic diagnostic aid; radiopaque medium.

ty·ros·a·mine (tye·ros'uh·meen) *n.* TYRAMINE.

tyro·sin·ase (tye'ro·sin·ace, ·aze, tirr'o·) *n.* A copper-containing enzyme found in plants, molds, crustaceans, mollusks, and some bacteria. In the presence of oxygen, it causes the oxidation of monophenols and polyphenols with the introduction of —OH groups and/or formation of quinones.

ty·ro·sine (tye'ro·seen, ·sin) *n.* [Gk. *tyros,* cheese, + *-ine*]. β-*p*-Hydroxyphenylalanine, $C_9H_{11}NO_3$, an amino acid widely distributed in proteins; a precursor of epinephrine, thyroxine, and melanin.

tyro·sin·emia, tyro·si·nae·mia (tye"ro·si·nee'mee·uh) *n.* [*tyrosine* + *-emia*]. An inborn error of metabolism in which there is a deficiency of *p*-hydroxyphenylpyruvic acid oxidase with abnormally high blood levels of tyrosine and sometimes methionine, increased urinary excretion of *p*-hydroxyphenylpyruvic, acetic, and lactic acids and sometimes methionine; manifested clinically by hepatic cirrhosis, mild generalized aminoaciduria, renal glycosuria, and renal rickets. See also *tyrosinosis.*

ty·ro·sin·osis (tye"ro·si·no'sis) *n.* [*tyrosine* + *-osis*]. 1. Excretion in the urine of unusual amounts of tyrosine and of its first oxidation products. 2. A transient deficiency of the enzyme *p*-hydroxyphenylpyruvic oxidase in early life, resulting in tyrosinuria as a part of a generalized aminoaciduria; clinically similar to phenylketonuria; the infant may exhibit seizures, gastrointestinal disturbances, failure to thrive, and unless treated by diet, mental retardation. See also *tyrosinemia.*

tyro·sin·uria (tye"ro·sin·yoo'ree·uh) *n.* [*tyrosine* + *-uria*]. The presence of tyrosine in the urine.

tyro·syl (tye'ro·sil) *n.* The univalent radical, *p*-$HOC_6H_4CH_2$-$CH(NH_2)CO$—, of the amino acid tyrosine.

ty·ro·thri·cin (tye"ro·thrigh'sin) *n.* A polypeptide mixture produced by the growth of *Bacillus brevis* and consisting of the antibiotic substances gramicidin and tyrocidine; used as an antibacterial applied locally in infections due to gram-positive organisms.

Ty·son's glands [E. *Tyson,* English physician and anatomist, 1649–1708]. Sebaceous glands of the prepuce which secrete the smegma.

Tyzine. Trademark for tetrahydrozoline, a vasoconstrictor used as the hydrochloride salt for relief of nasal congestion.

Tyz·zer's disease [L. E. *Tyzzer,* U.S. pathologist, 1875–1965]. A fatal infection of animals due to *Actinobacillus piliformis* (*Bacillus piliformis*) originally described in Japanese waltzing mice.

Tzanck test (tsa^hn'k) [A. *Tzanck,* Russian dermatologist, 1886–1954]. The demonstration of degenerative changes in epidermal cells in bullae of pemphigus by microscopic examination of a smear made from the base of an early intact bulla and stained with Giemsa stain.

U

U 1. Symbol for uranium. 2. *In molecular biology,* a symbol for uracil.

U. Abbreviation for *unit.*

uber·ty (yoo'bur·tee) *n.* [L. *ubertas,* from *uber,* fertile]. Fertility; productiveness. **—uber·ous** (·us) *adj.*

ubi·qui·none (yoo·bick'wi·nohn, yoo''bi·kwi·nohn') *n.* Any of a group of lipid-soluble compounds that have a 2,3-dimethoxy-5-methylbenzoquinone nucleus with a variable substituent containing 1 to 10 terpene-like units and that function as electron carriers in the mitochondrial electron transport system. Syn. *coenzyme Q, mitoquinone.*

ud·der, *n.* The mammary gland of the cow and other animals.

UDPG–glycogen transglucosidase. Uridine diphosphate glucose–glycogen glucosyl transferase, an enzyme important in the metabolism of glycogen that catalyzes the reaction nUDP-glucose $\rightleftharpoons$ (glucose)n + n(UDP). Syn. *glycogen synthetase.*

UDP-glucose. URIDINE DIPHOSPHOGLUCOSE.

Uf·fel·mann's test (ōōf'el·mahn) [J. A. C. *Uffelmann,* German physician, 1837–1894]. A test for lactic acid in which a reagent consisting of ferric chloride solution and phenol is added to gastric juice. Lactic acid produces a canary yellow color, whereas hydrochloric acid decolorizes the reagent.

Uhl's anomaly [H.S.M. *Uhl,* U.S. internist, b. 1921]. Marked congenital hypoplasia of the right atrial and ventricular myocardium. Syn. *parchment heart.*

¹ul-, ule-, ulo- [Gk. *oulē*]. A combining form meaning *scar.*

²ul-, ule-, ulo- [Gk. *oulon*]. A combining form meaning *gums, gingival.*

ula (yoo'luh) *n.pl.* [Gk. *oula,* pl. of *oulon,* gum]. GINGIVA.

ul·cer (ul'sur) *n.* [L. *ulcus, ulceris*]. An interruption of continuity of an epithelial surface, with an inflamed base.

ul·cer·ate (ul'sur·ate) *v.* [L. *ulcerare,* to make sore]. To become converted into, or affected with, an ulcer.

ul·cer·a·tion (ul''sur·ay'shun) *n.* [L. *ulceratio*]. The process of formation of an ulcer.

ul·cer·a·tive (ul'sur·uh·tiv) *adj.* Pertaining to, or characterized by, ulceration.

ulcerative blepharitis. Marginal blepharitis with ulceration of the eyelids.

ulcerative colitis. An inflammatory disease of unknown etiology involving primarily the mucosa and submucosa of the colon. It is peculiar to man and not contagious; manifested clinically by abdominal pain, diarrhea, and rectal bleeding. Compare *granulomatous colitis.*

ulcerative stomatitis. Stomatitis characterized by the formation of ulcers and necrosis of oral tissues.

Ulcerban. A trademark for sucralfate, an antiulcerative.

ulcero-. A combining form meaning *ulcer, ulcerous.*

ul·cero·gen·ic (ul''sur·o·jen'ick) *adj.* [*ulcero-* + *-genic*]. Tending to produce ulcers.

ul·cero·glan·du·lar (ul''sur·o·glan'dew·lur) *adj.* [*ulcero-* + *glandular*]. Tending to produce ulcers and involve lymph nodes; said of one form of tularemia.

ul·cero·mem·bra·nous (ul''sur·o·mem'bruh·nus) *adj.* [*ulcero-* + *membranous*]. Pertaining to, or characterized by, ulceration, and accompanied by fibrinous inflammation with accompanying formation of a false membrane.

ulceromembranous gingivitis. NECROTIZING ULCERATIVE GINGIVITIS.

ul·cer·ous (ul'sur·us) *adj.* Characterized by or pertaining to ulcers.

ul·cus (ul'kus) *n.,* pl. **ul·cera** (·sur·uh) [L.]. ULCER.

ulcus can·cro·sum (kang·kro'sum). 1. CANCER. 2. BASAL CELL CARCINOMA.

ulcus cru·ris (kroo'ris). Indolent ulcer of the leg.

ulcus ex·e·dens (eck'se·denz). BASAL CELL CARCINOMA.

ulcus in·du·ra·tus (in·dew·ray'tus). CHANCRE.

ulcus mol·le (mol'ee). CHANCROID.

ulcus ro·dens (ro'denz). BASAL CELL CARCINOMA.

ulcus ser·pens (sur'penz). 1. SERPIGINOUS ULCER. 2. An irritating, purulent ulcer of the cornea, often caused by pneumococci.

ulcus tu·ber·cu·lo·sum (tew·bur''kew·lo'sum). LUPUS VULGARIS.

ulcus ve·ne·re·um (ve·neer'ee·um). 1. CHANCRE. 2. CHANCROID.

ulcus ven·tric·u·li (ven·trick'yoo·lye). GASTRIC ULCER.

ulcus vul·vae acu·tum (vul'vee a·kew'tum). A condition of one or more erosive ulcers on the external genitalia of young girls. The cause is not known; *Bacillus crassus* is implicated by some. Aphthae, herpes simplex, and erythema multiforme enter into the differential diagnosis.

ul·da·ze·pam (ul·day'ze·pam) *n.* 2-[(Allyloxy)amino]-7-chloro-5-(*o*-chlorophenyl)-3*H*-1,4-benzodiazepine, $C_{18}H_{15}Cl_2N_3O$, a tranquilizer.

ule-. See *ul-.*

ule·gy·ria (yoo''le·jye'ree·uh) *n.* [*ule-,* scar, + *gyr-* + *-ia*]. Shrinkage and sclerosis of individual gyri or groups of gyri, with preservation of the general convolutional pattern of the cerebral cortex. Characteristically, there is destruction of the lower parts of the walls of the convolution, with relative sparing of the crown.

uler·y·the·ma (yoo·lerr''i·theem'uh) *n.* [*ul-,* scar, + *erythema*]. An erythematous skin disease marked by the formation of cicatrices.

ulerythema cen·trif·u·gum (sen·trif'yoo·gum). LUPUS ERYTHEMATOSUS.

ulerythema oph·ry·og·e·nes (off·ree·oj'e·neez). Ulerythema of the eyebrows with loss of hair.

ulerythema sy·co·si·for·me (sigh·ko''si·for'mee). KELOID SYCOSIS.

ulet·ic (yoo·let'ick) *adj.* [*ule-* + *-ic*]. Pertaining to the gums.

ulex·ine (yoo·leck'seen) *n.* CYTISINE.

uli·tis (yoo·lye'tis) *n.* [*ul-*, gums, + *-itis*]. A generalized inflammation of the gums.

Ull·rich-Turner syndrome (ŏŏl'rikh) [O. *Ullrich* and H. H. *Turner*]. Webbing of the neck, short stature, cubitus valgus, and hypogonadism in the male. Syn. *male Turner's syndrome.*

ul·mus (ul'mus) *n.* [L., elm]. The inner bark of *Ulmus fulva* (slippery elm); mucilaginous and demulcent; has been used mainly in folk medicine.

ul·na (ul'nuh) *n.*, L. pl. & genit. sing. **ul·nae** (·nee) [L., elbow, forearm (rel. to Gk. *ōlenē* and OE. *eln*boga → *el*bow)] [NA]. The bone on the inner side of the forearm, articulating with the humerus and the head of the radius above and with the radius below. See also Table of Bones in the Appendix and Plate 1. —**ul·nar** (ul'nur) *adj.*

ulnar bursa. The synovial sheath of the tendons of the flexor digitorum superficialis and profundus muscles. NA *vagina synovialis communis musculorum flexorum.*

ulnar carpal collateral ligament. The ulnar collateral ligament of the wrist. See *ulnar collateral ligament.*

ulnar collateral artery. Either of the two branches of the brachial artery which pass through a portion of the upper arm to the rete olecrani; the superior ulnar collateral artery (NA *arteria collateralis ulnaris superior*) or the inferior ulnar collateral artery (NA *arteria collateralis ulnaris inferior*). See also Table of Arteries in the Appendix.

ulnar collateral ligament. 1. (of the elbow:) A triangular ligament on the medial side of the elbow joint attached to the medial epicondyle of the humerus, with an anterior band of fibers passing to the coronoid process of the ulna, a posterior band to the olecranon, and a transverse band connecting the olecranon and the coronoid process. NA *ligamentum collaterale ulnare.* 2. (of the wrist:) A ligament passing from the styloid process of the ulna to the pisiform and triquetral bones. NA *ligamentum collaterale carpi ulnare.*

ulnar eminence of the wrist. EMINENTIA CARPI ULNARIS.

ulnar notch or **incisure.** A depression on the medial surface of the lower end of the radius for articulation with the head of the ulna. NA *incisura ulnaris.*

ul·no·car·pal (ul''no·kahr'pul) *adj.* Of or pertaining to the ulna and the carpus, or wrist.

ul·no·car·pe·us (ul''no·kahr'pee·us) *n.* FLEXOR CARPI ULNARIS BREVIS.

ulo-. See *ul-.*

Ulo. Trademark for chlophedianol, an antitussive drug.

uloc·a·ce (yoo·lock'uh·see) *n.* [*ulo-*, gums, + *-cace*]. Ulcerative inflammation of the gums.

ulo·der·ma·ti·tis (yoo''lo·dur'muh·tye'tis) *n.* [*ulo-* + *dermatitis*]. Inflammation of the skin with formation of cicatrices.

uloid (yoo'loid) *adj.* [*ul-*, scar, + *-oid*]. Scarlike.

ulor·rha·gia (yoo''lo·ray'jee·uh) *n.* [*ulo-*, gums, + *-rrhagia*]. Bleeding from the gums.

ulo·sis (yoo·lo'sis) *n.* [Gk. *oulōsis*, from *oulē*, scar]. CICATRIZATION.

Ulo·so·nia par·vi·cor·nis (yoo''lo·so'nee·uh pahr·vi·kor'nis). A beetle that may act as an intermediate host of *Hymenolepis diminuta*, the rat tapeworm.

ulot·ic (yoo·lot'ick) *adj.* [*ulo-*, scar, + *-ic*]. Pertaining to, or tending toward, cicatrization.

ulot·o·my (yoo·lot'uh·mee) *n.* [*ulo-*, gums, + *-tomy*]. Incision into the gum.

ul·ti·mate (ul'ti·mut) *adj.* [ML. *ultimare, ultimatus*, to come to an end, from L. *ultimus*, final, last]. 1. Final, farthest, extreme. 2. Elemental, basic.

ultimate analysis. Analysis of a compound to determine the proportion of its constituent elements.

ultimate cause. The remote cause which initiated a set of events, such as may culminate in an illness. Contr. *primary cause.*

ul·ti·mo·bran·chi·al (ul''ti·mo·brank'ee·ul) *adj.* [L. *ultim*us, last, + *branchial*]. Pertaining to the caudal pharyngeal or branchial pouch derivatives.

ultimobranchial bodies. Bodies considered by some to be rudimentary fifth pharyngeal pouches, by others, to be lateral thyroid primordia and fourth pouch derivatives. They are the source of the cells in the thyroid gland which produce calcitonin. Syn. *postbranchial bodies, lateral thyroids.*

ul·ti·mo·gen·i·ture (ul''ti·mo·jen'i·chur) *n.* [L. *ultim*us, last, + *genitura*, begetting]. The state of being the last born. —**ultimogeni·tary** (·terr·ee) *adj.*

ul·ti·mum mor·i·ens (ul'ti·mum mor'ee·enz) [L., last dying]. The right atrium, said to be the last part of the body to cease moving in death.

ultra- [L., beyond]. A prefix meaning *beyond, excess.*

ul·tra·brachy·ce·phal·ic (ul''truh·brack''ee·se·fal'ick) *adj.* [*ultra-* + *brachycephalic*]. Having an extremely high cephalic index.

ul·tra·brachy·cra·ni·al (ul''truh·brack''ee·kray'nee·ul) *adj.* [*ultra-* + *brachycranial*]. Having a cranial index of 90.0 or more.

ul·tra·cen·tri·fuge (ul''truh·sen'tri·fewj) *n.* [*ultra-* + *centrifuge*]. A high-speed centrifuge that will produce centrifugal fields up to several hundred thousand times the force of gravity; used for the determination of particle sizes, as in proteins or viruses, and for the analysis of such materials in complex fluids as blood plasma; may be equipped with instrumentation to permit optical observation of the sedimentation of substances in solution. —**ultra·cen·trif·u·gal** (·sen·trif'yoo·gul) *adj.*

ul·tra·di·an (ul·tray'dee·un) *adj.* [ultra- + L. *di*es, day]. Recurring in or manifesting cycles significantly more frequent than once a day. Contr. *circadian, infradian.*

ul·tra·dol·i·cho·cra·ni·al (ul''truh·dol''i·ko·kray'nee·ul) *adj.* [*ultra-* + *dolichocranial*]. Having a cranial index of 64.9 or less.

ul·tra·fil·ter (ul''truh·fil'tur) *n.* [*ultra-* + *filter*]. A filter that will separate colloidal particles from their dispersion mediums and from crystalloids.

ul·tra·fil·tra·tion (ul''truh·fil·tray'shun) *n.* [*ultra-* + *filtration*]. 1. The removal of all but the smallest particles, such as viruses, by filtration. 2. A method for the separation of colloids from their dispersion mediums and dissolved crystalloids by the use of ultrafilters.

ul·tra·mi·cro·scope (ul''truh·migh'kruh·skope) *n.* [*ultra-* + *microscope*]. A light microscope that is equipped to detect or resolve objects not detectable with the conventional light microscope, generally by means of dark-field microscopy. —**ultra·mi·cro·scop·i·cal** (·migh''kruh·skop'i·kul) *adj.*; **ultra·mi·cros·co·py** (·migh·kros'kuh·pee) *n.*

ul·tra·mi·cro·scop·ic (ul''truh·migh''kruh·skop'ick) *adj.* [*ultra-* + *microscopic*]. Undetectable by conventional light microscopy.

Ultran. Trademark for phenaglycodol, a mild neurosedative with muscle-relaxing action.

ul·tra·phago·cy·to·sis (ul''truh·fag''o·sigh·to'sis) *n.* [*ultra-* + *phagocytosis*]. COLLOIDOPEXY.

ul·tra·red (ul''truh·red') *n.* [*ultra-* + *red*]. INFRARED.

ul·tra·son·ic (ul''truh·son'ick) *adj.* [*ultra-* + *son-* + *-ic*]. A term, synonymous with supersonic but more commonly used than the latter in the health and life sciences, describing or pertaining to soundlike waves with a frequency above that of audible sounds, that is, above 20,000 Hz.

ultrasonic pulse. A pulse of ultrasonic energy. See also *ultrasonoscope.*

ultrasonic scaler. A scaler for removal of calculus and stain from the teeth that operates on the principle of high-frequency vibrations.

ultrasonic therapy. Therapy employing ultrasonic energy.

ul·tra·sono·gram (ul″truh·son′o·gram) *n.* [*ultra-* + *sono-* + *-gram*]. ECHOGRAM.

ul·tra·so·nog·ra·phy (ul″truh·so·nog′ruh·fee) *n.* [*ultra-* + *sono-* + *-graphy*]. PULSE-ECHO DIAGNOSIS.

ul·tra·sono·scope (ul″truh·son′o·skope) *n.* [*ultra-* + *sono-* + *-scope*]. An instrument used to detect and locate the position of regions of varying density in a medium by recording the echoes of ultrasonic waves reflected from these regions. The ultrasonic waves, modulated by pulsations, are introduced into the medium usually by means of a piezoelectric transducer. See also *pulse-echo diagnosis.*

ul·tra·sound (ul′truh·saownd″) *n.* [*ultra-* + *sound*]. The energy produced by pulsing a lead zirconate, quartz, or barium titanate crystal; utilized in medicine in three ways, depending on the power levels generated: power levels below 0.1 watt per sq cm are employed for diagnostic purposes using echo reflection techniques (echogram); power levels between 1 and 3 watts per sq cm are used in the physiotherapy of various joint and muscle disorders; power levels above 5 watts per sq cm are used to destroy tissue as in treatment of cancer. See also *pulse-echo technique.*

ultrasound diagnosis. PULSE-ECHO DIAGNOSIS.

ul·tra·struc·ture (ul′truh·struck″chur) *n.* [*ultra-* + *structure*]. Ultramicroscopic structure; the arrangement of ultramicroscopic particles.

ul·tra·vi·o·let (ul″truh·vye′uh·lit) *adj.* [*ultra-* + *violet*]. Of or pertaining to electromagnetic radiation having a wavelength shorter than that at the violet end of the visible spectrum and longer than that of any x-ray. Abbreviated, UV.

ultraviolet absorption histospectroscopy. Application of the quartz microscope to measurements of absorption spectra of cellular components in situ.

ultraviolet radiation. Radiation comprised of ultraviolet wavelengths.

ul·tra·vi·rus (ul′truh·vye″rus) *n.* [*ultra-* + *virus*]. A very small virus.

um·bel·lif·er (um·bel′i·fur) *n.* [L. *umbel*la, parasol, + *ferre,* to bear]. 1. A plant having flowers arranged in umbels. 2. A member of the Umbelliferae. **—um·bel·lif·er·ous** (um″be·lif′ur·us) *adj.*

Um·bel·lif·er·ae (um″buh·lif′ur·ee) *n.pl.* [NL., from *umbellifer*]. A family of plants comprising various medically significant genera. See also *Cicuta, Ferula, Eryngium, Daucus.*

um·ber (um′bur) *n.* [OF. (*terre d'*) *umbre,* Umbrian (earth)]. A native ferric hydroxide containing manganese dioxide and silicate; occurs as a dark-brown to brownish-red powder. Used as a pigment.

um·bi·lec·to·my (um″bi·leck′tuh·mee) *n.* [*umbil*icus + *-ectomy*]. 1. Excision of the umbilicus. 2. An operation for the relief of umbilical hernia.

um·bil·i·cal (um·bil′i·kul) *adj.* Of or pertaining to the umbilicus.

umbilical anus. An anomalous anus located in the umbilical region.

umbilical areola. A pigmented ring that surrounds the umbilicus in some individuals.

umbilical circulation. The circulation in the umbilical vessels between the fetus and the placenta.

umbilical cord. The long, cylindrical structure, invested by the amnion, containing the umbilical arteries and vein, and connecting the fetus with the placenta. NA *funiculus umbilicalis.*

umbilical cyst. VITELLOINTESTINAL CYST.

umbilical duct. VITELLINE DUCT.

umbilical fossa or **fissure.** A narrow groove on the visceral surface of the liver occupied by the round ligament of the liver (the left umbilical vein of the fetus). NA *sulcus venae umbilicalis.*

umbilical hernia. A hernia occurring through the umbilical ring, either early in life (infantile) from imperfect closure, or later (acquired) from diastasis of the rectus abdominis muscles, obesity, or muscular weakness. Syn. *annular hernia.* See also *omphalocele, hepatomphalocele.*

umbilical notch or **incisure.** A deep notch in the anterior border of the liver, marking the attachment of the falciform ligament. NA *incisura ligamenti teretis.*

umbilical plane. A horizontal plane passing through the umbilicus; this plane usually lies at the level of the intervertebral disk between the third and fourth lumbar vertebrae.

umbilical recess. A dilated portion of the left branch of the adult portal vein, marking the position of the left umbilical vein.

umbilical region. The middle of the three median abdominal regions, below the epigastric region and above the pubic region. NA *regio umbilicalis.*

umbilical ring. A dense fibrous ring surrounding the umbilicus at birth; normally the ring is obliterated by the formation of a mass of dense fibrous tissue. NA *anulus umbilicalis.*

umbilical souffle. FUNICULAR SOUFFLE.

umbilical vein. Originally one of paired veins conveying blood from the placenta to the sinus venosus; the proximal right umbilical vein disappears early in development, and the extraembryonic parts fuse to form a single vein in the umbilical cord. NA *vena umbilicalis sinistra.* See also Table of Veins in the Appendix.

umbilical vesicle. YOLK SAC.

um·bil·i·cate (um·bil′i·kut) *adj.* Having a depression like that of the navel.

um·bil·i·cat·ed (um·bil′i·kay·tid) *adj.* UMBILICATE.

um·bil·i·ca·tion (um·bil″i·kay′shun) *n.* 1. A depression like the navel. 2. The state of being umbilicated.

um·bil·i·cus (um·bil′i·kus, um″bi·lye′kus) *n.,* L. pl. & genit. sing. **umbili·ci** (·kigh, ·sigh) [L.] [NA]. The navel; the round, depressed cicatrix in the median line of the abdomen, marking the site of the aperture that in fetal life gave passage to the umbilical vessels. See also Plates 4, 23.

um·bo (um′bo) *n.,* pl. **um·bo·nes** (um·bo′neez), **umbos** [L., boss]. 1. A boss or bosselation. 2. Any central convex eminence.

umbo mem·bra·nae tym·pa·ni (mem·bray′nee tim′puh·nigh) [NA]. UMBO OF THE TYMPANIC MEMBRANE.

umbo of the tympanic membrane. The projection in the center of the lateral surface of the tympanic membrane. NA *umbo membranae tympani.*

um·bras·co·py (um·bras′kuh·pee) *n.* [L. *umbra,* shade, + *-scopy*]. RETINOSCOPY.

um·brel·la iris (um·brel′uh). IRIS BOMBÉ.

un-. A prefix meaning (a) *not, without;* (b) *to remove, deprive of.*

un·bal·ance (un·bal′unce) *n.* & *v.* 1. IMBALANCE. 2. To disturb any equilibrium, whether it is physical, physiological, or emotional.

un·bal·anced, *adj.* 1. Not in equilibrium. 2. EMOTIONALLY DISTURBED.

un·cal (unk′ul) *adj.* Pertaining to the uncus (2).

uncal herniation. TENTORIAL PRESSURE CONE.

un·cia (un′see·uh) *n.,* pl. **un·ci·ae** (·see·ee) [L.]. OUNCE.

un·ci·form (un′si·form) *adj.* & *n.* [L. *uncus,* hook, + *-iform*]. 1. Hook-shaped. 2. HAMATUM.

unciform process. The hamulus of the hamate bone.

Un·ci·nar·ia (un″si·nair′ee·uh) *n.* A generic name formerly applied to hookworms.

un·ci·na·ri·a·sis (un″si·na·rye′uh·sis) *n.* [*Uncinar*ia + *-iasis*]. ANCYLOSTOMIASIS.

un·ci·nate (un′si·nate) *adj.* [L. *uncinatus,* from *uncinus,* hook, barb]. 1. Hooked. 2. Pertaining to the uncus (2).

uncinate epilepsy. A form of epilepsy characterized by recurrent uncinate fits.

uncinate fasciculus of the hemisphere. Long association fibers that lie beneath the limen insulae and connect the orbital frontal gyri and part of the inferior and middle frontal gyri with anterior portions of the temporal lobe. NA *fasciculus uncinatus.*

uncinate fit or **seizure.** A form of psychomotor or temporal lobe seizure announced by an aura of olfactory hallucinations that are often disagreeable, such as of something burning, and frequently followed by disturbances of consciousness and automatisms, such as smacking of the lips; usually associated with irritative lesions of the uncus and hippocampus. Compare *gustatory fit.*

uncinate gyrus. UNCUS (2).

uncinate process of the ethmoid bone. A hooklike projection from the inferior portion of either labyrinth; it articulates with the ethmoid process of the inferior turbinate bone. NA *processus uncinatus ossis ethmoidalis.*

uncinate process of the pancreas. An extension from the head of the pancreas to the left behind the superior mesenteric vessels. NA *processus uncinatus pancreatis.*

uncinate seizure. UNCINATE FIT.

un·ci·pi·si·for·mis (un″si·pye″si·for′mis) *n.* An occasional band of muscle running from the pisiform to the hamulus of the hamate.

un·com·pen·sat·ed (un·kom′pun·say·tid) *adj.* [*un-* + *compensated*]. Not compensated.

uncompensated acidosis. Acidosis in which the physiologic compensatory mechanisms are unable to restore the reduced pH to its normal value.

uncompensated alkalosis. Alkalosis in which the physiologic compensatory mechanisms are unable to restore the elevated pH to its normal value.

un·com·pet·i·tive inhibition. Enzyme inhibition in which the inhibitor binds to the enzyme-substrate complex, preventing further reaction to give the normal products. Contr. *competitive inhibition, noncompetitive inhibition.*

un·con·di·tioned (un″kun·dish′und) *adj.* [*un-* + *conditioned*]. Not dependent on learning or conditioning.

unconditioned reflex. A precise invariable response to a stimulus, inherited and not acquired by association. Contr. *conditioned reflex.*

un·con·ju·gat·ed bile acid (un·kon′joo·gay·tid). The residual cholic acid remaining when glycine or taurine is removed from the bile acid.

unconjugated bilirubin. Bilirubin in a form that is not combined as a glucuronate or sulfate.

un·con·scious (un·kon′shus) *adj.* & *n.* [*un-* + *conscious*]. 1. *In psychiatry,* pertaining to behavior or experiences not controlled by the conscious ego. 2. Insensible; in a state lacking conscious awareness and with reflexes abolished. 3. The part of the mind, mental functioning, or personality not in the immediate field of awareness; the repository for data that may never have entered consciousness or which the individual may have become conscious of for a short time and then repressed. —**unconscious·ness** (·nus) *n.*

unconscious homosexuality. LATENT HOMOSEXUALITY.

unc·tion (unk′shun) *n.* [L. *unctio,* from *ungere,* to anoint]. 1. The act or process of anointing. 2. OINTMENT.

unc·tu·ous (unk′choo·us) *adj.* [ML. *unctuosus,* from *unctum,* ointment]. Greasy; oily.

un·cus (unk′us) *n.,* pl. & genit. sing. **un·ci** (un′sigh) [L., hook] [NA]. 1. HOOK. 2. The rostromedial protrusion of the gyrus parahippocampalis.

uncus gy·ri hip·po·cam·pi (jye′rye hip·o·kam′pye) [BNA]. UNCUS (2).

un·dec·yl (un·des′il) *n.* The univalent organic radical $CH_3(CH_2)_{10}$. Syn. *hendecyl.*

un·dec·y·len·ic acid (un·des″i·len′ick, ·lee′nick). 10-Undecenoic acid, $CH_2{=}CH(CH_2)_8COOH$, an unsaturated acid present in human sweat. It has fungistatic action and is used for the treatment of fungous infections.

un·de·fend·ed space of Pea·cock [T. B. *Peacock,* English physician, 1812–1882]. The thin membranous portion of the interventricular septum of the heart.

un·der·achiev·er (un″dur·uh·chee′vur) *n.* 1. A person who performs less well in specific areas than would be expected from certain known characteristics or a previous record. 2. Specifically, a student whose scholastic achievement falls below his measured aptitude or intelligence. Contr. *overachiever.* —**under·achieve** (·a·cheev′) *v.;* **underachieve·ment** (·munt) *n.*

un·der·cor·rec·tion of lens (un″dur·kuh·reck′shun). The spherical aberration that normally exists in a simple lens. Rays from the outer zones of the source are brought to a focus closer to the lens than the rays from the central portion.

un·der·wa·ter exercise. Prescribed exercises carried out in a pool or tub where buoyancy permits or facilitates the movements of weak muscles.

un·der·weight (un″dur·wate′, un′dur·wate″) *adj.* Below the normal weight range for age and height.

Un·der·wood's disease [M. *Underwood,* English physician, 1737–1820]. SCLEREMA NEONATORUM.

un·de·scend·ed ovaries. A rare congenital anomaly in which the ovaries fail to descend to normal position, accompanied by amenorrhea, poorly developed secondary sexual characters, and limitation of growth. The other genitalia may be developed normally, and the body configuration is female.

undescended testis. The condition in which a testis is either in the abdomen or in the inguinal canal. See also *cryptorchism, pseudocryptorchism.*

un·dif·fer·en·ti·at·ed (un″dif″ur·en′shee·ay·tid) *adj.* Not differentiated.

undifferentiated-cell leukemia. STEM CELL LEUKEMIA.

undifferentiated type of schizophrenia. A form of schizophrenia with mixed symptomatology, unclassifiable as one of the more distinct types. It includes all early, as yet undifferentiated, forms at the first attack, and may be acute, appearing suddenly and disappearing within a brief period though often recurring; or chronic, not classifiable as of another type.

un·dine (un·deen′, un′dine) *n.* [L. *unda,* water, wave]. A glass container for irrigating the eye.

un·din·ism (un′di·niz·um) *n.* [L. *und*a, water, wave, + *-ism*]. Sexual excitation aroused by running water, urine, or micturition.

un·do·ing, *n. In psychiatry,* a defense mechanism, particularly characteristic of the obsessive-compulsive neurosis, in which one performs a symbolic act, often repeatedly, to undo or annul in some magic way the possible effects of one's unrecognized impulses or of some act for which one has unconscious guilt.

un·du·lant (un′dew·lunt) *adj.* [L. *undulans,* from *undulare,* to undulate]. Fluctuating; rising and falling like waves.

undulant fever. BRUCELLOSIS.

un·du·lat·ing (un′dew·lay·ting) *adj.* Having a wavy outline.

undulating membrane. A membrane projecting laterally from certain protozoa, especially seen in trypanosomes.

un·du·la·tion (un″dew·lay′shun) *n.* [L. *undulare,* to undulate, from *undula,* dim. of *unda,* wave]. A wavelike motion.

un·du·la·to·ry (un′dew·luh·to″ree) *adj.* Moving like waves.

un·equal (un·ee′kwul) *adj.* [*un-* + *equal*]. Differing in size, amount, or degree.

unequal cleavage. Cleavage producing blastomeres of unequal size.

unequal segmentation. Segmentation producing blastomeres of unequal size, those of the animal pole being smaller and more numerous than those of the vegetal pole.

unequal stereoblastula. AMPHIMORULA.

unequal twins. Twins in which only one of the pair is fully developed.

ung. Abbreviation for *unguentum,* ointment.

un·gual (ung'gwul) *adj.* [*ungu*is + *-al*]. Pertaining to the nails.

ungual phalanx. The terminal phalanx.

ungual tuberosity. The expanded distal end of a terminal phalanx. NA *tuberositas phalangis distalis.*

un·guen·tum (ung·gwen'tum) *n.* [L.]. OINTMENT. Abbreviated, ung.

un·guis (ung'gwis) *n.,* pl. **un·gues** (·gweez) [L. (rel. to Gk. *onyx*)] [NA]. A fingernail or toenail.

unguis in·car·na·tus (in·kahr·nay'tus). Ingrowing nail; onychocryptosis.

un·gu·la (ung'gew·luh) *n.,* pl. **un·gu·lae** (·lee) [L., hoof, claw]. 1. An instrument for extracting a dead fetus. 2. A hoof; a claw.

un·gu·late (ung'gew·lut, ·late) *n. & adj.* [L. *ungulatus,* from *ungula,* hoof]. 1. A hoofed mammal. 2. Hooved.

un·health·ful, *adj.* Injurious to health.

un·healthy (un·helth'ee) *adj.* 1. Lacking health; sickly. 2. *Colloq.* UNHEALTHFUL.

uni- [L. *unus*]. A combining form meaning *one.*

uni·ar·tic·u·lar (yoo''nee·ahr·tick'yoo·lur) *adj.* [*uni-* + *articular*]. Pertaining to a single joint.

uni·ax·i·al (yoo''nee·ack'see·ul) *adj.* [*uni-* + *axial*]. Pertaining to, on, or having one axis, as the uniaxial movement of a pivot joint.

uni·cam·er·al (yoo''ni·kam'ur·ul) *adj.* [*uni-* + *camer*a + *-al*]. Having only one cavity or chamber.

uni·cam·er·ate (yoo''ni·kam'ur·ut) *adj.* UNICAMERAL.

UNICEF (yoo'ni·sef). An acronym for *United Nations International Children's Emergency Fund.*

uni·cel·lu·lar (yoo''ni·sel'yoo·lur) *adj.* [*uni-* + *cellular*]. Composed of one cell.

unicellular gland. A gland consisting of a single cell.

uni·cen·tral (yoo''ni·sen'trul) *adj.* [*uni-* + *central*]. Having a single center.

uni·cen·tric (yoo''ni·sen'trick) *adj.* [*uni-* + *centr-* + *-ic*]. Having a single center.

uni·cor·nous (yoo''ni·kor'nus) *adj.* [L. *unicorn*is (from *cornu,* horn) + *-ous*]. Having one horn.

uni·cus·pid (yoo''ni·kus'pid) *adj.* [*uni-* + L. *cuspis, cuspidis*]. Having one cusp. Compare *cuspid, cuspidate.*

uni·fa·mil·ial (yoo''ni·fuh·mil'ee·ul) *adj.* [*uni-* + *familial*]. Pertaining to a single family.

uni·fi·lar (yoo''ni·fye'lur) *adj.* [*uni-* + *filar*]. Connected by one thread; furnished with one filament.

uni·grav·i·da (yoo''ni·grav'i·duh) *n.* [*uni-* + *gravida*]. A woman who is pregnant for the first time. Syn. *primigravida.*

uni·lat·er·al (yoo''ni·lat'ur·ul) *adj.* [*uni-* + *lateral*]. Pertaining to, or affecting, but one side.

unilateral anesthesia. Anesthesia of a lateral half of the body. Syn. *hemianesthesia.*

unilateral anophthalmia. MONOPHTHALMIA.

unilateral electroconvulsive therapy. Electroshock therapy with the electrodes applied only to the nondominant cerebral hemisphere.

unilateral fused kidney. SIGMOID KIDNEY.

unilateral harelip. SINGLE HARELIP.

unilateral hermaphroditism. The form of human hermaphroditism in which the following combinations are known: an ovary on one side and a testis, testis and ovary, or two ovotestes on the other; a testis on one side and an ovotestis on the other; no gonads on one side, with an ovary and a testis on the other.

unilateral nystagmus. MONOCULAR NYSTAGMUS.

uni·lo·bar (yoo''ni·lo'bur) *adj.* [*uni-* + *lobar*]. Having one lobe.

unilobar kidney. A kidney consisting of a single lobe, as in rats, dogs, and many other animals but not in man. Syn. *monopyramidal kidney.*

uni·loc·u·lar (yoo''ni·lock'yoo·lur) *adj.* [*uni-* + *locul*us + *-ar*]. Having but one loculus or cavity.

unilocular cyst. A cyst with a single cavity.

uni·mo·lec·u·lar reaction (yoo''ni·muh·leck'yoo·lur). FIRST-ORDER REACTION.

un·in·cised (un''in·size'd') *adj.* [*un-* + *incised*]. Uncut; unopened; undrained.

un·in·hib·it·ed bladder (un''in·hib'i·tid). An abnormal urinary bladder that shows only a variable loss of cerebral inhibition over reflex bladder contractions, representing, of all neurogenic bladders, the least variance from normal. The vesical reflex is intact, and micturition can be initiated and interrupted voluntarily. It is seen normally in infants and abnormally in the adult enuretic, and in patients with subtotal destruction of the cerebral cortex or cortical regulatory system.

uni·nu·cle·ar (yoo''ni·new'klee·ur) *adj.* [*uni-* + *nuclear*]. Having a single nucleus.

uni·oc·u·lar (yoo''nee·ock'yoo·lur) *adj.* [*uni-* + *ocular*]. MONOCULAR.

un·ion (yoon'yun) *n.* [L. *unio,* from *unus,* one]. 1. A joining. 2. A coming or growing together into one; specifically, the consolidation of bone fractures or the healing of a wound.

uni·oval (yoo''nee·o'vul) *adj.* [*uni-* + *ov*um + *-al*]. Formed from one ovum; uniovular.

uni·ovu·lar (yoo''nee·ov'yoo·lur) *adj.* [*uni-* + *ovular*]. Pertaining to or derived from one egg.

uniovular twins. Twins arising from a single ovum.

unip·a·ra (yoo·nip'uh·ruh) *n.* [*uni-* + *-para*]. A woman who has borne but one child.

uni·par·i·ens (yoo''ni·păr'ee·enz) *adj.* [NL.]. UNIPAROUS.

unip·a·rous (yoo·nip'uh·rus) *adj.* [*uni-* + *-parous*]. Bearing one offspring, or producing one ovum, at a time.

Unipen. Trademark for the sodium salt of nafcillin, a semisynthetic penicillin antibiotic.

uni·pen·nate (yoo''ni·pen'ate) *adj.* [*uni-* + *pennate*]. Comparable in structure to the arrangement of barbs on one side of a feather shaft. Contr. *bipennate.*

unipennate muscle. A muscle whose fibers are inserted obliquely into one side of a tendon. NA *musculus unipennatus.*

uni·po·lar (yoo''ni·po'lur) *adj.* [*uni-* + *polar*]. 1. Having but one pole or process. 2. Pertaining to one pole.

unipolar cell. A nerve cell with one major process, as a cell of the dorsal root ganglions.

unipolar lead. An electrocardiographic lead with the negative, or indifferent, electrode at zero potential and the voltage determined by the positive, or exploring, electrode. See also *unipolar limb lead, precordial lead.*

unipolar limb lead. *In electrocardiography,* a limb lead with the negative, or indifferent, electrode at zero potential on the right foot and the positive, or exploring, electrode on another limb, designated VR (right arm), VL (left arm), or VF (left foot). Contr. *standard limb lead.*

unip·o·tent (yoo·nip'o·tunt) *adj.* [*uni-* + *potent*]. Giving rise to only one cell or tissue type; said of embryonic or multiplying cells. —**uni·po·ten·cy** (yoo''ni·po'ten·see) *n.;* **uni·po·ten·tial** (·po·ten'chul) *adj.*

uni·sex·u·al (yoo''ni·seck'shoo·ul) *adj.* [*uni-* + *sexual*]. Provided with the sexual organs of one sex only.

unit, *n.* [*unity,* from L. *unitas,* from *unus,* one]. 1. A single thing or person or a group considered as a whole. 2. A standard weight or measurement. Abbreviated, U. 3. A molecule or distinctive portion of a larger molecule.

uni·tar·i·an (yoo''ni·tăr'ee·un) *adj.* UNITARY (1).

unitarian theory. A theory of blood-cell formation which supposes that all blood cells come from a single parental blood cell, the hemocytoblast or hematopoietic stem cell. Syn. *monophyletic theory of hemopoiesis.*

unitarian theory of antibodies. The theory opposed to the belief that each different serologic reaction is based on a separate antibody, maintaining to the contrary that the same antibody can perform all or most of these functions.

uni·tary (yoo'ni·terr"ee) *adj.* 1. Pertaining to, or having the qualities of, a unit. 2. Pertaining to monsters having the organs of a single individual.

unit character. One of a pair of sharply contrasted traits that are inherited according to the Mendelian law of segregation.

United Nations International Children's Emergency Fund. An organization, often identified by the acronym UNICEF and created by and dependent on the General Assembly of the United Nations, which deals with rehabilitation of children in war-ravaged countries, with maternal and child welfare, and, where necessary, with development of a technical and health program particularly as applied to children.

United States Pharmacopeia. The pharmacopeia of the United States of America, officially recognized by the Federal Food, Drug, and Cosmetics Act. Abbreviated, U.S.P.

United States Public Health Service. The agency concerned with the development of a public-health program and the handling of health problems within the jurisdiction of the federal government. Abbreviated, USPHS.

Unitensen. Trademark for cryptenamine, a mixture of antihypertensive alkaloids from *Veratrum viride,* used as the acetate or tannate salts.

unit membrane. The trilaminar structure of the plasma and intracellular membranes of cells, approximately 75 Å in thickness, seen in the electron microscope as having outer darker lines 20 Å in width; composed of a fluid matrix of protein and lipid.

unit of energy. UNIT OF WORK.

unit of force. The dyne; the force which, when acting for one second, will give to one gram a velocity of one centimeter per second.

unit of heat. The calorie or B.T.U.

unit of work. The erg; the work done by a force of one dyne acting through a distance of one centimeter in the direction of the force. Syn. *unit of energy.*

uni·va·lent (yoo"ni·vay'lunt, yoo·niv'uh·lunt) *adj.* [*uni-* + *valent*]. 1. Having a valence of one. 2. Of vaccines: effective against one specific pathogenic agent. Contr. *polyvalent.*

uni·ver·sal, *adj.* [L. *universalis,* from *universus,* whole]. 1. Generalized, widespread. 2. Relatively unrestricted in application.

universal adenitis. Widespread induration of the lymph nodes, associated with primary syphilis.

universal calcinosis. CALCINOSIS UNIVERSALIS.

universal congenital atrichia. ALOPECIA CONGENITALIS.

universal donor. A blood donor of group O.

universal infantilism. Generalized retarded physical development associated with absence of secondary sex characters.

universal recipient. An individual of AB blood group.

universal stain. STRUMIA'S UNIVERSAL STAIN.

un·load·ing reflex. Sudden removal of an external load against which a muscle is contracted normally produces a biphasic electromyographic response, the first phase showing reduced or even absent action potentials, and the second phase, greatly increased potentials which may be larger than those seen before unloading. In paretic limbs, the second phase also shows markedly reduced or absent action potentials.

un·mod·i·fied insulin. AMORPHOUS INSULIN.

un·my·e·li·nat·ed (un·migh'e·li·nay·tid) *adj.* Lacking a myelin sheath; especially, never having formed one. Compare *demyelinated.*

Un·na bodies or **cells** (ŏŏn'ah) [P. G. *Unna,* German dermatologist, 1859–1929]. RUSSELL BODIES.

Unna's paste boot [P. G. *Unna*]. A sheath or casing for the leg used in treating varicose ulcers and veins by relieving venous hydrostatic pressure. A paste of zinc oxide (Unna's), gelatin, and glycerin is applied to the leg, and a bandage is placed over the paste.

Unna's plasma cell [P. G. *Unna*]. PLASMA CELL.

Unna-Thost syndrome [P. G. *Unna*]. Symmetrical hyperkeratosis of the palms and soles; congenital or when acquired preceded by hyperhidrosis.

un·num·bered hospital. In U.S. Army medicine, a fixed hospital designed normally for operation in the continental United States or any of its possessions. All such hospitals are assigned names such as U.S. Army Hospital, Fort Belvoir, or in case of a general type hospital, Letterman Army Hospital.

un·of·fi·cial, *adj.* [*un-* + *official*]. Describing a drug or remedy that is not included in the United States Pharmacopeia or National Formulary.

un·or·ga·nized, *adj.* [*un-* + *organized*]. 1. Without organs. 2. Not arranged in the form of an organ or organs.

unorganized ferment. EXTRACELLULAR ENZYME.

un·paired allosome. MONOSOME.

un·re·al·i·ty, *n. In psychiatry,* the distorted picture that a patient may have of a situation or event of life. What he sees is not in keeping with an interpretation of the same facts by an independent observer, but has been altered by his feelings or preconceptions.

un·re·duced dislocation. A dislocation in which the dislocated bone has not been replaced in normal position.

un·re·solved pneumonia. ORGANIZING PNEUMONIA.

un·rest, *n.* A state of uneasiness characterized by general body and mental tension, and sometimes excessive body activity.

un·sat·u·rat·ed (un·satch'uh·ray"tid) *adj.* 1. Not saturated. 2. Characterizing an organic compound having double or triple bonds.

unsaturated hydrocarbon. A hydrocarbon that has one or more double or triple bonds between carbon atoms.

un·sex, *v.* [*un-* + *sex*]. To remove the testes in male, or the ovaries in female, animals.

unslaked lime. CALCIUM OXIDE.

un·sound, *adj.* Unhealthy, diseased, or not properly functioning. —**un·sound·ness,** *n.*

unsoundness of mind. Incapacity to govern one's affairs.

un·spec·i·fied, *adj.* Not specific.

unspecified mental retardation. Subnormal general intellectual functioning which has not been nor cannot be defined more precisely, but which is clearly recognized to be below average.

un·sta·ble (un·stay'bul) *adj.* [*un-* + *stable*]. 1. Movable, not fixed in position, irregular, unsteady, vacillating. 2. Insecure; changeable; specifically, characterized by emotional lability, alterations of mood, or a volatile temperament. See also *cyclothymic.* 3. Readily decomposing, said of chemical compounds.

unstable colon. IRRITABLE COLON.

un·stri·at·ed (un·strye'ay·tid) *adj.* Not striated.

unstriated fibers. SMOOTH MUSCLE FIBERS.

unstriated muscle. SMOOTH MUSCLE.

un·striped (un·stripe't') *adj.* Not striped or striated.

unstriped fibers. SMOOTH MUSCLE FIBERS.

unstriped muscle. SMOOTH MUSCLE.

un·thrift·y, *adj.* Of a domestic animal: not thriving; low in body weight for its age. —**unthrift·i·ness,** *n.*

un·unit·ed (un"yoo·nigh'tid) *adj.* [*un-* + *united*]. Not joined.

ununited fracture. A fracture in which, after the normal period, there is failure of union.

Un·ver·richt-Lund·borg disease (ŏŏn'feʰ·rikht, luend'borʸ) [H. *Unverricht,* German physician, 1853–1912; and H. *Lundborg*]. PROGRESSIVE FAMILIAL MYOCLONIC EPILEPSY.

Unverricht's disease or **syndrome** [H. *Unverricht*]. PROGRESSIVE FAMILIAL MYOCLONIC EPILEPSY.

Unverricht's familial myoclonus [H. *Unverricht*]. PROGRESSIVE FAMILIAL MYOCLONIC EPILEPSY.

un·well, *n.* [*un-* + *well*]. 1. Ill; sick. 2. *Obsol. colloq.* Menstruating.

unwinding protein. A protein involved in the replication of DNA which acts by attaching to the double helix and helping to separate the strands, thus permitting duplication.

up-beat nystagmus. Nystagmus in which the fast component is upward; a common finding with lesions of the brainstem, particularly at the level of the vestibular nuclei, and in various types of drug intoxication.

UPI Abbreviation for *uteroplacental insufficiency.*

up·per, *adj.* Situated relatively high in physical position.

upper brachial plexus paralysis. Paralysis due to a lesion of the fifth and sixth cervical nerve roots, commonly from birth injury, and affecting chiefly the functions of the biceps, deltoid, brachialis, and brachioradialis muscles, with loss of abduction and external rotation of the arm and weak forearm flexion and supination. Sensation over the deltoid and radial surfaces of the arm and forearm may be impaired. The paralysis may be transient or permanent, depending on the degree of injury. Syn. *Erb-Duchenne paralysis.* Contr. *lower brachial plexus paralysis.*

upper extremity. The shoulder girdle, arm, forearm, wrist, and hand. NA *membrum superius.* See also Plates 7, 9, 16.

upper horizontal plane. SUBCOSTAL PLANE.

upper motor neuron. Any efferent neuron having its cell body in the motor cortex and connecting with the motor nuclei of the brainstem and anterior horns of the spinal cord. Contr. *lower motor neuron.*

upper motor neuron lesion. An injury to the cell body or axon of an upper motor neuron, resulting in spastic paralysis of the muscle involved, hyperactive deep reflexes but diminished or absent superficial reflexes, little or no muscle atrophy, absence of reaction of degeneration, and the presence of pathological reflexes and signs. Lesions may be located in the cerebral cortex, internal capsule, cerebral peduncles, brainstem, or spinal cord, and may be due to various causes. Contr. *lower motor neuron lesion.*

upper urinary tract. The kidneys and the ureters; the urinary system above the ureteral insertion into the bladder.

upper uterine segment. The upper and major portion of the uterine musculature, which actively contracts and thickens during labor. See also *retraction ring.*

up·right·ing, *n.* An orthodontic tipping movement to place teeth in a more vertical axial inclination.

upside-down stomach. The inverted appearance sometimes seen when a considerable portion of the stomach is herniated through the diaphragm into the thoracic cavity, especially when the abnormality is an organoaxial volvulus of the stomach through a parahiatal diaphragmatic hernia.

[1]ur-, uro-. A combining form meaning *urine, urinary.*

[2]ur-, uro- [Gk. *oura, tail*]. A combining form meaning (a) *caudal;* (b) *tail, tail-like.*

urachal fossa. RETROPUBIC SPACE.

ura·chus (yoor'uh·kus) *n.* [Gk. *ourachos*] [NA]. An epithelial tube or cord connecting the apex of the urinary bladder with the allantois, regarded as the stalk of the allantois or as the degenerate apex of the primitive bladder. Its connective tissue forms the median umbilical ligament. See also Plate 25. —**ura·chal** (·kul) *adj.*

ura·cil (yoor'uh·sil) *n.* 2,4(1*H*,3*H*)-Pyrimidinedione, $C_4H_4N_2O_2$, a pyrimidine base important mainly as a component of ribonucleic acid. Symbol, U

uracil mustard. 5-[Bis(2-chloroethyl)amino]uracil, $C_8H_{11}Cl_2N_3O_2$, a compound similar to nitrogen mustard (mechlorethamine hydrochloride); useful for palliative treatment of certain neoplastic diseases.

ura·cra·sia (yoor"uh·kray'see·uh, ·zee·uh) *n.* [*ur-* + Gk. *akrasia,* incontinence]. Incontinence of urine; enuresis.

ura·cra·tia (yoor"uh·kray'shee·uh) *n.* [*ur-* + Gk. *akrateia,* incontinence]. URACRASIA.

uraemia. UREMIA.

ura·gogue (yoor'uh·gog) *n.* [Gk. *ouragōgos*]. A diuretic. —**ura·gog·ic** (yoor"uh·goj'ick) *adj.*

uran-, urano- [Gk. *ouranos,* sky; roof, palate]. A combining form meaning *palate, palatal.*

ura·nal (yoor'uh·nul) *adj.* [*uran-* + *-al*]. Pertaining to the palate.

uranal angle. The angle determined by connecting the point that lies in the sagittal curvature of the hard palate by straight lines with the premaxillary point and the posterior nasal spine, respectively. The less arched the palate, the greater is this angle.

ura·nal·y·sis (yoor"uh·nal'i·sis) *n.* [*ur-* + *analysis*]. URINALYSIS.

ura·nin (yoo'ruh·nin) *n.* The sodium derivative of fluorescein; fluorescein sodium.

uran·i·nite (yoo·ran'i·nite) *n.* PITCHBLENDE.

ura·nis·co·plas·ty (yoor"uh·nis'ko·plas·tee) *n.* [*uraniscus* + *-plasty*]. URANOPLASTY.

ura·nis·cor·rha·phy (yoor"uh·nis·kor'uh·fee) *n.* [*uraniscus* + *-rrhaphy*]. Suture of a palatal cleft; staphylorrhaphy.

ura·nis·cus (yoor"uh·nis'kus) *n.* [Gk. *ouraniskos*]. PALATE.

ura·nism (yoor'uh·niz·um) *n.* [Gk. *Ourania,* an epithet of Aphrodite]. HOMOSEXUALITY. Contr. *dionism.*

ura·ni·um (yoo·ray'nee·um) *n.* [after the planet *Uranus*]. U = 238.03. A heavy metallic element, atomic weight 92, density 19.05, of the radium group; occurs as silver-white, lustrous, radioactive crystals or powder. As concentrated from its ores uranium contains 99.3% of the isotope weighing 238, 0.7% of the 235 isotope, and a negligible amount of the 234 isotope. Uranium 235 may be made to undergo fission with the release of a large amount of energy. Uranium 238 can absorb a neutron to produce uranium 239; this spontaneously loses a beta particle to form neptunium, which, in turn, loses another beta particle to form plutonium, the last also being fissionable.

uranium fission. NUCLEAR FISSION.

uranium rays. BECQUEREL RAYS.

urano-. See *uran-.*

ura·no·col·o·bo·ma (yoor"uh·no·kol"uh·bo'muh) *n.* [*urano-* + *coloboma*]. Cleft hard palate, not involving the alveolar process.

ura·no·plas·ty (yoor'uh·no·plas"tee) *n.* [*urano-* + *-plasty*]. A plastic operation for the repair of cleft palate. —**ura·no·plas·tic** (yoor"uh·no·plas'tick) *adj.*

ura·no·ple·gia (yoor"uh·no·plee'jee·uh) *n.* [*urano-* + *-plegia*]. Paralysis of the muscles of the soft palate.

ura·nor·rha·phy (yoor"uh·nor'uh·fee) *n.* [*urano-* + *-rrhaphy*]. Suture of a cleft palate; staphylorrhaphy.

ura·nos·chi·sis (yoor"uh·nos'ki·sis) *n.* [*urano-* + *-schisis*]. 1. Cleft hard palate. See *cleft palate.* 2. Cleft hard palate and alveolar process. Syn. *gnathopalatoschisis.*

uran·o·schism (yoo·ran'o·skiz·um) *n.* URANOSCHISIS.

ura·no·schis·ma (yoor"uh·no·skiz'muh) *n.* URANOSCHISIS.

ura·no·staph·y·lo·plas·ty (yoor"uh·no·staf'i·lo·plas"tee) *n.* [*urano-* + *staphylo-* + *-plasty*]. URANOPLASTY.

ura·no·staph·y·lor·rha·phy (yoor"uh·no·staf"i·lor'uh·fee) *n.* [*urano-* + *staphylo-* + *-rrhaphy*]. Repair of a cleft in both the hard and soft palates.

ura·nyl (yoo'ruh·nil) *n.* The bivalent uranium radical UO_2^{2+}, which forms salts with many acids, as, for example uranyl acetate, $UO_2(C_2H_3O_2)_2.2H_2O$.

ura·ro·ma (yoor"uh·ro'muh) *n.* Aromatic odor of urine.

urase (yoor'ace, ·aze) *n.* UREASE.

urate (yoor'ate) *n.* A salt of uric acid. —**urat·ic** (yoo·rat'ick) *adj.*

ura·te·mia, ura·tae·mia (yoor"uh·tee'mee·uh) *n.* [*urate* + *-emia*]. The presence of urates in the blood.

urate oxidase. URICASE.

ura·tu·ria (yoor″uh·tew′ree·uh) *n.* [*urate* + *-uria*]. The presence of urates in the urine.

urban typhus. MURINE TYPHUS.

urban yellow fever. Yellow fever transmitted from man to man by the bite of the mosquito *Aëdes aegypti.*

urea (yoo·ree′uh) *n.* [NL., from F. *urée,* from Gk. *ouron,* urine]. Carbamide, $CO(NH_2)_2$, a product of protein metabolism; formerly used externally to treat infected wounds but now used mainly as a diuretic, administered orally or intravenously. **—ure·al** (·ul) *adj.*

urea clearance test. A test for kidney function in which the excretory efficiency of the kidneys is tested by the amount of blood cleared of urea in 1 minute as determined by the ratio of the blood urea to the amount of urea excreted in urine during a fixed time.

urea cycle. A cyclic reaction pathway in the formation of arginine and urea. The sequence involves the conversion of ornithine to citrulline to arginine, which, in the presence of the enzyme arginase, forms urea and ornithine. Syn. *Krebs-Henseleit cycle.*

ure·am·e·ter (yoor″ee·am′e·tur) *n.* [*urea* + *-meter*]. An apparatus for determining the amount of urea in a liquid by measuring the volume of nitrogen evolved.

ure·am·e·try (yoo″ree·am′e·tree) *n.* [*urea* + *-metry*]. The determination of the amount of urea in a liquid.

urea nitrogen. The nitrogen of urea, as distinguished from the nitrogen in the form of protein or other nitrogenous substances.

ure·ase (yoor′ee·ace, ·aze) *n.* An enzyme, obtained from jack bean, that catalyzes hydrolysis of urea to ammonia and carbon dioxide and is used in the estimation of urea.

urec·chy·sis (yoo·reck′i·sis) *n.* [*ur-* + Gk. *ekchysis,* outflow]. Extravasation of urine into the tissues.

Urecholine Chloride. Trademark for bethanechol chloride, a cholinergic drug.

ure·de·ma, uroe·de·ma (yoor″e·dee′muh) *n.* [*ur-* + *edema*]. Swelling of tissues from extravasation of urine.

ure·depa (yoor″e·dep′uh) *n.* Ethyl [bis(1-aziridinyl)phosphinyl]carbamate, $C_7H_{14}N_3O_3P$, an antineoplastic agent.

ured·o·fos (yoo·red′o·fos) *n.* Diethyl [thio[*o*-[3-(*p*-tolylsulfonyl)ureido]phenyl]carbamoyl]phosphoramidate, $C_{19}H_{25}N_4O_6P$, a veterinary anthelmintic.

ure·he·pat·ic syndrome (yoor″e·he·pat′ick). HEPATORENAL SYNDROME.

ure·ide (yoor′ee·ide) *n.* A compound of urea and an acid radical.

ure·mia, urae·mia (yoo·ree′mee·uh) *n.* [*ur-* + *-emia*]. A complex biochemical abnormality occurring in kidney failure; characterized by azotemia, chronic acidosis, anemia, and a variety of systemic and neurologic symptoms and signs. **—ure·mic, urae·mic** (·mick) *adj.*

uremic acidosis. Metabolic acidosis due to decreased renal ability to excrete acids; seen in chronic kidney disease.

uremic amblyopia. Loss of vision without disease of the retina, sometimes accompanying an attack of uremia.

uremic convulsion. Convulsion associated with uremia.

uremic frost. A whitish appearance of the skin due to dried urea aggregates; seen in advanced renal failure.

uremic medullary cystic disease. MEDULLARY CYSTIC DISEASE OF THE KIDNEY.

uremic sponge kidney. MEDULLARY CYSTIC DISEASE OF THE KIDNEY.

ure·om·e·ter (yoor″ee·om′e·tur) *n.* UREAMETER.

ure·om·etry (yoor″ee·om′e·tree) *n.* UREAMETRY.

ure·o·tel·ic (yoor″ee·o·tel′ick) *adj.* [*urea* + *tel-* + *-ic*]. Characterizing an animal in which urea is the principal compound of nitrogenous waste, as in mammals. Compare *uricotelic.* **—ureotel·ism** (·iz·um) *n.*

ur·er·y·thrin (yoor·err′i·thrin) *n.* UROERYTHRIN.

ure·si·es·the·sia, ure·si·aes·the·sia (yoo·ree″see·es·theezh′uh, ·theez′ee·uh) *n.* [*uresis* + *esthesia*]. The feeling of a need to urinate.

ure·sis (yoo·ree′sis) *n.* [Gk. *ourēsis*]. URINATION.

-uret [NL. *-uretum,* from F. *-ure* (as in *sulfure,* sulfide)]. *Obsol.* -IDE.

ure·ter (yoo·ree′tur, yoor′e·tur) *n.* [Gk. *ourētēr*] [NA]. Either of the long, narrow tubes conveying the urine from the pelvis of each kidney to the urinary bladder. See also Plates 8, 14, 24, 25, 26. **—ure·ter·al** (yoo·ree′tur·ul), **ure·ter·ic** (yoor″e·terr′ick) *adj.*

ureteral obstruction. Any hindrance to the flow of urine through the ureter to the bladder.

ure·ter·ec·ta·sis (yoo·ree″tur·eck′tuh·sis, yoor″e·tur·) *n.* [*ureter* + *ectasis*]. Dilatation of a ureter.

ure·ter·ec·to·my (yoo·ree″tur·eck′tuh·mee, yoor″e·tur·) *n.* [*ureter* + *-ectomy*]. Excision of a ureter.

ureteric bud. A dorsomedial outgrowth of a mesonephric duct; the anlage of a ureter, a renal pelvis and its calyxes, and the collecting tubules of a kidney.

ureteric plica. BAR OF THE BLADDER.

ure·ter·itis (yoo·ree″tur·eye′tis, yoor″e·tur·) *n.* [*ureter* + *-itis*]. Inflammation of a ureter.

ureteritis cys·ti·ca (sis′ti·kuh). A form of chronic ureteral inflammation in which minute cysts are formed in the epithelium.

uretero-. A combining form meaning *ureter, ureteral.*

ure·tero·cele (yoo·ree′tur·o·seel) *n.* [*uretero-* + *-cele*]. A cyst-like dilatation at the termination of a ureter; of congenital origin or due to a narrowing of the terminal orifice.

ure·tero·ce·lec·to·my (yoo·ree″tur·o·se·leck′tuh·mee) *n.* [*ureterocele* + *-ectomy*]. Surgical removal of a ureterocele.

ure·tero·co·los·to·my (yoo·ree″tur·o·ko·los′tuh·mee) *n.* [*uretero-* + *colo-* + *-stomy*]. Implantation of a ureter, severed from the urinary bladder, into the colon.

ure·tero·cys·tic (yoo·ree″tur·o·sis′tick) *adj.* [*uretero-* + *cystic*]. Pertaining to a ureter and the urinary bladder.

ure·tero·cys·tos·to·my (yoo·ree″tur·o·sis·tos′tuh·mee) *n.* [*uretero-* + *cyst-* + *-ostomy*]. The surgical formation of a communication between a ureter and the urinary bladder.

ure·tero·en·ter·ic (yoo·ree″tur·o·en·terr′ick) *adj.* [*uretero-* + *enteric*]. Pertaining to, or connected with, a ureter and adjacent bowel.

ure·tero·en·ter·os·to·my (yoo·ree″tur·o·en″tur·os′tuh·mee) *adj.* [*uretero-* + *entero-* + *-stomy*]. Surgical formation of a passage from a ureter to some portion of the intestine.

ure·ter·og·ra·phy (yoo·ree″tur·og′ruh·fee) *n.* [*uretero-* + *-graphy*]. Radiography of the ureters after the injection of a radiopaque substance, usually through a ureteral catheter.

ure·tero·hemi·ne·phrec·to·my (yoo·ree″tur·o·hem″ee·ne·freck′tuh·mee) *n.* [*uretero-* + *heminephrectomy*]. Surgical removal of a portion of a kidney and its ureter in cases of reduplication of ureter, pelvis, or the entire upper urinary tract.

ure·tero·hy·dro·ne·phro·sis (yoo·ree″tur·o·high″dro·ne·fro′sis) *n.* [*uretero-* + *hydro-* + *nephrosis*]. Distention of a ureter and the pelvis of its kidney, due to distal obstruction to outflow of urine.

ure·tero·il·e·al (yoo·ree″tur·o·il′ee·ul) *adj.* [*uretero-* + *ileal*]. Pertaining to a ureter and the ileum.

ureteroileal neocystostomy. A surgical procedure in which an isolated segment of the ileum is used for a portion of a ureter.

ure·tero·in·tes·ti·nal (yoo·ree″tur·o·in·tes′ti·nul) *adj.* [*uretero-* + *intestinal*]. Pertaining to the ureter and the intestine.

ureterointestinal anastomosis. Surgical implantation of a ureter into the small or large intestine.

ure·tero·lith (yoo·ree′tur·o·lith) *n.* [*uretero-* + *-lith*]. A calculus in a ureter.

ure·tero·li·thi·a·sis (yoo·ree″tur·o·li·thigh′uh·sis) *n.* [*uretero-* + *lithiasis*]. The presence or formation of a calculus in a ureter.

ure·tero·li·thot·o·my (yoo·ree″tur·o·li·thot′uh·mee) *n.* [*ure-*

tero- + *lithotomy*]. Incision of a ureter for removal of a calculus.

ure·ter·ol·y·sis (yoo·ree″tur·ol′i·sis) *n.* [*uretero-* + *-lysis*]. Surgical mobilization of a ureter to relieve obstruction due to kinking or external compression.

ure·tero·meg·a·ly (yoo·ree″tur·o·meg′uh·lee) *n.* [*uretero-* + *-megaly*]. Abnormal enlargement, chiefly circumferential, of the ureter.

ure·tero·neo·cys·tos·to·my (yoo·ree″tur·o·nee″o·sis·tos′tuh·mee) *n.* [*uretero-* + *neo-* + *cystostomy*]. Surgical reimplantation of the upper end of a divided ureter into the urinary bladder.

ure·tero·neo·py·elos·to·my (yoo·ree″tur·o·nee″o·pye″e·los′tuh·mee) *n.* [*uretero-* + *neo-* + *pyelostomy*]. Suturing the distal end of a severed ureter into a new opening in the pelvis of the kidney.

ure·tero·ne·phrec·to·my (yoo·ree″tur·o·ne·freck′tuh·mee) *n.* [*uretero-* + *nephrectomy*]. Surgical removal of a kidney and its ureter.

ure·tero·pel·vic (yoo·ree″tur·o·pel′vick) *adj.* [*uretero-* + *pelvic*]. Pertaining to a ureter and renal pelvis.

ureteropelvic junction. The point at which the renal pelvis becomes the ureter proper.

ure·tero·pel·vio·plas·ty (yoo·ree″tur·o·pel′vee·o·plas·tee) *n.* [*uretero-* + *pelvi-* + *-plasty*]. A surgical procedure aimed at the correction of abnormalities of a ureter and renal pelvis.

ure·tero·plas·ty (yoo·ree′tur·o·plas″tee) *n.* [*uretero-* + *-plasty*]. A plastic operation on a ureter.

ure·tero·py·eli·tis (yoo·ree″tur·o·pye″e·lye′tis) *n.* [*uretero-* + *pyel-* + *-itis*]. Inflammation of a ureter and the pelvis of a kidney.

ure·tero·py·elog·ra·phy (yoo·ree″tur·o·pye″e·log′ruh·fee) *n.* [*uretero-* + *pyelo-* + *-graphy*]. Radiographic visualization of the upper urinary tract by the injection of a contrast medium, usually through a ureteral catheter.

ure·tero·py·elo·ne·os·to·my (yoo·ree″tur·o·pye″e·lo·nee·os′tuh·mee) *n.* [*uretero-* + *pyelo-* + *neo-* + *-stomy*]. Surgical formation of a new passageway from the pelvis of a kidney to its ureter.

ure·tero·py·elo·ne·phri·tis (yoo·ree″tur·o·pye″e·lo·ne·frye′tis) *n.* [*uretero-* + *pyelo-* + *nephritis*]. Inflammation of a ureter and its kidney and pelvis.

ure·tero·py·elo·ne·phros·to·my (yoo·ree″tur·o·pye″e·lo·ne·fros′tuh·mee) *n.* [*uretero-* + *pyelo-* + *nephro-* + *-stomy*]. Surgical anastomosis of the ureter with the pelvis of its kidney.

ure·tero·py·elo·plas·ty (yoo·ree″tur·o·pye′e·lo·plas·tee) *n.* [*uretero-* + *pyelo-* + *plasty*]. Any plastic operation involving the upper portion of a ureter and the adjacent pelvis of the kidney.

ure·tero·py·elos·to·my (yoo·ree″tur·o·pye″e·los′tuh·mee) *n.* [*uretero-* + *pyelostomy*]. Surgical excision of part of a ureter and implantation of the remaining part into a new aperture made into the pelvis of the kidney. Compare *dismembered pyeloplasty.*

ure·ter·or·rha·gia (yoo·ree″tur·o·ray′jee·uh) *n.* [*uretero-* + *-rrhagia*]. Hemorrhage from a ureter.

ure·ter·or·rha·phy (yoo·ree″tur·or′uh·fee) *n.* [*uretero-* + *-rrhaphy*]. Surgical suture of a ureter.

ure·tero·sig·moid·os·to·my (yoo·ree″tur·o·sig″moy·dos′tuh·mee) *n.* [*uretero-* + *sigmoid* + *-stomy*]. Surgical implantation of a ureter, severed from the urinary bladder, into the sigmoid colon.

ure·ter·os·to·my (yoo·ree″tur·os′tuh·mee) *n.* [*uretero-* + *-stomy*]. Transplantation of a ureter to the skin; the formation of an external ureteral fistula.

ure·tero·the·cal shunt (yoo·ree″tur·o·theek′ul). ARACHNOID-URETEROSTOMY.

ure·ter·ot·o·my (yoo·ree″tur·ot′uh·mee) *n.* [*uretero-* + *-tomy*]. Surgical incision of a ureter.

ure·tero·ure·ter·al (yoo·ree″tur·o·yoo·ree′tur·ul) *adj.* [*uretero-* + *ureteral*]. Pertaining to both ureters, or to two parts of one ureter, as ureteroureteral anastomosis.

ure·tero·ure·ter·os·to·my (yoo·ree″tur·o·yoo·ree″tur·os′tuh·mee) *n.* [*uretero-* + *uretero-* + *-stomy*]. Surgical formation of a passage between the ureters or between different parts of the same ureter.

ure·tero·uter·ine (yoo·ree″tur·o·yoo′tur·ine) *adj.* [*uretero-* + *uterine*]. Pertaining to the ureters and the uterus.

ure·tero·va·gi·nal (yoo·ree″tur·o·vaj′i·nul, ·va·jye′nul) *adj.* [*uretero-* + *vaginal*]. Pertaining to the ureters and the vagina.

ure·tero·ves·i·cal (yoo·ree″tur·o·ves′i·kul) *adj.* [*uretero-* + *vesica*]. Pertaining to the ureters and the urinary bladder.

ure·tero·ves·i·co·pexy (yoo·ree″tur·o·ves′i·ko·peck″see) *n.* [*uretero-* + *vesico-* + *-pexy*]. Fixation of the distal ureter along and outside the posterior wall of the urinary bladder, for correction of vesicoureteral reflux in children.

ure·than (yoor′e·than) *n.* 1. Ethyl carbamate, $NH_2COOC_2H_5$; has been used as a hypnotic and as a neoplastic suppressant drug. 2. Any ester of carbamic acid.

ure·thane (yoor′e·thane) *n.* URETHAN.

urethr-, urethro-. A combining form meaning *urethra, urethral.*

ure·thra (yoo·ree′thruh) *n.*, L. pl. & genit. sing. **ure·thrae** (·three) [Gk. *ourēthra*, from *ourein*, to urinate]. The canal through which the urine is discharged, extending from the neck of the urinary bladder to the external urethral orifice, divided in the male into the prostatic portion, the membranous portion, and the spongy or penile portion, and 8 to 9 inches long. (See Plate 25.) In the female, it is about 1½ inches in length. (See Plates 23, 24.) —**ure·thral** (·thrul) *adj.*

urethra fe·mi·ni·na (fem·i·nigh′nuh) [NA]. The female urethra.

urethral bulb. BULB OF THE URETHRA.

urethral carina. A continuation of the anterior column of the vagina in the vestibule as far as the external orifice of the urethra. NA *carina urethralis vaginae.*

urethral caruncle. A small, red, benign, inflammatory, tender mass on the posterior wall of the female urethral meatus.

urethral crest. CRISTA URETHRALIS URETHRAE MASCULINAE.

urethral erotism. *In psychoanalysis,* erotism focused on the urethra and urination, first appearing at a stage of psychosexual development between the anal and the phallic stages.

urethral fold. One of a pair of folds flanking the urethral groove on the caudal surface of the genital tubercle or phallus.

urethral glands. Small, branched, tubular mucous glands in the mucous membrane of the urethra. Syn. *Littré's glands.* NA *glandulae urethrales.*

urethral groove. A groove on the caudal surface of the genital tubercle or phallus, bounded by the urethral folds and urethral membrane. Syn. *urogenital groove, genital fossa.*

urethral lacunae. Pitlike depressions in the mucous membrane of the penile urethra into which open the ducts of the urethral glands (of Littré). NA *lacunae urethrales.*

urethral meatus. MEATUS URETHRAE.

urethral membrane. UROGENITAL MEMBRANE.

urethral plate. A solid plate of endodermal cells, derived from the endoderm of the urogenital membrane, that temporarily obliterates the cavity of the phallic part of the urogenital sinus and later forms a large part of the penile urethra.

urethral profile. A graphic demonstration of transmural urethral pressure; useful in assessing urinary obstruction problems. Compare *urethrograph.*

urethral ring. Anulus urethralis; a mass of smooth muscle around the internal urethral orifice of the urinary bladder.

urethral sound. An elongated steel instrument, usually

slightly conical, for examination and dilatation of the urethra.

urethral sphincter. SPHINCTER URETHRAE MEMBRANACEAE.

urethral synovitis. *Obsol.* Gonorrheal arthritis.

urethral syringe. A syringe adapted to force liquid into the male urethra.

urethra mas·cu·li·na (mas·kew·lye′nuh) [NA]. The male urethra.

urethra mu·li·e·bris (mew·lee·ee′bris) [BNA]. URETHRA FEMININA.

urethrascope. URETHROSCOPE.

urethra vi·ri·lis (vi·rye′lis) [BNA]. URETHRA MASCULINA.

ure·threc·to·my (yoor″e·threck′tuh·mee) *n.* [*urethr-* + *-ectomy*]. Surgical excision of the urethra or portion of it.

ure·thri·tis (yoor″e·thrye′tis) *n.*, pl. **ure·thrit·i·des** (·thrit′i·deez) [*urethr-* + *-itis*]. Inflammation of the urethra.

urethritis cys·ti·ca (sis′ti·kuh). Urethral inflammation characterized by submucosal cyst formation.

urethritis or·i·fi·cii ex·ter·ni (or·i·fish′ee·eye eck·stur′nigh). Inflammation of the urethra at the meatus, usually characterized by superficial ulceration about the glans penis; most often seen in male infants.

urethritis ve·ne·rea (ve·neer′ee·uh). *Obsol.* GONORRHEA.

ure·thro·bul·bar (yoo·ree″thro·bul′bur) *adj.* [*urethro-* + *bulbar*]. Pertaining to the urethra and the bulb of the corpus spongiosum penis.

ure·thro·cele (yoo·ree′thro·seel) *n.* [*urethro-* + *-cele*]. A urethral protrusion or diverticulum occurring, usually, in the female urethra.

ure·thro·cu·ta·ne·ous (yoo·ree″thro·kew·tay′nee·us) *adj.* [*urethro-* + *cutaneous*]. Pertaining to the urethra and the skin.

ure·thro·cys·ti·tis (yoo·ree″thro·sis·tye′tis) *n.* [*urethro-* + *cystitis*]. Inflammation of the urethra and urinary bladder.

ure·thro·cys·to·cele (yoo·ree″thro·sis′to·seel) *n.* [*urethro-* + *cysto-* + *-cele*]. A herniation of the urethra and urinary bladder into the vagina.

ure·thro·gram (yoo·ree′thro·gram) *n.* [*urethro-* + *-gram*]. A radiographic visualization of the urethra by the use of a contrast medium.

ure·thro·graph (yoo·ree′thro·graf) *n.* [*urethro-* + *-graph*]. A recording urethrometer.

ure·throg·ra·phy (yoor″e·throg′ruh·fee) *n.* [*urethro-* + *-graphy*]. Radiography of the urethra employing an opaque contrast substance.

ure·throm·e·ter (yoor″e·throm′e·tur) *n.* [*urethro-* + *-meter*]. An instrument for determining the caliber of the urethra or for measuring the lumen of a urethral stricture.

ure·thro·per·i·ne·al (yoo·ree″thro·perr″i·nee′ul) *adj.* [*urethro-* + *perineal*]. Pertaining to, or involving, both the perineum and the urethra.

ure·thro·phy·ma (yoo·ree″thro·figh′muh) *n.* [*urethro-* + *phyma*]. A urethral tumor.

ure·thro·plas·ty (yoo·ree′thro·plas″tee) *n.* [*urethro-* + *-plasty*]. A plastic operation upon the urethra; surgical repair of the urethra.

ure·thro·pros·tat·ic (yoo·ree″thro·pros·tat′ick) *adj.* [*urethro-* + *prostatic*]. Relating to the urethra and the prostate.

ure·thro·rec·tal (yoo·ree″thro·reck′tul) *adj.* [*urethro-* + *rectal*]. Involving both the urethra and the rectum.

ure·thror·rha·phy (yoo″re·thror′uh·fee) *n.* [*urethro-* + *-rrhaphy*]. Surgical restoration of the continuity of the urethra.

ure·thror·rhea, ure·thror·rhoea (yoo·ree″thro·ree′uh) *n.* [*urethro-* + *-rrhea*]. A discharge from the urethra.

urethrorrhea ex li·bi·di·ne (ecks li·bid′i·nee). The normal mucous secretion occurring during sexual excitement preparatory to coitus.

ure·thro·scope (yoo·ree′thruh·skope) *n.* [*urethro-* + *-scope*]. An instrument for inspecting the interior of the urethra. Compare *panendoscope.* —**ure·thro·scop·ic** (yoo·ree″thruh·skop′ick) *adj.*

ure·thros·co·py (yoor″e·thros′kuh·pee) *n.* [*urethro-* + *-scopy*]. Inspection of the urethra with the aid of the urethroscope.

ure·thro·spasm (yoo·ree′thro·spaz·um) *n.* [*urethro-* + *spasm*]. Spasmodic contraction of the urethral sphincter.

ure·thro·ste·no·sis (yoo·ree″thro·ste·no′sis) *n.* [*urethro-* + *stenosis*]. Stricture of the urethra.

ure·thros·to·my (yoor″e·thros′tuh·mee) *n.* [*urethro-* + *-stomy*]. A fistula created between the penile or perineal skin with some portion of the anterior urethra.

ure·thro·tome (yoo·ree′thruh·tome) *n.* [*urethro-* + *-tome*]. An instrument used for performing an internal urethrotomy.

ure·throt·o·my (yoor″e·throt′uh·mee) *n.* [*urethro-* + *-tomy*]. The operation of cutting a stricture of the urethra.

ure·thro·tri·go·ni·tis (yoo·ree″thro·trye″go·nigh′tis) *n.* [*urethro-* + *trigonitis*]. Inflammation of the trigone of the urinary bladder, usually the anterior segment, and the adjacent urethra.

ure·thro·va·gi·nal (yoo·ree″thro·vaj′i·nul, ·va·jye′nul) *n.* [*urethro-* + *vaginal*]. Pertaining to the urethra and the vagina.

ure·thro·ves·i·cal (yoo·ree″thro·ves′i·kul) *adj.* [*urethro-* + *vesical*]. Pertaining to the urethra and the urinary bladder.

ure·thro·ves·i·co·va·gi·nal (yoo·ree″thro·ves″i·ko·va·jye′nul, ·vaj′i·nul) *adj.* [*urethro-* + *vesico-* + *vaginal*]. Pertaining to the urethra, urinary bladder, and vagina.

ur·gen·cy (ur′jun·see) *n.* Urgent desire to empty the urinary bladder.

Ur·gin·ea (ur·jin′ee·uh) *n.* A genus of the Liliaceae, which includes *Urginea maritima,* and *U. indica,* sources of squill.

ur·hi·dro·sis (yoor″hi·dro′sis) *n.* [*ur-* + *hidrosis*]. Excretion in the sweat of some of the constituents of the urine, chiefly urea, in excess of normal, as in uremia.

-uria [*ur-* + *-ia*]. A combining form designating (a) *a* (specified) *condition of urine;* (b) *the presence of a* (specified) *substance in urine.*

uric (yoor′ick) *adj.* Pertaining to the urine.

uric-, urico-. A combining form meaning *uric acid.*

uric acid. 2,6,8-Trioxypurine, $C_5H_4N_4O_3$, a product of protein metabolism; present in blood and urine. See also Table of Chemical Constituents of Blood in the Appendix.

uric·ac·i·de·mia, uric·ac·i·dae·mia (yoor″ick·as″i·dee′mee·uh) *n.* [*uric acid* + *-emia*]. HYPERURICEMIA.

uric acid reagent of Fo·lin and Den·is [O. K. O. *Folin* and W. G. *Denis*]. An aqueous solution of sodium tungstate, phosphoric acid, and alcohol added to a solution of lithium carbonate and phosphoric acid; used in the determination of uric acid in the blood.

uric·ac·i·du·ria (yoor″ick·as″i·dew′ree·uh) *n.* [*uric acid* + *-uria*]. The presence of excessive amounts of uric acid in the urine.

uricaemia. Uricemia (= HYPERURICEMIA).

uri·can·i·case (yoor″i·kan′i·kace, ·kaze) *n.* An enzyme in the liver that catalyzes conversion of urocanic acid to *l*-glutamic acid.

uri·case (yoor′i·kace, ·kaze) *n.* An enzyme present in the liver, spleen, and kidney of most mammals except man. In the presence of gaseous oxygen, it converts uric acid to allantoin. Syn. *urate oxidase.*

uri·ce·mia, uri·cae·mia (yoor″i·see′mee·uh) *n.* [*uric-* + *-emia*]. HYPERURICEMIA.

urico-. See *uric-.*

uri·col·y·sis (yoor″i·kol′i·sis) *n.* [*urico-* + *-lysis*]. The disintegration of uric acid.

uri·co·su·ria (yoor″i·ko·sue′ree·uh) *n.* [*urico-* + *-uria*]. Urinary excretion of uric acid.

uri·co·su·ric (yoo″ri·ko·sue′rick) *adj.* & *n.* [*uric-* + *-uric*]. 1. Promoting or relating to uricosuria. 2. A drug or substance that promotes uricosuria.

uri·co·tel·ic (yoor″i·ko·tel′ick) *adj.* [*urico-* + *tel-*, end, + *-ic*]. Characterizing an animal in which uric acid is the principal compound of nitrogenous waste, as in birds, snakes, and lizards. Compare *ureotelic.* —**uricotel·ism** (·iz·um) *n.*

uri·dine (yoor′i·deen, ·din) *n.* Uracil riboside, $C_9H_{12}N_2O_6$, a nucleoside composed of one molecule each of uracil and

D-ribose. One of the four main riboside components of ribonucleic acid.

uridine di·phos·pho·glu·cose (dye·fos″fo·gloo′koce, ·koze). A nucleotide sugar derivative consisting of one molecule of D-glucose esterified to the terminal phosphate residue of uridine disphosphate; it functions as the donor of glucose residues in the biosynthesis of glycogen. Abbreviated, *UDP-glucose.*

uridine monophosphate. URIDYLIC ACID.

uri·dro·sis (yoor″i·dro′sis) *n.* URHIDROSIS.

uri·dyl·ic acid (yoor″i·dil′ick). A mononucleotide component, $C_9H_{13}N_2O_9P$, of ribonucleic acid which yields uracil, D-ribose, and phosphoric acid on complete hydrolysis.

urin-, urino-. A combining form meaning *urine.*

uri·nal (yoor′i·nul) *n.* [*urin-* + *-al*]. A vessel for receiving urine.

uri·nal·y·sis (yoor″i·nal′i·sis) *n.* [*urin-* + an*alysis*]. Analysis of the urine; in routine examination, this involves chemical, physical, and microscopical tests.

uri·nary (yoor′i·nerr·ee) *adj.* 1. Of or pertaining to urine. 2. Pertaining to, part of, in, or associated with the urinary system.

urinary abscess. An abscess resulting from extravasation of urine.

urinary bladder. BLADDER (2).

urinary calculus. A calculus situated in any part of the urinary system.

urinary cyst. A retention cyst in the kidney.

urinary fistula. An abnormal tract from any portion of the urinary system; discharges urine through an opening on the skin or into an organ, viscus, or cavity.

urinary infiltration. Passage of urine into tissue spaces, as into tissues of the perineum following rupture of the urethra or the urinary bladder.

urinary meatus. The external opening of the urethra. NA *ostium urethrae externum.*

urinary obstruction. Any hindrance to the passage of urine through the urinary system, specifically to the evacuation of urine from the bladder.

urinary reflex. VESICAL REFLEX.

urinary sediment. Sediment consisting of the formed elements in urine, including casts, epithelial cells, erythrocytes, leukocytes, mucous threads, and spermatozoa.

urinary stammering. *Obsol.* STAMMERING BLADDER.

urinary stuttering. *Obsol.* STAMMERING BLADDER.

urinary system. The system made up of the kidneys, ureters, urinary bladder, and urethra, whose function is the elaboration and excretion of urine.

urinary tract. The passage for the urine, including the kidneys, renal pelves, ureters, urinary bladder, and urethra.

uri·nate (yoor′i·nate) *v.* [ML. *urinare, urinatus*]. To discharge urine from the bladder. **—uri·na·tion** (yoor″i·nay′shun) *n.*

uri·na·tive (yoor′i·nay″tiv) *n.* A drug that stimulates the flow of urine; a diuretic.

urine (yoor′in) *n.* [L. *urina*]. The fluid excreted by the kidneys. In health, urine has an amber color, a slightly acid reaction, a faint odor, a saline taste, and a specific gravity of 1.005 to 1.030. The quantity excreted in 24 hours varies with the amount of fluids consumed but averages between 1,000 and 1,500 ml. The amount of solids in the urine varies with the diet, more being excreted on a high-protein, high-salt diet. Normally between 40 to 75 g of solids are present in the 24-hour urine, of which approximately 25% is urea, 25% chlorides, 25% sulfates and phosphates, and the remainder organic substances including organic acids, pigments, neutral sulfur, hormones. The most important abnormal constituents present in disease are protein, sugar, blood, pus, acetone, diacetic acid, fat, chyle, tube casts, various cells, and bacteria.

uri·nif·er·ous (yoor″i·nif′ur·us) *adj.* [*urin-* + *-iferous*]. Carrying or conveying urine.

uriniferous tubule. One of the numerous winding tubules of the kidney. See also *nephron.*

uri·nif·ic (yoor″i·nif′ick) *adj.* Excreting or producing urine.

uri·nip·a·rous (yoor″i·nip′uh·rus) *adj.* [*urin-* + *-parous*]. Producing urine.

urino-. See *urin-.*

uri·no·cry·os·co·py (yoor″ri·no·krye·os′kuh·pee) *n.* [*urino-* + *-cryoscopy*]. Cryoscopy of the urine.

uri·no·gen·i·tal (yoor″i·no·jen′i·tul) *adj.* [*urino-* + *genital*]. UROGENITAL.

uri·nog·e·nous (yoor″i·noj′i·nus) *adj.* [*urino-* + *-genous*]. UROGENOUS.

uri·nol·o·gy (yoor″i·nol′uh·jee) *n.* [*urino-* + *-logy*]. The science of diagnosis of disease by means of urinary analysis.

uri·no·ma (yoor″i·no′muh) *n.*, pl. **urinomas, urinoma·ta** (·tuh) [*urin-* + *-oma*]. A cyst containing urine.

uri·nom·e·ter (yoor″i·nom′e·tur) *n.* [*urino-* + *-meter*]. A hydrometer for measuring the specific gravity of urine.

uri·nom·e·try (yoor″i·nom′e·tree) *n.* [*urino-* + *-metry*]. The determination of the specific gravity of urine.

uri·nos·co·py (yoor″i·nos′kuh·pee) *n.* [*urino-* + *-scopy*]. UROSCOPY. **—uri·no·scop·ic** (·no·skop′ick) *adj.*

uri·nose (yoor′i·noce, ·noze) *adj.* URINOUS.

uri·nous (yoor′i·nus) *adj.* [*urin-* + *-ous*]. Having the characteristics of urine.

urinous abscess. An abscess containing urine mingled with the pus.

uri·po·sia (yoor″i·po′see·uh) *n.* [*ur*ine + Gk. *pos*is, drink, drinking, + *-ia*]. The drinking of urine.

uri·sol·vent (yoor″i·sol′vunt) *adj.* Dissolving uric acid.

uri·tis (yoo·rye′tis) *n.* [L. *ur*ere, to burn, + *-itis*]. Inflammation following a burn.

ur·ning (oor′ning) *n.* [Ger., from *Uranismus,* uranism]. A male homosexual.

uro-. See *ur-.*

uro·ac·i·dim·e·ter (yoor″o·as″i·dim′e·tur) *n.* [*uro-* + *acid* + *-meter*]. An instrument for measuring the acidity of urine.

uro·an·the·lone (yoor″o·anth′e·lone) *n.* Anthelone derived from urine.

uro·azo·tom·e·ter (yoor″o·az″o·tom′e·tur) *n.* [*uro-* + *azoto-* + *-meter*]. An apparatus for quantitative estimation of the nitrogenous substances in urine.

uro·ben·zo·ic acid (yoor″o·ben·zo′ick). HIPPURIC ACID.

uro·bi·lin (yoor″o·bye′lin, ·bil′in) *n.* A bile pigment produced by reduction of bilirubin by intestinal bacteria, with intermediate formation of urobilinogen, and excreted by the kidneys or removed by the liver.

uro·bi·lin·emia, uro·bi·lin·aemia (yoor″o·bye″li·nee′mee·uh, ·bil″i·) *n.* [*urobilin* + *-emia*]. The presence of urobilin in the blood.

uro·bi·lin·ic·ter·us (yoo″ro·bye″li·nick′tur·us) *n.* [*urobilin* + *icterus*]. Jaundice associated with urobilinemia.

uro·bi·lino·gen (yoor″o·bye·lin′o·jen) *n.* A chromogen, formed in feces and present in urine, from which urobilin is formed by oxidation.

uro·bi·lino·gen·uria (yoor″o·bye·lin″o·je·new′ree·uh) *n.* [*urobilinogen* + *-uria*]. 1. An excess of urobilinogen in the urine. 2. Urobilinogen in the urine.

uro·bi·lin·oi·din (yoor″o·bye″li·noy′din) *n.* A form of urinary pigment derived from hematin and resembling urobilin though not identical with it.

urobilin test. 1. SCHLESINGER'S TEST. 2. SCHMIDT'S TEST.

uro·bi·lin·uria (yoor″o·bye″li·new′ree·uh, ·bil″i·) *n.* [*urobilin* + *-uria*]. The presence of an excess of urobilin in urine.

uro·can·ic acid (yoor″o·kan′ick). 4-Imidazoleacrylic acid, $C_6H_6N_2O_2$, found in dog's urine as a product of deamination of histidine.

uroch·e·ras (yoo·rock′ur·us) *n.* [*uro-* + Gk. *cherades,* gravel]. Gravel in urine.

uro·che·sia (yoor″o·kee′zhuh, ·zee·uh) *n.* [*uro-* + Gk. *chez*ein, to defecate, + *-ia*]. Discharge of urine through the anus.

uro·chlo·ral·ic acid (yoor″o·klo·ral′ick). 2,2,2-Trichloroethyl β-D-glucosiduronic acid, $C_8H_{11}Cl_3O_7$, a metabolic product of chloral hydrate excreted in urine. It gives a false positive copper reduction test for sugar.

uro·chrome (yoor'o·krome) *n.* [*uro-* + *-chrome*]. A yellow pigment in urine.

uro·chro·mo·gen (yoor"o·kro'muh·jen) *n.* A substance occurring in tissues, which is oxidized to urochrome.

uro·clep·sia (yoor"o·klep'see·uh) *n.* [*uro-* + Gk. *kleptein*, to do secretly, to steal, + *-ia*]. Involuntary or unconscious urination.

uro·cris·ia (yoor"o·kriz'ee·uh, ·kris'ee·uh) *n.* [*uro-* + Gk. *krisis*, judgment, determining, + *-ia*]. Diagnosis by means of urinary examination and analysis.

uro·cri·sis (yoo"ro·krye'sis) *n.* [*uro-* + *crisis*]. 1. Painful spasms of the urinary tract in tabes dorsalis. 2. The critical stage of a disease distinguished by the excretion of a large volume of urine.

uro·cy·a·nin (yoor"o·sigh'uh·nin) *n.* [*uro-* + *cyan-* + *-in*]. UROGLAUCIN.

uro·cy·an·o·gen (yoor"o·sigh·an'o·jin) *n.* [*uro-* + *cyano-* + *-gen*]. A blue pigment found in urine.

uro·cy·a·nose (yoor"o·sigh'uh·noce, ·noze) *n.* UROCYANOGEN.

uro·cy·a·no·sis (yoor"o·sigh"uh·no'sis) *n.* [*uro-* + *cyan-* + *-osis*]. Blue discoloration of the urine, usually from the presence of excess amounts of indican oxidized to indigo blue; also from drugs such as methylene blue.

uro·de·um, uro·dae·um (yoo"ro·dee'um) *n.* [NL., from *ur-* + Gk. *hodaion*, on the way]. The portion of the cloaca into which the urogenital ducts open.

uro·dy·nam·ics (yoor"o·dye·nam'icks) *n.* [*uro-* + *dynamics*]. The study of the forces responsible for moving urine along the urinary tract; urinary tract hydrodynamics.

uroedema. UREDEMA.

uro·en·ter·one (yoor"o·en'tur·ohn) *n.* UROGASTRONE.

uro·er·y·thrin (yoor"o·err'i·thrin) *n.* [*uro-* + *erythr-* + *-in*]. A red pigment found in urine.

uro·fla·vin (yoor"o·flay'vin) *n.* [*uro-* + *flav-* + *-in*]. A fluorescent compound of unknown structure, with properties similar to riboflavin, excreted in the urine along with the vitamin, following ingestion of riboflavin.

uro·fus·cin (yoor"o·fus'in) *n.* [*uro-* + L. *fuscus*, dark, + *-in*]. A pigment found occasionally in urine in cases of porphyrinuria.

uro·fus·co·hem·a·tin, uro·fus·co·haem·a·tin (yoor"o·fus"ko·hem'uh·tin) *n.* A red pigment derived from hematin, occurring in the urine.

uro·gas·trone (yoor"o·gas'trone) *n.* A substance extracted from urine which inhibits gastric secretion.

uro·gen·i·tal (yoor"o·jen'i·tul) *adj.* [*uro-* + *genital*]. Pertaining to the urinary and genital organs.

urogenital aperture. The external opening of the embryonic urogenital sinus.

urogenital canal. UROGENITAL TUBE.

urogenital cloaca. An abnormal common opening of the urethra and vagina due to a defective urethrovaginal septum.

urogenital diaphragm. The sheet of tissue stretching across the pubic arch, formed by the deep transverse perineal and the sphincter urethrae muscles. Syn. *triangular ligament, trigonium urogenitale.* NA *diaphragma urogenitale.*

urogenital duct. 1. The male urethra from the orifices of the ejaculatory ducts to the fossa navicularis. 2. In certain vertebrates, the mesonephric duct.

urogenital fissure. *In embryology,* the cleft between the genital folds forming the aperture of the urogenital sinus.

urogenital fold or **ridge.** A fold or swelling of the dorsal coelomic wall containing the mesonephros and its duct and, later, the gonad and paramesonephric duct.

urogenital groove. URETHRAL GROOVE.

urogenital membrane. The part of the cloacal membrane cranial or ventral to the urorectal (cloacal) septum; it forms the floor of the urethral groove of the phallus.

urogenital sinus. 1. DEFINITIVE UROGENITAL SINUS. 2. PRIMITIVE UROGENITAL SINUS.

urogenital system. The combined urinary and genital systems, which are intimately related embryologically and anatomically. NA *apparatus urogenitalis.* See also Plates 24, 25.

urogenital tract. The chain of organs that constitutes the urogenital system.

urogenital triangle. A triangle with the base between the two ischial tuberosities (tubers) and the apex below the symphysis pubis.

urogenital tube. *In embryology,* the ventral part of the cloaca after division by the urorectal septum. It comprises the vesicourethral primordium and the urogenital sinus. Syn. *urogenital canal.*

urog·e·nous (yoo·roj'e·nus) *adj.* [*uro-* + *-genous*]. Producing urine; derived from urine.

uro·glau·cin (yoor"o·glaw'sin) *n.* [*uro-* + Gk. *glaukos*, bluish-green, + *-in*]. A blue pigment sometimes occurring in urine.

uro·gram (yoor'o·gram) *n.* [*uro-* + *-gram*]. A radiograph or radiographic visualization of the urinary tract made after intravenous or retrograde injection of an opaque contrast medium.

urog·ra·phy (yoo·rog'ruh·fee) *n.* [*uro-* + *-graphy*]. Radiographic visualization of the urinary tract by the use of a contrast medium.

uro·gra·vim·e·ter (yoor"ro·gra·vim'e·tur) *n.* [*uro-* + *gravimeter*]. URINOMETER.

uro·hem·a·tin, uro·haem·a·tin (yoor"o·hem'uh·tin, ·hee'muh·tin) *n.* Hematin in the urine.

uro·hem·a·to·ne·phro·sis, uro·haem·a·to·ne·phro·sis (yoor"ro·hem"uh·to·ne·fro'sis, ·hee"muh·to·) *n.* [*uro-* + *hemato-* + *nephrosis*]. Distention of the pelvis of a kidney with blood and urine.

uro·hem·a·to·por·phy·rin, uro·haem·a·to·por·phy·rin (yoor"ro·hem"uh·to·por'fi·rin, ·hee"muh·to·) *n.* Hematoporphyrin, occasionally occurring in urine in certain pathologic states.

uro·hy·per·ten·sin (yoo"ro·high"pur·ten'sin) *n.* [*uro-* + *hypertension* + *-in*]. A substance or substances derived from urine that increase blood pressure when injected intravenously.

uro·ki·nase (yoor"o·kigh'nace, ·kin'aze) *n.* An enzyme, present in human urine, that catalyzes conversion of plasminogen to the active proteolytic enzyme plasmin. It produces lysis of blood clots and has therapeutic utility as a thrombolytic (fibrinolytic) agent.

uro·ki·net·ic (yoor"o·ki·net'ick, ·kigh·net'ick) *adj.* [*uro-* + *kinetic*]. Caused by a reflex from the urinary system; generally denotes indigestion secondary to irritation or disease of the urinary tract.

Urokon. Trademark for sodium acetrizoate, a radiodiagnostic agent.

uro·leu·kin·ic acid (yoor"o·lew·kin'ick). An acid found in the urine in alkaptonuria.

uro·lite (yoor'o·lite) *n.* UROLITH.

uro·lith (yoor'o·lith) *n.* [*uro-* + *-lith*]. A calculus occurring in urine. —**uro·lith·ic** (yoor"o·lith'ick) *adj.*

uro·li·thi·a·sis (yoor"o·li·thigh'uh·sis) *n.* [*urolith* + *-iasis*]. 1. The presence of, or a condition associated with, urinary calculi. 2. The formation of urinary calculi.

uro·li·thot·o·my (yoor"o·li·thot'uh·mee) *n.* [*uro-* + *lithotomy*]. Removal of a calculus from anywhere in the urinary tract.

urol·o·gist (yoo·rol'uh·jist) *n.* A person skilled in urology; a specialist in the diagnosis and treatment of diseases of the urogenital tract in the male and the urinary tract in the female. Syn. *genitourinary surgeon.*

urol·o·gy (yoo·rol'uh·jee) *n.* [*uro-* + *logy*]. 1. The branch of medical science embracing the study and treatment of the diseases and the abnormalities of the urogenital tract in the male and the urinary tract in the female. 2. The scientific study of the urine. —**uro·log·ic** (yoor″o·loj′ick) *adj.*

uro·lu·te·in (yoor″o·lew′tee·in) *n.* [*uro-* + *lute-* + *-in*]. A yellow pigment sometimes found in urine.

uro·man·cy (yoor′o·man″see) *n.* [*uro-* + Gk. *manteia,* divination]. *Obsol.* Diagnosis by observation of the urine.

uro·man·tia (yoo″ro·man′shee·uh) *n. Obsol.* UROMANCY.

uro·mel·a·nin (yoo″ro·mel′uh·nin) *n.* [*uro-* + *melan-* + *-in*]. A black pigment that sometimes appears in urine as a decomposition product of urochrome.

urom·e·lus (yoo·rom′e·lus) *n.* [NL., from Gk. *oura,* tail, + *melos,* limb]. SYMPUS MONOPUS.

urom·e·ter (yoo·rom′e·tur) *n.* URINOMETER.

uron-, urono- [Gk. *ouron*]. A combining form meaning *urine, urinary.*

uro·ne·phro·sis (yoor″o·ne·fro′sis) *n.* [*uro-* + *nephrosis*]. HYDRONEPHROSIS.

uron·ic acid (yoo·ron′ick). Any group of monobasic sugar acids obtained when the primary alcohol group of an aldose is oxidized to carboxyl, without oxidizing the aldehyde group.

urono-. See *uron-.*

uro·nol·o·gy (yoor″o·nol′uh·jee) *n.* [*urono-* + *-logy*]. UROLOGY.

uron·on·com·e·try (yoor″on·ong·kom′e·tree) *n.* [*uron-* + *onco-* + *-metry*]. Measurement of the quantity of urine passed or excreted in a definite period, as 24 hours.

uro·nos·co·py (yoor″o·nos′kuh·pee) *n.* [*urono-* + *-scopy*]. Examination of urine by inspection and use of the microscope.

urop·a·thy (yoo·rop′uth·ee) *n.* [*uro-* + *-pathy*]. Any disease involving the urinary tract.

uro·pep·sin (yoor″o·pep′sin) *n.* [*uro-* + *pepsin*]. The urinary end product of the secretion of pepsinogen into the bloodstream by gastric cells, followed by transport to the kidneys and excretion in urine.

uro·phe·in (yoor″o·fee′in) *n.* [*uro-* + *pheo-* + *-in*]. A gray pigment found in urine.

uro·pit·tin (yoor″o·pit′in) *n.* [*uro-* + Gk. *pitta,* pitch, + *-in*]. A resinous decomposition product of urochrome.

uro·pla·nia (yoor″o·play′nee·uh) *n.* [*uro-* + *-plania*]. The presence of urine elsewhere than in the urinary organs; discharge of urine from an orifice other than the urethra.

uro·poi·e·sis (yoor″o·poy·e′sis) *n.* [*uro-* + *-poiesis*]. The production of urine.

uro·por·phy·rin (yoor″o·por′fi·rin) *n.* Any of several isomeric, metal-free porphyrins, occurring in small amounts in normal urine and feces, characterized by having as substituents four acetic acid (—CH_2COOH) and four propionic acid (—CH_2CH_2COOH) groups.

uro·psam·mus (yoor″o·sam′us) *n.* [NL., from *uro-* + Gk. *psammos,* sand]. Urinary gravel or sediment.

uro·pyg·i·al (yoor″o·pij′ee·ul) *adj.* [*uro-* + Gk. *pygē,* rump, + *-al*]. Pertaining to the uropygium, the fleshy and bony posterior prominence that supports the tail feathers of a bird.

uropygial gland. A large bilobed sebaceous gland found dorsal to the last sacral vertebra of fowl. Its oily secretion reaches the surface of the skin by way of a short duct. Syn. *preen gland.*

uro·rec·tal (yoor″o·reck′tul) *adj.* [*uro-* + *rectal*]. Pertaining to the urinary organs and the rectum.

urorectal plicae. The lateral folds that fuse to form the urorectal septum of the embryo.

urorectal septum. The embryonic horizontal connective-tissue septum that divides the cloaca into the rectum and primary urogenital sinus. Syn. *cloacal septum, Douglas' septum.*

uro·ro·se·in (yoor″o·ro′zee·in) *n.* [*uro-* + L. *roseus,* rosy, + *-in*]. A urinary pigment that does not occur preformed in the urine, but is present in the form of a chromogen, indoleacetic acid, which is transformed into the pigment upon treatment with a mineral acid. It is said to be identical with urorrhodin.

uror·rha·gia (yoor″o·ray′jee·uh) *n.* [*uro-* + *-rrhagia*]. Excessive discharge of urine, as in diabetes insipidus.

uror·rho·din, uro·rho·din (yoor″o·ro′din) *n.* [*uro-* + *rhod-* + *-in*]. A red pigment found in urine and derived from uroxanthin.

uror·rho·dino·gen (yoor″o·ro·din′uh·jen) *n.* The chromogen which by decomposition produces urorrhodin.

uro·ru·bin (yoor″o·roo′bin) *n.* [*uro-* + L. *ruber,* red, + *-in*]. A red pigment found in urine, seen only in disease.

uro·sa·cin (yoo·ro′suh·sin) *n.* [*ur-* + L. *rosaceus,* of roses, + *-in*]. URORRHODIN.

uros·che·sis (yoo·ros′ke·sis) *n.* [*uro-* + Gk. *schesis,* stationary condition, retention]. Urinary retention.

uros·co·pist (yoo·ros′kuh·pist) *n.* A person who makes a specialty of urinary examinations; a technician who examines urine for evidence of disease.

uros·co·py (yoo·ros′kuh·pee) *n.* [*uro-* + *-scopy*]. Examination of urine; URONOSCOPY. —**uro·scop·ic** (yoor″o·skop′ick) *adj.*

uro·se·in (yoo·ro′see·in) *n.* [*ur-* + L. *roseus,* rose-colored, + *-in*]. URORRHODIN.

uro·se·mi·ol·o·gy (yoor″o·sem″ee·ol′uh·jee) *n.* [*uro-* + *semiology*]. Examination of the urine as an aid to diagnosis.

uro·sep·sis (yoor″o·sep′sis) *n.* [*uro-* + *sepsis*]. Systemic toxicity from extravasated urine.

uro·spec·trin (yoor″o·speck′trin) *n.* [*uro-* + L. *spectrum,* image, + *-in*]. A pigment of normal urine.

uro·ste·a·lith (yoor″o·stee′uh·lith) *n.* [*uro-* + *stear-* + *-lith*]. A fatlike substance occurring in some urinary calculi.

uro·the·li·um (yoor″o·theel′ee·um) *n.* [*uro-* + *-thelium*]. The epithelium of the urinary tract. —**urotheli·al** (·ul) *adj.*

uro·tox·ia (yoor″o·tock′see·uh) *n.* UROTOXY.

uro·tox·ic (yoor″o·tock′sick) *adj.* [*uro-* + *toxic*]. 1. Pertaining to poisonous substances eliminated in urine. 2. Pertaining to poisoning by urine or some of its constituents.

uro·tox·ic·i·ty (yoor″o·tock·sis′i·tee) *n.* [*uro-* + *toxicity*]. The toxic properties of urine.

uro·tox·in (yoor″o·tock′sin) *n.* [*uro-* + *toxin*]. A poisonous or toxic constituent of urine.

uro·toxy (yoor′o·tock″see) *n.* The unit of toxicity of urine; the amount necessary to kill a kilogram of living substance.

Urotropin. A trademark for methenamine.

Urov disease. KASHIN-BECK DISEASE.

uro·xan·thin (yoor″o·zan′thin) *n.* [*uro-* + *xanth-* + *-in*]. A yellow pigment in human urine which yields indigo blue on oxidation.

ur·rho·din (yoor′o·din, yoo·ro′din) *n.* URORRHODIN.

ur·sol·ic acid (ur·sol′ick). A triterpene acid, $C_{30}H_{48}O_3$, occurring in the waxlike coating of the skin or cuticle of fruits and in the leaves of certain plants. Used as an emulsifying agent in the manufacture of pharmaceuticals and food products.

ur·ti·ca (ur′ti·kuh, ur·tye′kuh) *n.* [L.]. 1. A plant of the genus *Urtica;* a nettle. 2. WHEAL.

ur·ti·cant (ur′ti·kunt) *n.* Something that produces urticaria.

ur·ti·car·ia (ur″ti·kăr′ee·uh) *n.* [NL., from L. *urtica,* nettle]. Hives or nettle rash. A skin condition characterized by the appearance of intensely itching wheals or welts with elevated, usually white, centers and a surrounding area of erythema. They appear in crops, widely distributed over the body surface, tend to disappear in a day or two, and usually are unattended by constitutional symptoms. —**urticar·i·al** (·ee·ul) *adj.*

urticaria bul·lo·sa (buh·lo′suh, bŏŏl·o′suh). Urticaria with the formation of fluid-filled vesicles or bullae on the surface of the wheals.

urticaria fac·ti·tia (fack·tish′ee·uh). DERMOGRAPHIA.

urticaria hem·or·rhag·i·ca (hem″o·raj′i·kuh). A type of urticaria bullosa in which the vesicles contain bloody fluid.

urticarial fever. Schistosomiasis caused by *Schistosoma japonicum.*

urticaria med·i·ca·men·to·sa (med″i-kuh-men-to′suh). Urticaria due to the ingestion of a drug to which the individual is allergic.

urticaria pap·u·lo·sa (pap″yoo-lo′suh). An intensely pruritic skin eruption seen in children, characterized by recurrent crops of erythematous patches and papules on the extensor surfaces of the extremities; it is related to insect bites. Syn. *lichen urticatus, prurigo simplex.*

urticaria pig·men·to·sa (pig″men-to′suh). A disease involving mast cells and occurring in several different forms. There are cutaneous manifestations of urticaria in a form affecting children and one affecting adults, and there is a systemic form usually without skin lesions. The skin manifestations have a variety of appearances, ranging from innumerable brown macules to solitary red-brown nodules; urtication occurs on stroking the lesions.

urticaria so·la·ris (so-lair′is). Urticaria occurring in certain individuals due to exposure to sunlight.

ur·ti·car·io·gen·ic (ur″ti-kăr″ee-o-jen′ick) *adj.* [*urticaria* + *-genic*]. Producing urticaria.

ur·ti·cate (ur′ti-kate, -kut) *adj. & v.* [L. *urticatus,* from *urticare,* to sting]. 1. Characterized by the presence of wheals. 2. To produce urticaria or urtication (1).

ur·ti·ca·tion (ur″ti-kay′shun) *n.* [ML. *urticatio,* from L. *urticare,* to sting]. 1. A sensation as if one had been stung by nettles. 2. Production of wheals.

uru·shi·ol (uh-roo′shee-ol) *n.* [Jap. *urushi,* lacquer, + *-ol*]. The irritant fraction of poison ivy and poison oak, consisting of derivatives of catechol with an unsaturated 15-carbon side chain.

-us [L., nominative masculine singular suffix]. A suffix designating *an individual characterized by a* (specified) *trait or anomaly.*

USAN *U*nited *S*tates *A*dopted *N*ames, a cooperative nomenclature program for selecting nonproprietary names for new drugs early in the course of their investigation as potential therapeutic agents.

us·ne·in (us′nee-in) *n.* USNIC ACID.

us·nic acid (us′nick). An antibacterial phenolic substance, $C_{18}H_{16}O_7$, found in lichens, as in *Usnea barbata.*

us·nin·ic acid (us-nin′ick). USNIC ACID.

U.S.P. Abbreviation for *United States Pharmacopeia.*

USPC United States Pharmacopeial Convention.

USPHS Abbreviation for *United States Public Health Service.*

us·ti·lag·i·nism (us″ti-laj′i-niz-um) *n.* [*Ustilago* + *-ism*]. A condition resembling ergot poisoning; caused by eating corn containing the fungus *Ustilago maydis.*

Us·ti·la·go (us″ti-lay′go) *n.* [L.]. A genus of parasitic fungi; the smuts.

us·tion (us′chun) *n.* [L. *ustio,* a burning, from *urere, ustus,* to burn]. *In surgery,* CAUTERIZATION.

uta (oo′tuh) *n.* [Sp.]. A form of American mucocutaneous leishmaniasis, consisting of single or multiple skin ulcers of the nose and lips. It occurs in cool climates and at altitudes over 600 m. The etiologic agent is *Leishmania brasiliensis.*

uter-, utero-. A combining form meaning *uterus, uterine.*

uter·al·gia (yoo″tur-al′jee-uh) *n.* [*uter-* + *-algia*]. Pain in the uterus.

uter·ine (yoo′tur-in, yoo′tuh-rine) *adj.* [L. *uterinus*]. Pertaining to the uterus.

uterine apoplexy. Massive infiltration of blood into the myometrium of the pregnant uterus, subsequent to premature separation of the placenta.

uterine appendages. The ovaries and oviducts.

uterine artery. A large branch of the internal iliac artery, supplying the uterus and uterine tube, the round and broad ligaments of the uterus, and a portion of the vagina; the homologue in the female of the deferential artery. NA *arteria uterina.*

uterine canal. CAVITY OF THE UTERUS.

uterine cervix. CERVIX OF THE UTERUS.

uterine croup. Inflammation of the endometrium with pseudomembrane formation.

uterine displacement. Any change in position of the uterus from the accepted normal. See also *anteversion, prolapse, retroversion.*

uterine dysmenorrhea. Dysmenorrhea caused by uterine disease.

uterine fibroid. LEIOMYOMA UTERI.

uterine glands. Glands of the endometrium. NA *glandulae uterinae.*

uterine inertia. *In obstetrics,* the diminution or cessation of uterine contractions during labor.

uterine isthmus. ISTHMUS UTERI.

uterine milk. A white fluid found between the placental villi of the pregnant uterus.

uterine plexus. 1. A venous plexus on the walls of the uterus and extending into the broad ligament. NA *plexus venosus uterinus.* 2. A visceral nerve plexus supplying the uterus.

uterine relaxing factor. LUTUTRIN.

uterine sinus. A venous sinus in the wall of the gravid uterus.

uterine souffle. A soft, blowing sound, synchronous with the maternal heart, heard over the abdomen at the sides of the uterus. The sound is due to the circulation of the blood in the large uterine arteries and veins. Its value as a diagnostic sign of pregnancy is doubtful.

uterine sound. A graduated probe for measurement of the uterine cavity.

uterine tube. The oviduct in mammals. Syn. *fallopian tube.*

uterine veil. A cap fitted over the cervix uteri to prevent the entrance of semen.

uter·is·mus (yoo″tur-iz′mus) *n.* [*uter-* + *-ismus*]. Uterine contraction of a spasmodic and painful character.

uter·i·tis (yoo″tur-eye′tis) *n.* [*uter-* + *-itis*]. Inflammation of the uterus; METRITIS.

utero-. See *uter-.*

utero·ab·dom·i·nal (yoo″tur-o-ab-dom′i-nul) *adj.* Pertaining to the uterus and the abdomen.

uteroabdominal pregnancy. Gestation with one fetus in the uterus and another within the peritoneal cavity.

utero·ad·nex·al (yoo″tur-o-ad-neck′sul) *adj.* [*utero-* + *adnexal*]. Pertaining to the uterus and its tubes and ovaries.

utero·cer·vi·cal (yoo″tur-o-sur′vi-kul) *adj.* [*utero-* + *cervical*]. Pertaining to the uterus and the cervix of the uterus.

uterocervical canal. The canal of the cervix of the uterus. NA *canalis cervicus uteri.*

utero·co·lic (yoo″tur-o-ko′lick, -kol′ick) *adj.* [*utero-* + *colic*]. Pertaining to the uterus and the colon.

utero·en·ter·ic (yoo″tur-o-en-terr′ick) *adj.* [*utero-* + *enteric*]. UTEROINTESTINAL.

utero·fix·a·tion (yoo″tur-o-fick-say′shun) *n.* [*utero-* + *fixation*]. HYSTEROPEXY.

utero·ges·ta·tion (yoo″tur-o-jes-tay′shun) *n.* Gestation within the cavity of the uterus; normal pregnancy.

uter·og·ra·phy (yoo″tur-og′ruh-fee) *n.* [*utero-* + *-graphy*]. Radiographic visualization of the uterine cavity by means of contrast medium injected therein through the cervical canal; metrography, hysterography.

utero·in·tes·ti·nal (yoo″tur-o-in-tes′ti-nul) *adj.* Pertaining to the uterus and the intestine.

utero·ma·nia (yoo″tur-o-may′nee-uh) *n.* [*utero-* + *-mania*]. Mental disorder associated with uterine disorder.

uter·om·e·ter (yoo″tur-om′e-tur) *n.* [*utero-* + *-meter*]. An instrument used to measure the uterus.

utero-ovar·i·an (yoo″tur-o-o-văr′ee-un) *adj.* [*utero-* + *ovarian*]. Pertaining to the uterus and the ovaries.

utero-ovarian pregnancy. Gestation with one fetus in the uterus and another in the ovary.

utero-ovarian varicocele. A varicose condition of the veins of the pampiniform plexus in the broad ligament.

utero·pa·ri·e·tal (yoo″tur-o-puh-rye′e-tul) *adj.* [*utero-* + *pari-*

etal]. Pertaining to the uterus and the abdominal wall.
utero·pel·vic (yoo″tur·o·pel′vick) *adj.* Pertaining to the uterus and the pelvic ligaments.
utero·pex·ia (yoo″tur·o·peck′see·uh) *n.* HYSTEROPEXY.
utero·pexy (yoo′tur·o·peck″see) *n.* [*utero-* + *-pexy*]. HYSTEROPEXY.
utero·pla·cen·tal (yoo″tur·o·pluh·sen′tul) *adj.* [*utero-* + *placental*]. Pertaining to the uterus and the placenta.
uteroplacental apoplexy. COUVELAIRE UTERUS.
uteroplacental insufficiency. A condition in which uterine and placental function fails to meet fetal needs. Abbreviated, UPI
utero·plas·ty (yoo′tur·o·plas″tee) *n.* [*utero-* + *-plasty*]. A plastic operation on the uterus.
utero·rec·tal (yoo″tur·o·reck′tul) *adj.* [*utero-* + *rectal*]. Pertaining to the uterus and the rectum.
utero·sa·cral (yoo″tur·o·say′krul) *adj.* [*utero-* + *sacral*]. Pertaining to the uterus and the sacrum.
uterosacral ligament. A concentric band of connective tissue covered with peritoneum that passes backward from the cervix of the uterus on either side of the rectum to the posterior wall of the pelvis.
utero·sal·pin·gog·ra·phy (yoo″tur·o·sal″pin·gog′ruh·fee) *n.* [*utero-* + *salpingo-* + *-graphy*]. HYSTEROSALPINGOGRAPHY.
utero·scope (yoo′tur·o·skope) *n.* [*utero-* + *-scope*]. A uterine speculum.
uter·ot·o·my (yoo″tur·ot′uh·mee) *n.* [*utero-* + *-tomy*]. HYSTEROTOMY.
utero·ton·ic (yoo″tur·o·ton′ick) *adj.* [*utero-* + *tonic*]. Increasing muscular tone of the uterus.
utero·trac·tor (yoo″tur·o·track′tur) *n.* [*utero-* + *tractor*]. 1. A uterine tenaculum or volsella forceps. 2. A wide, heavy, sharp-toothed retractor used to make continuous traction on the anterior portion of the cervix of the uterus during surgery.
utero·tu·bal (yoo″tur·o·tew′bul) *adj.* [*utero-* + *tubal*]. Pertaining to the uterus and the oviducts.
uterotubal pregnancy. Gestation with one fetus in the uterus and another in an oviduct.
utero·va·gi·nal (yoo″tur·o·va·jye′nul, ·vaj′i·nul) *adj.* [*utero-* + *vaginal*]. Pertaining to the uterus and vagina.
uterovaginal canal. 1. The common canal formed by the uterus and vagina. 2. *In embryology,* the single cavity formed by fusion of the paramesonephric ducts.
uterovaginal plexus. 1. A visceral nerve plexus on each side of the uterine cervix, composed of the pelvic part of the hypogastric plexus and the third and fourth sacral nerves. NA *plexus uterovaginalis.* 2. The uterine and vaginal plexuses considered as a single venous plexus.
utero·ven·tral (yoo″tur·o·ven′trul) *adj.* [*utero-* + *ventral*]. Pertaining to the uterus and the abdomen.
utero·ves·i·cal (yoo″tur·o·ves′i·kul) *adj.* [*utero-* + *vesical*]. Pertaining to the uterus and the urinary bladder.
uterovesical pouch. VESICOUTERINE EXCAVATION.
uter·us (yoo′tur·us) *n.*, pl. & genit. sing. **uteri** (yoo′tur·eye) [L.] [NA]. The womb; the organ of gestation which receives and holds the fertilized ovum during the development of the fetus, and becomes the principal agent in its expulsion during parturition. See also Plates 23, 24.
uterus acol·lis (a·kol′is). A uterus in which the vaginal part of the cervix is abnormally small or absent.
uterus ar·cu·a·tus (ahr·kew·ay′tus). A subvariety of uterus bicornis in which there is merely a vertical depression in the middle of the fundus uteri.
uterus bi·cor·nis (bye·kor′nis). 1. A human uterus divided into two horns or compartments due to an arrest of development. 2. The normal uterus in many mammals, as carnivores.
uterus bi·loc·u·la·ris (bye·lock″yoo·lair′is). UTERUS SEPTUS.
uterus di·del·phys (dye·del′fis). UTERUS DUPLEX.
uterus du·plex (dew′plecks). A uterus that is double from failure of the paramesonephric ducts to unite.
uterus mas·cu·li·nus (mas·kew·lye′nus). UTRICLE (2).
uterus par·vi·col·lis (pahr·vi·kol′is). A malformation in which the vaginal portion of the uterus is small but the body is normal.
uterus sep·tus (sep′tus). A uterus in which a median septum more or less completely divides the lumen into halves.
uterus uni·cor·nis (yoo·ni·kor′nis). A uterus having but a single lateral half with usually only one uterine tube; it is the result of faulty development.
uti·li·za·tion time (yoo″ti·li·zay′shun). *Obsol.* The period of time during which a given stimulus is effective in causing excitation of a tissue.
utri·cle (yoo′tri·kul) *n.* [L. *utriculus,* dim. of *uter,* leather bag]. 1. A delicate membranous sac communicating with the semicircular canals of the ear. 2. The uterus masculinus, or prostatic utricle; a vestigial blind pouch in the colliculus seminalis opening into the prostatic urethra. The homolog of a part of the female vagina; derived from the fused distal ends of the paramesonephric ducts. Syn. *utriculus masculinus, sinus pocularis.* NA *utriculus prostaticus.* See also Plate 25. —**utric·u·lar** (yoo·trick′yoo·lur) *adj.*
utricular duct. UTRICULOSACCULAR DUCT.
utricular recess. ELLIPTICAL RECESS.
utric·u·li·tis (yoo·trick″yoo·lye′tis) *n.* [*utriculus* + *-itis*]. 1. Inflammation of the prostatic utricle. 2. Inflammation of the utricle of the ear.
utric·u·lo·am·pul·lary (yoo·trick″yoo·lo·am′puh·lair″ee) *adj.* Pertaining to the utricle and ampullae of the internal ear.
utriculoampullary nerve. NA *nervus utriculoampullaris.* See Table of Nerves in the Appendix.
utric·u·lo·sac·cu·lar (yoo·trick″yoo·lo·sack′yoo·lur) *adj.* [*utriculus* + *saccular*]. Pertaining to the utricle and saccule of the ear.
utriculosaccular duct. A membranous tube uniting the utricle and the saccule; from it arises the endolymphatic duct. NA *ductus utriculosaccularis.*
utri·cu·lus (yoo·trick′yoo·lus) *n.*, pl. **utricu·li** (·lye) [L.] [NA]. UTRICLE.
utriculus mas·cu·li·nus (mas·kew·lye′nus). UTRICLE (2).
utriculus pro·sta·ti·cus (pros·tat′i·kus) [NA]. UTRICLE (2).
UV Abbreviation for *ultraviolet.*
uva-ur·si (yoo′vuh ur′sigh) *n.* [L., bear's grape]. The dried leaves of *Arctostaphylos uva-ursi* or its varieties *coactylis* and *adenotricha.* Contains, besides tannic and gallic acids, quercetin, the glucosides arbutin (ursin) and methylarbutin, ursolic acid (urson), isoquercitrin, and hydroquinone; has been used in the treatment of inflammations of the urinary tract.
uvea (yoo′vee·uh) *n.* [ML., from L. *uva,* grape]. The pigmented, vascular layer of the eye, the iris, ciliary body, and choroid. —**uve·al** (·ul) *adj.*
uveal tract. The iris, ciliary body, and choroid.
uve·itis (yoo″vee·eye′tis) *n.* [*uvea* + *-itis*]. Inflammation of the uvea. —**uve·it·ic** (·it′ick) *adj.*
uveo·en·ceph·a·li·tis (yoo″vee·o·en·sef″uh·lye′tis) *n.* UVEOMENINGOENCEPHALITIS.
uveo·me·nin·go·en·ceph·a·li·tis (yoo″vee·o·me·nin″go·en·sef″uh·lye′tis) *n.* [*uvea* + *meningo-* + *encephalitis*]. A syndrome of unknown cause, characterized by severe bilateral nontraumatic uveitis, meningoencephalitis of varying severity with increased cells and protein in the cerebrospinal fluid, poliosis and patchy vitiligo most often distributed symmetrically, and dysacousia in a high percentage of patients; usually observed in young adults. Syn. *Vogt-Koyanagi-Harada syndrome.*
uveo·neur·ax·i·tis (yoo″vee·o·newr″ack·sigh′tis) *n.* [*uvea* + *neuraxitis*]. UVEOMENINGOENCEPHALITIS.
uveo·par·otid (yoo″vee·o·puh·rot′id) *adj.* Pertaining to the uvea and the parotid gland.
uveoparotid fever. A manifestation of sarcoidosis consisting of uveitis, parotitis, and fever. Syn. *Heerfordt's disease, uveoparotitis.*

uveo·par·o·ti·tis (yoo″vee·o·păr″o·tye′tis) *n.* [*uvea* + *parotitis*]. UVEOPAROTID FEVER.

uvul-, uvulo-. A combining form meaning *uvula.*

uvu·la (yoo′vew·luh) *n.*, genit. **uvu·lae** (·lee) [L., dim. of *uva*, grape, bunch of grapes]. The conical appendix hanging from the free edge of the soft palate, containing the uvular muscle covered by mucous membrane. —**uvu·lar** (·lur) *adj.*

uvula ce·re·bel·li (serr·e·bel′eye). UVULA VERMIS.

uvu·lae (yoo′vew·lee) *n.* [short for *musculus uvulae*]. The muscle of the uvula. NA *musculus uvulae.* See also Table of Muscles in the Appendix.

uvula fis·sa (fis′uh). CLEFT UVULA.

uvula pa·la·ti·na (pal·uh·tye′nuh) [NA]. UVULA.

uvu·lap·to·sis (yoo″vew·lap·to′sis) *n.* [*uvula* + *-ptosis*]. UVULOPTOSIS.

uvulatome. UVULOTOME.

uvu·lat·o·my (yoo″vew·lat′uh·mee) *n.* [*uvula* + *-tomy*]. UVULECTOMY.

uvula ver·mis (vur′mis) [NA]. The most caudally situated lobule of the vermis of the cerebellum. It is separated from the flocculonodular lobe by the posterolateral fissure.

uvula ve·si·cae (ve·sigh′see) [NA]. A longitudinal ridge on the trigone of the urinary bladder directed toward the urethral opening.

uvu·lec·to·my (yoo″vew·leck′tuh·mee) *n.* [*uvul-* + *-ectomy*]. Surgical resection of the uvula.

uvu·li·tis (yoo″vew·lye′tis) *n.* [*uvul-* + *-itis*]. Inflammation of the uvula.

uvulo-. See *uvul-.*

uvu·lo·nod·u·lar (yoo″vew·lo·nod′yoo·lur) *adj.* [*uvulo-* + *nodulus* + *-ar*]. Pertaining to the uvula and the nodulus of the cerebellum.

uvulonodular sulcus. A groove separating the uvula from the nodulus of the cerebellum. Syn. *posterolateral fissure.*

uvu·lop·to·sis (yoo″vew·lop·to′sis, ·lop′tuh·sis) *n.* [*uvulo-* + *-ptosis*]. A relaxed and pendulous condition of the uvula.

uvu·lo·tome, uvu·la·tome (yoo′vew·luh·tome) *n.* [*uvulo-* + *-tome*]. An instrument used in uvulotomy.

uvu·lot·o·my (yoo″vew·lot′uh·mee) *n.* [*uvulo-* + *-tomy*]. UVULECTOMY.

U wave of the electrocardiogram. A deflection, usually of low amplitude, following the T wave. It is often absent normally; its cause and significance are not certain.

V

V Symbol for vanadium.

v Abbreviation for *volt.*

vac·cin (vack'sin) *n.* VACCINE.

vac·ci·na (vack·sigh'nuh) *n.* VACCINIA.

vac·ci·na·ble (vack'si·nuh·bul) *adj.* Susceptible of successful vaccination.

vac·ci·nal (vack'si·nul) *adj.* Pertaining to vaccination or to vaccine.

vaccinal fever. Fever following vaccination.

vac·ci·nate (vack'si·nate) *v.* 1. To administer vaccine to produce immunity. 2. To inoculate to produce immunity to smallpox.

vac·ci·na·tion (vack''si·nay'shun) *n.* 1. Inoculation with the virus of vaccinia in order to protect against smallpox. 2. The inoculation or ingestion of organisms or antigens to produce immunity in the recipient.

vaccination rash. A skin eruption which sometimes follows vaccination; it is usually transitory but sometimes assumes an eczematous or erythematous form.

vac·cine (vack'seen, vack·seen') *n.* [L. *vaccinus,* of cows, from *vacca,* cow]. 1. Originally, a suspension of cowpox virus used to produce immunity against smallpox. 2. A preparation administered to induce immunity in the recipient; may be a suspension of living or dead organisms or a solution of either pollens or viral or bacterial antigens.

vaccine lymph. The virus of vaccinia as obtained from the calf.

vaccine therapy. The attempt to produce active immunity against disease by the use of specific antigens. See also *vaccination.*

vaccine virus. VACCINIA VIRUS.

vac·cin·ia (vack·sin'ee·uh) *n.* [NL., from L. *vaccinus,* of cows]. An acute infectious disease caused by smallpox vaccination or by accidental contact of abraded skin with vaccinia virus. It is characterized by the development of a localized lesion that progresses from papule to vesicle to pustule to crust. The infection stimulates the production of antibodies that are protective against smallpox.

vaccinia gan·gre·no·sa (gang''gre·no'suh). PROGRESSIVE VACCINIA.

vac·cin·i·al (vack·sin'ee·ul) *adj.* 1. Pertaining to or characteristic of vaccinia. 2. Resembling vaccinia.

vaccinia ne·cro·sum (ne·kro'sum). PROGRESSIVE VACCINIA.

vaccinia virus. A pox virus, *Poxvirus officinale,* related to, but distinct from, the viruses of smallpox (*Poxvirus variolae*) and cowpox (*Poxvirus bovis*) used primarily for vaccination against smallpox.

vac·cin·i·form (vack·sin'i·form) *adj.* Resembling vaccinia.

vac·ci·noid (vack'si·noid) *adj.* Resembling vaccinia.

vac·ci·no·pho·bia (vack''si·no·fo'bee·uh) *n.* [*vaccinate* + *-phobia*]. Abnormal fear of vaccination.

vac·ci·no·style (vack'si·no·stile) *n.* [*vaccinate* + *style,* pointed instrument]. A small, metallic lance formerly used in smallpox vaccination.

vac·ci·no·ther·a·py (vack''si·no·therr'uh·pee) *n.* The therapeutic use of vaccine.

vacua. A plural of *vacuum.*

vac·u·o·lar (vack''yoo·o'lur, vack'yoo·uh·lur) *adj.* Pertaining to or characterized by vacuoles.

vac·u·o·late (vack'yoo·o·late) *adj.* Having, or pertaining to, vacuoles.

vac·u·o·lat·ed (vack'yoo·o·lay''tid) *adj.* Containing one or more vacuoles; said of a cell or cytoplasm.

vac·u·o·la·tion (vack''yoo·o·lay'shun) *n.* The formation of vacuoles; the state of being vacuolated.

vac·u·ole (vack'yoo·ole) *n.* [F., dim. of L. *vacuum,* empty space]. 1. A clear space in a cell. 2. A cavity bound by a single membrane; usually a storage area for fat, glycogen, secretion precursors, liquid, or debris, in contradistinction to the artifacts induced by technical manipulation.

vac·u·ol·iza·tion (vack''yoo·o·li·zay'shun) *n.* VACUOLATION.

vac·u·ome (vack'yoo·ome) *n.* [*vacuole* + *-ome*]. GOLGI APPARATUS.

vac·u·um (vack'yoo·um) *n.,* pl. **vacuums, vac·ua** (·yoo·uh) [L., from *vacare,* to be empty]. A space from which most of the air has been exhausted.

vacuum extractor. An obstetrical instrument employing suction rather than forceps in the second stage of labor.

vacuum tube. A highly evacuated glass tube containing electrodes, which is variously used in electronic circuitry and for production of beta and x-rays.

vag-, vago-. A combining form meaning *vagus, vagal.*

vag·a·bond·age (vag'uh·bon·dij) *n.* [F.]. Uncontrollable desire to wander from home.

vag·a·bond neurosis (vag'uh·bond). VAGABONDAGE.

vagabond's disease. Pigmentation and lichenification of the skin due to chronic scratching associated with long-standing cases of pediculosis corporis.

va·gal (vay'gul) *adj.* Pertaining to the vagus nerve.

vagal accessory nerve. INTERNAL RAMUS OF THE ACCESSORY NERVE.

vagal arrhythmia. PHASIC SINUS ARRHYTHMIA.

vagal attack. VASOVAGAL ATTACK.

vagal nuclei. Dorsal motor nucleus of the vagus, dorsal sensory nucleus of the vagus, nucleus ambiguus, nucleus of the tractus solitarius.

vagal triangle or **trigone.** TRIGONUM NERVI VAGI.

vagi. Plural and genitive singular of *vagus.*

vagin-, vagino-. A combining form meaning *vagina, vaginal*.

va·gi·na (va·jye'nuh) *n.*, L. pl. & genit. sing. **vagi·nae** (·nee), E. pl. **vaginas** [L., sheath, scabbard]. 1. SHEATH (2). 2. [NA] The musculomembranous canal from the vulvar opening to the cervix of the uterus. See also Plates 23, 24.

vagina bul·bi (bul'bye) [NA]. The connective tissue surrounding the posterior part of the eyeball.

vagina ca·ro·ti·ca fas·ci·ae cer·vi·ca·lis (ka·rot'i·kuh fash'ee·ee sur·vi·kay'lis) [NA]. CAROTID SHEATH.

vagina den·tis (den'tis). The fleshy sheath surrounding the fang in venomous snakes.

vaginae fi·bro·sae di·gi·to·rum ma·nus (figh·bro'see dij·i·to'rum man'us) [NA]. The fibrous tendon sheaths of the muscles of the hand.

vaginae fibrosae digitorum pe·dis (ped'is) [NA]. The fibrous tendon sheaths of the muscles of the foot.

vaginae mu·co·sae di·gi·to·rum ma·nus (mew·ko'see dij·i·to'rum man'us) [BNA]. VAGINAE SYNOVIALES DIGITORUM MANUS.

vaginae mucosae digitorum pe·dis (ped'is) [BNA]. VAGINAE SYNOVIALES DIGITORUM PEDIS.

vaginae ner·vi op·ti·ci (nur'vye op'ti·sigh) [BNA]. The sheaths (external and internal) of the optic nerve: VAGINA EXTERNA NERVI OPTICI and VAGINA INTERNA NERVI OPTICI.

vaginae sy·no·vi·a·les di·gi·to·rum ma·nus (si·no·vee·ay'leez dij·i·to'rum man'us) [NA]. The synovial sheaths of the digits of the hand.

vaginae synoviales digitorum pe·dis (ped'is) [NA]. The synovial sheaths of the digits of the foot.

vaginae synoviales ten·di·num di·gi·to·rum ma·nus (ten'di·num dij·i·to'rum man'us) [NA]. The synovial sheaths of the tendons of the digits of the hand.

vaginae synoviales tendinum digitorum pe·dis (ped'is) [NA]. The synovial sheaths of the tendons of the digits of the foot.

vaginae ten·di·num di·gi·ta·les ma·nus (ten'di·num dij·i·tay'leez man'us) [BNA]. VAGINAE SYNOVIALES TENDINUM DIGITORUM MANUS.

vaginae tendinum digitales pe·dis (ped'is) [BNA]. VAGINAE SYNOVIALES TENDINUM DIGITORUM PEDIS.

vagina ex·ter·na ner·vi op·ti·ci (ecks·tur'nuh nur'vye op'ti·sigh) [NA]. The outer dense fibrous sheath of the optic nerve, continuous with the dura mater.

vagina fi·bro·sa ten·di·nis (figh·bro'suh ten'di·nis) [NA]. A fibrous sheath surrounding the tendon of a muscle and usually confining the tendon in a bony groove. Each sheath may be given the specific name of the tendon it surrounds.

vagina in·ter·na ner·vi op·ti·ci (in·tur'nuh nur'vye op'ti·sigh) [NA]. The inner delicate fibrous sheath of the optic nerve continuous with the pia mater.

va·gi·nal (va·jye'nul, vaj'i·nul) *adj.* [*vagin-* + *-al*]. 1. Pertaining to or resembling a vagina or sheath. 2. Pertaining to or affecting the vagina.

vaginal ballottement. The rebound of the fetus against a finger inserted into the vagina. Syn. *internal ballottement*.

vaginal bulb. 1. One of the solid epithelial bulbs forming the lower part of the fetal vagina, regarded as of paramesonephric duct origin. 2. BULB OF THE VESTIBULE.

vag·i·na·lec·to·my (vaj''i·nuh·leck'tuh·mee) *n.* VAGINECTOMY (2).

vaginal gland. One of the mucous glands found exceptionally in the mucous membrane of the fornices of the vagina.

vaginal hernia. A perineal hernia that follows the course of the vagina after leaving the abdomen, and which may enter the labium majus; resembles a labial inguinal hernia.

vaginal hysterectomy. Hysterectomy in which the removal is effected through the vagina.

vaginal jelly. Any one of a group of substances introduced into the vagina for the treatment of disease or for contraceptive purposes.

vaginal ligament. A fibrous band occasionally present in the spermatic cord, which represents the remains of the vaginal process of the peritoneum. NA *vestigium processus vaginalis*.

vaginal lithotomy. Lithotomy in which the incision is made through the anterior vaginal wall.

vaginal ovariocele. Displacement of the vaginal wall by one or both ovaries.

vaginal plexus. 1. A nerve network supplying the walls of the vagina. 2. A plexus of veins near the entrance to the vagina. NA *plexus venosus vaginalis*.

vaginal plug. A portion of the coital ejaculate of the male of several species, including rodents and nonhuman primates, which coagulates in the vagina following copulation to form a temporary fibrous plug.

vaginal process of the peritoneum. A tube of peritoneum which evaginates through the inguinal canal into the scrotum (or labium majus) during embryonic life. In the male, the distal portion persists as the tunica vaginalis testis. In the female, a portion occasionally persists, forming the canal of Nuck. NA *processus vaginalis peritonei*.

vaginal process of the sphenoid bone. A projection from the inferior surface of the body of the sphenoid bone, running horizontally inward from near the base of the medial pterygoid plate. NA *processus vaginalis ossis sphenoidalis*.

vaginal process of the styloid. VAGINAL PROCESS OF THE TEMPORAL BONE.

vaginal process of the temporal bone. A sheathlike plate of bone extending backward from carotid canal to mastoid process; it separates behind into two laminas enclosing the styloid process. Syn. *vaginal process of the styloid*.

vaginal proctocele. RECTOCELE.

vaginal sac. VAGINAL PROCESS OF THE PERITONEUM.

vaginal sphincter. The bulbospongiosus muscle in the female.

vaginal touch. Digital examination of the genital organs through the vagina.

vagina mas·cu·li·na (mas·kew·lye'nuh). UTRICLE (2).

vagina mu·co·sa in·ter·tu·ber·cu·la·ris (mew·ko'suh in·tur·tew·bur·kew·lair'is) [BNA]. VAGINA SYNOVIALIS INTERTUBERCULARIS.

vagina mus·cu·li rec·ti ab·do·mi·nis (mus'kew·lye reck'tye ab·dom'i·nis) [NA]. SHEATH OF THE RECTUS.

va·gi·na·pexy (va·jye'nuh·peck''see) *n.* [*vagina* + *-pexy*]. COLPOPEXY.

vagina pro·ces·sus sty·loi·dei (pro·ses'us stye·loy'dee·eye) [NA]. A ridge of bone on the temporal bone partially surrounding the base of the styloid process.

vagina sy·no·vi·a·lis com·mu·nis mus·cu·lo·rum flex·o·rum (si·no·vee·ay'lis kom·yoo'nis mus·kew·lo'rum fleck·so'rum) [NA]. ULNAR BURSA.

vagina synovialis in·ter·tu·ber·cu·la·ris (in·tur·tew·bur·kew·lair'is) [NA]. The synovial sheath surrounding the tendon of the long head of the biceps brachii muscle as it lies in the intertubercular groove; the sheath is a continuation of the joint capsule.

vagina synovialis mus·cu·li ob·li·qui su·pe·ri·o·ris (mus'kew·lye ob·lye'kwye sue·peer·ee·o'ris) [NA]. A synovial sheath surrounding the tendon of the superior oblique muscle where the tendon passes around its trochlea.

vagina synovialis mus·cu·lo·rum fi·bu·la·ri·um com·mu·nis (mus·kew·lo'rum fib·yoo·lair'ee·um kom·yoo'nis) [NA alt.]. The synovial sheath of the peroneus longus and brevis muscle tendons. NA alt. *vagina synovialis musculorum peroneorum communis*.

vagina synovialis musculorum pe·ro·ne·o·rum com·mu·nis (perr·o·nee·o'rum kom·yoo'nis) [NA]. The synovial sheath of the peroneus longus and brevis muscle tendons. NA alt. *vagina synovialis musculorum fibularium communis*.

vagina synovialis ten·di·nis (ten'di·nis) [NA]. A double-layered sheath lined with synovial membrane which surrounds the tendon of a muscle where the tendon passes over a bony prominence or beneath a retinaculum. Each sheath is given the specific name of the tendon or tendons it surrounds.

vagina synovialis tendinis mus·cu·li flex·o·ris car·pi ra·di·a·lis (mus'kew·lye fleck·so'ris kahr'pye ray·dee·ay'lis) [NA]. The synovial sheath of the tendon of the flexor carpi radialis muscle.

vagina synovialis tendinis musculi flexoris hal·lu·cis lon·gi (hal'yoo·sis long'guy, lon'jye) [NA]. The synovial sheath of the tendon of the flexor hallucis muscle.

vagina synovialis tendinis musculi ti·bi·a·lis pos·te·ri·o·ris (tib·ee·ay'lis pos·teer·ee·o'ris) [NA]. The synovial sheath of the tendon of the tibialis posterior muscle.

vagina ten·di·nis mus·cu·li ex·ten·so·ris car·pi ul·na·ris (ten'di·nis mus'kew·lye ecks·ten·so'ris kahr'pye ul·nair'is) [NA]. The synovial sheath of the tendon of the extensor carpi ulnaris muscle.

vagina tendinis musculi extensoris di·gi·ti mi·ni·mi (dij'i·tye min'i·migh) [NA]. The synovial sheath of the tendon of the extensor digiti minimi muscle.

vagina tendinis musculi extensoris hal·lu·cis lon·gi (hal'yoo·sis long'guy, lon'jye) [NA]. The synovial sheath of the tendon of the extensor hallucis longus muscle.

vagina tendinis musculi extensoris pol·li·cis lon·gi (pol'i·sis long'guy, lon'jye) [NA]. The synovial sheath of the tendon of the extensor pollicis longus muscle.

vagina tendinis musculi fi·bu·la·ris lon·gi (fib·yoo·lair'is long'guy, lon'jye) [NA alt.]. The synovial sheath of the tendon of the peroneus longus muscle. NA alt. *vagina tendinis musculi peronei longi.*

vagina tendinis musculi flex·o·ris hal·lu·cis lon·gi (fleck·so'ris hal'yoo·sis long'guy, lon'jye) [NA]. The synovial sheath of the tendon of the flexor hallucis longus muscle.

vagina tendinis musculi flexoris pol·li·cis lon·gi (pol'i·sis long'guy, lon'jye) [NA]. RADIAL BURSA.

vagina tendinis musculi pe·ro·naei lon·gi (perr'o·nee·eye long'guy, lon'jye) [BNA]. VAGINA TENDINIS MUSCULI PERONEI LONGI.

vagina tendinis musculi pe·ro·nei lon·gi (perr'o·nee·eye long'guy, lon'jye) [NA]. The synovial sheath of the tendon of the peroneus longus muscle. NA alt. *vagina tendinis musculi fibularis longi.*

vagina tendinis musculi ti·bi·a·lis an·te·ri·o·ris (tib·ee·ay'lis an·teer·ee·o'ris) [NA]. The synovial sheath of the tendon of the tibialis anterior muscle.

vagina tendinis musculi tibialis pos·te·ri·o·ris (pos·teer·ee·o'ris) [BNA]. VAGINA SYNOVIALIS TENDINIS MUSCULI TIBIALIS POSTERIORIS.

vagina ten·di·num mus·cu·li ex·ten·so·ris di·gi·to·rum pe·dis lon·gi (ten'di·num mus'kew·lye ecks·ten·so'ris dij·i·to'rum ped'is long'guy, lon'jye) [NA]. The synovial sheath of the tendons of the extensor digitorum longus muscle of the foot.

vagina tendinum musculi flex·o·ris di·gi·to·rum pe·dis lon·gi (fleck·so'ris dij·i·to'rum ped'is long'guy, lon'jye) [NA]. The synovial sheath of the tendons of the flexor digitorum longus muscle of the foot.

vagina tendinum mus·cu·lo·rum ab·duc·to·ris lon·gi et ex·ten·so·ris bre·vis pol·li·cis (mus·kew·lo'rum ab·duck·to'ris long'guy et ecks·ten·so'ris brev'is pol'i·sis) [NA]. The synovial sheath of the tendons of the long abductor and short extensor muscles of the thumb.

vagina tendinum musculorum ex·ten·so·ris di·gi·to·rum et ex·ten·so·ris in·di·cis (ecks·ten·so'ris dij·i·to'rum et ecks·ten·so'ris in'di·sis) [NA]. The synovial sheath of the tendons of extensors of the fingers and extensor of the index finger.

vagina tendinum musculorum ex·ten·so·rum car·pi ra·di·a·li·um (ecks·ten·so'rum kahr'pye ray·dee·ay'lee·um) [NA]. The synovial sheath of the tendons of the long and short extensor carpi radialis muscles.

vagina tendinum musculorum flex·o·rum com·mu·ni·um (fleck·so'rum kom·yoo'nee·um) [BNA]. Vagina synovialis communis musculorum flexorum (= ULNAR BURSA).

vagina tendinum musculorum pe·ro·nae·o·rum com·mu·nis (pe·ro·nee·o'rum kom·yoo'nis) [BNA]. VAGINA SYNOVIALIS MUSCULORUM PERONEORUM COMMUNIS.

vagina va·so·rum (vay·so'rum, va·) [BNA]. A general term for a fibrous sheath surrounding certain vessels.

vag·i·nec·to·my (vaj"i·neck'tuh·mee) *n.* [*vagin-* + *-ectomy*]. 1. Excision of the vagina or a portion of it. 2. Excision of the tunica vaginalis.

vag·i·nic·o·line (vaj"i·nick'uh·line) *adj.* [*vagin-* + L. *col*ere, to inhabit, + *-ine*]. Of, or pertaining to, microorganisms that inhabit the vagina.

vag·i·nif·er·ous (vaj"i·nif'ur·us) *adj.* [*vagin-* + *-iferous*]. Producing, or bearing, a sheath.

vag·i·nis·mus (vaj"i·niz'mus) *n.* [*vagin-* + *-ismus*]. Painful spasm of the vagina.

vag·i·ni·tis (vaj"i·nigh'tis) *n.* [*vagin-* + *-itis*]. 1. Inflammation of the vagina. 2. Inflammation of a sheath.

vagino-. See *vagin-*.

vag·i·no·cele (vaj'i·no·seel) *n.* [*vagino-* + *-cele*]. COLPOCELE.

vag·i·no·dyn·ia (vaj"i·no·din'ee·uh) *n.* [*vagin-* + *-odynia*]. Neuralgic pain of the vagina.

vag·i·no·fix·a·tion (vaj"i·no·fick·say'shun) *n.* [*vagino-* + *fixation*]. Fixation of the uterus to the vagina.

vag·i·no·my·co·sis (vaj"i·no·migh·ko'sis) *n.* [*vagino-* + *mycosis*]. A fungous infection of the vagina, usually by *Candida albicans.*

vag·i·no·plas·ty (vaj'i·no·plas"tee) *n.* [*vagino-* + *-plasty*]. A plastic operation on the vagina.

vag·i·no·scope (vaj'i·nuh·scope) *n.* [*vagino-* + *-scope*]. A vaginal speculum.

vag·i·nos·co·py (vaj"i·nos'kuh·pee) *n.* [*vagino-* + *-scopy*]. Inspection of the vagina.

vag·i·not·o·my (vaj"i·not'uh·mee) *n.* [*vagino-* + *-tomy*]. 1. Incision of the vagina; COLPOTOMY. 2. Incision of a tendon sheath.

va·gi·tus (va·jye'tus) *n.* [L., from *vagire,* to cry]. The cry of an infant.

vagitus ute·ri·nus (yoo·te·rye'nus). The cry of a child while still in the uterus.

vagitus va·gi·na·lis (vaj·i·nay'lis). The cry of a child while the head is still in the vagina.

vago-. See *vag-*.

va·go·ac·ces·so·ry (vay"go·ack·ses'uh·ree) *adj.* Pertaining to the vagus and spinal accessory nerves.

vagoaccessory-hypoglossal paralysis. JACKSON'S SYNDROME.

vagoaccessory syndrome. Ipsilateral paralysis of the soft palate, pharynx, and larynx, with flaccidity and atrophy of the sternocleidomastoid and part of the trapezius muscle of the same side, due to a lesion of the nucleus ambiguus and nucleus of the spinal accessory nerve or their root fibers. Syn. *Schmidt's syndrome.*

va·go·gram (vay'go·gram) *n.* [*vago-* + *-gram*]. ELECTROVAGOGRAM.

va·go·lyt·ic (vay'go·lit'ick) *adj. & n.* [*vago-* + *-lytic*]. 1. Having the effect of inhibiting the vagus nerve. 2. Any agent that inhibits the vagus nerve.

va·go·pres·sor reflex (vay"go·pres'ur). Reflex rise in blood pressure by vasoconstriction, resulting from the stimulation of afferent fibers of the vagus nerve in the right atrium by decrease in venous pressure.

va·got·o·mized (vay·got'uh·mize'd) *adj.* Pertaining to a person or animal whose vagus nerves have been severed for therapeutic or experimental purposes.

va·got·o·my (vay·got'uh·mee) *n.* [*vago-* + *-tomy*]. 1. Surgical division of vagus nerves. 2. Specifically, section of thoracic and abdominal vagal branches, usually for treatment of peptic ulcer; described as selective when only gastric branches are divided and as highly selective or superselective when only the gastric fundus and corpus are denervated, leaving the antrum and pylorus unaffected.

vagotomy shock. A hypotensive state due to depression of the local reflex mechanism when the vagus nerves are cut.

va·go·to·nia (vay″go·to′nee·uh) *n.* [*vago-* + *-tonia*]. A condition due to overaction of the vagus nerves and modification of functions in organs innervated by them. —**vago·ton·ic** (·ton′ick) *adj.*

va·got·o·nin (vay·got′uh·nin, vay″go·to′nin) *n.* [*vago-* + *tone* + *-in*]. A substance derived from the pancreas that stimulates the parasympathetic system.

va·go·tro·pic (vay″go·tro′pick) *adj.* [*vago-* + *-tropic*]. Having an effect upon, or influencing, the vagus nerve.

va·go·va·gal (vay″go·vay′gul) *adj.* Due to both the afferent and efferent impulses of the vagus nerve.

vagovagal syncope. Syncope of reflex origin in which the entire reflex arc is within the vagal system. Syncope is due to reflex cardiac asystole and is associated with distention of the esophagus, bronchus, etc.; it can be inhibited by anticholinergic agents such as atropine.

va·grant (vay′grunt) *adj.* [OF. *waucrant*]. Wandering, as a vagrant cell.

va·gus (vay′gus) *n.*, pl. & genit. sing. **va·gi** (·guy, ·jye) [L., wandering]. The tenth cranial nerve; a mixed nerve whose voluntary motor fibers arise in the nucleus ambiguus and are distributed to the muscles of larynx and pharynx; parasympathetic fibers from the dorsal motor nucleus of the vagus are widely distributed to autonomic ganglia to function in the regulation of motor and secretory activities of the abdominal and thoracic viscera. Somatic sensory fibers go to the skin of the external auditory meatus and the meninges, and visceral sensory fibers reach the pharynx, larynx, and thoracic and abdominal viscera. Syn. *pneumogastric nerve.* NA *nervus vagus.* See also Table of Nerves in the Appendix.

vagus shock. VAGOTOMY SHOCK.

va·gus·stoff (vay′gus·shtof, vah′gōōs·) *n.* [*vagus* + Ger. *Stoff*, substance]. A substance liberated at the terminations of the fibers of the vagus nerve which depresses heart action; now believed to be acetylcholine.

Valbazen. A trademark for albendazole, an anthelmintic.

va·lence (vay′lunce) *n.* [L. *valentia*, power, capacity, from *valere*, to be strong]. 1. The capacity of an atom to combine with other atoms in definite proportions. 2. By analogy, also applied to radicals and atomic groups. Valence is measured with the combining capacity of a hydrogen atom taken as unity. —**va·lent** (·lunt) *adj.*

va·len·cy (vay′lun·see) *n.* VALENCE.

Val·en·tine's position [F. C. *Valentine*, U.S. surgeon, 1851–1909]. A position used in ureteral irrigation. With the patient supine, the hips are flexed by means of a double inclined plane.

Va·len·tin's bodies or **corpuscles** (vah′len·teen) [G. G. *Valentin*, Swiss physiologist, 1810–1883]. Small amyloid bodies in nerve tissue.

Valentin's ganglion [G. G. *Valentin*]. A gangliform enlargement at the junction of the middle and posterior branches of the superior dental plexus; PSEUDOGANGLION.

valer-, valero-. A combining form meaning *valeric.*

val·er·ate (val′ur·ate) *n.* A salt of valeric acid.

va·le·ri·an (va·leer′ee·un) *n.* The dried rhizome and roots of *Valeriana officinalis;* contains volatile oil and, possibly, alkaloids. It has been used in treatment of hysteria, hypochondriasis, and similar emotional states.

va·le·ri·a·nate (va·leer′ee·uh·nate) *n.* VALERATE.

va·le·ri·an·ic acid (va·leer″ee·an′ick). VALERIC ACID.

va·le·ric acid (va·lerr′ick, va·leer′ick). $C_5H_{10}O_2$. Four isomeric modifications of this acid are known: Normal valeric or propylacetic acid, $CH_3(CH_2)_3COOH$; isovaleric or isopropylacetic acid, $(CH_3)_2CHCH_2COOH$, the valeric acid of commerce; methylethylacetic acid, $CH_3(C_2H_5)CHCOOH$; and trimethylacetic acid, $(CH_3)_3CCOOH$.

valero-. See *valer-.*

val·e·tham·ate bromide (val·e·tham′ate). 2-Diethylaminoethyl 3-methyl-2-phenylvalerate methylbromide, $C_{19}H_{32}BrNO_2$, an anticholinergic drug used in the treatment of hypermotility and spasm of the gastrointestinal, genitourinary, and biliary tracts.

val·e·tu·di·nar·i·an (val″e·tew″di·nerr′ee·un) *adj.* [L. *valetudinarius*, sickly, from *valetudo*, state of health, ill health]. INVALID.

val·e·tu·di·nar·i·an·ism (val″e·tew″di·nerr′ee·an·iz·um) *n.* [*valetudinarian* + *-ism*]. Feeble or infirm state due to invalidism.

val·gus (val′gus) *adj.* [L., bent outward, bowlegged]. Usually, indicating an abnormal turning away from the midline of the body, as in talipes valgus. Contr. *varus.*

val·ine (val′een, ·in, vay′leen, ·lin) *n.* α-Aminoisovaleric acid, $C_5H_{11}NO_2$, an amino acid constituent of many proteins. It is considered essential to man, as well as to certain animals.

val·i·no·my·cin (val″i·no·migh′sin) *n.* An antibiotic which acts to transport potassium ions across mitochondrial and other membranes; useful in experiments on ion transport functions.

Valium. Trademark for diazepam, a tranquilizer.

valla. Plural of *vallum.*

val·late (val′ate) *adj.* [L. *vallare, vallatus*, to surround with a rampart, from *vallum*, palisade, rampart]. Surrounded by a walled depression; cupped.

vallate papilla. One of the large, flat papillae, each surrounded by a trench, in a group anterior to the sulcus terminalis of the tongue. Syn. *circumvallate papilla.*

val·lec·u·la (va·leck′yoo·luh) *n.*, pl. **vallecu·lae** (·lee) [L., dim. of *valles*, valley]. A shallow groove or depression.

vallecula ce·re·bel·li (serr·e·bel′eye) [NA]. The depression between the cerebellar hemispheres.

vallecula epi·glot·ti·ca (ep·i·glot′i·kuh) [NA]. A depression between the lateral and median glossoepiglottic folds on each side.

vallecula lin·guae (ling′gwee). VALLECULA EPIGLOTTICA.

vallecula un·guis (ung′gwis). VALLUM UNGUIS.

Val·leix's points (vahⁿ·lecks) [F. L. I. *Valleix*, French physician, 1807–1855]. PAINFUL POINTS.

Vallestril. Trademark for methallenestril, an orally effective, nonsteroid estrogen.

Val·let's mass. FERROUS CARBONATE MASS.

val·ley fever. COCCIDIOIDOMYCOSIS.

val·lum (val′um) *n.*, pl. **val·la** (·uh) [L.]. WALL.

vallum un·guis (ung′gwis) [NA]. The depression in the skin for the root of the nail.

Valmid. Trademark for ethinamate, a central depressant drug with short duration of action.

val·noc·ta·mide (val·nock′tuh·mide) *n.* 2-Ethyl-3-methylvaleramide, $C_8H_{17}NO$, a tranquilizer.

Valpin. Trademark for the parasympatholytic agent anisotropine methylbromide.

val·pro·ate sodium (val·pro′ate). Sodium 2-propylvalerate, $C_8H_{15}NaO_2$, an anticonvulsant.

val·pro·ic acid (val·pro′ick). 2-Propylvaleric acid, $C_8H_{16}O_2$, an anticonvulsant; also used as the sodium salt, valproate sodium.

Val·sal·va maneuver (vahˡ·sahˡ′vahʰ) [A. M. *Valsalva*, Italian anatomist, 1666–1723]. Forcible exhalation against the closed glottis, increasing intrathoracic pressure and impeding venous return to the heart.

Valsalva's antrum [A. M. *Valsalva*]. MASTOID ANTRUM.

Valsalva's sinus [A. M. *Valsalva*]. AORTIC SINUS.

Valsalva's test [A. M. *Valsalva*]. A maneuver to test the patency of the auditory tubes. While the nose and mouth are kept closed, forcible expiratory efforts are made; if the auditory tubes are patent, air should pass into the tympanic cavities.

Val·su·a·ni's disease (vahˡ·soo·ah′nee) [E. *Valsuani*, Italian physician, 19th century]. Progressive pernicious anemia in pregnant and lactating women.

val·va (val'vuh) *n.*, pl. & genit. sing. **val·vae** (·vee) [L.]. VALVE.
valva aor·tae (ay·or'tee) [NA]. AORTIC VALVE.
valva at·rio·ven·tri·cu·la·ris dex·tra (ay''tree·o·ven·trick·yoo·lair'is decks'truh) [NA]. TRICUSPID VALVE. NA alt. *valva tricuspidalis.*
valva atrioventricularis si·nis·tra (si·nis'truh) [NA]. MITRAL VALVE. NA alt. *valva mitralis.*
valva ileo·ce·ca·lis (il·ee·o·see·kay'lis) [NA]. ILEOCECAL VALVE.
valva mi·tra·lis (mi·tray'lis) [NA alt.]. MITRAL VALVE. NA alt. *valva atrioventricularis sinistra.*
valva tri·cus·pi·da·lis (trye·kus·pi·day'lis) [NA alt.]. TRICUSPID VALVE. NA alt. *valva atrioventricularis dextra.*
valva trun·ci pul·mo·na·lis (trun'sigh pul·mo·nay'lis, trunk'eye) [NA]. PULMONARY VALVE.
valve, *n.* [L. *valva,* leaf of a door]. A device in a vessel or passage which prevents reflux of its contents.
valve of the navicular fossa. GUÉRIN'S FOLD.
valve of the sinus venosus. One of the right and left folds of the opening of the sinus venosus into the right atrium found in the embryonic heart. The right disappears. The left forms the crista terminalis and portions of the valve of the inferior vena cava and of the valve of the coronary sinus.
valve of Vieussens [R. de *Vieussens*]. SUPERIOR MEDULLARY VELUM.
valves of Kerckring [T. *Kerckring*]. CIRCULAR FOLDS.
valves of Morgagni [G. B. *Morgagni*]. ANAL VALVES.
val·vot·o·my (val·vot'uh·mee) *n.* [*valve* + *-tomy*]. Surgical incision into a valve. Syn. *diclidotomy.* See also *valvulotomy.*
valvul-, valvulo-. A combining form meaning *valve, valvular.*
val·vu·la (val'vew·luh) *n.*, pl. & genit. sing. **valvu·lae** (·lee) [NL., dim. of *valva*]. VALVE.
valvula bi·cus·pi·da·lis (bye·kus·pi·day'lis) [BNA]. Valva atrioventricularis sinistra (= MITRAL VALVE).
valvula co·li (ko'lye) [BNA]. Valva ileocecalis (= ILEOCECAL VALVE).
valvulae ana·les (ay·nay'leez) [NA]. ANAL VALVES.
valvulae con·ni·ven·tes (kon·i·ven'teez). CIRCULAR FOLDS.
valvulae se·mi·lu·na·res aor·tae (sem·ee·lew·nay'reez a·or'tee) [BNA]. Valva aortae (= AORTIC VALVE).
valvulae semilunares ar·te·ri·ae pul·mo·na·lis (ahr·teer'ee·ee pul·mo·nay'lis) [BNA]. Valva trunci pulmonalis (= PULMONARY VALVE).
valvula fo·ra·mi·nis ova·lis (fo·ram'i·nis o·vay'lis) [NA]. A ridge on the interatrial septum which is the remains of the primary septum of the foramen ovale in the fetus. NA alt. *falx septi.*
valvula fos·sae na·vi·cu·la·ris (fos'ee na·vick·yoo·lair'is) [NA]. GUÉRIN'S FOLD.
valvula lym·pha·ti·ca (lim·fat'i·kuh) [NA]. A valve in a lymphatic vessel.
valvula pro·ces·sus ver·mi·for·mis (pro·ses'us vur·mi·for'mis) [BNA]. A fold of mucous membrane at the opening of the vermiform appendix into the cecum.
valvula py·lo·ri (pye·lo'rye) [BNA]. PYLORIC VALVE.
val·vu·lar (val'vew·lur) *adj.* 1. Pertaining to a valve. 2. Resembling a valve.
valvular pneumothorax. A type of open pneumothorax in which a margin of the wound acts as a valve. Air enters the pleural space with an inhalation, and is prevented by the valve from escaping during exhalation. Therefore, the air tension in the pleural space increases. Syn. *tension pneumothorax.*
valvula se·mi·lu·na·ris an·te·ri·or ar·te·ri·ae pul·mo·na·lis (sem·ee·lew·nair'is an·teer'ee·or ahr·teer'ee·ee pul·mo·nay'lis) [BNA]. VALVULA SEMILUNARIS ANTERIOR TRUNCI PULMONALIS.
valvula semilunaris anterior trun·ci pul·mo·na·lis (trun'sigh pul·mo·nay'lis) [NA]. The anterior semilunar cusp of the valve of the pulmonary trunk.
valvula semilunaris dex·tra aor·tae (decks'truh ay·or'tee) [BNA]. VALVULA SEMILUNARIS DEXTRA VALVAE AORTAE.
valvula semilunaris dextra ar·te·ri·ae pul·mo·na·lis (ahr·teer'ee·ee pul·mo·nay'lis) [BNA]. VALVULA SEMILUNARIS DEXTRA VALVAE TRUNCI PULMONALIS.
valvula semilunaris dextra val·vae aor·tae (val'vee ay·or'tee) [NA]. The right semilunar cusp of the aortic valve.
valvula semilunaris dextra valvae trun·ci pul·mo·na·lis (trun'sigh pul·mo·nay'lis) [NA]. The right semilunar cusp of the valve of the pulmonary trunk.
valvula semilunaris posterior aor·tae (ay·or'tee) [BNA]. VALVULA SEMILUNARIS POSTERIOR VALVAE AORTAE.
valvula semilunaris posterior val·vae aor·tae (val'vee ay·or'tee) [NA]. The posterior semilunar cusp of the aortic valve.
valvula semilunaris si·nis·tra aor·tae (si·nis'truh ay·or'tee) [BNA]. VALVULA SEMILUNARIS SINISTRA VALVAE AORTAE.
valvula semilunaris sinistra ar·te·ri·ae pul·mo·na·lis (ahr·teer'ee·ee pul·mo·nay'lis) [BNA]. VALVULA SEMILUNARIS VALVAE TRUNCI PULMONALIS.
valvula semilunaris sinistra val·vae aor·tae (val'vee ay·or'tee) [NA]. The left semilunar cusp of the aortic valve.
valvula semilunaris sinistra valvae trun·ci pul·mo·na·lis (trun'sigh pul·mo·nay'lis) [NA]. The left semilunar cusp of the valve of the pulmonary trunk.
valvula si·nus co·ro·na·rii (sigh'nus kor·o·nair'ee·eye) [NA]. CORONARY VALVE.
valvula sinus coronarii [The·be·sii] (the·bee'zee·eye) [BNA]. Valvula sinus coronarii (= CORONARY VALVE).
valvula spi·ra·lis [Heis·te·ri] (spye·ray'lis high'stur·eye) [BNA]. Plica spiralis (= SPIRAL VALVE).
valvula tri·cus·pi·da·lis (trye·kus·pi·day'lis) [BNA]. Valva atrioventricularis dextra (= TRICUSPID VALVE).
valvula ve·nae ca·vae in·fe·ri·o·ris (vee'nee kay'vee in·feer·ee·o'ris) [NA]. CAVAL VALVE.
valvula venae cavae inferioris [Eu·sta·chii] (yoo·stay'kee·eye) [BNA]. Valvula venae cavae inferioris (= CAVAL VALVE).
valvula ve·no·sa (vee·no'suh) [NA]. A general term for any valve in a vein.
val·vu·lec·to·my (val''vew·leck'tuh·mee) *n.* [*valvul-* + *-ectomy*]. Surgical excision of a valve, usually a heart valve.
val·vu·li·tis (val''vew·lye'tis) *n.* [*valvul-* + *-itis*]. Inflammation of a valve, especially of a cardiac valve.
valvulo-. See *valvul-.*
val·vu·lo·plas·ty (val'vew·lo·plas''tee) *n.* [*valvulo-* + *-plasty*]. Plastic surgical repair of a valve, usually a heart valve.
val·vu·lo·tome (val'vew·lo·tome) *n.* [*valvulo-* + *-tome*]. An instrument designed especially for incising the valves of the heart.
val·vu·lot·o·my (val''vew·lot'uh·mee) *n.* [*valvulo-* + *-tomy*]. The surgical incision of a valve of the heart, as in mitral stenosis.
val·yl (val'il) *n.* The univalent radical, $(CH_3)_2CHCH(NH_2)CO$—, of the amino acid valine.
vam·pire, *n.* [Hungarian *vampir,* from Slavic, prob. from Tatar *ubyr,* witch]. 1. In worldwide folk belief, a living corpse that rises from its grave at night and sucks the blood of the living. 2. A bloodsucking bat, belonging to the family Phyllostomidae, found in South and Central America and along the southern border of the United States.
vam·pir·ism (vam'pi·riz·um) *n.* [*vampire* + *-ism*]. 1. Belief in vampires (1). 2. The acts or practice of vampires; blood sucking. 3. NECROPHILISM.
van·a·date (van'uh·date) *n.* A salt of vanadic acid.
va·na·di·um (vuh·nay'dee·um) *n.* [NL., from ON. *Vanadīs,* a goddess]. V = 50.9415. A rare metallic element, atomic number 23, density 6.11.
va·na·di·um·ism (vuh·nay'dee·um·iz·um) *n.* [*vanadium* + *-ism*]. A chronic form of intoxication due to the absorption

of vanadium; occurs in workers using the metal or its compounds.

van Bo·gaert–Ber·trand disease (Flemish vahn bo'gh hært, French vahn boh·gähr'; behr·trahn') [L. *van Bogaert,* Belgian neuropathologist, 20th century; and I. *Bertrand,* Belgian neuropathologist, 20th century]. SPONGY DEGENERATION OF INFANCY.

van Bogaert–Canavan disease or **spongy degeneration** [L. *van Bogaert* and M. M. *Canavan*]. SPONGY DEGENERATION OF INFANCY.

van Bogaert–Nyssen disease [L. *van Bogaert* and R. *Nyssen*]. A familial form of metachromatic leukodystrophy appearing in adult life and characterized clinically by schizophrenic symptoms.

van Bogaert's subacute sclerosing leukoencephalitis [L. *van Bogaert*]. SUBACUTE SCLEROSING PANENCEPHALITIS.

Vancocin. Trademark for vancomycin, an antibiotic substance useful for treatment of severe staphylococcic infections.

van·co·my·cin (van"ko·migh'sin) *n.* A complex antibiotic substance produced by *Streptomyces orientalis;* useful for treatment of severe staphylococcic infections.

van Cre·veld–von Gierke's disease (vahn krey'velt) [S. *van Creveld,* Dutch pediatrician, b. 1894; and E. *von Gierke*]. VON GIERKE'S DISEASE.

van Deen's test (vahn deyn') [I. A. *van Deen,* Dutch physiologist, 1804–1869]. A guaiac test for occult blood.

Van de Graaff generator [R. J. *Van de Graaff,* U.S. physicist, 1901–1967]. A high-voltage electrostatic generator using a high-speed belt as a charge conveyer. Such generators are used for research in nuclear physics and as a source of high-voltage x-rays and cathode rays for radiation therapy, food sterilization, and industrial radiography.

van den Bergh's method (vahn den berrgh', de berr'ugh) [A. A. H. *van den Bergh,* Dutch physician, 1869–1943]. The indirect form of van den Bergh's test.

van den Bergh's test or **reaction** [A. A. H. *van den Bergh*]. Either of the two tests for serum bilirubin. In the direct test, diluted serum is added to diazo reagent. A bluish-violet color becoming maximal in 10 to 30 seconds is an immediate direct reaction supposedly indicating conjugated bilirubin and therefore the presence of obstructive jaundice. A red color beginning after 1 to 15 minutes and gradually turning to violet is a delayed direct reaction, indicating impaired liver function. A red color appearing at once and changing to violet is a biphasic direct reaction. In the indirect test, alcohol is added to serum which is then centrifuged. The diazo reagent is added to the supernatant fluid. An immediate violet-red color supposedly indicates nonconjugated bilirubin and signifies a hemolytic jaundice. The tests are now used as a modification in which diazotized serum or plasma is compared with a standard solution of diazotized bilirubin.

van der Hoe·ve's syndrome (Dutch vahn dur hoo'vuh). Osteogenesis imperfecta with blue sclerae and conductive hearing loss.

van der Waal's forces. Attractive forces that operate on all molecules when they are close together.

van Ge·huch·ten's cell (vahn ghe·hœkh'ten) [A. *van Gehuchten,* Belgian neurologist, 1861–1914]. GOLGI CELL, type II.

Van Gie·son's stain [I. *van Gieson,* U.S. neuropathologist, 1865–1913]. Selective staining of connective tissue with a picric acid-fuchsin solution.

van Han·se·mann's cells. Large multinuclear epithelioid cells with basophilic inclusions, seen in malakoplakia.

va·nil·la (vuh·nil'uh) *n.* [Sp. *vainilla,* dim. of *vaina,* sheath, from L. *vagina*]. The cured, full-grown, unripe fruit of *Vanilla planifolia,* or *V. tahitensis.* The fresh fruit possesses none of the pleasant odor commonly associated with the fruit. Two enzymes, under the influence of gentle heat and moisture, produce vanillin from two of three glycosides, and perhaps another aromatic substance from a third glycoside. Vanilla is used solely as a flavoring agent. Syn. *vanilla bean.*

vanilla-worker's itch. Acarodermatitis urticarioides caused by *Tyroglyphus siro.*

va·nil·lic acid (vuh·nil'ick). 3-Methoxy-4-hydroxybenzoic acid, $C_8H_8O_4$, the crystalline solid resulting from oxidation of vanillin.

va·nil·lin (va·nil'in, van'i·lin) *n.* 3-Methoxy-4-hydroxybenzaldehyde, $C_8H_8O_3$; used as a flavoring agent in place of vanilla.

va·nil·lism (vuh·nil'iz·um) *n.* A form of contact dermatitis characterized by marked itching; occurring among vanilla workers.

va·nil·lyl·man·del·ic acid (van"i·lil·man·del'ick, va·nil"il·). 3-Methoxy-4-hydroxymandelic acid, $C_9H_{10}O_5$, a major degradation product of adrenal medullary catecholamines excreted in the urine, where its measurement is used as a test for pheochromocytoma. Abbreviated, VMA

van·ish·ing lungs. Thin-walled abnormal air spaces, which develop under the effect of chemotherapy when the disease process in the lungs resolves.

Van Slyke and Cullen's method [D. D. *Van Slyke,* U.S. biochemist, 1883–1971]. A test for alkali reserve in which fresh oxalated plasma is brought into equilibrium with expired air so that it combines with as much carbon dioxide as it is able to hold under normal tension. The plasma is then acidified and the carbon dioxide given off is measured.

Van Slyke and Kirk method [D. D. *Van Slyke*]. A nitrous acid procedure for determining the α-amino acid nitrogen content of urine.

Van Slyke and Neill method [D. D. *Van Slyke*]. A manometric method of analysis of gases in blood and other solutions.

Van Slyke and Palmer method [D. D. *Van Slyke*]. A test for organic acids in urine in which carbonates and phosphates are precipitated and the filtrate is titrated with acid from pH 8 to pH 2.7. In diabetes this titration approximates closely the amount of β-hydroxybutyric and acetoacetic acids in the urine.

Van Slyke apparatus [D. D. *Van Slyke*]. A graduated glass buret connected with a mercury leveling bulb, used in volumetric determination of blood gases.

Van Slyke, MacFadyen, and Hamilton Ninhydrin method [D. D. *Van Slyke*]. A method for amino acid nitrogen in urine in which the urine sample, previously freed from urea by treatment with urease, is heated at 100°C in a closed reaction vessel with ninhydrin. Amino acids present yield carbon dioxide quantitatively under these conditions.

Van Slyke's method [D. D. *Van Slyke*]. 1. A method for acetone bodies in urine based on a combination of Shaffer's oxidation of β-hydroxybutyric acid to acetone and Denigès' precipitation of acetone as a basic mercuric sulfate compound. Glucose and certain other interfering substances are removed by precipitation with copper sulfate and calcium hydroxide. Preservatives other than toluene or copper sulfate should not be used. 2. A method for chlorides in blood in which proteins are oxidized and chlorides precipitated with silver nitrate. Excess silver is titrated with thiocyanate.

Van Slyke titration method [D. D. *Van Slyke*]. A method for plasma bicarbonates in which plasma is treated with an excess of standard acid which is titrated back with standard alkali to the original pH of the plasma as drawn.

van't Hoff's factor i [J. H. *van't Hoff,* Dutch physical chemist, 1852–1911]. A factor correcting for dissociation of an electrolyte in solution used in calculating osmotic pressure according to van't Hoff's law.

van't Hoff's law [J. H. *van't Hoff*]. The osmotic pressure of a dilute solution, at constant temperature, is proportional to the concentration of solution; at constant concentration, the osmotic pressure is proportional to the temperature.

van't Hoff's principle of mobile equilibrium [J. H. *van't Hoff*]. Any change of the temperature of a system in equilibrium is followed by a reverse thermal change within the system.

va·po·cau·ter·i·za·tion (vay"po·kaw"tur·i·zay'shun) *n.* [*vapor* + *cauterization*]. Cauterization by live steam.

va·por (vay'pur) *n.* [L.]. A gas, especially the gaseous form of a substance which at ordinary temperatures is liquid or solid.

vapor bath. A bath in which the bather is exposed to moist vapors.

va·po·res ute·ri·ni (va·po'reez yoo"tur·eye'nigh) [L.]. *Obsol.* HYSTERIA.

va·por·ish (vay'pur·ish) *adj.* 1. Of the nature of vapor. 2. Given to periods of depression or hysteria.

va·por·iza·tion (vay"pur·i·zay'shun) *n.* The conversion of a solid or liquid into a vapor. —**va·por·ize** (vay'pur·ize) *v.*

va·por·iz·er (vay'pur·eye"zur) *n.* 1. ATOMIZER. 2. A device for converting a substance, usually a liquid, into vapor.

vapor pressure. The pressure of a liquid, solid, or solution which is exerted by a vapor when a state of equilibrium has been reached between the liquid, solid, or solution and its vapor.

va·pors (vay'purz) *n.pl. Obsol.* Lowness of spirits; HYSTERIA.

va·po·ther·a·py (vay"po·therr'uh·pee) *n.* [*vapor* + *therapy*]. The therapeutic employment, as in respiratory diseases, of medicated or nonmedicated vapor, steam, or spray.

Va·quez's disease (vah·kez') [L. H. *Vaquez*, French physician, 1860–1936]. POLYCYTHEMIA VERA.

vari·abil·i·ty, *n.* Differences among members of a species resulting from genetic or environmental causes.

vari·able, *adj & n.* 1. Inconstant; subject to variation. 2. A quantity or magnitude which may vary in value under differing conditions. See also *curve* (2).

variable region. A region of the immunoglobulin molecule consisting of sequences of amino acids in the light and the heavy chains which vary from one antibody to another, are involved in the region which binds antigen, and are therefore believed to confer specificity on antibody molecules. Contr. *constant region.*

vari·ance (văr'ee·unce) *n.* The square of the standard deviation. The second moment when deviations are taken from the mean.

var·i·ant (văr'ee·unt) *n. & adj.* [L. *varians*, varying, from *variare*, to vary]. 1. *In bacteriology*, a colony which differs in appearance from the parent colony grown on the same medium; MUTANT. 2. Exhibiting or constituting variation.

var·i·a·tion (văr"ee·ay'shun) *n.* [L. *variatio*, from *variare*, to vary]. 1. Deviation from a given type as the result of environment, natural selection, or cultivation and domestication. 2. Diversity in characteristics among related objects.

varic-, varico-. A combining form meaning *varix, varicose.*

var·i·ca·tion (văr"i·kay'shun) *n.* 1. The formation of a varix. 2. A system of varices.

var·i·ce·al (văr"i·see'ul, va·ris'ee·ul) *adj.* Of or pertaining to a varix or varices.

var·i·cec·to·my (văr"i·seck'tuh·mee) *n.* [*varic-* + *-ectomy*]. Excision of a varix or varicose vein, as distinguished from avulsion of a vein.

var·i·cel·la (văr"i·sel'uh) *n.* [NL., dim. of *variola*]. CHICKENPOX.

varicella gan·grae·no·sa (gang·gre·no'suh). Varicella in which the eruption leads to a gangrenous ulceration.

varicella in·oc·u·la·ta (i·nock·yoo·lay'tuh). Vaccination of susceptibles with the clear vesicular fluid from varicella lesions.

var·i·cel·la·tion (văr"i·se·lay'shun) *n.* Preventive inoculation with the virus of chickenpox (varicella).

varicella-zoster virus. A virus of the herpesvirus group causing chickenpox and herpes zoster infections in man; the viruses for these diseases have been considered identical as they are physically and immunologically indistinguishable.

var·i·cel·li·form (văr"i·sel'i·form) *adj.* [*varicella* + *-iform*]. Characterized by vesicles resembling those of chickenpox (varicella).

var·i·cel·loid (văr"i·sel'oid) *adj.* [*varicella* + *-oid*]. Resembling chickenpox (varicella).

varices. Plural of *varix.*

var·ic·i·form (va·ris'i·form, văr'i·si·) *n.* [*varic-* + *-iform*]. Having the form of a varix; VARICOSE.

varico-. See *varic-.*

var·i·co·bleph·a·ron (văr"i·ko·blef'uh·ron) *n.* [*varico-* + *blepharon*]. Varicose veins of an eyelid.

var·i·co·cele (văr'i·ko·seel) *n.* [*varico-* + *-cele*]. Dilatation of the veins of the pampiniform plexus of the spermatic cord, forming a soft, elastic, often uncomfortable swelling.

var·i·co·ce·lec·to·my (văr"i·ko·se·leck'tuh·mee) *n.* [*varicocele* + *-ectomy*]. Surgical excision of dilated spermatic veins for relief of varicocele.

var·i·cog·ra·phy (văr"i·kog'ruh·fee) *n.* [*varico-* + *-graphy*]. Radiographic visualization of the course and extent of a collection of varicose veins.

var·i·coid (văr'i·koid) *adj.* [*varic-* + *-oid*]. Resembling a varix.

var·i·com·pha·lus (văr"i·kom'fuh·lus) *n.* [*varic-* + *omphalus*]. A varicosity at the navel.

var·i·co·phle·bi·tis (văr"i·ko·fle·bye'tis) *n.* [*varico-* + *phlebitis*]. Inflammation of a varicose vein or veins.

var·i·cose (văr'i·koce, ·koze) *adj.* [L. *varicosus*, from *varix*]. 1. Characterizing blood vessels that are dilated, knotted, and tortuous. 2. Due to varicose veins.

varicose aneurysm. An arterovenous aneurysm in which the blood is carried into the vein through a connecting pulsating sac; the associated veins also may be dilated and pulsating.

varicose ulcer. STASIS ULCER.

varicose veins. Veins that have become abnormally dilated and tortuous, because of interference with venous drainage or weakness of their walls.

var·i·co·sis (văr"i·ko'sis) *n.*, pl. **varico·ses** (·seez) [*varic-* + *-osis*]. An abnormal dilatation of the veins.

var·i·cos·i·ty (văr"i·kos'i·tee) *n.* 1. The state of exhibiting varices or being varicose. 2. VARICOSE VEIN.

var·i·cot·o·my (văr"i·kot'uh·mee) *n.* [*varico-* + *-tomy*]. Surgical excision of a varicose vein.

va·ric·u·la (va·rick'yoo·luh) *n.*, pl. **varicu·lae** (·lee) [NL., dim. of *varix*]. A varix of the conjunctiva.

Varidase. Trademark for a purified mixture of streptokinase and streptodornase, enzymes elaborated by hemolytic streptococci. The mixed enzymes cause liquefaction and removal of necrotic tissue and thickened or clotted exudates resulting from wounds or inflammatory processes, thereby promoting normal repair of tissue.

var·ie·gat·ed position effect (văr'ee·e·gay"tid). The phenomenon whereby the expression of a gene depends on its position with respect to adjacent chromosomal material.

var·ie·gate porphyria (văr'ee·e·gate). PORPHYRIA CUTANEA TARDA HEREDITARIA.

va·ri·ety, *n.* [L. *varietas*, diversity]. A subdivision of a species; a stock, strain, breed.

var·i·form (văr'i·form) *adj.* [L. *varius*, diverse, + *-form*]. Having diversity of form.

va·ri·o·la (va·rye'o·luh) *n.* [ML., perhaps from L. *varus*, pimple]. SMALLPOX.

variola minor. A mild form of smallpox due to a less virulent strain. Syn. *alastrim.*

va·ri·o·lar (va·rye'o·lur) *adj.* [*variola* + *-ar*]. Pertaining to or characterized by smallpox.

var·i·o·late (văr'ee·o·late) *v.* [from *variola*]. To inoculate with smallpox virus. —**var·i·o·la·tion** (văr"ee·o·lay'shun) *n.*

variola ve·ra (veer'uh). True smallpox as distinguished from varioloid.

var·i·ol·ic (văr″ee·ol′ick) *adj.* VARIOLAR.

var·i·ol·i·form (văr″ee·o′li·form, ·ol′i·form) *adj.* [*variola* + *-iform*]. Resembling smallpox.

var·i·o·li·za·tion (văr″ee·uh·li·zay′shun) *n.* VARIOLATION.

var·i·o·loid (văr′ee·o·loid) *adj. & n.* [*variola* + *-oid*]. 1. Resembling smallpox. 2. A mild form of smallpox in persons who have been successfully vaccinated or who previously had the disease.

va·ri·o·lous (va·rye′o·lus) *adj.* VARIOLAR.

variolous erythema. The initial eruption of variola.

va·ri·o·lo·vac·cine (va·rye″o·lo·vack′seen, ·vack·seen′) *n.* [*variola* + *vaccine*]. A vaccine obtained from the lymph in lesions produced in a heifer inoculated with smallpox virus. The virus may also be cultivated in a chick embryo by chorioallantoic inoculation.

va·ri·o·lo·vac·cin·ia (va·rye″o·lo·vack·sin′ee·uh) *n.* [*variola* + *vaccinia*]. A form of vaccinia or cowpox induced in a heifer by inoculating it with smallpox virus.

var·ix (văr′icks) *n.*, pl. **var·i·ces** (·i·seez) [L.]. 1. A dilated and tortuous vein. 2. A tortuous, enlarged artery or lymphatic vessel.

varix lym·phat·i·cus (lim·fat′i·kus). Dilatation of the lymphatic vessels, especially that due to *Wuchereria bancrofti.*

va·rus (vair′us) *adj.* [L., bent, stretched, or grown outwards or awry]. Usually, denoting an abnormal turning inward toward the midline of the body, as in talipes varus and coxa vara; occasionally, as in genu varus (bowleg), denoting an abnormal turning outward. Contr. *valgus.*

vas (vas) *n.*, pl. **va·sa** (vay′suh, ·zuh), genit. pl. **va·so·rum** (vay·so′rum) [L.]. VESSEL.

vas-, vasi-, vaso- [L. *vas*]. A combining form meaning (a) *vessel, vascular;* (b) *ductus deferens;* (c) *vasomotor.*

vasa aber·ran·tia he·pa·tis (ab·e·ran′shee·uh hep′uh·tis) [BNA]. Remnants of the bile ducts in atrophied liver substance sometimes persisting from fetal life, in the left lobe of the liver.

vasa af·fe·ren·tia lym·pho·glan·du·lae (af·e·ren′shee·uh lim·fo·glan′dew·lee) [BNA]. VASA AFFERENTIA NODI LYMPHATICI.

vasa afferentia no·di lym·pha·ti·ci (no′dye lim·fat′i·sigh) [NA]. The afferent lymphatic vessels of a lymph node.

vasa au·ris in·ter·nae (aw′ris in·tur′nee) [NA]. A collective term for the vessels of the inner ear.

vasa bre·via (brev′ee·uh), sing. **vas bre·ve** (brev′ee). The short gastric arteries. See Table of Arteries in the Appendix.

vasa deferentia. Plural of *vas deferens.*

vasa ef·fe·ren·tia lym·pho·glan·du·lae (ef·e·ren′shee·uh lim·fo·glan′dew·lee) [BNA]. VASA EFFERENTIA NODI LYMPHATICI.

vasa efferentia no·di lym·pha·ti·ci (no′dye lim·fat′i·sigh) [NA]. The efferent lymphatic vessels of a lymph node.

vas af·fe·rens ar·te·ri·ae in·ter·lo·bu·la·ris (af′e·renz ahr·teer′ee·ee in·tur·lob·yoo·lair′is) [NA]. The afferent branch of an interlobular artery to a glomerulus of the kidney.

vas afferens glo·me·ru·li re·na·lis (glo·merr′yoo·lye re·nay′lis) [BNA]. VAS AFFERENS ARTERIAE INTERLOBULARIS.

vasa lym·pha·ti·ca (lim·fat′i·kuh) [NA]. Plural of *vas lymphaticum.*

vasa lymphatica pro·fun·da (pro·fun′duh) [NA]. The deep lymphatic vessels.

vasa lymphatica su·per·fi·ci·a·lia (sue·pur·fish·ee·ay′lee·uh) [NA]. The superficial lymphatic vessels.

vas ana·sto·mo·ti·cum (a·nas·to·mot′i·kum) [NA]. An anastomotic vessel.

vasa ner·vo·rum (nur·vo′rum). The blood vessels supplying nerves.

vasa prae·via (pree′vee·uh). Presentation of the velamentous vessels across the lower uterine segment, seen with a low implantation of the placenta.

vasa rec·ta (reck′tuh), sing. **vas rec·tum** (reck′tum) [L., straight vessels]. The thin-walled channels that carry blood to the renal medulla and originate from the efferent arterioles of the juxtamedullary glomeruli.

vasa san·gui·nea re·ti·nae (sang·gwin′ee·uh ret′i·nee) [NA]. A collective term for the blood vessels of the retina.

vasa va·so·rum (vay·so′rum) [NA]. The blood vessels supplying the walls of arteries and veins having a caliber greater than 1 mm. See also Plate 6.

vas ca·pil·la·re (kap·i·lair′ee) [NA]. CAPILLARY (2).

vas col·la·te·ra·le (ko·lat·e·ray′lee) [NA]. A collateral vessel.

vascul-, vasculo-. A combining form meaning *vascular.*

vas·cu·lar (vas′kew·lur) *adj.* [L. *vasculum* (dim. of *vas,* vessel) + *-ar*]. Consisting of, pertaining to, or provided with, vessels.

vascular arborization. A treelike branching of blood vessels.

vascular bed. The total blood supply—arteries, capillaries, and veins—of an organ or region.

vascular bundle sheath. PHLOEM SHEATH.

vascular circle of the optic nerve. A complete or incomplete circle of two or more short ciliary arteries within the sclera adjacent to the optic nerve. Syn. *circle of Haller, circle of Zinn.* NA *circulus vasculosus nervi optici.*

vascular cone. LOBULE OF THE EPIDIDYMIS.

vascular dysmenorrhea. CONGESTIVE DYSMENORRHEA.

vascular epithelium. ENDOTHELIUM.

vascular flap. A pedicle flap that includes an artery and vein in its base.

vascular fold. A fold of peritoneum containing vessels.

vascular foramen. Any small opening, especially on the surface of a bone, for the passage of a blood vessel.

vascular headache. A throbbing headache due to painful dilatation and distention of branches of the external carotid artery.

vascular hemophilia. A bleeding disorder associated with increased bleeding time and low factor VIII activity.

vas·cu·lar·i·ty (vas″kew·lăr′i·tee) *n.* The quality of being vascular.

vas·cu·lar·iza·tion (vas″kew·lur·i·zay′shun) *n.* 1. The process of tissues becoming vascular. 2. The formation and extension of vascular capillaries within and into tissues. —**vas·cu·lar·ize** (vas′kew·lur·ize) *v.*

vascular polyp. A pedunculated angioma.

vascular reflex. VASOMOTOR REFLEX.

vascular retinopathy. Retinal manifestations of such diseases as arterial hypertension, chronic nephritis, eclampsia, and advanced arteriosclerosis, characterized by various combinations and degrees of hemorrhages, exudates, vascular sclerosis, and sometimes by papilledema (malignant hypertension).

vascular system. CARDIOVASCULAR SYSTEM.

vas·cu·la·ture (vas′kew·luh·chur) *n.* The distribution or arrangement of blood vessels in an organ or part.

vas·cu·li·tis (vas″kew·lye′tis) *n.*, pl. **vascu·lit·i·des** (·lit′i·deez) [*vascul-* + *-itis*]. Inflammation of a vessel; ANGIITIS.

vasculitis-hypersensitivity syndrome. ALLERGIC VASCULITIS SYNDROME.

vasculo-. See *vascul-.*

vas·cu·lo·gen·e·sis (vas″kew·lo·jen′e·sis) *n.* [*vasculo-* + *-genesis*]. The formation of the vascular system.

vas·cu·lo·tox·ic (vas″kew·lo·tock′sick) *adj.* Chemically damaging to blood vessels.

vas·cu·lum (vas′kew·lum) *n.*, pl. **vascu·la** (·luh) [L.]. A small blood or lymph vessel.

vas de·fe·rens (def′ur·enz), pl. **vasa de·fe·ren·tia** (def·e·ren′chee·uh). DUCTUS DEFERENS.

vas·ec·to·my (vas·eck′tuh·mee) *n.* [*vas* deferens + *-ectomy*]. Surgical division or resection of the ductus deferens; used to produce male sterility for birth control.

vas ef·fe·rens ar·te·ri·ae in·ter·lo·bu·la·ris (ef′e·renz ahr·teer′ee·ee in·tur·lob·yoo·lair′is) [NA]. The efferent blood vessel from a glomerulus of the kidney.

vas efferens glo·me·ru·li re·na·lis (glo·merr′yoo·lye re·nay′lis) [BNA]. VAS EFFERENS ARTERIAE INTERLOBULARIS.

vasi-. See *vas-*.
vas·i·cine (vas'i·seen, ·sin) *n.* PEGANINE.
vas·i·fac·tion (vas''i·fack'shun) *n.* [*vasi-* + L. *facere*, to make]. VASOFORMATION.
vas·i·for·ma·tion (vas''i·for·may'shun) *n.* [*vasi-* + *formation*]. The process by which a structure assumes the appearance of a vessel or duct.
vas·i·tis (vas·eye'tis) *n.* [*vas* deferens + *-itis*]. Inflammation of the ductus deferens.
vas lym·pha·ti·cum (lim·fat'i·kum), pl. **vasa lymphati·ca** (·kuh) [NA]. LYMPHATIC (2).
vaso-. See *vas-*.
va·so·ac·tive (vay''zo·ack'tiv) *adj.* Effecting the reactivity of blood vessels.
vaso·con·stric·tion (vay''zo·kun·strick'shun, vas''o·) *n.* [*vaso-* + *constriction*]. The constriction of blood vessels; particularly, functional narrowing of the arteriolar lumen.
vaso·con·stric·tive (vay''zo·kun·strick'tiv, vas''o·) *adj.* [*vaso-* + *constrictive*]. Promoting, stimulating, or characterized by constriction of blood vessels.
vaso·con·stric·tor (vay''zo·kun·strick'tur, vas''o·) *n. & adj.* [*vaso-* + *constrictor*]. 1. A nerve or an agent that causes constriction of blood vessels. 2. Causing vasoconstriction.
vasoconstrictor center. The pressor area of the vasomotor center.
vasoconstrictor fibers. Nerve fibers which, upon stimulation, produce constriction of blood vessels.
vasoconstrictor nerves. The nerves which cause constriction of blood vessels. See also *vasomotor nerves*.
va·so·cu·ta·ne·ous (vas''o·kew·tay'nee·us) *adj.* Pertaining to the vas deferens and the skin.
vaso·den·tin (vay''zo·den'tin, vas''o·) *n.* [*vaso-* + *dentin*]. A type of dentin in which blood vessels lie in anastomosing canals, found in the teeth of some fishes.
vaso·den·tine (vay''zo·den'teen, vas''o·) *n.* VASODENTIN.
vaso·de·pres·sor (vay''zo·de·pres'ur, vas''o·) *n. & adj.* [*vaso-* + *depressor*]. 1. An agent that produces vasomotor depression. 2. Lowering blood pressure or causing vasomotor depression.
vasodepressor syncope. VASOVAGAL SYNCOPE.
vaso·dil·a·ta·tion (vay''zo·dil''uh·tay'shun, dye''luh·tay'shun, vas''o·) *n.* [*vaso-* + *dilatation*]. Dilatation of the blood vessels, particularly functional increase of the arteriolar lumen.
vaso·di·la·tion (vay''zo·dye·lay'shun, vas''o·) *n.* [*vaso-* + *dilation*]. VASODILATATION.
vaso·di·la·tive (vay''zo·dye·lay'tiv, vas''o·) *adj.* Promoting, stimulating, or characterized by vasodilatation.
vaso·di·la·tor (vay''zo·dye·lay'tur, vas''o·) *n. & adj.* [*vaso-* + *dilator*]. 1. A nerve or agent that causes dilatation of blood vessels. 2. Pertaining to the relaxation of the smooth muscle of the vascular system. 3. Producing dilatation of blood vessels.
vasodilator center. The depressor area of the vasomotor center.
vasodilator fibers. Nerve fibers whose function is to dilate blood vessels.
vasodilator nerves. The nerves which cause dilatation of blood vessels. See also *vasomotor nerves*.
vaso·epi·did·y·mos·to·my (vaz''o·ep''i·did''i·mos'tuh·mee, vas''o·) *n.* [*vaso-* + *epididymo-* + *-stomy*]. Anastomosis of a ductus deferens with its epididymal duct.
vaso·for·ma·tion (vay''zo·for·may'shun, vas''o·) *n.* [*vaso-* + *formation*]. The process in which blood vessels are produced or formed.
vaso·for·ma·tive (vay''zo·for'muh·tiv, vas''o·) *adj.* [*vaso-* + *formative*]. Forming or producing vessels.
vasoformative cell. A cell which forms blood vessels.
vaso·gen·ic (vay''zo·jen'ick, vas''o·) *adj.* [*vaso-* + *-genic*]. 1. Pertaining to the development of blood or lymph vessels. 2. Vascular in origin.
vasogenic shock. Peripheral circulatory failure due to arteriolar and capillary vasodilatation.
va·sog·ra·phy (vay·zog'ruh·fee, vas·og') *n.* [*vaso-* + *-graphy*]. Radiography of blood vessels.
vaso·hy·per·ton·ic (vay''zo·high''pur·ton'ick, vas''o·) *adj.* [*vaso-* + *hypertonic*]. VASOCONSTRICTOR (2).
vaso·hy·po·ton·ic (vay''zo·high''po·ton'ick, vas''o·) *adj.* [*vaso-* + *hypotonic*]. VASODILATOR (2, 3).
vaso·in·hib·i·tor (vay''zo·in·hib'i·tur, vas''o·) *n.* [*vaso-* + *inhibitor*]. A drug or agent tending to inhibit the action of the vasomotor nerves. —**vasoinhibi·to·ry** (·to·ree) *adj.*
vaso·li·ga·tion (vay''zo·lye·gay'shun, vas''o·) *n.* [*vaso-* + *ligation*]. Surgical ligation of a ductus deferens.
vaso·mo·tion (vay''zo·mo'shun, vas''o·) *n.* [*vaso-* + *motion*]. The rhythmic increase or decrease of the caliber of a blood vessel, especially precapillary sphincters.
vaso·mo·tor (vay''zo·mo'tur, vas''o·) *adj.* [*vaso-* + *motor*]. 1. Pertaining to or regulating the contraction (vasoconstriction) and expansion (vasodilatation) of blood vessels. 2. VASOCONSTRICTOR (2).
vasomotor center. A large, diffuse area in the reticular formation of the lower brainstem, extending from just below the obex to the region of the vestibular nuclei, and from the floor of the fourth ventricle almost to the pyramids; stimulation of the rostral and lateral portions of this center (pressor area) causes a rise in blood pressure and tachycardia, and stimulation of a smaller portion around the obex (depressor area) results in a fall in blood pressure and bradycardia. It is now thought that variations in the interaction between the two areas, with excitatory fibers from the pressor area and inhibitory fibers from the depressor area converging on vasoconstrictor nerves, control vasomotor activity.
vasomotor headache. CLUSTER HEADACHE.
vasomotor nerves. 1. The nerves concerned with controlling the caliber of blood vessels: those which cause constriction (vasoconstrictor nerves) and those which cause dilatation (vasodilator nerves). 2. VASOCONSTRICTOR NERVES.
vasomotor neurosis. ANGIONEUROSIS.
vasomotor paralysis. Paralysis of the vasomotor mechanism with resultant atony and dilatation of the blood vessels.
vasomotor reflex. Constriction or dilatation of a blood vessel in response to stimulation. Syn. *vascular reflex*.
vasomotor rhinitis or **catarrh**. ALLERGIC RHINITIS.
vasomotor syncope. VASOVAGAL SYNCOPE.
vasomotor system. The nerve supply of the blood vessels.
vaso·mo·tric·i·ty (vay''zo·mo·tris'i·tee, vas''o·) *n.* The qualities of vasomotor action.
vaso·neu·ro·sis (vay''zo·new·ro'sis, vas''o·) *n.* [*vaso-* + *neur-* + *-osis*]. ANGIONEUROSIS.
vaso·or·chid·os·to·my (vas''o·or''kid·os'tuh·mee, vay''zo·) *n.* [*vaso-* + *orchido-* + *-stomy*]. Surgical anastomosis of a ductus deferens with any portion of its testis.
vaso·pa·ral·y·sis (vay''zo·puh·ral'i·sis, vas''o·) *n.* [*vaso-* + *paralysis*]. VASOMOTOR PARALYSIS.
vaso·pa·re·sis (vay''zo·puh·ree'sis, ·păr'e·sis, vas''o·) *n.* [*vaso-* + *paresis*]. A partial vasomotor paralysis.
vaso·pres·sin (vay''zo·pres'in, vas''o·) *n.* ANTIDIURETIC HORMONE.
vaso·pres·sor (vay''zo·pres'ur, vas''o·) *n.* [*vaso-* + *pressor*]. Any substance that causes contraction of the smooth muscle of vessels. See also *arteriopressor, venopressor*.
vaso·punc·ture (vay''zo·punk'chur, vas''o·) *n.* [*vaso-* + *puncture*]. Surgical puncture of a ductus deferens.
vaso·re·lax·a·tion (vay''zo·re·lack·say'shun, vas''o·) *n.* [*vaso-* + *relaxation*]. Diminution of vascular tension.
vas·or·rha·phy (vaz·or'uh·fee) *n.* [*vaso-* + *-rrhaphy*]. End-to-end or end-to-side suture of a ductus deferens or of a blood vessel.
vas·os·cil·la·tor bed (vay·zos'si·lay''tur, vaz·os'). A bed that may be tipped to provide postural vascular exercise. See also *oscillating bed*.

vaso·sec·tion (vay″zo·seck′shun, vaz″o·) *n.* [*vaso-* + *section*]. Severing of a ductus deferens.

vaso·spasm (vay′zo·spaz·um, vaz″o·) *n.* [*vaso-* + *spasm*]. VASOCONSTRICTION; ANGIOSPASM.

vaso·spas·tic (vay″zo·spas′tick, vaz″o·) *adj.* [*vaso-* + *spastic*]. ANGIOSPASTIC.

vasospastic syndrome. RAYNAUD'S PHENOMENON.

vaso·stim·u·lant (vay″zo·stim′yoo·lunt, vaz″o·) *adj. & n.* [*vaso-* + *stimulant*]. 1. Inducing or exciting vasomotor action. 2. Any agent that promotes vasomotor action.

vas·os·to·my (va·zos′tuh·mee) *n.* [*vaso-* + *-stomy*]. The surgical establishment of an artificial opening into a ductus deferens.

vas·ot·o·my (va·zot′uh·mee) *n.* [*vaso-* + *-tomy*]. Surgical incision of a ductus deferens.

vaso·ton·ic (vay″zo·ton′ick, vas″o·) *adj. & n.* [*vaso-* + *tonic*]. 1. Pertaining to the tone or degree of vasoconstriction of the blood vessels. 2. VASOSTIMULANT (2).

vaso·to·nin (vay″zo·to′nin, vas″o·) *n.* [*vasoto*nic + *-in*]. A vasoconstrictor substance present in the blood.

vaso·tribe (vay′zo·tribe, vas″o·) *n.* [*vaso-* + *-tribe*]. ANGIOTRIBE.

vaso·troph·ic (vay″zo·trof′ick, vas″o·) *adj.* [*vaso-* + *-trophic*]. Concerned in the nutrition of blood vessels.

vaso·va·gal (vay″zo·vay′gul, vas″o·) *adj.* [*vaso-* + *vagal*]. Pertaining to the blood vessels and vagus nerve.

vasovagal attack (of Gowers) [W. R. *Gowers*]. Anxiety, pallor, bradycardia, hypotension, sweating, nausea, precordial and respiratory distress, often culminating in syncope; due to excessive vagal effect on the vascular system. Compare *vasovagal syncope.* See also *angina pectoris vasomotoria, carotid sinus syncope.*

vasovagal reflex. Reflex vagal stimulation from peripheral blood vessels.

vasovagal syncope. The common faint, occurring as a response to sudden emotional stress, pain, or injury; characterized by hypotension, pallor, sweating, hyperventilation, bradycardia, and loss of consciousness from excessive vagal effect on the vascular system. Syn. *vasodepressor syncope.* Compare *vasovagal attack.*

vaso·vas·os·to·my (vay″zo·va·zos′tuh·mee, vas″o·) *n.* [*vaso-* + *vaso-* + *-stomy*]. Surgical anastomosis of one portion of a ductus deferens to another.

vaso·ve·sic·u·lec·to·my (vay″zo·ve·sick″yoo·leck′tuh·mee, vas″o·) *n.* [*vaso-* + *vesicul-* + *-ectomy*]. Surgical excision of a ductus deferens and seminal vesicle.

Vasoxyl. Trademark for methoxamine, a peripheral vasoconstrictor used as the hydrochloride salt for management of hypotension during surgery.

vas pro·mi·nens (pro′mi·nenz, prom′i·) [NA]. One of the capillary loops in the ridge of connective tissue that lies above the line of attachment of the lamina basilaris to the spiral ligament of the cochlea and extends throughout the cochlear duct.

vas rectum. Singular of *vasa recta.*

vas spi·ra·le (spye·ray′lee) [NA]. The largest of the blood vessels that lie in the connective tissue on the under surface of the lamina basilaris of the cochlear duct.

vas·tus muscles (vas′tus) [L., immense]. The vastus intermedius (NA *musculus vastus intermedius*), vastus lateralis (NA *musculus vastus lateralis*), and vastus medialis (NA *musculus vastus medialis*) muscles; combined with the rectus femoris muscle, they make up the quadriceps femoris, the extensor muscle of the thigh. See also Table of Muscles in the Appendix.

Vatensol. Trademark for guanoclor, an antihypertensive drug used as the sulfate salt.

Va·ter-Pa·ci·ni corpuscle (fah′tur, pa^h·chee′nee) [A. *Vater*, German anatomist, 1684–1751; and F. *Pacini*]. LAMELLAR CORPUSCLE.

Vater's ampulla [A. *Vater*]. The hepatopancreatic ampulla, where the common bile duct and main pancreatic duct empty.

vault, *n.* [OF. *vaute,* from L. *volvere, volutus,* to turn, roll]. 1. An arched structure, as a dome. 2. Specifically, the vault of the skull; CALVARIA.

V2 carcinoma. A poorly differentiated transplantable carcinoma of the rabbit which originally occurred as the result of malignant transformation in a Shope papilloma.

V.C.G. Abbreviation for *vectorcardiogram.*

VD Abbreviation for *venereal disease.*

V.D.H. Valvular disease of the heart.

Veau's operation (vo) [V. *Veau,* French surgeon, b. 1871]. A modification of Dieffenbach's operation for the repair of cleft palate.

ve·cor·dia (ve·kor′dee·uh) *n.* [L., from *vecors,* senseless, mad]. Any mental disorder.

vec·tion (veck′shun) *n.* [L., *vectio,* carrying, conveyance, from *vehere,* to carry]. The conveyance of disease germs from sick to well persons.

vec·tis (veck′tis) *n.* [L., bar, lever]. An instrument similar to the single blade of a forceps, used in hastening the delivery of the fetal head in labor.

vec·tor (veck′tur) *n.* [L., carrier, from *vehere,* to carry]. 1. An arthropod or other agent that carries microorganisms from an infected person to some other person. 2. A quantity involving both magnitude and direction, as velocity, force, momentum, which may be represented by a straight line of suitable length and direction. —**vec·to·ri·al** (veck·to′ree·ul) *adj.*

vec·tor·car·dio·gram (veck″tur·kahr′dee·o·gram) *n.* [*vector* + *cardiogram*]. The part of the pathway of instantaneous vectors during one cardiac cycle, consisting of P, QRS, and T loops. Abbreviated, V.C.G. Syn. *monocardiogram.*

vec·tor·car·dio·graph (veck″tur·kahr′dee·o·graf *n.* [*vector* + *cardiograph*]. An apparatus for recording a vectorcardiogram.

vec·tor·car·di·og·ra·phy (veck″tur·kahr″dee·og′ruh·fee) *n.* [*vector* + *cardiography*]. A method of recording the direction and magnitude of the instantaneous cardiac vectors. Continuous loops are recorded in the frontal, horizontal, and sagittal planes.

veg·an (vej′an″) *n.* A vegetarian who excludes from his diet all protein of animal origin.

veg·e·ta·ble, *adj.* [ML. *vegetabilis,* capable of growing, from *vegetare,* to grow, thrive]. Of or pertaining to plants.

vegetable albumin. Albumin found in plant or vegetable matter.

vegetable amylase. DIASTASE.

vegetable casein. A protein of plant origin resembling the casein of milk, as legumin conglutin. Syn. *gluten casein.*

vegetable diastase. DIASTASE.

vegetable insulin. GLUCOKININ.

veg·e·tal (vej′e·tul) *adj.* [ML. *vege*tare, to grow, + *-al*]. 1. VEGETABLE. 2. Pertaining to the basic functions shared by both plants and animals such as metabolism, respiration, reproduction, and growth.

vegetal pole. The relatively inactive, yolk-laden pole of an ovum. Syn. *vegetative pole, antigerminal pole.* Contr. *animal pole.*

veg·e·ta·tion, *n.* [ML. *vegetatio,* growth]. 1. An excrescence on a cardiac valve or other portion of the heart, composed of platelets, fibrin, and often bacteria, and resembling a plant in general shape; seen in bacterial endocarditis and other diseases. 2. Any plant-shaped abnormal structure.

veg·e·ta·tive (vej″e·tay′tiv) *adj.* 1. Involved in, or pertaining to, growth and nutrition rather than reproduction. 2. Functioning involuntarily or unconsciously; pertaining to the autonomic nervous system. 3. Pertaining to vegetation, or a pathologic growth.

vegetative dermatitis. DERMATITIS VEGETANS.

vegetative nervous system. AUTONOMIC NERVOUS SYSTEM.

vegetative neurosis. PSYCHOPHYSIOLOGIC DISORDERS.

vegetative pole. VEGETAL POLE.

ve·hi·cle (vee'i·kul) *n.* [L. *vehiculum,* conveyance, from *vehere,* to convey]. A liquid or solid substance, generally inactive therapeutically, employed as a medium or carrier for the active component of a medicine.

veil, *n.* [L. *velum,* veil, covering]. CAUL (1).

Veil·lo·nel·la (vay''yo·nel'uh) *n.* [A. *Veillon,* French bacteriologist, 1864–1931]. A genus of microorganisms belonging to the family Neisseriaceae; they are small, gram-negative, anaerobic cocci.

Veillonella al·ca·les·cens (al''kuh·les'enz). A species found in the saliva of man and other animals.

Veillonella dis·coi·des (dis·koy'deez). A species found in the buccal cavity.

Veillonella or·bi·cu·lus (or·bick'yoo·lus). A species found in the intestinal tract; of unknown pathogenicity.

Veillonella par·vu·la (pahr'vew·luh). A species found in the mouth and digestive tract of man and other animals.

Veillonella ren·i·for·mis (ren·i·for'mis). A species found in the urogenital tract; of unknown pathogenicity.

Veil·lon's tube (veh·yoh$^{n'}$) [A. *Veillon*]. A glass tube for use in making bacterial cultures. One end is fitted with a rubber stopper, the other with a cotton plug.

vein, *n.* [OF. *veine,* from L. *vena*]. A blood vessel carrying blood from the tissues toward the heart. Veins, like arteries, have three coats, but the media is less well developed; many also possess valves. For veins listed by name, see Table of Veins in the Appendix. See also Plates 9, 10.

vein of Lab·bé (la^{h}·be$^{y'}$) [L. *Labbé,* French surgeon, 1832–1916]. An inferior anastomotic vein that connects the superficial middle cerebral vein with the transverse sinus.

vein of Tro·lard (tro^{h}·lăhr') [P. *Trolard,* French anatomist, 1842–1910]. A superior anastomotic vein that connects the superficial middle cerebral vein with the superior longitudinal sinus.

vein retractor. An instrument with a small, smooth, flanged blade, used to retract blood vessels without injury to them.

vein stripper. A long-handled surgical instrument, used to remove varicose veins, usually introduced intraluminally throughout the involved length of vein.

vela. Plural of *velum.*

ve·la·men (ve·lay'mun) *n.,* pl. **ve·lam·i·na** (·lam'i·nuh) [L., covering]. A veil or covering membrane.

velamentous insertion. The insertion of the umbilical cord, which first attaches to fetal membranes and then passes on to the placenta.

velamentous placenta. A placenta with the umbilical cord arising from the outer border.

vel·a·men·tum (vel''uh·men'tum, vee''luh·) *n.,* pl. **velamen·ta** (·tuh) [L., covering]. A veil, or covering membrane. —**velamen·tous** (·tus) *adj.*

velamen vul·vae (vul'vee). HOTTENTOT APRON.

ve·lar (vee'lur) *adj.* [*vel*um + *-ar*]. 1. Of or pertaining to a velum, especially the velum palatinum. 2. Of consonant sounds: formed with the back of the tongue touching or almost touching the soft palate or the back part of the hard palate, as *g* in gut, *k* in talk, or *ch* in Bach.

Velban. Trademark for vinblastine, an antineoplastic drug used as the sulfate salt.

veldt or **veld sore** (velt). Chronic shallow ulcers of exposed parts of the body, noted particularly in subtropical hot desert regions of Australia, Africa, and the Middle East; of uncertain, but possibly diphtheritic, etiology.

ve·li·ger (vee'li·jur, vel'i·jur) *n.* [L., sail-bearing, from *velum,* sail]. A larval mollusk with a velum.

vel·li·cate (vel'i·kate) *v.* [L. *vellicare,* from *vellere,* to pluck at]. To twitch spasmodically.

vel·li·ca·tion (vel''i·kay'shun) *n.* [L. *vellicatio*]. Spasmodic twitching of muscular fibers.

vel·lus (vel'us) *n.* [L., fleece]. The fine, downy hair that appears on all parts of the human body except the palms and soles and those parts, such as the scalp, where terminal hair grows. Compare *lanugo.* Contr. *terminal hair.*

ve·loc·i·ty (ve·los'i·tee) *n.* [L. *velocitas,* from *velox,* swift]. RATE; change per unit of time.

ve·lo·pha·ryn·geal (vee''lo·fuh·rin'jee'ul, ·jul) *adj.* Pertaining to the velum and the pharynx.

Vel·peau's bandage (vel·po') [A. A. L. M. *Velpeau,* French surgeon, 1795–1867]. A bandage that fixes the arm against the side, with the forearm flexed at an angle of 135°, the palm resting upon the midclavicular region opposite. By successive turns about the body, the bandage envelops the shoulder, arm, forearm, and hand.

Velpeau's deformity [A. A. L. M. *Velpeau*]. The deformity that occurs in fractures of the lower end of the radius (Colles' fracture).

ve·lum (vee'lum) *n.,* genit. **ve·li** (·lye), pl. **ve·la** (·luh) [L., sail; veil, covering]. 1. A veil or veil-like structure. 2. A band of cilia in front of the mouth, seen in certain larval stages of various mollusks.

velum in·ter·po·si·tum rhom·ben·ce·pha·li (in·tur·poz'i·tum rhom·ben·sef'uh·lye). The choroid plexus in the roof of the third ventricle of the brain.

velum me·dul·la·re an·te·ri·us (med·uh·lair'ee an·teer'ee·us) [BNA]. Velum medullare superius (= SUPERIOR MEDULLARY VELUM).

velum medullare in·fe·ri·us (in·feer'ee·us) [NA]. INFERIOR MEDULLARY VELUM.

velum medullare pos·te·ri·us (pos·teer'ee·us) [BNA]. Velum medullare inferius (= INFERIOR MEDULLARY VELUM).

velum medullare su·pe·ri·us (sue·peer'ee·us) [NA]. SUPERIOR MEDULLARY VELUM.

velum pa·la·ti (pa·lay'tye). VELUM PALATINUM.

velum pa·la·ti·num (pal·uh·tye'num) [NA]. The posterior portion of the soft palate.

velum pen·du·lum pa·la·ti (pen'dew·lum pa·lay'tye). VELUM PALATINUM.

velum ter·mi·na·le (tur·mi·nay'lee). LAMINA TERMINALIS.

ven-, vene-, veni-, veno-. A combining form meaning *vein, venous.*

ve·na (vee'nuh) *n.,* pl. & genit. sing. **ve·nae** (·nee) genit. pl. **ve·na·rum** (vee·nair'um) [L.] [NA]. VEIN.

vena ana·sto·mo·ti·ca inferior (a·nas·to·mot'i·kuh) [NA]. The inferior anastomotic vein. See Table of Veins in the Appendix.

vena anastomotica superior [NA]. The superior anastomotic vein. See Table of Veins in the Appendix.

vena an·gu·la·ris (ang·gew·lair'is) [NA]. The vein accompanying the angular artery.

vena ap·pen·di·cu·la·ris (ap·en·dick·yoo·lair'is) [NA]. The vein or veins draining from the vermiform appendix.

vena aquae·duc·tus ve·sti·bu·li (ack·we·duck'tus ves·tib'yoo·lye) [BNA]. VENA AQUEDUCTUS VESTIBULI.

vena aque·duc·tus co·chle·ae (ack·we·duck'tus cock'lee·ee) [NA]. The vein draining the aqueduct of the cochlea.

vena aqueductus ve·sti·bu·li (ves·tib'yoo·lye) [NA]. The vein draining the aqueduct of the vestibule.

vena au·ri·cu·la·ris posterior (aw·rick·yoo·lair'is) [NA]. The vein accompanying the posterior auricular artery.

vena ax·il·la·ris (ack·si·lair'is) [NA]. The vein or veins accompanying the axillary artery.

vena azy·gos (az'i·gos) [NA]. AZYGOS VEIN.

vena ba·sa·lis (ba·say'lis) [NA]. BASAL VEIN.

vena basalis com·mu·nis (kom·yoo'nis) [NA]. The vein formed by the union of the superior and inferior basal veins of the left and right inferior pulmonary veins.

vena basalis inferior [NA]. The inferior basal vein draining into the common basal vein of the left and right inferior pulmonary veins.

vena basalis [Ro·sen·tha·li] (ro·zun·tah'lye) [BNA]. Vena basalis (= BASAL VEIN).

vena basalis superior [NA]. The superior basal vein draining into the common basal vein of the left and right inferior pulmonary veins.

vena ba·si·li·ca (ba·sil'i·kuh) [NA]. BASILIC VEIN.

vena bron·chi·a·les an·te·ri·o·res (bronk·ee·ay'leez an·teer·ee·o'reez) [BNA]. VENAE BRONCHIALES.

vena bul·bi pe·nis (bul'bye pee'nis) [NA]. The vein draining the bulb of the penis.

vena bulbi ves·ti·bu·li (ves·tib'yoo·lye) [NA]. The vein draining the bulb of the vestibule.

vena ca·na·li·cu·li coch·le·ae (kan·uh·lick'yoo·lye kock'lee·ee) [NA]. The vein draining the canaliculus of the cochlea.

vena ca·na·lis pte·ry·goi·dei (ka·nay'lis terr·i·goy'dee·eye) [NA]. The vein of the pterygoid canal.

vena canalis pterygoidei [Vi·dii] (vid'ee·eye) [BNA]. VENA CANALIS PTERYGOIDEI.

vena ca·va (kay'vuh, kav'uh), pl. **ve·nae ca·vae** (vee'nee kay'vee). Either of the two veins which empty into the right atrium; the vena cava inferior or the vena cava superior.

vena cava inferior [NA]. INFERIOR VENA CAVA.

vena cava superior [NA]. SUPERIOR VENA CAVA.

vena cen·tra·lis glan·du·lae su·pra·re·na·lis (sen·tray'lis glan'dew·lee sue·pruh·re·nay'lis) [NA]. CENTRAL VEIN OF THE SUPRARENAL GLAND.

vena centralis re·ti·nae (ret'i·nee) [NA]. The central vein of the retina.

vena ce·pha·li·ca (se·fal'i·kuh) [NA]. CEPHALIC VEIN.

vena cephalica ac·ces·so·ria (ack·se·so'ree·uh) [NA]. The accessory cephalic vein.

vena ce·re·bri anterior (serr'e·brye) [NA]. The anterior cerebral vein.

vena cerebri mag·na (mag'nuh) [NA]. The great cerebral vein. See Table of Veins in the Appendix.

vena cerebri magna [Ga·le·ni] (ga·lee'nigh) [BNA]. VENA CEREBRI MAGNA.

vena cerebri me·dia (mee'dee·uh) [BNA]. VENA CEREBRI MEDIA SUPERFICIALIS.

vena cerebri media pro·fun·da (pro·fun'duh) [NA]. The deep medial cerebral vein, a tributary of the basal vein.

vena cerebri media su·per·fi·ci·a·lis (sue·pur·fish·ee·ay'lis) [NA]. The superficial medial cerebral vein. Syn. *Sylvian vein.*

vena cer·vi·ca·lis pro·fun·da (sur·vi·kay'lis pro·fun'duh) [NA]. The deep cervical vein.

vena cho·ri·oi·dea (ko·ree·oy'dee·uh) [BNA]. VENA CHOROIDEA.

vena cho·roi·dea (ko·roy'dee·uh) [NA]. The vein draining the choroid plexus of the lateral ventricle.

vena cir·cum·flexa ilii pro·fun·da (sur·kum·fleck'suh il'ee·eye pro·fun'duh) [NA]. The vein accompanying the deep circumflex iliac artery.

vena circumflexa ilii su·per·fi·ci·a·lis (sue·pur·fish·ee·ay'lis) [NA]. The vein accompanying the superficial circumflex iliac artery.

vena co·li·ca dex·tra (kol'i·kuh decks'truh) [NA]. The vein accompanying the right colic artery.

vena colica me·dia (mee'dee·uh) [NA]. The vein accompanying the middle colic artery.

vena colica si·nis·tra (si·nis'truh) [NA]. The vein accompanying the left colic artery.

vena co·mi·tans (kom'i·tanz), pl. **ve·nae co·mi·tan·tes** (vee'nee com·i·tan'teez) [NA]. Any vein accompanying an artery of the same name.

vena comitans ner·vi hy·po·glos·si (nur'vye high·po·glos'eye) [NA]. The vein accompanying the hypoglossal nerve.

vena cor·dis mag·na (kor'dis mag'nuh) [NA]. The great cardiac vein. See Table of Veins in the Appendix.

vena cordis me·dia (mee'dee·uh) [NA]. The middle cardiac vein. See Table of Veins in the Appendix.

vena cordis par·va (pahr'vuh) [NA]. The small cardiac vein. See Table of Veins in the Appendix.

vena co·ro·na·ria ven·tri·cu·li (kor·o·nair'ee·uh ven·trick'yoo·lye) [BNA]. The coronary vein of the stomach; the combined right and left gastric veins (vena gastrica dextra and vena gastrica sinistra).

vena cu·ta·nea (kew·tay'nee·uh) [NA]. A cutaneous vein.

vena cys·ti·ca (sis'ti·kuh) [NA]. The vein draining blood from the gallbladder.

vena di·plo·i·ca fron·ta·lis (di·plo'i·kuh fron·tay'lis) [NA]. The diploic vein of the frontal bone.

vena diploica oc·ci·pi·ta·lis (ock·sip·i·tay'lis) [NA]. The diploic vein of the occipital bone.

vena diploica tem·po·ra·lis anterior (tem·po·ray'lis) [NA]. The diploic vein of the adjacent parts of the frontal and parietal bones.

vena diploica temporalis posterior [NA]. The diploic vein of the posterior part of the parietal bone.

vena dor·sa·lis cli·to·ri·dis (dor·say'lis kli·tor'i·dis) [BNA]. VENA DORSALIS CLITORIDIS PROFUNDA.

vena dorsalis clitoridis pro·fun·da (pro·fun'duh) [NA]. The deep dorsal vein of the clitoris.

vena dorsalis pe·nis (pee'nis) [BNA]. VENA DORSALIS PENIS PROFUNDA.

vena dorsalis penis pro·fun·da (pro·fun'duh) [NA]. The deep dorsal vein of the penis.

venae. Plural and genitive singular of *vena.*

venae ano·ny·mae dex·tra et si·nis·tra (a·non'i·mee decks'truh et si·nis'truh) [BNA]. VENAE BRACHIOCEPHALICAE DEXTRA ET SINISTRA.

venae ar·ci·for·mes re·nis (ahr·si·for'meez ree'nis) [BNA]. Venae arcuatae renis (= ARCUATE VEINS).

venae ar·cu·a·tae re·nis (ahr·kew·ay'tee ree'nis) [NA]. ARCUATE VEINS.

venae ar·ti·cu·la·res man·di·bu·lae (ahr·tick·yoo·lair'eez man·dib'yoo·lee) [BNA]. VENAE ARTICULARES TEMPOROMANDIBULARES.

venae articulares tem·po·ro·man·di·bu·la·res (tem''po·ro·man·dib·yoo·lair'eez) [NA]. The veins related to the temporomandibular joint.

venae au·di·ti·vae in·ter·nae (aw·di·tye'vee in·tur'nee) [BNA]. VENAE LABYRINTHI.

venae au·ri·cu·la·res an·te·ri·o·res (aw·rick·yoo·lair'eez an·teer·ee·o'reez) [NA]. The anterior auricular veins.

venae ba·si·ver·te·bra·les (bay''si·vur·te·bray'leez) [NA]. The basivertebral veins. See Table of Veins in the Appendix.

venae bra·chi·a·les (bray·kee·ay'leez) [NA]. The veins accompanying the brachial artery.

venae bra·chio·ce·pha·li·cae dex·tra et si·nis·tra (bray·kee·o·se·fal'i·see decks'truh et si·nis'truh) [NA]. The brachiocephalic veins. See Table of Veins in the Appendix.

venae bron·chi·a·les (bronk·ee·ay'leez) [NA]. The vessels which drain blood from the larger branches of the principal bronchi.

venae bronchiales pos·te·ri·o·res (pos·teer·ee·o'reez) [BNA]. VENAE BRONCHIALES.

venae ca·ver·no·sae pe·nis (kav·ur·no'see pee'nis) [NA]. The veins draining the corpora cavernosa of the penis.

venae cen·tra·les he·pa·tis (sen·tray'leez hep'uh·tis) [NA]. CENTRAL VEINS OF THE LIVER.

venae ce·re·bel·li in·fe·ri·o·res (serr·e·bel'eye in·feer·ee·o'reez) [NA]. The veins draining the inferior portions of the cerebellum.

venae cerebelli su·pe·ri·o·res (sue·peer·ee·o'reez) [NA]. The veins draining the superior portion of the cerebellum.

venae ce·re·bri (serr'e·brye) [NA]. Any of the veins draining blood from the brain.

venae cerebri in·fe·ri·o·res (in·feer·ee·o'reez) [NA]. The veins draining the inferior surface and base of the brain.

venae cerebri in·ter·nae (in·tur'nee) [NA]. The veins that drain blood from the basal ganglia and adjacent structures.

venae cerebri su·pe·ri·o·res (sue·peer·ee·o'reez) [NA]. The veins that drain the superficial surface of the brain.

venae cho·roi·de·ae ocu·li (ko·roy'dee·ee ock'yoo·lye) [NA alt.]. VENAE VORTICOSAE.

venae ci·li·a·res (sil·ee·air'eez) [NA]. The veins that drain blood from the ciliary body and adjacent structures.

venae ciliares an·te·ri·o·res (an·teer·ee·o'reez) [BNA]. The anterior ciliary veins. See *venae ciliares.*

venae ciliares pos·te·ri·o·res (pos·teer·ee·o'reez) [BNA]. The posterior ciliary veins. See *venae ciliares.*

venae cir·cum·flex·ae fe·mo·ris la·te·ra·les (sur·kum·fleck'see fem'o·ris lat·e·ray'leez) [NA]. The veins accompanying the lateral femoral circumflex artery.

venae circumflexae femoris me·di·a·les (mee·dee·ay'leez) [NA]. The veins accompanying the medial femoral circumflex artery.

venae co·li·cae dex·trae (kol'i·see decks'tree) [BNA]. VENA COLICA DEXTRA.

venae comitantes. Plural of *vena comitans.*

venae con·junc·ti·va·les (kon·junk·ti·vay'leez) [NA]. The veins of the conjunctiva.

venae conjunctivales an·te·ri·o·res (an·teer·ee·o'reez) [BNA]. VENAE CONJUNCTIVALES.

venae conjunctivales pos·te·ri·o·res (pos·teer·ee·o'reez) [BNA]. VENAE CONJUNCTIVALES.

venae cor·dis (kor'dis) [NA]. The veins of the heart.

venae cordis an·te·ri·o·res (an·teer·ee·o'reez) [NA]. The anterior cardiac veins. See Table of Veins in the Appendix.

venae cordis mi·ni·mae (min'i·mee) [NA]. The smallest of the cardiac veins, opening into the cavities of the heart.

venae cos·to·ax·il·la·res (kos''to·ack·si·lair'eez) [BNA]. The veins draining the costal wall of the axilla.

venae di·gi·ta·les com·mu·nes pe·dis (dij·i·tay'leez kom·yoo'neez ped'is) [BNA]. VENAE DIGITALES DORSALES PEDIS.

venae digitales dor·sa·les pe·dis (dor·say'leez ped'is) [NA]. The superficial veins of the dorsal surfaces of the toes.

venae digitales pal·ma·res (pal·mair'eez) [NA]. The veins of the palmar aspect of the fingers.

venae digitales pe·dis dor·sa·les (ped'is dor·say'leez) [BNA]. VENAE DIGITALES DORSALES PEDIS.

venae digitales plan·ta·res (plan·tair'eez) [NA]. The veins of the plantar surface of the toes.

venae digitales vo·la·res com·mu·nes (vo·lair'eez kom·yoo'neez) [BNA]. The common palmar digital veins.

venae digitales volares pro·pri·ae (pro'pree·ee) [BNA]. The proper palmar digital veins.

venae di·plo·i·cae (di·plo'i·see) [NA]. DIPLOIC VEINS.

venae dor·sa·les cli·to·ri·dis su·per·fi·ci·a·les (dor·say'leez kli·tor'i·dis sue·pur·fish·ee·ay'leez) [NA]. The superficial dorsal veins of the clitoris.

venae dorsales lin·guae (ling'gwee) [NA]. The veins of the dorsal part of the tongue.

venae dorsales pe·nis sub·cu·ta·ne·ae (pee'nis sub·kew·tay'nee·ee) [BNA]. VENAE DORSALES PENIS SUPERFICIALES.

venae dorsales penis su·per·fi·ci·a·les (sue·pur·fish·ee·ay'leez) [NA]. The superficial dorsal veins of the penis.

venae du·o·de·na·les (dew·o·de·nay'leez) [BNA]. The veins draining blood from the duodenum.

venae em·is·sa·ri·ae (em·i·sair'ee·ee) [NA]. EMISSARY VEINS.

venae epi·gas·tri·cae su·pe·ri·o·res (ep·i·gas'tri·see sue·peer·ee·o'reez) [NA]. The veins accompanying the superior epigastric artery.

venae epi·scle·ra·les (ep·i·skle·ray'leez) [NA]. The veins lying superficial to the sclera.

venae eso·pha·ge·ae (ee·so·faj'ee·ee) [NA]. The vessels which drain blood from the esophagus.

venae eth·moi·da·les (eth·moy·day'leez) [NA]. The veins accompanying the anterior and posterior ethmoidal arteries.

venae fi·bu·la·res (fib·yoo·lair'eez) [NA alt.]. VENAE PERONEAE.

venae fron·ta·les (fron·tay'leez) [BNA]. VENAE SUPRATROCHLEARES.

venae gas·tri·cae bre·ves (gas'tri·see brev'eez) [NA]. The veins accompanying the short gastric arteries.

venae ge·nus (jen'us) [NA]. The veins accompanying the genicular arteries.

venae glu·tae·ae in·fe·ri·o·res (gloo'tee·ee in·feer·ee·o'reez, gloo·tee'ee) [BNA]. VENAE GLUTEAE INFERIORES.

venae glutaeae su·pe·ri·o·res (sue·peer·ee·o'reez) [BNA]. VENAE GLUTEAE SUPERIORES.

venae glu·te·ae in·fe·ri·o·res (gloo'tee·ee in·feer·ee·o'reez, gloo·tee'ee) [NA]. The veins accompanying the inferior gluteal artery.

venae gluteae su·pe·ri·o·res (sue·peer·ee·o'reez) [NA]. The veins accompanying the superior gluteal artery.

venae hae·mor·rhoi·da·les in·fe·ri·o·res (hem·o·roy·day'leez in·feer·ee·o'reez) [BNA]. VENAE RECTALES INFERIORES.

venae he·pa·ti·cae (he·pat'i·see) [NA]. HEPATIC VEINS.

venae hepaticae dex·trae (decks'tree) [NA]. The right hepatic veins draining into the inferior vena cava.

venae hepaticae me·di·ae (mee'dee·ee) [NA]. The middle hepatic veins draining into the inferior vena cava.

venae hepaticae si·nis·trae (si·nis'tree) [NA]. The left hepatic veins draining into the inferior vena cava.

venae in·ter·ca·pi·ta·les (in·tur·kap·i·tay'leez) [NA]. The veins in the clefts between the fingers.

venae in·ter·ca·pi·tu·la·res ma·nus (in·tur·ka·pit·yoo·lair'eez man'us) [BNA]. VENAE INTERCAPITALES.

venae intercapitulares pe·dis (ped'is) [BNA]. The veins in the clefts between the toes.

venae in·ter·cos·ta·les (in·tur·kos·tay'leez) [BNA]. See *venae intercostales anteriores, venae intercostales posteriores.*

venae intercostales an·te·ri·o·res (an·teer·ee·o'reez) [NA]. The veins accompanying the anterior intercostal arteries.

venae intercostales pos·te·ri·o·res [IV-XI] (pos·teer·ee·o'reez) [NA]. The veins accompanying the posterior intercostal arteries.

venae in·ter·lo·ba·res re·nis (in·tur·lo·bair'eez ree'nis) [NA]. INTERLOBAR VEINS.

venae in·ter·lo·bu·la·res he·pa·tis (in·tur·lob·yoo·lair'eez hep'uh·tis) [NA]. The interlobular veins of the liver. See *interlobular veins.*

venae interlobulares re·nis (ree'nis) [NA]. The interlobular veins of the kidney. See *interlobular veins.*

venae in·ter·ver·te·bra·les (in·tur·vur·te·bray'leez) [BNA]. VENA INTERVERTEBRALIS.

venae in·tes·ti·na·les (in·tes·ti·nay'leez) [BNA]. VENAE JEJUNALES ET ILEI.

venae je·ju·na·les et ilei (je·joo·nay'leez et il'ee·eye) [NA]. The veins accompanying the jejunal and ileal branches of the superior mesenteric artery.

venae la·bi·a·les an·te·ri·o·res (lay·bee·ay'leez an·teer·ee·o'reez) [NA]. The veins draining the anterior portions of the labia majora and minora.

venae labiales in·fe·ri·o·res (in·feer·ee·o'reez) [NA]. The veins of the lower lip.

venae labiales pos·te·ri·o·res (pos·teer·ee·o'reez) [NA]. The veins draining the posterior portions of the labia majora and minora.

venae la·by·rin·thi (lab·i·rin'thigh) [NA]. The small veins draining the inner ear.

venae lum·ba·les (lum·bay'leez) [BNA]. See *venae lumbales [I et II], venae lumbales [III et IV].*

venae lumbales [I et II] [NA]. The veins accompanying the first and second lumbar arteries.

venae lumbales [III et IV] [NA]. The veins accompanying the third and fourth lumbar arteries.

venae mas·se·te·ri·cae (mas·e·terr'i·see) [BNA]. The veins draining the region of the masseter muscle.

venae max·il·la·res (mack·si·lair'eez) [NA]. The veins draining the structures adjacent to the maxilla.

venae me·di·as·ti·na·les (mee·dee·as·ti·nay'leez) [NA]. The small vessels which drain blood from the anterior mediastinum.

venae mediastinales an·te·ri·o·res (an·teer·ee·o'reez) [BNA]. VENAE MEDIASTINALES.

venae me·nin·ge·ae (me·nin'jee·ee) [NA]. The veins draining blood from the dura mater.

venae meningeae me·di·ae (mee'dee·ee) [NA]. The veins accompanying the middle meningeal artery.

venae me·ta·car·pe·ae dor·sa·les (met·uh·kahr'pee·ee dor·say'leez) [NA]. The veins of the dorsum of the hand.

venae metacarpeae pal·ma·res (pal·mair'eez) [NA]. The veins of the palm of the hand.

venae metacarpeae vo·la·res (vo·lair'eez) [BNA]. VENAE METACARPEAE PALMARES.

venae me·ta·tar·se·ae dor·sa·les pe·dis (met·uh·tahr'see·ee dor·say'leez ped'is) [NA]. The veins of the dorsum of the foot.

venae metatarseae plan·ta·res (plan·tair'eez) [NA]. The veins of the sole of the foot.

vena emis·sa·ria (em''i·sair'ee·uh) [NA]. EMISSARY VEIN.

vena emissaria con·dy·la·ris (kon·di·lair'is) [NA]. CONDYLOID EMISSARY VEIN.

vena emissaria mas·toi·dea (mas·toy'dee·uh) [NA]. MASTOID EMISSARY VEIN.

vena emissaria oc·ci·pi·ta·lis (ock·sip·i·tay'lis) [NA]. OCCIPITAL EMISSARY VEIN.

vena emissaria pa·ri·e·ta·lis (pa·rye·e·tay'lis) [NA]. PARIETAL EMISSARY VEIN.

venae mus·cu·la·res (mus·kew·lair'eez) [BNA]. The veins draining blood from the extrinsic muscles of the eyeball.

venae mus·cu·lo·phre·ni·cae (mus·kew·lo·fren'i·see) [NA]. The veins accompanying the musculophrenic artery.

venae na·sa·les ex·ter·nae (nay·say'leez ecks·tur'nee) [NA]. The small veins draining the outer surface of the nose.

venae ob·tu·ra·to·ri·ae (ob·tew·ruh·to'ree·ee) [NA]. The veins accompanying the obturator artery.

venae oe·so·pha·ge·ae (ee·so·faj'ee·ee) [BNA]. VENAE ESOPHAGEAE.

venae pal·pe·bra·les (pal·pe·bray'leez) [NA]. The veins of the eyelids.

venae palpebrales in·fe·ri·o·res (in·feer·ee·o'reez) [NA]. The veins of the lower eyelids.

venae palpebrales su·pe·ri·o·res (sue·peer·ee·o'reez) [NA]. The veins of the upper eyelids.

venae pan·cre·a·ti·cae (pan·kree·at'i·see) [NA]. The vessels which drain blood from the pancreas into the splenic and the superior mesenteric veins.

venae pan·cre·a·ti·co·du·o·de·na·les (pan·kre·at''i·ko·dew·o·de·nay'leez) [NA]. The veins that drain blood from the adjacent areas of the duodenum and pancreas.

venae pa·ra·um·bi·li·ca·les (păr·uh·um·bil·i·kay'leez) [NA]. PARAUMBILICAL VEINS.

venae pa·ro·ti·de·ae (pa·rot·i·dee'ee, păr·o·tid'ee·ee) [NA]. The veins that drain blood from the parotid region.

venae parotideae an·te·ri·o·res (an·teer·ee·o'reez) [BNA]. RAMI PAROTIDEI VENAE FACIALIS.

venae parotideae pos·te·ri·o·res (pos·teer·ee·o'reez) [BNA]. VENAE PAROTIDEAE.

venae par·um·bi·li·ca·les [Sap·peyi] (păr·um·bil·i·kay'leez sa·pay'eye) [BNA]. Venae paraumbilicales (= PARAUMBILICAL VEINS).

venae pec·to·ra·les (peck·to·ray'leez) [NA]. The veins that drain blood from the pectoral area.

venae per·fo·ran·tes (pur·fo·ran'teez) [NA]. The veins that accompany the perforating branches of the femoral artery.

venae pe·ri·car·di·a·cae (perr·i·kahr·dye'uh·see) [NA]. The veins that drain blood from the parietal pericardium.

venae pe·ri·car·di·a·co·phre·ni·cae (perr·i·kahr·dye''uh·ko·fren'i·see) [NA]. The veins accompanying the pericardiacophrenic artery.

venae pe·ro·nae·ae (perr·o·nee'ee) [BNA]. VENAE PERONEAE.

venae pe·ro·ne·ae (perr·o·nee'ee) [NA]. The veins accompanying the peroneal artery. NA alt. *venae fibulares.*

venae pha·ryn·ge·ae (fa·rin'jee·ee) [NA]. The veins draining blood from the pharynx.

venae phre·ni·cae in·fe·ri·o·res (fren'i·see in·feer·ee·o'reez) [NA]. The veins accompanying the inferior phrenic artery.

venae phrenicae su·pe·ri·o·res (sue·peer·ee·o'reez) [NA]. The veins accompanying the superior phrenic artery.

vena epi·gas·tri·ca inferior (ep·i·gas'tri·kuh) [NA]. The vein accompanying the inferior epigastric artery.

vena epigastrica su·per·fi·ci·a·lis (sue·pur·fish·ee·ay'lis) [NA]. The vein accompanying the superficial epigastric artery.

vena epigastrica superior [BNA]. Singular of *venae epigastricae superiores.*

venae po·pli·te·ae (pop·lit'ee·ee) [BNA]. Plural of *vena poplitea.*

venae pro·fun·dae cli·to·ri·dis (pro·fun'dee kli·tor'i·dis) [NA]. The deep veins of the clitoris.

venae profundae fe·mo·ris (fem'o·ris) [NA]. The veins accompanying the deep femoral artery.

venae profundae pe·nis (pee'nis) [NA]. The deep veins of the penis.

venae pu·den·dae ex·ter·nae (pew·den'dee ecks·tur'nee) [NA]. The veins accompanying the external pudendal artery.

venae pul·mo·na·les (pul·mo·nay'leez) [NA]. The pulmonary veins.

venae pulmonales dex·trae (decks'tree) [NA]. The veins bringing back blood from the right lung to the left atrium.

venae pulmonales si·nis·trae (si·nis'tree) [NA]. The veins bringing back blood from the left lung to the left atrium.

venae ra·di·a·les (ray·dee·ay'leez) [NA]. The veins accompanying the radial artery.

venae rec·ta·les in·fe·ri·o·res (reck·tay'leez in·feer·ee·o'reez) [NA]. The inferior rectal veins accompanying the inferior rectal artery.

venae rectales me·di·ae (mee'dee·ee) [NA]. The veins draining the middle portion of the rectum.

venae re·na·les (re·nay'leez) [NA]. The veins accompanying the renal artery.

venae re·nis (ree'nis) [NA]. The veins within the kidney itself.

venae sa·cra·les la·te·ra·les (sa·kray'leez lat·e·ray'leez) [NA]. The veins accompanying the lateral sacral artery.

venae scro·ta·les an·te·ri·o·res (skro·tay'leez an·teer·ee·o'reez) [NA]. The veins draining the anterior portion of the scrotum.

venae scrotales pos·te·ri·o·res (pos·teer·ee·o'reez) [NA]. The veins draining the posterior portion of the scrotum.

venae sig·moi·de·ae (sig·moy'dee·ee) [NA]. The veins accompanying the sigmoid branches of the inferior mesenteric artery.

venae spi·na·les (spye·nay'leez) [NA]. The veins draining blood from the spinal cord.

venae spinales ex·ter·nae an·te·ri·o·res (ecks·tur'nee an·teer·ee·o'reez) [BNA]. The veins draining blood from the anterior part of the pia mater of the spinal cord.

venae spinales externae pos·te·ri·o·res (pos·teer·ee·o'reez) [BNA]. The veins draining blood from the posterior part of the pia mater of the spinal cord.

venae spinales in·ter·nae (in·tur'nee) [BNA]. The veins draining blood from the substance of the spinal cord.

venae stel·la·tae (stel·ay'tee) [BNA]. STELLATE VEINS.

venae sub·cu·ta·ne·ae ab·do·mi·nis (sub·kew·tay'nee·ee ab·dom'i·nis) [NA]. The veins of the subcutaneous tissues of the abdomen.

venae su·pra·re·na·les (sue·pruh·re·nay'leez) [BNA]. See *vena suprarenalis dextra, vena suprarenalis sinistra.*

venae su·pra·troch·le·a·res (sue·pruh·trock·le·ay'reez) [NA]. The veins of the forehead.

venae tem·po·ra·les pro·fun·dae (tem·po·ray'leez pro·fun'dee) [NA]. The veins that drain blood from the region of the temporal muscle.

venae temporales su·per·fi·ci·a·les (sue·pur·fish·ee·ay'leez) [NA]. The veins that drain blood from the superficial temporal region.

venae The·be·sii (the·bee'zee·eye). VENAE CORDIS MINIMAE.

vena eth·moi·da·lis (eth·moy·day'lis). Singular of *venae ethmoidales.*

vena ethmoidalis anterior [BNA]. The anterior ethmoidal vein.

vena ethmoidalis posterior [BNA]. The posterior ethmoidal vein.

venae tho·ra·ci·cae in·ter·nae (tho·ray'si·see in·tur'nee) [NA]. The veins that accompany the internal thoracic artery.

venae tho·ra·co·epi·gas·tri·cae (tho''ruh·ko·ep·i·gas'tri·see) [NA]. The superficial veins of the lateral wall of thorax and abdomen.

venae thy·mi·cae (thigh'mi·see) [NA]. The veins that drain blood from the thymus.

venae thy·re·oi·de·ae in·fe·ri·o·res (thigh·ree·oy'dee·ee in·feer·ee·o'reez) [BNA]. The vena thyroidea inferior and the venae thyroideae mediae.

venae thyreoideae su·pe·ri·o·res (sue·peer·ee·o'reez) [BNA]. The veins accompanying the superior thyroid artery.

venae thy·roi·de·ae me·di·ae (thigh·roy'dee·ee mee'dee·ee) [NA]. The veins that drain blood from the middle portion of each thyroid lobe.

venae ti·bi·a·les an·te·ri·o·res (tib·ee·ay'leez an·teer·ee·o'reez) [NA]. The veins accompanying the anterior tibial artery.

venae tibiales pos·te·ri·o·res (pos·teer·ee·o'reez) [NA]. The veins accompanying the posterior tibial artery.

venae tra·che·a·les (tray·kee·ay'leez) [NA]. The veins that drain blood from the trachea.

venae trans·ver·sae col·li (trans·vur'see kol'eye) [NA]. The veins accompanying the transverse artery of the neck.

venae tym·pa·ni·cae (tim·pan'i·see) [NA]. The veins that drain blood from the middle ear.

venae ul·na·res (ul·nair'reez) [NA]. The veins that accompany the ulnar artery.

venae ute·ri·nae (yoo·te·rye'nee) [NA]. The veins that accompany the uterine artery.

venae ve·si·ca·les (ves·i·kay'leez) [NA]. The veins that drain blood from the urinary bladder.

venae ves·ti·bu·la·res (ves·tib·yoo·lair'eez) [NA]. The veins that drain blood from the vestibule of the inner ear.

venae vor·ti·co·sae (vor·ti·ko'see) [NA]. The stellate veins of the choroid coat of the eyeball. NA alt. *venae choroideae oculi.*

vena fa·ci·a·lis (fay·shee·ay'lis) [NA]. The facial vein. See Table of Veins in the Appendix.

vena facialis anterior [BNA]. The anterior facial vein. See *facial* in the Table of Veins in the Appendix.

vena facialis com·mu·nis (kom·yoo'nis) [BNA]. The common facial vein. See *facial* in the Table of Veins in the Appendix.

vena facialis posterior [BNA]. The posterior facial vein. See *retromandibular* in the Table of Veins in the Appendix.

vena fa·ci·ei pro·fun·da (fay·shee·ee'eye pro·fun'duh) [NA]. The vein draining blood from the deep structures of the face.

vena fe·mo·ra·lis (fem·o·ray'lis) [NA]. FEMORAL VEIN.

vena fe·mo·ro·po·pli·tea (fem·o·ro·pop·lit'ee·uh) [BNA]. A superficial vein of the lower posterior portion of the superficial thigh.

vena Ga·le·ni (ga·lee'nigh). The great cerebral vein. See Table of Veins in the Appendix.

vena gas·tri·ca dex·tra (gas'tri·kuh decks'truh) [NA]. The vein accompanying the right gastric artery.

vena gastrica si·nis·tra (si·nis'truh) [NA]. The vein accompanying the left gastric artery.

vena gas·tro·epi·plo·i·ca dex·tra (gas''tro·ep·i·plo'i·kuh decks'truh) [NA]. The vein accompanying the right gastroepiploic artery.

vena gastroepiploica si·nis·tra (si·nis'truh) [NA]. The vein accompanying the left gastroepiploic artery.

vena hae·mor·rhoi·da·lis me·dia (hem·o·roy·day'lis mee'dee·uh) [BNA]. VENA RECTALIS MEDIA.

vena haemorrhoidalis superior [BNA]. VENA RECTALIS SUPERIOR.

vena he·mi·azy·gos (hem·ee·az'i·gos) [NA]. HEMIAZYGOS VEIN.

vena hemiazygos ac·ces·so·ria (ack·se·so'ree·uh) [NA]. The accessory hemiazygos vein. See Table of Veins in the Appendix.

vena hy·po·gas·tri·ca (high·po·gas'tri·kuh) [BNA]. VENA ILIACA INTERNA.

vena ileo·co·li·ca (il·ee·o·kol'i·kuh) [NA]. The vein accompanying the iliocecal artery.

vena ili·a·ca com·mu·nis (i·lye'uh·kuh kom·yoo'nis) [NA]. The vein accompanying the common iliac artery.

vena iliaca ex·ter·na (ecks·tur'nuh) [NA]. The vein accompanying the external iliac artery.

vena iliaca in·ter·na (in·tur'nuh) [NA]. The vein accompanying the internal iliac artery.

vena ilio·lum·ba·lis (il''ee·o·lum·bay'lis) [NA]. The vein accompanying the iliolumbar artery.

vena in·ter·cos·ta·lis su·pe·ri·or dex·tra (in·tur·kos·tay'lis sue·peer'ee·or decks'truh) [NA]. A vein draining the upper intercostal spaces on the right into the azygos vein.

vena intercostalis superior si·nis·tra (si·nis'truh) [NA]. The vein draining the upper intercostal spaces on the left into the brachiocephalic vein.

vena intercostalis su·pre·ma (sue·pree'muh) [NA]. The vein draining the posterior portion of the first intercostal space.

vena in·ter·ver·te·bra·lis (in·tur·vur·te·bray'lis) [NA]. Any one of the veins traversing an intervertebral canal.

vena ju·gu·la·ris anterior (jug·yoo·lair'is) [NA]. The anterior jugular vein. See Table of Veins in the Appendix.

vena jugularis ex·ter·na (ecks·tur'nuh) [NA]. The external jugular vein. See Table of Veins in the Appendix.

vena jugularis in·ter·na (in·tur'nuh) [NA]. The internal jugular vein. See Table of Veins in the Appendix.

vena la·bi·a·lis inferior (lay·bee·ay'lis) [BNA]. The vein of the lower lip.

vena labialis superior [NA]. The vein of the upper lip.

vena la·cri·ma·lis (lack·ri·may'lis) [NA]. The vein draining blood from the region of the lacrimal gland.

vena la·ryn·gea inferior (la·rin'jee·uh) [NA]. The vein draining blood from the lower part of the larynx.

vena laryngea superior [NA]. The vein draining blood from the upper part of the larynx.

vena li·e·na·lis (lye·e·nay'lis) [NA]. The vein accompanying the splenic artery.

vena lin·gua·lis (ling·gway'lis) [NA]. The vein accompanying the lingual artery.

vena lum·ba·lis ascen·dens (lum·bay'lis a·sen'denz) [NA]. ASCENDING LUMBAR VEIN.

vena mam·ma·ria in·ter·na (ma·mair'ee·uh in·tur'nuh) [BNA]. VENA THORACICA INTERNA.

vena me·di·a·na an·te·bra·chii (mee·dee·ay'nuh an·te·bray'kee·eye) [NA]. A superficial vein of the middle of the anterior surface of the forearm.

vena mediana an·ti·bra·chii (an·ti·bray'kee·eye) [BNA]. VENA MEDIANA ANTEBRACHII.

vena mediana ba·si·li·ca (ba·sil'i·kuh) [NA]. A vein occasionally present as a branch of the median antebrachial vein to the basilic vein.

vena mediana ce·pha·li·ca (se·fal'i·kuh) [NA]. A vein occasionally present as a branch of the median antebrachial vein to the cephalic vein.

vena mediana col·li (kol'eye) [BNA]. A vein occasionally present in the anterior midline of the neck formed by a union of the anterior jugular veins.

vena mediana cu·bi·ti (kew'bi·tye) [NA]. The median cubital vein. See Table of Veins in the Appendix.

vena me·sen·te·ri·ca inferior (mes·en·terr'i·kuh) [NA]. The vein draining blood from the area supplied by the inferior mesenteric artery.

vena mesenterica superior [NA]. The vein accompanying the superior mesenteric artery.

vena na·so·fron·ta·lis (nay·zo·fron·tay'lis) [NA]. A vein draining blood from the forehead into the superior ophthalmic veins.

vena ob·li·qua atrii si·nis·tri (ob·lye'kwuh ay'tree·eye si·nis' trye) [NA]. OBLIQUE VEIN OF THE LEFT ATRIUM.

vena obliqua atrii sinistri [Mar·shal·li] (mahr·shal'eye) [BNA]. Vena obliqua atrii sinistri (= OBLIQUE VEIN OF THE LEFT ATRIUM).

vena oc·ci·pi·ta·lis (ock·sip·i·tay'lis) [NA]. The vein accompanying the occipital artery.

vena oph·thal·mi·ca inferior (off·thal'mi·kuh) [NA]. The inferior ophthalmic vein. See Table of Veins in the Appendix.

vena ophthalmica superior [NA]. The superior ophthalmic vein. See Table of Veins in the Appendix.

vena oph·thal·mo·me·nin·gea (off·thal''mo·me·nin'jee·uh) [BNA]. A small meningeal vein draining into the superior ophthalmic vein or into the superior petrosal sinus.

vena ova·ri·ca (o·vair'i·kuh) [BNA]. See *vena ovarica dextra, vena ovarica sinistra.*

vena ovarica dex·tra (decks'truh) [NA]. The vein draining blood from the right ovary into the inferior vena cava.

vena ovarica si·nis·tra (si·nis'truh) [NA]. The vein draining blood from the left ovary into the left renal vein.

vena pa·la·ti·na (pal·uh·tye'nuh) [BNA]. VENA PALATINA EXTERNA.

vena palatina ex·ter·na (ecks·tur'nuh) [NA]. A vein draining blood from the tonsillar region into the facial vein.

vena phre·ni·ca inferior (fren'i·kuh) [BNA]. Any of the veins that accompany the inferior or superior phrenic arteries. See also *venae phrenicae inferiores, venae phrenicae superiores.*

vena po·pli·tea (pop·lit'ee·uh) [NA]. The vein accompanying the popliteal artery.

vena por·tae (por'tee) [NA]. The portal vein. See Table of Veins in the Appendix.

vena posterior ven·tri·cu·li si·nis·tri (ven·trick'yoo·lye si·nis' trye) [NA]. The posterior vein of the left ventricle. See Table of Veins in the Appendix.

vena pre·py·lo·ri·ca (pree·pye·lo'ri·kuh) [NA]. The prepyloric vein. See Table of Veins in the Appendix.

vena pro·fun·da fe·mo·ris (pro·fun'duh fem'o·ris) [NA]. The vein accompanying the deep femoral artery.

vena profunda lin·guae (ling'gwee) [NA]. The deep lingual vein.

vena pu·den·da in·ter·na (pew·den'duh in·tur'nuh) [NA]. The vein accompanying the internal pudendal artery.

vena pul·mo·na·lis in·fe·ri·or dex·tra (pul·mo·nay'lis in·feer' ee·or decks'truh) [NA]. The inferior right pulmonary vein. See Table of Veins in the Appendix.

vena pulmonalis inferior si·nis·tra (si·nis'truh) [NA]. The inferior left pulmonary vein. See Table of Veins in the Appendix.

vena pulmonalis superior dex·tra (decks'truh) [NA]. The superior right pulmonary vein. See Table of Veins in the Appendix.

vena pulmonalis superior si·nis·tra (si·nis'truh) [NA]. The superior left pulmonary vein. See Table of Veins in the Appendix.

vena rec·ta·lis me·dia (reck·tay'lis mee'dee·uh). Singular of *venae rectales mediae.*

vena rectalis superior [NA]. The vein accompanying the superior rectal artery.

vena re·tro·man·di·bu·la·ris (ret''ro·man·dib·yoo·lair'is) [NA]. The retromandibular vein. See Table of Veins in the Appendix.

vena sa·cra·lis me·dia (sa·kray'lis mee'dee·uh) [BNA]. VENA SACRALIS MEDIANA.

vena sacralis me·di·a·na (mee·dee·ay'nuh) [NA]. The vein accompanying the middle sacral artery.

vena sa·phe·na ac·ces·so·ria (sa·fee'nuh ack·se·so'ree·uh) [NA]. An occasional vein in the thigh medial to the great saphenous vein.

vena saphena mag·na (mag'nuh) [NA]. The great saphenous vein. See Table of Veins in the Appendix.

vena saphena par·va (pahr'vuh) [NA]. The small saphenous vein. See Table of Veins in the Appendix.

vena sca·pu·la·ris dor·sa·lis (skap·yoo·lair'is dor·say'lis) [NA]. The vein draining the dorsal scapular region.

vena sep·ti pel·lu·ci·di (sep'tye pe·lew'si·dye) [NA]. A vein draining the septum pellucidum.

vena sper·ma·ti·ca (spur·mat'i·kuh) [BNA]. See *vena testicularis dextra, vena testicularis sinistra.*

vena spi·ra·lis mo·di·o·li (spye·ray'lis mo·dye'o·lye) [NA]. A small vein in the spiral modiolus.

vena ster·no·clei·do·mas·toi·dea (stur''no·klye''do·mas·toy' dee·uh) [NA]. The vein draining blood from the region of the sternocleidomastoid muscle.

vena stri·a·ta (strye·ay'tuh) [NA]. The vein draining blood from the region of the corpus striatum.

vena sty·lo·mas·toi·dea (stye·lo·mas·toy'dee·uh) [NA]. The vein accompanying the stylomastoid artery.

vena sub·cla·via (sub·klay'vee·uh) [NA]. The vein accompanying the subclavian artery.

vena sub·cos·ta·lis (sub·kos·tay'lis) [NA]. The vein accompanying the subcostal artery.

vena sub·lin·gua·lis (sub·ling·gway'lis) [NA]. The vein accompanying the sublingual artery.

vena sub·men·ta·lis (sub·men·tay'lis) [NA]. The vein accompanying the submental artery.

vena su·pra·or·bi·ta·lis (sue·pruh·or·bi·tay'lis) [NA]. The vein of the medial portion of the forehead draining into the angular vein.

vena su·pra·re·na·lis dex·tra (sue·pruh·re·nay'lis decks'truh) [NA]. The vein draining blood from the right suprarenal vein into the inferior vena cava.

vena suprarenalis si·nis·tra (si·nis'truh) [NA]. The vein draining blood from the left suprarenal gland into the left renal vein.

vena su·pra·sca·pu·la·ris (sue·pruh·skap·yoo·lair'is) [NA]. The vein accompanying the suprascapular artery.

vena tem·po·ra·lis me·dia (tem·po·ray'lis mee'dee·uh) [NA]. A vein draining blood from the temporal muscle into the superficial temporal vein.

vena ter·mi·na·lis (tur·mi·nay'lis) [BNA]. VENA THALAMOSTRIATA.

vena tes·ti·cu·la·ris (tes·tick·yoo·lair'is) [BNA]. See *vena testicularis dextra, vena testicularis sinistra.*

vena testicularis dex·tra (decks'truh) [NA]. The vein draining blood from the right testis into the inferior vena cava.

vena testicularis si·nis·tra (si·nis'truh) [NA]. The vein draining blood from the left testis into the left renal vein.

vena tha·la·mo·stri·a·ta (thal''uh·mo·strye·ay'tuh) [NA]. The vein draining blood from the region of the thalamus and corpus striatum.

vena tho·ra·ca·lis la·te·ra·lis (tho·ruh·kay'lis lat·e·ray'lis) [BNA]. VENA THORACICA LATERALIS.

vena tho·ra·ci·ca in·ter·na (tho·ray'si·kuh in·tur'nuh). Singular of *venae thoracicae internae.*

vena tho·ra·ci·ca la·te·ra·lis (tho·ray'si·kuh lat·e·ray'lis) [NA]. The vein accompanying the lateral thoracic artery.

vena tho·ra·co·acro·mi·a·lis (tho''ruh·ko·a·kro·mee·ay'lis) [NA]. The vein accompanying the thoracoacromial artery.

vena thy·re·oi·dea ima (thigh·ree·oy'dee·uh eye'muh) [BNA]. An occasional vein draining blood from the thyroid gland into the left brachiocephalic vein.

vena thyreoidea superior [BNA]. VENA THYROIDEA SUPERIOR.

vena thy·roi·dea inferior (thigh·roy'dee·uh) [NA]. The vein accompanying the inferior thyroid artery.

vena thyroidea superior [NA]. The vein accompanying the superior thyroid artery.

ve·na·tion (vee·nay'shun) *n.* 1. Distribution of venous circulation of a part or organ. 2. *In botany,* the pattern of the veins of leaves.

vena trans·ver·sa fa·ci·ei (trans·vur'suh fay·shee·ee'eye) [NA]. The transverse facial vein.

vena transversa sca·pu·lae (skap'yoo·lee) [BNA]. VENA SUPRASCAPULARIS.

vena um·bi·li·ca·lis (um·bil·i·kay'lis) [BNA]. Vena umbilicalis sinistra (= UMBILICAL VEIN).

vena umbilicalis si·nis·tra (si·nis'truh) [NA]. UMBILICAL VEIN.

vena ver·te·bra·lis (vur·te·bray'lis) [NA]. The vein accompanying the vertebral artery in the neck.

vena vertebralis ac·ces·so·ria (ack·se·so'ree·uh) [NA]. An accessory vertebral vein passing through the transverse foramen of the seventh cervical vertebra.

vena vertebralis anterior [NA]. An anterior tributary of the vertebral vein.

vene-. See *ven-.*

ve·nec·to·my (ve·neck'tuh·mee) *n.* [*ven-* + *-ectomy*]. Surgical excision of a vein or a portion of one.

ve·neer crown (ve·neer'). A full crown in which a window is prepared in the facial aspect to be filled with a tooth-colored material for esthetic reasons.

ve·nene (ve·neen') *n.* VENIN.

ven·e·nif·er·ous (ven"e·nif'ur·us) *adj.* [L. *venenifer,* from *venenum,* poison]. Conveying poison.

ven·e·no·sa (ven"e·no'suh) *n.pl.* [L. *venenosus,* full of poison]. The venomous snakes.

venepuncture. VENIPUNCTURE.

ve·ne·re·al (ve·neer'ee·ul) *adj.* [L. *venereus,* of Venus, goddess of love]. Pertaining to, or produced by, sexual intercourse.

venereal adenitis. LYMPHOGRANULOMA VENEREUM.

venereal collar. COLLAR OF VENUS.

venereal disease. A contagious disease generally acquired during sexual intercourse, including gonorrhea, syphilis, chancroid, granuloma inguinale, and lymphogranuloma venereum. Abbreviated, VD.

venereal lymphogranuloma. LYMPHOGRANULOMA VENEREUM.

venereal lymphogranulomatosis. LYMPHOGRANULOMA VENEREUM.

venereal sore. CHANCRE (1).

venereal spirochetosis. A venereal disease of rabbits caused by *Treponema cuniculi.* Syn. *pallidoidosis.*

venereal ulcer. CHANCROID.

venereal verruca. CONDYLOMA ACUMINATUM.

venereal wart. CONDYLOMA ACUMINATUM.

ve·ne·re·ol·o·gist (ve·neer"ee·ol'uh·jist) *n.* An expert in venereal diseases.

ve·ne·re·ol·o·gy (ve·neer"ee·ol'uh·jee) *n.* [*venere*al + *-logy*]. The study of venereal diseases.

ve·ne·reo·pho·bia (ve·neer"ee·o·fo'bee·uh) *n.* [*venere*al + *-phobia*]. Abnormal fear of getting a venereal disease.

ven·ery (ven'ur·ee) *n.* [ML. *veneria,* from *Venus,* goddess of love]. Indulgence in sexual activities.

vene·sec·tion, veni·sec·tion (ven"i·seck'shun, vee"ni·) *n.* [*vene-* + *section*]. PHLEBOTOMY.

vene·su·ture, veni·su·ture (ven"i·sue'chur) *n.* [*vene-* + *suture*]. The suturing of a vein.

Ven·e·zue·lan equine encephalitis. Equine encephalomyelitis due to Venezuelan virus.

Venezuelan virus. An immunologically distinct type of arbovirus originally recovered from the brains of Venezuelan horses affected with equine encephalomyelitis. Infection of man is generally less serious with this strain.

veni-. See *ven-.*

Ven·ice treacle. THERIACA.

ven·in (ven'in) *n.* A mixture of the venom of various poisonous snakes; once used in neurasthenia, hysteria, chorea.

veni·punc·ture (ven'i·punk"chur) *n.* [*veni-* + *puncture*]. The surgical puncture of a vein.

venisection. Venesection (= PHLEBOTOMY).

venisuture. VENESUTURE.

veno-. See *ven-.*

ve·no·atri·al (vee"no·ay'tree·ul) *adj.* Pertaining to a vein and an atrium; specifically, to the vena cava and the right atrium of the heart.

ve·no·au·ric·u·lar (vee"no·aw·rick'yoo·lur) *adj.* [*veno-* + *-auricular*]. VENOATRIAL.

ven·oc·clu·sive (veen"uh·klew'siv) *adj.* Pertaining to or characterized by vein blocking.

ve·noc·ly·sis (ve·nock'li·sis) *n.,* pl. **venocly·ses** (·seez) [*veno-* + Gk. *klysis,* injection]. Injection of a nutritive solution or of drugs into a vein.

ve·no·fi·bro·sis (vee"no·figh·bro'sis) *n.* [*veno-* + *fibrosis*]. An increase in fibrous connective tissue in a vein wall, usually at the expense of muscular and elastic elements.

ve·no·gram (vee'no·gram) *n.* [*veno-* + *-gram*]. A radiograph of veins following the injection of a contrast medium. Syn. *phlebogram.*

ve·nog·ra·phy (vee·nog'ruh·fee) *n.* [*veno-* + *-graphy*]. Radiographic examination of veins following injection of a contrast medium.

ven·om (ven'um) *n.* [OF. *venim,* from L. *venenum*]. Poison, especially a poison secreted by certain reptiles and arthropods.

venom leukocytolysis. Destruction of leukocytes by the action of venom.

ven·o·mo·sal·i·vary (ven"uh·mo·sal'i·verr·ee) *adj. In zoology,* designating the salivary glands of certain animals that secrete venom instead of saliva.

ve·no·mo·tor (vee"no·mo'tur) *adj.* [*veno-* + *motor*]. Causing veins to contract.

ven·om·ous (ven'uh·mus) *adj.* [*venom* + *-ous*]. POISONOUS.

ve·no·peri·to·ne·os·to·my (vee"no·perr"i·to·nee·os'tuh·mee) *n.* [*veno-* + *peritoneo-* + *-stomy*]. *Obsol.* Surgical implantation of a divided greater saphenous vein into the peritoneal cavity for drainage of ascites. Syn. *Ruotte's operation.*

ve·no·pres·sor (vee"no·pres'ur) *adj.* [*veno-* + *pressor*]. Tending to raise the blood pressure in the veins. See also *vasopressor.*

ve·no·scle·ro·sis (vee"no·skle·ro'sis) *n.* [*veno-* + *sclerosis*]. Induration of veins; PHLEBOSCLEROSIS.

ve·nos·i·ty (ve·nos'i·tee) *n.* 1. A condition in which arterial blood shows characteristics of venous blood. 2. An excess of blood in the venous system. 3. A large number of blood vessels in a part.

ve·nos·ta·sis (ve·nos'tuh·sis, vee"no·stay'sis) *n.* [*veno-* + *-stasis*]. Retardation or prevention of the return flow of the blood to the heart, as by compression of veins, obstruction, or varicosities.

ve·no·throm·bot·ic (vee"no·throm·bot'ick) *adj.* [*veno-* + *thrombotic*]. Having the property of producing venous thrombosis.

ve·not·o·my (ve·not'uh·mee) *n.* [*veno-* + *-tomy*]. PHLEBOTOMY; surgical incision of a vein.

ve·nous (vee'nus) *adj.* [*ven-* + *-ous*]. Pertaining to the veins.

venous artery. An artery carrying venous blood, as a pulmonary artery.

venous blood. The blood in the vascular system from the point of origin of the small venules in tissues to the capillary beds in the lungs where free carbon dioxide is released into the alveoli and oxygen taken up; includes the blood in the pulmonary arteries. Contr. *arterial blood.*

venous capillary. The terminal part of a capillary network, opening into a venule. Syn. *postcapillary.*

venous circle of the mammary gland. An anastomosis of veins around the nipple.

venous claudication. Lameness due to venous stasis. Syn. *angiosclerotic paroxysmal myasthenia.*

venous hemangioma. A vascular hamartoma whose component vessels have the characteristics of veins.

venous hum. A continuous blowing or singing murmur heard on auscultation in the neck veins, normally in children and also in states of high cardiac output. Syn. *humming-top murmur, bruit de diable.*

venous plexus. Any network of interconnecting veins.

venous pressure. The tension of the blood within the veins.

venous pulse. A pulse observed in a vein arising from phasic changes in venous pressure.

venous sinus of the sclera. A canal in the sclera close to the sclerocorneal junction running circularly around the periphery of the cornea. It gives rise to the anterior ciliary veins. Syn. *Schlemm's canal.* NA *sinus venosus sclerae.*

ve·no·ve·nos·to·my (vee″no·ve·nos'tuh·mee) *n.* [*veno-* + *veno-* + *-stomy*]. The anastomosing of two veins.

vent, *n. & v.* [alteration of *fent,* slit, opening, from MF. *fente,* from *fendre,* to split]. 1. Any aperture or outlet. 2. VENTILATE (3).

ven·ter (ven'tur) *n.* [L.]. 1. BELLY; ABDOMEN. 2. BELLY OF A MUSCLE. 3. The cavity of the abdomen.

venter anterior mus·cu·li di·gas·tri·ci (mus'kew·lye dye·gas' tri·sigh) [NA]. The anterior belly of the digastric muscle. See *digastric* in the Table of Muscles in the Appendix.

venter fron·ta·lis mus·cu·li oc·ci·pi·to·fron·ta·lis (fron·tay'lis mus'kew·lye ock·sip·i·to·fron·tay'lis) [NA]. The frontal part of the occipitofrontalis muscle.

venter inferior musculi omo·hy·oi·dei (o·mo·high·oy'dee·eye) [NA]. The inferior belly of the omohyoid muscle. See *omohyoid* in the Table of Muscles in the Appendix.

venter mus·cu·li (mus'kew·lye) [NA]. BELLY OF A MUSCLE.

venter oc·ci·pi·ta·lis mus·cu·li oc·ci·pi·to·fron·ta·lis (ock·sip·i·tay'lis mus'kew·lye ock·sip″i·to·fron·tay'lis) [NA]. The occipital part of the occipitofrontalis muscle. See *occipitofrontalis* in the Table of Muscles in the Appendix.

venter posterior musculi di·gas·tri·ci (dye·gas'tri·sigh) [NA]. The posterior belly of the digastric muscle. See *digastric* in the Table of Muscles in the Appendix.

venter superior musculi omo·hy·oi·dei (o·mo·high·oy'dee·eye) [NA]. The superior belly of the omohyoid muscle. See *omohyoid* in the Table of Muscles in the Appendix.

ven·ti·late, *v.* [L. *ventilare,* to wave in the air, from *ventus,* wind]. 1. To renew the air in a place. 2. To oxygenate the blood in the capillaries of the lungs. 3. To air or discuss (one's feelings and emotional problems).

ven·ti·la·tion, *n.* [L. *ventilatio,* from *ventilare,* to wave in the air]. 1. The act or process of supplying fresh air, i.e., air whose partial pressure of oxygen is higher and of carbon dioxide lower than in the air being replaced. 2. The act or process of purifying the air of a place. 3. *In psychiatry,* the ready verbal expression of an individual's emotional problems, whether in a psychotherapeutic setting or in a conversation with another person in whom the person confides.

ven·ti·lom·e·ter (ven″ti·lom'e·tur) *n.* [*ventil*ate + *-meter*]. An apparatus used to measure the volume of air breathed in and out per unit time under different environmental conditions; applied particularly to the measurement of tidal volume, vital capacity, inspiratory and expiratory reserve volume, minute volume, and maximum breathing capacity.

ven·ti·lom·e·try (ven″ti·lom'e·tree) *n.* PNEUMATOMETRY.

ven·trad (ven'trad) *adv.* [*ventr-* + *-ad*]. In a dorsal-to-ventral direction. Compare *anteriad.* Contr. *dorsad.*

ven·tral (ven'trul) *adj.* [*vent*er + *-al*]. Situated on or relatively near the "belly side" of the trunk or of the body as a whole; in human anatomy: ANTERIOR. Contr. *dorsal* (1).

ventral aorta. The arterial trunk or trunks between the heart and the first aortic arch in embryos or lower vertebrates.

ventral cornu. CORNU ANTERIUS MEDULLAE SPINALIS.

ventral corticospinal tract. ANTERIOR CORTICOSPINAL TRACT.

ventral hernia. A hernia of any part of the abdominal wall not involving the inguinal, femoral, or umbilical openings. Three varieties occur: median, lateral, and postincision. Syn. *abdominal hernia.*

ventral horn. CORNU ANTERIUS MEDULLAE SPINALIS.

ventral median fissure. ANTERIOR MEDIAN FISSURE.

ventral mesentery. *In embryology,* the peritoneal fold, extending from the ventral border of the cranial portion of the gut to the ventral body wall. See also *lesser omentum, gastrohepatic ligament, hepatoduodenal ligament, ventral mesogaster.*

ventral mesocardium. A ventral mesentery of the heart; not formed in human development.

ventral mesogaster. The ventral mesentery of the stomach.

ventral nucleus of the thalamus. A nucleus of the thalamus which may be subdivided into three separate nuclei: the ventral posterior nucleus, which relays specific sensory impulses to cortical regions, and the ventral anterior and ventral lateral nuclei, which relay impulses from the basal ganglia and cerebellum.

ventral pancreas. The embryonic pancreas arising as a diverticulum of the common bile duct; it forms a part of the adult organ.

ventral pancreatic duct. The duct of the ventral embryonic pancreas which arises as a diverticulum from the floor of the primitive duodenum. It usually persists as the proximal portion of the main pancreatic duct.

ventral root. A bundle of efferent nerve fibers emerging from the anterior part of the spinal cord and joining with the dorsal root to form a spinal nerve. NA *radix ventralis nervorum spinalium.*

ventral sacroiliac ligament. Any of numerous thin bands of fibers connecting the lateral part of the sacrum to the adjacent margin of the ilium on the ventral side of the sacroiliac articulation. NA (pl.) *ligamenta sacroiliaca ventralia.*

ventral spinocerebellar tract. ANTERIOR SPINOCEREBELLAR TRACT.

ventral spinothalamic tract. ANTERIOR SPINOTHALAMIC TRACT.

ventral supraoptic decussation or **commissure.** The more ventral fibers that cross dorsal to and slightly behind the optic chiasma. The connections of these fibers are not definitely known. Syn. *Gudden's commissure.* See also *commissurae supraopticae.*

ventral tegmental decussation. The decussation of the rubrospinal tracts in the midbrain. Syn. *tegmental decussation of Forel.*

ventral white commissure. WHITE COMMISSURE.

ventri-, ventro- [L. *venter, ventris,* belly]. A combining form meaning (a) *abdomen;* (b) *ventral.*

ven·tri·cle (ven'tri·kul) *n.* [L. *ventriculus,* dim. of *venter,* belly]. A small cavity or pouch.

ventricle of Arantius [G. C. *Arantius*]. ARANTIUS'S VENTRICLE.

ventricle of Morgagni [G. B. *Morgagni*]. LARYNGEAL VENTRICLE.

ventricle of the larynx. LARYNGEAL VENTRICLE.

ventricles of the brain. Cavities in the interior of the brain, comprising the two lateral ventricles and the third and fourth ventricles.

ven·tric·u·lar (ven·trick'yoo·lur) *adj.* Of or pertaining to a ventricle.

ventricular block. Block of one or both of the interventricular foramens, the cerebral aqueduct, or the lateral and medial apertures of the fourth ventricle; interfering with the flow of cerebrospinal fluid from the brain ventricles and causing obstructive hydrocephalus.

ventricular complex. The QRS complex (ventricular depolarization complex) and T wave (ventricular repolarization complex) of the electrocardiogram.

ventricular congenital laryngocele. An abnormally deep pocket between the true and false vocal folds.

ventricular depolarization complex. QRS COMPLEX OF THE ELECTROCARDIOGRAM.

ventricular escape. Temporary assumption of pacemaker function by the ventricular myocardium, due to absence or abnormal slowing of impulses from the sinoauricular and atrioventricular nodes.

ventricular extrasystole. PREMATURE VENTRICULAR CONTRACTION.

ventricular fibrillation. A cardiac arrhythmia characterized by rapid, irregular, uncoordinated ventricular excitation without effective ventricular contraction and cardiac output; direct-current defibrillation is the emergency treatment of choice.

ventricular filling sound. THIRD HEART SOUND.

ventricular fold. VESTIBULAR FOLD.

ventricular fusion beat. FUSION BEAT.

ventricular gallop. A low-pitched series of heart sounds heard with the stethoscope in early diastole at the end of rapid ventricular filling. Syn. *S_3 gallop, filling gallop, protodiastolic gallop.* See also *third heart sound.*

ventricular gradient. *In electrocardiography,* the vectorial sum of the mean QRS (Â QRS) and T (Â T) vectors; this relationship between the electrical sequence of depolarization and repolarization provides a means of differentiating primary from secondary T wave changes. Symbol, G, Ĝ, g, ĝ.

ventricular grooves. Two furrows, one on the anterior, one on the posterior surface of the heart; they indicate the interventricular septum.

ventricular ligament. VESTIBULAR LIGAMENT.

ventricular plexus. A nerve plexus found in the ependyma of the ventricles of the brain. It has been described in the cat and the monkey.

ventricular premature beat. PREMATURE VENTRICULAR CONTRACTION.

ventricular preponderance. Relative increase in the weight of one cardiac ventricle as compared to the other.

ventricular puncture. The introduction of a hollow needle into one of the ventricles of the brain, almost always one of the lateral ones, for diagnostic or therapeutic purposes.

ventricular repolarization complex. T WAVE OF THE ELECTROCARDIOGRAM.

ventricular rhythm. IDIOVENTRICULAR RHYTHM.

ventricular septal defect. A defect, usually congenital, of the septum between the ventricles of the heart. Syn. *maladie de Roger.*

ventricular septum. INTERVENTRICULAR SEPTUM.

ventricular strain. A nonspecific electrocardiographic term describing QRS and T changes presumed related to right and left ventricular hypertrophy, respectively; at present there is disagreement as to the electrocardiogram patterns and their significance.

ventricular tachycardia. A serious cardiac arrhythmia characterized by rapid regular, or only slightly irregular beats, originating in the ventricle at the rate of 150 to 200 per minute; the QRS complex of the electrocardiogram is widened and slurred and is completely unrelated to the normal atrial complex (P wave).

ventriculi. Plural and genitive singular of *ventriculus.*

ven·tric·u·li·tis (ven·trick″yoo·lye′tis) *n.* [*ventricul*us + *-itis*]. Inflammation of the ependymal lining of the ventricles of the brain.

ventriculo-. A combining form meaning *ventricle, ventricular.*

ven·tric·u·lo·atri·al (ven·trick″yoo·lo·ay′tree·ul) *adj.* [*ventriculo-* + *atrial*]. Concerning a cerebral ventricle and a cardiac atrium; usually refers to shunting of cerebrospinal fluid to the heart through a ventriculoatriostomy.

ventriculoatrial shunt. Surgical communication between a lateral cerebral ventricle to just above the right atrium by means of a plastic tube for the relief of hydrocephalus. See also *ventriculovenous shunt.*

ven·tric·u·lo·atri·os·to·my (ven·trick″yoo·lo·ay″tree·os′tuh·mee) *n.* [*ventriculo-* + *atrio-* + *-stomy*]. Surgical creation of a shunt from a cerebral ventricle to the right cardiac atrium, by means of a catheter containing a one-way valve; used to drain away excess cerebrospinal fluid in the treatment of hydrocephalus.

ven·tric·u·lo·cis·ter·nos·to·my (ven·trick″yoo·lo·sis″tur·nos′tuh·mee) *n.* [*ventriculo-* + *cistern* + *-stomy*]. Surgical establishment of communication between the ventricles of the brain and the subarachnoid cisterns; it may be performed by a third ventriculostomy or by the Torkildsen procedure in which communication is established between a lateral ventricle and the cisterna magna.

ven·tric·u·lo·cor·dec·to·my (ven·trick″yoo·lo·kor·deck′tuh·mee) *n.* [*ventriculo-* + *cord* + *-ectomy*]. *Obsol.* Surgical excision of the wall of the laryngeal ventricle and part of the vocal folds, for the relief of laryngeal stenosis, as from bilateral abductor paralysis of the vocal folds. Syn. *Chevalier Jackson's operation.*

ven·tric·u·lo·gram (ven·trick′yoo·lo·gram) *n.* [*ventriculo-* + *-gram*]. A radiograph of the brain after the direct introduction of gas or an opaque medium into the cerebral ventricles.

ven·tric·u·log·ra·phy (ven·trick″yoo·log′ruh·fee) *n.* [*ventriculo-* + *-graphy*]. A method of demonstrating the ventricles of the brain by radiography after the ventricular fluid has been replaced by gas or by an opaque medium injected directly into the ventricular system. See also *pneumoventriculography.*

ven·tric·u·lo·jug·u·lar (ven·trick″yoo·lo·jug′yoo·lur) *adj.* [*ventriculo-* + *jugular*]. Of or pertaining to a cerebral ventricle and a jugular vein.

ventriculojugular shunt. VENTRICULOVENOUS SHUNT.

ven·tric·u·lo·mas·toid·os·to·my (ven·trick″yoo·lo·mas″toy·dos′tuh·mee) *n.* [*ventriculo-* + *mastoid* + *-stomy*]. A surgical treatment of hydrocephalus in which the temporal horn of a lateral ventricle is connected to the ipsilateral mastoid antrum, usually by a piece of polyethylene tubing.

ven·tric·u·lom·e·try (ven·trick″yoo·lom′e·tree) *n.* [*ventriculo-* + *-metry*]. Measurement of the intraventricular (intracranial) pressure.

ven·tric·u·lo·peri·to·ne·al (ven·trick″yoo·lo·perr″i·to·nee′ul) *adj.* [*ventriculo-* + *peritoneal*]. Pertaining to a cerebral ventricle and the peritoneal cavity.

ventriculoperitoneal shunt. Surgical communication between a lateral cerebral ventricle and the peritoneal cavity by means of a plastic or rubber tube, for the relief of hydrocephalus.

ven·tric·u·lo·pleur·al (ven·trick″yoo·lo·ploor′ul) *adj.* [*ventriculo-* + *pleural*]. Pertaining to a cerebral ventricle and the pleural cavity.

ventriculopleural shunt. Surgical connection between a lateral cerebral ventricle and the pleural cavity by means of a plastic tube, for the relief of hydrocephalus.

ven·tric·u·lo·punc·ture (ven·trick″yoo·lo·punk′chur) *n.* [*ventriculo-* + *puncture*]. VENTRICULAR PUNCTURE.

ven·tric·u·lo·scope (ven·trick′yoo·lo·skope) *n.* [*ventriculo-* + *-scope*]. An instrument for inspecting the interior of the cerebral ventricles and for electrocoagulation of the choroid plexus.

ven·tric·u·los·co·py (ven·trick″yoo·los′kuh·pee) *n.* [*ventriculo-* + *-scopy*]. Examination of the ventricles of the brain by means of an endoscope.

ven·tric·u·los·to·my (ven·trick″yoo·los′tuh·mee) *n.* [*ventriculo-* + *-stomy*]. The surgical establishment of drainage of cerebrospinal fluid from the ventricles of the brain.

ven·tric·u·lo·sub·arach·noid (ven·trick″yoo·lo·sub″uh·rack′noid) *adj.* [*ventriculo-* + *subarachnoid*]. Of or pertaining to the subarachnoid space and the ventricles of the brain.

ven·tric·u·lo·ve·nous (ven·trick″yoo·lo·vee′nus) *adj.* [*ventriculo-* + *venous*]. Pertaining to a cerebral ventricle and the venous system.

ventriculovenous shunt. Surgical connection between a lateral ventricle and the venous system, usually a jugular vein which drains into the superior vena cava, by means of a plastic tube for the relief of hydrocephalus. See also *ventriculoatrial shunt.*

ven·tric·u·lus (ven·trick′yoo·lus) *n.*, pl. & genit. sing. **ventricu·li** (·lye) [L.]. 1. GIZZARD. 2. VENTRICLE. 3. [NA] STOMACH.

ventriculus ce·re·bri (serr′e·brye). VENTRICLE OF THE BRAIN.

ventriculus cor·dis (kor′dis) [NA]. A ventricle of the heart.

ventriculus dex·ter (decks′tur) [NA]. RIGHT VENTRICLE OF THE HEART.

ventriculus la·ryn·gis (la·rin′jis) [NA]. LARYNGEAL VENTRICLE.

ventriculus laryngis [Mor·ga·gnii] (mor·gah′nee·eye) [BNA]. Ventriculus laryngis (= LARYNGEAL VENTRICLE).

ventriculus la·te·ra·lis (lat·e·ray′lis) [NA]. LATERAL VENTRICLE.

ventriculus me·di·us (mee′dee·us). THIRD VENTRICLE.

ventriculus op·ti·cus (op′ti·kus). The lumen of the embryonic optic vesicle, continuous with that of the diencephalon.

ventriculus quar·tus (kwahr′tus) [NA]. FOURTH VENTRICLE.

ventriculus si·nis·ter (si·nis′tur) [NA]. LEFT VENTRICLE OF THE HEART.

ventriculus ter·mi·na·lis (tur·mi·nay′lis) [NA]. TERMINAL VENTRICLE.

ventriculus ter·ti·us (tur′shee·us) [NA]. THIRD VENTRICLE.

ven·tri·cum·bent (ven″tri·kum′bunt) *adj.* [*ventri-* + recum*bent*]. PRONE.

ven·tri·duc·tion (ven″tri·duck′shun) *n.* [*ventri-* + L. *ducere,* to lead]. Drawing a part toward the abdomen.

ven·tri·lat·er·al (ven″tri·lat′ur·ul) *adj.* [*ventri-* + *lateral*]. At the side of the ventral surface.

ven·tri·me·sal (ven″tri·mee′sul) *adj.* [*ventri-* + *mes-* + *-al*]. In the middle in front.

ventro-. See *ventri-*.

ven·tro·cys·tor·rha·phy (ven″tro·sis·tor′uh·fee) *n.* [*ventro-* + *cysto-* + *rrhaphy*]. The suturing of an incised cyst, or bladder, to an opening in the abdominal wall. See also *marsupialization.*

ven·tro·fix·a·tion (ven″tro·fick·say′shun) *n.* [*ventro-* + *fixation*]. The stitching of a displaced viscus to the abdominal wall; specifically, the operative attachment of the uterus to the anterior abdominal wall for prolapse or displacement.

ven·tro·hys·tero·pexy (ven″tro·his′tur·o·peck″see) *n.* [*ventro-* + *hysteropexy*]. Ventrofixation of the uterus.

ven·tro·lat·er·al (ven″tro·lat′ur·ul) *adj.* [*ventro-* + *lateral*]. Pertaining to or directed toward the ventral and lateral aspects of the body or a part.

ventrolateral sulcus. ANTEROLATERAL SPINAL SULCUS.

ventrolateral sulcus of the medulla. ANTEROLATERAL SULCUS OF THE MEDULLA OBLONGATA.

ven·tro·me·di·al (ven″tro·mee′dee·ul) *adj.* [*ventro-* + *medial*]. Pertaining to or directed toward the anterior aspect and toward the midline.

ventromedial hypothalamic nucleus. The larger of two cell groups of the medial hypothalamic area. NA *nucleus ventromedialis hypothalami.*

ven·tro·me·di·an (ven″tro·mee′dee·un) *adj.* [*ventro-* + *median*]. At the middle of the ventral surface.

ven·trop·to·sis (ven″trop·to′sis) *n.* [*ventro-* + *-ptosis*]. GASTROPTOSIS.

ven·tros·co·py (ven·tros′kuh·pee) *n.* [*ventro-* + *-scopy*]. PERITONEOSCOPY.

ven·trose (ven′troce) *adj.* [L. *ventrosus,* from *venter,* belly]. Having a belly, or a swelling like a belly (potbelly).

ven·tros·i·ty (ven·tros′i·tee) *n.* OBESITY.

ven·tro·sus·pen·sion (ven″tro·sus·pen′shun) *n.* [*ventro-* + *suspension*]. The operation of correcting a displacement of the uterus by shortening the round ligaments or attaching them to the anterior abdominal wall.

ven·tro·ves·i·co·fix·a·tion (ven″tro·ves″i·ko·fick·say′shun) *n.* Suturing of the uterus to the urinary bladder and abdominal wall.

Ven·tu·ri effect (ven·too′ree) [G. B. *Venturi,* Italian physicist, 1746–1822]. As the velocity of flow of a fluid through a constricted section of a tube increases, the pressure decreases, a principle used to measure flow of a fluid.

ven·tu·ri·me·ter (ven·tew′ri·mee·tur) *n.* [G. B. *Venturi* + *-meter*]. A differential pressure flowmeter.

Venturi waves [G. B. *Venturi*]. Negative systolic waves, recorded at cardiac catheterization distal to a stenotic pulmonic valve, ascribed to the conversion of pressure energy into velocity energy as the blood passes the narrowed orifice or the sucking action of the stream on the fluid column in the cardiac catheter facing downstream.

ve·nu·la (ven′yoo·luh) *n.*, pl. **venu·lae** (·lee) [L.] [NA]. VENULE.

venulae rec·tae (reck′tee) [NA]. The straight venules of the kidney.

venulae stel·la·tae (stel·ay′tee) [NA]. The stellate venules of the kidney.

venula ma·cu·la·ris inferior (mack·yoo·lair′is) [NA]. The venule draining the inferior portion of the macula of the retina.

venula macularis superior. [NA]. The venule draining the superior portion of the macula of the retina.

venula me·di·a·lis re·ti·nae (mee·dee·ay′lis ret′i·nee) [NA]. The venule draining the central portion of the retina.

venula na·sa·lis re·ti·nae inferior (na·say′lis ret′i·nee) [NA]. The venule draining the lower portion of the nasal part of the retina.

venula nasalis retinae superior [NA]. The venule draining the upper portion of the nasal part of the retina.

venula tem·po·ra·lis re·ti·nae inferior (tem·po·ray′lis ret′i·nee) [NA]. The venule from the lower portion of the temporal part of the retina.

venula temporalis retinae superior [NA]. The venule from the upper portion of the temporal part of the retina.

ven·ule (ven′yool) *n.* [L. *venula,* dim. of *vena,* vein]. A small vein. NA *venula.* —**ven·u·lar** (·yoo·lur) *adj.*

ve·nus (vee′nus) *n.* [L., goddess of love]. 1. Sexual intercourse. 2. Alchemic name for copper.

vera·ce·vine (verr″uh·see′veen, ·vin) *n.* A nonketonic base, obtained from veratrum viride, believed to be one of the original alkanolamine bases of veratrum viride alkaloids.

Veracillin. Trademark for the sodium salt of dicloxacillin, a semisynthetic penicillin antibiotic.

ve·ra·pa·mil (ve·rah′pa·mil) *n.* 5-[(3,4-Dimethoxyphenethyl)-methylamino]-2-(3,4-dimethoxyphenyl)-2-isopropylvaleronitrile, $C_{27}H_{38}N_2O_4$, a coronary vasodilator.

ve·rat·ri·dine (vuh·rat′ri·deen, ·din) *n.* An alkaloid, $C_{36}H_{51}NO_{11}$, isolated from both sabadilla seed and veratrum viride.

ver·a·trine (verr′uh·treen, ·trin) *n.* 1. CEVADINE. 2. A mixture of alkaloids from veratrum viride.

ve·rat·ro·sine (ve·rat′ro·seen, ·sin) *n.* A glucoside isolated from veratrum viride, which on hydrolysis yields D-glucose and veratramine.

ve·ra·trum (ve·ray′trum) *n.* [L., hellebore]. The dried rhizome and roots of green hellebore (*Veratrum viride*) or white hellebore (European hellebore, *Veratrum album*).

veratrum vir·i·de (virr′i·dee). The dried rhizome and roots of green hellebore (*Veratrum viride*); contains a number of hypotensive alkaloids, including protoveratrine A and protoveratrine B. Certain of its alkaloids and alkaloidal extracts are used in the treatment of acute hypertensive states. Syn. *green hellebore, American hellebore.*

ver·bal (vur′bul) *adj.* [L. *verbalis,* from *verbum,* word]. 1. Pertaining to words. 2. Pertaining to speech or discourse.

verbal agraphia. Inability to write words, although single letters can be written.

verbal aphasia. In the classification of Henry Head, BROCA's APHASIA.

verbal asynergy. VOCAL ASYNERGY.

Ver·bas·cum (vur·bas′kum) *n.* [L.]. A genus of plants of the family Scrophulariaceae. The leaves and flowers of *Verbascum thapsus* have been used as a demulcent.

ver·big·er·a·tion (vur·bij″ur·ay′shun) *n.* [L. *verbigerare,* to talk, chat, from *verbum,* word, + *gerere,* to carry on, bring forth]. The frequent and obsessional repetition of the same word, phrase, or even sound without reference to its meaning. Compare *autoecholalia.*

Vercyte. Trademark for pipobroman, a cytotoxic drug used for treatment of polycythemia vera and chronic granulocytic leukemia.

verd-, verdo- [OF. *verd,* green]. A combining form meaning *green-colored.*

ver·di·gris (vur′di·gree, ·gris) *n.* [OF. *vert de Grice,* green of Greece]. 1. A mixture of basic copper acetates. 2. A deposit upon copper, from the formation of cupric salts.

verdo-. See *verd-.*

ver·do·glo·bin (vur″do·glo′bin) *n.* [*verdo-* + *globin*]. CHOLEGLOBIN.

ver·do·he·min (vur″do·hee′min) *n.* [*verdo-* + *hemin*]. A green-colored bile pigment; a derivative of hemin in which the porphyrin ring has opened, rendering the iron labile.

ver·do·nych·ia (vur″do·nick′ee·uh) *n.* [*verd-* + *onych-* + *-ia*]. Green discoloration of the nails.

ver·do·per·ox·i·dase (vur″do·pur·ock′si·dace, ·daze) *n.* [*verdo-* + *peroxidase*]. MYELOPEROXIDASE.

ver du Cayor [F.]. *CORDYLOBIA ANTHROPOPHAGA.*

ver·gence (vur′junce) *n. In ophthalmology,* a disjunctive reciprocal movement of the eyes, as convergence, divergence.

ver·gens (vur′jenz) *adj.* [L., from *vergere,* to bend, incline]. Inclining.

verg·er prism (vur′jur). A prism used in the testing and training of the ability of the eyes to converge, diverge, or supraverge.

ver·ge·ture (vur′je·tewr) *n.* [F.]. The presence of lineae albicantes on the abdomen.

Ver·hoeff's stain [F. H. *Verhoeff,* U.S. ophthalmologist, 1874–1969]. A hematoxylin-ferric chloride-potassium iodide stain for elastin fibers.

Veriloid. Trademark for the fraction of veratrum viride alkaloids known by the generic name alkavervir.

ver ma·caque (vair mah·kahk′) [F.]. A club-shaped larval form of the tropical warble fly, *Dermatobia hominis.*

vermes. Plural of *vermis.*

vermi- [L. *vermis*]. A combining form meaning *worm.*

ver·mi·ci·dal (vur″mi·sigh′dul) *adj.* [*vermi-* + *-cide* + *-al*]. Destructive of worms.

ver·mi·cide (vur′mi·side) *n.* [*vermi-* + *-cide*]. An agent that destroys worms.

ver·mic·u·lar (vur·mick′yoo·lur) *adj.* [ML. *vermicularis,* from *vermiculus,* small worm]. Wormlike.

vermicular contraction. Peristaltic contraction.

vermicular motion or **movement.** PERISTALSIS.

vermicular pulse. A small, rapid pulse imitating the movement of a worm.

vermicular sulcus. The groove between the vermis and a cerebellar hemisphere.

ver·mic·u·late (vur·mick′yoo·lut, ·late) *adj.* [L. *vermiculari,* to be wormy]. Resembling or shaped like a worm.

ver·mic·u·la·tion (vur·mick″yoo·lay′shun) *n.* [L. *vermiculatio,* worminess]. A wormlike motion; peristaltic motion.

ver·mi·cule (vur′mi·kewl) *n.* [L. *vermiculus,* dim. of *vermis,* worm]. A small worm.

ver·mic·u·lose (vur·mick′yoo·loce) *adj.* [L. *vermiculosus*]. 1. VERMIFORM; VERMICULAR. 2. Infested with worms or larvae.

ver·mic·u·lous (vur·mick′yoo·lus) *adj.* VERMICULOSE.

ver·mic·u·lus (vur·mick′yoo·lus) *n.* [L., dim. of *vermis,* worm]. A little worm or grub.

ver·mi·form (vur′mi·form) *adj.* [ML. *vermiformis,* from L. *vermis,* worm]. Worm-shaped.

vermiform appendix. The small, blind gut projecting from the cecum. NA *appendix vermiformis.*

vermiform process. VERMIFORM APPENDIX.

ver·mi·fuge (vur′mi·fewj) *n.* [*vermi-* + *-fuge*]. Any agent that kills or expels intestinal worms. —**ver·mif·u·gal** (vur·mif′yoo·gul, vur″mi·few′gul) *adj.*

ver·mi·lin·gual (vur″mi·ling′gwul) *adj.* [*vermi-* + *lingual*]. Having a worm-shaped tongue.

ver·mil·ion border (vur·mil′yun). The mucocutaneous junction of the lips.

ver·mil·ion·ec·to·my, ver·mil·lion·ec·to·my (vur·mil″yun·eck′tuh·mee) *n.* [*vermilion* border + *-ectomy*]. Surgical removal of the vermilion border of the lips.

ver·min (vur′min) *n.* [OF., from a variant of L. *vermis,* worm]. Animals that are obnoxious or harmful to man, especially those infesting his person, domesticated animals, or buildings, as flies, lice, rats, or mice.

ver·mi·na·tion (vur″mi·nay′shun) *n.* Infestation with vermin or worms. The multiplication of parasitic vermin by breeding.

ver·min·ous (vur′min·us) *adj.* Infested with, or pertaining to, vermin.

verminous abscess. An abscess containing worms.

ver·mi·pho·bia (vur″mi·fo′bee·uh) *n.* [*vermi-* + *-phobia*]. Abnormal fear of worms or of infection by worms.

ver·mis (vur′mis) *n.,* pl. **ver·mes** (·meez) [L., worm (rel. to Gmc. *wurmiz* → E. *worm*)]. 1. WORM. 2. [NA] The median lobe of the cerebellum, between the hemispheres, or lateral lobes.

vermis syndrome. Cerebellar dysfunction marked chiefly by disturbances in gait and the tendency to lose balance while sitting or standing, due to disease involving the vermis.

ver·nal (vur′nul) *adj.* [L. *vernalis,* from *ver,* spring]. 1. Occurring in the spring. 2. Pertaining to the spring.

vernal conjunctivitis. A form of conjunctivitis, allergic in origin, recurring each spring or summer and disappearing with frost. Syn. *conjunctivitis catarrhalis aestiva, spring catarrh, spring conjunctivitis.*

Ver·net's rideau phenomenon (vehr·neh′) [M. *Vernet,* French neurologist, b. 1887; F. *rideau,* curtain]. Constriction of the posterior wall of the pharynx in saying "ah," like drawing a curtain; absent in glossopharyngeal paralysis.

Vernet's syndrome [M. *Vernet*]. JUGULAR FORAMEN SYNDROME.

Ver·neuil's disease or **bursitis** (vehr·nœy′) [A. A. S. *Verneuil,* French surgeon, 1823–1895]. SYPHILITIC BURSITIS.

Verneuil's neuroma [A. A. S. *Verneuil*]. PLEXIFORM NEUROFIBROMA.

ver·ni·er (vur′nee·ur) *n.* [P. *Vernier,* French physicist, 1580–1637]. A device attached to the graduated scale of various instruments which permits subdividing and measuring the smallest unit of this scale into tenths or other fractions.

vernier acuity. The ability of the eye to perceive a break in contour; the aligning discrimination of the eye, accurate on an average to a few seconds of arc (3.0 to 3.5), or less than the diameter of a single foveal cone.

ver·nine (vur′neen) *n.* GUANOSINE.

Vernitest. Trademark for quinaldine blue, a diagnostic stain used in obstetrics.

ver·nix ca·se·o·sa (vur′nicks kay″see·o′suh) [L., cheeselike varnish]. A cheesy deposit on the surface of the fetus derived from the stratum corneum, sebaceous secretion, and remnants of the epitrichium.

Ver·no·nia (vur·no′nee·uh) *n.* [W. *Vernon,* English botanist, 17th century]. A genus of plants of the Carduaceae; certain species have been used medicinally.

Ve·ro·cay bodies (beh·ro·kigh′) [J. *Verocay,* Uruguayan pathologist, 1876–1927]. Small whorls of fibrils, surrounded by radially arranged elongated cells, seen in neurofibromas.

ve·ro·di·gen (ve·ro′di·jen) *n.* GITALIN.

Veronal. Trademark for barbital, a barbiturate sedative and hypnotic.

ver·ru·ca (ve·roo′kuh) *n.* [L.]. WART.

verruca acu·mi·na·ta (a·kew″mi·nay′tuh). CONDYLOMA ACUMINATUM.

verruca dig·i·ta·ta (dij″i·tay′tuh). A soft, warty papule usually seen on the scalp or in the beard with fingerlike projections and a horny cap.

verruca fi·li·for·mis (fye″li·for′mis). A soft, slender, soft-pointed, threadlike warty papule usually seen on the face and neck.

verruca nec·ro·gen·i·ca (neck″ro·jen′i·kuh). TUBERCULOSIS VERRUCOSA.

verruca pe·ru·a·na (pe·roo·ah′nuh) [erroneous hybrid of Sp. *verruga peruana* and NL. *verruca peruviana*]. VERRUGA PERUANA.

verruca pe·ru·vi·a·na (pe·roo·vee·ay′nuh) [NL.] VERRUGA PERUANA.

verruca pla·na ju·ve·ni·lis (play′nuh joo″ve·nigh′lis). A smooth, flat, small type of wart seen most often in children on the back of the hands and face, often arranged in lines.

verruca plan·ta·ris (plan·tair′is). Verruca vulgaris occurring on the sole of the foot as a painful, callus-covered papule. Syn. *plantar wart.*

verruca se·ni·lis (se·nigh′lis). SEBORRHEIC KERATOSIS.

verruca vul·ga·ris (vul·gair′is). The common wart, a viral disease producing hard hyperkeratotic papules, most commonly on the fingers.

ver·ru·ci·form (ve·roo′si·form) *adj.* [*verruca* + *-iform*]. Wart-like.

ver·ru·coid (verr′uh·koid) *adj.* [*verruca* + *-oid*]. Resembling a wart.

ver·ru·cose (verr′uh·koce, ve·roo′) *adj.* [L. *verrucosus,* from *verruca,* wart]. Warty; covered with or having warts.

verrucose mycotic dermatitis. BLASTOMYCOSIS.

ver·ru·cous (ve·roo′kus) *adj.* VERRUCOSE.

verrucous aortitis. Warty deformity of the aortic intima.

verrucous carcinoma. A low-grade malignant tumor of squamous epithelial cells presenting a grossly warty appearance.

verrucous endocarditis. Small thrombotic nonbacterial wart-like lesions on the heart valves and endocardium. Occurs frequently in systemic lupus erythematosus; may occur terminally, with or without clinical symptoms, in a variety of illnesses.

verrucous nevus. NEVUS VERRUCOSUS.

ver·ru·ga (ve·roo′guh) *n.* [Sp.]. Verruca (= WART).

verruga pe·ru·a·na (pe·roo·ah′nuh) [Sp., Peruvian wart]. The benign form of bartonellosis (Carrión's disease), endemic in the mountainous areas of northwestern South America, characterized by a skin eruption of purpuric vascular papules interspersed with nodular elements, the proliferation of epithelial cells, and the presence in the lesions of the causative agent, *Bartonella bacilliformis,* usually in the cytoplasm of endothelial cells. It is related etiologically and immunologically to Oroya fever, but the two diseases differ greatly in their clinical picture.

Versapen. Trademark for hetacillin, a semisynthetic penicillin antibiotic.

Versene. A trademark for various synthetic amino acids and their salts, as ethylenediaminetetraacetic acid and its salts; the substances are used as chelating and sequestering agents.

ver·si·col·or (vur′si·kul″ur) *adj.* [L., from *vertere, versus,* to turn, change]. 1. Many-colored, variegated. 2. Iridescent, changing in color.

ver·sion (vur′zhun) *n.* [ML., turn, turning, from L. *vertere,* to turn]. 1. Turning; manipulation during delivery to alter the presentation of the fetus. 2. Movement of both eyes in conjugate gaze. 3. The condition of an organ or part being turned or placed away from its normal position.

vertebr-, vertebro-. A combining form meaning *vertebrae, vertebral.*

ver·te·bra (vur′te·bruh) *n.,* L. pl. & genit. sing. **verte·brae** (·bree), genit. pl. **ver·te·bra·rum** (vur″te·brair′um) [L., joint, vertebra, from *vertere,* to turn] [NA]. One of 33 bones forming the spinal or vertebral column. A typical vertebra consists of a body and an arch, the latter being formed by two pedicles and two laminas. The arch supports seven processes—four articular, two transverse, and one spinous. See also Table of Bones in the Appendix and Plates 1, 14.

vertebra den·ta·ta (den·tay′tuh). AXIS (2).

ver·te·bra·dym·ia (vur″te·bruh·dim′ee·uh) *n.* [*vertebra* + *-dymia*]. SPONDYLODIDYMIA.

vertebrae cer·vi·ca·les (sur·vi·kay′leez) [NA]. CERVICAL VERTEBRAE.

vertebrae coc·cy·ge·ae (kock·sij′ee·ee) [NA]. The vertebrae forming the coccyx.

vertebrae lum·ba·les (lum·bay′leez) [NA]. LUMBAR VERTEBRAE.

vertebrae sa·cra·les (sa·kray′leez) [NA]. The vertebrae forming the sacrum.

vertebrae tho·ra·ca·les (tho·ruh·kay′leez) [BNA]. Vertebrae thoracicae (= THORACIC VERTEBRAE).

vertebrae tho·ra·ci·cae (tho·ray′si·see) [NA]. THORACIC VERTEBRAE.

ver·te·bral (vur′te·brul) *adj.* Of or pertaining to a vertebra or vertebrae.

vertebral aponeurosis. A thin aponeurotic lamina extending along the whole length of the back part of the thoracic region, serving to bind down the sacrospinalis muscle and separating it from those muscles that unite the spine to the upper extremity.

vertebral arch. An arch formed by the paired pedicles and laminas of a vertebra; the posterior part of a vertebra which together with the anterior part, the body, encloses the vertebral foramen in which the spinal cord is lodged. NA *arcus vertebrae.*

vertebral arteriography. Radiography of the vertebral artery and its branches by the injection of a radiopaque medium.

vertebral artery. See Table of Arteries in the Appendix.

vertebral arthropathy. Arthropathy associated with depressions and rugosities of the vertebrae.

vertebral–basilar artery insufficiency syndrome. BASILAR ARTERY INSUFFICIENCY SYNDROME.

vertebral body. A short column of bone forming the anterior, weight-bearing segment of a vertebra.

vertebral canal. A canal formed by the foramens of the vertebrae; it contains the spinal cord and its meninges. NA *canalis vertebralis.*

vertebral column. The flexible supporting column of the body made up of vertebrae separated by intervertebral disks and bound together by ligaments. Syn. *spinal column.* NA *columna vertebralis.*

vertebral foramen. The space included between the body and arch of a vertebra, passage to the spinal cord and its appendages. NA *foramen vertebrale.*

vertebral formula. A formula used to indicate the number and arrangement of the vertebrae.

vertebral groove. The groove formed by the laminas of the vertebrae and the sides of the spinous processes; it lodges the deep muscles of the back.

vertebral incisure or **notch.** One of the notches above and below the pedicles of the vertebrae; in the articulated vertebral column, the notches of contiguous pairs of bones form the intervertebral foramens. See also *inferior vertebral incisure, superior vertebral incisure.*

vertebral pedicle. The portion of bone projecting backward from each side of the body of a vertebra, and connecting the lamina with the body. NA *pediculus arcus vertebrae.*

vertebral plexus. 1. A sympathetic nerve plexus surrounding the vertebral and basilar arteries. NA *plexus vertebralis.* 2. A plexus of large veins associated with the vertebral column throughout its length. It may be subdivided into the anterior and posterior external (NA *plexus venosi vertebrales externi anterior et posterior*) and the anterior and posterior internal vertebral plexuses (NA *plexus venosi vertebrales interni anterior et posterior*).

vertebral process. One of the processes projecting from a vertebra, as the transverse process, the superior articular process, the inferior articular process, or the spinous process.

vertebral region. The area over the vertebral column. NA *regio vertebralis.*

vertebral sinus. VERTEBRAL PLEXUS (2).

vertebral spine. SPINOUS PROCESS OF A VERTEBRA.

vertebral tubercles. Three elevations, the superior, inferior, and lateral, subdividing the transverse process of the twelfth thoracic vertebra; similar rudimentary prominences are found on the transverse processes of the tenth and eleventh thoracic vertebrae.

vertebral veins. The plexus of thin-walled valveless veins situated about the spinal cord within the vertebral canal. Syn. *meningorachidian veins.*

vertebral venous system. A group of venous anastomoses that pass through the intervertebral foramens to connect the veins of the pelvic cavity, the pelvic girdle, the shoulder girdle, and the body wall with the vertebral veins and thus with the sinuses of the dura mater. Syn. *system of Batson.*

vertebra mag·na (mag'nuh). SACRUM.

vertebra pla·na (play'nuh). A vertebra that has been reduced in vertical height owing to a collapse of the vertebral body.

vertebra pro·mi·nens (prom'i·nenz) [NA]. The seventh cervical vertebra, so called because its spinous process projects beyond the others.

ver·te·brar·te·ri·al (vur''te·brahr·teer'ee·ul) *adj.* [*vertebr-* + *arterial*]. Giving passage to the vertebral artery, as the transverse foramens in the transverse processes of the cervical vertebrae.

vertebrarterial foramen. FORAMEN TRANSVERSARIUM.

Ver·te·bra·ta (vur''te·brah'tuh, ·bray'tuh) *n.pl.* [NL.]. A major group in the animal kingdom, commonly classified as a subphylum of the Chordata, and comprising the mammals, birds, reptiles, amphibians, and fishes. They are characterized by a spinal column, which develops in embryonic life about a notochord, composed of bony or, in certain fishes, cartilaginous vertebrae, and which contains the spinal cord that connects with a brain enclosed in a skull.

ver·te·brate (vur·te·brut) *adj. & n.* [L. *vertebratus,* jointed, articulated]. 1. Having a vertebral column; belonging to the Vertebrata. 2. Resembling a vertebral column in flexibility, as a vertebrate catheter. 3. A member of the Vertebrata.

ver·te·brat·ed (vur'te·bray·tid) *adj.* VERTEBRATE (1, 2).

ver·te·brec·to·my (vur''te·breck'tuh·mee) *n.* [*vertebr-* + *-ectomy*]. Surgical excision of a portion of a vertebra.

vertebro-. See *vertebr-.*

ver·te·bro·chon·dral (vur''te·bro·kon'drul) *adj.* [*vertebro-* + *chondral*]. Pertaining to, or involving, a vertebra and a costal cartilage.

vertebrochondral ribs. The highest three false ribs on each side; they are united in front by their costal cartilages.

ver·te·bro·cos·tal (vur''te·bro·kos'tul) *adj.* [*vertebro-* + *costal*]. Pertaining to or involving a vertebra and a rib.

vertebrocostal triangle. LUMBOCOSTAL TRIANGLE OF BOCHDALEK.

ver·te·bro·di·dym·ia (vur''te·bro·di·dim'ee·uh) *n.* [*vertebro-* + Gk. *didymos,* twin]. Conjoined twins united by vertebrae.

ver·tex (vur'tecks) *n.,* L. pl. **ver·ti·ces** (vur'ti·seez) [L., top, crown of the head]. 1. *In craniometry,* the highest point, in the sagittal plane, on the outer surface of a skull oriented on the Frankfort horizontal plane. 2. [NA] The crown of the head. 3. The center of a lens surface; the point on either lens surface which lies on the principal axis.

vertex cor·ne·ae (kor'nee·ee) [NA]. The central, most prominent point of the cornea.

vertex presentation. *In obstetrics,* the most usual type of presentation, with the occiput the presenting part.

vertex ve·si·cae (ve·sigh'see) [BNA]. APEX VESICAE URINARIAE.

ver·ti·cal (vur'ti·kul) *adj.* [L. *verticalis,* from *vertex,* top]. 1. Pertaining to the vertex. 2. Pertaining to the position of the long axis of the human body in the erect posture.

vertical axis. 1. The long axis of the body. 2. A vertical line passing through the center of the eyeball.

vertical concomitant strabismus. A squint in which one eye turns up, the deviation remaining constant in all fields of vision.

vertical diameter. The distance between the foramen magnum and the vertex.

vertical diameter of the cranium. An imaginary line from the basion to the bregma.

vertical dimension. *In prosthetic dentistry,* the distance between any two selected points in a vertical plane of the upper and lower jaws when the teeth, artificial dentures, or other devices are in occlusion.

vertical hemianopsia. HOMONYMOUS HEMIANOPSIA.

vertical illumination. Microscopical illumination in which a beam of light is thrown on the object from above, or from the direction of observation. Syn. *direct illumination.*

vertical index. The ratio of the vertical diameter of the skull to the maximum anteroposterior diameter, multiplied by 100.

vertical lingual muscle. The vertical muscle fibers of the intrinsic musculature of the tongue. NA *musculus verticalis linguae.* See also Table of Muscles in the Appendix.

vertical nystagmus. Involuntary, rhythmic up-and-down oscillation of the eyes.

vertical strabismus. Squint in the vertical direction, called sursumversion when involving both eyes upward, deorsumduction when downward, and right or left hypertropia according to the higher eye. See also *vertical concomitant strabismus.*

vertical transmission. Transmission (of a disease) from one generation to the next, genetically or otherwise congenitally. Contr. *horizontal transmission.*

vertices. A plural of *vertex.*

ver·ti·cil (vur'ti·sil) *n.* [L. *verticillus,* whorl of a spindle]. A whorl; a circle of leaves, tentacles, hairs, organs, or processes radiating from an axis on the same horizontal plane. —**ver·ti·cil·late** (vur''ti·sil'ate) *adj.*

ver·tig·i·nous (vur·tij'i·nus) *adj.* [L. *vertiginosus*]. Resembling or affected with vertigo.

vertiginous aura. Dizziness announcing an epileptic seizure.

ver·ti·go (vur'ti·go) *n.,* pl. **vertigoes, ver·tig·i·nes** (vur·tij'i·neez) [L.]. 1. The sensation that the outer world is revolving about oneself (objective vertigo) or that one is moving in space (subjective vertigo). 2. Any subjective or objective illusion of motion or position.

vertigo par·a·ly·sant (păr''uh·lye'zunt, F. pa^{h}·ra^{h}·lee·zah$^{n'}$). PARALYTIC VERTIGO.

ver·tig·ra·phy (vur·tig'ruh·fee) *n.* [L. *vertere,* to turn, change, + *-graphy*]. SECTIONAL RADIOGRAPHY.

ver·u·mon·ta·ni·tis (verr''yoo·mon''tuh·nigh'tis) *n.* [*verumontanum* + *-itis*]. Inflammation of the colliculus seminalis.

ver·u·mon·ta·num (verr''yoo·mon·tay'num) *n.* [L. *veru,* spit, dart, + *montanum,* of a mountain or mound]. COLLICULUS SEMINALIS.

ver·vet (vur'vit) *n.* A monkey of the species (or species group) *Cercopithecus aethiops;* especially, one belonging to the southern and eastern subspecies, *C. aethiops pygerythrus.*

vervet monkey disease. GREEN MONKEY FEVER.

Ve·sa·lius' bone (ve·say'lee·us) [A. *Vesalius,* Flemish anatomist, 1514–1564]. OS VESALII.

Vesalius' foramen [A. *Vesalius*]. FORAMEN OF VESALIUS.

Vesalius' ligament [A. *Vesalius*]. INGUINAL LIGAMENT.

Vesalius' vein [A. *Vesalius*]. An emissary vein passing through Vesalius' foramen.

ve·sa·nia (ve·say'nee·uh) *n.* [L., from *vesanus,* insane, from *sanus,* sound, sane]. Unsoundness of mind. —**vesa·nic** (·nick) *adj.*

ve·si·ca (ve·sigh'kuh, ves'i·kuh) *n.,* pl. & genit. sing. **vesi·cae** (·see, ·kee) [L.]. BLADDER.

vesica bi·par·ta (bye·pahr'tuh). A urinary bladder that is incompletely reduplicated by partial frontal or sagittal septa.

vesica du·plex (dew'plecks). Reduplication of the urinary bladder.

vesicae. Plural and genitive singular of *vesica.*

vesica fel·lea (fel'ee·uh) [NA]. GALLBLADDER.

ves·i·cal (ves'i·kul) *adj.* [*vesica* + *-al*]. Of or pertaining to a bladder, especially the urinary bladder.

vesical blind spot. *In urology,* the area or areas of the anterior urinary bladder wall which cannot be visualized in cystoscopic examination.

vesical calculus. A calculus in the urinary bladder.

vesical crisis. Paroxysmal attack of bladder pain, with difficulty in urination, seen in tabes dorsalis.

vesical diverticulum. A diverticulum of the urinary bladder.

vesical ectopia. Exstrophy of the urinary bladder.

vesical fistula. An abnormal opening from the urinary bladder communicating externally with the skin or internally with another pelvic organ.

vesical hernia. Hernia of the urinary bladder.

vesical plexus. 1. An autonomic nerve plexus surrounding the vesical arteries. NA *plexus vesicalis.* 2. A venous plexus about the lower part of the urinary bladder and base of the prostate gland. NA *plexus venosus vesicalis.*

vesical reflex. The reflex or automatic response of the urinary bladder to empty itself, induced by distention of the organ to a certain capacity or degree, normally controlled by voluntary inhibition and release. Syn. *urinary reflex, vesicourethral reflex.*

vesical trigone. TRIGONE (2).

ves·i·cant (ves'i·kunt) *n.* [L. *vesica,* bladder, blister, + *-ant*]. 1. A blistering agent. 2. *In military medicine,* BLISTER GAS.

ves·i·ca·tion (ves''i·kay'shun) *n.* [L. *vesica,* bladder, blister]. The formation of a blister; a blister. —**ves·i·cate** (ves'i·kate) *v.*

ves·i·ca·to·ry (ves'i·kuh·tor·ee) *adj.* & *n.* 1. Blistering; causing blisters. 2. A blistering agent.

vesica um·bi·li·ca·lis (um·bil·i·kay'lis). The umbilical vesicle, or yolk sac, of mammals.

vesica uri·na·ria (yoor·i·nair'ee·uh) [NA]. URINARY BLADDER.

ves·i·cle (ves'i·kul) *n.* [L. *vesicula,* dim. of *vesica,* bladder]. 1. A small bladder; especially a small sac containing fluid. 2. A small bulla, as seen in herpes simplex or chickenpox.

vesico- [L. *vesica,* bladder]. A combining form meaning (a) *bladder;* (b) *vesicle* or *blister.*

ves·i·co·ab·dom·i·nal (ves''i·ko·ab·dom'i·nul) *adj.* Pertaining to the urinary bladder and the abdomen.

vesicoabdominal fistula. A fistula extending from the urinary bladder through the abdominal wall and opening externally onto the skin of the abdomen.

ves·i·co·bul·lous (ves''i·ko·bul'us) *adj.* VESICULOBULLOUS.

ves·i·co·cele (ves'i·ko·seel) *n.* [*vesico-* + *-cele*]. CYSTOCELE.

ves·i·co·cer·vi·cal (ves''i·ko·sur'vi·kul) *adj.* [*vesico-* + *cervical*]. Pertaining to the urinary bladder and the uterine cervix.

ves·i·co·en·ter·ic (ves''i·ko·en·terr'ick) *adj.* [*vesico-* + *enteric*]. VESICOINTESTINAL.

ves·i·co·fix·a·tion (ves''i·ko·fick·say'shun) *n.* [*vesico-* + *fixation*]. CYSTOPEXY.

ves·i·co·in·tes·ti·nal (ves''i·ko·in·tes'ti·nul) *adj.* [*vesico-* + *intestinal*]. Pertaining to the urinary bladder and the intestinal tract.

ves·i·co·li·thot·o·my (ves''i·ko·li·thot'uh·mee) *n.* [*vesico-* + *lithotomy*]. CYSTOLITHOTOMY.

ves·i·co·pros·tat·ic (ves''i·ko·pros·tat'ick) *adj.* [*vesico-* + *prostatic*]. Pertaining to the prostate gland and the urinary bladder.

ves·i·co·pu·den·dal (ves''i·ko·pew·den'dul) *adj.* [*vesico-* + *pudendal*]. Of or pertaining to both the urinary bladder and the pudendum.

vesicopudendal plexus. The vesical and pudendal venous plexuses, collectively.

ves·i·co·pus·tule (ves''i·ko·pus'tewl) *n.* A vesicle which is developing into a pustule. —**vesicopus·tu·lar** (·tew·lur) *adj.*

ves·i·co·rec·tal (ves''i·ko·reck'tul) *adj.* [*vesico-* + *rectal*]. Pertaining to the urinary bladder and the rectum.

ves·i·co·rec·to·va·gi·nal (ves''i·ko·reck''to·va·jye'nul, ·vaj'i·nul) *adj.* [*vesico-* + *recto-* + *vaginal*]. Pertaining to the urinary bladder, rectum, and vagina.

vesicorectovaginal cloaca. A cavity in the pelvis into which rectum, urinary bladder, and vagina all open; it may be congenital or due to trauma, infections, tumors, or irradiation damage.

ves·i·co·sig·moid (ves''i·ko·sig'moid) *adj.* [*vesico-* + *sigmoid*]. Pertaining to the urinary bladder and the sigmoid colon.

ves·i·cos·to·my (ves''i·kos'tuh·mee) *n.* [*vesico-* + *-stomy*]. CYSTOSTOMY.

ves·i·cot·o·my (ves''i·kot'uh·mee) *n.* [*vesico-* + *-tomy*]. Surgical incision of the urinary bladder; CYSTOTOMY (1).

ves·i·co·um·bil·i·cal (ves''i·ko·um·bil'i·kul) *adj.* Pertaining to the urinary bladder and the umbilicus.

vesicoumbilical ligament. MEDIAN UMBILICAL LIGAMENT.

ves·i·co·ure·ter·al (ves''i·ko·yoo·ree'tur·ul) *adj.* Pertaining to the urinary bladder and to a ureter or to the ureters.

ves·i·co·ure·thral (ves''i·ko·yoo·ree'thrul) *adj.* Pertaining to the urinary bladder and the urethra.

vesicourethral canal or **anlage.** The part of the primitive urogenital sinus, cephalad to the openings of the mesonephric ducts, which develops into the urinary bladder and primary urethra.

vesicourethral reflex. VESICAL REFLEX.

ves·i·co·ure·thro·va·gi·nal (ves''i·ko·yoo·ree''thro·va·jye'nul, ·vaj'i·nul) *adj.* [*vesico-* + *urethro-* + *vaginal*]. Pertaining to the urinary bladder, urethra, and vagina.

ves·i·co·uter·ine (ves''i·ko·yoo'tur·in, ·yoo'tuh·rine) *adj.* [*vesico-* + *uterine*]. Pertaining to the urinary bladder and the uterus.

vesicouterine excavation or **pouch.** The part of the peritoneal cavity between the anterior suface of the uterus and the urinary bladder. NA *excavatio vesicouterina.*

ves·i·co·utero·va·gi·nal (ves''i·ko·yoo''tur·o·va·jye'nul, ·vaj'i·nul) *adj.* [*vesico-* + *utero-* + *vaginal*]. Pertaining to the urinary bladder, uterus, and vagina.

vesicouterovaginal fistula. An abnormal opening connecting the vagina, urinary bladder, and uterine cavity.

ves·i·co·va·gi·nal (ves''i·ko·va·jye'nul, ·vaj'i·nul) *adj.* [*vesico-* + *vaginal*]. Pertaining to the urinary bladder and the vagina.

vesicovaginal fistula. An abnormal tract between the urinary bladder and the vagina.

vesicovaginal septum. A sheet of connective tissue which has been described as existing between the urinary bladder and the anterior wall of the vagina.

vesicul-, vesiculo-. A combining form meaning *vesicle, vesicular.*

ve·si·cu·la (ve·sick'yoo·luh) *n.,* pl. **vesicu·lae** (·lee) [L.]. VESICLE.

vesicula fel·lea (fel'ee·uh). GALLBLADDER.

vesicula oph·thal·mi·ca (off·thal'mi·kuh) [NA]. OPTIC VESICLE.

vesicula op·ti·ca in·ver·sa (op'ti·kuh in·vur'suh). The optic vesicle after it has invaginated to form the optic cup.

vesicula pro·sta·ti·ca (pros·tat'i·kuh). The prostatic utricle; UTRICLE (2).

ve·sic·u·lar (ve·sick'yoo·lur) *adj.* [*vesicul-* + *-ar*]. 1. Pertaining to, or composed of, vesicles. 2. Produced in air vesicles.

3. *In cytology,* pertaining to nuclei whose chromatin is widely dispersed, with or without a thin nuclear membrane.

vesicular appendix. Vestigial remnants of cranial mesonephric tubules, located in the distal end of the mesosalpinx or adjacent broad ligament. NA (pl.) *appendices vesiculosae.*

vesicular bronchiolitis. BRONCHOPNEUMONIA.

vesicular emphysema. Emphysema characterized pathologically by enlarged, deformed air spaces involving the alveoli, alveolar ducts, and respiratory bronchioles.

vesicular exanthema. An acute febrile virus disease of swine characterized by the presence of vesicles on the nose, feet, and mucous membrane of the mouth.

vesicular follicle. The stage in the development of an ovarian follicle at which it has developed a fluid-filled vesicle. See *ovarian follicle.*

vesicular mole. HYDATIDIFORM MOLE.

vesicular morula. BLASTULA.

vesicular rale. CREPITANT RALE.

vesicular resonance. The normal pulmonary resonance dependent on the air-containing lung vesicles.

vesicular respiration. Soft breath sounds heard over the normal lung, with inspiratory sounds of higher pitch, louder and longer in duration than expiratory sounds.

vesicular stomatitis. BEDNAR'S APHTHAE.

vesicular supporting tissue. *Obsol.* PSEUDOCARTILAGE.

vesicular transport. CYTOPEMPSIS.

vesicula se·mi·na·lis (sem-i-nay'lis) [NA]. SEMINAL VESICLE.

ve·sic·u·late (ve-sick'yoo-late, -lut) *adj. & v.* 1. Like a vesicle. 2. Covered with or composed of vesicles. 3. To produce, or be transformed into, vesicles.

ve·sic·u·lat·ed (ve-sick'yoo-lay-tid) *adj.* VESICULATE (2).

ve·sic·u·la·tion (ve-sick"yoo-lay'shun) *n.* The formation of vesicles; the state of becoming vesiculated.

ve·sic·u·lec·to·my (ve-sick"yoo-leck'tuh-mee) *n.* [*vesicul-* + *ectomy*]. Surgical resection, complete or partial, of the seminal vesicles.

ve·sic·u·li·tis (ve-sick"yoo-lye'tis) *n.* [*vesicul-* + *-itis*]. Inflammation of the seminal vesicles.

vesiculo-. See *vesicul-.*

ve·sic·u·lo·bron·chi·al (ve-sick"yoo-lo-bronk'ee-ul) *adj.* Having vesicular and bronchial characteristics.

vesiculobronchial respiration. BRONCHOVESICULAR RESPIRATION.

ve·sic·u·lo·bul·lous (ve-sick"yoo-lo-bul'us) *adj.* [*vesiculo-* + *bull*a + *-ous*]. Characterized by both vesicles and bullae at the same time.

ve·sic·u·lo·cav·ern·ous (ve-sick"yoo-lo-kav'ur-nus) *adj.* [*vesiculo-* + *cavernous*]. Having vesicular and cavernous characteristics.

vesiculocavernous respiration. Respiration that is both vesicular and cavernous.

ve·sic·u·lo·gram (ve-sick'yoo-lo-gram) *n.* [*vesiculo-* + *-gram*]. A radiograph of the seminal vesicles, following injection of a radiopaque medium by way of the ejaculatory ducts or the ductus deferens.

ve·sic·u·log·ra·phy (ve-sick"yoo-log'ruh-fee) *n.* [*vesiculo-* + *-graphy*]. Radiography of the seminal vesicles with the injection of a contrast medium. Syn. *seminal vesiculography.*

ve·sic·u·lo·pap·u·lar (ve-sick"yoo-lo-pap'yoo-lur) *adj.* [*vesiculo-* + *papular*]. 1. Consisting of vesicles and papules. 2. Having characteristics of both vesicles and papules.

ve·sic·u·lo·pus·tu·lar (ve-sick"yoo-lo-pus'tew-lur) *adj.* [*vesiculo-* + *pustular*]. 1. Consisting of vesicles and pustules. 2. Having characteristics of both vesicles and pustules.

ve·sic·u·lot·o·my (ve-sick"yoo-lot'uh-mee) *n.* [*vesiculo-* + *-tomy*]. Surgical incision of a seminal vesicle.

Vesprin. Trademark for triflupromazine, a phenothiazine tranquilizer used, as the hydrochloride salt, to treat various psychiatric disorders and psychoses and also employed as an antiemetic.

ves·sel (ves'ul) *n.* [OF., from L. *vascellum,* dim. of *vas*]. A receptacle for fluids, especially a tube or canal for conveying blood or lymph. Comb. form *vascul(o)-.*

ves·sig·non (ves'ig-non, ves'i-nyon) *n.* [F., from *vessie,* bladder, vesicle]. A tumor within the synovial membrane of the hock of a horse.

vestibula. Plural of *vestibulum.*

ves·tib·u·lar (ves-tib'yoo-lur) *adj.* 1. Pertaining to a vestibule. 2. Particularly, pertaining to the vestibular part of the eighth cranial nerve, concerned with equilibrium.

vestibular apparatus. The anatomical parts concerned with the vestibular portion of the eighth cranial nerve, including the saccule, utricle, semicircular canals, vestibular nerve, and vestibular nuclei. Syn. *vestibulolabyrinthine apparatus.*

vestibular aqueduct. AQUEDUCT OF THE VESTIBULE.

vestibular area. A triangular area, lateral to the sulcus limitans, beneath which lie the terminal nuclei of the vestibular nerve.

vestibular bulb. BULB OF THE VESTIBULE (of the vagina).

vestibular cecum. The blind sac at the beginning of the cochlear duct in the vestibule of the internal ear. NA *cecum vestibulare.*

vestibular covering layer. The connective-tissue layer covering the upper surface of the basilar membrane of the cochlea.

vestibular fold. A fold of mucous membrane on either side of the larynx enclosing a vestibular ligament and forming one boundary of the rima vestibuli. Syn. *false vocal cord, ventricular fold.* NA *plica vestibularis.*

vestibular fossa of the vagina. The part of the vestibule of the vagina which lies posterior to the vaginal orifice. NA *fossa vestibuli vaginae.*

vestibular ganglion. The ganglion of the vestibular part of the eighth cranial nerve, located in the auditory meatus. NA *ganglion vestibulare.*

vestibular glands. Glands of the vestibule of the vagina, comprising the compound tubuloalveolar major vestibular glands (of Bartholin), one in each lateral wall (NA *glandula vestibularis major*), and the minor vestibular glands (NA *glandulae vestibulares minores*), which are several small branched tubular mucous glands around the urethral orifice.

vestibular lamina. The vertical sheet of oral ectoderm that splits to form the vestibule of the mouth. Syn. *lip furrow band.*

vestibular ligament. The portion of the quadrangular membrane which lies in the vestibular fold of the larynx. NA *ligamentum vestibulare.*

vestibular lip. The lower margin of the internal spiral sulcus in the cochlea.

vestibular membrane of Reissner [E. *Reissner*]. PARIES VESTIBULARIS DUCTUS COCHLEARIS.

vestibular nerve. The portion of the vestibulocochlear nerve concerned with the sense of equilibrium. NA *pars vestibularis nervi octavi.* See Table of Nerves in the Appendix.

vestibular neuronitis. A benign disorder of unknown cause mainly affecting young adults and characterized by a transient attack of vertigo, absent response to caloric stimulation on one side, nystagmus with the quick component to the opposite side, and normality of auditory function.

vestibular nuclei. Lateral vestibular nucleus, medial vestibular nucleus, spinal vestibular nucleus, and superior vestibular nucleus.

vestibular nystagmus. Nystagmus due to a disorder of the vestibulolabyrinthine apparatus.

vestibular paralysis. Loss of vestibular function, as may be caused by certain antibiotics, manifested by vertigo, tinnitus, nausea, and vomiting, followed by disturbances of gait, posture, and impaired response to the caloric stimulation of the tympanic membranes.

vestibular reaction. The response of the labyrinth to sound vibrations.

vestibular reflexes. 1. The responses to strong stimulation of the vestibular apparatus: pallor, nausea, vomiting, and postural changes. 2. Static and statokinetic reflexes that maintain bodily posture against the force of gravity and during walking and other forms of voluntary muscular activity.

vestibular seizure. A brief epileptic episode in which the excitatory source is presumably in the receptors of the labyrinth.

vestibular system. VESTIBULAR APPARATUS.

vestibular vertigo. Vertigo that is presumed to arise from a disorder of the vestibular nerve or from the vestibular nuclei and their immediate connections.

vestibular window. An oval opening in the medial wall of the middle ear, closed by the foot plate of the stapes. Syn. *oval window*. NA *fenestra vestibuli*. See also Plate 20.

ves·ti·bule (ves'ti·bewl) *n.* [F., from L. *vestibulum*]. An approach; an antechamber.

vestibule of the ear. The oval cavity of the internal ear, which forms the entrance to the cochlea. NA *vestibulum auris internae*. See also Plate 20.

vestibule of the larynx. The portion of the cavity of the larynx above the vocal folds. NA *vestibulum laryngis*.

vestibule of the mouth. The space bounded internally by the teeth and gums, externally by the lips and cheeks. NA *vestibulum oris*.

vestibule of the nose. The skin-lined portion of each nasal cavity, between the naris and the limen nasi. NA *vestibulum nasi*.

vestibule of the vagina. The portion of the vulva bounded by the minor lips. NA *vestibulum vaginae*.

vestibulo-. A combining form meaning *vestibule, vestibular*.

ves·tib·u·lo·cer·e·bel·lar (ves·tib"yoo·lo·serr"e·bel'ur) *adj.* [*vestibulo-* + *cerebellar*]. Pertaining to vestibular fibers and the cerebellum.

vestibulocerebellar tract. A nerve tract of vestibular root fibers and secondary vestibular fibers that reach the fastigial nuclei in the cerebellum by way of the inferior cerebellar peduncle.

ves·tib·u·lo·coch·le·ar (ves·tib"yoo·lo·kock'lee·ur) *adj.* 1. Pertaining to the vestibule and the cochlea of the internal ear. 2. Pertaining to or comprising the vestibular and cochlear nerves.

vestibulocochlear ganglion. ACOUSTIC GANGLION.

vestibulocochlear nerve. The common trunk of the vestibular and cochlear nerves. Syn. *acoustic nerve, eighth cranial nerve*. NA *nervus vestibulocochlearis*. See also Table of Nerves in the Appendix.

vestibulolabyrinthine apparatus. VESTIBULAR APPARATUS.

ves·tib·u·lo·oc·u·lar (ves·tib"yoo·lo·ock'yoo·lur) *adj.* Pertaining to the vestibular and the ocular nerves.

vestibuloocular reflex. An acceleratory reflex, observed as a rotation of the eyes in the opposite direction when the head is quickly rotated, stimulating the semicircular canals. It can also be evoked by irrigation of external auditory meatus by hot or cold water.

vestibuloocular tract. A tract of homolateral and contralateral nerve fibers arising mainly from the superior and medial vestibular nuclei, which ascends in the medial longitudinal fasciculus to the nuclei of the oculomotor, trochlear, and abducent nerves; it mediates reflex movements of head and eyes.

ves·tib·u·lo·spi·nal (ves·tib"yoo·lo·spye'nul) *adj.* Pertaining to vestibular and spinal regions of the central nervous system.

vestibulospinal tract. A nerve tract that originates principally from the lateral vestibular nucleus and descends in the anterior funiculus of the spinal cord; it mediates impulses concerned with static equilibrium. NA *tractus vestibulospinalis*.

ves·tib·u·lot·o·my (ves·tib"yoo·lot'uh·mee) *n.* [*vestibulo-* + *-tomy*]. A surgical opening into the vestibule of the labyrinth.

ves·ti·bu·lum (ves·tib'yoo·lum) *n.*, genit. **vestibu·li** (·lye), pl. **vestibu·la** (·luh) [L.]. VESTIBULE.

vestibulum au·ris in·ter·nae (aw'ris in·tur'nee) [NA]. VESTIBULE OF THE EAR.

vestibulum bur·sae omen·ta·lis (bur'see o·men·tay'lis) [NA]. Vestibule of the omental bursa, the portion adjacent to the epiploic foramen.

vestibulum la·by·rin·thi os·sei (lab·i·rin'thigh os'ee·eye) [BNA]. Vestibulum auris internae (= VESTIBULE OF THE EAR).

vestibulum la·ryn·gis (la·rin'jis) [NA]. VESTIBULE OF THE LARYNX.

vestibulum na·si (nay'zye) [NA]. VESTIBULE OF THE NOSE.

vestibulum oris (o'ris) [NA]. VESTIBULE OF THE MOUTH.

vestibulum va·gi·nae (va·jye'nee) [NA]. VESTIBULE OF THE VAGINA.

ves·tige (ves'tij) *n.* [F., from L. *vestigium*, footprint]. A trace or remnant of something formerly present or more fully developed; a vestigium. —**ves·tig·ial** (ves·tij'ee·ul) *adj.*

vestigial fold of Marshall [J. *Marshall*]. LIGAMENT OF THE LEFT VENA CAVA.

vestigial muscle. A muscle that is rudimentary in man but well developed in lower animals.

ves·tig·i·um (ves·tij'ee·um) *n.*, pl. **vestig·ia** (·ee·uh) [L.]. An anatomic relic of fetal or embryonic life.

vestigium pro·ces·sus va·gi·na·lis (pro·ses'us vaj·i·nay'lis) [NA]. VAGINAL LIGAMENT.

Vestran. A trademark for prazepam, a muscle relaxant.

vest suture. A two-layer traction suture employed to anchor the urinary bladder neck or prostate to the perineum following radical prostate surgery or avulsion injuries of the membranous urethra.

Vesulong. Trademark for the antibacterial sulfonamide sulfazamet.

ve·ta (vay'tah, vee'tah) *n.* [Sp.]. ALTITUDE SICKNESS.

vet·er·i·nar·i·an (vet"ur·i·nerr'ee·un) *n.* A person who practices veterinary medicine.

vet·er·i·nary (vet'ur·i·nerr"ee) *adj. & n.* [L. *veterinarius*, from *veterinae*, beasts of burden]. 1. Pertaining to the practice of medicine with animals, especially domesticated animals. 2. VETERINARIAN.

veterinary ambulance. An ambulance designed to transport sick or injured animals.

veterinary dispensary. *In U.S. Army medicine*, an establishment providing for the care and treatment of animals not requiring hospitalization.

veterinary hospital. 1. A hospital for the care of animals. 2. *In military medicine*, a permanent animal hospital established at a military station and designed to serve only the needs of that hospital.

veterinary medicine. The branch of medical practice which treats of the diseases and injuries of animals.

veterinary surgeon. A person whose practice is limited to the treatment of domestic large and small animals, or to meat and food inspections on behalf of the national or state governments.

veterinary surgery. The surgery of animals.

V factor. A thermolabile factor found in blood, which is necessary for the growth of *Hemophilus influenzae*, and identified as diphosphoridine nucleotide, triphosphoridine nucleotide, or nicotinamide nucleoside.

V genes. Genes coding for the variable regions of immunoglobulin molecules. Contr. *C genes*.

vi·a·ble (vye'uh·bul) *adj.* [F., from *vie*, life]. Capable of living; likely to live. —**vi·a·bil·i·ty** (vye"uh·bil'i·tee) *n.*

Viadril. Trademark for sodium hydroxydione succinate, a steroid with hypnotic, mild analgesic, and, possibly, some amnesic action.

vi·al (vye'ul) *n.* [ME. *viole,* variant of *fiole,* phial, from Gk. *phialē*]. A small glass bottle.

Vi antigen (vee eye) *n.* [*vi*rulent]. One of the sheath or envelope antigens of enterobacteria, such as the *Salmonella,* which inhibit the agglutination of the organisms in O (somatic) antiserums.

vi·bes·ate (vye'bes·ate, vib'es·) *n.* A modified polyvinyl plastic applied in solution as a liquid spray to form an occlusive surgical dressing for burns, wounds, and other lesions.

vi·bex (vye'becks) *n.,* pl. **vi·bi·ces** (·bi·seez) [L., mark of a blow]. A linear hemorrhage giving the appearance that it was caused by a whiplash.

ví·bo·ra de la cruz (vee'bo·rah deh lah krooce') [Sp., lit., viper of the cross]. *Bothrops alternata,* a pit viper of southern South America.

Vibramycin. Trademark for doxycycline, a tetracycline antibiotic.

vi·bra·tile (vye'bruh·til, ·tile) *adj.* Characterized by an oscillating movement; vibratory.

vibrating epithelium. CILIATED EPITHELIUM.

vi·bra·tion (vye·bray'shun) *n.* [L. *vibratio,* from *vibrare,* to shake, quiver]. Oscillation; a rapid fluctuation; a periodic movement in alternately opposite directions from a position of equilibrium. **—vi·brate** (vye'brate) *v.;* **vi·brat·ing** (vye'bray·ting) *adj.*

vibration treatment. Massage by rapid shaking of the body or a part, maintained by a mechanical machine or oscillator.

vi·bra·tor (vye'bray·tur) *n.* A device for conveying mechanical vibration to a part.

vi·bra·to·ry (vye'bruh·tor·ee) *adj.* Characterized by vibrations.

vibratory massage. Light, rapid percussion either by hand or by an electric apparatus.

vibratory sense. A composite sensation, comprising touch and rapid alterations of deep pressure sense. Its conduction depends upon both cutaneous and deep afferent fibers that ascend in the dorsal columns of the cord. It is elicited by placing a vibrating tuning fork over the bony prominences of the body.

Vib·rio (vib'ree·o) *n.* [NL., from L. *vibrare,* to shake, quiver]. A genus of bacteria of the family Spirillaceae; being typically short, bent, motile rods, single or united end to end in spirals. Many species liquefy gelatin.

vibrio, *n.* 1. Any bacterium of the genus *Vibrio.* 2. Any curved, motile microorganism.

Vibrio chol·e·rae (kol'e·ree). The causative organism of cholera. Formerly called *Vibrio comma.*

Vibrio com·ma (kom'uh). *VIBRIO CHOLERAE.*

Vibrio fe·tus (fee'tus). The species of bacteria that causes vibriosis.

vi·bri·on sep·tique (vee·bree·ohn sep·teek') [F.]. *CLOSTRIDIUM SEPTICUM.*

vi·bri·o·sis (vib''ree·o'sis) *n.,* pl. **vibrio·ses** (·seez) [*Vibrio* + *-osis*]. An infectious disease, primarily of cattle, sheep, and goats, caused by *Vibrio fetus* and characterized by abortion, retained placenta, and metritis; occasionally a disease in humans, primarily infants, including enteritis and bacteremia.

vi·bris·sa (vye·bris'uh, vi·) *n.,* pl. **vibris·sae** (·ee) [L. *vibrissae,* hairs in the nose, from *vibrare,* to quiver]. 1. One of the hairs in the vestibule of the nose. 2. One of the long, coarse hairs on the face of certain animals, such as the whiskers of a cat.

vi·bro·car·dio·gram (vye''bro·kahr'dee·o·gram) *n.* [L. *vibr*are, to shake, + *cardiogram*]. The graphic display of heart sound vibrations.

vi·bro·mas·sage (vye''bro·muh·sahj') *n.* VIBRATORY MASSAGE.

vi·bur·num opu·lus (vye·bur'num op'yoo·lus). The dried bark of *Viburnum opulus,* preparations of which have been used empirically in various menstrual disorders. Syn. *high-bush cranberry bark, true cramp bark.*

viburnum pru·ni·fo·li·um (proo''ni·fo'lee·um) [L., the wayfaring tree]. The dried bark of the root or stem of *Viburnum prunifolium* or *V. rufidulum,* preparations of which have been used to treat various uterine disorders and as a general antispasmodic. Syn. *blackhaw.*

vi·car·i·ous (vye·kăr'ee·us) *adj.* [L. *vicarius,* from *vice,* in place of, instead]. Taking the place of something else; said of a habitual discharge occurring in an abnormal situation.

vicarious menstruation. The discharge of blood at the time of menstruation from some place other than the vagina, as in endometriosis.

vice, *n.* [OF., from L. *vitium*]. 1. A physical defect. 2. Depravity. 3. Immorality. **—vi·cious** (vish'us) *adj.*

Vi·chy water (vish'ee, F. vee·shee'). A mildly laxative and antacid mineral water obtained from Vichy, France.

vi·ci·a·nose (vis'ee·uh·noce) *n.* A disaccharide, $C_{11}H_{20}O_{10}$, which, on hydrolysis, yields *l*-arabinose and dextrose.

vi·cious (vish'us) *adj.* [OF., from L. *vitiosus*]. Faulty, defective, badly formed.

vicious union. The healing of a fracture in improper position, with resulting deformity.

Vicq d'Azyr's bundle or **fasciculus** (veek daʰ·zeer') [F. *Vicq D'Azyr,* French anatomist, 1748–1794]. MAMILLOTHALAMIC TRACT.

Vicq d'Azyr's foramen [F. *Vicq D'Azyr*]. FORAMEN CECUM (2).

Vicq d'Azyr's tract [F. *Vicq D'Azyr*]. MAMILLOTHALAMIC TRACT.

Vicryl. A trademark for polyglactin, an absorbable suture material.

Vic·to·ria blue. A basic triphenylmethane dye used for staining viruses and other plant and animal tissues.

vid·ar·a·bine (vid·ăr'uh·been) *n.* ADENINE ARABINOSIDE.

vid·e·og·no·sis (vid''ee·og·no'sis) *n.* [*video,* from L. *videre,* to see, + *-gnosis*]. Television transmission of x-ray pictures; makes possible long-distance consultation and diagnosis.

Vid·i·an artery (vid'ee·un) [V. *Vidius* (Guido Guidi), Italian physician, 1500–1569]. The maxillary artery. See Table of Arteries in the Appendix.

Vidian canal [V. *Vidius*]. PTERYGOID CANAL.

Vidian nerve [V. *Vidius*]. The nerve of the pterygoid canal.

Vi·en·na green. PARIS GREEN.

Vier·ordt's hemotachometer (feer'ort) [K. *Vierordt,* German physiologist, 1818–1884]. An apparatus for blood flow measurement.

Vieus·sens' annulus (vyœh·sahⁿss') [R. *Vieussens,* French anatomist, 1641–1716]. ANNULUS OVALIS.

Vieussens' ansa [R. *Vieussens*]. ANSA SUBCLAVIA.

Vieussens' centrum ovale [R. *Vieussens*]. CENTRUM OVALE.

vi·fil·con A (vye·fil'kon). a copolymer of methacrylic acid, 2-hydroxyethyl methacrylate, ethylene dimethacrylate, and 1-vinyl-2-pyrrolidinone, a hydrophilic contact lens material.

vig·il (vij'il) *n.* [L. *vigilia,* from *vigil,* watchful, wakeful]. Watchful wakefulness; a period of sleeplessness.

vig·il·am·bu·lism (vij''il·amb'yoo·liz·um) *n.* [*vigil* + L. *ambulare,* to walk, + *-ism*]. Ambulatory automatism in the waking state.

vig·i·lance (vij'i·lunce) *n.* [L. *vigilantia*]. The state of being awake, alert.

Villaret's syndrome [N. *Villaret,* French neurologist, 1877–1946]. Ipsilateral paralysis of the ninth, tenth, eleventh, and twelfth cranial nerves and of the cervical sympathetic fibers (Horner's syndrome) due to a lesion in the posterior retroparotid space. Similar to the Collet-Sicard syndrome.

villi. Plural of *villus.*

villi in·tes·ti·na·les (in·tes·ti·nay'leez) [NA]. INTESTINAL VILLI.

vil·lik·i·nin (vi·lick'i·nin) *n.* A substance, present in acid extracts of intestinal mucosa, that produces strong movements of the intestinal villi.

villi pleu·ra·les (ploo·ray'leez) [BNA]. Occasional small appendages of pleura from the inferior border of the lung or in the costomediastinal sinus.

villi sy·no·vi·a·les (si·no·vee·ay'leez) [NA]. SYNOVIAL VILLI.

vil·li·tis (vi·lye'tis) *n.* [*vill*us + *-itis*]. Inflammation of the laminas of the corium of a horse's hoof.

vil·lo·si·tis (vil''o·sigh'tis) *n.* [L. *villos*us, shaggy, villous, + *-itis*]. Inflammation of the villous surface of the placenta.

vil·lous (vil'us) *adj.* [*vill*us + *-ous*]. Pertaining to a villus; covered with villi; characterized by villus-like projections.

villous adenoma. A slow-growing potentially malignant neoplasm of the intestinal, usually colonic, mucosa; may be clinically manifested by bleeding and large volumes of mucoid diarrhea with high potassium content.

villous carcinoma. A type of papillary carcinoma in which the papillae are exceptionally long and grossly of velvety appearance.

villous synovitis. A type of synovitis in which villous growths develop within the articular cavity.

villous tenosynovitis. A chronic inflammatory reaction of a tendon sheath producing thickening of the lining with the formation of redundant folds and villi.

vil·lus (vil'us) *n.*, pl. **vil·li** (·eye) [L., shaggy hair]. A minute, elongated projection from the surface of a mucous membrane or other membrane.

vil·lus·ec·to·my (vil''us·eck'tuh·mee) *n.* [*villus* + *-ectomy*]. Synovectomy; surgical excision of a hypertrophied fold of the synovial membrane of a joint.

vi·lox·a·zine (vi·lock'suh·zeen) *n.* 2-[(*o*-Ethoxyphenoxy)-methyl]morpholine, $C_{13}H_{19}NO_3$, an antidepressant, used as the hydrochloride salt.

vin·bar·bi·tal (vin·bahr'bi·tol, ·tal) *n.* 5-Ethyl-5-(1-methyl-1-butenyl)barbituric acid, $C_{11}H_{16}N_2O_3$, a barbituate with intermediate duration of action; used also as the sodium derivative.

vin·blas·tine (vin·blas'teen) *n.* An alkaloid, $C_{46}H_{58}N_4O_9$, from the periwinkle plant, *Vinca rosea;* an antineoplastic drug, used as the sulfate salt. Syn. *vincaleukoblastine.*

vin·ca·leu·ko·blas·tine (vink''uh·lew''ko·blas'teen) *n.* VINBLASTINE.

Vin·cent's angina (væⁿ·sahⁿ', angl. vin'sunt) [J. H. *Vincent,* French bacteriologist, 1862–1950]. 1. VINCENT'S INFECTION, involving the pharyngeal and tonsillar tissues. 2. VINCENT'S INFECTION, in general.

Vincent's gingivitis [J. H. *Vincent*]. NECROTIZING ULCERATIVE GINGIVITIS.

Vincent's infection or **disease** [J. H. *Vincent*]. A noncontagious infection principally of the oral mucosa, characterized by ulceration and formation of a gray pseudomembrane. Fusiform bacteria *(Fusobacterium fusiforme)* and spirochetes (principally *Borrelia vincenti),* always in association with other microorganisms, are present in abundance but are not known to be causally involved. See also *Vincent's angina, necrotizing ulcerative gingivitis.*

Vincent's stomatitis [J. H. *Vincent*]. An extension of necrotizing ulcerative gingivitis to other oral tissues. See also *Vincent's angina.*

vin·co·fos (vin'ko·fos) *n.* 2,2-Dichlorovinyl methyl octyl phosphate, $C_{11}H_{21}Cl_2O_4P$, an anthelmintic.

vin·cris·tine (vin·kris'teen) *n.* An alkaloid, $C_{46}H_{56}N_4O_{10}$, from the periwinkle plant, *Vinca rosea;* an antineoplastic drug, differing from vinblastine in its spectrum of activity, used as the sulfate salt. Syn. *leurocristine.*

vincula. Plural of *vinculum.*

vincula lin·gu·lae ce·re·bel·li (ling'gew·lee serr·e·bel'eye) [BNA]. Prolongations from the lingula of the cerebellum.

vincula ten·di·num di·gi·to·rum ma·nus (ten'di·num dij·i·to'rum man'us) [NA]. The slender tendinous filaments that connect the phalanges with the flexor tendons of the fingers.

vincula tendinum digitorum pe·dis (ped'is) [NA]. The slender tendinous filaments that connect the phalanges with the flexor tendons of the toes.

vin·cu·lum (vink'yoo·lum) *n.*, pl. **vincu·la** (·luh) [L., bond, cord, from *vincire,* to bind, restrain]. A ligament or frenum.

vinculum bre·ve (brev'ee) [NA]. A short vinculum or a short filament.

vinculum lon·gum (long'gum) [NA]. A long vinculum or long filament.

vinculum ten·di·num (ten'di·num) [BNA]. VINCULA TENDINUM DIGITORUM MANUS.

vin·de·sine (vin'de·seen) *n.* 3-Carbamoyl-4-deacetyl-3-di-(methoxycarbonyl)vincaleukoblastine, $C_{43}H_{55}N_5O_7$, an antineoplastic.

Vine·berg operation or **procedure** [A. *Vineberg,* Canadian surgeon, 20th century]. Implantation of the internal thoracic artery and vein into the ventricular myocardium; a procedure for myocardial revascularization in severe coronary atherosclerotic heart disease.

vin·e·gar, *n.* [OF. *vinaigre,* from *vin,* wine, + *aigre,* sour]. 1. A weak (approximately 6%) solution of acetic acid containing coloring matter and other substances (esters, mineral matter, etc.) formed by fermentation of alcoholic liquids and commonly obtained from fruit juices or other sugar-containing liquids that have first undergone alcoholic fermentation. The process involves the oxidation of ethyl alcohol, forming acetic acid as the final product. 2. A pharmaceutical preparation obtained by macerating a drug with diluted acetic acid and filtering.

Vine·land social maturity scale. A psychologic test designed to measure social maturity, based on the presence or absence of certain common social behaviors characteristic of specified age groups; used with children and with other individuals when more sophisticated psychologic tests cannot be carried out.

vin·gly·cin·ate (vin·glye'si·nate) *n.* Deacetylvincaleukoblastine 4-(*N,N*-dimethylglycinate), $C_{48}H_{63}N_5O_9$, an antineoplastic agent; used as the sulfate salt. Compare *vinblastine.*

vin·leu·ro·sine (vin·lew'ro·seen) *n.* An alkaloid, derived from *Vinca rosea,* Linn., that has antineoplastic activity; used as the sulfate salt.

vin·ro·si·dine (vin·ro'si·dine) *n.* An alkaloid, derived from *Vinca rosea,* Linn., that has antineoplastic activity; used as the sulfate salt.

Vinson-Plummer syndrome [P. P. *Vinson,* U.S. physician, 1890–1959; and H. S. *Plummer*]. PLUMMER-VINSON SYNDROME.

vi·nyl (vye'nil, vin'il) *n.* The univalent organic radical $H_2C{=}CH{-}$.

vi·nyl·ene (vye'ni·leen) *n.* The bivalent organic radical $-CH{=}CH-$.

vinyl ether. Divinyl ether, $(CH_2{=}CH{-})_2O$, a volatile liquid used as a general anesthetic for short operative procedures and as an adjunct to other anesthetics when the operation is of longer duration.

vi·nyl·i·dene (vye·nil'i·deen) *n.* The bivalent organic radical $H_2C{=}C{=}$.

Viocin. A trademark for viomycin, an antibiotic used as the sulfate salt for the treatment of tuberculosis.

Vioform. Trademark for iodochlorhydroxyquin, a local anti-infective agent.

vi·o·la·ceous (vye''o·lay'shus) *adj.* Violet; said of a discoloration, usually of the skin.

vi·o·la·quer·ci·trin (vye''o·luh·kwur'si·trin) *n.* RUTIN.

vi·o·la·tion (vye''uh·lay'shun) *n.* [L. *violatio,* from *violare,* to outrage]. 1. RAPE; the act of violating or ravishing. 2. *In legal medicine,* the act of coitus without violence or force but by means of deception, by the influence of alcohol or drugs, or by intimidation.

vi·o·let blindness. AMIANTHINOPSY.

vi·o·my·cin (vye''o·migh'sin) *n.* A polypeptide antibiotic substance or a mixture of substances produced by strains of *Streptomyces griseus* var. *purpureus* (more commonly called *Streptomyces puniceus*); used as the sulfate salt, intramuscularly administered, for treatment of tuberculosis resistant to other therapy.

vi·os·ter·ol (vye·os′tur·ole, ·ol) *n.* Vitamin D_2 or CALCIFEROL; now officially designated ergocalciferol.

Vio-Thene. A trademark for oxyphencyclimine, an anticholinergic drug used as the hydrochloride salt.

vi·per (vye′pur) *n.* [L. *vipera*]. Any of various poisonous snakes of the family Viperidae.

Vi·pera (vye′pur·uh) *n.* [L.]. A genus of the family Viperidae or true vipers.

Vipera rus·sel·lii (ruh·sel′ee·eye). One of the most important species of venomous snakes of Asia. Syn. *ticpolonga, daboia.*

Vi·per·i·dae (vye·perr′i·dee) *n. pl.* A family of venomous snakes possessing long, curved, movable front fangs which can be erected when striking. Some Viperidae are: *Vipera berus,* the European viper; *V. russellii,* Russell's viper; *Bitis gabonica,* Gaboon viper; *B. lachesis,* puff adder; *B. nasicornis,* rhinoceros viper; *Echis carinatus,* saw-scaled viper; night adders of the genus *Causus; Aspis cornutus,* horned viper.

Vira-A. A trademark for vidarabine, an antiviral.

viraemia. VIREMIA.

vi·ral (vye′rul) *adj.* [*vir*us + *-al*]. Belonging to, caused by, or involving a virus.

viral gastroenteritis or **enteritis.** An acute sporadic epidemic self-limited infectious gastroenteritis with negative bacteriologic studies, characterized by diarrhea, nausea, vomiting, and variable systemic symptoms. Various viruses have been implicated, including echoviruses and parvoviruses.

viral hepatitis. See *infectious hepatitis, serum hepatitis.*

Virazole. A trademark for ribavirin, an antiviral.

Vir·chow cell (firr^{k}h′o, virr^{k}h′o) [R. L. K. *Virchow,* German pathologist, 1821–1902]. LEPRA CELL.

Virchow-Robin spaces [R. L. K. *Virchow* and C. P. *Robin*]. PERIVASCULAR SPACES OF VIRCHOW-ROBIN.

Virchow's angle [R. L. K. *Virchow*]. The angle formed by the union of a line joining the nasofrontal suture and the most prominent point of the lower edge of the superior alveolar process with a line joining the same point and the superior border of the external auditory meatus.

Virchow's crystals [R. L. K. *Virchow*]. HEMATOIDIN CRYSTALS.

Virchow's law [R. L. K. *Virchow*]. All cells are derived from preexisting cellular elements.

Virchow's line [R. L. K. *Virchow*]. A line from the root of the nose to the lambda.

Virchow's node [R. L. K. *Virchow*]. SIGNAL NODE.

Virchow's spaces [R. L. K. *Virchow*]. PERIVASCULAR SPACES OF VIRCHOW-ROBIN.

vi·re·mia, vi·rae·mia (vye·ree′mee·uh) *n.* [*vir*us + *-emia*]. The presence of a virus in the bloodstream.

vires. Plural of *vis.*

vir·gin (vur′jin) *n.* [L. *virgo, virginis*]. 1. A female who has never experienced sexual intercourse as normally understood; medicolegally, perforation of the hymen need not have occurred for loss of virginity. 2. A person of either sex who has not experienced sexual intercourse. —**virgin·al** (·ul) *adj.*; **vir·gin·i·ty** (vur·jin′i·tee) *n.*

vir·gin·ia·my·cin (vur·jin″yuh·mye′sin) *n.* An antibiotic consisting of two factors, M_1 and S_1, produced by *Streptomyces virginiae;* used as a veterinary food additive.

vir·i·dans streptococci (virr′i·danz). A group of streptococci including strains not causing beta hemolysis, although many members cause alpha hemolysis; they do not elaborate a C substance and therefore cannot be classified by the Lancefield method. Both pathogenic and saprophytic organisms are involved, the former often being isolated in conditions such as subacute bacterial endocarditis, bronchopneumonia, urinary-tract infections, and focal inflammations.

vi·rid·o·ful·vin (vi·rid″o·ful′vin) *n.* An antibiotic, derived from *Streptomyces viridogriseus,* that has antifungal activity.

vir·ile (virr′il) *adj.* [L. *virilis,* manly, from *vir,* man]. Pertaining to, or characteristic of, the male.

virile reflex. 1. PENILE REFLEX. 2. A sudden downward movement of the penis when the prepuce or glans of the relaxed organ is pulled upward.

vir·i·les·cence (virr″i·les′unce) *n.* The acquiring of characters more or less like those of the male.

vir·i·lism (virr′i·liz·um) *n.* [*virile* + *-ism*]. 1. Masculinity; the development of male traits or characteristics in the female. 2. FEMALE PSEUDOHERMAPHRODITISM.

vir·i·lis·mus (virr″i·liz′mus) *n.* VIRILISM.

vi·ril·i·ty (vi·ril′i·tee) *n.* [L. *virilitas*]. 1. The condition of being virile. 2. Sexual potency.

vir·il·iza·tion (virr″i·li·zay′shun) *n.* The assumption or appearance of male secondary sexual characters.

vir·il·iz·ing (virr″i·lye′zing) *adj.* 1. Producing male secondary sex characters. 2. Producing virility.

virilizing lipoid-cell tumor. ADRENOCORTICOID ADENOMA OF THE OVARY.

vi·ri·on (vye′ree·on) *n.* The complete, mature virus particle, identical to the infectious unit.

vi·rip·o·tent (vi·rip′o·tunt, vye·) *adj.* [L. *vir,* man, + *potens,* powerful]. Of the human male, sexually mature.

vi·ro·cyte (vye′ro·site) *n. Obsol.* An atypical lymphocyte resembling those seen in infectious mononucleosis, present in some cases of viral diseases, such as influenza, infectious hepatitis, and acute respiratory disease.

vi·rol·o·gist (vi·rol′o·jist, vye·) *n.* A person who studies viruses and virus diseases.

vi·rol·o·gy (vi·rol′o·jee, vye·) *n.* [*vir*us + *-logy*]. The study of viruses and virus diseases.

vi·ro·pex·is (vye″ro·peck′sis) *n.* [*vir*us + *pexis*]. The mechanism by which animal viruses enter the host cell intact, thought to be through phagocytosis into vacuoles.

Viroptic. A trademark for trifluridine, an ophthalmic antiviral.

vir·tu·al (vur′choo·ul) *adj.* [ML. *virtualis,* from L. *virtus,* virtue, capacity]. 1. Being a specified kind of thing in effect, or by way of function, but not in fact, as a virtual focus. 2. Formed of virtual foci, as a virtual image.

virtual focus. The point at which divergent rays would meet if prolonged in a backward direction. Syn. *negative focus.*

virtual image. The image of an object, such as that seen in a plane mirror, formed of diverging rays which are prolonged backward until they meet at a point. An image formed of virtual foci.

vi·ru·ci·dal (vye″ruh·sigh′dul) *adj.* [*virus* + *cidal*]. Having a destructive effect upon a virus or viruses.

vi·ru·ci·din (vye″ruh·sigh′din, virr″yoo·) *n.* [*virus* + *-cide* + *-in*]. An agent capable of destroying a virus.

vir·u·lence (virr′yoo·unce) *n.* [L. *virulentia,* from *virulentus,* poisonous]. Malignancy; noxiousness; infectiousness. The disease-producing power of a microorganism. —**viru·lent** (·lunt) *adj.*

vi·rus (vye′rus) *n.* [L., poison]. Any of a vast group of minute structures, in the range of 250 to 10 nm, composed of a sheath of protein encasing a core of nucleic acids (deoxyribonucleic or ribonucleic acids), capable of infecting almost all members of the animal and plant kingdoms, including bacteria (bacteriophage), characterized by a total dependence on living cells for reproduction, and lacking independent metabolism. Heterogeneous in form and function, viruses may be considered as either living objects or inert chemicals, and a growing number have been crystallized.

vi·rus·cyte (vye′rus·site) *n.* [*virus* + *-cyte*]. VIROCYTE.

virus meningitis. Aseptic meningitis caused by a virus, such as nonparalytic poliomyelitis, Coxsackie, echo, and mumps viruses.

virus of Car·re′ (ka^{h}·re^{y}′). The virus originally described by

Carré in 1905 as the primary cause of canine distemper.
virus pneumonia. Pneumonia caused by one of a number of viruses, such as influenza viruses, adenovirus, and respiratory syncytial virus.
vi·ru·stat·ic (vye″ruh·stat′ick) *adj.* [*virus* + *-static*]. Having a disruptive effect upon a virus or viruses.
virus vac·ci·num (vack·sigh′num). SMALLPOX VACCINE.
vis (vis) *n.*, pl. **vi·res** (vye′reez) [L.]. Force; energy; power.
vis a fron·te (a fron′tee) [L.]. 1. A force that attracts or a force pulling from the front. 2. The factors promoting return of blood to the right side of the heart.
vis·am·min (vis·am′in) *n.* KHELLIN.
vis a ter·go (a tur′go) [L.]. 1. A force that pushes something before it, or a force that pushes from behind. 2. The function of the left ventricular pump in returning blood to the right side of the heart.
viscera. Plural of *viscus.* See also Plates 13, 14, 25.
vis·cer·al (vis′ur·ul) *adj.* Pertaining to a viscus or to the viscera.
visceral arch. 1. One of the series of mesodermal ridges covered by epithelium bounding the lateral wall of the oral and pharyngeal region of vertebrates; embryonic in higher forms, they contribute to the formation of the face and neck. 2. The skeleton of a visceral arch. 3. In gill-bearing vertebrates, one of the first two arches as opposed to the remaining or branchial arches.
visceral brain. LIMBIC LOBE.
visceral cleft. An embryonic fissure between the visceral arches, produced by rupture of the closing plate between a pharyngeal pouch and its corresponding external visceral groove.
visceral cranium. The portion of the skull which forms the face and jaws.
visceral crisis. Lightning pains referable to a viscus, seen in tabes dorsalis. See also *gastric crisis, nephralgic crisis, clitoris crisis, rectal crisis, vesical crisis.*
visceral ectopia. A congenital hernia into the umbilical cord.
visceral epilepsy. CONVULSIVE EQUIVALENT.
vis·cer·al·gia (vis″ur·al′jee·uh) *n.* [*viscera* + *-algia*]. Pain in a viscus.
visceral groove. The external groove or furrow between two embryonic visceral arches, lined by ectoderm. Syn. *branchial groove, pharyngeal groove.*
visceral larva migrans. 1. The migration of nematode larvae, especially ascarids such as *Toxocara canis* and *Toxocara cati* through the kidney, brain, eye, or other tissues of the host species. 2. A disease of young children, calves, and puppies produced by the migration of ascarid larvae through various body tissues.
visceral leishmaniasis. KALA AZAR.
visceral lymphomatosis. A form of the avian leukosis complex affecting primarily the liver and kidney and to a lesser extent all organs of the body.
visceral muscle. 1. A muscle of a viscus. 2. A muscle associated with the visceral skeleton.
visceral nerve. Any nerve supplying a visceral structure.
visceral nervous system. AUTONOMIC NERVOUS SYSTEM.
visceral pericardium. EPICARDIUM.
visceral pleura. PULMONARY PLEURA.
visceral pouch. PHARYNGEAL POUCH.
visceral reflex. Any reflex induced by a stimulus applied to an internal organ.
visceral sensation. Any crude sensation appreciated as coming from the internal organs or viscera, such as pain or a feeling of distention or fullness.
visceral skeleton. The part of the skeleton that encloses pelvic and thoracic viscera: the pelvis, ribs, and sternum.
viscero-. A combining form meaning *viscus, viscera, visceral.*
vis·cero·car·di·ac (vis″ur·o·kahr′dee·ack) *adj.* [*viscero-* + *cardiac*]. Pertaining to the viscera and the heart.
viscerocardiac reflex. Alteration in the activity of the heart in response to stimulation of an internal organ.
vis·cero·cep·tor (vis″ur·o·sep′tur) *n.* [*viscero-* + *receptor*]. INTEROCEPTOR.
vis·cero·in·hib·i·to·ry (vis″ur·o·in·hib′i·tor·ee) *adj.* Inhibiting the movements of viscera.
vis·cero·meg·a·ly (vis″ur·o·meg′uh·lee) *n.* [*viscero-* + *megaly*]. SPLANCHNOMEGALY.
visceromotor reflex. Tensing of skeletal muscles evoked by stimuli originating in the viscera, especially the contraction of the muscles of the abdominal wall resulting from visceral pain.
vis·cer·op·to·sis (vis″ur·op·to′sis) *n.* [*viscero-* + *-ptosis*]. Prolapse of a viscus, especially of the intestine; downward displacement of the intestine in the abdominal cavity; once considered clinically significant.
vis·cero·sen·so·ry (vis″ur·o·sen′suh·ree) *adj.* [*viscero-* + *sensory*]. Pertaining to sensation in the viscera.
viscerosensory reflex. A form of referred pain in which stimuli within the viscera cause a painful sensation when touch or pressure is applied to some superficial region of the body.
vis·cero·tome (vis′ur·o·tome) *n.* [*viscero-* + *-tome*]. 1. An instrument used only in postmortem examinations to secure specimens of the liver or other internal organ. 2. The areas of the viscera supplied with sensory fibers from a single spinal nerve.
vis·cer·ot·o·my (vis″ur·ot′uh·mee) *n.* [*viscero-* + *-tomy*]. The process of cutting out a piece of liver or other internal organ with the viscerotome.
vis·cero·to·nia (vis″ur·o·to′nee·uh) *n.* [*viscero-* + *-tonia*]. The behavioral counterpart of component I (endomorphy) of the somatotype, manifested predominantly by a desire for assimilation and the conservation of energy through sociability, relaxation, and love of food. —**viscero·ton·ic** (·ton′ick) *adj.*
vis·cero·troph·ic (vis″ur·o·trof′ick) *adj.* Pertaining to trophic changes induced by visceral conditions.
vis·cero·tro·pic (vis″ur·o·tro′pick, ·trop′ick) *adj.* [*viscero-* + *-tropic*]. Attracted to or seeking the viscera.
vis·cid (vis′id) *adj.* [L. *viscidus*]. Adhesive; glutinous.
vis·cid·i·ty (vi·sid′i·tee) *n.* The quality or state of being viscid.
vis·co·liz·er (vis′ko·lye″zur) *n.* [L. *viscosus,* sticky]. A machine used in reduction of size of fat particles, or in homogenization of a mixture or tissue. See also *homogenizer.*
vis·com·e·ter (vis·kom′e·tur) *n.* VISCOSIMETER.
vis con·ser·va·trix (kon·sur·vay′tricks). The natural strength of an organism to resist disease or injury.
vis·co·sim·e·ter (vis″ko·sim′e·tur) *n.* [*viscosity* + *-meter*]. An apparatus for determining the degree of viscosity of a fluid.
vis·cos·i·ty (vis·kos′i·tee) *n.* [ML. *viscositas,* from L. *viscosus,* viscous]. The resistance that a liquid exhibits to the flow of one layer over another. The property of offering resistance to a change of form, arising from the molecular attraction between the molecules of a liquid.
viscosity-effusion meter. An instrument for determining the concentration of anesthetic gases during surgical anesthesia.
vis·cous (vis′kus) *adj.* Glutinous; sticky; semifluid; having high viscosity.
vis·cus (vis′kus) *n.*, pl. **vis·cera** (vis′ur·uh) [L.]. Any one of the organs enclosed within one of the four great cavities, the cranium, thorax, abdomen, or pelvis; especially an organ within the abdominal cavity. See also Plates 13, 14, 25.
vis for·ma·ti·va (for·muh·tye′vuh). Energy manifesting itself in the formation of new tissue to replace that which has been destroyed.
vis·i·bil·i·ty limit. 1. The maximum distance to which prominent objects, such as trees or houses, located in a definite direction and viewed against the horizon sky, are visible to an observer of normal eyesight under existing conditions of atmosphere, light, etc. For an object to be regarded as visible, it must be recognized by the observer, who has

previous knowledge of its character from having seen it on occasions when the atmosphere was clear. 2. *In physiologic optics,* minimum visible or minimal separable acuity.

vis·i·ble spectrum. The wavelengths of light between the range of 400 to 750 nm.

vis in·er·ti·ae (i·nur'shee·ee). The force by virtue of which a body at rest tends to remain at rest.

vis in situ. Intrinsic force due to position.

vi·sion (vizh'un) *n.* [L. *visio,* from *videre,* to see]. 1. The act of seeing; sight. 2. The capacity or ability to see. 3. Loosely, visual acuity. 4. A mental image. 5. *In psychiatry,* a hallucinatory phenomenon in which the patient sees something not actually present. 6. A dream.

vision test. Any test for visual acuity, as the Abridged A. O. color vision test, afterimage test, color threshold test, Holmgren test, Ishihara's test, Nagel's test, Pugh's test, red lens test, or Snellen test.

vis·it·ing nurse. A nurse working for an official or voluntary community health agency who provides care to families in their homes.

visiting staff. ATTENDING STAFF.

visiting surgeon. A surgeon whose duties require regular attendance at a hospital or dispensary as well as emergency visits to operate upon or care for patients himself or to supervise the care given by house surgeons.

Visken. A trademark for pindolol, a vasodilator.

vis me·di·ca·trix na·tu·rae (med·i·kay'tricks na·tew'ree). The healing power of nature apart from medicinal treatment.

vis·na (vis'nuh) *n.* A chronic disease of the central nervous system of sheep, observed in Iceland and caused by a conventional RNA virus with a long incubation period, during which the animal appears well. It was in relation to this disease that Sigurdsson first used the term "slow infection."

Vistaril. Trademark for the tranquilizer hydroxyzine pamoate.

vi·su·al (vizh'yoo·ul) *adj.* [L. *visualis,* from *visus,* sight, vision, from *videre,* to see]. 1. Pertaining to sight. 2. Producing mental images.

visual acuity. The measured central vision, dependent upon the clarity of the retinal focus, integrity of the nervous elements, and cerebral interpretation of a given stimulus at a given distance as tested with a Snellen or similar chart; the result is usually expressed as a fraction with the numerator the distance at which the test was performed and the denominator the distance at which the symbol (letter, picture, E) should be seen by a normal eye. In the U.S.A. using Snellen's letter chart at 20 feet, normal visual acuity is 20/20.

visual agnosia. A condition characterized by inability to name a seen object or to indicate its use by gesture, despite intactness of vision, clarity of mind, and absence of aphasia. See also *visual object agnosia, visual verbal agnosia.*

visual allesthesia. Displacement of an image to the opposite half of the visual field; seen in patients with gross unilateral field defects and diffuse brain disease, but also in severe psychotic states and in migraine.

visual alternans. *Obsol.* Pulsation of the aorta and left ventricle with alternating weak and strong displacement when viewed fluoroscopically.

visual amnesia. VISUAL APHASIA; the patient recognizes the object by sight but cannot name it.

visual angle. The angle at the eye subtended by the extremities of the object viewed. Syn. *optic angle.*

visual aphasia. A condition which was described and named by C. S. Freund in 1889, and which consists of an inability to name an object clearly seen until it has been perceived through some other sense, such as tactile, auditory, or olfactory. The patient recognizes the object by sight but cannot name it. Syn. *optic aphasia, intercortical sensory aphasia of Starr.*

visual area, center, or **cortex.** 1. The visual projection area and visuopsychic area of the cerebral cortex. 2. Sometimes applied to include the lateral geniculate bodies and the superior colliculi.

visual aura. The initial event of a seizure which consists either of unformed visual images, such as flashes or balls of light, suggesting an occipital lobe origin, or of formed visual images, such as persons, suggesting a temporal lobe origin.

visual axis. The line of vision; a line connecting the fixation point and fovea and passing through the nodal point of the eye. Compare *geometrical axis.*

visual cell. One of the rods or cones of the retina.

visual field. FIELD OF VISION.

visual fixation. FIXATION (3).

visual hearing. The understanding of speech by means of visual impulses. See also *lip reading.*

vi·su·al·iza·tion (vizh''yoo·ul·i·zay'shun) *n.* 1. Perceiving images in the mind with such distinctness that they seem to be seen by the eyes. 2. The act of making visible or of becoming visible, as by means of a microscope, x-ray photograph, otoscope, or other indirect means.

visual line. VISUAL AXIS.

visual-motor, *adj.* VISUOMOTOR.

visual-motor gestalt test. BENDER GESTALT TEST.

visual object agnosia. The inability to recognize objects by sight in spite of adequate vision; may be total or may pertain only to inanimate objects, to all animate objects, to a person's body or any part or side of it, or to the attributes, such as form, color, or dimensions of objects; lesions in the visuopsychic area are considered to be responsible. Syn. *nonsymbolic visual agnosia.*

visual plane. A plane that passes through the axis of vision of both eyes.

visual pragmatagnosia. VISUAL AGNOSIA.

visual pragmatamnesia. 1. Inability to recall the visual image of an object. 2. VISUAL AGNOSIA.

visual projection area. The cortical receptive center for visual impulses, located in the walls and margins of the calcarine sulcus of the occipital lobe, characterized by the stripe (stria) of Gennari. Syn. *Brodmann's area 17, striate area.*

visual purple. RHODOPSIN.

visual receptive aphasia. VISUAL APHASIA.

visual seizure. VISUAL AURA.

visual sensory aphasia. VISUAL APHASIA.

visual verbal agnosia. The inability to recognize words or fractions of words (agnostic alexia), musical symbols, or numbers and other mathematical symbols, in spite of adequate vision, usually due to a lesion in the angular gyrus or connections thereof with other cortical regions such as Wernicke's and Broca's areas. Syn. *symbolic visual agnosia.*

visual violet. IODOPSIN.

visual white. LEUKOPSIN.

visual yellow. An intermediary substance formed in the retina from rhodopsin after exposure to light first results in a transient orange, which then is converted into an indicator yellow before finally breaking up into retinene (vitamin A aldehyde) and vitamin A.

visuo-. A combining form meaning *vision, visual.*

vi·suo·au·di·to·ry (vizh''yoo·o·aw'di·tor·ee) *adj.* [*visuo-* + *auditory*]. Pertaining to hearing and seeing, as visuoauditory nerve fibers, which connect the visual and auditory centers.

visuoauditory revival. Psychiatric treatment in which soldiers suffering from combat neuroses are made to view moving pictures of actual battle scenes with appropriate sound effects; each individual, as he relives his emotional experiences, becomes conscious of the similar behavior of others and realizes that his reactions are not unique.

vi·su·og·no·sis (vizh''yoo·og·no'sis) *n.* [*visuo-* + *-gnosis*]. Appreciation and recognition of visual impressions.

vi·suo·mo·tor (vizh″yoo·o·mo′tur) *adj.* [*visuo-* + *motor*]. 1. Pertaining to seeing and the performance of skilled voluntary movements, as in the ability to copy a simple design or writing. 2. Of or pertaining to the connections between the visual and the motor cortex.

vi·suo·psy·chic (vizh″yoo·o·sigh′kick) *adj.* [*visuo-* + *psychic*]. Pertaining to the visuopsychic area.

visuopsychic area or **cortex.** The visual association areas of the occipital cortex surrounding the visual projection area; the parastriate area and the peristriate area, collectively.

vi·suo·sen·so·ry (vizh″yoo·o·sen′sur·ee) *adj.* [*visuo-* + *sensory*]. Pertaining to the visual projection area of the occipital cortex, Brodmann's area 17.

visuosensory area or **cortex.** VISUAL PROJECTION AREA.

vi·sus (vye′sus) *n.* [L., from *videre,* to see]. VISION.

visus bre·vi·or (brev′ee·or). MYOPIA.

visus co·lo·ra·tus (kol·o·ray′tus). CHROMATOPSIA.

visus de·bil·i·tas (de·bil′i·tas). ASTHENOPIA.

visus de·co·lo·ra·tus (dee·kol·o·ray′tus). ACHROMATOPSIA.

visus di·mi·di·a·tus (dim·i·dye·ay′tus). HEMIANOPSIA.

visus di·ur·nus (dye·ur′nus). HEMERALOPIA.

visus du·pli·ca·tus (dew·pli·kay′tus). DIPLOPIA.

visus he·be·tu·do (heb·e·tew′do). AMBLYOPIA.

visus ju·ve·num (joo′ve·num). MYOPIA.

visus lu·ci·dus (lew′si·dus). PHOTOPSIA.

visus mus·ca·rum (mus·kair′um). Specks before the eyes.

visus se·ni·lis (se·nigh′lis). PRESBYOPIA.

vis vi·tae (vye′tee). VITAL FORCE.

vi·tal (vye′tul) *adj.* [L. *vitalis,* from *vita,* life]. Pertaining to life.

vital activity or **action.** The physiologic activity or functioning, as of the heart, lungs, and vital centers of the brain and spinal cord, that is necessary for maintenance of life.

vital affinity. According to vitalist doctrines, the power of tissues to select their particular required nutrients.

vital capacity. The volume of air that can be expelled from the lungs by the most forcible expiration after the deepest inspiration. It is the maximum stroke volume of the thoracic pump and is affected by any factor restricting either the amount of filling or emptying of the lungs. A timed vital capacity is a measure of rate of emptying of the lungs and aids greatly in determining the maximum ventilatory capacity. A normal individual can exhale three-fourths or more of his vital capacity in one second.

vital capacity test. A test for pulmonary function. See *vital capacity.*

vital dye. A dye suitable for staining living tissues within the whole living body.

vital force. The energy or power characteristic of living organisms.

vi·tal·ism (vye′tul·iz·um) *n.* [*vital* + *-ism*]. The theory that the activities of a living organism are under the guidance of a special form of energy, force, or agency which has none of the attributes of matter or energy. —**vital·ist** (·ist) *n.,* **vital·ist·ic** (·ist′ick) *adj.*

vi·tal·i·ty (vye·tal′i·tee) *n.* [L. *vitalitas,* from *vitalis,* vital]. The power to grow, develop, perform living functions; vigor.

vi·tal·ize (vye′tul·ize) *v.* To endow with the capacity to grow or develop as a living thing.

Vitallium. Trademark for an alloy of cobalt, chromium, and molybdenum used in certain surgical appliances and procedures.

vi·ta·lom·e·ter (vye″tuh·lom′e·tur) *n.* [*vital* + *-meter*]. An electrical instrument used to determine the vitality of a dental pulp.

vital red. An acid disazo dye used in the determination of plasma and blood volumes.

vi·tals (vye′tulz) *n. pl.* The organs essential to life.

vital sensibilities. The sensations that are of prime importance in self-preservation.

vital stain. INTRAVITAL STAIN.

vital statistics. The data concerning births, marriages, and deaths; a branch of biostatistics.

vi·ta·mer (vye′tuh·mur) *n.* [*vita*min + *-mer*]. Any of a group of chemically related substances that possess a specific vitamin activity, as the D vitamers, or the K vitamers.

vi·ta·min, vi·ta·mine (vye′tuh·min) *n.* [L. *vita,* life, + *amine*]. Any of a group of organic compounds present in variable, minute quantities in natural foodstuffs, required for the normal growth and maintenance of the life of animals, including man, who, as a rule, are unable to synthesize these compounds. They are effective in small amounts and do not furnish energy, but are essential for transformation of energy and for the regulation of the metabolism in the organism.

vitamin A. 3,7-Dimethyl-9-(2,6,6-trimethyl-1-cyclohexen-1-yl)-2,4,6,8-nonatetraen-1-ol, $C_{20}H_{29}OH$, a component of liver oils that may be obtained also from certain carotenoids and produced by synthesis. It is a component of pigments concerned with visual accommodation to light and color vision; is essential for development, maturation, and metabolism of epithelial cells; and may have a role in promotion of growth and in synthesis of glucocorticoids. Used medicinally in the form of the alcohol or one of its esters with edible fatty acids. One unit of vitamin A is the biological activity of 0.30 microgram of the alcohol form of vitamin A. Syn. *retinol, vitamin* A_1, *vitamin A alcohol, anti-infective vitamin, antixerophthalmic vitamin.*

vitamin A acid. RETINOIC ACID.

vitamin A alcohol. VITAMIN A.

vitamin A aldehyde. RETINENE.

vitamin B_1. Thiamine, occurring naturally as the hydrochloride and pyrophosphate, and used medicinally principally as the hydrochloride and nitrate salts.

vitamin B_2. RIBOFLAVIN.

vitamin B_2 phosphate. RIBOFLAVIN-5′-PHOSPHATE.

vitamin B_6. 1. PYRIDOXINE. 2. A group name for pyridoxal, pyridoxamine, and pyridoxine, or any member of the group.

vitamin B_{12}. The anti-pernicious-anemia factor, present in liver, essential for normal hemopoiesis; identical with cyanocobalamin. Syn. *extrinsic factor.*

vitamin B_{17}. A misnomer for Laetrile.

vitamin B_c. FOLIC ACID.

vitamin B_T. A factor required for growth and survival of the mealworm, *Tenebrio molitor,* identified as carnitine.

vitamin B_x. PARA-AMINOBENZOIC ACID.

vitamin B complex. A group of water-soluble vitamins, occurring in various foods, that include thiamine (vitamin B_1), riboflavin (vitamin B_2), niacin (nicotinic acid), pyridoxine (vitamin B_6), pantothenic acid, inositol, *p*-aminobenzoic acid, biotin, folic acid, and vitamin B_{12}.

vitamin C. ASCORBIC ACID.

vitamin D. Any one of several sterols having antirachitic activity, as ergocalciferol (vitamin D_2, calciferol) and cholecalciferol (vitamin D_3). Vitamin D occurs in fish liver oils (principally D_3) and is also obtained by irradiating ergosterol (D_2). It is essential for normal deposition of calcium and phosphorus in bones and teeth. Deficiency leads to rickets in children, osteomalacia in adults. Syn. *antirachitic vitamin.*

vitamin D milk. Cow's milk fortified by the direct addition of vitamin D, by exposure to ultraviolet rays, or by feeding irradiated yeast to the animals.

vitamin D–refractory rickets. Rickets that develops despite nutritional doses of vitamin D and that fails to respond to therapeutic amounts. See also *familial hypophosphatemia.*

vitamin D–resistant rickets. VITAMIN D–REFRACTORY RICKETS.

vitamin E. 5,7,8-Trimethyltocol, $C_{29}H_{50}O_2$, commonly known as α-tocopherol (alpha tocopherol), biologically the most active of a series of related compounds called tocopherols. Vitamin E occurs in wheat germ and other oils, and is also produced by synthesis. Its deficiency in rats may produce reproductive sterility, muscular dystrophy, and degeneration. It is believed to be needed in human physiological processes, but its role is not understood. One international unit is equivalent to 1 mg of *dl-α-*tocopheryl acetate.

vitamin F. A term formerly used for essential fatty acids, as linoleic acid ($C_{18}H_{32}O_2$), linolenic acid ($C_{18}H_{30}O_2$), and arachidonic acid ($C_{20}H_{32}O_2$).

vitamin G. Vitamin B_2; RIBOFLAVIN.

vitamin H. A water-soluble component of the vitamin B complex identical with biotin (coenzyme R).

vitamin H'. PARA-AMINOBENZOIC ACID.

vitamin K. Any one of at least three naphthoquinone derivatives, vitamin K_1, vitamin K_2, and vitamin K_3. Vitamin K is essential for formation of prothrombin. In vitamin-K deficiency, the blood clotting time is markedly prolonged and hemorrhages result. Syn. *antihemorrhagic vitamin, prothrombin factor.*

vitamin K_1. PHYTONADIONE.

vitamin K_2. 2-Methyl-3-difarnesyl-1,4-naphthoquinone ($C_{41}H_{56}O_2$) isolated from putrefied fish meal; occurs in microorganisms.

vitamin K_3. MENADIONE.

vitamin K_5. 2-Methyl-4-amino-1-naphthol, $C_{11}H_{11}NO$, a vitamin K compound used as the water-soluble hydrochloride.

Vitamin K Analogue. A trademark for menadiol sodium diphosphate, a water-soluble prothrombinogenic compound with the actions and uses of menadione.

vitamin-K test. A liver-function test in which 2 mg of menadione is administered intramuscularly. If the prothrombin level rises more than 20 percent in 24 hours, liver function is normal.

vitamin M. *Obsol.* FOLIC ACID.

vitamin P [*p*ermeability]. *Obsol.* A collective term for substances, such as citrin or one or more of its components, believed to be concerned with maintenance of the normal state of the walls of small blood vessels, and that have been used for the treatment of conditions characterized by increased capillary permeability and fragility.

vitamin P-P. NIACIN.

vitamin V. PARA-AMINOBENZOIC ACID.

vitel·lary (vit'i-lerr"ee, vye'ti·) *adj.* Pertaining to the vitellus; vitelline.

vi·tel·li·cle (vi·tel'i·kul, vye·) *n.* The yolk sac or umbilical vesicle.

vi·tel·li·form (vi·tel'i·form) *adj.* [*vitel*lus + *-form*]. Yolklike.

vitelliform macular dystrophy. BEST'S DISEASE.

vi·tel·lin (vi·tel'in, vye·) *n.* [*vitel*lus + *-in*]. A phosphoprotein in egg yolk.

vi·tel·line (vi·tel'in, ·een, ·ine) *adj.* [ML. *vitellinus*]. Pertaining to the vitellus or yolk.

vitelline ansa. The yolk-sac vein uniting with the umbilical vein in young embryos. Syn. *ansa vitellina.*

vitelline artery. An artery passing from the yolk sac to the primitive aorta of the embryo. Syn. *omphalomesenteric artery.*

vitelline circulation. The circulation between embryo and yolk sac via the vitelline or omphalomesenteric vessels.

vitelline disk. CUMULUS OOPHORUS.

vitelline duct. The constricted part of the yolk sac opening into the midgut in the region of the future ileum. Syn. *omphalomesenteric duct, umbilical duct, yolk stalk.*

vitelline membrane. A structureless cytoplasmic membrane on the surface of the ovum.

vitelline sac. YOLK SAC.

vitelline space. PERIVITELLINE SPACE.

vitelline sphere. The mulberry-like mass of cells that results from the fission of the substance of the ovum after fertilization. Syn. *yolk sphere.*

vitelline veins. OMPHALOMESENTERIC VEINS.

vi·tel·li·rup·tive (vi·tel"i·rup'tiv) *adj.* Characterized by vitelliform lesions and ruptures or hemorrhages, as: vitelliruptive macular degeneration.

vitelliruptive macular degeneration. BEST'S DISEASE.

vi·tel·lo·in·tes·ti·nal cyst (vi·tel"o·in·tes'ti·nul). A localized cystic dilatation of a part of the persistent vitelline duct.

vi·tel·lo·lu·te·in (vi·tel"o·lew'tee·in) *n.* [*vitel*lus + L. *lute*us, yellow, + *-in*]. A yellow pigment of yolk.

vi·tel·lo·mes·en·ter·ic (vi·tel"o·mes"en·terr'ick) *adj.* [*vitel*lus + *mesenteric*]. OMPHALOMESENTERIC.

vi·tel·lo·ru·bin (vi·tel"o·roo'bin) *n.* [*vitel*lus + L. *rub*er, red, + *-in*]. A reddish pigment obtained from the yolk of egg.

vi·tel·lus (vi·tel'us, vye·tel'us) *n.* [L.]. YOLK.

vitellus ovi (o'vye). The yolk of an egg.

vi·ti·a·tion (vish"ee·ay'shun) *n.* [L. *vitiatio,* from *vitiare,* to spoil, from *vitium,* defect, vice]. A change that lessens utility or efficiency or neutralizes an action.

vit·i·lig·i·nes (vit"i·lij'i·neez) *n.pl.* [plural of *vitiligo*]. Depigmented areas in the skin, as the lineae albicantes and the variously shaped foci of vitiligo.

vit·i·li·go (vit"i·lye'go) *n.* [L., a kind of tetter]. A skin disease characterized by an acquired achromia in areas of various sizes and shapes. There is an almost complete lack of pigment with hyperpigmented borders. Lesions are more marked in areas exposed to sun. **—viti·lig·i·nous** (·lij'i·nus) *adj.*

vitiligo cap·i·tis (kap'i·tis). ALOPECIA AREATA.

vit·i·li·goi·dea (vit"i·lye·goy'dee·uh) *n.* XANTHOMA.

vitiligo iri·dis (eye'ri·dis). MUELLER'S SPOTS.

vitreal cavity. VITREOUS CHAMBER.

vit·re·in (vit'ree·in) *n.* A complex protein, of the collagen-gelatin type, present in small amounts in the vitreous humor of the eye.

vit·reo·den·tin (vit"ree·o·den'tin) *n.* [L. *vitre*us, of glass, + *dentin*]. A variety of dentin with but few dentinal tubules.

vit·reo·den·tine (vit"ree·o·den'teen, ·tin) *n.* VITREODENTIN.

vit·re·ous (vit'ree·us) *adj. & n.* [L. *vitreus,* from *vitrum,* glass]. 1. Glassy; hyaline. 2. VITREOUS BODY.

vitreous body. The transparent, gelatin-like substance filling the greater part of the eyeball. NA *corpus vitreum.* See also Plate 19.

vitreous chamber. The portion of the eyeball posterior to the crystalline lens and anterior to the retina, which is filled by the vitreous humor. NA *camera vitrea bulbi.*

vitreous degeneration. HYALINE DEGENERATION.

vitreous floaters. FLOATERS.

vitreous humor. 1. VITREOUS BODY. 2. The more fluid portion of the vitreous body enmeshed in the more fibrous portion. NA *humor vitreus.* Contr. *aqueous humor.*

vitreous membrane. HYALOID MEMBRANE.

vitreous stroma. The more fibrous portion of the vitreous body. NA *stroma vitreum.* Contr. *vitreous humor* (2).

vi·tres·cence (vi·tres'unce) *n.* The condition of becoming hard and transparent like glass.

vit·re·um, *n.* VITREOUS BODY.

vit·ric (vit'rick) *adj.* Pertaining to glass or any vitreous substance.

vi·tri·na (vi·trye'nuh) *n.* VITREOUS HUMOR.

vitrina au·di·to·ria (aw·di·to'ree·uh). ENDOLYMPH.

vitrina au·ris (aw'ris). ENDOLYMPH.

vitrina ocu·la·ris (ock·yoo·lair'is). VITREOUS HUMOR.

vit·ri·ol (vit'ree·ul) *n.* [OF., from ML. *vitriolum,* from L. *vitrum,* glass]. 1. Any substance having a glassy fracture or appearance. 2. SULFURIC ACID. 3. Any crystalline salt of sulfuric acid. **—vit·ri·o·lat·ed** (vit'ree·o·lay"tid), **vit·ri·ol·ic** (vit"ree·ol'ick) *adj.*

vitriolic acid. SULFURIC ACID.

vi·tri·tis (vi·trye'tis) *n.* [L. *vitr*um, glass, + *-itis*]. *Obsol.* GLAUCOMA.

vit·ro·den·tin, vit·ro·den·tine (vit"ro·den'tin) *n.* 1. Calcified tissue allegedly occurring on or in the scales or teeth of certain lower fishes. 2. *Erron.* VITREODENTIN.

vit·ro·pres·sion (vit″ro·presh′un) *n.* [L. *vitrum*, glass, + *-pression* as in impression, compression]. Pressure with a glass slide on the skin to aid in study and diagnosis of skin lesions.

vit·rum, *n.* [L.]. GLASS.

Vivactil. Trademark for protriptyline, an antidepressant drug used as the hydrochloride salt.

vi·var·i·um (vye·văr′ee·um) *n.*, pl. **vivar·ia** (·ee·uh), **vivariums** [L.]. A place where live animals are kept.

vi·vax malaria (vye′vacks). Malaria caused by *Plasmodium vivax*, characterized by typical paroxysms occurring every two or three days, typically every second day. Syn. *benign tertian malaria, tertian malaria.*

vivi- [L. *vivus*]. A combining form meaning *alive, living.*

vivi·dif·fu·sion (viv″i·di·few′zhun) *n.* [*vivi-* + *diffusion*]. The passage of diffusible substances from blood of a living animal flowing through collodion tubes into a surrounding medium.

viv·i·fi·ca·tion (viv″i·fi·kay′shun) *n.* The act of making alive or of converting into living tissue.

vi·vip·a·rous (vye·vip′uh·rus, vi·) *adj.* [L. *viviparus*, from *vivus*, living, + *parere*, to bring forth]. Bringing forth the young alive. Contr. *oviparous.* —**vivi·par·i·ty** (vye″vi·păr′i·tee) *n.*

vivi·sec·tion (viv″i·seck′shun) *n.* [*vivi-* + *section*]. The cutting of a living individual; especially, a surgical procedure upon an anesthetized animal for research purposes. —**vivi·sect** (viv′i·sekt) *v.*

vivi·sec·tion·ist (viv″i·seck′shun·ist) *n.* A person who practices or defends vivisection or experimental work on animals.

vivi·sec·tor (viv′i·seck″tur) *n.* A person who practices vivisection.

V lead. Abbreviation for *voltage lead.*

Vleminckx's solution or **lotion.** SULFURATED LIME SOLUTION.

VMA Abbreviation for *vanillylmandelic acid.*

VMC Abbreviation for *von Meyenburg complex.*

vo·cal (vo′kul) *adj.* [L. *vocalis*, from *vox*, voice]. Pertaining to the voice or the organs of speech.

vocal asynergy. Faulty coordination of the muscles of the larynx, as in chorea.

vocal cord. VOCAL FOLD.

vocal fold. In the larynx, either the right or left fold bounding the rima glottidis. Each is covered by mucous membrane which is supported anteriorly by a vocal ligament, posteriorly by the vocal process of an arytenoid cartilage. NA *plica vocalis.*

vocal fremitus. The sounds of the voice transmitted to the ear when it is applied to the chest of a person speaking.

vo·ca·lis (vo·kay′lis) *n.* The muscle lying beneath the true vocal folds. NA *musculus vocalis.* See also Table of Muscles in the Appendix.

vocal ligament. The thickened margin of the elastic cone of the larynx which supports the mucous membrane of the anterior part of a vocal fold. NA *ligamentum vocale.*

vocal lip. Either of the shelflike projections into the cavity of the larynx whose edges constitute the vocal cords or folds.

vocal node or **nodule.** SINGER'S NODE.

vocal process. The anterior process of an arytenoid cartilage. NA *processus vocalis.*

vocal resonance. The sound of the spoken voice transmitted through the lungs and the chest wall and heard on auscultation. Abbreviated, V.R.

Vo·ges-Pros·kauer test or **reaction** (fo′gus, pro^h^s′kaow·ur) [O. *Voges*, German physician, b. 1867; and B. *Proskauer*, German bacteriologist, 1851–1915]. A test for the formation of acetylmethylcarbinol from glucose by various microorganisms, especially useful in the differentiation of the aerogenes group (V.P. positive) from the coliforms (V.P. negative). To an appropriate culture, potassium hydroxide, creatine, and distilled water are added. A slowly developing red color indicates a positive reaction. Abbreviated, V.P. test. Syn. *acetylmethylcarbinol test.*

Vogt disease or **syndrome** (fohkt) [Cécile *Vogt*, 1875–1962; and O. *Vogt*, 1870–1959, German neurologists]. STATUS MARMORATUS.

Vogt-Ko·ya·na·gi-Ha·ra·da syndrome [C. *Vogt*; Y. *Koyanagi*, Japanese, b. 1880; and E. *Harada*]. UVEOMENINGOENCEPHALITIS.

Vogt-Koyanagi syndrome [C. *Vogt* and Y. *Koyanagi*]. UVEOMENINGOENCEPHALITIS.

Vogt-Spielmeyer disease. SPIELMEYER-VOGT DISEASE.

Vogt's point (fohkt) [P. F. E. *Vogt*, German surgeon 1847–1885]. A point selected for trephining and arresting traumatic meningeal hemorrhage; found by taking a horizontal line two fingerbreadths above the zygomatic arch, and a vertical line a thumb's breadth behind the sphenofrontal process of the zygoma, the intersection of the two marking the point.

voice, *n.* [OF. *vois*, from L. *vox*]. The sounds produced by the vibration of the vocal folds and modified by the resonance organs, especially as used in speaking or singing.

void, *v.* [OF. *voider*, from a derivative of L. *vacuus*, empty]. To evacuate, emit, discharge (especially excrement).

Voil·le·mier's point (vwah·l^e^m·ye^y^′) [L. C. *Voillemier*, French urologist, 20th century]. A point on the linear alba 6 to 7 cm below a line drawn between the two anterior superior spines of the ilium; suprapubic puncture of the urinary bladder is made at this point in fat or edematous individuals.

vol. %. Abbreviation for *volume percent.*

vo·la (vo′luh) *n.* [L.]. The palm of the hand or the sole of the foot. —**vo·lar** (·lur) *adj.*

vola ma·nus (man′us) [BNA]. PALMA MANUS.

volar arches. See *deep palmar arch* and *superficial palmar arch.*

volar carpal ligament. PALMAR CARPAL LIGAMENT.

volar intercarpal ligament. The palmar intercarpal ligament. See *intercarpal ligament.*

vol·a·tile (vol′uh·til) *adj.* [L. *volatilis*, flying, from *volare*, to fly]. Readily vaporizing; evaporating. —**vol·a·til·iza·tion** (vol″uh·til·i·zay′shun) *n.*; **vol·a·til·ize** (vol′uh·til·ize) *v.*

volatile alkali. 1. AMMONIA. 2. AMMONIUM CARBONATE.

volatile oil. Oil characterized by volatility, variously obtained from tissues of certain plants, particularly odoriferous ones. The oil may exist as such in the plant or may be formed during the process of obtaining it, as by hydrolytic or pyrolytic action. Volatile oils may contain a variety of chemical compounds, for example hydrocarbons, alcohols, ethers, aldehydes, ketones, acids, phenols, esters, and sulfur and nitrogen compounds. Syn. *essential oil.*

vol·az·o·cine (vol·az′o·seen, vo·lay′zo·seen) *n.* 3-(Cyclopropylmethyl)-1,2,3,4,5,6-hexahydro-*cis*-6,11-dimethyl-2,6-methano-3-benzazocine, $C_{18}H_{25}N$, an analgesic.

vole, *n.* Any ratlike rodent belonging to the genus *Microtus.*

vole bacillus. A bacillus closely allied to *Mycobacterium tuberculosis* and causing a disease in voles resembling tuberculosis and rat leprosy. It is highly pathogenic for rats. Syn. *Mycobacterium tuberculosis* var. *muris.*

vo·le·mic (vo·lee′mick) *adj.* [*vol*ume + *hem-* + *-ic*]. Pertaining to volume of blood or plasma.

Vol·hard-Ar·nold method (fo^h^l′hart) [F. *Volhard*, German physician 1872–1950]. A method for chlorides in urine in which the urine is acidified with nitric acid and the chlorides are precipitated with a measured excess of standard silver nitrate solution. The silver chloride formed is filtered off and in the filtrate the excess silver nitrate is titrated with standard ammonium thiocyanate solution. Ferric ammonium sulfate is used as an indicator.

Volhard-Harvey method [F. *Volhard*]. A method for chlorides in urine which differs from the Volhard-Arnold method in that the excess of silver nitrate is titrated directly without filtering and hence in the presence of the silver chloride. The procedure is thus more rapid, but the end point is more difficult to determine.

Volhard's and Fahr's test [F. *Volhard;* and K. T. *Fahr,* German physician, 1877–1945]. 1. A test of the kidney's ability to concentrate urine when fluids are withheld for a prolonged period. A specific gravity persistently below 1.025 is considered abnormal. 2. A test of the kidney's ability to secrete dilute urine after the fasting patient drinks 1,500 ml of water. A specific gravity persistently above 1.003 is considered abnormal.

Vol·hyn·ia fever (vol·hin'ee·uh, vo·lin'ee·uh) [*Volhynia* (*Volyn*), a region in the western Ukraine]. TRENCH FEVER.

vo·li·tion (vo·li'shun) *n.* [ML. *volitio,* from L. *velle,* to wish, want]. The conscious will or determination to act. —**volition·al** (·ul) *adj.*

volitional facial palsy or **paralysis.** A form of supranuclear paralysis of the facial nerve in which the involvement is most marked on voluntary contraction, such as when the patient tries to show his teeth or retract the corners of his mouth. Emotional facial movements are preserved or even exaggerated. The lesion may be located either in the lower third of the precentral convolution controlling facial movements or in the pathway between this area and the motor nucleus of the facial nerve. Compare *amimia.*

Volk·mann's canals (fohlk'mahn) [A. W. *Volkmann,* German physiologist, 1800–1877]. In compact bone, the vascular channels that lack the concentric lamellae of haversian systems. The term is commonly erroneously applied to nutrient canals in compact bone, whether haversian or Volkmann's.

Volkmann's contracture [R. von *Volkmann,* German surgeon, 1830–1889]. Ischemic muscular contracture of the arm and hand resulting from pressure injury or a tight cast; often accompanied by muscle degeneration and ultimate extensive fibrosis and claw hand.

Volkmann's paralysis [R. von *Volkmann*]. The paralysis that accompanies Volkmann's contracture.

Volkmann's splint [R. von *Volkmann*]. Two lateral supports and a foot piece, used in fractures of the lower extremity.

vol·ley, *n.* [MF. *volee,* from *voler,* to fly]. Approximately simultaneous discharges, as nerve impulses that travel simultaneously in different axons of a nerve or that are discharged simultaneously from groups of central neurons.

Voll·mer patch test [H. *Vollmer,* U.S. pediatrician, b. 1896]. A tuberculin test in which gauze saturated with tuberculin is applied to an intact skin surface under adhesive plaster.

vol·sel·la (vol·sel'uh) *n.* [variant of *vulsella*]. A forceps having one or more hooks at the end of each blade.

vol·sel·lum (vol·sel'um) *n.* VOLSELLA.

volt, *n.* [A. *Volta,* Italian physicist, 1745–1827]. The unit of electromotive force and electric potential; the electromotive force that, steadily applied to a conductor whose resistance is one ohm, will produce a current of one ampere. Abbreviated, v

volt·age, *n.* Electromotive force measured in volts.

voltage lead. A unipolar precordial lead. Abbreviated, V lead.

vol·ta·ic (vol·tay'ick) *adj.* [A. *Volta* + *-ic*]. Of or pertaining to A. Volta or to voltaism; GALVANIC.

voltaic current. GALVANIC CURRENT.

voltaic electricity. GALVANIC ELECTRICITY.

vol·ta·ism (vol'tuh·iz·um) *n.* [*volta*ic + *-ism*]. GALVANISM.

volt-ammeter, *n.* An instrument for measuring both voltage, or potential, and amperage, or amount of current.

volt-ampere, *n.* The power developed in an electric circuit when the current is one ampere and the potential one volt; equivalent in a direct current to a watt.

Vol·ter·ra method. A method for phenols in urine in which the urine is distilled from slightly alkaline solution to obtain the free volatile phenols in the distillate. After acidification, a second distillate is obtained; this represents the conjugated volatile phenols present. Ether extraction of the remaining fluid separates the aromatic hydroxy acids from "residual phenols." Each fraction, after proper preparation, is treated with the phosphotungstic-phosphomolybdic acid color reagent of Folin and Ciocalteu and the resulting color compared with that obtained from a standard phenol solution.

volt·me·ter (vohlt'mee"tur) *n.* [*volt* + *meter*]. An instrument for measuring voltage, or electromotive force.

Vol·to·li·ni's disease (vohl"to·lee'nee) [F. E. R. *Voltolini,* German otolaryngologist, 1819–1889]. Chronic suppurative otitis media.

volume curve. A recording of volume variations; particularly, that of ventricular volume during the cardiac cycle.

volume dose. *In radiation therapy,* the total energy absorbed by an entire irradiated volume of tissue. See also *integral dose.*

volume index. The relation of the volume of the red corpuscles to their number.

volume percent. The number of milliliters of a substance contained in 100 ml of medium. Usually refers to gas (O_2 or CO_2) contained in blood. Symbol, vol. %.

vol·u·met·ric (vol"yoo·met'rick) *adj.* [*vol*ume + *metric*]. Pertaining to measurement by volume.

volumetric analysis. Quantitative determination of an element or constituent by titration with a standardized volumetric solution.

volumetric solution. A standard solution generally containing 1, ½, or ⅒ gram-equivalent of a substance in 1,000 ml of solution. Used in volumetric analysis. Abbreviated, V.S.

vol·un·tary, *adj.* [L. *voluntarius,* from *voluntas,* will]. Under control of the will; performed by an exercise of the will.

voluntary muscle. A muscle directly under the control of the will; SKELETAL MUSCLE.

vol·u·tin granules (vol'yoo·tin) [(*Spirillum*) *volut*ans, a species of bacterium, + *-in*]. Granules found in the cytoplasm of many bacterial and yeast cells, composed chiefly of complex salts of metaphosphoric acid polymers and staining red with methylene blue or toluidine blue. Syn. *metachromatic granules.*

vol·vu·lo·sis (vol·vew·lo'sis) *n.* [(*Onchocerca*) *volvul*us + *-osis*]. ONCHOCERCIASIS.

vol·vu·lus (vol'vew·lus) *n.* [NL., from L. *volvere,* to roll, to turn]. A twisting of the bowel upon itself so as to occlude the lumen and, in severe cases, compromise its circulation. It occurs most frequently in the sigmoid flexure.

vo·mer (vo'mur) *n.* [L., plowshare] [NA]. The thin plate of bone which is situated vertically between the nasal cavities, and which forms the posterior portion of the septum of the nose. See also Table of Bones in the Appendix.

vo·mer·ine (vo'muh·reen, vom'uh·reen, ·rine) *adj.* Pertaining to or involving the vomer.

vom·ero·na·sal (vom"ur·o·nay'zul, vo"mur·o·) *adj.* [*vomer* + *nasal*]. Pertaining to the vomer and the nasal cavity.

vomeronasal cartilage. A strip of hyaline cartilage extending from the anterior nasal spine upward and backward on either side of the septal cartilage of the nose and attached to the anterior margin of the vomer. NA *cartilago vomeronasalis.*

vomeronasal organ. A slender tubule ending in a blind sac; situated in the anteroinferior part of the nasal septum; vestigial in humans. NA *organum vomeronasale.*

vom·it, *v.* & *n.* [L. *vomitum,* from *vomere,* to vomit]. 1. To expel from the stomach by vomiting. 2. Matter expelled from the stomach by vomiting.

vom·it·ing, *n.* The forcible ejection of the contents of the stomach through the mouth. Compare *regurgitation* (2).

vomiting center. A region located dorsolaterally in the reticular formation of the medulla oblongata at the level of the olivary nuclei; it includes the tractus solitarius and its nucleus of termination; the region is also concerned in associated activities such as salivation and respiratory movement.

vomiting gas. A chemical agent that causes coughing, sneezing, pain in nose and throat, nasal discharge, sometimes tears, often followed by headache and vomiting; as, for example, adamsite. Syn. *irritant smoke (obsol.).* See also *sternutator.*

vomiting reflex. Vomiting induced by tickling or touching the fauces or pharynx.

vom·i·tive (vom'i·tiv) *adj.* EMETIC.

vó·mi·to ne·gro (vom'i·to nay'gro) [Sp., black vomit]. Hematemesis in yellow fever.

vom·i·to·ry (vom'i·to·ree) *n.* [L. *vomitorium*]. 1. Any agent that induces emesis. 2. A vessel used to receive vomited material.

vom·i·tu·ri·tion (vom''i·tew·rish'un) *n.* RETCHING.

vom·i·tus (vom'i·tus) *n.* [L.]. VOMIT (2).

vomitus cru·en·tes (kroo·en'teez). Bloody vomit.

vomitus ma·ri·nus (ma·rye'nus). SEASICKNESS.

vomitus ma·tu·ti·nus (ma·tew·tye'nus). MORNING SICKNESS.

vomitus ni·ger (nigh'jur). BLACK VOMIT.

von Al·dor's test. A test for proteoses in which phototungstic acid is added to urine, the precipitate is washed with absolute alcohol and dissolved in potassium hydroxide, and a test for protein is applied.

von Berg·mann's incision (fo^h^n be^h^rk'ma^h^n) [E. *von Bergmann,* German surgeon, 1836–1907]. An oblique incision in the flank to expose the kidney. Syn. *Bergmann's incision.*

von den Vel·den's method (fo^h^n d^e^n fel'd^e^n) [R. *von den Velden,* German physician, 1880–1941]. Treatment of cardiac arrest by intracardiac injection.

von Eco·no·mo's disease (fo^h^n e^y^·ko·no'mo) [C. *von Economo,* Austrian neurologist, 1876–1931]. ENCEPHALITIS LETHARGICA.

Vonedrine. Trademark for phenylpropylmethylamine, a vasoconstrictor applied topically, as the hydrochloride salt, to relieve nasal congestion.

von Eu·len·burg's disease (fo^h^n oy'l^e^n·boork) [A. *von Eulenburg,* German physician, 1840–1917]. PARAMYOTONIA CONGENITA.

von Gier·ke's disease (fo^h^n geer'ke^h^) [E. *von Gierke,* German pathologist, 1877–1945]. A form of glycogenosis characterized by marked diminution in, or absence of, hepatic glucose 6-phosphatase resulting in hepatic glycogenosis, hypoglycemia, and acidosis. Syn. *glycogen storage disease, hepatic glycogenosis, type I of Cori, van Creveld–von Gierke's disease.*

von Grae·fe's knife (fo^h^n gre^y^'fe^h^) [F. W. *von Graefe,* German ophthalmologist, 1828–1870]. A small knife with a long, narrow blade, used in ophthalmic surgery.

von Graefe's sign [F. W. *von Graefe*]. Lid lag in hyperthyroidism.

von Hippel–Lindau disease [E. *von Hippel* and A. *Lindau*]. HIPPEL-LINDAU DISEASE.

von Hippel's disease [E. *von Hippel*]. Angiomatosis of the retina. See also *Hippel-Lindau disease.*

von Jaksch–Pollak test [R. *von Jaksch*]. A test for detecting the presence of melanin in urine in which ferric chloride is added to urine. If melanin is present, there develops a gray color and a dark precipitate of phosphates and adhering melanin.

von Jaksch's anemia or **disease** (fo^h^n ya^h^ksh') [R. *von Jaksch,* Czechoslovakian physician, 1855–1947]. A nonspecific symptom complex of childhood consisting of severe anemia, extreme leukocytosis with lymphocytosis, lymphadenopathy, and hepatosplenomegaly in response to rickets, congenital syphilis, malnutrition, gastrointestinal disturbances, and a wide variety of other conditions and infections.

von Kós·sa's stain (fo^h^n ko'sho^h^) [J. *von Kóssa,* Austro-Hungarian pathologist]. A histologic technique using silver nitrate to demonstrate ground substance involved in calcification, thereby providing indirect evidence of the presence of calcium.

von Mey·en·burg complex (fo^h^n migh'^e^n·boork) [H. *von Meyenburg,* 20th century]. Multiple clusters of intrahepatic bile ducts in a collagenous stroma, presumed to represent persistence of fetal structures; suggested as possible antecedents to polycystic disease of the liver. Syn. *bile-duct hamartoma, multiple bile-duct adenoma, multiple microhamartoma of liver.*

von Noor·den treatment (fo^h^n nohr'd^e^n) [C. H. *von Noorden,* German physician, 1858–1944]. A former diabetic diet with protein restriction and the limitation of carbohydrate intake to oatmeal.

von Pir·quet test (fo^h^n peer·ke^h^') [C. P. *von Pirquet,* Austrian physician, 1874–1929]. A tuberculin test in which the substance is applied to a superficial abrasion of the skin.

von Reck·ling·hausen's disease (fo^h^n rek·ling·haow'z^e^n) [F. D. *von Recklinghausen,* German pathologist, 1833–1910]. 1. NEUROFIBROMATOSIS. 2. HEMOCHROMATOSIS. 3. Generalized osteitis fibrosa cystica.

von Recklinghausen's hemofuscin [F. D. *von Recklinghausen*]. A brown, iron-negative, granular pigment occurring in intestinal and arterial smooth muscle in cases of true hemochromatosis; now often regarded as lipofuscin or chromolipid.

von Stein's test (fo^h^n shtine) [S. A. F. *von Stein,* Russian otologist, b. 1855]. 1. A test for body equilibrium, in which the patient with disturbances of the labyrinthine or cerebellar pathways is unable to stand or hop on one foot when his eyes are closed. 2. A test for body equilibrium in which the patient is placed upon a platform that is slowly tilted. Equilibrium is considered normal if the patient can sustain a forward inclination of the platform of 35 to 40 degrees before falling forward, and a backward inclination of 25 to 30 degrees before falling backward. Wide variation in the physiological range makes the test of little practical value. Syn. *goniometer test.*

Vontrol. Trademark for diphenidol, an antiemetic drug.

von Wil·le·brand's disease (fo^h^n vil'e^h^·bra^h^nt) [E. A. *von Willebrand,* German-Finnish physician, 1870–1949]. VASCULAR HEMOPHILIA.

Voor·hees bag [J. D. *Voorhees,* U.S. obstetrician, 1869–1929]. A hydrostatic rubber bag used occasionally to dilate the uterine cervix for the induction of labor.

vo·ra·cious (vo·ray'shus) *adj.* [L. *vorax, voracis,* from *vorare,* to devour]. Having an insatiable appetite or desire for food.

Vo·ro·noff's operation [S. *Voronoff,* Russian physiologist, 1866–1951]. Testicular implantations in the hope of effecting rejuvenation.

-vorous [from L. *vorare,* to devour, + *-ous*]. A combining form meaning *eating, feeding on.*

vor·tex (vor'tecks) *n.,* pl. **vor·ti·ces** (·ti·seez) [L., a whirl, from *vertere,* to turn]. A structure having the appearance of being produced by a rotary motion about an axis.

vortex coc·cy·ge·us (kock·sij'ee·us) [BNA]. The point of convergence of the lanugo hairs over the coccyx.

vortex cor·dis (kor'dis) [NA]. VORTEX OF THE HEART.

vortex len·tis (len'tis). LENS STAR.

vortex of the heart. The region at the apex of the heart where the superficial layer of muscle of both ventricles (vortex fibers) passes into the deep layer of the ventricles. NA *vortex cordis.*

vortices. Plural of *vortex.*

vortices pi·lo·rum (pi·lo'rum) [NA]. Hair whorls.

vor·ti·cose (vor'ti·koce) *adj.* Whirling; having a whorled appearance.

Vos·sius cataract or **ring** (fo^h^s'yoos) [A. *Vossius,* German ophthalmologist, 1855–1925]. PIGMENTED CATARACT.

vox (vocks) *n.* [L.]. VOICE.

vox ab·scis·sa (ab·sis'uh) [NL.]. Loss of voice.

vox cap·i·tis (kap'i·tis) [NL.]. The upper register of the voice; falsetto voice.

vox cho·ler·i·ca (ko·lerr'i·kuh) [NL.]. A peculiar, faint voice noted in the last stage of cholera.

vox rau·ca (raw'kuh) [L.]. Hoarse voice.

vo·yeur (vwah·yur') *n.* [F., from *voir,* to see]. A person, usually a male, who obtains sexual gratification from witnessing the sexual acts of others or from viewing persons in the nude. —**voyeur·ism** (·iz·um) *n.*

V patterns or **syndromes.** See *A-V patterns.*

VPB Abbreviation for *ventricular premature beat.*

V.P. test. Abbreviation for *Voges-Proskauer test.*

V.R. Abbreviation for *vocal resonance.*

Vro·lik's disease [W. *Vrolik,* Dutch physician, 1801–1863]. OSTEOGENESIS IMPERFECTA CONGENITA.

V.S. Abbreviation for *volumetric solution.*

vu·e·rom·e·ter (vew''ur·om'e·tur) *n.* [F. *vue,* sight, + *-meter*]. An apparatus for determining the interpupillary distance.

vul·can·ize (vul'kuh·nize) *v.* [*Vulcan,* the fire god]. To subject rubber to a process wherein it is treated with sulfur at a high temperature, and thereby rendered either flexible or very hard.

vul·ner·a·ble (vul'nur·uh·bul) *adj.* [L. *vulnerabilis,* from *vulnus, vulneris,* injury]. Susceptible to injury of any kind.

vul·nus (vul'nus) *n.* [L.]. WOUND.

Vul·pian effect or **phenomenon** (vu^el·pya^n') [E. F. A. *Vulpian,* French physician, 1826–1887]. In hemiparalysis of the tongue, sudden dilatation of the tongue and slow movements of the paralyzed side, occurring when the ipsilateral chorda tympani is stimulated; considered to be due to stimulation of the mesencephalic root of the trigeminal nerve with liberation of acetylcholine. See also *Vulpian-Heidenhain-Sherrington phenomenon.*

Vulpian-Heidenhain-Sherrington phenomenon [E. F. A. *Vulpian,* R. P. H. *Heidenhain,* and C. S. *Sherrington*]. Stimulation of intact sensory nerve fibers in atrophic muscles may produce enough antidromic impulses generating sufficient acetylcholine to cause a slow, small, maintained contraction.

Vulpian reaction [E. F. A. *Vulpian*]. On immersion of fresh adrenal tissue in ferric chloride solution, the medulla colors green. This is a general reaction of the catechol group and is given by catechol, pyrogallol, dopa, epinephrine, and norepinephrine.

Vulpian's atrophy [E. F. A. *Vulpian*]. A form of progressive spinal muscular atrophy affecting the muscles of the scapulohumeral region.

vul·sel·la (vul·sel'uh) *n.* [L., tweezers, from *vellere, vulsus,* to pluck]. VOLSELLA.

vul·sel·lum (vul·sel'um) *n.*, pl. **vulsel·la** (·luh). VOLSELLA.

vulv-, vulvo-. A combining form meaning *vulva, vulvar.*

vul·va (vul'vuh) *n.*, genit. **vul·vae** (·vee) [L., covering, womb]. The external genital organs in woman. NA *pudendum femininum.* —**vul·var** (·vur), **vul·val** (·vul) *adj.*

vulva con·ni·vens (ko·nye'venz). A form of vulva in which the labia majora are in close apposition.

vul·vae acu·tum ul·cus (vul'vee a·kew'tum ul'kus). ULCUS VULVAE ACUTUM.

vulva hi·ans (high'anz) [NL., gaping vulva, from *hiare,* to gape]. The form of vulva in which the labia majora are gaping.

vulvar anus. An anomalous condition in which the anus is imperforate, the rectum opening into the vulva.

vulvar atresia. VULVAR FUSION.

vulvar fusion. Cohesion of the labia minora occluding all or part of the vestibule; it may be congenital, but is more generally acquired following irritation.

vul·vec·to·my (vul·veck'tuh·mee) *n.* [*vulv-* + *-ectomy*]. Surgical excision of the vulva.

vul·vis·mus (vul·viz'mus) *n.* [*vulv-* + *-ismus*]. VAGINISMUS.

vul·vi·tis (vul·vye'tis) *n.* [*vulv-* + *-itis*]. Inflammation of the vulva.

vulvo-. See *vulv-.*

vul·vo·va·gi·nal (vul''vo·va·jye'nul, ·vaj'i·nul) *adj.* [*vulvo-* + *vaginal*]. Of or pertaining to both the vulva and vagina.

vul·vo·vag·i·ni·tis (vul''vo·vaj''i·nigh'tis) *n.* [*vulvo-* + *vagin-* + *-itis*]. Inflammation of the vulva and of the vagina existing at the same time.

Vvedenski, Vvedensky. See *Wedensky.*

v wave. 1. The positive-pressure wave in the atrial or venous pulse due to caval and atrial filling during ventricular systole. 2. The giant positive-pressure wave in the atrial or venous pulse, produced by fusion of the regurgitant wave with the c and v waves, obliterating the negative x wave and producing a venous pulse wave similar to that found in the ventricles.

V-Z virus. VARICELLA-ZOSTER VIRUS.

W

W 1. Symbol for wolfram (= TUNGSTEN). 2. Abbreviation for *watt.*

Wa·chen·stein-Zak method (va^{k}h′^{e}n·shtine) [M. *Wachenstein,* Austrian-U. S. pathologist and chemist, 1905–1965]. A histochemical method for bismuth based on the oxidation of bismuth sulfide, the form occurring in tissues, to sulfate by hydrogen peroxide and conversion of the sulfate to orange-red brucine iodide salt.

Wa·da test [J. *Wada,* Japanese neurosurgeon in Canada, 20th century]. The intracarotid injection of 10% amobarbital for lateralization of the speech center. The method has also been applied to the lateralization of the primary epileptic focus.

wad·ding, *n.* [F. *ouate*]. 1. Carded cotton or wool, used for surgical dressings, generally not of the first quality. 2. Cotton batting, sometimes glazed to render it nonabsorbent.

waddling gait. The gait, resembling that of a duck, seen in various muscular dystrophies, due to difficulty in fixing the pelvis. It is also seen in association with dislocation of the hips.

wa·fer, *n.* A thin sheet made by heating moistened flour and formerly used to enclose powders that are taken internally. Syn. *cachet.*

Wag·ner-Jau·regg treatment (vahg′nur yaow′reck) [J. *Wagner* von *Jauregg,* Austrian physician, 1857–1940]. Treatment of central nervous system syphilis by fever of artificially induced malaria.

Wagner's corpuscles [R. *Wagner,* German physician, 1805–1864]. TACTILE CORPUSCLES.

Wagner's operation [W. *Wagner,* German surgeon, 1848–1900]. An osteoplastic resection of the skull.

Wag·staffe's fracture [W. W. *Wagstaffe,* English surgeon, 1843–1910]. Fracture with separation of the medial malleolus.

Wahl's sign (vahl) [E. von *Wahl,* German surgeon, 1833–1890]. A sign of intestinal obstruction, in which there is local meteorism or distention proximal to the point of obstruction.

waist, *n.* The narrowest portion of the trunk between the hips and the ribs.

waist·line, *n.* The circumference of the waist.

wake·ful·ness, *n.* 1. A physiologic state in which the organism is alert and aware or conscious of itself and its responses to internal and external stimuli. 2. INSOMNIA.

wak·ing dream (way′king). An illusion or hallucination.

Walcher's position [G. A. *Walcher,* German gynecologist, 1856–1935]. The posture of a patient lying on the back with the thighs and legs hanging over the edge of the table. Used during a difficult delivery to lengthen the true conjugate.

Wal·den·ström's disease (va^{h}l′d^{e}n·strœm) [J. H. *Waldenström,* Swedish surgeon, b. 1877]. OSTEOCHONDRITIS DEFORMANS JUVENILIS.

Waldenström's hypergammaglobulinemic purpura. A syndrome of purpura and polyclonal hypergammaglobulinemia, usually occuring in middle-aged women.

Waldenström's macroglobulinemia. A syndrome related to multiple myeloma in which a malignant clone of lymphocytes produces a monoclonal paraprotein (M component) composed of IgM. Syn. *macroglobulinemia.*

Wal·dey·er's epithelium (va^{h}l′digh·ur) [H. W. G. *Waldeyer*-Hartz, German anatomist, 1836–1921]. GERMINAL EPITHELIUM.

Waldeyer's fascia [H. W. G. *Waldeyer*-Hartz]. The portion of the pelvic fascia surrounding the pelvic portion of each ureter.

Waldeyer's fossae [H. W. G. *Waldeyer*-Hartz]. The inferior duodenal and superior duodenal fossa and the paraduodenal recess.

Waldeyer's glands [H. W. G. *Waldeyer*-Hartz]. Modified sweat glands at the border of the tarsal plates of the eyelids.

Waldeyer's tonsillar ring [H. W. G. *Waldeyer*-Hartz]. A ring of lymphatic tissue formed by the two palatine tonsils, the pharyngeal tonsil, and smaller groups of lymphatic follicles at the base of the tongue and behind the posterior pillars of the fauces.

Walk·er carcinosarcoma 256. A transplantable malignant tumor that may grow in a sarcomatous pattern, a carcinomatous pattern, or a mixture of the two; originally the tumor arose spontaneously in the mammary gland region of a pregnant albino rat.

Walker-Reisinger method. A capillary tube microcolorimetric adaptation of the Sumner dinitrosalicylic acid method of determining the amount of reducing substances in blood or urine.

Walker sarcoma. WALKER CARCINOSARCOMA 256.

walk·ing caliper. CALIPER SPLINT.

walking iron or **splint.** A metal support attached to a splint, shoe, or plaster cast designed to permit walking without the sole of the foot coming in contact with the ground, used in ambulatory treatment of fractures of the lower leg.

walking ventilation. A test of breathing response to mild exercise. The patient walks at a rate of 2 miles per hour on level ground, and after 4 minutes the expired air is collected and measured.

walking wounded. *In military medicine,* a sick or wounded person who can walk from the place where he became a casualty to the place where he can receive medical treatment; an ambulant case.

wall, *n.* [L. *vallum,* rampart]. The bounding side or inside surface of a natural or artificial cavity or vessel.

Wal·lace-Di·a·mond method [G. B. *Wallace,* U.S. pharmacologist, b. 1874; and J. R. *Diamond*]. A screening test for excesses and deficiencies of urobilinogen in the urine, using Ehrlich's reagent and serial dilution of the urine.

Wallace loop. A modification of the ileal conduit in which the two distal ureters are joined together and hooked end to end to the proximal end of the defunctionalized ileal segment. See also *Bricker's loop.*

Wal·len·berg's syndrome (vaʰl'ᵉn·beʰrk) [A. *Wallenberg,* German physician, 1862–1949]. A neurovascular syndrome involving the lateral portion of the medullary tegmentum. It is usually due to occlusion of the vertebral artery, sometimes to occlusion of the posterior inferior cerebellar artery or one of the lateral medullary arteries. It is characterized by ipsilateral fifth, ninth, and eleventh cranial nerve palsies, Horner's syndrome and cerebellar ataxia, and contralateral loss of pain and temperature sense. Syn. *lateral medullary syndrome.*

wal·le·ri·an degeneration (wah·lirr'ee·un) [A. V. *Waller,* English physician, 1816–1870]. A basic pathologic process affecting peripheral nerves, in which there is degeneration of the axis cylinder and myelin distal to the site of axonal interruption, associated with central chromatolysis.

wallerian law [A. V. *Waller*]. Transection of a nerve produces changes in the myelin sheath that are associated with degeneration of the axons distal to the lesion.

wall·eye (wawl'eye) *n.* 1. LEUKOMA (1). 2. EXOTROPIA. —**wall·eyed** (·ide) *adj.*

wal·nut brain. *Informal.* The severely atrophic brain, observed post mortem in patients with advanced Alzheimer's or ¹Pick's disease, which has been likened in appearance to a shelled walnut.

Wal·thard's inclusions, islets, or **rests** (vaʰl'tart) [M. *Walthard,* Swiss gynecologist, 1867–1933]. Groups of epithelial cells found in the superficial part of the ovaries, uterine tubes, and ligaments.

Wal·ther's ganglion (vaʰl'tur) [A. F. *Walther,* German anatomist, 1688–1746]. COCCYGEAL GANGLION.

Walther's ligament [A. F. *Walther*]. The posterior tolofibular ligament.

Wal·ton's operation [A. J. *Walton,* English surgeon, 1881–1955]. 1. An operation for the relief of hourglass stomach due to ulcer of the lesser curvature. 2. An operation for reconstructing the common bile duct.

wan·der·ing, *adj.* 1. Moving about. 2. Abnormally movable.

wandering abscess. An abscess in which the pus has traveled along the connective-tissue planes and points at some locality distant from its origin. Syn. *abscessus per decubitum.*

wandering atrial pacemaker. WANDERING SUPRAVENTRICULAR PACEMAKER.

wandering cell. *In histology,* any of various mobile cells of the lymphocytic series, such as lymphoid cells, free macrophages, eosinophils, plasma cells, and mast cells, found in varying numbers in loose connective tissue.

wandering erysipelas. A form of erysipelas in which the erysipelatous process successively disappears from one part of the body to appear subsequently in another part.

wandering kidney. FLOATING KIDNEY.

wandering nystagmus. OCULAR NYSTAGMUS.

wandering rash. BENIGN MIGRATORY GLOSSITIS.

wandering spleen. FLOATING SPLEEN.

wandering supraventricular pacemaker. Shifting of the cardiac impulse formation from the sinus node to the atrium or atrioventricular node; recognizable on the electrocardiogram.

Wang·en·steen's apparatus [O. H. *Wangensteen,* U.S. surgeon, b. 1898]. A suction apparatus connected with a Wangensteen or Miller-Abbott tube, which provides and maintains constant gentle aspiration, used for relief of gastric and intestinal distention, and in the treatment of obstruction.

Wangensteen tube [O. H. *Wangensteen*]. A long slender catheter, passed through the nose into the stomach or duodenum to provide continuous drainage.

Wang's test (wahng) [*Wang* Chung Tik, Chinese physician, 1889–1931]. Indican, if present, is converted into indigosulfuric acid and titrated with potassium permanganate solution.

war·ble fly (wor'bul). A fly of the family Oestridae, the cause of warbles.

war·bles, *n.* The disease produced by infestation of domestic animals and man with the larva of the warble fly or botfly. See also *bot.*

War·burg apparatus (vahr'bŏŏrk) [O. H. *Warburg,* German biochemist, b. 1883]. An apparatus, used in studies of cellular respiration and metabolism and also of enzymatic reactions, consisting of one or more reaction chambers maintained at constant temperature in which utilization of oxygen and production of carbon dioxide by small portions of tissue or other test material are measured manometrically.

ward, *n.* [OE. *weard,* watch, guarding]. A division or large room of a hospital.

War·dell method (wawr·del') [Emma Louise *Wardell,* U.S. biochemist, b. 1886]. MYERS AND WARDELL METHOD.

War·drop's disease [J. *Wardrop,* English surgeon, 1782–1869]. ONYCHIA MALIGNA.

Ward's triangle. An area of relative weakness in the neck of the femur produced by the pattern of the trabeculae; a vulnerable site for fracture.

warfarin embryopathy. A syndrome of nasal hypoplasia, optic atrophy, epiphyseal stippling, and delayed psychomotor development, in offspring of mothers who were treated with warfarin anticoagulant during pregnancy.

war·fa·rin sodium (wahr'fuh·rin) [*W*isconsin *A*lumni *R*esearch *F*oundation]. 3-(α-Acetonylbenzyl)-4-hydroxycoumarin sodium, $C_{19}H_{15}NaO_4$, an anticoagulant drug.

war fever. EPIDEMIC TYPHUS.

war gas. A chemical agent which, in field concentrations, produces a toxic or strongly irritant effect. May be a finely dispersed liquid or solid as well as a true gas. Based on physiologic action, five classes of war gases, or chemical warfare agents, are recognized: lacrimators, sternutators, lung irritants, vesicants, systemic poisons.

war injury. Any wound or trauma caused by small-arms or artillery fire, bomb burst, or other war weapons, incurred during battle action or during the disposition of military or naval forces in a theater of operations.

warm-blooded, *adj.* Having a relatively high and constant body temperature, as birds and mammals; HOMEOTHERMIC. Syn. *hematothermal.* Contr. *cold-blooded.*

war medicine. MILITARY MEDICINE.

War·ner's hand. The posture of the hand seen in Sydenham's chorea in which, when the arms are held extended in front of the body, the wrists are sharply flexed and the fingers hyperextended at the proximal and terminal phalanges.

war neurosis. A gross stress reaction to combat, and sometimes to the war situation in general, resulting in a transient situational personality disturbance usually accompanied by somatic complaints and conversion symptoms.

War·ren's incision [J. C. *Warren,* U.S. surgeon, 1842–1927]. A pear-shaped cut encircling the breast for mastectomy.

Warren's operation [J. M. *Warren,* U.S. surgeon, 1811–1867]. A form of uranoplasty.

wart (wort) *n.* 1. VERRUCA VULGARIS. 2. Any rough-surfaced skin papule.

War·ten·berg's disease [R. *Wartenberg,* U.S. neurologist, 1887–1956]. CHEIRALGIA PARESTHETICA.

Wartenberg's sign [R. *Wartenberg*]. 1. Of facial palsy: diminution of palpebral vibration of the upper lid on the affected side when light pressure is exerted against both closed eyes. 2. Of ulnar paralysis: the little finger is maintained in a position of abduction. 3. In lesions of the corticospinal tract, flexion of the fingers against resistance results in abduction, flexion, and opposition of the thumb on the affected side; similar to Hoffmann's sign. 4. Pendulousness of the leg sign: decreased swinging of the leg or legs affected by parkinsonism after the patient's legs are placed so that they can swing freely and are caused to do so.

Wartenberg's wheel [R. *Wartenberg*]. A pinwheel used for testing pain sensation.

War·thin-Fin·kel·dey giant cells [A. S. *Warthin,* U.S. pathologist, 1866–1931; and W. *Finkeldey*]. Multinucleated giant cells found in lymphoid tissue in patients with measles. They contain many small, moderately vesicular nuclei closely clumped together and relatively scanty cytoplasm. The nuclei may number 100 in a cell and give the so-called mulberry outline.

Warthin's sign [A. S. *Warthin*]. A sign of acute pericarditis in which pulmonary sounds are exaggerated.

Warthin-Starry method [A. S. *Warthin*]. A silver nitrate stain for spirochetes in sections of human and animal tissue.

Warthin's tumor [A. S. *Warthin*]. A benign salivary gland tumor, usually of the parotid gland, composed of lymphoid interstitial tissue arranged in papillary processes and covered by a layer of epithelium. Syn. *adenocystoma lymphomatosum.*

wash, *n.* Any of a class of liquid medicinal preparations, usually solutions but sometimes suspensions, for local application without friction or rubbing.

washed sulfur. Sublimed sulfur that has been washed with a dilute solution of ammonia to remove traces of acid. It is the preferred form for internal administration.

wash·er·wom·an's itch. Dermatitis of the hands, a general term for various eruptions, usually a fungus infection or contact dermatitis; seen in those who have their hands frequently in water.

washing soda. A hydrous form of sodium carbonate, $Na_2CO_3.10H_2O$.

wasp waist. A very slender waist caused by atrophy of the trunk muscles, as seen in muscular dystrophy.

Was·ser·mann antibody (vahs'ur·mahn) [A. P. von *Wassermann,* German bacteriologist, 1866–1925]. Antibody which reacts with cardiolipin in serological tests for syphilis.

Wassermann-fast, *adj.* [A. P. von *Wassermann*]. SERORESISTANT.

Wassermann's test [A. P. von *Wassermann*]. A complement-fixation test for syphilis currently utilizing sensitized lipid extracts of beef heart as antigen in order to detect reagin.

waste, *n. & v.* [OF., variant of *guaste,* from L. *vastare,* to lay waste]. 1. Useless matter. 2. Material of no metabolic utility. 3. EXCREMENT. 4. To become thin; to pine away. —**wast·ing,** *adj.*

wast·er (way'stur) *n.* 1. A child suffering from marasmus. 2. An animal affected with tuberculosis, usually bovine types.

wasting palsy. Any progressive muscular atrophy.

watch·mak·er's cramp. 1. An occupational neurosis characterized by painful cramps of the muscles of the hands. 2. Spasm of the orbicularis oculi muscle, due to holding a jeweler's lens.

wa·ter, *n.* 1. The liquid consisting of molecules of the composition H_2O, or aggregates thereof. 2. *In pharmacy,* any saturated aqueous solution of a volatile oil or other aromatic or volatile substance. Syn. *aromatic water.*

water balance. FLUID BALANCE.

water bath. *In chemistry,* an apparatus utilizing the heat of boiling water for drying solids containing moisture or for evaporating fluids without subjecting them to heat that will cause decomposition.

water bed. A bed provided with a water mattress. Syn. *hydrostatic bed.*

water blister. A blister with watery contents.

water brash. PYROSIS.

water-braxy (waw'tur·brack"see) *n.* BRAXY.

water-clear cell. CLEAR CELL (1).

water-drinking test or **tonography.** A provocative test for open-angle glaucoma in which the patient drinks water. Increase in ocular pressure of more than 6 mmHg when the initial tension is 30 mm, or of more than 9 mmHg when initial tension is less than 30 mm, is indicative of a positive reaction. Osmotic changes in blood serum are responsible for the change in ocular tension.

water farcy. FARCY.

water for injection. U.S.P. title for water purified by distillation and that contains no added substance; intended for use as a solvent for preparation of parenteral solutions. See also *bacteriostatic water for injection, sterile water for injection.*

water-gurgle test. A test for esophageal stricture in which the swallowing of water causes a gurgling sound heard on auscultation.

water-hammer pulse. A pulse characterized by a rapid forceful ascent or upstroke. See also *Corrigan pulse.*

Wa·ter·house-Fri·de·rich·sen syndrome [R. *Waterhouse,* English physician, 1872–1958; and C. *Friderichsen*]. The association of bacteremia, particularly acute meningococcemia, massive skin hemorrhage, shock, and acute adrenal hemorrhage and insufficiency.

water intoxication. Cramps, dizziness, headache, vomiting, convulsions, and coma, produced by excessive administration of water or hypotonic solutions, or from water retention, resulting in hemodilution; may occur after administration of tap water enemas, especially to small children, or after head trauma, encephalitis, or from hypothalamic tumors or administration of drugs or anesthetics which result in inappropriate secretion of antidiuretic hormone.

water itch. 1. SCHISTOSOME DERMATITIS. 2. ANCYLOSTOMIASIS.

water mattress. A large, mattress-shaped, leak-proof bag which, when filled with water, conforms to the patient's body with uniform pressure, and supports his weight without excessive pressure on tissues overlying bony prominences.

water moccasin. 1. COTTONMOUTH MOCCASIN. 2. *Erron.* Any of various harmless North American water snakes.

water of crystallization. Water that is coordinated, bound, or held in a lattice position in a crystal in definite molecular proportion and is essential for the characteristic form of the crystal. It may often be removed by heating, with resultant physical disruption of the crystal.

water of hydration. Water that may be variously combined in a substance in definite molecular proportion and that may be expelled by heating without essentially altering the physical form of the substance or changing its chemical identity.

water on the brain. HYDROCEPHALUS.

water-pitressin test. A combination of water intoxication induced by forced liquid intake, with administration of pitressin to detect the existence of epilepsy in a patient. A seizure will be produced in about 50% of all persons predisposed to convulsions. Since the test is positive in a high percentage of normal individuals, and does not rule out epilepsy if negative, it is no longer used, although it was extensively employed around World War I.

wa·ters, *n.pl.* AMNIOTIC FLUID.

wa·ter·shed, *n. In neurology,* the territory at the distal extent of any major arterial supply, and particularly the region at the junction between the terminal branches of two major cerebral arteries, such as the anterior and middle cerebral.

Waters' projection [C. A. *Waters,* U.S. radiologist, 1888–

1961]. A PA x-ray of the face taken with the chin positioned on the film and the nose raised off the film 2 to 3 cm. Designed to demonstrate the maxillae, zygomata, orbits, and nasal passages.

water-sterilizing bag. LYSTER BAG.

water test. A test for Addison's disease based on the fact that patients with this disease do not have a normal diuresis following the rapid intake of a large quantity of water. After a water load any hourly urine volume will not exceed the total night urine volume in a patient with Addison's disease.

water-vomiting disease. EPIDEMIC VOMITING.

wa·tery eye. EPIPHORA.

Wat·son-Crick model [J. D. *Watson,* U.S. geneticist, b. 1928; and F. H. C. *Crick,* English biophysicist, b. 1916]. The model illustrating the double helical complementary structure of deoxyribonucleic acid.

Watson-Schwartz test [C. J. *Watson,* U.S. physician, b. 1900; and S. *Schwartz,* U.S. physician, b. 1916]. A test for porphobilinogen in the urine; used to diagnose acute porphyria.

Watson's method [B. P. *Watson,* U.S. obstetrician, b. 1880]. Induction of labor by the successive use of castor oil, quinine, and pituitrin.

Watson's operation [E. M. *Watson,* U.S. surgeon, 20th century]. A method of urethral reconstruction, in which the gap between the severed ends of the posterior urethra is bridged by urethral flaps.

watt, *n.* [J. *Watt,* Scottish engineer, 1736–1819]. A unit of power, in the meter-kilogram-second system, that produces energy at the rate of one joule per second. It is the power required to cause an unvarying current of one ampere to flow between points differing in potential by one volt. Abbreviated, W.

watt·age (wot'ij) *n.* Consumption or output of an electric device in watts.

wat·tle, *n.* One of the pendulous, erythematous skin folds situated ventral to the larynx in galliform birds. Syn. *lappet.*

watt·me·ter (wot'mee"tur) *n.* [*watt* + *-meter*]. An instrument for measuring electric power or activity in watts.

Waugh-Rud·dick test. A procedure reputed to test a tendency toward thromboembolic disease in which the clotting time of a mixture of whole blood and serial dilutions of heparin is measured.

wave, *n.* 1. A uniform movement in a body which is propagated with a continuous motion, each part of the body vibrating through a fixed path. 2. The course traced by a lever or a beam of light on a surface moving at right angles to the direction of lever or beam. 3. A curve or undulation traced by a recording device, as an electrocardiograph or electroencephalograph, and reflecting alterations in electrical activity or in pressure of a part.

wave-and-spike. SHARP AND SLOW WAVE COMPLEX.

wave front. A surface at which all vibratory motion is of like phase concurrently.

wave·length, *n.* The distance in the line of advancement between two points of a sine wave such that the two points are in the identical phase of the wave cycle. Differences in wavelength distinguish visible light, roentgen rays, and gamma rays from one another. Frequency and wavelength are related by the equation, $C = f\lambda$, where C is the velocity of wave propagation, f is the frequency of the waves, and λ is their wavelength. Abbreviated, wl. Symbol, λ.

wave number. The number of waves or cycles of light flux or radiant energy. measured through a distance of 1 cm.

wax, *n.* Any substance, of plant, animal, or mineral origin, consisting of a mixture of one or more of the following constituents: high molecular weight fatty acids, high molecular weight monohydric alcohols, esters of the fatty acids and alcohols, and solid hydrocarbons. Waxes are usually hard, brittle solids that become pliable on warming and melt on further heating.

wax bougie. A bougie made of linen or gauze impregnated with melted wax.

wax-bulb catheter. A catheter having a waxed tip, which, on being passed into the ureter, indicates the presence of nonopaque calculi by scratches on the wax.

waxy, *adj.* 1. Resembling or covered with wax. 2. Affected with amyloid degeneration or amyloidosis.

waxy cast. A tubal renal cast composed of translucent, usually amyloid, material.

waxy degeneration. 1. AMYLOID DEGENERATION. 2. ZENKER'S DEGENERATION.

waxy flexibility. *In psychiatry,* a form of stereotypy in which the patient maintains a posture in which he was placed with waxlike rigidity for a much longer period than is normally tolerable; typical of the catatonic type of schizophrenia. Compare *catalepsy.*

waxy infiltration. AMYLOID DEPOSITION.

waxy kidney. A kidney which is the seat of amyloidosis.

waxy liver. A liver that is the seat of amyloidosis.

waxy spleen. LARDACEOUS SPLEEN.

WBC Abbreviation for (a) *white blood cell;* (b) *white blood count.*

weak foot. Chronic eversion of the foot, due usually to faulty walking habits associated with loss of muscular tone. Frequently confused with flatfoot.

weak sight. ASTHENOPIA.

wean, *v.* To cease to suckle or nurse offspring at a period when the latter is capable of taking substantial food from sources other than the breast. —**wean·ing,** *n.*

wean·ling, *n.* A child or an animal that has been newly weaned.

weanling brash. Diarrhea in a nursing infant given food other than mother's milk.

wear-and-tear pigments. Pigments such as hemofuscin, hemosiderin, and lipochrome, observed in increased amounts in tissues of older individuals.

weav·er's bottom. LIGHTERMAN'S BOTTOM.

web, *n.* A membranelike structure; especially, the skin and underlying tissue between the bases of fingers or toes. See also *pterygium* (3). —**webbed,** *adj.*

webbed fingers or **toes.** Connection of adjacent fingers or toes at the lateral aspects by interdigital tissue; a form of syndactyly.

webbed neck. A condition in which a thick triangular fold of loose skin extends from each lateral side of the neck across the upper aspect of the shoulder, as seen in gonadal dysgenesis. Syn. *pterygium colli.*

webbed penis. A marked chordee associated with penoscrotal hypospadias, in which the penis is integral with the scrotum.

Weber-Christian disease [F. P. *Weber,* British physician, 1863–1962; and H. A. *Christian,* U.S. physician, 1876–1951]. Febrile, relapsing, nodular nonsuppurative panniculitis.

Weber-Fechner law. FECHNER'S LAW.

Weber's crossed paralysis [H. D. *Weber,* British physician, 1823–1918]. WEBER'S SYNDROME.

Weber's disease [F. P. *Weber*]. STURGE-WEBER DISEASE.

We·ber's glands (vey'bur) [E. H. *Weber,* German anatomist and physiologist, 1795–1878]. Racemose glands situated in the posterior portion of the tongue.

Weber's law [E. H. *Weber*]. To excite a series of sensations differing by equal increments, the stimuli must increase in geometric proportion.

Weber's organ or **vesicle** [M. I. *Weber,* German anatomist, 1795–1875]. UTRICLE (2).

Weber's syndrome [H. D. *Weber*]. A form of crossed paralysis caused by a lesion in the upper brainstem involving the cerebral peduncle and oculomotor nerve, characterized by partial or complete third nerve paralysis on the same side and contralateral spastic hemiplegia including the lower two-thirds of the face. Compare *Millard-Gubler syndrome.*

Weber's test [F. E. *Weber*-Liel, German otologist, 1832-1891]. A hearing test in which the vibrations from a tuning fork placed on the forehead of a normal patient are referred to the midline and heard equally in both ears; in unilateral middle-ear deafness, the sound is heard in the diseased ear; in deafness due to disease of the auditory nerve on one side, it is heard better in the normal ear.

Web·ster's operation [J. C. *Webster,* Canadian gynecologist, 1863-1950]. BALDY-WEBSTER OPERATION.

Webster's test [J. *Webster,* English chemist, 1878-1927]. A method for detecting trinitrotoluene in urine.

Wechs·ler-Belle·vue intelligence scale [D. *Wechsler,* U.S. psychologist, b. 1896; and *Bellevue* Hospital, New York City]. A verbal and performance test for persons aged 16 to 64 years, comprising 11 subtests: information, comprehension, arithmetical reasoning, digit memory, similarities, vocabulary, picture arrangement, picture completion, block design, object assembly, and digit symbol.

We·den·sky facilitation (vvʸe·dʸen'skee) [N. I. *Wedensky (Vvedenski)* Russian neurologist, b. 1884]. An effect resembling facilitation across a nerve block, observed when two stimuli are applied in succession to the motor nerve of a curarized muscle, involving the summation of the end-plate potentials which, on reaching a critical intensity, results in muscular contraction.

Wedensky inhibition or **phenomenon** [N. I. *Wedensky*]. Total or partial block to nerve conduction when successive stimuli fall in the refractory period resulting from a previous stimulus.

wedged vertebra. A deformed vertebral body resembling a wedge, usually due to compressive forces acting on normal or diseased bone.

wedge pressure. Pulmonary capillary pressure, measured at cardiac catheterization by wedging the cardiac catheter in the most distal pulmonary artery branch; it reflects mean left atrial pressure. Syn. *pulmonary artery wedge pressure.*

weep·ing, *adj. & n.* 1. Exuding, as a raw or excoriated surface bathed with a moist discharge. 2. LACRIMATION. 3. Exudation or leakage of a fluid.

weeping eczema. EXUDATIVE ECZEMA.

weeping sinew. GANGLION (2).

We·ge·ner's granulomatosis (veʸ'guh·nur) [F. *Wegener*]. A rare disease of unknown causation characterized by necrotizing granulomas in the air passages, necrotizing vasculitis, and glomerulitis.

Weg·ner's disease (veʸg'nur) [F. R. G. *Wegner,* German pathologist, 1843-1917]. Osteochondritic epiphyseal separation in congenital syphilis.

Weich·sel·baum's coccus (vike'sᵉl·baowm) [A. *Weichselbaum,* Austrian pathologist, 1845-1920]. *NEISSERIA MENINGITIDIS.*

Wei·del reaction (vye'dᵉl) [H. *Weidel,* Austrian chemist, 1849-1899]. A test for xanthine in which a small amount of the substance to be tested is brought into solution in bromine water. It is evaporated to dryness, and ammonia fumes are allowed to come into contact with the dry residue. The presence of xanthine is shown by development of a red color.

Weigert-Meyer law. A urological maxim which states that in cases of reduplication of the upper urinary tract, the lower ureteral orifice belongs to the upper pelvis (Weigert), or in cases where the two orifices are located side by side, the medial orifice belongs to the upper pelvis (Meyer).

Wei·gert's law (vigh'gurt) [C. *Weigert,* German pathologist, 1845-1904]. Loss of an animal part may be followed by overproduction of the part during repair.

Weigert's method [K. *Weigert,* German pathologist, 1843-1904]. A technique for staining myelin sheaths with hematoxylin.

Weigert's stain. A fuchsin-resorcin-ferric chloride stain for elastin.

weight, *n.* The force with which a body is attracted by the earth. For weights listed by name, see Tables of Weights and Measures in the Appendix.

weight traction. The traction exerted by means of a weight, connected to the injured limb.

Weil-Fe·lix reaction (vile, fee'licks) [E. *Weil,* Austrian physician, 1880-1922; and A. *Felix,* British bacteriologist, 1887-1956]. The agglutination of certain strains of *Proteus vulgaris* (OX 19, OX 2, OX K) by the serums of patients with certain rickettsial infections, probably due to the presence of similar antigens in both *Proteus* and *Rickettsia.*

Weil-Felix test. An agglutination test based on the Weil-Felix reaction; used in the diagnosis of certain rickettsial diseases.

Weill-Mar·che·sa·ni syndrome (veʰl, mar''ke·zah'nee) [G. Weill, French, 20th century; and O. *Marchesani,* German ophthalmalogist, 1900-1952]. A heritable disorder of connective tissue manifested by short stature, brachydactylia, and spherophakia with associated myopia and glaucoma. Syn. *Marchesani syndrome.*

Weil method. A titrimetric method for trypsin based on the employment of casein as the substrate and enterokinase as the activator, the addition of formol, and titration with tetramethylammonium hydroxide.

Weil's disease [A. *Weil,* German physician, 1848-1916]. A severe form of leptospirosis, characterized by jaundice, oliguria, circulatory collapse, and hemorrhagic tendencies. Syn. *icterohemorrhagic fever, leptospirosis icterohemorrhagica, spirochetal jaundice.*

Weil's method or **stain** [A. *Weil,* U.S. neuropathologist, b. 1887]. An iron hematoxylin method for myelin sheaths which may be used for sections embedded either in paraffin or collodion.

Weil's test [R. *Weil,* U.S. physician, 1876-1917]. A test for syphilis based on the observation that hemolysis does not occur if the erythrocytes of a syphilitic patient are mixed with a solution of dried cobra venom.

Wein·bach method [A. P. *Weinbach,* U.S. biochemist, b. 1911]. A method for determining the sodium content in blood. After deproteinization, the sodium in the filtrate is precipitated in alcoholic medium as the triple salt, uranyl zinc sodium acetate, which is washed, dissolved in water, and titrated with standard sodium hydroxide.

Wein·grow's heel reflex. In corticospinal tract lesions, tapping of the midplantar region of the foot or the base of the heel is followed by plantar flexion and fanning of the toes.

Weir's incision (weer) [R. F. *Weir,* U.S. surgeon, 1838-1927]. A lumbar incision for nephrectomy.

Weir's operation [R. F. *Weir*]. 1. A procedure for correction of hallux valgus. 2. APPENDICOSTOMY.

Weis·bach's angle (vice'baᵏh) [A. W. *Weisbach,* Austrian anthropologist, 1837-1914]. An angle formed by lines starting from the basion and from the middle of the frontal suture and meeting at the alveolar point.

Weis·mann's theory (vice'maʰn) [A. F. L. *Weismann,* German biologist, 1834-1914]. A doctrine stating that hereditary material or germ plasm is distinct from the somatoplasm; that there is a continuity of germ plasm from generation to generation; that a change in the somatoplasm or body cannot affect the germ plasm, which renders it impossible for acquired characteristics to be inherited; and that during development the heredity determiners are sorted out to the parts of the body where they give rise to hereditary characteristics. Compare *pangenesis.* See also *blastogenesis.*

Weiss's sign (vice) [N. *Weiss,* Austrian physician, 1851-1883]. CHVOSTEK'S SIGN.

Weisz test. A test for urochromogen in urine in which a 1% solution of potassium permanganate is added to dilute urine. In the presence of urochromogen, a yellow tint will appear due to the oxidation of the urochromogen.

Welch bacillus [W. H. *Welch,* American pathologist, 1850–1934]. CLOSTRIDIUM PERFRINGENS.

Wells' facies [T. S. *Wells,* English gynecologist, 1818–1897]. The anxious drawn expression of the face in the presence of large cystic tumors of the ovary.

Wells-Stenger test. STENGER TEST.

Welt·mer·ism (welt'mur·iz·um) *n.* [C. E. *Weltmer,* U.S. faith healer, b. 1880]. Suggestion therapy based on a theory of harmony between mind and body.

wen, *n.* A sebaceous cyst. The term is commonly used when the lesion occurs on the scalp.

Wenck·e·bach phenomenon (venk'eʰ·bakʰ) [K. F. *Wenckebach,* Dutch physician, 1864–1940]. A form of second-degree atrioventricular block with progressive prolongation of the P-R interval, resulting finally in a nonconducted P wave; at this point the P-R interval shortens and the sequence recurs. See also *atrioventricular block.*

Werd·nig-Hoff·mann atrophy, disease, paralysis, or **syndrome** (veʰrt'nik, hoʰf'mahn) [G. *Werdnig,* Austrian neurologist, b. 1862; and J. *Hoffmann*]. INFANTILE SPINAL MUSCULAR ATROPHY.

Werl·hof's disease (veʰrl'hofe) [P. G. *Werlhof,* German physician, 1699–1767]. IDIOPATHIC THROMBOCYTOPENIC PURPURA.

Wer·mer's syndrome. Type I of multiple endocrine adenomatosis, in which there is a grouping of tumors or hyperplasia of the parathyroids, islets of the pancreas, and pituitary gland, frequently accompanied by the Zollinger-Ellison syndrome.

Wer·ne·kinck's commissure (veʰr'neʰ·kink) [F. C. G. *Wernekinck,* German anatomist, 1798–1835]. Decussating fibers of the middle cerebellar peduncle.

Wer·ner-His disease or **syndrome** (veʰr'nur, hiss) [H. *Werner,* German physician, 1874–1946; and W. *His,* Jr.]. TRENCH FEVER.

Werner's disease [H. *Werner*]. TRENCH FEVER.

Werner's syndrome [C. W. O. *Werner,* German physician, 20th century]. A multisystem disorder, probably of autosomal recessive inheritance, characterized by premature senescence, diminished body growth (dwarfism), cataracts, scleroderma-like skin changes, osteoporosis, and multiglandular dysfunction, particularly hypogonadism. Compare *Hutchinson-Gilford syndrome.*

Wernicke hemianopic pupillary reaction or **reflex.** WERNICKE'S SIGN.

Wer·ni·cke-Mann paralysis (veʰr'ni·keʰ, angl. vur'ni·kee, wur') [K. *Wernicke,* German neurologist, 1848–1905; and L. *Mann*]. A partial hemiplegia of the extremities characterized by a typical dystonic posture of the arm and hand and disorder of gait.

Wernicke's aphasia [K. *Wernicke*]. A classical division of aphasia including those sensory aphasias characterized by volubility of speech with paraphasia and often jargon, and loss of comprehension of spoken and written words; due, as a rule, to a lesion in the posterior perisylvian region.

Wernicke's area [K. *Wernicke*]. The posterior portion of the left superior temporal gyrus, Brodmann's areas 41 and 42, destruction of which gives rise to a loss of comprehension of spoken language.

Wernicke's encephalopathy [K. *Wernicke*]. A disease of acute onset, characterized clinically by nystagmus, abducens and conjugate gaze palsies, ataxia of gait, mental confusion, and, in patients who recover, by an amnesic (Korsakoff's) psychosis; pathologically there are symmetrical areas of necrosis in the paraventricular regions of the thalamus and hypothalamus, the mamillary bodies, the periaqueductal region of the midbrain, floor of the fourth ventricle, and the superior vermis. The disease is usually observed in alcoholics and is due to nutritional deficiency, more specifically a deficiency of thiamine.

Wernicke's sign [K. *Wernicke*]. A reaction obtained in some cases of hemianopsia in which a pencil of light thrown on the blind side of the retina gives rise to no movement in the iris, but, when thrown upon the normal side, produces contraction of the iris. It indicates that the lesion producing the hemianopsia is situated at or anterior to the geniculate bodies.

Wernicke's syndrome [K. *Wernicke*]. 1. WERNICKE'S ENCEPHALOPATHY. 2. PRESBYOPHRENIA.

Wert·heim-Schau·ta operation (vehrt'hime, shaow'tah) [E. *Wertheim,* Austrian gynecologist, 1864–1920; and F. *Schauta*]. An operation for cystocele.

Wertheim's operation [E. *Wertheim*]. A radical total hysterectomy for carcinoma of the uterine cervix.

Werth's tumor. PSEUDOMYXOMA PERITONEI.

Wes·ter·gren method (ves'tur·greʸn'') [A. *Westergren,* Swedish physician, b. 1891]. A method to determine the blood sedimentation rate in which normal for men is 0 to 15 and for women is 0 to 20 mm in 1 hour.

West Nile fever. An acute febrile disease clinically resembling dengue fever and occurring principally in the Near East, caused by the West Nile virus. Syn. *Mediterranean dengue.*

West Nile virus [*West Nile,* a region in northwestern Uganda]. A group B arbovirus, widespread in Africa and southern Asia, producing a very mild encephalitis similar to the St. Louis and Japanese B encephalitides. In the Near East it causes West Nile fever.

West·phal maneuver (vest·fahl) [C. F. O. *Westphal,* German neurologist, 1833–1890]. Brief sweeping movements of the eyes, or of the head and neck, to trace letters, whereby alexic or dyslexic patients derive kinesthetic clues for the recognition of letters.

Westphal nucleus [C. F. O. *Westphal*]. AUTONOMIC NUCLEUS OF THE OCULOMOTOR NERVE.

Westphal-Pilcz reflex [A. K. O. *Westphal,* German neurologist, 1863–1941; and A. *Pilcz*]. PUPILLARY REFLEX (4).

Westphal's disease or **neurosis** [C. F. O. *Westphal*]. HEPATOLENTICULAR DEGENERATION.

Westphal's pupillary reflex [A. K. O. *Westphal*]. PUPILLARY REFLEX (4).

Westphal's sign [C. F. O. *Westphal*]. Absence of the knee jerk, particularly in patients with tabes dorsalis.

Westphal-Strümpell pseudosclerosis [C. F. O. *Westphal* and E. A. G. G. *Strümpell*]. HEPATOLENTICULAR DEGENERATION.

West's syndrome [W. J. *West,* English physician, 19th century]. A clinical triad consisting of infantile spasms, psychomotor regression, and EEG abnormalities, most often hypsarrhythmia. In most cases West's syndrome appears in infants already suffering from some form of brain damage or disease.

wet-and-dry-bulb thermometer. A device for determining the relative humidity. It consists of two thermometers, the bulb of one of which is kept saturated with water vapor. The evaporation of water vapor has a cooling effect which depresses the temperature. The temperature difference between the two thermometers depends upon the relative humidity.

wet brain. Edema of the brain.

wet-bulb temperature. The temperature indicated when a current of air is passed over a thermometer bulb which is enclosed by a wet jacket. Evaporation of water from the jacket lowers temperature, the degree of lowering being inversely related to the humidity of the atmosphere. Contr. *dry-bulb temperature.*

wet cup. A cup for abstracting blood through incisions in the skin.

wet cupping. The abstraction of blood after scarification.

wet dream. Seminal emission during sleep, generally accompanying an erotic dream.

wet gangrene. MOIST GANGRENE.

wet nurse. A woman who furnishes breast feeding to an infant not her own.

wet pack. A blanket wrung out of warm or cold water.

wetting agent. A substance, commonly a synthetic organic compound, that causes a liquid to spread more readily upon a solid surface, chiefly through reduction of surface tension. Wetting agents are either ionic or nonionic, the former being further classified as cationic or anionic, depending on whether the characteristic activity is inherent in the cation or anion.

Wet·zel's grid [N. C. *Wetzel,* U.S. pediatrician, b. 1897]. A precision control chart for measuring and guiding growth and development of children from 5 to 18 years. Body build, maturation, nutritional grade, metabolic rate, and caloric intake are all determined by this graphic method.

We·ver-Bray effect or **phenomenon** [E. G. *Wever,* U.S. psychologist, b. 1902; and C. W. *Bray,* U.S. psychologist, b. 1904]. The microphonic response of the cochlea, so called because of resemblance to the electrical phenomena produced by sound waves in microphones. It consists of electrical potentials caused by the stimulation of the cochlea by sound.

Weyl's test (vile) [T. *Weyl,* German chemist, 1851-1913]. A test for creatinine in which a ruby-red color, then yellow, results when a solution containing creatinine is treated with sodium nitroprusside and sodium hydroxide.

W factor. BIOTIN.

Whar·ton's duct [T. *Wharton,* English anatomist, 1614-1673]. SUBMANDIBULAR DUCT.

Wharton's jelly [T. *Wharton*]. The mucoid connective tissue that constitutes the matrix of the umbilical cord.

wheal, *n.* A primary lesion of the skin that is a pruritic, circumscribed, edematous, usually transitory elevation that varies in size from a pin-head to that of the palm or larger, occurring classically in urticaria but also after insect bites, animal bites, trauma, or even as an effect of such physical agents as heat, cold, or sunlight. Syn. *pomphus, urtica.*

wheal-and-flare response. CUTANEOUS ANAPHYLAXIS.

wheat bug. A mite of the genus *Pediculoides.*

wheat-germ oil. An oil obtained from the embryo of choice *Triticum vulgare.* A group of chemically related substances have been separated from this oil, to which were given the name tocopherols; they possess the activity of vitamin E. One of these, α-tocopherol, is especially active biologically.

Wheat·stone bridge [C. *Wheatstone,* British physicist, 1802-1875]. An electric circuit containing four resistances in branches or arms. When the bridge is suitably adjusted or balanced, any one resistance can be calculated in terms of the other three.

Wheel·house operation [C. G. *Wheelhouse,* English surgeon, 1826-1909]. An external urethrotomy for stricture.

wheel rotation of Helm·holtz [H. L. F. von *Helmholtz*]. The rotations of the eyeball around the line of fixation causing the iris to roll around like a wheel.

wheeze, *n.* A whistling or sighing noise produced in the act of breathing, often audible only on stethoscopic examination.

whet·stone crystal. A type of uric acid found in acid urine.

whey (whay) *n.* The liquid part of milk separating from the curd.

whip bougie. A variety of filiform bougie.

whip catheter. FILIFORM CATHETER.

whip cell. A flagellated cell.

whip·lash injury. A syndrome, including headache, pain and tenderness of the occipitonuchal muscles and other supporting structures of the head and neck, related to the sudden extension or flexion of the neck which may occur in automobile occupants when their car is struck from behind or from the front.

Whip·ple operation [A. O. *Whipple,* U.S. surgeon, 1881-1963]. Radical pancreaticoduodenectomy for carcinoma of the ampullary area and pancreatic head.

Whip·ple's disease [G. H. *Whipple,* U.S. pathologist, b. 1878]. A generalized disease associated with an intracellular bacterium and characterized by infiltration of the intestinal wall and lymphatics by glycoprotein-filled macrophages; there is steatorrhea, lymphadenopathy, arthritis, polyserositis, emaciation, and lipophagic intestinal granulomatosis. Syn. *intestinal lipodystrophy.*

Whipple's triad [A. O. *Whipple*]. The three conditions which together are diagnostic of hyperinsulinism: attacks invariably occur while fasting; fasting blood sugar is below 50 mg/dl; immediate recovery from an acute attack occurs upon administration of glucose.

whip·worm, *n.* *TRICHURIS TRICHIURA.*

whirl·pool bath. A bath in which an arm, or a leg, or the greater part of the body is immersed in hot water which is agitated by a whirling or churning current of equally hot water mixed with air.

whis·key nose. RHINOPHYMA.

whis·per, *n.* A low, sibilant sound produced by the passage of the breath through the glottis without vibrating the vocal folds.

whispered pectoriloquy. The transmission of whispered voice sounds through the chest wall, heard stethoscopically; indicates consolidation near a large air passage.

whis·tling face syndrome. CRANIOCARPOTARSAL DYSPLASIA.

white, *adj.* Having a color produced by reflection of all the rays of the spectrum; opposed to black.

white, *n.* Any white substance, as white of egg.

white arsenic. ARSENIC TRIOXIDE.

white beeswax. Bleached yellow wax; WHITE WAX.

white blood cell. LEUKOCYTE. Abbreviated, WBC.

white blood count. The calculation of the number of white blood cells per volume of blood or the determination of the percentages of each type of leukocyte. Abbreviated, WBC.

white cinnamon. CANELLA.

white comb. COMB DISEASE.

white commissure. 1. A band of myelinated nerve fibers in the spinal cord separating the anterior gray commissure from the bottom of the anterior median fissure. Syn. *anterior white commissure.* NA *commissura alba medullae spinalis.* 2. See *white commissure* (1) (= anterior white commissure), *posterior white commissure.*

white corpuscle. LEUKOCYTE.

white diarrhea of chicks. PULLORUM DISEASE.

white fat. Ordinary adipose tissue as distinguished from brown fat; characterized by unilocular cells and white or yellow color.

white fibers. COLLAGENOUS FIBERS.

white fibrous tissue. FIBROUS CONNECTIVE TISSUE.

white-grained mycetoma. A form of mycetoma, caused by any of eleven different etiological agents, in which the grains discharged in the exudate or on unstained tissue sections are white.

white head. WITKOP.

White·head's operation [W. *Whitehead,* English surgeon, 1840-1913]. 1. Treatment of hemorrhoids by total excision of the hemorrhoidal area. 2. Excision of the tongue through the mouth, using scissors only.

White·horn's method [J. C. *Whitehorn,* U.S. biochemist, b. 1894]. A method for determining blood chlorides in which chlorides from the blood filtrate are precipitated with silver nitrate, and the excess silver is titrated with a standard thiocyanate solution.

white infarct. An infarct in which the hemorrhage is slight, or the blood and blood pigments have been removed so that the infarct has become decolorized.

white leprosy. VITILIGO.

white line. LINEA ALBA.

white line of Fraen·kel (frenk'ul) [E. *Fraenkel,* German anatomist and pathologist, 1853–1925]. In scurvy, the zone of calcified cartilage at the end of the diaphysis which appears more opaque than usual by radiography because of the increased radiolucency of the other portions of the bone.

white lotion. A lotion prepared by interaction of zinc sulfate and sulfurated potash; used in the treatment of various types of skin diseases for which sulfur is employed.

white matter. WHITE SUBSTANCE.

White method. LEE-WHITE METHOD.

white muscle. Skeletal muscle that appears paler in the fresh state than red muscle; it has more myofibrils and less sarcoplasm in its fibers.

white-muscle disease. A degenerative process of skeletal or cardiac muscle affecting cattle and chickens and thought to result from at least three causes: vitamin E deficiency, selenium deficiency, and the toxic effect of certain poisonous plants.

white noise. WHITE SOUND.

white petrolatum. Petrolatum wholly or nearly decolorized. Used as an ointment base and a protectant.

white pine. The dried inner bark of *Pinus strobus;* has been used as an ingredient in cough syrups. Syn. *white pine bark.*

white·pox, *n.* A mild form of smallpox.

white precipitate. AMMONIATED MERCURY.

white pulp. The lymphocytic portion of the spleen consisting of B and T lymphocyte zones and associated arterial vasculature and lymphatics; the site of antibody formation in the spleen. Contr. *red pulp.*

white ramus communicans. A communicating nerve connecting the sympathetic trunk with the dorsal and ventral roots of a spinal nerve. Syn. *preganglionic ramus.*

whites, *n.* LEUKORRHEA.

white sa·po·ta (sa·po'tuh). *CASIMIROA EDULIS.*

White's method [C. *White,* English surgeon, 1728–1813]. A method of reducing dislocation of the shoulder, in which the unbooted heel is placed in the axilla and traction is exerted on the arm. Syn. *Cooper's method.*

white softening. *Obsol.* Softening of nerve substance in which the affected area presents a whitish color due to fatty degeneration following anemia.

White's operation [J. W. *White,* U.S. surgeon, 1850–1916]. An operation in which the testes are removed for hypertrophy of the prostate.

white sound. 1. A noise made up of pure tones, harmonics, and discordants throughout the range of human hearing in equal parts and at equal intensities. It is used as a background noise in speech intelligibility tests. 2. The noise component in audio analgesia.

white-sponge nevus of mucosa. NEVUS SPONGIOSUS ALBUS.

white spots. Gray or yellowish-white elevated spots, 2 to 15 mm in diameter, of varying shape and distinctness of outline, often occurring on the ventricular surface of the anterior leaflet of the mitral valve.

white substance or **matter.** The part of the central nervous system composed of myelinated nerve fibers. NA *substantia alba.* Contr. *gray substance.*

white substance of Schwann [F. T. *Schwann*]. MYELIN.

white swelling. In orthopedics, enlargement of a joint or part without increased local heat or redness; usually due to tuberculosis.

white thrombus. A thrombus composed principally of a deposit of fibrin.

white vitriol. ZINC SULFATE.

white wax. Bleached yellow wax. See also *yellow wax.*

Whit·field's ointment [A. *Whitfield,* English dermatologist, 1867–1947]. An ointment used in treatment of superficial fungous infections of the skin. It contains 6% benzoic acid, and 3% salicylic acid in a petrolatum or polethylene glycol ointment base.

whit·low (whit'lo) *n.* [ME. *whitflawe,* from *whit,* white, + *flawe,* flaw]. Suppurative inflammation of the end of a finger or toe. See also *felon, paronychia.*

Whit·man's operation [R. *Whitman,* U.S. orthopedist, 1857–1946]. A type of excision of the talus for relief of talipes calcaneus.

Whit·ten effect. The simultaneous induction of estrus in a group of female mice by the introduction of a male, following group housing of the females to synchronize the occurence of anestrus.

WHO Abbreviation for *World Health Organization.*

whole-body counter. A device, with heavy shielding to keep out background radiation and with ultrasensitive scintillation detectors and electronic equipment, used to identify and measure the radiation in the body of humans and animals.

whole endotoxic O antigen. ENDOTOXIN.

whoop (hoop, whoop) *n.* The inspiratory crowing sound that precedes or occurs during a coughing paroxysm.

whoop·ing cough (hoop'ing). PERTUSSIS.

Whytt's disease (white) [R. *Whytt,* Scottish physician, 1714–1766]. 1. Tuberculous meningitis in children. 2. OBSTRUCTIVE HYDROCEPHALUS.

Whytt's reflex [R. *Whytt*]. 1. LIGHT REFLEX. 2. PUPILLARY REFLEX (1).

Wick·ham's striae [L.-F. *Wickham,* French dermatologist, 1861–1913]. A network of delicate bluish-white lines associated with the characteristic lesions of lichen planus.

wick·ing, *n.* Loosely twisted unspun cotton or gauze, employed in packing cavities; a gauze wick.

Wi·dal's syndrome (vee·dahl') [G. F. I. *Widal,* French physician, 1862–1929]. ACQUIRED HEMOLYTIC ANEMIA.

Widal test [G. F. I. *Widal*]. A microscopic or macroscopic agglutination test for the diagnosis of typhoid fever and other Salmonella infections. Living cultures may be used specially prepared to preserve the Vi antigen; killed bacterial suspensions may be prepared with formalin to preserve the flagellar (H) antigen or with alcohol to preserve the somatic (O) antigen.

wide-angle glaucoma. OPEN-ANGLE GLAUCOMA.

wide-field oculars. Oculars with a wide field of view, now used especially in biobjective dissecting microscopes.

Wi·gand's manuever (vee'gahnt) [J. H. *Wigand,* German obstetrician and gynecologist, 1766–1817]. Extraction of the aftercoming head by pressure above the symphysis with the second hand, the first being under the infant's body.

Wil·bur and Ad·dis method. A spectroscopic procedure for the determination of urobilinogen.

Wild·bolz's reaction (vilt'bohlts) [H. *Wildbolz,* Swiss urologist, 1873–1940]. In tuberculous patients, the intradermal injection of a small amount of the patient's urine produces an extensive local inflammatory reaction.

wild cherry. The stem bark of *Prunus serotina;* it contains an enzyme, emulsin, which acts on a cyanogenetic glycoside to form hydrocyanic acid. Used as a flavoring agent, especially for cough syrups.

Wil·der test [R. M. *Wilder,* U.S. physician, b. 1885]. CUTLER-POWER-WILDER TEST.

Wil·der·muth's ear (vil'dur·moot) [H. A. *Wildermuth,* German psychiatrist, 1852–1907]. A congenital deformity of the ear characterized by a prominent anthelix and a turned-down or maldeveloped helix.

Wilde's incision [W. R. W. *Wilde,* Irish surgeon, 1815–1876]. An incision for the relief of mastoid periostitis made about half an inch behind the pinna and parallel to it.

wildfire rash. MILIARIA.

wild ginger. ASARUM.

Wil·hel·mi's method. FRAME, RUSSELL, AND WILHELMI'S METHOD.

Wilks' disease [S. *Wilks,* English physician, 1824–1911]. 1. Subacute glomerulonephritis. 2. VERRUCA NECROGENICA.

Wilks' syndrome or **symptom complex** [S. *Wilks*]. MYASTHENIA GRAVIS.

will, *n. In psychology,* the faculty by which the mind chooses its ends and directs action in carrying out its purpose.

Wil·lems' method or **treatment** [C. *Willems,* Belgian surgeon, 20th century]. A method of treating acute suppurative arthritis by arthrotomy and immediate mobilization.

Wil·liam·son's test [R. T. *Williamson,* English physician, 1862–1937]. Blood from a diabetic patient decolorizes a boiling solution of methylene blue and potassium hydroxide.

Williamson's test or **sign** [O. K. *Williamson,* English physician, 1866–1941]. A sign of pleural effusion or pneumothorax in which the leg blood pressure is lower than the arm blood pressure on the same side.

Willi-Prader syndrome. PRADER-WILLI SYNDROME.

Wil·lis forceps [D. A. *Willis,* U.S. surgeon, 1900–1952]. A forceps, designed for foreign body removal, attached to an electric battery and lamp, the forceps blades being insulated from each other. Upon contact with a metallic object, the circuit is completed and the lamp glows.

Willis salt flotation method. FLOTATION METHOD.

Willis's circle [T. *Willis,* English anatomist, 1621–1675]. CIRCLE OF WILLIS.

Willis's disease [T. *Willis*]. DIABETES MELLITUS.

Willis's glands [T. *Willis*]. CORPORA ALBICANTIA.

Willis's nerve [T. *Willis*]. The ophthalmic branch of the trigeminal nerve.

Willis's paracusis [T. *Willis*]. PARACUSIA WILLISII.

Willis's pouch [T. *Willis*]. OMENTAL BURSA.

will to power. *In Adlerian psychology,* the neurotic and excessive aggressiveness of an individual compensating for feelings of inferiority and insecurity.

Wilms's or **Wilms' tumor** (vilmss) [M. *Wilms,* German surgeon, 1867–1918]. A malignant mixed mesodermal tumor of the kidney, usually affecting infants and children.

Wilpo. Trademark for phentermine, an anorexigenic drug used as the hydrochloride salt in sustained release dosage form.

Wil·son central terminal. *In electrocardiography,* an indifferent electrode of near zero potential obtained by connecting the three limbs of the subject to a central terminal through resistances of 5,000 ohms each.

Wilson-Mikity syndrome [M. G. *Wilson,* U.S. pediatrician, b. 1922; and V. G. *Mikity,* U.S. radiologist, b. 1919]. Progressive pulmonary insufficiency with dyspnea, tachypnea, rib retraction, and cyanosis, coming on at or soon after birth in very premature infants, whose chest radiographs characteristically show numerous small radiolucent cystlike lesions of the lungs.

Wilson's disease [S. A. K. *Wilson,* U.S. neurologist, 1877–1937]. HEPATOLENTICULAR DEGENERATION.

Wilson's pronator sign [S. A. K. *Wilson*]. In Sydenham's chorea, on extension of the arms above the head, the forearms are inadvertently pronated so that the palms face outward.

Wilson's sign [S. A. K. *Wilson*]. Corectopia as evidence of mesencephalic disease of any type.

Wilson's test [K. M. *Wilson,* U.S. obstetrician, b. 1885]. A test for pregnancy in which urine is injected into a female rabbit, the test being positive if the rabbit ovaries develop corpora hemorrhagica.

Wim·berg·er's line. A zone of increased calcification is seen in roentgenograms ringing the epiphyses of long bones in rickets. Compare *Wimberger's sign.*

Wimberger's sign. Bilateral metaphyseal defects on the upper medial aspect of the tibias seen radiographically in congenital syphilis and other conditions. Compare *Wimberger's line.*

Winck·el's disease (vink'el) [F. K. L. W. von *Winckel,* German physician, 1837–1911]. Sepsis of the newborn associated with acute hemolytic anemia, hemoglobinuria, jaundice, and often neurologic symptoms. Syn. *epidemic hemoglobinuria.*

wind·age (win'dij) *n.* Compression of air by the passage of a missile, shell, etc., near the body, causing blast injury.

Win·daus digitonin test (vin'daowss) [A. *Windaus,* German chemist, 1876–1959]. A histochemical method for 3β-OH sterols, such as cholesterol, vitamin-D compounds, and isoandrosterone, using digitonin solution to produce needle-shaped birefringent crystals observed under the polarizing microscope.

wind-broken, *adj.* Affected with expiratory dyspnea; said especially of horses.

wind colic. BLOAT (2).

wind·gall (wind'gawl) *n.* A soft tumor or synovial swelling in the region of the fetlock joint of the horse.

wind·kes·sel (wind'kes·ul, vint') *n.* [Ger., air chamber, compression chamber]. Compression chamberlike action of the aorta and its immediate branches in buffering pressure and flow changes during the cardiac cycle. This function of the large capacity and elastic walls of the vessels converts pulsatile flow to nearly continuous flow.

wind·lass (wind'lus) *n.* [ON. *vindāss,* from *vinda,* to wind, + *āss,* pole]. A device for providing traction. The rope or strap to be pulled is wound around a cylindrical part of the apparatus which is turned by means of a crank. Considerable mechanical advantage is usually gained thereby.

windlass traction. A method of exerting traction on an extremity of the body. Extension straps, attached to the skin by means of adhesive tape or to bone by means of a pin passed through it, are wound upon a specially designed windlass. Turning the device produces the desired amount of pull and facilitates subsequent adjustment of degree of traction with minimal disturbance to the patient.

wind·mill murmur. CONTINUOUS MURMUR.

win·dow, *n.* [ON. *vindauga,* lit., wind-eye]. *In anatomy,* a small aperture in a bone or other unyielding tissue. See also *fenestra* and Plate 20.

wind·pipe, *n.* TRACHEA.

wind-puff, *n.* WINDGALL.

wind·stroke, *n.* Acute spinal paralysis of a horse.

wind sucking. CRIBBING (2).

wine·glass, *n.* A measure of nearly two fluidounces, or 60 ml.

wine spot. PORT-WINE NEVUS.

wing, *n.* ALA.

wing cell. The polyhedral cells of the epidermis.

winged scapula. Projection of the scapula posteriorly, particularly noticeable when the arm is extended and pressed against a fixed object in front of the patient, due to weakness or paralysis of the serratus anterior muscle.

Wi·ni·war·ter's operation (vin'i·vah^r''tur) [A. von *Winiwarter,* Austrian surgeon, 1848–1917]. A cholecystojejunostomy in two stages.

wink, *v.* 1. To close and open one eye voluntarily. 2. To blink.

wink·ing reflex. Sudden closure of the eyelids in response to the unexpected appearance of any object within the field of vision. Contr. *blink reflex.*

winking spasm. Spasmodic twitching or blinking of the eyelids. May be a habit tic or be associated with irritative conditions of the eye or of the trigeminal or facial nerve. Syn. *spasmus nictitans.*

wink response. ANAL REFLEX.

Wins·low's foramen [J. B. (Jacobus Benignus) *Winslow,* French anatomist, 1669–1760]. EPIPLOIC FORAMEN.

Winslow's pancreas [J. B. *Winslow*]. UNCINATE PROCESS OF THE PANCREAS.

Winslow's stars [J. B. *Winslow*]. Capillary whorls that form the beginning of the vorticose veins of the choroid.

Winstrol. Trademark for stanozolol, a steroid anabolic androgen.

Win·ter·bot·tom's sign [T. M. *Winterbottom,* British physician, 1765–1859]. Enlargement of the posterior cervical lymph nodes in trypanosomiasis (sleeping sickness).

win·ter cough. Chronic bronchitis recurring every winter.

win·ter·green, *n.* GAULTHERIA.

wintergreen oil. TEABERRY OIL.

Win·ter·nitz phenomenon. Hemorrhage into an atherosclerotic plaque producing coronary occlusion.

Win·ter·stei·ner's compound F. CORTISONE.

winter vomiting disease. NONBACTERIAL GASTROENTERITIS.

Win·trich's sign (vin'trikh) [A. *Wintrich,* German physician, 1812–1882]. A sign for cavitation of the lungs in which there is a change in percussion note when the mouth is closed or open.

Win·trobe-Lands·berg method [M. M. *Wintrobe,* U.S. internist, b. 1901; and J. W. *Landsberg*]. A blood sedimentation rate technique in which a single tube is used for sedimentation rate and hematocrit determination.

Wintrobe method [M. M. *Wintrobe*]. An acid hematin method for hemoglobin using a special hemometer with a yellow glass standard.

wire loop lesion. A thickened portion of the glomerular capillary basement membrane occasionally seen in the nephropathies of systemic lupus erythematosus.

wir·ing, *n.* Securing in position, by means of wire, fragments of a broken bone.

Wir·sung's canal or **duct** (virr'zoŏng) [J. G. *Wirsung,* German anatomist, 1600–1643]. PANCREATIC DUCT.

wiry, *adj.* Resembling wire; tough and flexible.

wiry pulse. A small, rapid, tense pulse, which feels like a cord.

wis·dom tooth. The third molar tooth in man. NA *dens serotinus.*

wish fulfilment. The discharge of psychologic or emotional tension by imagining a satisfactory solution or satisfying situation which reduces anxiety; a central theme in psychoanalytic theory, serving to explain the manifestation of repressed wishes in the form of neurotic symptoms, common errors, and (normally) dreams; a partial substitute for the forbidden or unattainable satisfaction.

wish·ful thinking. A thinking process, superficially logical, but guided more by a person's desires and wishes than by his realistic consideration of the facts.

Wis·kott-Al·drich syndrome [R. A. *Aldrich,* U.S. pediatrician, 20th century]. A familial, sex-linked recessive disease, characterized by thrombocytopenia, bleeding diathesis, chronic eczema, recurrent infections (especially of ears), leukopenia with decreased lymphocytes in lymph nodes and spleen but not in the bone marrow, decreased gamma-A and gamma-M globulins, and deficient thymic maturation. Incomplete forms may exist.

Wis·tar rat. 1. An albino rat belonging to a strain kept at the Wistar Institute in Philadelphia. 2. Any albino rat with ancestry traceable to a Wistar rat.

witch meal. LYCOPODIUM.

witch's milk. Milk sometimes secreted from the breasts of a newborn infant.

Wi·teb·sky's substances. GROUP-SPECIFIC SUBSTANCES.

with·draw·al, *n.* 1. The taking away or removal of anything. 2. The discontinuance of a drug or medication. 3. COITUS INTERRUPTUS. 4. *In psychiatry,* a pattern of behavior in which an individual removes himself from conflicts by retreating from people and the world of reality; seen in its most pathologic form in schizophrenics.

withdrawal syndrome or **symptoms.** The complex of physical and psychological disturbances observed in addicts upon withdrawal of the addicting agent. Severity of the autonomic and psychomotor disturbances varies with the agent, length of addiction, and size of dosage.

with·ers (wi*th*'urz) *n.pl.* The ridge above the shoulders of the horse, formed by the spinous processes of the first eight or ten thoracic vertebrae.

wit·kop (wit'kop) *n.* [Afrikaans, white head]. A noncontagious favoid condition of the scalp characterized by white, hard, dry, friable, confluent, firmly adherent crusts which give the appearance of a tightly fitting, white skull cap, seen only in prenatal syphilis in natives of South Africa. Syn. *dikwakwadi, white head.*

Witt·maak-Eck·bom syndrome. RESTLESS LEGS.

Wit·zel's operation (vit'sel) [F. O. *Witzel,* German surgeon, 1856–1925]. A method of temporary gastrostomy.

wit·zel·sucht (vit'sul·zoŏkht) *n.* [Ger., lit., joking mania]. A mental condition characterized by silly behavior, shallow facetiousness, and unstable mood; regarded as a symptom of frontal lobe disease such as brain tumor.

wl Abbreviation for *wavelength.*

Wohl·fahr·tia (vohl·fahr'tee·uh) *n.* [P. *Wolfart,* German medical writer, d. 1726]. A genus of flesh flies. See also *Sarcophagidae.*

Wohlfahrtia mag·nif·i·ca (mag·nif'i·kuh). The Old World flesh fly; the larvae are deposited in cutaneous lesions or in one of the body openings.

Wohlfahrtia mei·geni (migh'ge·nigh). A North American flesh fly.

Wohlfahrtia vig·il (vij'il). A North American flesh fly.

Wohl·fart-Ku·gel·berg-We·lan·der disease (vohl'fahrt) [G. *Wohlfart,* E. *Kugelberg,* and L. *Welander*]. A heredofamilial form of spinal muscular atrophy which becomes clinically manifest in early childhood or later, sometimes not until early adulthood, and progresses slowly, permitting survival into adulthood and sometimes into old age; affects the proximal muscles of the limbs predominantly; can be inherited as a dominant, a sex-linked recessive, or an autosomal recessive trait. Syn. *proximal spinal muscular atrophy, chronic proximal spinal muscular atrophy.*

Wohl·ge·muth method (vohl'ge·moot) [J. *Wohlgemuth,* German physician, b. 1874]. A method for the quantitative determination of amylase in feces.

Woil·lez' disease [E. J. *Woillez,* French physician, 1811–1882]. Acute idiopathic pulmonary hyperemia and edema. See also *pulmonary edema.*

Wol·fen·den's position [R. N. *Wolfenden,* English laryngologist, 1854–1925]. *Obsol.* A prone position with the head and arms hanging over the edge of the bed, used to induce swallowing when it is impeded by ulceration of the epiglottis.

Wolff-Eis·ner test (vohlf ice'nur) [A. *Wolff-Eisner,* German serologist, 1877–1948]. CALMETTE TEST.

Wolff·ian (wŏol'fee·un, vol') *adj.* Described by or named after K. F. Wolff, German anatomist, 1733–1794.

Wolffian adenoma. ADRENOCORTICOID ADENOMA OF THE OVARY.

Wolffian body. MESONEPHROS.

Wolffian cyst. A cyst of mesonephric origin, usually near the ovary or uterine tube.

Wolffian duct. MESONEPHRIC DUCT.

Wolffian rests. MESONEPHRIC RESTS.

Wolffian ridge. UROGENITAL FOLD.

Wolffian tubules. The functional tubules of the mesonephros.

Wolff method. A procedure for determining the protein concentration of the gastric contents.

Wolff-Parkinson-White syndrome [L. *Wolff,* U.S. physician, 20th century; John *Parkinson,* English physician, 19th century; and P. D. *White,* U.S. physician, 20th century]. A disorder of activation of the heart due to accelerated conduction between the atria and ventricles and an abnormal excitation of the ventricles; characterized electrocardiographically by a short PR interval and a wide abnormal QRS complex, and clinically often by paroxysmal supraventricular tachycardia. Abbreviated, W-P-W syndrome. Syn. *pre-excitation syndrome.*

Wolff's law [J. *Wolff,* German surgeon, 1836–1902]. Every change in the use or static relations of a bone leads not only to a change in its internal structure and architecture but also to a change in its external form and function.

wolf·jaw, *n.* Bilateral cleft of the lip, jaw, and palate.

Wölf·ler's operation (vœlf'lur) [A. *Wölfler,* Bohemian surgeon, 1850–1917]. Anterior gastroenterostomy for pyloric obstruction.

wolf·ram (wŏŏl'frum) *n.* [Ger.]. TUNGSTEN.

Wolf·ring's glands (voʰlf'ring) [E. F. von *Wolfring,* Polish ophthalmologist, 1832–1906]. Mucosal glands situated in the eyelids, particularly behind the superior tarsal plate.

wolfs·bane (wŏŏlfs'bane) *n.* 1. ACONITE. 2. Any plant of the genus *Aconitum,* especially *A. lycoctonum.*

wolf's claw. LYCOPODIUM.

Wol·hyn·ia fever (vol·hin'ee·uh, wol·) [after *Wolhynia (Volhynia),* a region of the northwestern Ukraine]. TRENCH FEVER.

Wol·las·ton's doublet [W. H. *Wollaston,* English physician and physicist, 1766–1828]. Two planoconvex lenses placed in the eyepiece of a microscope for correction of chromatic aberration.

Wol·man's disease [M. *Wolman,* Israeli neuropathologist, 20th century]. A rare, autosomal recessive, inborn error of lipid metabolism in which large amounts of cholesteryl esters and triglycerides accumulate in the liver and other organs.

Wolt·man-Ker·no·han syndrome [H. W. *Woltman,* U.S. neurologist, b. 1889; and W. *Kernohan*]. CRUS PHENOMENON.

womb (woom) *n.* UTERUS.

Wong's method [S. Y. *Wong,* Chinese biochemist, b. 1894]. A method for determining the iron content in blood in which the blood is treated with sulfuric acid and potassium persulfate. The proteins are removed with tungstic acid, and the iron in the filtrate is determined colorimetrically.

wood, *n.* The hard fibrous part of trees; the part within the bark.

wood alcohol. METHYL ALCOHOL.

wood charcoal. Charcoal prepared by incomplete combustion of wood.

wood·en, *adj.* 1. Resembling wood in stiffness. 2. Made of wood.

wooden tongue. A disease of the tongue of cattle caused by a gram-negative rod, *Actinobacillus lignieresi;* formerly confused with actinomycosis.

wood·fern. *DRYOPTERIS.*

wood oil. GURJUN BALSAM.

Wood's light, filter, or **lamp** [R. W. *Wood,* U.S. physicist, 1868–1955]. A light filter, made of glass containing nickel oxide, which transmits only ultraviolet rays; has been used in the diagnosis of infections by fungi, such as tinea capitis, which fluoresce when radiated with ultraviolet light.

Wood's muscle [J. *Wood,* English surgeon, 1825–1891]. EXTENSOR CARPI RADIALIS INTERMEDIUS.

wood spirit. METHYL ALCOHOL.

wood sugar. XYLOSE.

wood tick. *DERMACENTOR ANDERSONI.*

wood vinegar. Vinegar obtained by the dry distillation of wood.

woody thyroiditis. RIEDEL'S DISEASE.

wool fat. The purified, anhydrous, fatlike substance from the wool of sheep, *Ovis aries;* chiefly composed of esters of high molecular weight alcohols, as cholesterol and lanosterol, with fatty acids. Used as an ointment base. Syn. *anhydrous lanolin.*

woolly monkey. A large, prehensile-tailed South American monkey of the genus *Lagothrix,* inhabiting rain forests in the Amazon basin and adjacent mountain slopes.

Wool·ner's tip [T. *Woolner,* English sculptor, 1825–1892]. The apex of the helix of the ear.

wool-skein test. HOLMGREN'S TEST.

wool soap. SUINT.

wool·sort·er's disease. Anthrax brought on by inhalation of anthrax bacilli found in woolen particles.

word blindness. ALEXIA.

word deafness. AUDITORY VERBAL AGNOSIA.

word sal·ad. Meaningless words or neologisms emitted by psychotic patients, particularly with schizophrenia. Syn. *schizophasia.* Compare *jargon aphasia.*

Wo·rin·ger-Ko·lopp disease [F. *Woringer* and P. *Kolopp*]. A variety of mycosis fungoides with a special affinity for involvement and destruction of the epidermis. Syn. *epidermotropic reticulosis, pagetoid reticulosis.*

work hypertrophy. Muscular hypertrophy due to increased work; a form of adaptive hypertrophy.

work·ing distance. *In microscopy,* the distance between the object and the objective.

working side. In mandibular movements, the side towards which the mandible moves during lateral excursions.

working through. *In psychoanalysis,* repetition, extension, and deepening of interpretation in order to overcome resistances that persist after the initial interpretation of repressed instinctual impulses and thus to bring about insight and produce significant and lasting change in the patient.

work therapy. OCCUPATIONAL THERAPY.

work-up, *n.*The results of investigation of a patient's illness, including history, physical examination, and laboratory and x-ray studies.

work up, *v.*To investigate a patient's illness by a variety of means.

World Health Organization. A specialized agency of the United Nations Organization whose broad purposes in the international health field are primarily to assist governments upon request in the field of health; to promote standards, provide information, and foster research in the field of health; to promote cooperation among scientific and professional groups; to promote and foster activities in the field of maternal and child health and of mental health; and to study and report on administrative and social techniques as relating to preventive medicine. It has authority to make sanitary and quarantine regulations, to regulate morbidity and mortality nomenclature, and to set standards for purity and potency of biological and pharmaceutical products. Abbreviated, WHO.

worm, *n.* A member of the phyla Annelida, Nemathelminthes, or Platyhelminthes. The medically important forms belong to the last two phyla.

worm abscess. VERMINOUS ABSCESS.

Wor·mi·an bone (wur'mee·un) [O. *Worm,* Danish anatomist, 1588–1654]. SUTURAL BONE.

worm·seed, *n.* SANTONICA.

wormseed oil. CHENOPODIUM OIL.

wound (woond) *n.* The disruption of normal anatomical relationships, or loss of tissue, resulting from surgery or physical injury.

wound clip. SKIN CLIP.

wound diphtheria. SURGICAL DIPHTHERIA.

wound hormones. Substances that can stimulate growth by resumption of division in mature cells.

wound shock. HYPOVOLEMIC SHOCK.

W-P-W syndrome. Abbreviation for *Wolff-Parkinson-White syndrome.*

Wre·den operation (vrʸeʰ'dʸin) [R. R. *Wreden,* Russian surgeon, 20th century]. STONE OPERATION.

Wreden's sign or **test** [R. R. *Wreden,* Russian otologist, 1837–1893]. The lack of mucoid material in the middle ear of a newborn child as evidence that the child had been born alive.

Wreden-Stone operation. STONE OPERATION.

Wright's stain [J. H. *Wright,* U.S. pathologist, 1870–1928]. A specially prepared polychrome methylene blue stain used to color the formed elements of blood in smears.

Wright's syndrome [I. S. *Wright,* U.S. physician, b. 1901]. A neurovascular syndrome produced by prolonged hyperabduction of the arms causing occlusion of the subclavian artery and stretching of the trunks of the brachial plexus, which produces paresthesias, numbness, and tingling, followed by ulcers in the fingertips in protracted cases.

wrin·kles, *n.pl.* Minute crevices or furrows in the skin sometimes caused by habitual frowning, but particularly by old age, due to dehydration and atrophy of the corium.

Wris·berg's cartilage (vris'beʰrk) [H. A. *Wrisberg,* German anatomist, 1739–1808]. CUNEIFORM CARTILAGE.

Wrisberg's ganglion [H. A. *Wrisberg*]. CARDIAC GANGLION.

Wrisberg's ligament [H.A. *Wrisberg*]. The posterior meniscofemoral ligament. See *meniscofemoral ligament.*

Wrisberg's nerve [H. A. *Wrisberg*]. 1. NERVUS CUTANEUS BRACHII MEDIALIS. 2. NERVUS INTERMEDIUS.

Wrisberg's pars intermedius [H. A. *Wrisberg*]. NERVUS INTERMEDIUS.

wrist, *n.* 1. The part of the upper limb at which the hand joins the forearm. NA *carpus.* 2. WRIST JOINT.

wrist drop, wrist-drop. Inability to extend the hand at the wrist due to paralysis of the extensor muscles of the forearm and hand.

wrist extension reflex. CARPOPHALANGEAL REFLEX (2).

wrist flexion reflex. Flexion of the fingers induced by percussion of the flexor tendons of the wrist on the palmar surface of the forearm when the hand is in supination and the fingers are slightly flexed.

wrist joint. The joint in which the proximal row of carpal bones articulates with the radius and the articular disk of the distal radioulnar joint. NA *articulatio radiocarpea.* See also Table of Synovial Joints and Ligaments in the Appendix.

writer's cramp or **paralysis.** An occupational spasm affecting a hand.

writing hand. A peculiar position assumed by the hand in parkinsonism, with an exaggerated flexion of the metacarpophalangeal joints and an extension of the fingers.

wry-head, *n.* PLAGIOCEPHALY.

wry·neck, *n.* TORTICOLLIS.

w.s. Abbreviation for *water soluble.*

Wu·cher atrophy [Ger. *Wucherung,* proliferation]. Subcutaneous fat atrophy following a nonspecific inflammatory exudate.

Wuch·er·er·ia (voo''kur·err'ee·uh, wooch·ur·eer'ee·uh) *n.* [O. *Wucherer,* German physician, 1820–1873]. A genus of filarial worms found in all the warm regions of the world. The larva or microfilaria must be ingested by a mosquito for metamorphosis to take place.

Wuchereria ban·crof·ti (ban·krof'tye). A species of filaria of worldwide distribution. Man is the only known definitive host.

Wuchereria ma·layi (may·lay'eye). *BRUGIA MALAYI.*

wuch·er·e·ri·a·sis (wooch''ur·e·rye'uh·sis, vook''ur·) *n.* [*Wuchereria* + *-iasis*]. Infection with worms of the genus *Wuchereria.* See also *filariasis, elephantiasis.*

Wun·der·lich's curve or **law** (voon'dur·liᵏʰh) [C. R. A. *Wunderlich,* German physician, 1815–1877]. The fever oscillations in typhoid fever, representing the course of the disease.

Wundt's tetanus (voont) [W. M. *Wundt,* German physiologist, 1832–1920]. A prolonged tetanic contraction induced in a frog's muscle by injury or the closure of a strong, direct electric current.

w/v Weight in volume; indicating that a weighed quantity of a solid substance is contained in solution in a measured volume of liquid.

Wyamine. Trademark for mephentermine, a sympathomimetic amine used as the base and the sulfate salt to produce vasoconstriction.

Wycillin. A trademark for preparations containing crystalline procaine penicillin G.

Wydase. A trademark for hyaluronidase, a spreading factor.

Wy·eth pins [J. A. *Wyeth,* U.S. surgeon, 1845–1922]. Twelve-inch steel pins designed to hold a tourniquet in place in amputation at the hip or shoulder.

Wy·lie's operation [W. G. *Wylie,* U.S. gynecologist, 1848–1923]. Shortening of the round ligaments of the uterus for relief of retroflexion.

X

X. Symbol for the decimal scale of potency or dilution; used by homeopaths.

xa·nox·ate (za·nock'sate) *n.* 7-Isopropoxy-9-oxoxanthene-2-carboxylate, $C_{17}H_{14}O_5$, a bronchodilator, used as the sodium salt.

xanth-, xantho- [Gk. *xanthos*]. A combining form meaning *yellow.*

xan·thate (zan'thate) *n.* A salt of xanthic acid.

xan·the·las·ma (zanth"e·laz'muh) *n.* [*xanth-* + Gk. *elasma,* plate]. Yellowish raised plaques occurring around the eyelids, resulting from lipid-filled cells in the dermis.

xan·the·las·moi·dea (zanth"e·laz·moy'dee·uh) *n.* [NL., from *xanthelasma* + *-oid*]. URTICARIA PIGMENTOSA.

xan·thene (zan'theen) *n.* 1. Dibenzopyran, $C_{13}H_{10}O$, a three-ring heterocyclic compound resulting from the joining of two benzene rings by a methylene (CH_2) and also an oxygen bridge. Certain derivatives are medicinally important. 2. Any of several derivatives of xanthene (1).

xan·thic (zan'thick) *adj.* [*xanth-* + *-ic*]. 1. Yellow. 2. Pertaining to xanthine.

xan·thine (zan'theen, ·thin) *n.* 2,6(1*H*,3*H*)-Purinedione, or 2,6-dioxopurine, $C_5H_4N_4O_2$, found in plant and animal tissues; an intermediate product in the transformation of adenine and guanine into uric acid. See also *hypoxanthine.*

xanthine calculi. Brown to red, hard and laminated calculi; rare and found in the urinary bladder.

xanthine oxidase. A flavoprotein enzyme catalyzing the oxidation of certain purines.

xan·thi·nol ni·a·cin·ate (zan'thi·nol nigh"uh·sin'ate). 7-{2-Hydroxy-3-[(2-hydroxyethyl)methylamino]propyl}theophylline, compound with nicotinic acid, $C_{13}H_{21}N_5O_4.C_6H_5NO_2$, a peripheral vasodilator.

xan·thi·nu·ria (zan"thi·new'ree·uh) *n.* [*xanthine* + *-uria*]. The presence of xanthine in urine.

xan·thi·uria (zan"thi·yoo'ree·uh) *n.* [*xanthi*ne + *-uria*]. XANTHINURIA.

xantho-. See *xanth-.*

xan·tho·chroia (zan"tho·kroy'uh) *n.* [Gk. *xanthochroos,* yellow-skinned, + *-ia*]. A yellow discoloration of the skin.

xan·tho·chro·mat·ic (zan"tho·kro·mat'ick) *adj.* [*xantho-* + *chromatic*]. Yellow-colored.

xan·tho·chro·mia (zan"tho·kro'mee·uh) *n.* [*xantho-* + *-chromia*]. 1. A yellow discoloration of the skin. 2. The yellow discoloration of the cerebrospinal fluid, diagnostic of hemorrhage in the spinal cord, brain, or subarachnoid or subdural space. **—xanthochro·mic** (·mick) *adj.*

xan·thoch·ro·ous (zan·thock'ro·us) *adj.* [Gk. *xanthochroos,* from *xanthos,* yellow, + *chroa,* complexion]. Yellow-skinned.

xan·tho·cy·a·no·pia (zan"tho·sigh"uh·no'pee·uh) *n.* [*xantho-* + *cyan-* + *-opia*]. A defect of color vision in which yellow and blue are perceived, while red and green are not.

xan·tho·cy·a·nop·sia (zan"tho·sigh"uh·nop'see·uh) *n.* XANTHOCYANOPIA.

xan·tho·cyte (zan'tho·site) *n.* [*xantho-* + *-cyte*]. A cell containing a yellow pigment.

xan·tho·der·ma (zan"tho·dur'muh) *n.* [*xantho-* + *-derma*]. A yellow discoloration of the skin.

xan·tho·fi·bro·ma the·co·cel·lu·la·re (zan"tho·figh·bro'muh theek"o·sel·yoo·lair'ee). LUTEOMA.

xan·tho·gran·u·lo·ma (zan"tho·gran"yoo·lo'muh) *n.* [*xantho-* + *granuloma*]. JUVENILE XANTHOGRANULOMA. **—xantho·granu·lom·a·tous** (·lom'uh·tus) *adj.*

xan·tho·gran·u·lo·ma·to·sis (zan"tho·gran"yoo·lo"muh·to'sis) *n.* [*xantho-* + *granuloma* + *-osis*]. HAND-SCHÜLLER-CHRISTIAN SYNDROME.

xanthogranulomatous pyelonephritis. A rare, chronic, inflammatory renal disease characterized by diminished or absent renal function, high fever, renal enlargement, staghorn calculi, and replacement of the kidney with fat-filled macrophages.

xan·tho·ky·an·o·py (zanth"o·kigh·an'o·pee) *n.* XANTHOCYANOPIA.

xan·tho·ma (zan·tho'muh) *n.*, pl. **xanthomas, xanthoma·ta** (·tuh) [*xanth-* + *-oma*]. A collection of lipid-filled histiocytes, appearing grossly as a yellow mass, and usually found in the subcutaneous tissue, often around tendons.

xanthoma cell. FOAM CELL.

xanthoma di·a·bet·i·co·rum (dye"uh·bet"i·ko'rum). Xanthomas occurring in hyperlipemic diabetic patients.

xanthoma dis·sem·i·na·tum (di·sem"i·nay'tum). Xanthomas appearing as papules or plaques diffusely distributed chiefly over the face, flexor surfaces, and often the mucous membranes.

xanthoma pal·pe·bra·rum (pal·pe·brair'um). XANTHELASMA.

xan·tho·ma·to·sis (zan·tho"muh·to'sis) *n.* [*xanthoma* + *-osis*]. A condition marked by the deposit of a yellow or orange lipid material in the reticuloendothelial cells, the skin, and the internal organs. See also *lipidosis.*

xan·tho·ma·tous (zan·tho'muh·tus, ·thom'uh·) *adj.* Of the nature of, or affected with, xanthoma.

xanthomatous cirrhosis. Intrahepatic biliary cirrhosis complicated by high blood lipid levels and xanthomatous deposits in various tissues and organs.

xanthomatous giant-cell tumor of the tendon sheath. A benign, usually well-defined tumor composed of vacuolated macrophages and multinucleated giant cells set in a collagenic stroma, which varies greatly in amounts.

xanthoma tu·ber·o·sum (tew"bur·o'sum). Xanthomas appearing as papules, nodules, plaques, or linear lesions on the extensor surfaces, usually grouped together and often found about the joints. Tendon sheaths or other internal structures may be involved, giving various and bizarre symptoms.

xanthoma tuberosum mul·ti·plex (mul'ti·plecks). FAMILIAL HYPERBETALIPOPROTEINEMIA.

xan·thone (zan'thone) *n.* 1. Dibenzopyrone, 9-xanthenone, or benzophenone oxide, $C_{13}H_8O_2$, obtained when the CH_2 bridge of xanthene is oxidized to CO. Certain dyes and some yellow flower pigments are derivatives of xanthone. 2. Any of several derivatives of xanthone (1).

xan·tho·phane (zan'tho·fane) *n.* [*xantho-* + Gk. *phainein,* to appear]. A yellow pigment found in the retinal cones.

xan·tho·phore (zan'tho·fore) *n.* [*xantho-* + *-phore*]. A yellow chromatophore.

xan·tho·phose (zanth'o·foze) *n.* [*zantho-* + *-phose*]. A yellow phose.

xan·tho·phyll (zan'tho·fil) *n.* [*xantho-* + *-phyll*]. A dihydroxy-α-carotene, $C_{40}H_{56}O_2$, a yellow pigment widely distributed in nature. Syn. *lutein.* Contr. *anthocyanin.*

xan·tho·pia (zan·tho'pee·uh) *n.* [*xanth-* + *-opia*]. XANTHOPSIA.

xanthoproteic acid. The characteristic yellow substance resulting when proteins containing tyrosine are treated with concentrated nitric acid.

xanthoproteic reaction or **test.** A test for proteins based on treatment with concentrated nitric acid. The yellow color that develops changes to deep orange on alkalization with ammonia.

xan·tho·pro·tein (zanth"o·pro'tee·in, ·teen) *n.* [*xantho-* + *protein*]. A yellowish derivative formed by the action of concentrated nitric acid on proteins. —**xantho·pro·te·ic** (·pro·tee'ick) *adj.*

xanthoprotein reaction. XANTHOPROTEIC REACTION.

xan·thop·sia (zan·thop'see·uh) *n.* [*xanth-* + *-opsia*]. Yellow vision; the condition in which objects look yellow; sometimes occurring in jaundice.

xan·thop·sin (zan·thop'sin) *n.* [*xanth-* + *opsin*]. Visual yellow, produced by the action of light on rhodopsin.

xan·thop·sy·dra·cia (zan·thop"si·dray'shee·uh) *n.* [*xantho-* + Gk. *psydrak*ion, pimple, + *-ia*]. The occurrence on the skin of yellow papules or pustules.

xan·thop·ter·in (zan·thop'tur·in) *n.* 2-Amino-4,6-dihydroxypteridine, $C_6H_5N_5O_2$, a yellow pigment, widely distributed in animal organisms and representing an element of the structure of folic acid; it may have a role in hemopoiesis.

xan·tho·rham·nin (zan"tho·ram'nin) *n.* The 3-rhamninoside, $C_{34}H_{42}O_{20}$, of rhamnetin, obtained from the berries of *Rhamnus infectoria* (*tinctoria*) and other *Rhamnus* species. On hydrolysis it yields rhamninose and the aglycone rhamnetin.

xan·thor·rhea, xan·thor·rhoea (zan"tho·ree'uh) *n.* [*xantho-* + *-rrhea*]. An acrid, purulent, yellow discharge from the vagina.

xan·tho·sine (zanth'o·seen, ·sin) *n.* A nucleoside made up of xanthine and ribose.

xan·tho·sis (zan·tho'sis) *n.* [*xanth-* + *-osis*]. A reversible discoloration of the skin due to a deposit of carotenoid pigment; occurs from eating quantities of carrots, squash, sweet potatoes, etc. A similar dicoloration results from taking quinacrine over a period of time.

xanthosis fun·di di·a·bet·i·ca (fun'dye dye·uh·bet'i·kuh). A condition, seen in diabetic retinopathy, in which the retinal vessels are extremely well defined and the retina in the posterior part of the eye has a peculiar orange-yellow color.

xan·thous (zanth'us) *adj.* [*xanth-* + *-ous*]. Having a yellow coloration.

xan·thox·y·lum (zan·thock'si·lum) *n.* [NL., from *xantho-* + Gk. *xylon,* wood]. The dried bark and fruit of *Zanthoxylum americanum,* or of *Z. clavaherculis;* have been used for treatment of various ailments. Syn. *prickly ash bark, prickly ash berries.*

xan·thu·re·nic acid (zan"thew·ree'nick). 4,8-Dihydroxyquinaldic acid, $C_{10}H_7NO_4$, excreted in the urine of pyridoxine-deficient animals following ingestion of tryptophan.

xan·thu·ria (zan·thew'ree·uh) *n.* XANTHINURIA.

xan·thy·drol (zan·thigh'drol) *n.* Xanthen-9-ol, $C_{13}H_{10}O_2$, used for the detection of urea.

xanthydrol method. A histochemical method for urea based on fixation of tissue in xanthydrol in acetic acid to precipitate dixanthylurea which is birefringent under the polarizing microscope.

xan·thyl·ic (zan·thil'ick) *adj.* Pertaining to xanthine.

X^g blood group. An erythrocyte antigen defined by its reaction to anti-X^g antiserum, found in the blood of a multiply transfused patient. It is the only known sex-linked blood group, being located on the X chromosome (hence its designation).

X chromosome. A sex-determining factor in ovum and approximately one-half of sperm. Ova fertilized by spermatozoa having the X chromosome give rise to female offspring.

X chromosome inactivation. According to Lyon's hypothesis, random inactivation of one X chromosome which occurs in early embryogenesis in somatic cells of females.

x descent or **wave.** The negative pressure wave in the atrial and jugular venous pulse tracing which occurs during ventricular systole; it is due primarily to downward motion of the atrioventricular valves, although atrial relaxation may contribute to the initial portion of the x descent.

x-disease. 1. A condition characterized by idiopathic malaise, cardiac arrhythmia, digestive disturbances, and cold intolerance. 2. A viral dermatitis of cattle characterized by hyperkeratosis.

Xe Symbol for xenon.

xen-, xeno- [Gk. *xenos,* foreign, stranger, guest, host]. A combining form meaning (a) *different, foreign;* (b) *alien, intrusive;* (c) *host,* as in relation to parasites.

xe·no·di·ag·no·sis (zen"o·dye"ug·no'sis, zee"no·) *n.* [*xeno-* + *diagnosis*]. The procedure of using a suitable arthropod to transfer an infectious agent from a patient to a susceptible laboratory animal.

xe·no·ge·ne·ic (zeen"o·je·nay'ick, zen"o·je·nee'ick) [*xeno-* + *-geneic,* from Gk. *genos, geneos,* race, breed, species (rel. to L. *genus*)]. *adj.* Of transplanted organs or tissues: originally belonging to an organism of a different species. Compare *heterogenous.* See also *xenograft.*

xe·no·gen·e·sis (zen"o·jen'e·sis, zee"no·) *n.* [*xeno-* + *-genesis*]. 1. HETEROGENESIS. 2. The hypothetical production of offspring completely unlike the parent. —**xenogen·ic** (·ick) *adj.*

xe·no·graft (zen'o·graft, zee"no·) *n.* [*xeno-* + *graft*]. A transplant from one species to another, especially one involving a wider genetic or species disparity than a heterograft.

xe·nol·o·gy (ze·nol'uh·jee) *n.* [*xeno-* + *-logy*]. The study of the host relationship of parasites, as of intermediary and definitive hosts.

xe·no·me·nia (zen"o·mee'nee·uh, zee"no·) *n.* [*xeno-* + *men-* + *-ia*]. VICARIOUS MENSTRUATION.

xe·non (zee'non, zen'on) *n.* [Gk. *xenos,* strange, + *-on*]. Xe = 131.30. An inert gaseous element, atomic number 54, found in the atmosphere.

xe·no·pho·bia (zen"o·fo'bee·uh, zee"no·) *n.* [*xeno-* + *-phobia*]. An abnormal fear of strangers.

xe·no·plas·ty (zee'no·plas"tee, zen'o·) *n.* [*xeno-* + *-plasty*]. HETEROPLASTY. —**xeno·plas·tic** (zee"no·plas'tick, zen"o·) *adj.*

Xen·op·syl·la (zen"op·sil'uh, zen"o·) *n.* [*xeno-* + Gk. *psylla,* flea]. A genus of fleas of the family Pulicidae.

Xenopsylla che·o·pis (kee·o'pis). The tropical rat flea; found chiefly in tropical and subtropical regions. A vector for bubonic plague and *Hymenolepis diminuta,* a tapeworm.

This flea attacks man and other mammals, in addition to the rat, its natural host. It transmits the organism of murine typhus, *Rickettsia mooseri*, from rat to rat and from rat to man.

Xen·o·pus (zen'o·pus) *n.* A genus of African toad belonging to the Pipidae, used in laboratory tests for pregnancy.

***Xenopus* pregnancy test.** A pregnancy test in which urine containing chorionic gonadotropin is injected into a female African clawed toad (*Xenopus laevis*). If five or more eggs are deposited by the toad within 12 hours after injection, the test is positive.

-xenous [Gk. *xenos*]. A combining form meaning *host*.

xer-, xero- [Gk. *xēros*]. A combining form meaning *dry*.

xe·ran·tic (ze·ran'tick) *adj.* [Gk. *xērantikos*, from *xērainein*, to dry up]. Having desiccative properties; drying. —**xeran·sis** (·sis) *n.*

xe·ra·sia (ze·ray'zee·uh, ·zhuh) *n.* [Gk. *xērasia*, dessication, dryness, from *xēros*, dry]. A disease of the hair marked by cessation of growth and excessive dryness.

xe·ro·der·ma (zeer"o·dur'muh) *n.* [NL., from Gk. *xēroder-mos*, dry-skinned, from *xēros*, dry, + *derma*, skin]. A condition of excessively dry skin.

xeroderma pig·men·to·sum (pig·men·to'sum). A genodermatosis characterized by premature degenerative changes in the form of keratoses, malignant epitheliomatosis, and hyper- and hypopigmentation.

xe·ro·der·mos·te·o·sis (zeer"o·dur"mos·tee·o'sis) *n.* [*xero-* + *derm-* + *oste-* + *-osis*]. SJÖGREN'S SYNDROME.

xe·ro·ma (ze·ro'muh) *n.* [*xer-* + *-oma*]. XEROPHTHALMIA.

xe·ro·mam·mo·gram (zeer"o·mam'o·gram) *n.* [*xero-* + *mammogram*]. A xeroradiographic depiction of the breast.

xe·ro·mam·mog·ra·phy (zeer"o·ma·mog'ruh·fee) *n.* [*xero-* + *mammography*]. Xeroradiography of the breast.

xe·ro·me·nia (zeer"o·mee'nee·uh) *n.* [*xero-* + *men-* + *-ia*]. The presence of the usual constitutional disturbances at the menstrual period but without the menstrual flow of blood.

xe·ro·myc·te·ria (zeer"o·mick·teer'ee·uh) *n.* [*xero-* + Gk. *myktēr*, nostril, + *-ia*]. Lack of moisture in the nasal passages.

xe·ron·o·sus (ze·ron'o·sus) *n.* [NL., from *xero-* + Gk. *nosos*, disease]. A condition of dryness of the skin.

xe·ro·pha·gia (zeer"o·fay'jee·uh) *n.* [*xero-* + *-phagia*]. The habitual eating of dry or desiccated food.

xe·roph·a·gy (ze·rof'uh·jee) *n.* [*xero-* + *-phagy*]. XEROPHAGIA.

xe·roph·thal·mia (zeer"off·thal'mee·uh) *n.* [Gk. *xērophthalmia*, dry blepharitis, from *xēros*, dry, + *ophthalmos*, eye]. A dry and thickened condition of the conjunctiva, sometimes following chronic conjunctivitis, disease of the lacrimal apparatus, or vitamin-A deficiency. See also *xerosis*.

xe·ro·ra·di·og·ra·phy (zeer"o·ray"dee·og'ruh·fee) *n.* [*xero-* + *radiography*]. A rapid method of recording a roentgen image by a dry process. A powdered surface of an electrically charged selenium plate records the roentgen image. —**xeroradi·o·graph·ic** (·o·graf'ick) *adj.*

xe·ro·sis (ze·ro'sis) *n.*, pl. **xero·ses** (·seez) [*xer-* + *-osis*]. Abnormal dryness of a tissue, as of the skin, eye, or mucous membranes.

xerosis con·junc·ti·vae (kon·junk·tye'vee). A condition marked by silver-gray, shiny, triangular spots on both sides of the cornea, within the region of the palpebral aperture, consisting of dried epithelium, flaky masses, and microorganisms. The spots are observed in some cases of hemeralopia. See also *xerophthalmia*.

xerosis in·fan·ti·lis (in·fan'ti·lis). Xerophthalmia marked by a lusterless, grayish white, foamy, greasy, very persistent deposit on the conjunctiva. Syn. *keratitis sicca*.

xe·ro·sto·mia (zeer"o·sto'mee·uh) *n.* [*xero-* + *-stomia*]. Dry mouth, caused by insufficient secretion of saliva.

xe·ro·tes (zeer'o·teez) *n.* [Gk. *xērotēs*, dryness]. Dryness of the body.

xe·rot·ic (ze·rot'ick) *adj.* Pertaining to or characterized by xerosis.

xerotic keratitis. KERATOMALACIA.

xe·ro·to·cia (zeer"o·to'shee·uh) *n.* [*xero-* + Gk. *tokos*, childbirth, + *-ia*]. DRY LABOR.

xe·ro·trip·sis (zeer"o·trip'sis) *n.* [*xero-* + Gk. *tripsis*, a rubbing]. Dry friction.

X factor. A heat-stable product of blood identified as hematin, generally required as a growth factor of the genus *Hemophilus*.

xip·a·mide (zip'uh·mide) *n.* 4-Chloro-5-sulfamoyl-2′, 6′-salicyloxylidide, $C_{15}H_{15}ClN_2O_4S$, a diuretic, antihypertensive.

xiph-, xiphi-, xipho-. A combining form meaning *xiphoid*.

xiphi·ster·nal (zif"i·stur'nul) *adj.* [*xiphisternum* + *-al*]. Pertaining to the body and xiphoid process of the sternum.

xiphisternal crunch or **sound.** A crunching sound of unknown cause heard over the junction of the xiphoid process and sternum; not apparently associated with disease.

xiphi·ster·num (zif"i·stur'num) *n.* XIPHOID PROCESS.

xipho·cos·tal (zif"o·kos'tul) *adj.* [*xipho-* + *costal*]. Pertaining to the xiphoid process and to the ribs.

xiphocostal ligament. COSTOXIPHOID LIGAMENT.

xi·phod·y·mus (zi·fod'i·mus) *n.* [*xipho-* + *-dymus*]. Conjoined twins with two heads, two thoraces, four arms, abdominal and pelvic regions in common, with two legs or occasionally a rudimentary third leg. See also *dicephalus tetrabrachius*.

xiph·o·dyn·ia (zif"o·din'ee·uh) *n.* [*xiph-* + *-odynia*]. Pain in the xiphoid process.

xiph·oid (zif'oid, zye'foid) *adj.* & *n.* [Gk. *xiphoeidēs*, from *xiphos*, sword]. 1. Sword-shaped; ensiform. 2. Pertaining to the xiphoid process. 3. XIPHOID PROCESS.

xiphoid angle. The angle formed by the costal margins at the lower end of the xiphoid process.

xiphoid appendix or **cartilage.** XIPHOID PROCESS.

xiph·oid·itis (zif"oid·eye'tis) *n.* [*xiphoid* + *-itis*]. Inflammation of the xiphoid process.

xiphoid process. The elongated process projecting caudad from the lower end of the sternum between the cartilages of the seventh ribs. Cartilaginous in early life, it usually becomes osseous after the age of 50. Syn. *ensiform process*. NA *processus xiphoideus*.

xi·phop·a·gus (zi·fop'uh·gus, zye·) *n.* [*xipho-* + *-pagus*]. Conjoined twins united at the inferior end of the sternum; a type of thoracopagus.

xipho·ster·nal (zif"o·stur'nul) *adj.* XIPHISTERNAL.

xiphosternal crunch. XIPHISTERNAL CRUNCH.

xipho·um·bil·i·cal (zif"o·um·bil'i·kul) *adj.* Pertaining to or extending between the xiphoid process and the umbilicus.

X-linkage. The usual case of sex-linkage in which a gene is physically located on the X chromosome. An X-linked recessive trait will be expressed in all males but only in homozygous females.

X-linked. Of a genetically determined trait: caused or controlled by a gene on the X chromosome.

XO syndrome. GONADAL DYSGENESIS.

x-ray, X-ray, *n.* 1. Any electromagnetic radiation having a wavelength in the approximate range of 0.1 to 100 angstroms, usually produced by bombarding a metal target with fast electrons in a highly evacuated tube and that has a spectrum characteristic of the target metal. X-rays penetrate various thicknesses of solids, strongly ionize tissues, affect photographic plates, and cause certain substances to fluoresce. Syn. *roentgen ray*. 2. Any photograph taken with x-rays.

x-ray burn. RADIATION BURN.

x-ray diffraction. When x-rays are passed through crystals, they are diffracted in a manner similar to light rays passed through a ruled diffraction grating. A study of the diffraction of x-rays gives information on the crystal structure.

x-ray kymograph. A device, usually consisting of a special grid and film cassette, one of which moves with x-ray

exposures timed to record motions of organs sequentially.
x-ray kymography. Kymography using x-ray techniques.
x-ray pelvimetry. Measurement of the pelvis and fetal head by radiography. A number of methods are utilized, all of which are concerned with correcting the distortion and magnification which occur with the technique. Syn. *pelvioradiography.*
x-ray photograph. RADIOGRAPH (1).
x-ray photography. RADIOGRAPHY.
x-ray service. The professional service in a medical institution performing, supervising in the performance of, and consulting in regard to x-ray diagnosis and radiation therapy.
x-ray therapy. Therapy with x-rays.
x-ray unit. Any assemblage of equipment primarily for diagnostic or therapeutic use of x-rays.
x wave. X DESCENT.
XXXX syndrome. A variant of Klinefelter's syndrome, in which mental retardation is more characteristic.
XXXXY syndrome. A syndrome of male phenotype but sometimes ambiguous genitalia, characterized by small stature, moderate to severe mental retardation, characteristic facies, radioulnar synostosis and occasionally congenital heart disease.
xyl-, xylo- [Gk. *xylon*]. A combining form meaning *wood.*
xy·lam·i·dine (zye·lam'i·deen) *n.* *N*-[2-(*m*-Methoxyphenoxy)propyl]-2-*m*-tolylacetamidine, $C_{19}H_{24}N_2O_2$, an antiserotonin compound; used as the *p*-toluenesulfonate (tosylate) salt.
xy·lan (zye'lan) *n.* A hemicellulose of the pentosan type, occurring in woody tissue, such as corncobs, peanut shells, straw. On hydrolysis it yields xylose.
xy·la·zine (zye'luh·zeen) *n.* 5,6-Dihydro-2-(2,6-xylidino)-4*H*-1,3-thiazine, $C_{12}H_{16}N_2S$, a veterinary analgesic and muscle relaxant.
xy·lem (zye'lum) *n.* [Ger., from Gk. *xylon,* wood]. *In botany,* the inner or woody portion of a vascular bundle of a plant. Contr. *phloem.*
xy·lene (zye'leen) *n.* Dimethylbenzene, $C_6H_4(CH_3)_2$, a colorless, mobile, flammable liquid. The xylene of commerce is a mixture of the three isomerides: *ortho-, meta-,* and *para-*xylenes. Has many industrial uses, and is used as a solvent and clearing agent in microscopy. Syn. *xylol.*
xy·le·nol (zye'le·nol) *n.* Dimethylphenol, $(CH_3)_2C_6H_3OH$, existing in six isomeric forms, all crystalline and slightly soluble in water; used in the preparation of coal-tar disinfectants.
xylidine ponceau. PONCEAU 2R.
xylo-. See *xyl-.*
Xylocaine. Trademark for lidocaine, a local amide anesthetic used as the hydrochloride salt.
xy·lol (zye'lol) *n.* XYLENE.
xy·lo·me·taz·o·line (zye"lo·me·taz'o·leen, ·met"uh·zo'leen) *n.* 2-(4-*tert*-Butyl-2,6-dimethylbenzyl)-2-imidazoline, $C_{16}H_{24}N_2$, a vasoconstrictor used topically to reduce swelling and congestion of the nasal mucosa; employed as the hydrochloride salt.
xy·lo·pho·bia (zye"lo·fo'bee·uh) *n.* [*xylo-* + *-phobia*]. An abnormal fear of trees, wooded plants, or forests.
xy·lose (zye'loce) *n.* Wood sugar, $C_5H_{10}O_5$, obtained from vegetable fibers; used medicinally as a diabetic food.
xylose excretion test. The measurement of the urinary excretion of D-xylose for 5 hours following ingestion of a given load of which normally 65% is absorbed in the small intestine, as a screening test for malabsorption syndromes, in which smaller than normal amounts are excreted.
xy·lo·ther·a·py (zye"lo·therr'uh·pee) *n.* [*xylo-* + *therapy*]. Treatment of disease by the application of certain woods to the body.
xy·lyl (zye'lil) *n.* 1. The univalent radical $CH_3C_6H_4CH_2$—. 2. The univalent radical $(CH_3)_2C_6H_3$—.
xylyl bromide. Methylbenzylbromide, $CH_3C_6H_4CH_2Br$, existing as *ortho-, meta-,* and *para-* forms. The mixed isomers are a lacrimatory poison "gas."
xyphoid, *adj. & n.* XIPHOID.
xy·ro·spasm (zye'ro·spaz·um) *n.* [Gk. *xyron,* razor, + *spasm*]. Spasm of the wrist and forearm muscles; an occupational disease of barbers.
xys·ma (ziz'muh) *n.* [Gk., shavings, scraps]. The flocculent pseudomembrane sometimes seen in the stools in diarrhea.
xys·ter (zis'tur) *n.* [Gk. *xystēr,* scraper, from *xyein,* to scrape]. A surgeon's raspatory or scraping instrument.
XYY male. An aneuploid state in which affected males with an extra Y chromosome are taller than usual and are regarded by some as having a tendency to sociopathic behavior.
x zone. ANDROGENIC ZONE.

Y

Y Symbol for yttrium.

-y [F. *-ie,* from L. and Gk. *-ia*]. A noun suffix meaning a *state, condition,* or *quality.* See also *-ia.*

Yaba virus. A poxvirus which produces self-limiting cutaneous histiocytomas in monkeys and other primates, including humans.

yawn, *v.* To perform the act of yawning.

yawn·ing, *n.* The often involuntary act of opening the mouth widely, accompanied by deep inspiration, and frequently stretching of the arms, shoulders, and chest to assist in the inspiratory act followed by relaxation of the muscles involved, usually performed when sleepy or bored.

yaws (yawz) *n.* An infectious tropical disease caused by *Treponema pertenue;* manifested by a primary cutaneous lesion followed by a granulomatous skin eruption, and occasionally late destructive lesions of the skin and bones.

Y axis. The line joining the sella turcica and the gnathion.

Yb Symbol for ytterbium.

Y chromosome. A sex-determining factor in the spermatozoon giving rise to male offspring.

y descent or **wave.** The negative wave of the atrial and jugular venous pulse pressure tracing in early ventricular diastole, produced by ventricular relaxation and atrioventricular valve opening with rapid ventricular filling.

yeast, *n.* The name applied to cells of various species of *Saccharomyces.* Certain of these, in dried form, are employed nutritionally as a source of protein and members of the B-complex group of vitamins.

yeast adenylic acid. Adenosine 3′-monophosphate. See *adenosine monophosphate.*

yeast meningitis. Meningitis caused by yeasts such as *Cryptococcus neoformans* or *Blastomyces dermatitidis.*

yeast nucleic acid. RIBONUCLEIC ACID.

yellow baboon. *Chaeropithecus* (or *Papio*) *cynocephalus,* the common baboon of East Africa and of central Africa south of the equatorial rain forests.

yellow blindness. A rare form of tritanopia in which there is inability to distinguish yellow or shades of yellow. See also *blue blindness.*

yellow body. CORPUS LUTEUM.

yellow cartilage. ELASTIC CARTILAGE.

yellow elastic tissue. ELASTIC TISSUE.

yellow enzyme. Any one of a group of enzymes containing a specific protein combined with isoalloxazine mononucleotide or isoalloxazine-adenine dinucleotide, and involved in certain biologic oxidations. See also *flavoprotein.*

yellow fat. Ordinary adipose tissue as distinguished from brown fat; characterized by unilocular cells and white or yellow color.

yellow fever. An acute viral disease transmitted to man by mosquitoes and characterized by fever, icterus, bradycardia, proteinuria, and a bleeding tendency. See also *urban yellow fever, sylvan yellow fever.*

yellow fibers. ELASTIC FIBERS.

yellow hepatization. The gross yellow appearance of the lungs in lobar pneumonia when a purulent exudate complicates the disease. Compare *red hepatization.*

yellow jack. YELLOW FEVER.

yellow jasmine root. GELSEMIUM.

yellow lead oxide. LEAD MONOXIDE.

yellow marrow. Marrow that consists largely of fat cells, which impart a yellow color. Few hemopoietic cells are present. NA *medulla ossium flava.* Contr. *red marrow.*

yellow mercuric oxide. MERCURIC OXIDE, YELLOW.

yellow ointment. An official oleaginous ointment base containing 5% yellow wax and 95% petrolatum.

yellow petrolatum. PETROLATUM.

yellow precipitate. MERCURIC OXIDE, YELLOW.

yel·low·root, *n.* HYDRASTIS.

yellow spot. MACULA LUTEA.

yellow wax. The purified wax from the honeycomb of the bee, *Apis mellifera.* It consists chiefly of myricin (myricyl palmitate); also contains cerotic acid (cerin), melissic acid, and about 6% hydrocarbons of the paraffin series. Used in the formulation of ointments, cerates, plasters, suppositories, and surgical dressings in which it acts mechanically, either giving stiffness or serving to repel water. Syn. *beeswax.*

Yemen ulcer. TROPICAL ULCER.

Yer·sin·ia (yur·sin′ee·uh, yerr.) *n.* [A. *Yersin,* French bacteriologist, 1863–1943]. A genus of small, aerobic or facultatively anaerobic non-spore-forming, gram-negative bacilli, all of which can produce disease in man and animals.

Yersinia en·tero·co·lit·i·ca (en″tur·o·ko·lit′i·kuh). A relatively large gram-negative coccobacillus infecting both man and animals; may cause acute mesenteric lymphadenitis or enterocolitis.

Yersinia pes·tis (pes′tis) [L., of plague]. The coccobacillus that causes sylvatic, bubonic, and pneumonic plague. Formerly called *Pasteurella pestis.*

Yersinia pseu·do·tu·ber·cu·lo·sis (sue″do·tew·bur″kew·lo′sis). A gram-negative coccobacillus that causes pseudotuberculosis in animals and lymphadentis in man. Formerly called *Pasturella pseudotuberculosis.*

Y factor. PYRIDOXINE.

-yl [from Gk. *hylē,* wood, matter]. A combining form meaning (a) a *univalent chemical radical,* as in ethyl and hydroxyl; (b) a *radical containing oxygen,* as in antimonyl and carbonyl; (c) a *radical of organic acids,* as in acetyl and formyl.

ylang-ylang oil (ee′lahng ee′lahng). A volatile perfume oil obtained from the flowers of *Cananga odorata,* a southern Asiatic tree.

Y ligament. ILIOFEMORAL LIGAMENT.

Y-linkage. A special case of sex linkage in which a gene is physically located on the Y chromosome. Y-linked traits can only be expressed in males.

-yne. A suffix designating an *unsaturated straight-chain hydrocarbon having one triple bond.*

Yodoxin. A trademark for diiodohydroxyquin, an antiamebic and antitrichomonal drug.

yo·him·bé, yo·him·bi (yo·him′bee) *n.* The rubiaceous tree *Corynanthe yohimbi (Pausinystalia yohimbe)* growing in the southern Cameroons district in Africa. The bark contains several alkaloids of which the most important is yohimbine; both bark and yohimbine have been employed for reputed aphrodisiac effect.

yo·him·bine (yo·him′been) *n.* The principal alkaloid, $C_{21}H_{26}N_2O_3$, of yohimbé, identical with quebrachine. Has been used as an aphrodisiac and also in treating angina pectoris and arteriosclerosis.

yoked muscles. Muscles that act equally at the same time in opposite eyes, as the medial rectus of one eye and the lateral rectus of the other.

yolk, *n.* The nutritive part of an ovum. See also *deuteroplasm.*

yolk granules. The elements composing the yolk.

yolk plug. The mass of yolk protruding into the blastopore of amphibian gastrulas as a result of epiboly.

yolk sac. An extraembryonic membrane composed of endoderm and splanchnic mesoderm. It encloses the yolk mass in reptiles, birds, and monotremes, or a cavity in higher mammals. It is also the site of the formation of the primitive blood cells.

yolk-sac entoderm. The epithelial lining of the yolk sac, continuous with that of the gut.

yolk-sac placenta. OMPHALOCHORION.

yolk sphere. VITELLINE SPHERE.

yolk stalk. VITELLINE DUCT.

Yomesan. Trademark for niclosamide, an anthelmintic.

Yo·shi·da tumor. A transplantable poorly differentiated malignant tumor that developed originally in an albino rat fed *o*-aminoazotoluol and painted with potassium arsenite; it grows in both solid and ascitic forms.

Young·burg and Fo·lin method. A method for determining urea in urine in which diluted urine is treated with an alcoholic urease solution to convert urea into ammonia, and the ammonia present is then determined by direct nesslerization.

young female syndrome. AORTIC ARCH SYNDROME.

young monocyte. PROMONOCYTE (1).

Young's method [H. H. *Young,* U.S. urologist, 1870–1945]. A procedure for reconstruction of the posterior urethra.

Young's operation [H. H. *Young*]. 1. PERINEAL PROSTATECTOMY. 2. Total excision of the seminal vesicles and partial excision of the ejaculatory ducts, using a suprapubic incision. 3. Plastic operation for epispadias, in which a new tube is formed from the skin of the groove.

Young's punch [H. H. *Young*]. A cautery punch for removal of prostatic obstruction transurethrally.

Young's rule [T. *Young,* English physician, 1773–1829]. A rule to determine dosage of medicine for children; specifically, dose = child's age in years, multiplied by adult dose, divided by the sum of the child's age plus 12.

youth, *n.* The period between childhood and maturity.

yper·ite (ee′pur·ite) *n.* [*Ypres,* Belgium]. Bis(2-chloroethyl)-sulfide, $(C_2H_4Cl)_2S$, so-called mustard gas, a vesicant liquid that has been used in chemical warfare.

yp·sil·i·form (ip·sil′i·form) *adj.* [Gk. *upsilon,* twentieth letter of the Greek alphabet, + *-iform*]. Resembling the Greek letter Υ; Y-shaped.

Yt Alternate symbol for yttrium.

yt·ter·bi·um (i·tur′bee·um) *n.* [NL., after *Ytterby,* Sweden]. Yb = 173.04. A rare metallic element, atomic number 70, density 7.0.

yt·tri·um (it′ree·um) *n.* Y = 88.9059. A rare metallic element, atomic number 39, density 4.34.

Yuge's syndrome. UVEOMENINGOENCEPHALITIS.

Yvon's coefficient (ee·vohⁿ′) [P. *Yvon,* French physician, 1848–1913]. The ratio between urinary urea and phosphates (1:8).

Yvon's test [P. *Yvon*]. A test for acetanilid in which urine is extracted with chloroform and the residue heated with mercurous nitrate. A green color indicates acetanilid.

y wave. Y DESCENT.

Z

Z [Ger. *z*usammen, together]. A stereo descriptor for geometric isomers indicating a configuration of atoms or groups on the same side of a theoretical plane intersecting the atoms causing the achiral center. Compare *trans, E.*

Z Symbol for (a) atomic number; (b) impedance.

Z. Abbreviation for *Zuckung,* contraction.

z. Abbreviation for *Z disk* (= INTERMEDIATE DISK).

Zactane. Trademark for ethoheptazine, an analgesic drug used as the citrate salt.

Zanchol. Trademark for florantyrone, a hydrocholeretic drug.

Zan·der's apparatus (sahn'dur) [J. G. W. *Zander,* Swedish physician, 1835–1920]. A special apparatus for passive exercise of a limb.

Zanosar. A trademark for streptozocin, an antibiotic.

zanthoxylum. XANTHOXYLUM.

Zap·pert's chamber (tsahp'urt) [J. *Zappert,* Austrian physician, 1867–1942]. A type of hemocytometer.

Zarontin. Trademark for ethosuximide, an anticonvulsant drug, primarily for absence attacks.

Z axis. The anteroposterior axis.

Z band. Z LINE.

Z disk [Ger. *Z*wischenscheibe]. INTERMEDIATE DISK.

zed·o·ary (zed'o·err·ee) *n.* [ML. *zedoaria,* from Per. *zedwār*]. The dried rhizome of species of *Curcuma;* resembles ginger.

Zeis's glands (tsice) [E. *Zeis,* German ophthalmologist, 1807–1868]. The sebaceous glands associated with the cilia.

Zel·ler's test (tsel'ur) [A. *Zeller,* German physician, 19th century]. A test for melanin in urine in which equal volumes of urine and bromine water are mixed. In the presence of melanin, a yellow precipitate will form and gradually become black.

Zell·we·ger's syndrome [H. *Zellweger,* U.S. pediatrician, 20th century]. CEREBROHEPATORENAL SYNDROME.

Zen·ker's degeneration (tsenk'ur) [F. A. *Zenker,* German pathologist, 1825–1898]. Necrosis and hyaline degeneration in striated muscle, seen especially in infectious disease.

Zenker's diverticulum or **pouch** [F. A. *Zenker,* German physician, 1825–1898]. A pulsion diverticulum of the esophagus.

Zenker's fixative or **fixing fluid** [K. *Zenker,* German pathologist, b. 1894]. A mixture of potassium bichromate, mercuric chloride, distilled water, and glacial acetic acid; used in numerous fixing techniques.

Zenker's hyaline degeneration or **necrosis.** ZENKER'S DEGENERATION.

Zenker's paralysis [F. A. *Zenker*]. Paralysis due to common peroneal nerve injury, usually manifested as foot drop.

ze·o·lite (zee'o·lite) *n.* [Gk. *zein,* to boil, + *lithos,* stone]. Any one of a group of hydrated aluminum and calcium or sodium silicates, of the type $Na_2O.2Al_2O_3.5SiO_2$ or $CaO.2Al_2O_3.5SiO_2$, certain of which may be used for water softening by an ion-exchange process.

Zephiran Chloride. A trademark for benzalkonium chloride, a quaternary antiseptic for topical application.

zer·a·nol (zerr'uh·nole) *n.* 3,4,5,6,7,8,9,10,11,12-Decahydro-7,14,16-trihydroxy-3-methyl-1*H*-2-benzoxacyclotetradecin-1-one, $C_{18}H_{26}O_5$, an anabolic agent.

ze·ro, *n.,* pl. **xeros, xeroes** [F. *zéro,* from ML. *zephirum,* from Ar. *ṣifr,* cipher]. 1. Any character denoting absence of quantity. 2. The point on thermometers from which temperatures are counted. Compare *absolute zero.*

zero threshold phenomenon. A situation in which there is no dose level which must be attained before there is an effect (for example, a gene mutation) and below which no change occurs.

ze·ta potential (zay'tuh). ELECTROKINETIC POTENTIAL.

Zettyn. Trademark for cetalkonium chloride, a local anti-infective compound.

z flap. A means of lengthening a linear contracted scar by transposing two triangular flaps of skin, the sutured incision having a z shape.

Zieh·en-Op·pen·heim's disease (tsee'un, ohp'en·hime) [G. T. *Ziehen,* German psychiatrist, b. 1862; and H. *Oppenheim*]. DYSTONIA MUSCULORUM DEFORMANS.

Ziehl-Neel·sen method or **stain** (tseel, neyl'zen) [F. *Ziehl,* German bacteriologist, 1859–1926; and F. K. A. *Neelsen*]. CARBOL-FUCHSIN STAIN.

Ziehl-Neelsen stain for tubercle bacilli [F. *Ziehl* and F. K. A. *Neelsen*]. A procedure for acid-fast staining of tubercle bacilli.

Ziems·sen's point (tseem'sen) [H. W. von *Ziemssen,* German physician, 1829–1902]. MOTOR POINT.

Zieve's syndrome [L. *Zieve,* U.S. internist, b. 1915]. Transient hyperlipemia, jaundice, hemolytic anemia, and abdominal pain occurring after drinking a large amount of ethyl alcohol.

zi·lan·tel (zi·lan'tel) *n.* Phosphonodithioimidocarbonic acid ethylene dibenzyl P,P,P',P-tetraethyl ester, $C_{26}H_{38}N_2O_6P_2S_4$, an anthelmintic.

Zim·mer·lin's type (tsim'ur·lin) [F. *Zimmerlin,* Swiss physician, 1858–1932]. SCAPULOHUMERAL MUSCULAR DYSTROPHY.

Zim·mer·mann reaction. A colorimetric procedure for the estimation of 17-ketosteroids. It involves treatment with *m*-dinitrobenzene and potassium hydroxide in an alcoholic solution.

zinc, *n.* [Ger. *Zink*]. Zn = 65.37. A bluish-white, lustrous, metallic element, atomic number 30, density 7.14. Salts of zinc are used as astringents and antiseptics.

zinc acetate. $Zn(C_2H_3O_2)_2.2H_2O$. White crystals or granules, freely soluble in water. Variously used as a topical astringent.

zinc chills. METAL FUME FEVER.

zinc chloride. $ZnCl_2$. White crystalline powder or granules, very soluble in water. Used topically as an astringent and desensitizer for dentin.

zinc·ite (zink'ite) *n.* 1. A native zinc oxide, orange-yellow to deep red. 2. Any ore of zinc.

zinc oxide. ZnO. Very fine, amorphous, white or yellowish-white powder, insoluble in water. Variously used in lotions, ointments, and pastes, as a topical astringent and protectant.

zinc phenolsulfonate. $Zn(HOC_6H_4SO_3)_2.8H_2O$. Colorless, transparent crystals, freely soluble in water. Has been used topically as an antiseptic and astringent, and internally as an intestinal antiseptic. Syn. *zinc sulfocarbolate.*

zinc pyr·i·thi·one (pirr''i·thigh'ohn). Bis [1-hydroxy-2(1*H*)-pyridinethionato] zinc, $C_{10}H_8N_2O_2S_2Zn$, an antibacterial, antifungal, and antiseborrheic compound.

zinc stearate. A compound of zinc with variable proportions of stearic and palmitic acids; a fine, white, bulky powder; insoluble in water and alcohol. Used in eczema and other cutaneous diseases, in the form of powder or made into an ointment.

zinc sul·fan·i·late (sul·fan'i·late). The zinc salt of *p*-aminobenzenesulfonic acid, $C_{12}H_{12}N_2O_6S_2Zn$, an antibacterial.

zinc sulfate. $ZnSO_4.7H_2O$. Colorless, transparent prisms or needles, or granular, crystalline powder, very soluble in water. Used topically as an astringent, and internally as an emetic in poisoning.

zinc sulfate turbidity test. A flocculation test for liver function, resembling the thymol turbidity test but using zinc sulfate as the precipitating agent and a buffer of lower ionic strength. It differentiates obstructive and hepatocellular jaundice in the early stages.

zinc sulfocarbolate. ZINC PHENOLSULFONATE.

zinc·um (zink'um) *n.* [NL.]. ZINC.

zinc un·dec·y·len·ate (un·des''i·len'ate). Zinc 10-undecenoate, $[CH_2{=}CH(CH_2)_8COO]_2Zn$, a fine white powder, practically insoluble in water. Used topically as a fungistatic agent.

zin·gi·ber (zin'ji·bur) *n.* GINGER.

Zinn's central artery (tsin) [J. G. *Zinn*, German anatomist, 1727–1759]. The central artery of the retina.

Zinn's circlet or **corona** [J. G. *Zinn*]. VASCULAR CIRCLE OF THE OPTIC NERVE.

Zinn's ligament, tendon, ring, or **annulus** [J. G. *Zinn*]. LIGAMENT OF ZINN.

Zinn's zonule [J. G. *Zinn*]. CILIARY ZONULE.

Zins·ser-Eng·man-Cole syndrome [F. *Zinsser*, 1865–1952; M. F. *Engman*, U.S. dermatologist, 1869–1953; and H. N. *Cole*]. DYKERATOSIS CONGENITA.

zir·co·ni·um (zur·ko'nee·um) *n.* [NL.]. Zr = 91.22. A metallic element, atomic number 40, density 6.53; resembles titanium and silicon.

zirconium dioxide. ZrO_2. A heavy, white powder, insoluble in water. Used topically in formulations for treatment of ivy poisoning; formerly employed as a radiopaque medium.

Z line. The Z disk (intermediate disk) viewed longitudinally.

Zn Symbol for zinc.

zo-, zoo- [Gk. *zōon*, living being, animal]. A combining form meaning *animal.*

zo·an·thro·py (zo·an'thruh·pee) *n.* [*zo-* + *anthrop-* + *-y*]. A delusional state in which the person imagines himself transformed into or inhabited by an animal.

-zoic [Gk. *zōikos*, of or pertaining to animals]. A combining form meaning *a* (specified) *mode of animal life.*

zo·la·mine (zo'luh·meen) *n.* 2-[[2-(Dimethylamino)ethyl](*p*-methoxybenzyl) amino]thiazole, $C_{15}H_{21}N_3OS$, an antihistaminic and topical anesthetic; used as the hydrochloride salt.

zo·ler·tine (zo'lur·teen) *n.* 1-Phenyl-4-(2-tetrazol-5-ylethyl)-piperazine, $C_{13}H_{18}N_6$, an antiadrenergic vasodilator; used as the hydrochloride salt.

Zollinger-Ellison syndrome [R. M. *Zollinger*, U.S. surgeon, b. 1903; and E. H. *Ellison*, U.S. surgeon, 1918–1970]. Gastric hypersecretion and hyperacidity, fulminating intractable atypical peptic ulceration, and hyperplasia of the islet cells of the pancreas.

zo·na (zo'nuh) *n.*, pl. & genit. sing. **zo·nae** (·nee) [L., from Gk. *zōnē*]. 1. ZONE; belt, or girdle. 2. HERPES ZOSTER.

zona ar·cu·a·ta (ahr·kew·ay'tuh). The inner zone of the lamina basilaris extending from the lower edge of the spiral groove of the cochlea to the external edge of the base of the outer pillars of Corti.

zona car·ti·la·gi·nea (kahr·ti·la·jin'ee·uh). LIMBUS OF THE SPIRAL LAMINA.

zona ci·li·a·ris (sil·ee·air'is). CILIARY ZONE.

zona co·lum·na·ris rec·ti (ko·lum·nair'is reck'tye). The portion of the anal canal in which lie the anal columns.

zona cu·ta·nea rec·ti (kew·ta'nee·uh reck'tye). The portion of the anal canal lined by skin.

zona den·ti·cu·la·ta (den·tick·yoo·lay'tuh). The inner zone of the lamina basilaris, together with the limbus of the spiral lamina.

zonae. Plural and genitive singular of *zona.*

zonaesthesia. Zonesthesia (= GIRDLE PAIN).

zona fas·ci·cu·la·ta (fa·sick·yoo·lay'tuh). The middle portion of the cortex of the suprarenal gland in which the cellular cords are radially disposed.

zona glo·me·ru·lo·sa (glo·merr·yoo·lo'suh). The outer zone of the adrenal cortex in which the cells are grouped in rounded masses.

zona he·mor·rhoi·da·lis (hem·o·roy·day'lis) [NA]. HEMORRHOIDAL RING.

zona in·cer·ta (in·sur'tuh) [NA]. The anterior portion of the reticular formation under the thalamus.

zona intermedia. The region of spinal gray matter that intervenes between the posterior and anterior gray horns, designated cytoarchitectonically as lamina VII of Rexed. It consists of a large number of internuncial neurons and well-defined cell columns (the dorsal nucleus of Clarke, intermediolateral nucleus, and intermediomedial nucleus) in certain regions.

zona in·ter·me·dia rec·ti (in·tur·mee'dee·uh reck'tye). The portion of the anal canal which lies between the cutaneous and columnar zones.

zona oph·thal·mi·ca (off'thal'mi·kuh). Herpes zoster along the course of the ophthalmic division of the fifth cranial nerve.

zona or·bi·cu·la·ris (or·bick·yoo·lair'is) [NA]. A thickening of the capsular ligament around the acetabulum.

zona pec·ti·na·ta (peck·ti·nay'tuh). The outer portion of the lamina basilaris, extending from the pillars of Corti to the spiral ligament.

zona pel·lu·ci·da (pe·lew'si·duh). The thick, solid, elastic envelope of the ovum. Syn. *oolemma.*

zona per·fo·ra·ta (pur·fo·ray'tuh). The lower edge of the spiral groove of the cochlea.

zona re·ti·cu·la·ris (re·tick·yoo·lair'is). 1. The inner zone of the adrenal cortex in which the cellular cords form a network. 2. RETICULAR LAYER.

zo·na·ry (zo'nuh·ree) *adj.* [L. *zonarius*, of a girdle]. 1. ZONAL; of or pertaining to a zone. 2. Arranged in a band. 3. Of a placenta, having zonary villi.

zonary villi. Villi restricted to an annular zone about the chorion, as in carnivores.

zona spon·gi·o·sa (spon·jee·o'suh). A thin zone of nerve cells and myelinated fibers, external to the substantia gelatinosa in the posterior column of the spinal cord.

zona tec·ta (teck'tuh). The inner portion of the lamina basilaris, bearing the spiral organ of Corti.

zone, *n.* [L. *zona,* girdle, zone, from Gk. *zōnē*]. A delimited area or region. **—zon·al** (zo'nul) *adj.*

zone of antibody excess. The zone at which there is complete precipitation of the antigen, with some residual unbound antibody in the supernatant.

zone of antigen excess. The zone in which the antigen-antibody complexes are soluble.

zone of equivalence. The zone at which the antigen and antibody have completely precipitated.

zone of inhibition. ZONE OF ANTIGEN EXCESS.

zone of Lissauer. DORSOLATERAL TRACT.

zone of Weil (vile) [L. A. *Weil,* German dentist, 19th century]. The cell-free layer found just inside the layer of odontoblasts in the dental pulp of the crown of a tooth.

zon·es·the·sia, zon·aes·the·sia (zo''nes·theezh'uh, ·theez'ee·uh) *n.* [Gk. *zōnē,* girdle, + *-esthesia*]. GIRDLE PAIN.

zone therapy. REFLEXOTHERAPY.

zo·nif·u·gal (zo·nif'yoo·gul) *adj.* [*zone* + *-fugal*]. Pertaining to the tendency to pass out of, or away from, a zone.

zo·nip·e·tal (zo·nip'e·tul) *adj.* [*zone* + *-petal*]. Pertaining to the tendency to pass into a zone from without.

zo·nu·la (zo'new·luh) *n.*, pl. **zonu·lae** (·lee). [L.]. ZONULE.

zonula ad·hae·rens, ad·he·rens (ad·heer'enz). *In electron microscopy,* the broader, innermost area of the terminal bar in which there is a small but distinct extracellular space.

zonula ci·li·a·ris (sil·ee·air'is) [NA]. CILIARY ZONULE.

zonula ciliaris [Zin·nii] (zin'ee·eye) [BNA]. Zonula ciliaris (= CILIARY ZONULE).

zonula oc·clu·dens (ock·lew'denz). *In electron microscopy,* the outermost area of the terminal bar at which there is a tight junction of the contiguous, lateral cell membranes.

zo·nu·lar (zo'new·lur) *adj.* [*zonule* + *-ar*]. Pertaining to a zonule.

zonular cataract. A partial, stationary cataract, which is bilateral and may be congenital or form in infancy, due to a disturbance of calcium metabolism; characterized by a grayish central disk surrounded by a clear lens substance. Syn. *lamellar cataract.*

zonular fibers. The fibers of the ciliary zonule. NA *fibrae zonulares.*

zonular keratitis. BAND KERATOPATHY.

zonular spaces. The spaces between the zonular fibers; a part of the posterior chamber of the eye. Syn. *canals of Petit.* NA *spatia zonularia.*

zo·nule (zo'newl, zon'yool) *n.* [L. *zonula,* dim. of *zona,* girdle, belt]. A small band.

zonule of Zinn [J. G. *Zinn*]. CILIARY ZONULE.

zo·nu·li·tis (zo''new·lye'tis, zon''yoo·) *n.* [*zonule* + *-itis*]. Inflammation of the ciliary zonule.

zo·nu·lol·y·sis (zo''new·lol'i·sis, zon''yoo·) *n.* ZONULYSIS.

zo·nu·lot·o·my (zo''new·lot'uh·mee, zon''yoo·) *n.* [*zonule* + *-tomy*]. The severing of the ciliary zonular fibers.

zo·nu·ly·sis (zo''new·lye'sis, zon''yoo·) *n.* [*zonule* + *-lysis*]. Enzymatic dissolution of the ciliary zonular fibers of the eye.

zoo-. See *zo-.*

zoo·der·mic (zo''o·dur'mick) *adj.* [*zoo-* + *dermic*]. Pertaining to, or taken from, the skin of some animal other than man; applied to a form of skin grafting.

zoo·eras·tia (zo''o·e·ras'tee·uh) *n.* [*zoo-* + Gk. *erastēs,* lover, + *-ia*]. Sexual intercourse with an animal.

zoo·ge·og·ra·phy (zo''o·jee·og'ruh·fee) *n.* [*zoo-* + *geography*]. The geography of animal life.

zoo·glea, zoo·gloea (zo''o·glee'uh, zo·og'lee·uh) *n.*, pl. **zoo·gleas, zoo·gle·ae, zoo·gloea** (·glee'ee) [NL., from *zoo-* + Gk. *gloia,* glue]. Microorganisms embedded in a jellylike matrix that has been formed as a result of their metabolic activities. **—zoo·gle·ic, zoo·gloe·ic** (·glee'ick) *adj.*

zo·og·o·ny (zo·og'uh·nee) *n.* [Gk. *zōogonia,* from *zōon,* animal, + *goneia,* generation, production]. The breeding of animals.

zoo·graft (zo'o·graft) *n.* [*zoo-* + *graft*]. A graft of tissue taken from an animal and transplanted to a human.

zo·oid (zo'oid) *adj.* & *n.* [Gk. *zōoeidēs,* from *zōon,* animal]. 1. Resembling an animal. 2. An individual member of a colonial form of animal life, such as coral.

zoo·lag·nia (zo''o·lag'nee·uh) *n.* [*zoo-* + Gk. *lagneia,* lust]. Sexual attraction toward animals.

zo·ol·o·gist (zo·ol'uh·jist) *n.* A scientist who studies animal life.

zo·ol·o·gy (zo·ol'uh·jee) *n.* [*zoo-* + *-logy*]. The scientific study of animals.

-zoon [Gk. *zōon,* animal]. A combining form meaning *living being, animal.*

zoo·no·sis (zo''o·no'sis, zo·on'o·sis) *n.*, pl. **zoono·ses** (·seez) [*zoo-* + Gk. *nosos,* disease (assimilated in form to the suffix *-osis*)]. A disease of lower animals transmissible to other vertebrate animals and man. **—zoo·not·ic** (·not'ick) *adj.*

Zoon's balanitis (zone) [J. J. *Zoon,* Dutch dermatologist, 20th century]. An inflammatory disease of the glans penis which clinically resembles Queyrat's erythroplasia.

zo·o·par·a·site (zo''o·păr'uh·site) *n.* [*zoo-* + *parasite*]. An animal parasite. **—zoo·par·a·sit·ic** (·păr''uh·sit'ick) *adj.*

zooparasitic cirrhosis. Cirrhosis resulting from the invasion of animal parasites or their ova, such as *Schistosoma.*

zo·oph·a·gous (zo·off'uh·gus) *adj.* [Gk. *zōophagos,* from *zōon,* animal, + *phagein,* to eat]. Subsisting on animal food.

zoo·phil·ia (zo''o·fil'ee·uh) *n.* ZOOPHILISM.

zo·oph·i·lism (zo·off'i·liz·um) *n.* [*zoo-* + *phil-* + *-ism*]. 1. The love of animals; it is usually immoderate, and toward certain animals. 2. *In psychiatry,* sexual pleasure from stroking or fondling animals.

zoo·pho·bia (zo''o·fo'bee·uh) *n.* [*zoo-* + *-phobia*]. Abnormal fear of animals.

zoo·phyte (zo'o·fite) *n.* [Gk. *zōophyton,* from *zōon,* animal + *phyton,* plant]. An invertebrate animal that superficially resembles a plant in appearance, as the sponges, hydroids, bryozoa.

zooplastic graft. ZOOGRAFT.

zoo·plasty (zo'o·plas''tee) *n.* [*zoo-* + *-plasty*]. The surgical transfer of zoografts; the transplantation of tissue from any of the lower animals to man. **—zoo·plas·tic** (zo''o·plas'tick) *adj.*

zo·op·sia (zo·op'see·uh) *n.* [*zo-* + *ops-* + *-ia*]. The seeing of animals, as an illusion or as a hallucination or in a dream; occurs commonly in delirium tremens.

zoo·spore (zo'o·spore) *n.* [*zoo-* + *spore*]. Motile spores occurring in algae and in lower fungi, such as the Phycomycetes. Syn. *swarm spore, swarm cell.*

zo·os·ter·ol (zo·os'tur·ol) *n.* [*zoo-* + *sterol*]. Any sterol of animal origin.

zo·ot·o·my (zo·ot'uh·mee) *n.* [*zoo-* + *-tomy*]. 1. Anatomy of animals other than man. 2. Dissection of animals.

zoo·tox·in (zo''o·tock'sin) *n.* [*zoo-* + *toxin*]. Any toxin or poison of animal origin.

zor·ba·my·cin (zor''buh·migh'sin) *n.* An antibiotic produced by a variant of *Streptomyces bikiniensis.*

zos·ter (zos'tur) *n.* [Gk. *zōstēr,* girdle]. HERPES ZOSTER.

zoster au·ri·cu·la·ris (aw·rick''yoo·lair'is). RAMSAY HUNT SYNDROME.

zoster bra·chi·a·lis (bray''kee·ay'lis). Herpes zoster affecting the arm or forearm.

zoster fa·ci·a·lis (fay·shee·ay'lis). Herpes zoster involving the sensory fibers of the trigeminal nerve distributed over the face. Any or all of the three branches may be involved.

zoster fem·o·ra·lis (fem·o·ray'lis). Herpes zoster occurring over the sacrum and extending down the thighs. The perineal region may be involved.

zos·ter·i·form (zos·terr'i·form) *adj.* [*zoster* + *-iform*]. Resembling herpes zoster.

zosteriform nevus. COBBLESTONE NEVUS.

zos·ter·oid (zos'tur·oid) *adj.* ZOSTERIFORM.

zoster oph·thal·mi·cus (off·thal'mi·kus). A herpes zoster eruption in the course of the ophthalmic division of the fifth nerve.

Z-plastic relaxing operation. An operation for the relaxation of scar contractures, effected by a Z-shaped incision, with transposition of the flaps.

Z-plas·ty (zee'plas·tee) *n.* Z-PLASTIC RELAXING OPERATION.

z point. 1. The lowest point on the atrial pressure tracing immediately following the a wave; it is produced by atrial relaxation and is interrupted by the c wave; it may also be identified in the jugular venous pulse tracing. 2. The lowest point on the left ventricular pressure tracing, which follows the atrial contribution to ventricular filling (a wave) and immediately precedes the isovolumetric rise of pressure.

Zr Symbol for zirconium.

zuck·er·guss (tsŏŏk'ur·gŏŏs) *adj.* [Ger.]. Sugar-coated; applied especially to hyaline thickening of the splenic capsule, but also to hyaline thickening of other mesothelial coverings.

zuckerguss spleen. ICED SPLEEN.

Zuck·er·kan·dl's bodies (tsŏŏk'ur·kahn''del) [E. *Zuckerkandl*, Austrian anatomist, 1849–1910]. PARAAORTIC BODIES.

Zuckerkandl's convolution [E. *Zuckerkandl*]. GYRUS PARATERMINALIS.

Zuckerkandl's tubercle [E. *Zuckerkandl*]. ADENOID.

zuck·ung (tsŏŏk'ŏŏng) *n.* [Ger.]. CONTRACTION; a term used in electrotherapeutics. Abbreviated, Z.

zu·clo·mi·phene (zoo·klo'mi·feen) *n.* (*Z*)-2-[*p*-Chloro-1,2-diphenylvinyl)phenoxy]triethylamine, $C_{26}H_{28}ClNO$, a gonad-stimulating agent.

Zwe·mer's test (zway'mur) [R. L. *Zwemer*, U.S. anatomist, b. 1902]. POTASSIUM TOLERANCE TEST.

zwit·ter·ion (tsvit'ur·eye''un) *n.* [Ger. *zwitter*, hybrid, + *ion*]. An ion that contains both a positive and a negative charge, but is neutral as a whole; a dipolar ion. Amino acids may form such ions by migration of a hydrogen ion from the carboxyl group to the basic nitrogen atom as, for example, when RNH_2COOH is thus converted to $RNH_3^+COO^-$.

zyg-, zygo- [Gk. *zygon*, yoke]. A combining form meaning (a) *yoke, joining;* (b) *union, fusion;* (c) *pair.*

zyg·apoph·y·sis (zig''uh·pof'i·sis, zye''guh·) *n.*, pl. **zygapophy·ses** (·seez) [*zyg-* + *apophysis*]. An articular process of a vertebra. —**zyg·apoph·y·se·al** (·uh·pof''i·see'ul, ·uh·po·fiz'ee·ul) *adj.*

zyg·ion (zig'ee·on, zij') *n.*, pl. **zyg·ia** (·ee·uh), **zygions.** *In craniometry,* a point at either end of the greatest bizygomatic diameter.

zy·go·dac·ty·ly (zye''go·dack'ti·lee) *n.* [*zygo-* + *-dactyly*]. SYNDACTYLY.

zy·go·ma (zye·go'muh, zi·go'muh) *n.*, pl. **zygoma·ta** (·tuh), **zygomas** [Gk. *zygōma*, from *zygoun*, to yoke, join together]. ZYGOMATIC BONE.

zy·go·mat·ic (zye''go·mat'ick) *adj.* & *n.* [*zygoma* + *-ic*]. 1. Of or pertaining to the zygomatic bone. 2. Either of two small subcutaneous muscles (NA *musculus zygomaticus major, musculus zygomaticus minor*) arising from, or in relation with, the zygomatic bone. See also Table of Muscles in the Appendix. 3. A somatic sensory nerve, a branch of the maxillary nerve which innervates the skin in the region of the zygomatic bone and temple. NA *nervus zygomaticus.* See also Table of Nerves in the Appendix.

zygomatic arch. The arch formed by the zygomatic process of the temporal bone, the zygomatic bone, and the temporal process of the zygomatic bone. NA *arcus zygomaticus.*

zygomatic bone. The bone that forms the prominence of the cheek. Syn. *cheekbone.* NA *os zygomaticum.* See also Table of Bones in the Appendix.

zygomatic fossa. INFRATEMPORAL FOSSA.

zygomatic margin. The anterior border of the great wing of the sphenoid; it articulates with the zygomatic bone and separates the orbital from the temporal surface. NA *margo zygomaticus alae majoris.*

zygomatico-. A combining form meaning *zygomatic bone.*

zy·go·mat·i·co·fa·cial (zye''go·mat''i·ko·fay'shul) *adj.* Pertaining to the zygomatic bone and the face.

zygomaticofacial nerve. NA *ramus zygomaticofacialis nervi zygomatici.* See Table of Nerves in the Appendix.

zy·go·mat·i·co·max·il·lary (zye''go·mat''i·ko·mack'si·lerr·ee) *adj.* [*zygomatico-* + *maxillary*]. Pertaining to the zygomatic bone and the maxilla.

zygomaticomaxillary suture. A suture between the line of junction between the maxillary border of the zygomatic bone and the zygomatic process of the maxilla. NA *sutura zygomaticomaxillaris.*

zy·go·mat·i·co·or·bit·al (zye''go·mat''i·ko·or'bi·tul) *adj.* [*zygomatico-* + *orbital*]. Pertaining to the zygomatic bone and the orbit.

zygomaticoorbital canal. A canal or canals in the orbital process of the zygomatic bone for the passage of the zygomaticofacial and zygomaticotemporal branches of the zygomatic nerve.

zy·go·mat·i·co·tem·po·ral (zye''go·mat''i·ko·tem'po·rul) *adj.* Pertaining to the zygomatic bone and the temporal bone or fossa.

zygomatic process of the frontal bone. A strong, prominent lateral projection from the supraorbital margin of the frontal bone which articulates with the zygomatic bone.

zygomatic process of the maxilla. A rough, triangular, serrated eminence which articulates with the maxillary process of the zygomatic bone. NA *processus zygomaticus maxillae.*

zygomatic process of the temporal bone. A long projection from the lower part of the squamous portion of the temporal bone, articulating with the zygomatic bone. NA *processus zygomaticus ossis temporalis.*

zygomatic reflex. Movement of the mandible toward the percussed side when the zygomatic bone is percussed; a modification of the jaw reflex.

zy·go·ma·ti·cus (zye''go·mat'i·kus) *n.* A muscle of facial expression associated with the zygoma; ZYGOMATIC (2).

zy·go·max·il·la·re (zy''go·mack''si·lair'ee) *n.* *In craniometry,* the point on the zygomaticomaxillary suture that lies most inferior to the horizontal plane.

Zy·go·my·ce·tes (zye''go·migh·see'teez) *n. pl.* [*zygo-* + *mycetes*]. A group of fungi characterized by sexual reproduction through the union of two similar gametes.

zy·go·my·co·sis (zye''go·migh·ko·sis) *n.* [*Zygomyc*etes + *-osis*]. MUCORMYCOSIS.

zy·go·ne·ma (zye''go·nee'muh) *n.* The chromonema when in the zygotene stage of meiosis.

zy·gos·i·ty (zye·gos'i·tee) *n.* The genetic state of the zygote, particularly with reference to identity (homozygosity) or nonidentity (heterozygosity) for one or more genes.

zy·go·spore (zye'go·spore) *n.* [*zygo-* + *spore*]. The spore resulting from the fusion of two similar gametes, as in certain algae and fungi.

zy·gote (zye'gote) *n.* [Gk. *zygōtos*, yoked]. 1. An organism produced by the union of two gametes. 2. The fertilized ovum before cleavage. —**zy·got·ic** (zye·got'ick) *adj.*

zy·go·tene (zye'go·teen) *n.* [*zygo-* + *-tene*]. The stage in the first meiotic prophase in which pairing of homologous chromosomes occurs. See also *diplotene, leptotene, pachytene.*

zygotic induction. *In bacteriology,* a type of transformation that occurs as a result of transfer of chromosomal material from one bacterium to another.

zygotic nucleus. SEGMENTATION NUCLEUS.

-zygous. A combining form meaning (a) *zygomatic;* (b) *zygotic.*

Zyloprim. Trademark for allopurinol, a suppressant for gout.

zym-, zymo- [Gk. *zymē*, leaven]. A combining form meaning (a) *fermentation, ferment;* (b) *enzyme.*

zy·mase (zye'mace) *n.* 1. ENZYME. 2. An enzyme mixture from yeast causing alcoholic fermentation.

zyme, *n.* [Gk. *zymē*, leaven]. ENZYME; FERMENT. **—zy·mic** (zye'mick) *adj.*

-zyme. A combining form meaning *enzyme.*

zymo-. See *zym-.*

zy·mo·gen (zye'mo·jen) *n.* [*zymo-* + *-gen*]. The inactive precursor of an enzyme which, on reaction with an appropriate kinase or other chemical agent, liberates the enzyme in active form.

zymogen granules. Secretion antecedent granules in gland cells, particularly those of the pancreatic acini and of the chief cells of the stomach, which are precursors of the enzyme secretion.

zy·mo·gen·ic (zye''mo·jen'ick) *adj.* [*zymo-* + *-genic*]. 1. Causing fermentation. 2. Pertaining to, or producing, a zymogen.

zymogenic cell. A cell that forms an enzyme, as that in a pancreatic acinus.

zy·mog·e·nous (zye·moj'e·nus) *adj.* ZYMOGENIC.

zy·mo·hex·ase (zye''mo·heck'sace) *n.* ALDOLASE.

zy·mo·hy·drol·y·sis (zye''mo·high·drol'i·sis) *n.* [*zymo-* + *hydrolysis*]. Hydrolysis produced by the action of an enzyme. Syn. *enzymatic hydrolysis.*

zy·moid (zye'moid) *adj.* [Gk. *zymoeidēs*]. Resembling an organized ferment.

zy·mol·o·gy (zye·mol'uh·jee) *n.* [*zymo-* + *-logy*]. The science of fermentation. **—zy·mo·log·ic** (zye''mo·loj'ick) *adj.*

zy·mol·y·sis (zye·mol'i·sis) *n.* [*zymo-* + *-lysis*]. FERMENTATION. **—zy·mo·lyt·ic** (zye''mo·lit'ick) *adj.*

zy·mo·lyte (zye'mo·lite) *n.* [*zymo-* + *-lyte*]. A material upon which an enzyme acts.

zy·mom·e·ter (zye·mom'e·tur) *n.* [*zymo-* + *-meter*]. An instrument for measuring fermentation.

zy·mo·nem·a·to·sis (zye''mo·nem''uh·to'sis) *n.* [*Zymonema* (a proposed genus including some of *Blastomyces*) + *-osis*]. BLASTOMYCOSIS.

zy·mo·phore (zye'mo·fore) *n.* [*zymo-* + *-phore*]. The active part or moiety of an enzyme which possesses its characteristic activity. **—zy·mo·pho·ric** (zye''mo·fo'rick) *adj.*

zy·mo·plas·tic (zye''mo·plas'tick) *adj.* [*zymo-* + *-plastic*]. Enzyme-producing.

zy·mo·pro·tein (zye''mo·pro'tee·in, ·teen) *n.* [*zymo-* + *protein*]. Any one of a class of proteins possessing catalytic powers.

zy·mo·sis (zye·mo'sis) *n.*, pl. **zymo·ses** (·seez) [Gk. *zymōsis*, fermentation, from *zymē*, leaven]. 1. FERMENTATION. 2. Any infectious or contagious disease. 3. The development or spread of an infectious disease. **—zy·mot·ic** (zye·mot'ick) *adj.*

zy·mos·ter·ol (zye·mos'tur·ole, ·ol) *n.* [*zymo-* + *sterol*]. A sterol from yeast.

zy·mur·gy (zye'mur·jee) *n.* [Gk. *zymourgos*, maker of leaven]. The branch of chemical technology dealing with the application of fermentation or enzymic action to any industrial process, as the curing of cheese, processing of leather, production of organic solvents.

Z.Z.Z. Increasing strengths of contraction.

Appendix

Tables

Name	Origin	Branches	Distribution
Accompanying median nerve	See *Median*		
Accompanying phrenic nerve	See *Pericardiacophrenic*		
Accompanying sciatic nerve	See *Sciatic*		
Acromiothoracic	See *Thoracoacromial*		
Alveolar, anterior superior (arteriae alveolares superiores anteriores [NA])	Infraorbital	Dental branches	Upper incisor and canine teeth; mucous membrane of maxillary sinus
Alveolar, inferior (arteria alveolaris inferior [NA])	Maxillary	Mental artery; dental and mylohyoid branches	Lower teeth; mandible and gums; mylohyoid muscle; buccal mucous membrane
Alveolar, posterior superior (arteria alveolaris superior posterior [NA])	Maxillary	Dental branches	Upper molar and premolar teeth and gums; mucous membrane of maxillary sinus; buccinator muscle
Angular (arteria angularis [NA])	Facial		Orbicularis oculi, nasalis, levator labii superioris, and procerus muscles; lacrimal sac; anastamoses with dorsal nasal branch of ophthalmic artery
Aorta, abdominal (aorta abdominalis [NA])	Continuation of descending aorta from level of lower border of twelfth thoracic vertebra	(1) Visceral celiac trunk superior mesenteric inferior mesenteric middle suprarenal renal testicular or ovarian (2) Parietal inferior phrenic lumbar (4 pairs) median sacral (3) Terminal common iliac	Diaphragm; body wall; abdominal and pelvic viscera; lower extremities
Aorta, abdominal (aorta abdominalis [NA])	Continuation of ascending aorta from upper border of right second costal cartilage to lower border of fourth thoracic vertebra	Brachiocephalic, left common carotid, left subclavian, lowest thyroid (occasionally)	
Aorta, ascending (aorta ascendens [NA])	Left ventricle	Left and right coronary	

Name	Origin	Branches	Distribution
Aorta, descending (aorta descendens [NA])	Continuation of arch of aorta. See *Aorta, abdominal; Aorta, thoracic*		
Aorta, thoracic (aorta thoracica [NA])	Portion of descending aorta in posterior mediastinum	Superior phrenic, posterior intercostal, subcostal arteries; bronchial, esophageal, mediastinal, and pericardial branches	Body wall; thoracic viscera; diaphragm
Appendicular (arteria appendicularis [NA])	Ileocolic		Vermiform appendix
Arch, deep palmar	See *Palmar arch, deep*		
Arch, plantar	See *Plantar arch*		
Arch, superficial palmar	See *Palmar arch, superficial*		
Arcuate of foot (arteria arcuata pedis [NA])	Dorsal pedal	Dorsal metatarsal, dorsal digital	Dorsal metatarsal portion of foot
Arcuate of kidney (arteriae arcuatae renis [NA])	Interlobar	Interlobular	Renal parenchyma
Auditory, internal	See *Labyrinthine*		
Auricular, deep (arteria auricularis profunda [NA])	Maxillary		Skin of external acoustic meatus; external surface of tympanic membrane
Auricular, posterior (arteria auricularis posterior [NA])	External carotid	Stylomastoid and posterior tympanic arteries; auricular, occipital, and stapedial branches	Digastric, stylohyoid, sternocleidomastoid, posterior auricular, occipitalis, and stapedius muscles; tympanic membrane and cavity; mastoid antrum; mastoid cells; semicircular canals; auricle; scalp; parotid gland
Axillary (arteria axillaris [NA])	Continuation of subclavian	Continues as brachial; highest thoracic, thoracoacromial, lateral thoracic, subscapular, anterior and posterior humeral circumflex	Muscles of upper arm, chest, and shoulder; mammary gland; shoulder joint; skin of pectoral region and shoulder; rete acromiale; head of humerus

Name	Origin	Branches	Distribution
Basilar (arteria basilaris [NA])	Formed by junction of two vertebral	Anterior inferior and superior cerebellar, labyrinthine, and posterior cerebral arteries; pontine branches	Pons; internal ear; cerebellum; pineal body; superior medullary velum; tela choroidea of third ventricle; temporal and occipital lobes of cerebrum
Brachial (arteria brachialis [NA])	Continuation of axillary	Deep brachial, inferior and superior ulnar collateral; terminates in radial and ulnar	Upper arm; elbow; forearm; hand
Brachial, deep (arteria profunda brachii [NA])	Brachial	Medial and radial collateral arteries; deltoid branch	Humerus; muscles of upper arm; radial nerve; rete olecrani
Brachiocephalic trunk (truncus brachiocephalicus [NA])	Arch of aorta	Right common carotid and right subclavian arteries; occasionally lowest thyroid artery, thymic and bronchial branches	Right side of neck and head; right shoulder girdle and arm; occasionally thymus gland, bronchus, inferior portion of thyroid gland
Buccal (arteria buccalis [NA])	Maxillary		Buccinator muscle; skin and mucous membrane of cheek; upper gums
Bulb of penis (arteria bulbi penis [NA])	Internal pudendal		Bulb of the penis; bulbourethral gland
Bulb of vestibule (of vagina) (arteria bulbi vestibuli [NA])	Internal pudendal		Bulb of the vestibule; major vestibular glands
Carotid, common (arteria carotis communis [NA])	Right from brachiocephalic, left from arch of aorta	External and internal carotid (terminal)	Region of neck and head
Carotid, external (arteria carotis externa [NA])	Common carotid	Superior thyroid, ascending pharyneal, lingual, facial (linguofacial trunk), occipital, posterior auricular, superficial temporal, maxillary	Anterior portion of neck; face; scalp; side of head; ear; dura mater
Carotid, internal (arteria carotis interna [NA])	Common carotid	Ophthalmic, posterior communicating, anterior cerebral, middle cerebral arteries; caroticotympanic and anterior choroid branches	Anterior portion of cerebrum; eye; forehead; nose; internal ear; trigeminal nerve; dura mater; hypophysis
Celiac (trunk) (truncus celiacus [NA])	Abdominal aorta	Left gastric, common hepatic, lienal, dorsal pancreatic	Esophagus; cardia and lesser curvature of stomach; liver; gallbladder; pylorus; duodenum; pancreas; greater omentum; spleen

TABLE OF ARTERIES (Continued)

Name	Origin	Branches	Distribution
Central of retina (arteria centralis retinae [NA])	Ophthalmic		Retina
Cerebellar, anterior inferior (arteria cerebelli inferior anterior [NA])	Basilar	Labyrinthine	Anterior portion of inferior surface of cerebellum
Cerebellar, posterior inferior (arteria cerebelli inferior posterior [NA])	Vertebral		Medulla; choroidplexus of fourth ventricle; inferior portion of cerebellum
Cerebellar, superior (arteria cerebelli superior [NA])	Basilar		Vermis and superior surface of cerebellum; pineal body; superior medullary velum; tela choroidea of third ventricle
Cerebral, anterior (arteria cerebri anterior [NA])	Internal carotid	Anterior communicating artery; cortical, central, orbital, frontal, and parietal branches	Cortex of frontal and parietal lobes; portion of basal ganglia
Cerebral, middle (arteria cerebri media [NA])	Internal carotid	Cortical, central, orbital, frontal, parietal, temporal, and striate branches	Corpus striatum; cortex of orbital, frontal, parietal, and temporal lobes
Cerebral, posterior (arteria cerebri posterior [NA])	Basilar	Cortical, temporal, occipital, parietooccipital, central, and posterior choroid branches	Thalamus; tela choroidea and choroid plexus of third ventricle, cortex of temporal and occipital bones
Cervical, ascending (arteria cervicalis ascendens [NA])	Inferior thyroid	Spinal branches	Muscles of neck; spinal cord and its membranes; vertebrae
Cervical, deep (arteria cervicalis profunda [NA])	Costocervical trunk		Deep neck muscles; spinal cord
Cervical, superficial (arteria cervicalis superficialis [NA])	Transverse cervical		Trapezius, levator scapulae, splenius cervicis, and splenius capitis muscles; posterior chain of lymph nodes
Cervical, transverse (arteria transversa colli [NA])	Thyrocervical trunk	Superficial cervical, descending scapular	Trapezius, levator scapulae, splenius, rhomboid, and latissimus dorsi muscles; posterior chain of lymph nodes

Name	Origin	Branches	Distribution
Choroid, anterior (arteria choroidea anterior [NA])	Internal carotid		Optic tract; cerebral peduncle; base of cerebrum; lateral geniculate body; tail of caudate nucleus; globus pallidus; internal capsule; choroid plexus of inferior horn of lateral ventricle.
Choroid, posterior (ramus choroideus arteriae cerebri posterioris [NA])	Posterior cerebral		Tela choroidea and choroid plexus of third ventricle
Ciliary, anterior (arteriae ciliares anteriores [NA])	Ophthalmic		Iris and conjunctiva
Ciliary, long posterior (arteriae ciliares posteriores longae [NA])	Ophthalmic		Ciliary muscle and iris
Ciliary, short posterior (arteriae ciliares posteriores breves [NA])	Ophthalmic		Choroid and ciliary processes
Circumflex, anterior humeral (arteria circumflexa humeri anterior [NA])	Axillary		Coracobrachialis, biceps brachii, and deltoid muscles; shoulder joint; head of humerus
Circumflex, deep iliac (arteria circumflexa ilium profunda [NA])	External iliac	Ascending branch	Abdominal muscles; psoas, iliacus, sartorius, and tensor fasciae latae muscles; skin over course of vessel
Circumflex, lateral femoral (arteria circumflexa femoris lateralis [NA])	Deep femoral	Ascending, descending, and transverse branches	Muscles of thigh
Circumflex, medial femoral (arteria circumflexa femoris medialis [NA])	Deep femoral	Deep, ascending, transverse, and acetabular branches	Muscles of thigh; hip joint
Circumflex, posterior humeral (arteria circumflexa humeri posterior [NA])	Axillary		Deltoid, teres minor, and triceps brachii muscles; posterior portion of shoulder joint; rete acromiale
Circumflex, scapular (arteria circumflexa scapulae [NA])	Subscapular		Subscapularis, infraspinatus, teres, deltoid, and triceps brachii muscles; scapula; shoulder joint
Circumflex, superficial iliac (arteria circumflexa ilium superficialis [NA])	Femoral		Sartorius, iliacus, and tensor fasciae latae muscles; inguinal lymph nodes; skin over course of vessel

TABLE OF ARTERIES (Continued)

Name	Origin	Branches	Distribution
Clitoris, deep of (arteria profunda clitoridis [NA])	Internal pudendal		Corpus cavernosum of the clitoris
Clitoris, dorsal of (arteria dorsalis clitoridis [NA])	Internal pudendal		Clitoris
Colic, left (arteria colica sinistra [NA])	Inferior mesenteric	Ascending and descending branches	Left portion of transverse colon; upper portion of descending colon; splenic flexure
Colic, middle (arteria colica media [NA])	Superior mesenteric	Left and right branches	Upper portion of ascending colon; hepatic flexure; right portion of transverse colon
Colic, right (arteria colica dextra [NA])	Superior mesenteric	Ascending and descending branches	Ascending colon
Collateral, inferior ulnar (arteria collateralis ulnaris inferior [NA])	Brachial		Triceps brachii, brachialis, and pronator teres muscles; rete olecrani
Collateral, middle or medial (arteria collateralis media [NA])	Deep brachial		Triceps brachii muscle; rete olecrani
Collateral, radial (arteria collateralis radialis [NA])	Deep brachial		Triceps brachii and brachioradialis muscle; rete olecrani
Collateral, superior ulnar (arteria collateralis ulnaris superior [NA])	Brachial		Triceps brachii muscle; elbow joint and rete olecrani
Communicating, anterior (arteria communicans anterior cerebri [NA])	Anterior cerebral		Anterior perforated substance
Communicating, posterior (arteria communicans posterior cerebri [NA])	Internal carotid		Optic chiasm; optic tract; tuber cinereum; mamillary body; hippocampal gyrus; internal capsule; cerebral peduncle; interpeduncular region; thalamus
Companion of sciatic nerve (arteria comitans nervi ischiadici [NA])	See *Sciatic*		
Conjunctival, anterior (arteriae conjunctivales anteriores [NA])	Ophthalmic		Conjunctiva
Conjunctival, posterior (arteriae conjunctivales posteriores [NA])	Ophthalmic		Conjunctiva

Name	Origin	Branches	Distribution
Coronary, left (arteria coronaria sinistra [NA])	Left posterior aortic sinus	Anterior interventricular, and circumflex branches	Left atrium; root of aorta and pulmonary artery; myocardium of both ventricles; interventricular septum
Coronary, right (arteria coronaria dextra [NA])	Anterior aortic sinus	Posterior interventricular branches	Right atrium; root of aorta and pulmonary artery; anterior wall of right ventricle; septal myocardium; left ventricle adjoining posterior interventricular sulcus
Costocervical trunk (truncus costocervicalis [NA])	Subclavian	Deep cervical, highest intercostal	First and second intercostal spaces; muscles of neck; spinal cord and its membranes
Cremasteric (arteria cremasterica [NA])	Inferior epigastric		Spermatic cord and cremaster muscle in the male (corresponds to artery of the round ligament of the uterus in the female)
Cystic (arteria cystica [NA])	Right hepatic branch of hepatic proper		Surface of gallbladder
Deferential (arteria ductus deferentis [NA])	Internal iliac	Ureteric branches	Seminal vesical; ductus deferens; epididymis
Dental	See *Alveolar*		
Digital, common palmar (arteriae digitales palmares communes [NA])	Superficial palmar arch	Proper palmar digital	Fingers
Digital, common plantar (arteriae digitales plantares communes [NA])	Plantar metatarsal	Proper plantar digital	Toes
Digital, dorsal (of foot) (arteriae digitales dorsales pedis [NA])	Arcuate		Dorsal areas of toes
Digital, dorsal (of hand) (arteriae digitales dorsales manus [NA])	Dorsal metacarpal		Dorsal areas of fingers
Digital, palmar proper (arteriae digitales palmares propriae [NA])	Common palmar digital		Fingers
Digital, plantar proper (arteriae digitales plantares propriae [NA])	Common plantar digital		Toes
Dorsal pedal (arteria dorsalis pedis [NA])	Anterior tibial	Lateral tarsal, medial tarsal, and arcuate arteries; deep plantar branch	Dorsal portion of foot and toes

Name	Origin	Branches	Distribution
Epigastric, deep	See *Epigastric, inferior*		
Epigastric, inferior (arteria epigastrica inferior [NA])	External iliac	Cremasteric or artery of round ligament of uterus; pubic and obturator branches	Skin and muscles of anterior abdominal wall; round ligament of uterus in the female, cremaster muscle and spermatic cord in the male; peritoneum
Epigastric, superficial (arteria epigastrica superficialis [NA])	Femoral		Skin of abdominal wall below umbilicus; superficial fascia; inguinal lymph nodes
Epigastric, superior (arteria epigastrica superior [NA])	Internal thoracic		Skin, fascia, muscles, and peritoneum of upper abdominal wall; diaphragm; falciform ligament of the liver
Episcleral (arteriae episclerales [NA])	Ophthalmic		Iris; ciliary processes; conjunctiva
Ethmoid, anterior (arteria ethmoidalis anterior [NA])	Ophthalmic	Anterior meningeal	Anterior and middle ethmoidal cells; dura mater of anterior cranial fossa; mucoperiosteum of middle nasal meatus; lateral wall and septum of nose; frontal air sinus; skin of dorsum of nose
Ethmoid, posterior (arteria ethmoidalis posterior [NA])	Ophthalmic		Posterior ethmoid cells; dura mater around cribriform plate; superior nasal meatus; superior nasal concha
Facial (arteria facialis [NA])	External carotid	Ascending palatine, submental, inferior and superior labial, angular arteries; tonsillar and glandular branches	Face; tonsil; auditory tube; root of tongue; submandibular gland
Facial, transverse (arteria transversa faciei [NA])	Superficial temporal		Masseter muscle; parotid gland; skin of face
Femoral (arteria femoralis [NA])	Continuation of external iliac	Continues as popliteal; superficial epigastric, superficial circumflex iliac, external pudendal, deep femoral, descending genicular	Skin of lower part of abdomen and groin; external genitalia; inguinal lymph nodes; muscles of medial, lateral, and anterior aspects of thigh; femur; knee joint

Name	Origin	Branches	Distribution
Femoral, deep (arteria profunda femoris [NA])	Femoral	Lateral and medial femoral circumflex, perforating	Muscles of thigh; hip joint; head and shaft of femur
Fibular (arteria fibularis [NA alternative])	See *Peroneal*		
Frontal	See *Supraorbital*		
Gastric, left (arteria gastrica sinistra [NA])	Celiac trunk	Esophageal branches	Lesser curvature and cardia of stomach; lower end of esophagus; occasionally left lobe of liver
Gastric, right (arteria gastrica dextra [NA])	Common hepatic		Pyloric portion of stomach
Gastric, short (arteriae gastricae breves [NA])	Lienal		Greater curvature of stomach
Gastroduodenal (arteria gastroduodenalis [NA])	Common hepatic	Superior, pancreaticoduodenal, right gastroepiploic	Pylorus; duodenum; pancreas; greater omentum; common bile duct
Gastroepiploic, left (arteria gastroepiploica sinistra [NA])	Lienal	Epiploic branches	Greater curvature of the stomach; greater omentum
Gastroepiploic, right (arteria gastroepiploica dextra [NA])	Gastroduodenal	Epiploic branches	Greater curvature of the stomach; greater omentum
Genicular, descending (arteria genus descendens [NA])	Femoral	Saphenous and articular branches	Knee joint; skin of medial distal portion of thigh; arterial retina on medial and lateral sides of knee; thigh muscles
Genicular, highest	See *Genicular, descending*		
Genicular, lateral inferior (arteria genus inferior lateralis [NA])	Popliteal		Knee joint
Genicular, lateral superior (arteria genus superior lateralis [NA])	Popliteal		Knee joint; thigh muscles
Genicular, medial inferior (arteria genus inferior medialis [NA])	Popliteal		Knee joint; proximal end of tibia; popliteus muscle
Genicular, medial superior (arteria genus superior medialis [NA])	Popliteal		Knee joint; patella; femur; vastus medialis muscle
Genicular, middle (arteria genus media [NA])	Popliteal		Knee joint; cruciate ligaments; patellar synovial and alar folds

Name	Origin	Branches	Distribution
Gluteal, inferior (arteria glutea inferior [NA])	Internal iliac	Sciatic	Buttock; hip joint; skin and muscles of back of upper thigh
Gluteal, superior (arteria glutea superior [NA])	Internal iliac	Superficial and deep branches	Buttock
Hemorrhoidal	See *Rectal*		
Hepatic, common (arteria hepatica communis [NA])	Celiac trunk	Right gastric, gastroduodenal, hepatic proper	Lesser and greater curvatures of stomach; pylorus; pancreas; greater omentum; gallbladder; liver
Hepatic, proper (arteria hepatica propria [NA])	Common hepatic	Cystic artery; right and left branches	Liver; gallbladder
Hypogastric	See *Iliac, internal*		
Ileal (arteriae ilei [NA])	Superior mesenteric		Ileum
Ileocolic (arteria ileocolica [NA])	Superior mesenteric	Appendicular artery; cecal branches	Ascending colon; cecum; vermiform process; lower part of ileum
Iliac, common (arteria iliaca communis [NA])	Abdominal aorta	Internal and external iliac	Psoas major muscle; peritoneum; fascia; pelvic viscera; external genitalia; gluteal region; lower limb
Iliac, external (arteria iliaca externa [NA])	Common iliac	Continues as femoral; inferior epigastric, deep circumflex iliac	Psoas major, iliacus, sartorius, tensor fasciae latae, cremaster, and abdominal wall muscles; external iliac lymph nodes; peritoneum; skin of lower abdominal wall; spermatic cord or round ligament of the uterus; lower limb
Iliac, internal (arteria iliaca interna [NA])	Common iliac	Iliolumbar, obturator, superior and inferior gluteal, inferior vesical, middle rectal, internal pudendal, umbilical (fetal), uterine or deferential	Pelvic wall and contents; gluteal region; medial portion of thigh; external genitalia; anal region
Iliolumbar (arteria iliolumbalis [NA])	Internal iliac	Lateral sacral arteries; lumbar, iliac, and spinal branches	Muscles and bones of pelvis; cauda equina

Name	Origin	Branches	Distribution
Infraorbital (arteria infraorbitalis [NA])	Maxillary	Anterior superior alveolar	Inferior rectus and inferior oblique muscles of the eye; orbicularis oculi muscle; lacrimal gland and sac; upper lip; anterior upper teeth; mucosa of maxillary sinuses
Innominate	See *Brachiocephalic*		
Intercostal, highest (arteria intercostalis suprema [NA])	Costocervical trunk	Posterior intercostal (I, II)	Posterior vertebral muscles; contents of first and second intercostal spaces; contents of vertebral canal
Intercostal, posterior (I, II) (arteriae intercostales posteriores I, II [NA])	Highest intercostal	Dorsal and spinal branches	First and second intercostal spaces
Intercostal, posterior (III–XI) (arteriae intercostales posteriores III–XI [NA])	Thoracic aorta	Dorsal, spinal, cutaneous, collateral, and mammary branches	Intercostal, pectoral, serratus anterior, iliocostalis, longissimus dorsi, multifidus spinae, and semispinalis dorsi muscles; abdominal wall; vertebrae; ribs; mammary gland; skin of body wall and back; contents of vertebral canal
Interlobar of kidney (arteriae interlobares renis [NA])	Renal	Arcuate of kidney	Renal lobes
Interlobular of kidney (arteriae interlobulares renis [NA])	Arcuate of kidney		Glomeruli of kidney
Interlobular of liver (arteriae interlobulares hepatis [NA])	Proper hepatic (right or left branch)		Lobules of liver
Interosseous, anterior (arteria interossea anterior [NA])	Common interosseous	Median artery	Deep anterior forearm
Interosseous, common (arteria interossea communis [NA])	Ulnar	Anterior and posterior interosseous	Forearm; rete olecrani
Interosseous, posterior (arteria interossea posterior [NA])	Common interosseous	Recurrent interosseous	Muscles and skin of posterior forearm; rete olecrani
Interosseous, recurrent (arteria interossea recurrens [NA])	Posterior interosseous		Supinator and anconeus muscles; rete olecrani
Interosseous, volar	See *Interosseous, anterior*		
Intestinal	See *Ileal; Jejunal*		

Name	Origin	Branches	Distribution
Jejunal (arteriae jejunales [NA])	Superior mesenteric		Jejunum
Labial, inferior (arteria labialis inferior [NA])	Facial		Mucous membrane, skin, muscles, and glands of lower lip
Labial, superior (arteria labialis superior [NA])	Facial		Mucous membrane, skin, muscles, and glands of upper lip; nasal septum; ala of nose
Labyrinthine (arteria labyrinthi [NA])	Basilar or anterior inferior cerebellar		Internal ear
Lacrimal (arteria lacrimalis [NA])	Ophthalmic		Lacrimal gland; superior and lateral rectus muscles; eyelids; conjunctiva; sclera; iris; ciliary processes; temporal fossa
Laryngeal, inferior (arteria laryngea inferior [NA])	Inferior thyroid		Constrictor pharyngis inferior muscle; mucous membrane of lower part of larynx
Laryngeal, superior (arteria laryngea superior [NA])	Superior thyroid		Muscles, mucous membrane, and glands of larynx
Lienal (arteria lienalis [NA])	Celiac trunk	Left gastroepiploic, short gastric, great pancreatic, dorsal pancreatic arteries; pancreatic and lienal branches	Pancreas; pancreatic duct; fundus and greater curvature of stomach; both surfaces of greater omentum; body of spleen
Lingual (arteria lingualis [NA])	External carotid	Sublingual and deep lingual arteries; suprahyoid and dorsal thyroid branches	Intrinsic and extrinsic muscles of tongue; mucous membrane of tongue and mouth; gums; sublingual gland; glossopalatine arch; tonsil; soft palate; epiglottis; frenulum of the tongue
Lingual, deep (arteria profunda lingualis [NA])	Lingual		Genioglossus muscle; intrinsic muscles of the tongue; mucous membrane of inferior surface of tongue
Linguofacial trunk	Combined facial and lingual arteries		
Lumbar (arteriae lumbales [NA])	Abdominal aorta	Dorsal and spinal branches	Muscles of back; lumbar vertebrae; fibrous capsule of the kidney

Name	Origin	Branches	Distribution
Lumbar, lowest (arteria lumbalis ima [NA])	Median sacral		Iliacus and gluteus maximus muscles; sacrum
Malleolar, anterior lateral (arteria malleolaris anterior lateralis [NA])	Anterior tibial		Lateral side of ankle
Malleolar, anterior medial (arteria malleolaris anterior medialis [NA])	Anterior tibial		Medial side of ankle
Mammary, external	See *Thoracic, lateral*		
Mammary, internal	See *Thoracic, internal*		
Masseteric (arteria masseterica [NA])	Maxillary		Masseter muscle
Maxillary (arteria maxillaris [NA])	External carotid	Deep auricular, anterior tympanic, inferior alveolar, middle meningeal, masseteric, buccal, deep temporal, posterior superior alveolar, infraorbital, artery of pterygoid canal, descending palatine, sphenopalatine, nasal	Jaws, teeth, and other deep structures of face; ear
Maxillary, external	See *Facial*		
Maxillary, internal	See *Maxillary*		
Median (arteria mediana [NA])	Anterior interosseous		Median nerve
Meningeal, anterior (arteria meningea anterior [NA])	Anterior ethmoid		Dura mater of anterior cranial fossa
Meningeal, middle (arteria meningea media [NA])	Maxillary	Accessory, meningeal, and petrous branches	Tensor, tympani muscle; semilunar ganglion; trigeminal nerve; dura mater of anterior and middle cranial fossae; skull; tympanic cavity; orbit; infratemporal fossa
Meningeal, posterior (arteria meningea posterior [NA])	Ascending pharyngeal		Dura mater of posterior and middle cranial fossae
Mental (arteria mentalis [NA])	Inferior alveolar		Lower lip and chin
Mesenteric, inferior (arteria mesenterica inferior [NA])	Abdominal aorta	Left colic, sigmoid, superior rectal	Transverse colon; splenic flexure; descending colon; sigmoid flexure; proximal portion of rectum

Name	Origin	Branches	Distribution
Mesenteric, superior (arteria mesenterica superior [NA])	Abdominal aorta	Inferior pancreatico-duodenal, jejunal, ileal, ileocolic, right colic, middle colic	Pancreas; duodenum; jejunum; ileum; mesentery; mesenteric lymph nodes; cecum; vermiform appendix; ascending colon; hepatic flexure
Metacarpal, dorsal (arteriae metacarpeae dorsales [NA])	Radial (dorsal carpal rete)	Dorsal digital	Dorsal areas of fingers
Metacarpal, palmar (arteriae metacarpeae palmares [NA])	Deep palmar arch		Interosseus and second, third, and fourth lumbrical muscles; metacarpal bones
Metacarpal, volar	See *Metacarpal, palmar*		
Metatarsal, dorsal (arteriae metatarseae dorsales [NA])	Arcuate of foot		Adjacent sides of toes
Metatarsal, plantar (arteriae metatarseae plantares [NA])	Plantar arch	Common digital arteries; perforating branches	Toes
Musculophrenic (arteria musculophrenica [NA])	Internal thoracic		Muscles of abdominal wall; diaphragm; lower six intercostal spaces
Nasal, dorsal (arteria dorsalis nasi [NA])	Ophthalmic		Dorsum of nose
Nasal, lateral posterior and septal posterior (arteriae nasales posteriores, laterales et septi [NA])	Maxillary		Nasal conchae, cavity, and septum
Nasopalatine	See *Sphenopalatine*		
Nutrient	A branch of any artery that supplies a bone. There may be a number of nutrient branches from any nearby artery		
Obturator (arteria obturatoria [NA])	Internal iliac	Pubic, acetabular, anterior, and posterior branches	Pelvic and thigh muscles (including obturators); pubis; hip joint; head of femur; bladder; ilium
Occipital (arteria occipitalis [NA])	External carotid	Mastoid, auricular, occipital, sternocleidomastoid, descending, and meningeal branches	Muscles of neck; posterior surface of auricle; mastoid cells; pericranium and scalp of posterolateral surface of the head

Name	Origin	Branches	Distribution
Ophthalmic (arteria ophthalmica [NA])	Internal carotid	Central retinal lacrimal, palpebral, ciliary, conjunctival, episcleral, supraorbital, ethmoid, meningeal, supratrochlear, dorsal nasal	Contents of orbit; diploë of frontal bone; mucous membrane of frontal sinus and ethmoidal cells; dura mater of anterior fossa of skull; superior nasal concha and meatus; lacrimal sac; skin of dorsum of nose
Ovarian (arteria ovarica [NA])	Abdominal aorta	Ureteric branches	Ovary; ureter; suspensory ligament of the ovary; broad ligament of the uterus; uterine tube; round ligament of the uterus; skin of labium majus and groin
Palatine, ascending (arteria palatina ascendens [NA])	Facial	Tonsillar branch	Styloglossus, stylopharyngeus, superior constrictor of pharynx, and levator veli palatini muscles; auditory tube; lateral wall of upper part of pharynx; soft palate; palatine tonsil
Palatine, descending (arteria palatina descendens [NA])	Maxillary	Greater and lesser palatine	Soft palate; palatine tonsil; mucous membrane of roof of mouth; gums; palatine glands; palatine bone; maxilla
Palatine, greater (arteria palatina major [NA])	Descending palatine		Mucous membrane of hard palate; gums; palatine glands; palatine bone; maxilla
Palatine, lesser (arteriae palatinae minores [NA])	Descending palatine		Soft palate; palatine tonsil
Palmar arch, deep (arcus palmaris profundus [NA])	Radial	Palmar metacarpal	Interossei and second, third, and fourth lumbrical muscles; metacarpals; joints of fingers
Palmar arch, superficial (arcus palmaris superficialis [NA])	Ulnar	Common palmar digital	Flexor tendons and tendon sheaths; joints and bones of fingers; skin of palm and fingers
Palpebral, lateral (arteriae palpebrales laterales [NA])	Ophthalmic	Superior palpebral arch, inferior palpebral arch	Upper and lower eyelids; conjunctiva

Name	Origin	Branches	Distribution
Palpebral, medial (arteriae palpebrales mediales [NA])	Ophthalmic	Superior palpebral arch, inferior palpebral arch	Upper and lower eyelids; conjunctiva; lacrimal caruncle; lacrimal sac
Pancreatic, dorsal (arteria pancreatica dorsalis [NA])	Lienal or celiac	Inferior pancreatic	Head and body of pancreas
Pancreatic, great (variable) (arteria pancreatica magna [NA])	Lienal		Posterior surface of pancreas, following course of pancreatic duct
Pancreatic, inferior (arteria pancreatica inferior [NA])	Dorsal pancreatic		Body and tail of pancreas
Pancreaticoduodenal, inferior (arteriae pancreaticoduodenales inferiores [NA])	Superior mesenteric		Head of pancreas; descending and inferior parts of duodenum
Pancreaticoduodenal, superior	Gastroduodenal	Pancreatic and duodenal branches	Second part of duodenum; common bile duct; pancreas
Pedal, dorsal	See *Dorsal pedal*		
Penis, deep (arteria profunda penis [NA])	Internal pudendal		Corpus cavernosum of the penis
Penis, dorsal (arteria dorsalis penis [NA])	Internal pudendal		Dorsum of penis; prepuce; glans; corpus cavernosum and its fibrous sheath
Perforating (arteriae perforantes [NA])	Deep femoral		Gluteus maximus, pectineus, adductor, biceps femoris, and posterior femoral muscles; shaft of femur
Pericardiacophrenic (arteria pericardiacophrenica [NA])	Internal thoracic		Phrenic nerve; pleura; pericardium; diaphragm
Perineal (arteria perinealis [NA])	Internal pudendal	Scrotal or labial branches	Perineum; posterior portion of scrotum or labium majus; subcutaneous structures in urogenital triangle
Peroneal (arteria peronea [NA])	Posterior tibial	Perforating, communicating, malleolar, and calcaneal branches	Soleus, tibialis posterior, flexor hallucis longus, peroneus, and extensor digitorum longus muscles; shaft of fibula; tibiofibular syndesmosis; ankle joint; dorsum of foot

Name	Origin	Branches	Distribution
Pharyngeal, ascending (arteria pharyngea ascendens [NA])	External carotid	Posterior meningeal and inferior tympanic arteries; pharyngeal branches	Pharynx; soft palate; palatine tonsil; auditory tube; cervical lymph nodes; tympanic cavity; dura mater of middle and posterior cranial fossae
Phrenic, inferior (arteriae phrenicae inferiores [NA])	Abdominal aorta	Superior suprarenal	Inferior surface of diaphragm; suprarenal gland; vena cava inferior; liver; esophagus; pericardium (from the right artery); spleen (from the left)
Phrenic, superior (arteriae phrenicae superiores [NA])	Thoracic aorta		Posterior surface of diaphragm
Plantar arch (arcus plantaris [NA])	Lateral plantar	Plantar metatarsal	Interosseous muscles; toes
Plantar, lateral (arteria plantaris lateralis [NA])	Posterior tibial	Plantar arch	Toes and related muscles; heel; skin on lateral side of foot
Plantar, medial (arteria plantaris medialis [NA])	Posterior tibial	Deep and superficial branches	Abductor hallucis and flexor digitorum brevis muscles; skin on medial surface of sole of foot
Popliteal (arteria poplitea [NA])	Continuation of femoral	Genicular, sural; anterior and posterior tibial	Knee and calf; muscles of thigh
Popliteal, lateral	See *Peroneal*		
Popliteal, medial	See *Tibial*		
Principal of thumb (arteria princeps pollicis [NA])	Radial	Radial index	Sides and palmar surface of thumb
Profunda brachii	See *Brachial, deep*		
Profunda femoris	See *Femoral, deep*		
Pterygoid canal, artery of (arteria canalis pterygoidei [NA])	Maxillary		Upper portion of pharynx; levator and tensor veli palatini muscles; auditory tube; tympanic cavity
Pudendal, external (arteriae pudendae externae [NA])	Femoral	Inguinal and anterior scrotal or labial branches	Scrotum or labium majus; skin of lower abdomen, of penis or clitoris, of scrotum or labium majus, and of perineum

Name	Origin	Branches	Distribution
Pudendal, internal (arteria pudenda interna [NA])	Internal iliac	Inferior rectal, perineal, urethral, artery of bulb of penis or of vestibule, dorsal and deep penile or clitoridal arteries; posterior scrotal or labial branches	External genitalia; perineum; anus and rectum
Pulmonary, left (arteria pulmonis sinistra [NA])	Pulmonary trunk	Branches to lobes and segments of left lung	Left lung
Pulmonary, right (arteria pulmonis dextra [NA])	Pulmonary trunk	Branches to lobes and segments of right lung	Right lung
Pulmonary trunk (truncus pulmonalis [NA])	Right ventricle	Left and right pulmonary	Lungs
Radial (arteria radialis [NA])	Brachial	Radial recurrent artery, principal artery of thumb, and deep palmar arch; dorsal and palmar carpal and superficial palmar branches	Muscles of forearm; radius; elbow, wrist, and carpal joints; skin of dorsum of hand and fingers; skin of palmar surface of thumb and lateral side of index finger
Radial of index finger (arteria radialis indicis [NA])	Principal artery of thumb		Lateral palmar aspect of index finger
Radial recurrent (arteria recurrens radialis [NA])	Radial		Supinator, brachialis, brachioradialis, and extensor carpi radialis brevis and longus muscles; elbow joints; rete olecrani
Ranine	See *Lingual, deep*		
Rectal, inferior (arteria rectalis inferior [NA])	Internal pudendal		Anal canal; levator ani and sphincter ani externus muscles; skin around anus and lower region of buttock
Rectal, middle (arteria rectalis media [NA])	Internal iliac		Rectum; ductus deferens; seminal vesicle; prostate gland
Rectal, superior (arteria rectalis superior [NA])	Inferior mesenteric		Muscular and mucous coats of the pelvic colon and proximal portion of the rectum; mucous coat of distal portion of rectum
Renal (arteria renalis [NA])	Abdominal aorta	Inferior suprarenal and interlobar arteries; ureteric branches	Suprarenal gland; upper end of ureter; kidney

Name	Origin	Branches	Distribution
Round ligament of the uterus, artery of (arteria ligamenti teretis uteri [NA])	Inferior epigastric		Round ligament of the uterus (corresponds to cremasteric artery in the male)
Sacral, lateral (arteriae sacrales laterales [NA])	Iliolumbar		Sacrum
Sacral, median (arteria sacralis mediana [NA])	Abdominal aorta	Lowest lumbar	Sacrum; rectum; coccyx
Scapular, circumflex	Subscapular		
Scapular, descending (arteria scapularis descendens [NA])	Transverse cervical		Muscles in the region of the medial border of the scapula
Scapular, transverse	See *Suprascapular*		
Sciatic (arteria comitans nervi ischiadici [NA])	Inferior gluteal		Sciatic nerve
Sigmoid (arteriae sigmoideae [NA])	Inferior mesenteric		Sigmoid colon and lower part of descending colon
Spermatic, external	See *Cremasteric*		
Spermatic, internal	See *Ovarian; Testicular*		
Sphenopalatine (arteria spheno-palatina [NA])	Maxillary		Nasal conchae and meati; mucous membrane of frontal, maxillary, sphenoidal, and ethmoidal air sinuses; posterior portion of nasal septum
Spinal, anterior (arteria spinalis anterior [NA])	Spinal branches of vertebral		Spinal cord and its coverings
Spinal, posterior (arteria spinalis posterior [NA])	Spinal branches of vertebral		Spinal cord and its coverings
Splenic	See *Lienal*		
Stylomastoid (arteria stylomastoidea [NA])	Posterior auricular		Mastoid cells; stapes; stepedius muscle and tendon; posterior portion of tympanic membrane

Name	Origin	Branches	Distribution
Subclavian (arteria subclavia [NA])	Left—arch of aorta Right—brachiocephalic	Continues as axillary; vertebral and internal thoracic arteries; thyrocervical and costocervical trunks	Muscles of neck and upper extremity; cervical vertebrae and canal; skull, brain, and meninges; pericardium; pleura; mediastinum; bronchi; sternum; skin over shoulder and anterior body wall; mammary gland; peritoneum
Subcostal (arteria subcostalis [NA])	Thoracic aorta	Dorsal and spinal branches	Quadratus lumborum, transversus abdominis, and obliquus abdominis internus muscles; lumbar vertebrae and contents of canal; skin of back
Sublingual (arteria sublingualis [NA])	Lingual		Mylohyoid,, geniohyoid, and genioglossus muscles; sublingual gland; frenulum of the tongue
Submental (arteria submentalis [NA])	Facial	Glandular branches	Mylohyoid, digastric, platysma, and depressor labii inferioris muscles; submandibular and sublingual glands
Subscapular (arteria subscapularis [NA])	Axillary	Thoracodorsal, scapular circumflex	Muscles of scapular and shoulder region; scapula; shoulder joint; axillary lymph nodes
Supraorbital (arteria supraorbitalis [NA])	Ophthalmic		Rectus superior and levator palpebrae superioris muscles; periosteum of root of orbit; diploë of frontal bone; mucous membrane of frontal sinus; trochlea of obliquus superior muscle; upper eyelid
Suprarenal, inferior (arteria suprarenalis inferior [NA])	Renal		Suprarenal gland
Suprarenal, middle (arteria suprarenalis media [NA])	Abdominal aorta		Suprarenal gland
Suprarenal, superior (arteria suprarenalis superior [NA])	Inferior phrenic		Suprarenal gland

Name	Origin	Branches	Distribution
Suprascapular (arteria suprascapularis [NA])	Thyrocervical trunk	Acromial branch	Clavicle; scapula; acromioclavicular and shoulder joints; muscles of these areas
Supratrochlear (arteria supratrochlearis [NA])	Ophthalmic		Anterior scalp
Sural (arteriae surales [NA])	Popliteal		Gastrocnemius, soleus, and plantaris muscles; skin and fascia of calf
Tarsal, lateral (arteria tarsea lateralis [NA])	Dorsal pedal		Extensor digitorum brevis muscle; navicular and cuboid bones and joint between them
Tarsal, lateral (arteria tarsea lateralis [NA])	Dorsal pedal		Skin of medial surface of foot; tarsal joints
Temporal, deep (arteriae temporales profundae [NA])	Maxillary		Temporal muscle; orbit; pericranium; skull
Temporal, middle (arteria temporalis media [NA])	Superficial temporal		Temporal muscle; temporal fascia
Temporal, superficial (arteria temporalis superficialis [NA])	External carotid	Transverse facial, middle temporal, zygomaticoorbital arteries; parotid, anterior auricular, frontal, and parietal branches	Temporal, masseter, frontalis, and orbicularis oculi muscles; parotid gland and duct; skin of face; external ear; external acoustic meatus; scalp
Testicular (arteria testicularis [NA])	Abdominal aorta	Ureteric branches	Testicle; ureter; epididymis
Thoracic, highest (arteria thoracica suprema [NA])	Axillary		Pectoral, intercostal, and serratus anterior muscles; thoracic wall
Thoracic, internal (arteria thoracica interna [NA])	Subclavian	Pericardiacophrenic, musculophrenic, and superior epigastric arteries; mediastinal, thymic, bronchial, sternal, perforating, mammary, and intercostal branches	Mediastinum and anterior thoracic wall
Thoracic, lateral (arteria thoracica lateralis [NA])	Axillary	Mammary branches	Pectoral, serratus anterior, and subscapularis muscles; axillary lymph nodes; mammary gland
Thoracic, twelfth	See *Subcostal*		

Name	Origin	Branches	Distribution
Thoracoacromial (arteria thoracoacromialis [NA])	Axillary	Acromial, clavicular, deltoid, and pectoral branches	Pectoral, deltoid, and subclavius muscles; mammary gland; sternoclavicular joint
Thoracodorsal (arteria thoracodorsalis [NA])	Subscapular		Latissimus dorsi, teres major, and serratus anterior muscles
Thyrocervical trunk (truncus thyrocervicalis [NA])	Subclavian	Inferior thyroid, suprascapular, transverse cervical	Muscles of neck, scapular region, and upper back; cervical spinal cord and vertebrae; larynx; trachea; esophagus; thyroid gland; pharynx
Thyroid, inferior (arteria thyroidea inferior [NA])	Thyrocervical trunk	Inferior laryngeal, and ascending cervical arteries; pharyngeal, esophageal, and tracheal branches	Esophagus; pharynx; larynx; trachea; posterior surface of thyroid gland; vertebrae; contents of vertebral canal; related muscles
Thyroid, lowest (inconsistent) (arteria thyroidea ima [NA])	Arch of aorta, brachiocephalic trunk or elsewhere		Lower part of thyroid gland
Thyroid, superior (arteria thyroidea superior [NA])	External carotid	Superior laryngeal artery; muscular, anterior, and posterior branches	Thyroid gland; esophagus; intrinsic muscles and mucous membrane of larynx; related muscles
Tibial anterior (arteria tibialis anterior [NA])	Popliteal	Tibial recurrent and malleolar arteries; malleolar branches	Knee, proximal tibiofibular, and ankle joints; muscles of lower leg; fascia and skin on front of leg
Tibial, anterior-recurrent (arteria recurrens tibialis anterior [NA])	Anterior tibial		Knee joint and overlying fascia and skin; tibialis anterior and extensor digitorum longus muscles
Tibial, posterior (arteria tibialis posterior [NA])	Popliteal	Plantar arteries; circumflex fibular branch	Shaft of tibia; shaft of fibula; sole of foot; muscles of lower leg; skin of medial and posterior part of leg and tarsus

Name	Origin	Branches	Distribution
Tibial, posterior recurrent (arteria recurrens tibialis posterior [NA])	Anterior tibial		Soleus, tibialis, posterior, flexor hallucis longus, flexor digitorum longus, and peroneus muscles; ankle joint; skin of medial and posterior part of leg and foot; sole of foot; shaft of tibia; shaft of fibula
Transverse facial	See *Facial, transverse*		
Tympanic, anterior (arteria tympanica anterior [NA])	Maxillary		Mucous membrane of tympanic cavity
Tympanic, inferior (arteria tympanica inferior [NA])	Ascending pharyngeal		Lining of medial wall of tympanic cavity
Tympanic, posterior (arteria tympanica posterior [NA])	Posterior auricular	Mastoid and stapedial branches	Tympanic membrane
Tympanic, superior (arteria tympanica superior [NA])	Middle meningeal	Frontal, parietal, and anastomotic branches	Tensor tympani muscle; lining of wall of tympanic cavity
Ulnar (arteria ulnaris [NA])	Brachial	Recurrent ulnar and common interosseous arteries; superficial palmar arch; dorsal carpal, deep palmar, and palmar carpal branches	Muscles of forearm; shafts of radius and ulna; median nerve; ulnar half of hand; carpal joints; skin over course of vessels
Ulnar, recurrent (arteria recurrens ulnaris [NA])	Ulnar	Anterior and posterior branches	Brachialis, pronator teres, flexor digitorum profundus, flexor digitorum sublimis, and flexor carpi ulnaris muscles; skin over medial cubital region; elbow joint; ulnar nerve
Umbilical (fetal) (arteria umbilicalis [NA])	Internal iliac		Ductus deferens; seminal vesicles; epididymis; ureter; bladder
Urethral (arteria urethralis [NA])	Internal pudendal		Urethra
Uterine (arteria uterina [NA])	Internal iliac	Vaginal artery; ovarian and tubal branches	Uterus; broad ligament of uterus; round ligament of uterus; uterine tube; portion of vagina
Vaginal (arteria vaginalis [NA])	Uterine		Vagina; fundus of bladder; rectum; vestibular bulb

Name	Origin	Branches	Distribution
Vertebral (arteria vertebralis [NA])	Subclavian	Basilar, anterior spinal, posterior spinal, and posterior inferior cerebellar arteries; meningeal branch	Muscles of neck; cervical vertebrae; cervical spinal cord and its membranes; intervertebral disks; bone and dura mater of posterior fossa of skull; falx cerebelli; cerebellum; medulla oblongata
Vesical, inferior (arteria vesicalis inferior [NA])	Internal iliac		Fundus of bladder; prostate gland; ductus deferens; seminal vesicle; lower part of ureter
Vesical, superior (arteriae vesicales superiores [NA])	Internal iliac (umbilical)		Lower part of ureter; upper part of bladder; ductus deferens; medial umbilical ligament
Vidian	See *Pterygoid canal, artery of*		
Volar arch	See *Palmar arch*		
Zygomaticoorbital (arteria zygomaticoorbitalis [NA])	Superficial temporal		Orbicularis oculi muscle; lateral portion of orbit

Name	Principal features	Bones with which articulation occurs and type of joint
Anvil	See *Incus*	
Astragalus	See *Talus*	
Atlas [NA]	First cervical vertebra; ringlike; lateral masses; anterior and posterior arches and tubercles; articular surfaces; vertebral and transverse foramens; sulcus for vertebral artery; ossifies in cartilage	Occipital bone, *bilateral gliding* Axis, 3 joints, *bilateral gliding* and *pivot* with dens
Axis [NA]	Second cervical vertebra; body; dens (odontoid process); laminae, pedicles; transverse processes and foramens; articular surfaces; thick spine; vertebral foramen; ossifies in cartilage	Atlas, 3 joints, *bilateral gliding* and *pivot* with dens Third cervical vertebra, *cartilaginous*
Calcaneum	See *Calcaneus*	
Calcaneus [NA]	Heel bone; largest tarsal bone; irregularly cuboid; tuber with medial and lateral processes; sustentaculum tali; trochlea; sinus tarsi; grooves for tendons of flexor hallucis longus and peroneal muscles; articular surfaces; ossifies in cartilage	Talus (3 facets), Cuboid } *gliding*
Calvaria [NA]	Skullcap or upper part of skull	
Calvarium	See *Calvaria*	
Capitate (os capitatum [NA])	Usually largest carpal bone; in distal row of carpal bones; occupies center of wrist; head; neck; body; ossifies in cartilage	Scaphoid Lunate Trapezoid Hamate Second, Third, Fourth } metacarpal } *gliding*
Carpus (ossa carpi [NA])	Consists of 8 short bones arranged in a proximal row (scaphoid; lunate; triquetrum; pisiform) and a distal row (trapezium; trapezoid; capitate; hamate)	
Central (os centrale [NA])	Occasional accessory bone of carpus; usually in man fuses with scaphoid but remains separate in many mammals	
Clavicle (clavicula [NA])	Collarbone; resembles the italic *"f"*; body; sternal and acromial extremities; conoid tubercle; trapezoid line; coracoid tuberosity; costal tuberosity; subclavian groove; first bone to ossify; ossifies partly in cartilage and partly in membrane	Sternum Scapula Cartilage of first rib } *gliding*
Coccyx (os coccygis [NA])	Last bone of vertebral column; usually composed of 4 small incomplete vertebrae fused together; base; apex; cornua; transverse processes; ossifies in cartilage	Sacrum, *cartilaginous*

Name	Principal features	Bones with which articulation occurs and type of joint
Concha, inferior nasal (concha nasalis inferior [NA])	Irregular scroll-shaped bone situated on lateral wall of nasal cavity; lacrimal, ethmoid, and maxillary processes; ossifies in cartilage	Ethmoid, Maxilla, Lacrimal, Palatine } *sutures*
Costal	See *Ribs*	
Coxal	See *Hipbone*	
Cranium [NA]	Braincase; composed of occipital, parietal (2), frontal, temporal (2), sphenoid, and ethmoid Sometimes cranium is used to designate entire skull without mandible	
Cuboid (os cuboideum [NA])	Roughly cubical bone in lateral part of tarsus; tuberosity; groove for tendon of peroneus longus	Calcaneus, Lateral cuneiform, Fourth and fifth metatarsals, Navicular } *gliding*
Cuneiform, inner	See *Cuneiform, medial*	
Cuneiform, intermediate (second cuneiform) (os cuneiforme intermedium [NA])	Wedge-shaped; smallest of the 3; articular surfaces; ossifies in cartilage	Navicular, Medial cuneiform, Lateral cuneiform, Second metatarsal } *gliding*
Cuneiform, lateral (third cuneiform) (os cuneiforme laterale [NA])	Wedge-shaped; articular surfaces; ossifies in cartilage	Navicular, Intermediate cuneiform, Cuboid, Second/Third/Fourth metatarsal } *gliding*
Cuneiform, medial (first cuneiform) (os cuneiforme mediale [NA])	Irregularly wedge-shaped; articular surfaces; largest of the 3; ossifies in cartilage	Navicular, Intermediate cuneiform, First and second metatarsals } *gliding*
Cuneiform, middle	See *Cuneiform, medial*	
Cuneiform, outer	See *Cuneiform, lateral*	
Epistropheus	See *Axis*	
Ethmoid (os ethmoidale [NA])	Irregular shape; situated in anterior part of base of skull and forming medial wall of each orbit and portion of roof and lateral wall of each nasal cavity; cribriform or horizontal plates; nasal slit; perpendicular plate; crista galli; alar processes; labyrinth with air cells; superior and middle nasal conchae, uncinate process; bulla; orbital plate; semilunar hiatus; ethmoid foramens; ossifies in cartilage	Sphenoid, Frontal, Nasal (2), Maxilla (2), Lacrimal (2), Palatine (2), Inferior nasal concha (2), Vomer } *sutures*

Name	Principal features	Bones with which articulation occurs and type of joint
Facial (ossa faciei [NA])	Bones of nose and jaws; maxilla, zygoma, nasal, lacrimal, palatine, inferior nasal concha, vomer, mandible, and parts of ethmoid and sphenoid	
Femur [NA]	Thighbone; largest, longest, and heaviest bone in the body; head; neck; greater and lesser trochanters; trochanteric fossa; quadrate tubercle; intertrochanteric line and crest; shaft; linea aspera and pectineal line; gluteal tuberosity; intercondylar line and fossa; medial and lateral condyles and epicondyles; adductor tubercle; articular surfaces; ossifies in cartilage	Hipbone, *ball-and-socket* Patella, *gliding* Tibia, combined *hinge* and *gliding*
Fibula [NA]	Splint bone; lateral bone of leg; head; body; medial crest; lateral malleolus; lateral malleolar fossa; articular surfaces; ossifies in cartilage	Tibia, *gliding* Talus with tibia and fibula, *hinge*
Flabella	Inconstant sesamoid bone occurring in lateral head of gastrocnemius muscle	
Foot	Composed of tarsus, metatarsus, and phalanges of foot	
Frontal (os frontale [NA])	Forehead bone; flat bone; frontal (squamous) part with eminences, glabella; superciliary arch, supraorbital margin and notch (foramen), zygomatic processes, temporal line, sagittal sulcus; orbital part forming upper portion of each orbit, anterior and posterior ethmoid foramens, spine or fovea for trochlea, fossa for lacrimal gland, frontal sinus; nasal part with spine; ossifies in membrane	Parietal (2) Sphenoid Ethmoid Nasal (2) Maxilla (2) Lacrimal (2) Zygoma (2) } *sutures*
Greater multangular	See *Trapezium*	
Hamate (os hamatum [NA])	Wedge-shaped; in distal row of carpal bones; hook-like process (hamulus); articular surfaces; ossifies in cartilage	Lunate Fourth and fifth metacarpals Triquetrum Capitate } *gliding*
Hammer	See *Malleus*	
Hand	Composed of carpus, metacarpus, and phalanges of hand	
Hipbone (os coxae [NA])	Large broad bone consisting of 3 parts; the ilium, ischium, and pubis; with its fellow forms pelvic girdle; with its fellow, sacrum and coccyx forms bony pelvis; acetabulum; obturator foramen; pubic arch; greater and lesser sciatic notches; articular surfaces; ossifies in cartilage	With its fellow of opposite side (symphysis pubis), *cartilaginous* Sacrum, *gliding*, very little movement Femur, *ball-and-socket*

Name	Principal features	Bones with which articulation occurs and type of joint
Humerus [NA]	Largest bone of upper limb; head; anatomic neck; greater and lesser tubercles; surgical neck; intertubercular sulcus; body; deltoid tuberosity; radial sulcus; condyle; capitulum; olecranon, coronoid, and radial fossae; trochlea; medial and lateral epicondyles; sulcus for ulnar nerve; articular surfaces; ossifies in cartilage	Scapula (glenoid cavity), *ball-and-socket* Ulna, *hinge* Radius, *gliding*
Hyoid (os hyoideum [NA])	U-shaped bone in front of neck; body; greater and lesser cornua; ossifies in cartilage	None
Ilium (os ilium [NA])	Broad expanded upper portion, the ala; body; crest; spines; gluteal lines; fossa; tuberosity; auricular surface; two-fifths (about) of acetabulum. See also *Hipbone*	
Incarial	See *Sutural*	
Incus [NA]	Resembles a premolar tooth with 2 roots; middle bone of auditory ossicles; body; long and short processes or crura; lenticular process; ossifies in cartilage	Malleus, Stapes } *gliding*
Inferior maxilla	See *Mandible*	
Inferior concha	See *Concha, inferior nasal*	
Inferior turbinate	See *Concha, inferior nasal*	
Innominate	See *Hipbone*	
Intermediate cuneiform	See *Cuneiform, intermediate*	
Ischium (os ischii [NA])	Heavy, posterior lower portion; body; tuber; ramus; spine; notches; lower boundary of obturator foramen; two-fifths (about) of acetabulum. See also *Hipbone*	
Lacrimal (os lacrimale [NA])	Small scale of bone resembling a fingernail; situated in the anterior medial wall of orbit; crest; descending process; hamulus; groove; ossifies in membrane	Frontal, Ethmoid, Maxilla, Inferior nasal concha } *sutures*
Lateral cuneiform	See *Cuneiform, lateral*	
Lesser multangular	See *Trapezoid*	
Lunate (os lunatum [NA])	One of proximal row of carpal bones; named from crescent-shaped articular facet; articular surfaces; ossifies in cartilage	Radius, *biaxial* Capitate, Hamate, Triquetrum, Scaphoid } *gliding*

Name	Principal features	Bones with which articulation occurs and type of joint
Magnum	See *Capitate*	
Malar	See *Zygoma*	
Malleus [NA]	Resembles a small hammer; head; neck; spur; crest; handle; anterior and lateral processes; ossifies in cartilage	Incus, *gliding*
Mandible (mandibula [NA])	Lower jaw; body, 2 rami; angle; coronoid and condyloid processes; symphysis; alveolar part; mental protuberance and tubercle; mylohyoid line and groove; mandibular and mental foramens; lingula; canal; articular surfaces; ossifies partly in membrane and partly in cartilage	Each temporal bone, combined *gliding* and *hinge*
Maxilla [NA]	Upper jaw; body with infraorbital foramen, sulcus, and canal, maxillary sinus, lacrimal groove, greater palatine sulcus, and foramen; zygomatic process; frontal process; ethmoid crest; alveolar process; maxillary tuber; palatine process; incisive crest, spine, and canal; nasal crest; maxillary hiatus; ossifies in membrane	Frontal, Ethmoid, Nasal, Zygoma, Lacrimal, Inferior nasal concha, Palatine, Vomer, Other maxilla } *sutures*
Medial cuneiform	See *Cuneiform, medial*	
Metacarpus (ossa metacarpalia I–V [NA])	Five bones of the hand proper; each with head, shaft, and base; numbered from 1 to 5 beginning on the thumb side; styloid process on lateral side of base of third; articular surfaces; each ossified in cartilage	Base of first with trapezium; Base of others with each other and with distal row of carpal bones } *gliding* Heads with corresponding phalanges, *ball-and-socket*
Metatarsus (ossa metatarsalia I–V [NA])	Five bones of foot proper; each with head, shaft, and base; numbered from 1 to 5 beginning on the great toe side; tuberosity on 1 and 5; articular surfaces; each ossifies in cartilage	Distal tarsal bones; Bases with each other } *gliding* Heads with corresponding phalanges, *ball-and-socket*
Middle turbinate	See *Ethmoid,* middle nasal concha (not a separate bone)	
Multangulum majus	See *Trapezium*	
Multangulum minus	See *Trapezoid*	
Nasal (os nasale [NA])	Rectangular plate; 2 form bridge of nose; ethmoid sulcus and crest; ossifies in membrane	Frontal, Ethmoid, Maxilla, Other nasal } *sutures*
Navicular (os naviculare [NA])	Boat-shaped; proximal articular facet markedly concave; tuberosity; articular surfaces; ossifies in cartilage	Talus, Three cuneiforms, Cuboid } *gliding*

Name	Principal features	Bones with which articulation occurs and type of joint
Navicular of hand	See *Scaphoid*	
Occipital (os occipitale [NA])	Posterior part and base of cranium; saucer-shaped; squamous part with internal and external protuberances, highest, superior, and inferior nuchal lines; sagittal and transverse sulci; lateral part with condyles, canal for hypoglossal nerve, condyloid canal, jugular notch, process and tubercle; basal part with pharyngeal tubercle and foramen magnum; squamous part ossifies in membrane, the rest in cartilage	Parietal (2), Temporal (2), Sphenoid } *sutures* Atlas, *bilateral gliding*
Os calcis [NA alternative]	See *Calcaneus*	
Os intercuneiforme	A very rare accessory ossicle of the foot situated between the medial and intermediate cuneiforms	
Os intermetatarseum	A very rare accessory ossicle of the foot situated between the bases of the first and second metatarsal bones	
Os magnum	See *Capitate*	
Os paracuneiforme	A very rare accessory ossicle of the foot situated between the navicular and medial cuneiform bones	
Ossa cranii [NA]	See *Cranium*	
Os vesalianum	See *Vesalian bone*, 1 and 2	
Ossicula auditus [NA]	See *Tympanic*	
Palatine (os palatinum [NA])	Forms portions of hard palate, orbits, and nasal cavities; irregularly L-shaped; horizontal part with nasal and palatine aspects, nasal and palatine crests, posterior nasal spine, lesser palatine foramens; perpendicular part with nasal and maxillary aspects, pyramidal, orbital, and sphenoid processes, conchal and ethmoid crests, greater palatine sulcus, and sphenopalatine notch; ossifies in membrane	Sphenoid, Ethmoid, Maxilla, Inferior nasal concha, Palatine (opposite), Vomer } *sutures*
Parietal (os parietale [NA])	Forms side and roof of cranium; quadrilateral plate of bone; superior and inferior temporal lines; parietal foramen; tubers; sulcus for superior sagittal sinus; sulcus for sigmoid sinus; ossifies in membrane	Parietal (opposite), Occipital, Frontal, Temporal, Sphenoid } *sutures*
Patella [NA]	Kneecap; triangular; largest sesamoid; ossifies in cartilage	Condyles of femur, *gliding*

Name	Principal features	Bones with which articulation occurs and type of joint
Pelvis [NA]	Bony pelvis composed of 2 hipbones, sacrum, and coccyx	
Phalanges (of foot) (ossa digitorum pedis [NA])	Two for great toe, 3 for each of others, 14 in all, usually fifth toe has only 2; each phalanx is a miniature long bone with head, shaft, and base; articular surfaces; tuberosity on distal phalanx; each ossifies in cartilage	Proximal row with corresponding metatarsal bones, *ball-and-socket* Interphalangeal joints, *hinge*
Phalanges (of hand) (ossa digitorum manus [NA])	Two for thumb, 3 for each finger, 14 in all; each phalanx is a miniature long bone with head, shaft, and base; articular surfaces; tuberosity on distal phalanx; each ossifies in cartilage	Proximal row with corresponding metacarpal bones, *ball-and-socket* Interphalangeal joints, *hinge*
Pisiform (os pisiforme [NA])	Most medial of proximal row of carpus; smallest carpal; resembles half a pea; articular surface; ossifies in cartilage	Triquetrum, *gliding*
Pubis (os pubis [NA])	Anterior lower portion; body; superior and inferior rami; tubercle; crest; pecten; upper boundary of obturator foramen, obturator crest and groove; one-fifth (about) of acetabulum. See also *Hipbone*	
Pyramidal	See *Triquetrum*	
Radius [NA]	Lateral bone of forearm; head; shaft; neck; tuberosity; styloid process; interosseous margin; ulnar notch; articular surfaces; ossifies in cartilage	Humerus, *gliding* Ulna, proximal, *pivot* Ulna, distal, *gliding* Lunate, Scaphoid, Triquetrum } *biaxial*
Ribs (costae [NA])	Twelve on each side; head; neck; body; tubercle; angle; costal groove; first is relatively broad and flat; second has tubercle; 11 and 12 are floating; each ossifies in cartilage	Head with vertebral bodies, Tubercle with transverse processes } *gliding* Sternum with first rib, Sternum with others } *cartilaginous*
Sacrum (os sacrum [NA])	Large triangular bone composed of 5 fused vertebrae; base; apex; intervertebral, pelvic, and dorsal foramens; articular processes; promontory; sacral crests; cornua; canal; hiatus; auricular facet; articular surfaces; ossifies in cartilage	Last lumbar vertebra, Coccyx } *cartilaginous* Hipbones, *gliding* (very little movement)
Scaphoid of foot	See *Navicular*	
Scaphoid (os scaphoideum [NA])	Largest bone of proximal row of carpal bones; comma-shaped; tubercle; articular surfaces; ossifies in cartilage	Trapezium, Trapezoid, Capitate, Lunate } *gliding* Radius, *biaxial*

Name	Principal features	Bones with which articulation occurs and type of joint
Scapula [NA]	Shoulder blade; flat, triangular bone of posterior part of shoulder; neck; spine; acromion; coracoid process; glenoid cavity; infraglenoid and supraglenoid tubercles; notch; subscapular, infraspinatus, and supraspinatus fossae; costal and dorsal aspects; medial, lateral, and superior margins; inferior, lateral, and superior angles; ossifies in cartilage	Humerus, *ball-and-socket* Clavicle, *gliding*
Semilunar	See *Lunate*	
Sesamoids (ossa sesamoidea [NA])	Small seed-like nodules of bone which develop in muscular tendons where they play against bone; patella, one in each tendon of insertion of flexor hallucis brevis muscle, and one in tendon of insertion of flexor pollicis brevis and of adductor pollicis are constant; others are variable; each develops in cartilage	
Skull	See *Cranium.* Sometimes used to include mandible as well	
Sphenoid (os sphenoidale [NA])	Forms anterior part of base of skull and portions of cranial, orbital, and nasal cavities; in shape resembles a butterfly with extended wings; body with air sinuses, sella turcica, hypophyseal fossa, dorsum sellae, posterior clinoid processes, clivus, chiasmatic groove, spine, carotid groove, crest, pterygoid fossa, rostrum; small wings each with optic canal, anterior clinoid process, superior orbital fissure; great wings each with foramen rotundum, foramen ovale, foramen spinosum, pterygoid processes, medial and lateral pterygoid plates, hamulus, scaphoid fossa, pterygoid canal; ossifies partly in membrane and partly in cartilage	Frontal Parietal (2) Occipital Temporal (2) Ethmoid Palatine (2) Zygoma (2) Vomer } *sutures*
Stapes [NA]	Resembles a stirrup; smallest of auditory ossicles; head; base; anterior and posterior crura; ossifies in cartilage	Incus Oval window } *gliding*
Sternum [NA]	Breastbone; dagger-shaped; manubrium; angle; body; xiphoid process; ossifies in cartilage	Clavicle (2), *gliding* First rib (2), *cartilaginous* Costal cartilages of ribs 2 to 7, *cartilaginous*
Stirrup	See *Stapes*	
Superior maxilla	See *Maxilla*	
Superior turbinate	See *Ethmoid,* superior nasal concha (not a separate bone)	

Name	Principal features	Bones with which articulation occurs and type of joint
Sutural (ossa suturarum [NA])	Irregular variable bones occasionally found along cranial sutures; most frequent in lambdoid suture	
Talus [NA]	Second largest bone of tarsus; head; neck; body; trochlea; lateral and posterior processes; medial and lateral tubercles; sulcus; articular surfaces; ossifies in cartilage	Tibia, Fibula } *hinge* Calcaneus (3 facets), Navicular } *gliding*
Tarsus (ossa tarsi [NA])	Posterior portion of foot; consists of 7 bones: calcaneus, talus, cuboid, navicular, and 3 cuneiforms	
Temporal (os temporale [NA])	Forms a portion of lateral aspect of skull and part of base of cranium; squamous part with zygomatic process, mandibular fossa, articular tubercle; tympanic part with external acoustic meatus, tympanic spine, styloid process and sheath, stylomastoid foramen, tympanic sulcus; mastoid part with air cells, notch, foramen, sigmoid sulcus; petrous part with apex, caroticotympanic and musculotubarial canals, jugular fossa, internal ear, carotid canal, internal acoustic meatus; articular surfaces; ossifies partly in membrane and partly in cartilage	Occipital, Parietal, Sphenoid, Zygoma } *sutures* Mandible, combined *gliding* and *hinge*
Tibia [NA]	Shinbone; large medial bone of leg; medial and lateral condyles; intercondylar eminence and intercondylar tubercles; tuberosity; body; soleal line; medial malleolus; articular surfaces; ossifies in cartilage	Femur, combined *hinge* and *gliding* Fibula, superior, Fibula, inferior } *gliding* Talus with fibula, *hinge*
Trapezium (os trapezium [NA])	In distal row of carpal bones; irregular bone with 6 surfaces; tubercle; articular surfaces; ossifies in cartilage	Scaphoid, Trapezoid, Second metacarpal } *gliding* First metacarpal, *saddle*
Trapezoid (os trapezoideum [NA])	Smallest bone in distal row of carpal bones; irregular bone with 6 surfaces; articular surfaces; ossifies in cartilage	Scaphoid, Second metacarpal, Trapezium, Capitate } *gliding*
Trigonal (os trigonum [NA])	Occasional extra tarsal bone; due to failure of center of ossification in lateral tubercle of talus to fuse with main center	
Triquetrum (os triquetrum [NA])	One of proximal row of carpal bones; wedge-shaped; articular surfaces; ossifies in cartilage	Lunate, Pisiform, Hamate } *gliding* Radius, *biaxial*
Turbinate, inferior	See *Concha, inferior nasal*	

TABLE OF BONES (Continued)

Name	Principal features	Bones with which articulation occurs and type of joint
Turbinate, middle	See *Ethmoid,* middle nasal concha (not a separate bone)	
Turbinate, superior	See *Ethmoid,* superior nasal concha (not a separate bone)	
Tympanic (ossicula auditus [NA])	Includes 3 auditory ossicles. See *Incus; Malleus; Stapes*	
Ulna [NA]	Medial bone of forearm; olecranon; coronoid process; radial and trochlear notches; tuberosity; body; head; styloid process; interosseous margin; supinator crest; articular surfaces; ossifies in cartilage	Humerus, *hinge* Radius, proximal, *pivot* Radius, distal, *gliding*
Unciform	See *Hamate*	
Vertebrae [NA]	Bones of vertebral column, 33 in all: cervical 7, thoracic 12, lumbar 5, sacrum 5 (fused), coccyx 4 (fused); each has body; arch; articular processes; transverse processes; spinous process; foramens; each vertebra ossifies in cartilage. See also *Atlas, Axis, Coccyx, Sacrum*	Between vertebral bodies, *cartilaginous* Between articular processes, *gliding*
Vesalian	(1) Occasional extra ossicle in carpus (2) Occasional extra ossicle at base of fifth metatarsal due to failure of separate center of ossification to fuse with main center	
Vomer [NA]	Forms posterior part of nasal septum; ala; ossifies in membrane	Sphenoid, Ethmoid, Maxilla (2), Palatine (2) } *sutures*
Wormian	See *Sutural*	
Wrist	See *Carpus*	
Zygoma (os zygomaticum [NA])	Cheekbone; forms cheek and lateral aspect of orbit; tubercle; temporal process; frontal process; foramens; ossifies in membrane	Frontal, Sphenoid, Temporal, Maxillary } *sutures*

Name	Origin	Insertion	Innervation	Function
Abductor accessorius digiti quinti	Rare variant of opponens digiti minimi of foot	Base of proximal phalanx of little toe	Lateral plantar	
Abductor digiti minimi of foot (musculus abductor digiti minimi [NA])	Medial and lateral tubercles of calcaneus and plantar fascia	Lateral surface of base of proximal phalanx of little toe	Lateral plantar	Supports lateral longitudinal arch and abducts little toe
Abductor digiti minimi of hand (musculus abductor digiti minimi [NA])	Pisiform and tendon of flexor carpi ulnaris	Medial surface of base of proximal phalanx of little finger	Ulnar	Abducts little finger
Abductor digiti quinti	See *Abductor digiti minimi of foot* or *of hand*			
Abductor hallucis (musculus abductor hallucis [NA])	Medial tubercle of calcaneus and plantar fascia	Medial surface of base of proximal phalanx of great toe	Medial plantar	Supports medial longitudinal arch; flexes great toe
Abductor indicis	See *Interossei, dorsal*			
Abductor ossis metatarsid quinti	Small variable portion of abductor digiti minimi of foot	Lateral side of base of fifth metatarsal	Lateral plantar	
Abductor pollicis brevis (musculus abductor pollicis brevis [NA])	Scaphoid, ridge of trapezium and flexor retinaculum	Lateral surface of base of proximal phalanx of thumb	Median	Abducts and flexes thumb
Abductor pollicis longus (musculus abductor pollicis longus [NA])	Posterior aspect of ulna, radius, and interosseous membrane	Lateral aspect of base of first metacarpal and trapezium	Dorsal interosseous of radial	Abducts and extends thumb
Accelerator urinae	See *Bulbospongiosus, male*			
Accessorius	See *Quadratus plantae; Iliocostalis thoracis*			
Accessorius ad flexorem carpi radialem	Variable additional slip of flexor carpi radialis			
Accessorius ad flexorem digitorum profundum	Variable additional slip of flexor digitorum profundus arising from coronoid process of ulna	Usually associated with tendons to middle and index fingers		
Accessorius ad flexorem pollicis longum	Variable extra part of flexor pollicis longus			

Name	Origin	Insertion	Innervation	Function
Accessorius of gluteus minimus	Occasional extra slip	Capsule of hip joint		
Accessory peroneal	Occasional variable extra slip of peroneus longus or brevis	Variable along lateral side of foot		
Accessory pterygoid	Occasional extra slip from body of sphenoid	Lateral pterygoid plate		
Adductor brevis (musculus adductor brevis [NA])	Pubis	Proximal part of linea aspera of femur and femur proximal to that line	Obturator	Adducts thigh
Adductor digiti secundi	Occasional extra part of oblique head of adductor of great toe			
Adductor hallucis (musculus adductor hallucis [NA])		Lateral aspect of base of proximal phalanx of great toe	Lateral plantar	Adducts great toe
(1) Oblique head (caput obliquum musculi adductoris hallucis [NA])	Plantar fascia and bases of second, third, and fourth metatarsals			
(2) Transverse head (caput transversum musculi adductoris hallucis [NA])	Transverse metatarsal ligament, and capsules of 4 lateral metatarsophalangeal joints			
Adductor hallucis transversus	See *Adductor hallucis, transverse head*			
Adductor longus (musculus adductor longus [NA])	Pubis	Linea aspera of femur	Obturator	Adducts thigh
Adductor magnus (musculus adductor magnus [NA])	(1) Inferior ramus of pubis and ramus of ischium	Linea aspera of femur	Obturator	Adducts thigh
	(2) Ischial tuber	Adductor tubercle of femur	Tibial	Extends thigh
Adductor minimus (musculus adductor minimus)	When present is a separate proximal portion of adductor magnus			

Name	Origin	Insertion	Innervation	Function
Adductor pollicis (musculus adductor pollicis [NA])		Medial aspect of base of proximal phalanx of thumb	Ulnar	Adducts and opposes thumb
(1) Oblique head (caput obliquum musculi adductoris pollicis [NA])	Trapezium, trapezoid, capitate, and bases of second, third, and fourth metacarpals			
(2) Transverse head (caput transversum musculi adductoris pollicis [NA])	Third metacarpal			
Adductor pollicis obliquus	See *Adductor pollicis, oblique head*			
Adductor pollicis transversus	See *Adductor pollicis, transverse head*			
Agitator caudae (variable)	Variable portion of gluteus maximus; sometimes arises separately from coccyx			
Amygdaloglossus (variable)	Scattered fibers of palatoglossus to tonsil			
Anconeus (musculus anconeus [NA])	Dorsal surface of lateral epicondyle of humerus	Olecranon of ulna	Radial	Extends elbow joint
Anconeus internus (variable)	See *Epitrochleo-olecranonis*			
Anconeus lateralis	See *Triceps brachii, lateral head*			
Anconeus longus	See *Triceps brachii, long head*			
Anconeus medialis	See *Triceps brachii, medial head*			
Antitragicus (vestigial) (musculus antitragicus [NA])	Lateral surface of antitragus	Anthelix and cauda helicis	Facial	
Arrectores pilorum (smooth) (musculi arrectores pilorum [NA])	Found in corium	Hair follicles	Sympathetic	Elevate hairs of skin

Name	Origin	Insertion	Innervation	Function
Articularis cubiti (musculus articularis cubiti [NA])	Posterior distal surface of humerus	Posterior aspect of elbow joint	Radial	Pulls capsule upward in extension of elbow joint
Articularis genus (musculus articularis genus [NA])	Distal fourth of anterior surface of femur	Synovial membrane of knee joint	Femoral	Draws synovial membrane proximally in extension of knee joint
Aryepiglotticus (inconstant) (musculus aryepiglotticus [NA])	Apex of arytenoid cartilage	Lateral margin of epiglottis	Recurrent laryngeal	Closes inlet of larynx
Arymembranous (inconstant)	Apex of arytenoid cartilage	Lateral margin of membranous part of aryepiglottic fold	Recurrent laryngeal	Closes inlet of larynx
Arytenoid				
(1) Oblique (musculus arytenoideus obliquus [NA])	Dorsal aspect of muscular process of arytenoid cartilage	Apex of opposite arytenoid cartilage	Recurrent laryngeal	Closes inlet of larynx
(2) Transverse (musculus arytenoideus transversus [NA])		Becomes continuous with thyroarytenoid		Approximates arytenoid cartilages
Aryvocalis (variable)	Variable slip of vocalis			
Atlantobasilaris internus (variable)	Occasional slip of longus capitis			
Attollens aurem (vestigial)	See *Auricular, superior*			
Attrahens aurem (vestigial)	See *Auricular, anterior*			
Auricular (vestigial)		Helix	Facial	Move auricle
(1) Anterior (musculus auricularis anterior [NA])	Galea aponeurotica			
(2) Inferior	Scattered fibers			
(3) Oblique (musculus obliquus auriculae [NA])	Scattered fibers over transverse sulcus of anthelix			
(4) Posterior (musculus auricularis posterior [NA])	Mastoid process			

Name	Origin	Insertion	Innervation	Function
Auricular (vestigial) (Continued)				
(5) Superior (musculus auricularis superior [NA])	Galea aponeurotica			
(6) Transverse (musculus transversus auriculae [NA])	Scattered fibers from concha to scapha			
Auriculofrontalis	Occasional slip of auricular anterior			
Axillary arches	Occasional slips of muscle in axillary fascia with various names			
Azygos uvulae	See *Uvulae*			
Biceps brachii (musculus biceps brachii [NA])		Tuberosity of radius and deep fascia of forearm	Musculocutaneous	Supinates and flexes forearm
(1) Long head (caput longum musculi bicipitis brachii [NA])	Supraglenoid tubercle of scapula			
(2) Short head (caput breve musculi bicipitis brachii [NA])	Tip of coracoid process of scapula			
Biceps femoris (musculus biceps femoris [NA])		Head of fibula, lateral condyle of tibia, and deep fascia on lateral aspect of knee		
(1) Long head (caput longum musculi bicipitis femoris [NA])	Ischial tuber		Tibial	Flexes knee joint and extends hip joint
(2) Short head (caput breve musculi bicipitis femoris [NA])	Linea aspera of femur		Peroneal	Flexes knee joint
Biceps flexor cruris	See *Biceps femoris*			
Biventer cervicis	See *Spinalis capitis*			
Biventer mandibulae	See *Digastric*			
Brachialis (musculus brachialis [NA])	Anterior aspect of humerus	Coronoid process of ulna	Musculocutaneous	Flexes elbow joint

Name	Origin	Insertion	Innervation	Function
Brachioradialis (musculus brachioradialis [NA])	Lateral supracondylar ridge of humerus	Lower end of radius	Radial	Flexes elbow joint
Bronchoesophageal (smooth) (musculus bronchoesophageus [NA])	Fibers from left bronchus to esophagus		Autonomic	
Buccinator (musculus buccinator [NA])	Alveolar process of maxilla and of mandible and pterygomandibular raphe	Blends about mouth with orbicularis oris	Facial	Compresses cheek and retracts angle of mouth
Buccopharyngeus (pars buccopharyngea musculi constrictoris pharyngis superioris [NA])	Portion of superior constrictor of pharynx			
Bulbocavernosus	See *Bulbospongiosus*			
Bulbospongiosus, male and female (musculus bulbospongiosus [NA])	Central part of perineum and median raphe of bulb in male	Fascia of perineum and of penis (clitoris)	Perineal	In male compresses urethra; in female contracts vaginal orifice and compresses bulb of vestibule
Caninus	See *Levator anguli oris*			
Cephalopharyngeus	Portion of superior constrictor of pharynx			
Ceratocricoid (musculus ceratocricoideus [NA])	Variable slip of posterior cricoarytenoid			
Ceratopharyngeus (pars ceratopharyngea musculi constrictoris pharyngis medii [NA])	Part of middle constrictor of pharynx			
Cervicalis ascendens	See *Iliocostalis cervicis*			
Chondroepitrochlearis (variable)	Occasional slip of muscle in axillary fascia			
Chondroglossus (variable portion of hyoglossus) (musculus chondroglossus [NA])	Lesser cornu of hyoid	Side of tongue	Hypoglossal	Depresses tongue

Name	Origin	Insertion	Innervation	Function
Chondrohumeralis	Occasional slip of muscle in axillary fascia			
Chondropharyngeus (pars chondropharyngea musculi constrictoris pharyngis medii [NA])	Portion of middle constrictor of pharynx			
Ciliary (smooth) (musculus ciliaris [NA])		Ciliary processes	Oculomotor; parasympathetic	Visual accommodation
(1) Meridional portion (fibrae meridionales musculi ciliaris [NA])	Scleral spur			
(2) Circular portion (fibrae circulares musculi ciliaris [NA])	Sphincter of ciliary body			
Ciliary (striate)	Portion of orbicularis oculi near lid margins		Facial	
Circumflexus palati	See *Tensor veli palatini*			
Cleidomastoid	Portion of sternocleidomastoid			
Cleidooccipital	Portion of sternocleidomastoid			
Coccygeofemoralis (variable)	Occasional slip of the gluteus maximus arising separately from coccyx			
Coccygeus (musculus coccygeus [NA])	Ischial spine and sacrospinous ligament	Lateral border of lower sacrum and upper coccyx	Sacral	Helps to form pelvic diaphragm
Complexus	See *Semispinalis capitis*			
Complexus minor	See *Longissimus capitis*			
Compressor bulbi proprius	Portion of bulbospongiosus, male			
Compressor hemispherium bulbi	Portion of bulbospongiosus, male			

TABLE OF MUSCLES (Continued)

Name	Origin	Insertion	Innervation	Function
Compressor labii	Portion of orbicularis oris			
Compressor naris	See *Nasalis, transverse part*			
Compressor nasi	See *Nasalis, transverse part*			
Compressor urethrae	See *Sphincter urethrae*			
Compressor vaginae	See *Bulbospongiosus, female*			
Compressor venae dorsalis (variable)	Portion of bulbospongiosus, male			
Constrictor of pharynx, inferior (musculus constrictor pharyngis inferior [NA])	Oblique line of thyroid cartilage, side of cricoid cartilage	Median raphe of posterior wall of pharynx	Pharyngeal plexus	Constricts pharynx
Constrictor of pharynx, middle (musculus constrictor pharyngis medius [NA])	Stylohyoid ligament and both cornua of hyoid	Median raphe of pharynx	Pharyngeal plexus	Constricts pharynx
Constrictor of pharynx, superior (musculus constrictor pharyngis superior [NA])	Medial pteryoid plate, pterygomandibular ligament, and mylohyoid line of mandible	Median raphe of pharynx	Pharyngeal plexus	Constricts pharynx
Constrictor radicis penis	Portion of bulbospongiosus, male			
Constrictor vaginae	See *Bulbospongiosus, female*			
Coracobrachialis (musculus coracobrachialis [NA])	Coracoid process of scapula	Medial aspect of shaft of humerus	Musculocutaneous	Flexes and adducts humerus
Coracobrachialis superior or brevis	Occasional proximal slip of coracobrachialis			
Corrugator cutis ani (smooth)	Found in skin about anus		Sympathetic	
Corrugator supercilii (musculus corrugator supercilii [NA])	Superciliary arch of frontal bone	Skin of forehead	Facial	Muscle of facial expression

Name	Origin	Insertion	Innervation	Function
Costalis	See *Iliocostalis thoracis*			
Costocervicalis	See *Iliocostalis cervicis*			
Costocoracoid (variable)	Occasional slip of muscle in axillary fascia			
Cremaster (musculus cremaster [NA])	Inferior margin of internal oblique abdominal muscle	Pubic tubercle	Genitofemoral	Elevates testis
Cricoarytenoid, lateral (musculus cricoarytenoideus lateralis [NA])	Lateral surface of cricoid cartilage	Muscular process of arytenoid cartilage	Recurrent laryngeal	Approximates vocal folds
Cricoarytenoid, posterior (musculus cricoarytenoideus posterior [NA])	Dorsal surface of cricoid cartilage	Muscular process of arytenoid cartilage	Recurrent laryngeal	Separates vocal folds
Cricopharyngeus (pars cricopharyngea musculi constrictoris pharyngis inferioris [NA])	Part of inferior constrictor of pharynx			
Cricothyroid (musculus cricothyroideus [NA])	Arch of cricoid cartilage	Lamina of thyroid cartilage	External branch of superior laryngeal	Tenses vocal folds
Crureus	See *Vastus intermedius*			
Cucullarius	See *Trapezius*			
Dartos (smooth) (tunica dartos [NA])	Found in skin and superficial fascia of scrotum		Sympathetic	Corrugates skin of scrotum
Deep transverse perineal (musculus transversus perinei profundus [NA])	Ramus of ischium	Central point of perineum	Perineal	Supports perineum
Deltoid (musculus deltoideus [NA])	Clavicle, acromion, and spine of scapula	Deltoid tuberosity of humerus	Axillary	Abducts humerus; anterior fibers flex and medially rotate humerus, posterior fibers extend and laterally rotate humerus
Depressor alae nasi	See *Nasalis, alar part*			

Name	Origin	Insertion	Innervation	Function
Depressor anguli oris (musculus depressor anguli oris [NA])	Mandible	Skin of angle of mouth	Facial	Muscle of facial expression
Depressor epiglottidis	Some fibers of thyroepiglottic			
Depressor labii inferioris (musculus depressor labii inferioris [NA])	Mandible	Skin of lower lip	Facial	Muscle of facial expression
Depressor septi nasi (musculus depressor septi [NA])	Maxilla	Septum of nose	Facial	Muscle of facial expression
Depressor supercilii (musculus depressor supercilii [NA])	A few fibers of orbicularis oculi	Eyebrow	Facial	Muscle of facial expression
Detrusor urinae	See *Detrusor vesicae*			
Detrusor vesicae (smooth)	In wall of urinary bladder		Autonomic	Empties urinary bladder
Diaphragm (diaphragma [NA])	Xiphoid cartilage, costal cartilages of ribs 5 to 9, lower ribs, and lumbar vertebrae	Central tendon	Phrenic	Acts as main muscle of inhalation; aids in expulsive actions such as sneezing and parturition
Digastric (musculus digastricus [NA])		Lesser cornu of hyoid via fascial sling		Elevates and fixes hyoid bone
(1) Anterior belly (venter anterior musculi digastrici [NA])	Inner surface of mandible near symphysis		Mylohyoid	
(2) Posterior belly (venter posterior musculi digastrici [NA])	Mastoid notch		Facial	
Dilator naris	See *Nasalis, alar part*			
Dilator pupillae (smooth) (musculus dilator pupillae [NA])	Circumference of iris	Margin of pupil	Sympathetic	Dilates pupil
Dilator tubae	See *Tensor veli palatini*			
Dorsoepitrochlearis (variable)	Occasional slip of muscle in axillary fascia			

Name	Origin	Insertion	Innervation	Function
Ejaculator urinae	See *Bulbospongiosus, male*			
Epicraniotemporalis	See *Auricular, anterior*			
Epicranius (musculus epicranius [NA])	See *Occipitofrontalis; Temporoparietalis*			
Epitrochlearis	See *Chondrohumeralis*			
Epitrochleo-olecranonis (variable)	Medial epicondyle of humerus	Olecranon	Radial	
Erector clitoridis	See *Ischiocavernosus*			
Erector penis	See *Ischiocavernosus*			
Erector pili	See *Arrectores pilorum*			
Erector spinae (musculus erector spinae [NA])	Composed of iliocostalis, longissimus, and spinalis			
Extensor carpi radialis accessorius (variable part of extensor carpi radialis brevis)				
Extensor carpi radialis brevior	See *Extensor carpi radialis brevis*			
Extensor carpi radialis brevis (musculus extensor carpi radialis brevis [NA])	Lateral epicondyle of humerus	Base of second and third metacarpals		Extends wrist
Extensor carpi radialis intermedius (variable part of extensor carpi radialis brevis)				
Extensor carpi radialis longior	See *Extensor carpi radialis longus*			
Extensor carpi radialis longus (musculus extensor carpi radialis longus [NA])	Lateral epicondyle of humerus	Base of second metacarpal	Radial	Extends wrist

Name	Origin	Insertion	Innervation	Function
Extensor carpi ulnaris (musculus extensor carpi ulnaris [NA])	Lateral epicondyle of humerus and dorsal margin of ulna	Base of fifth metacarpal	Radial	Extends wrist
Extensor coccygeus (vestigial)	See *Sacrococcygeus dorsalis*			
Extensor communis pollicis et indicis (variable)	Occasional extra slip of extensor pollicis longus			
Extensor digiti annularis (variable)	Occasional extra slip of muscle to ring finger			
Extensor digiti minimi (musculus extensor digiti minimi [NA])	Lateral epicondyle of humerus	Dorsum of proximal phalanx of little finger	Radial	Extends metacarpophalangeal joint of little finger
Extensor digitorum (musculus extensor digitorum [NA])	Lateral epicondyle of humerus	Tendon to dorsal aspect of each finger	Radial	Extends fingers at metacarpophalangeal joints
Extensor digitorum brevis (musculus extensor digitorum brevis [NA])	Dorsal surface of calcaneus	Extensor tendons of 4 medial toes	Deep peroneal	Dorsiflexes toes at metatarsophalangeal joints
Extensor digitorum brevis of hand (variable)	Carpal bones	Extensor tendons of metacarpals	Radial	Aids common extensor (extensor digitorum)
Extensor digitorum communis	See *Extensor digitorum*			
Extensor digitorum longus (musculus extensor digitorum longus [NA])	Anterior aspect of fibula, lateral aspect of lateral malleolus, and interosseous membrane	Common extensor tendons of 4 lateral toes	Deep peroneal	Dorsiflexes at metatarsophalangeal joints
Extensor hallucis brevis (most medial portion of extensor digitorum brevis) (musculus extensor hallucis brevis [NA])	Dorsal surface of calcaneus	Base of proximal phalanx of great toe	Deep peroneal	Dorsiflexes great toe at metatarsophalangeal joint
Extensor hallucis longus (musculus extensor hallucis longus [NA])	Medial surface of fibula and interosseous membrane	Base of proximal phalanx of great toe	Deep peroneal	Dorsiflexes ankle joint and great toe

Name	Origin	Insertion	Innervation	Function
Extensor indicis (musculus extensor indicis [NA])	Dorsal surface of ulna	Common extensor tendon of index finger	Dorsal interosseous	Extends metacarpophalangeal joint of index finger
Extensor medii digiti (variable)	Occasional extra slip of muscle to middle finger			
Extensor ossis metacarpi pollicis	See *Abductor pollicis longus*			
Extensor ossis metatarsi hallucis	Occasional separate slip of insertion of extensor hallucis longus into first metatarsal			
Extensor pollicis brevis (musculus extensor pollicis brevis [NA])	Dorsal surface of radius and interosseous membrane	Dorsal surface of proximal phalanx of thumb	Dorsal interosseous	Extends metacarpophalangeal joint of thumb
Extensor pollicis longus (musculus extensor pollicis longus [NA])	Dorsal surface of radius and interosseous membrane	Dorsal surface of proximal phalanx of thumb	Dorsal interosseous	Extends metacarpophalangeal joint of thumb
Extensor primi internodii longus hallucis	Occasional extra slip of insertion of extensor hallucis longus into proximal phalanx of great toe			
Extensor primi internodii pollicis	See *Extensor pollicis brevis*			
Extensor secundi internodii pollicis	See *Extensor pollicis longus*			
External oblique of abdomen	See *Oblique, external abdominal*			
External thyroarytenoid (lateral part of thyroarytenoid)				
Fibularis brevis (musculus fibularis brevis [NA alternative])	See *Peroneus brevis*			
Fibularis longus (musculus fibularis longus [NA alternative])	See *Peroneus longus*			

Name	Origin	Insertion	Innervation	Function
Fibularis tertius (musculus fibularis tertius [NA alternative])	See *Peroneus tertius*			
Fibulocalcaneus (variable)	Occasional extra slip of quadratus plantae or of flexor digitorum longus			
Fibulotibialis (variable)	Occasional extra slip of popliteus			
Flexor accessorius (musculus flexor accessorius [NA alternative])	See *Quadratus plantae*			
Flexor carpi radialis (musculus flexor carpi radialis [NA])	Medial epicondyle of humerus	Base of second metacarpal	Median	Flexes wrist joint
Flexor carpi radialis brevis (variable)	Lateral surface of distal half of radius	Variable into carpus or index finger	Median	Flexes wrist joint
Flexor carpi ulnaris (musculus flexor carpi ulnaris [NA])	Medial epicondyle of humerus	Pisiform, hamulus of hamate, and proximal end of fifth metacarpal	Ulnar	Flexes wrist joint
Flexor carpi ulnaris brevis (variable)	Distal one-fourth of palmar surface of ulna	Pisiform, hamulus of hamate, and proximal end of fifth metacarpal	Ulnar	Flexes wrist joint
Flexor digiti minimi brevis of foot (musculus flexor digiti minimi brevis [NA])	Base of fifth metatarsal and plantar fascia	Lateral side of proximal phalanx of little toe	Lateral plantar	Flexes little toe at metatarsophalangeal joint
Flexor digiti minimi brevis of hand (musculus flexor digiti minimi brevis [NA])	Hamulus of hamate and flexor retinaculum	Medial side of proximal phalanx of little finger	Ulnar	Flexes metacarpophalangeal joint of little finger
Flexor digitorum accessorius (musculus flexor accessorius [NA alternative])	See *Quadratus plantae*			
Flexor digitorum brevis (musculus flexor digitorum brevis [NA])	Medial tubercle of calcaneus and plantar aponeurosis	Four tendons, one to middle phalanx of each of 4 lateral toes	Medial plantar	Flexes toes at metatarsophalangeal and proximal interphalangeal joints

Name	Origin	Insertion	Innervation	Function
Flexor digitorum longus (musculus flexor digitorum longus [NA])	Posterior aspect of tibia	Four tendons, one to base of distal phalanx of each of 4 lateral toes	Tibial	Flexes toes at metatarsophalangeal and interphalangeal joints
Flexor digitorum profundus (musculus flexor digitorum profundus [NA])	Medial and anterior aspects of ulna and interosseous membrane	Four tendons, one to base of distal phalanx of each finger	Ulnar to medial portion, median to lateral portion	Flexes fingers primarily at distal interphalangeal joints; aids in flexing at wrist and other joints of fingers
Flexor digitorum sublimis	See *Flexor digitorum superficialis*			
Flexor digitorum superficialis (musculus flexor digitorum superficialis [NA])	Medial epicondyle of humerus, coronoid process of ulna, and anterior process of radius	Four tendons, one to base of middle phalanx of each finger	Median	Flexes fingers primarily at proximal interphalangeal joints; aids in flexing wrist and metacarpophalangeal joints
Flexor hallucis brevis (musculus flexor hallucis brevis [NA])	Plantar aspect of cuboid and plantar fascia	Base of proximal phalanx of great toe	Medial plantar	Flexes metatarsophalangeal joint of great toe
Flexor hallucis longus (musculus flexor hallucis longus [NA])	Posterior aspect of fibula	Base of distal phalanx of great toe	Tibial	Flexes great toe; plantar flexes foot; supports arches of foot
Flexor ossis metacarpi pollicis	See *Opponens pollicis*			
Flexor pollicis brevis (musculus flexor pollicis brevis [NA])	Flexor retinaculum and ridge of trapezium	Base of proximal phalanx of thumb	Median	Flexes metacarpophalangeal joint of thumb
Flexor pollicis longus (musculus flexor pollicis longus [NA])	Anterior aspect of radius and interosseous membrane	Base of distal phalanx of thumb	Median	Flexes thumb
Frontalis	See *Occipitofrontalis*			
Gastrocnemius (musculus gastrocnemius [NA])		Posterior surface of calceneus via calcaneal tendon	Tibial	Plantar flexes ankle joint; flexes knee joint
(1) Lateral head (caput laterale musculi gastrocnemii [NA])	Lateral condyle of femur			
(2) Medial head (caput mediale musculi gastrocnemii [NA])	Medial condyle of femur			

TABLE OF MUSCLES (Continued)

Name	Origin	Insertion	Innervation	Function
Gemellus, inferior (musculus gemellus inferior [NA])	Tuber of ischium	Greater trochanter of femur	Nerve to quadratus femoris	Rotates femur laterally
Gemellus, superior (musculus gemellus superior [NA])	Spine of ischium	Greater trochanter of femur	Nerve to obturator internus	Rotates femur laterally
Genioglossus (musculus genioglossus [NA])	Upper mental tubercle of mandible	Hyoid and lateral side of tongue	Hypoglossal	Protrudes and depresses tongue
Geniohyoglossus	See *Genioglossus*			
Geniohyoid (musculus geniohyoideus [NA])	Lower mental tubercle of mandible	Body of hyoid	Superior ramus of ansa cervicalis	Elevates and draws hyoid forward
Geniopharyngeus (variable)	Occasional slip of genioglossus to superior constrictor of pharynx			
Glossopalatinus	See *Palatoglossus*			
Glossopharyngeus (pars glossopharyngea musculi constrictoris pharyngis superioris [NA])	Part of superior constrictor of pharynx			
Gluteus maximus (musculus gluteus maximus [NA])	Lateral surface of ilium, posterior surface of ischium and coccyx, and sacrotuberous ligament	Gluteal tuberosity and iliotibial tract	Inferior gluteal	Extends hip joint; extends trunk on legs when raising body from a seated position
Gluteus medius (musculus gluteus medius [NA])	Lateral surface of ilium	Greater trochanter	Superior gluteal	Abducts femur
Gluteus minimus (musculus gluteus minimus [NA])	Lateral surface of ilium	Greater trochanter	Superior gluteal	Abducts and medially rotates femur
Gluteal, small anterior (variable) (gluteal, fourth)	Occasional accessory slip of gluteus minimus			
Gracilis (musculus gracilis [NA])	Pubis	Medial surface of tibia	Obturator	Adducts femur; flexes knee joint
Hamstrings	Semimembranosus, semitendinosus, and biceps femoris as a group			

Name	Origin	Insertion	Innervation	Function
Helicis major (vestigial) (musculus helicis major [NA])	Spina helicis	Ascending part of helix	Facial	
Helicis minor (vestigial) (musculus helicis minor [NA])	Spina helicis	Crux of helix	Facial	
Hyoglossus (musculus hyoglossus [NA])	Body and greater cornu of hyoid	Side of tongue	Hypoglossal	Depresses tongue
Hyopharyngeus	See *Constrictor of pharynx, middle*			
Iliacus (musculus iliacus [NA])	Iliac fossa and sacrum	Lesser trochanter	Femoral	Flexes hip joint and trunk on lower extremity
Iliacus minor (variable) (musculus psoas minor [NA])	Occasional separate lateral part of iliacus			
Iliocapsulotrochantericus (variable)	Occasional separate slip of iliacus			
Iliococcygeus (musculus iliococcygeus [NA])	Part of levator ani			
Iliocostalis (lateral part of erector spinae) (musculus iliocostalis [NA])			Posterior rami of spinal	Extends vertebral column and assists in lateral movements of trunk
(1) Cervicis (musculus iliocostalis cervicis [NA])	Upper 6 ribs	Posterior tubercles of transverse processes of fourth, fifth, and sixth cervical vertebrae		
(2) Lumborum (musculus iliocostalis lumborum [NA])	Iliac crest, lumbar vertebrae, sacrum, and lumbodorsal fascia	Lower 6 ribs		
(3) Thoracis (musculus iliocostalis thoracis [NA])	Lower 6 ribs	Upper 6 ribs		
Iliocostalis dorsi	See *Iliocostalis thoracis*			
Iliocostocervicalis	See *Iliocostalis cervicis; Iliocostalis thoracis*			

Name	Origin	Insertion	Innervation	Function
Iliopsoas (musculus iliopsoas [NA])	Combined iliacus and psoas			
Incisive, of lower lip (musculi incisivi labii inferioris)	Portion of orbicularis oris			
Incisive, of upper lip (musculi incisivi labii superioris)	Portion of orbicularis oris			
Inferior constrictor of pharynx	See *Constrictor of pharynx, inferior*			
Inferior lingual	See *Longitudinalis of tongue*			
Inferior oblique	See *Oblique, inferior*			
Inferior rectus	See *Rectus inferior bulbi*			
Inferior tarsal	See *Tarsal*			
Infraclavicularis (variable)	Occasional slip of pectoralis major passing over clavicle			
Infracostals	See *Subcostals*			
Infraspinatus (musculus infraspinatus [NA])	Infraspinous fossa of scapula	Greater tubercle of humerus	Suprascapular	Rotates humerus laterally
Interarytenoideus	See *Arytenoid*			
Intercostal, external (musculi intercostales externi [NA])	Lower border of rib above	Superior border of rib below	Anterior rami of thoracic	Accessory muscles of respiration (inhalation)
Intercostal, innermost (musculi intercostales intimi [NA])	Lower border of rib above	Superior border of rib below	Anterior rami of thoracic	Accessory muscles of respiration (exhalation)
Intercostal, internal (musculi intercostales interni [NA])	Lower border of rib above	Superior border of rib below	Anterior rami of thoracic	Accessory muscles of respiration (exhalation)
Internal oblique of abdomen	See *Oblique, internal abdominal*			
Interossei, dorsal (of foot) (4) (musculi interossei dorsales [NA])	Each by 2 heads from sides of adjacent metatarsals	Extensor tendon of each of 4 lateral toes	Lateral plantar	Abduct toes; aid in flexion at metatarsophalangeal joints and in extension at interphalangeal joints

Name	Origin	Insertion	Innervation	Function
Interossei, dorsal (of hand) (4) (musculi interossei dorsales [NA])	Each by 2 heads from sides of adjacent metacarpals	Extensor tendons of second, third, and fourth fingers	Ulnar	Abduct fingers; aid in flexion at metacarpophalangeal joints and in extension at interphalangeal joints
Interossei, palmar (3) (musculi interossei palmares [NA])	Medial side of second and lateral side of fourth and fifth metacarpals, respectively	Extensor tendons of second, third, and fourth fingers	Ulnar	Adduct second, fourth, and fifth fingers and assist dorsal interossei
Interossei, plantar (3) (musculi interossei plantares [NA])	Medial side of third, fourth, and fifth metatarsals, respectively	Extensor tendons of third, fourth, and fifth toes	Lateral plantar	Adduct toes and assist dorsal interossei
Interossei, volar	See *Interossei, palmar*			
Interspinales (musculi interspinales [NA])			Dorsal rami of spinal	Rotate and extend the vertebral column
(1) Cervicis (musculi interspinales cervicis [NA])	Spine of vertebra below	Spine of vertebra above		
(2) Lumborum (musculi interspinales lumborum [NA])	Spine of vertebra below	Spine of vertebra		
(3) Thoracis (musculi interspinales thoracis [NA])	Spine of vertebra below	Spine of vertebra above		
Intertransversales	See *Intertransverse*			
Intertransverse (musculi intertransversarii [NA])			Anterior rami of spinal for lateral portions; posterior rami of spinal for medial portions	Lateral movements of vertebral column
(1) Cervical (a) Anterior (musculi intertransversarii anteriores cervicis [NA])	Transverse process of cervical vertebra	Transverse process of contiguous cervical vertebra		
(b) Posterior (musculi intertransversarii posteriores cervicis [NA])				

Name	Origin	Insertion	Innervation	Function
Intertransverse (musculi intertransversarii [NA]) (Continued)				
(2) Lumbar (a) Lateral (musculi intertransversarii laterales lumborum [NA])	Transverse process of lumbar vertebra	Transverse process of contiguous lumbar vertebra		
(b) Medial (musculi intertransversarii mediales lumborum [NA])				
(3) Thoracic (variable) (musculi intertransversarii thoracis [NA])	Transverse process of thoracic vertebra	Transverse process of contiguous thoracic vertebra		
Invertor femoris (variable)	Occasional extra slip of gluteus minimus			
Ischiobulbosus (variable)	Ischium	Perineal raphe	Perineal	Assists bulbospongiosus
Ischiocavernosus (musculus ischiocavernosus [NA])	Ischium	Crus of penis (clitoris)	Perineal	Assists in erection
Ischiococcygeus	See *Coccygeus*			
Ischiofemoralis (variable)	Occasional extra slip of gluteus maximus arising from ischial tuber			
Ischiopubicus (variable)	Portion of sphincter of urethra			
Laryngopharyngeus	See *Constrictor of pharynx, inferior*			
Lateral cricoarytenoid	See *Cricoarytenoid, lateral*			
Lateral rectus	See *Rectus lateralis*			
Latissimocondyloid (variable)	Occasional slip of latissimus dorsi to olecranon			
Latissimus colli	See *Platysma*			

Name	Origin	Insertion	Innervation	Function
Latissimus dorsi (musculus latissimus dorsi [NA])	Spines of lower 6 thoracic vertebrae, spines of lumbar vertebrae, lumbodorsal fascia, crest of ilium, lower ribs, and inferior angle of scapula	Intertubercular sulcus of humerus	Thoracodorsal	Adducts and extends humerus; used to pull body upward in climbing; accessory muscle of respiration
Latissimus thoracis	See *Latissimus dorsi*			
Levator anguli oris (musculus levator anguli oris [NA])	Maxilla	Skin of angle of mouth	Facial	Muscle of facial expression
Levator anguli scapulae	See *Levator scapulae*			
Levator ani (musculus levator ani [NA])			Anterior rami of third and fourth sacral, and perineal	Supports pelvic viscera
(1) Iliococcygeus (musculus iliococcygeus [NA])	Pelvic surface of ischial spine and pelvic fascia	Central point of perineum, anococcygeal raphe, and coccyx		
(2) Levator prostatae (musculus levator prostatae [NA])		Some fibers inserted into the prostate		
(3) Pubococcygeus (musculus pubococcygeus [NA])	Pubis and pelvic fascia			
(4) Puborectalis (musculus puborectalis [NA])	Pubis	Some fibers that form a sling around the lower part of the rectum		
Levator claviculae (variable)	Occasional slip of levator scapulae inserted into clavicle			
Levator epiglottiidis (variable)	Occasional slip of genioglossus to epiglottis			
Levator glandulae thyroideae (variable) (musculus levator glandulae thyroideae [NA])	Hyoid	Isthmus of thyroid gland		
Levator labii superioris (musculus levator labii superioris [NA])	Maxilla	Skin of upper lip	Facial	Muscle of facial expression

Name	Origin	Insertion	Innervation	Function
Levator labii superioris alaeque nasi (musculus levator labii superioris alaeque nasi [NA])	Maxilla	Skin of upper lip and ala of nose	Facial	Muscle of facial expression
Levator menti	See *Mentalis*			
Levator palati	See *Levator veli palatini*			
Levator palpebrae superioris (musculus levator palpebrae superioris [NA])	Roof of orbit	Skin of upper eyelid and superior tarsus	Oculomotor	Raises upper eyelid
Levator prostatae	See *Levator ani*			
Levator scapulae (musculus levator scapulae [NA])	Transverse process of upper cervical vertebrae	Medial margin and superior angle of scapula	Dorsal scapular and anterior rami of third and fourth cervical	Elevates shoulder; rotates inferior angle of scapula medially
Levator veli palatini (musculus levator veli palatini [NA])	Apex of petrous part of temporal bone and cartilaginous part of auditory tube	Aponeurosis of soft palate	Pharyngeal plexus	Raises soft palate
Levatores costarum (12 pairs) (musculi levatores costarum [NA])	Transverse process of vertebra (seventh cervical to eleventh thoracic)	Angle of rib below	Anterior rami of thoracic	Aid in raising ribs
(1) Breves (musculi levatores costarum breves [NA])				
(2) Longi (musculi levatores costarum longi [NA])				
Longissimus (middle part of erector spinae) (musculus longissimus [NA])			Posterior rami of spinal	Extends vertebral column and assists in rotation and lateral movements of trunk
(1) Capitis (musculus longissimus capitis [NA])	Transverse processes of upper 6 thoracic vertebrae and articular processes of lower 4 cervical vertebrae	Mastoid process of temporal bone		
(2) Cervicis (musculus longissimus cervicis [NA])	Transverse processes of upper 6 thoracic vertebrae	Transverse processes of second to sixth cervical vertebrae		

Name	Origin	Insertion	Innervation	Function
Longissimus (middle part of erector spinae) (musculus longissimus [NA]) (Continued)				
(3) Thoracis (musculus longissimus thoracis [NA])	Iliac crest, sacroiliac ligament, spines of lumbar and sacral vertebrae	Ribs and transverse processes of thoracic and upper lumbar vertebrae		
Longissimus dorsi	See *Longissimus thoracis*			
Longitudinalis of tongue	Base of tongue	Tip of tongue	Hypoglossal	Alters shape of tongue
(1) Inferior (musculus longitudinalis inferior [NA])				
(2) Superior (musculus longitudinalis superior [NA])				
Longus capitis (musculus longus capitis [NA])	Transverse processes of third and sixth cervical vertebrae	Basal portion of occipital bone	Anterior rami of upper 4 cervical	Flexes head
Longus cervicis	See *Longus colli*			
Longus colli (musculus longus colli [NA])			Anterior rami of cervical	Flexes vertebral column
(1) Inferior oblique portion	Bodies of first 3 thoracic vertebrae	Anterior tubercles of fifth and sixth cervical vertebrae		
(2) Superior oblique portion	Transverse processes of third to fifth thoracic vertebrae	Anterior tubercle of atlas		
(3) Vertical portion	Bodies of last 3 cervical and first 3 thoracic vertebrae	Bodies of second to fourth cervical vertebrae		
Lumbricals of fingers (4) (musculi lumbricales [NA])	Tendons of flexor digitorum profundus muscle	One to extensor tendon of each finger	Two lateral by median and 2 medial by ulnar	Flex at metacarpophalangeal joints and extend at interphalangeal joints
Lumbricals of toes (4) (musculi lumbricales [NA])	Tendons of flexor digitorum longus	One to extensor tendon of each of 4 lateral toes	Medial one by medial plantar, others by lateral plantar	Flex at metatarsophalangeal joints and extend at interphalangeal joints
Masseter (musculus masseter [NA])	Arch of zygoma	Ramus and angle of mandible	Mandibular	Muscle of mastication; closes mouth and clenches teeth

Name	Origin	Insertion	Innervation	Function
Mentalis (musculus mentalis [NA])	Incisor fossa of mandible	Skin of chin	Facial	Muscle of facial expression
Middle constrictor of pharynx	See *Constrictor of pharynx, middle*			
Multifidus (part of transverse spinal) (musculi multifidi [NA])	Sacrum, sacroiliac ligament, mammillary processes of lumbar vertebrae, transverse processes of thoracic vertebrae, articular processes of lower 4 cervical vertebrae	Spines of vertebrae	Posterior rami of spinal	Extends and rotates vertebral column
Mylohyoid (musculus mylohyoideus [NA])	Mylohyoid line of mandible	Hyoid	Nerve to mylohyoid	Elevates hyoid and supports floor of mouth
Mylopharyngeal (pars mylopharyngea musculi constrictoris pharyngis superioris [NA])	Portion of superior constrictor of pharynx			
Nasalis (musculus nasalis [NA])			Facial	
(1) Alar part (pars alaris musculi nasalis [NA])	Maxilla	Ala of nose		Widens nasal opening
(2) Transverse part (pars transversa musculi nasalis [NA])	Maxilla	Bridge of nose		Depresses nasal cartilage
Oblique arytenoid	See *Arytenoid, oblique*			
Oblique, auricular	See *Auricular, oblique*			
Oblique, external abdominal (musculus obliquus externus abdominis [NA])	Lower 8 ribs	Xiphoid, linea alba, crest of ilium, pubis	Lower 6 thoracic	Supports abdominal viscera; flexes vertebral column
Oblique, inferior of eye (musculus obliquus inferior bulbi [NA])	Medial aspect of floor of orbit	Sclera	Oculomotor	Rotates eyeball upward and outward
Oblique, inferior of head (musculus obliquus capitis inferior [NA])	Spine of axis	Transverse process of atlas	Posterior ramus of first cervical	Aids in extension and lateral movements of head

Name	Origin	Insertion	Innervation	Function
Oblique, internal abdominal (musculus obliquus internus abdominis [NA])	Lumbodorsal fascia, iliac crest, inguinal ligament	Lower 3 ribs, linea alba, xiphoid, pubis	Lower 6 thoracic and iliohypogastric	Supports abdominal viscera; flexes vertebral column
Oblique, superior of eye (musculus obliquus superior [NA])	Margin of optic canal	Sclera	Trochlear	Rotates eyeball downward and outward
Oblique, superior of head (musculus obliquus capitis superior [NA])	Transverse process of atlas	Occipital bone	Posterior ramus of first cervical	Aids in extension and lateral movements of head
Obturator externus (musculus obturatorius externus [NA])	Pubis, ischium, and superficial surface of obturator membrane	Trochanteric fossa of femur	Obturator	Rotates femur laterally
Obturator internus (musculus obturatorius internus [NA])	Pubis, ischium, and deep surface of obturator membrane	Greater trochanter of femur	Nerve to obturator internus	Rotates femur laterally
Occipitalis	See *Occipitofrontalis*			
Occipitalis minor (variable)	See *Transverse nuchal*			
Occipitofrontalis (musculus occipitofrontalis [NA])			Facial	
(1) Frontal part (venter frontalis musculi occipitofrontalis [NA])	Galea aponeurotica	Skin of forehead		Elevates eyebrows and draws scalp forward
(2) Occipital part (venter occipitalis musculi occipitofrontalis [NA])	Superior nuchal line of occipital bone	Galea aponeurotica		Draws scalp backward
Occipitoscapular (variable)	Occasional extra slip of rhomboideus major			
of Aeby	See *Depressor labii inferioris*			
of Albinus	See *Risorius; Scalene, least*			
of Bell	Smooth muscle of urinary bladder running forward from each ureteric orifice			

Name	Origin	Insertion	Innervation	Function
of Bochdalak	See *Triticeoglossus*			
of Bowman	See *Ciliary*			
of Boyden	See *Sphincter of common bile duct*			
of Brücke	See *Ciliary, meridional portion*			
of Chassaignac	One of the axillary arch muscles			
of Gantzer	See *Accessorius ad flexorem digitorum profundum; Accessorius ad flexorem carpi radialem; Accessorius ad flexorem pollicis longum*			
of Gegenbauer	See *Auriculofrontalis*			
of Gruber	See *Peroneocalcaneus externus*			
of Guthrie	See *Sphincter urethrae*			
of Hall	See *Ischiobulbosus*			
of Henle	See *Auricular, anterior*			
of Hilton	See *Aryepiglotticus*			
of Horner	See *Orbicularis oculi, lacrimal part*			
of Houston	See *Compressor venae dorsalis*			
of incisure of helix (variable)	Bridges incisure of helix			
of Jung	See *Pyramidal of ear*			
of Klein	See *Compressor labii*			
of Langer	One of axillary arch muscles			
of Landström	Smooth fibers in orbital fascia			
of Ludwig	See *Aryvocalis*			
of Macallister	See *Fibulocalcaneus*			

Name	Origin	Insertion	Innervation	Function
of Merkel	See *Ceratocricoid*			
of Müller	See *Orbital; Tarsal; Ciliary, circular portion*			
of Oddi	See *Sphincter of hepatopancreatic ampulla*			
of Raux	See *Rectourethralis*			
of Riolan	See *Orbicularis oculi, ciliary part*			
of Rouget	See *Ciliary, circular portion*			
of Santorini	See *Risorius*			
of Treitz	See *Rectococcygeus; Suspensory of duodenum*			
of Wilson	See *Sphincter urethrae*			
of Wood	See *Extensor carpi radialis intermedius*			
Omohyoid (musculus omohyoideus [NA])			Ansa cervicalis	Depresses hyoid
(1) Inferior belly (venter inferior musculi omohyoidei [NA])	Superior margin of scapula	Intermediate tendon		
(2) Superior belly (venter superior musculi omohyoidei [NA])	Intermediate tendon	Hyoid		
Opponens digiti minimi of foot	See *Opponens digiti quinti of foot*			
Opponens digiti minimi of hand (musculus opponens digiti minimi [NA])	Flexor retinaculum and hamulus of hamate	Medial aspect of fifth metacarpal	Ulnar	Deepens palm
Opponens digiti quinti of foot (variable) (musculus opponens digiti quinti)	Occasional insertion of part of flexor digiti minimi brevis into fifth metatarsal			

Name	Origin	Insertion	Innervation	Function
Opponens digiti quinti of hand	See *Opponens digiti minimi of hand*			
Opponens hallucis (variable)	Occasional insertion of some fibers of flexor hallucis brevis into shaft of first metatarsal			
Opponens pollicis (musculus opponens pollicis [NA])	Ridge of trapezium and flexor retinaculum	First metacarpal	Median	Opposes thumb
Orbicularis oculi (musculus orbicularis oculi [NA]) (1) Ciliary part (2) Lacrimal part (pars lacrimalis musculi orbicularis oculi [NA]) (3) Orbital part (pars orbitalis musculi orbicularis oculi [NA]) (4) Palpebral part (pars palpebralis musculi orbicularis oculi [NA])	Medial aspect of orbit	Skin about eyelids	Facial	Closes lids; muscle of facial expression
Orbicularis oris (musculus orbicularis oris [NA]) (1) Labial part (pars labialis musculi orbicularis oris [NA]) (2) Marginal part (pars marginalis musculi orbicularis oris [NA])	Lies in skin about mouth		Facial	Closes lips; muscle of facial expression
Orbicularis palpebrarum	See *Orbicularis oculi*			
Orbital (smooth) (musculus orbitalis [NA])	Bridges inferior orbital fissure		Sympathetic	
Palatoglossus (musculus palatoglossus [NA])	Inferior surface of soft palate	Side of tongue	Accessory	Elevates tongue and constricts fauces

Name	Origin	Insertion	Innervation	Function
Palatopharyngeus (musculus palatopharyngeus [NA])	Soft palate and auditory tube	Aponeurosis of pharynx	Accessory	Aids in swallowing
Palmaris brevis (musculus palmaris brevis [NA])	Palmar aponeurosis	Skin of medial border of hand	Ulnar	Deepens palm
Palmaris longus (variable) (musculus palmaris longus [NA])	Medial epicondyle of humerus	Flexor retinaculum and palmar aponeurosis	Median	Flexes wrist joint
Papillary (cardiac) (musculi papillares [NA])	Ventricles of heart		Autonomic	Contract in systole of heart
(1) Anterior of left ventricle (musculus papillaris anterior ventriculi sinistri [NA])				
(2) Anterior of right ventricle (musculus papillaris anterior ventriculi dextri [NA])				
(3) Posterior of left ventricle (musculus papillaris posterior ventriculi sinistri [NA])				
(4) Posterior of right ventricle (musculus papillaris posterior ventriculi dextri [NA])				
(5) Septal of right ventricle (musculi papillares septales [NA])				
Pectinate (cardiac) (musculi pectinati [NA])	Auricles of heart		Autonomic	Contract in systole of heart
Pectineus (musculus pectineus [NA])	Pubis	Femur distal to lesser trochanter	Femoral (occasionally obturator)	Adducts femur and flexes hip joint
Pectoralis major (musculus pectoralis major [NA])	Clavicle, sternum, first 6 ribs, aponeurosis of external oblique abdominal muscle	Intertubercular sulcus of humerus, lateral side	Medial and lateral anterior thoracic	Adducts and medially rotates humerus; flexes shoulder joint; depresses shoulder girdle

Name	Origin	Insertion	Innervation	Function
Pectoralis minor (musculus pectoralis minor [NA])	Third to fifth ribs	Coracoid process of scapula	Medial and lateral anterior thoracic	Draws shoulder forward
Pectorodorsalis (variable)	Occasional slip of muscle in axillary fascia			
Peroneocalcaneus externus (variable)	Occasional slip of insertion of peroneus brevis or longus into calcaneus			
Peroneocalcaneus internus (variable)	Occasional extra slip of tibialis posterior			
Peroneocuboideus (variable)	Occasional slip of insertion of peroneus brevis or longus into cuboid			
Peroneotibialis (variable)	Occasional extra slip of popliteus			
Peroneus accessorius (variable)	Occasional extra slip of peroneus brevis or longus			
Peroneus brevis (musculus peroneus brevis [NA])	Lateral surface of fibula	Base of fifth metatarsal	Superficial peroneal	Everts and plantar flexes foot
Peroneus longus (musculus peroneus longus [NA])	Lateral condyle of tibia and lateral surface of fibula	First cuneiform and first metatarsal	Superficial peroneal	Everts and plantar flexes foot; supports arches
Peroneus tertius (musculus peroneus tertius [NA])	Medial surface of fibula	Fifth metatarsal	Deep peroneal	Everts and dorsiflexes foot
Petropharyngeus (variable)	Occasional slip from petrous part of temporal bone to pharynx			
Petrosalpingostaphylinus	See *Levator veli palatini*			
Petrostaphylinus	See *Levator veli palatini*			
Pharyngopalatinus (musculus pharyngopalatinus)	See *Palatopharyngeus*			

Name	Origin	Insertion	Innervation	Function
Piriformis (musculus piriformus [NA])	Second to fifth sacral vertebrae, ilium, and sacrotuberous ligament	Greater trochanter of femur	Anterior rami of first and second sacral	Rotates femur laterally
Plantaris (variable) (musculus plantaris [NA])	Lateral condyle of femur	Calcaneus	Tibial	Flexes knee joint; plantar flexes foot
Platysma (platysma [NA])	Fascia of neck	Mandible and skin about mouth	Facial	Muscle of facial expression
Platysma myoides	See *Platysma*			
Pleuroesophageal (smooth) (musculus pleuroesophageus [NA])	Fibers from left mediastinal pleura to esophagus		Autonomic	
Popliteus (musculus popliteus [NA])	Lateral condyle of femur	Back of tibia	Tibial	Rotates tibia medially; flexes knee joint
Popliteus minor	Part of popliteus inserted into back of capsule of knee joint			
Posterior cricoarytenoid	See *Cricoarytenoid, posterior*			
Procerus (musculus procerus [NA])	Skin over nose	Skin of forehead	Facial	Muscle of facial expression
Pronator pedis	See *Quadratus plantae*			
Pronator quadratus (musculus pronator quadratus [NA])	Anterior surface of ulna	Anterior surface of radius	Palmar interosseous	Pronates forearm
Pronator radii teres	See *Pronator teres*			
Pronator teres (musculus pronator teres [NA])	(1) Medial epicondyle of humerus (2) Coronoid of ulna	Lateral aspect of radius	Median	Pronates forearm
Psoas magnus	See *Psoas major*			
Psoas major (part of iliopsoas) (musculus psoas major [NA])	Lumbar vertebrae and fascia	Lesser trochanter of femur	Anterior rami of second and third lumbar	Flexes hip joint and trunk on lower extremity
Psoas minor (variable) (musculus psoas minor [NA])	Last thoracic and first lumbar vertebrae	Iliopectineal eminence	Anterior ramus of first lumbar	Flexes trunk on pelvis

Name	Origin	Insertion	Innervation	Function
Psoas parvus	See *Psoas minor*			
Pterygoid, external	See *Pterygoid, lateral*			
Pterygoid, internal	See *Pterygoid, medial*			
Pterygoid, lateral (musculus pterygoideus lateralis [NA])	(1) Sphenoid (2) Lateral pterygoid plate	Neck of mandible and capsule of temporomandibular joint	Mandibular	Muscle of mastication; protrudes mandible
Pterygoid, medial (musculus pterygoideus medialis [NA])	(1) Lateral pterygoid plate (2) Tubercle of maxilla	Medial surface of angle of mandible	Mandibular	Muscle of mastication; clenches teeth
Pterygopharyngeus (pars pterygopharyngea musculi constrictoris pharyngis superioris [NA])	Portion of superior constrictor of pharynx			
Pterygospinous (variable)	Occasional slip from spine of sphenoid to medial pterygoid plate			
Pubocavernosus (variable)	Occasional slip of ischiocavernosus arising from pubis			
Pubococcygeus (musculus pubococcygeus [NA])	Portion of levator ani			
Puboprostatic (smooth) (musculus puboprostaticus [NA])	Fibers in pelvic fascia between pubis and prostate		Autonomic	
Puborectalis (musculus puborectalis [NA])	Part of levator ani			
Pubovaginalis (musculus pubovaginalis [NA alternative])	Part of levator ani; in female corresponds to levator prostatae in male			
Pubovesicalis (smooth) (musculus pubovesicalis [NA])	Fibers in pelvic fascia between pubis and urinary bladder		Autonomic	
Pyramidal, abdominal (variable) (musculus pyramidalis [NA])	Pubis	Linea alba	Anterior ramus of twelfth thoracic	Supports abdominal viscera

Name	Origin	Insertion	Innervation	Function
Pyramidal of ear (vestigial) (musculus pyramidalis auriculae [NA])	Part of tragicus			
Pyramidalis nasi	See *Procerus*			
Quadratus femoris (musculus quadratus femoris [NA])	Ischial tuber	Quadrate tubercle of femur	Nerve to quadratus femoris	Adducts and laterally rotates femur
Quadratus labii inferiores	See *Depressor labii inferioris*			
Quadratus labii superioris	See *Levator labii superioris*			
Quadratus lumborum (musculus quadratus lumborum [NA])	Iliac crest, lumbodorsal fascia, and lumbar vertebrae	Last rib	Anterior rami of first 3 lumbar	Assists in lateral movements of vertebral column
Quadratus menti	See *Depressor labii inferioris*			
Quadratus plantae (musculus quadratus plantae [NA])	Calcaneus and plantar fascia	Tendons of flexor digitorum longus	Lateral plantar	Assists in flexion of toes
Quadriceps extensor	See *Quadriceps femoris*			
Quadriceps femoris (musculus quadriceps femoris [NA])	Combined rectus femoris and vastus muscles			
Radialis externus brevis	See *Extensor carpi radialis brevis*			
Radialis externus longus	See *Extensor carpi radialis longus*			
Radialis internus	See *Flexor carpi radialis*			
Radiocarpeus (variable)	See *Flexor carpi radialis brevis*			
Rectococcygeus (smooth) (musculus rectococcygeus [NA])	Fibers in pelvic fascia between coccyx and rectum		Autonomic	
Rectourethralis (smooth) (musculus rectourethralis [NA])	Fibers in pelvic fascia between rectum and membranous urethra of male		Autonomic	

Name	Origin	Insertion	Innervation	Function
Rectouterine (smooth) (musculus rectouterinus [NA])	Fibers in pelvic fascia between rectum and cervix of uterus		Autonomic	
Rectovesical (smooth) (musculus rectovesicalis [NA])	Fibers in pelvic fascia between rectum and urinary bladder		Autonomic	
Rectus abdominis (musculus rectus abdominis [NA])	Pubis	Xiphoid, fifth to seventh costal cartilages	Anterior rami of lower 6 thoracic	Supports abdominal viscera; flexes vertebral column
Rectus capitis anterior (musculus rectus capitis anterior [NA])	Lateral portion of atlas	Occipital bone	Anterior rami of first and second cervical	Flexes head
Rectus capitis anticus major	See *Longus capitis*			
Rectus capitis anticus minor	See *Rectus capitis anterior*			
Rectus capitis lateralis (musculus capitis lateralis [NA])	Transverse process of atlas	Occipital bone	Anterior ramus of first cervical	Assists in lateral movements of head
Rectus capitis posterior major (musculus rectus capitis posterior major [NA])	Spine of axis	Occipital bone	Posterior ramus of first cervical	Extends head
Rectus capitis posterior minor (musculus rectus capitis posterior minor [NA])	Posterior tubercle of atlas	Occipital bone	Posterior ramus of first cervical	Extends head
Rectus capitis posticus major	See *Rectus capitis posterior major*			
Rectus capitis posticus minor	See *Rectus capitis posterior minor*			
Rectus externus oculi	See *Rectus lateralis bulbi*			
Rectus femoris (musculus rectus femoris [NA])		Patella and ultimately into tubercle of tibia	Femoral	
(1) Reflected head	Dorsum ilii			Flexes hip joint
(2) Straight head	Anterior inferior spine of ilium			Extends knee joint

Name	Origin	Insertion	Innervation	Function
Rectus inferior bulbi (musculus rectus inferior bulbi [NA])	Lower border of optic canal	Sclera	Oculomotor	Rotates eyeball downward and somewhat inward
Rectus inferior oculi	See *Rectus inferior bulbi*			
Rectus internus oculi	See *Rectus medialis bulbi*			
Rectus lateralis bulbi (musculus rectus lateralis bulbi [NA])	Lateral border of optic canal	Sclera	Abducent	Rotates eyeball laterally
Rectus lateralis oculi	See *Rectus lateralis bulbi*			
Rectus medialis bulbi (musculus rectus medialis bulbi [NA])	Medial border of optic canal	Sclera	Oculomotor	Rotates eyeball medially
Rectus medialis oculi	See *Rectus medialis bulbi*			
Rectus superior bulbi (musculus rectus superior bulbi [NA])	Upper border of optic canal	Sclera	Oculomotor	Rotates eyeball upward and somewhat inward
Rectus superior oculi	See *Rectus superior bulbi*			
Rectus thoracis (variable)	Occasional separate slip associated with sternalis			
Retrahens aurem (vestigial)	See *Auricular, posterior*			
Rhomboideus major (musculus rhomboideus major [NA])	Spines of second to fifth thoracic vertebrae	Medial margin of scapula	Dorsal scapular	Draws scapula backward and aids in rotating inferior angle medially
Rhomboideus minor (musculus rhomboideus minor [NA])	Spines of seventh cervical and first thoracic vertebrae	Medial margin of scapula	Dorsal scapular	Same as rhomboideus major
Rhomboatloideus (variable)	Occasional extra slip of rhomboideus major to atlas			
Rhombooccipitalis	Occipitoscapular			
Risorius (musculus risorius [NA])	Fascia over masseter	Skin at angle of mouth	Facial	Muscle of facial expression

TABLE OF MUSCLES (Continued)

Name	Origin	Insertion	Innervation	Function
Rotatores (part of transversospinalis) (musculi rotatores [NA])			Posterior rami of spinal	Extend and rotate vertebral column
(1) Cervicis (musculi rotatores cervicis [NA])	Transverse processes of cervical vertebrae	Laminae of vertebrae above		
(2) Lumborum (musculi rotatores lumborum [NA])	Transverse processes of lumbar vertebrae	Laminae of vertebrae above		
(3) Thoracis (musculi rotatores thoracis [NA])	Transverse processes of thoracic vertebrae	Laminae of vertebrae above		
Rotatores breves (musculi rotatores breves)	Transverse process of vertebrae below	Laminae of vertebrae above	Posterior rami of spinal	Extend and rotate vertebral column
Rotatores longi (musculi rotatores longi)	Transverse processes of vertebrae	Laminae of vertebrae second above	Posterior rami of spinal	Extend and rotate vertebral column
Sacrococcygeus anterior (musculus sacrococcygeus anterior)	See *Sacrococcygeus ventralis*			
Sacrococcygeus dorsalis (vestigial) (musculus sacrococcygeus dorsalis [NA])	Dorsal aspect of sacrum	Coccyx	Posterior rami of sacral	
Sacrococcygeus posterior	See *Sacrococcygeus dorsalis*			
Sacrococcygeus ventralis (vestigial) (musculus sacrococcygeus ventralis [NA])	Ventral aspect of sacrum	Coccyx	Anterior rami of sacral	
Sacrolumbalis	See *Iliocostalis lumborum*			
Sacrospinalis (musculus sacrospinalis)	See *Erector spinae*			
Salpingopharyngeus (musculus salpingopharyngeus [NA])	Portion of palatopharyngeus arising from auditory tube			
Sartorius (musculus sartorius [NA])	Anterior superior iliac spine	Tibia	Femoral	Flexes hip and knee joints; rotates femur laterally

Name	Origin	Insertion	Innervation	Function
Scalene, anterior (musculus scalenus anterior [NA])	Transverse processes of third to sixth cervical vertebrae	Tubercle of first rib	Anterior rami of third and fourth cervical	Flexes vertebral column laterally; accessory muscle of respiration (inhalation)
Scalene, least (variable) (musculus scalenus minimus [NA])	Occasional extra slip of posterior scalene			
Scalene, middle (musculus scalenus medius [NA])	Transverse processes of second to sixth cervical vertebrae	First rib	Anterior rami of third and fourth cervical	Flexes vertebral column laterally; accessory muscle of respiration (inhalation)
Scalene, posterior (musculus scalenus posterior [NA])	Tubercles of fourth to sixth cervical vertebrae	Second rib	Anterior rami of third and fourth cervical	Flexes vertebral column laterally; accessory muscle of respiration (inhalation)
Scalenus anticus	See *Scalene, anterior*			
Scalenus minimus	See *Scalene, least*			
Scalenus posticus	See *Scalene, posterior*			
Scansorius (variable)	Occasional extra slip of gluteus minimus			
Semimembranosus (musculus semimembranosus [NA])	Ischial tuber	Medial condyle of tibia	Tibial	Flexes knee joint and extends hip joint
Semispinalis (part of transversospinalis) (musculus semispinalis [NA])			Posterior rami of spinal	
(1) Capitis (musculus semispinalis capitis [NA])	Transverse processes of upper 6 thoracic and articular processes of lower 4 cervical vertebrae	Occipital bone		Extends head
(2) Cervicis (musculus semispinalis cervicis [NA])	Transverse processes of upper 6 thoracic and lower 4 cervical vertebrae	Spines of second to fifth cervical vertebrae		Extends and rotates vertebral column
(3) Thoracis (musculus semispinalis thoracis [NA])	Transverse processes of lower 6 thoracic vertebrae	Spines of last 2 cervical and first 4 thoracic vertebrae		
Semispinalis colli	See *Semispinalis cervicis*			

Name	Origin	Insertion	Innervation	Function
Semispinalis dorsi	See *Semispinalis thoracis*			
Semitendinosus (musculus semitendinosus [NA])	Ischial tuber	Medial aspect of proximal portion of tibia	Tibial	Flexes knee joint and extends hip joint
Serratus anterior (musculus serratus anterior [NA])	Upper 8 or 9 ribs	Medial border of scapula	Long thoracic	Draws scapula forward; draws inferior angle laterally
Serratus anticus	See *Serratus anterior*			
Serratus magnus	See *Serratus anterior*			
Serratus posterior inferior (musculus serratus posterior inferior [NA])	Lumbodorsal fascia, spines of lowest thoracic and upper lumbar vertebrae	Last 4 ribs	Lower thoracic	Accessory muscle of respiration
Serratus posterior superior (musculus serratus posterior superior [NA])	Ligamentum nuchae, spines of seventh cervical and upper thoracic vertebrae	Second to fifth ribs	Second and third thoracic	Accessory muscle of respiration
Serratus posticus inferior	See *Serratus posterior inferior*			
Serratus posticus superior	See *Serratus posterior superior*			
Soleus (musculus soleus [NA])	Fibula, popliteal fascia, and tibia	Calcaneus	Tibial	Plantar flexes foot
Sphenosalpingostaphylinus	See *Tensor veli palatini*			
Sphincter ani externus (divided into subcutaneous, superficial, and deep portions) (musculus sphincter ani externus [NA])	Tip of coccyx	Surrounds anus	Pudendal	Closes anus
Sphincter ani internus (smooth) (musculus sphincter ani internus [NA])			Autonomic	
Sphincter of Boyden	See *Sphincter of common bile duct*			
Sphincter of common bile duct (smooth) (musculus sphincter ductus choledochi [NA])	Sphincter in distal part of common duct		Autonomic	

Name	Origin	Insertion	Innervation	Function
Sphincter of hepatopancreatic ampulla (smooth) (musculus sphincter ampullae hepatopancreaticae [NA])	Sphincter of major duodenal papilla		Autonomic	
Sphincter of Oddi	See *Sphincter of hepatopancreatic ampulla*			
Sphincter pupillae (smooth) (musculus sphincter pupillae [NA])	Circular fibers of iris		Parasympathetic (oculomotor)	
Sphincter of pylorus (smooth) (musculus sphincter pylori [NA])	Sphincter of pylorus of stomach		Autonomic	
Sphincter of urinary bladder (smooth) (musculus sphincter vesicae [NA])	Outlet of urinary bladder		Autonomic	
Sphincter oris	See *Orbicularis oris*			
Sphincter urethrae (musculus sphincter urethrae [NA])	Ramus of pubis	Median raphe	Perineal	Compresses urethra
Sphincter vaginae	See *Bulbospongiosus, female*			
Spinalis (medial part of erector spinae) (musculus spinalis [NA])			Posterior rami of spinal	
(1) Capitis (variable) (musculus spinalis capitis [NA])	Spines of upper thoracic and lowest cervical vertebrae	Occipital bone		Extends head
(2) Cervicis (variable) (musculus spinalis cervicis [NA])	Spines of lower cervical and upper thoracic vertebrae	Spines of second to fourth cervical vertebrae		Extends and assists in rotation and lateral movements of trunk
(3) Thoracis (musculus spinalis thoracis [NA])	Spines of lower 2 thoracic and upper 2 lumbar vertebrae	Spines of fourth to eighth thoracic vertebrae		
Spinalis colli	See *Spinalis cervicis*			
Spinalis dorsi	See *Spinalis thoracis*			

Name	Origin	Insertion	Innervation	Function
Splenius capitis (musculus splenius capitis [NA])	Ligamentum nuchae, spines of last cervical and upper thoracic vertebrae	Mastoid process	Posterior rami of spinal	Extends head
Splenius cervicis (musculus splenius cervicis [NA])	Ligamentum nuchae, spines of last cervical and upper thoracic vertebrae	Transverse processes of upper cervical vertebrae	Posterior rami of spinal	Extends vertebral column
Splenius colli	See *Splenius cervicis*			
Stapedius (musculus stapedius [NA])	Pyramidal process	Neck of stapes	Facial	Draws base of stapes toward tympanic cavity
Staphylinus externus	See *Tensor veli palatini*			
Staphylinus internus	See *Levator veli palatini*			
Staphylinus medius	See *Uvulae*			
Sternalis (variable) (musculus sternalis [NA])	Fascia of chest wall		Anterior thoracic	
Sternochondroscapular (variable)	Occasional slip of muscle in axillary fascia			
Sternoclavicularis (variable)	Small extra slip of subclavius occasionally arising from sternum			
Sternocleidomastoid (musculus sternocleidomastoideus [NA])	Manubrium of sternum and clavicle	Mastoid process	Accessory	Flexes head
Sternocostalis	See *Transverse thoracic*			
Sternofascialis (variable)	Occasional slip from manubrium of sternum to fascia of neck			
Sternohyoid (musculus sternohyoideus [NA])	Manubrium of sternum	Hyoid	Ansa cervicalis	Depresses hyoid
Sternothyroid (musculus sternothyroideus [NA])	Manubrium of sternum	Thyroid cartilage	Ansa cervicalis	Depresses larynx

Name	Origin	Insertion	Innervation	Function
Styloauricularis (variable)	Occasional slip from styloid process to cartilage of external ear			
Styloglossus (musculus styloglossus [NA])	Styloid process	Side of tongue	Hypoglossal	Elevates tongue
Stylohyoid (musculus stylohyoideus [NA])	Styloid process	Hyoid	Facial	Elevates hyoid
Stylopharyngeus (musculus stylopharyngeus [NA])	Styloid process	Lateral wall of pharynx	Glossopharyngeal	Pulls up pharynx
Subanconeus	See *Articularis cubiti*			
Subclavius (musculus subclavius [NA])	First costal cartilage and first rib	Clavicle	Nerve to subclavius	Depresses lateral end of clavicle
Subcostals (variable) (musculi subcostales [NA])	Lower ribs	Chest wall	Thoracic	Muscles of respiration
Subcrureus	See *Articularis genus*			
Subcutaneous colli	See *Platysma*			
Subscapular (musculus subscapularis [NA])	Subscapular fossa	Lesser tubercle of humerus	Subscapular	Rotates humerus medially
Superficial transverse of perineum (musculus transversus perinei superficialis [NA])	Tuber of ischium	Central point of perineum	Perineal	Supports perineum
Superior lingual	See *Longitudinalis of tongue*			
Superior oblique	See *Oblique, superior*			
Supinator (musculus supinator [NA])	Lateral epicondyle of humerus, fascia about elbow joint, and shaft of ulna	Radius	Dorsal interosseous of forearm	Supinates forearm
Supinator longus	See *Brachioradialis*			
Supinator radii brevis	See *Supinator*			

Name	Origin	Insertion	Innervation	Function
Supraclavicularis (variable)	Occasional slip from manubrium to clavicle			
Supraspinalis (variable)	Occasional slips between tips of spines of cervical vertebrae			
Supraspinatus (musculus supraspinatus [NA])	Supraspinous fossa	Greater tubercle of humerus	Suprascapular	Abducts humerus
Suspensory of duodenum (smooth) (musculus suspensorius duodeni [NA])	Scattered fibers in suspensory ligament of duodenum		Autonomic	
Tarsal (smooth) (musculus tarsalis inferior et superior [NA])	Smooth muscle in eyelids		Sympathetic	
Temporal	See *Temporalis*			
Temporalis (musculus temporalis [NA])	Temporal fossa	Coronoid process of mandible	Mandibular	Closes mouth; clenches teeth; retracts lower jaw
Temporoparietalis (musculus temporoparietalis [NA])	Part of epicranius			
Tensor fasciae latae (musculus tensor fasciae latae [NA])	Iliac crest	Iliotibial tract and ultimately into tibia	Superior gluteal	Abducts lower extremity; flexes hip joint; extends knee joint
Tensor fasciae suralis (variable)	Occasional slip of biceps femoris into fascia of calf			
Tensor palati	See *Tensor veli palatini*			
Tensor tarsi	Part of orbicularis oculi			
Tensor tympani (musculus tensor tympani [NA])	Cartilaginous portion of auditory tube	Manubrium of malleus	Mandibular	Tenses tympanic membrane
Tensor vaginae femoris	See *Tensor fasciae latae*			
Tensor veli palatini (musculus tensor veli palatini [NA])	Scaphoid fossa of sphenoid and wall of auditory tube	Aponeurosis of soft palate	Mandibular	Tenses soft palate and opens auditory tube

Name	Origin	Insertion	Innervation	Function
Teres major (musculus teres major [NA])	Lateral margin of scapula	Intertubercular sulcus of humerus	Subscapular	Adducts and medially rotates humerus
Teres minor (musculus teres minor [NA])	Lateral margin of scapula	Greater tubercle of humerus	Axillary	Laterally rotates humerus
Thyroarytenoid (musculus thyroarytenoideus [NA])	Lamina of thyroid cartilage	Muscular process of arytenoid cartilage	Recurrent laryngeal	Relaxes vocal folds; closes vestibule of larynx
Thyroarytenoid, external	See *Thyroarytenoid*			
Thyroarytenoid, internal	See *Vocalis*			
Thyroarytenoid, superior (variable)	See *Ventricular*			
Thyroepiglottic (musculus thyroepiglotticus [NA])	Lamina of thyroid cartilage	Epiglottis	Recurrent laryngeal	Closes inlet of larynx
Thyrohyoid (musculus thyrohyoideus [NA])	Thyroid cartilage	Hyoid	Ansa cervicalis	Draws hyoid and thyroid cartilages toward each other
Thyropharyngeus (pars thyropharyngea musculi constrictoris pharyngis inferioris [NA])	Portion of inferior constrictor of pharynx			
Tibialis anterior (musculus tibialis anterior [NA])	Tibia and interosseous membrane	First cuneiform and first metatarsal	Deep peroneal	Dorsiflexes and inverts foot
Tibialis anticus	See *Tibialis anterior*			
Tibialis gracilis	See *Plantaris*			
Tibialis posterior (musculus tibialis posterior [NA])	Fibula, tibia, and interosseous membrane	Bases of metatarsals and all tarsal bones except talus	Tibial	Plantar flexes and inverts foot; supports arches of foot
Tibialis posticus	See *Tibialis posterior*			
Tibialis secundus (variable)	Back of tibia	Capsule of ankle joint		
Tibioaccessorius	See *Quadratus plantae*			

Name	Origin	Insertion	Innervation	Function
Tibiofascialis (variable)	Occasional extra slip of tibialis anterior inserted into fascia of dorsum of foot			
Trachealis (smooth) (musculus trachealis [NA])	Transverse fibers in dorsal wall of trachea	Tracheal cartilages	Autonomic	Lessens caliber of trachea
Trachelomastoid	See *Longissimus capitis*			
Tragicus (vestigial) (musculus tragicus [NA])	Crosses tragus		Facial	
Transversalis abdominis	See *Transverse abdominal*			
Transversalis colli	See *Longissimus cervicis*			
Transverse abdominal (musculus transversus abdominis [NA])	Costal cartilages of lower 6 ribs, lumbodorsal fascia, iliac crest, and inguinal ligament	Xiphoid, linea alba, inguinal ligament, and pubis	Anterior rami of lower 6 thoracic and iliohypogastric	Supports abdominal viscera and flexes vertebral column
Transverse arytenoid	See *Arytenoid*			
Transverse auricular (vestigial)	See *Auricular*			
Transverse of neck	See *Longissimus cervicis*			
Transverse lingual (musculus transversus linguae [NA])	Median septum of tongue	Dorsum and sides of tongue	Hypoglossal	Alters shape of tongue
Transverse mental (musculus transversus menti [NA])	Part of depressor anguli oris			
Transverse nuchal (variable) (musculus transversus nuchae [NA])	Occasional extra slip of occipitofrontalis			
Transverse of foot	See *Adductor hallucis*			
Transverse pedis	See *Adductor hallucis, transverse head*			
Transverse, deep of perineum	See *Deep transverse perineal*			

Name	Origin	Insertion	Innervation	Function
Transverse, superficial perineal	See *Superficial transverse of perineum*			
Transverse spinal	Multifidus, rotatores, and semispinales as a group			
Transverse thoracic (musculus transversus thoracis [NA])	Mediastinal surface of xiphoid and body of sternum	Second to sixth costal cartilages	Anterior rami of thoracic	
Transverse urethral	Part of sphincter urethrae			
Transverse vaginal	Part of sphincter of urethra of female			
Transversospinalis (musculus transversospinalis [NA])	Composed of multifidus, rotatores, and semispinales			
Transversus colli	See *Longissimus cervicis*			
Trapezius (musculus trapezius [NA])	Occipital bone, ligamentum nuchae, spines of seventh cervical and all thoracic vertebrae	Clavicle, acromion, and spine of scapula	Accessory	Rotates inferior angle of scapula laterally; raises shoulder; draws scapula backward
Triangularis	See *Depressor anguli oris*			
Triangularis labii inferioris	See *Depressor anguli oris*			
Triangularis labii superioris	See *Levator anguli oris*			
Triangularis sterni	See *Transverse thoracic*			
Triceps brachii (musculus triceps brachii [NA])		Olecranon of ulna	Radial	Extends elbow joint; long head also aids in adducting humerus
(1) Long head (caput longum musculi tricipitis brachii [NA])	Infraglenoid tubercle			
(2) Lateral head (caput laterale musculi tricipitis brachii [NA])	Shaft of humerus			

Name	Origin	Insertion	Innervation	Function
Triceps brachii (musculus triceps brachii [NA]) (Continued)				
(3) Medial head (caput mediale musculi tricipitis brachii [NA])	Shaft of humerus			
Triceps surae (musculus triceps surae [NA])	Combined gastrocnemius and soleus			
Triticeoglossus (variable)	Occasional slip from base of tongue to triticeous cartilage			
Trochlear	See *Oblique, superior of eye*			
Ulnaris externus	See *Extensor carpi ulnaris*			
Ulnaris internus	See *Flexor carpi ulnaris*			
Uvulae (musculus uvulae [NA])	Posterior nasal spine	Aponeurosis of soft palate	Accessory	
Vastus crureus	See *Vastus intermedius*			
Vastus externus	See *Vastus lateralis*			
Vastus intermedius (musculus vastus intermedius [NA])	Anterior and lateral aspect of femur	Patella and ultimately into tubercle of tibia	Femoral	Extends knee joint
Vastus internus	See *Vastus medialis*			
Vastus lateralis (musculus vastus lateralis [NA])	Capsule of hip joint and lateral aspect of femur	Patella and ultimately into tubercle of tibia	Femoral	Extends knee joint
Vastus medialis (musculus vastus medialis [NA])	Medial aspect of femur	Patella and ultimately into tubercle of tibia	Femoral	Extends knee joint
Ventricular (musculus ventricularis)	Lateral fibers of thyroarytenoid		Vagus	
Vertical lingual (musculus verticalis linguae [NA])	Dorsal aspect of tongue	Sides and base of tongue	Hypoglossal	Alters shape of tongue

Name	Origin	Insertion	Innervation	Function
Vocalis (musculus vocalis [NA])	Medial fibers of thyroarytenoid, internal		Vagus	
Zygomatic	See *Zygomatic, major*			
Zygomatic, major (musculus zygomaticus major [NA])	Zygoma	Skin about mouth	Facial	Muscle of facial expression
Zygomatic, minor (musculus zygomaticus minor [NA])	Zygoma	Skin about mouth	Facial	Muscle of facial expression

Name	Central attachment	Components*	Branches	Distribution
Abducens (sixth cranial) (nervus abducens [NA])	Brainstem at inferior border of pons	Motor	Muscular filaments	Lateral rectus muscle of eyeball
Accessory (eleventh cranial) (nervus accessorius [NA])				
(1) Bulbar part (cranial) (radices craniales [NA])	Lateral aspect of medulla oblongata	Motor	Internal ramus to vagus	Striate muscles of larynx and pharynx
(2) Spinal part (radices spinales [NA])	Upper 5 or 6 cervical segments of cord	Motor	External ramus to cervical plexus	Trapezius and sternocleidomastoid muscles
Accessory obturator	See *Obturator, accessory*			
Accessory phrenic (nervi phrenici accessorii [NA])	Occasional branch from fifth cervical which arises with the subclavian		Joins phrenic	Diaphragm
Acoustic	See *Vestibulocochlear*			
Alveolar, anterior superior (rami alveolares superiores anteriores nervi infraorbitalis [NA])	Infraorbital	Somatic sensory	Filaments	Upper incisor and cuspid teeth, mucosa of nasal floor
Alveolar, inferior (nervus alveolaris inferior [NA])	Mandibular	Somatic sensory	Mental and filaments	Lower teeth, skin of lower lip and chin
		Motor	Mylohyoid	Mylohyoid and anterior belly of digastric muscles
Alveolar, middle superior (ramus alveolaris superior medius nervi infraorbitalis [NA])	Maxillary	Somatic sensory	Filaments	Upper premolar teeth
Alveolar, posterior superior (rami alveolares superiores posteriores nervi infraorbitalis [NA])	Maxillary	Somatic sensory	Filaments	Upper molar teeth and mucosa of maxillary sinus
Alveolar, superior (nervi alveolares superiores [NA])	See *Alveolar, anterior superior, middle superior,* and *posterior superior*			

*Nerves to muscles contain proprioceptive sensory fibers in addition to motor fibers; muscular branches of third, fourth, sixth, and twelfth cranial nerves may be exceptions.

Name	Central attachment	Components*	Branches	Distribution
Ampullary, anterior (nervus ampullaris anterior [NA])	Vestibular	Sensory (movement of head in space—dynamic)	Filaments	Ampulla of anterior semicircular duct
Ampullary, inferior	See *Ampullary, posterior*			
Ampullary, lateral (nervus ampullaris lateralis [NA])	Vestibular	Sensory (movement of head in space—dynamic)	Filaments	Ampulla of lateral semicircular duct
Ampullary, posterior (nervus ampullaris posterior [NA])	Vestibular	Sensory (movement of head in space—dynamic)	Filaments	Ampulla of posterior semicircular duct
Anastomotic, peroneal	See *Peroneal, anastomotic*			
Anococcygeal (nervi anococcygei [NA])	Fourth and fifth sacral and coccygeal segments of cord	Somatic sensory	Filaments	Skin in vicinity of coccyx
Ansa cervicalis (ansa cervicalis [NA])	By a superior and an inferior ramus from first, second, and third cervical segments of spinal cord	Motor	Filaments	Omohyoid, sternohyoid, and sternothyroid muscles
Auditory	See *Vestibulocochlear*			
Auricular (ramus auricularis nervi vagi [NA])	Vagus	Somatic sensory	Filaments	Skin of auricle and external acoustic meatus
Auricular, anterior (nervi auriculares anteriores [NA])	Mandibular	Somatic sensory	Filaments	Skin anterior to external ear
Auricular, great (nervus auricularis magnus [NA])	Second and third cervical segments (cervical plexus)	Somatic sensory	Auricular, facial, and mastoid branches	Skin about ear
Auricular, posterior (nervus auricularis posterior [NA])	Facial	Motor	Filaments	Occipital and intrinsic muscles of auricle, stylohyoid and posterior belly of digastric muscles
Auriculotemporal (nervus auriculotemporalis [NA])	Mandibular	Somatic sensory	Filaments	Skin of scalp and temple, temporomandibular joint
Axillary (nervus axillaris [NA])	Fifth and sixth cervical segments of cord (brachial plexus)	Motor	Muscular, articular, and cutaneous branches	Deltoid and teres minor muscles
		Somatic sensory	Lateral cutaneous of arm	Skin of lateral aspect of shoulder and arm

Name	Central attachment	Components*	Branches	Distribution
Bigeminus	Old name for third sacral nerve			
Buccal (nervus buccalis [NA])	Mandibular	Somatic sensory	Filaments	Skin and mucosa of cheek
Buccinator	See *Buccal*			
Calcaneal (rami calcanei laterales nervi suralis [NA])	Sural	Somatic sensory	Filaments	Skin of heel
Cardiac, inferior cervical (nervus cardiacus cervicalis inferior [NA])	Inferior cervical ganglion	Sympathetic. Visceral sensory	To cardiac plexuses	Heart
Cardiac, inferior or thoracic (nervus cardiacus inferior)	Vagus	Parasympathetic. Visceral sensory	To cardiac plexuses	Heart
Cardiac, middle (nervus cardiacus medius)	Vagus	Parasympathetic. Visceral sensory	To cardiac plexuses	Heart
Cardiac, middle cervical (nervus cardiacus cervicalis medius [NA])	Middle cervical ganglion	Sympathetic. Visceral sensory	To cardiac plexuses	Heart
Cardiac, superior (nervus cardiacus superior)	Vagus	Parasympathetic. Visceral sensory	To cardiac plexuses	Heart
Cardiac, superior cervical (nervus cardiacus cervicalis superior [NA])	Superior cervical ganglion	Sympathetic. Visceral sensory	To cardiac plexuses	Heart
Cardiac, thoracic (nervi cardiaci thoracici [NA])	Second to fifth thoracic ganglia	Sympathetic. Visceral sensory	To cardiac plexuses	Heart
Caroticotympanic (nervi caroticotympanici [NA])	Branches between tympanic plexus and internal carotid plexus			
(1) Inferior				
(2) Superior				
Carotid, external (nervi carotici externi [NA])	Superior cervical ganglion	Sympathetic	Plexuses on external carotid artery and its branches	Filaments to smooth muscle and glands of head
Carotid, internal (nervus caroticus internus [NA])	Superior cervical ganglion	Sympathetic	Plexus on internal carotid artery and its branches	Filaments to smooth muscle and glands of head

Name	Central attachment	Components*	Branches	Distribution
Cavernous of penis or clitoris (nervi cavernosi penis, nervi cavernosi clitoridis [NA])	Pelvic plexus	Autonomic	Filaments	Corpora cavernosa of penis or clitoris
Cervical, first (dorsal ramus)	First cervical segment of cord	Motor	Muscular	Deep muscles of back of neck
Cervical, first (ventral ramus)	First cervical segment of cord	Motor	To cervical plexus	Neck muscles
Cervical, second (dorsal ramus)	Second cervical segment of cord	Motor. Somatic sensory	Greater occipital	Deep muscles of back of neck and skin of back of neck
Cervical, second (ventral ramus)	Second cervical segment of cord	Motor. Somatic sensory	To cervical plexus	Neck muscles and skin
Cervical, third (dorsal ramus)	Third cervical segment of cord	Motor. Somatic sensory	Third occipital	Neck muscles and skin
Cervical, third (ventral ramus)	Third cervical segment of cord	Motor. Somatic sensory	To cervical plexus	Neck muscles and skin
Cervical, fourth to eighth (dorsal rami)	Fourth to eighth cervical segments of cord	Motor. Somatic sensory	Muscular and cutaneous	Deep muscles of neck and upper portion of back, skin of upper back
Cervical, fourth (ventral ramus)	Fourth cervical segment of cord	Motor. Somatic sensory	To cervical plexus	Neck muscles, diaphragm
Cervical, fifth to eighth (ventral rami)	Fifth to eighth cervical segments of cord	Motor. Somatic sensory	To brachial plexus	Muscles and skin of upper extremity
Cervical, descending	See *Ansa cervicalis, inferior ramus*			
Cervical, superficial	See *Transverse of neck*			
Chorda tympani [NA])	Intermedius	Parasympathetic	Filaments via lingual	Submandibular and sublingual salivary glands
		Sensory (taste)	Filaments via lingual	Taste buds of anterior two-thirds of tongue
Ciliary, long (nervi ciliares longi [NA])	Nasociliary	Somatic sensory	Filaments	Eyeball
Ciliary, short (nervi ciliares breves [NA])	Ciliary ganglion	Parasympathetic	Filaments	Ciliary muscle and constrictor fibers of iris
	Nasociliary	Somatic sensory	Filaments	Eyeball
Circumflex	See *Axillary*			
Cluneal, inferior (nervi clunium inferiores [NA])	Posterior cutaneous nerve of thigh	Somatic sensory	Filaments	Skin of lower gluteal region

TABLE OF NERVES (Continued)

Name	Central attachment	Components*	Branches	Distribution
Cluneal, medial (nervi clunium medii [NA])	First, second, and third sacral (dorsal rami)	Somatic sensory	Filaments	Skin of medial gluteal region
Cluneal, superior (nervi clunium superiores [NA])	First, second, and third sacral (dorsal rami)	Somatic sensory	Filaments	Skin of upper gluteal region
Clunial	See *Cluneal*			
Coccygeal (nervus coccygeus [NA])	Coccygeal segment of cord	Somatic sensory	Filaments	Skin over coccyx
Cochlear (cochlear part of eighth cranial—vestibulocochlear) (pars cochlearis nervi octavi [NA])	Brainstem at lower border of pons	Somatic sensory	Filaments	Spiral organ (of Corti) of internal ear
Common peroneal	See *Peroneal, common*			
Crural, anterior	See *Femoral*			
Cutaneous, abdominal anterior	Iliohypogastric	Somatic sensory	Filaments	Skin over lower anterior abdomen
Cutaneous, antebrachial, lateral (nervus cutaneus antebrachii lateralis [NA])	Musculocutaneous	Somatic sensory	Filaments	Skin of lateral aspect of forearm
Cutaneous, antebrachial, medial (nervus cutaneus antebrachii medialis [NA])	Brachial plexus	Somatic sensory	Filaments	Skin of medial aspect of forearm
Cutaneous, antebrachial, posterior (nervus cutaneus antebrachii posterior [NA])	Radial	Somatic sensory	Filaments	Skin of posterior aspect of forearm
Cutaneous, antibrachial	See *Cutaneous, antebrachial*			
Cutaneous, brachial, lateral inferior (nervus cutaneus brachii lateralis inferior [NA])	Radial	Somatic sensory	Filaments	Skin of lower lateral aspect of arm
Cutaneous, brachial, lateral superior (nervus cutaneus brachii lateralis superior [NA])	Axillary	Somatic sensory	Filaments	Skin of lateral aspect of arm

Name	Central attachment	Components*	Branches	Distribution
Cutaneous, brachial, medial (nervus cutaneus brachii medialis [NA])	Brachial plexus	Somatic sensory	Filaments	Skin of medial aspect of arm
Cutaneous, brachial, posterior (nervus cutaneus brachii posterior [NA])	Radial	Somatic sensory	Filaments	Skin of posterior aspect of arm
Cutaneous colli	See *Transverse of neck*			
Cutaneous, femoral, medial (anterior internal of thigh)	Femoral	Somatic sensory	Filaments	Skin of medial aspect of thigh
Cutaneous, femoral, middle (anterior middle of thigh)	Femoral	Somatic sensory	Filaments	Skin of anterior middle aspect of thigh
Cutaneous, femoral, lateral (nervus cutaneus femoris lateralis [NA])	Lumbar plexus	Somatic sensory	Filaments	Skin of lateral aspect of thigh
Cutaneous, femoral, posterior (nervus cutaneus femoris posterior [NA])	Sacral plexus	Somatic sensory	Filaments	Skin of posterior aspect of thigh
Cutaneous of arm	See *Cutaneous, brachial*			
Cutaneous of calf	See *Cutaneous, sural*			
Cutaneous of foot				
(1) Cutaneous, dorsal intermediate (nervus cutaneus dorsalis intermedius [NA])	Superficial peroneal	Somatic sensory	Filaments	Skin of dorsum of foot
(2) Cutaneous, dorsal lateral (nervus cutaneus dorsalis lateralis [NA])	Sural	Somatic sensory	Filaments	Skin of dorsolateral part of foot
(3) Cutaneous, dorsal medial (nervus cutaneus dorsalis medialis [NA])	Superficial peroneal	Somatic sensory	Filaments	Skin of dorsomedial part of foot
Cutaneous of forearm	See *Cutaneous, antebrachial*			

Name	Central attachment	Components*	Branches	Distribution
Cutaneous of hand				
(1) Cutaneous, dorsal (ramus dorsalis nervi ulnaris [NA])	Ulnar	Somatic sensory	Filaments	Skin of medial dorsal part of hand
(2) Cutaneous, palmar, lateral (ramus palmaris nervi mediani [NA])	Median	Somatic sensory	Filaments	Skin of lateral part of palm
(3) Cutaneous, palmar, medial (ramus palmaris nervi ulnaris [NA])	Ulnar	Somatic sensory	Filaments	Skin of medial part of palm
Cutaneous of leg	See *Cutaneous, sural*			
Cutaneous of neck	See *Transverse of neck*			
Cutaneous of thigh	See *Cutaneous, femoral*			
Cutaneous, sural, lateral (nervus cutaneus surae lateralis [NA])	Common peroneal	Somatic sensory	Filaments	Skin of lateral part of calf
Cutaneous, sural, medial (nervus cutaneus surae medialis [NA])	Tibial	Somatic sensory	Filaments	Skin of medial part of calf
Cutaneous, perforating (variable)	Pudendal plexus	Somatic sensory	Filaments	Skin of posterior aspect of buttocks
Deep peroneal	See *Peroneal, deep*			
Deep temporal	See *Temporal, deep*			
Dental	See *Alveolar*			
Descendens cervicis	See *Ansa cervicalis, inferior ramus*			
Descendens hypoglossi	See *Ansa cervicalis, superior ramus*			
Digital of fingers				
(1) Dorsal radial (nervi digitales dorsales nervi radialis [NA])	Radial	Somatic sensory	Filaments	Skin of dorsum of lateral fingers
(2) Dorsal ulnar (nervi digitales dorsales nervi ulnaris [NA])	Ulnar	Somatic sensory	Filaments	Skin of dorsum of medial fingers and tips of fingers
(3) Palmar common median (nervi digitales palmares communes nervi mediani [NA])	Median	Somatic sensory	Proper palmar	

Name	Central attachment	Components*	Branches	Distribution
Digital of fingers (Continued)				
(4) Palmar common ulnar (nervi digitales palmares communes nervi ulnaris [NA])	Ulnar	Somatic sensory	Proper palmar	
(5) Palmar proper median (nervi digitales palmares proprii nervi mediani [NA])	Common palmar median	Somatic sensory	Filaments	Palmar surface of lateral fingers
(6) Palmar proper ulnar (nervi digitales palmares proprii nervi ulnaris [NA])	Common palmar ulnar	Somatic sensory	Filaments	Palmar surface of medial fingers
Digital of toes				
(1) Dorsal (nervus cutaneus dorsalis intermedius [NA])	Intermediate dorsal cutaneous of foot	Somatic sensory	Filaments	Dorsal aspect of toes
(2) Dorsal of lateral side of great toe and medial side of second toe (nervi digitales dorsales hallucis lateralis et digiti secundi medialis [NA])	Deep peroneal	Somatic sensory	Filaments	Adjacent sides of great and second toes
(3) Plantar common lateral (nervi digitales plantares communes nervi plantaris lateralis [NA])	Lateral plantar	Somatic sensory	Proper plantar	
(4) Plantar common medial (nervi digitales plantares communes nervi plantaris medialis [NA])	Medial plantar	Somatic sensory	Proper plantar	
(5) Plantar proper lateral (nervi digitales planteres proprii nervi plantaris lateralis [NA])	Common lateral plantar	Somatic sensory	Filaments	Plantar aspect of lateral toes
(6) Plantar proper medial (nervi digitales plantares proprii nervi plantaris medialis [NA])	Common medial plantar	Somatic sensory	Filaments	Plantar aspect of medial toes
Dorsal of penis or clitoris (nervus dorsalis penis, nervus dorsalis clitoridis [NA])	Pudendal	Somatic sensory	Filaments	Penis (clitoris)

TABLE OF NERVES (Continued)

Name	Central attachment	Components*	Branches	Distribution
Dorsal scapular (nervus dorsalis scapulae [NA])	Brachial plexus	Motor	Filaments	Major and minor rhomboids, levator scapulae
Erigent (nervi erigentes [NA alternative])	See *Splanchnic, pelvic*			
Ethmoid, anterior (nervus ethmoidalis anterior [NA])	Nasociliary	Somatic sensory	Filaments, external nasal	Mucosa of nasal cavity and anterior ethmoid air cells
Ethmoid, posterior (nervus ethmoidalis posterior [NA])	Nasociliary	Somatic sensory	Filaments	Mucosa of sphenoid and posterior ethmoid air cells
Facial (seventh cranial) (nervus facialis [NA])	Brainstem at level of inferior border of pons	Motor	Stapedial, auricular, temporal, zygomatic, buccal, mandibular, and cervical branches	Stapedius, stylohyoid, posterior belly of digastric, and muscles of facial expression
		Parasympathetic. Sensory (taste) See *Intermedius*		
Femoral (nervus femoralis [NA])	Lumbar plexus	Motor. Somatic sensory	Muscular, articular, saphenous, and cutaneous of thigh	Pectineus, quadriceps femoris, sartorius, iliacus, and skin
Fibular (nervus fibularis communis [NA alternative])	See *Peroneal*			
Fibular, communicating	See *Peroneal, anastomotic*			
Frontal (nervus frontalis [NA])	Ophthalmic	Somatic sensory	Supraorbital, supratrochlear	Skin of upper eyelid, forehead, and scalp
Furcal (nervus furcalis)	Old term for fourth lumbar nerve, ventral ramus			
Genitocrural	See *Genitofemoral*			
Genitofemoral (nervus genitofemoralis [NA])	Lumbar plexus	Somatic sensory	Genital and femoral	Skin of thigh and scrotum (labium majus)
Glossopalatine	See *Intermedius*			

Name	Central attachment	Components*	Branches	Distribution
Glossopharyngeal (ninth cranial) (nervus glossopharyngeus [NA])	Lateral aspect of medulla oblongata	Motor	Muscular, pharyngeal, tonsillar, lingual, tympanic	Stylopharyngeus, and muscles of soft palate and pharynx via pharyngeal plexus
		Visceral sensory		Mucosa of posterior one-third of tongue, pharynx, middle ear and mastoid air cells
		Sensory (taste)		Taste buds of posterior one-third of tongue
		Parasympathetic		Parotid gland via otic ganglion
Gluteal (cutaneous)	See *Cluneal*			
Gluteal, inferior (nervus gluteus inferior [NA])	Sacral plexus	Motor		Gluteus maximus muscle
Gluteal, superior (nervus gluteus superior [NA])	Sacral plexus	Motor		Gluteus medius and minimus and tensor fasciae latae muscles
Hamstrings, nerve to (part of sciatic)	Sacral plexus	Motor		Biceps femoris, semitendinosus, semimembranosus, and part of adductor magnus muscles
Hemorrhoidal, inferior	See *Rectal, inferior*			
Hemorrhoidal, middle	Pudendal plexus	Sympathetic. Visceral sensory	Filaments	Rectum
Hemorrhoidal, superior	Hypogastric plexus	Sympathetic. Visceral sensory	Filaments	Rectum
Hypogastric (nervus hypogastricus [NA])	Superior hypogastric plexus (presacral)	Sympathetic. Visceral sensory	Inferior hypogastric or pelvic plexus	
Hypoglossal (twelfth cranial) (nervus hypoglossus [NA])	Medulla oblongata	Motor	Filaments	Intrinsic and extrinsic muscles of tongue
Iliohypogastric (nervus iliohypogastricus [NA])	Lumbar plexus	Motor. Somatic sensory	Filaments	Muscles and skin of anterior abdominal wall
Ilioinguinal (nervus ilioinguinalis [NA])	Lumbar plexus	Motor. Somatic sensory	Anterior scrotal (labial)	
Infraorbital (nervus infraorbitalis [NA])	Maxillary	Somatic sensory	Alveolar, palpebral, nasal, labial	Upper teeth, mucosa of nasal floor, skin of face

TABLE OF NERVES (Continued)

Name	Central attachment	Components*	Branches	Distribution
Infratrochlear (nervus infratrochlearis [NA])	Nasociliary	Somatic sensory	Filaments	Skin of eyelids and root of nose
Intercostobrachial (nervi intercostobrachiales [NA])	Second thoracic segment ventral ramus	Somatic sensory	Filaments	Skin of axilla and medial aspect of arm
Intermedius (part of seventh cranial) (nervus intermedius [NA])	Brainstem at inferior border of pons	Parasympathetic	Greater petrosal, chorda tympani	Glands of soft palate and nose via pterygopalatine ganglion submandibular and sublingual glands via submandibular ganglion
		Sensory (taste)		Taste buds of anterior two-thirds of tongue
Interosseous, anterior of forearm (nervus interosseus anterior [NA])	Median	Motor. Somatic sensory	Muscular and articular	Deep flexor muscles of forearm, articular
Interosseous, dorsal of forearm	See *Interosseous, posterior of forearm*			
Interosseous, posterior of forearm (nervus interosseus posterior [NA])	Radial	Motor. Somatic sensory	Muscular and articular	Deep extensor muscles of forearm, articular
Interosseous, crural (nervus interosseus cruris [NA])	Tibial	Somatic sensory	Filaments	Ankle joint
Interosseous, volar	See *Interosseous, anterior of forearm*			
Ischiatic (nervus ischiadicus [NA])	See *Sciatic*			
Jugular (nervus jugularis [NA])	Superior cervical ganglion	Sympathetic	Filaments	To glossopharyngeal and vagus nerves
Labial, anterior (nervi labiales anteriores [NA])	Ilioinguinal	Somatic sensory	Filaments	Labia majora and minora
Labial, inferior (rami labiales inferiores [NA])	Inferior alveolar	Somatic sensory	Filaments	Skin of lower lip
Labial, posterior (nervi labiales superiores [NA])	Pudendal	Somatic sensory	Filaments	Labia majora and minora
Labial, superior (rami labiales superiores [NA])	Superior alveolar	Somatic sensory	Filaments	Skin of upper lip

Name	Central attachment	Components*	Branches	Distribution
Lacrimal (nervus lacrimalis [NA])	Ophthalmic	Somatic sensory	Filaments	Lacrimal gland and skin about lateral commissure of eye
Laryngeal, external (ramus externus nervi laryngei superioris [NA])	Superior laryngeal	Motor	Filaments	Cricothyroid muscle
Laryngeal, inferior (nervus laryngeus inferior [NA])	Recurrent laryngeal	Motor	Filaments	Intrinsic muscles of larynx
Laryngeal, internal (ramus internus nervi laryngei superioris [NA])	Superior laryngeal	Visceral sensory	Filaments	Mucosa of larynx
Laryngeal, recurrent (nervus laryngeus recurrens [NA])	Vagus	Motor. Parasympathetic	Inferior laryngeal, cardiac	Heart
Laryngeal, superior (nervus laryngeus superior [NA])	Vagus	Motor. Visceral sensory	Internal and external laryngeal	
Lingual (nervus lingualis [NA])	Mandibular	Somatic sensory	Filaments, sublingual	Mucosa of floor of mouth and anterior two-thirds of tongue
Long thoracic	See *Thoracic, long*			
Lumbar (5 pairs) (nervi lumbales [NA])	Lumbar segments of cord	Motor. Somatic sensory. Visceral sensory. Sympathetic (upper segments only)	Ventral and dorsal rami	Dorsal rami to skin and deep muscles of lower back, ventral rami to lumbar plexus
Lumboinguinal	See *Genitofemoral*			
Malar	See *Zygomaticofacial*			
Mandibular (nervus mandibularis [NA])	Trigeminal	Motor (masticator nerve). Somatic sensory	Masseteric, temporal, pterygoid, buccal, auriculotemporal, inferior alveolar, mylohyoid, meningeal, lingual	Tensor tympani, tensor veli palatini, mylohyoid, anterior belly of digastric and muscles of mastication; lower teeth and adjacent mucosa, anterior two-thirds of tongue, cheek, lower face, meninges
Masseteric (nervus massetericus [NA])	Mandibular	Motor	Filaments	Masseter muscle
Masticator	Motor part of mandibular			

TABLE OF NERVES (Continued)

Name	Central attachment	Components*	Branches	Distribution
Maxillary (nervus maxillaris [NA])	Trigeminal	Somatic sensory	Middle meningeal, pterygopalatine, zygomatic, infraorbital, superior alveolar	Skin of upper part of face, upper teeth, mucosa of nose and palate, meninges
Meatal, external acoustic (nervus meatus acustici externi [NA])	Auriculotemporal	Somatic sensory	Filaments	External acoustic meatus
Median (nervus medianus [NA])	Brachial plexus	Motor. Somatic sensory	Articular, muscular, anterior interosseous, digital	Flexor muscles of forearm, small muscles of thumb, two lateral lumbricals, skin of hand, hand joints
Meningeal	Vagus	Somatic sensory	Filaments	Meninges
Meningeal, middle (ramus meningeus medius nervi maxillaris [NA])	Maxillary	Somatic sensory	Filaments	Meninges
Mental (nervus mentalis [NA])	Inferior alveolar	Somatic sensory	Filaments	Skin of lower lip and chin
Musculocutaneous (of lower extremity)	See *Peroneal, superficial*			
Musculocutaneous (of upper extremity) (nervus musculocutaneous[NA])	Brachial plexus	Motor. Somatic sensory	Muscular, lateral cutaneous of forearm	Coracobrachialis, brachialis and biceps brachii muscles, skin of lateral aspect of forearm
Musculospiral	See *Radial*			
Mylohyoid (nervus mylohyoideus [NA])	Inferior alveolar	Motor	Filaments	Mylohyoid and anterior belly of digastric muscles
Nasal, anterior	See *Nasal, external*			
Nasal, external (rami nasales externi nervi infraorbitalis [NA])	Infraorbital	Somatic sensory	Filaments	Skin of side of nose
Nasal, external (rami nasalis externus nervi nasociliaris [NA])	Nasociliary	Somatic sensory	Filaments	Skin of lower half of nose and tip of nose
Nasal, internal	See *Ethmoid, anterior*			
Nasal, lateral (rami nasales laterales nervi nasociliaris [NA])	Nasociliary	Somatic sensory	Filaments	Mucosa of lateral wall of nasal cavity

Name	Central attachment	Components*	Branches	Distribution
Nasal, medial (rami nasales mediales nervi nasociliaris [NA])	Nasociliary	Somatic sensory	Filaments	Mucosa of nasal septum
Nasal, posterior inferior lateral (rami nasales posteriores inferiores laterales [NA])	Greater palatine	Somatic sensory	Filaments	Mucosa of inferior nasal concha
Nasal, posterior superior lateral (rami nasales posteriores superiores laterales [NA])	Maxillary via pterygopalatine ganglion	Somatic sensory	Filaments	Mucosa of superior and middle nasal conchae
Nasociliary (nervus nasociliaris [NA])	Ophthalmic	Somatic sensory	Long ciliary, ethmoid, infratrochlear	Eyeball, skin and mucosa of eyelids and nose, mucosa of ethmoid air cells
Nasopalatine (nervus nasopalatinus [NA])	Maxillary via pterygopalatine ganglion	Somatic sensory	Nasal rami	Mucosa of nose and hard palate
Obturator (nervus obturatorius [NA])	Lumbar plexus	Motor. Somatic sensory	Muscular, cutaneous and articular	Adductor, gracilis, obturator externus muscles, skin of medial aspect of thigh, hip and knee joints
Obturator, accessory (variable)	Lumbar plexus	Motor	Filaments	Pectineus muscle
Obturator internus (variable)	Sacral plexus	Motor	Filaments	Obturator internus and superior gemellus muscles
Occipital, greater (nervus occipitalis major [NA])	Second cervical segment dorsal ramus	Somatic sensory	Filaments	Skin of posterior portion of scalp
Occipital, lesser (nervus occipitalis minor [NA])	Cervical plexus	Somatic sensory	Filaments	Skin of lateral part of scalp and posterior aspect of auricle
Occipital, third (variable) (nervus occipitalis tertius [NA])	Third cervical segment, dorsal ramus	Somatic sensory	Filaments	Skin of posterior aspect of neck and scalp
Octavus (nervus octavus [NA alternative])	See *Vestibulocochlear*			
Oculomotor (third cranial) (nervus oculomotorius [NA])	Brainstem in region of posterior perforated substance	Motor	Filaments	Levator palpebrae superioris, medial, lateral and inferior rectus, inferior oblique muscles
		Parasympathetic	Via ciliary ganglion	Ciliary and sphincter pupillae muscles

Name	Central attachment	Components*	Branches	Distribution
of Andersch	See *Tympanic*			
of Arnold	See *Auricular*			
of Bell	See *Thoracic, long*			
of Eisler	See *Cutaneous, perforating*			
of Jacobson	See *Tympanic*			
of Vidius	See *Pterygoid canal, nerve of*			
of Wrisberg	See *Intermedius*			
Olfactory (first cranial) (nervi olfactorii [NA])	Olfactory bulb	Sensory (smell)	Filaments	Olfactory mucosa
Ophthalmic (nervus ophthalmicus [NA])	Trigeminal	Somatic sensory	Lacrimal, frontal, nasociliary, infratrochlear	Skin of forehead, upper eyelids, anterior part of scalp, orbit and eyeball, meninges, mucosa of nose and air sinuses
Optic (second cranial) (nervus opticus [NA])	Optic tracts	Sensory (vision)	Filaments	Retina
Orbital (rami orbitales [NA])	Maxillary via pterygopalatine ganglion	Somatic sensory	Filaments	Orbit
Orbital	See *Zygomatic*			
Palatine, anterior	See *Palatine, greater*			
Palatine, greater (nervus palatinus major [NA])	Maxillary via pterygopalatine ganglion	Somatic sensory	Filaments	Mucosa of hard and soft palates
Palatine, lesser (nervi palatini minores [NA])	Maxillary via pterygopalatine ganglion	Somatic sensory	Filaments	Mucosa of soft palate, uvula, and palatine tonsil
Palatine, middle	See *Palatine, lesser*			
Palatine, posterior	See *Palatine, lesser*			
Palpebral, inferior (rami palpebrales inferiores [NA])	Infraorbital	Somatic sensory	Filaments	Lower eyelid
Palpebral, superior (rami palpebrales superiores [NA])	Lacrimal, frontal, and nasociliary	Somatic sensory	Filaments	Upper eyelid
Pathetic	See *Trochlear*			

Name	Central attachment	Components*	Branches	Distribution
Pectoral, lateral (nervus pectoralis lateralis [NA])	Brachial plexus	Motor	Filaments	Pectoralis major and minor muscles
Pectoral, medial (nervus pectoralis medialis [NA])	Brachial plexus	Motor	Filaments	Pectoralis major and minor muscles
Pelvic splanchnic	See *Splanchnic, pelvic*			
Perineal (nervi perineales [NA])	Pudendal	Motor. Somatic sensory	Filaments	Muscles of perineum, skin of root of penis and scrotum (labium majus)
Peroneal, anastomotic (variable) (ramus communicans peroneus nervi peronei communis [NA])	Common peroneal	Somatic sensory	Filaments	Skin of lateral aspect of leg
Peroneal, common (nervus peroneus communis [NA])	Sciatic (sacral plexus)	Motor. Somatic sensory	Lateral sural cutaneous, superficial and deep peroneal	Short head of biceps femoris, knee joint
Peroneal, deep (nervus peroneus profundus [NA])	Common peroneal	Motor. Somatic sensory	Dorsal digital, muscular, cutaneous and articular rami	Muscles of anterior compartment of leg, skin between first and second toes
Peroneal, superficial (nervus peroneus superficialis [NA])	Common peroneal	Motor. Somatic sensory	Dorsal cutaneous of foot, muscular and cutaneous rami	Peroneus longus and brevis, skin of lateral aspect of leg and dorsum of foot
Petrosal, deep (nervus petrosus profundus [NA])	Internal carotid plexus	Sympathetic	To nerve of pterygoid canal	
Petrosal, greater (nervus petrosus major [NA])	Geniculate ganglion	Visceral sensory. Parasympathetic	Via nerve of pterygoid canal to pterygopalatine ganglion	Mucosa and glands of palate and nose
Petrosal, greater superficial	See *Petrosal, greater*			
Petrosal, lesser (nervus petrosus minor [NA])	Tympanic plexus	Parasympathetic	To otic ganglion	Parotid gland
Petrosal, lesser superficial	See *Petrosal, lesser*			
Petrosal, small deep	See *Caroticotympanic*			

Name	Central attachment	Components*	Branches	Distribution
Phrenic (nervus phrenicus [NA])	Cervical plexus	Motor	Filaments	Diaphragm
Phrenic, accessory	See *Accessory phrenic*			
Piriformis, nerve to	Sacral plexus	Motor	Filaments	Piriformis muscle
Plantar, lateral (nervus plantaris lateralis [NA])	Tibial	Motor. Somatic sensory	Muscular, cutaneous, and articular rami	Quadratus plantae, adductor hallucis, small muscles of little toe, and lateral 3 lumbrical muscles of foot, skin of lateral aspect of sole, foot joints
Plantar, medial (nervus plantaris medialis [NA])	Tibial	Motor. Somatic sensory	Muscular, cutaneous, and articular rami	Abductor hallucis, flexor digitorum brevis, flexor hallucis brevis, and first lumbrical of foot, skin of medial aspect of sole, foot joints
Pneumogastric	See *Vagus*			
Popliteal, external	See *Peroneal, common*			
Popliteal, internal	See *Tibial*			
Popliteal, lateral	See *Peroneal, common*			
Popliteal, medial	See *Tibial*			
Presacral (nervus presacralis [NA])	The superior hypogastric plexus			
Pterygoid, external	See *Pterygoid, lateral*			
Pterygoid, internal	See *Pterygoid, medial*			
Pterygoid, lateral (nervus pterygoideus lateralis [NA])	Mandibular	Motor	Filaments	Lateral pterygoid muscle
Pterygoid, medial (nervus pterygoideus medialis [NA])	Mandibular	Motor	Filaments	Medial pterygoid muscle
Pterygoid canal, nerve of (nervus canalis pterygoidei [NA])	Greater and deep petrosal	Parasympathetic. Sympathetic	Filaments along branches from pterygopalatine ganglion	Glands of nose, palate, and pharynx
Pterygopalatine (nervi pterygopalatini [NA])	Maxillary	Somatic sensory	Filaments	Mucosa of palate and nose

Name	Central attachment	Components*	Branches	Distribution
Pudendal (nervus pudendus [NA])	Pudendal plexus	Motor. Somatic sensory	Rectal, perineal, scrotal (labial)	Muscles and skin of perineal region
Quadratus femoris, nerve to	Sacral plexus	Motor. Somatic sensory	Filaments	Quadratus femoris and inferior gemellus muscles, hip joint
Radial (nervus radialis [NA])	Brachial plexus	Motor. Somatic sensory	Cutaneous, interosseous, muscular, superficial and deep rami	Extensor muscles of forearm and hand, brachioradialis, skin of posterior aspect of arm, forearm and wrist, elbow, carpal, and hand joints
Rectal, inferior (nervi rectales inferiores [NA])	Pudendal	Motor. Somatic sensory	Filaments	External anal sphincter, skin about anus
Recurrent	See *Laryngeal, recurrent*			
Recurrent	See *Spinosal*			
Recurrent	See *Tentorial*			
Rhomboids, nerve to	See *Dorsal scapular*			
Saccular (nervus saccularis [NA])	Vestibular of eighth cranial	Sensory (position of head in space)	Filaments	Macula sacculi
Sacral (5 pairs) (nervi sacrales [NA])	Sacral segments of cord	Motor. Somatic sensory. Visceral sensory. Parasympathetic	Dorsal and ventral rami	Dorsal rami to deep muscles of lower back and overlying skin, ventral rami to sacral and pudendal plexuses, pelvic viscera
Saphenous (nervus saphenus [NA])	Femoral	Somatic sensory	Filaments	Skin of medial aspect of leg and foot, knee joint
Scapular, dorsal	See *Dorsal scapular*			
Scapular, posterior	See *Dorsal scapular*			
Sciatic (nervus ischiadicus [NA])	Sacral plexus	Composed of tibial and common peroneal		
Sciatic, small	See *Cutaneous, femoral posterior*			
Scrotal, anterior (nervi scrotales anteriores [NA])	Ilioinguinal	Somatic sensory	Filaments	Skin of pubic area and scrotum
Scrotal, posterior (nervi scrotales posteriores [NA])	Pudendal	Somatic sensory	Filaments	Skin of scrotum

Name	Central attachment	Components*	Branches	Distribution
Serratus anterior	See *Thoracic, long*			
Spermatic, external (ramus genitalis nervi genitofemoralis [NA])	Genitofemoral	Somatic sensory	Filaments	Skin of scrotum and skin near subcutaneous inguinal ring
Sphenopalatine	See *Pterygopalatine*			
Sphenopalatine, long	See *Nasopalatine*			
Sphenopalatine, short	See *Nasal, posterior superior lateral*			
Spinal accessory	See *Accessory*			
Spinosal (ramus meningeus nervi mandibularis [NA])	Mandibular	Somatic sensory	Filaments	Meninges
Splanchnic, greater (nervus splanchnicus major [NA])	Fifth to ninth or tenth thoracic sympathetic ganglia	Sympathetic. Visceral sensory	Filaments	Cardiac, pulmonary, esophageal, and celiac plexuses
Splanchnic, least (variable) (nervus splanchnicus imus [NA])	Lowest thoracic sympathetic ganglion	Sympathetic. Visceral sensory	Filaments	Renal plexus
Splanchnic, lesser (nervus splanchnicus minor [NA])	Ninth and tenth thoracic sympathetic ganglia	Sympathetic. Visceral sensory	Filaments	Celiac plexus
Splanchnic, lumbar (nervi splanchnici lumbales [NA])	Lumbar sympathetic ganglia	Sympathetic. Visceral sensory	Filaments	Celiac, mesenteric and hypogastric plexuses
Splanchnic, pelvic (nervi splanchnici pelvini [NA])	Second to fourth sacral segments of cord	Parasympathetic. Visceral sensory	Filaments in pelvic plexus	Pelvic viscera
Splanchnic, sacral (nervi splanchnici sacrales [NA])	Sacral sympathetic ganglia	Sympathetic. Visceral sensory	Filaments	Pelvic plexus
Stapedius, nerve to (nervus stapedius [NA])	Facial	Motor	Filaments	Stapedius muscle
Statoacoustic	See *Vestibulocochlear*			
Subclavius, nerve to (nervus subclavius [NA])	Brachial plexus	Motor	Filaments	Subclavius muscle
Subcostal (nervus subcostalis [NA])	Ventral ramus of twelfth thoracic	Motor. Somatic sensory	Muscular and cutaneous rami	Muscles and skin of anterior abdominal wall

Name	Central attachment	Components*	Branches	Distribution
Sublingual (nervus sublingualis [NA])	Lingual	Somatic sensory	Filaments	Area of sublingual gland
Suboccipital (nervus suboccipitalis [NA])	Dorsal ramus of first cervical	Motor	Muscular	Deep muscles of back of neck
Subscapular (nervus subscapularis [NA])	Brachial plexus	Motor	Muscular	Subscapular and teres major muscles
Subscapular, long	See *Thoracodorsal*			
Supraacromial	See *Supraclavicular, lateral*			
Supraclavicular, anterior	See *Supraclavicular, medial*			
Supraclavicular, intermediate (nervi supraclaviculares intermedii [NA])	Cervical plexus	Somatic sensory	Filaments	Skin of lower anterior aspect of neck and anterior chest wall
Supraclavicular, lateral (nervi supraclaviculares laterales [NA])	Cervical plexus	Somatic sensory	Filaments	Skin of lateral aspect of neck and shoulder
Supraclavicular, medial (nervi supraclaviculares mediales [NA])	Cervical plexus	Somatic sensory	Filaments	Skin of lower anterior aspect of neck and anterior chest wall, sternoclavicular joint
Supraclavicular, middle	See *Supraclavicular, intermediate*			
Supraclavicular, posterior	See *Supraclavicular, lateral*			
Supraorbital (nervus supraorbitalis [NA])	Frontal	Somatic sensory	Filaments	Skin of upper eyelid and forehead
Suprascapular (nervus suprascapularis [NA])	Brachial plexus	Motor	Filaments	Supraspinatus and infraspinatus muscles
Suprasternal	See *Supraclavicular, medial*			
Supratrochlear (nervus supratrochlearis [NA])	Frontal	Somatic sensory	Filaments	Skin of medial aspect of forehead, root of nose, and upper eyelid
Sural (variable) (nervus suralis [NA])	Combined medial and lateral sural cutaneous			

TABLE OF NERVES (Continued)

Name	Central attachment	Components*	Branches	Distribution
Sural, lateral	See *Cutaneous, sural, lateral*			
Sural, medial	See *Cutaneous, sural, medial*			
Temporal	See *Zygomaticotemporal*			
Temporal, deep (nervi temporales profundi [NA])	Mandibular	Motor	Filaments	Temporal muscle
Temporomalar	See *Zygomatic*			
Tensor tympani, nerve to (nervus tensoris tympani [NA])	Mandibular via otic ganglion	Motor	Filaments	Tensor tympani muscle
Tensor veli palatini, nerve to (nervus tensoris veli palatini [NA])	Mandibular via otic ganglion	Motor	Filaments	Tensor veli palatini muscle
Tentorial (ramus tentorii nervi ophthalmici [NA])	Ophthalmic	Somatic sensory	Filaments	Meninges
Terminal (nervi terminales [NA])	Medial olfactory tract	Not known	Filaments	
Thoracic (12 pairs) (nervi thoracici [NA])	Thoracic segments of cord	Motor. Somatic sensory. Visceral sensory. Sympathetic	Dorsal and ventral rami	Dorsal rami to deep muscles of back and skin of back, ventral rami to brachial plexus and intercostal nerves, sympathetic and visceral sensory to viscera and blood vessels
Thoracic, internal anterior	See *Pectoral, medial*			
Thoracic, lateral anterior	See *Pectoral, lateral*			
Thoracic, long (nervus thoracicus longus [NA])	Brachial plexus	Motor	Filaments	Serratus anterior muscle
Thoracic, medial anterior	See *Pectoral, medial*			
Thoracic, posterior	See *Thoracic, long*			
Thoracodorsal (nervus thoracodorsalis [NA])	Brachial plexus	Motor	Filaments	Latissimus dorsi muscle

Name	Central attachment	Components*	Branches	Distribution
Tibial (nervus tibialis [NA])	Sciatic	Motor. Somatic sensory	Interosseous crural, cutaneous, sural, plantar	Muscles of back of leg and sole of foot, skin of back of leg and sole, knee and foot joints
Tibial, anterior	See *Peroneal, deep*			
Tibial, posterior	Posterior division of tibial			
Tibial, recurrent	Common peroneal	Motor. Somatic sensory	Muscular and articular rami	Tibialis anterior muscle, knee joint
Transverse of neck (nervus transversus colli [NA])	Cervical plexus	Somatic sensory	Filaments	Skin of neck
Trifacial	See *Trigeminal*			
Trigeminal (fifth cranial) (nervus trigeminus [NA])	Brainstem at inferior surface of pons. See *Ophthalmic; Maxillary; Mandibular*			
Trochlear (fourth cranial) (nervus trochlearis [NA])	Dorsal surface of midbrain	Motor	Filaments	Superior oblique muscle of eye
Tympanic (nervus tympanicus [NA])	Glossopharyngeal	Visceral sensory. Parasympathetic	Filaments	Mucosa of middle ear and mastoid air cells, to parotid gland via otic ganglion
Ulnar (nervus ulnaris [NA])	Brachial plexus	Motor. Somatic sensory	Muscular, cutaneous and articular	Flexor carpi ulnaris, flexor digitorum profundus, adductor pollicis, muscles of hypothenar eminence, interossei, medial 2 lumbricals, skin of medial part of hand, joints of hand
Utricular (nervus utricularis [NA])	Vestibular	Somatic sensory (position of head in space—static)	Filaments	Macula utriculi
Utriculoampullary (nervus utriculoampullaris [NA])	Vestibular	Combined utricular and ampullary		
Vaginal (nervi vaginales [NA])	Pelvic plexus	Sympathetic. Parasympathetic	Filaments	Vagina

TABLE OF NERVES (Continued)

Name	Central attachment	Components*	Branches	Distribution
Vagus (tenth cranial) (nervus vagus [NA])	Lateral aspect of medulla oblongata	Motor	Pharyngeal and laryngeal	Muscles of pharynx and larynx
		Parasympathetic	Cardiac, esophageal, and abdominal	Heart, smooth muscle of thoracic and abdominal viscera
		Somatic sensory taste	Auricular	Ear, meninges, tongue
		Visceral sensory	Pharyngeal, laryngeal, thoracic, and abdominal (anterior and posterior vagal trunks)	Mucosa of pharynx and larynx; thoracic and abdominal viscera
Vertebral (nervus vertebralis [NA])	First thoracic sympathetic ganglion (cervicothoracic ganglion)	Sympathetic	Vertebral plexus	
Vestibular (vestibular part of eighth cranial)	Brainstem at lower border of pons	Somatic sensory (position of head in space—dynamic)	Ampullary, utricular, saccular	Ampullae of semicircular canals, macula sacculi and macula utriculi
Vestibulocochlear (eighth cranial) (nervus vestibulocochlearis [NA])	See *Cochlear; Vestibular*			
Volar	See *Digital, palmar*			
Zygomatic (nervus zygomaticus [NA])	Maxillary	Somatic sensory	Filaments	Skin over zygoma and temple
Zygomaticofacial (ramus zygomaticofacialis nervi zygomatici [NA])	Zygomatic	Somatic sensory	Filaments	Skin over zygoma
Zygomaticotemporal (ramus zygomaticotemporalis nervi zygomatici [NA])	Zygomatic	Somatic sensory	Filaments	Skin of temple

Name	Type	Named* ligaments
Acromioclavicular (articulatio acromioclavicularis [NA])	Gliding	Articular disk Coracoclavicular (1) Conoid (2) Trapezoid Acromioclavicular
Ankle (articulatio talocruralis [NA])	Hinge	Medial (1) Anterior tibiotalar (2) Posterior tibiotalar (3) Tibiocalcaneal (4) Tibionavicular Anterior talofibular Posterior talofibular Calcaneofibular
Astragalocalcaneal	See *Subtalar*	
Atlantoaxial	See *Lateral atlantoaxial; Median atlantoaxial*	
Atlantooccipital (articulatio atlantooccipitalis [NA])	Gliding	Anterior atlantooccipital membrane Posterior atlantooccipital membrane Anterior oblique (lateral) atlanto-occipital ligament
Calcaneocuboid (articulatio calcaneocuboidea [NA])	Gliding	Dorsal calcaneocuboid Long plantar Plantar calcaneocuboid Calcaneocuboid
Calcaneonavicular	See *Talocalcaneonavicular*	
Carpal	See *Intercarpal; Mediocarpal; Pisiform*	
Carpometacarpal of thumb (articulatio carpometacarpea pollicis [NA])	Saddle	
Carpometacarpal of fingers (articulationes carpometacarpeae [NA])	Gliding	Dorsal carpometacarpal Interosseous carpometacarpal Palmar carpometacarpal
Central atlantoepistropheal	See *Median atlantoaxial*	
Costotransverse (upper 10 ribs only) (articulatio costotransversaria [NA])	Gliding	Costotransverse Superior costotransverse Lateral costotransverse Lumbocostal
Cuboideometatarsal	Gliding	Dorsal tarsometatarsal Plantar tarsometatarsal

* Each synovial joint has an articular capsule.

Name	Type	Named* ligaments
Cuboideonavicular (inconstant)	Gliding	Dorsal cuboideonavicular Interosseous cuboideonavicular Plantar cuboideonavicular
Cuneocuboid	Gliding	Dorsal cuneocuboid Interosseous cuneocuboid Plantar cuneocuboid
Cuneometatarsal	Gliding	Dorsal tarsometatarsal Interosseous cuneometatarsal Plantar tarsometatarsal
Cuneonavicular (articulatio cuneonavicularis [NA])	Gliding	Dorsal cuneonavicular and plantar cuneonavicular
Distal radioulnar (articulatio radioulnaris distalis [NA])	Gliding	Articular disk
Distal tibiofibular (syndesmosis tibiofibularis [NA])	Frequently contains an extension of the ankle joint	Anterior tibiofibular Posterior tibiofibular Interosseous membrane of the leg
Ear ossicles (articulationes ossiculorum auditus [NA])	See *Incudomalleolar; Incudostapedial*	
Elbow (articulatio cubiti [NA])		Annular radial Quadrate
(1) Humeroradial (articulatio humeroradialis [NA])	Gliding	Oblique cord Radial collateral
(2) Humeroulnar (articulatio humeroulnaris [NA])	Hinge	Ulnar collateral
(3) Proximal radioulnar (articulatio radioulnaris proximalis [NA])	Pivot	Interosseous membrane of forearm
Foot (articulationes pedis [NA])	See *Ankle; Calcaneocuboid; Interphalangeal of toes; Metatarsophalangeal; Subtalar; Talocalcaneonavicular; Tarsometatarsal*	
Hand (articulationes manus [NA])	See *Carpometacarpal of fingers; Carpometacarpal of thumb; Intercarpal; Interphalangeal of fingers; Metacarpophalangeal; Pisiform; Wrist*	
Head of rib (articulatio capitis costae [NA])	Combined hinge and gliding	Intraarticular of head of rib Radiate of head of rib
Hip (articulatio coxae [NA])	Ball-and-socket	Iliofemoral Ischiofemoral Pubofemoral Acetabular Transverse acetabular Ligament of head of femur

Name	Type	Named* ligaments
Humeroradial	See *Elbow* (1)	
Humeroulnar	See *Elbow* (2)	
Incudomalleolar (articulatio incudomallearis [NA])	Gliding	
Incudostapedial (articulatio incudostapedia [NA]	Gliding	
Intercarpal (articulationes intercarpeae [NA]) (1) Distal (between 4 bones of distal row) (2) Proximal (between 3 bones of proximal row excluding pisiform)	Gliding. See also *Mediocarpal, Pisiform*	Interosseous intercarpal Transverse carpal (=flexor retinaculum) Dorsal carpal (=extensor retinaculum) Dorsal intercarpal Palmar intercarpal
Intercuneiform	Gliding	Dorsal intercuneiform Interosseous intercuneiform Plantar intercuneiform
Intermediate tarsometatarsal	See *Cuneometatarsal*	
Intermetacarpal (4 medial metacarpal bases) (articulationes intermetacarpeae [NA])	Gliding	Dorsal metacarpal Interosseous metacarpal Palmar metacarpal
Intermetatarsal (articulationes intermetatarseae [NA])	Gliding	Dorsal metatarsal Interosseous metatarsal Plantar metatarsal Deep transverse metatarsal
Interphalangeal of fingers (articulationes interphalangeae manus [NA])	Hinge	Collateral Palmar
Interphalangeal of toes (articulationes interphalangeae pedis [NA])	Hinge	Collateral Plantar
Intertarsal (articulationes intertarseae [NA])	See *Calcaneocuboid; Cuboideonavicular; Cuneocuboid; Cuneonavicular; Intercuneiform; Subtalar; Talocalcaneonavicular; Transverse tarsal*	
Intervertebral (between articular facets of vertebrae—2 superior and 2 inferior for each) (juncturae zygapophyseales [NA])	Gliding	

Name	Type	Named* ligaments
Knee (articulatio genus [NA])	Combined hinge and gliding	Alar folds Anterior cruciate Anterior meniscofemoral Arcuate popliteal Coronary Fibular collateral Infrapatellar synovial fold Lateral meniscus Lateral patellar retinaculum Medial meniscus Medial patellar retinaculum Oblique popliteal Patellar Posterior cruciate Posterior meniscofemoral Tibial collateral Transverse
Lateral atlantoaxial (articulatio antlantoaxialis lateralis [NA])	Gliding	Accessory atlantoaxial Anterior atlantoaxial Posterior atlantoaxial
Lateral atlantoepistropheal	See *Lateral atlantoaxial*	
Lateral tarsometatarsal	See *Cuboideometatarsal*	
Mandibular	See *Temporomandibular*	
Medial tarsometatarsal	Gliding	Dorsal tarsometatarsal Interosseous tarsometatarsal Plantar tarsometatarsal
Median atlantoaxial (articulatio atlantoaxialis mediana [NA])	Pivot	Alar Apical of dens Cruciform atlantal Transverse atlantal Longitudinal bundles Tectorial membrane
Mediocarpal (articulatio mediocarpea [NA])	Gliding, ball-and-socket	Radiate carpal
Metacarpophalangeal (articulationes metacarpophalangeae [NA])	Ball-and-socket	Collateral Palmar Deep transverse metacarpal
Metatarsophalangeal (articulationes metatarsophalangeae [NA])	Ball-and-socket	Collateral Plantar Deep transverse metatarsal
Midtarsal	See *Transverse tarsal*	
Pisiform (articulatio ossis pisiformis [NA])	Gliding	Pisohamate Pisometacarpal
Pisotriquetral	See *Pisiform*	

Name	Type	Named* ligaments
Proximal radioulnar	See *Elbow* (3)	
Proximal tibiofibular (articulatio tibiofibularis [NA])	Gliding	Anterior of head of fibula Posterior of head of fibula
Radiocarpal	See *Wrist*	
Radioulnar	See *Elbow* (3); *Distal radioulnar*	
Sacroiliac (articulatio sacroiliaca [NA])	Gliding	Ventral sacroiliac Interosseous sacroiliac Dorsal sacroiliac
Shoulder (articulatio humeri [NA])	Ball-and-socket	Coracohumeral Inferior glenohumeral Middle glenohumeral Superior glenohumeral Transverse humeral Glenoid lip
Sternocostal (articulationes sternocostales [NA])	Gliding	Interarticular sternocostal Radiate sternocostal Costoxiphoid Internal and external intercostal membranes
Sternoclavicular (articulatio sternoclavicularis [NA])	Gliding	Articular disk Anterior sternoclavicular Costoclavicular Interclavicular Posterior sternoclavicular
Subtalar (articulatio subtalaris [NA])	Gliding	Interosseous talocalcaneal Lateral talocalcaneal Medial talocalcaneal
Talocalcaneal	See *Subtalar*	
Talocalcaneonavicular (articulatio talocalcaneonavicularis [NA])	Gliding	Calcaneonavicular Talonavicular Plantar calcaneonavicular or spring
Talocrural	See *Ankle*	
Talonavicular	See *Talocalcaneonavicular*	
Tarsal	See *Calcaneocuboid; Cuboideonavicular; Cuneonavicular; Cuneocuboid; Intercuneiform; Subtalar; Talocalcaneonavicular; Transverse tarsal*	

Name	Type	Named* ligaments
Tarsometatarsal (articulationes tarsometatarseae [NA])	See *Cuboideometatarsal; Cuneometatarsal; Medial tarsometatarsal*	
Temporomandibular (articulatio temporomandibularis [NA])	Combined gliding and hinge	Articular disk Sphenomandibular Stylomandibular Lateral
Tibiofibular	See *Distal tibiofibular, Proximal tibiofibular*	
Transverse tarsal (articulatio tarsi transversa [NA])	Combined calcaneocuboid and talocalcaneonavicular	
Wrist (articulatio radiocarpea [NA])	Biaxial	Dorsal radiocarpal Radial collateral of wrist Articular disk of distal radioulnar joint Ulnar collateral of wrist Palmar radiocarpal Palmar ulnocarpal

The following list includes only those veins and venous sinuses and plexuses which have no accompanying artery of the same name, or which differ considerably from the accompanying artery. For all other veins—for example, the deep veins of the upper and lower extremity, or of the body wall—see the Table of Arteries for the accompanying vein of the same name; these veins have tributaries with the same distribution as the branches of the accompanying arteries.

Name	Region or tributary drained	Location	Drains into:
Accessory hemiazygos (vena hemiazygos accessoria [NA])	3 or 4 upper left intercostal spaces	Left side of vertebral column	Either azygos or hemiazygos
Accompanying hypoglossal nerve (vena comitans nervi hypoglossi [NA])	Digastric triangle	Accompanies the hypoglossal nerve	Retromandibular
Anterior cardiac (venae cordis anteriores [NA])	Front of right ventricle	Front of right ventricle	Right atrium
Anterior facial	See *Facial*		
Anterior jugular (vena jugularis anterior [NA])	Anterior part of neck	Near midline of neck	External jugular or subclavian
Ascending lumbar (vena lumbalis ascendens [NA])	Lumbar area	Lumbar spinal column	Azygos on right, hemiazygos on left
Azygos (vena azygos [NA])	Right chest wall; begins from ascending lumbar vein	Right side of vertebral column	Superior vena cava
Basal (vena basalis [NA])	Anterior perforated substance	Base of brain	Internal cerebral
Basilar plexus (plexus basilaris [NA])	Both inferior petrosal sinuses	Basilar part of occipital bone	Anterior part of internal vertebral plexus
Basilic (vena basilica [NA])	Ulnar side of hand and forearm	Medial side of biceps brachii muscle	Joins brachial to form axillary
Basivertebral (venae basivertebrales [NA])	Bodies of vertebrae	Bodies of vertebrae	External vertebral plexuses
Brachiocephalic (venae brachiocephalicae dextra et sinistra [NA])	Internal jugular and subclavian	Root of neck	Superior vena cava
Cavernous sinus (sinus cavernosus [NA])	Superior ophthalmic	Lateral to sella turcica	Superior and inferior petrosal sinuses
Cephalic (vena cephalica [NA])	Radial side of hand and forearm	Lateral side of arm	Axillary
Common facial	See *Facial*		
Confluence of sinuses (confluens sinuum [NA])	Occipital area (inner surface)	Occipital bone	Variable connection between transverse sinuses

Name	Region or tributary drained	Location	Drains into:
Coronary of stomach	Combined right and left gastric veins		
Coronary sinus (sinus coronarius [NA])	Most of the veins of the heart	Posterior part of coronary sulcus	Right atrium
Cubital (vena mediana cubiti [NA])	Palmar forearm	Cubital area	Basilic
Deep cerebral	See *Internal cerebral*		
Diploic (venae diploicae [NA])	Diploë of cranium	Inside the frontal, temporal, parietal, and occipital bones	Either internally into the dural sinuses or externally into superficial veins, such as the occipital or supraorbital
Ductus venosus (ductus venosus [NA])	Embryonic bypass from umbilical vein to inferior vena cava		
Emissary (venae emissariae [NA])	Venous sinuses inside cranium	Small foramens in skull, such as parietal, mastoid, condylar, occipital, and postcondylar	Veins external to the skull, as the posterior auricular or occipital
External jugular (vena jugularis externa [NA])	Posterior auricular and posterior part of facial	Side of neck	Subclavian
External vertebral plexuses, anterior and posterior (plexus venosi vertebrales externi [NA])	Vertebra and surrounding muscles	Anterior and posterior to the vertebral column	Basivertebral and intervertebral veins
Facial (vena facialis [NA])	Continuation of angular	Anterior side of face	Retromandibular or internal jugular
Great cardiac (vena cordis magna [NA])	Anterior aspect of ventricles	Anterior interventricular sulcus of heart	Coronary sinus
Great cerebral (vena cerebri magna [NA])	Internal cerebral veins	Below and behind the splenium of the corpus callosum	Straight sinus
Great saphenous (vena saphena magna [NA])	Medial side of leg and thigh	Medial side of leg and thigh	Femoral
Hemiazygos (vena hemiazygos [NA])	Left ascending lumbar	Left side of vertebral column	Azygos
Hemorrhoidal plexus	See *Rectal plexus*		
Hepatic (venae hepaticae [NA])	Substance of liver	Converge to the sulcus of the inferior vena cava	Inferior vena cava

Name	Region or tributary drained	Location	Drains into:
Inferior anastomotic (venae anastomotica inferior [NA])	Interconnect middle superficial cerebral vein and transverse sinus		
Inferior cerebral (venae cerebri inferiores [NA])	Base of brain	Beneath base of hemispheres	Various sinuses
Inferior ophthalmic (vena ophthalmica inferior [NA])	Lower part of orbit	Floor of orbit	Pterygoid plexus and cavernous sinus
Inferior petrosal sinus (sinus petrosus inferior [NA])	Cavernous sinus	Inferior petrosal sulcus	Internal jugular
Inferior pulmonary, left (vena pulmonalis inferior sinistra [NA])	Apical and basal	Lower lobe of left lung	Left atrium
Inferior pulmonary, right (vena pulmonalis inferior dextra [NA])	Apical and basal	Lower lobe of right lung	Left atrium
Inferior sagittal sinus (sinus sagittalis inferior [NA])	Falx cerebri	Lower edge of falx cerebri	Straight sinus
Inferior vena cava (vena cava inferior [NA])	Common iliac veins, blood from lower extremities and abdomen	In front of vertebral column to the right of the aorta	Right atrium
Innominate	See *Brachiocephalic*		
Intercavernous sinuses, anterior and posterior (sinus intercavernosi [NA])	Connect the cavernous sinuses		
Internal cerebral (venae cerebri internae [NA])	Terminal and choroid veins	Beneath splenium of corpus callosum	Great cerebral
Internal jugular (vena jugularis interna [NA])	Brain, face, and neck; transverse sinus	Side of neck	Brachiocephalic
Internal vertebral plexuses, anterior and posterior (plexus venosi vertebrales interni [NA])	Vertebrae and meninges	Within the vertebral canal, anterior and posterior to the spinal cord	Intervertebral veins
Jugular	See *Anterior jugular; External jugular; Internal jugular*		
Least cardiac (venae cordis minimae [NA])	Walls of heart	Walls of heart	Each chamber of heart

Name	Region or tributary drained	Location	Drains into:
Long saphenous	See *Great saphenous*		
Median cubital (vena mediana cubiti [NA])	Palmar forearm	Cubital area, between cephalic and basilic	
Middle cardiac (vena cordis media [NA])	Posterior aspect of heart	Posterior interventricular septum	Coronary sinus
Oblique vein of left atrium (vena obliqua atrii sinistri [NA])	Left atrium	Back of left atrium	Coronary sinus
Occipital sinus (sinus occipitalis [NA])	Region around foramen magnum	Attached margin of falx cerebelli	Confluence of sinuses
of Galen	See *Great cerebral*		
of Marshall	See *Oblique vein of left atrium*		
of Sappey	See *Paraumbilical*		
of Vieussens	See *Anterior cardiac*		
Pampiniform plexus (plexus pampiniformis [NA])	Testis or ovary	Surrounding distal part of testicular or ovarian artery	Testicular or ovarian
Paraumbilical (venae paraumbilicales [NA])	Around umbilicus	Round ligament of the liver	Portal
Portal (vena portae [NA])	Superior mesenteric and lienal	Lesser omentum	Sinusoids of liver
Posterior facial	See *Retromandibular*		
Posterior vein of left ventricle (vena posterior ventriculi sinistri [NA])	Left ventricle	Posterior aspect of left ventricle	Coronary sinus
Prepyloric (vena prepylorica [NA])	Pylorus	On ventral surface of junction of stomach and pylorus	Gastric veins
Prostatic plexus (plexus prostaticus [NA])	Prostate	Fascial sheath of prostate	Internal iliac veins
Pterygoid plexus (plexus pterygoideus [NA])	Veins corresponding to branches of maxillary artery	Between pterygoid muscles	Maxillary
Ranine	See *Accompanying hypoglossal nerve*		
Rectal plexus (plexus venosus rectalis)	Rectum	Wall of rectum	Superior, middle, and inferior rectal veins
Retromandibular (vena retromandibularis [NA])	Superficial temporal and maxillary	In parotid gland	Facial

Name	Region or tributary drained	Location	Drains into:
Saphenous	See *Great saphenous; Small saphenous*		
Short saphenous	See *Small saphenous*		
Sigmoid sinus (sinus sigmoideus [NA])	Transverse sinus	Groove on temporal bone	Internal jugular
Small cardiac (vena cordis parva [NA])	Back of right atrium and ventricle	Coronary sulcus	Coronary sinus
Small saphenous (vena saphena parva [NA])	Leg and foot	Back of leg	Popliteal
Sphenoparietal sinus (sinus sphenoparietalis [NA])	Meninges	Small wing of sphenoid	Cavernous sinus
Straight sinus (sinus rectus [NA])	Inferior sagittal sinus and great cerebral vein	Junction of falx cerebri and tentorium cerebelli	Transverse sinus
Superior anastomotic (vena anastomotica superior [NA])	Interconnects middle superficial cerebral vein and superior sagittal sinus		
Superior cerebral (venae cerebri superiores [NA])	Cortex of brain	Surface of brain	Superior sagittal sinus
Superior ophthalmic (vena ophthalmica superior [NA])	Tributaries corresponding to branches of ophthalmic artery	Orbit	Cavernous sinus
Superior petrosal sinus (sinus petrosus superior [NA])	Cavernous sinus	Superior petrosal sulcus of temporal bone	Transverse sinus
Superior pulmonary, left (vena pulmonalis superior sinistra [NA])	Apicoposterior, anterior, and lingual	Upper lobe of left lung	Left atrium
Superior pulmonary, right (vena pulmonalis superior dextra [NA])	Anterior, posterior, and vein from middle lobe	Upper and middle lobes of right lung	Left atrium
Superior sagittal sinus (sinus sagittalis superior [NA])	Superior cerebral veins and diploic veins	Attached margin of falx cerebri	Confluence of sinuses and transverse sinus
Superior vena cava (vena cava superior [NA])	Head, chest wall, and upper extremities	Right upper mediastinum	Right atrium
Thebesian	See *Least cardiac*		
Transverse sinus (sinus transversus durae matris [NA])	Usually the right is a continuation of the superior sagittal and the left of the straight sinus	Attached margin of tentorium cerebelli	Sigmoid sinus

TABLE OF VEINS (Continued)

Name	Region or tributary drained	Location	Drains into:
Umbilical (vena umbilicalis sinistra [NA])	Embryonic vein from placenta to fetus		
Vesical plexus (plexus venosus vesicalis [NA])	Pudendal and prostatic plexuses	Around base of urinary bladder	Internal iliac
Vorticose (venae vorticosae [NA])	Veins of eyeball	Eyeball	Superior ophthalmic veins

Acetone, serum: 0.3–2.0 mg/100 ml
Albumin, serum: 3.5–5.5 g/100 ml
Aldolase: 0–8 IU/liter
Alpha-amino nitrogen, plasma: 3.0–5.5 mg/100 ml
Ammonia, whole blood, venous: 30–70 μg/100 ml
Amylase, serum (Somogyi): 60–180 units/100 ml; 0.8–3.2 IU/liter
Arterial blood gases:
  HCO_3^-: 21–28 meq/liter
  Pco_2: 35–45 mmHg
  pH: 7.38–7.44
  Po_2: 80–100 mmHg
Ascorbic acid, serum: 0.4–1.0 mg/100 ml
  Leukocytes: 25–40 mg/100 ml
Barbiturates, serum: 0
  "Potentially fatal" level (Schreiner) phenobarbital: Approx. 8 mg/100 ml
  Most short-acting barbiturates: 3.5 mg/100 ml
Base, total, serum: 145–155 meq/liter
Bilirubin, total, serum (Mallory-Evelyn): 0.3–1.0 mg/100 ml
  Direct, serum: 0.1–0.3 mg/100 ml
  Indirect, serum: 0.2–0.7 mg/100 ml
Bromides, serum: 0
  Toxic levels: Above 17 meq/liter; 150 mg/100 ml
Bromsulphalein, BSP (5 mg/kg body weight. IV): 5% or less retention after 45 min
Calcium, ionized: 2.3–2.8 meq/liter; 4.5–5.6 mg/100 ml
Calcium, serum: 4.5–5.5 meq/liter; 9–11 mg/100 ml
Carbon dioxide—combining power, serum (sea level): 21–28 meq/liter; 50–65 vol%
Carbon dioxide content, plasma (at sea level): 21–30 meq/liter; 50–70 vol%
Carbon dioxide tension, arterial blood (sea level): 35–45 mmHg
Carbon monoxide content, blood: Symptoms with over 20% saturation of hemoglobin
Carotenoids, serum: 50–300 μg/100 ml
Ceruloplasmin, serum: 27–37 mg/100 ml
Chlorides, serum (as Cl): 98–106 meq/liter
Cholesterol:
  Total, serum (Man-Peters method): 180–240 mg/100 ml
  Esters, serum: 100–180 mg/100 ml
Cholesterol ester fraction of total cholesterol, serum: 68–72%
Complement, serum, total hemolytic (CH_{50}): 150–250 units/ml
Copper, serum (mean ± 1 SD): 114 ± 14 μg/100 ml
Corticosteroids, plasma (Porter-Silber)(mean ± 1 SD): 13 ± 6 μg/100 ml at 8:00 A.M.
Cortisol (competitive protein binding): 5–20 μg/100 ml at 8:00 A.M.
Creatine phosphokinase, serum:
  Females: 5–25 U/ml
  Males: 5–35 U/ml
Creatinine, serum: 1–1.5 mg/100 ml
Dilantin, plasma:
  Therapeutic level, 10–20 μg/ml
  Toxic level, >30 μg/ml
Ethanol, blood:
  Mild to moderate intoxication: 80–200 mg/100 ml
  Marked intoxication: 250–400 mg/100 ml
  Severe intoxication: Above 400 mg/100 ml
Fatty acids, serum: 380–465 mg/100 ml
Fibrinogen, plasma: 160–415 mg/100 ml
Folic acid, serum: 6–15 ng/ml
Gastrin, serum: 40–150 pg/ml
Globulins, serum: 2.0–3.0 g/100 ml
Glucose (fasting):
  Blood (Nelson-Somogyi): 60–90 mg/100 ml
  Plasma: 75–105 mg
Hemoglobin, blood (sea level):
  Males: 14–18 g/100 ml
  Females: 12–16 g/100 ml
Immunoglobulins, serum:
  IgA: 90–325 mg/100 ml
  IgG: 800–1,500 mg/100 ml
  IgM: 45–150 mg/100 ml
Iodine: See Table A
Iron, serum:
  Males and females (mean ± 1 SD): 107 ± 31 μg/100 ml
Iron-binding capacity, serum (mean ± 1 SD): 305 ± 32 μg/100 ml
  Saturation: 20–45%
Ketones, total: 0.5–1.5 mg/100 ml
Lactic acid, blood: 0.6–1.8 meq/liter
Lactic dehydrogenase, serum:
  200–450 units/ml (Wrobleski)
  60–100 units/ml (Wacker)
  25–100 IU/liter
Lead, serum: <20 μg/100 ml
Lipase, serum (Cherry-Crandall): 1.5 ml *N*/20 NaOH (upper limit of normal). (However, values above 1.0 should be regarded with suspicion.)
Lipids, total, serum: 500–600 mg/100 ml
Lipids, triglyceride, serum: 50–150 mg/100 ml
Magnesium, serum: 1.5–2.5 meq/liter; 2–3 mg/100 ml
Nitrogen, nonprotein, serum: 15–35 mg/100 ml
5′-Nucleotidase, serum: 0.3–2.6 Bodansky units/100 ml
Nutrients, various: See Table B
Osmolality, serum: 280–300 mOsm/kg serum water
Oxygen content:
  Arterial blood (sea level): 17–21 vol %
  Venous blood, arm (sea level): 10–16 vol %
Oxygen percent saturation (sea level):
  Arterial blood: 97%
  Venous blood, arm: 60–85%
Oxygen tension, blood: 80–100 mmHg
pH blood: 7.38–7.44
Phosphatase, acid, serum:
  Bessey-Lowry method: 0.10–0.63 unit
  Bodansky method: 0.5–2.0 units
  Fishman-Lerner (tartrate sensitive): <0.6 unit/100 ml (up to 0.15/100 ml)
  Gutman method: 0.5–2.0 units

International units: 0.2–1.8
King-Armstrong method: 1.0–5.0 units
Shinowara method: 0.0–1.1 units
Phosphatase, alkaline, serum:
Bessey-Lowry method: 0.8–2.3 units (3.4–9)*
Bodansky method: 2.0–4.5 units (3.0–13.0)*
Gutman method: 3.0–10.0 units
International units: 21–91 U/liter at 37°C incubation
King-Armstrong method: 5.0–13.0 units (10.0–20.0)*
Shinowara method: 2.2–8.6 units
Phospholipids, serum: 150–250 mg/100 ml (as lecithin)
Phosphorus, inorganic, serum: 1–1.5 meq/liter; 3–4.5 mg/100 ml
Potassium, serum: 3.5–5.0 meq/liter
Proteins, total, serum: 5.5–8.0 g/100 ml
Protein fractions, serum:
Albumin: 3.5–5.5 g/100 ml (50–60%)
Globulin: 2.0–3.5 g/100 ml (40–50%)
α_1: 0.2–0.4 g/100 ml (4.2–7.2%)
α_2: 0.5–0.9 g/100 ml (6.8–12%)
β: 0.6–1.1 g/100 ml (9.3–15%)
γ: 0.7–1.7 g/100 ml (13–23%)
Pyruvic acid, serum: 0–0.11 meq/liter
Salicylate, plasma: 0
Therapeutic range: 20–25 mg/100 ml
Toxic range: over 30 mg/100 ml
Sodium, serum: 136–145 meq/liter
Steroids: See Table C
Transaminase, serum glutamic oxalacetic (SGOT): 10–40 Karmen units/ml; 6–18 IU/liter
Transaminase, serum glutamic pyruvic (SGPT): 10–40 Karmen units/ml; 3–26 IU/liter
Urea nitrogen, whole blood: 10–20 mg/100 ml
Uric acid, serum:
Males: 2.5–8.0 mg/ml
Females: 1.5–6.0 mg/ml
Vitamin A, serum: 50–100 μg/100 ml
Vitamin B_{12}, serum: 200–600 pg/ml
Zinc, serum: 120 ± 20 μg/100 ml

*SOURCE: G. W. Thorn et al.: Harrison's Principles of Internal Medicine, 8th ed. Copyright © 1977 by McGraw-Hill, Inc. Used by permission of McGraw-Hill Book Company.

TABLE A. COMPARATIVE VALUES COMMONLY OBTAINED FOR TESTS OF THYROID FUNCTION IN VARIOUS CLINICAL SITUATIONS

Diagnostic and clinical status	24-h ^{131}I uptake, %	Serum PBI,* μg/100 ml	Serum T4† μg/100 ml	BMR, % normal standard	Resin T3‡ uptake, % normal control
Euthyroidism:					
Normal values	15–50	4–8	4–11	−15–+15	85–115
Pregnancy	Normal/high	High	High	+20–+25	Low
Iodide deficiency	High	Normal/low	Normal/low	Normal/low	Normal/low
Iodide therapy, 3.0 mg/day	Low	High	Normal	Normal	Normal
Thyroid, USP, >120 mg/day	Low	Normal/high	Normal/high	Normal/high	Normal/high
L-Thyroxine, >0.4 mg/day	Low	Normal/high	Normal/high	Normal/high	Normal/high
L-Triiodothyronine, >0.1 mg/day	Low	Low	Low	Normal/high	Normal/high
Congestive heart failure	Variable	Normal/low	Normal/low	Variable	Normal/high
Hyperthyroidism:					
Untreated	50–100	7–20	11–20	High	115–160
Pregnancy	High	High	High	High	Normal/high
Iodide therapy, >2.0 mg/day	Low	>20	5–15	High/normal	High/normal
Thyroid, USP, >120 mg/day	>20	High	High	High	High
L-Thyroxine, 0.4 mg/day	>20	High	High	High	High
L-Triiodothyronine, 0.1 mg/day	>20	High	High	High	High
Antithyroid drug therapy (euthyroid)	Variable	Normal	Normal	Normal	Normal
Thyroiditis (acute):	Low	Normal/high	Normal/high	Normal/high	Normal/high
Myxedema (primary):					
Untreated	0–15	0–4	0–4	−20–−50	Low‡
Thyroid, USP, 120 mg/day (euthyroid)	Low	Normal¶	Normal¶	Normal	Normal
L-Thyroxine, 0.4 mg/day-euthyroid	Low	Normal/high	Normal/high	Normal	Normal/high
L-Triiodothyronine, 0.1 mg/day (euthyroid)	Low	Low	Low	Normal	Normal

TABLE B. BIOCHEMICAL AIDS IN DIAGNOSING NUTRITIONAL DEFICIENCY

Nutrient	Test	Level suggesting nutritional disorder	Normal range
Protein	Plasma total protein	<6.0 g%	6.5–8.0 g%
	Serum albumin	<3.5 g%	4.0–5.2 g%
	Plasma essential amino acid/ total amino acid	<0.3	0.3–0.5
Vitamin A and carotene	Plasma vitamin A	<20 μg%	50–100 μg%
	Plasma carotenoids	<30 μg%	100–200 μg%
	Response to 200,000 IU Vitamin A	Plasma level increases ×2	< ×1
Vitamin D	Serum Ca	<35 meq/L	4.5–6 meq/L
	Serum P	<0.8 meq/L	1.0–1.5 meq/L
	Serum alkaline phosphatase	>15 units—adults	5–13 K-A units
		>20 units—children	10–20 K-A units
Vitamin C	Whole blood	<0.20 mg%	0.4–1.0 mg%
	Buffy coat	<10 mg%	25–40 mg%
Thiamine	Blood lactate	>15 mg%	9–15 mg%
	Plasma pyruvate	>2.0 mg%	0.8–2.0 mg%
	Transketolase (TK) RBC	<850 μg hexose/ml/hr	900–1500 μg hexose/ml
	Thiamine pyrophosphate effect on TK	>15%	<15%
	Urinary thiamine	<50 μg/g creatinine	100–500 mg/g creatinine
Riboflavin	Plasma flavin adenine dinucleotide	<1.5 μg	2–3 μg%
	Urinary riboflavin	<50 μg/g creatinine	100–500 μg/g creatinine
Pyridoxine	Urinary xanthurenic acid after 10 g *dl*-tryptophane	>50 mg/24 hr	trace
Vitamin B_{12}	Plasma B_{12} level (*Euglena gracilis* in serum)	<100 μμg/ml	200–900 μμg/ml
	Schilling test	<8% ^{60}Co B_{12}	>8% nucleide following 1 mg B_{12} I.M.
Pantothenic acid	Serum	<50 mμ g/ml	100 mμ g/ml
Folic acid	Serum level (*L. casei*)	<5 mμg/ml	5–20 mμg/ml serum
	Formiminoglutamic acid (Figlu) after 20 g histidine HCl p.o.	>75 mg/12 h in urine	0–55 mg/12 h
Iron	Serum iron	<60 μg/100 ml	60–190 μg%
	Serum iron-binding capacity	>400 μg	250–400 μg%
Magnesium	Serum	<1.5 meq/L	1.5–3.0 meq/L
Copper	Serum	<85 μg%	114 μg%
Zinc	Plasma	<80 μg%	120 μg%
Vitamin K	Plasma prothrombin time	>20 s	10–15 s
Tocopherol	Plasma	<0.4 mg%	0.5–2.0 mg%
Sodium	Serum	<132 meq/L	132–142 meq/L
Potassium	Serum	<3.5 meq/L	3.5–5.0 meq/L

*The presence in serum of trace quantities of mercurial salts will render values for the PBI and BEI factitiously low by the usual methods. Normal values for the serum butanol-extractable iodine (BEI) and the serum T4 by column are 3.2 to 6.5 μg%.

†Serum T4 designates values obtained by the binding displacement method of Murphy and Pattee (J. Clin. Endoc. 26: 247, 1966).

‡The Resin-T3 values listed here are for the resin sponge method (Triosorb, Abbott) expressed as a percent of a standard control serum. This test is also expressed as an absolute percent uptake with normal values ranging from 25 to 35 percent (See JAMA 202: 135, 1967). The Resin-T3 test is not generally diagnostic of hypothyroidism because of excessive overlap of values in the low normal range with those in hypothyroidism.

¶The PBI and serum T4 values may be lower than normal in patients receiving some lots of desiccated thyroid, USP, or thyroglobulin (Proloid).

TABLE C. PLASMA AND URINE STEROIDS

Steroid	Plasma	Urine
17-hydroxycorticoids	9–24 μg/100 ml (8 A.M.)	2–10 mg/24 h (Porter-Silber) 5–23 mg/24 h (ketonic)
17-ketosteroids		7–25 mg/24 h (male) 4–15 mg/24 h (female)
Testosterone	0.37–1.0 μg/100 ml (male) 0–0.1 μg/100 ml (female)	47–156 μg/24 h (male) 0–15 μg/24 h (female)
Aldosterone	0.015 μg/100 ml	2–10 μg/24 h

TABLE OF COMMON RADIOACTIVE PHARMACEUTICALS

Name of preparation	Radioactive half-life	Principal radiation: type and energy*	Principal uses
Iodinated I 125 serum albumin	^{125}I 60 days	Beta (none) Gamma (0.035)	Determination of blood volume and cardiac output
Iodinated I 131 serum albumin	^{131}I 8.08 days	Beta (0.608) Gamma (0.364)	Determination of blood volume and cardiac output
Chlormerodrin Hg 197 injection	^{197}Hg 64.8 hours	Beta (none) Gamma (0.077)	Brain tumor localization
Chlormerodrin Hg 203 injection	^{203}Hg 46.6 days	Beta (0.21) Gamma (0.279)	Brain tumor localization
Cyanocobalamin Co 57 capsules Cyanocobalamin Co 57 solution	^{57}Co 270 days	Beta (none) Gamma (0.122)	Diagnosis of pernicious anemia
Cyanocobalamin Co 60 capsules Cyanocobalamin Co 60 solution	^{60}Co 5.27 years	Beta (0.306) Gamma (1.17, 1.33)	Diagnosis of pernicious anemia
Gold Au 198 injection	^{198}Au 2.70 days	Beta (0.97) Gamma (0.411)	Neoplastic suppressant (by intracavitary injection)
Sodium Chromate Cr 51 injection	^{51}Cr 27.8 days	Beta (none) Gamma (0.32)	Determination of blood volume, red cell volume, red cell survival time
Sodium iodide I 125 solution	^{125}I 60 days	Beta (none) Gamma (0.035)	Determination of thyroid function
Sodium iodide I 131 capsules Sodium iodide I 131 solution	^{131}I 8.08 days	Beta (0.608) Gamma (0.364)	Neoplastic suppressant; determination of thyroid function
Sodium iodohippurate I 131 injection	^{131}I 8.08 days	Beta (0.608) Gamma (0.364)	Determination of renal function
Sodium phosphate P 32 solution	^{32}P 14.3 days	Beta (1.71) Gamma (none)	Neoplastic and polycythemic suppressant; tumor localization
Sodium rose bengal I 131 injection	^{131}I 8.08 days	Beta (0.608) Gamma (0.364)	Determination of hepatic function
Technetium Tc 99m (sodium pertechnetate Tc 99m solution)	^{99m}Tc 5.997 hours	Beta (none) Gamma (0.140)	Brain tumor localization

*The energy of the radiation is given in million electron volts (mev).

ELY'S TABLE OF THE DURATION OF PREGNANCY

Explanation: In the upper horizontal row of numbers, find the date of last menstruation; the number beneath, set in *italics*, will show the expiration of 280 days or ten months of 28 days each.

January	1	2	3	4	5	6	7	8	9	10	11	12	13	14	15	16	17	18	19	20	21	22	23	24	25	26	27	28	29	30	31	
October	*8*	*9*	*10*	*11*	*12*	*13*	*14*	*15*	*16*	*17*	*18*	*19*	*20*	*21*	*22*	*23*	*24*	*25*	*26*	*27*	*28*	*29*	*30*	*31*	*1*	*2*	*3*	*4*	*5*	*6*	*7*	*November*
February	1	2	3	4	5	6	7	8	9	10	11	12	13	14	15	16	17	18	19	20	21	22	23	24	25	26	27	28				
November	*8*	*9*	*10*	*11*	*12*	*13*	*14*	*15*	*16*	*17*	*18*	*19*	*20*	*21*	*22*	*23*	*24*	*25*	*26*	*27*	*28*	*29*	*30*	*1*	*2*	*3*	*4*	*5*				*December*
March	1	2	3	4	5	6	7	8	9	10	11	12	13	14	15	16	17	18	19	20	21	22	23	24	25	26	27	28	29	30	31	
December	*6*	*7*	*8*	*9*	*10*	*11*	*12*	*13*	*14*	*15*	*16*	*17*	*18*	*19*	*20*	*21*	*22*	*23*	*24*	*25*	*26*	*27*	*28*	*29*	*30*	*31*	*1*	*2*	*3*	*4*	*5*	*January*
April	1	2	3	4	5	6	7	8	9	10	11	12	13	14	15	16	17	18	19	20	21	22	23	24	25	26	27	28	29	30		
January	*6*	*7*	*8*	*9*	*10*	*11*	*12*	*13*	*14*	*15*	*16*	*17*	*18*	*19*	*20*	*21*	*22*	*23*	*24*	*25*	*26*	*27*	*28*	*29*	*30*	*31*	*1*	*2*	*3*	*4*		*February*
May	1	2	3	4	5	6	7	8	9	10	11	12	13	14	15	16	17	18	19	20	21	22	23	24	25	26	27	28	29	30	31	
February	*5*	*6*	*7*	*8*	*9*	*10*	*11*	*12*	*13*	*14*	*15*	*16*	*17*	*18*	*19*	*20*	*21*	*22*	*23*	*24*	*25*	*26*	*27*	*28*	*1*	*2*	*3*	*4*	*5*	*6*	*7*	*March*
June	1	2	3	4	5	6	7	8	9	10	11	12	13	14	15	16	17	18	19	20	21	22	23	24	25	26	27	28	29	30		
March	*8*	*9*	*10*	*11*	*12*	*13*	*14*	*15*	*16*	*17*	*18*	*19*	*20*	*21*	*22*	*23*	*24*	*25*	*26*	*27*	*28*	*29*	*30*	*31*	*1*	*2*	*3*	*4*	*5*	*6*		*April*
July	1	2	3	4	5	6	7	8	9	10	11	12	13	14	15	16	17	18	19	20	21	22	23	24	25	26	27	28	29	30	31	
April	*7*	*8*	*9*	*10*	*11*	*12*	*13*	*14*	*15*	*16*	*17*	*18*	*19*	*20*	*21*	*22*	*23*	*24*	*25*	*26*	*27*	*28*	*29*	*30*	*1*	*2*	*3*	*4*	*5*	*6*	*7*	*May*
August	1	2	3	4	5	6	7	8	9	10	11	12	13	14	15	16	17	18	19	20	21	22	23	24	25	26	27	28	29	30	31	
May	*8*	*9*	*10*	*11*	*12*	*13*	*14*	*15*	*16*	*17*	*18*	*19*	*20*	*21*	*22*	*23*	*24*	*25*	*26*	*27*	*28*	*29*	*30*	*31*	*1*	*2*	*3*	*4*	*5*	*6*	*7*	*June*
September	1	2	3	4	5	6	7	8	9	10	11	12	13	14	15	16	17	18	19	20	21	22	23	24	25	26	27	28	29	30		
June	*8*	*9*	*10*	*11*	*12*	*13*	*14*	*15*	*16*	*17*	*18*	*19*	*20*	*21*	*22*	*23*	*24*	*25*	*26*	*27*	*28*	*29*	*30*	*1*	*2*	*3*	*4*	*5*	*6*	*7*		*July*
October	1	2	3	4	5	6	7	8	9	10	11	12	13	14	15	16	17	18	19	20	21	22	23	24	25	26	27	28	29	30	31	
July	*8*	*9*	*10*	*11*	*12*	*13*	*14*	*15*	*16*	*17*	*18*	*19*	*20*	*21*	*22*	*23*	*24*	*25*	*26*	*27*	*28*	*29*	*30*	*31*	*1*	*2*	*3*	*4*	*5*	*6*	*7*	*August*
November	1	2	3	4	5	6	7	8	9	10	11	12	13	14	15	16	17	18	19	20	21	22	23	24	25	26	27	28	29	30		
August	*8*	*9*	*10*	*11*	*12*	*13*	*14*	*15*	*16*	*17*	*18*	*19*	*20*	*21*	*22*	*23*	*24*	*25*	*26*	*27*	*28*	*29*	*30*	*31*	*1*	*2*	*3*	*4*	*5*	*6*		*September*
December	1	2	3	4	5	6	7	8	9	10	11	12	13	14	15	16	17	18	19	20	21	22	23	24	25	26	27	28	29	30	31	
September	*7*	*8*	*9*	*10*	*11*	*12*	*13*	*14*	*15*	*16*	*17*	*18*	*19*	*20*	*21*	*22*	*23*	*24*	*25*	*26*	*27*	*28*	*29*	*30*	*1*	*2*	*3*	*4*	*5*	*6*	*7*	*October*

TABLE OF ELEMENTS*

The following values apply to elements as they exist in materials of terrestrial origin and to certain artificial elements. When used with due regard to the footnotes, they are considered reliable to ±1 in the last digit, or ±3 if that digit is in small type.

Based on the assigned relative atomic mass of carbon-12

Name	Symbol	Atomic no.	Atomic wt. (1969)
Actinium	Ac	89	
Aluminum	Al	13	26.9815[a]
Americium	Am	95	
Antimony	Sb	51	121.7_5
Argon	Ar	18	39.94_8[b,c,d,g]
Arsenic	As	33	74.9216[a]
Astatine	At	85	
Barium	Ba	56	137.3_4
Berkelium	Bk	97	
Beryllium	Be	4	9.01218[a]
Bismuth	Bi	83	208.9806[a]
Boron	B	5	10.81[c,d,e]
Bromine	Br	35	79.904[c]
Cadmium	Cd	48	112.40
Calcium	Ca	20	40.08
Californium	Cf	98	
Carbon	C	6	12.011[b,d]
Cerium	Ce	58	140.12
Cesium	Cs	55	132.9055[a]
Chlorine	Cl	17	35.453[c]
Chromium	Cr	24	51.996[c]
Cobalt	Co	27	58.9332[a]
Copper	Cu	29	63.54_6[c,d]
Curium	Cm	96	
Dysprosium	Dy	66	162.5_0
Einsteinium	Es	99	254
Erbium	Er	68	167.2_6
Europium	Eu	63	151.96
Fermium	Fm	100	
Fluorine	F	9	18.9984[a]
Francium	Fr	87	
Gadolinium	Gd	64	157.2_5
Gallium	Ga	31	69.72
Germanium	Ge	32	72.5_9
Gold	Au	79	196.9665[a]
Hafnium	Hf	72	178.4_9
Helium	He	2	4.00260[b,c]
Holmium	Ho	67	164.9303[a]
Hydrogen	H	1	1.008_0[b,d]
Indium	In	49	114.82
Iodine	I	53	126.9045[a]
Iridium	Ir	77	192.2_2
Iron	Fe	26	55.84_7
Krypton	Kr	36	83.80
Lanthanum	La	57	138.905_5[b]
Lawrencium	Lr	103	
Lead	Pb	82	207.2[d,g]
Lithium	Li	3	6.94_1[c,d,e]
Lutetium	Lu	71	174.967
Magnesium	Mg	12	24.305[c]
Manganese	Mn	25	54.9380[a]
Mendelevium	Md	101	
Mercury	Hg	80	200.5_9
Molybdenum	Mo	42	95.9_4

TABLE OF ELEMENTS* (Continued)

Name	Symbol	Atomic no.	Atomic wt. (1969)
Neodymium	Nd	60	144.2_4
Neon	Ne	10	20.17_9[c]
Neptunium	Np	93	237.0482[b,f]
Nickel	Ni	28	58.7_1
Niobium	Nb	41	92.9064[a]
Nitrogen	N	7	14.0067[b,c]
Nobelium	No	102	
Osmium	Os	76	190.2
Oxygen	O	8	15.999_4[b,c,d]
Palladium	Pd	46	106.4
Phosphorus	P	15	30.9738[a]
Platinum	Pt	78	195.0_9
Plutonium	Pu	94	
Polonium	Po	84	
Potassium	K	19	39.10_2
Praseodymium	Pr	59	140.9077[a]
Promethium	Pm	61	
Protactinium	Pa	91	231.0359[a,f]
Radium	Ra	88	226.0254[a,f,g]
Radon	Rn	86	
Rhenium	Re	75	186.2
Rhodium	Rh	45	102.9055[a]
Rubidium	Rb	37	85.467_8[c]
Ruthenium	Ru	44	101.0_7
Samarium	Sm	62	150.4
Scandium	Sc	21	44.9559[a]
Selenium	Se	34	78.9_6
Silicon	Si	14	28.08_6[d]
Silver	Ag	47	107.868[c]
Sodium	Na	11	22.9898[a]
Strontium	Sr	38	87.62[g]
Sulfur	S	16	32.06[d]
Tantalum	Ta	73	180.947_9[d]
Technetium	Tc	43	98.9062[f]
Tellurium	Te	52	127.6_0
Terbium	Tb	65	158.9254[a]
Thallium	Tl	81	204.3_7
Thorium	Th	90	232.0381[a,f]
Thulium	Tm	69	168.9342[a]
Tin	Sn	50	118.6_9
Titanium	Ti	22	47.9_0
Tungsten	W	74	183.8_5
Uranium	U	92	238.029[b,c,e]
Vanadium	V	23	50.941_4[b,c]
Wolfram	W	74	183.8_5
Xenon	Xe	54	131.30
Ytterbium	Yb	70	173.0_4
Yttrium	Y	39	88.9059[a]
Zinc	Zn	30	65.3_7
Zirconium	Zr	40	91.22

*Source: 1969 Table of Atomic Weights from the Commission on Atomic Weights of the International Union of Pure and Applied Chemistry.

[a] Mononuclidic element.

[b] Element with one predominant isotope (about 99 to 100% abundance).

[c] Element for which the atomic weight is based on calibrated measurements.

[d] Element for which variation in isotopic abundance in terrestrial samples limits the precision of the atomic weight given.

[e] Element for which users are cautioned against the possibility of large variations in atomic weight due to inadvertent or undisclosed artificial isotopic separation in commercially available materials.

[f] Most commonly available long-lived isotope.

[g] In some geological specimens this element has a highly anomalous isotopic composition, corresponding to an atomic weight significantly different from that given.

TABLE OF THE MORE COMMON LATIN AND GREEK TERMS AND ABBREVIATIONS USED IN PRESCRIPTION WRITING

Term or abbreviation	Latin or Greek	Translation
$\bar{aa}$, $\bar{a}a$	ana	of each
a.c.	ante cibum	before meals
ad	ad	to; up to
ad lib.	ad libitum	at pleasure
alternis horis	alternis horis	every other hour
ante	ante	before
aq.	aqua	water
aq. dest.	aqua destillata	distilled water
b.i.d.	bis in die, bis in dies	twice daily
bis	bis	twice
$\bar{c}$, c	cum	with
caps.	capsula	a capsule
chart.	charta	a paper
collyr.	collyrium	an eyewash
divid.	divide	divide (thou)
d.t.d. No. iv	dentur tales doses No. iv	let 4 such doses be given
elix.	elixir	an elixir
enem.	enema	an enema
et	et	and
fldxt.	fluidextractum	fluidextract
ft.	fac; fiat; fiant	make (thou); let it be made; let them be made
ft. chart. vi	fiant chartulae vi	let 6 powders be made
ft. pulv. et div. in char. xii	fiat pulvis et divide in chartulas xii; *or,* fiat pulvis in chartulas xii dividenda	let 12 powders be made
gtt.	gutta(e)	drop(s)
H.	hora	an hour
hor. som., H.S.	hora somni	at bedtime
in d.	in dies	from day to day; daily
inf.	infusum	an infusion
inject.	injectio	an injection
inter	inter	between
lin.	linimentum	a liniment
liq.	liquor	a solution
lot.	lotio	a lotion
M.	misce	mix (thou)
m.	minimum	a minim
min.	minimum	a minim
mist.	mistura	a mixture
no.	numero, numerus	number
noctis	noctis	of the night
non	non	not
non rep.	non repetatur	do not repeat
O.D.	oculus dexter	the right eye
O.L.	oculus laevus	the left eye
omn. hor.	omni hora	every hour
omni nocte	omni nocte	every night
p.c.	post cibos; post cibum	after eating; after food
pil.	pilula(e)	pill(s)
p.r.n.	pro re nata	as occasion arises; occasionally
pulv.	pulvis; pulveres; pulveratus	powder; powders; powdered
q.h.	quaque hora	each hour; every hour

TABLE OF THE MORE COMMON LATIN AND GREEK TERMS AND ABBREVIATIONS USED IN PRESCRIPTION WRITING (Continued)

Term or abbreviation	Latin or Greek	Translation
q. 2 h.	quaque secunda hora	every 2 hours
q.i.d.	quater in die	4 times a day
q.s.	quantum sufficit; quantum sufficiat; quantum satis	a sufficient quantity; as much as is sufficient
S.	signa; signetur	write (thou); let it be written; label (thou)
S.A.	secundum artem	according to art
sig.	signa; signetur	write (thou); let it be written; label (thou)
sine	sine	without
sol.	solutio	a solution
sp.	spiritus	spirit
ss, $\overline{ss}$	semis	a half
suppos.	suppositorium	a suppository
syr.	syrupus	syrup
tabel.	tabella (dim. of *tabula,* a table)	a lozenge
talis	talis	such; like this
t.d.	ter die	3 times a day
t.i.d.	ter in die	3 times a day
tinct.	tinctura	a tincture
tr.	tinctura	a tincture
ung.	unguentum	an ointment
ut dict.	ut dictum	as directed

āā, āa	of each
C′	complement
E_0	electroaffinity
F_1	first filial generation
F_2	second filial generation
L_+	limes death
L_0	limes zero
Q_{O_2}	oxygen consumption
m-	meta-
o-	ortho-
p-	para-
℞	[*L. recipe*]. Take
S.	[*L. signa*]. Write
c̄, c	[*L. cum*]. With
s̄s̄, ss	[*L. semis*]. One-half
~~m~~, ~~M~~	[*L. misce*]. Mix
O.	[*L. octarius*]. Pint
C.	[*L. congius*]. Gallon
°	degree
♏	minim
℈	scruple
ʒ	dram (apothecaries')
fʒ	fluidram
oz.	ounce (avoirdupois)
℥	ounce (troy)
f℥	fluidounce
μ	micron
μμ	micromicron
mμ	millimicron, micromillimeter
σ	$^1/_{1000}$ of a second
π	3.1416—ratio of circumference of a circle to its diameter
lb.	pound (avoirdupois)
℔.	pound (apothecaries')
®	registered trademark status
mg %	milligrams per cent
vol. %	volume per cent
μg	microgram
□, ♂	male
○, ♀	female
*	birth
†	death
−	negative; levorotatory
+	positive; dextrorotatory
±	either positive or negative; not definite; racemic
	denotes a reversible reaction
#	number
∧	value considered as a vector in electrocardiography
w/v	weight in volume

TABLE OF THERMOMETRIC EQUIVALENTS*

Celsius to Fahrenheit Scales

$\frac{9}{5}$C.° + 32 = F.°

C.°	F.°	C.°	F.°	C.°	F.°	C.°	F.°	C.°	F.°
−20	−4.0	21	69.8	61	141.8	101	213.8	141	285.8
−19	−2.2	22	71.6	62	143.6	102	215.6	142	287.6
−18	−0.4	23	73.4	63	145.4	103	217.4	143	289.4
−17	1.4	24	75.2	64	147.2	104	219.2	144	291.2
−16	3.2	25	77.	65	149.	105	221.	145	293.
−15	5.	26	78.8	66	150.8	106	222.8	146	294.8
−14	6.8	27	80.6	67	152.6	107	224.6	147	296.6
−13	8.6	28	82.4	68	154.4	108	226.4	148	298.4
−12	10.4	29	84.2	69	156.2	109	228.2	149	300.2
−11	12.2	30	86.	70	158.	110	230.	150	302.
−10	14.	31	87.8	71	159.8	111	231.8	151	303.8
− 9	15.8	32	89.6	72	161.6	112	233.6	152	305.6
− 8	17.6	33	91.4	73	163.4	113	235.4	153	307.4
− 7	19.4	34	93.2	74	165.2	114	237.2	154	309.2
− 6	21.2	35	95.	75	167.	115	239.	155	311.
− 5	23.	36	96.8	76	168.8	116	240.8	156	312.8
− 4	24.8	37	98.6	77	170.6	117	242.6	157	314.6
− 3	26.6	38	100.4	78	172.4	118	244.4	158	316.4
− 2	28.4	39	102.2	79	174.2	119	246.2	159	318.2
− 1	30.2	40	104.	80	176.	120	248.	160	320.
0	32.	41	105.8	81	177.8	121	249.8	161	321.8
1	33.8	42	107.6	82	179.6	122	251.6	162	323.6
2	35.6	43	109.4	83	181.4	123	253.4	163	325.4
3	37.4	44	111.2	84	183.2	124	255.2	164	327.2
4	39.2	45	113.	85	185.	125	257.	165	329.
5	41.	46	114.8	86	186.8	126	258.8	166	330.8
6	42.8	47	116.6	87	188.6	127	260.6	167	332.6
7	44.6	48	118.4	88	190.4	128	262.4	168	334.4
8	46.4	49	120.2	89	192.2	129	264.2	169	336.2
9	48.2	50	122.	90	194.	130	266.	170	338.
10	50.	51	123.8	91	195.8	131	267.8	171	339.8
11	51.8	52	125.6	92	197.6	132	269.6	172	341.6
12	53.6	53	127.4	93	199.4	133	271.4	173	343.4
13	55.4	54	129.2	94	201.2	134	273.2	174	345.2
14	57.2	55	131.	95	203.	135	275.	175	347.
15	59.	56	132.8	96	204.8	136	276.8	176	348.8
16	60.8	57	134.6	97	206.6	137	278.6	177	350.6
17	62.6	58	136.4	98	208.4	138	280.4	178	352.4
18	64.4	59	138.2	99	210.2	139	282.2	179	354.2
19	66.2	60	140.	100	212.	140	284.	180	356.
20	68.								

*Courtesy, *The United States Pharmacopeia*

TABLE OF THERMOMETRIC EQUIVALENTS (Continued)

Fahrenheit to Celsius Scales

$(F.° - 32) \times 5/9 = C.°$

F.°	C.°	F.°	C.°	F.°	C.°	F.°	C.°	F.°	C.°
0	−17.78	51	10.56	101	38.33	151	66.11	201	93.89
1	−17.22	52	11.11	102	38.89	152	66.67	202	94.44
2	−16.67	53	11.67	103	39.44	153	67.22	203	95.
3	−16.11	54	12.22	104	40.	154	67.78	204	95.56
4	−15.56	55	12.78	105	40.56	155	68.33	205	96.11
5	−15.	56	13.33	106	41.11	156	68.89	206	96.67
6	−14.44	57	13.89	107	41.67	157	69.44	207	97.22
7	−13.89	58	14.44	108	42.22	158	70.	208	97.78
8	−13.33	59	15.	109	42.78	159	70.56	209	98.33
9	−12.78	60	15.56	110	43.33	160	71.11	210	98.89
10	−12.22	61	16.11	111	43.89	161	71.67	211	99.44
11	−11.67	62	16.67	112	44.44	162	72.22	212	100.
12	−11.11	63	17.22	113	45.	163	72.78	213	100.56
13	−10.56	64	17.78	114	45.56	164	73.33	214	101.11
14	−10.	65	18.33	115	46.11	165	73.89	215	101.67
15	−9.44	66	18.89	116	46.67	166	74.44	216	102.22
16	−8.89	67	19.44	117	47.22	167	75.	217	102.78
17	−8.33	68	20.	118	47.78	168	75.56	218	103.33
18	−7.78	69	20.56	119	48.33	169	76.11	219	103.89
19	−7.22	70	21.11	120	48.89	170	76.67	220	104.44
20	−6.67	71	21.67	121	49.44	171	77.22	221	105.
21	−6.11	72	22.22	122	50.	172	77.78	222	105.56
22	−5.56	73	22.78	123	50.56	173	78.33	223	106.11
23	−5.	74	23.33	124	51.11	174	78.89	224	106.67
24	−4.44	75	23.89	125	51.67	175	79.44	225	107.22
25	−3.89	76	24.44	126	52.22	176	80.	226	107.78
26	−3.33	77	25.	127	52.78	177	80.56	227	108.33
27	−2.78	78	25.56	128	53.33	178	81.11	228	108.89
28	−2.22	79	26.11	129	53.89	179	81.67	229	109.44
29	−1.67	80	26.67	130	54.44	180	82.22	230	110.
30	−1.11	81	27.22	131	55.	181	82.78	231	110.56
31	−0.56	82	27.78	132	55.56	182	83.33	232	111.11
32	0.	83	28.33	133	56.11	183	83.89	233	111.67
33	0.56	84	28.89	134	56.67	184	84.44	234	112.22
34	1.11	85	29.44	135	57.22	185	85.	235	112.78
35	1.67	86	30.	136	57.78	186	85.56	236	113.33
36	2.22	87	30.56	137	58.33	187	86.11	237	113.89
37	2.78	88	31.11	138	58.89	188	86.67	238	114.44
38	3.33	89	31.67	139	59.44	189	87.22	239	115.
39	3.89	90	32.22	140	60.	190	87.78	240	115.56
40	4.44	91	32.78	141	60.56	191	88.33	241	116.11
41	5.	92	33.33	142	61.11	192	88.89	242	116.67
42	5.56	93	33.89	143	61.67	193	89.44	243	117.22
43	6.11	94	34.44	144	62.22	194	90.	244	117.78
44	6.67	95	35.	145	62.78	195	90.56	245	118.33
45	7.22	96	35.56	146	63.33	196	91.11	246	118.89
46	7.78	97	36.11	147	63.89	197	91.67	247	119.44
47	8.33	98	36.67	148	64.44	198	92.22	248	120.
48	8.89	99	37.22	149	65.	199	92.78	249	120.56
49	9.44	100	37.78	150	65.56	200	93.33	250	121.11
50	10.								

Troy Weight

1 pound = 22.816 cubic inches of distilled water at 62°F.

Grains gr.		*Pennyweights* dwt.		*Ounces* oz.		*Pound* ℔.
24	=	1		—		
480	=	20	=	1		
5760	=	240	=	12	=	1

Avoirdupois Weight

1 pound = 1.2153 pounds troy

Grains gr.		*Drams* dr.		*Ounces* oz.		*Pound* lb.
27.34375	=	1				
437.5	=	16	=	1		
7000	=	256	=	16	=	1

Apothecaries' Weight

Grains gr.		*Scruples* ℈		*Drams* ʒ		*Ounces* ℥		*Pound* ℔.
20	=	1						
60	=	3	=	1				
480	=	24	=	8	=	1		
5760	=	288	=	96	=	12	=	1

Apothecaries' Measure

Minims ♏		*Fluidrams* fʒ		*Fluidounces*		*Pints* O.		*Gallon* C.
60	=	1						
480	=	8	=	1				
7,680	=	128	=	16	=	1		
61,440	=	1024	=	128	=	8	=	1

Metric Weights

1 gram = 1 cubic centimeter of distilled water at 4°C.

		Grams		*Grains*		*Av. Ounces*
Milligram	=	0.001	=	0.01543		
Centigram	=	0.01	=	0.15432		
Decigram	=	0.1	=	1.54324		
Gram	=	1.	=	15.43248	=	.03528
Decagram	=	10.	=		=	.3528
Hectogram	=	100.	=		=	3.52758
Kilogram	=	1,000.	=		=	35.2758

Comparative Values of Standard and Metric Measures of Length

Inches	*Centimeters*	*Inches*	*Millimeters*
1	2.54	1/25	1.00
2	5.08	1/12	2.12
3	7.62	1/8	3.18
4	10.16	1/4	6.35
5	12.70	1/3	8.47
6	15.24	1/2	12.70
7	17.78	5/8	15.88
8	20.32	2/3	16.93
9	22.86	3/4	19.05
10	25.40	5/6	21.16
11	27.94	7/8	22.22
12	30.48	11/12	23.28

Comparative Values of Avoirdupois and Metric Weights

Av. Ounces	*Grams*	*Av. Pounds*	*Grams*
1/16	1.772	1	453.59
1/8	3.544	2	907.18
1/4	7.088	2.2	1000.00
1/2	14.175	3	1360.78
1	28.350	4	1814.37
2	56.699	5	2267.96
3	85.049	6	2721.55
4	113.398	7	3175.15
5	141.748	8	3628.74
6	170.097	9	4082.33
7	198.447	10	4535.92
8	226.796		
9	255.146		
10	283.495		
11	311.845		
12	340.194		
13	368.544		
14	396.893		
15	425.243		

Comparative Values of Apothecaries' and Metric Liquid Measures

Minims	*Cubic Centimeters*	*Fluidrams*	*Cubic Centimeters*	*Fluidounces*	*Cubic Centimeters*
1	0.06	1	3.70	1	29.57
2	0.12	2	7.39	2	59.15
3	0.19	3	11.09	3	88.72
4	0.25	4	14.79	4	118.29
5	0.31	5	18.48	5	147.87
6	0.37	6	22.18	6	177.44
7	0.43	7	25.88	7	207.01
8	0.49			8	236.58
9	0.55			9	266.16
10	0.62			10	295.73
11	0.68			11	325.30
12	0.74			12	354.88
13	0.80			13	384.45
14	0.86			14	414.02
15	0.92			15	443.59
16	0.99			16	473.17
17	1.05			17	502.74
18	1.11			18	532.31
19	1.17			19	561.89
20	1.23			20	591.46
25	1.54			21	621.03
30	1.85			22	650.60
35	2.16			23	680.18
40	2.46			24	709.75
45	2.77			25	739.32
50	3.08			26	768.90
55	3.39			27	798.47
				28	828.04
				29	857.61
				30	887.19
				31	916.76
				32	946.33
				48	1419.49
				56	1656.08
				64	1892.66
				72	2129.25
				80	2365.83
				96	2839.00
				112	3312.16
				128	3785.32

Metric Linear Measure

		Meter		U. S. Inches		Feet		Yards		Miles
Millimeter	=	.001	=	.03937	=	.00328				
Centimeter	=	.01	=	.3937	=	.03280				
Decimeter	=	.1	=	3.937	=	.32808	=	.10936		
Meter	=	1.	=	39.37	=	3.2808	=	1.0936		
Decameter	=	10.	=		=	32.808	=	10.936		
Hectometer	=	100.	=		=	328.08	=	109.36	=	.062137
Kilometer	=	1,000.	=		=	3,280.8	=	1,093.6	=	.62137

Comparative Values of Metric Liquid and Apothecaries' Measures

Cubic Centi-meters	Minims	Cubic Centi-meters	Flui-drams	Cubic Centi-meters	Fluid-ounces
0.05	0.81	5	1.35	30	1.01
0.07	1.14	6	1.62	50	1.69
0.09	1.46	7	1.89	75	2.54
1	16.23	8	2.17	100	3.38
2	32.5	9	2.43	200	6.76
3	48.7	10	2.71	300	10.15
4	64.9	25	6.76	400	13.53
				473	16.00
				500	16.91
				600	20.29
				700	23.67
				800	27.05
				900	30.43
				1000	33.82

Table for Converting Metric Weights into Apothecaries' Weights

Grams	Exact Equivalents in Grains	Grams	Exact Equivalents in Grains
0.01	0.1543	12.0	185.189
0.02	0.3086	13.0	200.621
0.03	0.4630	14.0	216.054
0.04	0.6173	15.0	231.486
0.05	0.7716	16.0	246.918
0.06	0.9259	17.0	262.351
0.07	1.0803	18.0	277.783
0.08	1.2346	19.0	293.216
0.09	1.3889	20.0	308.648
0.1	1.543	21.0	324.080
0.2	3.086	22.0	339.513
0.3	4.630	23.0	354.945
0.4	6.173	24.0	370.378
0.5	7.716	25.0	385.810
0.6	9.259	26.0	401.242
0.7	10.803	27.0	416.674
0.8	12.346	28.0	432.107
0.9	13.889	29.0	447.538
1.0	15.432	30.0	462.971
2.0	30.865	31.0	478.403
3.0	46.297	32.0	493.835
4.0	61.730	40.0	617.294
5.0	77.162	45.0	694.456
6.0	92.594	50.0	771.618
7.0	108.027	60.0	925.942
8.0	123.459	70.0	1080.265
9.0	138.892	80.0	1234.589
10.0	154.324	90.0	1388.912
11.0	169.756	100.0	1543.236

Table for Converting Apothecaries' Weights into Metric Weights

Grains	Grams	Grains	Grams
1/50	0.00130	50	3.240
1/32	0.00202	51	3.305
1/20	0.00324	52	3.370
1/18	0.00360	53	3.434
1/16	0.00405	54	3.499
1/15	0.00432	55	3.564
1/12	0.00540	56	3.629
1/10	0.00648	57	3.694
1/8	0.00810	58	3.758
1/6	0.01080	59	3.823
1/5	0.01296	60	3.888
1/4	0.01620	61	3.953
1/3	0.02160	62	4.018
1/2	0.03240	63	4.082
3/4	0.04860	64	4.147
1	0.0648	65	4.212
2	0.1296	66	4.277
3	0.1944	67	4.342
4	0.2592	68	4.406
5	0.3240	69	4.471
6	0.3888	70	4.536
7	0.4536	71	4.601
8	0.5184	72	4.666
9	0.5832	73	4.730
10	0.6480	74	4.795
11	0.7128	75	4.860
12	0.7776	76	4.925
13	0.8424	77	4.990
14	0.9072	78	5.054
15	0.9720	79	5.119
16	1.037	80	5.184
17	1.102	81	5.249
18	1.166	82	5.314
19	1.231	83	5.378
20	1.296	84	5.443
21	1.361	85	5.508
22	1.426	86	5.573
23	1.490	87	5.638
24	1.555	88	5.702
25	1.620	89	5.767
26	1.685	90	5.832
27	1.749	91	5.897
28	1.814	92	5.962
29	1.879	93	6.026
30	1.944	94	6.091
31	2.009	95	6.156
32	2.074	96	6.221
33	2.138	97	6.286
34	2.203	98	6.350
35	2.268	99	6.415
36	2.333	100	6.480
37	2.398	120	7.776
38	2.462	150	9.720
39	2.527	180	11.664
40	2.592	200	12.958
41	2.657	480	31.103
42	2.722	500	32.396
43	2.786	600	38.875
44	2.851	700	45.354
45	2.916	800	51.833
46	2.981	900	58.313
47	3.046	960	62.207
48	3.110	1000	64.799
49	3.175		

Metric Doses with Approximate Apothecary Equivalents

The approximate dose equivalents in the following table represent the quantities that would be prescribed, under identical conditions, by physicians using, respectively, the metric or the apothecary system of weights and measures. When prepared dosage forms, such as tablets, capsules, pills, etc., are prescribed in the metric system, the pharmacist may dispense the corresponding approximate equivalent in the apothecary system, and vice versa. However, this does not authorize the alternative use of the approximate dose equivalents given below for specific quantities on a prescription that requires compounding, nor in converting a pharmaceutical formula from one system of weights or measures to the other system; for such purposes exact equivalents must be used.

Liquid Measures		Weights	
Metric	*Approximate Apothecary Equivalents*	*Metric*	*Approximate Apothecary Equivalents*
1000 ml	1 quart	30 g	1 ounce
750 ml	1-1/2 pints	15 g	4 drams
500 ml	1 pint	10 g	2-1/2 drams
250 ml	8 fluidounces	7.5 g	2 drams
200 ml	7 fluidounces	6 g	90 grains
100 ml	3-1/2 fluidounces	5 g	75 grains
50 ml	1-3/4 fluidounces	4 g	60 grains (1 dram)
30 ml	1 fluidounce	3 g	45 grains
15 ml	1/2 fluidounce (4 fluidrams)	2 g	30 grains (1/2 dram)
10 ml	2-1/2 fluidrams	1.5 g	22 grains
8 ml	2 fluidrams	1 g	15 grains
5 ml	75 minims (1-1/4 fluidrams)	0.75 g	12 grains
4 ml	1 fluidram	0.6 g	10 grains
3 ml	45 minims	0.5 g	7-1/2 grains
2 ml	30 minims	0.45 g	7 grains
1 ml	15 minims	0.4 g	6 grains
0.75 ml	12 minims	0.3 g	5 grains
0.6 ml	10 minims	0.25 g	4 grains
0.5 ml	8 minims	0.2 g	3 grains
0.3 ml	5 minims	0.15 g	2-1/2 grains
0.25 ml	4 minims	0.12 g	2 grains
0.2 ml	3 minims	0.1 g	1-1/2 grains
0.1 ml	1-1/2 minims	75 mg	1-1/4 grains
0.06 ml	1 minim	60 mg	1 grain
		50 mg	3/4 grain
		40 mg	2/3 grain
		30 mg	1/2 grain
		25 mg	3/8 grain
		20 mg	1/3 grain
		15 mg	1/4 grain
		12 mg	1/5 grain
		10 mg	1/6 grain
		8 mg	1/8 grain
		6 mg	1/10 grain
		5 mg	1/12 grain
		4 mg	1/15 grain
		3 mg	1/20 grain
		2 mg	1/30 grain
		1.5 mg	1/40 grain
		1.2 mg	1/50 grain
		1 mg	1/60 grain
		0.8 mg	1/80 grain
		0.6 mg	1/100 grain
		0.5 mg	1/120 grain
		0.4 mg	1/150 grain
		0.3 mg	1/200 grain
		0.25 mg	1/250 grain
		0.2 mg	1/300 grain
		0.15 mg	1/400 grain
		0.1 mg	1/600 grain

NOTE: A milliliter (ml) is for all practical purposes equivalent to a cubic centimeter (cc).

A SELECTION OF MEDICAL WORD-FORMING ELEMENTS (Continued from inside front cover) listed according to their plain English translations

Prefixes are identified by a hyphen at the end: DYS-, HYPER-; suffixes and stem-suffix combinations, by a hyphen at the beginning: -IA, -ITIS; and stems alone (most of which occur in various positions in words), by a hyphen both at the beginning and at the end: -HEPAT-, -PATH-, -VENTR-.

Equivalent Latin- and Greek-derived elements are identified as such: -OCUL- [L.], -OPHTHALM- [Gk.]. The Latin word elements combine preferentially with other Latin elements (as in *oculomotor*) and Greek with Greek (as in *ophthalmoplegic*), but there are many exceptions.

This list includes only forms that differ considerably from the corresponding plain English words, thus excluding such items as -ARTERI- (*artery*), -BILI- (*bile*), and excluding -CAV- at *cavity* but including it at *hollow*.

The stems and affixes listed here, plus hundreds more, are entered at their own alphabetical places in the body of the dictionary where their forms, meanings, and origins are treated in greater detail.

navel	-UMBILIC- [L.], -OMPHAL- [Gk.]
near, next to	-PROXIM-, AD-, JUXTA-
neck	-CERVIC-, -COLL- [L.], -TRACHEL- [Gk.]
needle	-ACU-
nerve	-NEUR-
next (to)	JUXTA-
nipple	-THEL- [Gk.], -MAMILL- [L.]
non-, not	A(N)- [Gk.], IN- [L.]
normal	-ORTH-, -EU-
nose	-(R)RHIN- [Gk.], -NAS- [L.]
nourish(ment)	-TROPH-[Gk.], -nutri- [L.]
nucleus	-KARY-
oil	-OLE- [L.], -ELE- [Gk.]
old (age)	-GER(ONT)- [Gk.], -SEN(EC)- [L.]
on, upon	HYPER- [Gk.], SUPRA- [L.]
one, single	-UN(I)- [L.], -MON(O)- [Gk.]
opening	-STOM-, -TREMA(T)-
opposite, opposing	ANT(I)- [Gk.], CONTR(A)- [L.]
origin, original	-PROT-, -ARCH(E)-
other	-ALL(O)-
outer, superficial	EPI-, ECT(O)-
outside (part of)	ECT(O)-
outside, beyond	EXTR(A)-
ovary	-OOPHOR-
over, above	HYPER- [Gk.], SUPER-, SUPRA- [L.]
over, covering	EPI-
ovum	-O(O)-
own, individual	-IDI(O)-
pain	-ALG-, -ODYN- [Gk.], -DOL(OR)- [L.]
paralysis	-PLEG(IA)
part	-MER-
peculiar, unique	-IDI(O)-
perspire, perspiration	-HIDR-
pelvis (renal)	-PYEL-
physician	-IATR-
place	-TOP- [Gk.], -LOC- [L.]
poison	-TOX(I)-
pregnant, pregnancy	-GRAVID-, -GEST(A)- [L.], -CYESIS [Gk.]
pressure	-BAR- [Gk.], -TENS(I)- [L.]
process	-OSIS, -ESIS
producing, production	-GEN-, -GENESIS
prolapse	-PTOT-, -PTOSIS
pulse	-SPHYGM-
puncture	-CENT(E)-
pus	-PY(O)- [Gk.], -PUR(U)- [L.]
pupil	-COR-

quick, fast	-TACH(Y)-
quick, quicken	-OXY-
rapid(ity)	-TACH(Y)-
ray	-RADI- [L.], -ACTIN- [Gk.]
record, recording	-GRAM
recording instrument	-GRAPH
rectum	-PROCT-
red	-RUBR- [L.], -ERYTHR- [Gk.]
reduce, contract	-MEI(O)-
repair	-PLASTY ("moulding"), -(R)RHAPHY ("sewing")
respiration	-PNEA
rib	-COST-
ring	-AN(N)UL- [L.], -CYCL- [Gk.]
root	-RADIC- [L.], -(R)RHIZ- [Gk.]
saliva	-PTYAL-, -SIAL-
same	-HOM(O)- [Gk.], -IPS(I)- [L.]
scale, scaly	-SQUAM-
self	-AUT(O)-
sewing up, suturing	-(R)RHAPHY
sharp	-OXY- [Gk.], -ACUT- [L.]
sheath	-VAGIN- [L.], -LEMM- [Gk.]
short	-BREV- [L.], -BRACH(Y)-, -MICR- [Gk.]
shoulder	-OM- [Gk.], -HUMER- [L.]
shoulderblade	-SCAPUL-
sick(ness), ill(ness)	See *disease*
side	-LATER-
single, simple	-UN(I)- [L.], -MON(O)-, -HAPL- [Gk.]
skin	-CUT(I)- [L.], -DERM- [Gk.]
sleep	-SOMN- [L.] ,-HYPN-, -NARC- [Gk.]
slow	-BRADY- [Gk.], -TARD-, -LENT- [L.]
smooth	-LEI(O)-
soft, softening	-MALAC- [Gk.], -MOLL-, -LEN- [L.]
solid	-STER(E)-
sole	-PLANT-
sore	-ULCER- [L.], -HELC- [Gk.]
sound	-PHON-
speak, speech	-GLOSS-, -GLOTT-, -PHAS-, -LOG-
spindle	-FUS(I)-
spine, spinal column	-(R)RHACHI(D)-
spleen	-LIEN-
split, divided	-SCHIZ-, -SCHIST- [Gk.], -FISS- [L.]
stand, standstill	-STAT-, -STAS-
starch	-AMYL-
stomach	-GASTR-
stone, concretion	-LITH- [Gk.], -CALCUL- [L.]
straight	-RECT- [L.], -ORTH- [Gk.]
strength	-STHEN-